FOURTH EDITION

CIVETTA, TAYLOR, & KIRBY'S CRITICAL CARE

FOURTH EDITION

CIVETTA, TAYLOR, & KIRBY'S

CRITICAL CARE

Edited by

Andrea Gabrielli, MD, FCCM
Professor of Anesthesiology and Surgery
Division of Critical Care Medicine
Section Head, NeuroCritical Care
University of Florida College of Medicine;
Medical Director, Cardiopulmonary Service and Hyperbaric Medicine
Shands Hospital at the University of Florida
Gainesville, Florida

A. Joseph Layon, MD, FACS
Professor of Anesthesiology, Surgery, and Medicine
Chief, Division of Critical Care Medicine
University of Florida College of Medicine;
Medical Director, Surgical Critical Care
Shands Hospital at the University of Florida;
Medical Director, Gainesville Fire Rescue Service
Gainesville, Florida

Mihae Yu, MD, FACS
Professor of Surgery
University of Hawaii John A. Burns School of Medicine
Vice Chair of Education of
University of Hawaii Surgical Residency Program
Program Director of Surgical Critical Care Fellowship Program
Director of Surgical Intensive Care,
The Queen's Medical Center
Honolulu, Hawaii

Wolters Kluwer Health | Lippincott Williams & Wilkins
Philadelphia • Baltimore • New York • London
Buenos Aires • Hong Kong • Sydney • Tokyo

Acquisitions Editor: Brian Brown
Managing Editor: Nicole Dernoski
Project Manager: Rosanne Hallowell
Manufacturing Manager: Kathleen Brown
Marketing Manager: Angella Panetta
Design Coordinator: Teresa Mallon
Cover Designer: Larry Didona
Production Services: Aptara, Inc.

Fourth Edition
© 2009 by Lippincott Williams & Wilkins, a Wolters Kluwer Business
530 Walnut Street
Philadelphia, PA 19106
LWW.com

Printed in the United States

Library of Congress Cataloging-in-Publication Data

Civetta, Taylor, & Kirby's critical care / edited by Andrea Gabrielli, A. Joseph Layon, Mihae Yu. — 4th ed.
p. ; cm.
Rev. ed. of: Critical care / [edited by] Joseph M. Civetta, Robert W. Taylor, Robert R. Kirby. 3rd ed. c1997.
Includes bibliographical references and index.
ISBN 978–0–7817–6869–6 (alk. paper)
1. Critical care medicine. I. Gabrielli, Andrea. II. Layon, A. Joseph. III. Yu, Mihae. IV. Civetta, Joseph M. V. Taylor, Robert W. (Robert Wesley), 1949– VI. Kirby, Robert R. VII. Critical care. VIII. Title: Civetta, Taylor, and Kirby's critical care. IX. Title: Critical care.
[DNLM: 1. Critical Care. 2. Intensive Care Units. WX 218 C582 2009]
RC86.7.C69 2009
616.02′8—dc22

2008040424

---

10 9 8 7 6 5 4 3 2 1

To the memory of my father, Pietro:
He would have been proud to see the results of my efforts.
To my dear mother Giuliana for her unconditional support.
To my brother Marco, the *real* smart guy of the family.
To my students, friends, and colleagues world wide.
To our patients:
Our inspiration for compassionate care.
—Andrea Gabrielli

To my children Maria, Nicolas, and Daniel—who teach me about unconditional love and humility.
To my best friend and partner Susana E. Picado—who taught me to be better.
To my green-eyed kid sister Serena M. Layon, 1954–2008—who taught me that suffering and dignity were reconcilable.
To those for whom I am honored to care.
To those who struggle for justice and peace—as Brecht noted, these are irreplaceable
—A. Joseph Layon

To my Dad, General Jae Hung Yu & the Seventh Division for their sacrifices and changing history for the better.
To my Mom, the late Esang Yoon who was the wind beneath our wings.
To the late Dr. Thomas J. Whelan Jr. who continues to mentor me in the practice of Surgery and Code of conduct.
To Joe and Judy Civetta who sparked my continuing love for Critical Care and being the guiding light for all Peepsters.
And to my daughter Pearl (&CD) who has the Master Key to All...
—Mihae Yu

CONTENTS

CONTRIBUTING AUTHORS

Patricia L. Abbitt, MD
Professor of Radiology and Section Chief, Body Imaging
Department of Radiology
University of Florida College of Medicine
Gainesville, Florida

Steven G. Achinger, MD
Texas Diabetes Institute
University Center for Community Heath Dialysis West
San Antonio, Texas

Gareth Adams, MD
Department of Neurosurgery
Baylor College of Medicine
Ben Taub General Hospital
Houston, Texas

Olufemi Akindipe, MD
Assistant Professor
Division of Pulmonary and Critical Care Medicine
Department of Medicine
University of Florida College of Medicine
Gainesville, Florida

Serge Alpandari, MD, MSc
Infectious Diseases and Infection Control Senior Physician
Intensive Care Unit
Hopital G. Chatiliez
Tourcoing, France

Adrian Alvarez, MD
Staff Anesthesiologist
Department of Anesthesiology
Hospital de Clinicas, General San Martin
Faculty of Medicine, University of Buenos Aires
Ciudad Autonoma de Buenos Aires, Argentina

Marcelo Amato, MD
Faculdade de Medicina
Universidade de São Paulo
São Paulo, Brazil

Giuditta Angelini
Assistant Professor of Anesthesiology and Medicine
University of Wisconsin-Madison School of Medicine and Public Health
Madison, Wisconsin

Djillali Annane, MD, PhD
Professor in Medicine
General Intensive Care Unit
University of Versailles Saint Quentin, UniverSud Paris
Versailles
Chief
General Intensive Care Unit
Raymond Poincaré Hospital–Assistance Publique Hôpitaux de Paris
Garches, France

Massimo Antonelli, MD
Professor
Department of Anesthesiology and Intensive Care
Università Cattolica del Sacro Cuore
Chief
Department of Anesthesiology and Intensive Care
Policlinico-Universitario—A. Gemelli
Rome, Italy

Veena B. Antony, MD
Professor of Medicine, Molecular Genetics and Microbiology
Department of Medicine, College of Medicine
University of Florida
Chief, Division of Pulmonary Critical Care and Sleep Medicine
Department of Medicine
University of Florida Shands Hospital
Gainesville, Florida

Lennox K. Archibald, MD, FRCP, DTM&H
Hospital Epidemiologist
Department of Medicine, Division of Infectious Diseases
College of Medicine, University of Florida
Shands Hospital at the University of Florida
Gainesville, Florida

Juan Carlos Ayus, MD, FACP, FASN
Director of Clinical Research
Nephrology
Renal Consultants of Houston
Houston, Texas

Keri A. Baacke, MD
Maternal Fetal Medicine Fellow
University of Florida
Department of Maternal Fetal Medicine
Gainesville, Florida

Mariona Badia, MD, PhD
Associate Professor
Department de Medicina
Universidad de Lleida
Intensive Care Unit
Hospital Universitario Arnau de Vilanova
Lleida, Spain

Sean M. Bagshaw, MD, MSc, FRCPC
Department of Intensive Care and Department of Medicine
Austin & Hospital
Melbourne, Victoria, Australia

Michael J. Banner, PhD
Professor
Department of Anesthesiology
University of Florida College of Medicine
Gainesville, Florida

Philip S. Barie, MD, MBA, FCCM, FACS
Professor of Surgery
Chief of Division of Critical Care and Trauma
Department of Surgery
Weill Cornell Medical College
New York, New York

Cody B. Barnett, MD
Assistant Clinical Professor
University of South Alabama College of Medicine
Internal Medicine Center
Mobile, Alabama

Claudia L. Barthold, MD
Assistant Professor/Assistant Residency Director
Emergency Medicine
University of Nebraska
Assistant Medical Director
Nebraska Regional Poison Center
Nebraska Medical Center
Omaha, Nebraska

Robert H. Bartlett, MD
Professor of Surgery, Emeritus
Department of Surgery
University of Michigan
Ann Arbor, Michigan

Miho K. Bautista, MD
Staff Physician
Geriatric Research, Education, and Clinical Center
North Florida / South Georgia Veterans Health System
Clinical Assistant Professor
Division of Career Development and Education;
Department of Aging & Geriatrics
University of Florida College of Medicine
Gainesville, Florida

Maher A. Baz, MD
Associate Professor of Medicine
Department of Medicine
University of Florida
Medical Director, Lung Transplant Program
Shands Hospital
Gainesville, Florida

Elizabeth Cordes Behringer, MD
Anesthesiologist-Intensivist
Department of Anesthesiology
Cedars Sinai Medical Center
Los Angeles, California
Clinical Professor of Anesthesiology
University of California, Irvine
Orange, California

Giuseppe Bello, MD
Research Fellow
Department of Anesthesiology and Intensive Care
Università Cattolica del Sacro Cuore
Senior Staff
Department of Anesthesiology and Intensive Care
Policlinico Universitario—A. Gemelli
Rome, Italy

Rinaldo Bellomo, MBBS, MD, FRACP, FJFICM
Professor
Division of Medicine
Melbourne University
Director of Research
Department of Intensive Care
Austin Hospital
Melbourne, Australia

Howard Belzberg, MD, FCCM
Associate Professor of Surgery
University of Southern California
School of Medicine
Chief of Critical Care
Los Angeles County – USC Medical Center
Los Angeles, California

Jeffrey A. Bennett, MD
Assistant Professor of Neuroradiology
Department of Radiology
University of Florida
Gainesville, Florida

Eugene V. Beresin, MD
Professor
Department of Psychiatry
Harvard Medical School
Director of Child and Adolescent Psychiatry
Residency Training
Department of Psychiatry and Child Psychiatry Services
Massachusetts General Hospital
Boston, Massachusetts

Ira M. Bernstein, MD
Professor and Vice Chair for Obstetrics
Department of Obstetrics and Gynecology
University at Vermont College of Medicine
Attending Physician and Director of Maternal Fetal Medicine
Women's Health Care Service
Fletcher Allen Health Care
Burlington, Vermont

Rebecca J. Beyth, MD
Physician Researcher
Geriatric Research, Education, and Clinical Center
North Florida / South Georgia Veterans Health System
Associate Professor and Chief
Division of Career Development and Education;
Department of Aging and Geriatrics
University of Florida College of Medicine
Gainesville, Florida

Indermeet S. Bhullar, MD
Director of Trauma ICU
Department of Surgery
Sacred Heart Hospital
Pensacola, Florida

Luca M. Bigatello, MD
Associate Professor of Anesthesia
Harvard Medical School
Director, Critical Care
Department of Anesthesia and Critical Care
Massachusetts General Hospital
Boston, Massachusetts

Umberto Bivona, PhD
Psychologist Consultant
Post-Coma Unit
IRCCS Santa Lucia Foundation
Rome, Italy

Thomas J. J. Blanck, MD, PhD
Professor and Chairman
Department of Anesthesiology
Professor, Physiology and Neuroscience
New York University
Chairman
Department of Anesthesiology
NYU Medical Center
New York, New York

Paul B. Blanch, BA, RRT
Courtesy Assistant
Department of Anesthesiology
University of Florida College of Medicine, Shands Hospital
Equipment Specialist
Department of Respiratory Care
Gainesville, Florida

Thomas P. Bleck, MD, FCCM
Professor of Neurology, Neurological Surgery, and Medicine, and
Vice-Chairman for Academic Programs
Northwestern University Feinberg School of Medicine
Chicago, Illinois
The Ruth Cain Ruggles Chairman
Department of Neurology
Evanston Northwestern Healthcare
Evanston, Illinois

Ernest F. J. Block, MD, MBA
Clinical Associate Professor of Surgery
Department of Surgery
University of Florida
Gainsville, Florida
Director, Trauma Services
Department of Surgical Education
Orlando Regional Medical Center
Orlando, Florida

Eric L. Bloomfield, MD
Assistant Professor of Anesthesiology
Mayo Clinic College of Medicine
Rochester, Minnesota

Karen L. Booth, MD
Clinical Assistant Professor
Department of Pediatrics
Stanford University
Attending Pediatric Cardiologist
Department of Pediatrics
Lucile Packard Children's Hospital
Palo Alto, California

Karen Bordson, DO
Research Instructor, Volunteer Faculty
Department of Obstetrics and Gynecology
The University of Kansas School of Medicine
Kansas City, Kansas
Staff Physician
Department of Obstetrics and Gynecology
North Kansas City, Missouri

Adrien Bougle, MD
Fellow in Anesthesiology and Critical Care Medicine
University of Versailles Saint Quentin,
UniverSud Paris Versaille,
Garches, France

Philip Boysen, MD
Professor of Anesthesiology and Medicine
Executive Associate Dean for Graduate Medical Education
The University of North Carolina at Chapel Hill
Chapel Hill, North Carolina

John F. Burke, MD
Professor of Surgery
Department of Surgery
Harvard Medical School
Chief, Trauma, Emergency Surgery, and Surgical Critical Care
Department of Surgery
Massachusetts General Hospital
Boston, Massachusetts

Frederick M. Burkle, Jr., MD, MPH, DTM
Senior Fellow
Harvard Humanitarian Initiative
Harvard University
Cambridge, Massachusetts

James E. Calvin, Jr., MD
James B. Herrick Professor of Medicine
Rush University
Section Director, Section of Cardiology
Department of Medicine
Rush University Medical Center
Chicago, Illinois

Morgan Camp, MD
Resident
Department of Radiology - College of Medicine - University of Florida
Gainesville, Florida

William G. Cance, MD
Professor
Department of Surgery
University of Florida
Gainesville, Florida

Lawrence J. Caruso, MD
Associate Professor
Department of Anesthesiology and Surgery
University of Florida
Associate Chief
Division of Critical Care Medicine
Shands Hospital Gainesville, FL

Salvatore Cassese, MD
Resident in Cardiology
Division of Cardiology
Federico II University
Naples, Italy

Jorge H. Castro, MD
Surgical Critical Care Clinical Fellow
Critical Care Department
University of Pittsburgh/ UPMC
Pittsburgh, Pennsylvania

Juan C. Cendan, MD
Assistant Professor
Department of Surgery
University of Florida
Gainesville, Florida

Cherylee W. J. Chang, MD, FACP
Associate Clinical Professor
Departments of Medicine and Surgery
University of Hawaii at Manoa, John A. Burns School of Medicine
Medical Director
Neuroscience Institute/Neurocritical Care
The Queen's Medical Center
Honolulu, Hawaii

Michael D. Christian, MD, FRCPC
Lecturer
Department of Medicine
University of Toronto
Attending Physician
Critical Care & Intectious Diseases
Mount Sinai Hospital & University Health Network
Toronto, Canada

Marianne E. Cinat, MD, FACS
Associate Professor of Surgery
University of California Irvine Medical Center
Orange, California

Maria Paola Ciurli, PhD
Senior Staff Member Post-Coma Unit
Department of Neuropsychological Diagnosis and Therapy
Rome, Italy

Cornelius J. Clancy, MD
Associate Professor of Medicine
Director, Mycology Research Unit
Department of Medicine
University of Pittsburgh
Staff Physician
Department of Medicine
VA Medical Center
Pittsburgh, Pennsylvania

Michael Coburn, MD
Vice Chairman and Residency Program Director
Scott Department of Urology
Baylor College of Medicine
Chief of Urology, Ben Taub General Hospital
Houston, Texas

Jonathan B. Cohen, MD
Anesthesiology / Critical Care Medicine
Tampa General Hospital
Tampa, Florida

Giorgio Conti, MD
Associate Professor
Department of Anesthesiology and Intensive Care
Università Cattolica del Sacro Cuore
Chief
Paediatric Intensive Care Unit
Policlinico Universitario—A. Gemelli
Rome, Italy

Jamie B. Conti, MD, FACC, FHRS
Professor and Interim Chief
Division of Cardiovascular Medicine
Department of Medicine
Director
Clinical Cardiac Electrophysiology
University of Florida
Gainesville, Florida

Timothy J. Coons, RRT, MBA
Director, Cardiopulmonary and Neurological Services
Shands Hospital at the University of Florida
Gainesville, Florida

Mark S. Cooper, BM, BCh, PhD
Senior Lecturer in Endocrinology
Division of Medical Sciences
University of Birmingham
Consultant Endocrinologist
Department of Medicine
University Hospital Birmingham
Birmingham, United Kingdom

C. Clay Cothren, MD, FACS
Assistant Professor of Surgery
Department of Surgery
University of Colorado School of Medicine
Program Director
Trauma and Acute Care Surgery Fellowship
Department of Surgery
Denver Health Medical Center
Denver, Colorado

Douglas B. Coursin, MD
Professor
Departments of Anesthesiology and Internal Medicine
University of Wisconsin School of Medicine and Public Health
University of Wisconsin Hospitals and Clinics
Madison, Wisconsin

Claudia Crimi, MD
Research Fellow
Department of Anaesthesia and Critical Care
Harvard Medical School
Boston, Massachusetts

Ettore Crimi, MD
Resident in Anesthesia
Department of Anesthesia and Critical Care
Massachusetts General Hospital,
Harvard Medical School
Boston, Massachusetts

Kristina Crothers, MD
Assistant Professor
Section of Pulmonary and Critical Care
Department of Internal Medicine
Yale University School of Medicine
Staff Physician
Yale New Haven Hospital
New Haven, Connecticut

Gohar H. Dar, MD
Staff
Departments of Cardiothoracic Anesthesiology
and Critical Care Medicine
Cleveland Clinic
Cleveland, Ohio

Rabih O. Darouiche, MD
VA Distinguished Service Professor
Department of Medicine and Physical Medicine
and Rehabilitation
Baylor College of Medicine
Staff Physician
Department of Medicine and Spinal Cord Injury Care Lines
Michael E. Debakey Veterans Affairs Medical Center
Houston, Texas

Elizabeth Lee Daugherty, MD, MPH
Fellow
Division of Pulmonary and Critical Care Medicine
Department of Medicine
Johns Hopkins University School of Medicine
Baltimore, Maryland

David A. Decker, MD
Vascular Neurology Fellow
Department of Neurology
University of Florida College of Medicine
McKnight Brain Institute
Gainesville, Florida

Harakh V. Dedhia, MBBS, FACP, FCCP, FCCM
Professor
Department of Medicine and Anesthesiology
Section of Pulmonary—CCM
West Virginia University Health Science Center
Medical Director, Medical ICU and Respiratory Care
Department of Medicine
West Virginia University Hospital
Morgantown, West Virginia

Giuseppe De Luca, MD, PhD
Assistant Professor
Clinical and Experimental Medicine
Eastern Piedmont University
Chief
Interventional Cardiology, Clinical Cardiology
Ospedale Maggiore Della Carita
Novara, Italy

Leonardo De Luca, MD
Medical Staff
Department of Cardiovascular Sciences
European Hospital
Rome, Italy

Demetrios Demetriades, MD, PhD, FACS
Professor of Surgery and Emergency Medicine,
Director of Trauma and Surgical Intensive Care Unit
Los Angeles County - USC Medical Center
University of Southern California
School of Medicine
Los Angeles, California

Clifford S. Deutschman, MS, MD, FCCM
Professor of Anesthesiology and Critical Care and Surgery
Department of Anesthesiology and Critical Care
University of Pennsylvania School of Medicine
Attending Physician, Surgical Critical Care Service
Department of Anesthesiology and Critical Care
Hospital of the University of Pennsylvania
Philadelphia, Pennsylvania

Hector D. Dini, MD
Staff
Department of Anesthesia
Hospital Britanico de Buenos Aires
Buenos Aires, Argentina

Jack A. Di Palma, MD
Professor and Director
Division of Gastroenterology
University of South Alabama College of Medicine
Mobile, Alabama

Karen E. Doucette, MD, MSc
Assistant Professor
Division of Infectious Diseases, Department of Medicine
University of Alberta
Edmonton, Alberta, Canada

Jonathan D. Dreier, MD
Anesthesia Critical Care Fellow
Department of Anesthesia and Critical Care Medicine
University of South Florida College of Medicine
Tampa, Florida

David J. Dries, MSE, MD
Assistant Medical Director
Surgical Care
Health Partners Medical Group
University of Minnesota
Minneapolis, Minnesota

Quan-Yang Duh, MD
Professor
Department of Surgery
University of California, San Francisco
Attending Surgeon
Department of Surgery
VA Medical Center
San Francisco, California

Stephanie H. Dunlap, DO
Medical Director, Heart Transplant Program
Rush University Medical Center
Chicago, Illinois

Herbert L. DuPont, MD
Director, Center for Infectious Diseases
The University of Texas–Houston School of Public Health
Chief, Internal Medicine
St. Luke's Episcopal Hospital
Vice-Chairman, Department of Medicine
Baylor College of Medicine
Houston, Texas

Soumitra Eachempati, MD, FACS
Department of Surgery and Public Health
Weill Cornell Medical College
New York Presbyterian Hospital
New York, New York

Rodney K. Edwards, MD, MS
Associate Director
Phoenix Perinatal Associates
Obstetrix Medical Group
Phoenix, Arizona

A. Ahsan Ejaz, MD
Clinical Associate Professor
Division of Nephrology, Hypertension & Transplantation
University of Florida
Director of Inpatient Nephrology Services
Division of Nephrology, Hypertension, and Transplantation
UF & Shands Hospital
Gainesville, Florida

Elamin M. Elamin, MD, MSx, FACP, FCCP
Associate Professor
Anesthesiology Department
University of Florida
Associate Professor
Department of Anesthesiology
Shands Hospital
Gainesville, FL

Timothy C. Fabian, MD, FACS
Harwell Wilson Professor and Chairman
Department of Surgery
University of Tennessee Health Science Center
Memphis, Tennessee

Samir Fakhry, MD, FACS
Professor of Surgery
Department of Surgery
Virginia Commonwealth University, Inova Campus
Chief, Trauma and Surgical Critical Care
Department of Trauma Services
Inova Fairfax Hospital
Falls Church, Virginia

Kevin J. Farrell, MD
Assistant Professor of Surgery
Department of Surgery
Emory University School of Medicine
Atlanta, Georgia

Robert J. Feezor, MD
Assistant Professor
Division of Vascular Surgery and Endovascular Therapy
Department of Surgery
University of Florida College of Medicine
Gainsville, Florida

Joseph Feldschuh, MD, FACC
Clinical Associate Professor Emeritus
Departments of Medicine and Pathology
New York Medical College
New York, New York
Attending
Departments of Medicine and Cardiology
Montefiore Hospital and Medical Center
Bronx, New York

Niall D. Ferguson, MD, FRCPC, MSc
Assistant Professor
Department of Medicine & Interdepartmental Division of Critical Care Medicine
University of Toronto
Research Director
Department of Critical Care Medicine
University Health Network
Toronto, Ontario, Canada

Sebastian Fernandez-Bussy, MD
Clinical Assistant Professor
Lung Transplant Program
University of Florida
Gainsville, Florida

Joseph Ferreira BS, CPTC, CTOP II
Director of Clinical Operations
Life Alliance Organ Recovery Agency
University of Miami Miller School of Medicine
Miami, Florida

Henry E. Fessler, MD
Associate Professor
Department of Pulmonary and Critical Care Medicine
Johns Hopkins School of Medicine
Director, Fellowship Training Program in Pulmonary and Critical Care
Department of Medicine
Johns Hopkins Hospital
Baltimore, Maryland

Rhonda S. Fishel, MD, MBA, FACS
Associate Professor of Surgery
Department of Surgery
Johns Hopkins School of Medicine
Associate Chief of Surgery
Director of Surgical Critical Care
Department of Surgery
Sinai Hospital of Baltimore
Baltimore, Maryland

Jay A. Fishman, MD
Associate Professor
Department of Medicine
Harvard Medical School
Director
Transplant Infectious Disease Program
Associate Director, Transplant Center
Infectious Disease Division
Massachusetts General Hospital
Boston, Massachusetts

Kathleen E. Fitzgerald, RN, BSN
Staff Nurse, Surgical ICU
Shands Hospital at the University of Florida
Gainesville, Florida

Timothy C. Flynn, MD
Professor of Surgery
Department of Surgery
Senior Associate Dean
University of Florida College of Medicine
Gainesville, Florida

Rita Formisano, MD, PhD
Director of Neuro-Rehabilitation Department
Post-Coma Unit
I.R.C.C.S. Santa Lucia Foundation
Rome, Italy

Cory M. Franklin, MD
Retired Director of the Division of Critical Care
Cook County Hospital (Stroger)
Chicago, Illinois

Michael A. Frölich, MD, MS
Associate Professor
Department of Anesthesiology
University of Alabama at Birmingham
Birmingham, Alabama

Brian Fuehrlein, PhD
MD PhD Student
College of Medicine and Department of Biomedical Engineering
University of Florida
Gainesville, Florida

W. Craig Fugate, MD
Director
Florida Division of Emergency Management
State of Florida
Tallahassee, Florida

Andrea Gabrielli, MD, FCCM
Professor of Anesthesiology and Surgery
Division of Critical Care Medicine
Section Head, NeuroCritical Care
University of Florida College of Medicine;
Medical Director, Cardiopulmonary Service and Hyperbaric Medicine
Shands Hospital at the University of Florida
Gainesville, Florida

Robert Peter Gale, MD
Counselor
International Bone Marrow Transplant Registry
University of Wisconsin
Milwaukee, Wisconsin

George D. Garcia, MD
Trauma Surgery and Surgical Critical Care Fellow
University of Miami -Jackson Memorial Hospital
The DeWitt Daughtry Family Department of Surgery
Division of Trauma, Surgical Critical Care & Burns
Leonard M. Miller School of Medicine
Miami, Florida

A. Joseph Garcia, MD
Senior Staff Physician
Departments of Emergency Medicine and Critical Care Medicine
Henry Ford Hospital
Detroit, Michigan

Cynthia Wilson Garvan, PhD
Research Assistant Professor
Division of Biostatistics
College of Medicine
University of Florida
Gainesville, Florida

Achille Gaspardone, MD, Mphil
Aggregate Professor of Cardiology
Department of Medicine
Tor Vergata University
Chief
Division of Cardiology
Ospedale S. Eugenio
Rome, Italy

Georges A. Ghacibeh, MD
Northeast Regional Epilepsy Group
Hackensack, New Jersey

Dany E. Ghannam, MD
Fellow
Department of Infectious Diseases
UT/MD Anderson Cancer Center
Houston, Texas
Fellow
Department of Critical Care Medicine
Stanford University of Medicine
Stanford, CA

Lewis R. Goldfrank, MD
Professor and Chair,
Department of Emergency Medicine
New York University School of Medicine
New York, New York

Shankar P. Gopinath, MD
Department of Neurosurgery
Baylor College of Medicine
Ben Taub General Hospital
Houston, Texas

Dietrich Gravenstein, MD
Associate Professor of Anesthesiology
Department of Anesthesiology
University of Florida College of Medicine
Associate Professor
Department of Anesthesiology
Shands Hospital at the University of Florida
Gainesville, Florida

J. S. Gravenstein, MD
Graduate Research Professor, Emeritus
Department of Anesthesiology
University of Florida College of Medicine
Gainesville, Florida

David M. Greer, MD, MA
Asssistant Professor of Neurology
Department of Neurology, Neurocritical Care and Stroke Group
Massachusetts General Hospital
Boston, Massachusetts

Jeffrey S. Groeger, MD
Professor
Department of Medicine
Weill Medical College of Cornell University
Chief, Urgent Care Service
Department of Medicine
Memorial Sloan Kettering Cancer Center
New York, New York

Jonathan Haft, MD
Department of Surgery
University of Michigan Health System
Ann Arbor, Michigan

Stephen B. Hanauer, MD
Professor
Department of Medicine and Clinical Pharmacology
University of Chicago
Chief
Gastroenterology, Heptalogy and Nutrition
University of Chicago Medical Center
Chicago, Illinois

Ikram U. Haque, MD
Assistant Professor
Department of Pediatrics
University of Florida College of Medicine
Attending Physician
Shands Children's Hospital at the University of Florida
Gainesville, Florida

Cathleen Harris, MD
Assistant Professor
Department of Obstetrics and Gynecology
University of Vermont
Fletcher Allen Health Care
Burlington, Vermont

Holger H. Hasselbring, MD
Dr.Med. And Chairman
Department of Anesthesiology and Critical Care Medicine
Teaching Hospital of Ruhr-University
Director
Department of Anesthesiology and Critical Care Medicine
Augusta-Kranken-Anstalt
Bochum, Germany

Kevin W. Hatton, MD
Fellow
Division of Critical Care Medicine
Department of Anesthesiology
University of Florida College of Medicine
Gainesville, Florida

George Hatzakis, MSc, PhD
Division of Trauma and Critical Care
Los Angeles County - USC Medical Center
Los Angeles, California

William Hayden, MD
Professor of Pediatrics
Director of Pediatric Intensive Care Unit
Rush University School of Medicine
Chicago, Illinois

Stephen O. Heard, MD
Professor
Departments of Anesthesiology and Surgery
University of Massachusetts Medical School
Chairman
Department of Anesthesiology
UMass Memorial Medical Center
Worcester, Massachusetts

Bryce A. Heese, MD, MA
Assistant Professor
Department of Pediatrics
University of Florida
Department of Pediatrics
Shands Hospital
Gainesville, Florida

Marcelo E. Heinig, MD
Division of Nephrology, Hypertension and Transplantation
University of Florida College of Medicine
Gainesville, Florida

Alan W. Hemming, MD, MSc
Professor
Department of Surgery
University of Florida
Chief
Division of Transplantation & Hepatobiliary Surgery
Department of Surgery
Shands at the University of Florida
Gainesville, Florida

Dean R. Hess, PhD, RRT
Associate Professor
Department of Anesthesia
Harvard Medical School
Assistant Director
Department of Respiratory Care
Massachusetts General Hospital
Boston, Massachusetts

Zoltan G. Hevesi, MD
Associate Professor
Department of Anesthesiology and Surgery
University of Wisconsin
Director of Transplant Anesthesiology
Department of Anesthesiology and Surgery
University of Wisconsin Hospital and Clinics
Madison, Wisconsin

Thomas L. Higgins, MD, MBA
Professor of Medicine; Assistant Professor of Anesthesia
Departments of Medicine and Anesthesiology
Tufts University School of Medicine
Boston, Massachusetts
Chief, Critical Care Division
Critical Care/Department of Medicine
Baystate Medical Center
Springfield, Massachusetts

Hao Chih Ho, MD
Assistant Professor
Department of Surgery
University of Hawaii
Medical Director
Trauma Division
The Queen's Medical Center
Honolulu, Hawaii

Jamie Hochman, MS, CRT
Systems Administrator
Sinai Hospital of Baltimore
Baltimore, Maryland

Maureane Hoffman, MD, PhD
Professor
Department of Pathology
Duke University
Director
Blood Bank and Hematology Laboratories
Durham VA Medical Center
Durham, North Carolina

Brian L. Hoh, MD
Assistant Professor
Department of Neurological Surgery
University of Florida College of Medicine
Gainesville, Florida

M. Barbara Honnebier, MD, PhD
Pediatric and Adult Plastic and Reconstructive Surgery
Cranio-Maxillo-Facial Surgery
The Queens' Medical Center and Kapiolani
Medical Center for Women and Children
Honolulu, Hawaii

Charles W. Hoopes, MD
Assistant Professor
Department of Surgery
University of California, San Francisco
Section Chief
Cardiopulmonary Transplantation
University of California, San Francisco
San Francisco, California

Ramona O. Hopkins, PhD
Chair, Psychology Department
Associate Professor, Psychology and Neuroscience
Psychology Department
Brigham Young University
Provo, Utah
Department of Critical Care Medicine
Pulmonary and Critical Care Division
Intermountain Medical Center
Murray, Utah
Department of Critical Care Medicine
Pulmonary and Critical Care Division
LDS Hospital
Salt Lake City, Utah

David B. Hoyt, MD, FACS
Professor and Chair
Department of Surgery
University of California, Irvine
Chief of Surgery
Department of Surgery
University of California, Irvine Medical Center
Orange, California

Laurence Huang, MD
Professor
Department of Medicine
University of California, San Francisco
Chief, AIDS Chest Clinic
Department of Medicine, HIV/AIDS Division
and Division of Pulmonary and Critical Care Medicine
San Francisco General Hospital
San Francisco, California

Thomas S. Huber, MD, PhD
Professor of Surgery
Department of Surgery
University of Florida College of Medicine
Shands Hospital–The University of Florida
Gainesville, Florida

Ahamed H. Idris, MD
Professor of Surgery and Medicine
Department of Surgery
University of Texas Southwestern Medical Center at Dallas
Senior Attending Physician
Emergency Medicine
Parkland Memorial Hospital
Dallas, Texas

Steven R. Insler, DO
Staff Anesthesiologist and Critical Care Physician
Departments of Cardiac Anesthesia and Critical Care Medicine
The Cleveland Clinic Foundation
Cleveland, Ohio

Felicia A. Ivascu, MD
Trauma Surgery and Surgical Critical Care Fellow
University of Miami -Jackson Memorial Hospital
The DeWitt Daughtry Family Department of Surgery
Division of Trauma, Surgical Critical Care & Burns
Leonard M. Miller School of Medicine
Miami, Florida

James C. Jackson, PsyD
Division of Allergy/Pulmonary/Critical Care Medicine
Center for Health Services Research
Department of Psychiatry
Vanderbilt University School of Medicine
Nashville, Tennessee

J. Michael Jaeger, PhD, MD
Department of Anesthesiology
Division of Critical Care Medicine
Co-Medical Director, TCV-PO
University of Virginia Health System
Charlottesville, Virginia

Sridivya Jaini, MD, MS
Jacobi Medical Center
Department of Medicine
Bronx, New York

Michael A. Jantz, MD, FCCP
Associate Professor of Medicine
Department of Pulmonary, Critical Care, and Sleep Medicine
University of Florida
Associate Professor of Medicine
Pulmonary, Critical Care, and Sleep Medicine
Shands Hospital
Gainesville, Florida

Edgar J. Jimenez, MD, FCCM
Associate Professor
Department of Medicine
University of Florida and Florida State University
Director, Medical Critical Care
Critical Care Medicine
Orlando Regional Medical Center
Orlando, Florida

Aaron Joffee, MD
Clinical Assistant Professor of Medicine
University of Wisconsin School of Medicine and Public Health
Madison, Wisconsin

Raja Kandaswamy, MD
Associate Professor
Department of Transplant Surgery
University of Minnesota
Transplant and General Surgeon
Department of Transplant Surgery
University of Minnesota Medical Center, Fairview
Minneapolis, Minnesota

Scott R. Karlan, MD
Assistant Clinical Professor of Surgery
Department of Surgery
University of California, Los Angeles
Associate Director of Trauma
Department of Surgery
Cedars-Sinai Medical Center
Los Angeles, California

Paraskevi A. Katsaounou, MD
Lecturer in Pulmonary Medicine
Department of Critical Care and Pulmonary Services
University of Athens Medical School
Evangelismos Hospital
Athens, Greece

Eileen H. Kim, MIA, MD
Post-Doctoral Fellow
Phoebe R. Berman Bioethics Institute
Johns Hopkins University
Baltimore, Maryland
Attending Physician
Critical Care Medicine
Mercy Hospital of Philadelphia
Philadelphia, Pennsylvania

Robin D. Kim, MD
Assistant Professor of Surgery
Division of Transplantation & Hepatobiliary Surgery
University of Florida College of Medicine
Gainesville, Florida

Craig S. Kitchens, MD
Professor of Medicine
Department of Medicine
University of Florida
Associate Chief of Staff (Education)
Medical Service
Malcolm Randall VA Medical Center
Gainesville, Florida

Orlando C. Kirton, MD, FACS, FCCM, FCCP
Professor of Surgery/Associate Program
Director Integrated General Surgery Residency
Program
Vice Chairman, Department of Surgery
University of Connecticut, School of Medicine
Farmington, Connecticut

Charles T. Klodell, MD
Assistant Professor
Department of Surgery
University of Florida
Gainesville, Florida

Marin H. Kollef, MD
Professor of Medicine
Department of Pulmonary and Critical Care Medicine
Washington University School of Medicine
Director
Medical Intensive Care Unit
Barnes-Jewish Hospital
St. Louis, Missouri

Meghavi S. Kosboth, DO
Clinical Fellow
Division of Rheumatology and Clinical Immunology
University of Florida
Gainesville, Florida

Andreas H. Kramer, MD, FRCPC
Assistant Professor
Departments of Critical Care and Clinical Neurosciences
University of Calgary
Calgary, Alberta, Canada

Christopher J. Krebs, MD
Neuroradiology Fellow
Department of Radiology
University of Florida College of Medicine
Gainesville, Florida

Anand Kumar, MD
Associate Professor of Medicine
Departments of Medicine, Medical Microbiology
and Pharmacology/Therapeutics
University of Manitoba, Winnipeg, MB Canada
Department of Medicine
University of Medicine and Dentistry, New Jersey
Camden, New Jersey
Attending Physician
Department of Critical Care Medicine
Health Sciences Centre/St. Boniface Hospital
Winnipeg, Manitoba, Canada

Aseem Kumar, PhD
Associate Professor
Canada Research Chair in Biomolecular Science
Laurentian University
Department of Chemistry and Biochemistry
Sudbury, Ontario, Canada

Franco Laghi, MD
Professor of Medicine
Department of Pulmonary and Critical Care Medicine
Loyola University of Chicago, Stritch School of Medicine
Maywood, Illinois
Staff Physician
Pulmonary and Critical Care Medicine
Edward Hines Jr. VA Hospital
Hines, Illinois

A. Joseph Layon, MD, FACS
Professor of Anesthesiolosy, Surgery, and Medicine
Chief, Division of Critical Care Medicine
University of Florida College of Medicine;
Medical Director, Surgical Critical Care
Shands Hospital at the University of Florida;
Medical Director, Gainesville Fire Rescue Service
Gainesville, Florida

Aimée C. LeClaire, PharmD
Clinical Assistant Professor
College of Pharmacy
University of Florida
Clinical Pharmacy Specialist, Surgical Critical Care
Department of Pharmacy
Shands at the University of Florida
Gainesville, Florida

Marc Leone, MD, PhD
Departement d'Anesthesie et de Reanimation
Centre Hospitalier Universitaire Nord
Chemin des Bourrely, France

Olivier Y. Leroy, MD
Chief
Intensive Care Unit
Hopital Guy Chatiliez
Tourcoing, France

David M. Levi, MD
Associate Professor
Department of Surgery
University of Miami
Surgeon
Department of Surgery
UM/Jackson Memorial Medical Center
Miami, Florida

John G. Lieb, II, MD
Fellow in Gastroenterology
Division of Gastroenterology
Department of Medicine
University of Florida
Gainesville, Florida

Jack J. M. Ligtenberg, MD
Internist-Intensivist
Intensive & Respiratory Care Unit (ICB)
University Medical Center Groningen (UMCG)
Netherlands

John Paul M. Longphre, MD, MPH
Chief Resident
Division of Occupational and Environmental Medicine
Duke University
Durham, North Carolina
Associate Medical Director
Workcare, Inc. and Workplace Group, LLC
Greensboro, North Carolina

Lawrence Lottenberg, MD, FACS
Associate Professor of Surgery and Anesthesiology
Department of Surgery
University of Florida College of Medicine
Trauma Medical Director
Acute Care Surgery
Shands Hospital at the University of Florida
Gainesville, Florida

Michele A. Lorand, MD, FAAP
Chair, Division of Child Protective Services
Department of Pediatrics
John H. Stroger, Jr. Hospital of Cook County
Chicago, Illinois

Harrinarine Madhosingh, MD
Clinical Assistant Professor,
Division of Infectious Diseases
Department of Medicine
University of Florida
Gainesville, Florida

John W. Mah, MD
Assistant Professor
Department of Surgery
University of Connecticut School of Medicine
Medical Director, Surgical ICU
Department of Surgery/Critical Care
Hartford Hospital
Hartford, Connecticut

Michael E. Mahla, MD
Professor of Anesthesiology & Neurosurgery
Department of Anesthesiology
University of Florida
College of Medicine
Gainesville, Florida

Patrick T. Mailloux, DO
Assistant Professor of Medicine
Department of Medicine
Tufts University School of Medicine
Boston, Massachusetts
Attending Physician/Intensivist
Critical Care Division/Department of Medicine
Baystate Medical Center
Springfield, Massachusetts

Elizabeth Manias RN, M.Pharm, NNursStud, PhD
Associate Professor and Associate Head of Research Training
Equity and Staff Development Coordinator
School of Nursing and Social Work
The University of Melbourne
Carlton, Victoria, Australia

Edward M. Manno, MD
Associate Professor
Department of Neurology
Mayo Clinic
Medical Director
Neurological Intensive Care Unit
Saint Mary's Hospital
Rochester, Minnesota

Daniel R. Margulies, MD, FACS
Director of Trauma and Surgical Critical Care
Department of Surgery
Cedars-Sinai Medical Center
Los Angeles, California

Paul E. Marik, MD, FCCm, FCCP
Professor of Medicine
Chief, Division of Pulmonary and Critical Care Medicine
Thomas Jefferson University
Philadelphia, Pennsylvania

John J. Marini, MD
Director of Translational Research
HealthPartners Research Foundation
Professor of Medicine
University of Minnesota
Minneapolis, Minnesota

Paolo Marino, MD
Chief and Professor of Cardiology
Eastern Piedmont University
Clinical Cardiology
Department of Clinical and Experimental Medicine
Azienda Ospedaliera Universitaria
Maggiore della Carta
Novara, Italy

Claude Martin, MD
Professor
Department of Intensive Care
Marseille Medical School
Chief
Intensive Care Unit
Nord Hospital
Marseille, France

Larry C. Martin, MD
Professor of Surgery
Department of Surgery
Division Director, Acute Care Surgery
University of Florida College of Medicine
Gainesville, Florida

Elizabeth Martinez, MD, MHS
The Johns Hopkins University School of Medicine
Department of Anesthesiology & Critical Care Medicine
Baltimore, Maryland

Mali Mathru, MD
Professor
Department of Anesthesiology
University of Alabama at Birmingham School of Medicine
Director, Division of Critical Care
and Perioperative Medicine
Department of Anesthesiology
University of Alabama at Birmingham Hospital
Birmingham, Alabama

Benjamin M. Matta, BS
PhD Candidate
Departments of Surgery and Immunology
University of Pittsburgh
Pittsburgh, Pennsylvania

S. Anjani D. Mattai, MD
Instructor in Medicine
Department of Medicine
Weill Medical College of Cornell University
Assistant Attending Physician
Department of Medicine
Memorial Sloane-Kettering Cancer Center
New York, New York

Maria Matteis, PhD
Senior Staff Member
Post-Coma Unit
IRCCS Santa Lucia Foundation
Rome, Italy

Kristin L. Mekeel, MD
Fellow
Transplantation and Hepatobiliary Surgery
Department of Surgery
University of Florida
Shands Hospital at University of Florida
Gainesville, Florida

Richard J. Melker, MD, PhD
Professor
Anesthesiology, Biomedical Engineering and Pediatrics
University of Florida College of Medicine
Gainesville, FL

Scott T. Micek, PharmD
Clinical Pharmacist
Critical Care
Department of Pharmacy
Barnes-Jewish Hospital
St. Louis, Missouri

William M. Miles, MD
Professor of Medicine
Division of Cardiovascular Medicine
University of Florida College of Medicine
Gainesville, Florida

Andrew C. Miller, MD
Departments of Emergency Medicine and Internal Medicine
The State University of New York Downstate Medical
Center and
Kings County Hospital Center
Brooklyn, New York

Toshiki Mizobe, MD
Associate Professor
Department of Anesthesiology
Kyoto Prefectrual University of Medicine
Kyoto, Japan

Taro Mizutani, MD, PhD
Professor and Chair
Department of Emergency and Critical Care Medicine
University of Tsukuba (Institute of Clinical Medicine)
Chief
Department of Emergency and Critical Care Medicine
University of Tsukuba Hospital
Tsukuba, Japan

Jerome H. Modell, MD
Emeritus Professor
Department of Anesthesiology
University of Florida College of Medicine
Gainesville, Florida

Ismaël Mohammedi, MD
Universite Claude Bernard
Service d' Anesthesie-Reanimation
Hopital Edouard Herriot
Lyon, France

Lyle L. Moldawer, PhD
Professor and Vice-Chairman (Research)
Department of Surgery
University of Florida College of Medicine
Gainesville, Florida

Wilma E. Monteban-Kooistra, MD
Internist - Intensivist
Intensive & Respiratory Care Unit (ICB)
University Medical Center Groningen (UMCG)
Groningen, The Netherlands

Richard E. Moon, MD, CM, FACP, FCCP, FRCPC
Professor
Departments of Anesthesiology and Medicine
Duke University
Anesthesiologist and Medical Director
Center for Hyperbaric Medicine & Environmental Physiology
Department of Anesthesiology
Duke University Medical Center
Durham, North Carolina

Ernest E. Moore, MD
Vice Chairman and Professor of Research
Department of Surgery
University of Colorado at Denver
Bruce Rockwell Distinguished Chair of Trauma Surgery
Department of Surgery
Denver Health
Denver, Colorado

Frederick A. Moore, MD, FACS
Chief
Surgical Critical Care & Acute Care Surgery
Department of Surgery
The Methodist Hospital
Houston, Texas

Sharon E. Moran, MD
Assistant Professor
Division of Surgical Critical Care
Department of Surgery
University of Hawaii
The Queens Medical Center
Honolulu, Hawaii

Jan S. Moreb, MD
Professor
Department of Medicine
University of Florida
Department of Medicine
Shands Hospital
Gainesville, Florida

Alison Morris, MD, MS
Assistant Professor
Department of Medicine
University of Pittsburgh
Pittsburgh, Pennsylvania

Thomas C. Mort, MD
Associate Professor of Surgery and Anesthesiology
Department of Anesthesiology
University of Connecticut School of Medicine
Senior Anesthesiologist
Medical Director, Simulation Center
Associate Director, Surgical ICU
Department of Anesthesiology
Hartford Hospital
Hartford, Connecticut

David W. Mozingo, MD, FACS
Professor of Surgery and Anesthesia
Department of Surgery
University of Florida
Director, Shands Burn Center
Department of Surgery
Shands at the University of Florida
Gainesville, Florida

Ronald A. Mudry, MD
Assistant Professor
Department of Medicine
West Virginia University
Associate Fellowship Director
Section of Pulmonary/CCM
Ruby Memorial Hospital
Morgantown, WV

Susanne Muehlschlegel, MD
Assistant Professor of Neurology, Anesthesiology and Critical Care Surgery
Neurocritical Care Service
UMass Memorial Medical Center, University Campus
University of Massachusetts Medical School
Worcester, Massachusetts

Deane Murfin, MBBCh, DA(SA), FCA(SA)
Consultant Anaesthetist
Department of Anaesthesia
University of the Witwatersrand
Chris Hani Baragwanath Hospital
Johannesburg, South Africa

Michael J. Murray, MD, PhD
Professor of Anesthesiology
Department of Anesthesiology
Mayo Clinic College of Medicine
Rochester, Minnesota
Consultant in Anesthesiology
Department of Anesthesiology
Mayo Clinic
Phoenix, Arizona

Neil A. Mushlin, DO
Fellow
Division of Pulmonary and Critical Care Medicine
Thomas Jefferson University
Philadelphia, Pennsylvania

Matthew Musulin, MD
Fellow in Clinical Neurophysiology
Department of Neurology
University of Florida College of Medicine
Gainesville, Florida

Ece A. Mutlu, MD, MBA
Assistant Professor of Medicine
Section of Digestive Diseases
Rush University Medical Center
Chicago, Illinois

Gökhan M. Mutlu, MD
Associate Professor of Medicine
Division of Pulmonary and Critical Care Medicine
Northwestern University Feinberg School of Medicine
Attending Physician
Division of Pulmonary and Critical Care Medicine
Northwestern Memorial Hospital
Chicago, Illinois

Bhiken I. Naik, MBBCh(Wits), DA(SA)
Lecturer
Department of Anaesthesiology
University of Witwatersrand
Senior Specialist
Department of Anaesthesiology
Chris Hani Baragwanath Hospital
Gauteng, South Africa

Minh-Hong Nguyen, MD
Professor of Medicine
Department of Medicine
University of Pittsburgh
Director, Transplant Infectious Diseases
Director, Antimicrobial Management Program
Department of Medicine
University of Pittsburgh Medical Center
Pittsburgh, Pennsylvania

Minh-Ly Nguyen, MD
Assistant Professor of Medicine
Department of Medicine
Emory University School of Medicine
Staff Physician
Department of Medicine
Grady Health System
Atlanta, Georgia

Jennifer A. Oakes, MD
Assistant Professor
Emergency Medicine
University of Nebraska
Medical Director Nebraska Regional Poison Center
Nebraska Medical Center
Omaha, Nebraska

Juan B. Ochoa, MD, FACS
Associate Professor
Department of Surgery
University of Pittsburgh Medical School
Medical Director of Trauma Division
Department of Surgery
Presbyterian University Hospital
Pittsburgh, Pennsylvania

Ronnie Otero, MD
Wayne State University
Department of Emergency Medicine and Surgery
Henry Ford Hospital
Detroit, Michigan

Cristina Palacio, JD
Associate General Counsel
Legal Services
Shands Healthcare
Gainesville, Florida

Nimisha K. Parekh, MD, MPH
Assistant Clinical Professor of Medicine
University of California, Irvine
School of Medicine
Orange, California

Robert I. Parker, MD
Professor and Vice Chair for Academic Affairs
Department of Pediatrics
State University of New York at
Stony Brook School of Medicine
Director, Pediatric Hematology/Oncology
Associate Director and Director of Clinical Trials
Stony Brook University Cancer Center
Stony Brook University Medical Center
Stony Brook, New York

David A. Paulus, MD
Professor
Department of Anesthesiology
University of Florida
Anesthesiologist
Department of Anesthesiology
Shands Hospital at the University of Florida
Gainesville, Florida

V. Ram Peddi, MD
Director
Kidney Transplant Research
Department of Transplantation
California Pacific Medical Center
Transplant Nephrologist
California Pacific Medical Center
San Francisco, California

John F. Perry, Jr, MD
Professor
Department of Surgery
University of Minnesota
Minneapolis, Minnesota

Kevin Y. Pei, MD
Fellow
University of Hawaii
Department of Surgery
Division of Surgical Critical Care
The Queens Medical Center
Honolulu, Hawaii

Carl W. Peters, MD
Clinical Associate Professor
Department of Anesthesiology
University of Florida
Staff Intensivist
Anesthesiology
Division of Critical Care Medicine
Shands Hospital at the University of Florida
Gainesville, Florida

Keith R. Peters, MD
Associate Professor
Department of Radiology
University of Florida
Associate Professor
Department of Radiology
Shands Hospital
Gainesville Florida

Matthew James Peterson, ME
Graduate Research Assistant in Biomedical Engineering and Anesthesiology
J. Cravton Pruitt Family Department of Biomedical Engineering
University of Florida
Gainesville, Florida

Scott W. Peterson, MD
Department of Radiology
University of Florida
College of Medicine
Gainesville, Florida

Frederic M. Pieracci, MD, MPH
Departments of Surgery and Public Health
Weill Cornell Medical College
NewYork-Presbyterian Hospital
New York, New York

Michael R. Pinsky, MD, CM, Drhc, FCCP, FCCM
Professor
Department of Critical Care Medicine
University of Pittsburgh Medical Center
Staff Intensivist
Department of Critical Care Medicine
University of Pittsburgh Medical Center
Pittsburgh, Pennsylvania

F. Elizabeth Poalillo, RN, MSN, ARNP, CCRN
Nursing Operations Manager, MICU, SICU, NSICU
Orlando Regional Medical Center
Orlando, Florida

Andrew N. Pollak, MD
Chief, Orthopedic Trauma
R. Adams Cowley Shock Trauma Center
Associate Professor of Orthopedics
University of Maryland School of Medicine
Baltimore, Maryland

Petar J. Popovic, MD, PhD
Assistant Professor
Department of Surgery
University of Pittsburgh Medical School
Pittsburgh, Pennsylvania

David T. Porembka, DO, FCCM
Professor of Anesthesiology, Surgery, Internal Medicine (Cardiology)
Adjunct Professor of United States Air Force Aerospace Medicine
Director of Perioperative Echocardiography
Associate Director of Intensive Care Medicine
University of Cincinnati College of Medicine
Cincinnati, Ohio

Raymond O. Powrie, MD, FRCP, FACP
Associate Professor
Department of Medicine, Obstetrics and Gynecology
The Warren Alpert Medical School at Brown University
Senior Vice President for Quality and Clinical Effectiveness
Women & Infants' Hospital of Rhode Island
Providence, Rhode Island

Ernesto A. Pretto, Jr., MD, MPH
Professor
Department of Anesthesiology
University of Miami School of Medicine
Chief
Division of Solid Organ Transplant
Department of Anesthesiology
Jackson Memorial Medical Hospital
Miami, Florida

Peter Pronovost, MD, PhD
Professor
Department of Anesthesiology and Critical Care, Surgery, and Health Policy and Management
The Johns Hopkins University School of Medicine
Medical Director, Center for Innovations in Quality Patient Care
Director Quality and Safety Research Group
Baltimore, Maryland

Ludwig J. Pyrtek, MD
Chair in Surgery
Director of Surgery/Chief Division of General Surgery
Department of Surgery
Hartford Hospital
Hartford, Connecticut

Issam I. Raad, MD
Professor and Chairman
Infectious Disease/Infection Control
University of Texas M.D. Anderson Cancer Center
Houston, Texas

Alejandro A. Rabinstein, MD
Department of Neurology
Mayo Clinic College of Medicine
Rochester, Minnesota

Amin Rahemtulla, PhD, FRCP
Counselor
International Bone Marrow Transplant Registry
University of Wisconsin
Milwaukee, Wisconsin

S. Sujanthy Rajaram, MD
Assistant Professor of Medicine
Department of Medicine
Division of Critical Care
Robert Wood Johnson Medical School UMDNJ
Camden, New Jersey

H. David Reines, MD
Professor
Department of Surgery
Virginia Commonwealth University
Richmond, Virginia
Vice Chair Surgery
Department of Surgery
Inova Fairfax Hospital
Falls Church, Virginia

Konrad Reinhart, MD, PhD
Wayne State University
Department of Emergency Medicine and Surgery
Henry Ford Hospital
Detroit, Michigan

Zaccaria Ricci, MD
Staff Anesthesiologist
Department of Pediatric Cardiac Surgery
Bambino Gesu Hospital
Rome, Italy

Winston T. Richards, MD
Clinical Assistant Professor
Department of Surgery
The University of Florida
Faculty Member, Division of Acute Care Surgery
Shands Hospital
Gainesville, Florida

Emmanuel P. Rivers, MD, MPH, IOM
Clinical Professor
Department of Emergency Medicine
Wayne State University
Vice Chairman and Research Director
Department of Emergency Medicine and Surgery
Henry Ford Hospital
Detroit, Michigan

Claudia S. Robertson, MD
Professor
Department of Neurosurgery
Baylor College of Medicine
Director
Neurosurgical ICU
Department of Neurosurgery
Ben Taub General Hospital
Houston, Texas

Steven A. Robicsek, MD, PhD
Assistant Professor
Department of Anesthesiology
University of Florida
Shands Hospital at University of Florida
Gainesville, Florida

Jose Rodriguez-Paz, MD
The Johns Hopkins University
School of Medicine
Department of Anesthesiology & Critical Care Medicine
Baltimore, Maryland

Claudio Ronco, MD
Chief
Department of Nephrology, Dialysis, and Transplantation
San Bortolo Hospital
Vicenza, Italy

Amy F. Rosenberg, PharmD
Department of Pharmacy Services
Shands Hospital at the University of Florida
Gainesville, Florida

Stephen J. Roth, MD, MPH
Associate Professor
Department of Pediatrics
Stanford University School of Medicine
Medical Director
Cardiovascular ICU
Lucile Salter Packard Children's Hospital
Palo Alto, California

Daniel T. Ruan, MD
Instructor of Surgery
Department of Surgery
University of California, San Francisco
San Francisco, California

Lewis Rubinson, MD, PhD
Disaster Medicine Director
Healthcare Coalition
Public Health Seattle King County
Seattle, Washington

Steven Sandoval, MD
Department of Surgery
Department of Surgery, Trauma and Critical Care, and Burns
SUNY Stony Brook
University Hospital at Stony Brook
Stony Brook, New York

Stephanie A. Savage, MD
Fellow
Trauma and Surgical Critical Care
University of Tennessee Health Science Center
Memphis, Tennessee

Sherry J. Saxonhouse, MD
Assistant Professor of Medicine
Division of Cardiovascular Medicine
University of Florida College of Medicine
Gainesville, Florida

Thomas M. Scalea, MD
Francis X. Kelly Professor of Trauma Surgery
Trauma Department
University of Maryland School of Medicine
Physician-in-Chief
R Adams Cowley Shock Trauma Center
Baltimore, Maryland

Denise Schain, MD
Associate Professor
Division of Infectious Diseases
Department of Medicine
University of Florida College of Medicine
Gainesville, Florida

Michael Schlame, MD
Associate Professor
Department of Anesthesiology
New York University School of Medicine
Attending Anesthesiologist
Department of Anesthesiology
NYU Medical Center
New York, New York

Carsten M. Schmalfuss, MD
Adjunct Clinical Assistant Professor
Division of Cardiovascular Medicine
University of Florida
Staff Cardiologist
Section of Cardiology
Malcolm Randall VA Medical Center
Gainesville, Florida

Eran Segal, MD
Director, General ICU
Department of Anesthesiology and Intensive Care
Sheba Medical Center
Ramat-Gan, Israel

Allen M. Seiden, MD, FACS
Professor of Otolaryngology
Department of Otolaryngology—Head and Neck Surgery
University of Cincinnati Academic Health Center
Cincinnati, Ohio

Steven A. Seifert, MD, FACMT, FACEP
Professor
Emergency Medicine
University of New Mexico School of Medicine
Medical Director
New Mexico Poison and Drug Information Center
University of New Mexico Health Sciences Center
Albuquerque, New Mexico

Hani Seoudi, MD
Assistant Professor
Department of Surgery
Virginia Commonwealth University, Inova Campus
Attending Surgeon
Department of Trauma Services
Inova Fairfax Hospital
Falls Church, Virginia

Donald R. Sessions, ETMP
Special Operations Chief
Gainesville Fire Rescue Department
Gainesville, Florida

Daniel I. Sessler, MD
Chair
Department of Outcomes Research
The Cleveland Clinic
Director, Outcomes Research Institute
and Weakley Professor of Anesthesiology, University of Louisville
Department of Outcomes Research
The Cleveland Clinic
Cleveland, Ohio

Christoph N. Seubert, MD, PhD
Associate Professor
Department of Anesthesiology
University of Florida College of Medicine
Chief
Division of Neuroanesthesia
Director
Intraoperative Neurophysiologic Monitoring Laboratory
Shands at the University of Florida
Gainesville, Florida

David Shade BA, JD
Division of Pulmonary and Critical Care Medicine
Johns Hopkins University School of Medicine
Baltimore, Maryland

Stephen D. Shafran, MD, FRCPC
Professor and Director
Division of Infectious Diseases
Department of Medicine
University of Alberta
Head
Section of Infectious Diseases
Department of Medicine
University of Alberta Hospital
Edmonton, Alberta
Canada

Jack D. Shannon, MD
Assistant Professor
Department of Anesthesiology
Texas Tech University Health Sciences Center
Lubbock, Texas

Marc J. Shapiro, MD, MS, FACS, FCCM
Professor of Surgery and Anesthesiology
Department of Surgery
SUNY Stony Brook
Chief of General Surgery, Trauma, Critical Care, and Burns
Department of Surgery
University Hospital at Stony Brook
Stony Brook, New York

Takeru Shimizu, MD, PhD
Assistant Professor
Department of Anesthesiology and Critical Care Medicine
University of Tsukuba
Tsukuba, Japan

William C. Shoemaker, MD
Professor of Clinical Surgery
Division of Trauma/ICU
Department of Surgery
University of Southern California
Attending Surgeon
Department of Surgery
Los Angeles County Hospital
Los Angeles, California

Avner Sidi, MD
Associate Professor
Department of Anesthesiology and Intensive Care
Tel Aviv University
Tel Aviv, Israel
Vice Chairman
Head of PACU
Department of Anesthesiology
Sheba Medical Center
Ramat-Gan, Israel

Marc A. Simon, MD, MS, FACC
Assistant Professor
Department of Medicine
University of Pittsburgh
Staff Cardiologist, Heart Failure and Cardiac Transplant Program
Cardiovascular Institute
University of Pittsburgh Medical Center
Pittsburgh, Pennsylvania

Jennifer A. Sipos, MD
Assistant Professor
Division of Endocrinology
University of Florida
Gainesville, Florida

Christopher Lee Sistrom, MD, MPH
Associate Professor
Radiology Department
University of Florida
Gainesville, Florida

Lee P. Skrupky, Pharm.D., BCPS
Critical Pharmacy Specialist, Critical Care
Department of Pharmacy
Barnes-Jewish Hospital
St. Louis, Missouri

Robert N. Sladen, MBChB, MRCP(UK), FRCP(C), FCCM
Professor and Vice-Chair of Anesthesiology
Chief, Division of Critical Care Medicine
Director, Cardiothoracic and Surgical Intensive Care Units
Department of Anesthesiology
College of Physicians and Surgeons of Columbia University
New York, New York

Matthew S. Slater, MD
Associate Professor
Department of Surgery
Oregon Health and Sciences University
Attending Surgeon
Cardiothoracic Surgery
Portland Veterans Administration Medical Center
Portland, Oregon

Danny Sleeman, MD, FACS, FRCS
Professor of Surgery
Department of Surgery
University of Miami
Staff Surgeon
General Surgery
Jackson Memorial Hospital
Miami, Florida

Wendy I. Sligl, MD
Assistant Clinical Professor
Divisions of Infectious Diseases and Critical Care Medicine
University of Alberta
Edmonton, Alberta
Canada

Arthur S. Slutsky, MD
Professor of Medicine, Surgery and Biomedical Engineering
Director, Interdepartmental Division of Critical Care Medicine
Department of Medicine
University of Toronto
Vice President, Research
Department of Medicine and Critical Care Medicine
Keenan Research Center at the Li Ka Shing Knowledge Institute of St. Michael's Hospital
Toronto, Ontario, Canada

David V. Smullen, MD, MSEE
Assistant Professor of Neuroradiology
Department of Radiology
University of Florida College of Medicine
Gainesville, Florida

Eric S. Sobel, MD, PhD
Associate Professor
Department of Medicine
University of Florida
Clinical Faculty Member
Shands Hospital at the University of Florida
Gainesville, Florida

Howard K. Song, MD, PhD
Assistant Professor
Department of Surgery
Oregon Health and Science University
Staff Physician
Department of Surgery
Oregon Health & Science University Hospital
Portland, Oregon

Edward D. Staples, MD
Department of Surgery
Division of Thoracic and Cardiovascular Surgery
University of Florida College of Medicine
Gainesville, Florida

John K. Stene, MD, PhD
Professor
Departments of Anesthesiology and Neurosurgery
Penn State Milton S. Hershey Medical Center
Attending
Neuro Science Intensive Care Unit
Penn State Milton S. Hershey Medical Center
Hershey, Pennsylvania

Deborah M. Stern, MD, MPH
Director of Neurotrauma ICU
R. Adams Cowley Shock Trauma Center
Assistant Professor of Surgery
University of Maryland School of Medicine
Baltimore, Maryland

Andrew Stolbach, MD
Assistant Professor
Department of Emergency Medicine
Johns Hopkins University
Attending Physician
Department of Emergency Medicine
Johns Hopkins Hospital
Baltimore, Maryland

R. Todd Stravitz, MD, FACP, FACG
Associate Professor of Medicine
Hepatology Section
Virginia Commonwealth University
Department of Internal Medicine
Virginia Commonwealth University Medical Center
Richmond, Virginia

Arturo Suarez, MD
Wayne State University
Department of Surgery and Emergency Medicine
Henry Ford Hospital
Detroit, Michigan

Kathirvel Subramaniam, MD
Clinical Assistant Professor
Department of Anesthesiology
University of Pittsburgh
Clinical Cardiac Anesthesiologist
Department of Anesthesiology
University of Pittsburgh Medical Center Presbyterian Hospital
Pittsburgh, Pennsylvania

Murat Sungur, MD
Assistant Professor
Department of Anesthesiology, Critical Care Medicine
University of Florida
Shands Hospital
Gainesville, Florida

David E. R. Sutherland, MD, PhD
Professor of Surgery
John S. Najarian Surgical Chair in Clinical Transplant
Chief, Division of Transplantation
University of Minnesota
Minneapolis, Minnesota

Maria Suurna, MD
Resident in Otolaryngology
Department of Otolaryngology—Head and Neck Surgery
University of Cincinnati Academic Health Center
Cincinnati, Ohio

Sankar Swaminathan, MD
Associate Professor of Medicine
Division of Infectious Diseases
Department of Medicine
University of Florida
Co-Director, Program in Cancer Genetics, Epigenetics and Tumor Virology
UF Shands Cancer Center
Gainesville, Florida

Michael Sydow, MD, PhD
Professor
Department of Anesthesiology, Emergency and Intensive Care Medicine
University of Goettinger
Goettinger, Germany
Chief
Department of Anesthesiology and Intensive Care Medicine
St. Johannes Hospital
Dortmund, Germany

Danny M. Takanishi, Jr., MD, FACS
Associate Professor and Chairman
Department of Surgery
University of Hawaii
Director of Surgical Clinical Research
Department of Surgery
The Queen's Medical Center
Honolulu, Hawaii

Christopher D. Tan, Pharm.D, BCPS
Adjunct Professor
Pharmacy Practice (UCP)/Pharmacy (USC)
University of the Pacific/University of Southern California
Clinical Pharmacist
Department of Pharmacy
Queens Medical Center
Honolulu, Hawaii

Jamie Taylor, MD
Department of Anesthesiology and Critical Care
University of Pennsylvania
School of Medicine
Philadelphia, Pennsylvania

Lisa Thannikary, MD
Lecturer
Department of Anaesthesiology
University of Witwatersrand
Specialist
Department of Anaesthesiology
Chris Hani Baragwanath Hospital
Gauteng, South Africa

S. Rob Todd, MD, FACS
Medical Director
Surgical Intensive Care Unit
Associate Program Director
Surgical Critical Care and Acute Care Surgery
Department of Surgery
The Methodist Hospital
Houston, Texas

Jose Javier Trujillano, MD, PhD
Associate Professor
Department de Ciencies Mediques Basiques
Universidad de Lleida
Intensive Care Unit
Hospital Universitario Arnau de Vilanova
Lleida, Spain

Krista L. Turner, MD
Department of Surgery
The Methodist Hospital
Houston, Texas

Andreas G. Tzakis, MD, PhD
Professor of Surgery
Department of Surgery
University of Miami School of Medicine
Director, Miami Transplant Institute
Department of Surgery
Jackson Memorial Medical Center
Miami, Florida

Kimi R. Ueda, PharmD
Kidney/Pancreas Transplant Pharmacist
Barry S. Levin, MD, Department of Transplantation
California Pacific Medical Center
San Francisco, California

Craigan T. Usher, MD
Assistant Professor
Child and Adolescent Psychiatry
Oregon Health & Science University
Portland, Oregon

Kürsat Uzun, MD
Professor of Medicine
Department of Pulmonary and Critical Care Medicine
Meram Medical School
Selcuk University
Konya, Turkey

Edward Valenstein, MD
Professor and Chair
The William L. and Janice M. Neely Professor of Neurology
Department of Neurology
University of Florida College of Medicine
Attending Neurologist
Shands Hospital at the University of Florida
Gainesville, Florida

Johannes H. van Oostrom, PhD
Associate Professor
Department of Anesthesiology
University of Florida
Associate Chair for Graduate Education
Department of Biomedical Engineering
University of Florida
Gainesville, Florida

Joseph Varon, MD, FACP, FCCP, FCCM
Clinical Professor of Medicine
The University of Texas Health Science Center
Professor of Acute and Continuing Care
St. Luke's Episcopal Hospital
Houston, Texas

Thomas C. Vary, PhD
Distinguished Professor
Cellular and Molecular Physiology
Penn State University College of Medicine
Hershey, Pennsylvania

Theodoros Vassilakopoulos, MD
Associate Professor
Department of Critical Care
University of Athens Medical School
Attending Physician
Department of Critical Care
Evangelismos Hospital
Athens, Greece

George Velmahos, MD, PhD, MSEd
Professor of Surgery
Chief, Division of Trauma, Emergency Surgery, and Surgical Critical Care
Harvard Medical School
Boston, Massachusetts

Nicholas Verne, MD
Professor and Chief
Division of Gastroenterology, Hepatology, and Nutrition
The Ohio State University
Columbus, Ohio

David B. Waisel, MD
Associate Professor of Anaesthesia, Harvard Medical School
Senior Associate in Anaesthesia,
Department of Anesthesiology, Perioperative and Pain Medicine
Children's Hospital Boston
Boston, Massachusetts

Howard Waitzkin, MD, PhD
Distinguished Professor
Departments of Sociology, Family & Community Medicine, and Internal Medicine
University of New Mexico
Albuquerque, New Mexico

J. Matthias Walz, MD
Assistant Professor
Department of Anesthesiology
University of Massachusetts Medical School
Anesthesiologist
SICU Attending
Department of Anesthesiology
UMass Memorial Medical Center
Worcester, Massachusetts

Hsiu-Po Wang, MD
Associate Professor of Internal Medicine
College of Medicine
National Taiwan University
Chief, Endoscopy Division
Chief, Department of Internal Medicine
National Taiwan University Hospital, Yun-Lin Branch
Taipei, Taiwan

Michael F. Waters, MD, PhD
Director, Stroke Program
Assistant Professor of Neurology and Neuroscience
University of Florida College of Medicine
McKnight Brain Institute
Gainesville, Florida

Kenneth Waxman, MD
Director of Trauma and Surgical Education
Department of Surgical Education
Santa Barbara Cottage Hospital
Santa Barbara, California

Christian Waydhas, MD
Associate Professor
Department of Trauma Surgery
University of Duisburg—Essen
Head of Trauma—ICU
Department of Trauma Surgery
University Hospital Essen
Essen, Germany

Carl P. Weiner, MD, MBA, FACOG
Chairman, Department Obstetrics and Gynecology
University of Kansas - Kansas City
Kansas City, Kansas

Dale H. Whitby, PharmD, BCPS
Senior Editor
Department of Clinical Pharmacology
Gold Standard, Inc.
Tampa, Florida
Clinical Staff Pharmacist
Kentucky Children's Hospital
University of Kentucky Health Care
Lexington, Kentucky

Eelco F. M. Wijdicks, MD
Professor of Neurology
Department of Neurology
Chair, Division of Critical Care
Mayo College of Medicine
Rochester, Minnesota

Robert D. Winfield, MD
Resident
Department of Surgery
University of Florida
Gainesville, Florida

William E. Winter, MD
Professor
Departments of Pathology, Immunology & Laboratory Medicine
Pediatrics, and Molecular Genetics & Microbiology
University of Florida, College of Medicine
Clinical Chemist
Shands Hospital
Gainesville, Florida

Charles C. J. Wo, BS
Department of Surgery
Division of Trauma, Critical Care
Los Angeles County — USC Medical Center
Los Angeles, California

Linda L. Wong, MD
Professor
Department of Surgery
University of Hawaii John A. Burns School of Medicine
Director of Liver Transplant
Department of Surgery
Hawaii Medical Center East
Honolulu, Hawaii

Gregory W. Woo, MD
Division of Cardiovascular Medicine
University of Florida
College of Medicine
Gainesville, Florida

Kenneth E. Wood, DO
Professor of Medicine and Anesthesiology
Department of Medicine and Anesthesiology
University of Wisconsin School of Medicine
Senior Director of Medical Affairs
Director of Critical Care Medicine and Respiratory Care
University of Wisconsin Hospital and Clinics
Madison, Wisconsin

Jean-Pierre Yared, MD
Staff
Outcomes Research
Medical Director
Cardiovascular ICU
Department of Cardiothoracic Anesthesiology
Cleveland Clinic
Cleveland, Ohio

Mihae Yu, MD, FACS
Professor of Surgery
University of Hawaii John A. Burns School of Medicine
Vice Chair of Education of
University of Hawaii Surgical Residency Program
Program Director of Surgical Critical Care Fellowship Program
Director of Surgical Intensive Care
The Queen's Medical Center
Honolulu, Hawaii

Yakov Yusim, MD
Instructor
Anesthesiology and Intensive Care
Tel-Aviv University, Sackler Faculty of Medicine
Tel Aviv, Israel
Staff Anesthesiologist
Department of Anesthesiology
Sheba Medical Center
Ramat-Gan, Israel

Arno L. Zaritsky, MD
Executive Medical Director
Children's Hospital of The King's Daughters
Norfolk, Virginia

R. Zafonte, DO
Physical Medicine & Rehabilitation
University of Pittsburgh Medical Center
Pittsburgh, Pennsylvania

Janice L. Zimmerman, MD
Head, Critical Care Division and Director, Medical ICU
Department of Medicine
The Methodist Hospital
Houston, Texas

Roberto T. Zori, MD
Professor
Division of Genetics and Metabolism (Department of Pediatrics)
University of Florida
Chief
Division of Genetics and Metabolism (Department of Pediatrics)
University of Florida
Gainesville, Florida

FOREWORD

The first edition of this textbook was published in 1988. The three of us (JMC, RWT, and RRK) requested Dr. Robert Zeppa, then Chairman of the Department of Surgery at the University of Miami, to draft the first Foreword. He did so in a succinct and beautifully articulated fashion, noting that Dr. Civetta was recruited in 1972 to manage the SICU at (then) Jackson Memorial Hospital. Dr. Zeppa's expressed purpose was to "provide a classroom for the teaching of applied pharmacology and abnormal physiology to house officers." Although this concept is well accepted nowadays, in many institutions during the 1970s and 1980s it was a radical departure from traditional care and was not always greeted with unbridled enthusiasm and good grace by other physicians. The synergy of the operating surgeons and the on-the-spot intensivists was effective in Miami and we believed that the model was worth promulgating for use elsewhere. The three of us became fast friends and colleagues. One of the results of these relationships was the publishing of *Critical Care*, an early attempt to meld the specialties of surgery, internal medicine, and anesthesiology into the still rather new specialty of critical care medicine. If anyone actually read it, we hoped that the collaborative model of critical care would also be fostered.

Four years later in 1992 we had been persuaded to publish a second edition of *Critical Care*. The second edition contained 1,998 pages compared to the first edition's 1,769 pages. Since the number of chapters was essentially the same, we liked to think that the extra 200+ pages represented an increase in knowledge concerning the topics covered. We wrote "that the revisions tended to provide greater documentation and less opinion, as if it took visualization as an actual textbook chapter to stimulate conversion from a personal, generalized manner of thinking to a more defined and documented presentation designed to impart information." Do we feel the same way today when electronic publishing supersedes much of the traditional textbook? We're not sure, but with the publishing of the fourth edition, we expect to find out!

In 1995 the publishers, pleased by the previous two editions we assumed, prevailed upon us to generate a third edition, which appeared two years later in 1997. This edition was dedicated by us to Dr. Zeppa who had died in 1993. We commented that "His visions and his love for patients, students, and residents will live on in the minds and memories of his disciples and associates." The book was one means by which this rather lofty goal might be achieved. The page count had increased to 2,363. We hoped that the additional pages reflected improved clinical applications of increased knowledge rather than superfluous verbiage.

In 2004, a fourth edition was requested, but this time we demurred and suggested that new editors would bring a fresh approach and an improved knowledge base compared to the old (literally and figuratively) editors. After a rather extensive search to find the best and the brightest, Drs. Mihae Yu, A. Joseph Layon, and Andrea Gabrielli were first recruited and then recommended enthusiastically by us. They were just as enthusiastically accepted by the publishers to plot the course of the new version. In keeping with the earlier editions, the specialties of surgery (Dr. Yu), internal medicine (Dr. Layon), and anesthesiology (Drs. Layon and Gabrielli) were once again represented. They have both kept the book the same (it is organized to help at the bedside right now) and radically revised it (new concepts, new chapters, and new authors). There are about 25 new chapters—reflecting the state of the world, not just the critical care world, today. Section XX contains four of the new chapters: Chapter 175, Mass Casualty Incidents: Organizational and Triage Management Issues Which Impact Critical Care; Chapter 176, Bioterrorism; Chapter 177, Emergent Pandemic Infections and Critical Care; and Chapter 178, Disaster Response. Half of the remaining chapters are totally new and almost all the rest (mostly those which must be there in every text, such as electrolytes, physiology of diseases of systems, shock and its subdivisions, and technical procedures) have new authors. The added authors range from well-known names who "own" the topic to the up-and-comers, whom we have always loved to choose. The chapters range from Chapter 12, The Virtual ICU and Telemedicine: Computers, Electronics, and Data Management; Chapter 133, High-Frequency Ventilation: Lessons Learned and Future Directions; and Chapter 4, Breaking Bad News to Patients; to Chapter 13, Universal Precautions: Protecting the Practitioner; Chapter 30, Intensive Care Unit Point of Care Testing; and Chapter 52, Gene Therapy in Critical Illness: Past Applications and Future Potential. In fact, there are only a few of the original chapters with the original authors, including Chapter 137, Extracorporeal Circulation for Respiratory or Cardiac Failure by Robert Bartlett, and Chapter 20, Bedside Assessment and Monitoring of Pulmonary Function and Power of Breathing in the Critically Ill by Michael J. Banner.

Suffice it to say, however, that our confidence in these editors and their accomplishments with the publishing of this edition knows no bounds. We look forward to reading all the new material with as much enthusiasm as we did our own earlier versions, perhaps even more so since we no longer will fear the possible slings and arrows of exuberant (read: outrageous) critics. We know these editors well, having worked with them and participated in their education in their formative years. They are superbly qualified to carry on the tradition of this publication. In nautical terms, we wish them fair winds and a following sea.

Joseph M. Civetta, MD
Robert W. Taylor, MD
Robert R. Kirby, MD

PREFACE

A preface is the remarks made before speaking or writing, from the Latin *prae*, in front of or before, and *far*, to say. It precedes or heralds whatever is coming—in this case, a book with 178 chapters. As such, it is our last chance to tell the readers the story behind this work.

First of all, without the help, guidance, forbearance, and pluck of Ms. Hope Olivo, whose full-time job as an Editor in the Department of Anesthesiology at the University of Florida College of Medicine is to help the likes of Doctor Gabrielli and me with our writing and pursuits in publications, our book might not have made it to the publisher.

Second, our colleagues at Lippincott Williams & Wilkins—Brian Brown, Nicole Dernoski, Rosanne Hallowell, Kathleen Brown, Angela Panetta, Teresa Mallon, and Larry Didona—and the production services group, Aptara—Max Leckrone and his associates-kept us on time (more or less) and provided us the encouragement needed as we headed into the last 5 miles of our marathon. Our colleagues and families have put up with us—quite an achievement and, for this, we thank them.

Third, as editors and writers, we tried to ensure that this book has an international flavor, which represents Critical Care Medicine today. As such, it is not an American book, but a text written by colleagues from throughout the world that deals with common issues, whether one practices in America, Asia, Europe, Antarctica, Africa, or Oceania.

Fourth, we have added a handful of new chapters to address additional issues: financing intensive care medicine, collaborative care, decision making, breaking bad news to our patients and their families, quality and safety in critical care medicine, computers and the remote intensive care unit, skin care and the prevention of pressure sores, genetics, pandemic infections, triage, disaster response, bioterrorism, and ethics, among others. Given our recent history, it is not by accident that the last two chapters are juxtaposed.

We wanted to provide for our colleagues an accessible, reader-friendly, and, as much as possible, a complete and up-to-date reference for the intensive care unit, although the readers need to keep in mind that Critical Care Medicine is a rapidly changing field as research gallops forward. It has been our intention that practitioners at various levels of training could use this book; whether we have succeeded will be judged by our readers.

In the last book by Nico Kazantzakis, *Report to Greco*, as the main character dies, he gives a summary of his life to his metaphorical grandfather, the painter, El Greco. His grandfather says to him, "Report!" And the character of the book says, "Grandfather, I have done what I can. I have done the best I can."

El Greco replies, "That is not good enough."

"Grandfather, I have done *more* than I could," says the main character. And with this, El Greco is satisfied.

You be the judge. Have we succeeded? Let us know.

Lastly, of course—as is often said and remains true—success has a thousand parents, failure only one. Whatever mistakes of omission or commission are found herein are ours and ours alone. We three editors share a friendship, have given each other guidance and moral support, and will share any failures and successes of our travail.

A. Joseph Layon
(layon@ufl.edu)
Gainesville, Florida

Andrea Gabrielli
(agabrielli@anest.ufl.edu)
Gainesville, Florida

Mihae Yu
(mihaey@hawaii.edu)
Honolulu, Hawaii

SECTION I ■ INTRODUCTION/GENERAL CONCEPTS

CHAPTER 1 ■ NATIONAL HEALTH SYSTEMS AND THE PLACE OF INTENSIVE CARE MEDICINE: WHICH MODEL?

HOWARD WAITZKIN • A. JOSEPH LAYON

INTRODUCTION

Barriers to access and the financial burden of health care, no longer problems in many economically developed nations, have emerged as major concerns in the United States. Over the past century, initiatives to resolve barriers to access, as well as legislative and administrative maneuvers to rein in cost, have failed. New investigative techniques in health services research, based largely on the cost-effectiveness model, have entered into the evaluation of technology and clinical practices, including those in critical care medicine. In this chapter we will place critical care in the context of the U.S. health system characterized—especially—by access and cost problems; offer an interpretation that traces problems of costs to underlying social contradictions and social structures within and outside the health system; and consider how these issues might change under varying models of a national health program.

While we provide a discussion of possible organizational and financing methods for a health system, the reader should understand that our viewpoint of a potentially optimal system is clearly expressed; while some of our colleagues will disagree with this view, we welcome the needed debate.

BARRIERS TO ACCESS: THE HUMAN EXPERIENCE

Barriers to health care access have become pervasive in the United States. These barriers not only prevent a sizeable number of our fellow citizens from receiving needed services—the number is approximately 57 to 59 million without access (1) at *some point* during a year (Fig. 1.1 and Table 1.1) and 47 million (16% of our population) without access throughout the year (2, 3)—but also impose fundamental ethical problems for physicians and other health workers who find themselves unable to solve problems that may lead to patients' morbidity or even mortality.

We will detail the global picture in a later section. However, below we wish to use the following summaries to depict the experiences of patients seen personally by one of us (HW), a practitioner of general internal medicine, and teacher of residents and students at community health centers and public hospitals. Although these examples do not comprehensively depict all the barriers to access that patients experience in the United States, they do give a human face to the troubling statistical data on access barriers. Some of the patients experienced problems that required critical care; others might well have required critical care if primary care practitioners had not intervened. The stories also provide a context for the policy analyses and recommendations for change that follow.

Fellow Citizens Suffering from Cutbacks and Increased Copayments under Medicaid

The first two patients illustrate problems of access for patients covered under Medicaid, the joint state–national program that aims to ensure access to care for eligible, low-income people. Medicaid covers individuals with dependent children, those who are disabled, and many people in nursing homes. To be eligible, a person must earn a monthly income falling below the level of poverty determined by state and federal governments.

- A 31-year-old diabetic and legally blind man began to experience severe unilateral headaches but could not afford a computed tomography (CT) scan of the head because his monthly deductible under Medicaid, which he was required to pay out of pocket each month, increased from $50 to $250. He later was brought delirious to the emergency room, where an emergency CT scan revealed a brain tumor with poor prognosis. After several days in the intensive care unit, he died. At his death, his physicians felt that the tumor may have been resected successfully if he had received attention earlier, when his severe headaches first began.
- A 56-year-old man with metastatic soft tissue sarcoma could not afford follow-up visits, medications, visiting nurse, or hospice, because his deductible under Medicaid had increased to $350 per month. This patient died in pain and without adequate nursing support in his home because of financial barriers.

Fellow Citizens Facing Restrictions due to Policies of a County-administered Medically Indigent Adult Program

The next group of patients did not receive needed care despite eligibility for medical benefits under the county government's

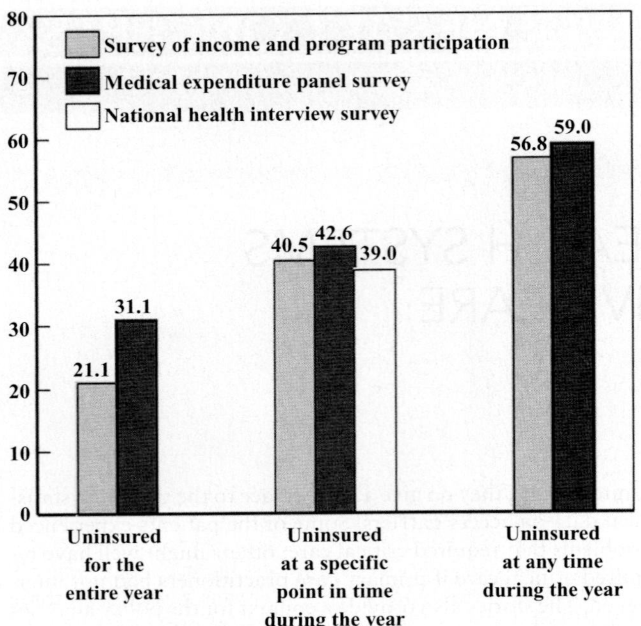

FIGURE 1.1. Estimated number of nonelderly people without health insurance at defined periods of 1998. Numbers in millions. Source: Congressional Budget Office.

program for medically indigent adults (MIAs). This program covers adults who are not eligible under the Medicaid program, but whose income is below the state-defined poverty limit. To reduce costs, many states decentralized MIA programs to county governments during the early 1980s. Counties vary widely in services provided and in copayments required from patients.

- A 63-year-old man with hypertension, renal insufficiency, and prostatic hypertrophy causing urinary obstruction could not gain approval from the county's MIA program for a prostatectomy, because it was considered an elective procedure. His urinary obstruction and renal function gradually worsened. Eventually, he was admitted to an intensive care unit with renal failure and severe hypertension. At that point, because he required dialysis, he became eligible for federal Medicare benefits. The very significant costs of dialysis—more than $100,000 per year—were likely avoidable had he been allowed to undergo the prostatectomy when initially indicated.
- A 52-year-old man developed unstable angina after a myocardial infarction, for which he was admitted to a coronary care unit. The MIA program disapproved funding for elective coronary angiography, even though national standards of cardiologic practice required its being performed under these circumstances.

Abandonment due to Inability to Pay

Many patients in the United States have established relationships with physicians who follow them for many years until, either because of job loss, a company's decision not to provide insurance as a fringe benefit, divorce or death of a spouse, geographic relocation, or other changes in circumstances, they lose their insurance. While some physicians will continue to care for a patient with whom they have an established relationship, others, at the time that their patient loses insurance, may decline to continue to follow the patient, because of the patient's inability to pay full fees. "Abandonment" is a legal principle, by which the physician is prevented from declining to see a patient whom he or she previously has followed unless a suitable substitute is arranged and the patient agrees to this arrangement (4). Nevertheless, neither governmental agencies nor professional organizations enforce these principles in cases when patients lose insurance.

TABLE 1.1

SOME CONSEQUENCES OF BEING UNINSURED IN THE UNITED STATES

Health care indicators for eight countries	Australia	Canada	France	Germany	Japan	New Zealand	United Kingdom	United States
Health expenditures per capita ($)	2,876	3,165	3,159	3,005	2,249	2,083	2,546	6,102
Life expectancy at age 60[a]	18.2	17.7	18.4	17.5	19.6	17.1	16.9	16.6
Deaths amenable to medical care/100,000 population	88	92	75	106	81	109	130	115
Access problems (%)[b]	34	26	n/a	28	n/a	38	13	51
Breast cancer 5-year survival (%)	80.0	82.0	79.7	78.0	79.0	79.0	80.0	88.9
Myocardial infarction 30-day hospital mortality (%)	8.8	12.0	8.0	11.9	10.3	10.9	11.0	14.8
Deaths from surgical or medical mishaps/100,000 population (2004)[a]	0.4	0.5	0.5	0.6	0.2	n/a	0.5	0.7

[a]Average of male and female healthy life expectancies. [b]Percentage of adults with health problems who did not fill prescription or skipped doses, had a medical problem but did not visit doctor, or skipped test, treatment, or follow-up in the past year because of costs.
From Davis K. Uninsured in America – Problems and possible solutions. *Br Med J*. 2007;334:346.

- A 63-year-old man with hypertension, renal insufficiency, and prostatic enlargement causing urinary obstruction, described above, had worked for many years as a custodian for a small health maintenance organization (HMO). While he worked there, one of the HMO's physicians saw him informally for his high blood pressure. Because the HMO did not provide health care as a fringe benefit for its own nonprofessional employees, these visits generally were provided as a free service by the physician, who believed that an employee with a major health problem should receive at least some needed care. After a cutback, however, the HMO laid off this patient from his job, and the physician decided that he no longer could justify offering free services. As a result, the patient spent several months with severe hypertension, until he could be seen at a local community health center.
- A 44-year-old unemployed woman was followed by her physician for about 8 years because of reflex sympathetic dystrophy, a very painful condition of her legs and feet that periodically required low doses of a narcotic and a tranquilizer for symptom relief. When the patient went through a divorce, she lost her husband's insurance coverage. Shortly thereafter, her long-time physician informed her that, because she now lacked insurance, he could no longer see her. Several months passed during which she could not receive needed treatment, until a physician at a community health center agreed to see her.

Treatment Delay because of Noninsured Status and Early Death

One of the most troubling effects of access barriers in the United States involves deaths that could be prevented if people were able to obtain required care. In our experience, such tragedies arise most commonly when patients cannot find appropriate services for the diagnosis and treatment of cancer. When symptoms of cancer arise, such patients experience critical delays, with a deleterious impact on the eventual outcome of their disease. Problems in cancer services arise for patients who face access barriers despite coverage by public insurance, as noted previously. Barriers become especially grim, however, when patients lack insurance altogether.

- A 48-year-old Japanese American woman ran her own small landscape gardening business. Because of the high cost of individual health insurance policies, she decided to remain uninsured. After noticing a breast lump, she delayed seeking care because she did not have a regular doctor and because she feared the expenses of care; she hoped the mass would disappear. When the mass continued to grow after 3 months, she began to seek care from private physicians, who declined to see her due to lack of insurance. After 6 months, she eventually was able to find care at a community health center. Evaluation for metastatic disease was arranged by special request with a nuclear medicine facility at a university hospital; without the personal intervention of her physicians and the donation of specialty services, the appropriate scan would not have been done. The scan revealed extensive metastatic cancer. Her chemotherapy also was delayed because of access barriers. At one point, she was admitted to an intensive care unit with life-threatening complications of metastatic cancer. Within 6 months, the patient died.

Lack of Medical Care to the Homeless Threatening the Health of the General Community

Other social problems in U.S. society heighten the impact of barriers to health care access; among these problems, homelessness is of great significance. Despite their poverty, homeless people experience difficulty in obtaining needed care under public insurance programs. For instance, many programs require an address to ensure that the expenses of care are assigned to the correct county or other governmental unit. Because they may not be able to provide an address, the homeless frequently cannot obtain public coverage. In addition, they tend to be more vulnerable to access barriers even when covered.

- A 38-year-old uninsured, homeless man was admitted to a university hospital from the emergency room because of active pulmonary tuberculosis. He had come to the emergency room because of hemoptysis. During a week of hospitalization, including 2 days in the medical intensive care unit because of respiratory insufficiency, he was treated with three antibiotics, until his sputum was free of organisms. Due to financial problems, the hospital recently had initiated a policy that outpatient prescriptions would not be filled unless they were paid for directly by the patient or were chargeable to public or private insurance. For this reason, the patient was asked to travel after discharge to the county health department for his outpatient prescriptions to continue necessary treatment for tuberculosis. However, the patient did not find transportation and consequently did not receive his outpatient medications. Four weeks later, he again developed bloody sputum and respiratory distress, and was readmitted to the intensive care unit for active tuberculosis; this time, his treatment became more complicated since he had developed a medication-resistant organism because of the interruption in antibiotics.

Undocumented Immigrants

Another patient group experiencing major barriers to access is undocumented immigrants, who are not covered under most public programs. These individuals contribute substantially to the economic productivity of the United States, especially in the Southwest and Southeast regions, and pay much more in taxes than they receive in public benefits (5). Although they tend to be healthier and to utilize health care services less than age-matched U.S. citizens (6), they have few options for care when ill.

- A 31-year-old undocumented man from Mexico presented with carpal tunnel syndrome of his right hand, interfering with his work as a tailor. He had worked and had taxes deducted from his pay at a local clothing factory for the past 18 years. Acromegaly associated with a pituitary tumor was diagnosed, but radiation therapy or neurosurgery could not be arranged because of financial impediments. After waiting nearly 3 months for care, the patient was lost to follow-up when he returned to Mexico.
- A 22-year-old undocumented woman from Mexico with systemic lupus erythematosus was admitted to the intensive care unit because of delirium associated with end-stage renal

failure and, after emergency dialysis, was stabilized. Hospital administrators decided not to permit long-term dialysis because of an anticipated cost of about $100,000 per year and the patient's lack of insurance. As a result, she was discharged from the hospital. Two weeks later she died at home.

The Working Poor

The following two patients show the special problems of working people who lose their insurance because of job loss. They also illustrate issues that are especially important for work in health services research and policy, described below.

- A 55-year-old man who served as office worker in a small horticultural company lost his job after 25 years with the same firm. One month later, he lost his health insurance, which had been provided as a fringe benefit of employment. After another month, he suddenly passed out and was taken to a county hospital's intensive care unit because his private physician refused to see him without insurance. Upper gastrointestinal hemorrhage from a bleeding duodenal ulcer, with resulting loss of consciousness, was diagnosed. After treatment with transfusions and medications, the patient slowly recovered. Nearly 1 year after losing his job, the patient found employment again as an office worker, received insurance coverage, and returned to his former physician for care.
- A 53-year-old woman, who had worked as a receptionist and clerical worker, was not working partly because of symptoms of pain and limited mobility associated with premature osteoporosis. She relied on the insurance coverage of her husband. About 3 months after he lost his job, she fell and fractured her forearm and wrist. Her private physician would not see her, due to lack of insurance coverage. She was taken to the county hospital, where resident physicians tried to realign the fractures, but she was left with a deformity.

These last two patients have been particularly influential for one of us (HW), as they were his parents. These individuals were proud people, who worked hard throughout their lives and were very reluctant to avail themselves of public welfare or insurance programs. As such, they viewed their problems as their own responsibility. At various times, they expressed the view that they somehow deserved the misfortunes that befell them, because they had not found a way to attend college during and after the Great Depression.

These cases illustrate two central themes regarding barriers to health care access in the United States. First, these barriers involve fundamental issues of personal dignity. The difficulties faced by each of these fellow humans degrade the individuals and families involved, at a time when they are most in need. Personal dignity requires more from social policy than we have yet achieved in the United States.

Second, such problems can happen to anyone, largely as a matter of bad luck. Severe illness, often requiring access to critical care medicine, can strike people who have lived their lives in accord with the mainstream standards of their communities. When misfortune arises, the United States does not provide a "safety net" ensuring access to basic medical services. Further, these problems do not only affect poor people and members of minority groups, although their impact is particularly severe for such individuals and families. Indeed, the barriers alluded to above—and detailed below—can exert unpredictable and devastating effects for a large part of the U.S. population, including a substantial part of the middle class.

THE NATIONAL PROBLEMS OF ACCESS AND COSTS

Having described barriers to access at the level of individual, flesh-and-blood patients who suffer from these problems, we now turn to the national level. The United States remains the only economically developed country in the world without a national health program that ensures universal access to health care services. Barriers to access and escalating costs of care have created a chronic crisis, which will continue as a target of policy during coming years.

Access

As of 2005, approximately 47 million people in the United States lacked health insurance (3). This number, representing about 16% of the population, has increased by more than 13 million persons during the past decade; most of the uninsured are working people (Fig. 1.2). Uninsured workers are spread across company size, as both large and small businesses frequently do not pay for health insurance as a fringe benefit of employment.

In addition to the uninsured, approximately 50 million people are underinsured (7). These are persons who, even though they hold health insurance policies, would be bankrupted by a major illness. Indeed, illness is currently the most frequent cause of personal bankruptcy in the United States (8). The underinsured include many elderly people, as well as a substantial part of the so-called middle class. For instance, Medicare pays for less than half of the medical expenses of senior citizens 65 years of age or older, and elderly people spend more money out of pocket on health care, in inflation-controlled dollars, than they did before the enactment of Medicare in 1965 (7). Many more millions of people cannot use their

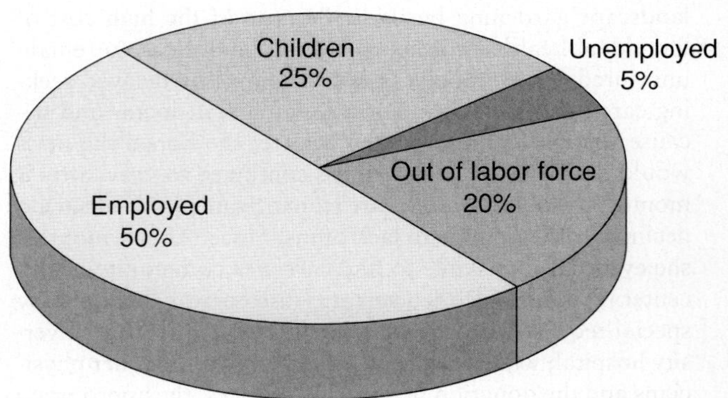

FIGURE 1.2. Who are the uninsured? Out of labor force = students older than 18 years, homemakers, the disabled, and early retirees. Source: Himmelstein DU, Woolhandler S. Available at: www.pnhp.org. Accessed March 15, 2007.

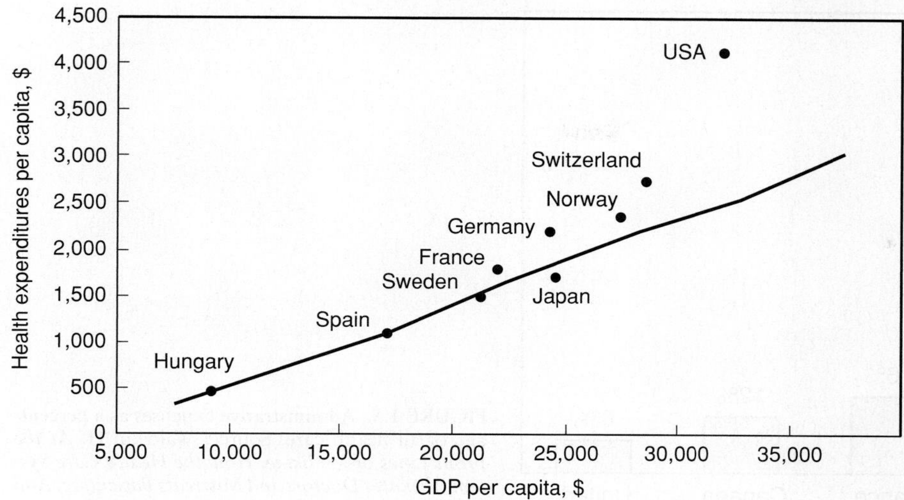

FIGURE 1.3. Health expenditures and gross domestic product (GDP) per capita, 1998. Source: Bodenheimer T. High and rising health care costs. Part 1: seeking an explanation. *Ann Intern Med.* 2005;142:84.

insurance because of copayments, deductibles, exclusions, or pre-existing medical conditions that disqualify them from coverage. U.S. private insurance ironically excludes those who need it most: People with pre-existing illness.

Public programs do not adequately protect people who experience such barriers. For example, the national Medicaid program, which was initiated to provide needed care for poor people, has proven insufficient and has deteriorated over time. States have varied widely in the proportion of the population below the poverty level who are covered by Medicaid, and on average the proportion of the poor population eligible for Medicaid benefits has declined markedly since 1980. Indeed, our own experience at public, state-supported teaching hospitals suggests that some states work very hard not to pay for the services their citizens need. For example, at the University of Florida Health Science Center, patients from southern Georgia—often covered by Georgia Medicaid—are cared for. Interestingly, the state of Georgia Medicaid office often will not only not pay for the services provided their citizens, but also will not take calls from the Faculty Group Practice—the billing arm of the medical school—to determine what needs be done so payment from Georgia will be made. Caught in the middle, as one might expect, are the children of Georgia whose medical care is provided by University of Florida physicians, and whose expenses are covered by Georgia Medicaid.

Costs

In spite of these access problems, the costs of health care in the United States have continued to grow. Uncontrolled costs have become the second major component of the nation's health crisis. In 2005, these costs totaled more than $2 trillion annual, or about 16% of the gross national product (9). Between 1985 and 1992, health spending grew exponentially, despite explicit policies to control costs, including the expansion of managed care, the initiation of Medicare's program of diagnosis-related groups, and the spread of mandated utilization review. Although costs to corporations that purchased health insurance for employees moderated during the mid-1990s, these costs began to increase again during the late 1990s; costs for consumers continued to rise, as corporate employers passed on a greater proportion of their costs to employees (10).

The costs of health care in the United States far exceed those of any other country. For instance, on both an absolute and per capita basis, the United States spends much more on health care than any of the economically developed nations of Europe, Canada, and Japan (Fig. 1.3). All these other countries, despite their lower health care costs, have initiated national health programs that provide universal access to needed services (11).

Although uncontrolled costs comprise a multifaceted problem, administrative waste deserves special emphasis (12). Figure 1.4 shows the growth of physicians and administrators in the U.S. health care system since 1970. As can be seen, administrators represent the fastest-growing sector of the health care labor force, expanding at three times the rate of physicians and other clinical personnel. The United States spends more on administration than any other economically developed country, with approximately 25% of health care costs going to this area. This figure compares unfavorably to all countries with national health programs, which spend between 6% and 14%

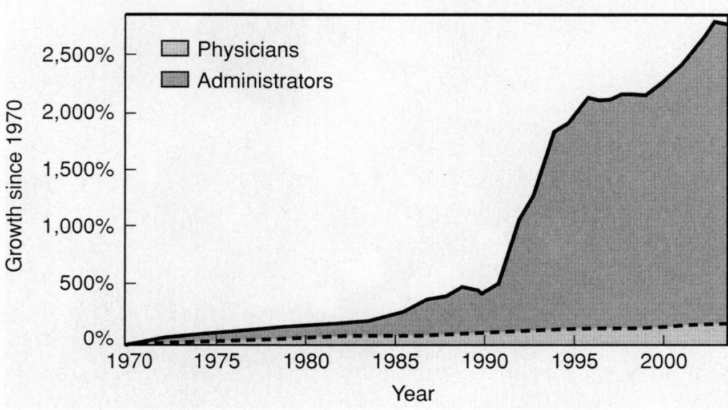

FIGURE 1.4. Growth of physicians and administrators, 1970–2004. Source: Himmelstein DU, Woolhandler S. Available at: www.pnhp.org. Accessed March 15, 2007.

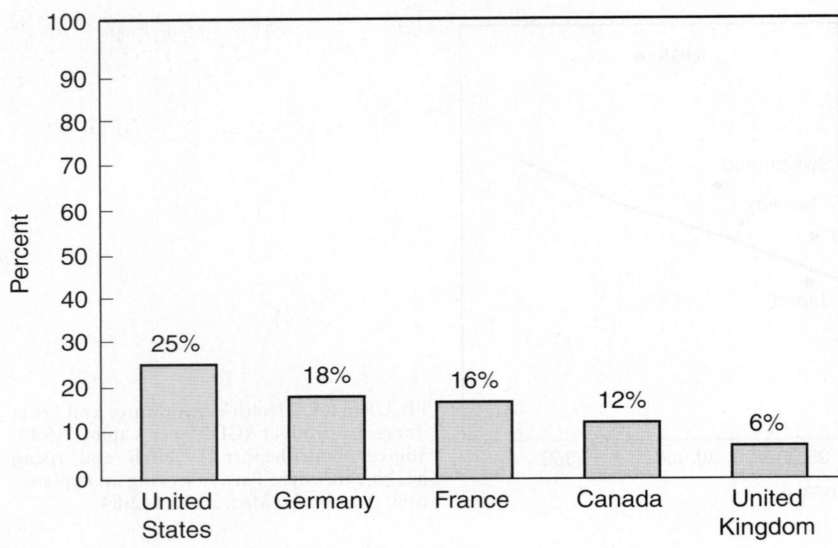

FIGURE 1.5. Administrative expenses as a percentage of all health care. Source: Waitzkin H. *At the Front Lines of Medicine: How the Health Care System Alienates Doctors and Mistreats Patients... And What We Can Do About It.* Lanham, MD: Rowman and Littlefield; 2004.

of health care costs on administration (Fig. 1.5). If the United States could reduce administrative spending to a proportion comparable to that of countries with national health programs, the savings—currently about 10% of total expenditures of $2 trillion, or about $200 billion—would be adequate to provide universal access to health services without additional spending (9,13).

How might administrative savings be achieved to help control costs? To answer this question, let us discuss the intensive care unit nurse shown in Figure 1.6. As judged by the spots on her uniform, this nurse suffers from a common hospital-acquired infection: "billing sticker-itis." These stickers come from the sources shown in Figure 1.7. In most U.S. hospitals, each intravenous line, each medication, each gown, each

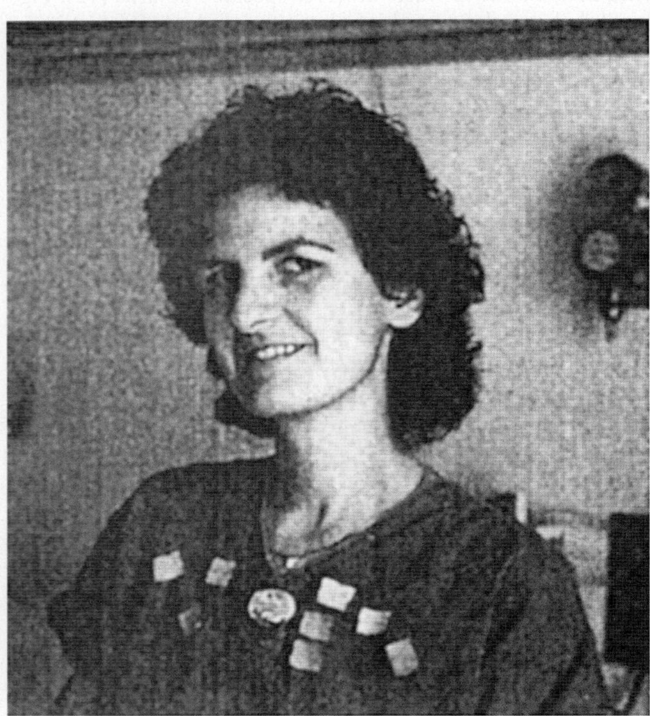

FIGURE 1.6. A nurse suffering from a hospital-acquired infection Source: Waitzkin H. *At the Front Lines of Medicine: How the Health Care System Alienates Doctors and Mistreats Patients... And What We Can Do About It.* Lanham, MD: Rowman and Littlefield; 2004.

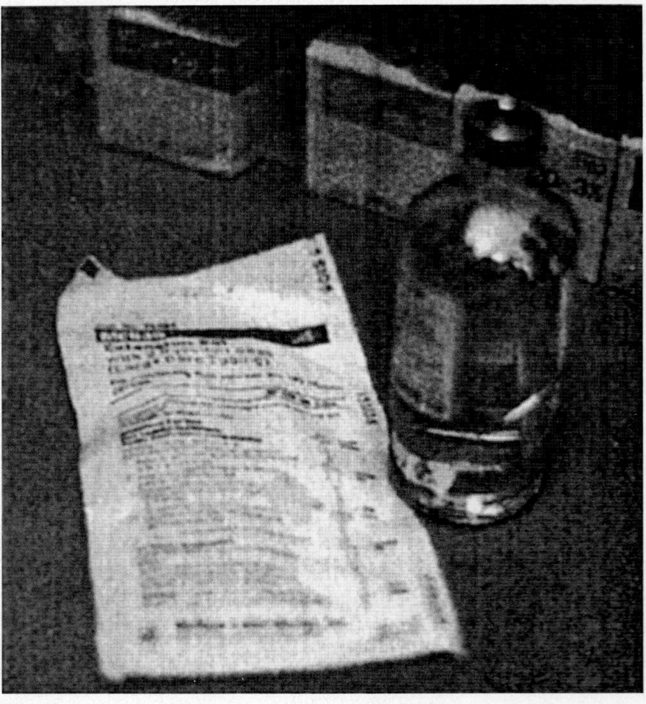

FIGURE 1.7. Source of the nurse's hospital-acquired infection, "billing sticker-itis." Source: Waitzkin H. *At the Front Lines of Medicine: How the Health Care System Alienates Doctors and Mistreats Patients... And What We Can Do About It.* Lanham, MD: Rowman and Littlefield; 2004.

surgical instrument, and each toothbrush has a billing sticker attached to it. A typical nurse like this one spends between 10% and 30% of his or her time gathering these stickers and on related administrative functions. The billing stickers are converted to cards or other pieces of paper and sent to the hospital's billing department, where—in a typical urban hospital—more than 100 employees computerize the charges and prepare separate bills for the more than 1,000 insurance companies that process private and public insurance claims. These companies differ widely in their reporting requirements, billing procedures, copayments, deductibles, exclusions, and other policies. Such different provisions greatly increase the administrative costs of submitting bills by hospitals and practitioners.

A national health program in the United States could drastically reduce such wasteful administrative practices by eliminating the need for billing in hospitals. As in Canada and several European countries, hospitals could be funded through global annual budgets negotiated with the national health program, rather than the present costly and cumbersome billing apparatus. From the standpoint of insurance companies, administrative overhead comprises a rapidly growing component of costs. Overall, insurance overhead has increased to 11.7%, as compared to about 1.3% in Canada (12).

An additional component of administrative waste arises from the intense marketing and advertising of medical products. U.S. pharmaceutical and supply firms annually spend more than $10 billion on advertising and "detailing" of drugs and other medical products; this figure exceeds the total costs for teaching medical students in the United States. Such promotional activities are intended to influence physicians' prescribing habits. Patients and/or insurers bear the costs of these promotional activities through higher than necessary drug prices. Again, such wasteful practices could be restricted under a national health program that would provide needed medications and supplies, but at a lower overall cost.

In summary, we face a cruel contradiction in the United States. On the one hand, at least a third of our population face barriers to health care access because of lack of insurance, underinsurance, or insurance that cannot be used to meet existing needs. On the other hand, we spend more money on health care than any other economically developed nation, and the costs of care continue to rise at a rate that threatens our economic security. Paradoxically, the numbers of uninsured in the United States have increased roughly in parallel to increases in spending.

THE FAILURE OF PAST POLICIES

At the heart of the health policy debate in the United States has been a very basic question: Is health care a basic human right, one that each of our citizens should have *simply because* they are citizens? Or should health care be treated like other commodities, such as cars, houses, and food—if one has the resources, one can obtain them; otherwise, one cannot? On the individual level is the issue of the inherent value of each person, and whether that value entitles one to health care. The concept of a right to needed services is not new to this country. For example, the constitutional right to legal representation guarantees that all individuals are entitled to basic services. However, the U.S. Constitution does not provide for a clear right to health care, in contrast to the constitutions of many other countries (14).

Policy Options

Competitive Strategies

Since the 1980s, competitive strategies have achieved prominence in health policy circles. Such proposals aim to foster competition among providers, and thus to lower costs (15). Competitive strategies culminated in "managed competition," a policy option favored initially by the Clinton Administration (1992–2000) and whose elements appear in many recent proposals for a national health program. The basic assumption is that, by allowing competitive forces of the market to control health care delivery, competitive policies would result in a high-quality, cost-effective system.

Competitive strategies have received major criticism. Forces of competition generally have not controlled health care costs, as illustrated by the rise in overall costs at a rate higher than general inflation and by higher costs in regions with greater competition among health care providers (16). Further, medical services have never shown the characteristics of a competitive market, since government pays for more than 40% of health care, and the insurance, pharmaceutical, and medical equipment industries all manifest monopolistic tendencies that inhibit competition. Hospitals and physicians maintain political–economic power through professional organizations that reduce the impact of competitive strategies. Physicians also affect the demand for services through recommendations about referrals, diagnostic studies, and treatment. Analytically, the effects of competition on costs are difficult to separate from other important changes, especially the effects of general inflation, the requirement of major copayments by patients, and the impact of prepayment. Additionally, competitive strategies do not curtail administrative waste, as noted above.

Such competitive strategies in public programs also have led to major dislocations and gaps in services (17). For example, competitive contracting and prospective reimbursement under Medicaid have worsened the financial crises of hospitals with a large proportion of indigent clients. The resultant disruption in services due to underfunding of Medicaid has led to a measurable worsening of some patients' medical conditions. In some states, competitive health plans have suffered severe and unpredicted financial problems, and patients have encountered major barriers to access, including direct refusal of care by providers.

Several ethical issues have also arisen with competitive strategies. On an individual level, autonomy may be compromised through elimination of a patient's free choice of physicians and hospitals. Increased out-of-pocket costs may further impair autonomy by restricting access to care, especially among the poor. A multitiered system remains in place, as the working poor and unemployed receive more limited coverage than the middle class, who receive care different from that received by the wealthy and our national elected officials.

Corporate Involvement in Health Care

Various policies have encouraged corporate expansion in the medical field. By the mid-1970s, private insurance companies, pharmaceutical firms, and medical equipment manufacturers had already achieved prominent positions in the medical marketplace. In the 1980s and 1990s, multinational corporations took over community hospitals in all regions of the country, acquired and/or managed many public hospitals, bought or built teaching hospitals affiliated with medical schools, and gained control of ambulatory care organizations (18).

Corporate profitability in health care has encountered few obstacles, despite declines in profit margins for some corporations during the late 1990s. For instance, in 2006, profits as a percentage of revenues for the seven largest pharmaceutical corporations were between 14% and 21%—the highest among U.S. industrial groups (19). Nationally, for-profit chains came to control about 15% of all hospitals, but in some states—for example, California, Florida, Tennessee, and Texas—the chains operate between one third and one half of hospitals. Ownership of nursing homes by corporate chains has increased by more than 30%. For-profit corporations have enrolled over 70% of all HMO subscribers throughout the country.

While proponents perceive several economic advantages of corporate involvement in health care, substantiation of such claims is limited. For example, it is argued that tough-minded managerial techniques increase efficiency, enhance quality, and decrease costs, although several studies have shown that for-profit health care organizations perform worse or no better on these criteria than nonprofit ones (20). Similarly, research on corporate management has not supported the claim that corporate takeover can alleviate the financial problems of hospitals serving indigent clients (7).

Corporate involvement in health care has also raised ethical questions. For instance, there is concern that corporate strategies lead to reduced services for the poor. While some corporations have established endowments for indigent care, the ability of such funds to ensure long-term access is doubtful, especially when cutbacks occur in public-sector support. Other ethical concerns have focused on physicians' conflicting loyalties to patients versus their corporate employers, the implications of physicians' referrals of patients for services to corporations in which the physicians hold financial interests, and the unwillingness of for-profit hospitals to provide unprofitable, but needed, services, such as trauma programs. Such observations lead to doubts about the wisdom of policies that encourage corporate penetration of health care.

Public-sector Programs

Policies enacted since 1980 have greatly reduced public-sector health programs. Cutbacks have occurred in the Medicaid and Medicare programs, block grants for maternal and child health, migrant health services, community health centers, birth control services, health planning, educational assistance for medical students and residents (affecting especially minority recruitment), the National Health Service Corps, the Indian Health Service, and the National Institute of Occupational Safety and Health. Many federally sponsored research programs have also been cut. During this same time period, some measures of health and well-being in the United States either stopped improving or actually became worse. For example, a marked slowing in the rate of decline in infant mortality coincided with cutbacks in federal prenatal and perinatal programs; indeed, in several low-income urban areas, infant mortality increased. Among African Americans, postneonatal and maternal mortality rates stopped falling after decades of steady decline, many African American women did not receive adequate prenatal care, and overall mortality rates for African Americans, especially men, remained much worse than those for Caucasians (7). These reversals in health status and health services, emerging as direct manifestations of changes in federal policies, have been unique among economically developed countries.

Alongside these programmatic cutbacks, bureaucratization and regulation in the health care system have grown rapidly. A distinction between the rhetoric of reduced government, versus the reality of greater government intervention, is nowhere clearer than in the Medicare diagnosis-related group (DRG) program. Intended as a cost-control device, DRGs introduced unprecedented complexity and bureaucratic regulation. By providing reimbursement to hospitals at a fixed rate for specific diagnoses, DRGs encouraged hospitals to limit the length of stay, as well as services provided during hospitalization. Hospitals responded to DRG regulations with an expansion of their own bureaucratic staffs and data-processing operations, more intensive utilization review, and a tendency to discharge patients with unstable conditions. Private hospitals admitting a small proportion of indigent patients profited under DRGs; public and university hospitals that served a higher percentage of indigent and multiproblem patients faced an unfavorable case mix within specific DRGs and, thus, fared poorly. The extensive utilization review that DRGs encouraged focused on cost cutting, rather than ensuring quality of care. Moreover, DRGs' contribution to cost control remained unclear, in comparison to other factors such as reduced inflation in the economy as a whole.

THE PLACE OF CRITICAL CARE MEDICINE IN A HEALTH SYSTEM

Any health system, however organized, will have need for subspecialty care, including critical care medicine services. Even in a system in which primary and preventive services are emphasized, there will be traumatic injuries, perforated colons, and massive hemorrhages resultant from surgical interventions, all requiring intensive care services. In the United States 27% of Medicare spending is for end-of-life care, and 46% of all Medicare charges occur in the last year of life, most in the last 60 days of life (21, 22). This is a significant portion of national health spending—encompassing about $91 billion in 2001 (0.9% of the gross domestic product) (23)—and one might ask if there is value generated by this spending.

While, in general, life-saving therapy costing less than or equal to US $100,000 per quality adjusted life year (QALY) saved is considered "cost effective" (i.e., is of "value"), there are some technical problems with this method of determining usefulness, or cost effectiveness of different therapies. For example, QALY is a mathematically derived *value* of the health-related quality of life during a given time period during which survival has occurred. One QALY may not be equal to another and, in fact, it has been suggested that this is not the case (24). When considering terminally or critically ill patients, cost per QALY may not be useful for several reasons: (a) in physician–patient interactions, decisions are not frequently made based on this parameter; (b) data and methodologic uncertainties inherent in the generation of this metric are not easily handled, making the analysis appear mathematically rigorous when it is in fact not; and (c) the metric does not answer the question of how one treatment compares with another (24).

Finally, although palliative care—as appropriate—has been suggested as a means to decrease the use of health resources, including use of critical care services, it appears that this would impact only about 10% of spending during the last year of life (22).

Thus, for better or for ill, in the system of care in the United States, 33% to 50% of individuals spend time in an intensive care unit (ICU) during their last year of life. Approximately 20% of those who die do so in an ICU. The use of ICU services incurs significant costs of between approximately $2,000 and $3,000 per day; this is about sixfold higher than a non-ICU day. Although the ICU accounts for only 8% of total hospital beds, 20% of hospital expenditures are incurred while patients are in the ICU (23, 25). While these numbers apply to the United States, other industrialized countries have similar issues, although ICUs may represent, in these countries, a smaller portion of the health system.

So if in any health system, no matter whether organized under capitalist (United States), social democratic (Norway), or socialist (Cuba) principles, ICUs will make up a component of the system, at least part of the duty of those in charge of these units must be to ensure that the social resources are efficiently utilized (23, 25). Table 1.2 details some of the techniques that may be put in place in an attempt to ensure the quality of ICU services. And how might we define *quality*? Simply put, the services provided are those that are needed; they are provided humanely; the services follow—at minimum—best practice, evidence-based medicine; the services utilized are provided with technical excellence; and, finally, the principle of the "commons"—that these resources are social and that they need be distributed with fairness—is observed. The fact that the health system of the United States is the most expensive of the industrialized countries, while ranking 37th in performance and 72nd in population health, is suggestive of what we ought to try to change (23). Figures 1.8 through 1.10 detail some of this information.

TABLE 1.2

PARAMETERS ENHANCING QUALITY OF INTENSIVE CARE UNIT (ICU) CARE

Open vs. closed ICU structure
24-h intensivist presence
Length of shifts for intensivists
Weekend cross-coverage by intensivists
Remotely located intensivist (telemedicine)
Length of shifts for house officers
Nighttime cross-coverage by house officers
Use of a daily goals sheet for each patient
Mobile ICU team to assess unstable ward patients
Formation of a ventilator team
Computerized nighttime cross-coverage signouts
Role of the ICU medical director
Availability of an intermediate care unit
Pharmacist participation in ICU rounds
Role of advanced nurse practitioners
Nurse/patient ratio
Supplying cost information to ordering physicians
Disallowing standing orders for diagnostic testing
Infection control processes
Automated early identification of clustered infections
Dissemination of clinical performance data
Family visiting hours
Palliative and end-of-life care
Nurse–physician communication and other aspects of ICU "culture"

From: Garland A. Improving the ICU—part 2. *Chest.* 2005;127: 2165–2179.

WHERE TO FROM HERE?

With increasing discontent among the general public and practitioners, health policy debates have taken on a certain urgency. While an ethical perspective tells us that basic health care for all is an individual right and a societal obligation, the burgeoning costs of the U.S. system hamper domestic economic growth and stability, and meanwhile, millions of people face major access barriers. Is there a better way to handle this problem? What are some of the models from which we might draw inspiration?

Change in health policies to address these problems doubtless will occur, but the specifics of change remain difficult to predict in the complex political terrain of the United States. The last part of this chapter examines local and national actions to correct the difficult problems of access and costs. There is no justification for the continuing and needless suffering experienced by human beings such as those whose stories are summarized earlier in this chapter. In this rich and powerful country, we deserve better.

Perspectives from Other Countries

Planning for a national health program in the United States requires open-minded consideration of the strengths and weaknesses of presently existing national health programs around the world. For instance, most countries in Western Europe and the Scandinavian area have initiated national health program structures, permitting private practice in addition to a strong public sector. Canada has achieved universal entitlement to health care through a national health program that depends on private practitioners, private hospitals, and strong planning and coordinating roles for the national and provincial governments. Thus, we must not condemn ourselves to the fallacy that thinking and planning for a national health care system must, by definition, remove some of what is most loved about our health system today: The intimate, one-on-one personal interaction between physician and patient.

National health programs vary widely in the degree to which the national government employs health professionals and owns health institutions. For example, the national health programs of the United Kingdom, Denmark, and the Netherlands[1] contract with self-employed general practitioners for primary care; Canadian private practitioners receive public insurance payments on a mainly fee-for-service basis; and in

[1] Although the Dutch have recently embarked upon a managed care system comprised of a partnership between the government and private insurance. See Enthoven AC: Going Dutch – Managed Competition Health Insurance in the Netherlands. *N Engl J Med.* 2007;357:2421.

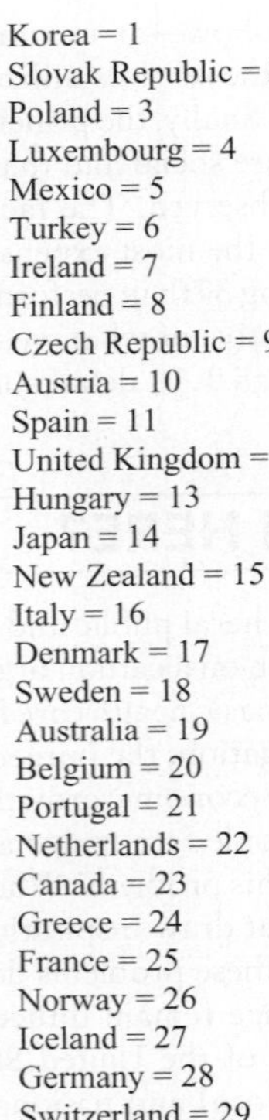

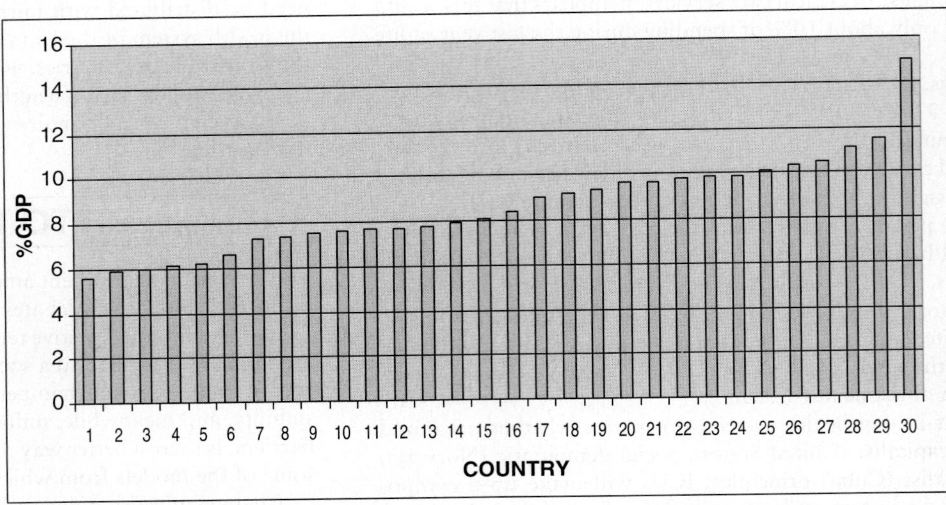

FIGURE 1.8. Percent gross domestic product (GDP) expended on health—world—2003. Source: www.irdes.fr/ecosante/OCDE/500.html.

Finland and Sweden a high proportion of practicing doctors work as salaried employees of government agencies. In the United Kingdom, the national government owns most hospitals; regional or local governments own many hospitals in Sweden, Finland, and other Scandinavian countries; and Canada's system depends on governmental budgeting for both public and private hospitals.

The Canadian system is very pertinent to the United States, because of geographic proximity and cultural similarity. Canada ensures universal entitlement to health services

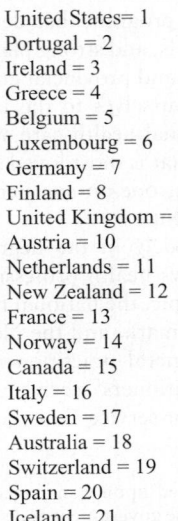

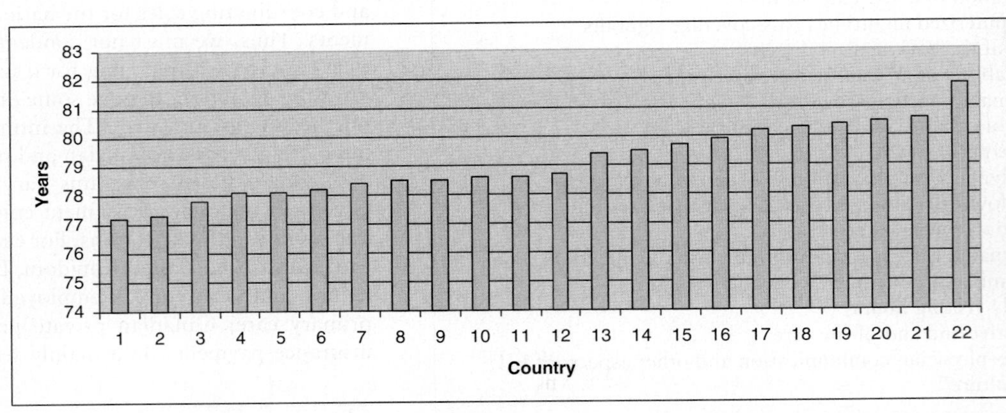

FIGURE 1.9. Life expectancy at birth—world. Source: www.irdes.fr/ecosante/OCDE/111000.html.

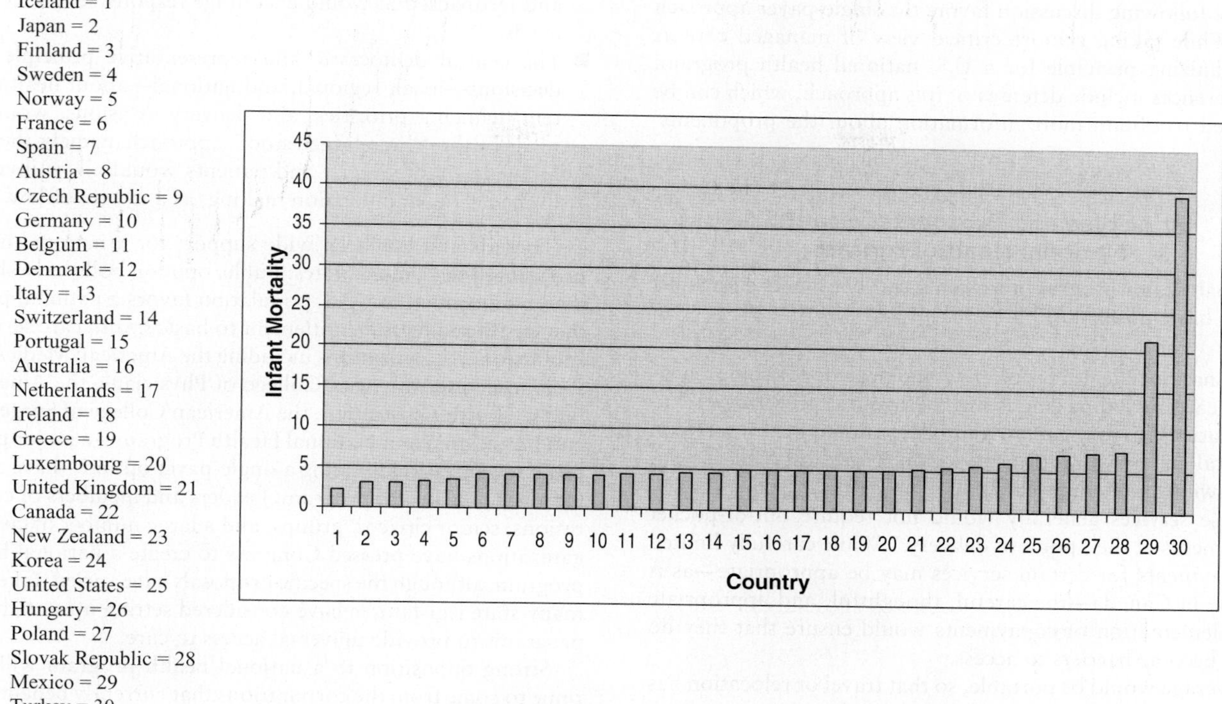

FIGURE 1.10. Infant mortality: Deaths per 1,000 live births—world—2002. Source: www.irdes.fr/ecosante/OCDE/500.html.

through a combination of national and provincial insurance programs. Doctors generally receive public insurance payments on a fee-for-service arrangement. Hospitals obtain public funds through prospectively negotiated contracts, eliminating the need to bill for specific services. Progressive taxation finances the Canadian system, and the private insurance industry does not play a major role in the program's administration. Most Canadian provinces have initiated policies that aim to correct remaining problems of access based on geographic maldistribution. Cost controls in Canada depend on contracted global budgeting with hospitals, limitations on reimbursements to practitioners—a policy that remains controversial for physicians in some provinces—and markedly lower administrative expenses because of reduced eligibility, billing, and collection procedures.

Because of the commonly expressed concern about costs in the United States, the experiences of existing national health programs are instructive. U.S. health care expenditures, already the highest in the world, account for approximately 16% of the gross domestic product. The presumption that a national health program would increase costs is not necessarily correct; depending on how it is organized, costs might well fall to below their prior level. First, a major savings would come from reduced administrative overhead for billing, collection procedures, eligibility determinations, and other bureaucratic functions that no longer would be necessary. In the Canadian national health program, for instance, global budgeting for hospitals has greatly reduced administrative costs, and a much smaller role for the private insurance industry has lowered costs even further by restricting corporate profit. A classic but still accurate analysis by the U.S. General Accounting Office showed that, due to savings from reduced administrative functions and entrepreneurialism, a single-payer national health program like Canada's, if introduced in the United States, would lead to negligible added costs despite achieving universal access to care (13).

A National Health Program for the United States

Because of the deepening crisis created by the problems of access and costs, both locally and nationally, a national health program for the United States has cycled on and off the policy agenda for many years. Unsuccessful proposals for such a program span three quarters of a century of U.S. history (26), so the pace of passage and implementation remains in doubt. During the first years of the Clinton Administration, another cycle of intense debate occurred, but proposals again suffered defeat. As a result, the United States remains the only economically developed country without a national health program that provides universal entitlement to health care services. Yet because the underlying problems of access and costs have persisted, and have actually continued to worsen in many respects, the need for a national health program still remains recognized by broad segments of the U.S. population.

Although policy debates change quickly and often focus on much more limited reforms, two options have remained as the most prominent proposals for a national program: Those based on managed care versus those based on a "single-payer" system modeled broadly along the lines of Canada's national health program. At the outset, we wish to make clear that one of us (HW) helped develop the single-payer proposal, and that the following discussion favors the single-payer approach (27). While taking a more critical view of managed care as an organizing principle for a U.S. national health program, the references include defenses of this approach, which can be reviewed to obtain more information about the proponents' views.

Principles and Prospects for a U.S. National Health Program

National health program proposals can be appraised against several basic principles:

- The national health program would provide for comprehensive care, including diagnostic, therapeutic, preventive, rehabilitative, environmental, and occupational health services; dental and eye care; transportation to medical facilities; social work; and counseling.
- These services generally would not require out-of-pocket payments at the "point of delivery." While carefully limited copayments for certain services may be appropriate—as is done in Canada—the careful, thoughtful, and appropriate implementation of copayments would ensure that they do not become barriers to access.
- Coverage would be portable, so that travel or relocation has no effect on a person's ability to obtain health care.
- Financing for the national health program would come from a variety of sources, including continued corporate taxation, "health taxes" on cigarettes and alcoholic beverages, "conservation taxes" on fossil fuels and other energy sources, "pollution taxes" on known sources of air and water pollution, and a restructured individual tax. Taxation would be progressive, in that individuals and corporations with higher incomes would pay taxes at a higher rate.
- The national health program would reduce administrative costs, private profit, and wasteful procedures in the health care system. A national commission would establish a generic formulary of approved drugs, devices, equipment, and supplies. A national trust fund would disburse payments to private and public health facilities through global and prospective budgeting. Profit to private insurance companies and other corporations would be closely restricted.
- Professional associations would negotiate the fee structures for health care practitioners regionally. Financial incentives would encourage cost-control measures through health maintenance organizations, community health centers, and a plurality of practice settings.
- To improve geographic maldistribution of health professionals, the national health program would subsidize education and training in return for required periods of service by medical graduates in underserved areas.
- The national health program would initiate programs of prevention that emphasize individual responsibility for health, risk reduction—including programs to reduce smoking, alcoholism, and substance abuse—nutrition, maternal and infant care, occupational and environmental health, long-term services for the elderly, and other efforts to promote health.
- Elected community representatives would work with providers' groups in local advisory councils. These councils would participate in quality assurance efforts, planning, and feedback that would encourage responsiveness to local needs.
- The central democratic and representative principle that decisions—local, regional, and national—about health system financing priorities, and delivery decisions, would be made by the "three-legged stool" approach; namely, the government, practitioners, and patients would all be involved in the debate and decision making, as a matter of law.

There is and has been wide support for a national health program in the United States. Public opinion polls have shown that a majority of the U.S. population favors a national policy that ensures universal entitlement to basic health care services. Professional organizations including the American Medical Association,[2] the American College of Physicians, the American Public Health Association, the American College of Surgeons,[3] and Physicians for a National Health Program—a major physicians' organization favoring a single-payer option—have called for a national health program. Leaders and members of corporations, senior citizens' groups, and a large number of civic organizations have pressed Congress to create a national health program, although the specific proposals have varied. Likewise, many state legislatures have considered setting up state health programs to provide universal access to care.

Strong opposition to a national health program will continue to come from the corporations that currently benefit from the lack of an appropriate national policy: The private insurance industry, pharmaceutical and medical equipment firms, and the for-profit health care chains. While corporate resistance should not be underestimated, there is also support for a national health program from the corporate world. The costs of private sector medicine have become a major burden to many nonmedical companies that provide health insurance as a fringe benefit to employees. Corporations that do not directly profit from health care have influenced public policy in the direction of cost containment. In Canada, Western Europe, and Scandinavia, corporations have come to look kindly on the cost controls and services that national health programs provide, even when corporate taxation contributes to the programs' financing.

A National Health Program Based on Managed Care

Proposals for managed care as the basis of a national health program have been complex and have changed over time. The Clinton Administration presented a lengthy proposal that received wide attention during the mid-1990s but was ultimately defeated by a broad coalition of interest groups. Although Clinton did not pursue this proposal in the later years of his

[2]However, the "prescription made by the AMA" consists of a series of relatively standard approaches, including relying on incentives and voluntary approaches; building upon the employer-based system and not weakening incentives for employers to offer coverage; using a combination of public and private approaches to expand coverage; recognizing the budget challenges facing most states; and recognizing the importance of consumer outreach and education on health coverage options. A single-payer plan is explicitly excluded by this branch of organized medicine. See http://www.ama-assn.org/ama1/pub/upload/mm/450/hccu-final.pdf.

[3]The American College of Surgeons stated that the single-payor approaches probably provide the best assurance that patients would be able to seek care from the physician of their choice. Russell TR. From my perspective. *Bull Am Coll Surg.* 2003;88:3–4.

presidency, its framework has remained the basis of other proposals, and the managed care approach likely will persist in future proposals. For instance, elements of the managed care approach appeared in the proposals of candidates entering the 2008 presidential campaign. Our purpose here is to summarize the key features of managed care as the central principle of a national health program and some of the concerns that have been raised about this approach.

Managed care, although difficult to define simply since it encompasses diverse organizational structures, generally refers to administrative control over the organization and practice of health services, through large corporate entities. Historically, managed care has included such prepaid approaches as HMOs, preferred provider organizations (PPOs), and proposals for national programs organized on principles of administrative control and market competition. Managed care assumes that quality of care is ensured through administrative control and through competition in the marketplace.

The first proposals for a national health program based on managed care appeared during the 1970s. In 1977, Alain Enthoven, an economist whose prior career had focused on military policy analysis at the U.S. Department of Defense and corporations serving as military contractors, offered to the Carter Administration a proposal for a "Consumer Choice Health Plan," based on "regulated competition in the private sector." This proposal was built in part on prior initiatives by Paul Ellwood for a national "health maintenance strategy" and by Scott Fleming for "structured competition within the private sector" (28). Although Carter rejected the plan, Enthoven soon afterward published the proposal in the medical literature (29) and in a separate monograph (30). This plan, which presented the basic conceptual structure of all subsequent proposals for national health programs based on managed care, contained important concepts from the military policy work that Enthoven had spearheaded a few years earlier at the Pentagon (31).

During the 1980s, Enthoven collaborated with Ellwood, other proponents of HMOs, corporate executives, and officers of private insurance companies in developing refinements of the proposal. An emphasis on "managed competition" arose during the mid-1980s, in response to concerns raised by economists and business leaders that the original proposal conveyed free-market assumptions requiring modification through closer "management" of the program (32). After publication of a revised proposal in 1989 (33), the coalition supporting managed competition broadened to include officials of the largest U.S. private insurance companies that were diversifying into managed care. These business leaders entered into continuing meetings with Enthoven and other proponents of managed competition at Ellwood's Wyoming home, as part of the so-called "Jackson Hole group." The managed care sector of the private insurance industry provided major funding for the Jackson Hole group, as well as financial and logistic support for the Clinton presidential campaign and consultation for the Presidential Health Care Task Force.

Although most proposals for managed competition have emerged from this intellectual tradition, certain proposals have suggested modifications in the conceptual structure outlined by Enthoven and colleagues. For instance, although managed competition traditionally has encouraged employer-sponsored plans with participation by private insurance companies, other proposals have separated employment from insurance through the creation of a single, tax-financed, globally budgeted public fund, which would contract with private plans for a minimum benefit package (34). All managed competition proposals, however, incorporate concepts initiated by Enthoven and colleagues, and all of them call for large-scale changes in how professionals practice medicine, and how physicians and consumers make choices.

There are four essential features of managed competition. The first element involves large organizations of health care providers. As described in the Clinton proposal, these "accountable health partnerships" (AHPs) are large, integrated organizations of insurers and providers that would offer health plans competitively. Large businesses would participate in these partnerships. The AHPs would operate much as do current managed care organizations (MCOs) and would drastically reduce medical practice based on fee-for-service reimbursement. Instead, physicians and hospitals would be largely absorbed into MCOs. In principle, this shift in the organization of medical practice would allow more stringent management of practice conditions by high-level managers, whose responsibility would be to control costly and potentially self-interested actions by physicians and hospitals.

A second major element of the proposal involves large organizations of purchasers. The Clinton proposal referred to these organizations as "health insurance purchasing cooperatives" (HPICs); similar proposals have used somewhat different terminology. Such organizational purchasers would buy health plans from the large organizations of health care providers (AHPs in the Clinton plan). Organized mainly by state governments, these large purchasers would represent small employers and individuals, including both self-employed and unemployed people. In theory, these large, "intelligent purchasers" would make informed decisions about costs and quality of services. Under managed competition, Medicaid and possibly Medicare eventually would be privatized and converted to sponsorship by state-organized purchasers.

A uniform benefits package, referred to as "uniform effective health benefits" (UEHBs) in the Clinton proposal, is the third essential component of a national health program based on managed care. This benefits package would be extended to the entire population. An appointed national health board would define the minimum benefits contained in the package. This board's decisions about coverage would rely mainly on research about the outcomes and effectiveness of health services.

Tax code changes comprise the fourth essential element of a national health program based on managed care. These changes would restrict the ability of corporations and individuals to claim tax deductions for health care expenditures. Specifically, corporations and individuals could not claim tax deductions for coverage that exceeds the basic coverage provided by the minimum benefits package. Although corporations and individuals could buy additional coverage without tax deductions, these changes in tax code would provide incentives to purchase less expensive coverage overall.

Advocates of a managed care approach to a national health program claim several advantages of this approach. First, it would expand access to health services while still preserving a major role for the private insurance industry. Insurance companies, for instance, could run large managed care programs as fundamental parts of AHPs. As a result, this approach would create less drastic changes in the U.S. health system than a single-payer plan and thus, proponents argue, would stand a better chance of passage in Congress. Because managed care would rely on market forces for cost containment, according to advocates, it would prove more consistent with mainstream political and economic values. Competition, from this view, would lead to improved quality, since managed care plans would have to compete with one another for patients. In selecting among competitive plans, consumers also would need to become more informed about cost-effective care, partly because they would be required to pay copayments for most services.

Several unknowns have persisted in such proposals, and the Congressional debate on the Clinton Administration proposal was unable to fully clarify these issues. The extent of the basic benefits to be covered under a national program remained to be worked out. Details of how a national program based on managed care would be financed, in particular the tax increases to be borne by families and corporations, were not clearly specified. This latter question about the specifics of projected tax code changes, of course, was important, since estimates of the additional costs of a national health program based on managed care ranged from $30 billion to $100 billion per year. Whether overall health care expenditures would be capped through a global budgeting mechanism remained ambiguous. How transition would occur from the present system was not clarified. Further, the degree to which state governments would enjoy flexibility to enact varying forms of coverage and organization remained under debate.

Both supporters and opponents have raised major concerns about managed care as the basis of a national health program. Demographic limitations would restrict its impact, since about 30% of the U.S. population live outside metropolitan areas that could support three or more competing managed care plans. Proponents of managed care have emphasized these demographic limitations to the success of a national health program based on managed care principles (35). Whether managed care could control costs remains unclear; states with the most extensive managed care programs have shown costs as high, or higher, than elsewhere. Administrative costs, already more than 25% of overall health care expenditures, likely would increase still further, since managed care is administratively intensive and new organizational sponsors would introduce additional managerial layers. Despite intent to use research on effectiveness and outcomes to define the uniform minimum benefits package and to assess quality of care, such research has produced verified data about only a small number of medical conditions and procedures.

Several practical questions also have arisen concerning acceptability of a national health program based on managed care to providers and consumers. While expanding the decision-making power of large insurance companies, such a program probably would reduce consumers' freedom to choose practitioners, and micromanagement of clinical decisions likely would increase. Because the ability to buy additional coverage beyond the basic benefits package would depend on income, this provision would perpetuate unequal, multitiered coverage. Whether a national program would succeed in curbing insurance companies' selection or exclusion of patients by risk of costly illness remains in doubt. Managed care likely would create higher out-of-pocket payments and taxes for a substantial part of the population who currently are insured. Furthermore, several polls have shown less public support for managed care as a basis for a national health program than for other alternatives. Evidence that managed care would solve the access problem while controlling costs remains uncertain. Importantly, it is not clear whether a national health program could address successfully the problems and tensions that managed care has introduced into the patient–doctor relationship.

Finally, the place of academic medicine, especially in the context of continuous and ongoing funding needed for education, research, and quality improvement, is unclear in this system.

We look to our system of university-based health science centers not just for scientific and technical advances, but for the creation of the next generation of practitioners: Physicians, nurses, respiratory therapists, occupational and physical therapists, laboratory technicians, and so forth. How will the alteration in funding impact the education of these individuals? How will the altered organization of health care affect the already precarious financial position of the academic medical center? Such questions remained unanswered under managed care proposals for a national health program.

The powerful coalition built up around managed care as the basis for a national program did not succeed in enacting this policy. Although it addressed some of the concerns raised about managed care, the Clinton team did not agree to change the basic structure of the proposal. This reluctance to consider other options seriously may have stemmed partly from the support that the Clinton campaign received from the managed care sector of the private insurance industry, as well as a perception that simpler and more popular options, including a single-payer approach, were unlikely to pass Congress.

Failure to achieve a workable national health program generated great disappointment, as well as financial waste. Some analysts believed that failure of managed care was a necessary step toward adoption of a simpler approach such as a single-payer option. A less sanguine view holds that the Clinton failure led to retrenchment, cutbacks, and reinforcement for the paradox of pervasive access barriers coupled with high costs.

A Single-payer National Health Program

This option would provide universal entitlement to needed health care while controlling costs through a single-payer financing system. A single-payer, or "monopsony," financial structure has achieved substantial savings by reducing administrative waste in the national health programs of Canada, Sweden, and Australia. While none of these programs is without problems, all have minimized barriers to access while controlling costs.

The following features of a single-payer option are based on the proposals of Physicians for a National Health Program (PNHP), of which one of us (HW) is a founding member. The summary provided here leaves out details contained in national publications to which many colleagues have contributed (28, 36–38). From its initiation in 1985, PNHP has grown as a national organization to include more than 13,000 members, who are physicians and other health professionals spanning all specialties, states, age groups, and practice settings. Participants in PNHP have come together with a common perception that the problems of access and costs are intolerable and a belief that a single-payer national health program will remove barriers to access while controlling costs. Although supported by a substantial proportion of the U.S. population in polls, a

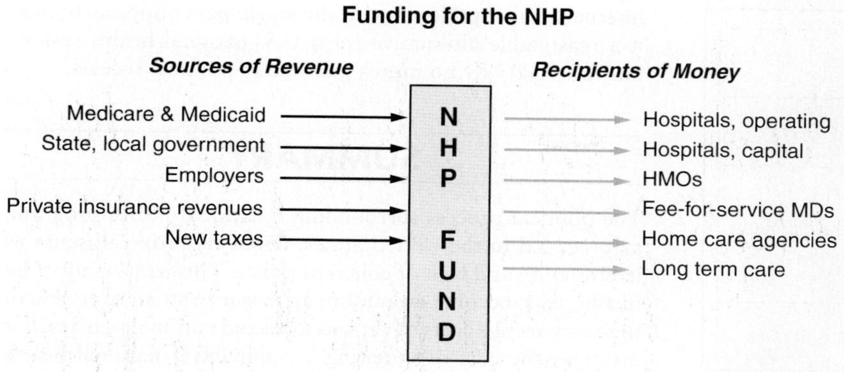

Funding for the NHP

Sources of Revenue		*Recipients of Money*
Medicare & Medicaid →	N	→ Hospitals, operating
State, local government →	H	→ Hospitals, capital
Employers →	P	→ HMOs
Private insurance revenues →		→ Fee-for-service MDs
New taxes →	F	→ Home care agencies
	U	→ Long term care
	N	
	D	

FIGURE 1.11. Funding for a national health program (NHP) under the single-payer proposal. HMO, health maintenance organizations.

single-payer system was not the option proposed by the Clinton Administration. On the other hand, a single-payer approach did emerge as one of the two options for a national health program under consideration in the U.S. Congress.

Coverage under the single-payer proposal would be universal—everyone would be covered. The national health program would provide comprehensive coverage for all medically necessary care, including long-term care. Under this plan, there would be no out-of-pocket costs or copayments for needed services. Copayments are not preferred since they have been found to be substantial disincentives to needed care among low-income patients. Further, copayments would not be necessary because costs would be controlled by a single, publicly financed plan that would greatly curtail administrative waste and would achieve cost reductions through monopsony financing. A single-payer national health program would eliminate competing private insurance. This approach would facilitate cost control and would discourage multiple tiers of care for different income groups, but of course would engender opposition from the wealthy and powerful private insurance industry.

Under a single-payer national health program, hospitals would receive payment through a global budgeting system. The very costly billing apparatus, which is responsible for unnecessary administrative costs in hospitals under the present system, would be eliminated. Instead, hospitals would negotiate an annual global budget for all operating costs. It is important to note that hospitals would remain privately owned and run, rather than becoming part of a nationalized ownership structure. To reduce overlapping and duplicative facilities that increase overall costs, capital purchases and expansion would be budgeted separately, based on regional health planning goals. Regional health planning boards, with members elected by consumers and providers, would make these decisions about capital expenditures and expansion.

The national health program would collect and disburse virtually all payments for health services (Fig. 1.11). This single-payer structure would provide the major overall source of cost control. Total expenditures would be capped at the proportion of the gross domestic product spent for health services during the year prior to implementation of the national health program. Initially, during a transition period of approximately 3 years, funding would come from existing sources to minimize economic disruption: Medicare and Medicaid, state and local governments, employers, and private insurance premiums. After the transition period, the collection of payments would be converted to a simplified process based on taxation, in which the average company, individual, and family would pay approximately the same in taxes as was previously paid in insurance premiums, deductibles, copayments, and other out-of-pocket spending.[4] The national health program would distribute payments for services to hospitals, MCOs, physicians, home care agencies, and long-term care agencies.

Payment for physicians and ambulatory care would occur under one of three options. First, physicians could choose to be paid on a fee-for-services basis. Under this option, state medical associations would negotiate a simplified fee schedule for the range of covered services; practitioners would accept fees as payment in full and would not bill patients separately, except for a small number of uncovered services such as purely cosmetic surgery. As a second option, the national health program would provide capitation payments to MCOs employing salaried physicians. However, provisions of this option would protect against possible abuses seen under prior managed care programs; for instance, free disenrollment privileges would be required, and MCOs would be prohibited from selective enrollment of healthier patients. Capitation fees would cover operating costs only, rather than capital purchases, profits, or physician incentives. Under the capitation option, global budgeting would apply to inpatient care. The third option for physician payment would involve salaries received from globally budgeted institutions, such as hospitals, community clinics, and home care agencies.

The national health program would cover all needed drugs and medical supplies. An expert board would develop a national formulary based on principles of generic drug substitution and assurance of high standards of biologic quality. As far as possible, reimbursement procedures would encourage the use of less expensive generic alternatives. This provision would reduce the excessive costs incurred from the promotion and detailing of new drugs without greater demonstrated efficacy than less expensive formulations.

How would the national health program look from the patient's point of view? First, universal access to comprehensive care would remove barriers to access. There would be no out-of-pocket costs, and patients would have free choice of doctors and hospitals. Hassles in using and processing private or public insurance would be reduced through the implementation of a single program for everyone.

From the practitioner's point of view, conditions of practice would improve considerably, especially because the wallet

[4]A PNHP publication provides further details about these financing mechanisms (37).

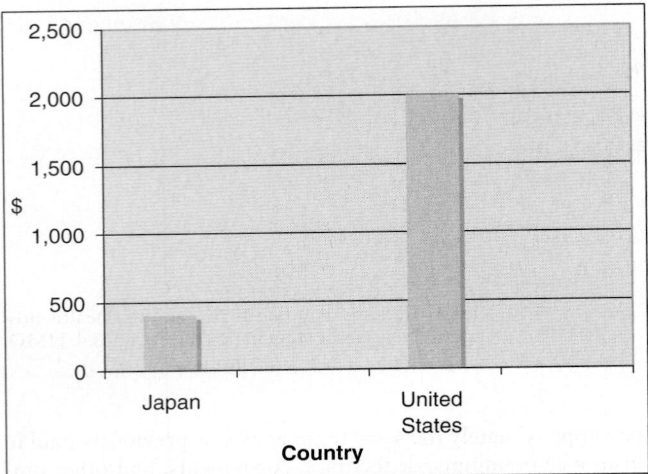

FIGURE 1.12. Cost of health insurance in a new car, by country of production. Source: Waitzkin H. *At the Front Lines of Medicine: How the Health Care System Alienates Doctors and Mistreats Patients... And What We Can Do About It.* Lanham, MD: Rowman and Littlefield; 2004.

biopsy—that emotionally and ethically degrading procedure that physicians often must use before deciding how to diagnose or treat a patient—no longer would be necessary. Instead, the national health program would cover fully all needed services. Doctors would most likely experience greater clinical freedom and less intrusive micromanagement by administrators. In addition, physicians would be free to choose from a variety of practice settings. Overall, there would be little change in anticipated income; as in Canada, practitioners in the primary care specialties could anticipate equal or somewhat greater earnings than previously, and only the highest paid surgical subspecialists could expect to see a fall in income.

From the corporate viewpoint, companies would experience stabilization in costs of health care. Those corporations that currently provide health insurance as a fringe benefit of employment likely will see a reduction in health care expenses; projections for automobile manufacturers like Ford or Chrysler indicate that costs will decline more than $4,000 per employee per year. Companies that do not currently provide health insurance as a fringe benefit will experience higher costs, but the single-payer national health program will provide subsidies for small businesses that are at greatest financial risk. Economic competitiveness of U.S. corporations overall will increase, since companies will incur health care costs more in line with those of their international competitors. Figure 1.12 depicts the international disadvantage for U.S. automakers, which spend much more per car on health care than do their competitors in countries with national health programs.

In summary, a single-payer national health program would provide universal, comprehensive coverage, without out-of-pocket payments. Hospitals would be paid a global, "lump sum" operating budget, to be negotiated annually. Capital budgets for hospitals would be negotiated based on regional health planning goals. Physicians and ambulatory care would be paid through one of three options: Fee for service, capitation in HMOs, or salary in globally budgeted institutions. A single, public payer would control costs and achieve public accountability while minimizing administrative waste. Simplicity and international experience with the single-payer approach make it a reasonable alternative for a U.S. national health system, but rationality by no means guarantees political success.

SUMMARY

The political process surrounding a national health program, as practiced in the United States, conveys an overall sense of irrationality and lack of coherent policy. This irrationality and incoherence become even more apparent from an overview of the comparative costs of various local and national policies. For instance, the cost of initiating a single-payer national health program that would solve the access problem while controlling costs would consume very little additional expenditures, certainly an order of magnitude less than current expenditures on possibly outdated or unnecessary military systems like the Stealth bomber, as well as public support of the private financial sector in such efforts as savings and loan bailouts. On the other hand, as estimated by the U.S. Congressional Budget Office, a national health program based on managed care would represent a substantial increase in expenditures, on the order of $80 billion per year (39).

For better or worse, the lack of a national health program will continue to plague the United States. Patients and practitioners, including those who specialize in critical care medicine, will continue to experience this unpleasant reality until we, as a country, finally correct the problem through concerted action. The chronic crisis of U.S. health policy gives reasons for pessimism but also clarifies some of the opportunities that await us in trying to construct a more humane society and a more humane health care system.

References

1. Congressional Budget Office. *How Many People Lack Insurance and for How Long?* Washington, DC: Congressional Budget Office; 2003.
2. DeNavas-Walt C, Proctor BD, Lee CH. U.S. Census Bureau: Current Population Reports. In: *Income, Poverty, and Health Insurance Coverage in the United States: 2005.* Washington, DC: U.S. Government Printing Office; 2006.
3. Davis K. Uninsured in America—problems and possible solutions. *Br Med J.* 2007;334:346.
4. American Medical Association. Ending the patient-physician relationship. Available at: http://www.ama-assn.org/ama/pub/category/4609.html. Accessed March 13, 2007.
5. Berk ML, Schur CL, Chavez LR, et al. Health care use among undocumented Latino immigrants. *Health Aff (Millwood).* 2000;19:51.
6. Goldman DP, Smith JP, Sood N. Immigrants and the cost of medical care. *Health Aff (Millwood).* 2006;25:17
7. Waitzkin H. *At the Front Lines of Medicine: How the Health Care System Alienates Doctors and Mistreats Patients... And What We Can Do About It.* Lanham, MD: Rowman and Littlefield; 2004.
8. Himmelstein DU, Warren E, Thorne D, et al. Illness and injury as contributors to bankruptcy. *Health Aff (Millwood).* 2005;Suppl Web Exclusives:W5-63-W5-73.
9. Centers for Medicare and Medicaid Services. National health expenditure data. Available at: http://www.cms.hhs.gov/NationalHealthExpendData/02_NationalHealthAccountsHistorical.asp. Accessed March 31, 2007.
10. Kuttner R. The American health care system: health insurance coverage. *N Engl J Med.* 1999:340.
11. Bodenheimer T. High and rising health care costs. Part 1: seeking an explanation. *Ann Intern Med.* 2005;142:84.
12. Woolhandler S, Campbell T, Himmelstein DU. Costs of health care administration in the United States and Canada. *N Engl J Med.* 2003;349:768.
13. U.S. General Accounting Office. *Canadian Health Insurance: Lessons for the United States.* Washington, DC: Government Printing Office (GAO Publ. No. GAO/HRD-91-90; B-244081); 1991.

14. Fuenzalida-Puelma HL, Hernán L, Connor SS. *The Right to Health in the Americas: A Comparative Constitutional Study.* Washington, DC: Pan American Health Organization; 1989.
15. Enthoven A, Kronick R. Universal health insurance through incentives reform. *JAMA.* 1991;265:2532.
16. Robinson JC. Consolidation and the transformation of competition in health insurance. *Health Aff (Millwood).* 2004;23:11.
17. Waitzkin H, Schillaci M, Willging CE. Multi-method evaluation of health policy change: An application to Medicaid managed care in a rural state. *Health Services Research.* 2008; in press.
18. Callahan D, Wasunna AA. *Medicine and the Market: Equity v. Choice.* Baltimore: Johns Hopkins University Press; 2006.
19. Fortune 500 ranking of America's largest corporations, 2006. Available at: http://money.cnn.com/magazines/fortune/fortune500/industries/Pharmaceuticals/2.html. Accessed March 31, 2007.
20. McCormick D, Himmelstein DU, Woolhandler S, et al. Relationship between low quality-of-care scores and HMOs' subsequent public disclosure of quality-of-care scores. *JAMA.* 2002;288:1484.
21. Pronovost P, Angus DC. Economics of end-of-life care in the intensive care unit. *Crit Care Med.* 2001;29(Suppl):N46–N51.
22. Emanuel EJ. Cost savings at the end of life—what do the data show? *JAMA.* 1996;275:1907–1914.
23. Garland A. Improving the ICU—part 1. *Chest.* 2005;127:2151–2164.
24. Eccles M, Mason J. How to develop cost-conscious guidelines. *Health Technol Assess.* 2001;5:16.
25. Garland A. Improving the ICU—part 2. *Chest.* 2005;127:2165–2179.
26. Committee on the Costs of Medical Care. *Medical Care for the American People: The Final Report of the Committee on the Costs of Medical Care* (adopted October 31, 1932). New York: Arno Press; 1972.
27. Himmelstein DU, Woolhandler S, the Writing Committee of the Working Group on Program Design, Physicians for a National Health Program. A national health program for the United States: a physicians' proposal. *N Engl J Med.* 1989;320:102.
28. Enthoven AC. *Theory and Practice of Managed Competition in Health Care Finance.* Amsterdam: North-Holland; 1988.
29. Enthoven AC. Consumer-choice health plan. *N Engl J Med.* 1978;298:650, 709.
30. Enthoven AC. *Health Plan: The Only Practical Solution to the Soaring Cost of Medical Care.* Reading, MA: Addison-Wesley; 1980.
31. Waitzkin H. The strange career of managed competition: military failure to medical success? *Am J Public Health.* 1994;84:482.
32. Enthoven AC. Managed competition in health care and the unfinished agenda. *Health Care Fin Rev.* 1986;Suppl:105.
33. Enthoven AC, Kronick F. A consumer-choice health plan for the 1990's. *N Engl J Med.* 1989;320:29, 94.
34. Starr P, Zelman WA. A bridge to compromise: competition under a budget. *Health Aff (Millwood).* 1993;12(Suppl):7.
35. Kronick R, Goodman DC, Wennberg J, et al. The marketplace in health care reform: the demographic limitations of managed competition. *N Engl J Med.* 1993;328:148.
36. Grumbach K, Bodenheimer T, Himmelstein DU, et al. Liberal benefits, conservative spending: the Physicians for a National Health Program proposal. *JAMA.* 1991;265:2549.
37. Harrington C, Cassel C, Estes CL, et al. A national long-term care program for the United States: a caring vision. *JAMA.* 1991;266:3023.
38. Physicians for a National Health Program. Single-payer resources. Available at: http://www.pnhp.org/facts/single_payer_resources.php. Accessed April 2, 2007.
39. Congressional Budget Office. *An Analysis of the Managed Competition Act.* Washington, DC: Government Printing Office; 1994.

CHAPTER 2 ■ LIFE AND DEATH IN THE ICU: ETHICAL CONSIDERATIONS

DAVID B. WAISEL

"Death in the ICU is not always preventable and should neither be unduly hastened nor delayed" (1).

Approximately 20% of all deaths in the United States—roughly 500,000 patients annually—occur in, or after a stay in, the intensive care unit (ICU) (2). The principles guiding end-of-life care center on the desire to have patients receive appropriate, carefully chosen, intensive therapy with comfort, dignity, security from fear, and the chance to be with loved ones. Doing this in a technology-driven and death-denying health care system requires incorporating the principles of palliative care throughout the intensive care practice (3–5).

A BRIEF HISTORY OF END-OF-LIFE CARE

The modern history of end-of-life care began with demands of patients to refuse treatments. In 1974, the American Medical Association asserted that "the purpose of cardiopulmonary resuscitation is the prevention of sudden unexpected death. Cardiopulmonary resuscitation is not indicated in cases of terminal irreversible illness where death is not unexpected" (6). Limiting resuscitation in patients with terminal illness was becoming acceptable (7–9).

In the renowned 1976 case of Karen Ann Quinlan, the courts upheld the right to refuse potentially life-sustaining care when they permitted the ventilator to be disconnected from the supposed ventilator-dependent Quinlan (10). The *Quinlan* decision was based on the general constitutional right to privacy. After mechanical ventilation was discontinued, Quinlan lived for nearly a decade, sustained by nasogastric feedings. The 1984 case of *Bartling* established the right for a competent person to refuse potentially life-sustaining care (11). For 6 months, Bartling, a competent adult patient with an incurable disease, received mechanical ventilation against his clear wishes, declaring, at one point, "While I have no wish to die, I find intolerable the living conditions forced upon me . . . " (11). Similar in reasoning to *Quinlan*, the appellate court supported the right of a competent patient to refuse medical treatment based on the constitutional right to privacy.

The 1990 case of *Cruzan* brought about a crucial change in the right to refuse treatment (12). Several years before an incapacitating accident, Cruzan had expressed to a friend a desire not to live in a state of diminished capacity. Cruzan's surrogates wanted to withdraw treatment, but the Supreme Court of Missouri mandated continued care because Cruzan's informal statements did not meet Missouri's evidentiary standard of "clear and convincing evidence" of a patient's wish to terminate potentially life-sustaining care. The case was appealed to the United States Supreme Court, but unlike *Quinlan* and *Bartling*, the Supreme Court grounded the right of a competent patient to refuse treatment in the more powerful liberty interest of the Fourteenth Amendment, which states, "No State shall make or enforce any law which shall abridge the privileges or immunities of citizens of the United States; nor shall any State deprive any person of life, liberty or property . . . " The decision upheld the rights of states to determine the standards for the level of certainty required, permitting Missouri to use the "clear and convincing evidence" standard, but also permitting other states to use different standards (12–14).

Intensive care unit practices may also lead surrogates to demand care for their loved ones. An archetypical case involves Helga Wanglie, an 86-year-old patient in a persistent vegetative state who was receiving mechanical ventilation. The medical center believed that further therapy would be futile for Mrs. Wanglie and wanted to withdraw mechanical ventilation. When Mr. Wanglie refused the medical center request to stop mechanical ventilation, the medical center sought appointment of an independent guardian to supplant Mr. Wanglie as her guardian. The Court declared that Mr. Wanglie was best able to be Mrs. Wanglie's surrogate (15,16).

Competent patients have a right to refuse potentially life-sustaining medical treatment (17). The modifier "potentially" is used before life-sustaining medical treatment to acknowledge that although physicians may *believe* that a therapy is life sustaining, there is rarely certainty that the intervention *will* be life sustaining. For the incompetent patient, three hierarchical levels of judgment direct the decision-making process for end-of-life care. The once competent patient's previously expressed preferences for end-of-life care should be followed as is best possible. When the patient's declared preferences are not known, *substituted judgment*, the surrogate's intimate knowledge of the patient's attitudes and beliefs, may be used to direct care. While these are two distinct categories, both levels require the surrogate to sufficiently know the patient to appropriately choose or interpret the patient's preferences. These standards put significant burdens on decision makers who may have legitimate doubts about the appropriateness of their decisions. When a surrogate has to make decisions for a patient who has never been competent, such as a young child or a mentally disabled adult, substituted judgment is impossible, and the surrogate must rely on the *best interests standard*. The best interests standard requires the surrogate to make decisions based on the surrogate's view of what is best for the patient.

ADVANCED CARE PLANNING

Advanced care planning permits patients to declare preferences for medical treatment if they become incapacitated. Respecting these preferences is how physicians honor the ethical principle of respect for autonomy, in which patients have the right to make substantially informed decisions about medical therapy and the resultant trajectory of their lives.

Advanced directives are designed to minimize the likelihood of undesired overtreatment and undertreatment of the patient. Partially as a result of *Cruzan*, the Patient Self-Determination Act (PSDA) was introduced in 1991 to increase the use of advance directives. The PSDA requires health care institutions—hospitals, nursing homes, and hospice programs—to notify individuals about their rights regarding advanced directives. The two types of advanced directives are living wills and health care proxies; the latter are also known as a durable power of attorney for health care decisions. Although living wills allow patients to declare the extent of desirable interventions, they are often unable to directly address the subtleties that characterize clinical situations. Nonetheless, some generalizations can be made. A willingness to accept highly invasive treatment suggests a willingness to accept less invasive treatment, and a willingness to accept therapy in a more impaired state suggests a willingness to accept therapy in a less impaired state. Similarly, a willingness to forgo therapy in a less impaired state suggests a willingness to forgo therapy in a more impaired state (18). Notwithstanding these generalizations, the difficulty of applying living wills to clinical situations lead some to prefer the greater flexibility provided by the health care proxy, in which the surrogate decision maker can consider the specific details when making clinical decisions. Health care proxies permit patients to designate surrogate decision makers—including nonfamily members—to make decisions for them should they become unable to make such decisions for themselves. If the patient does not assign surrogacy, most jurisdictions have a hierarchy for doing so. Surrogacy is not always effective, particularly for patients who do not make their preferences clearly known to the surrogate before losing their decision-making capacity (19). Given the strengths and weaknesses of each approach, a combination of the two (a designated proxy with some written form of preferences) may be the best option.

Advanced care documents are only somewhat effective. Typically, advanced directives are inadequately discussed, documented, disseminated, and followed (Table 2.1) (19–26). Inadequate use of advanced directives may be due to concerns about the stability of declared preferences, although about 75% of preferences remain stable over a several-year period (27–29). Preferences were most stable when the preference was to refuse treatment, and decisions were about the most and least serious issues (27). A worsening in functional status resulted in a greater interest in refusing care (27). Because preferences tend to trend toward what may be considered conventional preferences, intensivists should be less skeptical of conventional preferences and more curious and inquisitive about unusual preferences (27). Gender and educational level seem to have minimal effect on the stability of preferences (29,30).

Intensivists should not assume that the advanced directive will be an authoritative map of preferences (31). Instead, the advanced directive should be used in conjunction with an ongoing alliance with family and friends to consider future care. Although discussions about end-of-life care in the intensive care unit appear likely to be less successful because of the forced short-term relationship, the frequent, intense meetings to consider end-of-life issues aid in the development of a functional relationship (24). Successful conversations focus on advanced care planning as an ongoing process and are designed to help guide the decision-making of patients and surrogates (32). Discussion of defined questions permit intensivists to highlight the

TABLE 2.1

WHY ADVANCED DIRECTIVES FAIL

- **Not done**
  - ☐ Patients radically overestimate their 6-month survival and thus avoid advanced care planning or favor more aggressive care than if they had known their true likelihood of survival.
  - ☐ People defer advanced care planning because they think they are too young to need it or because they do not want to contemplate it.
- **Inauthentic preferences**
  - ☐ Default responses ("Please check 'no' if you do not want intubation") tend to be chosen more frequently than if the question is phrased neutrally and requires a forced choice ("Please check 'yes' if you want intubation or check 'no' if you do not want intubation").
  - ☐ Patients may not know their "authentic" preferences and, even if they do, a one-time assessment may not reveal them.
  - ☐ Physicians may be inadequately trained or have insufficient time to successfully elicit values or attitudes about end-of-life care.
  - ☐ Advanced directives rarely cover specific situations, and few patients successfully communicate their treatment preferences to their families.
- **Unavailable documents**
  - ☐ Because the term *advanced directive* is unfamiliar, people may not realize what clinicians are requesting when clinicians ask if the patient has such a document. People are more familiar with the terms *health care proxy*, *DNR* (do not resuscitate), and *living will*.
  - ☐ Patients falsely assume that doctors and hospitals have copies of their advanced directives.
  - ☐ There is inadequate communication and sharing of documents among health care providers (although there is a rising presence of Web-based national systems).
- **Inadequate application**
  - ☐ Surrogates correctly predicted patients' preferences for treatment 68% of the time. Prior discussion did not necessarily improve the correct rate of prediction.
  - ☐ Advanced directives may be ignored when they defy the physician's goals.
  - ☐ Physician–patient discussion of treatment preferences did not improve physicians' understanding of the patient preferences.

Sources: Shalowitz DI, Garrett-Mayer E, Wendler D. The accuracy of surrogate decision makers: a systematic review. *Arch Intern Med.* 2006;166:493–497; Danis M, Southerland LI, Garrett JM, et al. A prospective study of advanced directives for life-sustaining care. *N Engl J Med.* 1991;324:882–888; Forrow L. The green eggs and ham phenomena. *Hastings Cen Rep* 1994;24:S29–32; Freer JP, Eubanks M, Parker B, et al. Advanced directives: ambulatory patients' knowledge and perspectives. *Am J Med.* 2006;119:1088 e9–13; Haidet P, Hamel MB, Davis RB, et al. Outcomes, preferences for resuscitation, and physician-patient communication among patients with metastatic colorectal cancer. SUPPORT Investigators. Study to Understand Prognoses and Preferences for Outcomes and Risks of Treatments. *Am J Med.* 1998;105:222–229; Schneiderman LJ, Kronick R, Kaplan RM, et al. Effects of offering advanced directives on medical treatments and costs. *Ann Intern Med.* 1992;117:599–606; Teno JM, Fisher ES, Hamel MB, et al. Medical care inconsistent with patients' treatment goals: association with 1-year Medicare resource use and survival. *J Am Geriatr Soc.* 2002;50:496–500; Hammes BJ, Rooney BL. Death and end-of-life planning in one midwestern community. *Arch Intern Med.* 1998;158:383–390; and Kressel LM, Chapman GB, Leventhal E. The influence of default options on the expression of end-of-life treatment preferences in advanced directives. *J Gen Intern Med.* 2007;22:1007–1010.

inherent uncertainties of prognostication in medicine and the value of speaking in likelihoods.

While competent patients may modify their previously declared preferences, demented patients who previously made an informed choice to limit certain therapy may express an interest in receiving that therapy (33). If a patient manifests evidence of decision-making capacity, such as being able to provide internally coherent reasoning, their wishes to receive therapy should be honored. However, the process of resolving this situation in a patient without decision-making capacity, and with almost no likelihood of *regaining* decision-making capacity, is more complex. It would be quite easy to simply provide therapy; however, that is unlikely to reflect their true desires if they had the capacity. In this situation, it is better to choose therapy based on multiple sources, including significant others, documentation, and the best interests standard.

FUTILITY

The concept of futile care has undergone several changes over the past decade (34). Previously, attempts were made to define futile care based on a specific percentage of the likelihood of achieving a certain outcome; for example, cardiopulmonary resuscitation is futile when the likelihood of a patient with this disease process being discharged from the hospital is less than 1% with 95% confidence. This approach failed, in large part because it was difficult to know the likelihood of success in the individual patient. Policies based on this approach inappropriately de-emphasized the importance of individual values and preferences such as the willingness to atypically undertake extensive burdens for relatively minor or highly unlikely benefits (35).

A clearer way to think about futility is to delineate treatments that will not accomplish their intended goals from treatments that have a very low likelihood of accomplishing their goals. Thus, in this sense, therapy may be labeled futile when it cannot accomplish its intended specific goal, for example, when mechanical ventilation cannot accomplish pulmonary gas exchange. In this sense, questions about futile care are infrequent.

The ability to resolve differences of opinions about applying treatments with low likelihoods of success is important. Such treatments may be considered inadvisable because of the burden to the patient, cost, or uncertain benefit, but they are not futile. As discussed above, policies based on definitional approaches are hard to apply and do not respect individual values. A policy based on a procedural approach, in which the process for resolving conflict is described, is more practical. Good policies are public, reflect the moral values of the community, and include processes for identifying stakeholders, initiating and conducting the policy, commencing appellate mechanisms, and determining relevant information (35). Discussions about inadvisable treatment should bear in mind qualitative and quantitative considerations. The qualitative aspects define the goals of the treatment, and the quantitative aspects state the likelihood of achieving a defined result. When offering likelihoods of a result, physicians should be clear whether the information used to form the estimation is from intuition, clinical experience, or rigorous scientific studies. Scoring systems useful for population-level predictions should be considered as contributory but not determinative for decision making for individuals.

Recently, Texas has enacted a legislative approach to resolving disputes about appropriate care. Physicians are permitted to unilaterally withhold or withdraw treatments they regard as futile, provided they obtain the agreement of the hospital ethics committee. The impact of this questionable strategy for conflict resolution is being closely monitored (36–38).

CARE OF THE DYING PATIENT

"End-of-life care seems too early until it is too late—too often" (39).

Management of symptoms, pain, dyspnea, sleep, and other distressing physical and psychological symptoms, including depression and discomfort from catheters and suctioning, needs to be integrated into the routine of intensive care (40–42). The goal is to provide patients and families the best of intensive therapy and palliative care, because physicians cannot predict which path the patient's course will take. By aggressively providing medical, emotional, psychological, and spiritual care, the patient is more able to focus on decision making and related matters. Poor-quality end-of-life care harms more than just the patient. One third of family members who had relatives die in the intensive care unit had posttraumatic stress syndrome (43).

Good end-of-life care requires successful communication between nurses and physicians to improve patient care and minimize the stress of clinical practice (44). Dissimilar training and experiences of nurses and physicians lead to differences that can hinder communication and collaboration. By virtue of their profession, nurses spend more time with patients and families, take a more holistic view, and may feel more frustrated by conflicting opinions. In the ICU, nurses tend to feel ignored and that their opinions are not respected (45). While physicians tend to think that nurses have a great deal of influence, many nurses would like a more active role in end-of-life decisions (46). Physicians in the United States lag behind those in European countries in terms of involving nurses in end-of-life decision-making. Nurses involved in providing such aspects of care felt greater satisfaction and were more committed to a successfully operating unit (47).

Good-quality end-of-life care also requires effective communication among families and clinicians. In one study, 10% of family members in the ICU believed they received contradictory information, and more than half of family members did not know the roles for each clinician (48). Factors that improve communication among the clinicians and between the clinicians and family include minimizing hierarchy, implementing protocols for multidisciplinary communication, and using team training to improve communication skills and diminish the effects of differences in training (45,49–52). Extensive communication involving a weekly team meeting, which included a physician leader, a nurse, a chaplain, and a social worker, decreased discord and length of ICU stay, but it did not affect mortality rate (53). Implementing daily medical updates by the intensivist and adding physician support personnel, such as a social worker and a clinical nurse specialist to elaborate and provide further information, decreased length of stay, mortality, and costs (54). Daily goal worksheets requiring active acknowledgment from providers improved understanding of the goals of the interventions and tasks, decreased length of ICU stay, and improved workflow (52). A "proactive end-of-life conference and a brochure" with a focused communication strategy improved the response to bereavement (55). The communication strategy with family members was based on the mnemonic VALUE: "to Value and appreciate what the family members said, to Acknowledge the family members' emotions, to Listen, to ask questions that would allow the caregiver to Understand who the patient was as a person, and to Elicit questions from the family members (55)." Given the variety of successes, it would not be unreasonable to suggest that communication can be improved by simply having a reasonable protocol.

Self-imposed attitudinal barriers affect end-of-life care (Table 2.2) (45,56,57). In Western society, individuals tend to assume immortality while intensive care physicians tend to view death as a failure rather than as a natural end to life (39). Prognostic uncertainty fosters this death-denying attitude. Thus, the most commonly adopted attitude is to hold out for the most beneficial possibility—no matter how unlikely—rather than critically analyzing likely outcomes (39). This view may push physicians to wait for proof of failure of therapy, rather than to instigate timely escalation of palliative care. The "siloing"

TABLE 2.2

BARRIERS TO END-OF-LIFE CARE

- Cultural
  - Denial of death
  - Prognostic uncertainty
  - Siloing of professional activity
  - Emotional overtones of withdrawal of therapy, particularly mechanical ventilation
- Unwarranted optimism
  - Unrealistic patient, family, and/or clinician expectations about prognosis or effectiveness of treatment
  - Disagreement among physicians and nurse about prognoses, which may slow initiation of good end-of-life care; these disagreements were greater in sicker patients and patients with longer intensive care unit stays
- Communication
  - Perception of inadequate communication between nurses and physicians
  - Perception of inadequate communication between training physicians and attending physicians
  - Lack of multidisciplinary approach to communication
- Insufficient training of intensivists in palliative medicine
- Inadequate financing and insurance coverage for palliative care

Sources: Nelson JE. Identifying and overcoming the barriers to high-quality palliative care in the intensive care unit. *Crit Care Med.* 2006;34:S324–331; Reader TW, Flin R, Mearns K, et al. Interdisciplinary communication in the intensive care unit. *Br J Anaesth.* 2007;98:347–352; Estfan B, Mahmoud F, Shaheen P, et al. Respiratory function during parenteral opioid titration for cancer pain. *Palliat Med.* 2007;21:81–86; Frick S, Uehlinger DE, Zurcher Zenklusen RM. Assessment of former ICU patients' quality of life: comparison of different quality-of-life measures. *Intensive Care Med.* 2002;28:1405–1410; and Frick S, Uehlinger DE, Zuercher Zenklusen RM. Medical futility: predicting outcome of intensive care unit patients by nurses and doctors–a prospective comparative study. *Crit Care Med.* 2003;31:456–461.

of surgeons, internists, subspecialist consultants, nurses, and specialty nurses, often with relevant prognostic and treatment information, results in poor communication, to the patient's detriment (39,58).

Race is a barrier to good end-of-life care. Difficulties associated as a member of a minority group include inadequate access to care secondary to finances, geography, and language differences. Family members of African Americans were more likely to report concerns about being adequately informed and were more likely to report financial hardships than whites (59). In addition, due to historical abuses, some African Americans and members of other minority groups may mistrust the health care establishment. This mistrust may lead to family/surrogate decisions, such as the desire to attempt every therapy and to forgo palliative care, that are not necessarily in the best interests of the patient because of the fear that the motivation for suggesting that the patient forego certain therapies is not made in the patient's best interests.

Critical care medicine can improve practices surrounding end-of-life care by viewing it as a clinical state to be studied, with emphasis on legitimizing research, assessing the needs of families of dying patients, providing guidelines-based professional support for withdrawal of care, assessing interventions, and modeling of good end-of-life care (1,60). One of the most influential studies of end-of-life care was the SUPPORT study (61).[1]

What is defined as good care is often determined by what is measured. The information in this section needs to be tempered with the knowledge that there are issues with measurements used to define quality care. Process measurements, based on whether a task is performed—such as occurrence of multidisciplinary discussions, the frequency of caregiver/family meetings, chaplaincy visits, attendance at unit educational programs, and presence of policies—are easy to measure and collect (62,63). However, isolated process measurements are, at best, indirect measurements of improvements in care, even when there is evidence supporting a process-to-outcome link. Outcome measurements are patient-related results, such as length of stay, patient or family member symptoms, or satisfaction of care (63). Outcome measurements can be misunderstood or too inexact. For example, having fewer days per admission due to inappropriate transfer of patients to the ward is not the same as having fewer days per admission due to improved care. Some outcome measurements—for example, pain management—are hard to characterize and may be reduced to using less reliable surrogate characteristics for interpretation, such as behavioral cues for pain management.

[1]The SUPPORT study was a multimillion dollar, 9,100-patient two-phased study designed to assess end-of-life care. In the observational phase, trained individuals followed patients near the end of life to identify problems in their care. They asked patients about preferences for interventions such as mechanical ventilation and pain medication and the importance of various outcomes, such as being able to interact with others. In the following interventional phase, these trained individuals sought to improve communication of patient preferences to the clinicians. The study found many of the problems discussed in this chapter, such as insufficient use of documented preferences, inadequate pain management, inconsistent communication among clinicians, and an overestimation of medicine's ability to deny death. Although the intervention phase of the study did not improve end-of-life care, the knowledge gained from the SUPPORT study's many analyses and publications has shaped nearly all subsequent research in end-of-life care.

WITHDRAWAL OF CARE

While ethically equivalent, there is an emotional difference between withdrawing care and withholding care (60). But in fact because withdrawal of therapy permits a trial of the therapy in question, it is superior to the withholding of therapy, because if therapy is withheld, the patient will never know if the therapy could be applied with an acceptable benefit-to-burden ratio. Intensivists are more likely to fulfill a patient's wishes by implementing a trial of therapy and reviewing it at specific intervals for appropriateness (64). A physician's willingness to withdraw therapy is affected by a prediction of poorer cognitive function, a prediction of a less than 10% chance of survival, and patient preferences (1,65).

Practices of withdrawal of mechanical ventilation vary in hope of maximizing patient comfort during this process. Some intensivists prefer a slow terminal wean while others prefer more rapid extubation (66). Either way, neuromuscular blockade should not be initiated after the decision to withdraw life support has been made. Neuromuscular blockade does not provide sedation or pain relief for the patient and impairs the ability of the intensivist to assess the comfort of the patient. Although some may argue that neuromuscular blockade minimizes the trauma to the family witnessing the withdrawal of life support, that argument does not outweigh the potential harm to the patient (67). Explaining to the family the reasons to avoid neuromuscular blockade may make it more tolerable for them to be present through the dying process.

Physicians should aggressively treat discomfort when withdrawing therapy, even if treatment may hasten death. The doctrine of double effect emphasizes the intention of the clinician in cases in which actions may have both good and bad effects. Consider the intensivist seeking to provide comfort to terminally ill patients. Although two possible effects of the opioids are recognized and foreseen—relief of pain followed by respiratory depression—only the good effect, pain relief, is intended, and thus the intensivist is not held morally culpable if respiratory depression and a sooner death should occur (68). If the intensivist uses far more opioids than necessary to make the patient comfortable, or if the intensivist chooses an agent without pain-relieving properties—for example, intravenous potassium—then the intensivist can no longer plausibly claim that the intention was solely to relieve pain and suffering. The doctrine of double effect oversimplifies the concept of intentionality, particularly by assuming that clinical intentions are unambiguous and recognizable to the actor. More important, it centers the justification of the action on the physician's intent rather than on the patient's authorization.

Withdrawal of implantable cardiac defibrillator shock therapy presents an interesting problem for clinicians (69). Painful defibrillations prolong life. In a patient near the end of life, the discomfort of the shocks may no longer be worth the benefit. The continuation of implantable cardiac defibrillator therapy should be based on the benefits and burdens. In one study comparing patients in which one group had the defibrillator turned off and the other group did not, continuing defibrillator therapy did not extend life, suggesting little benefit in exchange for the discomfort of continued defibrillation (69).

DISTRIBUTIVE JUSTICE AND RATIONING IN THE ICU

Distributive justice refers to an equitable allocation of resources. Distributive justice can be viewed as a substantive request, such as determining a fundamental and inviolable level of health care for all members of a society. Distributive justice can also be viewed as a process for achieving justice, using approaches including queuing and potential benefit to determine valid distribution. These approaches belie simplicity; consider the different interpretations of benefit, such as quality-adjusted life years, functional status, or the fair innings approach, which aims to level the playing field for characteristics such as gender that are not under control of the individual (3,70,71).

Because critical care services account for more than 1% of the gross domestic product in the United States, hospitals, intensive care units, and critical care physicians are under pressure to control costs (72). An argument sometimes made for invoking futility as a reason not to perform a therapy is that futile care is a waste of health care dollars. This statement implies rationing, in that money is a scarce resource that could be better used elsewhere. The Task Force on Values, Ethics, and Rationing in Critical Care defined rationing as the "allocation of healthcare resources in the face of limited availability, which necessarily means that beneficial interventions are withheld from some individuals" (72). Rationing may be viewed more optimistically as a means of using resources wisely to minimize inequities and maximize population health (70).

It is helpful to consider three taxonomic categories of rationing (72). The first is the limited availability due to external constraints, such as not giving a medication that is not on a formulary or diverting ambulances from an emergency department of an overfull hospital. This form of rationing is beyond the physician's control.

A second category of rationing occurs from following clinical guidelines. For example, local hospital policies may define pathways for evaluation of certain diseases, such as requiring a specific radiologic study before proceeding to a more costly study. Rationing from clinical guidelines may also, for example, limit the use of certain antibiotics to control emergence of resistant organisms. Deviations from clinical guidelines should be based on patient characteristics and scientific literature, not on personal idiosyncrasies.

The third category of rationing is based on clinical judgment. Clinical judgment is used when it is unclear how guidelines should be applied or when guidelines do not exist. Clinical judgment is imperfect. Decisions about therapy are influenced by a patient's race, pre-illness employment status, the intensivist's interest in rationing, and the political power of clinical services (73–76).

For rationing polices to be fair, there should be public access to decision-making policies and rationale, a framework for principled decision making as a means for resolving dispute, and an appeals process (3). When considering rationing, one should recognize the difference between the statistical patient and the individual, or identifiable, patient. Clinical guidelines are developed in reference to the statistical patient, which is the ideal and abstract future patient. It is easier and more proper to discuss rationing for the statistical patient, such as whether society should spend dollars on preventive care, primary care, or tertiary care. When participating in those debates on a macro level, physicians may wish to consider their obligation to their patient community as well as to society as a whole.

Clinical judgment refers to the known individual patient. When faced with an identifiable patient whose situation does not align precisely with guidelines or studies, it is improper for a physician to determine and implement rationing based on distributive justice at the bedside (3). When caring for the individual patient, physicians are required to maximize use of resources while ensuring that care remains focused on patients (3).

Triaging is a special consideration of distributive justice. The utility principle encourages actions that maximize "the greatest good for the greatest number" and is at the heart of permitting unequal outcomes as long as overall health is maximized. It is by this principle that, for example, physicians in the midst of a mass casualty will choose to provide discrete, rapid, and potentially life-sustaining care—chest tubes, tracheal intubation, and so forth—to many patients before devoting these resources to the treatment of a single resource-intensive head injury (77). Implicit in the utility principle is that like patients are treated similarly, without regard to other factors, such as socioeconomic status. The utility principle is suitable for a mass casualty situation in which all patients are equally unknown and no prior relationship with the patient has been established. It may, however, be less suitable for considering distribution of an absolute scarce resource, such as ECMO (extracorporeal membrane oxygenation). In this case, many would suggest that the presence of a patient–physician relationship, current use of the resource, the appropriateness of the claim to the resource, and the idea that every person should have an equal chance to potentially life-sustaining resources should weigh heavily in these complicated balancing-act decisions. It is helpful to have considered relevant factors and a potential process to resolving these dilemmas before confronting them.

PHYSICIAN-ASSISTED SUICIDE, VOLUNTARY EUTHANASIA, AND PHYSICIAN AID IN DYING

The term *physician-assisted suicide* means that the physician makes a lethal dose of medicine available to the patient, but that the patient must perform the act of ingestion. The term *voluntary euthanasia* means that the physician administers the medication directly on a patient's request (78). While there may be a distinction between making the medication available and actually administering it, the distinction may not be ethically significant, as both require effort and contribution from the physician. Similarly, while requiring the patient to perform the final act may protect against abuses, psychological pressure may defeat safeguards inherent in requiring the patient to self-ingest. For purposes of this discussion, unless otherwise specified, voluntary euthanasia and physician-assisted suicide will be considered together and the term *physician aid in dying* (PAD) used to denote both. *Nonvoluntary euthanasia* is distinct from PAD and means that the physician administers the medication, but there has been no formal request by the patient. Arguments surrounding PAD center on the interpretations of the principles of respect for autonomy and beneficence, as well as the possible ramifications of legalization (Table 2.3) (79).

TABLE 2.3

PAD: ARGUMENTS FOR AND AGAINST LEGALIZING PHYSICIAN AID IN DYING

	For	Against
AUTONOMY *Individuals have the right to make informed choices about their lives.*	■ Individuals should be permitted to decide whether the burdens of being alive outweigh the benefits.	■ Requests for PAD are false expressions of autonomy because inadequate control of suffering—including pain, discomfort, loss of dignity, depression, the feeling of being a personal and financial burden, and "tiredness of life"—lead to poorly informed and forced choices.
BENEFICENCE *The obligation to do good for our patients.*	■ Doing good means physicians are obligated to help patients have a good death (as defined by the patient).	■ Doing good means doing a better job of maintaining patients' comfort and dignity.
Nonmalfeasance *The obligation to "do no harm."*		■ Physicians do not cause death.
LEGALIZATION	■ Legal safeguards and public oversight (such as the yearly reporting by the Oregon Department of Human Services on the Death with Dignity Act) will prevent abuses.	■ There will be concerns that clinicians may offer, feel pressure to offer, or be perceived to offer PAD for inappropriate reasons (e.g., race/gender/socioeconomic status). ■ Permitting PAD will discourage physicians from aggressively addressing the problems surrounding end-of-life care. ■ Permitting PAD will devalue the sanctity of life, thus further nudging society down the psychological slippery slope toward nonvoluntary euthanasia.

In European countries that have not decriminalized PAD, surveys indicate that voluntary euthanasia accounted for 0.05% to 0.46% of deaths and nonvoluntary euthanasia accounted for 0.11% to 2.26% of all deaths (80). Patients wished to hasten death when they considered themselves a burden to others, when they worried about suffering and receiving a substandard quality of care in the future, and when they were depressed, hopeless, and without adequate social support (81–83).

Some countries have legalized PAD. Although the Dutch had been practicing PAD for several decades, in 1993 the Dutch parliament granted physicians immunity from prosecution, provided that proper procedures were followed (Table 2.4) (84,85). In 2002, PAD was explicitly legalized in the Netherlands. Four nationwide investigations (in 1990, 1995, 2001, and 2005) have been conducted into the Dutch practice of PAD and nonvoluntary euthanasia (86–88). The 1990 Remmelink study found that 1.7% of all deaths were as a result of euthanasia. The 1995 and 2001 studies showed an increase in euthanasia as a percent of all deaths to 2.4% and 2.6%, respectively, and in the 2005 study the rate returned to 1.7%. Deaths from assisted suicide decreased from 0.2% of all deaths for the first three studies to 0.1% for the 2005 study. The decreases in the 2005 study may be from epidemiologic changes or the use of other techniques to alleviate symptoms, such as terminal sedation. Deaths from nonvoluntary euthanasia decreased from 0.8% of all deaths in 1990 to 0.4% in 2005. Reporting improved from less than 20% of PAD cases in 1990 to nearly 80% in 2005. In 2005, physicians chose not to report because they did not believe they were ending life (76% of nonreports), because they were concerned about whether criteria had been met (9.7% of nonreports), and because they viewed euthanasia as a private matter between the patient and physician. Nearly all the patients who received PAD appeared to have had a short life expectancy, with approximately 45% of granted requests for euthanasia or assisted suicide having a life expectancy of 1 week.

TABLE 2.4

COMMON CRITERIA FOR PATIENT ELIGIBILITY FOR PAD

1. The patient must clearly, voluntarily, and repeatedly request to die.
2. The patient's judgment must not be distorted.
3. The patient must have an incurable condition associated with severe, unrelenting, and intolerable suffering.
4. The physician is obligated to ensure the request is not made out of inadequate comfort care.
5. PAD should be done in context of a physician–patient relationship.
6. Consultation with other experts should be made to review and verify the facts about prognosis and current comfort management.
7. Document above and fulfill reporting requirements.

Sources: Quill TE, Cassel CK, Meier DE. Care of the hopelessly ill. Proposed clinical criteria for physician-assisted suicide. *N Engl J Med.* 1992;327:1380–1384; and Vincent JL. End-of-life practice in Belgium and the new euthanasia law. *Intensive Care Med.* 2006;32:1908–1911.

TABLE 2.5

QUALITY END-OF-LIFE CARE

Honor patient wishes.

- Have a system for continually evaluating and communicating end-of-life preferences.
- Review therapies at specified intervals to assess whether they are legitimate and consistent with the patient's desires.
- Treat iatrogenic events by outcome and not by etiology.
- Consider whether care guidelines apply to the specific patient.

Address needs of clinicians.

- Commit to a multidisciplinary practice that leads to respectful and productive collaboration and communication.
- Provide ongoing education about palliative care and cultural beliefs.
- Provide opportunities for bereavement, debriefing, and psychological support.
- Provide time and space for professional conversations and personal reflections.

Address needs of the family.

- Have a presentable senior team member inform family of bad news in private using non-technical language.
- Help families find meaning in the death of their loved one.
- Accept, support, and comfort the family.
- Assure family of patient comfort.
- Enable family to be with and help the patient.
- Clarify roles of clinicians to family.

Quality End-of-Life Care

Incorporate palliative care into intensive care.

- Reassess advanced care planning continuously and by focusing on the patient.
- Initiate end-of-life discussions early.
- Withdraw ventilatory therapy in a manner that permits recognition of distress; aggressively treat discomfort with opioids and sedatives.

Hold regular meetings with family and team to clarify intermediate and long-term goals.

- Identify objectives.
- Review medical facts and options for treatment.
- Agree on a care plan and on criteria to define success or failure of a plan.
- Understand and respect the narratives and perspectives of others.
- Seek out perspectives on dying, dependence, and loss of function.
- Use multidisciplinary approach to keep family informed.
- Provide sufficient time for questions.

Work to improve end-of-life care.

- Perform end-of-life research.
- Measure and assess end-of-life care.
- Promote a change in attitude toward end-of-life care.
- Maintain knowledge of end-of-life law.
- Maintain knowledge of end-of-life guidelines and care.

In 1997, the State of Oregon in the United States legalized the Oregon Death with Dignity Act, which permitted terminally ill patients to receive prescriptions in lethal quantities for the purpose of self-administration. It does not permit any other forms of PAD, such as another person administering the medication. From 1998 through 2006, 292 patients used 456 prescriptions authorized by this law. The most common diseases for patients choosing to ingest a lethal dose of medication were malignant neoplasms (81% of patients), amyotrophic lateral sclerosis (8% of patients), and chronic lower respiratory tract diseases (4% of patients) (89). Of the 23 patients receiving prescriptions in 1998, 21 had used the prescriptions and 2 were alive in 1999 (90). In 2006, 40 physicians wrote 65 prescriptions. Of those 65 patients, 35 used the prescriptions, 19 died of their underlying disease, and 11 lived throughout the year (89). The financial and educational status of patients did not seem to play a role in the request for PAD.

In 2003, Belgium passed a law permitting euthanasia (85). In the first 15 months after passage of the law, euthanasia represented 0.2% of all deaths. This appeared to be a decrease in euthanasia when compared with studies performed in 1998 and 2001 (91).

Interpretation of this information is not straightforward. The consistency of the data from the Netherlands and Oregon indicate that these two societies are not sliding down a slippery slope to increased misuse (92). Another view, however, is that not enough time has passed to see if this slide will occur (93).

Doc, Will You Help Me Die?

In a national survey of U.S. physicians, 18% reported receiving a request for assistance with suicide and 11% received a request for euthanasia (94). The majority of both sets of physicians received multiple requests (94). About 6.4% of physicians honored at least one request for PAD, with their last case split between physician-assisted suicide and euthanasia. In the survey, 4.7% of all physicians had performed lethal injection and 3.3% had participated in physician-assisted suicide (94). For these reasons, it is important for physicians to have a practiced approach to managing patient requests for PAD (95) (Table 2.5).

Depression should be assessed to determine (a) if the patient is able to make rational decisions, (b) whether the depression is treatable, and (c) whether treating the depression would change the circumstances (95). Physicians should explore what patients mean by requesting aid in dying and should overtly focus on patient dignity and comfort. Because patients may request PAD as prevention against future abandonment and suffering, physicians should emphasize that they will be actively involved throughout the end-of-life period (95). Given that survey data indicate that some physicians honor requests for PAD, physicians should clarify their position on participating in PAD for themselves and to their patients.

ETHICS CONSULTATION IN THE ICU

The goals of ethics consultation services are to "protect patient rights, diffuse real or imagined conflicts and cause a change in patient care that improves quality" (96). Ethics consultation can help address treatment conflicts, reduce costs without diminishing quality, and limit inappropriate nonbeneficial or unwanted interventions (97). In a randomized controlled trial, individuals who received ethics consultation in the ICU were not more likely to die than individuals who did not receive consultation (98). ICU ethics consultations proved to be valuable across a range of populations (99).

Much of the information about ethics consultation services in the United States comes from a 2000 survey. Most ethics consultation services use a small group, typically about three people, to perform consults, although some use the full ethics committees or a single individual to perform consults. Various individuals performed ethics consultation, including physicians, nurses, social workers, chaplains, administrators, and lay people. Most ethics consultation services have been practicing between 5 and 10 years. Three common characteristics of ethics consultation services were that they

1. permitted anyone to request an ethics consultation,
2. required notification—not permission—of the patient, surrogate, and attending physician prior to performing a consult, and
3. made recommendations that are wholly voluntary.

PEARLS

- Treat patients and families in the manner you would want you and your family to be treated—that is, with respect for personal values, feelings, and preferences.
- Know common approaches and forms for advance directives in your jurisdiction.
- Intensivists should focus end-of-life discussions with surrogate decision makers on what the patient would have wanted, not what they would want for the patient.
- Know local policies regarding dispute resolution.
- End-of-life decision making is a dynamic process requiring frequent reconsideration of therapy and goals and communication among the clinicians, the patient surrogates, and, if available, the patient.
- Attitudes on the unit are infectious.
- Actively root out personal presumptions and biases in health care, and challenge them so they do not affect the care provided.
- Recognize the benefits of trials of therapy in terms of maximizing the likelihood of fulfilling the patient's desires for end-of-life care. It is one thing to presume that the burdens of therapy are not worth the benefits; it is more ethically stout to test that assumption and then withdraw therapy when it is shown that the burdens outweigh the benefits.
- Withdrawing potentially life-sustaining therapy requires active clinical assessment and treatment to minimize harm to the patient and family.
- Just as intensivists seek consultation for diagnosing and treating subspecialty medical problems, intensivists should seek consultation for diagnosing and treating intricate ethical dilemmas.

References

1. Cook D, Rocker G, Giacomini M, et al. Understanding and changing attitudes toward withdrawal and withholding of life support in the intensive care unit. *Crit Care Med.* 2006;34:S317–23.

2. Angus DC, Barnato AE, Linde-Zwirble WT, et al. Use of intensive care at the end of life in the United States: an epidemiologic study. *Crit Care Med.* 2004;32:638–643.
3. Smith GP 2nd. Distributive justice and health care. *J Contemp Health Law Policy.* 2002;18:421–430.
4. Carlet J, Thijs LG, Antonelli M, et al. Challenges in end-of-life care in the ICU. Statement of the 5th International Consensus Conference in Critical Care: Brussels, Belgium, April 2003. *Intens Care Med.* 2004;30:770–784.
5. Thompson BT, Cox PN, Antonelli M, et al. Challenges in end-of-life care in the ICU: statement of the 5th International Consensus Conference in Critical Care: Brussels, Belgium, April 2003: executive summary. *Crit Care Med* 2004;32:1781–1784.
6. Standards for cardiopulmonary resuscitation (CPR) and emergency cardiac care (ECC). *JAMA.* 1974;227(Suppl):833–868.
7. Optimal care for hopelessly ill patients. A report of the Clinical Care Committee of the Massachusetts General Hospital. *N Engl J Med.* 1976;295:362–364.
8. Fried C. Terminating life support: out of the closet! *N Engl J Med.* 1976;295:390–391.
9. Rabkin MT, Gillerman G, Rice NR. Orders not to resuscitate. *N Engl J Med.* 1976;295:364–366.
10. *In the Matter of Karen Quinlan*, 70 N. J. 10,335 A.2d 647, cert. denied, 429 U.S. 922 (1976).
11. *Bartling v Superior Court*, 163 Cal.App.3d 186 [209 Cal. Rptr. 220] (1984).
12. *Cruzan v Director, Missouri Department of Health*, 110 S. Ct. 2841 (1990).
13. Emanuel EJ. Securing patients' right to refuse medical care: in praise of the *Cruzan* decision. *Am J Med.* 1992;92:307–312.
14. Bioethicists' statement on the U. S. Supreme Court's Cruzan decision. *N Engl J Med.* 1990;323:686–687.
15. *In re the conservatorship of Helga M. Wanglie*, No. PX-91-283, District Probate Division, 4th Judicial district of the County of Hennepin, State of Minnesota (1993).
16. Angell M. The case of Helga Wanglie - a new kind of "right to die" case. *N Engl J Med.* 1991;325:511–512.
17. Council on Ethical and Judicial Affairs, American Medical Association. Decisions near the end of life. *JAMA.* 1992;267:2229–2233.
18. Pearlman RA, Cain KC, Starks H, et al. Preferences for life-sustaining treatments in advance care planning and surrogate decision making. *J Palliat Med.* 2000;3:37–48.
19. Shalowitz DI, Garrett-Mayer E, Wendler D. The accuracy of surrogate decision makers: a systematic review. *Arch Intern Med.* 2006;166:493–497.
20. Danis M, Southerland LI, Garrett JM, et al. A prospective study of advance directives for life-sustaining care. *N Engl J Med.* 1991;324:882–888.
21. Forrow L. The green eggs and ham phenomena. *Hastings Cen Rep.* 1994;24:S29–32.
22. Freer JP, Eubanks M, Parker B, et al. Advance directives: ambulatory patients' knowledge and perspectives. *Am J Med.* 2006;119:1088 e9-13.
23. Haidet P, Hamel MB, Davis RB, et al. Outcomes, preferences for resuscitation, and physician-patient communication among patients with metastatic colorectal cancer. SUPPORT Investigators. Study to Understand Prognoses and Preferences for Outcomes and Risks of Treatments. *Am J Med.* 1998;105:222–229.
24. Prendergast TJ. Advance care planning: pitfalls, progress, promise. *Crit Care Med.* 2001;29:N34–39.
25. Schneiderman LJ, Kronick R, Kaplan RM, et al. Effects of offering advance directives on medical treatments and costs. *Ann Intern Med.* 1992;117:599–606.
26. Teno JM, Fisher ES, Hamel MB, et al. Medical care inconsistent with patients' treatment goals: association with 1-year Medicare resource use and survival. *J Am Geriatr Soc.* 2002;50:496–500.
27. Ditto PH, Smucker WD, Danks JH, et al. Stability of older adults' preferences for life-sustaining medical treatment. *Health Psychol.* 2003;22:605–615.
28. Emanuel LL, Emanuel EJ, Stoeckle JD, et al. Advance directives: stability of patients' treatment choices. *Arch Intern Med.* 1994;154:209–217.
29. Carmel S, Mutran EJ. Stability of elderly persons' expressed preferences regarding the use of life-sustaining treatments. *Soc Sci Med.* 1999;49:303–311.
30. Danis M, Garrett J, Harris R, et al. Stability of choices about life-sustaining treatments. *Ann Intern Med.* 1994;120:567–573.
31. Teno JM. Advance directives: time to move on. *Ann Intern Med.* 2004;141:159–160.
32. Hammes BJ, Rooney BL. Death and end-of-life planning in one midwestern community. *Arch Intern Med.* 1998;158:383–390.
33. Woien S. Conflicting preferences and advance directives. *Am J Bioeth.* 2007;7:64-65; discussion W4-6.
34. Consensus statement of the Society of Critical Care Medicine's Ethics Committee regarding futile and other possibly inadvisable treatments. *Crit Care Med.* 1997;25:887–891.
35. Tomlinson T, Czlonka D. Futility and hospital policy. *Hastings Cent Rep.* 1995;25(3):28–35.
36. Truog RD. Tackling medical futility in Texas. *N Engl J Med.* 2007;357: 1–3.
37. Paris JJ, Billinngs JA, Cummings B, et al. *Howe v MGH* and *Hudson v Texas Children's Hospital*: two approaches to resolving family-physician disputes in end-of-life care. *J Perinatol.* 2006;26:726–729.
38. Fine RL, Mayo TW. Resolution of futility by due process: early experience with the Texas Advance Directives Act. *Ann Intern Med.* 2003;138:743–746.
39. Nelson JE. Identifying and overcoming the barriers to high-quality palliative care in the intensive care unit. *Crit Care Med.* 2006;34:S324–31.
40. Lynn J, Teno JM, Phillips RS, et al. Perceptions by family members of the dying experience of older and seriously ill patients. SUPPORT Investigators. Study to Understand Prognoses and Preferences for Outcomes and Risks of Treatments. *Ann Intern Med.* 1997;126:97–106.
41. Bergbom-Engberg I, Haljamae H. Patient experiences during respirator treatment–reason for intermittent positive-pressure ventilation treatment and patient awareness in the intensive care unit. *Crit Care Med.* 1989;17:22–25.
42. Teno JM, Clarridge BR, Casey V, et al. Family perspectives on end-of-life care at the last place of care. *JAMA.* 2004;291:88–93.
43. Azoulay E, Pochard F, Kentish-Barnes N, et al. Risk of post-traumatic stress symptoms in family members of intensive care unit patients. *Am J Respir Crit Care Med.* 2005;171:987–994.
44. Puntillo KA, McAdam JL. Communication between physicians and nurses as a target for improving end-of-life care in the intensive care unit: challenges and opportunities for moving forward. *Crit Care Med.* 2006;34:S332–340.
45. Reader TW, Flin R, Mearns K, et al. Interdisciplinary communication in the intensive care unit. *Br J Anaesth.* 2007;98:347–352.
46. Ho KM, English S, Bell J. The involvement of intensive care nurses in end-of-life decisions: a nationwide survey. *Intensive Care Med.* 2005;31:668–673.
47. Ferrand E, Lemaire F, Regnier B, et al. Discrepancies between perceptions by physicians and nursing staff of intensive care unit end-of-life decisions. *Am J Respir Crit Care Med.* 2003;167:1310–1315.
48. Azoulay E, Pochard F, Chevret S, et al. Meeting the needs of intensive care unit patient families: a multicenter study. *Am J Respir Crit Care Med.* 2001;163:135–139.
49. Leonard M, Graham S, Bonacum D. The human factor: the critical importance of effective teamwork and communication in providing safe care. *Qual Saf Health Care.* 2004;13(Suppl 1):i85–90.
50. Sexton JB, Thomas EJ, Helmreich RL. Error, stress, and teamwork in medicine and aviation: cross sectional surveys. *BMJ.* 2000;320:745–749.
51. Undre S, Sevdalis N, Healey AN, et al. Teamwork in the operating theatre: cohesion or confusion? *J Eval Clin Pract.* 2006;12:182–189.
52. Pronovost P, Berenholtz S, Dorman T, et al. Improving communication in the ICU using daily goals. *J Crit Care.* 2003;18:71–75.
53. Lilly CM, De Meo DL, Sonna LA, et al. An intensive communication intervention for the critically ill. *Am J Med.* 2000;109:469–475.
54. Ahrens T, Yancey V, Kollef M. Improving family communications at the end of life: implications for length of stay in the intensive care unit and resource use. *Am J Crit Care.* 2003;12:317–323.
55. Lautrette A, Darmon M, Megarbane B, et al. A communication strategy and brochure for relatives of patients dying in the ICU. *N Engl J Med.* 2007;356:469–478.
56. Estfan B, Mahmoud F, Shaheen P, et al. Respiratory function during parenteral opioid titration for cancer pain. *Palliat Med.* 2007;21:81–86.
57. Frick S, Uehlinger DE, Zurcher Zenklusen RM. Assessment of former ICU patients' quality of life: comparison of different quality-of-life measures. *Intensive Care Med.* 2002;28:1405–1410.
58. Byock I, Twohig JS, Merriman M, et al. Promoting excellence in end-of-life care: a report on innovative models of palliative care. *J Palliat Med.* 2006;9:137–151.
59. Welch LC, Teno JM, Mor V. End-of-life care in black and white: race matters for medical care of dying patients and their families. *J Am Geriatr Soc.* 2005;53:1145–1153.
60. Tallgren M, Klepstad P, Petersson J, et al. Ethical issues in intensive care–a survey among Scandinavian intensivists. *Acta Anaesthesiol Scand.* 2005;49:1092–1100.
61. The SUPPORT Principal Investigators. A controlled trial to improve care for seriously ill hospitalized patients. The study to understand prognoses and preferences for outcomes and treatments (SUPPORT). *JAMA.* 1995;274:1591–1598.
62. Curtis JR, Engelberg RA. Measuring success of interventions to improve the quality of end-of-life care in the intensive care unit. *Crit Care Med.* 2006;34:S341–347.
63. Clarke EB, Curtis JR, Luce JM, et al. Quality indicators for end-of-life care in the intensive care unit. *Crit Care Med.* 2003;31:2255–2262.
64. Rocker G, Dunbar S. Withholding or withdrawal of life support: the Canadian Critical Care Society position paper. *J Palliat Care.* 2000;16(Suppl):S53–62.
65. Cook D, Rocker G, Marshall J, et al. Withdrawal of mechanical ventilation in anticipation of death in the intensive care unit. *N Engl J Med.* 2003;349:1123–1132.
66. Faber-Langendoen K. The clinical management of dying patients receiving mechanical ventilation. A survey of physician practice. *Chest.* 1994;106:880–888.
67. Truog RD, Burns JP, Mitchell C, et al. Pharmacologic paralysis and

withdrawal of mechanical ventilation at the end of life. *N Engl J Med.* 2000;342:508–511.
68. Quill TE, Dresser R, Brock DW. The rule of double effect - a critique of its role in end-of-life decision making. *N Engl J Med.* 1997;337:1768–1781.
69. Lewis WR, Luebke DL, Johnson NJ, et al. Withdrawing implantable defibrillator shock therapy in terminally ill patients. *Am J Med.* 2006;119:892–896.
70. Williams A. The 'fair innings argument' deserves a fairer hearing! Comments by Alan Williams on Nord and Johannesson. *Health Econ.* 2001;10:583–585.
71. Francis LP, Battin MP, Jacobson JA, et al. How infectious diseases got left out–and what this omission might have meant for bioethics. *Bioethics.* 2005;19:307–322.
72. Truog RD, Brock DW, Cook DJ, et al. Rationing in the intensive care unit. *Crit Care Med.* 2006;34:958–963.
73. Whittle J, Conigliaro J, Good CB, et al. Racial differences in the use of invasive cardiovascular procedures in the department of veterans affairs medical system. *N Engl J Med.* 1993;329:621–627.
74. Guyatt G, Cook D, Weaver B, et al. Influence of perceived functional and employment status on cardiopulmonary resuscitation directives. *J Crit Care.* 2003;18:133–141.
75. Cassell J, Buchman TG, Streat S, et al. Surgeons, intensivists, and the covenant of care: administrative models and values affecting care at the end of life–updated. *Crit Care Med.* 2003;31:1551–1557; discussion 7–9.
76. Marshall MF, Schwenzer KJ, Orsina M, et al. Influence of political power, medical provincialism, and economic incentives on the rationing of surgical intensive care unit beds. *Crit Care Med.* 1992;20:387–394.
77. Moskop JC, Iserson KV. Triage in medicine, II: underlying values and principles. *Ann Emerg Med.* 2007;49:282–287.
78. Emanuel EJ. Euthanasia: historical, ethical and empiric processes. *Arch Intern Med.* 1994;154:1890–1901.
79. Waisel DB, Truog RD. The end-of-life sequence. *Anesthesiology.* 1997;87:676–686.
80. Seale C. National survey of end-of-life decisions made by UK medical practitioners. *Palliat Med.* 2006;20:3–10.
81. Kelly B, Burnett P, Pelusi D, et al. Terminally ill cancer patients' wish to hasten death. *Palliat Med.* 2002;16:339–345.
82. Breitbart W, Rosenfeld B, Pessin H, et al. Depression, hopelessness, and desire for hastened death in terminally ill patients with cancer. *JAMA.* 2000;284:2907–2911.
83. Wilson KG, Scott JF, Graham ID, et al. Attitudes of terminally ill patients toward euthanasia and physician-assisted suicide. *Arch Intern Med.* 2000;160:2454–2460.
84. Quill TE, Cassel CK, Meier DE. Care of the hopelessly ill. Proposed clinical criteria for physician-assisted suicide. *N Engl J Med.* 1992;327:1380–1384.
85. Vincent JL. End-of-life practice in Belgium and the new euthanasia law. *Intens Care Med.* 2006;32:1908–1911.
86. van der Maas PJ, van Delden JJM, Pijnenborg L, et al. Euthanasia and other medical decisions concerning the end of live. *Lancet.* 1991;338:669–674.
87. van der Maas PJ, van der Wal G, Haverkate I, et al. Euthanasia, physician-assisted suicide, and other medical practices involving the end of life in the Netherlands, 1990–1995. *N Engl J Med.* 1996;335:1699–1705.
88. van der Heide A, Onwuteaka-Philipsen BD, Rurup ML, et al. End-of-life practices in the Netherlands under the Euthanasia Act. *N Engl J Med.* 2007;356:1957–1965.
89. Oregon Department of Human Services. Oregon's Death with Dignity Act. Portland, OR: March 8, 2007.
90. Chin AE, Hedberg K, Higginson GK, et al. Legalized physician-assisted suicide in Oregon–the first year's experience. *N Engl J Med.* 1999;340:577–583.
91. Bilsen J, Stichele RV, Mortier F, et al. The incidence and characteristics of end-of-life decisions by GPs in Belgium. *Fam Pract.* 2004;21:282–289.
92. Onwuteaka-Philipsen BD, van der Heide A, Koper D, et al. Euthanasia and other end-of-life decisions in the Netherlands in 1990, 1995, and 2001. *Lancet.* 2003;362:395–329.
93. Cohen-Almagor R. Non-voluntary and involuntary euthanasia in The Netherlands: Dutch perspectives. *Issues Law Med.* 2003;18:239–257.
94. Meier DE, Emmons CA, Wallenstein S, et al. A national survey of physician-assisted suicide and euthanasia in the United States. *N Engl J Med.* 1998;338:1193–1201.
95. Quill TE. Doctor, I want to die. Will you help me? *JAMA.* 1993;270:870–873.
96. Fox E, Myers S, Pearlman RA. Ethics consultation in United States hospitals: a national survey. *Am J Bioeth.* 2007;7:13–25.
97. Schneiderman LJ, Gilmer T, Teetzel HD. Impact of ethics consultations in the intensive care setting: a randomized, controlled trial. *Crit Care Med.* 2000;28:3920–3924.
98. Schneiderman LJ, Gilmer T, Teetzel HD, et al. Effect of ethics consultations on nonbeneficial life-sustaining treatments in the intensive care setting: a randomized controlled trial. *JAMA.* 2003;290:1166–1172.
99. Gilmer T, Schneiderman LJ, Teetzel H, et al. The costs of nonbeneficial treatment in the intensive care setting. *Health Aff.* 2005;24:961–971.
100. Kressel LM, Chapman GB, Leventhal E. The influence of default options on the expression of end-of-life treatment preferences in advance directives. *J Gen Intern Med.* 2007;22:1007–1010.
101. Frick S, Uehlinger DE, Zuercher Zenklusen RM. Medical futility: predicting outcome of intensive care unit patients by nurses and doctors–a prospective comparative study. *Crit Care Med.* 2003;31:456–461.

CHAPTER 3 ■ UNDERSTANDING REACTIONS OF PATIENTS AND FAMILIES

CRAIGAN T. USHER • EUGENE V. BERESIN

So profound was the isolation in which I was then operating that it did not occur to me that for the mother of a patient to show up at the hospital wearing blue cotton scrubs could only be viewed as a suspicious violation of boundaries.

Joan Didion, The Year of Magical Thinking

UNDERSTANDING ODD OR DISRUPTIVE PATIENT–DOCTOR INTERACTIONS

Critical care medicine is a high stakes endeavor, one that requires broad medical knowledge, diagnostic acumen, procedural precision, team maintenance skills, and an empathic approach to patients and families. Maintaining a balance of these duties can be taxing under ideal conditions, but can grow frustrating when ventilators fail to operate properly, laboratory reports lag sluggishly behind, or staff members become overwhelmed. Similarly, it can be puzzling to physicians and nurses when patients and family members who, under extreme stress, act in somewhat bizarre ways, such as showing up in scrubs as Joan Didion describes in her heart-wrenching *The Year of Magical Thinking*. Also bewildering to intensive care unit (ICU) staff, who typically deal with adults, is how to provide comfort and support to families who want to have children visit critically ill loved ones.

Meanwhile, demanding, "entitled," or rudely behaving patients and families are troubling—even infuriating—to many physicians, nurses, and ICU staff. Occasionally, these difficult staff–patient exchanges arise from problems with the care providers themselves; factors such as depression, anxiety, overwork, sleep deprivation, longstanding interpersonal rigidity, and the cumulative effects of stress (1,2) may cause some physicians and nurses to fail to adequately address the emotional needs of their patients and patients' families (3,4). At other times, patients and families with markedly impaired abilities to negotiate interpersonal relationships become overwhelmed and subsequently act in ways that are extremely problematic. The judgment of these families and patients can become clouded by longing, shame, rage, and despair, making reasoning with them almost impossible. In this chapter, we endeavor to relieve the critical care practitioner of some of the fury that problematic patient and difficult family member encounters engender, offer some reason where none seems to exist, and provide suggestions for less alarming, routine ICU interactions. Herein, we pose—and offer practical answers to—the following questions:

- What is the psychological impact of critical illness and ICU treatment on patients and families?
- Why are some patients and families so taxing to deal with and others so easily treated, soothed, and able to be active team members?
- How should one approach problematic interactions with patients?
- What are some tips for enhancing communication between staff and family members?
- What are some ways to handle family requests for children to visit the ICU?

INITIAL STEPS

The psychological impact of critical illness and ICU treatment on patients and their families can be very powerful. Although problematic patient–doctor interactions are often due to emotional or relationship factors, there are many steps (Table 3.1) that can be taken before focusing on these factors. First, whenever one encounters a problematic patient, the initial questions should be: "Do I feel safe?" and "Are the other patients and staff feeling safe?" Physicians are taught to override their sense of danger. As medical students and interns, they begin placing catheters and doing lumbar punctures, charging through their fears. This sometimes translates to physicians overriding their inner sense of "danger" when managing potentially violent patients, a situation possibly leading to injury. It is thus important for physicians and nurses to "tune in" (5) to their sense of alarm and, when necessary, to call on security personnel, administer calming medications, or apply temporary physical restraint. The principle also applies to angry or threatening family members. If one feels in imminent danger, then contacting security—before examining the roots of the conflict and attempting to reason with family members—is key.

Next, medical causes of disruptive behavior should be ruled out. ICU patients acting in a bizarre or agitated manner often do so as part of a delirium. This may entail suffering persecutory delusions that staff members are torturing them or hallucinations that are arrestingly frightening. Since delirium can be lethal (6), it is very important to first discover and treat the underlying causes of delirium and to administer treatment for agitation, which may include a bedside sitter or use of calming pharmacotherapy, including neuroleptics. A full discussion of delirium is provided in Chapter 150 of this textbook.

TABLE 3.1

A HIERARCHY OF QUESTIONS TO ADDRESS WHEN CONFRONTED WITH DIFFICULT PATIENT–DOCTOR INTERACTIONS IN THE INTENSIVE CARE UNIT (ICU)

SAFETY Are staff and other patients safe? If not, how can we secure the safety of the unit?
DELIRIUM Is the patient suffering delirium? If so, is the etiology of this delirium being effectively addressed?
PSYCHIATRIC ILLNESS Does the patient have an anxiety, mood, or psychotic disorder or another psychiatric illness? If so, is adequate treatment for these conditions being given?
INTOXICATION AND WITHDRAWAL Is the patient intoxicated with alcohol and/or other substances? Is the patient withdrawing from alcohol or other substances? Are we addressing the untoward effects of withdrawal?
PSYCHOSOCIAL STRESSORS Can we reduce pain, sleeplessness, isolation, and other stressors related to being in the ICU?
PERSONALITY PROBLEMS What is the patient's predominant mode of coping? How can we best manage this patient's uniquely taxing mechanisms of defense and have a different type of relationship with the patient than the one we are having now?

Adapted from Usher CT. Problematic behavior of patients, family and staff in the intensive care unit. In: Irwin RS, Rippe JM, eds. *Irwin and Rippe's Intensive Care Medicine.* 6th ed. Philadelphia: Lippincott Williams & Wilkins; 2008.

In addition, a number of patients come to the ICU with established psychiatric diagnoses, including major depression, anxiety disorders, substance abuse, and schizophrenia. Occasionally, discontinuation of a patient's outpatient psychopharmacologic medication is performed purposefully (7). In other instances, admitting physicians fail to review the outpatient medication lists, and unintended disruptions (8) in the proper treatment of a patient's psychiatric illness ensue. This can lead to some patients suffering panic attacks, and cause others psychotic exacerbation with paranoia and hallucinations. Some patients experience discontinuation phenomena, such as the fatigue and myalgias associated with abrupt cessation of serotonin reuptake inhibitors (SRIs), or outright withdrawal syndromes specifically related to sudden discontinuation of alcohol, stimulants, narcotics, or sedative medications. Hence, on admission, it is important to learn about a patient's psychiatric and substance abuse history, and to find out what medications, if any, have been useful in the past in treating their illness or potential withdrawal. At any point in this evaluation process, psychiatric consultation may be helpful.

Finally, before examining psychological factors leading to problematic ICU staff–patient relationships, it is important to maximize patient comfort. Remember, staff in the ICU grow very accustomed to their workspace. They may enjoy laughs with colleagues, coffee and doughnuts in the break room, or other comforts, while most patients are miserable with pain, endotracheal tube discomfort, ICU noise, sleeplessness, and isolation (9,10). Working hard to minimize these factors by providing adequate analgesia, effective sleep agents, uninterrupted time with family and loved ones, and efficient use of tubes and catheters may reduce some of the patient discomfort that drives disruptive behavior.

EXISTENTIAL CONCERNS OF PATIENTS AND FAMILIES IN THE INTENSIVE CARE UNIT

Being an ICU patient, or having a loved one who is critically ill, is intensely stressful (11,12). Studies indicate that 3 months after patients are treated in the ICU, approximately one third of caregivers and family members are at risk for depression (13) and posttraumatic stress disorder (14). Patients' most prominent concern early in their ICU stays involves how they feel physically. Pain, hunger, restless exhaustion, the irritation of tubes and catheters, and isolation are the predominate focus of the acutely ill individual; it is usually not until the convalescent or subacute period in the patient's hospital course that larger, existential crises and psychological problems come to the forefront (15).

Critical illness raises many existential concerns for patients and loved ones. Looming in the minds of patients and family members of ICU patients is the prospect of death, with critically ill individuals often reflecting on their lives. Confronting death may fill them with guilt, regret, and wishes that they could have accomplished more. In others, this may be a time of contentment and reflecting on lives well lived. Amazingly, this can occur even in a delirious patient. For example, one 80-year-old gentleman who had undergone emergency cardiac bypass surgery happily shared that, amid his postoperative delirious days, he "went on a train trip in my head, with stops along the way involving each stage of my life. My marriage, the birth of my children, the child we lost, the different businesses I had run, everything was in there." Family members also reflect on the lives of their ill loved ones and their relationships with them. For many, fond memories and experiences will abound; for others, traumatic memories may arise, leading to some surprising interactions with staff that may seem to come from out of the blue.

Thoughts about not only the past, but also the future, arise in critically ill patients and their family members. Patients often worry about how they will function once discharged from the ICU and hospital. Depending on the nature of their injury, patients may ponder such questions as: Will I ever have to live in a nursing home? Will I ever be free of dialysis? Will I ever walk unassisted again, or visit Paris? Although excited that their loved ones will survive, friends and family must often confront concerns about the future. Loved ones wonder how they will financially and emotionally shoulder the often heavy burden of caring for their mother, father, husband, wife, partner, or friend after hospitalization. Ambivalence and tension between, on the one hand, being excited that the ICU patient has survived and, on the other hand, concern about his or her quality of life and how to handle extreme medical problems in the long term cause many patients and family members psychological suffering.

There are pressing concerns about the present as well. Most patients are treated in the ICU because their bodies fail to handle the most fundamental tasks of life. Whether involving breathing on their own, feeding themselves, or handling secretions, urination, and bowel movements, ICU patients are often dependent on others. This leads many patients to feel loathsomely dependent. Still others may long for exceeding amounts of attention, reacting to the loss of autonomy with complete resignation. Loved ones, particularly those who are caretakers of chronically ill individuals, also feel the sting of this loss of autonomy. For example, one woman who, for several years, had taken care of her husband suffering end-stage Parkinson disease tenderly commented: "It's not just that my husband's sick; it's that I have to trust you doctors and nurses to take care of him. That's *my* job."

COPING IN THE INTENSIVE CARE UNIT

It is difficult to bear the intense feelings of pain, love, loss, regret, and hope that being treated in the ICU, or having a loved one treated for critical illness, engenders. Families and patients vary in their ability to tolerate these emotions. To an amazing extent, most families and patients are able to muster inner strength, gain security from each other or draw on outside resources, and cope well in times of adversity. While such families and patients may continue to suffer stress and depressive symptoms, their mature psychological coping mechanisms (Table 3.2) allow them to work smoothly with ICU staff.

On the other hand, some families and patients are extremely difficult to manage in the ICU. Such individuals typically fall into two categories: (a) those with personality disorders, whose personal and professional lives were replete with problems before they entered the ICU; and (b) those who have simply regressed, utilizing primitive coping mechanisms that, outside the ICU, would be less apparent.

Personality disorders refer to severe, pervasive exaggerations of normal personality traits—styles of dealing with the world (15). As the focus of intensive care medicine is on the here and now, and major psychosocial investigations of a patient or family member's life outside the unit are inappropriate, distinguishing between the two categories is unnecessary in this chapter. Also, for the sake of convenience, we refer only to the "personality-disordered patient"; however, please note that the descriptions provided may also characterize family members. Note also that these descriptions also encompass the more rare, "easy-going" family member or patient who is simply pushed to his or her psychological limit, and hence appears personality-disordered.

All patients with personality disorders have difficulty tolerating affect, or emotion. They also demonstrate impaired reasoning, thus compromising their ability to subdue intense feelings. Further complicating matters, they often have difficulty distinguishing what others are feeling and their own motives and tendencies (15). Without their awareness, and to the

TABLE 3.2

MECHANISMS OF DEFENSE EMPLOYED BY PATIENTS, FAMILY, AND STAFF IN THE INTENSIVE CARE UNIT (ICU)

Defense	Description	ICU-relevant examples
NARCISSISTIC DEFENSES		
Denial	Failing to be aware of some aspect of reality in order to avoid the painful consequences of this, despite otherwise intact reality testing	A patient denies that she has cancer, refusing to talk about hospital aftercare, convinced that: "It's just a cough. I'm fine."
Distortion	Molding reality to fit one's need to feel superior, attractive, or powerful	A patient protects against feeling ill and romantically unappealing by convincing himself that: "My doctor always smiles at me seductively. I bet on the outside we'd go out on a date."
Projection	Placing one's unacceptable inner urges and affects outside the self, often projecting them (like a movie projector) onto the screen of another individual	A patient with many regrets says: "I bet my wife and kids wish they had treated me more nicely."
IMMATURE DEFENSES		
Acting out	Giving into an impulse to relieve inner tension, gratifying this wish without regard for the consequences	An anxious son lights up a cigarette at his father's bedside, sending the ICU into a panic.
Passive-aggressive action	The use of procrastination, failing to do something, and other devices that cause disruption to either the individual or others but appear benign	An intern neglects to dictate a transfer summary for a patient whom the day before she admitted she found "totally obnoxious."
Regression	Reverting to an earlier developmental stage using the strategies from that developmental era to tackle a stressful event or set of emotions	A 24-year-old college senior admitted after a motor vehicle collision feels that her friends, family, and she are quite vulnerable. She thus cradles a teddy bear and uses "baby talk," eliciting paternal/maternal responses from the ICU staff and bringing to mind the security she felt as a child.
Somatization	Converting psychological stress into physical symptoms	After hip replacement, a patient who "can't stand" her physical therapist refuses to get out of bed for this treater because her leg legitimately throbs with pain whenever the therapist enters the room.
NEUROTIC DEFENSES		
Controlling	Scheduling or managing aspects of a painful event or problem in order to alleviate anxiety	A patient's daughter routinely demands a review of his medication, medication doses, lab test results, and imaging studies.
Displacement	Transferring overwhelming emotions and thoughts related to one entity to another, which shares similar features	A woman whose husband has emphysema is disappointed with him for not quitting cigarettes; in displacement, she yells at her adult son who is eating a cheeseburger and fries in the hospital cafeteria, saying: "You need to lose weight and eat more healthy foods!"
Intellectualization	Much like controlling, involves excessive focus on the intellectual aspects of illness or hospitalization	A physician is very anxious about her husband's spine surgery and convalescence and asks questions ad nauseam about the surgeon's approach and the materials used rather than sitting at her husband's bedside.
MATURE DEFENSES		
Anticipation	Realistically looking at the future and making management plans for upcoming challenges	A father, whose wife is dying in the ICU, asks the patient's social worker for a referral to a grief support network for her daughter and himself, saying: "Right now I can't even think straight, but I know this is going to be hard and we'll need help."
Humor	Utilizing comedy to help oneself and others acknowledge and tolerate painful aspects of reality	While rolling to the operating room for leg amputation, an elderly woman drolly comments to the medical student: "You think my pedicures will be half-price?"
Sublimation	Accepting that one's impulse is socially unacceptable, adapting it into one that is useful and gratifying	A college student visiting a friend hates how emotionally sterile the ICU environment is and would like to scream at the doctors and nurses. Instead, she becomes determined to go to medical school and become a warm, empathic physician.
Suppression	Consciously delaying focusing on a painful topic or aspect of reality, saving it for later	A family who desperately wanted their grandmother to be part of a wedding service is concerned that she will not survive a subdural bleed. Wisely, the bride's mother counsels: "This is upsetting, but let's just cross that bridge when we come to it. For now, let's work on taking good care of grandma."

Adapted from Sadock BJ, Sadock VA. *Kaplan & Sadock's Synopsis of Psychiatry.* 9th ed. Philadelphia: Lippincott Williams & Wilkins; 2003:207. Blackman JS. *101 Defenses: How the Mind Shields Itself.* New York: Brunner-Routledge; 2004.

surprise of their caretakers, such individuals consistently employ defense mechanisms, which cause disruptions that take on a life of their own. To examine this more closely, let us examine a simple hypothetical, toxic hospital interaction:

> A nurse's aide asked a nondelirious middle-aged litigator recovering from back surgery what he wanted for the following day's meals. The man handed this caretaker his menu and barked: "I want some decent food, not the crap you serve here!" Caught off-guard, the nurse's aide picked up the menu, but distracted by the man's rudeness, left it by the sink after she left the room. The next day, when the wrong cuisine arrived on the man's tray, he derided this attractive and typically savvy staff member as "ugly," "incompetent," and "worthless." He complained bitterly to everyone who entered his room about this woman and the "dietary travesty" for the rest of the day.

Some may argue that clinicians simply need to work with a patient's overt behavior: "What you see is what you get. Deal with it!" Accordingly, these people argue that our job in the ICU is not to delve into the motivations driving a patient's actions or feelings. Such folks may simply dismiss the attorney's behavior as rude and note that he had a finicky palate. Alternatively, we contend that investigating the emotions and inner conflicts underlying the man's rudeness offers a deeper, more sympathetic version of what occurred. We can first speculate that this man, a powerful lawyer outside the hospital accustomed to getting his own lunch and going to the bathroom without the aid of a bedpan, felt extremely "incompetent." Perhaps used to knowing every aspect of his client's cases and his staff's work, he also loathed the idea of the medical and surgical staff knowing more about his magnetic resonance imaging (MRI) scan, labs, and even his lunch time than he did. Finally, he may also have been quite attracted to the nurse's aide and, pale, unshaven, and sitting in bed wearing a hospital johnny, felt that he himself looked very ugly. Through his brief comment, the man was able to redirect his intolerable feelings. He turned his sadness into hostility and *projected* his feelings of incompetence onto the nurse's aide. She, in turn, felt flustered and perhaps angrily, "accidentally" (passively aggressively) left his menu by the sink. He was also able to defend against his concern of not knowing what is supposed to happen in the hospital, by pointing out that he knows he was getting the wrong meals, and was able to engage his doctors and nurses in a discussion about his food as opposed to his medical treatment. Thus, the man's defenses took on a life of their own with conflict over a breakfast tray, thereby distracting from his chief psychological troubles. In this case, the man's behavior falls in the "narcissistic" category, which represents one of the four main, difficult patterns of interpersonal behavior we have identified (16). Below we describe each personality type and offer management advice on treating the narcissistic, obsessive, dependent, and overly dramatic patient (Table 3.3).

The Narcissistic Patient

Patients in the ICU lose autonomy. In almost every way, they are at the mercy of ICU staff and visitors, leading many patients to feel infantilized. For most patients, then, regaining a sense of control over their lives is important. Meanwhile, for the narcissistic patient, this need takes on an overwhelming, life-or-death urgency. Narcissistic patients approach the world in a grandiose fashion with an exaggerated sense of self-importance. They typically believe they are special and unique, requiring excessive admiration. They have significant problems with empathy and feel a strong sense of entitlement for care, concern, or special treatment (17). If they fail to receive these "entitlements," they attack, sometimes ruthlessly. It should be noted that these traits often are responses to underlying feelings of insecurity, low self-esteem, ineffectiveness, and profound feelings of deprivation—typically stemming from neglectful interactions in their childhood. Despite their overt demonstrations of strength and power, in reality they feel weak and fragile; it is crucial to recognize that they are not in touch with these underlying feelings, and that if confronted, they will fiercely deny and reject that they have them.

Occasionally, as the example above demonstrates, the narcissist's need for control and special care may take the form of scathing critique concerning the health care staff. These patients often deride nurses ("That's the wrong bandage!"), belittle housestaff ("You must be new at this, Doogie"), and drop names ("Dr. Thompson, the world famous nephrologist, is a buddy of mine from college; he never allows patients to be treated like this") to demonstrate their "connections." Staff reactions to such patients include rage and revulsion when they are the subject of derision, or, more commonly in more junior house officers, nurses, or staff, feelings of inadequacy or inferiority when a patient presents as an entitled, very important patient (VIP).

Insofar as possible, it is best to collaborate with—rather than confront—this type of patient. To avoid caustic exchanges ending in both the patient and physician feeling hurt or enraged, one must choose to have a different relationship with the patient, which can be accomplished by avoiding authoritarian condescension and appealing to the patient's narcissism. Remember, when narcissistic patients examine their surroundings in the ICU, all they see are their inadequacy, inability, and incapacity. The nasogastric tube attached to the churning pump reminds them that they cannot nourish themselves; the ventilator brings to mind that they cannot breathe on their own; the bedpan is a glaring reminder that they cannot even relieve themselves independently. When a physician or nurse uses a tone of voice that conveys respect, and chooses words that remind patients that, despite their infirmities, they are still valuable people, he or she is able to meet patients' needs, offering them the respect they so desperately crave. This may entail calling patients "sir," "ma'am," "Mr.," "Ms.," "Dr.," or "Professor" as appropriate. It is also useful to ask narcissistic patients about their lives before they came down with the debilitating illness. This promotes the notion that you think of these patients as vital, able-bodied individuals who happen to be suffering severe infirmity, as opposed to thinking of them as fragile nonentities—a patient's worst fear.

Narcissistic patients appreciate gaining as much control as possible. Hence, even controlling their light switch and TV, using patient-controlled analgesia, or being able to choose to "go first" or "go last" when the phlebotomist performs rounds helps patients feel like more of a collaborator in their care. Finally, avoiding power struggles with narcissistic patients is of the utmost importance. For example, a psychologically minded ICU nurse who was typically well liked by staff and patients was being bossed around by a VIP, who eventually asked for a different nurse. Rather than be offended, the nurse simply exchanged patients with a colleague. She offered: "Hey, when I was young I would have been offended and told him '*I* am *your* nurse and *you* are stuck with me.' But he's not in the ICU

TABLE 3.3

COMMON PROBLEMATIC PERSONALITY STYLES ENCOUNTERED IN THE INTENSIVE CARE UNIT (ICU)

Personality type	Core deficit	Characteristic behavior	Suggested response
Dependent	Hypersensitive to abandonment, inadequacy, and aloneness—poor "object constancy"; defended against isolation	■ Unending need for nurturance and support ■ Demands special care ■ Childlike; cries easily and complains of abandonment and insufficient care	■ Schedule exam and rounding times. ■ Anticipate nursing staff changes, physician care shifts, and transfer to floor. ■ Validate patient's plight and offer to help within reason. ■ Enlist family members for support. ■ Support nurses and colleagues who may need to spend extra time with these patients.
Narcissistic	Hypersensitive to loss of control and stature; defended against looking weak	■ Denies severity of illness ■ Shows bravado ■ Critical of ICU staff and care	■ Acknowledge patient's stature. ■ Enlist patient as active partner in care and decision making.
Obsessive	Hyperaware of loss of control; defended against the unknown; craving mastery	■ Excessive focus on medical facts and minutiae ■ Rigid, with restricted affect; not apt to "show emotional cards"	■ Schedule patient and family meetings. ■ Have a set amount of information to share with patient and family. ■ Provide factual, as opposed to nuanced, explanations of data. ■ Avoid emotional commentary or inquiry and avoid authoritarian approach.
Dramatic	Difficulty feeling cared for or thought of except within emotionally extreme exchanges; minor insults felt deeply	■ Engaging and charming to some staff, denigrating and caustic to others ■ May have multiple allergies and phobias ■ May "fire" some staff, take exceptions to rules, and seek intimate connections with others	■ Acknowledge patient's positive attributes. ■ Validate patient's plight and offer to help within reason. ■ Discuss patient with colleagues and set limits, as necessary, as a team.

Adapted from Kahana RJ, Bibring GL. Personality types in medical management. In: Zinberg NE, ed. *Psychiatry and Medical Practice in a General Hospital.* New York: International Universities Press; 1965:108. Usher CT. Problematic behavior of patients, family and staff in the intensive care unit. In: Irwin RS, Rippe JM, eds. *Irwin and Rippe's Intensive Care Medicine.* 6th ed. Philadelphia: Lippincott Williams & Wilkins; 2008.

for me to be his nurse. He's here because he's sick and needs help. So I just found another nurse to take care of him."

The Dependent Patient

Dependent patients are hypersensitive to being alone and suffer intense anxiety. These individuals feel empty and isolated, often because they came from families that never provided adequate caretaking. They cling tenaciously to clinicians or family members, often engendering feelings of disdain and aversion. Clinicians are typically idealized and considered endowed with superhuman powers. Such patients have an inability to hold onto the comforting feelings they receive from ICU staff, friends, or relatives when those people are not actively helping them. In psychiatric terms, we would state that, similar to the early toddler, the dependent patient has poor object permanence, unable to conjure a mental image of his mother when she's out of sight (18). Thus, these patients demand urgent assistance with nearly every aspect of ICU life. Often these entreaties are the same as one would expect any hospitalized person would want: Better food, more analgesia, softer pillows, more frequent visits and doctor reports, enhanced light, nicer views, gentler exams, and fewer tubes and catheters. However, for the dependent patient, these concerns take on an overwhelming urgency, often driving ICU staff to distraction.

Addressing—as opposed to avoiding—the relationship needs of the dependent patient involves frequent visits and keeping the patient informed. Nurses and doctors should let such patients know when they plan to come back into the room, when rounds might take place in the morning, when transfer to another ward will happen, and when tests will take place. For many dependent patients, this basic information will not be enough to soothe their demands for instant anxiety relief. In these situations, the nurse–patient or physician–patient relationship can be transformed by (a) validating that the patient's concerns are real, (b) communicating to the patient that his or her request is understood, and (c) explaining to the patient that the staff will do everything in their power to help, but that it may not be possible to provide everything the patient demands.

These three tasks are accomplished through statements that include two words: "I wish." For example, an exceedingly dependent patient in the ICU whimpered to her young house officer: "Doctor, I'm so scared. Please, please keep checking on me!" The savvy resident responded: "Mrs. D, your illness is severe and I am certain very frightening. While *I wish* I could stop by every hour, I have a lot to do in the hospital today. I promise, though, to check in with you this evening around 5 p.m." With the woman's fear and anxiety validated—believing that her physician would keep her and her problems in mind throughout the day and actually stop in for a visit (which the resident did with all of her patients)—this patient felt comforted and acted less demanding.

The Obsessive Patient

Obsessive individuals are emotionally constricted and rigid. They tend to focus on minute details and lose the big picture. They are compelled to make the "right" or "perfect" decision based on "facts" and never feel that they—or their caregivers—have all the information to provide optimal treatment. Consequently, they are intensely frustrating to providers, who feel assaulted by endless questions and devalued, as the provider never has the patient's confidence in treatment decisions (15). Caring for the patient or family member who pays obsessive attention to detail and routine can be very taxing. By clinging to the "rules of medicine" as a 7- to 10-year-old child might adhere to the rules of a board game, the obsessive patient can irritate physicians and nurses. In contrast to narcissistic patients who regain control over their surroundings via denial, distortion, and bullying behavior, obsessive individuals defend against feelings of helplessness by focusing on medical minutiae. The obsessive logic goes: "a place for each thing and each thing in its place" (19). Of course, everything in the ICU is out of place; patients do not know what their radiographs show right away; their labs are a mystery to them for several hours, even days; and the meaning of the blips and bleeps of monitors buzzing around them is not understood. So, with often very rudimentary medical knowledge, the obsessive patient or family member works hard to gain mastery over these details. Losing the forest for the trees, the obsessive patient asks incessant questions. For example, one woman with Guillain-Barré syndrome demanded to know why she was not being transfused when she saw an "L" marked next to her "HCT" of 32.3%. When her nurse sat down next to her bed, summarized her lab report, and explained the team's management rationale, the patient felt knowledgeable and was soothed. Again, dealing with this type of difficult patient interaction takes extra time and a firm decision on the practitioner's part to have a different relationship with the patient. Obsessive patients cannot stand the paternalistic, authoritarian approach, and the practitioner who is not flexible will get into fruitless standoffs with these patients. Statements such as "you just rest and let us take care of you" are intensely irritating to the obsessive patient. Instead, offering the obsessive individual a set amount of information, with a satisfying but not overwhelming amount of detail, can be key. This may mean showing the obsessive patient or family member a chest radiograph or reviewing their "lytes" at bedside. Second, the obsessive patient, like all patients, appreciates routine. Announcing and, insofar as possible, keeping to a schedule in which nurses and physicians will visit are important. Finally, scientific, deductive reasoning ("if your labs show X, then we'll respond by doing Y") curbs the obsessive patient's anxiety.

The Dramatic Patient

Linked to many instances in early childhood trauma and because they have intense difficulty identifying their own affective state, in distinguishing how they think and feel from how others think and feel (20), dramatic patients fail to recognize subtlety. They thus engage in highly volatile relationships. In the hospital, these patients—many of whom suffer borderline personality disorder in the official psychiatric nomenclature (17)—engage their physicians and nurses in relationships that are intensely intimate or staggeringly conflictual. The dramatic patient often seduces some staff members and alienates others. This leaves ICU personnel at odds, with some having had a very positive experience with the patient, using phrases like "lovely," "charming," and "delightful" to describe the patient, and others considering the patient obstreperous or toxic. When clinicians who have such divergent experiences with a dramatic patient convene, there is often a conflict over how to manage the patient's demands. This experience is dubbed "splitting" and can create tremendous tension. The deleterious effects of splitting, which include mistreating the patient and high staff tension, are minimized when physicians and nurses acknowledge that they have had much different emotional experiences with a patient. Once this is done, limits can be set in a manner that both soothes the patient and settles the staff (Table 3.4).

Dramatic patients are also notorious for their hypersensitivity to physical pain and perceived slight and threat of abandonment by physicians and nurses. Similar to the dependent

TABLE 3.4

PRINCIPLES OF EFFECTIVE LIMIT SETTING IN THE INTENSIVE CARE UNIT (ICU)

- **Validate:** Acknowledge the patient's real struggles.
- **Explain:** Provide limits in a clear and concise manner and avoid overly euphemistic statements such as: "Refrain from unsafe behavior." Instead, say: "Please stop throwing things!"
- **Be flexible:** Before speaking with the patient, discuss as a team what the patient may ask for and what the ICU team can be flexible in offering. For example, can a patient begging for a cigarette be administered nicotine gum or a transdermal patch?
- **Determine consequences:** Know in advance how to handle transgression of limits; these do not necessarily need to be shared with the patient or his or her family, but can give the ICU team a sense of security.
- **Avoid arguments:** Long, drawn-out battles of wit or reason are rarely useful. Leaving the patient's bedside in order to cool down, think of a new strategy, or consult a colleague is better than acting impulsively.

Adapted from Usher CT. Problematic behavior of patients, family and staff in the intensive care unit. In: Irwin RS, Rippe JM, eds. *Irwin and Rippe's Intensive Care Medicine*. 6th ed. Philadelphia: Lippincott Williams & Wilkins; 2008.

patient, validating the very dramatic patient's feelings is key. Although the clinical staff may believe that dramatic patients are "exaggerating" or "faking" their symptoms, even if these assessments may be accurate, it is futile to believe that these concerns can be managed by approaches that entail feelings such as "I hope that they will just go away or stop if I ignore them." One must have an explicit plan to improve the relationship with a patient. As one of our (CU) senior residents at Walter-Reed Army Medical Center once intoned, "Sir, hope is not a course of action!" It can be immensely soothing to dramatic patients if you convey your understanding of their struggles and let them know that you are aware of many of the problems they are facing. Furthermore, asking, "Are there some problems that I've missed that we need to make certain we are helping with?", can lead to further improvement in your relationship.

COMMUNICATING WITH FAMILIES IN THE INTENSIVE CARE UNIT

The ear says more
Than any tongue.

W.S. Graham, "The Hill of Intrusion"

Family members and friends are not mere visitors to the ICU (21). They are often charged, sometimes reluctantly (22), with understanding a patient's diagnosis, prognosis, and treatment options, in addition to making informed decisions when their loved one is unable to express his or her own medical care preferences. Family members also play an integral role in encouraging their critically ill spouses, siblings, aunts, and uncles. In addition, they may help nurses provide care, and often spend much time on the phone or e-mailing, communicating progress and problems to relatives and friends of the patient who cannot visit the ICU. A study by Pochard et al. found that the prevalence of depression in family members of intensive care unit patients was 69%, while 35% suffered marked anxiety (12). These symptoms may make it very hard for family members and loved ones to function in their roles as caretakers, nurturers, communicators, and decision makers while on the unit; moreover, it impacts their abilities as mothers, fathers, and employees outside the unit.

Quality communication between ICU staff and family members of ICU patients is central to:

- Reducing family stress and dissatisfaction (23)
- Minimizing conflict surrounding end-of-life decisions (24)
- Decreasing futile interventions (25)
- Reducing friction between ICU staff and families (26)

Again, while some families may utilize maladaptive coping strategies or appear very similar to the personality profiles listed in Table 3.3, ICU staff committed to communicating with families stand the best chance of promoting patient and family security and alleviating suffering.

While each family and critical care situation is unique, following some general guidelines (Table 3.5) for interacting with families can be helpful. These include being clear and concise when explaining the medical information; asking to make certain the data are understood; scheduling appointments for family meetings; listening more and talking less; tuning in to those things that make the patient and family special (27); and providing early diagnostic and prognostic information, even if this involves admitting uncertainty (28). Keep in mind that most families rate the clinician's ability to communicate above their clinical prowess (29).

TABLE 3.5

CORE PRINCIPLES OF COMMUNICATION WITH FAMILIES IN THE INTENSIVE CARE UNIT (ICU)

CLEAR Provide family members and loved ones with clear, concise descriptions of the patient's condition and avoid jargon. Frequently ask if there are any questions and provide more detail as necessary.
ON TIME Schedule appointments for family meetings or treatment updates. Try, as best as possible, to be on time. If you will be late or unavailable, send a representative.
RESPECT THE PATIENT'S UNIQUENESS These appointments are as much about what you say as how well you listen. Focus carefully on what makes the patient special and try to learn the names of the people who are important to the patient.
EARLY DIAGNOSIS AND PROGNOSIS Even if it means saying, "I'm not sure," try to inform the family early in the ICU stay.

Adapted from Usher CT. Problematic behavior of patients, family and staff in the intensive care unit. In: Irwin RS, Rippe JM, eds. *Irwin and Rippe's Intensive Care Medicine.* 6th ed. Philadelphia: Lippincott Williams & Wilkins; 2008.

Despite early, open dialogue between ICU clinicians and patients' families, problems nevertheless will arise. Owing to stress, depression, and anxiety, some families may not want to participate in the decision-making process regarding their loved one's care (22). Referral to unit support staff, including social workers who are able to assess the needs of family members, can be very helpful.

At times, the family members' judgment may be clouded by anger toward the patient. For example, the relatives of a patient who is being treated in the ICU following a suicide attempt may be upset at the patient for "wanting to leave them behind," and hence may make decisions out of anger, frustration, and disappointment (30). If one senses that this is the case, bringing these feelings out into the open—what psychotherapists term "making the implicit explicit"—can help families consider treatment decisions more thoughtfully.

Breakdowns in understanding and communication between clinicians and families occur when, wrought with guilt or a profound sense of duty, family members demand that staff "do everything possible" for the patient, even when aggressive care is futile. One scenario in which this occurs involves the distant son or daughter who has played a minimal role in his or her parent's life and feels overwhelming guilt. Alternatively, family members may feel they "need" a relative so badly that losing him or her would be psychologically devastating. This may impair their reasoning to the point that they overinterpret subtle cues as signs that their loved ones can hear them, appreciate their presence, or "want to keep on fighting." Sometimes these wishful perceptions cause family members to make decisions counter to what the patient requested before he or she was incapacitated. In these cases, it can be transformative when the clinician conveys an understanding of what the patient means to his or her family members and also offers a solution that preserves the family members' views of themselves and of the patient.

For example, after a prolonged battle with cancer, a war veteran was admitted to an ICU in respiratory failure. The patient's daughter was made aware that this man had little chance of making a meaningful recovery; yet in family meetings, she foreclosed any discussion of withdrawing ventilator support. "He's a fighter; he's made it this far and he's gonna keep fighting," she protested. In response, a very empathic intensivist explored how much this woman's father meant to her, learning that this patient being a "fighter" inspired his daughter to battle with her own illness. The ICU physician described back to this woman what an inspirational life her father had lived, conveying an understanding what "being a fighter" meant in their family. Upon hearing these words—that the physician "got it" and was still recommending a full discussion of treatment options—the patient's daughter relaxed her stance and was willing to discuss end-of-life care options with the ICU team and the rest of her family.

A family's spoken language and cultural understanding of health, illness, and dying play crucial roles in their ability to meaningfully communicate with ICU staff members. Both literally and figuratively, it is important for families to sense that ICU physicians and staff members are working hard to "speak the family's language." Translated literally, this means that ICU staff must ensure that families can understand the content of what the staff are conveying. For families who may not enjoy a medically rich vocabulary, this means avoiding the use of technical terms and medical jargon, and frequently asking if there are questions. Meanwhile, for families for whom English is not their first language, offering and utilizing medical interpreters is extremely important (31). Family members should not be used as interpreters, as it places a major burden on these individuals to remain intellectually engaged in understanding and conveying material and to emotionally cope with the information they are processing. Family members who become the "go-to" person in terms of interpreting may also emphasize certain facts to loved ones in order to influence their decisions or can reluctantly become primary decision makers based solely on their fluency, but not out of a desire to lead the family in making medical decisions.

All families hold explanations for illness embedded in a cultural identity. To physicians steeped in the Western allopathic medical tradition, some culturally bound beliefs—often stemming from a family or individual's religious, spiritual, ethnic identity—may seem strange such that a meaningful dialogue about a patient's medical condition seems impossible. As one puzzled intern intoned after a troubling family meeting, "I was talking about heart failure, while his wife kept talking about spirits. It was weird, I was like, 'Are we having the same conversation?'." In order to prevent such Babelic dialogue, physicians can benefit from being openly curious about the way a family member will integrate the information he or she has to share. Thus, it may be helpful to open a family meeting by asking family members what their understanding of the situation is and, perhaps, why they believe their loved one is experiencing the problems he or she is. This helps set the stage for a more fruitful conversation, by establishing that the physician hopes to offer information that will be integrated into, but not supplant, a family's perspective. One can also suggest to families that they invite a trusted friend, priest, shaman, or other culturally esteemed individual to family meetings with medical staff, or offer to review the information with that person.

Of course, despite the best efforts of clinicians and family members, standstills sometimes occur. In those situations where family members linger at odds with each other or with ICU staff regarding medical decisions, an ethics consultation is helpful.

PROMOTING UNDERSTANDING AND COMMUNICATION WITH CHILDREN AND TEENAGERS IN THE INTENSIVE CARE UNIT

If the behavior of ICU patients and their family members and loved ones can be perplexing and irritating to critical care physicians and nurses, then understanding the reactions of children visiting the ICU can be downright bewildering. Still, parents often ask if their son or daughter should visit a parent or loved one in the ICU and, if so, how to facilitate these visits. Thus, it behooves the physician or nurse interested in practicing whole-family care to keep in mind a few developmental principles.

The first issues to consider when a family asks about a child visiting in the ICU are whether it is appropriate for the developmental level of the child and whether the child could visit the unit and feel safe, as well as ascertaining the motivation for the visit. It is thus most important to ask: Whose idea is it for the child to visit, and why? Occasionally, when the staff inquires who the child's visit is for, revelations about the individual's own experience are revealed. For example, one man who was quite emotionally distraught wanted his 4-year-old son to visit his grandmother, who was on a ventilator and likely to pass away. This preschool-aged boy had experienced little contact with his grandmother prior to her illness and had clearly stated he did not want to go. Yet, his father explained to the ICU social worker: "Well, I just think he *ought* to see grandma. I always wanted to see my grandma and regret it, so I think my son should see his." Having made that statement, the man realized that his desire to have his son come to the ICU was a projection of his own wishes to relieve guilty feelings about failing to visit his own grandmother. With the help of the unit social worker, the gentleman and his wife instead opted to have their son stay at home, but were able to learn some simple phrases to explain to this youngster what was going on with his grandmother.

Meanwhile, there are very good reasons for children to visit loved ones in the ICU: To promote attachment and understanding; to reduce fears, hopelessness, and guilt; and to fulfill a mutual desire on the part of the patient and child to see one another (32). For example, when a child's parent is hospitalized but likely to recover, the child's fears of his mother or father dying or going through immeasurable torment may be assuaged by visiting. The visit may have a dual positive purpose—it may buoy the spirits of the hospitalized parent.

In addition to gauging emotional factors when helping families decide whether a child should visit the ICU, safety factors must also be considered. For example, the child who becomes overwhelmingly anxious, even dangerously hyperactive, is not a great candidate for visiting the ICU. Also, given their undeveloped immunocompetence, it is typically considered inappropriate for infants under 9 months to visit the hospital.

Finally, children, adolescents, and families need to be prepared for an ICU visit. This is best done by having a staff member meet with the child and an accompanying adult family member to provide guidance about the experience. They need both an appreciation of what may be seen, felt, and understood in the ICU, and what consequences may require attention after a visit. Providing information and explanations to the child and family member must take into account the cognitive and emotional level of the child. The information that follows may be helpful to staff when taking these developmental considerations into account.

Preschoolers (3- to 6-year-olds)

There are three features of preschool-aged children that are central to their visiting the ICU: The fact that they are egocentric, they employ magical thinking, and they are keenly focused on body integrity. Regarding the first two points, children often believe they are responsible for their own illnesses or the illnesses of loved ones. For example, one little girl believed her mother was in the ICU because the same day her mother was hit by a car, she had "said a swear." With great effort, this little girl's father assuaged her guilt and explained the nature of the car accident. Meanwhile, remember that children of this age are very concerned with body integrity; they love bandages, often believing that "boo-boos" that are not properly covered will ooze out the life force. Hence, when children see tubes and catheters, blood-smeared intravenous sites, or wounds, they can become tremendously fearful. They may also reason that these things are what is keeping the patient in the ICU and making him or her ill, as opposed to thinking that the ICU is keeping the patient there to provide loved ones the necessary care to keep him or her alive. Providing children with pictures of what they will see in the ICU—such as showing them an IV pole, a stretcher, a monitor, and a puppet play about what the ICU will be like before they visit—can be key to helping them gain a sense of mastery over their ICU visit. For example, after taking a tour of an empty ICU room and being told what to expect, one proud 6-year-old commented: "My dad was connected to this bag (IV fluids) on this pole and this machine, 'cuz his lither and his kid knees aren't working, but it was okay, these machines were helping."

School-aged Children (7- to 11-year-olds)

Around the age of 7, children begin developing a more sophisticated world view based on logic. They have a voracious appetite for knowledge and understanding the "rules" of a system. For example, first-graders love board games. However, this desire for understanding is balanced with not wanting to look "dumb," so school-aged children will often not ask questions. The key to preparing children of this age for visits with critically ill relatives and family friends is to provide basic details about illness and frequently ask if they have any questions. Too much information can overwhelm children of this age, who may still find the internal organ "goings on" of an ill individual quite mysterious. Helping children gain a sense of mastery by buying books and using diagrams or models to explain what is happening to a relative may be very helpful. Finally, giving children something to do, such as filling a water pitcher or vase, opening cards, or presenting a gift, can help alleviate boredom and promote a sense of accomplishment—they will feel like they have been helpful to the loved one. One last note on children of this age is that early in the school-age developmental era, children gain a sense that death is permanent. This may bring about a profound anxiety. Exploring children's thoughts on the matter and reassuring them that their life routines and schedules will continue despite the possible loss of a loved one can be very reassuring.

Preteens and Adolescents (12+ Years)

Teenagers have a much stronger sense of medical reality and, with this understanding, more robust, emotional responses. Some adolescents may throw themselves into the caretaker role, wanting to operate on the level of adult family members that are visiting. Others may choose to avoid the hospital, finding the experience too overwhelming. Helpful measures can be taken such as being nonjudgmental, laying out the pros and cons of visiting relatives, and avoiding "guilt trips" such as "this may be the last time you ever get to see your uncle so you'd better go." Also, when providing adolescents with information before they come to the hospital, they may be quite offended when they are "spoken down to"; hence, a very nonauthoritarian, open discussion of what is happening to their relative or loved one is the best approach. Finally, it is helpful when communicating with anxious teenagers to ask, in an open-ended manner, if there is anything they are worried about. Most teenagers loathe comments such as "I can see you're worried. Just admit it," which can lead to painful arguments during the drive to and from the hospital. Particularly with teenagers, but also with younger children, in family conferences, it is important for doctors and nurses to look them in the eye, shake their hand, and ask if they have any questions—treating them as full members of the family.

SUMMARY

> Mindful practitioners attend in a non-judgmental way to their own physical and mental processes during ordinary, everyday tasks. This critical self-reflection enables physicians to listen attentively to patients' distress, recognize their own errors, refine their technical skills, make evidence-based decisions, and clarify their values so that they can act with compassion, technical competence, presence and insight.
>
> *Ronald Epstein (33)*

Care in the ICU requires highly specialized knowledge and skill on the part of all health professionals. However, the technical skills required for optimal care may be severely compromised by the emotional reactions of patients and families. Physicians in the ICU should see themselves not only in a capacity to cure or stabilize illness, but also in a unique position to heal. Healing involves more than applying current scientific knowledge, diagnostic procedures, and therapeutic technique. Beyond these critical factors, it requires providing comfort, reassurance, open and honest communication, respect, and empathy (34). Too often, care is compromised by the interference of the patient and/or families in the therapeutic process. When the clinician can appreciate the types of personalities and reactions of patients and families in crisis situations, understand the underlying psychological processes that engender them, and maintain an acute awareness of his or her own responses to them, he or she will be fully able to provide the best possible care in the ICU.

Working in the ICU is, of necessity, a multidisciplinary team-based enterprise. As such, there is no substitute for discussion by team members of both the medical aspects of their patients' conditions and their emotional reactions, especially as they impact individual clinician and team functioning. Being mindful pertains not only to the individual, but also to the team, and taking some time for distance from the patient, communication, and reflection is often clarifying and rejuvenating. Moreover, the ICU staff should welcome the assistance of consultants and mentors with extensive experience in their management of difficult patients and families.

References

1. Coomber S, Todd C, Park G, et al. Stress in UK intensive care unit doctors. *Br J Anaesth.* 2002;89:873.
2. Fischer JE, Calame A, Dettling AC, et al. Experience and endocrine response in neonatal and pediatric critical nurses and physicians. *Crit Care Med.* 2000;28:3281.
3. Krebs EE, Garrett JM, Konrad TR. The difficult doctor? Characteristics of physicians who report frustration with patients: an analysis of survey data. *BMC Health Serv Res.* 2006;6:128.
4. Rincon HG, Granados M, Unutzer J, et al. Prevalence, detection, and treatment of anxiety, depression, and delirium in the adult critical care unit. *Psychosomatics.* 2001;42:391.
5. Trenoweth S. Perceiving risk in dangerous situations: risk of violence among mental health inpatients. *J Adv Nurs.* 2003;42:278.
6. Ely EW, Shintani A, Truman B, et al. Delirium as a predictor of mortality in mechanically ventilated patients in the intensive care unit. *JAMA.* 2004;291:1753.
7. Pronovost P, Weast B, Schwarz M, et al. Medication reconciliation: a practical tool to reduce the risk of medication errors. *J Crit Care.* 2003;18:201.
8. Vira T, Colquhoun M, Etchells E. Reconcilable differences: correcting medication errors at hospital admission and discharge. *Qual Saf Health Care.* 2006;15:122.
9. Biancofiore G, Bindi ML, Romanelli AM, et al. Stress-inducing factors in ICUs: what liver transplant recipients experience and what caregivers perceive. *Liver Transpl.* 2005;11:967.
10. van de Leur JP, van der Schans CP, Loef BG, et al. Discomfort and factual recollection in intensive care unit patients. *Crit Care.* 2004;8(6):R467–473.
11. Richter JC, Waydhas C, Pajonk FG. Incidence of posttraumatic stress disorder after prolonged surgical intensive care unit treatment. *Psychosomatics.* 2006;47:223.
12. Pochard F, Azoulay E, Chevret S, et al. Symptoms of anxiety and depression in family members of intensive care unit patients: ethical hypothesis regarding decision-making capacity. *Crit Care Med.* 2001;29:1893.
13. Im K, Belle SH, Schulz R, et al. Prevalence and outcomes of caregiving after prolonged (> or =48 hours) mechanical ventilation in the ICU. *Chest.* 2004;125:597.
14. Azoulay E, Pochard F, Kentish-Barnes N, et al. Risk of post-traumatic stress symptoms in family members of intensive care unit patients. *Am J Respir Crit Care Med.* 2005;171:987.
15. Groves JE, Beresin EV. Difficult patients, difficult families. *New Horizons.* 1998;6(4):331.
16. Bibring GL, Kahana RJ. *Lectures in Medical Psychology: An Introduction of the Care of Patients.* New York: International Universities Press; 1968.
17. American Psychiatric Association. *Diagnostic and Statistical Manual of Mental Disorders.* 4th ed., Text Revision (DSM-IV-TR). Washington, DC: American Psychiatric Association Press; 1994.
18. Greenberg JR, Mitchell SA. *Object Relations in Psychoanalytic Theory.* Cambridge, MA: Harvard University Press; 1983.
19. Dor J. *The Clinical Lacan.* New York: Other Press; 1999.
20. Fonagy P. Attachment and borderline personality disorder. *J Am Psychoanal Assoc.* 2000;48:1129.
21. Molter NC. Families are not visitors in the critical care unit. *Dimens Crit Care Nurs.* 1994;13:2.
22. Azoulay E, Pochard F, Chevret S, et al. Half the family members of intensive care unit patients do not want to share in the decision-making process: a study in 78 French intensive care units. *Crit Care Med.* 2004;32:1832.
23. Malacrida R, Bettelini R, Molo C, et al. Reasons for dissatisfaction: a survey of relatives of intensive care patients who died. *Crit Care Med.* 1998;26:1187.
24. Lilly CM, De Meo DL, Sonna LA, et al. An intensive communication intervention for the critically ill. *Am J Med.* 2000;109:469.
25. Rivera S, Kim D, Garone S, et al. Motivating factors in futile clinical interventions. *Chest.* 2001;119:1944.
26. Fins JJ, Solomon MZ. Communication in intensive care settings: the challenge of futility disputes. *Crit Care Med.* 2001;29(Suppl 2):10.
27. McDonagh JR, Elliot TB, Engleberg RA, et al. Family satisfaction with family conferences about end-of-life care in the intensive care unit. *Crit Care Med.* 2004;32:1484.
28. Leclaire MM, Oakes JM, Weinert CR. Communication of prognostic information for critically ill patients. *Chest.* 2005;128:1728.
29. Curtis JR, Patrick DL, Shannon SE, et al. The family conference as a focus to improve communication about end-of-life care in the intensive care unit: opportunities for improvement. *Crit Care Med.* 2001;29(Suppl 2):26.
30. Wasserman D. Passive euthanasia to attempted suicide. One form of aggressiveness of relatives. *Acta Psychiatr Scand.* 1989;79:460.
31. Karliner LS, Jacobs EA, Chen AH, et al. Do professional interpreters improve clinical care for patients with limited English proficiency? A system review of the literature. *Health Serv Res.* 2007;42:727–754.
32. Clarke C, Harrison D. The needs of children visiting on adult intensive care units: a review of the literature and recommendations for practice. *J Adv Nurs.* 2001;34:61.
33. Epstein RM. Mindful practice. *JAMA.* 1999;282:833.
34. Novak DH, Epstein RM, Paulsen RH. Toward creating physician-healers: fostering medical students' awareness, personal growth, and well-being. *Acad Med.* 1999;74:516.

CHAPTER 4 ■ BREAKING BAD NEWS TO PATIENTS

RHONDA S. FISHEL • JAMIE HOCHMAN

Case History

November 1, 2005: The patient is a 50-year-old Caucasian female who has had a 3-month history of intermittent left suprapubic pain, nausea, and fever; the episodes last 24 to 48 hours. Her past history is significant for mild hypothyroidism for which she takes levothyroxine. Her last menses was 2 years ago, and she has been followed for a uterine leiomyoma. She does not smoke or drink. The patient is a surgeon and an intensivist. Physical exam is remarkable for a 6-cm uterine mass, which is not fixed. Ultrasonography demonstrates an irregular uterine mass, which does not have increased blood flow. The study is interpreted as a likely growth of a previously benign fibroid. On October 31, 2005, she undergoes a total abdominal hysterectomy and bilateral salpingo-oophorectomy; frozen section shows large areas of uterine necrosis but does not demonstrate malignant cells. On postoperative day 1, the permanent pathology is interpreted as a 9-cm high-grade uterine sarcoma. Her gynecologist, also a colleague, sits at the patient's bedside and delivers this diagnosis. That evening, the patient has a computed tomography (CT) scan of the chest, which shows a pulmonary metastasis. Some months later, the gynecologist reveals to the patient that he was so distraught from giving her bad news that night that he developed laryngitis for the next several days.

Practitioners who choose a career in critical care medicine—or other emergent fields—will soon realize that a significant focus of their practice will be delivering and processing bad news. The excitement of applying bold clinical skills, using advanced technology, and making life-or-death decisions in the most critical patients will be tempered by the need to participate in the most somber of discussions. Giving bad news is not easy, thrilling, or glamorous—but it is essential. Done appropriately, it will provide the patient and family solace in a time of pain; done poorly, it is injury added to illness.

In this chapter, we will consider cultural, professional, and clinical barriers to effective communication. A framework will be provided to help the practitioner who must have these difficult conversations. This will include suggestions and scenarios based on our (RF and JH) experiences—both good and bad—as clinicians for over 25 years. We have learned immensely from our mentors, nurses, respiratory therapists, and social workers; from readings of others' words of wisdom; and from those that we have supervised.

Each country's health system and group of providers are sited in a cultural and social milieu. This siting determines, to a greater or lesser extent, some of the myriad ways with which we respond to the communication difficulties we detail below. As citizens of the United States, we realize that the discussion we bring to bear below is at least partially a result of our social and cultural setting, among other factors. Other of our colleagues, in the west and the east, might approach this issue somewhat differently. This is our approach.

Finally, it is a common misconception among physicians that they are the sole purveyors of the conversations surrounding the delivery of bad news. Nothing could be further from the truth. Physicians may initiate the conversations, but the aftermath is frequently laid on the doorstep of other practitioners—most especially our nurse and social worker colleagues. They must often decipher, interpret, elaborate, and provide emotional support for the patient and family, long after the physician has left.

BARRIERS TO EFFECTIVE COMMUNICATION

Influences from American culture and our professional training can be impediments to the effective delivery of bad news (Table 4.1). In the new millennium, communication has become increasingly truncated. Inundation with cell phones, e-mails, and text messaging has generated an ABS (abbreviation-based society), and time is—or at least appears to be—of the essence. We call others when we know that they are not at home, so that we can leave a message on their answering machine. We do not have time for the nuances and articulated detail of spoken or written conversation.

Our society has carried the winner or loser mentality from the battlefield to the gridiron to popular television shows. Contestants must be winners or be banished; there is no middle ground. We watch media coverage and re-enactment of medical miracles, which we accept as expected outcomes. We forget that miracle is defined as an "extraordinary event taken as a sign of divine intervention in human affairs" (Webster's New Explorer Dictionary [published 2000]). In our society, bad events and outcomes must be accompanied by the assessment of blame. "Let bygones be bygones" would not be an apt description of our litigious society. This societal Trifecta, when applied to the medical field, suggests that we are losers if our patients do not get better, and we are to blame. Many intensivists will tell you that in America, the last rites are cardiopulmonary resuscitation. Untoward outcomes from these societal influences may include intimidation of the practitioner, thus preventing a frank conversation with a patient or a family. Perhaps worse, the practitioner comes to see the battle as being between him or her and the disease, with the patient suffering as collateral damage.

Aspects of training, particularly of physicians in certain specialties, have encouraged traits that are the antithesis of the compassionate communicator. A majority of practicing physicians have reported having received no formal training in effectively communicating bad news (1). For example, surgeons are taught to be self-reliant, resilient, and tough. Emotions must be

TABLE 4.1

BARRIERS TO EFFECTIVE COMMUNICATION

American society	Physician training
■ Communicates in small sound bites	■ Personality issues
■ Has a winner or loser mentality	■ Training and indoctrination
■ Is constantly bombarded with shows about miracles	■ Time constraints
■ Believes the last rite is cardiopulmonary resuscitation	■ Fatigue
■ Believes the quicker the better	■ Fear of failure if patient dies

checked at the operating room door as surgeons prepare to be the master of the ritual. The sentiment reflected in the admonition given to young residents preparing to begin night duty—"call me if you need me, need me if you call me, and remember, it is a sign of weakness"—is not ambiguous. How do you then get them to flip the switch to something kinder and gentler? Many high-pressure specialties—certainly surgery, critical care medicine, and anesthesiology—attract a personality type that is driven, action-oriented, and without the patience to communicate effectively.

For those in training and in practice, the efficient use of time is an ongoing challenge. Further, the new work hour limitation for house staff compounds this stress. How does one accomplish all the tasks in the allowable time period? Unfortunately, the delivery of bad news cannot be neatly fit into a schedule, and may be quite time consuming. Finally, if the caregiver is exhausted, it may be hard to muster the energy needed to do this task well. The results from a questionnaire study completed by 167 physicians at the 1999 annual meeting of the American Society of Clinical Oncology noted that a majority of responding physicians felt that they did not have enough time to engage in difficult conversations with patients (2).

Giving patients and families devastating news takes its toll on the sender as well as the recipient. Each practitioner will need to develop two preservation strategies. The first is to have the ability to compartmentalize and be able to move on to a subsequent task. The second is to consider yourself an emotional filter, of which you need to determine the "porosity." If you are moved to tears and incapacitated every time you deliver bad news, burn-out may be in your near future. On the other hand, if you feel nothing as you give your patient the diagnosis of leukemia, you have lost the reason to be in clinical medicine. Naturally, the "porosity" of our filters will differ with the clinical scenario, and a portion of it will be out of our control.

The Institute for Professionalism and Ethical Practice at Children's Hospital, Boston, developed a workshop named Program to Enhance Relational and Communication Skills (PERCS) to prepare health care professionals for engaging in difficult conversations. The workshop participants commented that to become competent in delivering bad news, one must leave his or her badge at the door, be genuine, invite colleagues from other disciplines into the conversation, and attend to the emotional needs of the patient. It is also important to avoid insensitive and careless terms such as "incompetent cervix" or "harvesting organs" (3).

THE BEST WAY TO GIVE THE WORST NEWS

Every practitioner will develop his or her own style of speaking with families and, particularly, a style of how to break bad news. Table 4.2 provides some guidelines for these discussions.

Begin by preparing what you will say. It is very important to consider the context in which the patient/family will be hearing your message. They have or will form an opinion about you that may or may not have merit. You may appear too young, or be of the wrong demographic for them to trust what you say. They may have had a bad experience in your hospital or have emotional dysfunction that impairs their ability to listen to and accept the information you are preparing to present. In these situations, it is good to have another member of the care team with you, both to increase your credibility and to bear witness.

Unlike many communications in our e-mail, text-messaging, sound-bite society, this one must be a conversation. Your goals at the end of this conversation are to have the patient or family understand your message and to feel that you have acted responsibly and professionally. The best ways to accomplish this goal are by paying respect to the situation and by encouraging and watching their responses. Everyone should be sitting, as much as is possible, and pagers and cell phones should be turned off or given to others to hold. Speak directly, make eye contact, and watch the family members'/patient's reaction. Are they listening to you? Are they understanding you? Do you need to slow down, ask if they understand what you say, or repeat some of the information? This advice is simple but crucial to effective communication.

If a patient spoke only Spanish, we would not have a conversation with him in English. In our training, we learned the language of medicine, to which we added common abbreviations and idioms. Whether intentional or not, we speak to our patients in this language, much to their bewilderment. Figure 4.1 provides an example of an intensive care unit (ICU) assessment given to a family in medical language (A) and in English (B).

TABLE 4.2

GUIDELINES FOR EFFECTIVE CONVERSATIONS

- ■ Prepare what you are going to say in advance.
- ■ Take a colleague with you.
- ■ Engage in a two-way conversation with patients and families.
- ■ Watch for verbal and nonverbal cues.
- ■ Speak directly and maintain eye contact.
- ■ Avoid slang and jargon.
- ■ Be patient and give patients and families time to absorb information.
- ■ Be empathetic.

A. Physician speak:
Your father has a pleural effusion and we will probably need to perform a thoracentesis. His ejection fraction has deteriorated and we may need to float a pulmonary artery occlusion catheter. His BUN and creatinine have increased and we are worried that he is becoming coagulopathic. This clinical picture may represent SIRS or sepsis or this could be adrenal insufficiency. Further laboratory analysis is needed. A cortisol stimulation is pending.

B. Physician speak revised:
Your father has fluid on his lung and we may need to drain the fluid. We do this at the bedside and he will be given medication so it doesn't hurt. His heart is not pumping as well as it should and we may need to put in a special IV so we can follow this closely. His kidneys are also a little worse but we think we can fix it. His blood does not clot properly. If you put this all together, it may be that he is fighting a bad infection that makes his whole body sick. Sometimes all of this happens because a little gland above the kidneys is not working right. We are going to do some tests to figure this out.

FIGURE 4.1. An intensive care unit assessment given to a family in medical language (A) and in English (B).

We should not assume that our patients will question what they do not understand. They may not want to appear ignorant in our "temple." It is more important to sound intelligible than intelligent. One should avoid "inadvertent disempowering behavior" (Caroline Pace, personal communication, 2006), where the patient or family members, already at a disadvantage because of illness, now must feel inadequate because they do not understand the communication.

It is not necessary to feel sorry for patients, but it is crucial to have empathy for their situations. Though perhaps irrational, upon the receipt of bad news, there is a sense of isolation from others not afflicted. Patients hope that you can acknowledge, if not relate, to their feelings. There are practitioners—some of you reading these words now—young or fortunate enough not to have experienced loss or tragedy. Empathy is a quality of humanity and is not well faked. It has been said that "empathy is my pain in your heart" (4).

We may become frustrated when a family member or a patient seems slow to grasp what is so obvious to us as health care providers. For example, we may view a patient with a ruptured cerebral aneurysm, approaching brain death, as a straightforward fatality. However, the family members, seeing a relatively healthy-looking patient on the ventilator, may wonder when he will wake up. Remember, they lack your perspective and may have only had a few hours or a few days to process their family tragedy.

The traditional relationship between physician and patient has often been patriarchal. The physician was held on a pedestal (at least outwardly) by the remainder of the care team, so there was a natural comfort in surrendering one's fate to an omnipotent healer. Dr. Rachel Remen, in *My Grandfather's Blessing*, challenged this paradigm. Dr. Remen, who has struggled with the complications of Crohn disease since her late teens, counsels those with chronic or terminal illness, as well as the physicians and nurses who care for those patients. Her book suggests that the relationship between caregiver and patient is that of equals, with each bringing their strengths and weaknesses to the fore. This defines the important concept of service, which she describes with the comment:

> I have served impeccably with parts of myself of which I am ashamed.

Implicit in this admission is the acknowledgment that weaknesses may be strengths in difficult settings. However, she warns that the stress of caring for chronically ill and dying patients will take its toll on the provider, particularly if that stress is not recognized and defused (5).

Baile and Buckman described a simple mnemonic to help practitioners convey bad news (6) (Table 4.3). The SPIKES protocol emphasizes the critical features of this type of communication. A small, laminated copy of this protocol may be a good addition to the stethoscope and penlight in the ICU house officer's armamentarium.

TABLE 4.3

SPIKES PROTOCOL

Setting: Establish patient rapport by creating an appropriate setting that provides for privacy, patient comfort, uninterrupted time, sitting at eye level, and inviting significant other(s) (if desired).
Perception: Elicit the patient's perception of his or her problem.
Invitation: Obtain the patient's invitation to disclose the details of the medical condition.
Knowledge: Provide knowledge and information to the patient. Give information in small chunks, check for understanding, and frequently avoid medical jargon.
Empathize: Empathize and explore emotions expressed by the patient.
Summary and strategy: Provide a summary of what you said and negotiate a strategy for treatment or follow-up.

From Baile WF, Kudelka AP, Beale EA, et al. Communication skills training in oncology: description and preliminary outcomes of workshops on breaking bad news and managing patient reactions to illness. *Cancer.* 1999;86:887–897. Baile et al.'s protocol was adapted from Buckman R. *How to Break Bad News: A Guide For Healthcare Professionals.* Baltimore: Johns Hopkins University Press; 1992.

CLINICAL SCENARIOS

There are many specific scenarios in which bad news is given. In the critical care setting, these consist primarily of sudden catastrophic events and end-of-life issues.

Sudden Catastrophic Events

A sudden catastrophic event is usually the unexpected death of a family member, but may also include situations where the patient or family member has sustained an adverse, life-changing event, such as a traumatic injury with quadriplegia, a massive myocardial infarction, or severe stroke. Seasoned health care professionals are easily able to identify clinical scenarios that result in poor outcomes. "Just as medications need to be dispensed with consideration for choice, dosage, and timing, so, too, should clinical information be communicated with regard to the choice of what to communicate, the degree of detail that is preferred by the family, and at a time that is most appropriate to the family's needs" (7). As you enter the room, remember the suggestions listed above. Have another member of the team with you, sit down, turn off cell phones and pagers, and introduce the members of your team.

You have the solemn task of giving information that in some cases will change the listeners' lives forever. Give the news directly, particularly when the patient has died, and get to the point within a few sentences:

> Your son was in a head-on collision. He had massive injuries; we tried everything we could to save his life, but I am sorry to tell you that he died.

It is unkind to put the family through the ups and downs of what transpired during an hour-long resuscitation. Use the term *dead* or *died*; the message should not have more than one possible interpretation. One should not be cruel but, rather than stating that the patient has "moved on" or "passed away," one should state that he or she is dead. As that news is heard, the family will react, sometimes verbally, sometimes physically, and sometimes in silence. During this time, your input will not be heard. When the family members return their gaze in your direction, you can give more information or ask if there are further questions. Occasionally, families will turn their anger toward you and imply that the patient would still be alive if he or she had received competent care. Stay calm and reiterate that the injuries were severe—perhaps with some detail—and that everything possible was done for the patient. End by giving your condolences. Provide the family members a means by which they can contact the team if they have questions a day, a week, or a month later, and leave a team member behind to answer any questions that they may not have wanted to ask you. In addition, the family may need to ask another person to verify and thus validate your comments.

End-of-life Issues

On television and in the movies, characters will be critically ill or sustain horrific trauma. They must either die or be well by the end of the show. Unfortunately, this fantasy forms the perception of most of the public, and thus presents a constant challenge for the critical care provider, who must guide patients and families through the process of illness and—in some cases—dying. We believe that the most important priorities are the care and advocacy for the patient and the relationship with the family. The clinical aspects of care are well represented in this textbook and will not be covered here.

TABLE 4.4

THE INITIAL INTENSIVE CARE UNIT FAMILY MEETING

- Meet with the family as soon as possible.
- If possible, include the patient in the conversation.
- Determine if the patient has a living will or advanced directive, and the identity of the decision maker.
- Begin the clinical discussion with a review of the patient's illness.
- Emphasize the influence of comorbidities on the outcome of illness.
- If the prognosis is particularly dismal, one should "hang crepe."
- Be leery of giving statistics.
- Inquire about the family's level of religious and/or spiritual beliefs.
- Outline the goals of treatment and how we measure whether the patient is meeting those goals.

As early as possible in the patient's ICU course, the critical care provider should meet with the family (Table 4.4). If the patients are coherent and competent, they should be included in the conversation, as they are the decision makers. However, in the ICU, patients with end-of-life issues are often not sufficiently awake to participate in this discussion. Determine if the patient has a living will or advanced directive, and the identity of the decision maker. This accomplished, the clinical discussion should begin with a review of the patient's illness, as well as the important topic of the patient's pre-existing state of health. The influence of comorbidities on the outcome of illness needs to be emphasized. If the prognosis is particularly dismal, one should "hang crepe," that is, set the stage for the likelihood of further bad news. Be leery of giving statistics; make sure that the family and patient understand that statistics are primarily of predictive value and may not deal with their particular situation. Inquire about the family's level of religious and/or spiritual beliefs. This can be a powerful source of comfort in a time of crisis and loss. Many faiths believe that life does not end with death, which can facilitate acceptance. Whether or not the critical care provider's beliefs match those of the patient and family *is not relevant* in these discussions. It is important for all concerned to remember that there are aspects of the patient's course that we cannot control. Finally, the provider should outline what the goals of treatment will be, and how we measure whether the patient is meeting those goals.

If the information includes unexpected and catastrophic news, such as a patient who went to the operating room for an elective colon resection and is found to have extensive metastatic disease, it should be delivered similarly to news of a sudden death. The recipient will need to process this information and may be unresponsive, or even turn pale for a moment. Judge when to continue the discussion, but remember that you are unlikely to successfully convey important details during this conversation. Speak broadly, offer a later detailed discussion, and give the patient hope to recover from the acute phase of this disease. Patients want the truth to be balanced with hope. Specifically, oncology patients wish for information to be presented honestly, but not too bluntly as to destroy hope. Physicians need to emphasize what *can* be done, not focus on concerns that cannot be fixed (8).

As the patient's ICU stay continues, members of the care team should give regular progress reports. A feature of the daily rounds should be an assessment of the patient's condition. All viewpoints must be heard, but in the end, the team should decide on a uniform message for the patient and the family. Their situation is stressful and confusing enough without receiving mixed messages, as might occur in a large teaching institution with several services caring for the patient. Further, dysfunctional or suspicious families may use discordant assessments as verification of their belief that "one hand doesn't know what the other hand is doing." The report given to the family will include how the patient is doing in relation to the goals that were set. The daily or regular meetings give the family and the patient time to adjust to the situation. Critical care providers will often encounter family denial of clinical deterioration. While we tend to view denial disparagingly, it can also be a circuit breaker (or surge protector) from the overwhelming effect of the message. In these instances, give the information incrementally. Emily Dickinson understood this phenomenon:

> Tell all the Truth but tell it slant—
> Success in circuit lies
> Too bright for our Infirm Delight
> The Truth's superb surprise
> As Lightning to the Children eased
> With explanation kind
> The Truth must dazzle gradually
> Or every man be blind
>
> Emily Dickinson

In addition to the daily assessment of the condition of the patient, the team should consider if care has become futile. If the patient's clinical course continues to decline or fails to improve—with little hope that it will—it is likely time for a conversation about withdrawal of care. Occasionally, families request to withdraw care from a patient, but generally this topic is broached by the critical care team. If possible, have members of the multidisciplinary team present; again, it provides cohesion of message. Review the patient's course up to this point and how goals have not been met. Although we express that our purpose in the ICU is to prolong life, there comes a point when we are actually prolonging death. That point may not be clear as we approach it, but is recognized after we pass it. The conundrum of ICU care in the new millennium is that there are patients whom we can keep alive but cannot make well.

When asking families to agree to withdrawal of care or comfort care orders, the provider should consider his or her choice of words very carefully. Family members should not be made to feel like the executioner of their loved one. We prefer an approach such as the following:

> You know your father much better than we do. Oftentimes, as people get older or have suffered for a long time with a chronic illness, they are not as afraid of death as they are of the prolonged process of dying. As much as you want him to remain alive, he has counted on you to convey his wishes. Our best attempts to battle his illness have failed; we cannot save him, but I promise that we can make him comfortable.

TABLE 4.5

PROGRESSION OF HOPE

- Hope for cure
- Hope for long remission
- Hope for short remission
- Hope for comfort
- Hope for a good death
- Hope for a legacy

From Dunn G. What in the world is comfort care? Presented at the American College of Surgeons Meeting, New Orleans, October 9, 2007.

Lautrette et al. emphasized several other aspects of a good end-of-life discussion with the family. Repeat back what families have said; do not present treatment options as equally practical; and learn to tolerate periods of silence. Most importantly, make sure the family understands that good care will be given, even if all possible treatments are not applied (9).

Sometimes various members of the family will have differing opinions on withdrawal of care. Good communication during frequent family meetings was found to result in less psychological stress, anxiety, and depression for families dealing with the loss of a loved one (10). Though decision making usually rests with only one person, achieving a consensus is desirable to prevent subsequent recriminations.

CONCLUSION

As critical care providers, we are on a first-name basis with death, tragedy, and sorrow. On a daily basis, we must find the balance to serve and stay true to our values. Irrespective of your belief in a higher power—even if you do not have such a belief—consider the insightful words of the Serenity Prayer:

> The Serenity Prayer
>
> God grant me the serenity
> to accept the things I cannot change;
> courage to change the things I can;
> and wisdom to know the difference.
>
> Reinhold Niebuhr

Dunn described the stages of hope (Table 4.5), which illustrate the importance of perspective (11). We must remember that a death with dignity is not a failure. In the end, the words of Dr. Edward Livingstone Trudeau ring true:

To cure sometimes, to relieve often, to comfort always (12).

Case History (Continued)

The patient undergoes resection of the lung metastasis. Six weeks later, she has numerous metastatic lesions in both lungs. She begins weekly treatment consisting of chemotherapy and biologic agents. Unable to operate during that time, the patient and her friend develop a lecture entitled "Giving and Receiving Bad News—Lessons I Learn" to educate her audiences by sharing her experiences as both a clinician and as a patient. A positron emission tomography/CT scan obtained 4 months later shows that her tumor is in remission. She returns to patient care and remains in remission 14 months later.

The patient (RF) and the friend (JH) are the authors of this chapter.

References

1. Rosenbaum M, Ferguson K, Lobas J. Teaching medical students and residents skills for delivering bad news: a review of strategies. *Acad Med.* 2004;79(2):107–115.
2. Baile W, Lenzi R, Parker RB, et al. Oncologist's attitudes toward and practices in giving bad news: an exploratory study. *J Clin Oncol.* 2002;20(8):2189–2196.
3. Browning D, Meyer E, Truog R, et al. Difficult conversations in health care: cultivating relational learning to address the hidden curriculum. *Acad Med.* 2007;82(9):905–912.
4. Komarnicki JW, ed. *How to Teach Towards Character Development.* Conshohocken, PA: Infinity Publisher; 2004:101.
5. Remen N. *My Grandfather's Blessing.* New York: The Berkley Publishing Group; 2000.
6. Baile WF, Kudelka AP, Beale EA, et al. Communication skills training in oncology: description and preliminary outcomes of workshops on breaking bad news and managing patient reactions to illness. *Cancer.* 1999;86:887–897. Baile et al.'s protocol was adapted from Buckman R. *How to Break Bad News: A Guide For Health care Professionals.* Baltimore: Johns Hopkins University Press; 1992.
7. Truog R, Christ G, Browning D, et al. Sudden traumatic death in children "We did everything, but your child didn't survive." *JAMA.* 2006;295(22):2646–2654.
8. Evans W, Tulsky J, Back A, et al. Communication at times of transitions: how to help patients cope with loss and re-define hope. *Cancer J.* 2006;12(5):417–424.
9. Lautrette A, Ciroldi M, Ksibi H, et al. End of life conferences: rooted in the evidence. *Crit Care Med.* 2006;43(11 Suppl):s364–s372.
10. Cordts G, Grant M, Sevransky J. Palliative care in the intensive care unit. *Contemp Crit Care.* 2007;4(12):1–12.
11. Dunn G. What in the world is comfort care? Presented at the American College of Surgeons Meeting, New Orleans, October 9, 2007.
12. Strauss MB. *Anonymous: Familiar Medical Quotations.* Boston: Little Brown and Company; 1968:410.

CHAPTER 5 ■ INFORMED CONSENT

EILEEN H. KIM • MICHELE A. LORAND • WILLIAM HAYDEN • CORY M. FRANKLIN

Informed consent is the process of providing patients with information about the risks, benefits, and potential alternatives to the care they are offered. Informed consent is an essential part of the therapeutic discussion and is central to the relationship created between patient and physician (1,2).

The roots of the informed consent doctrine can be traced as far back as the Magna Carta, but its practical basis was established in the early 20th century in the 1914 New York case *Schloendorff v New York Hospital* concerning a patient with a fibroid uterine tumor. The patient agreed to an abdominal evaluation under anesthesia but specifically refused any surgery (3). Despite this refusal, the surgeon removed the tumor while the patient was anesthetized. This resulted in the modern foundation for informed consent, authored by Judge Benjamin Cardozo (later to become a famous Justice of the U.S. Supreme Court),

> "Every human being of adult years and sound mind has a right to determine what shall be done with his own body. . . " (3)

Ironically, today *Schloendorff* is nearly synonymous with patient autonomy and informed consent, but at the time there was no specific mention of informed consent as an actual principle. The case did not address issues such as what amount or type of information is necessary for a patient to make appropriate care decisions, nor did it result in damage recovery.

The process of informed consent did not become an established part of American medical practice until the late 20th century. Two historical tragedies proved instrumental in the creation of the informed consent doctrine as we know it today. The first event was the Nuremberg Code (1946–1949), which was developed as a result of the notorious Nazi medical experiments at Dachau during World War II (4). This code provided that "voluntary consent of the human subject is absolutely essential" and "the person involved. . . should have sufficient knowledge and comprehension of the elements of the subject matter as to enable him to make an understanding and enlightened decision" (5).

The Tuskegee Syphilis Study (1932–1972), conducted under the direction of the United States government, marked the second event. The study resulted in the deliberate withholding of syphilis treatment from several hundred rural African American males so that investigators could gain information regarding the serious complications of late-stage syphilis. When the facts surrounding this experiment finally became public, it raised the consciousness about the rights of patients and of research subjects regarding what information doctors must disclose (6).

Unfortunately, a wide gap still persists between the idealized elements of informed consent and what is commonly observed in clinical practice today. Too often, "informed consent" is simply another shopworn phrase of internal contradictions along the lines of "rush hour," "United Nations," or "reliable software." Simply put, when a harried medical student, nurse, or ward clerk hurries into a patient's room with a boilerplate form, the patient is expected to sign immediately. Informed consent is thus often neither informed nor consent. Having a signed informed consent form is not the same as *getting* informed consent.

This chapter will discuss the current status of informed consent in the intensive care unit (ICU). It will stress the principles of sharing information, making good faith attempts to understand patient values and decision-making processes, and finally, avoiding manipulation and coercion of the vulnerable ICU patient.

THE ETHICAL FOUNDATIONS OF INFORMED CONSENT

The ethical foundations of informed consent encompass the classic principles of autonomy, beneficence, and justice. These three virtues provide the moral framework for informed consent and present guidelines for appropriate clinical action (7).

Autonomy

Autonomy, from the Greek words for self *(auto)* and rule (*nomos*), refers to the capacity for self-governing and the patient's right to self-determination. This includes the right to select a course of medical therapy that best reflects individual values and preferences. A prerequisite of autonomy is that an individual maintains the right to hold certain beliefs and to exercise independent thought. From these principles arise the ability to choose a certain course of action, to act according to this preference, and to accept the subsequent consequences of that decision. For this to occur, an individual must have access to relevant information and must also possess freedom from both internal and external constraints.

Practically speaking, before patients can reasonably form an opinion regarding available therapeutic options, they must first appreciate the nature of their medical condition, recognize the range of possible interventions, and understand the possible risks, benefits, and consequences associated with each option. This is essentially the mental checklist the physician should perform when speaking with the patient. It is the physician's duty to ensure that the patient understands the medical diagnosis, the details of the proposed therapy, the available alternatives, and the consequences of refusal. Although the responsibility to provide this information lies with the physician, it is the patient who must ultimately integrate the facts and determine the most appropriate course of action.

Generally, autonomous action requires that individuals enter into the physician–patient relationship voluntarily and remain free to accept or refuse treatment without feeling coerced or intimidated. This is often not the case in the ICU. Patients frequently arrive in the ICU in a vulnerable condition, often admitted without their consent or knowledge. The additional stresses of critical illness leave them susceptible to fear, pain, or anxiety. With these factors in mind, the ICU physician must maintain a balance between talking to the patient and making prompt therapeutic decisions. Given the emergent nature of developments in the ICU, it may be impractical to engage in an extensive discussion regarding every procedure or therapy, but whenever possible, it is essential to provide patients with sufficient information to let them guide the overall course of their care. The balance between acting and letting the patient act characterizes the essence of informed consent in the ICU (8).

Beneficence

Beneficence (doing good), and its associated principle, nonmaleficence (not doing harm) affirm the physician's obligation to provide benefit while refraining from committing harm. Beneficence compels the physician to treat illness, provide other appropriate therapy, and relieve pain. Nonmaleficence compels the physician to avoid causing pain and to refrain from committing unnecessary harm. It would be unreasonable to state that physicians must avoid all risks in treating patients. Obviously, many ICU therapies and interventions pose considerable risk to the patient and may also cause pain. The therapeutic relationship in the ICU represents a working relationship between physician and patient, which balances potential benefits against potential harms whenever possible. Physicians are not neutral observers and, as long as they avoid coercive techniques, it is certainly acceptable—and some would argue mandatory—for them to provide their professional recommendation based on their clinical experience (9).

Justice

The third principle, justice, is generally not a source of conflict between the individual physician and patient in matters of informed consent. Ideally, the rules of informed consent serve to motivate the social virtue of justice; when conflicts do occur, they relate more commonly to societal versus individual claims and thus do not involve the physician–patient relationship. An exception is organ transplantation, a situation in which the transplant surgeon's primary duty is directed to the proper allocation of organs rather than to a specific patient (10). Implicit in the relationship of justice to informed consent is the specific involvement of society's instrument of justice: the court.

LEGAL FOUNDATIONS OF INFORMED CONSENT

The progression of legal opinions during the past century illustrates the evolution of the currently recommended standards of informed consent. The term *informed consent* was first used in 1957 by an unheralded attorney named Paul Gebhard, drawing on his experience in labor law negotiations (11). In *Salgo v Leland Stanford Jr. University,* Gebhard used the term in a friend-of-the-court brief on behalf of the American College of Surgeons to refer to the requirement that a physician must disclose to a patient the relevant risks and benefits of a procedure (12).

Determining the acceptable limits of appropriate treatment that a physician can offer is essential to understanding the legal considerations of informed consent. *Schloendorff* established the precedent that a physician performing nonemergent surgery without the patient's authorization constituted a form of battery, "a touching that is not consented to" (3). Judge Cardozo opined that "a surgeon who performs an operation without his patient's consent commits an assault." Since *Schloendorff* addressed only issues of self-determination and autonomy, appropriate standards for adequate consent remained unaddressed for decades.

Canterbury v Spence (1972) later served to establish a minimum standard of information disclosure. The case concerned a patient who underwent a laminectomy for back pain (13). While recovering from surgery, the patient fell out of bed and suffered partial paralysis. After an initial trial failed to establish medical negligence, the argument shifted to the surgeon's failure to fully disclose all known risks associated with the surgical procedure. At the time, laminectomy carried an approximately 1% risk of paralysis, a risk that the surgeon openly admitted he did not disclose to the patient. The surgeon stated that he felt communication of that risk to the patient is not good medical practice because it might deter patients from undergoing needed surgery (13). The court rejected this position and found negligence in the failure to disclose the risk of paralysis. It further emphasized that a physician's obligations extended beyond merely diagnosing and offering treatment. Inherent in the duty to heal exists an obligation to communicate risks and benefits so that patients receive the information necessary to formulate an educated decision:

> True consent to what happens to one's self is the informed exercise of a choice, and that entails an opportunity to evaluate knowledgeably the options available and the risks attendant upon each (13).

By establishing the physician's duty to disclose the relevant risks of surgery, *Canterbury v Spence* carved out an obligation on the part of the physician to present patients with adequate disclosure for any intervention. In *Cobbs v Grant* (1972), the California Supreme Court found a physician did not need to provide a "lengthy polysyllabic discourse on all possible complications" or a "minicourse of medical science." The court required disclosure of "such information as a skilled professional would provide" (14). This introduced the concept of a medical community standard for informed consent disclosure, further codified in *Truman v Thomas (15)*.

Whereas previous cases had merely emphasized obtaining patient permission and providing sufficient information prior to performing an intervention, *Truman* extended the obligations of the physician. A 30-year-old patient who ultimately died of cervical cancer had seen her physician regularly over numerous years, during which time she repeatedly refused to undergo a pap smear. When her cervical cancer was diagnosed, the mass was no longer operable, and she died shortly thereafter. The court, referencing principles previously established by *Canterbury v Spence*, ruled the physician had negligently failed in his duty to provide adequate disclosure because he did not specifically emphasize death as a potential consequence of refusing a pap smear. Citing *Cobbs v Grant,* the court concluded,

> A patient must be apprised not only of the risks inherent in the procedure [prescribed, but also] the risk of a decision not to undergo the treatment, and the probability of a successful outcome of the treatment.

This case became the first to consider the consequences of refusing a medical therapy. It represents the transition from medical paternalism toward a more interactive discussion between physician and patient that recognizes the patient's right to self-determination. Our current models of informed consent have all developed as a result of that transition (16).

CURRENT ETHICAL MODELS OF THE PHYSICIAN–PATIENT RELATIONSHIP

The models of informed consent, which propose strategies for presenting information to patients and discussing alternatives, arose originally from the paternalistic Hippocratic tradition. In the *physician-centered model*—alternatively known as the paternalist, parental, or priestly model—the physician is the authority figure and guardian (17). In prioritizing the principle of beneficence (or doing good), the physician engages the patient in decision making only to provide relevant information and encourage acceptance of the proposed therapy. Historically, Hippocrates advocated "concealing most things from the patient while you are attending to him." Similarly, in 1871, Oliver Wendell Holmes asserted, "Your patient has no more right to all the truth you know than he has to all the medicine in your saddlebags... He should get only just so much as is good for him" (18).

In time, greater emphasis on patient self-determination emerged, along with a higher priority on patient autonomy. Consequently, the *informative model*—also known as the scientific, engineering, consumer, or independent choice model—emerged as an alternative patient-centered strategy. It minimized physician bias and value judgment while recognizing the physician as technician and source of information. This provided the patient with options regarding the range of medical choices, along with the risks and benefits of potential alternatives. In contrast to the physician-centered model, the informative model asserts the physician's duty to provide facts and medical knowledge without expressing bias toward any particular treatment strategy. Ultimately, it is only the patient who determines which course of action best suits his or her values and goals.

By minimizing physician input, this departure from paternalism represented an attempt to achieve complete patient autonomy. Nevertheless, this remained an unsatisfactory strategy for achieving informed consent. True informed consent requires an interactive process between physician and patient. In clinical practice, the physician–patient relationship is a collaborative process by which both sides take equal responsibility for participation with the shared goal of enhanced understanding. Clearly, the physician must be more than a technical adviser. The ICU is where the physician's training, knowledge, and experience are most important in providing interpretive guidance about diagnosis and treatment. This means that the patient may on occasion request and receive a great deal of information; other times this will be impossible, and the physician will be the primary decision maker.

Two current models of shared decision making propose strategies for mutual understanding through an interactive process. The first, the *interpretive model*, focuses on clarifying the patient's values and determining preferences regarding the goals of therapy. The physician may help the patient recognize and express his preferences by serving as a counselor who provides information and engages the patient in a joint process to achieve understanding. A discussion of treatment options allows the patient to recognize his or her own priorities and to determine which option may best realize these values. The physician's guidance allows the patient to demonstrate his or her autonomy and self-understanding.

The second model of shared decision making, the *deliberative model*, requires the physician to provide clinical information and then elicit information from the patient regarding his or her understanding and goals. In representing an idealized interaction between physician and patient, the physician integrates medical information with the patient's values. In this model, the physician should express opinions and preferences regarding appropriate therapy. Patient autonomy is preserved through the patient's moral understanding and action.

These idealized models of the physician–patient relationship recognize that informed consent is a *process* of shared decision making. Examining the values of both the patient and the physician contributes to decisions regarding treatment benefits or risks (19). The optimal model for the physician–patient relationship is one that achieves a level of interactive and shared decision making, thereby prioritizing patient autonomy while still engaging the participation of a concerned physician (20).

CURRENT LEGAL STANDARDS OF INFORMED CONSENT

Considerable uncertainty and debate remain regarding how much information a physician should reasonably provide so that a patient can adequately appreciate the risks associated with any particular therapeutic intervention (21). The perpetual dilemma of informed consent in the ICU is that, in extreme situations, both of benefit and risk, a greater obligation lies on the physician to adhere strictly to the guiding principles of informed consent. At the same time, the ICU patients, because of their weakened condition, may be less able to comprehend and make decisions. In any discussion of possible risks, a physician should routinely disclose to the patient the complications that would most commonly occur; a reasonable figure would be a complication with a probability of at least 1% to 5%. If the potential risk is particularly serious or potentially fatal, it seems obvious that even rare complications with less than a 1% probability should be mentioned (e.g., the vascular complications of routine central venous catheter placement). However, some may argue that the occasional one-in-a-million fatal complication is not the appropriate standard for disclosure (to say nothing of the fact that some physicians may not be aware of these rare complications). Because opinions differ, there is no uniform legal standard that defines the level of information required to meet the standard of adequate disclosure (22). Consequently, three standards of disclosure have been developed and currently exist: the professional community standard, the reasonable patient standard, and the individual patient standard (23,24).

Standards of Disclosure

The Professional Community Standard

The professional community standard was, for decades, the traditional standard for informed consent. According to this standard, a physician should provide the level of information that physicians in the community would communicate to patients in comparable situations. Courts would assess physician disclosure based on the standard practices of other physicians with similar training and experience working under similar circumstances. Because of the imprecise definition of "professional community," the professional standard was used to justify a broad range of interpretations, albeit without solid grounding in clinical criteria. The community could range from very specific practice locations to a broad geographic region or otherwise could refer to a level of specialized training or experience. In some circumstances, even the opinions of a "respectable minority" of physicians would constitute an appropriate practice standard. As such, the expectation of what the physician would tell the patient was notoriously imprecise. It was difficult to define which specific surgical or procedure risks a physician should appropriately disclose to a patient. Furthermore, physicians often invoked the concept of therapeutic privilege, which permitted them to withhold *all* information if they thought it would be injurious to the patient. This doctrine has fallen out of favor both clinically and legally (13).

Critics cited not only the imprecision but also the paternalistic nature of the professional community standard. According to this standard, the physician ultimately determined the threshold of risk that should be disclosed to the patient. The obvious problem with this model was that if the community standard did not include the disclosure of a potential complication or other information that patients may reasonably want to know, the physician was not obligated to disclose it. For example, physicians might prescribe penicillin, and, while a potentially lethal anaphylactic reaction to the drug was possible, because it was rare it would not necessarily be mentioned as one of the complications. Although physicians could not be expected to divulge every possible complication of a procedure or adverse reaction to a drug, many still felt it unacceptable that the standard for providing information rested solely in the hands of the physician.

The Reasonable Patient Standard

In response to this paternalistic standard, and in concert with the trend toward greater emphasis on the patient's right to self-determination, American courts began recognizing an alternative reasonable patient standard to judge the adequacy of risk disclosure. Since it was unreasonable to expect a physician to disclose every potential risk associated with a particular treatment, the reasonable patient standard required the physician to disclose all information a reasonable person would need to make an informed decision. This new standard deemed that even rare complications should be explained to the patient if the consequences (death, severe injury) were such that a reasonable person would want to know them.

However, there are also problems with this model. For one, the physician must divine what a reasonable person would want to know. (Would a reasonable person want to know about anaphylactic responses to penicillin?) Second, the ICU, a setting in which life and death decisions are commonplace, may not lend itself to the enforced neutrality of a reasonable person standard. The physician would be performing a grave disservice by simply reciting the potential complications of endotracheal intubation to a patient in respiratory distress, and thus, a different standard was needed.

The Individual Patient Standard

In the ICU, the physician's input is critical to good decision making, which is why the optimal model for physician–patient relationships is one of interactive and shared decision making. The individual patient standard addresses this relationship. Based on the interaction with the patient and an understanding of the patient's beliefs, the physician should disclose specific information so the patient can reach a decision consistent with his or her principles. The distinction between the different standards is subtle but significant. Under the professional community standard, the physician asks, "What should I tell the patient?" Under the reasonable person standard, the physician asks, "What does a reasonable person want to know?" Under the individual person standard, the physician asks, "What does *this* patient want to know?" Obviously, the most idealized standard of disclosure, the individual person standard, is ultimately the most difficult to achieve. Courts may not require such an idealized standard in all cases, but when questions of informed consent arise, this is the standard that courts are most likely to favor.

Adjustments of Standards

In discussing these legal standards, a note of caution is in order: These models represent guidelines for medical encounters where both parties—patient and physician—can interact. In the ICU, patient situations are constantly changing, life and death decisions are commonplace, and emergencies sometimes make the search for an ideal physician–patient relationship impractical. Unlike the long-term relationship between the patient and the primary physician, the intensivist is often meeting the patient for the first time under conditions of extreme duress (25). For the patient, admission to the ICU is almost always a stressful and potentially overwhelming situation in which critical illness creates an unusual dependence and power imbalance. The patient may be unable to comprehend or express his or her wishes (see Competence and Decision-Making Capacity, later). Other times, an autonomous patient may choose to relinquish medical decision making at the physician's discretion when acute care is required (26).

It is also important that physicians use language the patient can understand when explaining the risks and benefits of any intervention. This means not only adequate translation for patients who do not speak English but also making the explanation as nontechnical as possible. Even in the best of situations, patients may have difficulty extracting important information from discussions with physicians. When physicians lapse into technical jargon, the anxious, frightened patient may have little or no opportunity to process what is being said. It is important that in the appropriate situations, physicians make use of translators, family members, and other intermediaries.

An extensive discussion regarding the risks and benefits of care are the desired standard, but in the ICU, less is sometimes more. In an emergency, the necessity of keeping the patient informed sometimes becomes a luxury that time and circumstance may not permit. Emergency circumstances, in which a patient lacks decisional capacity and no proxy decision maker is identifiable, do not realistically allow for voluntary consent from a medically incompetent patient. In truly emergent situations, if the patient lacks capacity, no proxy decision maker is available, and the potentially lifesaving intervention must be administered immediately, the "emergency exception" to informed consent permits the physician to intervene without obtaining formal informed consent. In these situations, the intensivist should document the emergent nature of the situation and the difficulty in obtaining informed consent. (See When Consent Cannot Be Obtained.)

COMPETENCE AND DECISION-MAKING CAPACITY

Hospitalized patients, especially the critically ill, often suffer from impairments in their ability to comprehend, process, or analyze information. Under the influence of pain medication, sedation, or the physical and mental stresses of illness, even the healthiest ICU patient may not fully appreciate or be able to actively participate in health care decisions, as the emotional stresses of critical illness may temporarily compromise their decisional capacity (27). As one study noted, for very sick patients, the ability to perform simple cognitive tasks is impaired to the point that an adult patient may temporarily function at the level of a 10-year-old child (28). This presents a unique challenge for critical care practitioners when discussing medically complex issues.

Definition of Terms: Competence versus Capacity

"Competence" and "capacity" both refer to the patient's ability to make decisions. Although the terms are often used interchangeably, their legal and medical definitions differ. Strictly speaking, *competence* refers to a legal determination and does not refer specifically to the patient's ability to make appropriate health care decisions (29). A court decides whether or not a person is legally competent, and generally, when "competence" is used as a legal term, it refers to patients' ability or inability to conduct their personal affairs, not necessarily to make health care decisions. It is unusual (but not unheard of) for petitioners to go to court specifically to ask that the court declare a patient incompetent to make medical care decisions. More often than not, this legal determination regarding who decides care for a patient remains in limbo and is left to the patient's family and doctors.

If the courts are not involved with a patient's ability to make decisions, health care providers commonly invoke the term "medical competence," but they are really referring to the patient's *capacity*. Decision-making capacity is a clinical judgment in contrast to legal competence, which specifically describes the patient's ability to make health care decisions. The need to assess capacity by the physician arises when there is reason to question whether the patient can make decisions about care (30). When assessing the patient's capacity, i.e., what most observers refer to imprecisely as whether the patient is competent to consent to care, the examining physician must determine whether the patient understands the five basic elements of capacity (31) (see Table 5.1). During an interview, if a patient demonstrates satisfactory understanding of these five facts, it can reasonably be inferred that the patient possesses adequate decision-making capacity.

TABLE 5.1

THE FIVE ELEMENTS PATIENTS MUST UNDERSTAND TO DETERMINE THEIR CAPACITY

1. The diagnosis
2. The proposed therapy
3. The risks and benefits of the proposed therapy
4. The alternative options
5. The risks and benefits of refusal

Source: Franklin C, Rosenbloom B. Proposing a new standard to establish medical competence for the purpose of critical care intervention. *Crit Care Med.* 2000;28:3035.

Informal Assessments

Informal assessments of a patient's cognitive abilities occur regularly throughout physician–patient interactions; in the critically ill patient, mental status may fluctuate during the course of hospitalization or even during the course of the day. Unless presented with evidence to suspect otherwise, the treating physician should assume that the patient remains capable of independent choice; this is the default position, unless the patient's decision-making capacity is questioned. If this is the case, the health care provider is obliged to demonstrate that the patient cannot make medical decisions. If the clinical situation suggests the patient is not capable of independent choice, a more formal evaluation may be initiated (32).

Physicians may be more likely to doubt a patient's mental capacity if the patient's choices appear unreasonable or contradict the physician's personal values. The patient who refuses a relatively low-risk, high-benefit intervention, or a terminally ill patient who insists on pursuing a painful intervention with little proven benefit, are both scenarios that may prompt a physician to question the patient's decision-making capacity. In these situations, the physician must first attempt to decipher whether the patient's seemingly illogical behavior actually follows a rational thought process. A critically hemorrhaging patient who refuses a blood transfusion may be medically frustrating to care for, but this refusal becomes understandable once it is revealed that the patient is a Jehovah's Witness. Similarly, the patient with end-stage metastatic cancer who has failed multiple rounds of chemotherapy may seem irrational for insisting on pursuing invasive experimental procedures. This seemingly irrational insistence may become more understandable in the context of an upcoming family event, anniversary, or graduation.

External and Emotional Factors

In the ICU, external factors, including sundowning, sedation, pain medication, or altered sleep patterns, may contribute to transient, reversible episodes of incapacity. Whenever possible, attempts should be made to minimize the impact of these influences and optimize the patient's cognitive status prior to making a capacity assessment. The patient's judgment is often compromised by emotional factors, e.g., anger, fear, denial, depression, or pain; this is especially true in the ICU (and in the emergency room). The common scenario of the 50-year-old executive with crushing substernal chest pain who denies he is having a heart attack and wants to sign out of the hospital is an example of how denial may compromise a patient's judgment.

Health care providers should recognize that the patient's decisions under those conditions may not be those they would choose in a less stressful environment. The physician must attempt to ensure that external factors do not unduly influence the patient. True informed consent requires the patient's unhindered judgment. When the patient's judgment appears to be unduly compromised, the physicians should use appropriate measures such as family intervention, psychiatric consultation, or medication aimed at treating the specific problem. The frightened patient who refuses necessary medical care is often grateful if, after appropriate intervention, proper care is provided.

For particularly high-risk interventions or close calls, a second physician, generally someone with expertise in this area, such as a psychiatrist or neurologist, may be called to evaluate the patient. In such cases, the physician should inform the consultant in advance about the situation so the consultant can conduct a focused interview and provide the necessary information.

Legal Interventions

In rare circumstances, questioning a patient's capacity means seeking a court determination of legal incompetence. In practice, resorting to the court is rarely necessary. Rather than deferring to the court system, most states recognize the authority of a spouse, family member, or friend to make decisions in the best interest of the patient. However, when family members and health care providers cannot agree about the most appropriate course of action after attempts at resolution, a legal opinion may be the only option. Courts are generally reluctant to get involved in health care decisions, so this should generally be the last option.

SURROGATE DECISION MAKING

In the United States in 1990, a landmark piece of legislation, The Patient Self-Determination Act, established a patient's right to a name a legal, durable power of attorney for health care if that person should lose decision-making capacity. Most states have their own statutes governing advanced directives. These statutes regulate the authority of a health care proxy decision maker and establish rules that balance the authority of a surrogate decision maker with the patient's preferences. In the absence of a durable power of attorney for health care decisions, an increasing number of states currently recognize the authority of family and friends to act as legal surrogate decision makers, with the limits and scope of this authority varying by state (33). A detailed discussion of the role of surrogate decision makers, specifically concerning end-of-life decisions, is discussed elsewhere in this textbook. (See Chapter 2: Life and Death in the ICU: Ethical Considerations.)

The authority of potential decision makers generally gives priority to family members with closer blood ties. A typical ranking of default surrogate decision makers might be as follows:

1. spouse
2. adult children
3. parents
4. adult siblings
5. other relatives.

If multiple surrogate decision makers are identified (e.g., more than one adult child or adult sibling), some statutes require consensus among all family members, whereas others accept a majority decision. If no blood relative can be identified, several states also include "close friend" in the list of acceptable surrogates, generally giving them the lowest priority. In most states, however, any interested party can challenge the authority of the presumed decision maker, with court appointed guardians generally having top priority.

It has been shown that sometime during their ICU stay, approximately 50% to 75% of patients lack decision-making capacity (34). At least one study found that advanced directives are infrequently used and seldom effective. This suggests a very real need for the participation of family and friends in critical care decision making. At the same time, when determining the most appropriate course of action, the decision maker should select the options that are consistent with the patient's previously demonstrated behavior and values. Guidelines for proxy decision making have recommended *substituted judgment*, by which proxy decision makers refer to past interactions, experiences, or conversations with the patient and draw on these experiences to select the course of action the patient would have preferred. Physicians should present the same level of information to health care proxies that would have been provided to the patient to help them arrive at the best decision.

The shared, interactive, decision-making process between physician and patient extends to the proxy decision maker. Surrogate decision makers, in turn, serve as an extension of the patient, attempting to communicate the choices and concerns the patient would have expressed. If no advanced directive exists, and family or friends cannot comfortably infer the incapacitated patient's likely preferences, the most appropriate guide for proxy decision making is what they believe to be in the patient's best interests. When substituted judgment is not possible, the presumption remains that family members, sharing similar cultural background and upbringing, are most likely to reflect the patient's preferences (35).

Even though most patients trust that designated family members and physicians would accurately anticipate their preferences, several studies have questioned whether proxy decision makers misjudge patient preferences (36). Evidence suggests proxy decision makers correctly predict patient preferences approximately two thirds of the time when presented with hypothetical scenarios regarding end-of-life decisions (37). In general, proxy decision makers tended to pursue treatment more aggressively than patients would have chosen for themselves (38). This discrepancy possibly reflects a tendency of surrogates to select interventions that they would choose for themselves rather than accurately representing the preferences of the incapacitated patients (39). Current data remain inconclusive regarding whether explicit patient–surrogate discussion improves the accuracy of proxy decision making.

The inadequacies inherent in surrogate decision making highlight the problem of shared decision making in critical care medicine. Despite the questionable accuracy of substituted judgment, however, family members are the most appropriate surrogate decision makers. In spite of the demonstrated inaccuracy of proxy decision makers, most patients nevertheless indicate that they would prefer that a family member make medical decisions regarding their care (35). The participation of interested participants—including patient, family, friends, clinicians, attending physician, consulting physicians, and nurses—is a necessary but complex process in determining the most appropriate treatment for a patient who cannot decide.

WHEN CONSENT CANNOT BE OBTAINED

In certain situations in the ICU, it is impossible to obtain consent from the patient. Family members may on occasion be available to provide surrogate consent, but often they are either not present or, for various reasons, are unable to give consent. Currently, no standardized guidelines exist to direct the most appropriate course of action in those cases. When an emergency exists—defined as any situation where delay in providing care would endanger the patient's life or substantially affect his or her health adversely—health care providers can then assume implied consent and proceed with essential treatment (22). The treating physician must determine situations of implied consent in an emergency. Most authorities believe there are three major areas of clinical incompetence for which implied consent permits treatment:

1. the patient who cannot communicate (e.g., unconsciousness);
2. the patient who is unable to understand the situation (e.g. delirium, mental retardation, or language barrier); and
3. the patient who has attempted suicide (e.g., the patient who takes an overdose or shoots himself or herself) but now refuses care.

In these cases, the physician should proceed immediately with any treatment considered lifesaving.

The intent of implied consent is to protect seriously ill impaired patients at risk of imminent death. The general rule is when life or limb is imminently threatened, disclosure can be more limited. The health care provider must balance the urgency of the situation with the time it takes to obtain consent from a surrogate.

Procedures not considered immediately lifesaving that would otherwise require consent, such as central venous access, arterial and pulmonary artery catheters, or diagnostic bronchoscopy, can provide significant benefit in emergencies but do carry risks. Performing these procedures without consent may theoretically violate a patient's autonomy, but electing to forego them because consent cannot be obtained denies patients the benefit of these interventions. In most emergencies, these interventions should be performed without consent, as they represent the best interests of the patient. Diagnostic tests and procedures presenting minimal risk, including blood draws or peripheral IV placement, generally do not require formal consent, nor do noninvasive diagnostic modalities, including radiographs or computerized tomographic scans.

Implied consent gives critical care practitioners a great deal of latitude. However, there are limitations to the discretion afforded. More careful disclosure is mandated, even in emergencies, if the therapy is elective or in borderline situations when reasonable alternatives exist. For example, the patient with a potential intra-abdominal infection may not understand the need for immediate exploratory laparotomy. If the patient is stable and surgery is merely one diagnostic option, computerized tomographic scans and frequent observation may provide information equivalent to a laparotomy. In selected situations such as described, the treating physician should remain flexible when possible.

SIGNING OUT OF THE HOSPITAL AGAINST MEDICAL ADVICE

One of the most difficult situations for the ICU staff is the extremely uncooperative, combative patient. In most cases, these patients are reacting to fear, pain, illicit drug ingestion, or alcohol withdrawal. Usually, care can be delivered after appropriate sedation or analgesia, although, occasionally, a patient must be physically restrained. The indication for physical restraint is when patients present a risk to themselves or to others. In rare circumstances, despite the best efforts of the staff, a patient may refuse all treatment and demand to leave the hospital. The staff is then forced to reconcile the conflict between respecting the patient's rights and their duty to care for and protect the patient from harm. There may be no easy resolution of this problem.

The right to leave the hospital against medical advice is the prerogative of the competent patient. If the patient meets the general test of medical competence (as described in the five basic elements of capacity [31] [Table 5.1]), the patient must be allowed to leave the hospital, even if the staff disagrees with the decision or the decision seems irrational. However, all decisions by patients to leave against medical advice should be scrutinized by senior staff to ensure the patient truly is competent. Those decisions that appear irrational should be scrutinized with even more care. A classic example is the aforementioned 50-year-old male with an acute myocardial infarction, otherwise competent but who, in a fit of denial, demands to sign out of the hospital. All avenues should be used to get the patient to stay, including a detailed discussion of the situation and an appeal to family or friends who accompany the patient to the hospital. Ultimately, however, if the patient refuses to listen, because he is competent, he must be permitted to leave. In such situations—very trying ones, indeed—health care providers must attempt to provide any appropriate care or workup before the patient leaves. Staff should avoid recriminations, and the patient should also be reassured he or she can return for care at any time.

Other situations are not so clear-cut. In many cases, the patient's competence is in question. Possible physiologic causes for the patient's condition, e.g., hypoxemia, electrolyte disturbances, sepsis, should be identified. If the patient cannot be deemed competent, staff may decide to institute treatment over the objection of the patient, which might even entail physical restraint. Failure to restrain when indicated carries a significant risk to both patient and health care providers. The classic counterpoint to the aforementioned myocardial infarction patient is the patient in a motor vehicle accident who appears intoxicated but wants to sign out of the hospital. If the physician suspects that the patient is intoxicated, based on clinical observation even before confirmation of blood alcohol concentration, the patient should not be allowed to leave until appropriate radiologic assessment of the head and neck have been performed.

Some health care providers are overly concerned with the liability they may incur by treating a patient against his or her wishes. When competence cannot be established with certainty, if the staff decides to restrain the patient, they may theoretically open themselves to charges of battery. Such an outcome is extremely unlikely, and almost certainly less likely than the alternative of being charged with negligent discharge. The consequences of being responsible for the negligent death of unrestrained patients are far more serious than the responsibility for holding patients against their will for several hours. When the staff's actions are medically reasonable, they are acting in good faith, and if they document their decision (see next section), the likelihood of successful litigation against them is remote.

TABLE 5.2

DOCUMENTATION OF PATIENTS WHO LEAVE THE HOSPITAL AGAINST MEDICAL ADVICE

Description of the patient's condition
The basic questions used to assess the patient's competence
Risks, benefits, and alternatives of treatment
Urgency of the situation
Any attempts to contact family members or other potential surrogates (detail who, when, and what interaction occurred)

Documentation

All situations of implied consent or decisions to leave the hospital against medical advice require *scrupulous* and *detailed* documentation. The information that should be included in the medical record is listed in Table 5.2.

Specialty consultations with neurology or psychiatry are not mandatory but may be useful in assessing the patient and documenting the situation. In difficult cases, it may be necessary to involve a representative of the hospital's administration or legal counsel.

PATIENT COMPREHENSION OF CONSENT FORMS

Currently there is no medical or legal consensus regarding which procedures require formal consent. As a general guideline, there is a greater need to discuss the risks and benefits more formally for procedures that carry greater risk (16). This standard results in consent policies that vary significantly from hospital to hospital. One survey of informed consent practices found that, while over 90% of hospitals surveyed required formal consent for gastrointestinal endoscopy, fiberoptic bronchoscopy, or medical research, fewer than 10% required consent for nasogastric intubation or bladder catheterization (40). Of note, requirements for consent varied between medical and surgical services, even within the same institution.

Achieving satisfactory informed consent may not always be possible, even when physicians explain the procedures to patients. In one study of patients who consented to moderately invasive bedside procedures (thoracentesis, paracentesis, bone marrow aspirate, or lumbar puncture), 90% of the patients surveyed reported that the physician had explained the indication for the procedure, although only 70% could correctly recall the reason for the procedure. Although 86% of patients reported that the physician had informed them of the risks of the procedure, only 57% could later name any of the risks (41). This raises the question of how effectively information is communicated to patients, as well as how accurately patients understand and recall information presented to them.

To anticipate patient needs and to simplify the consent process, many institutions use standardized consent forms that include essential information regarding particular procedures or interventions. The use of a standardized ICU admission consent package, describing and requesting consent for the most commonly performed procedures, can enhance the informed consent process (42). Standardized forms, however, do not necessarily guarantee clear communication. As a response to defensive medicine concerns, standardized consent forms may describe all possible adverse consequences instead of actually trying to inform the patient (43). Moreover, standardized lists of complications may not communicate the risks most relevant to any particular patient, especially in the ICU, where a patient's changing medical condition can present a dynamic series of risks and benefits. The risk of an iatrogenic pneumothorax from central venous catheter placement during mechanical ventilation carries different implications than a similar complication when the catheter is simply placed for fluid replacement.

Despite these caveats, standardized consent forms for common procedures may be useful in initiating dialogue between patient and physician. Standardized consent forms may also be necessary for especially complex ICU surgical procedures such as organ transplantation or experimental surgery. In these situations, a detailed informational document provides patient and health care providers a ready reference. The language of such forms should be reviewed periodically to ensure simplicity and reader-friendly, understandable language. Even when standardized forms are used, health care providers should write a note in the patient's medical record detailing the conversation between the patient and physician.

RESEARCH CONSENT IN THE ICU

Like every specialty, critical care medicine has achieved progress through research involving the participation of volunteers (44). Critically ill patients represent a particularly vulnerable population, which raises concerns about their ability to give voluntary, autonomous consent to participate in clinical research (45). Ongoing critical care research recognizes a corresponding obligation to protect this vulnerable population. Requesting consent for voluntary participation in research differs fundamentally from discussing informed consent for therapeutic interventions. When discussing the risks, benefits, and alternatives of any therapeutic or diagnostic intervention, both the clinician and patient seek a course of action that would maximally benefit the patient. In contrast, the goal of research is to generate information that may benefit *future* patients but does not necessarily benefit the individual research participant (46). This creates a potential conflict of interest between researcher and patient, and thus, researchers must exercise particular caution in protecting the rights of patients. Federal regulations, known as "the common rule," have been designed to protect this vulnerable population of research participants (47).

Patients participating in clinical research may misunderstand or overestimate the individual benefits of participation; alternatively, they may not fully recognize the potential risks. Although the possibility for personal benefit does exist, a patient might be randomized to a nontreatment arm of a trial or may alternatively receive experimental therapy with unexpected, hazardous side effects (48,49). Researchers are obligated to ensure that research participants recognize the additional risks and benefits of participation. Occasionally, this means a researcher may ask a research participant to accept a disproportionate share of risk, with no prospect of additional individual gain. The exact limits of risk a vulnerable patient may be asked to accept have not been specifically defined (50).

The research consent process should clearly delineate the nature of the research and structure of the trial, specifically including details on any randomization process (46). In contrast to therapeutic interventions, informed consent for research represents a process that continues throughout the course of a clinical study, and thus routine updates for the patient may be necessary. Standardized consent forms may be useful in communicating the relevant information, and the physician must ensure that information is clearly explained. Clinical research consent forms may be used as reference documents during the study. Because of concerns regarding literacy and language comprehension, the complexity of language should generally target comprehension for no higher than a sixth-grade reading level.

Since few patients are likely to have voiced their preferences regarding research participation, proxy decision makers for patients who lack decision-making capacity are left to infer the most appropriate actions in certain situations (51). Emergency situations in which patients cannot consent and surrogates cannot be located raise concerns about the ethics of conducting research in these cases. Although regulations have sought to protect potential research subjects, they acknowledge that denying research participation to patients who cannot give consent may also deny them potentially beneficial therapy. A 1996 amendment to the Code of Federal Regulations for the Protection of Human Subjects permits emergency research with certain provisions if consent cannot be obtained (52). Clinical trials describe waivers of consent based on implied consent (53). Delayed consent is another mechanism that has been used for clinical trials that compared two clinically acceptable therapies (54).

THE ETHICAL CARE OF CHILDREN IN AN INTENSIVE CARE UNIT

The same basic principles of ethical decision making outlined throughout this chapter apply when treating children, with the understanding that the surrogate decision makers in most pediatric cases are the child's parents. However, dilemmas can arise, and when they do, can prove to be distressing to all involved. These issues arise in the care of critically ill children as well as in the care of the general pediatric population (55–57).

A basic concept in caring for a critically ill child is the age of responsibility, i.e., when children can decide for themselves. Our society affords adults certain rights that it does not allow to children, such as voting, driving, and purchasing alcohol or tobacco. Included among these is the right to make decisions regarding one's own medical care. The age of responsibility, and therefore the age at which a young person can consent to medical care, is a complex dilemma in medical ethics. There is no standardized answer as to when minor patients should be able to make decisions regarding their treatment. The factors to be considered include not only the children's age, but also their reasoning skills, level of understanding, experience, severity of illness, and the type of procedure or treatment being offered. In most states, 18 years is the age when a person becomes an adult and can make his or her own health care decisions. This is known as the age of majority. However, there are numerous consent statutes or rules of common law that the critical care physician should be aware of that allow medical treatment of a minor younger than 18 years of age without parental consent (58).

The Emergency Exception

A minor can seek emergency medical care without parental consent. Emergencies are generally defined the same way they would be for adults (see When Consent Cannot Be Obtained).

The Emancipated Minor Exception

Emancipated minors are children younger than 18 years of age (or whatever the age of majority is in the state of residence) who can decide their own medical care. The specific criteria for emancipated minors vary from state to state, but generally pertain to minors who are either married, pregnant, a parent, in the military, financially independent and living apart from their parents, or those who have been legally declared emancipated by the court. Pediatric critical care practitioners should be familiar with laws concerning the age of majority and emancipated minors in the state where they practice.

The Mature Minor Exception

This concept involves minors generally 14 years of age or older deemed capable of providing informed consent. In certain cases, if minors are sufficiently mature and possess the intelligence to understand and appreciate the benefits, risks, and alternatives to the proposed treatment, and can make voluntary and rational choices, they can decide their own care. States differ in how much weight they give to the concept of mature minors and, again, practitioners should be familiar with laws concerning mature minors in the state in which they practice.

Exceptions Based on a Specific Medical Condition

The minor who seeks care for certain conditions can give consent without parental involvement. These conditions generally include mental health services, pregnancy and contraceptive services, testing or treatment for human immunodeficiency virus infection or AIDS, sexually transmitted or communicable disease testing and treatment, drug or alcohol dependency counseling and treatment, or care for a crime-related injury.

Exceptional Situations

There are several other situations involving consent for minors that the critical care specialist may encounter; these are described in the sections that follow.

When Parents Cannot Be Reached or Are Absent

Parents are generally the best surrogate decision makers for their children. Custom and practice dictate that surrogate decision makers are generally ranked in the following order: parents, health care professionals, courts, and finally, social/governmental agencies. Unfortunately, there are occasions when these principles do not apply, and disagreement may arise regarding who best represents the concerns of the minor patient. When parents are absent and cannot be reached in emergency situations, critical care practitioners may use their best medical judgment in instituting treatment. Physicians should seek the support of their decision from other practitioners, as well as clearly documenting that good faith attempts have been made to reach the parents. Documentation should ensure that medical criteria for the particular intervention have been met and should include the circumstances surrounding the inability to contact the parents.

When Abuse and/or Neglect Is Suspected

The law is clear that whenever child abuse or neglect is suspected, medical practitioners are mandated reporters. They are required to report their suspicions to state or local authorities in accordance with the child abuse reporting laws in the state where they practice (59,60). In most states, the practitioner is allowed to proceed with the initial diagnosis and stabilization of the suspected abused child, even in the absence of parental consent. It is obviously best to engage the parent in a straightforward manner concerning the medical decision-making process and obtain consent; however, there may be situations in which the parent is unavailable or unwilling to participate. In these cases, the practitioner should consult the local state child abuse laws and either take protective custody of the child or begin custody proceedings with the appropriate authorities. Most major children's hospitals have child abuse teams with experience in cases of suspected child abuse, along with knowledge of the procedures related to parental consent in these difficult situations. Critical care practitioners should consult these teams early in such cases. Generally, a physician or social worker with expertise in child abuse can work with a family to secure the best interests of the child.

When Parents' Religious Beliefs Interfere with Lifesaving Medical Care

The most common religious issue encountered in pediatric critical care is the child who needs a blood transfusion but cannot obtain it due to the refusal of the parents, who are perhaps Jehovah's Witnesses, to provide consent because it is forbidden by their faith. In some jurisdictions, these cases can be pursued as neglect, but in other jurisdictions, exemptions to child abuse and neglect laws prevent legal repercussions when the alleged abuse or neglect has occurred in the name of religion. However, there is ample precedent to support the decision to administer blood if a child's life is in danger, although this action generally requires legal intervention and hospital involvement (61). Most hospitals have ethics committees or consultants to help practitioners and surrogates work out the critical issues. Depending on the hospital model, ethics committees can be either informational, ensuring that all parties have the same facts and understand the issues and options, or act as decision makers to whom the clinicians can defer. It is both prudent and fair to the child and family to involve a medical ethicist or hospital ethics committee before proceeding with the medical treatment needed. Furthermore, these actions will demonstrate an effort to preserve the relationship between doctor, patient, and family so that all parties have access to the advocates available to discuss the issue. Surreptitious action to institute treatment is *never* indicated.

When the Parents or Surrogate and Health Care Team Disagree on the Care of a Critically Ill Child

This situation arises most commonly in end-of-life situations regarding the propriety and timing of providing care (62,63). These are obviously emotionally wrenching circumstances if health care professionals and parents or surrogates disagree. Health care providers may anticipate the termination of ventilator support in a severely brain-injured patient or a terminal cancer patient days, or even weeks, before parents or surrogates reach an understanding that this is the proper decision. Parents or surrogates may hold out unreasonable hope, however understandable, in the face of a child's impending death. Patience is usually the best approach. Time and reasoned discussion generally resolve these issues. This strategy requires the understanding that those involved may be at different stages of acceptance. Collegial communication eventually brings the concerned parties to an acceptable conclusion. It is imperative that critical care practitioners offer parents or surrogates sufficient opportunity to discuss their feelings and emotions. A distant, emotionally detached approach by the critical care provider is inappropriate and complicates the delivery of care.

When there is neither common ground nor hope of agreement between the critical care provider and parents or surrogates, the final resort is to take the issue to the courts. Practitioners should not undertake formal legal action lightly. Experience has shown that in most cases, attorneys, courts, and judges, rather than hearing such cases, prefer resolution outside the courtroom. Besides being expensive, the legal process requires time and energy, both physical and emotional, on the part of all involved. In this adversarial process between the critical care provider and parents or surrogates involving end-of-life decisions, medical professionals should keep in mind that, in some cases, courts have ruled against the medical team who originally instituted the proceedings (64). Whenever pediatric critical care practitioners consider going to court for resolution, they should consult the hospital's legal staff and ethics committee to explore other options and coordinate an optimal strategy for all parties involved. They should remember that the best interests of the pediatric patient are their paramount concern.

SUMMARY

A traditional attitude in medicine has been to equate informed consent with obtaining a patient's signature on a boilerplate document. However, informed consent has evolved significantly from that approach so that today, it means much more than simply a signed form. It is now understood as a process intended to create trust between the critical care practitioner and patients. The physician has an obligation to explain the therapy, complications, alternatives, and the risks of alternatives to the patient. There is no simple answer to define exactly how or what the physician must tell the patient. The approach to disclosing information will vary, depending on the goals of care, the urgency of the situation, and the relationship that develops between the patient and critical care provider. There will never be an ideal single standard of informed consent.

Depending on the clinical situation, the requirements for informed consent disclosure lie along a continuum. In life-threatening emergencies where a patient may lack the capacity to decide, limited disclosure is acceptable and, in some cases, the only option. At the other end of the spectrum is the heightened level of disclosure required when asking patients to participate in critical care research. The *sine qua non* of medical research is the guarantee of the patient's complete understanding and voluntary consent. In those cases, instead of a 5-minute discussion with the patient, obtaining informed consent may require several sessions and considerable effort. Between these two extremes are the quotidian clinical situations in which mutual trust becomes the watchword. Regardless of the complication rate of a particular procedure, or which legal standard the physician seeks to meet when informing the patient, informed consent is optimal when the physician has earned the patient's trust and is comfortable with the patient's understanding of the clinical situation.

There is a belief among some learned but cynical observers that true informed consent represents an impossible goal, because patients will never have the same knowledge base or level of clinical understanding as their critical care physician, and hence, the conclusion that detailed explanations are merely an exercise in futility. Such cynicism misses the point. It is precisely because of that imbalance of knowledge and power between physician and patient that when health care providers seek to obtain informed consent, they redouble their efforts not only to inform patients, but also to earn their trust.

References

1. Beauchamp T, Faden R. *A History and Theory of Informed Consent*. New York, NY: Oxford University Press; 1986.
2. Katz J. *The Silent World of Doctor and Patient*. Baltimore, MD: Johns Hopkins University Press; 2002.
3. *Schloendorff v Society of New York Hospital*, 211 NY 125, 105 NE 92 (1914).
4. Meisel A. Legal and ethical myths about informed consent. *Arch Intern Med*. 1996;156:2521.
5. *Trials of War Criminals before the Nuremberg Military Tribunals*. Vols I and II. The Medical Case. Washington, DC: U.S. Government Printing Office; 1948.
6. Jones J. *Bad Blood*. New York, NY: The Free Press; 1981.
7. Menikoff J. *Law and Bioethics*. Washington, DC: Georgetown University Press; 2001.
8. Cook D. Patient autonomy versus paternalism. *Crit Care Med*. 2001;29(2 Suppl):N24.
9. Quill TE, Brody H. Physician recommendations and patient autonomy: finding a balance between physician power and patient choice. *Ann Intern Med*. 1996;125:763.
10. Franklin C. Organ transplants: a doctor's dilemma. *New York Times*. January 3, 2000:A18.
11. P.G. Gebhard, 69, Developer of the term 'informed consent' [obituary]. *New York Times* August 26, 1997:A13.
12. *Salgo v Leland Stanford Jr. Univ. Bd. Of Trustees*, 154 Cal App. 2d 560, 317 P.2d 170 (1957).
13. *Canterbury v Spence*, 464 F2d 772 (DC Cir 1972), cert denied, 409 US 1064 (1972).
14. *Cobbs v Grant*, 8 Cal. 3d 229, 104 Cal Rptr. 505, 502 P.2d 1 (1972).
15. *Truman v Thomas*, 611 P.2d902 (Cal. 1980).
16. Dagi TF. Changing the paradigm for informed consent. *J Clin Ethics*. 1994;5:246.
17. Emanuel EJ, Emanuel LL. Four models of the physician-patient relationship. *JAMA*. 1992;267:2221.
18. Laine C. Patient-centered medicine. A professional evolution. *JAMA*. 1996;275:152.
19. Brock DW. The ideal of shared decision making between physicians and patients. *Kennedy Inst Ethics J*. 1991;1:28.
20. Whitney SN, McGuire AL, McCullough LB. A typology of shared decision making, informed consent, and simple consent. *Ann Intern Med*. 2004;140:54.

21. Bernat JL, Peterson LM. Patient-centered informed consent in surgical practice. *Arch Surg.* 2006;141:86.
22. Sprung CL. Informed consent in theory and practice: legal and medical perspectives on the informed consent doctrine and a proposed reconceptualization. *Crit Care Med.* 1989;17:1346.
23. Karlawish JH. Shared decision making in critical care: a clinical reality and an ethical necessity. *Am J Crit Care.* 1996;5:391.
24. Piper A Jr. Truce on the battlefield: a proposal for a different approach to medical informed consent. *J Law Med Ethics.* 1994;22:301.
25. Schweickert W, Hall J. Informed consent in the intensive care unit: ensuring understanding in a complex environment. *Curr Opin Crit Care.* 2005;11:624.
26. Lidz CW, Meisel A, Osterweis M, et al. Barriers to informed consent. *Ann Intern Med.* 1983;99:539.
27. Marzuk PM. The right kind of paternalism. *N Engl J Med.* 1985;313:1474.
28. Cassell EJ, Leon AC, Kaufman SG. Preliminary evidence of impaired thinking in sick patients. *Ann Intern Med.* 2001;134:1120.
29. Berg JW, Appelbaum PS, Grisso T. Constructing competence: formulating standards of legal competence to make medical decisions. *Rutgers Law Rev.* 1996;48:345.
30. Brody H. Shared decision making and determining decision-making capacity. *Prim Care.* 2005;32:645.
31. Franklin C, Rosenbloom B. Proposing a new standard to establish medical competence for the purpose of critical care intervention. *Crit Care Med.* 2000;28:3035.
32. Appelbaum PS, Grisso T. Assessing patients' capacities to consent to treatment. *N Engl J Med.* 1988;319:1635.
33. Menikoff JA, Sachs GA, Siegler M. Beyond advance directives: health care surrogate laws. *N Engl J Med.* 1992;327:1165.
34. Burchardi H. A surrogate for decision-making in the ICU. *Intensive Care Med.* 2001;27:1243.
35. Arnold RM, Kellum J. Moral justifications for surrogate decision making in the intensive care unit: implications and limitations. *Crit Care Med.* 2003;31(5 Suppl):S347.
36. Seckler AB, Meier DE, Mulvihill M, et al. Substituted judgment: how accurate are proxy predictions? *Ann Intern Med.* 1991;115:92.
37. Shalowitz DI, Garrett-Mayer E, Wendler D. The accuracy of surrogate decision makers: a systematic review. *Arch Intern Med.* 2006;166:493.
38. Suhl J, Simons P, Reedy T, et al. Myth of substituted judgment: surrogate decision making regarding life support is unreliable. *Arch Intern Med.* 1994;154:90.
39. Sulmasy DP, Terry PB, Weisman CS, et al. The accuracy of substituted judgments in patients with terminal diagnoses. *Ann Intern Med.* 1998;128:621.
40. Manthous CA, DeGirolamo A, Haddad C, et al. Informed consent for medical procedures: local and national practices. *Chest.* 2003;124:1978.
41. Sulmasy DP. Patients' perceptions of the quality of informed consent for common medical procedures. *J Clin Ethics.* 1994;5:189.
42. Davis N, Pohlman A, Gehlbach B, et al. Improving the process of informed consent in the critically ill. *JAMA.* 2003;289:1963.
43. Hopper KD, TenHave TR, Tully DA, et al. The readability of currently used surgical/procedure consent forms in the United States. *Surgery.* 1998;123:496.
44. Drazen JM. Volunteers at risk. *N Engl J Med.* 2006;355:1060.
45. Luce JM, Cook DJ, Martin TR, et al.: American Thoracic Society. The ethical conduct of clinical research involving critically ill patients in the United States and Canada: principles and recommendations. *Am J Respir Crit Care Med.* 2004;170:1375.
46. Silverman HJ, Luce JM, Lanken PN, et al. NHLBI Acute Respiratory Distress Syndrome Clinical Trials Network (ARDSNet). Recommendations for informed consent forms for critical care clinical trials. *Crit Care Med.* 2005;33:867.
47. Karlawish JH. Research involving cognitively impaired adults. *N Engl J Med.* 2003;348:1389.
48. Dunn LB. Enhancing informed consent for research and treatment. *Neuropsychopharmacology.* 2001;24:595.
49. Suntharalingam G. Cytokine storm in a phase 1 trial of the anti-CD28 monoclonal antibody TGN1412. *N Engl J Med.* 2006;355:1018.
50. Weijer C. The ethical analysis of risk in intensive care unit research. *Crit Care.* 2004;8:85.
51. Bigatello LM, George E, Hurford WE. Ethical considerations for research in critically ill patients. *Crit Care Med.* 2003;31(3 Suppl):S178.
52. Luce JM. Is the concept of informed consent applicable to clinical research involving critically ill patients? *Crit Care Med.* 2003;31(3 Suppl):S153.
53. Fisher M. Ethical issues in the intensive care unit. *Curr Opin Crit Care.* 2004;10:292.
54. Finfer S. A comparison of albumin and saline for fluid resuscitation in the intensive care unit. *N Engl J Med.* 2004;350:2247.
55. Zawistowski CA. Ethical problems in pediatric critical care: Consent. *Crit Care Med.* 2003;31(5 Suppl):S407.
56. Cooke RW. Good practice in consent. *Semin Fetal Neonatal Med.* 2005;10:63.
57. Nelson RM. Ethics in the intensive care unit. Creating an ethical environment. *Crit Care Clin.* 1997;13:691.
58. Committee on Pediatric Emergency Medicine, American Academy of Pediatrics. Consent for emergency medical services for children and adolescents. *Pediatrics.* 2003;111:703.
59. Child Abuse Prevention and Treatment Act (CAPTA), 1974. U.S. Department of Health and Human Services.
60. Keeping Children and Families Safe Act of 2003 (P.L. 108-36). U.S. Department of Health and Human Services, Administration for Children and Families.
61. American Academy of Pediatrics, Committee on Bioethics. Religious objections to medical care. *Pediatrics.* 1997;99:279.
62. *In re Karen Quinlan.* 70 N.J. 10 (1976)—Supreme Court of New Jersey.
63. Illinois Health Care Surrogate Act of 1998. 755 ILCS 40.
64. *Matter of Hofbrauer,* 65 App. Div. 2d 108, 411 N.Y.S. 2d 416 (App. Div. 1978); 47 NY 2nd 648,419 NYS 2d 936, 393 NE 2d 1009 (1979).

CHAPTER 6 ■ JUDICIAL INVOLVEMENT IN END-OF-LIFE DECISIONS

CRISTINA PALACIO

Treatment decisions are made by patients in consultation with their physicians every day. For incapacitated patients, these decisions are made either through written or oral advance directives or by their surrogates. As discussed in Chapter 5 and below, the concepts of informed consent and self-determination provide the underpinnings for these dialogues and decisions. The process of consultation and informed decision making should be essentially the same regardless of whether the decision is to treat or not to treat—even when the decision is made in an end-of-life context. The fact that private end-of-life dialogues occur daily in hospitals has long been recognized by our courts. In 1981, New York Court of Appeals Judge Jones stated:

> There is reliable information that for many years physicians and members of patients' families . . . have in actuality been making decisions to withhold or to withdraw life support procedures from incurably ill patients incapable of making the critical decisions for themselves. While of course, there can be no categorical assurance that there have been no erroneous decisions thus reached, or even that in isolated instances death has not been unjustifiably hastened

for unacceptable motives, at the same time there is no empirical evidence that either society or its individual members have suffered significantly in consequence of the absence of active judicial oversight. There is no indication that the medical profession whose members are most closely aware of current practices senses the need for or desires judicial intervention (1).

Notwithstanding the court's opinion, there is a significant body of case law in the last three decades indicating that there are, indeed, circumstances in which the medical profession looks to the judiciary for direction. Moreover, there are many cases indicating that, regardless of the medical profession's desire or need, patients or their representatives seek judicial intervention. "Beginning with the case of Karen Ann Quinlan in 1976, patients, their family members and health care providers have come to the courts on several thousand occasions seeking guidance and resolution of disputes involving termination of life support" (2).

The purpose of this chapter is to present cases that have had significant impact on the development of legal reasoning in end-of-life treatment decisions and that demonstrate the circumstances under which judicial intervention has been sought. These cases provide guidance for physicians in the critical care setting, as they establish general principles that are relied on by many jurisdictions. However, the law regarding judicial intervention in treatment decisions varies from state to state; when in doubt as to how to proceed in any particular circumstance, a provider should be aware of the individual case law and statutory requirements of her or his jurisdiction.

SCHIAVO: FULL CIRCLE, NEW TREND, OR ABERRATION?

Undoubtedly, one of the first cases that comes to mind today when discussing judicial intervention in treatment decisions is the case of Theresa (Terri) Marie Schiavo. The Schiavo case arguably represents the epitome of judicial intervention in treatment decisions. From the first trial on Michael Schiavo's January 2000 petition for authorization to discontinue artificial nutrition and hydration of Terri Schiavo (3), to Terri Schiavo's death on March 31, 2005, the Schiavo case generated numerous opinions and orders from the Sixth Judicial Circuit Court of Florida (4), four opinions from the Florida Second District Court of Appeals (5), one from the Florida Supreme Court (6), a U.S. District Court opinion (7), and two U.S. Court of Appeals opinions (8). What were the issues in the Schiavo case that resulted in such extensive judicial (not to mention legislative and even executive) intervention? Were they unique in some way?

In February 1990, at the age of 27, Terri Schiavo suffered cardiac arrest. She was resuscitated by paramedics, but never regained consciousness. Almost 9 years later, her husband, Michael Schiavo, petitioned the court to authorize removal of her feeding tube. In describing Terri's medical condition, the court noted that "[s]ince 1990, Theresa has lived in nursing homes with constant care. She is fed and hydrated by tubes.... She has had numerous health problems, but none have been life threatening. The evidence is overwhelming that Theresa is in a permanent or persistent vegetative state.... She is not asleep. She has cycles of apparent wakefulness and apparent sleep without any cognition or awareness. As she breathes, she often makes moaning sounds. Theresa has severe contractures of her hands, elbows, knees, and feet" (9).

It is striking how similar this description is to that of Karen Quinlan provided by the New Jersey Supreme Court almost 30 years earlier in the seminal case of *In the Matter of Karen Quinlan:*

> The ... medical consensus was that Karen in addition to being comatose is in a chronic and persistent 'vegetative' state, having no awareness of anything or anyone around her and existing at a primitive reflex level. Although she does have some brain stem function ... and has other reactions one normally associates with being alive, such as moving, reacting to light, sound and noxious stimuli, blinking her eyes and sounds and chewing motions ... Karen remains in the intensive care unit ..., receiving 24-hour care .... She is nourished by feeding by way of a nasal-gastro tube.... The result is that her condition is considered remarkable under the unhappy circumstances involved.... Her posture is described as fetal-like and grotesque; there is extreme flexion-rigidity of the arms, legs and related muscles and her joints are severely rigid and deformed (10).

Like the Schiavo case, the Quinlan case garnered national attention. Karen Ann Quinlan, like Terri Schiavo, suffered a sudden, unexpected anoxic event one evening; she was 21. Like Terri, Karen never regained consciousness (11).

The *Quinlan* case is one of the most significant right-to-die cases, cited in opinions from many different jurisdictions in the last 30 years (although notably absent in any *Schiavo* opinion, which relied on Florida case law) (12). It was the first ruling in the United States permitting the withdrawal of life-sustaining treatment from a permanently incapacitated patient. "From the fight mounted by Julia and Joe Quinlan have come decisions and actions with far-reaching impact, including the development of the living will and the advance directive and the establishment of ethics committees in every hospital in the United States" (13). The outcome in both cases was ultimately the same—the courts authorized both Quinlan's and Schiavo's guardians to withdraw life-sustaining treatment (ventilator support and feeding tube, respectively). Unlike Schiavo, the Quinlan case did not involve a prolonged entanglement with the judiciary; Quinlan had two decisions, both within 1 year (14). Does Schiavo represent a new trend in judicial intervention, or is it an aberration? To answer that question, it is useful to review the development and trends in the case law regarding the right to refuse medical treatment, and life-sustaining or prolonging treatments more specifically.

THE UNDERLYING PREMISE: TREATMENT DECISIONS LIE WITH THE PATIENT

The Concept of Informed Consent

An analysis of judicial intervention in treatment decisions must begin with a discussion on who holds the right to make a treatment decision. As was discussed in Chapter 5, the decision to accept proposed treatment lies with the patient or her or his surrogate decision maker. In *Cruzan v. Director, Missouri Department of Health,* the first U.S. Supreme Court case to explore the federal right of an incapacitated patient to refuse life-prolonging treatment, the Court began its analysis by stating the legal reasoning supporting the basic premise of informed consent: "At common law, even the touching of one person by another without consent and without legal justification was a battery.... This notion of bodily integrity has been embodied in the requirement that informed consent is generally required for medical treatment" (15).

As noted by the *Cruzan* court, this was not the first time it had emphasized the fundamental notion of bodily integrity that underlies the doctrine of informed consent. One hundred years earlier, the Supreme Court considered the action brought by Clara L. Botsford, who was injured while riding in a Union Pacific Railway Company train sleeping car. Shortly before trial, Union Pacific petitioned the court for an order to require Botsford to undergo a surgical examination by a physician other than her own surgeon, alleging that the company would otherwise be without its own witnesses to testify on her condition. In rejecting the company's petition, the Supreme Court observed that "no right is held more sacred, or is more carefully guarded, by the common law, than the right of every individual to the possession and control of his own person, free from all restraint or interference of others, unless by clear and unquestionable authority of law" (16). A few decades later, in 1914, the highly regarded Justice Benjamin Cardozo (17) reviewed a claim by Mary E. Schloendorff that her surgeon had performed an operation for which she had not consented, resulting, she alleged, in gangrene of her left arm and finger amputations. In his opinion Justice Cardozo stated: "In the case at hand, the wrong complained of is not merely negligence. It is trespass" (18). Cardozo went on to scribe a passage that is oft quoted in cases involving end-of-life treatment decisions: "Every human being of adult years and sound mind has a right to determine what shall be done with his own body; and a surgeon who performs an operation without his patient's consent, commits an assault, for which he is liable in damages" (19).

Thus, the concept of informed consent originated within the common-law framework of assault and battery—an action for injury based on nonconsensual touching. While the common-law analysis remains viable, many jurisdictions have found that the right to consent is also embodied in a constitutional right to privacy. For example, in 1977 the Supreme Judicial Court of Massachusetts stated that:

> [t]here is implicit recognition in the law of the Commonwealth, as elsewhere, that a person has a strong interest in being free from nonconsensual invasion of his bodily integrity.... One means by which the law has developed in a manner consistent with the protection of this interest is through the development of the doctrine of informed consent.
>
> ***
>
> Of even broader import, but arising from the same regard for human dignity and self-determination, is the unwritten constitutional right of privacy found in the penumbra of specific guaranties of the Bill of Rights (20).

(As discussed later, however, in *Cruzan* the U.S. Supreme Court subsequently analyzed the right to refuse treatment within the context of the constitutionally protected liberty interest, not privacy [21].)

In more recent times, the doctrine of informed consent has transitioned from the common-law 'intentional' tort of assault and battery to the tort of negligence. Thus, most actions based on informed consent today are brought as claims of medical malpractice or negligence (*i.e.*, failure to meet the medical standard of care). Some states have codified the concept of informed consent as negligence in statute or regulations (22).

The Right to Refuse Treatment

Thus, it has long been established that a physician cannot provide treatment or perform a procedure without a patient's (or the patient's surrogate's) consent. It would seem to follow that a physician cannot provide treatment or perform a procedure when a patient (or the patient's surrogate) refuses. If a patient has a right to consent to medical treatment, the logical corollary is that a patient also has the right to refuse medical treatment. Without the right to refuse, the right to consent would be illusory, as demonstrated by the circumstances in a clinical case frequently cited in the refusal of treatment ethics literature—the case of Dax Cowart (23).

In July 1973, 26-year-old Dax Cowart and his father were enveloped in a fiery explosion as they started their car, which they unknowingly parked near a large, leaking propane gas transmission line. Cowart's father died on the way to the hospital. Cowart suffered severe burns to his face and body, and corneal damage to both eyes, leaving him blind. Over a period of 9 months in Dallas' Parkland Hospital he underwent repeated skin grafting, enucleation of his right eye, surgical closing of his left eye in order to protect it from infections, and amputation of the distal parts of his fingers on both hands. He was then transferred to the University of Texas Medical Branch in Galveston, where he was bathed daily in a Hubbard tank (a very large stainless steel tank filled with temperature-controlled water) to control infections over his body and legs (24).

In the beginning, while Cowart consistently stated that he did not want to live, he accepted treatment. Two days after his transfer, however, he refused to consent to further corrective surgery on his hands. He insisted that he be allowed to leave the hospital and return home to die (the expected outcome of discontinuing the daily tanking that controlled infection). The tanking was continued over his objections. In response to his frequent periods of anger and despair, and hours of arguments with his mother regarding his wish to leave the hospital, a psychiatric consult was requested (25). In reviewing the case, his psychiatrist Dr. Robert B. White wrote: "Donald's wish [to discontinue treatment] seemed in great measure logical and rational; as my psychiatric duties brought me to know him well, I could not escape the thought that if I were in his position I would feel as he did. I asked two other psychiatric colleagues to see the patient, and they came to the same conclusion" (26,27). Nevertheless, his "logical and rational" (i.e., capacitated) wish to terminate treatment was not respected. Instead, his psychiatrist helped him obtain legal assistance, agreeing that if a court ruled that Cowart had the right to refuse further treatment, all life-sustaining treatment would be stopped (28). However, a hearing was never held as, shortly after an attorney agreed to represent him, Cowart agreed to continue treatment. He was discharged from the hospital 5 months later. After discharge, Cowart attempted suicide at least two times before accepting his new life circumstances (29).

Since *Dax,* the courts have recognized that "[t]he purpose underlying the doctrine of informed consent is defeated somewhat if, after receiving all information necessary to make an informed decision, the patient is forced to choose only from alternative methods of treatment and precluded from foregoing all treatment whatsoever.... [T]he doctrine of informed consent—a doctrine borne of the common-law right to be free from nonconsensual physical invasions—permits an individual to refuse medical treatment" (30).

Like the doctrine of informed consent, the right to refuse to consent has also been found to be supported not only by the common-law principles of assault and battery, but also by state and/or federal constitutionally protected rights (31). Similarly, the right to refuse treatment has been codified to some extent in all states in the form of statutes relating to advance directives (32).

THE DEVELOPMENT OF JUDICIAL ANALYSIS IN CRITICAL CARE/END-OF-LIFE DECISIONS

Prior to *Quinlan* in 1976, there were relatively few cases involving a patient's right to refuse care (33). However, as mentioned earlier, *Quinlan* heralded the proliferation of a new line of cases, prompted by technological advancements in medicine that made it possible to sustain life (or, alternatively stated, prolong dying) through artificial means. In 1987, the Arizona Supreme Court wrote: "Not long ago the realms of life and death were delineated by a bright line. Now this line is blurred by wondrous advances in medical technology—advances that until recent years were only ideas conceivable by such science-fiction visionaries as Jules Verne and H.G. Wells. Medical technology has effectively created a twilight zone of suspended animation where death commences while life, in some form, continues" (34). As the Arizona court notes, the rub is that "[s]ome patients, however, want no part of a life sustained only by medical technology. Instead, they prefer a plan of medical treatment that allows nature to take its course and permits them to die with dignity" (35).

Generally speaking, it is the exercise of this "fundamental" right to refuse treatment that is at the center of most judicial intervention in treatment decisions. Even though the right to refuse treatment is recognized as the obvious extension of the right to consent, and even though it has been held to be a constitutionally protected right, it is not an absolute right. As with other constitutionally protected "fundamental" rights, the right to refuse treatment is circumscribed under certain conditions through judicial and legislative action. Additionally, the exercise of the right may result in disagreements between patients, surrogates, family, and/or providers that often lead to judicial intervention (36).

Quinlan Sets the Stage

In 1973, Dax Cowart was caught at the cusp of the transition from a time when "the realms of life and death were delineated by a bright line" to a time when that line "is blurred by wondrous advances in medical technology" (37). Six months after Cowart's discharge, his psychiatrist noted: "Had Donald been burned a few years ago, before our increasingly exquisite medical and surgical technology became available, none of the moral, humanitarian, medical, or legal questions his case raised would have had time to occur; he would simply have died. But Donald lived... [and] [h]e has imposed upon us the responsibility to explore the questions he has asked.... 'What gives a physician the right to keep alive a patient who wants to die?'"(38). In 1976, the New Jersey Supreme responds that, at least for a patient who has no hope of recovery, a physician does not in fact have that right.

Just 2 years after Dax Cowart's accident, 22-year-old Karen Quinlan stopped breathing for at least two 15-minute periods. Three days after admission, she was diagnosed as comatose and required a respirator to assist her breathing. After a while, she progressed from a coma to a persistent vegetative state. Attempts to wean her from the respirator were unsuccessful. Her treating physicians believed that she would not live long without respirator support, and that removal would also risk further brain damage and increase risk of infection. Additionally, as described earlier, Quinlan was nourished through a nasogastric tube. At the time that the New Jersey Supreme Court considered the case, which was less than one year after her anoxic event, Quinlan had lost at least 40 pounds, and was in a permanent fetal-like position with her joints severely rigid and deformed (39). Joseph Quinlan, believing that his daughter would not want to continue to live in this condition, requested the withdrawal of life support. Her physician refused, believing that the standard of care at that time prohibited withdrawal (40). In *Quinlan,* the court considered her father's petition to be declared her guardian and authorized to have her respirator removed (41).

The court's own description of the case denotes its groundbreaking importance:

> [This] litigation has to do, in final analysis, with [Karen's] life, – its continuance or cessation, – and the responsibilities, rights and duties, with regard to a fateful decision concerning it, of her family, her guardian, her doctors, the hospital, the State through its law enforcement authorities, and finally the courts of justice.
>
> ***
>
> The matter is of transcendent importance, involving questions related to the definition and existence of death; the prolongation of life through artificial means developed by medical technology undreamed of in past generations.... [T]he impact of durationally indeterminate and artificial life prolongation on the rights of the incompetent, her family and society in general; the bearing of constitutional right and the scope of judicial responsibility... (42).

The court provides an extensive review of Karen's condition, juxtaposing her persistent vegetative state to the conditions recognized under the traditional definition of death, including brain death, which it finds "obfuscated" by developments in medical technology (43). Additionally, the court cites a statement of Bishop Lawrence B. Casey, reproduced in an amicus brief filed by the New Jersey Catholic Conference, to describe the existing gap in the law on these matters:

> In the present public discussion of the case of Karen Ann Quinlan it has been brought out that responsible people involved in medical care, patients and families have exercised the freedom to terminate or withhold certain treatments as extraordinary means in cases judged to be terminal... in accord with the expressed or implied intentions of the patients themselves. To whatever extent this has been happening it has been without sanction in civil law.
>
> ***
>
> It is both possible and necessary for society to have laws and ethical standards which provide freedom for decisions... to terminate or withhold extraordinary treatment in cases which are judged [by

> physicians] to be hopeless.... Indeed, to accomplish this, it may simply be required that courts and legislative bodies recognize the present standards and practices of [physicians] who have been doing what the parents of Karen Ann Quinlan are requesting authorization to have done for their beloved daughter (44).

With its analysis of the constitutional and legal issues at the heart of the case, the *Quinlan* court takes initial steps in filling in the "gap" perceived by Bishop Casey and the court itself.

First, the court analyzes the argument that Joseph Quinlan's right to refuse life-prolonging treatment for his daughter is supported by his constitutional right to free exercise of religion. As alluded to earlier, no constitutional right is absolute. But, interference with such a right is strictly limited and generally requires a "compelling state interest." With respect to religious beliefs, the New Jersey court outlines cases where religious freedom is curtailed; for example, "for the sake of life" courts had sometimes ordered blood transfusions for Jehovah's Witnesses and prohibited the handling of venomous snakes or ingestion of poison as part of religious ceremonies (45). In this case, however, the court does not recognize Joseph Quinlan's assertion of an independent parental right of religious freedom to support his request to terminate life support. The court then turns to the argument that keeping Karen alive violates her Eighth Amendment right against cruel and unusual punishment. Consistent with other courts that had considered Eighth Amendment claims unrelated to criminal sanctions, the *Quinlan* court holds that while an "accident of fate and nature" may have caused Karen to be in a condition that was in fact cruel and unusual, it could not be said to be "punishment" in the constitutional sense.

The third, and persuasive, constitutional right advanced by Joseph Quinlan on behalf of his daughter was the right of privacy. Relying on the right of privacy found in the New Jersey Constitution and in the penumbra of the Bill of Rights by the Supreme Court in *Griswold v. Connecticut* (46), the court decides that:

> no external compelling interest of the State could compel Karen to endure the unendurable, only to vegetate a few measurable months with no realistic possibility of returning to any semblance of cognitive or sapient life. We perceive no thread of logic distinguishing between such a choice on Karen's part and a similar choice which, under the evidence in this case, could be made by a competent patient, terminally ill, riddled with cancer and suffering great pain; such a patient would not be resuscitated or put on a respirator [as testified by an expert neurologist in the case] and *a fortiori* would not be kept *against his will* on a respirator (47).

The court notes that its affirmation of Karen's right to refuse treatment is based upon an analysis that assumes competency to assert a right of choice. In trying to determine what her wishes would have been were she capacitated, the court found that statements she had allegedly made were insufficient evidence of her desires. Nevertheless, the *Quinlan* court believed that if a decision to refuse life-prolonging treatment is a "valuable incident" of the right of privacy, then it should not be "discarded" merely because a patient's condition prevents the conscious exercise of the choice (48). (It is interesting to note that the court makes no references to cases holding that a capacitated patient has the right to refuse life-prolonging treatment, but uses the testimony of a physician to support the "unwritten and unspoken standard of medical practice" [49].) Consequently, the *Quinlan* court establishes the right of an incapacitated terminally ill or "incurable" patient to refuse procedures that prolong the dying process, granting her father the ability to make the decision for her, based on his "best judgment" of what her choice would be (50).

Having found there was no compelling state interest to support interference with Karen's right to refuse life-prolonging treatment, the court addressed the contention that discontinuation of life-supporting treatment for Karen was inconsistent with the prevailing medical standards (51). In discussing the relevant considerations, the court asks "What justification is there to remove [care and treatment decisions] from the control of the medical profession and place it in the hands of the courts?" (52). The court notes the "agitation of the medical community in the face of modern life prolongation technology and its search for definitive policy" regarding the continuation of extraordinary life-prolonging treatment to the incurably dying patient, agitation caused by the uncertainty regarding potential civil and criminal liability for openly practicing the evolving medical standard of withholding or withdrawing such treatment (53). The *Quinlan* court wanted to "free physicians, in the pursuit of their healing vocation, from possible contamination by self-interest or self-protection concerns, which would inhibit their independent medical judgments" (54), and permit decisions to be made within the patient/family–doctor relationship, without fear of liability and without the need to turn to the court for confirmation. However, the court was reluctant to propose that physicians be granted total immunity. Its solution was to suggest that physicians seek input from hospital ethics committees. Finally, with very little analysis, the court finds that the termination of life support in circumstances such as Karen Quinlan's would not lead to criminal liability, concluding that while the state has the power to punish the taking of human life, that power does not extend to an individual's exercise of their privacy right to refuse medical treatment, and by extension, to a third party exercising that right for the patient.

In summary, the *Quinlan* court clearly articulates for the first time the principle that an incapacitated patient has the same right to refuse life-prolonging treatment as a terminally ill capacitated patient. While not using the term "substituted judgment," the court sets the stage for the development of that standard by directing Karen's father to use his "best judgment" of what *her* choice would be. In addressing the issue of potential criminal liability, *Quinlan* helped to remove that fear from a medical profession concerned with application of a changing standard of care. It did not, however, establish clear guiding standards for analysis of this evolving area. Instead, it suggests an interdisciplinary approach to assure oversight of physician practice by encouraging the referral of such cases to hospital ethics committees. While the court states that it "consider[s] . . . a practice of applying to a court to confirm such decisions [to be] generally inappropriate, not only because that would be gratuitous encroachment upon the medical profession's field of competence, but because it would be impossibly cumbersome," its approach left significant room for continuing judicial intervention (55).

Saikewicz Develops a Standard Approach

The State Interest Test

Shortly after *Quinlan*, the Supreme Court of Massachusetts tackled a similar (though somewhat more complex) case in *Belchertown v. Saikewicz* (56). In April 1976 (1 month after the *Quinlan* decision), the superintendent of the Belchertown State School petitioned the Hampshire County Probate Court for appointment of a guardian ad litem with the power to make medical treatment decisions for Joseph Saikewicz, a resident of the school. Saikewicz, a 67-year-old man with the mental age of a $2^1/_2$-year-old, was diagnosed with acute myeloblastic monocytic leukemia. After reviewing the medical information, including the recommendation of Saikewicz's attending physicians that he not receive chemotherapy, the guardian ad litem recommended to the Probate Court that Saikewicz go untreated, letting his disease run its natural course. The Probate Court agreed, but given the import and novelty of its decision, the Probate Court itself asked for appellate review of the case.

The *Saikewicz* court was presented with expert testimony indicating that acute myeloblastic monocytic leukemia was, at that time, incurable and inevitably fatal. Regardless, most capacitated patients chose to have chemotherapy, enduring its significantly unpleasant side effects even though the potential for remission was only 30% to 50%, and when it did occur remission typically lasted for only 2 to 13 months. Thus, while chemotherapy was the normal medically indicated course of treatment, it could only provide the possibility of some uncertain and limited extension of life. The court was also presented with testimony indicating that patients over the age of 60 had more difficulty tolerating chemotherapy, and were less likely to have even a temporary remission. Given Saikewicz's age and condition, the court was informed that left untreated, he would live for a matter of weeks or, at most, several months. Juxtaposed to this information, the court considered testimony regarding the difficulty that Saikewicz would have undergoing chemotherapy. Difficulty not just because of the toxic side effects, the cause of which he would be unable to comprehend, nor because he could not appreciate the potential benefit; but also because Saikewicz's mental age would have made it impossible for him to cooperate with administration of the chemotherapy without restraint, which would cause him mental and physical anguish and could also lead to complications such as pneumonia.

Balancing the factors in favor of chemotherapy (the chance of lengthening his life and that most capacitated individuals chose treatment, even against the odds) against those factors mitigating against chemotherapy (limited benefit of treatment for a patient of Saikewicz's age and condition, his inability to cooperate with treatment, the possible toxic side effects, and other adverse effects associated with his inability to cooperate), the *Saikewicz* court ordered that no treatment be provided, except as needed to reduce his suffering or discomfort during the natural course of the disease. The court issued its order on July 9, 1976. Saikewicz died on September 4, due to bronchial pneumonia. On November 28, 1977, the *Saikewicz* court issued an opinion intended to provide comprehensive guidance in the review of cases related to the withholding of critical care in end-of-life situations, both for capacitated and incapacitated patients.

As a prelude to its analysis of the broader issues, the court recognized the importance of its task and succinctly outlined the critical questions raised by cases involving the refusal of life-prolonging treatments:

> We recognize at the outset that this case presents novel issues of fundamental importance that should not be resolved by mechanical reliance on legal doctrine. Our task of establishing a framework in the law on which the activities of health care personnel and other persons can find support is furthered by seeking the collective guidance of those in health care, moral ethics, philosophy, and other disciplines.... [T]he principal areas of determination are: A. The nature of the right of any person, competent or incompetent, to decline potentially life-prolonging treatment. B. The legal standards that control the course of decision whether or not potentially life-prolonging, but not life-saving, treatment should be administered to a person who is not competent to make the choice. C. The procedures that must be followed in arriving at that decision (57).

The *Saikewicz* court begins its analysis of the nature of the right of a person to decline life-prolonging treatment with a look at the current medical ethics, which it finds well expressed by the view that "we should not use *extraordinary* means of prolonging life or its semblance when, after careful consideration, consultation and the application of the most well conceived therapy it becomes apparent that there is no hope for the recovery of the patient. Recovery should not be defined simply as the ability to remain alive; it should mean life without intolerable suffering" (58). This ethos was also recognized by the *Quinlan* court, which observed that "physicians distinguish between curing the ill and comforting and easing the dying;... they refuse to treat the curable as if they were dying or ought to die, and... they have sometimes refused to treat the hopeless and dying as if they were curable" (59). Additionally, the court reviewed the established principle that a person has a fundamental right to be free from nonconsensual invasion of her or his bodily integrity as recognized by the U.S. Supreme Court in *Botsford*, and the concept of self-determination as embodied in the right to privacy recognized by the U.S. Supreme Court in *Griswold* and by the New Jersey Supreme Court in *Quinlan*. Based on the fact, as mentioned above, that no constitutional right is totally absolute, the court conducts a survey of recent decisions from various states addressing patients' rights to decline extraordinary life-prolonging or -preserving treatments, and formulates a concise summary list of the "state interests" to be weighed against the individual's fundamental right to privacy and self-determination: 1. the preservation of life, 2. the protection of the interests of innocent third parties, 3. the prevention of suicide, and 4. maintaining the ethical integrity of the medical profession (60). This four-pronged test has been widely adopted by the courts in determining when an individual patient's ability to exercise her or his constitutional right to refuse treatment can be circumscribed (Table 6.1).

In applying the state interest test to Saikewicz's situation (albeit in retrospect, after Saikewicz had died), the court concludes that the most significant state interest enumerated was the preservation of life. It finds, however, that such interest must be weighed against the traumatic cost of prolongation of life to the patient, stating that "[t]here is a substantial distinction in the State's insistence that human life be saved where the affliction is curable, as opposed to the State interest where, as here, the issue is not whether, but when, for how long, and at what cost to the individual that life may briefly extended" (61). The second element of the test, the protection of innocent third parties, is inapplicable to Saikewicz's case (62). Likewise, the third state interest, the prevention of suicide, is not applicable to Saikewicz's plight (63). The court nevertheless notes that a competent adult's refusal of medical treatment that would result in death is not equivalent to suicide, as even if death was the patient's intent, the patient's medical condition was not of her or his own making. Moreover, the court distinguishes the

TABLE 6.1

STATE INTERESTS ANALYSES

State interest	Potential use
Preservation of life	Historically, this argument has not been very successful in supporting the state's authority to override refusal of care for an incapacitated patient. The state would most likely have to show that the incapacitated patient was likely to regain capacity or significant physical/mental function, that is, that the patient is "curable." It is more likely to be successful in overriding refusal of life-sustaining treatment for a nonterminal capacitated patient. As demonstrated by many Jehovah Witness cases, however, even in those instances it may not prove a strong enough state interest.
Protection of the interests of innocent third parties	Cases seem to indicate that this argument would only be successful if the state could show a total abandonment of a person legally responsible for the care/well-being of the third party, for example, that the third party would become a ward of the state.
Prevention of suicide	Like the preservation of life, this state interest is most likely to be raised in cases involving refusal of life-saving treatment by capacitated patients who are not terminal, but perhaps suffering from depression or other mental health issues indicating suicidal ideation, even if there are significant "quality of life" issues.
Maintaining the ethical integrity of the medical profession	While this argument was used by the state early in the development of the right-to-die jurisprudence to deny a patient's refusal of care, today it would most likely be proposed by counsel for the physician, supporting her or his reluctance to continue treatment deemed to be not only medically futile, but also ethically repugnant to continue to impose on a dying patient.

state interest in the prevention of "irrational self-destruction" from a right to intervene in a "rational decision to refuse treatment when death is inevitable and the treatment offers no hope of cure or preservation of life" (64). When deciding whether or not a patient's wishes to forgo treatment will be honored, the last state interest to be considered is the maintenance of the ethical integrity of the medical profession. In reviewing the applicability of this standard to Saikewicz, the court agrees with the *Quinlan* court's finding that the prevailing medical ethical ethos at that time recognized that the dying were frequently more in need of comfort than treatment. The court also notes the testimony of Saikewicz's own attending physicians, who recommended against treatment. Additionally, the court relied on the *Botsford* principles that a patient has the right to bodily integrity, and on the doctrines of informed consent and right to privacy. The court concludes that the state interest in maintaining the ethical integrity of the medical profession is not threatened by the decision to permit Saikewicz to forgo chemotherapy.

The Substituted Judgment Standard

In addition to articulating the four state interests to be used in determining when a patient's fundamental right to refuse life-prolonging medical treatment may be denied, the *Saikewicz* court addresses the important question regarding the rights of an *incompetent* patient to forgo such treatment. The court poses two distinct questions: "First, does a choice exist? That is, is it the unvarying responsibility of the State to order medical treatment in all circumstances involving the care of an incompetent person? Second, if a choice does exist under certain conditions, what considerations enter into the decision-making process?" (65). The court finds the first question relatively easy to answer. Since it is recognized that a person has the right to refuse medical treatment in appropriate circumstances, then "the principles of equality and respect for all individuals" dictate that the right extends to incompetent as well as competent individuals. In so finding, the court recognizes the state's *parens patriae* responsibility to protect the "best interests" of incompetent persons, interpreted by courts to mandate the provision of medical treatment for incompetent patients to prevent immediate and severe danger to life. But the court distinguishes the state's responsibility to provide life-saving treatment from its obligation to provide treatment under other circumstances (66). Consequently, the court finds that "[t]o protect the incompetent person within its power, the State must recognize the dignity and worth of such person and afford to that person the same panoply of rights and choices it recognizes in competent persons" (67).

Having concluded that an incompetent patient possesses the same right to refuse treatment as a competent patient, the *Saikewicz* court set out to establish how a court can assure that the incompetent patient's right is exercised in a manner that provides the "fullest possible expression to the character and circumstances" of the individual patient (68). The court uses the *Quinlan* decision as a starting point for its analysis, but gives significant weight to the difference between Karen Quinlan's and Joseph Saikewicz's circumstances. While the *Quinlan* court was unable to ascertain conclusively the decision Karen herself would have made in her situation, it was nonetheless clear that she *could* have made an informed decision prior to her incapacity. It made sense, then, that her father could use his "best judgment," based on his knowledge of her preferences and life philosophy, to determine what Karen would have wanted for herself. Saikewicz never had capacity; consequently, the court found the best judgment standard unsuitable. While the court saw some value in an "objective" viewpoint based on what a majority of people would do in like circumstances, akin to the "reasonable person" inquiry used in negligence, it rejected that standard. Instead, the court opined that the critical goal is to determine, as accurately as possible, the wants and needs of the individual involved, regardless of whether or not it is what the reasonable or prudent person would do, and despite the difficulty of making that determination for the developmentally disabled. The court therefore adopted a "substituted judgment" standard. In analyzing the specific pros and cons of chemotherapy for Saikewicz, as discussed above, the court found that the decision to withhold care was in fact based on a regard for Saikewicz's actual interest and preferences. After *Saikewicz,* the "substituted judgment" doctrine becomes the primary legal standard for asserting an incapacitated patient's right to refuse life-prolonging treatment.

Procedures for Appropriate Review of Decision

Finally, the *Saikewicz* court reviews the issue of procedural safeguards applicable to withholding life-prolonging procedures from incapacitated patients. The court focuses on procedures of the Massachusetts Probate Court. However, in discussing the type of information relevant to an appropriate process, the *Saikewicz* court specifically "reject[s] the approach adopted by the New Jersey Supreme court in the *Quinlan* case of entrusting the decision whether to continue artificial life support to the patient's guardian, family, attending doctors, and hospital 'ethics committee'" (69). Rather than considering "judicial resolution of this most difficult and awesome question—whether potentially life-prolonging treatment should be withheld from a person incapable of making his own decision—as constituting a 'gratuitous encroachment' on the domain of medical expertise," as stated in *Quinlan*, the *Saikewicz* court suggests that "such questions of life and death seem . . . to require the process of detached but passionate investigation and decision that forms the ideal on which the judicial branch of government was created" (70). Thus, the New Jersey and Massachusetts Supreme Courts express significantly different views regarding the degree of judicial intervention necessary or appropriate in end-of-life treatment decisions for the incapacitated.

Clear and Convincing Standard of Proof for Substituted Judgment

Incapacitated Adults

In 1981, the Court of Appeals of New York (71) reviewed two separate cases in *In the Matter of Storar* (72) where the guardians of incapacitated patients objected to the continued use of life-prolonging treatments for two terminally ill patients. In one case the court held that the guardian's wish should have been followed; in the other, the court found that treatment should have been provided (73). What circumstances led to the different outcomes?

In the first case, the patient was 83-year-old Brother Joseph Fox, who was in excellent health until he had an operation for a hernia he sustained while moving flower tubs. During the procedure, Brother Fox suffered cardiac arrest and substantial brain damage. He was placed on a respirator, and remained in a persistent vegetative state. Father Philip Eichner, president of the school for which Fox had worked during the 9 years prior to the operation, asked that the respirator be disconnected. Fox had previously made it known that he would not have wanted to be maintained on a respirator in his present condition. He had first made this view known during formal religious discussions on the moral implications of the *Quinlan* case. The hospital refused to disconnect the respirator without court authorization, resulting in a petition to the court by Father Eichner.

In the second case, John Storar, a profoundly developmentally disabled 52-year-old man who resided in a state facility, was diagnosed with cancer of the bladder after blood was noticed in his urine. His mother, who was his court-appointed guardian, consented to a 6-week course of radiation therapy, after which his disease went into remission. Six months later, after blood was again found in his urine, Storar was diagnosed with terminal bladder cancer. Despite the prognosis for a very limited lifespan, the facility physicians requested consent for blood transfusions, to permit Storar to remain energetic and maintain his daily activities (feeding himself, showering, taking walks, and running). Similar to Saikewicz, Storar did not like the transfusions, as he could not understand the purpose. But unlike the case in *Saikewicz,* there was no evidence of excessive pain, discomfort, or mental anguish presented. While Storar's mother initially consented, after a month she withdrew her consent (74), whereupon the facility director asked for judicial intervention. While the trial court agreed with the guardians' requests in both cases, the Court of Appeals agreed with Father Eichner, but not with Storar's mother.

In the Eichner case, the District Attorney intervened, asserting that the state's interest in preserving life outweighs a patient's right to refuse medical treatment. The court begins its analysis by citing Justice Cardozo's finding in *Schloendorff* that a surgeon who performs a procedure on a patient without her or his consent is liable for assault. While recognizing that other state courts had found a constitutional right to privacy supporting the right to refuse treatment, citing both *Quinlan* and *Saikewicz*, the *Storar* court finds no need to address the constitutionality issue (noting that the U.S. Supreme Court had so far declined to address the question), finding the *Schloendorff* common-law principle of a right to bodily integrity sufficient (75). Responding to the District Attorney's assertion that preservation of life gave the state authority to intervene, the *Storar* court observed that "[a] State which imposes civil liability on a doctor if he violates the patient's right cannot also hold him criminally responsible if he respects that right. Thus a doctor cannot be held to have violated his legal or professional responsibilities when he honors the right of a competent adult patient to decline medical treatment" (76). But noting that Fox was competent at the time the matter was before the court, the District Attorney argues that whatever right to refuse treatment a patient has is personal and cannot be exercised by a third party on her or his behalf when she or he becomes incapacitated. Cognizant of the difficult questions presented by permitting one person to make an end-of-life decision for another, the court skirts the issue, finding that Brother Fox made the decision for himself *before* becoming incompetent. Testimony was presented regarding Brother Fox's statements on two occasions, 3 years before his hernia operation during discussions on the much publicized plight of Karen Quinlan and again shortly before the procedure. The court therefore finds "clear and convincing" evidence that the patient himself left instructions to terminate life-supporting procedures if he was in a terminal condition with no hope of recovery. While the court makes no reference to the "substituted judgment" standard developed in *Quinlan* and *Saikewicz*, the "clear and convincing evidence" standard articulated by the *Storar* court essentially establishes the burden of proof used to establish that a decision maker's exercise of an incapacitated patient's right to refuse life-prolonging procedures reflects what the patient would have done for her- or himself *i.e.*, substituted judgment.

Next the *Storar* court analyzes John Storar's situation, beginning with the observation that there can be no clear and convincing evidence of Storar's own decision, as Storar was never competent to make the decision. The court therefore refuses to apply the same reasoning it followed for *Fox*. Instead, it applies the law relating to the right of a parent or guardian to refuse medical treatment for an infant, relying on previous decisions that a parent cannot deny treatment to a child that threatens his or her life (77). In conclusion, and directly apposed to the *Saikewicz* finding, the *Storar* court holds that, even in light of Storar's terminal condition, life-prolonging treatment cannot be withheld because he was never capacitated. In essence, the *Storar* court finds that one must have had capacity at some time to apply the substituted judgment standard.

As with the *Quinlan* and *Saikewicz* courts, the *Storar* court also shares its general view on the role of the courts in end-of-life situations. Responding to the District Attorney's argument against Eichner's petition that courts should wait for the parties to act before considering whether liability exists, the court responds that "responsible parties who wish to comply with the law, in cases where the legal consequences of the contemplated action is uncertain, need not act at their peril. Nor is it inappropriate for those charged with the care of incompetent persons to apply to the courts for a ruling on the propriety of conduct which might seriously affect their charges." But the court emphasizes that seeking court intervention is optional, and that if in fact there is a desire to expand the court's role in cases regarding termination of life-prolonging treatment for incapacitated patients, the legislature should so mandate.

Minors

The question may be asked, How does the substituted judgment standard apply to minors? Under the *Saikewicz* analysis, it would be possible to have substituted judgment for a minor, but under the *Storar* analysis, since the minor has never had capacity, it would not be possible to ascertain with clear and convincing evidence what a minor's wishes would be.

In *In re Guardianship of Barry* (78), a Florida court considered the request of Mr. and Mrs. Barry, natural parents and appointed guardians for 10-month-old Andrew James Barry, to terminate his life support. Andrew was the second of twins, the first of which was stillborn. He was in a permanent vegetative state after suffering asphyxiation and seizures and was placed on a ventilator soon after birth. Diagnosed as having hypoxic ischemic encephalopathy with significant brain tissue destruction, Andrew was not expected to live much beyond 2 years, even with life support. The trial court approved the Barrys' request, based on the substituted judgment doctrine. The state appealed, arguing that the doctrine was wrongly applied since there could be no evidence of Andrew's intent. The appellate court found that for an adult a court could exercise substituted judgment even without evidence of the incapacitated patient's intentions; however, the doctrine could not be used in "the case of a child who has not reached maturity, . . . where . . . the court must be guided primarily by the judgment of the parents who are responsible for their child's well-being, provided, of course, that their judgment is supported by competent medical evidence" (79). After reviewing the medical condition of the child and considering the ethical and moral motivations (80), the appellate court found that the Barrys' decision was backed by uncontroverted medical evidence that Andrew was terminally ill and his condition was incurable and irreversible, and that their informed decision outweighed any state interest in prolonging Andrew's life through "extraordinary" measures. Moreover, like many courts before, the *Barry* court opines that "decisions of this character have traditionally been made within the privacy of the family relationship based on competent medical advice and consultation by the family with their religious advisors, if that be their persuasion" (81). Nevertheless, noting the continually increasing availability of advanced technology to artificially sustain life through "extraordinary" measures, and the lack of legislation or controlling judicial precedent (even in 1984, 8 years after *Quinlan*), the *Barry* court acknowledges the medical community's continuing discomfort in proceeding without judicial intervention, for fear of malpractice litigation or criminal prosecution. As in many of the cases since *Quinlan*, the *Barry* court expresses its views on the role of the courts in intervening in end-of-life decisions:

> Although judicial intervention need not be solicited as a matter of course, still the courts must always be open to hear these matters on request of the family, guardian, affected medical personnel, or the state. In cases where doubt exists, or there is a lack of concurrence among the family, physicians, and the hospital, or if an affected party simply desires a judicial order, then the court must be available to consider the matter (82).

As we have seen most recently with the case of Terri Schiavo, this is most certainly still the case.

In *Barry*, the Florida court addresses the issue of a child "who has not reached maturity." In *In re Swan,* the Maine Supreme Court considered the case of the "mature minor" (83). Like many states, Maine first considered the question of withdrawal of life-sustaining procedures from a permanently incapacitated—but not terminal—patient in the mid-1980s. Citing much of the reasoning discussed in *Botsford*, *Schloendorff*, *Saikewicz*, and *Storar*, the Maine court held in *In re Gardner* (84) that when there was clear and convincing evidence of an incapacitated patient's wishes not to be maintained by life-prolonging procedures, those wishes must be respected by his providers. A few years later in *Swan*, the court extended this principle to Chad Eric Swan, who was 17 years old when a tragic auto accident left him in a persistent vegetative state.

As in several cases discussed above, judicial involvement in *Swan* was initiated by his alternate decision makers, who filed for a declaratory judgment that neither the family, treating physicians, nor hospital would be civilly or criminally liable for a decision to terminate life-prolonging artificial nutrition and hydration. The District Attorney, representing the state's interests, argued that there was insufficient evidence of Chad's wishes, and that in any event, Chad's age reduced the legal significance of any statements he may have made. Evidence was presented that Chad had on two separate occasions had discussions regarding the status of two individuals. One was in a persistent vegetative state (and was coincidentally Gardner, of the case cited above, who was known by Chad's grandmother). The other was his brother's friend, who had been left in a permanent coma after a car accident. On each occasion, one a year before and one only 8 days before his own accident, Chad made specific statements that he would not want to be kept artificially alive under similar conditions. The *Swan* court found that these two statements presented clear and convincing evidence of Chad's wishes, and that the mere fact that he was not yet 18 at the time he made them did not negate their probative value: "The fact that Chad made these declarations as to medical treatment before he reached the age of 18 is at most a factor to be considered by the fact finder in assessing the seriousness and deliberativeness with which his declarations were made" (85). In so concluding, the court relied on the "well-recognized" principle that "[a] minor acquires capacity to consent to different kinds of invasions and conduct at different states of his development. Capacity exists when the minor has the ability of the average person to understand and weigh the risks and benefits" (86).

Consequently, the *Swan* court holds that there was clear and convincing evidence that Chad would have chosen to discontinue artificial life support measures, that his comments were in fact relevant despite his being a "minor" at the time of the declarations, and that his parents could exercise that decision on his behalf. (It is interesting to note that the court considered this decision to be made based on "Chad's own conclusion," not on a theory of substituted judgment; for this court the "substituted judgment" theory implies that there is not sufficient evidence of the patient's own desires.) While some states have adopted a "mature minor" doctrine permitting termination of life-prolonging procedures, many have not (87). Where not adopted, the *Barry* approach would be the most likely line of reasoning used in determining the appropriateness of life support withdrawal from a permanently incapacitated, but not terminal, minor patient.

A final interesting case to consider with regard to the incapacitated minor issue is the case of *In the Matter of Baby K* (88). Baby K was born with anencephaly; however, she was placed on a respirator at birth when she experienced difficulty breathing in order to permit her doctors to confirm the suspected diagnosis. After confirming the anencephaly, her physicians explained to her mother that most anencephalic children die within a few days. Their recommendation was that Baby K only be offered supportive care in the form of nutrition, hydration, and warmth. They also discussed the possibility of a "do not resuscitate" order. Baby K's mother and her treating physicians disagreed on the extent of care that was appropriate. While Baby K was able to breathe unaided at times, her mother insisted on the provision of mechanical ventilation to Baby K every time she had problems breathing on her own. Due to the disagreement, the hospital arranged for a transfer of Baby K to a nursing home. However, every time Baby K experienced breathing problems she was transferred back to the hospital emergency department for resuscitation and ventilation. After Baby K's third visit to the emergency room, the hospital (joined by Baby K's father) petitioned the court for a declaration that it was not required to continue to provide emergency medical treatment to Baby K, which it deemed medically and ethically inappropriate.

Baby K presents a different situation in that it is not the patient's representative who is advocating the termination of extraordinary life support measures, but the health care providers, thus invoking, one might argue, the fourth element of the *Saikewicz* state interest test *i.e.*, maintaining the ethical integrity of the medical profession (89). It is also unique in that the decision to withhold care was presented in the emergency room. As a result, rather than an analysis based on the end-of-life considerations expressed by many of the preceding decisions, the *Baby K* court analyzed the circumstances within the context of a hospital's Emergency Medical Treatment and Labor Act (EMTALA) (90) obligations. Pursuant to that analysis, the court finds that while the ER could not resolve Baby K's anencephaly, it could treat her respiratory failure, which was the emergency medical condition requiring stabilization under EMTALA. Thus, despite the discomfort of the medical team, the court holds that Baby K had to be resuscitated, regardless of her permanent incapacity and terminal condition, as long as she was brought to the emergency room for treatment. The court never addressed the question of withholding or withdrawal of treatment for Baby K in the event that the mother requested it, but under the EMTALA analysis, that would presumably no longer constitute a "request for . . . treatment" under the federal law (91).

The Terminally Ill Capacitated Patient

In the cases discussed previously, the courts relied on the widely accepted constitutional and/or common-law right of the capacitated patient to refuse medical treatment to support the incapacitated patient's right to refuse life-prolonging treatment. But yet, there has not yet been a case presented where the capacitated patient's right to refuse life-prolonging treatment is established. That case is represented by *Satz v. Perlmutter* (92).

In 1978, 73-year-old Abe Perlmutter lay in a hospital in Florida dying from amyotrophic lateral sclerosis (Lou Gehrig's disease). Perlmutter was on a respirator but was fully capacitated, and even able, albeit with difficulty, to speak. With no chance of recovery and little time left to live, Perlmutter requested to be disconnected from the respirator, and petitioned the court for an order permitting his physicians to do so. While the court's discussion doesn't specifically address why Perlmutter had to petition the court, it is reasonable to assume that his physicians were unwilling to comply with his wishes for fear of criminal prosecution, as in opposing the petition the State Attorney asserted not only that the state had a duty to preserve Perlmutter's life (as we have seen many states argue), but also that termination of life support by his family, medical personnel, or Perlmutter himself would be murder or manslaughter (93).

In reviewing Perlmutter's situation, the court relies on the rationale of *Saikewicz*, stating that "the pros and cons involved in such tragedies which bedevil contemporary society, mainly because of the incredible advancement in scientific medicine, are all exhaustively discussed in [*Saikewicz*]" (94). The court adopts the view of *Saikewicz* and the line of cases therein discussed, and finds that none of the state interests outlined in *Saikewicz* is sufficiently compelling to overcome Perlmutter's right to refuse or discontinue life-prolonging treatment under "the constitutional right to privacy . . . and expression of the sanctity of individual free choice and self-determination" (95).

It is somewhat ironic that the court asserts Perlmutter's rights as a capacitated patient based upon a decision relating to an incapacitated (and moreover, never capacitated) patient; yet the court takes care to limit its findings to the capacitated patient situation, stating, "[t]he problem is less easy of solution when the patient is incapable of understanding and we, therefore, postpone a crossing of that more complex bridge until such time as we are required to do so" (96). There is also a fascinating circularity, as *Saikewicz* and the other cases discussed previously relating to incapacitated patients are based on the presumed ability of a *capacitated* patient to make her or his own decision. Completing the circular approach, a few years after *Perlmutter*, in *John F. Kennedy Memorial Hospital v. Bludworth* (97), the Florida Supreme Court, citing extensively to its *Perlmutter* analysis, holds that a terminally ill *incapacitated* person has the same right to refuse life-prolonging treatment as a capacitated patient.

While adopting the District Court of Appeal's decision, the Florida Supreme Court extends the opinion by addressing the State Attorney's contention that the question of "death with dignity" is so complex that the courts should defer to the legislature to provide answers. Perlmutter's and his physician's attorneys, on the other hand, "maintain that it is an issue which cries out for judicial resolution in a comprehensive manner so that physicians, public officials, hospitals and other citizens of the state may be guided in their future conduct" (98). The court opines that the legislature is a more suitable forum for the detailed analysis and synthesis of the varied interested institutions and disciplines' viewpoints necessary for a comprehensive approach. "Nevertheless, preference for legislative treatment cannot shackle the courts when legally protected interests are at stake.... Legislative inaction cannot serve to close the doors of the courtrooms of [the] state to its citizens who assert cognizable constitutional rights" (99).

CODIFICATION OF JUDICIALLY DEVELOPED LAW

Not long after *Perlmutter*, Florida did in fact adopt legislation recognizing a competent person's right to refuse medical treatment, including life-prolonging treatment. Florida Statutes Chapter 765 on Health Care Advance Directives acknowledges that "[e]very competent adult has the fundamental right of self-determination regarding decisions pertaining to his or her own health, including the right to choose or refuse medical treatment. This right is subject to certain interests of society, such as the protection of human life and the preservation of ethical standards in the medical profession" (100). The statute also establishes guidelines for assuring that those rights are respected in the event of incapacity: "To ensure that such right is not lost or diminished by virtue of later physical or mental incapacity, the Legislature intends that a procedure be established to allow a person to plan for incapacity by executing a document or orally designating another person to direct the course of his or her medical treatment upon his or her incapacity" (101). Further, it sets forth the requirements for designating alternate decision makers or surrogates to make decisions for a patient in the event of incapacity, and provides a list of individuals who can be relied on to make decisions for an incapacitated patient who has not designated a surrogate. The statute "recognizes that for some the administration of life-prolonging medical procedures may result in only a precarious and burdensome existence" (102), and establishes procedures for the execution of living wills and the standards for withdrawing or withholding of life-prolonging procedures in the event that there is no living will. In so doing, Florida law codifies the "substituted judgment" standard established through *Saikewicz*, providing that the surrogate must make "only health care decisions for the principal which he or she believes the principal would have made under the circumstances if the principal were capable of making such decisions" (103). Moreover, the statute codifies the "clear and convincing" evidence requirement, providing that a proxy can only make a withholding or withdrawal decision if there is "clear and convincing" evidence that the decision would have been the one made by the patient were she or he capacitated (104). Finally, the Florida statute explicitly provides healthcare providers acting in good faith to fulfill patients' wishes regarding end-of-life care immunity from civil or criminal liability, thus removing the fear of litigation or prosecution that, as indicated in several cases discussed above, was a significant factor in the request for court involvement in refusal of care cases (105).

From the mid-1980s to the mid-1990s, most states adopted some form of legislation addressing procedures for withholding and withdrawing life-prolonging procedures; by 1994, 47 states had adopted some form of living will legislation, and all but two states had passed some form of health care agency act (106).

JUDICIAL INVOLVEMENT POSTLEGISLATION

The passage of legislation to address end-of-life situations helped to alleviate much of the uncertainty regarding the standards for reliance on patient and/or surrogate refusal of life-prolonging procedures, but it by no means eliminated the need for all judicial intervention. Continuing uncertainty regarding some of the terms of the legislation, and particularly disagreements among interested parties, still generate controversies that lead to judicial involvement.

In Arizona, the right to refuse life-prolonging treatment was first addressed by the state Supreme Court after the 1985 enactment of the Medical Treatment Decision Act (MTDA) (107) in *Rasmussen v. Fleming*. At age 70, Mildred Rasmussen had suffered three strokes and was suffering from a degenerative neural muscular disease and/or organic brain syndrome. Testimony from a court-appointed neurologist established that Rasmussen was in a persistent vegetative state. The question before the court was whether a guardian could exercise Rasmussen's right to refuse care (in this case through "do not resuscitate" and "do not hospitalize" orders).

The Arizona court began with an inquiry regarding whether Rasmussen had a *statutory* right to refuse medical treatment under the MTDA, which provided that "[a] person may execute a declaration directing the withholding or withdrawal of life-sustaining procedures in a terminal condition" (108). "Terminal condition" was defined as "an incurable or irreversible condition from which... death will occur without the use of life-sustaining procedures" (109). The court summarily found that Rasmussen did not have a statutory right to refuse care, as she never executed a living will, and secondly, she was not suffering from a terminal condition, as her physicians were not administering any life-sustaining procedures without which she would have died (110).

The statutory analysis, however, did not prove fatal to Rasmussen's guardian's request, as the court, finding no statutory support for Rasmussen's right to refuse care, turns to a more traditional analysis. Acknowledging that the U.S. Supreme Court had yet to address the issue of whether there was a federal constitutional right to refuse care embedded in the right to privacy, the Arizona court states that it "[agreed] with [her] sister states. The right to refuse medical treatment is a personal right sufficiently 'fundamental' or 'implicit in the concept of ordered liberty' to fall within the constitutionally protected zone of privacy" recognized by the Supreme Court (111).

Additionally the court finds that the Arizona constitution affords individuals a separate right to refuse medical treatment, as Article 2, § 8 expressly provides a right to privacy: "No person shall be disturbed in his private affairs, or his home invaded, without authority of law." While never previously applied to the refusal of medical treatment, the court finds the Arizona constitution provision applicable. Finally, citing *Botsford* and *Schloendorff* to assert the long-recognized law regarding an individual's right to be free from bodily invasion, the court holds that the common-law doctrine of informed consent permits an individual to refuse treatment as well (112).

As the cases reviewed before have shown, establishing the existence of the right is only the first step. "Whether emanating from constitutional penumbras or premised on common-law doctrine, the right to refuse medical treatment is not absolute" (113). Weighing Mildred Rasmussen's right to refuse care against the four state interests articulated in *Saikewicz*, the court finds that none of them outweigh Rasmussen's protected right under these circumstances. Of note, in deciding that the state's interest in preventing suicide does not outweigh Rasmussen's right to privacy, the court turns to the MDTA for support, as it provided that "[t]he withholding or withdrawal of life-sustaining procedures from a qualified patient in accordance with [the MTDA] does not, for any purpose, constitute a suicide" (114). Acknowledging that it had already held that the MTDA was inapplicable, the court contends that it would nonetheless be illogical to suggest that the state's interest in preventing suicide "magically disappears only when an individual becomes terminally ill and completes certain paper-work" (115).

Having established that Rasmussen had a right to refuse treatment, albeit not under the statute, and that such right was not outweighed by any of the four established state interests, the *Rasmussen* court then considers whether the right is retained if the patient is incapacitated and joins "[o]ther jurisdictions [that] have unanimously concluded that the right to refuse medical treatment is not lost merely because the individual has become incompetent and has failed to preserve the right" (116). Finally, the court addresses the issue of who may exercise the right for an incapacitated patient. In this case, no family member attempted to make decisions for Rasmussen. Instead, the Public Fiduciary was appointed her guardian. Thus, the court relies on Arizona statutes relating to the power of guardians, which provide that "a guardian may give any consents or approvals that may be necessary to enable the ward to receive medical or other professional care, counsel, treatment or service" (117). Finding that the right to consent to or approve the delivery of care must necessarily include the right to consent to or approve the delivery of *no* care, the court holds that Rasmussen's guardian has the statutory authority to exercise her right to refusal—but not with "unbridled" discretion. Based not on *Saikewicz*, but on a recommendation of the 1983 President's Commission for the Study of Ethical Problems in Medicine and Biomedical and Behavioral Research (118), the court opines that the "substituted judgment" standard is the most appropriate to apply in the case of an incapacitated patient. However, where there is no evidence of what the patient would have chosen, the court finds that the "best interests" standard is appropriate. (In Florida, this fallback standard has been codified in the Advance Directive statutes. The law may differ depending on the state.) Finally, the court finds that if there is a dispute regarding the substituted judgment or best interests of the incapacitated patient, the evidentiary standard must be that of "clear and convincing" evidence, as articulated by *Storar*.

As appears to be customary in these cases, the *Rasmussen* court could not conclude without stating its opinion regarding the role of the courts and the legislature in developing the law on refusal of life-prolonging treatments. "Last, but certainly not least, we address the degree to which judicial involvement is required in this type of case" (119). Observing that there have been differing points of view expressed, most notably those by the Massachusetts court in *Saikewicz* and the New Jersey Court in *Quinlan,* the Arizona court tends to agree with *Quinlan* that "judicial intervention in decisions of this nature can indeed be unduly cumbersome" (120), especially considering the fact that many opinions are written after the patient in question has died (121).

> A minimal amount of judicial involvement in an incompetent's affairs is unavoidable in cases such as this one . . . where guardianship is sought and an incompetency hearing is required . . . . Once the court resolves [those issues], however, its encroachment into the substantive decisions concerning medical treatment should be limited to resolving disputes among the patient's family, the attending physicians, an independent physician, the health care facility, the guardian, and the guardian ad litem . . . . Where, however, all affected parties concur in the proposed plan of medical treatment, court approval of the proposed plan of medical treatment is neither necessary nor required (122).

But, noting that this area continues to have many unresolved issues, the court also states that "[o]nly the Legislature has the resources necessary to gather and synthesize the vast quantities of information needed to formulate guidelines that will best accommodate the rights and interest of the many individuals and institutions involved in these tragic situations" (123).

In *In re Browning* (124), the issue was interpretation of statutory definitions. In 1984, Florida adopted the Life Prolonging Procedures Act (125), essentially codifying *Bludworth*, wherein the Florida Supreme Court held that a terminally ill incapacitated patient had the same right to refuse life-prolonging procedure as the court had established for a capacitated patient in *Perlmutter*. The act provided that any capacitated person could execute a living will directing the withholding or withdrawal of "life-prolonging procedures" in the event she or he should have a "terminal condition" (126). Life-prolonging procedures were defined to be mechanical or artificial means of sustaining, supplanting, or restoring any spontaneous vital function that, when applied to a person in a *terminal condition,* serves only to prolong the dying process, and specifically excluded nutrition and hydration (127). A terminal condition was defined as a condition from which there was no reasonable medical probability of recovery and from which death was *imminent* (128).

In 1985, Estelle Browning executed a living will, which, tracking the statutory language, stated: "If at any time I should have a terminal condition and if [it has been] determined that there can be no recovery from such condition and that my death is imminent, I direct that life-prolonging procedures be withheld or withdrawn when the application of such procedures would serve only to prolong artificially the process of dying" (129). Additionally, and inconsistent with the statute's definitions, Browning's living will stated that she did not want "nutrition and hydration . . . provided by gastric tube or intravenously" (130). One year later, at the age of 86, Browning suffered a stroke and massive hemorrhage in the left parietal lobe. After a short stay in the hospital, she was transferred to a nursing home. At first she received nutrition and hydration through a gastrostomy tube, which after a long series of complications and dislodging was replaced by a nasogastric tube. Nearly 2 years after her stroke, Browning's guardian filed a petition with the court to terminate the nasogastric feedings, in compliance with her living will. In addition to the living will, testimony was presented by friends and by her guardian, who had lived with Browning the years immediately preceding her stroke, that Browning had stated she never wanted to be maintained on life support if she were ever in her current condition.

The medical evidence indicated that Browning was in a persistent vegetative state, sustained only by virtue of the nutrition obtained through her nasogastric tube—presumably meeting the conditions for withdrawal stipulated in her living will. But, the applicable statute did not define hydration and nutrition as life-supporting measures, and testimony indicated that Browning could continue to live indefinitely, as long as she had the nasogastric tube. Medical evidence also indicated that while death would most certainly occur upon discontinuation of artificial nutrition and hydration, it would not do so immediately, but within 7 to 10 days. Thus, Browning's condition presented a number of problems from the statutory perspective. Since hydration and nutrition were not considered life-prolonging procedures, her persistent vegetative state could not be terminal, because so long as the gastric tube was in place, she could live indefinitely. Moreover, even if the gastric tube was removed, death would not occur for a week or more, raising the question of whether it was "imminent" enough to meet the definition of terminal. The trial court denied Browning's guardian's petition, concluding that Browning's death was not imminent and that therefore withdrawal was not permitted under the statute. While the district court of appeal agreed, it found that despite the inapplicability of the statute, Florida constitution's right to privacy protection entitled Browning to refuse life-prolonging procedures, even though she was not in a terminal condition, as defined by the statute (131). The Florida Supreme Court agreed with the district court of appeal, providing an extensive analysis that included reviews of *Rasmussen*, *Schloendorff*, *Cruzan*, *Perlmutter*, *Bludworth,* and *Barry* regarding their findings that (a) both capacitated and incapacitated persons have a right to privacy that includes the right to refuse life-prolonging treatments; (b) a surrogate may make a decision on behalf of an incapacitated patient through substituted judgment, established with clear and convincing evidence and without judicial approval; and (c) there must be a compelling state interest to override the right of refusal. The Florida Supreme Court concluded that "without prior judicial approval, a surrogate or proxy... may exercise the constitutional right of privacy for one who has become incompetent and who, while competent, expressed his or her wishes orally or in writing. We also determine that there is no legal distinction between gastrostomy or nasogastric feeding and any other means of life support" (132). In essence, the court effectively found that Florida law's exclusion of artificial nutrition and hydration from life-prolonging procedures, and of persistent vegetative state as a terminal condition, was inconsistent with the right to privacy as interpreted by previous decisions; moreover, the statute's parameters were not supported by the requisite compelling state interest to overcome the right. Shortly after *Browning*, Florida law was amended, defining terminal to include persistent vegetative state, no longer excluding artificial nutrition and hydration as a life-prolonging procedure, and eliminating the requirement that death be "imminent" before a condition is considered terminal. Today, the statute also expressly allows withholding and withdrawal for patients who have an "end stage condition," defined as an "irreversible condition... which has resulted in progressively severe and permanent deterioration and which, to a reasonable degree of medical probability, treatment of the condition would be ineffective" (133).

Despite the fact that many of the previously referenced state court decisions infer that the right to refuse medical care was a recognized component of a right to privacy embedded in the penumbra of the Bill of Rights, it was not until 1990 (14 years after *Quinlan*) that the Supreme Court actually declared that the U.S. Constitution grants a "right to die" in *Cruzan v. Director, Missouri Department of Health* (134), a case relating to Missouri law addressing living wills.

In January 1983, 29-year-old Nancy Cruzan lost control of her car and was discovered in a ditch—not breathing and without a heartbeat. It was estimated that she was anoxic for 12 to 14 minutes before paramedics were able to resuscitate her. Cruzan never regained consciousness, and progressed from a coma to a persistent vegetative state (135). She was not on a ventilator. Although she was able to orally ingest some nutrition, it was insufficient; therefore, to ease feeding and promote her recovery, a gastrostomy feeding and hydration tube was implanted with the consent of her husband. Rehabilitative efforts failed, and when it became apparent that she had no medically reasonable chance of recovery, her parents (who were her court-appointed guardians) requested that the hospital terminate artificial nutrition and hydration measures. Even though this was 14 years after *Quinlan*, and with all the intervening cases noted previously, the hospital refused to comply with the parents' request without a court order.

The Missouri Supreme Court analyzed the Cruzans' request in light of the parameters established by Missouri statutes, which like Florida statutes prior to *Browning*, defined a "death-prolonging procedure" to exclude "the performance of any procedure to provide nutrition or hydration" (136). Also similar to pre-*Browning* Florida law, statutes defined "terminal condition" as "an incurable or irreversible condition that, without the administration of life-sustaining treatment, will... result in death within a relatively short time" (137). Thus, any living will referring to the withholding of death-prolonging (or life-prolonging) procedures would be interpreted under Missouri law to exclude the withholding or withdrawing of nutrition and/or hydration through artificial means. The Missouri Supreme Court found that Cruzan's right to refuse life-prolonging treatment, regardless of whether it was based in the constitutional right of privacy or in a common-law right to refuse, was outweighed by Missouri's statutorily expressed policy favoring preservation of life (138). Moreover, it held that even if Cruzan did in fact have a right to refuse treatment, there was not clear and convincing evidence to support the parents' claim that they were exercising substituted judgment for their daughter. The case was appealed to the U.S. Supreme Court based on the parents' claim that the Missouri law imposed impermissible limitations on Nancy Cruzan's constitutional rights.

As had many of the other courts, the U.S. Supreme Court began its analysis by discussing the fundamental premise of bodily integrity and the right to informed consent (referring back to its own decision in *Botsford* and the much cited Justice Cardozo quote from *Schloendorff*) and the logical corollary—the right to refuse treatment. Similar to many of the other courts facing these issues for the first time, the Supreme Court comments that prior to *Quinlan*, there were relatively few cases addressing the right to refuse life-prolonging treatment and opines that the dramatic increase of cases since *Quinlan* (139) can be attributed (still in 1990, 14 years after Quinlan) to "the advance of medical technology capable of sustaining life well past the point where natural forces would have brought certain death in earlier times" (140). The *Cruzan* court does an extensive review of the post-*Quinlan* cases, concluding that most jurisdictions based the right to refuse treatment on the common-law right to informed consent and/or a constitutional privacy right. But *Cruzan* represents the first case in which the U.S. Supreme Court directly addresses the issue of whether the U.S. Constitution protects an individual's right to refuse medical treatment even when exercise of that right will inevitably result in death—*i.e.*, a right to die (141).

Prior to *Cruzan,* numerous Supreme Court decisions seemed to indicate that the Fourteenth Amendment's prohibition against the state "[depriving] any person of life, liberty or property, without due process of law" protects an individual's life and/or liberty interest in refusing unwanted medical treatment. Cruzan's parents relied on those cases to successfully assert that the forced administration of life-sustaining medical treatment, including artificial hydration and nutrition, violates a competent individual's constitutionally protected liberty interest. However, the question remained whether this constitutionally protected right to refuse life-prolonging treatment extended to Nancy Cruzan, who was not competent to make her own refusal. More specifically, the question presented to the Supreme Court was whether Missouri's statutory requirement that an incapacitated patient's wishes to have life-prolonging procedures withdrawn be supported by clear and convincing evidence (the *Storar* standard) impermissibly restricted the exercise of her Fourteenth Amendment right to refuse unwanted medical treatment.

The Supreme Court answers no; the clear and convincing standard developed through the analyses of *Quinlan*, *Saikewicz*, and *Storar*, and codified by Missouri, is not unconstitutional. While the Supreme Court finds that an incapacitated patient does have a Fourteenth Amendment liberty interest in refusing life-prolonging treatment, it holds that Missouri established a constitutionally permissible "procedural safeguard to assure that the action of the surrogate conforms as best it may to the wishes expressed by the patient while competent" (142).

SCHIAVO

Returning to the question raised at the beginning of this chapter, does *Schiavo* represent a new trend in judicial intervention, or is it an aberration? As the previous cases indicate, while *Schiavo* may have been particularly drawn-out litigation, ultimately it presented no new issues, nor groundbreaking legal analysis or precedent. Schiavo's circumstances were extremely similar to Quinlan's, Cruzan's, and Browning's (143). In fact, *Browning* is cited repeatedly in the *Schiavo* trial and appellate court decisions (144). The issue in *Schiavo* was not whether an incapacitated patient had the right to refuse life-prolonging procedures. Rather, Schiavo was a disagreement between family members regarding who should speak for Terri Schiavo and what she in fact would want—in other words, who was her appropriate surrogate, and whether there was clear and convincing evidence of her wishes.

While Michael Schiavo, Terri's husband, was her court-appointed guardian, who under *Browning* and Florida statutes had authority to exercise Terri's right to refuse life-prolonging procedures, he petitioned the court for intervention because he knew that he and Terri's parents had significantly differing views about his wife's end-of-life wishes. The court found

TABLE 6.2

CASES ESTABLISHING SIGNIFICANT CONCEPTS

Case	Significance
Union Pacific Railway Co v. Botsford (1891)	U.S. Supreme Court sets foundation for informed consent doctrine and right-to-die debate, stating "no right is held more sacred or is more carefully guarded, by the common law, than the right of every individual to the possession and control of his own person, free from all restraint or interference of others, unless by clear and unquestionable authority of law."
Schloendorff v. Society of New York Hospital (1914)	Articulates the concept of self-determination that lies at heart of the right to refuse life-prolonging treatment: "Every human being of adult years and sound mind has a right to determine what shall be done with his own body."
In the Matter of Quinlan (1976)	First U.S. ruling permitting withdrawal of life-sustaining treatment from a permanently incapacitated patient.
Belchertown v. Saikewicz (1977)	Summarizes previous cases to establish concise four "state interests" test for use in determining when it is appropriate to override patient refusal of critical care and articulates substituted judgment standard for incapacitated patients.
Satz v. Perlmutter (1978)	Clearly establishes right of capacitated patient with terminal illness to refuse treatment.
In the Matter of Storar (1981)	Adopts clear and convincing evidence as standard of proof for establishing substituted judgment.
Cruzan v. Director, Missouri Department of Health (1990)	First U.S. Supreme Court case to specifically address the right to die as protected by the U.S. Constitution's Fourteenth Amendment.

that there was clear and convincing evidence that Terri Schiavo would choose to refuse life-prolonging nutrition and hydration in her condition, and that her husband was an appropriate guardian. Her parents, while continuing to debate that finding, then argued that Terri was not, despite all the expert medical testimony to the contrary, in a persistent vegetative state. They were convinced that she was actually cognizant and interactive, and simply in need of the right rehabilitative therapy (145). When this argument failed to convince the trial and appellate courts, Terri Schiavo's parents went as far as accusing Michael Schiavo of abusing their daughter, and even raised implications of his having something to do with her initial anoxic event.

The Schiavo case resulted in extensive judicial review, extraordinary legislative intervention, and even executive orders, an amount of activity and level of governmental involvement unprecedented in any previous "right-to-die" case. Nevertheless, the court decisions were all consistent with established judicial precedent and Florida statutory provisions. In 2005, shortly after Schiavo's death, the *New York Times* reported:

> Experts say that unlike the Quinlan case, which established the concept that families can prevail over the state in end-of-life decisions, the Schiavo case created no major legal precedents. But it could well lead to new laws. Already, some states are considering more restrictive end-of-life measures like preventing the withdrawal of a feeding tube without explicit written directions. That troubles some medical ethicists and doctors (146).

Dr. Diane Meier, an end-of-life care expert in New York, stated about Schiavo: "I am concerned about the erosion of a very hard-won multiple-decade process of agreeing that these decisions belong inside families....We've always said that autonomy and self-determination does trump the infinite value of an individual life, that people have the right to control what is done to their own body. I think that is at risk" (147). Fortunately, we have not in fact seen any such shift occur. The case of Terri Schiavo was a tragic family disagreement. While it may have been particularly acrimonious, it nevertheless indicates the kind of case that is likely to come before a court today. As the appellate court stated in *Schiavo*, "It may be unfortunate that when families cannot agree, the best forum we can offer for this private, personal decision is a public courtroom and the best decision-maker we can provide is a judge with no prior knowledge of the ward, but the law currently provides no better solution that adequately protects the interests of promoting the value of life" (148). In *Schiavo*, the courts decided that there was clear and convincing evidence that Terri Schiavo "would wish to permit a natural death process to take its course" (149), consistent with the legal precedents set forth in all the cases discussed previously in this chapter. (See Table 6.2 for summary of cases.)

References

1. *In the Matter of Storar*, 52 N.Y.2d 363, dissent at 385 (1981).
2. Diane E. Hoffman, *Mediating Life and Death Decisions*, 36 Ariz. L. Rev. 821 (1994).
3. *In re the Guardianship of Theresa Marie Schiavo*, Order of Judge George W. Greer, Circuit Court for Pinellas County, Florida, Probate Division, File No. 90-2908GD-003 (2000).
4. *See generally*, Cerminara K. and Goodman K., *Key events in the case of Theresa Marie Schiavo*. http://www6.miami.edu/ethics/schiavo/terri_schiavo_timeline.html. Accessed October 13, 2006.
5. *In re Guardianship of Schiavo*, 780 So. 2d 176 (Fla. 2dD.C.A. 2001) (*Schiavo I*); *In re Guardianship of Schiavo*, 792 So. 551 (Fla. 2d D.C.A. 2001) (*Schiavo II*); *In re Guardianship of Schiavo*, 800 So. 2d 640 (Fla. 2d D.C.A. 2001) (*Schiavo III*); *In re Guardianship of Schiavo*, 851 So. 2d 182 (Fla. 2d D.C.A. 2003) (*Schiavo IV*).
6. *Bush v. Schiavo*, 885 So. 2d 321 (Fla. 2004).
7. *Schiavo ex rel. Schindler v. Schiavo*, 375 F. Supp. 2d 1378 (M.D. Fla. 2005).
8. *Schiavo ex rel. Schindler v. Schiavo*, 403 F. 3d 1223 (11th Cir. 2005), 403 F. 3d 1289 (11th Cir. 2005).
9. *Schiavo I*, n.5 at 177.
10. *In the Matter of Karen Quinlan*, 355 A.2d 647, 655 (N.J. 1976).
11. It is an interesting coincidence that the date of Terri Schiavo's death, March 31, is also the date (in 1976) that the New Jersey Supreme Court ruled that Karen Ann Quinlan could be disconnected from her respirator. Quinlan remained in a persistent vegetative state without respirator support until her death in 1985.
12. *See, e.g., In re Browning*, 543 So. 2d 258 (Fla. 2d D.C.A. 1989), aff'd 568 So. 2d 4 (Fla. 1990); *Bouvia v. Los Angeles*, 195 Cal. App. 3d 1075 (1987); *Storar*, 52 N.Y. 2d 363.
13. Columbia University/Fathom Knowledge Network Inc. End-of-Life Decisions Seminar, 2000. http://www.fathom.com/course/10701024/contributors.html. Accessed November 29, 2006.
14. *In re Quinlan*, 137 N.J. Super. 227 (Ch. Div. 1975); *In the Matter of Karen Quinlan*, 355 A. 2d 647 (N.J.1976).
15. *Cruzan v. Director, Missouri Department of Health*, 497 U.S. 261, 269 (1990).
16. *Union Pacific Railway Company v. Botsford*, 141 U.S. 250, 251 (1891).
17. Justice Benjamin Cardozo served on the New York Court of Appeals from 1914 to 1932, when he was appointed to the U.S. Supreme Court, where he served until his death in 1938. "Benjamin Cardozo remains one of the most influential and respected jurists of the twentieth century. His decisions in tort law and fiduciary responsibility defined many standards that continue today." *The Historical Society of the Courts of the State of New York*. http://www.courts.state.ny.us/history/Cardozo.htm. Accessed November 29, 2006.
18. *Schloendorff v. Society of New York Hospital*, 211 N.Y. 125, 129 (1914).
19. *Id.* at 130; cited, *e.g.*, in *Cruzan*, 497 U.S. at 269; *Browning*, 568 So.2d 4 at10; *Rasmussen v. Fleming*, 154 Ariz. 207, 216 (1987).
20. *Belchertown State School v. Saikewicz*, 373 Mass 728, 738-739 (1977), referring to *Griswold v. Connecticut*, 381 U.S. 479 (1965), the landmark case holding that the right to contraception is a privacy right found in the penumbra of the constitution, and *Roe v. Wade*, 410 U.S. 113 (1973), holding that a woman's right to an abortion is also a privacy right.
21. *Cruzan*, 497 U.S. 261.
22. *See, e.g.*, Florida Statutes §766.103, Florida Medical Consent Law, providing that "No recovery shall be allowed...against any physician...in an action brought for treating, examining, or operating on a patient without his or her informed consent when...[t]he action of the physician...in obtaining the consent...was in accordance with an accepted standard of medical practice...."
23. *See, e.g.*, Ben A. Rich, *Medical Paternalism v. Respect for Patient Autonomy: The More Things Change the More They Remain the Same*, 10 Mich. St. J. of Med. & Law 87 (2006), "One of the most exhaustively analyzed and discussed clinical cases is that of Dax Cowart...."
24. Howard University College of Medicine, Clinical Ethics Course, Spring 2002, Case Materials. *Refusal of Life-sustaining Treatment and Euthanasia, A Demand to Die*. http://www.med.howard.edu/ethics/cases/demand_die.htm. Accessed December 1, 2006.
25. *Id.*
26. Dax Cowart's birth name was Donald; he changed it after his discharge from the hospital following the accident because he felt that the person he was before the accident no longer existed. *See* Ben A. Rich, *The Values History: A New Standard of Care*, 40 Emory L. J. 1109, note 82 (1991).
27. *Refusal of Life-sustaining Treatment and Euthanasia, A Demand to Die*. http://www.med.howard.edu/ethics/cases/demand_die.htm, at "Dax's Case commentary" by Robert B. White [from hereinafter "Dax's Case Commentary"].
28. *Id.*
29. Today Dax Cowart is a plaintiff's attorney in Corpus Christi. While he asserts that he is happy to be alive, he maintains that his refusal at that time should have been honored. *See* Ben A. Rich, 40 Emory L. J. 1109, at note 80; *see also* Loretta M. Kopelman, AMA (Virtual Mentor) Medical Education *On Distinguishing Justifiable from Unjustifiable Paternalism* (2005). http://www.ama-assn.org/ama/pub/category/11857.html#3. Accessed December 1, 2006; Kayhan Parsi, AMA (Virtual Mentor), Through the Patients Eyes, Sept. 2001, *Conversation with a Famous Patient*. http://www.ama-assn.org/ama/pub/category/6268.html. Accessed December 1, 2006.
30. *Rasmussen v. Fleming*, 154 Ariz. 207, 216; *See also*, *Barber v. Superior Court* 147 Cal. App. 3d 1006, 1015 (2d A.D., 1983) ("A long line of cases, approved by the [California] Supreme Court...have held that where a doctor performs treatment in the absence of an informed consent, there is an actionable battery. The obvious corollary to this principle is that a competent adult patient has the legal right to refuse medical treatment.")
31. *See, e.g., Rasmussen*, 154 Ariz. at 215 ("The right to refuse medical treatment is a personal right sufficiently 'fundamental' or 'implicit in the concept

of ordered liberty' to fall within the constitutionally protected zone of privacy contemplated by the Supreme Court."); *See also, Fosmire v. Nicoleau,* 75 N.Y.2d 218, 226 (Ct. of App. 1990) ("We have recently held that this 'fundamental common-law right is coextensive with the patient's liberty interest protected by the due process clause of our State Constitution'....") and *Cruzan,* 497 U.S. at 278 ("The principle that a competent person has [under the Fourteenth Amendment] a constitutionally protected liberty interest in refusing unwanted medical treatment may be inferred from our prior decisions.")

32. *See, e.g.* Find Law for the Public. http://estate.findlaw.com/estate-planning/living-wills/estate-planning-law-state-living-wills.html. Accessed November 29, 2006.
33. Cruzan, 497 U.S. at 270, citing to Karnezis, *Patient's Right to Refuse Treatment Allegedly Necessary to Sustain Life,* 93 A.L.R.3d 67 (1979), and Cantor, *A Patient's Decision to Decline Life-Saving Medical Treatment: Bodily Integrity Versus the Preservation of Life,* 26 Rutgers L. Rev. 228, 229 and n.5 (1973).
34. *Rasmussen,* 15 Ariz., at 211.
35. *Id.*
36. "Where... all affected parties concur in the proposed plan of medical treatment, court approval of the proposed plan of medical treatment is neither necessary nor required." *Rasmussen,* 15 Ariz. at 224.
37. *Id.* at 211.
38. *"Dax's Case Commentary."*
39. *Quinlan,* 355 A. 2d at 655.
40. *Id.* "It seemed to be the consensus not only of the treating physicians but also of the several qualified experts who testified in the case, that removal from the respirator would not conform to medical practices, standards and traditions."
41. *Quinlan* was initiated when Joseph Quinlan sought an adjudication of incompetency for his daughter Karen and an appointment as her guardian, with the express authority to discontinue life support. Because of the extraordinary nature of this latter request, the treating physicians and the hospital were included in Quinlan's complaint, to assure that they could not interfere should he be granted the requested authority. Additionally, the Prosecutor of Morris County was joined, to assure that the issue of potential criminal sanctions was addressed. Finally, the Attorney General of New Jersey intervened, in order to assert the state's interests in the preservation of life.
42. Quinlan, 355 A.2d at 651-652.
43. *Id.* at 655-656.
44. *Id.* at 659-660.
45. *Id.* at 661.
46. *Griswold v. Connecticut,* 381 U.S. 479 (1965).
47. *Quinlan,* 355 A.2d at 663, emphasis in original.
48. *Id.* at 664.
49. *Id.* at 657.
50. The court takes care in its analysis to distinguish Karen's situation from that of Delores Heston, a severely injured young Jehovah's Witness woman who was incapacitated due to shock and who required surgery and a blood transfusion to save her life and return her to "vibrant health." *Quinlan* at 663, citing its decision in *Kennedy Memorial Hospital v. Heston,* 58 N.J. 576 (1971).
51. The court "almost" takes judicial notice that in fact, physicians had been making decisions to withhold resuscitative or maintenance therapy for terminal bedridden patients, especially with family consent. *Id.* at 667.
52. *Id.* at 665, quoting Judge Muir from lower court *Quinlan* decision 137 N.J. Super. 227, 259 (Ch. Div. 1975).
53. *Id.* at 666.
54. *Id.* at 668.
55. In fact, the court itself did not expect that ethics committees would eliminate the need for court intervention: "[The suggestion for review by ethics committees] is not to say that in the case of an otherwise justifiable controversy access to the courts would be foreclosed; we speak rather of a general practice and procedure." *Id.* at 669.
56. *Superintendent of Belchertown State School v. Joseph Saikewicz,* 373 Mass. 728 (1977).
57. *Id.* at 736.
58. *Id.* at 738 quoting Lewis, Machine medicine and its relation to the fatally ill, 206 *JAMA.* 387 (1968). Emphasis in original.
59. *Quinlan,* 355 A. 2d at 667.
60. *Saikewicz,* 373 Mass. at 741.
61. *Id.* at 742.
62. This test is significant in cases involving a parent's refusal of life-sustaining treatment, for example, the refusal of blood transfusions by parents who are Jehovah's Witnesses. *See, e.g., Dade County v. Wons,* 541 So. 2d 96 (Fla.1989); *In re Matter of Dubreuil,* 692 So. 2d 819 (Fla. 1994); *St. Mary's Hospital v. Mark Ramsey,* 465 So. 2d 666 (Fla. 4th D.C.A. 1985); and *Fosmire,* 75 NY 2d 218, none of which found the state's interest in the protection of innocent third parties (minor children) sufficiently compelling to override the patient's (parent's) privacy and/or religious right to refuse blood transfusion.
63. If Dax had made it to the courts, however, there is little doubt that the state's interest in preventing suicide would have been a significant consideration, as that is how his own physicians characterized his desire to discontinue treatment: "I... told [Dax] that I and the other doctors involved could not accede immediately to his demand to leave; we could not participate in his suicide." "Dax's Case Commentary."
64. *Saikewicz,* 373 Mass. at 744.
65. *Id.* at 745.
66. *See, e.g., Green Appeal,* 448 Pa. 338 (1972), wherein the Pennsylvania Supreme Court reviewed a Jehovah's Witness's mother's refusal to consent to her child's surgery to correct paralytic scoliosis due to the high risk of the procedure, and more specifically, to the planned transfusion in connection with the surgery. The Pennsylvania court held that "the state does not have an interest of sufficient magnitude outweighing a parent's religious beliefs when the child's life is *not immediately imperiled* by his physical condition." Emphasis in original.
67. *Saikewicz,* 373 Mass. at 747.
68. *Id.*
69. *Id.* at 758.
70. *Id.* at 759.
71. In New York, the Court of Appeals is equivalent to the Supreme Court of other states *i.e.,* it is the highest court; the New York Supreme Court is the trial court.
72. *In the Matter of Storar,* 52 N.Y.2d 363 (1981).
73. In *Storar,* both patients had died by the time the case reached the Court of Appeals.
74. While not very relevant to the court's analysis, it is important to note, for practical purposes, that there was evidence presented indicating that Mrs. Storar was not provided with information regarding the consequences of not giving her son transfusions. She therefore was presumably unaware that he would die sooner without the transfusions. She only knew that he disliked them and tried to avoid them, and so believed he would want them stopped. Thus, it could not be said that Mrs. Storar had made an "informed refusal."
75. *But see Fosmire,* 75 N.Y. 2d 218, wherein the same court later finds the right to refuse medical treatment to be protected by the state constitution's due process clause.
76. *Storar,* 52 N.Y. 2d at 377. In a footnote to this quote, the court does allude to the possibility that the state interests in protecting third parties or prevention of suicide could be the basis for intervention.
77. *See, e.g., Custody of a Minor,* 375 Mass. 733, 737 (1978), and *M.N. and V.N. v. Southern Baptist,* 648 So. 2d 769, 770 (Fla. 1st D.C.A. 1994). The dissent opinion in *Storar,* 52 N.Y. 2d, however, quotes a recent article written by the Chief Justice of the World Court of Human Rights, stating that "doctors at the Yale University School of Medicine willingly acknowledged that they had quietly allowed 43 severely deformed infants to die by withholding treatment after the parents agreed there was little chance for 'meaningful life.' The doctors disclosed this in hopes of breaking down 'a major social taboo.'" *Storar,* 52 N.Y. 2d at 386, citing Kutner, *Euthanasia: Due Process for Death With Dignity; The Living Will,* 54 Ind. L.J. 201, 223.
78. *In re Guardianship of Andrew James Barry,* 445 So.2d 365 (Fla. 2d D.C.A. 1984).
79. *Id.* at 371.
80. The court mentions that the Barrys sought consult with several priests to assure that their position was consistent with the Catholic doctrine and morality. It was also noted that there was no financial motivation, as all of Andrew's medical expenses were covered by insurance.
81. *Barry,* 445 So. 2d at 371.
82. *Id.* at 372.
83. *In re Chad Eric Swan,* 569 A.2d 1202 (Me. 1990).
84. *In re Gardner,* 534 A.2d 947 (Me. 1987).
85. *Swan,* 569 A. 2d at 1205.
86. *Id.* at 1205, quoting Prosser and Keaton on Torts § 18 at 115 (5th ed. 1984).
87. *See generally* Ann Eileen Driggs, The mature minor doctrine: do adolescents have the right to die? *Case Western Reserve University Health Matrix: Journal of Law-Medicine,* 11 Health Matrix 687 (Summer 2001).
88. *In the Matter of Baby K,* 16 F.3d 590 (4th Cir. 1994).
89. While not directly addressing the issue of the ethical integrity of the medical profession, this case could be read to reject the viability of "medical futility," as the argument was raised by the hospital in asserting that providing treatment to Baby K was "futile" and against the prevailing standard of care for infants with anencephaly. The court rejected this argument. This is interesting given that Virginia arguably codified the concept of medical futility in Section 54.1-2990 of its Health Care Decisions Act, which the court noted as providing that nothing in the Virginia advance directive statute could be construed "to require a physician to prescribe or render medical treatment to a patient that the physician determines to be medically or ethically inappropriate." Whether this was meant to apply to the futility argument was not addressed, but regardless, the court found that to any extent that statute might be argued to apply to Baby K's situation, it was pre-empted by the EMTALA requirement.
90. 42 U.S.C.A. §§1395dd (b) (1) (A), (e) (3) (A) (Supp. 1991).
91. 42 U.S.C.A. §1395dd (a) (2006).
92. *Satz v. Perlmutter,* 362 So. 2d 160 (Fla. 4th D.C.A.., 1978), approved, 379 So. 2d 359 (Fla. 1980).

93. *See also Barber v. Superior Court,* 147 Cal.App.3d 1006 (2d Appellate District, 1983), wherein two physicians were charged with murder and conspiracy to commit murder for terminating intravenous nutrition and hydration life support measures on a patient in a permanent vegetative state at the request of the patient's wife, based on comments the patient had made regarding Karen Ann Quinlan's circumstances. The court found it was not murder, there was no requirement to have the court approve treatment withdrawal, and that the wife was the proper person to act on behalf of the patient.
94. *Satz,* 362 So. 2d at 162.
95. *Id.* at 162 quoting *Saikewicz,* 373 Mass. at 742.
96. *Id.* at 162.
97. In *John F. Kennedy Memorial Hospital v. Bludworth* (Fla. 1984), Francis B. Landy was in a permanent coma. Fearing liability for affecting a withdrawal based on Landy's living will, the hospital filed for declaratory relief from the court to determine its liability and responsibilities. The Florida Supreme Court ruled that there was no need for court approval.
98. *Perlmutter,* 379 So.2d at 360.
99. *Id.* at 360; *but see* Charles Baron, Life and death decision making: judges v. legislators as sources of law in bioethics, 1 *Journal of Health & Biomedical Law* 107 (2004), for a discussion of advantages to court review of these issues.
100. Florida Statutes ("F.S.") §765. 102 (2005).
101. *Id.*
102. *Id.*
103. F.S. §765. 205 (2005).
104. F.S. §765.401 (2005).
105. F.S. §765.109.
106. Baron, *Life and Death Decision Making,* at 122.
107. Arizona Revised Statutes (A.R.S.) §§ 36-3201–3210 (Supp. 1986).
108. *Rasmussen,* 15 Ariz., at 214, citing to A.R.S. § 36-3202(A) (Supp. 1986).
109. *Id.* citing A.R.S. § 36-3201(6) (Supp. 1986). The current statute no longer provides a definition of terminal; instead, the statute provides a model living will that allows life-prolonging treatment to be withheld or withdrawn if a person is in a terminal condition, irreversible coma, or persistent vegetative state. A.R.S. § 36-3262 (2007).
110. Rasmussen had at one time had a nasogastric tube, but it had to be removed and it was discovered that she could swallow, although the food had to be placed in her mouth.
111. *Rasmussen,* 15 Ariz. at 215.
112. *See Rasmussen* quote cited at note 30.
113. *Rasmussen,* 15 Ariz. at 216.
114. A.R.S. §§ 36-3208(Supp. 1986).
115. *Rasmussen,* 15 Ariz. at 218.
116. *Id.* at 219.
117. *Id.* at 220, citing A.R.S. § 14-5312(A) (3) (Supp. 1986).
118. *Deciding to Forego Life-sustaining Treatment,* President's Commission for the Study of Ethical Problems in Medicine and Biomedical and Behavioral Research (1983).
119. *Rasmussen,* 15 Ariz. at 223.
120. *Id.* at 224.
121. Rasmussen died prior to the Arizona Supreme Court decision, as did Storar and Fox.
122. *Rasmussen,* 15 Ariz. at 224.
123. *Id.* at 225.
124. *In re Guardianship of Browning,* 568 So.2d 4 (Fla.1990), affirming 543 So. 2d 258 (Fla. 2d D.C.A. 1989).
125. Chapter 765, Florida Statutes.
126. F.S. §765.04(1) (1987).
127. F.S. §765.03(3) (1987).
128. F.S. §765.03(6) (1987) 129.
129. *Browning,* 568 So. 2d at 8.
130. *Id.*
131. *In re Guardianship of Browning* 543 So.2d 258 (Fla. 2d D.C.A. 1989).
132. *Browning,* 568 So. 2d at 17.
133. F. S. § 765.101(4) (2006).
134. *Cruzan,* 497 U.S. 261.
135. Cruzan's condition was described as "oblivious to her environment except for reflexive responses to sound and perhaps painful stimuli;...[having] a massive enlargement of the ventricles filling with cerebrospinal fluid in the area where the brain has degenerated and [her] cerebral cortical atrophy is irreversible, permanent, progressive and ongoing;...her highest cognitive brain function is exhibited by her grimacing perhaps in recognition of ordinarily painful stimuli, indicating the experience of pain and apparent response to sound;...her four extremities are contracted with irreversible muscular and tendon damage to all extremities." *Cruzan v. Harmon,* 760 S.W. 2d 408, 411 (M.O. 1989). Compare this to Schiavo description.
136. *Id.* at 420 (M.O. 1988), citing Missouri Revised Statutes, §459.010(3), Revised 1986.
137. *Id.* at 420 citing §459.010(6), RSMo1986.
138. The Massachusetts Supreme Court's view is well stated in the following passage: "Prior to *Quinlan*, the common law preferred to err on the side of life. Choices for incompetents were made to preserve life, not hasten death. *Quinlan* changed the calculus. Moving from the common law's prejudice in favor of life, *Quinlin* (sic) subtly recast the state's interest in life as an interest in the quality of life (cognitive and sapient), struck a balance between quality of life and Karen Quinlan's right to privacy and permitted the termination of life sustaining procedure. By rhetorical device of replacing a concern for life with quality of life, the court managed 'to avoid affronting previously accepted norms' in reaching its decision. [Cite omitted.] *** As we previously stated however, the state's interest is not in quality of life. The state's interest is an unqualified interest in life." *Cruzan v. Harmon,* 760 S.W. 2d at 422.
139. The Missouri Supreme Court's survey of reported state court cases between 1976 (Quinlan) and 1988 indicated 54 decisions from 17 states. *See Cruzan v. Harmon,* 760 S.W.2d at 412 n. 4.
140. *Cruzan,* 497 U.S. at 270.
141. In *Quinlan* the New Jersey Supreme Court found a U.S. constitutionally protected right, and other state supreme courts had so held, but the U.S. Supreme Court did not itself address this until *Cruzan.*
142. *Cruzan,* 497 U.S. at 280. The U.S. Supreme Court also found that "a State may properly decline to make judgments about the 'quality' of life that a particular individual may enjoy, and simply assert an unqualified interest in the preservation of human life to be weighed against the constitutionally protected interests of the individual." *Id.* at 282.
143. It is interesting to note that Estelle Browning's guardian's attorney George Felos was also Michael Schiavo's attorney.
144. *See, e.g.,* Order of Circuit Judge George W. Greer, *In Re: The Guardianship of Teresa Marie Schiavo,* Pinellas County, Florida, Probate Division File No 90-2908GD-003, 2/11/2000. "This court is called upon to apply the law as set forth in *In re: Guardianship of Estelle M. Browning*...to the facts of this case."
145. While the Medical Examiner's autopsy report evaded a direct answer to the question of whether Terri Schiavo was in a persistent vegetative state, stating that PVS is a "clinical diagnosis arrived at through physical examination of living patients," the neuropathologist's findings included in the autopsy report indicated that Terri Schiavo's brain was "grossly abnormal" and weighed only 615 grams—less than half of the expected weight for a woman her age. It was noted that Karen Ann Quinlan's brain weighed 835 grams at the time of her death, after 10 years in a similar state (Terri was in a persistent vegetative state for 15 years.) Report of Autopsy, Medical Examiner, District Six, Jon R. Thogmartin, M.D. Chief Medical Examiner, Case #5050439, June 13, 2005.
146. Sheryl Gay Stolberg, Schiavo's case may reshape American law. *New York Times,* April 1, 2005. http://www.nytimes.com/2005/04/01/politics/01legacy.html?ex=1168146000&en=fa93a9fdd67891f1&ei=5070. Accessed November 25, 2006.
147. *Id.,* quoting Dr. Diane E. Meier.
148. *Schiavo IV, 851* So. 2d at 187.
149. *Schiavo I,* 780 So. 2d at 180.

CHAPTER 7 ■ COLLABORATIVE CARE: PHYSICIAN AND NURSING INTERACTIONS AND THE FOUNDATION OF A SUCCESSFUL UNIT

ELIZABETH MANIAS

This chapter will discuss collaborative care in terms of four major areas: (a) definition of collaborative care, (b) the makeup of the critical care team and ancillary health professionals, (c) forms of communication, and (d) team effort. The first examines the meanings associated with collaborative care, with particular reference to the critical care context. The various interdisciplinary health professionals who make up the critical care team, including medical personnel, nurses, pharmacists, respiratory therapists, social workers, occupational therapists, physical therapists, and nutritionists, are described in the second area. The third area considers the forms of communication that take place in critical care settings, including critical care rounds, nursing handover between nurses, and admission and discharge practices. The fourth area focuses on functioning as a team and involves orientation of new team members, patient monitoring and observation, and communication with patients' families.

MEANINGS ASSOCIATED WITH COLLABORATION

For health professionals to collaborate, it is important to understand how collaborative care is interpreted. Collaborative care involves communicating information, opinions, and feelings; sharing decision making, tasks, and goals; negotiating power to enable more equitable participation and mutual respect; and facilitating the uptake of effective treatment (1–3). Henneman et al. (4) described collaborative care as a joint venture with two or more health professionals working together to achieve a common goal. It is a cooperative endeavor in which individuals contribute willingly in planning and organizing patient care. Health professionals offer their expertise and share responsibility for final outcomes while other individuals acknowledge their involvement in the venture. These interpretations of collaborative care assume that professional relations between interacting individuals are equal—that is, power relations are equal.

BALANCE OF POWER

However, it is also important to acknowledge that sometimes power relations between individuals may be unequal, thereby affecting the quality of collaboration that takes place (5). Unequal power relations can be influenced by perceived knowledge and expertise attributed to various health professionals, miscommunication, different goals of care developed for patients, and different designated roles or titles. Such an acknowledgment challenges health professionals to critically analyze how they carry out their work to enable greater opportunities for collaboration to occur (3).

BENEFITS AND AIM OF CARE

The ultimate aim of collaborative care is to produce positive outcomes for patients. Some of the positive outcomes associated with improving collaboration include the following: a decline in nosocomial infections (6), improved patients' quality of life (7), lower mortality rates (8), reduced length of hospital or critical care stay (9,10), reduced cost of care (6,9), and reduced adverse events such as oversedation and readmission to critical care (6). Other outcomes have been related to the effects of collaboration on the health professional, the health care team, and the organization (11–14). Benefits of collaboration for the health professional include feelings of self-worth, competence, and importance. For the health care team, collaboration is seen to create opportunities for clarification of interactive roles and to enhance respect for, and collegiality between, individuals of various disciplines. For the organization, collaboration is understood to promote productivity, retention, and satisfaction of employees (4).

MEMBERS OF THE CRITICAL CARE TEAM: THE NEED FOR INTERDEPENDENT WORKING RELATIONSHIPS

The critical care setting is a complex organizational system comprising various health professionals who need to function as an interdependent team (Fig. 7.1). These health professionals have particular roles and functions to bring about high-quality patient care and support. The challenge is to understand how these roles and functions fit with those of other professions, with the aim of developing solid working relationships (15,16). For example, physicians are trained to take charge and assume the role of leadership in health care and responsibility for decisions. For them, learning to share in an interprofessional team is a challenge since they may assume or be expected by other team members to take on the leadership role (13,16). Other health professionals, such as nurses and social workers, may

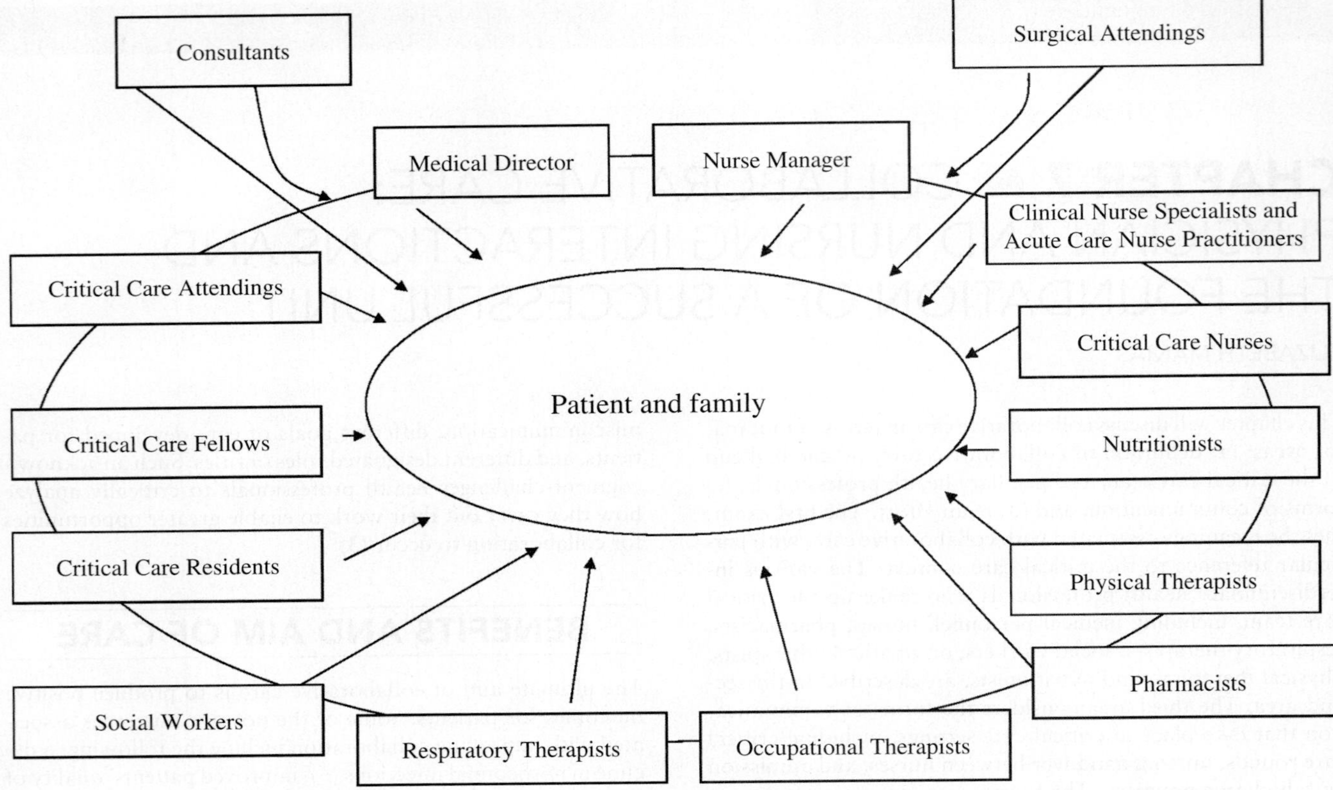

FIGURE 7.1. Interrelationships of health professionals involved with providing collaborative care in the critical care unit.

place greater emphasis on patients' and families' accounts of the patient's health, rather than relying on objective data as much as is done by physicians. As a result, physicians may not place much weight on accounts of patients and families provided by nurses and social workers, preferring instead to see numeric data to address a situation. Since expectations about roles and functions are largely unspoken, they create obstacles that are not readily identified by team members who experience difficulties with collaboration. The solution involves ensuring that professional expectations are made apparent to all involved. Success in achieving collaborative care depends on committed interdisciplinary work that is incremental, continuous, and sustained (17–20).

HEALTH PROFESSIONALS WITHIN THE CRITICAL CARE UNIT

Various medical professionals have an input in patient care within critical care, including the critical care medical director, critical care unit attending physicians, critical care unit fellows, and critical care unit residents. Medical professionals from outside the critical care unit also play an important role and include consultants, surgical attendings (21,22), residents, and other ancillary personnel.

Critical Care Director

The critical care unit is overseen by a director with demonstrated competence in the provision of critical care services. The director manages the administrative aspects of the unit, including the development and implementation of policies and procedures, review of the appropriate use of critical care resources, and education of unit staff. Together with the nurse manager of the critical care unit, the medical director assumes ultimate responsibility for the safety and appropriateness of services provided in the setting. Consequently, the medical director plays an important role in guiding patient care during unstable clinical situations that require careful titration of therapy, such as multiorgan failure and resuscitation procedures. This responsibility includes the need to communicate regularly with other health professionals and the family about current and future patient goals of treatment. Usually, the medical director has final authority over admission and discharge practices of the critical care unit.

Critical Care Attending Physicians

Critical care attending physicians are primarily accountable for the day-to-day unit and patient management responsibilities. These individuals have expert knowledge in pathophysiology, physiology, pharmacology, and the technical aspects of monitors and invasive equipment, as well as competence in managing critically ill patients. Critical care attending physicians provide a leading role in dealing with the sensitivities associated with dying patients and their families. Also important are attributes related to the latest research and quality improvement activities, as well as facilitating education among health professionals in the unit. In the absence of the medical director, it is the critical care attending physicians who make decisions relating to the admissions and discharges of patients.

Critical Care Fellows

Fellows are required to undertake a specified period of the critical care experience, usually a 1-year fellowship in which they work at least 9 months in a critical care environment (e.g., a neurologic or medical intensive care unit), with the remaining 3 months involving either allocation to a clinical area (e.g., respiratory care or trauma service) or conducting research relevant to critical care. Fellows have comprehensive knowledge about the medical histories, surgical and diagnostic procedures, and laboratory data and medications relating to all patients in the critical care unit. In association with the critical care resident, they provide this information on ward round presentations and in discussions with other health professionals, including consultants, surgeons, and nurses. Fellows are required to review the assessment charts of complicated patients with residents and are expected to guide residents in managing patients with respect to issues such as setting mechanical ventilation parameters, providing hemodynamic support and invasive monitoring, prescribing antibiotics, and managing adverse events. Critical care attending physicians assist fellows in making appropriate patient care decisions and providing them with greater input at the beginning of their training compared to later in the training year, at which point fellows are expected to make more independent decisions.

Critical Care Residents

Residents are junior members of the medical staff who rotate through the critical care unit to learn the fundamental principles of treating critically ill patients. They collaborate with critical care fellows in collecting patient assessment data and formulating a management plan. During their rotation in the critical care unit, they develop beginning level competencies in regard to treating patients with complex health care needs. Residents give patient presentations during ward rounds, where they are provided with feedback on their comprehension and understanding of patient assessment, management, and evaluation of care.

Critical Care Nurses

Critical care nurses provide comprehensive skilled care to critically ill patients by maintaining a continual presence at the bedside. Their extensive knowledge and expertise enable them to recognize changes in patients' clinical manifestations and implement strategies aimed at preventing worsening conditions and minimizing complications. They support patients and families by acting as their advocates and play an integral role in the decision-making process with the health care team. In the United States, critical care nurses may be certified through the American Association of Critical Care Nursing by undertaking specialized education and testing and are recognized as critical care registered nurses (CCRNs). In other countries such as Australia and the United Kingdom, critical care nurses may complete specialized postgraduate critical care qualifications at a university.

A nurse manager of the critical care unit provides clear lines of authority for critical care nurses and is accountable for the delivery of good-quality patient care from the nursing staff. This health professional must have the ability to ensure that critical care nursing practices address key standards of care. Aside from expertise in current advances in the field of critical care nursing, the nurse manager also has experience with health information systems, risk management, and health care economics.

Advanced practice roles within the critical care unit include acute care nurse practitioners and clinical nurse specialists. Clinical nurse specialists undertake roles that involve education, consultation, research, and management. Acute care nurse practitioners undertake direct patient care activities and research (23), most often in conjunction with the critical care medicine team. Both clinical nurse specialists and acute care nurse practitioners continue to perform many of the interventions involved with conventional nursing practice. They also function autonomously and in collaboration with other health professionals in an effort to produce optimal patient outcomes. Compared to other critical care nurses, those in advanced practice roles require a greater depth and breadth of knowledge and a greater understanding in interpreting patient data and undertaking complex interventions. Clinical nurse specialists and acute care nurse practitioners are also required to have completed additional postgraduate work, usually at a master's level.

CONSULTANTS OUTSIDE THE CRITICAL CARE UNIT

Consultants of services outside the critical care unit are specialists who provide important information about a particular facet of patient management to the critical care team. Their role is to answer specific questions, as noted by a critical care health professional in the patient's medical record. To ensure time is used appropriately and constructively, the critical care team should discuss the issue of concern beforehand and provide a rational argument in seeking a consultant's referral. It is usually the attending physician's role to write the consultant referral. Any suggestions provided by consultants should be discussed with the critical care team before treatment is implemented.

Surgical Attendings

Surgical attendings are surgeons who play an important role in the management of surgical procedures required by critically ill patients. They interact with patients and their families in relation to preoperative, intraoperative, and postoperative care, as well as long-term follow-up in terms of ensuring optimal recovery from surgery. Although surgical attendings conduct daily rounds in the critical care unit, specific aspects of patient management usually reside with the critical care team. In the context of the surgical team, surgical residents play much the same role as do critical care residents.

Pharmacists

Pharmacists are integral to patient care in a way that extends beyond their traditional role of supplying and distributing medications. With the increasing sophistication of medications available, their role encompasses the education of physicians, nurses, and other health professionals in prescribing, administering, and monitoring the practices and preparation of medications for critical care patients. They have extensive knowledge about pharmacokinetics and pharmacodynamic principles associated with severe illness, poisoning and drug intoxication, sedation practices, pain relief, and antibiotic use.

Pharmacists also make up various medicinal preparations. For critical care units, these preparations commonly include total parenteral nutrition and the incorporation of cytotoxics, antibiotics, potassium, or opioids into intravenous fluids. These preparations are made up in laminar flow cabinets of hospital pharmacy departments under sterile conditions.

One of the most important tasks of pharmacists is to ensure medications are administered in a manner that promotes therapeutic efficacy and minimizes adverse outcomes. More specifically, they help physicians and nurses by coordinating the development, implementation, and evaluation of medication protocols or guidelines. For this reason, pharmacists attend ward rounds and team meetings to familiarize themselves with patients' medical conditions and how these affect medication therapy. The Society of Critical Care Medicine has released a position paper about the scope and practice of critical care pharmacy practice and service (24).

Respiratory Therapists

Respiratory therapists work with physicians and nurses and are involved with maintaining ventilation equipment and monitoring the airway management of critically ill patients. Airway management may include the provision of oxygen therapy, mechanical ventilation, and aerosol medication therapy. They also play a role in titrating ventilation parameters to suit the breathing and hemodynamic patterns of patients, formulating weaning procedures, and providing patient and family education. Although respiratory therapists are well established in North America, they rarely exist in the United Kingdom, Europe, Australia, or Asia, countries or continents in which nurses are responsible for the patients' respiratory equipment and clinical management of respiratory function in collaboration with physician consultation.

Social Workers

Social workers work with the health care team to provide a conduit between management plans for the critical care patient and family members. They possess specialized knowledge about health policies and services, social welfare systems, and community resources. With this information to guide their practice, social workers act as important advocates for critically ill patients and families. Examples of activities conducted by social workers include assisting in the adjudication of family–patient–health care team disagreements, leading team discussions in root cause analyses of ICU-related problems, locating temporary accommodation for family members during patients' stay in hospital, and providing resources to help cover health care costs.

Occupational Therapists

Occupational therapists are educated to conduct a complete evaluation of the impact of illness on the activities of critically ill patients at home, in work situations, and during recreational situations. They work synergistically with other disciplines of the health care team to reduce the physical and psychological disability of patients. Before patients are discharged, occupational therapists often visit the home environment to make comprehensive assessments of the current facilities and changes required to accommodate the patient's needs.

Physical Therapists

Physical therapists assess and treat critically ill patients with a temporary or permanent physical disability, with the aim of achieving the highest degree of recovery. Treatment modalities used by physical therapists include exercise, mobilization and manipulation, massage, splinting, the application of hot and cold compresses, suctioning of respiratory secretions, and electrical stimulation. Conditions treated include birth deformities, fractures, back strain, spinal injuries, strokes, and multiple sclerosis. Rehabilitation after surgery, such as open heart, orthopedic, and abdominal surgery, is another area of responsibility.

Nutritionists

Qualified nutritionists are a vital part of the health care team who consult with physicians, nurses, pharmacists, and family members in the critical care unit. The aim of nutritionists is to improve the nutritional health and promote the recovery of the critical care patient. Nutritionists possess detailed knowledge of the food principles that apply to health and disease states; the biochemical properties of food; the mechanisms underlying food absorption, metabolism, digestion, and elimination; and the indications for nutritional support. They also have an in-depth understanding of the interactions of particular food products with medications commonly used in critical care.

Nutritionists play an important role in the decision to introduce parenteral or enteral feeding or other forms of nutrient supplementation for critically ill patients. Critically ill patients are susceptible to malnutrition as they undergo invasive procedures and diagnostic tests, and disease states may alter the digestive process of nutrients. In collaboration with physicians and nurses, nutritionists determine the precise requirements for energy, protein, vitamins, minerals, essential fatty acids, electrolytes, and water to be administered through parenteral or enteral feeding. Enteral feeds are usually made in a hospital diet kitchen, the process of which is supervised by nutritionists. Conversely, critical care pharmacists prepare parenteral nutrition solutions using sterile laminar flow environments.

FORMS OF COMMUNICATION

Health professionals interact with each other using different forms of communication, depending on the intended purpose. These forms of communication include critical care ward rounds, nursing handovers, and communication concerning admission to and discharge of patients from critical care units. The effective collaboration within these forms of communication is essential to the overall function of critical care units, which significantly affects the patient's risk-adjusted mortality and length of stay (25–27).

Critical Care Ward Rounds

Critical care ward rounds are recognized as an important forum for various health professionals to come together and discuss the daily goals of care. The goals of care serve various functions, which include recognizing patient problems, sharing information, initiating treatment, evaluating the effectiveness of changes in treatment, and increasing learning opportunities for the critical care staff (28). Ineffective patient care and decision making can occur if the goals of care are not communicated clearly, leading to increased costs and the possibility of medical errors (27).

Critical care rounds should be multidisciplinary and include various personnel in addition to the critical care physicians: the nurse unit manager, the specific nurse assigned to each patient, the pharmacist, the respiratory therapist, and others such as the social worker and dietitian. Although some part of the ward round may be undertaken away from the bedside to prevent interruptions adversely affecting decision making, the health care team must also be present at the bedside, since direct patient assessment is integral to identifying problems. Such problems may include inappropriate ventilation settings, patient agitation and confusion, an incorrectly positioned endotracheal tube, and pain as shown by abdominal guarding and inappropriate breathing.

Usually, it is the role of the critical care fellow to present each patient with feedback provided by the critical care attending physician. In this manner, the ward round provides a formalized process of education and training for less experienced medical personnel. It is also an opportunity for other health professionals to provide their feedback on various perspectives of the patients' care, including wound management, nutrition, and medication management. The critical care physician is then able to direct discussions and debates for the planning of patient care (5).

The ward round should be a structured process occurring at a formally designated time each day. Scheduled ward rounds allow physicians, nurses, and other health professionals to plan their attendance despite unexpected situations that can occur. Organizing the ward round as a haphazard process, where it is conducted at different times of day, may mean that certain health professionals will not be able to attend (29). A lack of representation at ward rounds by particular disciplines may adversely affect the range of opinions and possible therapies for patients. A well-organized ward round is more likely to become a creative space in which health professionals of different disciplines can contribute to developing strategic plans for patient care and to sharing openly their clinical activities with other individuals.

The patient presentation should be concise and clear without redundant and irrelevant information, such as unrelated details about the patients' past medical history or superfluous explanations of daily activities. There are several steps that should be followed to ensure the patient presentation functions smoothly (Table 7.1).

TABLE 7.1

STEPS TO TAKE FOR AN EFFECTIVE WARD ROUND

- Know who the patient is in terms of the patient's name, age, sex, and reason for admission to critical care.
- Summarize past medical treatments since admission in terms of when they happened, where they happened, and patient response. It may help to document information in the form of clear, concise points to which you can refer during the presentation. This process will enable you to update your colleagues quickly without having to look for information in voluminous medical histories.
- Assess current patient problems in an organized manner using a body systems approach.
- Discuss the plans for the day, including anticipated patient response.
- Ensure the patient's medical record and radiographs are readily available.
- Be sure that all medication orders and observation charts are readily accessible at the bedside.
- All key pathology investigation results should be available. The pathology laboratory may need to be contacted before the round commences to obtain all necessary results.
- Use the presentation as a time to seek information from members of the health care team to find out more about your patient's needs (e.g., social workers, physical therapists).
- Ensure the relevant health professionals know about changes made to treatment and the role played by the individual in this process.
- Determine if the patient's family members need to be contacted either during or following the ward round in relation to treatment decisions. Make arrangements to contact the family members for consultation or consent for procedures if needed.

To improve the quality of care, a daily goals sheet can be used during ward rounds, with input from nurses, physicians, and other health professionals. A daily goals sheet is a document that is completed during ward rounds and posted at the bedside of each patient. It summarizes the plan of prioritized activities for a patient during the course of a day. Information recorded on the goals sheet depends on specific characteristics of the unit (Table 7.2). Because each sheet is a work in progress, it is usually discarded the day after use and not included in the patient's medical record. Information contained in the goals sheet can serve as a guide to assist physicians, nurses, and other health professionals in documenting their progress. Past research has shown a significant reduction in the length of intensive care stay of patients from 6.4 days to 4.3 days after introduction of a daily goals sheet. The understanding of the goals of care by nurses and physicians, as well as communication between them, had also improved (27).

Nursing Handover Between Nurses

The nursing handover is a verbal form of communication involving nurses from one working shift communicating with those of the oncoming working shift. The purpose of the

TABLE 7.2

SAMPLE DAILY GOALS SHEET

Name: .... ID No.:	Bed No.: .... Date: ....
Pathology tests and diagnostic procedures	Invasive lines, drains, catheters
Haemodynamic parameters	External specialist consultation
Medications (new prescriptions, changes to current medications)	Patient mobilization
Sedation, analgesia, muscle paralysis	Nutrition
Ventilation support	Family discussion, consent for procedures
Transfer to other units	Other
House staff team	

handover is to ensure continuity of patient care between nurses. Beyond its use as a mode of transferring information about patients, the handover is a complex form of communication that encompasses social and environmental contexts (30,31).

Manias and Street (30) conducted an observational study of handover practices in a critical care unit through the use of participant observation, individual interviews, focus groups, and professional journaling. In their study, the charge nurse of the previous shift gave a "global" handover of all patients to oncoming nurses of the next shift. Oncoming nurses then proceeded to a bedside handover, where bedside nurses from the previous shift focused on a patient's individual needs. The

TABLE 7.3

STEPS TO ENSURE AN EFFECTIVE NURSING HANDOVER

- Be on time for the nursing handover and come prepared with paper and pen.
- Take notes about changes in patient status and particular activities that need to be performed during the course of the shift.
- Ask questions of the nurse giving the handover, especially if you are unfamiliar with or unclear about particular issues.
- Be respectful of the patients and families you are discussing. Avoid use of judgmental language, labeling or stereotyping patients, or making negative comments about them.
- Use correct terminology and professional language in describing patient diagnosis and treatment. Use only easily understood abbreviations that are typical of the critical care setting.
- Avoid repetition and irrelevant information.

global handover functioned mainly as a form of communication between charge nurses of the oncoming and previous shifts. During this time, the charge nurses often directed comments to each other and did not involve other oncoming nurses in their discussions. At the bedside handover, nurses from the previous shift regarded requests from oncoming nurses for patient information as a form of criticism of their own clinical practices, and they sometimes expressed fear and anxiety about the process. Nurses from the previous shift were concerned with demonstrating that they were in control of their environment, as evidenced by a tidy bedside area, a patient whose vital signs were stable, and the completion of all set tasks. They needed to fit into the expected norm of a busy, efficient, and effective nurse—essentially, a nurse who was in control of the bedside area. This need to maintain control impeded effective communication during the nursing handover.

Charge nurses of working shifts need to acknowledge the interests of all oncoming nurses when presenting patient information in the global handover. The global handover needs to be perceived as an opportunity for *all* nurses to openly discuss the care plans of various patients, rather than merely as a forum in which only charge nurses communicate with each other. Nurses should not expect themselves to fit into an expected norm of a busy and tidy nurse who is always in control of the bedside area. Instead, an appreciation of the inherent messiness of a critical care setting will help facilitate supportive and collaborative communication during the nursing handover. The nursing handover is then more likely to be a time in which nurses can develop strategic plans for patient care and can share their clinical activities openly. Several steps (Table 7.3) should be followed to ensure that the nursing handover process functions smoothly and effectively (32).

Admission and Discharge Practices of Critical Care Units

Consensus guidelines have been developed to provide general information about criteria and procedures for admission and discharge practices (33,34). These guidelines detail objective clinical parameters to assist health professionals in their decision making about patient flow to and from the unit. Aside from consensus guidelines, organizational factors, which are closely linked to collaborative care, have drawn attention and been examined for associations between admission and discharge practices of critical care settings and patient mortality.

OPEN AND CLOSED SYSTEMS

An organizational factor that has been examined in terms of admission and discharge practices is the open or closed system of care (22). In the *open system*, various health professionals are present in the unit, but physicians directing patient care have obligations at a site separate from the critical care setting, such as the operating room or inpatient or outpatient areas. A physician with expertise in critical care may or may not be involved to assist with management of care in an open system arrangement. In a *closed system*, care is provided by a critical care–based team of physicians, nurses, pharmacists, respiratory therapists, and other health professionals.

In a prospective cohort study, the effect of changing from an open to a closed critical care unit was examined in terms of clinical outcomes (35). A consecutive sample of 124 patients admitted under an open system was compared to that of 121 patients admitted after changing to a closed system. In the closed system, the ratio of actual mortality (31.4%) to predicted mortality (40.1%) was 0.78. In the open system, the ratio of actual mortality (22.6%) to predicted mortality (25.2%) was 0.90. Notably, 52% of house staff in the closed system rated their level of experience in managing critically ill patients as "very experienced" compared with 15% in the open system. Nurses commented that they were very confident about the clinical decisions made by physicians in the closed system compared to the open system (41% vs. 7%, $p < 0.01$). The authors suggested the results may be an indication of the improved communication between physicians and nurses in the closed system.

TIME OF DAY

Another organizational factor identified as being important in relation to admission and discharge practices is time of day, with specific attention to weekdays versus weekends and daytime versus nighttime. A cohort study of all 23,134 emergency admissions over a 3 1/2-year period showed that weekend critical care admissions were associated with an increased adjusted mortality compared with weekday admissions (odds ratio [OR] 1.20, 95% confidence interval [CI] 1.01–1.43) (36). The adjusted mortality was similar for admissions made after business hours compared with those made during business hours (OR 0.98, CI 0.85–1.13). On the other hand, the adjusted risk of death was higher after business hours as compared with during business hours (OR 6.89, CI 5.96–7.96). The time of discharge from the critical care unit was not associated with additional hospital mortality. These findings provide evidence of the importance played by the organization of critical care services. It is also possible that there are more opportunities for collaborative care in planning and managing patient flow during times when there are greater numbers of health professionals and greater availability of more experienced staff (35).

FUNCTIONING AS A TEAM

The integral functioning of a critical care team goes beyond the interactions of health professionals during the specified forums of communication elucidated previously. It also involves developing an understanding of unpredictable events that can lead to clinical crises. Providing support for new team members, monitoring and observing patients for changes in clinical outcomes, and facilitating the involvement of family members are crucial facets for the foundation of a successful collaborative unit.

New Team Members

Specialized health care requires a tailored form of orientation for health professionals entering the critical care setting. Experienced clinicians in critical care are faced with the challenge of how to deliver important information to new team members to facilitate effective learning. This challenge is compounded by the difficulty associated with a shortage of appropriately trained nurses and physicians. Comprehensive preparation through orientation programs has been shown to be a vital component for retaining health professionals (37). In a recent survey of the American Association of Critical Care Nurses, the nurse managers of 300 critical care units (52.1% response rate) provided information about staffing, professional advancement, staff satisfaction, orientation, and quality indicators (38). Eighty percent of responding nurse managers had a standardized orientation program. The responding nurse managers also indicated that graduate nurses were actively employed and trained to work in the critical care setting.

Orientation of newly employed health professionals to critical care departments should be viewed as a shared responsibility among senior health professionals, educators, and new staff members. The sharing of responsibilities improves the effectiveness of the orientation process because it allows more efficient completion of activities associated with the orientation, promotes collegial relationships, and links knowledge with practice. Orientation should occur through a structured program with defined goals that are agreed on by all individuals concerned.

The new staff member needs to be matched with a primary mentor and a secondary mentor, based on their discipline backgrounds, past experiences, attitudes, and learning styles. This matching process should be a strategic rather than a random choice to stimulate critical thinking, encourage open communication, and stimulate further professional development. The designation of a mentor based on random choice often leads to the use of multiple mentors, leading to inconsistent and confusing messages being conveyed (39).

Learning opportunities should be structured using a combined learner-led, theoretical, and clinical program (37). Such a model facilitates the transfer of knowledge to the practice setting. Theoretical reference material provided to the new staff member should include information about unit policies and protocols, roles and responsibilities of various members of the health care team, and the pathophysiology, assessment, and treatment relating to common patient conditions observed in the unit.

Although new staff members are very likely to have a rich array of experiences, experienced mentors are also influenced by the critical care culture in which they are positioned. As a result, new staff members and experienced mentors could be accustomed to performing activities their own way, which may lead to conflict. New staff members may feel that their learning needs and past experiences are not adequately recognized while mentors may feel that their advice is being ignored. By identifying potential problems from the outset, the orientation process can be more individually adapted to the team member's specific needs, the focus of which is becoming part of the unit. Developing a sense of belonging can help to solidify collaboration between the new staff member and other health professionals.

Monitoring and Observation of Critically Ill Patients

Most patients in critical care require constant monitoring and observation, such as patients with multisystem organ failure, multiple trauma, and adult respiratory distress syndrome. The nurse:patient ratio in many parts of the world is generally 1:2 (21). However, in Australia, the nurse:patient ratio for carrying out nursing activities in critical care units is 1:1. As nurses maintain a constant presence at the bedside, they play a critical role in undertaking regular monitoring of patients, assist in the early diagnosis of impending problems, and recommend appropriate interventions to be administered.

Patients in critical care require clinical parameters to be measured hourly or more frequently if these parameters change quickly. Also important is the close observation of patients through physical methods of inspection, palpation, percussion, and auscultation. Comprehensive judgment should be used in interpreting the significance of information obtained to avoid the complacency that could occur with repetitious documentation of clinical parameters and observations.

Nurses' knowledge in conducting patient monitoring and observation is largely constructed by their ongoing experiences and education in the critical care context. On the other hand, medical residents and critical care fellows who work in critical care for a limited period have to rely on past experiences and knowledge as their major sources of information, which may not necessarily be compatible with the types of decisions required in critical care. As an illustration, in an ethnographic study on professional relationships (5), a critical care fellow with previous experience in anesthetics was confronted by a situation involving a patient who had gone to the operating room for a duodenal ulcer repair and returned to the critical care setting. Within an hour of the patient's return, the bedside nurse, who was a clinical nurse specialist, reported to the fellow that the patient was restless, cold, and not breathing well with the ventilator. Based on his past anesthetic experience, the fellow advised the nurse to extubate the patient. The nurse drew on her knowledge of similar patients in critical care and believed that the patient needed additional sedative and analgesic treatment rather than removal of the endotracheal tube. She presented the situation to the critical care attending who agreed with her view and requested that the patient receive further analgesic and sedative medications (5).

Critical care attending physicians are ultimately responsible for less experienced medical personnel; however, these more experienced physicians may be present in the unit only during discrete times of the day. Due to their lack of availability, the critical care attending physician may be able to address only a small portion of the educational needs of junior medical team members in explaining the significance of a patient's clinical parameters and observations. Instead, due to their constant presence in the environment, nurses provide a substantive component of the educational needs of critical care fellows and residents in interpreting data obtained from patient monitoring and observation.

Nurses and physicians collectively provide valuable knowledge in making decisions about information obtained from patient data. It is therefore important that any rigid role boundaries between them are broken down. Maintaining rigid role boundaries creates distrust and disrespect between nurses and physicians, thereby hindering future progression of informed decision making. In effect, nurses need to be accepted as the "eyes and ears" of all levels of the critical care medical team to extend their perceptual capabilities.

Communication with Family Members

The admission of a critically ill patient is a stressful time for families, especially in the current health care environment of advanced technology, greater sophistication of interventional treatment, and multiple health professionals providing care. This critical care event can adversely affect the functioning of family members and their ability to communicate and understand complex information (40). If miscommunication is allowed to occur, the likely outcomes are care fragmentation, family alienation, and the development of distrustful relationships between family members and health professionals, and among health professionals themselves. Such disagreements can result in poor-quality patient care. Collaboration among health professionals is required for the comprehensive support and involvement of family members. As nurses are continuously present at the bedside, they need to interact regularly with other health professionals involved in direct patient care to synthesize information in a way that can be easily communicated to family members (41).

In a descriptive study involving interviews with family members, and observations of interactions between family members and intensive care staff, Söderström et al. (40) found that initial impressions had a sustained effect on family members and influenced future interactions. Family members who understood explicit information and implicit messages were open in their interactions with staff, adjusted well to the critical care environment and were more accepting of the situation (40). In other words, a mutual understanding existed between these family members and critical care staff. Explicit information involved details about the rules and policies of the unit, the condition of the patient, and how to behave in front of the patient. There were also implicit messages inherent in the information. For example, the message "you can visit the patient freely" meant "as long as you do not disturb us in our work." In addition, the message "you can ask questions freely" was conveyed "as long as we find them relevant" (40). Unfortunately, some family members did not fully understand either the explicit information or the implicit messages, and consequently either became withdrawn and quiet or more vocal in their communication by asking many questions. For these individuals, there was a mutual misunderstanding with staff. These family members did not adjust well to the environment and were either ignored or insulted by critical care staff.

It is important that nurses and physicians reflect on how they communicate with family members at initial meetings and in future interactions. Mutual understanding is more likely to occur if information is presented in a clear and unambiguous way. Family members need to have questions answered honestly, and they require regular communication about the patient's progress and prognosis, treatment received, and changes in patient condition (42). They need to be reassured that health professionals care about the patient and support family members in their coping strategies. Family members should be able to speak with the physician and bedside nurse daily, have flexible visiting hours, be able to assist with simple patient care if desired, and have a place where they can be alone.

SUMMARY

Underlying a health care system that is facing pressure to improve efficiency are critical care services, which are predicted to become more important as the population ages, as the boundaries within hospital areas and between health professionals become blurred, and as more specialized technology develops over time. Health professionals need to examine how to adapt their approach to collaborative care in a complex and ever-changing health care climate. By themselves, sophisticated technology and treatment are not sufficient to address the needs of patients and families—positive and conducive relationships are the critical drivers for improved care.

PEARLS

- Health professionals need to acknowledge that sometimes power relations between individuals may be unequal, thereby affecting the quality of collaboration that takes place.
- Collaborative care can bring about positive outcomes for patients, their families, health professionals, the health care team, and the health care organization.
- The critical care setting is a complex organizational system comprising various health professionals who need to function as an interdependent team. The challenge is to understand how their roles and functions fit with those of other professions, with the aim of developing solid working relationships.
- The ward round needs to function as a structured process, occurring at a formally designated time every day.
- A daily goals sheet should be used during ward rounds, with input from nurses, physicians, and other health professionals to summarize the plan of prioritized activities for a patient during the course of a day.
- The nursing handover should be considered a time in which nurses can develop strategic plans for patient care and share openly their clinical activities with each other.

- Organizational factors such as the presence of an open or closed unit and time of day can impact on collaborative care. These factors can influence patient outcomes in relation to critical care admission and discharge.
- Comprehensive preparation through orientation programs has been shown to be a vital component for retaining newly employed health professionals in the critical care unit and bringing about collaborative care.
- Due to their constant presence, nurses provide a substantive component of the educational needs of critical care fellows and residents in interpreting data obtained from patient monitoring and observation.
- Collaboration among health professionals is required for the comprehensive support and involvement of family members of patients.

References

1. Leonard M, Graham S, Bonacum D. The human factor: the critical importance of effective teamwork and communication in providing safe care. *Qual Saf Health Care.* 2004;13(Suppl 1):i85.
2. Thomas EJ, Sexton JB, Helmreich RL. Translating teamwork behaviours from aviation to healthcare: development of behavioural markers for neonatal resuscitation. *Qual Saf Health Care.* 2004;13(Suppl 1):i57.
3. Zwarenstein M, Bryant W. Interventions to promote collaboration between nurses and doctors. Cochrane Database of Syst Rev. 2000;(2):CD000072. Review.
4. Henneman EA, Lee JL, Cohen JI. Collaboration: a concept analysis. *J Adv Nurs.* 1995;21:103.
5. Manias E, Street A. The interplay of knowledge and decision making between nurses and doctors in critical care. *Int J Nurs Stud.* 2001;38:129.
6. Jain M, Miller M, Belt D, et al. Decline in ICU adverse events, nosocomial infections and cost through a quality improvement initiative focusing on teamwork and culture change. *Qual Saf Health Care.* 2006;15:235.
7. Eubanks P. Quality improvement key to changing nurse–MD relations. *Hospitals.* 1991;65:26.
8. Wheelan SA, Burchill CN, Tilin F. The link between teamwork and patients' outcomes in intensive care units. *Am J Crit Care.* 2003;12:527.
9. Curley C, McEachern JE, Speroff T. A firm trial of interdisciplinary rounds on the inpatient medical wards. *Med Care.* 1998;36(8 Suppl):AS4.
10. Schneiderman LJ, Gilmer T, Teetzel HD, et al. Effect of ethics consultations on nonbeneficial life-sustaining treatments in the intensive care setting: a randomized controlled trial. *JAMA.* 2003;290:1166.
11. Boyle DK, Miller PA, Forbes-Thompson SA. Communication and end-of-life care in the intensive care unit. *Crit Care Nurs Q.* 2005;28:302.
12. Miller PA. Nurse-physician collaboration in an intensive care unit. *Am J Crit Care.* 2001;10:341.
13. Shirey MR. Authentic leaders creating healthy work environments for nursing practice. *Am J Crit Care.* 2006;15:256.
14. Vazirani S, Hays RD, Shapiro MF, et al. Effect of a multidisciplinary intervention on communication and collaboration among physicians and nurses. *Am J Crit Care.* 2005;14:71.
15. Gerardi D. Using mediation techniques to manage conflict and create healthy work environments. *AACN Clin Issues.* 2004;15:182.
16. Hall P. Interprofessional teamwork: professional cultures as barriers. *J Interprofessional Care.* 2005;19(Suppl 1):188.
17. Curtis JR, Cook DJ, Wall RJ, et al. Intensive care unit quality improvement: a 'how to' guide for the interdisciplinary team. *Crit Care Med.* 2006;34:211.
18. Day L. Advocacy, agency, and collaboration. *Am J Crit Care.* 2006;15:428.
19. LeTourneau B. Physicians and nurses: friends or foes? *J Healthcare Manage.* 2004;49:12.
20. Thomas EJ, Sexton JB, Helmreich RL. Discrepant attitudes about teamwork among critical care nurses and physicians. *Crit Care Med.* 2003;31:956.
21. Brilli RJ, Spevetz A, Branson RD, et al. Critical care delivery in the intensive care unit: defining clinical roles and the best practice model. *Crit Care Med.* 2001;29:2007.
22. Haupt MT, Bekes CE, Brilli RJ, et al. Guidelines on critical care services and personnel: recommendations based on a system of categorization of three levels of care. *Crit Care Med.* 2003;31:2677.
23. Howie JN, Erickson M. Acute care nurse practitioners: creating and implementing a model of care for an inpatient general medical service. *Am J Crit Care.* 2002;11:448.
24. Rudis M, Brandi K. Position paper on critical care pharmacy services. *Crit Care Med.* 2000;28:3746.
25. Baggs JG, Schmitt MH, Mushlin AI, et al. Association between nurse-physician collaboration and patient outcomes in three intensive care units. *Crit Care Med.* 1999;27:1991.
26. Knaus WA, Wagner DP, Zimmerman JE, et al. Variations in mortality and length of stay in intensive care units. *Ann Int Med.* 1993;118:753.
27. Narasimthan M, Eisen LA, Mahoney CD, et al. Improving nurse-physician communication and satisfaction in the intensive care unit with a daily goals worksheet. *Am J Crit Care.* 2006;15:217.
28. Manias E, Street A. Nurse-doctor interactions during critical care ward rounds. *J Clin Nurs* 2001;10:442.
29. Manias E, Aitken R, Dunning T. Graduate nurses' communication with health professionals when managing patients' medications. *J Clin Nurs.* 2005;14:354.
30. Manias E, Street A. The nursing handover: uncovering the hidden practices of nurses. *Int Crit Care Nurs.* 2000;16:373.
31. Philpin S. 'Handing over': transmission of information between nurses in an intensive therapy unit. *Nurs Crit Care.* 2006;11:86.
32. Levett-Jones T, Bourgeois S. *The Clinical Placement.* Marrickville, Australia: Elsevier, 2007.
33. Smith G, Nielsen M. ABC of intensive care: criteria for admission. *BMJ.* 1999;318:1544.
34. Society of Critical Care Medicine. Guidelines for ICU admission, discharge and triage. *Crit Care Med.* 1999;27:633.
35. Carson S, Stocking C, Podsadecki T, et al. Effects of organizational change in the medical intensive care unit of a teaching hospital: a comparison of 'open' and 'closed' formats. *JAMA.* 1996;276:322.
36. Uusaro A, Kari A, Ruokonen E. The effects of ICU admission and discharge times on mortality in Finland. *Int Care Med.* 2003;29:2144.
37. Thomason TR. ICU nursing orientation and postorientation practices: a national survey. *Crit Care Nurs Q.* 2006;29:237.
38. Kirchhoff KT, Dahl N. American Association of Critical-Care Nurses' national survey of facilities and units providing critical care. *Am J Crit Care.* 2006;15:13.
39. Hardy R, Smith R. Enhancing staff development with a structural preceptor program. *J Nurs Care Qual.* 2001;15:9.
40. Söderström I-M, Saveman B-I, Benzein E. Interactions between family members and staff in intensive care units—an observation and interview study. *Int J Nurs Stud.* 2006;43:707.
41. Tracy MF, Ceronsky C. Creating a collaborative environment to care for complex patients and families. *AACN Clin Issues.* 2001;12:383.
42. Norton SA, Tilden VP, Tolle SW, et al. Life support withdrawal: communication and conflict. *Am J Crit Care.* 2003;12:548.

CHAPTER 8 ■ CLINICAL DECISION MAKING

JONATHAN B. COHEN • JONATHAN D. DREIER

Decision making is a complex process that involves not only interpersonal aspects but influences from recognized and unrecognized outside sources. The psychology behind decision making seems to be just as important as the quality of the evidence the decisions should be based on. In this chapter, we discuss the factors that influence the clinician's decision-making process.

IDENTIFICATION OF THE PROBLEM

For a physician to solve a problem, it must first be correctly and succinctly identified. The identification of the problem relies on gathering data from the medical history and physical exam, laboratory, and radiographic and other diagnostic testing. From this, a problem is identified and a question is posed. This question may relate to either diagnosis (i.e., in the patient with electrocardiogram [ECG] changes and complaints of chest pain, has this patient suffered a myocardial infarction?) or treatment (i.e., in this patient who has unequivocally suffered an ischemic stroke, what is the best treatment for him or her?). Figure 8.1 outlines the scope of what physicians attempt to accomplish when confronted with a clinical problem.

Clinical Knowledge

After the appropriate diagnostic or therapeutic question has been raised, the process for determining the solution is undertaken. The information required by the clinician to solve a particular problem has many different origins. Some of this information comes from our own requisite knowledge and is termed *background knowledge*. *Foreground knowledge*, in contrast, is obtained through the analysis of clinical investigations and research.

It is unarguable that medical training is a lifelong process. As training is begun, the vast majority of our total knowledge of how to solve a problem is composed of background knowledge. This background knowledge consists of material retained from reading pathophysiology textbooks and attending lectures and that taught to us directly by our professors. The personal experiences and biases of those who write the texts, give the lectures, and lead clinical teaching rounds enter into, and become part of, this background knowledge.

Foreground knowledge is much more specific than background knowledge. The information is typically much more focused and answers a very particular question. This type of knowledge increases during a physician's career, as research is conducted and reading systematic reviews replaces the reading of standard textbooks. Evidence-based medicine (EBM) makes up the largest component of foreground knowledge and has been cited as the "major revolution" in foreground knowledge (1). EBM has been described as the integration of research, clinical expertise, and patient values (2).

At varying times during her or his career, the physician innately has varying levels of both background and foreground knowledge (Fig. 8.2) (2). In practice, both types are necessary to answer a clinical question, but the acquisition of knowledge is simply not enough. Application of the knowledge gained is necessary to formulate a clinical decision (Fig. 8.3).

Analysis and Application

Most clinical scenarios with which the physician is confronted are something that she or he has previously seen. The clinician compares the history and physical examination along with preliminary laboratory data to the previous clinical experiences and makes a diagnosis. This type of process is most frequently referred to as *pattern recognition*. The benefits to pattern recognition are that it is rapid, efficient, and usually correct. It allows the clinician to make a diagnosis without the prolonged considerations of differential diagnosis (3). Typically, these patterns take the form of illness scripts. An *illness script* is a combination of textbook knowledge of a disease as well as the way that it has manifested itself to the clinician based on past experience (4). The primary fault with pattern recognition is the same as its primary benefit: It is very unsophisticated. It has the potential to lure the clinician into the simplistic realm of pattern recognition when the medical problem itself may be very complex (5).

When a physician is confronted with a situation not previously experienced—that is, no pattern or illness script exists—analytic reasoning is needed to reach a proper diagnosis. Analytic reasoning is more complex and time consuming. It involves the asking of several questions that allow the clinician to reach a more thoughtful conclusion. How much a physician relies on pattern recognition and on analytic reasoning to arrive at a diagnosis depends on the physician's experience. A seasoned physician has a larger database of patterns from which to recognize a disorder as compared to, for example, a medical resident. Physicians at tertiary-care facilities have different databases of patterns as compared to country physicians. Nonetheless, when the physician arrives at a diagnosis, a new pattern is generated that may be used in the future (Fig. 8.4).

On arrival at a diagnosis, the clinician frequently reflects on it. He or she reconfirms that the diagnosis accurately fits with the available information from the history, physical examination, laboratory data, and other diagnostic studies. She or he decides that other diagnoses from the differential diagnostic list have been reasonably excluded as likely causes. The principle of Occam's razor is often taught in clinical diagnosis classes

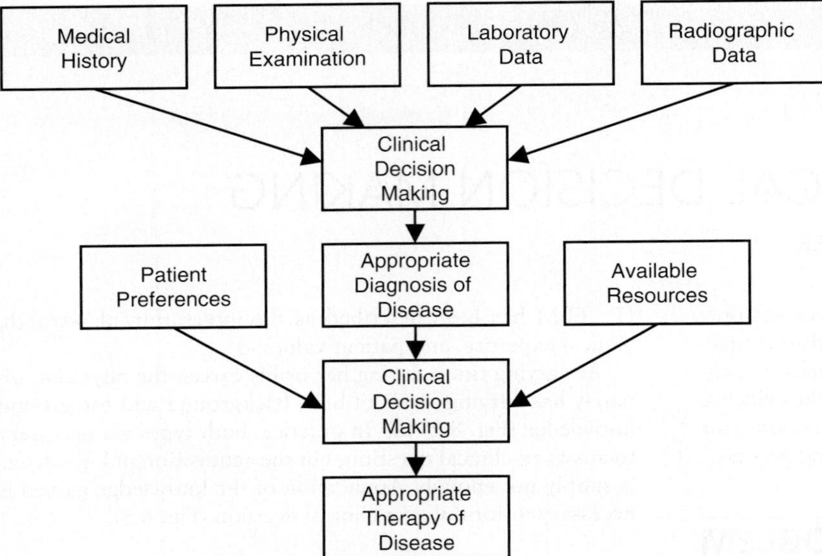

FIGURE 8.1. Clinical decision making in the diagnosis and therapy of a disease.

in medical school. Paraphrased, it states that "All other things being equal, the simplest solution is the best." The premise of the Occam's razor principle is important in that a diagnostic theory that introduces the smallest number of uncertainties is likely to be most valid. Although the concept of Occam's razor is elegant and attractive, much like pattern recognition, it can make complex situations too simplistic and should be used with caution. Both Hickam's dictum and Saint's triad (6) have attempted to issue cautionary warnings to clinicians about the failure to consider concomitant diseases. Certainly, a patient is far more likely to have several common diseases, rather than one rare disease, to explain a group of symptoms. As populations age, the likelihood of patients having multiple medical conditions increases, and the likelihood of having more than one condition that explain a particular set of symptoms also increases.

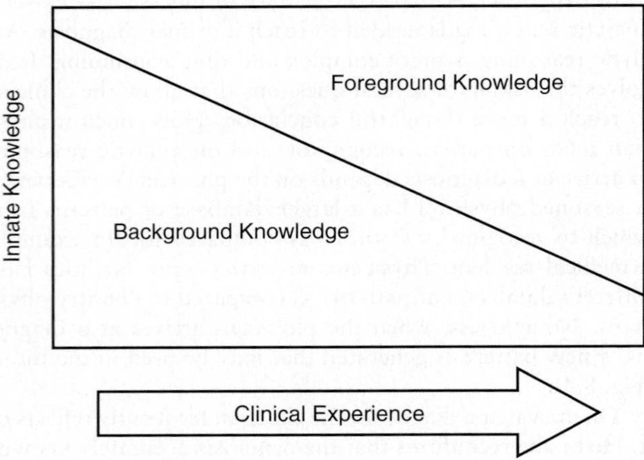

FIGURE 8.2. Changes in foreground and background knowledge as clinical experience increases. (From: Sackett DL, Straus SE, Richardson WS, et al. *Evidence-based Medicine. How to Practice and Teach EBM*. 2nd ed. Edinburgh, Scotland: Churchill Livingstone; 2000, with permission.)

TOOLS FOR HELPING CLINICIANS MAKE DECISIONS

Heuristics

The simplest definition of a heuristic is that it represents a rule of thumb. The use of heuristics typically leads to a rapid and efficient solution to a problem (7–9). Some of the more popular heuristics in medicine are "treat the patient and not the number," and "when you hear hoofbeats, think horses, not zebras" (10). Evidence shows that heuristics are used extensively by experienced physicians (11). The use of heuristics is fraught with bias, however. The most commonly occurring biases are discussed below.

Anchoring or Focalism

Clinicians start with an implicit reference point, the most likely in the list of differential diagnoses or anchor; they then make adjustments to its likelihood of being the most correct diagnosis based on further data. This heuristic describes the common human tendency to rely too heavily—or anchor—on one piece of information when making clinical decisions. In other words, the clinician is reluctant to discard the initial diagnosis despite mounting evidence that refutes it.

Availability

In this case, the physician bases his or her prediction of the likelihood of a patient having a disease on how easily an example can be brought to mind. For example, a physician assigns a diagnosis to a patient based on the diagnosis that a recent patient had with the same set of symptoms.

Denial

If the outcome or diagnosis is too upsetting, the clinician may rate the likelihood of the patient having the diagnosis as less likely than what its true prevalence would be.

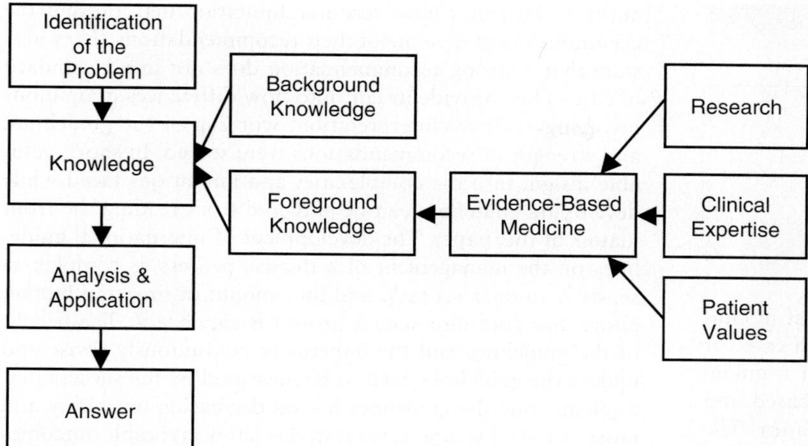

FIGURE 8.3. The steps in clinical decision making.

Representativeness

This bias results when commonality between patients with similar symptoms is assumed. In this heuristic, the likelihood that a patient has a particular disease because she or he matches a pattern or illness script increases even though the disease itself may be infrequent. Several other heuristics have been postulated (Table 8.1). The above are the most frequently cited in psychological literature.

Standards and Guidelines

When issued by an officiating agency, a standard is a rule. The American Society of Anesthesiologists (ASA) considers a standard to be the minimum requirements for clinical practice. Standards are generally accepted principles for patient management (12) and may be modified only under extreme circumstances. The ASA has developed standards in three areas:

1. Preanesthesia care
2. Postanesthesia care
3. Basic anesthetic monitoring

A standard of care is uniform throughout medical practice but case specific and time specific, and thus necessarily will change over time (13). The American College of Medical Quality states that medical standards reflect both the art (consensus of opinion of clinical judgment) and science (published peer-reviewed literature) of medicine (13). Deviations from standards result in both underuse and overuse of medical resources. Standards are sometimes also referred to as *standard operating procedures*.

Standard operating procedures (SOPs), more specifically, are detailed written instructions to achieve uniformity of the performance of a specific function (14). A clinical guideline, sometimes called a medical guideline or clinical protocol, is a

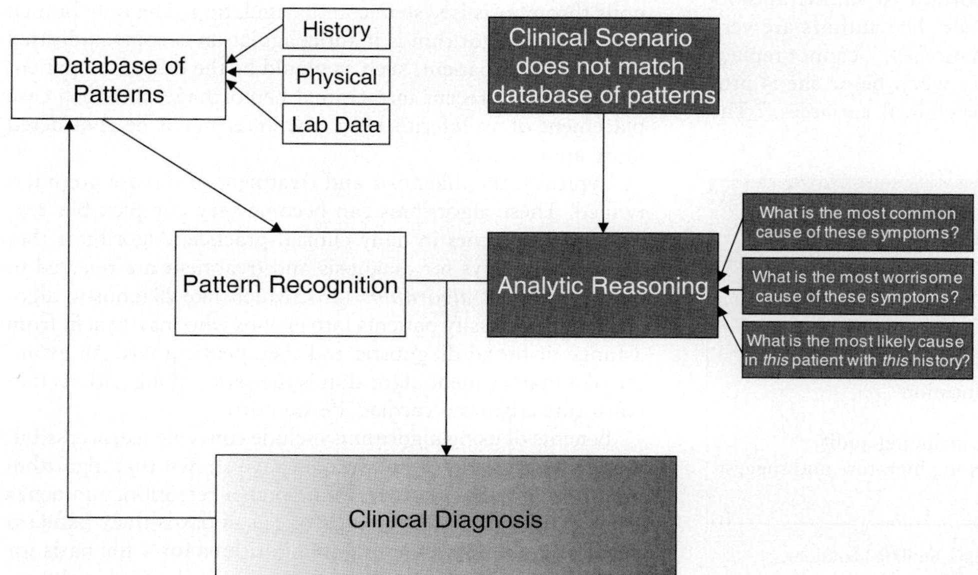

FIGURE 8.4. Pattern recognition and analytic reasoning in the development of a clinical diagnosis.

TABLE 8.1

LESSER-KNOWN TYPES OF HEURISTICS

Affect heuristics
Effort heuristic
Familiarity heuristic
Fluency heuristic
Recognition heuristic

systematically developed statement designed to assist in clinician and patient decisions about appropriate health care for specific clinical circumstances (15). The content of a guideline contains recommendations that are evidence based and obtained from systematic reviews of the medical literature. The purposes of clinical guidelines are noted in Table 8.2.

Some argue that the term *clinical protocol* should be reserved for a more detailed and specific set of steps for the management of a single condition (16,17). Clinical guidelines are somewhat more flexible than standards. Deviation from guidelines to accommodate differences between patients is acceptable, whereas a standard (or standard operating procedure) should be applied uniformly to all patients. Certain characteristics have been identified that contribute to guideline use:

1. Inclusion of specific recommendations
2. Sufficient supporting evidence
3. A clear structure
4. An attractive layout (18)

Perhaps the disease process that has received the most significant amount of attention in terms of guideline development has been sepsis. The Surviving Sepsis Campaign has just released its 2008 guidelines for the management of severe sepsis and septic shock (19). Sepsis is a devastatingly common disease with a high mortality. The speed and appropriateness of therapy in the initial hours after presentation are likely to influence outcome (19). For these reasons, the development of easy-to-follow guidelines for clinicians, which summarize best practices, is very important and would be expected to have an effect on the morbidity and mortality of those suffering from sepsis. At the beginning of this important paper, the authors of the guidelines address certain issues. The authors are very careful to state that their recommendations "... cannot replace clinician's decision-making capability when he or she is provided with a patient's unique set of clinical variables." The authors warn that local resource limitation may prevent the accomplishment of some of their recommendations. They also state that a strong recommendation does not imply standard of care. They provide insight into how differences in opinions involving evidence interpretation, wording of the guidelines, and strength of recommendations were solved. In short, valuable insight into the complexities and limitations faced while developing guidelines can be gathered from reading the front matter of this paper. The development of international guidelines on the management of a disease process as complex as sepsis is an onerous task, and the amount of time and human effort that goes into such a project is significant. The benefit of the guidelines and the impetus to continuously revise and update the guidelines need to be measured by the success that implementing the guidelines has on decreasing morbidity and mortality. At this time, several studies show favorable outcomes to the implementation of the Surviving Sepsis Campaign guidelines (20,21). One study that found no statistically significant decrease in mortality was inadequately powered to do so (22).

TABLE 8.2

PURPOSES OF DEVELOPING CLINICAL GUIDELINES

To describe appropriate care based on the best available scientific evidence and broad consensus
To reduce inappropriate variation in practice
To provide a more rational basis for referral
To provide a focus for continuing education
To promote efficient use of resources
To act as a focus for quality control, including audit
To highlight shortcomings of the existing literature and suggest appropriate future research
From http://www.openclinical.org/guidelines.html#fieldandlohr.

Algorithms

An algorithm is a guideline that has been placed into a flowchartlike format. This allows for a linear approach to clinical information. At various points (nodes) during the algorithm, input from the clinician is required in the form of observations to be made, decisions to be considered, and actions to be taken. Answers at each of the decision-making points determines the further development of the diagnosis. The goal at each branching point is to further classify the disease state of the patient. As the algorithm progresses, the testing to confirm the diagnosis typically gets more complex, invasive, and costly. An example of this may be the diagnostic evaluation of chest pain. The initial evaluation begins with a thorough history and physical exam, and then may progress through electrocardiography, evaluation of cardiac enzymes, echocardiography, and, finally, coronary angiography.

Treatment algorithms are typically less complex than diagnostic algorithms since they are necessarily more focused to a single diagnosis. For example, the standard treatment of a venous thrombosis is systemic anticoagulation. The only branch point in this algorithm is if anticoagulation is contraindicated in a particular patient, such as would be the case if the patient had suffered a recent intracranial hemorrhage, in which case placement of an inferior vena cava filter might be considered more appropriate.

Typically, the diagnosis and treatment of disease are intertwined. These algorithms can become very complex but represent what occurs in daily clinical practice. Algorithms that contain pathways for diagnosis and treatment are referred to as *management algorithms* (23). Much like diagnostic algorithms, they classify patients into groups who may benefit from a range of broad diagnostic and therapeutic goals. An example of a management algorithm is the series of algorithms that constitute advanced cardiac life support.

Benefits of using algorithms include convenience, accessibility, and ease of use. Some studies have shown that algorithm use has resulted in faster learning, higher retention, and better compliance with established practice standards than standard prose text (24–27). In addition, algorithms form the basis for the programming behind computer-assisted decision making.

Algorithms also have been criticized (23). One criticism is that the format of the algorithm is too rigid. Patients do not always present with concrete signs and symptoms. In addition, patients are variable in their personal preferences to modalities of treatments. The Agency for Health Care Policy and Research (AHCPR) clinical guideline program attempts to address this latter limitation by inserting branching points in algorithms that recognize the importance of, and allow for, patient preference in decision making.

Another criticism challenges the clinical validity of the algorithms used in practice; however, this challenge is not unique to algorithms and also is a valid criticism for the use of some guidelines. Hardon (23) recommends the annotation of the nodes in the algorithm with links to the literature that, in turn, validates the basis of the algorithm's recommendations. This would allow the clinician to further research different points of the algorithm, allowing for more precise definitions, additional clinical detail, and identification of important gaps in the literature.

Algorithms may lack specificity. For example, a node in an algorithm may state, "Obtain cardiac output measurement." Cardiac output obviously may be obtained from several methods of variable invasiveness. This may reflect a lack of consensus on the best method, or the best method under a particular set of circumstances, for determination of cardiac output. Nodes involving the gathering of information from the patient (i.e., the quality of pain) or other subjective information (i.e., the level of agitation of a patient) may result in user bias. Conversely, algorithms may be too specific. It is easy to imagine how a management algorithm meant to address a symptom, such as chest pain, can develop into a flowchart with over 100 nodes. The clutter can be distracting and counterproductive to the use of the algorithm. Simplicity and standardization have been advocated for successful algorithm development by the Society for Medical Decision Making (28).

In summary, algorithms are a method of representing guidelines for care consisting of nodes where observations, decisions, and actions occur. Depending on the input of the user, different pathways are taken to classify and identify a disease process, treat a disease, or both. Management algorithms allow for the simultaneous diagnosis and treatment of a disease process. Although many benefits to the use of algorithms exist, so do the drawbacks. Nonetheless, they play a central role in computer-based decision models. Medal (29) is a collection of over 11,000 algorithms that may be useful to clinicians or biomedical researchers.

Clinical Pathways

Clinical pathways are multidisciplinary plans of care designed to support the implementation of guidelines and protocols. They support clinical management, clinical and nonclinical resource management, and clinical audit, as well as financial management (30). Clinical pathways have four main components:

1. A timeline
2. The categories of care or activities and their interventions
3. Intermediate and long-term outcome criteria
4. The variance record (31,32)

Clinical pathways differ from guidelines, protocols, and algorithms, as they are used by a multidisciplinary team and their focus lies on the quality and coordination of care after clinical decisions have already been made to begin the therapy or diagnostic evaluation (30,33).

Bundles

A bundle is a group of interventions related to a disease process that, when executed together, result in better outcomes than when implemented individually. It is a structured way of improving the processes of care and patient outcomes: A small, straightforward set of practices, generally three to five, that, when performed collectively and reliably, have been proven to improve patient outcomes (34). All practices set forth in a bundle must be completed; they have been designed such that each practice can be completed on an all-or-none scale. That is, a practice cannot be almost completed—it either is completed or it is not completed. The practices are scientifically robust, rigorously scrutinized, and based on the highest level of evidence available at the time they are released. The goal of the Institute for Healthcare Improvement (IHI) when releasing the bundles was for the focus of clinicians to be on the *implementation* of the elements of the bundle as opposed to the *content* of the elements of the bundle. The key elements of a bundle are that it is made up of very few (but very important) practices, the accountability for its completion lies with an identified person or team, and the completion of the bundle in its entirety improves outcomes. Bundles that have been assembled by the IHI are noted in Table 8.3.

Guidelines from the Institute for Healthcare Improvement

Formed in 1991, the Institute for Healthcare Improvement (IHI) has worked to improve the delivery and execution of health care services for over a decade. Owing to the groundbreaking work of Deming, Juran, and Crosby (35–37), they have spearheaded a model for improvement over the past 17 years to assist health care systems in process and quality improvement.

Any discussion regarding quality improvement (QI) must first focus on the historical framework. QI is defined as a planned approach to transform organizations by evaluating and improving systems to achieve better outcomes. Intrinsic to this definition is the specification of program/production/service components, measurement, and identification of outcomes criteria; these consist of a number of components. Deming, Juran, and Crosby had slightly different ideas about

TABLE 8.3

INSTITUTE FOR HEALTHCARE IMPROVEMENT (IHI) BUNDLES

Sepsis resuscitation bundle
Sepsis management bundle
Central line bundle
Surgical site bundle
Ventilator-associated pneumonia bundle

TABLE 8.4

COMPONENTS TO QUALITY

Deming's 14 Points	Juran's Quality Planning	Crosby's Implementation Program
Create constancy of purpose for improvement of product and service	Establish the infrastructure needed to establish and maintain the quality improvement (QI) program	Management commitment: Make it clear where management stands on quality
Adopt the new philosophy	Identify the specific needs for improvement—the QI projects	QI teams: Create QI teams
Cease dependence on mass inspection	For each project, establish a team with clear responsibility for bringing the project to conclusion	Measurement: Create quality measurement to provide for objective evaluation and corrective action
End the practice of awarding business on price tag alone	Provide the resources, training, and support needed by the team	Cost of quality: Define the ingredients of the cost of quality
Improve constantly and forever the system of production and service	Determine who the customers are: The vital few and useful many	Quality awareness: Increase awareness and commitment to quality by all employees
Institute training	Determine the needs of the customer	Corrective action: Provide a systematic approach to resolving problems
Institute leadership	Develop product features that respond to customer needs	Zero defects: Identify activities that must be conducted to implement a zero defects program
Drive out fear	Develop processes that are able to produce what the customer needs/wants	Supervisor training: Prepare supervisors to implement the quality program
Break down barriers between staff areas	Transfer the resulting plans to the operating forces	Zero defects day: Initiate the zero defects program
Eliminate slogans, exhortations, and targets for the workforce	Keep the planned process in its planned state	Goal setting: Work teams establish goals
Eliminate numeric quotas	Evaluate actual quality performance	Error-cause removal: Employees identify obstacles to achieving goals and producing quality goods or services
Remove barriers to pride of workmanship	Compare actual performance to quality goals	Recognition: To appreciate those who contribute in the quality effort
Institute a vigorous program of education and training	Measure: Statistical significance, economic significance, and trends	Quality councils: To coordinate the organization's quality program
Take action to accomplish the transformation	Act on the differences	Do it over again: To emphasize the QI program is continuous

QI; however, there were similarities between each of these quality innovators, which are exemplified in Table 8.4 (35–37).

IHI promotes a strategy of "changing health care together" and embodies this approach through their philosophy of "all teach, all learn." This system reinforces the idea that committed individuals and organizations can, through collaboration, more quickly and efficiently improve health care delivery than any single individual or corporate entity. Figure 8.5 embodies IHI's strategy for transforming health care. At the core of their work is innovation, the creation and testing of new ideas and concepts for improving patient care. Here, they work intensely with cutting-edge organizations on a project basis to test new solutions to old problems. Once a promising change concept has been successfully developed in one setting, it will require being fully vetted and piloted in other settings.

Strategic Relationships. IHI has developed various closely aligned, strategic relationships with dozens of organizations that test and deploy these changes. These high-level partnerships focus on transforming entire systems of care by concentrating on strategic objectives and system-level improvement. IHI has accomplished this at the global level, consulting with health care organizations and countries throughout the world. It is accomplished through multiple methods including developing strategic partnerships as previously discussed and their IMPACT network, where health care organizations come together to achieve dramatic improvement results in clinical outcomes, patient and provider satisfaction, and financial performance, as well as in learning and innovation communities. Learning and innovation communities are collaborative change laboratories focused on front-line improvement. Participating organizations work with each other and with IHI faculty to rapidly test and implement meaningful, sustainable change within a specific topic area. Learning and innovation communities are the next-generation evolution of the Breakthrough Series, IHI's traditional methodology for collaborative improvement.

For example, the improving outcomes for high-risk critically ill patients community focuses on identifying and rescuing patients whose condition is clinically worsening; providing

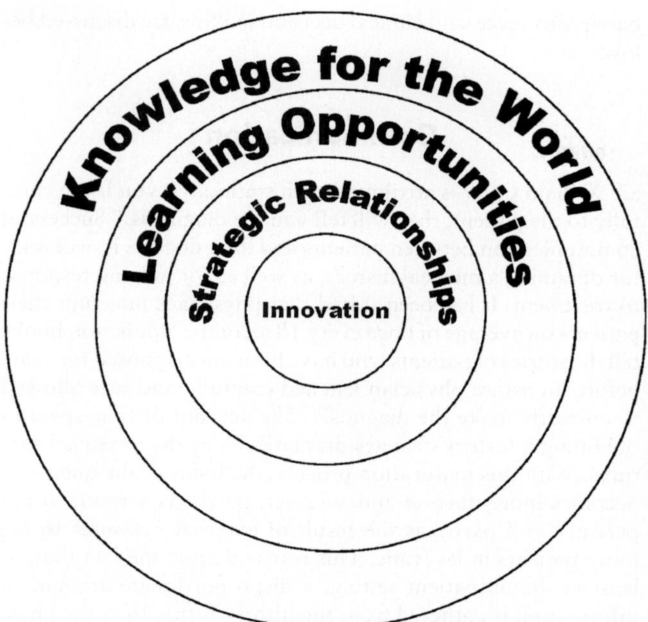

FIGURE 8.5. The Institute for Healthcare Improvement's strategy for transforming health care.

appropriate, reliable, and timely care to high-risk and critically ill patients using evidence-based therapies; creating a highly effective multidisciplinary team; integrating patient and family into care so they receive the care they want; and the development of an infrastructure that promotes quality care. Specific interventions include ventilator and central venous access bundles, rapid-response teams, glucose control both inside and outside of the ICU, sepsis resuscitation and management bundles, multidisciplinary rounds and daily goals, handoffs, and a palliative care team to assist with end-of-life care. As a result of focusing on these areas, the IHI predicts that hospital organizations will be able to decrease raw mortality by greater than 25%, intensive care unit (ICU) mortality by 20%, and ICU length of stay by 20%.

Learning opportunities, the next layer of the IHI strategy, offers a wide variety of learning opportunities for health care professionals from expert faculty and experienced colleagues around the world. This is accomplished through seminars and Web-based and professional development programs that create opportunities for organizations and individuals to learn and implement best-practice ideas online. These programs are designed for leaders who seek to gain a particular set of skills that are required for an organization to succeed in its improvement agenda. Programs offered by IHI include training for board members, patient safety officers, improvement advisors, and operations managers, as well as personnel in other critical roles.

The final step in the IHI learning system is the broad dissemination of best-practice improvement knowledge, knowledge for the world. This is accomplished primarily through campaigns, the IHI Web site, professional education, and fellowship programs (38).

The Institute for Healthcare Improvement may be best known for its 100,000 Lives Campaign. The goal of the campaign, besides the saving of the lives of 100,000 hospitalized patients, was the building of a reusable national infrastructure

TABLE 8.5

THE INSTITUTE FOR HEALTHCARE IMPROVEMENT (IHI) CAMPAIGNS

Goals of the 100,000 Lives Campaign:

- Deploy rapid response teams at the first sign of patient decline
- Deliver reliable, evidence-based care for acute myocardial infarction to prevent deaths from heart attack
- Prevent adverse drug events (ADEs) by implementing medication reconciliation
- Prevent central line infections by implementing a series of interdependent, scientifically grounded steps
- Prevent surgical site infections by reliably delivering the correct perioperative antibiotics at the proper time
- Prevent ventilator-associated pneumonia by implementing a series of interdependent, scientifically grounded steps

Goals of the 5 Million Lives Campaign

- Prevent pressure ulcers by reliably using science-based guidelines for their prevention
- Reduce methicillin-resistant *Staphylococcus aureus* (MRSA) infection by reliably implementing scientifically proven infection control practices
- Prevent harm from high-alert medications starting with a focus on anticoagulants, sedatives, narcotics, and insulin
- Reduce surgical complications by reliably implementing all of the changes in care recommended by the Surgical Care Improvement Project (SCIP)
- Deliver reliable, evidence-based care for congestive heart failure to reduce readmissions
- Get Boards on Board defining and spreading the best-known leveraged processes for hospital Boards of Directors, so that they can become far more effective in accelerating organizational progress toward safe care

From www.ihi.org/campaign.

for the implementation of evidence-based change. The IHI proclaimed at the conclusion of its campaign that 122,300 lives were actually saved by the implementation of their six interventions (Table 8.5). Criticism was generated relating to the statistical analysis that lead to calculation of the number of lives saved by the initiative, as well as the evidence that showed a benefit to rapid-response teams (39). At the conclusion, however, even the toughest critics believe that the campaign did save lives and was worthy of implementation (40).

Perhaps the most important accomplishment of the campaign was its ability to unite clinicians, allied health care workers, and hospital administrators across the country in support of evidence-based guidelines with the purpose of reducing harm to patients. Currently, the IHI is in the middle of its 5 Million Lives Campaign, with six new interventions designed to eliminate five million cases of patient injury.

Computerized Decision Support/Fuzzy Logic

Intensive care medicine frequently involves making rapid decisions on the basis of a large and disparate array of often incomplete information. Intensivists typically rely on conventional wisdom, evidence, and personal experience to arrive at subjective assessments and judgments. Due to an increased focus on outcomes, physicians are being asked to adhere to explicit guidelines and bundles that have been agreed on by the medical community at large (41). A vast majority of these guidelines have an inherent logical structure and therefore make them suitable for computer implementation. As a result, there has been increasing interest in computer-based support tools to automate certain aspects of the medical decision-making process in the intensive care unit (42). Compared with the human brain, computers are well suited to make rapid calculations, allowing the creation of decision networks that support near-limitless complexity. The variable nature of disease and patient characteristics makes it difficult to decide what should be done in every conceivable set of circumstances. In these situations, physicians must depend on intuitive decision making, sometimes defined as the art of medicine; intuitive decision making is usually described as being unsuitable to computerization.

Subjective judgments generally defy description in terms of the kinds of deterministic mathematical equations that computers are well suited to solve. The methods of fuzzy logic are suited to this kind of task and can lead to algorithms that emulate the nonexplicit nature of clinical decision making (43,44). Fuzzy logic was first introduced by Zadeh in the 1960s (45) and is now a well-established engineering discipline (46,47). Given that fuzzy logic is particularly advantageous in areas where a precise mathematical description of the control process(es) is impossible makes it especially suited to support medical decision making.

Fuzzy logic has been successfully tested in areas of medicine that include the ICU (48). Nemoto et al. (48) were able to create a fuzzy logic controller to facilitate weaning on pressure support mechanical ventilation using patient vital signs and respiratory mechanics such as peak inspiratory and mean airway pressures. Huang et al. (49) created a fuzzy logic controller to control intracranial pressure using propofol sedation. Finally, models for treatment of septic shock have also been created (50). Fuzzy logic provides a means for encapsulating the subjective decision-making process in an algorithm suitable for computer implementation. It appears to be eminently suited to aspects of medical decision making. Further development using fuzzy logic in the ICU is underway, and FDA-approved, commercially available products are on the horizon.

COMPLEXITIES IN DECISION MAKING

In actuality, decision making is much more complex than the search for knowledge and the application of answers. Most of the original research into the study of how humans make decisions focused on economics (51). The process of decision making in critical care medicine is unique from many decision-making processes in business for one major reason: Decisions may be acutely time sensitive. As hypoxia is progressing, one does not have the luxury of multiple diagnostic tests, obtaining a complete history, and a prolonged analysis of the data. If a working diagnosis and appropriate therapeutic measures cannot be instituted quickly, the patient may perish. Several other barriers to successful clinical decision making are discussed below.

Communication

Sir William Osler is attributed with stating, "If you listen carefully to the patient, they will tell you the diagnosis." Successful communication between patients and their doctors is necessary for obtaining a medical history, as well as for judging response to treatment. It has been stated that physicians interrupt their patients on average of once every 18 seconds. Nonfiction books tell the stories of patients who have been misdiagnosed for years before an astute physician listened carefully and was allowed to correctly make the diagnosis. The amount of time spent in obtaining a history changes dramatically as the physician matures. With this maturation process, the focus of the questions becomes more narrow and succinct, partly as a result of experience and partly as the result of external pressures to see more patients in less time. This is true despite the fact that, at least in the outpatient setting, a disproportionate amount of information is gathered from the history rather than the physical examination or laboratory data (52). In fact, allowing for 90 seconds of spontaneous conversation at the beginning of an outpatient consult—the so-called 90-second rule—has been advocated (53).

Communication in the intensive care unit is quite different. Many of the patients are unable to communicate effectively as a result of severe illness and subsequent neurologic disability, sedative and analgesic medications, and the presence of an endotracheal tube or tracheostomy. This makes communication even more difficult, since the patient may not respond, for example, to abdominal pain on physical examination until it becomes quite severe. Communication may rely on gathering information from the first responders on the scene and the paramedic run sheets subsequently generated. Studies of paramedical personnel show that they can relatively adequately diagnosis cerebral vascular accidents (54), acute myocardial infarction (55), and those with difficulty breathing (56), even though there is a tendency toward overdiagnosis. Although one might think it somewhat better to overdiagnose than underdiagnose, the reliability of information gathered by the first responders may not always be reliable. Information gathered from spouses or next of kin may be variable as well. In the outpatient setting, a history given by the surrogates was accurate in terms of medical history and medication use (57), cigarette and coffee use (58), but not concerning alcohol use (58) or dietary data (59); knowledge of drug use or other illicit activities is more poorly correlated between the patient and a family member (60). In the above-mentioned studies, the information for comparison was gathered in an outpatient setting. The distress of having a loved one acutely and severely ill may affect the ability to recall details of the patient's medical history necessary for diagnosis and treatment. In practice, revisiting the patient's medical history with the family after the initial admission to the intensive care unit may be more fruitful.

Language Barriers

A gap in understanding between patients and health care workers can become quite problematic. Language has been cited as the most common barrier in any health care setting and has been found to be a risk factor to adverse outcomes (61). Interestingly, a recent study determined that nursing staff versus physicians found a language barrier to be more stressful (97% vs. 78%, respectively) and more of an impediment to the delivery of quality care (95% vs. 88%, respectively) (62). Also of note, adherence to medication regimens are more frequently a problem for non-English speakers (63). These data can likely be extrapolated to adherence with nonmedication regimens that have been advised by health care providers as well, although no specific studies have elucidated this point. As immigration continues to rise in the United States, we will be faced with, perhaps, more non-English-speaking patients than in previous years. Although a language barrier should not be a reason for inequities of care provided in a health care setting, there is no universally accepted solution to address this. Each hospital must develop its own resources for dealing with non-English-speaking patients. One method that is exceedingly popular is to have bilingual nurses translate for physicians. In a study evaluating the efficacy of nurse-translators in an ambulatory setting and comparing them to the videotaped interaction, which was translated by blinded medical interpreters, misinterpretations resulting in physician misunderstanding occurred in about 50% of cases (64). In many of these settings, the problems included nurses' further interpretation of the patients' words to become more consistent with the clinical picture and the use of cultural metaphors that did not translate accurately to English. This study demonstrates that even with a language as common as Spanish, misinterpretation that affects the clinician's ability to formulate an accurate diagnosis is still prone to occur. Speaking a nondominant language in a country that tends to be monolingual may also lead to medical interventions that are possibly unnecessary. Despite similar mechanisms of injury, the degree of hypotension during resuscitation, injury severity score (ISS), illicit substance use, alcohol use, and a higher Glasgow coma scale (GCS) score, Spanish-speaking trauma patients were more likely to be endotracheally intubated than their English-speaking counterparts (65).

Resource Limitation

Adherence to recommended guidelines may be well beyond the control of the physician if she or he does not have access to adequate resources or a referral network, and decision making may be affected. It has been suggested that the lack of the immediate availability of an anesthesiologist may interfere with the ability to adhere to consensus guidelines, decreasing the rate of elective cesarean deliveries (66,67). Guidelines aimed at reducing the risk of central venous catheter infections have been available since 1996 (68,69). Yet in 2003, less than 10% of American internists acknowledged using chlorhexidine gluconate for skin preparation prior to insertion. The major factor that determined the use of the antiseptic agent was its availability at the institution (70). Furthermore, lack of appropriate equipment was associated with lack of adherence to guidelines.

Fear of Litigation

The practice of defensive medicine involves using diagnostic and therapeutic measures as a safeguard, or self-protection, in case charges of medical malpractice are levied at some time in the future. Defensive medicine may result in additional, unnecessary testing and/or referrals to other health care providers, or it may result in the practitioner's refusal to treat certain groups of high-risk patients (71). In a 2005 survey, 93% of 824 physicians in Pennsylvania reported practicing defensive medicine (71). The most frequent form of defensive medicine practiced was ordering expensive imaging studies. A study of Israeli otolaryngologists determined that almost 80% of surgeons varied from the American Academy of Otolaryngology–Head and Neck Surgery recommendations regarding coagulation screening tests before tonsillectomy and adenoidectomy. Most of those surgeons that deviated from the practice guidelines stated that the reason for this behavior was the practice of defensive medicine (72). In a study of Illinois neonatologists, many perceived a "gray zone" of resuscitative practices related to the gestational age at which resuscitation would be used or withheld (73). At less than 25 weeks' gestation, the neonatologists were significantly more fearful of litigation should they not resuscitate. The conclusion of this study was that external influences may affect delivery room resuscitation practices. The practice of defensive medicine is not simply the harmless addition of a few unnecessary diagnostic tests. It contributes to the skyrocketing costs of health care and, in some instances, can worsen the expected clinical outcome of patients (74).

Personal Biases and Interindividual Differences

Physicians may make their future decisions biased by their previous experiences. Practicing medicine in the same manner as one's instructors was, and still is, commonplace. The emergence of evidence-based practice is attempting to exchange personal bias for objective scientifically based practice. A previously missed diagnosis may sort to the top of the differential diagnosis list when the physician is confronted with a subsequent patient with a similar presentation; this may be especially true if a bad outcome or medicolegal issue occurred with the previous patient. Although this is frequently assumed to occur, at least one study disagrees with this philosophy, suggesting that physicians with greater malpractice experience showed no systematic differences in initial management choice or subsequent test recommendations (75).

Several studies have examined the differences of the clinical decision-making process between individuals. Although the methods themselves are similar, some differences do exist. It has been found that the more expert diagnosticians ask fewer questions, consider less in their differential diagnoses, and arrive at the correct diagnosis in less time (3,76,77). Although the accumulation of medical knowledge, vast experience, and an excellent memory undoubtedly helps a clinician become a master diagnostician, simply attaining these three qualities does not guarantee diagnostic superiority. Ongoing research is focusing on how these qualities are individually and collectively used by clinicians.

Clinical Inertia

Clinical inertia refers to the practice of *not* intensifying treatments of patients who are not yet at goals defined by evidence-based medicine. Clinical inertia has been called a leading cause of potentially preventable adverse events, disability, death, and excess medical care costs. Traditionally, the focus of clinical inertia has been on chronic illnesses, such as diabetes, hypertension, and hypercholesterolemia. It appears, however, that clinical inertia is readily present in the ICU as well.

Intensivists in Germany, when polled, claimed that 91.6% used lung-protective strategies suggested by ARDSnet (acute respiratory distress syndrome network), 67.4% used intensive insulin therapy, and 79% used low-dose hydrocortisone therapy for septic shock. When the ICUs were actually surveyed, it was found that only 4.2% of patients were ventilated with ARDSnet-suggested strategies, only 8.8% had tight glucose control, and only 30.6% of patients with septic shock were, in fact, treated with low-dose hydrocortisone (78). Clinical inertia represents a specific phenomenon differing from lack of resources; in clinical inertia, the resources exist and are available—they are simply not used. Multiple causes have been proposed, including fallacious reasoning and overall complexity (79).

Inability to Locate Pertinent Information

Almost 20 years ago, Greenes (80) astutely observed that physicians were faced not with data overload, but information underload. That is, data is available from a multitude of sources, but the navigation through these sources to find relevant information is a harrowing task. It is well recognized that some, if not much, of the information contained in textbooks is outdated by the time the book is put into print. Bias can exist anywhere and everywhere within experimental design and execution, which can result in less-than-conclusive results (Table 8.6). If the data are collected and analyzed, and a manuscript is submitted, the research is subject to publication bias. Several factors have been identified as influencing rates of publication, including sample size, funding, quality, and prestige (81). It has long been felt that authors of smaller studies can boost their chance of publication by showing a stronger effect of their intervention. One answer to solving some of the publication bias is the creation of meta-analyses; however, significant problems can arise from combining studies that have different criteria for enrollment. As an example, consider the early studies conducted on patients suffering with acute respiratory distress syndrome (ARDS). ARDS had been known previously as shock lung, stiff lung, wet lung, and white lung. Prior to the 1994 American-European Consensus Conference on ARDS, different studies identified what we now commonly call ARDS by different criteria. This resulted in drastically different outcomes observed in response to similar treatment strategies. For a meta-analysis to have significance, the disease process must be understood and the definitions for patients included in the studies must be universal.

TABLE 8.6

TYPES OF BIAS THAT CAN EXIST IN RESEARCH

Referral bias
Nonrespondent bias
Insensitive measure bias
Expectation bias
Recall bias
Attention bias
Verification bias
Contamination bias
Cointervention bias
Compliance bias
Withdrawal bias
Proficiency bias

A final problem is that no study may exist regarding the best treatment when patients have two disease processes with competing treatment goals—for example, the treatment of the patient with cerebral edema and concomitant cerebral vasospasm. The goals of therapy for each of those processes are evidence-based and well published. The appearance of a patient who is suffering from both processes at the same time is not infrequent, but the literature on the treatment of such a patient is nonexistent at the time of the writing of this chapter.

It should be noted that the limitations of searching computer databases have not been addressed. Identifying all possible search parameters prior to conducting a database search is necessary. For example, searching an online computer database such as PubMed for literature dealing with the treatment of retinopathy of prematurity and for that dealing with retrolental fibroplasia generates different results despite the fact that these represent the same clinical entity. Keeping current with changes in medicine is also important. Searching for treatments for *Stenotrophomonas* infections produces different results from those produced when searching for treatments for *Xanthomonas* infections. These bacteria are the same, but the name change is a result of a reinterpretation of the taxonomic position, which occurred in the early 1980s (82). Searching databases for synonyms for the same disease process can yield up to a tenfold difference in results! Although lack of information is definitely problematic, too much information may also be a problem. In one study, the introduction of additional options increased the difficulty of the physician to make decisions. In one scenario, the uncertainty in deciding between two similar treatment options led some physicians to avoid this decision altogether and recommend not starting either treatment regimen for the patient (83).

Fatigue

It has long been felt that stress has a profound impact on clinical judgment and medical decision making. Research into the role that stress and fatigue have on clinical performance is actively ongoing.

Libby Zion's tragic death on March 4, 1984—a result of complications due to serotonin syndrome—drew public attention to the conditions under which resident physicians work. Although a grand jury exonerated the physicians, it was discovered that residents were working consistently more than 100 hours per week, sometimes continuously for 30 to 40 hours, and with minimal supervision. Although other factors contributed to Ms. Zion's death, the role that fatigued physicians played was seen as a serious potential danger. In March 1987, the New York State Commissioner of Health appointed Doctor Bertrand Bell to oversee a committee to evaluate the findings of the grand jury. The Bell Committee, as it was later called, handed down recommendations for the limitation of resident work hours. These limitations, also referred to as the Libby Law, were initially instituted in New York, but were eventually adopted elsewhere. On July 1, 2003, the Accreditation Council for Graduate Medical Education (ACGME) instituted standards for all accredited residency programs, limiting the work week to 80 hours; this has been adopted by all residency programs to maintain accreditation. One study found that 35.9% more serious medical errors were made—including 56.6% more nonintercepted serious errors—during a traditional call schedule (one-in-three) than during the intervention schedule that limited call hours to those recommended by the Bell Committee (84). Decline in cognitive performance has been specifically reported in ECG interpretation (85), monitoring during anesthesia (86), and surgical performance. One report suggested that surgical complication rates were 45% higher among residents who had been on call the previous night (87).

One study found that staying awake for 24 hours continuously impairs cognitive performance to a similar degree as having a 0.1% blood alcohol level (88). One of the first qualities to be impaired by alcohol intoxication is insight, which may lead some to assume that insight is equally impaired by those who are sleep deprived. That is, they do not fully appreciate how much their practice is impaired by sleep deprivation. Although insight may be impaired, interestingly, subjective ratings of high pressure in the workplace and insufficient sleep are associated with an increase in self-reported omissions in patient care (89). Thus, it seems that the sleep-deprived physician may realize she or he is taking less than optimal care of a patient but does nothing about it.

Has the ACGME limitation of work hours resulted in decreased morbidity and mortality? A recent study indicates that it may have, noting that there was a decreased short-term mortality among high-risk medical patients in teaching hospitals, but no difference was seen among surgical patients (90). Similar results were found in another study performed in Veterans Administration Hospitals (91), finding a decrease in the mortality of medical patients but no associations with surgical patients.

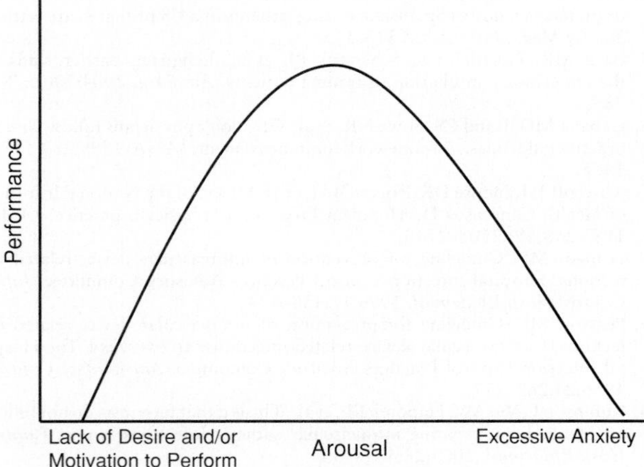

FIGURE 8.6. Performance versus arousal plot of the Yerkes-Dodson law. (From Yerkes RM, Dodson JD. The relation of strength of stimulus to rapidity of habit-formation. *J Comp Neurol Psychol.* 1908; 18(5):459–482, with permission.)

Stress

Although stress and fatigue are inherently related, and too much of either is not beneficial, some degree of stress, or arousal, is necessary to perform well and make sound decisions and judgments. This idea was proposed by psychologists Robert M. Yerkes and J.D. Dodson in 1908 (92) (Fig. 8.6). Different tasks may require different levels of arousal. For example, intellectually demanding tasks may require a lower level of arousal so that concentration may be facilitated; on the other hand, tasks demanding stamina or persistence may be performed better with higher levels of arousal (to increase motivation). Excessive arousal, anxiety, or stress results in diminished performance in clinical scenarios as seen on the downward portion of the graph.

SUMMARY

In many ways, clinical decision making resembles the practice of medicine as a whole; there is an artistic and a scientific component to both. How physicians acquire knowledge is well known. Knowledge gained from books is constantly supplanted by knowledge gained from critical reviews of the medical literature. How physicians apply that knowledge to arrive at a clinical decision is not as well understood and varies greatly between clinicians. Physicians use standards, guidelines, algorithms, clinical pathways, and bundles to assist in the provision of rapid, evidence-based care. Organizations such as the Institute for Healthcare Improvement assist in the identification and dispersion of best practices. As technology advances and information is shared both more readily and more rapidly, standardization of the practice of medicine will continue to increase. Although critics exist who fear the evolution of cookbook medicine, outcomes support the benefit conferred by the application of standards, bundles, and guidelines. The application of fuzzy logic and computerized decision support to the medical field is very exciting and has almost limitless utility at the bedside of the critically ill patient. One, of course, must realize that nothing can replace clinical judgment.

In the day-to-day practice of medicine, decision making is affected by other influences as well. Communication and language barriers, fatigue and stress, and the inability to locate pertinent information all impede a physician's ability to make accurate and efficient decisions. Nonetheless, hundreds of thousands of medical decisions are made in hospitals across the world on a daily basis that affect the lives of our patients. We have just begun to understand all the components involved in making those decisions.

References

1. Del Mar C, Doust J, Glasziou P. *Clinical Thinking: Evidence, Communication and Decision-Making.* Malden, MA: Blackwell; 2006.
2. Sackett DL, Straus SE, Richardson WS, et al. *Evidence-based Medicine. How to Practice and Teach EBM.* 2nd ed. Edinburgh, Scotland: Churchill Livingstone; 2000.
3. Dhaliwal G. Clinical decision-making: understanding how clinicians make a diagnosis. In: Saint S, Drazen J, Solomon C, eds. *Clinical Problem Solving.* New York, NY: McGraw-Hill; 2006.
4. Feltovich PJ, Barrows HS. Issues of generality in medical problem solving. In: Schmidt HG, De Volder ML, eds. *Tutorials in Problem-based Learning: a*

New Direction in Teaching the Health Professions. Assen, the Netherlands: Van Gorcum; 1984:128–142.
5. Leape LL. Error in medicine. *JAMA.* 1994;272:1851–1857.
6. Hilliard AA, Weinberger SE, Tierney LM Jr, et al. Clinical problem-solving. Occam's razor versus Saint's Triad. *N Engl J Med.* 2004;350(6):599–603.
7. Tversky A, Kahneman D. Availability: a heuristic for judging frequency and probability. *Cogn Psychol.* 1973;5:207–232.
8. Tversky A, Kahneman D. Judgment under uncertainty: heuristics and biases. *Science.* 1974;185:1124–1130.
9. Tversky A, Kahneman D. Evidential impact of base rates. In: Kahneman D, Slovic P, Tversky A, eds. *Judgment under Uncertainty: Heuristics and Biases.* Cambridge, England: Cambridge University Press; 1982.
10. McDonald CJ. Medical heuristics: the silent adjudicators of clinical practice. *Ann Intern Med.* 1996;124:56–62.
11. Patel VL, Kaufman DR, Arocha JF. Emerging paradigms of cognition in medical decision-making. *J Biomed Inform.* 2002;35:52–75.
12. http://www.asahq.org/publicationsAndServices/standards/01.pdf. Accessed January 1, 2008.
13. http://www.acmq.org/policies /policies3and4.pdf. Accessed January 1, 2008.
14. U.S. Department of Health and Human Services Food and Drug Administration Center for Drug Evaluation and Research (CDER) Center for Biologics Evaluation and Research (CBER) Guidance for Industry E6 Good Clinical Practice: Consolidated Guidance April 1996, ICH.
15. Field MJ, Lohr KN, eds. *Clinical Practice Guidelines: Directions for a New Program, Institute of Medicine.* Washington, DC: National Academy Press; 1990.
16. http://www.openclinical.org/guidelines.html#fieldandlohr. Accessed January 1, 2008.
17. Delamothe T. Wanted: guidelines that doctors will follow [editorial]. *BMJ.* 1993;307:218.
18. Wollersheim H, Burgers J, Grol R. Clinical guidelines to improve patient care. *Neth J Med.* 2005;63(6):188–192.
19. Delinger RP, Levy MM, Carlet MD, et al. Surviving Sepsis Campaign: international guidelines for the management of severe sepsis and septic shock: 2008. *Crit Care Med.* 2008;36:296–327.
20. Hurtado FJ, Nin N. The role of bundles in sepsis care. *Crit Care Clin.* 2006; 22(3):521–529.
21. Kortgen A, Niederprum P, Bauer M. Implementation of an evidence-based "standard operating procedure" and outcome in septic shock. *Crit Care Med.* 2006;34(4):943–949.
22. Shapiro NI, Howell MD, Talmor D, et al. Implementation and outcomes of the Multiple Urgent Sepsis Therapies (MUST) protocol. *Crit Care Med.* 2006;34(4):1025–1032.
23. Hadorn C. Use of algorithms in clinical guideline development in clinical practice guideline development: methodology perspectives. AHCPR Pub. No. 95-0009. Rockville, MD: Agency for Health Care Policy and Research; January, 1995:93–104.
24. Grimm RK, Shimoni K, Harlon W, et al. Evaluation of patient-care protocol use by various providers. *N Engl J Med.* 1975;292:507–511.
25. Komaroff AL, Black WL, Flatley M, et al. Protocols for physicians' assistants: management of diabetes and hypertension. *N Engl J Med.* 1974;290:307–312.
26. Sox HC. Quality of patient care by nurse practitioners and physician's assistants: a ten year perspective. *Ann Intern Med.* 1979;91:459–468.
27. Sox HC, Sox CH, Tompkins RK. The training of physician's assistants: the use of a clinical algorithm system for patient care, audit of performance and education. *N Engl J Med.* 1973;288:818–824.
28. Proposal for clinical algorithm standards. Society for Medical Decision Making Committee on Standardization of Clinical Algorithms. *Med Decis Making.* 1992;12:149–154.
29. www.medal.org.
30. http://www.openclinical.org/clinicalpathways.html. Accessed January 1, 2008.
31. Hill M. The development of care management systems to achieve clinical integration. *Adv Pract Nurs Q.* 1998;4(1):33–39.
32. Hill M. CareMap and case management systems; evolving models designed to enhance direct patient care. In: Blancett SS, Flarey DL, eds. *Reengineering Nursing & Health Care: Handbook for Organizational Transformation.* Boston, MA: Jones and Bartlett; 1995.
33. http://www.oqp.med.va.gov/cpg/faqs.asp. Accessed January 1, 2008.
34. http://www.ihi.org/IHI/Topics/CriticalCare/IntensiveCare/Improvement Stories/WhatIsaBundle.htm, Accessed January 1, 2008.
35. W. Edwards Deming Institute (2008). http://www.deming.org/. Accessed January 1, 2008.
36. Juran Institute (2008). http://www.juran.com/. Accessed January 1, 2008.
37. Phillip Crosby Associated (2008). http://www.philipcrosby.com/pca/index.html. Accessed January 1, 2008.
38. Institute of Healthcare Improvement (2008). http://www.ihi.orh/ihi. Accessed January 12, 2008.
39. Wachter RM, Pronovost PJ. The 100,000 Lives Campaign: a scientific and policy review. *Jt Comm J Qual Patient Saf.* 2006;32(11):621–627.
40. Robeznieks A. IHI campaign draws more fire. Article questions methodology, rapid-response teams. *Mod Healthc.* 2006;36(49):14–15.
41. Kohn L, Corrigan J, Donaldson M, eds. *To Err Is Human: Building. A safer health care system.* Committee on Quality of Health Care in America, Institute of Medicine. Washington, DC: National Academy Press. 2000;63:101–107.
42. Hanson CW, Marshall BE. Artificial intelligence applications in the intensive care unit. *Crit Care Med.* 2001;29:427–435.
43. Steimann F. On the use and usefulness of fuzzy sets in medical AI. *Artif Intell Med.* 2001;21:131–137.
44. Helgason CM, Jobe TH. Causal interactions, fuzzy sets and cerebrovascular 'accident': the limits of evidence-based medicine and the advent complexity-based medicine. *Neuroepidemiology.* 1999;18:64–67.
45. Zadeh LA. Fuzzy sets. *Inf Control.* 1965;8:338–352.
46. Cox E. Fuzzy fundamentals. *IEEE Spectrum.* 1992;Oct:58.
47. Hess J. Fuzzy logic and medical device technology. *Med Device Technol.* 1992;6(8):37–46.
48. Nemoto T, Hatzakis GE, Thorpe CW, et al. Automatic control of pressure support mechanical ventilation using fuzzy logic. *Am J Respir Crit Care Med.* 1999;160:550–556.
49. Huang SJ, Shieh JS, Fu M, et al. Fuzzy logic control for intracranial pressure via continuous propofol sedation in a neurosurgical intensive care unit. *Med Eng Phys.* 2006;28(7):639–647.
50. Paetz J. Knowledge-based approach to septic shock patient data using a neural network with trapezoidal activation functions. *Artif Intell Med.* 2003;28(2):207–230.
51. von Neumann J, Morgenstern O. Theory of Games and Economic Behavior. Princeton, NJ: Princeton University Press; 1944.
52. Hampton JR, Harrison MJ, Mitchell JR, et al. Relative contributions of history taking, physical examination, and laboratory investigation to diagnosis and management of medical outpatients. *BMJ.* 1975;2:486–489.
53. Langewitz W, Denz M, Keller A, et al. Spontaneous taking time at start of consultation in outpatient clinic cohort study. *BMJ.* 2002;325:682–683.
54. Zweifler RM, York D, U TT, et al. Accuracy of paramedic diagnosis of stroke. *J Stroke Cerebrovasc Dis.* 1998;7(6):446–448.
55. Bright H, Pocock J. Prehospital recognition of acute myocardial infarction. *CJEM.* 2002;4(3):212–214.
56. Ackerman R, Waldron RL. Difficulty breathing: agreement of paramedic and emergency physician diagnoses. *Prehosp Emerg Care.* 2006;10(1):77–80.
57. Lipworth L, Fryzek JP, Fored CM, et al. Comparison of surrogate with self-respondents regarding medical history and prior medication use. *Int J Epidemiol.* 2001;30(2):303–308.
58. McLaughlin JK, Mandel JS, Mehl ES, et al. Comparison of next-of-kin with self-respondents regarding questions on cigarette, coffee, and alcohol consumption. *Epidemiology.* 1990;1(5):408–412.
59. Fryzek JP, Lipworth L, Signorello LB, et al. The reliability of dietary data for self- and next-of-kin respondents *Ann Epidemiol.* 2002;12(4):278–283.
60. Fernández Hermida JR, Secades Villa R, Vallejo Seco G, et al. Evaluation of what parents know about their children's drug use and how they perceive the most common family risk factors. *J Drug Educ.* 2003;33(3):337–353.
61. Aboul-Enein FH, Ahmed F. How language barriers impact patient care: a commentary. *J Cult Divers.* 2006;13(3):168–169.
62. Bernard A, Whitaker M, Ray M, et al. Impact of language barrier on acute care medical professionals is dependent upon role. *J Prof Nurs.* 2006;22(6):355–358.
63. Westberg SM, Sorensen TD. Pharmacy-related health disparities experienced by non-English-speaking patients: impact of pharmaceutical care. *J Am Pharm Assoc (2003).* 2005;45(1):48–54.
64. Elderkin-Thompson V, Silver RC, Waitzkin H. When nurses double as interpreters: a study of Spanish-speaking patients in a US primary care setting. *Soc Sci Med.* 2001;52(9):1343–1358.
65. Bard MR, Goettler CE, Schenarts PJ, et al. Language barrier leads to the unnecessary intubation of trauma patients. *Am Surg.* 2004;70(9):783–786.
66. Cabana MD, Rand CS, Powe NR, et al. Why don't physicians follow clinical practice guidelines? A framework for improvement. *JAMA.* 1999;282:1458–1465.
67. Kosecoff J, Kanouse DE, Rogers WH, et al. Effects of the National Institutes of Health Consensus Development Program on physician practice. *JAMA.* 1987;258(19):2708–2713.
68. Pearson ML. Guideline for prevention of intravascular device-related infections. Hospital Infection Control Practices Advisory Committee. *Infect Control Hosp Epidemiol.* 1996;17:438–473.
69. Pearson ML. Guideline for prevention of intravascular device-related infections, I: intravascular device-related infections: an overview. The Hospital Infection Control Practices Advisory Committee. *Am J Infect Control.* 1996;24:262–277.
70. Rubinson L, Wu AW, Haponik EE, et al. Why is it that internists do not follow guidelines for preventing intravascular catheter infections? *Infect Control Hosp Epidemiol.* 2005;26:525–533.
71. Studdert DM, Mello MM, Sage WM, et al. Defensive medicine among high-risk specialist physicians in a volatile malpractice environment. *JAMA.* 2005;293(21):2609–2617.
72. Toker A, Shvarts S, Perry ZH, et al. Clinical guidelines, defensive medicine, and the physician between the two. *Am J Otolaryngol.* 2004;25(4):245–250.

73. Weiss AR, Binns HJ, Collins JW Jr, et al. Decision-making in the delivery room: a survey of neonatologists. *J Perinatol.* 2007;27(12):754–760. Epub 2007 Aug 30.
74. DeKay ML, Asch DA. Is the defensive use of diagnostic tests good for patients, or bad? *Med Decis Making.* 1998;18(1):19–28.
75. Glassman PA, Rolph JE, Petersen LP, et al. Physicians' personal malpractice experiences are not related to defensive clinical practices. *J Health Polit Policy Law.* 1996;21(2):219–241.
76. Elstein AS, Shulman LS, Sprafka SA. *Medical Problem Solving: An Analysis of Clinical Reasoning.* Cambridge, MA: Harvard University Press; 1978.
77. Neufeld VR, Norman GR, Freightner JW, et al. Clinical problem-solving by medical students: a cross-sectional and longitudinal analysis. *Med Educ.* 1981;15:315–322.
78. Brunkhorst FM, Engel C, Jaschinsky U, et al, and the German Competence Network Sepsis (SepNet). Treatment of severe sepsis and septic shock in Germany: the gap between perception and practice—results from the German Prevalence Study. *Infection.* 2005;33(Suppl 1):49.
79. Miles RW. Fallacious reasoning and complexity as root causes of clinical inertia. *J Am Med Dir Assoc.* 2007;8:349–354.
80. Greenes RA. "Desktop knowledge"—a new focus for medical education and decision support. *Methods Inf Med.* 1989;28(4):332–339.
81. Fouque D. Producing systematic reviews of best quality: a prerequisite for evidence-based nephrology. *J Nephrol.* 1999;12:314–317.
82. Palleroni NJ, Bradbury JF. *Stenotrophomonas*, a new bacterial genus for *Xanthomonas maltophilia* (Hugh 1980) Swings et al. 1983. *Int J Syst Bacteriol.* 1993;43(3):606–699.
83. Redelmeier DA, Shafir E. Medical decision-making in situations that offer multiple alternatives. *JAMA.* 1995;273:302–305.
84. Landrigan CP, Rothschild JM, Cronin JW, et al. Effect of reducing interns' work hours on serious medical errors in intensive care units. *N Engl J Med.* 2004;351(18):1838–1848.
85. Friedman RC, Bigger JT, Kornfeld DS. The intern and sleep loss. *N Engl J Med.* 1971;285:201–203.
86. Denisco RA, Drummond JN, Gravenstein JS. The effect of fatigue on the performance of a simulated anesthetic monitoring task. *J Clin Monit.* 1987;3:22–24.
87. Marcus A. "Doctors Blunder When Lacking Slumber." HealthDayNews, 2002.
88. Dawson D, Reid K. Fatigue, alcohol and performance impairment. *Nature.* 1997;388:235.
89. Feddock CA, Hoellein AR, Wilson JF, et al. Do pressure and fatigue influence resident job performance? *Med Teach.* 2007;29(5):495–497.
90. Shetty KD, Bhattacharya J. Changes in hospital mortality associated with residency work-hour regulations. *Ann Intern Med.* 2007;147:73–80.
91. Volpp KG, Rosen AK, Rosenbaum PR, et al. Mortality among patients in VA hospitals in the first 2 years following ACGME resident duty hour reform. *JAMA.* 2007;298(9):984–992.
92. Yerkes RM, Dodson JD. The relation of strength of stimulus to rapidity of habit-formation. *J Comp Neurol Psychol.* 1908;18(5):459–482.

CHAPTER 9 ■ HOW TO READ A MEDICAL JOURNAL AND UNDERSTAND BASIC STATISTICS

CHRISTOPHER LEE SISTROM • CYNTHIA WILSON GARVAN

"All men by nature desire to know."

Aristotle, Metaphysics

The practice of medicine has long been characterized as a combination of art and science. The exploration into the interactions of art and science in modern critical care medicine is a worthwhile endeavor, because it informs how we acquire knowledge and apply it in practice. With respect to the so-called "art of medicine," we believe that a better way to express this concept is with the term *expertise*. This is an essential quality that is manifest in individuals or small groups. Readers who have worked in an intensive care unit (ICU) will immediately recognize the importance of the individual as well as the collective expertise of teams of nurses and doctors in caring for acutely ill patients. Experts are often prepared with comprehensive formal education about their specialty. However, didactic instruction and reading alone are not sufficient to acquire practical expertise. The key to expertise is extensive and involves ongoing, direct experience in performing the activity in question. Expert practitioners learn from personal—sometimes bitter—experience about what works and what fails in their setting. This helps explain the growing popularity of "hospitalists" and "intensivists" during the past decade (1,2).

In this chapter, we will discuss some fundamentals integral to understanding the science of statistics and its application to medical research. We acknowledge that many of the ideas we present are not readily explained in a single book chapter. However, we hope that we will stimulate the reader to both seek expert assistance initially and pursue further study. We have provided a number of our favorite resources as suggested references. To make our explanations as concrete as possible, we cite several papers from core journals that deal with the problem of ventilator-associated pneumonia (VAP) since the problem of VAP is a common concern of all critical care practitioners. VAP serves as a useful example of a disease process with a specific definition, straightforward epidemiology, clearly articulated prevention strategies, and simple treatment options (i.e., various antibiotics). The study designs reported in these papers will include cross-sectional, cohort, and randomized clinical trials, and will illustrate various didactic points covered in the body of the chapter.

FROM INFORMATION TO KNOWLEDGE

So how does science inform expertise in ICU work and how should practitioners use the "product" of science—journal articles—to improve care? First, it is helpful to define science as a collaborative process for acquiring, validating, and disseminating knowledge. The last part of our definition—knowledge—deserves some elaboration. A common definition of knowledge is *justified true belief* (JTB) (3), which serves quite well for our purposes. It should be self-evident that to know something (we'll refer to it as "P") means that one must believe P, and that P must be true. A harder concept to understand is that true belief must be justified in order to qualify as knowledge. To put it succinctly, true belief without justification is simply a "lucky guess." This leads right back to defining the scientific method as an ongoing process for justification through empirical verification of shared belief. The goals of science are distinct from the method, and explicate the uses (applications) for the knowledge once it is acquired and corroborated. Most classic descriptions of scientific purpose include description, explanation, prediction, and control of the phenomena under consideration (3). Medicine is certainly an applied science, and the four goals are directly applicable when the phenomena of interest are human health and disease.

Journal articles and presentations at meetings are the main mechanisms for scientists in any field to advance, debunk, or corroborate various theories and hypotheses (i.e., advance and test knowledge claims). Critical care medicine is no exception, and this means that one ought to view individual papers that describe results and make claims from original research as part of a large work in progress, rather than any kind of established truth. Literature reviews, meta-analyses, and texts such as this one are written with the implicit acknowledgment of the contingent and dynamic nature of medical science and the knowledge it produces. A wonderful example of this dynamic is found in the controversy surrounding a clinical trial of ventilator settings for acute respiratory distress syndrome (ARDS) patients that was halted after an interim analysis, the results of which were released in advance of publication by the *New England Journal of Medicine* (4). Within weeks, rather intense and quite public criticism of the results and conduct of the trial was forthcoming from research subject advocacy groups as well as from within the academic community. These critics took issue with the trialist's choice of treatment arms, claiming that they "excluded the middle" in comparing tidal volumes of 6 versus 12 mL/kg when most practitioners generally used an intermediate setting (8–10 mL/kg).

Effective reading of the medical literature requires an understanding of the role that journal articles play in scientific progress as described above. Equally important is a facility for critical thinking, tempered by a healthy dose of skepticism. By critical thinking, we mean being able to make and understand logical arguments consisting of premises and conclusions. In medical literature, these premises are often descriptions of empiric evidence that are made in quantitative terms (i.e., statistics). The key to critical reading—and effective writing—of medical literature is to not get lost in the numbers and to focus on assertions of evidence—methods and results—and how they are used to support conclusions in the abstract and discussion sections. Skepticism may be restated as having an active bullshit (BS) detector. We use this term in all seriousness and with due deference to the philosophical work of Harry Frankfurt (5). He asserts that BS is increasingly common in modern society and proposes a quite simple and useful conceptual framework to handle it. Frankfurt articulates three distinct ways that people relate to the truth in what they say and write. These include telling the truth, lying, and BS. The difference between lying and BS is crucial and relates to the motives of the speaker/writer. Deliberately stating something that one believes to be untrue (i.e., a lie) implies an understanding and concern for what is actually true. In contrast, BS is produced with little or no regard for the truth status, coherence, or relevance of its content. To be successful, BS only has to be formulated and stated so as to sound good to the audience. By Frankfurt's definition, under the pressure of publish or perish, medical literature has its fair share of BS—and readers would do well to keep this in mind.

We firmly believe that readers of this text are principled and ethical professionals who would never knowingly make or condone untrue (or BS) statements concerning any aspect of patient care. Unfortunately, a few members of the industries associated with the practice of medicine have deliberately told partial truths and sometimes even outright falsehoods. This may occur during overzealous marketing of drugs and medical devices to both physicians and patients. Perhaps more difficult for the average reader of peer-reviewed medical journals to guard against is the undue influence of a large and increasing amount of industry sponsorship of clinical research. Editors of biomedical journals and local research oversight committees both share a growing concern about this issue and have policies in place to ensure disclosure of potential conflicts of interest. A growing social phenomenon, closely related to BS, is that of deliberate ignorance about potentially difficult truths in some industries. Dr. Robert N. Proctor from Stanford has even coined a name for the study of organizational ignorance: *Agnotology* (6). U.S. corporate culture has recently suffered from its tendency to ignore accounting and other structural problems until they threaten the existence of the company and land top executives in prison. Closer to home, we find high-profile cases of pharmaceutical companies brought to task for apparently ignoring or downplaying evidence of significant adverse events related to highly profitable drugs. By way of contrast, the physician culture seeks to expose difficult truths and learn from adverse events in the form of morbidity and mortality conferences. Another quite valuable kind of "afteraction" review can occur during a formal autopsy where the explicit question is, What actually happened to this patient? coupled with an implicit query about how things could have been done better. However, the tradition of postmortem examination and review of care seems well on its way to being abandoned (7).

In describing the nature of expertise in critical care medicine, we emphasized the importance of extensive personal experience by practitioners in learning how to make complex patient care decisions, and to quickly and effectively execute them. To acquire and maintain such expertise in critical care also requires general training about basic concepts of pathophysiology and therapeutics, as well as more discrete technical knowledge. A relatively new theory about optimizing and standardizing medical care holds that practitioners should routinely consult published evidence and/or official guidelines derived from research results. This is, of course, evidence-based medicine (EBM). Despite repeated claims that EBM is a new paradigm for medical practice, physicians have always used empirical observation supplemented with published evidence to acquire knowledge about the nature of illness, the probable course, and sequelae of disease, as well as the likely results of various treatment options. The assertion made by EBM proponents is that individual clinical experience is merely anecdote with limited power to explain, predict, or control the patient's medical problems. It should be noted that the EBM movement itself is subject to sharp criticism, though a relatively small amount has found its way into the mainstream clinical literature (8–10). One thread of this criticism argues that EBM purports to be a superior strategy for informing of clinical decisions, yet we have no randomized trials of care rendered under the EBM model versus more traditional (expertise-based) methods (11–13). As we will discuss below, there is a complementary "middle way" between anecdotal (single-case) evidence and meta-analysis of clinical trials to learn what works in a local practice.

Zealots of EBM may overemphasize the value of published clinical trials and meta-analyses at the expense of local evidence for guiding practice. It is important to distinguish regularly and systematically recorded local empirical evidence from personal anecdote. The former requires considerable resources, interdisciplinary cooperation, careful planning, and consistent execution to be useful. Anecdote is, by definition, based on singular events in the context of individual cases. We have already discussed the value of "afteraction" review in the form of morbidity/mortality conferences and formal autopsy. Another example of systematic local evidence is a database of critical care patients that allows clinicians and managers to have a snapshot of current case mix and clinical status. This same database can be retrospectively mined for quality indicators, clinical trends, and outcomes. As electronic medical records systems and computerized critical care management applications gain traction, some of the clinical data collection and storage will be automatically performed. In the meantime, we encourage intensivists to create, maintain, and routinely consult a robust database of clinical information about all of their patients. Simply sharing information among a critical care team about such things as rates of ventilator-associated pneumonia and skin breakdown stimulate both formal and informal efforts to standardize interventions and improve outcomes. Such local analyses can also help to focus reading of current literature as it emerges, as well as guide searches for published evidence, to answer specific clinical questions. Payers, regulators, and accreditation bodies are increasingly asking hospitals to report "quality indicators" that require exactly the sort of hospital-based process and outcomes analysis that we recommend above.

In subsequent sections of this chapter, we will describe and illustrate some basic principles of study design and statistical analysis. One purpose of this explanation is to provide readers with tools to critically analyze the published literature pertaining to medical practice in the ICU setting. Some readers engaged in or planning a career in critical care or related research will undoubtedly find this material to be rather rudimentary. However, in keeping with our proposed "middle way," where intensivists routinely collect data about their own patients, simple analytic methods can be quite useful. These include calculating rates, proportions, incidence, prevalence, and risk as well as simple bivariate statistics from cohorts of critical care patients.

THE BAYESIAN–FREQUENTIST DIALECTIC

Empirical observation about almost anything we encounter can be predicated in one of three ways: Always, never, or sometimes. Our experience in medicine—and, indeed, most things—is generally of the "sometimes" variety. Thus, to make sense of complex and varying evidence over time, it was necessary to start recording, counting, and tabulating things and events. It can be argued that this is the main reason humans developed methods of counting, numbers to represent the results, and eventually mathematics. Quantifying observations, incorporating the resulting numbers into premises, and using normative methods for making and validating inferential conclusions are the *raison d'etre* of probability theories and related statistical methods. Using these tools, enumerative inductions can be quantified with increasing sophistication. Over the past three centuries, western scientific methods have been spectacularly successful at describing, explaining, predicting, and sometimes controlling natural phenomena including human disease, disability, and death. During this time, two separate ways of conceptualizing about and calculating with quantitative empirical data have been articulated. These are, of course, the frequentist and Bayesian paradigms. What follows will draw on concepts from several fields including philosophy of science, biostatistics, and medical decision making. Experts in these disciplines may feel that we are oversimplifying or distorting some of these concepts and, for that, we apologize.

The *frequentist paradigm* is related to scientific realism, a view which holds that the universe is deterministic. Theories are further from, or closer to, some absolute reality, and accepting a theory implies belief that it actually is true. Population parameters are defined as being real, fixed, and singular (i.e., they are constants rather than variables). Causal and correlative relationships are likewise fixed and uniform. Any variance or error in our estimations of parameters and relationships between them come from only three sources: Sampling, unobserved factors, and measurement. In this view, if one could "simply" measure the right things precisely and often enough, a complete understanding of a "clockwork" universe would be attained. This translates into a very particular way to view the results of experiments and statistical inference. Hypotheses are tested by calculating the probability of observing the results of an experiment or sample measurement given a specific answer or parameter value. A clinical trial of drug treatment for a particular disease is a classic example. The assumption is that there actually is a fixed and immutable answer to a question of the form, Does drug A work better than placebo in treating disease X? Analyzing the trial produces a single yes/no answer to that question, and the uncertainty is expressed as the chance that the answer would be wrong if we could repeat the experiment over and over (type I and type II error).

Clinicians function in a largely frequentist world. They make dichotomous (yes/no) decisions about disease status and categoric (choice between types) decisions about treatment based on what they believe to be definitive diagnoses. The basic logic behind clinical decisions parallels that of frequentist hypothesis tests: "I am going to make a choice under uncertainty about the disease that my patient has and how to treat it. I know that I will be wrong some of the time and seek to minimize that frequency but will never eliminate it." The relative frequency of making the wrong diagnosis or selecting the wrong treatment is analogous to frequentist type I and type II errors.

The *Bayesian paradigm* is related to empiricism. This philosophic view holds that all we can ever know about is what we have observed. There is absolutely no way of knowing whether the data-generating process is deterministic, stochastic, or chaotic. Further, for any given set of observations, there is an infinite set of theories that could explain it—this is called *underdetermination*. In selecting theories, the main criteria is that they are empirically adequate (agree with the data). Belief in a theory in any absolute sense simply because it agrees with observations is never justified. Population parameters are viewed as not necessarily fixed or even ever knowable. Formal Bayesian theory holds that parameters have distributions of possible values. In contrast, the frequentist theory relies on fixed parameters and only allows samples to have distributions. Under Bayesian reasoning, hypothesis testing takes the form of calculating the probability that the parameter takes a certain value given the observed data and our past experience. Note that this is exactly opposite to the frequentist ordering where we take the population parameter as given and ask questions about the probability of observing the data.

The Bayesian world view is often represented as being incompatible with frequentist thinking. Modern Bayesians advocate a revolutionary paradigm shift in biostatistics and medical decision making (14,15). This is modeled after Thomas Kuhn's description of scientific revolutions exemplified by heliocentric replacing geocentric cosmology, and Einstein's relativity versus Newtonian physics (16). In fact, Bayes introduced the concepts of prior and posterior probabilities about a century before Fisher and Pearson struggled over frequentist methods for analyzing agricultural experiments (17). One reason that frequentist methods for statistical testing initially became popular was that the required calculations were relatively easy to perform by hand. With the advent of powerful computers in the late 20th century, Bayesian statistics became possible to compute, and their conceptual advantages could be realized in practice. The ideas behind Bayesian decision making seem to be more understandable to most physicians, as evidenced by the common misapprehension of frequentist core principles such as the p value and confidence intervals (18,19).

Most physicians are familiar with a small subset of the Bayesian paradigm, though it is known by the deceptively inclusive name of "Bayes Theorem." The theorem quantifies how prior probability for disease X is modified by a Bayes factor (the likelihood ratio) derived from knowledge about test performance and the current patient's test result (20). The product of this operation is the posterior probability of disease X in our patient, given the test result (positive or negative). The posterior probability is known as the positive or negative predictive value of the test. To illustrate the Bayes Theorem, consider the following example taken from Armitage (21). From genetic theory, it is known that a woman with a hemophiliac brother has a probability of being a carrier of a hemophiliac gene. A recombinant DNA diagnostic probe test provides information that contributes toward discriminating between carriers and noncarriers of a hemophiliac gene. The prior probability of the woman being a carrier for the gene is 0.50. This probability will be modified after the DNA test result is known, resulting in the posterior probability that the woman is a carrier given either a negative or positive test result.

MOTIVATIONS FOR READING MEDICAL LITERATURE

There are many reasons for reading medical literature. Patients and family members often desire to educate themselves in order to become better advocates. Medical students and residents read articles for problem-based learning sessions and journal clubs. Physicians read articles in order to "keep up" with the medical literature and also to learn more about treating an individual patient. Physician researchers stay abreast of their research fields by regularly reading journals in their area of expertise. Physician researchers may also read articles in a peer review process. Finally, policy makers at various levels (e.g., government, payers, hospital, ICU directors) read and synthesize medical research in order to write guidelines and make informed policy decisions. Various reasons for reading medical literature will determine the extent of statistical expertise and rigor required for critical assessment. Herein we will touch on basic statistical concepts, discuss common study designs, and provide guidelines for critical reading of medical literature. *Interpreting the Medical Literature* (22) is a useful resource for many consumers of medical journal articles. We also recommend *The Handbook of Research Synthesis* by Cooper and Hedges (23) for more detail on methodology for in-depth medical literature reviews including meta-analysis.

Basic Statistical Concepts

Statistics is the science of collecting, describing, and analyzing data. It is the science that provides the analytical framework for transforming information into knowledge. Of course, this knowledge is imperfect unless, perhaps, a biologic mechanism is identified that completely explains a phenomenon. Statistical methods quantify the imperfection of knowledge by providing results with an associated measure of error (e.g., level of significance, p value, margin of error).

There are statistical concepts underpinning nearly every aspect of research, a process that includes the following six steps:

1. Pose a research question and formulate into statistical terms
2. Design a study
3. Collect data
4. Describe data
5. Analyze data using statistical inference
6. Answer the research question

Basic statistical concepts in the research process will be outlined below, but first, we give some vocabulary:

- *Population*—entire group of individuals of interest
- *Sample*—a subset of the population

TABLE 9.1

NOMENCLATURE AND SYMBOLS OF STANDARD PARAMETERS AND ASSOCIATED STATISTICS

Characteristic	Population parameter	Statistic
Mean	μ	$\overline{X}$
Median	η	$\widetilde{X}$
Variance	σ^2	S^2
Standard deviation	σ	S
Proportion	π	p
Correlation	ρ	r
Regression coefficient	β	b

- *Data element*—a measurement or observation on an individual
- *Population parameter*—a summarizing characteristic of all possible data values such as a population mean or proportion (the value of a population parameter is usually the object of a research question)[1]
- *Statistic*—any quantity calculated from data
- *Inference*—process of extending or generalizing information known about a sample to the entire population
- *Probability distribution*—assignment of probability to the possible values of data that could be observed
- *Sampling distribution*—assignment of probability to the possible values of a statistic that could be observed

Table 9.1 gives the notation for common population parameters and the corresponding statistics that estimate them. Figure 9.1 shows the relationship between a probability distribution (represented by the dotted line) and a histogram. The probability distribution of a set of all possible values of a measure (e.g., all possible ages, all possible values of the PaO_2/FiO_2 ratio, all possible plateau airway pressures, etc.) is conceptual and not observable, whereas a histogram can be graphed from sample data. We have insight into the actual shape of the probability distribution from observing the outline of the sample histogram; the more data we have, the more refined our histogram is, and the true shape of the probability distribution of the data emerges more clearly.

In the "big picture" view, the science of statistics turns information into knowledge by connecting the object of a research question (an unobservable population parameter) into evidence provided by a research study (observable data) through statistical theory. Here we will assume the frequentist paradigm. For example, an investigator asks a research question such as the following: "What is the incidence of ventilator-associated pneumonia?" The research question is then "translated" statistically into a question about a population parameter. The "incidence of ventilator-associated pneumonia" is a population proportion (i.e., π). A research study will be designed, and data from a sample will be collected. To analyze the data, an inference will be made. In other words, information from the sample will be generalized to the entire population. Figure 9.2 illustrates a hypothetic population and sample. Each circle represents an individual in a critical care setting. Dark

[1] *Population* generally refers to the group of individuals of interest, but in the term *population parameter*, population refers to the "population" of all possible values of a measure (i.e., data element).

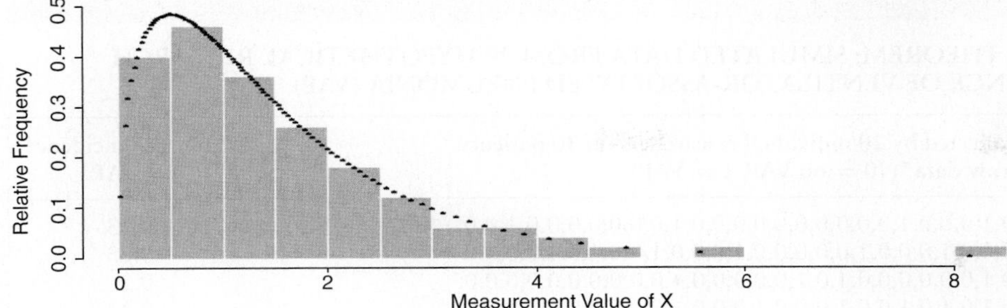

FIGURE 9.1. The "measurement value of X" represents numerical data, such as PaO_2/FiO_2 ratio. A histogram of sample data is graphed with bars indicating the relative frequency of observations in a given interval. The population of measurements is distributed according to a probability density curve (*dashed line*).

circles are patients who have VAP. As Figure 9.2 indicates, a valid inference depends on obtaining data from a sample that fairly represents the population of interest—hence, the concept of random sample, a sample free from systematic bias in the way it is chosen or retained in a study.

Valid inference also depends on the selection of an appropriate statistical method to analyze data. Statistical methods are based on statistical and mathematical theory. They all assume certain conditions (e.g., random sample, large sample size, normally distributed data, etc.) in order to provide valid results. Researchers (typically a team of physicians and biostatisticians) are responsible for choosing appropriate statistical methods and checking that no violations of assumptions have occurred. Statistical methods work like this: My research question is about a *population parameter* (e.g., incidence of VAP, a population proportion, π). Using my data, I can compute a *statistic* that estimates the unknown population parameter (e.g., incidence of VAP in my sample, a sample proportion, p). I will then apply the correct *theory* that will connect the statistic I have observed to the population parameter of interest. The theoretical connection occurs through the mathematical knowledge of the sampling distribution of a statistic. To better understand the idea of sampling distribution, refer to Table 9.2.

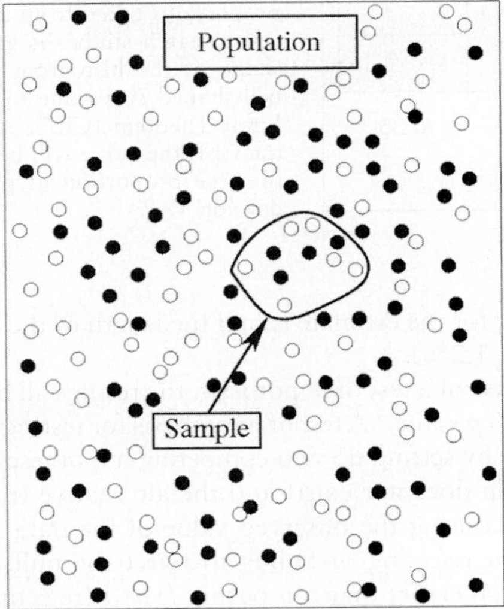

FIGURE 9.2. Each circle represents an individual in a critical care setting. Dark circles are patients who have ventilator-associated pneumonia (VAP). When statistical inference is conducted, information from the sample is extended (or generalized) to the population of interest. Thus, the proportion of patients with VAP would be estimated to be 40% $\pm$ a margin of error based on the sample data.

Suppose that 20 research teams are interested in estimating the incidence of VAP, and each team can observe 30 patients. Table 9.2 contains the raw data and the sample proportion (i.e., observed incidence of VAP) obtained in each study. In this conceptual framework, we can think of the statistic (e.g., sample proportion, p) as having a probability distribution (i.e., sampling distribution). I can visualize the probability shape of the sample proportion by graphing a histogram (Fig. 9.3).

In the case of a sample proportion, the Central Limit Theorem (CLT) tells us that under certain conditions (i.e., random sample and large sample size), the shape of the sampling distribution will be normal, centered at the value "π." Note that the histogram in Figure 9.3 has an approximately normal shape. The CLT also tells us that the center of the normal curve is "π," the true incidence rate of VAP. Here is the power of the statistical method; even if we do not know the probability shape of the original data, under conditions that are not too difficult to achieve, we (approximately) know the probability shape of the statistic and its connection to the population parameter of interest. We can then use this connecting theory to conduct inference. This "central" idea (hence the namesake of the Central Limit Theorem) is depicted in Figure 9.4 for the case of numerical data—say, the ages of patients who develop VAP in a critical care unit. In this case, the CLT tells us that the shape of the sampling distribution of the sample mean ($\overline{X}$) will be normal, centered at the value "μ"—the population mean—even though the probability distribution of the original data is not normal.

The theory underlying statistical methods generally requires the understanding of probability and calculus, and thus is something of a "black box" for many. For a more in-depth discussion about statistical inference, see Cox (24).

There are three basic goals of statistical inference:

1. Estimation
2. Test of hypothesis
3. Prediction

In the *estimation* type of inference, the research question is concerned with estimating some characteristic or feature of a population of measurements (e.g., what is the incidence of VAP?). In the *test of hypothesis* type of inference, the research question is concerned with testing a relationship (e.g., does protocol-driven weaning reduce the incidence of VAP?). Finally, the *prediction* inference type of research question estimates a characteristic or feature of a population of measurements that will be observed in the future (e.g., what will be the incidence of VAP in 10 years' time?). The form of statistical results will depend on the inference goal. In the case of estimation, the result will be reported in terms of a confidence interval. A confidence

TABLE 9.2

ILLUSTRATION OF CENTRAL LIMIT THEOREM: SIMULATED DATA FROM 20 HYPOTHETICAL RESEARCH STUDIES AND CALCULATED INCIDENCE OF VENTILATOR-ASSOCIATED PNEUMONIA (VAP)

Research team identifier	Data collected by 20 individual researchers on 30 patients (i.e., "raw data") (0 = no VAP, 1 = VAP)	Observed incidence of VAP
1	0,0,0,0,1,0,0,0,1,0,0,0,0,0,0,0,0,0,0,1,0,0,0,0,0,0,0,1,0,0	0.13
2	0,1,0,0,0,0,1,0,0,0,1,0,0,0,0,0,1,0,0,0,1,0,0,1,0,1,0,0,0,0	0.23
3	1,0,1,0,1,0,0,0,0,0,0,1,0,1,0,0,0,0,0,0,1,0,0,0,0,0,0,0,0,0	0.2
4	1,0,0,0,1,0,1,0,1,0,0,1,0,0,0,1,0,0,0,1,0,0,0,0,0,0,0,0,0,0	0.23
5	0,1,0,0,0,0,0,0,0,0,0,0,0,0,0,0,0,0,0,0,0,0,0,0,1,0,0,0,0,0	0.07
6	1,1,0,0,0,0,1,0,1,0,1,1,0,0,0,1,0,0,0,0,0,0,0,0,0,1,0,0,0,0	0.27
7	0,0,0,1,1,0,0,0,0,0,0,0,0,0,1,1,0,0,0,1,0,0,0,0,0,0,0,0,0,1	0.2
8	0,0,1,0,0,0,1,0,1,0,0,1,0,0,1,0,0,0,0,1,0,1,0,1,0,0,0,0,0,1	0.3
9	1,0,0,0,1,0,0,0,0,0,0,1,0,0,0,0,0,1,0,1,0,0,0,0,0,0,0,0,0,0	0.17
10	0,0,1,0,1,0,0,0,0,0,0,0,0,0,0,0,0,1,0,0,0,0,0,1,0,0,0,0,0,0	0.13
11	1,0,1,0,0,0,1,0,0,0,0,1,0,0,1,0,0,1,0,0,0,1,0,0,0,0,0,0,0,0	0.23
12	0,0,0,0,1,0,1,0,1,0,0,1,1,0,0,0,0,0,0,1,0,1,1,0,0,0,0,1,0,1	0.33
13	1,0,1,0,1,0,1,0,0,0,0,1,0,1,1,0,0,0,0,1,0,0,0,0,0,0,0,0,0,0	0.27
14	0,1,0,0,0,1,0,0,0,0,1,0,0,0,0,0,0,0,0,0,0,0,1,0,0,0,0,0,0,0	0.13
15	0,1,1,0,1,0,1,0,1,0,0,0,0,0,1,0,0,0,0,1,0,0,0,0,0,0,1,0,0,1	0.3
16	0,0,1,0,0,0,1,0,0,0,0,1,0,0,1,0,1,0,1,0,0,0,0,1,0,0,0,0,0,0	0.23
17	1,1,0,0,1,0,1,0,1,0,0,0,0,0,0,0,0,0,0,0,0,1,0,0,0,0,1,0,0,0	0.23
18	1,0,0,0,1,0,1,0,1,0,0,1,0,0,1,0,1,0,0,1,1,0,0,0,1,0,0,0,1,1	0.4
19	0,0,1,0,0,0,0,0,0,0,0,0,1,0,0,1,1,0,0,0,0,1,0,0,0,0,0,1,1,0	0.23
20	0,0,1,0,1,0,1,0,1,0,0,1,0,0,1,0,0,0,0,1,0,1,0,0,0,0,0,0,1,1	0.33

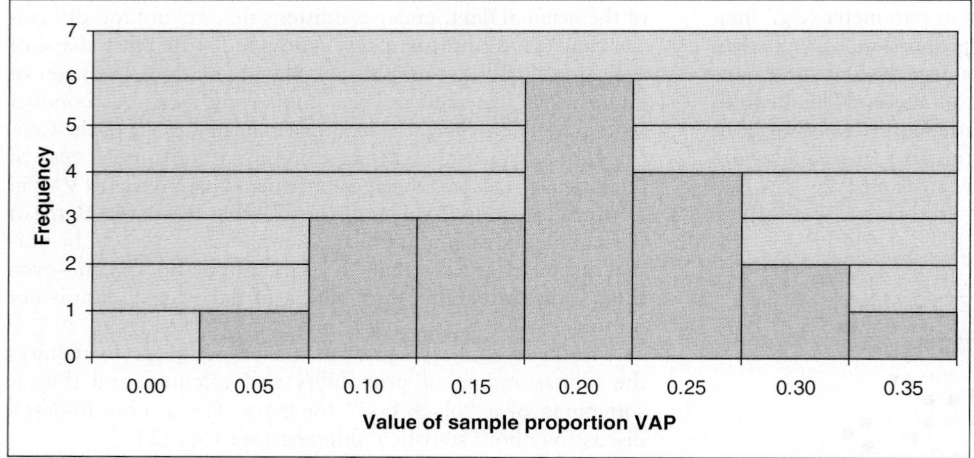

FIGURE 9.3. The histogram of ventilator-associated pneumonia (VAP) proportions taken from 20 hypothetical research studies is graphed. The shape of the histogram resembles a bell-shaped curve due to the Central Limit Theorem (CLT). According to the CLT, the curve will be centered at the true proportion of patients who develop VAP.

interval gives a plausible range of values for a population parameter such as a mean, a proportion, or an odds ratio, along with a measure of method success (i.e., the confidence). Tejerina et al. found that VAP was present in 439 out of 2,897 patients, 13.2%. Based on these data, a 95% exact confidence interval (CI) for VAP is given by (12.0%, 14.4%) (25). This means that in 95 out of 100 studies, the true value of VAP incidence would be captured in the constructed confidence interval.[2] The margin of error for the estimate is half the length of the confidence interval (or 1.2%).

In the case of a test of hypothesis, the result will be reported in terms of a *p* value.[3] A test of hypothesis for testing a relationship works by setting up two competing hypotheses—the null (relationship does not exist) and the alternative (relationship exists)—and using the observed value of the data to provide evidence for rejecting or failing to reject the null. There are two potential errors that can occur: *Type I* (rejecting the null hypothesis when it is true) and *type II* (failing to reject the null

[2]A 95% confidence interval does not mean that there is a 95% probability that the true value of the population parameter falls in the interval. In the frequentist paradigm the population parameter is considered a fixed, absolute value. The probability that this value falls inside the confidence interval is either 0% or 100% (i.e., it either falls inside or outside).

[3]A *p* value is the probability of the observed data (or data showing a more extreme departure from the null hypothesis) when the null hypothesis is true.

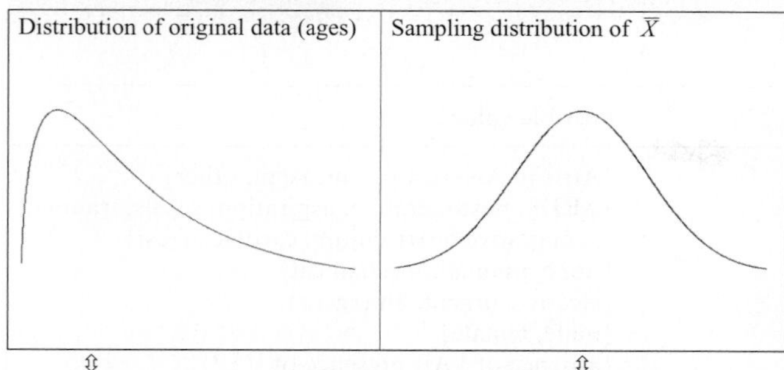

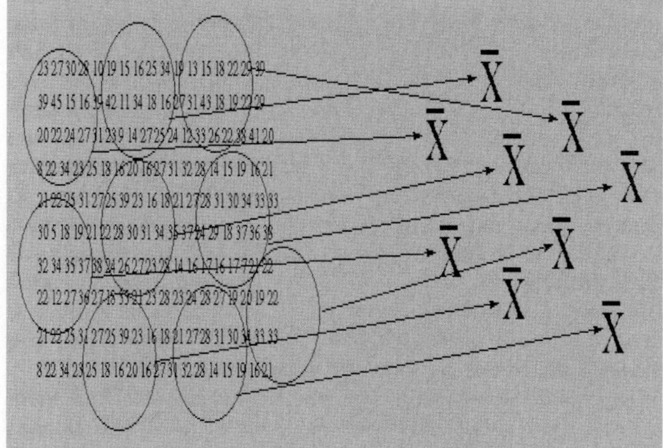

FIGURE 9.4. Data is sampled from a probability distribution of any shape. In this illustration the original data comes from a distribution that is skewed right. Suppose multiple studies are conducted and for each study the statistic $\overline{X}$ is calculated from the sample data. The Central Limit Theorem posits that the distribution of the statistic is normal with mean μ, the population mean of the original data.

hypothesis when it is false). The *power* of a test is the probability of rejecting the null hypothesis when it is false (the reverse of the probability of type I error). The observed value of the data (i.e., the value of the test statistic) provides a p value that is compared to a predetermined level of significance, also known as alpha (α) or the probability of type I error. When the p value is smaller than the set level of significance (typically set at 0.05), there is evidence for rejecting the null hypothesis and concluding that a relationship exists between two factors. When the p value is larger than the set level of significance, then the test conclusion is to fail to reject null hypothesis. Evidence for concluding that there is no relationship between two factors depends on designing a study with adequate power to detect a "meaningful" relationship.

Tejerina et al. conducted a series of tests of hypotheses to test the relationship of factors thought to be associated with the development of VAP (e.g., gender, neuromuscular disease, sepsis, type of ventilation). They found a number of factors that were significantly related to VAP at the 0.05 level of significance. For example, sepsis was significantly associated with development of VAP (p value less than 0.001). The odds ratio of sepsis and VAP (estimate of the strength of association) was given as 19.9 with 95% CI as (15.7, 25.4). This means that the odds of developing VAP in patients with sepsis were 19.9 times higher than the odds of developing VAP in patients who did not have sepsis. The 95% confidence interval gives a plausible range of values indicating that a feasible range for the odds ratio is as low as 15.7 and as high as 25.4. In 95 out of 100 studies the true value of the odds ratio will be captured in the 95% CI.

In the case of inference where prediction is the goal, the result will be reported in terms of a prediction interval. A prediction interval is analogous to a confidence interval but will be calculated in such a way to reflect the additional source of variation due to estimating future values. Estimating the incidence of VAP in 10 years' time would be an example of inference with prediction as its goal.

After collecting the data, we use two main tools to describe it: graphs and summary statistics. A list of summary statistics is given in Table 9.1. In the analysis step, we will use a statistical method that can generally be classified as a univariate, bivariate, or multivariate[4] method, according to the number of data elements involved in the research question. For example, estimating VAP involves one data element and would be considered a univariate analysis. Investigating the relationship of type of ventilation and VAP would be a bivariate analysis. Analyses involving more than two data elements are commonly referred to as "multivariate." The choice of statistical method will depend on the inference goal, the number of data elements in the analysis (i.e., univariate, bivariate, and multivariate), and the data type(s).

There are five data types:

1. Categorical nominal
2. Categorical ordinal
3. Binary
4. Numerical discrete
5. Numerical continuous

Data types are determined by the possible values a data element can have. Categorical data have values that are names or categories and not meaningful numbers. The categorical ordinal data type has values that can be ordered. The categorical nominal data type has values that have no natural ordering. Binary data have two values. Numerical discrete data when graphed are isolated points on a number line, while numerical continuous data have values that can be conceptually viewed as an interval on the number line. Table 9.3 gives examples of data types from the critical care literature. Table 9.4 lists the most common statistical methods with a brief description of each. For more detail about statistical methods, see Motulsky (26), Armitage et al. (21), and D'Agostino et al. (27). Understanding how statistical methods are applied is crucial to understanding the "evidence" that EBM generates. As Gauch wrote, "Method precedes results; method affects results. Method matters" (28).

The sixth and final step of the research process—answering the research question—is of paramount importance. Researchers present results in the form of technical reports, abstracts, posters, oral or platform presentations, manuscripts, and books. Writing and presenting results clearly is an art form in and of itself. The research is not complete unless important patterns are summarized, the specific aims of a study are addressed, methods are described clearly, and the "story" of the

[4]In technically precise terms, a multivariate analysis involves the analysis of outcome data that is multidimensional (e.g., cluster analysis, factor analysis, principal components, etc.). A common usage of "multivariate analysis," though, is an analysis that includes more than two variables (e.g., multiple regression, logistic regression, etc.).

TABLE 9.3

VARIABLE TYPES

Data type	Examples	Possible values
Categorical nominal	* Race	{African American, Caucasian, other}
	* Causes of acute respiratory failure	{ARDS, postoperative, aspiration, sepsis, trauma, congestive heart failure, cardiac arrest}
Categorical ordinal	* Ventilation type	{none, manual, mechanical}
	* Type of surgery	{elective, urgent, emergent}
Binary	* Gender	{male, female}
	* VAP	{absence of VAP, presence of VAP}
Numerical discrete	* Number of prior surgeries	{0, 1, 2, 3...}
	* Number of central venous lines	{0, 1, 2, 3, ...}
Numerical continuous	* Age	{0 to 100+ years of age}
	* PaO_2	{80 to 100 mm Hg}

ARDS, acute respiratory distress syndrome; VAP, ventilator-associated pneumonia.

data is told. For more on writing about the results of statistical analyses, see *The Chicago Guide to Writing about Numbers* and *The Chicago Guide to Writing about Multivariate Analysis*, both by Jane Miller (29,30).

Types of Research Studies

The statistical methods used to analyze research data depend on how the study that gave rise to that data was conducted. There are four basic types of study designs used in clinical research:

1. Cross-sectional
2. Case control
3. Cohort
4. Experimental (clinical trials)

For the following discussion about these study designs, we need to clarify some terms that are commonly used to describe medical research and epidemiologic findings. These may have different meanings depending on the context they are used in. These terms include sample, outcome, factor, exposure, treatment, and control.

TABLE 9.4

STANDARD STATISTICAL TECHNIQUES, TESTS, AND TOOLS

Statistical method	Scenario
z-test, t-test, Wilcoxon signed rank test	Inference about population mean from one population
z-test	Inference about population proportion from one population
z-test, t-test, Wilcoxon rank sum test	Inference about difference of population means, two independent populations
Paired t-test, Wilcoxon signed rank test	Inference about difference of population means, paired data
z-test, chi-square test	Inference about comparing two population proportions, independent populations
McNemar's test of paired categorical data	Inference about comparing row and column marginal frequencies
Pearson correlation, Spearman correlation	Inference about correlation of bivariate numerical data
chi-square test	Inference about bivariate categorical data
ANOVA, Krukal Wallis test	Inference about population means of independent groups
Repeated measures, ANOVA	Inference about population means of independent groups in the case of repeated measures
Multiple regression	Inference about relationship of numerical response and set of categorical and/or numerical explanatory variables
Logistic regression	Inference about relationship of binary response and set of categorical and/or numerical explanatory variables
Longitudinal analysis	Inference about data arising from a vector of measurements representing the same variable observed at a number of different time points
Survival analysis	Inference about "time until event" data
Hierarchical linear model	Inference about data arising from a "nested" or "multilevel" design where one or more factors are subsampled within one or more other factors in such a way as to restrict certain combinations (e.g., for a study of surgery patient outcome, "doctor" as a factor is nested within "hospital" as a factor)

ANOVA, analysis of variance.

TABLE 9.5

COMPARISON OF FOUR STUDY DESIGN TYPES

	Cross-sectional	Case control	Cohort	Experimental
Sample selection	One sample selected without regard to outcome or factor status	Multiple samples selected based on outcome status: Outcome present (cases) and outcome absent (controls)	Multiple samples selected based on factor exposure status	One sample selected with outcome status identical Sample randomized to treatment or control group
What is measured	Status of both outcome and factor(s)	Status of factor(s) in case and control groups	Status of outcome in exposed and unexposed groups	Status of outcome in treated and control groups
Time reference	Present look at time	Backward look in time	Forward look in time	Forward look in time
Example reference	*J Crit Care* 2002;17(3):161	*Chest* 2002;122(6):2115	*J Crit Care* 2006;21(1):56	*Am J Resp Crit Care Med* 2006;173(12):1348

- The term *sample* refers to the subjects being studied in the research. This reminds us that we are looking at a subset of a population of interest and that the purpose of the research is to apply what we find out about the sample to the population.
- The *outcome* of any research is handled in statistical analysis as the independent variable. The outcome is what we are primarily interested in understanding, treating, or preventing. In medical research, the outcome often relates to some disease or condition, with the simplest results being present or absent. In the following critical care–related examples, VAP (present or absent) will serve as the outcome. Defining and determining outcome (disease) status in clinical research and epidemiology is a large subject in itself. We will stipulate that there is an unambiguous and agreed upon way to measure the outcome status in the following discussion and examples.
- A *factor* is measured along with the outcome to determine if there is a correlation between them. In statistical parlance, factors are referred to as independent variables while the outcome is the dependent variable. The structure of relationships between factors and outcome is often quite complex, which, under the philosophy of scientific realism, reflects some underlying causal structure. In our example of VAP, factors that have positive association with VAP are considered to be risk factors. On the other hand, a protective factor has a negative association with the outcome (VAP). Note that we avoid directly asserting that an association between factor and outcome implies that the factor causes or prevents the outcome in deference to the old—and still true today—saying that correlation does not prove causation.
- With respect to a factor, *exposure* simply refers to the status (or level) of the factor in a particular subject. In the case of VAP (outcome), we would say that a patient in a coma is exposed to the risk factor of obtundation. Perhaps the best known example to both professional and lay public is lung cancer (outcome) with a risk factor of tobacco use to which a person is exposed if he or she is a smoker.
- In any clinical research, factors and outcomes are things that we seek to observe, measure, and record, but not influence. In contrast, a *treatment* (or intervention) is something that is actively controlled by the investigator. Conveniently, statistical terminology uses the term *treatment* in the same spirit as implied in clinical research. That is to say, treatment is an experimentally manipulated factor whose influence on the outcome we are interested in knowing.
- In experimental studies, the term *control* group refers to subjects that do not receive any treatment. In case control studies (described further below), *control* subjects are those who do not have the outcome in question.

Table 9.5 summarizes the features of the four types of clinical research designs in their simplest forms, and they are each described below in more detail. We also include an example from current core literature in critical care medicine to illustrate the principles. It would be useful for readers to obtain copies of these papers and review them along with our explanations. Please note that these studies often used more complex and involved methods of statistical analysis including secondary outcome measures. However, we will focus only on primary outcomes, factors, or treatments, and simple relationships between them. The order in which we present the design types reflects increasing cost, time, and potential risk or inconvenience for patients. Thus, observational and retrospective studies (cross-sectional and case control) are discussed first, followed by prospective cohort studies and clinical trials.

Cross-sectional

A cross-sectional study does not involve the passage of time. A single sample is selected without regard to outcome or risk factor exposure status. Information on outcome and exposure status is determined with data collected at a single time point. The status of the outcome can be compared between exposed and unexposed groups. It is important to understand that even though we may define one attribute as the "outcome" and others as "factors," there is no logical way to determine anything other than the current relationship between them. Without additional information, there is no valid way to infer even the temporal order of factor levels and outcome status, let alone any causal connection.

Our example comes from the *Journal of Critical Care* (31). It is titled "Prevention of ventilator-associated pneumonia: current practice in Canadian intensive care units." In this study, Heyland et al. wanted to know the current status of VAP prevention strategies in Canadian ICUs prior to disseminating a new set of clinical guidelines. There is not really a defined "outcome" in this study; rather, a number of factors of interest were simultaneously measured. Such a study design is sometimes called a "snapshot." In this case, dietitians recruited by the investigators directly observed VAP prevention strategies in ICUs throughout Canada on a single date (April 18, 2001). Since the 66 observers recorded data for every patient currently in their assigned ICU, the unit of analysis was a single patient (N = 702). The investigators followed up the initial observations by manually abstracting the medical chart entries from April 18, 2001, for each of the 702 patients. Again, the unit of observation was a single patient. Finally, surveys were filled out by 66 ICU directors that asked questions about the regular practices relating to VAP prevention on their unit; thus, the unit of observation for this part of the study was an individual ICU (N = 66). These three methods are good examples of the various ways that cross-sectional data can be gathered and aggregated.

From the many results presented in this paper, we present a few examples of the sorts of statistics that are typically reported in cross-sectional studies. From the survey of ICU directors, we get results like university affiliation (29/66 = 44%) and number of beds (mean = 13.9). From the observations and chart abstractions, authors report patient gender (women = 299/702 for 43% and men = 403/702 for 57%), intubated and ventilated (403/702 for 57%), and patient age (mean = 63.5 years). As for VAP prevention strategies from direct observation, we have elevation of head of bed (mean = 30 degrees) and kinetic bed therapy (22/702 for 3%). From the survey of unit directors, 61 of 66 (92%) responded that they never used special endotracheal tubes that allowed subglottic secretion drainage, and none stated that they used prophylactic antibiotics. This example is typical of cross-sectional studies in that only descriptive statistics (as just described) are necessary and usually suffice. Additional methods that might be used in analyzing a cross-sectional study such as this one would be simple statistics to quantify relationships (correlation) between measured factors (none was reported in the paper). For example, at the ICU level, authors could have used survey results to look for a relationship between university affiliation and VAP strategies such as subglottic secretion drainage. This would be done by cross-tabulating the two variables into a 2 × 2 table in this case. The appropriate statistical method to test for a significant relationship between two categoric variables is a chi-square test (or the Fisher exact test in the case of sparse cell sizes).

Case Control

In a case control study, the investigator compares individuals who have a positive outcome status (the cases) and individuals who do not have the outcome (the controls). In the simplest implementation of the case control method, one or more control patients (outcome negative) are chosen for each case (outcome positive). When the outcome being studied is relatively rare, there are often more available candidates for controls than for cases in the sample available for study. A subsample of available controls is usually selected to match the cases on characteristics (factors) that might be related to the outcome but are not of primary interest to the research question. For example, it is common to match on gender and age by finding a single control subject with same gender and similar age for each case. This is called 1:1 (control:case) matching. When there are many more outcome-negative (control) candidates, investigators may use 2:1, 3:1, or greater (control:case) matching ratios while still maintaining similarity between each case and its controls (e.g., gender and age).

Investigators look backward in time (i.e., retrospectively) to collect information about risk or protective factors for both cases and controls by examining past records, interviewing the subject, or in some other way. Unlike with a cross-sectional study, we can get an indication of whether the factor status predated the development of the outcome by asking the questions carefully. However, case control studies are subject to well-known bias in assessing presence and timing of risk/protective factors. It is very important to understand that in a case control study, the outcome frequency is fixed in the design, which means that we cannot directly estimate risk of the outcome. We can estimate relative risk of the outcome between different status levels of the factors by calculating the odds ratio between cases and controls for each factor. This estimate of relative risk will be biased, depending on the actual prevalence of the outcome in the population of interest and the relative numbers of cases and controls. For example, in a 1:1 case control study, the outcome frequency is, by definition, 50%. If the actual frequency of the outcome in the population is less than 10%, the odds ratios will severely overestimate the relative risk increase or reduction. The raw odds ratios may be corrected for this bias to form a better estimate of relative risk, though this is rarely done in practice.

An example of a case control study looking at factors associated with VAP can be found in *Chest* (32). It is titled "Epidemiology and outcomes of ventilator-associated pneumonia in a large US database" and was written by Rello et al. The investigators used information from a large (750,000/year) database of inpatient hospital (N = 100) admission abstracts (MediQaul-Profile Database) for 18 months beginning in January of 1998. They first identified 9,080 patients having at least 1 day of mechanical ventilation in the ICU during their hospitalization without an admission diagnosis of pneumonia. Of these, 842 (9.3%) developed pneumonia after initiation of ventilation, thus meeting criteria for VAP. From one to three controls (VAP negative, N = 2,243) were selected to match each case (VAP positive, N = 842) on duration of ventilation, severity of illness on admission, and age. It is important to note that after this step, none of the matched factors can be meaningfully evaluated because their distributions were forced to be in direct proportion to each other during the process of matching.

Investigators calculated odds ratios between cases and controls for several factors that might alter risk of developing VAP in practice; these included gender, race, obtundation, and type of ICU admission (trauma, medical, surgical) among others. As an example of how such results are evaluated, the numbers of males and females in VAP-positive cases were 540 (64%) and 302 (36%) and for VAP-negative controls were 4,262 (52%) and 3,976 (48%), respectively. The odds ratio male:female is calculated by (540)(3,976)/(302)(4,262) = 1.67. This can be interpreted by stating that the odds of VAP in males are 67% greater than for females, which can be used as an estimate of the relative risk of VAP in males compared with females. Note that in the original sample of patients, the frequency of VAP was 9.3%, whereas in the case:control sample used to estimate relative risk in males, it was 27%. Thus, the estimate of relative risk should be revised downward by methods that are beyond the scope of this chapter.

Cohort

A cohort is a group of individuals. The term comes from Roman military tradition where legions of the army were divided into ten cohorts, and each in turn divided into centuries. These cohorts "march forward together" in time. In a typical prospective cohort study, investigators follow subjects after study inception to collect information about development of the outcome (disease). In a retrospective study, outcome status is determined from records produced prior to beginning the study. The cohorts are articulated based on information about risk factors predating the outcome determination. In both types, initially outcome-negative (disease-free) subjects are divided into groups (cohorts) based on exposure status with respect to a risk factor. Cumulative incidence (the proportion that develops the outcome in a specified length of time) can be computed and compared for the exposed and unexposed cohorts. The main difference between prospective and retrospective cohort studies is whether the time period in question is before (retrospective) or after (prospective) the study is begun. In terms of bias and error in measuring outcome and risk factors, the retrospective cohort design is more problematic because we must rely entirely on historical records to know that subjects were initially outcome negative, what their risk factor status was, and the subsequent outcome status over time.

Despite logistical difficulty and expense, prospective cohort studies are very attractive to investigators because they allow direct estimation of absolute risk for the outcome of interest as well as differences in outcome based on various risk (or protective) factors (relative risk). In general, outcomes that develop quickly are easier to evaluate prospectively since the study will be finished sooner, with less chance for subjects to drop out or be lost to follow-up. Critical care medicine lends itself quite well to prospective cohort studies for this reason.

An example of a multinational and quite complex cohort study comes from the *Journal of Critical Care* (25). The title of this paper is "Incidence, risk factors, and outcome of ventilator-associated pneumonia" and Tejerina et al. report results of a study encompassing 361 ICUs in 20 countries. The cohort in question included 2,897 consecutive ICU patients who were mechanically ventilated for more than 2 days, with reason for admission not being pneumonia. These patients were a subset from a larger (N = 5,183) and already completed prospective study. Even though the authors analyzed existing data, they properly labeled their study as prospective because the patients were entered into the original study at time of admission to ICU, and all information was sequentially recorded in a database as the research progressed.

The outcome of VAP was strictly defined using Centers for Disease Control and Prevention (CDC) criteria prior to study inception and measured for each patient on a daily basis as yes/no. Though it may seem a trivial point, it is important to note that all patients had a VAP status of "no" on the first day of their ICU stay. Multiple baseline and clinical factors were measured. In the results section, the authors first considered the entire sample as a single cohort and reported the incidence of VAP as 439/2,897 (15%). There is not a meaningful hypothesis for the simple question of VAP incidence in the whole cohort, and we are instead making an estimate of VAP incidence in the population. Because of the large sample size, the authors were able to place 95% confidence intervals on this estimate of 14% to 16%.

In reading the rest of the results, it is helpful to think of each separate factor as dividing the entire study group (N = 2,897) into "subcohorts." For example, gender would give two cohorts (male = 1,809 and female = 1,088) for which VAP incidence was 293 (16%) for the males and 142 (13%) for the females. When considering the factor of problem type (medical = 1,911 and surgical = 986), the VAP incidence was 322 (17%) for medical and 117 (12%) for surgical. The null hypothesis in each of these "subcohort" studies is that VAP incidence is equal between the factor levels (male/female and medical/surgical). In these two examples, the null hypothesis was rejected for each of the factors (gender $p = 0.02$ and problem $p < 0.001$). Below, we give an example of a randomized trial with a sample size in each of three groups of about 130. The percentages of VAP are similar in magnitude as are the intergroup differences (roughly 18%, 10%, and 13%). However, because of the smaller sample size, the results do not reach statistical significance (at the 0.05 level).

There are two problems with doing multiple separate tests for simultaneously measured factors in a big study such as this one. First, the measured factors quite probably interact with each other in a complex way in their combined effect on VAP development. Thus, in any single (univariate) analysis such as with gender and VAP, the calculated relationship may be confounded with one or more other factors, and therefore biased away from the actual effect. Second, it is problematic to look at the same set of data repeatedly using different factor combinations because by sheer chance, 1 in 20 such tests will be "significant" at the 0.05 level. The optimal solution to both these problems is to perform multivariable regression analysis where the joint effect of all variables is tested simultaneously. The authors of this paper did such analyses, though the details are beyond the scope of this chapter. Suffice it to say, gender showed no significant effect on VAP after accounting for all other factors while problem still did. Finally, it is important to note that multivariable analysis cannot rescue a study from being confounded by unmeasured factors. The only certain way to avoid confounding is through the random assignment of factor levels prior to measuring the outcome (i.e., an experimental study).

Experimental (Clinical Trial)

In an experimental study (called a clinical trial in medical research), the investigator selects a sample of subjects with the same outcome status and randomly assigns each to a treatment (or intervention) condition. Subjects are followed in time, and the status of the outcome is measured and compared between the treatment groups. Thus, experiments and clinical trials are, by definition, prospective. As described above, the term *control group* is used for subjects that do not receive any treatment or intervention. Sometimes patients who are given "standard" treatment are said to be in the control group. A randomized experiment is the only way to definitively establish causality by empirical means. Similarly, for testing medical treatments and interventions, randomized trials are the only sure way to determine clinical efficacy. Both necessary and sufficient conditions to establish causality between a factor or treatment and outcome status are met in a randomized trial. These include unambiguous temporal association of cause before effect and elimination of any potential confounding factors (measured or unmeasured) that might affect the outcome. This helps to explain what may seem to be near-worship of the "prospective randomized clinical trial" in many discussions about medical research.

A good example of a randomized clinical trial comes from the *American Journal of Respiratory and Critical Care Medicine* (33). The title of this paper is "Oral decontamination with chlorhexidine reduces the incidence of ventilator-associated pneumonia," which nicely describes the research question and the result. The investigators, Koeman et al., wanted to determine if two oral decontamination regimens would reduce incidence of VAP in intubated patients. They performed a classic double-blinded, placebo-controlled clinical trial where 385 eligible patients were randomized to three treatment arms. These included chlorhexidine 2% (CHX), chlorhexidine 2% and colistin 2% (CHX/COL), and water (PLAC). During the ICU stay, all patients got mouth swabbing at identical intervals with the type of solution unknown to those caring for the patients. The primary outcome was carefully defined and evaluated using chart abstraction by a team of physicians who did not know the treatment assignment. These two design elements satisfy the definition of a double-blinded study because neither patients and providers nor those determining the outcome knew what the treatment assignments were. The first table in the results (their Table 1) shows baseline characteristics grouped by treatment assignment. Such a table is always included in any complete report of a randomized trial. The baseline characteristics are measured and presented because they might also influence the outcome (VAP). We are always reassured to see relative equality of the baseline characteristics because it shows us that "randomization works." Note that the true power of randomized treatment assignment lies in the fact that we know that any other factors or characteristics that were not anticipated and/or measured will, by definition, also be equally distributed between the treatment arms. Some might rightfully observe that such baseline characteristic tables are superfluous to the core logic of a randomized trial. We carry on presenting them because they are reassuring and otherwise informative.

The outcome can be most simply expressed as an incidence of VAP during the ICU stay with individuals having a yes/no answer. When tabulated, the results (VAP/total) were PLAC = 23/130 (17.7%), CHX = 13/127 (10.2%), and CHX/COL = 16/128 (12.5%). The trialists performed sophisticated statistical techniques using days to onset of VAP and survival analysis, as well as interim analyses to allow early termination of the trial. These are beyond the scope of this brief chapter. The null hypothesis in this study is that the incidence (hazard in survival analysis) of VAP was identical among all three treatment arms. The alternate hypothesis is that one or more of the treatment groups had significantly different incidence (hazard) of VAP. A chi-square test on the simple incidence of VAP between the treatment groups gives a p value at 0.20, which indicates that the null hypothesis cannot be rejected. However, using survival analysis, authors found that both CHX ($p = 0.012$) and CHX/COL ($p = 0.030$) reduced the hazard of VAP compared with PLAC.

This is a good example of how the type of outcome variable analyzed affects the power of a study to detect differences. For simple counting of VAP incidence, the outcome variable is dichotomous (yes/no), while for survival analysis, the outcome variable is quantitative (days to development of VAP). In general, outcomes that are defined and measured numerically have "more information," and thus greater power to detect small differences, than categoric or dichotomous ones. In the paper cited above, the authors did not report the results of the simple chi-square test, which failed to reject the null hypothesis. We can speculate that if the chi-square statistic on simple VAP incidence had shown significant differences, the authors would have reported it. Finally, we recall the results of our cohort study example with similar VAP percentage differences but much larger sample size. In that study, the achieved p values were much lower, reflecting the greater power of large samples to demonstrate small effects.

CRITICAL READING OF THE MEDICAL LITERATURE

Articles in the medical literature generally follow a prescribed structure consisting of the following components: (a) title, (b) author list, (c) keywords, (d) funding source, (e) abstract, (f) objective and hypothesis, (g) background, (h) methods (includes study design, measures, and data analysis), (i) description of sample, (j) presentation of findings and results, (k) discussion and conclusions, and (l) references.

Statistical aspects permeate a large number of articles in the medical literature. Miller (30) describes the similarity of writing about statistical analysis to the presentation of a legal argument. She writes:

> In the opening statement, a lawyer raises the major questions to be addressed during the trial and gives a general introduction to the characters and events in question. To build a compelling case, he then presents specific facts collected and analyzed using standard methods of inquiry. If innovative or unusual methods were used, he introduces experts to describe and justify those techniques. He presents individual facts, then ties them to other evidence to demonstrate patterns or themes. He may submit exhibits such as diagrams or physical evidence to supplement or clarify the facts. He cites previous cases that have established precedents and standards in the field and discusses how they do or do not apply to the current case. Finally, in the closing argument he summarizes conclusions based on the complete body of evidence, restating the critical points but with far less detail than in the evidence portion of the trial.

Good scholarly writing should resemble a good legal argument. Good writing in the medical literature should also provide transparency of method in sufficient detail to allow for results to be replicated. Research quality is difficult to evaluate but integral to the process of "taking information to knowledge"—the ultimate goal for reading medical literature. Evaluation of literature and judging research quality is itself an academic discipline within the larger science of literature review. In broad strokes, we can group indicators of quality that are relevant to statistical considerations into the following categories: sampling and participation, measurement, data management, analytic framework (includes study design and statistical analysis), and reporting of results. Below we outline the structure of an article and point out quality indicators to look for in the "anatomy" of a research article.

Title, Author List, Keywords, and Funding Source

A good title can convey important information about the topic of a manuscript and can let readers know what is new or different about the work. For example, in a classic paper published in the journal *Intensive Care Medicine* (34), the title speaks eloquently of the content: "Prevention of nosocomial pneumonia in intubated patients: respective role of mechanical subglottic secretion drainage and stress ulcer prophylaxis." Much has been written about the content and ordering of author lists for scientific journal articles and it should suffice to say that "honesty is the best policy." Keywords are popular and certainly useful, though they represent the author's subjective decisions about what is important. Ultimately, the National Library of Medicine staff does an excellent job of generating structured abstracts (e.g., MESH terms) from biomedical journal articles using the whole paper to do so. These PubMed database entries have become the dominant means by which the scientific community searches through the medical literature. Given the discussion above concerning the influence of corporate support on the conduct of research, it is vital that funding sources and author conflicts of interest be clearly and completely stated in any published paper. In the case of public or nonprofit research support, virtually all such agreements require authors to acknowledge the funding source in any related publications.

Abstract

Although we know that we should spend time in analyzing the medical literature, it is clear that, given the pressures of everyday life and the journals that appear with seemingly increasing frequency on our desks each month, we are often tempted to read only the title and the abstract. One final caveat: There may be important disparities among the results, discussion, and abstract. One memorable report compared two forms of fluid resuscitation. Three patients in one group had been given from two to three times the amount specified in the protocol. With exclusion of these patients properly in the data analysis, *as noted* in the results section, there were *no* differences between the two groups. With inclusion of patients with protocol violations, there was a "statistically significant" difference. The abstract cited the "statistically significant" analysis without any reference to the patients who should have been excluded. The authors' conclusion of a statistically significant difference in treatment modalities was, in fact, denied by their own results. If you are in a hurry, do not just read the abstract and move on; come back and read the article properly when you have enough time.

Objective and Hypothesis

Obviously, the most pertinent starting point is an understanding of the investigator's objective. The investigator has the obligation to state clearly and specifically the purpose of the study conducted, but this may be difficult to discern. In such cases, we may question whether the author had, indeed, a clear objective. "Fishing expeditions," that is, extensive data collection projects with the intention of exploring and identifying important relationships, achieve success when the captain knows where the fish are. In other words, the so-called gold mine of data does not guarantee that statistical search will lead to "pay dirt" and reveal important new relationships. The author, or we as researchers, must formulate specific objectives and a clear-cut hypothesis for testing. Lack of an understanding of objectives handicaps the reader and the author in any assessment or interpretation of the results.

A more specific and somewhat more subtle question in assessing objectives is classification of a study as descriptive and exploratory versus analytic. Using epidemiologic terminology, descriptive studies are those that "describe" diseases, characterize disease patterns, and explore relationships, particularly in regard to person, place, and time. Such studies mainly serve the purpose of "hypothesis generation." The specific hypothesis can then be tested by an analytic study, one whose primary objective involves the test of a specific hypothesis.

To illustrate this distinction, a descriptive study reported the use of high-level positive end-expiratory pressure (PEEP) in acute respiratory insufficiency in patients who developed severe, progressive, acute respiratory insufficiency despite aggressive application of conventional respiratory therapy (35). Later, the term *optimal PEEP,* introduced in the first study, was updated in another descriptive study of 421 patients reported in 1978 (36). The second study entailed treatment of a large group with respiratory failure using titration of PEEP in conjunction with intermittent mandatory ventilation, but using cardiovascular interventions to support cardiac function until a preselected end point of 15% shunt could be achieved. The first study represented a description of the development of a treatment regimen; in the second study, refinements in this treatment regimen were applied to a broader population. Later, a hypothesis was constructed to test whether, in moderate arterial hypoxemia, there was any improvement in patient outcome or resource utilization using "optimal PEEP" compared with similar modalities of therapy, with an end point defined as achievement of nearly complete arterial oxygen saturation at nontoxic inspired oxygen fractions.

The hypothesis that PEEP titration to achieve an intrapulmonary shunt of less than 20% would have a better outcome or would achieve faster resolution of the disease process could not be substantiated in the analytic study (37). The two descriptive studies (35,36) identified a specific hypothesis that the third or analytic study tested.

Background

The background is generally an introduction with rationale on why the research that is being presented is important. This section should also contain a literature review and argument to show how the current research fills a gap in previous work. Sufficient detail on how the literature review was conducted should be reported so that it can be reproduced. The background should also reference seminal papers in the research area.

Methods: Study Design

The reader should consider carefully the definitions of the groups studied and the population to which the investigators intend to refer their findings. For instance, in the three PEEP studies quoted, the reader might assume that the failure to prove the hypothesis in the third study invalidated the findings of the two earlier descriptive studies. The third, an analytic study, however, involved only patients with early and moderate arterial hypoxemia. The original group of patients that was studied specifically excluded these patients and concentrated on developing therapy for those who had persistent hypoxemia despite aggressive application of conventional respiratory therapy. Thus, a technique that reversed hypoxemia in patients who were refractory to the then "conventional therapy" of acute respiratory insufficiency was found not to be useful in another population that had only moderate hypoxemia and did not have true adult respiratory distress syndrome. If the authors do not state clearly the populations with which they are dealing, the readers can easily lose this important distinction. This has even greater importance in review articles that may omit the important qualifiers or modifiers found in the original reports. The fact that a particular form of therapy useful in advanced disease has no particular advantage in patients with mild disease indicates that therapy should be restricted to patients who can benefit from treatment, rather than arrive at some alternative conclusion that titration of PEEP to preselected end points has no advantage.

The reader should examine carefully the methods section for a description of the study design, a definition of inclusion/exclusion criteria, and information about data management. A sample size justification should be given in the methods section that indicates the expected precision when the objective of a study is to estimate an unknown quantity or a power analysis when the objective of a study is a test of hypothesis, such as testing the relationship of groups (e.g., treatment group vs. control group) on a certain measure.

Epidemiologically, there are two major classifications of study design: experimental and observational. Loosely defined, an experimental study is one in which the investigator has control over or can manipulate the major factor under study. The epitome of the experimental study is the randomized controlled trial in which the investigator demonstrates "control" over the factor under study by randomizing patients to various regimens. Many prophylactic and therapeutic studies tend to be experimental in design. It cannot be assumed that just because a study was experimental and the investigator may have randomized patients that the study was well done and its conclusions are valid. Experimental studies are prone to various sources of bias and to poor execution. The label *randomized* is not equivalent to assurance of high quality, nor does it alone add validity to the study. Thus, randomized studies also need careful assessment of their design, methods, analyses, and conclusions. One other factor, *blinding,* is often viewed as an attribute of the highest-quality studies. If subjective elements are used to judge the effectiveness of treatment, there is a compelling rationale to blind the investigators. If there are subjective assessments of the patients' response, there is a compelling rationale to blind the subjects. If all of the outcome variables are objective, blinding, strictly speaking, is unnecessary. Thus, in the assessment of a new medication to relieve pain, double blinding (both subjects and investigators) is necessary.

When the investigators cannot manipulate the major factor under study, they must rely on what has been observed; this study is an observational study. We should not view observational studies as being inferior to experimental studies. Clearly, a tight, well-designed, well-executed experimental study carries the greatest strength of evidence, but observational studies can also provide substantial, sound medical evidence. In fact, a well-planned and well-executed observational study can be much more informative than a weakly designed and poorly executed randomized study. There are various approaches to the design of observational studies, such as cross-sectional, case control, prospective cohort, and retrospective cohort. The interested reader should consult basic epidemiology or statistics textbooks for further descriptions of these various design strategies and for the relative strengths and weaknesses of each design format (38,39).

With respect to observational studies, the reader should determine whether the data collection was prospective or retrospective. The principal advantage of prospective data collection is that the researchers, having clearly identified the objectives, can ensure collection of this relevant information in a manner that they can determine. Retrospective analysis of medical records depends on what happens to appear in the record, often with no indication of the manner in which the information was obtained. For example, gender, age, and hospital outcome (survival or death) are key data elements that may not appear for *every patient* in a retrospective chart review. Clearly, without a specified protocol, the researcher cannot anticipate that a daily blood gas, serum creatinine, or any other intermittent measurement dependent on a specific order will appear in the chart. Everyone should attempt a retrospective study (at least once) to learn the pitfalls and the impossibility of obtaining a complete database. This would enable each of the then-frustrated researchers to read other retrospective studies both with a great deal of deserved skepticism and with empathy for the difficulties with such research.

Selection of the study group is another important step. The researcher should look for possible sources of selection that would make the sample atypical or nonrepresentative. A sample selected by a random selection mechanism is generally more representative than a "convenience" sample; however, this is difficult to achieve. Allocation of treatments by a random mechanism is more achievable, but even such seemingly "random" allocation of cases such as alternate days may introduce an unappreciated bias. For instance, the Trauma Service at the University of Miami/Jackson Memorial Medical Center had two separate teams that alternated coverage every 24 hours. Patients admitted on alternate days, therefore, are cared for by different teams of physicians. A study that entailed alternate-day assignment to treatment groups would entail, as well, the factor of differences in physician practice style, a factor that could not be disentangled in analysis of study results.

We must also consider the nature of the control group or standard of comparison. We frequently encounter the "historical control" group that usually has a "poorer" result than the contemporary group. The problem, of course, is that the basic assumption that the modality of treatment under investigation is the only cause for the difference in results is clearly erroneous. It has been tempting to ascribe the remarkable reduction in wartime mortality from World War II to Korea to Vietnam to the marked diminution in delay between injury and treatment. However, the entire surgical training experience changed during that time, an almost completely new pharmacopoeia was available in Vietnam, and, most assuredly, many other variables are yet unaccounted for between the two eras. In fact, the principal reason for randomization in a study is to attempt to distribute the unknown and potentially important variables equally among groups to avoid selection bias. We may also see this effect if subjects accrue slowly and the study thus runs over many years. Other aspects of therapy may change and have a greater impact on outcome than the original variable selected for study.

Two aspects of clinical research that sometimes perplex beginning researchers and inexperienced readers are validity and generalizability. *Validity* deals with the ability of a study to give a scientifically sound answer to the question posed. Insofar as possible, this answer should be free from bias, uninfluenced by the effects of other related or confounding variables and with good statistical precision. Only then is there a basis for a *valid* study result.

Generalizability deals with extrapolation of study findings to a larger population or to other groups. Assessment of generalizability depends on the degree to which the study subjects are representative of some larger target population and how well the selection of study subjects simulates the process of drawing a random sample from a population.

The ideal is for studies to be both valid and generalizable. In practice, this is rarely the case. In the design of clinical research, investigators face many situations in which they must choose between validity and generalizability. When faced with a choice, undoubtedly they should opt for validity. Without a valid study, an investigator has little or nothing of scientific merit. The investigator may have actually drawn a random sample from a larger population and have virtually ideal generalizability. But, if in the process validity was threatened or compromised, the findings are worthless. With findings of questionable or doubtful validity, there is nothing of value to generalize. Generalizability plays a subordinate role and, in fact, should not surface until validity has been firmly established. Often the reader must assume the onus of assessment of generalizability and of whether findings can be extrapolated to other populations.

Methods: Measures

In the reporting of research results, clarity in the definitions of the terms and measurements made has great importance. The more clearly the authors (or we as potential researchers) define the terms, including diagnostic criteria, measurements made, and the criteria of outcome, the more likely it is that we, the readers, can interpret the findings correctly and gain a proper perspective. For instance, in the field of invasive catheter-related infection, terms such as *colonization, contamination,* and *infection of the catheter* abound. Authors often use these terms differently, leading to great difficulty in interpretation and synthesis of results from different studies. Furthermore, a "positive culture" may represent different bacteriologic methodologies: Some authors use a semiquantitative culture of an intracutaneous catheter segment (40), whereas others use blood cultures aspirated through the catheter (41). Clearly, results from one methodology may not be comparable to another, and interpretations based on differing methodologies may lead to different conclusions.

We must also try to evaluate the methods of classification or of measurement. The essential question is to assess whether inconsistencies in observation or evaluation could have sufficient impact to influence materially the results of the study. We also must evaluate the reliability and reproducibility of the observations; this is more difficult to assess. Frequently, some clues inform the reader of the author's concern with and awareness of reproducibility and reliability. When a subjective element enters into an assessment, an author often refers to and sometimes provides data on the results of evaluations by independent observers and their degree of agreement. *Interrater reliability* refers to the ability of two or more independent raters to make the same observations. *Intrarater reliability* refers to an observation made by the same rater over two or more different times. With respect to abstracting information from charts, interrater and intrarater reliability is usually in the range of only 80% to 90%. An author who devotes some attention to issues concerning measurement or laboratory error seemingly would be cognizant of the importance of reproducibility and reliability. It is well to be suspicious of results from a study that seems entirely devoid of concern with these elements, especially if some subjective element is clearly involved in diagnosis, observation, or assessment of outcome.

Methods: Data Analysis

In reality, the first question we, as readers, should ask is, Are the data worthy of statistical analysis? We must then examine the methods of statistical analysis to determine whether they were appropriate to the source and nature of the data and whether the analysis was correctly performed and interpreted. These questions are difficult to answer. However, we recognize that this is an entire field to itself for which this chapter should stimulate the reader to pursue more vigorous study.

One of the first issues that should cross the reader's mind is to ask whether the observed and reported finding could result simply from chance, the luck of the draw, or sampling variation. An arsenal of statistical methodology is available ranging from simple (e.g., t-test, chi-square test) to sophisticated (multiple logistic regression, Cox proportional hazards model) to examine the role of chance in the analysis of study results. Each medical reader may not have sufficient expertise to assess whether the investigators have chosen their methodology appropriately and have correctly performed the statistical analyses. Authors should provide rationale and references for innovative or unusual methods. A discussion of loss to follow-up, detection of outliers, item nonresponse, and possible imputation of missing data should be included in the data analysis section. Authors should clearly describe the analytic framework of a research study. Readers should beware when multiple analyses (i.e., "data fishing") are conducted without appropriate adjustments. We hope that the journal's peer review process has included some form of assessment of the statistical aspects of the report. Until we, the readers, learn enough, we must solicit expert biostatistical assistance. A biostatistician can evaluate more complex issues in addition to assessing the appropriateness of statistical methods. These include model diagnostics such as fit indices and the results of sensitivity analysis (if performed).

Description of the Sample

The CONSORT statement (http://www.consort-statement.org) is an important research tool that has been endorsed by prominent medical journals such as *The Lancet, Annals of Internal Medicine,* and the *Journal of the American Medical Association.* The CONSORT guidelines offer a standard way for researchers to report clinical trials that is appropriate for adaptation by other types of research studies. Authors should provide readers with a clear picture of the progress of all study participants, from the time they are assessed for enrollment until the end of their involvement. Information about reasons for loss to follow-up should be clearly stated. When authors describe the sample, sociodemographic and other descriptive information relevant to the study (e.g., medical history, disease severity and duration) should be clearly reported.

Presentation of Findings or Results

Authors must walk the fine line of clear and concise data presentation in the results section without editorializing or drawing conclusions from the data they presented. Remember, the facts should speak for themselves. The author must still detour into enough necessary detail for the reader to judge the importance of the data. Important findings require proper documentation. If a small number of subjects are presented, a table listing the important demographic characteristics is useful so that the reader has a clear understanding of the population studied.

It is surprising how often numerical inconsistencies are contained within reports published in even the most reputable medical journals. This may be partly caused by the many drafts and revisions compounded by textual proofreading, computational and tabular proofreading, and other processes. Because of the frequency of these errors, the reader may wish to use some quick checks: Columns and rows should add up to their indicated totals; percentages of mutually exclusive categories should add up to 100%; numbers in tables and figures should agree with those in the text; and totals in various tables describing the same population should agree. With the ubiquitous presence of hand-held calculators and personal computers, we can even run some of our own statistical tests, especially when the reported results appear incompatible with our quick mental assessment or even personal bias!

Clarity and precision are important criteria to judge the overall scientific validity of an article. Assessments, comparisons, and judgments belong in the discussion section. However, when these are enthusiastically included in the results section, they strongly suggest bias in the author's approach. Strictly speaking, investigators should undertake an analytic study when they can wholeheartedly support affirmation or rejection of the hypothesis under test. Thus, inclusion of subjective opinions (e.g., "markedly improved outcome") in the results section may be a subtle indication that the investigators performed the study to confirm their pre-existing personal views.

However, three points should be remembered. First, it is the author's responsibility to provide the reader with information on the specific statistical analysis used in assessing the role of chance. Second, whatever the level of significance reported, no matter how small the p value, we can never rule out chance with certainty. An exceedingly small p value (1 instance in 1,000) denotes that chance is an unlikely explanation of the result, but the possibility remains, although unlikely, that this is indeed that 1 instance in 1,000. The third point is that a statistically significant result is not necessarily important or indicative of a real effect, only that an effect of chance has been ruled out with some reasonable certainty.

As clinicians, we know that measurements of pulmonary artery occlusion pressure (PAOP) differ among observers. For instance, estimation of PAOP from a visual inspection of the

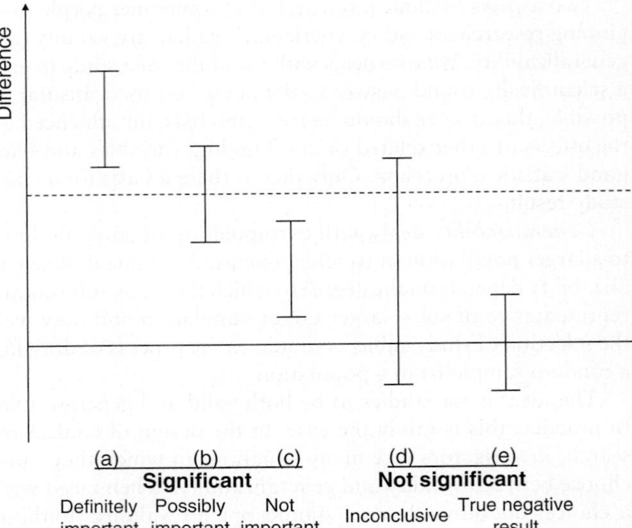

FIGURE 9.5. Suppose two groups are compared on a numerical measure and the confidence interval for the mean difference between groups is calculated. The threshold that corresponds to a meaningful difference between the groups is indicated by the *dashed line*. Five results are possible. Confidence intervals in cases (a), (b), and (d) capture or fall above the "importance" threshold, and thus are candidates for practical importance or "clinical significance." Cases (a) and (b) are statistically significant since they do not contain zero (confidence intervals containing zero indicate no difference between groups). Case (c) is statistically significant but not practically important. Case (e) is neither statistically nor clinically significant. (From Berry G. Statistical significance and confidence intervals. *Med J Aust.* 1986;144:618–619; reprinted in *J Clin Pract.* 1988;42:465–468.)

oscilloscope tracing may be 3 to 4 mm Hg different from the results calculated electronically and displayed in digital form on the monitor. In reviewing the effects of a drug, however, some investigators may interpret a change of the same magnitude (3–4 mm Hg) as an "effect" of the therapy. Thus, in addition to deciding whether a particular result is "statistically significant," that is, if it represents a real event (or results from chance), we must decide whether it has any real clinical, biologic meaning. Figure 9.5, adapted from Berry (42), illustrates five possible relationships between statistically significant and clinically significant results. Confidence intervals depicted in the figure are intervals that give plausible ranges of the difference between two groups. Confidence intervals in cases (a), (b), and (d) capture or fall above the "importance" threshold, and thus are candidates for practical importance or "clinical significance." Cases (a) and (b) are statistically significant since they do not contain zero (confidence intervals containing zero indicate no difference between groups). Case (c) is statistically significant but not practically important. Case (e) is neither statistically nor clinically significant.

Furthermore, in our interpretation of study results we must, with reasonable certainty, rule out the possibility of *bias* and *confounding*. A result may be highly significant statistically but the study design and conduct could lead to a substantially biased result, or there may be some other related variable that also explains statistically significant results.

Confounding refers to effects of one or more related variables. In its strict epidemiologic definition, a confounding variable is one that is associated with both the "exposure" (independent variable) and the "outcome" (dependent variable) under study. For example, in an observational study comparing the mortality experience of two modalities of treatment for head injuries, an obvious "confounding" variable would be the severity of the injury. Clearly, the severity of the injury relates to the dependent variable under study: Mortality. The injury severity, however, may also have an association with the independent variable: The choice of the particular modality of treatment. Thus, any finding of a difference in mortality between modalities of treatment, even if statistically significant, might be explained by the confounding effects of the severity of injury.

The important point is to judge whether the authors have considered all of the pertinent known confounding variables in their analyses and have taken proper steps to account for their effects. The reader, without substantive knowledge of the particular field of study, may be unable to delineate what pertinent potential confounding variables should have been considered. We (authors and readers) must cautiously proceed with forming conclusions.

Bias refers to a systematic departure from the truth. Bias may exist in many forms, and many statistical and epidemiologic adjectives can precede the word "bias" to denote some specific hazard or snag that can lead to a departure from the truth. Sackett (43) provides a useful compendium of the various biases that lurk to ensnare the unwary investigator, and the unwary reader, in the conduct of biomedical research. We shall use the three adjectives: selection, observation, and analysis.

Selection bias refers to how subjects were entered into the study. Is the manner of selection of persons for study such that the study will result in substantial distortion of the truth? As a simple example, consider a study comparing outcome of surgery in patients who agree and volunteer to undergo the operation with those who refuse. Those who choose surgery may be better operative risks (at least from their own perception), probably with less comorbid disease than that found in the nonsurgical group. Of course, other factors may have influenced the other group to refuse surgery. Still, the difference in the outcome of surgery might be more likely to result from the selective nature of the groups rather than from any real effect of the surgical procedure.

Observation bias refers to the methodology for handling and evaluating subjects during the course of the study. If a therapeutic intervention group receives more attention, more supportive therapy, and more intense scrutiny than a control group, an observed difference in outcome might more likely be explained by observation bias rather than by any real effects of the intervention. Retrospective studies are particularly prone to observation bias.

Analysis bias refers to fallacies that exist in the choice of statistical methods to analyze data. An example is the "average age at death" fallacy. Calculation of average age at death among decedents does *not* measure longevity; it reflects mainly the age composition of the total members of the groups, mostly those who are alive. For example, consider a newspaper report of a study that compared the average age at death of U.S. professional football players with professional baseball players (44). The report stated that football players died, on average, 7 years earlier than baseball players. It would be erroneous to conclude that this differential reflects the more hazardous and traumatic aspects of professional football compared with professional baseball. In fact, professional football is a much newer sport (dating from the mid-1920s) than professional baseball (dating from the 1860s). Consequently, the total group of professional baseball players is considerably older than the total group of professional football players. As an extreme example of this average-age-at-death bias, consider the result anticipated in a comparison of the average age at death in a children's hospital with that in a retirement community hospital.

When, in the assessment of a study, we can rule out with reasonable certainty that the finding does *not* result from chance, bias, or confounding, we are well on the road to determining a real and meaningful effect. Finally, it is important to emphasize that the interpretation of *statistical significance* does not in and of itself connote medical or biologic importance.

Discussion and Conclusions

In the discussion section, the author provides an interpretation of findings. Here the author can attach clinical relevance to the reported statistically significant findings. The findings may be compared with those of other studies and interpretations. Possible explanations for results can be postulated and differences from other reports in the literature explained. Hopefully the author bases the conclusions on the findings. This is not always the case. When we discuss the results, we should consider whether they have any meaning in the real world of bedside practice. A "significant" but relatively small difference in cardiac performance discovered only in carefully controlled circumstances has little resemblance to the constantly changing status of the critically ill patient in whom such a finding may not have any real import. We must ask ourselves whether the demonstrated result is important in influencing or directing bedside practice. We must retain our skepticism and use it to balance enthusiasm.

This section should contain a discussion of limitations. Authors who conclude that results would have been statistically significant if only a larger sample had been available display their lack of foresight and preparation; clearly, the time to discover the proper sample size is at the outset, the study-planning phase. Rather, it would be refreshing to encounter conclusions that forthrightly admitted that the hypothesis was incorrect, that the study showed that therapy did not lead to improvement, or that the investigator headed off on the wrong track. Negative reports of this sort will prevent other investigators from pursuing ideas that turn out to be flawed and can also direct investigators, including themselves, along more fruitful pathways.

The reporting of negative studies has been addressed from an editorial standpoint (45). Angell states, "... it is widely believed that reports of negative studies are less likely to be published than those of positive studies and some data have been put forth to support this belief.... It is assumed that editors and reviewers are biased against negative studies, considering them less inherently interesting than positive studies. However, a bias against publishing negative studies would distort the scientific literature" (45). Although she believes that the *New England Journal of Medicine* publishes fewer negative reports than positive ones, it is not a matter of policy. She asks, "Does it deal with an important question? Is the information new and interesting? Was the study well done?.... We feel a particular obligation to publish a negative study when it contradicts an earlier study we have published and is of a similar or superior quality. When a good study addresses an important question, the answer is interesting and the work deserves publication whether the result is positive or negative" (45).

Finally, we should consider whether the conclusions are relevant to the questions posed by the investigators. Far too many reports begin with "unwarranted assumptions" in the introduction, end with "foregone conclusions" in the discussion, and contain in between a mass of barely relevant data. If we care to spend the time necessary to review published reports and, in particular, to do the preparation necessary before we embark on our own clinical investigations, such discouraging assessments will occur much less frequently.

LITERATURE REVIEW AND RESEARCH SYNTHESIS

Practicing physicians, researchers, patients, and family members are inundated with unmanageable amounts of information; the need exists for literature to "efficiently integrate valid information and provide a basis for rational decision making" (46). Systematic literature reviews (SLRs) assemble, critically appraise, and synthesize the results of primary investigations addressing a topic of concern (23). Systematic reviews contain a summary of all past research on an area of interest using a methodology incorporating explicit methods in limiting bias (systematic errors) and reducing chance effects, thus providing more reliable results upon which to draw conclusions and make decisions (47). The steps of the systematic literature review guide the researcher through the process of systematically evaluating the existing literature in light of a predetermined research question (48). Meta-analysis is often conducted as part of an SLR.

The Cochrane Collaboration is an international not-for-profit and independent organization, dedicated to making up-to-date, accurate information about the effects of health care readily available worldwide through the methodology of systematic literature reviews. It produces and disseminates systematic reviews of health care interventions and promotes the search for evidence in the form of clinical trials and other studies of interventions. More information can be found on their Web site, http://www.cochrane.org. A search of the Cochrane library for ventilator-associated pneumonia gave this title: "Prevention of ventilated associated pneumonia in critically ill patients treated for stress ulcers."

SUMMARY

In *De Anima*, Aristotle declared that "it is necessary, while formulating the problems of which in our further advance we are to find the solutions, to call into council the views of those of our predecessors who have declared any opinion on this subject, in order that we may profit by whatever is sound in their suggestions and avoid their errors." This wisdom still holds today. In order to "council the views" of medical researchers, physicians must develop a competency for reading the medical literature and understanding basic statistical concepts. We humbly accept that a book chapter can only provide an introduction of topics, and we encourage the reader to seek out additional educational opportunities. The National Institutes of Health (NIH) has made the paradigm of interdisciplinary research a cornerstone of the NIH Roadmap (http://nihroadmap.nih.gov). We advocate, whenever and wherever possible, collaboration among physicians, nurses, biostatisticians, data managers, and support professionals to form research groups (informal or formal). We believe, as does the NIH, that such efforts have great potential for increasing the quality and efficiency of both conducting and consuming research. The ultimate goal is, of course, improved cost-effective care and quality of life for patients and their families.

ACKNOWLEDGEMENTS

Joseph M. Civetta, Theodore Colton, Renee Parker-James, and Huang Teng-Yu

References

1. Fuchs RJ, Berenholtz SM, Dorman T. Do intensivists in ICU improve outcome? *Best Pract Res Cli Anaesthesiol.* 2005;19(1):125–135.
2. Young MP, Birkmeyer JD. Potential reduction in mortality rates using an intensivist model to manage intensive care units. *Eff Clin Pract.* 2000;3(6):284–289.
3. Rosenberg A. *Philosophy of Science.* New York: Routledge; 2000.
4. ARDS Net. Ventilation with lower tidal volumes as compared with traditional tidal volumes for acute lung injury and the acute respiratory distress syndrome. The Acute Respiratory Distress Syndrome Network. *N Engl J Med.* 2000;342(18):1301–1308.
5. Frankfurt HG. *On Bullshit.* Princeton, NJ: Princeton University Press; 2005.
6. Arenson KW. What organizations don't want to know can hurt. *New York Times.* August 22, 2006.
7. Hill RB, Anderson RE. The autopsy crisis reexamined: the case for a national autopsy policy. *Milbank Q.* 1991;69(1):51–78.
8. Grahame-Smith D. Evidence-based medicine: Socratic dissent. *BMJ.* 1995;310:1126–1127.
9. Anon. Evidence-based medicine, in its place (editorial). *Lancet.* 1995;346:785.
10. Goodman NW. Who will challenge evidence-based medicine? *J R Coll Physicians Lond.* 1999;33(3):249–251.
11. Shahar E. A Popperian perspective of the term 'evidence-based medicine.' *J Eval Clin Pract.* 1997;3(2):109–116.
12. Couto JS. Evidence-based medicine: a Kuhnian perspective of a transvestite non-theory. *J Eval Clin Pract.* 1998;4(4):267–275.
13. Sehon SR, Stanley DE. A philosophical analysis of the evidence-based medicine debate. *BMC Health Serv Res.* 2003;3(1):14.
14. Goodman SN. Toward evidence-based medical statistics. 2: The Bayes factor. *Ann Intern Med.* 1999;130(12):1005–1013.
15. Bland JM, Altman DG. Bayesians and frequentists. *BMJ.* 1998;317(7166):1151–1160.
16. Kuhn TS. *The Structure of Scientific Revolutions.* 3rd ed. Chicago: University of Chicago Press; 1996.
17. Bayes T. An essay toward solving a problem in the doctrine of chances. *Philos Trans Roy Soc London.* 1764;53:370–418.
18. Goodman SN. Toward evidence-based medical statistics. 1: the P value fallacy. *Ann Intern Med.* 1999;130(12):995–1004.
19. Agresti A, Min Y. Frequentist performance of Bayesian confidence intervals for comparing proportions in 2×2 contingency tables. *Biometrics.* 2005;61(2):515–523.
20. Black WC, Armstrong P. Communicating the significance of radiologic test results: the likelihood ratio. *Am J Roentgenol.* 1986;147(6):1313–1318.
21. Armitage P, Berry G, Matthews JNS. *Statistical Methods in Medical Research.* 4th ed. Malden, MA: Blackwell Publishing; 2002.
22. Gehlbach S. *Interpreting the Medical Literature.* New York: McGraw Publishing; 2002.
23. Cooper H, Hedges LV. *The Handbook of Research Synthesis.* New York: Russell Sage Foundation; 1994.
24. Cox DR. *Principles of Statistical Inference.* New York: Cambridge University Press; 2006.
25. Tejerina E, Frutos-Vivar F, Restrepo MI, et al. Incidence, risk factors, and outcome of ventilator-associated pneumonia. *J Crit Care.* 2006;21(1):56–65.
26. Motulsky H. *Intuitive Biostatistics.* New York: Oxford University Press; 1995.
27. D'Agostino RB, Sullivan LM, Beiser AS. *Introductory Applied Biostatistics.* Belmont, CA: Duxbury Publications; 2006.

28. Gauch HG. *Scientific Method in Practice*. New York: Cambridge University Press; 2003.
29. Miller J. *The Chicago Guide to Writing about Numbers*. Chicago: The University of Chicago Press; 2004.
30. Miller J. *The Chicago Guide to Writing about Multivariate Analyses*. Chicago: The University of Chicago Press; 2005.
31. Heyland DK, Cook DJ, Dodek PM. Prevention of ventilator-associated pneumonia: current practice in Canadian intensive care units. *J Crit Care*. 2002; 17(3):161–167.
32. Rello J, Ollendorf DA, Oster G, et al. Epidemiology and outcomes of ventilator-associated pneumonia in a large US database. *Chest* 2002;122(6): 2115–2121.
33. Koeman M, van der Ven AJ, Hak E, et al. Oral decontamination with chlorhexidine reduces the incidence of ventilator-associated pneumonia. *Am J Respir Crit Care Med*. 2006;173(12):1348–1355.
34. Mahul P, Auboyer C, Jospe R, et al. Prevention of nosocomial pneumonia in intubated patients: respective role of mechanical subglottic secretion drainage and stress ulcer prophylaxis. *Intens Care Med*. 1992;18:20–25.
35. Kirby RR, Downs JB, Civetta JM, et al. High level positive end-expiratory pressure (PEEP) in acute respiratory insufficiency. *Chest*. 1975;67: 156.
36. Gallagher TJ, Civetta JM, Kirby RR. Terminology update: optimal PEEP. *Crit Care Med*. 1978;6:323.
37. Nelson LD, Civetta JM, Hudson-Civetta JA. Titrating positive end-expiratory pressure therapy in patients with early, moderate arterial hypoxemia. *Crit Care Med*. 1987;15:14.
38. Colton T. *Statistics in Medicine*. Boston: Little, Brown; 1974.
39. Hennekeus CH, Buring J. *Epidemiology in Medicine*. Boston: Little, Brown; 1987.
40. Hudson-Civetta JA, Civetta JM, Martinez OV, et al. Risk and detection of pulmonary catheter-related infection in septic surgical patients. *Crit Care Med*. 1987;15:29.
41. Applefeld JJ, Caruthers TE, Reno DJ, et al. Assessment of the sterility of the long term cardiac catheterization using the thermodilution Swan-Ganz catheter. *Chest*. 1978;74:377.
42. Berry G. Statistical significance and confidence intervals. *Med J Aust*. 1986; 144:618–619; reprinted in *J Clin Pract*. 1988;42:465–468.
43. Sackett DL. Biases in analytic research. *J Chronic Dis*. 1979;32:51.
44. *Real Paper*. 1978.
45. Angell M. Negative studies. *N Engl J Med*. 1989;321:464.
46. Mulrow CD. Rationale for systematic reviews. *BMJ*. 1994;309:597–599.
47. Oxman AD, Guyatt GH. The science of reviewing research. *Ann NY Acad Sci*. 1993;703:125–133.
48. Classen S, Garvan CW, Awadzi K, et al. Systematic literature review and structural model for older driver safety. *Topics Geriatr Rehab*. 2006;22(2): 87–98.

CHAPTER 10 ■ QUALITY ASSURANCE, SAFETY, AND OUTCOMES

ELIZABETH MARTINEZ • JOSE RODRIGUEZ-PAZ • PETER PRONOVOST

Several Institute of Medicine (IOM) reports raised the nation's awareness about a significant problem with patient safety in health care (1,2). These reports stated that the number of deaths attributed to medical errors per year is between 44,000 and 98,000, and highlighted that the systems in which patients receive care were to blame rather than frontline caregivers. While many efforts have been made to improve patient safety, there is still little evidence showing systematic improvements in safety since these IOM reports (3). However, efforts have been severely limited by a scarce understanding of the science of patient safety and a lack of rigorous methodologies to design and implement changes and monitor progress.

Patient safety is a broad and relatively new area of research that cannot be covered in one chapter. Thus, regulatory strategies and details of error reporting will not be covered herein. The goal of this chapter is to present a practical framework infused with an evidence-based medicine approach that health care professionals may use to implement patient safety improvement efforts. To accomplish this goal, we will begin by explaining the science of patient safety, which is the foundation for understanding why errors occur and how to identify the factors contributing to these errors. After presenting this foundation, we will review a model with four measures to help evaluate our progress in improving patient safety. In the last section of this chapter, we describe a framework of strategies to guide the implementation of improvement efforts.

SCIENCE OF PATIENT SAFETY

Similar to any field of investigation, there is a science to patient safety that warrants understanding in order to effectively and efficiently research safety in health care organizations. A summary of the tenets of the science of safety includes that humans are fallible, broken systems—rather than individuals—allow errors and leaders have the power to fix broken systems (Table 10.1). For this science, a system is a set of interdependent elements that interact to achieve a shared aim. There are two human elements that interact within a system: The frontline staff, who does the work, and management, who has the power to design, control, and redesign the work. In order to fix a broken system, we must first identify the failure(s). Over a decade ago, James Reason, among others, introduced the human factor's analysis and classified system failures as either active or latent (4). *Active failures* are actions involving direct patient contact by frontline staff that have an immediate adverse effect on patients. These failures occur closest to the patient and are not a reflection of a health care worker's professional ability. *Latent failures* are managerial or organizational in nature in which the adverse event is not immediately evident. Frontline caregivers are often aware of active and latent failures, but the avenues to communicate these failures for system redesign either are not known or are not available.

TABLE 10.1

PRINCIPLES OF THE SCIENCE OF SAFETY

The science of safety teaches that:
■ Fallibility is part of the human condition.
■ We cannot change the human condition.
■ Harm is the result of a cascade of broken systems.
■ Therefore, in order to improve safety, the system must be the focus, rather than individuals who make errors.
■ Individuals can change the systems under which people work
■ We must focus on interpersonal communication, and accept the responsibility for the system in which we work
■ Leaders control the potential to change systems

There are safety mechanisms inherently built into health care by nature of its purpose—to improve an individual's health. For example, medications are used to relieve symptoms or resolve an illness. Patients may have a medication allergy—the presence and nature of which is a ubiquitous question of every health care professional—with red-flag documentation in the patient's history and in pharmacy records. This is a system designed to provide safer patient care. With this in mind, most medical errors occur when multiple failures in a system align. Reason's "Swiss cheese" model (Fig. 10.1) illustrates how multiple failures, though singularly insufficient in allowing harm to reach the patient, can align and cause an adverse event. Below is an explanation of the adverse event illustrated in this figure.

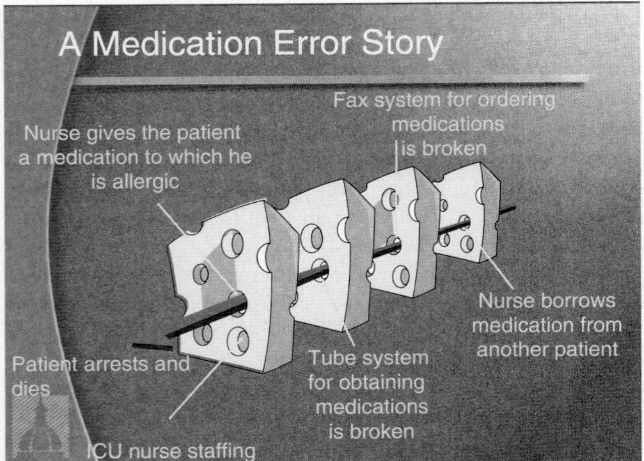

FIGURE 10.1. The "Swiss cheese" model of a medical error. The events leading up to an adverse event involving a medication error are illustrated. The Swiss cheese model is a concept originating from the work of James Reason, in which he proposes that the alignment of multiple system failures allows harm to reach a patient. His premise is that system failures occur often, with health care professionals and other systems built in to catch a failure (e.g., final safety check at the pharmacy to catch medication allergies). Couched in this way, it takes the alignment of several failures or defects to occur to pass by and harm a patient. (Adapted from Reason J. Understanding adverse events: human factors. In: Vincent C, ed. *Clinical Risk Management*. London: BMJ Publications; 1995.)

A Medication Error

Brief Description

A patient is administered ampicillin despite a documented allergy to penicillins. On cursory review, the physician who wrote the order and the nurse who administered the medication are at fault because they failed to remember, or check for, any medication allergies. Further, multiple caregivers *not* involved in the event condemned the negligent actions of these bedside caregivers.

Detailed Investigation

However, the event needed a more in-depth investigation with appropriate lenses to identify the system failures that resulted in this error. First, let us review the circumstances leading up to the error through the eyes of the caregivers involved.

The patient was exhibiting signs of pneumonia. The bedside nurse knew that administering an antibiotic within 1 hour would dramatically improve the patient's outcome, and timely antibiotic administration a core measure for pneumonia therapy mandated by the Joint Commission on Accreditation of Healthcare Organizations (JCAHO). On further discussion with the staff, investigators uncovered that the nurse's concern over administering the antibiotic quickly was perpetuated by a broken fax machine and tube system. This was troubling because orders were faxed to pharmacy, and medications were sent from the pharmacy through a tube system for a quick turnaround. In addition, the person employed to run errands had been cut to save money. Because the system to obtain medications quickly failed, the nurse borrowed the ampicillin from another patient.

Analysis

This case illustrates how each step aligned to achieve a catastrophic outcome. Unfortunately, by borrowing the antibiotic from another patient, the pharmacy was bypassed and a crucial safety check of potential medications allergies was missed. This example is powerful because:

- It demonstrates the frontline caregiver's commitment to quality and patient safety (i.e., timely antibiotic administration for pnemonia).
- It uncovers the real defects that resulted in the event (i.e., broken fax, broken tube system, runner abolished, pharmacy safety check bypassed).
- It provides obvious solutions to fix the problem (i.e., fix the fax machine and tube system, and consider reinstating the runner position).

It is important to recognize that fixing broken systems often takes resources. Health care organizations must consider the marginal costs and benefits of implementing—as well as not implementing—patient safety initiatives. Thus, it is important to have a system to prioritize where the greatest hazards exist. Indeed, in the real world, correcting one problem may introduce new hazards (unintended consequences) or—due to the consumption of scarce resources—result in *not* correcting another. As such, organizations should ensure that the impact of their patient safety improvement efforts is evaluated.

As illustrated in the above example, systems in health care are exceedingly complex. Efforts to improve a system are often difficult to implement and can introduce new hazards.

Frontline caregivers are not the only individuals that are blamed for mistakes. Bad outcomes are often blamed on a patient's medical condition or age (e.g., too old or too young), complexity of an operation (e.g., multiple-procedure operation), or devices in place that are sources of infection (e.g., ventilator). Nevertheless, the science of safety has taught us that many bad outcomes traditionally attributed to patients may be caused by system factors that influence the organization and delivery of care. For example, intensive care unit (ICU) physician and nurse staffing, teamwork, and communication have been shown to impact patient mortality (5,6).

Pearls for Quality and Safety Initiatives

Through our efforts to improve safety in health care, we have learned many lessons:

- First, experiences from large health care organizations have taught us that the context in which care is delivered (culture) is a key element in making safety a reality.
- Second, safety interventions must be goal directed and patient centered. Small-scale efforts that target a particular unit and subpopulation of patients (e.g., ICU) are more often successful than large-scale efforts that try to improve care throughout a health system.
- Third, frontline caregivers must understand the science of safety and evaluate safety risks with lenses that see hazardous systems, and not incompetent people.
- Fourth, the efforts of frontline staff must be concrete and goal oriented, with a measurable intervention or outcome.
- Fifth, local leaders need to understand the science and culture of safety and support the efforts of frontline caregivers.

HOW TO EVALUATE PROGRESS IN PATIENT SAFETY

Measuring Safety

The first step toward improving patient safety is the ability to *measure* progress to improve patient safety. Health care currently has few scientifically sound or feasible measures or the tools required to accomplish this task. We have borrowed tools from other disciplines—for example, organizational psychology, sociology, and human-factors engineering—that have developed basic safety-related principles. As Brennan et al. noted in a recent article (7), health care has borrowed the basic science of safety from other disciplines, but needs to further develop the science of safety and its application in the complex systems of health care (8–13).

To quantify improvement one must measure and remeasure to show positive change. Unfortunately, patient safety efforts cannot always be evaluated with a valid rate. To be valid as a rate, a measure must have a clearly defined numerator (i.e., the defect), denominator (i.e., population at risk), and method of surveillance in which bias is minimized. With safety, most events are rare, what we are measuring is not clearly defined, and our surveillance systems are poorly developed; all of these introduce bias (14).

Moreover, the variables that we do try to measure coexist with other variables that also affect patient safety and make isolation more difficult. For example, measuring caregiver compliance with effective use of briefings before critical tasks can be affected by teamwork, communication, or the culture of safety (15). Consequently, health care has turned to the Donabedian model of quality to measure safety (16). This model evaluates structure (i.e., organization of care), its connection to process (i.e., what is done), and influence on outcomes. We have added safety culture (i.e., the context in which care is delivered) to this model because of its importance in effectively implementing any interventions. While most measures of quality focus on process or outcomes, many patient safety measures focus on the structure (e.g., staffing) and culture (e.g., staff perceptions of safety) in which the process of care occurs. In addition, cultural variables, such as communication and teamwork, are doubly important, given that both are leading contributing factors in all sentinel events (www.jointcommission.org).

The IOM expressed the need to address culture, and the National Quality Forum (www.qualityforum.org) recommended that health care organizations measure culture annually (1). The Safety Attitudes Questionnaire (SAQ) is a valid and reliable instrument that assesses the frontline caregiver's perceptions of safety culture (17). Furthermore, results from SAQ administrations at the Johns Hopkins Hospital and in over 70 hospitals in the Michigan Keystone ICU project (18) found that better perceptions of teamwork and safety in a clinical area can be achieved through specific interventions (19,20). In addition, these interventions (e.g., daily goals checklist, care bundles, and the Comprehensive Unit-based Safety Program) have been associated with lower rates of nurse turnover, catheter-related bloodstream infection (CRBSI), decubitus ulcer, and in-hospital mortality (21,22).

To move forward with patient safety efforts, a measurement model is needed to determine whether patients are safer. The model described below is adapted from Donabedian, with the addition of a safety culture parameter. Researchers at the School of Medicine at Johns Hopkins University developed and tested this model in over 200 ICUs across the United States as part of ongoing collaborative projects (18,23).

How Do We Know That We Are Safer?

The key question to reliably answer, particularly as we implement improvement interventions, is whether patients are safer. Despite all of the publicity generated by IOM reports on patient safety and all of the efforts made to improve patient safety, many question the empiric evidence claiming that safety has improved (7,14,24,25). With a few exceptions, most efforts to date do not provide a clear answer as to whether patients are safer now than at the start of the patient safety movement. This deficiency is partly due to the relative novelty of safety as a science, as well as the methodologic challenges of rigorous measurement and data collection.

Measuring compliance with process measures (e.g., four therapies known to reduce ventilator-associated pneumonia) or monitoring outcomes (e.g., decreased CRBSI rates) is the most advanced methodology to evaluate whether or not we are safer. However, not all safety interventions can be measured as rates, and evaluating "changes made" can be difficult. In this section, we will outline a model that uses two rate-based measures and two measures that cannot produce valid rates of patient safety; all four are equally important.

The model we developed focuses on measures of safety rather than broader measures of quality. It has been used at the Johns Hopkins Hospital and in over 100 ICUs in the state of Michigan (23). Four methodologically validated questions are the basic outline for this model and cover the domains of health care that affect safety (i.e., structure, process, outcomes, and culture).

How Often Do We Harm Patients? (Outcome Measure, Valid Rate)

Understandably, patient outcomes have been a ubiquitous focus in health care for centuries. When measuring harm, however, it is important to make sure that the harm you are measuring is preventable with appropriate interventions. If you measure an inevitable outcome, your data will not be reliable or valid (26). A good example—and possibly the only valid measure of harm at this time—is catheter-related bloodstream infections, because most are preventable. In addition, a solid infrastructure is in place to reliably measure harm rates (i.e., hospital infection control departments and Centers for Disease Control and Prevention guidelines) and significantly reduce infections (22,27,28).

How Often Do We Do What We Should? (Process Measure, Valid Rate)

A process measure is an indicator of whether patients reliably receive *evidence-based* interventions *known* to prevent complications in the targeted outcome. For example, washing your hands and applying chlorhexidine to sterilize the site before a catheter line insertion are two of five sterilization processes known to reduce bloodstream infections. When measuring processes, it is essential to remember that patient factors, bias in measurement, and interventions that *might* prevent a complication all play a role in complications. Unfortunately, existing process measures only capture acute myocardial infarction, congestive heart failure, and pneumonia; in many hospitals, this accounts for a small percentage of discharges (29). It will be extremely important to focus research efforts on more scientifically sound process measures since "what we do" directly impacts care, and the closer a mistake is in proximity to the patient, the higher the risk for harm.

How Do We Know We've Learned from Our Defects/Mistakes? (Structural Measure, Nonrate)

In our patient safety efforts, whether we have learned from our previous defects has received the least attention. Structural interventions, however, can have a profound impact on patient safety. For example, intensivist staffing in critical care has been associated with a 30% relative reduction in hospital mortality (5). In addition, structure and process measures work together to produce an outcome.

The use of validated tools, such as the Learning from Defect (LFD) tool, can help hospitals evaluate how care is organized and delivered to evaluate whether interventions are improving safety. Defects can be identified through various venues (e.g., morbidity and mortality conferences, incident reporting systems). The main goal of the LFD tool is to extensively investigate a small number of defects and make significant system changes based on the findings—dig an inch wide and a mile deep. To assess if a hospital, department, or clinical area has learned from a defect investigation, measure whether the recommendations made to avoid harm were actually implemented.

How Well Have We Created a Culture of Safety? (Cultural Measure, Nonrate)

As we discussed earlier, safety culture in health care is the context in which care is delivered. The beliefs, values, and opinions of the organizations' leaders and managers strongly influence safety culture. Safety culture is a measure of how caregivers communicate and interact, and strongly influences patient outcomes (www.jointcommission.org) (30). Validated tools, such as the SAQ (17), assess the caregiver's perceptions of safety climate in his or her clinical area. The SAQ includes six domains that affect culture: Teamwork climate, safety climate, perceptions of management, stress recognition, job satisfaction, and working conditions. Culture should be measured annually and is best administered at the clinical care area level rather than hospitalwide, given the variation in assessments among clinical areas within a single hospital. Scores are most interpretable when presented as the percent of staff in a clinical area reporting positive culture scores. A good indication that a clinical area is safe is to have at least 80% of staff in that area reporting a positive safety culture.

FRAMEWORK FOR IMPROVING PATIENT SAFETY

There are two strategies in this framework to improve patient safety. One strategy focuses on the rate-based measures we discussed and the other addresses the non–rate-based measures. The rate-based measures will be described in the context of collaborative projects, because such projects or interventions involve reorganizing the delivery of care (i.e., process, or what we do) to improve patient outcomes. The non–rate-based measures will be described in the Comprehensive Unit-based Safety Program (CUSP) because CUSP focuses on the structure of an organization and its culture. Before describing a collaborative, we should mention that a single institution can implement this project.

Collaboratives

A collaborative involves the participation of multiple health care organizations in a structured program with a shared goal of improving an aspect of clinical care. For our patient safety framework, this also means the involvement of a multidisciplinary team from each patient care area or hospital participating in the collaborative. Teams will implement and evaluate interventions with support from other frontline staff in their care area. To succeed, organizations designing collaboratives should do the following:

- Identify one important clinical outcome for improvement (e.g., eliminate CRBSI).
- Assemble a team to manage the project, particularly data collection and coordination with the collaborative's core research center.
- Educate all caregivers in the patient care areas participating in the best practices of care for their outcome, and measure compliance with the interventions at baseline.

- Give teams suggestions to reach their goals, but encourage them to adapt implementation of the interventions to fit their culture and resources.
- Limit time to implementation of an intervention.

As with all care improvement projects that are successful, measurement of baseline compliance and change over time are key data points to collect.

Collaboratives are successful when sites network to share existing knowledge and accomplish a common goal. Through group meetings and conference calls, teams can learn about best practices and innovative methods used by other teams to approach a problem or succeed. In addition, collaboratives bring a shared momentum that can increase sustainability (31,32).

There are, of course, pitfalls to any project in a multicenter or single hospital setting. Some problems to consider and rectify, or adjust for, are:

- Inadequate resources
- Poor leadership support
- Vague expectations and objectives for team members
- Poor communication
- Complex study plans
- Inadequate management of data collection and data quality
- Wasted efforts to "reinvent the wheel" rather than adopt the practices proven effective by others

Designing a Collaborative to Improve Health Care Safety

Considering the benefits and pitfalls outlined above, designing a collaborative requires a culture (i.e., the set of values, attitudes, and beliefs of the group) with a shared consensus of safety, and an understanding of the science (i.e., the technical components of how care is organized and delivered) of patient safety. The following intervention design incorporates both components in simple and reproducible steps to improve patient safety; it has been validated in several large collaborative efforts (22,33):

- Identify evidence-based interventions associated with an improved outcome through review of peer-reviewed publications.
- Select goal-oriented interventions that have the biggest impact on outcomes and transform them into behaviors. For example, we identified five behaviors in the literature that reduce CRBSI: Handwashing, cleaning of the skin with chlorhexidine, use of full barrier precautions, avoidance of the femoral site, and removal of unnecessary lines. In selecting behaviors, the focus should be on interventions with the strongest treatment effect (i.e., lowest number needed to treat) and the lowest barrier to use. One would not, for example, start with controversial or burdensome interventions that most caregivers have not yet accepted.
- Develop and implement measures that evaluate either the outcome or use of the behaviors or interventions.
- Measure baseline performance and establish databases to facilitate accurate data management and timely feedback to teams.
- Ensure that patients receive evidence-based interventions through four basic phases: Engagement, education, execution, and evaluation (Table 10.2).

This framework to improve patient safety has been applied with previously designed tools and interventions in the Michigan collaborative previously mentioned. This project implemented the five evidence-based behaviors to reduce CRBSI, as outlined above, as an intervention and achieved dramatic reductions in infection rates (22). This intervention also included a component to *reduce complexity* and introduce a *redundant safety check*. To decrease complexity, a line cart was introduced, which centralized, in one place, all of the supplies required to place a central catheter. In addition, a checklist of questions stayed with the cart to ensure compliance with the best practices for central catheter placement. The checklist is typically completed by a nurse and is added assurance that the operator washed his or her hands appropriately and draped the entire patient; used sterile gloves, mask, and gown; and maintained a sterile field while placing the catheter. *The*

TABLE 10.2

CHANGE MODEL: HOW TO ENSURE PATIENTS RECEIVED EVIDENCE-BASED INTERVENTIONS

Steps	What do you do?	Catheter-related bloodstream infection (CRBSI) as example
ENGAGE	Make the problem real.	Share local CRBSI infection rates.
EDUCATE	Develop an educational plan to reach *all* members of the caregiver team.	Present evidence-based practices at grand rounds, multidisciplinary team meetings, etc. Present information on how you will improve care, and measure that behavior or outcome.
EXECUTE	Develop a safety culture. Reduce complexity of the processes.	Develop a culture of intolerance of CRBSI. Make certain that all equipment to do it right is easily available to the provider; put everything in one place (i.e., a line cart).
	Introduce redundancy in processes.	Introduce checklists that identify the key steps to reduce CRBSI.
	Have regular team meetings.	Develop a project plan focusing on one to two tasks a week. Identify who owns each step of the process.
EVALUATE	Measure and give feedback.	Develop a data collection plan and database to facilitate tracking of progress. Provide real-time feedback. Post progress in highly visible locations for all staff to see. Identify causes of defects.

nurse is empowered to stop the procedure if a sterile technique is compromised. This intervention resulted in a 66% reduction in the overall CRBSI rate, with a median rate reduced from 2.7 per 1,000 catheter days prior to the intervention to 0 by month 3 and through month 18 of the postintervention.

Comprehensive Unit-based Safety Program: A Strategy to Learn from Mistakes and Improve Culture (Nonrate Measures)

The CUSP is a six-step program that has been tested and successfully used to improve the quality and safety in ICUs (Table 10.3) (10,21). It provides a structured approach to improve safety culture by educating staff about the science of safety, including staff in the process of identifying and mitigating hazards, partnering the unit with a leader who can make change happen, and providing tools to learn from defects and improve the organization of work (21).

The Comprehensive Unit-based Safety Program in Detail

Safety culture is assessed in the first step of the CUSP and reassessed about 1 year after the CUSP is under way to evaluate the impact of the program on safety culture. The initial measure is a baseline assessment of staff perceptions of safety culture in their clinical area and their perceptions of the organization's commitment to patient safety. The Safety Attitudes Questionnaire is the instrument used, and is perceived as the most valid, reliable, and widely used survey to measure culture (34). Education is a crucial next step since it provides staff with a new set of lenses to identify hazards and recommend system changes to improve care—knowledge fosters awareness. In the third step, the frontline staff identifies patient safety hazards in their clinical area and suggests interventions for improvement. There are other sources to identify hazards, such as patient safety reporting systems, morbidity and mortality conferences, or liability claims. However, the most powerful method of incident reporting is to ask staff how they think the next patient will be harmed, and how it can be prevented from happening.

In step four, a senior executive builds a partnership with a unit or clinical area. This involves monthly rounds on the

TABLE 10.3

STEPS IN THE COMPREHENSIVE UNIT-BASED SAFETY PROGRAM (CUSP)

	Step	Description
1	Measure safety climate (baseline).	Assess safety culture in each clinical area through Safety Attitudes Questionnaire (SAQ) administered to all staff.
2	View educational material.	Educate all staff about the science of safety through lectures and other educational materials.
3	Complete forms identifying patient safety issues.	■ Ask all staff the following: □ Think about the last patient who would have been harmed without the staff intervening. □ How will the next patient be harmed? □ How can this harm be prevented or mitigated? ■ Establish incident reporting system.
4	A senior executive should be responsible for application of the CUSP in the intensive care unit.	Have a monthly meeting of all staff in the clinical area with a senior executive to: ■ Help prioritize safety efforts ■ Remove barriers for system changes ■ Provide resources ■ Demonstrate hospital commitment to patient safety ■ Foster relationship between senior leadership and staff
5	Implement projects/improvements.	■ Select two to three safety issues to focus on at one time (based on step 3). ■ Simple goals: □ Reduce complexity in a process. □ Create independent redundancies to ensure that appropriate critical steps are done (i.e., have two or more staff check independent of one another). ■ Example: Medication reconciliation, an independent redundancy done at patient discharge to recheck appropriateness of orders
6	Repeat measure of safety culture.	Remeasure safety culture to see if the CUSP has been successful (i.e., scores improve).

Adapted from Pronovost PJ, King J, Holzmueller CG, et al. A Web-based tool for the Comprehensive Unit-based Safety Program (CUSP). *Jt Comm J Qual Saf.* 2006;32(3):119–129; and Pronovost P, Weast B, Rosenstein B, et al. Implementing and validating a comprehensive unit-based safety program. *J Pat Saf.* 2005;1(1):33–40.

unit with staff to help them prioritize safety efforts, ensure they have the resources to implement improvements, and hold them accountable for evaluating whether safety has improved. In the fifth step, we ask staff to learn from one defect a month, and implement one tool designed to improve care delivery per quarter (e.g., daily goals or morning briefing) to improve communication and teamwork (11,13).

Implementing the Comprehensive Unit-based Safety Program

To implement the CUSP, start by choosing one patient care area, such as the ICU. Next, assemble a patient safety team using staff from that clinical area; they will be responsible for oversight of the program. To be most effective, this team should include the ICU director or an ICU physician safety champion, the nurse manager, another ICU physician and nurse, a risk manager or patient safety officer, and a senior executive from the institution. We have found that the program works best if the physician and nurse who will lead the program have at least 20% of their time devoted to improving patient safety. The first unit will be your beta site; subsequent teams from other clinical areas should learn from its successes and failures. The ultimate goal is to have every area in your hospital organize and manage safety through the CUSP.

Evidence of Comprehensive Unit-based Safety Program Benefits

The CUSP has been associated with significant improvements in safety culture. For example, the percent of staff reporting a positive safety climate increased from 35% before the CUSP to 60% after the CUSP (21). In addition, teams identified and mitigated several specific hazards through the CUSP. For example, as a result of asking staff how the next patient will be harmed, and using the LFD tool, the ICU created a dedicated ICU transport team, implemented point-of-care pharmacists, implemented the daily goals sheet, labeled epidural catheters to prevent inadvertent IV connection, and standardized the equipment in transvenous pacing kits (35). Moreover, the use of the CUSP was also associated with a reduced length of stay and nurse turnover.

In summary, the CUSP has several benefits worthy of repeating:

- Improving safety culture is necessary for staff compliance in implementing any safety intervention or project.
- It is malleable enough to add improvement tools.
- It is a venue to introduce rigorous research methods.
- It is a learning laboratory to identify and mitigate hazards.
- It provides the potential to improve patient outcomes.

Improvement Tools

Through our efforts to improve patient safety, tools have been developed to reorganize the way care is delivered. For example, five interventions known to decrease morbidity, mortality, or duration of ventilator support were assembled in a ventilator bundle to improve care for mechanically ventilated patients (36). These interventions include:

- Elevating head of bed to greater than or equal to 30 degrees
- Utilization of appropriate sedation (i.e., patient able to follow simple commands)
- Appropriate stress ulcer prophylaxis (i.e., received medication)
- Appropriate deep vein thrombosis prophylaxis (i.e., received mechanical devices or medications for prevention)
- Daily assessment for extubation (i.e., evaluate with rapid shallow breathing index or trial of spontaneous ventilation)

We have organized our tools into a Patient Safety Toolbox, and provide an example of several tools in our ICU collaboratives (Table 10.4).

Learning from Defects

While patient safety reporting systems have been advocated as a strategy to improve safety, their benefits lie in the rich information reported about the incidents (14,35). We must learn from these incidents. The LFD tool is designed to guide in the investigation of an incident or defect (23). This tool guides the investigators to evaluate system defects (e.g., computer malfunction for physician order entry), offers a structured approach to share what went wrong, and outlines a plan to improve the defects and follow-up (i.e., close the loop) to evaluate whether care is safer. If the loop is not closed, the error will be repeated.

The LFD process is a condensed root cause analysis (RCA);[1] however, the LFD can be implemented with fewer resources, can investigate near-misses that rarely trigger a hospital-level RCA, and can be done more frequently by more clinical areas or departments. The LFD tool is part of the CUSP, but can also be used to investigate liability claims, incidents reported to patient safety reporting systems, and incidents brought up at morbidity and mortality conferences. This is a one-page tool, divided into four sections that ask the following:

- What happened?
- What factors contributed or minimized the risk of patient harm?
- What actions can be taken to reduce the likelihood of a similar incident?
- How do we know that our actions improved safety?

One of the major advantages of the LFD is that it allows ICUs to analyze in real time any incident and produce a plan to improve safety. Examples of the LFD tool have been previously published (35). This tool has been used successfully in morbidity and mortality meetings, as well as performance improvement meetings, to structure discussions around the system failures that resulted in the defects and away from the traditional focus on health care provider inadequacies.

Improving Teamwork and Communication

Effective teamwork and communication are essential for high-quality and safe delivery of care to our patients. Teamwork and communication failures are the most common contributing factors for adverse events in the ICU, and a root cause of sentinel events throughout the health care system[2] (37–39).

---

[1] (http://www.jointcommission.org/SentinelEvents/Policyand Procedures/)

[2] (http://www.jointcommission.org/NR/rdonlyres/FA465646–5F5F-4543-AC8F-E8AF6571E372/0/root_cause_se.jpg)

TABLE 10.4

INTENSIVE CARE UNIT (ICU) PATIENT SAFETY TOOL BOX

Tool	Problem	Purpose	Who should use	How to use
Improving communication **Daily goal sheet (DGS)**	Communication failures have resulted in patient harm, increased length of stay, and provider dissatisfaction.	Improve communication among care team and family members regarding the patient's care plan	All health care providers involved in patient care (physician, nurse, nutritionist, respiratory therapist, etc.)	During morning rounds, the "team" reviews the days' goals for each patient. The patient's nurse keeps the DGS at the bedside. The form is revisited during the day as the care plan changes.
Learning from a Defect (LFD) tool	Health care organizations can improve the way they evaluate and learn from defects.	Provide a structured approach to identify systems that contributed to the defect, and take action to fix the defect	All staff involved in the delivery of care; can be used to investigate incident reports, in morbidity and mortality conferences, etc.	Complete on at least one defect per month. Review different defects from different sources. Take action to resolve the defect and follow up to ensure safety has improved.
Care improvement **Bloodstream infection checklist**	Catheter-related bloodstream infections (CRBSIs) are associated with increased morbidity, mortality, and cost of care.	Improve teamwork Comply with infection control practices Eliminate CRBSIs	Nurse at the bedside	Checklist to be completed by nurse. If operator fails to complete a step, the nurse will stop the process. Completed checklist is turned in to unit leader.
Ventilator bundle	Mechanical ventilation increases risk of complications (e.g., ventilator-associated pneumonia [VAP]), length of stay, and death. VAP incidence in ICU ranges from 10% to 60%	Eliminate VAP Reduce length of stay Reduce the risk of death	All staff involved in the delivery of care	Complete five interventions (described in text). Check off on DGS to ensure this is done daily.

Adapted from the Johns Hopkins Quality and Safety Research Group. Patient safety toolbox. Available at: http://www.safetyresearch.jhu.edu/QSR/Safety/toolbox/. Accessed August 1, 2007.

Team training has the potential to improve teamwork and communication in health care, and has been used effectively in other high-risk industries (e.g., commercial aviation, nuclear power). While there are guidelines in the medical literature regarding methods to train effective teams, there are few programs in health care to improve teamwork and communication. Implementing team training in health care will take time and resources to design and implement a curriculum and evaluate the effectiveness of the curriculum on team interactions. To implement teamwork training, health care organizations must commit to a long-term plan to integrate team training into their existing curriculum, including the use of interdisciplinary simulation that will be discussed later in this chapter (40).

Other methods to improve communication and teamwork that fit more easily into daily work are a daily goals sheet, briefing and debriefing tools, and multidisciplinary rounds, which are well known to intensivists (8,9,13,20,41). These tools are relatively new, but the evidence supporting the benefits is increasing, and they all provide a method to standardize communication. We have demonstrated that improvements in teamwork culture, measured with the SAQ, were associated with decreased medication errors, ventilator-associated pneumonia and CRBSI rates, and ICU length of stay (13,22,36,42,43).

Daily Goals Sheet

The daily goals sheet has been used since July 2001 during multidisciplinary rounds in the ICUs at Johns Hopkins to improve communication (13). This tool is a one-page checklist that is completed every morning to document the establishment of the care plan, set goals, and review potential safety risks for each patient. The goals sheet stays with the patient, is updated as needed, and is used as an information sheet for all staff involved in the patient's care. While its history of use has been in the ICU, this checklist can be modified for use on regular floor units and during operating room (OR) sign-out or emergency department rounds.

The ICU version of the daily goals sheet includes the following (13):

- What needs to be done to move the patient closer to transfer or discharge?
- What is the patient's greatest safety risk?
- What are the plans for pain management, cardiovascular management, and respiratory management?
- Is it appropriate to evaluate the patient's rapid shallow breathing index?
- Is there any planned diuresis and nutritional support?
- Are any antibiotic levels needed?
- Can any lines, tubes, or drains be discontinued?
- Are any tests or procedures planned? Have consents and ordering been completed?
- Consider key local safety initiatives, including family updates, or implementation of local protocols.

To evaluate the impact of the daily goals sheet, all care team members should answer two simple questions after rounding at each patient's bedside: Do you understand the patient's goals for the day? and Do you understand what work needs to be accomplished on this patient today? These questions were the impetus behind the development of this checklist. When asked initially, less than 10% of the residents and nurses at the time actually knew the care plan for the day. Traditional bedside rounds tended to focus as much or more on teaching staff about the disease than what work needed to occur to treat the patient. About 4 weeks after implementing the daily goals sheet, 95% of the residents and nurses understood the goals for each patient (13). Moreover, after implementing the daily goals sheet, length of stay in a surgical ICU at Johns Hopkins decreased from a mean of 2.2 days to just 1.1 days (13).

Briefings and Debriefings

Similar to the daily goals sheet, briefing and debriefing tools are designed to promote effective interdisciplinary communication and teamwork. Both have been used in the operating rooms, in sign-out from the ICU nursing staff to the intensivist, and between OR nursing and anesthesia coordinators (8,9,11). A briefing is a structured review of the case at hand among all team members before any task is undertaken with the patient. A debriefing occurs after a procedure or situation in which the team reviews what worked well, what failed, and what can be done better in the future.

The following is an example of an OR briefing. The first step is to introduce first names and roles of all team members. Next, confirm the correct patient, site/side, and procedure (JCAHO "time-out"), and make sure all team members understand the procedure and what is required to ensure its success. A check of all necessary equipment (e.g., electrocautery) and medications (e.g., appropriate antibiotic) is done. Finally, staff should consider, If something were to go wrong, what would it be? and discuss plans to mitigate the hazard.

While a briefing will typically focus on a critical procedure, it can also focus on unit management. For example, each morning, an ICU attending and nurse meet to discuss (a) events that happened overnight, (b) admissions and discharges for the day, and (c) potential hazards that may occur during the day. This morning briefing organizes the ICU team and prioritizes the workflow for the unit, allocates resources, and mitigates potential hazards (11).

Other Tools to Improve Safety

Protocols

Protocols are common for the management of routine interventions or procedures. For example, many ICUs have recently implemented a protocol for tight glycemic control in postoperative patients based on increasing evidence that it decreases the risk of surgical site infections and improves outcomes. While protocols are copious in health care, they are only effective if staff are aware of them and implement them appropriately. Thus, health care organizations should evaluate whether all team members are aware that the protocol exists, whether the protocol is appropriately used, and whether the protocol actually improves care. To evaluate a protocol's effectiveness will require defining the parameters to be followed and balancing the burden of data collection with these measures.

Testing Knowledge and Ability: Beyond See One, Do One, Teach One

Testing the knowledge and ability of health care workers will take coordination and resources. To more formally evaluate clinician knowledge, some institutions have a hospitalwide intranet site for clinical care issues (e.g., protocols, guidelines for equipment use, knowledge and competency testing) that staff visit regularly. For example, to decrease CRBSIs in an ICU, frontline caregivers were required to complete an online training session and pass the assessment. Simulation offers a strategy to evaluate a trainee or staff's ability or skill.

Simulation

Simulation is a powerful tool/technique that has been used in high-risk industries to improve safety and reduce errors (44,45). The benefits of simulation in health care have been described as follows (46):

- Frequent training for emergencies (crisis resource management [CRM])
- Teamwork training (a weak link in the whole process of patient safety)
- Skills training and evaluation of competency before a trainee touches a patient
- Testing of new procedures and usability of new devices

Health care takes place in a complex, high-stress environment that impacts human performance and patient outcomes. High-fidelity simulation allows us to not only examine human performance, but also analyze system-based problems. Although most of medical simulation is still new, it provides an opportunity to reorganize our "see one, do one, teach one" method of clinical training and better prepare trainees before they practice medicine. We need a more thorough evaluation of the impact of simulation on patient safety, but like other industries, the face validity of this tool is likely to drive change and impact outcome. This impact will be especially apparent in the training domain, both for technical and nontechnical or behavioral skills (communication skills, leadership, task management, teamwork, situational awareness, and decision making) (47,48). These behavioral skills are common contributors that underlie critical events in health care (49), although organizations have not developed methods to incorporate these needed skills in current training practices. Simulation allows trainees to practice in an environment that is safe for the trainee and the patient. In addition, trainees are exposed to common, rare, and crisis situations, and can practice learned competencies and receive immediate feedback about their performance (50,51).

SUMMARY

Patient safety as a science is a relatively new and broad field of research in health care that draws upon many disciplines. Many health care organizations have made concerted efforts to address the hazards that plague safety. Over the past several years, most of our efforts have investigated causes and executed interventions to improve patient safety. Only now are researchers beginning to discuss how to evaluate these interventions and determine if patients are indeed safer. To evaluate our program—and reliably answer whether patients are safer—will require valid measures and the ability to know whether we mitigated hazards, an area that is currently underdeveloped. Yet, the measurement model we describe in this chapter should move us in the right direction in developing new measures of safety.

To begin to improve patient safety we can implement collaborative projects and the Comprehensive Unit-based Safety Program. The CUSP fosters a culture of safety in that staff will learn why patient safety is important, how to identify system failures in their workplace, and whom they can turn to in their efforts to make changes that improve safety. Indeed, staff feel valued for their opinions and recognized when senior leaders listen. Once a more solid safety culture is established, interventions can be implemented more effectively through collaborative projects. The CUSP also provides feasible and reliable tools to implement improvements in communication, teamwork, and adverse-event investigations. We have provided information on several, but not all, tools used in our safety efforts. For example, medication reconciliation can decrease medication errors in discharge or transfer orders if the tool is truly used as an independent check (52,53).

Collaborative projects are important because multiple sites that share the same goal can network to share successes and correct failures. There is a shared momentum that increases sustainability, which is typically a problem for a project or intervention. There can be pitfalls to large collaboratives, including inadequate resources, poor leadership, inadequate management of data collection and quality, and vague expectations and objectives for team members. These major issues must be addressed before a collaborative is initiated.

Any safety program should provide a practical, goal-oriented set of tools that improve culture and lead to measurable improvements in patient safety, using the principles described in this article as a guide. Further research is necessary to identify other effective safety interventions. Links must be developed between the structural elements of health care delivery and patient safety outcomes. Some of these structural elements might include intensivist staffing models, presence of pharmacists, use of the CUSP, improved nurse-to-patient ratio, and implementation of patient safety reporting systems. Given the data to date, it seems reasonable that all ICUs should be routinely assessing their culture of safety.

Although work is necessary at the organizational level, the question of whether our patients are safer can be meaningfully answered. Significant and very exciting improvements are beginning to be implemented throughout the United States. The critical care community must continue to develop the science of safety and, to a certain extent, create it, but many of the foundations have clearly already been laid.

References

1. Kohn L, Corrigan J, Donaldson M, eds. *Institute of Medicine. To Err Is Human: Building a Safer Health System.* Washington, DC: National Academies Press; 1999.
2. Institute of Medicine. *Crossing the Quality Chasm: A New Health System for the 21st Century.* Washington, DC: National Academies Press; 2001.
3. Leape LL, Berwick DM. Five years after to err is human: what have we learned? *JAMA.* 2005;293(19):2384–2390.
4. Reason J. Understanding adverse events: human factors. *Qual Health Care.* 1995;4(2):80–89.
5. Pronovost PJ, Angus DC, Dorman T, et al. Physician staffing patterns and clinical outcomes in critically ill patients: a systematic review. *JAMA.* 2002;288(17):2151–2162.
6. Pronovost PJ, Jenckes MW, Dorman T, et al. Organizational characteristics of intensive care units related to outcomes of abdominal aortic surgery. *JAMA.* 1999;281(14):1310–1317.
7. Brennan T, Gawande A, Thomas E, et al. Accidental deaths, saved lives, and improved quality. *N Engl J Med.* 2005;353(13):1405–1409.
8. Makary MA, Holzmueller CG, Sexton JB, et al. Operating room debriefings. *Jt Comm J Qual Saf.* 2006;32(7):407–410.
9. Makary MA, Holzmueller CG, Thompson DA, et al. Operating room briefings: working on the same page. *Jt Comm J Qual Saf.* 2006;32(6):351–355.
10. Pronovost PJ, King J, Holzmueller CG, et al. A Web-based tool for the Comprehensive Unit-based Safety Program (CUSP). *Jt Comm J Qual Saf.* 2006; 32(3):119–129.
11. Thompson DA, Holzmueller CG, Cafeo CL, et al. A morning briefing: setting the stage for a clinically and operationally good day. *Jt Comm J Qual Saf.* 2005;31(8):476–479.

12. Pronovost PJ, Hobson DB, Earsing K, et al. A practical tool to reduce medication errors during patient transfer from an intensive care unit. *J Clin Outcomes Manage.* 2004;11(1):26,29–33.
13. Pronovost P, Berenholtz S, Dorman T, et al. Improving communication in the ICU using daily goals. *J Crit Care.* 2003;18(2):71–75.
14. Pronovost PJ, Miller MR, Wachter RM. Tracking progress in patient safety: an elusive target. *JAMA.* 2006;296(6):696–699.
15. Sexton JB, Thomas E, Pronovost PJ. The context of care and the patient care team: the safety attitudes questionnaire. In: Reid PP, Compton WD, Grossman JH, et al., eds. *Building a Better Delivery System. A New Engineering Health Care Partnership.* Washington, DC: National Academies Press; 2005:119–123.
16. Donabedian A. The quality of care. How can it be assessed? *JAMA.* 1988; 260(12):1743–1748.
17. Sexton JB, Helmreich RL, Neilands TB, et al. The safety attitudes questionnaire: psychometric properties benchmarking data, and emerging research. *BMC Health Serv Res.* 2006;6(44) (doi:10.1186/1472-6963-6-44).
18. Pronovost PJ, Goeschel C. Improving ICU care: it takes a team. *Healthcare Exec.* 2005;14–22.
19. Thomas EJ, Sexton JB, Neilands TB, et al. The effect of executive walk rounds on nurse safety climate attitudes: a randomized trial of clinical units. *BMC Health Serv Res.* 2005;5(1):28 (doi:10.1186/1472-6963-5-28).
20. Defontes J, Surbida S. Preoperative safety briefing project. *Permanente J.* 2004;8(2):21–27.
21. Pronovost P, Weast B, Rosenstein B, et al. Implementing and validating a comprehensive unit-based safety program. *J Pat Saf.* 2005;1(1):33–40.
22. Pronovost P, Needham D, Berenholtz S, et al. An intervention to decrease catheter-related bloodstream infections in the ICU. *N Engl J Med.* 2006; 355(26):2725–2732.
23. Pronovost PJ, Holzmueller CG, Sexton JB, et al. How will we know patients are safer? An organization-wide approach to measuring and improving patient safety. *Crit Care Med.* 2006;34(7):1988–1995.
24. Altman D, Clancy C, Blendon R. Improving patient safety—five years after the IOM report. *N Engl J Med.* 2004;351(20):2041–2043.
25. Wachter R. The end of the beginning: patient safety five years after "to err is human." *Health Aff (Millwood).* 2004;(Supp Web Exclusives W4):534–545.
26. Hayward R, Hofer T. Estimating hospital deaths due to medical errors; preventability is in the eye of the reviewer. *JAMA.* 2004;286(4):415–420.
27. Berenholtz SM, Pronovost PJ, Lipsett PA, et al. Eliminating catheter-related bloodstream infections in the intensive care unit. *Crit Care Med.* 2004;32 (10):2014–2020.
28. Centers for Disease Control and Prevention. National nosocomial infections surveillance (NNIS) system report, data summary from January 1992 through June 2004. *Am J Infect Control.* 2004;32:470–485.
29. Jha A, Li Z, Orav E, et al. Care in U.S. hospitals–the Hospital Quality Alliance program. *N Engl J Med.* 2005;353(3):265–274.
30. Sexton JB, Thomas EJ, Helmreich RL. Error, stress and teamwork in medicine and aviation. A cross-sectional study. *Chirurg.* 2000;71(6 suppl):138–142.
31. Mills PD, Weeks WB. Characteristics of successful quality improvement teams: lessons from five collaborative projects in the VHA. *Jt Comm J Qual Saf.* 2004;30(3):152–162.
32. Ovretveit J, Bate P, Cleary P, et al. Quality collaboratives: lessons from research. *Qual Saf Health Care.* 2002;11:345–351.
33. Pronovost PJ, Berenholtz SM, Goeschel CA, et al. Creating high reliability in healthcare organizations. *Health Serv Res.* 2006;41(4):1599–1617.
34. Colla J, Bracken A, Kinney L, et al. Measuring patient safety climate: a review of surveys. *Qual Saf Health Care.* 2005;14:364–366.
35. Pronovost PJ, Holzmueller CG, Martinez E, et al. A practical tool to learn from defects in patient care. *Jt Comm J Qual Saf.* 2006;32(2):102–108.
36. Berenholtz SM, Milanovich S, Faircloth A, et al. Improving care for the ventilated patient. *Jt Comm J Qual Saf.* 2004;30(4):195–204.
37. Pronovost P, Wu AW, Dorman T, et al. Building safety into ICU care. *J Crit Care.* 2002;17(2):78–85.
38. Pronovost PJ, Wu AW, Sexton JB. Acute decompensation after removing a central line: practical approaches to increasing safety in the intensive care unit. *Ann Intern Med.* 2004;140(12):1025–1033.
39. Leonard M, Graham S, Bonacum D. The human factor: the critical importance of effective teamwork and communication in providing safe care. *Qual Saf Health Care.* 2004;13(Suppl 1):i85–90.
40. Hamman WR. The complexity of team training: what we have learned from aviation and its applications to medicine. *Qual Saf Health Care.* 2004; 13(Suppl 1):i72–79.
41. Pronovost PJ, Holzmueller CG, Clattenburg L, et al. Team care: beyond open and closed intensive care units. *Curr Opin Crit Care.* 2006;12(6):604–608.
42. Sexton JB, Makary MA, Tersigni AR, et al. Teamwork in the operating room: frontline perspectives among hospitals and operating room personnel. *Anesthesiology.* 2006;105(5):877–884.
43. Jain M, Miller L, Belt D, et al. Decline in ICU adverse events, nosocomial infections and cost through a quality improvement initiative focusing on teamwork and culture change. *Qual Saf Health Care.* 2006;15(4):235–239.
44. Fowlkes J, Dwyer DJ, Oser RL, et al. Event-based approach to training. *Int J Aviation Psychology.* 1998;8:209–221.
45. Gaba D. Structural and organizational issues in patient safety: a comparison of health care to other high-hazard industries. *Calif Manage Rev.* 2000;43: 83–102.
46. Cooper J. The role of simulation in patient safety. In: Dunn WF, ed. *Simulators in Critical Care and Beyond.* Des Plaines, IL: Society of Critical Care Medicine; 2004:20–24.
47. Fletcher G, Flin R, McGeorge P, et al. Anaesthetists' Non-Technical Skills (ANTS): evaluation of a behavioural marker system. *Br J Anaesth.* 2003; 90(5):580–588.
48. Reader T, Flin R, Lauche K, et al. Non-technical skills in the intensive care unit. *Br J Anaesth.* 2006;96(5):551–559.
49. Patey R, Flin R, Fletcher G, et al. Anaesthetists' nontechnical skills (ANTS). In: Hendricks K, ed. *Advances in Patient Safety: From Research to Implementation.* Washington, DC: Agency for Healthcare Research and Quality; 2005:325–326.
50. Grenvik A, Schaefer JJ 3rd, DeVita MA, et al. New aspects on critical care medicine training. *Curr Opin Crit Care.* 2004;10(4):233–237.
51. Salas E, Wilson KA, Burke CS, et al. Using simulation-based training to improve patient safety: what does it take? *Jt Comm J Qual Saf.* 2005;31(7): 363–371.
52. Holzmueller CG, Hobson D, Berenholtz SM, et al. Medication reconciliation: are we meeting the requirement? *J Clin Outcomes Mgt.* 2006;13(8):441–444.
53. Pronovost P, Weast B, Schwarz M, et al. Medication reconciliation: a practical tool to reduce the risk of medication errors. *J Crit Care.* 2003;18(4):201–205.
54. Reason JT. *Human Error.* New York: Cambridge University Press; 1990.
55. Reason J. Understanding adverse events: human factors. In: Vincent C, ed. *Clinical Risk Management.* London: BMJ Publications; 1995.

CHAPTER 11 ■ EXTERNAL COMPLIANCE ORGANIZATIONS AND MEASURES

DANNY M. TAKANISHI JR.

The Institute of Medicine in 1999 published a landmark treatise, *To Err Is Human: Building a Safer Health System* (1). This document served as a solemn reminder to all involved in the delivery of health care that safeguards were vital in order to realize much needed improvements in patient safety. Public awareness further fortified the impetus toward the establishment of a systems approach and external evaluation measures to address this need through multiple mechanisms, at both local and national levels.

The Joint Commission on Accreditation of Healthcare Organizations (JCAHO); the Agency for Healthcare Research and Quality (AHRQ); VHA (not an abbreviated word), Inc.; the

Centers for Medicare and Medicaid Services; and the Leapfrog Group are a few examples of organizations that have focused attention on improving the quality of patient care (2–10). Despite shared vision, implementation has proved to be a challenge. The definition of reliable measures of quality continues to be debated, the sustainability of implemented programs is also being questioned, and the impact of measures formulated to improve patient safety is still unclear (2,4,5,7,8,11–21).

The intensive care unit (ICU) is fertile ground to test implementation of quality initiatives. More than 5 million patients are admitted to ICUs in the United States annually (2). This accounts for only 8% to 10% of the acute care beds but comprises 20% to 30% of all acute care hospital costs (19). Notwithstanding, 10% of these patients will die and innumerable others will encounter preventable adverse events (5). Giraud et al. found that iatrogenic complications occur in up to 31% of patients and can be severe in 13% (19). It has been estimated that integration of quality standards and best practices can save more than 100,000 lives and $5.4 billion in costs annually (2).

CHRONICLE OF PERFORMANCE IMPROVEMENT INITIATIVE

In 2000, the Institute of Medicine grimly reported that up to 98,000 deaths annually in the United States were preventable, all resulting from medical errors. A recommendation was made to establish as a national priority a center for patient safety. This report further justified the development of mandatory and voluntary reporting systems, essential components in the evolution of a culture of safety and quality improvement (1). In parallel, 1 year prior, at the behest of the President's Advisory Commission on Consumer Protection and Quality in the Health Care Industry, the not-for-profit National Quality Forum (NQF) was established (15). The mission of this entity was to promote improvement in health care by the establishment of national benchmarks to measure health care quality and reporting of performance. This organization formulated 30 standards directed at improving patient safety, and published this in 2003 (22). A number are applicable to the ICU setting.

Notwithstanding, JCAHO has been an active participant in the process driving improvements in patient safety. This organization originated under the auspices of the American College of Surgeons in 1917, becoming an independent group in 1951. This entity was solely driven by health care professionals and served the function of assisting hospitals to improve quality of care and staff recruitment, and for accreditation of graduate medical education programs (4). Then, in 1965, the federally funded Medicare program was established by Congress. Statutorily, under the Social Security Amendments of 1965, a category called "deemed status" was established, which declared that any hospital accredited by JCAHO was also eligible to participate in the Medicare program. This was emblematic of the changes that were gradually occurring, as use of accreditation as an external quality improvement evaluation mechanism was expanding beyond the health care sector. Now there was governmental influence, soon to be followed by the public's use of accreditation as a means to evaluate the safety of health care delivery. JCAHO currently accredits almost 15,000

TABLE 11.1

JCAHO NATIONAL QUALITY FORUM MEASURES FOR THE INTENSIVE CARE UNIT (ICU)

Measure set	Performance measure
ICU-1	Ventilator associated-pneumonia (VAP) prevention: patient positioning
ICU-2	Stress ulcer disease (SUD) prophylaxis
ICU-3	Deep vein thrombosis (DVT)
ICU-4	Central line–associated primary bloodstream infection (further subcategorized a–k)

From the Joint Commission on Accreditation of Healthcare Organizations (JCAHO). National Hospital Quality Measures—ICU. Available at: http://www.jointcommission.org/Performance Measurement/MeasureReserveLibrary/Spec+Manual+--+ICU.htm. Accessed July 1, 2007.

health care organizations in the United States and over 96% of hospital beds in the United States are in accredited hospitals (3,4). This organization in July 2005 had instituted a reporting provision for four ICU core measures, based on the 2003 report by the NQF. These measures include ventilator-associated pneumonia prevention; patient positioning; stress ulcer prophylaxis; deep venous thrombosis prophylaxis; and central catheter-associated bloodstream infection (Table 11.1). Additionally, two test measures have also been recommended: ICU length of stay (risk adjusted) and hospital mortality for ICU patients (15).

There are other organizations and agencies involved in the external evaluation of health care institutions. This list includes the National Committee for Quality Assurance (NCQA), the American Medical Accreditation Program (AMAP), the American Accreditation Healthcare Commission/Utilization Review Accreditation Commission (AAHC/URAC), and the Accreditation Association for Ambulatory Healthcare (AAAHC). Other agencies, such as the Foundation for Accountability (FACCT), AHRQ, Institute for Healthcare Improvement (IHI), the National Coalition on Health Care (NCHC), and the Leapfrog Group also carry out unique roles in the assurance of safe, quality health care delivery (10). Each of these entities has differing missions and structures, and some are therefore better positioned to impact the ICU. Most of the accrediting agencies have in common, however, tenets established by JCAHO at its inception as an accrediting body: (a) accreditation is a voluntary process, (b) the evaluation of quality represents a cross-sectional analysis of the institution at the time of evaluation, (c) the accreditation is based on previously defined standards and indicators of quality, and (d) the process of accreditation must occur periodically based on a fixed number of years (8).

THE JOINT COMMISSION ON ACCREDITATION OF HEALTH CARE ORGANIZATIONS

The role of JCAHO, the oldest accrediting body for health care worldwide and the largest hospital regulator in the United

States, has evolved significantly since it was first conceived as a standing committee of the American College of Surgeons in 1917 (4,7). This organization's role in the external accreditation process broadened in response to the dynamic changes that the health care environment experienced in the 1970s and 1980s. The escalating costs of health insurance threatened businesses in the globally competitive marketplace, resulting in the drive for cost containment and the eventual implementation of managed care and capitation payments. Concomitantly, rising costs of health insurance were continually passed on to employees, who were then responsible for copayments for health care services in addition to a rising proportion of employer-subsidized health insurance. In parallel, health care institutions were financially pressured to restructure and to reorganize in order to meet the challenge of providing efficient, safe, and quality health care. Hence, it was a rational direction that this external accrediting agency took, in assisting the purchasers of health care services to make informed decisions regarding choice of health plans and providers, through the accreditation process. Finally, in response to public demand for representation in policy development and in the establishment of standards, JCAHO added public members to its board and to its advisory committees in 1982 (4). This was also followed by the development of an Office of Quality Monitoring, which provides a mechanism to address public complaints pertaining to an institution's alleged noncompliance with standards, and by the disclosure of performance reports detailing the accreditation status of an institution, and their performance in each of the standards, on the JCAHO Web site.

The accreditation process is still voluntary, as it was when this organization was first conceptualized in the early 1900s. It is noteworthy that approximately 50% of the JCAHO standards have direct relevance on patient safety, although the remaining standards all possess some relationship to patient safety indirectly (23,24). Therefore, the public, employers, insurers, and governmental agencies all tend to share the common belief that those institutions with accreditation provide higher-quality professional care. Available data do not disagree with this presumption.

It is worth pointing out that the definition of quality and the best measures and outcomes to assess quality and safety in the ICU setting are still not clear and many investigators have attempted to define these variables (12,25,26). Conceptually, quality measures must be validated as reliable tools that impact performance improvement and allow for standardization, so that comparisons of quality and safety can be readily made between all ICUs. Equally important is the a priori establishment of meaningful objective goals that will translate into measurable changes in quality improvement (12,16). To this end, JCAHO has recommended for national implementation four core measures and proposed two test measures. The quality benchmarks targeted include measuring the percentage of patients with central venous catheter bloodstream infections, the percentage of patients with ventilator-associated pneumonia, the percentage of patients with stress ulcers and use of prophylaxis, and the percentage of patients with deep venous thrombosis and use of prophylaxis (3). The test measures include ICU length of stay and hospital mortality. The nuances of these measures, particularly in terms of data collection, enforcement, and shortcomings and controversy as indices of quality, are discussed elsewhere (7,15,17,18).

INSTITUTE FOR HEALTHCARE IMPROVEMENT

The not-for-profit, Boston-based IHI was founded in 1991, as a by-product of the National Demonstration Project on Quality Improvement in Healthcare. Their Web site provides guidelines and tools for tracking change in practice, in addition to outcomes (9). This organization has released a report in conjunction with the NCHC, *Care in the ICU: Teaming Up to Improve Quality*. The basic premise is that improvements in ICU care that promote safety and quality are achievable now, based on evidence-based literature. This organization has proposed the use of care "bundles" (e.g., for patients on ventilators, or those with central lines), "rapid response teams," the implementation of multidisciplinary rounds with daily goals assessment, and implementing the "intensivist-led model" of ICU care. The IHI defines a "bundle" as a "structured way of improving the processes of care and patient outcomes: a small, straightforward set of practices—generally three to five—that, when performed collectively and reliably, have been proven to improve patient outcomes" (9,21). The initiatives of the IHI are closely aligned with JCAHO, particularly in terms of the four critical care JCAHO core measures discussed earlier.

LEAPFROG GROUP

This agency was founded in November 2000, after a group of employers in 1998 began the process of determining how best to approach the challenge of purchasing affordable, quality health care for their employees. Notably, this came on the heels of the Institute of Medicine's report *To Err Is Human: Building a Safer Health System*, which had recommended that large employers provide reinforcement for the provision of safe, quality health care through market pressure. This group comprises a number of Fortune 500 corporations and spans a broad range of purchasers of health care representing more than 34 million individuals (2,7). The Centers for Medicare and Medicaid Services is supporting this group in the propagation of information-identifying facilities achieving established standards. The Leapfrog Group had proposed a tripartite approach to address the patient safety initiative, and it estimated that this would save up to 58,300 lives and prevent more than 500,000 medication errors annually. The three recommendations included use of computerized physician order entry, increased evidence-based hospital referrals, and improved ICU physician staffing.

In common with proposals put forth by other organizations and agencies vested in patient safety and quality care in the ICU environment, the Leapfrog Group has conducted its own surveys to determine the degree to which institutions have been able to implement their recommendations. Significantly, some insurers have established incentives for health care facilities that integrate Leapfrog Group initiatives into their programs. The results have been promising, but not without the ire of certain constituencies of the health care system. The American Hospital Association has questioned whether standards promulgated by outside, or external, agencies should be embraced by hospitals, and the costs to implement and to sustain programs for computerized order entry or to employ qualified intensivists already in short supply have also been challenged.

PAY FOR PERFORMANCE

The quest for quality in health care has garnered tremendous interest during the past decade. One development is the concept of pay for performance, which is predicated on providing financial incentives to health care providers (both physicians and hospitals) who meet predetermined quality benchmarks prospectively established by insurers. A component of many iterations of this concept is public disclosure of health care provider results, in order to allow for a more informed decision in securing quality care (27). A number of organizations have provided input, such as the American Medical Association and JCAHO (28,29). Central to all models of pay for performance, both organizations concur that measurements should be "credible, reliable, and valid," in addition to being "measurable and transparent" and evidence based.

There has been a paucity of studies done to evaluate these models, in order to determine their effectiveness on the provision of quality care. The Integrated Healthcare Association and the Center for Medicare and Medicaid Services have validated their pay-for-performance models in terms of demonstrable improvement in quality care, and the considerable physician interest and involvement. Effective July 1, 2007, those participating in the Medicare program were provided the opportunity to voluntarily report their performance data (selected from 74 performance measures) to the Centers for Medicare and Medicaid Services and receive a bonus payment of up to 1.5% of allowed charges on all Medicare claims from July 1, 2007, through December 31, 2007, as part of the Physician Quality Reporting Initiative (PQRI). This followed the federal Centers' Physician Voluntary Reporting Program, which was not associated with a financial incentive. This information will not be made public, but the mechanism was devised to provide physicians with experience reporting quality data.

SUMMARY

Improving patient safety and delivering high-quality care to the critically ill patient is a universal goal. The ICU retains a prominent role in hospitals, given the complex nature of patients cared for and the contribution of this care to the escalating costs experienced by the health care system in the United States. A number of initiatives are in place to implement processes to improve care in this environment. To this end, external organizations are playing a crucial role in establishing policy for patient safety and the delivery of quality care through both regulatory (accreditation) and financial incentives. Correspondingly, a number of agencies are actively conducting research that will likely translate into improved patient safety, as results of these studies become incorporated into the regulatory process (supported by financial remuneration) to effect needed change (6,30).

References

1. Institute of Medicine. *To Err Is Human: Building A Safer Health System.* Available at: http://www.iom.edu/CMS/8089/5575.aspx. Accessed July 1, 2007.
2. Simmons JC. Focusing on quality and change in intensive care units. *The Quality Letter.* October 2002.
3. Joint Commission on Accreditation of Healthcare Organizations (JCAHO). National Hospital Quality Measures—ICU. Available at: http://www.jointcommission.org/PerformanceMeasurement/MeasureReserveLibrary/Spec+Manual+-+ICU.htm. Accessed July 1, 2007.
4. Schyve PM. The evolution of external quality evaluation: observations from the Joint Commission on Accreditation of Healthcare Organizations. *Int J Qual Health Care.* 2000;12:255.
5. Marinelli AM. Can regulation improve safety in critical care? *Crit Care Clin.* 2005;21:149–162.
6. Meyer GS, Battles J, Hart JC, et al. The US agency for health care research and quality's activities in patient safety research. *Int J Qual Health Care.* 2003; 15(Suppl I):i25.
7. Angus DC, Black N. Improving care of the critically ill: institutional and health-care system approaches. *Lancet.* 2004;363:1314.
8. Gallesio AO, Ceraso D, Palizas F. Improving quality in the intensive care unit setting. *Crit Care Clin.* 2006;22:547.
9. Institute for Healthcare Improvement. Intensive care: changes. Available at: http://www.ihi.org/IHI/Topics/CriticalCare/IntensiveCare/Changes. Accessed July 1, 2007.
10. Viswanathan HN, Salmon JW. Accrediting organizations and quality improvement. *Am J Manag Care.* 2000;6:1117.
11. Randolph AG, Pronovost P. Reorganizing the delivery of intensive care could improve efficiency and save lives. *J Eval Clin Pract.* 2002;8:1.
12. Zimmerman JE, Alzola C, von Rueden KT. The use of benchmarking to identify top performing critical care units: a preliminary assessment of their policies and practices. *J Crit Care.* 2003;18:76.
13. Halm EA, Siu AL. Are quality improvement messages registering? *Health Serv Res.* 2005;40:311.
14. Curtis JR, Cook DJ, Wall RJ, et al. Intensive unit quality improvement: a "how-to" guide for the interdisciplinary team. *Crit Care Med.* 2006;34: 211.
15. McMillan TR, Hyzy RC. Bringing quality improvement into the intensive care unit. *Crit Care Med.* 2007;35(Suppl):S59.
16. Pronovost PJ, Berenholtz SM, Ngo K, et al. Developing and pilot testing quality indicators in the intensive care unit. *J Crit Care.* 2003;18: 145.
17. Marik PE, Hedman L. What's in a day? Determining intensive care unit length of stay. *Crit Care Med.* 2000;28:2090.
18. Weissman C. Analyzing intensive care unit length of stay data: problems and possible solutions. *Crit Care Med.* 1997;25:1594.
19. Garland A. Improving the ICU: part 1. *Chest.* 2005;127:2151.
20. Garland A. Improving the ICU: part 2. *Chest.* 2005;127:2165.
21. Stockwell DC, Slonim AD. Quality and safety in the intensive care unit. *J Intensive Care Med.* 2006;21:199.
22. Safe Practices for Better Healthcare: A Consensus Report, 2003. Available at: http://www.qualityforum.org/projects/completed/safe_practices. Accessed July 1, 2007.
23. Saufl NM, Fieldus MH. Accreditation: a "voluntary" regulatory requirement. *J Perianesth Nurs.* 2003;18:152.
24. Catalano K. JCAHO's national patient safety goals 2006. *J Perianesth Nurs.* 2006;21:6.
25. Berenholtz SM, Dorman T, Ngo K, et al. Qualitative review of intensive care unit quality indicators. *J Crit Care.* 2002;17:1.
26. Osler T, Horne L. Quality assurance in the surgical intensive care unit. Where it came from and where it's going. *Surg Clin North Am.* 1991;71: 887.
27. Spinelli RJ, Fromknecht JM. Pay for performance: improving quality care. *Health Care Manag.* 2007;26:128.
28. American Medical Association. Guidelines for pay for performance programs. February 24, 2005. Available at: http://www.ama-assn.org/ama1/pub/upload/mm/368/guidelines4pay62705.pdf. Accessed July 1, 2007.
29. Joint Commission on Accreditation of Healthcare Organizations (JCAHO). Principles for the construct of pay-for-performance. Available at: http://www.jointcommission.org/PublicPolicy/pay.htm. Accessed July 1, 2007.
30. Dean Beaulieu N, Epstein AM. National committee on quality assurance health-plan accreditation: predictors, correlates of performance, and market impact. *Med Care.* 2002;40:325.

CHAPTER 12 ■ THE VIRTUAL ICU AND TELEMEDICINE: COMPUTERS, ELECTRONICS, AND DATA MANAGEMENT

ERAN SEGAL

Although there are numerous models of ICU design, the approach of most intensivists is that a physician-led, multidisciplinary team in a closed unit format is best in terms of quality and outcome. It has been estimated that implementation of ICU staffing and organization in this manner can save more than 50,000 lives a year in the United States (1). Several studies show that a dedicated intensivist can improve use of intensive care beds and also decrease mortality (2–4). However, the number of patients requiring critical care is rapidly growing, and research has shown that in a few years, the shortage of pulmonologists and intensivists will lead to dramatic reductions in the ability of critically ill patients to be cared for by dedicated intensivists (5). Recent recommendations by the Leapfrog Group have called for increased staffing of adult ICUs, the compliance of which will be very difficult for many institutions despite the very real possibilities of improved finances and quality. Provonost et al. (6) used a model to show a yearly savings of up to US $13 million in a 6- to 18-bed ICU if staffing recommendations were attained. The shortage of ICU clinicians and the explosion of information collected while caring for the critically ill patient lends itself to applying sophisticated information technology to improve ICU care.

Computerized systems can improve ICU work on many levels, from replacing the flow sheet filled with the patients' continual record of vital signs, to systems that allow all documentation to be entered, manipulated, and archived electronically. The systems available today allow vital signs to be collected automatically; physicians' and nurses' notes entered into the system; and information from the admitting and discharge system regarding all patient demographics provided in the record. Laboratory results are another layer of information that can be automatically entered into the patient's electronic record. The computerized patient record can be linked to other systems such as the radiology, echocardiography, or microbiology systems. An extremely important feature is the potential for added patient safety, a significant benefit of electronic systems.

IMMEDIATE CONCERNS

The vast, unwieldy amount of data collected on each patient in the ICU requires the use of computerized systems. It is very difficult for clinicians to use all the information obtained from monitors, ventilators, and laboratories without computerized support. Advantages of storing patient data on computerized systems include the following:

- Computerized physician order entry (CPOE) can decrease errors in prescription and in executing drug orders. This may lead to substantial error prevention and improved outcome.
- Computerized systems allow recording and manipulating data to optimize decision making.
- Complex rules and decision support tools are available to improve clinical decision making and reduce errors.
- Computerized systems can improve adherence to protocols, thus leading to improved quality and outcomes.
- Computerized systems can be used to improve monitoring and care of patients remotely (the remote ICU or e-ICU) using monitoring and audiovisual tools that enable experienced clinicians to improve care in ICUs that do not have full-time staffing.

Although implementing a computerized system can greatly improve patient care, there are potential risks due to our increased reliance on these systems, which will be discussed later in this chapter.

CLASSIFICATION OF INFORMATION TECHNOLOGY (IT) SOLUTIONS FOR CRITICAL CARE

Electronic Charting

The most basic application of computerized systems is the electronic chart. The information on flow sheets in critical care includes, almost universally, the recording of all physiologic data including hemodynamic data, information from ventilators, and other electronic devices such as syringe pumps, specific stand-alone monitors, dialysis and hemofiltration machines, and information from central hospital systems such as pathology, imaging, hospital information systems, and echocardiography.

The presentation of this information, composed of different types of data—numeric, analog, images—with different time stamps and rates of refreshing the data, is quite complex. Some elements need to be updated at very rapid rates such as the physiologic parameters from the monitors and ventilators, whereas information from the microbiology laboratory—type of bacteria, specific identification, and sensitivities—should be updated as the information develops, although the time stamp of the

Dr. Segal is a consultant of IMDsoft Inc.

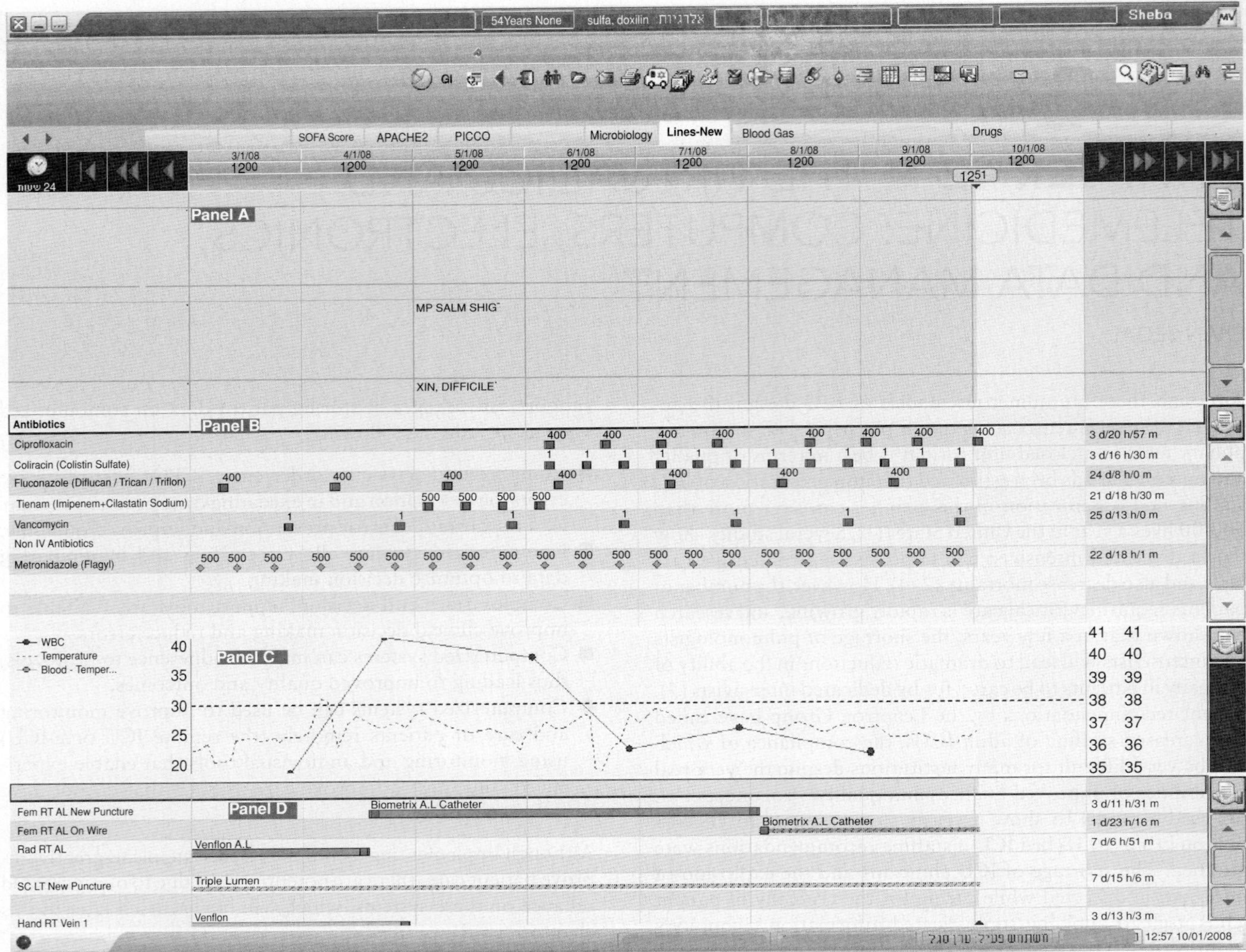

FIGURE 12.1. A screen shot of the computerized system demonstrating the use of different information sources to provide a clinical picture. In this screen, information from the microbiology lab (**panel A**), antibiotic administration (**panel B**), temperature and white blood cell count (**panel C**), and a Gantt chart of duration of intravenous lines (**panel D**) are reported together to enable easier assessment of the patient's infectious status. This and other kinds of data presentations can be customized by the clinicians at the ICU, hospital, or enterprise level.

acquisition of the sample is equally as important as the time of availability of the additional information (Fig. 12.1).

Drug administration and standing orders also need to be part of the flow sheet and require a different type of presentation of the information. Very often, a Gantt type of chart—showing a horizontal bar with start to end times of different processes—is a good way of presenting this type of data. Data should be made available electronically in different types of formats to optimize its usefulness in various types of situations. Tables, graphs, Gantt charts, and combinations of all of these are critical for a convenient and user-friendly presentation. When deciding on a computerized system, clinicians should be aware that data collected within a 24-hour period such as from a foldable paper flow sheet or an A3 paper sheet cannot conveniently fit on a single computer screen, so instruction on the techniques of scrolling in the specific program should be provided. At the same time, information from many weeks or days can be presented very rapidly and easily with one or two mouse clicks—for example, the lactate or white blood cell count (WBC) values of the patient for the duration of even the longest admission. This kind of ability is not available when using paper charting.

Undoubtedly, a most important aspect of deploying a computerized system is the ability to customize it to the unit's specific needs and requirements. Clinical work should not be changed due to implementation of a computerized system, but rather the system should be adaptable to the mode of operation in a particular ICU. Despite the similarities in critical care throughout the world, there are significant differences between ICUs in different institutions and ICUs within the same institution, and thus, a computerized system should be adaptable and customizable in any ICU.

Customization

Customizing the electronic medical record can produce a visual spectrum of work flow, depending on how the information is entered into the system, to the way data are presented.

Computing capabilities allow different users who log onto the system to view different types of information and in a presentation more suitable for their needs. Thus, an infectious disease consultant may wish to see pertinent information regarding cultures, white count, and fever on the same screen, whereas a nephrologist may want to be presented with electrolyte and metabolic data, as well as fluid balance initially. With a customizable system, complex order sets can be created and easily prescribed according to unit, procedure, or surgeon's protocol. The use of protocols and routine prescriptions may improve standardization and compliance with evidence-based procedures.

Complex Alerts

Computerized alerts can improve needed clinical activity. Paltiel et al. (7) showed that an alert presented by computers throughout the hospital for a low potassium level could reduce the time to treatment of hypokalemia. We looked at the impact of an electronic alert in a computerized patient record, and showed that when implementing this alert, the proportion of blood glucose measurements within the desired range significantly increased whereas the proportion of elevated glucose measurements decreased. This was achieved without an increase in the proportion of hypoglycemic episodes (8). We also showed that an alert that notifies the clinicians of a low potassium level reduces the time to treat the patient. There are programs designed to deal with specific topics and clinical problems. Juneja et al. (9) showed that a program dedicated to treating patients who require insulin while in the ICU to maintain tight glucose control led to better results compared to the situation before the program was implemented.

Decision support can improve the use of various resources. Perez et al. (10) used decision support to reduce the use of blood products in an intensive care unit. Rood et al. (11) showed that using an alert system designed to improve glycemic control in an ICU improved the time to achieving desired glucose control (Fig. 12.2). In fact, a computerized system can enable the application of many types of alerts. In our ICU, the computerized system alerts staff when a patient is receiving vancomycin and a blood level has not been drawn; when a patient's PaO_2 is high

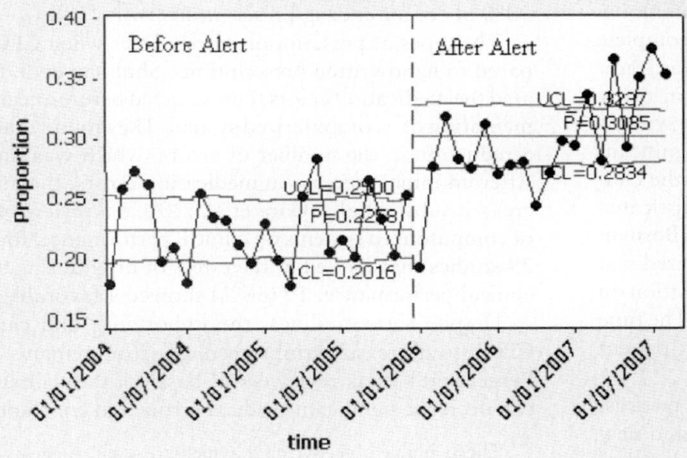

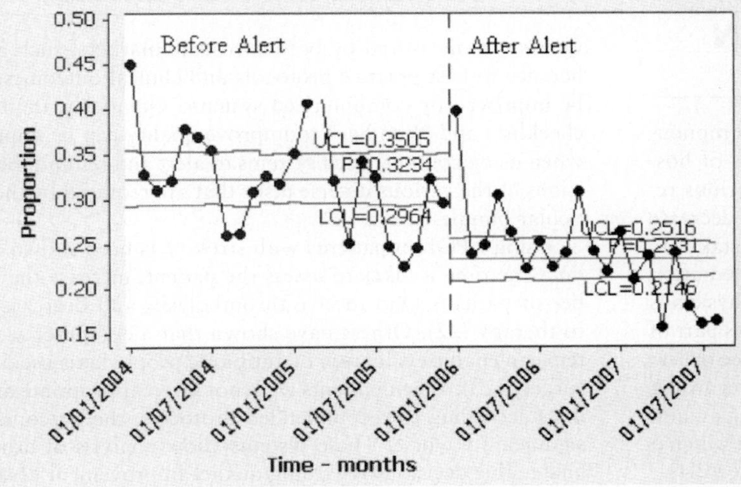

FIGURE 12.2. Effect of implementation of an electronic alert regarding glucose measurement on the incidence of optimal (**top panel**) versus high (**bottom panel**) glucose measurements. When an alert was implemented, proportion of optimal glucose levels increased and proportion of high glucose levels decreased significantly. (Modified from Segal E, Haviv-Yadid Y, Livingstone D, et al. An electronic alert to improve glucose control in a general ICU. *Intensive Care Med.* 2007;33[Suppl 2]:S234.)

when the FiO_2 is greater than 0.3; and if a patient has not had a bowel movement in 3 days. All of these alerts are relevant to our daily clinical practice and help decrease variability in our work.

Alerts can be provided to clinicians in various ways. In a surgical ICU, a wireless system sent pages to the respective physicians, notifying them of abnormal physiological and laboratory results. The alerting system identified patients with a higher risk of death and longer stay in the ICU (12). The ability to identify high-risk patients and alert clinicians to critical events may enable earlier intervention and improved outcome.

EFFECTS ON WORKLOAD

The implementation of a computerized system may generate concern over the increased workload associated with the transition. Certainly an initial effort at customizing the system to fit the local clinical work flow is required, which may vary for different commercial systems. The time required for training of staff should also be considered when deciding on a computerized system. Even when the system is in place, there are clinicians who feel uncomfortable working with a keyboard and mouse rather than with pen and paper. These concerns, however, are decreasing as work with computers increases in everyday life, as well as the fact that computers are commonly used even in ICUs that have not yet implemented a complete electronic patient record. Hospital information systems, radiology, and laboratories are often computerized, but in many ICUs, clinicians still copy results from these various systems onto a paper flow sheet. In a computerized system, significant portions of the charting workload are eliminated for the clinicians, and thus more time is available for more sophisticated charting and reporting and also for direct patient care. Bosman et al. (13) showed that implementation of a computerized system decreased the time nurses spent on charting information on critically ill patients following cardiothoracic surgery. The time saved by the computerized system was spent on direct patient care, increasing the time at the bedside.

When clinicians work with computerized patient records, there are changes in the characteristics of the work, and new types of distractions may occur. An observational study of clinicians working with a computerized order entry system showed that there are distractions in working with the computer that may, in some cases, lead to potentially significant errors (14).

COMPUTERIZED PHYSICIAN ORDER ENTRY (CPOE)

Despite the evidence regarding the advantages of computerized provider order entry systems, only 5% to 10% of hospitals in the United States use them, according to various reports (15,16). CPOE has been proposed as a tool to decrease prescription errors due to handwriting legibility, mistakes in dosage, incompatibility, and allergy alerts. The implementation of CPOE can significantly impact the daily work of physicians and nurses (17). The use of a computerized database as part of the prescription process can lead to improvement, since orders can be evaluated by the database and provide alerts regarding drug–drug interaction, double prescription, drug allergies, and effects of disease processes on drug dose. This is true when a decision support capability is part of the CPOE (Table 12.1).

TABLE 12.1

TYPES OF ERRORS THAT SHOULD BE PREVENTED BY CPOE WITH DECISION SUPPORT

Drug allergy: For same drug, drug class, or vehicle component
Dose limits: According to age, weight, disease, and laboratory result
Double prescription: Overlap of the same drug or drug class to an existing order
Maximal dose: Both for single administration or cumulative dose
Drug–drug interaction: Significant interactions of various drugs or drug families
Order verification: Alert for orders requiring double signature or specific identification (e.g., blood products)
Test requirement: Drugs requiring drug level measurements (e.g., antibiotics, anticonvulsants)

There are more basic forms of electronic information systems. Computerized systems that do not have decision support as part of the available tools will only provide information regarding the drug–drug administration and dosage, but may not be able to alert when prescriptions have mistakes in them. The Leapfrog Group designed a Web-based test for CPOE and requires hospitals to prove that their CPOE can detect at least 50% of common drug prescription errors (18).

The types of prescription errors differ when CPOE is compared to handwritten prescriptions. Shulman et al. (19) evaluated the medication errors that occurred before and after implementation of a computerized system. They found that there was a reduction in the number of errors, which was time-related. After an initial increase in medication errors, the numbers decreased substantially. Garg et al. (20), in a review of the effect of computerized systems on clinical performance, found that of 29 studies that looked at the effect of drug dosing systems on clinical performance, 19 (66%) showed a favorable outcome.

Despite these findings, the importance and capability of CPOE to decrease harmful medical errors remains debatable. Berger and Kichak reviewed the basis for the claim that CPOE can decrease significant medical errors and concluded that:

> The available objective data, which are scant, suggest that, at best, there is a potential for these systems to decrease ADEs (adverse drug events) and their additional medical costs (21).

QUALITY IMPROVEMENT

Quality, as measured by both surrogate markers, such as adherence to best practice protocols and clinical outcomes, may be improved by computerized systems. Obviously, the use of checklists and "bundles" to improve quality can be improved when using computerized systems to alert and remind the clinicians of the various diverse tasks that are required by the particular bundle.

Using CPOE in patients with stroke has been shown to reduce the time it takes to assess the patient, increase the number of patients who receive thrombolysis, and decrease time to therapy (22). Others have shown that a computerized system can enable evaluation of antibiotic prophylaxis use during surgery (23). When patients were not given appropriate antibiotics according to recommended protocols, the outcome was significantly worse. These systems allow analysis of drug use and enable decisions regarding quality improvement (24).

ERRORS AND THEIR PREVENTION

Errors are a major issue in intensive care medicine and are reported to occur 1.7 times a day per patient in an ICU (25). The impact of medical errors on patient outcomes was emphasized in the famous "To err is human" report by the Institute of Medicine (26). The use of computerized systems has a potential of reducing error by improving standardization and reviewing databases of information about the patient's baseline diseases, drug allergies, previous procedures, and tests. There is also an advantage to improving compliance with protocols and unit procedures, which computerized systems can enable.

Drug errors range from illegible prescriptions to mistakes in patient identification and lapses in knowledge of patient allergies, drug–drug interactions, and dosing considerations. Many of these types of errors can be reduced or completely eliminated using computerized systems. Vardi et al. (27) showed that using CPOE as part of an electronic patient record can completely eliminate drug order mistakes in a pediatric ICU when they applied it to resuscitation orders, which, in pediatrics, are particularly prone to mistakes because of the diversity in patient size and the urgency of the situation.

THE REMOTE ICU

The requirements for physician staffing of ICUs calls for 24-hour coverage by trained physicians. The ICU should be directed by a dedicated trained intensivist who is in-house during the day, available for answering pages within 5 minutes, and able to provide physician or physician extender presence within the requirement for intensivist coverage of all critically ill patients as recommended by the Leapfrog Group. Coupled with the increasing shortage of intensive care clinicians, the desire for ICU coverage by trained intensivists has led to an interest in remote systems that enable direction of patient care in remote ICUs. These kinds of systems allow for a central hospital or critical care physicians group to assume responsibility for patients who are cared for in a peripheral ICU. There are reports of improved clinical outcomes, including mortality and length of stay, while caring for a higher-severity population of patients (28). Breslow et al. (29) described their experience with a remote ICU that was involved in the care of patients in two adult ICUs and provided 19 hours per day of monitoring by physicians and physician extenders. During the period of remote ICU work, they observed a reduction in ICU mortality, a decreased length of stay, and cost reduction, which more than compensated for the costs of the system; the effectiveness of this technology has been shown (30).

Vespa et al. (31) used a robotic telepresence system to respond to nursing pages in a neuro-ICU. They showed that during use of the robot system, the time for an attending face-to-face response to nursing page was significantly decreased for all types of calls. More than that, they had a decrease in length of stay of 2 days for patients with subarachnoid hemorrhage (SAH) and 1 day for patients with head trauma. ICU occupancy increased by 11%, with a substantial cost savings.

Tang et al. (32) recently described their experience with a remote ICU with respect to physician and nurse work flow. They found that the clinical team providing remote support used most of the time for monitoring and integration of monitored data. There were many interruptions during the routine work due to the need for observing or dealing with an unstable patient or due to a request for intervention from the local team. They also found that while physicians attended to specific problems that were primarily self-initiated, the nurses were alerted by automatic alarms in 80% of the cases. Also, nurses were required to spend a significant portion of their time recording bedside notes into the remote ICU chart. They conclude that when implementing these technologies, the different work flows of physicians and nurses have to be considered.

RISKS OF COMPUTERIZED SYSTEMS

Dangers of IT implementation in critical care may be due to several factors (33). There may be complaints regarding increased workload, required changes in clinical work flow, persistence of paper components, and some emotional issues and problems with communications. There may also be issues related to blind dependence on the computer, so that if a default dose of drug was incorrectly customized into the drug database, clinicians might not be aware and prescribe the inappropriate dose. This has led to the creation of the term "e-Iatrogenesis" (34).

Han et al. (35) published a worrisome report of an increase in mortality—from 2.8% to 6.6%—in a pediatric ICU following implementation of CPOE. This may have been due to problems with the integration of pharmacy and clinical work flow into the system using the CPOE. For example, drugs could not be provided even in extreme situations unless prescribed through the CPOE. Other investigators have not found this phenomenon (36); in fact, a group from Seattle found a reduction in mortality as well as in risk-adjusted mortality, although these effects were not statistically significant. Keene et al. (37) also did not find an increase in mortality after implementing CPOE in a pediatric ICU.

RETURN ON INVESTMENT

A significant question raised when considering the purchase and implementation of a computerized system is that of cost. These systems are not inexpensive, and thus their economic utility needs to be analyzed. On the one hand, costs of the system include not only the hardware and software of a system, but also the burden of time invested in customizing the system, training of personnel, and the maintenance required. It is unrealistic to expect a computerized system to run perfectly "right out of the box." To achieve optimal results, a local "champion" of the system must be identified and appointed, with involvement of all components of the ICU team in the process. On the hospital level, when implementing a computerized system, pertinent management officials and IT quality and risk management should all take part in the assessment, customization, and follow-up.

The potential financial rewards of a computerized system (Table 12.2) range from an improvement in standardization of care, which may lead to better clinical outcomes, to a reduction in errors and adverse events, with a consequent decrease in malpractice litigation. Moreover, the ability to defend against malpractice claims may be improved with an accurate record that is easily retrievable, and therefore should lead to improved risk-management activities. Smaller but not inconsequential cost savings may be due to the lower cost of archiving

TABLE 12.2

POTENTIAL COST SAVINGS WITH COMPUTERIZED RECORDS

Improved adherence to protocols
- Reduced complications
- Decreased length of stay

Decrease in drug prescription errors
Encouragement of using less costly—but equally effective—drugs
Better information regarding the use of medications and equipment
Improved billing
Improved risk management
Improved record keeping and ability to contest medical malpractice claims
Decreased cost of archiving records

computerized records versus paper charts. Additionally, adherence to protocols that suggest use of more cost-effective procedures can decrease use of unnecessary more-expensive drugs.

Billing is probably improved by the use of a computerized system and may contribute to return on investment (ROI). The bottom line of ROI is difficult to prove, but many clinicians agree that there is a potential for computerized systems to decrease costs and, at the same time, improve quality.

SUMMARY

With advances in information technology and in design of computerized systems for critical care, the significance of these systems for clinical care and for impacting patient outcome is increasing. There is no doubt that the use of computerized systems in critical care will increase in the coming years. The implementation of systems should be focused on improving the information at the clinician's fingertips to reduce errors, improve adherence to protocols, and provide better clinical outcomes.

References

1. Pronovost PJ, Waters H, Dorman T. Impact of critical care physician workforce for intensive care unit physician staffing. *Curr Opin Crit Care.* 2001; 7(6):456–459.
2. Reynolds HN, Haupt MT, Thill-Baharozian MC, et al. Impact of critical care physician staffing on patients with septic shock in a university hospital medical intensive care unit. *JAMA.* 1988;260(23):3446–3450.
3. Brown JJ, Sullivan G. Effect on ICU mortality of a full-time critical care specialist. *Chest.* 1989;96(1):127–129.
4. Pollack MM, Katz RW, Ruttimann UE, et al. Improving the outcome and efficiency of intensive care: the impact of an intensivist. *Crit Care Med.* 1988;16(1):11–17.
5. Angus DC, Kelley MA, Schmitz RJ, et al. Caring for the critically ill patient. Current and projected workforce requirements for care of the critically ill and patients with pulmonary disease: can we meet the requirements of an aging population? *JAMA.* 2000;284(21):2762–2770.
6. Pronovost PJ, Needham DM, Waters H, et al. Intensive care unit physician staffing: financial modeling of the Leapfrog standard. *Crit Care Med.* 2006;34(3 Suppl):S18–24.
7. Paltiel O, Gordon L, Berg D, et al. Effect of a computerized alert on the management of hypokalemia in hospitalized patients. *Arch Intern Med.* 2003;163(2):200–204.
8. Segal E, Haviv-Yadid Y, Livingstone D, et al. An electronic alert to improve glucose control in a general ICU. *Intensive Care Med.* 2007;33(Suppl 2):S234.
9. Juneja R, Roudebush C, Kumar N, et al. Utilization of a computerized intravenous insulin infusion program to control blood glucose in the intensive care unit. *Diabetes Technol Ther.* 2007;9(3):232–240.
10. Perez ER, Winters JL, Gajic O. The addition of decision support into computerized physician order entry reduces red blood cell transfusion resource utilization in the intensive care unit. *Am J Hematol.* 2007;82(7):631–633.
11. Rood E, Bosman RJ, van der Spoel JI, et al. Use of a computerized guideline for glucose regulation in the intensive care unit improved both guideline adherence and glucose regulation. *J Am Med Inform Assoc* 2005;12(2):172–180.
12. Major K, Shabot MM, Cunneen S. Wireless clinical alerts and patient outcomes in the surgical intensive care unit. *Am Surg.* 2002;68(12):1057–1060.
13. Bosman RJ, Rood E, Oudemans-van Straaten HM, et al. Intensive care information system reduces documentation time of the nurses after cardiothoracic surgery. *Intensive Care Med.* 2003;29(1):83–90.
14. Collins S, Currie L, Patel V, et al. Multitasking by clinicians in the context of CPOE and CIS use. *Medinfo.* 2007;12(Pt 2):958–962.
15. Usage of CPOE steadily increasing, Leapfrog says. *Healthcare Benchmarks Qual Improv.* 2006;13(3):33–34.
16. Jha AK, Ferris TG, Donelan K, et al. How common are electronic health records in the United States? A summary of the evidence. *Health Aff (Millwood).* 2006;25(6):w496–507.
17. Popernack ML. A critical change in a day in the life of intensive care nurses: rising to the e-challenge of an integrated clinical information system. *Crit Care Nurs Q.* 2006;29(4):362–375.
18. Kilbridge PM, Welebob EM, Classen DC. Development of the Leapfrog methodology for evaluating hospital implemented inpatient computerized physician order entry systems. *Qual Saf Health Care.* 2006;15(2):81–84.
19. Shulman R, Singer M, Goldstone J, et al. Medication errors: a prospective cohort study of hand-written and computerised physician order entry in the intensive care unit. *Crit Care.* 2005;9(5):R516–521.
20. Garg AX, Adhikari NKJ, McDonald H, et al. Effects of computerized clinical decision support systems on practitioner performance and patient outcomes: a systematic review. *JAMA.* 2005;293:1223–1238.
21. Berger RG, Kichak JP. Computerized physician order entry: helpful or harmful? *J Am Med Inform Assoc.* 2004;11(2):100–103.
22. Nam HS, Han SW, Ahn SH, et al. Improved time intervals by implementation of computerized physician order entry-based stroke team approach. *Cerebrovasc Dis.* 2007;23(4):289–293.
23. Hartmann B, Sucke J, Brammen D, et al. Impact of inadequate surgical antibiotic prophylaxis on perioperative outcome and length of stay on ICU in general and trauma surgery. Analysis using automated data collection. *Int J Antimicrob Agents.* 2005;25(3):231–236.
24. Hartmann B, Junger A, Brammen D, et al. Review of antibiotic drug use in a surgical ICU: management with a patient data management system for additional outcome analysis in patients staying more than 24 hours. *Clin Ther.* 2004;26(6):915–924; discussion 904.
25. Donchin Y, Gopher D, Olin M, et al. A look into the nature and causes of human errors in the intensive care unit. *Crit Care Med.* 1995;23(2):294–300.
26. *IOM: To Err Is Human: Building a Safer Health System.* Washington, DC: National Academy Press; 1999.
27. Vardi A, Efrati O, Levin I, et al. Prevention of potential errors in resuscitation medications orders by means of a computerised physician order entry in paediatric critical care. *Resuscitation.* 2007;73(3):400–406.
28. Zawada ET Jr, Kapaska D, Herr P, et al. Prognostic outcomes after the initiation of an electronic telemedicine intensive care unit (eICU) in a rural health system. *S D Med.* 2006;59(9):391–393.
29. Breslow MJ, Rosenfeld BA, Doerfler M, et al. Effect of a multiple-site intensive care unit telemedicine program on clinical and economic outcomes: an alternative paradigm for intensivist staffing. *Crit Care Med.* 2004;32(1):31–38.
30. Rosenfeld BA, Dorman T, Breslow MJ, et al. Intensive care unit telemedicine: alternate paradigm for providing continuous intensivist care. *Crit Care Med.* 2000;28(12):3925–3931.
31. Vespa PM, Miller C, Hu X, et al. Intensive care unit robotic telepresence facilitates rapid physician response to unstable patients and decreased cost in neurointensive care. *Surg Neurol.* 2007;67(4):331–337.
32. Tang Z, Weavind L, Mazabob J, et al. Workflow in intensive care unit remote monitoring: a time-and-motion study. *Crit Care Med.* 2007;35(9):2057–2063.
33. Campbell EM, Sittig DF, Ash JS, et al. Types of unintended consequences related to computerized provider order entry. *J Am Med Inform Assoc.* 2006; 13:547–556.
34. Weiner JP, Kfuri T, Chan K, et al. "e-Iatrogenesis": the most critical unintended consequence of CPOE and other HIT. *J Am Med Inform Assoc.* 2007;14(3):387–388; discussion 389.
35. Han YY, Carcillo JA, Venkataraman ST, et al. Unexpected increased mortality after implementation of a commercially sold computerized physician order entry system. *Pediatrics.* 2005;116(6):1506–1512.
36. Del Beccaro MA, Jeffries HE, Eisenberg MA, et al. Computerized provider order entry implementation: no association with increased mortality rates in an intensive care unit. *Pediatrics.* 2006;118(1):290–295.
37. Keene A, Ashton L, Shure D, et al. Mortality before and after initiation of a computerized physician order entry system in a critically ill pediatric population. *Pediatr Crit Care Med.* 2007;8(3):268–271.

CHAPTER 13 ■ UNIVERSAL PRECAUTIONS: PROTECTING THE PRACTITIONER

HARRINARINE MADHOSINGH • DENISE SCHAIN

INTRODUCTION

Infection control is a key factor in reducing the transmission of nosocomial infections. It involves the use of specific measures in an attempt to reduce the spread of infectious agents from health care workers (HCWs) and the hospital environment to the patient, and from the patient back into the hospital environment to other patients and to HCWs. Increased length of stay and total hospital cost have been associated with nosocomial methicillin-resistant *Staphylococcus aureus* (MRSA) infections (1,2). Through prevention, costs associated with treating these infections, as well as length of hospitalization, can be reduced. In this chapter, we will take a brief look at the history of infection control, define the various infection control measures, and explore the application of these measures as they apply to common bacterial and viral agents in the health care setting.

HISTORICAL PERSPECTIVE

One of the pioneers of infection control measures was undoubtedly the Hungarian obstetrician Ignaz Semmelweis (3). Bored with his study of law, Semmelweis switched to medicine and graduated from the Second Vienna Medical School in 1844. After his graduation, he worked on the obstetric wards at Allegemeines Krankenhaus in Vienna. It was there that he became alarmed by the high rates of puerperal sepsis ("childbed fever"). It was noted that infection rates were much lower on the teaching ward for midwives compared to that of the medical students and physicians. Semmelweis postulated that women likely became infected when cared for by medical students and physicians who were often coming directly to the obstetric ward after performing autopsies on women who had died of puerperal fever. The death of Jacob Kolletschka, a friend of Semmelweis, who sustained a scalpel injury while performing an autopsy on a patient who died of childbed fever, cemented the association between autopsies and puerperal fevers, especially with the autopsy of his friend showing similar pathologic features to those patients who had died of puerperal fever. Semmelweis then implemented a simple measure by asking the medical students and physicians to wash their hands with a chlorine solution after performing autopsies prior to attending to patients. With this simple measure of handwashing, the rates of puerperal fever drastically dropped on the obstetric teaching ward for the women cared for by the medical students and physicians. Semmelweis' methods failed to gain favor due to a combination of several factors, not the least of which was that chlorine solution was not gentle on the hands. It was not until much later that Semmelweis got credit for his astute observation and intervention. Another pioneer of infection control was the British surgeon Joseph Lister (4). Lister used the results of earlier experiments done by Louis Pasteur, who had used an animal model to demonstrate transmission of infection by microbes, and then applied these to humans. He showed that chemicals could be used to prevent infection, and used carbolic acid spray on wounds to prevent gangrene, also spraying it on surgical instruments and incisions, thus achieving lower infection rates. Lister also encouraged his surgical colleagues to use a 5% solution of carbolic acid on their hands before and after operations. Further improvements and modifications were made to these early advances and ultimately led to the modern era of infection control.

PRECAUTIONS

There are several types of precautions for use in patient care settings that have been described; making sense of them and knowing when to implement each can be confusing. The Centers for Disease Control and Prevention (CDC) has published guidelines outlining the recommended approach to infection control, as well as the definition and application of the various precautions. It is noteworthy that implementation of standard precautions (previously termed *universal*) does not negate the need for further specialized infection control precautions if necessary, such as droplet precautions for influenza, airborne isolation for pulmonary tuberculosis, or contact isolation for MRSA. There are four types of precautions recommended in the CDC guidelines (5):

1. Standard (previously termed *universal*)
2. Contact
3. Droplet
4. Airborne

Standard Precautions

Standard precautions are those that are applied to which the practitioner comes into contact, regardless of the diagnosis. Standard precautions include handwashing before and after contact with every patient, and between anatomic sites on the same patients. Based on the clinical task and setting, additional precautions may be required to care for patients who do not have a diagnosis requiring other specific categories of isolation. These precautions apply to blood and body fluids (including secretions and excretions, excluding sweat), broken skin, and mucous membranes. If indicated, the HCW may also require use of (a) gloves; (b) mask, eye protection, and face shield; and/or (c) gowning.

Other considerations include special handling of patient care equipment, including sharps and other instruments, and environmental control with correct disposal and cleaning of linen and other contaminated items. It is important to note that, while not all of these additional precautions apply in every circumstance and are only used if indicated, the standard precaution of handwashing is truly universal and must be done before and after every patient contact.

Handwashing

Hands must be washed before and after every patient contact, even in clinical situations where there has been no visual contamination with blood, body fluids, secretions, excretions, and contaminated items. Further, hands must be washed immediately after gloves are removed if they were worn. In addition, washing hands should be done whenever indicated to avoid transfer of microorganisms to other patients and the environment, such as after contact with IV tubing or a monitor even when there has been no direct patient contact. A plain, nonantimicrobial soap could be used for routine handwashing. An antimicrobial soap or a waterless antiseptic agent can be used for specific circumstances, such as control of outbreaks or hyperendemic infections, or may be chosen by some facilities to be used on a daily basis in all patient areas. Alcohol-based hand sanitizers have been shown to be more convenient, faster, and more efficient than handwashing (6,7), and many institutions have these available throughout patient care areas. However, alcohol-based regimens are not recommended in all situations.

Gloves

Clean, nonsterile gloves are appropriate when contact with blood, body fluids, secretions, excretions, and contaminated items is expected. In addition, clean gloves should be used if there is expected contact with broken skin or mucous membranes. Recommendations also include changing of gloves between tasks and procedures on the same patient if contact with material containing a high concentration of microorganisms is made. Further, it has been recommended that gloves be changed between contact with different anatomic sites on the same patient. Gloves should be removed immediately after use and before contact with the environment to avoid surfaces and items becoming contaminated. Proper disposal of gloves prior to going to another patient should be ensured. It is essential to change gloves between patient contacts, as the failure to do so is an infection control hazard (8).

Handwashing or use of a hand sanitizer should always be performed after removal of gloves and prior to seeing the next patient. According to published CDC guidelines, the use of gloves does not replace the need for handwashing. The rationale is that gloves may have small, inapparent defects or may be torn during use, and hands can become contaminated during removal of gloves (8).

Mask, Eye Protection, and Face Shield

Many procedures can generate aerosols or droplets and may create splashes or sprays of blood or other body fluids. The mucous membranes of the HCW, including those of the eyes, nose, and mouth, are at risk for exposure when performing procedures or patient care tasks that may generate aerosols or droplets. Masks, goggles (eye protection), or face shields are universally available and should be worn to protect the mucous membranes of the HCW. Bronchoscopy, suctioning, and intubation are examples of procedures that may generate aerosols.

Gown

Gowns should be worn if there is expected direct contact with an infected patient or environment during procedures or routine patient care. A clean, nonsterile gown is adequate for protecting skin and preventing soiling of clothing during such procedures and patient care activities. Gowns should be removed immediately after patient contact and should not be worn outside of the patient's room. Hands should be washed after removal of gowns to avoid contamination of the environment or other patients.

Patient Care Equipment

Patient care equipment soiled with blood, body fluids, secretions, and excretions should be handled in a manner that prevents skin and mucous membrane exposures, contamination of clothing, and transfer of microorganisms to other patients and environments. Multiuse equipment should be appropriately cleaned or processed prior to being used for the care of another patient. Single-use items should be disposed of in the appropriate manner, including use of a puncture-resistant sharps container if indicated.

Environmental Control and Linen

Adequate procedures for the routine care, cleaning, and disinfection of environmental surfaces, beds, bedrails, bedside equipment, and other frequently touched surfaces should be used. Soiled linen should be handled and transported in a manner that prevents skin and mucous membrane exposure and contamination of clothing (5).

Patient Placement

Patients who may contaminate an environment or who do not—or cannot be expected to—assist in maintaining appropriate hygiene or environmental control should be placed in a private room.

Occupational Health and Bloodborne Pathogens

Handling of sharps (needles, scalpels, and other sharp instruments or devices) during use, cleaning, or disposal should be done with extreme care to avoid percutaneous injury. Many institutions have training programs for new staff in order to avoid such injuries. These involve directions on never recapping used needles, avoiding manipulation using both hands, or using other techniques that involve the point of a needle being directed toward any part of the user's body. Used needles should not be removed from disposable syringes by hand, and bending or breaking, or otherwise manipulating used needles by hand, should not be done. Used disposable syringes and needles, scalpel blades, and other sharp items should be placed in an appropriate puncture-resistant container, which should be located as close as practical to the area in which the items are used. Reusable sharps can be placed in a puncture-resistant container for transport to the reprocessing area. Many facilities, based on CDC recommendations, have converted to needleless or self-covering sharps.

Contact Precautions

Contact precautions are designed to reduce the risk of transmission of epidemiologically important microorganisms such as antibiotic-resistant Gram-positive or Gram-negative organisms. Transmission of these organisms may take place either by direct or indirect contact. Direct contact transmission from patient to staff includes physical transfer of microorganisms to the HCW from an infected or colonized patient. This usually takes place via skin-to-skin contact. Activities that are a risk for direct contact include turning and bathing patients, assisting patients with personal hygiene, or performing patient transfers, dressing changes, or other patient care activities that require physical contact. Direct contact transmission can also occur between two patients sharing common areas in the same room, such as sinks and chairs.

Indirect contact transmission involves contact of a susceptible host or HCW with a contaminated intermediate object, usually inanimate, in the patient's environment. These inanimate objects can harbor pathogenic microorganisms, and thus serve as agents of transmission; they are referred to as *fomites*. Fomites have been described as sources of MRSA, vancomycin-resistant enterococcus (VRE), and Gram-negative organisms such as *Pseudomonas* and *Acinetobacter* because these organisms can potentially survive for months (9).

Contact precautions are applied to patients with known or suspected infection or colonization (presence of microorganism in or on patient but without clinical signs and symptoms of infection) with epidemiologically important microorganisms that can be transmitted by direct or indirect contact. Contact precautions involve patient placement, gloves and handwashing, gowning, and precautions with patient transport and patient care equipment. Patients should be placed in a private room if possible; however, the door to the room may be left open. When a private room is not available, the patient can be placed in a room with a patient who has colonization or active infection with the same microorganism but no other infection (*cohorting*). If a private room is not available and cohorting is not achievable, the epidemiology of the microorganism should be considered and the patient population taken into consideration when determining patient placement. An example of this would include the avoidance of placing an immunocompromised patient in the same room as a patient with a resistant organism.

Gloves and handwashing should be used as with standard precautions, and gowns should be used if there will be substantial contact with the patient, environmental surfaces, or items in a patient's room. A gown should also be worn if the patient is incontinent, has diarrhea, or has an ileostomy, colostomy, or wound drainage not covered or contained by a dressing. Patient transport should be limited only to essential purposes, and if the patient is transferred out of the room, precautions should be taken to ensure minimal risk of transmission to other patients and environmental surfaces or equipment. Patient care equipment such as stethoscopes, thermometers, and IV pumps should be dedicated to a single patient (or cohort) to avoid sharing between patients, leading to transfer of organisms.

Droplet Precautions

Droplet precautions aim to reduce the risk of spreading infectious agents by droplet transmission. Transmission in this manner involves contact between the conjunctiva and other mucous membranes (nose, mouth) of either a patient or HCW with large droplets (greater than 5 μm in size) containing microorganisms generated from a person who is either infected or colonized. Droplets can be generated in various ways including coughing, sneezing, or talking and during procedures such as suctioning or bronchoscopy. Transmission via large particle droplets requires close contact between source and recipient persons, as droplets do not remain suspended in the air and generally travel only short distances—usually less than 3 feet (5). According to CDC recommendations, because droplets do not remain suspended in the air, special air handling and ventilation are not required to prevent droplet transmission, and the door to the patient's room may remain open.

Droplet precautions apply to any patient known or suspected to be infected with epidemiologically important pathogens that can be transmitted by infectious droplets, such as MRSA, meningococcal infection, and *Acinetobacter* pneumonia. Invasive *Haemophilus influenzae* type B, influenza, mycoplasma pneumonia, and parvovirus B19 also require droplet precautions. In addition to the standard precautions, patients should be placed in a private room or cohorted. If cohorting is not possible, spatial separation of at least 3 feet between other patients and visitors should be maintained. A mask should be worn if working within 3 feet of the patient, and transport should be limited to essential purposes only. If transport becomes necessary, the patient should be masked to minimize dispersal by droplets.

Airborne Precautions

Airborne precautions are designed to reduce the risk of airborne transmission of infectious agents. Airborne transmission occurs by dissemination of either airborne droplet nuclei—small particle residue, 5 μm or smaller in size, of evaporated droplets that may remain suspended in the air for long periods of time—or dust particles containing the infectious agent. Microorganisms carried in this manner can be dispersed widely by air currents or may travel long distances through ventilation systems. They may be inhaled by a susceptible host within the same room or by a patient several rooms or floors away from the source patient. Therefore, special air handling and ventilation are required to prevent airborne transmission. Airborne precautions apply to patients known or suspected to be infected with epidemiologically important pathogens such as tuberculosis or varicella zoster virus (10) that can be transmitted by the airborne route. The patient should be placed in a private room that has (a) monitored negative air pressure in relation to the surrounding areas, (b) 6 to 12 air exchanges per hour, and (c) appropriate discharge of air outdoors or monitored high-efficiency filtration of room air before the air is circulated to other areas in the hospital. The room door should be kept closed and the patient should be kept in the room.

If a private room is not available, the patient should be placed in a room with a patient who has an active infection

TABLE 13.1

RECOMMENDED ISOLATION PRECAUTIONS FOR SELECTED PATHOGENS

Organism	Recommended precaution/isolation
Methicillin-resistant *Staphylococcus aureus*	Contact
Vancomycin-resistant enterococcus	Contact
Clostridium difficile	Contact
Multidrug-resistant Gram-negative infections	Consider contact
Varicella-zoster virus	Contact/airborne
Influenza	Droplet
Tuberculosis	Airborne
Neisseria meningitides	Droplet

with the same microorganism, unless otherwise recommended, but with no other infection. When a private room is not available and cohorting is not possible, consultation with infection control professionals is advised before patient placement. Respiratory protection should be worn; the N95 respiratory mask provides an adequate barrier to various airborne organisms including tuberculosis (11,12). Susceptible persons should not enter the room of patients known or suspected to have rubeola (measles) or varicella (chickenpox) if other immune caregivers are available. If susceptible persons must enter the room of a patient known or suspected to have measles or chickenpox, they should wear adequate respiratory protection—the N95 respirator; persons immune to measles or chickenpox need not wear respiratory protection. Patient transport should be limited to the movement and transport of the patient from the room for essential purposes only. If transport or movement is necessary, minimize patient dispersal of droplet nuclei by placing an N95 mask on the patient. A summary of the recommended precautions is provided in Table 13.1.

VIRUSES

The major viruses of concern in the health care setting are human immunodeficiency virus (HIV), influenza virus, and the hepatitis viruses, hepatitis B and C (HBV, HCV). Nosocomial outbreaks of herpes simplex virus I (HSV type I), pneumonia (13), and varicella zoster virus have been reported (14–16); however, these events are generally rare (17). We will discuss HIV first and then move on to a discussion of the hepatitides. The herpes viruses will be briefly discussed with specific regard to precautions. Again, the application of standard (universal) precautions is recommended in all patients, regardless of the etiology of infection.

HIV

HIV is the virus that causes acquired immunodeficiency syndrome (AIDS). Two species of HIV—HIV-1 and HIV-2—infect humans. These are thought to have originated in southern Cameroon as a species-jumping event from wild chimpanzees (HIV-1) and an old-world monkey, the Sooty Magabey (HIV-2), to humans. The virus was first discovered in France in 1983 and named the lymphadenopathy-associated virus (LTAV). However, U.S. scientists later confirmed the discovery, naming the virus human T-cell lymphotropic virus 3 (HTLV-3). In 1986, the name was changed to HIV. The AIDS epidemic was documented to begin in the early 1980s when the CDC reported a cluster of *Pneumocystis jiroveci* (formerly *carinii*) pneumonia in homosexual men. The virus is a single-stranded RNA virus classified in the genus Lentivirus of the family Retroviridae. Upon entry into the cell, the virus uses reverse transcriptase to convert its genome into a double-stranded DNA that then integrates itself into host nuclear DNA for transcription of its genome using host cellular machinery. The transcribed virus then enters the cytoplasm where it undergoes translation and later, under the influence of the enzyme protease, becomes cleaved to be incorporated into mature virions.

HIV is transmitted primarily by exposure to blood and other body fluids. The three primary methods of transmission are (a) via unprotected sexual intercourse, (b) vertical transmission (mother to child), and (c) with contaminated needles (either occupational exposure or with the use of IV drugs). Blood products are now screened routinely for HIV, and transfusion-associated transmission has been, for the most part, eliminated. Animal models of mucosal transmission have shown that after initial exposure, HIV replicates within dendritic cells of the skin and mucosa. The virus later spreads via lymphatics, infecting CD4$^+$ cells, and the process ultimately becomes a chronic disseminated infection. The delay in systemic spread leaves a "window of opportunity" for postexposure prophylaxis (PEP) using antiretroviral drugs designed to block replication of HIV. PEP aims to inhibit the replication of the initial inoculum of virus and thereby prevent establishment of chronic HIV infection. Several studies have investigated the rates of exposure in HCWs, and nurses have been found to be at highest risk. The most common exposure was via percutaneous injury. Several other types of exposures among HCWs have been described and include (a) mucous membrane exposure, (b) nonintact skin exposure, and (c) bites resulting in blood exposure.

Studies have assessed the average risk of HIV transmission to HCWs after a percutaneous injury and estimated the risk to be approximately 0.3% (95% confidence interval [CI], 0.2%–0.5%) (18,19) and after a mucous membrane exposure to be 0.09% (95% CI, 0.006%–0.5%) (20). Transmission of HIV via nonintact skin exposure has been documented (21); however, the average risk for transmission via this route is much less than for mucous membrane exposures (22). The risk for transmission after exposure to fluids or tissues other than HIV-infected blood also has not been quantified but is also considerably lower than for blood exposures.

Several factors may affect the risk of HIV transmission after an occupational exposure. Increased risk was associated with (a) a larger quantity of blood from the source, (b) a procedure that involves placing a needle directly into a vein or artery, (c) a deep tissue injury, and (d) blood exposure from a patient with terminal disease, as there is usually a higher viral load in AIDS. Studies have shown that more blood is transferred by deeper injuries and hollow-bore needles, which support the observation that risk is related to blood quantity.

Postexposure Management

Postexposure prophylaxis for HIV has been investigated with various regimens. However, the administration of antiretroviral medications is the only active outcome of postexposure evaluation. One approach to postexposure prophylaxis has been published by the AIDS Education and Training Center (AETC). The initial step is prompt treatment of the exposure site including washing wounds and skin sites with soap and water, and flushing mucous membranes with water. This should be followed by immediate reporting to facilitate rapid evaluation of the HCW, including testing for HIV and hepatitis B and C, evaluation of the source patient, and initiation of medications for the HCW if indicated. The use of local antiseptics at the injury site is not contraindicated, although there is no evidence of efficacy. The types of exposure, as outlined above, as well as the type and amount of fluid/tissue should be assessed. Potentially infectious fluids include blood and blood-containing fluids; fluids from other sites such as semen, vaginal secretions, and cerebrospinal fluid (CSF); and synovial, pleural, peritoneal, pericardial, and amniotic fluids. The source patient also needs to be evaluated, including serologic studies for HIV using antibody testing, hepatitis B surface antigen, and hepatitis C antibody. Direct viral assays, usually polymerase chain reaction (PCR), for routine screening of source patients are not recommended. If the source patient is not found to be infected with a bloodborne pathogen, further testing of the HCW may not be warranted. However, if the infection status of the source remains unknown, the comorbidities, clinical symptoms, and high-risk behaviors of the source patient should be considered. If the source patient is considered high risk, postexposure prophylaxis should be initiated.

Both basic and expanded PEP regimens have been described. Ideally, PEP regimens should be started within hours of exposure. If there is a question regarding which regimen—basic or expanded—to use, the basic regimen should be started in order to avoid delay. The exact course duration of PEP has not been determined. However, 4 weeks is recommended for HCWs and other occupational exposures, such as law enforcement encounters. PEP has been shown to be protective in animal studies. A basic regimen consists of two nucleoside reverse transcriptase inhibitors (NRTIs). Examples of basic regimens include a combination of lamivudine or emtricitabine with either stavudine or tenofovir. Combivir (zidovudine and lamivudine) or Truvada (tenofovir and emtricitabine) have also been recommended. Expanded regimens include the addition of another drug class such as protease inhibitors (PIs) or nonnucleoside reverse transcriptase inhibitors (NNRTIs). The preferred expanded regimen is one that includes the PI lopinavir/ritonavir (Kaletra) with two NRTIs.

The AETC has published algorithms derived from the U.S. Public Health Service guidelines for management of occupational exposures to HIV, hepatitis B, and hepatitis C (5) (Figs. 13.1 and 13.2). HIV-positive class 1 is defined as a source patient with asymptomatic HIV infection or known low viral load. HIV-positive class 2 refers to a source patient with symptomatic HIV infection, AIDS, acute seroconversion syndrome, or known high viral load.

Influenza Virus

Influenza viruses are RNA viruses belonging to the family Orthomyxoviridae. Infection with these viruses causes an acute febrile illness usually occurring during the winter months and characterized by sudden onset of high fever, headache, myalgia, arthralgia, and cough. Those at risk for more severe disease include young children, the elderly, and immunocompromised patients. Although the infection can be self-limited, it may also result in severe prostration in elderly patients, primary influenza pneumonia, and secondary bacterial pneumonia. Transmission of the virus occurs person to person via large virus-laden droplets. Therefore, droplet precautions are used

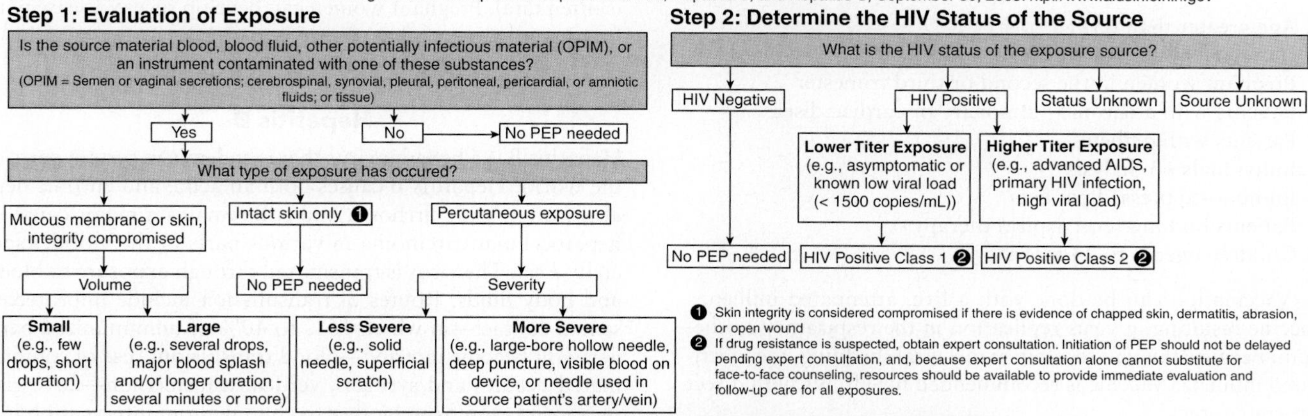

Exposure Type	HIV Positive Class 1	HIV Positive Class 2
Percutaneous - Less Severe	Recommend Basic Regimen	Recommend Expanded Regimen
Percutaneous - More Severe	Recommend Expanded Regimen	Recommend Expanded Regimen
Mucous Membrane/Nonintact Skin - Small Volume	Consider Basic Regimen	Recommend Basic Regimen
Mucous Membrane/Nonintact Skin - Large Volume	Recommend Basic Regimen	Recommend Expanded Regimen

3. Source of unknown HIV status: PEP generally not warranted; consider basic regimen for source with HIV factors
Unknown source: PEP generally not warranted; consider basic regimen where exposure to HIV-infected person likely

FIGURE 13.1. HIV postexposure prophylaxis (PEP) algorithm for health care workers. (From U.S. Public Health Service Guidelines for the Management of Occupational Exposures to HIV, Hepatitis B, and Hepatitis C, September 30, 2005. Available at: www.aidsinfo.nih.gov. Accessed November, 2006.)

Post-Exposure Prophylaxis for Hepatitis B Virus

Updated U.S. Public Health Service Guidelines for the Management of Occupational Exposure to HBV, HCV, and HIV and Recommendations for Postexposure Prophylaxis – June 29, 2001. Available online at www.aidsinfo.gov

Management of Exposures to HBV

- Any blood or body fluid exposure to an unvaccinated person should lead to the initiation of the hepatitis B vaccine series
  - Recombivax HB® 10 mcg or Energix-B® 20 mcg IM at 0, 1, and 6 months
- When Hepatitis B Immune Globulin (HBIG) is indicated, it should be administered as soon as possible after the exposure (preferably withih 24 hours, but is recommended up to 1 week following an occupational exposure)
  - Hepatitis B vaccine can be administered simultaneously with HBIG but at a separate site
- Test for anti-HBs 1-2 months after last dose of vaccine[5]

Vaccination/Ab response of worker	Treatment		
	Source HBsAg (+)	Source HBsAg (–)	Source unknown or not available for testing
Unvaccinated	HBIG (0.06 mL/kg IM) × 1 and vaccinate	Vaccinate	Vaccinate
Vaccinated-responder[5]	No PEP	No PEP	No PEP
Vaccinated-nonresponder	HBIG (0.06 mL/kg IM) × 1 and revaccinate or HBIG (0.06 mL/kg IM) × 2 (at time of exposure and 1 month after exposure)	No PEP	If known high risk treat as HBsAg (+)
Vaccinated-Ab response unknown	Test exposed person for anti-HBs 1. If adequate, no PEP necessary 2. If adequate, administer HBIG × 1 and vaccinate booster	No Treatment	Test exposed person for anti-HBs 1. If adequate, no PEP necessary 2. If inadequate, give vaccine booster and recheck titer in 1-2 months

5. Adequate anti-HBs ≥ 10 mIU/mL

Post-Exposure Management for Hepatitis C Virus

Updated U.S. Public Health Service Guidelines for the Management of Occupational Exposures to HBV, HCV, and HIV and Recommendations for Postexposure Prophylaxis – June 29, 2001. Available online at www.aidsinfo.gov

Management of Exposures to HCV

- Perform testing for anti-HCV for the source
- Perform baseline testing for anti-HCV and ALT activity for the exposed person
- Perform follow-up testing
  - Anti-HCV and ALT activity at 4-6 months or
  - HCV RNA by PCR at 4-6 weeks for earlier detection
- Confirm anti-HCV results reported positive by enzyme immunoassay with supplemental test [e.g. recombinant immunoblast assay (RIBA) or HCV RNA by PCR]

Post-Exposure Management for HCV

- No regimen proven beneficial for PEP
- Early identification of chronic disease and referral for management
- Immediately refer HCW to hepatitis C specialist for management

FIGURE 13.2. Postexposure recommendations for hepatitis B and hepatitis C in health care workers. (From U.S. Public Health Service Guidelines for the Management of Occupational Exposures to HIV, Hepatitis B, and Hepatitis C, September 30, 2005. Available at: www.aidsinfo.nih.gov. Accessed November, 2006.)

for patients who are admitted to the hospital with active or suspected influenza infection. While droplet precautions prevent spread, the mainstay of disease prevention is annual immunization of both HCWs and the at-risk patient population, which is defined as:

- Age greater than 65
- Residents of nursing homes or long-term care facilities
- Pregnant women in the second or third trimester
- Patients with a chronic pulmonary or cardiac disease
- Patients with diabetes
- Individuals on dialysis
- Immunosuppressed patients
- Patients on long-term aspirin therapy
- Children aged 6 to 23 months

Vaccination can be done with a live, attenuated influenza vaccine resulting in virus replication in the respiratory epithelium. Because this can result in active viral shedding, the inactivated influenza vaccine is recommended for HCWs with direct patient contact.

Hepatitides

Several hepatitis viruses have been described, including hepatitis A, B, C, D, E, and G. Hepatitis A is caused by a picornavirus and is transmitted by the oral–fecal route, usually by contaminated food. It causes only an acute form of hepatitis that is generally self-limited and confers immunity to future infections. Hepatitis A is not usually a concern in the health care setting. Hepatitis D is caused by a delta virus and can only replicate in the presence of hepatitis B. Hepatitis E is like hepatitis A in that it causes an acute, usually self-limited hepatitis and is also transmitted via the oral–fecal route. In a small percent of cases, hepatitis E can develop into an acute severe liver disease that is often fatal. Pregnant women can develop severe disease with fulminant hepatic failure due to hepatitis E. By far, hepatitis B and C pose the greatest threat to health care workers.

Hepatitis B

Hepatitis B is a hepadnavirus that is endemic in certain parts of the world. Hepatitis B causes both an acute and chronic hepatitis, often with cirrhosis, and still remains a major cause of hepatocellular carcinoma in various parts of the world, especially Asia. The virus is transmitted through exposure to blood and body fluids. Routes of transmission include unprotected sexual contact—in which 16% to 40% of unimmunized partners will become infected—blood transfusions, use of contaminated needles and syringes, vertical transmission—20% risk of transmission from mother to child without intervention in a hepatitis B surface antigen (HBsAg)-positive mother—and occupational exposure including needlesticks. As with many viral infections, the risk of transmission from a bloodborne exposure is closely related to the volume of blood exposure and the number of copies of virus present in the blood of the source.

Per the CDC guidelines, risk of transmission of hepatitis B is also related to the hepatitis B envelope antigen (HBeAg) status of the source patient. In patients who were both HBsAg and HBeAg positive, the risk of developing clinical hepatitis from a needle injury was 22% to 31%. The risk of developing serologic evidence of infection was 36% to 62%. If the source patient was HBsAg positive with a negative HBeAg, the risk of developing clinical hepatitis from a needle injury was 1% to 6%, and the risk of developing serologic evidence of hepatitis B infection was 23% to 37% (23). Blood exposure and percutaneous injuries with contaminated blood are among the most efficient modes of transmitting hepatitis B since blood has the highest titers of hepatitis B compared to other body fluids. Interestingly, some studies suggest that most infected HCWs could not recall a percutaneous injury but rather recalled caring for a patient who was HBsAg positive when investigations of outbreaks were performed (24–27). Hepatitis B has been shown to survive in dried blood at room temperature for at least 1 week (28) and it is possible that contact with environmental surfaces is a potential risk for hepatitis B transmission, as has been shown in patients and staff of hemodialysis units (29–31).

The key factor in preventing hepatitis B infection in the health care setting is vaccination, and most facilities require that employees who come into direct contact with patients or with risk of exposure to blood and body fluids undergo the hepatitis B vaccination series. In fact, hepatitis B vaccination is part of the routine immunization schedule for children in the United States; by the age of 18 months, children who are up to date on their vaccinations have been fully immunized for hepatitis B. As with childhood vaccination, the protocol for adult immunization consists of three doses of the vaccine. For those whose hepatitis B vaccination series is interrupted, there is no need to restart. Vaccination can resume based on where in the series the patient was at the time of the interruption.

In the event that a health care worker is not immunized, postexposure prophylaxis (Fig. 13.2) is available in the form of hepatitis B immune globulin (HBIG). When indicated, HBIG should be given as soon as possible, preferably within 24 hours. Data on efficacy when HBIG was given after 7 days are not available. However, multiple doses of HBIG within 1 week of exposure are 75% effective in preventing hepatitis B infection. Postexposure hepatitis B vaccination is recommended in addition to HBIG because unimmunized HCWs continue to be at risk for exposure. In addition, data derived from vertical transmission regarding concurrent vaccination and HBIG administration show a better rate of prevention—85% to 95% with combined therapy as opposed to either therapy alone—70% to 75%.

Hepatitis C

Hepatitis C is an RNA virus in the family Flaviviridae. The virus replicates mainly in the hepatocytes after binding to specific receptors and entering the cells. Like hepatitis B, hepatitis C causes both acute and chronic hepatitis and is a risk factor for development of hepatocellular carcinoma. The virus is transmitted by direct contact with blood and body fluids containing blood. Various routes of transmission have been identified. Of note, IV drug abusers seem to have the highest incidence of developing hepatitis C due to the sharing of contaminated needles. While sexual transmission is possible, it is largely due to the possibility of blood contact and not other body fluids such as semen or vaginal secretions. Vertical transmission is also possible, although this occurs infrequently. In the health care setting, hepatitis C is not transmitted efficiently through occupational exposure to blood, and thus has a low incidence after accidental percutaneous exposure. Mucous membrane or skin exposures, both intact and nonintact, rarely result in transmission of hepatitis C. To date, there is no available vaccine for hepatitis C, and studies have shown no beneficial effect of giving immune globulin. Instead, postexposure management is aimed at the early detection of hepatitis C infection and the development of chronic disease for which treatment can be given.

The risk of acquiring hepatitis C also varies depending on the nature of exposure. After accidental percutaneous exposure from a known HCV-positive source, the incidence of seroconversion is 1.8% (32). Transmission from mucous membranes rarely occurs, and no cases of transmission in health care workers have been described from intact or nonintact skin exposures to blood (33,34). Furthermore, the risk of transmission from exposure to fluids other than blood has not been determined, but is postulated to be low. Although data are limited on the survival of HCV in the environment, one study has suggested that HCV-RNA is resistant to drying at room temperature for at least 48 hours (35).

Herpes Viruses

Human herpes viruses (HHVs) are DNA viruses that cause a variety of diseases in humans. Several human herpes viruses have been described including HHV-1 (also known as herpes simplex virus [HSV-1]), HHV-2 (herpes simplex virus [HSV-2]), HHV-3 (varicella-zoster virus [VZV]), HHV-4 (Epstein-Barr virus [EBV]), HHV-5 (cytomegalovirus [CMV]), HHV-6 (Roseolovirus), HHV-7, and HHV-8 (Kaposi sarcoma–associated virus). The seroprevalence of CMV is relatively high by adolescence (36) and has been documented to be up to 60% to 90% in adult populations. EBV generally causes a self-limited mild disease, but can cause infectious mononucleosis in teenagers and young adults. Thus, the herpes viruses of most importance in the health care setting are HSV-1, HSV-2, and VZV.

HSV-1 and HSV-2 cause blisters or sores either in the oral or genital area and can be transmitted to the health care worker by direct contact with the lesions, when they are present, and when appropriate use of precautions is forgone. VZV is the causative agent of chickenpox as well as shingles. Like other herpes viruses, VZV lies dormant in the dorsal root ganglia of the nervous system and can reactivate to produce zoster ("shingles"). VZV can be transmitted both by direct contact with a patient who has active skin lesions (vesicles) as well as via respiratory secretions in which the virus is shed during active infection, such as disseminated zoster. The recommended approach to patients with varicella-zoster disease includes both contact and airborne isolation.

One issue that arises in the clinical setting is the exposure of the nonimmune pregnant HCW to patients with CMV or VZV disease, as primary infection with either virus during pregnancy can be devastating to both mother and child. Some studies have shown that up to 50% of pregnant women are seropositive for CMV (37). In addition, the incidence of primary CMV during pregnancy is 1% to 4%, depending on certain variables. The transmission of CMV requires prolonged or recurrent close contact and can also be transmitted sexually. Since there are no effective therapies for treatment of CMV in pregnancy, prevention is the best method to avoid the complications of disease. Vaccines for CMV are available and, although there has been no change in the rate of CMV infection, there has been a reduction in disease severity in those who are vaccinated prior to primary infection. While there have been no conclusive recommendations regarding the precautions to be used by nonimmune pregnant HCWs with respect to patients with CMV, it would seem prudent to identify patients with active CMV infection so that these HCWs can be aware of the risk or be assigned to another patient. It must be recognized, however, that any patient can actively shed CMV without clinical signs or symptoms. This is the foundation for the CDC's strong recommendation of meticulous adherence to handwashing before and after patient care as the best way to prevent disease transmission in *all* settings. In patients with proven or suspected CMV pneumonitis, mask and eye protection may be a consideration in the nonimmune or seronegative pregnant HCW. As with CMV, a vaccine is available for VZV. The vaccine is a live, attenuated vaccine that is given in two doses spaced 4 to 8 weeks apart; it is 70% to 90% effective in preventing infection and 95% effective in preventing severe disease up to 10 years after administration. The vaccine is recommended for nonpregnant women of childbearing age and is not recommended for pregnant women, with a further stipulation being that women should not become pregnant for at least 1 month after each dose of the vaccine. In the event that a pregnant HCW who is nonimmune becomes exposed to VZV, postexposure prophylaxis is available. Varicella-zoster immunoglobulin is recommended within 96 hours of exposure and has been reported be up to 90% effective in preventing severe disease (38). It is recommended that nonimmune HCWs be vaccinated, especially female HCWs of childbearing age. If a pregnant HCW is not immune and has had exposure to VZV, prophylaxis should be instituted. In addition, contact and airborne precautions should be used at all times in patients with VZV disease.

Bacteria

Having discussed the major viruses of importance in the health care setting, we will now turn to a discussion of bacterial organisms including MRSA, VRE, *Clostridium difficile*, selected Gram-negative organisms, and *Mycobacterium tuberculosis*. Standard precautions are recommended for all patients, but additional precautions include contact precautions (MRSA, VRE, *C. difficile*) and airborne precautions (tuberculosis).

Methicillin-resistant *Staphylococcus aureus*

Methicillin-resistant *S. aureus* has become a major problem both in hospital-acquired (HA-MRSA) infections as well as community-acquired (CA-MRSA) infections. MRSA infections in the hospital are associated with both longer stays and higher costs. Data from the U.S. National Nosocomial Infections Surveillance Systems indicate that MRSA accounts for 55% of *S. aureus*–related infections in the intensive care setting in the United States. CA-MRSA is a microbiologically distinct isolate with a specific sensitivity pattern and the presence of the Panton-Valentine leukocidin (PVL) exotoxin. While it was previously thought that the PVL exotoxin was the virulence factor for CA-MRSA, studies in PVL-negative and PVL-positive mice failed to support this assertion; thus, the factor responsible for the virulence of CA-MRSA remains uncharacterized. Methicillin resistance is related to the acquisition of a staphylococcal cassette chromosome (SCC) that is known as the *mecA* gene. CA-MRSA can be distinguished from hospital-acquired MRSA by the presence of type 4 SCC (39). Expression of the *mecA* gene leads to an altered penicillin-binding protein, PBP2a, which has a reduced affinity for β-lactam rings.

CA-MRSA has been associated with significant skin and soft tissue infections, often requiring surgical drainage, usually in hospital emergency departments, as well as more severe infections such as necrotizing pneumonia, necessitating hospital admission. Nosocomial infections with HA-MRSA include catheter-related bacteremia, postsurgical wound infections, postoperative neurosurgical meningitis, ventilator-associated pneumonia, and device and graft infections. Risk factors for MRSA infection include patients with open wounds or pressure ulcers, invasive devices—such as catheter, tracheostomy, gastrostomy, nasogastric tube, and indwelling bladder catheter—recent antibiotic therapy, hospitalization or significant health care contact within the past 6 months, increased age, and male gender. Knowing the MRSA infection status of patients is helpful in determining who should be isolated or cohorted. While nasal swabs for MRSA culture are a way to identify those who are colonized, the time delay in identifying these patients based on cultures makes this option less useful. PCR has been proposed as a means of rapid identification of MRSA-colonized patients; however, this may not be cost effective. Although there are differences in the ways that hospitals approach the issue of screening patients for MRSA, once it is isolated from a culture, the patient should be immediately placed on contact precautions.

While there are antibiotic options available to treat MRSA infections, as well as to decolonize carriers of MRSA, prevention of spread is the most important method in combating MRSA infections. Patients with MRSA infection in the hospital should be placed on contact precautions. However, handwashing remains a critical factor in preventing spread. Health care workers must wash their hands before and after any contact with a patient, even when gloves are worn as part of MRSA contact precautions. Recommendations for preventing the spread of MRSA also include cohorting of patients if isolation in a single room is not possible. Contact precautions should be observed meticulously, especially with any anticipated contact with an open wound or ulcer, mucous membranes, or any blood or body fluid contact. Mask and eye protection are indicated if exposure to aerosols generated by the coughing patient is likely or when irrigating wounds. Precautions for MRSA-infected or -colonized patients remain the same regardless of the strain (HA-MRSA or CA-MRSA).

Fomites have been implicated in the transmission of MRSA. Environmental surfaces that have been described as vectors of MRSA transmission include a plastic patient chart (survived 11 days), a laminated tabletop (survived 12 days), and a cloth curtain (survived 9 days) (40). Further, even in the outpatient setting, studies have shown that environmental surfaces are important sources of transmission including a patient examination table, a computer keyboard, a pulse oximeter, and multiple patient chairs located in the triage station, the waiting room, and the examination room (41). Daily routine cleaning should be done with a disinfectant and performed in a sanitary manner as is done in all rooms regardless of the presence of MRSA. Equipment should be routinely cleaned, disinfected, or sterilized per institution policy.

Clostridium difficile

Members of the genus *Clostridium* are Gram-positive rods that are anaerobic and spore forming. *C. difficile* is the causative organism of pseudomembranous colitis and *C. difficile*–associated diarrhea (CDAD), which occurs with the use of antibiotics that eradicate normal gut flora. The organism produces two toxins, enterotoxin (toxin A) and cytotoxin (toxin B), which are responsible for diarrhea and inflammation. While growing *C. difficile* in culture is the gold standard for diagnosis, enzyme-linked immunosorbent assay (ELISA) testing for toxin A or B has a high sensitivity and specificity when performed on three separate stool specimens. In addition to watery diarrhea, computed tomography (CT) scan of the abdomen demonstrating colonic wall thickening is a key finding. Complications of untreated infection include toxic megacolon and bowel perforation. A major risk factor for the development of *C. difficile* diarrhea is the use of antibiotics—especially penicillins, clindamycin, and cephalosporins, particularly third-generation cephalosporins. Repeated enemas, prolonged nasogastric tube insertion, and gastrointestinal surgery also increase the risk of developing a disease.

The disease is spread from person to person by spores that are shed in the stool. Such spores can survive up to 70 days in the environment and can be carried on the hands of health care workers, who then have direct contact with uninfected patients or with environmental surfaces—floors, bedpans, toilets—thus contaminating them with *C. difficile*.

The treatment of *C. difficile* colitis includes oral metronidazole or oral vancomycin. A newer agent, nitazoxanide, has not received Food and Drug Administration (FDA) approval for this indication, but shows promise in small clinical trials. As with MRSA, longer hospital stays and increased costs have been directly related to infection with *C. difficile*. Recommendations for preventing spread include standard precautions as well as contact precautions if soiling of clothes is likely. It is important to note that handwashing is the only method to be used in preventing spread of *C. difficile*, as the alcohol substitutes do not kill the spores. However, the mechanical action of applying the hand sanitizer may eliminate some spores from the hand of the HCW. Waste material should also be handled in a proper way. Furthermore, limiting the use of inappropriate antibiotics is central to lowering the risk of developing *C. difficile*–associated diarrhea.

Vancomycin-resistant Enterococcus

Enterococci are Gram-positive, facultatively anaerobic organisms that colonize the gastrointestinal tract. Two species, *Enterococcus faecalis* (90% to 95%) and *Enterococcus faecium* (5% to 10%), are commensal in the intestines of humans. While the organism is not highly invasive, infections caused by enterococci include catheter-related bacteremia, urinary tract infections, diverticular abscess, cholangitis, and endocarditis. While many strains of enterococci remain susceptible to ampicillin, penicillin, and vancomycin, there has been an alarming increase in the incidence of VRE, which has implications both for therapy and prevention. In addition, there is concern regarding resistance in other bacteria, such as *S. aureus*, as VRE appears to have an enhanced ability to pass resistant genes (such as vanA) to other Gram-positive organisms.

Risk factors for VRE colonization and infection have not been clearly identified, although there seems to be a higher incidence in patients who are immunosuppressed—transplant and chemotherapy patients in an intensive care setting who have renal insufficiency. In addition, a higher risk of colonization and infection is logically associated with intra-abdominal surgery or gastrointestinal tract manipulation such as endoscopic retrograde cholangiopancreatography (ERCP), indwelling urinary catheters, enteral feeding tubes, and central venous catheters, as these are all—with the exception of the central venous catheter—associated with the natural reservoir of the organism. Patients on broad-spectrum antibiotics, and especially those who have received oral vancomycin, are also at higher risk for colonization or infection with a VRE species. The use of intravenous vancomycin is associated to a lesser extent with VRE colonization and infection.

Transmission generally occurs from a colonized or infected patient to the HCW via direct contact with either the patient or contaminated environmental surfaces (fomites), such as toilets, doorknobs, and even Yankauer suction devices (42). In general, the lack of proper hand hygiene appears to be the major factor in the spread of VRE from patient to HCW and back to other patients. Studies have shown a dramatic decrease in the incidence of VRE with the enforcement of proper hand hygiene, either with alcohol-based solutions or with routine handwashing (43). Proper environmental cleaning has been shown to also decrease the transmission of VRE (44). Patients who are known to be colonized or infected with VRE should be placed in contact isolation to prevent spread of the organism.

As with MRSA, the issue of screening for VRE has been addressed by several studies. One study has shown advantage in a clinical active surveillance strategy (culture of a rectal swab on admission, weekly while the patient was in the intensive care unit [ICU], and at discharge) with a cost savings ranging from $56,258 to $303,334 per month (45). A decision should be made at the institutional level regarding the cost effectiveness of a screening program. The available data support strong consideration for a routine screening program with resultant preventive measures (contact isolation) to help control the spread of VRE.

Tuberculosis

Mycobacterium tuberculosis (MTB) is the causative agent of all forms of tuberculosis—pulmonary, central nervous system (CNS), and disseminated. The disease is spread by aerosol droplets from persons with active infection when they cough, sneeze, speak, or spit. Infectious droplets are 0.5 to 5 μm in diameter; about 40,000 can be produced in a single sneeze and 3,000 in a single cough. The probability of transmission from person to person depends on several factors, including (a) quantity of infectious droplets expelled, (b) effectiveness of ventilation, (c) duration of exposure, and (d) the virulence of the Mycobacterial strain. Persons who are in direct contact with an infected patient, either frequently or for a prolonged time, have the highest risk of developing tuberculosis, with an estimated infection rate of 22%. A person with untreated, active tuberculosis can infect 10 to 15 people per year. Others at risk for infection include persons living in endemic areas—some parts of Asia, Haiti, and South America; immunocompromised patients—those with HIV/AIDS and those on immunosuppressive medications; health care workers serving high-risk patients; and IV drug abusers. Single males, alcoholics, the urban poor—especially the homeless—migrant farm workers, and prison inmates have been associated with a higher frequency of tuberculosis.

The rate of tuberculosis in the United States has steadily declined since a resurgence between 1985 and 1992 that correlated with the AIDS epidemic prior to the development of highly active antiretroviral therapy. Since then, the majority of MTB cases in the United States are now diagnosed in persons who are immigrants from endemic areas. There has been a recent deceleration in the yearly percentage of decline, from an average of 7.1% per year (1993 through 2000) to 3.8% per year (2001 through 2005). This has raised concerns regarding the progress toward the goal of eliminating MTB in the United States. According to the most recent CDC data, a total of 14,093 cases of TB were reported in the United States in 2005, which was down from 14,516 in 2004; this decrease represents the smallest decline in over a decade. A CDC study has also shown racial/ethnic disparities, as well as a disparity between U.S.-born and foreign-born MTB rates. In 2005, Hispanics, African Americans, and Asians were respectively 7.3, 8.3, and 19.6 times more likely than Caucasians to become infected with the disease. Furthermore, MTB rates were 8.7 times higher for foreign-born individuals as compared to their U.S. counterparts. More than half of foreign-born cases were reported in patients from Mexico, the Philippines, Vietnam, India, and China. The more alarming data from the most recent CDC report is the finding of higher rates of multidrug- and extended drug-resistant tuberculosis. In developing countries, rates of tuberculosis have been increasing in concordance with the rise of HIV as well as the neglect of TB control programs.

The most effective way to prevent the spread of tuberculosis to the HCW is to identify patients at high risk of active infection, which includes an assessment of symptoms—for example, fever, night sweats, shortness of breath, hemoptysis, and weight loss—as well as demographic factors including questioning about immigration from an endemic area, recent incarceration, and contact with patients known to have tuberculosis, and then isolating these patients. The patient must be placed in a negative pressure isolation room with airborne precautions. Patients should have three expectorated or induced sputum specimens sent for acid-fast staining and culture for acid-fast bacilli (AFB). Patients with suspected MTB infection cannot be removed from isolation until three adequate sputum specimens—or an equivalent, such as specimens obtained by bronchoscopy or bronchoalveolar lavage—have been obtained and are negative for AFB by smear. AFB culture may take up to 6 weeks to grow organisms, and is therefore not used to decide on discontinuation of isolation unless there is a very high index of suspicion. Newer diagnostic techniques including MTB DNA PCR can be used on a variety of AFB-negative body fluids or can be used to determine if early growth of AFB in liquid media is MTB or a nontuberculous mycobacteria.

Gram-Negative Organisms

Recently, the incidence of multidrug-resistant, Gram-negative infections has stirred debate as to whether isolation precautions such as those in place for resistant Gram positives should be instituted. The National Nosocomial Infections Surveillance System has reported increases in the prevalence of multidrug-resistant Gram-negative infections including *Pseudomonas*, *Enterobacter*, and *Klebsiella*, as well as extended-spectrum β-lactamase (ESBL)–producing organisms. In addition, some institutions have reported outbreaks of highly resistant *Acinetobacter baumannii* infections (46,47). Furthermore, interest in *Acinetobacter* is growing now that the organism has been found in soldiers returning from Iraq and Afghanistan.

A recent review of the data related to *Pseudomonas*, Enterobacteriaceae (*Escherichia coli* and *Klebsiella*) and *Acinetobacter baumannii* infection led the authors to conclude that there was not sufficient evidence to determine that infection control measures would be effective in controlling the spread of multidrug-resistant Gram-negative bacteria (48). However, outbreaks of resistant Gram-negative infections have become all too common and have been associated with catheters (49) and other intravascular devices (50), including one report of *Stenotrophomonas* prosthetic valve endocarditis (51). In addition, fatalities have been reported with certain outbreaks (52). Control of outbreaks has included both antibiotic restriction as well as institution of contact isolation. When dealing with multidrug-resistant, virulent, Gram-negative organisms, especially in such settings as the ICU, contact isolation should be strongly considered for use in colonized and infected patients as suggested by CDC guidelines (5).

References

1. Cosgrove SE, Qi Y, Kaye KS, et al. The impact of methicillin resistance in *Staphylococcus aureus* bacteremia on patient outcomes: mortality, length of stay, and hospital charges. *Infect Control Hosp Epidemiol.* 2005;26:166–174.
2. Chaix C, Durand-Zaleski I, Alberti C, et al. Control of endemic methicillin-resistant *Staphylococcus aureus*: a cost-benefit analysis in an intensive care unit. *JAMA.* 1999;282:1745–1751.
3. Wiklicky H, Skopec M. Ignaz Philipp Semmelweis, the prophet of bacteriology. *Infect Control.* 1983;4(5):367–370.
4. Herr HW. Ignorance is bliss: the Listerian revolution and education of American surgeons. *J Urol.* 2007;177(2):457–460.
5. Centers for Disease Control and Prevention. Guidelines for the management of occupational exposures to hepatitis B, hepatitis C, and HIV and recommendations for postexposure prophylaxis. *MMWR Morb Mortal Wkly Rep.* 2001;50(RR11):1–42. Available at http://www.cdc.gov/ncidod/dhqp/gl_occupational.html.
6. Widmer AF, Conzelmann M, Tomic M, et al. Introducing alcohol-based hand rub for hand hygiene: the critical need for training. *Infect Control Hosp Epidemiol.* 2007;28(1):50–54. Epub 2006 Dec 29.
7. Boyce JM, Pittet D. Guideline for hand hygiene in health-care settings. Recommendations of the healthcare infection control practices advisory committee and the ICPAC/SHEA/APIC/IDSA Hand hygiene task force. *MMWR Recomm Rep.* 2002;51:1–45.
8. Garner JS, Hospital Infection Control Practices Advisory Committee. Guidelines for Isolation Precautions in Hospitals, *Am J Infect Control.* 1996;24:24–31.
9. Kramer A, Schwebke I, Kampf G. How long do nosocomial pathogens persist on inanimate surfaces? A systematic review. *BMC Infect Dis.* 2006;16:130.
10. Menkhaus NA, Lanphear B, Linnemann CC. Airborne transmission of varicella-zoster virus in hospitals. *Lancet.* 1990;336(8726):1315.
11. Li Y, Wong T, Chung J, et al. In vivo protective performance of N95 respirator and surgical facemask. *Am J Ind Med.* 2006;49(12):1056–1065.
12. Fennelly KP. Personal respiratory protection against Mycobacterium tuberculosis. *Clin Chest Med.* 1997;18(1):1–17.
13. Mohan S, Hamid NS, Cunha BA. A cluster of nosocomial herpes simplex virus type 1 pneumonia in a medical intensive care unit. *Infect Control Hosp Epidemiol.* 2006;27(11):1255–1257. Epub 2006 Oct 17.
14. Gustafson TL, Lavely GB, Brawner ER, et al. An outbreak of airborne nosocomial varicella. *Pediatrics.* 1982;70(4):550–556.
15. Hyams PJ, Stuewe MC, Heitzer V. Herpes zoster causing varicella (chickenpox) in hospital employees: cost of a casual attitude. *Am J Infect Control.* 1984;12(1):2–5.
16. Gustafson TL, Shehab Z, Brunell PA. Outbreak of varicella in a newborn intensive care nursery. *Am J Dis Child.* 1984;138(6):548–550.
17. Daubin C, Vincent S, Vabret A, et al. Nosocomial viral ventilator-associated pneumonia in the intensive care unit: a prospective cohort study. *Intens Care Med.* 2005;31(8):1116–1122. Epub 2005 Jul 6.
18. Bell DM. Occupational risk of human immunodeficiency virus infection in healthcare workers: an overview. *Am J Med.* 1997;102(suppl 5B):9–15.
19. Henderson DK, Fahey BJ, Willy M, et al. Risk for occupational transmission of human immunodeficiency virus type 1 (HIV-1) associated with clinical exposures: a prospective evaluation. *Ann Intern Med.* 1990;113:740–746.
20. Ippolito G, Puro V, De Carli G. Italian Study Group on Occupational Risk of HIV Infection. The risk of occupational human immunodeficiency virus in health care workers. *Arch Int Med.* 1993;153:1451–1458.
21. Centers for Disease Control and Prevention. Update: human immunodeficiency virus infections in health-care workers exposed to blood of infected patients. *MMWR Morb Mortal Wkly Rep.* 1987;36:285–289.
22. Fahey BJ, Koziol DE, Banks SM, et al. Frequency of nonparenteral occupational exposures to blood and body fluids before and after universal precautions training. *Am J Med.* 1991;90:145–153.

23. Werner BG, Grady GF. Accidental hepatitis-B-surface-antigen-positive inoculations: use of e antigen to estimate infectivity. *Ann Intern Med.* 1982;97: 367–369.
24. Garibaldi RA, Hatch FE, Bisno AL, et al. Nonparenteral serum hepatitis: report of an outbreak. *JAMA.* 1972;220:963–966.
25. Rosenberg JL, Jones DP, Lipitz LR, et al. Viral hepatitis: an occupational hazard to surgeons. *JAMA.* 1973;223:395–400.
26. Callender ME, White YS, Williams R. Hepatitis B virus infection in medical and health care personnel. *BMJ.* 1982;284:324–326.
27. Chaudhuri AKR, Follett EAC. Hepatitis B virus infection in medical and health care personnel [Letter]. *BMJ.* 1982;284:1408.
28. Bond WW, Favero MS, Petersen NJ, et al. Survival of hepatitis B virus after drying and storage for one week [Letter]. *Lancet.* 1981;1:550–551.
29. Hennekens CH. Hemodialysis-associated hepatitis: an outbreak among hospital personnel. *JAMA.* 1973;225:407–408.
30. Garibaldi RA, Forrest JN, Bryan JA, et al. Hemodialysis-associated hepatitis. *JAMA.* 1973;225:384–389.
31. Snydman DR, Bryan JA, Macon EJ, et al. Hemodialysis-associated hepatitis: a report of an epidemic with further evidence on mechanisms of transmission. *Am J Epidemiol.* 1976;104:563–570.
32. Alter MJ. The epidemiology of acute and chronic hepatitis C. *Clin Liver Dis.* 1997;1:559–568.
33. Sartori M, La Terra G, Aglietta M, et al. Transmission of hepatitis C via blood splash into conjunctiva [Letter]. *Scand J Infect Dis.* 1993;25:270–271.
34. Ippolito G, Puro V, Petrosillo N, et al. Simultaneous infection with HIV and hepatitis C virus following occupational conjunctival blood exposure [Letter]. *JAMA.* 1998;280:28.
35. Piazza M, Borgia G, Piccioto L, et al. HCV-RNA survival as detected by PCR in the environment. *Boll Soc Ital Biol Sper.* 1994;70(5-6):167–170.
36. Staras SA, Dollard SC, Radford KW, et al. Seroprevalence of cytomegalovirus infection in the United States, 1988–1994. *Clin Infect Dis.* 2006;43(9):1143–1151. Epub 2006 Oct 2.
37. Griffiths PD, Baboonian C, Rutter D. Congenital and maternal cytomegalovirus infection in a London population. *Br J Obstet Gynaecol.* 1991;98: 135–140.
38. Enders G. Management of varicella-zoster contact and infection in pregnancy using a standardized varicella-zoster ELISA test. *Postgrad Med J.* 1985;61:23.
39. Kowalski TJ, Berbari EF, Osmon DR. Epidemiology, treatment, and prevention of community-acquired methicillin-resistant Staphylococcus aureus infections. *Mayo Clin Proc.* 2005;80(9):1201–1207.
40. Huang R, Mehta S, Weed D, et al. Methicillin-resistant Staphylococcus aureus survival on hospital fomites. *Infect Control Hosp Epidemiol.* 2006; 27(11):1267–1269. Epub 2006 Sep 28.
41. Johnston CP, Cooper L, Ruby W, et al. Epidemiology of community-acquired methicillin-resistant Staphylococcus aureus skin infections among healthcare workers in an outpatient clinic. *Infect Control Hosp Epidemiol.* 2006;27(10):1133–1136. Epub 2006 Aug 31.
42. Brown M, Willms D. Colonization of Yankauer suction catheters with pathogenic organisms. *Am J Infect Control.* 2005;33(8):483–485.
43. Gordin FM, Schultz ME, Huber RA, et al. Reduction in nosocomial transmission of drug-resistant bacteria after introduction of an alcohol-based handrub. *Infect Control Hosp Epidemiol.* 2005;26(7):650–653.
44. Hayden MK, Bonten MJ, Blom DW, et al. Reduction in acquisition of vancomycin-resistant enterococcus after enforcement of routine environmental cleaning measures. *Clin Infect Dis.* 2006;42(11):1552–1560. Epub 2006 Apr 27.
45. Shadel BN, Puzniak LA, Gillespie KN, et al. Surveillance for vancomycin-resistant enterococci: type, rates, costs, and implications. *Infect Control Hosp Epidemiol.* 2006;27(10):1068–1075. Epub 2006 Sep 21.
46. Longo B, Pantosti A, Luzzi I, et al. An outbreak of Acinetobacter baumannii in an intensive care unit: epidemiological and molecular findings. *J Hosp Infect.* 2006;64(3):303–305. Epub 2006 Sep 14.
47. Bogaerts P, Naas T, Wybo I, et al. Outbreak of infection by carbapenem-resistant Acinetobacter baumannii producing the carbapenemase OXA-58 in Belgium. *J Clin Microbiol.* 2006;44(11):4189–4192. Epub 2006 Sep 6.
48. Harris AD, McGregor JC, Furuno JP. What infection control interventions should be undertaken to control multidrug-resistant gram-negative bacteria? *Clin Infect Dis.* 2006;43(Suppl 2):S57–61.
49. Wolfenden LL, Anderson G, Veledar E, et al. Catheter-associated bloodstream infections in 2 long-term acute care hospitals. *Infect Control Hosp Epidemiol.* 2007;28(1):105–106.
50. Siegman-Igra Y, Golan H, Schwartz D, et al. Epidemiology of vascular catheter-related bloodstream infections in a large university hospital in Israel. *Scand J Infect Dis.* 2000;32(4):411–415.
51. Mehta NJ, Khan IA, Mehta RN, et al. Stenotrophomonas maltophilia endocarditis of prosthetic aortic valve: report of a case and review of literature. *Heart Lung.* 2000;29(5):351–355.
52. Niu MT, Knippen M, Simmons L, et al. Transfusion-transmitted Klebsiella pneumoniae fatalities, 1995 to 2004. *Transfus Med Rev.* 2006;20(2):149–157.

CHAPTER 14 ■ INTRAHOSPITAL TRANSPORT OF CRITICALLY ILL PATIENTS

ISMAËL MOHAMMEDI

The transportation of critically ill patients may be divided into specific categories:

- *Primary transport* (prehospital care) is the transfer of patients from site of illness or injury to first hospital contact.
- *Secondary transport* is the transfer of the patient from one hospital to another for continuing clinical care (interhospital transfer) or between departments within the same hospital (intrahospital transfer).

Technological developments have dramatically improved the information available from diagnostic testing such as computed tomography (CT), magnetic resonance imaging (MRI), angiography, cardiac catheterization, and nuclear imaging, as well as various interventions that can be done using these tools. As a result, critically ill patients are, with increasing frequency, moving not only between the intensive care unit (ICU) and the operating room (OR), but often on longer journeys to remote locations throughout the hospital. However, the safest place for the critically ill patient remains his or her room in the ICU, connected to ventilator and other life-support equipment, with complete monitoring installed—and with a physician–nurse team present to provide care. Transfer of critically ill patients to another location always involves some degree of risk. Therefore, the decision to transport must be based on a careful assessment of the potential benefits weighed against the potential risks. If transport is justified, it should be undertaken in a manner that does not jeopardize the level and quality of care being given. Indeed, lack of monitoring and inappropriately trained staff leading to a significant number of adverse events have been widely reported. These findings resulted in the publication of guidelines by professional organizations on how the transfer of the critically ill should be conducted (1–6).

TRANSPORT SCENARIOS

Vigilance and anticipation are basic attributes of critical care medicine, and are vital in the safe conduct of each transport. Differences exist, however, in the physiologic status of patients likely to be encountered, as well as the expected stressors imposed by the move. Therefore, organization and logistics should be adapted to each specific transfer. In developing a rational approach, we may consider four different common scenarios for intrahospital transport, as defined by Venkataraman and Orr (7).

Transfer from Critical Care Areas (to Ward)

Individuals transferring out of a critical care area no longer need the extensive monitoring they had in the ICU. They should not be experiencing cardiovascular or respiratory instability and may be expected to continue a process of improvement. Major concerns are alterations in level of consciousness and development of airway problems.

Transfer to Critical Care Areas (from Emergency Department or Ward)

Patients moving to critical care areas present a different set of challenges. Physiologic status may change rapidly, as in the patient with sepsis who has deteriorated on the ward, or the trauma victim who is being resuscitated in the emergency department (ED). In this setting, the potential for adverse events or secondary insults likely will increase through the transport process, and the breadth of monitoring and preparation required is increased. Clearly, the data in head-injured patients point out the importance of vigilance in this scenario. Andrews et al. (8) studied 50 head-injured patients who required intrahospital transfer; 35 were transported from the ICU (to CT scan or OR) and 15 from the ED (to CT scan and then to ICU or OR). They found insults in a greater proportion in patients transferred from ED than in the ICU patients, despite similar injury severity scores. Although these authors did not clearly explain this finding—66% versus 80% patients with insults after transport—it may be that in such patients optimal preparation, monitoring, and resuscitation are more easily obtained with neuro-ICU-trained physicians than ED physicians.

Round-trip Transfer from Critical Care to Noncritical Care Areas (i.e., to CT Scan)

This is probably the most neglected part of intrahospital transport and perhaps one of the most dangerous. Critically ill patients journey outside of the ICU for various diagnostic and therapeutic interventions and for an undetermined period of time. Adverse events or mishaps during transport may be related to physiologic changes or to technical or equipment problems (Table 14.1). Minor changes in heart rate or blood pressure may have little impact; however, unplanned extubation of the airway or loss of intravenous access for pressor support can have lethal consequences. Problems may occur and must be anticipated for any organ system. Early detection of such changes and rapid intervention are critically important to outcome.

Transfer between Critical Care Areas

The transfer of patients between critical care areas (from the OR to ICU or from the ICU to OR) are unlikely to isolate patients in remote areas of the hospital with limited resources. Issues involving the transport process itself are still relevant, however, and the nature of events leading to such transports puts these patients at significant risk. Much as Insel et al. (9) demonstrated hemodynamically significant changes in adults during transfer from the OR to ICU, Venkataraman and Orr (7) described major cardiorespiratory changes in children going from the OR to the ICU. Many of them required significant interventions such as ventilator changes or vasoactive infusions for stabilization (10–14). Petre et al. (15) noted that patients undergoing complex cardiothoracic procedures could leave the OR with multiple inotropic or vasoactive infusions, invasive monitors, pacemakers, and even intra-aortic balloon pumps or ventricular assist devices, but all required monitoring and adjustment during the transport process. They observed that patients were frequently unstable when they arrived in the ICU.

The same potential for physiologic deterioration is present when patients are transferred from the ICU to the OR, frequently compounded by the fact that these transfers are urgent or emergent. The transport and transfer process may be thought of as an extension of our care and clearly places patients at risk for physiologic changes that are at least as great as in the areas between which they are being transported.

ADVERSE EFFECTS

Deterioration in respiratory, cardiovascular, and other physiologic systems is a potential complication of any patient transport. This may be due to the movement of the patient or may be related to equipment dysfunction. Apart from physiologic changes, problems may arise from organizational and system efficiencies.

Overall Complications during Intrahospital Transport

Studying factors related to mishaps, Smith et al. (13) prospectively followed a series of 125 intrahospital transports from the ICU. Mishaps were defined as events having a detrimental effect on patient stability (e.g., ventilator disconnection, tracheal extubation, intravenous catheter infiltration or disconnection, vasoactive infusion disconnection, invasive monitor or catheter-related mishap, or monitor failure). Twenty-four percent of patients were believed to be less stable on return to the ICU. Eleven percent of transports had multiple misadventures, and more than one third involved at least one mishap. This series revealed several interesting trends. Transports to the CT scanner were more likely to involve mishaps than any other destination, particularly if any delays occurred at the site. Contributing factors were believed to include the physical isolation

TABLE 14.1

POTENTIAL COMPLICATIONS DURING TRANSPORT

Physiologic	Technical
CARDIOVASCULAR	
Hypertension	ECG lead disconnect or artifact
Hypotension	Monitor failure
Hypervolemia	Arterial catheter/central venous catheter disconnect
Hypovolemia/bleeding	Vasoactive drug infusion error or disconnect
Arrhythmias	Pacer malfunction
Congestive heart failure/pulmonary edema	IABP malfunction
Decreased cardiac output/inadequate tissue perfusion	Inability to fit IABP into elevator or ancillary location
Ischemia/Infarction	Loss of invasive monitoring catheters
Compromise of vascular anastomoses/grafts/bypasses	
RESPIRATORY	
Hypoxemia/desaturation	Loss of unprotected airway
Hypercapnia/respiratory acidosis	Extubation/endotracheal tube obstruction
Hypocapnia/respiratory alkalosis	Loss of gas supply
Tachypnea	Inability to match bedside ventilator mode
Bronchospasm	Ventilator malfunction
Loss of functional residual capacity	Lack of house gas lines at remote or diagnostic locations
Increased airway pressures/hemodynamic compromise	Chest tube occlusion or loss
Pneumothorax	
Aspiration	
NEUROLOGIC	
Increased ICP	ICP monitor loss or malfunction
Decreased cerebral perfusion pressure	Inability to maintain adequate head-up positioning
Inadequate cerebral blood flow	Errors with pentobarbital infusion during induced coma
Excessive cerebral blood flow	Loss of electrophysiologic monitoring capabilities
Seizures	Difficulty in temperature control
Cerebral edema	
Hemorrhage	
Stroke	
Herniation	
OTHER	
Metabolic acidosis/alkalosis	Pulled nasogastric or feeding tube
Hyperglycemia/hypoglycemia	Pulled Foley catheter
Hyperthermia/hypothermia	Pulled surgical drain/catheter
Oliguria/polyuria	Tangled infusion and monitoring catheters
	Loss of hyperalimentation source
	Compression stocking malfunction
	Bed malfunction
	Transport elevator malfunction

ECG, electrocardiogram; IABP, intra-aortic balloon pump; ICP, intracranial pressure.

of the patient during the procedure and the transfer of the patient from the bed to the scanner and back. Overall, 75% of mishaps occurred at the remote study site. Surprisingly, emergent transports were not more likely to have mishaps, nor was a correlation observed between the number of catheters and monitors and the incidence of mishaps.

Indeck et al. (16) reported, in a prospective evaluation of 103 consecutive transports carried out for diagnostic studies, that 68% of all transports experienced serious physiologic changes and that each of these required increased levels of support to the patient. These investigators also found that only 24% of the transports resulted in a change in patient management within 48 hours. They concluded that the decision to transport patients must be weighed carefully in the face of a 75% chance that the study result will not alter management.

Changes in patient management amounted to 39% in the experience of Hurst et al. (17), who studied a group of 81 surgery/trauma patients transported for a total of 100 diagnostic procedures. The examination with the highest efficiency included angiography and abdominal CT scanning, which resulted in therapeutic consequences in 57% and 51% of patients, respectively. They also found that physiologic changes—defined as a blood pressure ± 20 mm Hg, heart rate ± 20 beats per minute, respiratory rate ± 5 breaths per minute, or oxygen saturation ± 5% for 5 minutes duration—occurred in 66% of transported patients. These authors further demonstrated that while physiologic changes are frequent during transport, they are also frequent in ICU patients as a consequence of the severity of illness. They concluded that, if appropriate monitoring and ventilatory support are provided during transport, the frequency of life-threatening complications is quite small.

This is confirmed by the study of Szem et al. (18), who studied 203 intrahospital transports. They reported only 12 serious complications, including marked hypoxemia, cardiac arrest, hypotension, cerebral infarction, pneumothorax requiring chest tube placement, and rupture of an infected arteriovenous fistula, without any transport-related deaths.

It could be thus concluded that, even though intrahospital transport of the critically ill patient is associated with increased complications, the large variation of their incidence (ranging from 6% to 68% in the literature) may be attributed to differences in patient population and/or to definitions used.

Specific Complications during Intrahospital Transport

Cardiocirculatory Events

Cardiovascular changes seem to be common. Insel et al. (9) studied patients being transferred from the OR to the ICU after either major general or vascular surgery, carotid endarterectomy, or coronary artery bypass, comparing them to ICU patients undergoing transport for diagnostic or other nonoperative procedures. In the major postoperative groups, significant lability in blood pressure and pulse were noted. Despite continuous arterial blood pressure monitoring, 20% of patients in the major vascular and general surgery group required vigorous fluid resuscitation for hypotension on arrival to the ICU, whereas 36% required either nitroglycerin or nitroprusside for control of hypertension.

A prospective study of medical patients monitored, in addition to the standard electrocardiogram monitor, with a continuous 12-lead ST-segment analysis, showed that cardiac events that cannot be seen with the usual monitoring may occur (19).

It has been reported that the accuracy of noninvasive blood pressure monitoring is limited (20). Direct intra-arterial pressure measurements were taken in 44 transported patients as a gold standard and were compared with readings from four portable automatic oscillotonometers—the Dinamap 8100, Lifestat 100, Propaq 102, and Takeda UA711. All underread systolic pressure (by 13%, 21%, 19%, and 13%, respectively) and overread diastolic pressure (by 15%, 5%, 27%, and 15%, respectively) as compared to direct pressure measurement.

Respiratory Events

It has been noted that O_2 saturation can drop significantly when sedated patients are moved to and from the operating room (OR) or postanesthesia care unit (PACU). Hensley et al. (21) found that 60% of patients prepared for coronary bypass surgery became hypoxemic, with a SpO_2 less than 90%, during placement of invasive monitors after a standard premedication with morphine and scopolamine on their way to the OR, despite normal mental status. Tyler et al. (22) report that in a series of adult patients recovering from anesthesia, 12% desaturated to a SpO_2 of less than 85% and fully 35% of patients to a SpO_2 of less than 90% during transport from the OR to the PACU.

Healthy pediatric patients are no less at risk. Despite administering 100% oxygen for 3 minutes after surgery, Kataria et al. (23) found a significant age-related fall in SpO_2 during a 120 to 180 second transfer to the PACU, with the mean SpO_2 being 88% in children younger than 6 months of age. Studying healthy children with American Society of Anesthesiologists physical status I or II, Tomkins et al. (24) found that 24% became hypoxemic (SpO_2 less than 90%) during the first 10 minutes after termination of anesthesia. Significantly, clinical signs of respiratory compromise such as cyanosis or upper airway obstruction correlated poorly with measured hypoxemia.

For nonoperative mechanically ventilated patients, similar results have been shown. Waydhas et al. (25) found, in a study of 49 trips for 28 patients, that the arterial partial pressure of oxygen (PaO_2 /fraction of inspired oxygen (FiO_2) ratio dropped more than 20% after 21 of the transports. For ten of the patients studied, changes in the PaO_2/FiO_2 persisted for more than 24 hours.

Because the possibilities for treatment are reduced during the transfer period, two studies were undertaken to evaluate predictors that could identify patients whose respiratory function might deteriorate to allow the weighing of the benefit against the hazards of transfer before the actual transport takes place. Marx et al. (26) investigated 98 mechanically ventilated patients. In 54 transports (55% of studied patients), there was a decrease in the PaO_2/FiO_2 ratio, and a decrease of more than 20% from baseline was noted in 23 of the transferred patients (24%). Predictors for respiratory deterioration included age greater than 43 years and a required FiO_2 greater than 0.5. In a second study, 88 intrahospital transports involving 62 patients were analyzed (27). In 56 transports (64%), the PaO_2/FiO_2 ratio decreased by more than 20% from baseline. A high pretransfer PaO_2/FIO_2 ratio (greater than 200) was the only factor predictive for respiratory deterioration in multivariate analysis. Neither Marx et al. (26) nor Mohammedi et al. (27) have found a relationship between the duration of transfer and respiratory deterioration.

Manual bag ventilation of ICU patients transported to OR, or to other hospital locations, appears to be common. Small, older studies showed that such manual positive pressure ventilation is reasonable for short-term transit care, such as transferring an ICU patient to the OR just down the corridor. Weg and Has (28) compared parameters among 20 patients transported either with a mechanical ventilator or ventilated by bag mask. They found no significant hemodynamic changes and only transient variations in $PaCO_2$ between the two groups. Gervais et al. (12) compared manual ventilation with and without spirometry for tidal volume monitoring, and mechanical ventilation with a portable device that allowed tidal volume to be set but had no capacity for measurement. Both groups without spirometry developed significant decreases in $PaCO_2$ and increases in pH. When manual ventilation with tidal volume monitoring was used to approximate the minute ventilation patients received in the ICU, no significant changes were observed. By way of contrast, in a prospective study of ventilator-dependent patients who underwent procedures outside the ICU, Braman et al. (11) examined changes in arterial blood gas partial pressures and hemodynamic parameters in two treatment groups. Group 1 was ventilated manually during transport, and group 2 was ventilated by a portable volume-limited ventilator (with settings matched to the bedside ventilator). Significant changes in $PaCO_2$ (greater than 10 mm Hg) and pH were common in both groups, as was hypotension. However, the rate of occurrence was clearly greater in the manually ventilated group (75% vs. 44%), and two of the group 1 patients developed new cardiac arrhythmias. Blood gas deterioration correlated strongly with the development of hypotension and new arrhythmias. A similar but more recent study confirms these findings. After transport, 5 of 11 patients in the manually ventilated group, compared to 1 of 11 patients in a mechanically ventilated group, showed a significant deterioration in the PaO_2/FiO_2 ratio. The mean tidal volume and positive end-expiratory pressure in the manually ventilated group showed significantly larger variation than in the mechanically ventilated group (29). The authors concluded that the use of a transport ventilator provides more stable ventilatory support than does manual ventilation.

However, only a few comparative studies regarding portable ventilators have been published. Zanetta et al. (30) reported, in a bench model, that the performance of five transport ventilators, and three ICU ventilators that can be used for this purpose, set in a volume-controlled mode and submitted to various combinations of resistive and elastic loads, were very inhomogeneous.

Although many data have accumulated with respect to mishaps during transport, less is known about adverse long-term effects. Kollef et al. (31) found that, in a group of 273 ventilated patients who were transported, the incidence of ventilator-associated pneumonia was 24.4% compared with 4.4% in 248 nontransported patients with a similar severity of illness. A risk-adjusted matched cohort study showed a ventilator-associated pneumonia (VAP) rate of 26% in transported patients compared with 10% in the matched nontransported patients (32). This study was designed to examine the impact of intrahospital transport (IHT) on the occurrence of VAP, not to explore its mechanism. However, the authors proposed some explanations: the supine position during IHT, the frequent manipulations of the ventilator circuits needed during IHT that increase the risk of aspiration of gastric content or of contaminated secretions, and the fact that technical difficulties are often encountered when suction of airways is needed during transport. However, the ICU mortality rate was similar in both groups of patients.

Neurological Events

The population of transported patients in whom physiologic variation poses the greatest clinical threat are those with head trauma, which requires tight regulation of oxygenation, blood pressure, and intracranial pressure (33). Secondary insults such as hypoxia, hypotension, or decreased cerebral perfusion pressure are devastating in head-injured patients. Gentleman and Jennett (34) found that "suboptimum care" was responsible for most avoidable deaths after head trauma, and that more than one third of deaths in neurotrauma patients had avoidable factors. In a large audit of head-injured patients, these investigators report compromised airways in over 25% of victims arriving in the neurosurgical unit, with 15% to 22% demonstrating hypoxemia. Andrews et al. (8) report secondary insults occurring in 47% of neurotrauma patients during transport from the ER and that fully 80% of patients had insults within the first 4 hours after transfer.

CONTRIBUTING FACTORS

In a cross-sectional analysis of intrahospital transfer incidents reported to the Australian Incident Monitoring Study in Intensive Care system, Beckmann et al. (35) identified 176 reports of 191 incidents relating to intrahospital transportation from 37 ICUs. Clinical management errors accounted for 61% of the problems (the most common patient/staff management issues identified were communication and liaison issues between the ICU and sites of destination or origin), with equipment failure responsible for the remainder. Factors contributing to the incident were classified as system-based factors (work practices, equipment, physical environment structure) in 46%, and human-based factors (knowledge-based, rules-based, skills-based, or technical error) in 54%. Many of these human-based contributing factors suggest that personnel involved may not have had adequate training. From these data, the authors developed recommendations for intrahospital transport and a checklist for documenting the processes of care before, during, and after the transfer period, which are further discussed.

The Three Phases of Transport

Preparation begins with careful evaluation of the risks and benefits of the transport. The decision to move a patient should be made by the senior medical practitioner of the critical care team. The transport may be broken down into three phases: the preparatory phase, the transfer phase, and posttransport stabilization.

Preparatory Phase

This is probably the most important stage. Adequate attention to this first phase minimizes problems in the other two.

1. Stabilization of the patient before transport is an obvious goal, although overruling priorities may make this impossible. As a rule, all anticipated procedures should be performed in the critical care area before transport. Careful assessment of the patient's airway is critical, and adequate oxygenation and ventilation must be ensured. In patients who are combative or show decreased levels of consciousness for whatever reason, careful consideration should be given to electively securing the airway before transport. Similarly, elective intubation should be entertained in patients with significant burn injuries (especially inhalational injury), chest trauma, or respiratory distress. An apparently insignificant pneumothorax can progress rapidly—particularly if the patient is receiving positive pressure ventilation—and tube thoracostomy should be considered. Once in place, chest tubes may be transported under water seal, and then, ideally, reattached to suction during any therapeutic or diagnostic procedure. If necessary, vasoactive infusions should be addressed to obtain a steady state before any elective transport. Intravascular volume resuscitation should be well under way in patients with shock caused by trauma, and large-bore vascular access catheters should be in place before

movement. When blood pressure cannot be stabilized, surgical exploration and control of bleeding must take precedence over any further diagnostic procedures.

2. Communication and coordination are essential to the safe conduct of transport. When a patient is transferred to or from the critical care area, or between critical care areas, information should be passed from physician to physician and nurse to nurse regarding the patient's condition, treatment, and management. Timing of arrival and procedures should be confirmed with personnel at the patient's destination, especially when CT, angiography, or nuclear medicine are involved; this is of particular importance as mishaps are more likely when delays occur in these areas. Ideally, patient escort or security may arrange to clear the transport route and to have elevators standing by. If the responsible physician does not accompany the patient, the physician must at least be aware when the transport is taking place. The reasons for the transport should be documented in the patient's chart. It is of critical importance that the patient "handoff" be carried out in a flawless manner and that documentation be complete.
3. Resuscitative and scheduled medications, fluids, monitors, life-support equipment, and adequate personnel need to be assembled. Airway supplies, including equipment for intubation and ventilation and an oxygen supply, are essential. A checklist should be used to assist in preparation.

Transport Phase

The goal during the transport phase is to maintain the same level of care as the patient had in the critical care area. As much as possible, we should strive to achieve the following:

1. Maintain patient stability through monitoring.
2. Continue the present ongoing management.
3. Avoid iatrogenic mishaps.
4. Reduce to a minimum transfer duration.

In transports from the ICU to and from ancillary locations, every attempt should be made to return monitoring and care to the ICU level during the procedure. Modalities such as pulmonary artery pressure, which may be difficult to follow in a moving patient, can again be monitored in a stationary location. By adhering to the principles of thorough preparation and minimizing time spent during the transport phase, we should decrease the potential for complications.

Posttransport Stabilization

When a patient returns to the ICU, no less attention should be paid to the posttransport stabilization phase than to other components of the process. Patients may continue to be at increased risk of secondary insults through the first 4 hours after return (34). Additional issues may arise, and communication is thus essential. The primary team may be unaware of *all* of the problems that began in the OR/ED or during the transport, or important new findings may follow from a diagnostic procedure. The transport team members must review these issues with the full critical care team, including the nurses who will be working with the patient. This communication is especially important for the trauma patients, who may have physicians from several disciplines involved in their care.

MINIMUM STANDARDS

Accompanying Personnel

Adequate and appropriate personnel should be gathered to accompany the patient, including a minimum of two people, one of whom is the patient's critical care nurse. Nursing care plays a vital role in the ICU and must be continued throughout the transport process to ensure proper administration of scheduled medications, titration of vasoactive infusions, and accurate record keeping. A trained physician must accompany any unstable patient who requires extensive acute interventions. This dedicated team should be available for the entire duration of the transport and needs to be familiar with all equipment.

Equipment

A standard set of equipment should be available for most critical care transports. Basic resuscitation drugs such as epinephrine, atropine, and antiarrhythmic agents, along with a cardiac monitor and defibrillator, are appropriate for most transfers to or between critical care areas. Airway support supplies, including a self-inflating resuscitation bag (to allow ventilation in the event that a temporary interruption of the compressed gas source occurs), masks, oral airways, and a functioning laryngoscope with appropriate blades and endotracheal tubes, are mandatory. An adequate oxygen supply should allow full support during the anticipated duration outside the ICU, with a 30-minute reserve time. Intravenous fluids should include maintenance requirements, as well as isotonic crystalloids, colloids, and blood products as indicated for resuscitation. Medications given by infusion should be continued by battery-operated volumetric pumps to avoid unnecessary interruption of life-supporting drugs (e.g., vasopressors). All scheduled and anticipated medications (e.g., insulin, antibiotics, sedatives, and muscle relaxants) also should accompany the patient.

All battery-operated transport equipment should have charge indicators and backup batteries. Regular servicing and checking of transport equipment is essential.

A trolley or bed attachment to carry all equipment and drugs above is highly recommended.

Monitoring

Perhaps more than any other patients, the critically ill demand that we individualize monitoring schemes, support systems, and the transport process. Guidelines have been set as the minimum acceptable standards (task force):

- Continuous monitoring with periodic documentation of electrocardiogram and pulse oximetry
- Intermittent measurement and documentation of blood pressure, respiratory rate, and pulse rate

In addition, selected patients, based on clinical status, may benefit from monitoring by the following:

- Capnography
- Continuous intra-arterial pressure, pulmonary arterial pressure, and intracranial pressure

- Intermittent measurements of central venous pressure, pulmonary artery occlusion pressure, and cardiac output

Intubated patients receiving mechanical ventilation should have airway pressure monitored. If a transport ventilator is used, it should have alarms to indicate disconnects or excessively high airway pressures.

SPECIAL CIRCUMSTANCES

Hemodynamically Unstable Patients

The importance of stabilization before transport cannot be overemphasized. Adequate large-bore venous access, resuscitation fluids, and blood products must be available throughout the transport. One person may need to be assigned the sole task of managing blood and fluid administration, especially if any significant amount of time is to be spent at an ancillary location. Patients with cardiovascular collapse may require multiple vasopressor and inotropic infusions that must be available for adjustment during transport and may, at times, be moved to the OR with cardiopulmonary resuscitation in progress.

Neurotrauma Patients

Head injury is common in all age groups and remains a leading cause of morbidity and mortality in young adults. Once injured, the central nervous system has very small reserve for recovery. Although the primary injury cannot be reversed, secondary injuries are prevented by optimal cerebral perfusion pressure. These patients frequently require transport for diagnostic procedures not available in the ICU. However, transport can have an adverse impact on cerebral perfusion pressure by increasing intracranial pressure (ICP) or decreasing mean arterial pressure, or both, leading to secondary ischemic injuries. Patients with severe head injuries or other causes of increased ICP should be intubated to protect the airway and control ventilation. Management may include positioning with the head up 20 to 30 degrees, moderate hyperventilation, adequate hemodynamic management, and sedation. The ICP monitoring should not be interrupted during transport, and changes in posture of the patient should be avoided, but, if inevitable, very carefully performed.

Magnetic Resonance Imaging

MRI can provide invaluable diagnostic information but poses multiple management problems for the critically ill because of the effects of the magnetic field on monitoring and life-support equipment, physical isolation of the patient, and the frequently remote location of the scanner. If MRI is deemed necessary, careful planning is essential. With minor modification, most monitoring techniques are adaptable to the MRI suite. Because of patient isolation during the scan, particular attention should be paid to airway assessment.

SUMMARY

Intrahospital transport, a seemingly mundane event with a standard process, is actually one of the most risk-ridden actions we undertake in the ICU. As stated above, it is incumbent on us to ensure that these transports—needed to provide high-quality care—are indicated and carried out in the safest manner possible. The closest coordination between ICU nursing, the respiratory therapists, and the physicians is needed. Particular attention must be paid to monitoring. If these caveats are attended to, the transport can be carried out in the safest manner possible.

References

1. Warren J, Fromm RE Jr, Orr RA, et al; American College of Critical Care Medicine. Guidelines for the inter- and intrahospital transport of critically ill patients. *Crit Care Med.* 2004;32:256–262.
2. Ferdinande P. Recommendations for intra-hospital transport of the severely head injured patient. Working Group on Neurosurgical Intensive Care of the European Society of Intensive Care Medicine. *Intensive Care Med,* 1999; 25:1441–1443.
3. Australian and New Zealand College of Anaesthetists, Royal Australian College of Physicians, and Australian College for Emergency Medicine. Minimum standards for intrahospital transport of critically ill patients. Australian and New Zealand College of Anaesthetists, 2003.
4. American college of emergency physicians. Principles of appropriate patient transfer. *Ann Emerg Med.* 1990;19:337–338.
5. Société Française d'Anesthésie et de Réanimation. Recommandations concernant les transports médicalisés intrahospitaliers. Société Française Anesthésie et de Réanimation, 1994.
6. Chang DW; American Association for Respiratory Care (AARC). AARC Clinical Practice Guideline: in-hospital transport of the mechanically ventilated patient–2002 revision & update. *Respir Care.* 2002;47:721–723.
7. Venkataraman ST, Orr RA. Intrahospital transport of critically ill patients. *Crit Care Clin.* 1992;8:525–531.
8. Andrews PJ, Piper IR, Dearden NM, et al. Secondary insults during intrahospital transport of head-injured patients. *Lancet.* 1990;335:327–330.
9. Insel J, Weissman C, Kemper M, et al. Cardiovascular changes during transport of critically ill and postoperative patients. *Crit Care Med.* 1986;14:539–542.
10. Waddell G. Movement of critically ill patients within hospital. *Br Med J.* 1975;2:417–419.
11. Braman S, Dunn S, Amico C, et al. Complications of intrahospital transport in critically ill patients. *Ann Intern Med.* 1987;107:469–473.
12. Gervais H, Eberle B, Konietzke D, et al. Comparison of blood gases of ventilated patients during transport. *Crit Care Med.* 1987;15:761–763.
13. Smith I, Fleming S, Cernaianu A. Mishaps during transport from the intensive care unit. *Crit Care Med.* 1990;18:278–281.
14. Fromm R, Dellinger R. Transport of critically ill patients. *J Intensive Care Med.* 1992;7:223–233.
15. Petre J, Bazaral M, Estafanous F. Patient transport: an organized method with direct clinical benefits. *Biomed Instrum Technol.* 1989;23:100–107.
16. Indeck M, Peterson S, Smith J, et al. Risk, cost, and benefit of transporting ICU patients for special studies. *J Trauma.* 1988;28:1020–1025.
17. Hurst JM, Davis K Jr, Johnson DJ, et al. Cost and complications during in-hospital transport of critically ill patients: a prospective cohort study. *J Trauma.* 1992;33:582–585.
18. Szem JW, Hydo LJ, Fischer E, et al. High-risk intrahospital transport of critically ill patients: safety and outcome of the necessary "road trip." *Crit Care Med.* 1995;23:1660–1666.
19. Carson KJ, Drew BJ. Electrocardiographic changes in critically ill adults during intrahospital transport. *Prog Cardiovasc Nurs.* 1994;9:4–12.
20. Runcie CJ, Reeve WG, Reidy J, et al. Blood pressure measurement during transport. A comparison of direct and oscillotonometric readings in critically ill patients. *Anaesthesia.* 1990;45:659–665.
21. Hensley FA, Dodson DL, Martin DE, et al. Oxygen saturation during placement of invasive monitoring in the premedicated, unanesthetized cardiac patient. *Anesthesiology.* 1986;65:A22.
22. Tyler IL, Tantisira B, Winter PM, et al. Continuous monitoring of arterial oxygen saturation with pulse oximetry during transfer to the recovery room. *Anesth Analg.* 1985;64:1108–1112.
23. Kataria B, Harnik E, Mitchard R, et al. Postoperative arterial oxygen saturation in the pediatric population during transportation. *Anesth Analg.* 1988;67:280–282.
24. Tomkins D, Gaukroger P, Bentley M. Hypoxia in children following general anesthesia. *Anaesth Intensive Care* 1988;16:177–181.

25. Waydhas C, Schneck G, Duswald KH. Deterioration of respiratory function after intra-hospital transport of critically ill surgical patients. *Intensive Care Med.* 1995;21:784–789.
26. Marx G, Vangerow B, Hecker H, et al. Predictors of respiratory function deterioration after transfer of critically ill patients. *Intensive Care Med.* 1998;24:1157–1162.
27. Mohammedi I, Belkhouja K, Robert D. Risk factors of respiratory function deterioration after intrahospital transport in critically ill patients. *Ann Fr Anesth Reanim.* 2005;24:1314–1315.
28. Weg JG, Haas CF. Safe intrahospital transport of critically ill ventilator-dependent patients. *Chest.* 1989;96:631–635.
29. Nakamura T, Fujino Y, Uchiyama A, et al. Intrahospital transport of critically ill patients using ventilator with patient-triggering function. *Chest.* 2003;123:159–164.
30. Zanetta G, Robert D, Guerin C. Evaluation of ventilators used during transport of ICU patients—a bench study. *Intensive Care Med.* 2002;28:443–451.
31. Kollef MH, Von Harz B, Prentice D, et al. Patient transport from intensive care increases the risk of developing ventilator-associated pneumonia. *Chest.* 1997;112:765–773.
32. Bercault N, Wolf M, Runge I, et al. Intrahospital transport of critically ill ventilated patients: a risk factor for ventilator-associated pneumonia—a matched cohort study. *Crit Care Med.* 2005;33:2471–2478.
33. Yeguiayan JM, Lenfant F, Rapenne T, et al. Effects of intra-hospital transport of severely head injured patients on the parameters of cerebral perfusion. *Can J Anaesth.* 2002;49:890–891.
34. Gentleman D, Jennett B. Audit of transfer of unconscious head-injured patients to a neurosurgical unit. *Lancet.* 1990;335:330–334.
35. Beckmann U, Gillies DM, Berenholtz SM, et al. Incidents relating to the intra-hospital transfer of critically ill patients. An analysis of the reports submitted to the Australian Incident Monitoring Study in Intensive Care. *Intensive Care Med.* 2004;30:1579–1585.

CHAPTER 15 ■ INTERHOSPITAL TRANSPORT OF CRITICALLY ILL PATIENTS

JACK J.M. LIGTENBERG • WILMA E. MONTEBAN-KOOISTRA

IMMEDIATE CONCERNS

> It is a wet, cold Friday night. Lights flash in the distance. The sound of a siren approaches. An ambulance hurtles through the night carrying a critically ill patient. The nurse and doctor, both inexperienced and sincerely wishing they weren't there, watch the monitor anxiously. They have left the security of one hospital for that of another; like in a circus trapeze act, they hang suspended for a moment. For at that instant the sickest patient in the region is travelling at over 100 km/hour down an unknown highway. Will they catch the trapeze, or will they fall?
>
> *Citation from Philip Haji-Michael (1)*

There appears to be little awareness of the problems/adverse events of interfacility movement of critically ill patients. Both national and international guidelines are in place, but appear not to be followed in a considerable number of transfers. Aeromedical transport of patients may have advantages, depending on the distance and the condition of the patient, but also has its specific drawbacks. Interhospital transport of critically ill patients has changed from volunteer work to a specific skill of emergency and intensive care medicine. The intensive care unit (ICU) patient deserves appropriate medical care during the road trip or in the air. Health authorities should be made aware of the fact that an organizational structure guaranteeing safe critical care transferrals requires extensive financial and human investments.

INTERHOSPITAL TRANSPORT OF INTENSIVE CARE UNIT PATIENTS

The number of interhospital transports of critically ill patients gradually expands. Conservative estimates mention more than 11,000 transfers per year in the United Kingdom (2). There are various reasons for this increase, partly due to local or national circumstances such as shortage of ICU beds or insurance motives, but also caused by centralization of patient groups in specialized centers, specific treatment options, second opinions, and new and established services covering extensive areas with people living in remote locations (3,4).

The primary goal of interhospital transport is to get the right patient, with the right personnel and the right equipment, to the right place in the right amount of time (5). This secondary transport should only occur if it is likely to improve the patient's clinical outcome. The transport itself, at least, has to be as safe as possible and should add no extra risk to the patient. Circulatory or ventilatory problems may arise in the ambulance as well as during transportation in the air (6–8). Monitoring possibilities are limited during transportation, access to the patient may be limited, and fewer—and sometimes less skilled—"hands" are available compared to the ICU environment. Necessary interventions, if the patient deteriorates, may be difficult during the road or air trip, as may be the physical examination (9).

GROUND TRANSPORT USING A STANDARD AMBULANCE OR MOBILE INTENSIVE CARE UNIT

In a recent study evaluating 100 consecutive interhospital transfers of ICU patients over the road, adverse events occurred in more than 30%: Approximately half of these events were graded as being of vital importance (Table 15.1). Recommendations for safe transport made by the intensivist of the receiving ICU were ignored in a considerable number of cases. It is quite worrisome that there appeared to be

The authors have no competing financial or other interests.

TABLE 15.1

EXAMPLES OF RECORDED ADVERSE EVENTS DURING INTERHOSPITAL TRANSPORT

Transfer characteristics	Adverse event	Severity (grade 1–3)[a]
Pulmonary embolus	PaO_2 on departure 4.2 kPa[b]; not intubated; PaO_2 on arrival 4.7 kPa	3
Esophageal bleeding	Only one peripheral intravenous line; no accompanying physician; active bleeding; PaO_2 on arrival 6.7 kPa	3
Sepsis; rhabdomyolysis	RI; shock on arrival	2
Imminent RI; Wegener granulomatosis	No blood pressure measured on the road (160 km); PaO_2 on arrival 6.7 kPa; SO_2 86%	1
Pulmonary embolus	No accompanying physician; RI on arrival	2
ARDS; MOF	SO_2 93% at departure; 69% on arrival	3
Streptococcus pneumoniae sepsis; imminent RI	Not intubated (despite advice); norepinephrine via peripheral intravenous line	3
Sleep apnea syndrome; RI	PaO_2 on departure 6.9 kPa; during transport SO_2 ↓ 74% and cardiac ischemia; no physician	3
Hemorrhagic shock; mechanical ventilation	No accompanying physician; active bleeding; 3 units packed cells on the road; oxygenation problems	3
Infectious endocarditis; mechanical ventilation	No physician; hemodynamically unstable on the road	1
Septic shock; imminent respiratory insufficiency	Not intubated (despite advice); RI on arrival	3
Septic shock; MOF	Norepinephrine via peripheral intravenous line	2
Suicide attempt (benzodiazepine)	Deep coma; not intubated; apnea en route; cyanotic on arrival	3
Postsurgical; mechanical ventilation	Oxygen supply breakdown before arrival	3
COPD, pneumonia	Shortage of oxygen before arrival	3
Hemodialysis postsurgical	No blood pressure measured on the road	1
Active bleeding digestive tract	Only one peripheral intravenous line	1
ARDS; mechanical ventilation	Ambulance breakdown; 40-min delay	1

RI, respiratory insufficiency, (imminent) need for mechanical ventilation; ARDS, acute respiratory distress syndrome; MOF, multiple organ failure; COPD, chronic obstructive pulmonary disorder.
[a]Grade of severity. Grade 1: Deviation from guidelines/protocol. Grade 2: Of vital importance; immediate action needed on arrival. Grade 3: Of vital importance; immediate action needed on arrival; probably avoidable.
[b]Conversion from kPa to mm Hg: Multiply by 7.5.
From Ligtenberg JJ, Arnold LG, Stienstra Y, et al. Quality of interhospital transport of critically ill patients: a prospective audit. *Crit Care.* 2005;9: R446–R451.

little awareness of the problems/adverse events that may occur during transportation. A substantial part of the adverse events could have been avoided simply by adhering to protocols. Interestingly, few events were caused by technical problems during transport, such as shortage of oxygen. Other important points for improvement, emerging from several studies, are (a) transparent pretransport communication between professionals; (b) feedback about adverse events; (c) careful preparation of the patient; and, in selected transfers, (d) the utilization of a specialist retrieval team eventually using a mobile intensive care unit (MoICU). Several positive experiences have been described working with specialist retrieval teams (10,11). In the study of Bellingan et al., transports by a specialist retrieval team, compared to standard ambulance with a doctor from the referring hospital, resulted in more stable transports and a reduction in mortality in the first 12 hours from 7.7% to 3% (10). Based on such data, it seems logical to use a specialist retrieving team for critically ill patients (12). However, such a team of specialists will not be available always and at every location. Furthermore, it appears to be difficult to predict which patients will deteriorate during transfer and, therefore, may benefit most from a specialist team (6). It is strongly recommended, in any event, that each referring and tertiary institution have a plan using locally available resources if the referring facility is not able to conduct the transfer. This plan has to address (a) pretransport coordination and communication, (b) transport personnel, and (c) transport equipment and monitoring during transport (13) (Table 15.2). Several excellent papers with practical guidelines for safe ICU transfers that can help in making such a plan have been published (11,13–15).

AIR MEDICAL TRANSPORT OF CRITICALLY ILL PATIENTS

The optimal way of transporting critically ill patients remains controversial. Aeromedical transport (AMT) of patients from the scene or between hospitals may offer advantages but also has its specific drawbacks. The overall benefits of aeromedical services, measured by sound data, remain uncertain and anecdotal, although ample efforts have been made to describe the value of aeromedical transportation to the health system (16). The European HEMS and Air Rescue Committee (EHAC) has put forward the collection of information related to the operation of air ambulances worldwide as a point of interest.

TABLE 15.2

EQUIPMENT RECOMMENDATIONS FOR THE MOBILE INTENSIVE CARE UNIT

Oxygen with flows up to 25 L/min for greater than 3 h, with backup oxygen supply of greater than 1 h capability
Airway management equipment: Laryngoscope, tubes, cricothyrotomy set, bag-valve mask
Mechanical ventilator with—at minimum—a mandatory volume and a pressure mode of ventilation; a backup ventilator system, which should be able to deliver at least 5 cm of PEEP
ECG monitoring
Invasive hemodynamic monitoring: Arterial pressure, PAP, and ICP
Pulse oximetry with backup
Capnometry with backup
Capability for up to six infusion pumps
Adequate suction, with backup (stomach, chest tubes, and endotracheal suction, simultaneously)
Pharmacy (sedatives, analgesics, vasoactives, volume expanders, paralytics, antiarrhythmics)
Defibrillator, transcutaneous cardiac pacemaker
Backup batteries
Adequate communication equipment

PEEP, positive end-expiratory pressure; ECG, electrocardiogram; PAP, pulmonary artery pressure; ICP, intracranial pressure.
Modified from Gebremichael M, Borg U, Habashi NM, et al. Interhospital transport of the extremely ill patient: the mobile intensive care unit. *Crit Care Med.* 2000;28:79–85.

The use of AMT differs greatly between various countries, depending, among other things, on health care financing, distances to tertiary hospitals, and the presence of large rural areas. It is difficult to get an overview of AMT in different countries. In the 1990s, for example, there were already more than 170 air medical programs in operation in the United States (17). In the United States, 28% of helicopter transports are scene calls, whereas the remaining 72% are interhospital transfers. In Australia, where experience with AMT is widespread, patients are transported between intensive care units by land ambulance in the metropolitan areas, by helicopter for journeys of less than 400 km, and by fixed wing aircraft for longer distances (18). In Germany more than 50 AMT helicopters are available, having already performed, in the first quarter of 2006, more than 3,000 intensive care transports [source: Allgemeiner Deutscher Automobil Club (ADAC)]. In 1998, in the southern part of Germany, AMT was used in 14% of interhospital transports, ground transport using a MoICU in 16%, and standard ambulance with physician in 59% of cases (19). Table 15.3 shows the top ten patient categories using AMT in the United States. Table 15.4 describes patient categories using helicopter transport in Germany.

TABLE 15.3

TOP TEN PATIENT CATEGORIES USING AIR MEDICAL SERVICES IN THE UNITED STATES

Group	Number of flights	Percentage of total transports per patient
Trauma/burn/emergency	222	22%
Pediatrics, newborn	221	23%
Medicine, coronary	135	4%
Congenital heart	129	15%
General pediatrics, ICU	117	31%
Medicine, critical care	93	17%
Pediatrics, surgery	74	9%
Thoracic cardiac surgery	68	8%
Neurosurgery adult	60	6%
Surgery transplant	35	6%

ICU, intensive care unit.
Source: UMHS Data Warehouse, United States. Modified from Rosenberg BL, Butz DA, Comstock MC, et al. Aeromedical service: how does it actually contribute to the mission? *J Trauma.* 2003;54: 681–688.

SPECIFIC BENEFITS AND DRAWBACKS OF MEDICAL AIR TRANSPORT

Air medical transport can be divided into two categories: Fixed wing or airplane, and rotor wing or helicopter transport. The most important advantage of helicopter transport is that it is time saving, resultant from the aircraft speed and the ability to avoid traffic delays and ground obstacles. This time benefit must be balanced against organizational delays, flight time from the helicopter base to the referring hospital, and transfer

TABLE 15.4

INTERHOSPITAL TRANSPORT USING AIR MEDICAL HELICOPTER SERVICES IN GERMANY: PER PATIENT CATEGORY

Cardiac/cardiac surgery	33%
Neurosurgery, adult	22%
Trauma	18%
Neurology	7%
Medicine, critical care	5%
Vascular surgery	5%
Surgery	3%

Source: W. Wyrwich, Airmed 1996, Germany.

between vehicles/ambulances at the beginning and end (14,20). However, helicopters provide a less comfortable environment than road ambulances or airplanes. Cramped compartments, noise, and turbulence may interfere with patient examination, monitoring, and therapy (21). Helicopters have a poorer safety record compared to ground ambulances and fixed-wing aircrafts (14). The National Transportation Safety Board identified poor weather as the greatest hazard to helicopter air medical transport. Other risk factors of helicopter flights are nighttime flights, disorientation from the lack of visual clues, and pressure to make the flight (22). Airplanes provide increased range, greater speed, and more room for the patient(s), crew, and equipment than helicopters. Less cabin noise and turbulence result in fewer problems, and pressurization can be set in the desired range. Airplane operations are limited, however, to areas that have appropriate runways. Furthermore, airplane patient transfers require multiple means of transportation (i.e., hospital to ambulance to airplane) (21).

Other aspects that must be dealt with during AMT are as follows:

1. Boyle's law, the impact of which is that with increased altitude and decreasing atmospheric pressure, the volume of a gas expands. This can affect any body cavity or piece of equipment that contains a gas. For this reason, patients with a pneumothorax should have an unclamped chest tube. Similarly, other drains should also be unclamped and monitored. Intravenous bags rather than bottles should be used (air in a bottle will expand) and intravenous lines are best placed on pumps. Endotracheal tube cuffs will also expand, so the cuff pressure should be monitored and adjusted, as needed (8). The cuff can be filled with water, but it has been noted that there may still be a rise in pressure (23).
2. Additional stress of flight: Acceleration/deceleration, dehydration, noise, vibration, anxiety, and motion sickness are frequently encountered in helicopters and small airplanes (24).
3. Hypoxemia: As pressure is reduced, the quantity of oxygen available also decreases at altitude. Although oxygen still constitutes 21% of the atmospheric pressure, each breath brings fewer oxygen molecules to the lungs, resulting in hypoxia. Cabin pressurization has eliminated this problem in most airplanes. Patients with impaired pulmonary function are more at risk for hypoxemia.

Patients who might benefit from AMT are those with a time-dependent disorder, because air transport might save time (25). Good clinical studies defining the benefits of AMT for specific patient groups are needed (26). For some patient categories, for example, acute myocardial infarction and traumatic brain injury, the advantages of AMT seem clear (8,27). For other patient groups, data are lacking. Many investigators try to establish the ideal distance in which air medical transport may be beneficial (28). Helicopter air medical transport can be considered for journeys from about 80 to 400 km or over 2 hours. Airplane medical transport tends to be a more efficient process for patients more distant than approximately 400 km from care (18). On the other hand, interhospital ground transport with a dedicated team, proper patient stabilization before transport, and a transport vehicle with intensive care facilities has been proven to be safe over long distances (29,30).

APPROACH TO THE INTERHOSPITAL TRANSPORT OF THE CRITICALLY ILL PATIENT

Indication for the Transfer

A decision to transfer should be made after communication between professionals of the referring and receiving hospital. It must be clear who is responsible for the preparation and transportation of the patient, following existing local and/or international guidelines.

Mode of Transportation, Accompanying Staff, and Necessary Equipment

Each referring and tertiary institution must have a standard plan using locally available resources if the referring facility is not able to conduct the transfer. This plan has to address mode of transportation (standard ambulance, MoICU, air medical transport), transport personnel (intensive care physician and nurse of the referring or receiving ICU, specialist retrieval team), transport equipment, and monitoring during transport.

Guidelines for Transportation

In the literature, several excellent papers have been published with guidelines for equipment, ambulance requirements, and staffing (13–15). Strict adherence to simple protocols and guidelines will increase the quality of transports and minimize the risk for the patient.

Emphasizing the Importance of Safe Transport among Medical Professionals, and Hospital Administrators

This is a very important subject in increasing the quality of interhospital transports, since there appears to be little awareness of the problems/adverse events among medical professionals (6). Interhospital transport of critically ill patients requires specific skills of emergency and intensive care medicine. Health authorities should be made aware of the fact that safe critical care transferrals require extensive financial investments.

References

1. Haji-Michael P. Critical care transfers—a danger foreseen is half avoided. *Crit Care.* 2005;9:343–344.
2. Mackenzie PA, Smith EA, Wallace PG. Transfer of adults between intensive care units in the United Kingdom: postal survey. *BMJ.* 1997;314:1455–1456.
3. Green A, Showstack J, Rennie D, et al. The relationship of insurance status, hospital ownership, and teaching status with interhospital transfers in California in 2000. *Acad Med.* 2005;80:774–779.
4. Whitelaw AS, Hsu R, Corfield AR, et al. Establishing a rural emergency medical retrieval service. *Emerg Med J.* 2006;23:76–78.
5. Schneider C, Gomez M, Lee R. Evaluation of ground ambulance, rotor-wing, and fixed-wing aircraft services. *Crit Care Clin.* 1992;8:533–564.
6. Ligtenberg JJ, Arnold LG, Stienstra Y, et al. Quality of interhospital transport of critically ill patients: a prospective audit. *Crit Care.* 2005;9:R446–R451.

7. Beckmann U, Gillies DM, Berenholtz SM, et al. Incidents relating to the intra-hospital transfer of critically ill patients. An analysis of the reports submitted to the Australian Incident Monitoring Study in Intensive Care. *Intens Care Med.* 2004;30:1579–1585.
8. Essebag V, Halabi AR, Churchill-Smith M, et al. Air medical transport of cardiac patients. *Chest.* 2003;124:1937–1945.
9. Gray A, Bush S, Whiteley S. Secondary transport of the critically ill and injured adult. *Emerg Med J.* 2004;21:281–285.
10. Bellingan G, Olivier T, Batson S, et al. Comparison of a specialist retrieval team with current United Kingdom practice for the transport of critically ill patients. *Intens Care Med.* 2000;26:740–744.
11. Gebremichael M, Borg U, Habashi NM, et al. Interhospital transport of the extremely ill patient: the mobile intensive care unit. *Crit Care Med.* 2000;28:79–85.
12. Manji M, Bion JF. Transporting critically ill patients. *Intens Care Med.* 1995;21:781–783.
13. Warren J, Fromm RE Jr, Orr RA, et al. Guidelines for the inter- and intra-hospital transport of critically ill patients. *Crit Care Med.* 2004;32:256–262.
14. Wallace PG, Ridley SA. ABC of intensive care. Transport of critically ill patients. *BMJ.* 1999;319:368–371.
15. Shirley PJ, Bion JF. Intra-hospital transport of critically ill patients: minimising risk. *Intens Care Med.* 2004;30:1508–1510.
16. Rosenberg BL, Butz DA, Comstock MC, et al. Aeromedical service: how does it actually contribute to the mission? *J Trauma.* 2003;54:681–688.
17. Fromm RE Jr, Varon J. Air medical transport. *J Fam Pract.* 1993;36:313–318.
18. Shirley PJ. Australia has considerable experience of transporting critically ill patients. *BMJ.* 1999;319:1137.
19. Lackner CK, Reith MW, Gross S, et al. Arzbegleiteteter patiententransporte 1998 in Bayern. *Notfall Rettungsmedizin.* 2000;3:407–418.
20. Svenson JE, O'Connor JE, Lindsay MB. Is air transport faster? A comparison of air versus ground transport times for interfacility transfers in a regional referral system. *Air Med J.* 2006;25:170–172.
21. Rodenberg R, Blumen IJ. Air medical transport. In: *Rosen's Emergency Medicine. Concepts and Clinical Practice.* 6th ed. Philadelphia: Mosby Inc.; 2006.
22. National Transportation Safety Board. NTSB calls for stricter regulation of air ambulance flights. *Internet.* Accessed 2006.
23. Henning J, Sharley P, Young R. Pressures within air-filled tracheal cuffs at altitude–an in vivo study. *Anaesthesia.* 2004;59:252–254.
24. Demmons LL, Cook EW III. Anxiety in adult fixed-wing air transport patients. *Air Med J.* 1997;16:77–80.
25. Clemmer TP, Thomas F. Transport of the critically ill. *Crit Care Med.* 2000;28:265–266.
26. Varon J, Fromm RE Jr, Marik P. Hearts in the air: the role of aeromedical transport. *Chest.* 2003;124:1636–1637.
27. Davis DP, Peay J, Serrano JA, et al. The impact of aeromedical response to patients with moderate to severe traumatic brain injury. *Ann Emerg Med.* 2005;46:115–122.
28. Diaz MA, Hendey GW, Winters RC. How far is that by air? The derivation of an air: ground coefficient. *J Emerg Med.* 2003;24:199–202.
29. Takala J, Kurola J. Initial evaluation of eastern Finland rescue helicopter benefit. *Int Care Med.* 1999;25:S112.
30. Arfken CL, Shapiro MJ, Bessey PQ, et al. Effectiveness of helicopter versus ground ambulance services for interfacility transport. *J Trauma.* 1998;45:785–790.

CHAPTER 16 ■ INVASIVE PRESSURE MONITORING: GENERAL PRINCIPLES

ELIZABETH LEE DAUGHERTY • DAVID SHADE • HENRY E. FESSLER

The sophistication of bedside intensive care unit (ICU) monitoring equipment and the precision of its displayed values may tempt clinicians to accept these data without question. However, critically ill patients place substantial demands on these measurement technologies. Although the technology is governed by rigorous industry standards, it is not foolproof. To ensure accuracy and recognize and correct sources of error, the practicing intensivist must be aware of key technical aspects of pressure transduction.

This chapter reviews the basic principles of vascular pressure measurement, including principles of wave transmission, transduction, signal processing, and recording. Clinical aspects of measuring vascular pressure, such as its indications and interpretation of findings, are covered in other chapters. The goal of this chapter is to equip the practicing clinician to select the appropriate measurement tool, optimize its performance, and recognize and correct its shortcomings.

WAVE TRANSMISSION

The technical demands for recording an accurate systemic or pulmonary arterial pressure are much more stringent than for venous pressures. In order to discern fine details within a venous pressure, such as the a and v waves, high fidelity is needed, but even a simple water manometer can measure a central venous pressure. Therefore, this chapter will focus on the measurement of arterial pressure.

Cardiac contraction generates a pressure wave that travels at wave speed, much faster than the propulsion of the stroke volume through the arteries. This pressure wave must travel down the arterial tree and through a catheter, stopcocks, tubing, and a flush device, until finally terminating at the transducer. The pressure wave signal is invariably altered along the way. Modifications that are due to vascular characteristics often convey important biologic information. However, other modifications may be introduced by the external connecting tubing, catheters, and stopcocks. These changes can obscure important findings or mislead the clinician. These external connections are usually the weakest link between the patient and the bedside monitor, and every effort should be made to minimize the degradation of the signal occurring between the blood vessel and the transducer. Some familiarity with the vocabulary and physics of wave transmission is necessary to discuss how this goal can be achieved.

Natural Frequency

A pressure wave travels down the conducting tubing and deflects the transducer diaphragm, which rebounds and generates a reflected wave. When this reflected wave reaches the tip of the catheter, another reflected wave travels back toward the transducer. The oscillatory behavior of this system is determined by certain physical properties of its components (1–4). The *natural frequency* (f_n) of a system is the frequency at which a signal, such as a change in pressure, will oscillate in a uniform, frictionless tube. This frequency is measured in hertz (Hz), cycles per second. As will be seen, a higher f_n is desirable in a high-fidelity measuring device. Natural frequency decreases with increasing tube length, since at any given wave speed, a round trip in a longer tube simply takes more time. Natural frequency increases with wave speed, which in turn increases with tube radius and tube wall stiffness and decreases with the density of the conducting medium (5). Thus, short, wide, rigid tubing; a stiff transducer; and dense conducting media (e.g., saline rather than air) yield a higher f_n.

Damping

Pressure waves would reverberate forever in the absence of friction. However, friction is present in the pressure monitoring system due the movement of the waves in the conducting tubing. Although there is no net flow in the system, minute amounts of the medium shift to and fro during wave transfer. The friction generated by the movement of the conducting medium decreases the amplitude of the reflected wave, or *damps* it. Stiffer transducer diaphragms and stiffer conducting tubing will result in less damping since smaller volumes are required to displace them. Damping is also influenced by the mass of the conducting medium since wave transmission requires acceleration and deceleration of that medium. Finally, tubing resistance, which impedes the minute amount of reciprocative flow needed for pressure wave transmission, causes dissipation of energy from the pressure wave and increases damping. The damping coefficient, zeta (ζ), is therefore calculated from the determinants of mass of the system, the tubing's length and radius, the density of the conducting medium, and the resistance of the system as calculated from Poiseuille's Law:

$$\zeta = \frac{4\mu}{r^3}\sqrt{\frac{\rho L}{\pi E}} \qquad [1]$$

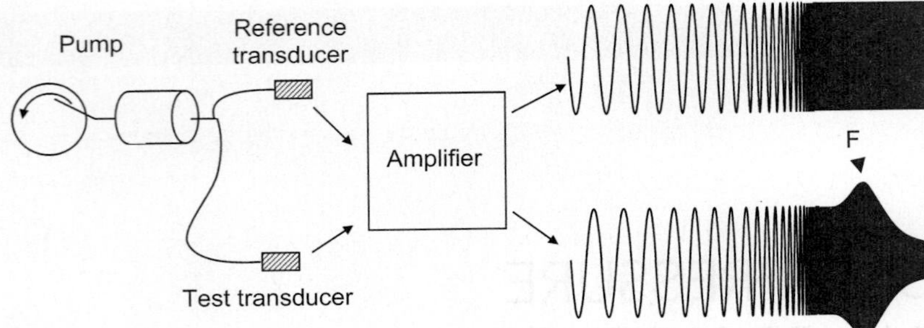

FIGURE 16.1. A device for bench testing the frequency response of pressure transducers and tubing. A pump generates a sinusoidal pressure through a range of frequencies. These are applied simultaneously to a high-fidelity reference transducer and the test transducer–tubing system. The output from the test transducer increases to a maximal amplitude at its natural frequency, designated *F*.

where E = stiffness coefficient of the transducer and tubing ($\Delta P/\Delta V$), ρ = density of conducting fluid, μ = viscosity of conducting fluid, r = tube radius, and L = tube length. Note that both natural frequency, f_n, and damping, ζ, are influenced by some of the same factors, but in opposite directions.

Since friction and inertia cannot be eliminated in real systems, one cannot measure the undamped f_n of a pressure wave but instead measures the wave's damped natural frequency, f_d. The f_d and ζ define the performance capacity of a catheter–tubing–transducer system, which must be adequate to accommodate the signal it is transducing, the pulse.

The complex pulse wave is composed of a group of simple sine waves of varied amplitude and frequency. The highest-amplitude sine wave component of the pulse wave has a frequency equal to the heart rate. The pulse wave is reproduced by summing this component and a series of *harmonics*, each with a smaller amplitude and a frequency that is some multiple of the primary frequency (second harmonic = 2 × primary frequency, etc.). Combining the first six to ten harmonics results in a close representation of the actual pulse contour. Thus, a recording system must be able to capture a frequency at least six to ten times the pulse rate with good fidelity to be able to faithfully record an arterial pressure tracing.

When the frequency of the harmonics that contribute meaningfully to the contour of the pulse wave approach the f_d of the recording system, considerable errors can occur. This effect is analogous to pushing a pendulum at its f_d, where a small, well-timed repetitive push can cause a large amplitude oscillation. The effect of this phenomenon in a transducer system can be demonstrated using a test system like that illustrated in Figure 16.1. A pressure wave of a given amplitude is generated and simultaneously recorded by a high-fidelity reference transducer and by the tubing–transducer system being tested. As the range of pressure wave frequencies is varied, one can observe and compare the output recorded by both devices. The amplitude of the test transducer peaks at its damped natural frequency, when the input wave frequency is perfectly in phase with the reflected wave oscillating in the transducer system. Because adequate measurement demands that f_d exceed the pulse rate by six to ten times, to appropriately record pressure in a patient with a pulse of 120 (2 Hz; Hz = heart rate/60), f_d should exceed 12 to 20 Hz. Transducer–tubing systems commonly found in clinical use often meet this criterion by only a narrow margin (6).

In the same way that a pendulum pushed at its f_n in the absence of friction would spin continuously around its axis, a completely undamped transducer stimulated at its f_n would record a pressure of infinite amplitude. The relationship between the amplitudes of output and input signals is expressed in the *amplitude ratio*. When the amplitude ratio equals one, the transducer is reproducing the wave exactly. When it is greater than one, the transducer is amplifying the wave, and when it is less than one, the wave is being damped. Standard engineering equations can be used to calculate the amplitude ratio and the effects of different degrees of damping at varying frequencies, as is illustrated in Figure 16.2. In this figure, frequency ratios represent the relationship between the input frequency and the damped natural frequency of the system. When the frequency ratio equals one, the input wave is at exactly the transducer's natural frequency. In a system with little damping

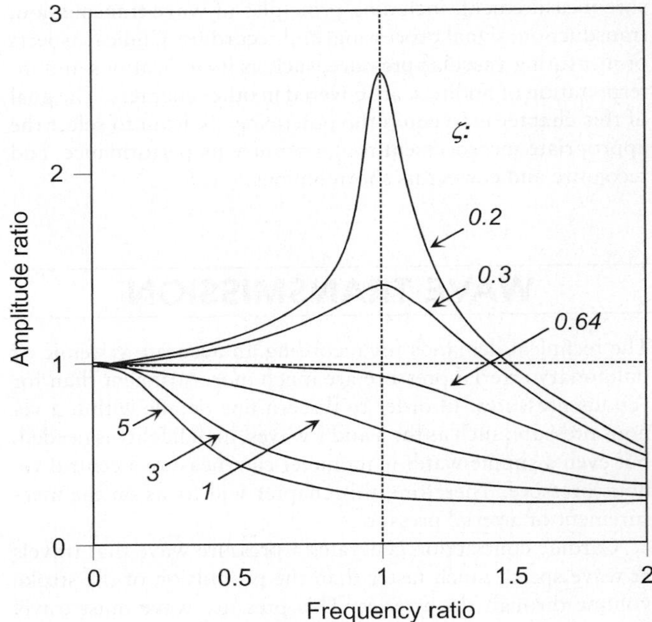

FIGURE 16.2. Effects of damping on transducer output. The frequency ratio is the ratio between the frequency at which the transducer is being stimulated and its natural frequency. The amplitude ratio is the ratio between the amplitudes of input to output signals. Different degrees of damping, zeta (ζ), are shown. With little damping, the output greatly amplifies the input over a wide range of frequencies and reaches maximum at the natural frequency. With extensive damping, the output amplitude falls at relatively low frequencies. At ζ of approximately 0.64, damping is critical (i.e., this is the lowest ζ where the amplitude ratio never exceeds one). However, this damping does not yield the broadest usable bandwidth. If one considers an amplitude ratio from 0.85 to 1.15 as reasonably accurate, then a ζ of 0.4 to 0.5 provides a greater bandwidth. This would mean that harmonics near the natural frequency would be amplified by up to 15%, and above the natural frequency they would be attenuated. However, if the natural frequency is high enough relative to the wave being studied, this will still yield acceptable accuracy.

(low values of ζ), one sees a significant rise in the amplitude ratio when input frequencies approach f_d. When a system is "overdamped," the recorded system output drops significantly below the true amplitude at frequencies that are well below the natural frequency. *Critical damping* is the least amount of damping resulting in an amplitude ratio no greater than one and an output signal that is never amplified (7).

When choosing the ideal damping for a clinical transducer system, one targets the level of damping that extends the usable frequency range or band width to the greatest degree. The most useful damping for a clinical transducer system is less than critical damping, or slight underdamping. Although the amplitude ratio is slightly greater than one near f_d (6,8), the amplification of the highest-frequency harmonics of a pulse wave does not generally result in clinically important errors.

There is an important relationship between the f_d and ζ necessary to accurately record a vascular pressure. If the f_d is well above six to ten times the pulse, the system can accurately reproduce that wave over a wide range of zetas. High harmonics that will be distorted are of such minute amplitude that their amplification or attenuation will not distort the reproduced wave. Conversely, when f_d approaches important frequencies in the pulse wave, the values of ζ that allow for high fidelity recording are more limited. Gardner evaluated this relationship in a variety of commercially available transducers and found many of those systems to be barely adequate for pressure measurements in those critically ill patients with tachycardia and a hyperdynamic heart (6). Further, pulmonary artery waveforms have more high-frequency components than do systemic arterial waveforms. For this reason, careful selection of f_d and ζ are especially important in systems intended to measure pulmonary pressures, where any small errors may be clinically significant.

Standardized industry guidelines (9) ensure that the transducers themselves are appropriate for ICU use. Either the transducer's f_d or its usable bandwidth will be listed in the technical specifications. Bandwidths are generally described in terms of Hz either as "flat to X Hz," or "+/– 15% to X Hz," indicating little distortion in the amplitude ratio up to the designated frequency. Guidelines require a frequency response range up to 200 Hz for typical external strain gage pressure transducers (9), and catheter tip micro transducers may have a useable bandwidth up to 20,000 Hz (10,11).

TRANSDUCTION

Transducer Properties

For our purposes, transduction is the conversion of a pressure signal to an electrical one. Accurate conversion of signals requires several key system characteristics, including stability, linearity, adequate frequency response, lack of hysteresis, and freedom from noise.

Stability implies that the characteristics of the system remain constant over time. Both a system's gain and its baseline may be influenced by instability, or drift, resulting in errors. Baseline refers to the electrical signal corresponding to atmospheric pressure, and gain is the relationship between a change in pressure and a change in electrical signal. If the baseline of a system drifts from a pressure of zero to 10 mm Hg, the application of 100 mm Hg would be recorded as 110. In this case the applied pressure is measured accurately, but the starting point requires correction. If the gain has drifted, the starting point is correct, with a zero reading being equal to atmospheric pressure, but application of 100 mm Hg would result in an incorrect electrical signal measuring 110 mm Hg. A change in baseline is more easily detected and corrected, by rezeroing the transducer, than is instability in gain.

Linearity indicates that electrical output remains linearly proportional to input throughout the range of measurement. Linear signals can be calibrated with few data points and linear amplifiers for such signals are relatively easy to design. With computer-based signal processing, linearity has become less important. Although most unprocessed output of pressure transducers is nonlinear, this problem may be corrected either through electronic processing or by setting the limits of a transducer's useable range to include only its most linear portion.

Frequency response describes a system's outputs in response to input signals of varying frequencies, usually in terms of *amplitude distortion* and *phase distortion*. Amplitude distortion refers to a change in the output ratio at different frequencies, as previously described. *Phase distortion* refers to the phase shift between input and output pressure waves that results from time lag. For example, the pulse displayed on the bedside display lags behind cardiac contraction by the momentary time it took for the pulse to travel down the arterial tree and external tubing. A constant phase shift is not problematic, as long as correction is made for this phenomenon when attempting to precisely synchronize events such as the electrocardiogram (ECG) and pulse. However, phase shift can be a significant problem in systems that cause different degrees of shift for inputs of varying frequency. Such a system would allow a different, frequency-dependent phase shift for the various components of a complex biologic wave and would produce a slurred output waveform.

Transducers should be free of *hysteresis*, in which the output signal varies with the system's recent history. That is, as it passes through the same pressure, a system with hysteresis will indicate a different value on the way down than on the way up. This characteristic would distort instantaneous recording of pulsatile signals.

Finally, a transducer should also introduce minimal *noise*. Both mechanical and electrical noise may influence vascular pressure measurement. Interference from patient movement, mechanical ventilation, fluorescent lighting, and nearby electronics should be minimized as much as possible.

Transducer Design

Several authors have reviewed the theory of transducer design (1,2,4,12,13). Manufacturers have utilized varying ways to address the four elements of transducer design we have discussed above. The most commonly used design is known as a Wheatstone bridge. This design uses four strain sensors whose resistance changes when they are stretched or compressed. The bridge is designed such that all resistances are equal when no strain is applied to the transducer. When pressure is applied, two of the resistors are stretched and the others are compressed. The measured pressure is determined from the resulting imbalance of resistance between the pairs of resistors.

The strain sensors of most clinical transducers are etched from silicon. With this technology, transducers can be inexpensive enough to make them appropriate for single use. This decreases processing costs and also limits their potential role in nosocomial infection. The transducers are durable and small, require minimal power and simple electronics, and are manufactured with a degree of uniformity that eliminates the need for tedious manual calibration of each transducer (14). Silicon's substantial changes in resistance with minimal changes in length give these strain gauges a high degree of sensitivity (15). This small requirement for volume displacement optimizes f_d and ζ. The Association for the Advancement of Medical Instrumentation and the American National Standards Institute have published manufacturing standards that dictate accuracy and safety characteristics for clinical transducers (9).

THE TUBING SYSTEM

Tubing

Although the fidelity of recorded pressures cannot exceed the capabilities of the transducer, performance is usually degraded below that optimal potential by other components between the transducer and the patient. Therefore, the most accurate waves can be recorded from micro-transducer–tipped catheters that are inserted directly in a blood vessel. For external transducers, every element added between the blood vessel and the transducer is a potential problem. The problems are minimized by designs that reduce ζ or increase f_d. Because damping is proportional to resistance, smaller intravascular catheters (16), clot, or kinking of the catheter will increase damping. Because the mass of fluid in the catheter also increases damping, catheter and tubing length should be minimized. Longer tubing systems have decreased f_d and reduce the usable bandwidth. Thus, if very long connecting tubes are used between the patient and transducer, more errors are likely than if the transducer is in close proximity to the blood vessel (17). Wave speed increases in stiffer tubes, so compliant tubing will also decrease f_d (12,16,18). Because air is compressible, bubbles increase the compliance of the system, both increasing damping and decreasing f_d. As an extreme illustration of this phenomenon, removing microscopic air bubbles by boiling the liquid used to fill the connecting tubing can double the f_d of a transducer system (8). Warmer room temperature can also alter f_d by softening tubing and expanding air bubbles (19).

Flush Systems

In the flush device, resistance reduces high pressure in the flush bag to <1 mm Hg at the transducer, while maintaining a continuous flow of solution to prevent clots (20,21). Depressing a lever or plunger bypasses the resistance, exposes the transducer to a square wave of pressure, and generates rapid flow into the patient. This can displace small clots or, as will be seen, can be used to test the intact recording system. Drip chambers should not be used in the tubing from the flush bag, or should be purged of air prior to use to eliminate risk of air embolization from turbulence during rapid flushes (21,22). Air dissolved under pressure in the flush bag can also form bubbles when decompressed in the tubing downstream from the flush device (19). These gradually collect and coalesce at stopcocks or connections and can impair the fidelity of recorded waveforms.

SIGNAL PROCESSING

Electronic Filtration

Transducer output may be electronically filtered to minimize noise, electrical interference, respiratory artifact, and other sources of error. Filtering can be applied either to the raw electrical signal with electronic circuits or after digital conversion with computer algorithms. Forms of filtration include low-pass filters, which attenuate high-frequency components; high-pass filters, which attenuate low-frequency components; and band-pass filters, which allow a frequency range to pass unaltered and attenuate frequencies surrounding the band. Filters can vary in their cutoff frequencies, their extent of attenuation, and the sharpness of the transition from passage to blockage.

By first separating a pulse wave into systolic and diastolic portions, different filters may be applied to the regions to suit each component's anticipated characteristics. Although the manufacturer specifies a default set of filters, the clinician may select other options based on observation of the waveform. If the catheter–tubing–transducer combination has f_d that is sufficient for the measured waveform, a low-pass filter with a cutoff frequency just below f_d will attenuate excessive high-frequency noise without distorting the true waveform. Such selective filtering, like appropriate mechanical damping, extends the usable bandwidth.

Analog-to-digital Conversion

Electrical transducer output is transmitted to a digital computer for further processing, analysis, recording, and display. Digital processors are binary devices, meaning they only recognize the absence or presence of a voltage level, as designated by a 0 or 1. The total number available to a binary device is equal to 2^n, where n is the number of digit positions. Each digit position is referred to as a "bit." Thus, an eight-bit quantity, a byte, can assume 256 different values ($2^8 = 256$).

To process an electrical signal, a computer must convert the voltage to a number, analog-to-digital (A/D) conversion. The analog input voltage may assume any of the infinite continuous values within its range, such as 0 to 5 volts. The digital output, however, must be a discrete number whose possible output values are finite and depend on the A/D converter resolution. A/D converter resolution is specified in bits. Thus, an 8-bit A/D converter's output must assume 1 of just 256 possible values, while the output of a 12-bit converter may assume any 1 of 4,096 values ($2^{12} = 4{,}096$).

The input voltage is linearly mapped to the output numbers. An 8-bit A/D converter with an input of 0 volts will therefore have an output of 0, 2.5 volts will convert to an output of 128, and 5 volts an output of 256. Each different value of the A/D converter's output represents a range of (5.00/256) or 19.5 millivolts. Any voltage falling within a range of 19.5 millivolts is rounded up or down to the nearest digital output value. If the full-range input voltage is calibrated to represent 0 mm Hg to 300 mm Hg (so that 0 volts = 0 mm Hg and 5 volts = 300 mm Hg), then the finest resolution of the A/D converter is 1.2 mm Hg. This resolution can be increased by increasing the bits in the output. A 12-bit A/D converter with a 0- to 300-mm Hg pressure transducer has a resolution of 0.07 mm Hg

($2^{12} = 4{,}096$; $300/4{,}096 = 0.073$). The A/D resolution sets the resolution limit for the displayed waveform and any derived pressures calculated after conversion. However, even an eight-bit converter should be adequate for most clinical decisions.

The digitization process is also influenced by the *sampling rate*. The continuous analog transducer voltage output is sampled as a series of "snapshots," reducing the digital output signal to a series of points. The points are constrained in the *y* plane, pressure, by the A/D resolution. They are also constrained in the *x* plane, time, by the sampling rate. If one represented a circle using increasing numbers of dots, three equidistant dots would look like a triangle; four like a square; five like a pentagon. As more dots are added, the representation will look increasingly circular. Analogously, a sufficient sampling rate of an input waveform is essential to adequately represent the wave in digital form. Representation of a sine wave of frequency *f* requires sampling at a frequency of 2**f*, known as the Nyquist sampling rate. Complex waveforms like the pulse must be sampled at a frequency at least twice that of the highest-frequency component of interest. For a pulmonary arterial pressure input whose highest significant frequency components can reach 20 Hz, an A/D converter must sample at a minimum of 40 Hz. After sampling, curve-fitting algorithms are also applied to reduce the potentially jagged appearance of a wave on the bedside display.

Digital Display

The pressure waveform is processed further to display parameters such as systolic pressure, mean pressure, or pulmonary artery occlusion pressure as numerical values. This software has substantially evolved and improved. Early digital displays simply used the highest and lowest pressures within a certain time window as systolic and diastolic. They displayed values that fluctuated erratically with minor patient or transducer movement. Later electronics timed the calculation of systolic and diastolic values to the ECG. This change reduced sensitivity to random artifact, but still captured substantial beat-to-beat variation. Low-pass filtering of the analog signal was added to obtain mean pressure. Alternatively, the digitized values within a time window including several complete heart beats may be averaged (a moving average). The window duration and filtration frequency represent a compromise between rapid response to sudden changes and stability of the displayed values. Short windows produce more variability and more false monitor alarms, while long windows may delay the recognition of important changes. More complicated algorithms can be used to select the peak systolic and nadir diastolic values and display their moving averages.

Simple averages or ECG-gated values, however, do not anticipate known sources of error. Vascular pressures change physiologically with the respiratory cycle. Vascular pressure measurements recorded within the thorax, such as pulmonary artery pressure, vary due to the changes in pleural pressure and respiration-induced changes in vascular filling. In vessels with low pressures, and particularly when pleural pressure changes are exaggerated due to disease or effort, the respiratory variation may confound clinical decisions. As a reflection of the state of cardiac filling, one is generally interested in the *transmural* pressure of intrathoracic vessels. However, the pressure on their surface is usually unmeasurable. Therefore, by convention, these vascular pressures are measured at end-expiration. Barring significant recruitment of expiratory muscles, pressure on the surface of vessels within the thorax is likely to be close to atmospheric pressure at end-expiration. For systemic arterial pressures, this rationale is less compelling. Mean arterial pressure, integrating pressures through the respiratory cycle, represents the average pressure driving arterial flow. Nevertheless, systolic and diastolic arterial pressures are also conventionally recorded at end-expiration.

More advanced processing algorithms attempt to display digital values timed to end-expiration. Simply searching for the highest or lowest value within a time window (e.g., highest systolic value) is insufficient, because the phase difference between the respiratory cycle and the associated changes in vascular pressure differs when the patient is on positive pressure ventilation or breathing spontaneously. That is, pleural pressure falls during spontaneous ventilation, rises during positive pressure ventilation, and changes biphasically during assisted ventilation. The highest systolic value will occur at end-expiration in the spontaneously breathing patient but not in patients on other modes.

Therefore, more complicated logic is necessary. The waveform is divided into individual beats, and separate filters are applied to systolic and diastolic phases and the mean pressure to reduce artifact. Systolic, diastolic, and mean pressures are calculated individually for each cardiac cycle. A *weighted* moving average is then computed, in which each heartbeat contributes to the average in inverse proportion to its variance from the previous average. For example, a systolic pressure from a heartbeat that is close to the average systolic pressure is weighted more heavily than one that is far from the previous average. This yields approximately end-expiratory values as follows: Inspiration is generally more rapid and of shorter duration than expiration. Therefore, vascular pressures under the influence of pleural pressure will change rapidly during inspiration, and slowly during late expiration. The algorithm weights the calculated pressure toward the slowly changing, end-expiratory values. Note, however, that this logic will fail with patients receiving inverse ratio ventilation and patients with both rapid respiratory rates and slow heart rates. For the measurement of pressures where accuracy is critical (such as the pulmonary artery wedge pressure), one should not rely on the displayed numerical pressure. End-expiration must be determined by inspecting the patient, and the simultaneous pressure measured directly from the waveform. An electronic cursor, placed manually or automatically and inspected for proper positioning, should be used to ensure end-expiratory values.

TROUBLESHOOTING

Simplicity and uniformity in transducer and catheter setup is key to minimizing opportunity for errors. Tubing should be stiff tubing designed for pressure monitoring, used with a minimum length and few stopcocks and connectors.

Zeroing

A common source of error is the zero reference level for pressure measurement. All pressures are measured relative to the horizontal plane at which the transducer is set to zero. When the transducer is connected to a fluid-filled catheter, any hydrostatic pressure imposed by the catheter will be sensed by the transducer. The recorded pressure will rise as the transducer is lowered, and vice versa. This continues to occur when the catheter is attached to a patient.

Most agree that vascular pressure should be referenced to the level of the heart; that is, the recording system should read zero pressure when the open end of a transduced fluid-filled tube is held at the horizontal plane of the heart. The optimal external anatomic landmark representing this plane remains a subject of debate. Many suggest the midaxillary line (23,24), but others have recommended estimation of the uppermost boundary of the heart (25). For simplicity and uniformity, the midaxillary line is best for general use. More complicated systems invite errors in practice, even if their perfect application could theoretically improve accuracy.

This anatomic reference level should be on the same horizontal plane, not of the transducer diaphragm, but of the port or stopcock that is opened to atmospheric pressure when the electronics are zeroed. The transducer itself could be in any convenient location. The amplifier will add or subtract the hydrostatic pressure of the fluid between the zero point and transducer. After zeroing, however, the height of the transducer relative to the zero level must remain fixed. For this reason, the zero reference level should be dictated by a unitwide policy, and proper zero positioning should be confirmed prior to recording vascular pressure. If the transducer height moves, the zero reference level will change, resulting in erroneous readings. A parallel change in all the vascular pressures measured with the same transducer (e.g., central venous, pulmonary arterial, and wedge pressures), in a clinically stable patient, suggests a change in transducer level.

One simple way to provide consistency is to secure the transducer to the patient's arm near the heart and zero it using the port molded into the transducer body. This will allow fewer errors than attaching the transducer to an IV pole, in which case elevating the bed or sitting the patient up will change his or her horizontal relationship to the zero point. However, rezeroing to the cardiac level will be needed when patient orientation is changed (such as lateral decubitus or prone positions). Care must also be taken that the transducer has not rotated to a dependent position on the arm, or slipped to the elbow in a patient who is anything but completely flat.

Calibration

Modern disposable transducers are generally accurate to ±3% (26) and do not require calibration. Transducer accuracy can be compromised by mechanical trauma, overpressurization during assembly, or fluid entry on the ambient pressure side of the transducer diaphragm. Accuracy of a clinical transducer can be verified by calibration against a mercury manometer. For older, expensive, reusable transducers, this step was essential, since the gain had to be adjusted for each transducer. Most contemporary bedside monitors do not even allow gain adjustment, and an inaccurate transducer is best simply replaced.

Testing the Frequency Response

Intensive care units, operating rooms, and other monitoring settings combine various components from various manufacturers into their systems for vascular pressure measurement. The parts may vary between units or perhaps even from patient to patient or nurse to nurse, and will change as suppliers change over time. The performance specifications of individual components such as transducers and amplifiers are provided in their user manuals, but the performance of the integrated system is usually untested.

Fortunately, the catheter–tubing–transducer system allows simple bedside study. By using the flush device, one can apply a near square-wave pressure signal, and the features of the recorded output can be examined. When the flush device resistor is bypassed, a high-pressure signal is produced, which goes off-scale on the bedside monitor. When the lever is released, however, a square-wave low-pressure signal is generated, which falls within the range of the display. Proper functioning is indicated when this signal rapidly reverberates a few times and then decays back to the underlying vascular pressure.

If one records the effects of such a fast flush, those results may also be assessed quantitatively. The time between peaks of the oscillating signal is the roundtrip travel time of the pressure wave to the catheter tip and back. It is equal to $1/f_d$. The decrease in amplitude of consecutive oscillations is from damping. ζ can be calculated from the amplitude ratio of consecutive oscillations A_1 and A_2 (1,6):

$$\zeta = -\ln \frac{\left(\frac{A_2}{A_1}\right)}{\sqrt{\pi^2 + \left[\ln\left(\frac{A_2}{A_1}\right)\right]^2}} \qquad [2]$$

Using this equation, clinical engineers can evaluate their hospital's complete catheter–transducer subsystem. A related bench technique uses a "pop test," in which a balloon attached to a transducer and catheter system is popped with a needle to produce the square wave of pressure. The Association for the Advancement of Medical Instrumentation publishes a comprehensive manual to guide the evaluation of pressure transducer systems by clinical engineering departments (19).

Overdamping Errors

Overdamping is a common problem that causes errors in the measurement of systolic and diastolic pressure. Overdamping is suggested during a bedside flush test by a gradual pressure decay or an undershoot and slow return to baseline without any oscillation (27). The effect of overdamping on the waveform is to first cause the wave to lose details such as the dicrotic notch and a brisk systolic upstroke, or the a, v, and c waves of a venous pressure. With more damping, the wave will appear sinusoidal, systolic pressure will fall, and diastolic pressure rise toward the mean arterial pressure. Even with extreme overdamping, the mean pressure remains accurate.

Numerous problems in the catheter–tubing–transducer subsystem can cause overdamping. These include air bubbles, blood clots or fibrin within the catheter or tubing, catheter tips abutting a vessel wall, or kinks or partially closed stopcocks. Flushing or changing the tubing and obsessively purging air bubbles solves many overdamping problems. If the damped waveform is associated with kinking or thrombosis of the catheter, poor blood return, or sensitivity to minor catheter movement, it may need replacement.

Underdamping Errors

In tachycardic, hyperdynamic patients, excessive oscillation may be apparent in the pulse recording, especially at peak systole. This problem occurs when important harmonics of the pulse approach the transducer system's f_d. Underdamping causes systolic and diastolic pressure to be over- and underestimated, respectively. The excessive oscillations will also interfere with the algorithms used to calculate a digital display of systolic and diastolic pressure. Even manual estimation of these pressures from the bedside oscilloscope or printed record is inaccurate, since the pulse pressure is exaggerated.

The characteristics of the transducer system can be studied and optimized to reduce underdamping errors. During observation of a fast flush, oscillations that are widely spaced indicate a low f_d, which may poorly suit a patient whose pulse is dynamic with upper harmonics of high amplitude. Natural frequency is reduced by lengthy or compliant tubing or by bubbles. Removing unneeded tubing extensions and diligently clearing bubbles will bring the flush test oscillations closer together, and the waveform will show more detail with greater accuracy.

The reverberations in the pulse can be smoothed away by injecting a tiny bubble of air into the transducer or catheter. However, this practice is not recommended. While the air bubble will increase the damping, it also decreases f_d. The waveform will be made to appear more normal, but may be no more accurate. If larger bubbles are introduced, the excessive damping causes the pulse pressure to narrow toward the mean arterial pressure. The effects of adding a bubble of increasing size on a flush test and arterial pressure tracing is shown in Figure 16.3. Note that a small bubble (middle panel) yields a wave that looks appropriate, but the widely spaced oscillations after the fast flush indicate the reduced f_d.

One would like to increase the damping of the system without decreasing its natural frequency. This effect can be achieved by reducing the amplifier high-pass filtration frequency just enough to eliminate the reverberations, as is outlined in most monitoring equipment user's manuals. Too much electronic damping will degrade the waveform just as would excess mechanical damping. Filtering should generally not be reduced below 12 Hz to avoid removing the higher-order harmonics contributing to the systolic waveform. There are also mechanical devices that attach to a stopcock near the transducer and increase damping. These devices are designed to match the transducer impedance to that of the tubing, decreasing wave reflections without altering f_d (6,12).

Artifact that appears similar to underdamping can also occur when long, flexible catheters are vibrated by high-velocity blood flow, termed "catheter whip." This phenomenon should be suspected when long intravascular catheters are used in high-flow vessels of much larger diameter, such as long femoral or pulmonary artery catheters. Contributions of underdamping to the waveform appearance can be ruled out by inspecting the fast flush and optimizing the external tubing system. Artifact due to movement of the catheter tip is difficult to eliminate. In the pulmonary artery, stabilizing the catheter tip by inflating the balloon to measure a pulmonary artery occlusion pressure will remove the "whip." Measurement of mean pressures will also remain accurate.

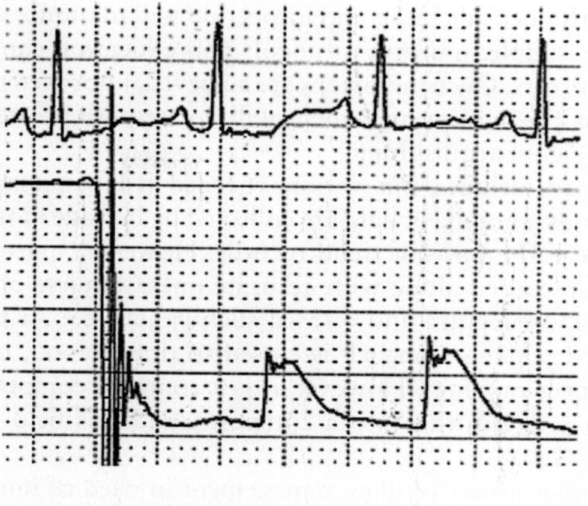

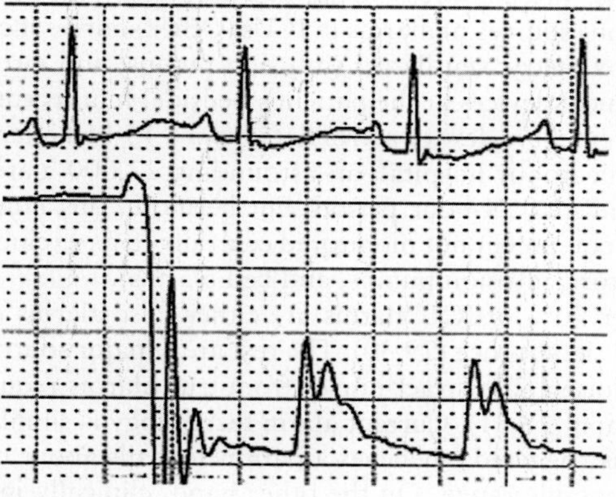

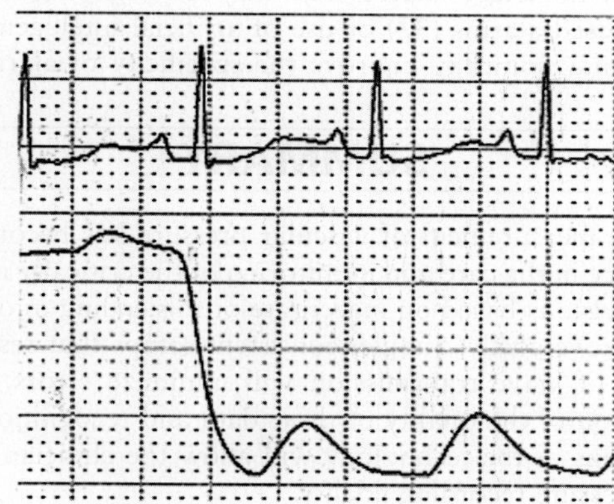

FIGURE 16.3. Effects of adding a bubble of increasing size to a transducer–catheter system recording an arterial pressure waveform and recording of a "fast flush." The upper panel shows the waveform with no bubble. The flush oscillates rapidly, and the pulse shows a brisk hyperdynamic upstroke and slight overshoot. In the middle panel, a small (<0.1 mL) bubble decreases the natural frequency of the system. This is shown by the wider spacing of the oscillations following the fast flush, and increases the peak systolic overshoot. The bottom panel shows the effects of a slightly larger bubble. The return from the flush is now delayed and does not oscillate, and the pulse waveform is lacking in detail with a reduced amplitude.

FUTURE DIRECTIONS

Fifty years of engineering refinement have produced transducers that are many times more accurate than needed for most clinical decisions in critical care medicine. Basic knowledge of the physics of wave transmission and transduction and thoughtful bedside setup and inspection will minimize artifact. Further, simple, uniform protocols and education can reduce human errors. Once there steps are achieved, improved invasive vascular pressure measurement will not require greater accuracy in signal acquisition.

Instead, technical innovation is needed in data management. Enormous amounts of data are collected by bedside monitoring systems in the form of trend records. However, spurious values are recorded along with accurate ones. A nurse or doctor can easily recognize and discard such values (e.g., a pressure recorded while a stopcock is closed to draw blood, or while a patient is moving). However, it is a complex computational task to program this into a computer, and this field is in its infancy (28).

Another aspect of data management in need of innovation is alarms. Vascular pressure monitoring systems are only one of numerous sources of alarms in ICUs. Other sources include the ECG, oximetry, ventilators, infusion pumps, and virtually all mechanical devices at the patient's bedside. In a recent quality improvement review of alarm data from a 15-bed intermediate care unit in our hospital, an astounding 27,000 alarms were recorded in a 24-hour period. Furthermore, this number excluded equipment not monitored centrally (e.g., excluded were ventilators, infusion pumps, and bed alarms).

Over 90% of ICU alarms are either false alarms or of no clinical significance (29,30). The rest are a major source of ambient noise and distract nurses from true alarms requiring intervention (28,31). Current alarm technology is simplistic. An alarm is triggered whenever a parameter falls above or below an acceptable range. On the other hand, clinically important trends do not trigger alarms until they fall outside of the range. Trend-based alarms (32) or use of artificial intelligence algorithms may someday improve the specificity of alarms (28).

SUMMARY

Invasive measurement of vascular pressure has become commonplace in the care and monitoring of the critically ill. However, decisions based on inaccurate or misleading information could prove costly. Simple, consistent setups that respect the physics of wave transmission will minimize errors. Critical evaluation of the quality of these data and recognition of the limitations of the technology will allow the clinician to optimize pressure recording fidelity.

PEARLS

- *Natural frequency* is the frequency at which a wave oscillates in a tubing system.
- *Damping* is the attenuation of a wave due to friction.
- Natural frequency and damping characteristics set the performance limits of a system of a transducer and all its attached tubing and connectors.
- The pulse is a complex waveform whose accurate recording requires a system with adequate natural frequency and damping.
- Clinical pressure recording systems are optimized with proper setup, flushing, and zeroing.
- Use of the fast-flush device on a pressure transducer can diagnose potential sources of error.

References

1. Fry DL. Physiologic recording by modern instruments with particular reference to pressure recording. *Physiol Rev.* 1960;40:753–788.
2. van der Tweel LH. Some physical aspects of blood pressure, pulse wave, and blood pressure measurements. *Am Heart J.* 1957;53(1):4–17.
3. Kleinman B. Understanding natural frequency and damping and how they relate to the measurement of blood pressure. *J Clin Monit.* 1989;5(2):137–147.
4. Hansen AT, Warburg E. The theory for elastic liquid-containing membrane manometers. *Acta Physiol Scand.* 1950;19:306–332.
5. Wilson TA, Hyatt RE, Rodarte JR. The mechanisms that limit expiratory flow. *Lung.* 1980;158(4):193–200.
6. Gardner RM. Direct blood pressure measurement–dynamic response requirements. *Anesthesiology.* 1981;54(3):227–236.
7. Fessler H, Shade D. Measurement of vascular pressure. In: Tobin MJ, ed. *Principles and Practice of Intensive Care Monitoring.* New York: McGraw-Hill; 1997:91–106.
8. Shapiro GG, Krovetz LJ. Damped and undamped frequency responses of underdamped catheter manometer systems. *Am Heart J.* 1970;80(2):226–236.
9. *Blood Pressure Transducers.* 2nd ed. Arlington, VA: Association for the Advancement of Medical Instrumentation; 1994.
10. Nichols WW, Walker WE. Experience with the Millar PC-350 catheter-tip pressure transducer. *Biomed Eng.* 1974;9(2):58–60.
11. Millar HD, Baker LE. A stable ultraminiature catheter-tip pressure transducer. *Med Biol Eng.* 1973;11(1):86–89.
12. Allan MW, Gray WM, Asbury AJ. Measurement of arterial pressure using catheter-transducer systems. Improvement using the Accudynamic. *Br J Anaesth.* 1988;60(4):413–418.
13. Geddes LA. *The Direct and Indirect Measurement of Blood Pressure.* Chicago: Year Book Medical Publishers; 1970.
14. Bailey RH, Bauer JH, Yanos J. Accuracy of disposable blood pressure transducers used in the critical care setting. *Crit Care Med.* 1995;23(1):187–192.
15. Geddes LA, Athens W, Aronson S. Measurement of the volume displacement of blood-pressure transducers. *Med Biol Eng Comput.* 1984;22(6):613–614.
16. Heimann PA, Murray WB. Construction and use of catheter-manometer systems. *J Clin Monit.* 1993;9(1):45–53.
17. Miller GS, Zbilut JP. Practical evaluation of catheter-transducer coupling systems for artifact. *Heart Lung.* 1983;12(2):156–161.
18. Hunziker P. Accuracy and dynamic response of disposable pressure transducer-tubing systems. *Can J Anaesth.* 1987;34(4):409–414.
19. *Evaluation of Clinical Systems for Invasive Blood Pressure Monitoring.* Arlington, VA: Association for the Advancement of Medical Instrumentation; 1992.
20. Gardner RM, Warner HR, Toronto AF, et al. Catheter-flush system for continuous monitoring of central arterial pulse waveform. *J Appl Physiol.* 1970;29(6):911–913.
21. Gardner RM, Bond EL, Clark JS. Safety and efficacy of continuous flush systems for arterial and pulmonary artery catheters. *Ann Thorac Surg.* 1977;23(6):534–538.
22. Soule DT, Powner DJ. Air entrapment in pressure monitoring lines. *Crit Care Med.* 1984;12(6):520–522.
23. Pedersen A, Husby J. Venous pressure measurement. I. Choice of zero level. *Acta Med Scand.* 1951;141(3):185–194.
24. Yang SS. *From Cardiac Catheterization Data to Hemodynamic Parameters.* 3rd ed. Philadelphia: Davis; 1988.
25. Courtois M, Fattal PG, Kovacs SJ Jr, et al. Anatomically and physiologically based reference level for measurement of intracardiac pressures. *Circulation.* 1995;92(7):1994–2000.
26. Gardner RM. Accuracy and reliability of disposable pressure transducers coupled with modern pressure monitors. *Crit Care Med.* 1996;24(5):879–882.
27. Morris AH, Chapman RH, Gardner RM. Frequency of technical problems encountered in the measurement of pulmonary artery wedge pressure. *Crit Care Med.* 1984;12(3):164–170.
28. Imhoff M, Kuhls S. Alarm algorithms in critical care monitoring. *Anesth Analg.* 2006;102(5):1525–1537.
29. Tsien CL, Fackler JC. Poor prognosis for existing monitors in the intensive care unit. *Crit Care Med.* 1997;25(4):614–619.
30. Chambrin MC, Ravaux P, Calvelo-Aros D, et al. Multicentric study of monitoring alarms in the adult intensive care unit (ICU): a descriptive analysis. *Intens Care Med.* 1999;25(12):1360–1366.
31. Edworthy J, Hellier E. Alarms and human behaviour: implications for medical alarms. *Br J Anaesth.* 2006;97(1):12–17.
32. Schoenberg R, Sands DZ, Safran C. Making ICU alarms meaningful: a comparison of traditional vs. trend-based algorithms. *Proc AMIA Symp.* 1999;379–383.

CHAPTER 17 ■ NONINVASIVE CARDIOVASCULAR MONITORING

WILLIAM C. SHOEMAKER • HOWARD BELZBERG • CHARLES C.J. WO • GEORGE HATZAKIS • DEMETRIOS DEMETRIADES

DEFINITION OF THE PROBLEM

Research in acute life-threatening emergencies has clearly shown that early recognition and vigorous therapy of shock facilitated by monitoring in acute life-threatening emergencies are the keys to successful resuscitation, because delayed therapy increases mortality and morbidity (1–8). Acute critical illness and shock from trauma, hemorrhage, high-risk surgery, sepsis, burns, stroke, and cardiac emergencies are circulatory problems that can be described by hemodynamic monitoring. There were significantly reduced mortality and morbidity in prospective randomized trials of optimal hemodynamic goals when they were achieved early, that is, <24 hours after emergency department (ED) admission and before onset of organ failure (1–4). However, outcome was not improved when optimal goals were accomplished late, defined as >24 hours after ED admission or after the onset of organ failure (3,4). The central focus of hemodynamic monitoring used is to provide appropriate therapy as determined by the adequacy of tissue perfusion and oxygenation. Recent experiences have demonstrated that early intervention is associated with improved outcome. Identification of the adequacy of perfusion is a function of balancing oxygen delivery with oxygen demand. Invasive monitoring requires time and technology, often leading to delays that reduce the potential benefit of the information gathered. In addition to the need for rapid monitoring, the challenge of continuous data collection and analysis as opposed to intermittent static observations is of major concern in the selection of monitoring techniques.

Pulmonary artery catheters (PACs) or Swan-Ganz catheters provide the maximum circulatory data at the bedside to describe the hemodynamic status in a wide variety of clinical states, emergencies, and other acute conditions (1–18). However, PACs require intensive care unit (ICU) environments, and by the time the patient gets an ICU bed, it is often too late for early therapy. Since circulatory diseases are the leading cause of acute death, it is appropriate to develop and test hemodynamic methods and concepts for early use in emergencies and acute illnesses.

The principal difference between noninvasive monitoring compared with invasive PAC monitoring with blood gases taken at intervals is that the former provides online, real-time visual displays of multiple hemodynamic patterns describing cardiac, pulmonary, and tissue perfusion functions and their interrelationships (5–7). By contrast, invasive monitoring is taken once or at intervals as a set of static values and is primarily used to describe departures from the normal range as well as thresholds for circulatory disorders. For example, cardiac index (CI) <2.0 L/minute/m^2, systolic blood pressure (SBP) <90 mm Hg, or mean arterial pressure (MAP) <70 mm Hg is used to define shock. However, noninvasive monitoring uniquely displays early hemodynamic patterns of acute illnesses that may underlie circulatory mechanisms (8–10). These patterns are not like static signposts, but are patterns of curves that may resemble biphasic or U waves. Stress responses may initially elevate CI, heart rate (HR), and MAP values, but initially high values are not sustained in the presence of hypovolemia, anemia, or impaired cardiac function and subsequently they rapidly fall to low levels along with arterial saturation of oxygen (SpO_2) and transcutaneous partial pressure of oxygen/fraction of inspired oxygen ($PtcO_2/FiO_2$) values (see below). These sequential hemodynamic patterns provide new descriptive dimensions to understand the process of acute circulatory problems and resuscitation. Moreover, noninvasive patterns with information systems can predict outcome and support therapeutic decision making (16–18).

Noninvasive hemodynamic monitoring was found to be safe for patients and staff, convenient, inexpensive, reasonably accurate, and available anywhere in the hospital, doctors' offices, or prehospital areas. Early recognition of abnormal hemodynamic or incipient shock patterns allows therapy to be given earlier, more vigorously, and with greater effectiveness (6–10). Timing of treatment is as essential as the therapy itself in achieving good outcome.

There are a variety of modalities that have been developed to provide for hemodynamic monitoring by invasive, minimally invasive, and noninvasive methods. Many of these methods are presented in detail elsewhere in this textbook, but are mentioned here to emphasize their interrelationships. These methods can be grouped by their basic technologies, including Doppler ultrasound techniques, transcutaneous/transmucosal sensors of gases, monitors of hemoglobin saturation, expired gases, and a variety of dilution techniques. Each of these methods has its own strengths and weaknesses; taken together they have the potential to create a robust multidimensional picture of patients' hemodynamic states and their responses to therapeutic interventions. When only one method is used, its limitations may obscure the real problem and limit clinical usefulness.

NONINVASIVE HEMODYNAMIC MONITORING

Conventional Vital Signs

Conventional vital signs include heart rate and mean arterial pressure; heart rate may be automatically derived from the electrocardiogram (ECG), and the systolic, diastolic, and mean arterial pressure measured directly or automated by DynaMAP (Tampa, FL), or from an indwelling arterial catheter if one is already in place.

Arterial Hemoglobin Oxygen Saturation by Pulse Oximeter

The standard pulse oximeter (Nellcor, Pleasanton, CA) is routinely used for continuous hemoglobin saturation (SpO_2) monitoring (16). Two different wavelengths of infrared light are reflected from the capillaries to identify and evaluate the oxygen saturation of the arterial component. Sudden changes in the arterial hemoglobin saturation are useful in assessing changes in pulmonary function. This has had a major impact on clinical practice both inside and outside the operating room. Unfortunately, arterial oxygen saturation by itself does not indicate the oxygen delivery (DO_2) or the oxygen consumption/demand (VO_2), and is not a reliable measure of tissue oxygenation/perfusion or the hemodynamic status.

Cardiac Output Monitoring by Thoracic Electric Bioimpedance

In thoracic electric bioimpedance (TEB) methods, pairs of noninvasive disposable prewired hydrogel electrodes consisting of an outer injecting electrode and an inner sensing electrode are positioned on the anterior thoracic skin surface at the levels of the lung apex and the base; ECG leads are also placed on the precordium and shoulders (6,7,11,19–32). The outer pairs of electrodes pass a small-amplitude (0.2–5.0 mA) alternating current at 40 to 100 kHz through the patient's thorax to produce an electrical field. The injected electrical signals travel predominantly down the aorta, which has lower electrical resistance than aerated lung. Each ventricular contraction propels the stroke volume down the aorta, increasing aortic blood volume and aortic flow and lowering impedance. The impedance is sensed by the inner recording electrodes that capture the baseline impedance (Zo), the first derivative of the impedance waveform (dZ/dt), and the ECG (6,7,19). Changes in aortic blood flow throughout the cardiac cycle are quantitatively related to changes in the electrical impedance.

We have routinely used two TEB devices, PhysioFlow (VasoCOM, Bristol, PA) and IQ 101 (Noninvasive Medical Technologies, Las Vegas, NV), which were applied to the patient as soon as possible after arrival into the ED (5–7,19). When clinically indicated, the PAC was inserted in the operating room (OR) or ICU and was used to validate the noninvasive TEB method. Both of these TEB instruments gave satisfactory results when compared with the cardiac output values measured by the thermodilution (COtd) method using PACs. In 907 simultaneous pairs of TEB and thermodilution measurements in 267 patients, r was 0.92, r^2 was 0.84, and p was <0.001 (11). The IQ 101 recently has been taken off the market for revisions and re-engineering.

In paired simultaneous TEB and COtd or other hemodynamic measurements, studies have reported satisfactory agreement between the methods (6,7,28–41). Raaijmakers et al. (25) found general agreement between several TEB systems reported over the past three decades, particularly in recent models using improved technology and algorithm. Simultaneous CI measurements by TEB and COtd during cardiac evaluation were satisfactorily correlated at rest ($r = 0.83$) and during exercise for cardiology workup ($r = 0.86$) (42,43). Reported errors between TEB systems and COtd were usually within twice the average difference in successive COtd estimations. We reported an average difference of 9.7% between TEB and COtd and an average difference of 9.5% between rapidly repeated COtd measurements in the same patient (6,7). Therefore, we routinely take four or five measurements and delete the most aberrant values. Some of the older systems such as the NCOM3 (BoMED, San Diego, CA) and its successor BioZ (CardioDynamics, San Diego, CA) had satisfactory correlations in many patients, but wide variations in about one fourth of patients, resulting in an overall average error of 25%.

Thoracic Electric Bioimpedance Applications

TEB cardiography was found to be helpful for diagnosis and therapy in the initial ED resuscitation since it is difficult clinically to detect early (occult) shock from BP and HR alone (13,23,24,33). In clinical trials, the diagnosis differed in 12 (13%) patients and the treatment changed in 35 (39%) patients after TEB results became available (33). Using TEB did not adversely affect defibrillation, resuscitation, or survival in patients during out-of-hospital cardiac arrest treated with biphasic waveform defibrillators (26). Ambulatory TEB provided useful values in both supine and tilt positions compared with Doppler cardiography (27). TEB has been used in the home, OR, ED, and ICU for thoracic fluid status monitoring after resuscitation from acute circulatory problems and for pacemaker optimization (6,7,28–41).

TEB provides a reasonably accurate, cost-effective, and noninvasive system that can replace PAC monitoring for various types of acute ED patients as well as for coronary care unit patients, those with pulmonary hypertension, intra- and postoperative coronary artery bypass, pediatric cardiac conditions (44,45), and diagnostic evaluation (46,47) and therapeutic responses (31–39). This technology may be used for healthy outpatient settings as well (46). For example, the effect of 1 unit of blood donation in 197 healthy volunteers demonstrated that stroke volume index values decreased from a baseline of 47.0 $\pm$ 6.9 (standard deviation [SD]) mL/m^2 to 43.9 $\pm$ 7.3 mL/m^2 after blood donation (32). Several groups reported that TEB was a feasible and accurate method for noninvasive monitoring of stroke index and cardiac index (44–47). Pianosi (44,45) measured exercise cardiac output by thoracic impedance in healthy children and with cystic fibrosis.

Use of Thoracic Electric Bioimpedance in Various Cardiac Conditions

The annual heart failure costs are about $56 billion, with two thirds of the cost consumed in the management of acutely decompensated patients. Systolic blood pressure alone did not reliably reflect the cardiac output status in 245 outpatient visits for heart failure (39–41,48). TEB may provide an outpatient tool to evaluate cardiomyopathies, heart failure, and pulmonary edema in the early and late stages (49,50) and also guide vasodilation therapy (49).

TEB has been used to assess cardiovascular status in hypertensive heart disease and to provide more complete physiologic characterization for effective targeted drug management in the ED (51). Physicians' clinical assessments were compared with measured TEB values in 186 patients. Diagnosis changed in 51% with more incidence of changed diagnosis in patients with a low CI (52). In another study, TEB and COtd values were compared with physicians' clinical judgments, assessed as high, medium, or low, and clinical judgment was incorrect 58% of the time (53).

TEB was found to be reliable for chronic fluid management in 33 patients diagnosed as New York Heart Association class III or IV. Of the ten patients hospitalized for fluid overload on 25 occasions in 20 months, TEB cardiac output identified patients in pulmonary edema who were subsequently hospitalized with PAC monitoring for fluid overload and PAC measurements reflected TEB values (54). TEB measurements were reproducible in both intra- and interday values in stable coronary artery disease patients (55), and diagnosed chronic heart failure and severity of cardiac dysfunction in ED patients with dyspnea (56). Other cardiac functions presented in the bioimpedance technology include velocity index, thoracic fluid content, and the left ventricular ejection time (57,58), and these values correlated well with outcome in 52 hypertensive patients who eventually demonstrated a 33% mortality (59).

Thoracic Electric Bioimpedance Combined with Other Noninvasive Methods for Comprehensive Monitoring: Transcutaneous Oxygen and Carbon Dioxide for Evaluation of Tissue Perfusion

TEB combined with conventional vital signs (MAP and HR), pulse oximetry (SpO_2), and transcutaneous O_2 and CO_2 tensions and organized at the bedside of emergency patients in the ED, OR, or ICU provides the maximum noninvasive physiologic information previously only available by the PAC (5–7,18). Noninvasive variables were chosen to reflect (a) cardiac function by CI, MAP, and HR; (b) changes in respiratory function by SpO_2; and (c) tissue perfusion reflected by transcutaneous pressure of CO_2 (mm Hg) ($PtcCO_2$) and transcutaneous pressure of O_2 (mm Hg) indexed to the fractional inspired O_2 concentration ($PtcO_2/FiO_2$) (6,7). These noninvasive hemodynamic data were continuously displayed online in real time beginning shortly after ED admission. The values were continuously monitored, recorded by an interfaced personal computer, and filed directly into a database to describe sequential hemodynamic patterns related to survival or death (6,7,11,18). Martin et al. (20) used TEB with SpO_2, and tissue perfusion by $PtcO_2/FiO_2$ values in pediatric trauma patients to predict outcome and track their hospital course.

$PtcO_2$ reflects delivery of oxygen to the local area of skin; it also parallels the mixed venous oxygen tension. It uses the same Clark polarographic oxygen electrode routinely used in standard blood gas analyses. Oxygen tensions are determined in a representative area of the skin surface heated to 44°C to increase emissivity of oxygen across the stratum corneum, and to prevent vasoconstriction in the local area being measured. Transcutaneous CO_2 tensions are continuously monitored by a standard Stowe-Severinghaus electrode in the O_2 sensor unit.

Whole Body Electrical Bioimpedance

Whole body electrical bioimpedance (WBEB) uses proprietary electrodes arranged in a wrist-to-ankle configuration (43,60–62). An alternating current of 30 kHz, 1.4 mA is delivered through the two electrodes, and the bioimpedance fluctuations are measured. The ECG is used to measure HR. CI by WBEB compared satisfactorily with the COtd in 28 patients with bypass grafts (60).

Echocardiography: Transesophageal and Transtracheal Cardiography

Two-dimensional (2-D) Doppler echocardiography maps the anatomic relations of the heart by ultrasonic wave pulses sent out from transducers placed on the chest wall, esophageal tube, or endotracheal tube. The sound waves are bounced off the walls and valves of the heart and are captured by sensors as echoes that are electronically plotted to produce images corresponding to anatomic features of the heart, including the right and left atrium, the atrial septum, valves, pulmonary vessels, and the thoracic duct.

Transesophageal echocardiography (TEE) is useful in evaluating heart valve abnormalities, tumors, blood clots, dissecting aortic aneurysms, and congenital defects. Doppler techniques are for diagnostic imaging rather than a continuous hemodynamic assessment tool; the images may be distorted by obesity, chronic obstructive pulmonary disease (COPD), hyperinflation of the lungs, chest trauma, and surgical dressings. Doppler echocardiology favorably compared with TEB in 16 normal subjects; the mean differences in CI between both methods were relatively small ($r = 0.87$) (43).

Doppler techniques are able to provide some qualitative information about flow through vessels, but are limited by the need for expert interpretation of the images and the need for very sensitive transducer placement. These factors provide for a useful diagnostic tool, but limit the reproducibility of the measurements and their use for continuous monitoring.

Lithium Dilution Cardiac Output Measurements

Lithium chloride, 0.3 mmol, is used as the indicator for calculation of cardiac output by the standard indicator dilution technique (63). The system requires an intravenous catheter for rapid infusion of the lithium indicator and a disposable lithium-selective electrode in the arterial catheter tubing with an attached battery-operated roller pump to withdraw blood through the lithium sensor.

Pulse Contour Cardiac Output System

The pulse contour method analyzed the systolic part of the arterial pressure waveform based on a complex analysis of waveform harmonics (64,65). The disadvantage of this approach is that it requires calibration by invasive methods, and the calibration lasts only as long as the patient's arterial vasoactive status remains constant. This is a major limitation for unstable postoperative patients.

Noninvasive Partial CO_2 Rebreathing Cardiac Output Measurement

Noninvasive partial CO_2 rebreathing cardiac output (NICO) measurement is a cardiac output monitoring system based on CO_2 elimination measured by the direct Fick principle. The system measures CO_2 on a breath-by-breath basis to provide a continuous estimation of metabolic demand, with precise tidal volume and flow analyses (flow/volume). The cardiac output is proportional to the changes in CO_2 elimination divided by the change in end-tidal CO_2 measured by a CO_2 sensor, which periodically adds a rebreathing volume into the ventilatory circuit (NICO, Novametrics Medical Systems, Wallingford, CT). The system also provides compliance assessments that facilitate adjustment of ventilatory parameters to optimize compliance with positive end-expiratory pressure (PEEP) and tidal volume settings. Three NICO values averaged over 1 minute were compared with 418 paired thermodilution measurements in 122 patients during cardiac catheterization prior to cardiac surgery. The overall correlation was $r = 0.89$ with a small bias (66–68).

The NICO system was prospectively compared with thermodilution in 122 patients (a) during cardiac catheterization; (b) before, during, and after coronary bypass surgery; and (c) during treatment for acute congestive heart failure (CHF). The authors concluded that NICO provided an accurate noninvasive measurement of CI (67,68). The system is minimally invasive but it requires the patient to have tracheal intubation, a closed ventilatory circuit, and mechanically assisted ventilation.

These techniques share the shortcomings of thermodilution with PACs in that they give only episodic sets of measurements, require critical care conditions, and need frequent recalibration.

Gastric Transmucosal Oxygen and Carbon Dioxide Tensions

By positioning a balloon against the stomach wall and allowing for gas to equilibrate between the gastric mucosa and the lumen of the balloon, O_2 and CO_2 tensions in tissue adjacent to the probe may be extrapolated to assess the degree of anaerobic metabolism. Some investigators have found this technique useful in titrating resuscitation in shock. The difficulty with this is the limited tissue bed assessed and the assumption that perfusion of the monitored tissue reflects the other tissues. Details of this technology are described in other chapters.

Near-infrared Spectroscopy

Near-infrared spectroscopy (NIRS) is used to measure tissue myoglobin oxygen saturation (StO_2) of the hypothenar space as an alternative to transcutaneous O_2 and CO_2 to assess regional tissue perfusion (69–71). Regional perfusion markers have been extrapolated to estimate the overall tissue perfusion status. These measurements were reported to be reliable for resuscitation and monitoring, but their role remains to be defined throughout in the clinical environment. NIRS feasibility studies were undertaken in 46 ED patients, six of whom were hospitalized for heart failure with one death (69).

TABLE 17.1

HEMODYNAMIC VALUES IN TRAUMA PATIENTS BY INVASIVE AND NONINVASIVE MONITORING

	Invasive		Noninvasive	
Variable, unit	Survivors ($N = 178$) Mean ± SEM	Nonsurvivors ($N = 89$) Mean ± SEM	Survivors ($N = 592$) Mean ± SEM	Nonsurvivors ($N = 69$) Mean ± SEM
CI, L/min/m^2	4.31 ±0.06	3.72 ± 0.07[a]	4.10 ± 0.04	3.67 ± 0.10[a]
MAP, mm Hg	98 ± 1	90 ± 1[a]	89 ± 1	78 ± 2[a]
HR, beat/min	109 ± 1	105 ± 1[b]	103 ± 1	114 ± 2[a]
SpO_2, %	99 ± 0.4	95 ± 1[a]	98 ± 0	96 ± 0.2[a]
CVP, cm H_2O	11.5 ± 0.3	12.5 ± 0.3[b]	—	—
SvO_2, %	74 ± 0.4	72 ± 0.6[a]	—	—
DO_2, mL/min/m^2	640 ± 9	522 ± 9[a]	617 ± 10	487 ± 21[a]
VO_2, L/min/m^2	158 ± 2	130 ± 3[a]	—	—
$PtcCO_2$, torr	—	—	47 ± 1	62 ± 7[a]
$PtcO_2/FiO_2$	—	—	230 ± 5	107 ± 9[a]
Hct,%	33 ± 0.2	33 ± 0.33	4 ± 1	30 ± 1
SP, %	—	—	89 + 0.1	75 + 0.2[a]

SEM, standard error of means; CI, cardiac index; MAP, mean arterial pressure; HR, heart rate; SpO_2, arterial hemoglobin saturation by pulse oximetry; $PtcCO_2$, transcutaneous CO_2 tension; $PtcO_2/FiO_2$, transcutaneous O_2 tension indexed to FiO_2; SP, survival probability.
[a]$p < 0.01$; [b]$p < 0.05$, comparing survivors with their corresponding nonsurvivors using unpaired Student's t-test.

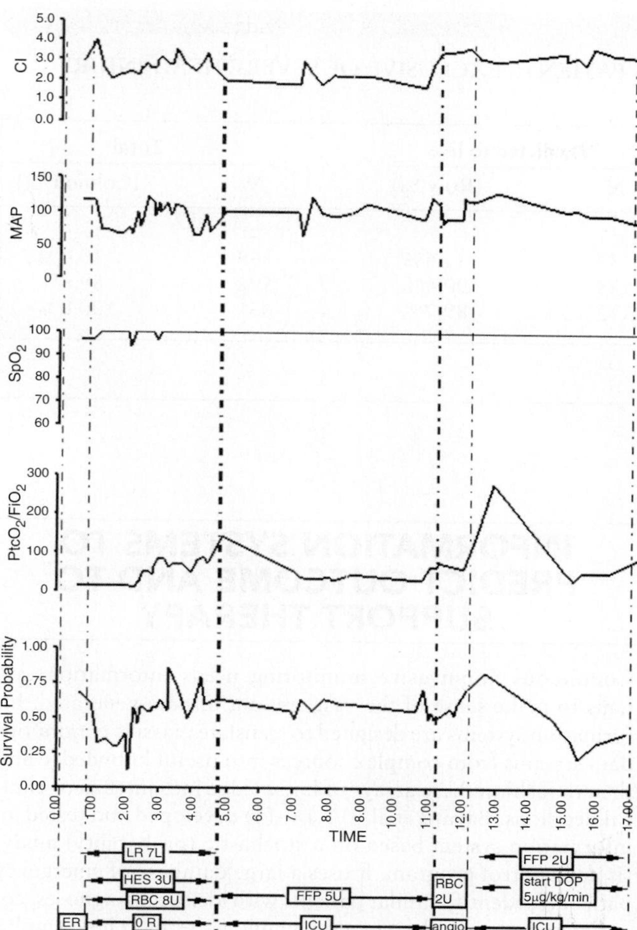

FIGURE 17.1. Data from a 66-year-old man who was involved in a motor vehicle accident and sustained lacerations of the spleen and descending aorta, hemothorax, and multiple rib fractures. The injury severity score was 59, the Glasgow coma scale was 9, and he sustained an estimated initial blood loss of 4,000 mL. He was operated on between 1 and 5 hours after emergency department (ED) admission (splenectomy and repair of thoracic aortic laceration). He was given 7 liters of Ringer lactate, 8 units of packed red cells, and 1,500 mL starch in the operating room (OR) followed by 5 units of fresh frozen plasma in the intensive care unit (ICU) and 2 more units of packed red cells and 2 units of fresh frozen plasma (lowest section of the graph). *Upper row:* Cardiac index (CI). *Second row:* Mean arterial pressure (MAP). *Third row:* Pulse oximetry (SpO_2). *Fourth row:* $PtcO_2/FiO_2$. *Lowest row:* Survival probability. Time, in hours from ED admission, is noted below the bottom horizontal line. Therapies are outlined in boxes: FFP, fresh frozen plasma; HES, hydroxyethyl starch; RBC, packed red blood cell transfusion; DOP, dopamine; LR, lactated Ringer solution, which was given at the rate 150 mL/hr postoperatively. Time and place of resuscitation (ER, OR, ICU) indicated at lowest line. Note: The CI fell to around 2 L/min/m^2 throughout most of the intraoperative and immediate postoperative period, the MAP fell to around 60 to 70 mm Hg, the $PtcO_2/FiO_2$ was less than 100 torr throughout most of the course, and the SP was less than 50% throughout most of the course. Despite this evidence of hypovolemia, the operating surgeon was reluctant to give more fluids for fear of disrupting the repaired aortic laceration. The patient developed acute respiratory distress syndrome (ARDS), sepsis, cardiac failure, and renal failure. He died 31 days after admission.

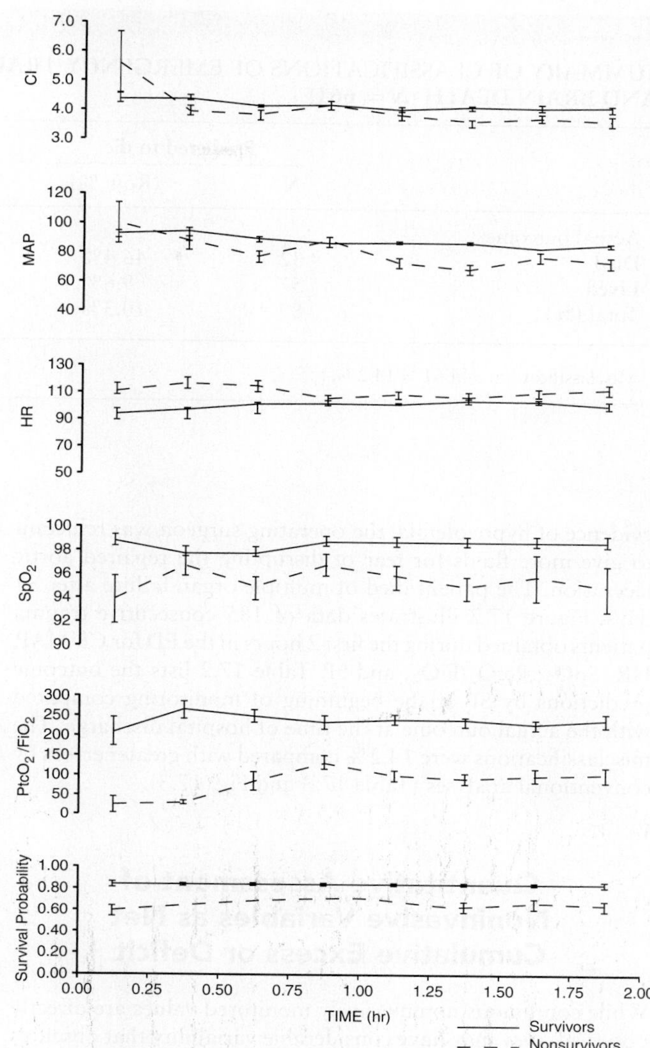

FIGURE 17.2. Survivors' (*solid line*) and nonsurvivors' (*dashed line*) temporal patterns are shown for the first 48 hours after their emergency department (ED) admission. Mean values ± standard error of means (SEM) are shown for cardiac index (CI) in mL/min/m^2, heart rate (HR), mean arterial pressure (MAP), pulse oximetry (SpO_2), transcutaneous oxygen tension indexed to the fractional inspired oxygen concentration ($PtcO_2/FiO_2$), and survival probability (SP). All values are keyed to at the time of admission to the ED. Note that the survivors' cardiac index, MAP, SpO_2, $PtcO_2/FiO_2$, and SP values were generally higher than those of the nonsurvivors. The mean survivors' SP values were significantly higher than the mean nonsurvivors' SP values in this observation period.

Summary of Survivors' and Nonsurvivors' Data by Invasive and Noninvasive Monitoring

Table 17.1 summarizes the monitored data of 661 surviving and nonsurviving trauma patients. Survivors had greater CI, MAP, SpO_2, $PtcO_2/FiO_2$, DO_2, VO_2, and survival probability (SP) values. Figure 17.1 illustrates data of a 66-year-old man who sustained an auto accident with lacerations of the spleen, thoracic aorta, and multiple rib fractures with an estimated initial blood loss of over 4,000 mL. Despite the data and other

TABLE 17.2

SUMMARY OF CLASSIFICATIONS OF EMERGENCY TRAUMA PATIENTS EXCLUSIVE OF SEVERE HEAD INJURY AND BRAIN DEATH ($N = 661$)

	Predicted to die		Predicted to live		Total	
	N	(Row %)	*N*	(Row %)	*N*	(Column %)
Actual outcome						
Died	32	46.4%	37	53.6%	69	10.4%
Lived	57	9.6%	535	90.4%	592	89.6%
Total (%)	89	10.3%	572	89.7%	661	100.0%

Misclassification: 94/661 = 14.2%.

evidence of hypovolemia, the operating surgeon was reluctant to give more fluids for fear of disrupting the repaired aortic laceration. The patient died of multiple organ failure after 31 days. Figure 17.2 illustrates data of 185 consecutive trauma patients obtained during the first 2 hours in the ED for CI, MAP, HR, SpO_2, $PtcO_2/FiO_2$, and SP. Table 17.2 lists the outcome predictions by SP at the beginning of monitoring compared with the actual outcome at the time of hospital discharge. The misclassifications were 14.2% compared with greater errors by conventional analyses (Table 17.3 and Fig. 17.3).

Quantitative Assessment of Noninvasive Variables as Net Cumulative Excess or Deficit

While continuous noninvasively monitored values are directly observed, they may have considerable variability that obscures the underlying patterns. To overcome this problem, we calculated the net cumulative excess or deficit of physiologic variables by integrating the areas between the curves of monitored data and normal values to provide a quantitative measure of the overall net cumulative deficit in cardiac, pulmonary, and tissue perfusion functions.

INFORMATION SYSTEMS TO PREDICT OUTCOME AND TO SUPPORT THERAPY

Continuous noninvasive monitoring needs information systems to make sense of the vast amount of data generated. Information systems are designed to translate massive continuous data streams from complex sources into useful knowledge and then to fashion these arrays of knowledge into intelligent clinical decisions. Bayard et al. (11,16–18) developed and tested an information system based on a stochastic (probability) analysis and control program. It uses a large database of emergency patients to identify similar patients with identical diagnoses, covariates, and very close hemodynamic patterns. These similar patients, defined as "nearest neighbors," are used as surrogates to compute in real time the SP of newly admitted study patients. A patient's SP for a given state is calculated by first extracting from the database 40 or more "nearest neighbors" whose clinical and hemodynamic patterns most closely resemble those of the study patient. Then the SP is calculated as the fraction of nearest neighbors that survived. The SP predicts outcome and is also a digitized measure of severity of illness; low SP values are quantitatively related to the likelihood of death and reflect illness severity (11,17,18).

TABLE 17.3

MISCLASSIFICATIONS IN PREDICTION BY VARIOUS OUTCOME PREDICTORS

Method	Criteria	Misclassification rate
Initial heart rate	S <95, NS >96 beats/min	(70/159) 45%
Initial MAP	S >85, NS <70 mm Hg	(76/159) 47%
Lowest MAP	S >50, NS <50 mm Hg	(83/159) 52%
Initial cardiac index	S >3.8, NS <3.8 L/min/m^2	(72/159) 43%
APACHE II	S <27, NS >27	(30/97) 31%
Survival probability, present study	S >82%, NS <82%	(94/661) 14.2%

MAP, mean arterial pressure; S, survivors; NS, nonsurvivors.

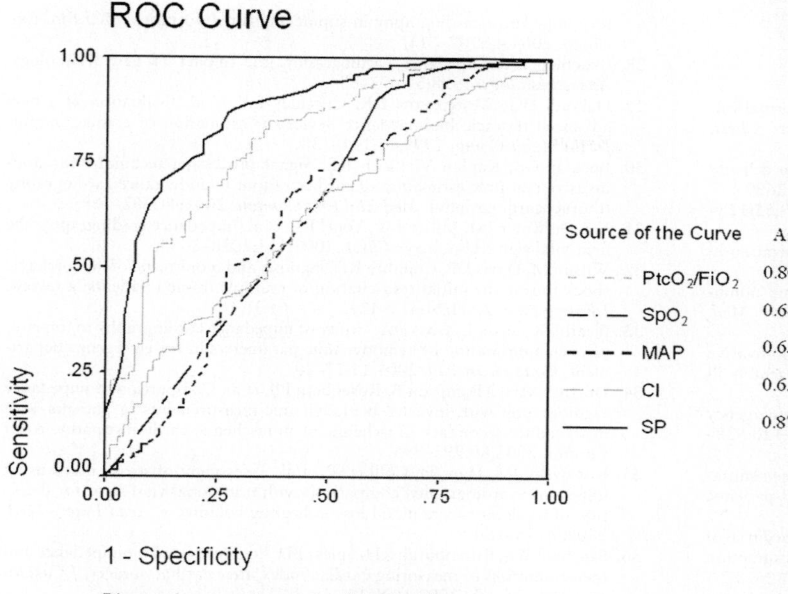

FIGURE 17.3. Receiver operating characteristic (ROC) curves calculated for data collected in trauma patients over the first 24-hour period after emergency department (ED) admission. The area under the curves represents the sensitivity and specificity for each variable: 1.00 represents 100% correct, 0.50 represents no correlation. These areas under the ROC curve were 0.85 for survival probability (SP), 0.81 for transcutaneous oxygen tension indexed to the fractional inspired oxygen concentration ($PtcO_2/FiO_2$), 0.64 for pulse oximetry (SpO_2), 0.61 for mean arterial pressure (MAP), and 0.59 for cardiac index (CI).

The therapeutic decision support program uses the study patient's nearest neighbors' responses to various therapies that were given to them and recorded in the database. The likely responses of the study patient are suggested by the nearest neighbors' responses known from the database (11,17). This approach includes the following characteristics: (a) the patient's course is described by a three-dimensional trajectory; (b) the first derivative of the initial vector projects the patient's course if there are no inherent changes or external influences; (c) the second derivative tracks changes in the patient's course from either internal compensations, further deterioration, spontaneous improvement, or external influences such as changes in therapy; and (d) the integral sums up the total influences. Methods of machine learning (37,38), and dynamic programming for stochastic control (39,40) motivated the program.

MINIMALLY INVASIVE MONITORING

Noninvasive Hemodynamic Monitoring with Central Venous Pressure Catheters and Oximeters

Rivers et al. (10) used noninvasive hemodynamic monitoring and central venous pressure (CVP) catheters with attached oximeters at their tips to guide resuscitation of septic and septic shock patients in the ED. They showed significantly improved survival in septic patients with early goal-directed therapy started in the ED based on minimally invasive monitoring. They identified their septic patients in the first hour after ED admission; this was followed by 6 hours of goal-directed therapy in the ED in protocol patients, and compared for a similar period with standard therapy in the control group. Then, the patients were sent to the appropriate in-hospital department without the knowledge of whether the patient had been randomized to the protocol or the control group (10). The treatment administered in the first 6 hours impacted outcomes. This demonstrates that the following are important: early treatment, and resuscitation to a flow-related goal rather than the traditional blood pressure goal.

SUMMARY

Noninvasive systems are able to continuously display variables online, in real time throughout the patient's hospital course, and with information systems to predict outcome and support therapeutic decision making. Because they are simple, safe, easy to use, inexpensive, reasonably accurate, and available anywhere in the hospital, some form of noninvasive hemodynamic monitoring with an appropriate information system will replace invasive monitoring for acutely ill patients.

PEARLS

1. One-dimensional monitoring with one type of monitor may obscure the real problem. Therefore, it is essential to monitor cardiac, pulmonary, and tissue perfusion/oxygenation functions and their interrelationships to show the whole picture.
2. Comprehensive noninvasive hemodynamic monitoring with an information system will predict outcome and guide therapy.
3. Continuous, online, real-time visual displays of hemodynamic patterns are safer for both patient and staff, are inexpensive, are user friendly, approximate PAC values, and may be used throughout the hospital and prehospital areas.
4. There is no single magic number for optimal blood flow, because the microcirculation needed for tissue perfusion/oxygenation must also be adequate, just as rush hour traffic may greatly affect flow in main arteries, or side streets, or both. It is necessary to optimize both total blood flow and tissue perfusion/oxygenation.

References

1. Shoemaker WC, Appel PL, Kram HB. Prospective trial of supranormal values of survivors as therapeutic goals in high risk surgical patients. *Chest.* 1988;94:1176.
2. Boyd O, Grounds M, Bennett D. Preoperative increase of oxygen delivery reduces mortality in high risk surgical patients. *JAMA.* 1993;270:2699.
3. Boyd O, Hayes M. The oxygen trail: the goal. *Brit Med Bull.* 1999;55:125–139.
4. Kern JW, Shoemaker WC. Meta-analysis of hemodynamic optimization in high-risk patients. *Crit Care Med.* 2002;30:1686–1692.
5. Shoemaker WC, Appel PL, Kram HB, et al. Multicomponent noninvasive physiologic monitoring of circulatory function. *Crit Care Med.* 1988;16:482–490.
6. Shoemaker WC, Belzberg H, Wo CCJ, et al. Multicenter study of noninvasive monitoring systems as an alternative to invasive monitoring of acutely ill emergency patients. *Chest.* 1998;114:1643–1652.
7. Shoemaker WC, Wo CCJ, Chan L, et al. Outcome prediction of emergency patients by noninvasive hemodynamic monitoring. *Chest.* 2001;120:528–537.
8. Bishop MW, Shoemaker WC, Appel PL, et al. Relationship between supranormal values, time delays and outcome in severely traumatized patients. *Crit Care Med.* 1993;21:56.
9. Bishop MH, Shoemaker WC, Kram HB, et al. Prospective randomized trial of survivor values of cardiac index, oxygen delivery, and oxygen consumption as resuscitation endpoints in severe trauma. *J Trauma.* 1995;38:780–787.
10. Rivers E, Nguyen B, Havsted S, et al. Early goal-directed therapy in the treatment of severe sepsis and septic shock. *N Engl J Med.* 2002;345:1368–1377.
11. Shoemaker WC, Wo CCJ, Cheien L-C, et al. Evaluation of invasive and noninvasive hemodynamic monitoring in trauma patients. *J Trauma.* 2006;60:82–90.
12. Moore FA, Haemel JB, Moore EE, et al. Incommensurate oxygen consumption in response to maximal oxygen availability predicts postinjury oxygen failure. *J Trauma.* 1992;33:58.
13. Yu M, Levy MM, Smith P, et al. Effect of maximizing oxygen delivery on mortality and morbidity rates in critically ill patients: a prospective randomized control study. *Crit Care Med.* 1993;21:830–838.
14. Creamer JE, Edwards JD, Nightingale P. Hemodynamic and oxygen transport variables in cardiogenic shock secondary to acute myocardial infarction. *Am J Cardiol.* 1990;65:1287.
15. Rady MY, Edwards JD, Rivers EP, et al. Measurement of oxygen consumption after uncomplicated acute myocardial infarction. *Chest.* 1993;103:886–895.
16. Bayard DS, Botnen A, Shoemaker WC, et al. Stochastic analysis of therapeutic modalities using a database of patient responses. *IEEE Symposium on Computer Based Medical Systems (CBMS).* 2001;11:439–444.
17. Shoemaker WC, Wo CCJ, Botnan A, et al. Development of a hemodynamic database in severe trauma patients to define optimal goals and predict outcome. *IEEE Symposium on Computer Based Medical Systems (CBMS).* 2001;11:445–452 .
18. Shoemaker WC, Bayard DS, Botnen A, et al. Mathematical program for outcome prediction and therapeutic support for trauma beginning within 1 hr of admission: a preliminary report. *Crit Care Med.* 2005;33:1499–1506.
19. Charloux A, Lonsdorfer-Wolf E, Richard R, et al. A new impedance cardiograph device for the noninvasive evaluation of cardiac output at rest and during exercise: comparison with the "direct" Fick method. *Eur J Appl Physiol.* 2000;82:313–320.
20. Martin M, Brown C, Bayard DS, et al. Continuous noninvasive monitoring of cardiac performance and tissue perfusion in pediatric trauma. *J Pediatr Surg.* 2005;40:1957–1963.
21. Shoemaker WC, Appel PL, Kram HB. Role of oxygen debt in the development of organ failure, sepsis and death in high-risk surgical patients. *Chest.* 1992;102:208–215.
22. Shoemaker WC, Wo CCJ, Bishop MH, et al. Multicenter trial of a new thoracic electrical bioimpedance device for cardiac output estimations. *Crit Care Med.* 1994;22:1907–1912.
23. Summers RL, Vogel J, Emerman CE. Impact of impedance cardiography on diagnosis and therapy of emergent dyspnea: the ED-IMPACT trial. *Acad Emerg Med.* 2006;13:365–371.
24. Summers RL, Shoemaker WC, Peacock WF, et al. Bench to bedside: electrophysiologic and clinical principles of noninvasive hemodynamic monitoring using impedance cardiography. *Acad Emerg Med.* 2003;10:669–680.
25. Raaijmakers E, Faes TJ, Scholten RJ, et al. A meta-analysis of three decades of validating thoracic impedance cardiography. *Crit Care Med.* 1999;27:1203–1213.
26. White RD, Blackwell TH, Russell JK, et al. Transthoracic impedance does not affect defibrillation, resuscitation or survival in patients with out-of-hospital cardiac arrest treated with a non-escalating biphasic waveform defibrillator. *Resuscitation.* 2005;64:63–69.
27. Cybulski G, Michalak E, Kozluk E, et al. Stroke volume and systolic time intervals: beat-to-beat comparison between echocardiography and ambulatory impedance cardiography in supine and tilted positions. *Med Biol Eng Comp.* 2004;42:707–711.
28. Critchley LA. Impedance cardiography: the impact of new technology. *Anaesthesiology.* 1998;53:677–684.
29. Haryadi DG, Westenskow DR, Critchley LA, et al. Evaluation of a new advanced thoracic bioimpedance device for estimation of cardiac output. *J Clin Monit Comp.* 1999;15:131–138.
30. Bucklar GB, Kaplan V, Bloch KE. Signal processing technique for non-invasive real-time estimation of cardiac output by inductance cardiography (thoracocardiography). *Med Biol Eng Comput.* 2003;41:302–309.
31. Van De Water JM, Miller TW, Vogel RL, et al. Impedance cardiography: the next vital sign technology? *Chest.* 2003;123:2028–2033.
32. Wilson M, Davis DP, Coimbra R. Diagnosis and monitoring of hemorrhagic shock during the initial resuscitation of multiple trauma patients: a review. *J Emerg Med.* 2003;24:413–422.
33. Neath SX, Lazio L, Guss DA. Utility of impedance cardiography to improve physician estimation of hemodynamic parameters in the emergency department. *Cong Heart Fail.* 2005;11:17–20.
34. Drazner MH, Thompson B, Rosenberg PB, et al. Comparison of impedance cardiography with invasive hemodynamic measurements in patients with heart failure secondary to ischemic or nonischemic cardiomyopathy. *Am J Cardiol.* 2002;89:993–995.
35. Kosowsky JM, Han JH, Collins SP, et al. Assessment of stroke index using impedance cardiography: comparison with traditional vital signs for detection of moderate acute blood loss in healthy volunteers. *Acad Emerg Med.* 2002;9:775–780.
36. Sageman WS, Riffenburgh RH, Spiess BD. Equivalence of bioimpedance and thermodilution in measuring cardiac index after cardiac surgery. *J Cardiothor Vasc Anesth.* 2002;16:8–14.
37. Richard R, Lonsdorfer-Wolf E, et al. Non-invasive cardiac output evaluation during a maximal progressive exercise test, using a new impedance cardiograph device. *Euro J Appl Physiol.* 2001;85:202–207.
38. Engoren M, Barbee D. Comparison of cardiac output determined by bioimpedance, thermodilution, and the Fick method. *Am J Crit Care.* 2005;14:40–45.
39. Albert NM, Hail MD, Li J, et al. Equivalence of the bioimpedance and thermodilution methods in measuring cardiac output in hospitalized patients with advanced, decompensated chronic heart failure. *Am J Crit Care.* 2004;13:469–479.
40. Imhoff M, Lehner JH, Lohlein D. Noninvasive whole-body electrical bioimpedance cardiac output and invasive thermodilution cardiac output in risk surgical patients. *Crit Care Med.* 2000;28:2812–2818.
41. Barin E, Haryadi DG, Schookin SI, et al. Evaluation of a thoracic bioimpedance cardiac output monitor during cardiac catheterization. *Crit Care Med.* 2000;28:698–702.
42. Smit HJ, Vonk Noordegraaf A, Marcus JT, et al. Determinants of pulmonary perfusion measured by electrical impedance tomography. *Euro J Appl Physiol.* 2004;92:45–49.
43. Cotter G, Moshkovitz Y, Kaluski E, et al. Accurate, noninvasive continuous monitoring of cardiac output by whole-body electrical bioimpedance. *Chest.* 2004;125(4):1431–1440.
44. Pianosi PT. Measurement of exercise cardiac output by thoracic impedance in healthy children. *Euro J Appl Physiol.* 2004;92:425–430.
45. Pianosi PT. Impedance cardiography accurately measures cardiac output during exercise in children with cystic fibrosis. *Chest.* 1997;111:333–337.
46. Scherhag A, Kaden JJ, Kentschke E, et al. Comparison of impedance cardiography and thermodilution-derived measurements of stroke volume and cardiac output at rest and during exercise testing. *Cardiovasc Drug Ther.* 2005;19:141–147.
47. Weiss SJ, Ernst AA, Godorov G, et al. Bioimpedance-derived differences in cardiac physiology during exercise stress testing in low-risk chest pain patients. *South Med J.* 2003;96:1121–1127.
48. Parrott CW, Quale C, Lewis DL, et al. Systolic blood pressure does not reliably identify vasoactive status in chronic heart failure. *Am J Hypertens.* 2005;18(Pt 2):82S–86S.
49. Bhalla V, Isakson S, Bhalla MA, et al. Diagnostic ability of B-type natriuretic peptide and impedance cardiography: testing to identify left ventricular dysfunction in hypertensive patients. *Am J Hypertens.* 2005;18(Pt 2):73S–81S.
50. Yancy C, Abraham WT. Noninvasive hemodynamic monitoring in heart failure: utilization of impedance cardiography. *Congest Heart Fail.* 2003;9:241–250.
51. Ventura HO, Taler SJ, Strobeck JE. Hypertension as a hemodynamic disease: the role of impedance cardiography in diagnostic, prognostic, and therapeutic decision making. *Am J Hypertens.* 2005;18(Pt 2):26S–43S.
52. Van De Water JM, Dalton ML, Parish DC, et al. Cardiopulmonary assessment: is improvement needed? *World J Surg.* 2005;29(Suppl 1):S95–98.
53. Veale WN Jr, Morgan JH, Beatty JS, et al. Hemodynamic and pulmonary fluid status in the trauma patient: are we slipping? *Am Surgeon.* 2005;71:621–626.
54. Yu CM, Wang L, Chau E, et al. Intrathoracic impedance monitoring in patients with heart failure: correlation with fluid status and feasibility of early warning preceding hospitalization. *Circulation.* 2005;112:841–848.

55. Treister N, Wagner K, Jansen PR. Reproducibility of impedance cardiography parameters in outpatients with clinically stable coronary artery disease. *Am J Hypertens.* 2005;18(Pt 2):44S–50S.
56. Barcarse E, Kazanegra R, Chen A, et al. Combination of B-type natriuretic peptide levels and non-invasive hemodynamic parameters in diagnosing congestive heart failure in the emergency department. *Cong Heart Fail.* 2004;10:171–176.
57. Packer M, Abraham WT, Mehra MR, et al. Utility of impedance cardiography for the identification of short-term risk of clinical decompensation in stable patients with chronic heart failure. *J Am Coll Cardiol.* 2006;47:2245–2252.
58. Sanford T, Treister N, Peters C. Use of noninvasive hemodynamics in hypertension management. *Am J Hypertens.* 2005;8(Pt 2):87S–91S.
59. Ramirez MF, Tibayan RT, Marinas CE, et al. Prognostic value of hemodynamic findings from impedance cardiography in hypertensive stroke. *Am J Hypertens.* 2005;18(Pt 2):65S–72S.
60. Kaukinen S, Koobi T, Bi Y, et al. Cardiac output measurement after coronary artery bypass grafting using bolus thermodilution, continuous thermodilution, and whole-body impedance cardiography. *J Cardiothor Vasc Anesth.* 2003;17:199–203.
61. Kauppinen PK, Koobi T, Hyttinen J, et al. Segmental composition of whole-body impedance cardiogram estimated by computer simulations and clinical experiments. *Clin Physiol.* 2000;20:106–113.
62. Koobi T, Kaukinen S, Turjanmaa VM, et al. Whole-body impedance cardiography in the measurement of cardiac output. *Crit Care Med.* 1997;25:779–785.
63. Linton RA, Band DM, Haire KM. A new method for measuring cardiac output using lithium dilution. *Br J Anaesth.* 1993;71:262–266.
64. Nichols WW, O'Rourke MF. *MacDonald's Blood Flow in Arteries.* 5th ed. London: Hodder Arnold Publication; 2005.
65. Linton NWP, Linton RAF. Estimation of changes in cardiac output from the arterial blood pressure waveform in the upper limb. *Br J Anaesth.* 2001;86:486–494.
66. Capek JM, Roy RJ. *IEEE Trans BME.* 1988:653–661.
67. Jaffe MB:. Partial CO2 rebreathing cardiac output: operating principles of the NICO system. *J Clin Monit.* 1999;15:387–401.
68. Tordi N, Mourot L, Matusheski B, et al. Measurements of cardiac output during constant exercises: comparison of two non-invasive techniques. *Int J Sports Med.* 2004;25:145–149.
69. Beilman GJ, Groehler KE, Lazaron V, et al. Near infrared spectroscopy measurement of regional tissue oxyhemoglobin saturation during hemorrhagic shock. *Shock.* 1999;12:196–200.
70. Cohn SM, Crookes BA, Proctor KG. Near-infrared spectroscopy in resuscitation. *J Trauma.* 2003;54(5):S199–S202.
71. Myers DE, Anderson LD, Seifert RP, et al. Noninvasive method for measuring local hemoglobin oxygen saturation in tissue using wide gap second derivative near-infrared spectroscopy. *J Biomed Optics.* 2005;10(3):1–18.

CHAPTER 18 ■ HEMODYNAMIC MONITORING: ARTERIAL AND PULMONARY ARTERY CATHETERS

SHARON E. MORAN • KEVIN Y. PEI • MIHAE YU

Since the introduction of the pulmonary artery catheter (PAC) in the 1970s, initial enthusiasm has been tempered by allegation that the use of PAC may cause harm (1). Several academic societies have convened expert panels to review the literature and discuss important issues regarding PAC utilization (2). For most critical care practitioners, the benefits of using PACs has warranted continued use in high-risk patients, but controversy remains.

Inherent in the use of the PAC is the assumption that flow-related variables such as cardiac output/cardiac index (CO/CI) and oxygen delivery (DO_2) to the tissues are important for survival. Shoemaker et al. popularized this concept when they observed that the differentiating parameters between survivors and nonsurvivors were flow-related variables such as DO_2, oxygen consumption (VO_2), and CO instead of the traditional values of blood pressure (BP), heart rate (HR), urine output, and arterial oxygen tension (PaO_2) (3,4). In addition, Bihari et al. (5) reported that as DO_2 was augmented in critically ill patients, oxygen consumption of the tissues increased, suggesting that a supply dependency existed. The biggest criticism of the supply dependency concept was the mathematical coupling between DO_2 and VO_2 since cardiac output is on both sides of the equation. In a study using independent measurement of VO_2, Yu et al. (6) demonstrated that some but not all critically ill patients showed an increase in VO_2 as DO_2 improved. The theory of supply dependency and titrating DO_2 until the VO_2 slope flattens is an attractive concept but is not practical. Some patients may not demonstrate a plateau; furthermore, a patient's VO_2 is constantly changing secondary to variations in activity (turning, suctioning), temperature, vasoactive agents, and nutritional support. An easier clinical end point of resuscitation is the mixed venous oxygen saturation (SvO_2), which reflects the balance between DO_2 and VO_2 (see below) (7).

Review of all the literature studying resuscitation to CI, DO_2, and SvO_2 goals (both pro and con) is beyond the scope of this chapter but is summarized in the practice guidelines for PAC (2). The controversy is NOT whether DO_2 is important to tissues but rather *how much* is necessary to meet the demands of individual tissues. It is also clear that global values of DO_2 may not translate into transport of oxygen to the individual tissue beds, but until we have a tool to measure all tissue oxygenation states (or one tissue bed that is a surrogate marker for the rest of the body), the amount of oxygen delivery necessary for tissue perfusion will remain controversial.

Over the decades, clinicians have progressed from treatment of BP, HR, and urine output to markers of anaerobic metabolism such as lactic acid and base deficit, and then to flow-related variables such as DO_2, VO_2, and SvO_2. What we currently need is an easy, noninvasive method to measure tissue oxygenation and the energy state of the cells. This would allow "titration" of DO_2 to meet tissue demands rather than aiming for a single global survival value of DO_2 and SvO_2 (3,4). We consider these end points of resuscitation to be NOT mutually exclusive, but to complement each other into what we call "tiers" of resuscitation. Instead of discarding the value of DO_2 manipulation, we should seek better measurements of end points of resuscitation, and search for treatment modalities to improve oxygen transport into the cells.

While literature on use of PAC is vast and confusing, it is important for readers to critically evaluate the studies by asking the following questions:

1. What patient population was chosen for the study and was that an appropriate choice of patients?
2. Were the patients chosen early in the course of illness, or after they developed multisystem organ failure (MSOF)? Was there a time specified to reach the goal? Timing of resuscitation is essential for successful outcome. Studies stressing early resuscitative efforts (7–10) demonstrate better outcomes with DO_2 and SvO_2 goals than studies with no time specification (11,12). Given that early resuscitation improves outcome, studies that demonstrate lack of benefit from PAC may be flawed if enrollment occurs within 48 hours of respiratory failure since resuscitation should be completed by 24 hours (13).
3. What were the deletion criteria? Studies excluding patients with acute cardiac or pulmonary problems would be deleting patients who would most benefit from PAC use. One study that deleted patients who already had a PAC, chronic obstructive pulmonary disease (COPD), renal failure, acute myocardial infarct, and liver disease reported no advantage of PAC use (13).
4. Did patients with good cardiac function and ability to respond to increased metabolic demands "negate" the average differences in DO_2 between the control and treated groups; that is, did the study enroll patients with good cardiac function who reached their hemodynamic goals with minimum intervention? These patients tend to do well with low mortality. There are two studies that deleted patients with good cardiac function, but these studies had conflicting outcome results, most likely due to differences in treatment and timing of goal achievement (12,14).
5. What were the hemodynamic goals of the study: CI, DO_2, or SvO_2, or any one or combination of these? Our preference has been to use oxygen delivery indexed (DO_2I) rather than CI since the acceptable CI would vary with hemoglobin levels (15,16).
6. How was the treatment administered? Were fluids given to reach a certain pulmonary artery occlusion pressure (PAOP)? Is left ventricular stroke work index (LVSWI) an appropriate end point for fluid administration since a high BP would lead to an elevated LVSWI without an adequate preload (12)? How were fluid and blood given? What were the dosages of inotropes and did large amounts of inotropes (i.e., 200 μg/kg/minute of dobutamine) possibly contribute to negative outcome (12)?
7. What percent of study patients did not reach the goals? Was failure to reach goals due to inadequate effort by the treating team or due to the inherent inability of the patient's myocardium to respond to treatment? We demonstrated that in the initial phases of our prospective randomized trials, failure to reach DO_2I of $\geq$600 mL/minute/m^2 occurred 46% of the time but decreased to 19% in the second part of the trial (14). High failure rates (>70%) to reach hemodynamic goals have been reported in some studies with negative outcomes (12,17).

Differences in study design and treatment algorithm may have contributed to the confusion. Nevertheless, our therapeutic regimen is limited, and as clinicians, we continue to optimize DO_2 with the hope of delivering oxygen to the tissues.

PEARLS

- Identify patients who may benefit from PAC insertion (Table 18.1), and identify what hemodynamic information is needed to guide treatment.
- Insert the PAC early. The best treatment for MSOF is prevention. The majority of successful outcome studies suggest that timing is of the essence.
- Ensure proper readings. *No* information is better than *wrong* information leading to erroneous treatment. Studies have demonstrated an alarming degree of user error (18–20). A corollary is that infrequent use of PAC may lead to more error (both nursing and physician related).

TABLE 18.1

INDICATIONS FOR PULMONARY ARTERY CATHETER INSERTION

PRECAUTIONARY REASONS
For prevention of multisystem organ failure in high-risk patients (perforated viscus)
For preoperative assessment of high-risk patients with cardiac, pulmonary, and renal dysfunction
For management of high-risk patients postoperatively (major hemorrhage)
For patients with expected large fluid shifts: sepsis, bleeding, multiple trauma, burns, and cirrhosis
TREATMENT OF SHOCK
Hypotension not relieved with fluid
Suspected cardiac event or cardiac compromise contributing to shock
Oliguria not responding to fluid
Patients with multiple organ dysfunction
For continuous SvO_2 monitoring
TO GUIDE TREATMENT IN PULMONARY DYSFUNCTION
To differentiate cardiogenic causes of hypoxia from acute respiratory distress syndrome and guide fluid management
For monitoring cardiac output in patients requiring high positive end-expiratory pressure ($\geq$15 cm H_2O)
TREATMENT OF CARDIAC DYSFUNCTION
Complicated myocardial infarction
Congestive heart failure with poor response to afterload reduction and diuretic therapy
Suspected tamponade or contusion from blunt chest injury
Pulmonary hypertension with myocardial dysfunction

- Have a specific goal for the patient (i.e., DO_2, SvO_2). The goal may vary depending on the type of disease, and also as the patient's clinical condition changes (16). For example, the preoperative patients may have a modest DO_2 goal (21) compared to shock patients (10,22). Older patients (>75 years of age) may have lower metabolic rates and need less DO_2 to meet tissue demands (6,14).
- Use of the PAC requires judgment. The "optimum" PAOP may vary as the patient's condition (compliance of the heart, degree of ventilator support) changes. The optimum DO_2 may vary as the patient's course of illness changes.
- Instead of using single values of DO_2 or CI as end points of resuscitation, individualize DO_2 to achieve normal values of traditional parameters (BP, HR, urine output), lactate levels, and SvO_2 levels. Additional monitoring of peripheral tissues is currently available such as gastrointestinal tonometry (23), transcutaneous pressure of O_2 ($PtcO_2$) and CO_2 ($PtcCO_2$) (24–26), and near-infrared spectroscopy (27). While orthogonal polarization spectral imaging of oral capillaries holds promise (28,29), further validation studies are needed.
- Do not expect information that the PAC was not designed to give. Central pressure may not give accurate information about the intravascular volume (30). Central and global values such as DO_2 and SvO_2 may not reflect adequate oxygenation state or cellular viability and function in all the tissue beds.

INDICATIONS FOR PULMONARY ARTERY CATHETER INSERTION

Indications for PAC insertion (Table 18.1) have been broadly categorized to (a) precautionary measures in high-risk patients, (b) shock states, (c) pulmonary problems, and (d) cardiac dysfunction.

Preoperative intervention of high-risk surgical patients using PACs remains a controversial area and recommendations are vague in the American College of Cardiology/American Heart Association (ACC/AHA) guidelines (2,31). The key points are as follows: insert the PAC with enough time to achieve the hemodynamic goals (usually the day before), communicate with the anesthesiologist regarding the information obtained while in the intensive care unit (ICU), and monitor the patient in the ICU beyond 24 hours to allow for fluid shifts to occur.

The goals of preoperative invasive monitoring are to (a) optimize preload (plot the Starling curve, see below); (b) optimize CI and stroke volume index (SVI) by adjusting preload, afterload, and contractility (possibly by using inotropes); (c) maintain DO_2 to perfuse the rest of the body and prevent MSOF; (d) perfuse the coronaries by maintaining coronary perfusion pressure (CPP) and DO_2; (e) decrease myocardial work and myocardial oxygen consumption (MVO_2) by keeping systolic blood pressure and heart rate normal; and (f) prevent myocardial infarct by avoiding wide swings (>15%) in heart rate and blood pressure (21,32,33). Further details in utilization of PACs for treatment of high-risk patients, shock, and cardiopulmonary failure are covered in other chapters.

The PAC is inserted to obtain information beyond the physical exam. Clinical predictors of hemodynamic status in the critically ill patient, such as chest radiograph, jugulovenous distention, and urine output, are inaccurate (1,34). Physicians are correctly able to predict PAOP and CI only 30% to 70% of the time. With insertion of the PAC, four types of information may be obtained:

1. Central pressures in relationship to the right ventricle (i.e., central venous pressure [CVP] or right atrial [RA] pressure); central pressures in relationship to the left ventricle (i.e., PAOP to estimate left ventricular end-diastolic pressure [LVEDP])
2. Cardiac function measured as cardiac output and presented as cardiac index
3. SvO_2
4. Intrapulmonary shunt (Qs/Qt)

General Considerations

The technical aspects of PAC insertion are presented in "Vascular Cannulation." It is essential that the catheter be positioned and transduced properly, and a knowledgeable clinician must be able to correctly interpret the data (18,35,36). Physicians should understand the basic physical principles involved in catheterization, know the design of the catheter, and be able to recognize and remedy technical errors.

Although the modern PAC has features that weren't available when it was introduced, the general principles of placement have not changed. If the PAC has fiberoptic bundles at the tip for continuous SvO_2 monitoring, external *in vitro* calibration is done prior to removing the catheter tip from the casing. The PAC is then flushed to assess the patency of its lumens and to fill the catheter with a noncompressible column of fluid capable of transmitting pressures. There is a distal port for monitoring the pulmonary artery pressures (PAPs) and a central port approximately 30 cm from the tip that will lie in the right atrium in the average-size heart. For cardiac output monitoring, a thermistor is located proximal to the tip to measure temperature changes (discussed below). The catheter is placed through the protective sheath and the balloon is checked for integrity prior to insertion. The transducer is placed at the level of the patient's midaxillary line and zeroed to atmospheric pressure (phlebostatic point). If the transducer elevates above the patient level, the readings will be falsely low. Conversely, if the transducer falls below the patient level, the readings will be falsely high. This is typically noted in beds that are designed to rotate patients.

PRESSURE MEASUREMENTS

Normal hemodynamic values are presented in Table 18.2.

Pressure changes in the heart or vessels cause movement of the catheter, which is then converted to an electrical signal by a transducer (37). Electrical noise is filtered and the signal is amplified and displayed as a tracing on a monitor. Before insertion, the function of the system is checked by shaking the catheter and seeing good waveforms on the monitor. If the waveform is dampened, the system should be flushed to rid the catheter and tubings of all air bubbles, and all connections should be tightened. After inserting the PAC 15 to 20 cm into the introducer in the vein, the balloon is inflated and the catheter is gently advanced. The natural flow of blood from the vena cava

TABLE 18.2

NORMAL HEMODYNAMIC VALUES

Hemodynamic parameter	Normal range
Systolic blood pressure	100–140 mm Hg
Diastolic blood pressure	60–90 mm Hg
Mean arterial pressure (MAP)	70–105 mm Hg
Heart rate	60–100 beats/min
Right atrial (RA) or central venous pressure (CVP)	0–8 mm Hg
Right ventricle systolic pressure	15–30 mm Hg
Right ventricular diastolic pressure	0–8 mm Hg
Pulmonary artery (PA) systolic pressure	15–30 mm Hg
PA diastolic pressure	4–12 mm Hg
Mean PA	9–16 mm Hg
Pulmonary artery occlusion pressure (PAOP, wedge)	6–12 mm Hg
Left atrial pressure (LAP)	6–12 mm Hg
Cardiac output (L/min)	Varies with patient size
Cardiac index (L/min/m^2)	2.8–4.2 L/min/m^2
Right ventricular ejection fraction (RVEF)	40%–60%
Right ventricular end-diastolic volume indexed to body surface area (RVEDVI)	60–100 mL/m^2
Hemoglobin	12–16 g/dL
Arterial oxygen tension (PaO_2)	70–100 mm Hg
Arterial oxygen saturation	93%–98%
Mixed venous oxygen tension (PvO_2)	36–42 mm Hg
Mixed venous oxygen saturation (SvO_2)	70%–75%

through the heart and to the lungs guides the catheter to the pulmonary vasculature (38). While passing from the vena cava to a branch of the pulmonary artery, characteristic waveforms are displayed on the monitor (Fig. 18.1). Once the catheter is advanced to the "wedged" position, the balloon is deflated and the catheter adjusted until 1.25 to 1.5 mL of inflation is needed to produce the PAOP tracing. The balloon should only be inflated long enough to record a measurement in order to avoid rupture of the artery or infarction of the downstream segment of lung. The balloon should always be deflated when withdrawing the catheter to avoid vascular and valvular injury. The catheter should coil gently in the right ventricle (RV) and sit in a larger branch of the pulmonary artery (Fig. 18.2).

A chest radiograph is done to assess for pneumothorax and may help to confirm proper position. If there is not an obvious wedge tracing, blood may be sampled from the distal port with the balloon inflated, after discarding about 15 mL from the distal port. The sample should have a higher PaO_2 and pH with a lower PCO_2 than blood aspirated when the balloon is deflated (39). Proper placement is also indicated by the SvO_2 signal quality (if using a fiberoptic catheter), which is displayed in different ways by different manufacturers. The quality of the signal may be altered by a fibrin clot at the tip of the catheter or by placement of the tip against a vessel wall and may suggest that the catheter is in too far or that the patient is hypovolemic with collapse of the vessel wall around the catheter tip. If the

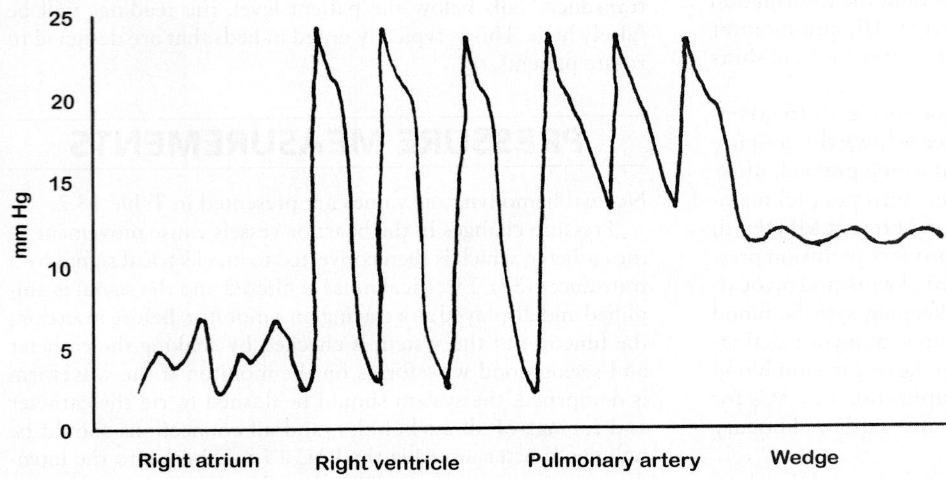

FIGURE 18.1. Waveforms seen during pulmonary artery catheter insertion.

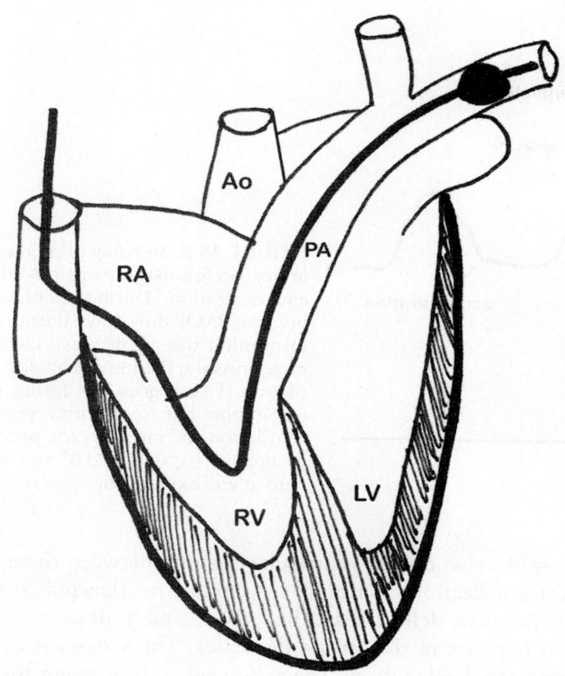

FIGURE 18.2. Proper position of the pulmonary artery catheter. RA, right atrium; RV, right ventricle; PA, pulmonary artery; LV, left ventricle; AO, aorta.

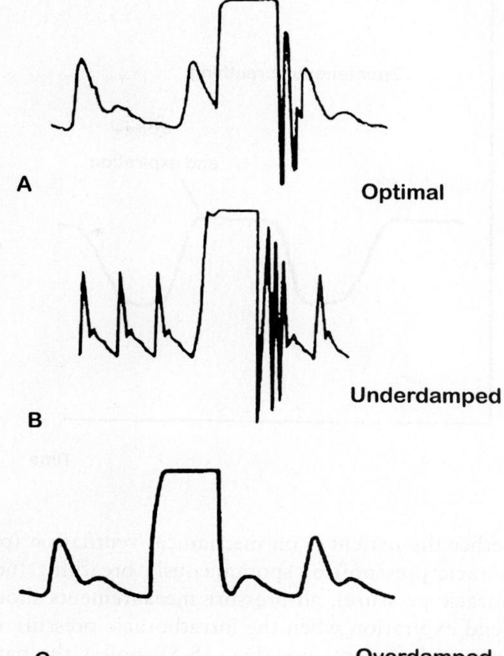

FIGURE 18.4. Checking transducer reliability by the "fast flush square wave testing."

catheter is in too far, the PAOP tracing will continue to elevate and is called "overwedging" (Fig. 18.3). If this occurs, the balloon should be deflated and the catheter pulled back (≅1 cm) and the balloon inflated again until a good tracing is seen with 1.25 to 1.5 mL of balloon inflation.

Because there is a tendency for materials to oscillate at their natural frequencies, the pressure signal may be distorted (40). This effect may be reduced by using stiff, noncompliant tubing and the shortest length (<4 feet) in the setup of the catheter and monitoring system. The loss of transmitted signal is referred to as damping, and catheters may be over- or underdamped. The degree of damping can be determined by a "fast flush" device (Fig. 18.4). When the catheter is rapidly flushed, a square wave is produced, followed by a series of oscillations before the tracing returns to the baseline pressure reading (41). The appearance of the oscillations demonstrates the degree of damping. Underdamping, which occurs more frequently, is identified by several sharp oscillations and produces higher systolic pressure readings (Fig. 18.4B). Overdamping results in a rounded oscillation and results in lower readings, and may be due to clots, air bubbles, or kinking in the catheter (Fig. 18.4C). Another factor that may interfere with the signal is catheter whip, which results from contraction of the heart. The tracing will show high-frequency distortion. This may be minimized by a high-frequency filter built into the transducer system (40).

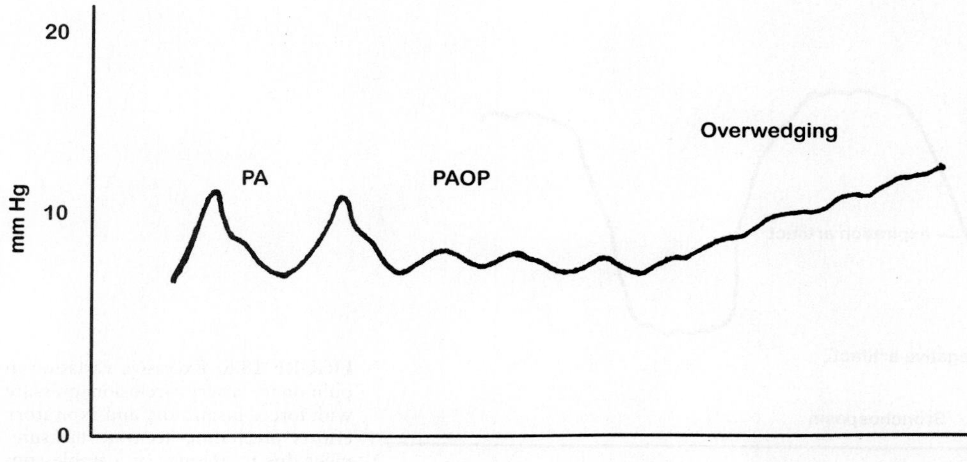

FIGURE 18.3. Overwedged tracing. PA, pulmonary artery; PAOP, pulmonary artery occlusion pressure.

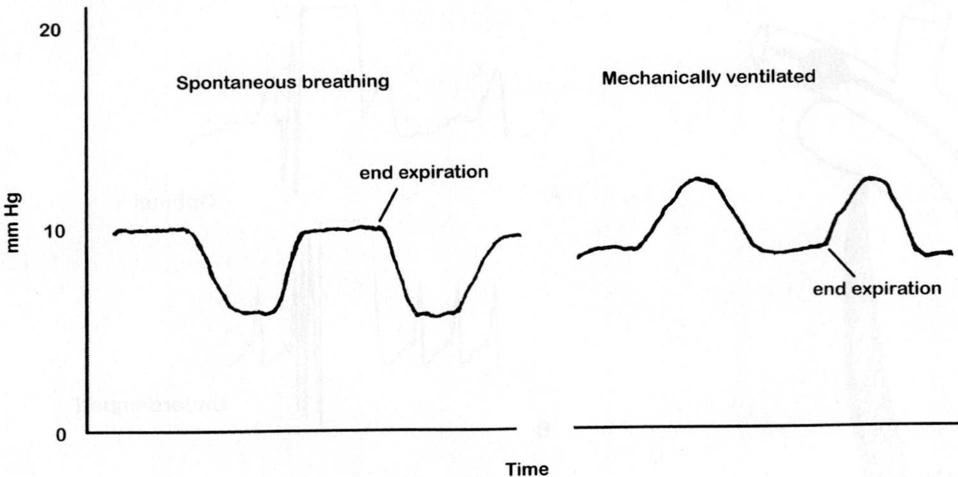

FIGURE 18.5. Reading of pulmonary artery occlusion pressure (PAOP) at end expiration. During spontaneous breaths, PAOP dips down during peak inspiration due to negative intrathoracic pressure. During mechanical ventilation, PAOP goes up during peak inspiration due to positive pressure ventilation and intrathoracic pressure. In both situations, PAOP should be read at end expiration.

Whether the patient is on mechanical ventilation (positive intrathoracic pressure) or spontaneously breathing (negative intrathoracic pressure), all pressure measurements should occur at end expiration when the intrathoracic pressure is closest to atmospheric pressure (Fig. 18.5) (unless the patient is on higher levels of positive end-expiratory pressure [PEEP]). This point can be determined by watching the patient's respiratory movements or displaying the airway pressure tracing on the same monitor where the pulmonary artery pressure is displayed. If respiratory variation is so pronounced that there is no flat end expiration, then it is best NOT to record a number (Fig. 18.6). In this situation, patients may need to be sedated, or if getting a PAOP is crucial, even paralyzed. What is unacceptable is to "guess" what the number may be, leading to wrong conclusions and wrong treatment. *No* information is better than *wrong* information.

The first characteristic waveform seen when inserting a PAC is the right atrium (RA) tracing (Fig. 18.7). The tracing can be seen while inserting the catheter or by transducing the right atrial pressure once the PAC is in position. There are two main positive pressure deflections, called the a and v waves. The a wave follows the P wave of the electrocardiogram and is due to the pressure increase during atrial systole (Figs. 18.7 and 18.8). The v wave results from atrial filling against a closed tricuspid valve during ventricular systole. Between these two positive deflections is a small c wave due to tricuspid closure. Two negative deflections called the x and y descents occur when pressure in the atrium decreases. The x descent occurs during atrial relaxation. The y descent is seen when the tricuspid valve opens and blood flows from the atrium to the ventricle.

The best estimate of CVP and PAOP is at end diastole when the atrium contracts. For CVP, where the c wave emerges from the a wave (also called the z-point) is the optimum reading point. If this point is not clear, read the pressure at the middle of the x descent. Certain patterns in the RA tracing may be seen in disease states (Fig. 18.7). a waves may not be seen in patients with atrial fibrillation. Sawtoothed a waves will be present during atrial flutter. Large a, or "cannon" waves occur during atrioventricular (A-V) dissociation when the atrium contracts against a closed valve, or during complete heart block. A steep y descent is seen in tricuspid regurgitation and the x descent is not apparent. Both descents are prominent in RV infarction. Tamponade tends to cause loss of the y descent due to impairment of ventricular filling. In pericarditis, sharp a and v waves are followed by steep x and y descents. Large v waves are seen in mitral regurgitation, congestive heart failure, and ventricular septal defect due to the increase in atrial pressure. Recognizing

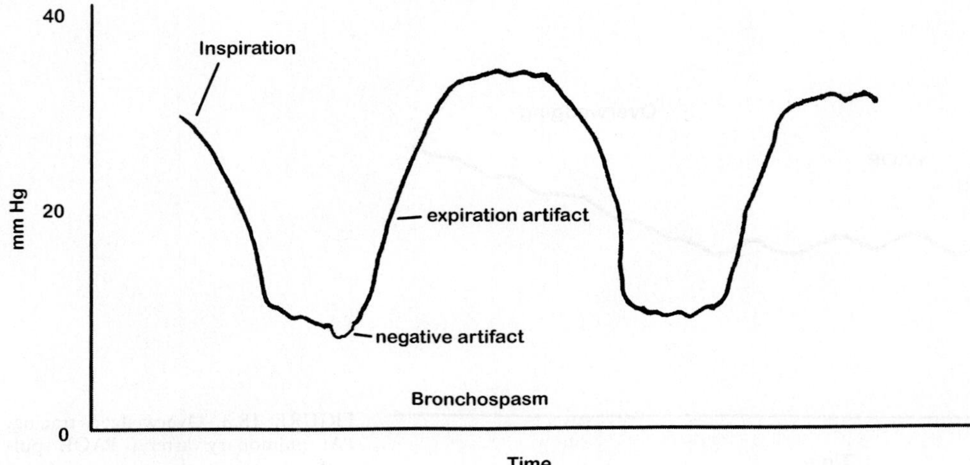

FIGURE 18.6. Excessive variation in pulmonary artery occlusion pressure with forced inspiratory and expiratory efforts precluding accurate measurement due to absence of a stable end-expiratory point.

A) Atrial Fibrillation

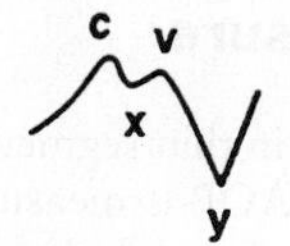

B) Atrial Flutter

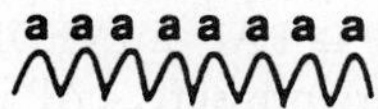

C) Complete AV Block

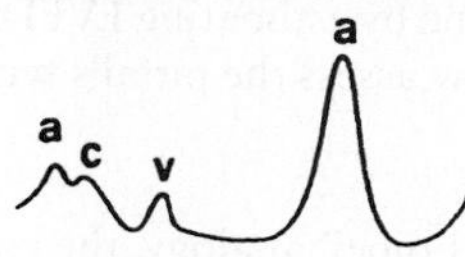

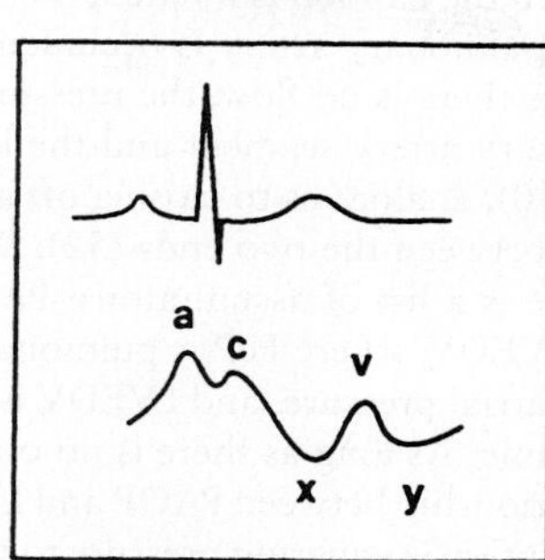

D) Tricuspid Regurgitation

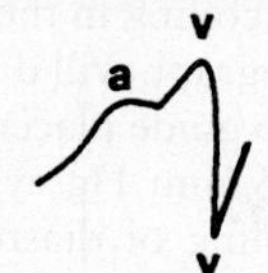

E) Pericardial Tamponade

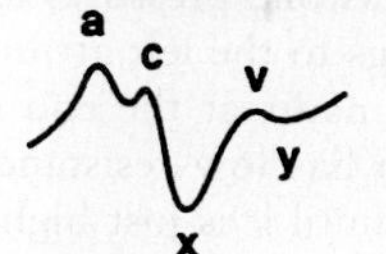

F) Constrictive Pericarditis

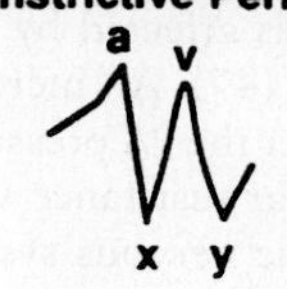

FIGURE 18.7. Pressure tracings from the right atrial port in normal and pathologic conditions (refer to text).

these patterns may help to suggest a diagnosis before a confirmatory echocardiogram is obtained.

The pressures observed in the right atrium range from 0 to 8 mm Hg. Higher pressures may not necessarily mean fluid overload, but reflect the volume of the right heart and the ability of the ventricle to eject that volume. There is little relationship between CVP and PAOP or left heart pressures in patients with valvular or coronary artery disease or when pulmonary artery pressures are elevated (42,43). It is in these situations of right heart failure, severe pulmonary disease, and in most of the critically ill patients when monitoring the CVP only (and not the PAOP) would be misleading.

The next waveform seen is that of the right ventricle (Fig. 18.1). The pressures here are higher with a wider difference between systolic and diastolic. If no RV waveform is seen after inserting the catheter 30 cm from the internal jugular or subclavian vein entry site, the catheter may be curling in the atrium or passing into the inferior vena cava. The catheter should be quickly advanced through the ventricle both to avoid dysrhythmias and to keep the catheter from warming and losing its stiffness. The RV systolic pressures generally range from 15 to 30 mm Hg and diastolic pressures from 4 to 12 mm Hg. In right heart failure, the RV diastolic pressures may be high enough that the waveform mimics the PA. Low RV pressures will be seen in hypovolemic shock and they will also be close to PA pressures. One concern at this point of insertion is causing a right bundle branch block (RBBB), or even complete heart block in patients with pre-existing left bundle branch block (LBBB) (44). However, the incidence of complete heart block appears to be no greater in patients with LBBB than without (45).

Once the catheter enters the pulmonary artery, the waveform shows an increase in diastolic pressure while the systolic pressure remains about the same as in the ventricle, sometimes referred to as the "step up" (Fig. 18.1). This transition may be difficult to discern when there is hypovolemia, tamponade,

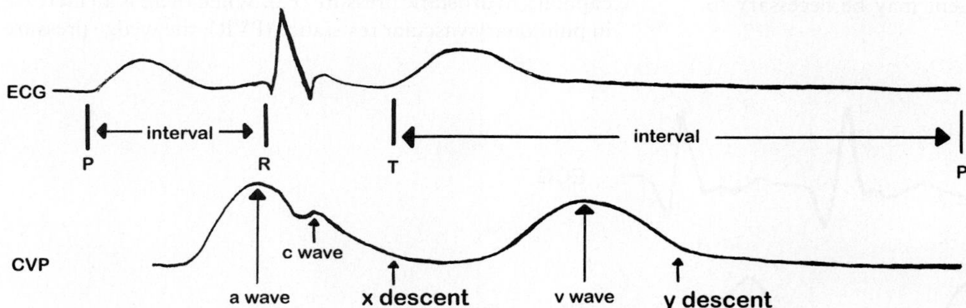

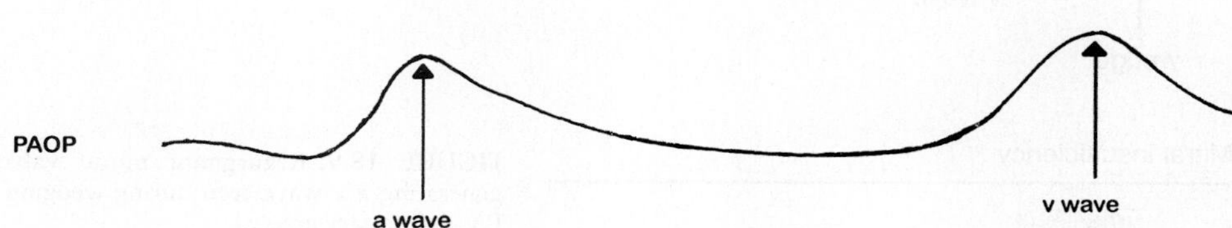

FIGURE 18.8. Reading of central venous pressure (CVP) and pulmonary artery occlusion pressure (PAOP) in relationship to the cardiac cycle (electrocardiogram).

RV failure, or catheter whip. If there is no change in waveform after inserting the catheter 50 cm, it may be coiling in the ventricle and is at risk of knotting. A chest radiograph will discern the problem and fluoroscopy may be used to guide placement. Normal PA pressures range from 15 to 25 mm Hg systolic over 8 to 15 mm Hg diastolic. The beginning of diastole is marked by a dicrotic notch on the PA tracing, corresponding to the closure of the pulmonic valve (46). This incisura distinguishes the PA from the RV when RV diastolic pressures are elevated. As blood flows through the lungs to the left atrium, the PA pressure drops until it reaches a nadir at the end of diastole. Since the pulmonary circulation has low resistance, the diastolic pressure is able to decrease until it is just higher than PAOP. The highest PA systolic pressure occurs during the T wave of the corresponding electrocardiogram (ECG). The pulmonary circulation is very dynamic and is affected by acidosis, hypoxia, sepsis, and vasoactive drugs (47). An increase in CO may also seemingly paradoxically lower the PA pressures by a reflexive decrease in pulmonary vascular resistance with fluid resuscitation and decreased sympathetic nervous system discharge (48).

The transition to the wedge position is noted by a drop in mean pressure from the PA. The PAOP usually ranges from 6 to 12 mm Hg in normal states. PAOP most closely reflects LVEDP after atrial contraction and before ventricular contraction (Fig. 18.8). There are often no clear a, c, or v waves. The point 0.05 seconds after onset of QRS of the ECG is where the pressure best estimates LVEDP (49). When v waves are prominent such as in mitral insufficiency, the bottom of the v wave or the a wave may be used to measure the PAOP (Fig. 18.9). A prominent v wave may fool the novice into thinking that the catheter is not wedging. It is important to note the change in wave form from PA to v wave tracing (although the two waves may look remarkably similar). One way of differentiation is that the v wave occurs later in the ECG cycle after the T wave while the PA wave occurs right after QRS (Fig. 18.9). There may be large a waves secondary to a decrease in left ventricle compliance (50); the point 0.05 seconds after initiation of QRS again best reflects LVEDP. Even though the measurements are correlated with the ECG and are done during end expiration, the PAOP may be exaggerated by respiratory muscle activity, especially during active or labored exhalation. Once the patient is adequately sedated, a short-acting paralyzing agent may be necessary to eliminate this effect (51) (Fig. 18.6).

Principles of Measuring Pulmonary Artery Occlusion Pressure

When the balloon is inflated, the blood flow in that segment of the pulmonary artery is occluded and the PAOP is measured. Since there is no flow, the pressure between the occluded pulmonary artery segment and the left atrium will equalize (Fig. 18.10), analogous to closing off a pipe with pressures equalizing between the two ends (52). With the closed pipe analogy, there is a list of assumptions: PAOP ≅ PcP ≅ LAP ≅ LVEDP ≅ LVEDV, where PcP is pulmonary capillary pressure, LAP is left atrial pressure, and LVEDV is left ventricular end-diastolic volume. As long as there is no obstruction in this conduit, the relationship between PAOP and LVEDP may hold. The final assumption is equating pressure to volume by estimating LVEDV or "preload" with LVEDP. We will now assess the pitfalls with each one of these assumptions.

1. PAOP ≅ PcP ≅ LAP. In the "closed pipe" analogy, the column of blood between the catheter tip and the left atrium should be patent and not narrowed by alveolar pressures. This occurs in the dependent areas of the lung, where the pressures from blood flow in the right atrium and pulmonary artery are greater than the alveolar pressure, or zone 3 in the West classification (53). In other areas of the lung (zone 1 or 2), the pulmonary arteries may collapse from higher alveolar pressures and the wedge pressure may partially reflect alveolar pressure (Fig. 18.11). Because the PAC is directed by blood flow, it is more likely to pass into zone 3, where pulmonary arterial and venous pressures exceed alveolar pressures. This is especially true when the patient is supine, since there is greater volume of lung located in a dependent position (54). When pulmonary artery diastolic pressure is lower than the PAOP, this implies incorrect positioning of the PAC (i.e., blood cannot flow in reverse direction), and may be due to transmission of alveolar pressures on the PAOP in non–zone 3 catheter position. Other factors that may cause errors in estimation of PAOP to LAP are pulmonary venous obstruction and respiratory variation as well as high ventilator support (PAOP reads higher than LAP).

   The PAOP usually closely approximates the pulmonary capillary hydrostatic pressure (Pc). When there is an increase in pulmonary vascular resistance (PVR), the wedge pressure

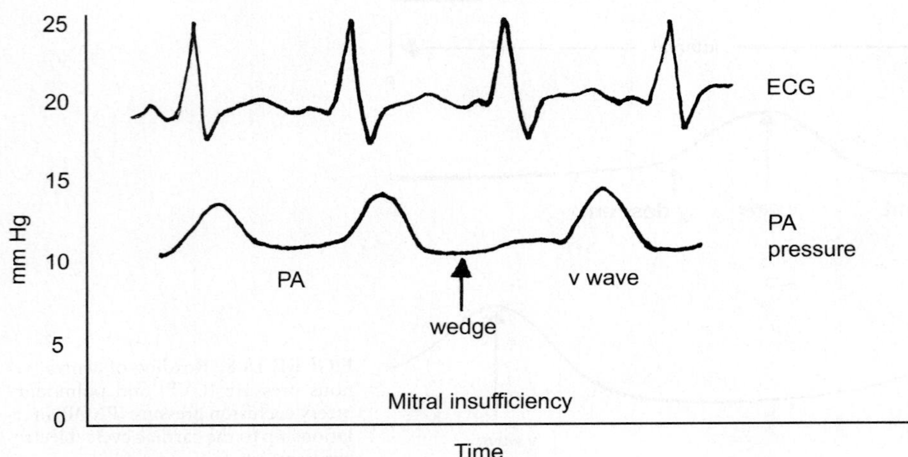

FIGURE 18.9. Regurgitant mitral valve generating a v wave seen during wedging. PA, pulmonary artery.

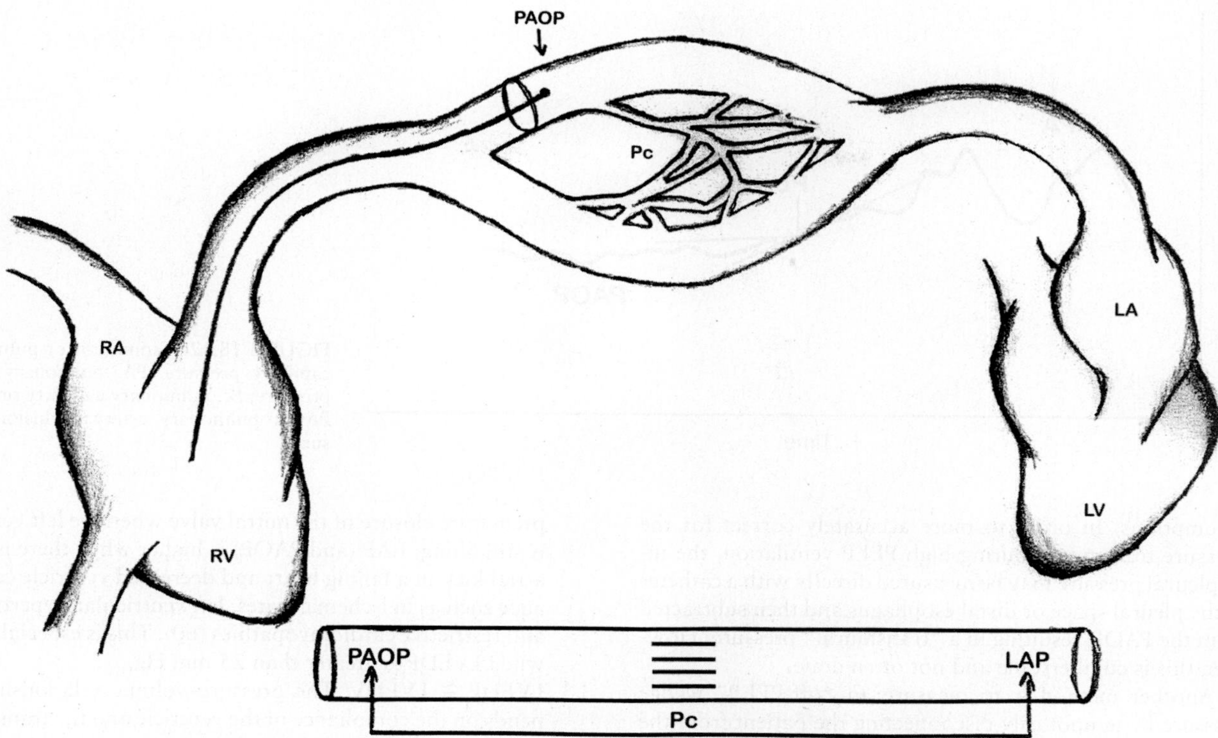

FIGURE 18.10. Closed pipe analogy: blocking of flow by the balloon with theoretical equalization of pressure in the conduit. RA, right atrium; RV, right ventricle; PAOP, pulmonary artery occlusion pressure; Pc, pulmonary capillary; LAP, left atrial pressure; LV, left ventricle.

underestimates Pc. A difference of 2 to 3 mm Hg between the PAOP and pulmonary artery diastolic (PAD) pressure is a clue that there may be a discrepancy between PAOP and Pc (35). Hydrostatic pulmonary edema may therefore occur at lower wedge pressures. A method of calculating the Pc has been described by recording the rapid drop in pressure decline when the catheter balloon is inflated in the wedge position (55). The point where the rapid decline transitions to a more gradual slope before reaching the PAOP is the Pc (Fig. 18.12).

Increased intrathoracic pressure secondary to respiratory failure and the addition of PEEP in ventilated patients affects pulmonary vascular pressures. Up to about 15 cm H_2O, PAOP closely correlates with LAP (56). During higher PEEP states, the PAOP may not reflect the true filling pressure of the heart (i.e., pressure outside minus pressure inside the heart). Although the heart is seeing the high PEEP support at all times, on-PEEP PAOP is *not* giving the information that we need from the PAOP, which is the cardiac filling pressure. In general, 5 cm H_2O of PEEP is said to raise the measured PAOP by 1 mm Hg, but a greater effect is seen in hypovolemic patients or when the catheter is not in West zone 3 (57). High PEEP may also turn zone 3 status to zone 2 or 1 by compressing the pulmonary artery and/or pulmonary vein. Another formula predicts that 50% of PEEP is transmitted to the pleural space (54). However, in noncompliant lungs, such as in the acute respiratory distress syndrome, the alveolar pressure is not effectively transmitted to the vasculature. Also, pulmonary disease is not homogeneous. In complicated cases, it is best to avoid formulas or

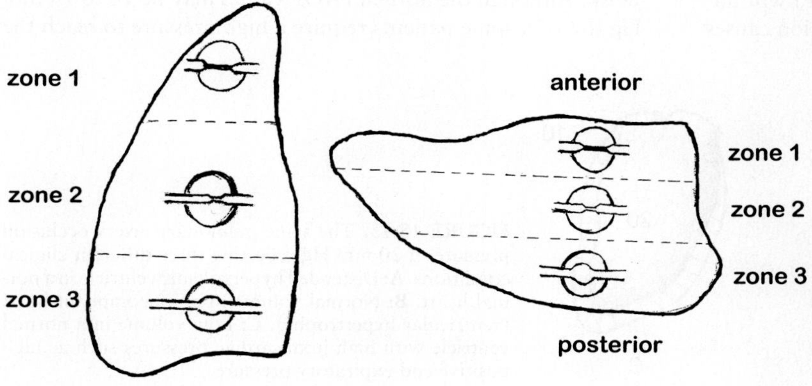

FIGURE 18.11. West's lung zones. PAP, pulmonary arterial pressure; PalvP, pulmonary alveolar pressure; PvP, pulmonary venous pressure. Zone 1: PAP <PalvP> PvP (there is no blood flow across the collapsed pulmonary capillary bed). Zone 2: PAP > PalvP > PvP (there is some flow since PAP is greater than PalvP). Zone 3: PAP > PalvP < PvP (pulmonary arteries are patent).

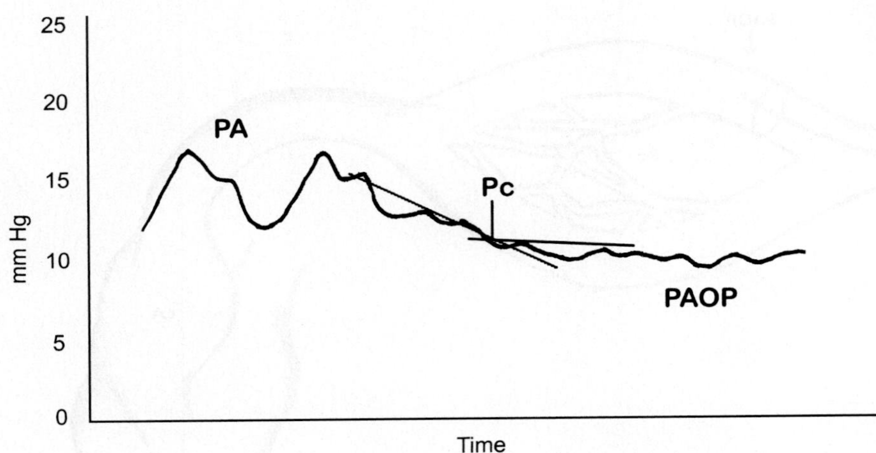

FIGURE 18.12. Estimation of pulmonary capillary pressure. PA, pulmonary artery pressure; Pc, pulmonary capillary pressure; PAOP, pulmonary artery occlusion pressure.

assumptions. In order to more accurately correct for the pressure transmitted during high PEEP ventilation, the intrapleural pressure may be measured directly with a catheter in the pleural space or distal esophagus and then subtracted from the PAOP, resulting in a "transmural" pressure. However, this is cumbersome and not often done.

Another method is to measure an "off-PEEP" wedge pressure by temporarily disconnecting the patient from the ventilator circuit and recording the nadir of the tracing (58). This nadir pressure better reflects LAP than the on-PEEP PAOP. The discontinuation should be brief (<1 second) so that a decrease in PaO_2 from derecruitment of alveoli does not occur (59). The brief off-PEEP state will not change physiologic conditions such as venous return and cardiac function. The procedure should be coordinated and done by trained personnel only when the PAOP is needed to make a clinical decision. The balloon is inflated first to ensure good position, then deflated. The FiO_2 may be increased temporarily for patient safety, the balloon reinflated, and at end expiration, the patient is disconnected from the ventilator for 1 second and then reconnected while the PAOP tracing is being recorded. The drop in PAOP upon ventilator disconnection is the off-PEEP PAOP (58). When done properly, it is extremely rare to cause hypoxia.

2. LAP ≅ LVEDP. LAP (and thus PAOP) will overestimate LVEDP if there is an obstruction between the left atrium and the left ventricle such as a myxoma or mitral stenosis. Mitral valve regurgitation also causes the PAOP to read higher than the true LVEDP because of the additional pressure of the retrograde flow of blood across the valve resulting in a large v wave (see above). LAP (and thus PAOP) will underestimate LVEDP when severe aortic regurgitation causes premature closure of the mitral valve when the left ventricle is still filling. LAP (and PAOP) is higher when there is a left atrial kick in a failing heart and decreased ventricle compliance such as in ischemic states, left ventricular hypertrophy, and restrictive cardiomyopathies (60). This is especially true when LVEDP is greater than 25 mm Hg.
3. LVEDP ≅ LVEDV. The pressure–volume relationship depends on the compliance of the ventricle and the transmural ventricular distending force. The compliance of the ventricles will change with ischemia, infarct, and hypertrophy. A stiff heart (myocardial hypertrophy) will need higher pressures to obtain the same amount of volume as a normal heart (Fig. 18.13). The transmural ventricular distending force (intracavitary pressure minus juxtacardiac pressure) will depend on the pressure inside and outside the heart. External forces elevating juxtacardiac pressures may be high ventilator support or pericardial tamponade, which may cause elevation of PAOP but may not reflect ventricular filling pressure.

Clinical Use of the Pulmonary Artery Occlusion Pressure

As long as the previously mentioned assumptions regarding the relationship between PAOP, LAP, and LVEDP have been evaluated, the PAOP may be used as an estimate of LAP with reasonable correlation (52,61). The optimum wedge pressure depends on the patient, but has been defined as the pressure where there is minimal increase in stroke volume or left ventricular stroke work. Although the normal PAOP values may be 10 to 14 mm Hg (62,63), some patients require a high pressure to reach the

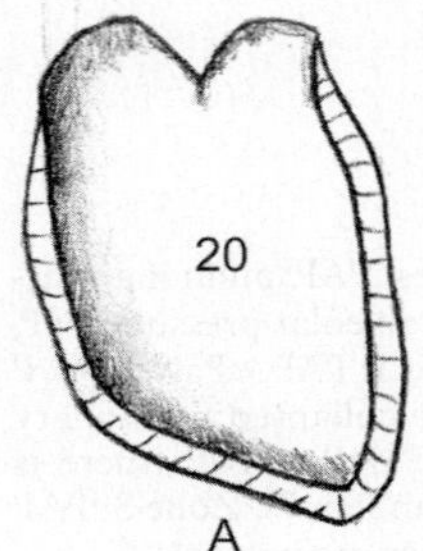

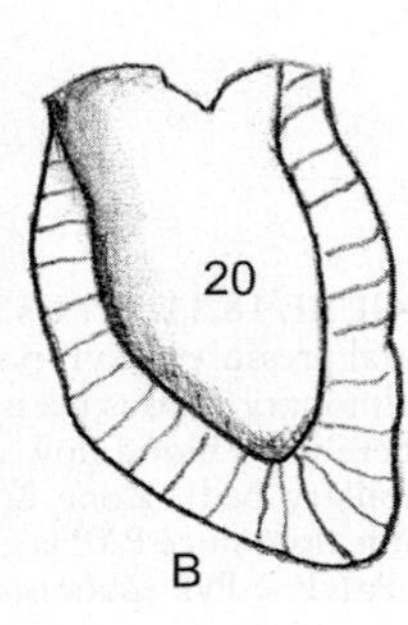

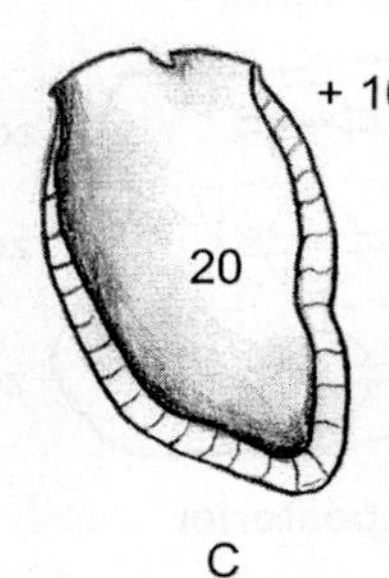

FIGURE 18.13. The same pulmonary artery occlusion pressure of 20 mm Hg reflecting three different clinical conditions. **A:** Distended hypervolemic ventricle in a normal heart. **B:** Normal volume in a noncompliant heart (ventricular hypertrophy). **C:** Low volume in a normal ventricle with high juxtacardiac pressures such as high positive end-expiratory pressure.

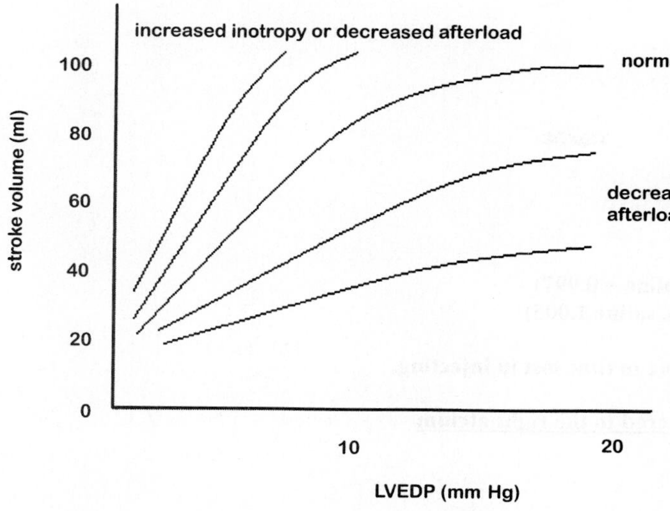

FIGURE 18.14. Frank-Starling curves (family of curves) showing the relationship between left ventricular end-diastolic pressure (LVEDP) to stroke volume (SV, mL/beat). Augmenting preload increases LVEDP with a concomitant increase in SV (up to a certain point). The effects of manipulating preload, afterload, and contractility and shifting to another curve can be seen.

optimum stroke volume (Fig. 18.14). The Starling curve plotting stroke volume index to PAOP (as an estimate of LVEDP) may help identify the optimum wedge but some patients may have a flat curve. If vasoactive agents are started, the heart may now be on a different curve requiring new assessment of the optimum PAOP. The optimum PAOP varies not only from patient to patient, but also temporally within the same patient as the clinical condition changes (such as vasoactive agents, myocardial compliance, and external forces around the heart). There are no set numbers to treat to, but each patient must be individually assessed and assessed *repeatedly,* making the PAC a highly user-dependent tool.

Elevated wedge pressures may help differentiate hydrostatic pulmonary edema from that caused by increased permeability. A PAOP of 24 mm Hg or higher is associated with a tendency for hydrostatic edema (64). Lower pressures may imply increased capillary permeability and traditionally, a PAOP of <18 mm Hg has implied a pulmonary (or noncardiogenic) cause of lung edema. When there is an increase in PVR, the wedge pressure underestimates Pc and hydrostatic pulmonary edema may therefore occur at lower wedge pressures (see Fig. 18.12).

Volumetric PACs are designed with the ability to measure right ventricular ejection fraction (RVEF), from which the right ventricular end-diastolic volume indexed (RVEDVI) to body surface area (BSA) is calculated. Traditionally, the right heart function was deemed unimportant and thought to merely act as a conduit to get blood to the left ventricle. However, right heart dysfunction with septal deviation may impact LV compliance and contractility, and the function of RV is important when pulmonary artery pressures are elevated. The volumetric PACs have two additional electrodes that provide continuous measurement of the ECG and a thermistor with a rapid response. From beat-to-beat change in temperature, the ejection fraction (EF) is calculated. EF (%) = SVI/EDVI × 100, where SVI is stroke volume indexed and EDVI is end-diastolic volume indexed to BSA. CI/HR = EDVI – ESVI, where ESVI is end-systolic volume indexed to BSA (65). RVEDVI has been shown to be a more accurate measure of cardiac preload than pressure measurements in certain patient populations (66,67). The measurement of RVEF has been validated by comparisons with transesophageal echocardiography (68). The RVEDVI in healthy individuals falls between 60 and 100 mL/m^2. The information obtained from the volumetric catheter has been used to predict response to fluid challenge when the values are relatively low (<90 mL/m^2) (66). The validity of the RVEF measurement is compromised by tachycardia (pulse >120 beats per minute) and atrial fibrillation (irregular heart rate) (69).

CARDIAC OUTPUT

The ability of the heart to meet increasing tissue oxygen demand is perhaps the single most important determinant in oxygen delivery and tissue perfusion. The evolution of cardiac output measurement started with Adolf Fick, who in the 1870s proposed that uptake or release of a substance by an organ is the product of blood flow through that organ and the difference between arterial and venous values of that substance. The original "dye" was oxygen and the organ studied was the lung. Fick's equation stated: $CO = VO_2/(CaO_2 - CvO_2)$, where VO_2 is oxygen consumption, CaO_2 is arterial content of O_2, and CvO_2 is mixed venous content of O_2.

This principle is widely accepted as an accurate though invasive assessment of cardiac output since a pulmonary artery catheter must be placed to obtain accurate mixed venous oxygen content. Its practical use is limited by the cumbersome measurement of oxygen consumption. Stewart (1897) and Hamilton (1932) utilized the concept but used a known amount of dye injected into central circulation followed by serial peripheral arterial measurements of dye concentration (i.e., change in dye concentration over time), and calculated the flow. The area under the curve after plotting time (x axis) versus dye concentration (y axis) reflected the cardiac output using the following equation: Cardiac output = Amount of dye injected/integral (dye concentration × function of time). The next revolutionary step in cardiac output measurement was using temperature as the dye. Crystalloid solution (usually 10 mL, but 5 mL may be used in volume-restricted patients) is injected into the RA port at similar parts of the respiratory cycle (end expiration), within 4 seconds in a smooth manner (70). The thermistor near the tip of the PAC detects the change in temperature,

Modified Stewart-Hamilton equation

$$Q = \frac{VI\,(TB - TI) \times SI \times CI \times 60 \times CT \times K}{SB \times CB \quad {}_0^{\infty}\int \Delta TB \; dt}$$

Q = Cardiac Output
VI = volume of injectate
TI = injectate temperature
TB = blood temperature
CI = specific heat of the injectate (D5W = 0.965, saline = 0.997)
SI = specific gravity of the injectate (D5W = 1.018, saline 1.005)
60 = seconds/minute
CT = correction factor (loss of thermal indicator due to time lost in injecting, catheter length, patient's temperature)

$$= \frac{\text{TB – mean temperature of the injectate delivered to the right atrium}}{\text{TB – TI (pre-injectate temperature)}}$$

SB = specific gravity of blood (1.045)
CB = specific heat of the blood (0.87)

${}_0^{\infty}\int \Delta TB \; dt$ = integral of blood temperature change

$$\text{Computation constant (K)} = \frac{SI \times CI \times 60 \times CT \times VI}{SB \times CB} = \text{changes with VI}$$

FIGURE 18.15. The modified Stewart-Hamilton equation for estimating cardiac output.

and the change in blood temperature over time is proportional to the blood flow from the ventricle. Several measurements (three to five) should be taken and the average of the values (within 10% of each other) used. Principles of the modified Stewart-Hamilton equation calculate the cardiac output (Fig. 18.15).

Although initial studies used iced solutions as injectates, ambient temperature injectate is now the standard solution used with excellent reproducibility and correlation with iced injection (71) and has less likelihood of reflexive bradycardia (72). It is important to note that iced injectates (0°C to 5°C) are associated with higher reproducibility and the highest signal-to-noise ratio (73) and may be necessary in hypothermic patients. Falsely low CO will occur if an error in the system increases the change in temperature (which is in the denominator of the Stewart-Hamilton equation): the temperature probe reading the injectate is cooler than the actual injectate (or the solution is warmer than the temperature reading of the injectate), more than allotted "dye" amount is injected (>10 mL fluid), there is too rapid an injection, or the injection occurs during positive pressure ventilation. Falsely high CO may occur if the temperature probe measuring injectate reads warmer than the actual injectate (if the solution is cooler than the temperature reading of the injectate), less than the allotted amount of "dye" (<10 mL) is used, or the catheter has migrated distally with less change in temperature difference. Most institutions use temperature probes at the site of injection (RA port) so that variations in injectate temperature should not contribute to errors in CO measurements.

Another development in the evolution of measuring CO is the PAC with continuous cardiac output (CCO) monitoring (74,75). A heat element is embedded in the PAC to deliver small pulsations of heat, which is detected by a rapid-response thermistor placed distally to the heat source. The change in temperature detected is then used to calculate cardiac output. Although there is no gold standard for measuring CO at the bedside, CCO values are reproducible and close to manual CO measurements, although discrepancies are observed at extremely low-flow states (74). Unlike the manual injection of crystalloid, the measurements are done at random parts of the respiratory cycle and are less subject to human error, which may account for some of the differences in the two techniques. A word of caution is that the CCO value may not change instantly when the cardiac output changes (e.g., with titration of inotropes), but the effect of treatment can be seen in seconds if using a continuous SvO_2 monitor. Due to the heat-generating wire coil in the distal end, these catheters must be removed before magnetic resonance imaging.

Starling Curves (Fig. 18.14)

Drs. Frank and Starling described the relationship between myocardial stretch and contractility. Myocardial stretch is an independent determinant of stroke work and the actin–myosin interaction has a linear correlation with the strength of systolic contraction up to a certain point. Given the heart's dynamic environment, a family of curves is more representative of the true preload–to–stroke volume relationship. Increasing afterload or decreasing contractility shifts the curve down and to the right (i.e., more stretch is necessary to produce a similar difference in stroke volume). One cannot stress enough the importance of reassessment after each therapy. For example, initiating afterload reduction may put the heart on a different Starling curve (to the left and up, Fig. 18.14), but may decrease the preload. Unless more fluid is given to optimize the LVEDP (i.e., PAOP), the best stroke volume may not be achieved.

MIXED VENOUS OXYGEN SATURATION (SEE CHAPTER ON VENOUS OXIMETRY)

Specialized PACs with the ability to measure mixed venous oxygen saturation (SvO_2) continuously using principles of reflection spectrophotometry are available (Fig. 18.16). Oxygen saturation is the ratio of hemoglobin bound to O_2 divided by total hemoglobin, and when measured at the tip of the PAC, reflects mixing of deoxygenated blood from superior and inferior vena cavae and coronary vessels. The SvO_2 value indicates the balance between oxygen delivery to the tissues and the amount consumed by the tissues before returning to the heart.

Rearranging the Fick Equation

$$SvO_2(\%) =$$

$$SaO_2 - \frac{VO_2}{CO\,(L/min) \times Hgb\,(g/dL) \times 1.36\,(mLO_2/g\,Hgb) \times 10}$$

Four factors determine the SvO_2 value: three parameters contributing to oxygen delivery (CO, hemoglobin, and SaO_2), and one parameter for O_2 consumption. Low SVO_2 suggests insufficient O_2 delivery or increased O_2 consumption. SVO_2 is also a harbinger of shock and may decrease before overt shock is apparent (14,15,25,76). Mixed venous oxygen saturation has also regained popularity as an end goal of resuscitation with decreased mortality (7,77–79). Inadequate oxygen delivery can be the result of decreased cardiac output, low hemoglobin, or low oxygen saturation. Increased consumption may occur due to activity, fever, hyperthyroid state, or repayment of oxygen debt. High SvO_2 suggests low cellular consumption such as in late sepsis, arteriovenous shunts (cirrhosis), or excessive inotrope use. Hypothermia, sedation, paralysis, anesthesia, hypothyroidism, and cyanide poisoning can also reduce VO_2. The catheter should also be checked to ensure that distal migration has not occurred leading to sampling of pulmonary capillary blood that is normally highly saturated (~100%). Inflating the balloon (wedging) should determine that the catheter is in too far if the PAOP tracing is seen with <1.25 mL of air.

Calibration by lab oximeter on a daily basis is important to check for drifting and whenever the values do not seem to correlate with the patient's clinical condition. Even if the PAC does not have continuous SvO_2 monitoring, SvO_2 can be checked by sending a blood sample from the distal PA port (by drawing slowly at the rate of 1 mL over 20 seconds to prevent sampling of pulmonary capillary blood) and sending it to the lab for oximeter analysis (direct saturation measurement and not arterial blood gas [ABG] analysis). If the PAC has continuous SvO_2 monitoring, a signal quality indicator is generated. If the signal intensity suggests poor quality, errors include (a) that PAC is in too far, (b) there are fibrin clots around the tip, (c) the catheter is touching the vessel wall, or (d) the patient may be hypovolemic. Repositioning the PAC or flushing the PA port may resolve this issue.

INTRAPULMONARY SHUNT (QS/QT)

Shunt refers to the portion (in %) of blood that flows (CO) from the right side of the heart to the left completely deoxygenated (Fig. 18.17). We will not discuss cardiac shunts in this chapter. Physiologic shunt = Anatomic shunt + Intrapulmonary shunt. Anatomic shunt refers to the direct drainage of the venous system to the left ventricle through the bronchial, thebesian, and pleural veins (~2%–5% of CO). Intrapulmonary shunt (Qs/Qt) is expressed as the % of cardiac output passing through completely collapsed alveoli with no or little gas exchange so that the ventilation-to-perfusion ratio is zero (i.e., $V/Q = 0$).

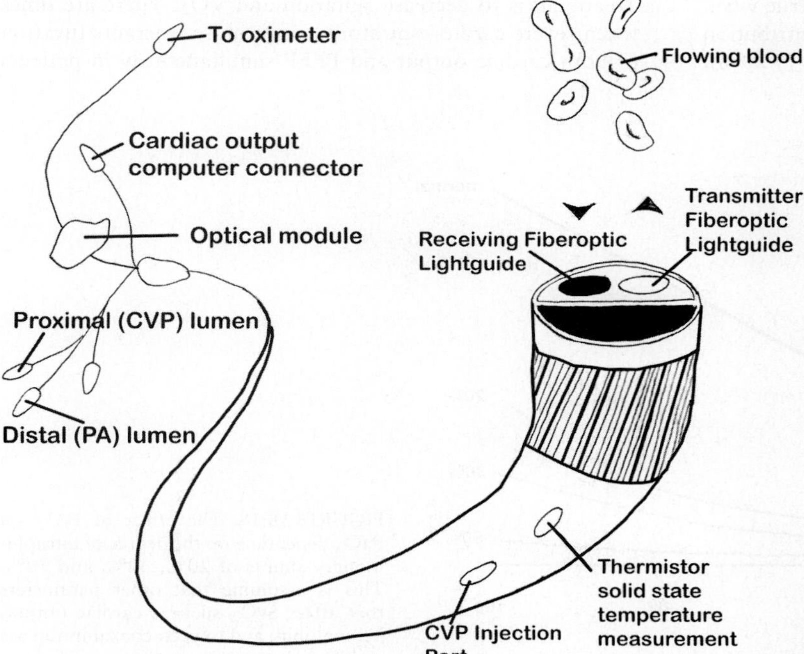

FIGURE 18.16. Fiberoptic catheter using principles of spectrophotometry.

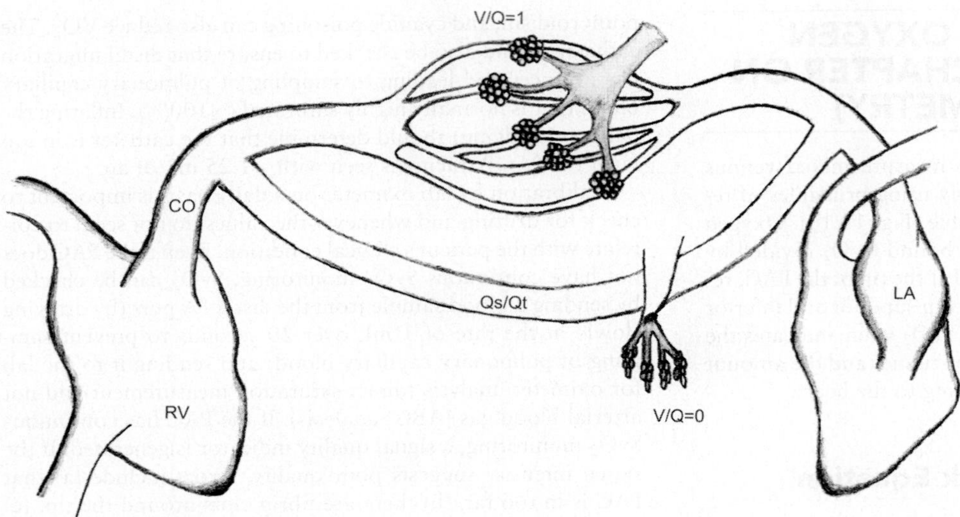

FIGURE 18.17. Intrapulmonary shunt (Qs/Qt) is the percent of cardiac output (CO) not involved with gas exchange (goes through collapsed alveoli), with ventilation/perfusion V/Q = O. LA, left atrium; RV, right ventricle.

Venoarterial admixture or shuntlike states refer to blood flow passing through partially open alveoli (i.e., V/Q <1). Acute shunt will not respond to FiO_2 and the treatment is PEEP to open the alveoli and make them responsive to FiO_2. Venous admixture will demonstrate some response to FiO_2. If the shunt is minimal (normal condition), there is almost a linear relationship between FiO_2 and PaO_2, but as the shunt increases, FiO_2 no longer affects PaO_2 in a linear fashion (Fig. 18.18). This is an important concept as one cannot improve hypoxemia by increasing FiO_2 alone, but needs to open the alveoli with PEEP. If the shunt equation is calculated on a FiO_2 of <1.0, both the shunt and venous admixture will be captured in the equation. Intrapulmonary shunt (Qs/Qt) is calculated as $(CcO_2 - CaO_2)/(CcO_2 - CvO_2)$, where CcO_2 is the pulmonary capillary content of O_2, CaO_2 is the arterial content of O_2, and CvO_2 is the mixed venous content of O_2 (Table 18.3). Since pulmonary capillary blood cannot be sampled, the saturation is assumed to be 100%, which usually holds true when the FiO_2 is 1.0. It is important to understand the contribution of a low SvO_2 to PaO_2 if there is a moderate shunt (>20%). Any decrease in SvO_2 in a patient with >20% shunt will allow more deoxygenated blood to go into the arterial circulation, resulting in a lower PaO_2. This is called nonpulmonary cause of hypoxia. For example, if a patient with a 20% intrapulmonary shunt and a hemoglobin of 15 g/dL has an acute cardiac event, and the CO decreases from 5 to 3 L/minute, the PaO_2 will decrease from ~80 to 65 mm Hg (Fig. 18.19). In the exact same scenario, if the patient's hemoglobin is 10 g/dL, the PaO_2 will decrease from 70 to 55 mm Hg. This demonstrates the importance of low SvO_2 contributing to lower PaO_2. If the PEEP had been increased in this patient to treat a low PaO_2, a further decrease in CO would have resulted in worsening SvO_2 and PaO_2. Treatment in this case is to optimize CO first to see if PaO_2 improves. Another example: If a patient is agitated and the arterial saturation decreases, this may be due to increased oxygen consumption and low SvO_2 in a patient with a moderate intrapulmonary shunt, and not from an acute pulmonary event. Treatment is to decrease agitation and VO_2. There are times when severe cardiorespiratory compromise warrants titration of both cardiac output and PEEP simultaneously in patients

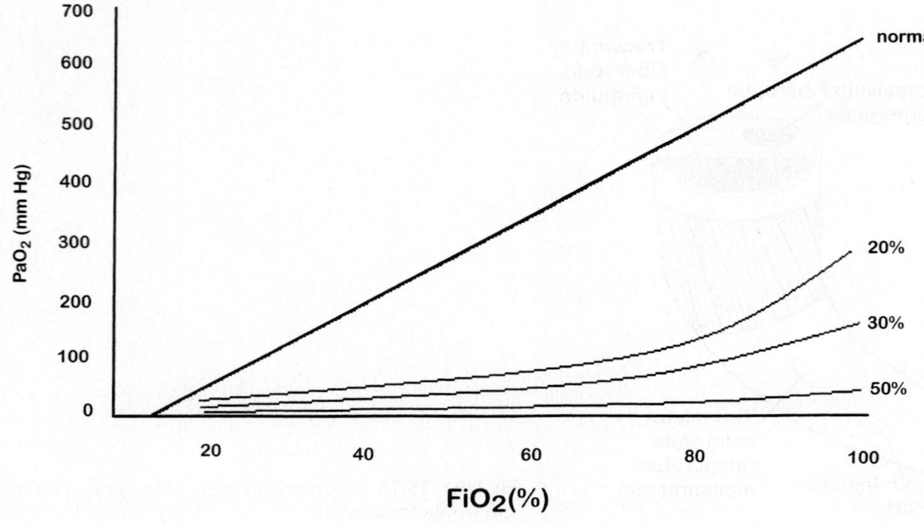

FIGURE 18.18. The effect of FiO_2 on PaO_2 depending on the degree of intrapulmonary shunts of 20%, 30%, and 50%. This is assuming that other parameters that affect SvO_2 such as cardiac output, hemoglobin, and oxygen consumption are remaining constant.

TABLE 18.3

DERIVED CALCULATIONS (ALL ARE INDEXED TO BODY SURFACE AREA)

Parameter	Equation	Key points	Normal range	Units
Stroke volume indexed (SVI)	CI/HR or EDVI – ESVI	Amount of blood ejected with each contraction (per m^2)	30–65	mL/beat/m^2
Left ventricular stroke work index (LVSWI)	SVI × (MAP – PAOP) × 0.0136	External work for the left ventricle in 1 beat	43–61	g · m/m^2
Right ventricular stroke work index (RVSWI)	SVI × (MPAP – CVP) × 0.0136	External work for the right ventricle in 1 beat	7–12	g · m/m^2
Pulmonary vascular resistance indexed (PVRI)	$\frac{(MPAP - PAOP) \times 80}{CI}$	Resistance for right ventricle; 80 converts mm Hg/min/L to dynes · sec/cm^5	255–285	dynes · sec/cm^5
Systemic vascular resistance (SVR)	$\frac{(MAP - CVP) \times 80}{CI}$	Resistance for left ventricle	1,970–2,390	dynes · sec/cm^5/m^2
Arterial oxygen content of blood (CaO_2)	(Hgb × 1.36 mL O_2/gHgb × SaO_2) + (0.0031 × PaO_2)	Amount of oxygen in arterial blood, majority is carried by Hgb (1.36 mL of O_2/g of Hgb if blood is 100% saturated), very little is dissolved (0.0031 × PaO_2)	16–22	mL O_2/dL blood
Mixed venous oxygen content of blood (CvO_2)	(Hgb × 1.36 mL O_2/gHgb × SvO_2) + (0.0031 × PvO_2)	Amount of oxygen in mixed venous blood (sampled at the pulmonary artery)	12–17	mL O_2/dL blood
Arterial-mixed venous oxygen content difference ($AVDO_2$)	CaO_2–CvO_2	How much O_2 was consumed by the tissues before returning to the heart	3–5	mL O_2/dL blood
Delivery of oxygen indexed (DO_2I)	CaO_2 × CI × 10	Primary determinant of organ perfusion	500–600	mL O_2/min/m^2
Oxygen consumption indexed (VO_2I)	(CaO_2 – CvO_2) × CI × 10	Oxygen consumed by the tissues	120–160	mL O_2/min/m^2
Intrapulmonary shunt (Qs/Qt)	(CcO_2 – CaO_2)/(CcO_2 – CvO_2) CcO_2 = (Hgb × 1.36 × 100% saturation) + (0.0031 × PAO_2) PAO_2 = FiO_2 × [(760 mm Hg – 47 mm Hg)] – ($PaCO_2$/RQ)	% of CI that is not involved with gas exchange and goes to the arterial side deoxygenated; >20% usually requires ventilator support. Since pulmonary capillary blood cannot be sampled, 100% saturation is assumed. 760 is atmospheric pressure at sea level; 47 is water vapor pressure.	3–5	% of cardiac output
Coronary perfusion pressure (CPP)	CPP = DBP – PAOP	The major determinant of flow in a fixed, diseased conduit is the pressure difference.	50–60	mm Hg

CI, cardiac index (mL/min/m^2); HR, heart rate (beats/min); EDVI, end-diastolic volume index (mL/m^2); ESVI, end-systolic volume index (mL/m^2); MAP, mean arterial pressure; DBP, diastolic blood pressure (mm Hg); PAOP, pulmonary artery occlusion pressure (mm Hg); CVP, central venous pressure; Hgb, hemoglobin (g/dL); CcO_2, pulmonary capillary content of oxygen; PAO_2, partial pressure of oxygen in the alveoli; RQ, respiratory quotient VCO_2/VO_2 is 0.8 for a mixed fuel diet.

with life-threatening hypoxia. It is important to understand the interaction of one organ on the other and the relationship between PaO_2, hemoglobin, and cardiac output (Fig. 18.19).

DERIVED VARIABLES

See Table 18.3 for the equations and normal values. Once the flow and pressure variables have been obtained from the PAC, further hemodynamic calculations may be done to obtain complete information. Most bedside monitors are capable of calculating and displaying the numbers, but clinicians must understand the significance and pitfalls of these values.

Stroke volume index (SVI) is the quantity of blood ejected from the ventricle with each contraction (i.e., the difference between end-diastolic and end-systolic volumes). SVI accounts for the effect of the heart rate's contribution to CI, and is an important variable because one does not want to augment CI by causing tachycardia (Fig. 18.14). SVI varies with preload, afterload, and contractility. Preload is the theoretical stretch of ventricles at end diastole.

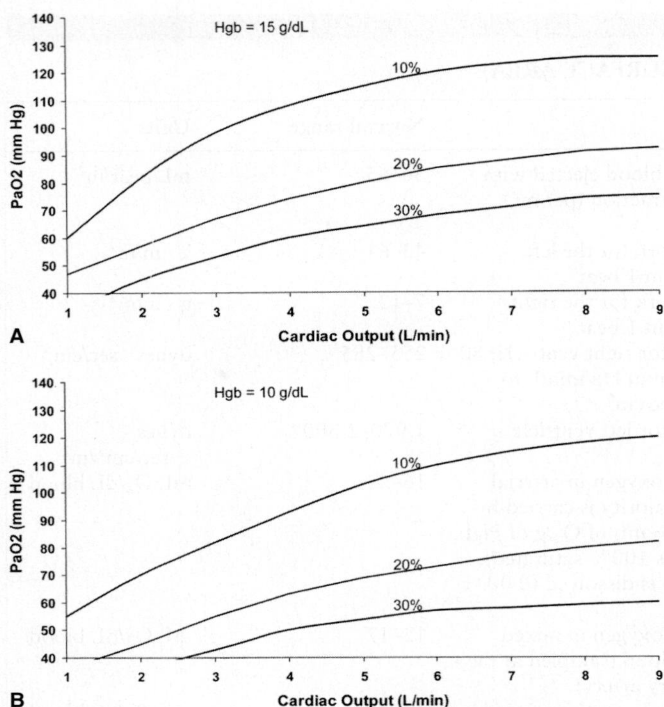

FIGURE 18.19. Relationship between PaO_2, cardiac output, and three different intrapulmonary shunt states (10%, 20%, and 30%) for patients with a hemoglobin of 15 g/dL and 10 g/dL. This graph demonstrates "nonpulmonary" causes for PaO_2 changes where a low cardiac output or low hemoglobin will impact PaO_2 depending on the degree of shunt.

According to Frank and Starling, the stretch of myocardium augments contractility to a certain point, and then cardiac output is negatively affected by further increases (80). Afterload is the interplay between aortic compliance, peripheral vascular resistance, viscosity of blood, aortic impedance, and aortic wall resistance. Afterload is therefore the force that myocytes must overcome during each contraction. Contractility is the maximum velocity of myocardial fiber contraction; it is the myocytes' inherent ability, independent of preload. All these parameters are extremely dynamic and require frequent reassessment.

Left ventricular stroke work index (LVSWI) estimates the work of the left ventricle in one beat. Work is the product of force and distance. Physiologically, this translates to the product of change in pressure and change in volume. Current technology does not allow continuous measurements of both ventricular volumes at the bedside. Stroke work index is low in cardiogenic and hypovolemic shock. In trauma patients, it has been suggested that high LVSWI is associated with decreased mortality (81,82). It should be noted that not all work is alike since "good work" is associated with large volume change with little pressure, and "bad work" is associated with large pressure change with little volume movement.

Right ventricular stroke work index (RVSWI) is the right heart's ability to produce forward flow against the pulmonary circulation and estimates external work for the RV in one beat. The work generated by RV is markedly less than LV due to a relatively low pulmonary pressure system. In patients with pulmonary hypertension and consequent right heart failure, the RVSWI must compensate accordingly (discussed below).

Pulmonary vascular resistance index (PVRI) is the resistance for the right ventricle. Resistance to blood flow is analogous to electrical circuit resistance defined by Ohm's Law. Resistance = Pressure/Flow. Physiologically, the pressure change between two vascular beds drives the flow (i.e., cardiac index). PVRI reflects resistance in the pulmonary vasculature. Pulmonary hypertension exists when systolic PAP is >35 mm Hg or mean PAP is >25 mm Hg (83,84). In critically ill patients, the most common causes for elevated PAP are acute respiratory distress syndrome, acute LV dysfunction, and pulmonary embolism (83,85–89). Patients with comorbid conditions such as chronic pulmonary hypertension may suffer from interstitial lung disease, COPD, or liver or cardiac disease. The right ventricle is exquisitely sensitive to increases in afterload and lacks the ability to overcome pulmonary hypertension with PAP >40 mm Hg (84). Subsequent decrease in cardiac output is due to the combination of decreased RVSWI and decreased filling of the left ventricle as a result of interventricular septal deviation (90). Since cardiac output is indexed to BSA, PVR should also be indexed and presented as PVRI.

Systemic vascular resistance index (SVRI) is the resistance for the left ventricle. In the context of hyperdynamic states with high cardiac index and decreased SVRI, the patient may be in distributive shock. Patients with low cardiac index and high SVRI are in hypovolemic or cardiogenic shock. It is important to recognize that SVRI represents the interplay of vascular diameter and viscosity, of which neither variable is easily measured. SVRI is calculated; therefore error is introduced if any of its subcomponents carries inaccuracy. Since CO is indexed to BSA, SVR should also be indexed and presented as SVRI.

Arterial oxygen content of blood (CaO_2) is the amount of oxygen carried in arterial blood. When evaluating delivery of oxygen, the CaO_2 is of critical importance. Each gram of hemoglobin carries 1.36 to 1.39 mL of oxygen if it is 100% saturated. Oxygen is poorly soluble in plasma and the dissolved oxygen contribution to arterial oxygen content is negligible. Therefore, saturation (SaO_2) plays a more important role than pressure of oxygen (PaO_2).

Mixed venous oxygen content of blood (CvO_2) is the amount of oxygen carried in the mixed venous blood. Low mixed venous oxygen content has similar clinical implications as low SvO_2 and suggests decreased oxygen delivery or increased oxygen consumption (see above). Since the blood is sent for oximeter analysis for saturation value and not PvO_2, the PvO_2 value in the equation (Table 18.3) is usually substituted with the normal PvO_2 value of 40 mm Hg since the amount dissolved is so small that a PvO_2 substitution of 0 to 70 mm Hg will not make a difference in the calculation of CvO_2.

Delivery of oxygen indexed to BSA (DO_2I) is the amount of oxygen delivered to the tissues by hemoglobin, arterial saturation, and flow (CI) (i.e., the product of cardiac index and arterial oxygen content of blood). The survival benefit of titrating to a specific DO_2I value has been extensively studied as an end point of resuscitation with conflicting results. The controversy surrounding DO_2 augmentation is discussed in the beginning of this chapter (10,14,21,22,25,32,91–93).

Oxygen consumption indexed (VO_2I): There are two methods of assessing oxygen consumption: Fick's principle and indirect calorimetry (94). Fick's principle states that the rate of diffusion of a known indicator (oxygen) is proportional to the product of concentration gradient and flow. Physiologically, this translates to the difference between arterial and mixed venous oxygen content multiplied by the cardiac output. Consumption can also be assessed by indirect calorimetry and is typically 3.5 mL of oxygen/kg (95). Indirect calorimetry compares the difference between inspired and expired oxygen to carbon dioxide ratios. There is usually a discrepancy (either way) of up to 11% between Fick's principle and indirect calorimetry, partially explained by Fick's method not accounting for pulmonary oxygen consumption (96–99). Shoemaker first noted that a higher VO_2I of >160 mL/minute/m^2 was associated with survival (3,4). It may reflect cells' ability to increase metabolic rate and utilize oxygen during stressed states. The concept of "critical DO_2I" where VO_2 becomes delivery dependent has been described in certain disease states with values occurring at DO_2 of <450 mL oxygen/minute/m^2 (100–102). Although the concept is attractive, it is difficult to use VO_2 as a therapeutic end point since VO_2 varies constantly depending on sedation, temperature, paralysis, loop diuretics, complete mechanical ventilation, vasoactive agents, and the progress of the underlying disease process (6,15).

Coronary perfusion pressure (CPP): In compliant vessels, flow to the coronary arteries can be augmented via coronary artery dilation. However, in patients with coronary artery disease with fixed vessels, flow depends on the pressure gradient between the two ends. Due to high LV pressures, coronaries feeding the LV fill during diastole, and maintenance of diastolic pressure is important. In patients undergoing preoperative optimization, nitroglycerin can be used to preferentially dilate nondiseased coronary vessels, thereby augmenting oxygen delivery to the myocytes. Generally CPP >50 mm Hg is desired, but there is individual variation.

SPECIAL COMMENT ON OBESITY AND DERIVED PARAMETERS

The validity of derived parameters indexed to body surface area has been questioned in morbidly obese patients. Several studies have demonstrated that derived parameters indexed to body surface area are appropriate and closely approximate indexing to body mass index. The large body surface area in the obese patient does not affect these measurements (103–105).

COMPLICATIONS OF PULMONARY ARTERY INSERTION

Pulmonary artery catheter insertion is an invasive procedure and carries inherent risks (106–108). Complications related to central venous access are discussed in other chapters. The overall complication rate associated with PACs can be as high as 25%. The procedural risks are pneumothorax, hemothorax, and knotting of catheters. Multiple prospective and retrospective studies have reported the most common complications including infection, thrombosis, arrhythmias, new bundle branch blocks, and pulmonary artery rupture (109,110). Serious complications (PA rupture and cardiac perforation with tamponade) are infrequent, but they can be fatal if unrecognized. Although reports of PAC-related infection are up to 22%, consequential bacteremia is relatively rare (0.7%–2.2%) (111). Catheters inserted for greater than 3 days may be associated with more infectious and thrombotic complications (112,113). Arrhythmias were relatively common, occurring in up to 75% of insertions. However, clinically significant arrhythmias requiring treatment were rare; 3% developed new bundle branch blocks, but this complication was not associated with increased mortality (109,110). Pulmonary artery rupture is exceedingly rare with a reported incidence of 0.031% (114) but usually occurs in patients with pulmonary hypertension and can be fatal due to high pulmonary pressures. Slow inflation of the balloon with immediate abortion if there is too much resistance or the waveform shows overwedging are important preventive maneuvers. Placement of pulmonary artery catheters requires skilled operators who are trained to troubleshoot and recognize complications when they occur. As discussed earlier in this chapter, perhaps the most dangerous complication of pulmonary artery catheters is the misinterpretation of information.

ARTERIAL LINES

Indications for invasive pressure monitoring are (a) hypodynamic states including all forms of shock and (b) frequent blood sampling for blood gas analysis and labs. Other indications include monitoring of response to vasoactive agents and severe peripheral vascular disease precluding noninvasive blood pressure monitoring. There are no true absolute contraindications.

Arterial cannulation is relatively safe with nonocclusive thrombosis and hematoma being the most common complications (115). Selection of anatomic site is an important consideration; percutaneous arterial catheters can be introduced in the radial, brachial, axillary, femoral, and dorsalis pedis arteries. Placement in brachial arteries is ill advised; it is an end artery and patients may develop ipsilateral hand ischemia in up to 40% of insertions (116,117). The radial artery remains the most popular placement site due to its ease of access and relatively low complication rates. A preprocedure Allen test assesses the patency of collateral arteries, but this test has poor correlation with distal flow and likelihood of hand ischemia (118,119).

Pressure Measurement

Continuous measures of systolic blood pressure (SBP), diastolic blood pressure (DBP), and mean arterial pressure (MAP) are displayed with invasive arterial catheters. Four elements must be considered in direct pressure measurement: (a) energy content, (b) transformation of pressure pulse, (c) reflection of pressure wave, and (d) recording system. Each element can introduce error in invasive blood pressure monitoring rendering the often large discrepancy between cuff and invasive pressures. The SBP is determined by the ventricular ejection velocity and volume. This pulse wave meets increasing impedance as the caliber of vessels decrease. Additionally, pulse amplification is proportional to distance from aorta; consequently, the radial artery pressure tends to be higher than aortic pressure.

Volume and velocity of left ventricular ejection, peripheral resistance, distensibility of arterial wall, and viscosity of blood determine the peak SBP. Usage of long tubing (≥4 feet) or microbubbles in the closed system can result in inaccurate measurements, specifically underdamping and falsely high SBP. Underdamping produces characteristic waveforms with sharp and overshooting upstroke and small, artifact pressure waves along the waveform. Overdamped tracings are caused by kinking, macrobubbles, or mechanical obstruction of tubing. Overdamped waveforms are characteristically diminished in their upstroke and exhibit loss of the dicrotic notch. The dynamic response of arterial monitoring circuits is assessed by a fast flush square wave test (Fig. 18.4). A properly calibrated system produces one overdamped waveform followed by several oscillating overshoot waves (120).

Waveform analysis (Fig. 18.20) demonstrates the typical points associated with (a) systolic upstroke, (b) systolic peak, (c) systolic decline, (d) dicrotic notch, (e) diastolic runoff, and (f) end diastole. Examination of the arterial waveform provides useful information regarding a patient's clinical status. Left ventricular ejection produces the first, sharp upstroke at

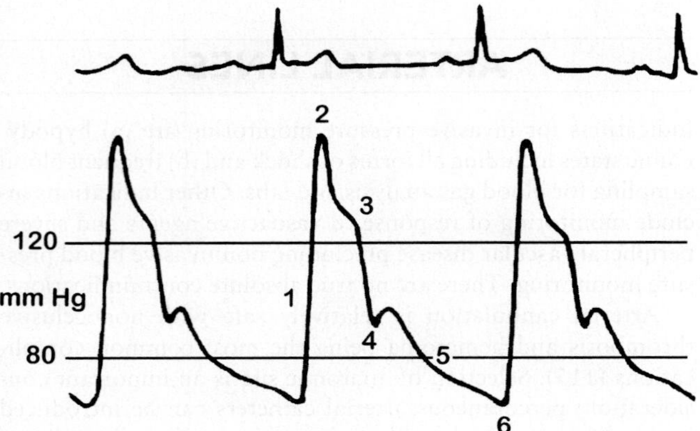

FIGURE 18.20. Arterial waveform analysis (see text for explanation of points 1–6).

the beginning of aortic valve opening (Fig. 18.20, points 1 and 2). As the ventricular flow is dispersed peripherally, the waveform declines (point 3); this is also when the heart is in isovolumetric relaxation and diastolic filling. Just prior to closure of the aortic valve and as a result of isovolumetric relaxation, there is a slight drop in pressure known as the incisura (at the aorta) or dicrotic notch (at the periphery) (point 4). Further decrease in the pressure waveform reflects the runoff to distal arterioles (points 5 and 6). More peripheral arteries exhibit narrower waveforms and higher systolic pressures and wider pulse pressures, although the mean arterial pressure remains similar to central vessels. The etiology of varying pulse contours in the periphery is related to the elasticity, amplification, and distortion of smaller arteries (121). Various cardiac conditions produce characteristic arterial waveforms. In aortic stenosis, narrow waveform and loss of the dicrotic notch secondary to diseased valve are seen. Aortic regurgitation may exhibit widened pulse pressures and a sharp upstroke, sometimes accompanied by two peaks.

Systolic pressure variation (SPV): Variations in systolic blood pressure and ventricular stroke volume are of greater magnitude in hypovolemic states (122). Theories on the etiology of this phenomenon relate to the characteristics unique to hypovolemia and include (a) the superior vena cava is more easily collapsible, (b) there is an increased effect of transmural pressures in the right atrium, and (c) the preload and stroke volume relationship is on the steep portion of the Frank-Starling curve. Usually, a decrease in left ventricular stroke volume occurs with inspiration due to the positive pressure ventilation. Originally, Perel described SPV as two components (Fig. 18.21)—delta up (Δup) and delta down (Δdown)—while emphasizing the strong correlation between Δdown and hypovolemic states (123–125). Δup is the difference between maximum SBP and a reference SBP (usually at expiratory pause during mechanical ventilation). Δdown is similarly the difference between minimum SBP and reference SBP and represents a decrease in stroke volume during expiration. SPV >10 mm Hg indicates hypovolemia and suggests responsiveness to fluid challenge (126). SPV also has significant correlation with the left ventricular end-diastolic area by echocardiogram (127) and PAOP (128). Note that SPV, like stroke volume variation, may be sensitive to changes in volume status, but may not necessarily equate to actual intravascular blood volume.

Stroke volume variation (SVV): Arterial pressure variation during the respiratory cycle is a well-documented phenomenon (122). Pulsus paradoxicus describes falls in arterial pressures (>10 mm Hg) during inspiration and rises in pressures during expiration in spontaneously breathing patients. Reverse pulsus paradoxicus occurs in ventilated patients. Proprietary algorithms in new monitor devices analyze the pulse-to-pulse variation in a semi-continuous fashion with updates at 20-second intervals. SVV is not a measurement of absolute preload; rather, it is an assessment of response to fluid resuscitation (128–131). SVV >9.5% to 15% is associated with fluid responsiveness. SVV is only approved for use in sedated, mechanically ventilated patients who are in sinus rhythm (rhythm must be regular or the variation may be due to irregular rate rather than volume status).

$$\text{SVV} = (\text{SV maximum} - \text{SV minimum}) / [(\text{SV maximum} + \text{SV minimum})/2] \times 100$$

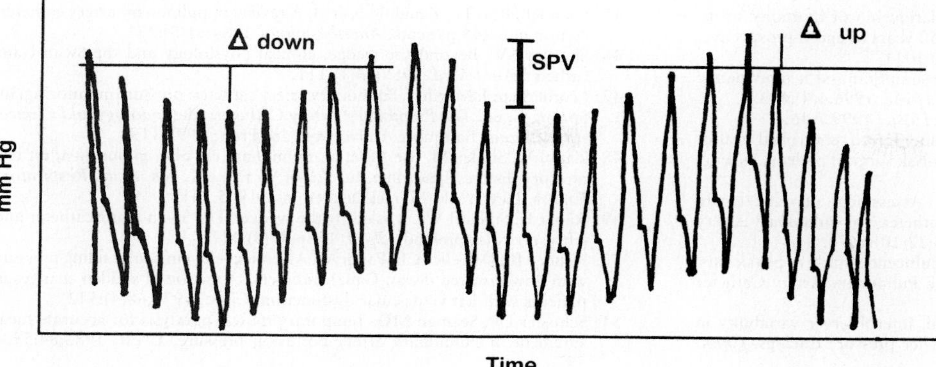

FIGURE 18.21. Systolic pressure variation (SPV). See text.

Available technology on the market: Several companies market continuous arterial catheter cardiac output monitoring with several important distinctions. The main difference between the aforementioned technologies is that Lidco analyzes areas under a concentration curve, whereas Flotrac analyzes stroke volume based on pulse pressure variances.

LidcoPlus (Lidco, Cambridge, UK): LidcoPlus combines the previously validated Lidco lithium indicator dilution calibration procedure with continuous pulse contour analysis for real-time cardiac output assessment (132). A small amount of lithium chloride is injected in a vein and the concentration of arterial sampling over time produces a concentration-time curve. The area under this curve provides the cardiac output by integral mathematics. The manufacturer recommends calibration every 8 hours. Studies have shown that LidcoPlus provides similar cardiac output results as traditional pulmonary artery catheters over a wide range of hemodynamic states (133,134).

FloTrac (Edwards Lifesciences, Irvine, CA, USA) features continuous cardiac output and stroke volume variation without need for calibration utilizing an existing arterial catheter. Assumptions are made regarding the patient's vascular compliance given his or her age, weight, and height. Proprietary software analyzes waveform contours beat to beat and evaluates cardiac output based on the concept that stroke volume is related to beat-to-beat pressure changes. The algorithm also takes into account the dynamic changes in vascular compliance by assessing the characteristic changes associated with alterations in vascular tone. Preliminary studies have demonstrated similar cardiac output results compared to intermittent, bolus thermodilution techniques (135). Although the use of SVV has only been validated in heavily sedated patients without spontaneous respirations and in sinus rhythm, preliminary data confirm that SVV may be utilized in spontaneously breathing patients with quiet respirations.

SUMMARY

The value of any monitoring system is to impact outcomes. Although surrounded by controversy, there remains a group of patients who may benefit from invasive monitoring. It is imperative that technology is used by trained personnel who understand both the benefits and the limitations of the devices. Equally important is the concept of early resuscitation before the onset of multisystem organ failure. The next quantum leap in hemodynamic monitoring will come when we are able to treat patients with noninvasive technology with the goal of delivering oxygen to every tissue bed. It is also conceivable that if we can constantly measure with minimally invasive devices cardiac output and cardiac preload, intravascular blood volume status, central SvO_2, and tissue oxygenation (see chapters on noninvasive cardiovascular monitoring, monitoring tissue perfusion, blood volume, and venous saturation monitoring), the PAC could become obsolete in the future. Until that time, it has been difficult to reproduce the continuous reliable information obtained from the PAC.

References

1. Connors AF Jr, Speroff T, Dawson NV, et al. The effectiveness of right heart catheterization in the initial care of critically ill patients. SUPPORT Investigators. *JAMA.* 1996;276(11):889.
2. Practice guidelines for pulmonary artery catheterization: an updated report by the American Society of Anesthesiologists Task Force on Pulmonary Artery Catheterization. *Anesthesiology.* 2003;99(4):988.
3. Shoemaker WC, Elwyn DH, Levin H, et al. Use of nonparametric analysis of cardiorespiratory variables as early predictors of death and survival in postoperative patients. *J Surg Res.* 1974;17(5):1.
4. Shoemaker WC, Montgomery ES, Kaplan E, et al. Physiologic patterns in surviving and nonsurviving shock patients. Use of sequential cardiorespiratory variables in defining criteria for therapeutic goals and early warning of death. *Arch Surg.* 1973;106(5):630.
5. Bihari D, Smithies M, Gimson A, et al. The effects of vasodilation with prostacyclin on oxygen delivery and uptake in critically ill patients. *N Engl J Med.* 1987;317(7):397.
6. Yu M, Burchell S, Takiguchi SA, et al. The relationship of oxygen consumption measured by indirect calorimetry to oxygen delivery in critically ill patients. *J Trauma.* 1996;41(1):41.
7. Rivers E, Nguyen B, Havstad S, et al. Early goal-directed therapy in the treatment of severe sepsis and septic shock. *N Engl J Med.* 2001;345(19):1368.
8. Moore FA, Haenel JB, Moore EE, et al. Incommensurate oxygen consumption in response to maximal oxygen availability predicts postinjury multiple organ failure. *J Trauma.* 1992;33(1):58.
9. Bishop MH, Shoemaker WC, Appel PL, et al. Relationship between supranormal circulatory values, time delays, and outcome in severely traumatized patients. *Crit Care Med.* 1993;21(1):56.
10. Fleming A, Bishop M, Shoemaker W, et al. Prospective trial of supranormal values as goals of resuscitation in severe trauma. *Arch Surg.* 1992;127(10):1175.
11. Gattinoni L, Brazzi L, Pelosi P, et al. A trial of goal-oriented hemodynamic therapy in critically ill patients. SvO2 Collaborative Group. *N Engl J Med.* 1995;333(16):1025.
12. Hayes MA, Timmins AC, Yau EH, et al. Elevation of systemic oxygen delivery in the treatment of critically ill patients. *N Engl J Med.* 1994;330(24):1717.
13. Wheeler AP, Bernard GR, Thompson BT, et al. Pulmonary-artery versus central venous catheter to guide treatment of acute lung injury. *N Engl J Med.* 2006;354(21):2213.

14. Yu M, Burchell S, Hasaniya NW, et al. Relationship of mortality to increasing oxygen delivery in patients > or = 50 years of age: a prospective, randomized trial. *Crit Care Med.* 1998;26(6):1011.
15. Yu M. Invasive and noninvasive oxygen consumption and hemodynamic monitoring in elderly surgical patients. *New Horiz.* 1996;4(4):443.
16. Yu M. Oxygen transport optimization. *New Horiz.* 1999;7:46.
17. Sandham JD, Hull RD, Brant RF, et al. A randomized, controlled trial of the use of pulmonary-artery catheters in high-risk surgical patients. *N Engl J Med.* 2003;348(1):5.
18. Iberti TJ, Daily EK, Leibowitz AB, et al. Assessment of critical care nurses' knowledge of the pulmonary artery catheter. The Pulmonary Artery Catheter Study Group. *Crit Care Med.* 1994;22(10):1674.
19. Iberti TJ, Fischer EP, Leibowitz AB, et al. A multicenter study of physicians' knowledge of the pulmonary artery catheter. Pulmonary Artery Catheter Study Group. *JAMA.* 1990;264(22):2928.
20. Komadina KH, Schenk DA, LaVeau P, et al. Interobserver variability in the interpretation of pulmonary artery catheter pressure tracings. *Chest.* 1991;100(6):1647.
21. Berlauk JF, Abrams JH, Gilmour IJ, et al. Preoperative optimization of cardiovascular hemodynamics improves outcome in peripheral vascular surgery. A prospective, randomized clinical trial. *Ann Surg.* 1991;214(3): 289.
22. Shoemaker WC, Kram HB, Appel PL, et al. The efficacy of central venous and pulmonary artery catheters and therapy based upon them in reducing mortality and morbidity. *Arch Surg.* 1990;125(10):1332.
23. Gutierrez G, Palizas F, Doglio G, et al. Gastric intramucosal pH as a therapeutic index of tissue oxygenation in critically ill patients. *Lancet.* 1992;339(8787):195.
24. Shoemaker WC, Bayard DS, Wo CC, et al. Outcome prediction in chest injury by a mathematical search and display program. *Chest.* 2005; 128(4):2739.
25. Yu M, Chapital A, Ho HC, et al. A prospective randomized trial comparing oxygen delivery versus transcutaneous pressure of oxygen values as resuscitative goals. *Shock.* 2007;27(6):615.
26. Yu M, Morita SY, Daniel SR, et al. Transcutaneous pressure of oxygen: a non-invasive and early detector of peripheral shock and outcome. *Shock.* 2006;26(5):450.
27. Cohn SM, Nathens AB, Moore FA, et al. Tissue oxygen saturation predicts the development of organ dysfunction during traumatic shock resuscitation. *J Trauma.* 2007;62(1):44.
28. De Backer D, Creteur J, Preiser JC, et al. Microvascular blood flow is altered in patients with sepsis. *Am J Respir Crit Care Med.* 2002;166(1):98.
29. Boerma EC, Mathura KR, van der Voort PH, et al. Quantifying bedside-derived imaging of microcirculatory abnormalities in septic patients: a prospective validation study. *Crit Care.* 2005;9(6):R601.
30. Yamauchi H, Biuk-Aghai E, Yu M, et al. Circulating blood volume measurements in crtically ill surgical patients correlate poorly with pulmonary artery catheter measurements. *Hawaii Med J.* 2008;67(1):8–11.
31. ACC/AHA guideline for perioperative cardiovascular evaluation for noncardiac surgery–executive summary. *Circulation.* 2002;105:1257.
32. Boyd O, Grounds RM, Bennett ED. A randomized clinical trial of the effect of deliberate perioperative increase of oxygen delivery on mortality in high-risk surgical patients. *JAMA.* 1993;270(22):2699.
33. Wilson RJ, Woods I. Cardiovascular optimization for high-risk surgery. *Curr Opin Crit Care.* 2001;7(3):195.
34. Eisenberg PR, Jaffe AS, Schuster DP. Clinical evaluation compared to pulmonary artery catheterization in the hemodynamic assessment of critically ill patients. *Crit Care Med.* 1984;12(7):549.
35. Tuman KJ, Carroll GC, Ivankovich AD. Pitfalls in interpretation of pulmonary artery catheter data. *J Cardiothorac Anesth.* 1989;3(5):625.
36. Connors AF Jr, McCaffree DR, Gray BA. Evaluation of right-heart catheterization in the critically ill patient without acute myocardial infarction. *N Engl J Med.* 1983;308(5):263.
37. Civetta JM. Pulmonary artery catheter insertion. In: Sprung C, ed. *The Pulmonary Artery Catheter: Methodology and Clinical Application.* Baltimore: University Park Press; 1983:21.
38. Swan HJ, Ganz W, Forrester J, et al. Catheterization of the heart in man with use of a flow-directed balloon-tipped catheter. *N Engl J Med.* 1970;283(9):447.
39. Morris AH, Chapman RH. Wedge pressure confirmation by aspiration of pulmonary capillary blood. *Crit Care Med.* 1985;13(9):756.
40. Kett D, Schein R. Techniques for pulmonary artery catheter insertion. In: Sprung C, ed. *The Pulmonary Artery Catheter: Methodology and Clinical Applications.* Baltimore: University Park Press; 1993:43.
41. Daily EK, Schroeder JS. Principles and hazards of monitoring equipment. In: *Techniques in Bedside Hemodynamic Monitoring.* St. Louis: The C.V. Mosby Company; 1989:34.
42. Sarin CL, Yalav E, Clement AJ, et al. The necessity for measurement of left atrial pressure after cardiac valve surgery. *Thorax.* 1970;25(2):185.
43. Civetta JM, Gabel JC. Flow directed-pulmonary artery catheterization in surgical patients: indications and modifications of technic. *Ann Surg.* 1972;176(6):753.
44. Thompson I, Dalton B, Lappas D. Right bundle-branch block and complete heart block caused by the Swan-Ganz catheter. *Anesthesiology.* 1979; 51:359.
45. Shah KB, Rao TL, Laughlin S, et al. A review of pulmonary artery catheterization in 6,245 patients. *Anesthesiology.* 1984;61(3):271.
46. Sharkey SW. Beyond the wedge: clinical physiology and the Swan-Ganz catheter. *Am J Med.* 1987;83(1):111.
47. Leatherman J, Marini J. Pulmonary artery catheter: pressure monitoring. In: Sprung C, ed. *The Pulmonary Artery Catheter: Methodology and Clinical Applications.* Baltimore: University Park Press; 1993:119.
48. Zapol W, Snider M, Rie M, et al. Pulmonary circulation during adult respiratory distress syndrome. In: Zapol W, Falke K, eds. *Acute Respiratory Failure.* New York: Marcel Dekker, Inc.; 1985:241.
49. Raper R, Sibbald WJ. Misled by the wedge? The Swan-Ganz catheter and left ventricular preload. *Chest.* 1986;89(3):427.
50. Fisher ML, De Felice CE, Parisi AF. Assessing left ventricular filling pressure with flow-directed (Swan-Ganz) catheters. Detection of sudden changes in patients with left ventricular dysfunction. *Chest.* 1975;68(4):542.
51. Schuster DP, Seeman MD. Temporary muscle paralysis for accurate measurement of pulmonary artery occlusion pressure. *Chest.* 1983;84:593–597.
52. Lappas D, Lell WA, Gabel JC, et al. Indirect measurement of left-atrial pressure in surgical patients–pulmonary-capillary wedge and pulmonary-artery diastolic pressures compared with left-atrial pressure. *Anesthesiology.* 1973;38(4):394.
53. West JB, Dollery CT, Naimark A. Distribution of blood flow in isolated lung; relation to vascular and alveolar pressures. *J Appl Physiol.* 1964;19:713.
54. O'Quin R, Marini JJ. Pulmonary artery occlusion pressure: clinical physiology, measurement, and interpretation. *Am Rev Respir Dis.* 1983; 128(2):319.
55. Cope DK, Allison RC, Parmentier JL, et al. Measurement of effective pulmonary capillary pressure using the pressure profile after pulmonary artery occlusion. *Crit Care Med.* 1986;14(1):16.
56. Lozman J, Powers SR Jr, Older T, et al. Correlation of pulmonary wedge and left atrial pressures. A study in the patient receiving positive end expiratory pressure ventilation. *Arch Surg.* 1974;109(2):270.
57. Civetta JM. Invasive catheterization. In: Shoemaker W, Thompson W, eds. *Critical Care: State of the Art.* Fullerton, CA: Society of Critical Care Medicine; 1980:1.
58. Carter RS, Snyder JV, Pinsky MR. LV filling pressure during PEEP measured by nadir wedge pressure after airway disconnection. *Am J Physiol.* 1985;249(4 Pt 2):H770.
59. De Campo T, Civetta JM. The effect of short-term discontinuation of high-level PEEP in patients with acute respiratory failure. *Crit Care Med.* 1979;7(2):47.
60. Rahimtoola SH. Left ventricular end-diastolic and filling pressures in assessment of ventricular function. *Chest.* 1973;63(6):858.
61. Longman J, Powers S, Older T, et al. Correlation of pulmonary wedge and left atrial pressures. *Arch Surg.* 1974;109:270.
62. Parker JO, Case RB. Normal left ventricular function. *Circulation.* 1979;60(1):4.
63. Packman MI, Rackow EC. Optimum left heart filling pressure during fluid resuscitation of patients with hypovolemic and septic shock. *Crit Care Med.* 1983;11(3):165.
64. Guyton AC, Lindsey AW. Effect of elevated left atrial pressure and decreased plasma protein concentration on the development of pulmonary edema. *Circ Res.* 1959;7(4):649.
65. Zwissler B, Briegel J. Right ventricular catheter. *Curr Opin Crit Care.* 1998;4:177.
66. Diebel L, Wilson RF, Heins J, et al. End-diastolic volume versus pulmonary artery wedge pressure in evaluating cardiac preload in trauma patients. *J Trauma.* 1994;37(6):950.
67. Durham R, Neunaber K, Vogler G, et al. Right ventricular end-diastolic volume as a measure of preload. *J Trauma.* 1995;39(2):218.
68. Chang MC, Black CS, Meredith JW. Volumetric assessment of preload in trauma patients: addressing the problem of mathematical coupling. *Shock.* 1996;6(5):326.
69. European Society of Intensive Care Medicine. Expert panel: the use of the pulmonary artery catheter. *Intensive Care Med.* 1991;17(3):I.
70. Conway J, Lund-Johansen P, Thermodilution method for measuring cardiac output. *Eur Heart J.* 1990;11(Suppl I):17.
71. Olsson B, Pool J, Vandermoten P, et al. Validity and reproducibility of determination of cardiac output by thermodilution in man. *Cardiology.* 1970;55(3):136.
72. Harris AP, Miller CF, Beattie C, et al. The slowing of sinus rhythm during thermodilution cardiac output determination and the effect of altering injectate temperature. *Anesthesiology.* 1985;63(5):540.
73. Elkayam U, Berkley R, Azen S, et al. Cardiac output by thermodilution technique. Effect of injectate's volume and temperature on accuracy and reproducibility in the critically ill patient. *Chest.* 1983;84(4): 418.
74. Le Tulzo Y, Belghith M, Seguin P, et al. Reproducibility of thermodilution cardiac output determination in critically ill patients: comparison between bolus and continuous method. *J Clin Monit.* 1996;12(5):379.
75. Seguin P, Colcanap O, Le Rouzo A, et al. Evaluation of a new semi-continuous cardiac output system in the intensive care unit. *Can J Anaesth.* 1998;45(6):578.

76. Burchell SA, Yu M, Takiguchi SA, et al. Evaluation of a continuous cardiac output and mixed venous oxygen saturation catheter in critically ill surgical patients. *Crit Care Med.* 1997;25(3):388.
77. Rivers E. The outcome of patients presenting to the emergency department with severe sepsis or septic shock. *Crit Care.* 2006;10(4):154.
78. Rivers EP, Nguyen HB, Huang DT, et al. Early goal-directed therapy. *Crit Care Med.* 2004;32(1):314.
79. Otero RM, Nguyen HB, Huang DT, et al. Early goal-directed therapy in severe sepsis and septic shock revisited: concepts, controversies, and contemporary findings. *Chest.* 2006;130(5):1579.
80. Katz AM. Ernest Henry Starling, his predecessors, and the "Law of the Heart." *Circulation.* 2002;106(23):2986.
81. Chang MC, Mondy JS, Meredith JW, et al. Redefining cardiovascular performance during resuscitation: ventricular stroke work, power, and the pressure-volume diagram. *J Trauma.* 1998;45(3):470.
82. Martin RS, Norris PR, Kilgo PD, et al. Validation of stroke work and ventricular arterial coupling as markers of cardiovascular performance during resuscitation. *J Trauma.* 2006;60(5):930.
83. Barst RJ, McGoon M, Torbicki A, et al. Diagnosis and differential assessment of pulmonary arterial hypertension. *J Am Coll Cardiol.* 2004;43(12 Suppl S):40S.
84. Chin KM, Kim NH, Rubin LJ. The right ventricle in pulmonary hypertension. *Coron Artery Dis.* 2005;16(1):13.
85. Benza RL, Park MH, Keogh A, et al. Management of pulmonary arterial hypertension with a focus on combination therapies. *J Heart Lung Transplant.* 2007;26(5):437.
86. Girgis RE, Mathai SC. Pulmonary hypertension associated with chronic respiratory disease. *Clin Chest Med.* 2007;28(1):219.
87. O'Callaghan D, Gaine SP. Combination therapy and new types of agents for pulmonary arterial hypertension. *Clin Chest Med.* 2007;28(1):169.
88. Oudiz RJ. Pulmonary hypertension associated with left-sided heart disease. *Clin Chest Med.* 2007;28(1):233.
89. Ryu JH, Krowka MJ, Pellikka PA, et al. Pulmonary hypertension in patients with interstitial lung diseases. *Mayo Clin Proc.* 2007;82(3):342.
90. Zamanian RT, Haddad F, Doyle RL, et al. Management strategies for patients with pulmonary hypertension in the intensive care unit. *Crit Care Med.* 2007;35(9):2037.
91. Fenwick E, Wilson J, Sculpher M, et al. Pre-operative optimisation employing dopexamine or adrenaline for patients undergoing major elective surgery: a cost-effectiveness analysis. *Intensive Care Med.* 2002;28(5):599.
92. Kern JW, Shoemaker WC. Meta-analysis of hemodynamic optimization in high-risk patients. *Crit Care Med.* 2002;30(8):1686.
93. Yu M, Takanishi D, Myers SA, et al. Frequency of mortality and myocardial infarction during maximizing oxygen delivery: a prospective, randomized trial. *Crit Care Med.* 1995;23(6):1025.
94. Hanique G, Dugernier T, Laterre PF, et al. Evaluation of oxygen uptake and delivery in critically ill patients: a statistical reappraisal. *Intensive Care Med.* 1994;20(1):19.
95. Brandi LS, Bertolini R, Calafa M. Indirect calorimetry in critically ill patients: clinical applications and practical advice. *Nutrition.* 1997;13(4):349.
96. Peyton PJ, Robinson GJ. Measured pulmonary oxygen consumption: difference between systemic oxygen uptake measured by the reverse Fick method and indirect calorimetry in cardiac surgery. *Anaesthesia.* 2005;60(2):146.
97. Bizouarn P, Blanloeil Y, Pinaud M. Comparison between oxygen consumption calculated by Fick's principle using a continuous thermodilution technique and measured by indirect calorimetry. *Br J Anaesth.* 1995;75(6):719.
98. Oudemans-van Straaten HM, Scheffer GJ. Oxygen consumption after cardiopulmonary bypass–different measuring methods yield different results. *Intensive Care Med.* 1994;20(6):458.
99. Smithies MN, Royston B, Makita K, et al. Comparison of oxygen consumption measurements: indirect calorimetry versus the reversed Fick method. *Crit Care Med.* 1991;19(11):1401.
100. Lorente JA, Renes E, Gomez-Aguinaga MA, et al. Oxygen delivery-dependent oxygen consumption in acute respiratory failure. *Crit Care Med.* 1991;19(6):770.
101. Appel PL, Shoemaker WC. Relationship of oxygen consumption and oxygen delivery in surgical patients with ARDS. *Chest.* 1992;102(3):906.
102. Schumacker PT, Cain SM. The concept of a critical oxygen delivery. *Intensive Care Med.* 1987;13(4):223.
103. Beutler S, Schmidt U, Michard F. Hemodynamic monitoring in obese patients: a big issue. *Crit Care Med.* 2004;32(9):1981.
104. Collis T, Devereux RB, Roman MJ, et al. Relations of stroke volume and cardiac output to body composition: the strong heart study. *Circulation.* 2001;103(6):820.
105. Stelfox HT, Ahmed SB, Ribeiro RA, et al. Hemodynamic monitoring in obese patients: the impact of body mass index on cardiac output and stroke volume. *Crit Care Med.* 2006;34(4):1243.
106. Hadian M, Pinsky MR. Evidence-based review of the use of the pulmonary artery catheter: impact data and complications. *Crit Care.* 2006;10(Suppl 3):S8.
107. Carrico CJ, Horovitz JH. Monitoring the critically ill surgical patient. *Adv Surg.* 1977;11:101.
108. McNally JB. Invasive monitoring with the Swan-Ganz catheter. *Ariz Med.* 1974;31(6):421.
109. Sprung CL, Elser B, Schein RM, et al. Risk of right bundle-branch block and complete heart block during pulmonary artery catheterization. *Crit Care Med.* 1989;17(1):1.
110. Sprung CL, Pozen RG, Rozanski JJ, et al. Advanced ventricular arrhythmias during bedside pulmonary artery catheterization. *Am J Med.* 1982;72(2):203.
111. Payen D, Gayat E. Which general intensive care unit patients can benefit from placement of the pulmonary artery catheter? *Crit Care.* 2006;10(Suppl 3):S7.
112. Sise MJ, Hollingsworth P, Brimm JE, et al. Complications of the flow-directed pulmonary artery catheter: a prospective analysis in 219 patients. *Crit Care Med.* 1981;9(4):315.
113. Rosenwasser RH, Jallo JI, Getch CC, et al. Complications of Swan-Ganz catheterization for hemodynamic monitoring in patients with subarachnoid hemorrhage. *Neurosurgery.* 1995;37(5):872.
114. Kearney TJ, Shabot MM. Pulmonary artery rupture associated with the Swan-Ganz catheter. *Chest.* 1995;108(5):1349.
115. Slogoff S, Keats AS, Arlund C. On the safety of radial artery cannulation. *Anesthesiology.* 1983;59(1):42.
116. Mortensen JD. Clinical sequelae from arterial needle puncture, cannulation, and incision. *Circulation.* 1967;35(6):1118.
117. Barnes RW, Petersen JL, Krugmire RB Jr, et al. Complications of brachial artery catheterization: prospective evaluation with the Doppler ultrasonic velocity detector. *Chest.* 1974;66(4):363.
118. Mangar D, Thrush DN, Connell GR, et al. Direct or modified Seldinger guide wire-directed technique for arterial catheter insertion. *Anesth Analg.* 1993;76(4):714.
119. Barone JE, Madlinger RV. Should an Allen test be performed before radial artery cannulation? *J Trauma.* 2006;61(2):468.
120. Gardner RM. Direct blood pressure measurement–dynamic response requirements. *Anesthesiology.* 1981;54(3):227.
121. O'Rourke MF, Yaginuma T. Wave reflections and the arterial pulse. *Arch Intern Med.* 1984;144(2):366.
122. Michard F. Changes in arterial pressure during mechanical ventilation. *Anesthesiology.* 2005;103(2):419.
123. Perel A. The value of delta Down during haemorrhage. *Br J Anaesth.* 1999;83(6):967.
124. Perel A. Assessing fluid responsiveness by the systolic pressure variation in mechanically ventilated patients. Systolic pressure variation as a guide to fluid therapy in patients with sepsis-induced hypotension. *Anesthesiology.* 1998;89(6):1309.
125. Perel A. Arterial pressure waveform analysis during hypovolemia. *Anesth Analg.* 1996;82(3):670.
126. Rick JJ, Burke SS. Respirator paradox. *South Med J.* 1978;71(11):1376.
127. Coriat P, Vrillon M, Perel A, et al. A comparison of systolic blood pressure variations and echocardiographic estimates of end-diastolic left ventricular size in patients after aortic surgery. *Anesth Analg.* 1994;78(1):46.
128. Preisman S, Kogan S, Berkenstadt H, et al. Predicting fluid responsiveness in patients undergoing cardiac surgery: functional haemodynamic parameters including the Respiratory Systolic Variation Test and static preload indicators. *Br J Anaesth.* 2005;95(6):746.
129. Michard F, Teboul JL. Predicting fluid responsiveness in ICU patients: a critical analysis of the evidence. *Chest.* 2002;121(6):2000.
130. Berkenstadt H, Friedman Z, Preisman S, et al. Pulse pressure and stroke volume variations during severe haemorrhage in ventilated dogs. *Br J Anaesth.* 2005;94(6):721.
131. Berkenstadt H, Margalit N, Hadani M, et al. Stroke volume variation as a predictor of fluid responsiveness in patients undergoing brain surgery. *Anesth Analg.* 2001;92(4):984.
132. Linton R, Band D, O'Brien T, et al. Lithium dilution cardiac output measurement: a comparison with thermodilution. *Crit Care Med.* 1997;25(11):1796.
133. Kurita T, Morita K, Kato S, et al. Lithium dilution cardiac output measurements using a peripheral injection site comparison with central injection technique and thermodilution. *J Clin Monit Comput.* 1999;15(5):279.
134. Linton RA, Jonas MM, Tibby SM, et al. Cardiac output measured by lithium dilution and transpulmonary thermodilution in patients in a paediatric intensive care unit. *Intensive Care Med.* 2000;26(10):1507.
135. McGee WT, Horswell JL, Calderon J, et al. Validation of a continuous, arterial pressure-based cardiac output measurement: a multicenter, prospective clinical trial. *Crit Care.* 2007;11(5):R105.

CHAPTER 19 ■ MONITORING TISSUE PERFUSION AND OXYGENATION

KENNETH WAXMAN

Shock occurs when tissue oxygen delivery is inadequate to meet metabolic demands, and cellular dysfunction results. Since a primary goal of treating shock is elimination of cellular hypoxia, it logically follows that detecting and treating shock would best be monitored by measuring the state of tissue perfusion and cellular oxygenation. To this end, many devices that have the capability of monitoring tissue perfusion and oxygenation have been developed. However, to date, none of these devices has gained widespread acceptance in clinical practice. Why is this? This chapter will outline underlying principles of tissue perfusion and oxygenation and review the complexities of making clinically useful measurements with existing monitoring approaches.

There are multiple components of the circulation that contribute to cellular oxygenation, each of which is related to monitoring of tissue perfusion and oxygenation. As shown in Figure 19.1, tissue perfusion is determined by cardiac output, the distribution of cardiac output to regional tissue beds, and the state of the microcirculation. Tissue oxygenation is determined by perfusion as well as by arterial oxygenation, nutritional blood flow, and cellular extraction of oxygen. This is a complex system, which is highly dynamic: Alteration of any component has physiologic impact upon other components. Moreover, there is enormous heterogeneity within the circulation, both between organs and within organs. Hence tissue perfusion and oxygenation is never uniform between organs, nor even in particular tissue beds. Nonetheless, despite these complexities, there are several principles that allow useful monitoring to occur:

1. Peripheral perfusion and oxygenation monitors are not replacements for other commonly used monitors, but instead provide unique physiologic information.
2. A measured decrease in peripheral tissue perfusion may provide a significant and early warning of circulatory insufficiency.
3. In low-flow shock states (such as hemorrhagic or cardiogenic shock), there is a characteristic redistribution of regional blood flow, such that blood flow to the heart and brain is preserved, while peripheral blood flow is decreased. Blood flow to the skin decreases very early in this process; hence, monitoring skin perfusion is a very sensitive indicator of circulatory shock. Blood flow to other tissues such as the intestinal tract also decreases relatively early in shock, making the gut an alternative sensitive monitoring site. Unfortunately, in high-flow shock states (such as septic shock), the distribution of regional blood flow is less predictable, and interpretation of peripheral perfusion data becomes more complex.
4. A measured decrease in peripheral tissue oxygenation may be a significant warning of decreased tissue perfusion, decreased hemoglobin concentration, arterial oxygenation, or increased cellular utilization of oxygen. Sorting out these alternative explanations for abnormal tissue oxygenation can lead to prompt diagnosis and treatment of the underlying problem.
5. Monitors of tissue perfusion and oxygenation can be used in several ways. They can serve as early sensitive but nonspecific warning devices to alarm when decreases of blood flow or oxygenation occur. In addition, these monitoring approaches can be used as components of a system of monitoring, such that their specificity is enhanced. For example, combining tissue oxygen monitoring with pulse oximetry can indicate that a decreased tissue oxygen value is not due to arterial hypoxemia.
6. Monitoring changes of tissue oxygenation in response to changes in cardiac output or arterial oxygen may provide meaningful clinical information. The use of these devices in response to physiologic challenges adds another dimension to their potential value

MONITORING TECHNIQUES

Pulse Oximetry

Pulse oximeters are designed to monitor arterial oxygen saturation, not tissue perfusion or oxygenation. In fact, the technology of pulse oximetry is precisely designed to detect oxyhemoglobin saturation, even when blood flow is greatly reduced. Estimation of arterial oxygen saturation is thus of great benefit in monitoring arterial oxygenation, but of little value in assessing the circulation. A patient in shock may have 100% arterial oxygen saturation, and pulse oximetry will reflect this regardless of the state of the circulation, as long as the probe can detect pulsation. When pulsations can no longer be detected, the monitor ceases to function. Hence, it is only the absence of a signal that indicates very low flow, and this absence is both insensitive and nonspecific. Pulse oximetry is, however, useful in combination with tissue oxygen monitors to indicate whether low tissue oxygenation is due to arterial hypoxemia or to inadequate circulation.

Transcutaneous Oxygen

In 1956 Clark developed a practical polarographic electrode to measure oxygen tension, using a semipermeable polyethylene membrane-covered platinum cathode (1). The Clark electrode has become the standard for blood gas analysis. Subsequently,

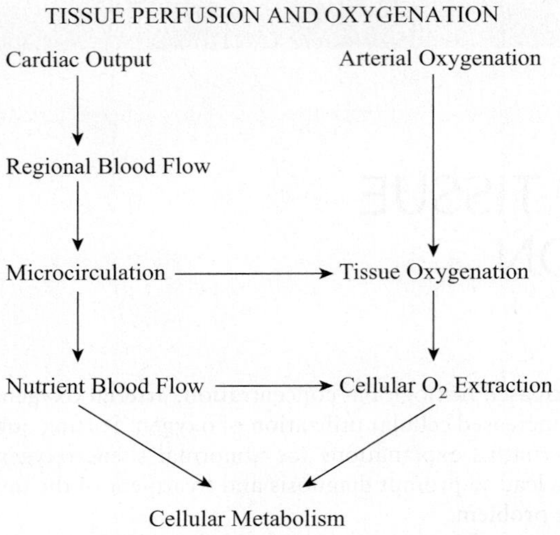

FIGURE 19.1. Tissue perfusion and oxygenation is determined by a complex interaction of systemic and regional blood flow and oxygenation, as well as by the state of the microcirculation and by cellular metabolism.

the Clark electrode was placed into a heated probe, and utilized for transcutaneous oxygen monitoring. Heating of the skin by the transcutaneous electrode is necessary to allow diffusion of oxygen across the stratum corneum. This occurs because heating the skin to 44°C or higher rapidly (over minutes) melts the lipoprotein barrier to oxygen diffusion. Heating the skin, however, also affects this tissue, dilating the underlying vessels and increasing local blood flow. In addition, heating decreases oxygen solubility, shifting the oxyhemoglobin dissociation curve to the right (2). Initial measurements must be delayed for up to 5 minutes for the skin to heat. Moreover, transcutaneous oxygen tension ($PtcO_2$) values may be site specific, sometimes with lower values in the extremities of patients with peripheral vascular disease. For critical care monitoring, most studies utilize the torso. Despite these confounding issues, transcutaneous oxygen monitoring provides useful physiologic data that are meaningfully related to tissue oxygenation.

Experimental studies have shown that transcutaneous oxygen monitoring is sensitive to arterial oxygen tension during normal cardiac output, but is more sensitive to perfusion in low-flow shock (3). In adult patients, $PtcO_2$ is approximately 80% of the arterial oxygen tension (PaO_2) during normal hemodynamic conditions. However, when blood flow is diminished, $PtcO_2$ also decreases. $PtcO_2$ is therefore related to both perfusion and oxygenation. When perfusion is normal, $PtcO_2$ varies with arterial oxygenation. When perfusion is inadequate, $PtcO_2$ varies with cardiac output. Hence, a normal $PtcO_2$ value indicates that both oxygenation and perfusion are relatively normal. A low $PtcO_2$ indicates that either oxygenation and/or cardiac output are inadequate. If arterial oxygenation is normal (as indicated by blood gases or pulse oximetry), low $PtcO_2$ indicates low-flow shock (4).

The relationship between $PtcO_2$ and PaO_2 can be quantitated, utilizing the $PtcO_2$ index, which is simply defined as $PaO_2/PtcO_2$. In a study that simultaneously measured cardiac index, $PtcO_2$, and PaO_2 in a large number of critically ill surgical patients, it was found that when cardiac output was relatively normal (cardiac index >2.2 L/minute/m^2), the $PtcO_2$ index averaged 0.79 ± 0.12. In individual patients with these normal cardiac outputs, $PtcO_2$ varied linearly with PaO_2. When cardiac output decreased, however, the $PtcO_2$ index decreased as well. For patients with a cardiac index between 1.5 and 2.2 L/minute/m^2, the $PtcO_2$ index averaged 0.48 ± 0.07. For patients with a cardiac index below 1.5 L/minute/m^2, the $PtcO_2$ index was 0.12 ± 0.12 (4). These data confirm that when blood flow is relatively normal, $PtcO_2$ varies with arterial oxygenation. However, with low-flow shock, $PtcO_2$ becomes very sensitive to changes in cardiac output.

Clinical studies have demonstrated the usefulness of trans cutaneous oxygen monitoring in detecting shock. When $PtcO_2$ monitors are placed during acute emergency resuscitation, low $PtcO_2$ values detect both hypoxemia and hemorrhagic shock. Moreover, the response of $PtcO_2$ during fluid infusion is a sensitive indicator of the efficacy of shock resuscitation (5,6).

Transcutaneous oxygen monitoring thus has benefit both as an early detector of shock and as a monitor to titrate resuscitation to a physiologic end point. It is noninvasive and inexpensive, and is therefore widely applicable for patients at risk, such as during emergency resuscitation of trauma and acute surgical emergencies, in the perioperative and postanesthesia period, and in the intensive care unit (ICU). However, while end points of successful resuscitation utilizing transcutaneous oxygen monitoring have been suggested, such values have not been validated in large prospective studies. The only risk of transcutaneous oxygen monitoring is minor skin burn beneath the probe if probe temperatures exceed 44°C or if the device is left in place for excessive periods of time.

Tissue Oxygen Monitors

In addition to transcutaneous oxygen probes, alternative direct tissue oxygen monitoring techniques have been developed. An advantage of such tissue probes is that heating of the skin is not necessary. In addition, specific tissues can be monitored to provide organ-specific information. Probes may be placed into the subcutaneous tissue, which is very sensitive to low flow. They may also be placed into muscle, which is perhaps less sensitive to low flow, but more rapidly responsive to resuscitation. Probes may also be placed directly into organs. For example, specific probes are now available for placement in the brain to provide a measure of cerebral oxygenation.

Two techniques for direct tissue oxygen monitoring are available. Polarographic electrodes incorporated into needles have been most widely utilized. In addition, a technique utilizing the phenomenon of fluorescence quenching is available. Tissue oxygen probes contain a fluorescent compound that is O_2 sensitive, such that its fluorescent emission is diminished in direct proportion to the amount of O_2 present. Energy from the monitor is transmitted through fiberoptic elements to the florescent compound in the probe, resulting in the emission of light, which is then measured by sensors in the tissue probe. The intensity of the emitted light is inversely proportional to the tissue pO_2 (7).

Another method of tissue oxygen monitoring is transconjunctival. The conjunctiva of the eye does not have a stratum corneum, so oxygen is freely diffusable. Transconjunctival probes are placed against the eye, and allow continuous tissue oxygen monitoring without heating; the technology has been utilized both during anesthesia and shock (8).

Direct tissue oxygen monitoring devices offer alternatives to transcutaneous monitoring, with the potential advantages of more rapid initial readings, a variety of monitoring sites, and no heating necessary. However, there are little clinical data to determine the relative sensitivities and specificities of these various techniques.

Near-infrared Spectroscopy

Near-infrared spectroscopy (NIS) has been developed as a noninvasive measure of tissue oxygenation (9–12). NIS measures the ratio of oxygenated hemoglobin to total hemoglobin (StO_2) in the microcirculation of the underlying muscle by measuring the absorption and reflectance of light. Using cutaneous probes placed upon the thenar eminence, values of 87% ± 6% have been measured in normal volunteers. Early clinical experience suggests that StO_2 values decrease during shock and increase with successful resuscitation. A recent multicenter trial in trauma patients suggested that a StO_2 value of 75% may be a therapeutic goal. This monitoring approach has potential value, as it provides convenient, continuous, noninvasive measurements. However, clinical data are limited. Tissue edema may be a confounding factor, as the distance between the probe and the underlying muscle affects measurements. Again, the sensitivity and specificity of this device compared to other tissue oxygen monitoring devices has not been studied. NIS has been demonstrated to have a close relationship to base deficit in critically injured patients (13) as well as predicting development of organ failure in traumatic shock patients (14).

NIS has also been utilized as a cerebral oximeter. By passing light through the scalp and skull, this technology provides a noninvasive measure of cerebral oxygenation.

Gastric Tonometry

The mesenteric circulatory bed, particularly the gut mucosa, is prone to hypoperfusion and ischemia during shock. Tonometry has been developed as a technique to detect adequacy of gastrointestinal mucosal perfusion (14). The technique is based upon calculation of the gastrointestinal intramucosal pH (pHi). The basis of this measurement is that the gastrointestinal mucosal pCO_2 equilibrates with the gastric luminal pCO_2. Measurement of luminal pCO_2 was originally accomplished by placing a tube with an attached balloon into the stomach, allowing time for the CO_2 to diffuse; measuring pCO_2 in the balloon, assuming that luminal pCO_2 equals mucosal pCO_2; and then calculating pHi by the Henderson-Hasselbalch equation as follows:

$$\text{pHi} = 6.1 + \log(\text{HCO}_3^-)/(\text{pCO}_2) \times 0.031$$

Gastric pHi monitoring has recently been improved by utilizing gas tonometry without the need for balloons, utilizing capnography. This improvement decreases the lag time necessary for equilibration of carbon dioxide, and allows for more continuous measurements.

The potential usefulness of gastric tonometry has been suggested in clinical studies, in which pHi has been reported to reflect the severity of shock and to increase during successful resuscitation (14). However, the technique has not gained widespread acceptance, in part because the accuracy of the pHi measurement has been questioned. Utilization of arterial bicarbonate as an estimate of mucosal bicarbonate concentrations may be inaccurate. Measurements can be also be altered by gastric acid secretion, because buffering of gastric acid by bicarbonate can produce CO_2 in the gastric lumen, which will confound the estimate of mucosal pCO_2. Enteral feeding may also affect pHi, although this effect is variable. To minimize these errors, it has been suggested that gastric feeding be withheld and antacid medication given prior to pHi monitoring. However, the variation and inaccuracies of gastric tonometry have limited its widespread application. Moreover, clear treatment end points have not been validated.

Several alternatives to gastric tonometry have been studied. Sublingual capnography is a less invasive technique, which shows promise as a sensitive indicator of tissue acidosis in shock models and in early clinical reports (15). This device was recalled in 2004 for infectious complications and may be reinstated in the future. Alternative luminal monitoring sites, such as the small intestine, rectum, and bladder, have also been proposed as monitoring sites for pHi monitoring (16).

Transcutaneous and End-tidal Carbon Dioxide

Transcutaneous carbon dioxide may be measured using the Severinghaus carbon dioxide electrode. Because CO_2 is more diffusible than is O_2, heating of the probe is not necessary. In analogy with $PtcO_2$ monitoring, transcutaneous CO_2 parallels arterial values when cardiac output is relatively normal, although transcutaneous values are normally 10 to 30 mm Hg higher than arterial. During low-flow shock, transcutaneous pCO_2 is increased, due to accumulation of carbon dioxide in the tissues due to inadequate perfusion (2). Increased transcutaneous pCO_2 may thus be utilized as an indicator of inadequate circulation, particularly if arterial pCO_2 is normal. In combination with low $PtcO_2$, increased transcutaneous pCO_2 gives additional evidence of circulatory shock. End-tidal CO_2 may also be utilized as a measure of perfusion; end-tidal CO_2 is decreased during low-flow states due to decreased pulmonary flow (17). Decreased end-tidal CO_2 values in combination with increased transcutaneous pCO_2 and normal arterial pCO_2 values are strong evidence of circulatory shock. This is an example of how combining noninvasive monitoring data can provide additional information.

TISSUE BLOOD FLOW

Measuring tissue blood flow can provide an indication of the adequacy of both cardiac output and regional blood flow. In critical illness, blood flow measurement has the particular potential to be combined with tissue oxygen monitoring to help determine if inadequate tissue oxygenation is due to perfusion deficits. Hence, a reliable tissue perfusion monitor has great appeal.

Many technologies have been developed to measure tissue perfusion. The best studied of these is laser Doppler. Laser Doppler utilizes analysis of scattering of light to determine quantitative blood flow in a small area around the probe (18). A variety of probes have been developed, which can be placed noninvasively onto the skin, or into tissues with needle probes. Laser Doppler measurements have been shown to be useful in detecting changes in blood flow under many experimental conditions. However, clinical utility has been limited due to the large variation in blood flow within tissues (19). Because of these variations, no normal values, no optimal values, and no therapeutic goal values for blood flow have been determined.

Numerous alternative approaches to monitoring tissue perfusion have also been developed. Measurement of local blood flow by thermal diffusion has been developed as an alternative to light scattering, and implantable probes using this technology are available. In addition, magnetic resonance imaging, positron emission tomography, and contrast-enhanced ultrasonography have been used to measure tissue perfusion, although these are not available as continuous monitoring devices. Fluorescence microangiography has also been developed to provide both visual imaging of the microcirculation and measurements of local blood flow (20,21). As with laser Doppler monitoring, validated clinical applications for these technologies have yet to be defined.

The Oxygen Challenge Test

An approach to utilize tissue oxygen monitoring in a more dynamic manner was proposed by Dr. Hunt's group in San Francisco (22). Endeavoring to assess adequacy of tissue perfusion in postoperative patients, they measured subcutaneous pO_2 before and after patients breathed high inspired O_2 concentrations. The expected response in well-perfused patients was a rapid increase in tissue pO_2. Many postoperative patients failed to demonstrate this response, which was, however, restored with intravenous fluid infusion. A physiologic explanation for the responses of tissue pO_2 to inspired O_2 is interesting. If there is no cellular O_2 deficit, then additional dissolved O_2 supplied after breathing O_2 is not required nor utilized by cells, and therefore results in increased tissue pO_2. However, if there is a cellular O_2 deficit (shock), then any additional dissolved O_2 would be rapidly utilized, and would thus not result in increased tissue pO_2. The tissue pO_2 response to inspired O_2 may then be a relatively rapid and minimally invasive method to detect cellular hypoxia. This approach, named the oxygen challenge test, was evaluated in trauma patients (22,23) (Table 19.1). The O_2 challenge test had 100% sensitivity and specificity in detecting flow-dependent O_2 consumption in invasively monitored patients in the intensive care unit. It also appeared to be a very sensitive indicator of shock during acute resuscitation. This method, utilizing either transcutaneous or direct tissue O_2 monitors, has potential to detect which patients require fluid resuscitation, to provide a physiologic end point for resuscitation, and to detect the patients in whom initial resuscitation is inadequate and who therefore require additional monitoring and therapy. Using a noninvasive transcutaneous ($PtcO_2$) monitor, Yu et al. have studied the O_2 challenge test in patients in the intensive care unit and have validated the sensitivity and specificity of the test in identifying patients in occult shock. In addition, their data has defined an increase in $PtcO_2$ of greater than 20 to 25 mm Hg in response to a FiO_2 of 1.0 as a therapeutic endpoint (24,25). In a prospective randomized trial using the oxygen challenge test as an end point of resuscitation compared to the oxygen delivery variables from the pulmonary artery catheter, an improved survival was reported (25). The skin is the first to vasoconstrict (even before the gastrointestinal tract) and the last to perfuse in shock states, and the use of the $PtcO_2$ monitor may give an early warning signal of occult shock. The same authors used the oxygen challenge test to identify patients who may benefit from activated protein C (26). Monitoring and treating the peripheral tissue oxygenation state does not exclude utilization of central hemodynamic parameters such as cardiac output and oxygen delivery (DO_2), but does allow manipulation of DO_2 to reach a specific goal of tissue perfusion rather than aiming for a general DO_2 value.

TABLE 19.1

OXYGEN CHALLENGE TEST

1. Select patients who have baseline arterial O_2 saturation over 90% on FiO_2 <0.6–0.8.
2. Obtain baseline transcutaneous (or tissue) pO_2 value.
3. Increase FiO_2 to 1.0.
4. After 5 min, repeat transcutaneous (or tissue) pO_2 measurement.
5. If transcutaneous (or tissue) pO_2 increases >20–25 torr, patient can be assumed to have no flow-dependent oxygen consumption.
6. If transcutaneous (or tissue) pO_2 increases <20 torr, provide therapy to increase oxygen delivery until step 5 is met.

From Waxman K, Annas C, Daughters K, et al. A method to determine the adequacy of resuscitation using tissue oxygen monitoring. *J Trauma*. 1994;36:852–858; Yu M, Morita SY, Daniel SR, et al. Transcutaneous pressure of oxygen: a non-invasive and early detector of peripheral shock and outcome. *Shock*. 2006;26:450–456; and Yu M, Chapital A, Ho HC, et al. A prospective randomized trial comparing oxygen delivery versus transcutaneous pressure of oxygen values as resuscitative goals. *Shock*. 2007;27:615–622.

SUMMARY

Monitoring tissue perfusion and oxygenation provides important physiologic information. However, there is currently no consensus on how to utilize these devices. Great potential exists to develop noninvasive systems utilizing these devices, which will provide sensitive and specific indications both of the severity of shock and end points for resuscitation. Such systems would provide a minimally invasive approach to improve the treatment of shock. To achieve acceptance and application of such systems will require quality clinical studies to determine and validate optimal treatment goals.

PEARLS

1. A decreased transcutaneous oxygen value may be an early warning of decreased arterial oxygenation, decreased hemoglobin, or decreased cardiac output.
2. The ratio of transcutaneous oxygen to arterial oxygen may be utilized as an end point of resuscitation, with a goal of 0.8.
3. Near-infrared spectroscopy devices placed on the thenar eminence provide a measure of tissue oxygenation, with a normal value of 87% ± 6% saturation. Values less than 75% may indicate shock.

4. Sublingual tonometry is a less invasive alternative to gastric tonometry, but this technology needs to be reinstated since it has been recalled.
5. Increased transcutaneous pCO_2 is an indicator of tissue acidosis.
6. The presence of decreased end-tidal pCO_2 in the face of normal arterial pCO_2 is an indicator of low cardiac output.
7. The response of transcutaneous or tissue oxygen monitors to an increased FiO_2 is an indication of the presence or absence of flow-dependent oxygen consumption. An increase in tissue oxygen of greater than 24 torr may be utilized as an end point of resuscitation.

References

1. Clark LC. Measurement of oxygen tension: a historical perspective. *Crit Care Med.* 1981;9:694–702.
2. Tremper KK, Waxman K. Transcutaneous monitoring of respiratory gases. In: Nochomovitz M, Cherniack NS, eds. *Non-Invasive Respiratory Monitoring.* New York: Churchill Livingstone; 1985:1–28.
3. Tremper KK, Waxman K, Shoemaker WC. Effects of hypoxia and shock on transcutaneous pO2 values in dogs. *Crit Care Med.* 1979;7:526–531.
4. Tremper KK, Shoemaker WC. Transcutaneous oxygen monitoring of critically ill adults, with and without low flow shock. *Crit Care Med.* 1981;9:706–711.
5. Waxman K, Sadler R, Eisner M, et al. Transcutaneous oxygen monitoring of emergency department patients. *Am J Surg.* 1983;146:35–38.
6. Tatevossian RG, Wo CCJ, Velmahos GC, et al. Transcutaneous oxygen and CO_2 as early warning of tissue hypoxia and hemodynamic shock in critically ill emergency patients. *Crit Care Med.* 2000;28:2248–2253.
7. Shaw AD, Zheng L, Thomas Z, et al. Assessment of tissue oxygen tension: comparison of dynamic fluorescence quenching and polarographic electrode technique. *Crit Care.* 2002;6:76–80.
8. Abraham E, Smith M, Silver S. Conjunctival and transcutaneous monitoring during cardiopulmonary arrest and cardiopulmonary resuscitation. *Crit Care Med.* 1984;12:419–423.
9. Beilman GJ, Groehler KE, Lazaron V, et al. Near-infrared spectroscopy measurement of regional tissue oxyhemoglobin saturation during hemorrhagic shock. *Shock.* 1999;12:196–200.
10. Taylor JH, Mulier KE, Myers DE, et al. Use of near-infrared spectroscopy in early determination of irreversible hemorrhagic shock. *J Trauma.* 2005;58:1119–1125.
11. Crooks BA, Cohn SM, Bloch S. Can near-infrared spectroscopy identify the severity of shock in trauma patients. *J Trauma.* 2005;58:806–813.
12. Ikossi DG, Knudson MM, Morabito DJ, et al. Continuous muscle tissue oxygenation in critically injured patients: a prospective observational study. *J Trauma Injury Infect Crit Care.* 2006;61:780–790.
13. Cohn SM, Nathens AB, Moore FA, et al. Tissue oxygenation saturation predicts the development of organ dysfunction during traumatic shock resuscitation. *J Trauma.* 2007;62:44–55.
14. Guzman JA, Kruse JA. Continuous assessment of gastric intramucosal pCO2 and pH in hemorrhagic shock using capnometric recirculating gas tonometry. *Crit Care Med.* 1997;25:533–537.
15. Creteur J. Gastric and sublingual capnometry. *Curr Opin Crit Care.* 2006;12:272–277.
16. Walley KR, Friesen BP, Humer MF, et al. Small bowel tonometry is more accurate than gastric tonometry in detecting gut ischemia. *J Appl Physiol.* 1998;85:1770–1777.
17. Falk JL, Rackow EC, Weil MH. End-tidal carbon dioxide concentration during cardiopulmonary resuscitation. *N Eng J Med.* 1988;318:607–611.
18. Johnson JM, Taylor WF, Shepherd AP, et al. Laser-Doppler measurement of skin blood flow: comparison with plethysmography. *J Appl Physiol.* 1984;56:798–803.
19. Chang N, Goodson WH, Gottrup F, et al. Direct measurement of wound and tissue oxygen tension in postoperative patients. *Ann Surg.* 1983;197:470–478.
20. Waxman K, Formosa P, Soliman H. Laser Doppler velocimetry in critically ill patients. *Crit Care Med.* 1987;15:780–783.
21. Mcveigh ER. Emerging imaging techniques. *Circ Res.* 2006;14:879–886.
22. Littooy F, Fuchs R, Hunt TK, et al. Tissue oxygen as a real-time measure of oxygen transport. *J Surg Res.* 1976;20:321–325.
23. Waxman K, Annas C, Daughters K, et al. A method to determine the adequacy of resuscitation using tissue oxygen monitoring. *J Trauma.* 1994;36:852–858.
24. Yu M, Morita SY, Daniel SR, et al. Transcutaneous pressure of oxygen: a non-invasive and early detector of peripheral shock and outcome. *Shock.* 2006;26:450–456.
25. Yu M, Chapital A, Ho HC, et al. A prospective randomized trial comparing oxygen delivery versus transcutaneous pressure of oxygen values as resuscitative goals. *Shock.* 2007;27:615–622.
26. Chapital A, Yu M, Ho H. Transcutaneous pO_2 as a selection criteria for activated protein C use. *J Trauma.* 2008;65:30–33.

CHAPTER 20 ■ BEDSIDE ASSESSMENT AND MONITORING OF PULMONARY FUNCTION AND POWER OF BREATHING IN THE CRITICALLY ILL

MICHAEL J. BANNER

IMMEDIATE CONCERNS

Major Problems

Work of breathing per minute, or *power of breathing* (POB), reflects the balance between patient spontaneous breathing demand (driven by metabolic and neural factors) and the support provided by the ventilator. Increases in respiratory muscle loading and, thus, POB result primarily from increased physiologic elastance and resistance. Because compliance is the reciprocal of elastance, as total compliance (lungs and chest wall) decreases, elastic loading of the respiratory muscles increases. The total resistive load is affected by physiologic airways and breathing apparatus resistances. Elastance, resistance, or both can significantly increase the POB or load on the respiratory muscles, predisposing to muscle fatigue (loss of the force-generating capacity of the muscles), carbon dioxide retention, and hypoxemia.

Ventilatory support may be applied to partially or totally unload respiratory muscles. High levels of ventilatory support totally unload the muscles and, if applied for too long a period, may lead to atrophy. Conversely, too little support risks muscle fatigue. Unfortunately, in either case, the duration of mechanical ventilation may be needlessly prolonged for reconditioning/training if respiratory muscle atrophy is present or to provide needed rest if the muscles are fatigued. Optimization of ventilatory support to each patient's unique needs requires information of the load on the respiratory muscles as well as gas exchange. This manuscript will focus on POB measurements as my approach to assess the load on the muscles and to provide a quantitative and goal-oriented method for appropriately setting pressure support ventilation (PSV).

STRESS POINTS

1. Respiratory muscles are force generators, and the diaphragm accounts for 70% of normal tidal volume (V_T).
2. The diaphragm has high endurance capability well suited to low-tension, high-repetition activity (breathing). However, it can be readily fatigued by increased air flow resistance and duration of respiratory muscle contraction.
3. Imposed POB against a highly resistant ventilator circuit and endotracheal tube leads to fatigue. Patients with an already increased physiologic POB because of respiratory disease tolerate such increases poorly.
4. Bedside measurement of POB, including breath-by-breath analysis, and separation into its component parts are possible with a commercially available bedside monitor.
5. Inaccurate assessments of respiratory muscle loads by using parameters like respiratory muscle pressure (Pmus) may result because of failure to assess chest wall compliance and its contributions.
6. Factors that load the respiratory muscles include increases of inspiratory flow rate and minute ventilation, physiologic dead space volume–to–tidal volume ratio (V_D/V_T), intrinsic positive end-expiratory pressure (PEEP), breathing apparatus resistance, and the ventilator response time. Many of these factors can be altered favorably by careful adjustment and replacement of highly resistant elements of the circuit (particularly the endotracheal tube).
7. Respiratory muscle fatigue results from an imbalance of energy supply and demand.
8. Inferences as to POB, such as increased spontaneous breathing frequency (f) and tidal volume (V_T) *alone* can be misleading.
9. Successful weaning from mechanical ventilation often requires a decrease in the imposed POB to a tolerable level. PSV is uniquely capable to decrease or eliminate this workload when titrated in accordance with measured POB.

ESSENTIAL DIAGNOSTIC TESTS AND PROCEDURES

1. Most patients can be followed by conventional assessment. However, when weaning, extubation, or both are difficult or seemingly impossible, measurements of airway pressures, V_T, and POB with its component parts may be useful in assessing the patient and guiding ventilatory therapy.
2. Spontaneous and breathing patterns (f and V_T), as well as the use of accessory respiratory muscles such as the sternocleidomastoid (SCM) muscle, should be continuously monitored, but their limitations for predicting and assessing diaphragmatic fatigue, as detailed in this chapter, should be well understood.

INITIAL THERAPY

1. Decrease the imposed POB to zero using PSV as the first step. This workload is of no value for muscle conditioning and predisposes to fatigue.
2. Add additional PSV as necessary to reduce the physiologic workload (elastance and resistance) to clinically acceptable levels (i.e., POB of approximately 5–10 joules/minute).
3. Use the largest internal diameter endotracheal tube that is unlikely to result in airway damage. A 1.0-mm increase of the inside diameter is associated with significantly less resistive imposed work (parenthetically to be noted is that less air is needed for cuff inflation with larger tubes, thereby decreasing the risk of cuff-induced tracheal damage).
4. Do not reduce PSV below the level that eliminates imposed POB. To do so reloads the respiratory muscles, predisposing to fatigue.
5. In difficult cases, use clinical parameters to supplement—but not to replace—direct noninvasively measured POB.

RESPIRATORY MUSCLES

Respiratory muscles are the *force generators* that drive the respiratory system (1). Regarded as the primary inspiratory muscle, the diaphragm accounts for approximately 70% of normal V_T exchange. Other inspiratory muscles that account for the balance of tidal ventilation are the external intercostals, parasternals, and scalenes (2). The SCM muscles are major *accessory* inspiratory muscles that have a predominantly pump-handle action on the rib cage, elevating the first ribs and sternum (Fig. 20.1). During quiet breathing, they are usually inactive, but are always active during exercise and conditions of respiratory muscle loading.

The internal intercostal and abdominal muscles are involved with exhalation. On contraction, the internal intercostal muscles lower the ribs, thus deflating the lungs. The external abdominal oblique, internal abdominal oblique, transverse abdominis, and rectus abdominis (1,2) (Fig. 20.1) are the most important and powerful expiratory muscles. When these muscles contract, the abdominal wall is pulled inward, causing increased intra-abdominal pressure that forces the diaphragm cephalad into the thoracic cavity (3). Concomitantly, the lower ribs are pulled downward and medially. The net effect of these actions is deflation of the rib cage. Normally, exhalation is a passive process and the abdominal muscles are inactive. With increased muscle loads (e.g., increased airway resistance), however, the abdominal muscles are recruited and exhalation becomes an active, energy-consuming process.

THE DIAPHRAGM

Because the diaphragm is the primary muscle of inspiration, the physiologic characteristics and responses of this muscle during conditions of loaded and unloaded breathing are described.

Muscle Fiber Types

The adult diaphragm is composed of three types of skeletal muscle fibers: Type 1 (≤60%), type 2A (≤20%), and type 2B (≤20%) (4). Skeletal muscle fibers are differentiated on the basis of (a) velocity of shortening (fast and slow fibers), and (b) the major pathway to form adenosine triphosphate (ATP) (oxidative and glycolytic fibers) (5). In general, muscle fibers are composed of two contractile protein filaments: Myosin (thick filament) and actin (thin filament). Fibers containing myosin with high ATPase activity (enzyme that catalyzes the hydrolysis of ATP to adenosine diphosphate [ADP], releasing chemical energy stored in ATP) are classified as *fast fibers;* those containing myosin with lower ATPase activity are *slow fibers.* In general, the more energy that is available for contraction, the greater is the velocity of muscle fiber shortening.

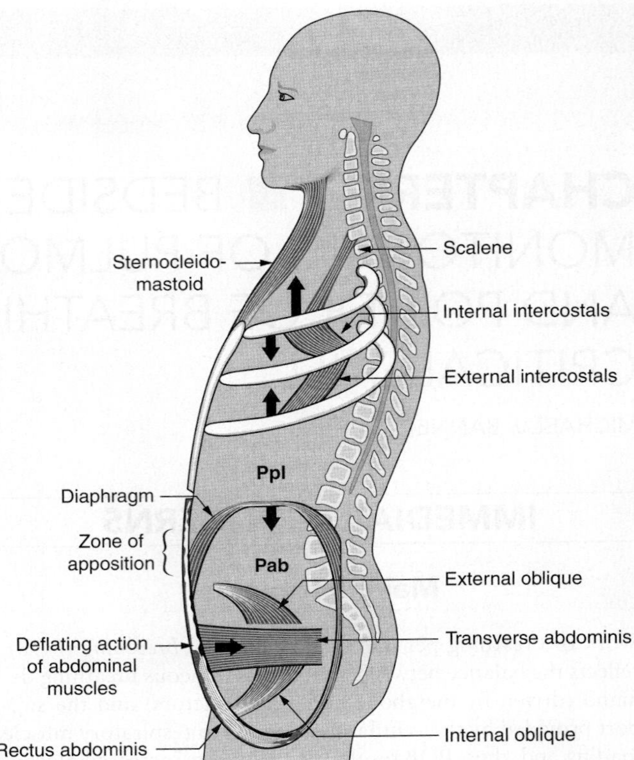

FIGURE 20.1. Diagrammatic representation of inspiratory and expiratory muscles; arrows indicate direction of action. Pab, abdominal pressure; Ppl, intrapleural pressure. (Modified from Roussos C. *Chest.* 1985;88:S125.)

Force Generation and Fatigue

Muscle fibers differ in terms of size and force development. Glycolytic fibers are larger in diameter than oxidative fibers. A greater force or tension can be developed by a large-diameter muscle fiber. Consequently, a type 2B fiber (strength oriented) can generate more force than a type 1 fiber during contraction (4,5). Fibers also differ in their ability to resist fatigue (muscle fails as a force generator). Type 2B fibers fatigue rapidly, whereas type 1 fibers are resistant to fatigue (endurance oriented), a characteristic that allows them to maintain contractile activity for long periods. Type 2A fibers have an intermediate capacity to resist fatigue (4,6).

Endurance and Strength

In general, the diaphragm is an endurance-oriented (low-tension, high-repetition activity), not strength-oriented (high-tension, low-repetition activity), muscle because most of the muscle mass is composed of type 1, slow oxidative fibers. In fact, it is capable of impressive feats of endurance. An Olympic marathon runner can maintain high minute ventilation of approximately 50 L/minute several hours per day for many days in succession. Despite this endurance performance, the diaphragm can be fatigued in a matter of minutes by an increased resistance to flow rate or increased duration of muscle contraction (4).

The duration of diaphragmatic contraction is the duty cycle of the breath taken as the ratio of inspiratory time to total respiratory cycle time (T_I/T_{tot}). Normally, the T_I/T_{tot} ratio is approximately 0.33 (7). The diaphragm, although contracting rhythmically from minute to minute, requires time to recover before contraction resumes. Impingement on this recovery time by an increase in respiratory rate, duration of contraction, or both predisposes to respiratory muscle fatigue. An increase in respiratory rate, as in acute respiratory failure, causes a greater reduction in expiratory time than inspiratory time, thus increasing T_I/T_{tot} and contributing to the development of fatigue (6,7). In patients with severe respiratory muscle loading, we have measured T_I/T_{tot} ratios as high as 0.50 to 0.60.

Measurement of Work of Breathing

The load on the respiratory muscles is a reverse force that opposes the contractile force of the muscles and may be assessed by measuring the work of breathing per breath, that is, by integrating the change in esophageal pressure (Pes) and V_T (8,9).

$$\text{Work} = \int \text{Pes}\, V_T$$

POB, the rate at which work is done, is a better assessment of respiratory muscle loads than work per breath because it is a measure over time, not for an individual breath. Because of wide variations in breath-to-breath work measurements, at times this method of assessing respiratory muscle workloads is difficult to interpret. POB is determined by averaging work per breath data over 1 minute.

The total respiratory muscle work performed by a spontaneously breathing, intubated patient connected to a mechanical ventilator includes *imposed* and *physiologic* components (Table 20.1). Imposed POB (work per minute performed by the patient to breathe spontaneously through the endotracheal tube, ventilator breathing circuit, and demand-flow system) is an additional flow-resistive workload superimposed on the physiologic work (10–12). Imposed POB may equal or exceed the physiologic work under some conditions (13–15).

Imposed POB of the ventilator and endotracheal tube, a series resistance, is assessed by integrating the change in pressure measured at the carinal end of the endotracheal tube and V_T (16). Pressure at the carinal or tracheal end of the tube is measured by inserting a narrow (1-mm outside diameter), air-filled catheter through the tube and positioning it at the carinal end. V_T is measured by integrating the flow signal from a miniature flow sensor (pneumotachograph) positioned between the Y piece of the breathing circuit and the endotracheal tube.

TABLE 20.1

WORK PER BREATH TO DETERMINE POWER OF BREATHING PERFORMED BY A SPONTANEOUSLY BREATHING, INTUBATED PATIENT (SEE FIG. 20.3)

Total work per breath
Physiologic work
Elastic and flow resistive
Imposed work
Resistive work imposed by breathing apparatus (endotracheal tube, breathing circuit, demand-flow system, exhalation valves)

These data are, in turn, averaged over 1 minute to determine imposed POB (Fig. 20.2). Imposed POB should be nullified to zero by using appropriate levels of PSV (Fig. 20.2A).

Physiologic work per minute or power of breathing includes elastic (work required to overcome the elastic forces of the respiratory system during inflation) and flow-resistive (work required to overcome the resistance of the airways and tissues to the flow of gas) components, and is approximately 4 to 8 joules/minute (8,17). Based on studying over 500 adults in a 10-year span, a clinically acceptable range for *total* POB appears to be about 5 to 10 joules/minute.

The Campbell Diagram

POB performed by the patient on the respiratory system (physiologic power of breathing) and the ventilator and endotracheal tube (imposed power of breathing) during spontaneous ventilation is calculated by integrating the changes in esophageal pressure (indirect measurement of intrapleural pressure) and volume. Intraesophageal pressure is measured with a balloon catheter positioned in the middle to lower third of the esophagus. Correct position is confirmed using an occlusion test as described by Baydur et al. (18) (i.e., after occlusion of the airway opening, the *change* in pressure at the airway opening and in the esophagus are nearly the same during spontaneous inspiratory efforts). V_T is measured as described previously. Data from these measurements and measurement of chest wall compliance are processed and the work of breathing calculated using the Campbell diagram (9,19,20) (Fig. 20.3). Work per breath measurements are then averaged over 1 minute to compute POB.

Chest Wall Influence on Power of Breathing Measurements

To calculate work of breathing so as to determine POB using the Campbell diagram, chest wall compliance must first be measured. Accuracy in measuring chest wall compliance requires a relaxed and mechanically ventilated patient. To measure chest wall compliance, one approach is to administer adequate sedation (1–2 mg of intravenous midazolam) or induce pharmacologic paralysis to induce relaxation, and then the mechanical ventilator rate is increased transiently to approximately 10 to 12 breaths/minute. Under conditions of

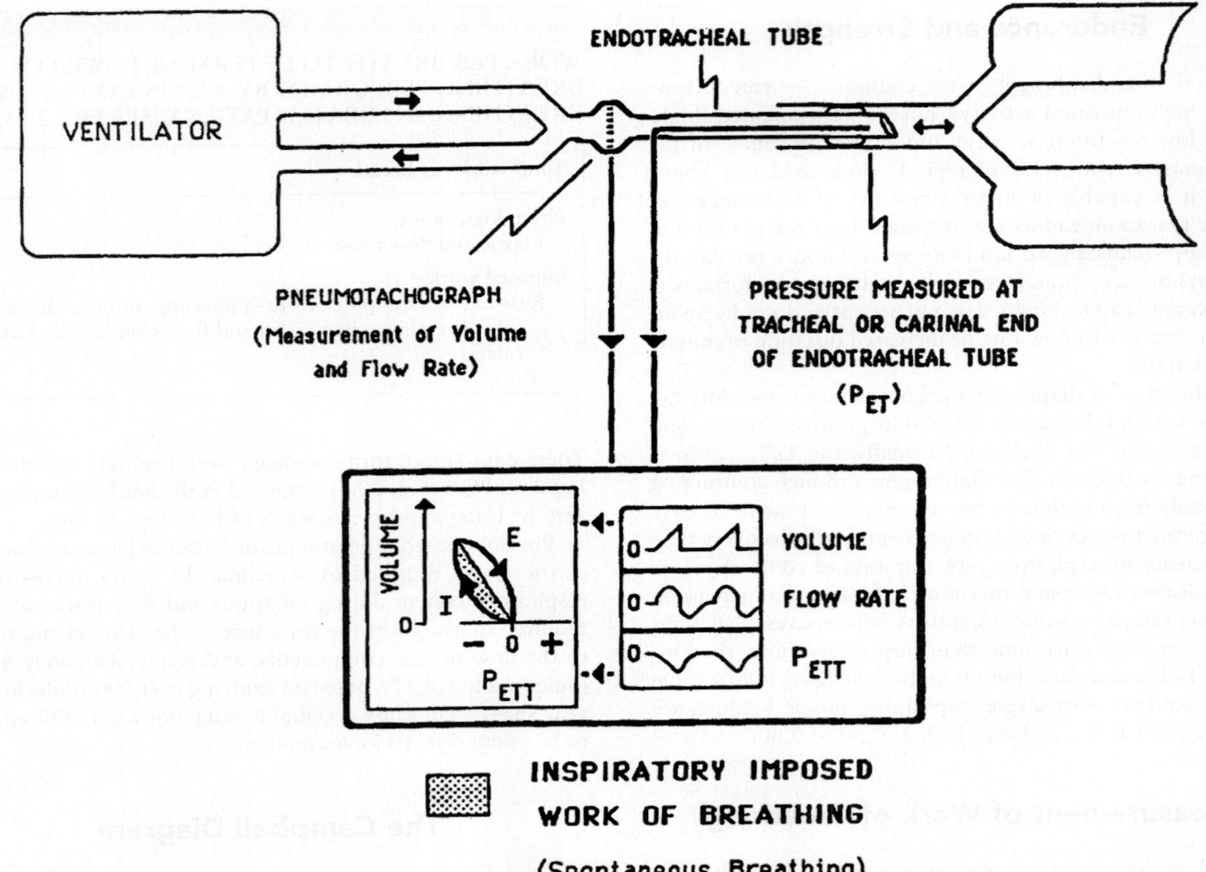

FIGURE 20.2. Work imposed by the breathing apparatus is determined during spontaneous breathing by measuring change in pressure at the tracheal or carinal end of the endotracheal tube (P_{ET}) and change in volume (tidal volume) between the Y piece of the ventilator breathing circuit and the endotracheal tube. P_{ET} and the change in volume are directed to a respiratory monitor and are integrated to display a pressure–volume (work) loop and provide real-time calculations of the inspiratory imposed work of breathing (i.e., the shaded area of the loop). I, inhalation; E, exhalation (see Fig. 20.2A). (*continued*)

mechanical inflation with a preselected V_T and a relaxed patient, esophageal pressure increases. The changes in esophageal pressure and volume are integrated to produce a pressure–volume loop that moves in a counterclockwise direction. The slope of this pressure–volume loop is interpreted as chest wall compliance. Measured chest wall compliance values for adult patients who were diagnosed with acute respiratory failure averaged 0.109 ± 0.037 L/cm H_2O (21). Subsequently, when the patient resumes breathing spontaneously, total POB (physiologic plus imposed) is then computed using the Campbell diagram as previously described.

Alternative Measurements

Measurement of the area enclosed within an esophageal pressure–volume loop during spontaneous breathing *underestimates* the work per breath, and thus POB, because the area of the loop includes only the resistive work (physiologic plus imposed) and a small portion of the elastic work (see Fig. 20.3). Some investigators fitted a right triangle to the esophageal pressure–volume loop to infer elastic work; however, this approach also underestimates elastic work of breathing (22). Measurement of the pressure change at the Y piece of the ventilator breathing circuit tubing or at the carinal end of the endotracheal tube and the change in volume during spontaneous breathing allows calculation *only* of the work imposed by the ventilator and ventilator plus the endotracheal tube, respectively (11,16). Thus, accurate measurement of the total POB (physiologic plus imposed) requires monitoring equipment with appropriate hardware and software to use the Campbell diagram.

Using Pmus, the sum of elastic pressure (V_T divided by respiratory system compliance) and resistive pressure (flow rate times total resistance, which is respiratory system resistance plus endotracheal tube resistance) alone to predict work per breath via a conversion factor has been advanced (23). However, in our experience this is an inaccurate method of predicting work of breathing per breath. This method does not take into consideration the effects of decreased chest wall compliance on increasing elastic work and, thus, total work per breath.

We measured total work per breath (imposed plus physiologic work) with an esophageal balloon catheter using the Campbell diagram, as well as calculating POB on over 200 adults receiving PSV while simultaneously calculating Pmus.

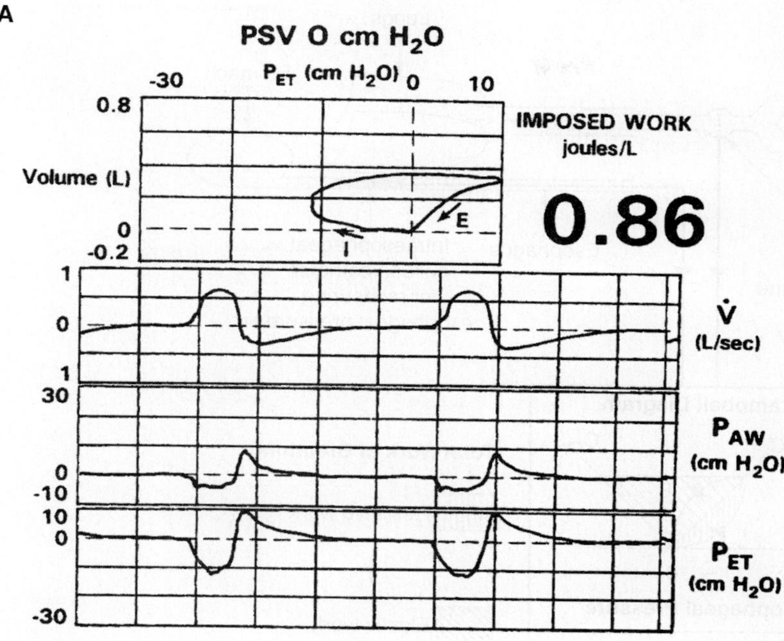

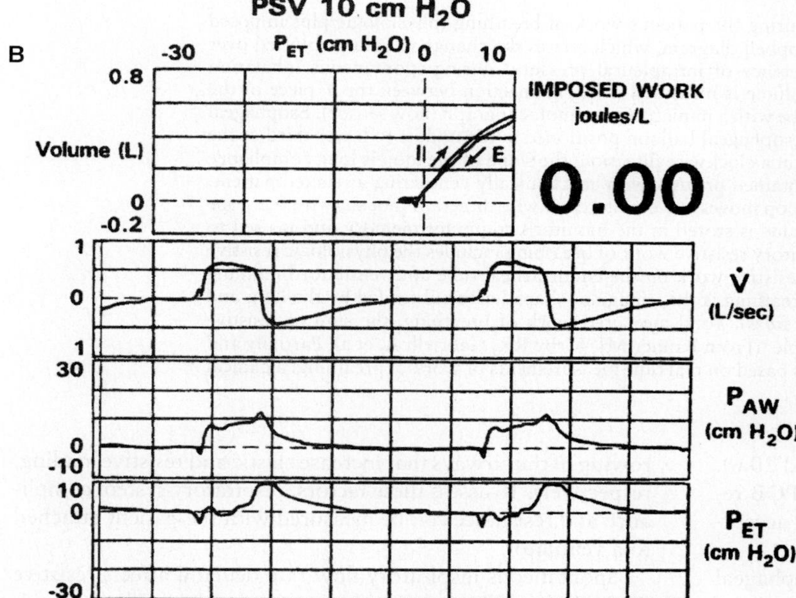

FIGURE 20.2. (*Continued*) Recordings of imposed work of breathing obtained by integrating the changes in pressure at the tracheal or carinal end of the endotracheal tube (P_{ET}) and volume at the Y piece of the ventilatory breathing circuit for a patient intubated with an 8.5-mm internal diameter endotracheal tube and connected to a ventilator (7200a, Puritan-Bennett) while breathing spontaneously with zero end-expiratory pressure. Inspiratory flow rate ($\dot{V}$) and airway pressure (P_{AW}) are measured at the Y piece of the breathing circuit (see Fig. 20.2). The pressure–volume loop moves in a clockwise direction during inhalation (I) and exhalation (E), and the area circumscribed within the loop to the left of zero pressure is imposed work. **A:** No pressure support ventilation (PSV) is applied. Notice the value of imposed work and that P_{ET} decreases by a greater amount than P_{AW} during spontaneous inhalation because of the resistance of the endotracheal tube. **B:** PSV of 10 cm H_2O is applied, and imposed work decreases to zero. P_{AW} increases to a greater level, and P_{ET} does not decrease during inhalation compared with A. Notice that volume increases from approximately 0.35 L in A to 0.50 L in B as a result of PSV. A *minimal* level of PSV is that which corresponds to *zero* imposed work of breathing.

We found that Pmus was a poor predictor of work per breath ($r^2 = 0.42$). Because this approach resulted in both over- and underestimations of the work of breathing per breath, it is not recommended for use in clinical practice for patients attached to life-support ventilators.

Noninvasive Measurement of Power of Breathing

Power of breathing can be calculated noninvasively (POB_N) with reasonable clinical accuracy for patients receiving ventilatory support by using an artificial neural network (ANN) (24). An ANN is a contemporary computational tool used for predicting, as in predicting a physiologic parameter for example. In one clinical study (24), data from an esophageal balloon catheter and airway pressure/flow sensor were used to measure POB invasively as defined above. A pretrained ANN provided real-time calculation of POB_N. The ANN used five parameters, each readily determined from pressure and flow tracings obtained at the airway opening of an individual patient to predict POB (i.e., spontaneous minute ventilation, intrinsic positive end-expiratory pressure [PEEPi], inspiratory pressure trigger depth, inspiratory flow rise time, and Pmus) (Fig. 20.4). Invasive POB and POB_N were measured at various levels of PSV, ranging from 5 to 25 cm H_2O. POB_N was highly correlated

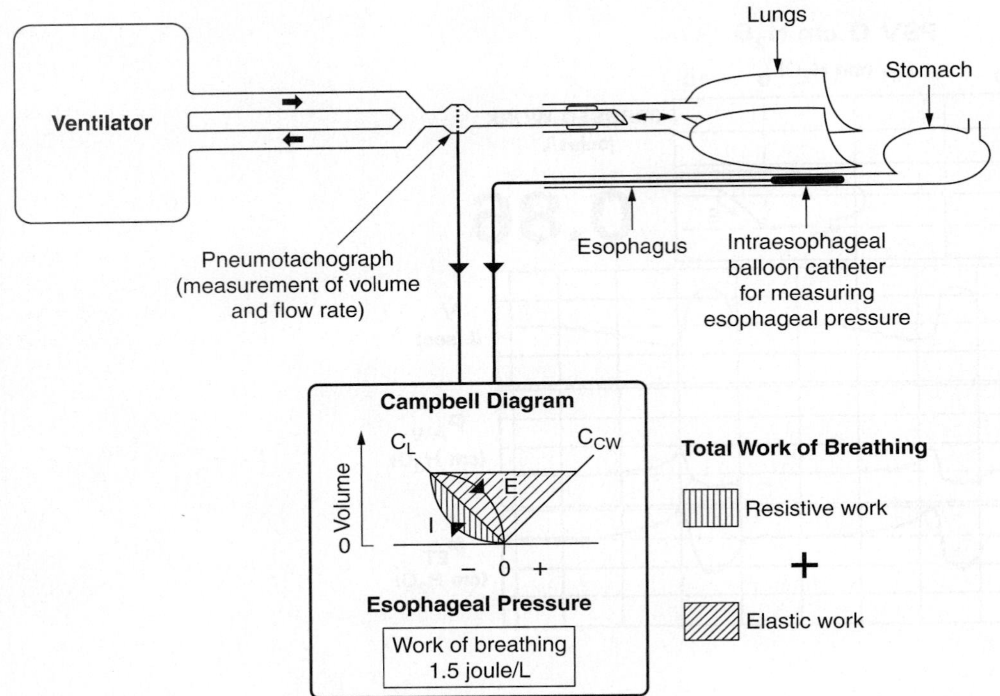

FIGURE 20.3. Clinical method of measuring the patient's work of breathing (physiologic plus imposed work). Work is computed using the Campbell diagram, which relates the change in volume plotted over the change in esophageal pressure (inference of intrapleural pressure) during spontaneous inhalation (I) and exhalation (E). The change in volume is measured at the connection between the Y piece of the breathing circuit and the endotracheal tube with a miniature pneumotachograph (flow sensor). Esophageal pressure (Pes) is measured with an intraesophageal balloon positioned in the middle to lower third of the esophagus. The Pes–volume loop moves in a clockwise direction; the slope of the loop is lung compliance (C_L). Chest wall compliance (C_{CW}) is obtained previously by mechanically ventilating a relaxed patient. Under these conditions the Pes–volume loop moves in a counterclockwise direction (not shown); the slope of the loop is C_{CW}. (This compliance value is stored in the monitor's computer memory and is used to construct the Campbell diagram.) Inspiratory resistive work of breathing includes the physiologic resistive work on the airways and the imposed resistive work on the endotracheal tube and ventilator breathing circuit (*vertical lines*). Elastic work of breathing is the triangular-shaped area subtended by the lung and chest wall compliance curves (*diagonal lines*). Total measured work of breathing, the sum of resistive and elastic work, is 1.5 J/L in this example. (From Banner MJ, Kirby RR, Gabrielli A, et al. Partially and totally unloading the respiratory muscles based on real time measurements of work of breathing: a clinical approach. *Chest.* 1994;106:1835.)

with invasive POB ($r = 0.91$, $p < 0.002$) (Figs. 20.5 and 20.6). A Bland–Altman plot comparing POB_N and invasive POB revealed that bias was zero and precision was clinically acceptable at 2.2.

This method obviates the need for inserting an esophageal balloon catheter, and thus greatly simplifies measurement of power of breathing. It could be fully automated into mechanical ventilators. POB_N may be a clinically useful tool for consideration when setting PSV to unload the respiratory muscles.

LOADING FACTORS

For healthy, asymptomatic individuals, the load on the respiratory muscles results from normal impedance (compliance and resistance) and ventilation loads (25). Increases in respiratory muscle loading result from a variety of physiologic and breathing apparatus factors. Physiologic factors include decreases in lung or chest wall compliance, or both, secondary to pulmonary abnormalities (Figs. 20.7 and 20.8, and Table 20.2) or bronchoconstriction, leading to peripheral, widespread narrowing of the airways that increase elastic and resistive loading, respectively. To assess these factors, respiratory system compliance and resistance can be measured with the patient attached to a ventilator.

Spontaneous inspiratory flow rate demand affects resistive POB directly. This relationship can be explained by an analogy of the Ohm Law of electricity (i.e., change in pressure equals inspiratory flow rate demand multiplied by airway resistance). Assuming a fairly constant airway resistance over a range of flow rates, increases in the patient's peak inspiratory flow rate demand result in greater changes in pressure. Because work $= \int Pes\ V_T$, a greater change in pressure with the same change in volume produces greater work per breath, and thus POB (17).

Minute Ventilation

Increases in the V_D/V_T ratio and minute ventilation also are forms of respiratory muscle loading that lead to increased POB (25). Under both conditions, the respiratory muscle pump is

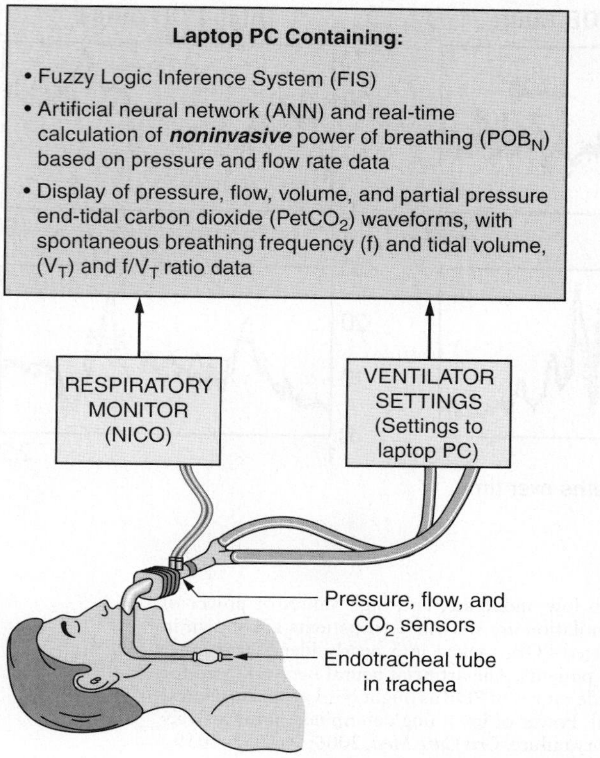

Laptop PC Containing:
- Fuzzy Logic Inference System (FIS)
- Artificial neural network (ANN) and real-time calculation of ***noninvasive*** power of breathing (POB_N) based on pressure and flow rate data
- Display of pressure, flow, volume, and partial pressure end-tidal carbon dioxide ($PetCO_2$) waveforms, with spontaneous breathing frequency (f) and tidal volume, (V_T) and f/V_T ratio data

RESPIRATORY MONITOR (NICO)

VENTILATOR SETTINGS (Settings to laptop PC)

Pressure, flow, and CO_2 sensors

Endotracheal tube in trachea

FIGURE 20.4. Schematic representation of a patient with acute respiratory failure attached to a ventilator and connected to respiratory monitoring equipment (NICO, Respironics) containing an artificial neural network (ANN) for the noninvasive determination of power of breathing (POB_N).

forced to work harder per minute (power) to meet the metabolic demands and maintain appropriate oxygen and carbon dioxide exchange. Assuming no change in oxygen consumption and carbon dioxide minute production, an increase in V_D/V_T from 0.3 to 0.5, typical of adults with acute respiratory failure in my experience, requires the respiratory muscle pump to work proportionately harder by increasing exhaled minute ventilation by 50% to maintain the same alveolar minute ventilation and appropriate carbon dioxide elimination to control $PaCO_2$ (Table 20.3).

Intrinsic Positive End-expiratory Pressure

Increased levels of PEEPi, or auto PEEP, as a result of increased expiratory airway resistance, inadequate exhalation time, or both, is another form of respiratory muscle loading. PEEPi must be counterbalanced by an equivalent change in alveolar pressure before air can flow into the lungs (26). Consider a patient with dynamic hyperinflation and a PEEPi level of 5 cm H_2O breathing room air spontaneously. Intra-alveolar pressure must decrease by at least 6 cm H_2O (instead of 1 cm H_2O under normal conditions) so that alveolar pressure falls below ambient pressure. A pressure gradient between the mouth and alveoli must occur for air to flow into the lungs. Under these conditions, a greater decrease in pleural pressure is required than normal, and a greater POB results.

Breathing Apparatus

Several breathing apparatus factors affect the imposed work of breathing. *The endotracheal tube is probably the most significant resistor in the breathing apparatus* (11,12,27–29). Breathing through a narrow internal diameter endotracheal tube attached to a highly resistive demand-flow continuous positive airway pressure (CPAP) system requires a large change in pressure to move a specific volume. An increased resistive workload is imposed by the apparatus (30,31) (Fig. 20.9).

Ventilator Response Time and Automatic and Variable Inspiratory Pressure Assist

The response time of the ventilator (time delay from the initiation of spontaneous inhalation to the onset of flow in the airway) directly affects the imposed POB. It is partly affected by the method of triggering the system "on," and partly by the ventilator's sensitivity/trigger setting. The response characteristics of a ventilator's demand-flow CPAP system are improved by moving the pressure-measuring/triggering site physically closer to the respiratory muscles (i.e., at the tracheal or carinal end of the endotracheal tube) (32). Significantly less imposed work results from pressure-triggering the system on at

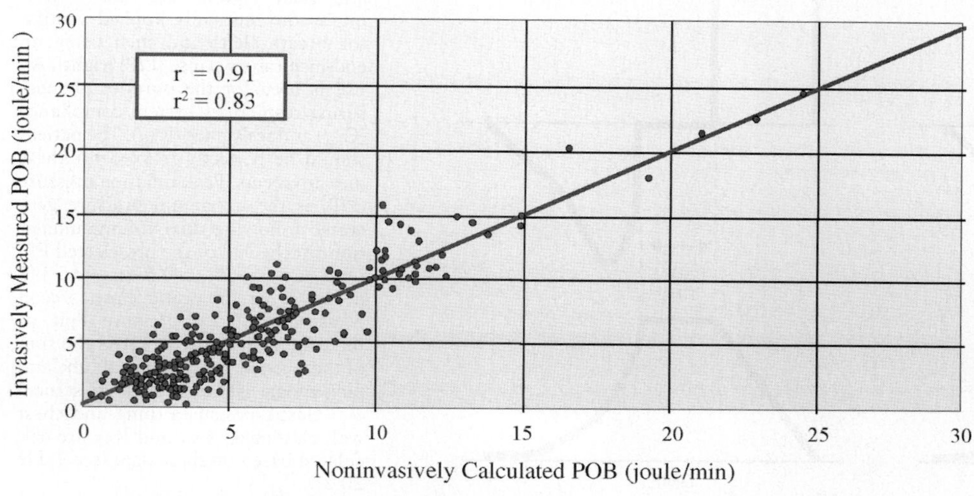

FIGURE 20.5. Relationship between directly or invasively measured power of breathing requiring the use of an intraesophageal balloon catheter (*y* axis) and noninvasively predicted/calculated power of breathing (POB) (*x* axis) using the nonlinear multilayer Perceptron artificial neural network model is shown. A highly significant correlation (r = 0.91, $p < 0.002$) between the two was found. The model was a *very good predictor of POB* as evidenced by the high value for the coefficient of determination, $r^2 = 0.83$, $p < 0.002$. (From Banner MJ, Euliano NR, Brennan V, et al. Power of breathing determined noninvasively using an artificial neural network in patients with respiratory failure. *Crit Care Med.* 2006;34:1052–1059.)

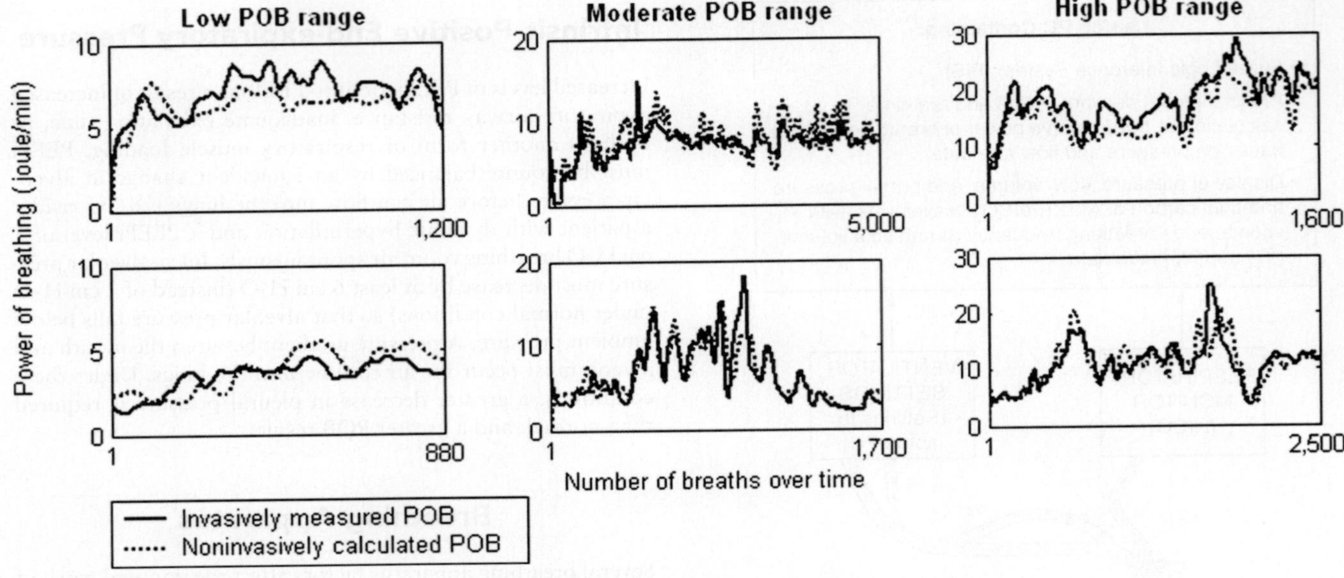

FIGURE 20.6. Examples of trend plots of patients with low, moderate, and high values of power of breathing (POB) while treated with pressure support ventilation are shown. Two patients are shown in each category. Note that noninvasively predicted/calculated POB tracked in a nearly identical manner with invasively measured POB for all three categories of patients. The artificial neural network used for predicting/calculating POB appears to be accurate over wide ranges of POB as might be expected in clinical practice. (From Banner MJ, Euliano NR, Brennan V, et al. Power of breathing determined noninvasively using an artificial neural network in patients with respiratory failure. *Crit Care Med.* 2006;34:1052–1059.)

the carinal end of the endotracheal tube compared with the conventional method of pressure-triggering from inside the ventilator or using flow-by (flow-triggered) initiation (33,34). During spontaneous inhalation, *automatic and variable* inspiratory pressure assist results when using tracheal pressure rather than breathing-circuit Y-piece pressure to control the operation of the ventilator, which, in turn, acts to decrease imposed resistive work of breathing to nearly zero (35). This is described as a closed-loop tracheal pressure ventilator control system (Figs. 20.10 and 20.11).

With pressure-triggering from inside the ventilator or with flow-by triggering, an initial pressure drop across the

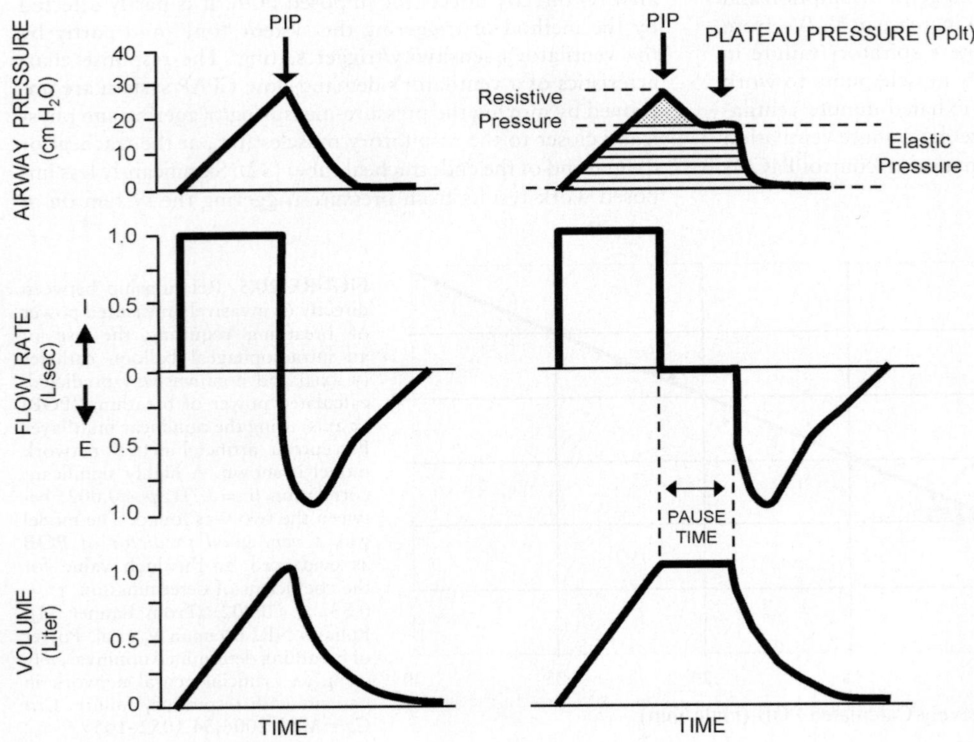

FIGURE 20.7. Pressure at the Y piece of the breathing circuit, referred to as "airway pressure"; flow rate during inhalation (I) and exhalation (E); and tidal volume are shown during a conventionally applied ventilator breath (**left**) and then using an end-inspiratory pause (EIP) (**right**). An EIP is used for the purpose of measuring respiratory system compliance (C_{RS}) and resistance (R_{RS}). The patient should be perfectly relaxed for these measurements. Peak inflation pressure (PIP) is the maximum pressure generated following tidal volume inhalation. At the end of the preselected EIP time, usually about 0.5 seconds, PIP decreases to the static elastic recoil pressure or plateau pressure (Pplt) of the respiratory system. PIP is the sum of the resistive (endotracheal tube and physiologic airways series resistance) and elastic pressures (lung and chest wall elastance). C_{RS} and R_{RS} are calculated based on these data (see Table 20.2).

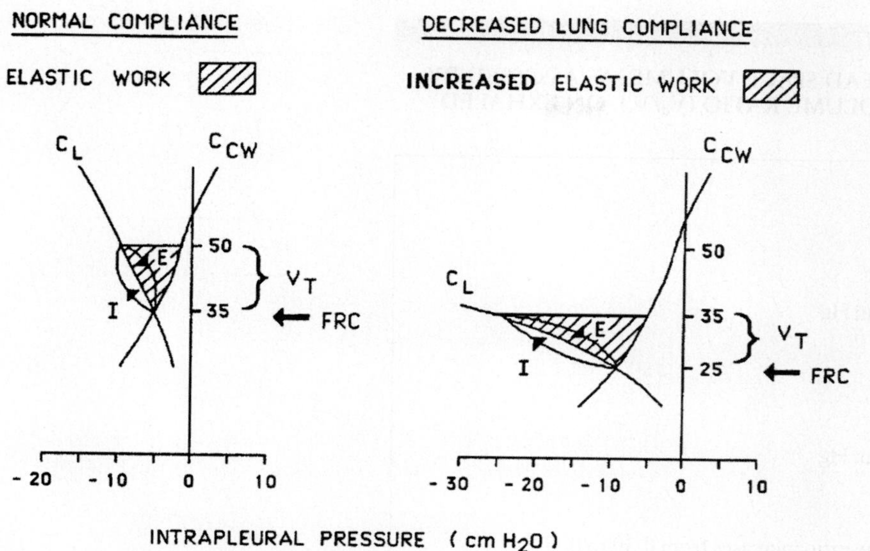

FIGURE 20.8. Elastic work of breathing varies inversely with lung compliance (C_L). Functional residual capacity (FRC) is defined as the intersection of the lung and chest wall compliance (C_{CW}) curves. Under conditions of normal lung compliance (**left**), a change in intrapleural pressure occurs accompanied by a change in tidal volume (V_T) during spontaneous inhalation (I) and exhalation (E). The pressure–volume loop moves in a *clockwise* direction. Elastic work of breathing is the area indicated by the diagonal lines. Decreases in C_L result in increased elastic work of breathing; notice flattened C_L curve and increased elastic work area (*diagonal lines*) (**right**). In addition to decreased lung volume (decreased FRC), a greater change in intrapleural pressure is required to exchange a smaller tidal volume, a characteristic of acute respiratory failure.

endotracheal tube must be generated by the patient before flow is initiated. This effort results in significant increases in imposed work. By contrast, pressure-triggering at the carinal end of the endotracheal tube effectively decreases the resistance by the endotracheal tube during spontaneous inhalation, thus decreasing the imposed POB.

The sensitivity/trigger setting on the ventilator directly affects the imposed POB. At a higher setting, a greater change in pressure is required to trigger the system on, thereby increasing the POB (35).

CLINICAL IMPLICATIONS OF RESPIRATORY MUSCLE LOADING

Fatigue

Increased respiratory muscle loading results in increases in the force and duration of diaphragmatic contraction, and leads to an increased tension-time index of the diaphragm (TTdi) (7). TTdi is the product of transdiaphragmatic pressure over the maximum transdiaphragmatic pressure (Pdi_{max}) and the ratio of inspiratory time to total cycle time ($TTdi = Pdi/Pdi_{max} \times T_I/T_{tot}$). The TTdi is similar to the tension-time index for the heart and gives a useful approximation of muscle energy demands (6,7). During spontaneous breathing, the change in transdiaphragmatic pressure is normally about 10 cm H_2O and the T_I/T_{tot} ratio is 0.33, effecting a TTdi of 0.03 (TTdi = 10 cm H_2O/100 cm $H_2O \times 0.33$). With increased respiratory muscle loading, Pdi may increase to 30 cm H_2O and T_I/T_{tot} to about 0.5, resulting in a TTdi of 0.15. Breathing patterns with a TTdi of about 0.15 to 0.20 are called *fatiguing* to indicate that the diaphragm will, in time, fail (6,7). Presumably, when the demand of the diaphragm exceeds 0.15 to 0.20, sufficient energy supplies are not available (6,7). This threshold TTdi is related to the limitation of blood perfusion and oxygen delivery to the muscle (Fig. 20.12).

TABLE 20.2

CALCULATIONS OF RESPIRATORY SYSTEM COMPLIANCE AND RESISTANCE (SEE FIG 20.7)

$$^a\text{Respiratory system compliance} = \frac{\text{Tidal volume}}{\text{Inspiratory plateau pressure} - \text{PEEP}}$$

$$0.05\ \text{L/cm H}_2\text{O} = \frac{1\ \text{L}}{20\ \text{cm H}_2\text{O} - 0\ \text{cm H}_2\text{O}}$$

$$^b\text{Respiratory system resistance} = \frac{\text{Peak inflation pressure} - \text{Inspiratory plateau pressure}}{\text{Inspiratory flow rate}}$$

$$10\ \text{cm H}_2\text{O/L/sec} = \frac{30\ \text{cm H}_2\text{O} - 20\ \text{cm H}_2\text{O}}{1\ \text{L/sec}}$$

[a] Reflects elastic work of spontaneous breathing; that is, the *lower* the respiratory system compliance, the *greater* the elastic work of breathing, and vice versa (see Fig. 20.8).
[b] Reflects resistive work of spontaneous breathing; that is, the greater the respiratory system resistance (physiologic + imposed resistances), the greater the resistive work of breathing, and vice versa.

TABLE 20.3

EFFECT OF INCREASED PHYSIOLOGIC DEAD SPACE VOLUME, AS ASSESSED BY THE DEAD SPACE VOLUME TO TIDAL VOLUME RATIO (V_d/V_t), ON EXHALED MINUTE VENTILATION (V_E)

$$PaCO_2 = \frac{VCO_2}{V_E(1 - V_D/V_T)} \times 760\ \text{mm Hg}$$

A. $V_D/V_T = 0.30$ (normal)

$$PaCO_2 = \frac{200\ \text{mL/min}}{6{,}000\ \text{mL/min}\ (1 - 0.30)} \times 760\ \text{mm Hg}$$

$PaCO_2 = 36$ mm Hg

B. $V_D/V_T = 0.50$ (increased)

$$PaCO_2 = \frac{200\ \text{mL/min}}{9{,}000\ \text{mL/min}\ (1 - 0.50)} \times 760\ \text{mm Hg}$$

$PaCO_2 = 34$ mm Hg

As physiologic dead space volume to tidal volume ratio increases from 0.30 to 0.50, spontaneous minute ventilation increases from 6,000 mL/min to 9,000 mL/min (50% increase in respiratory muscle loading) to maintain the same alveolar minute ventilation and essentially the same $PaCO_2$, assuming no change in VCO_2.

VCO_2, carbon dioxide minute production.

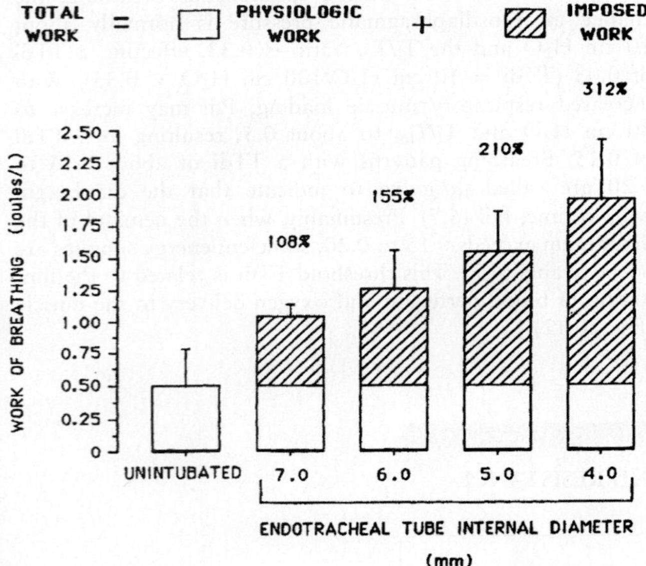

FIGURE 20.9. Influence of endotracheal tube size on imposed and total work of breathing. Before intubating a group of piglets ($N = 8$; weight, approximately 10 kg), the mean physiologic work, as measured using the method described by Campbell, was 0.5 J/L. Subsequently, all animals breathed through endotracheal tubes of 7-, 6-, 5-, and then 4-mm internal diameter, which were sequentially inserted into their tracheas. Imposed work of the endotracheal tube (*diagonally striped columns*) is superimposed on the physiologic work (*open columns*), yielding the total work of breathing on the respiratory muscles. The narrower the endotracheal tube was, the greater the imposed and, thus, total work of breathing. Total work increased by 312% with the narrowest internal diameter endotracheal tube, predisposing to respiratory muscle fatigue. (From Widner L, Banner MJ. A method of decreasing the imposed work of breathing associated with pediatric endotracheal tubes [abstract]. *Crit Care Med.* 1992;20;S82.)

Energy Supply and Demand

Respiratory muscle fatigue develops for the same reasons that one develops angina pectoris: *Demand for energy exceeds the supply of energy* (6,36). Energy supply refers to the proportion of cardiac output, blood perfusion, oxygen, and nutrients to the respiratory muscles that directly affect the synthesis of ATP. Respiratory muscle fatigue develops when ATP hydrolysis exceeds ATP synthesis as a result of an imbalance between energy supply and demand. Under conditions of increased muscle loading, respiratory muscle energy demands increase. Increases in muscle blood flow demand and oxygen consumption predispose to the development of muscle ischemia, fatigue, and respiratory failure (36,37). V_T decreases and increases in dead space to V_T ratio, and arterial carbon dioxide levels result when the respiratory muscles fail as force generators. Clinically, diaphragmatic fatigue is associated with abdominal paradox (abnormal inward movement of the diaphragm during spontaneous inhalation) and respiratory alternans (Fig. 20.13).

Breathing Pattern

Frequency

When pulmonary mechanics deteriorate, the respiratory muscles are loaded and POB increases. As a result, the breathing pattern changes (Table 20.4). These changes are vagally mediated by afferent or sensory fibers (load sensors) in the lungs and respiratory tract. Three types of afferent fibers modulate the breathing pattern: (a) slowly adapting receptors (SARs); (b) rapidly adapting receptors (RARs) (also termed *deflation, cough,* or *irritant receptors*), both of which are pulmonary stretch or mechanoreceptors; and (c) chemosensitive or C-fiber endings (38). SARs are found in the bronchial smooth muscle

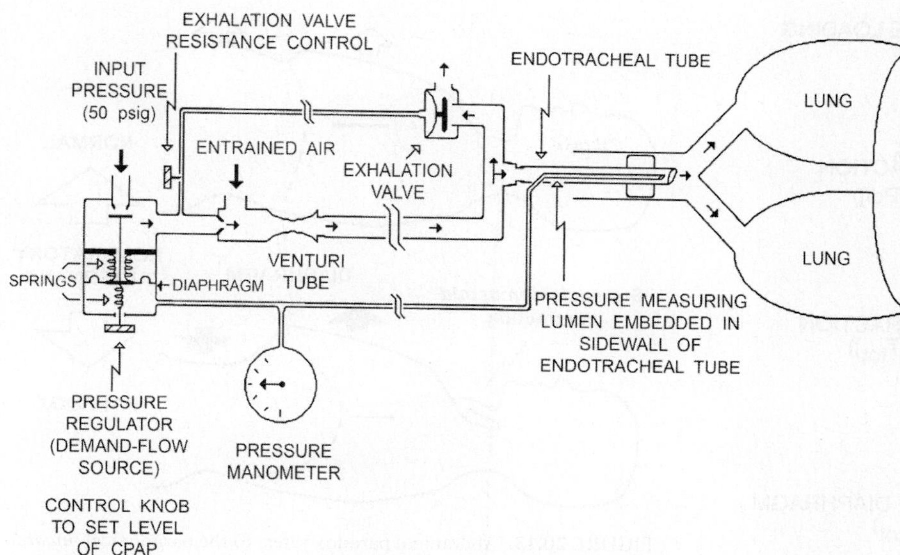

FIGURE 20.10. Pneumatically powered tracheal pressure control (TPC) system employs *closed-loop* feedback control by using *tracheal* pressure from the carinal or distal end of the endotracheal tube to control system operation during spontaneous breathing. Inspiratory assist pressure provided at the Y piece of the breathing circuit is *automatic and variable* on demand during spontaneous inhalation. That is, the greater the patient's inspiratory effort demand-flow is, the lower the tracheal pressure signal, the more the pressure regulator (demand-flow valve) opens, and the greater the inspiratory pressure assist measured at the Y piece of the breathing circuit. The greater the pressure assist or pressure support ventilation–like effect is, the greater the work by the system to minimize imposed resistive work of breathing (see Fig. 20.11). Note: The exhalation valve closes during inhalation and opens partly during exhalation to function as a threshold resistor so as to maintain the preselected level of continuous positive airway pressure (CPAP).

fibers, RARs are situated in the superficial layers of the respiratory tract mucosa, and C fibers are found in the airway epithelium (38).

Central Nervous System Modulation

The mechanoreceptors monitor changes in pulmonary mechanics and thoracic gas volume (functional residual capacity) (39,40). After a decrease in lung compliance (increase in respiratory muscle load), an increase in discharge activity occurs. Similar responses result after increases in total resistance. C-fiber endings are activated by many substances produced in the lungs such as histamine, bradykinin, and some prostaglandins. Some sympathetic afferents also may be activated in response to increases in mechanical loads. Afferent discharge signals from the sensory fibers are directed by the vagus nerve to the central respiratory controllers in the central nervous system (CNS), modifying their output signals, which in turn modify the breathing pattern (3).

Stimulation of these receptors produces patterns of rapid, shallow breathing and an optimal breathing frequency to minimize large changes in intrapleural pressure (41). Patients with loaded respiratory muscles breathe at a faster rate and a smaller V_T to minimize the POB, the so-called "minimal POB" or "least average force" concept, producing the most energy-efficient combination of breathing frequency and V_T (17,41,42). When the frequency is too low, much elastic work is required to produce large V_Ts; when the frequency is too high, much resistive work is required (as well as useless work to ventilate the dead space with each breath) (17) (Fig. 20.14). This mechanism also functions to protect the respiratory muscles from exhaustive, fatiguing contractions that can lead to muscle fiber splitting, hemorrhage, and self-destruction (3).

Inferred Work of Breathing

Spontaneous breathing frequency and tidal volume are used as inferences of the POB (43). An abnormal adult respiratory muscle workload is inferred when the spontaneous respiratory rate is greater than 25 to 30 breaths/minute; a breathing rate of 15 to 25 breaths/minute is inferred to mean that workload is tolerable and in a more normal range. These inferences,

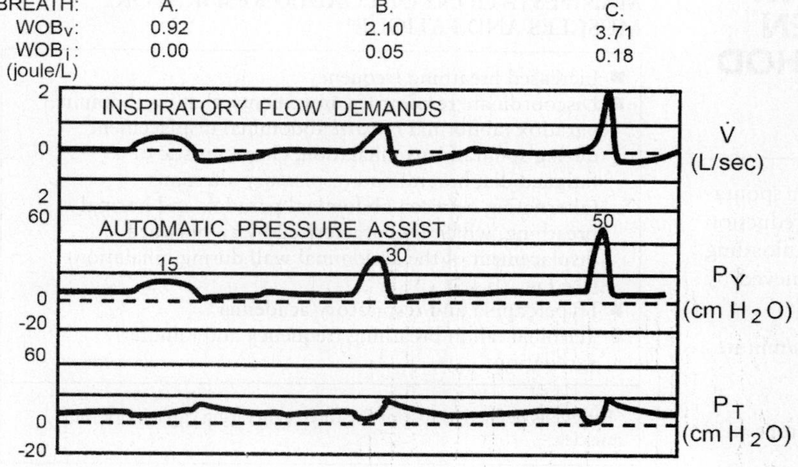

FIGURE 20.11. Operation of the tracheal pressure control (TPC) system as shown in Figure 20.10 illustrates the *automatic and variable* inspiratory pressure assist to minimize imposed resistive work of breathing (WOBi). Data for work of breathing by the ventilator assisting inhalation (WOBv) are also shown. Peak inspiratory flow rate demands for breaths "A," "B," and "C" are 0.5, 1.0, and 2 L/second, respectively. TPC responds automatically by providing inspiratory assist in proportion with the demands at 15, 30, and 50 cm H_2O, respectively, to decrease WOBi to nearly zero for all conditions. Breathing circuit pressure measured at the Y piece (P_Y), not pulmonary airway pressure as reflected by tracheal pressure (P_T), is increased. The greater the patient's inspiratory flow rate demand is, the greater the inspiratory pressure assist to minimize WOBi, and vice versa.

INCREASED RESPIRATORY MUSCLE LOADING

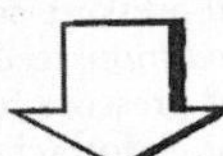

INCREASED FORCE OF CONTRACTION
(Transdiaphragmatic Pressure [Pdi])

AND

INCREASED DURATION OF CONTRACTION
(Inspiratory time/total cycle time [T_I/T_{tot}])

INCREASED TENSION-TIME INDEX OF DIAPHRAGM
($Pdi/Pdi_{max} \times T_I/T_{tot}$)

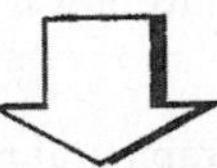

INCREASED RESPIRATORY MUSCLE ENERGY DEMANDS
(Blood flow, O_2, Nutrients)

$$\text{FATIGUE} \propto \frac{\text{DEMAND (Work of Breathing-Afterload)}}{\text{SUPPLY (Blood flow, } O_2\text{, nutrients)}}$$

FIGURE 20.12. Increased respiratory muscle loading and the subsequent effects leading to fatigue are shown. Fatigue is defined as loss of the *force-generating* capacity of the respiratory muscles.

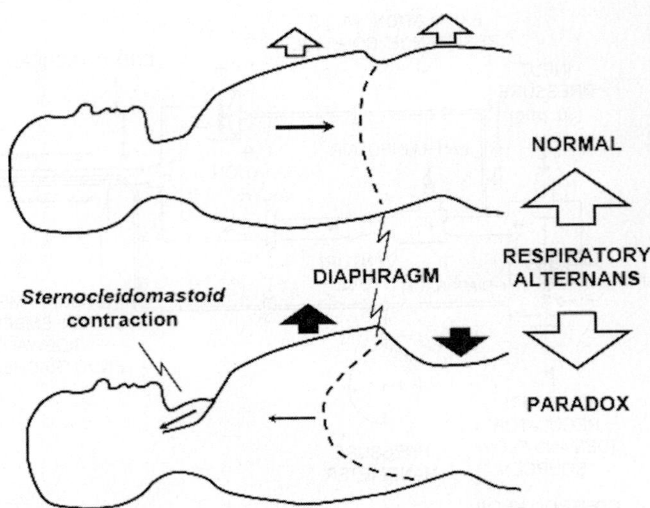

FIGURE 20.13. Abdominal paradox refers to the paradoxical *inward* movement of the abdomen during spontaneous inhalation (**bottom**). Normally, the abdomen moves outward during inhalation, like the chest (**top**). As diaphragmatic fatigue occurs (diaphragm fails as force generator), the diaphragm is no longer able to contract and move downward to displace the abdominal viscera and move the abdomen outward. The inward abdominal movement during inhalation is a response to the passive and cephalad diaphragmatic movement due to the negative intrathoracic pressure induced by contraction of accessory respiratory muscles like the sternocleidomastoid muscles, for example. *Respiratory alternans* is the manifestation of the alternating activity of the diaphragm and the intercostals and accessory respiratory muscles. When the diaphragm, working against a fatiguing load, fails, the accessory respiratory muscles assume a greater share of the work of breathing. Subsequently, when these muscles in turn fail, the diaphragm, now rested, resumes its activity and the cycle repeats. Hence, respiratory alternans is characterized by normal alternating with paradoxical breathing. These signs with tachypnea reflect early diaphragmatic fatigue and may actually precede acute hypercapnia.

however, seem to be inaccurate and misleading with regard to the POB (44,45). Although patients breathing between 15 and 25 breaths/minute often demonstrate an apparently acceptable breathing pattern, the respiratory muscle workloads may vary from fatiguing to normal to zero (44,45).

INAPPROPRIATE RESPIRATORY MUSCLE UNLOADING WHEN USING CONVENTIONAL METHOD FOR SETTING PRESSURE SUPPORT VENTILATION

A primary goal of mechanical ventilatory support for spontaneously breathing patients with respiratory failure is reduction of excessive POB. Appropriate respiratory muscle unloading to decrease power of breathing is thought to be achieved by setting PSV using the following conventional method:

- Spontaneous breathing frequency 15 to 25 breaths/minute
- Tidal volume 6 to 8 mL/kg ideal body weight
- Absence of SCM contraction
- Appearance of breathing comfortably and no apparent anxiety or adverse cardiovascular effects

We evaluated the effects on respiratory muscle workloads using this method of applying PSV in 115 adults (55 males, 60 females, weight 81 ± 18 kg, age 55 ± 11 years) with varying degrees of respiratory failure from various etiologies (e.g., pneumonia, sepsis, trauma, congestive heart failure) (institutional review board [IRB] approved). A combined

TABLE 20.4

MANIFESTATIONS OF LOADED RESPIRATORY MUSCLES AND FATIGUE[a]

- Increased breathing frequency
- Discoordinate respiratory movements, that is, abdominal paradox (abnormal *inward* abdominal displacement during spontaneous inhalation, characteristic of a fatigued diaphragm) and respiratory alternans (alternating between abdominal paradox and normal breathing, which is characterized by an outward displacement of the abdominal wall during inhalation) (see Fig. 20.13)
- Hypercapnia and respiratory academia
- Terminal fall in breathing frequency and minute ventilation

[a]Fatigue is defined as loss of the force-generating capacity of the muscles.

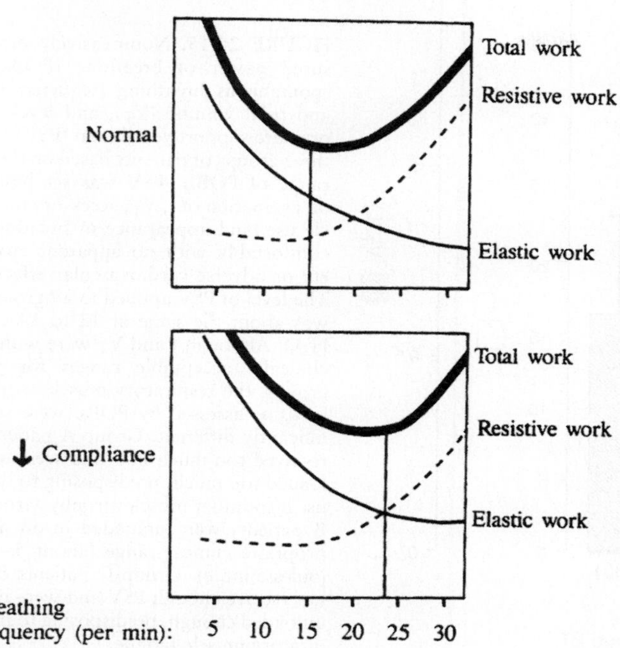

FIGURE 20.14. Minimal work of breathing (WOB): Optimal breathing frequency concept as described by Otis (17) and Sant' Ambrogio and Sant' Ambrogio (41). Total WOB (*thick line*) consists of resistive (*dashed line*) and elastic work (*thin line*). Under normal conditions (**top**), patients adopt a breathing frequency and tidal volume combination, which corresponds to minimal total WOB; that is, for adults, an optimal breathing frequency and tidal volume are approximately of 12 to 15/minute and 500 mL, respectively. Elastic work is excessive at lower breathing frequencies and higher tidal volumes. Conversely, resistive work increases at higher breathing frequencies and lower tidal volumes. The body adopts a motion that strains it the least. Under conditions of decreased compliance (increased elastance), the respiratory muscles are loaded (**bottom**), and a breathing frequency of 12/minute and tidal volume of 500 mL are no longer optimal because elastic work, and thus total WOB, are increased. The optimal breathing frequency and tidal volume combination corresponding to minimal total WOB are a frequency of approximately 25/minute and a tidal volume of about 250 mL. Thus, a rapid, shallow breathing pattern is a compensatory, energy-efficient breathing strategy to minimize WOB.

pressure/flow sensor, positioned between the endotracheal tube and Y piece of the ventilator, was directed to a respiratory monitor (NICO, Respironics and Convergent Engineering). The following were measured continuously after using the aforementioned method for setting PSV: POB_N, spontaneous f and V_T, and level of PSV. Patients were monitored for their entire time they were on ventilatory support. The intensive care unit (ICU) staff were blinded to measurements. POB_N respiratory monitors were continuously checked by a research respiratory therapist who did not intervene with clinical management decisions. PSV was combined with intermittent mandatory ventilation (IMV) (6 ± 3/minute), PEEP (8 ± 4 cm H_2O), and FIO_2 (0.55 ± 0.15).

Patients were divided into three respiratory muscle workload groups: Group A: $POB_N < 5$ joules/minute; group B: $POB_N > 5$ and < 10 joules/minute; and Group C: $POB_N > 10$ joules/minute. Data were analyzed using analysis of variance (ANOVA); α was set at 0.05. (Group A represents patients whose workload is negligible, predisposing to respiratory muscle disuse atrophy. Group B represents patients in a clinically appropriate range based on studying over 500 adults. Group C represents patients whose workload per minute may be in a fatiguing range.)

It was revealed that approximately the *same* level of PSV was applied to all groups (i.e., 12–14 cm H_2O by setting PSV using the conventional method as previously defined). Although f and V_T were in appropriate ranges most of the time for all groups, group A was unloaded too much, predisposing to the development of disuse atrophy (largest group); group C was not unloaded enough, predisposing to muscle fatigue; and group B (only 12% of patients) was unloaded appropriately (Fig. 20.15). For 66% of our patients ($N = 76$) whose level of PSV was set based on the conventional method of inferring workloads, the respiratory muscles were either unloaded too much or not unloaded enough. These findings support the need to include both respiratory muscle load (POB_N) and tolerance (f, V_T) measurements to ensure appropriate unloading when using PSV (i.e., a combined load and tolerance strategy is advocated).

We contend that the breathing pattern *alone* is not an accurate predictor of POB. The breathing pattern reflects tolerance for the load on the respiratory muscles, where POB_N reflects the magnitude of the load. Both breathing pattern and POB_N data should be used in a complementary manner when selecting a level of PSV to unload the respiratory muscles.

Data also suggest that the perceived inspiratory effort sensation during spontaneous breathing (how the patient feels, degree of comfort) is not related to the presence of fatiguing or nonfatiguing diaphragmatic contractions (46).

DECREASING RESPIRATORY MUSCLE LOADS (POWER OF BREATHING)

Therapeutic Objectives

Objectives of therapy for loaded or fatigued muscles include the following: (a) decrease energy demand (POB), and (b) increase energy supply (oxygen, blood flow, and nutrient delivery) to the respiratory muscles. PSV is advocated to unload the respiratory muscles, decrease the POB, and decrease the energy demands of patients with decreased compliance and increased resistance (47,48). It also augments spontaneous breathing by potentially decreasing the work imposed by the resistance of the breathing apparatus to zero (10,28).

In the PSV mode, the ventilator is patient-triggered on, and an abrupt rise in airway pressure to a preselected positive pressure limit results from a variable flow rate of gas from the ventilator. As long as the patient maintains an inspiratory effort, airway pressure is held constant at the preselected level. Gas flow rate from the ventilator ceases when the patient's inspiratory flow rate demand decreases to a predetermined percentage of the initial peak mechanical inspiratory flow rate (e.g., 25%). The ventilator is thus flow-cycled "off" in the PSV mode.

Once the preselected inspiratory pressure limit is set, the patient interacts with the pressure-assisted breath and retains

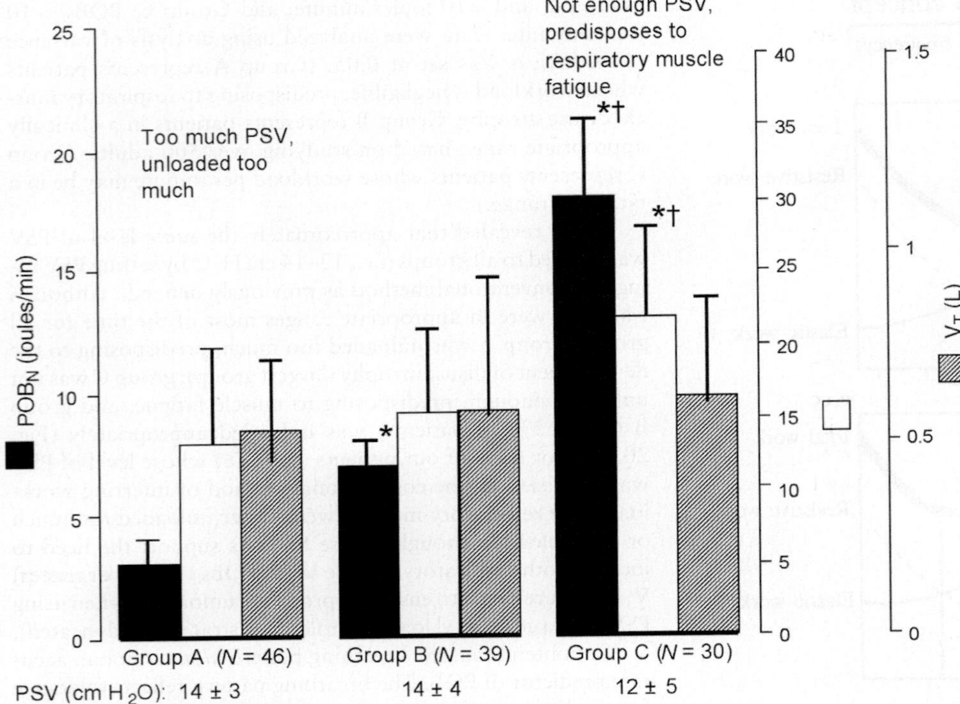

FIGURE 20.15. Noninvasively measured power of breathing (POB_N), spontaneous breathing frequency (f) and tidal volume (V_T), and level of pressure support ventilation (PSV) for three groups of patients based on their range of POB_N. PSV was set based on evaluation of f, V_T, accessory muscle use, and appearance of breathing comfortably with no apparent anxiety or adverse cardiovascular effects. The level of PSV applied to all groups was about the same at 12 to 14 cm H_2O. Although f and V_T were within clinically acceptable ranges for all groups, the respiratory muscle workloads as assessed by POB_N were significantly different. Group A patients received too much PSV and were unloaded too much, predisposing to disuse respiratory muscle atrophy. Group B patients were unloaded in an appropriate clinical range (about 5–10 joules/minute). Group C patients did not receive enough PSV and were not unloaded enough, predisposing to respiratory muscle fatigue.

control over inspiratory time and flow rate, expiratory time, breathing rate, V_T, and minute volume (Fig. 20.16). Patient work decreases, and ventilator work increases at incremental levels of PSV (21,27). Decreasing the load on a muscle to an appropriate level decreases the force and duration of muscle contraction (tension-time index) (6), energy demand, muscle ischemia, and fatigue. For a patient with increased respiratory muscle load or POB (e.g., 15 joules/minute), a clinician may also unload the respiratory muscles to a more appropriate range, which appears to be about 5 to 10 joules/minute using PSV. This range is based on studying over 500 adults treated with PSV.

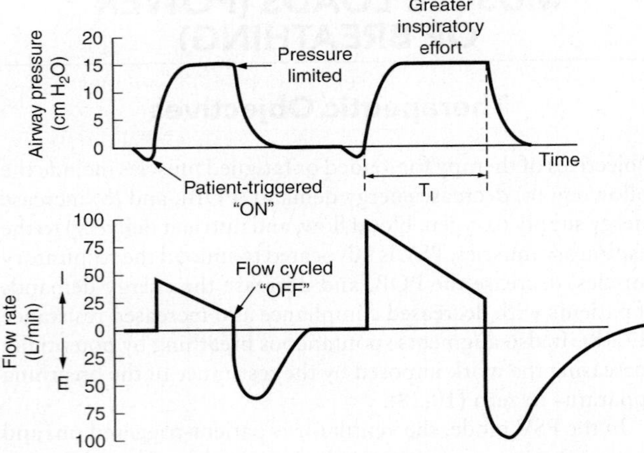

FIGURE 20.16. Airway pressure and flow waveforms are depicted for pressure support ventilation (PSV). After the ventilator is patient-triggered "on," an abrupt rise in pressure ensues to a preselected limit, and a decelerating inspiratory flow waveform results. When the inspiratory flow rate decreases to a predetermined percentage of the initial peak inspiratory flow rate (e.g., 25%), the ventilator flow cycles "off." On the right, a greater inspiratory effort, a longer inspiratory time (T_I), and higher peak inspiratory flow rate demand are illustrated at the same level of PSV. The clinician sets the level of PSV, while the patient *interacts* with the pressure-supported breath and retains control over breathing rate, T_I, flow rate, and tidal volume.

Partial and Total Respiratory Muscle Unloading

The level of PSV may be set to partially or totally unload the respiratory muscles (21,48,49). During partial unloading, PSV is increased until the patient's POB is decreased to a tolerable range. My goal usually is 5 to 10 joules/minute, an appropriate range for physiologic POB. During inhalation with PSV, positive pressure actively assists lung inflation. A portion of the POB is provided, relieving and unloading the respiratory muscles of the increased workload, and decreasing the force and duration of muscle contraction. Work is performed in part by the patient and in part by the ventilator (i.e., a work-sharing approach). Partial respiratory muscle unloading is appropriate to provide a nonfatiguing workload and promote muscle conditioning.

Titration of Pressure Support Ventilation

The level of PSV may be set to provide appropriate, or optimal, respiratory muscle loads. The exact level of this load is not known, but some authorities suggest that near-normal workloads are well tolerated (21,50). In a carefully done study, Brochard et al. (50) report that at a PSV of approximately 15 cm H_2O, an optimal muscle load corresponded to a patient work of breathing of 0.52 ± 0.12 joules/L. (This is proportional to a POB range of 5–10 joules/minute.) An optimal load was defined as that which maintained maximal diaphragmatic electrical activity without fatigue (specifically, the lowest level of PSV at which no reduction in the ratio of high- to low-frequency components of the diaphragm's electromyographic signal occurred). A reduction of 80% or less of the initial high/low ratio is defined as incipient diaphragmatic fatigue (51).

Patient Characteristics

Physiologic patient characteristics should also be considered. Weak, malnourished, and chronically ill patients will not tolerate normal workloads as well as physically powerful individuals with short-term illness. The latter patients may be able to generate twice the normal work range without developing fatigue. Because the tolerance may vary, setting the level of PSV so that the POB is in an appropriate range of 5 to 10 joules/minute is a reasonable initial guideline (24).

Available evidence suggests that total unloading, allowing fatigued respiratory muscles to rest and recover, is appropriate (4,6,52). The time for respiratory muscle recovery after chronic fatigue is estimated to be at least 24 hours (6). A reasonable approach is to totally unload the respiratory muscles of such patients for approximately 24 hours by using high levels of PSV (e.g., >30 cm H_2O). Subsequently, when appropriate, PSV may be decreased so that the patient POB is in a normal, tolerable range and the respiratory muscles are partially unloaded (27).

My experience and that of others (14) suggests that all intubated, spontaneously breathing patients in respiratory failure should receive a minimal level PSV that reduces imposed POB to zero (Figs. 20.2 and 20.2A) (10). Additional PSV may be required to decrease the abnormally high physiologic work associated with the disease process to a normal level (21). Subsequently, as the patient's respiratory status improves, PSV may be decreased while ensuring that the POB is in a nonfatiguing range. PSV should not be decreased to zero or below the level required to decrease imposed work to zero. To do so functionally reloads the respiratory muscles and risks fatigue. Extubation at the level of PSV results in zero imposed POB; that is, about 10 cm H_2O for most adults seems reasonable.

POWER OF BREATHING AS A CRITERION FOR EXTUBATION

POB, the rate at which work is done per minute, is a better assessment of respiratory muscle workload than work of breathing per breath because it is a measure over time, not for an individual breath. Spontaneous breathing f, V_T, f/V_T ratio, minute ventilation (MV), PaO_2/FIO_2 ratio, $PaCO_2$, and SCM use are used typically when evaluating a patient's readiness for extubation. We hypothesized that POB may be another parameter for predicting successful extubation. To test this hypothesis, we studied adults with respiratory failure who were candidates for extubation.

We evaluated 25 adults (15 males, 10 females, age 56 ± 19 years, weight 80 ± 25 kg) in an IRB-approved study where POB was measured in real time and noninvasively (POB_N), without the need of an esophageal balloon, using a monitor (NICO, Respironics, Convergent Engineering) (1). Data from a combined pressure/flow sensor, positioned between the endotracheal tube (sizes ranged from 6–8 mm internal diameter) and ventilator circuit, were directed to the monitor. All patients were studied immediately prior to extubation using minimal ventilator settings (intermittent mandatory ventilation 0 per minute, pressure support ventilation 10 cm H_2O, continuous positive airway pressure 5 cm H_2O, and FIO_2 0.4). An arterial blood gas was obtained. Data were analyzed using a Mann-Whitney U test; α was set at 0.05 for statistical significance.

It was found that POB_N ranged from 2 to 10 joules/minute for patients successfully extubated ($N = 20$) and 10 to 23 joules/minute for those failing extubation ($N = 5$), requiring reintubation and ventilatory support. POB_N was significantly lower, and related breathing parameters were significantly different for patients successfully extubated (Table 20.5).

POB_N values >10 joules/minute were associated with failed extubation. *A critical value for POB_N to predict successful extubation may be about 10 joules/minute* (53). A larger sample size is needed to thoroughly evaluate these pilot data findings for determining a critical value. POB_N data coincided with typically used breathing parameters for assessing readiness for extubation; that is, when f, V_T, f/V_T ratio, PaO_2/FIO_2 ratio, and $PaCO_2$ data were clinically acceptable, and in the absence of SCM activity, patients were successfully extubated. It appears that POB_N may be a parameter to consider for predicting extubation from ventilatory support.

TABLE 20.5

NONINVASIVE POWER OF BREATHING (POB_N) IN RELATION TO TYPICAL VARIABLES USED WHEN CONSIDERING EXTUBATION AND REMOVAL FROM VENTILATORY SUPPORT

	POB_N	f	V_T	f/V_T	MV	PaO_2/FIO_2	$PaCO_2$	SCM
Successful extubation	6.1[a] ±2.9	16[a] ±5	0.53[a] ±0.1	34[a] ±12	8.9[a] ±3.5	300[a] ±78	40[a] ±6	No
Failed extubation	14.8 ±5	33 ±9	0.35 ±0.1	109 ±50	11 ±2.5	225 ±70	45 ±5	Yes for most patients

[a] $p < 0.05$.

Data are mean ± standard deviation. POB_N (joules/min), spontaneous breathing frequency (f) (per minute), tidal volume (V_T) (L), f/V_T (breaths/min/L), minute ventilation (MV) (L/min), sternocleidomastoid contraction (SCM).

Noninvasive Power of Breathing for Weaning

Maintaining patients in a normal POB_N range may be appropriate when the decision to "wean to extubation" is *not* contemplated and spontaneous ventilation is allowed. Under this ventilatory support condition, PSV can be applied to maintain POB_N in a normal range and low IMV rates are applied, assuming the patient is hemodynamically stable. Still others may need to have their respiratory muscles totally unloaded, requiring high levels of PSV (>20 cm H_2O).

When the decision is made to "wean to extubation," a patient's respiratory muscle endurance and ventilatory reserve need to be probed. The PSV level may be set to maintain POB_N at about 5 to 10 joules/minute so as to assess the patient's workload tolerance. It is not so much the amount of POB_N performed; rather, a patient's ability to *tolerate* a specific respiratory muscle workload is the important concept. When assessing workload tolerance, it has been reported that breathing pattern parameters (f, V_T, f/V_T ratio, MV, accessory respiratory muscle use) do not always correlate, and are not good predictors of work of breathing. It is not implied that breathing pattern parameters should be ignored. On the contrary, these parameters provide useful diagnostic information and should be used. POB_N and breathing pattern data should be used in a complementary manner when assessing respiratory muscle workload tolerance (54).

The aforementioned range of POB_N levels appears appropriate for patients with acute forms of respiratory failure and need to be evaluated in patients with chronic forms of respiratory failure, as in chronic obstructive pulmonary disease (COPD).

Multiple Noninvasive Power of Breathing Range Concept

1. Initial phases of ventilatory support
   A. Maintain POB_N in a low range (0–2 joules/minute) for patients whose respiratory muscles are fatigued—total unloading (about 24 hours) promotes respiratory muscle rest and recovery.
   B. Maintain POB_N in a normal range (5–10 joules/minute) when allowing spontaneous breathing—use when the patient is weak and still has substantial pulmonary disorders.
2. Weaning phase of ventilatory support

Probe the patient's reserve by maintaining POB_N at a higher range (up to 12 joules/minute). This allows for a relatively prolonged assessment of a patient's respiratory muscle tolerance and endurance.

SUMMARY

Respiratory muscle loads of intubated patients receiving ventilatory support may be visualized as a continuum; muscles at one end are highly loaded and at the other end are totally unloaded, predisposing to fatigue and atrophy, respectively. The terms, *nosocomial respiratory failure* and *iatrogenic ventilator dependency* (14), describe the inappropriate prolongation of ventilatory support. This problem may result from respiratory muscle fatigue (caused by increased muscle loading from breathing through a highly resistive apparatus, increased physiologic work, or insufficient ventilatory support) or muscle atrophy (as a result of total unloading of respiratory muscles by too high levels of PSV) (14).

With either fatigue or atrophy, the respiratory muscles become weak, failing as force generators. Hypoventilation, hypercapnia, and failure to wean often result, thus prolonging the need for ventilatory support. Fatigue or atrophy can occur, in part, from lack of assessing and adjusting respiratory muscle afterload, thereby failing to perceive their often subtle onset. Measurement of the POB_N provides objective and tested data that can be used to set ventilator modes such as PSV to prevent either occurrence, and may expedite eventual weaning and extubation.

References

1. Roussos C, Macklem P. The respiratory muscles. *N Engl J Med.* 1982;307:786.
2. De Troyer A. Respiratory muscles. In: Crystal RG, West JB, eds. *The Lung: Scientific Foundations.* New York: Raven Press; 1991:869.
3. Roussos C. Function and fatigue of respiratory muscles. *Chest.* 1985;88:5124.
4. Braun NMT, Faulkner J, Hughes RL. When should respiratory muscles be exercised? *Chest.* 1983;84:76.
5. Vander AJ, Sherman JH, Luciano DS. *Human Physiology.* 5th ed. New York: McGraw-Hill; 1992:283.
6. Grassino A, Macklem PT. Respiratory muscle fatigue and ventilatory failure. *Ann Rev Med.* 1984;35:625.
7. Jenkins FH, Olsen GN. Chronic obstructive lung disease and acute respiratory failure. In: Klein EF, ed. *Acute Respiratory Failure: Problems in Critical Care.* Vol 1, no 3. Philadelphia: JB Lippincott; 1987:466.
8. Milic-Emili J. Work of breathing. In: Crystal RG, West JB, eds. *The Lung: Scientific Foundations.* New York: Raven Press; 1991:1065.
9. Banner MJ, Jaeger MJ, Kirby RR. Components of the work of breathing and implications for monitoring ventilator-dependent patients. *Crit Care Med.* 1994;22:515.
10. Banner MJ, Kirby RR, Blanch PB. Decreasing imposed work of the breathing apparatus to zero using pressure support ventilation. *Crit Care Med.* 1993;21:1333.
11. Bersten All, Rutten AJ, Vedig AE. Additional work of breathing imposed by endotracheal tubes, breathing circuits, and intensive care ventilators. *Crit Care Med.* 1989;17:671.
12. Bolder PM, Healy EJ, Bolder AR. The extra work of breathing through adult endotracheal tubes. *Anesth Analg.* 1986;65:853.
13. Kirton O, Banner MJ, Axelrod A. Detection of unsuspected imposed work of breathing: case reports. *Crit Care Med.* 1993;21:790.
14. Civetta JM. Nosocomial respiratory failure or iatrogenic ventilator dependency. *Crit Care Med.* 1993;21:171.
15. Kirton OC, DeHaven B, Morgan J, et al. Endotracheal tube flow resistance and elevated imposed work of breathing masquerading as ventilator weaning intolerance [abstract]. *Chest.* 1993;104S:133S.
16. Banner MJ, Kirby RR, Blanch PB. Site of pressure measurement during spontaneous breathing with continuous positive airway pressure: effect on calculating imposed work of breathing. *Crit Care Med.* 1992;20:528.
17. Otis AB. The work of breathing. In: Fenn WO, Rahn H, eds. *Handbook of Physiology: A Critical, Comprehensive Presentation of Physiological Knowledge and Concepts. Section 3: Respiration.* Washington, DC: American Physiological Society; 1964:463.
18. Baydur A, Behrakis P, Zin WA. A simple method for assessing the validity of the esophageal balloon technique. *Am Rev Respir Dis.* 1982;126:788.
19. Campbell EJM. *The Respiratory Muscles and the Mechanics of Breathing.* Chicago: Year Book Medical Publishers; 1958.
20. Agostoni E, Campbell EJM, Freedman S. Energetics. In: Campbell EJM, Agostoni E, Davis JN, eds. *The Respiratory Muscles: Mechanics and Neural Control.* Philadelphia: WB Saunders; 1970:115.
21. Banner MJ, Kirby RR, Gabrielli A, et al. Partially and totally unloading the respiratory muscles based on real time measurements of work of breathing: a clinical approach. *Chest.* 1994;106:1835.
22. Zapletal A, Samanek M, Paul T. *Lung Function in Children and Adolescents.* New York: S Karger Publishers; 1987.
23. Nelcor. *Puritan Bennett 840 Operations and Technical Reference Manual.* Addendum, PAV+ option. Carlsbad, CA: Nelcor; 2006:20–23.
24. Banner MJ, Euliano NR, Brennan V, et al. Power of breathing determined

non-invasively using an artificial neural network in patients with respiratory failure. *Crit Care Med.* 2006;34:1052–1059.

25. MacIntyre NR, Leatherman NE. Mechanical loads on the ventilatory muscles. *Am Rev Respir Dis.* 1989;139:968.
26. Marini JJ. Breathing effort and work of breathing during mechanical ventilation. In: Banner MJ, ed. *Positive-Pressure Ventilation: Problems in Critical Care.* Vol. 4, no. 2. Philadelphia: JB Lippincott; 1990:184.
27. Brochard L, Rua F, Lorino H. Inspiratory pressure support compensates for the additional work of breathing caused by the endotracheal tube. *Anesthesiology.* 1991;75:739.
28. Fiastro JF, Habib MP, Quan SF. Pressure support compensates for inspiratory work due to endotracheal tubes and demand continuous positive airway pressure. *Chest.* 1988;93:499.
29. Shapiro M, Wilson RK, Casar G. Work of breathing though different sized endotracheal tubes. *Crit Care Med.* 1986;14:1028.
30. LeSouef PN, England SJ, Bryan AC. Total resistance of the respiratory system in preterm infants with and without an endotracheal tube. *J Pediatr.* 1984;104.
31. Widner L, Banner MJ. A method of decreasing the imposed work of breathing associated with pediatric endotracheal tubes [abstract]. *Crit Care Med.* 1992;20:S82.
32. Kacmarek RM, Shimada Y, Ohmura A. Optimizing mechanical ventilatory assist tube. *J Pediatr.* 1984;104:108.
33. Banner MJ, Blanch PB, Kirby RR. Imposed work of breathing and methods of triggering a demand-flow, continuous positive airway pressure system. *Crit Care Med.* 1993;21:183.
34. Messinger G, Banner MJ, Gabrielli A, et al. Tracheal pressure triggering a demand-flow CPAP system decreases work of breathing [abstract]. *Anesthesiology.* 1994;81:A272.
35. Banner MJ, Blanch PB. Gabrielli A. Tracheal pressure control provides automatic and variable inspiratory pressure assist to decrease imposed resistive work of breathing. *Crit Care Med.* 2002;30:1106–1111.
36. Tobin MJ, Skorodin M, Alexis CG. Weaning from mechanical ventilation. In: Taylor RW, Shoemaker WC, eds. *Critical Care: State of the Art.* Vol. 12. Fullerton, CA: Society of Critical Care Medicine; 1991:373.
37. Bellemare F, Wight D, Lavigne CM, et al. Effect of tension and timing of contraction on blood flow of the diaphragm. *J Appl Physiol.* 1983;54:1597.
38. Cohen CA, Zagelbaumm G, Gross D, et al. Clinical manifestations of inspiratory muscle fatigue. *Am J Med.* 1982;73:308.
39. Barnes PJ. Neural control of airway smooth muscle. In: Crystal RG, West JB, eds. *The Lung: Scientific Foundations.* New York: Raven Press; 1991:903.
40. Sant' Ambrogio G, Sant' Ambrogio FB. Reflexes from the airway, lung, chest wall, and limbs. In: Crystal RG, West JB, eds. *The Lung: Scientific Foundations.* New York: Raven Press; 1991:1383.
41. Sant' Ambrogio G. Information arising from the tracheobronchial tree of mammals. *Physiol Rev.* 1982;62:531.
42. Otis AB, Fenn WO, Rahn HL. Mechanics of breathing in man. *J Appl Physiol.* 1950;2:592.
43. MacIntyre NR. Weaning from mechanical ventilatory support: volume-assisting intermittent breaths versus pressure-assisting every breath. *Respir Care.* 1988;33:121.
44. Banner MJ, Kirby RR, Kirton OC, et al. Breathing frequency and pattern are poor predictors of work of breathing in patients receiving pressure support ventilation. *Chest.* 1995;108:1338.
45. Kirton O, Banner MJ, DeHaven CB, et al. Respiratory rate and related assessments are poor inferences of patient work of breathing [abstract]. *Crit Care Med.* 1993:S242.
46. Silas SL, Simpson SQ, Levy H. Rapid shallow breathing index does not correlate with airway occlusion pressure or work of breathing [abstract]. *Chest.* 1993;104:1305.
47. Bradley TD, Chartrand DA, Fitting JW, et al. The relation of inspiratory effort sensation to fatiguing patterns of the diaphragm. *Am Rev Respir Dis.* 1986;134:1119.
48. MacIntyre NR. Respiratory function during pressure support ventilation. *Chest.* 1986;89:677.
49. MacIntyre NR, Nishimura M, Usada Y. The Nogoya conference on system design and patient-ventilator interactions during pressure support ventilation. *Chest.* 1990;97:1463.
50. Brochard L, Had A, Lorino H. Inspiratory pressure support prevents diaphragmatic fatigue during weaning from mechanical ventilation. *Am Rev Respir Dis.* 1989;139:513.
51. Gross D, Grassino A, Ross WRD, et al. Electromyogram pattern of diaphragmatic fatigue. *J Appl Physiol.* 1979;46:1.
52. Murciano D, Aubier M, Lecoguie Y, et al. Effects of theophylline on diaphragmatic strength and fatigue in patients with chronic obstructive pulmonary disease. *N Engl J Med.* 1984;311:349.
53. Bonett S, Banner MJ, Euliano NR, et al. Power of breathing as a predictor of for extubation from ventilatory support [abstracted]. *Respir Care.* 2005; 50:1521.
54. Gabrielli A, Lyon AJ, Euliano N, et al. Respiratory monitor recommends appropriate pressure support ventilation settings to unload respiratory muscles [abstracted]. *Crit Care Med.* 2006;33:A113.

CHAPTER 21 ■ PULSE OXIMETRY AND PLETHYSMOGRAPHY

JOHANNES H. VAN OOSTROM • BRIAN FUEHRLEIN • RICHARD J. MELKER

Pulse oximetry is a standard of care and is ubiquitous in operating rooms, inpatient hospital wards, physicians' offices, and emergency medical service (EMS) transport units. Obtaining an oxygen saturation noninvasively from a pulse oximeter probe is often the first step in the decision-making process of caring for a patient.

HISTORY

Stokes (1) reported that the colored substance in blood carries oxygen. This was followed by Hoppe-Seyler (2), who first crystallized this substance and coined the term *hemoglobin*. Additionally, it was shown that the pattern of light absorption changes when shaken with air (2).

Hertzman (3) described using photoelectric plethysmography of fingers and toes as a dynamic analysis of the peripheral circulation. The device consisted of a beam of light directed from an ordinary automobile headlight bulb on the finger or toe placed above a shielded photoelectric cell of the photoemissive type, purchased from the radio trade. The photoelectric oscillations with variations in the blood content of the digit were recorded by a string galvanometer or suitable oscillograph after amplification. Movements of the arm were minimized as transmission to the finger would compromise the reading; a comfortable saddle or sling was necessary to secure the arm to achieve the desired muscle relaxation that affects finger volume. This method was also used over the nasal septum, and the values were compared.

Millikan et al. (4) first coined the term *oximeter* and described a method for the continuous measurement of arterial saturation. A small unit placed over the shell of the ear contained a lamp, two color filters, and two barrier-type, light-sensitive cells, with which the transmission of either green or red light was measured. The green reading was dependent on how much total hemoglobin was between the lamp and the photocell, and was used to measure the degree of vasodilation, or "blood thickness" in the ear. This enabled one to choose the correct direct reading calibration scale for the estimation of arterial oxygen saturation, as measured in the red reading. This method has an accuracy of 5% in the top half of its range and 8% in the bottom half. In 1942, Goldie (5) developed a device for the continuous measurement of oxygen saturation of circulating blood in humans.

These devices led to Wood and Geraei (6), who improved upon these to develop a method for photoelectric determination of arterial oxygen saturation in humans. Prior instruments were required to be preset to known arterial saturation values, and could not be conveniently used in patients who had arterial hypoxia, nor could they be used for the actual determination of arterial oxygen saturation. The older devices could only be used for qualitative changes in saturation. As a result of these shortcomings, Wood and Geraei (6) developed a device that could measure, and follow continuously, the absolute value of arterial oxygen saturation from a pickup unit attached to the pinna of the human ear. This new design consisted of a photoelectric earpiece that allowed simultaneous measurement of the transmission of red and near-infrared light through either the normal heat-flushed ear or the bloodless ear. Then, by calculation, the light transmission of the blood alone in these spectral regions could be determined, and in turn the percentage of oxygen saturation of this blood content could be derived. While this device was used in clinical physiologic laboratories, its use did not spread.

After this promising beginning, oximetry research went dormant until 1972, when Aoyagi (7) began his work. Aoyagi and his group wanted to build upon the theories and success of the Wood oximeter, and created a dye densitometry method in which two wavelengths of light were used; the ratio of the two optical densities was calculated to obtain a dye curve. This curve was expected to correspond to dye concentrations in blood. It was during this series of experiments that the importance of the pulsatile variations was first reported. After investigating the effect of this pulsatile component, using mathematical analysis of the Beer-Lambert law, it was concluded that calculating the ratio of two optical densities compensates for the pulsations. It was at this point that Aoyagi derived three main conclusions:

1. If the optical density of the pulsating portion is measured at two appropriate wavelengths and the ratio of the optical densities is obtained, the result must be equivalent to Wood's ratio.
2. With this method, arterial blood is selectively measured, and the venous blood does not affect the measurement. Therefore, the probe site is not restricted to the ear.
3. With this method, the reference for optical density calculation is set for each pulse. Therefore, an accidental shift of probe location introduces a short artifact and quick return to normal measurements.

Continuing his work on oximeters until 1975, Aoyagi had, by 1975, developed a technique very similar to modern-day pulse oximeters. Two wavelengths of light, 630 nm and 900 nm, were chosen. From the transmitted light intensity data, the pulsation amplitude (AC) and the total intensity (DC) were obtained, and the ratio, AC/DC, was calculated. This ratio was obtained at both wavelengths of light to create a ratio of ratios that corresponded to SaO_2.

In 1980, Minolta developed OXIMET using two optical fibers and precision optics. They adopted the finger as the probe site and proved that pulse oximetry was accurate (7). Nellcor followed this in 1983 with development of the N-100. This was a convenient pulse oximeter that used high-performance light-emitting diodes (LEDs), a highly sensitive and accurate photodiode, and a microcomputer. These technologic advances led to the widespread clinical use of pulse oximeters in the 1980s.

As pulse oximeters have continued to improve, active research is being conducted in several key areas:

- Accuracy as it relates to optimum alarm-level setting
- A quick response time to desaturation
- Eliminating the problems associated with weakened pulses
- Eliminating motion artifact (7)

THEORY

Oximetry is based on the Beer-Lambert law of optical wavelength-dependent absorption of light energy. The Beer-Lambert law describes that light intensity (I) decreases exponentially when transmitted through a measurement compartment. The rate of the exponential decrease depends on the concentration of material inside the measurement compartment (C) and a wavelength-dependent absorption coefficient (a). In addition, the decrease depends on the optical pathlength (L) of the compartment:

$$I = I_o e^{-aLC} \quad [1]$$

For simplicity, we can define absorbance (A) as:

$$A = -\ln(I/I_o) = aLC \quad [2]$$

The wavelength-dependent absorption coefficient (a) varies by wavelength of the emitted light, and depends on the material the light is transmitted through. Since we are interested in oxygenated hemoglobin and reduced hemoglobin, we can study the magnitude of those absorption coefficients. Figure 21.1 shows these data.

If we define C_o as the relative concentration of oxygenated hemoglobin (compared to the total amount of hemoglobin) and C_r as the relative concentration of reduced hemoglobin, we can then define the total absorbance of light at a given wavelength as:

$$A = WL(a_o C_o + a_r C_r) \quad [3]$$

where W is the weight of hemoglobin per unit volume. Note that $C_o + C_r = 1.0$.

In Figure 21.1, it is seen that at a wavelength of 805 nm, the coefficient for oxygenated hemoglobin (a_r) equals the coefficient for reduced hemoglobin (a_r). A measurement at this wavelength will give us a value for WL:

$$WL = A_{805}/a_{805} \quad [4]$$

If we now measure at any other wavelength, we can solve an equation for the relative concentration of oxygenated hemoglobin (C_o):

$$C_o = \frac{a_{805}}{a_o - a_r}\frac{A}{A_{805}} - \frac{a_r}{a_o - a_r} \quad [5]$$

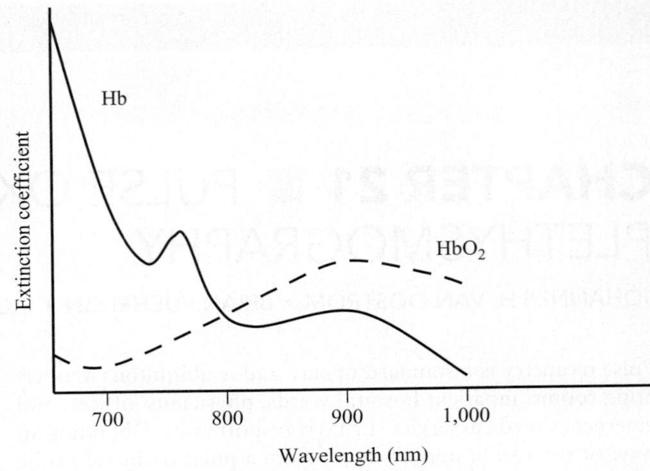

FIGURE 21.1. Absorption versus wavelength changes for oxygenated hemoglobin (HbO_2) and reduced hemoglobin (Hb)

All the absorption coefficients a are constants that depend on the physical media and wavelength. We can thus group those together and rewrite this equation as:

$$C_o = x\frac{A}{A_{805}} + y \quad [6]$$

This shows that we can measure the relative concentration of oxygenated hemoglobin by looking at the ratio of the absorbance (which we can measure) and adjusting with some known constants.

While in the laboratory setting we can tightly control the pathlength, L, and use a laser light at exactly 805 nm, this is not true in an *in vivo* setting. If we want to apply this method to a sensor that emits light through a finger or earlobe, there are significant issues to consider.

For example, if we use a finger as our measurement compartment, Eq. 2 will generally hold, but we need to add the absorption of other materials in the finger:

$$A_{total} = A_{arterial} + A_{venous} + A_{other\ tissues} \quad [7]$$

Since we are only interested in $A_{arterial}$, the other absorbance values need be eliminated. This can be done by taking the time derivative of A_{total}. The time derivative of the venous and tissue components will be zero. The pulsatile part of A_{total} is the arterial component, and the time derivative will be nonzero; this is where the "pulse" in pulse oximetry comes from: It analyzes only the pulsatile portion of the absorbance.

When using a finger sensor, we do not have the ability to choose any wavelength we want. Generally, LEDs are used, which can only be made in a limited number of wavelengths. Wavelengths that are typically used are 660 nm (red light) and 910 nm (infrared light). We can then define a ratio, R, as the ratio of the derivative of absorbances at two different wavelengths:

$$R = \frac{dA_1/dt}{dA_2/dt} \quad [8]$$

Applying similar logic as in the 805-nm case, we can derive an equation for C_o:

$$C_o = \frac{k_1 + k_2 R}{k_3 + k_4 R} \quad [9]$$

where constants k are a combination of the (oxygenated and reduced) absorption coefficients a at the two wavelengths. While these coefficients are only dependent on the physical optical properties of hemoglobin, in practice, the constants k in Eq. 9 are determined empirically by pulse oximeter manufacturers, and are generally unpublished.

REASONS FOR ERRORS

Pulse oximetry fundamentally relies upon adequate perfusion of the vascular bed being monitored. Without sufficient blood flow, oxygen content cannot be adequately analyzed. Decreased perfusion may be caused by a variety of factors including hypotension, medications, ambient temperature, poor circulation, and so forth. Clinicians will often search multiple fingers, toes, and earlobes for a site that can provide a saturation value. Decreased perfusion, leading to the inability of the pulse oximeter to provide a saturation value, is very common. While central site probes may never be ubiquitous, their utility in patients with poor peripheral perfusion cannot be understated. Since these central sites reflect carotid artery flow, they will rarely experience errors due to poor perfusion of the vascular bed.

Pulse oximeters are calibrated using saturation curves of healthy adult volunteers. They are, therefore, the most accurate at high saturation levels and less so at low saturation levels. Unfortunately, from the clinical standpoint, the low saturation levels are where they are the most useful to us. Nonetheless, this is rarely of major consequence, as the clinical difference between a saturation of 83% and 80% is usually very minimal.

It is clinically important to be able to detect rapid hemoglobin desaturation with minimal delay. There is often, regrettably, a delay in this detection. The calculation of oxygenation is a moving average of user-preset length. The delayed response time problem for pulse oximetry–detected desaturations can be partially overcome by reducing the average setting to the shortest duration, usually 2 seconds (8). However, because of an increased likelihood of false alarms and artifact, this is seldom done clinically. To overcome the problem of delayed response time, it is necessary to develop processing algorithms sensitive enough to detect changes quickly, while allowing for artifact rejection and avoiding false alarms; this is an area of active research.

Other sources of error have been explored by Trivedi et al. (9). The researchers looked at very common sources of error, including ambient light and motion artifact. Error rates with excess ambient light were as high as 63% for heart rate and 57% for saturation. For motion artifact, simulated with 2-Hz and 4-Hz tremors, all tested pulse oximeters showed clinically significant error rates in saturation with both movement artifact rates. Error rates were low in the 2-Hz motion for heart rate calculations; however, all devices failed at 4-Hz motion. Other investigators have also reported on the errors and false alarms associated with movement artifact (10–13). Additional sources of error include darkly pigmented skin (14), nail polish, thermal injuries to fingers and/or toes, and inaccessibility of the extremities.

Another very common problem encountered is the lack of compatibility between probes and devices of the various manufacturers. van Oostrom and Melker (15) compared the accuracy of nonproprietary probes designed for use with a variety of pulse oximeters with that of their corresponding proprietary probes. A controlled signal was used on the Human Patient Simulator to simulate apnea. Statistical significance was not found in most of the comparisons, but in some instances the proprietary probes were closer to arterial oxygen than the nonproprietary probes. Whether or not the manufacturer of the probe is the same as the manufacturer of the pulse oximeter may have importance. Table 21.1 summarizes the various reasons for errors (16).

As can be seen from Eq. 2, the intensity of light measured at the detector varies by pathlength changes caused by the arterial pulsations. All other parameters in the equation are constant

TABLE 21.1

REASONS FOR ARTIFACTUAL MEASUREMENT IN PULSE OXIMETRY

VOLUME ARTIFACTS	
Motion	Causes blood volume changes at the measurement site, resulting in difficulties calculating the saturation (23,44)
Low perfusion	Vasoconstriction, an inflated blood pressure cuff, etc., will cause the pulsatile portion of the plethysmogram to be small, causing difficulties calculating saturation (9)
NOISE	
Light interference	Caused by other light sources, such as fluorescent lights, and other ambient light sources (9)
Electrical interference	Powerful radio-frequency signals can cause voltage fluctuations on the detector signal from the pulse oximeter probe (45)
PATIENT-RELATED INTERFERENCE	
Presence of carboxyhemoglobin and/or methemoglobin in blood	Will cause inaccurate calculation of saturation (46)
Dyes present in blood	Depending on the dye, inaccurate saturation calculation will result (47)
Skin pigmentation	Will cause a filtering of the light emitted by the pulse oximeter probe, and cause inaccurate saturation calculations (48)

(at least within several minutes). As pathlength changes are caused by volume changes at the sensor site, it is for this reason that volume artifacts are a frequent problem. Other errors can be caused by light interference from sources outside of the measurement system or electrical interference, and will typically show up in the plethysmogram as additional waveform fluctuations. The effects of this noise are a distorted plethysmogram and can cause incorrect heart rates and saturations to be calculated. One last source of errors is the patient him- or herself: Carboxyhemoglobin present in the blood can cause an inaccurate calculation of saturation.

ALTERNATE-SITE PROBES

The standard location to measure pulse oximetry is the finger. Such probes are common and work well for most normal cases, but other sites are also possible. The *nasal septum* was explored as a possible monitoring site in 1937 (17). Groveman et al. (18) also explored the nasal septum, believing that it represents a constant picture of the internal carotid circulation and reflected cerebral flow. Cucchiara and Messick (19) showed that plethysmography from the nasal septum failed to estimate cerebral blood flow during carotid occlusion. In 1991, the nasal septum was explored during hypothermia (20). Fourteen patients were monitored every 20 minutes during major abdominal procedures. The nasal septum probe was superior to the finger probe in detecting a pulse during hypothermia. The authors concluded that monitoring at the nasal septum was more reliable than monitoring at the finger in hypothermic patients. They acknowledged several limitations, including use during nasal intubation, in patients with extremely small nostrils, or in the presence of a nasogastric tube.

Buccal probes have been evaluated as an alternative probe site. They were prepared by taping a malleable metal bar securely over the back of a disposable Nellcor finger probe and bending the metal bar and probe around the corner of a patient's mouth (21). It was determined that buccal SpO_2 was greater than finger SpO_2 and agreed more closely with SaO_2. The authors determined that buccal pulse oximetry is a viable alternative to the finger. Limitations included longer preparation time, difficult placement, and possible dislodgement during airway maneuvers.

Awad et al. (22) demonstrated that the *ear plethysmographic waveform* is relatively immune to vasoconstriction. They also determined that the photoplethysmographic width has a good correlation to cardiac output. They concluded that the ear is more suitable for monitoring hemodynamic changes than the finger.

Generally, any site that has an arterial bed and is thin enough to safely transmit red and infrared light through can be used for pulse oximetry. Several monitoring locations have become standard of care, including the fingers and toes. A flexible earlobe probe is also used quite frequently when the fingers and toes are inaccessible. Since finger probes work quite well for the majority of patients, it is unlikely that alternate-site probes will ever become ubiquitous. Since the nasal septum, nares, cheek, and ear measure oxygenation from central sites and reflect the blood flow of the carotid arteries, their potential for measuring other physiologic parameters is only beginning to be explored.

OVERCOMING LIMITATIONS

Errors and interference on pulse oximetry can largely be eliminated or prevented. Volume/movement artifact can be reduced by ensuring that the measurement site is kept in place or moved slowly. Massimo developed probes that use a third light source (23); with this additional measurement, it is possible to estimate nonarterial volume changes due to movement artifact. This allows for compensation for those artifacts and creates a more stable signal that is not as susceptible to motion artifact. Light interference can largely be eliminated by covering the measurement site by using a properly sized probe, or by external means such as towels or other covers. Patient-related artifacts can be reduced by fully understanding the patient's physiology, and by proper selection of the measurement site.

PHOTOPLETHYSMOGRAPHY

Photoplethysmography is the measurement of volume changes with light transmission. The photoplethysmograph (PPG) is displayed on most pulse oximeter devices; however, it is frequently ignored as oxygen saturation and pulse rate are the numbers of interest. There is an abundance of physiologic information that can potentially be extracted from this rarely used and noninvasively obtained signal.

Fundamentals

There are two main frequencies of variation in the value of light hitting the photodiode, and both are affected by absorption of the light by blood and various tissues. The low-frequency component (LFC)—or nonpulsatile component—represents the baseline amount of light hitting the detector. This value is affected by the total path traveled by the light. Skin, bone, cartilage, adipose, blood, and so forth, all absorb light, and it is this relatively constant path that results in a baseline amount of light hitting the detector. This baseline amount fluctuates at a lower frequency than the heart rate. Since the biologic tissues in the path of the light are constant, with the exception of venous and arterial blood, the changes in the LFC correspond to changes in baseline blood volume in the path of the light. The majority of this baseline blood resides in the venous system.

The pulsatile cardiac component (PCC) corresponds to changes in the arterial blood volume with each heartbeat. The magnitude of change of the PCC with each heartbeat is related to stroke volume, and the area under the curve of each heartbeat is related to the volume of blood entering the vascular bed with each beat (24). The PCC is therefore a representation of flow into a vascular bed while the LFC is a representation of changes in venous volume (Fig. 21.2A).

The typical pulse oximeter displays a processed waveform (Fig. 21.2B). Since the raw data collected by the device correspond to light hitting the photodiode, which is inversely related to blood volume, the waveform must be inverted to resemble an arterial pressure waveform. If the PPG was displayed as raw data and not inverted, point A would represent increasing light hitting the photodiode, corresponding to a decrease in blood volume, and point B would correspond to the point of

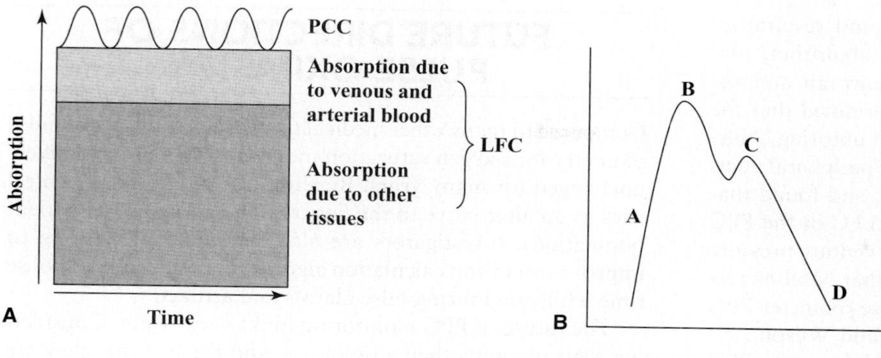

FIGURE 21.2. **A:** A graphic representation of the low-frequency component (LFC) and pulsatile cardiac component (PCC) from a typical finger probe. The PCC is typically less than 5% of the total signal acquired. **B:** A typical display of a processed pulse oximeter waveform. *A* represents the rate of maximum volume increase, *B* represents the point of maximum volume, *C* is the "dicrotic notch," and *D* is the minimal basal volume.

maximum light hitting the photodiode, or the point of least blood in the vascular bed being monitored. The steepness of the flow of the inflow phase A may be used as an indicator of ventricular contraction, and the amplitude of the phase may be used as an indicator of stroke volume (24). The vertical position of the dicrotic notch can be used as an indicator of vasomotor tone. Under most circumstances, the notch descends to the baseline during increasing vasodilation and climbs toward the apex with vasoconstriction (24).

Signal Processing

Prior to the advent of powerful personal computers, many researchers printed the PPG waveform and measured various parameters with a ruler; more recent efforts involve elaborate mathematical and signal processing models. Bhattacharya et al. (25) employed a novel concept aimed at detection of the dominant nonsinusoidal period and the extraction of the associated periodic component. This detection and extraction was performed with a moving window to accommodate the variations of the physiologic oscillations. They also characterized the system with a nonlinear dynamic system.

Goldman et al. (23) from the Masimo Corporation published a detailed description of their signal extraction for error reduction. Massimo Signal Extraction Technology (SET) uses a new conceptual model of light absorption for pulse oximetry and employs discrete saturation transformed to isolate individual saturation components in the optical pathway. Johansson (26) processed the PPG signal using a 16th-order bandpass Bessel filter and a 5th-order bandpass Butterworth filter; a neural network analysis was then performed. Nilsson et al. (27) employed three separate methods for the evaluation of the PPG (called the blood volume pulse) for changes caused by exercise. First, they derived a single parameter from the distribution found in the average histogram of the time-aligned beats. Their second approach analyzed the ratio observed between the first harmonic and higher harmonics in the signal. The third approach evaluated the dicrotic notch depth directly from the PPG waveform. The significance of these findings will be elaborated below.

Uses of the Photoplethysmograph

The PPG is a noninvasively obtained window into many physiologic parameters. Since a pulse oximeter probe can be placed by those with minimal or no training and are found in virtually every aspect of medical care, there are many active research projects exploring the potential uses of the PPG.

Several researchers have attempted to construct mathematical relationships between the PPG and various indices of arterial mechanics. Kato et al. (28) measured the PPG from a finger pulse oximeter and pressure at the ipsilateral radial artery simultaneously. The authors concluded that a four-element, two-compartment model can be applied to the PPG to determine peripheral vascular wall mechanics. Chowienczyk et al. (29) determined that PPG assessment may provide a useful method to examine vascular reactivity. Millasseau et al. in 2002 (30) concluded that contour analysis of the digital volume pulse (DVP) provides a simple, reproducible, noninvasive measure of large artery stiffness, and in 2003 (31) determined that indices of pressure wave reflection and large artery stiffness can be used as an index of vascular aging. Bortolotto et al. (32) concluded that the second derivative of the PPG and the pulse wave velocity can both be used to evaluate vascular aging in hypertensives.

Other researchers are exploring the use of the PPG for noninvasively determining respiratory rate. Changes in intrathoracic pressure during the respiratory cycle displace venous blood, affecting the LFC. These changes also affect cardiac return, changing the amplitude of the PCC. During spontaneous breathing, subatmospheric pressure during inspiration draws air and blood together into the lungs; blood is drawn from the vena cava into the right heart and pulmonary vascular bed. A minor decrease in peripheral venous pressure (PVP) ensues. Soon thereafter, the expiratory pressure normalizes the system. During positive pressure ventilation, the inspiration is drawn by positive pressure, which raises intrathoracic pressure and reduces venous return to the right heart. Simultaneously, and very briefly, blood forced from the low-pressure pulmonary vascular bed increases return to the left heart as well as stroke volume (33). This is followed by a decrease in cardiac output as venous return into the central circulation drops off. The extent of the fluctuations caused by positive pressure ventilation depends on the state of filling of the peripheral vascular bed, the intrathoracic pressure changes, peripheral vasoconstrictor activity, and central blood volume (24). Since positive pressure ventilation often accompanies general anesthesia, which causes vasodilation and damped vasomotor response, respiratory fluctuations are emphasized. It was also discovered that early hypovolemia may be reflected in an exaggerated respiratory wave before other more classic signs of decreased urine output, tachycardia, or hypotension (24).

Nilsson et al. (34) extracted the cardiac and respiratory related components, applied a mathematic algorithm, and developed a new PPG device for monitoring heart rate and respiratory rate simultaneously; their study determined that the PPG has the potential for respiratory rate monitoring. Nilsson et al. (27) hypothesized that the filling of peripheral veins is a major mechanism behind the LFC signal, and found that a correlation exists in the amplitudes of the LFC in the PPG and the respiratory variations in peripheral venous pressure ($p < 0.01$). Leonard et al. (35,36) concluded that baseline respiratory rate was easily identified from a pulse oximeter PPG using wavelet transforms. The study of Foo and Wilson (37) determined that the respiratory rate obtained from the PPG was significantly related to that estimated by a calibrated air pressure transducer during tidal breathing in the absence of motion artifact ($p < 0.05$). Nilsson et al. (27) concluded that respiration can be monitored by the PPG with high sensitivity and specificity regardless of anesthesia and ventilatory mode. Leonard et al. (38) continued their work by developing a fully automated algorithm for the determination of respiratory rate from the PPG.

Researchers have also been exploring the relationship between the PPG and volume status. Perel et al. (39) found that the difference between systolic pressure at end-expiration and the lowest value during the respiratory cycle (d-Down) correlated to the degree of hemorrhage. It also correlated with the cardiac output and the pulmonary capillary wedge pressure. Thus, the changes in systolic pressure with respiration, as demonstrated by arterial pressure waveforms (systolic pressure variation [SPV]) and its d-Down component, are accurate indicators of hypovolemia in ventilated dogs subjected to hemorrhage. Rooke et al. (40) also concluded that SPV and the d-Down appear to follow shifts in intravascular volume in relatively healthy, mechanically ventilated humans under isoflurane anesthesia. Building on this principle, Partridge (41) attempted to use pulse oximetry as a noninvasive method to assess intravascular volume status. The study showed that the PPG correlated with the systolic pressure variation ($r = 0.61$), which was previously shown to be a sensitive indicator of hypovolemia. Shamir et al. (42) investigated ventilation-induced changes in the PPG after removing and reinfusing 10% of the estimated blood volume in 12 anesthetized patients. The plethysmographic SPV was measured as the vertical distance between maximal and minimal peaks of waveforms during the ventilatory cycle and expressed as a percentage of the amplitude of the PPG signal during apnea. This was measured during five consecutive mechanical breaths before apnea and the mean value was obtained for analysis. The 10% loss of estimated blood volume resulted in increased heart rate without changes in mean arterial pressure. Both the PPG waveform changes and the SPV from the arterial blood pressure tracing increased significantly after blood withdrawal ($p < 0.01$). The changes in the PPG correlated with the changes in the SPV. After volume replacement, heart rate decreased while arterial pressure remained unchanged. There were no significant changes in the PPG waveform or the SPV with volume replacement. Fuehrlein et al. (43) investigated the use of PPG for volume status changes during blood donation and hemodialysis. They concluded that the PPG could be used to detect changes in volume status and vascular instability during hemodialysis and blood donation.

FUTURE DIRECTIONS OF PULSE OXIMETRY

Compared to many other medical technologies, the use of pulse oximetry for oxygen saturation monitoring has been relatively unchanged for many years. Researchers are exploring central sites as an alternative to the fingers or toes for specific patient populations. Investigators are also continuously working to improve saturation calculation algorithms to improve response time while minimizing false alarms and artifact.

The future of PPG monitoring looks very bright. Considering their ubiquity, their ease of use, and the fact that they are noninvasive, the medical community would embrace new pulse oximetry technology. Research projects are currently focused on the use of the PPG for arterial mechanics, respiratory rate, and volume status measurements.

References

1. Stokes G. On the reduction oxygenation of the colouring matter of the blood. *Philosoph Mag.* 1864;28:391.
2. Hoppe-Seyler F. Uber die chemischen und optischen Eigenschaffen des Blutfarbstoffs. *Arch Pathol Anat Physiol.* 1864;29:233–251.
3. Hertzman A. Photoelectric plethysmography of the fingers and toes in man. *Proc Soc Exp Biol Med.* 1937;37:529.
4. Millikan G, Papenheimer J, Rawson A. Continuous measurement of oxygen saturation in man. *Am J Physiol.* 1941;133:390.
5. Goldie E. Device for continuous indication of oxygen saturation of circulating blood in man. *J Sci Instrument.* 1942;19:23–25.
6. Wood E, Geraei J. Photoelectric determination of arterial saturation in man. *J Lab Clin Med.* 1949;34:387–401.
7. Aoyagi T. Pulse oximetry: its invention, theory and future. *J Anesth.* 2003;17: 259–266.
8. Grace R. Pulse oximetry: gold standard or false sense of security? *Med J Austr.* 1994;160(10):638–644.
9. Trivedi N, Ghouri A, Shah N, et al. Effects of motion, ambient light and hypoperfusion on pulse oximeter function. *J Clin Anesth.* 1997;9:179–183.
10. Reich D, Timcenko A, Bodian C, et al. Predictors of pulse oximetry data failure. *Anesthesiology.* 1996;84:859–864.
11. Moller J, Johannessen N, Espersen K, et al. Randomized evaluation of pulse oximetry in 20,802 patients: 1. Design, demography, pulse oximetry failure rate and overall complication rate. *Anesthesiology.* 1993;78:436–444.
12. Runciman W, Webb R, Barker L, et al. The Australian Incident Monitoring Study: the pulse oximeter: applications and limitations: an analysis of 2000 incident reports. *Anesth Intens Care.* 1993;21:543–550.
13. Lawless S. Crying wolf: false alarms in a pediatric intensive care unit. *Crit Care Med.* 1994;22:981–985.
14. Jubran A. Pulse oximetry. *Crit Care.* 1999;3:R11–17.
15. van Oostrom J, Melker R. Comparative testing of pulse oximeter probes. *Anesth Analg.* 2004;98:1354–1358.
16. van Oostrom JH, Mahla ME, Gravenstein D. The Stealth Station Image Guidance System may interfere with pulse oximetry. *Can J Anaesth.* 2005; 52(4):379–382.
17. Hertzman A. Photoelectric plethysmography of the nasal septum in man. *Proc Soc Exp Biol Med.* 1937;37:290.
18. Groveman J, Cohen D, Dillon J. Rhinoplethysmography: pulse monitoring at the nasal septum. *Anesth Analg.* 1966;45(1):63–68.
19. Cucchiara R, Messick J. The failure of nasal plethysmography to estimate cerebral blood flow during carotid occlusion. *Anesthesiology.* 1981;55(5): 585–586.
20. Ezri T, Lurie S, Konichezky A, et al. Pulse oximetry from the nasal septum. *J Clin Anesth.* 1991;3:447–450.
21. O'Leary R, Landon M, Benumof J. Buccal pulse oximeter is more accurate than finger pulse oximeter in measuring oxygen saturation. *Anesth Analg.* 1992;75:495–498.
22. Awad A, Stout R, Ghobashy M, et al. Analysis of the ear pulse oximeter waveform. *J Clin Monit Comp.* 2006;20(3):175–184.
23. Goldman J, Petterson M, Kopotic R, et al. Masimo Signal Extraction in pulse oximetry. *J Clin Monit Comp.* 2000;16:475–483.
24. Murray W, Foster A. The peripheral pulse wave: information overlooked. *J Clin Monit.* 1996;12:365–377.
25. Bhattacharya J, Kanjilal P, Muralidhar V. Analysis and characterization of the photo-plethysmographic signal. *IEEE Trans Biomed Eng.* 2001;48(1): 5–11.

26. Johansson A. Neural network for photoplethysmographic respiratory rate monitoring. *Med Biol Eng Comp.* 2003;41:424–428.
27. Nilsson L, Johansson A, Kalman S. Respiratory variations in the reflection mode photoplethysmographic signal. Relationships to peripheral venous pressure. *Med Biol Eng Comp.* 2003;41:149–154.
28. Kato R, Sato J, Iuchi T, et al. Quantitative determination of arterial wall mechanics with pulse oximetric finger plethysmography. *J Anesth.* 1999;13: 197–204.
29. Chowienczyk P, Kelly R, MacCallum H, et al. Photoplethysmographic assessment of pulse wave reflection: blunted response to endothelium-dependent beta2-adrenergic vasodilation in type II diabetes mellitus. *J Am Coll Cardiol.* 1999;34(7):2007–2014.
30. Millasseau S, Kelly R, Ritter J, et al. Determination of age-related increases in large artery stiffness by digital pulse contour analysis. *Clin Sci.* 2002;103:371–377.
31. Millasseau S, Kelly R, Ritter J, et al. The vascular impact of aging and vasoactive drugs: comparison of two digital volume pulse measurements. *Am J Hypertens.* 2003;16:467–472.
32. Bortolotto L, Blacher J, Kondo T, et al. Assessment of vascular aging and atherosclerosis in hypertensive subjects: second derivative of photoplethysmogram versus pulse wave velocity. *Am J Hypertens.* 2000;13:165–171.
33. Pinsky M, Summer W. Cardiac augmentation by phasic high intra-thoracic pressure support in man. *Chest.* 1983;84:370–375.
34. Nilsson L, Johansson A, Kalman S. Monitoring of respiratory rate in postoperative care using a new photoplethysmographic technique. *J Clin Monit Comp.* 2000;16:309–315.
35. Leonard P, Beattie T, Addison P, et al. Standard pulse oximeters can be used to monitor respiratory rate. *Emerg Med J.* 2003;20(6):524–525.
36. Leonard P, Grubb N, Addison P, et al. An algorithm for the detection of individual breaths from the pulse oximeter waveform. *J Clin Monit Comp.* 2004;18:309–312.
37. Foo J, Wilson S. Estimation of breathing interval from the photoplethysmographic signals in children. *Physiol Measure.* 2005;26(6):1049–1058.
38. Leonard P, Douglas J, Grubb N, et al. A fully automated algorithm for the determination of respiratory rate from the photoplethysmogram. *J Clin Monit Comp.* 2006;20(1):33–36.
39. Perel A, Pizov R, Cotev S. Systolic blood pressure variation is a sensitive indicator of hypovolemia in ventilated dogs subjected to graded hemorrhage. *Anesthesiology.* 1987;67(4):498–502.
40. Rooke G, Schwid H, Shapira Y. The effect of graded hemorrhage and intravascular volume replacement on systolic pressure variation in humans during mechanical and spontaneous ventilation. *Anesth Analg.* 1995;80:925–932.
41. Partridge B. Use of pulse oximetry as a noninvasive indicator of intravascular volume status. *J Clin Monit.* 1987;3:263–268.
42. Shamir M, Eidelman LA, Floman Y, et al. Pulse oximetry plethysmographic waveform during changes in blood volume. *Br J Anaeth.* 1999;2:178–181.
43. Fuehrlein B, Melker R, Ross E. Alar photoplethysmography: a new methodology for monitoring fluid removal and carotid circulation during hemodialysis. *J Clin Monit Comp.* 2007;4:211–218.
44. Jopling MW, Mannheimer PD, Bebout DE. Issues in the laboratory evaluation of pulse oximeter performance. *Anesth Analg.* 2002;94(1 Suppl):S62–68.
45. Block FE Jr, Detko GJ Jr. Minimizing interference and false alarms from electrocautery in the Nellcor N-100 pulse oximeter. *J Clin Monit.* 1986;2(3):203–205.
46. Barker SJ, Tremper KK, Hyatt J. Effects of methemoglobinemia on pulse oximetry and mixed venous oximetry. *Anesthesiology.* 1989;70(1):112–117.
47. Vokach-Brodsky L, Jeffrey SS, Lemmens HJ, et al. Isosulfan blue affects pulse oximetry. *Anesthesiology.* 2000;93(4):1002–1003.
48. Ralston AC, Webb RK, Runciman WB. Potential errors in pulse oximetry. III: effects of interferences, dyes, dyshaemoglobins and other pigments. *Anaesthesia.* 1991;46(4):291–295.

CHAPTER 22 ■ CAPNOGRAPHY

J.S. GRAVENSTEIN • DAVID A. PAULUS

Capnometry refers to the measurement of carbon dioxide, regardless of the method used. Capnography describes the method of obtaining a capnogram, that is, a tracing of carbon dioxide concentration as a function of time or volume. A capnograph is the instrument used to generate a capnogram. Capnometry has become the minimal standard of practice for the American Society of Anesthesiologists whenever a patient's airway is breached with an endotracheal tube, a laryngeal mask airway, or an esophageal tracheal airway. If carbon dioxide can be detected breath after breath after placing the artificial airway, the clinician has the first and best—if not the only—indication that the artificial airway is ventilating the patient's lungs rather than the esophagus and stomach.

The delivery of carbon dioxide to the exhaled gas is the final step in a complex system. Metabolism generates carbon dioxide, which is absorbed upon tissue perfusion, at which point venous blood flow delivers the CO_2 to the heart, which powers pulmonary perfusion, and delivers it to the lungs and, via ventilation, gathers it from the alveoli when a breath finally pushes it to the outside. Thus, the discovery of carbon dioxide after intubation of the patient's airway, while essential, is but the tip of the proverbial iceberg. In this chapter, we provide a clinician's overview of capnometry and its applications in the perioperative period and the intensive care unit.

HISTORY

Carbon dioxide and its measurement have enjoyed a colorful history (1). Jan Baptista van Helmont (1579–1644) recognized a spirit escaping from burning wood and called it gas sylvester (from Latin *silva* = wood and *silvester* = woody). The recognition that a gas could reside in something solid found expression in the term "fixed air" introduced by J. Black in 1755. He discovered the gas to be a constituent of carbonated alkali. Later, Antoine-Laurent de Lavoisier (1743–1794) showed the gas to be an oxide of carbon. What an extraordinary circumstance: Carbon (of coal and diamonds) connected with oxygen was a gas! John Tyndall (1820–1893) spoke of "perfectly colorless and invisible gases and vapors" such as carbonic acid (now called carbon dioxide) that could well absorb radiant energy. This insight enabled him to detect carbon dioxide in the exhaled gas. However, before capnography based on physical methods could gain a foothold in clinical practice, a chemical method described by John Scott Haldane (1860–1936) became the gold standard. He caused a precisely measured volume of gas to be drawn into a closed system that made it possible to expose the gas to absorbents such as sodium or potassium hydroxide. These agents removed the carbon dioxide from the sample; the vanished volume was attributed to the absorbed carbon dioxide. Refinements of this method were widely used, yet the methods were time consuming. Chemical methods in general destroy the gas to be measured and allow only snapshots of respiratory carbon dioxide.

A number of methods exploited the physics of energy absorption. August Hermann Pfund (1879–1949), professor of optics in Baltimore, measured the effects of interposing more or less carbon dioxide between a heat source and a temperature sensor. Karl Friedrich Luft (1900–1999) employed infrared energy beamed through cells with and without carbon dioxide, thus enabling the measurements of the energy absorbed by the gas in question. Later generations of this same principle gave rise to the currently most widely used infrared spectroscopic method of capnography.

Two other methods deserve brief mention, as both of them entered the market without gaining a firm foothold. One of them became known as Raman scattering, a technique that exploits the power of laser energy to affect the amplitude of molecular vibration. Another method made use of mass spectrometry, in which charged particles are separated by their mass, thus enabling the identification and concentration of different gases.

SITES OF MEASUREMENT

Capnography, herein examined, focuses on the detection and monitoring of carbon dioxide in the exhaled gases. That carbon dioxide can also be lost and consequently collected and measured from the skin (2), from the stomach (3), sublingually (4), and even from the rectum (5) deserves mention but will not be discussed in this chapter.

STEADY OR UNSTEADY STATE

With modern methods, continuous readings of exhaled carbon dioxide tensions and volumes can be obtained. We speak of steady state when the tension is exerted by carbon dioxide in different tissue and organ compartments and blood and alveolar gas have reached equilibrium, and when the input of carbon dioxide from metabolism equals the output of carbon dioxide via ventilation and, to a small extent, via skin, flatus, feces, and urine. A steady state can exist with high, normal, or low arterial, alveolar, or end-tidal carbon dioxide tension ($PaCO_2$, $PACO_2$, or $PETCO_2$). However, all too often, we do not have a steady state: Tissue depleted of carbon dioxide can absorb liters of carbon dioxide from blood until tissue PCO_2 and blood PCO_2 reach equilibrium; conversely, such tissue stores can contribute CO_2 to that generated by metabolism. For example, prolonged hyperventilation can exhaust tissue stores of carbon dioxide and bicarbonate. Under these conditions, the maintenance of a normal $PaCO_2$ requires less than normal ventilation because some of the metabolic carbon dioxide filters back into the tissues instead of being exhaled. Conversely, high tissue stores of carbon dioxide (e.g., after a cardiac and respiratory arrest) will call for greater than normal ventilation until steady state is once again reached. A depressed respiratory center (e.g., under the influence of an opiate) will lead to an imbalance of input and output as the tissues take up some of the carbon dioxide while the rest leaves the body in the exhaled gas. Once the tissues and blood reach equilibrium, steady state will once again supervene in the presence of elevated levels of $PaCO_2$, $PACO_2$, and $PETCO_2$. Renal compensation of metabolic acidosis or alkalosis will also lead to an unsteady state that can last for many hours. The point: Capnograms can hide as much as they reveal, and thus the interpretation of capnograms calls for discerning clinicians.

CONVENTIONS OF MEASUREMENTS

Before describing the different methods of capnography, the conventions of reporting the tension or concentration of CO_2 present in the exhaled gas must be discussed. The tension of the gas can be reported in mm Hg (same as torr), with normal end-tidal values between 35 mm Hg and 45 mm Hg, which translates into 4.67 kPa and 6.0 kPa, respectively. The amount of carbon dioxide present in a gas sample can also be reported in percent or as a fraction of the volume of gas. Here caution needs to be exercised: 5.0% end-tidal PCO_2 (equal to the end-tidal fraction, Fet, 0.05) at a barometric pressure at sea level of 760 mm Hg (101 kPa) would amount to 38 mm Hg (5.05 kPa). However, many millions of people live in cities at altitude. Assume, for example, Mexico City with an ambient pressure of perhaps 550 mm Hg (73 kPa). Here, 5.0% end-tidal CO_2 would represent only 27.5 mm Hg (3.65 kPa). The influence of the pressure exerted by water vapor (47 mm Hg or 6.26 kPa at 37), which is not affected by barometric pressure but rises and falls as a function of temperature, also plays an important

TABLE 22.1

CARBON DIOXIDE AND BAROMETRIC PRESSURE AT 37°C

Barometric pressure	End-tidal PCO_2	End-tidal percent or fraction of volume	Alveolar partial pressure of water vapor	Alveolar percent or fraction of water vapor
Sea level at 760 mm Hg	38 mm Hg or 5.05 kPa	5.0% or fe 0.05	47 mm Hg or 6.26 kPa	6.2% or fe H_2O 0.06
Elevation[a] 550 mm Hg	27.5 mm Hg or 3.65 kPa	5.0% or fe 0.05	47 mm Hg or 6.26 kPa	8.5% or fe H_2O 0.08

[a] At altitude assuming hyperventilation to an end-tidal PCO_2 of 27.5 mm Hg.
While hyperventilation can reduce the volume of carbon dioxide in the alveoli, it cannot reduce the tension of water vapor, which, as long as the temperature stays at 37°C, will remain at 47 mm Hg. Some capnometers offer readings that assume dry or wet gas at 37°C.
f stands for fraction where 1 = 100% and f 0.05 = 5%.

role at altitude (Table 22.1). As we wish to correlate alveolar gas tension with the tension of gases in blood (reported in mm Hg or kPa), we prefer to report gaseous carbon dioxide not in percent, but as PCO_2 in mm Hg or kPa.

METHODOLOGIES

Chemical

Carbon dioxide goes into solution, combines with water to form carbonic acid, and establishes an equilibrium between dissolved CO_2 and bicarbonate. This reaction, which changes the pH, gives rise to chemical methods using pH indicators for the estimation of carbon dioxide concentration in moist gas, or colorimetric $EtCO_2$ (Fig. 22.1).

Changes in temperature and the addition or removal of H^+ ions, in turn, affect the ratio of bicarbonate to carbonic acid, and dissolved CO_2, therefore, plays a crucial role in the acid-based equilibrium of blood, which is assessed by measuring pH and PCO_2 and calculating bicarbonate in blood. This is discussed in detail elsewhere in this book, as is the importance of buffers (primarily hemoglobin) and carbonic anhydrase, which accelerate the reaction:

$$CO_2 + H_2O \leftrightharpoons H_2CO_3 \leftrightharpoons HCO_3^- + H^+$$

Sidestream and Mainstream (On-airway) Capnography: Time-based Methods

The gas to be analyzed has to be collected from the patient under conditions that prevent contamination of the gas with ambient air. Ideally, we would like to sample tracheal gas; that is rarely possible. A cuffed endotracheal tube with a port close to the mouth offers the next best opportunity to collect exhaled gas from the patient before it mixes with gas from the outside or the breathing circuit. First, we will a look at the sidestream method.

Sidestream

On its way to the analyzer through a capillary, the gas cools (from body to room temperature) and the water vapor condenses, forming droplets. Two measures minimize the potential problem of having water obstruct the flow of gas or confound the spectroscopic analysis: Collecting capillaries made out of Nafion tubing enables the water vapor in the tube to equilibrate with the water vapor in air surrounding the tube. This leads to a reduction of water vapor in the capillary. The second, a more prosaic method, consists of a water trap situated close to the analyzer.

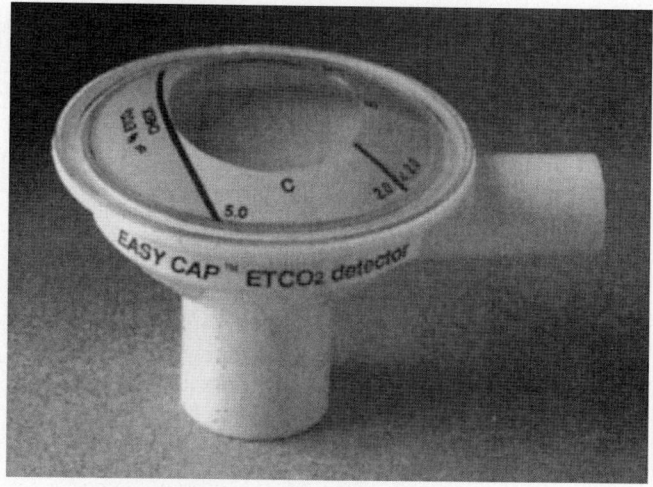

FIGURE 22.1. A device that detects CO_2 by chemically induced color change (Nellcor, Inc.).

Figure 22.2 shows a typical time-based capnogram obtained under ideal conditions. Here we plot the tension of carbon dioxide in the ordinate and time in the abscissa. Observe the angles α and β, both of which in a healthy individual approach 90 degrees. A respiratory pause at the end of exhalation will cause the plateau phase to become horizontal.

With the sidestream method, the costly analyzer can be kept out of the way; a thin, long aspirating capillary presents no encumbrance to the clinical team; and aspirated gas can be analyzed for carbon dioxide as well as other gases. Furthermore, gas can be aspirated from nasal prongs with minimal annoyance to a conscious patient. Commercial configurations are available that enable the simultaneous aspiration of gas from one nostril while delivering oxygen to the other nostril or

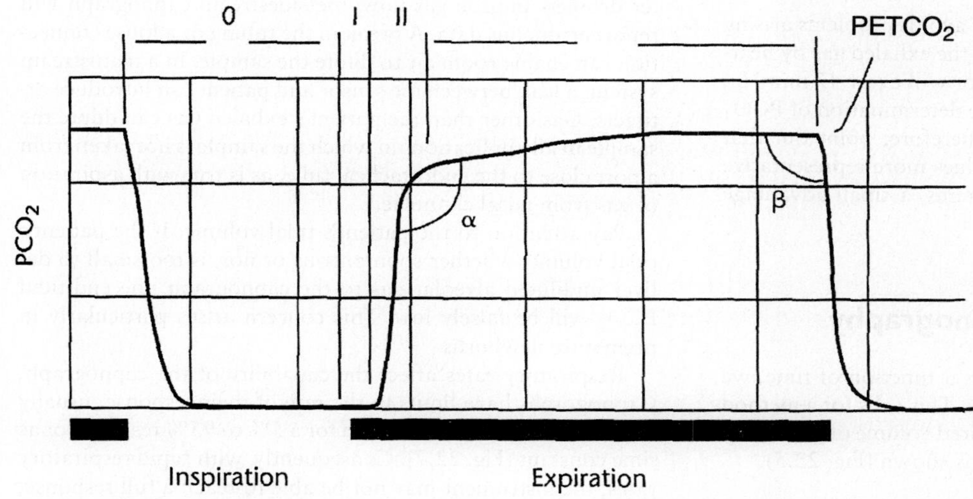

FIGURE 22.2. Capnogram showing exhaled PCO_2 versus time. Expiration shows phase I (dead space gas free of CO_2), phase II (rapid appearance of CO_2), and phase III (plateau). The α angle describes the transition from phase II to III and the β angle that from phase III to phase 0, the beginning of inspiration.

to the mouth. However, in that application, contamination of the aspirated gas with room air or oxygen is possible, although several studies have shown clinically satisfactory results with these arrangements. At a minimum, such a system can provide evidence of ventilation and enable the recording of respiratory rates.

The sidestream method has two well-recognized drawbacks. The longer the capillary is, the longer the travel time for the gas from the patient to the analyzer. That causes the capnogram to be out of phase with simultaneously recorded flow or pressure tracings. The long travel also gives the leading edge of a gas a chance to mix with the gas it is replacing in the tubing, which produces slurring of the capnogram, particularly noticeable with rapid respiratory rates (Fig. 22.3).

Many sidestream capnometers aspirate up to 200 mL gas per minute into the analyzer. Premature newborns, with their small tidal volumes and high respiratory rates, will then develop capnograms that show false low end-tidal and false high inspiratory PCO_2 values. Two mechanisms contribute to these conditions: On the one hand, the tiny patient's tidal volume might be so low as to cause the capnograph to aspirate gas from the breathing tube, thus diluting the exhaled gas from the patient. On the other hand, the time constant of the capnograph may be too long to respond adequately to rapid breaths. Modern capnographs offer low rates of aspiration (30–50 mL/minute) and short time constants (6).

Mainstream

Instead of aspirating a sample of respired gas with a sidestream system, it is possible to determine the concentration of carbon dioxide close to the patient's mouth in a "mainstream" or "on-airway" method (Fig. 22.4). The method eliminates two weaknesses of the sidestream system: Without a need to transport the gas through a capillary to the analyzer, mainstream capnograms show no slurring of the capnographic tracings. Of course, these advantages come with a (tolerable) cost: The carbon dioxide sensor must be brought close to the patient's mouth, which adds weight to the breathing circuit/endotracheal tube; in this position, the sensor is exposed to potential damage, and obtaining gas samples from a spontaneously breathing, nonintubated patient is more difficult than would be true from a sidestream system. Nevertheless, mainstream systems have been adapted for capnography even in nonintubated infants.

The mainstream, on-airway system avoids problems arising out of condensation of water vapor in the exhaled gas by heating of the sensor. At 37°C, water vapor will exert 47 mm Hg, thus affecting—if not powerfully—the determination of PCO_2 in sidestream systems. Purists will, therefore, point out that mainstream capnography will give values more representative of alveolar gases than sidestream systems, a small advantage with no clinical significance.

Volume-based Capnography

Instead of plotting the respired gas as a function of time, we can also plot it as a function of volume. This calls for a method to measure, breath by breath, the respired volume of gas. Commonly, only the exhaled tidal volume is shown (Fig. 22.5).

Observe on Figure 22.5:

A: The tracing starts with the beginning of exhalation, which consists of dead space free of CO_2.

B: As the dead space is cleared, gas from the sequentially smaller and smaller airways, and finally alveoli, will be exhaled. A steeply rising concentration of carbon dioxide over volume reflects this phase. The phase ends in a distinctive knee and then transitions into a more or less horizontal phase.

C: The gently rising horizontal phase adds volume from distant lung segments.

D: The end-tidal value, normally about 40 mm Hg, represents alveolar gas if lung function and tidal volume are normal.

E: The inspiratory limb of the breath is not recorded, as is the custom with volume-based capnograms.

The measurement of the exhaled volume presents challenges. Not only is the flow rate not uniform over the entire exhaled volume, but also the presence of water vapor, barometric pressure, composition of the exhaled gas (imagine the presence of helium!), configuration of the sensor, and response time of the flow meter can all affect the accuracy of the measurement (7).

Observe in Figure 22.5 the gap between the end-tidal value and the arterial carbon dioxide tension; thus, together with an arterial blood gas, the single breath method enables the clinician to estimate the volume of carbon dioxide in the exhaled breath (X), the volume of the alveolar dead space (Y), and the volume of the anatomic dead space (Z). Fletcher adopted an estimation of the "efficiency" of ventilation by drawing a horizontal line through the end-tidal concentration of carbon dioxide (8) (Fig. 22.6).

Check of Capnograph

Before accepting the data provided by capnographs, check the technical details of the instruments, whether sidestream or mainstream and whether time or volume based. Calibration can be accomplished with a test gas, with references built into the instrument, and for mainstream systems with cells that mimic the presence of a known carbon dioxide concentration. When in doubt, the user can test his or her own exhaled gas. However, this will not test the linearity of the instrument.

For sidestream systems, check for a properly connected sampling system and patent tubing. When secretions or water droplets impede gas flow, the sidestream capnograph will report erroneous data. A break in the tubing or a loose connection can enable room air to dilute the sample. In a mainstream system, a leak between the sensor and patient can introduce artifacts. Gas other than the patient's exhaled gas can dilute the sample in all applications in which the sample is not taken from a port close to the endotracheal tube, as is true with aspiration of gas from nasal cannulae.

Pay attention to the patient's tidal volume. If the patient's tidal volume, whether spontaneous or not, is too small to deliver undiluted alveolar gas to the capnograph, the end-tidal PCO_2 will be falsely low. This concern arises particularly in premature newborns.

Respiratory rates affect the capability of the capnograph. Capnographs have limits to the rate of their response, usually expressed either as time needed for a 5% to 95% response or as time constant (Fig. 22.7). Consequently, with rapid respiratory rates, the instrument may not be able to reach a full response,

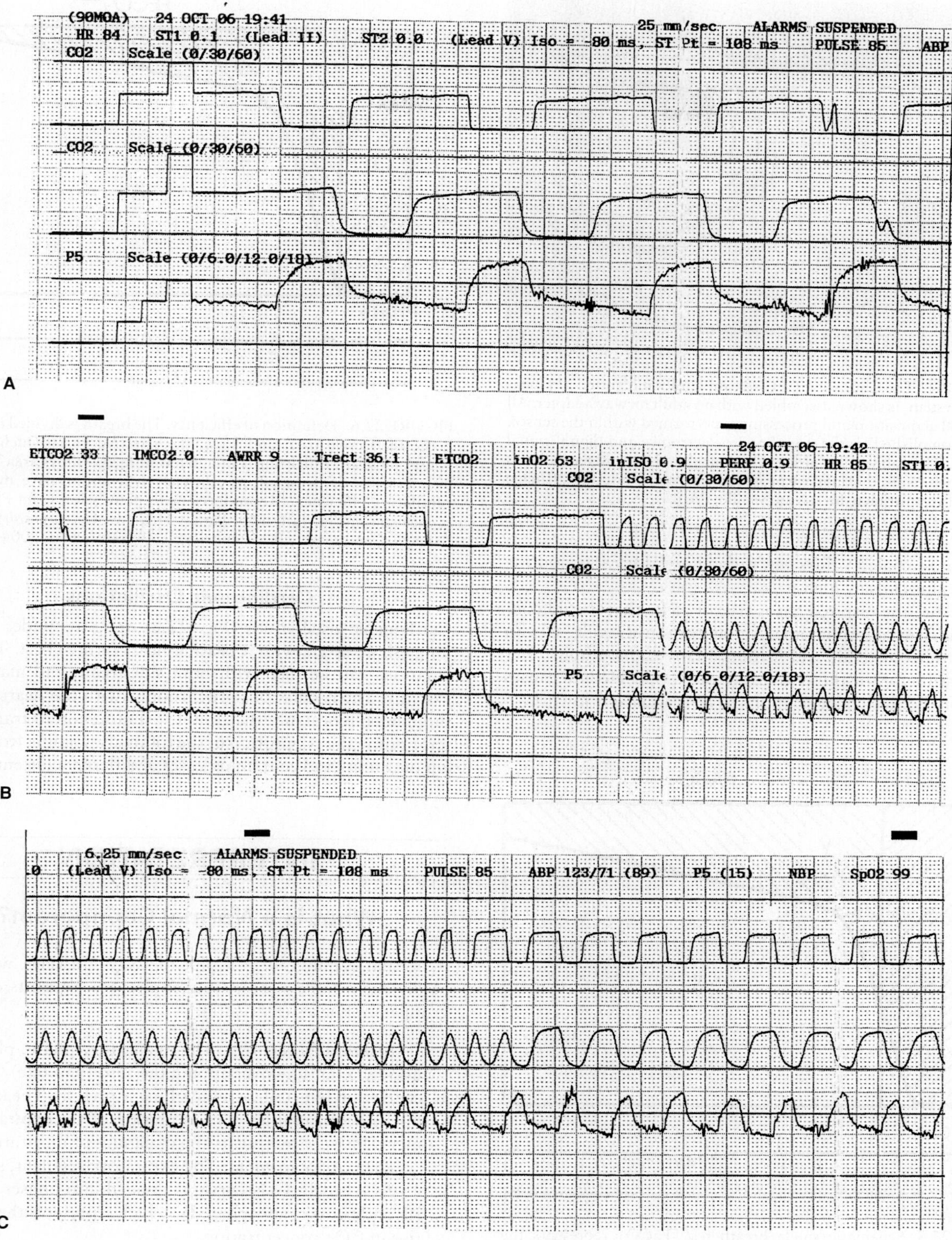

FIGURE 22.3. **A:** The top capnogram derives from an on-airway sampling location. The middle tracing is a capnogram from a sidestream device. Notice the on-airway waveform is a little more crisp than that from the sidestream device. The data were collected from a patient during mechanical ventilation. The increase in airway pressure is associated with the sudden disappearance of CO_2 and the drop in airway pressure signals exhalation. Travel time of gas in the capillary of the sidestream capnogram causes the on-airway curve to lag behind the pressure tracings. **B:** Increasing respiratory rate briefly to 60 breaths per minute eliminates the plateau in the sidestream-derived waveform with reduced end-tidal CO_2, while the on-airway device still shows a plateau. **C:** Dropping the rate to 30 breaths per minute results in the plateau reappearing in the on-airway device.

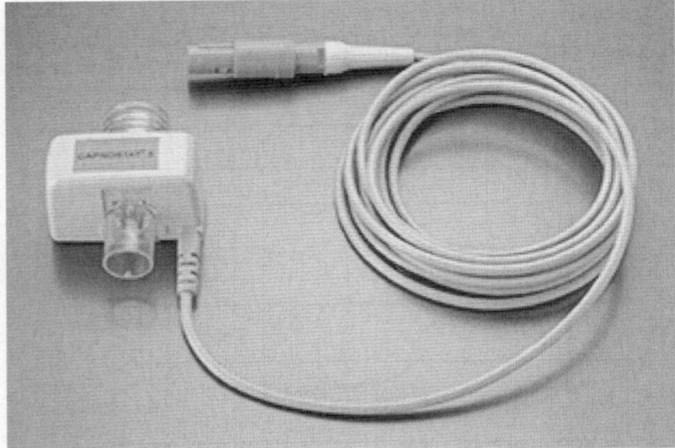

FIGURE 22.4. The Capnostat CO_2 sensor, a fully integrated gas measurement system, is shown assembled with an adult airway adapter. All of the signal acquisition and processing is performed within the sensor. This is accomplished by the use of microelectronics and digital signal processing. The capnogram along with calculated parameters such as end-tidal and inspired values are provided via a serial interface. (Image courtesy of Respironics, Inc., Murrysville, PA.)

and the end-exhaled values can present as falsely low and the inspired values falsely high.

Make sure the respired gas is free of gases that would confound the spectrographic analysis of carbon dioxide, as can be true of nitrous oxide and helium. Many capnographs offer compensation for the presence of nitrous oxide. Helium causes the carbon dioxide concentrations to be read falsely low (9).

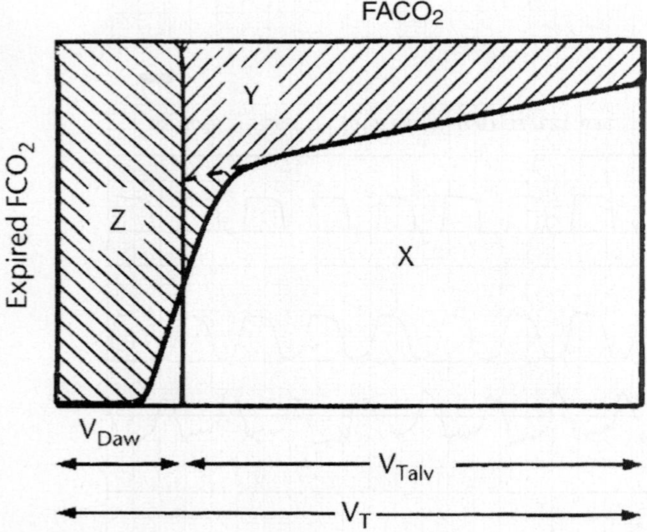

FIGURE 22.5. Schematic single breath test. $FaCO_2$ represents the FCO_2 of a gas in equilibrium with arterial blood. Area X represents the volume of CO_2 in the breath. Area Y represents the alveolar dead space. The alveolar dead space fraction is given by Y/(X + Y). V_{Talv} is the alveolar tidal volume. The physiologic dead space fraction is represented by areas (Y + Z)/(X + Y + Z). Note that fractions are used, rather than partial pressures, in order that the areas may represent CO_2 volumes, actual or notional. Observe the horizontal line of an invasively obtained $FaCO_2$. (Reproduced with permission from Fletcher R. In Gravenstein JS, Jaffe MB, Paulus DA, eds. *Capnography, Clinical Aspects*. Cambridge, UK: Cambridge University Press; 2004:381.)

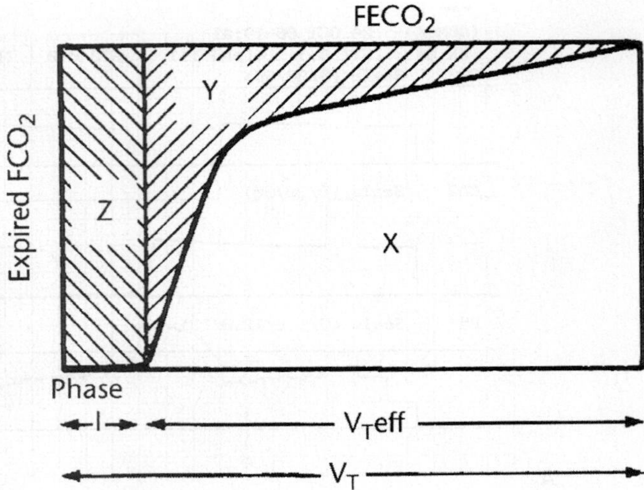

FIGURE 22.6. Definition of efficiency. The breath is divided into phase I, the ineffective part, and V_{Teff}, the effective part (which contains phases I and II). Efficiency is calculated from 100 times area X divided by areas (X + Y). In effect, efficiency is a noninvasive measure of ventilatory efficiency. (Reproduced with permission from Fletcher R. In Gravenstein JS, Jaffe MB, Paulus DA, eds. *Capnography, Clinical Aspects*. Cambridge, UK: Cambridge University Press; 2004:382.)

Cardiogenic Oscillations

Cardiogenic oscillations (Fig. 22.8) are a reminder that the lungs share space with a beating heart in the chest. These oscillations can be seen with both sidestream and mainstream systems. The oscillations synchronous with the heart beat are thought to represent "the complex summation of transient alterations in the proportion of the total flow coming from different lung units and containing gases of different concentrations" (10).

INTERPRETATION

What Is a Normal Capnogram?

A normal capnogram is a plot of CO_2 and time, which can be divided into inspiratory and expiratory segments, each one grouped in phases (Fig. 22.2).

Inspiratory segment: The inspiratory phase, phase 0, is usually a flat line overlapping the zero (baseline) CO_2 concentration line, unless rebreathing is present. The latter part of the horizontal baseline is phase I of the expiratory segment. Phase 0 represents the dynamics of inspiration.

Expiratory segment: The expiratory segment, similar to a single breath CO_2 curve, is divided into phases I, II, and III, and occasionally phase IV, which represents the terminal rise in CO_2 concentration.

Phase I: Phase I represents CO_2-free gas from the apparatus and anatomic dead space.

Phase II: Phase II consists of a rapid S-shaped upswing on the tracing due to mixing of dead space gas with alveolar gas.

α Angle: The angle between phases II and III has been referred to as the α angle, and increases as the slope of phase III increases. Changes of the α angle correlate with

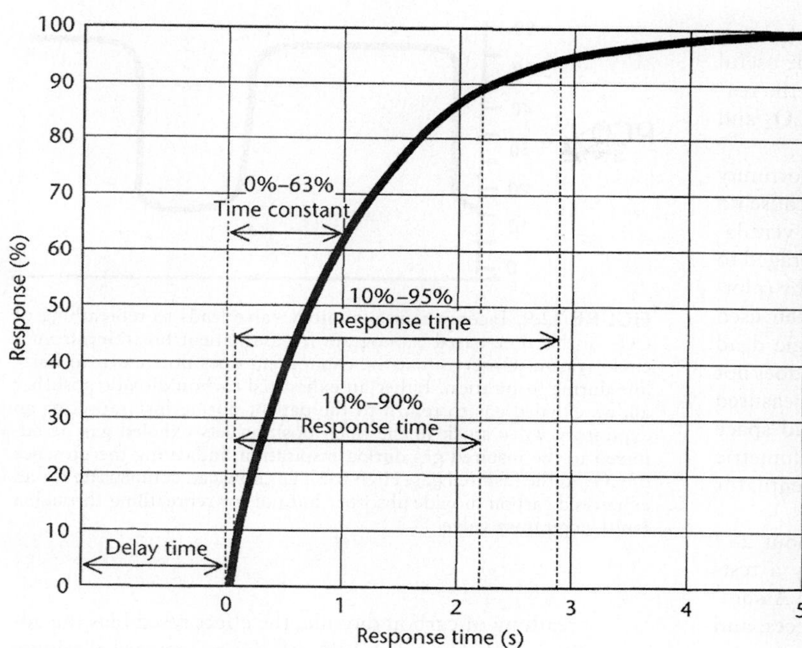

FIGURE 22.7. For sidestream sampling, total response time is equal to the delay or transit time in the sampling catheter plus the measurement rise time, which is expressed different ways. (Reproduced from Gravenstein JS, Paulus DA, Hayes TJ. *Capnography in Clinical Practice.* 2nd ed. Boston: Butterworth-Heinemann, 1989.)

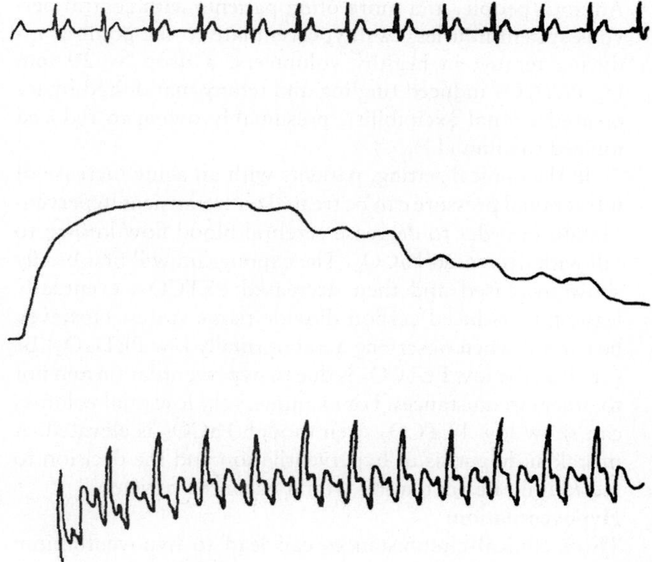

FIGURE 22.8. Simultaneous electrocardiogram and capnogram with cardiogenic oscillations and pneumotachygraph. Cardiogenic oscillations in this capnogram (**middle tracing**) were generated from a healthy volunteer who breathed into a mouthpiece, to which a pneumotachygraph (set at high sensitivity) and sidestream capnograph sampling connector were attached. An electrocardiogram (**top tracing**) was recorded simultaneously. Oscillations appeared on the capnogram only on the down-slope. The oscillation occurred at the same rate as the heartbeat, but 2 to 3 seconds after the pneumotachygraph because of the travel time of the gas in the sidestream capnograph. In order to generate a pneumotachygraph, the subject kept his glottis open after an exhalation was completed.

sequential emptying of alveoli. In general, the more heterogeneous are functional units of the lung, and the wider one is the α angle.

Phase III: Phase III is the link between the α angle and the $PETCO_2$. Its slope increases with ventilation/perfusion (V/Q) mismatch, and it is determined by the gas-emptying sequence of the alveolar units. If the units empty synchronously, the CO_2 expired results in a smooth flat or slightly upsloping phase III. In patients with severe V/Q scatter and longer time constants, CO_2 emptying is sequential, resulting in a steeper rising slope of phase III. In general, the more severe the mismatch is, the steeper the slope. Factors such as changes in cardiac output, CO_2 production, airway resistance, breathing pattern (tachypnea), and low functional residual capacity (FRC) may further affect the V/Q status of the various units in the lung, and thus influence the height or the slope of phase III.

An incompetent expiratory valve resulting in rebreathing may affect the α angle and up-slope the phase III of the capnograph. A simultaneous recording of flow rate waveforms is potentially used to differentiate this technical problem from an abnormal plateau of phase III of the capnograph. For a healthy, spontaneously breathing adult or with optimal mechanical ventilation, the α angle should show a smooth curve (see Fig. 22.2), end-tidal values of 35 to 45 mm Hg, and an arterial $PaCO_2$ of only 3 to 4 mm Hg higher than the end-tidal values. There would be no carbon dioxide in the inspired air.

How can we be sure that ventilation is normal when we don't have arterial blood gas analyses available? A stethoscope would be helpful in confirming normal breath sounds left and right. A spontaneously breathing patient should be breathing regularly, without a tracheal tug during inspiration; the left and right chest should rise equally and evenly during inspiration; and during expiration, the abdominal muscles should not contract. If clinical findings raise doubts about the adequacy of ventilation, even with a normal-appearing capnogram, the arterial blood gas should be analyzed. Should $PETCO_2$ fail reasonably to reflect $PaCO_2$, capnography can still provide useful trend data, but the clinician will now need to identify the reason for a larger than normal difference between $PETCO_2$ and $PaCO_2$.

The volume-based method provides a valuable opportunity to estimate the volume of carbon dioxide exhaled. Because no single breath equals the next, even with mechanical ventilation, several to many breaths need be sampled and averaged to arrive at a reasonable estimate. Volumetric capnography (plotting CO_2 concentration over expired volume) has been used for real-time calculations of anatomic and physiologic dead space ventilation. Since anatomic dead space generally does not change rapidly, alterations of physiologic dead space measured in real time can indicate changes in the alveolar dead space component. While the information obtained from volumetric capnography could be theoretically useful to titrate ventilator parameters, its use is currently not widespread.

Normally, we expect 200 to 250 mL/minute (about 2–3 mL/kg/minute) of carbon dioxide to be produced by a resting, healthy, normothermic adult of average weight. Assuming steady state (ignoring small losses through skin, feces, and urine), the volume exhaled would represent the volume produced. Diet can change the respiratory quotient (RQ = carbon dioxide production/oxygen consumption), usually assumed to be around 0.8.

What Are the Signs of an Abnormal Capnogram?

For a valid measurement of the tidal volume during mechanical ventilation, the exhaled rather than the inspired volume must be measured. Positive pressure during inspiration can cause gas to escape through a leak or around the endotracheal tube; such loss is less likely during passive expiration.

Equipment Related

Ventilator-related Failures or Gas Leaks

1. **Leaks:** With mechanical ventilation, leaks in the breathing circuit are likely to spill gas during inspiration when the pressure in the system is high, and thus can lead to hypoventilation despite a properly calculated (but not measured) minute ventilation.
2. **Inspired CO_2**
   In the absence of intentionally added carbon dioxide, three mechanisms can lead to the appearance of inspired carbon dioxide:
   a. **Exhausted carbon dioxide absorber:** With a circle system, as used in anesthesia, an exhausted carbon dioxide absorber will cause rebreathing.
   b. **Incompetent expiratory valve:** An incompetent expiratory valve will lead to rebreathing of the carbon dioxide deposited in the expiratory limb of the breathing circuit.
   The two conditions described above, however, can be distinguished by simply raising the fresh gas flow to exceed minute ventilation: That will prevent rebreathing owing to an exhausted carbon dioxide absorber, but will not prevent rebreathing through a defective (stuck in the open position) expiratory valve. Whether an exhausted carbon dioxide absorber or a defective valve causes rebreathing of carbon dioxide, the effect resembles the addition of dead space, which calls for an increase of minute ventilation lest carbon dioxide retention leads to rising $PACO_2$, $PaCO_2$, and $PETCO_2$ (Fig. 22.9).
   c. **Incompetent inspiratory valve:** Malfunction of the inspiratory valve generates a typical capnogram (Fig. 22.10).

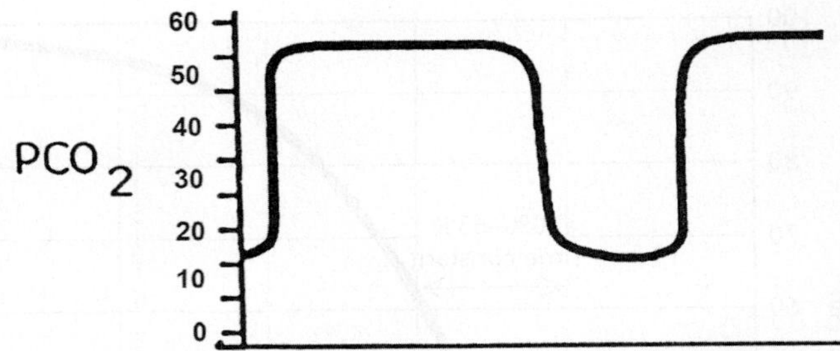

FIGURE 22.9. Incompetent expiratory valve leads to rebreathing of CO_2 in this time-based capnogram from a patient breathing from a circle system. Observe that the capnogram does not return to baseline during inspiration. Either an exhausted carbon dioxide absorber allows exhaled gas to return to the patient during inspiration or an expiratory valve stuck in the open position lets exhaled gas be admixed to the inspired gas during inspiration, indicating the presence of CO_2 in the inspired gas. High fresh gas flow can compensate for an exhausted carbon dioxide absorber but not for rebreathing through a faulty expiratory valve.

3. **Abnormal capnograms with normal production of carbon dioxide**

Hyperventilation:
Anxious people, and more often patients with central nervous system injuries, can hyperventilate to the point of inducing tetany; in healthy volunteers, a drop by 20 mm Hg $PETCO_2$ induced tingling and tetany manifested by increased axonal excitability, presumably owing to reduced ionized calcium (11).

In the clinical setting, patients with an acute increase of intracranial pressure can be treated with transient hyperventilation in order to decrease cerebral blood flow known to fall with decreased $PaCO_2$. The capnogram will first briefly show increased and then decreased $PETCO_2$, eventually leading to reduced carbon dioxide tissue stores. However, be careful when observing an abnormally low $PETCO_2$! Be sure that the low $PETCO_2$ is due to hyperventilation and not to other circumstances. For example, very low tidal volumes can show low $PETCO_2$ even though $PaCO_2$ is elevated. A mistaken diagnosis of hyperventilation and the decision to reduce minute ventilation would harm the patient.

Hypoventilation:
Three clinical circumstances can lead to hypoventilation: Drug- or disease-induced depression of the respiratory center, drug- or disease-induced muscle weakness, and airway obstruction. With the onset of hypoventilation, less carbon dioxide appears in the exhaled gas, carbon dioxide accumulates in the tissues, and venous PCO_2 rises. Eventually, the retained carbon dioxide levels reach a new equilibrium after renal compensation has reached its peak. There will be higher than normal levels of body stores of carbon dioxide, $PaCO_2$, $PACO_2$, and $PETCO_2$. Once a new steady state has been reached, and assuming unchanged metabolism, the amount of carbon dioxide exhaled per minute will be the same as before the perturbation; however, the end-expired

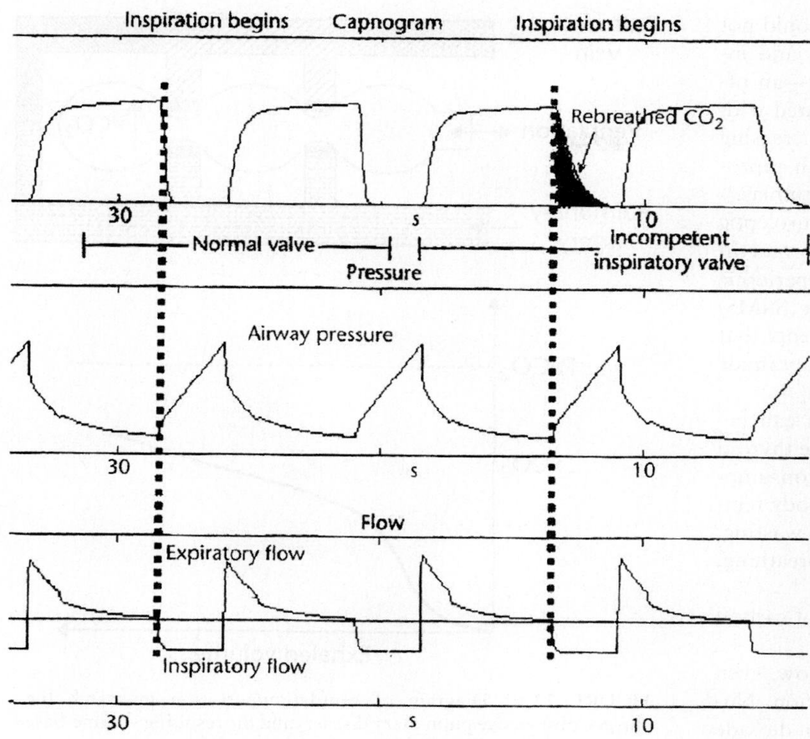

FIGURE 22.10. Illustration of the difference between normally functioning and incompetent inspiratory valves. Note that the CO_2 tracing in the normal capnogram rapidly drops to baseline at the start of inspiration (marked by increase in airway pressure **[center tracing]** and inspiratory flow **[bottom tracing]**). When the inspiratory valve is incompetent, exhaled CO_2 from the previous breath enters the inspiratory limb of the circle breathing system, and is rebreathed at the next breath. The presence of CO_2 in the inspiratory limb is evident from the widened capnogram (*shaded area*). (Generated with BreathSim software from Goldman JM, Ward DR, Daniel L. BreathSim, a mathematical model-based simulation of the anesthesia breathing circuit, may facilitate testing and evaluation of respiratory gas monitoring equipment. *Biomed Sci Instrum.* 1996;32:293–298.)

values will be elevated. Instituting hyperventilation at this point will bring end-tidal values back toward "normal," at which point continued hyperventilation will result in respiratory alkalosis. In patients with elevated $PETCO_2$ on mechanical ventilation, clinicians should resist the temptation to increase minute ventilation without first going through a differential diagnosis of an elevated $PETCO_2$ lest they delay the treatment of an underlying process.

4. **Abnormal capnograms with increased production of carbon dioxide**

Exogenous CO_2 production:

Bicarbonate infusion: Bicarbonate infused in the treatment of metabolic acidosis will dissociate under most clinical conditions (carbonic anhydrase being available) and liberate carbon dioxide, perhaps as much as 1 L/50 mmol (Fig. 22.11).

Carbon dioxide insufflation: Carbon dioxide insufflation during laparoscopic (etc.) procedures burdens the body with many extra liters (at times >40 L in adults) of carbon dioxide. Cardiac output and buffering capacity of blood will influence the rate of gas release. The blood carries much of the gas to the lungs, where increased ventilation is needed to maintain normal arterial gas values. Fortunately, after releasing the gas from the abdominal cavity, arterial blood gas values return toward normal over about an hour (12). Some surgeons like to flood the surgical field with carbon dioxide. In case of venous aspiration of gas, the aspirate would be the readily absorbed carbon dioxide rather than air containing close to 80% of poorly absorbed nitrogen (13).

Endogenous CO_2 production:

Shivering, as seen in patients with severe nervous system injuries or when emerging from anesthesia, can double the consumption of oxygen and thus the production of carbon dioxide. Fever triggered by the liberation of pyrogens from infectious agents, toxins, or inflammation is the most common cause of increased CO_2 production. Much rarer is malignant hyperthermia (MH), an autosomal dominant inherited disorder of skeletal muscle that sends carbon dioxide production into overdrive. In susceptible patients, halothane—and, to a lesser degree, other halogenated anesthetics—and succinylcholine can trigger the syndrome.

A rising $PETCO_2$ provides the first warning many minutes before increasing blood or body temperature can be detected. While the syndrome arises usually during anesthesia, it sometimes becomes manifest hours later. The syndrome

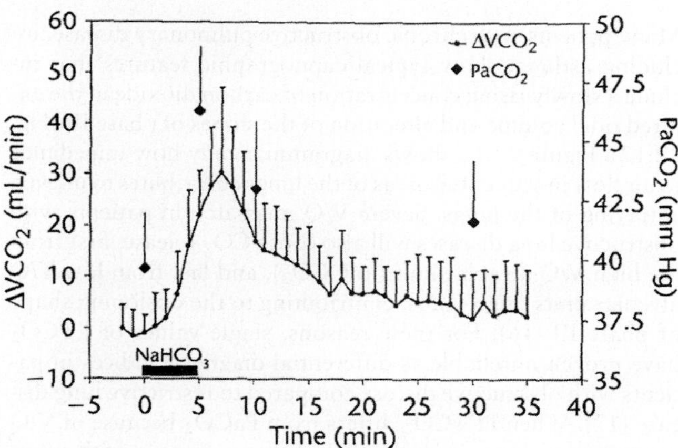

FIGURE 22.11. Time course of the changes in VCO_2 (ΔVCO_2) and $PaCO_2$ in 16 artificially ventilated critically ill patients during and after the infusion of 1/5 mmol/kg sodium bicarbonate over 5 minutes. (Reproduced with permission from Levraut J, Garcia P, Jiunti C, et al. The increase in CO_2 production induced by N_aHCO_3 is affected by blood albumin and hemoglobin concentrations. *Intens Care Med.* 2000;26:558.)

provides a telling example of why the clinician should not simply blame rising $PETCO_2$ on hypoventilation and increase minute ventilation without ruling out MH—an often fatal condition if not detected in time and treated with dantrolene. Of course, in the treatment of MH, increasing minute ventilation becomes necessary, together with appropriate treatment of fever, hyperkalemia, and arrhythmias.[1]

Rarely, the syndrome is triggered by neuroleptic drugs such as prochlorperazine (Compazine), promethazine (Phenergan), clozapine (Clozaril), and risperidone (Risperdal). This neuroleptic malignant syndrome (NMS) has also been associated with nonneuroleptic agents that block central dopamine pathways (e.g., metoclopramide [Reglan], amoxapine [Asendin], and lithium) (14).

High metabolic activity with hyperthyroidism can become symptomatic after infection or trauma to the thyroid gland. Tachycardia, markedly increased oxygen consumption and carbon dioxide production, and raised body temperature characterize the syndrome. When muscle wasting, particularly in elderly hyperthyroid men, affects breathing, capnography can be misleading.

5. **Abnormal capnograms with reduced production of carbon dioxide**
If production of carbon dioxide is abnormally low, even "normal" ventilation will represent hyperventilation. Numerous conditions can lead to a decrease of carbon dioxide production. Currently, the most common circumstance is iatrogenically decreased body temperature (e.g., as induced during cardiopulmonary bypass). Submersion in cold water, hypothyroidism, and several mitochondrial diseases can also decrease metabolism (15). Often the clinician will need to consider arterial blood gas values in order to correctly interpret normal and low $PETCO_2$.

CAPNOGRAPHY: CLINICAL APPLICATIONS

Obstructive Lung Diseases

Many patients with chronic obstructive pulmonary disease, including asthma, show typical capnographic features that include a slowly rising concentration of carbon dioxide in the expired tidal volume and alteration of the slopes of phase III (Fig. 22.12). Figure 22.12 shows diagrammatically how impedance to air flow in sequential areas of the lungs contributes to uneven emptying of the lungs. Severe V/Q mismatch in patients with obstructive lung diseases will also cause CO_2 release, first from the high V/Q alveolar unit (low CO_2), and last from low V/Q alveolar units (high CO_2), contributing to the upsloping shape of phase III (16). For these reasons, single values of $ETCO_2$ have proven unreliable as differential diagnosis indices in patients with obstructive disease compared to restrictive lung disease (17). When $PETCO_2$ differs from $PaCO_2$ because of V/Q mismatching, changes in the $PETCO_2$ may be seen with a corresponding increase, decrease, or no change in $PaCO_2$. In these cases, a direct measurement of dead space ventilation with volumetric capnography can be useful to predict the relationship between $PaCO_2$ and $PETCO_2$.

$ETCO_2$ during weaning from mechanical ventilation has been used with success to prevent dangerous, and frequently unrecognized, hypercapnia in patients with increased dead space ventilation (18). Unfortunately, in many cases, relevant hypercapnic episodes (increases of $ETCO_2$ of greater than 3 mm Hg) can only be detected with a sensitivity of 82% and a specificity of 76%, making arterial sampling during weaning a frequent necessity. Despite these limitations, capnography may substantially reduce the number of arterial blood gas analyses necessary during weaning from mechanical ventilations (19). One can describe the degree of flattening by reporting an α angle as shown in Figure 22.13.

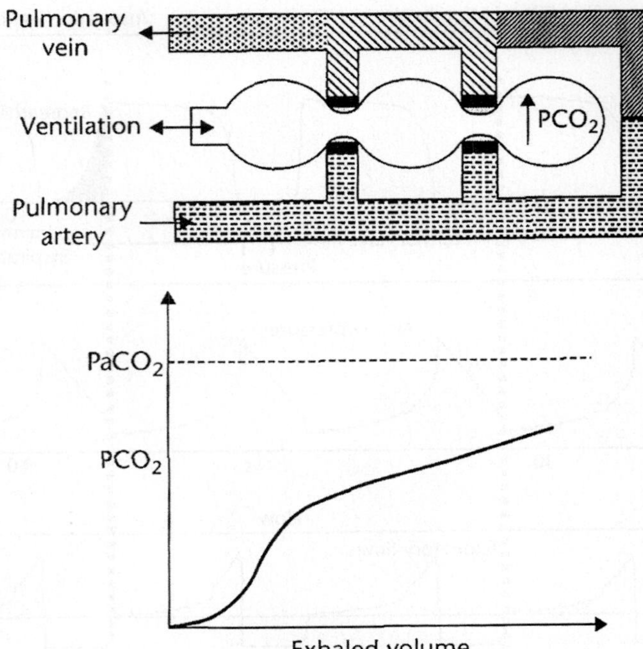

FIGURE 22.12. Diagram of ventilation/perfusion mismatch (i.e., chronic obstructive pulmonary disease) and the resulting volume-based capnogram. The diagram shows the narrowed air passages resulting in decreased ventilation of distal alveoli. (Reproduced with permission from Anderson JT. In Gravenstein JS, Jaffe MB, Paulus DA, eds. *Capnography, Clinical Aspects.* Cambridge, UK: Cambridge University Press; 2004:192.)

Ventilation/Perfusion Mismatch

In healthy individuals, the ventilation-to-perfusion ratio comes close to 1:1. Under the influence of gravity, the lower lungs are favored with perfusion over ventilation as compared to the upper lungs. Any pathologic condition that disturbs this balance can result in a mismatch. Under physiologic conditions, we expect the arterial CO_2 tension to be 3 to 5 mm Hg higher than the end-tidal CO_2 tension. In general, neither end-tidal nor arterial CO_2 can exceed venous PCO_2. A conspiracy of ventilation/perfusion inequalities can raise or decrease arterial to alveolar PCO_2 differences depending on the patient's disease, position, ventilatory pattern and pulmonary perfusion pressure, and flow. Acute respiratory distress syndrome (ARDS) is an example of severe V/Q scatter. Low lung compliance and an increase in resistance imply longer time constants and sequential CO_2 emptying, resulting in a steeper rising slope of phase III of a time-based capnogram. Such a ventilatory

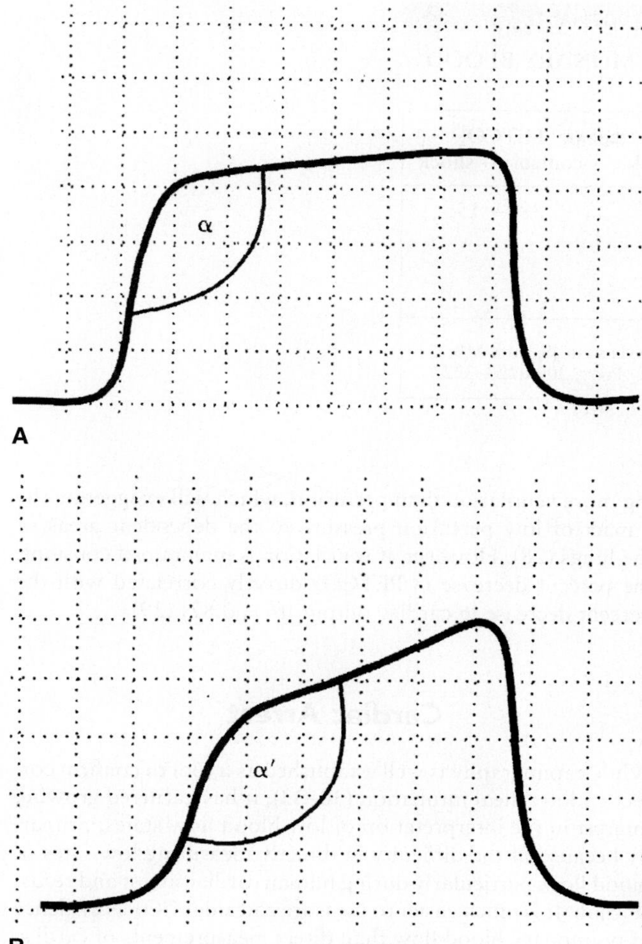

FIGURE 22.13. **A:** Normal capnogram showing α of 105 degrees. **B:** Capnogram during acute bronchospasm showing α' of 140 degrees.

disturbance in ARDS can be monitored with a real-time capnograph. However, when a significantly widened $PaCO_2$–$PETCO_2$ difference is observed, it is likely that coexisting significant dead space ventilation occurs. In these cases, direct measurement of dead space ventilation with volumetric capnography confirms the suspected diagnosis.

Recent reports in pediatric populations suggest that a dead space volume–to–tidal volume (V_D/V_T) ratio of 60% is a critical ratio for lack of reliability of $PETCO_2$ in patients with increased extravascular lung water (20). In this subset of patients with a particularly poor prognosis, a V_D/V_T ratio more than 65% identifies patients at risk for respiratory failure following extubation (20). This observation mirrors our personal experience in adult ARDS patients, whereas a V_D/V_T ratio more than 60% identifies patients with grave pulmonary dysfunction (21) and increased risk of death (22).

The $PaCO_2$–$PETCO_2$ difference in ARDS patients has recently found another interesting application. It has been theorized that the narrowing of this difference, while positive end-inspiratory pressure is applied, indicates the best possible recruitment of unstable alveoli without overdistension (23). In other words, calculating the V_D/V_T ratio in patients with a wide $PaCO_2$–$PETCO_2$ difference could be strategically useful to optimize positive end-expiratory pressure, thereby limiting promotion of excessive "West zone 1" in the lung.

Bronchial Intubation as an Example of a Shunt

With intubation of usually the right, mainstem bronchus, a classic example of a large shunt develops: One lung is perfused but not ventilated. About half of the cardiac output is shunted past the lung, and its desaturated blood is mixed with the saturated blood coming from the other lung. The mixing effect of the shunt is more pronounced for oxygen (46 mm Hg O_2 venous blood into 100 mm Hg pO_2 arterial blood) than for carbon dioxide (46 mm Hg CO_2 venous blood into 40 mm Hg PCO_2 arterial blood). The initial reduction of exhaled CO_2 results in a reduced $PETCO_2$ value until the system comes back into equilibrium. A partial and variable compensation for such a large shunt is caused by hypoxic pulmonary vasoconstriction, limiting the $PaCO_2$–$PETCO_2$ gap.

Pulmonary Embolism as an Example of Dead Space Ventilation

A typical example of dead space ventilation occurs when an embolus blocks perfusion such that lung tissue is ventilated but not perfused. Depending on the tidal volume of the nonperfused lung segment, the dead space being ventilated can substantially dilute the $PETCO_2$, leading to large differences between $PaCO_2$ and $PETCO_2$ (Fig. 22.14). In the same patient, the plateau of the CO_2 volume capnograph flattens

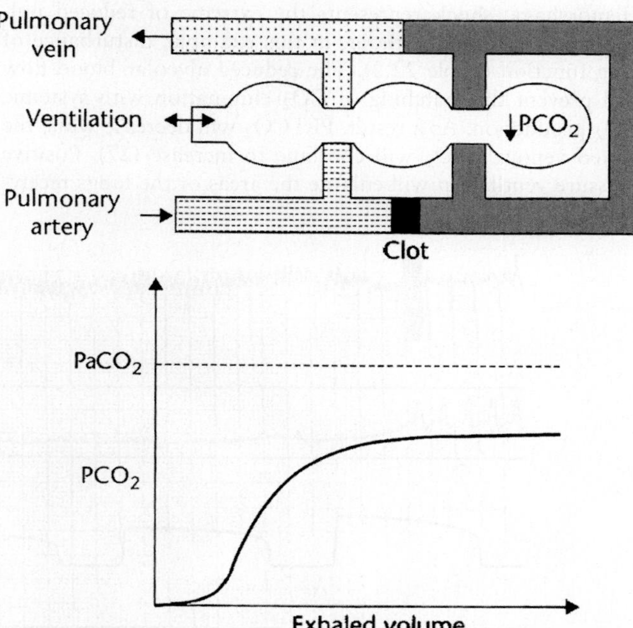

FIGURE 22.14. Diagram of ventilation/perfusion mismatch (i.e., chronic obstructive pulmonary disease) secondary to a clot (pulmonary embolus) on ventilated but not perfused alveoli and volume-based capnogram. (Reproduced with permission from Anderson JT. In Gravenstein JS, Jaffe MB, Paulus DA, eds. *Capnography, Clinical Aspects.* Cambridge, UK: Cambridge University Press; 2004:192.)

TABLE 22.2

THE EFFECT OF HEMORRHAGIC SHOCK AND REDUCED PULMONARY BLOOD FLOW ON THE ELIMINATION OF CARBON DIOXIDE

	Tissue control → shock	Venous control → shock	Arterial control → shock	$PETCO_2$ control → shock
$PETCO_2$				38 → 15
PCO_2	50 →	45 → 96	40 →	
PO_2	45 →	40 → 15	97 →	
SO_2	65 →	70 → 20	99 →	

Modified from Ward, KR. The basis for capnometric monitoring in shock. In: Gravenstein JS, Jaffe MB, Paulus DA. *Capnography, Clinical Aspects*. Cambridge, UK: Cambridge University Press; 2004:223–322.)

(24). If the patient's respiratory drive is intact, alveolar hypoxia and increased alveolar dead space will result in increased minute ventilation with resultant low end-tidal PCO_2 values.

With ablation of this compensation, as in a patient who is chemically paralyzed, heavily sedated, or anesthetized, the $PaCO_2$ always increases from baseline, and the (a-ET)PCO_2 gap widens (25). The pulmonary artery angiogram, spiral chest computerized tomography, and scintillation V/Q lung scan remain the gold standards for diagnosing pulmonary embolism. Unfortunately, while capnography has the advantage of being noninvasive and practical at the bedside, it lacks specificity (26).

Low Cardiac Output State

Hemorrhagic shock represents the extreme of reduced pulmonary blood flow without, in this example, disturbance of lung function (Table 22.2). The reduced alveolar blood flow will prevent the matching of CO_2 elimination with systemic CO_2 production. As a result, $PETCO_2$ will decrease while the mixed venous PCO_2 will continue to increase (27). Positive pressure ventilation will enlarge the areas of the lungs receiving more ventilation than perfusion, which will exaggerate the impact of low perfusion pressure to the dependent areas of the lungs (28). However, if ventilation is maintained constant, the percent decrease in $PETCO_2$ directly correlated with the percent decrease in cardiac output ($r^2 = 0.82$) (29).

Cardiac Arrest

While capnography is well established as a tool to confirm correct endotracheal intubation (30–33), it has garnered growing interest in the interpretation of low blood flow states, primarily because of the difficulty in directly measuring low rates of blood flow, particularly during human cardiac arrest and resuscitation. It is much easier to measure end-tidal CO_2 as evidence of pulmonary blood flow than direct measurements of cardiac output.

With sudden cardiac standstill, the capnogram shows quickly vanishing carbon dioxide levels in the exhaled gas. Thus, continued ventilation will wash the carbon dioxide out of the unperfused lungs. After three or four time constants, there will be very little carbon dioxide left in the unperfused lungs (Fig. 22.15).

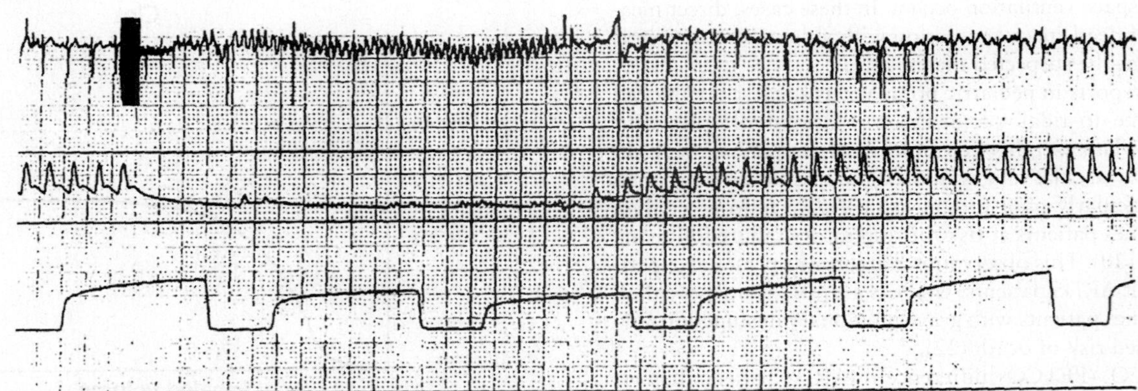

FIGURE 22.15. A patient undergoing the implantation of an automatic internal cardiac defibrillator was monitored with electrocardiogram (ECG; **top**), radial artery pressure (**middle**), and mainstream capnography (**bottom**). Induced ventricular fibrillation (*black area* in ECG) and defibrillation are apparent in the ECG tracing. Observe decay of arterial pressure. During absent pulmonary blood flow, the patient's lungs were ventilated and with two breaths the end-tidal PCO_2 fell from 35 mm Hg before fibrillation to 22 mm Hg.

Conversely, with re-establishment of circulation, the reappearance of carbon dioxide provides welcome evidence of pulmonary perfusion. During cardiac arrest, carbon dioxide will have accumulated in tissue and, because of acidosis development during shock and arrest, the addition of hydrogen ions will cause bicarbonate to be converted to carbon dioxide. A number of recent studies have shown that end-tidal CO_2 varies directly with cardiac output during cardiac arrest (34,35) and provides a useful indicator of the efficacy of resuscitation efforts. The relative effect of pharmacologic intervention during cardiopulmonary resuscitation (CPR) can also be assessed by the $ETCO_2$. For example, following the administration of epinephrine, the prior relationships of end-tidal CO_2 may be altered due to the changes in pulmonary and peripheral vascular resistance and preferential redirection of blood flow (36). In some instances, epinephrine may cause decreased pulmonary blood flow and end-tidal CO_2, while at the same time coronary perfusion pressure increases because of increased peripheral vascular resistance (37).

Investigators have used end-tidal CO_2 as a substitute for the measurement of blood flow in studies of CPR techniques (38,39). Because end-tidal CO_2 is directly related to cardiac output when minute ventilation is held constant, it is a useful tool for bedside real-time evaluation of effectiveness of chest compression. Unfortunately, if ventilation is not constant in any low state, including cardiac arrest, then end-tidal carbon dioxide levels are unreliable.

CAPNOGRAPHY STANDARDS IN THE INTENSIVE CARE UNIT

The American Association of Respiratory Care (AARC) strongly recommends the use of capnography in patients who are mechanically ventilated in the intensive care unit (ICU). However, when capnography is used as an indirect monitor of $PaCO_2$ in the critically ill patient, one has to consider limitations that can affect the accuracy of this technology, as listed below:

1. The composition of the respiratory gas mixture may affect the capnogram, such as the use of high O_2 concentrations in critically ill patients (40).
2. The breathing frequency may alter the slope of phase III and the $PETCO_2$ measured value (41).
3. The presence of Freon, used as a propellant in metered-dose inhalers, can cause an artificial increase of the $PETCO_2$ reading (42).
4. Contamination of the monitor or sampling system by secretions or condensate, a sample tube of excessive length, a sampling rate that is too high, or obstruction of the sampling chamber can lead to unreliable results.
5. Use of filters can lead to falsely low $PETCO_2$ readings (43).
6. Small tidal volume delivery, especially in neonates and pediatric patients, with low continuous flow rates that leak into the ventilator circuit, around the tracheal tube cuffs, or as a result of uncuffed tubes can result in a factitiously low $PETCO_2$ value (44).
7. A low cardiac output state may result in an artificially low $PETCO_2$ value.
8. In the presence of a carbonated beverage in the stomach, one may see several breaths with a factitiously elevated $PETCO_2$ value (45).

REVERSAL OF THE $PaCO_2$–$PETCO_2$ DIFFERENCE

A $PETCO_2$ higher than $PaCO_2$ or "reversed gradient" has been occasionally observed in pregnant and obese patients (46,47). The mechanisms for the reversals remain to be elucidated. However, this phenomenon has been appreciated only when phase III has a steep slope or when a terminal "step-up knee" of the waveform is present. As seen in Figure 22.16, a host of circumstances can be associated with large arterial to

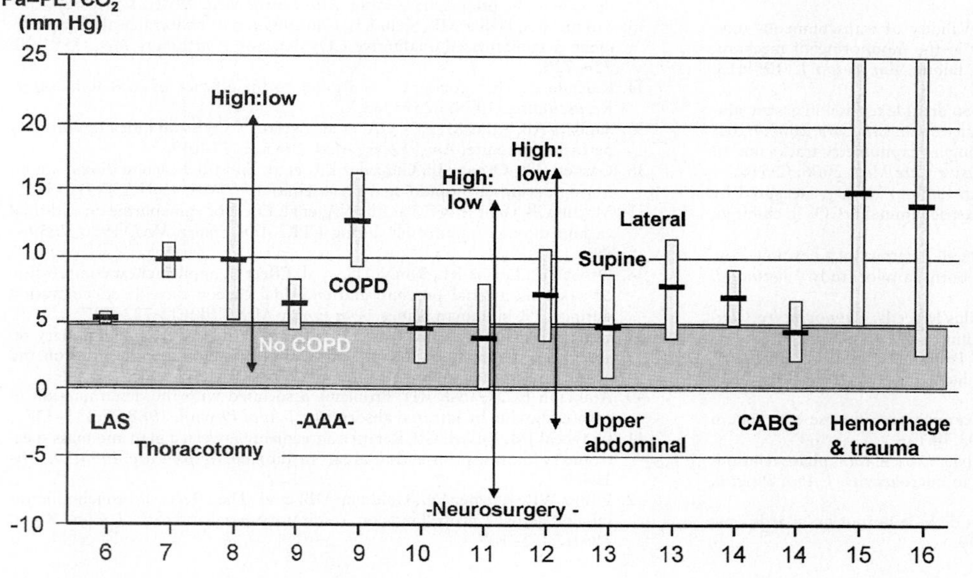

FIGURE 22.16. Intraoperative values of the arterial–end-tidal PCO_2 differences. The means ± standard deviation of the differences reported in 12 different articles are shown as vertical bars. The numbers on the horizontal axis are the references. The stippled area is the presumed "normal" value of 0 to 5 mm Hg. The surgical procedure is identified. Note that surgical position, major diseases, and unstable cardiovascular status increase the difference. Note also the reported high and low values (*arrows*). COPD, chronic obstructive pulmonary disease; LAS, lower abdominal surgery; AAA, abdominal aortic aneurysmectomy; CABG, coronary artery bypass grafting. (Reproduced with permission from Wahba RWM, Tessler MJ. Misleading end-tidal CO_2 tensions. Brief review. *Can J Anaesth.* 1996;43:862.)

alveolar PCO_2 differences, rarely attributable to a single mechanism (47).

CONFIRMATION OF BRAIN DEATH

The diagnosis of brain death must meet many conditions, one of which is the unresponsiveness of the brainstem to rising carbon dioxide tensions in the absence of drug effects. In 2006, the Stroke Service of the Massachusetts General Hospital (48) presented a detailed description of apnea testing. Key features include, but are not limited to, criteria for body temperature and blood pressures, and call for an arterial pH of 7.35 to 7.45, preoxygenation, and a $PaCO_2$ of 35 to 45 mm Hg for at least 20 minutes prior to discontinuation of mechanical ventilation. After discontinuation of ventilation, apnea is said to exist if $PaCO_2$ increases from 40 mm Hg up to 60 mm Hg, or a 20 mm Hg or greater increase from the pretest baseline. (See the original document for important details.)

SUMMARY

The attention of physiologists and physicians has been recently focused on time and volume capnography to monitor the dynamics of CO_2 in critically ill patients as the result of respiratory and/or cardiovascular derangement. Therefore, capnographic features need to be interpreted in view of the clinician's knowledge of either factors. Despite its limitations, capnography can provide significant and clinically useful information, and may often allow life-saving diagnostic and therapeutic alterations. As capnographic technology improves and clinical experience of the intensivist accumulates, we anticipate more widespread use of this monitoring modality in the future.

References

1. Jaffe MB. Brief history of time and volumetric capnography. In: Gravenstein JS, Jaffe MB, Paulus DA, eds. *Capnography, Clinical Aspects.* Cambridge, UK: Cambridge University Press; 2004:341–354.
2. Rosner V, Hannhart B, Chabot F, et al. Validity of transcutaneous oxygen/carbon dioxide pressure measurement in the monitoring of mechanical ventilation in stable chronic respiratory failure. *Eur Respir J.* 1999;13:1044.
3. Groeneveld ABJ. Tonometry of partial carbon dioxide tension in gastric mucosa: use of saline, buffer solutions, gastric juice or air. *Crit Care.* 2000;4:201.
4. Creteur J, De Backer D, Sakr Y, et al. Sublingual capnometry tracks microcirculatory changes in septic patients. *Intensive Care Med.* 2006;32:516.
5. Weiss M, Schmitz A, Salgo B, et al. Rectal luminal $PrCO_2$, measured by automated air tonometry, does not reflect gastric luminal $PrCO_2$ in children. *J Anesth.* 2006;20:243.
6. Hagerty JJ, Kleinman ME, Zurakowski D, et al. Accuracy of a new low-flow sidestream capnography technology in newborns: a pilot study. *J Perinatol.* 2002;22:219.
7. Jaffe MB. In: Gravenstein JS, Jaffe MB, Paulus DA, eds. *Capnography, Clinical Aspects.* Cambridge, UK: Cambridge University Press; 2004:413–421.
8. Fletcher R. In: Gravenstein JS, Jaffe MB, Paulus DA, eds. *Capnography, Clinical Aspects.* Cambridge, UK: Cambridge University Press; 2004:381–384.
9. Ball JA, Grounds RM. Calibration of three capnographs for use with helium and oxygen gas mixtures. *Anaesthesia.* 2003;58:156.
10. Lauzon A, Elliott AR, Paiva M, et al. Cardiogenic oscillation phase relationships during single-breath tests performed in microgravity. *J Appl Physiol.* 1998;84:661.
11. Kazama T, Ikeda K, Kato T, et al. Carbon dioxide output in laparoscopic cholecystectomy. *Br J Anaesth.* 1996;76:530.
12. O'Connor BR, Kussman BD, Park KW. Severe hypercarbia during cardiopulmonary bypass: a complication of CO_2 flooding of the surgical field. *Anesth Analg.* 1998;86:264.
13. Adnet P, Lestavel P, Krivosic-Horber R. Neuroleptic malignant syndrome. *Br J Anaesth.* 2000;85:129.
14. Macefield G, Burke D. Paresthesia and tetany induced by voluntary hyperventilation increased excitability of human cutaneous and motor axons. *Brain.* 1991;114:527.
15. Morey TE. Carbon dioxide production and anesthesia. In: Gravenstein JS, Jaffe M, Paulus DA, eds. *Clinical Capnography: Clinical Aspects. Carbon Dioxide Over Time and Volume.* Cambridge, UK: Cambridge University Press; 2004:257–268.
16. Strömberg NOT, Gustafsson PM. Ventilation inhomogeneity assessed by nitrogen washout and ventilation-perfusion mismatch by capnography in stable and induced airway obstruction. *Pediatr Pulmonol.* 2000;29:94–102.
17. Brown LH, Gough JE, Seim RH. Can quantitative capnometry differentiate between cardiac and obstructive causes of respiratory distress? *Chest.* 1998;113:323–326.
18. Saura P, Blanch L, Lucangelo U, et al. Use of capnography to detect hypercapnic episodes during weaning from mechanical ventilation. *Intensive Care Med.* 1996;22:374–381.
19. Niehoff J, DelGuercio C, LaMorte W, et al. Efficacy of pulse oximetry and capnometry in postoperative ventilatory weaning. *Crit Care Med.* 1988;16:701–705.
20. Hubble CL, Gentile MA, Tripp DS, et al. Deadspace to tidal volume ratio predicts successful extubation in infants and children. *Crit Care Med.* 2000;28:2034–2040.
21. Gabrielli A, Euliano N, Layon AJ, et al. Deadspace volume-to-tidal volume ratio for classifying pulmonary dysfunction in respiratory failure, abstracted. *Anesthesiology.* 2007;107:A1520.
22. Nuckton TJ, Alonso JA, Kallet RH, et al. Pulmonary dead-space fraction as a risk factor for death in the acute respiratory distress syndrome. *N Engl J Med.* 2002;346:1281–1286.
23. Murray IP, Modell JH, Gallagher TJ, et al. Titration of PEEP by the arterial minus end-tidal carbon dioxide gradient. *Chest.* 1984;85:100–104.
24. Schreiner MS, Leksell LG, Gobran SR, et al. Microemboli reduce phase III slopes of CO_2 and invert phase II slopes of infused SF6. *Respir Physiol.* 1993;91:137–154.
25. Nikodymova L, Daum S, Stiksa J, et al. Respiratory changes in thromboembolic disease. *Respiration.* 1968;25:51–66.
26. Patel MM, Rayburn DB, Browning JA, et al. Neural network analysis of the volumetric capnogram to detect pulmonary embolism. *Chest.* 1999;116:1325–1332.
27. Weil MH, Bisera J, Trevino RP, et al. Cardiac output and end-tidal carbon dioxide. *Crit Care Med.* 1985;13:907–909.
28. Ward KR. The basis for capnometric monitoring in shock. In: Gravenstein JS, Jaffe MB, Paulus DA. *Capnography, Clinical Aspects.* Cambridge, UK: Cambridge University Press; 2004:223–222.
29. Leigh MD, Jones JC, Motley HL. The expired carbon dioxide as a continuous guide of the pulmonary and circulatory systems during anesthesia and surgery. *J Thorac Cardiovasc Surg.* 1961;41:597–610.
30. Bhende MS, Thompson AE, Cook DR. Validity of a disposable end-tidal CO_2 detector in verifying endotracheal tube position in infants and children. *Ann Emerg Med.* 1990;19:483.
31. Mickelson KS, Sterner SP, Ruiz E. Exhaled PCO_2 as a predictor of endotracheal tube placement. *Ann Emerg Med.* 1986;15:657.
32. Ornato JP, Shipley JB, Racht EM, et al. Multicenter study of end-tidal carbon dioxide in the prehospital setting. *Ann Emerg Med.* 1992;21:518–523.
33. Vukmir RB, Heller MB, Stein KL. Confirmation of endotracheal tube placement: a miniaturized qualitative CO_2 detector. *Ann Emerg Med.* 1991;20:726–729.
34. Kalenda Z. The capnogram as a guide to the efficacy of cardiac massage. *Resuscitation.* 1978;6:259–263.
35. Sanders AB, Atlas M, Ewy GA, et al. Expired CO_2 as an index of coronary perfusion pressure. *Am J Emerg Med.* 1985;3:147–149.
36. Garnett AR, Ornato JP, Gonzalez ER, et al. End-tidal carbon dioxide monitoring during cardiopulmonary resuscitation. *JAMA.* 1987;257:512–515.
37. Martin GB, Gentile NT, Paradis NA, et al. Effect of epinephrine on end-tidal carbon dioxide monitoring during CPR. *Ann Emerg Med.* 1990;19:396–398.
38. Ornato JP, Levine RL, Young DS, et al. Effect of applied chest compression on systemic arterial pressure and end-tidal carbon dioxide concentration during CPR in human beings. *Ann Emerg Med.* 1989;18:732–737.
39. Ornato JP, Gonzalez ER, Garnett AR, et al. Effect of cardiopulmonary resuscitation compression rate on end-tidal carbon dioxide concentration and arterial pressure in man. *Crit Care Med.* 1988;16:241–245.
40. Ammann EC, Galvin RD. Problems associated with the determination of carbon dioxide by infrared absorption. *J Appl Physiol.* 1968;25:333–335.
41. Graybeal JM, Russell GB. Relative agreement between a man and mass spectrometry for measuring end-tidal carbon dioxide. *Respir Care.* 1994;39:190–194.
42. Elliott WR, Raemer DB, Goldman DB, et al. The effects of bronchodilator-inhaler aerosol propellants on respiratory gas monitors. *J Clin Monit.* 1991;7:175–180.

43. Hardman JG, Curran J, Maharan RP. End-tidal carbon dioxide measurement and breathing system filters. *Anaesthesia.* 1997;52:646–648.
44. Branson RD. The measurement of energy expenditure: instrumentation, practical considerations, and clinical application. *Respir Care.* 1990;35:640–656.
45. Li J. Capnography alone is imperfect for endotracheal tube placement confirmation during emergency intubation. *J Emerg Med.* 2001;20:223–229.
46. Shankar KB, Moseley H, Kumar Y, et al. Arterial to end tidal carbon dioxide tension difference during caesarean section anaesthesia. *Anaesthesia.* 1986;41:698.
47. Wahba RWM, Tessler MJ. Misleading end-tidal CO_2 tensions. Brief review. *Can J Anaesth.* 1996;43:862.
48. Stroke Service of the Massachusetts General Hospital. http://www.massgeneral.org/stopstroke/protocolBrainDeath.asp. Accessed.

CHAPTER 23 ■ ECHOCARDIOGRAPHY

DAVID T. POREMBKA

Echocardiography is a vital diagnostic modality for the intensivist. Numerous investigations using transesophageal echocardiography (TEE), yet not all-inclusive in the intensive care setting ($n = 2{,}738$), have shown its merit. The diagnostic capability varies (43%–99%), but most vital and interactive information obtained with beneficial results typically approaches 75%. As a result of TEE, the therapeutic implications for appropriate interventions (medical and surgical) are as high as 69%. Compared to the surface examination (transthoracic echocardiography, or TTE), TEE—because of improved imaging windows—essentially doubles the benefits of the aforementioned data (1–22). Furthermore, echocardiography lessens the potential for physician misdiagnosis and misadventures. Because this mode is useful in indicating the most appropriate medical/surgical interventions, outcomes can be potentially improved (1–22).

Significant cognitive skills and knowledge are required when using surface or esophageal echocardiography (23–25). Echocardiography is an extension of the physical examination and data obtained from the use of invasive monitoring, and encompasses handheld or portable echocardiography (TTE), TEE, three-dimensional reconstruction, stress echocardiography, contrast echocardiography, intravascular ultrasound (IVUS), and intracardiac echocardiography. Several guidelines and recommendations are available in the medical literature (11,23,24,26).

Although controversy on the appropriate level of training between our cardiology experts and intensivists still exists, a selective "training curriculum" is now being provided in selected subspecialties such as Emergency Medicine (27–29). In a recent *Critical Care Medicine* supplement, a suggested limited curriculum for intensivists was presented in detail for consideration (30,31) (Tables 23.1–23.4). Despite the current trend to allow the intensivist to independently interpret basic echocardiography features, the importance of consulting with an expert in TEE for difficult cases cannot be overemphasized. By doing so, a bilateral dynamic exchange in learning, teaching, research, and clinical care can only improve and lead to better outcomes and a probable decrease in overall cost to health care and to the patient. Intensive care physicians should totally embrace echocardiography as an integral complement in the care of the critically ill and injured patient (32,33).

This chapter will review the benefits and the efficacy of echocardiography (TTE, TEE) in the critical care setting.

INDICATIONS AND CONTRAINDICATIONS

Indications

The indications are straightforward but will vary with the type of intensive care setting (cardiac, cardiothoracic, surgery, trauma, or medical), the individual's expertise (fellow, resident, vs. faculty), and the institution's commitment to providing resources on a 24/7 service to assist in the diagnosis of these critically ill and injured patients (Table 23.3). Timely and accurate diagnoses are crucial in numerous situations (e.g., penetrating or blunt trauma-related cardiac structural damage or the presence of cardiac tamponade, aortic dissection/aneurysm or traumatic injury, or shock not responding to conventional treatment). The typical indications for echocardiography include but are not limited to the following:

- Ventricular performance and/or hemodynamic instability (ventricular failure, systolic and/or diastolic failure)
- Hypovolemia
- Pericardial diseases including cardiac tamponade
- Pulmonary embolism
- Complications following myocardial injury
- Complications following cardiothoracic surgery
- Aortic pathology
- Acute valvular dysfunction
- Infective endocarditis (IE) and associated complications
- Unexplained hypoxemia (intracardiac right-to-left shunts)

The benefit of TEE compared to the surface examination includes these prime indications and others because of better imaging quality to assess aortic pathology, cardiac valve endocarditis, and the presence of thrombi in the atrial appendage. TEE is also used as a guide in patients with atrial fibrillation undergoing electrical cardioversion. Another major benefit of imaging characteristics with TEE is that it allows visualization of a good cardiac acoustic window, even in

TABLE 23.1

GENERAL COGNITIVE AND TECHNICAL ECHOCARDIOGRAPHY KNOWLEDGE

Indications and applications of TTE in critically ill patients
Indications and contraindications to the use of TEE
Knowledge of appropriate alternative diagnostic modalities
Ultrasound physics
Principles of M-mode echocardiography
Principles of 2-dimensional echocardiography
Principles of Doppler echocardiography and the Doppler examination
Color-flow imaging
Imaging techniques
Standard transducer positions
Standard cardiac views
Imaging platforms
"Knobology" of various platforms
Image acquisition and storage
Recognizing normal anatomy visualized by TTE and TEE
Recognizing common structural abnormalities
Ability to communicate the result of the examination to the patient and other physicians, and produce a written report

TTE, transthoracic echocardiography; TEE, transesophageal echocardiography
Reproduced with permission from Mazraeshahi et al.[30]

patients with skin tapes, chest tubes, dressings, pneumothoraces, surgical wounds, severe obesity, and emphysema. A classic indication for TEE in the intensive care unit (ICU) is the acute evaluation of ventricular performance in conflicting clinical and pulmonary artery catheter (PAC) presentations. For example, the presence of hypovolemia can be demonstrated by the presence of turbulence in the left ventricular outflow tract (LVOT) via color flow Doppler, or by the appearance of systolic cavitary obliteration and inward movement of the distal anterior mitral valve leaflet that may cause obstruction. A fundamental use of TEE is the assessment of enlarged end-systolic and end-diastolic ventricular volumes in patients with normal or high cardiac output and stroke volume index. In a patient with shock, the clinician echocardiographer can determine with a quick look if there is inadequate ventricular systolic function or hypovolemia. Divergent therapies can be implemented immediately from the echocardiographic hemodynamic findings (31,34–41). Finally, the use of echocardiography, particularly TEE, in cardiac arrest situations and once an artificial airway is secured is a prime indication to assess various abnormalities during and after cardiopulmonary resuscitation (CPR) (34,35,42,43).

TABLE 23.2

PROCEDURAL COMPETENCY ASSESSMENT BASED ON SUCCESSFUL INTERROGATION OF CARDIAC PATHOLOGIC CONDITIONS

Mitral valvular disease	20
Aortic valvular disease	20
Ventricular performance, RWMA or ischemic heart disease, volume assessment, and/or ventricular interactions	30
Aortic dissection and aneurysms	10
Aortic debris	10
Aortic trauma	30
Pericardial disease and pericardial tamponade	10
Endocarditis and complications	20
Identification of right-heart failure and pulmonary embolism	10
Intracardiac and extracardiac masses	10
Normal examinations	10
Esophageal intubations	10
RWMA, regional wall motion abnormality	10

Reproduced with permission from Mazraeshahi et al.[30]

Contraindications

Contraindications for echocardiography in the surface mode are nil and are limited only by obtaining views sufficiently adequate so an accurate diagnosis can be secured. With any limited acoustic windows or in cases when the diagnosis is in question, one should proceed to TEE. A relative contraindication for TEE is any known or suspected esophageal or gastric pathology, including recent esophageal or gastric surgery, esophageal varices in patients with portal hypertension, and suspected or known cervical spine injury. An uncooperative patient whose airway is not artificially secured is a relative contraindication unless adequate topical anesthesia is provided, or sedation even to the point of total control of the patient's airway and general anesthesia (34–41). A penetrating esophageal injury, suspected or known by the mechanism of injury, remains an absolute contraindication to TEE.

EXAMINATION

The examination for surface echocardiography and TEE will be briefly presented. Adequate texts and atlases on this topic can be easily accessed. With recent improvements in echocardiographic technologies, and two-dimensional and color flow Doppler echocardiography, excellent views can be obtained. At present with the surface approach, one can obtain three- or four-dimensional imaging; in the near future, TEE will be a standard modality in all the platforms.

For the surface examination, there are four major positions or approaches to the heart on the thorax:

1. Parasternal position with long-axis (left ventricular [LV] in sagittal section, LV inflow, and right ventricular [RV] outflow) and short-axis views (LV apex, papillary muscles [midlevel], mitral valve [basal level], aortic valve/RV outflow, and pulmonary trunk bifurcation)
2. Apical position including the four-chamber view
3. Five-chamber or two-chamber views, suprasternal notch position; involving the long-axis aorta and short-axis pulmonary artery
4. Subcostal position interrogating the RV outflow, the RV and LV inflow, and the inferior vena cava and hepatic vein (31,34–41,43) (Figs. 23.1–23.15).

In the esophageal approach, the imaging obtained is markedly improved, allowing more extensive pathologies to be diagnosed and interrogated due to the ability of this approach to visualize the structures (cardiac and extracardiac) with better resolution (lower frequency) (Figs. 23.15 and 23.16).

TABLE 23.3

CLINICAL INDICATION FOR THE USE OF ECHOCARDIOGRAPHY IN THE ICU

HYPOTENSION/SHOCK
1. Assessment of LV systolic function
   i. Global assessment of LV function
   ii. Recognizing decreased LV function
   iii. Defining overall contractility and ejection fraction
2. Assessment of RV function
   i. Recognizing signs of RV failure, including decreased RV systolic function, dilated RV, and dilated IVC
3. Global assessment of volume status including
   i. Recognizing hyperdynamic small LV
   ii. Estimation of central venous pressure
   iii. Measurement of IVC size and respiratory variation
4. Identification of pericardial effusion and tamponade
   i. Understanding tamponade physiology
   ii. Recognizing signs of tamponade, including diastolic collapse of the RV free wall and RA wall

HEMODYNAMIC ASSESSMENT
1. Measurement of cardiac output
   i. Understanding Doppler techniques for calibration of stroke volume
   ii. Calculation of ejection fraction
   iii. Calculation of stroke volume and cardiac output
2. Measurement of cardiac chambers size including
   i. LV size
   ii. RV size
   iii. LA size
   iv. RA size
3. Estimating intracardiac pressures including
   i. RA pressure
   ii. RV systolic pressure
   iii. LA pressure
4. Evaluation of preload by
   i. Measurement of LV and RV end-diastolic area and volume
   ii. Measurement of IVC size and respiratory variation
   iii. Estimation of central venous pressure
5. Understanding echocardiographic signs of diastolic dysfunction
6. Global assessment of valvular function and integrity with Doppler

MYOCARDIAL INFARCTION COMPLICATIONS
1. Recognizing regional wall motion abnormalities
2. Recognizing rupture of free wall and septum
3. Recognizing acute mitral regurgitation
4. Identifying LV thrombus
5. Identifying pericardial effusion/tamponade
6. Recognizing echocardiographic signs of RV infarct

POSTOPERATIVE (CARDIOTHORACIC SURGERY) COMPLICATIONS
1. Identifying LV and RV dysfunction
2. Identifying acute valvular dysfunction
3. Recognizing prosthetic valve dysfunction
4. Identifying pericardial effusion and tamponade

RV DYSFUNCTION AND PULMONARY HYPERTENSION
1. Identifying echocardiographic signs of RV failure, RV dilation, and acute cor pulmonale
2. Measurement of central venous, RA, and RV systolic pressure

VALVULAR DYSFUNCTION
1. Understanding the role of Doppler echocardiography in valvular dysfunction
2. Recognizing echocardiographic signs of aortic stenosis
3. Recognizing echocardiographic signs of aortic regurgitation
4. Recognizing echocardiographic signs of mitral regurgitation
5. Recognizing echocardiographic signs of tricuspid regurgitation

PERICARDIAL DISEASES
1. Identifying the presence of pericardial effusion and its location
2. Identifying echocardiographic signs of tamponade

ENDOCARDITIS
1. Identifying valvular vegetation or oscillating intracardiac mass
2. Recognizing valvular regurgitation
3. Recognizing prosthetic-valve dysfunction

DISEASES OF AORTA
1. Understanding the role of echocardiography in diagnosis of aortic dissection and aortic aneurysm
2. Measurement of aortic diameter in ascending aortic arch and abdominal aorta

INTRACARDIAC SHUNTS
1. Understanding the role of contrast echocardiography with the use of agitated saline for finding intracardiac shunts

LV, left ventricle; RV, right ventricle; IVC, inferior vena cava; RA, right atrium; LA, left atrium.
Reproduced with permission from Mazraeshahi et al.[30]

VENTRICULAR PERFORMANCE (SYSTOLIC AND DIASTOLIC FUNCTION)

The incidence and prevalence of systolic (SHF) and diastolic heart failure (DHF) is considerable, and is rising, probably due to the increasing aging population. Consequently, much experience with this group has been gained and has led to a better understanding of caring for these marginal patients (44–47). The reported incidences for SHF in the ICU are 61% to 68% and for DHF 16% to 39%. Overall, when a patient is described with a syndrome of heart failure, echocardiographic investigations reveal the presence of DHF to vary from 40% to 71% (47).

Systolic Function

Determination of systolic function in ICU patients is constantly debated among clinicians, even when echocardiography is not

TABLE 23.4

SUMMARY OF ACC/AHA RECOMMENDATIONS FOR PHYSICIANS IN ECHOCARDIOGRAPHY

Level of expertise	Duration (mo)	Number of studies performed	Cumulative number of studies interpreted	Annual studies to maintain competence
1	3	75	150	
2	6	150	300	300
3	12	300	750	500
Stress echo		100		100
TEE		50		25–50

TEE, transesophageal echocardiography.
Reproduced from Otto CM. *Textbook of Clinical Echocardiography.* 3rd ed. Philadelphia, PA: WB Saunders; 2004, with permission.

used at the bedside. Echocardiography remains an extension of the clinical examination and the patients' clinical signs and symptoms, but the use of portable handheld echocardiography as part of the physician's armamentarium should be encouraged. The comparison of echocardiography to the pulmonary catheter (PAC) is still significantly controversial; PAC has not been validated in prospective peer-reviewed investigations, and thus should not be considered the gold standard. In concert, when one refers to a patient's ejection fraction (EF) while obtaining an echocardiographic examination, clinical decisions are limited, and intuitive assumptions and interventions are still being entertained (48). This latter LV function parameter (EF) is load dependent (as well as fractional shortening, systolic time tissue velocity of the mitral annulus, and regional wall motional analysis) and often used as an index of myocardial performance, far better in accuracy than PAC-related parameters such as stroke volume, stroke volume index, and cardiac index. Recently, the strain and strain rate via echocardiography has been gaining favor as a useful parameter to evaluate load independently from indices of cardiac performance (49). The physician's capability to construct and interpret pressure/volume loops for the determination of contractility is a controversial issue, particularly in the clinical setting of septic shock. How to intervene in the ventricular performance or optimization? What is preload? What are the goals of resuscitation and their end points (50–57)? These are all reasonable questions, and why echocardiography is not part of the standard of management of these critically ill patients is yet to be investigated.

Even though left ventricular ejection fraction (LVEF) is a limited myocardial performance index, it is a strong predictor of clinical outcome in most cardiac abnormalities (58–60). Of interest, EF is more reliable as a general predictor of mortality, second only to age, than when used to quantify the extent of coronary artery disease or degree of perfusion defects (61,62). Surface approach echocardiography by the use of the modified Simpson rule is superior to estimating either intracardiac volumes or LVEF (63,64). In fact, TEE in this situation underestimates volume by foreshortening the LV view with less incorporation of apex. Volumetric measurements should be objectively quantified:

$$LVEF = (LVEDV - LVESV)/LVEDV$$

where LVEDV refers to left ventricular end-diastolic volume and LVESV to left ventricular end-systolic volume. LVEF may also be calculated from LV dimensions measured with M-mode echocardiography at the midventricular level (65,66) (Figs. 23.17 and 23.18).

Other methods for approximating ventricular volumes are color kinesis and acoustic quantification (67,68) (Fig. 23.19).

Three-dimensional echocardiography is currently the best practice technique for estimating volumes and EF with greater accuracy by minimizing the inherent problems of not being able to always obtain orthogonal foreshortened, short-axis, and four-chamber views. Excellent comparative investigations with magnetic resonance imaging (MRI) and computed tomography (CT) with echocardiography reveal its accuracy as far as quantitative determinations (69,70).

The Doppler measure of systolic function is now a standard methodology in the interrogation of systolic function (71,72); acceleration (dV/dT) is easily measured by using

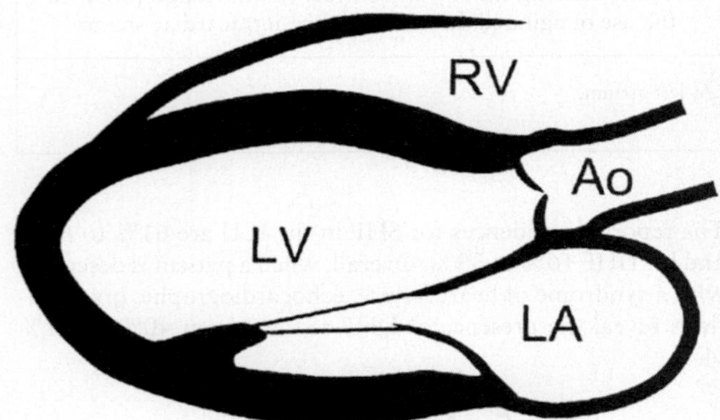

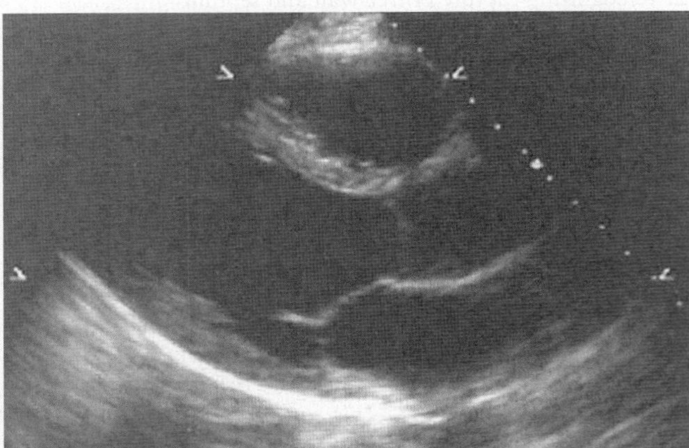

FIGURE 23.1. The parasternal long-axis view is shown. Ao, aorta; LA, left atrium; LV, left ventricle; RV, right ventricle. (From Feigenbaum H, Armstrong WF, Ryan T, eds. *Feigenbaum's Echocardiography.* 6th ed. Philadelphia, PA: Lippincott Williams & Wilkins; 2005, with permission.)

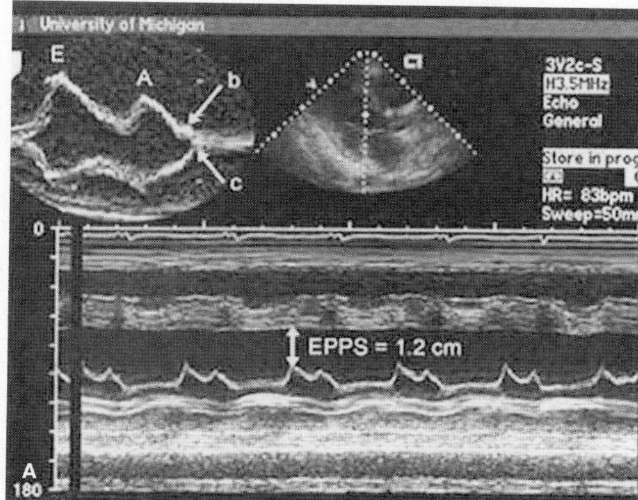

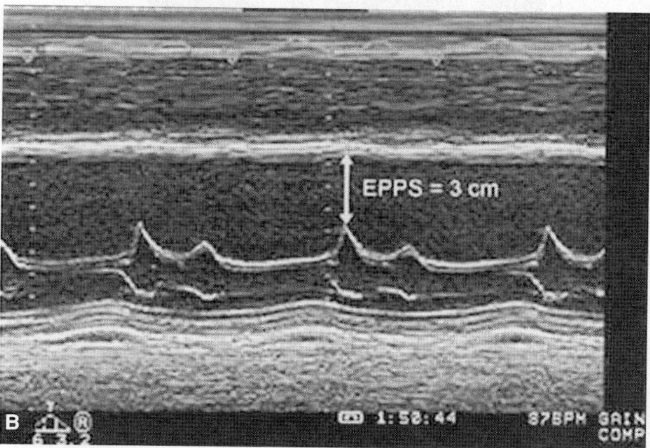

FIGURE 23.13. M-mode echocardiograms recorded in two patients with significant systolic dysfunction. **Top:** An E-point septal separation (EPSS) of 1.2 cm (normal M6 mm). **Bottom:** Recording in a patient with more significant left ventricular systolic dysfunction in which the EPSS is 3.0 cm. Also note the interrupted closure of the mitral valve with a B bump (**top**), indicating an increase in the left ventricular end-diastolic pressure. (From Feigenbaum H, Armstrong WF, Ryan T, eds. *Feigenbaum's Echocardiography.* 6th ed. Philadelphia, PA: Lippincott Williams & Wilkins; 2005, with permission.)

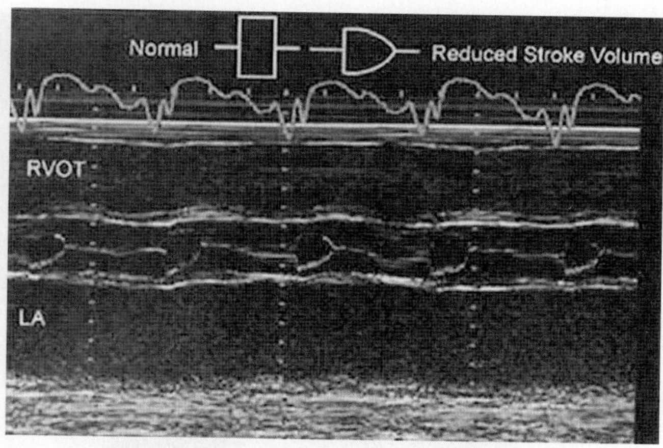

FIGURE 23.14. M-mode echocardiogram recorded through the aortic valve in a patient with reduced cardiac function and decreased forward stroke volume. Note the rounded closure of the aortic valve, indicating decreasing forward flow at the end of systole. Normal and abnormal aortic valve opening patterns are noted in a schematic superimposed on the figure. (From Feigenbaum H, Armstrong WF, Ryan T, eds. *Feigenbaum's Echocardiography.* 6th ed. Philadelphia, PA: Lippincott Williams & Wilkins; 2005, with permission.)

the clinical symptoms and hemodynamic presentations may appear similar, the primary function and myocardial structural derangements are quite distinctive. There are marked advancements for treatment of systolic heart failure, but treatment for diastolic failure is still empiric. Echocardiography can serially follow and evaluate the treatment management of these patients (112), and in so doing, prognostic indicators can be detected (129,143). Therefore, the use of echocardiography in the syndromes of heart failure is crucial for enhancement of patient care and outcome. Even in sepsis, bedside evaluation of the ventricular function with echocardiography is a proven imaging tool (144).

Left ventricular morphologic and functional characteristics in primary systolic and diastolic heart failure compared with controls and their follow-up changes are represented in tables 23.8 and 23.9.

PERICARDIAL DISEASE AND PERICARDIAL TAMPONADE

Echocardiography is an ideal technique to detect pericardial maladies such as pericardial effusions leading toward tamponade (acute vs. chronic), restrictive versus constrictive pericardial disease processes, and infiltrative processes, infective or not (congenital, neoplastic, metabolic, radiation induced, iatrogenic, and traumatic) (35,41,43).

Pericardial effusions can readily be identified by either the surface or esophageal approach. When the effusion is posterior and/or loculated (regional), the surface image may bypass its presence. Regional tamponade is not securely identified but may be juxtaposed to either ventricle and/or may involve the right atrium, vena cava, or pulmonary veins. The detection of a pericardial effusion ensures the diagnosis of a pericarditis. However, a patient with fibrinous acute pericarditis may often present with a normal echocardiogram. When fluid is detected, the clinician may proceed to drain it and determine if it is of an infectious cause (exudative), a complication of congestive heart failure (transudative), or traumatic in nature (hemorrhagic) (145).

In the syndrome of congestive heart failure (14%), myocardial infarction (15%), and valvular heart disease (21%), pericardial effusion is relatively common and may proceed to a tamponade syndrome (146,147). In cardiac surgical patients, the vast majority will have an effusion that presents usually on the second postoperative day and maximizes toward the tenth day (148). Fortunately, cardiac tamponade is unusual in these surgical patients, typically averaging 1% of the cases, with the exception of the cardiac transplanted patient in whom a higher frequency can result from repeated mediastinal procedures or rejection (149,150). Of interest, female gender, valvular intervention, and/or anticoagulants are predisposing factors (151).

An asymptomatic patient with chronic effusive pericarditis can present with a large effusion (152). Etiologic factors

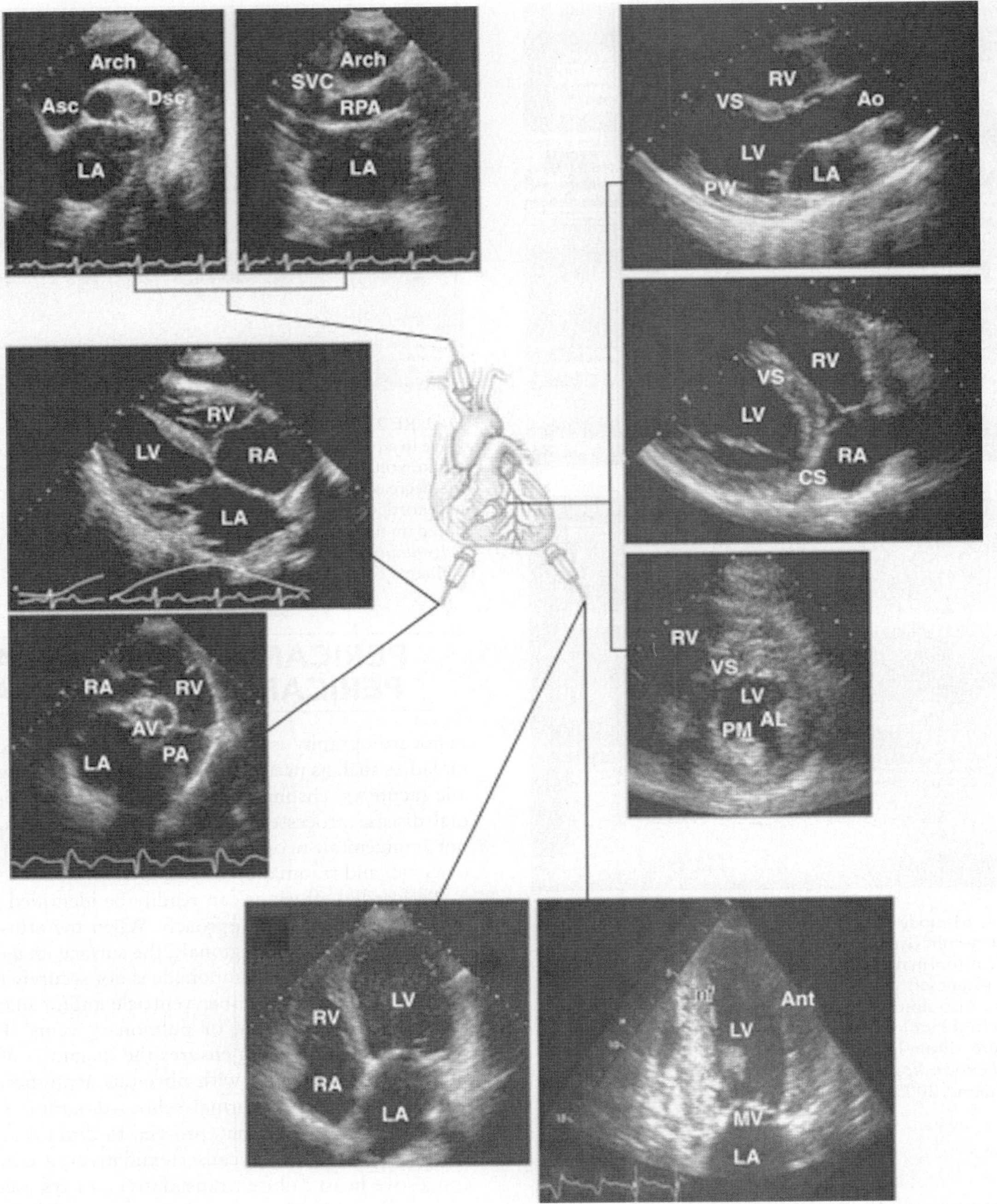

FIGURE 23.15. Diagram of cardiac structures from standard tomographic planes: parasternal long-axis view (*left*), parasternal short-axis view (*upper right*), and apical four-chamber view (*lower right*).

of this chronic process include uremia, neoplasm, tuberculosis (knobbed calcified pericardium), and connective tissue disorders (127,153). Typically, extensive effusion without any inflammatory disorders can be associated with a malignancy (127,152,154).

Echocardiography easily characterizes the relative contributions of cardiac enlargement or encroachment on the atrial/ventricular chambers and their ventricular and atrial performance, identifying underlying physiologic hemodynamic aberrations (35,41,43). Via M-mode echocardiography, one will see an echo-free space between the visceral and parietal pericardium dynamically throughout the cardiac cycle (Fig. 23.24).

If during systole there is a prominent separation, the fluid extent is deemed important. This modality is quite sensitive, as is two-dimensional echocardiography, which can detect either small (less than 5 mm), moderate (5–10 mm), or large (greater than 10 mm) fluid amounts, as well as its global or regional involvement. As stated earlier, as the fluid volume increases, it will extend from the posterobasilar LV apically and then anteriorly, subsequently lateral and posterior to the LA (Fig. 23.25).

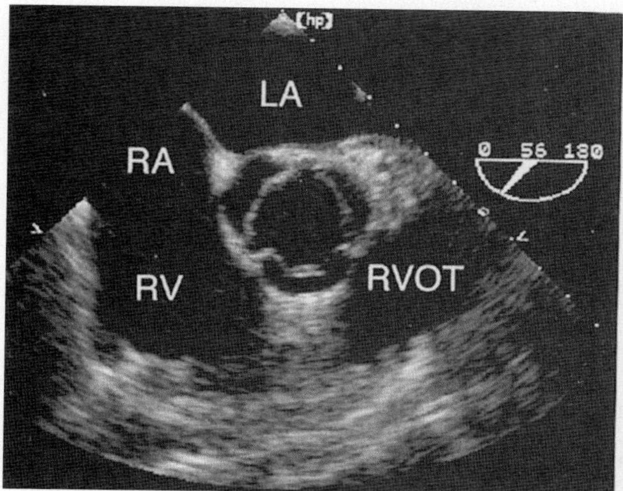

FIGURE 23.16. From the esophagus, the probe can be flexed to yield a basal short-axis projection. LA, left atrium; RA, right atrium; RV, right ventricle; RVOT, right ventricular outflow tract. (From Feigenbaum H, Armstrong WF, Ryan T, eds. *Feigenbaum's Echocardiography.* 6th ed. Philadelphia, PA: Lippincott Williams & Wilkins; 2005, with permission.)

Drainage is performed for diagnostic purposes (e.g., infectious pathogens, cancer) or therapeutic reasons (hemodynamic compromise or pericardial tamponade) (35,41,43,151,155, 156).

In regard to the end of this dynamic progression of fluid involvement, cardiac tamponade becomes a life-threatening event that must be correctly identified, diagnosed, and relieved in an expeditious fashion (157,158). Dynamic tamponade presentation depends on several physiologic considerations: the underlying ventricular performance; the rate of its development (increasing pericardial pressures in contrast to the intracardiac pressures with elevating venous pressures and decreasing to negative transmural pressures); the inherent intracardiac pressures, particularly of the ventricles; and the presenting intravascular volume or preload, especially in a hemorrhagic condition. If the patient has pre-existing right ventricular afterload and/or pulmonary artery hypertension, the echocardiographic findings will be delayed because of the abnormal RV loading conditions. Normally, the diastolic collapse of the RV—depicted as abnormal posterior motion of the anterior RV wall during diastole—indicates that the pericardial pressure is exceeding the early diastolic RV pressure. In other words, the RV diastolic transmural pressure is negative (159). In contrast, if the patient's underlying left ventricular systolic dysfunction is impaired, the echocardiographic characteristics of tamponade will present earlier in the hemodynamic "fluid" progression with smaller volumes (160).

The echocardiographic indicators of pericardial tamponade include the following:

- Decrease in end-systolic and end-diastolic dimensions
- Relative increase in RV dimensions during spontaneous ventilation (inspiration) as compared to an increase in LV dimension
- Right atrial diastolic collapse
- Left ventricular diastolic inversion
- Greater than 50% decrease in transmitral inflow
- Decrease in aortic flow velocities during inspiration.

A large pericardial effusion (greater than 10 mm) may reveal a "swinging" heart throughout the cardiac cycle. In contrast, flow across the tricuspid valve and pulmonary flow velocities (PVF) increase dramatically during inspiration, primarily in the systolic component of the PVF (161). Even though RV diastolic collapse is a sensitive indicator of tamponade, different loading conditions with varied ventricular performance will lower its specificity. Right atrial (RA) diastolic volume is an even more sensitive (100%) marker for tamponade but, again, its specificity is not the best (162).

Of note, if the duration of RA diastolic collapse exceeds one third of the cardiac cycle, the specificity increases (162). LA collapse is not usually detected (25%), but when it does exist, the specificity is markedly higher. LV diastolic collapse is much less common, probably due to the ventricular chamber properties (163–165). As in any dynamic hemodynamic setting, clinical conditions may vary, and pericardiocentesis is not necessary in every case of pericardial effusion. The absence of any chamber inversion has a high negative predictive value (92%), with the positive predictive value reaching 58%. Abnormal right-sided venous flows carry 82% and 88% positive and negative predictive values, respectively, for pericardial effusion (166).

If the pericardial fluid increases rapidly, the patient may initially have no prominent symptoms or may have only shortness of breath, with or without chest pain. Shortly thereafter, the patient will deteriorate to systolic hypotension, venous hypertension (distended jugular veins), and pulsus paradoxus. In the volume-depleted patient, these findings might not be initially present until rapid repletion of preload unmasks these characteristics (35,41,43,167).

Diastolic filling is also limited in constrictive pericarditis. Normal thickness of the pericardium does not preclude this diagnosis, which can be surgically confirmed in 28% of the cases of a negative series (168). The observed venous patterns of constrictive pericarditis from tamponade are characteristic. Because the ventricular chambers are fixed in volume by the pericardium, venous return is unimpeded during ejection, thereby ablating the normal venous surge during systole. Cardiac compression at end systole does not occur, so when the tricuspid valve opens the return of flow into the ventricle, it is of higher velocity, resulting in a biphasic venous return with a diastolic component faster than the systolic component (145). In contrast with tamponade, during inspiration in constrictive pericarditis, the decrease in intrathoracic pressure is not transmitted to the heart, and venous return does not fall (125,145,169). TEE measurement of the LV wall is markedly better than the surface approach (170,171).

The echocardiographic findings of this type of pericarditis include the flattening of the LV posterior wall, abnormal posterior septal motion in early diastole, rapid atrial filling, and the occasional premature opening of the pulmonic valve due to elevation of the RV pressure above the pulmonary artery pressure. Via the M-mode modality, there may be notching of the ventricular septum during early diastole or atrial systole secondary to a transient reversal of ventricular septal transmural pressure gradient (172). The above findings are not highly sensitive, yet a normal examination essentially excludes the diagnostic presence of constrictive pericarditis (173). Via two-dimensional echocardiography, the sonographer will detect dilation or lack of collapse of the hepatic veins and inferior vena cava, biatrial distention, and an abnormal contour between the LA and LV posterior walls. LV performance may be

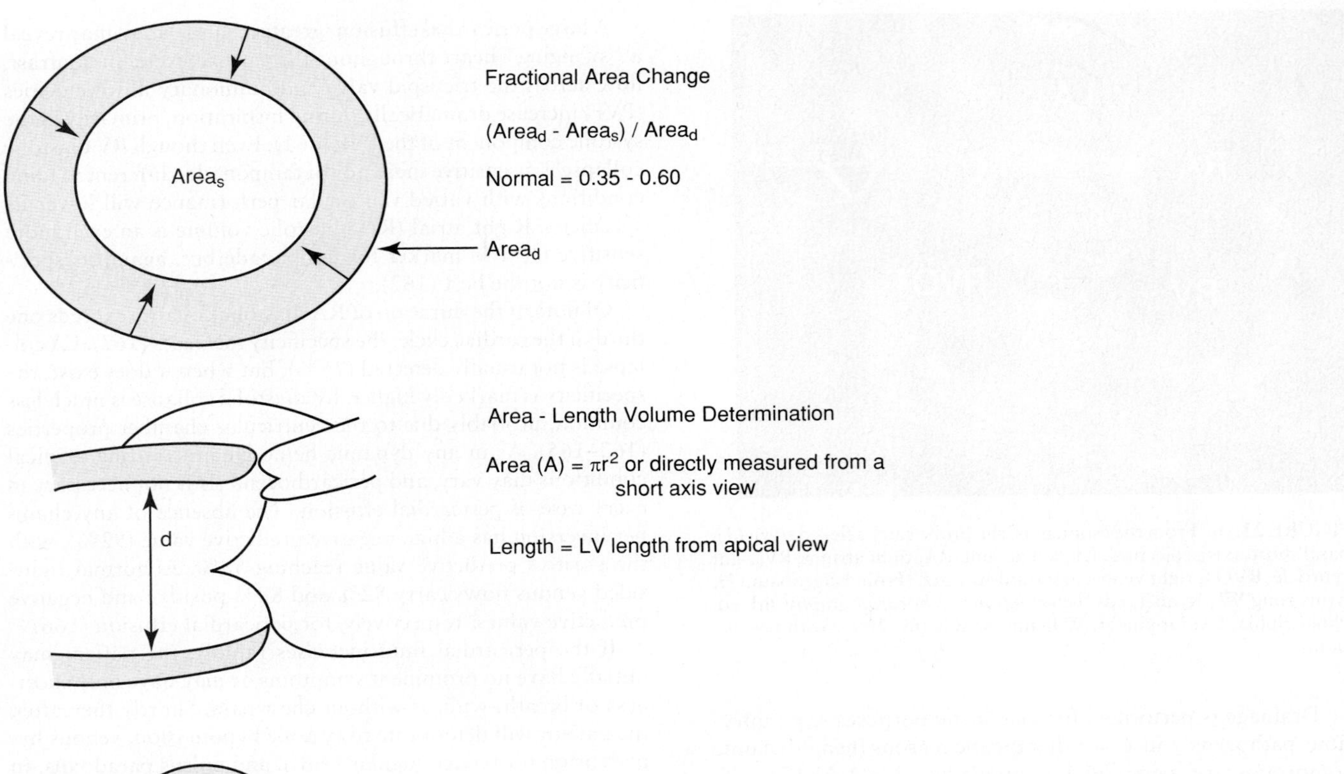

FIGURE 23.17. Schematic representation of two-dimensionally derived measurements of left ventricular systolic function. **Top:** The methodology for determining fractional area change, which is defined by the formula in the figure. **Middle** and **bottom:** Using the geometric assumption that the left ventricular cavity represents a cylinder and cone configuration, the volume of each separate component can be calculated as noted. The overall left ventricular volume equals the sum of the two volumes. See text for further details. (From Feigenbaum H, Armstrong WF, Ryan T, eds. *Feigenbaum's Echocardiography.* 6th ed. Philadelphia, PA: Lippincott Williams & Wilkins; 2005, with permission.)

preserved unless there is a mixed pattern of restrictive–constrictive physiology (174,175). By applying Doppler techniques, the E velocities and E/A ratios on LV and RV inflow increase (due to the abnormal rapid early diastolic filling-restrictive pattern). In constrictive pericarditis, there is a prominent early diastolic velocity Ea when interrogated by tissue Doppler. The linear response to LA pressure increases, and the ratio of E/Ea is inverted (176).

When evaluating propagation velocity with color M-mode Doppler, the early diastolic transmitral flow is greater than 45 cm/second (176). These findings are counterintuitive to restrictive pathology and filling with reduced Ea (less than 8 cm/second) (177,178). A classic characteristic of constrictive pericarditis is when the mitral inflow velocity decreases up to 40% while flow through the tricuspid valve is greatly enhanced in the first cardiac cycle after inspiration. In concert, the respiratory variation in PVF is markedly influenced (179,180). When there is coexisting elevated LA pressure, this exaggerated transmitral inflow velocity may not be apparent (179,181). Even though there is an increased velocity in the PVF, especially during expiration, the ratio of S/D is reduced even further by affecting the diastolic component (182). Figure 23.26 describes in detail the comparisons and dissimilarities in the restrictive and constrictive pathologies (145).

Penetrating cardiac injury should be briefly presented here considering that it is a unique pathology with life-threatening lesions that are not always obvious by routine clinical examination (183). If the patient arrives at a definitive tertiary care setting alive, immediate control of the hemorrhage should be attempted, at times with an immediate thoracotomy in the emergency department or in the operating room (184,185). A bloody effusion may be contained in the pericardial space

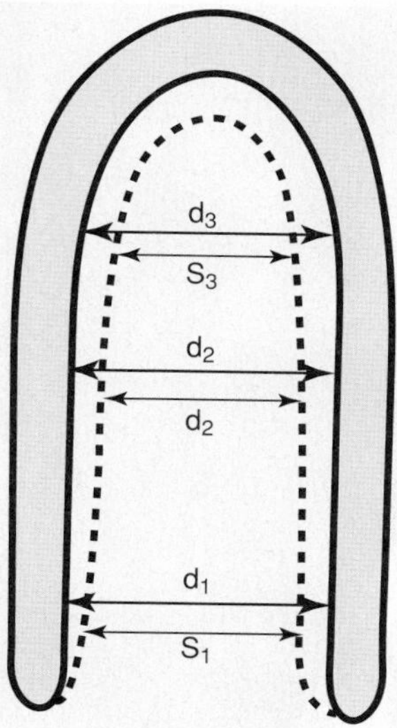

$$EF = K_{apex} + [(d_3^2 - S_3^2) + (d_2^2 - S_2^2) + (d_1^2 + S_1^2)]$$

$$K_{apex} = -5\%, 0, +5\%, +10\% \text{ or } +15\%$$

FIGURE 23.18. Schematic representation of a simplified method for determining the left ventricular ejection fraction from three separate minor-axis dimensions at the base, mid, and distal portion of the left ventricle in an apical view. The contribution of the apex is expressed as a constant (K_{apex}) ranging from −5% to +15%. (From Feigenbaum H, Armstrong WF, Ryan T, eds. *Feigenbaum's Echocardiography.* 6th ed. Philadelphia, PA: Lippincott Williams & Wilkins; 2005, with permission.)

(if there is a contiguous pathway to the thorax) or extend externally, followed by profound shock and rapid death by exsanguination. The lesions have multiple configurations, ranging from a ventricular mural wound to small, irregular, and multiple lesions. In obvious cases, surface echocardiography may identify pericardial tamponade and/or large lesions (ventricular septal defect [VSD]). Following resuscitation, the clinician should further investigate the clinical picture via TEE, since small lesions—yet significant and potentially fatal—may be missed, including VSD, defects through valve leaflets, intracardiac thrombi, or regional tamponade (186,187). One of the largest studies to date on this topic is by Degiannis et al. (188). In a 32-month period, 117 patients with penetrating injuries of the mediastinum were evaluated retrospectively. A 17% mortality by stabbing was observed, whereas victims with gunshot wounds (GSW) revealed an expected higher mortality of 81% (158). Another series revealed a 7% occult injury, with a similar mortality rate contrast between GSW and stab wounds (185). The clinician should always keep in mind that these patients are a complex challenge and that hemodynamic stability does not preclude an unexpected malady. Complacency should not occur (186,187).

ASSESSMENT OF MYOCARDIAL PERFORMANCE

In extrapolating the information reviewed in the sections of LV performance and pericardial disease, echocardiography is found to be an extremely useful diagnostic tool that can be used in a timely manner to delineate the cause of the shock state, whether hypovolemia, hyperdynamic derangements—type B metabolic lactic acidosis (sepsis, septic shock, liver failure, heavy metal poisoning)—and myocardial injury. An echocardiographic examination is easily performed, and the information obtained can avoid the placement of a PAC. The initial echocardiographic observation evaluates LV function and volume. In a hypovolemic condition, the ventricle exhibits systolic cavitary obliteration, with turbulence in the left ventricular outflow tract (LVOT) seen via color flow Doppler. In extreme hypovolemia, the distal anterior leaflet of the anterior mitral valve in systole will cause obstruction to flow (39,40,189). This condition is amplified if relative hypovolemic states and tachycardia are observed in patients with hypertrophic obstructive cardiomyopathy (HOCM) (40). Some of these echocardiographic indicators of a decreased preload state may be observed in patients who appear clinically normovolemic, regardless of baseline ventricular function (39,189).

Ventricular performance and ventricular interactions and loading conditions are quite complex in sepsis, SIRS (systemic inflammatory response syndrome), and septic shock (115,119–124). Echocardiography may clarify the effects of medical and/or pharmacologic interventions in these profoundly critically ill patients. However, often their physiologic effects are affected by the inherent (premorbid) chamber physical properties (pressure/volume characteristics) or fluid dynamics. A paradoxical response between survivors and nonsurvivors can be observed when a Frank-Starling curve is plotted against volume load in an animal model. The greater the end-systolic and end-diastolic volumes, the better the chance for survival (190). Furthermore, a paradoxical decrease in the slope of isovolumetric/pressure line (an index of contractility that is load independent) is associated with a decrease in cardiac compliance but increase in survival (191).

The effect of sepsis cardiomyopathy may result in a lower ejection fraction (which is load dependent) with high cardiac output, tachycardia, higher stroke volume, and elevated mixed venous saturation. As the patient deteriorates, hypotension occurs, impairment of cellular function follows, and the global ventricular volume response to resuscitation and fluid becomes ineffective (192–195). If there is no normalization of the above parameters within 48 to 72 hours, the chance for survival greatly diminishes. Persistent tachycardia is a marker of death (49). An apparent sympathovagal imbalance increases heart rate variability in the adult and pediatric patient populations. Atrial dysrhythmia and dysfunction is common in the clinical presentation and the progression of sepsis. TEE is obviously a valuable diagnostic tool for evaluating atrial function and volume by reviewing the left atrial appendage flow characteristics in concert with analysis of ventricular function and volume, ventricular interaction of dependency, transmitral inflow velocities, and pulmonary venous flow patterns (195,196).

In sepsis or SIRS, the right ventricle responds to fluid loading, but at some unknown end point, when the volume and pressure are exceedingly high, the compensatory response is no longer beneficial and mortality dramatically rises. A transitory increase of pulmonary artery pressure appears to be associated with increased mortality, but no serial investigations have been completed (197,198). In a clinical investigation by Poelaert et al. (22) based on transmitral inflow velocities and pulmonary venous flow patterns, patients with a decreased transmitral

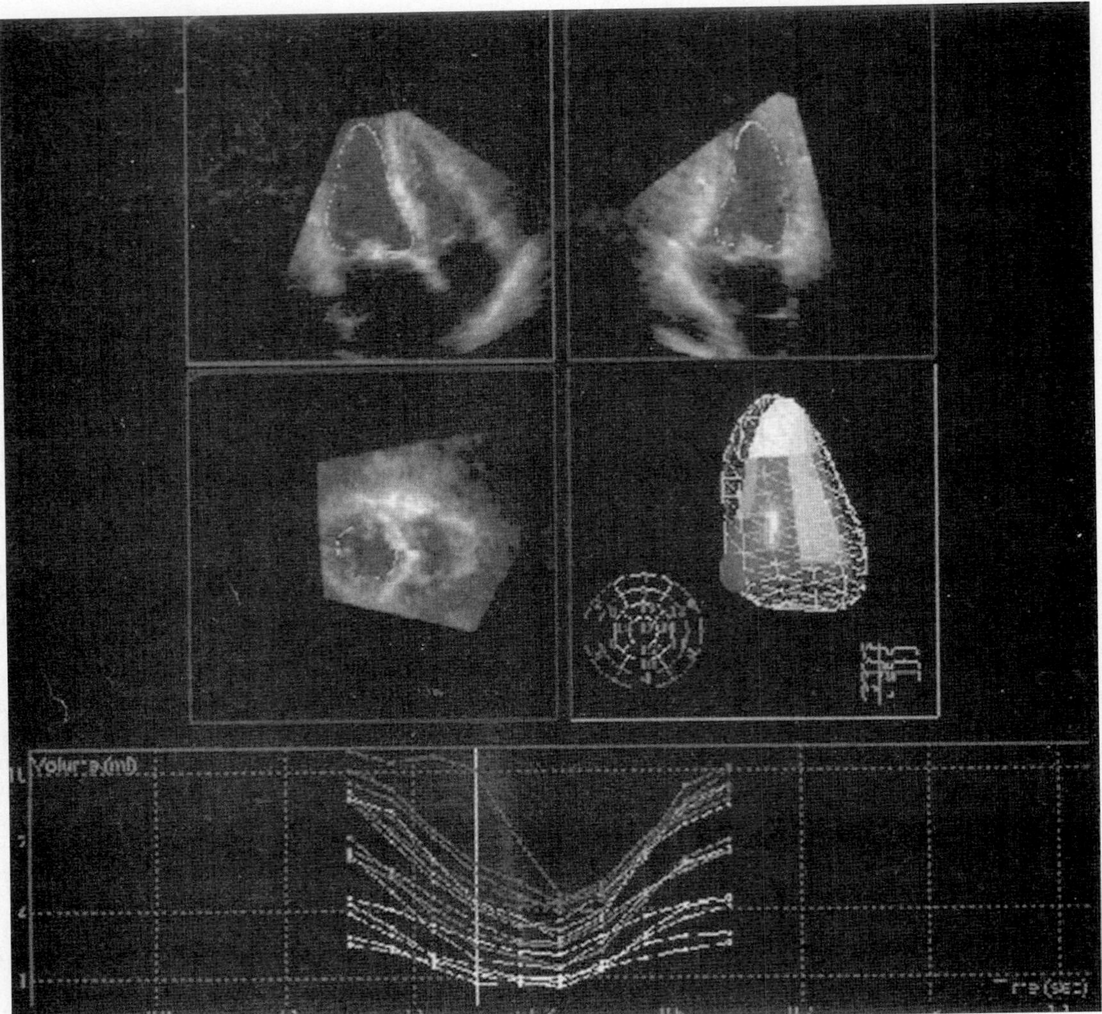

FIGURE 23.19. The left ventricular volume cast (lower right) was created from 3D echocardiography imaging. Regional left ventricular volume changes are shown in the plot at the bottom. The color of each line corresponds to the segment of the same color in the left ventricular cast. (From Oh JK, Seward JB, Tajik AJ. *The Echo Manual.* 3rd ed. Philadelphia, PA: Lippincott Williams & Wilkins; 2006. Used with permission of Mayo Foundation for Medical Education and Research.)

inflow velocity, abnormal pulmonary venous flow, and decrease in fractional area contraction are more likely to die as compared to two other subgroups. This pattern is particularly seen in older patients.

The hyperdynamic circulatory response of sepsis was earlier associated with a myocardial depressant factor (199) and presently is related to various mediators, cytokines, and humoral factors that are all related and intertwined (200). Interestingly, it is now known that there is a protective effect of early exposure to some of these mediators/cytokines that can induce the reversal of myocardial depression (192,194,201,202).

In summary, appreciating cardiac function in septic shock patients will assist in the determination of the pharmacologic interventions, fluid augmentation, and other modalities (203–205). It is intuitive reasoning that if the baseline cardiac junction is poor, the volume should be instilled judiciously and adjunct pharmacologic measures should be administered earlier and more aggressively. Echocardiography is a useful tool to initially identify and follow all hemodynamic variables. This diagnostic tool alone might suffice, but until further data are available, using it in conjunction with invasive monitoring is crucial (192,194,201,206).

PULMONARY EMBOLISM

One of the most catastrophic cardiovascular events that can occur that is either underdiagnosed or overdiagnosed is pulmonary embolism (PE) (207–212). A low cardiac output and RV failure post PE presages mortality. Early identification of these derangements may assist in managing these critically ill patients by providing prognostic indicators, stratification for more intensive surveillance, and any necessary interventions (213). Even appropriate anticoagulation may not eliminate a PE. Several diagnostic tests are available, including a 64-cut chest computed tomography, magnetic resonance imaging,

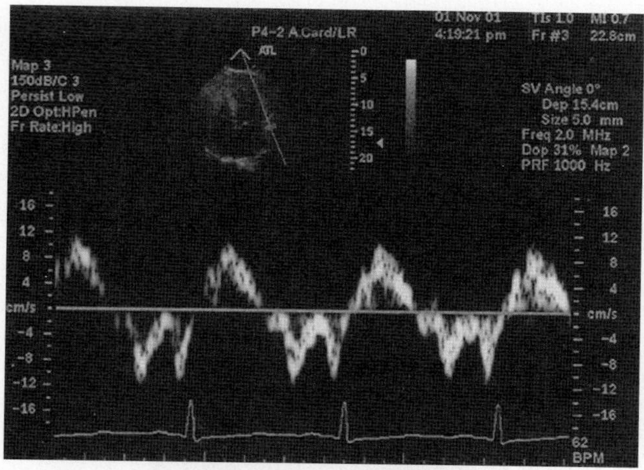

FIGURE 23.20. Normal spectral tissue Doppler. (From Dittoe N, Stulz D, Schwartz BP, et al. Quantitative left ventricular systolic function: from chamber to myocardium. *Crit Care Med.* 2007;35(8):S330, with permission.)

pulmonary angiography, and echocardiography (207) (Table 23.10).

The classic echocardiographic signs for a PE are the following:

- Dilation of the chamber and thinning of the right ventricle wall with global hypokinesis
- Pulmonic insufficiency
- Tricuspid insufficiency
- Right atrial dilatation with decreased atrial function
- Septal flattening or paradoxical motion of the ventricular septum
- Increased RV/LV dimensions
- Pulmonary artery hypertension
- Dilation of the pulmonary artery
- Identification of thrombi.

If the patient's RV function is normal until the event, these echocardiographic events would occur acutely, and catastrophic events would result when 75% of the pulmonary

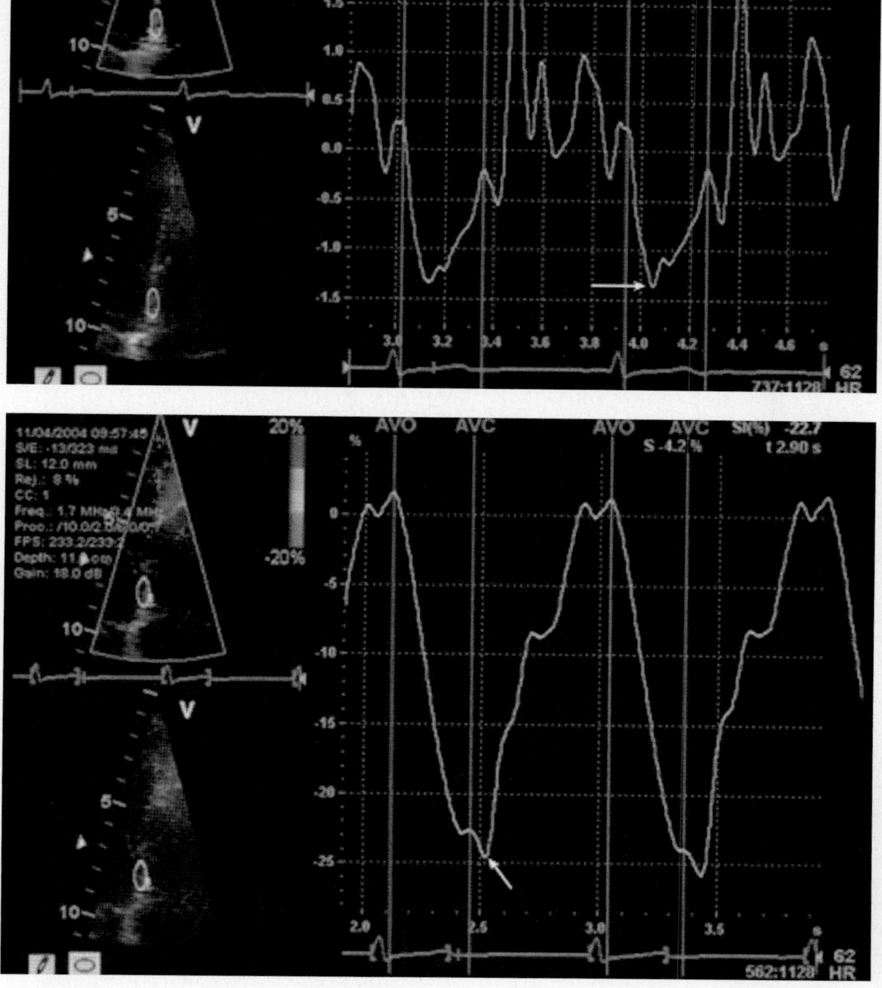

FIGURE 23.21. Recording of strain rate, which represents the rate of deformation; the peak negative strain rate (*arrow*) was −1.3/s. (From Oh JK, Seward JB, Tajik AJ. *The Echo Manual.* 3rd ed. Philadelphia, PA: Lippincott Williams & Wilkins; 2006. Used with permission of Mayo Foundation for Medical Education and Research.)

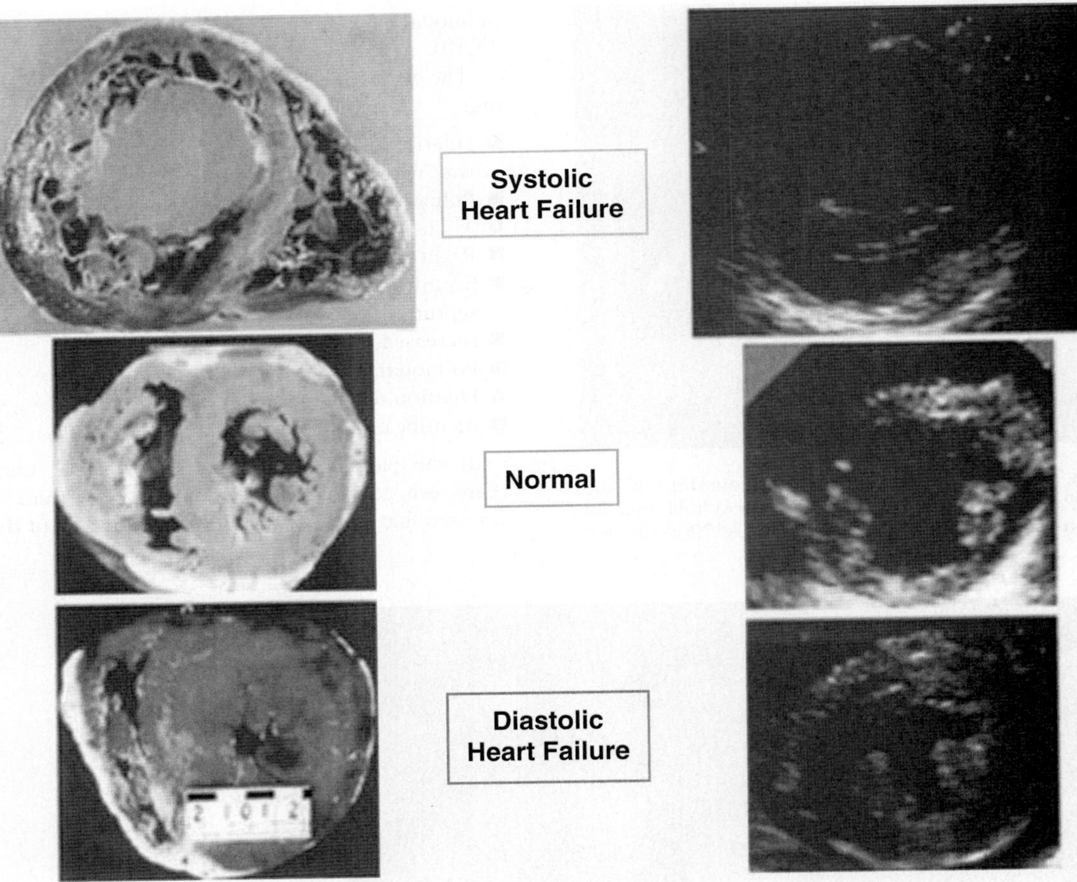

FIGURE 23.22. Ventricular remodeling in systolic and diastolic heart failure. **Left:** Autopsy examples. **Right:** Cross-sectional 2-dimensional echocardiographic views of systolic and diastolic heart failures compared with normals are illustrated. In systolic heart failure, the left ventricular cavity is markedly dilated and wall thickness is not increased. In diastolic heart failure, the cavity size is normal or decreased and wall thickness is markedly increased. (Reprinted from Konstam MA. Systolic and diastolic dysfunction in heart failure? Time for a new paradigm. *J Card Fail.* 2003;9:1–3, with permission.)

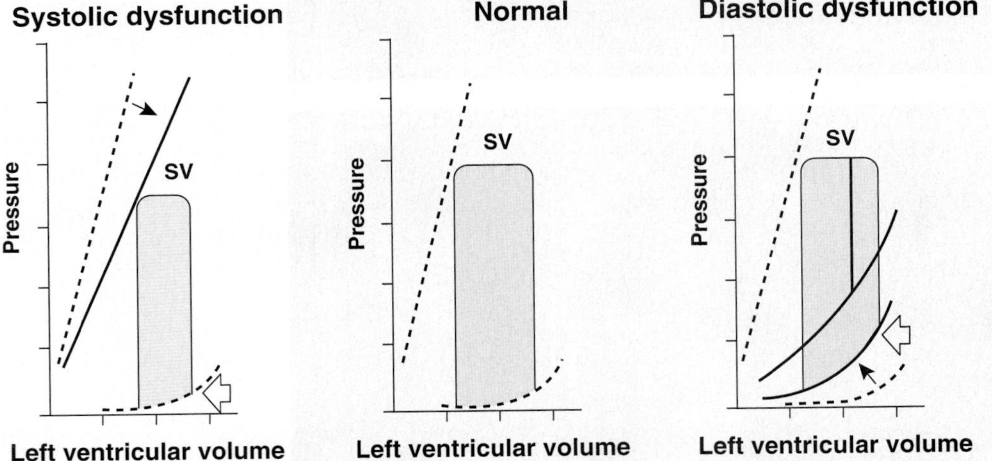

FIGURE 23.23. Schematic diagram of pressure–volume relations in normals, systolic and diastolic heart failure. In systolic heart failure, a downward and rightward shift of the end-systolic pressure–volume line indicates decreased contractile function, which is the principal cause of reduced ejection fraction and forward stroke volume (SV). In primary diastolic heart failure, diastolic pressure–volume relation (*dashed line*) shifts upward and to the left, indicating a disproportionate and a greater increase in diastolic pressures for any increase in diastolic volumes. If there is also a decrease in end-diastolic volume, then a decrease in stroke volume also occurs. (Reprinted from Aurigemma GP, Gassach WH. Diastolic heart failure. *N Engl J Med.* 2004;35:1097–1105, with permission.)

TABLE 23.5

FACTORS INFLUENCING THE LEFT VENTRICULAR END-DIASTOLIC PRESSURE–VOLUME RELATION (CHAMBER STIFFNESS)

Left ventricular physical properties
- Left ventricular chamber volume and mass
- Composition of the left ventricular wall
- Viscosity, stress relaxation, creep

Factors intrinsic to the left ventricle
- Myocardial relaxation
- Coronary turgor

Factors extrinsic to the left ventricle
- Pericardial restraint
- Atrial contraction
- Right ventricular interaction
- Pleural and mediastinal pressure

Reproduced from Hoit BD. Left ventricular diastolic function. *Crit Care Med.* 2007;35:5340–5347, with permission.

vasculatures are obstructed. Earlier signs may manifest with as little as a 25% obstruction of the pulmonary vasculature (214). According to the International Cooperative Pulmonary Embolism registry, the presence of RV hypokinesis is associated with increased mortality at 30 days even with a systolic systemic pressure greater than 90 mm Hg (215).

If the patient exhibits pre-existing chronic pulmonary artery hypertension with RV hypertrophy, thrombosis of the right-sided circulation may be initially better tolerated. Eventually, RV failure will ensue and dominate the cardiovascular presentation (211,216). Morris-Thurgood and Frenneaux (217) describe RV and RA pressures with reversal of the transseptal diastolic pressure gradient when intravascular volume replacement is attempted to enhance diastolic ventricular interaction. In the situations where other diagnostic tests may fail, echocardiography is a useful diagnostic tool to determine right ventricular afterload and associated hemodynamic findings significant for PE (207–211,215).

AORTIC PATHOLOGY: ATHEROSCLEROTIC DEBRIS, TRAUMA, ANEURYSM AND DISSECTION, SINUS OF VALSALVA ANEURYSM

Atherosclerotic Debris

Prior to the advent of enhanced diagnostic imaging techniques, clinicians routinely underappreciated the prevalence and importance of diseases affecting the aorta, particularly in patients following cardiac surgery and the general population in the critical care setting (218–229). Adverse events, such as a cryptogenic stroke, could previously not be explained until advancements were made for better resolution in head CT, MRI, carotid ultrasound with color flow and Doppler capabilities, and TEE (228). Cardiac-originating embolism accounts for 15% to 30% of ischemic strokes in the general population. In the SPARC (Stroke Prevention Assessment of Risk in a Community) study, the incidence of detecting a plaque greater than 4 mm in the aorta of 588 randomly chosen patients (average age 66.9 years) was 43.7% (230). Of these, 29.9% presented lesions either in the arch or ascending portions of the thoracic aorta. The presence of a protruding debris or plaque greater than 4 mm approached 7.6% in the ascending aorta and 2.4% both in the arch and ascending portion (220,221,231). In an earlier investigation, an atheromatous plaque greater than 4 mm was regarded as an independent risk factor for a central event (232). Because of the excellent acoustic window to the heart and thoracic aorta, TEE is considered to be one of the first diagnostic tools to evaluate the potential source for the embolic phenomenon (233–239). Although it remains insensitive to detecting smaller and irregular cardiac emboli and intraaortic debris (240), it is a far superior diagnostic tool than TTE (241,242). TEE can easily identify the cause for a cerebral infarction, especially in the ascending aorta and its arch (243). Even if patients' underlying rhythm is sinus, patients with atherosclerotic plaques are at risk for stroke (244–246).

TABLE 23.6

MORPHOLOGIC AND FUNCTIONAL CHANGES IN DIASTOLIC VS. SYSTOLIC HEART FAILURE

Parameters	Diastolic heart failure	Systolic heart failure
Left ventricular cavity, size	Normal or decreased	Increased
Left ventricular mass	Increased	Increased
Mass/cavity	Increased	Normal or decreased
Wall thickness	Increased	Decreased
End-diastolic stress	Increased	Increased
End-systolic stress	Normal	Increased
End-diastolic volume	Normal	Increased
End-systolic volume	Normal or decreased	Increased
Ejection fraction	Normal	Decreased
Mechanical dyssynchrony	May be present	May be pesent
Left ventricular shape and geometry	Usually remains unchanged	Spherical

Reproduced from Chatterjee K, Massie B. Systolic and diastolic heart failure: differences and similarities. *J Card Fail.* 2007;13:569–576, with permission.

TABLE 23.7

CLASSIFICATION OF LEFT VENTRICULAR FILLING PATTERNS

	Normal	Abnormal relaxation	Pseudonormalization	Restriction
E/A ratio	1–1.5	<1	1–1.5	>2
DT, ms	160–240	≥240	160–240	≤150
IVRT, ms	60–100	≥110	60–100	<60
PV S/D ratio	~1[a]	>1	<1	<1
A_r duration	<A	>A	>A	>A
A_r vel, cm/s	<20	<35	>35	>25[b]
Ea, cm/s	>8	<8	<8	<8
Vp, cm/s	>45	<45	<45	<45

E/A, mitral E/A ratio; DT, decelerating time; IVRT, isovolumic relaxation time; PV S/D, pulmonary vein systolic and diastolic flow; Ar, atrial reversal flow of pulmonary vein; A, mitral A duration; vel, velocity; Ea, early mitral annular longitudinal tissue velocity; Vp, velocity of transmitral flow propagation.
[a]Young patients and athletes may have values of <1.
[b]If atrial contractile failure is present, the value will be <25 cm/s.
Reproduced from Hoit B. Left ventricular diastolic function. *Crit Care Med.* 2007;35:5340–5347, with permission.

Unfortunately, in the presence of pre-existing atrial fibrillation, the chance for such an embolic event greatly increases (196). If there is associated atherosclerotic debris, particularly protruding, pedunculated, and free-flowing debris, the issue of anticoagulation does not reduce the problem (247,248). In addition to atrial fibrillation, if there is concurrent presence of a patent foramen ovale (PFO), the risks continue to rise (249). The existence of an atrial septal aneurysm increases the incidence for paradoxical embolism and stroke to 8.8% (250–252).

Aortic Trauma

The identification and pathogenesis of aortic trauma is better understood since TEE was added to the arsenal of the acute care physician. A vast number of these patients will succumb in the field due to extensive comorbid conditions, exsanguination, or tamponade. As expected, a significant number of patients (13% to 20%) will have been identified with this fatal injury (253), usually at postmortem; these deaths are second in frequency only to traumatic brain injury (TBI). A vast majority (75%) of blunt aortic injuries are due to motor vehicular crashes (253). If the patient arrives to the hospital trauma bay with vital signs, the presence of an aortic injury may be hidden or occult, considering that the physician is concentrating on the other life-threatening conditions (e.g., TBI, intraabdominal hemorrhage, pelvic injury, chest trauma, or pneumothoraces) (254). Of the patients who arrive to the hospital alive (33%), about a third of them will rapidly become hemodynamically unstable (255–259). Unless the clinician interrogates the aorta at the time of admission, this injury may be missed (220,222). Autopsy series reveal that the site of injury (acceleration-deceleration) is usually located near the aortic isthmus (54% to 65%), and

TABLE 23.8

ECHOCARDIOGRAPHIC LEFT VENTRICULAR MORPHOLOGIC AND FUNCTIONAL CHARACTERISTICS IN PRIMARY SYSTOLIC AND DIASTOLIC HEART FAILURE COMPARED WITH CONTROLS

	Controls	Systolic heart failure	Diastolic heart failure
LVEDV (mL)	102 + 12	192 + 10[a]	87 + 10
LVESV (mL)	46 + 11	137 + 9[a]	37 + 9
LVEF %	54 + 2	31+ 2[a]	60 + 2[b]
LV mass (g)	125 + 12	232 + 9[a]	160 + 9[b]
LV mass/volume	1.49 + 0.17	1.22 + 0.14	2.12 + 0.14[c]
NE pg/mL	169	287	306; $p = 0.007$
BNP pg/mL	3	28	56; $p = 0.02$

LVEDV, left ventricular end-diastolic volume; LVESV, left ventricular end-systolic volume; LVEF, left ventricular ejection fraction; LV, left ventricle; NE, norepinephrine; BNP, B-type natriuretic peptide.
[a]Systolic heart failure vs. controls, $p < 0.001$
[b]Diastolic heart failure vs. controls, $p < 0.001$
[c]Diastolic heart failure vs. controls, $p < 0.002$
Published with permission from Chatterjee K, Massie B. Systolic and diastolic heart failure: differences and similarities. *J Card Fail.* 2007;13:569–576.

TABLE 23.9

CHANGES IN LEFT VENTRICULAR END-DIASTOLIC VOLUMES (LVEDV) AND PRESSURES (LVEDP), EJECTION FRACTION (LVEF), AND LEFT VENTRICULAR STIFFNESS MODULUS (STIFF-MOD) DURING 64 + 9 MONTHS IN PATIENTS WITH DIASTOLIC HEART FAILURE

	Initial	End of follow-up
LVEDV mL/m^2	68 + 9	76 + 8
LVEF %	67 + 3	60 + 4
LVEDP mm Hg	14 + 3	26 + 2[a]
Stiff-Mod kN/m^2	3.4 + 0.6	6.3 + 0.9[a]

[a] $p < 0.05$ follow-up vs. initial.
Reprinted from Handoko ML, et al. Does diastolic heart failure evolve to systolic heart failure?: (abstract). *Circulation.* 2006; 114(Suppl II):816, with permission.

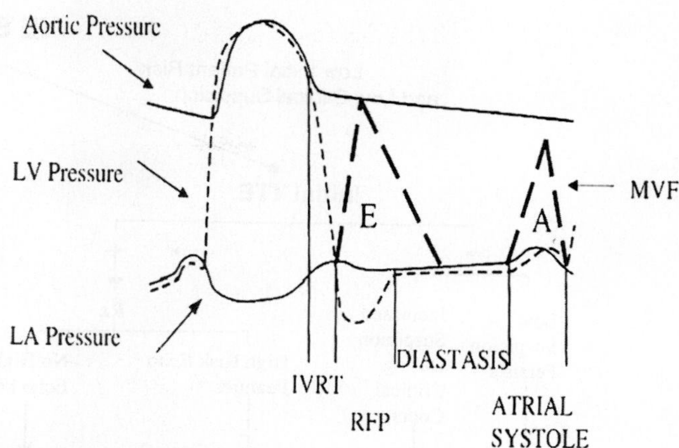

FIGURE 23.25. The four phases of diastole are schematically shown and include the isovolumic relaxation time (*IVRT*), which begins with aortic valve closure and extends to mitral valve opening, rapid early filling (*RFP*), diastasis, and atrial systole. Doppler E and A waves are superimposed. Note the points of left atrial-left ventricular (*LA-LV*) crossover and their relation to the mitral filling waves (*MVF*).

multiple sites may be involved in extreme physical forces. In vertical acceleration-deceleration, the injury may occur at the root of the aortic valve (253,255,256,260). Aortography is not the gold standard, and the addition of TEE complements helical CT. If the patient is hemodynamically stable, high-definition (356-cut) computed tomography may be the gold standard followed by TEE (220,222,224) (Tables 23.11 and 23.12). At present, if the patient is hemodynamically stable, CT angiography or a 64-cut chest CT should be performed initially, with TEE used to complement the diagnostic imaging modality (261). In these imaging schemes, most of the aorta is visualized. The benefit of TEE is its capability to visualize the aortic valve, the presence of aortic insufficiency, and the LV function and preload in real time, as well as identify pericardial effusions, especially when they are smaller, posterior, and loculated. These latter findings are typically not seen in the emergent FAST (focused assessment with sonography for trauma) examination commonly used in the trauma bay. Another benefit of TEE is color flow Doppler identification of differential flow and/or turbulence as a sign of a potential injury (transection, subadventitial tear, intimal flap, intraluminal defect, or thrombus formation) (35,36,220,262–267). The detection of a periaortic hematoma or mediastinal hematoma may lead the physician to suspect an aortic injury (Table 23.13). The major disadvantages for echocardiography are reverberation artifacts, limited access to the superior ascending thoracic aorta, and the inability to adequately define the great vessels. However, in reviewing TEE investigations in aortic trauma, it is clear that the operator experience, training, and its availability are crucial to uniformly identifying or excluding aortic injury (268).

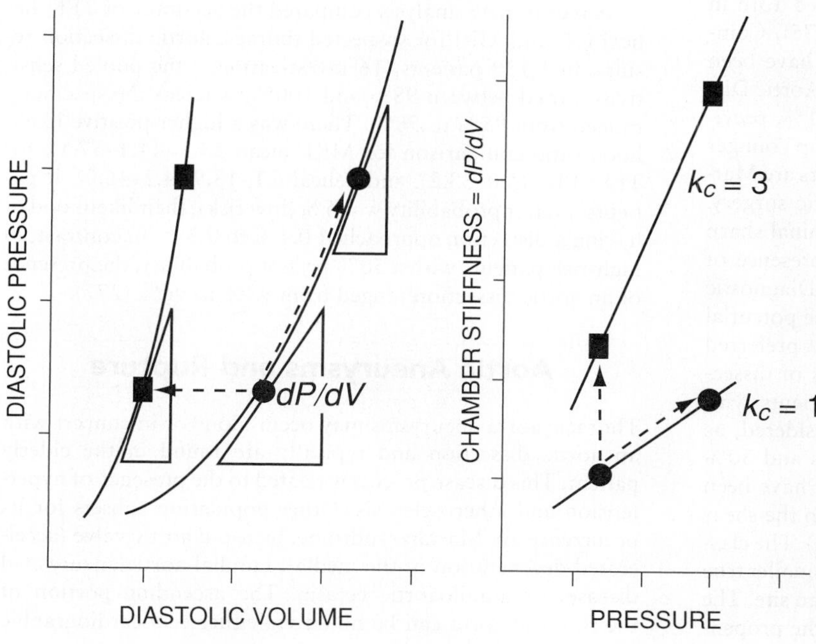

FIGURE 23.24. Left: End-diastolic pressure–volume in two ventricles with differing passive diastolic properties. Chamber stiffness is dP/dV at any point on the end-diastolic pressure–volume relation. The stiffer chamber on the left has a steeper overall slope. **Right:** Same data plotted as pressure vs. chamber stiffness. Because of the exponential nature of the end-diastolic pressure–volume relation, the relation between chamber stiffness and pressure is a straight line whose slope is the chamber stiffness constant (k_c) that characterizes the overall slope of the end-diastolic pressure–volume relation. A similar relationship holds for stress and strain. (Reproduced from LeWinter MM, Osol G. Normal physiology of the cardiovascular system. In: *Hurst's The Heart.* 11th ed. New York, NY: McGraw-Hill; 2004:S342, with permission.)

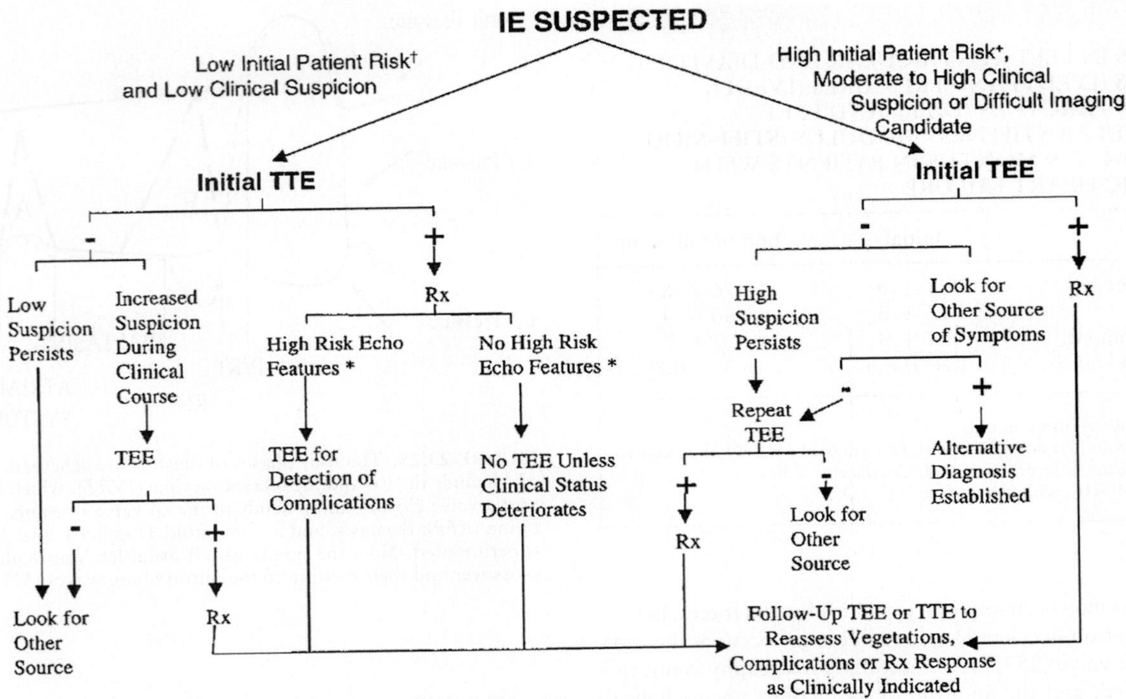

FIGURE 23.26. Approach to diagnostic use of echocardiography. TTE, transthoracic echocardiography; TEE, transesophageal echocardiography; IE, infective endocarditis. (Reproduced from Bayer AS, Bolger AF, Taubert KA, et al. Diagnosis and management of infective endocarditis and its complications. *Circulation.* 1998;98:2936–2948, with permission.)

Thoracic Aortic Dissection

Thoracic aortic dissection is another potentially life-threatening event that can be detected by TEE. Besides TEE, other imaging techniques following the historical use of angiography, which continue to gain acceptance, are 64-slice chest CT and MRI (particularly for chronic evaluation), or a combination of the above (41,220,269–271). The incidence for aortic dissection approaches 4.5/1,000 and is ranked 13th in cause of death in Western societies (41,220,253–275). Common predisposing conditions are well known and have been documented in the IRAD (International Registry of Aortic Dissection) (e.g., hypertension 72%, atherosclerosis 31%, previous cardiac surgery 18%). In the population subgroup younger than 40 years of age, the predominant etiologic factors are Marfan syndrome, bicuspid aortic valve, or prior aortic surgery. Symptoms can range from chest pain and/or abdominal sharp constant tearing pain, back pain, syncope to the presence of tachycardia, hypotension, or hypertension (269). Diagnostic imaging needs to be urgently performed to assess the potential for immediate surgery, as well as to determine the preferred surgical approach. There are several classifications of dissections: type A or B, De Bakey, or Stanford. In patients with acute proximal aortic involvement, surgery is considered, as the mortality with this group is 20% by 24 hours and 30% by 48 hours (269). Most type B dissections (73%) have been managed medically with pharmacotherapy to lessen the shear forces and flow and distention of the aorta (269,276). The classic echocardiographic depiction for a dissection is a smaller true lumen, larger false lumen, and an intimal flap with an site. The presence of a thrombus in the false lumen reveals the propensity for a lower morbidity and mortality. These lesser untoward events are seen in patients when the flow is minimal or unidirectional versus bidirectional from the true to false lumens. At times, there may be several entry sites, and flow may not be limited to one area of the thoracic aorta. TEE visualizes the integrity or involvement of the aortic valve leaflets in type A dissections, and allows the evaluation of LV performance and regional wall motion analysis (RWMA) and the detection of a pericardial effusion or tamponade.

A recent meta-analysis compared the accuracy of TEE, helical CT, and MRI for suspected thoracic aortic dissection results. In 1,139 patients (16 investigations), the pooled sensitivity varied between 98% and 100%, whereas the specificity ranged from 95% to 98%. There was a higher positive likelihood ratio comparison for MRI: mean 25.3 (11.1–57.1); for TEE, 14.1 (6.0–33.2); and helical CT, 13.9 (4.2–46.0). If patients' pretest probability was 5% (low risk), their likelihood of having a dissection approached 0.1% to 0.3%. In contrast, in high-risk patients with a 50% pretest probability, the presence of an aortic dissection ranged from 93% to 96% (277).

Aortic Aneurysms and Rupture

Thoracic aorta aneurysms may occur alone or in concert with an aortic dissection and typically are found in the elderly patient. This disease process is related to the presence of hypertension and atherosclerosis. Other population subsets for its occurrence are Marfan syndrome, bicuspid aortic valve (accelerated degeneration of the media), familial aortic aneurysmal disease, or annuloaortic ectasia. The ascending portion of the thoracic aorta can be noted via either echocardiographic

TABLE 23.10

IMAGING AND BIOMARKER FINDINGS SUGGESTIVE OF HIGHER RISK IN PE PATIENTS

Source	Subjects, no.	Diagnostic finding	Outcome	Sensitivity, % (95% CI)	Specificity, % (95% CI)	Positive predictive value, % (95% CI)	Negative predictive value, % (95% CI)
Echocardiography							
Ten Wolde et al. (214) 2004	310	RV dysfunction	Hospital mortality		58‡	5‡	
Kucher et al. (215) 2005	1035	RV hypokinesis	30-day mortality	52.4 (43.7–61.0)	62.7 (59.5–65.8)	16.1 (12.8–19.9)	90.6 (88.1–92.7)
Contrast-enhanced CT							
Schoepf et al. (327) 2004	454	RV/LV diameter >0.9	30-d mortality	78.2 (65.6–87.9)‡	38.0 (33.3–43.0)‡	15.6 (11.8–20.3)‡	92.3 (87.0–95.5)‡
van der Meer et al. (328) 2005	120	RV/LV diameter >1.0	PE-related 90 day mortality	100‡	45.1‡	10.1 (2.9–17.4)	100 (94.3–100)
Troponin							
Pruszczyk et al. (329) 2003	64	cTnT >0.01 ng/mL	Hospital mortality	100 (62.9–100)	57.0 (44.1–69.0)	25.8 (13.9–42.6)	98.5 (87.0–99.8)
Mehta et al. (330) 2003	38	cTnI >0.04 ng/mL	Cardiogenic shock	85.7 (48.7–99.3)	61.3 (43.8–76.3)	33.3 (16.3–56.3)	95.0 (76.4–99.7)
Punukollu et al. (331) 2005	33	cTnI >0.04 ng/mL	RV dysfunction	66.7 (43.7–83.7)	73.3 (48.0–89.1)	75.0 (50.5–89.8)	64.7 (41.3–82.7)
BNP							
Pruszczyk et al. (329) 2003	79	NT-proBNP >600 pg/mL	Hospital mortality	100‡	33‡	22.7‡	100‡
Kucher et al. (332) 2003	73	BNP >50 pg/mL	Combined end point*	95 (76–99)	60 (47–72)	48 (33–63)	97 (81–99)
Combined testing							
Binder et al. (333) 2005	111	NT-proBNP >1,000 pg/mL and RV dysfunction	Combined end point†	61.1 (38.6–79.7)	79.6 (70.3–86.5)	36.7 (21.9–54.5)	91.4 (83.2–95.8)
Scridon et al. (334) 2005	141	cTnI >0.1 ng/mL and RV/LV diameter > 0.9	30-d mortality	60.7 (42.4–76.4)	75.2 (66.5–82.3)	37.8 (25.1–52.4)	88.5 (80.6–93.2)

*Combined end point of death, cardiopulmonary resuscitation, mechanical ventilation, vasopressors, thrombolytics, catheter fragmentation, surgical embolectomy.
†Combined end point of cardiopulmonary resuscitation, mechanical ventilation, vasopressors, thrombolytics.
‡Other values and CIs not reported.

TABLE 23.11

TRANSESOPHAGEAL ECHOCARDIOGRAPHY (TEE) AND ANGIOGRAPHY (AORTOGRAPHY OR CONTRAST-ENHANCED SPIRAL COMPUTED TOMOGRAPHY FOR TRAUMATIC AORTIC IMAGING (TAI)

	Sensitivity, %	Specificity, %	NPV, %	PPV, %
Minor TAI ($n = 7$)				
TEE ($n = 208$)	100	100	100	100
Angiography ($n = 206$)	84	100	97	100
Major TAI ($n = 33$)				
TEE ($n = 208$)	97	100	99	100
Angiography ($n = 206$)	97	100	99	100
All TAI ($n = 41$)				
TEE ($n = 208$)	98	100	99	100
Angiography ($n = 206$)	83	100	96	100

NPV, negative predictive value; PPV, positive predictive value.
Reproduced with permission from Khalil et al. (220).

modality, although TEE is the preferred choice. The aortic size is well characterized by gender and age. Once the dilatation reaches greater than 5 cm, there is an increased risk of rupture, and replacement is generally considered. After the size of the aorta expands past 6.0 cm, the risk for rupture and dissection reaches greater than 6.9% per year, with a mortality rate of 11.8% annually (278). TEE can assist in the decision process for root replacement or placement of a prosthetic device and reimplantation of the coronary arteries. In patients with bicuspid aortic pathology, greater than 50% of the patients will have root dilatation and aortic insufficiency (41,220,272,278–281).

The localized absence of the media in the aortic wall will result in possible rupture of the sinus of Valsalva. Usually, it will rupture into adjacent structures such as the cardiac chambers (RV or RA) or through the ventricular septum. TEE invariably will visualize the aneurysm (ventricular side of the aortic valve), particularly of the ventricular septum. The apical long

TABLE 23.12

TEE AND HELICAL CHEST CT FOR THE IDENTIFICATION OF TRAUMATIC ARTERIAL INJURIES IN SEVERE BLUNT TRAUMA

	Sensitivity (%)	Specificity (%)	NPV (%)	PPV (%)
Multiplane				
TEE ($n = 106$)	93 (68–100)	100 (96–100)	99 (94–100)	100 (77–100)
Helical CT ($n = 99$)	73 (45–92)	100 (96–100)	95 (89–99)	100 (71–100)

TEE, transesophageal echocardiography; CT, computed tomography; NPV, negative predictive value; PPV, positive predictive value.
Reproduced with permission from Vignon et al. (314).

TABLE 23.13

AORTIC PATHOLOGY: COMPUTED TOMOGRAPHY FOR TRAUMA

Parameter	Hematoma direct signs	Periaortic direct signs	Direct signs
No. patients	1,346	1,346	1,346
TN	671	1,258	1,299
FP	656	69	28
NPV, %	100	100	99.9
Sensitivity, %	100	100	95
Specificity, %	50	95	98
TAI	19	19	19
TP	19	19	18
PPV, %	3	22	39
FN	0	0	1

TN, true negative; FP, false positive; NPV, negative predictive value; TAI, traumatic aortic injury; TP, true positive; PPV, positive predictive value; FN, false negative.
Reproduced with permission from Khalil et al. (220).

and parasternal views may discriminate between this pathology and a membranous septum. In a nonruptured sinus of Valsalva aneurysm, echocardiography will visualize thinning of the wall that is larger than the other sinuses. The intensivist needs to be aware that this situation can be associated with endocarditis, syphilis, a potentially fatal rupture, a source of emboli, and fistulae communicating with ventricular chambers. In the latter case, a significant left-to-right shunting can be demonstrated by using color flow Doppler echocardiography, with a continuous turbulent jet within the ruptured aneurysm into the receiving chamber (41,220,282–288). If the aneurysm communicates with the right atrium, the flow is continuous during systole and diastole. An increase in size of either the RA or RV will eventually occur (225,287,289–292).

Intramural Hematoma

A subpopulation of trauma patients will present with intramural hematoma (IMH), which arises from rupture of the vasa vasorum in the aortic medial wall layers, and is characterized by blood in the aortic wall in the absence of an intimal tear. IMH may be a precursor for the progression to a dissection. The associated prevalence is 10% to 30% of patients with a pre-existing dissection (274). Surgery is usually contemplated for type A dissection whereas intervention is warranted for a type B. The comparative mortality rates (medical vs. surgical), respectively, for types A and B are 36% versus 14% and 20% versus 14% (269,293).

INFECTIVE ENDOCARDITIS

Infective endocarditis (IE) is a challenge to all disciplines, particularly for intensive care physicians who have to analyze how IE factors into the differential diagnosis of a fever of unknown origin. Recurrent positive blood cultures while the patient is on antibiotics may provide a clue to its existence, especially if the pathogens are *Staphylococcus aureus*, streptococci, and enterococci. However, there is an increasing incidence of culture-negative IE that includes such

TABLE 23.14

DEFINITION OF INFECTIVE ENDOCARDITIS (IE) ACCORDING TO THE MODIFIED DUKE CRITERIA

PATHOLOGIC CRITERIA

Micro-organisms demonstrated by culture or histologic examination of a vegetation, a vegetation that has embolized, or an intracardiac abscess specimen; or

Pathologic lesions; vegetation or intracardiac abscess confirmed by histologic examination showing active endocarditis

CLINICAL CRITERIA

2 major criteria; or

1 major criterion and 3 minor criteria; or

5 minor criteria

POSSIBLE IE

1 major criterion and 1 minor criterion; or

3 minor criteria

REJECTED

Firm alternative diagnosis explaining evidence of IE; or

Resolution of IE syndrome with antibiotic therapy for <4 days; or

No pathologic evidence of IE at surgery or autopsy, with antibiotic therapy for <4 days; or

Does not meet criteria for possible IE as above

Reprinted with permissions from Li et al. (326).

TABLE 23.15

DEFINITION OF TERMS USED IN THE MODIFIED DUKE CRITERIA FOR THE DIAGNOSIS OF INFECTIVE ENDOCARDITIS (IE)

MAJOR CRITERIA

Blood culture positive for IE

Typical micro-organisms consistent with IE from 2 separate blood cultures: viridans streptococci, *Streptococcus bovis*, HACEK group, *Staphylococcus aureus;* or community-acquired enterococci in the absence of a primary focus;

or

Micro-organisms consistent with IE from persistently positive blood cultures defined as follows: At least 2 positive cultures of blood samples drawn >12 h apart; or all of 3 or a majority of 4 separate cultures of blood (with first and last sample drawn at least 1 h apart)

Single positive blood culture for *Coxiella burnetii* or antiphase IgG antibody titer >1:800

Evidence of endocardial involvement

Echocardiogram positive for IE (TEE recommended for patients with prosthetic valves, rated at least "possible IE" by clinical criteria, or complicated IE [paravalvular abscess]; TTE as first test in other patients) defined as follows: oscillating intracardiac mass on valve or supporting structures, in the path of regurgitant jets, or on implanted material in the absence of an alternative anatomic explanation; or abscess; or new partial dehiscence of prosthetic valve; new valvular regurgitation (worsening or changing or pre-existing murmur not sufficient)

MINOR CRITERIA

Predisposition, predisposing heart condition, or IDU

Fever, temperature >38°C

Vascular phenomena, major arterial emboli, septic pulmonary infarcts, mycotic aneurysm, intracranial hemorrhage, conjunctival hemorrhage, and Janeway lesions

Immunologic phenomena: glomerulonephritis, Osler nodes, Roth spots, and rheumatoid factor

Microbiologic evidence: positive blood culture but does not meet a major criterion as noted above[a] or serologic evidence of active infection with organism consistent with IE

Echocardiographic minor criteria eliminated

TEE, transesophageal echocardiography; TTE, transthoracic echocardiography; IDU, intravenous drug user.

[a]Excludes single positive cultures for coagulace-negative staphylococci and organisms that do not cause endocarditis.

Reprinted with permissions from Li et al. (326).

fastidious agents as *Coxiella burnetii, Tropheryma whipplei, Legionella pneumophila, Bartonella* spp., the HACEK group *(Haemophilus* spp., *Actinomycetemcomitans, Cardiobacterium hominis, Eikenella corrodens, Kingella* spp.), and fungi (including *Candida, Histoplasma*, and *Aspergillus* spp.) (294,295). The classic patient presentation with Janeway lesions, Osler nodes, Roth spots, and petechiae and history of rheumatic heart disease is not seen in the developed world (296). However, in the industrial world, the risks are related to age, degenerated valvular disease, prosthetic valves, and the increasing incidence of nosocomial infections. Besides in HIV infection patients where it can be present in up to 90% of the cases, IE can be found increasingly in the younger population, with social trends such as body piercing and self intravenous injection of recreational drugs, including HIV infection (40%–90%) (294,295) (Tables 23.14 and 23.15).

Identification of Vegetations

Perhaps more important than clinical findings, echocardiography is very useful for the identification of vegetations. Two fundamental predisposing factors are associated with the development of IE: cardiac endothelial injury and a microbiologic source. In endothelial injury, there is aberrant flow with a high-velocity jet directed onto the endothelial surface or increased shear stress through a narrow orifice. In the latter, there is a propensity for bacterial deposits downstream of the constriction via a Venturi effect. The detection of vibratory oscillations of vegetation or associated disruptive cardiac structures (torn leaflet, rupture of chordae tendineae) may indicate the presence of IE, as well as noting diastolic vibrations of the aortic valve or systolic vibrations of the mitral valve (M-mode echocardiography). Other characteristic findings involve structures that are in the path of a high-velocity jet as seen in valve regurgitation; these include motion of the valve that is chaotic and independent; texture that is gray scale in relation to the myocardium; an amorphous shape; the presence of a fistula or abscess; and new onset of regurgitation for either native or prosthetic valves. There may be associated obstructions, perivalvular leaks, or dehiscence. With these findings, there are stringlike mobile strands of vegetations or degenerative areas adjacent to the prosthetic device. In the mitral valve position, if there is a prosthetic device, TEE will easily identify these maladies. However, TTE is a better tool for visualizing the mechanical valve in the aortic position. Overall, TEE is a better diagnostic modality to visualize vegetations and associated complications. The sensitivities for TTE and TEE are 60% to 90% and 85% to 95%, respectively, while the specificities for both techniques (TTE and TEE) are far better: 90% to 98% (295,297–305). In the context of a negative TEE, the negative predictive value is only 90%; thus, maintaining good clinical judgment with clinical correlation is always a necessity (306–308). An algorithm proposed by Bayer et al. (309) can be used by the echocardiographer intensivist for this diagnostic dilemma (295,309).

Indications for Surgery

The most prominent indications for surgery are hemodynamic compromise or collapse from valve destruction, a persistent fever despite antibiotic treatment, and development of a fistula or abscess due to perivalvular spread of infection. Other indications are the presence of highly resistant organisms or aggressive pathogens, perioperative prosthetic valvular endocarditis, and large vegetations (greater than 10 mm). This latter indication is of particular concern given that the increasing size of the vegetation is associated with embolic events (294,295). A task force that includes input from the American Heart Association and the American College of Cardiology recently corroborated this last indication (310).

MYOCARDIAL INJURY

In patients with acute myocardial infarction, echocardiography is a crucial tool in the diagnosis and exclusion of myocardial injury, especially in patients with chest pain and nondiagnostic electrocardiographic (ECG) findings. Other roles for echocardiography are evaluating the extent of myocardium at risk and involvement after reperfusion; evaluating viable myocardium; assessing patients with hemodynamic instability and related complications following infarction; and risk stratification (102).

Echocardiography is also commonly used for evaluating acute coronary syndromes (ACS) by measuring intraventricular dyssynchrony by tissue velocity and strain imaging (41) (Fig. 23.27).

Resting and stress echocardiography are modalities for detecting ACS and complications of myocardial injury by prognostication using analysis of regional wall motion abnormalities (RWMA) scoring, as well as assessing diastolic dysfunction and stress-induced alterations (311). All LV wall segments can be seen from the apical, parasternal, and occasionally subcostal views. The American Society of Echocardiography proposes a standard for this RWMA scoring by using either a 16- or 17-segment model (43,312). The benefit of observing RWMA is that the patient may be asymptomatic and hemodynamically may not exhibit any aberrations. However, not all RWMAs are related to myocardial ischemia, such as loading conditions applied to the heart, paced rhythms, and conduction delays. Typically, after reperfusion, there may be persistent RWMA representing a delayed return of normal function, which is described as a stunned myocardium. This physiology, as well as the existence of global transitory dysfunction such as hibernating myocardium, must be put into the clinical context of the patient's condition.

In patients with acute ST-elevation myocardial infarction (STEMI), the affected myocardium becomes an akinetic or dyskinetic segment. Following interventions (reperfusion), there is usually improvement in the afflicted segments within 24 to 48 hours, and echocardiography can be used serially to assess these patients for improvements or extension of the injury. Contrast echocardiography, low-dose dobutamine infusion, or strain imaging can also assess viability (49,313).

Complications

Numerous complications follow an acute myocardial infarction. Echocardiography is a mainstay in assessing these problems, which range from rupture of papillary muscle and ventricular septal defects (VSD) to cardiopulmonary resuscitation (41,314).

Rupture

Acute free wall rupture also occurs less frequently in the postinterventional period (1.0%). About half of the ruptures will result in out-of-hospital sudden deaths. Following myocardial injury, the mortality of free wall rupture varies between 8% and 17%, with a significant number (40%) occurring within the first 24 hours and 85% after 1 week (266,315,316). Besides hemodynamic collapse or cardiac arrest, there may be severe bradycardia. Some patients may experience syncope, chest pain, or emesis. In these dire situations, echocardiography (TEE) is the diagnostic tool of choice. Pericardial effusions and/or cardiac tamponade may be found, keeping in mind that 25% of myocardial infarctions will have a pericardial effusion. Thrombus may exist, as well as the identification of flow via color flow Doppler (317). Also, a pseudoaneurysm may form following a free rupture that is contained in a limited portion of the pericardial space, most frequently the posterior wall. A pseudoaneurysm is traditionally characterized by a small neck communication between the LV and the aneurysmal cavity (ratio less than 0.5). Color flow Doppler may reveal flow, especially bidirectional (318).

Another cause for a new murmur is a ruptured papillary muscle (partial or complete) and mitral regurgitation (the extent of the murmur does not correlate with pathology). Extenuating circumstances for a new murmur may be LV regional or global remodeling, papillary muscle dysfunction with annular dilatation, or acute systolic anterior motion of the mitral valve. The latter cause is managed in a totally different way than with volume replacement, with primary intervention accomplished with beta-blockade and avoidance of vasodilators (319).

The most serious cause of new mitral regurgitation that must be acted on quickly is rupture of the posteromedial papillary segment. This acute problem may be even related to a small infarct corresponding to the circumflex or right coronary artery. The rupture may be complete or partial and is identified by color flow Doppler imaging. After papillary muscle rupture and its discovery by TEE, surgery is imminent for mitral valve replacement, with or without coronary revascularization. In a series by Moursi et al. (320), in 65% of the patients with TEE, the head of the papillary muscle was observed in the LA.

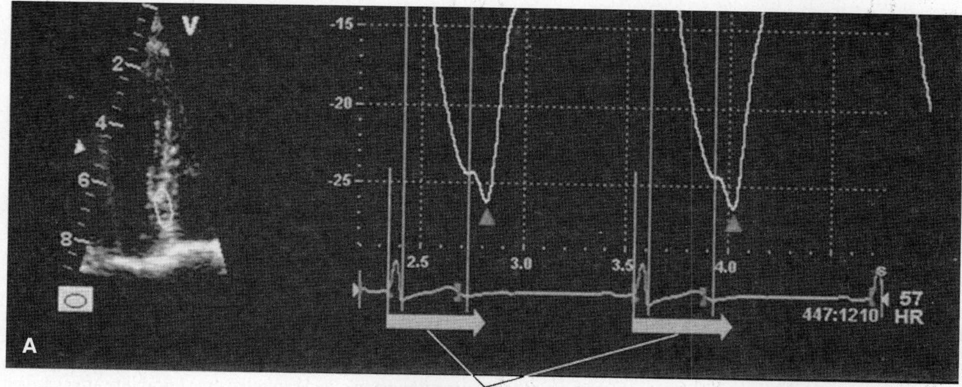

Time to peak systolic strain

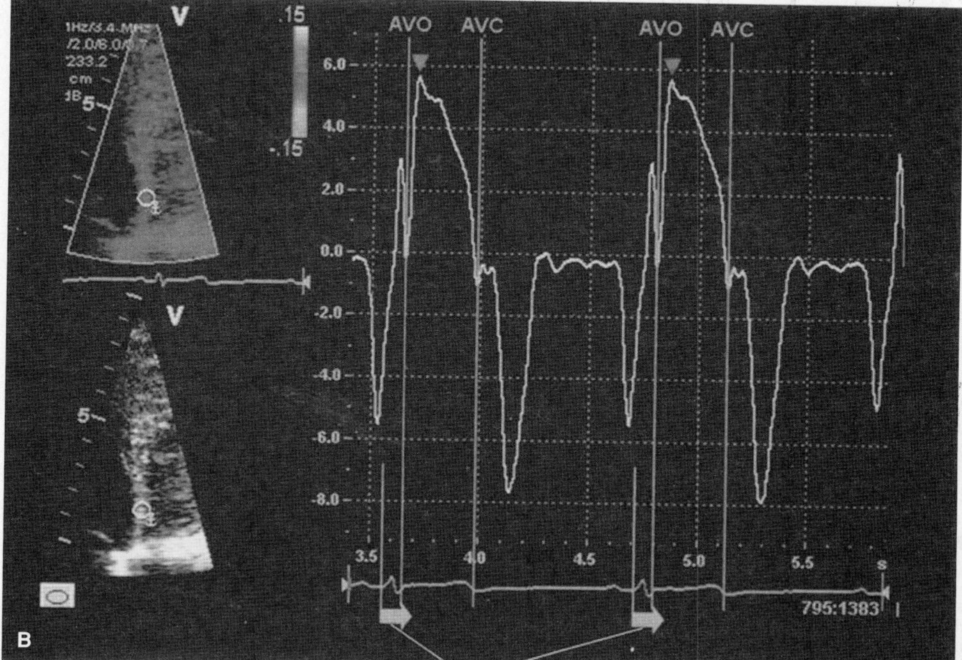

Time to peak tissue velocity

FIGURE 23.27. Measurement of intraventricular dyssynchrony by tissue velocity and strain imaging. **A:** Recording of strain from the basal segment of the ventricular septum from the apical four-chamber view. Time to peak systolic strain is measured from onset of QRS to the peak negative value including the postsystolic shortening. The timing of the peak negative strain is when shortening of the myocardium is maximum. **B:** Recording of tissue velocity from the basal segment of the ventricular septum. Peak systolic velocity is the positive wave during the ejection period. Time to peak tissue velocity is from onset of QRS to the positive peak velocity. The time interval is determined from 2 to 12 segments to measure intraventricular dyssynchrony. (From Oh JK, Seward JB, Tajik AJ. *The Echo Manual.* 3rd ed. Philadelphia, PA: Lippincott Williams & Wilkins; 2006. Used with permission of Mayo Foundation for Medical Education and Research.)

Another characteristic finding seen in these patients (90%) was some erratic motion in the body of the LV (315,320–322).

Right Ventricular Infarction and Failure

Right ventricular infarction and/or failure is one of the most difficult clinical entities to support. Diagnosis of isolated failure or biventricular failure alters the management of these complex patients. Inferior myocardial infarction is associated with RV infarction (35%) (315,323). The subcostal view may visualize the RV easily. In suboptimal acoustic windows, TEE is considered. The classic findings are tricuspid regurgitation, a dilated thinned RV, severe global hypokinesis, reduced descent of the base of the RV free wall (apical four-chamber view), and plethora of the inferior vena cava without any respiratory variations in its diameter. In diastole, there is flattening of the ventricular septum and occasional paradoxical motion and, at times, bulging of the septum into the LV, indicative of a right-sided pressure/volume overload situation. The RA may reveal right atrial hypertension with displacement of the interatrial septum (315,323,324). If there is coexisting PFO in the presence of RV and/or RA afterload, a right-to-left shunt is possible through the atrial septum, resulting in hypoxemia and thus complicating the clinical presentation. The identification of a PFO is greatly enhanced by choosing TEE over the surface approach (325).

HEMODYNAMICS AND VALVE AREA CALCULATIONS

The intraoperative or perioperative physician expert in echocardiography must not only deal with the evaluation of ventricular function (global and regional), identification of aortic pathology, detection of masses, and visualization of normal abnormal pathology of native and prosthetic valves but must also be competent in the hemodynamic assessment of these patients. An appreciation of the basics of the hemodynamic calculations sets the stage for the building blocks of accurate detection of flow hemodynamics and physiology that may affect the patient's clinical care (medical or surgical). The calculation of pressure gradient determination uses the Bernoulli equation. Additional valve area calculations use the continuity equation, pressure half-time and deceleration time, proximal isovelocity surface area (PISA), and effective regurgitant orifice. Similarly, the determination of valvular area is complex and based on several echocardiographic and Doppler principles evaluating the continuity equation pressure half-time method, deceleration time method, and planimetry. An extensive review of these topics is beyond the scope of this chapter but is available in all major textbooks on echocardiography (31,41).

SUMMARY

The critical care physician should have at the bedside the availability and expertise to correctly use echocardiography as a first-line diagnostic and monitoring tool. Eventually, this field of critical care echocardiography should be encompassed in the training of the fellows in intensive care medicine. The implementation of training—basic skills versus full certification—is still being debated. Nevertheless, this imaging modality is crucial for timely medical and surgical interventions. Having a remote echocardiographic team may be helpful in this short term period, and the impact of echocardiography in critically ill and injured patients must not be minimized. A subset of the total field of echocardiography should include intensive care medicine. In the meantime, collaborating with our cardiology colleagues is the key for better understanding of echocardiographic findings in the setting of a critical illness.

References

1. Vignon P, Mentec H, Terre S, et al. Diagnostic accuracy and therapeutic impact of transthoracic and transesophageal echocardiography in mechanically ventilated patients in the ICU. *Chest.* 1994;106:1829–1834.
2. Albanese J, Leone M, Delmas A, et al. Terlipressin or norepinephrine in hyperdynamic septic shock: a prospective, randomized study. *Crit Care Med.* 2005;33:1897–1902.
3. Bruch C, Comber M, Schmermund A, et al. Diagnostic usefulness and impact on management of transesophageal echocardiography in surgical intensive care units. *Am J Cardiol.* 2003;91:510–513.
4. Chenzbraun A, Pinto FJ, Schnittger I. Transesophageal echocardiography in the intensive care unit: impact on diagnosis and decision-making. *Clin Cardiol.* 1994;17:438–444.
5. Colreavy FB, Donovan K, Lee KY, et al. Transesophageal echocardiography in critically ill patients. *Crit Care Med.* 2002;30:989–996.
6. Font VE, Obarski TP, Klein AL, et al. Transesophageal echocardiography in the critical care unit. *Cleve Clin J Med.* 1991;58:315–322.
7. Foster E, Schiller NB. The role of transesophageal echocardiography in critical care: UCSF experience. *J Am Soc Echocardiogr.* 1992;5:368–374.
8. Harris KM, Petrovic O, Davila-Roman VG, et al. Changing patterns of transesophageal echocardiography use in the intensive care unit. *Echocardiography.* 1999;16:559–565.
9. Heidenreich PA, Stainback RF, Redberg RF, et al. Transesophageal echocardiography predicts mortality in critically ill patients with unexplained hypotension. *J Am Coll Cardiol.* 1995;26:152–158.
10. Movsowitz HD, Levine RA, Hilgenberg AD, et al. Transesophageal echocardiographic description of the mechanisms of aortic regurgitation in acute type A aortic dissection: implications for aortic valve repair. *J Am Coll Cardiol.* 2000;36:884–890.
11. Patel MR, Spertus JA, Brindis RG, et al. ACCF proposed method for evaluating the appropriateness of cardiovascular imaging. *J Am Coll Cardiol.* 2005;46:1606–1613.
12. Khoury AF, Afridi I, Quinones MA, et al. Transesophageal echocardiography in critically ill patients: feasibility, safety, and impact on management. *Am Heart J.* 1994;127:1363–1371.
13. McLean AS. Transoesophageal echocardiography in the intensive care unit. *Anaesth Intensive Care.* 1998;26:22–25.
14. Oh JK, Seward JB, Khandheria BK, et al. Transesophageal echocardiography in critically ill patients. *Am J Cardiol.* 1990;66:1492–1495.
15. Pearson AC, Castello R, Labovitz AJ. Safety and utility of transesophageal echocardiography in the critically ill patient. *Am Heart J.* 1990;119:1083–1089.
16. Puybasset L, Saada M, Catoire P, et al. Contribution of transesophageal echocardiography in intensive care: a prospective assessment. *Ann Fr Anesth Reanim.* 1993;12:17–21.
17. Schmidlin D, Schuepbach R, Bernard E, et al. Indications and impact of postoperative transesophageal echocardiography in cardiac surgical patients. *Crit Care Med.* 2001;29:2143–2148.
18. Slama MA, Novara A, Van de Putte P, et al. Diagnostic and therapeutic implications of transesophageal echocardiography in medical ICU patients with unexplained shock, hypoxemia, or suspected endocarditis. *Intensive Care Med.* 1996;22:916–922.
19. Sohn DW, Shin GJ, Oh JK, et al. Role of transesophageal echocardiography in hemodynamically unstable patients. *Mayo Clin Proc.* 1995;70:925–931.
20. Wake PJ, Ali M, Carroll J, et al. Clinical and echocardiographic diagnoses disagree in patients with unexplained hemodynamic instability after cardiac surgery. *Can J Anaesth.* 2001;48:778–783.
21. Karski JM. Transesophageal echocardiography in the intensive care unit. *Semin Cardiothorac Vasc Anesth.* 2006;10:162–166.
22. Poelaert JI, Trouerbach J, De Buyzere M, et al. Evaluation of transesophageal echocardiography as a diagnostic and therapeutic aid in a critical care setting. *Chest.* 1995;107:774–779.
23. Mathew JP, Glas K, Troianos CA, et al. ASE/SCA recommendations and guidelines for continuous quality improvement in perioperative echocardiography. *Anesth Analg.* 2006;103:1416–1425.
24. Mathew JP, Glas K, Troianos CA, et al. American Society of Echocardiography/Society of Cardiovascular Anesthesiologists recommendations and guidelines for continuous quality improvement in perioperative echocardiography. *J Am Soc Echocardiogr.* 2006;19:1303–1313.
25. Quinones MA, Douglas PS, Foster E, et al. ACC/AHA clinical competence statement on echocardiography: a report of the American College of Cardiology/American Heart Association/American College of Physicians-American Society of Internal Medicine Task Force on clinical competence. *J Am Soc Echocardiogr.* 2003;16:379–402.
26. Quinones MA, Douglas PS, Foster E, et al. American College of Cardiology/American Heart Association clinical competence statement on echocardiography: a report of the American College of Cardiology/American Heart Association/American College of Physicians–American Society of Internal Medicine Task Force on clinical competence. *Circulation.* 2003;107:1068–1089.
27. Douglas PS, Khandheria B, Stainback RF, et al. ACCF/ASE/ACEP/ASNC/SCAI/SCCT/SCMR 2007 appropriateness criteria for transthoracic and transesophageal echocardiography. *J Am Coll Cardiol.* 2007;50:187–204.
28. Mandavia DP, Hoffner RJ, Mahaney K, et al. Bedside echocardiography by emergency physicians. *Ann Emerg Med.* 2001;38:377–382.
29. Moore CL, Rose GA, Tayal VS, et al. Determination of left ventricular function by emergency physician echocardiography of hypotensive patients. *Acad Emerg Med.* 2002;9:186–193.
30. Mazraeshahi RM, Farmer JC, Porembka DT. A suggested curriculum in echocardiography for critical care physicians. *Crit Care Med.* 2007;35:S431–433.
31. Otto CM. *Textbook of Clinical Echocardiography.* 3rd ed. Philadelphia, PA: WB Saunders; 2007.
32. Vieillard-Baron A, Slama M, Cholley B, et al. Echocardiography in the intensive care unit: from evolution to revolution? *Intensive Care Med.* 2008;34:243–249.
33. Price S, Nicol E, Gibson DG, et al. Echocardiography in the critically ill: current and potential roles. *Intensive Care Med.* 2006;32:48–59.
34. Porembka DT. Importance of transesophageal echocardiography in the critically ill and injured patient. *Crit Care Med.* 2007;35:S414–430.
35. Nanda NC, Domanski MJ, eds. *Atlas of Transesophageal Echocardiography.* 2nd ed. Philadelphia, PA: Lippincott Williams & Wilkins; 2006.
36. Vannan MA, Lang RM, Rabowski H, et al., eds. *Atlas of Echocardiography.* Current Medicine; 2005.
37. Feigenbaum H, Popp RL, Wolfe SB, et al. Ultrasound measurements of the left ventricle. A correlative study with angiocardiography. *Arch Intern Med.* 1972;129:461–467.
38. Weyman AE. The year in echocardiography. *J Am Coll Cardiol.* 2006;47:856–863.
39. Mingo S, Benedicto A, Jimenez MC, et al. Dynamic left ventricular outflow tract obstruction secondary to catecholamine excess in a normal ventricle. *Int J Cardiol.* 2006;112:393–396.
40. Araujo AQ, Arteaga E, Ianni BM, et al. Relationship between outflow obstruction and left ventricular functional impairment in hypertrophic cardiomyopathy: a Doppler echocardiographic study. *Echocardiography.* 2006;23:734–740.
41. Libby P, Braunwald E. *Braunwald's Heart Disease: A Textbook of Cardiovascular Medicine.* 8th ed. Philadelphia, PA: Elsevier Saunders; 2007.
42. Memtsoudis SG, Rosenberger P, Loffler M, et al. The usefulness of transesophageal echocardiography during intraoperative cardiac arrest in noncardiac surgery. *Anesth Analg.* 2006;102:1653–1657.

43. Oh JK, Seward JB, Tajik AJ. *The Echo Manual.* 3rd ed. Philadelphia, PA: Lippincott Williams & Wilkins; 2006.
44. Redfield MM, Jacobsen SJ, Burnett JC Jr, et al. Burden of systolic and diastolic ventricular dysfunction in the community: appreciating the scope of the heart failure epidemic. *JAMA.* 2003;289:194–202.
45. McMurray JJ, Pfeffer MA. Heart failure. *Lancet.* 2005;365:1877–1889.
46. Barker WH, Mullooly JP, Getchell W. Changing incidence and survival for heart failure in a well-defined older population, 1970–1974 and 1990–1994. *Circulation.* 2006;113:799–805.
47. Hogg K, Swedberg K, McMurray J. Heart failure with preserved left ventricular systolic function; epidemiology, clinical characteristics, and prognosis. *J Am Coll Cardiol.* 2004;43:317–327.
48. Pinsky MR, Vincent JL. Let us use the pulmonary artery catheter correctly and only when we need it. *Crit Care Med.* 2005;33:1119–1122.
49. Marwick TH. Measurement of strain and strain rate by echocardiography: ready for prime time? *J Am Coll Cardiol.* 2006;47:1313–1327.
50. Rivers EP, Kruse JA, Jacobsen G, et al. The influence of early hemodynamic optimization on biomarker patterns of severe sepsis and septic shock. *Crit Care Med.* 2007;35:2016–2024.
51. Huang DT, Clermont G, Dremsizov TT, et al. Implementation of early goal-directed therapy for severe sepsis and septic shock: a decision analysis. *Crit Care Med.* 2007;35:2090–2100.
52. Jones AE, Focht A, Horton JM, et al. Prospective external validation of the clinical effectiveness of an emergency department-based early goal-directed therapy protocol for severe sepsis and septic shock. *Chest.* 2007;132:425–432.
53. Nguyen HB, Smith D. Sepsis in the 21st century: recent definitions and therapeutic advances. *Am J Emerg Med.* 2007;25:564–571.
54. Roch A, Blayac D, Ramiara P, et al. Comparison of lung injury after normal or small volume optimized resuscitation in a model of hemorrhagic shock. *Intensive Care Med.* 2007;33:1645–1654.
55. Dellinger RP, Levy MM, Carlet JM, et al. Surviving sepsis campaign: international guidelines for management of severe sepsis and septic shock: 2008. *Intensive Care Med.* 2008;34(1):17–60.
56. O'Brien JM Jr, Ali NA, Aberegg SK, et al. Sepsis. *Am J Med.* 2007;120:1012–1022.
57. Bolli R. Preconditioning: a paradigm shift in the biology of myocardial ischemia. *Am J Physiol Heart Circ Physiol.* 2007;292:H19–27.
58. Dittoe N, Stultz D, Schwartz BP, et al. Quantitative left ventricular systolic function: from chamber to myocardium. *Crit Care Med.* 2007;35:S330–339.
59. Curtis JP, Sokol SI, Wang Y, et al. The association of left ventricular ejection fraction, mortality, and cause of death in stable outpatients with heart failure. *J Am Coll Cardiol.* 2003;42:736–742.
60. Wang TJ, Evans JC, Benjamin EJ, et al. Natural history of asymptomatic left ventricular systolic dysfunction in the community. *Circulation.* 2003;108:977–982.
61. Mock MB, Ringqvist I, Fisher LD, et al. Survival of medically treated patients in the coronary artery surgery study (CASS) registry. *Circulation.* 1982;66:562–568.
62. Sharir T, Germano G, Kavanagh PB, et al. Incremental prognostic value of post-stress left ventricular ejection fraction and volume by gated myocardial perfusion single photon emission computed tomography. *Circulation.* 1999;100:1035–1042.
63. Schiller NB, Shah PM, Crawford M, et al. Recommendations for quantitation of the left ventricle by two-dimensional echocardiography. American Society of Echocardiography Committee on Standards, Subcommittee on Quantitation of Two-Dimensional Echocardiograms. *J Am Soc Echocardiogr.* 1989;2:358–367.
64. Lang RM, Bierig M, Devereux RB, et al. Recommendations for chamber quantification: a report from the American Society of Echocardiography's Guidelines and Standards Committee and the Chamber Quantification Writing Group, developed in conjunction with the European Association of Echocardiography, a branch of the European Society of Cardiology. *J Am Soc Echocardiogr.* 2005;18:1440–1463.
65. Zamorano J, Cordeiro P, Sugeng L, et al. Real-time three-dimensional echocardiography for rheumatic mitral valve stenosis evaluation: an accurate and novel approach. *J Am Coll Cardiol.* 2004;43:2091–2096.
66. Teichholz LE, Kreulen T, Herman MV, et al. Problems in echocardiographic volume determinations: echocardiographic-angiographic correlations in the presence of absence of asynergy. *Am J Cardiol.* 1976;37:7–11.
67. Yvorchuk KJ, Davies RA, Chan KL. Measurement of left ventricular ejection fraction by acoustic quantification and comparison with radionuclide angiography. *Am J Cardiol.* 1994;74:1052–1056.
68. Bednarz J, Vignon P, Mor-Avi VV, et al. Color kinesis: principles of operation and technical guidelines. *Echocardiography.* 1998;15:21–34.
69. Sugeng L, Mor-Avi V, Weinert L, et al. Quantitative assessment of left ventricular size and function: side-by-side comparison of real-time three-dimensional echocardiography and computed tomography with magnetic resonance reference. *Circulation.* 2006;114:654–661.
70. Feigenbaum H, Armstrong WF, Ryan T, et al. *Feigenbaum's Echocardiography.* 6th ed. Philadelphia, PA: Lippincott Williams & Wilkins; 2005.
71. Nishimura RA, Tajik AJ. Evaluation of diastolic filling of left ventricle in health and disease: Doppler echocardiography is the clinician's rosetta stone. *J Am Coll Cardiol.* 1997;30:8–18.
72. Oh JK, Hatle L, Tajik AJ, et al. Diastolic heart failure can be diagnosed by comprehensive two-dimensional and Doppler echocardiography. *J Am Coll Cardiol.* 2006;47:500–506.
73. Sabbah HN, Khaja F, Brymer JF, et al. Noninvasive evaluation of left ventricular performance based on peak aortic blood acceleration measured with a continuous-wave Doppler velocity meter. *Circulation.* 1986;74:323–329.
74. Bauer F, Jones M, Shiota T, et al. Left ventricular outflow tract mean systolic acceleration as a surrogate for the slope of the left ventricular end-systolic pressure-volume relationship. *J Am Coll Cardiol.* 2002;40:1320–1327.
75. Nishimura RA, Tajik AJ. Quantitative hemodynamics by Doppler echocardiography: a noninvasive alternative to cardiac catheterization. *Prog Cardiovasc Dis.* 1994;36:309–342.
76. Bouchard A, Blumlein S, Schiller NB, et al. Measurement of left ventricular stroke volume using continuous wave Doppler echocardiography of the ascending aorta and M-mode echocardiography of the aortic valve. *J Am Coll Cardiol.* 1987;9:75–83.
77. Vinereanu D, Khokhar A, Fraser AG. Reproducibility of pulsed wave tissue Doppler echocardiography. *J Am Soc Echocardiogr.* 1999;12:492–499.
78. Dokainish H, Zoghbi WA, Lakkis NM, et al. Optimal noninvasive assessment of left ventricular filling pressures: a comparison of tissue Doppler echocardiography and B-type natriuretic peptide in patients with pulmonary artery catheters. *Circulation.* 2004;109:2432–2439.
79. Hsiao SH, Huang WC, Sy CL, et al. Doppler tissue imaging and color M-mode flow propagation velocity: are they really preload independent? *J Am Soc Echocardiogr.* 2005;18:1277–1284.
80. Oki T, Tabata T, Mishiro Y, et al. Pulsed tissue Doppler imaging of left ventricular systolic and diastolic wall motion velocities to evaluate differences between long and short axes in healthy subjects. *J Am Soc Echocardiogr.* 1999;12:308–313.
81. Mori K, Hayabuchi Y, Kuroda Y, et al. Left ventricular wall motion velocities in healthy children measured by pulsed wave Doppler tissue echocardiography: normal values and relation to age and heart rate. *J Am Soc Echocardiogr.* 2000;13:1002–1011.
82. Pela G, Bruschi G, Montagna L, et al. Left and right ventricular adaptation assessed by Doppler tissue echocardiography in athletes. *J Am Soc Echocardiogr.* 2004;17:205–211.
83. Oki T, Fukuda K, Tabata T, et al. Effect of an acute increase in afterload on left ventricular regional wall motion velocity in healthy subjects. *J Am Soc Echocardiogr.* 1999;12:476–483.
84. Nagueh SF, Bachinski LL, Meyer D, et al. Tissue Doppler imaging consistently detects myocardial abnormalities in patients with hypertrophic cardiomyopathy and provides a novel means for an early diagnosis before and independently of hypertrophy. *Circulation.* 2001;104:128–130.
85. Yu CM, Lin H, Yang H, et al. Progression of systolic abnormalities in patients with "isolated" diastolic heart failure and diastolic dysfunction. *Circulation.* 2002;105:1195–1201.
86. Wang M, Yip GW, Wang AY, et al. Peak early diastolic mitral annulus velocity by tissue Doppler imaging adds independent and incremental prognostic value. *J Am Coll Cardiol.* 2003;41:820–826.
87. Mankad S, Murali S, Kormos RL, et al. Evaluation of the potential role of color-coded tissue Doppler echocardiography in the detection of allograft rejection in heart transplant recipients. *Am Heart J.* 1999;138:721–730.
88. Dandel M, Hummel M, Muller J, et al. Reliability of tissue Doppler wall motion monitoring after heart transplantation for replacement of invasive routine screenings by optimally timed cardiac biopsies and catheterizations. *Circulation.* 2001;104:I184–1191.
89. Shan K, Bick RJ, Poindexter BJ, et al. Relation of tissue Doppler derived myocardial velocities to myocardial structure and beta-adrenergic receptor density in humans. *J Am Coll Cardiol.* 2000;36:891–896.
90. Galderisi M, Cattaneo F, Mondillo S. Doppler echocardiography and myocardial dyssynchrony: a practical update of old and new ultrasound technologies. *Cardiovasc Ultrasound.* 2007;5:28.
91. Edvardsen T, Gerber BL, Garot J, et al. Quantitative assessment of intrinsic regional myocardial deformation by Doppler strain rate echocardiography in humans: validation against three-dimensional tagged magnetic resonance imaging. *Circulation.* 2002;106:50–56.
92. Hoffmann R, Altiok E, Nowak B, et al. Strain rate measurement by Doppler echocardiography allows improved assessment of myocardial viability in patients with depressed left ventricular function. *J Am Coll Cardiol.* 2002;39:443–449.
93. Voigt JU, Exner B, Schmiedehausen K, et al. Strain-rate imaging during dobutamine stress echocardiography provides objective evidence of inducible ischemia. *Circulation.* 2003;107:2120–2126.
94. Yu CM, Fung JW, Zhang Q, et al. Tissue Doppler imaging is superior to strain rate imaging and postsystolic shortening on the prediction of reverse remodeling in both ischemic and nonischemic heart failure after cardiac resynchronization therapy. *Circulation.* 2004;110:66–73.
95. Gilman G, Khandheria BK, Hagen ME, et al. Strain rate and strain: a step-by-step approach to image and data acquisition. *J Am Soc Echocardiogr.* 2004;17:1011–1020.

96. Weidemann F, Jamal F, Kowalski M, et al. Can strain rate and strain quantify changes in regional systolic function during dobutamine infusion, B-blockade, and atrial pacing—implications for quantitative stress echocardiography. *J Am Soc Echocardiogr.* 2002;15:416–424.
97. Sutherland GR, Di Salvo G, Claus P, et al. Strain and strain rate imaging: a new clinical approach to quantifying regional myocardial function. *J Am Soc Echocardiogr.* 2004;17:788–802.
98. Teske AJ, De Boeck BW, Melman PG, et al. Echocardiographic quantification of myocardial function using tissue deformation imaging, a guide to image acquisition and analysis using tissue Doppler and speckle tracking. *Cardiovasc Ultrasound.* 2007;5:27.
99. Amundsen BH, Helle-Valle T, Edvardsen T, et al. Noninvasive myocardial strain measurement by speckle tracking echocardiography: validation against sonomicrometry and tagged magnetic resonance imaging. *J Am Coll Cardiol.* 2006;47:789–793.
100. Giglio V, Pasceri V, Messano L, et al. Ultrasound tissue characterization detects preclinical myocardial structural changes in children affected by Duchenne muscular dystrophy. *J Am Coll Cardiol.* 2003;42: 309–316.
101. Dutka DP, Donnelly JE, Palka P, et al. Echocardiographic characterization of cardiomyopathy in Friedreich's ataxia with tissue Doppler echocardiographically derived myocardial velocity gradients. *Circulation* 2000;102: 1276–1282.
102. Sengupta PP, Krishnamoorthy VK, Korinek J, et al. Left ventricular form and function revisited: applied translational science to cardiovascular ultrasound imaging. *J Am Soc Echocardiogr.* 2007;20:539–551.
103. Kolias TJ, Aaronson KD, Armstrong WF. Doppler-derived dP/dt and -dP/dt predict survival in congestive heart failure. *J Am Coll Cardiol.* 2000;36: 1594–1599.
104. Pai RG, Bansal RC, Shah PM. Doppler-derived rate of left ventricular pressure rise: its correlation with the postoperative left ventricular function in mitral regurgitation. *Circulation.* 1990;82:514–520.
105. Nixon JV, Murray RG, Leonard PD, et al. Effect of large variations in preload on left ventricular performance characteristics in normal subjects. *Circulation.* 1982;65:698–703.
106. Colan SD, Borow KM, Neumann A. Left ventricular end-systolic wall stress-velocity of fiber shortening relation: a load-independent index of myocardial contractility. *J Am Coll Cardiol.* 1984;4:715–724.
107. Carabello BA, Usher BW, Hendrix GH, et al. Predictors of outcome for aortic valve replacement in patients with aortic regurgitation and left ventricular dysfunction: a change in the measuring stick. *J Am Coll Cardiol.* 1987;10:991–997.
108. Yoshifuku S, Biro S, Ikeda Y, et al. Validation of TEI index in the estimation of cardiac function: an experimental study. *J Am Coll Cardiol.* 2002;39:372.
109. Tei C, Ling LH, Hodge DO, et al. New index of combined systolic and diastolic myocardial performance: a simple and reproducible measure of cardiac function–a study in normals and dilated cardiomyopathy. *J Cardiol.* 1995;26:357–366.
110. Miller D, Farah MG, Liner A, et al. The relation between quantitative right ventricular ejection fraction and indices of tricuspid annular motion and myocardial performance. *J Am Soc Echocardiogr.* 2004;17:443–447.
111. Hoit BD. Left ventricular diastolic function. *Crit Care Med.* 2007;35:S340–347.
112. Chatterjee K, Massie B. Systolic and diastolic heart failure: differences and similarities. *J Card Fail.* 2007;13:569–576.
113. Kitzman DW, Gardin JM, Gottdiener JS, et al. Importance of heart failure with preserved systolic function in patients > or = 65 years of age. CHS research group. cardiovascular health study. *Am J Cardiol.* 2001;87:413–419.
114. Vasan RS, Benjamin EJ, Levy D. Prevalence, clinical features and prognosis of diastolic heart failure: an epidemiologic perspective. *J Am Coll Cardiol.* 1995;26:1565–1574.
115. Merx MW, Weber C. Sepsis and the heart. *Circulation.* 2007;116:79–802.
116. Burns AT, Connelly KA, La Gerche A, et al. Effect of heart rate on tissue Doppler measures of diastolic function. *Echocardiography.* 2007;24:697–701.
117. Mirsky I, Pasipoularides A. Clinical assessment of diastolic function. *Prog Cardiovasc Dis.* 1990;32:291–318.
118. Weiss JL, Frederiksen JW, Weisfeldt ML. Hemodynamic determinants of the time-course of fall in canine left ventricular pressure. *J Clin Invest.* 1976;58:751–760.
119. Chopra M, Sharma AC. Distinct cardiodynamic and molecular characteristics during early and late stages of sepsis-induced myocardial dysfunction. *Life Sci.* 2007;81:306–316.
120. Rozenberg S, Besse S, Brisson H, et al. Endotoxin-induced myocardial dysfunction in senescent rats. *Crit Care.* 2006;10:R124.
121. Pirracchio R, Cholley B, De Hert S, et al. Diastolic heart failure in anaesthesia and critical care. *Br J Anaesth.* 2007;98:707–721.
122. Cinel I, Dellinger RP. Advances in pathogenesis and management of sepsis. *Curr Opin Infect Dis.* 2007;20:345–352.
123. Young JD. The heart and circulation in severe sepsis. *Br J Anaesth.* 2004; 93:114–120.
124. Rudiger A, Singer M. Mechanisms of sepsis-induced cardiac dysfunction. *Crit Care Med.* 2007;35:1599–1608.
125. Burkhoff D, Mirsky I, Suga H. Assessment of systolic and diastolic ventricular properties via pressure-volume analysis: a guide for clinical, translational, and basic researchers. *Am J Physiol Heart Circ Physiol.* 2005;289: H501–H512.
126. Zile MR, Tomita M, Ishihara K, et al. Changes in diastolic function during development and correction of chronic LV volume overload produced by mitral regurgitation. *Circulation.* 1993;87:1378–1388.
127. Appleton CP, Firstenberg MS, Garcia MJ, et al. The echo-Doppler evaluation of left ventricular diastolic function. A current perspective. *Cardiol Clin.* 2000;18:513–546, ix.
128. Oh JK, Appleton CP, Hatle LK, et al. The noninvasive assessment of left ventricular diastolic function with two-dimensional and Doppler echocardiography. *J Am Soc Echocardiogr.* 1997;10:246–270.
129. Ristow B, Ali S, Ren X, et al. Elevated pulmonary artery pressure by Doppler echocardiography predicts hospitalization for heart failure and mortality in ambulatory stable coronary artery disease: the Heart and Soul Study. *J Am Coll Cardiol.* 2007;49:43–49.
130. Garcia MJ, Rodriguez L, Ares M, et al. Myocardial wall velocity assessment by pulsed Doppler tissue imaging: characteristic findings in normal subjects. *Am Heart J.* 1996;132:648–656.
131. Miyatake K, Yamagishi M, Tanaka N, et al. New method for evaluating left ventricular wall motion by color-coded tissue Doppler imaging: in vitro and in vivo studies. *J Am Coll Cardiol.* 1995;25:717–724.
132. Dokainish H, Zoghbi WA, Lakkis NM, et al. Incremental predictive power of B-type natriuretic peptide and tissue Doppler echocardiography in prognoses of patients with congestive heart failure. *J Am Coll Cardiol.* 2005;45: 1223–1226.
133. Ommen SR, Nishimura RA, Appleton CP, et al. Clinical utility of Doppler echocardiography and tissue Doppler imaging in the estimation of left ventricular filling pressures: a comparative simultaneous Doppler-catheterization study. *Circulation.* 2000;102:1788–1794.
134. Nagueh SF, Middleton KJ, Kopelen HA, et al. Doppler tissue imaging: a noninvasive technique for evaluation of left ventricular relaxation and estimation of filling pressures. *J Am Coll Cardiol.* 1997;30:1527–1533.
135. Nagueh SF, Sun H, Kopelen HA, et al. Hemodynamic determinants of the mitral annulus diastolic velocities by tissue Doppler. *J Am Coll Cardiol.* 2001;37:278–285.
136. Takatsuji H, Mikami T, Urasawa K, et al. A new approach for evaluation of left ventricular diastolic function: spatial and temporal analysis of left ventricular filling flow propagation by color M-mode Doppler echocardiography. *J Am Coll Cardiol.* 1996;27:365–371.
137. Garcia MJ, Thomas JD, Klein AL. New Doppler echocardiographic applications for the study of diastolic function. *J Am Coll Cardiol.* 1998;32:865–875.
138. Gonzalez-Vilchez F, Ayuela J, Ares M, et al. Comparison of Doppler echocardiography, color M-mode Doppler, and Doppler tissue imaging for the estimation of pulmonary capillary wedge pressure. *J Am Soc Echocardiogr.* 2002;15:1245–1250.
139. Lawson WE, Brown EJ Jr, Swinford RD, et al. A new use for M-mode echocardiography in detecting left ventricular diastolic dysfunction in coronary artery disease. *Am J Cardiol.* 1986;58:210–213.
140. Hanrath P, Mathey DG, Siegert R, et al. Left ventricular relaxation and filling pattern in different forms of left ventricular hypertrophy: an echocardiographic study. *Am J Cardiol.* 1980;45:15–23.
141. Pritchett AM, Mahoney DW, Jacobsen SJ, et al. Diastolic dysfunction and left atrial volume: a population-based study. *J Am Coll Cardiol.* 2005;45: 87–92.
142. Dokainish H. Combining tissue Doppler echocardiography and B-type natriuretic peptide in the evaluation of left ventricular filling pressures: review of the literature and clinical recommendations. *Can J Cardiol.* 2007;23: 983–989.
143. Moller JE, Pellikka PA, Hillis GS, et al. Prognostic importance of diastolic function and filling pressure in patients with acute myocardial infarction. *Circulation.* 2006;114:438–444.
144. Vieillard-Baron A, Charron C, Chergui K, et al. Bedside echocardiographic evaluation of hemodynamics in sepsis: is a qualitative evaluation sufficient? *Intensive Care Med.* 2006;32:1547–1552.
145. Little WC, Freeman GL. Pericardial disease. *Circulation.* 2006;113:1622–1632.
146. Hoit BD. Pericardial disease and pericardial tamponade. *Crit Care Med.* 2007;35(Suppl):S355–364.
147. Maisch B. Pericardial disease with a focus on etiology, pathogenesis, pathophysiology, new diagnostic imaging methods, and treatment. *Curr Opin Cardiol.* 1994;9:379–388.
148. Weitzman LB, Tinker WP, Kranzon I, et al. The incidence and natural history of pericardial effusion after cardiac surgery: an echocardiography study. *Circulation.* 1984;69:506–511.
149. Kuvin JT, Harati NA, Pandian NG, et al. Postoperative cardiac tamponade in the modern surgical era. *Ann Thorac Surg.* 2002;74:1148–1153.
150. Ciliberto GR, Anjos MC, Gronda E. Significance of pericardial effusions after heart transplantation. *Am J Cardiol.* 1995;76:297–300.
151. Tsang TS, Barnes ME, Hayes SN, et al. Clinical and echocardiographic characteristics of significant pericardial effusions following cardiothoracic surgery and outcomes of echo-guided pericardiocentesis for management: Mayo Clinic experience, 1979–1998. *Chest.* 1999;116:322–331.

152. Imazio M, Trinchero R. Triage and management of acute pericarditis. *Int J Cardiol.* 2007;118:286–294.
153. Slobodin G, Hussein A, Rozenbaum M, et al. The emergency room in systemic rheumatic diseases. *Emerg Med J.* 2006;23:667–671.
154. Kobayashi M, Okabayashi T, Okamoto K, et al. Clinicopathological study of cardiac tamponade due to pericardial metastasis originating from gastric cancer. *World J Gastroenterol.* 2005;11:6899–6904.
155. Taguchi R, Takasu J, Itani Y, et al. Pericardial fat accumulation in men at risk for coronary artery disease. *Atherosclerosis.* 2001;157:203–209.
156. Iacobellis G, Leonetti F. Epicardial adipose tissue and insulin resistance in obese subjects. *J Clin Endocrinol Metab.* 2005;90:6300–6302.
157. Seferovic PM, Ristic AD, Imazio M, et al. Management strategies in pericardial emergencies. *Herz.* 2006;31:891–900.
158. Degiannis E, Loogna P, Doll D, et al. Penetrating cardiac injuries: recent experience in South Africa. *World J Surg.* 2006;30:1258–1264.
159. Leimgrubber PP, Klopfenstein HS, Wann LS, et al. The hemodynamic derangement associated with right ventricular diastolic collapse in cardiac tamponade: an experimental echocardiographic study. *Circulation.* 1983; 68:612–620.
160. Hoit BD, Gabel M, Fowler NO. Cardiac tamponade in left ventricular dysfunction. *Circulation.* 1990;82:1370–1376.
161. Hoit BD, Ramrakhyani K. Pulmonary venous flow in cardiac tamponade: influence of left ventricular dysfunction and the relation to pulsus paradoxus. *J Am Soc Echocardiogr.* 1991;4:559–570.
162. Gillam LD, Guyer DE, Gibson TC, et al. Hydrodynamic compression of the right atrium: a new echocardiographic sign of cardiac tamponade. *Circualtion.* 1983;68:294–301.
163. Maisch B, Seferovic PM, Ristic AD, et al. Guidelines on the diagnosis and management of pericardial diseases executive summary: the Task Force on the Diagnosis and Management of Pericardial Diseases of the European Society of Cardiology. *Eur Heart J.* 2004;25:587–610.
164. Reydel B, Spodick DH. Frequency and significance of chamber collapses during cardiac tamponade. *Am Heart J.* 1990;119:1160–1163.
165. Fussman B, Schwinger ME, Charney R, et al. Isolated of left-sided heart chambers in cardiac tamponade: demonstration by two-dimensional echocardiography. *Am Heart J.* 1991;121:613–616.
166. Merce J, Sagrista-Sauleda J, Permanyer-Miralda G, et al. Correlation between clinical and Doppler echocardiography findings in patients with moderate and large pericardial effusions: implications for the diagnosis of cardiac tamponade. *Am Heart J.* 1999;138:759–764.
167. Roy CL, Minor MA, Brookhart MA, et al. Does this patient with a pericardial effusion have cardiac tamponade? *JAMA.* 2007;297:1810–1818.
168. Talreja DR, Edwards WD, Danielson GK, et al. Constrictive pericarditis in 26 patients with histiologically normal pericardial thickness. *Circulation.* 2003;108(15):1852–1857.
169. Pinamonti B, Zecchin M, Di Lenarda A, et al. Persistence of restrictive left ventricular filling pattern in dilated cardiomyopathy: an ominous prognostic sign. *J Am Coll Cardiol.* 1997;29:604–612.
170. Ling LH, Oh JK, Tei C, et al. Pericardial thickness measured with transesophageal echocardiography: feasibility and potential clinical usefulness. *J Am Coll Cardiol.* 1997;29:1317–1323.
171. Cheitlin MD, Armstrong WF, Aurigemma GP, et al. ACC/AHA/ASE 2003 Guideline Update for the Clinical Application of Echocardiography: summary article. A Report of the American College of Cardiology/American Heart Association Task Force on Practice Guidelines (ACC/AHA/ASE Committee for the Clinical Application of Echocardiography). *J Am Soc Echocardiogr.* 2003;16:1091–1110.
172. Tei C, Child JS, Tanaka H, et al. Atrial systolic notch on the interventricular septal echogram: an echocardiographic sign of constrictive pericarditis. *J Am Coll Cardiol.* 1983;1:907–912.
173. Engel PJ, Fowler NO, Tei CW, et al. M-mode echocardiography in constrictive pericarditis. *J Am Coll Cardiol.* 1985;6:471–474.
174. Hoit BD. Imaging the pericardium. *Cardiol Clin.* 1990;8:587–600.
175. D'Cruz IA, Dick A, Gross CM, et al. Abnormal left ventricular-left atrial posterior wall contour: a new dimensional echocardiographic sign in constrictive pericarditis. *Am Heart J.* 1989;118:218–132.
176. Ha JW, Oh JK, Ling LH, et al. Annulus paradoxus: transmitral flow velocity to mitral annular velocity ratio is inversely proportional to pulmonary capillary wedge pressure in patients with constrictive pericarditis. *Circulation.* 2001;104:976–978.
177. Oh JK, Hatle LK, Sinak LJ, et al. Characteristic Doppler echocardiographic pattern of mitral inflow velocity in severe aortic regurgitation. *J Am Coll Cardiol.* 1989;14:1712–1717.
178. Rajagopalan N, Garcia MJ, Rodriguez L, et al. Comparison of new Doppler echocardiographic methods to differentiate constrictive pericardial heart disease and restrictive cardiomyopathy. *Am J Cardiol.* 2001;87:86–94.
179. Pozzoli M, Traversi E, Cioffi G, et al. Loading manipulations improve the prognostic value of Doppler evaluation of mitral flow in patients with chronic heart failure. *Circulation.* 1997;95:1222–1230.
180. Sun JP, Abdalla IA, Yang XS, et al. Respiratory variation of mitral and pulmonary venous Doppler flow velocities in constrictive pericarditis before and after pericardiectomy. *J Am Soc Echocardiogr.* 2001;14:119–126.
181. Oh JK, Tajik AJ, Appleton CP, et al. Preload reduction to unmask the characteristic Doppler features of constrictive pericarditis. *Circulation.* 1997; 95:796–799.
182. Troughton RW, Asher CR, Klein AL. Percarditis. *Lancet.* 2004;363:717–727.
183. Krug EG, Mercy JA, Dahlberg LL, et al. The world report on violence and health. *Lancet.* 2002;360:1083–1088.
184. Gao JM, Gao YH, Wei GB, et al. Penetrating cardiac wounds: principles for surgical management. *World J Surg.* 2004;28:1025–1029.
185. Burack JH, Kandil E, Sawas A, et al. Triage and outcome of patients with mediastinal penetrating trauma. *Ann Thorac Surg.* 2007;83:377–382; discussion 382.
186. Asensio JA, Soto SN, Forno W, et al. Penetrating cardiac injuries: a complex challenge. *Injury.* 2001;32:533–543.
187. Demetriades D, Charalambides C, Sareli P, et al. Late sequelae of penetrating cardiac injuries. *Br J Surg.* 1990;77:813–814.
188. Degiannis E, Loogna P, Doll D, et al. Penetrating cardiac injuries: recent experience in South Africa. *World J Surg.* 2006;30(7):1258–1264.
189. Aboulhosn J, Child JS. Left ventricular outflow obstruction: subaortic stenosis, bicuspid aortic valve, supravalvar aortic stenosis, and coarctation of the aorta. *Circulation.* 2006;114:2412–2422.
190. Cesar S, Potocnik N, Stare V. Left ventricular end-diastolic pressure-volume relationship in septic rats with open thorax. *Comp Med.* 2003;53:493–497.
191. Groban L, Dolinski SY. Transesophageal echocardiographic evaluation of diastolic function. *Chest.* 2005;128:3652–3663.
192. Azevedo LC, Janiszewski M, Soriano FG, et al. Redox mechanisms of vascular cell dysfunction in sepsis. *Endocr Metab Immune Disord Drug Targets.* 2006;6:159–164.
193. Bombardini T. Myocardial contractility in the echo lab: molecular, cellular and pathophysiological basis. *Cardiovasc Ultrasound.* 2005;3:27.
194. Assreuy J. Nitric oxide and cardiovascular dysfunction in sepsis. *Endocr Metab Immune Disord Drug Targets.* 2006;6:165–173.
195. Kumar A, Anel R, Bunnell E, et al. Pulmonary artery occlusion pressure and central venous pressure fail to predict ventricular filling volume, cardiac performance, or the response to volume infusion in normal subjects. *Crit Care Med.* 2004;32:691–699.
196. Donal E, Yamada H, Leclercq C, et al. The left atrial appendage, a small, blind-ended structure: a review of its echocardiographic evaluation and its clinical role. *Chest.* 2005;128:1853–1862.
197. Kortgen A, Niederprum P, Bauer M. Implementation of an evidence-based "standard operating procedure" and outcome in septic shock. *Crit Care Med.* 2006;34:943–949.
198. Krishnagopalan S, Kumar A, Parrillo JE, et al. Myocardial dysfunction in the patient with sepsis. *Curr Opin Crit Care.* 2002;8:376–388.
199. Parrillo JE, Burch C, Shelhamer JH, et al. A circulating myocardial depressant substance in humans with septic shock: septic shock with a reduced ejection fraction have a circulating factor that depresses in vitro myocardial cell performance. *J Clin Invest.* 1985;76:1539–1553.
200. Fischer UM, Radhakrishnan RS, Uray KS, et al. Myocardial function after gut ischemia/reperfusion: does NFkappaB play a role? *J Surg Res.* May 5, 2008 (Epub ahead of print).
201. Barth E, Radermacher P, Thiemermann C, et al. Role of inducible nitric oxide synthase in the reduced responsiveness of the myocardium to catecholamines in a hyperdynamic, murine model of septic shock. *Crit Care Med.* 2006;34:307–313.
202. Martins PS, Brunialti MK, da Luz Fernandes M, et al. Bacterial recognition and induced cell activation in sepsis. *Endocr Metab Immune Disord Drug Targets.* 2006;6:183–191.
203. Pinsky MR, Teboul JL. Assessment of indices of preload and volume responsiveness. *Curr Opin Crit Care.* 2005;11:235–239.
204. Poeze M, Solberg BC, Greve JW, et al. Monitoring global volume-related hemodynamic or regional variables after initial resuscitation: what is a better predictor of outcome in critically ill septic patients? *Crit Care Med.* 2005;33:2494–2500.
205. Pinsky MR. Protocolized cardiovascular management based on ventricular-arterial coupling. In: Pinsky MR, Payen D, eds. *Functional Hemodynamic Monitoring.* New York, NY: Springer-Verlag; 2005.
206. Axler O. Evaluation and management of shock. *Semin Respir Crit Care Med.* 2006;27:230–240.
207. Carlbom DJ, Davidson BL. Pulmonary embolism in the critically ill. *Chest.* 2007;132:313–324.
208. Kline JA, Hernandez-Nino J, Jones AE, et al. Prospective study of the clinical features and outcomes of emergency department patients with delayed diagnosis of pulmonary embolism. *Acad Emerg Med.* 2007;14: 592–598.
209. Raisinghani A, Ben-Yehuda O. Echocardiography in chronic thromboembolic pulmonary hypertension. *Semin Thorac Cardiovasc Surg.* 2006;18: 230–235.
210. Kucher N, Goldhaber SZ. Risk stratification of acute pulmonary embolism. *Semin Thromb Hemost.* 2006;32:838–847.
211. Cecconi M, Johnston E, Rhodes A. What role does the right side of the heart play in circulation? *Crit Care.* 2006;10(Suppl 3):S5.
212. Konstantinides SV. Acute pulmonary embolism revisited: thromboembolic venous disease. *Heart.* 2008;94:795–802.
213. Sanchez O, Trinquart L, Colobet I, et al. Prognostic value of right ventricular dysfunction in patients with haemodynamically stable pulmonary embolism: a systemic review. *Eur Heart J.* 2008;29:1569–1577.

214. ten Wolde M, Söhne M, Quak E, et al. Prognostic value of echocardiographically assessed right ventricular dysfunction in patients with pulmonary embolism. *Arch Intern Med.* 2004;164:1685–1689.
215. Kucher N, Rossi E, De Rosa M, et al. Prognostic role of echocardiography among patients with acute pulmonary embolism and a systolic arterial pressure of 90 mm Hg or higher. *Arch Intern Med.* 2005;165:1777–1781.
216. Jardin F, Dubourg O, Gueret P, et al. Quantitative two-dimensional echocardiography in massive pulmonary embolism: emphasis on ventricular interdependence and leftward septal displacement. *J Am Coll Cardiol.* 1987;10:1201–1206.
217. Morris-Thurgood JA, Frenneaux MP. Diastolic ventricular interaction and ventricular diastolic filling. *Heart Fail Rev.* 2000;5:307–323.
218. Bonomini F, Tengattini S, Fabiano A, et al. Atherosclerosis and oxidative stress. *Histol Histopathol.* 2008;23:381–390.
219. Mallika V, Goswami B, Rajappa M. Atherosclerosis pathophysiology and the role of novel risk factors: a clinicobiochemical perspective. *Angiology.* 2007;58:513–522.
220. Khalil A, Helmy T, Porembka DT. Aortic pathology: aortic trauma, debris, dissection, and aneurysm. *Crit Care Med.* 2007;35:S392–400.
221. Meissner I, Khandheria BK, Sheps SG, et al. Atherosclerosis of the aorta: risk factor, risk marker, or innocent bystander? A prospective population-based transesophageal echocardiography study. *J Am Coll Cardiol.* 2004; 44:1018–1024.
222. Nzewi O, Slight RD, Zamvar V. Management of blunt thoracic aortic injury. *Eur J Vasc Endovasc Surg.* 2006;31:18–27.
223. Baguley CJ, Sibal AK, Alison PM. Repair of injuries to the thoracic aorta and great vessels: Auckland, New Zealand 1995–2004. *ANZ J Surg.* 2005; 75:383–387.
224. Yu T, Zhu X, Tang L, et al. Review of CT angiography of aorta. *Radiol Clin North Am.* 2007;45:461–483.
225. Moustafa S, Mookadam F, Cooper L, et al. Sinus of valsalva aneurysms–47 years of a single center experience and systematic overview of published reports. *Am J Cardiol.* 2007;99:1159–1164.
226. Rustemli A, Bhatti TK, Wolff SD. Evaluating cardiac sources of embolic stroke with MRI. *Echocardiography.* 2007;24:301–308; discussion 308.
227. Sundt TM. Intramural hematoma and penetrating atherosclerotic ulcer of the aorta. *Ann Thorac Surg.* 2007;83:S835–841; discussion S846–850.
228. Sharifkazemi MB, Aslani A, Zamirian M, et al. Significance of aortic atheroma in elderly patients with ischemic stroke. A hospital-based study and literature review. *Clin Neurol Neurosurg.* 2007;109:311–316.
229. Bossone E, Evangelista A, Isselbacher E, et al. Prognostic role of transesophageal echocardiography in acute type A aortic dissection. *Am Heart J.* 2007;153:1013–1020.
230. Meissner L, Whisnant JP, Khandheria BK, et al. Prevalence of potential risk factors for stroke assessed by transesophageal echocardiography and carotid ultrasonography: the SPARC study. Stroke Prevention Assessment of Risk in a Community. *Mayo Clin Proc.* 1989;64:862–869.
231. Cardiogenic brain embolism. The second report of the Cerebral Embolism Task Force. *Arch Neurol.* 1989;46:727–743.
232. The French Study of Aortic Plaques in Stroke Group. Atherosclerotic disease of the aortic arch as a risk factor for recurrent ischemic stroke. *N Engl J Med.* 1996;19:1216–1221.
233. Pearson AC, Labovitz AJ, Tatineni S, et al. Superiority of transesophageal echocardiography in detecting cardiac source of embolism in patients with cerebral ischemia of uncertain etiology. *J Am Coll Cardiol.* 1991;17: 66–72.
234. Black IW, Hopkins AP, Lee LC, et al. Role of transoesophageal echocardiography in evaluation of cardiogenic embolism. *Br Heart J.* 1991;66:302–307.
235. Pop G, Sutherland GR, Koudstaal PJ, et al. Transesophageal echocardiography in the detection of intracardiac embolic sources in patients with transient ischemic attacks. *Stroke.* 1990;21:560–565.
236. DeRook FA, Comess KA, Albers GW, et al. Transesophageal echocardiography in the evaluation of stroke. *Ann Intern Med.* 1992;117:922–932.
237. Vandenbogaerde J, De Bleecker J, Decoo D, et al. Transoesophageal echo-Doppler in patients suspected of a cardiac source of peripheral emboli. *Eur Heart J.* 1992;13:88–94.
238. Lee RJ, Bartzokis T, Yeoh TK, et al. Enhanced detection of intracardiac sources of cerebral emboli by transesophageal echocardiography. *Stroke.* 1991;22:734–739.
239. Albers GW, Comess KA, DeRook FA, et al. Transesophageal echocardiographic findings in stroke subtypes. *Stroke.* 1994;25:23–28.
240. Sansoy V, Abbott RD, Jayaweera AR, et al. Low yield of transthoracic echocardiography for cardiac source of embolism. *Am J Cardiol.* 1995; 75:166–169.
241. Leung DY, Black IW, Cranney GB, et al. Prognostic implications of left atrial spontaneous echo contrast in nonvalvular atrial fibrillation. *J Am Coll Cardiol.* 1994;24:755–762.
242. Tunick PA, Rosenzweig BP, Katz ES, et al. High risk for vascular events in patients with protruding aortic atheromas: a prospective study. *J Am Coll Cardiol.* 1994;23:1085–1090.
243. Tunick PA, Kronzon I. Protruding atherosclerotic plaque in the aortic arch of patients with systemic embolization: a new finding seen by transesophageal echocardiography. *Am Heart J.* 1990;120:658–660.
244. Amarenco P, Cohen A, Tzourio C, et al. Atherosclerotic disease of the aortic arch and the risk of ischemic stroke. *N Engl J Med.* 1994;331:1474–1479.
245. Jones EF, Kalman JM, Calafiore P, et al. Proximal aortic atheroma: an independent risk factor for cerebral ischemia. *Stroke.* 1995;26:218–224.
246. Koren MJ, Bryant B, Hilton TC. Atherosclerotic disease of the aortic arch and the risk of ischemic stroke. *N Engl J Med.* 1995;332:1237; author reply 1237–1238.
247. Transesophageal echocardiographic correlates of thromboembolism in high-risk patients with nonvalvular atrial fibrillation. The Stroke Prevention in Atrial Fibrillation Investigators Committee on Echocardiography. *Ann Intern Med.* 1998;128:639–647.
248. Black IW, Hopkins AP, Lee LC, et al. Left atrial spontaneous echo contrast: a clinical and echocardiographic analysis. *J Am Coll Cardiol.* 1991;18:398–404.
249. Zenker G, Erbel R, Kramer G, et al. Transesophageal two-dimensional echocardiography in young patients with cerebral ischemic events. *Stroke.* 1988;19:345–348.
250. Lechat P, Mas JL, Lascault G, et al. Prevalence of patent foramen ovale in patients with stroke. *N Engl J Med.* 1988;318:1148–1152.
251. Webster MW, Chancellor AM, Smith HJ, et al. Patent foramen ovale in young stroke patients. *Lancet.* 1988;2:11–12.
252. Gallet B, Malergue MC, Adams C, et al. Atrial septal aneurysm—a potential cause of systemic embolism. An echocardiographic study. *Br Heart J.* 1985;53:292–297.
253. Feczko JD, Lynch L, Pless JE, et al. An autopsy case review of 142 nonpenetrating (blunt) injuries of the aorta. *J Trauma.* 1992;33:846–849.
254. Mattox KL, Wall MJ Jr. Historical review of blunt injury to the thoracic aorta. *Chest Surg Clin N Am.* 2000;10:167–182, x.
255. Fabian TC, Richardson JD, Croce MA, et al. Prospective study of blunt aortic injury: multicenter trial of the American Association for the Surgery of Trauma. *J Trauma.* 1997;42:374–80; discussion 380–383.
256. Dyer DS, Moore EE, Ilke DN, et al. Thoracic aortic injury: how predictive is mechanism and is chest computed tomography a reliable screening tool? A prospective study of 1,561 patients. *J Trauma.* 2000;48: 673–682; discussion 682–683.
257. Karmy-Jones R, Carter YM, Nathens A, et al. Impact of presenting physiology and associated injuries on outcome following traumatic rupture of the thoracic aorta. *Am Surg.* 2001;67:61–66.
258. Chirillo F, Totis O, Cavarzerani A, et al. Usefulness of transthoracic and transoesophageal echocardiography in recognition and management of cardiovascular injuries after blunt chest trauma. *Heart.* 1996;75:301–306.
259. Minard G, Schurr MJ, Croce MA, et al. A prospective analysis of transesophageal echocardiography in the diagnosis of traumatic disruption of the aorta. *J Trauma.* 1996;40:225–230.
260. Kodali S, Jamieson WR, Leia-Stephens M, et al. Traumatic rupture of the thoracic aorta. A 20-year review: 1969–1989. *Circulation.* 1991;84 (5 Suppl):III40–46.
261. Rivas LA, Munera F, Fishman JE. Multidetector-row computerized tomography of aortic injury. *Semin Roentgenol.* 2006;41:226–236.
262. Braunwald E, Zipes DP, Libby P, et al., eds. *Braunwald's Heart Disease: A Textbook of Cardiovascular Medicine.* 7th ed. Philadelphia, PA: WB Saunders; 2004.
263. Feigenbaum H, Armstrong WF, Ryan T, eds. *Feigenbaum's Echocardiography.* 6th ed. Philadelphi, PA: Lippincott Williams & Wilkins, 2005.
264. D'Cruz IA, ed. *Echocardiographic Anatomy: Understanding Normal and Abnormal Echocardiograms.* New York, NY: Mc-Graw-Hill/Appleton & Lange; 1995.
265. Porembka DT. Transesophageal echocardiography. *Crit Care Clin.* 1996; 12:875–918.
266. Fuster V, Alexander RW, O'Rourke RA, et al., eds. *Hurst's The Heart.* 11th ed. New York, NY: McGraw-Hill Professional; 2004.
267. Mathew J, Chakib A, eds. *Clinical Manual and Review of Transesophageal Echocardiography.* New York, NY: McGraw-Hill; 2005.
268. Cinnella G, Dambrosio M, Brienza N, et al. Transesophageal echocardiography for diagnosis of traumatic aortic injury: an appraisal of the evidence. *J Trauma.* 2004;57:1246–1255.
269. Ince H, Nienaber CA. Diagnosis and management of patients with aortic dissection. *Heart.* 2007;93:266–270.
270. Haidary A, Bis K, Vrachiolitis T, et al. Enhancement performance of a 64-slice triple rule-out protocol vs 16-slice and 10-slice multidetector CT-angiography protocols for evaluation of aortic and pulmonary vasculature. *J Comput Assist Tomogr.* 2007;31:917–923.
271. Iezzi R, Cotroneo AR, Marano R, et al. Endovascular treatment of thoracic aortic diseases: follow-up and complications with multi-detector computed tomography angiography. *Eur J Radiol.* 2008;65(3):365–376.
272. Nataf P, Lansac E. Dilation of the thoracic aorta: medical and surgical management. *Heart.* 2006;92:1345–1352.
273. Loewinger L, Budoff MJ. New advances in cardiac computed tomography. *Curr Opin Cardiol.* 2007;22:408–412.
274. Kamalakannan D, Rosman HS, Eagle KA. Acute aortic dissection. *Crit Care Clin.* 2007;23:779–800.
275. Erbel R, Alfonso F, Boileau C, et al. Diagnosis and management of aortic dissection. *Eur Heart J.* 2001;22:1642–1681.

276. Suzuki T, Mehta RH, Ince H, et al. Clinical profiles and outcomes of acute type B aortic dissection in the current era: lessons from the International Registry of Aortic Dissection (IRAD). *Circulation.* 2003;108(Suppl 1):II312–317.
277. Shiga T, Wajima Z, Apfel CC, et al. Diagnostic accuracy of transesophageal echocardiography, helical computed tomography, and magnetic resonance imaging for suspected thoracic aortic dissection: systematic review and meta-analysis. *Arch Intern Med.* 2006;166:1350–1356.
278. Davies RR, Goldstein LJ, Coady MA, et al. Yearly rupture or dissection rates for thoracic aortic aneurysms: simple prediction based on size. *Ann Thorac Surg.* 2002;73:17–27; discussion 27–28.
279. Isselbacher EM. Thoracic and abdominal aortic aneurysms. *Circulation.* 2005;111:816–828.
280. Nistri S, Basso C, Marzari C, et al. Frequency of bicuspid aortic valve in young male conscripts by echocardiogram. *Am J Cardiol.* 2005;96:718–721.
281. Ince H, Nienaber CA. Etiology, pathogenesis and management of thoracic aortic aneurysm. *Nat Clin Pract Cardiovasc Med.* 2007;4:418–427.
282. Greiss I, Ugolini P, Joyal M, et al. Ruptured aneurysm of the left sinus of Valsalva discovered 41 years after a decelerational injury. *J Am Soc Echocardiogr.* 2004;17:906–909.
283. Vereckei A, Vandor L, Halasz J, et al. Infective endocarditis resulting in rupture of sinus of Valsalva with a rupture site communicating with both the right atrium and right ventricle. *J Am Soc Echocardiogr.* 2004;17:995–997.
284. Vincelj J, Starcevic B, Sokol I, et al. Rupture of a right sinus of Valsalva aneurysm into the right ventricle during vaginal delivery: a case report. *Echocardiography.* 2005;22:844–846.
285. Vural KM, Sener E, Tasdemir O, et al. Approach to sinus of Valsalva aneurysms: a review of 53 cases. *Eur J Cardiothorac Surg.* 2001;20:71–76.
286. Shah RP, Ding ZP, Ng AS, et al. A ten-year review of ruptured sinus of valsalva: clinico-pathological and echo-Doppler features. *Singapore Med J.* 2001;42:473–476.
287. Smith RL, Irimpen A, Helmcke FR, et al. Ruptured congenital sinus of Valsalva aneurysm. *Echocardiography.* 2005;22:625–628.
288. Banerjee S, Jagasia DH. Unruptured sinus of Valsalva aneurysm in an asymptomatic patient. *J Am Soc Echocardiogr.* 2002;15:668–670.
289. Ott DA. Aneurysm of the sinus of Valsalva. *Semin Thorac Cardiovasc Surg Pediatr Card Surg Annu.* 2006: 165–176.
290. Patel ND, Williams JA, Barreiro CJ, et al. Valve-sparing aortic root replacement: early experience with the de paulis Valsalva graft in 51 patients. *Ann Thorac Surg.* 2006;82:548–553.
291. De Paulis R, Bassano C, Bertoldo F, et al. Aortic valve-sparing operations and aortic root replacement. *J Cardiovasc Med (Hagerstown).* 2007;8:97–101.
292. Ott DA. Aneurysm of the sinus of Valsalva. *Semin Thorac Cardiovasc Surg Pediatr Card Surg Annu.* 2006: 165–176.
293. Maraj R, Rerkpattanapipat P, Jacobs LE, et al. Meta-analysis of 143 reported cases of aortic intramural hematoma. *Am J Cardiol.* 2000;86:664–668.
294. Syed FF, Millar BC, Prendergast BD. Molecular technology in context: a current review of diagnosis and management of infective endocarditis. *Prog Cardiovasc Dis.* 2007;50:181–197.
295. Lester SJ, Wilansky S. Endocarditis and associated complications. *Crit Care Med.* 2007;35:S384–391.
296. Silverman ME, Upshaw CB Jr. Extracardiac manifestations of infective endocarditis and their historical descriptions. *Am J Cardiol.* 2007;100:1802–1807.
297. Erbel R, Rohmann S, Drexler M, et al. Improved diagnostic value of echocardiography in patients with infective endocarditis by transoesophageal approach. A prospective study. *Eur Heart J.* 1988;9: 43–53.
298. Mugge A, Daniel WG, Frank G, et al. Echocardiography in infective endocarditis: reassessment of prognostic implications of vegetation size determined by the transthoracic and the transesophageal approach. *J Am Coll Cardiol.* 1989;14:631–638.
299. Shively BK, Gurule FT, Roldan CA, et al. Diagnostic value of transesophageal compared with transthoracic echocardiography in infective endocarditis. *J Am Coll Cardiol.* 1991;18:391–397.
300. Daniel WG, Mugge A, Grote J, et al. Comparison of transthoracic and transesophageal echocardiography for detection of abnormalities of prosthetic and bioprosthetic valves in the mitral and aortic positions. *Am J Cardiol.* 1993;71:210–215.
301. Pedersen WR, Walker M, Olson JD, et al. Value of transesophageal echocardiography as an adjunct to transthoracic echocardiography in evaluation of native and prosthetic valve endocarditis. *Chest.* 1991;100: 351–356.
302. Reynolds HR, Jagen MA, Tunick PA, et al. Sensitivity of transthoracic versus transesophageal echocardiography for the detection of native valve vegetations in the modern era. *J Am Soc Echocardiogr.* 2003;16:67–70.
303. Alton ME, Pasierski TJ, Orsinelli DA, et al. Comparison of transthoracic and transesophageal echocardiography in evaluation of 47 Starr-Edwards prosthetic valves. *J Am Coll Cardiol.* 1992;20:1503–1511.
304. Zabalgoitia M, Herrera CJ, Chaudhry FA, et al. Improvement in the diagnosis of bioprosthetic valve dysfunction bytransesophageal echocardiography. *J Heart Valve Dis.* 1993;2:595–603.
305. Jaffe WM, Morgan DE, Pearlman AS, et al. Infective endocarditis, 1983–1988: echocardiographic findings and factors influencing morbidity and mortality. *J Am Coll Cardiol.* 1990;15:1227–1233.
306. Dodds GA, Sexton DJ, Durack DT, et al. Negative predictive value of the Duke criteria for infective endocarditis. *Am J Cardiol.* 1996;77:403–407.
307. Lowry RW, Zoghbi WA, Baker WB, et al. Clinical impact of transesophageal echocardiography in the diagnosis and management of infective endocarditis. *Am J Cardiol.* 1994;73:1089–1091.
308. Vieira ML, Grinberg M, Pomerantzeff PM, et al. Repeated echocardiographic examinations of patients with suspected infective endocarditis. *Heart.* 2004;90:1020–1024.
309. Bayer AS, Bolger AF, Taubert KA, et al. Diagnosis and management of infective endocarditis and its complications. *Circulation.* 1998;98:2936–2948.
310. American College of Cardiology/American Heart Association Task Force on Practice Guidelines, Society of Cardiovascular Anesthesiologists, Society for Cardiovascular Angiography and Interventions, et al. ACC/AHA 2006 guidelines for the management of patients with valvular heart disease: a report of the American College of Cardiology/American Heart Association Task Force on Practice Guidelines (writing committee to revise the 1998 Guidelines for the Management of Ppatients with Vlvular Heart Ddisease): developed in collaboration with the Society of Cardiovascular Anesthesiologists: endorsed by the Society for Cardiovascular Angiography and Interventions and the Society of Thoracic Surgeons. *Circulation.* 2006;114:e84–231.
311. Armstrong WF, Zoghbi WA. Stress echocardiography: current methodology and clinical applications. *J Am Coll Cardiol.* 2005;45:1739–1747.
312. Cerqueira MD, Weissman NJ, Dilsizian V, et al. Standardized myocardial segmentation and nomenclature for tomographic imaging of the heart. A statement for healthcare professionals from the Cardiac Imaging Committee of the Council on Clinical Cardiology of the American Heart Association. *Int J Cardiovasc Imaging.* 2002;18:539–542.
313. Voigt JU, Lindenmeier G, Exner B, et al. Incidence and characteristics of segmental postsystolic longitudinal shortening in normal, acutely ischemic, and scarred myocardium. *J Am Soc Echocardiogr.* 2003;16:415–423.
314. Vignon P. Hemodynamic assessment of critically ill patients using echocardiography Doppler. *Curr Opin Crit Care.* 2005;11:227–234.
315. Wilansky S, Moreno CA, Lester SJ. Complications of myocardial infarction. *Crit Care Med.* 2007;35:S348–354.
316. Raitt MH, Kraft CD, Gardner CJ, et al. Subacute ventricular free wall rupture complicating myocardial infarction. *Am Heart J.* 1993;126:946–955.
317. Mittle S, Makaryus AN, Mangion J. Role of contrast echocardiography in the assessment of myocardial rupture. *Echocardiography.* 2003;20: 77–81.
318. Bunch TJ, Oh JK, Click RL. Subepicardial aneurysm of the left ventricle. *J Am Soc Echocardiogr.* 2003;16:1318–1321.
319. Bybee KA, Kara T, Prasad A, et al. Systematic review: transient left ventricular apical ballooning: a syndrome that mimics ST-segment elevation myocardial infarction. *Ann Intern Med.* 2004;141:858–865.
320. Moursi MH, Bhatnagar SK, Vilacosta I, et al. Transesophageal echocardiographic assessment of papillary muscle rupture. *Circulation.* 1996;94: 1003–1009.
321. Birnbaum Y, Chamoun AJ, Conti VR, et al. Mitral regurgitation following acute myocardial infarction. *Coron Artery Dis.* 2002;13:337–344.
322. Hanlon JT, Conrad AK, Combs DT, et al. Echocardiographic recognition of partial papillary muscle rupture. *J Am Soc Echocardiogr.* 1993;6: 101–103.
323. Kinch JW, Ryan TJ. Right ventricular infarction. *N Engl J Med.* 1994;330: 1211–1217.
324. Goldberger JJ, Himelman RB, Wolfe CL, et al. Right ventricular infarction: recognition and assessment of its hemodynamic significance by two-dimensional echocardiography. *J Am Soc Echocardiogr.* 1991;4:140–146.
325. Manno BV, Bemis CE, Carver J, et al. Right ventricular infarction complicated by right to left shunt. *J Am Coll Cardiol.* 1983;1:554–557.
326. Li JS, Sexton DJ, Mick N, et al: Proposed modifications to the duke criteria for the diagnosis of infective endocarditis. *Clin Infect Dis.* 2000;30:633–638.
327. Schoepf UJ, Kucher N, Kipfmueller F, et al. Right ventricular enlargement on chest computed tomography: a predictor of early death in acute pulmonary embolism. *Circulation.* 2004;110:3276–3280.
328. van der Meer RW, Pattynama PM, van Strijen MJ, et al. Right ventricular dysfunction and pulmonary obstruction index at helical CT: prediction of clinical outcome during 3-month follow-up in patients with acute pulmonary embolism. *Radiology.* 2005;235:798–803.
329. Pruszczyk P, Bochowicz A, Torbicki A, et al. Cardiac troponin T monitoring identifies high-risk group of normotensive patients with acute pulmonary embolism. *Chest.* 2003;123:1947–1952.
330. Mehta NJ, Jani K, Khan IA. Clinical usefulness and prognostic value of elevated cardiac troponin I levels in acute pulmonary embolism. *Am Heart J.* 2003;145:821–825.

331. Punukollu G, Khan IA, Gowda RM, et al. Cardiac troponin I release in acute pulmonary embolism in relation to the duration of symptoms. *Int J Cardiol*. 2005;99:207–211.
332. Kucher N, Printzen G. Goldhaber SZ. Prognostic role of brain natriuretic peptide in acute pulmonary embolism. *Circulation*. 2003;107:2545–2547.
333. Binder L, Pieske B, Olschewski M, et al. N-terminal pro-brain natriuretic peptide or troponin testing followed by echocardiography for risk stratification of acute pulmonary embolism. *Circulation*. 2005;112:1573–1579.
334. Scridon T, Scridon C, Skali H, et al. Prognostic significance of troponin elevation and right ventricular enlargement in acute pulmonary embolism. *Am J Cardiol*. 2005;96:303–305.

CHAPTER 24 ■ TEMPERATURE MONITORING

TOSHIKI MIZOBE • DANIEL I. SESSLER

HISTORY

Well before the dawn of clinical thermometry, the temperature course of diseases such as malaria and enteric fever (typhoid and brucellosis) were well described in the *Corpus Hippocraticum* (circa 370–460 BC) (1). However, it wasn't until the 1590s when the astronomer Galileo invented the thermometer (or thermoscope) that humans could record temperature. His thermoscope was an open thermometer subject to atmospheric pressure. In 1612, Sanctorius of Justipolitanus at Padua first applied the thermometer to the human body. A major advance in temperature monitoring arrived in 1714 when Gabriel Fahrenheit invented the mercury thermometer (2). His scale, the Fahrenheit scale, was and remains commonly used in England and the United States. However, another scale, the Centigrade scale, invented by Anders Celsius in 1742, became popular in France and Germany. On the original Celsius scale, 0° was the temperature at which water boiled, while 100° was the temperature at which ice melted. Linnaeus reversed the scale in 1750.

Carl Reinhold Wunderlich developed the thermometer that was used clinically in medicine for over 130 years (3). It differed from previous ones in preserving the maximum temperature in any given session that, presumably, best represents core temperature. He published *Das Verhalten der Eigenwarme in Krankheiten* in 1868, in which he suggested that fever is not a disease, but rather a sign of disease. His thermometers were 22.5 cm long and took 20 minutes to register temperature. Measurements were made in the axilla with four to six daily observations made on patients with fever. After obtaining several million observations on approximately 25,000 patients, he established the fever patterns of diseases such as typhoid fever, various internal diseases, and pregnancy. He also established the average normal body temperature as 98.6°F (37°C). He concluded, "A physician who practiced medicine without employing the thermometer was like a blind man endeavoring to distinguish colors by feeling."

Wunderlich's findings were supported enthusiastically in Europe and in the United States. It was already recognized that thermometer use facilitated the recognition of diseases and allowed physicians to understand their natural progression. However, the curved and nonregistering thermometers then in use were so cumbersome that more portable instruments were required. With the size reduced by Wunderlich, clinical thermometry became a routine part of medical practice. By the 1860s, the axilla had become universally adopted as a convenient and reliable point of measurement. Once the use of alcohol and other germicidal agents became common in the late 1890s, sublingual placement replaced the axilla as the most popular measurement site.

In 1875 von Liebermeister first hypothesized that body temperature is regulated similarly in both healthy and ill people, but that fever occurs in illness because the body's internal thermostat is set to a higher temperature. Edward Seguin and William Draper introduced thermometry and patient charting in New York City hospitals in the mid-1860s. Medical thermometry quickly spread from hospitals to general practitioners, and from there to nurses and family. Mothers who could read a thermometer rendered invaluable service to their families in times of illness and provided important information for physicians. Seguin even concluded that thermometry is not only knowledge, but also social power.

TYPES OF THERMOMETERS

Mercury-in-glass Maximum

This familiar design consists of a mercury-filled bulb connected to a thin glass tube. As the body warms the mercury in the bulb, thermal expansion causes the mercury to move up the tube. After maximal thermal equilibrium is reached (which may require 4 minutes in the mouth and 10 minutes in the axilla), bulb temperature equals the body temperature. A constriction near the bulb holds the position of mercury when the thermometer is removed from the body, thus preserving the maximum temperature reading. After the thermometer is shaken to return mercury to the bulb, another measurement can be performed.

The advantages of mercury-in-glass thermometers are that they do not require electric power, accuracy is easily confirmed by calibration, and environmental conditions do not affect clinical measurements (4). The disadvantages of these thermometers include that they require a long equilibration time, they cannot be used orally except in cooperating adults, and they present a risk of mercury and glass exposure if damaged during storage and clinical use. For instance, about 1,600 glass thermometers were reported broken at a Glasgow Children's Hospital during a 6-month period. Spilled mercury disperses into tiny droplets that are difficult to see and easily become entrapped and emit a toxic vapor that can be inhaled or absorbed through the skin; the vapor may persist for months or even years (5).

Electronic Contact

A thermistor is an electrical resistor in which resistance changes rapidly in response to temperature fluctuation. In general, resistance decreases exponentially with increasing temperature. Electrical power is required for measuring the resistance and calibrating stored data in order to convert resistance data into temperature data. Thermocouples measure temperature by evaluating the tiny electrical potential (voltage) produced by the junction of two metals. Both thermistors and thermocouples are inexpensive, with a manufacturing cost as low as a few cents each, and are highly accurate. These thermometers are, by far, the most commonly used at present.

Most products display the maximum temperature and provide an audible tone when the temperature increase slows to 0.1°C in a preset time, generally in 8 seconds. Underreading occurs occasionally, especially when measuring axillary temperature where the dry skin requires a longer time to achieve thermal equilibrium with the sensor. Some devices provide a predictive mode that tracks the changing resistance to estimate the final temperature. This results in a rapid temperature reading within several seconds; however, accuracy is worse in the predictive mode than in the monitoring mode.

Infrared Aural Canal ("Tympanic")

Optical infrared emissions sensors can be used to measure surface temperature. Industrially, these devices are used to measure the temperature of objects that would be hard to otherwise measure, such as the temperature of molten steel. However, they are also used medically to measure skin temperature. The magnitude and spectrum of the infrared energy emitted depends on the local temperature, efficiency of the surface for radiating electromagnetic radiation (emissivity), filtering effect of any optical components, and sensor temperature. The resulting signal is converted into a temperature.

International standards permit a lower accuracy (±0.2°C) in laboratory testing of clinical infrared thermometers than the corresponding standards of conventional contact thermometers (±0.1°C). Even larger errors are permitted when the ambient temperature is out of normal room temperature, about 18°C to 26°C. Although rapid response is a major advantage of this type of device, users must ensure that the aural canal is not obscured by cerumen and that the ear canal is straightened by manipulating the ear lobe so that the sensor can point directly at deeper sections of the canal, which are nearer to the core temperature (6). Even though infrared aural canal thermometers are often labeled as "tympanic," they do not actually "see" the tympanic membrane but extrapolate tympanic or core temperature from the skin temperature in the aural canal.

SITES OF TEMPERATURE MEASUREMENT

The core thermal compartment is composed of well-perfused tissues with a temperature uniform and high compared with the rest of the body. Core temperature is considered the average temperature of the core compartment; it is not the highest temperature in the body, which is probably in the brain or liver. Core temperature can be evaluated in the pulmonary artery, distal esophagus, tympanic membrane, or nasopharynx. Even during rapid thermal perturbations (e.g., cardiopulmonary bypass), these temperature-monitoring sites remain reliable. Core temperature can be estimated with reasonable accuracy using oral, axillary, rectal, and bladder temperatures, except during extreme thermal perturbations (7,8).

1. Oral: The most common site of temperature measurement is probably under the tongue. Unfortunately, hot and cold drinks, open-mouth versus closed-mouth breathing, and tachypnea all affect oral temperature readings. However, nasogastric tubes do not interfere with oral temperature measurement (9–11). Carefully performed oral temperatures are reasonably accurate.
2. Axillary: Axillary temperature measurement is suited for intermittent monitoring, though the accuracy is worse than at other sites, probably due to probe positioning (7). Axillary measurements are, nonetheless, usually suitable if care is taken to position the probe over the axillary artery while keeping the arm at the patient's side.
3. Rectal: Rectal temperature measurement is most accurate when the sensor is placed more than 10 cm into the rectum. Rectal temperature correlates well with distal esophageal, bladder, and tympanic temperature, although it typically slightly exceeds core value. Also, it is the slowest to respond to rapid changes in body temperature (12). Consequently, rectal readings are often erroneous—sometimes by many degrees—during heat stroke, malignant hyperthermia, and other situations where core temperature changes rapidly. It is thus a poor choice when a purpose of monitoring is to detect rapid perturbations.
4. Tympanic: Actual tympanic membrane measurements, obtained with a thermocouple or thermistor, are highly accurate core temperatures (13). During induced hypothermia, tympanic temperature is much closer to brain temperature than other measurement sites (14).
5. Infrared aural canal: Infrared aural canal temperatures do not actually evaluate the tympanic membrane and are far less accurate. These measurements may be adequate when patients have wide ear canals (large circumference of the ear canal) and good visibility deep in the canal. However, values deviate considerably when hair or cerumen even partially occludes the canal—as is typical. Furthermore, fanning the face has been reported to lower the tympanic temperature. In general, infrared aural canal "tympanic" thermometers are insufficiently accurate for routine clinical measurements.
6. Distal esophageal: Distal esophageal temperature is an accurate monitoring site for core temperature when patients are anesthetized or sedated, particularly because this site is resistant to artifact (15). The most precise measurement is performed when the probe is 45 cm from the nose in adults. The temperature measurements taken in the proximal and midesophagus are influenced by the ambient air because they are near the trachea and bronchi. Transesophageal echocardiography (TEE) may affect the esophageal temperature because of the heat emitted by the probe.
7. Nasopharyngeal: Nasopharyngeal temperature monitoring is often performed during general anesthesia. The drawbacks of this site are that the measurements are affected by the probe position and that nasopharyngeal bleeding might occur. Nonetheless, it is an excellent site and usually

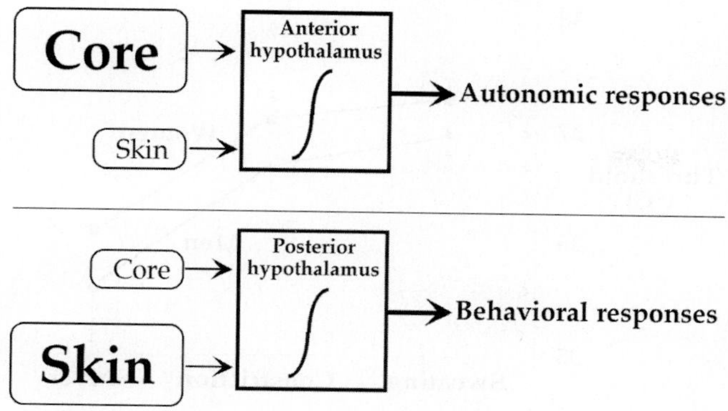

FIGURE 24.1. Control of autonomic and behavioral thermoregulatory defenses. Efferent defenses can be broadly divided into autonomic responses (e.g., sweating and shivering) and behavioral responses (e.g., closing a window, putting on a sweater). Autonomic responses depend largely on core temperature and are mediated largely by the anterior hypothalamus. In contrast, behavioral responses are mostly determined by skin temperature and are controlled by the posterior hypothalamus.

provides accurate and precise measurements of core temperature.

8. Urinary bladder: Urinary bladder temperature is measured by placing a probe in a Foley catheter. The measurement is affected by urinary flow during cardiopulmonary bypass and does not provide an accurate temperature measurement when urine flow is low (16). Under other circumstances, though, it is a reasonably accurate site.
9. Pulmonary artery: Pulmonary artery temperature is measured by a sensor located at the distal end of the balloon-tipped, flow-directed pulmonary artery catheter. It is generally considered the single, best core temperature measurement site, although obviously available in only a tiny fraction of patients. It is worth noting that brain temperature is slightly greater than pulmonary artery temperature, because core temperature at the pulmonary artery is the average value of the deep body structures. The gradient between core and brain temperatures tends to increase with fever and active cooling.

THERMOREGULATION

Precise control of core temperature is maintained by a powerful thermoregulatory system incorporating afferent inputs, central control, and efferent defenses. Efferent defenses can be broadly divided into autonomic responses (e.g., sweating and shivering) and behavioral responses (e.g., closing a window, putting on a sweater). Autonomic responses depend largely on core temperature and are mostly mediated by the anterior hypothalamus. In contrast, behavioral responses are roughly 50% determined by skin temperature and are controlled by the posterior hypothalamus (Fig. 24.1) (17,18).

Thermoregulation is maintained by feed-forward and feedback pathways. The signal from the cutaneous thermosensors detecting the change in environmental temperature is transmitted to the thermoregulatory center in the hypothalamus. The effectors receiving efferent signals from the thermoregulatory center control thermoregulatory homeostasis. Also, the deep thermosensors detecting the change in body temperature transmit the afferent signals to the center. Recent studies suggest that the feed-forward pathway may be more important than previously appreciated (Fig. 24.2).

Afferent Input

Dual detectors—cold sensors with myelinated A-delta fibers and warm sensors with unmyelinated C-fibers—exist in the subcutaneous layer of the skin. The peripheral temperature sensors are free nerve endings with no specialized structure. They differ in the temperature range over which they operate and in their responses to temperature change. The response curve of thermosensors for a constant temperature exhibits a maximal discharge frequency in the range of 25°C to 30°C for cold sensors and around 40°C for warm sensors (static response). Cold sensors react to cooling with a transient increase in activity (dynamic response) and are inhibited during warming (Fig. 24.3). Warm sensors demonstrate dynamic activation during a temperature increase and are inhibited during cooling.

The distribution density of cold sensors is several times greater than warm sensors in the skin. These peripheral sensors detect not only the body temperature, but also the environmental temperature. Most thermal input is conducted along the spinothalamic tracts, although both afferent and efferent thermal signals are diffusely distributed within the neuraxis. Interestingly, signals from nociceptive receptors are conducted along almost the same part of the spinothalamic tracts (19).

Thermosensors are also located in brain areas such as the hypothalamus, midbrain, and spinal cord, and in deep thoracic

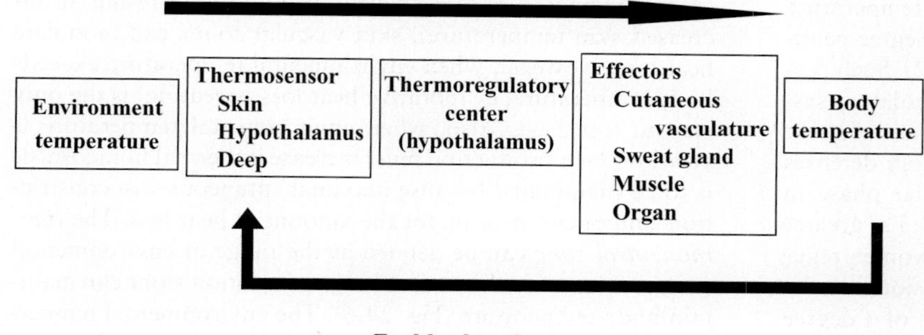

FIGURE 24.2. Signals from the cutaneous thermosensors detecting changes in environmental temperature are transmitted to the thermoregulatory center. The effectors that receive efferent signals control thermoregulatory homeostasis (feed-forward). Also, the deep thermosensors that detect changes in body temperature transmit the afferent signals to the central controller (feed-back).

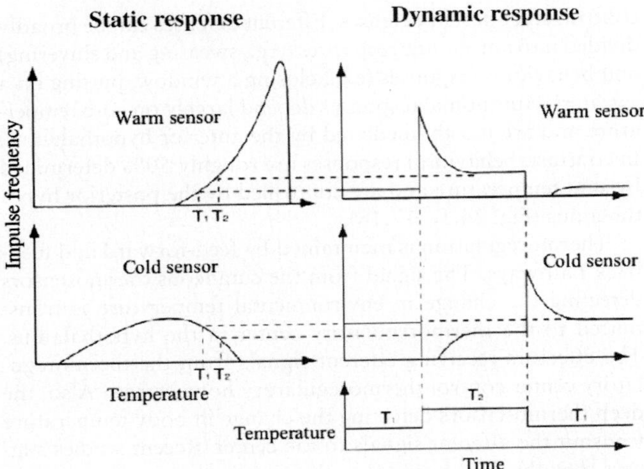

FIGURE 24.3. The response curve of thermosensors for a constant temperature exhibits a maximal discharge frequency in the range of 25°C to 30°C for cold sensors and around 40°C for warm sensors (static response). Cold sensors react to cooling with a transient increase in activity (dynamic response) and are inhibited during warming. Warm sensors demonstrate dynamic activation during a temperature increase and are inhibited during cooling (dynamic response). Change is seen in the impulse frequency while temperature turns from T1 to T2 and back to T1 again. (Modified from Hensel H. *Thermoreception and Temperature Regulation*. London: Academic Press; 1981.)

and abdominal tissues. These deep sensors detect core body temperature. The dynamic responses shown by peripheral thermosensors are not observed in the thermosensors in the brain. It is likely that there are also thermoreceptors in the thorax and abdomen, but their specific contributions in humans remain unknown.

Central Control

Thermal afferent signals are integrated at numerous levels within the neuraxis, including the spinal cord and brainstem. The hypothalamus is undoubtedly the dominant and most precise controller of body temperature, although the spinal cord dominates in birds. As there are few cold sensors in the hypothalamus, warm sensors are thought to send the stimulatory and inhibitory signals to the effectors.

Core temperature varies with a daily circadian rhythm (20). Normal temperature is altered slightly by factors such as age (0.5°C lower in the elderly), time of day (0.5°C higher in the afternoon), time of menstrual cycle in women (higher near ovulation), and exercise (21). Nonetheless, core temperature is normally controlled within a few tenths of a degree centigrade, virtually irrespective of the environment (22). Such precise control is maintained by a powerful thermoregulatory system incorporating afferent inputs, central control, and efferent defenses. The thresholds triggering thermoregulatory defenses are uniformly ~0.3°C greater during the follicular phase in women than in men (22), and are an additional ~0.5°C greater during the luteal phase (23). However, men and women regulate core body temperature with comparable precision, usually maintaining core temperature within a few tenths of a degree centigrade of the target temperature (Fig. 24.4).

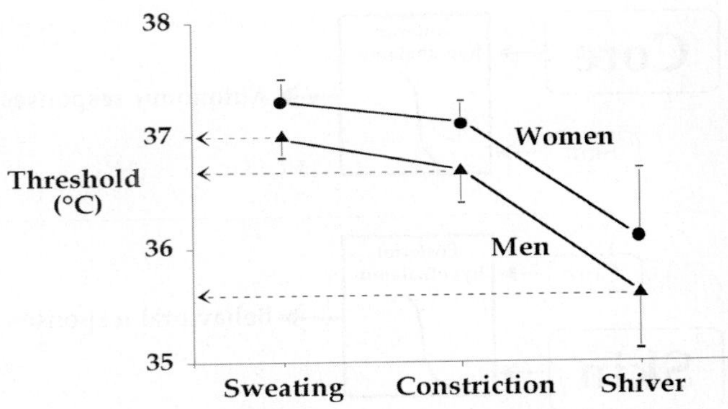

FIGURE 24.4. The thresholds (triggering core temperatures) for the three major autonomic thermoregulatory defenses: Sweating, vasoconstriction, and shivering. Temperatures between the sweating and vasoconstriction threshold define the interthreshold range (temperatures not triggering autonomic responses). The thresholds are uniformly about 0.3°C greater during the follicular phase in women than in men, and are an additional ≈0.5°C greater during the luteal phase. However, men and women regulate core body temperature with comparable precision. Results are presented as means ± standard deviation. (From Lopez M, Sessler DI, Walter K, et al. Rate and gender dependence of the sweating, vasoconstriction, and shivering thresholds in humans. *Anesthesiology.* 1994;80:780–788, with permission.)

Nonthermoregulatory cutaneous circulatory reflexes, including cardiopulmonary and arterial baroreceptor reflexes, modulate thermoregulatory vascular tone. The cardiopulmonary baroreceptor reflex controls peripheral vascular resistance in response to the change in blood volume through the central sympathetic nervous system and the renin–angiotensin pathway. The baroreceptor reflex is modified by the right atrial transmural pressure, which is the difference between central venous pressure and the intrathoracic pressure. Baroreflex loading by increased right atrial pressure in patients placed in the leg-up position results in an exaggeration of anesthesia-induced hypothermia because of attenuated peripheral vasoconstriction. In contrast, positive end-expiratory pressure (PEEP) ventilation decreases right atrial transmural pressure (RATP) and, as a consequence, attenuates perioperative hypothermia (Fig. 24.5) (24).

Efferent Responses

The balance between heat production and heat loss determines body temperature. Nonevaporative heat loss depends on the difference between skin temperature and environmental temperature. Given that skin blood flow is a primary determinant of skin temperature (e.g., increased blood flow results in increased skin temperature), skin vascular tonus can modulate heat loss. However, when environmental temperature exceeds body temperature, evaporative heat loss (sweating) is the only way to lose heat. Also, when environmental temperature is very low, heat production must increase if thermal homeostasis is to be maintained because maximal cutaneous vasoconstriction cannot compensate for the amount of heat loss. The *thermoneutral zone* can be defined as the range of environmental temperature over which cutaneous vasomotion alone can maintain body temperature (Fig. 24.6). The environmental temperature at which heat production increases—the lower critical

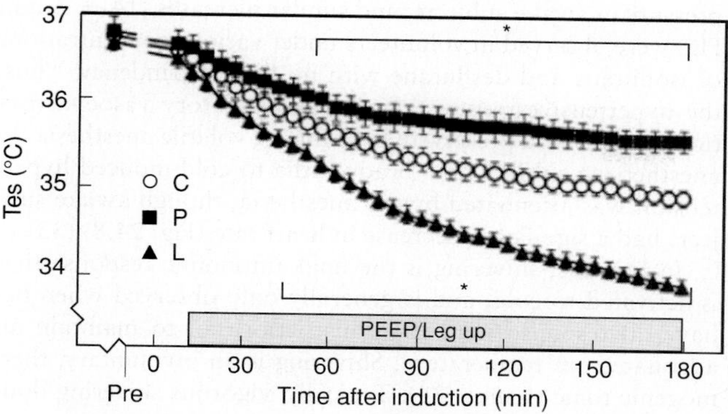

FIGURE 24.5. The esophageal temperature (Tes) after induction of anesthesia. Positive end-expiratory pressure (PEEP: 10 cm H_2O, P) or the leg-up position (*L*) was applied 10 minutes after induction of anesthesia. Baroreflex loading due to leg-up position exaggerates anesthesia-induced hypothermia because peripheral vasoconstriction is attenuated. Meanwhile, PEEP attenuated perioperative hypothermia because of stimulated vasoconstriction through baroreceptor unloading. Values are shown as mean ± standard of error. A significant difference compared with the control group (*C*). (From Nakajima Y, Mizobe T, Takamata A, et al. Baroreflex modulation of peripheral vasoconstriction during progressive hypothermia in anesthetized humans. *Am J Physiol Regul Integr Comp Physiol.* 2000;279:R1430–1436, with permission.)

temperature—is 29°C, while the temperature at which evaporative heat loss starts—the upper critical temperature—is 31°C.

Sweating is mediated by postganglionic cholinergic nerves that terminate on sweat follicles (25). These follicles apparently have no purpose other than thermoregulation. In this regard, they differ from most other thermoregulatory effectors that appear to have been co-opted by the thermoregulatory system but continue to play important roles, for example, vasomotion in blood pressure control or skeletal muscles in postural maintenance. Heat exposure can increase cutaneous water loss from trivial amounts to 500 mL per hour. Sweat loss in trained athletes can even exceed 1 L/hour. In a dry, convective environment, sweating can dissipate enormous amounts of heat—perhaps up to ten times the basal metabolic rate.

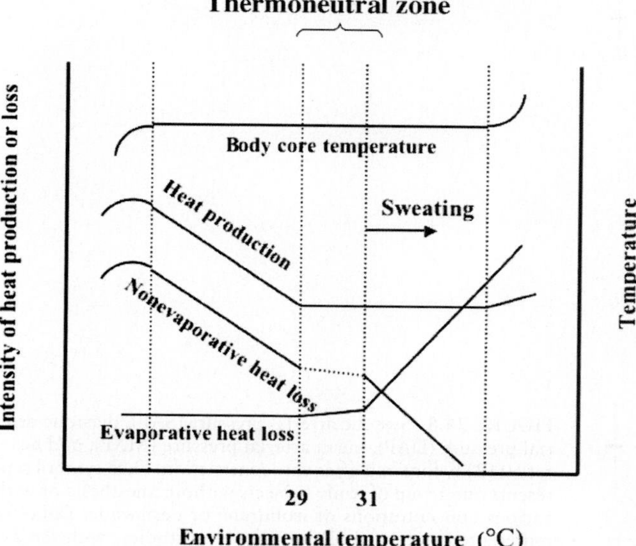

FIGURE 24.6. The thermoneutral zone is defined as the environmental temperature zone in which skin vascular tonus alone can maintain body temperature. The environmental temperature at which heat production increases (the lower critical temperature) is 29°C, while the temperature at which evaporative heat loss starts (the upper critical temperature) is 31°C.

As stated previously, sweating is the only mechanism by which the body can dissipate heat when environmental temperature exceeds core temperature. Fortunately, the process is remarkably effective, dissipating 0.58 kcal/g of evaporated sweat. Active precapillary vasodilation is mediated by a yet to be identified factor released from sweat glands and, thus, occurs synchronously with sweating. Recent evidence supports nitric oxide as the mediator of this response, although this theory remains controversial (26,27). Active dilation can increase cutaneous capillary flow enormously, perhaps to as much as 7.5 L/min (28). The purpose of this dilation, presumably, is to transport heat from muscles and the core to the skin surface where it can be dissipated to the environment by evaporation of sweat.

Cutaneous vasoconstriction is the first autonomic response to cold. Metabolic heat is lost primarily via convection and radiation from the skin surface, and vasoconstriction reduces this loss. Active arteriovenous shunt vasoconstriction is adrenergically mediated. The shunts are vessels 100 μm in diameter and convey 10,000 times as much blood as a comparable length of 10-μm capillaries (29). Anatomically, they are restricted to the fingers, toes, nose, and nipples. Despite this restriction, shunt vasoconstriction is among the most commonly used and important thermoregulatory defenses. The reason is that the blood traversing via shunts in the extremities must flow through the arms and legs, thus altering the heat content of these relatively large tissue masses. Local α-adrenergic sympathetic nerves mediate constriction in the thermoregulatory arteriovenous shunts, while *circulating* catecholamines only minimally affect flow. Roughly 10% of cardiac output traverses arteriovenous shunts; consequently, shunt vasoconstriction increases mean arterial pressure by approximately 15 mm Hg.

Thermoregulatory vasoconstriction reduces cutaneous heat loss. Although there is a major regional decrease in the distal extremities, these areas constitute a relatively small fraction of the body surface area. Nonetheless, heat loss does decrease throughout the extremities—including the proximal segments—because the entire limb cools when shunt flow is obliterated. In contrast, heat loss from the trunk decreases only slightly (Fig. 24.7). The overall reduction in heat loss that results from thermoregulatory vasoconstriction approximates 25%, which is similar to that provided by a single layer of most any insulator (30,31).

A major purpose of thermoregulatory vasoconstriction is to isolate core tissues from the environment, and thus restrict peripheral-to-core heat transfer. Normally, this is beneficial, but when patients are cooled therapeutically, thermoregulatory vasoconstriction slows transfer of heat from the skin surface to the core by trapping heat in peripheral tissues (32,33). The normal threshold (triggering core temperature) for vasoconstriction is approximately 36.5°C (22).

Thermoregulatory vasoconstriction affects blood pressure and heart rate. Vasoconstriction increases mean arterial

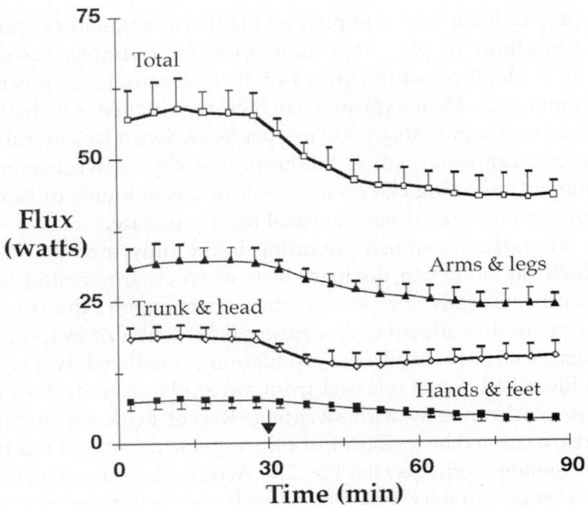

FIGURE 24.7. Cutaneous heat flux (heat loss) from the head and trunk (head, back, chest, and abdomen), legs and arms (upper arm, lower arm, thigh, and calf), and hands and feet. Total heat flux and flux from the arms and legs decreased about 25% after vasoconstriction was triggered by infusion of cold fluid at 30 elapsed minutes (*arrow*). Heat loss from the trunk and head decreased only 17%. In contrast, heat loss from the hands and feet decreased about 50%. Heat losses indicated in the lower three curves (arms and legs, trunk and head, hands and feet) comprise the total loss indicated at the top of the figure. Results are presented as means ± standard deviations. (From Sessler DI, Moayeri A, Støen R, et al. Thermoregulatory vasoconstriction decreases cutaneous heat loss. *Anesthesiology.* 1990;73:656–660.)

pressure in awake subjects, and similar increases (14 ± 5 mm Hg) were observed in volunteers under various concentrations of isoflurane and desflurane with no dose dependency. Thus, the hypertensive response to thermoregulatory vasoconstriction remains well preserved, even during volatile anesthesia. In anesthetized subjects, the bradycardia to cold-induced hypertension was attenuated by the anesthesia, though awake subjects had a significant decrease in heart rate (Fig. 24.8) (33).

In humans, shivering is the final autonomic response that is activated to cold, and is generally only observed when behavioral responses and vasoconstriction fail to maintain an adequate core temperature. Shivering is an involuntary, thermogenic tonic tremor (34). Typically, vigorous shivering doubles the metabolic rate (35,36), although greater increases can be sustained briefly. The shivering threshold is approximately 35.5°C (22), which is about 1°C less than the vasoconstriction threshold. The low shivering threshold suggests that this response is activated only under critical conditions, rather than being a preferred means of maintaining core temperature. Shivering begins with the pectoralis muscles, but most shivering thermogenesis occurs in the extremities where the largest muscles are located. The muscular activity of shivering does not perform any work, so all expended energy is converted into heat. However, the ability of shivering thermogenesis to protect core temperature is limited by two factors. The first is that active muscle must be supplied with oxygen and metabolic substrates, both of which are conveyed by blood. This need for blood flow in distal muscles counteracts the efforts of

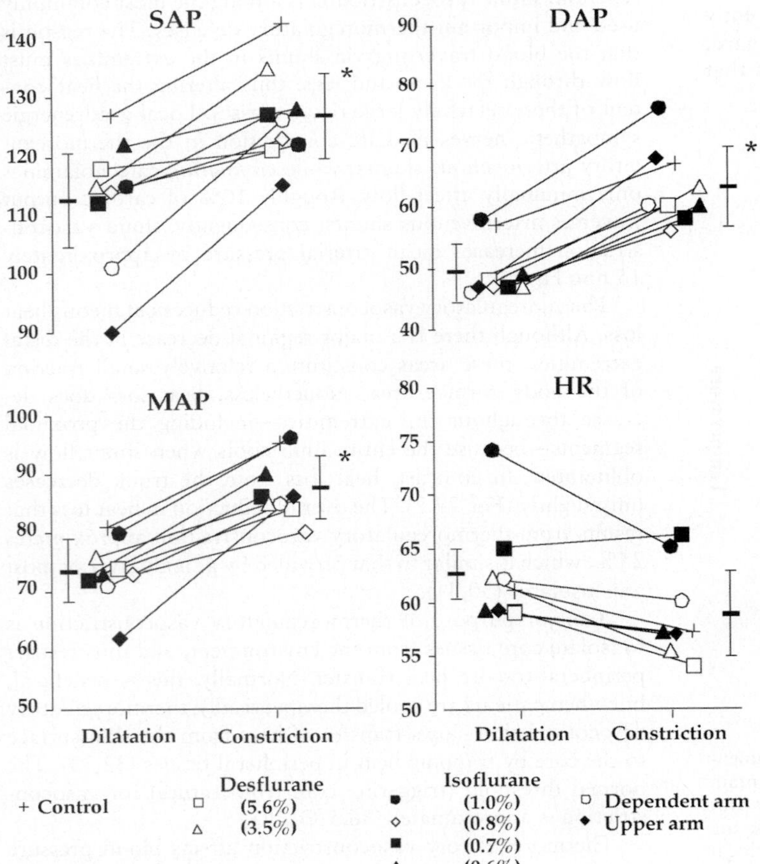

FIGURE 24.8. Systolic arterial pressure (SAP), diastolic arterial pressure (DAP), mean arterial pressure (MAP), and heart rate (HR) before and after vasoconstriction. Each symbol represents one group of study subjects without anesthesia or with various concentrations of isoflurane or desflurane. Data are represented as means of the individual studies, with the average and standard deviations for the entire study population also shown. Asterisks (∗) identify statistically significant differences from vasodilatation ($P < 0.001$). (From Greif R, Laciny S, Rajek A, et al. Blood pressure response to thermoregulatory vasoconstriction during isoflurane and desflurane anesthesia. *Acta Anaesthesiol Scand.* 2003;47:847–852, with permission.)

vasoconstriction to constrain metabolic heat to the core thermal compartment, and, thus, establishes a large core-to-peripheral tissue-temperature gradient. The second limitation of shivering is that most heat is generated peripherally, and thus easily dissipates to the environment.

An obvious consequence of shivering is increased metabolic rate. This increase, which is analogous to exercise, provokes a substantial adrenergic response. For example, a reduction in core temperature of only 0.7°C increases norepinephrine concentration by 400% and oxygen consumption by 30%. When core temperature decreases 1.3°C, norepinephrine concentration increases 700% and oxygen consumption doubles. As might be expected, shivering is associated with peripheral vasoconstriction and hypertension—although heart rate remains unchanged, as do plasma epinephrine and cortisol concentrations (37).

In general, energy-efficient effectors such as vasoconstriction are maximized before metabolically costly responses such as shivering are initiated. The interaction between thermal input, central control, and effector responses is shown in Figure 24.9; this figure also shows the normal values for the major autonomic response thresholds.

In the elderly, vasoconstriction in response to cold exposure is reduced (38), and it is likely that this is a clinically important observation because vasoconstriction is the primary autonomic response to cold exposure. Similarly, the shivering threshold is significantly reduced in the elderly (39). Interestingly, abnormally reduced thresholds were not apparent in subjects less than 80 years of age, and even then only occurred in a fraction of the population (Fig. 24.10). These data suggest that age-related thermoregulatory impairment may not be common in people younger than 80 years. The data further suggest that impairment is not a linear function of age, but instead occurs unpredictably in a fraction of the elderly population.

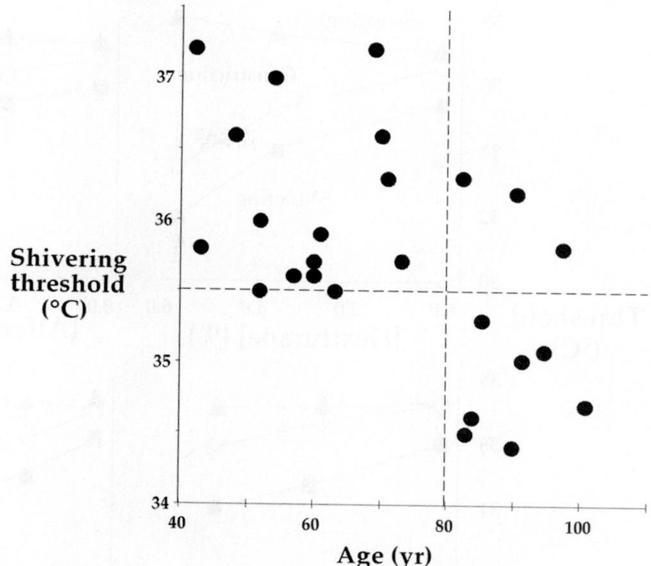

FIGURE 24.10. The effect of aging on the shivering threshold. Fifteen patients less than 80 years old (58 ± 10 years) (mean ± standard deviation) shivered at 36.1 ± 0.6°C; in contrast, ten patients aged 80 years or older (89 ± 7 years) shivered at a significantly lower mean temperature, 35.2 ± 0.8°C ($P < 0.001$). The shivering thresholds in seven of the ten patients 80 years or older was less than 35.5°C, whereas the threshold equaled or exceeded this value in all the younger patients. (From Vassilieff N, Rosencher N, Sessler DI, et al. The shivering threshold during spinal anesthesia is reduced in the elderly. *Anesthesiology.* 1995;83:1162–1166, with permission.)

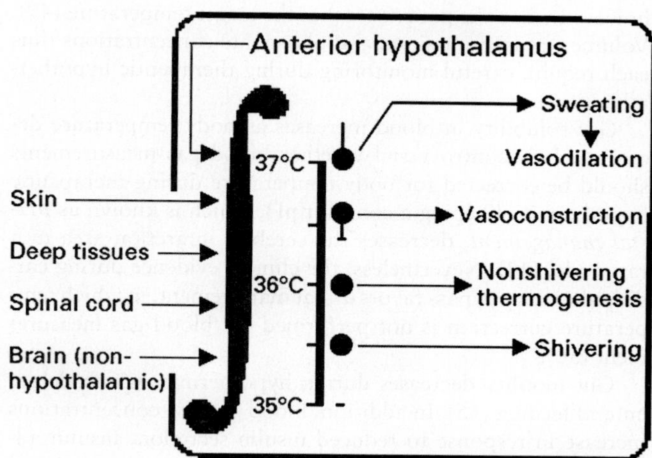

FIGURE 24.9. A schematic illustrating thermoregulatory control mechanisms. Mean body temperature is the integrated thermal input from a variety of tissues including the brain, skin surface, spinal cord, and deep core structures. These are shown entering the hypothalamus (*large square*) from the left. However, thresholds usually are expressed in terms of core temperature. A core temperature below the thresholds for response to cold provokes vasoconstriction, nonshivering thermogenesis, and shivering. Core temperature exceeding the hyperthermic thresholds produces active vasodilation and sweating. No thermoregulatory responses are initiated when core temperature is between these thresholds; these temperatures identify the interthreshold range. The interthreshold range in humans is usually only about 0.2°C. (Threshold data from Lopez M, Sessler DI, Walter K, et al. Rate and gender dependence of the sweating, vasoconstriction, and shivering thresholds in humans. *Anesthesiology.* 1994;80:780–788. Figure from Sessler DI. Perioperative hypothermia. *N Engl J Med.* 1997;336:1730–1737, with permission.)

The most powerful inhibitors of thermoregulation are general anesthetics. These drugs have been used to facilitate the induction of hypothermia for cardiac surgery and during neurosurgery. In sufficient doses, especially when combined with neuromuscular blockers, anesthetics can essentially obliterate defenses against hypothermia. Volatile anesthetics, such as desflurane and sevoflurane, have relatively little effect on sweating: Even full anesthetic doses increase the sweating threshold by only about 0.5°C. In contrast, anesthetic gases markedly reduce the vasoconstriction and shivering thresholds. Interestingly, the threshold for each major cold defense is reduced synchronously, as if they are similarly controlled (Fig. 24.11).

Neuromuscular blockers are not believed to have any effect on central control of thermoregulatory responses. However, they obviously cause paralysis and thus prevent shivering. It is equally obvious that muscle relaxants can only be given in the context of general anesthesia or substantial sedation, and that paralyzed patients require mechanical ventilation. Muscle relaxants are a suitable treatment for shivering in the intensive care unit (40), but are not a substitute for adequate sedation and appropriate thermal management.

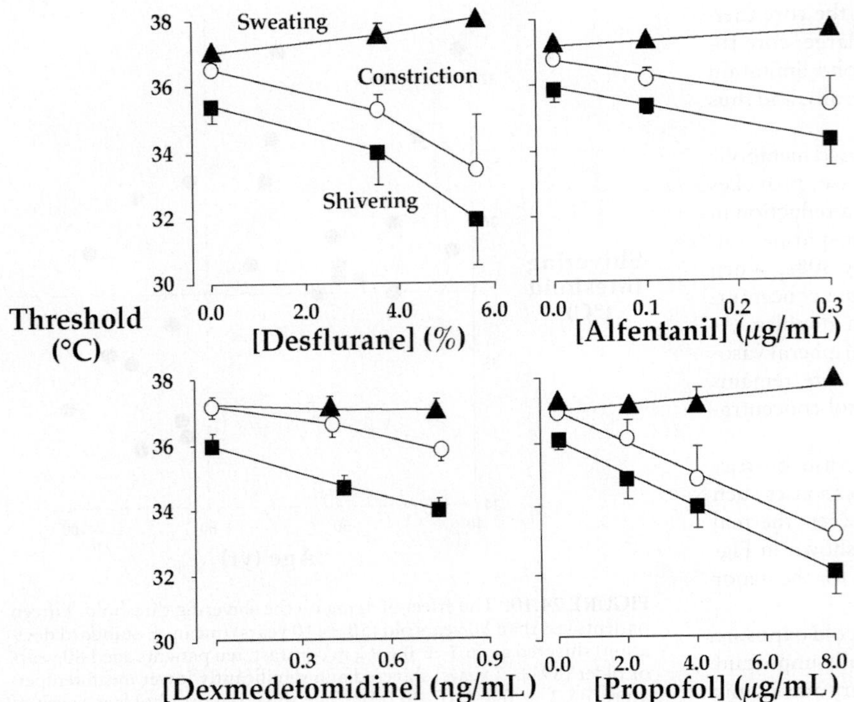

FIGURE 24.11. Concentration-dependent thermoregulatory inhibition by desflurane and isoflurane (halogenated volatile anesthetics), propofol (an intravenous anesthetic), and alfentanil (a μ-agonist opioid). General anesthetics are the most powerful known inhibitors of thermoregulatory control. The horizontal axis, in each case, spans a clinically relevant concentration range. The sweating (*triangles*), vasoconstriction (*circles*), and shivering (*squares*) thresholds are expressed in terms of core temperature at a designated mean skin temperature of 34°C. Anesthesia linearly, but slightly, increases the sweating threshold. In contrast, anesthesia produces substantial and comparable linear or nonlinear decreases in vasoconstriction and shivering thresholds. Typical anesthetic concentrations thus increase the interthreshold range (difference between the sweating and vasoconstriction thresholds) approximately 20-fold from its normal value near 0.2°C. Patients do not activate autonomic thermoregulatory defenses unless body temperature exceeds the interthreshold range; surgical patients are thus poikilothermic over a 3°C to 5°C range of core temperatures. Isoflurane 1% and desflurane 6% have comparable anesthetic potency. Error bars smaller than the data markers have been deleted. (From Sessler DI. Perioperative hypothermia. *N Engl J Med.* 1997;336:1730–1737, with permission.)

THERAPEUTIC HYPOTHERMIA

Systemic Consequences of Hypothermia

Patients undergoing mild hypothermia exhibit decreased heart rate, increased systemic vascular resistance, and normal stroke volume; consequently, mean arterial blood pressure in these patients remains normal (41). The electrocardiogram of hypothermic patients often displays a notch on the downstroke of the QRS complex (the Osborn wave) when core temperature reaches 33°C (42). However, cardiac arrhythmias are rarely seen during therapeutic hypothermia, even in patients with myocardial ischemia (43).

Overall, hypothermia has little effect on the respiratory system. Minute ventilation decreases during therapeutic hypothermia, but $PaCO_2$ remains normal since the metabolic rate decreases as well (44). Although pneumonia is listed as one of the major risk factors of hypothermia, it is relatively uncommon in adult patients subjected to short-term (12–24 hours) therapeutic hypothermia (43).

The number of leukocytes decreases and becomes less effective during hypothermia, a situation that could increase the incidence of infection, especially pneumonia (45). Prolonged hypothermia also decreases the number and function of platelets and delays clotting time, thus increasing the risk of hemorrhage (46).

During induction of therapeutic hypothermia, potassium shifts from the plasma into cells, resulting in hypokalemia. However, caution should be used in correcting this condition because during rewarming, the shift of potassium back into the plasma might lead to life-threatening hyperkalemia. Phosphate concentration decreases similarly (47,48). Urine output increases at induction of hypothermia as a result of decreased reabsorption in the ascending loop of Henle. It normalizes, however, when the patient reaches the target temperature (49). Volume status, potassium, and phosphate concentrations thus each require careful monitoring during therapeutic hypothermia.

Gas solubility in blood increases as body temperature decreases. It is controversial whether blood gas measurements should be corrected for body temperature during therapeutic hypothermia. Keeping a constant pH, which is known as *pH-stat management*, decreases the cerebral infarction area in a rat model (44). Nevertheless, the clinical evidence during cardiopulmonary bypass favors α-stat management, in which temperature correction is not performed for blood gas measurement (50).

Gut motility decreases during hypothermia, which delays enteral feeding (45). In addition, blood glucose concentrations increase in response to reduced insulin secretion. Insulin administration is recommended to correct hypothermia-induced hyperglycemia, and should probably be titrated to maintain a blood glucose concentration between 80 and 110 mg/dL (51,52).

Pathology of Cerebral Ischemia and Mechanism of Therapeutic Hypothermia

Cerebral injury occurs if inadequate blood flow to the brain occurs for more than 5 minutes (53). Cerebral ischemia produces a "whole-system failure" including adenosine triphosphate (ATP) energy depletion, ion pump failure, release of free radicals and excitotoxic neurotransmitters, and modulators such as

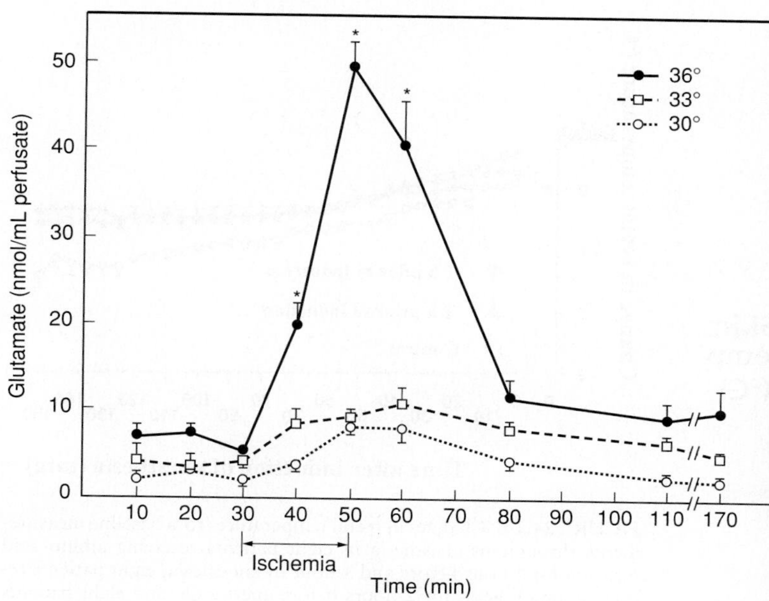

FIGURE 24.12. Time course of changes in striatal microdialysis-perfusate levels of glutamate in rats subjected to a 20-minute global forebrain ischemia by four-vessel occlusion at intraischemic brain temperatures of 30°C, 33°C, or 36°C. In normothermic rats, a massive extracellular release of glutamate was triggered by the ischemic insult, while in animals with hypothermic brain temperatures (33°C or 30°C), glutamate release was almost entirely suppressed. (From Busto R, Globus MY-T, Dietrich WD, et al. Effect of mild hypothermia on ischemia-induced release of neurotransmitters and free fatty acids in rat brain. *Stroke*. 1989;20:904–910, with permission.)

glutamate and calcium (54,55). The formation of free radicals and release of glutamate into the extracellular space are proportional to the intraischemic brain temperature (Fig. 24.12). Hyperthermia stimulates *N*-methyl-D-aspartate receptors, which increase intracellular calcium levels and enhance the free radicals resulting from the release of arachidonic acid (56,57).

Therapeutic Window

Anoxic brain injury is mainly proportional to the duration of ischemia, with death occurring within about 5 minutes of complete anoxia. Therefore, many physicians believe that hypothermia must be induced as early as possible. In other words, the earlier therapeutic hypothermia is started and the target temperature is reached, the greater the chance of a positive outcome (58,59).

The recommended duration for therapeutic hypothermia is 12 to 24 hours in the postresuscitation period. It is also reported that patients obtain best outcomes when therapeutic hypothermia is maintained between 48 and 72 hours (60,61). There is a consensus—although not evidence based—that patients should be very slowly rewarmed from therapeutic hypothermia.

FEVER

Hyperthermia is a generic term simply indicating a core body temperature exceeding normal values. In contrast, fever is a regulated increase in the core temperature targeted by the thermoregulatory system. Hyperthermia can result from a variety of causes and usually indicates a problem of sufficient severity that physician intervention is required. Fever is a special type of regulated hyperthermia that synchronously increases all thermoregulatory response thresholds. Fever thus represents an increase in the body's temperature set point. Fever is common among patients with neurologic injury and is associated with worse outcome from stroke, although fever probably improves infectious outcomes (62,63).

Normal body temperature is neither set nor maintained by circulating factors. In contrast, fever results when endogenous pyrogens increase the thermoregulatory target temperature ("set point"). Identified endogenous pyrogens include interleukin-1, tumor necrosis factor, interferon-α, and macrophage inflammatory protein-1 (64). Although it was initially believed that these factors acted directly on hypothalamic thermoregulatory centers, there is increasing evidence for a more complicated system involving vagal afferents. Most endogenous pyrogens have peripheral actions (e.g., immune system activation) in addition to their central generating capabilities (65,66).

Optimal treatment strategies for fever have yet to be established. Although active surface cooling of febrile patients makes intuitive sense, it is often either ineffective or counterproductive. This is principally because the febrile target set by the hypothalamus is in terms of *mean body* temperature, not core temperature. Weighted mean body temperature (for thermoregulatory purposes) is a linear combination of core and skin temperatures, with the skin contributing approximately 20% (67). A decreasing skin temperature of 4°C will thus *increase* the target core temperature by about 1°C. In intact patients, thermoregulatory defenses are more powerful than most types of surface cooling. The result is that active cooling fails to reduce core temperature, but does make patients highly uncomfortable, increases plasma catecholamine concentrations, augments metabolic rate, and provokes hypertension (Fig. 24.13) (68). However, in patients with restricted thermoregulatory defenses, surface cooling is an effective treatment for fever (69,70). The general strategy, then, is to distinguish active fever from passive hyperthermia. In the case of fever, treat the underlying fever source whenever possible because active cooling provokes considerable stress and usually is not particularly effective. In cases where hyperthermia appears passive or results from excessive heat production, simple cooling measures will usually be effective.

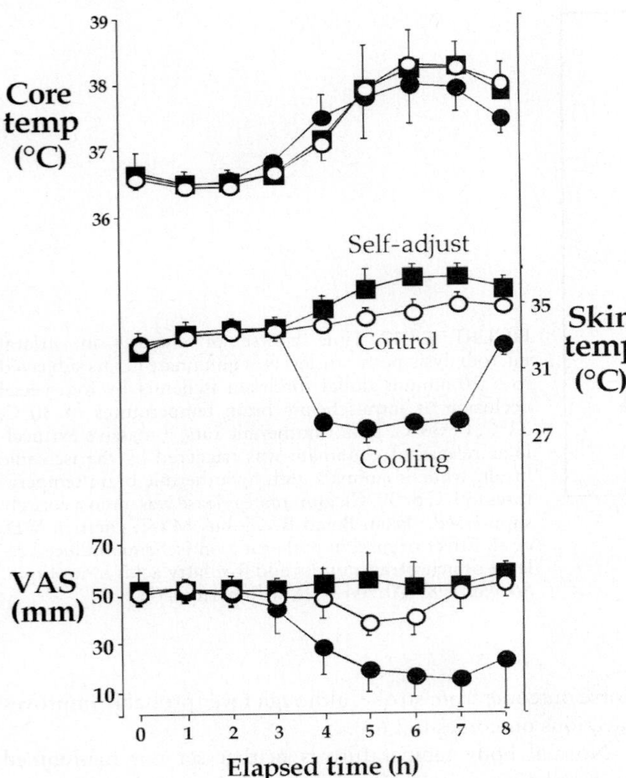

FIGURE 24.13. Change in core and skin temperature and thermal comfort after fever was induced by administration of interleukin-2, starting at elapsed time zero. The designated thermal management started after 3 elapsed hours and continued for 5 hours. This consisted of no treatment (control), self-adjustment per the subjects' comfort (self-adjust), and forced-air cooling (cooling). Thermal comfort is reported as millimeters on a visual analog scale (VAS), with 0 mm indicating the worst imaginable cold, 50 mm identifying thermoneutrality, and 100 mm being the worst imaginable heat. Active cooling made the subjects feel miserably cold, but did not reduce core temperature. Data are presented as means ± standard deviations. (From Lenhardt R, Negishi C, Sessler DI, et al. The effects of physical treatment on induced fever in humans. *Am J Med.* 1999;106:550–555, with permission.)

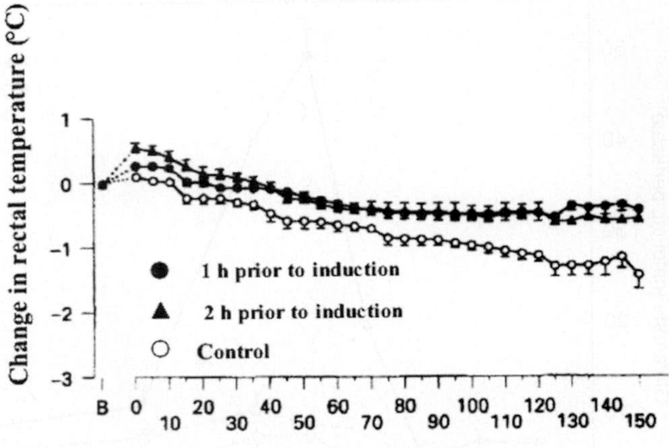

FIGURE 24.14. Changes in rectal temperature from baseline measurements throughout anesthesia in eight patients receiving amino acid infusion for 1 hour before and 1 hour of anesthesia, eight patients receiving amino acids for 2 hours before anesthesia, and eight patients receiving a nutrient-free saline solution for 1 hour before and 1 hour of anesthesia. Vertical bars = standard error of mean. (From Sellden E, Branstrom R, Brundin T. Preoperative infusion of amino acids prevent postoperative hypothermia. *Br J Anaesth.* 1996;76:227–234, with permission.)

DIET-INDUCED THERMOGENESIS

The increase in energy expenditure after the ingestion of a meal or infusion of nutrients has been referred to as dietary-induced or nutrient-induced thermogenesis. The thermogenesis induced by protein or amino acids is known to be largest and most prolonged. An intravenous infusion of 600 kJ (35 g) of amino acids increases energy expenditure in awake, healthy volunteers by 20%, and thus increases temperature of blood in the hepatic artery and vein by 0.3°C (71). In patients under general anesthesia for lower abdominal surgery, the continuous infusion of amino acids (240 kJ/hour) for 2 hours keeps core temperature about 0.3°C/hour greater than in patients not receiving the infusion (Fig. 24.14) (72). Furthermore, a continuous infusion at a rate of 4 kJ/kg/hour, for 2 hours before induction of spinal anesthesia, prevents hypothermia (Fig. 24.15) (73). Recently, a perioperative amino acid infusion at a rate of 4 kJ/kg/hour for 4 hours has been shown to increase the esophageal temperature at the end of surgery by 0.6°C, in addition to shortening the artificial ventilation period, intensive care unit (ICU) stay, and hospital stay after off-pump coronary artery bypass grafting (74).

Fructose is also known to elicit the greatest thermogenesis among the various carbohydrates that have been tested. Oral intake of 75 g fructose in awake healthy volunteers increases arterial blood temperature by more than 0.2°C (75). A continuous infusion of fructose, at a rate of 0.5 g/kg/hour for 4 hours in patients during general anesthesia for lower abdominal surgery, increased esophageal temperature at 3 hours after induction by 0.6°C. Fructose also increases the metabolic rate by approximately 20%, which is presumably the mechanism by which it increases body temperature (Fig. 24.16) (76).

SUMMARY

The signal from the cutaneous thermosensors detecting the change in environmental temperature is transmitted to the thermoregulatory center in the hypothalamus, which, in turn, controls efferent defenses. The thermoneutral zone can be defined as the range of environmental temperature over which cutaneous vasomotion alone can maintain body temperature, and ranges from roughly 29°C to 31°C.

Cutaneous vasoconstriction is the first autonomic response to cold. The normal threshold (triggering core temperature) for vasoconstriction is about 36.5°C. Shivering is the final autonomic response that is activated to cold and is generally only observed when behavioral responses and vasoconstriction fail to maintain an adequate core temperature. Vigorous shivering doubles the metabolic rate. The shivering threshold is approximately 35.5°C.

Patients undergoing mild hypothermia exhibit decreased heart rate, increased systemic vascular resistance, normal mean

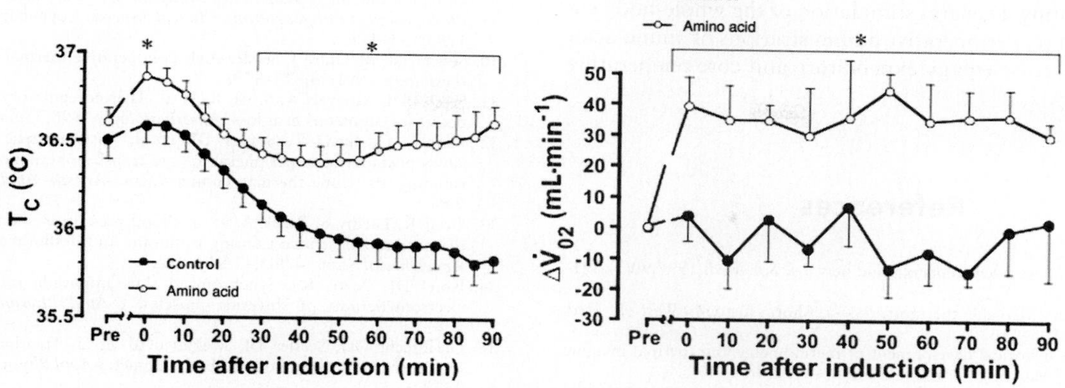

FIGURE 24.15. Change in tympanic membrane core temperature (Tc) during spinal anesthesia. Tc values at 0 minutes and after 30 minutes were significantly greater in the amino acid infusion group than the saline group. Data are presented as means ± standard error of mean. "Pre" indicates the period of pre–amino acid infusion. Asterisks (*) indicate a statistically significant difference between the groups ($P < 0.05$). (From Kasai T, Nakajima Y, Matsukawa T, et al. Effect of preoperative amino acid infusion on thermoregulatory response during spinal anaesthesia. *Br J Anaesth.* 2003;90:58–61, with permission.)

blood pressure, and stroke volume. Minute ventilation decreases during therapeutic hypothermia, but $PaCO_2$ remains normal because of the decreased metabolic rate. The number of leukocytes decreases. Prolonged hypothermia also decreases the number and function of platelets. During induction of therapeutic hypothermia, potassium shifts from the plasma into cells, resulting in hypokalemia. Conversely, during rewarming, the shift of potassium back into the plasma may lead to life-threatening hyperkalemia. Urine output increases at induction of hypothermia. Gut motility decreases during hypothermia, which delays enteral feeding. Blood glucose concentrations increase in response to reduced insulin secretion.

Thermoregulatory control is based on the integrated temperatures from tissues throughout the body, not just core temperature. Skin temperature contributes approximately 20% to thermoregulatory control. Decreasing skin temperature by 4°C will thus *increase* the target core temperature by about 1°C. In intact patients, thermoregulatory defenses are more powerful than most types of surface cooling. The result is that active cooling fails to reduce core temperature, but does make patients highly uncomfortable, increases plasma catecholamine concentrations, augments metabolic rate, and provokes hypertension. However, in patients with restricted thermoregulatory defenses, surface cooling is an effective treatment for fever.

Peripheral vasoconstriction plays a major role in the thermoregulatory response to reduced body temperature. The first response to cold is vasoconstriction, which reduces heat loss from the skin surface. Therefore, the change in cutaneous circulation in a nonthermoregulatory reflex, such as the baroreceptor reflex, interacts with the thermoregulatory vasoconstriction.

After the ingestion or infusion of nutrients, there is an increase in energy expenditure, which has been referred to as *dietary- or nutrient-induced thermogenesis*. This thermic effect of nutrition is divided into an obligatory component, representing the theoretically metabolic costs for the processing and

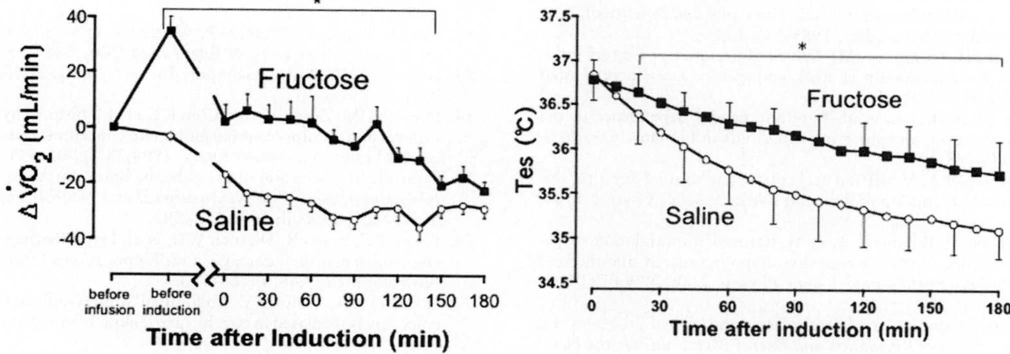

FIGURE 24.16. Core temperature measured at the distal esophagus (Tes) during surgery. Patients receiving the fructose infusion had significantly greater core temperatures than those receiving saline ($^*P = 0.001$), starting 20 minutes after induction of anesthesia until the end of the monitoring period (180 minutes after induction). Data are presented as mean ± standard deviation for ten patients in each group. (From Mizobe T, Nakajima Y, Ueno H, et al. Fructose administration increases intraoperative core temperature by augmenting both metabolic rate and the vasoconstriction threshold. *Anesthesiology.* 2006;104:1124–1130, with permission.)

storage of the nutrients ingested, and the facultative component, representing a general stimulation of the whole-body energy expenditure. Perioperative administrations of amino acids or fructose increase energy expenditure and core temperature during surgery.

References

1. Blumenthal I. Fever—concepts old and new. *J R Soc Med.* 1997;90(7):391–394.
2. Haller JS Jr. Medical thermometry—a short history. *West J Med.* 1985;142(1):108–116.
3. Ring EF. The historical development of thermometry and thermal imaging in medicine. *J Med Eng Technol.* 2006;30(4):192–198.
4. Smith LS. Reexamining age, race, site, and thermometer type as variables affecting temperature measurement in adults—a comparison study. *BMC Nurs.* 2003;2:1.
5. Blumenthal I. Should we ban the mercury thermometer? *J Royal Soc Med.* 1992;85:553.
6. Daanen HA. Infrared tympanic temperature and ear canal morphology. *J Med Eng Technol.* 2006;30(4):224–234.
7. Cork RC, Vaughan RW, Humphrey LS. Precision and accuracy of intraoperative temperature monitoring. *Anesth Analg.* 1983;62(2):211–214.
8. Bissonnette B, Sessler DI, LaFlamme P. Intraoperative temperature monitoring sites in infants and children and the effect of inspired gas warming on esophageal temperature. *Anesth Analg.* 1989;69(2):192–196.
9. Erickson R. Thermometer placement for oral temperature measurement in febrile adults. *Int J Nurs Stud.* 1976;13(4):199–208.
10. Heinz J. Validation of sublingual temperatures in patients with nasogastric tubes. *Heart Lung.* 1985;14(2):128–130.
11. Tandberg D, Sklar D. Effect of tachypnea on the estimation of body temperature by an oral thermometer. *N Engl J Med.* 1983;308(16):945–946.
12. Ramsey JG, Ralley FE, Whalley DG. Site of temperature monitoring and prediction of afterdrop after open heart surgery. *Can Anaesth Soc J.* 1985; 32:607–615.
13. Benzinger M. Tympanic thermometry in surgery and anesthesia. *JAMA.* 1969;209(8):1207–1211.
14. Shiraki K, Sagawa S, Tajima F, et al. Independence of brain and tympanic temperatures in an unanesthetized human. *J Appl Physiol.* 1988;65(1):482–486.
15. Crocker BD, Okumura F, McCuaig DI, et al. Temperature monitoring during general anaesthesia. *Br J Anaesth.* 1980;52(12):1223–1229.
16. Lilly JK, Boland JP, Zekan S. Urinary bladder temperature monitoring: a new index of body core temperature. *Crit Care Med.* 1980;8(12):742–744.
17. Satinoff E. Neural organization and evolution of thermal regulation in mammals—several hierarchically arranged integrating systems may have evolved to achieve precise thermoregulation. *Science.* 1978;201:16–22.
18. Satinoff E, Rutstein J. Behavioral thermoregulation in rats with anterior hypothalamic lesions. *J Comp Physiol Psychol.* 1970;71:77–82.
19. Kosaka M, Simon E, Walther O-E, et al. Response of respiration to selective heating of the spinal cord below partial transection. *Experientia.* 1969; 25:36–37.
20. Mistlberger T, Rusak B. Mechanisms and models of the circadian time keeping system. In: Kryger MH, Dement WC, eds. *Principles and Practice of Sleep Medicine.* Philadelphia: WB Saunders; 1989:141–152.
21. Crawford DC, Hicks B, Thompson MJ. Which thermometer? Factors influencing best choice for intermittent clinical temperature assessment. *J Med Eng Technol.* 2006;30(4):199–211.
22. Lopez M, Sessler DI, Walter K, et al. Rate and gender dependence of the sweating, vasoconstriction, and shivering thresholds in humans. *Anesthesiology.* 1994;80:780–788.
23. Stephenson LA, Kolka MA. Menstrual cycle phase and time of day alter reference signal controlling arm blood flow and sweating. *Am J Physiol.* 1985; 249:R186–191.
24. Nakajima Y, Mizobe T, Takamata A, et al. Baroreflex modulation of peripheral vasoconstriction during progressive hypothermia in anesthetized humans. *Am J Physiol Regul Integr Comp Physiol.* 2000;279(4):R1430–1436.
25. Brück K. Thermoregulation: control mechanisms and neural processes. In: Sinclair JC, ed. *Temperature Regulation and Energy Metabolism in the Newborn.* New York: Grune & Stratton; 1978:157–185.
26. Warren JB. Nitric oxide and human skin blood flow responses to acetylcholine and ultraviolet light. *FASEB J.* 1994;8:247–251.
27. Hall DM, Buettner GR, Matthes RD, et al. Hyperthermia stimulates nitric oxide formation: electron paramagnetic resonance detection of .NO-heme in blood. *J Appl Physiol.* 1994;77:548–553.
28. Detry J-MR, Brengelmann GL, Rowell LB, et al. Skin and muscle components of forearm blood flow in directly heated resting man. *J Appl Physiol.* 1972;32:506–511.
29. Hales JRS. Skin arteriovenous anastomoses, their control and role in thermoregulation. In: Johansen K, Burggren W, eds. *Cardiovascular Shunts: Phylogenetic, Ontogenetic and Clinical Aspects.* Copenhagen: Munksgaard; 1985:433–451.
30. Sessler DI, McGuire J, Sessler AM. Perioperative thermal insulation. *Anesthesiology.* 1991;74:875–879.
31. Sessler DI, Moayeri A, Støen R, et al. Thermoregulatory vasoconstriction decreases cutaneous heat loss. *Anesthesiology.* 1990;73:656–660.
32. Plattner O, Ikeda T, Sessler DI, et al. Postanesthetic vasoconstriction slows postanesthetic peripheral-to-core transfer of cutaneous heat, thereby isolating the core thermal compartment. *Anesth Analg.* 1997;85:899–906.
33. Greif R, Laciny S, Rajek A, et al. Blood pressure response to thermoregulatory vasoconstriction during isoflurane and desflurane anesthesia. *Acta Anaesthesiol Scand.* 2003;47:847–852.
34. Israel DJ, Pozos RS. Synchronized slow-amplitude modulations in the electromyograms of shivering muscles. *J Appl Physiol.* 1989;66:2358–2363.
35. Giesbrecht GG, Sessler DI, Mekjavic IB, et al. Treatment of immersion hypothermia by direct body-to-body contact. *J Appl Physiol.* 1994;76:2373–2379.
36. Horvath SM, Spurr GB, Hutt BK, et al. Metabolic cost of shivering. *J Appl Physiol.* 1956;8:595–602.
37. Frank SM, Higgins MS, Fleisher LA, et al. Adrenergic, respiratory, and cardiovascular effects of core cooling in humans. *Am J Physiol.* 1997;272:R557–R562.
38. Khan F, Spence VA, Belch JJF. Cutaneous vascular responses and thermoregulation in relation to age. *Clin Sci.* 1992;82:521–528.
39. Vassilieff N, Rosencher N, Sessler DI, et al. The shivering threshold during spinal anesthesia is reduced in the elderly. *Anesthesiology.* 1995;83:1162–1166.
40. Fahey MR, Sessler DI, Cannon JE, et al. Atracurium, vecuronium, and pancuronium do not alter the minimum alveolar concentration of halothane in humans. *Anesthesiology.* 1989;71:53–56.
41. Bernard SA, Gray TW, Buist MD, et al. Treatment of comatose survivors of out-of-hospital cardiac arrest with induced hypothermia. *N Engl J Med.* 2002;346(8):557–563.
42. Osborn JJ. Experimental hypothermia: respiratory and blood pH changes in relation to cardiac function. *Am J Physiol.* 1953;175:389–398.
43. Mild therapeutic hypothermia to improve the neurologic outcome after cardiac arrest. *N Engl J Med.* 2002;346(8):549–556.
44. Bernard SA, Buist M. Induced hypothermia in critical care medicine: a review. *Crit Care Med.* 2003;31(7):2041–2051.
45. Bernard SA, Mac CJB, Buist M. Experience with prolonged induced hypothermia in severe head injury. *Crit Care (Lond).* 1999;3(6):167–172.
46. Valeri CR, MacGregor H, Cassidy G, et al. Effects of temperature on bleeding time and clotting time in normal male and female volunteers. *Crit Care Med.* 1995;23(4):698–704.
47. Aibiki M, Kawaguchi S, Maekawa N. Reversible hypophosphatemia during moderate hypothermia therapy for brain-injured patients. *Crit Care Med.* 2001;29(9):1726–1730.
48. Machida S, Ohta S, Itoh N, et al. (Changes in tissue distribution of potassium during simple hypothermia). *Kyobu Geka.* 1977;30(5):413–418.
49. Zeiner A, Sunder-Plassmann G, Sterz F, et al. The effect of mild therapeutic hypothermia on renal function after cardiopulmonary resuscitation in men. *Resuscitation.* 2004;60(3):253–261.
50. Arrowsmith JE, Grocott HP, Reves JG, et al. Central nervous system complications of cardiac surgery. *Br J Anaesth.* 2000;84(3):378–393.
51. Curry DL, Curry KP. Hypothermia and insulin secretion. *Endocrinology.* 1970;87(4):750–755.
52. van den Berghe G, Wouters P, Weekers F, et al. Intensive insulin therapy in the critically ill patients. *N Engl J Med.* 2001;345(19):1359–1367.
53. Negovsky VA. Postresuscitation disease. *Crit Care Med.* 1988;16(10):942–946.
54. Illievich UM, Zornow MH, Choi KT, et al. Effects of hypothermic metabolic suppression on hippocampal glutamate concentrations after transient global cerebral ischemia. *Anesth Analg.* 1994;78(5):905–911.
55. Safar PJ. Resuscitation of the ischemic brain. In: Albin MS, ed. *Textbook of Neuroanesthesia: With Neurosurgical and Neuroscience Perspectives.* New York: McGraw-Hill; 1997:557–593.
56. Baena RC, Busto R, Dietrich WD, et al. Hyperthermia delayed by 24 hours aggravates neuronal damage in rat hippocampus following global ischemia. *Neurology.* 1997;48(3):768–773.
57. Coimbra CR, Plourde V. Abdominal surgery-induced inhibition of gastric emptying is mediated in part by interleukin-1 beta. *Am J Physiol.* 1996;270(3 Pt 2):R556–560.
58. Silfvast T, Tiainen M, Poutiainen E, et al. Therapeutic hypothermia after prolonged cardiac arrest due to non-coronary causes. *Resuscitation.* 2003; 57(1):109–112.
59. Tisherman SA. Suspended animation for resuscitation from exsanguinating hemorrhage. *Crit Care Med.* 2004;32(2 Suppl):S46–50.
60. Alzaga AG, Cerdan M, Varon J. Therapeutic hypothermia. *Resuscitation.* 2006;70(3):369–380.
61. Nolan JP, Hazinski MF, Steen PA, et al. Controversial topics from the 2005 International Consensus Conference on cardiopulmonary resuscitation and

emergency cardiovascular care science with treatment recommendations. *Resuscitation*. 2005;67(2–3):175–179.
62. Kluger MJ. Is fever beneficial? *Yale J Biol Med*. 1986;59:89–95.
63. Ginsberg MD, Busto R. Combating hyperthermia in acute stroke: a significant clinical concern. *Stroke*. 1998;29(2):529–534.
64. Davatelis G, Wolpe SD, Sherry B, et al. Macrophage inflammatory protein-1: a prostaglandin-independent endogenous pyrogen. *Science*. 1989;243(4894 Pt 1):1066–1068.
65. Blatteis CM. Role of the OVLT in the febrile response to circulating pyrogens. *Prog Brain Res*. 1992;91:409–412.
66. Blatteis CM, Sehic E. Fever: how may circulating pyrogens signal the brain? *News Physiol Sci*. 1997;12:1–9.
67. Cheng C, Matsukawa T, Sessler DI, et al. Increasing mean skin temperature linearly reduces the core-temperature thresholds for vasoconstriction and shivering in humans. *Anesthesiology*. 1995;82:1160–1168.
68. Lenhardt R, Negishi C, Sessler DI, et al. The effects of physical treatment on induced fever in humans. *Am J Med*. 1999;106:550–555.
69. Manthous CA, Hall JB, Olson D, et al. Effect of cooling on oxygen consumption in febrile critically ill patients. *Am J Resp Crit Care Med*. 1995;151:10–14.
70. Poblete B, Romand J-A, Pichard C, et al. Metabolic effects of i.v. propacetamol, metamizol or external cooling in critically ill febrile sedated patients. *Br J Anaesth*. 1997;78:123–127.
71. Brundin T, Wahren J. Effects of i.v. amino acids on human splanchnic and whole body oxygen consumption, blood flow, and blood temperatures. *Am J Physiol*. 1994;266(3 Pt 1):E396–402.
72. Sellden E, Branstrom R, Brundin T. Preoperative infusion of amino acids prevents postoperative hypothermia. *Br J Anaesth*. 1996;76(2):227–234.
73. Kasai T, Nakajima Y, Matsukawa T, et al. Effect of preoperative amino acid infusion on thermoregulatory response during spinal anaesthesia. *Br J Anaesth*. 2003;90(1):58–61.
74. Umenai T, Nakajima Y, Sessler DI, et al. Perioperative amino acid infusion improves recovery and shortens the duration of hospitalization after off-pump coronary artery bypass grafting. *Anesth Analg*. 2006;103(6):1386–1393.
75. Brundin T, Wahren J. Whole body and splanchnic oxygen consumption and blood flow after oral ingestion of fructose or glucose. *Am J Physiol*. 1993; 264(4 Pt 1):E504–513.
76. Mizobe T, Nakajima Y, Ueno H, et al. Fructose administration increases intraoperative core temperature by augmenting both metabolic rate and the vasoconstriction threshold. *Anesthesiology*. 2006;104(6):1124–1130.

CHAPTER 25 ■ BLOOD VOLUME MEASUREMENTS IN CRITICAL CARE

JOSEPH FELDSCHUH

Effective perfusion requires an optimal interplay between vascular volume and vasomotor tone. In the critical care setting, the blood volume and/or the vasomotor tone may be subject to rapid changes, and a patient may enter the critical care unit with pre-existing disturbances resulting from trauma, disease, or pharmacologic treatment. The intensivist must be able to recognize and treat acute and chronic blood volume disturbances in a manner that will optimize effective perfusion.

In this chapter, we will examine the role that radioisotopic blood volume measurement can play in the critical care unit. We will discuss the physiology of blood volume maintenance and blood volume disturbances, and then introduce the principles underlying radioisotopic blood volume measurement and some technical considerations required for accurate measurement. We will then discuss interpretation of blood volume measurement results in the critical care setting, including general guidelines for understanding blood volume status and several examples of how blood volume measurement can be applied in some common situations.

PHYSIOLOGY OF BLOOD VOLUME MAINTENANCE

The water in the body (total body water) is divided into two main compartments: The intracellular space (the water in the cells themselves) and the extracellular space. The extracellular space is further divided into the vascular space (the water in the blood) and the interstitial space (the water between the cells and outside the vascular space). Although red blood cells are cellular, they are considered part of the vascular space.

Blood volume, also referred to as circulating blood volume or intravascular volume, is the amount of blood in the vascular space—the vasculature and the chambers of the heart. This is the most important of fluid compartments and is the first to deplete into areas of injury, and the first to replete from intravenous infusion of fluid and blood. Plasma and red blood cells account for more than 99% of the blood volume, while white cells and platelets account for less than 1%. Blood normally comprises approximately 7% of an average adult's body weight, but it can range anywhere from 4% to 10% depending on a person's gender and body composition. Women on average have an 8% lower blood volume and 18% lower red cell volume than men of identical height and weight (1). Leaner people tend to have a higher percentage of blood, while more obese people tend to have a lower percentage.

Plasma Volume Maintenance

The amount of plasma in the circulation adjusts constantly to maintain perfusion, temperature, and hemodynamics. A prime goal of plasma volume maintenance is to maintain a normal whole blood volume and to optimize perfusion to the organs and cells. The albumin and the kidneys play particularly important roles in plasma volume maintenance.

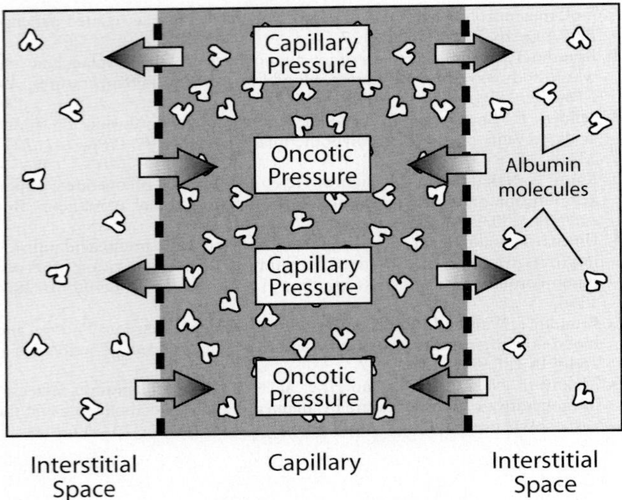

FIGURE 25.1. Dynamic equilibrium between hydrostatic (capillary) and oncotic pressure. Under normal conditions, there is a balance between the net hydrostatic pressure causing flux from the blood vessels into the interstitial space and the net oncotic pressure causing flux from the interstitial space into the blood vessels. The primary protein responsible for maintaining oncotic pressure is albumin, which occurs at a higher concentration in the blood vessels than in the interstitial space.

Albumin and Oncotic Pressure

The interstitial space functions in part as a reserve buffer of fluid, available as needed to provide additional fluid to the vascular space or accommodate excess fluid. Under normal circumstances, a constant flux of water across the capillary membranes between the vascular and interstitial spaces maintains a dynamic equilibrium. Hydrostatic pressure is higher in the vasculature than in the interstitial space, which causes water to flow out of the vascular space into the interstitial space. Counterbalancing this, the relatively higher concentration of albumin and other proteins in the vascular space results in a higher oncotic pressure, causing water to flow out of the interstitial space into the vascular space as described by Starling forces (Fig. 25-1).

Albumin is the primary protein responsible for maintaining oncotic pressure. A large enough total pool of albumin is needed to maintain the pressure gradient between the vascular and interstitial spaces, and a low enough capillary permeability is needed to keep albumin from transudating too quickly out of the circulation into the interstitial space. Normally, albumin transudates out of the plasma into the interstitial space at a rate of approximately 0.25% per minute, gets picked up by the lymphatic system, and eventually returns to the circulation via the lymphatic ducts. However, if too much albumin leaves the circulation too quickly, then the relative concentration of vascular albumin to interstitial albumin—and thus the oncotic pressure—decreases, causing a decrease in plasma volume.

The Kidneys and the Renin–Angiotensin–Aldosterone System

The kidneys are of particular importance in blood volume regulation. Under optimal circumstances, the kidneys' rate of excretion of sodium and water adjusts continually to maintain a normal whole blood volume.

When the kidneys receive decreased perfusion, the renin–angiotensin–aldosterone (RAA) system is activated. The RAA system includes both rapid- and slow-response mechanisms. The rapid response, a rise in blood pressure caused by angiotensin-mediated vasoconstriction, occurs almost immediately. The slower response, an increase in plasma volume caused by the actions of angiotensin II and aldosterone, can occur over the course of days.

The kidneys' response is essentially primitive—they respond to changes in perfusion without being able to differentiate the cause. Thus, while the kidneys ideally function to regulate blood volume, sometimes their responses are maladaptive. For example, if an individual has a normal blood volume but has renal artery stenosis or heart failure, the RAA system is activated, vasoconstriction increases, and excess plasma volume is retained even if the individual has a normal or even expanded blood volume.

The pituitary gland also plays a role in blood volume maintenance. It responds to increased concentration of solutes in plasma or decreased blood pressure by secreting antidiuretic hormone (ADH, also known as vasopressin), which stimulates water reabsorption in the kidneys, reducing urine output. Like the kidneys, the pituitary gland responds to indicators of decreased volume without being able to differentiate the cause.

Red Blood Cell Volume Maintenance

Red cell volume is primarily maintained through a balance of production (erythropoiesis) and destruction (hemolysis). Red blood cells are created in the bone marrow and, at the end of their life span, hemolyzed in the spleen or the liver. In the presence of normal bone marrow function, the rate of red cell production is controlled by the hormone erythropoietin, which is produced by the kidney, with the rate of production affected by indicators of blood oxygenation.

If red blood cells are lost (such as through hemorrhage), they can be replaced through the manufacture of new cells by the bone marrow. It can take days to months to replace lost red cells, depending on the amount lost and an individual's capacity for creating new red cells. A study of healthy males who donated 2 units of blood found that the subjects took a month to replace an average of 92% of the lost blood (2).

PEARLS

- Optimizing effective perfusion is a prime goal in managing critical care patients. Blood volume (plasma + red cell volume) and vasomotor tone both play key roles in perfusion.
- Clinical utilization of radioisotopic blood volume measurement promises to improve patient care by enabling fluid management decisions to be based on accurate quantification of blood volume, rather than on inaccurate estimates based on surrogate measurements or clinical assessment (see below).

Difficulties in Estimating Blood Volume

Many of the measurements available in a clinical setting are indicators or proxy measurements for perfusion (local or systemic), vasomotor tone (local or systemic), or blood volume. These measurements may include:

- Blood pressure and heart rate
- Blood gases, including pH, base deficit, and lactic acid as estimates of perfusion
- Hematocrit and hemoglobin as surrogate tests for red cell volume
- Blood urea nitrogen (BUN)/creatinine as an estimate of kidney function
- Urine output as an estimate of kidney function and/or perfusion
- Invasive procedures such as pulmonary artery catheterization for determination of intravascular pressures

None of these, however, is a direct measure of volume status. The physician in the critical care setting is faced with the difficult situation of administering or withholding fluids, blood, and blood components on the basis of these surrogate tests. In particular, hemoglobin and hematocrit are frequently inaccurate surrogate markers for blood volume. When using hematocrit or hemoglobin to estimate red cell volume, it is assumed that the whole blood volume remains normovolemic (euvolemic)—for example, that fluid replacement of lost red cells via plasma expansion is rapid and complete. This is frequently not the case. Review articles on fluid management discuss a variety of complex factors to consider when estimating a patient's volume status (3–5), and clinical estimation is frequently inaccurate. In a recent study, experienced cardiologists correctly estimated volume status only 51% of the time for 43 nonedematous, ambulatory heart failure patients (6).

Monitoring blood volume using clinical assessment and proxy measurements can be particularly misleading in the critical care setting, because compensatory responses to acute blood volume derangements occur at different rates. Changes in vasomotor tone may occur nearly instantaneously, while changes in plasma volume may occur over hours or days. Following acute blood loss, rapid changes in vasoconstriction, which can occur before any compensatory volume expansion takes place, may maintain a relatively normal peripheral blood pressure and hematocrit at the expense of organ perfusion. Administration of fluids, blood, or blood components can additionally complicate the picture.

Although no studies have explicitly evaluated clinical assessment against blood volume measurement in the critical care unit, a 2003 study (7) compared clinical estimates of intravascular volume with estimates obtained by determining corrected left ventricular flow time from transesophageal Doppler imaging. Clinical estimates agreed with Doppler imaging results only 30% of the time. It is not clear how accurate the Doppler imaging technique is for estimating blood volume, but in some ways this only emphasizes the uncertainty—not only do different methods of assessing volume status disagree, but we don't even know which surrogate methods are the most accurate.

It is a common intuitive assumption that achieving normovolemia facilitates effective perfusion and contributes to improved outcomes. There have, however, been few studies that specifically examined outcomes in relation to accurately measured blood volume with accurate norms. Some recent studies have provided suggestive evidence that achieving normovolemia is a valid goal in a number of clinical settings. In a heart failure study performed at Columbia Presbyterian Hospital, among 43 nonedematous patients, hypervolemic patients had a 2-year mortality rate of 55%, while normovolemic and slightly hypovolemic patients had a 2-year mortality rate of 0% (6). The American College of Cardiology has previously recommended assessment of volume status as an important factor in the diagnosis and treatment of heart failure, but this was the first study to provide a clear association between measured blood volume and patient outcome.

Recent studies have begun to explore how measuring blood volume in the surgical intensive care unit affects patient treatment and outcome (8). Blood volume measurement was performed 86 times for 40 patients with unclear volume statuses. Results led to a change in treatment 36% of the time, and in 42% of those cases, improvement was noted in one or more of the following parameters: Oxygenation, renal dysfunction, vasopressor use, and cardiac index. In the remaining 58% of cases, no improvement was noted, but no treatment changes were detrimental. Because this was a retrospective chart review, the results cannot be used to interpret how blood volume measurement affected outcomes. However, these studies provide preliminary evidence that incorporating blood volume measurement into critical care may impact a significant proportion of patients and may ultimately lead to improved treatment.

BLOOD VOLUME DISTURBANCES

Blood volume disturbances can occur in the red cell volume, the plasma volume, or both, and can occur to different degrees in each compartment (Fig. 25.2). Whole blood volume and red cell volume abnormalities are considered abnormal when they vary from their respective normal values. However, because homeostatic mechanisms are aimed at maintaining a normal whole blood volume, plasma volume disturbances are only abnormal when they fail to maintain a normal whole blood volume. For example, in a patient with red cell loss, a normal response is for plasma to expand to maintain a normal whole blood volume (Fig. 25.3). Conversely, if a patient has an expanded red cell mass, a contracted plasma volume is normal, although with severe red cell expansion, a balance between maintaining normovolemia and avoiding hemoconcentration occurs.

Blood volume abnormalities in the critical care unit may develop from a wide variety of causes. A patient may enter the critical care unit with existing blood volume disturbances and may experience rapid volume changes in response to acute conditions or volume-altering treatment. Comorbidities such as myocardial infarction, stroke, and diabetes may additionally affect blood volume, blood volume maintenance mechanisms, or response to treatment. Evidence of blood volume disturbances, such as hypotension, oliguria, or pulmonary edema, may or may not be present. Surrogate measurements, such as pressure measurements or hematocrit/hemoglobin measurements, often do not accurately reflect the patient's volume status.

While blood volume measurement will not, in itself, identify all of the factors contributing to a patient's blood volume disturbance, it will allow the physician to precisely quantify that disturbance and may help single out what underlying problems need most acutely to be treated. In addition, treating a patient to normovolemia may ease some of the patient's compensatory mechanisms and buy additional time until the underlying factors can be addressed.

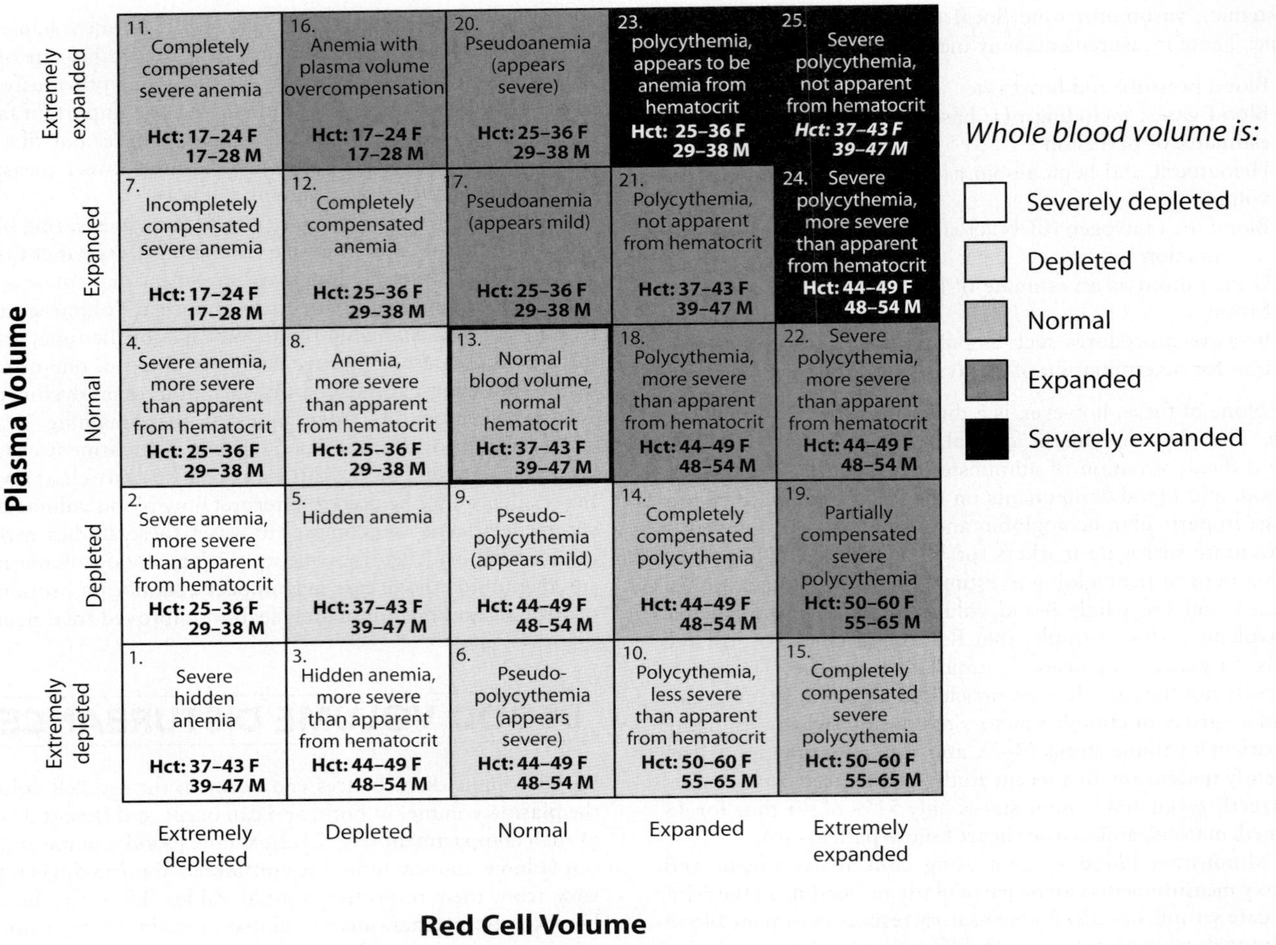

Plasma Volume \ Red Cell Volume	Extremely depleted	Depleted	Normal	Expanded	Extremely expanded
Extremely expanded	11. Completely compensated severe anemia **Hct: 17–24 F 17–28 M**	16. Anemia with plasma volume overcompensation **Hct: 17–24 F 17–28 M**	20. Pseudoanemia (appears severe) **Hct: 25–36 F 29–38 M**	23. polycythemia, appears to be anemia from hematocrit **Hct: 25–36 F 29–38 M**	25. Severe polycythemia, not apparent from hematocrit ***Hct: 37–43 F 39–47 M***
Expanded	7. Incompletely compensated severe anemia **Hct: 17–24 F 17–28 M**	12. Completely compensated anemia **Hct: 25–36 F 29–38 M**	17. Pseudoanemia (appears mild) **Hct: 25–36 F 29–38 M**	21. Polycythemia, not apparent from hematocrit **Hct: 37–43 F 39–47 M**	24. Severe polycythemia, more severe than apparent from hematocrit **Hct: 44–49 F 48–54 M**
Normal	4. Severe anemia, more severe than apparent from hematocrit **Hct: 25–36 F 29–38 M**	8. Anemia, more severe than apparent from hematocrit **Hct: 25–36 F 29–38 M**	13. Normal blood volume, normal hematocrit **Hct: 37–43 F 39–47 M**	18. Polycythemia, more severe than apparent from hematocrit **Hct: 44–49 F 48–54 M**	22. Severe polycythemia, more severe than apparent from hematocrit **Hct: 44–49 F 48–54 M**
Depleted	2. Severe anemia, more severe than apparent from hematocrit **Hct: 25–36 F 29–38 M**	5. Hidden anemia **Hct: 37–43 F 39–47 M**	9. Pseudo-polycythemia (appears mild) **Hct: 44–49 F 48–54 M**	14. Completely compensated polycythemia **Hct: 44–49 F 48–54 M**	19. Partially compensated severe polycythemia **Hct: 50–60 F 55–65 M**
Extremely depleted	1. Severe hidden anemia **Hct: 37–43 F 39–47 M**	3. Hidden anemia, more severe than apparent from hematocrit **Hct: 44–49 F 48–54 M**	6. Pseudo-polycythemia (appears severe) **Hct: 44–49 F 48–54 M**	10. Polycythemia, less severe than apparent from hematocrit **Hct: 50–60 F 55–65 M**	15. Completely compensated severe polycythemia **Hct: 50–60 F 55–65 M**

Whole blood volume is:
- Severely depleted
- Depleted
- Normal
- Expanded
- Severely expanded

FIGURE 25.2. Combinations of whole blood volume, red cell volume, and plasma volume disturbances. A number of distinct combinations of whole blood volume, red cell volume, and plasma volume status may be present in a given patient. Different combinations of volume status in each compartment can have different underlying causes, result in different complications, and require different treatment approaches. Considering the hematocrit or the volume in any single compartment alone does not provide sufficient information for fully understanding volume status. Hct, hematocrit.

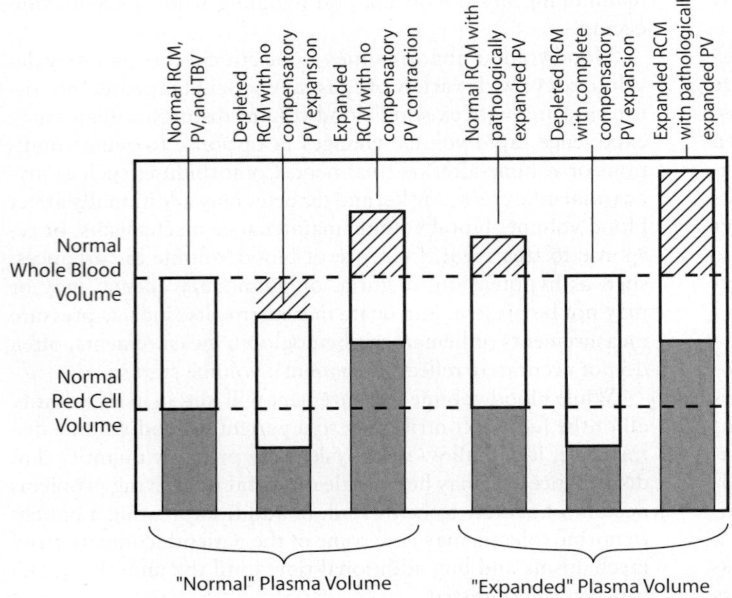

FIGURE 25.3. Plasma volume in relation to whole blood and red cell volume. Plasma volume must be interpreted in relation to red cell and whole blood volume. Among the left three bars, the "normal" plasma volume is only truly normal in the presence of a normal red cell and whole blood volume. Among the right three bars, the "expanded" plasma volume is in fact compensatory and normal when the red cell volume is depleted. RCM, red cell mass; PV, plasma volume; TBV, total blood volume.

BLOOD VOLUME MEASUREMENT

The earliest attempts to measure blood volume occurred in animals as early as the mid-1800s (9–12). In vivo blood volume measurement using the indicator dilution technique was first performed in humans around 1915 (13). This has remained the fundamental method underlying blood measurement.

The indicator dilution technique is based on the concept that the concentration of an indicator (or tracer) in an unknown volume is inversely proportional to that volume (Fig. 25.4). Roughly, blood volume measurement is performed as follows: A standard is prepared in which a known quantity of tracer is mixed in a known volume. The same quantity of tracer is injected into the circulation. After the tracer has mixed fully throughout the unknown volume, a sample is withdrawn, and the volume is calculated by comparing the concentration of tracer in the sample to the concentration of tracer in the standard. The gold standard for accurate measurement of blood volume is the indicator dilution technique using radioisotopic tracers. Blood volume measurement can provide information essential to understanding a patient's perfusion status. Although blood volume measurement has historically been infrequently used because of its complexity and length, recent semiautomated technology has enabled practical clinical application of this measurement (14,15).

Technical Considerations for Accurate Blood Volume Measurement

Many factors affect the accuracy and precision of blood volume measurement. The choice of indicator and details in measurement and correction factors can affect the accuracy of results. Because different investigators have used different tracers, sampling methods, and methods of calculation, it is difficult to compare results from different studies. Thus, when reviewing blood volume in the literature, attention should be paid to the reliability of the methods used by the investigators, as well as the methods used to predict each patient's normal blood volume.

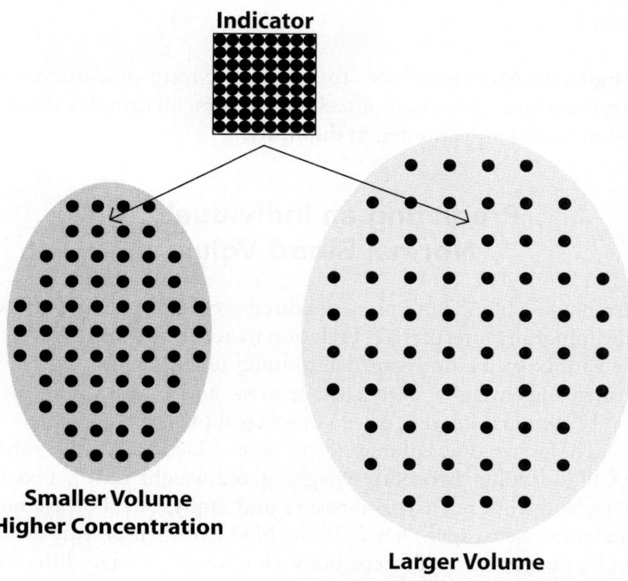

FIGURE 25.4. Indicator dilution. When a tracer (known amount in known volume) is injected into an unknown volume (i.e., intravascular space), the new concentration of the tracer is inversely related to the volume of the space it is injected into.

Optimal Tracers for Blood Volume Measurement

A prime consideration in blood volume measurement is the choice of indicator. An ideal indicator for blood volume measurement in humans should be harmless; remain unchanged when mixed in the vascular space; mix completely throughout the vascular space and not spread to any other spaces (such as interstitial fluid); and be accurately and precisely measurable.

The first indicators used for human patients were dyes (13,16–19). Evans blue dye (T-1824) has been one of the most widely studied and utilized dyes for measuring blood volume, and both Evans blue dye and indocyanine green are in current use.

Dyes fill many of the criteria required for a good indicator. They are largely innocuous and mix thoroughly in the plasma volume. However, in some situations, abnormality in the color or turbidity of the blood may lead to errors in measuring dye concentration. The primary drawback to dyes is that they are removed from the circulation at a rapid and variable rate. As with any marker that binds to plasma proteins, dye transudates into the interstitial space at a slow, steady rate. In addition, however, the liver reticuloendothelial cells remove dye rapidly. This disappearance of the dye through two different avenues is difficult to measure or accurately correct for. Additionally, dye can be cleared from the circulation in as little as 20 to 25 minutes. Since it can take 12 to 20 minutes for a tracer to mix completely in the blood volume, there is very little time after mixing is complete and before the dye is cleared from the circulation.

Radioisotopic tracers were introduced for human blood volume measurement in the late 1940s and early 1950s (20–22) and have essentially replaced dyes for most applications. Currently, chromium-51 (^{51}Cr) tagged red cells are used for red cell volume measurement, and radioactive iodine (^{131}I and ^{125}I) tagged albumin are used for plasma volume measurement.

Radioisotopic indicators mix more predictably in the vascular space and can be measured more precisely than dyes. Tagged red cells remain in the circulation for the life span of the cell or of the bond between the radioisotope and the cell. No loss of tagged red cells is expected during the 20 to 40 minutes of a blood volume measurement. Although some radioisotopically tagged albumin transudates into the interstitial space, under normal conditions more than 90% of the tracer remains in the circulation during blood volume measurement. Even with an abnormally high capillary permeability, more than 75% of the tagged albumin remains in the circulation after 40 minutes. The rate of transudation can be measured, and a correction performed to determine the true blood volume.

Double versus Single Labeling and the F Ratio

The current gold standard for blood volume measurement, as published by the International Council for Standardization in Hematology (ICSH) in 1980, is simultaneous measurement of red cell volume using radioisotopically tagged red cells and of plasma volume using radioisotopically tagged human serum albumin (23). One of the drawbacks of simultaneously measuring red cell and plasma volume is that it involves the preparation and administration of two radioisotopes, requiring a significant expenditure of time and involving many variables that are vulnerable to human error. In addition, red cell volume measurement requires reinfusion of the patient's own blood. Further, injecting two radioisotopes increases the patient's exposure to radioactivity, even though the exposure from each isotope is very small.

One alternative to double labeling is to precisely measure plasma volume and use the hematocrit to calculate the red cell volume. This procedure is less complicated and more rapid than double labeling, taking on average 90 minutes rather than 4 to 5 hours to complete (24). It is commonly used in research and clinical applications (25–30), but it has been controversial as to whether or not it is as accurate as double labeling (29,31–33).

One source of possible error arises from the use of the peripheral hematocrit. Because blood vessels throughout the body vary in size, the hematocrit in a large blood vessel (peripheral hematocrit) is higher than the average hematocrit of all the blood in the circulatory system (mean body hematocrit). The ratio of the mean body hematocrit to the peripheral hematocrit is known as the F ratio or F-cell ratio. The mean body hematocrit cannot be directly measured, but it can be calculated by multiplying the measured peripheral hematocrit by a previously determined value for the F ratio.

The F ratio can be measured by comparing the peripheral hematocrit with the ratio of measured red cell volume to whole blood volume. Most studies have found the average F ratio to be 0.91 (33–35), although some have found slightly different values (29,36). Some studies have found the F ratio to be consistent among a variety of patients (37,38), while others have found it to vary between subjects (31,32,37) or in the same subjects in response to different conditions (35,39). One difficulty in interpreting these results arises from the fact that different studies used different blood volume measurement methods. Depending on the accuracy and precision of the measurement methods, changes in F ratio may reflect physiologic changes or measurement error.

A more effective way to evaluate the accuracy of calculating whole blood and red cell volume from measured plasma volume and peripheral hematocrit is to compare blood volume results from both methods in the same patients. Few studies have done this. A recent study compared blood volume measurement using the ICSH-recommended method with a semiautomated plasma volume method (BVA-100, Daxor) (24). Measuring plasma volume alone provided results comparable to those from simultaneous measurement, even though there were minor differences in how plasma volume was measured between the two methods. The key advantage of the semiautomated method is that it provides results in 90 minutes and has the potential to provide preliminary results in as little as 20 to 30 minutes. This opportunity for rapid results makes blood volume measurement feasible for clinical use, particularly in acute situations.

Additional Technical Considerations

Mixing Time. Some blood subcircuits in the body, such as the skin, the spleen, and muscles at rest, have significantly slower circulation times than the average circulation time. For blood volume measurement to be complete, the tracer must mix with all the blood, including blood from these slower circuits. Withdrawing one or more samples before mixing is complete results in an erroneously high concentration of tracer, which will be reflected in an erroneously low blood volume. Although early studies erroneously thought that mixing was complete in 4 to 5 minutes, it normally requires 8 to 13 minutes for the radioisotope to fully mix with all the blood in the circulation. In patients with reduced cardiac output, such as with heart failure, up to 20 minutes may be required (40).

Multiple Sample Points. The two key variables that affect the accuracy of a blood volume—the mixing time and the transudation rate—require multiple samples for accurate measurement. With a single sample point, there is no way to determine if mixing is complete when the sample is withdrawn or to calculate the transudation rate and correct to true zero-time plasma volume. With two or three sample points, these key variables may be measured, but an error in a single point can greatly alter the results and cannot be readily detected. For reliable measurement, a minimum of four sample points—preferably five points to accommodate possible removal of erroneous points—should be taken at 6- to 8-minute intervals, beginning 10 to 12 minutes after injection (longer for patients known to have reduced cardiac output).

Plasma Packing. Failure to correct for plasma packing or for heparin used in the collection of samples can result in a false increase of the measured blood volume of 2% to 3% (41).

Accurate Hematocrit Measurement. Hematocrit should be measured using the most accurate currently available technology. Additionally, the hematocrit changes when a person moves from a standing to reclining position. In ambulatory patients, blood volume measurement should be initiated after the patient has been reclining for at least 15 minutes. (This is generally not a consideration for a patient in the intensive care unit, however.)

Duplicate Measurements. To ensure accurate measurements and improved detection of technical errors, all samples should be prepared and counted in duplicate.

Predicting an Individualized Normal Blood Volume

Even when blood volume is measured accurately, it can only be meaningfully interpreted in relation to accurate normal values. A variety of methods for determining normal blood volume, using body weight, body surface area, and (most accurately) body composition, have been developed (42).

The first blood volume norms were based on a fixed ratio of blood volume to body weight (fixed-weight ratio). Fixed-weight ratios are easy to measure and apply, but they are not accurate. Because fat has 2/35 the blood content of lean tissue (43), people with different body compositions have different normal blood volumes per unit of mass. An obese individual has a lower normal blood volume than a very lean individual of the same body weight. Fixed-weight ratio norms tend to systematically underestimate normal blood volume in obese individuals and overestimate it in lean individuals.

Some early studies attempted to develop more accurate norms by categorizing subjects based on body composition (44–46). While these studies proved that fixed-weight ratios are inaccurate for many patients, they did not offer viable alternatives, because their methods for evaluation of body composition were subjective and unreliable.

A number of studies have proposed body surface area as an alternative basis for norms (47–53), including, in 1995, the International Council on Standardization in Hematology (5). However, this method, while more accurate than fixed-weight ratio norms, does not reflect the physiology that underlies differences in blood volume norms. The ICSH paper, recognizing that the body surface area was not reliably accurate, recommended a broad normal range of ±25% from the predicted norm. This included 98% to 99% of the subjects studied, thus maximizing specificity. However, the authors acknowledged that an individual can have a significant blood volume abnormality within this "normal" range, resulting in limited clinical utility.

An easily measured, physiologically meaningful method for calculating normal blood volume had been presented in 1977 by Feldschuh and Enson (1). The authors utilized the Metropolitan Life height and weight tables, developed from over 100,000 measurements, which show the ideal weight for any given height based on mortality rates. Feldschuh and Enson hypothesized that individuals of the same deviation from ideal weight would have similar body compositions and hence similar normal blood volumes. They compared measured blood volume from 160 normal individuals of both sexes, with a wide range of height, weight, and body composition, to the subjects' percent deviation from ideal weight. These results were used to extrapolate a curve that described normal blood volume per unit mass in relation to percent deviation from ideal weight (Fig. 25.5). The subjects' blood volumes correlated well with this curve and did not show any systematic deviations based on weight, height, or deviation from ideal weight. In comparison,

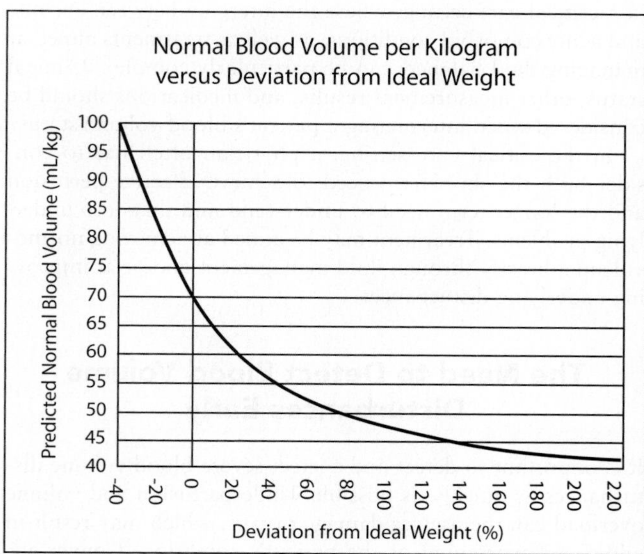

FIGURE 25.5. The deviation from ideal weight norm. Graph of blood volume norms at a given percent deviation from ideal weight for that height, as developed by Feldschuh and Enson (1).

fixed-weight ratio norms and body surface area norms showed systematic errors and/or wide scatter.

Based on these results, Feldschuh and Enson established a category system for interpreting the presence and severity of blood volume abnormalities. A normal blood volume was determined to be within 8% of the predicted normal, a mild hypo- or hypervolemia ±8% to ±16%, moderate ±16% to ±24%, severe ±24% to ±32%, and extreme more than ±32%. This classification scheme has lower specificity than the ICSH category but much higher sensitivity. Presentation of a patient's deviation from the predicted norm in combination with a classification of severity can provide a clinically useful balance between sensitivity and specificity. Milder deviations from normal may be identified more often, enabling earlier diagnosis and treatment, but a clinician can evaluate mild deviations in relation to the patient's specific situation and determine whether treatment or simply additional monitoring is needed. The use of incremental ranges of severity also reflects the fact that blood volume abnormalities may require different treatment approaches based on severity (54).

INTERPRETING BLOOD VOLUME MEASUREMENT RESULTS

Units of Measurement

In addition to absolute measurements, blood volume results for each compartment should be presented as the patient's deviation from his or her normal volume, as a percent deviation and in cubic centimeters. For example, a patient with a predicted normal blood volume of 2,500 mL and a measured blood volume of 2,000 mL has a blood volume depletion of –20% and –500 mL. The percentage indicates the severity of the patient's blood volume, and the absolute quantity of the depletion can help guide treatment. There are little data on the optimum blood volume associated with survival in critically ill patients, but due to expansion of intravascular space, a higher than normal value may be desirable (55).

Presentation of measured blood volume solely as an absolute value (such as 3,000 mL or 38 mL/kg) should be avoided, because it does not encourage interpretation of the measured volume in relation to the patient's norm.

Relationship between Whole Blood, Red Cell, and Plasma Volumes

When interpreting blood volume results, the whole blood volume should be considered first, with the red cell volume interpreted in relation to the whole blood volume, and the plasma volume interpreted in relation to both the whole blood and red cell volumes.

A normal whole blood volume may indicate that, even in the presence of anemia or polycythemia, the body's blood volume maintenance mechanisms are functioning appropriately. A depleted whole blood volume may indicate any of a number of disorders and/or maladaptive responses, including (but not limited to) recent acute blood loss, impairment in the kidneys' ability to regulate the blood volume, and iatrogenic causes such as overdiuresis. An expanded whole blood volume may indicate disorders and/or maladaptive responses including (but not limited to) heart failure, inappropriate activation of the RAA system, and iatrogenic causes such as overtransfusion.

The red cell volume should be interpreted in relation to the whole blood volume. For example, a 20% red cell deficit may occur with a normal whole blood volume (fully compensated anemia), a depleted whole blood volume (hypovolemic anemia), or an expanded whole blood volume (anemia with pathologic plasma volume expansion). Each of these is likely to result in markedly different peripheral hematocrits, have different underlying causes, and require different treatment approaches.

An additional tool for evaluating the red cell volume is the "normalized hematocrit," a ratio of the measured red cell volume to the patient's predicted normal whole blood volume. Unlike the peripheral hematocrit, which can provide a misleading estimate of red cell volume, the normalized hematocrit accurately reflects the red cell volume. Because it is presented in the same units as the peripheral hematocrit, the "normalized hematocrit" can be used in much the same way that hematocrit measurements are currently used (such as for evaluating the extent of anemia and determining transfusion triggers).

The plasma volume should always be considered in relation to the red cell and the whole blood volume. Because alterations in the plasma volume are part of the body's homeostatic mechanisms to maintain a normal blood volume, alterations in plasma volume may be beneficial or maladaptive. In general, if the whole blood volume is normal, then any changes in the plasma volume are compensatory and normal. If the whole blood volume is expanded or depleted, then the plasma volume is maladaptive. A plasma volume alteration may also be partially homeostatic and partially pathologic. For example, if a heart failure patient has anemia and an expanded whole blood volume, then some of the plasma volume is compensatory and some pathologic (see Fig. 25.3).

The Rate of Transudation

When five sample points are used to measure the plasma volume, the rate of decrease of radioisotope concentration over time is calculated in order to determine the true zero-time plasma volume. This rate of decrease reflects the rate of albumin transudation and may provide information about the patient's capillary permeability. The reliability of the transudation rate depends on the accuracy of the plasma volume measurement.

The normal rate of albumin transudation has not been fully established, but studies by Feldschuh and Enson (1) and others have found normal rates to range from a low of 0.05% per minute to a high of 0.45% to 0.50% per minute. Given an accurate blood volume measurement, a transudation rate above 0.50% per minute may be considered evidence of increased capillary permeability, and a rate between 0.45% and 0.50% per minute borderline. In such cases, possible causes of increased capillary permeability, including toxic damage, hypoalbuminemia, capillary leak syndrome, or other causes, should be evaluated and, if possible, treated. Patients with a high transudation rate may require a greater quantity of fluids in order to maintain a normal intravascular volume, and some amount of edema may be tolerated in order to avoid hypovolemia.

A normal transudation rate is not proof that a patient's capillary permeability is normal. An individual may accommodate increased capillary permeability by developing a larger ratio of interstitial to intravascular fluid (likely indicated by edema). The decreased ratio of intravascular to interstitial albumin allows for a normal transudation rate and a new homeostatic balance. This is common in hypoalbuminemia.

A transudation rate of less than 0.05% per minute, and especially a negative slope, is probably an indication of measurement error.

PEARLS

- **Whole blood, red cell,** and **plasma** volume measurements should each be presented as an absolute measurement and as a **deviation from the patient's predicted normal value.**
- The **normalized hematocrit** is the ratio of the measured red cell volume to the predicted normal whole blood volume. It is analogous to the peripheral hematocrit but is an accurate reflection of the red cell volume.
- The **slope** indicates how quickly albumin is transudating out of the circulation. A high slope (0.0050 or above) may indicate capillary leakage.
- The whole blood volume should be interpreted first, followed by the red cell volume and then plasma volume. Plasma volume should always be viewed in relation to red cell and whole blood volume disturbances, and homeostatic responses should be differentiated from maladaptive responses.

APPLICATIONS OF BLOOD VOLUME MEASUREMENT IN CRITICAL CARE

A number of comorbid conditions and other factors may underlie a patient's blood volume disturbance, and different factors may have opposing effects. This may be especially true in a critical care setting, where the interplay between chronic and acute comorbid conditions, as well as treatments aimed at managing fluid balance, can be particularly complex. Clinical status, other measurement results, and medications should be considered when interpreting a patient's blood volume status.

In the critical care setting, a physician often has to consider both the short-term need to achieve effective perfusion and the longer-term need to understand and diagnose underlying problems. Treatment may be aimed at achieving normovolemia directly through fluid management and/or at improving underlying disturbances.

The Need to Detect Blood Volume Disturbances Early

It is important to detect and correct severe blood volume disturbances as quickly as possible. Underperfusion and volume overload can themselves damage organs, which may result in additional worsening of the patient's condition. Conversely, maintaining normovolemia may improve perfusion and oxygen delivery to critical organs and buy time for successful treatment and recovery.

Undetected Hypovolemia

Early detection of hypovolemia is essential. By the time a patient becomes symptomatic, hypovolemia is often extreme, damage may have already occurred to critical organs (the gut and the kidneys are particularly susceptible), and deterioration may be rapid and unexpected (56).

In acute situations, the current primary measures used to track perfusion and evaluate fluid replacement requirements include pressure measurements (such as central venous pressure, intra-arterial or indirect auscultating blood pressure, and pulmonary artery catheter measurements) in conjunction with hematocrit/hemoglobin measurements. However, the body can respond to hypovolemia by initiating vasoconstrictive defense mechanisms, maintaining near-normal pressures even in the face of severe blood loss, and allowing the hypovolemia to remain undetected. A study of surgical intensive care unit patients demonstrated a weak correlation between blood volume results and pulmonary artery occlusion pressure, and no correlation between blood volume values and central venous pressure, cardiac index, and stroke volume index (57).

The patient's vasoconstrictive mechanisms are limited, and critical organs may experience hypoxia even when systemic pressures are near-normal—this situation can be termed "partially compensated shock." If hypovolemia progresses beyond the ability of the body's vasoconstrictive mechanisms to compensate, the blood pressure may suddenly collapse in disproportionate response to a small incremental decrease in blood volume, and the patient may enter an overt clinical crisis.

Hypovolemia is generally more dangerous and urgent than the same degree of hypervolemia, and sudden blood loss is more urgent than the same degree of chronic hypovolemia. A patient may tolerate a 40% increase in whole blood volume or an 80% increase in red cell volume for some time without suffering acute negative effects, but a 40% loss of blood or an 80% loss of red cells is an extreme medical emergency. A sudden loss of as little as 20% of the blood volume triggers an acute vasoconstrictive response, and a sudden 30% loss can lead to circulatory collapse. A rapid 40% to 45% loss is incompatible with life. Further, an already anemic or hypovolemic patient who experiences sudden blood loss will be less able to tolerate that loss than would a normovolemic or hypervolemic patient.

Even after fluid resuscitation (whether after partially compensated shock or circulatory collapse), damage to the gut and kidneys may result in severe complications. Reperfusion of infarcted bowels can lead to invasion of bacteria from the gut throughout the circulatory system. Hypoxia to the kidneys can damage the tubules, impairing their ability to reabsorb water.

Accurate blood volume measurement enables the treating physician to identify hypovolemia early—preferably before organ damage has occurred—and to place ongoing pressure measurements in context.

Undetected Hypervolemia

In the critical care unit, hypervolemia may be a result of comorbidities or iatrogenic causes such as overtransfusion. Hypervolemia usually develops slowly and is most frequently related to cardiac disease, particularly heart failure. Acute hypervolemia is almost always iatrogenic. Particular attention must be paid to patients who are oliguric or in renal shutdown, as these patients cannot remove excess fluid through urine output.

The hypervolemic patient is at risk for the development of pulmonary edema in response to increased pressure; hypoalbuminemia, which predisposes to pulmonary edema; and pulmonary hypertension as a maladaptive mechanism that may eventually lead to permanent pulmonary hypertension and worsening of heart failure.

It is often assumed that gross peripheral edema is an indication of hypervolemia. However, a hypervolemic patient may be nonedematous and remain undetected (6, 25), or an edematous patient may be normovolemic or hypovolemic in the important intravascular space. In the former case, a failure to recognize and treat hypervolemia may lead to the development of pulmonary hypertension or pulmonary edema. In the latter case, aggressive diuresis can precipitate hypovolemia and organ hypoperfusion. Clinical judgment using surrogate markers may not be consistently accurate (8).

Blood volume measurement can be used to accurately diagnose the presence and extent of hypervolemia. Treatment can vary depending on the severity of the patient's hypervolemia and the patient's kidney function and may include fluid restriction, diuretic therapy, hemodialysis if the patient is in kidney failure, or ultrafiltration.

PEARL

- Early detection and treatment of hypovolemia are essential to avoiding organ damage.

The Bleeding Patient: When to Perform Blood Volume Measurement

Bleeding, or more precisely evidence of blood loss, is common in the critical care setting. In blood volume measurement, it is assumed that the red cell volume remains constant during the course of the blood volume measurement. In a patient who is bleeding, this assumption does not hold true. Thus, it is important to evaluate the presence and rate of bleeding in order to determine when it is appropriate to perform a blood volume measurement.

If a patient is massively bleeding at a rate greater than 100 cm^3/hour, then blood volume measurement should not be performed. During the immediate stabilization process, fluid pressures should be the primary guide.

Blood volume measurement can be used as an estimate in patients who are losing blood at a rate of less than 100 cm^3/hour. A patient bleeding at this rate loses about 2.4 L/day, but only 50 to 60 cm^3 (approximately 1%–3% of the blood volume) during the 30 to 40 minutes of a blood volume measurement. While a blood volume measurement will be slightly less accurate, it will still provide a reasonable estimate. This is especially true for patients who have severe volume disturbances, as is common in the critical care setting. For example, if a patient is measured to have a blood volume depletion of –30%, even an uncertainty of $\pm 5\%$ does not alter the basic diagnosis of severe hypovolemia. Current practice of using hemoglobin/hematocrit value to guide red cell transfusion may not be addressing severe deviations in red cell volume (58). In a group of surgical intensive care unit patients, comparison of peripheral hematocrit with normalized hematocrit demonstrated a 95% confidence interval limit of agreement of ± 15.2 hematocrit % (58).

Tracking Changes in Blood Volume and Performing Follow-up Measurements

After an initial blood volume measurement, it is possible in a nonbleeding patient to track changes in blood volume with precise hematocrit measurements. If the patient's red cell volume remains stable, changes in the hematocrit reflect changes in blood volume as follows:

$$\text{Plasma volume} = \text{Red cell volume} \times (1 - \text{Hematocrit})/\text{Hematocrit}$$

$$\text{Whole blood volume} = \text{Red cell volume}/\text{Hematocrit}$$

For example, consider a patient who is found to have a measured red cell volume of 2,000 mL, plasma volume of 4,000 mL, and hematocrit of 33%. This patient is diuresed, and the hematocrit rises to 40%. The new volume is equal to:

$$\text{Plasma volume} = 2{,}000\text{ mL} \times (1 - 0.4)/0.4 = 3{,}000\text{ mL}$$

$$\text{Whole blood volume} = 2{,}000/0.4 = 5{,}000\text{ mL}$$

If a nonbleeding patient receives a transfusion, the volume response may be roughly estimated based on the type of fluid transfused and its expected effect on the hematocrit; a follow-up blood volume measurement may be needed for precise quantification. If a patient is bleeding or otherwise experiences a change in red cell volume that cannot be reasonably estimated, blood volume changes cannot be tracked with precision via changes in hematocrit. A follow-up blood volume measurement should be performed 24 to 48 hours after treatment is initiated.

In general, changes in blood volume may correlate with changes in symptoms, hemodynamic measurements, or clinical status, but these relationships are not necessarily straightforward. In one study of acute decompensated heart failure patients (59), after 24 to 48 hours of treatment blood volume correlated better with some hemodynamic measurements than did brain natriuretic peptide (BNP) levels. However, no measurements correlated closely enough with blood volume results for any hemodynamic measurement to serve as a surrogate measure for volume status, or vice versa.

BLOOD VOLUME MEASUREMENT IN SOME COMMON CRITICAL CARE SITUATIONS

Following are some examples of common situations in the critical care setting, with discussion of the roles blood volume and blood volume measurement may play in these situations.

Shock

The presentation of symptoms in shock may not be straightforward and can complicate assessment of the patient's volume status, especially in situations where several factors contribute to shock. Blood volume measurement can be of major importance in understanding the underlying cascade of events that precipitate shock and determining appropriate treatment. In a patient with hypovolemia, even in conjunction with other contributing factors, appropriate transfusion and fluid replacement are needed before severe multiorgan hypoperfusion and failure ensues.

For example, following a myocardial infarction, patients frequently become hypotensive. While cardiac damage usually plays a major, if not the predominant, role in the ensuing shock, blood volume derangements may play a significant additional role. A patient with a myocardial infarction may develop hypovolemia from severe vomiting, profuse sweating, or the use of anticoagulants. Sometimes blood loss secondary to gastrointestinal bleeding may trigger a myocardial infarction (MI). Because the blood loss may not be recognized as a precipitating factor in the MI, the patient may not be treated to restore volume. This may progress to renal or multiorgan damage. Accurate assessment of the volume status and prompt treatment of volume derangements are important for all types of shock, even those that do not appear on the surface to be volume related.

Acidosis

Acidosis frequently develops from hypoperfusion and a shift to anaerobic metabolism, resulting in increased lactic acid production. Under these circumstances, the body's metabolic defense mechanisms, which are strongly geared to maintain a pH of 7.4, may be overcome. At a pH of 7.0 to 7.1, major deterioration of all functions including cardiac metabolism occurs. At a pH of 6.85 to 6.9, the body's metabolic systems are so diminished that death is imminent.

Acidosis may also develop from other underlying causes. For example, in diabetic acidosis, ketoacidosis develops from hyperglycemia. Hypovolemia may be a contributing factor, though, because the severely dehydrated patient may have localized ischemia.

Blood volume measurement may be helpful in elucidating the underlying cause of acidosis and determining optimal therapy. If the acidosis is caused by hypoperfusion related to diminished blood volume, *aggressive and rapid* therapy is needed before irreversible deterioration occurs. In situations such as diabetic acidosis, therapy should also be directed at correcting the underlying condition (such as hyperglycemia) and correction of the electrolyte imbalance.

Hypoalbuminemia

Hypoalbuminemic patients, because of a shift in oncotic pressure, may be predisposed to edema formation in order to achieve a balance of hydrostatic and oncotic pressures that can maintain a normal blood volume. Rather than a normal ratio of 3:1 of extracellular to vascular volume, equilibrium between the two spaces may be reached at a ratio of 4:1 or 5:1. In such patients, the goal is to maintain a normal blood volume even if that means allowing an expanded extracellular volume. It is a common mistake to focus treatment on removal of obvious peripheral edema. Patients with hypoalbuminemia and/or capillary leak syndrome may require a larger volume of extracellular fluid in order to maintain a normal blood volume.

Hepatorenal Syndrome

In hepatorenal syndrome, the liver and kidneys fail simultaneously. Frequently, this syndrome originates with liver damage that progresses to cirrhosis and portal hypertension, causing edema and ascites. If the patient is overdiuresed to remove the edema, the patient becomes hypovolemic and the kidneys hypoperfused. If severe enough, this can lead to kidney failure, liver failure, and circulatory collapse. Hepatorenal syndrome is essentially part of a cascade of circulatory decompensation that, if not corrected, usually results in multiorgan failure and death.

Understanding the blood volume is essential to detecting and correcting this situation. It is usually not possible to diurese a patient with liver damage to completely remove edema, because diuresis does not correct the underlying imbalance between intravascular and interstitial volume. Instead, the reduced fluid simply redistributes throughout the vascular and extravascular space in the same ratio. This situation is similar when using paracentesis to treat ascites. Because paracentesis only removes ascitic fluid and does not address the underlying imbalance, the rapid removal of a large amount of ascitic fluid causes fluid to shift quickly from the vascular to the peritoneal space, resulting in hypovolemia, a drop in blood pressure, and collapse of the circulation.

Blood volume measurement can be performed on a patient with liver problems, edema, and/or ascites to determine what quantity of diuresis is possible without precipitating hypovolemia. A patient who is hypervolemic will be able to tolerate diuresis, and an edematous normovolemic patient should be diuresed only slowly and minimally, with careful follow-up. Some patients with edema and/or ascites may require a blood volume at the upper limit of normal in order to maintain adequate perfusion pressures. A patient who is hypovolemic should not be diuresed!

Oliguria

Oliguria may be an indication of impending renal shutdown resulting from renal hypoperfusion. After fluid is administered and urine flow is re-established, the physician must pay particular attention to urine output. Even a relatively short period of renal hypoperfusion may result in renal tubule damage that persists after reperfusion and impairs the ability of the tubules to reabsorb water and sodium.

Recovery from renal shutdown occurs in two phases—an oliguric phase and a natriuretic phase. In the oliguric phase, which occurs before resuscitation and persists until the kidneys begin to respond to reperfusion, the kidneys produce little to no urine. In this phase, it is important to monitor fluids so that the patient does not become hypervolemic. After the kidney begins to recover, the glomeruli may begin functioning again, but tubular damage may persist, leading to impairment in the kidneys' ability to reabsorb water and sodium. In this natriuretic phase, the patient may produce a large quantity of urine, which, if not replaced with enough fluid, may lead to hypovolemia and additional kidney hypoperfusion.

The transition from the oliguric to the natriuretic phase should be monitored in two main ways. The patient's urine output must be monitored in order to recognize the shift from the oliguric to the natriuretic phase, so that treatment can be altered as appropriate. Additionally, as long as the patient is not bleeding, baseline blood volume measurement followed by subsequent hematocrit measurements can help the physician track changes in the patient's blood volume. Ongoing evaluation of the fluid administration and volume relationship can help the physician more accurately determine the quantity and type of fluids and electrolytes required for the patient to maintain a normal blood volume.

Diuretic Resistance

The term *diuretic resistance* is frequently used when patients do not respond to relatively large quantities of IV diuretics. To some extent the term may be a misnomer, because diuretic resistance may be a reflection of severe hypoperfusion. A patient in renal shutdown will obviously not respond to diuretics, and occasionally aggressive use of diuretics precipitates renal shutdown. To differentiate true diuretic resistance from hypoperfusion of the kidneys, blood volume measurement in conjunction with renal tests can be helpful. This differentiation is particularly important because aggressive use of diuretics in a patient with marginal perfusion to the kidneys may precipitate renal shutdown.

Inappropriate Antidiuretic Syndrome and Renal Salt Wasting Syndrome: Differential Diagnosis

Hyponatremia, which is seen daily in the critical care unit, results in multiple disturbances at a metabolic level. Two of the primary causes of hyponatremia are syndrome of inappropriate secretion of antidiuretic hormone (SIADH) and renal salt-wasting syndrome. SIADH is often associated with head trauma, neurosurgery, or other neurologic disturbances in which the pituitary gland releases inappropriately high levels of antidiuretic hormone, resulting in the retention of water and the dilution of sodium in an expanded plasma volume. Excessive hypervolemia predisposes a patient to pulmonary hypertension and/or pulmonary edema, the latter of which may lead to sudden death.

In contrast, in renal salt-wasting syndrome the tubules do not reabsorb sufficient quantities of sodium, and too much salt is lost from the circulation into the urine. A particularly important cause of renal salt-wasting syndrome is damage to the tubules caused by hypoperfusion to the kidneys (such as may occur after even relatively short periods of hemorrhage). The tubules are particularly sensitive to damage from hypoperfusion, and when they experience anoxia, they may lose the ability to concentrate urine by reabsorbing sodium and water that has been filtered by the glomeruli. They also lose the ability to excrete acidic urine, which may result in a buildup of acid in the body. The low concentration of sodium contributes to a decrease in plasma volume, which can cause additional or continued hypovolemia, leading to further kidney hypoperfusion and complete renal shutdown.

Blood volume measurement can help differentiate between these two conditions. Given a normal amount of salt and fluid intake, a patient with SIADH will have an expanded blood volume, while a patient with renal salt-wasting syndrome will be hypovolemic. Other conditions, such as glomerular damage or overadministration of fluids, may also result in hyponatremia and an expanded plasma volume; these various diagnoses may be differentiated through results from other tests, such as plasma osmolality and urine and serum sodium, and the patient's clinical condition.

In both cases, it is important to treat the patient to normalize the blood volume and to restore a normal sodium concentration. For SIADH, this can include the administration of hypertonic sodium, fluid restriction, and possibly diuresis. For renal salt-wasting syndrome, this can include the administration of large quantities of fluids and sodium, in quantities sufficient not only to restore the already lost volume, but also to maintain intravascular volume and sodium in the face of continued losses. It is critically important to effectively differentiate between these two syndromes, because for each, treating with inappropriate fluid management can exacerbate the imbalance contributing to the hyponatremia and precipitate a clinical crisis, such as complete renal shutdown.

Cardiogenic and Noncardiogenic Pulmonary Edema: Differential Diagnosis

Cardiogenic pulmonary edema (caused by increased hydrostatic pressure in the alveoli), often secondary to hypervolemia, and noncardiogenic pulmonary edema (caused by damage to the membranes of the alveoli), also known as acute respiratory distress syndrome (ARDS), have different underlying causes and require different treatment approaches. The two conditions may present similar symptoms, and both are common in the critical care setting. When physical examination and noninvasive tests do not provide a definitive distinction, pulmonary capillary wedge pressure is often used to distinguish between the two, but results may be difficult to interpret in patients with pulmonary artery hypertension related to other conditions. Additionally, patients may have a combination of both conditions; increased hydrostatic pressure does not rule out damage to the alveoli. The relationship between blood volume and wedge pressures seems at best weak, with no correlation to central venous pressures (56).

Blood volume measurement, by detecting the presence or absence of hypervolemia, can be used in the differential diagnosis of cardiogenic and noncardiogenic pulmonary edema, especially in patients known to have pulmonary hypertension from other causes and in patients for whom invasive pulmonary artery catheterization is not desirable. Hypervolemia is more likely to be present in a patient with cardiogenic pulmonary edema, while noncardiogenic pulmonary edema may develop in a patient with normovolemia or hypovolemia. However, because both conditions may coexist, hypervolemia does not rule out ARDS. These conditions must also be reviewed in the context of evaluating albumin, as hypoalbuminemia by itself will predispose to pulmonary edema.

Diuretic therapy is a mainstay in the treatment of cardiogenic pulmonary edema. Aggressive diuretic therapy in hypovolemic patients is likely to worsen perfusion and may lead to renal and other organ damage. Hypovolemia can be readily identified with blood volume measurement. Even in patients with hypervolemia, especially if they also have alveolar damage, overly aggressive diuresis may result in hypovolemia and hypoperfusion. Evaluating the extent of hypervolemia and evaluating volume in relation to pressure measurements can help the physician determine how to diurese the patient safely. In a nonbleeding patient, once an initial blood volume is established, the hematocrit can be helpful in monitoring blood volume changes and tracking the patient's response to diuresis.

SUMMARY

While fluid resuscitation and blood volume management have long been mainstays in critical care, evaluation of blood volume has traditionally relied on assessment of the patient's clinical condition, which is often misleading, and surrogate measurements to estimate volume status, which are often inaccurate. Blood volume measurement has been a missing link in treating critically ill patients, and the clinical utilization of semiautomated radioisotopic blood volume measurement promises to complete that link.

On the simplest level, blood volume measurement results can be used to guide treatment more precisely; rather than relying on inaccurate surrogate measurements to estimate volume status, blood volume measurement results can be considered when making fluid management decisions. Additional tools such as the normalized hematocrit can be used as quickly understood, more accurate guides for determining when transfusion is required.

In addition, blood volume measurement, by providing an accurate, quantitative measurement of circulating blood volume, offers the opportunity to develop evidence-based approaches to treating volume derangements. Treatment algorithms with precise end points can be developed and tested, with an ultimate goal of developing a comprehensive, evidence-based approach to evaluating and treating blood volume derangements in the critical care setting.

References

1. Feldschuh J, Enson Y. Prediction of the normal blood volume. Relation of blood volume to body habitus. *Circulation.* 1977;56(4 Pt 1):605–612.
2. Valeri CR, Ragno G, Srey R. Restoration of red blood cell volume following 2-unit red blood cell apheresis. *Vox Sang.* 2003;85(2):85–87.
3. Gutierrez G, Reines HD, Wulf-Gutierrez ME. Clinical review: hemorrhagic shock. *Crit Care.* 2004;8(5):373–381. Epub 2004 Apr 2.
4. McGee S, Abernethy WB, Simel DL. Is this patient hypovolemic? *JAMA.* 1999;281:11.
5. Kreimeier U. Pathophysiology of fluid imbalance. *Crit Care.* 2000;4(Suppl 2):S3–7. Epub 2000 Oct 13.
6. Androne AS, Hryniewicz K, Hudaihed A, et al. Relation of unrecognized hypervolemia in chronic heart failure to clinical status, hemodynamics, and patient outcomes. *Am J Cardiol.* 2004;93(10):1254–1259.
7. Iregui MG, Prentice D, Sherman G, et al. Physicians' estimates of cardiac index and intravascular volume based on clinical assessment versus transesophageal Doppler measurements obtained by critical care nurses. *Am J Crit Care.* 2003;12(4):336–342.
8. Takanishi DM, Biuk-Aghai E, Yu M, et al. Availability of circulating blood volume alters fluid management in critically ill surgical patients. *Am J Surg.* In press.
9. Meek WJ, Glasser HS. Blood volume: a method for its determination with data for dogs, cats, and rabbits. *Am J Physiol.* 1918;47:302–317.
10. Dreyer G, Ray W. The blood volume of mammals as determined by experiments upon rabbits, guinea-pigs, and mice; and its relationship to the

body weight and to the surface area expressed in a formula. *Philos Tran R Soc.* 1911;201:133–160.
11. Sjostrand T. Blood volume. In: Hamilton WF, Dow P, eds. *Handbook of Physiology, Section 2: Circulation.* Vol. 1. Washington, DC: American Physiological Society; 1962:51–53.
12. Rasmussen AT, Rasmussen GB. The volume of blood during hibernation and other periods of year in the woodchuck (Marmatoa monax). *Am J Physiol.* 1917;44:132–148.
13. Keith NM, Rountree LG, Geraghty JT. A method for the determination of plasma and blood volume. *Arch Intern Med.* 1915;16:547.
14. Manzone TA, Dam HQ, Soltis D, et al. Blood volume analysis: a new technique and new clinical interest reinvigorate a classic study. *J Nucl Med Technol.* 2007;35(2):55–63.
15. Ertl AC, Diedrich A, Raj SR. Techniques used for the determination of blood volume. *Am J Med Sci.* 2007;334(1):32–36.
16. Smith HP. Blood volume studies II. Repeated determination of blood volume and short intervals by means of the dye method. *Am J Physiol.* 1920;51: 221.
17. Smith HP. The fate of an intravenously injected dye (brilliant vital red) with special reference to its use in blood volume determination. *Bull Johns Hopkins Hosp.* 1925;36:325.
18. Gergersen MI, Gibson JJ, Stead EA. Plasma volume determination with dyes, errors in colorometry: use of the blue dye T-1824. *Am J Physiol (Proc).* 1935;113:54.
19. Bradley EC, Barr JW. Determination of blood volume using indocyanine green (Cardio-Green) dye. *Life Sci.* 1968;7:1001–1007.
20. Hevesy G, Zerahn K. *Acta Physiol Scand.* 1942;4:376.
21. Gray SJ, Sterling K. The tagging of red cells and plasma proteins with radioactive chromium. *J Clin Invest.* 1950;29:1604–1613.
22. Storaasli JP, Kriefer H, Friedell HL, et al. *Surg Gynecol Obstet.* 1950;91: 458.
23. Recommended methods for measurement of red-cell and plasma volume: International Committee for Standardization in Haematology. *J Nucl Med.* 1980;21(8):793–800.
24. Dworkin H, Premo M, Dees S. Comparison of red cell and whole blood volume as performed using both chromium-51 tagged red cells and iodine-125 tagged albumin and using I-131 tagged albumin and extrapolated red cell volume. *Am J Med Sci.* 2001;334(1):32.
25. Androne AS, Katz SD, Lund L, et al. Hemodilution is common in patients with advanced heart failure. *Circulation.* 2003;107(2):226–229.
26. Mancini DM, Katz SD, Lang CC, et al. Effect of erythropoietin on exercise capacity in patients with moderate to severe chronic heart failure. *Circulation.* 2003;107(2):294–299.
27. Shevde K, Pagala M, Tyagaraj C, et al. Preoperative blood volume deficit influences blood transfusion requirements in females and males undergoing coronary bypass graft surgery. *J Clin Anesth.* 2002;14(7):512–517.
28. Alrawi SJ, Miranda LS, Cunningham JN Jr, et al. Correlation of blood volume values and pulmonary artery catheter measurements. *Saudi Med J.* 2002;23(11):1367–1372.
29. Fairbanks VF, Klee GG, Wiseman GA, et al. Measurement of blood volume and red cell mass: re-examination of 51Cr and 125I methods. *Blood Cells Mol Dis.* 1996;22(2):169–186; discussion 186a–186g.
30. Davy KP, Seals DR. Total blood volume in healthy young and older men. *J Appl Physiol.* 1994;76(5):2059–2062.
31. Balga I, Solenthaler M, Furlan M. Should whole-body red cell mass be measured or calculated? *Blood Cells Mol Dis.* 2000;26(1):25–31; discussion 32–36.
32. Nielsen S, Rodbro P. Validity of rapid estimation of erythrocyte volume in the diagnosis of polycythemia vera. *Eur J Nucl Med.* 1989;15(1):32–37.
33. Olmer M, Berland Y, Purgus R, et al. Determination of blood volume in nephrotic patients. *Am J Nephrol.* 1989;9(3):211–214.
34. Akira T, Tomoyuki I, Kazuhiro Y, et al. Effect of an exercise-heat acclimation program on body fluid regulatory responses to dehydration in older men. *Am J Physiol Regul Integr Comp Physiol.* 1999;277:R1041–R1050.
35. Lundvall J, Lindgren P. F-cell shift and protein loss strongly affect validity of PV reductions indicated by Hb/Hct and plasma proteins. *J Appl Physiol.* 1998;84:822–829.
36. Lee SMC, Williams WJ, Schneider SM. Role of skin blood flow and sweating rate in exercise thermoregulation after bed rest. *J Appl Physiol.* 2002;92:2026–2034.
37. Najean Y, Deschrywer F. The body/venous haematocrit ratio and its use for calculating total blood volume from fractional volumes. *Eur J Nucl Med.* 1984;9(12):558–560.
38. Chaplin H Jr, Mollison PL, Vetter H. The body/venous hematocrit ratio: its constancy over a wide hematocrit range. *J Clin Invest.* 1953;32(12):1309–1316.
39. Haller M, Brechtelsbauer H, Akbulut C, et al. Isovolemic hemodilution alters the ratio of whole-body to large-vessel hematocrit (F-cell ratio). A prospective, randomized study comparing the volume effects of hydroxyethyl starch 200,000/0.62 and albumin. *Infusions Ther Transfusion Med.* 1995; 22(2):74–80.
40. Jaenike JR, Schreiner BF Jr, Waterhouse C. The relative volumes of distribution of I131 tagged albumin and high molecular weight dextran in normal subjects and patients with heart disease. *J Lab Clin Med.* 1957;49:172–181.
41. Chaplin H Jr, Mollison PL. Correction for plasma trapped in red cell column of hematocrit. *Blood.* 1952;7:1227.
42. Feldschuh J, Katz S. The importance of correct norms in blood volume measurement. *Am J Med Sci.* 2007;334(1):41–46.
43. Jacobs DS, Demott WR, et al. *Laboratory Test Handbook.* 4th ed. Lexi-Comp Inc.; 1996:306.
44. Gregersen MI, Nickerson JL. Relation of blood volume and cardiac output to body type. *J Appl Physiol.* 1950;3(6):329–341.
45. Keys A, Brozek J, Henschel A, et al. *The Biology of Human Starvation.* Minneapolis: University of Minnesota Press; 1950.
46. Alexander JK, Dennis EW, Smight WG, et al. Blood volume, cardiac output, and distribution of systemic blood flow in extreme obesity. *Cardiovasc Res Cent Bull.* 1962-1963[Winter];1:39–44.
47. Samet P, Fritts HW Jr, Fishman AP, et al. The blood volume in heart disease. *Medicine (Baltimore).* 1957;36(2):211–235.
48. Baker RT, Kozoll DD, et al. The use of surface area as a basis for establishing normal blood volume. *Surg Gynecol Obstet.* 1957;104:183–189.
49. Wennesland R, Brown E, Hopper J, et al. Red cell, plasma and blood volume in healthy men measured by radiochromium (Cr51) cell tagging and hematocrit: influence of age, somatotype and habits of physical activity on the variance after regression of volumes to height and weight combined. *J Clin Invest.* 1959;38(7):1065–1077.
50. Nadler SB, Hidalgo JU, Bloch T. Prediction of blood volume in normal human adults. *Surgery.* 1962;51:224–232.
51. Retzlaff JA, Tause WN, Kielly JM. Erythrocyte volume, plasma volume and lean body mass in adult men and women. *Blood.* 1969;33:649–661.
52. Hurley PJ. Red cell and plasma volumes in normal adults. *J Nucl Med.* 1975;16:46–52.
53. Pearson TC, Guthrie DL, Simpson J, et al. Interpretation of measured red cell mass and plasma volume in adults: Expert Panel on Radionuclides of the International Council for Standardization in Haematology. *Br J Haematol.* 1995;89:748–756.
54. Lucas G. Approach to the multiple trauma patient (part I). *Hosp Med.* 1982; January.
55. Shoemaker WC, Montgomery ES, Kaplan E, et al. Physiologic patterns in surviving and nonsurviving shock patients. *Arch Surg.* 1973;106:630–636.
56. Chiara O, Pelosi P, Segala M, et al. Mesenteric and renal oxygen transport during hemorrhage and reperfusion: evaluation of optimal goals for resuscitation. *J Trauma.* 2001;51(2):356–362.
57. Yamauchi H, Biuk-Aghai EN, Yu M, et al. Circulating blood volume measurements in critically ill surgical patients correlate poorly with pulmonary artery catheter measurements. *HMJ.* 2007;66(12):318.
58. Takanishi DM, Yu M, Lurie D, et al. Peripheral blood hematocrit in critically ill surgical patients: an imprecise surrogate of true red cell volume. *Anesth Analg.* 2008;106:1808–1812.
59. James KB, Troughton RW, Feldschuh J, et al. Blood volume and brain natriuretic peptide in congestive heart failure: a pilot study. *Am Heart J.* 2005; 150(5):984.

CHAPTER 26 ■ VENOUS OXIMETRY

EMANUEL P. RIVERS • RONNY OTERO • A. JOSEPH GARCIA • KONRAD REINHART • ARTURO SUAREZ

IMMEDIATE CONCERNS

During initial management of the critically ill patient, physiologic variables such as blood pressure, heart rate, urine output, cardiac filling pressures, and cardiac output (CO) are used to guide resuscitative efforts. Despite normalization of these variables, significant imbalances between systemic oxygen delivery ($\dot{D}O_2$) and demand result in decreases in central ($Sc\bar{v}O_2$) and mixed ($S\bar{v}O_2$) venous oxygen saturation levels and global tissue hypoxia (1–3). This global tissue hypoxia, if left untreated, leads to anaerobic metabolism, lactate production, and oxygen debt. The magnitude and duration of oxygen debt have been implicated in the development of the inflammatory response, multisystem organ failure and increased mortality (4–8). Early restoration of global tissue normoxia aided by venous oxygen saturation monitoring has resulted in a reduction in inflammation, morbidity, mortality, and health care resource consumption (9,10). The purpose of this chapter is to review the physiologic principles and clinical utility of $S\bar{v}O_2$ in the management of the critically ill patient.

MAJOR PROBLEMS

Patient Selection for Continuous Venous Oximetry

Continuous venous oximetry is likely to be most useful in patients at greatest risk of developing global tissue hypoxia. This includes patients with significant acute or chronic cardiopulmonary disease undergoing major surgical procedures and undergoing therapy that may interfere with their ability to increase oxygen delivery during times of stress. It is also useful in patients who require hemodynamic and ventilator support (11).

Goals of Venous Oximetry Monitoring

The goals of continuous venous oximetry vary depending on the initial condition of the patient. Venous oximetry can be used as an end point in the early resuscitation or monitoring device for high risk patients at risk for developing global tissue hypoxia. The common goal is to ensure a balance between systemic oxygen delivery and demands. A stable and normal value for the $S\bar{v}O_2$ may indicate that further measurements are unnecessary. However, an abrupt decrease in $S\bar{v}O_2$ becomes a warning that investigation of oxygen delivery (CO, arterial oxygen saturation [SaO_2], and hemoglobin [Hgb] concentration), and systemic oxygen consumption [$\dot{V}O_2$] are needed so that specific therapy may be directed toward the underlying disorder (12).

STRESS POINTS

1. A normal $S\bar{v}O_2$ range is 65% to 75% (0.65 to 0.75) and suggests that the oxygen supply is meeting the demands of the tissues. Since $S\bar{v}O_2$ is a global value, a normal value does not guarantee absence of ischemic tissues.
2. There are four determinants of $S\bar{v}O_2$: CO, Hgb concentration, arterial oxygen content, and $\dot{V}O_2$. In the critically ill patient, an abrupt change in $S\bar{v}O_2$ indicates that a change in oxygen transport–demand balance has occurred but does not identify which determinant has changed.
3. A decrease in $S\bar{v}O_2$ may be caused by a decrease in CO, Hgb concentration, and arterial oxygen content or an increase in $\dot{V}O_2$.
4. An increase in $S\bar{v}O_2$ is more difficult to interpret. It may indicate distal migration of the catheter which is easy to check by determining catheter position (see below). Patients may have a high CO, $\dot{V}O_2$, or high arterial oxygen content, especially during anesthesia or mechanical ventilation where there is a larger amount of dissolved oxygen. If this is associated with persistent elevation of lactate levels, it is an ominous sign. In patients with cirrhosis, sepsis, and peripheral shunts, an abnormal distribution of peripheral blood flow may impair oxygen uptake so that $S\bar{v}O_2$ remains high. In cirrhosis, there is pathologic shunting between the arterial and venous system in the liver causing a high CO and high $S\bar{v}O_2$. The septic state is accompanied by a peripheral oxygen deficit, which can be partially reversed by maintaining an above-normal CO and $\dot{D}O_2$ (13). Higher-than-normal $S\bar{v}O_2$ may be required in sepsis to overcome the defect in peripheral oxygen use. Patients with anatomic shunts such as ventricular septal defects and arterial-venous fistulas for hemodialysis also may have abnormal mixing of arterial and venous blood leading to higher venous oxygen saturations.
5. Pulse oximetry and mixed venous oximetry can be combined into a tool of continuous cardiac and pulmonary monitoring.
6. The difference between arterial and venous saturation ($SaO_2 - S\bar{v}O_2$) is an estimation of arterial venous oxygen content difference and is inversely proportional to CO and directly proportional to oxygen consumption.
7. The ventilation/perfusion index ($\dot{V}/\dot{Q}$ I) gives an estimate of intrapulmonary shunt. Using saturation as an inference of oxygen content, respiratory dysfunction ($\dot{V}/\dot{Q}$ I) can be estimated from the equation $(1 - SaO_2)/(1 - S\bar{v}O_2)$.

ESSENTIAL TROUBLESHOOTING PROCEDURES

1. Continuous $S\bar{v}O_2$ measurements may drift and require daily calibration using laboratory co-oximetry.
2. Calibration should also be verified anytime the optical module is disconnected, or whenever the measurement is thought to be erroneous.
3. Distal migration of the pulmonary artery catheter (PAC) tip may cause a higher $S\bar{v}O_2$ reading due to proximity to pulmonary capillary blood, which is approximately 100% saturated. The catheter should be positioned in a large enough segment of the pulmonary artery to require $\leq$1.25 mL of air in the balloon to occlude that segment.
4. Infusion of fluids or blood through the distal port of the catheter may alter the light signal and the reading.
5. Decreased light intensity signal or damping of the pulmonary artery (PA) tracing may indicate migration distally or fibrin around the optic bundles. If irrigation of the catheter does not correct the artifact, the catheter should be withdrawn and repositioned.
6. A change in $S\bar{v}O_2$ of greater than 10% in either direction requires investigation.

INITIAL THERAPY

1. If $S\bar{v}O_2$ is low in association with a low CO, optimization procedures with fluids or inotropic agents should occur immediately. When titrating inotropic infusions, *a lack of response* ($S\bar{v}O_2$ does not increase) suggests inadequate therapy. CO should be reassessed and treatment augmented.
2. In cases of respiratory dysfunction, arterial saturation should respond to therapies such as increased fraction of inspired oxygen (FiO_2) and positive end-expiratory pressure (PEEP) within 8 to 10 minutes. If SaO_2 does not increase or if $S\bar{v}O_2$ decreases, either respiratory therapy has been ineffective or CO may be compromised.
3. After improvement in respiratory function, if the patient is receiving a high FiO_2, the FiO_2 may be decreased every 10 to 20 minutes if arterial and venous saturation remain stable. Increased difference in (SaO_2 minus $S\bar{v}O_2$) usually correlates with a sudden decrease in CO.
4. A decrease in A-V $S\bar{v}O_2$ difference that increase (SaO_2 minus $S\bar{v}O_2$) in response to measures CO indicates a successful intervention.

PHYSIOLOGY OF OXYGEN TRANSPORT

The process of oxygen transport includes loading oxygen into the red blood cells (hemoglobin) and delivering it to the tissue by the heart (cardiac output), as well as utilization of the oxygen in the periphery and the return of deoxygenated blood to the right side of the heart. Several terms must be defined to understand the components of oxygen transport (absolute values should be indexed to body surface area):

Oxygen delivery ($\dot{D}O_2$) is the volume of oxygen delivered (mL/minute) from the left ventricle each minute. $\dot{D}O_2 = CO \times CaO_2 \times 10$

Arterial content of oxygen (CaO_2) is the mL of O_2 in 100 mL of arterial blood.

$CaO_2 = (Hgb \times 1.34 \text{ to } 1.39 \text{ mL } O_2/\text{gm of Hgb} \times SaO_2) + (0.0031 \times PaO_2)$

Mixed venous content of oxygen ($C\bar{v}O_2$) is mL of O_2 in 100 mL of mixed venous blood. $C\bar{v}O_2 = (Hgb \times 1.34 \text{ to } 1.39 \text{ mL } O_2/\text{gm of Hgb} \times S\bar{v}O_2) + (0.0031 \times P\bar{v}O_2)$

Oxygen demand is the cellular oxygen requirement to avoid anaerobic metabolism. Oxygen demand is the amount of oxygen required by the body tissues to function under conditions of aerobic metabolism. Because oxygen demand is determined at the tissue level, it is difficult to quantify clinically.

Oxygen consumption ($\dot{V}O_2$) is the amount of oxygen consumed by the tissue, usually calculated by the Fick equation:

$$\dot{V}O_2 = (CaO_2 - C\bar{v}O_2) \times CO \times 10$$

$\dot{V}O_2$ is a mechanism by which the body "protects" the oxygen demand created at the tissue level. Increased $\dot{V}O_2$ in early stages of shock is associated with increased survival. Oxygen consumption may increase by increasing CO, widening the arterial-venous oxygen content difference, or both. In the normal state, both CO and arterial-venous oxygen difference may increase by about threefold, providing a total increase of $\dot{V}O_2$ during times of stress to about ninefold above the resting state. Normally, $\dot{V}O_2$ and oxygen demand are equal; however, in times of great oxygen demand or times in which either CO or arterial- venous oxygen content difference cannot increase to meet the oxygen demand of the cells, oxygen demand may exceed $\dot{V}O_2$. When this occurs, an oxygen debt accumulates and anaerobic metabolism and lactic acidosis ensue (14).

Oxygen uptake is the measured volume of oxygen removed from inspired gas each minute (using indirect calorimetry/metabolic gas monitor). Oxygen uptake differs slightly from $\dot{V}O_2$ in that the latter is a *calculated* value (from the Fick equation) and the former is the *measured* volume of oxygen taken up by the patient each minute. Oxygen uptake is measured by analyzing inspired and expired gas concentrations and inspired and expired volumes. Measurement of oxygen uptake may be useful for metabolic studies in assessing variations in $\dot{V}O_2$ as well as determining caloric needs.

Oxygen utilization coefficient (OUC) or extraction ratio (O_2ER) is the fraction of delivered oxygen that is consumed. OUC or $O_2ER = \dot{V}O_2/\dot{D}O_2$

Therefore, the oxygen utilization coefficient defines the balance between oxygen supply (delivery) and demand (consumption) (Fig. 26.1).

Oxygen transport is the processes contributing to oxygen delivery and oxygen consumption.

ASSESSMENT OF OXYGEN TRANSPORT BALANCE

Oxygen transport balance may be assessed on several levels. First, examination of the patient may reveal signs of hypoperfusion, including altered mentation, cutaneous

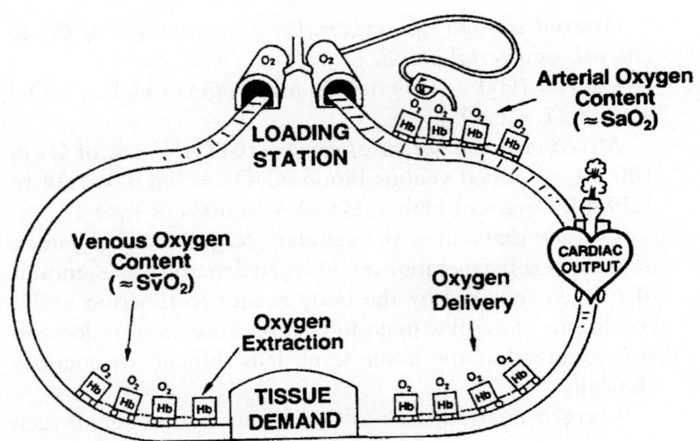

FIGURE 26.1. The physiology of oxygen transport and utilization.

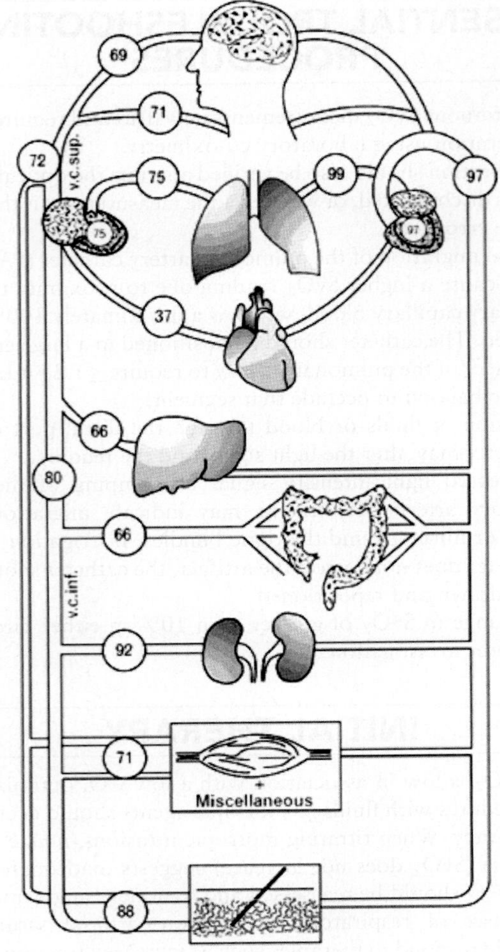

FIGURE 26.2. Venous oxygenation saturations of various organs. (From Reinhart K, Rudolph T, Bredle DL, et al. Comparison of central-venous to mixed-venous oxygen saturation during changes in oxygen supply/demand. *Chest.* 1989;95(6):1216–1221.)

hypoperfusion, oliguria, tachycardia, and, when all compensatory systems have failed, hypotension. Unfortunately, these clinical signs are often late, nonspecific, and at times uninterruptible in critically ill patients. A more physiologic approach is to assess the determinants of oxygen transport balance individually by using the Fick equation. The arterial-venous oxygen content difference may be used to assess the relative balance between CO and $\dot{V}O_2$. An increase in the arterial-venous oxygen content difference indicates that either flow is decreased or consumption is increased.

When the Fick equation is solved for $S\bar{v}O_2$ (Table 26.1), it becomes apparent that an inverse linear relation exists between $S\bar{v}O_2$ and oxygen utilization coefficient (11) if SaO_2 is maintained constant. $S\bar{v}O_2$ measured continuously is, therefore, an on-line indicator of the adequacy of the oxygen supply and of the demand in perfused tissues. The determinants of $S\bar{v}O_2$ are $\dot{V}O_2$, Hgb, CO, SaO_2, and, to a small degree, PaO_2. $S\bar{v}O_2$ represents the flow-weighted average of the venous oxygen saturations from all perfused tissues (Fig. 26.2). Therefore, tissues that have high blood flow but relatively low oxygen extraction (kidney) will have a greater effect on $S\bar{v}O_2$ than will tissues with low blood flow, although the oxygen extraction of these tissues may be high (myocardium) (15,16).

The interpretation of $S\bar{v}O_2$ requires consistent and intact vasoregulation (5). When vasoregulation is altered (such as in sepsis), oxygen uptake may be severely altered, causing a marked increase in $S\bar{v}O_2$. Septic patients can have a normal $S\bar{v}O_2$ while the hepatic venous saturation can be up to 15% lower (17,18). This reduced oxygen saturation was noted to arise from an increased regional metabolic rate rather than reduced perfusion. Flow-limited regional oxygen consumption may potentially exist despite the presence of a normal $S\bar{v}O_2$. Therefore, a normal $S\bar{v}O_2$ should not be considered as sole criteria to ensure optimal oxygen delivery in critically ill patients (19,20) (Fig. 26.3).

TABLE 26.1

DERIVATION OF $S\bar{v}O_2$ FROM FICK EQUATION

1. $\dot{V}O_2 = C(a-\bar{v})O_2 \times CO \times 10$	{Fick equation
2. $\dot{V}O_2/(CO \times 10) = C(a-\bar{v})O_2$	{Divide by CO × 10
3. $\dot{V}O_2/(CO \times 10) = CaO_2 - C\bar{v}O_2$	{Definition of $C(a-\bar{v})O_2$
4. $\dot{V}O_2/(CO \times 10) - CaO_2 = -C\bar{v}O_2$	{Subtract CaO_2
5. $C\bar{v}O_2 = CaO_2 - [\dot{V}O_2/(CO \times 10)]$	{Multiply by –l.
6. $C\bar{v}O_2 = 1 - \dot{V}O_2/(CO \times 10 \times CaO_2)$	{Divide by CaO_2
7. $C\bar{v}O_2/CaO_2 = 1 - \dot{V}O_2/\dot{D}O_2$	{Definition of $\dot{D}O_2$
8. $S\bar{v}O_2 = 1 - \dot{V}O_2/\dot{D}O_2$	{Definition of $S\bar{v}O_2$ if $SaO_2 = 1.0$

CO, cardiac output.

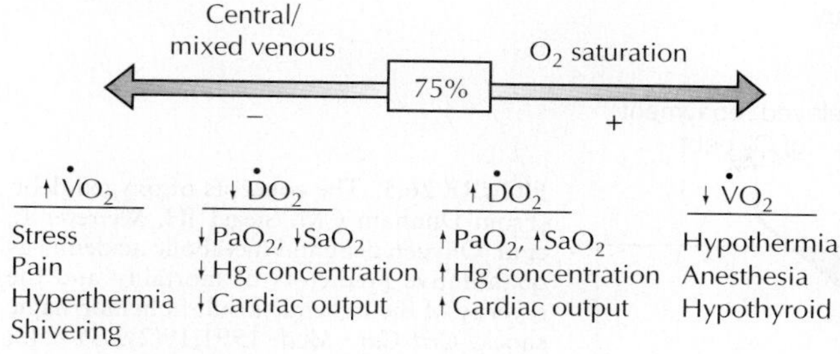

FIGURE 26.3. Variables that affect $S\bar{v}O_2$. (From Rivers EP, Ander DS, Powell D. Central venous oxygen saturation monitoring in the critically ill patient. *Curr Opin Crit Care.* 2001;7(3):204–211.)

Although oxygen demand cannot be measured, the relative balance between consumption and demand is best indicated by the presence of excess lactate in the blood. Lactic acidosis implies that demand exceeds consumption or oxygen supply dependency and anaerobic metabolism is present (14,21,22) (Fig. 26.4). The relative balance between oxygen supply and demand can be assessed by the oxygen utilization coefficient (1). Calculation of this coefficient, however, requires the measurement of CO, Hgb, SaO_2, PaO_2, $S\bar{v}O_2$, and mixed venous oxygen tension ($P\bar{v}O_2$). Mixed venous oxygen tension, a reflection of both PaO_2 and CO, is a better predictor of hyperlactatemia and death than either arterial PaO_2 or CO alone. A $P\bar{v}O_2$ below 28 mm Hg is usually associated with hyperlactatemia and increased mortality (23). Blood lactate concentrations greater than 4 mmol/L are unusual in normal and noncritically ill hospitalized patients and warrant concern. In hospitalized (non-ICU) nonhypotensive subjects, as well as in critically ill patients, a blood lactate concentration greater than 4 mmol/L may portend a poor prognosis (24). Since serum lactate is a global measurement, a normal lactate is not a guarantee that all tissue beds are adequately perfused.

ARTERIAL VENOUS OXYGEN CONTENT DIFFERENCE

From the Fick principle, we learned that CO was equal to oxygen consumption divided by arterial venous oxygen content difference ($CaO_2 - CvO_2$). Even in the critically ill patient, it is unlikely that Hgb or total body oxygen consumption can change sufficiently minute to minute to affect the calculations. Therefore, $(Ca - \bar{v})O_2$ usually reflects changes in cardiac output. In addition, immediate response to therapy—or lack thereof—can help tailor therapy more precisely and rapidly (25). Since the contribution of dissolved oxygen is minute (0.0031 × partial pressure of oxygen), and the factor (Hgb × 1.39 mL O_2/gm Hgb) occurs in both sides of the equation, $(Ca - \bar{v})O_2$ can be estimated by subtracting the values of pulse oximetry and continuous mixed venous oximetry ($SaO_2 - S\bar{v}O_2$).

INTRAPULMONARY SHUNT

Although PaO_2 is affected by changes in respiratory function (intrapulmonary shunt), PaO_2 is also affected by changes in CO if there is a moderate intrapulmonary shunt (≥20%). For example, if there is a 20% shunt (20% of CO is not involved with gas exchange) and blood goes to the left side of the heart deoxygenated, any decrease in $S\bar{v}O_2$ will decrease PaO_2. Thus, although no change in pulmonary function has occurred, a decrease in CO (or even any factor that decreases venous oxygen content) lowers PaO_2 and increases the alveolar-to-arterial oxygen tension gradient (26). This nonpulmonary effect on PaO_2 is important to understand since treatment of intrapulmonary shunt is to increase PEEP, which would be disastrous if low CO was the cause for low PaO_2. The equation for intrapulmonary shunt is as follows:

$$\dot{Q}sp/\dot{Q}t = \frac{Cc - Ca}{Cc - C\bar{v}}$$

where $\dot{Q}sp/\dot{Q}t$ is physiologic shunt (% of cardiac output), Cc is capillary oxygen content, Ca is arterial oxygen content, and $C\bar{v}$ is venous oxygen content. We can simplify the shunt equation by ignoring the calculation of Hgb-carried oxygen by dropping (Hgb × 1.39) and substituting saturations of 100% for the pulmonary capillary saturation, pulse oximetry for arterial saturation, and mixed venous oximetry for $S\bar{v}O_2$. The entire equation for pulmonary capillary content can be replaced by the term 1 (or 100% Hgb saturation). Because we have already substituted Sa for arterial content and $S\bar{v}$ for venous content, this estimation of physiologic shunt (the $\dot{V}/\dot{Q}$ I) can be

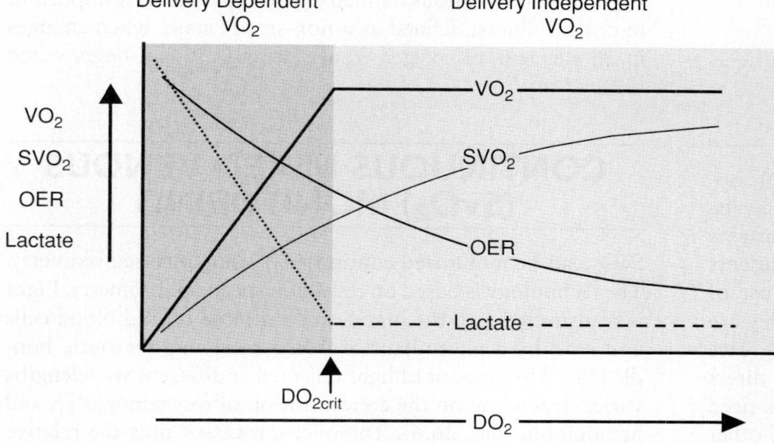

FIGURE 26.4. The relationship of oxygen transport variables and lactate levels.

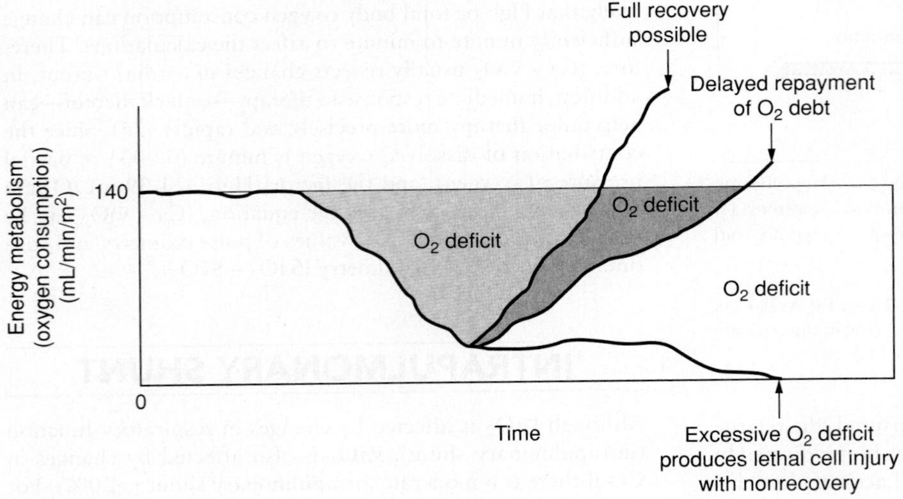

FIGURE 26.5. The concepts of oxygen debt. (From Dunham CM, Siegel JH, Weireter L, et al. Oxygen debt and metabolic acidemia as quantitative predictors of mortality and the severity of the ischemic insult in hemorrhagic shock. *Crit Care Med.* 1991;19(2):231–243; Rixen D, Siegel JH. Bench-to-bedside review: oxygen debt and its metabolic correlates as quantifiers of the severity of hemorrhagic and post-traumatic shock. *Crit Care.* 2005;9(5):441–453; and Siegel JH. The effect of associated injuries, blood loss, and oxygen debt on death and disability in blunt traumatic brain injury: the need for early physiologic predictors of severity. *J Neurotrauma.* 1995;12(4):579–590.)

represented by the equation (27):

$$\dot{V}/\dot{Q}I = \frac{1 - SaO_2}{1 - S\bar{v}O_2}.$$

For instance, if arterial saturation were 90% (or 0.9) and venous saturation were 60% (or 0.6), the Qs/Qt calculation would be

$$\frac{1 - 0.9}{1 - 0.6} = \frac{0.1}{0.4} = 25\%.$$

This estimation fails to reflect the severity of respiratory failure as judged by the need to use a FiO_2, and this equation needs to specify the FiO_2 of the patient to be meaningful.

THE CONSEQUENCES OF TISSUE HYPOXIA

When compensatory mechanisms such as increased systemic oxygen extraction are exceeded, tissue hypoxia results with pathologic significance not only *in vitro* (4), but also, low $S\bar{v}O_2$ is associated with the generation of inflammation and the mitochondrial impairment of oxygen use (28). The accumulation of global tissue hypoxia over time leads to oxygen deficits. The magnitude and duration of this oxygen debt has been associated with the generation of inflammatory biomarkers, morbidity, and mortality (8,28–32) (Fig. 26.5).

MONITORING OXYGEN TRANSPORT

Critically ill patients in the emergency department (ED), operating room (OR), and intensive care units (ICUs) may be grouped into three categories. Category 1 consists of patients requiring intensive observation or monitoring. These patients may have major risk factors or may be admitted because of the nature of their illness or the nature of the therapy they are receiving. Category 2 patients require intensive nursing care and often specialized technology and care facilities to direct therapy for major systemic illness. Category 3 patients need continuous physician intervention for hemodynamic and other instabilities. Continuous venous oximetry may have clinical applications in each of these broad classes of patients. The three major objectives of monitoring critically ill patients are (i) to ensure that the patient is stable, (ii) to provide an early warning system regarding untoward events, and (iii) to evaluate the efficiency and efficacy of interventions performed.

Category 1 patients undergoing hemodynamic and oxygen transport monitoring only because of underlying risk factors who have a normal and stable $S\bar{v}O_2$ have an intact balance between oxygen supply and demand. Further assessment of CO and arterial and mixed venous blood gas analysis to reach that conclusion can be eliminated, and there is "safety in no (other) numbers." If the patient becomes unstable as manifested by a decreasing $S\bar{v}O_2$, the monitoring system will meet the second objective by providing an early warning of the imbalance in oxygen supply and demand. In this situation, although an alert has been given, the cause of the oxygen transport imbalance is not necessarily clear. The change in $S\bar{v}O_2$ is sensitive but not specific. In this clinical situation, it may be necessary to measure CO, SaO_2, and Hgb. When the cause of the imbalance is identified, specific therapy may be instituted to restore the oxygen supply–demand balance. While interventions are applied, the continuous assessment of supply–demand balance may be used to evaluate the efficacy of the intervention with instant feedback. Continuous CO methodology should supplement but not supplant mixed venous oximetry. This is particularly important in critical illness, defined as a non-steady state, when changes in all elements of oxygen transport and use can be expected (32).

CONTINUOUS MIXED VENOUS ($S\bar{v}O_2$) MONITORING

$S\bar{v}O_2$ can be monitored continuously using infrared oximetry. The technology is based on reflection spectrophotometry. Light is transmitted into the blood, and reflected off red blood cells and read by a photodetector in the receiving fiberoptic bundle (11). The amount of light reflected at different wavelengths varies depending on the concentration of oxyhemoglobin and hemoglobin (Fig. 26.6). The microprocessor uses the relative

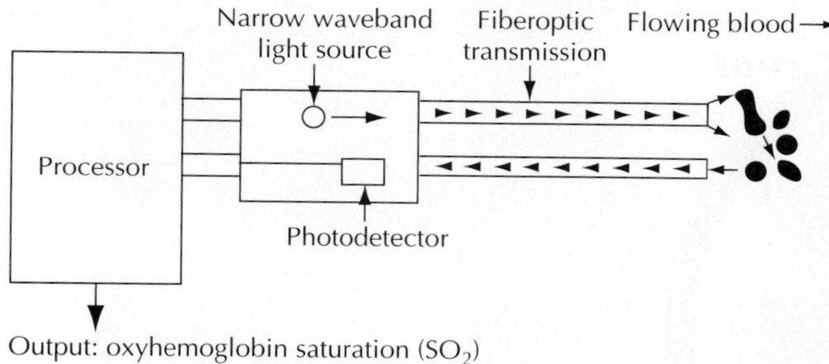

FIGURE 26.6. The technology of spectrophotometry. (From Rivers EP, Ander DS, Powell D. Central venous oxygen saturation monitoring in the critically ill patient. *Curr Opin Crit Care.* 2001;7(3):204–211.)

reflectances to calculate the oxyhemoglobin and total Hgb, the fraction of which represents $S\bar{v}O_2$. The catheter used to measure venous oxygen saturation can be a pulmonary artery or a modified central venous catheter.

The continuous oximetry system must be calibrated before use by a co-oximetry measured sample (33). This may be done *in vitro* by positioning the catheter tip next to a target that reflects the transmitted light in such a manner that the microprocessor can be calibrated. After *in vitro* calibration, the oxygen saturation of the central venous system, right atrium, right ventricle, and PA can be measured while the catheter is being floated into the proper position. These measurements during the insertion of the catheter may be useful to rule out intracardiac left-to-right shunts.

Once the PA catheter is in proper position, blood may be sampled through the distal port to calibrate or to verify the calibration of the system. The first *in vivo* calibration is usually done at 24 hours post–PAC insertion. A mixed venous sample is withdrawn and analyzed by laboratory co-oximetry. Blood drawn from the PA should be aspirated slowly (1 mL over 20 seconds) to prevent contamination by the highly oxygenated pulmonary capillary blood. The value obtained by the microprocessor at the time the blood sample is drawn is retained by the system. This may be compared against the value obtained from the laboratory sample, and, if a significant (greater than 2%) difference exists, the instrument may be recalibrated to the laboratory co-oximeter value. The calibration should be verified at any time the optical module is disconnected from the catheter, whenever the measurement is suspected of being erroneous, and every 24 hours to ensure stability of the system.

Because it is crucial that red blood cells be flowing past the tip of the catheter, proper positioning in the PA is necessary. Distal migration of the PA catheter tip is a common source of error. When the catheter tip advances into the distal segments of the PA, a high or increased $S\bar{v}O_2$, a decreased light intensity signal, or damping of the PA tracing may become evident. If these signs are encountered, the distal lumen of the catheter should be irrigated with flush solution to remove fibrin on the catheter tip. If the pressure waveform is not restored to a proper PA tracing by irrigation, the catheter should be slowly withdrawn until the PA pressure tracing is restored. At this point, the PA catheter balloon may be slowly inflated until the pulmonary artery occlusion pressure (PAOP) tracing is observed. If this tracing is not produced by inflation of the balloon to maximum volume (1.5 mL), the catheter should be slowly advanced until an occlusion pressure tracing is observed. At that point, the balloon can be deflated again and then slowly reinflated until a PAOP tracing occurs. The volume required to restore this tracing should be at least 75% of the total capacity of the balloon. Using the maximum balloon volume to attain a PAOP tracing ensures that the catheter is in the proximal section of the PA and is, in fact, a physiologic confirmation of the catheter tip position.

Distal migration of the PA catheter may cause artifactually high oxygen saturation because highly saturated (approximately 100%) pulmonary capillary blood is sampled. The catheter tip may be lodged against a vessel wall or bifurcation, causing an alteration in the light intensity received by the fiberoptic bundles. A low light intensity alarm must be corrected before the venous saturation measurement is considered reliable or before the system is recalibrated. Large fluctuations in the light intensity signal may indicate that the catheter tip is malpositioned but also may indicate a condition of intravascular volume deficit that allows compression or collapse of the pulmonary vasculature (especially during positive pressure ventilation) (34).

CONTINUOUS CENTRAL VENOUS ($Sc\bar{v}O_2$) MONITORING

Early management of the critically ill patient is frequently performed outside the intensive care unit. The time between the onset of critical illness and definitive ICU intervention can be significantly long and have outcome implications (35–37). Measurement of $S\bar{v}O_2$ requires placement of a pulmonary artery catheter, which may not be feasible early in the resuscitation of adult, pediatric, and neonatal patients. However, central venous assess can be obtained in both ICU and non-ICU settings making continuous $Sc\bar{v}O_2$ monitoring a convenient surrogate for $S\bar{v}O_2$.

Numerous animal and human models have examined the relationship between $S\bar{v}O_2$ and $Sc\bar{v}O_2$ obtained from the superior vena cava and right atria (Fig. 26.7). Superior venal caval (SVC) $Sc\bar{v}O_2$ is slightly lower and more accurately reflects $S\bar{v}O_2$ when patients were not in shock (38,39). Right atrial $Sc\bar{v}O_2$ has a better correlation than superior vena caval saturation and is not significantly different from $S\bar{v}O_2$ whether in shock or not in shock (38). In patients in shock a consistent reversal of this relationship occurs, the $Sc\bar{v}O_2$ is greater than $S\bar{v}O_2$, and this difference can range from 5% to 18% (38–40). Redistribution of blood flow away from the splenic, renal, and mesenteric bed toward the cerebral and coronary circulation including more desaturated blood (<30%) from the coronary sinus contribute to this observation (38). Thus, $Sc\bar{v}O_2$ will consistently overestimate the true $S\bar{v}O_2$ under shock conditions.

There has been considerable debate regarding whether $Sc\bar{v}O_2$ is a satisfactory substitute for $S\bar{v}O_2$, particularly in ranges above 65% (41–50). Although the absolute values of $Sc\bar{v}O_2$ and $S\bar{v}O_2$ differ, studies have shown close and consistent tracking of the two sites across a wide range of hemodynamic conditions (Figs. 26.8 and 26.9), thus making it clinically useful (43,51–62). The clinical utility or value of $S\bar{v}O_2/Sc\bar{v}O_2$ is in the lower ranges. The presence of a pathologically low $Sc\bar{v}O_2$ value (implying an even lower $S\bar{v}O_2$) is more clinically

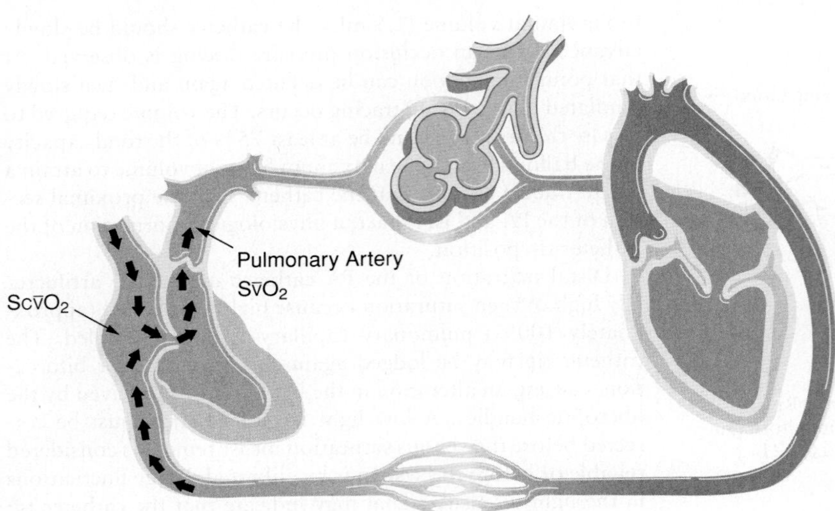

FIGURE 26.7. Central versus mixed venous oxygen saturation.

important than whether the values are equal. Goldman et al. (51) found that Sc$\bar{v}O_2$ <60% showed evidence of heart failure or shock or a combination of the two. Hyperdynamic septic shock ICU patients seldom exhibit S$\bar{v}O_2$ levels <60% to 65%, which, when sustained, is associated with increased mortality (12,63). Studies examining the clinical utility of Sc$\bar{v}O_2$ early in the course of disease presentation routinely encounter values less than 50%, which are considered critical (3,64,65). At these values, venous saturations are actually 5% to 18% lower in the pulmonary artery (38,40) and 15% lower in the splanchnic bed (19). Thus, although not numerically equivalent, these ranges of values have similar pathologic implications (51) and are associated with high mortality (23).

The clinical utility of an end point of resuscitation is determined by whether it changes clinical practice and morbidity/mortality. Irrespective of whether the Sc$\bar{v}O_2$ equals S$\bar{v}O_2$, the presence of a low Sc$\bar{v}O_2$ in early sepsis portends increased mortality and correcting this value by a treatment algorithm (66) improves morbidity and mortality. The concept of the approximately 5% numeric difference between S$\bar{v}O_2$ and Sc$\bar{v}O_2$ prompted the Surviving Sepsis Campaign to recommend reaching a S$\bar{v}O_2$ of 65% and/or Sc$\bar{v}O_2$ of 70% goal in the resuscitation portion of its severe sepsis and septic shock bundle (67,68).

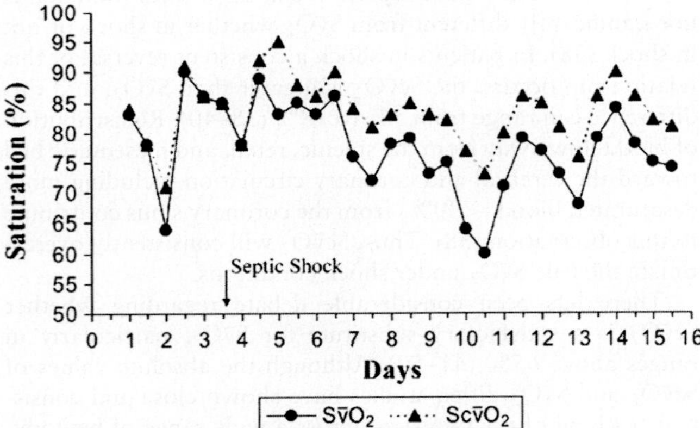

FIGURE 26.8. Central versus mixed venous oxygen saturation. (From Reinhart K, Rudolph T, Bredle DL, et al. Comparison of central-venous to mixed-venous oxygen saturation during changes in oxygen supply/demand. *Chest.* 1989;95(6):1216–1221.)

INTERPRETATION OF VENOUS OXYGEN SATURATION

The algorithm is presented in Figure 26.10. Mixed venous oxygen saturation values within the normal range (67%–75%) indicate a normal balance between oxygen supply and demand, provided that vasoregulation is intact and a normal distribution of peripheral blood flow is present. Values of S$\bar{v}O_2$ greater than 75% indicate an excess of $\dot{D}O_2$ over $\dot{V}O_2$ and are most commonly associated with syndromes of vasoderegulation such as cirrhosis and sepsis. High values also are seen in states of low $\dot{V}O_2$ (hypothermia, muscular paralysis, sedation, coma, hypothyroidism, or a combination of these factors), hyperoxygenation, high CO, inability to consume oxygen, and rarely, cyanide toxicity.

Uncompensated changes in any of the four determinants of S$\bar{v}O_2$ may result in a decrease in the measured value, but in complex, critically ill patients, the correlation between changes in S$\bar{v}O_2$ and changes in any of the individual determining factors is low (69). In a study of the patients in a surgical ICU, no statistical correlation existed between changes in either PaO_2 or SaO_2 and S$\bar{v}O_2$. Although there was a statistically significant correlation between changes in S$\bar{v}O_2$ and CO and $\dot{D}O_2$, the coefficients of determination (r^2) were too low to allow prediction of CO, oxygen consumption, or oxygen delivery from S$\bar{v}O_2$. Also, no statistical correlation existed between S$\bar{v}O_2$ and either arterial-venous oxygen content difference or calculated $\dot{V}O_2$. There was a significant inverse correlation between S$\bar{v}O_2$ and oxygen utilization coefficient, confirming the accuracy of the measurement and the reliability of S$\bar{v}O_2$ as an estimation of the oxygen utilization ratio—as long as arterial oxygen saturation is near 100%. The determinants of S$\bar{v}O_2$ are multifactorial, and, in critically ill patients, the degree of compensation for changes in one variable cannot be predicted (69). Patients with chronically impaired O_2 transport appear

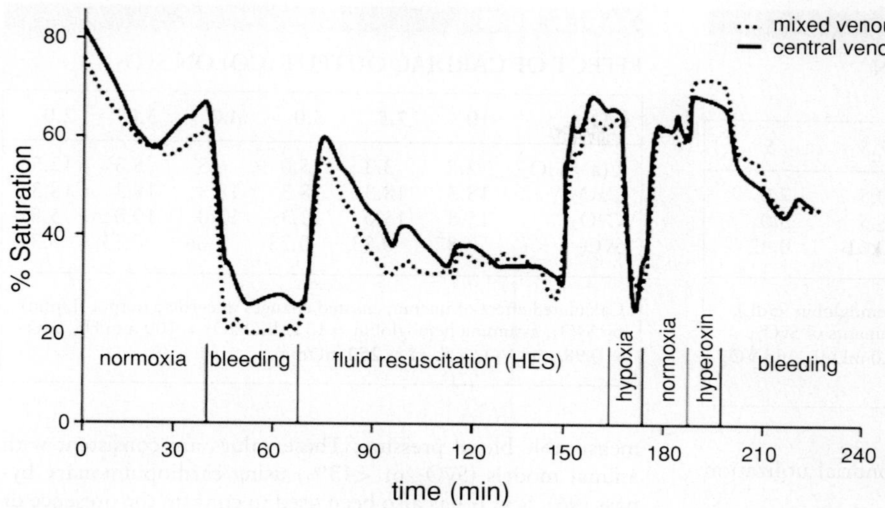

FIGURE 26.9. Central versus mixed venous oxygen saturation. HES, hydroxyethyl starch. (From Reinhart K, Rudolph T, Bredle DL, et al. Comparison of central-venous to mixed-venous oxygen saturation during changes in oxygen supply/demand. *Chest.* 1989;95(6):1216–1221.)

to tolerate very low $S\bar{v}O_2$ values better than acutely ill patients, presumably due to adaptive changes in the former group. Delayed lactate presentation may be seen in this group of patients (70,71).

It is useful, however, to appreciate the magnitude of change in $S\bar{v}O_2$ that would occur with an isolated change in any of the individual determinants. If no compensatory changes occur in $\dot{V}O_2$ or CO, Hgb must decrease by almost 50% (13 to 7.5 g/dl/L) before $S\bar{v}O_2$ decreases below the lower limit of the normal range (Table 26.2). The $S\bar{v}O_2$ changes would be even smaller because CO should increase in response to the acute anemia. However, if CO is fixed because of underlying cardiovascular disease, a decrease in Hgb will be reflected by a decrease in $S\bar{v}O_2$.

The effect of arterial oxygen tension on $S\bar{v}O_2$ in the absence of other compensatory changes is demonstrated in Table 26.3. As long as SaO_2 is maintained in a relatively normal range, the direct effect on $S\bar{v}O_2$ is minimal. However, when there is sufficient arterial hypoxemia to produce arterial desaturation, the $S\bar{v}O_2$ falls in direct proportion to the change in SaO_2. Similarly, changes in CO (Table 26.4) and $\dot{V}O_2$ (Table 26.5) may be shown to affect $S\bar{v}O_2$, although the magnitude of change in any of these individual parameters does not predict the magnitude of change in $S\bar{v}O_2$ because compensatory factors are usually involved. A decrease in $S\bar{v}O_2$ greater than 10% is likely to be clinically significant regardless of the initial value. A change from 70% to 60% may be associated with a large fractional change in CO if other factors did not change. On the other hand, a change from 60% to 50% is associated with a much smaller fractional change in CO but in the range of limited oxygen transport reserve and should raise more concern (Table 26.6).

When demand exceeds consumption, anaerobic metabolism must occur, and the eventual result is lactic acidosis. The lactate level, therefore, defines the balance between $\dot{V}O_2$ and oxygen demand. An elevated lactate implies either ongoing anaerobic metabolism (shock) or prior anaerobic metabolism and oxygen debt. A normal $S\bar{v}O_2$ implies the latter and a low $S\bar{v}O_2$, the former, in states of lactic acidosis, except in situations in

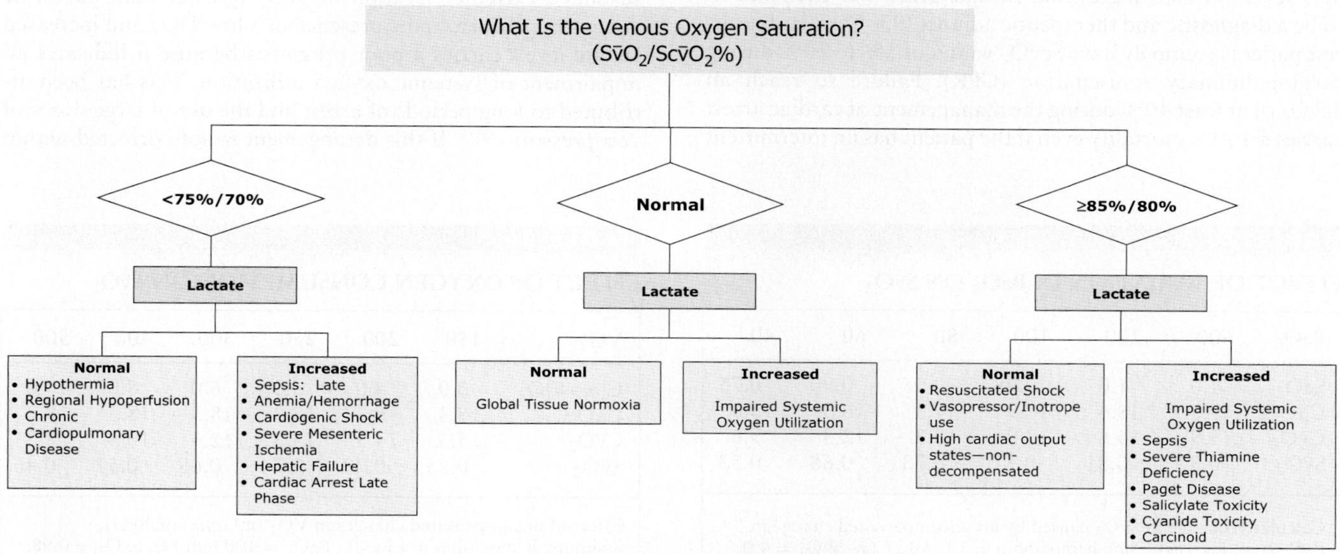

FIGURE 26.10. Diagnostic algorithm of $Sc\bar{v}O_2/S\bar{v}O_2$.

TABLE 26.2

EFFECT OF CHANGES IN HEMOGLOBIN CONCENTRATION ON $S\bar{v}O_2$

Hemoglobin	13	10	7.5	5
CaO_2	18.0	14.0	10.5	7.0
$C\bar{v}O_2$	14.0	10.0	6.5	3.0
$S\bar{v}O_2$	0.77	0.71	0.61	0.42

Calculated change in $S\bar{v}O_2$ caused by a change in hemoglobin (g/dL), assuming no compensatory changes in other determinants of $S\bar{v}O_2$; PaO_2 = 100 mm Hg, SaO_2 = 0.98, $C(a-\bar{v})O_2$ = 4.0 mL/dL, and $\dot{V}O_2$ and cardiac output are not changed.

TABLE 26.4

EFFECT OF CARDIAC OUTPUT (CO) ON $S\bar{v}O_2$

CO	10	7.5	5.0	4.0	3.0	2.0
$C(a-\bar{v})O_2$	2.5	3.3	5.0	6.3	8.3	12.5
CaO_2	18.3	18.3	18.3	18.3	18.3	18.3
$C\bar{v}O_2$	15.8	15.0	13.3	12.0	10.0	5.8
$S\bar{v}O_2$	0.87	0.83	0.73	0.66	0.55	0.31

Calculated effect of uncompensated changes in cardiac output (L/min) on $S\bar{v}O_2$, assuming hemoglobin = 13 g/dL, PaO_2 = 100 mm Hg, SaO_2 = 0.98, and $\dot{V}O_2$ is fixed at 250 mL/min.

which unloading cellular uptake or mitochondrial utilization are impaired.

CLINICAL USES OF $S\bar{v}O_2$ MONITORING

$S\bar{v}O_2$ values have been used extensively in various clinical scenarios in critically ill patients. These include during and after cardiac arrest (72,73), in cardiac surgery patients (74), during and after cardiac failure (75), shock (76), acute myocardial infarction (51,77), general medical ICU conditions (78–80), postoperative cardiovascular procedures (81), trauma (82–84), vascular surgery (85,86), septic shock (9,12,63), hypovolemia (87,88), pediatric surgery (75), in neonates (89), lung transplantation (90), and cardiogenic shock (91,92).

Cardiac Arrest

Management of the cardiac arrest patient by advanced cardiac life support (ACLS) guidelines include physical examination (i.e., palpation of a pulse) and electrocardiographic monitoring. $Sc\bar{v}O_2$ monitoring during cardiac arrest has been shown to be a diagnostic and therapeutic adjunct (93–95). Cardiac arrest patients routinely have $Sc\bar{v}O_2$ values of 5% to 20% during cardiopulmonary resuscitation (CPR). Failure to reach an $Sc\bar{v}O_2$ of at least 40% during the management of cardiac arrest carries a 100% mortality even if the patient has an intermittent measurable blood pressure. These values are consistent with animal models ($S\bar{v}O_2$ of <43%) using cardiopulmonary bypass (96). $Sc\bar{v}O_2$ has also been used to confirm the presence or absence of sustainable cardiac activity during electromechanical dissociation (EMD) or a pulseless idioventricular rhythm where over 35% of these patients have been shown to have spontaneous cardiac activity (pseudo-EMD) (97). If the $Sc\bar{v}O_2$ is greater than 60% during CPR, return of spontaneous circulation (ROSC) is likely, and the pulse should be frequently rechecked if EMD was present. Between $Sc\bar{v}O_2$ values of 40% and 72%, there is a progressive increase in the rate of ROSC. When an $Sc\bar{v}O_2$ greater than 72% is obtained, ROSC has likely occurred. Continuous $Sc\bar{v}O_2$ monitoring also provides an objective measure to confirm the adequacy or inadequacy of CPR in providing $\dot{D}O_2$.

Post–Cardiac Arrest Care

In the immediate postresuscitation period, patients are frequently hemodynamically unstable and have a high frequency of rearrest. Blood pressure (1,94) may be rendered insensitive in the measurement of cardiac output or oxygen delivery secondary to the high systemic vascular resistance of catecholamine therapy. An abrupt or gradual decrease in $S\bar{v}O_2$ (less than 40%–50%) indicates likelihood for rearrest. An $S\bar{v}O_2$ greater than 60% to 70% indicates hemodynamic stability. A sustained extreme elevation of $S\bar{v}O_2$ (greater than 80%), or venous hyperoxia, in the presence of a low $\dot{D}O_2$ and increased lactate levels carries a poor prognosis because it indicates an impairment of systemic oxygen utilization. This has been attributed to long periods of arrest and the use of large doses of vasopressors (98). If this derangement is not corrected within

TABLE 26.3

EFFECT OF VARIATION IN PaO_2 ON $S\bar{v}O_2$

PaO_2	600	200	100	80	60	40
SaO_2	1.0	1.0	0.98	0.95	0.90	0.75
CaO_2	19.8	18.6	17.9	17.3	16.3	13.6
$C\bar{v}O_2$	15.9	14.6	13.9	13.3	12.3	9.6
$S\bar{v}O_2$	0.87	0.81	0.77	0.73	0.68	0.53

Calculated change in $S\bar{v}O_2$ caused by an uncompensated change in PaO_2 (mm Hg), assuming hemoglobin = 13 g/dL, $C(a-\bar{v})O_2$ = 4.0 mL/dL, and $\dot{V}O_2$ and cardiac output are unchanged.

TABLE 26.5

EFFECT OF OXYGEN CONSUMPTION ON $S\bar{v}O_2$

$\dot{V}O_2$	150	200	250	300	400	500
$C(a-\bar{v})O_2$	3.0	4.0	5.0	6.0	8.0	10.0
CaO_2	18.3	18.3	18.3	18.3	18.3	18.3
$C\bar{v}O_2$	15.3	14.3	13.3	12.3	10.3	8.3
$S\bar{v}O_2$	0.85	0.79	0.74	0.68	0.57	0.46

Effect of uncompensated changes in $\dot{V}O_2$ (mL/min) on $S\bar{v}O_2$, assuming hemoglobin = 13 g/dL, PaO_2 = 100 mm Hg, SaO_2 = 0.98, and cardiac output is fixed at 5 L/min.

TABLE 26.6

PERCENTAGE OF ERROR RESULTING FROM ESTIMATION OF $P\bar{v}O_2$

Factor	Measured values of $S\bar{v}O_2$ 0.50	0.75	0.85
$C\bar{v}O_2$	1.2	0.8	0.7
$C(a-\bar{v})O_2$	1.2	2.6	4.8
$\dot{V}O_2$	1.2	2.6	4.8
$\dot{Q}_{sp}/\dot{Q}_t$	0.9	1.0	3.0

Theoretical maximum errors (%) in derived parameters if $P\bar{v}O_2$ is estimated at 20 and 50 mm Hg for each saturation value measured. Maximum error is 4.8% only at the extreme of estimating $P\bar{v}O_2$ to be 20 mm Hg when $S\bar{v}O_2$ is 0.85. The maximum error would be one half of this amount if $P\bar{v}O_2$ is estimated to be 35 mm Hg in all cases. These maximum predicted errors are not clinically significant.

the first 6 hours of the early postresuscitation period, the outcome is uniformly fatal (94). Venous hyperoxia can also be seen after acute myocardial infarction. Postexercise $S\bar{v}O_2$ overshoot and, hence, decreased systemic oxygen extraction during recovery represent a compensatory response of an enhanced peripheral vascular tone that maintains systemic arterial blood pressure in the setting of reduced cardiac output by linking central and peripheral blood flow (99).

Traumatic and Hemorrhagic Shock

The standards of Advanced Trauma Life Support focus on normalization of vital signs (100). Studies have shown that vital signs are insensitive end points of resuscitation and outcome predictors in hemorrhage and trauma resuscitation (1,101). Scalea et al. (101) and Kowalenko et al. (102) have shown that patients presenting with trauma and hemorrhage required additional resuscitation or surgical procedures if the $Sc\bar{v}O_2$ remained less than 65%. Kremzar et al. (82) examined whether maintaining normal levels of $S\bar{v}O_2$ in patients with multiple injuries is more relevant to survival than maintaining above-normal levels of oxygen transport. For patients with multiple injuries, maintaining normal $S\bar{v}O_2$ values and increasing $\dot{D}O_2$ only if required are more relevant for survival than routine maintenance of above-normal oxygen transport values. In a series of 10 seriously injured patients requiring resuscitation and definitive operative control of hemorrhage, Karzarian and Del Guercio (83) found that improvement of the $S\bar{v}O_2$ was associated with improved survival. In this study, mixed venous oxygen saturations were valuable predictors of survival and were a helpful parameter to monitor during the resuscitative, operative, and immediate postoperative periods.

Acute and Chronic Heart Failure and Pulmonary Hypertension

Cardiogenic shock is characterized by decreased $\dot{D}O_2$, decreased $S\bar{v}O_2$, increased O_2ER and evidence of tissue hypoxia (lactic acidosis, end-organ dysfunction) secondary to acute myocardial dysfunction (91,92). $S\bar{v}O_2$ has been shown to have therapeutic and prognostic utility in patients with acute myocardial infarction (77,92,103,104). Prospective outcome studies have not validated its clinical use in this patient population (105). Ander et al. (64) examined patients who presented with decompensated chronic severe heart failure (ejection fraction <30%) who were stratified into normal and elevated lactate (>2 mmol/L) groups. There was a significant prevalence of "occult cardiogenic shock" ($Sc\bar{v}O_2$ of 26.4%–36.8%) in the presence of normal vital signs. Using a goal-oriented approach of preload, afterload, contractility, coronary perfusion, and heart rate optimization, these patients required additional therapy compared to their counterparts with normal lactate levels. $Sc\bar{v}O_2$ and brain natriuretic peptide (BNP) level predict hemodynamics associated with lower survival rates and may be useful as noninvasive markers of prognosis in epoprostenol-treated pulmonary arterial hypertension (PAH) patients (106).

Severe Sepsis and Septic Shock

$S\bar{v}O_2$ in sepsis is commonly referred to as an end point of low impact in clinical decisions in sepsis because of the common perception that $S\bar{v}O_2$ is always increased in septic ICU patients. However, there are fundamental issues that render this modality clinically useful when applying it to the early stages of supply-dependent phase of sepsis (global tissue hypoxia) where saturation is low in both animal (107,108) and human models of sepsis (103). During this phase $S\bar{v}O_2$ is inversely correlated with lactate concentration ($r = -0.87$, $p < 0.001$). These data suggest that cellular oxygen utilization is largely maintained during rapidly fatal septic shock (109,110). Identifying sudden episodes of supply dependency in septic ICU patients (sudden decreases in $S\bar{v}O_2$) has diagnostic and prognostic significance (10,12,63). Previous studies have examined $S\bar{v}O_2$-guided goal-directed therapy after ICU admission and have found no outcome benefit in general ICU patients (79). However, in a study evaluating early goal-directed therapy (EGDT) using multiple hemodynamic end points including $S\bar{v}O_2$ in the most proximal stages of hospital admission, patients presenting with severe sepsis and septic shock were randomized to 6 hours of EGDT or standard therapy before ICU admission. Both groups were resuscitated to a central venous pressure (CVP) >8 mm Hg and mean arterial pressure (MAP) >65 mm Hg; however, the treatment group was resuscitated to a $Sc\bar{v}O_2$ >70% using additional therapies such as red cell transfusion, inotropes, and mechanical ventilation to reach this end point (Fig. 26.11). Over the initial 72 hours, there was a higher central venous O_2 saturation, lower lactate, lower base deficit, and higher pH in the EGDT versus the control group indicating more definitive resolution of global tissue hypoxia. Organ dysfunction, vasopressor use, duration of mechanical ventilation, and mortality were significantly reduced (9). This concept of EGDT has been reproduced in multiple studies and is one of the cornerstones of the resuscitation bundle recommended by the Surviving Sepsis Campaign (111).

Pulmonary Embolus

Patients with massive pulmonary embolism and obstructive shock usually require hemodynamic stabilization, thrombolytics, and mechanical interventions. Krivec et al. (112) examined

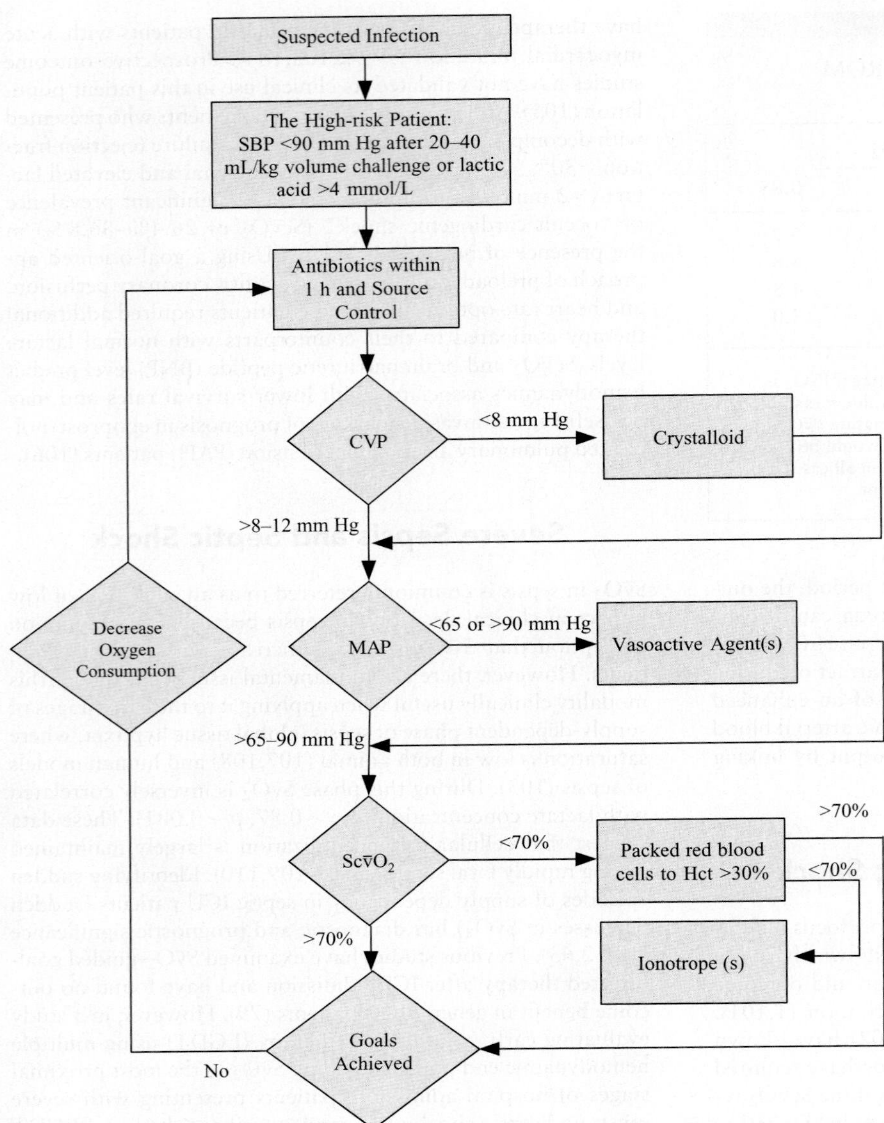

FIGURE 26.11. Early goal-directed therapy (EGDT) in severe sepsis and septic shock. CVP, central venous pressure; Hct, hematocrit; MAP, mean arterial pressure; SBP, systolic blood pressure; $Sc\bar{v}O_2$, central venous oxygen saturation. (From Rivers E, Nguyen B, Havstad S, et al. Early goal-directed therapy in the treatment of severe sepsis and septic shock. *N Engl J Med.* 2001;345(19):1368–1377.)

10 consecutive patients hospitalized in the ICU with obstructive shock following massive pulmonary embolism in a prospective observational study. During hemodynamic optimization and infusion of thrombolytics therapy, heart rate, CVP, mean pulmonary artery pressure, and urine output remained unchanged, but the relative change of $S\bar{v}O_2$ at hour 1 was higher than the relative changes of all other studied variables ($p < 0.05$). Serum lactate on admission and at 12 hours correlated to $S\bar{v}O_2$ ($r = -0.855$, $p < 0.001$). In obstructive shock after massive pulmonary embolism, $S\bar{v}O_2$ changes more rapidly than other standard hemodynamic variables.

Respiratory Failure

In nine of 13 patients with hypoxemic respiratory failure requiring positive end-expiratory pressure (PEEP), there was a strong correlation ($r = 0.88$) between $\dot{D}O_2$ and $S\bar{v}O_2$. Of the four patients not showing a good correlation, two had sepsis and two had nearly normal values of $S\bar{v}O_2$ and oxygen delivery at all levels of PEEP studied. Continuous measurement of $S\bar{v}O_2$ improves monitoring of patients, facilitates titration of respiratory therapies, detects abrupt changes in tissue oxygen consumption, and identifies levels of PEEP associated with greatest oxygen delivery (113).

Postoperative Thoracic and Cardiac Surgery Patients

Continuous $S\bar{v}O_2$ monitoring was examined in 19 patients as to its predictive value during the postoperative course after thoracotomy for a time period up to 60 hours. In all but one of the 10 patients with $S\bar{v}O_2$ less than 65% for at least one hour, complications occurred. A fall of $S\bar{v}O_2$ more than 5% or a value <60% predicted a period of hypotension in six patients. In two of them this coincided with a period of ventricular arrhythmias. In those with $S\bar{v}O_2$ below 65%, no postoperative complications such as arrhythmias, shock, respiratory dysfunction, or oliguria took place (76). Cardiac surgical patients are at risk of inadequate perioperative oxygen delivery caused by extracorporeal circulation and limited cardiovascular reserves (114,115). Four hundred and three elective cardiac surgical patients were enrolled in the study and randomly assigned to either the control or the protocol group. Goals of the protocol group were to maintain $S\bar{v}O_2$ >70% and a lactate concentration ≤2.0 mmol/L from ICU admission and up to 8 hours thereafter. The median hospital stay was shorter in the protocol group (6 vs. 7 days, $p < 0.05$), and patients were discharged faster from the hospital than those in the control group ($p < 0.05$). Discharge from the ICU was similar between groups ($p = 0.8$). Morbidity was less frequent at the time of hospital discharge in the protocol group (1.1% vs. 6.1%, $p < 0.01$) (116). Venous oximetry has also been shown to have clinical utility in weaning patients from ventricular assist devices (117,118).

Vascular Surgery

In 31 patients undergoing elective operations for aortic aneurysms ($n = 25$) and aortoiliac occlusive disease ($n = 6$), $S\bar{v}O_2$ was recorded throughout the operation. In all patients, unclamping the aorta resulted in a marked reduction of mean $S\bar{v}O_2$, with no change in the cardiac output or SaO_2. The unclamping of tube grafts was associated with a significant reduction in arterial pH ($p < 0.01$) and in $S\bar{v}O_2$ ($p < 0.001$) when compared with unclamping of bifurcation grafts. Despite a longer clamp time, unclamping the second limb of a bifurcation graft resulted in a smaller decrease in $S\bar{v}O_2$ when compared with that observed after unclamping the first limb (12% vs. 6%, $p < 0.01$). The change in $S\bar{v}O_2$ after unclamping the second limb was only 2% in aortobifemoral grafts and 9% in aortobi-iliac grafts. Reperfusion via extensive pelvic and lumbar collaterals in patients with aortoiliac occlusive disease reduces the degree of $S\bar{v}O_2$ decrease after aortic unclamping. Monitoring the changes in $S\bar{v}O_2$ during different types of aortic reconstruction helps to define precisely the physiologic alterations that occur in the course of these operations (85,86).

Postoperative High-Risk Patients

$Sc\bar{v}O_2$ and other biochemical, physiologic and demographic data were prospectively measured for 8 hours after major surgery. Data from 118 patients were analyzed; 123 morbidity episodes occurred in 64 of these patients. The optimal $Sc\bar{v}O_2$ cutoff value for morbidity prediction was 64.4%. In the first hour after surgery, significant reductions in $Sc\bar{v}O_2$ were observed, but there were no significant changes in cardiac index (CI) or oxygen delivery index during the same period. Significant fluctuations in $Sc\bar{v}O_2$ occur in the immediate postoperative period and are not always associated with changes in oxygen delivery, suggesting that oxygen consumption is also an important determinant of $Sc\bar{v}O_2$. Reductions in $Sc\bar{v}O_2$ are independently associated with postoperative complications (119–121).

Positioning Patients and Postural Changes

The effects of changes in positioning on $S\bar{v}O_2$ in critically ill patients with a low ejection fraction (≤30%) and the contribution of variables of oxygen delivery ($\dot{D}O_2$) and oxygen consumption ($\dot{V}O_2$) to the variance in $S\bar{v}O_2$ were examined. An experimental two-group repeated-measures design was used to study 42 critically ill patients with an ejection fraction of ≤30%. Patients were assigned randomly to one of two position sequences: supine, right lateral, left lateral; or supine, left lateral, right lateral. Data on $S\bar{v}O_2$ were collected at baseline, each minute after position change for 5 minutes, and at 15 and 25 minutes. A difference in $S\bar{v}O_2$ among the three positions across time was significantly different ($p < 0.0001$), with the greatest differences occurring within the first 4 minutes and in the left lateral position. $\dot{V}O_2$ accounted for a greater proportion of the variance in $S\bar{v}O_2$ with position change than did $\dot{D}O_2$ (122,123). Similar findings have been noted in $S\bar{v}O_2$ with orthostatic positioning and its superiority in reflecting central blood volume over central venous pressure (87).

Neonates and Pediatric Patients

$S\bar{v}O_2$ has been shown to be clinically useful in pediatric patients (124). However, the challenges of pulmonary artery catheterization make monitoring of the shock state with $S\bar{v}O_2$ limited, making $Sc\bar{v}O_2$ a convenient surrogate (75,89). In an experimental model of neonatal sepsis, $S\bar{v}O_2$ significantly correlates with right atrium oxygen saturation ($r^2 = 0.88$). Animal studies suggest that $Sc\bar{v}O_2$ at the right atrium can be a sure, efficient, and easy alternative for the neonatal patient (125), particularly during therapeutic interventions such as mechanical ventilation and intravascular volume resuscitation (126). Studies in patients have been less consistent. Simultaneous $Sc\bar{v}O_2$ and $S\bar{v}O_2$ values in children recovering from open heart surgery show $Sc\bar{v}O_2$ is consistently lower than $S\bar{v}O_2$. This difference may be secondary to residual intracardiac left-to-right shunting of blood or to altered distribution of systemic blood flow. The saturation difference between the two venous samples decreases during postoperative recovery, making a $Sc\bar{v}O_2$ blood sample an inadequate substitute for $S\bar{v}O_2$. Because $Sc\bar{v}O_2$ was frequently subnormal while $S\bar{v}O_2$ was in the normal range, monitoring of $S\bar{v}O_2$ could not be reliably used to rule out oxygen supply/demand imbalance during the early postoperative period in these patients (124,127). To overcome these clinical inconsistencies, a regression formula was derived: $S\bar{v}O_2 = 3 \times SVC + HIVC$ divided by 4, where SVC is superior vena cava saturation and HIVC is high inferior vena cava saturation (61). Validation of the clinical utility of $Sc\bar{v}O_2$ in children has the same challenges as in adults. A sepsis trial reported significant survival benefit when $Sc\bar{v}O_2$ was added to the pediatric model of septic shock. This study supports current recommendations by the American College of Critical Care Medicine for its use in neonatal and pediatric septic shock (Fig. 26.12) (128).

COST EFFECTIVENESS

Economic analysis of the technology of venous oximetry is complex. Because of its variable use in many clinical situations, the direct association with one single variable to outcome and health care resource consumption is not a simple one. In quantitating the economic impact, one must assess prevention of additional resource use such as venous blood gases and nursing time, hemodynamic life-threatening events, and decreased

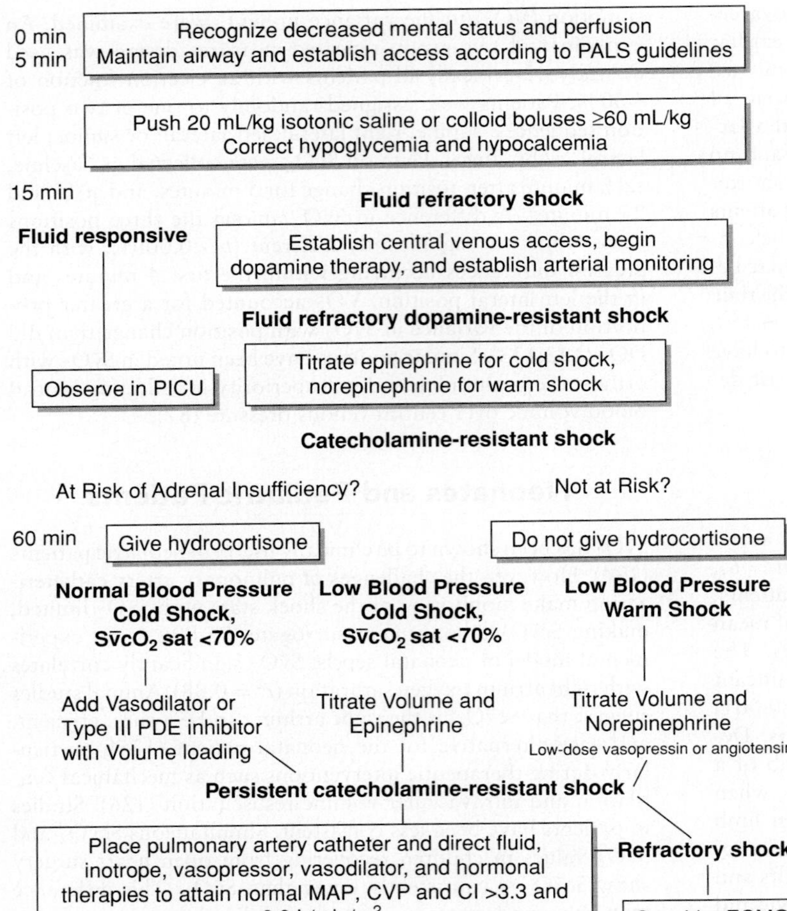

FIGURE 26.12. Pediatric advanced life support (PALS). Cl, chlorine; CVP, central venous pressure; ECMO; extracorporeal membrane oxygenation; MAP, mean arterial pressure; PDE, phosphodiesterase; PICU, pediatric intensive care unit; $Sc\bar{v}O_2$, central venous oxygen saturation. (From Carcillo JA, Fields AI. Clinical practice parameters for hemodynamic support of pediatric and neonatal patients in septic shock. *Crit Care Med.* 2002;30(6):1365–1378.)

health care resource consumption through improved morbidity and mortality. Significant reductions in the number of venous blood gas analyses, cardiac output measurement, and charges have been observed (113,129,130). Several studies have suggested that the increased cost of the fiberoptic catheter is not justifiable in terms of cost savings (131,132). However, in the treatment of sepsis and cardiothoracic patients, significant reductions in morbidity, mortality, and health care resource consumption have been observed with goal-directed algorithms using venous oximetry (116,133).

COMBINED VENOUS AND PULSE OXIMETRY

Pulse oximetry and continuous mixed venous oximetry can be combined into a useful tool if we understand the underlying physiology that allows certain inferences to be made as well as the limitations. The two devices together provide the capacity to evaluate simultaneous changes in the patient's cardiovascular and respiratory systems. Arterial oxygen tension and arterial oxygen saturation are related through the familiar oxyhemoglobin dissociation curve. SaO_2 values in the range of 70 to 95 reflect changes in PaO_2 and are useful in monitoring cardiorespiratory disease and directing therapy. Large changes in PaO_2 (80–600 mm Hg) can occur with minimum changes in SaO_2. To maintain arterial oxygen delivery, we keep SaO_2 values between 90% and 95%. Below 90%, desaturation diminishes arterial oxygen content and oxygen delivery; above 95%, SaO_2 values no longer track PaO_2 values. At a Hgb value of 13 g/dL, fully saturated Hgb would carry 18.07 mL of oxygen. If arterial PO_2 was 100 mm Hg, an additional 0.31 mL would be dissolved in plasma for a total oxygen content of 18.38 mL per 100 mL of blood. If PaO_2 fell to 75 mm Hg and SaO_2 concomitantly dropped to 95%, Hgb-carried oxygen would be 18.07 times 0.95, or 17.17 mL. The dissolved oxygen would be 75 times 0.003, or 0.23, and total oxygen content would be 17.4 mL in 100 mL of blood. In the first example, total oxygen content was 18.38 mL. If the second oxygen content, 17.4 mL, is divided by 18.38 mL, the quotient is 0.95; thus, total oxygen content changed the same amount as did the arterial saturation. We can obtain the same information by comparing changes in SaO_2 alone without following either PaO_2 or calculating total oxygen content. The same is true for $S\bar{v}O_2$ and mixed venous oxygen content (27,134,135).

APPLICABILITY

There are many valuable bedside uses for simultaneous oximetry. For instance, if a patient's respiratory function has improved, high FiO_2 may be weaned quickly. We have found that changes can be made every 5 minutes. This contrasts to the usual clinical scenario using blood gases where after a change in FiO_2 (15-minute equilibration period), drawing of blood is done. If patients have severely depressed oxygenation, PEEP therapy can be augmented much more rapidly by monitoring $S\bar{v}O_2$. In the case of cardiovascular collapse associated with low $S\bar{v}O_{2i}$ the response to blood and other fluid infusions as well as vasoactive drugs can be judged rapidly. If the intervention does not increase $S\bar{v}O_2$ quickly (within a few minutes), it probably has not been effective. Increased CO may result in increased oxygen consumption without a change in SaO_2 minus $S\bar{v}O_2$. This ability to judge the effectiveness of interventions quickly is certainly attractive and often gratifying to the clinician.

LIMITATIONS AND FUTURE QUESTIONS

In spite of studies questioning the value of $S\bar{v}O_2$ in ICU patients (94,127,132,136), there is considerable evidence that $Sc\bar{v}O_2$ may have a beneficial role in the early management of critically ill adults, children, and neonates (89,126). The ability to access this information earlier in the phases of critical illness is now a reality, and further studies are now in progress to confirm that early recognition and treatment of out-of-normal-range $Sc\bar{v}O_2$ values have significant outcome benefit.

CLINICAL EXAMPLES

Case 1

A 75-year-old male victim of a witnessed cardiac arrest presents to the emergency department. After bystander CPR was performed, emergency medical services (EMS) initiates advanced cardiac life support (ACLS) guidelines. He was found to be in ventricular fibrillation and was successfully defibrillated into normal sinus rhythm. He is admitted to the ICU.

Vital signs: Blood pressure (BP), 160/80; MAP, 106 mm Hg; heart rate (HR), 130 beats per minute; respiratory rate (RR), 16 (bag/valve/mask); temp, 36.4°C; SaO_2, 98% on 100% FiO_2; $Sc\bar{v}O_2$, 85%.

Arterial blood gas (ABG) (21%): pH, 7.20; $PaCO_2$, 31; PaO_2, 63; SaO_2, 93%; $NaHCO_3$, 18; base deficit, −5.

Complete blood count (CBC): White blood cells (WBC), 15.1; hemoglobin (Hb), 10.5; hematocrit (Hct), 31%; platelets (PLT), 400,000.

PA catheter: CI, 1.2/minute/m^2; PAOP, 22 cm/H_2O; CVP, 26 cm/H_2O; systemic venous resistance (SVR), 5,600 dynes/s · cm^5.

Baseline		Therapy		Result
$Sc\bar{v}O_2$(CPR) 15%		*Nitroglycerin*		60%
$S\bar{v}O_2$ 90%		*Rate control*		3.2
Lactate 8.4 (mmol/L)	→		→	
SaO_2 93%				100%
O_2ER 10%		*EEP 5*		40%

What's the Baseline?

This case (Fig. 26.13) illustrates several important elements. Namely, the interpretation of the $S\bar{v}O_2$ is limited without an arterial blood gas since a near-normal $S\bar{v}O_2$ value does not imply normal physiology. The oxygen extraction ratio (O_3ER) ($aO_2 - \bar{v}O_2$ difference/SaO_2) is only 10%. The value of $S\bar{v}O_2$ is also confounded by the presence of mild anemia. Hypoxemia and circulatory arrest with resultant hypoperfusion leads to anaerobic metabolism represented by the presence of lactic acidosis.

What's Happening?

The O_2ER is very low, and in the setting of cardiac arrest, can possibly relate to the vasoconstrictive effects of vasopressors used during ACLS or the cytotoxic damage of global tissue hypoxia and reperfusion. This impairment of systemic oxygen utilization is manifest as mixed venous hyperoxia. Global tissue hypoxia ensues as a consequence of decreased perfusion

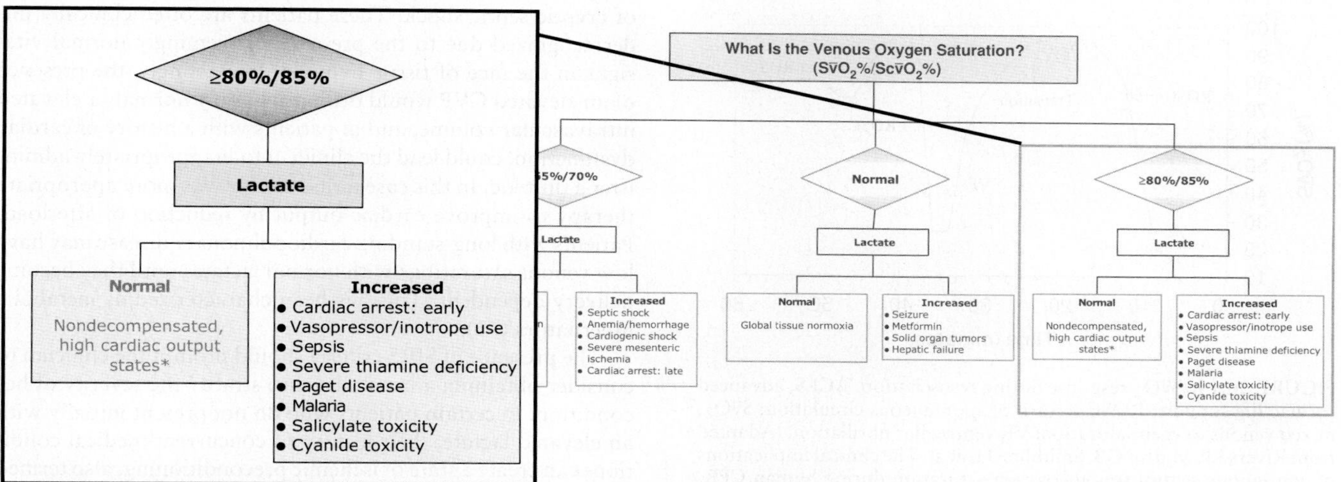

FIGURE 26.13. Baseline for Case 1.

and impaired tissue uptake resulting in lactic acidosis (73). It is notable that as treatment progresses with vasodilators, the O_2ER increases to 40% and lactate decreases.

What's the Interpretation?

The postresuscitative phase of cardiac arrest is characterized by a complex array of hemodynamic perturbations (Fig. 26.14). O_2ER can be up to 90% during cardiac arrest, and the failure to reach a $S\bar{v}O_2$ of 40% portends near 100% mortality (73). Once a return to spontaneous circulation (ROSC) is obtained, venous hyperoxia or an impaired O_2ER may be a temporary or permanent issue. The period immediately following multiple doses of vasopressors with ROSC is characterized by elevated circulating catecholamines and is termed the early postarrest phase. If efforts fail to decrease afterload, vasodilate the microcirculation, improve cardiac function to a $\dot{V}O_2$ above 90 mL/minute/m^2 within 6 hours after cardiac arrest and persistent lactic acidosis, death is imminent within 24 hours (73).

Similar scenarios to the early phase of cardiac arrest characterized by an elevated $S\bar{v}O_2$ and lactic acidosis can also be seen with vasopressor-dependent shock, sepsis, severe thiamine deficiency, severe Paget disease, malaria, salicylate toxicity, and cyanide toxicity. The later post-ROSC phase demonstrating low $S\bar{v}O_2$ and persistent lactic acidosis is comparable to hepatic failure, sepsis, anemia/hemorrhage, cardiogenic shock, and severe mesenteric ischemia.

Case 2

A 66-year-old female with a history of chronic obstructive lung disease (COPD) presents to the emergency department with a chief complaint of shortness of breath with fever for the past 4 days. She has had a cough productive of yellowish-greenish sputum and is tachypneic and in obvious respiratory distress.

Vital signs: BP, 140/80; HR, 118; RR, 24; temp, 38.0 C; pulmonary oxygen saturation (SpO_2), 88% on room air, 93% on 2 L/minute O_2

ED course: In the emergency department, the patient is noticeably more tachypneic and lethargic, so the patient is ultimately intubated for airway protection. Chest x-ray (CXR) study demonstrates a right lower lobe (RLL) infiltrate, consolidation, and airspace disease.

Hemodynamic monitoring in the ED: CVP, 16 cm/H_2O; $Sc\bar{v}O_2$, 44%; lactate, 1.9 mmol/L.

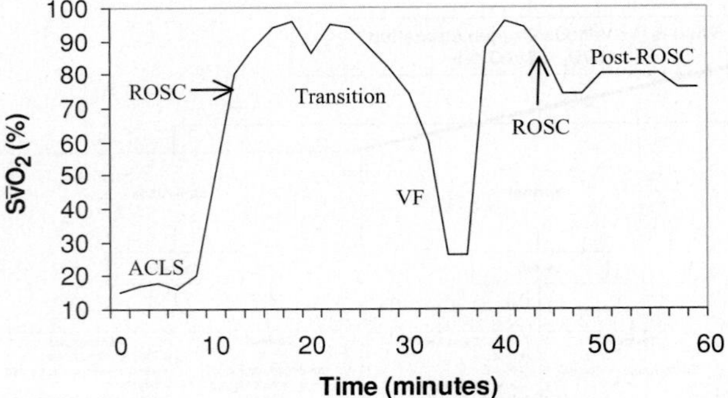

FIGURE 26.14. $S\bar{v}O_2$ response during resuscitation. ACLS, advanced cardiac life support; ROSC, return of spontaneous circulation; $S\bar{v}O_2$, mixed venous oxygen saturation; VF, ventricular fibrillation. (Adapted from Rivers EP, Martin GB, Smithline H, et al. The clinical implications of continuous central venous oxygen saturation during human CPR. *Ann Emerg Med.* 1992;21(9):1094–1101, with permission.)

About 1 minute after intubation, $Sc\bar{v}O_2$ monitoring begins to rise; $Sc\bar{v}O_2$ is now reading 58%. The patient is suctioned and copious thick sputum is removed. The patient's CVP improved to 8 cm H_2O after administration of a vasodilator. Repeat lactate reading increases 4.7 mmol/L.

Baseline		→	Therapy	→	Result
$Sc\bar{v}O_2$	44%		*Nitroglycerin*		58%
Lactate (mmol/L)	1.9		*Intubation*		4.7
SaO_2	88%				100%
O_2ER	50%				40%

What's the Baseline?

This patient has hypoxia, respiratory distress, and relatively stable vital signs (Fig. 26.15). The fever and clinical complaint in the presence of three systemic inflammatory response syndrome (SIRS) criteria makes pneumonia a likely inciting condition. The patient also exhibits hyperlactatemia and central venous hypoxia (low $Sc\bar{v}O_2$)

What's Happening?

The patient has symptoms consistent with pneumonia and hypoxemia with an O_2ER of 50%. This increased O_2ER despite a normal blood pressure with an elevated central venous pressure should alert the clinician of possible myocardial dysfunction.

What's the Interpretation?

The combination of three SIRS criteria and hyperlactatemia in the setting of infection heralds global hypoperfusion and organ dysfunction. The central venous hypoxemia reflects her oxygen delivery–dependent state. This illustrates the concept of cryptic septic shock. These patients are often clinically underrecognized due to the presence of seemingly normal vital signs in the face of tissue hypoxia. Interestingly, the presence of an elevated CVP would ordinarily imply normal or elevated intravascular volume, and in patients with a history of cardiac dysfunction, could lead the clinician to inappropriately administer a diuretic. In this case a vasodilator was more appropriate therapy to improve cardiac output by reduction of afterload. Patients with long-standing cardiopulmonary disease may have low venous saturations with normal lactates until they become delivery dependent. This has been characterized as metabolic hibernators (71).

The presence of SIRS criteria should prompt the clinician to consider obtaining a lactate level to stratify the severity of her condition. In certain patients who do not present initially with an elevated lactate, their history of concurrent medical conditions can create a state of ischemic preconditioning, also termed metabolic hibernation. This early recognition and treatment of

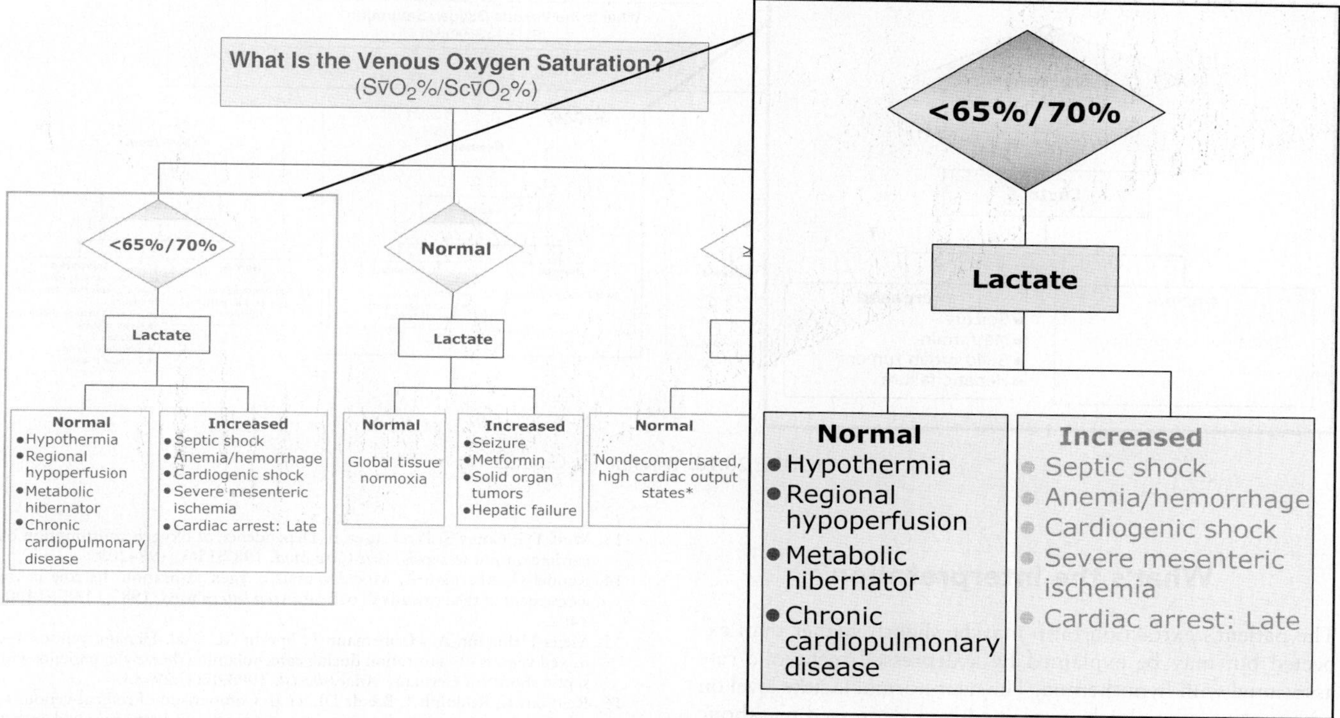

FIGURE 26.15. Baseline for Case 2.

the hypoperfused state was originally described by Rivers et al. where a protocolized approach to severe sepsis significantly improved morbidity and mortality. Similar hemodynamic conditions to this patient's *initial* presentation include hypothermia, a regional hypoperfused state, or congestive heart failure/cardiopulmonary disease.

Case 3

A 60-year-old male patient was brought to the emergency department from an assisted-living facility with a chief complaint of change in mental status. The patient has a past medical history significant for cerebral vascular accident (CVA), hypertension, schizophrenia, and diabetes. The patient was found slumped on a park bench.

Initially the patient is nonverbal and presents with the following vital signs: BP, 110/40; HR, 120; RR, 24; temp, 32°C; SaO_2, 96% on 2L O_2; Glasgow coma scale, 11.

Physical examination:

Patient receives 1-L bolus of crystalloids with mild increase in BP. The patient is taken to the monitored area of the ED because the nurse notices the patient is very slow to respond. The patient's bedside glucose is <50 mg/dL. The patient is given an amp of 50% dextrose. The patient's mental status immediately improves.

Labs: Na, 158; K, 5.2; Cl, 100; CO_2, 24; BUN, 90; creatinine, 1.8; glucose, 44; β-hydroxybutyrate, 8.0.

ABG: pH, 7.30; pCO_2, 44; paO_2, 100; SaO_2, 96%; HCO_3^-, 24; lactate, 2.0.

Hemodynamics: CVP, 1 cm H_2O, $Sc\bar{v}O_2$, 72%.
Hospital Course

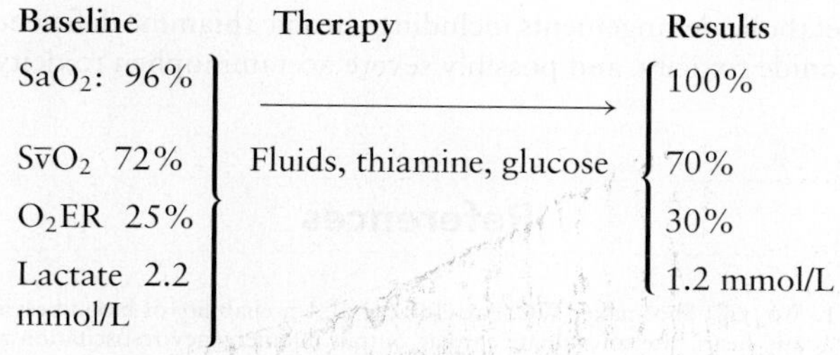

Baseline	Therapy	Results
SaO_2: 96%	→	100%
$S\bar{v}O_2$ 72%	Fluids, thiamine, glucose	70%
O_2ER 25%		30%
Lactate 2.2 mmol/L		1.2 mmol/L

What's the Baseline?

This patient's mental status is altered, probably due to the combination of hypoglycemia and hypothermia (Fig. 26.16). His initial presentation and hemodynamic measurements indicate severe volume depletion. The patient is maintaining a normal blood pressure but has evidence of progressing hemodynamic instability. Given his history, toxicologic and metabolic derangements may be responsible for his hemodynamic embarrassment.

What's Happening?

The patient is exhibiting evidence of anion gap metabolic acidosis (which may be due to ketonemia [β-hydroxybutyrate] and mild lactic acidosis) as well as abnormal chemistry and blood gas data. His O_2ER is 25%, which is in the normal range. The patient is hypothermic, which may account for the central venous oxygen saturation in the normal range. His mental status may be accounted for by hypoglycemia.

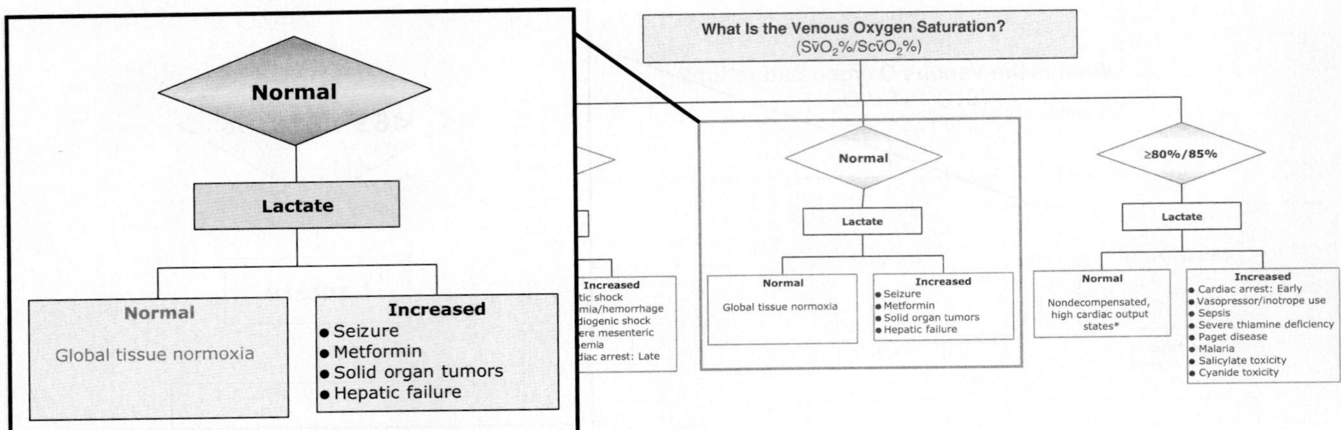

FIGURE 26.16. Baseline for Case 3.

What's the Interpretation?

The patient's extraction ratio may be slightly higher than expected but may be explained by a depressed metabolic rate associated with hypothermia. The near-normal lactate level on presentation may also be explained by a depressed metabolic rate despite the lack of substrate (glucose). The higher-than-expected O_2ER should be noted, and a search for disturbances of oxygen utilization should be considered. Entities that impair the tissues' ability to utilize oxygen consist of toxicologic and metabolic derangements including chronic thiamine deficiency, cyanide toxicity, and possibly severe acetaminophen toxicity.

References

1. Wo CC, Shoemaker WC, Appel PL, et al. Unreliability of blood pressure and heart rate to evaluate cardiac output in emergency resuscitation and critical illness. *Crit Care Med.* 1993;21(2):218–223.
2. Cortez A, Zito J, Lucas CE, Gerrick SJ. Mechanism of inappropriate polyuria in septic patients. *Arch Surg.* 1977;112(4):471–476.
3. Rady MY, Rivers EP, Nowak RM. Resuscitation of the critically ill in the ED: responses of blood pressure, heart rate, shock index, central venous oxygen saturation, and lactate. *Am J Emerg Med.* 1996;14(2):218–225.
4. Karimova A, Pinsky DJ. The endothelial response to oxygen deprivation: biology and clinical implications. *Intensive Care Med.* 2001;27(1):19–31.
5. Beal AL, Cerra FB. Multiple organ failure syndrome in the 1990s. Systemic inflammatory response and organ dysfunction. *JAMA.* 1994;271(3):226–233.
6. Bihari D, Smithies M, Gimson A, et al. The effects of vasodilation with prostacyclin on oxygen delivery and uptake in critically ill patients. *N Engl J Med.* 1987;317(7):397–403.
7. Bakker J, Gris P, Coffernils M, et al. Serial blood lactate levels can predict the development of multiple organ failure following septic shock. *Am J Surg.* 1996;171(2):221–226.
8. Rivers EP, Kruse JA, Jacobsen G, et al. The influence of early hemodynamic optimization on biomarker patterns of severe sepsis and septic shock. *Crit Care Med.* 2007;35(9):2016–2024.
9. Rivers E, Nguyen B, Havstad S, et al. Early goal-directed therapy in the treatment of severe sepsis and septic shock. *N Engl J Med.* 2001;345(19):1368–1377.
10. Varpula M, Tallgren M, Saukkonen K, et al. Hemodynamic variables related to outcome in septic shock. *Intensive Care Med.* 2005;31:1066–1071.
11. Nelson LD. Continuous venous oximetry in surgical patients. *Ann Surg.* 1986;203(3):329–333.
12. Krafft P, Steltzer H, Hiesmayr M, et al. Mixed venous oxygen saturation in critically ill septic shock patients. The role of defined events. *Chest.* 1993;103(3):900–906.
13. Wolf YG, Cotev S, Perel A, et al. Dependence of oxygen consumption on cardiac output in sepsis. *Crit Care Med.* 1987;15(3):198–203.
14. Kandel G, Aberman A. Mixed venous oxygen saturation. Its role in the assessment of the critically ill patient. *Arch Intern Med.* 1983;143(7):1400–1402.
15. Meier-Hellmann A, Hannemann L, Specht M, et al. Hepatic venous and mixed venous O_2 saturation during catecholamine therapy in patients with septic shock [in German]. *Anaesthesist.* 1993;42(1):29–33.
16. Reinhart K, Rudolph T, Bredle DL, et al. Comparison of central-venous to mixed-venous oxygen saturation during changes in oxygen supply/demand. *Chest.* 1989;95(6):1216–1221.
17. Takano H, Matsuda H, Kaneko M, et al. Hepatic venous oxygen saturation monitoring in patients with assisted circulation for severe cardiac failure. *Artif Organs.* 1991;15(3):248–252.
18. Ruokonen E, Takala J, Uusaro A. Effect of vasoactive treatment on the relationship between mixed venous and regional oxygen saturation. *Crit Care Med.* 1991;19(11):1365–1369.
19. Dahn MS, Lange MP, Jacobs LA. Central mixed and splanchnic venous oxygen saturation monitoring. *Intensive Care Med.* 1988;14(4):373–378.
20. Rivers EP, Ander DS, Powell D. Central venous oxygen saturation monitoring in the critically ill patient. *Curr Opin Crit Care.* 2001;7(3):204–211.
21. Bakker J, Vincent J-L. The oxygen supply dependency phenomenon is associated with increased blood lactate levels. *J Crit Care.* 1991;6:152–159.
22. Kruse JA, Haupt MT, Puri VK, et al. Lactate levels as predictors of the relationship between oxygen delivery and consumption in ARDS. *Chest.* 1990;98(4):959–962.
23. Kasnitz P, Druger GL, Yorra F, et al. Mixed venous oxygen tension and hyperlactatemia. Survival in severe cardiopulmonary disease. *JAMA.* 1976;236(6):570–574.
24. Aduen J, Bernstein WK, Khastgir T, et al. The use and clinical importance of a substrate-specific electrode for rapid determination of blood lactate concentrations. *JAMA.* 1994;272(21):1678–1685.
25. Wilson RF, Gibson D. The use of arterial–central venous oxygen differences to calculate cardiac output and oxygen consumption in critically ill surgical patients. *Surgery.* 1978;84(3):362–369.
26. Norwood SH, Civetta JM. Ventilatory support in patients with ARDS. *Surg Clin North Am.* 1985;65(4):895–916.
27. Rasanen J, Downs JB, Malec DJ, et al. Real-time continuous estimation of gas exchange by dual oximetry. *Intensive Care Med.* 1988;14(2):118–122.
28. Boulos M, Astiz ME, Barua RS, et al. Impaired mitochondrial function induced by serum from septic shock patients is attenuated by inhibition of nitric oxide synthase and poly(ADP-ribose) synthase. *Crit Care Med.* 2003;31(2):353–358.
29. Dunham CM, Siegel JH, Weireter L, et al. Oxygen debt and metabolic acidemia as quantitative predictors of mortality and the severity of the ischemic insult in hemorrhagic shock. *Crit Care Med.* 1991;19(2):231–243.
30. Rixen D, Siegel JH. Bench-to-bedside review: oxygen debt and its metabolic correlates as quantifiers of the severity of hemorrhagic and post-traumatic shock. *Crit Care.* 2005;9(5):441–453.
31. Siegel JH. The effect of associated injuries, blood loss, and oxygen debt on death and disability in blunt traumatic brain injury: the need for early physiologic predictors of severity. *J Neurotrauma.* 1995;12(4):579–590.
32. Snyder JV, Carroll GC. Tissue oxygenation: a physiologic approach to a clinical problem. *Curr Probl Surg.* 1982;19(11):650–719.
33. Nierman DM, Schechter CB. Mixed venous O_2 saturation: measured by co-oximetry versus calculated from PVO_2. *J Clin Monit.* 1994;10(1):39–44.

34. Nelson LD. Continuous monitoring of O_2 saturation. *Chest.* 1989;96(4): 956–957.
35. Varon J, Fromm RE Jr, Levine RL. Emergency department procedures and length of stay for critically ill medical patients. *Ann Emerg Med.* 1994;23(3):546–549.
36. Lundberg JS, Perl TM, Wiblin T, et al. Septic shock: an analysis of outcomes for patients with onset on hospital wards versus intensive care units. *Crit Care Med.* 1998;26(6):1020–1024.
37. Lefrant JY, Muller L, Bruelle P, et al. Insertion time of the pulmonary artery catheter in critically ill patients. *Crit Care Med.* 2000;28(2):355–359.
38. Lee J, Wright F, Barber R, Stanley L. Central venous oxygen saturation in shock: a study in man. *Anesthesiology.* 1972;36(5):472–478.
39. Scheinman MM, Brown MA, Rapaport E. Critical assessment of use of central venous oxygen saturation as a mirror of mixed venous oxygen in severely ill cardiac patients. *Circulation.* 1969;40(2):165–172.
40. Glamann DB, Lange RA, Hillis LD. Incidence and significance of a "step-down" in oxygen saturation from superior vena cava to pulmonary artery. *Am J Cardiol.* 1991;68(6):695–697.
41. Edwards JD, Mayall RM. Importance of the sampling site for measurement of mixed venous oxygen saturation in shock. *Crit Care Med.* 1998;26(8):1356–1360.
42. Martin C, Auffray JP, Badetti C, et al. Monitoring of central venous oxygen saturation versus mixed venous oxygen saturation in critically ill patients. *Intensive Care Med.* 1992;18(2):101–104.
43. Faber T. Central venous versus mixed venous oxygen content. *Acta Anaesthesiol Scand Suppl.* 1995;107:33–36.
44. Dongre SS, McAslan TC, Shin B. Selection of the source of mixed venous blood samples in severely traumatized patients. *Anesth Analg.* 1977;56(4):527–532.
45. Rigg JD, Nightingale PN, Faragher EB. Influence of cardiac output on the correlation between mixed venous and central venous oxygen saturation. *Br J Anaesth.* 1993;71(3):459.
46. Varpula M, Karlsson S, Ruokonen E, Pettila V. Mixed venous oxygen saturation cannot be estimated by central venous oxygen saturation in septic shock. *Intensive Care Med.* 2006;32(9):1336–1343.
47. Chawla LS, Zia H, Gutierrez G, et al. Lack of equivalence between central and mixed venous oxygen saturation. *Chest.* 2004;126(6):1891–1896.
48. Martin GB, Carden DL, Nowak RM, et al. Central venous and mixed venous oxygen saturation: comparison during canine open-chest cardiopulmonary resuscitation. *Am J Emerg Med.* 1985;3(6):495–497.
49. Pieri M, Brandi LS, Bertolini R, et al. Comparison of bench central and mixed pulmonary venous oxygen saturation in critically ill postsurgical patients [in Italian]. *Minerva Anesthesiol.* 1995;61(7–8):285–291.
50. Turnaoglu S, Tugrul M, Camci E, et al. Clinical applicability of the substitution of mixed venous oxygen saturation with central venous oxygen saturation. *J Cardiothorac Vasc Anesth.* 2001;15(5):574–579.
51. Goldman RH, Klughaupt M, Metcalf T, et al. Measurement of central venous oxygen saturation in patients with myocardial infarction. *Circulation.* 1968;38(5):941–946.
52. Reinhart K, Rudolph T, Bredle DL, et al. Comparison of central-venous to mixed-venous oxygen saturation during changes in oxygen supply/demand. *Chest.* 1989;95(6):1216–1221.
53. Schou H, Perez de Sa V, Larsson A. Central and mixed venous blood oxygen correlate well during acute normovolemic hemodilution in anesthetized pigs. *Acta Anaesthesiol Scand.* 1998;42(2):172–177.
54. Cohendy R, Peries C, Lefrant JY, et al. Continuous monitoring of the central venous oxygen saturation in surgical patients: comparison to the monitoring of the mixed venous saturation. *Acta Anaesthesiol Scand.* 1996;40(8 Pt 1):956.
55. Berridge JC. Influence of cardiac output on the correlation between mixed venous and central venous oxygen saturation. *Br J Anaesth.* 1992;69(4): 409–410.
56. Scalea TM, Holman M, Fuortes M, et al. Central venous blood oxygen saturation: an early, accurate measurement of volume during hemorrhage. *J Trauma.* 1988;28(6):725–732.
57. Davies GG, Mendenhall J, Symreng T. Measurement of right atrial oxygen saturation by fiberoptic oximetry accurately reflects mixed venous oxygen saturation in swine. *J Clin Monit.* 1988;4(2):99–102.
58. Herrera A, Pajuelo A, Morano MJ, et al. Comparison of oxygen saturations in mixed venous and central blood during thoracic anesthesia with selective single-lung ventilation [in Spanish]. *Rev Esp Anestesiol Reanim.* 1993;40(6):349–353.
59. Wendt M, Hachenberg T, Albert A, et al. Mixed venous versus central venous oxygen saturation in intensive medicine. *Anasth Intensivther Notfallmed.* 1990;25(1):102–106.
60. Emerman CL, Pinchak AC, Hagen JF, et al. A comparison of venous blood gases during cardiac arrest. *Am J Emerg Med.* 1988;6(6):580–583.
61. Weber H, Grimm T, Albert J. The oxygen saturation of blood in the venae cavae, right-heart chambers, and pulmonary artery, comparison of formulae to estimate mixed venous blood in healthy infants and children [in German (author's transl)]. *Z Kardiol.* 1980;69(7):504–507.
62. Ladakis C, Myrianthefs P, Karabinis A, et al. Central venous and mixed venous oxygen saturation in critically ill patients. *Respiration.* 2001;68(3):279–285.
63. Heiselman D, Jones J, Cannon L. Continuous monitoring of mixed venous oxygen saturation in septic shock. *J Clin Monit.* 1986;2(4):237–245.
64. Ander DS, Jaggi M, Rivers E, et al. Undetected cardiogenic shock in patients with congestive heart failure presenting to the emergency department. *Am J Cardiol.* 1998;82(7):888–891.
65. Rivers EP, Nguyen HB, Havstad S, et al. Early goal directed therapy in the treatment of severe sepsis and septic shock: an outcome evaluation [abstract]. *Chest.* 2000;118(4):87S.
66. Practice parameters for hemodynamic support of sepsis in adult patients in sepsis. Task Force of the American College of Critical Care Medicine, Society of Critical Care Medicine. *Crit Care Med.* 1999;27(3):639–660.
67. Dellinger RP, Carlet JM, Masur H, et al. Surviving Sepsis Campaign guidelines for management of severe sepsis and septic shock. *Intensive Care Med.* 2004;30(4):536–555.
68. Rivers E. Mixed vs central venous oxygen saturation may be not numerically equal, but both are still clinically useful. *Chest.* 2006;129(3):507–508.
69. Vaughn S, Puri VK. Cardiac output changes and continuous mixed venous oxygen saturation measurement in the critically ill. *Crit Care Med.* 1988;16(5):495–498.
70. Wiesemes R, Peters J. The role of mixed venous oxygen saturation in perioperative monitoring and therapy. A critical stock taking [in German]. *Anasthesiol Intensivmed Notfallmed Schmerzther.* 1993;28(5):269–278.
71. Rady M, Jafry S, Rivers E, et al. Characterization of systemic oxygen transport in end-stage chronic congestive heart failure. *Am Heart J.* 1994;128(4):774–781.
72. Rivers EP, Martin GB, Smithline H, et al. The clinical implications of continuous central venous oxygen saturation during human CPR. *Ann Emerg Med.* 1992;21(9):1094–1101.
73. Rivers EP, Rady MY, Martin GB, et al. Venous hyperoxia after cardiac arrest. Characterization of a defect in systemic oxygen utilization. *Chest.* 1992;102(6):1787–1793.
74. Waller JL, Kaplan JA, Bauman DI, Craver JM. Clinical evaluation of a new fiberoptic catheter oximeter during cardiac surgery. *Anesth Analg.* 1982;61(8):676–679.
75. de la Rocha AG, Edmonds JF, Williams WG, et al. Importance of mixed venous oxygen saturation in the care of critically ill patients. *Can J Surg.* 1978;21(3):227–229.
76. Krauss XH, Verdouw PD, Hughenholtz PG, et al. On-line monitoring of mixed venous oxygen saturation after cardiothoracic surgery. *Thorax.* 1975;30(6):636–643.
77. Muir AL, Kirby BJ, King AJ, et al. Mixed venous oxygen saturation in relation to cardiac output in myocardial infarction. *Br Med J.* 1970;4(730):276–278.
78. Birman H, Haq A, Hew E, et al. Continuous monitoring of mixed venous oxygen saturation in hemodynamically unstable patients. *Chest.* 1984;86(5):753–756.
79. Gattinoni L, Brazzi L, Pelosi P, et al. A trial of goal-oriented hemodynamic therapy in critically ill patients. SvO_2 Collaborative Group. *N Engl J Med.* 1995;333(16):1025–1032.
80. Bracht H, Hanggi M, Jeker B, et al. Incidence of low central venous oxygen saturation during unplanned admissions in a multidisciplinary intensive care unit: an observational study. *Crit Care.* 2007;11(1):R2.
81. Polonen P, Ruokonen E, Hippelainen M, et al. A prospective, randomized study of goal-oriented hemodynamic therapy in cardiac surgical patients. *Anesth Analg.* 2000;90(5):1052–1059.
82. Kremzar B, Spec-Marn A, Kompan L, et al. Normal values of SvO_2 as therapeutic goal in patients with multiple injuries. *Intensive Care Med.* 1997;23(1):65–70.
83. Kazarian KK, Del Guercio LR. The use of mixed venous blood gas determinations in traumatic shock. *Ann Emerg Med.* 1980;9(4):179–182.
84. Rady MY. Patterns of oxygen transport in trauma and their relationship to outcome. *Am J Emerg Med.* 1994;12(1):107–112.
85. Powelson JA, Maini BS, Bishop RL, et al. Continuous monitoring of mixed venous oxygen saturation during aortic operations. *Crit Care Med.* 1992;20(3):332–336.
86. Norwood SH, Nelson LD. Continuous monitoring of mixed venous oxygen saturation during aortofemoral bypass grafting. *Am Surg.* 1986;52(2):114–115.
87. Madsen P, Olesen HL, Klokker M, et al. Peripheral venous oxygen saturation during head-up tilt induced hypovolaemic shock in humans. *Scand J Clin Lab Invest.* 1993;53(4):411–416.
88. Madsen P, Iversen H, Secher NH. Central venous oxygen saturation during hypovolaemic shock in humans. *Scand J Clin Lab Invest.* 1993;53(1):67–72.
89. O'Connor TA, Hall RT. Mixed venous oxygenation in critically ill neonates. *Crit Care Med.* 1994;22(2):343–346.
90. Conacher ID, Paes ML. Mixed venous oxygen saturation during lung transplantation. *J Cardiothorac Vasc Anesth.* 1994;8(6):671–674.
91. Edwards JD. Oxygen transport in cardiogenic and septic shock. *Crit Care Med.* 1991;19(5):658–663.
92. Creamer JE, Edwards JD, Nightingale P. Hemodynamic and oxygen transport variables in cardiogenic shock secondary to acute myocardial infarction, and response to treatment. *Am J Cardiol.* 1990;65(20):1297–1300.

93. Snyder AB, Salloum LJ, Barone JE, et al. Predicting short-term outcome of cardiopulmonary resuscitation using central venous oxygen tension measurements. *Crit Care Med.* 1991;19(1):111–113.
94. Rivers EP, Rady MY, Martin GB, et al. Venous hyperoxia after cardiac arrest. Characterization of a defect in systemic oxygen utilization. *Chest.* 1992;102(6):1787–1793.
95. Nakazawa K, Hikawa Y, Saitoh Y, et al. Usefulness of central venous oxygen saturation monitoring during cardiopulmonary resuscitation. A comparative case study with end-tidal carbon dioxide monitoring. *Intensive Care Med.* 1994;20(6):450–451.
96. Osawa H, Yoshii S, Abraham SJ, et al. Critical values of hematocrit and mixed venous oxygen saturation as parameters for a safe cardiopulmonary bypass. *Jpn J Thorac Cardiovasc Surg.* 2004;52(2):49–56.
97. Paradis NA, Martin GB, Goetting MG, et al. Aortic pressure during human cardiac arrest. Identification of pseudo- electromechanical dissociation. *Chest.* 1992;101(1):123–128.
98. Rivers EP, Wortsman J, Rady MY, et al. The effect of the total cumulative epinephrine dose administered during human CPR on hemodynamic, oxygen transport, and utilization variables in the postresuscitation period. *Chest.* 1994;106(5):1499–1507.
99. Sumimoto T, Sugiura T, Takeuchi M, et al. Overshoot in mixed venous oxygen saturation during recovery from supine bicycle exercise in patients with recent myocardial infarction. *Chest.* 1993;103(2):514–520.
100. Deakin CD, Low JL. Accuracy of the advanced trauma life support guidelines for predicting systolic blood pressure using carotid, femoral, and radial pulses: observational study. *BMJ.* 2000;321(7262):673–674.
101. Scalea TM, Hartnett RW, Duncan AO, et al. Central venous oxygen saturation: a useful clinical tool in trauma patients. *J Trauma.* 1990;30(12):1539–1543.
102. Kowalenko T, Ander D, Hitchcock R, et al. Continuous central venous oxygen saturation monitoring during the resuscitation of suspected hemorrhagic shock [abstract]. *Acad Emerg Med.* 1994;1(2):A69.
103. Astiz ME, Rackow EC, Kaufman B, et al. Relationship of oxygen delivery and mixed venous oxygenation to lactic acidosis in patients with sepsis and acute myocardial infarction. *Crit Care Med.* 1988;16(7):655–658.
104. Verdouw PD, Hagemeijer F, Dorp WG, et al. Short-term survival after acute myocardial infarction predicted by hemodynamic parameters. *Circulation.* 1975;52(3):413–419.
105. Kyff JV, Vaughn S, Yang SC, et al. Continuous monitoring of mixed venous oxygen saturation in patients with acute myocardial infarction. *Chest.* 1989;95(3):607–611.
106. Chin KM, Channick RN, Kim NH, et al. Central venous blood oxygen saturation monitoring in patients with chronic pulmonary arterial hypertension treated with continuous IV epoprostenol: correlation with measurements of hemodynamics and plasma brain natriuretic peptide levels. *Chest.* 2007;132(3):786–792.
107. Griffel MI, Astiz ME, Rackow EC, et al. Effect of mechanical ventilation on systemic oxygen extraction and lactic acidosis during early septic shock in rats. *Crit Care Med.* 1990;18(1):72–76.
108. Hirschl RB, Heiss KF, Cilley RE, et al. Oxygen kinetics in experimental sepsis. *Surgery.* 1992;112(1):37–44.
109. Rackow EC, Astiz ME, Weil MH. Increases in oxygen extraction during rapidly fatal septic shock in rats. *J Lab Clin Med.* 1987;109(6):660–664.
110. Astiz ME, Rackow EC, Weil MH. Oxygen delivery and utilization during rapidly fatal septic shock in rats. *Circ Shock.* 1986;20(4):281–290.
111. Dellinger RP, Levy MM, Carlet JM, et al. Surviving Sepsis Campaign: international guidelines for management of severe sepsis and septic shock: 2008. *Intensive Care Med.* 2008;34(1):17–60. Epub 2007 Dec 4.
112. Krivec B, Voga G, Podbregar M. Monitoring mixed venous oxygen saturation in patients with obstructive shock after massive pulmonary embolism. *Wien Klin Wochenschr.* 2004;116(9–10):326–331.
113. Fahey PJ, Harris K, Vanderwarf C. Clinical experience with continuous monitoring of mixed venous oxygen saturation in respiratory failure. *Chest.* 1984;86(5):748–752.
114. Kirkeby-Garstad I, Sellevold OF, Stenseth R, et al. Marked mixed venous desaturation during early mobilization after aortic valve surgery. *Anesth Analg.* 2004;98(2):311–317, table of contents.
115. Tweddell JS, Ghanayem NS, Mussatto KA, et al. Mixed venous oxygen saturation monitoring after stage 1 palliation for hypoplastic left heart syndrome. *Ann Thorac Surg.* 2007;84(4):1301–1310; discussion 10–11.
116. Polonen P, Ruokonen E, Hippelainen M, et al. A prospective, randomized study of goal-oriented hemodynamic therapy in cardiac surgical patients. *Anesth Analg.* 2000;90(5):1052–1059.
117. Termuhlen DF, Swartz MT, Pennington DG, et al. Predictors for weaning patients from ventricular assist devices. *ASAIO Trans.* 1988;34(2):131–139.
118. Termuhlen DF, Swartz MT, Ruzevich SA, et al. Hemodynamic predictors for weaning patients from ventricular assist devices (VADs). *J Biomater Appl.* 1990;4(4):374–390.
119. Pearse R, Dawson D, Fawcett J, et al. Changes in central venous saturation after major surgery, and association with outcome. *Crit Care.* 2005;9(6):R694–699.
120. Shoemaker WC, Thangathurai D, Wo CC, et al. Intraoperative evaluation of tissue perfusion in high-risk patients by invasive and noninvasive hemodynamic monitoring. *Crit Care Med.* 1999;27(10):2147–2152.
121. Bland RD, Shoemaker WC, Abraham E, et al. Hemodynamic and oxygen transport patterns in surviving and nonsurviving postoperative patients. *Crit Care Med.* 1985;13(2):85–90.
122. Gawlinski A, Dracup K. Effect of positioning on SvO_2 in the critically ill patient with a low ejection fraction. *Nurs Res.* 1998;47(5):293–299.
123. Lewis P, Nichols E, Mackey G, et al. The effect of turning and backrub on mixed venous oxygen saturation in critically ill patients. *Am J Crit Care.* 1997;6(2):132–140.
124. Schranz D, Schmitt S, Oelert H, et al. Continuous monitoring of mixed venous oxygen saturation in infants after cardiac surgery. *Intensive Care Med.* 1989;15(4):228–232.
125. Baquero Cano M, Sanchez Luna M, Elorza Fernandez MD, et al. Oxygen transport and consumption and oxygen saturation in the right atrium in an experimental model of neonatal septic shock [in Spanish]. *An Esp Pediatr.* 1996;44(2):149–156.
126. Hirschl RB, Palmer P, Heiss KF, et al. Evaluation of the right atrial venous oxygen saturation as a physiologic monitor in a neonatal model. *J Pediatr Surg.* 1993;28(7):901–905.
127. Rasanen J, Peltola K, Leijala M. Superior vena caval and mixed venous oxyhemoglobin saturations in children recovering from open heart surgery. *J Clin Monit.* 1992;8(1):44–49.
128. Carcillo JA, Fields AI. Clinical practice parameters for hemodynamic support of pediatric and neonatal patients in septic shock. *Crit Care Med.* 2002;30(6):1365–1378.
129. Orlando R 3rd. Continuous mixed venous oximetry in critically ill surgical patients. 'High-tech' cost-effectiveness. *Arch Surg.* 1986;121(4):470–471.
130. Arnoldi D, Dechert R, Wise C. Use of continuous SvO_2 monitoring can decrease requirements for cardiac output determination in surgical ICU patients. *Crit Care Med.* 1995;23(1 Suppl):A22.
131. Pearson KS, Gomez MN, Moyers JR, et al. A cost/benefit analysis of randomized invasive monitoring for patients undergoing cardiac surgery. *Anesth Analg.* 1989;69(3):336–341.
132. Jastremski MS, Chelluri L, Beney KM, et al. Analysis of the effects of continuous on-line monitoring of mixed venous oxygen saturation on patient outcome and cost-effectiveness. *Crit Care Med.* 1989;17(2):148–153.
133. Huang DT, Angus DC, Dremsizov TT, et al. Cost-effectiveness of early goal-directed therapy in the treatment of severe sepsis and septic shock. *Crit Care.* 2003;7:S116.
134. Rasanen J, Downs JB, Hodges MR. Continuous monitoring of gas exchange and oxygen use with dual oximetry. *J Clin Anesth.* 1988;1(1):3–8.
135. Bongard FS, Leighton TA. Continuous dual oximetry in surgical critical care. Indications and limitations. *Ann Surg.* 1992;216(1):60–68.
136. Boutros AR, Lee C. Value of continuous monitoring of mixed venous blood oxygen saturation in the management of critically ill patients. *Crit Care Med.* 1986;14(2):132–134.

APPENDIX

APPENDIX 26.1

NORMAL RANGE, UNITS, AND DERIVATION FOR COMMON OXYGEN TRANSPORT TERMS

Parameter	Normal range	Units	Derivation
PaO_2	(Varies with FiO_2)	mm Hg	Measured
SaO_2	>0.92	(Fraction)	Measured
CaO_2	16–22	mL/dL	$(SaO_2 \times Hgb \times 1.38) + PaO_2 \times 0.0031)$
$P\bar{v}O_2$	35–45	mm Hg	Measured
$S\bar{v}O_2$	0.65–0.75	(Fraction)	Measured
$C\bar{v}O_2$	12–17	mL/dL	$(S\bar{v}O_2 \times Hgb \times 1.38) + (P\bar{v}O_2 \times 0.0031)$
$C(a - \bar{v})O_2$	3.5–5.5	mL/dL	$CaO_2 - C\bar{v}O_2$
$\dot{V}O_2$	180–280	mL/min	$C(a - \bar{v})O_2 \times CO \times 10$
$\dot{V}O_2$ indexed	120–160	mL/min/m^2	$C(a - \bar{v})O_2 \times CI \times 10$
$\dot{D}O_2$ indexed	500–600	mL/min/m^2	$CaO_2 \times CI \times 10$
$\dot{D}O_2$	700–1,400	mL/min	$CaO_2 \times CO \times 10$
OUC/O_2ER	0.23–0.32	(Fraction)	$\dot{V}O_2/\dot{D}O_2$

PaO_2, arterial oxygen tension; SaO_2, arterial oxygen saturation; CaO_2, arterial oxygen content; $P\bar{v}O_2$, mixed venous oxygen tension; $S\bar{v}O_2$, mixed venous oxygen saturation; $C\bar{v}O_2$, mixed venous oxygen content; $C(a - \bar{v})O_2$, arterial-venous oxygen content difference; $\dot{V}O_2$, oxygen consumption; $\dot{D}O_2$, oxygen delivery; OUC, oxygen utilization coefficient (extraction ratio); O_2ER, extraction ratio; FiO_2, fraction of inspired oxygen; Hgb, hemoglobin; CO, cardiac output.

Normal ranges are approximate and may vary between laboratories.

CHAPTER 27 ■ NEUROLOGIC MONITORING

CHRISTOPH N. SEUBERT • DIETRICH GRAVENSTEIN • STEVEN A. ROBICSEK • MICHAEL E. MAHLA

Neurologic monitoring in the intensive care unit (ICU) is used either in a general sense as part of a systems-based approach to assess one of the major bodily systems or with the specific intent to guide therapy and/or assess prognosis. Imaging studies of the central nervous system (CNS)—while not considered "monitoring" in the strict sense—play a central role in this assessment by establishing diagnoses and quantifying the extent of pathology. Important constraints for typical neuroradiologic imaging are presented in the first section below.

Many interventions in the ICU aimed at restoring or maintaining conditions that are favorable for recovery of the patient target normal brain and, by extension, affect the results of neurologic monitoring. Therefore, an understanding of the parameters that affect the state of the brain is necessary as the context for interpreting the results of neurologic monitoring. These are presented in the second section followed by a detailed discussion of available modalities for serial assessment or monitoring of the nervous system.

NEURORADIOLOGIC IMAGING

Routine imaging studies of the brain are important in the repeated assessment of a patient's neurologic status. Objective information, particularly about structural abnormalities, is essential to the clinical diagnosis. Neuroradiologic imaging studies typically take the form of computed tomography (CT) or magnetic resonance imaging (MRI). Although not considered "monitoring" per se, repeated studies or critically timed studies may provide important clues about the time course of a pathologic process (1). Typical imaging workup for various clinical diagnoses in critical care medicine is presented in Table 27.1.

To maximize the utility of an imaging study, the requesting physician needs to be aware of inherent strengths and weaknesses of the chosen imaging modality. The questions of contraindications to MRI, such as metal implants (see www.mrisafety.com), morbid obesity, claustrophobia, or the use of contrast agents, require special consideration. Whereas the quality of CT images is simply degraded by patient movement, MRI images acquired in an uncooperative, moving patient may contain "spurious pathology" because of misregistration of anatomic structures. The requesting physician needs to provide adequate details of the clinical history to the radiologist, so that the imaging protocol can be designed to maximize information. Finally, some thought should be given to the balance between the time spent obtaining the images and the risks to the patient from a reduced level of, or delay in, care during imaging and transport. Given the rapid development in MRI modalities or in postacquisition processing, such balance is frequently best achieved by consulting directly with the radiologist.

CT provides a map of the degree of radiographic absorption of intracranial structures. Generally, it is the test of choice for localizing blood and imaging bone. Newer helical CT scanners make image acquisition a comparatively fast process. This allows the two- and three-dimensional reconstruction of arterial anatomy from images during the first pass of radiocontrast administration to obtain a CT arteriogram.

MRI provides a map of the response of hydrogen nuclei to external magnetic fields. It is more versatile than CT, provides better imaging of posterior fossa contents, and is considerably more time consuming. T1 weighting enhances the detection of lipids, methemoglobin (e.g., as the subacute residual of a hemorrhage), and concentrated protein (e.g., in a colloid cyst). A radiofrequency pulse prior to T1 image acquisition can suppress the enhancement of lipids ("fat suppression") and is an example of a protocol change that affects the resulting image. T2 weighting enhances the detection of unbound water such as in cerebrospinal fluid (CSF) (Fig. 27.1). A radiofrequency pulse prior to T2 image acquisition (fluid attenuation inversion recovery [FLAIR] imaging) can suppress the enhancement of CSF and improve the detection of edema (Fig. 27.1). MRI can also be focused to detect moving elements such as in MR arteriography or venography or CSF flow studies. Axoplasmic motion of bulk water can be imaged with MRI to obtain a diffusion image (apparent diffusion coefficient [ADC] map). This axoplasmic motion stops shortly after brain ischemia; therefore, diffusion images provide the earliest radiographic evidence for the core zone of an ischemic stroke.

Contrast media distribute with the blood flow, and can therefore accentuate areas of increased vascularity such as in inflamed tissue or areas of tumor-induced angioneogenesis. Contrast media also distribute into—and thereby highlight—brain structures that are missing a blood–brain barrier such as the pineal gland or pituitary stalk, or brain areas where the blood–brain barrier has been disrupted. Brain perfusion can be imaged during a bolus administration of contrast medium either by MRI or by CT. The resulting map of the time to peak concentration of the contrast medium currently provides qualitative information on cerebral blood flow, although quantitative approaches are under development. Qualitative differences in cerebral blood flow can be used to identify the ischemic penumbra of a stroke.

CEREBRAL METABOLISM: FLOW–METABOLISM COUPLING

The cerebral metabolic rate for oxygen ($CMRO_2$) of the brain averages 3.0 to 3.8 mL O_2/minute/100 g. Although only 2% of body weight, the human adult brain accounts for 15% to 20% of the resting oxygen consumption and about 25% to

TABLE 27.1

TYPICAL IMAGING PROCEDURES FOR NEUROLOGIC DISEASES IN THEIR ACUTE PHASE

Neurologic disease	Initial imaging	Further workup/alternatives
Stroke	CT to rule out hemorrhage	Diffusion- and perfusion-weighted MRI to identify ischemic core and penumbra, respectively
Arteriovenous malformation	CT for hemorrhage	MR angiography or angiography as soon as possible
Intracerebral aneurysm	CT for subarachnoid hemorrhage	CT angiography or angiography to identify aneurysm; TCD for vasospasm
Brain tumor	MRI without and with contrast	
Traumatic brain injury	CT	MRI as indicated later
Multiple sclerosis	MRI without and with contrast	
Meningitis/encephalitis	CT without and with contrast	MRI without and with contrast after initial treatment
Intracranial abscess	CT without and with contrast	MRI without and with contrast even initially, if patient is stable
Granuloma	MRI without and with contrast	

CT, computed tomography; MRI, magnetic resonance imaging; TCD, transcranial Doppler ultrasonography.
Modified from Gilman S. Imaging the brain. First of two parts. *N Engl J Med.* 1998;338:812–820.

30% of the glucose consumption of the body. In order to meet this high demand for oxygen and glucose, the brain requires a high level of perfusion: 40 to 60 mL/minute/100 g of brain tissue. Cerebral blood flow is regulated by four primary factors: metabolic stimuli, chemical stimuli, perfusion pressure, and neural stimuli.

In the normal brain, an increase in cerebral metabolism is rapidly matched by local increases in cerebral blood flow (CBF). This is referred to as *regional flow–metabolism coupling* or *cerebral metabolic autoregulation* (2). CBF is thus linked to brain function and metabolism so that CBF varies in parallel with $CMRO_2$ (Fig. 27.2). Two compensatory responses to acute reductions in CBF have been established: Autoregulation and increased oxygen extraction (3–5). Oxygen extraction is able to vary within a narrow range. Misery perfusion occurs when oxygen extraction is increased as a response to increased $CMRO_2$, either when autoregulatory CBF compensation has been exceeded or uncoupling has occurred (6). As cerebral perfusion pressure (CPP) falls, cerebral blood flow is maintained initially by resistance arteriole vasodilation (7). Severe ischemia results as CPP is further reduced; the capacity of both CBF autoregulation and increased oxygen extraction is exhausted, and CBF falls as a function of pressure. Positron emission tomography (PET) studies indicate that this occurs with relatively preserved $CMRO_2$ in the penumbra of a focal ischemic area.

Several vasoactive metabolic mediators have been proposed for cerebral regulation, including hydrogen ion, potassium, CO_2, adenosine, glycolytic intermediates, phospholipid metabolites (2), and, more recently, nitric oxide (8). In humans, flow–metabolism coupling is evident during a variety of motor and cognitive tasks that can be mapped using CBF techniques (9).

The global relationship between CBF and $CMRO_2$ can be expressed by the Fick equation where $DajO_2$ is the arteriojugular difference in oxygen content:

$$CMRO_2 = DajO_2 \times CBF \quad \text{or} \quad DajO_2 = CMRO_2/CBF$$

In brain injury, during hypothermia, and under the influence of anesthetic agents, CBF and metabolism may become dissociated. In a series of 109 severe head injury patients, Bouma et al. reported that CBF measured within the first 6 hours after trauma was less than 18 mL/minute/100 g (i.e., the threshold for cerebral ischemia) in one third of the patients (10). Arterial vasospasm was an independent predictor of poor outcome (11). Secondary ischemic neurologic damage was associated with systemic factors, such as hypotension or hypoxemia, and local factors, such as intracranial hypertension, after the injury worsened outcome. Disruption of normal homeostatic mechanisms such as pressure autoregulation (see below) may also

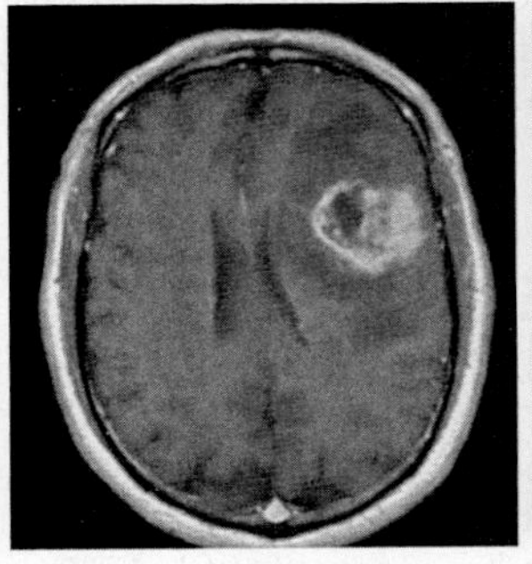

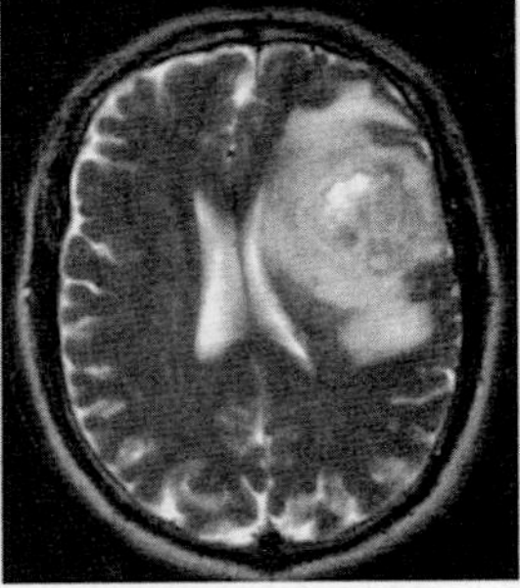

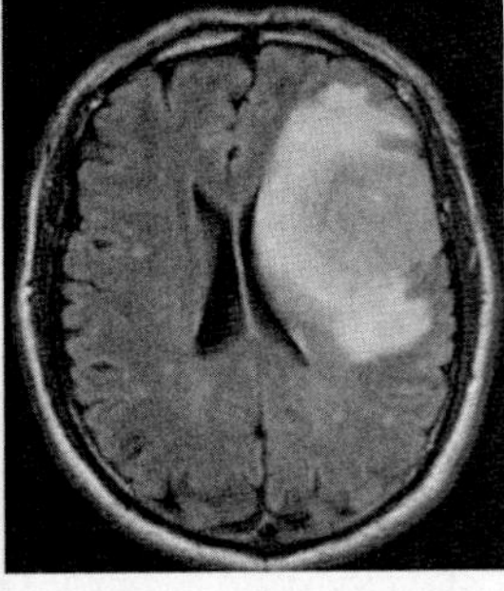

FIGURE 27.1. Magnetic resonance images from a patient with a glioblastoma multiforme. The axial, gadolinium-enhanced T1-weighted image demonstrates the enhancing tumor margin with its nonenhancing central necrosis. The axial, T2-weighted image shows water as a bright signal in perifocal edema and the central tumor necrosis, as well as in the cerebrospinal fluid, while the fluid attenuation inversion recovery image highlights only the edema around the tumor and suppresses the cerebrospinal fluid signal and the tumor necrosis. (Images courtesy of Ilona Schmalfuss, MD.)

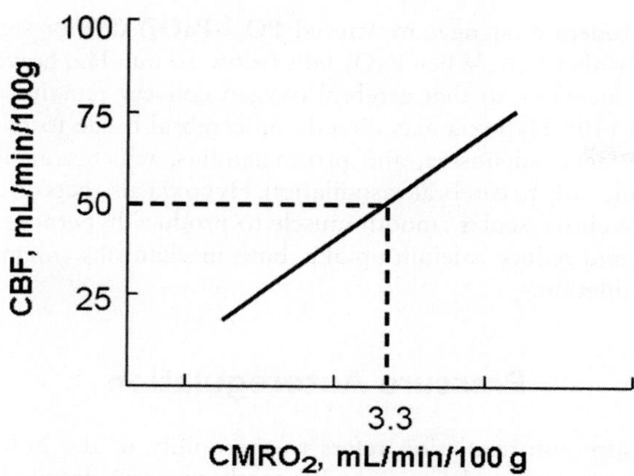

FIGURE 27.2. Flow–metabolism coupling in the central nervous system. As the metabolic needs of the brain—expressed as the cerebral metabolic requirement for oxygen ($CMRO_2$)—increases, cerebral blood flow (CBF) increases in parallel.

aggravate cerebral ischemia. Mechanical hyperventilation used to reduce intracranial pressure (ICP) may be deleterious by decreasing CBF, and may thus also lead to ischemia (12).

Hypothermia

Cerebral protection by hypothermia is commonly attributed to cerebral metabolic suppression. The temperature coefficient (Q_{10}) is the factor by which $CMRO_2$ is decreased by a 10°C decrease in temperature. Between 37°C and 27°C, the temperature coefficient is 2.23, but between 27°C and 17°C—a temperature range during which the electroencephalographic activity ceases—the temperature coefficient doubles to 4.53. Below 17°C, the Q_{10} returns to near 2.0 (Fig. 27.3). In the absence of electroencephalographic activity (e.g., during barbiturate coma), however, the Q_{10} remains near 2.0 over the entire temperature range. With moderate hypothermia (i.e., above 27°C), both CO_2 reactivity and autoregulation are intact while CBF and $CMRO_2$ remain coupled (13). Evidence suggests that there is a change in the coupling of blood flow and metabolism during deep cerebral hypothermia (below 25°C). Nonetheless, metabolic regulation remains a main determinant of CBF even during deep cerebral hypothermia (14).

Anesthetics

With the exception of ketamine, most intravenous and inhalational anesthetics depress cerebral metabolism (15,16), with consequent reductions in oxygen consumption ($CMRO_2$), CBF, and intracranial pressure (17). As $CMRO_2$ decreases, CBF is reduced proportionately because of flow–metabolism coupling. After the administration of propofol and thiopental, flow–metabolism coupling usually remains intact (17), and cerebral oxygen saturation is expected to either remain unaltered or improve. Etomidate, in contrast, can produce a rapid reduction in CBF accompanied by a slower reduction in $CMRO_2$, a finding first demonstrated in dogs and later replicated in humans (18,19). This mismatching of flow–metabolism coupling, with a greater reduction in flow than demand, may induce significant—albeit transient—cerebral oxygen desaturation.

Propofol is believed to maintain cerebral autoregulation, and even high doses of this drug do not obtund autoregulation or carbon dioxide reactivity (20). The effect of propofol on flow–metabolism coupling is more controversial, with at least one study demonstrating intact coupling (21). Both increased and decreased cerebral oxygen extraction have been demonstrated with propofol, suggesting CBF–$CMRO_2$ uncoupling (22,23). Despite the fact that normal flow–metabolism coupling is believed to be retained in only a proportion of head-injured patients, there is a paucity of data regarding the influence of propofol on flow–metabolism coupling after traumatic brain injury. It has been demonstrated that after traumatic brain injury, flow–metabolism coupling remains intact during a step increase in propofol infusion rates (24), as is the case in noninjured patients (25).

Benzodiazepines and opiates appear to have limited intrinsic effects on CBF, $CMRO_2$, and CBF–$CMRO_2$ coupling (26,27). Because of their sedative properties, they cause a decrease in CBF and intracranial pressure that parallels the sedation-induced decrease in $CMRO_2$. As with all anesthetics, the decreased sympathetic tone caused by the sedation, on the other hand, risks a decrease in mean arterial pressure that may in fact

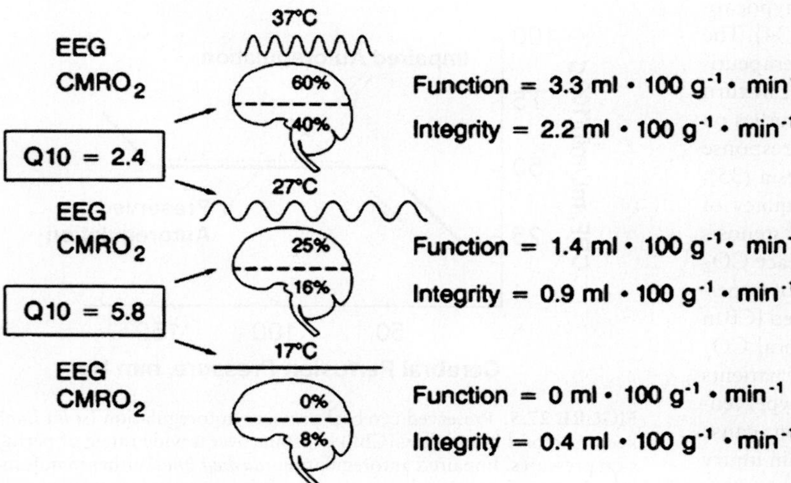

FIGURE 27.3. Theoretical interaction of temperature, brain function, metabolic requirements ($CMRO_2$), and calculated Q10 values. During temperature reduction from 37°C to 27°C, function is maintained, and metabolism devoted to both function and maintenance of integrity are presumed to be equally affected, with a slightly more than 50% reduction in $CMRO_2$ generating a Q10 value of 2.4. A further 10°C reduction in temperature to 17°C abolishes function, resulting in a step decrease in $CMRO_2$ such that the calculated Q10 value is 5.8. At this point, the total oxygen consumed by the brain is reduced to less than 8% of the normothermic value. (With permission from Black S, Michenfelder JD. Cerebral blood flow and metabolism. In: Cucchiara RF, Black S, and Michenfelder JD. *Clinical Neuroanesthesia*. 2nd ed. New York; Churchill Livingston. 1998:9.)

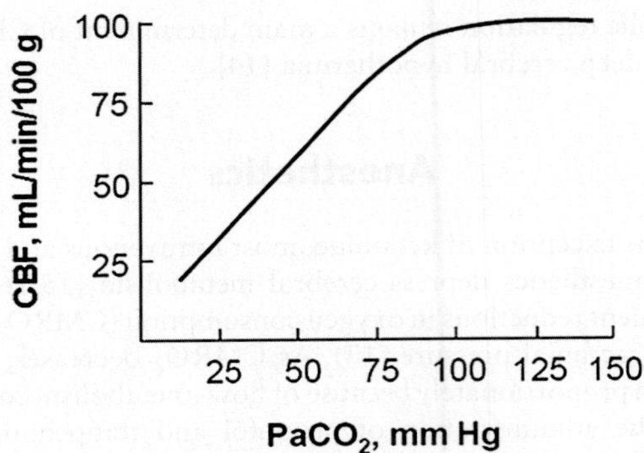

FIGURE 27.4. Effect of arterial CO_2 on cerebral blood flow (CBF).

diminish cerebral perfusion. Dexmedetomidine, an α_2-receptor agonist, is a recent and expensive sedative. Similar to opiates and benzodiazepines, its effects on cerebral physiology appear to be caused by the sedation (28). Limited experience in traumatic brain injury patients did not reveal adverse effects (29).

Arterial Blood Gases: Carbon Dioxide and Oxygen

Carbon dioxide is a potent cerebral vasodilator and thus a major determinant of CBF (Fig. 27.4) (30). At normotension, CBF increases almost linearly when the arterial partial pressure of carbon dioxide ($PaCO_2$) increases from 25 to 80 mm Hg. Global CBF varies 2% to 4% for each mm Hg change in $PaCO_2$ (31). The effects of $PaCO_2$ on the cerebral circulation are regulated by a complex and interrelated system of mediators. The initial stimulus of CO_2-induced vasodilation is a decrease in brain extracellular pH (32), further mediated by nitric oxide, prostanoids, cyclic nucleotides, potassium channels, and a decrease in intracellular calcium concentration as a final common pathway.

Arteriolar tone has an important influence on how $PaCO_2$ affects CBF. Moderate hypotension impairs the response of the cerebral circulation to changes in $PaCO_2$, while severe hypotension abolishes it altogether (33). Similarly, $PaCO_2$ modifies pressure autoregulation, and from hypercapnia to hypocapnia, there is a widening of the autoregulation plateau (34). The response of cerebral vessels to CO_2 can be used therapeutically by instituting hyperventilation to decrease CBF, in turn reducing cerebral blood volume and ICP. Numerous studies on CO_2 reactivity have generally demonstrated that the response is preserved during intravenous or inhalation anesthesia (35). CO_2 reactivity has also been used to assess the adequacy of brain perfusion in patients with internal carotid artery stenosis or cerebrovascular disease. In severe head injury, intact CO_2 vasoreactivity is a good predictor of the effectiveness of hyperventilation or barbiturate therapy in controlling elevated ICP in individual patients (36). Furthermore, impaired cerebral CO_2 vasoreactivity is associated with a poor outcome in patients with severe head injury (37). On the other hand, hyperventilation has been found to increase oxygen extraction, cause misery perfusion, and thereby promote secondary brain injury (12).

Moderate changes in arterial PO_2 (PaO_2) do not significantly alter CBF. When PaO_2 falls below 50 mm Hg, however, CBF increases so that cerebral oxygen delivery remains constant (30). Hypoxia acts directly on cerebral tissue to release lactic acid, adenosine, and prostaglandins, which contribute significantly to cerebral vasodilation. Hypoxia also acts directly on cerebrovascular smooth muscle to produce hyperpolarization and reduce calcium uptake, both mechanisms enhancing vasodilation.

Pressure Autoregulation

Pressure autoregulation refers to the ability of the brain to maintain total and regional CBF nearly constant despite large changes in systemic arterial blood pressure (Fig. 27.5), independently of flow–metabolism coupling (34). Autoregulation is generally expressed as the relationship between CBF and arterial blood pressure when cerebral venous and CSF pressures are low. It can be more precisely defined using the relationship between CBF and CPP that represents the difference between mean systemic arterial pressure and cerebral outflow pressure. Because the cerebral venous system is compressible and may act as a "Starling resistor" or waterfall phenomenon (38), outflow resistance is governed by whichever pressure is higher—CSF pressure (ICP) or venous outflow pressure (jugular bulb pressure).

The cerebral vascular resistance (R) can be expressed as:

$$R = CPP/CBF = (8/\pi) \times h \times (l/r^4)$$

where $(8/\pi)$ is a constant for calculation, h = blood viscosity, l = length, and r = radius of the vessel. Importantly, the radius enters to the fourth power in the equation, making it the most efficient means of controlling vascular resistance.

In adults under normal conditions, CBF remains constant between a CPP of roughly 60 and 150 mm Hg (34). The autoregulation curve is shifted to the right in hypertensive patients and to the left in neonates. At the lower limit of autoregulation, cerebral vasodilation is maximal, and below this level, CBF falls passively with CPP. Beyond the upper limit where vasoconstriction is maximal, the elevated intraluminal pressure may force the vessels to dilate, leading to an increase in CBF and damage

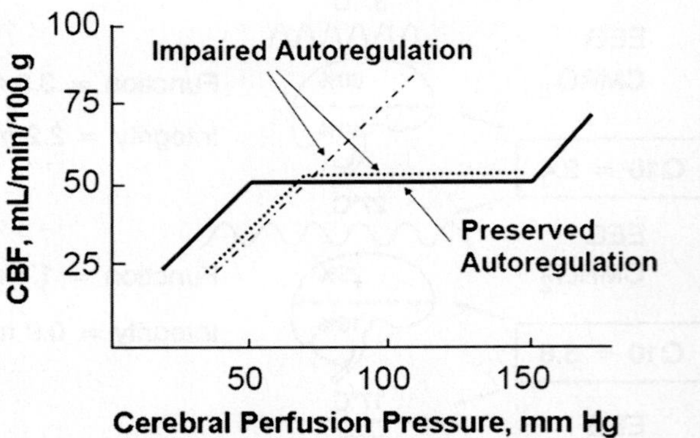

FIGURE 27.5. Preserved cerebral pressure autoregulation (*solid line*) keeps cerebral blood flow (CBF) constant over a wide range of perfusion pressures. Impaired autoregulation (*dashed lines*) either manifests as a shortened or even absent plateau of the autoregulation curve.

to the blood–brain barrier (34,39). Metabolic mediators, such as adenosine, can also be involved in the low-pressure range of autoregulation (39).

Pressure autoregulation can be impaired in many pathologic conditions, including brain tumor, subarachnoid hemorrhage, stroke, or head injury. A loss of CBF regulatory capacity can be attributed either to damage of the control system (e.g., cerebral vessels)—usually referred to as "paralysis" in the clinical literature (40)—or of the feedback mechanisms involved in the brain's hemodynamic control. Changes in the normal feedback mechanisms may include tissue acidosis, extracellular potassium increase, or alterations in cerebral neural pathways. Neurotransmitters can reach vasoactive levels in perivascular CSF as a result of synaptic overflow either during neuronal activation or in pathologic conditions.

Neurogenic Regulation

A major difference between other systemic circulations and the cerebral circulation is the relative lack of humoral and autonomic control on normal cerebrovascular tone. Hence, a maximal stimulation of the sympathetic or parasympathetic nerves alters CBF only slightly (41). Furthermore, there is considerable evidence that indicates the existence of age-related differences in cerebral resistance vessels to neural stimuli. For example, both in vivo and in vitro, cerebrovascular constrictor responses to noradrenaline or electrical transmural stimuli are greater in fetal and neonatal animals than in adult animals. The mechanism for the age-related decrease is unclear, but could be the result of such factors as loss of number or affinity of α-adrenergic receptors with development. However, changes in cerebrovascular sensitivity to α-adrenergic stimuli may not occur with age in all species. Electrical or reflex activation of sympathetic nerves reduces CBF in adult rabbits. Sympathetic stimulation may protect the cerebral circulation from hyperemia associated with even modest elevations in arterial blood pressure.

Other Factors Regulating Cerebral Blood Flow

Although cardiac output hardly influences CBF in normal conditions, it may significantly influence flow to ischemic regions (42,43). However, studies examining the possible relationship between changes in cardiac output and CBF have, for the most part, assessed the effect of drugs that increase cardiac output during either normotension or induced hypertension. Improving cerebral perfusion by volume loading is indirectly accomplished by improving blood rheology and directly accomplished by increasing systemic arterial pressure, and preventing occult decreases in systemic pressure in hypovolemic patients.

Since blood viscosity is a major determinant of vascular resistance, CBF is inversely related with hematocrit (44). Nevertheless, a continuing controversy questions whether CBF is purely rheologic or a function of changes in oxygen delivery to the tissue (45). Bouma and Muizelaar have claimed that viscosity directly participates in cerebral hemodynamic autoregulation, termed *viscosity autoregulation* (39).

CEREBRAL FUNCTION

Clinical Examination

Cerebral function can be monitored with instrumentation or assessed clinically. As the discussion of individual monitoring modalities below shows, each monitor offers only a small window into the state of the central nervous system. Even in combination, current monitors have significant limitations in spatial and/or temporal resolution. A neurologic examination of an alert patient, on the other hand, can comprehensively assess the function of the central nervous system. Furthermore, it can be repeated as often as needed and requires neither expensive technical equipment nor specialized technologists.

In clinical practice, however, the neurologic examination has important limitations. First, the patient's clinical status or underlying disease may limit the amount of information obtainable by a clinical examination. Second, the results and, by extension, the utility of a neurologic examination may be constrained by therapeutic interventions that are frequently used in the ICU. For example, in an intubated patient who is treated with neuromuscular blocking agents, the only evidence of recurrent generalized seizure activity may be increased intracranial pressure, while the postictal alteration of consciousness and the motor manifestations of the seizure go unnoticed. Finally, neurologic evaluations are performed intermittently and by examiners of variable skill, raising problems of reliability. Despite these limitations, the clinical examination forms the cornerstone of the neurologic assessment of ICU patients and typically directs further diagnostic or therapeutic interventions.

While a comprehensive discussion of a clinical neurologic examination is beyond the scope of this chapter, two aspects of the examination that are particularly pertinent to the ICU environment will be discussed in some detail. The first is the assessment of the level of consciousness, because of its ties to patient outcome for many different neurologic diseases. The second is the examination for assessing brain death, not only because it is a graded assessment of brainstem function, but also because it illustrates sources of error that may impact the results of the clinical neurologic examination in the ICU environment in general.

Level of Consciousness: Glasgow Coma Scale

The level of consciousness is typically assessed by the Glasgow coma scale (GCS). Numerical scores are assigned for best responses in the categories of eye opening, motor response, and verbal response (Table 27.2). The GCS was originally described more than 30 years ago for the continuous assessment of patients with traumatic brain injury after the initial period of stabilization (46). Because its assessment is quick, objective, and relatively reliable (47) and because the resulting score is easily documented and communicated, the GCS has gained widespread use in emergency medicine and critical care patients. It has been incorporated into the APACHE score (48) and the World Federation of Neurosurgical Societies (WFNS) grading of subarachnoid hemorrhage (49).

The level of consciousness is a reflection of the severity of many different disease states, and can be compromised not just by diseases of the central nervous system, but also at the extremes of a wide variety of other organ dysfunctions common in critical care. Not surprisingly, therefore, the scores from a tool

TABLE 27.2

GLASGOW COMA SCALE

Category	Grading		Comments
Eye opening	Spontaneous	4	Swelling may interfere with testing.
	To voice	3	
	To pain	2	
	None	1	
Motor response	Follows commands	6	Avoid description of flexion as decorticate and extension as decerebrate, because those terms denote an anatomic location of a lesion.
	Localizes pain	5	
	Withdraws to pain	4	
	Flexion to pain	3	
	Extension to pain	2	
	Flaccid	1	
Verbal response	Oriented	5	Impossible to assess in intubated patients. Some centers determine the response by inference and designate the final score with the subscript "T."
	Confused	4	
	Inappropriate	3	
	Incomprehensible	2	
	None	1	

The GCS score is the sum of the best attainable subscores in the categories of eye opening (E), motor (M), and verbal (V) responses. It ranges from 15 ($E_4 + M_6 + V_5$) to 3 ($E_1 + M_1 + V_1$).

such as the GCS that assesses the level of consciousness may be associated with prognosis and outcome. For the GCS, an association of lower scores with worsened outcome has been shown for traumatic brain injury (50), subarachnoid hemorrhage (51), brain abscess (52), survival after cardiac arrest (53,54), and septic encephalopathy (55). For example, in traumatic brain injury, a GCS score greater than 7 suggests a 90% likelihood of an outcome of moderate disability or better, whereas a score less than 7 suggests an increased risk of death or persistent vegetative state that approaches 60% to 90% for a GCS score of 3 (50,56,57). In aneurysmal subarachnoid hemorrhage, a GCS score less than 13 after initial treatment of increased intracranial pressure (i.e., WFNS grade 4 or 5) corresponds to a 60% to 90% chance of a poor functional outcome or death, while such outcomes only affect 14% of patients whose level of consciousness is unaffected (GCS 15, WFNS grade 1 or 2) (51).

Despite its widespread use and appeal, the GCS has several important limitations, even if applied correctly. One is the information loss inherent in reducing a graded assessment of three responses into a single number. The second is that mechanical problems such as swelling and endotracheal intubation may prevent proper assessment of eye opening and verbal response. In this setting, some clinicians assign the lowest component score, whereas others try to infer the "true" score from related neurologic findings, and still others add the subscript "T" to indicate an intubated patient. Third, sedatives and neuromuscular blocking agents affect the GCS score upon repeated assessment. Finally, although the degree of brainstem involvement may reflect the severity of coma, the GCS provides limited information about brainstem function.

Determination of Brain Death

The determination of brain death for purposes of organ donation or withdrawal of life support is an area that has brought both the merits and the limitations of the neurologic examination into clear focus. Because the clinical determination of brain death requires a comprehensive and methodical assessment of the patient (58), its steps may serve as a guide to the neurologic examination of a comatose patient. An algorithm for the determination of brain death is shown in Fig. 27.6. Given the gravity of the "therapeutic" consequences of the diagnosis of brain death, a prerequisite to its determination is a clinical picture, typically supported by imaging studies, that is consistent with the occurrence of brain death.

The first step in the neurologic examination for the determination of brain death is the determination of coma (i.e., lack of responsiveness to external stimuli due to unconsciousness as discussed above). Motor responses *elicited by the examination* need to be differentiated from spontaneous movements *during the examination*. The latter are typically brief, slow movements that originate from the spinal cord and do not become integrated into decerebrate or decorticate responses. Only rarely are they reproducible upon repeat testing. Reproducible partial eye opening that failed to reveal the iris has been described in response to a peripheral painful stimulus in a patient who fulfilled clinical criteria of brain death (59). Conditions that may confound the clinical diagnosis of brain death are listed in Table 27.3. In addition to considering such confounding conditions, the *diagnosis of brain death should be consistent with imaging studies and/or the overall clinical picture before the formal determination of brain death is considered.*

The next step in the neurologic examination is the assessment of brainstem function. As in the assessment of the level of consciousness, direct trauma to either afferent or efferent structures needs to be considered before any of the tests of brainstem function are interpreted as negative. Typical tests, their afferent and efferent pathways, and potentially interfering clinical conditions are summarized in Table 27.4.

To complete the diagnosis of brain death, an apnea test is performed to test the response to an acute decrease in the pH of CSF due to hypercarbia. Hypercarbia is induced by disconnecting mechanical ventilation, while continued oxygenation

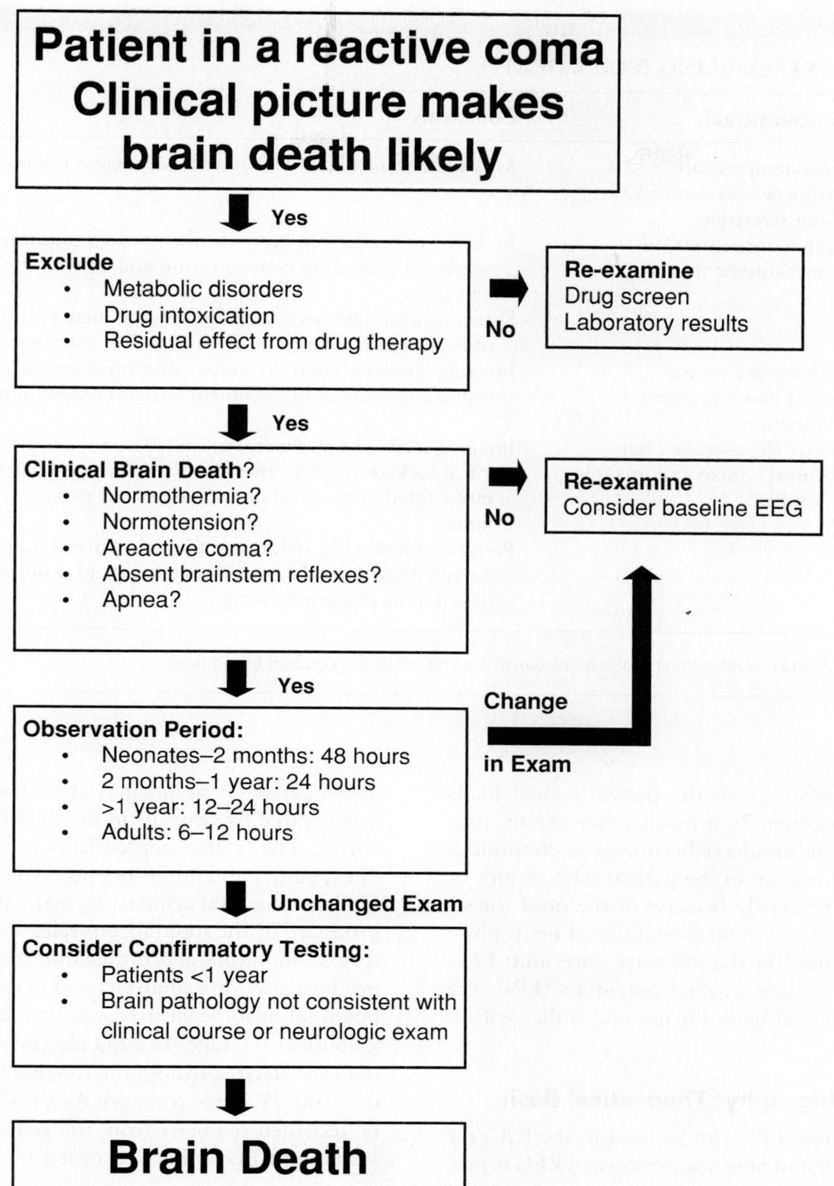

FIGURE 27.6.

is assured by both preoxygenation and apneic oxygenation. Absence of respiratory movements at an arterial PCO_2 of 60 mm Hg or after an increase in PCO_2 of 20 mm Hg is consistent with brain death. Apnea testing may be complicated by arterial hypotension due to loss of arterial and autonomic tone (60). While such hypotension corroborates the diagnosis of brain death, it makes the hemodynamic stability required for apnea testing difficult to attain. The apnea test may trigger movement responses, which reflect residual spinal activity (61).

Once all these criteria for brain death are met, either an observation period followed by repeat assessment or a confirmatory test is used to reach a final diagnosis (see Fig. 27.6). Cerebral angiography is the gold standard among confirmatory tests. Contrast media is injected into the aortic arch and distributes to the external carotid circulation, whereas the internal carotid and vertebral arteries fill only to the level of the skull base and atlanto-occipital junction, respectively. Similar findings can be obtained with magnetic resonance angiography or with single photon emission computed tomography 99mTc-HMPAO (SPECT). Electroencephalography and transcranial Doppler are also frequently used as confirmatory tests. Their role will be discussed in greater detail below.

Electrophysiologic Techniques

Neurophysiologic function testing has been used for more than 20 years as a diagnostic/prognostic tool in the intensive care unit (62–65). Snapshots of function of different parts of the nervous system have been used to predict the most likely long-term function of the nervous system. This information helps the intensivist determine whether continued aggressive

TABLE 27.3

NEUROLOGIC STATES RESEMBLING BRAIN DEATH

Disease state	Diagnostic aids	Comments
Hypothermia	Core temperature <32°C Osborne waves on ECG	May cause central nervous system depression up to clinical brain death
Acute poisoning	Drug screening Serum concentration measurements	In differentiating from brain death, consider antidote and/or document subtherapeutic drug concentration and/or wait for four elimination half-lives Direct central nervous system depressants may confound confirmatory testing of brain death because of $CMRO_2$–CBF coupling
Metabolic encephalopathy	Laboratory testing Intact lower brainstem function	Imaging studies should document structural central nervous system changes Imaging studies should document structural central nervous system changes
Akinetic mutism	Intact sleep–wake cycle	Imaging study shows frontal or mesencephalic brain lesion
Locked-in syndrome	Clinical course and imaging studies	Central locked-in syndrome: Corticobulbar and corticospinal tracts are interrupted at the level of the base of the pons; vertical eye movements are intact Peripheral locked-in syndrome: Guillain-Barré syndrome, advanced amyotrophic lateral sclerosis, neuromuscular blocking agents, organophosphate poisoning

ECG, electrocardiogram; $CMRO_2$, cerebral metabolic requirement for oxygen; CBF, cerebral blood flow.

intensive care is appropriate given the patient's most likely long-term neurologic outcome. To a much lesser extent, neurophysiologic testing modalities have been used as continuous monitors of neurologic function in the patient who cannot be assessed neurologically, primarily because of the need for sedation (66–68). There are two main modalities of neurophysiologic function testing used in the intensive care unit: Electroencephalography (EEG) and evoked potentials (EPs). For each modality, the theoretical basis for use and utility will be reviewed.

Electroencephalography: Theoretical Basis

In order to understand how EEG can be used in the ICU, the clinician must first understand how scalp-recorded EEG is produced and what factors may affect the recordings. EEG activity is generated by neurons in the pyramidal layer of the cerebral cortex. The scalp-recorded EEG is produced by a summation of excitatory and inhibitory postsynaptic potentials (EPSPs and IPSPs), not actual cellular depolarization. EPSPs and IPSPs are produced by the spontaneous release of small packets of excitatory or inhibitory neurotransmitters from a nerve terminal that produce only very small changes in the postsynaptic membrane potential, insufficient to cause depolarization. As a result, the amplitude (voltage) of EEG electrical activity is much smaller than the electrocardiogram, ranging from $<5\ \mu V$ in the elderly to $>100\ \mu V$ in the teenager. As a result, the EEG signal cannot be recorded remotely from the generator site, and practically speaking, EEG activity recorded from a single electrode only

TABLE 27.4

CLINICAL EXAMINATION OF THE BRAINSTEM DURING EVALUATION FOR BRAIN DEATH

Brainstem reflex	Afferent path	Efferent path	Caveats
Pupillary light reaction	II	III	Not confounded by systemic drugs; absence may be caused by prolonged administration of neuromuscular blocking agents
Ocular movements (oculocephalic reflex or caloric nystagmus)	VIII	III, VI	Confounded by damage from ototoxic drugs; cervical spine trauma may preclude testing of the oculocephalic reflex; voluntary ocular movements are sometimes the only finding that differentiates a "locked-in" syndrome from brain death
Corneal reflex/pressure on supraorbital nerve	V	VII	
Gag	IX	IX, X	May be difficult to assess in orotracheally intubated patient
Cough	X	X, cervical roots	Best tested by assessing the response to tracheal suctioning

reflects cortical activity directly beneath the recording site. In addition, because the EEG signal is so small, poor electrode contact with the scalp may result in significant loss of signal.

Maintenance of ion fluxes associated with the production of the EEG is an energy requiring process. Pharmacologic total suppression of the EEG will result in a 50% to 60% decrease in $CMRO_2$ (69,70). The decrease in oxygen requirement parallels the suppression of the EEG in cases of lesser suppression. An EEG that is merely slowed pharmacologically will be associated with a higher $CMRO_2$ than an EEG that is totally suppressed or flat.

The EEG is organized both spatially and temporally, but patterns of organization are much more difficult for the clinician to recognize, primarily because few clinicians have significant experience with normal EEG patterns, pathologic EEG patterns, or drug-induced EEG patterns. EEG patterns are described primarily in terms of frequency (how fast voltage oscillations occur) and amplitude (size or voltage). Slower frequency ranges include δ (3 Hz or slower) and θ (3.5–7.5 Hz). These frequencies are not seen in the normal awake adult but are commonly seen in the naturally asleep adult or in the adult who is receiving therapeutic doses of sedative-hypnotic and/or analgesic drugs. Faster frequency ranges include α (8–13 Hz) and β (>13 Hz). Alpha frequencies (8–13 Hz) tend to be present on the posterior part of the head and are most prominent with the eyes closed. Alpha activity disappears with attention and concentration, replaced with faster β activity. Beta frequencies are commonly seen more toward the front of the head and are associated with increased "function" of a particular part of the brain. In the neurologically abnormal patient, θ and δ frequencies may be focal, associated with a specific loss of function, or more global, associated with generalized neurologic dysfunction. Generally, the more severe the neurologic damage/dysfunction, the slower the recorded EEG activity will be. For example, a patient with a receptive and expressive aphasia will likely demonstrate EEG slowing (θ and δ waves) over the dominant temporal lobe.

Sedative-hypnotic drugs produce a change in neurologic function that is likewise paralleled by EEG changes. The EEG changes associated with sedative-hypnotic drugs are predictable, related both to the drug used and the dosage of drug given. The vast majority of sedative-hypnotic drugs used in the intensive care unit will produce identical, dose-related changes in the EEG. Table 27.5 shows EEG pattern changes associated with most drugs that would be used in the ICU environment. Limited information about dexmedetomidine, which is being increasingly used in the ICU for sedation, suggests that predictable EEG patterns do occur with this drug as with other sedatives and analgesics commonly used in the intensive care unit environment. Combinations of drugs, of course, will have different effects than when either drug is used alone. Specific data regarding the effect of combinations of drugs is limited and beyond the scope of this chapter. However, in general, both sedative and analgesic drugs will increase the primary effect of the drug being used in the higher dose as well as add effects of their own.

In summary, the scalp-recorded EEG reflects function of closely underlying neuronal tissue. Function may be altered

TABLE 27.5

SEDATIVE-HYPNOTIC AND ANALGESIC DRUGS AND THE ELECTROENCEPHALOGRAM (EEG)

Drug		Effect on EEG dominant frequency	Effect on EEG amplitude	Burst suppression
Barbiturates	Low dose	Fast frontal β activity	Slight ↑	Yes, with high doses
	Moderate dose	Frontal α frequency spindles	↑	
	High dose	Diffuse δ → burst suppression → silence	↑↑↑ → 0	
Etomidate	Low dose	Fast frontal β activity	↑	Yes, with high doses
	Moderate dose	Frontal α frequency spindles	↑	
	High dose	Diffuse δ → burst suppression → silence	↑↑ → 0	
Propofol	Low dose	Loss of α, ↑ frontal β	↑	Yes, with high doses
	Moderate dose	Frontal δ, waxing/waning α	↑	
	High dose	Diffuse δ → burst suppression → silence	↑↑ → 0	
Dexmedetomidine		Early appearance of high-amplitude δ frequency that increases with dose, similar to opiates	↑	No
Ketamine	Low dose	Loss of α, ↑ variability	↑↓	No
	Moderate dose	Frontal rhythmic delta	↑	
	High dose	Polymorphic δ, some β	↑↑ (β is low amplitude)	
Benzodiazepines	Low dose	Loss of α, increased frontal β activity	↑	No
	High dose	Frontally dominant δ and θ	↑	
Opiates	Low dose	Loss of β, α slows	↔↑	No
	Moderate dose	Diffuse θ, some δ	↑	
	High dose	δ, often synchronized	↑↑	

δ, <3-Hz frequency; θ, 3.5- to 7.5-Hz frequency; α, 8- to 13-Hz frequency; β, >13-Hz frequency.

by neurologic damage, pharmacologic means, normal changes in function associated with changes in alertness or sleep, or any combination of these factors. Thus, whether the EEG is used as a monitor or a diagnostic/prognostic tool, interpretation of data without a thorough knowledge of all factors that could influence recordings is not possible.

Diagnostic Electroencephalography: Clinical Utility in the Intensive Care Unit

Diagnostic EEG studies or EEG monitoring in the ICU is done primarily for one of three purposes: Brain death determination, monitoring for evidence of seizure activity or cerebral ischemia, and determination of drug effect for the purposes of titrating sedative and analgesic drugs or control of intracranial pressure.

Criteria for brain death vary from state to state, but in most states, a 16- to 32-channel isoelectric EEG on two consecutive recordings at least 24 hours apart can provide strong corroborating evidence for cessation of brain function (see Fig. 27.6). Because other factors affecting the EEG can produce an isoelectric EEG in the absence of brain death, the EEG cannot be used as the sole evaluation for brain death. While it is likely that drug levels (Table 27.5) will decline significantly over a 24-hour period, patients with massive drug overdose or impaired metabolic pathways may show an isoelectric EEG for much longer than 24 or 48 hours. In these cases, the neurologic examination may also not be useful since high drug levels may suppress even the most resistant reflex responses. Fortunately, other diagnostic testing methods, including other electrophysiologic and nonelectrophysiologic methods, may be helpful. Evoked potentials (see below), for example, are more resistant to drug effects than the EEG and can frequently be used to demonstrate brainstem and cortical function even in the face of an isoelectric EEG (71,72). In addition, EEG recorded immediately after cardiac arrest may show an isoelectric pattern that subsequently recovers (73). Cortical evoked potentials have also been demonstrated to be more reliable in assessing neurologic function immediately after an ischemic/anoxic insult (73). In summary, a scalp-recorded, 16- to 32-channel EEG is a helpful adjunct to the diagnosis of brain death, provided all other factors influencing the EEG are understood and controlled.

Continuous EEG monitoring in the ICU or, alternatively, sequential diagnostic EEG studies have been described for detection of nonconvulsive seizure (NCS) activity (or seizure activity in the pharmacologically paralyzed patient) and for detection of cerebral ischemia (66–68,74–76). This type of monitoring requires multiple channels of information to obtain adequate monitoring coverage of the entire brain. A highly trained technologist observes the patient simultaneously with the EEG recording, and operates the equipment and maintains recording electrodes during nursing care that will commonly dislodge them. The technologist also provides real-time neurophysiologic data to the clinicians caring for the patient. Processed EEG algorithms have been developed to facilitate detection of ischemia epileptiform and frank seizure activity during continuous EEG monitoring (77,78), but the technology has not yet evolved enough to eliminate the need for an on-site technologist with monitoring experience.

Continuous EEG monitoring in the ICU has demonstrated that NCSs are much more common than previously thought (75,76,79). NCSs have been reported following neurosurgical procedures, subarachnoid hemorrhage, CNS infection, head injury, and other conditions. In addition, there is evidence using neuron-specific enolase as a marker of neurologic injury that NCSs may produce neurologic damage and that seizure duration and time to diagnosis are significantly related to the extent of damage and long-term outcome. Without continuous EEG monitoring, NCSs cannot be detected, as they are not consistently and specifically associated with other findings such as hypertension and tachycardia (79).

The personnel and fiscal costs of continuous EEG monitoring have made it unfeasible except in the larger neurologic and neurosurgical intensive care units where many patients with conditions amenable to continuous monitoring require care (74). In addition, very little outcome data exist to demonstrate that such monitoring is overall cost effective. When considering real-time neurologic monitoring in the patient whose neurologic examination cannot be assessed, much work needs to be done to determine how continuous EEG monitoring will mesh with other neurologic monitoring modalities such as intracranial pressure, cerebral blood flow, brain tissue pO_2 monitoring, transcranial Doppler, and microdialysis monitoring. Theoretically and based on limited clinical data (74–79), there is much promise for continuous EEG monitoring when used as a part of a multimodality neurologic monitoring program.

Processed Electroencephalogram: Monitoring of Sedation

The use of the EEG to monitor the depth of sedation in patients in the ICU has been described extensively in the literature, and nearly all techniques utilize processed EEG rather than the unprocessed analog signal. Drug effect monitoring is generally accomplished using one or two channels of EEG information, generally recorded over the frontopolar region of the cerebral cortex. This location is chosen because application of surface recording electrodes is easy in this location (no hair) and most devices designed for this purpose have been validated using frontopolar recording locations. Usage of this smaller number of channels is based on the assumption that the drug effect will be similar in all areas of the brain. This assumption is generally valid except in the case of a patient with focal brain damage. In areas of damage, the drug effect will generally be greater than usual and must be interpreted in light of the abnormal baseline recording. None of the commercially available devices for monitoring drug effects on the EEG has been calibrated or validated appropriately for monitoring drug effects in the patient with the abnormal EEG, and relatively limited information is available on the use of EEG to monitor drug effects in neurologically damaged patients (80–83).

EEG drug effect monitoring is used most commonly for titrating sedative drugs, particularly in the pharmacologically paralyzed patient, but also for titration of barbiturate drugs used to control intracranial pressure (66–68,84,85). Devices used to monitor the drug effect either utilize unprocessed, raw analog EEG in a fashion similar to ECG monitoring in the ICU or utilize one of three signal processing techniques: Power spectrum analysis, bispectral analysis, or EEG entropy analysis. Examples of commercial monitors include the bispectral index (BIS), the patient state index, and entropy. Although the BIS has been used and studied most widely among these monitors, the concepts discussed below should apply to other EEG-based monitors of sedation as well.

BIS (Aspect Medical Systems, Inc., Natick, MA) monitoring has been used in the intensive care setting to guide dosing

TABLE 27.6

CLINICAL CONDITION EXPECTED WITH BISPECTRAL INDEX VALUES

100	Awake patient, amnesia unlikely
80	Sedated responsive patient, amnesia prominent unless significant event
70	Heavily sedated or unconscious patient, amnesia probable
60	General anesthesia, unresponsive to verbal stimuli
40	Deep hypnotic state
20	Burst suppression
0	Isoelectric electroencephalogram

of sedatives and reassure clinicians that paralyzed or agitated patients are amnestic but not excessively sedated (86). The BIS monitor processes EEG signals that are recorded from a self-adhesive electrode strip placed on the forehead. It calculates and displays a BIS value, a dimensionless number ranging from 0 to 100 that is derived from highly processed EEG data that includes EEG power, frequency, and bicoherence (87). Low BIS numbers indicate strong relationships among the EEG frequencies and reflect a condition consistent with a deep hypnotic state (Table 27.6). This relationship is valid despite the effects of age and infirmity on sensitivity to sedation (88,89).

Despite its obvious clinical utility, the aspects of imperfect performance of the BIS monitor are well known. For example, the BIS can decrease to numbers (20–50) consistent with deep general anesthesia during natural sleep without sedation (90). Moreover, although memory is less likely to form at lower BIS values, memory has been demonstrated even at a BIS in a range (40–60) associated with general anesthesia (91). Additionally, artifact from electromyographic (EMG), electro-oculographic (EOG) (92), or pacemaker generators (93) can produce significant but spurious BIS increases (from 50s to 80s). This raises the possibility of overdosing nonrelaxed or paced patients when attempting to maintain a given BIS range. BIS values can also be driven higher by medications that are CNS stimulants, such as ketamine, methylphenidate, or dexmedetomidine (94). In such cases, the BIS may not reflect the level of hypnosis or sedation experienced by the patient. Therefore, when the sedative dosages required to achieve a desired BIS range exceed normal expectations, the possibility of an artifactual interference deserves consideration.

Perhaps the most significant issue with BIS or other monitors of cortical anesthetic drug effect are their inability to differentiate deep sedation from cerebral ischemia. Both conditions cause loss of higher-frequency EEG waves (α and β slowing and δ and θ wave intrusion) and, in extreme states, both can produce burst suppression or isoelectric EEG patterns with a low BIS. When O_2 delivery decreases below a level sufficient to meet the $CMRO_2$, electrical function fails and BIS decreases. This may partly explain improved ICU outcomes when the BIS is maintained >60 (95). Therefore, the determination that sedation is adequate based on having achieved a target BIS value should only be made when one is confident that cerebral perfusion is adequate.

Interpretation of BIS or, for that matter, any EEG-based monitor of sedation is best accomplished when the patient's pharmacologic support remains stable in the face of changing CPP or, conversely, the CPP remains adequate and stable during pharmacologic adjustments and BIS changes. As a corollary, the BIS can assist with guiding therapy when the adequacy of O_2 supply to the CNS is in question (95).

In summary, other than for drug effect monitoring, use of the EEG in the ICU remains relatively limited, primarily because of personnel costs and difficulty in maintaining stable technical conditions for monitoring multiple channels of information. As our understanding of underlying mechanisms for neurologic injury improves, we may be able to learn which monitoring modalities are most useful for a given clinical scenario and which can more specifically target EEG monitoring to a smaller area of the brain. In addition, as computing power continues to improve, signal processing technology will likewise improve, and EEG monitoring equipment that recognizes artifact and self-corrects technical problems may reduce the need for the continuous presence of highly trained personnel to operate the EEG in the ICU environment.

Evoked Potentials

The EEG is a recording of the spontaneous electrical activity of the cerebral cortex. In contrast, EPs are recordings of the electrical activity from different parts of the nervous system produced by either sensory or motor stimuli applied to activated portions of the sensory and motor systems, respectively. With the exception of motor-evoked responses recorded from muscle, EPs are much smaller than background EEG or muscle electrical activity, and the responses from repetitive stimuli must be averaged in order to be able to discern the responses from other background biologic signals or environmental noise. Auditory responses are very small (generally <0.5 μV) and require as many as 1,000 to 2,000 averaged responses to clarify the signal. Somatosensory responses are larger (0.5–10 μV) and require fewer averages to clarify. EPs are described in terms of latency (time [msec] from stimulus application to onset or peak of response) and amplitude (μV) (Fig. 27.7). Conceptually, amplitude is the more important parameter for ICU studies because voltage is mainly related to the amount of functional neural tissue generating the response, and latency is related to the conduction time from the stimulus site to the generating site. This assumption, while usually true, is not always the case since a peripheral or cranial nerve injury may produce a nerve with fibers conducting at many different velocities. This situation would produce a desynchronized evoked response of

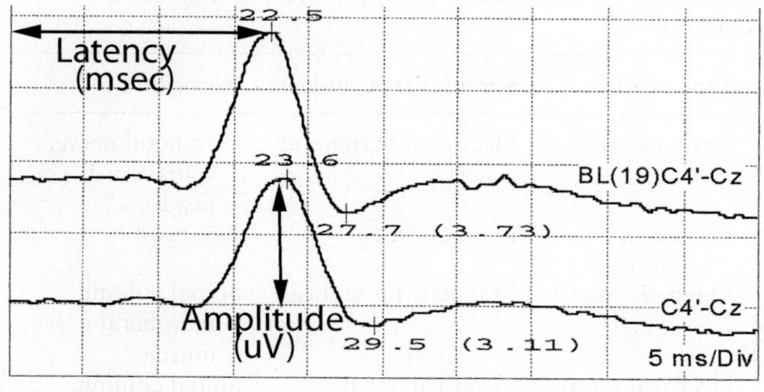

FIGURE 27.7. Latency is defined as the time from stimulus application to the onset or the peak of the response (peak latency shown here). Amplitude is the size (usually microvolts) of the evoked response.

smaller amplitude, even when the neural tissue generating the more rostral response is entirely normal.

In comparison with the EEG, EPs are much less susceptible to the effects of intravenous sedative-hypnotic drugs and not significantly affected by intravenous analgesics (96). Auditory EP responses will not be altered significantly by any sedating or analgesic regimen used in the ICU today. Notably, based on known effects of opiates and sedatives on brainstem auditory evoked potentials (BAEPs), patients admitted with opiate or sedative drug overdose and an isoelectric EEG will not show any significant abnormality of waves I through V related to the drug effect alone (71,72,96). Somatosensory EPs are somewhat more susceptible to the effects of sedative drugs. Subcortical somatosensory responses (see below) are resistant to drug effects to the same degree as the BAEP. Cortical somatosensory EPs do show significant increases in latency and decreases in amplitude with sedating medications (96), but generally they will not be completely abolished even by enough sedative medication to render the EEG isoelectric (71,72,96). This observation is also important for the patient with drug overdose.

Table 27.7 is a summary of the different types of evoked potentials that may be recorded or monitored in the ICU. In the ICU, EPs are most commonly utilized as diagnostic tests of neurologic function. The results of these tests are then frequently used as prognostic indicators of intermediate and long-term neurologic function. EPs may also be monitored continuously in the ICU but, like with the EEG, personnel and maintenance costs are very high, and only a few large neurologic or neurosurgical ICUs are able to provide real-time EP monitoring.

EPs reflect the function of nervous system tissue along the entire pathway involved with the stimulated system. For example, somatosensory EPs are recorded by applying an electrical stimulus to a distal peripheral nerve, recording from the peripheral nerve more centrally, recording over the spinal cord (usually cervical region), and recording over the cerebral cortex. Thus, function of *part* of the peripheral nervous system, spinal cord, brainstem, thalamus, internal capsule, and cerebral cortex is assessed with a single test. In contrast to EEG, EPs, therefore, are able to test the function of portions of the nervous system caudal to the cortex as well as a limited area of the cortex. Generally, when EPs are recorded or monitored in the ICU, the function of the tested or monitored pathway is assumed to reflect the function of the surrounding neural tissue,

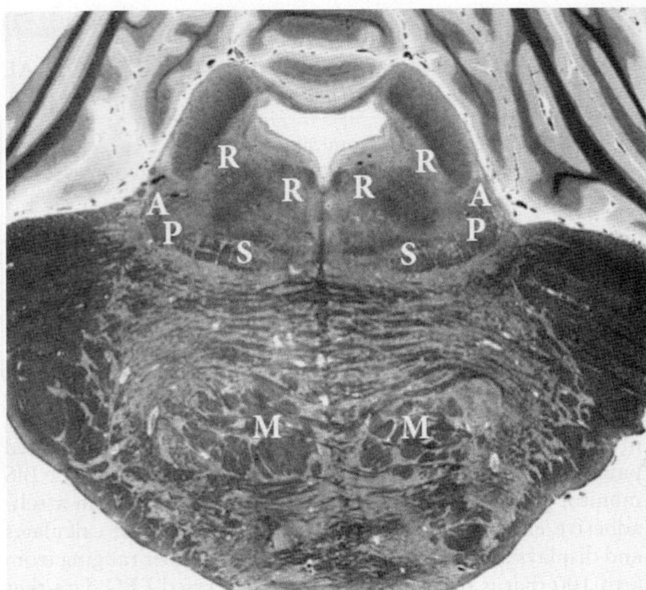

FIGURE 27.8. Section of the brainstem through the midpons. Note the relatively limited and separated territory of the brainstem actually monitored by evoked responses at this level. Function of the surrounding brain stem is assumed to be reflected by auditory and somatosensory function. Vital pathways and structures are near both the auditory and somatosensory pathways. A, auditory pathway; P, pain pathway; S, somatosensory pathway; R, reticular formation; M, descending motor pathway.

whether cortical, subcortical, or spinal cord (Fig. 27.8). This assumption concerning the surrounding neural tissue is clearly not always valid; however, considerable clinical evidence has demonstrated that EPs usually do reflect the function of the surrounding neural tissue and are very effective at detecting a developing injury and in prognosticating the long-term effects of an existing neurologic injury. This section of the chapter will examine BAEPs, somatosensory evoked potentials (SEPs), and transcranial motor evoked potentials (TcMEPs) and their use as diagnostic, prognostic, and monitoring tools in the ICU. While each modality will be considered separately, BAEPs and SEPs are most commonly recorded together to provide information about a larger portion of the nervous system. Because TcMEPs were only recently approved for use in humans, only limited information about the diagnostic, prognostic, and monitoring utility of TcMEPs in the ICU is available. Since only a few centers are able to provide continuous EP monitoring to detect ongoing function and developing injury, this section will focus on the diagnostic and prognostic uses of EPs.

TABLE 27.7

EVOKED POTENTIALS (EPs) IN THE INTENSIVE CARE UNIT

Type of EPs	Stimulus type and site	Recording sites
Somatosensory	Electrical, peripheral nerve	Peripheral nerve, spinal cord, head
Brainstem auditory	Loud click, ear	Ear, head
Magnetic motor	Magnetic pulse, head	Spinal column, peripheral nerve, muscle
Electrical motor	Electrical, head	Spinal column, peripheral nerve, muscle

Brainstem Auditory Evoked Potentials

The stimulus for the BAEP is a repetitive loud click applied either via headphone or via ear inserts. In order to interpret the information provided by BAEPs, the clinician must be aware of factors that may alter the ability to activate the auditory pathway with the click stimulus. For example, cerumen in the ear canal may muffle the applied stimulus. Trauma may anatomically disrupt the auditory apparatus (damage to the external auditory canal, tympanic membrane, middle ear apparatus). Aminoglycoside antibiotics may damage the inner ear transduction system. Fortunately, the eighth nerve itself produces a

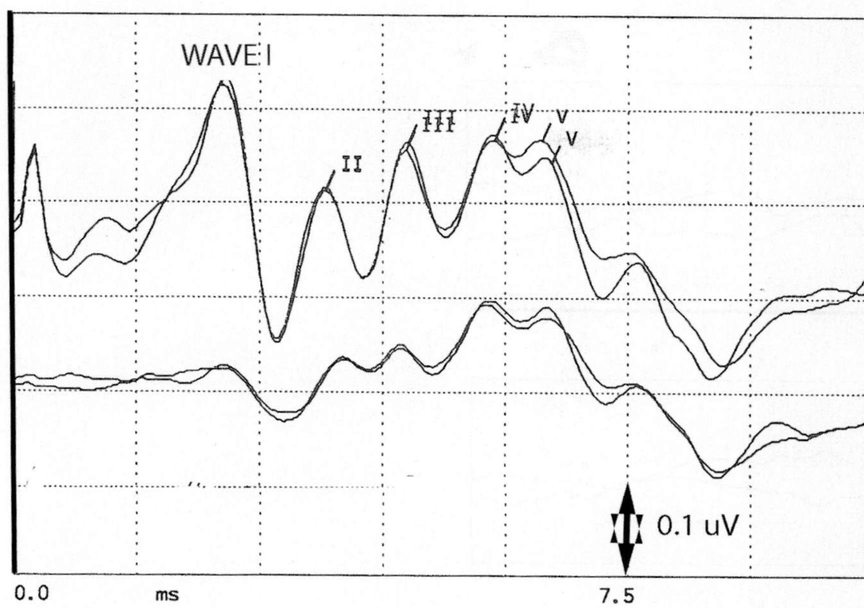

FIGURE 27.9. Normal brainstem auditory evoked response. Note the presence of wave I, the eighth nerve action potential, which confirms that the auditory apparatus is being properly stimulated.

recordable action potential (Fig. 27.9), and presence of this response confirms that the auditory stimulus has actually reached the nervous system. Without the presence of an eighth nerve action potential, no conclusions about the functioning of the more rostral auditory pathway can be made.

Figure 27.8 is a schematic representation of the auditory pathway in relationship to important brainstem and midbrain structures. The entire BAEP is generally completed within 10 msec of the stimulus application. Because the auditory pathway has multiple synapses that produce recordable responses from the lower pons through the midbrain, if the recorded response demonstrates abnormalities at any level, significant neurologic impairment of the patient is likely because of the functional significance of nearby motor, sensory, autonomic, cranial nerve, and reticular activating system structures. Based on results from multiple studies, if the BAEP beyond the cochlear nerve action potential (wave I) is absent bilaterally, the CNS prognosis is very grave and most patients will subsequently be determined to be brain dead by clinical and/or angiographic criteria (62,65,97–99). Figure 27.10 shows BAEP and SEP recordings from three different patients who were comatose following trauma or surgery and were being evaluated for CNS function with EP recordings in the surgical ICU. Patient A had absent BAEPs beyond wave I and absent SEPs, and was determined to be brain dead within 24 hours of the EP studies. Patient B had a normal recording of waves I through V, but SEPs were absent. This patient had a prolonged hospital course and never recovered any higher neurologic function. Patient C had normal BAEPs and SEPs despite a severely impaired neurologic examination and difficult to control seizures at the time of the SEP study. Subsequent EP studies continued to show intact BAEPs and SEPs despite abnormal posturing and difficult to control seizures. This patient went on to recover independent neurologic function after many months of rehabilitation (100). These three patients exemplify the most common usage of EPs in the ICU, and their studies and outcome reflect what is documented in the literature. In summary, absent BAEPs beyond wave I indicate a high likelihood of a brain death outcome. Intact and normal BAEPs may indicate a good outcome, especially in the face of normal SEPs. If SEPs are absent bilaterally, the best likely outcome is a chronic vegetative state, even with normal BAEP waves I through V.

The auditory pathway continues rostrally, and responses may be recorded that are generated in the auditory cortex (middle-latency auditory evoked responses). There are limited clinical data available that indicate that presence of a normal middle-latency auditory response is a good prognostic sign to the same degree as the SEP in the comatose patient.

The stimulus for the SEP is a repetitive electrical stimulus delivered to a peripheral nerve, most commonly the median nerve at the wrist or the posterior tibial nerve at the ankle, using surface electrodes or subdermal needle electrodes. The response (nerve action potential) is recorded proximally over the peripheral nerve or appropriate nerve plexus to be certain that the somatosensory stimulus is being appropriately delivered to the central nervous system (Fig. 27.11). The next recorded response is generated in the lower brainstem and recorded with a surface electrode placed over the upper cervical spine. The primary initial cortical response at the rostral end of the somatosensory pathway is recorded over the cortex on the opposite side from stimulus application, and usually occurs within 25 msec from stimulus application at the median nerve or 50 msec from stimulus application at the posterior tibial nerve. The normal SEP also contains responses that are later than the primary response. These responses, also generated by cortical neurons, are considered to be related to higher cognitive function. Most studies where SEPs are either monitored or used for diagnosis and prognosis only analyze the initial primary cortical response occurring prior to 25 msec. A few studies have also examined the prognostic significance of the later SEP or auditory responses (101,102), but the clinician should be aware that all of these later responses are highly influenced and easily abolished by any of the drugs used for sedation and analgesia in the ICU. In fact, later auditory responses have been used to gauge the depth of sedation in a fashion similar to the EEG bispectral index (102).

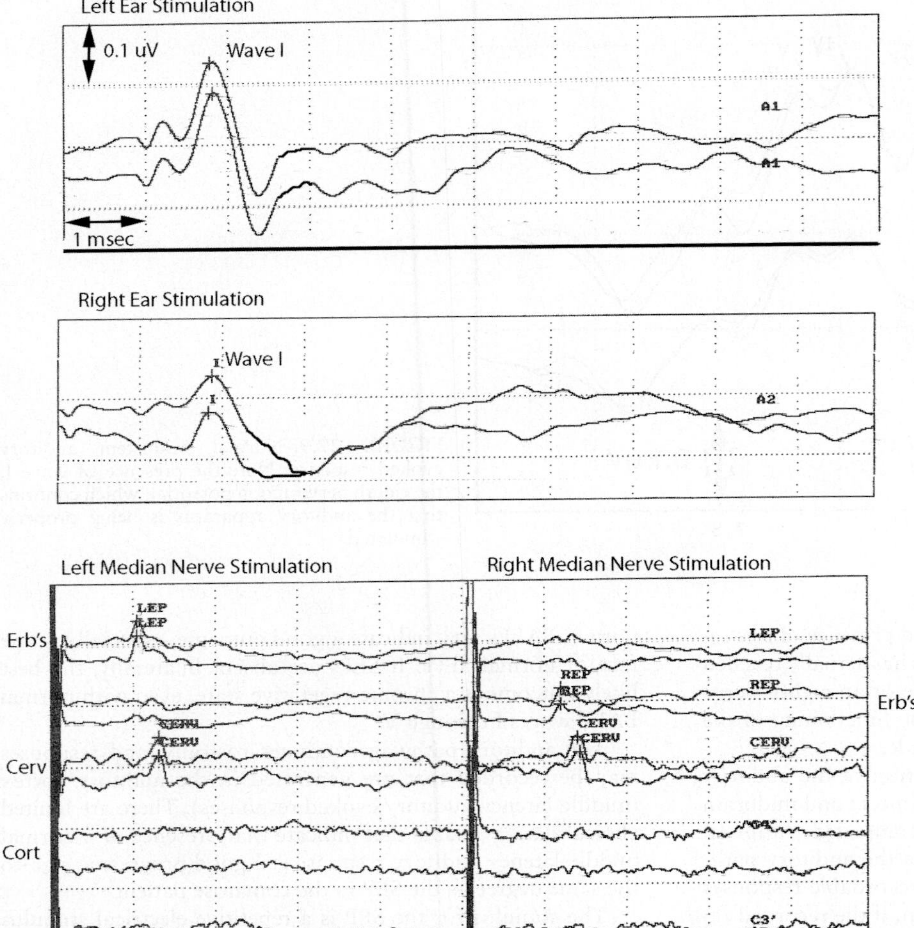

FIGURE 27.10. Neurophysiologic studies from three comatose patients. **A:** Brain-dead patient. This patient has no recordable evoked auditory response after wave I and no recordable somatosensory response after the cervical response. (*Continued*)

Figure 27.8 shows the somatosensory pathway schematically, together with the auditory pathway and nearby brainstem, midbrain, and cortical structures in a single slice through the pons. As shown in the figure, the auditory and somatosensory pathways are separated far enough to include multiple important structures in the territory between them. The anatomic locations of the two separated pathways explain why neurologic outcome is usually better when *both* evoked response modalities show a normal response. The presence of cortical responses to a peripheral stimulus indicates that the involved subcortical nervous pathway is intact and that cortical neurons are still functional to be activated and produce a measurable electrical response, both of which are necessary for a good long-term neurologic outcome.

In summary, the presence of normal SEPs bilaterally, based on all available literature, is an excellent prognostic sign. The absence of any SEP cortical response is a poor prognostic indicator. The degree of bad outcome can be predicted by the BAEP. Intact and normal BAEPs with absent cortical SEPs predict a best outcome of a chronic vegetative state. Outcome may be worse, however, as BAEPs commonly deteriorate later with rostral-to-caudal CNS deterioration. Absent BAEP responses beyond wave I predict a high likelihood of brain death. Present but abnormal SEPs are associated with intermediate outcomes between good/high function and a chronic vegetative state (62,64,65,97–99,102–105).

The motor pathway may be tested by transcranial stimulation of the motor cortex. The cortex may be activated by a magnetic or electrical stimulus. A descending response may then be recorded over the spinal cord at multiple levels: The peripheral nerve and (most commonly) the muscle. Cortical stimulation, either electrical or magnetic, commonly activates the motor cortex governing both the upper and lower extremities and produces a myogenic response that does not need to be averaged. The electrical stimulus intensity is quite high and is prohibitively painful in the awake subject. Thus, most of the limited work has been done using transcranial magnetic stimulation, which is much less painful and readily tolerated by the awake patient. What limited data are available indicate that results are mixed at best when using MEP testing as a prognostic indicator for long-term CNS outcome (106–109). Several carefully conducted studies also utilizing SEPs indicate that SEPs

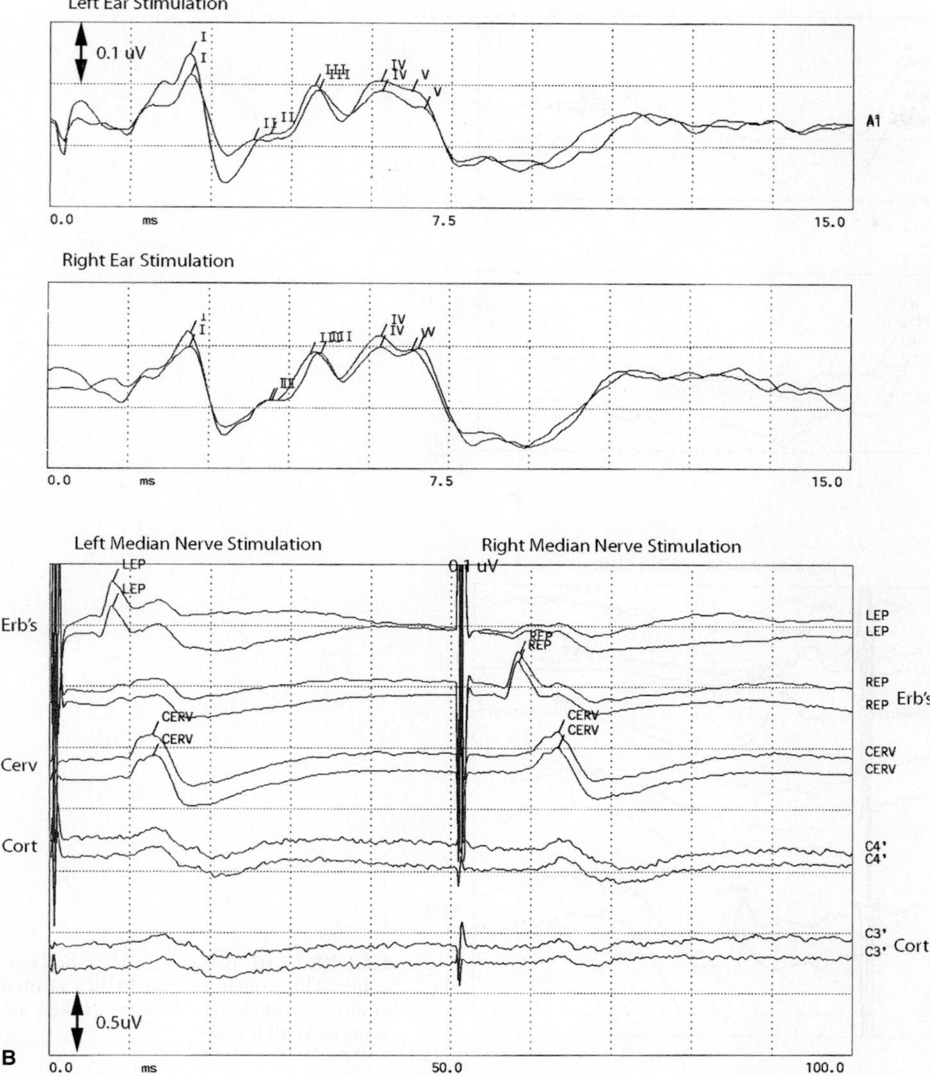

FIGURE 27.10. B: Chronic vegetative state. This patient has an intact auditory evoked response and no cortical somatosensory responses. (*Continued*)

are a much better prognostic indicator than MEPs (106,109). Much more work using MEPs needs to be done before any firm conclusions about their utility can be drawn.

Peripheral Nerve Stimulation

The rate of recovery from neuromuscular blocking (NMB) agents depends upon the NMB agent chosen, its dosing pattern (intermittent or continuous infusion), and numerous patient factors (e.g., pseudocholinesterase deficiency, hepatic or renal dysfunction, induced cytochrome P450 enzyme, organophosphate toxicity, among many others) (110). The suitability for extubation following prolonged neuromuscular blockade has traditionally relied upon functional strength testing, such as an ability to produce a negative inspiratory force or to sustain a head lift. Incomplete patient cooperation caused by sedation or confusion, among other reasons, can adversely affect these tests. Peripheral nerve stimulation (PNS) used for "muscle twitch" testing, or acceleromyography, complements such functional assessments by objectively revealing the condition of the neuromuscular junction, independent of patient participation.

Reliable interpretation of nerve stimulation requires uniform stimulation and placement parameters. Conventional PNS delivers current—adjustable up to 80 mA—in a train-of-four (TOF) series at 2 Hz as double-burst stimulation (DBS), as single shocks at 1.0 or 0.1 Hz, or by tetanic stimuli of 50 or 100 Hz. When tolerated, maximal current settings assure the best chance of delivering supra-threshold stimuli and activation of the greatest percentage of motor fibers despite changes of impedance or proximity, as can occur with electrode separation or desiccation, skin cooling, or peripheral edema. TOF and double-burst stimulation patterns do not require comparison to earlier responses for interpretation, and are therefore well suited for use in the ICU setting where recovery of neuromuscular function may take hours to days and may involve assessments by multiple providers.

Muscle twitch testing measures the force of muscle contractions in response to PNS. The ratio of the force between the last and first stimuli in a series (TOF or DBS) best defines the percentage of acetylcholine receptors occupied by *nondepolarizing* NMB agents in the neuromuscular junction, but is cumbersome to perform (111). Counting the loss of twitches

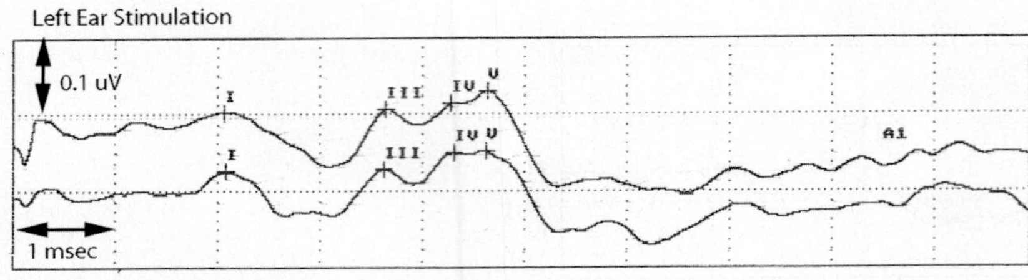

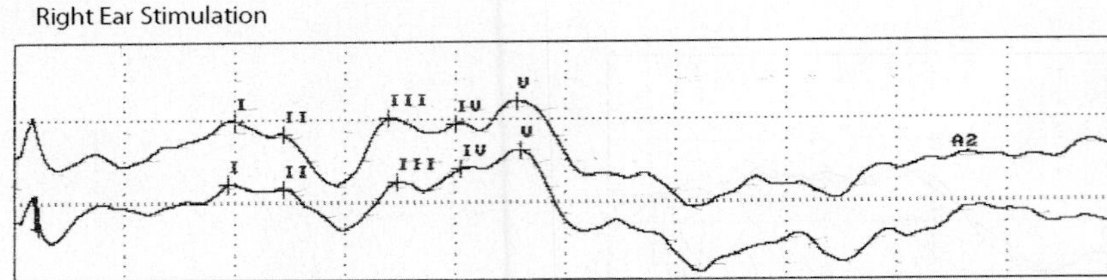

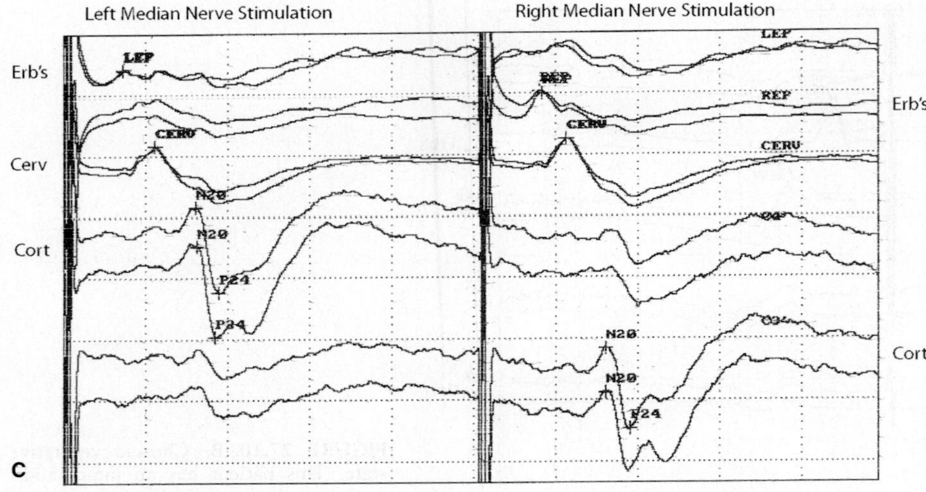

FIGURE 27.10. (*Continued*) **C:** Good outcome. This comatose patient has normal auditory and somatosensory evoked responses at all levels.

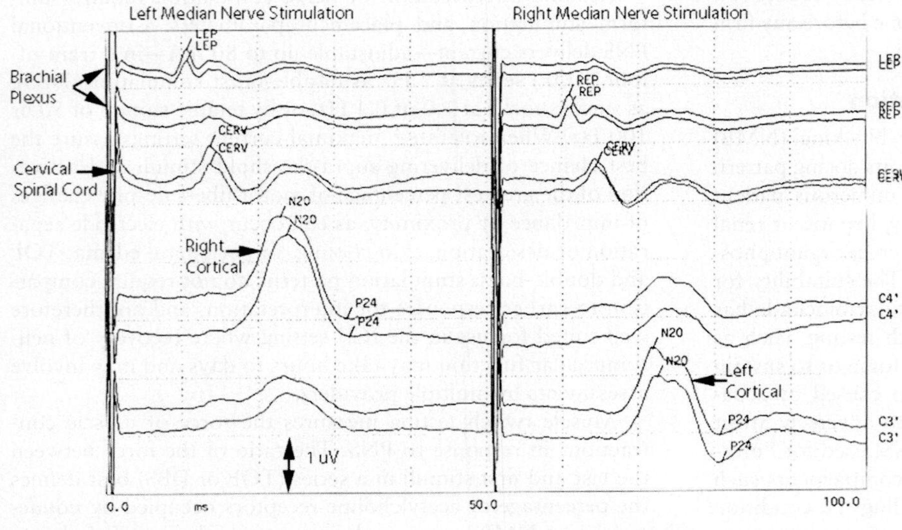

FIGURE 27.11. Normal median nerve somatosensory response. Reproducible responses at the brachial plexus and cervical levels confirm that a somatosensory stimulus is reaching the central nervous system. Without responses at both these levels, conclusions about cortical functions cannot be made.

TABLE 27.8

PERCENTAGE NEUROMUSCULAR JUNCTION BLOCKADE WITH NONDEPOLARIZING NEUROMUSCULAR BLOCKING AGENTS AND CORRESPONDING TRAIN-OF-FOUR AND CLINICAL RESPONSES

Response	% Blockade
Train-of-four 0/4	95
Train-of-four 1/4	90
Train-of-four 2/4	85
Train-of-four 3/4	80
Train-of-four 4/4	75
Sustained (≥5 sec) tetanus	50
Sustained (≥5 sec) head lift	25

in a TOF is a simpler method for assessing the level of block and has greater bedside utility (Table 27.8). In contrast, the TOF ratio does not change following the administration of a *depolarizing* NMB agent such as succinylcholine. When depolarizing NMB agents are used, the force of contraction diminishes equally across all stimuli and disappears altogether with sufficient dose. If an excessive depolarizing NMB agent is administered, a prolonged phase II block emerges. TOF responses during a phase II block behave similarly to responses obtained following nondepolarizing NMB agents.

The peripheral nerve stimulator is attached to a patient using two pregelled electrocardiogram electrodes, although needle electrodes can also be used. The electrodes should be placed closely (without the gels touching) to one another over a site where a nerve with motor function lies relatively superficial to the skin. Antegrade nerve conduction is improved if the positive lead is applied to the proximal electrode. The current path between electrodes should not contain the muscle whose movement is being monitored. Separation of electrodes beyond several centimeters increases the probability that the PNS current may depolarize muscle directly, causing movement unrelated to conduction through the neuromuscular junction and thus, misinterpretation of the level of neuromuscular blockade.

Common sites for electrode placement are over the course of the ulnar nerve at the medial aspect of the wrist or over the ulnar groove at the elbow. Stimulation of the ulnar nerve activates the m. adductor pollicis and twitches the thumb. Placement of the electrodes anterior to the tragus will stimulate the facial nerve, which innervates the m. corrugator supercilii and furrows the eyebrow. Stimulation of the posterior tibial nerve posterior to the medial malleolus causes the m. flexor hallucis brevis and great toe to move.

Cold will weaken muscle strength even in the absence of NMB agents, making PNS testing valuable in patients recovering from hypothermia (112). Patients who have had a stroke will experience an up-regulation of acetylcholine receptor density on the muscle membrane as the affected muscles denervate. As a result, PNS on an affected limb will produce a TOF response that exceeds the response seen from the same site PNS on a normal limb. To avoid overdosing or prematurely extubating a patient based on TOF testing, PNS should be performed on sites unaffected by prior nerve injury.

PNS is particularly helpful for monitoring the level of relaxation achieved during the infusion of NMB agents. PNS monitoring can help direct the rate of infusion and avoid excessive administration. Pharmacokinetic and pharmacodynamic models that illustrate the TOF response to PNS with succinylcholine and rocuronium NMB infusions can be found at http://vam.anest.ufl.edu/simulations/simulationportfolio.php.

CEREBRAL PERFUSION

All of the previously discussed monitors are monitors of nervous system function or imaging modalities of brain structures. When function fails, they do not necessarily give information about the *mechanism* of nervous system damage. One of the most common mechanisms of CNS damage is inadequate blood flow. The remainder of this chapter will examine those methods that are available to monitor the adequacy of CBF. These monitors provide information that is complementary to the functional assessment discussed above, because function only becomes altered when CBF decreases by more than half.

The most common clinical measure aimed at ensuring adequate CBF is to maintain the cerebral perfusion pressure above the lower limit of cerebral autoregulation. In cases of intracranial disease, the relevant pressure opposing adequate perfusion is the intracranial pressure.

Monitoring of Intracranial Pressure

ICP reflects the dynamic interaction of tissues and fluids within a fixed-volume, hard cranial shell of approximately 1,400 mL in an adult. Its contents can be divided into cerebral parenchyma, arterial and venous blood, and CSF components. The cerebral parenchyma accounts for 80% to 90% of the contents and includes both intra- and extracellular fluid as well as cellular membranes. The volume of the blood together with the CSF makes up the remaining 10% to 20%. The Monroe-Kellie doctrine, as modified by Cushing at the turn of the 19th century, states that any increase in volume of one intracranial component occurs at the expense of another. Normal intracranial pressure in adults is 8 to 15 mm Hg and in babies the pressure is 10 to 20 mm Hg (less when measured through a lumbar puncture). Compensatory mechanisms stabilize ICP in response to slight changes in CBF, as well as CSF production and absorption. In the absence of effective compensatory mechanisms, an increase in the volume of any one of the components will lead to an exponential increase in pressure, as illustrated by the pressure–volume relationship (Fig. 27.12) described by Langfitt (113). Compensation may be achieved by any of the following: (a) changes in the volume of CSF; (b) the slight distention of the dura; (c) changes in the intravascular volume, particularly in the venous channels; and (d) compression or swelling of the brain. The rate of change in the volume of intracranial contents is of importance. For example, a rapid increase in volume produced by an epidural hematoma may overwhelm the compensatory mechanisms and produce a rapid increase in ICP, whereas a slowly growing brain tumor may produce a gradual displacement of structures within the cranial vault without a significant increase in ICP.

ICP is not static. Pressure fluctuations occur with cardiac systole due to distention of the intracranial arteriolar tree and respiration (i.e., ICP falling with each inspiration and rising

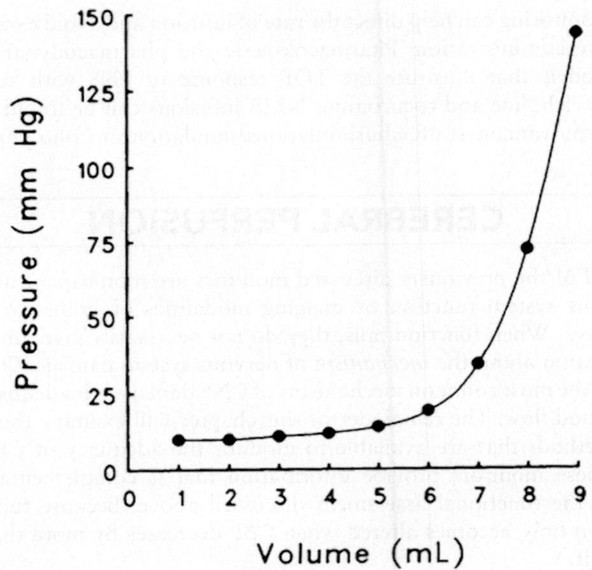

FIGURE 27.12. Pressure–volume relationship of the intracranial vault. Volume in milliliters (abscissa) of water added to a supratentorial extradural balloon in a monkey, 1 mL/hour. Pressure in millimeters of mercury (ordinate). (With permission from Langfitt TW. Increased intracranial pressure. *Clin Neurosurg.* 1969;16:43–71.)

with expiration). Straining or compression of neck veins can also cause a rise in pressure. A value in excess of 18 to 20 mm Hg is abnormal and must be treated.

As the ICP increases, the cerebral venous pressure increases in parallel so as to remain 2 to 5 mm Hg higher, or else the venous system would collapse. Because of this relationship, CPP can be satisfactorily estimated from mean arterial pressure minus ICP. Cerebral arterial circulation is normally autoregulated to maintain a constant CBF for a CPP between 60 and 150 mm Hg.

Clinical deterioration in neurologic status is widely considered a sign of increased ICP. Bradycardia, increased pulse pressure, and pupillary dilation are accepted as signs of increased ICP.

The five methods most commonly used to monitor ICP are (a) an intraventricular catheter, (b) a subarachnoid or subdural bolt, (c) a subdural catheter, (d) an intraparenchymal fiberoptic filament sensor, and (e) an extradural fiberoptic sensor. Each of these has its advantages and disadvantages. The intraventricular catheter is typically considered the gold standard. Its advantages include easy recalibration and a means to treat ICP elevations by removing CSF. On the other hand, placement may be difficult in the face of a distorting intracranial pathology. The other devices are easier to place, but the accuracy of the recorded values may be more difficult to verify. All ICP monitors are invasive and share a risk of infection of about 5%.

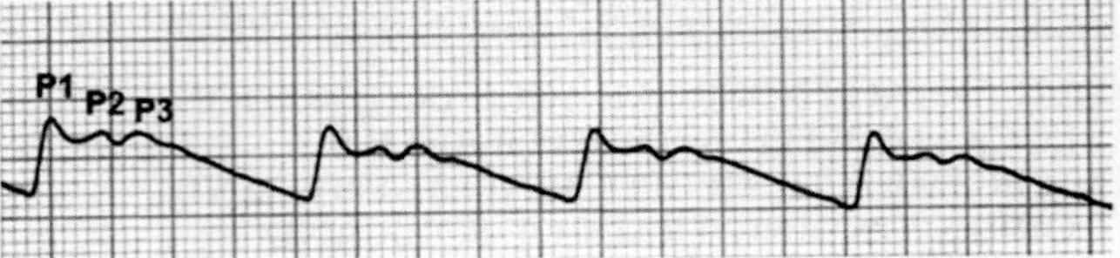

FIGURE 27.13. Intracranial pressure waveform showing the percussion wave (P1), tidal wave (P2), and dicrotic wave (P3). The timing of the peaks corresponds to the arterial pressure waveform. (Image courtesy of Integra Neurosciences, Inc.)

Patients who require ICP monitoring are generally considered to be those (a) with a closed head injury and a GCS less than or equal to 8; (b) in whom a CT scan shows significant brain distortion; (c) with worsening neurologic status; (d) in whom there is a need to sedate, paralyze, or operate in the context of an abnormal brain; (e) with postoperative complications; and (f) who are unconscious or in shock. The ICP data derived from such monitoring can serve as a useful therapeutic guide to clinical care.

Interpretation of Intracranial Pressure Waveforms

The normal ICP waveform has three characteristic peaks (P1, P2, and P3) of decreasing height that correlate with the arterial pulse waveform (Fig. 27.13). The P1 (or percussion) wave originates from arterial systole, and has a sharp peak and constant amplitude. The P2 (or tidal) wave is more variable and ends on the dicrotic notch. Elevation of the P2 component of the ICP waveform is thought to reflect decreased intracranial adaptive capacity and impaired autoregulation. However, sustained increases in ICP can occur without P2 elevation. The P3 (or dicrotic) wave follows the dicrotic notch and is venous in origin.

When consecutive ICP waveforms are observed over time, three distinct patterns—first described by Lundberg in 1960 as A, B, and C waves—may be observed (114). A waves, now more commonly referred to as plateau waves, are pathologic (Fig. 27.14). There is a rapid rise in ICP up to 50 to 100 mm Hg,

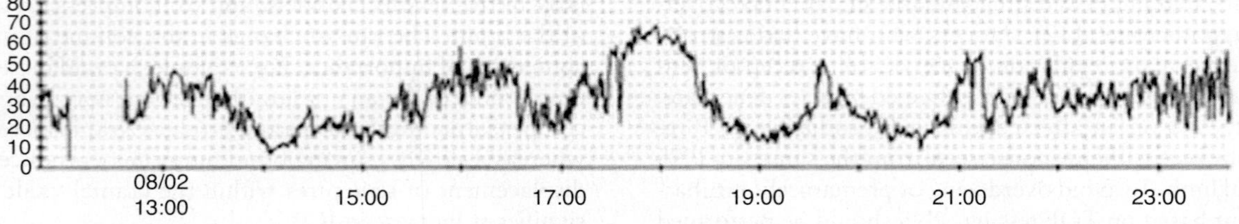

FIGURE 27.14. Lundberg plateau waves. The tracing of the intracranial pressure shows several pathologic increases of intracranial pressure, with plateaus lasting from 20 to 60 minutes. (Image courtesy Integra Neurosciences, Inc.)

TABLE 27.9

TECHNIQUES FOR MEASURING CEREBRAL BLOOD FLOW

Category	Technique	Resolution: Temporal	Resolution: Spatial	Invasiveness	Cost
Bedside	Kety-Schmidt	15 min	Hemispheric	Jugular catheter	+
	^{133}Xenon wash-out	3–15 min	3–4 cm	Jugular catheter, radiation	+
	Arteriovenous difference in oxygen content ($AVDO_2$), jugular venous oxygen saturation ($SJvO_2$)	<1 min	Global	Jugular catheter	+
	Double indicator dilution	3 min	Global	Jugular catheter, descending thoracic aortic catheter	+
	Near-infrared spectroscopy	<1 min	Local, bifrontal	No	+
	Thermal clearance probe	<1 min	Local, 1–2 cm	Exposed cortex	+
	Laser Doppler flow probe	<1 min	Local, 1–2 cm	Exposed cortex	+
Tomographic	Positron emission tomography (PET)	4–6 min/section	<1 cm	Radiation from positron emitter	+++++
	Stable Xenon computed tomography (CT)	4–6 min/section	<1 cm	Radiation from CT scan	+++
	Single photon emission tomography (SPECT)	4–6 min/section	<1 cm	Radiation from γ emitter	+++
	Magnetic resonance imaging (MRI)	4–6 min/section	<1 cm	No	+++

followed by a variable period during which the ICP remains elevated ("plateau"), followed by a rapid fall to the baseline. These plateau waves typically last from 5 to 20 minutes. They are generally seen in patients with already elevated ICP. During a series of plateau waves, both amplitude and duration may increase, leading to a "terminal" wave in which ICP may rise to levels that impede CBF. "Truncated" or atypical plateau waves that do not exceed 50 mm Hg are early indicators of neurologic deterioration. B and C waves are smaller fluctuations in ICP thought to be related to respiration and autonomic fluctuations in blood pressure (Traube-Hering-Mayer waves), respectively. They are of little clinical significance.

While a markedly decreased or elevated cerebral perfusion pressure may lead to ischemia or spontaneous hemorrhage, respectively, a normal cerebral perfusion pressure by no means ensures normal cerebral blood flow. Increased cerebrovascular resistance (e.g., because of carotid stenosis, cerebral vasospasm, or microcirculatory compromise) may cause ischemia despite normal cerebral perfusion pressure. Similarly, normal cerebral perfusion pressure may coexist with abnormally increased cerebral blood flow in settings such as posttraumatic vasoparalysis or normal perfusion pressure breakthrough after resection of an arteriovenous malformation.

Direct Cerebral Blood Flow Measurement

The ideal clinical method for CBF measurement in patients with intracranial pathology would be a noninvasive, inexpensive bedside procedure that is continuous or at least frequently repeatable, and provides good spatial resolution for superficial and deep structures of all vascular territories (115,116). No currently available method (Table 27.9) comes close to having all these characteristics. Nonetheless, determinations of CBF serve to validate other techniques of assessing cerebral perfusion and provide important insights into the pathophysiologic events in head injury or stroke.

Direct measurement of cerebral blood flow is possible by determining the kinetics of either wash-in or wash-out of an inert tracer compound, in a variation of the method originally described by Kety and Schmidt (117). The most widely used measurement involves the administration of a radioactive isotope of ^{133}Xe either per inhalation or intravenously, followed by measurement of the radioactivity wash-out, with γ detectors placed over specific areas of the brain. This method provides a spatial resolution of about 3 cm to 4 cm, depending on the number of detectors. In the normal brain, flow at different depths may be inferred from the early wash-out, which should reflect high-perfusion cortical gray matter, and low-perfusion deeper white matter. An important disadvantage of the technique is its lack of sensitivity for focal areas of hypoperfusion, which are obscured by adjacent areas of adequate flow—a phenomenon described as "look-through."

Radiologic methods like SPECT, PET, Xenon-enhanced CT or perfusion CT, or MRI provide excellent spatial resolution, but are not available at the bedside. Some are used clinically as confirmatory tests in the determination of brain death. SPECT and magnetic resonance angiography, for example, show a "hollow skull phenomenon" and absent intracranial flow, respectively. Xenon-enhanced CT, which can be combined with

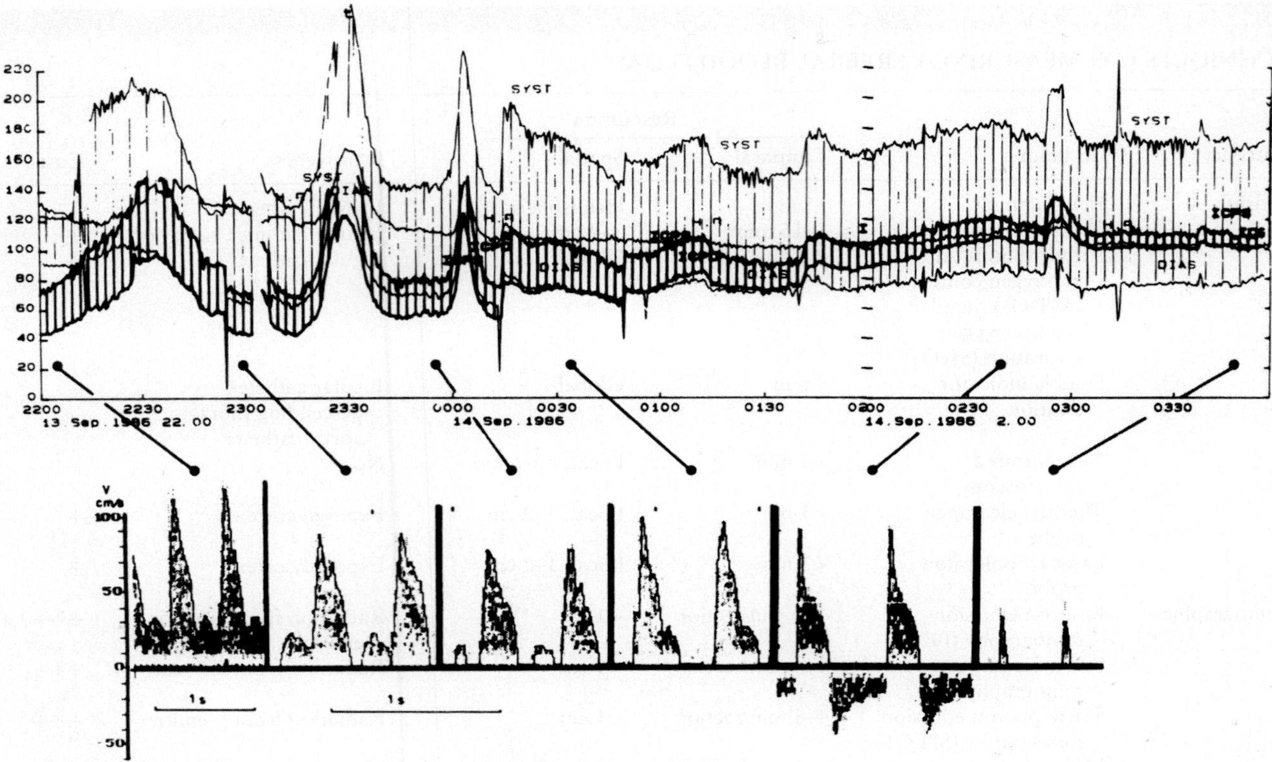

FIGURE 27.15. The flow velocity in intracerebral arteries shows a characteristic pattern of changes as intracranial pressure increases to the point of intracranial circulatory arrest and brain death. Initially, it resembles an arterial pressure wave form. (With permission from Hassler W, Steinmetz H, Gawlowski J. Transcranial Doppler ultrasonography in raised intracranial pressure and in intracranial circulatory arrest. *J Neurosurg*. 1988;68:745–751.)

standard CT scanning, has been used to obtain prognostic information and withhold unnecessarily aggressive therapy by assessing the severity of the decrease in CBF during stroke (118). Perfusion imaging allows the detection of a viable penumbra around areas of ischemia, which may be restored to normal function if the relative ischemia can be reversed.

Transcranial Doppler

An easy-to-apply, continuous, and noninvasive monitor of relative changes in CBF employs transcranial Doppler (TCD) ultrasound (119).

Theoretical Basis

Ultrasound waves are used to measure the velocity of blood flow in the basal arteries of the brain and the extracranial portion of the internal carotid artery. These waves are transmitted through the relatively thin temporal bone, the orbit, or the foramen magnum (120). When they contact moving red blood cells, they are reflected at a changed frequency through the brain and skull back to a detector. The change in frequency as blood cells move toward or away from the ultrasound transmitter and detector is an example of the Doppler effect, and is related to velocity and direction of flow. Velocity increases during systole and decreases during diastole; blood in the center of the lumen moves faster than that near the vessel wall, producing a spectrum of flow velocities. This spectrum resembles the shape of the waveform produced by an intra-arterial pressure transducer (Fig. 27.15). The TCD probe emits ultrasound waves as short pulses. Because ultrasound travels through tissue at a constant velocity, assessment of flow at different distances from the transducer becomes possible by varying the time window during which the reflected ultrasound waves are received. Thus, each arterial segment at the base of the brain has a distinct signature in terms of depth of insonation and direction of flow. TCD measurements are most commonly (and easily) made in the middle cerebral and internal carotid arteries, but may also be measured in other vessels, including the anterior cerebral, anterior communicating, posterior cerebral, posterior communicating, and basilar arteries. In approximately 10% of patients, particularly elderly females, technically satisfactory recordings cannot be obtained because of increased skull thickness (121).

Although TCD allows the interrogation of all arteries that supply the brain, it cannot provide a simple assessment of global or hemispheric CBF. In the setting of acute stroke or traumatic arterial dissection, the mere patency of a vessel is an important question that has diagnostic, therapeutic, and prognostic implications (120,121). For example, the presence of blood flow indicates recanalization of a vessel, and may be used to spare a patient the risks associated with thrombolytic therapy. Beyond the question of vessel patency, the link between TCD measurements and cerebral blood flow is indirect and subject to one technical limitation and two principal assumptions inherent in the link. The technical limitation is that the accuracy with which the flow velocity can be determined depends on the angle of insonation. Variability of repeated measurements can be minimized either by using a single examiner or by rigidly mounting the TCD probe on the patient's head with a headset, provided a shift in brain structures caused by a mass lesion does not displace the artery. The two principal assumptions that have to be met for TCD-measured blood flow velocity to correspond to CBF are as follows:

1. Flow and flow velocity are directly related only if the diameter of the artery remains constant.
2. Second, the blood flow in the basal arteries of the brain must be directly related to cortical CBF.

These assumptions likely represent an oversimplification and have not been supported adequately by evidence. Specifically, radioactive xenon-measured CBF does not correlate well with TCD-derived middle cerebral artery velocity during carotid endarterectomy or cardiopulmonary bypass (122–124). Likewise, normal variations in blood flow velocities are large (125). Despite this limitation, TCD has found many applications in the ICU, particularly in answering research questions in combination with other monitoring modalities that assess CBF. While these have contributed to our understanding, for example, the time course and mechanisms of secondary injury in brain trauma, their application is limited to a few centers (126–128).

Detection of Cerebral Vasospasm

TCD has been helpful in identifying vasospasm following aneurysmal subarachnoid hemorrhage (129–132). As the diameter of the arterial lumen decreases with vasospasm, the velocity of blood flowing through the narrowed vessel must increase if flow is to be maintained. Using absolute flow velocity alone, detection and documentation of the severity and duration of vasospasm are possible, with a specificity that approaches 100% but with limited sensitivity (125,133,134). Attempts have been made to improve the sensitivity by normalizing the flow velocity to that measured prior to the time of vasospasm (125) or to the flow velocity of the ipsilateral extracranial internal carotid artery (130). One important setting wherein absolute TCD flow velocity may underestimate the severity of vasospasm is that of increased ICP (135). Increases in ICP, however, lead to characteristic changes in the TCD waveform and increase the pulsatility index (see below).

Although TCD has contributed much to our understanding of the natural history of vasospasm following aneurysmal subarachnoid hemorrhage, most studies predate the current therapeutic approach of early exclusion of the aneurysm and supportive therapy with hypertensive-hypervolemic hemodilution and nimodipine. A recent advance in the treatment of vasospasm that highlights one limitation of TCD is the therapeutic dilation of stenotic arteries. TCD flow velocities may remain elevated despite successful dilation as a result of impaired autoregulation in the poststenotic vascular bed (136). Likewise, TCD cannot assess isolated distal vasospasm, which may account for as much as a third of all cases of vasospasm (137). Because of such specific limitations and some limitation in sensitivity (138,139), TCD is not universally used to assess patients with aneurysmal subarachnoid hemorrhage.

Assessment of Intracranial Pressure and Confirmation of Brain Death

The TCD-generated waveform exhibits sequential characteristic changes as intracranial pressure increases (Fig. 27.15) (140). As ICP increases, the systolic waveform becomes more peaked. As ICP nears diastolic blood pressure, diastolic flow diminishes and subsequently ceases. Once ICP exceeds diastolic blood pressure, TCD shows a pattern of to-and-fro movement of blood that indicates imminent intracranial circulatory arrest (Fig. 27.15). This change in waveforms can be used to calculate a pulsatility index by relating the difference between peak systolic and end-diastolic velocity either to the mean or to the systolic velocity. Such waveform analyses correlate well with the intracranial pressure (135,141), but cannot replace ICP monitoring because autoregulation, vasospasm, or proximal arterial stenosis may alter the TCD signal independent of the ICP (120).

Clinical brain death demonstrates a characteristic blood flow velocity pattern (Fig. 27.15) (142,143). There is a short systolic inflow of blood, followed by an exit of blood (flow direction reverses) from the cranium during diastole. TCD is a validated confirmatory test in the diagnosis of brain death, with a sensitivity that exceeds 90% and a specificity of 100% (144,145). While TCD can ascertain the diagnosis in most patients at the bedside, a large craniotomy or an inadequate bone window may preclude the complete examination necessary to confirm brain death.

Jugular Venous Oxygen Saturation Monitoring

Jugular venous oxygen saturation ($SjvO_2$) monitoring has been touted as an indicator of cerebral oxygen homeostasis. Changes in $SjvO_2$ from normal range (60%–70%) provide indirect information on the state of $CMRO_2$, and because blood flow is normally linked to $CMRO_2$, indirect information on CBF as well. Approximately 50% to 70% of patients with severe head trauma (GCS $\leq$8) will have an episode of desaturation ($SjvO_2$ <50%). Despite an ischemic threshold widely accepted to be $SjvO_2$ >50% during the early hyperemic conditions following head injury (146), the clinical utility of $SjvO_2$ monitoring remains unsettled.

The complexity of catheter placement, sample collection, and results interpretation may contribute to a mere 20% utilization of $SjvO_2$ monitoring in victims of moderate to severe head injury (147). $SjvO_2$ is preferentially measured from the flow-dominant internal jugular (IJ) vein (right 60%, left 25%, equal 15%) (148) to provide the best estimate of *whole* brain $CMRO_2$ conditions. Hemispheric dominance can be established by which side will, in response to unilateral compression of the IJ vein, produce the greater rise of intracranial pressure. Alternatively, IJ vein size seen by ultrasound provides a reasonable estimate of dominance, as does the relative size of the jugular foramina on CT scan of the head.

Cannulation of the jugular bulb for intermittent (standard catheters) or continuous (fiberoptic oximetry catheters) monitoring of jugular venous saturation is similar to internal jugular catheterization for central venous catheter placement; however, the needle, wire, and catheter are advanced in the cephalad direction. The risk of causing an intracranial vascular injury is reduced if the wire is not pushed into the jugular bulb. The catheter (hollow or oximetric) should be advanced slowly until resistance indicates it has reached the roof of the bulb. The catheter is then withdrawn 1 cm so that head movement cannot cause catheter-related vessel injury or thrombosis. It is recommended not to power-flush or administer infusions through this catheter.

An increase in $SjvO_2$ indicates either lowered $CMRO_2$ (less extraction) and/or increased or hyperemic CBF. A decrease in $SjvO_2$ (greater extraction) indicates increased $CMRO_2$, hypoxia/anemia, or oligemia. Observed changes in $SjvO_2$ might then help guide therapeutic interventions.

Abundant experience validates the association of jugular venous desaturation ($SjvO_2$ less than 50%) with worsened neurologic outcome. Conversely, mortality was reduced 66% when monitoring and managing the cerebral extraction of oxygen with $SjvO_2$ in conjunction with cerebral perfusion pressure than when cerebral perfusion pressure alone was managed (149). $CMRO_2$ increased in patients with elevated intracranial pressure (ICP $\geq$20 mm Hg) and normal to decreased cerebral extraction ("luxury perfusion") of oxygen with hyperventilation therapy. Elevated ICP associated with normal to increased cerebral extraction of oxygen was treated with mannitol, resulting in improved ICP and cerebral oxygenation.

Profound neurologic deterioration occurs with $SjvO_2$ desaturation to 30% or less (150). As cerebral circulatory arrest develops, the external carotid artery increasingly provides the blood sampled at the jugular bulb, and $SjvO_2$ then increases. In the clinical setting where brain death is expected, a ratio of mixed venous blood saturation to $SjvO_2$ less than 1 has been found to be highly sensitive (95%), specific (100%), and predictive (92%) for cerebral circulatory arrest (151).

The limitations with $SjvO_2$ monitoring may partly explain its low utilization. Admixture of extracranial blood through collateral venous drainage into the superior sagittal, sigmoid, and cavernous sinuses directly into the jugular bulb is believed to occur even when it is correctly placed into the jugular bulb (152). When samples are drawn faster than 2 mL/minute (153) or the catheter tip lies too short of the jugular bulb, extracranial blood may further contaminate the specimen and spuriously elevate $SjvO_2$. Even a "clean" $SjvO_2$ sample does not distinguish between lateralizing differences in flow, metabolism, or brain injury. Thus, because $SjvO_2$ reflects a global average from a variety of brain regions, marked regional hypoperfusion may not be reflected by a change in $SjvO_2$ (154). Although $SjvO_2$ and brain tissue oxygen pressure ($PbtO_2$), a measure of regional ischemia, usually track in the same direction, maintaining $SjvO_2$ above conventional thresholds did not reliably protect against the occurrence of regional ischemic insults. Consequently, $SjvO_2$ cannot be used alone to direct hyperventilation or to alert clinicians to evolving hypocapnia-induced regional cerebral ischemia. It is now clear that "acceptable" hyperventilation may cause harm that remains clinically undetected by $SjvO_2$ (155).

$SjvO_2$ monitoring may be most useful as a trend monitor in patients with diffuse global brain injury and when it identifies saturations below the ischemic threshold. Normal-range $SjvO_2$ can represent a "false-negative" measurement insofar as areas of regional ischemia may be present. Currently, the best technique for guiding therapy to a regional area of concern is with $PbtO_2$ monitoring.

Near-infrared Spectroscopy

Near-infrared spectroscopy (NIRS) utilizes the minimal absorption and greater penetration of wavelengths in this portion of the electromagnetic spectrum to evaluate changes in cerebral blood flow and cerebral oxygenation. Similar to pulse oximetry, NIRS compares differences in the absorption of hemoglobin (670–760 nm) to oxyhemoglobin (830 nm). In this manner, NIRS can be used for noninvasive assessment of brain oxygenation through an intact skull in human subjects by detecting changes in oxyhemoglobin concentrations associated with neural activity.

Application of straight-line photon transmission to oximetry was developed for clinical application in the early 1970s and reported by Jobsis in 1977 (156). A second type of NIRS—imaging of diffusion and scattering light—was developed by Kato et al. (157) and McCormick et al. (158) in 1991. NIRS utilizes light with a wavelength between 700 and 1,300 nm to penetrate the scalp, skull, and brain. A review of the development of the technique was recently published (159). NIRS offers the advantage of continuous, noninvasive monitoring of the cerebral cortex, and is typically done with one sensor each for the right and left hemisphere of the brain. Originally developed for monitoring neonates, the penetration in adults is significantly less compared to neonates. Additionally, extracranial changes in blood flow and oxygenation affect absorption values. NIRS may be as sensitive in detecting progressive cerebral hypoxia as EEG (160), but spatial resolution is limited by the number of detectors. Together with transcranial Doppler evaluation, it provides useful information in the hemodynamic evaluation of carotid artery occlusion (161), and in 2004 was described as a promising technique in the near future (162). At this time, clinical utility in the adult population remains limited.

Brain Oxygenation/Microdialysis

In contrast to most other techniques for evaluating brain oxygenation, tissue monitoring and microdialysis offer both the advantage and disadvantage of monitoring a very discrete region of tissue (163). Continuous brain tissue oxygen monitoring measures oxygen delivery and identifies cerebral hypoxia and ischemia in patients with brain injury, aneurysmal subarachnoid hemorrhage, or malignant stroke, or other patients at risk for secondary brain injury. Intraparenchymal direct oxygen partial pressure measurements ($PbrO_2$) have been shown to be of potential value in the management of cerebral perfusion and management of patients with traumatic brain injury (164,165).

In the 2007 Guidelines for the Management of Severe Head Injury (166), a brain tissue oxygenation threshold of less than 15 mm Hg was adopted as a level III recommendation. Based on many studies over the past decade (167–169), subthreshold levels of $PbrO_2$ have been associated with increased morbidity and mortality in patients with severe brain injury. Giri et al. described that increases in inspiratory oxygen has little effect on $PbrO_2$ in normal tissue, whereas in the injured brain, $PbrO_2$ is increased as long as blood flow is present (170). Stiefel et al. reported in 2005 a management strategy in severe traumatic brain injury that included $PbrO_2$ monitoring and therapy directed at maintaining brain oxygenation greater than

25 mm Hg (171). Using this multimodal approach, they observed reduced patient mortality compared to CPP-directed therapy.

Van den Brink et al. studied 101 comatose, nonpenetrating head injury patients, whose GCS score was greater than 8. Despite aggressive management of both ICP and CPP, brain tissue hypoxia frequently occurred (169). The depth and duration of tissue hypoxia was associated with an unfavorable outcome and death at 6 months after injury. In patients with severe injury in whom hyperventilation is considered, monitoring of brain oxygenation may be considered (172). The significance of local partial pressure of brain tissue oxygen continues to be debated; however, evidence for inclusion in multimodal monitoring is increasing.

Microdialysis is a technique that can be combined with brain tissue oxygen monitoring within the same highly localized probe (173,174). The intracerebral probe consists of a fluid path surrounded by a semipermeable membrane. This fluid path is perfused with a balanced salt solution that equilibrates with interstitial fluid from the brain. Therefore, the fluid returned from that fluid path contains substances from the brain in proportion to their local concentration, their specific membrane permeability, and the perfusate flow rate. Since the latter two do not change, the concentration of substances of interest can be followed over time. In the research context, this technique has been used to study topics as diverse as the role of excitotoxicity (175) or the proteomics of brain ischemia in stroke (176). The monitoring application closest to clinical utility, however, sets its sights considerably lower. It aims to determine the state of aerobic glucose utilization by following the ratio of metabolic intermediary products such as the pyruvate-to-lactate ratio. Ratiometric determinations of chemically similar molecules obviate the need to calibrate the probe based on the permeability of the substance(s) of interest. A decrease in the pyruvate-to-lactate ratio indicates an increase in anaerobic metabolism and/or mitochondrial dysfunction consistent with ischemia (173).

SUMMARY

Technologic advances in neurointensive care medicine have allowed successful treatment of severely injured patients. Early detection of the magnitude of the injury, damage control of coexisting diseases, prevention of secondary injury, and, ultimately, pharmacologic or surgical correction of the neurodisorders are all primary objectives of the focused neurointensive care team. Effective neuromonitoring techniques are fundamental tools to achieve these goals. As the field of neurocritical care continues to emerge as a subspecialty dedicated to the treatment of critically ill patients with neurologic diseases, the neuromonitoring level of sophistication will increase in parallel, and so will our ability to monitor cerebral physiology and pathophysiology in real time.

References

1. Gilman S. Imaging the brain. First of two parts. *N Engl J Med.* 1998;338: 812–820.
2. Lou HC, Edvinsson L, MacKenzie ET. The concept of coupling blood flow to brain function: revision required? *Ann Neurol.* 1987;22:289–297.
3. Derdeyn CP, Videen TO, Yundt KD, et al. Variability of cerebral blood volume and oxygen extraction: stages of cerebral haemodynamic impairment revisited. *Brain.* 2002;125:595–607.
4. Kety SS, King BD, Horvath SM, et al. The effects of an acute reduction in blood pressure by means of differential spinal sympathetic block on the cerebral circulation of hypertensive patients. *J Clin Invest.* 1950;29:402–407.
5. Boysen G. Cerebral hemodynamics in carotid surgery. *Acta Neurol Scand Suppl.* 1973;52:3–86.
6. Derdeyn CP, Yundt KD, Videen TO, et al. Increased oxygen extraction fraction is associated with prior ischemic events in patients with carotid occlusion. *Stroke.* 1998;29:754–758.
7. Rapela CE, Green HD. Autoregulation of canine cerebral blood flow. *Circ Res.* 1964;15(Suppl):205–212.
8. Buchanan JE, Phillis JW. The role of nitric oxide in the regulation of cerebral blood flow. *Brain Res.* 1993;610:248–255.
9. Petersen SE, Fox PT, Snyder AZ, et al. Activation of extrastriate and frontal cortical areas by visual words and word-like stimuli. *Science.* 1990; 249:1041–1044.
10. Bouma GJ, Muizelaar JP, Stringer WA, et al. Ultra-early evaluation of regional cerebral blood flow in severely head-injured patients using xenon-enhanced computerized tomography. *J Neurosurg.* 1992;77:360–368.
11. Lee JH, Martin NA, Alsina G, et al. Hemodynamically significant cerebral vasospasm and outcome after head injury: a prospective study. *J Neurosurg.* 1997;87:221–233.
12. Muizelaar JP, Marmarou A, Ward JD, et al. Adverse effects of prolonged hyperventilation in patients with severe head injury: a randomized clinical trial. *J Neurosurg.* 1991;75:731–739.
13. Michenfelder JD, Milde JH. The relationship among canine brain temperature, metabolism, and function during hypothermia. *Anesthesiology.* 1991;75:130–136.
14. Walter B, Bauer R, Kuhnen G, et al. Coupling of cerebral blood flow and oxygen metabolism in infant pigs during selective brain hypothermia. *J Cereb Blood Flow Metab.* 2000;20:1215–1224.
15. Stullken EH Jr, Milde JH, Michenfelder JD, et al. The nonlinear responses of cerebral metabolism to low concentrations of halothane, enflurane, isoflurane, and thiopental. *Anesthesiology.* 1977;46:28–34.
16. Alkire MT, Haier RJ, Barker SJ, et al. Cerebral metabolism during propofol anesthesia in humans studied with positron emission tomography. *Anesthesiology.* 1995;82:393–403; discussion 27A.
17. Michenfelder J. *Anesthesia and the Brain.* New York: Churchill Livingstone; 1988.
18. Milde LN, Milde JH, Michenfelder JD. Cerebral functional, metabolic, and hemodynamic effects of etomidate in dogs. *Anesthesiology.* 1985;63:371–377.
19. Edelman GJ, Hoffman WE, Charbel FT. Cerebral hypoxia after etomidate administration and temporary cerebral artery occlusion. *Anesth Analg.* 1997;85:821–825.
20. Matta BF, Lam AM, Strebel S, et al. Cerebral pressure autoregulation and carbon dioxide reactivity during propofol-induced EEG suppression. *Br J Anaesth.* 1995;74:159–163.
21. Doyle PW, Matta BF. Burst suppression or isoelectric encephalogram for cerebral protection: evidence from metabolic suppression studies. *Br J Anaesth.* 1999;83:580–584.
22. Ederberg S, Westerlind A, Houltz E, et al. The effects of propofol on cerebral blood flow velocity and cerebral oxygen extraction during cardiopulmonary bypass. *Anesth Analg.* 1998;86:1201–1206.
23. Nandate K, Vuylsteke A, Ratsep I, et al. Effects of isoflurane, sevoflurane and propofol anaesthesia on jugular venous oxygen saturation in patients undergoing coronary artery bypass surgery. *Br J Anaesth.* 2000;84:631–633.
24. Johnston AJ, Steiner LA, Chatfield DA, et al. Effects of propofol on cerebral oxygenation and metabolism after head injury. *Br J Anaesth.* 2003;91:781–786.
25. Heath KJ, Gupta S, Matta BF. The effects of sevoflurane on cerebral hemodynamics during propofol anesthesia. *Anesth Analg.* 1997;85:1284–1287.
26. Citerio G, Cormio M. Sedation in neurointensive care: advances in understanding and practice. *Curr Opin Crit Care.* 2003;9:120–126.
27. Rhoney DH, Parker D Jr. Use of sedative and analgesic agents in neurotrauma patients: effects on cerebral physiology. *Neurol Res.* 2001;23:237–259.
28. Prielipp RC, Wall MH, Tobin JR, et al. Dexmedetomidine-induced sedation in volunteers decreases regional and global cerebral blood flow. *Anesth Analg.* 2002;95:1052–1059.
29. Grille P, Biestro A, Farina G, et al. [Effects of dexmedetomidine on intracranial hemodynamics in severe head injured patients.] *Neurocirugia (Astur).* 2005;16:411–418.
30. Kety SS, Schmidt CF. The effects of altered arterial tensions of carbon dioxide and oxygen on cerebral blood flow and cerebral oxygen consumption of normal young men. *J Clin Invest.* 1948;27:484–492.
31. Reivich M. Arterial pCO_2 and cerebral hemodynamics. *Am J Physiol.* 1964;206:25–35.
32. Brian JE Jr. Carbon dioxide and the cerebral circulation. *Anesthesiology.* 1998;88:1365–1386.
33. Harper AM. Autoregulation of cerebral blood flow: influence of the arterial

blood pressure on the blood flow through the cerebral cortex. *J Neurol Neurosurg Psychiatry.* 1966;29:398–403.
34. Paulson OB, Strandgaard S, Edvinsson L. Cerebral autoregulation. *Cerebrovasc Brain Metab Rev.* 1990;2:161–192.
35. Eng C, Lam AM, Mayberg TS, et al. The influence of propofol with and without nitrous oxide on cerebral blood flow velocity and CO2 reactivity in humans. *Anesthesiology.* 1992;77:872–879.
36. Nordstrom CH, Messeter K, Sundbarg G, et al. Cerebral blood flow, vasoreactivity, and oxygen consumption during barbiturate therapy in severe traumatic brain lesions. *J Neurosurg.* 1988;68:424–431.
37. Berre J, Moraine JJ, Melot C. Cerebral CO2 vasoreactivity evaluation with and without changes in intrathoracic pressure in comatose patients. *J Neurosurg Anesthesiol.* 1998;10:70–79.
38. Luce JM, Huseby JS, Kirk W, et al. A Starling resistor regulates cerebral venous outflow in dogs. *J Appl Physiol.* 1982;53:1496–1503.
39. Bouma GJ, Muizelaar JP. Cerebral blood flow, cerebral blood volume, and cerebrovascular reactivity after severe head injury. *J Neurotrauma.* 1992;9(Suppl 1):S333–348.
40. Langfitt TW, Weinstein JD, Kassell NF. Cerebral vasomotor paralysis produced by intracranial hypertension. *Neurology.* 1965;15:622–641.
41. Thiel A, Zickmann B, Stertmann WA, et al. Cerebrovascular carbon dioxide reactivity in carotid artery disease. Relation to intraoperative cerebral monitoring results in 100 carotid endarterectomies. *Anesthesiology.* 1995;82:655–661.
42. Tranmer BI, Keller TS, Kindt GW, et al. Loss of cerebral regulation during cardiac output variations in focal cerebral ischemia. *J Neurosurg.* 1992; 77:253–259.
43. Todd MM, Weeks JB, Warner DS. The influence of intravascular volume expansion on cerebral blood flow and blood volume in normal rats. *Anesthesiology.* 1993;78:945–953.
44. Todd MM, Weeks JB, Warner DS. Cerebral blood flow, blood volume, and brain tissue hematocrit during isovolemic hemodilution with hetastarch in rats. *Am J Physiol.* 1992;263:H75–82.
45. Todd MM, Wu B, Maktabi M, et al. Cerebral blood flow and oxygen delivery during hypoxemia and hemodilution: role of arterial oxygen content. *Am J Physiol.* 1994;267:H2025–2031.
46. Teasdale G, Jennett B. Assessment of coma and impaired consciousness. A practical scale. *Lancet.* 1974;2:81–84.
47. Rowley G, Fielding K. Reliability and accuracy of the Glasgow Coma Scale with experienced and inexperienced users. *Lancet.* 1991;337:535–538.
48. Knaus WA, Draper EA, Wagner DP, et al. APACHE II: a severity of disease classification system. *Crit Care Med.* 1985;13:818–829.
49. Teasdale GM, Drake CG, Hunt W, et al. A universal subarachnoid hemorrhage scale: report of a committee of the World Federation of Neurosurgical Societies. *J Neurol Neurosurg Psychiatry.* 1988;51:1457.
50. Gennarelli TA, Champion HR, Copes WS, et al. Comparison of mortality, morbidity, and severity of 59,713 head injured patients with 114,447 patients with extracranial injuries. *J Trauma.* 1994;37:962–968.
51. Chiang VL, Claus EB, Awad IA. Toward more rational prediction of outcome in patients with high-grade subarachnoid hemorrhage. *Neurosurgery.* 2000;46:28–35; discussion 35–36.
52. Tseng JH, Tseng MY: Brain abscess in 142 patients: factors influencing outcome and mortality. *Surg Neurol.* 2006;65:557–562; discussion 562.
53. Edgren E, Hedstrand U, Kelsey S, et al. Assessment of neurological prognosis in comatose survivors of cardiac arrest. BRCT I Study Group. *Lancet.* 1994;343:1055–1059.
54. Niskanen M, Kari A, Nikki P, et al. Acute physiology and chronic health evaluation (APACHE II) and Glasgow coma scores as predictors of outcome from intensive care after cardiac arrest. *Crit Care Med.* 1991;19:1465–1473.
55. Eidelman LA, Putterman D, Putterman C, et al. The spectrum of septic encephalopathy. Definitions, etiologies, and mortalities. *JAMA.* 1996;275: 470–473.
56. Kuhls DA, Malone DL, McCarter RJ, et al. Predictors of mortality in adult trauma patients: the physiologic trauma score is equivalent to the Trauma and Injury Severity Score. *J Am Coll Surg.* 2002;194:695–704.
57. Massagli TL, Michaud LJ, Rivara FP. Association between injury indices and outcome after severe traumatic brain injury in children. *Arch Phys Med Rehabil.* 1996;77:125–132.
58. Wijdicks EF. *Brain Death.* Philadelphia: Lippincott Williams & Wilkins; 2001.
59. Santamaria J, Orteu N, Iranzo A, et al. Eye opening in brain death. *J Neurol.* 1999;246:720–722.
60. Goudreau JL, Wijdicks EF, Emery SF. Complications during apnea testing in the determination of brain death: predisposing factors. *Neurology.* 2000;55:1045–1048.
61. Saposnik G, Bueri JA, Maurino J, et al. Spontaneous and reflex movements in brain death. *Neurology.* 2000;54:221–223.
62. Facco E, Munari M, Baratto F, et al. Multimodality evoked potentials (auditory, somatosensory and motor) in coma. *Neurophysiol Clin.* 1993;23:237–258.
63. Fisher B, Peterson B, Hicks G. Use of brainstem auditory-evoked response testing to assess neurologic outcome following near drowning in children. *Crit Care Med.* 1992;20:578–585.
64. Pohlmann-Eden B, Dingethal K, Bender HJ, et al. How reliable is the predictive value of SEP (somatosensory evoked potentials) patterns in severe brain damage with special regard to the bilateral loss of cortical responses? *Intensive Care Med.* 1997;23:301–308.
65. Ruiz-Lopez MJ, Martinez de Azagra A, Serrano A, et al. Brain death and evoked potentials in pediatric patients. *Crit Care Med.* 1999;27:412–416.
66. Crippen D. Role of bedside electroencephalography in the adult intensive care unit during therapeutic neuromuscular blockade. *Crit Care.* 1997; 1:15–24.
67. Freye E. Cerebral monitoring in the operating room and the intensive care unit—an introductory for the clinician and a guide for the novice wanting to open a window to the brain. Part II: sensory-evoked potentials (SSEP, AEP, VEP). *J Clin Monit Comput.* 2005;19:77–168.
68. Hirsch LJ. Continuous EEG monitoring in the intensive care unit: an overview. *J Clin Neurophysiol.* 2004;21:332–340.
69. Hall R, Murdoch J. Brain protection: physiological and pharmacological considerations. Part II: The pharmacology of brain protection. *Can J Anaesth.* 1990;37:762–777.
70. Steen PA, Newberg L, Milde JH, et al. Hypothermia and barbiturates: individual and combined effects on canine cerebral oxygen consumption. *Anesthesiology.* 1983;58:527–532.
71. Drummond JC, Todd MM, U HS: The effect of high dose sodium thiopental on brain stem auditory and median nerve somatosensory evoked responses in humans. *Anesthesiology.* 1985;63:249–254.
72. Sutton LN, Frewen T, Marsh R, et al. The effects of deep barbiturate coma on multimodality evoked potentials. *J Neurosurg.* 1982;57:178–185.
73. Rothstein TL. Recovery from near death following cerebral anoxia: A case report demonstrating superiority of median somatosensory evoked potentials over EEG in predicting a favorable outcome after cardiopulmonary resuscitation. *Resuscitation.* 2004;60:335–341.
74. Kull LL, Emerson RG. Continuous EEG monitoring in the intensive care unit: technical and staffing considerations. *J Clin Neurophysiol.* 2005;22: 107–118.
75. Ronne-Engstrom E, Winkler T. Continuous EEG monitoring in patients with traumatic brain injury reveals a high incidence of epileptiform activity. *Acta Neurol Scand.* 2006;114:47–53.
76. Wartenberg KE, Mayer SA. Multimodal brain monitoring in the neurological intensive care unit: where does continuous EEG fit in? *J Clin Neurophysiol.* 2005;22:124–127.
77. Shi L, Agarwal R, Swamy MN. Model-based seizure detection method using statistically optimal filters. *Conf Proc IEEE Eng Med Biol Soc.* 2004;1:45–48.
78. Subasi A. Selection of optimal AR spectral estimation method for EEG signals using Cramer-Rao bound. *Comput Biol Med.* 2007;37:183–194.
79. Abou Khaled KJ, Hirsch LJ. Advances in the management of seizures and status epilepticus in critically ill patients. *Crit Care Clin.* 2006;22:637–659; abstract viii.
80. Deogaonkar A, Gupta R, DeGeorgia M, et al. Bispectral Index monitoring correlates with sedation scales in brain-injured patients. *Crit Care Med.* 2004;32:2403–2406.
81. Fabregas N, Gambus PL, Valero R, et al. Can bispectral index monitoring predict recovery of consciousness in patients with severe brain injury? *Anesthesiology.* 2004;101:43–51.
82. Schnakers C, Majerus S, Laureys S. Bispectral analysis of electroencephalogram signals during recovery from coma: preliminary findings. *Neuropsychol Rehabil.* 2005;15:381–388.
83. Schneider G, Heglmeier S, Schneider J, et al. Patient State Index (PSI) measures depth of sedation in intensive care patients. *Intensive Care Med.* 2004; 30:213–216.
84. Grindstaff RJ, Tobias JD. Applications of bispectral index monitoring in the pediatric intensive care unit. *J Intensive Care Med.* 2004;19:111–116.
85. Riker RR, Fraser GL, Wilkins ML. Comparing the bispectral index and suppression ratio with burst suppression of the electroencephalogram during pentobarbital infusions in adult intensive care patients. *Pharmacotherapy.* 2003;23:1087–1093.
86. Ozcan MS, Gravenstein D. The presence of working memory without explicit recall in a critically ill patient. *Anesth Analg.* 2004;98:469–470.
87. Rampil IJ. A primer for EEG signal processing in anesthesia. *Anesthesiology.* 1998;89:980–1002.
88. Ely EW, Truman B, Manzi DJ, et al. Consciousness monitoring in ventilated patients: bispectral EEG monitors arousal not delirium. *Intensive Care Med.* 2004;30:1537–1543.
89. Katoh T, Bito H, Sato S. Influence of age on hypnotic requirement, bispectral index, and 95% spectral edge frequency associated with sedation induced by sevoflurane. *Anesthesiology.* 2000;92:55–61.
90. Sleigh JW, Andrzejowski J, Steyn-Ross A, et al. The bispectral index: a measure of depth of sleep? *Anesth Analg.* 1999;88:659–661.
91. Lubke GH, Kerssens C, Phaf H, et al. Dependence of explicit and implicit memory on hypnotic state in trauma patients. *Anesthesiology.* 1999;90: 670–680.
92. Vivien B, Di Maria S, Ouattara A, et al. Overestimation of bispectral index in sedated intensive care unit patients revealed by administration of muscle relaxant. *Anesthesiology.* 2003;99:9–17.

93. Gallagher JD. Pacer-induced artifact in the bispectral index during cardiac surgery. *Anesthesiology.* 1999;90:636.
94. Johansen JW. Update on bispectral index monitoring. *Best Pract Res Clin Anaesthesiol.* 2006;20:81–99.
95. Dunham CM, Ransom KJ, McAuley CE, et al. Severe brain injury ICU outcomes are associated with cranial-arterial pressure index and noninvasive bispectral index and transcranial oxygen saturation: a prospective, preliminary study. *Crit Care.* 2006;10:R159.
96. Banoub M, Tetzlaff JE, Schubert A. Pharmacologic and physiologic influences affecting sensory evoked potentials: implications for perioperative monitoring. *Anesthesiology.* 2003;99:716–737.
97. Goodwin SR, Friedman WA, Bellefleur M. Is it time to use evoked potentials to predict outcome in comatose children and adults? *Crit Care Med.* 1991;19:518–524.
98. Morgalla MH, Bauer J, Ritz R, et al. [Coma. The prognostic value of evoked potentials in patients after traumatic brain injury.] *Anaesthesist.* 2006;55:760–768.
99. Nuwer MR. Electroencephalograms and evoked potentials. Monitoring cerebral function in the neurosurgical intensive care unit. *Neurosurg Clin N Am.* 1994;5:647–659.
100. Goodwin SR, Toney KA, Mahla ME. Sensory evoked potentials accurately predict recovery from prolonged coma caused by strangulation. *Crit Care Med.* 1993;21:631–633.
101. Lew HL, Dikmen S, Slimp J, et al. Use of somatosensory-evoked potentials and cognitive event-related potentials in predicting outcomes of patients with severe traumatic brain injury. *Am J Phys Med Rehabil.* 2003;82:53–61; quiz 62–64, 80.
102. Lew HL, Poole JH, Castaneda A, et al. Prognostic value of evoked and event-related potentials in moderate to severe brain injury. *J Head Trauma Rehabil.* 2006;21:350–360.
103. Carter BG, Butt W. Review of the use of somatosensory evoked potentials in the prediction of outcome after severe brain injury. *Crit Care Med.* 2001;29:178–186.
104. Carter BG, Butt W. Are somatosensory evoked potentials the best predictor of outcome after severe brain injury? A systematic review. *Intensive Care Med.* 2005;31:765–775.
105. Fischer C, Luaute J. Evoked potentials for the prediction of vegetative state in the acute stage of coma. *Neuropsychol Rehabil.* 2005;15:372–380.
106. Chistyakov AV, Hafner H, Soustiel JF, et al. Dissociation of somatosensory and motor evoked potentials in non-comatose patients after head injury. *Clin Neurophysiol.* 1999;110:1080–1089.
107. Mazzini L, Pisano F, Zaccala M, et al. Somatosensory and motor evoked potentials at different stages of recovery from severe traumatic brain injury. *Arch Phys Med Rehabil.* 1999;80:33–39.
108. Moosavi SH, Ellaway PH, Catley M, et al. Corticospinal function in severe brain injury assessed using magnetic stimulation of the motor cortex in man. *J Neurol Sci.* 1999;164:179–186.
109. Zentner J, Ebner A. Prognostic value of somatosensory- and motor-evoked potentials in patients with a non-traumatic coma. *Eur Arch Psychiatry Neurol Sci.* 1988;237:184–187.
110. Dhand UK. Clinical approach to the weak patient in the intensive care unit. *Respir Care.* 2006;51:1024–1040; discussion 1040–1041.
111. Hemmerling TM, Le N. Brief review: neuromuscular monitoring: an update for the clinician. *Can J Anaesth.* 2007;54:58–72.
112. Heier T, Caldwell JE. Impact of hypothermia on the response to neuromuscular blocking drugs. *Anesthesiology.* 2006;104:1070–1080.
113. Langfitt TW. Increased intracranial pressure. *Clin Neurosurg.* 1969;16:43–71.
114. Lundberg N. Continuous recording and control of ventricular fluid pressure in neurosurgical practice. *Acta Psychiatr Scand.* 1960;36:1–193.
115. Martin NA, Doberstein C. Cerebral blood flow measurement in neurosurgical intensive care. *Neurosurg Clin N Am.* 1994;5:607–618.
116. Steiner LA, Andrews PJ. Monitoring the injured brain: ICP and CBF. *Br J Anaesth.* 2006;97:26–38.
117. Kety SS and Schmidt CF. The nitrous oxide method for the quantitative determination of cerebral blood flow in man: theory, procedure, and normal values. *J Clin Invest.* 1948;27:476–493.
118. Firlik AD, Rubin G, Yonas H, et al. Relation between cerebral blood flow and neurologic deficit resolution in acute ischemic stroke. *Neurology.* 1998;51:177–182.
119. White H, Venkatesh B. Applications of transcranial Doppler in the ICU: a review. *Intensive Care Med.* 2006;32:981–994.
120. Ringelstein EB, Biniek R, Weiller C, et al. Type and extent of hemispheric brain infarctions and clinical outcome in early and delayed middle cerebral artery recanalization. *Neurology.* 1992;42:289–298.
121. Manno EM. Transcranial Doppler ultrasonography in the neurocritical care unit. *Crit Care Clin.* 1997;13:79–104.
122. Halsey JH, McDowell HA, Gelmon S, et al. Blood velocity in the middle cerebral artery and regional cerebral blood flow during carotid endarterectomy. *Stroke.* 1989;20:53–58.
123. Nuttall GA, Cook DJ, Fulgham JR, et al. The relationship between cerebral blood flow and transcranial Doppler blood flow velocity during hypothermic cardiopulmonary bypass in adults. *Anesth Analg.* 1996;82:1146–1151.
124. Weyland A, Stephan H, Kazmaier S, et al. Flow velocity measurements as an index of cerebral blood flow. Validity of transcranial Doppler sonographic monitoring during cardiac surgery. *Anesthesiology.* 1994;81:1401–1410.
125. Sloan MA, Haley EC Jr, Kassell NF, et al. Sensitivity and specificity of transcranial Doppler ultrasonography in the diagnosis of vasospasm following subarachnoid hemorrhage. *Neurology.* 1989;39:1514–1518.
126. Klingelhofer J, Sander D. Doppler CO2 test as an indicator of cerebral vasoreactivity and prognosis in severe intracranial hemorrhages. *Stroke.* 1992;23:962–966.
127. Martin NA, Patwardhan RV, Alexander MJ, et al. Characterization of cerebral hemodynamic phases following severe head trauma: hypoperfusion, hyperemia, and vasospasm. *J Neurosurg.* 1997;87:9–19.
128. Sander D, Klingelhofer J. Cerebral vasospasm following post-traumatic subarachnoid hemorrhage evaluated by transcranial Doppler ultrasonography. *J Neurol Sci.* 1993;119:1–7.
129. Grosset DG, Straiton J, du Trevou M, et al. Prediction of symptomatic vasospasm after subarachnoid hemorrhage by rapidly increasing transcranial Doppler velocity and cerebral blood flow changes. *Stroke.* 1992;23:674–679.
130. Lindegaard KF, Nornes H, Bakke SJ, et al. Cerebral vasospasm after subarachnoid haemorrhage investigated by means of transcranial Doppler ultrasound. *Acta Neurochir Suppl (Wien).* 1988;42:81–84.
131. Newell DW, Winn HR. Transcranial Doppler in cerebral vasospasm. *Neurosurg Clin N Am.* 1990;1:319–328.
132. Sekhar LN, Wechsler LR, Yonas H, et al. Value of transcranial Doppler examination in the diagnosis of cerebral vasospasm after subarachnoid hemorrhage. *Neurosurgery.* 1988;22:813–821.
133. Sloan MA, Burch CM, Wozniak MA, et al. Transcranial Doppler detection of vertebrobasilar vasospasm following subarachnoid hemorrhage. *Stroke.* 1994;25:2187–2197.
134. Wozniak MA, Sloan MA, Rothman MI, et al. Detection of vasospasm by transcranial Doppler sonography. The challenges of the anterior and posterior cerebral arteries. *J Neuroimaging.* 1996;6:87–93.
135. Klingelhofer J, Dander D, Holzgraefe M, et al. Cerebral vasospasm evaluated by transcranial Doppler ultrasonography at different intracranial pressures. *J Neurosurg.* 1991;75:752–758.
136. Giller CA, Purdy P, Giller A, et al. Elevated transcranial Doppler ultrasound velocities following therapeutic arterial dilation. *Stroke.* 1995;26:123–127.
137. Mizuno M, Nakajima S, Sampei T, et al. Serial transcranial Doppler flow velocity and cerebral blood flow measurements for evaluation of cerebral vasospasm after subarachnoid hemorrhage. *Neurol Med Chir (Tokyo).* 1994;34:164–171.
138. Sloan MA, Alexandrov AV, Tegeler CH, et al. Assessment: transcranial Doppler ultrasonography: report of the Therapeutics and Technology Assessment Subcommittee of the American Academy of Neurology. *Neurology.* 2004;62:1468–1481.
139. Lysakowski C, Walder B, Costanza MC, et al. Transcranial Doppler versus angiography in patients with vasospasm due to a ruptured cerebral aneurysm: a systematic review. *Stroke.* 2001;32:2292–2298.
140. Hassler W, Steinmetz H, Gawlowski J. Transcranial Doppler ultrasonography in raised intracranial pressure and in intracranial circulatory arrest. *J Neurosurg.* 1988;68:745–751.
141. Goraj B, Rifkinson-Mann S, Leslie DR, et al. Correlation of intracranial pressure and transcranial Doppler resistive index after head trauma. *AJNR Am J Neuroradiol.* 1994;15:1333–1339.
142. Newell DW, Grady MS, Sirotta P, et al. Evaluation of brain death using transcranial Doppler. *Neurosurgery.* 1989;24:509–513.
143. Petty GW, Mohr JP, Pedley TA, et al. The role of transcranial Doppler in confirming brain death: sensitivity, specificity, and suggestions for performance and interpretation. *Neurology.* 1990;40:300–303.
144. Ducrocq X, Hassler W, Moritake K, et al. Consensus opinion on diagnosis of cerebral circulatory arrest using Doppler-sonography: task force group on cerebral death of the Neurosonology Research Group of the World Federation of Neurology. *J Neurol Sci.* 1998;159:145–150.
145. Hadani M, Bruk B, Ram Z, et al. Application of transcranial Doppler ultrasonography for the diagnosis of brain death. *Intensive Care Med.* 1999;25:822–828.
146. The Brain Trauma Foundation. The American Association of Neurological Surgeons. The Joint Section on Neurotrauma and Critical Care. Guidelines for cerebral perfusion pressure. *J Neurotrauma.* 2000;17:507–511.
147. Stocchetti N, Paparella A, Bridelli F, et al. Cerebral venous oxygen saturation studied with bilateral samples in the internal jugular veins. *Neurosurgery.* 1994;34:38–43; discussion 43–44.
148. Hatiboglu MT, Anil A. Structural variations in the jugular foramen of the human skull. *J Anat.* 1992;180(Pt 1):191–196.
149. Cruz J. The first decade of continuous monitoring of jugular bulb oxyhemoglobin saturation: management strategies and clinical outcome. *Crit Care Med.* 1998;26:344–351.
150. Gopinath SP, Valadka AB, Uzura M, et al. Comparison of jugular venous oxygen saturation and brain tissue Po2 as monitors of cerebral ischemia after head injury. *Crit Care Med.* 1999;27:2337–2345.

151. Diaz-Reganon G, Minambres E, Holanda M, et al. Usefulness of venous oxygen saturation in the jugular bulb for the diagnosis of brain death: report of 118 patients. *Intensive Care Med.* 2002;28:1724–1728.
152. Shenkin GA, Harmel MH, Kety SS. Dynamic anatomy of the cerebral circulation. *Arch Neurol Psych.* 1948;60:12.
153. Matta BF, Lam AM. The rate of blood withdrawal affects the accuracy of jugular venous bulb. Oxygen saturation measurements. *Anesthesiology.* 1997;86:806–808.
154. Imberti R, Bellinzona G, Langer M. Cerebral tissue PO2 and SjvO2 changes during moderate hyperventilation in patients with severe traumatic brain injury. *J Neurosurg.* 2002;96:97–102.
155. Coles JP, Fryer TD, Coleman MR, et al. Hyperventilation following head injury: effect on ischemic burden and cerebral oxidative metabolism. *Crit Care Med.* 2007;35:568–578.
156. Jobsis FF. Noninvasive, infrared monitoring of cerebral and myocardial oxygen sufficiency and circulatory parameters. *Science.* 1977;198:1264–1267.
157. Kato T, Tokumaru A, O'Uchi T, et al. Assessment of brain death in children by means of P-31 MR spectroscopy: preliminary note. Work in progress. *Radiology.* 1991;179:95–99.
158. McCormick PW, Stewart M, Goetting MG, et al. Regional cerebrovascular oxygen saturation measured by optical spectroscopy in humans. *Stroke.* 1991;22:596–602.
159. Kato T. Principle and technique of NIRS-Imaging for human brain FORCE: fast-oxygen response in capillary event. *Int Congress Series.* 2004;1270:85–90.
160. Zauner A, Muizelaar JP. Measuring cerebral blood flow and metabolism. In: Reilly P, Bullock R, eds. *Head Injury.* London: Chapman & Hall; 1977:219–227.
161. Vernieri F, Tibuzzi F, Pasqualetti P, et al. Transcranial Doppler and near-infrared spectroscopy can evaluate the hemodynamic effect of carotid artery occlusion. *Stroke.* 2004;35:64–70.
162. Villringer A, Steinbrink J, Obrig H. Editorial comment–cerebral near-infrared spectroscopy: how far away from a routine diagnostic tool? *Stroke.* 2004;35:70–72.
163. Valadka AB, Furuya Y, Hlatky R, et al. Global and regional techniques for monitoring cerebral oxidative metabolism after severe traumatic brain injury. *Neurosurg Focus.* 2000;9:e3.
164. Manley GT, Hemphill JC, Morabito D, et al. Cerebral oxygenation during hemorrhagic shock: perils of hyperventilation and the therapeutic potential of hypoventilation. *J Trauma.* 2000;48:1025–1032; discussion 1032–1033.
165. Menzel M, Doppenberg EM, Zauner A, et al. Cerebral oxygenation in patients after severe head injury: monitoring and effects of arterial hyperoxia on cerebral blood flow, metabolism and intracranial pressure. *J Neurosurg Anesthesiol.* 1999;11:240–251.
166. Guidelines for the management of severe traumatic brain injury. X. Brain oxygen monitoring and thresholds. *J Neurotrauma.* 2007;24(Suppl 1):S65–70.
167. Bardt TF, Unterberg AW, Hartl R, et al. Monitoring of brain tissue PO2 in traumatic brain injury: effect of cerebral hypoxia on outcome. *Acta Neurochir Suppl.* 1998;71:153–156.
168. Valadka AB, Gopinath SP, Contant CF, et al. Relationship of brain tissue PO2 to outcome after severe head injury. *Crit Care Med.* 1998;26:1576–1581.
169. van den Brink WA, van Santbrink H, Steyerberg EW, et al. Brain oxygen tension in severe head injury. *Neurosurgery.* 2000;46:868–876; discussion 876–878.
170. Giri BK, Krishnappa IK, Bryan RM Jr, et al. Regional cerebral blood flow after cortical impact injury complicated by a secondary insult in rats. *Stroke.* 2000;31:961–967.
171. Stiefel MF, Spiotta A, Gracias VH, et al. Reduced mortality rate in patients with severe traumatic brain injury treated with brain tissue oxygen monitoring. *J Neurosurg.* 2005;103:805–811.
172. van Santbrink H, Maas AI, Avezaat CJ. Continuous monitoring of partial pressure of brain tissue oxygen in patients with severe head injury. *Neurosurgery.* 1996;38:21–31.
173. Hillered L, Vespa PM, Hovda DA. Translational neurochemical research in acute human brain injury: the current status and potential future for cerebral microdialysis. *J Neurotrauma.* 2005;22:3–41.
174. Hillered L, Persson L, Nilsson P, et al. Continuous monitoring of cerebral metabolism in traumatic brain injury: a focus on cerebral microdialysis. *Curr Opin Crit Care.* 2006;12:112–118.
175. Zauner A, Bullock R. The role of excitatory amino acids in severe brain trauma: opportunities for therapy: a review. *J Neurotrauma.* 1995;12:547–554.
176. Maurer MH, Berger C, Wolf M, et al. The proteome of human brain microdialysate. *Proteome Sci.* 2003;1:7.

CHAPTER 28 ■ RADIOGRAPHIC IMAGING AND BEDSIDE ULTRASOUND IN THE INTENSIVE CARE UNIT

PATRICIA L. ABBITT • MORGAN CAMP

Critically ill patients often require emergent and intensive use of imaging for diagnosis and guidance for surgical and supportive maneuvers. Complex surgical or trauma patients also need follow-up imaging for successful management during postoperative or posttraumatic hospitalization. Bedside drainage procedures guided by imaging are an important part of the care of the critically ill.

ANALYSIS OF THE CHEST RADIOGRAPH IN THE INTENSIVE CARE UNIT

Portable chest radiographs are the most common radiologic examination performed in patients in an intensive care unit (ICU). Chest radiographs of the ventilated patient are often used to monitor the clinical cardiopulmonary status as well as to evaluate placement of catheters and tubes. The position and any complication of placement of catheters and tubes that support the critically ill patient can be evaluated. Fluid overload, ventilator-associated pneumonia, lobar collapse, and pneumothorax are examples of parenchymal abnormalities detected and treated using the portable chest radiograph. The discussion that follows is meant to facilitate the correct interpretation of portable chest films for the intensivist.

Technical and Clinical Parameters Affecting Interpretation of the Portable Chest Radiograph

The portable AP chest radiograph taken of the critically ill patient is different from the standard upright PA and lateral chest radiograph. The portable radiograph is taken with the film relatively close to the radiographic source, which leads to enlargement of the cardiac blood vessels, and mediastinum, and can be misinterpreted as cardiomegaly, fluid overload, or a widened mediastinum. The critically ill patient is often sedated or has diminished alertness, leading to an underexpanded radiograph, which can result in small lung volumes and lower lobe volume loss or atelectasis (Fig. 28.1). Chest radiographs taken after extubation may appear "worse" when compared to films taken while the patient is receiving mechanical ventilatory support because the effects of positive pressure ventilation will be gone. Surgical procedures or disease processes affecting the upper abdomen can also contribute to elevation of the hemidiaphragms and predispose the patient to atelectasis, or even lobar collapse (Fig. 28.2). Pleural effusions develop related to fluid resuscitation with surgery or as sympathetic reactions to local inflammatory processes in the lung or upper abdomen. Pleural effusions will contribute to haziness at the lung bases and lead to nonvisualization of a diaphragm (Fig. 28.3). In the presence of a large pleural effusion, compressive atelectasis of the underlying lung will also occur.

The critically ill patient, with multiple support lines mental status and presents a challenge to the technologist filming the radiograph. Optimal positioning of the patient to include the entire lung fields and to avoid rotation of the patient on the film is quite difficult (Fig. 28.4). Cutoff of the lung apices or lung bases may occur as the technologist estimates their position. Radiographs taken in a lordotic position will accentuate the heart, making it appear larger and more globular than in standard positioning. Failure to minimize the intrusion of continuous electrocardiographic lead wires into the film will also magnify the interpretative difficulty. Interpretation of the portable chest radiograph in the intensive care unit must take into account these challenges, as well as the technical differences from the standard upright film, to provide an accurate interpretation.

Support Lines and Tubes

Multiple support lines and tubes are used to monitor and administer therapy to the ICU patient. Appropriate positioning of such support devices must be ensured devices by after placement performing a CXR to confirm placement and exclude complications such as a PRX or hematoma.

The presence of the endotracheal tube on a portable chest radiograph is indicative of ventilator support for a patient with respiratory insufficiency. The position of the endotracheal tube (ET) in most cases is determined by locating the radiopaque marker on the wall of the tube. The ET tube is ideally located in the trachea 2 to 4 cm above the carina or projected between the head of the clavicles and above the carina (Fig. 28.5). An ET that has been advanced too far into the airway may enter one of the two main bronchi, which can cause lobar collapse since the contralateral bronchial orifice would be blocked by the ET. Intubation of the right lower lobe bronchus can happen easily in an emergent or field

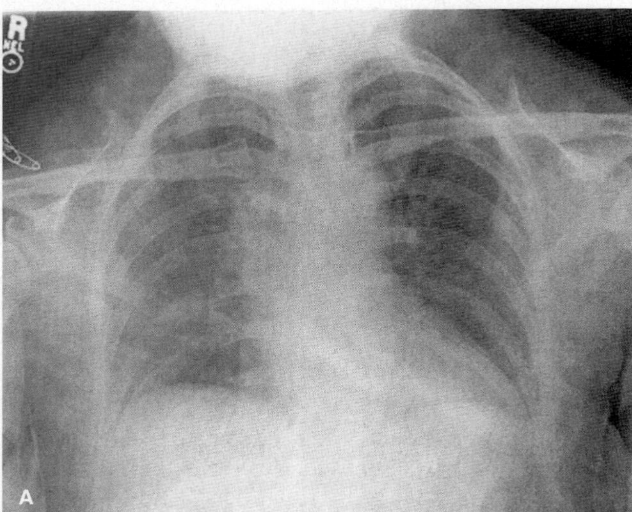

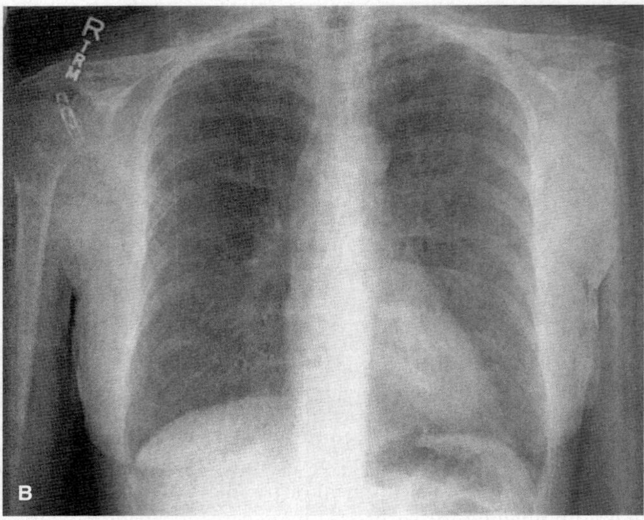

FIGURE 28.1. These two radiographs demonstrate the marked difference in the appearance of the chest when the film is taken (A) portably or (B) in the upright position. In the underexpanded portable chest film (A), the mediastinum looks wide, the heart looks bigger, and the vessels often look plumper. The diagnosis of fluid overload is erroneous as demonstrated by a radiograph taken minutes later (B) in the upright full inspiratory mode.

intubation because the trajectory of the right lower lobe bronchus is quite straight from the trachea (Fig. 28.6). Intubation of the right lower lobe bronchus may result in obstruction of the left bronchus, resulting in left lung collapse (Fig. 28.7) or right upper lobe bronchial obstruction with right upper lobe collapse. The inappropriate position of the ET leads to problems with patient ventilation until the endotracheal tube position is corrected.

Central Catheter Placement

Central venous catheters to be used for fluid, antibiotic administration, or parenteral nutrition may be placed into the subclavian or jugular veins with their tips projecting into the superior vena cava (SVC). The junction of the subclavian vein and jugular vein is usually located behind the medial head of the clavicle, so the course of the catheter in relation to the vessel should be evaluated. Most central catheters which are used

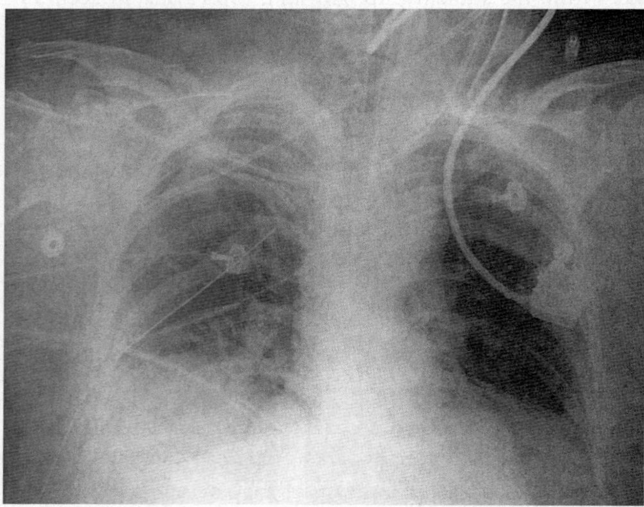

FIGURE 28.2. Lower lobe densities in this case are related to lobar collapse at the bases. The hemidiaphragms are elevated, and the heart is obscured by the densities caused by lower lobe collapse/volume loss. Lower lobe collapse can be differentiated from pleural effusions in this case because effusions would layer, causing haziness in the recumbent, critically ill patient.

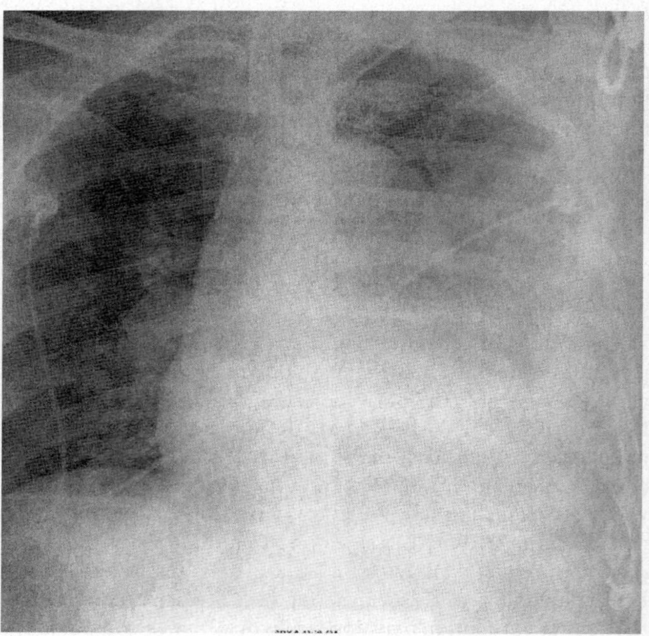

FIGURE 28.3. There is a sizable left pleural effusion that causes a gradient of density in the left chest and obscures the left hemidiaphragm, as opposed to the lucent right lung and clear diaphragm.

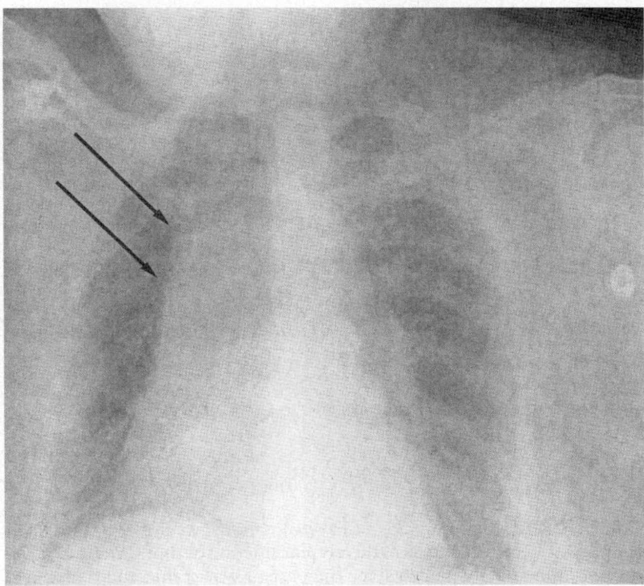

FIGURE 28.4. The mediastinum (*arrows*) is rotated to the right in this case, illustrating the difficulty of correctly positioning the critically ill patient on the film.

for central venous access are designed to terminate in the SVC, between the level of the clavicles and the carina, keeping the venous catheter above the reflection of the pericardium at the base of the great vessels (Fig. 28.8). This ensures that, if the superior vena cava is perforated by the catheter tip, bleeding into the pericardium will not occur. Therefore catheters that are advanced too far into the right heart or even into the inferior vena cava should be retracted, leaving the tip in the SVC. Some central venous access catheters, notably dialysis catheters, are designed to terminate in the right heart (Fig. 28.9).

When central venous catheters are placed into the chest, especially subclavian catheters, a postprocedural chest radiograph should be obtained to check catheter placement and to check for postprocedural complications, such as a pneumothorax. The apex of the lung is in close proximity to the puncture

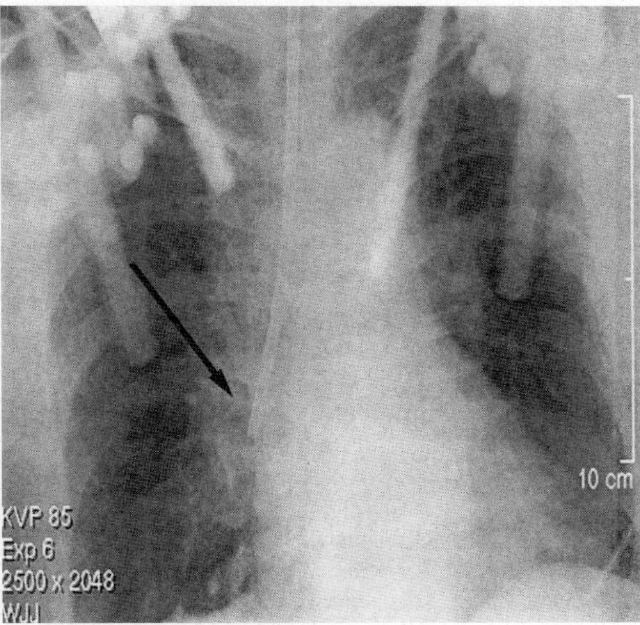

FIGURE 28.6. The small-bore tube changer used in this patient with cervical spinal traction has cannulated the right bronchus (*arrow*) reflecting its straight trajectory from the trachea. The tube changer can be used to maintain access to the airway in patients in whom reintubation may be necessary.

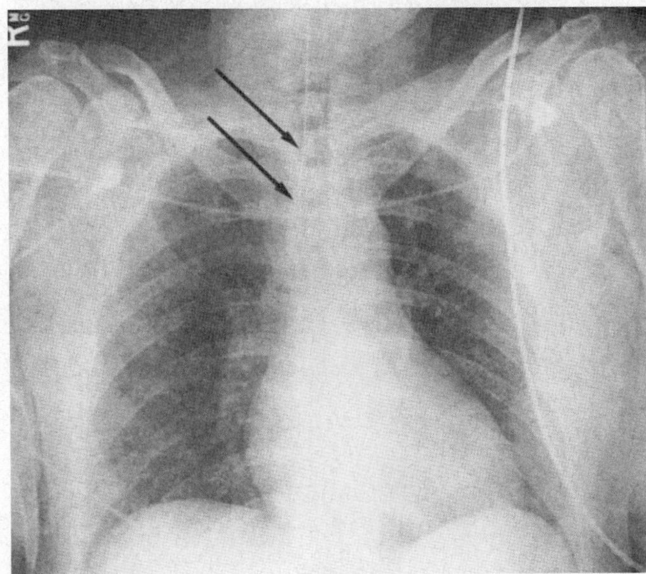

FIGURE 28.5. The endotracheal tube (*arrows*) is located in the trachea, between the clavicles and above the carina. The radiopaque marker is on one side of the tube to help identify its tip. Its position above the carina ensures equal ventilation to both lungs.

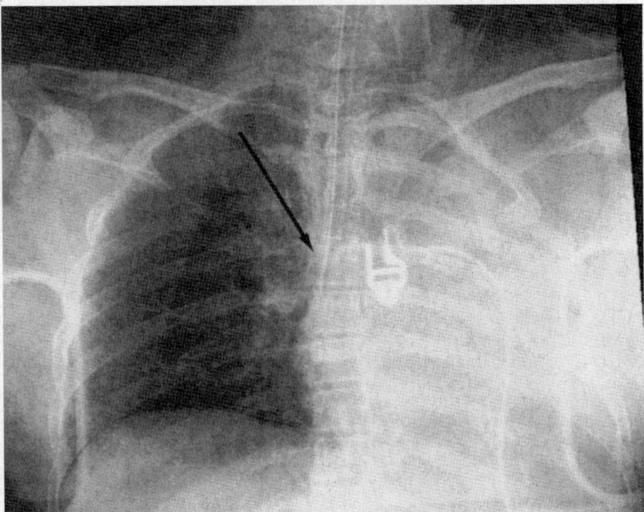

FIGURE 28.7. Emergent intubation has resulted in intubation of the bronchus intermedius. The left bronchus is blocked by the endotracheal tube. The entire left lung is collapsed, leading to an airless white left chest with shift of the mediastinum and heart to the left.

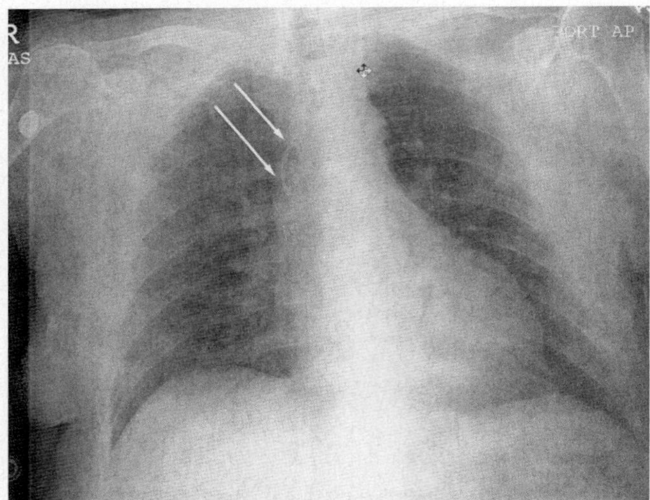

FIGURE 28.8. The tip of the central catheter (*arrows*) is in good position in the superior vena cava.

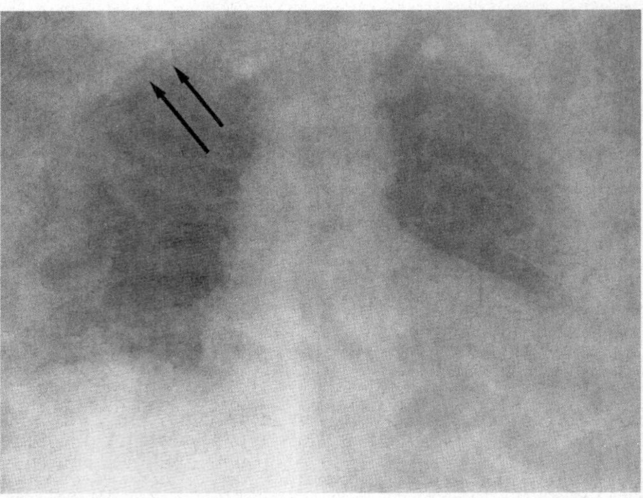

FIGURE 28.10. The lung edge (*arrows*) is noted at the right apex on this patient after a central catheter placement attempt. A chest tube was not immediately placed since the patient was stable and the pneumothorax was small.

site for a subclavian catheter and thus, is at risk for a pneumothorax. The proceduralist may expect to see a pneumothorax on the postprocedure chest film if the patient suddenly became short of breath, complained of chest pain, or if there was desaturation of oxygenation with catheter placement. A pneumothorax can also be asymptomatic.

A pneumothorax is recognized by visualization of the pleural interface inside the thoracic cavity where there is also an absence of lung markings, penpherally. Increased lucency (air) will surround the lung because of the extra air (Fig. 28.10). (Fig. 28.11). Tension pneumothorax may cause downward displacement on the diaphragm or contralateral mediastinal shift as the air accumulates within the pleural space (Fig. 28.12). The development of a tension pneumothorax may be correlated with sudden decompensation and require urgent intervention. A small pneumothorax in a patient on a ventilator may suddenly convert to a tension pneumothorax secondary to the presence of positive pressure ventilation. For this

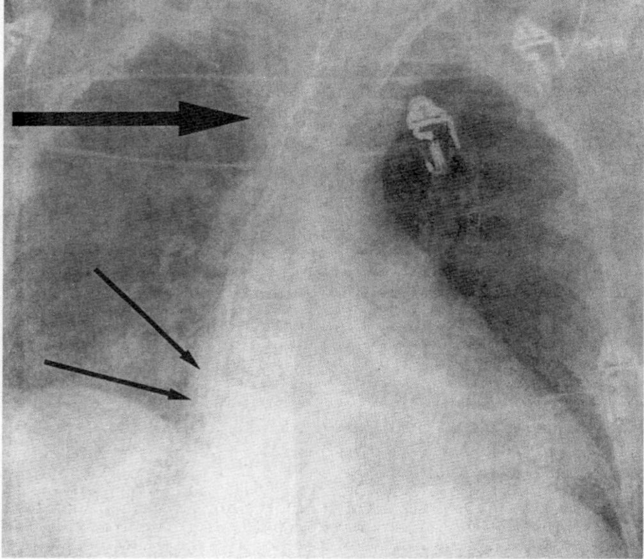

FIGURE 28.9. The tip of the larger-bore dialysis catheter is in the right atrium (*double arrows*), a deeper position than is expected for most standard central catheters. The introducer, a central catheter (*bold arrow*), is in good position in the SVC.

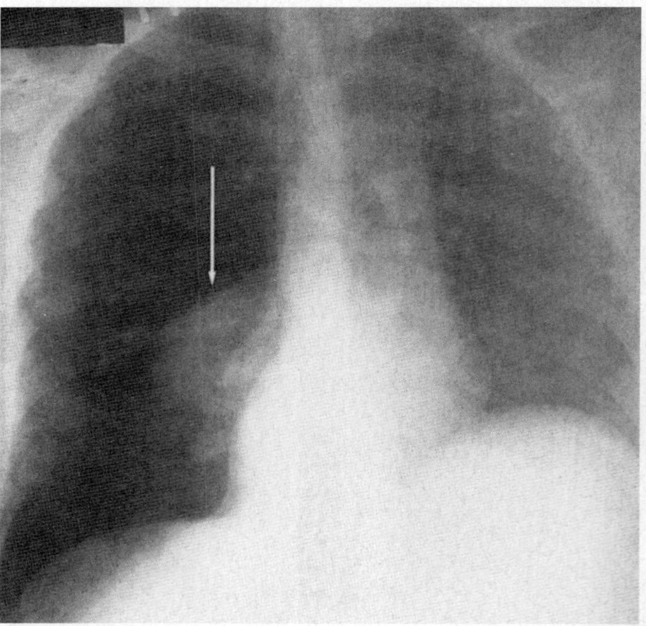

FIGURE 28.11. A large pneumothorax is present on the right. Air fills the right chest. There are no lung markings and the entire right lung has fallen centrally (*arrow*). The attempt at catheter placement was unsuccessful. No central venous catheter is noted. There is also a deep sulcus sign overlying the right diaphragm.

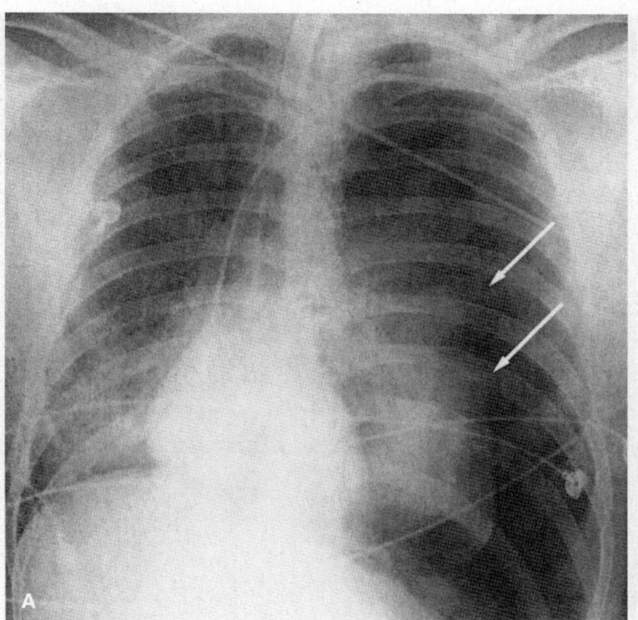

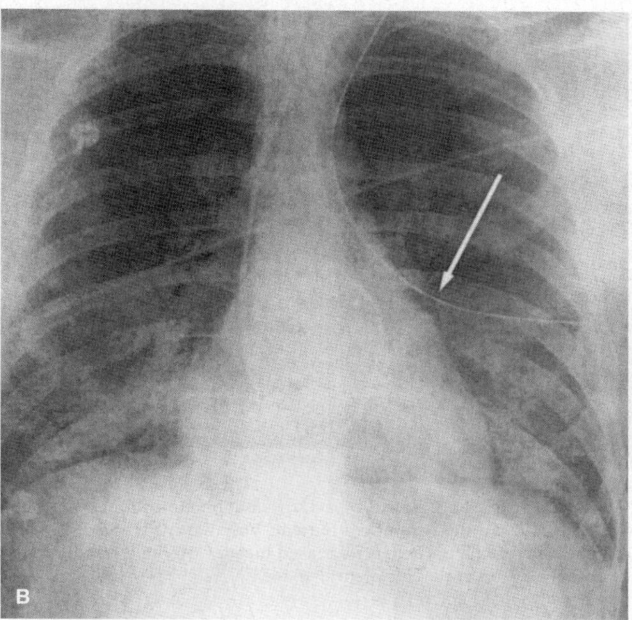

FIGURE 28.12. A: After catheter placement, a follow-up chest radiograph shows a large pneumothorax on the left. The lung edge is indicated by *arrows*. There is a shift of the mediastinum and depression of the left hemidiaphragm indicating a tension component. **B:** A chest tube (*arrow*) was inserted quickly to relieve the pneumothorax.

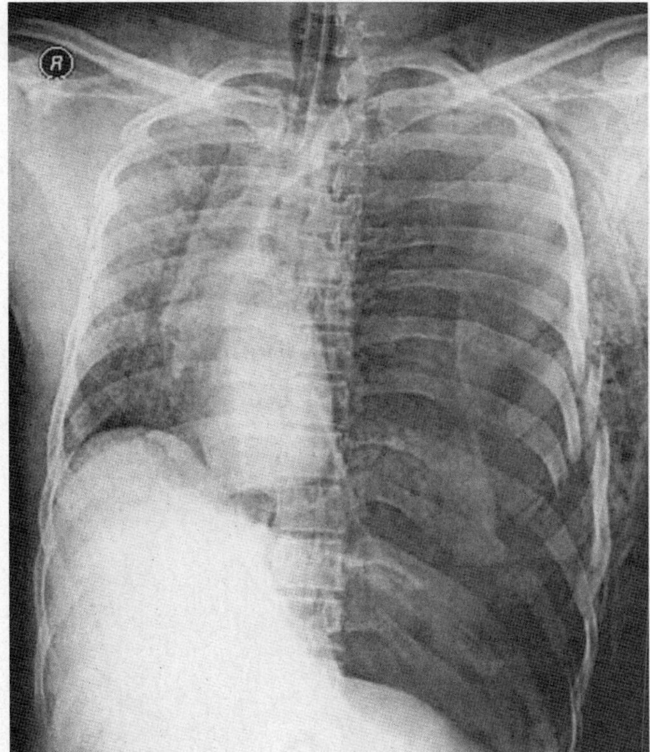

FIGURE 28.13. A tension pneumothorax is obvious, causing shift of the mediastinum toward the right. The left hemidiaphragm is depressed. Multiple left rib fractures are the cause of the tension pneumothorax in this case. Emergent left chest tube placement is necessary.

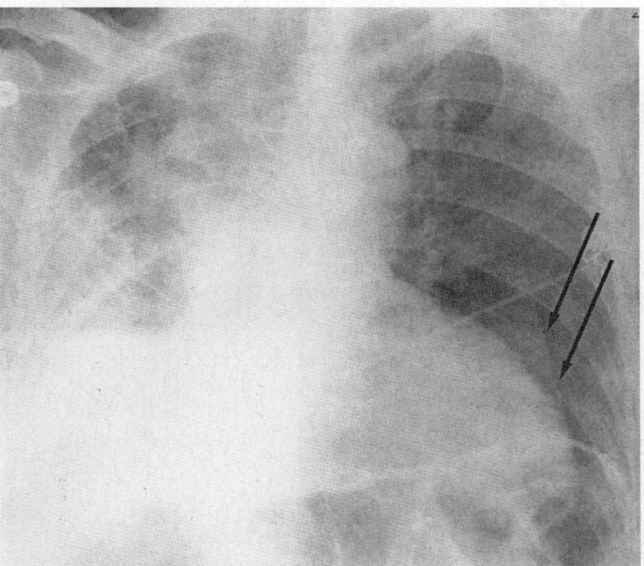

FIGURE 28.14. A skinfold (*arrows*) may be misinterpreted as a pleural catheter and lead to unnecessary chest tube placement. Recognizing the difference in appearance from the pleural edge and recognizing vascular markings peripheral to the skinfold will prevent an error from being made.

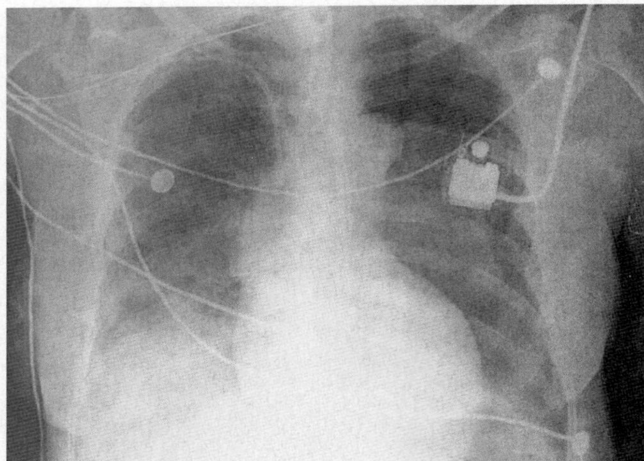

FIGURE 28.15. The presence of a large left pneumothorax may be hard to visualize in the recumbent patient. Vascular markings are lacking at the left apex, and there is increased lucency on the left indicating the presence of air in the left pleural space.

reason, patients on positive pressure ventilation who develop a pneumothorax will often be treated with a chest tube to avoid the development of a tension pneumothorax. Pneumothoraces are not only the result of central catheter placement but can be secondary to barotrauma with increasing ventilatory settings or secondary to chest trauma and rib fractures (Fig. 28.13).

The pleural interface that indicates the presence of a pneumothorax is not to be confused with a skinfold (Fig. 28.14). Skinfolds may be seen in older patients with redundant skin and can be misinterpreted as a pleural edge, or leading to misdiagnosis of a pneumothorax and inadvertant chest tube placement.

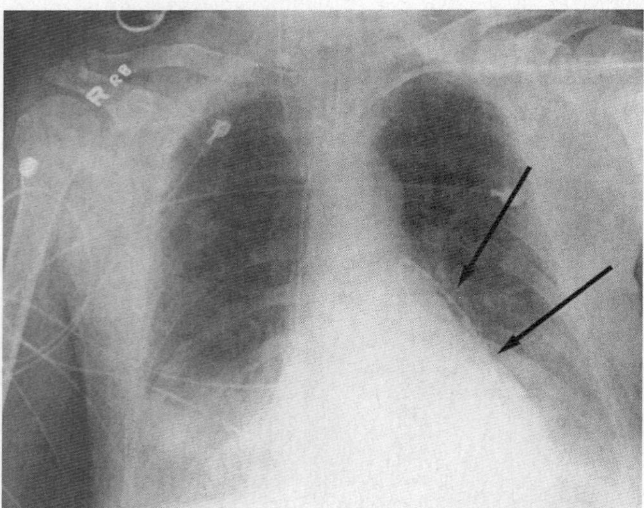

FIGURE 28.16. The tip of the pulmonary artery catheter (*arrows*) is well out of the left pulmonary artery. The catheter needs to be withdrawn several centimeters to be in optimal position with the tip of the catheter closer to the mediastinum.

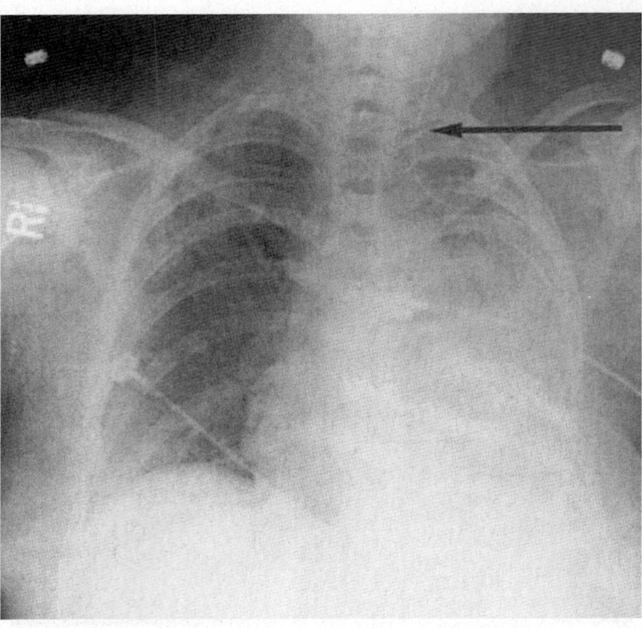

FIGURE 28.17. The left upper extremity PICC (*arrow*) extends into the left neck from the left arm and needs to be repositioned.

The critically ill patient is most often in the recumbent position after central catheter placement, which can make the recognition of a pneumothorax difficult (Fig. 28.15). A pneumothorax in the recumbent position may collect anteriorly, at the lung base, leading to the deep sulcus sign. The *deep*

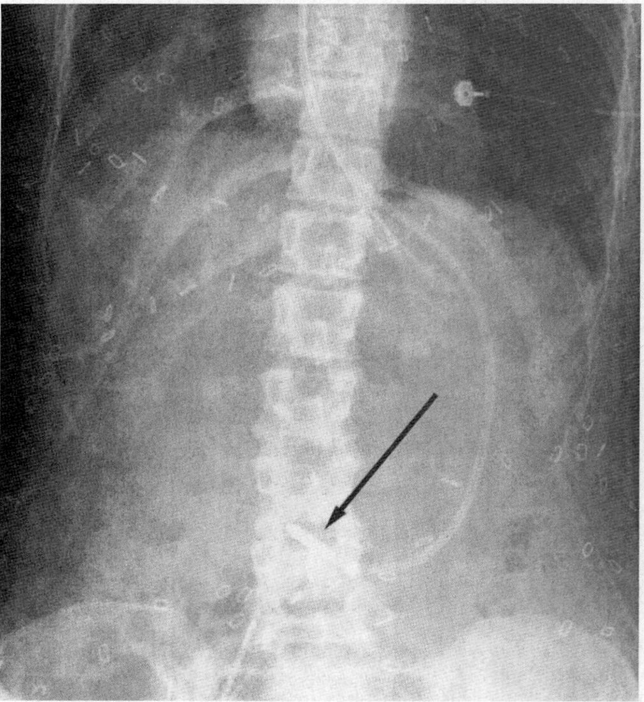

FIGURE 28.18. The tip of a weighted feeding tube is in the stomach (*arrow*).

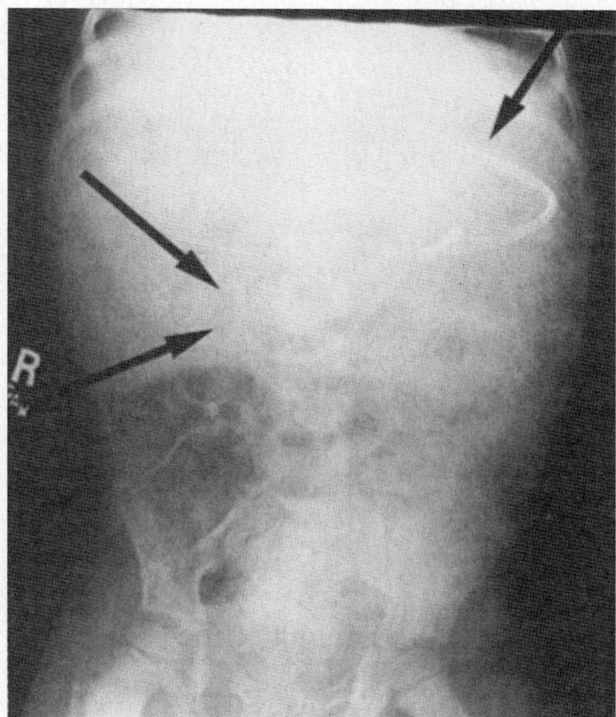

FIGURE 28.19. The feeding tube follows the gentle curvature of the stomach (*arrow*), descends in the duodenum (*double arrow*), and crosses back over the midline with the weighted tip at the level of the ligament of Treitz and in excellent position for feeding.

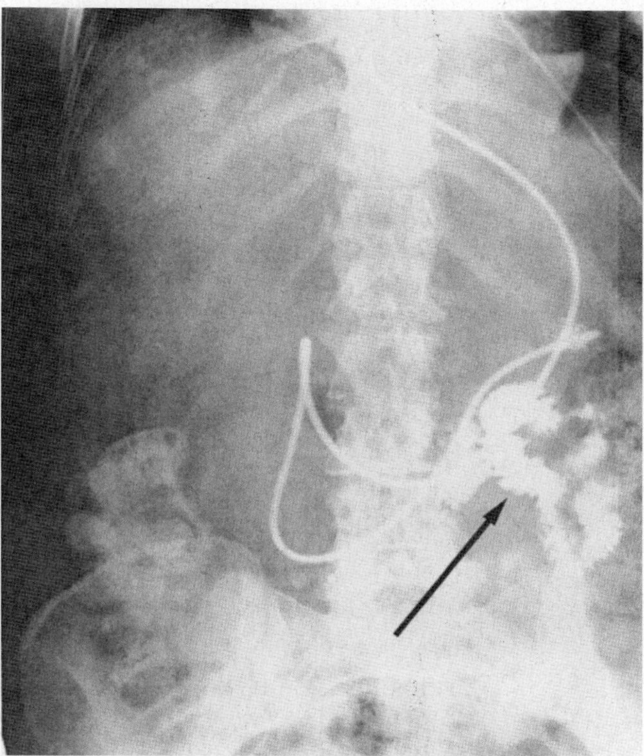

FIGURE 28.21. Contrast has been injected into the feeding tube to demonstrate that its tip is in the proximal jejunum and in excellent position for feeding. The small bowel folds are feathery in appearance (*arrow*). Contrast confirms that the tube is not coiled in the stomach.

sulcus sign is the lucency at the lung base caused by air trapped in the most anterior portion of the pleural space in a recumbent patient. This sign is a critical, yet subtle, finding that makes tremendous difference in a patients status. In critically ill patients who are difficult to position, the base of the lung may not be imaged, eliminating this diagnostic area on the film.

A pulmonary artery catheter (PAC) is usually placed via an introducer into the subclavian or jugular vein and advanced into either the right (most commonly) or left pulmonary artery

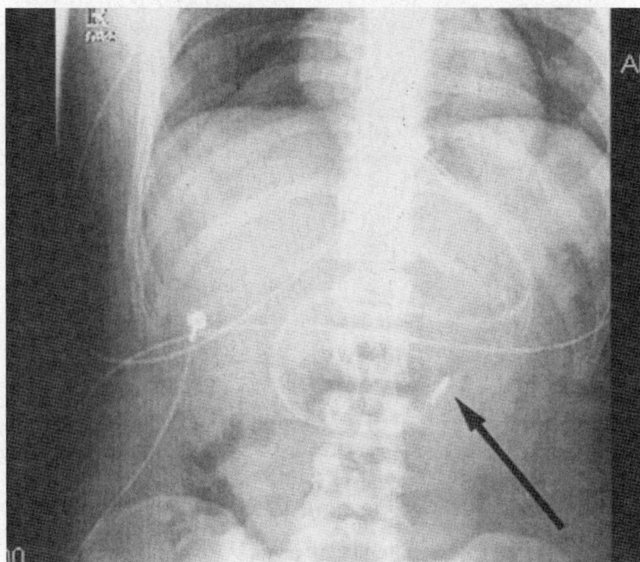

FIGURE 28.20. The tip of the feeding tube is in excellent position for feeding (*arrow*).

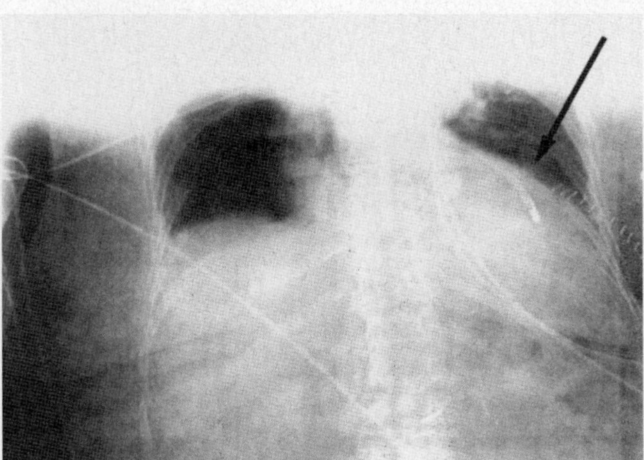

FIGURE 28.22. The feeding tube is not seen below the diaphragm. Its tip is seen above the diaphragm in the left lower lobe bronchus (*arrow*). If the tube's malposition is recognized and the tube is removed prior to feeding, no problems should ensue.

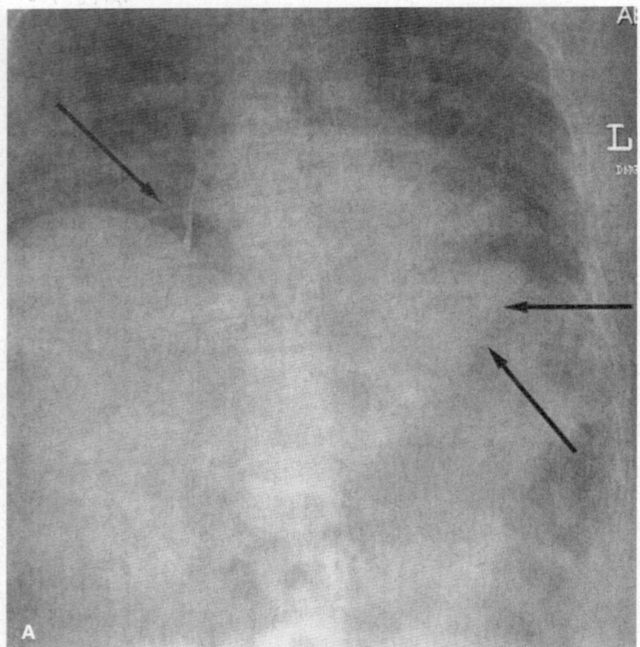

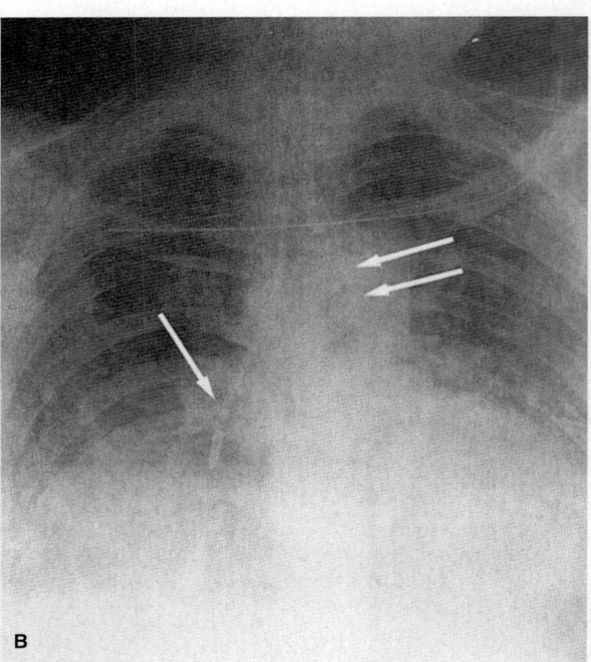

FIGURE 28.23. **A:** Tip of the weighted feeding tube (*arrow*) is in the bronchus to the right lower lobe, indicating the patient's inability to protect his airway. There is a nasogastric (NG) tube, indicated by the radiopaque stripe, coiled in the stomach (*double arrows*). **B:** Chest radiograph of the same patient showing the feeding tube in the right bronchus (*arrow*) and the NG tube in the esophagus (*double arrows*).

to facilitate its use as a monitor of cardiac function. The pulmonary artery catheter ideally should be positioned in the proximal right or left pulmonary artery. If the catheter is advanced too far distally, the balloon tip can cause pulmonary infarction (Fig. 28.16). If the pulmonary artery catheter is placed to be too proximal, as in the right ventricle, the catheter could trigger dysrhythmias and promote inaccurate measurements.

A peripherally inserted central catheter (PICC) is a long intravenous catheter, usually advanced from a peripheral upper extremity vein with optimal positioning of its tip in the SVC.

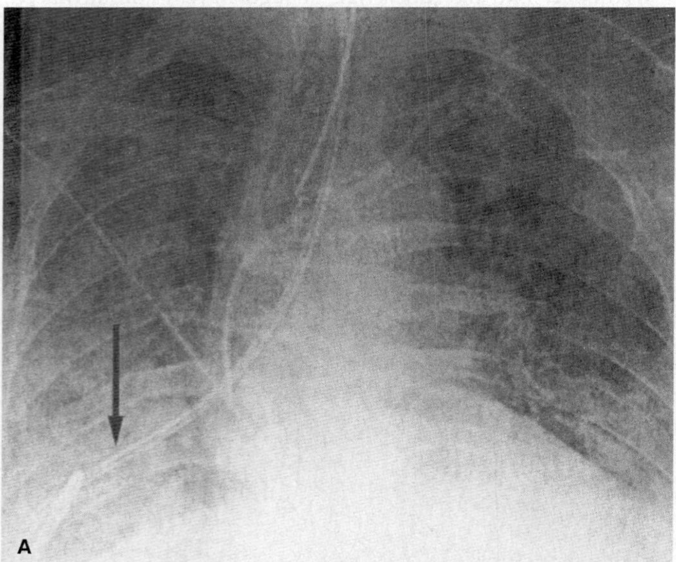

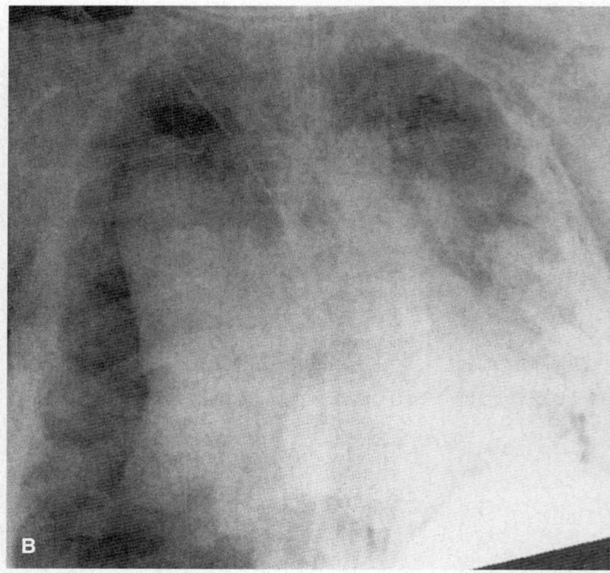

FIGURE 28.24. **A:** The feeding tube is coiled in the right lower lobe bronchus (*arrow*). **B:** After removal of the feeding tube, a tension pneumothorax became obvious on the right. The air, which is lucent in the pleural space, causes mass effect on the dense, noncompliant, wet right lung, which is unable to completely collapse. Prompt chest tube placement was necessary.

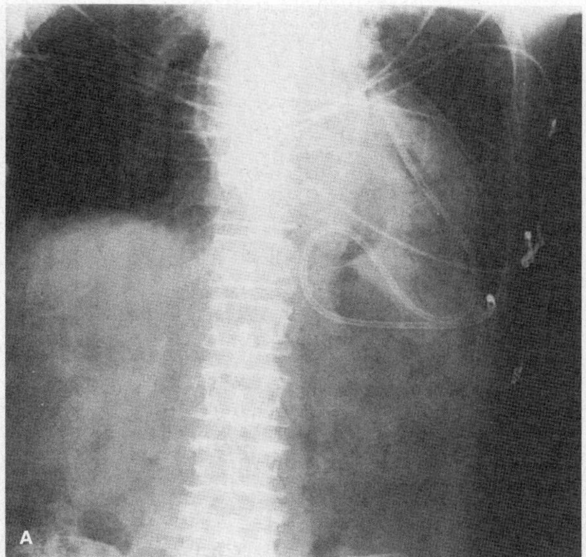

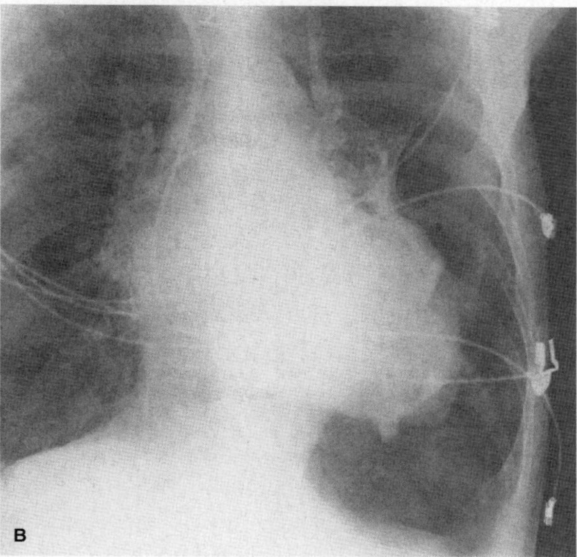

FIGURE 28.25. **A:** The feeding tube had been aggressively advanced into the left bronchus and was coiled in the left pleural space. **B:** Removal of the feeding tube led to the rapid development of a tension pneumothorax on the left, necessitating chest tube placement. Notice the lack of lung markings associated with the left pneumothorax.

A puncture of the lung and subsequent pneumothorax is not expected with PICC placement. The PICC is often hard to visualize on a radiograph since it is so small. Contrast instillation at the time of the radiograph may help in localizing the tip of a PICC. Peripherally inserted central catheters may be advanced too far into the heart, may coil in a vessel, or extend into the jugular vein from the subclavian vein (Fig. 28.17). In any of these situations, manipulation of the catheter will be necessary to optimize its placement. Some peripherally inserted central catheters cannot tolerate rapid injections of contrast agents necessary for CT scanning. The capabilities of the catheter for contrast injections are usually available from the product manufacturers on the product inserts.

The subclavian artery and vein course together, and plain radiographs of a PICC may not allow a distinction to be made of whether the catheter is in the vein or the artery. Clinical evaluation of catheter placement, either by transducing for a pressure reading or determining the oxygen saturation value of the blood, may be useful if there is concern that the catheter has been placed into the artery.

Feeding Tube Placement

A nasally or orally placed feeding tube is a commonly utilized in the critically ill patient. Feeding tube placement is considered optimal when the tip of the feeding tube is in the distal duodenum or proximal jejunum so that the risk of reflux of the administered feeds into the stomach will be minimized. Many of the commonly used enteral tubes have a weighted metallic tip to facilitate peristaltic movement into the small bowel. This weighted tip facilitates the recognition of the tube on the abdominal radiograph (Fig. 28.18). Some feeding tubes are placed surgically, and their appearance may be different (e.g. larger bore). Nasogastric (NG) tubes are meant to reside within the stomach for gastric decompression, administration of oral medications, and gastric pH monitoring. Most NG tubes have a radiopaque stripe marking the length of the tube with a side hole obvious as a break in the marker. The most proximal sidehole of the NG tube needs to reside in the stomach.

The ideal position for a feeding tube placed orally is with its tip at the ligament of Treitz or at least in the distal duodenum so reflux into the stomach and esophagus with feedings will not occur (Figs. 28.19–28.21). In patients with neurological injuries, or in heavily medicated patients, the inability to protect their airway may lead to cannulation of the bronchus with the feeding tube (Fig. 28.22). Similar to ETT placement, the right lower lobe bronchus may be cannulated by the enteric

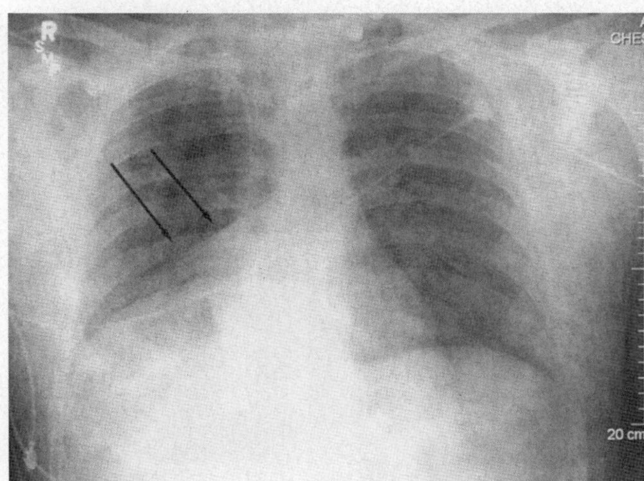

FIGURE 28.26. There is a triangular density at the right lung base (*arrows*) and shift of the heart toward the right, findings of right lower lobe collapse secondary to a mucus plug in the bronchus.

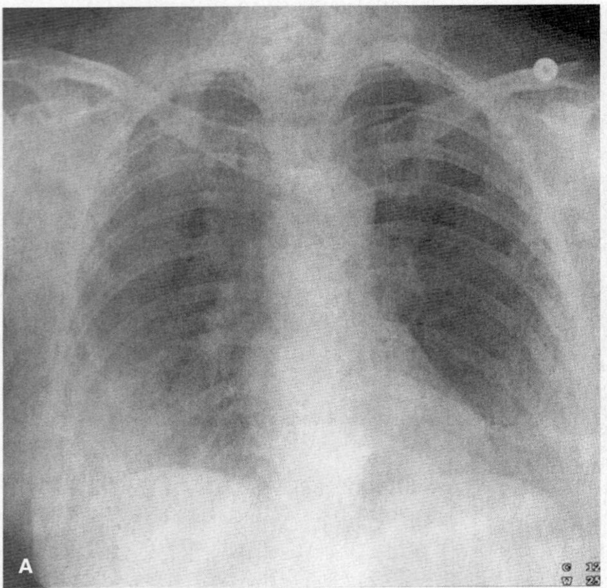

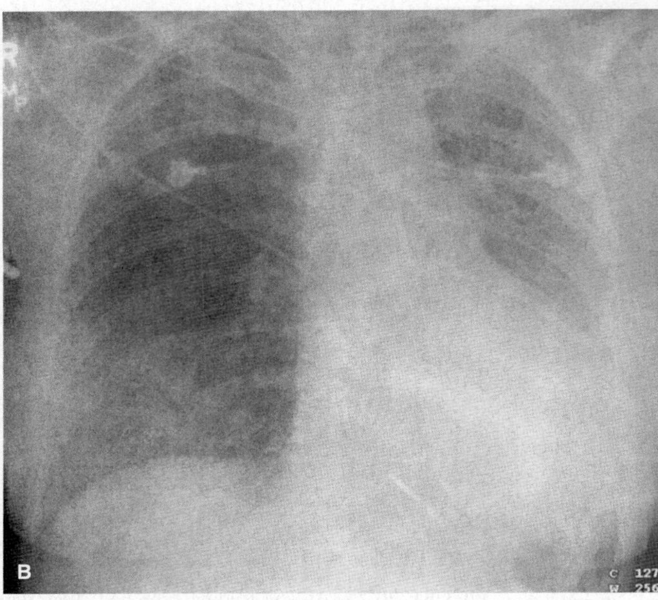

FIGURE 28.27. **A:** Preoperative chest radiograph shows excellent visualization of both hemidiaphragms and clear lungs. **B:** Postoperative (status post–median sternotomy) chest radiograph shows increased retrocardiac density, inability to see the left hemidiaphragm, inability to see through the heart, and shift of the heart toward the left—all findings of left lower lobe collapse.

tube because of its relatively straight course from the mouth (Fig. 28.23). Feeding tube malposition must be recognized to avoid the disastrous consequences of administering feeds into the lung.

A feeding tube that has been inadvertently placed into the bronchus and then advanced into the lung parenchyma may cause a sudden tension pneumothorax when the tube is removed from the lung because when such a tube is removed, the hole in the pleura and lung may result in a large gush of air and the development of a tension pneumothorax. (Figs. 28.24 and 28.25).

Parenchymal Abnormalities Seen on Chest Radiograph in the ICU

Collapsed Lung

Areas of collapsed lung are frequently seen on chest radiographs of the critically ill patient. Collapsed lung will be dense (white) on the chest film and will take up less room than a fully expanded, normally aerated lung (Fig. 28.26).

The most frequently encountered lobar collapse in the intensive care unit is left lower lobe collapse. Ventilator-dependent recumbent patients develop collapse in the left lower lobe,

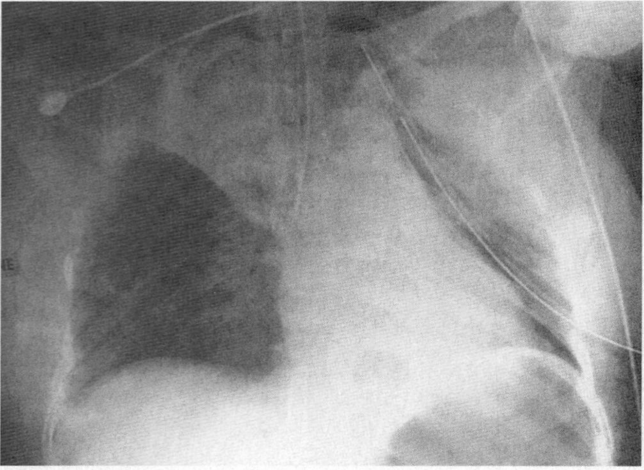

FIGURE 28.28. The triangular density in the right lung apex is right upper lobe collapse secondary to the low position of the endotracheal tube (ET) with obstruction of the right upper lobe bronchus. Retraction of the ET may allow re-expansion of the right upper lobe.

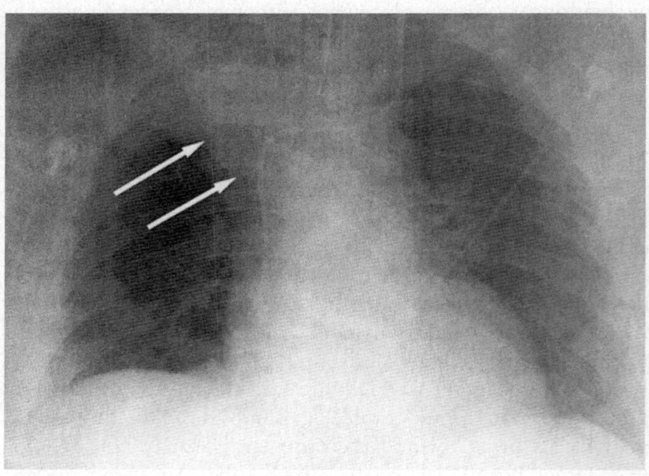

FIGURE 28.29. After pulmonary artery catheter placement, the triangular density of right upper lobe collapse (*arrows*) was noted.

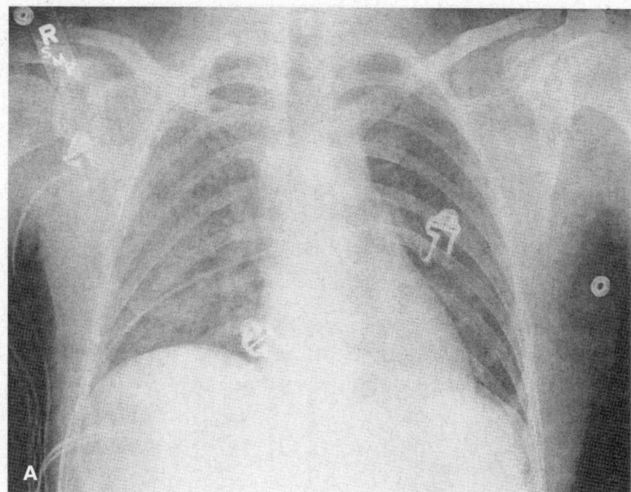

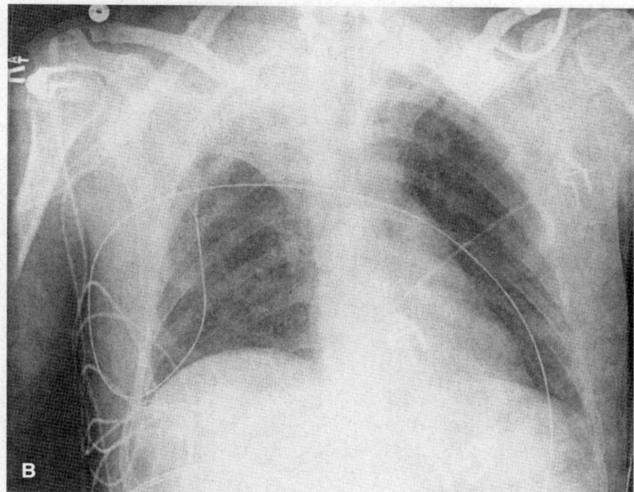

FIGURE 28.30. **A:** Normal preoperative radiograph. **B:** The triangular density of right upper lobe collapse is noted in this patient after fixation of the cervical spine.

usually secondary to diminished inspiratory effort, recumbent positioning, and the weight of the heart on the left lower lobe. On the chest film, left lower lobe collapse will result in increased density in the retrocardiac area. This is recognized by an inability to "see through" the heart to visualize the lower lobe pulmonary artery, and the left hemidiaphragm. The inability to visualize the hemidiaphragm on the left is secondary to the fact that the left lower lobe is airless. It is the air in the lower lobes that allows the diaphragm to be seen as a linear structure. In the patient with left lower lobe collapse, the heart and mediastinum with shift toward the left, since the collapsed left lower lobe is taking up less room than a normally expanded, fully aerated lobe (Fig. 28.27).

A malpositioned ET tube can lead to lobar or lung collapse by occluding the airway and preventing ventilation (Fig. 28.28). Repositioning of the ET tube may lead to complete re-expansion of the lung in some cases. Often, bronchoscopy is necessary to optimize ventilation by removing a mucous plug to improve ventilation.

Right upper lobe collapse causes a characteristic triangular density in the right lung apex. This characteristic triangular density should be recognized, as it might be encountered after intubation. Its appearance is characteristic and is not to be confused with a localized hemothorax, loculatal, pleural effusion, pneumothorax or pneumonia. The smooth inferior margin of the density is the minor fissure that sharply marginates the density and is pulled superiorly by the volume loss in the right upper lobe (Figs. 28.29 and 28.30). Right upper lobe collapse may respond to ET tube manipulation, bronchoscopy, or chest PT. Re-expansion of the right upper lobe can be documented by chest radiograph after such maneuvers (Fig. 28.31).

"White Out" of the Chest

A critically ill patient may present with clinical decompensation and a "white out" of one lung on the chest film. Careful analysis of the film is necessary to draw the correct conclusions, which will determine therapy.

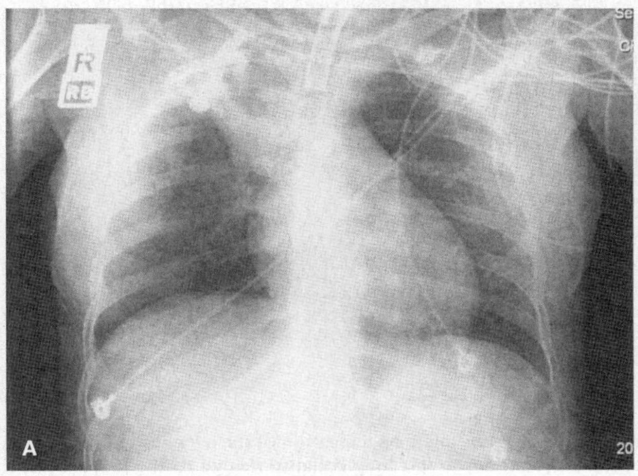

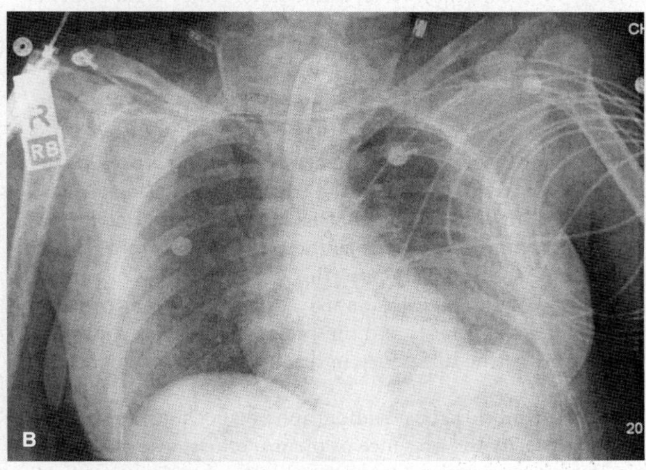

FIGURE 28.31. **A:** Right upper lobe collapse. **B:** Resolution after aggressive chest PT was administered.

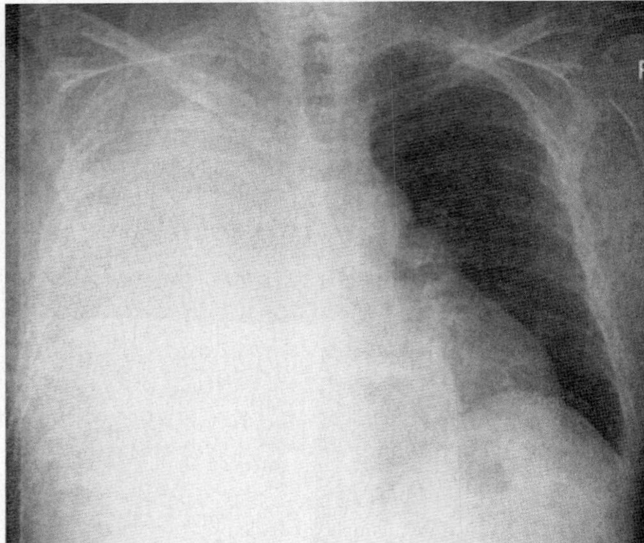

FIGURE 28.32. There is complete opacification of the right chest, and the heart is pushed away from the right chest, suggesting that there is something (fluid or mass) filling the right chest and having mass effect. CT scanning subsequently showed a large mass and effusion filling the right chest. There was associated compressive atelectasis or collapse of the right lung.

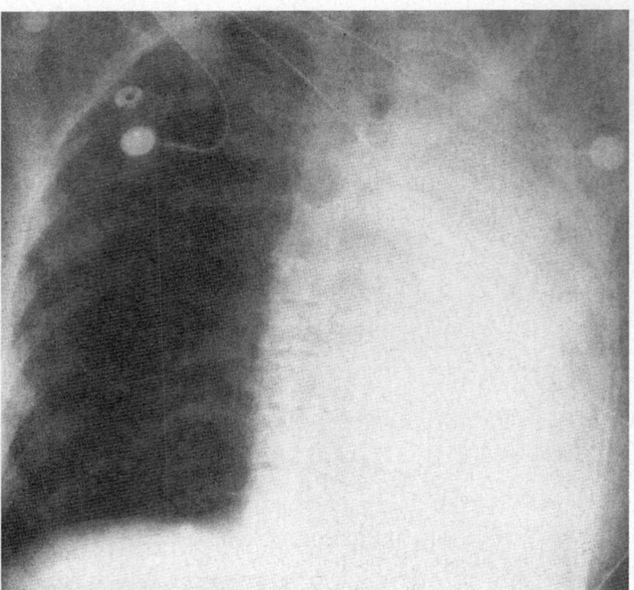

FIGURE 28.33. There is complete opacification of the left chest, and the heart is hidden in the density consistent with a completely collapsed left lung secondary to airway occlusion related to a mucus plug. No significant effusion is present, indicated by the fact that the heart is hidden in the density of the left chest rather than being shifted to the right. Bronchoscopy was necessary to remove the plug and allow re-expansion of the left lung.

A completely opacified hemithorax may be secondary to a large pleural effusion that fills the chest. The underlying lung may be compressed and surrounded by the large amount of fluid. When a large pleural effusion fills one hemithorax and the underlying lung is collapsed, the heart and mediastinum will be shifted *away* from the side filled with fluid (Fig. 28.32).

In some situations, the entire lung collapses secondary to mucus plugging or airway obstruction. In these circumstances in which there is no significant volume of pleural fluid, the mediastinum and heart will shift *toward* the side of collapse, which is also the side of airway obstruction (Fig. 28.33). This distinction of shift of the heart and mediastinum toward atelectatic lung, or away from a large effusion is critical because the observation leads to dramatically different therapies (bronchoscopy or chest tube) which immediately improve a patients ventilation (Fig. 28.34).

Pleural Effusions in the Intensive Care Unit

Pleural effusions that are large but do not completely fill the chest will, cause a gradient of haziness that obscures the hemidiaphragm and is worse at the lung base which gradually fades toward the lung apex. Pleural effusions in the recumbent patient do not cause a meniscus as they do in an upright patient because the effusion layers posteriorly in the supine patient. A large unilateral pleural effusion may cause an asymmetric density in the affected chest, and the presence of the effusion will be suggested by the difference in density in the two hemithoraces.

Lateral decubitus chest radiographs or bedside chest ultrasound may verify the presence of pleural effusion suspected on plain chest radiographs. Furthermore ultrasound of the chest, show the compressed underlying lung, and allow quantification of the pleural fluid (Fig. 28.35). Loculated fluid or internal septations within the fluid suggest that the pleural fluid is infected or hemorrhagic. Pleural fluid that is infected—that is, an empyema—needs drainage. Acute hematoma or an empyema may be difficult to drain with thoracentesis or small-bore chest

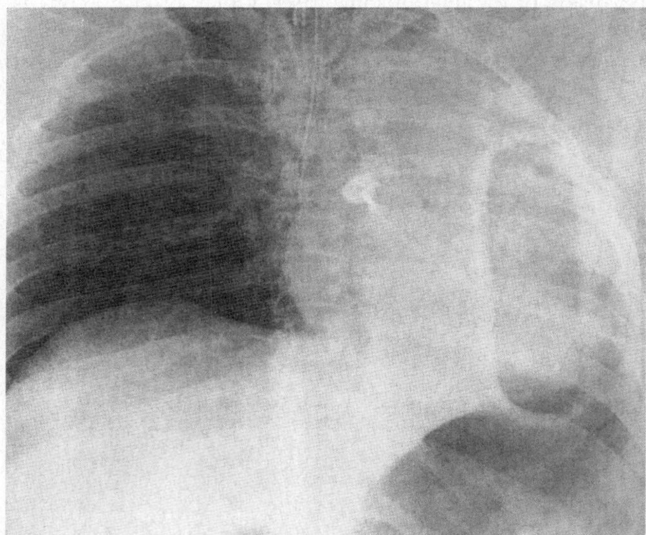

FIGURE 28.34. Complete opacification of the left chest in this trauma patient is secondary to left lung collapse related to the inappropriate endotracheal tube (ET) position. Retraction of the ET should aid left lung re-expansion.

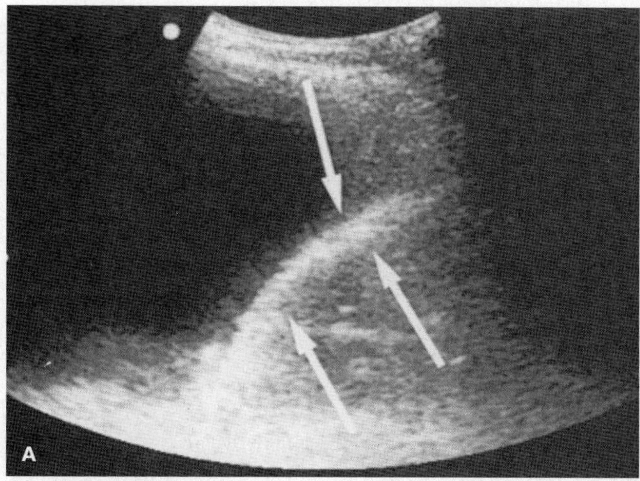

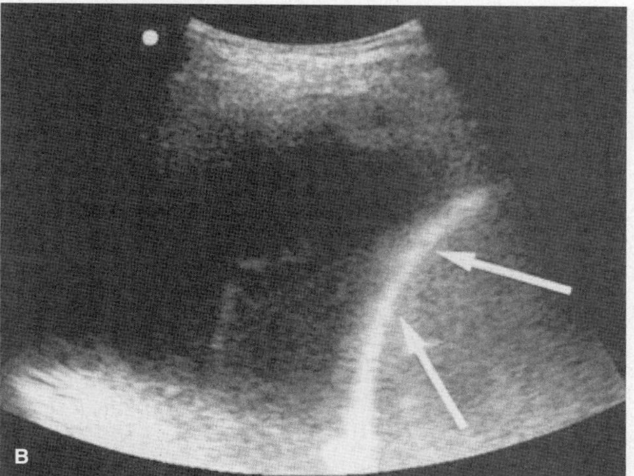

FIGURE 28.35. A and B: Ultrasound shows a large effusion (blank space) outlining the hemidiaphragm (*arrows*).

tubes, requiring either large-bore chest tubes or surgical decompression. Sometimes moderate to large effusions which cause the lung to collapse, can be drained to improve a patients ventilatory status to keep them from being intubated or to facilitate extubation (Fig. 28.36).

Airspace or Alveolar Opacification

Aspiration or ventilator-associated pneumonia (VAP) are two respiratory events that may complicate the clinical course of the patient in the ICU. Aspiration or VAP may prolong the stay in the ICU by contributing to respiratory failure and sepsis.

On a chest radiograph, VAP appreciated by an area of airspace opacification (cloud like) in the lung (Fig. 28.37). The region of VAP may begin in an area of lobar or segmental collapse. Air bronchograms may be seen, which are air-filled bronchi surrounded by infectious material in the alveoli of the lungs. Visualization of air bronchograms allows recognition that the process is a parenchymal or lung process, not a pleural effusion (Fig. 28.38). Patchy cloudlike opacification on the chest film is also indicative that the process is parenchymal.

The sudden onset of a large parenchymal consolidation, particularly in the lower lobes especially in the correct clinical scenario, may indicate that large volume bilaterally aspiration has occurred. Sometimes this can be confirmed at bronchoscopy

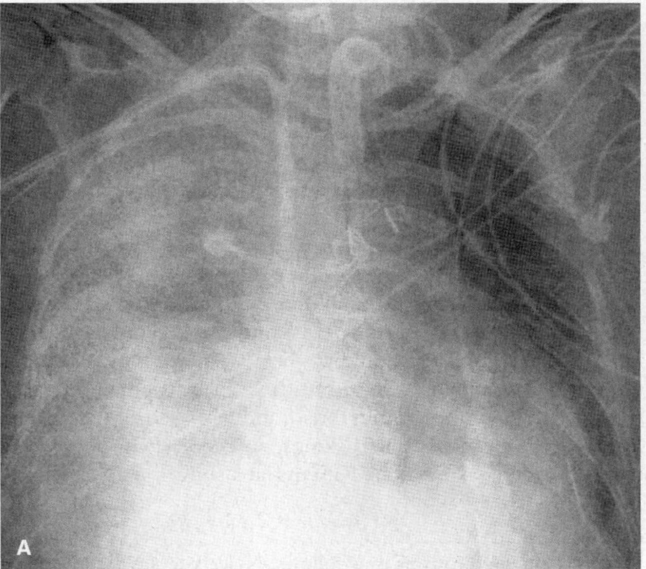

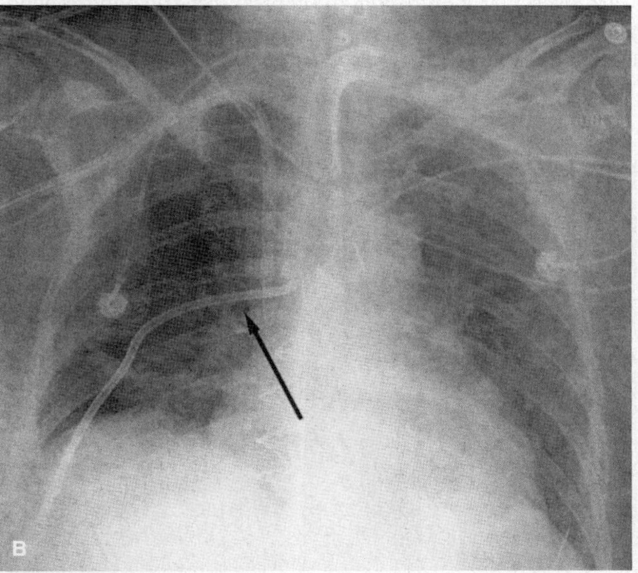

FIGURE 28.36. A: A large right pleural effusion causes diffuse opacification on the right. B: Placement of a pleural drain allowed normal aeration of the right lung. The pigtail pleural drainage catheter is indicated by the *arrow*. Note the resolution of the haziness and opacification of the right chest. The right hemidiaphragm is now visible.

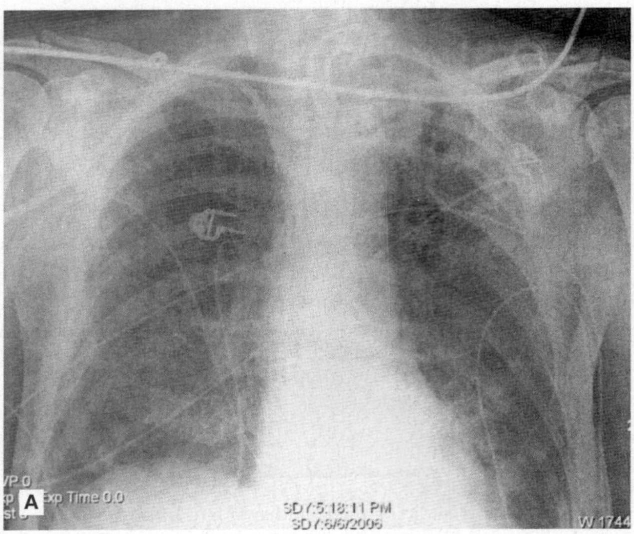

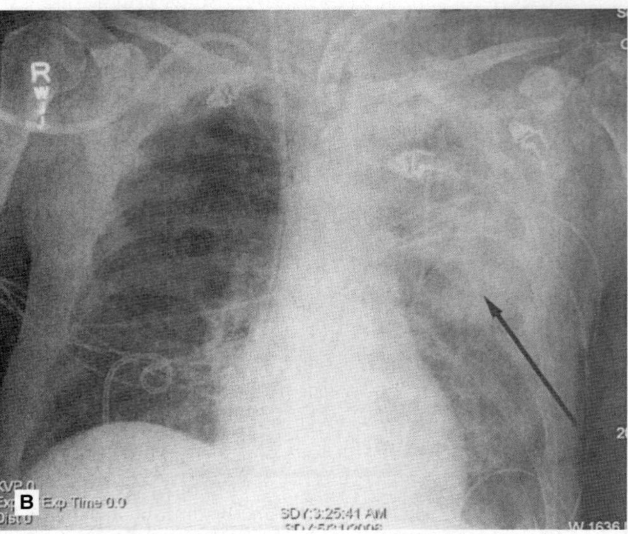

FIGURE 28.37. **A:** Tracheostomy tube noted in good position with clear lungs. **B:** Subsequently a large area of new left lung airspace opacification was noted on chest radiograph demonstrating interval development of ventilator-associated pneumonia (VAP).

when food particles are retrieved, substantiating the impression of aspiration (Figs. 28.39–28.41).

Fluid Overload Pattern

Massive fluid resuscitation is sometimes necessary in patients with trauma, during surgery, or as part of the management for sepsis. A fluid overload pattern may become obvious on a chest film with bilateral perihylar airspace opacification and bilateral pleural effusions. Patients with cardiogenic pulmonary edema and heart failure may have similar findings on a chest radiograph. Diffuse bilateral parenchymal opacification could also be seen in extensive pneumonia, pulmonary hemorrhage, or ARDS (acute respiratory distress syndrome). Cardiovascular monitoring, the clinical scenario and bronchoscopic results may be helpful in differentiating the various causes of the parenchymal opacification (Figs. 28.42–28.44).

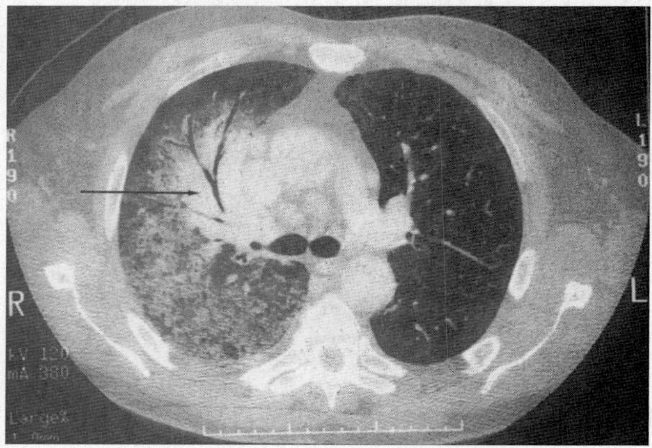

FIGURE 28.38. Aspiration pneumonia was documented on CT as a unilateral parenchymal process in the right lung. Air bronchograms are obvious (*arrow*).

CROSS-SECTIONAL IMAGING IN THE CRITICALLY ILL PATIENT

There are numerous medical or surgical situations that may result in an admission to the ICU. Cross-sectional imaging, often with CT, is instrumental in allowing rapid recognition of the correct diagnosis to facilitate care and follow-up in the critically ill patient.

CT scanning is the workhorse of diagnosis and imaging of the critically ill patient. Intravenous and oral contrast agents are used to optimize imaging, but their use may raise certain concerns. Intravenous contrast administration is especially helpful in vascular diagnoses such as aortic dissection or acute mesenteric thrombosis allowing recognition of an intimal flap in the aorta or embolus in mesenteric vessels. Intravenous contrast can be nephrotoxic in patients with renal insufficiency therefore. Pretreatment of such patients with fluid optimization, N-acetyl cysteine, and alkalinization[1] may minimize the effects of intravenous iodinated contrast agents. In some cases, intravenous contrast is not necessary for the particular question asked (e.g., "Is there free air?") and can be avoided. To administer intravenous contrast at a rapid rate for the scan, a well-placed venous access catheter is necessary.

Oral contrast is beneficial in many situations by delineating the GI tract from an abcess or mass and also to confirm a leak. However oral contrast should not be used in most emergent situations because it can delay a critical scan, or a patient cannot tolerate the volume of fluids. Also, iodine-based oral contrast agents are quite toxic to the lungs, so every effort should be made to avoid aspiration. Patients at aspiration risk should

[1]The formula used for this is as follows: N-acetyl cysteine, 1,200 mg IV for one dose, then 1,200 mg enterally or IV every 12 hours for three more doses. Additionally, into 1,000 mL of sterile H_2O is added 150 mEq NaH_2CO_3 and run in over 24 hours. A quantity of 250 mL is run in over the first 2 hours, then the rest is administered over the the remaining 22 hours.

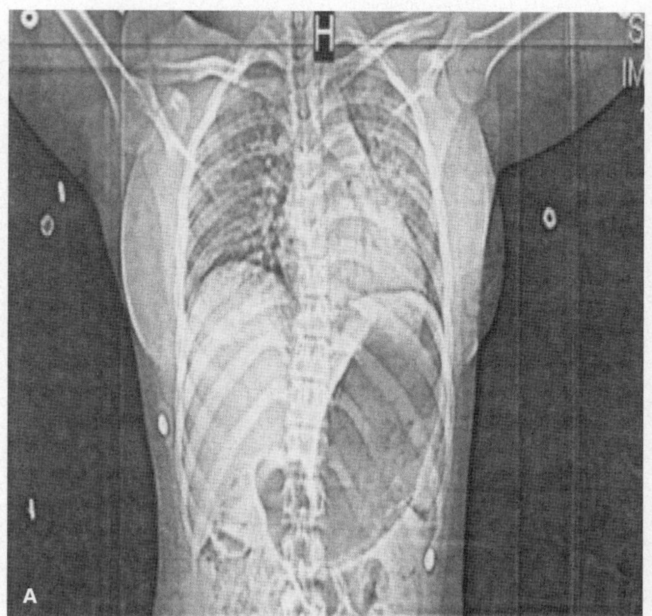

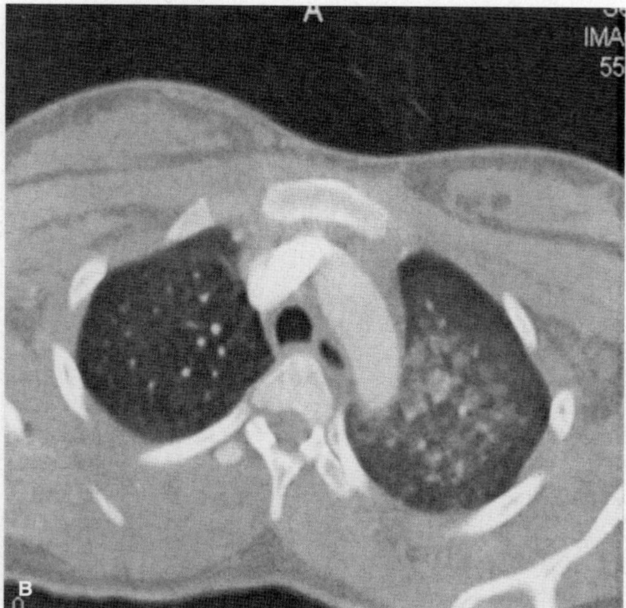

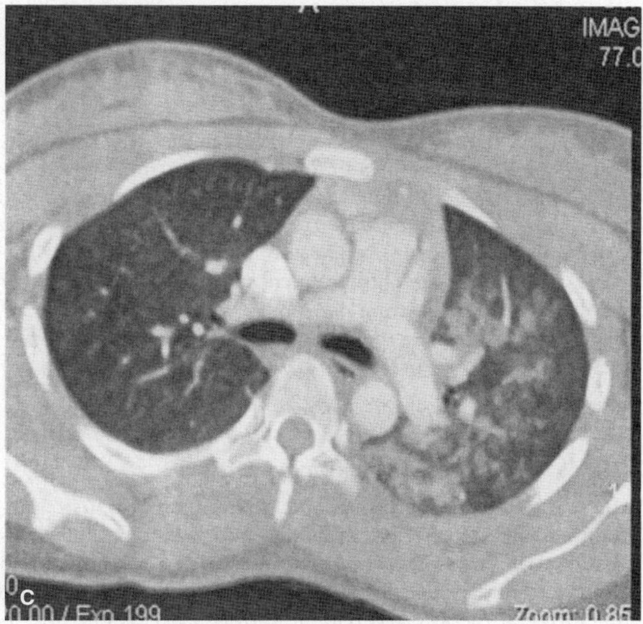

FIGURE 28.39. A–C: This young woman was witnessed to aspirate during an emergent delivery of a premature infant. CT images demonstrate the focal, unilateral airspace disease on the left.

be monitored as the oral contrast is administered and while the contrast is in the stomach. Administration of oral contrast into enteral tubes that are located beyond the stomach can be helpful.

Cross-Sectional Imaging in Certain Critical Situations

Aortic Aneurysm Rupture

Aortic aneurysm rupture is often seen in an older patient with atherosclerotic disease, which may present by severe back pain, hypotension, and cardiovascular collapse.

If the diagnosis is suspected, the most rapid recognition of an aortic aneurysm can be made by bedside ultrasound. Recognition of retroperitoneal hemorrhage accompanying aortic rupture may be limited with bedside ultrasound. CT allows visualization of the aortic aneurysm, with fluid and stranding in the retroperitoneum related to aortic leaking (Fig. 28.45). Immediate repair may be attempted by either open surgery or endoluminal stent placement. Emergent and massive resuscitation is often necessary in patients with aortic rupture.

Aortic Dissection

Aortic dissection typically causes severe back pain and can be confused clinically with myocardial infarction or pancreatitis (Fig. 28.46). Contrast enhanced CT or MR can be used in

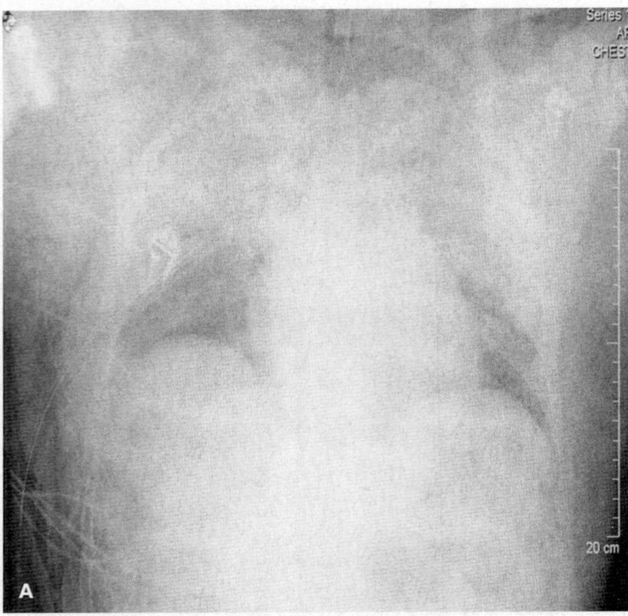

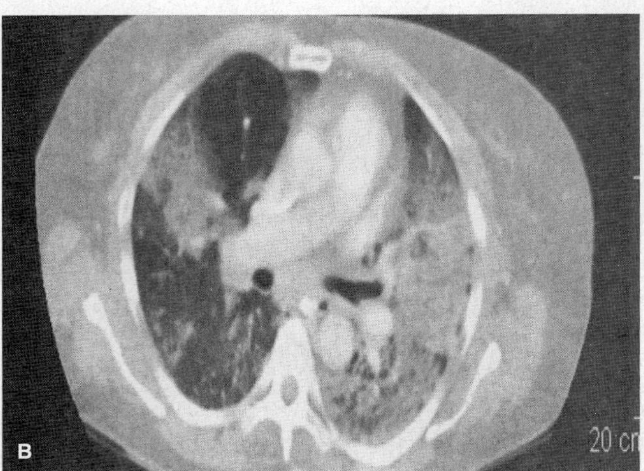

FIGURE 28.40. A trauma patient requiring prolonged extrication had extensive bilateral parenchymal opacification related to aspiration.

the emergent setting to make the diagnosis of aortic dissection as well as to define the extent of the dissection. Involvement of the aortic root or ascending aorta by a dissection is usually treated surgically to avoid or minimize complications of cardiac tamponade, myocardial infarction, or aortic valvular insufficiency. Aortic dissection that begins distal to the takeoff of the left subclavian artery may be treated medically with antihypertensive medications unless there are complicating factors such as mesenteric ischemia or renal dysfunction from aortic dissection. Endoluminal stents are increasingly being used in situations of aortic dissection.

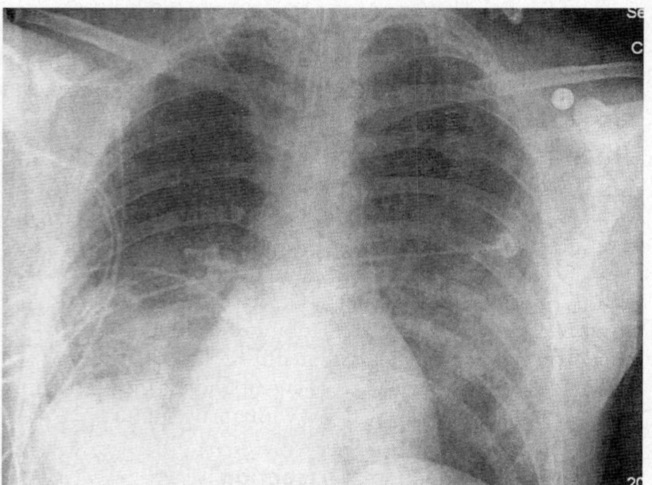

FIGURE 28.41. The postoperative radiograph shows the interval development of bibasilar airspace opacification, worse on the right. Clinically obvious aspiration occurred postoperatively.

Aortic Injury

Acute aortic injury occurs with significant chest trauma, particularly acute decelaration injuries, and is most often located near the embryonic attachment of the aorta to the pulmonary artery. Luminal irregularities at this site with surrounding mediastinal hematoma indicate a potentially unstable vascular injury. Either open surgical management or endoluminal stent grafting can be used for repair. Active arterial extravasation of contrast at the site of aortic injury does not have to be present to have an unstable aortic injury (Fig. 28.47).

Severe Pancreatitis

Pancreatitis has many causes, including alcohol abuse, gallstone passage, hypertriglyceridemia, and trauma. Acute pancreatitis from any cause can result in severe pain, nausea, and vomiting. Fluid resuscitation and electrolyte management are imperative in the affected patient and may necessitate an admission to the ICU. Peripancreatic fluid collections, which can become infected, often develop after a bout of severe pancreatitis. The severity of pancreatitis and complicating features like pseudoaneurysm formation, or splenic vein thrombosis can be elucidated by cross-sectional imaging (Fig. 28.48).

Trauma

Ultrasound of the trauma patient in the emergency department can detect free fluid, likely blood, related to organ injury. Subsequent CT scanning allows rapid evaluation of trauma to the head, chest, abdomen, and pelvis and any complicated extremity injuries. Three-phase imaging allows recognition of arterial bleeding, organ contusion or laceration, and urinary system injury. State-of-the-art scanners are rapid and can guide emergent surgical management or direct critical care monitoring.

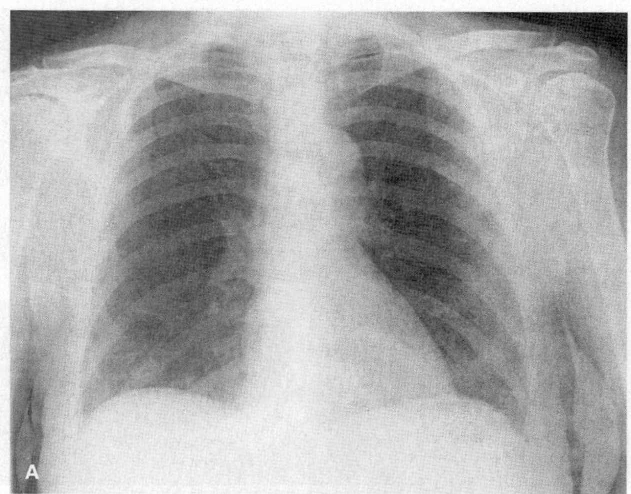

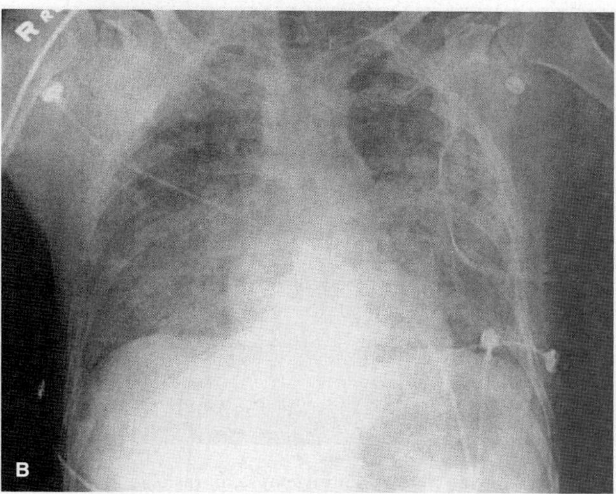

FIGURE 28.42. Preoperative (A) and postoperative (B) radiographs show the interval development of diffuse bilateral airspace opacification, consistent with pulmonary edema related to massive fluid resuscitation.

In the acute setting, arterial bleeding from organs or soft tissues must be managed immediately to prevent patient death. Blunt trauma can cause life-threatening hepatic, splenic, renal, or aortic trauma. Penetrating trauma likewise can result in arterial injury. Rapid surgery to stop bleeding or angiographic embolization are the two most common

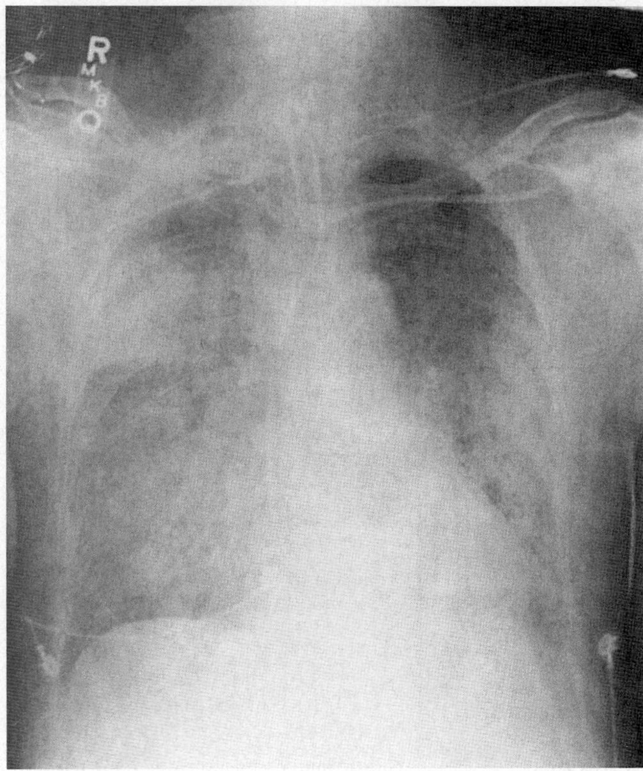

FIGURE 28.43. Pulmonary edema pattern with bilateral airspace opacification.

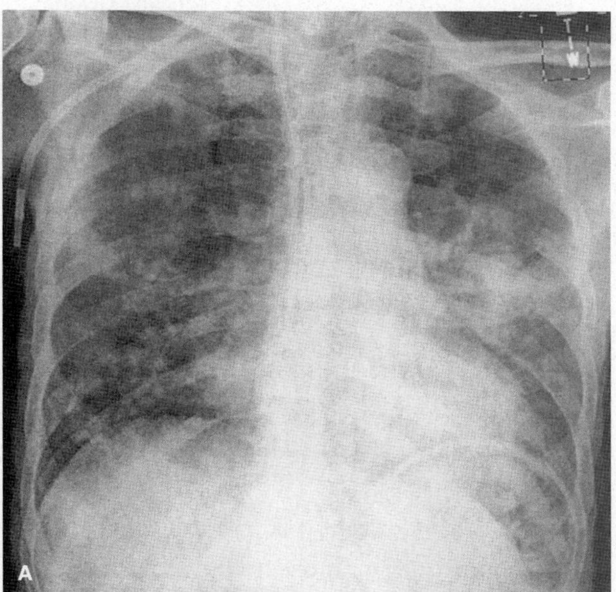

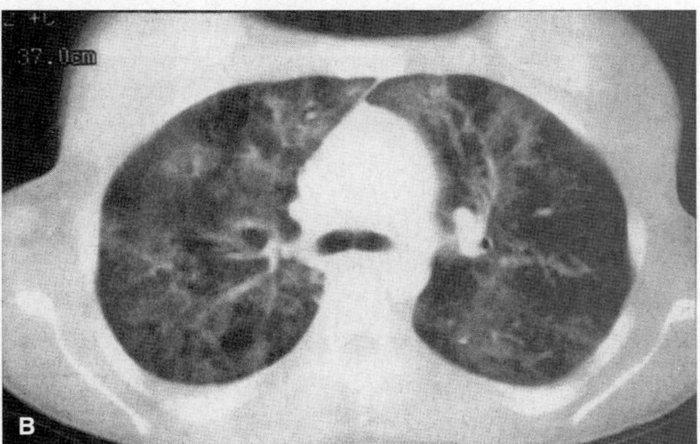

FIGURE 28.44. Chest radiograph and CT images of a patient with heart failure/fluid overload. Note the patchy bilateral parenchymal involvement.

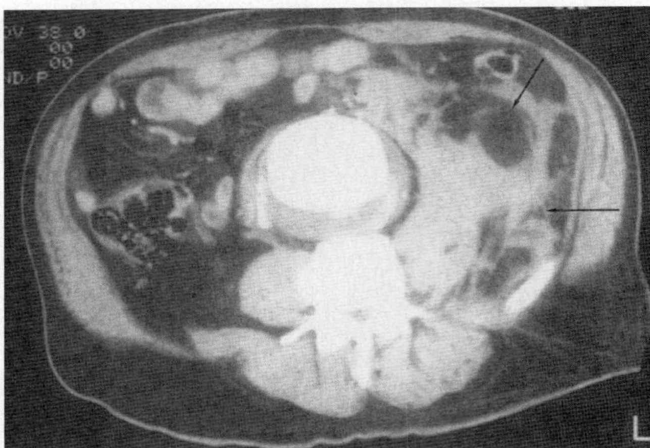

FIGURE 28.45. CT scan with intravenous contrast shows a large infrarenal aortic aneurysm and stranding (*arrows*) into the left retroperitoneum, indicating leakage around the aorta. This patient underwent emergent open repair.

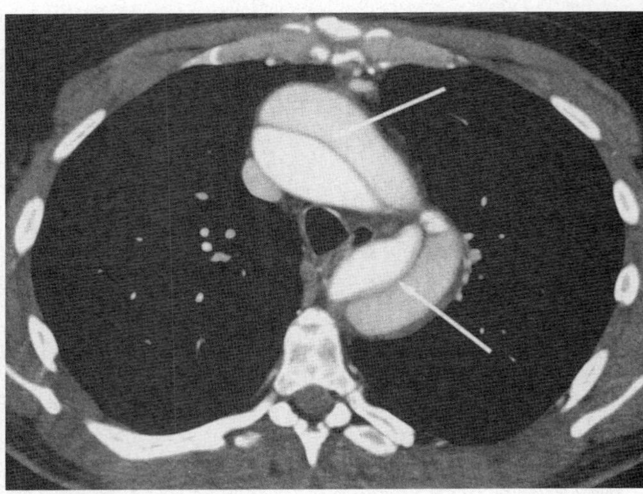

FIGURE 28.46. Aortic dissection is present in this case involving the ascending and descending thoracic aorta. The intimal flap separating the true and false lumen of the dissection is marked by *arrows*. Replacement of the aortic root and valve to minimize aortic insufficiency and cardiac tamponade was necessary.

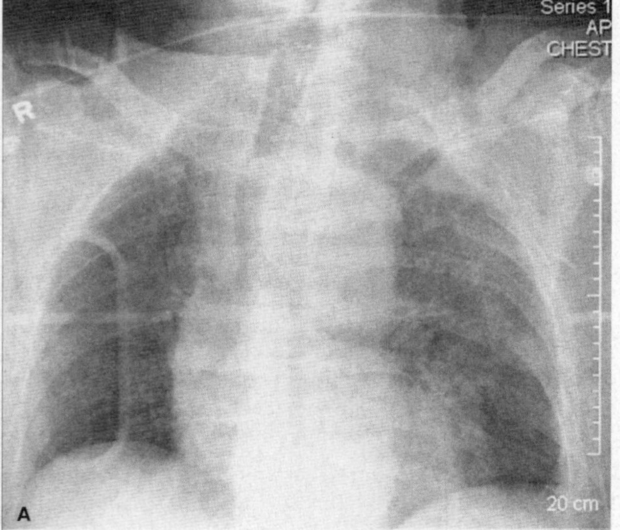

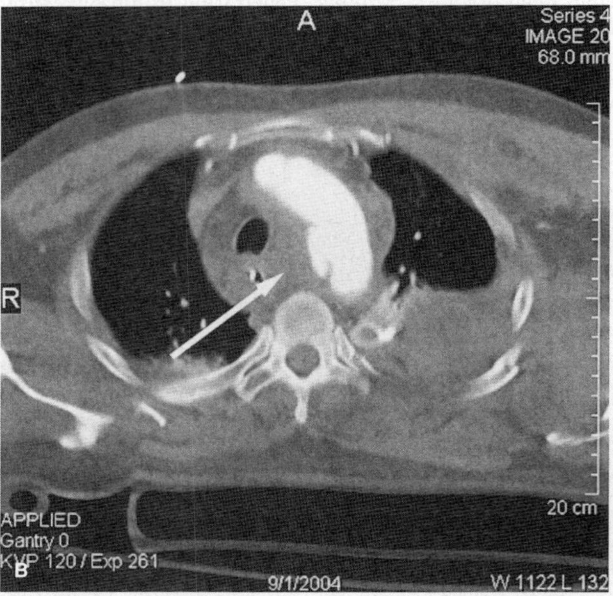

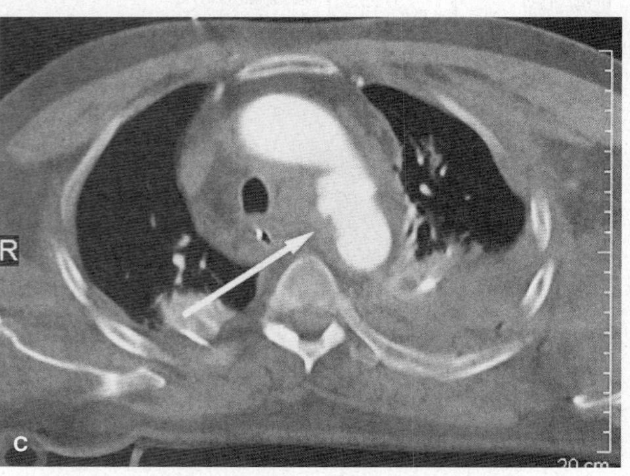

FIGURE 28.47. A–C: Acute aortic injury is identified here by recognition of the abnormal contour of the aorta (*arrows*) and the surrounding mediastinal hematoma. This is the typical site of aortic deceleration injury.

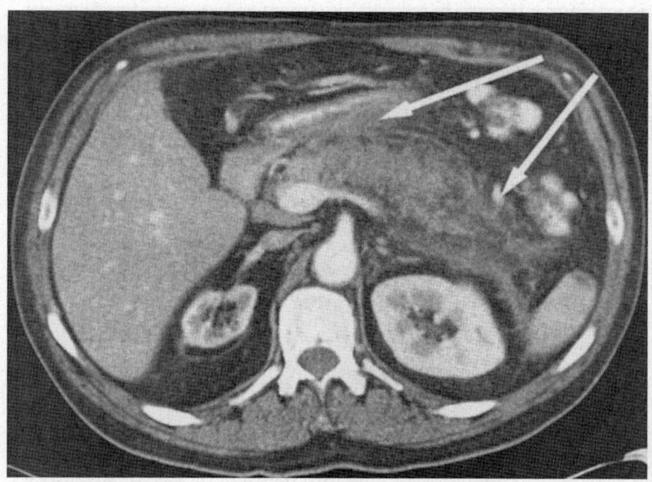

FIGURE 28.48. An acutely swollen edematous pancreas with peripancreatic stranding (*arrows*) is demonstrated in this case. Fluid resuscitation and electrolyte management were important features of this patient's care.

ways arterial bleeding is managed (Fig. 28.49). Critical neurological injuries that need emergent treatment are also evaluated during a trauma CT.

Postoperative Bleeding

Life-threatening hemorrhage may occur in an operative bed and result in rapid exsanguination. Immediate diagnostic imaging capabilities are essential in such cases to allow the diagnosis to be made and rapid repair efforts to occur (Fig. 28.50). Postoperative hemorrhage may be repaired by emergent surgery or embolization.

Sepsis/Septic Shock

Sepsis frequently occurs in ICU patients especially in the postoperative patient. CT scanning can identify sites of unsuspected abscess formation. Recognition and drainage of abscesses or fluid collections in the unstable septic patient can help treat the infection and improve a patients status (Fig. 28.51). Drainage procedures of the abscesses may be performed using percutaneous image-guided procedures or surgery. Some drainage procedures may be performed at the bedside on unstable

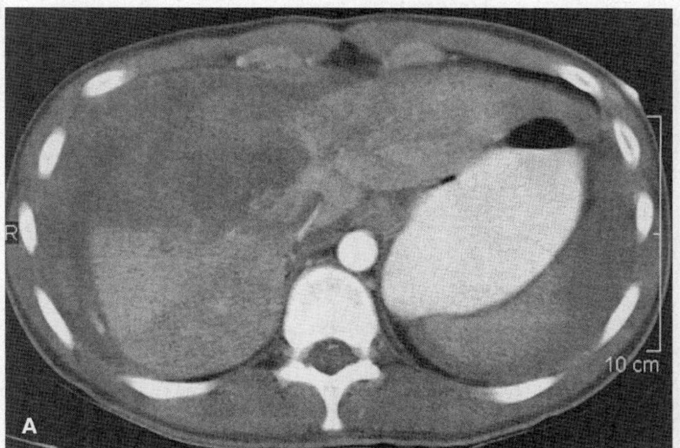

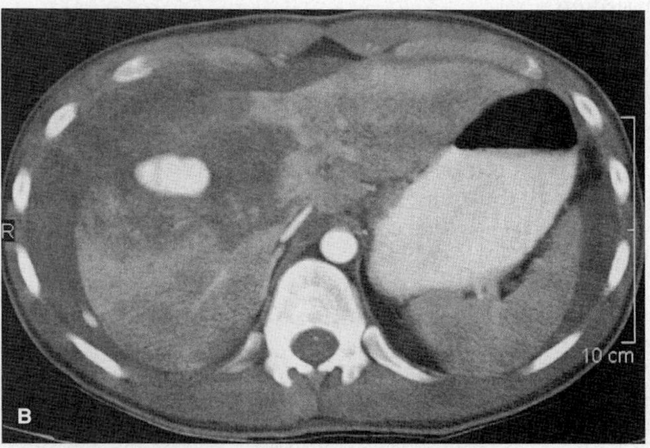

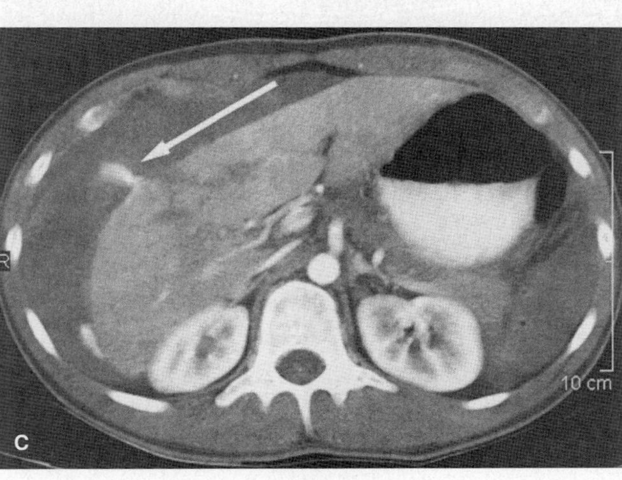

FIGURE 28.49. A–C: This 19-year-old man has a large liver laceration with active arterial extravasation. Contrast-laden blood is demonstrated squirting from the liver (*arrow*). Emergent surgery was necessary for control of the bleeding.

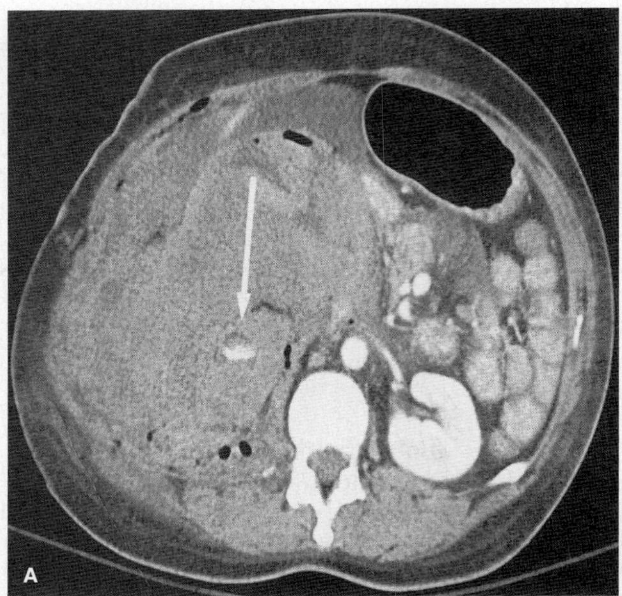

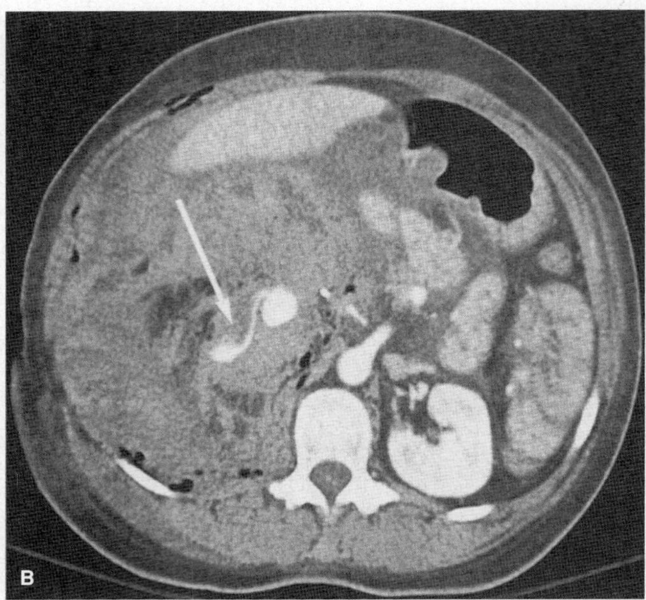

FIGURE 28.50. A and B: A large hematoma and active arterial extravasation (*arrows*) were obvious in this patient after radical nephrectomy for renal cell carcinoma. Arterial embolization was successful in halting the bleeding and stabilizing the patient.

patients using ultrasound. Other image-guided procedures require CT or fluoroscopy. Follow-up imaging after drainage will provide information regarding the efficacy of the drainage procedure.

Mesenteric Ischemia/Infarction

Patients with mesenteric ischemia may complain of severe abdominal pain, out of proportion to the clinical examination. Patients with mesenteric compromise may have elevated

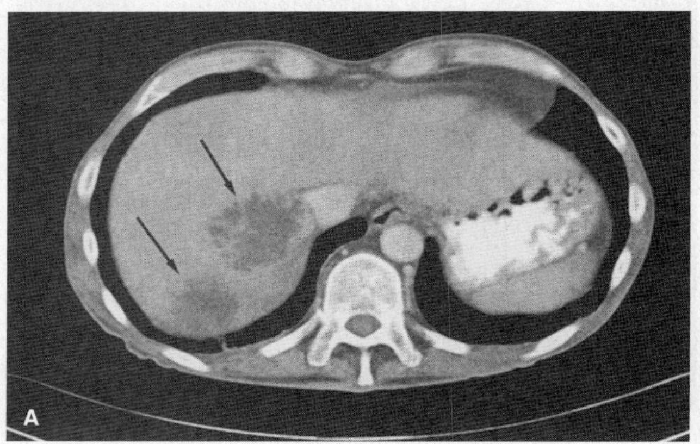

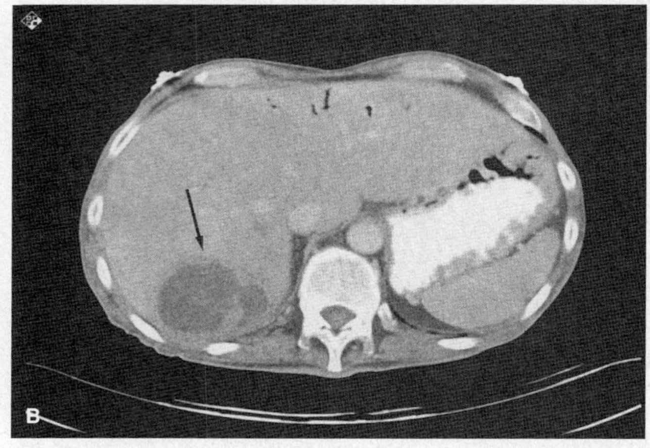

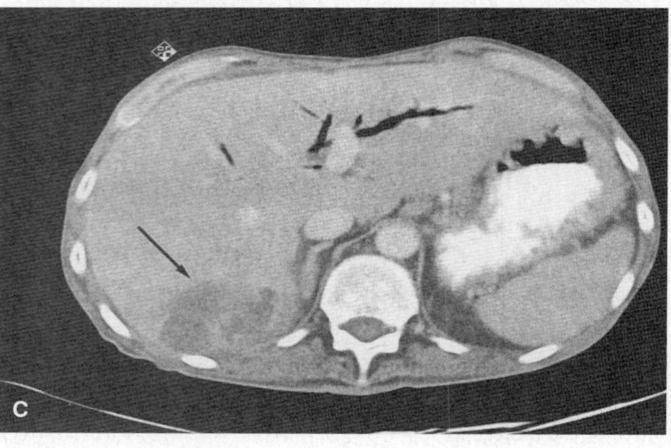

FIGURE 28.51. A–C: Multiple low-density liver lesions were identified (*arrows*) and eventually drained in this patient who presented with sepsis and hypotension related to cholangitis and liver abscesses.

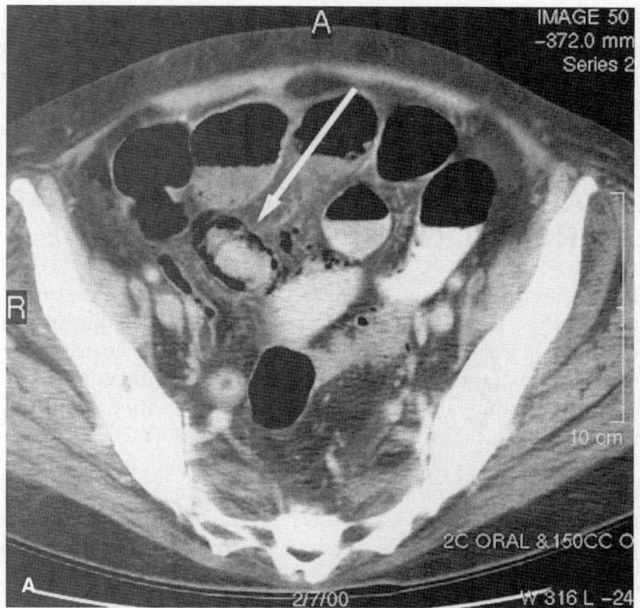

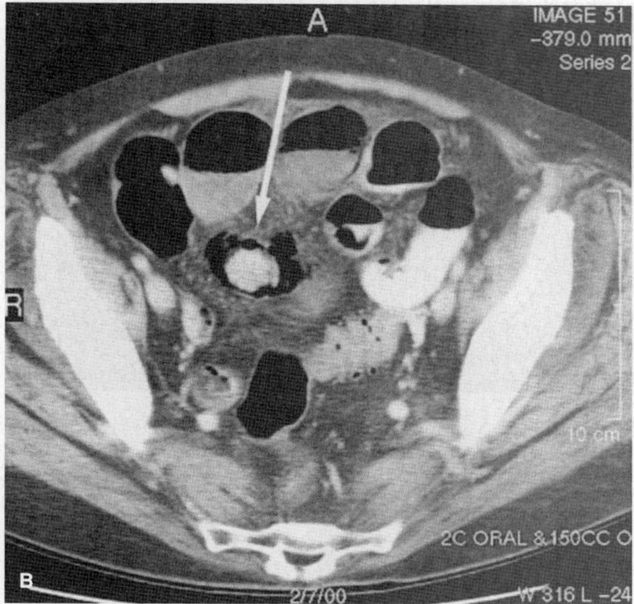

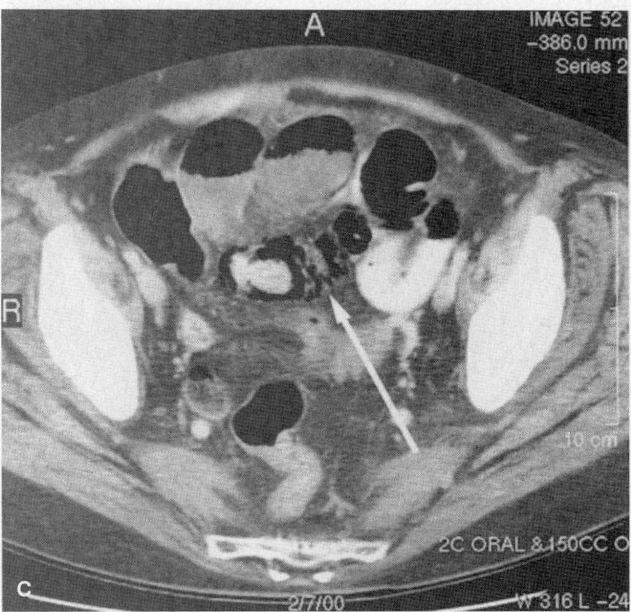

FIGURE 28.52. A–C: Multiple loops of small bowel are noted here to have air in the wall consistent with pneumatosis intestinalis (*arrows*). The patient's clinical status with septic parameters, hypotension, and elevated lactic acid levels made bowel ischemia likely. Necrotic bowel was resected at laparotomy.

lactic acid levels and elevated white blood cell counts. One often finds, in these cases, pre-existing risk factors such as severe atherosclerotic disease, emboli events secondary to atrial fibrillation, or profound episodes of global hypotension. Venous thrombosis is a less frequently encountered cause of mesenteric ischemia. Sometimes, vascular occlusion or an embolus can be seen in an artery of the gastrointestinal (GI) tract on contrast-enhanced CT. CT scanning may show pneumatosis intestinalis (air in the bowel wall), portal venous gas, or free air, all possible manifestations of bowel necrosis and infarction (Fig. 28.52). Patients with acute mesenteric ischemia do not necessarily show CT signs of bowel compromise and may benefit from surgical exploration to exclude mesenteric ischemia if the CT scan is unrevealing in the appropriate clinical setting. Pneumatosis intestinalis may be an innocuous finding, so correlation with the clinical situation should be made before the patient is taken to surgery.

Pulmonary Emboli

Significant emboli to the pulmonary arteries usually come from the legs or pelvis and may cause rapid patient decompensation. Many patients are at risk for the development of pulmonary emboli, especially after trauma, prolonged surgical procedures, and the hypercoagulability of malignancy. CT scanning of the chest with rapid infusion of intravenous contrast will allow the diagnosis and extent of pulmonary emboli to be evaluated so that appropriate therapy can be initiated (Figs. 28.53 and 28.54). Anticoagulation with heparin, low-molecular-weight heparinoids, and long-term Coumadin use are the most common ways pulmonary emboli are treated;

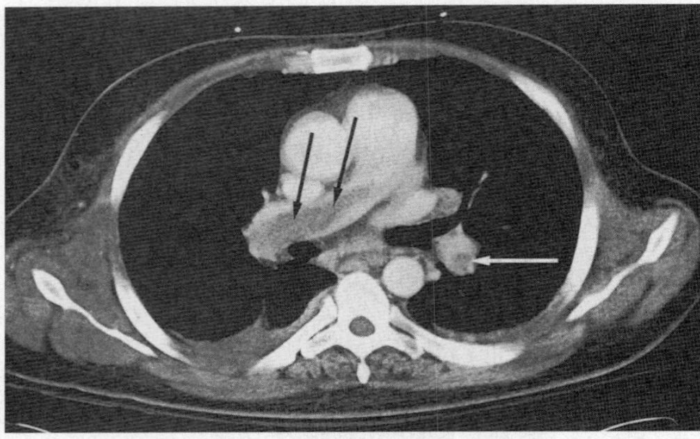

FIGURE 28.53. Multiple large filling defects (*arrows*) in the pulmonary arteries are present, consistent with pulmonary emboli. The patient's chest radiograph at this time was normal and clear.

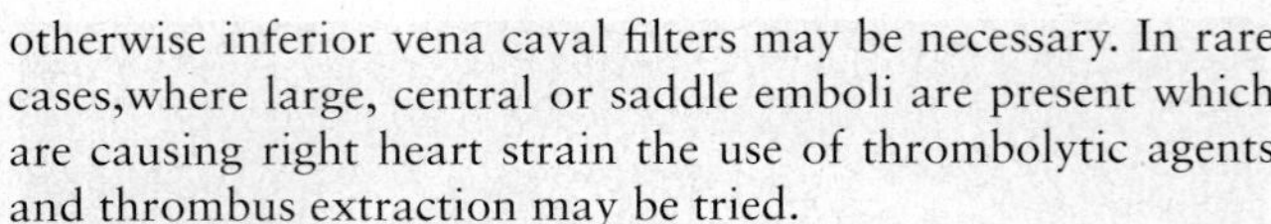

otherwise inferior vena caval filters may be necessary. In rare cases,where large, central or saddle emboli are present which are causing right heart strain the use of thrombolytic agents and thrombus extraction may be tried.

IMAGE-GUIDED INTERVENTIONAL PROCEDURES AT THE BEDSIDE

Image-guided procedures play a critical role in the care of patients in the ICU. Fluoroscopic or ultrasound decompression of the biliary tree or of an obstructed kidney may be necessary to manage a septic, obstructed patient. Some procedures will require that the patients be moved to the operative or fluoroscopic suite so that the procedure can be performed.

Bedside procedures to drain abscesses, fluid collections or chest tube placement can often be performed without moving the patient from the ICU. By keeping the patient in his or her bed, the critically ill patient remains surrounded by those who

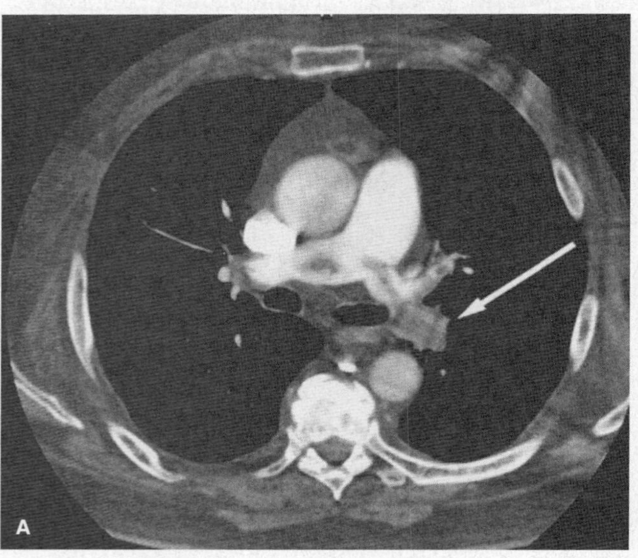

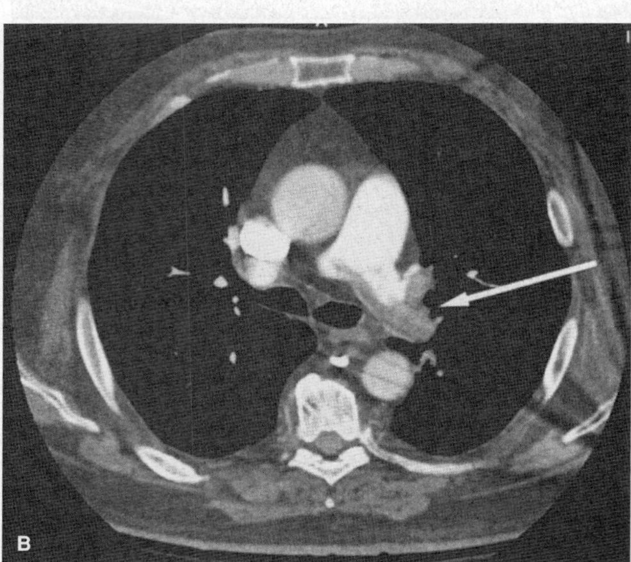

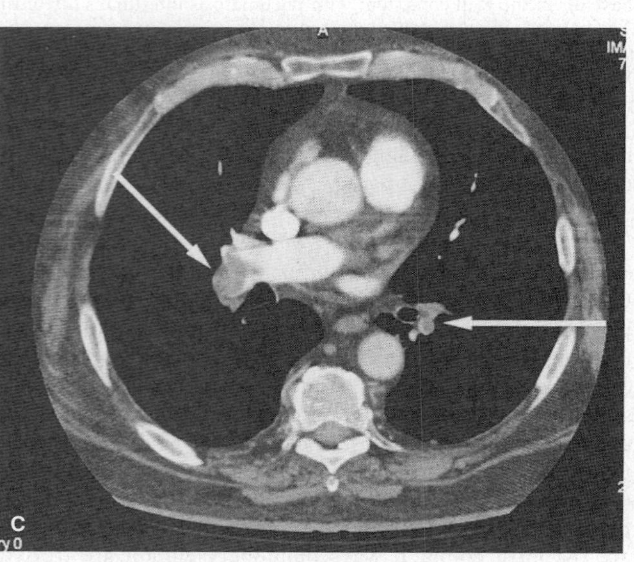

FIGURE 28.54. A–C: Another patient with massive pulmonary emboli (*arrows*).

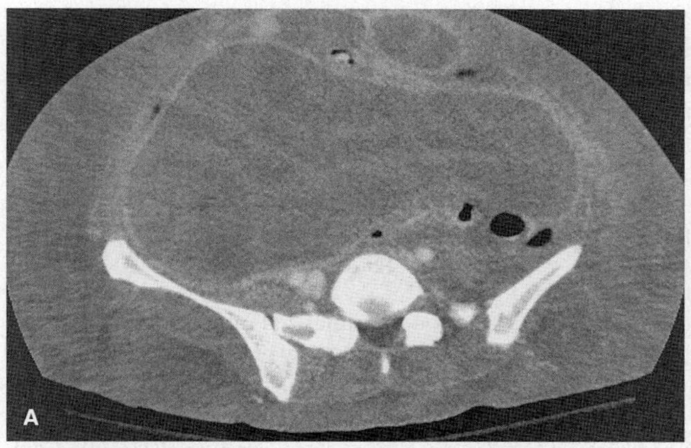

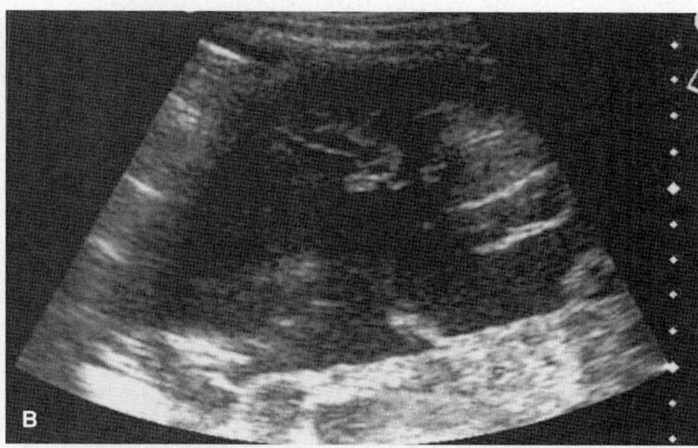

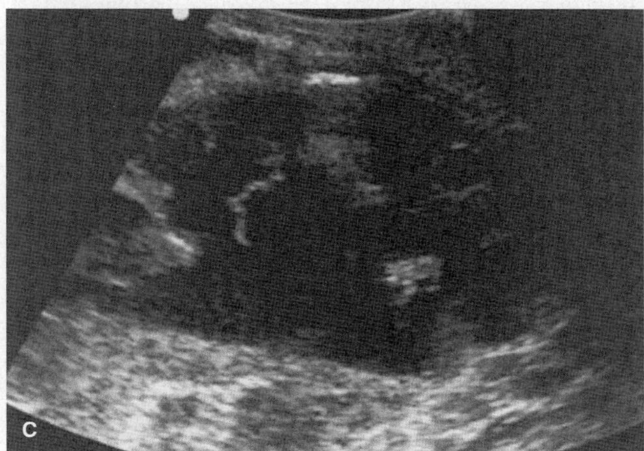

FIGURE 28.55. **A:** A large peripherally enhancing loculated collection was detected by CT but drained by ultrasound (**B** and **C**) in this unstable liver transplant recipient. Multiple septations and internal debris were present on ultrasound. Gram-negative rods were identified on Gram strain.

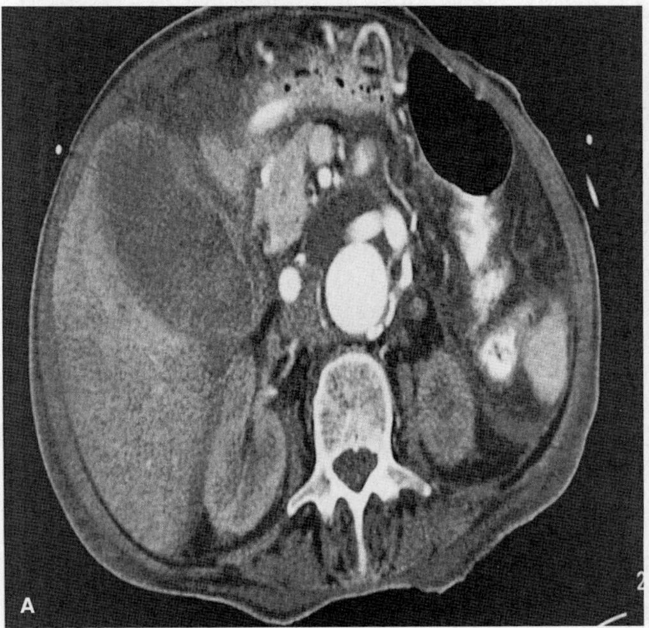

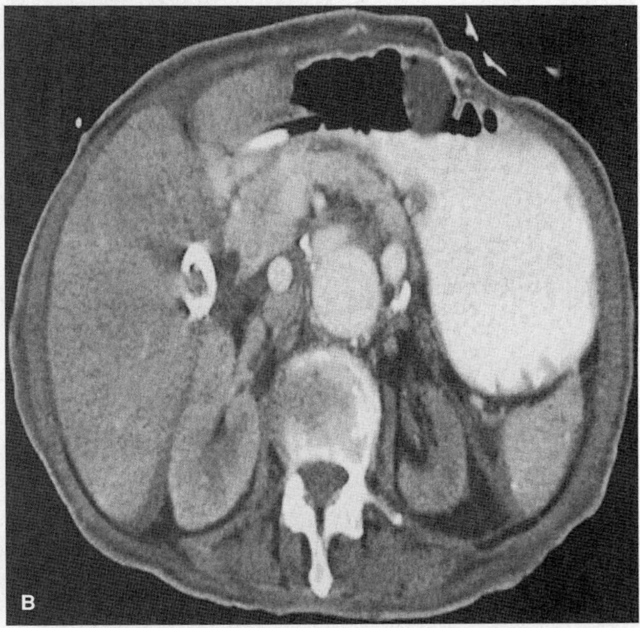

FIGURE 28.56. **A:** This postoperative patient became septic with positive blood cultures and elevation of white blood cell count. CT scanning showed a massively distended and sludge-filled gallbladder. Clinically, the gallbladder was palpable and tender. **B:** Postdrainage, the gallbladder is decompressed by a tube that goes through the liver. The material in the gallbladder was frankly purulent and grew *Staphylococcus aureus*.

know him medically the best—his nurses, respiratory therapists, and physicians. Any decompensation or change in patient status during the performance of the procedure can be dealt with by individuals familiar with the patient's care. Multiple transfers of the patient from bed to bed are eliminated if the patient remains in the unit. Dislodging important monitoring or support lines such as the endotracheal tube is less likely to occur if fewer transfers of the patient are made.

Bedside procedures on the critically ill patient are usually guided by ultrasound since it is a portable imaging modality. Ultrasound is ideal for localizing and draining large pleural effusions, large superficial fluid collections or abscesses, ascites, and gallbladder decompressions (Fig. 28.55). Air obscures the imaging efficacy of ultrasound, so pneumothorax, free air in the abdomen, or ileus with air-distended bowel makes ultrasound visualization limited. Some catheter placements deep in the pelvis or in posterior sites will require CT localization and will require the patient to be transported to the CT suite.

Ultrasound-guided procedures require that the patient be positioned to optimize visualization of the collection to be drained. The collection can be drained after it has been determined that the patient's coagulation factors are satisfactory (usually INR [international normalized ratio] of 1.5 or less and platelet count of 50,000 cells/microL or greater) and informed

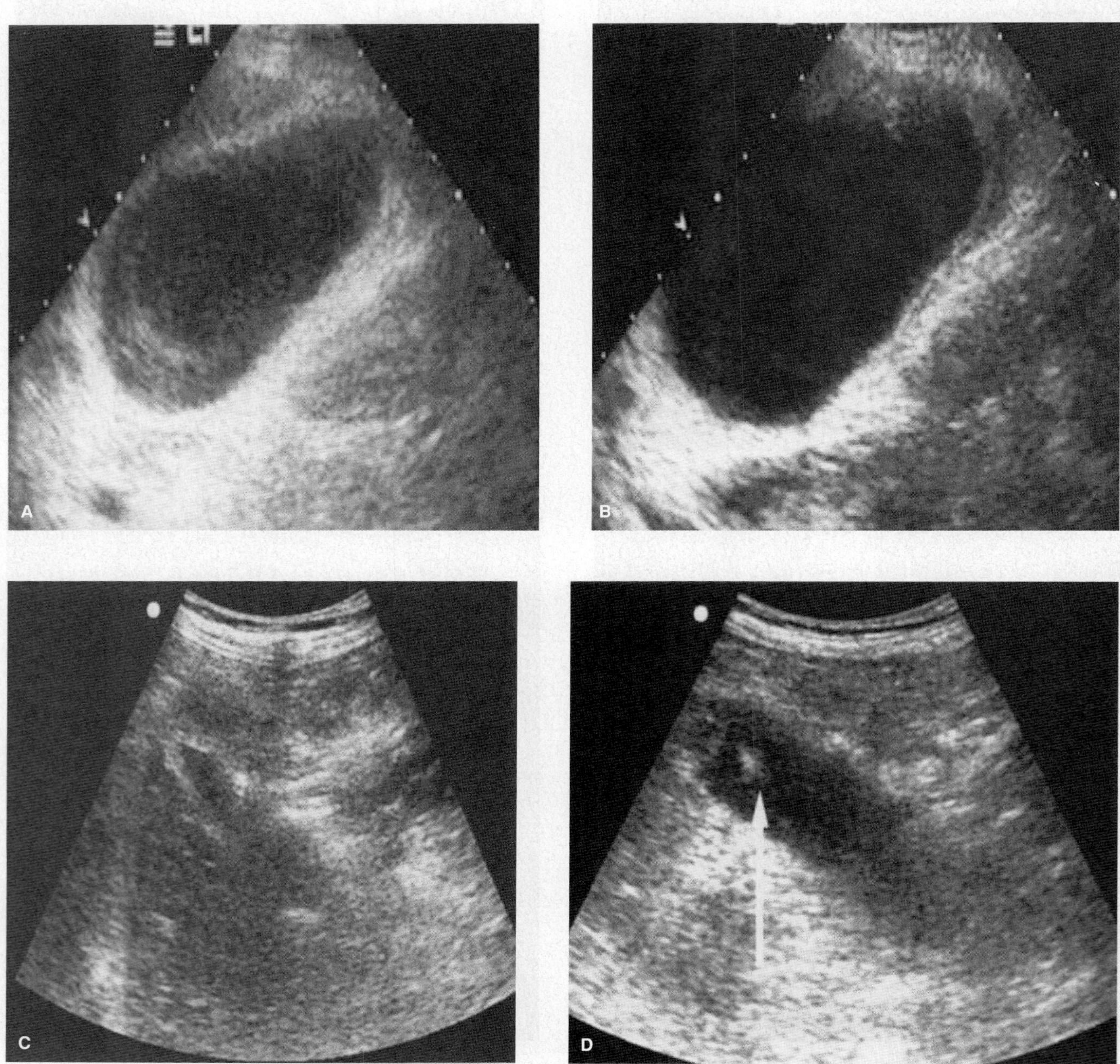

FIGURE 28.57. A distended gallbladder is visualized on bedside ultrasound (A and B). After the bedside drainage procedure (C and D), the gallbladder is decompressed and the drainage catheter is obvious within the lumen of the gallbladder (*arrow*). A small amount of liver has been traversed to place the drainage catheter.

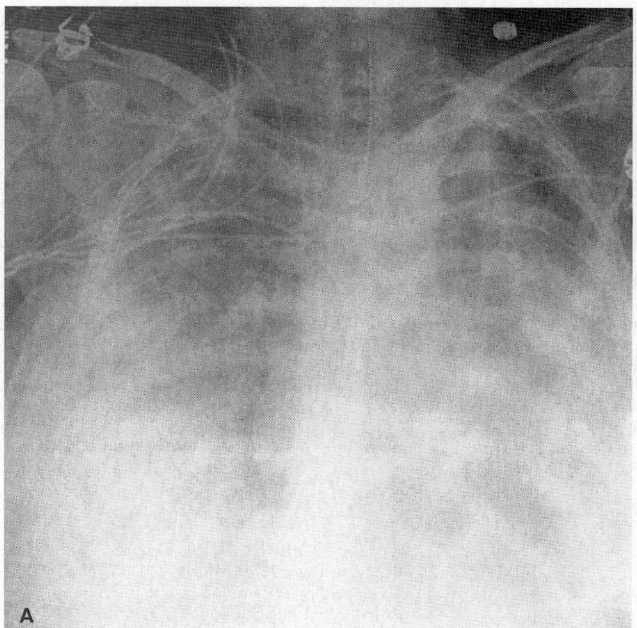

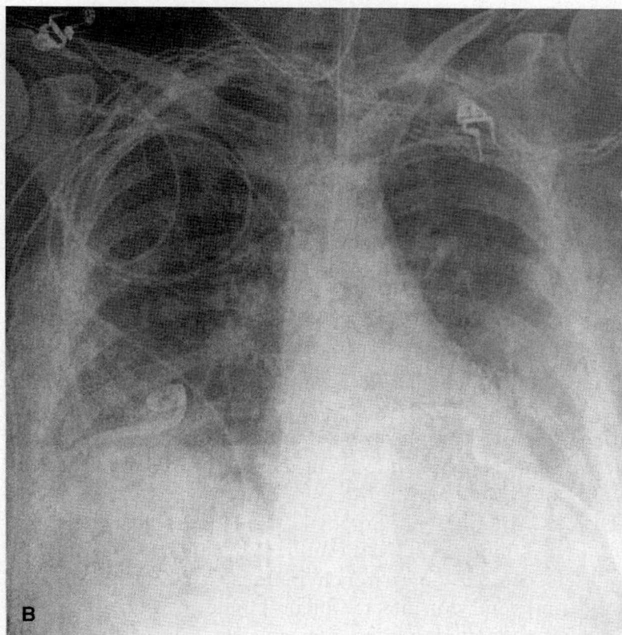

FIGURE 28.58. **A:** Large bilateral pleural effusions were successfully decompressed by placement of pleural drainage catheters. **B:** Note the resolution of the pleural densities with drainage. Catheter drainage helped ease the patient's respiratory distress.

consent is obtained. Collections are drained using the Seldinger technique. The collection is entered with a hollow needle, avoiding nearby vessels or organs. A guidewire is advanced into the collection. Several dilations are made over the guidewire, and a catheter is placed into the collection. Decompression of the collection is performed by manual withdrawal of the material. Jackson-Pratt suctioning is generally attached to the catheter for long-term suction. The material from the collection

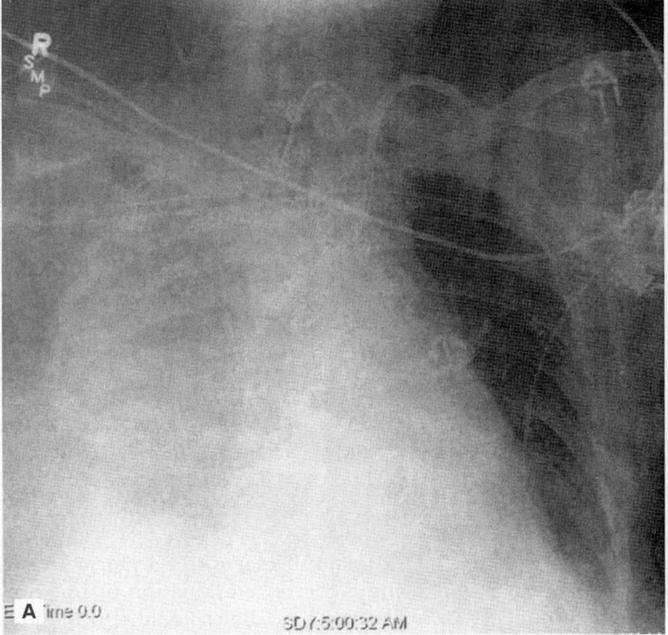

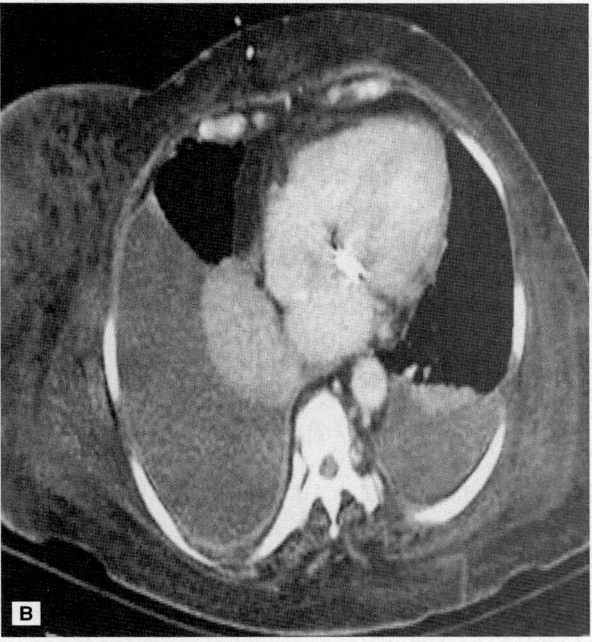

FIGURE 28.59. CT scanning showed a large pleural effusion with enhancement of the pleura consistent with an empyema, in a patient with fever and markedly elevated white blood cell count. Bedside drainage was performed and with the use of TPA and the percutaneous drainage catheter, 1,800 mL of serosanguineous fluid was withdrawn. Postprocedure chest radiograph showed remarkable clearing of the right chest. The infected fluid had a pH of less than 6.8. The patient's white blood cell count improved significantly after chest drainage.

can be sent for analysis, including Gram strain, culture and sensitivity, and chemistries such as amylase, lipase, and pH. Postprocedure imaging and clinical follow-up of the output of the drainage catheter will assess the efficacy of the drainage procedure.

Gallbladder decompression is generally performed on extremely ill, unstable, and septic patients with obstruction of their gallbladder either related to gallstones or acalculous cholecystitis. Gallbladder drainage is generally reserved for patients too unstable to undergo surgical removal of an obstructed and infected gallbladder who are thought to be septic with the gallbladder considered to be the source. Placement of gallbladder decompressive tubes should be through the liver into the gallbladder. The tube should be left in place for 6 to 8 weeks to minimize the chance of a bile leakage from the gallbladder. Possible complications of gallbladder drainage procedures include bile peritonitis, hemorrhage, or liver injury (Figs. 28.56 and 28.57).

Drainage of large pleural effusions may lessen the need for ventilatory support, allow the underlying lung to re-expand, and disclose underlying parenchymal disease (Figs. 28.58 and 28.59). Empyemas or infected pleural collections can be managed by image-guided tube placement to ensure complete drainage.

The critically ill patient in the ICU requires extensive and recurrent use of imaging to optimally diagnose and manage care. Diagnosis with portable chest radiographs or CT scans allow recognition of life-threatening conditions that require intervention. Bedside procedures usually with ultrasound guidance can not only be diagnostic but therapeutic as well.

Suggested Readings

Beaulieu Y, Marik PE. Bedside ultrasonography in the ICU: part 1. *Chest.* 2005; 128(2):881–895.

Beaulieu Y, Marik PE. Bedside ultrasonography in the ICU: part 2. *Chest.* 2005; 128(3):1766–1781. Review.

Bouhemad B, Zhang M, Lu Q, et al. Clinical review: bedside lung ultrasound in critical care practice. *Crit Care.* 2007;11(1):205.

Goodman LR, Putman CE. *Critical Care Imaging.* Philadelphia, PA: WB Saunders; 1992.

Hanley DF. Review of critical care and emergency approaches to stroke. *Stroke.* 2003;34(2):362–364.

Henschke CI, Yankelevitz DF, Wand A, et al. Accuracy and efficacy of chest radiography in the intensive care unit. *Radiol Clin North Am.* 1996;34(1):21–31.

Henschke CI, Yankelevitz DF, Wand A, et al. Chest radiography in the ICU. *Clin Imaging.* 1997;21(2):90–103.

Hobbs G, Mahajan R. *Imaging in Anaesthesia and Critical Care.* Philadelphia, PA: Churchill Livingstone; 2000.

Hopkins R, Peden C, Ghandi S. *Radiology for Anaesthesia and Intensive Care.* Greenwich Medical Media, 2002.

Imaging of the intensive care unit patient. *Clin Chest Med.* 1991;12(1):169–198.

Miller WT Jr, Tino G, Friedburg JS. Thoracic CT in the intensive care unit: assessment of clinical usefulness. *Radiology.* 1998;209(2):491–498.

Peruzzi W, Garner W, Bools J, et al. Pleural effusions in the critically ill: the evolving role of bedside ultrasound. *Crit Care Med.* 2005;33(8):1874–1875.

Peruzzi W, Garner W, Bools J, et al. Portable chest roentgenography and computed tomography in critically ill patients. *Chest.* 1988;93(4):722–726.

Primack S, Chiles C, Putman CE. Thoracic imaging in the intensive care unit. *Clin Intensive Care.* 1991;2(1):26–40.

Ravin CE, ed. *Imaging and Invasive Radiology in the Intensive Care Unit.* Philadelphia, PA: Churchill Livingstone; 1993.

Roddy LH, Unger KM, Miller WC. Thoracic computed tomography in the critically ill patient. *Crit Care Med.* 1981;9(7):515–518.

Singh V, McCartney JP, Hemphill JC 3rd. Transcranial Doppler ultrasonography in the neurologic intensive care unit. *Neurol India.* 2001;49(Suppl 1):S81–89.

Snow N, Bergin KT, Horrigan TP. Thoracic CT scanning in critically ill patients. Information obtained frequently alters management. *Chest.* 1990;97(6): 1467–1470.

Swensen SJ, Peters SG, LeRoy AJ, et al. Radiology in the intensive-care unit. *Mayo Clin Proc.* 1991;66(4):396–410.

Tocino I. Chest imaging in the intensive care unit. *Eur J Radiol.* 1996;23(1):46–57.

Trotman-Dickenson B. Radiology in the intensive care unit: part I. *J Intensive Care Med.* 2003;18(4):198–210.

Trotman-Dickenson B. Radiology in the intensive care unit: part 2. *J Intensive Care Med.* 2003;18(5):239–252.

Underwood GH Jr, Newell JD 2nd. Pulmonary radiology in the intensive care unit. *Med Clin North Am.* 1983;67(6):1305–1324.

Wiener MD, Garay SM, Leitman BS, et al. Computed tomography of the chest in the intensive care unit. *Crit Care Clin.* 1994;10(2):267–275.

CHAPTER 29 ■ NEUROIMAGING OF THE CRITICAL CARE PATIENT

JEFFREY A. BENNETT • CHRISTOPHER J. KREBS • DAVID V. SMULLEN

INTRODUCTION

Appropriate care of the critically ill patient depends on rapid, accurate diagnosis. The tremendous advances in computed tomography (CT) and magnetic resonance imaging (MRI) technology enable sophisticated studies to be performed swiftly and help to achieve this goal in patients who are often unable to provide a history or remain immobile for long periods. Software allows thin-section axial CT images to be reformatted in any plane, enabling a more complete evaluation of fractures and soft tissue abnormalities. Three-dimensional reformations of contrast-enhanced CT angiograms provide outstanding images of cerebral aneurysms and other vascular abnormalities, which can be rotated to match what will be seen from a surgical approach. Anatomic imaging can also be supplemented with physiologic data obtained with CT, MRI, and nuclear medicine. This provides information about phenomena such as cerebral blood flow, cerebrospinal fluid (CSF) flow, or the rate and direction of diffusion of water in soft tissues. This type of data can clarify diagnoses such as brain infarction or abscesses, and can be used to investigate the effects of hydrocephalus, vasospasm, and brain herniation. The images also provide valuable prognostic information.

The process of neuroradiologic interpretation is complex. Excellent image quality is essential, and, to this end, the examination should be tailored to the clinical indication, with an appropriate selection of imaging parameters such as field of view and timing of intravenous contrast injection. The accurate interpretation of the images obtained then depends on a thorough knowledge of anatomy, normal anatomic variations, and pathophysiology. A basic knowledge of medical physics is also required to understand the imaging characteristics of both normal and abnormal tissues. Excellent communication between the radiologist and clinician is essential, as all radiologic studies must be interpreted in clinical context. It should be kept in mind that the hardest thing for the radiologist to do in real-time practice is to label a study as *normal* with great confidence. The consequences of incorrectly classifying a study normal could be, obviously, very grave. This chapter does not attempt to teach the process of ruling out pathology, but rather serves as an introduction to the use of both standard and advanced imaging techniques as applied to the critically ill, neurologically compromised patient. The focus is on classic imaging findings of the brain, head and neck, and spine in the acute setting.

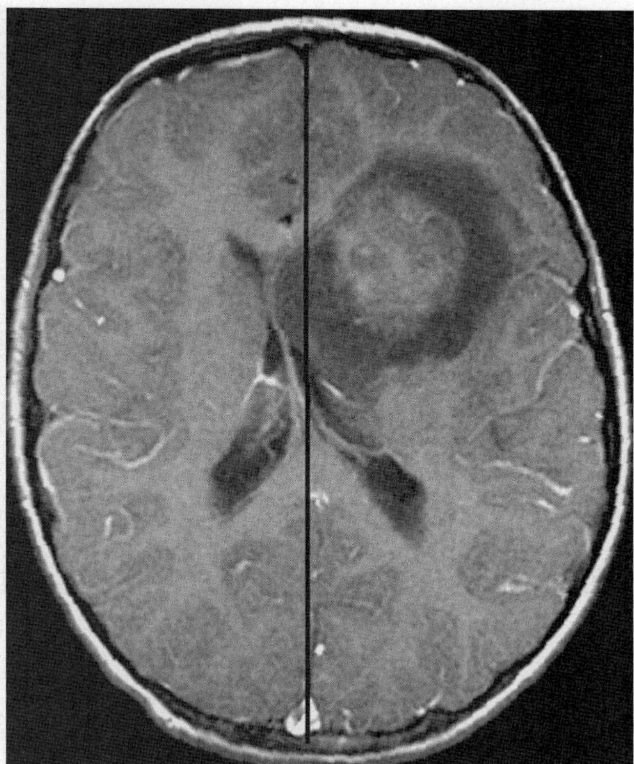

FIGURE 29.1. Postcontrast axial T1 magnetic resonance. A large left frontal mass results in subfalcine herniation with shift of the ventricles and septum pellucidum to the right across midline (*black line*).

HERNIATION SYNDROMES

A full description of any lesion includes location—for example, extra-axial, intra-axial, or intraventricular—size, density on CT or intensity on MRI with respect to normal tissue, the presence or absence of contrast enhancement, and the effect on surrounding structures. Many intracranial processes require immediate treatment to preserve brain function, and the urgency of any radiologic finding depends largely on the mass effect on normal neural tissue. This assessment must be made for all of the lesions subsequently described, and therefore is discussed first. The basic principle that allows this concept to be understood is that the brain and spinal cord are incompressible, and are contained in the confined space of the skull and spinal canal. Any abnormality, such as a hematoma, tumor, or edema, adds volume to this confined space and increases pressure, with the result that important normal structures are displaced. Initially, sulci in the region of the abnormality become compressed; with increasing mass effect, brain herniation occurs. Several distinct herniation syndromes have been described.

Subfalcine Herniation

This refers to brain that is shifted across the midline underneath the falx cerebri (Fig. 29.1). This tends to be more pronounced anteriorly, as the connections of the falx to the tentorium posteriorly are stronger and relatively immobile. There is compression of the ipsilateral lateral ventricle, and the contralateral temporal horn can become trapped and dilated as CSF continues to be produced there. This type of herniation can result in an anterior cerebral artery (ACA) territory infarct if the ACA is compressed against the dura. This is more likely to occur the more severe the midline shift, especially if greater than 1 cm.

Transtentorial Herniation

This can occur in two separate directions, downward or upward, with respect to the incisura, which is an opening in the dura through which the brainstem passes. The plane of the incisura can be approximated on midline sagittal images by drawing a line from the dorsum sella to the junction of the vein of Galen and straight sinus (Fig. 29.2A). This line should normally bisect the interpeduncular fossa and tectum. The splenium of the corpus callosum should lie above this line. When there is downward transtentorial herniation from a supratentorial mass, the optic chiasm will be displaced toward the sella, the interpeduncular fossa will be compressed, the brainstem will appear buckled, and the splenium of the corpus callosum will lie below the plane of the incisura (Fig. 29.2B). When there is upward transtentorial herniation, usually from a cerebellar mass, the brainstem will be compressed against the clivus, the fourth ventricle will be compressed, and brainstem structures will become superiorly displaced with respect to the plane of the incisura.

On axial images, transtentorial herniation can be assessed by evaluating the circum mesencephalic cisterns. With downward transtentorial herniation, the ambient cisterns and suprasellar cistern will become effaced (Fig. 29.3). When there is upward transtentorial herniation, the quadrigeminal plate

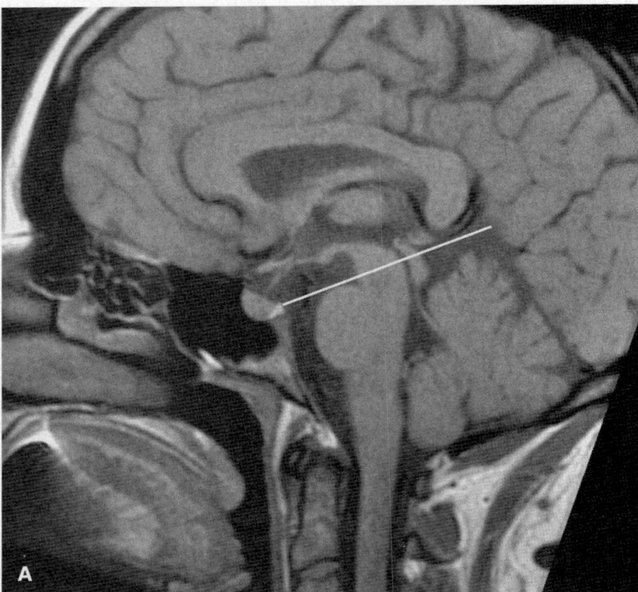

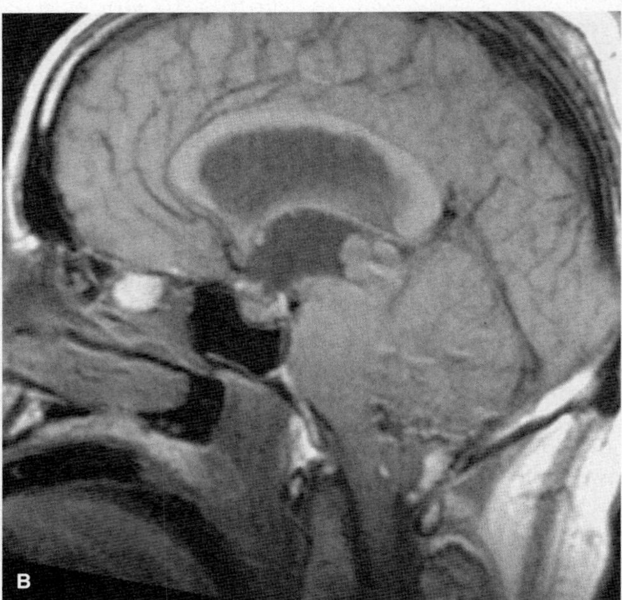

FIGURE 29.2. **A:** Normal midline sagittal T1 magnetic resonance (MR). The plane of the incisura (*white line*) runs from the posterior sella to the junction of the vein of Galen and the straight sinus. **B:** Sagittal T1 weighted MR. A large tectal mass resulting in hydrocephalus and downward transtentorial herniation. Here, a line drawn along the plane of the incisura would intersect the splenium of the corpus callosum and pass above the interpeduncular fossa.

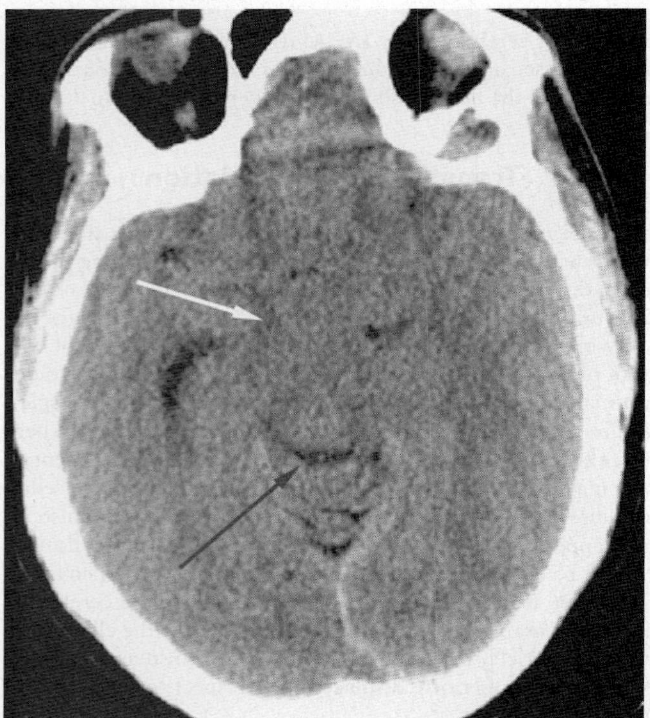

FIGURE 29.3. Axial computed tomography image in a patient with supratentorial mass effect resulting in downward transtentorial herniation. There is effacement of the suprasellar and ambient cisterns (*white arrow*) with preservation of the quadrigeminal plate cistern (*black arrow*).

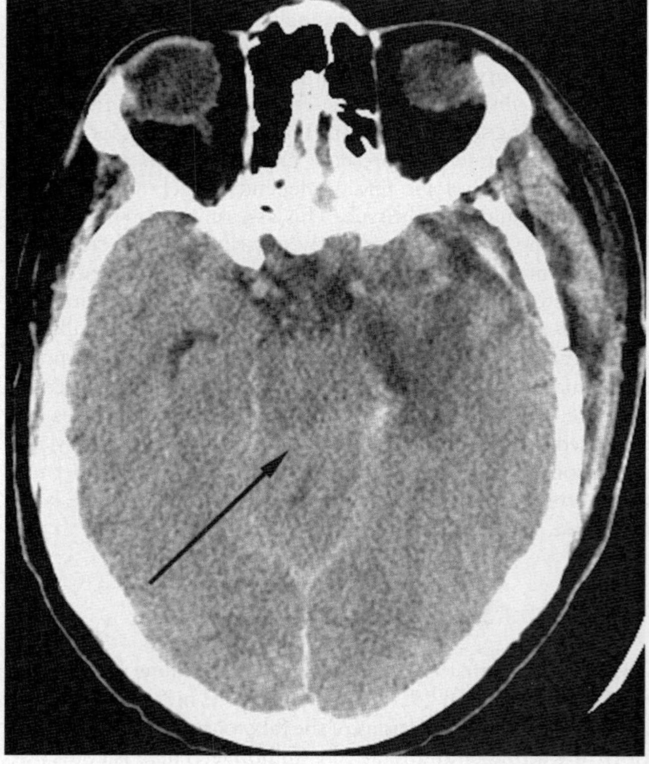

FIGURE 29.4. Axial computed tomography image in a patient with posterior fossa mass effect resulting in upward transtentorial herniation. Notice the effacement of the quadrigeminal plate cistern (*arrow*).

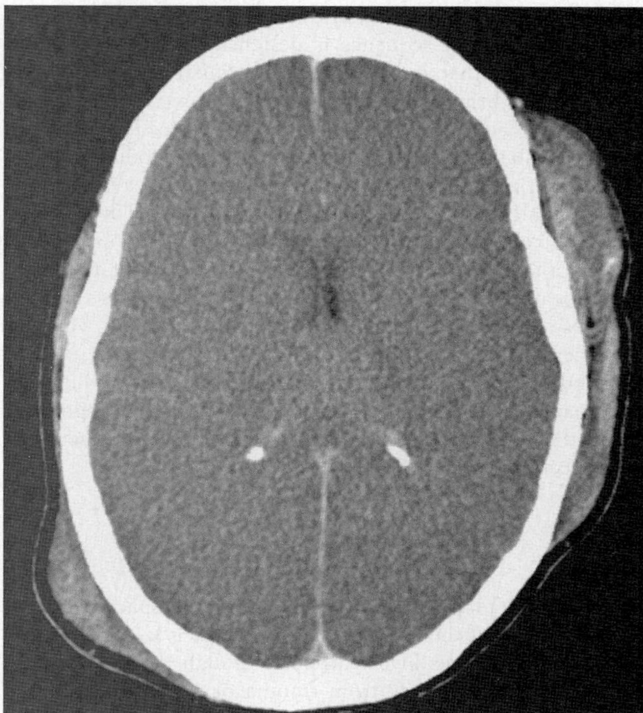

FIGURE 29.5. Axial noncontrast computed tomography. There is diffuse brain edema with loss of normal gray–white differentiation, effacement of the sulci, and compression of the ventricles.

cistern becomes effaced (Fig. 29.4). Uncal herniation, a subtype of downward transtentorial herniation, usually occurs as a result of a middle cranial fossa mass, and is recognized by the mesial portion of the temporal lobe, the uncus, displaced into the suprasellar cistern, causing effacement of the crural cistern.

Transtentorial herniation can cause vascular complications from compression of major arteries against the dura. Infarcts in both the anterior and posterior circulation can result. Postherniation hemorrhage can also occur when the mass effect resolves and the occluded vessel reperfuses. In the brainstem, these hemorrhages are referred to as *Duret hemorrhages*.

Tonsillar Herniation

This typically occurs as a result of a posterior fossa mass, and is recognized by the cerebellar tonsils being displaced through the foramen magnum. This can result in fourth ventricular outlet obstruction and hydrocephalus.

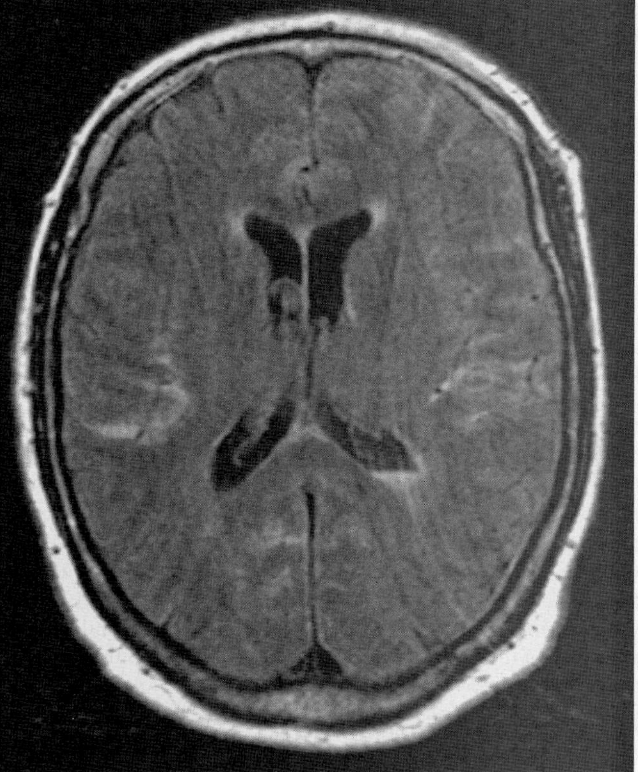

FIGURE 29.7. Axial fluid-attenuated inversion recovery magnetic resonance. Subarachnoid blood is present as bright signal in the sylvian fissures and sulci. A small amount of intraventricular hemorrhage is seen layering dependently in the left lateral ventricle.

BRAIN EDEMA

There are two types of brain edema, vasogenic and cytotoxic. *Cytotoxic edema* occurs with cell damage, as is seen with stroke. Cytotoxic edema is best detected with diffusion-weighted MR images. *Vasogenic edema* occurs with leakage of fluid into the extracellular space, and is a common finding associated with many lesions, including neoplasms and infection. Diffuse brain edema is recognized by loss of gray–white

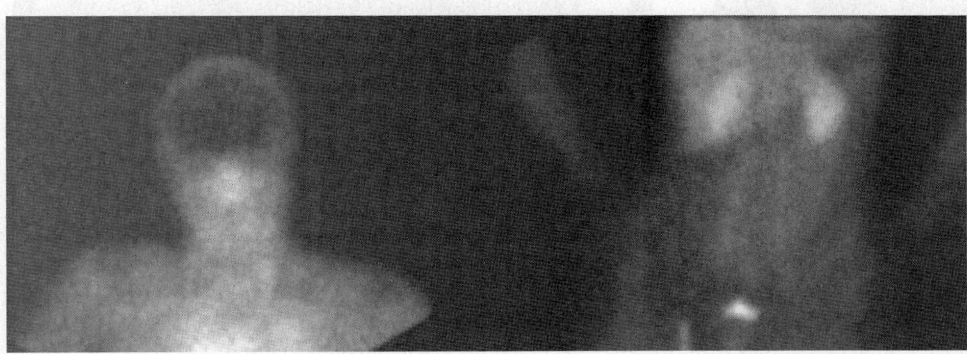

FIGURE 29.6. Tc-99m diethylene triamine penta-acetate brain death study. Projection images demonstrate no evidence of intracranial blood flow. There is increased activity over the nasal region (the "hot nose" sign commonly seen in brain death due to persistent external carotid arterial flow). Images from over the abdomen indicate perfusion of both kidneys, important information in a potential organ donor.

differentiation, effacement of sulci and cisterns, and slitlike ventricles (Fig. 29.5).

The intracranial vascular compartment, unlike the brain itself, is compressible, and so a mass within the confined space of the cranial vault that increases intracranial pressure will have a detrimental effect on the vascular compartment. Normally, there is a reserve volume and autoregulation ensures continued adequate blood flow to the brain despite increased intracranial pressure. However, this only works up to a point. Once intracranial pressure exceeds the capacity for blood to flow to the brain, brain death occurs. A nuclear medicine brain death study, often performed with Tc-99m diethylene triamine pentaacetate (DTPA), can be used to assess the presence of intracranial blood flow (Fig. 29.6).

INTRACRANIAL HEMORRHAGE

Noncontrast CT is the study of choice in the evaluation of acute intracranial hemorrhage, as it is a rapid, accessible test, which produces good contrast between the high-attenuating (bright) clot and the low-attenuating (dark) CSF. MRI is also very sensitive for the detection of blood products, and the appearance of the blood on different sequences can be used to date the hemorrhage. Fluid-attenuated inversion recovery (FLAIR) images provide good conspicuity of acute subarachnoid hemorrhage, as compared with conventional T1- and T2-weighted images. The FLAIR sequence is designed to suppress signal from the CSF so that it will appear dark. Subarachnoid hemorrhage appears bright on FLAIR images, and so becomes readily apparent (Fig. 29.7). The gradient recalled echo (GRE) sequence is also useful for the detection of blood products, as the hemoglobin affects the magnetic field in such a way as to decrease signal, the so-called *susceptibility artifact*. Thus, blood appears black on GRE images.

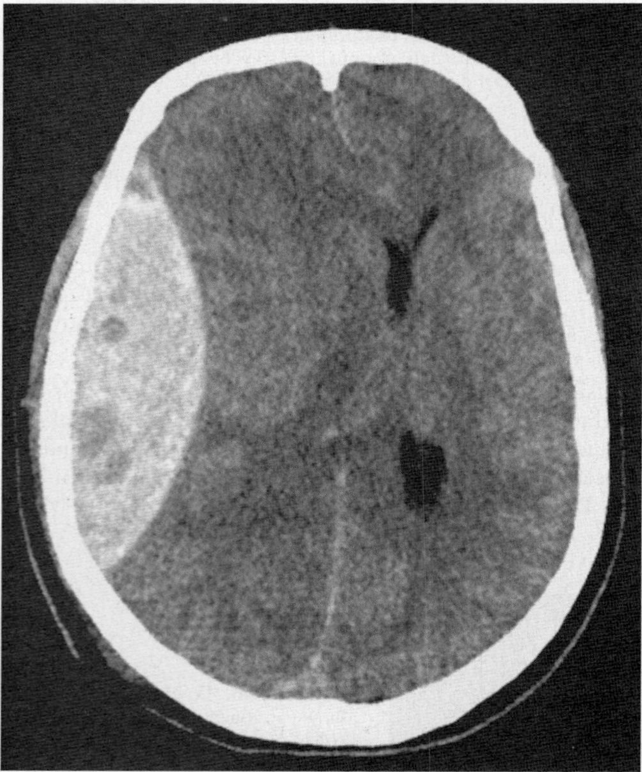

FIGURE 29.8. Axial noncontrast computed tomography. Large right epidural hematoma with significant mass effect resulting in subfalcine herniation. Note the classic biconvex shape as the blood is confined by the frontoparietal suture anteriorly and the parieto-occipital suture posteriorly. There was an associated parietal bone fracture (not visualized on this image).

As with all intracranial lesions, it is important to accurately localize hemorrhage on the imaging study, as this determines appropriate further workup and treatment. Moving from the outside in, this location can be extra-axial (i.e., epidural, subdural, or subarachnoid), intra-axial (i.e., involving the brain parenchyma itself), or intraventricular. The recognition of blood in each of these sites, and its implication, is discussed in this section.

Epidural Hematoma

An epidural hematoma occurs in the potential space between the inner table of the calvaria and the dura. It usually results from injury to a meningeal artery, although it can occur as a result of venous injury from trauma or surgery. The most common etiology is a skull fracture that crosses the middle meningeal artery, resulting in a temporal epidural hematoma. The arterial pressure is sufficient to separate the bone from the dura except at the sutures where the dura is very tightly adherent. This results in the classic biconvex shape of the

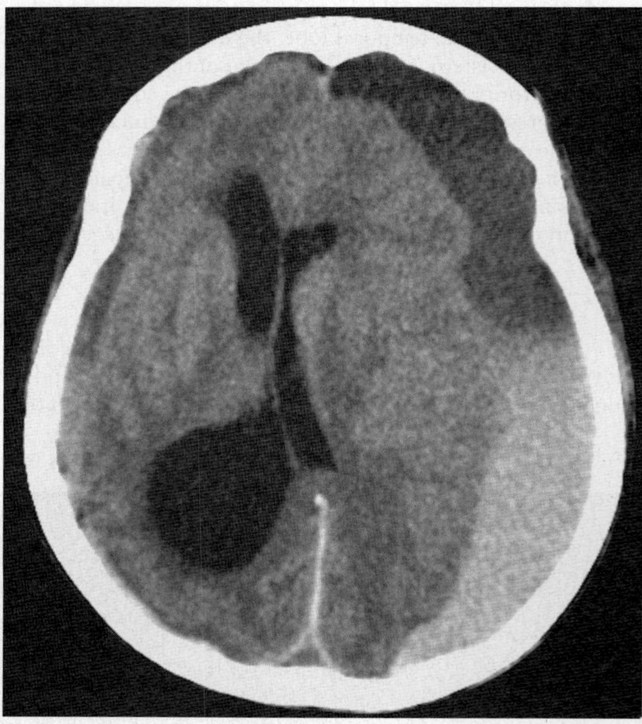

FIGURE 29.9. Axial noncontrast computed tomography. Bilateral subdural hematomas, left greater than right. There is a fluid–fluid level on the left secondary to settling out of the blood products as the patient was in a prolonged supine position.

hemorrhage, which is confined by suture lines (Fig. 29.8). An epidural hematoma can continue to expand and result in considerable mass effect, brain herniation, and death; it is, therefore, a surgical emergency.

Subdural Hematoma

A subdural hematoma is located between the dura mater and the arachnoid, and usually results from tearing of bridging veins that course from the cortex to the dura. It is differentiated from an epidural hematoma in that it crosses sutures and has a crescent shape (Fig. 29.9). The etiology can be trauma, especially when there is rotational shear injury, but may also be secondary to a coagulopathy. Subdural hematomas are more common in elderly patients, where atrophy has resulted in a stretching of the bridging veins, predisposing them to injury.

Subarachnoid Hemorrhage

The "worst headache of my life" should bring to mind a subarachnoid hemorrhage (SAH). This type of hemorrhage is located between the arachnoid and pia mater, and therefore is detected on imaging studies as blood filling the sulci and basilar cisterns (Fig. 29.10). Small-volume or subacute SAH may not be detectable with CT, and therefore a lumbar puncture to look for xanthochromia may still be warranted, although MRI can also be used to detect subtle SAH. Once an SAH has been diagnosed, an investigation of its cause is necessary. The leading cause is aneurysmal rupture. Arterial venous malformation (AVM) is a less common etiology. The most appropriate initial imaging study to search for a vascular abnormality is CT angiography (CTA). This is a minimally invasive study that requires a rapid injection of intravenous contrast at 4 to 6 mL/sec, and thin-section helical CT imaging in the arterial phase. A volume of data is produced that can be reformatted in any plane or in three dimensions, thus facilitating a thorough search for the location, size, and orientation of an aneurysm (Fig. 29.11), or an analysis of an AVM including feeding arteries, draining veins, and any associated flow-related aneurysms. Twenty percent of patients with an aneurysm will have more than one. The location of the SAH, as well as an irregular shape of an aneurysm, can help identify which aneurysm has ruptured and which one must therefore be secured first. If an underlying etiology cannot be identified, a conventional angiogram is warranted. If this also is negative, the patient should be reimaged in 1 week to look for possible recanalization of a thrombosed aneurysm. This can be done with CTA or digital subtraction angiography; in 10% of the cases no underlying etiology will be identified.

Patients with SAH need to be monitored for vasospasm. This typically first appears at 48 hours, peaks around 72 hours, and then decreases over the following 4 days. While vasospasm can occur as far as 2 weeks following the sentinel event, this is less common. Vasospasm is detected on CTA as constriction of vessels, often with compensatory physiologic dilatation of the more distal vessels. Studies still need to be performed to determine the percentage narrowing of vessels that should

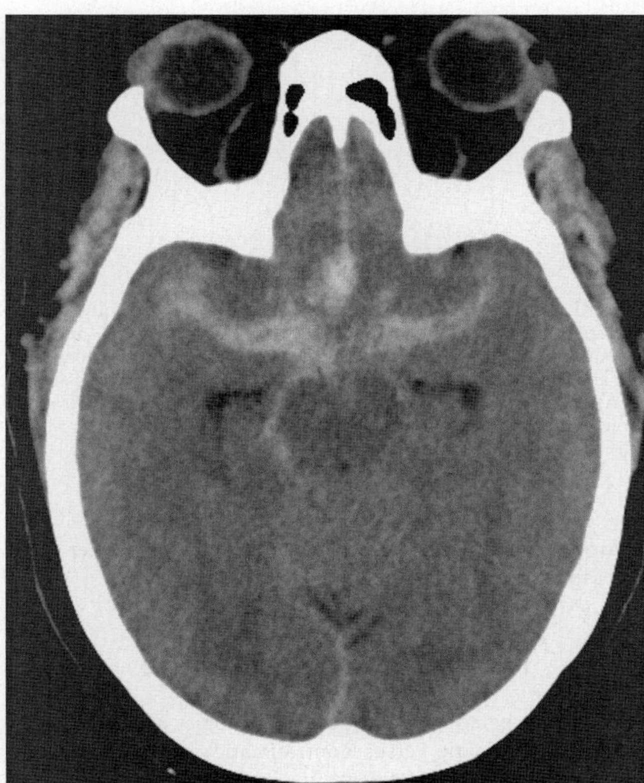

FIGURE 29.10. Axial noncontrast computed tomography. Diffuse subarachnoid blood products fill the anterior interhemispheric fissure and the basilar cisterns. This patient was found to have a ruptured anterior communicating artery aneurysm.

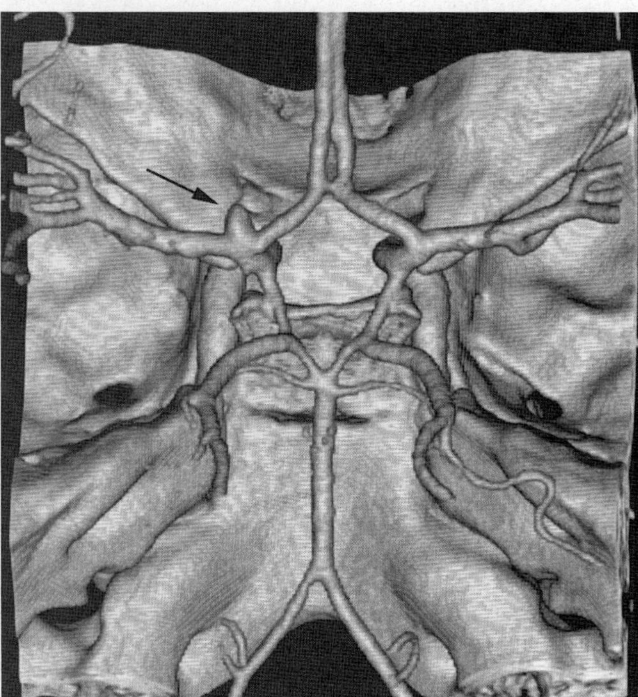

FIGURE 29.11. Volume surface-shaded rendering from a computed tomography angiogram. There is a small aneurysm projecting anterosuperiorly at the origin of the middle cerebral artery on the right.

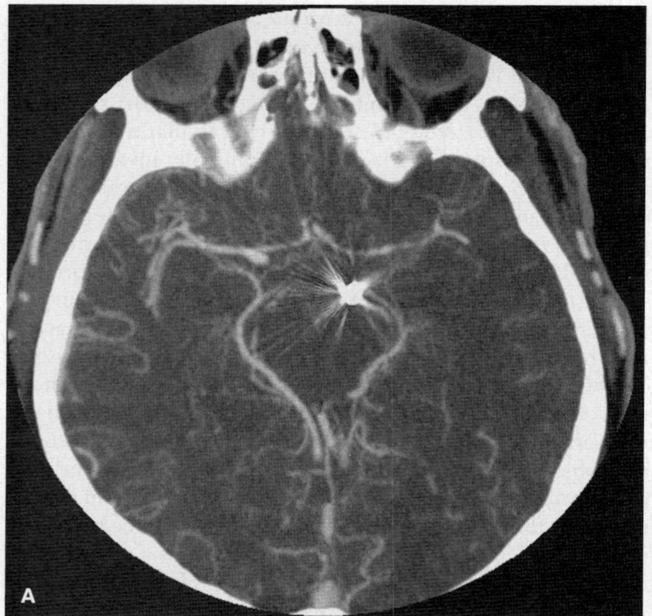

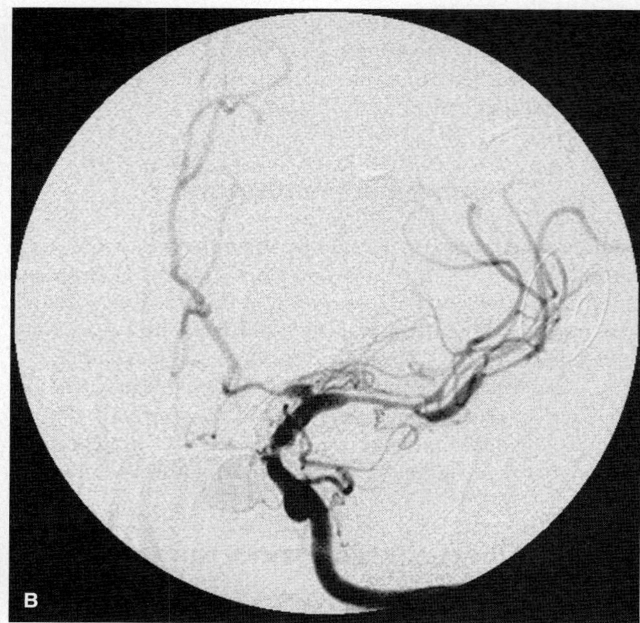

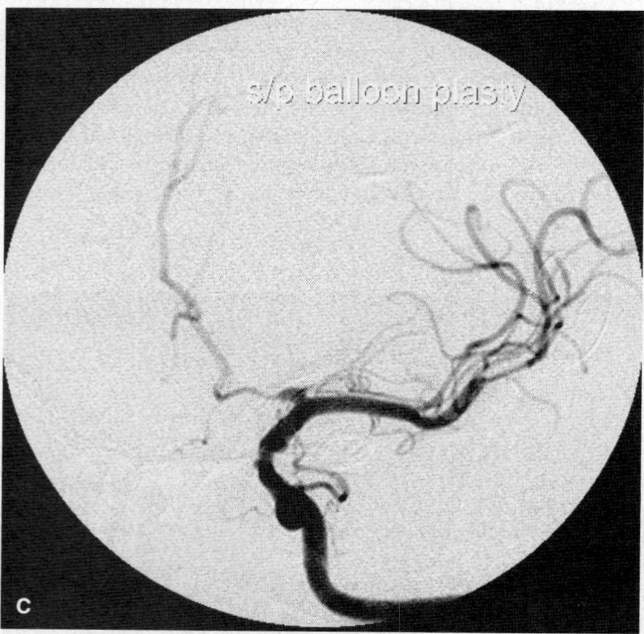

FIGURE 29.12. A: Axial computed tomography angiography image. Vasospasm affecting the left middle cerebral artery (MCA) and left posterior cerebral artery (PCA) following subarachnoid hemorrhage and aneurysm coiling. **B:** Frontal projection left internal carotid artery (ICA) angiogram also showing vasospasm in the left MCA. **C:** Frontal projection left ICA angiogram showing normal size of the left MCA following angioplasty for the vasospasm.

be deemed significant. Conventional angiography is a dynamic study and is a useful tool to visualize slow blood flow through a constricted vessel and delayed filling of capillary vessels. CT perfusion imaging can provide similar information by repeatedly imaging the brain during a rapid intravenous infusion of contrast. An analysis can then be made of the time it takes for maximum contrast enhancement of different vascular territories, the volume of contrast reaching a vascular territory, and the perfusion rate. A patient with vasospasm and compensatory blood flow through collaterals often just needs to be followed or treated with triple-H therapy (hypervolemia, hypertension, and hemodilution). A patient with vasospasm and decreased perfusion may need endovascular intervention, which can be performed with an intra-arterial calcium channel blocker such as verapamil or by angioplasty (Fig. 29.12).

Parenchymal Hemorrhage

Parenchymal hemorrhage has many etiologies and can be divided into traumatic versus nontraumatic causes. Traumatic causes include blunt and penetrating injuries resulting in a contusion, or rotational forces resulting in shear injury and diffuse axonal injury. Nontraumatic causes include hypertension (HTN), amyloid angiopathy, hemorrhagic stroke, hemorrhagic tumor, coagulopathy, and venous obstruction. In the setting of

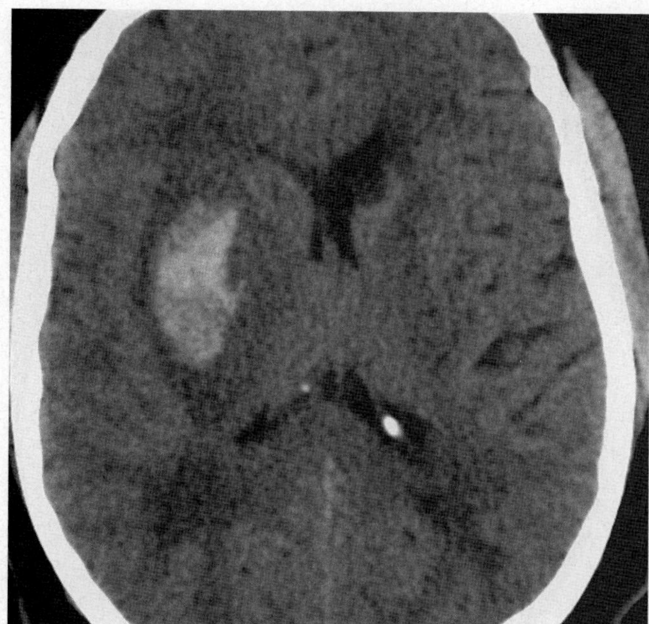

FIGURE 29.13. Axial noncontrast computed tomography. Hypertensive-related hemorrhage into the right basal ganglia.

nontraumatic injury, the underlying etiology may not be evident on CT or MRI and correlation with the clinical history is vital.

Parenchymal hemorrhage related to hypertension usually occurs with an acute elevation of blood pressure in the background of chronic hypertension. Chronic hypertension produces small-vessel disease that leads to lipohyalinosis. This affects the penetrating arteries such as the lenticulostriates and thalamoperforators, and explains why hypertensive hemorrhage most commonly occurs in the basal ganglia and thalamus (Fig. 29.13).

Amyloid angiopathy is deposition of β-amyloid in the media and adventitia of small- and midsized arteries of the leptomeninges and cortex. This leads to stenosis of the vessel lumen and weakening of the vessel wall, eventually resulting in the formation of microaneurysms. This predisposes patients to intraparenchymal—typically lobar—hemorrhages, which can be large and multiple. The most common locations are the frontal and parietal lobes.

Another nontraumatic source of intraparenchymal hemorrhage is venous obstruction. This has many causes, including hypercoagulable states, pregnancy, infection, malignancy, and birth control pills. The location of hemorrhage is dependent on the vascular territory of the occluded vein, and does not correspond to a typical arterial territory. Vascular congestion follows venous obstruction, which eventually leads to cell death and a venous infarct. This type of infarct tends to result in hemorrhage more frequently than arterial infarcts. The hemorrhage may also involve both cerebral hemispheres if there is occlusion of the superior sagittal sinus.

One important subset of patients with parenchymal hemorrhage is young patients with no history of trauma or other systemic disease. Special care should be given, and a careful search for an underlying vascular malformation such as AVM should be considered.

Intraventricular hemorrhage is usually secondary to extension from a parenchymal hemorrhage or has a traumatic etiology. Isolated intraventricular hemorrhage should raise the concern for an arterial venous malformation. Germinal matrix hemorrhage occurs in premature newborns and frequently extends into the ventricular system. Intraventricular hemorrhage is important to recognize because it can result in obstruction of CSF resorption and therefore hydrocephalus may ensue.

Parenchymal hemorrhage in the setting of trauma includes diffuse axonal injury (DAI) and contusion. DAI occurs secondary to rapid angular acceleration and deceleration, which results in disruption of axons and capillaries. The most common areas of involvement are the splenium of the corpus callosum, gray–white junction, and superior cerebellar peduncle. Only 20% of DAI cases are hemorrhagic, thus making MR more sensitive than CT. CT will show punctate areas of blood products surrounded by edema. MR demonstrates punctate areas of increased signal on FLAIR sequence and signal dropout on gradient echo sequence secondary to susceptibility artifact with hemorrhagic lesions. Nonhemorrhagic shear injury is detected by restricted diffusion on diffusion-weighted MR.

Brain contusion represents "bruising" of the brain cortex following multiple microhemorrhages. They can occur in a coup/contrecoup pattern. The underlying etiology is a combination of direct impact on the calvaria and the movement of the brain over bony ridges. The commonly involved areas are the frontal and temporal lobes. The temporal bones and roof of the orbit both have prominent bony ridges. The imaging hallmark of a brain contusion is a cortical hemorrhage with surrounding edema (Fig. 29.14).

STROKE

Stroke is the clinical term used to describe a permanent nontraumatic brain injury with resulting neurologic deficit. Strokes can be classified by their etiology as *ischemic,* secondary to hypoperfusion of an area of brain; *hemorrhagic,* rupture of a vascular structure leading to bleeding into the brain; or secondary to a substrate deficiency such as hypoglycemia. More than 75% of strokes are due to ischemia. A transient ischemic attack (TIA) is defined as transient neurologic symptoms or signs lasting less than 24 hours. An event that completely resolves after 24 hours is termed a reversible ischemic neurologic deficit (RIND).

Ischemic strokes can be thrombotic or embolic. In thrombotic strokes, clot forms locally on the wall of an artery, leading to decreased blood supply. In an embolic stroke, a clot becomes dislodged from the heart or an extracranial vessel, traveling to the brain and resulting in compromised blood supply. Both thrombotic and embolic strokes are secondary to blockage of arterial supply to an area of brain. However, in patients with a hypoperfusion state—hypotension, cardiac failure, dysrhythmia—decreased flow to the brain can result in damage to areas of brain with the least robust blood supply. This type of global hypoxic injury tends to occur first in the watershed areas of brain, for example, the anterior cerebral artery (ACA)–middle cerebral artery (MCA) or the MCA–posterior cerebral artery (PCA) watershed territories. Although far less common, stroke can also be the result of a venous occlusion. Predisposing factors include hypercoaguable states, pregnancy,

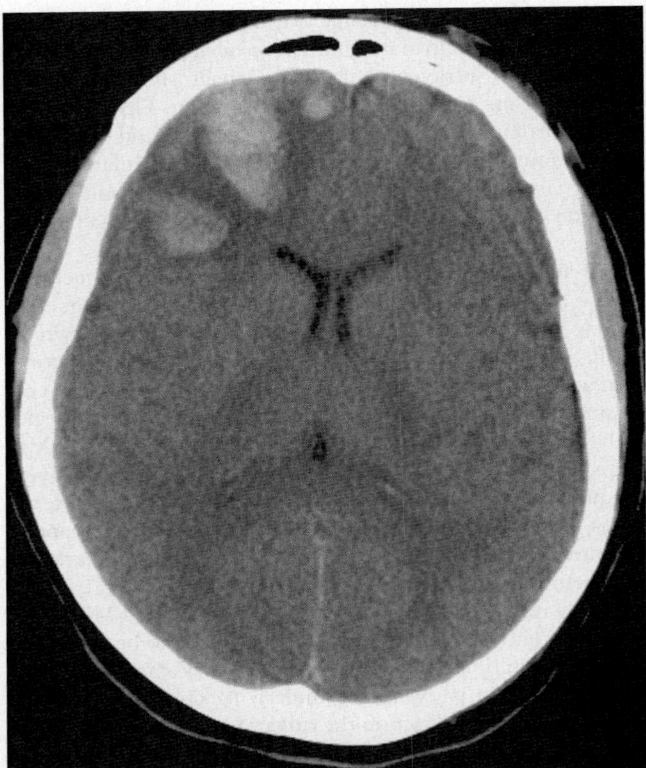

FIGURE 29.14. Axial noncontrast computed tomography. Posttraumatic contusion (intraparenchymal hemorrhage) in the right frontal polar region with surrounding vasogenic edema.

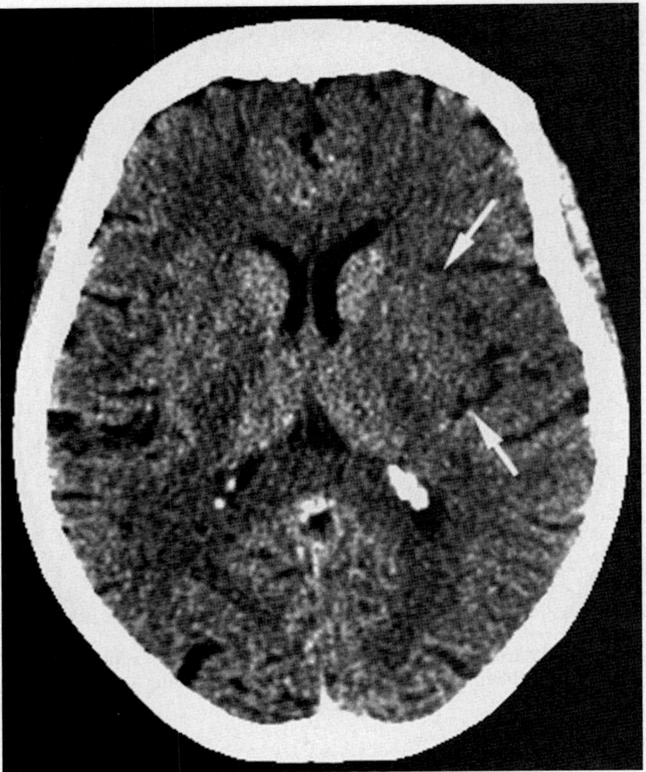

FIGURE 29.15. Axial noncontrast computed tomography. Subtle loss of gray–white differentiation along the insular cortex on the left (*arrows*), the so-called "insular ribbon sign."

meningitis, and sepsis. Blockage of venous outflow results in stasis of blood, which becomes deoxygenated, leading to subsequent neuronal death. Any venous structure can be involved, whether a cortical vein, a dural sinus, or the cavernous sinus. Venous infarcts should be considered in patients with ischemia affecting a nonarterial territory.

Noncontrast CT should be obtained as the initial imaging modality in patients with new neurologic deficits suspected of having a stroke. Noncontrast CT can rapidly identify patients with intracranial hemorrhage. Ischemic strokes will often show no discernible findings on noncontrasted study during the first 3 hours. Prior to 6 hours, only very subtle signs can be evident such as loss of gray–white matter distinction, haziness of the deep nuclei, or loss of the insular "ribbon" (Fig. 29.15). As time progresses, the patient will develop edema in the infarcted area, which can result in mass effect with shift of structures and potentially a herniation syndrome.

CT perfusion can often be rapidly obtained in evaluating patients for stroke. Perfusion CT produces color-coded maps of the brain at multiple levels showing differences in blood flow to areas of the brain. The color maps generated are mean transit time (MTT), cerebral blood flow (CBF), and cerebral blood volume (CBV) (Fig. 29.16). Mean transit time is the most sensitive measure to evaluate for any flow abnormality, but it is not specific. Flow will be prolonged in an area having a stroke, but also in areas with delayed flow for any reason, such as regions distal to a vascular stenosis. Decreased CBF is present in areas of the brain either at risk for or undergoing infarct. Cerebral blood volume is the most specific indicator of an area undergoing infarction. A low CBF with normal to increased CBV is an area at risk for ischemia but currently compensating for decreased flow by dilating vessels. Areas of brain with both decreased CBF and CBV are undergoing infarction. Limitations of perfusion CT include the need to administer intravenous contrast, long image acquisition times requiring often obtunded patients to hold completely still for 60 seconds, and the ability to only evaluate limited areas of the brain.

MRI with diffusion is currently the gold standard in acute stroke imaging. Once a hemorrhagic stroke has been excluded by CT, diffusion MR improves stroke detection to more than 95%. MR is much more sensitive for edema than CT. FLAIR sequences clearly demonstrate areas of edema not visible on CT (Fig. 29.17). Diffusion MR noninvasively detects ischemic changes within minutes of stroke onset. The technique sensitizes the images to detect microscopic—Brownian—motion of water molecules. The ability of water molecules to diffuse normally in an ischemic area rapidly decreases following onset of ischemia. Diffusion MR identifies areas of decreased water motion in regions of ischemia and displays them as bright areas (Fig. 29.17B). Since diffusion MR itself relies on T2-weighted sequences, some areas with high T2 signals that are not secondary to infarct-related edema can appear bright on diffusion imaging. Therefore, it is necessary to compare diffusion sequences with an apparent diffusion coefficient (ADC) map (Fig. 29.17C). Areas that are bright on diffusion and dark on ADC are consistent with acute infarct. Over time, the diffusion and ADC abnormalities will reverse as the stroke moves into a subacute phase. In evaluating for subacute stroke,

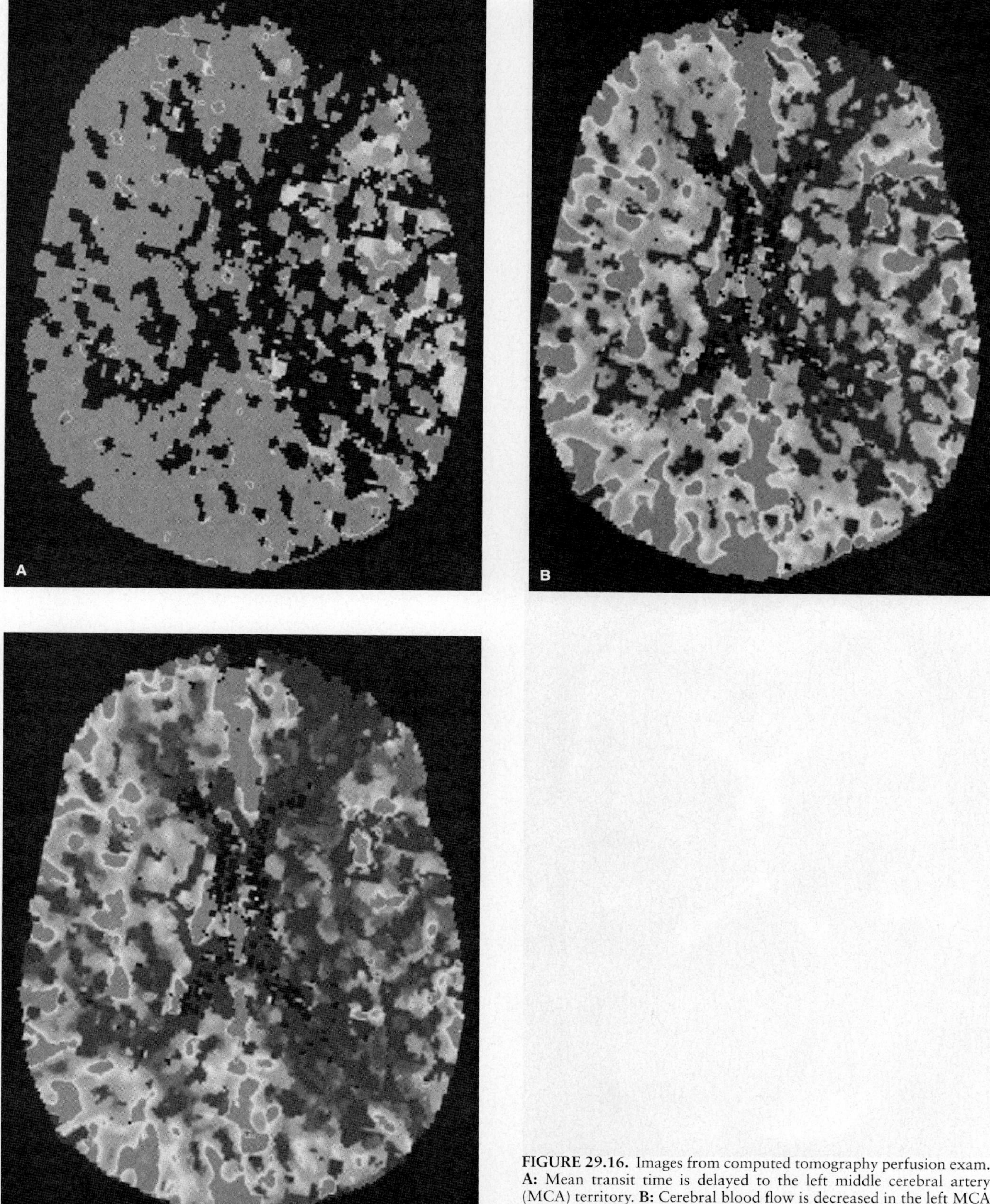

FIGURE 29.16. Images from computed tomography perfusion exam. A: Mean transit time is delayed to the left middle cerebral artery (MCA) territory. B: Cerebral blood flow is decreased in the left MCA territory. C: Cerebral blood volume is also decreased to the left MCA territory consistent with infarcting tissue.

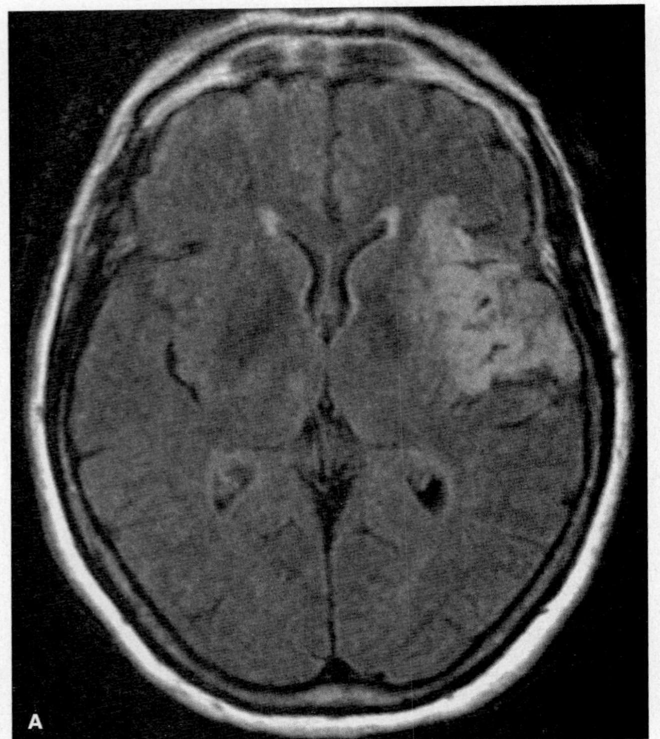

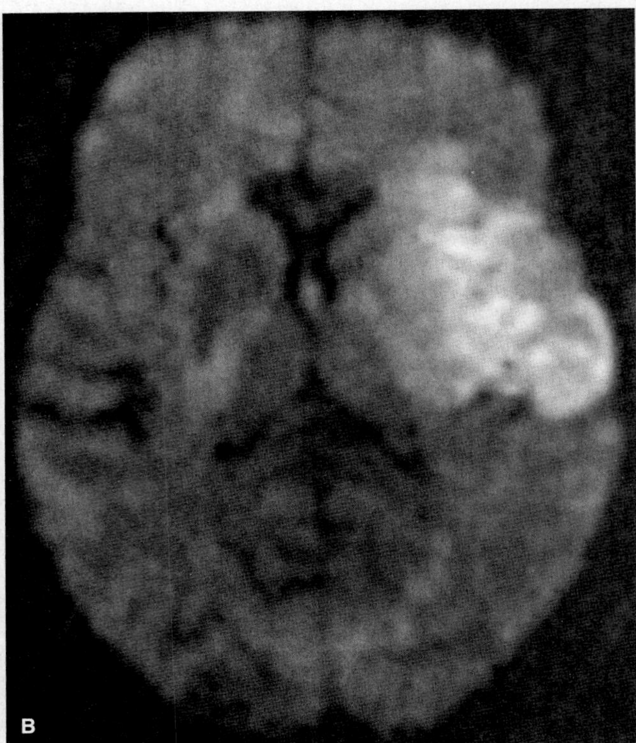

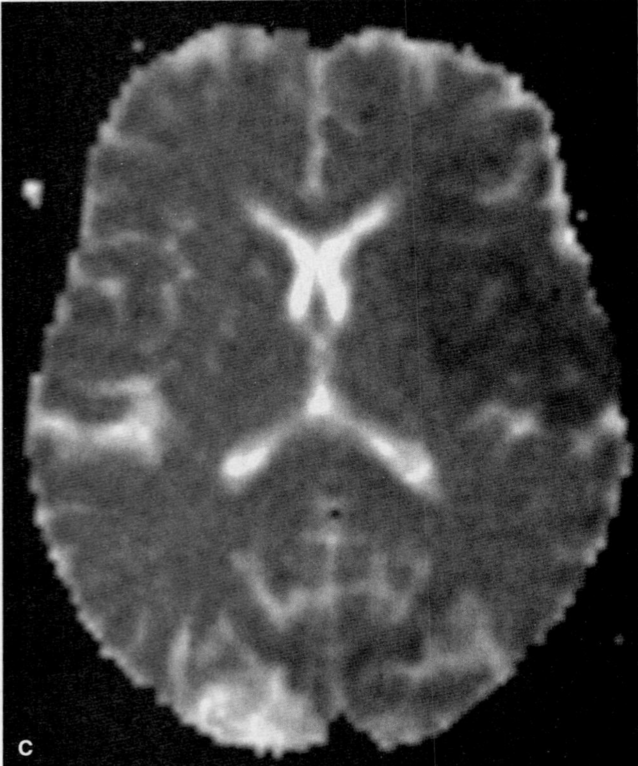

FIGURE 29.17. A: Axial fluid-attenuated inversion recovery magnetic resonance (MR). Cytotoxic edema is present as high signal in this patient with acute left middle cerebral artery (MCA) infarct. Axial diffusion-weighted MR (**B**) and axial apparent diffusion coefficient (ADC) map (**C**) showing high signal on the diffusion image and low signal on the ADC map in the left MCA territory consistent with diffusion restriction and acute infarct.

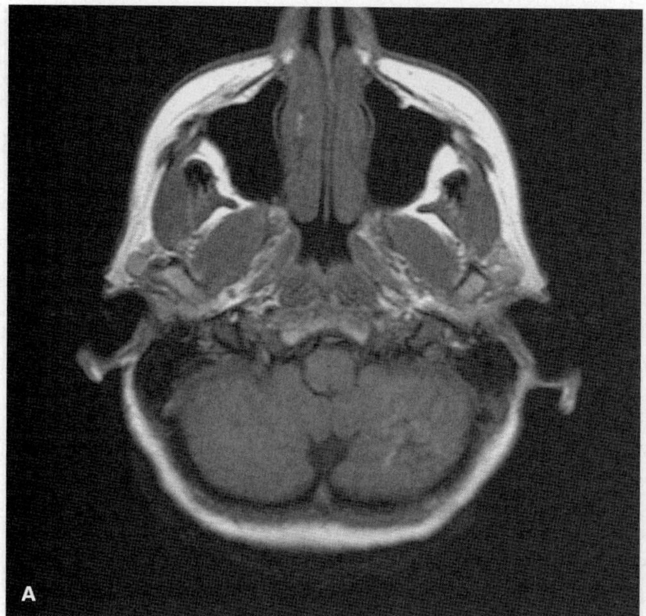

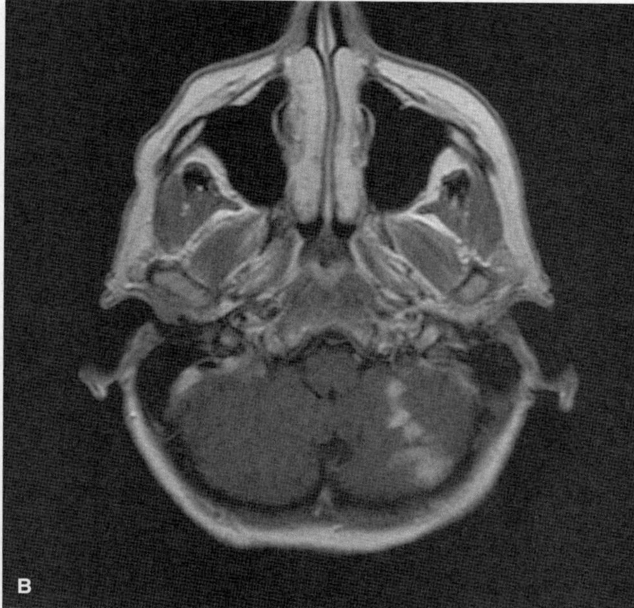

FIGURE 29.18. Pre- (A) and postcontrast (B) axial T1 magnetic resonance. Enhancing subacute infarct in the left posterior inferior cerebellar artery territory.

contrast-enhanced T1-weighted MR can show enhancement of a subacute infarct as soon as 2 to 3 days following the event. Contrast enhancement can persist for 8 to 10 weeks. The "2-2-2" rule is usually followed: The enhancement begins at 2 days, peaks at 2 weeks, and resolves by 2 months. Contrast enhancement is also seen with CT imaging of subacute stroke (Fig. 29.18).

INFECTION

Central nervous system (CNS) infections can progress rapidly, leading to stroke, hemorrhage, herniation, and death. Prompt recognition and initiation of therapy is therefore critical. Imaging can play an important role in evaluating for signs and complications of infection.

The discussion of CNS infection can take many different pathways, and may be divided into opportunistic and nonopportunistic infection, or specific pathogens can be studied individually. In the interest of simplicity, infection will be discussed anatomically. Noninfectious inflammatory disease will not be covered.

Leptomeningitis, commonly referred to as meningitis, is an inflammatory infiltration of the pia and arachnoid meninges that can be caused by bacterial, viral, or fungal agents. Most commonly, the infection occurs via hematogenous dissemination. It is important to initiate therapy quickly for patients suspected of having meningitis. Imaging is insensitive for early evidence of meningitis, as in early phases the brain most often appears normal. In fact, the most sensitive test for meningitis is a lumbar puncture, not an imaging exam. Imaging studies are more useful to evaluate for complications of meningitis. Noncontrast CT will often be relatively normal, but may show mild ventriculomegaly. Contrasted CT can show enhancing material within sulci and cisterns. CT angiography can show evidence of vasculitis, with multifocal areas of vessel irregularity.

MRI is a much more sensitive imaging modality for meningitis, though it, too, will often be unremarkable in the earliest stages of infection. FLAIR sequences can show high signal along the sulci from the proteinaceous material in the CSF (Fig. 29.19). Exudative material along the sulci will enhance in a serpiginous form on T1-weighted postcontrast images

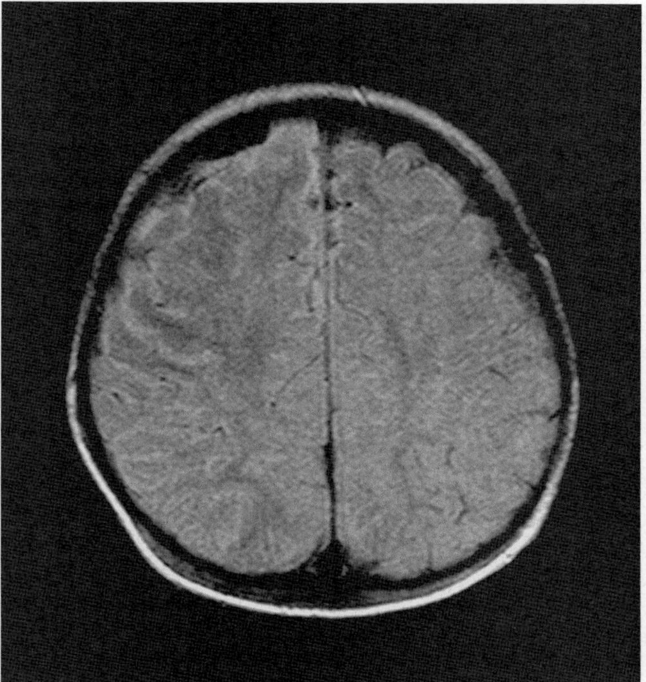

FIGURE 29.19. Axial fluid-attenuated inversion recovery magnetic resonance. High signal in a serpiginous pattern along the sulci representing the high-protein inflammatory exudates in bacterial meningitis.

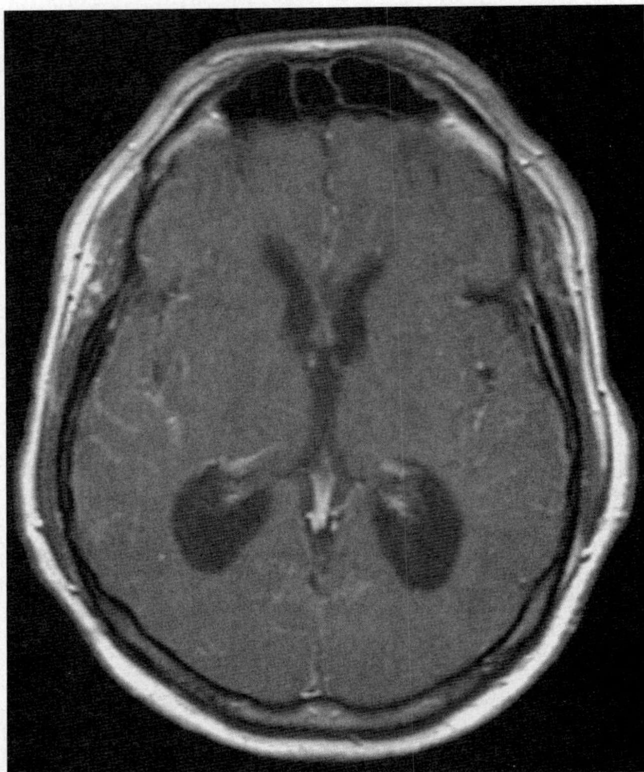

FIGURE 29.20. Postcontrast axial T1 magnetic resonance. Leptomeningeal enhancement in the characteristic serpiginous pattern along the sulci in a patient with bacterial meningitis.

(Fig. 29.20). MRI is also useful to evaluate for complications of meningitis such as ventriculitis, abscess, and infarcts. Infarcts are common complications of advanced meningitis. A vasculitis is caused by meningeal irritation, which potentially can progress to hinder arterial flow to brain. Additionally, venous infarcts can be seen secondary to septic venous thrombosis (Fig. 29.21).

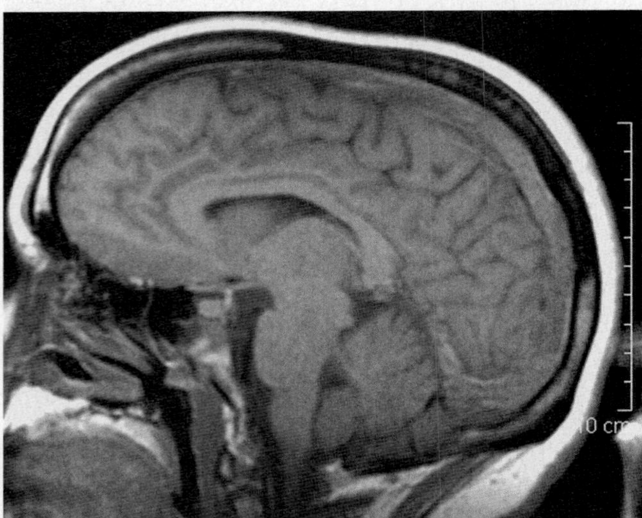

FIGURE 29.21. Sagittal T1 magnetic resonance. High signal is seen within the superior sagittal sinus representing thrombus.

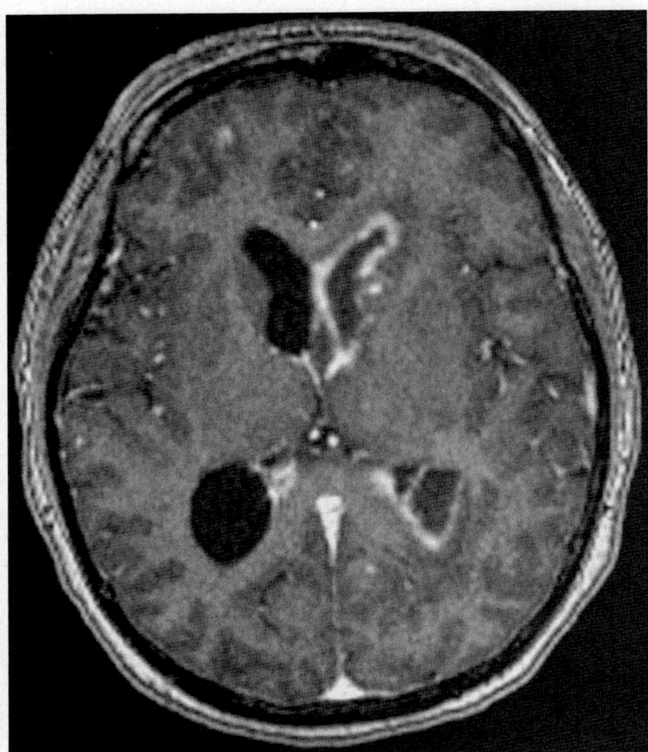

FIGURE 29.22. Postcontrast axial T1 magnetic resonance. Enhancement is present along the ependymal lining of the left lateral ventricle consistent with ventriculitis.

Ventriculitis, also called ependymitis, is a complication of meningitis or ventricular shunting. Again, MR is much more sensitive than CT, and will demonstrate enhancement along the ventricular margins (Fig. 29.22). There will often be increased FLAIR signal surrounding the ventricles, and the ventricles may appear enlarged. Keep in mind that this imaging appearance is not specific to infection; for example, in an immunocompromised individual, this can be seen in lymphoma.

Pachymeningitis, an infiltration of the dura, can be differentiated from leptomeningitis by its thick nodular enhancement pattern that closely approximates the calvaria and does not extend into the sulci. Pachymeningitis can be seen with tuberculosis and fungal infections, but noninfectious etiologies such as sarcoid and carcinomatosis should be considered as well.

Focal pyogenic infections of brain parenchyma lead to cerebritis. Cerebritis is brain inflammation usually secondary to hematogenous dissemination of bacteria. Fungal and parasitic etiologies are also possible, but less common. The most common areas affected are the territories supplied by the middle cerebral artery, specifically the frontal and parietal lobes. In early cerebritis, only MR imaging will demonstrate an abnormality, with FLAIR sequences showing an area of increased signal intensity. Later imaging features include an unencapsulated, poorly defined mass with patchy contrast enhancement on CT and MR. Untreated, over time, this infectious, inflammatory mass will develop a capsule, become more organized, and eventually develop as a brain abscess. The capsule rim will enhance on postcontrast CT and MR (Fig. 29.23A). FLAIR and T2-weighted imaging will often show prominent vasogenic

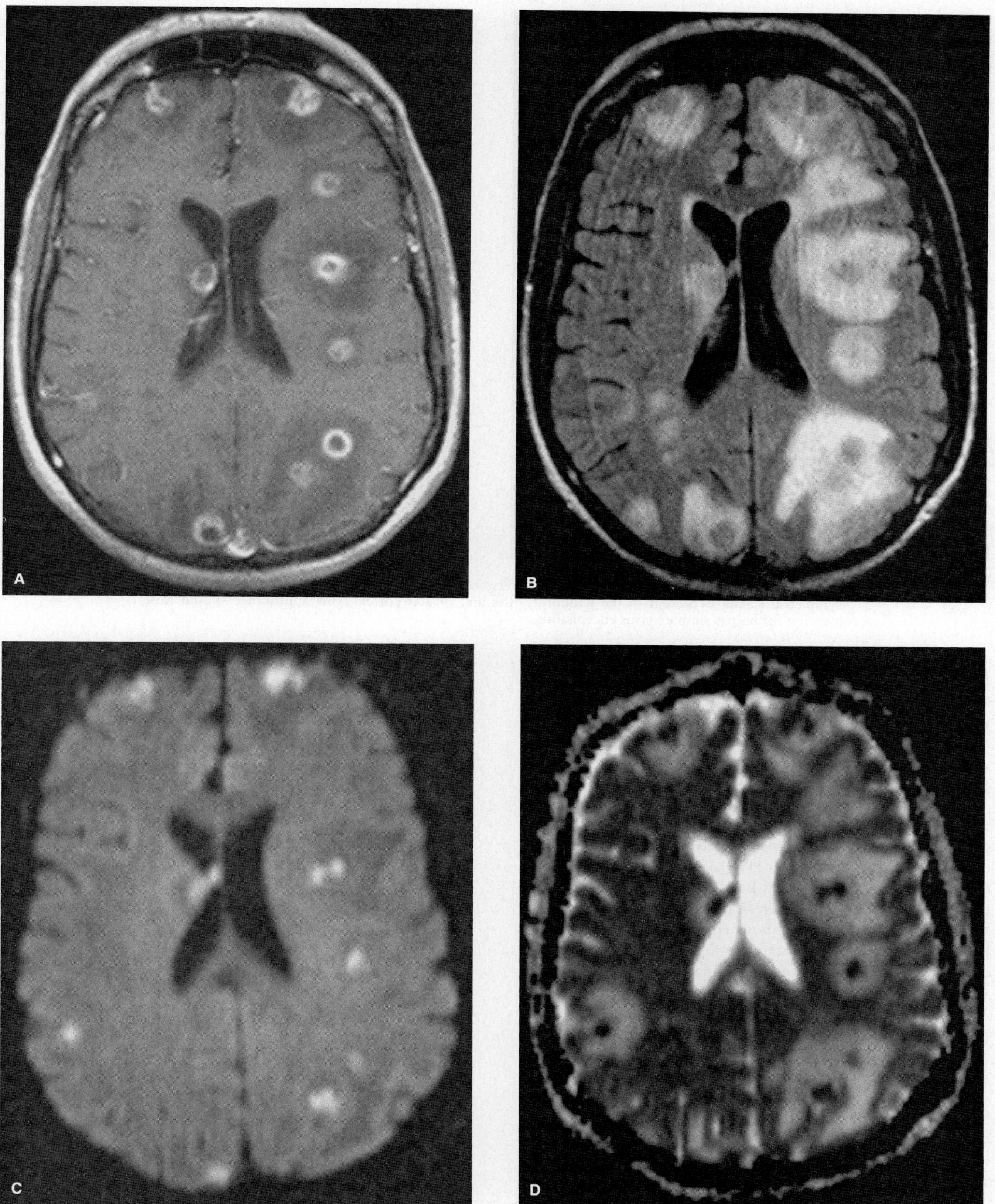

FIGURE 29.23. **A:** Postcontrast axial T1 magnetic resonance: Multiple rim-enhancing lesions. **B:** Axial fluid-attenuated inversion recovery magnetic resonance. Prominent vasogenic edema surrounding the lesions. Axial diffusion (**C**) and axial apparent diffusion coefficient magnetic resonance images (**D**) showing that the lesions demonstrate restricted diffusion, consistent with multiple brain abscesses. *Nocardia* was the causative agent in this patient.

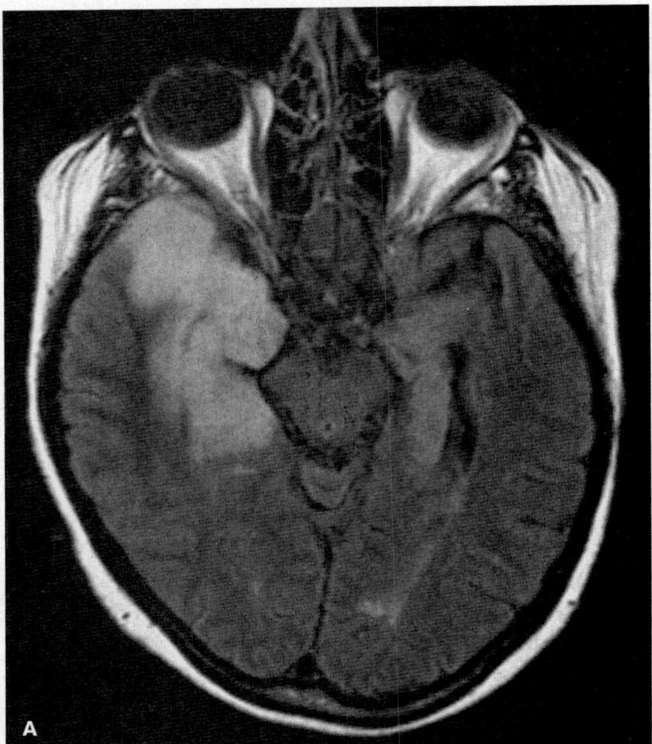

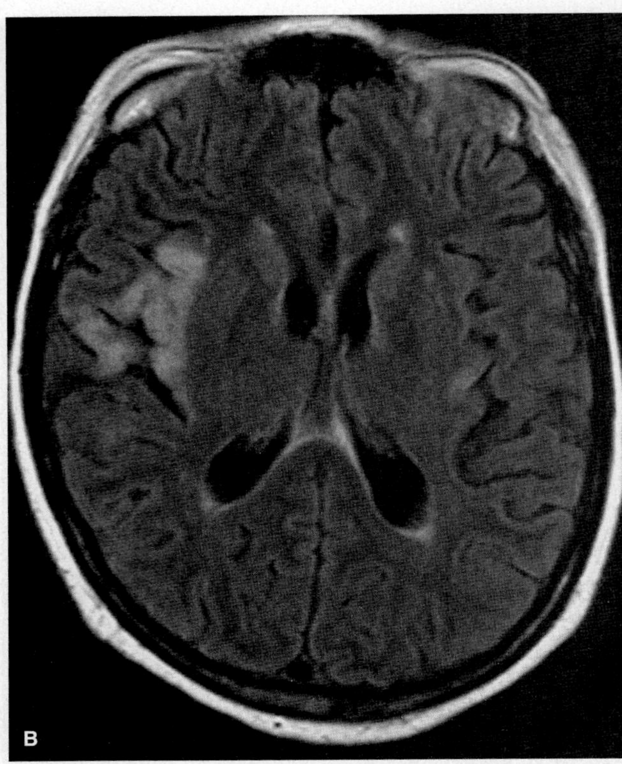

FIGURE 29.24. A, B: Axial fluid-attenuated inversion recovery magnetic resonance images. Bilateral asymmetric edema is present in the temporal lobes and insular cortex. This appearance should raise suspicion for herpes simplex virus encephalitis.

edema surrounding the abscesses (Fig. 29.23B). Often, the capsule will be thinnest on the ventricular side, which may help in distinguishing this ring-enhancing lesion from a malignancy. Additionally, brain abscesses will show restricted diffusion (Fig. 29.23C, D). The time course for the changes from cerebritis to abscess is approximately 2 weeks.

Encephalitis is brain inflammation caused by a viral infection or a hypersensitivity reaction to a foreign protein; approximately 2,000 cases are reported each year. Sources include herpes simplex virus (HSV), mosquito-borne viruses, cytomegalovirus, and Epstein-Barr virus. Herpes encephalitis progresses rapidly and can result in death without prompt recognition and therapy. It is usually due to reactivation of latent HSV-1 virus in an immunocompetent patient, which ascends into the brain via the trigeminal and olfactory nerves. Although CT is insensitive to early features of this disease, MRI will show findings within 2 days of onset. Initially, edema is seen in the medial temporal, insula, and inferior frontal lobes (Fig. 29.24A, B). Occasionally this is unilateral, but more often, asymmetric bilateral disease is present. Postcontrast imaging will show patchy vague enhancement in initial phases, progressing to gyriform enhancement within 1 week.

An empyema is a loculated collection of pus that can develop intracranially in either the subdural or epidural space. These are commonly referred to as subdural or epidural abscesses. These infections are considered a neurosurgical emergency and must be drained expediently. Most of these are supratentorial and present as an extra-axial collection. This fluid collection is often isodense to CSF on CT imaging, making MRI superior to CT in evaluating the extent and nature of this collection. On

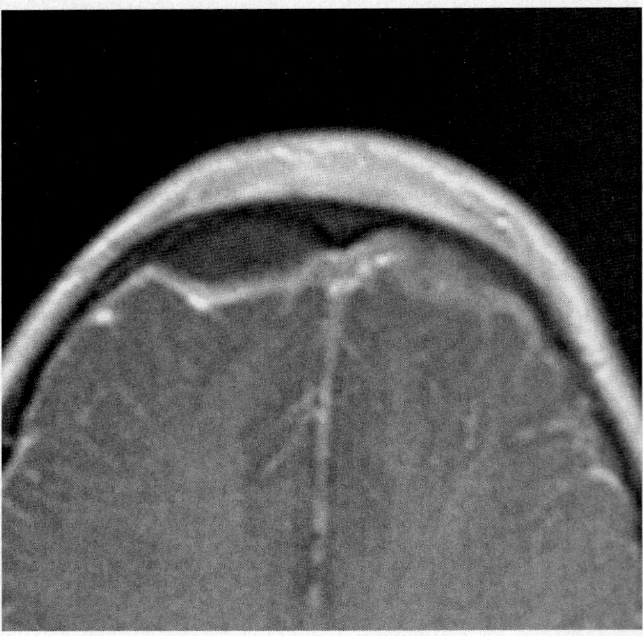

FIGURE 29.25. Axial postcontrast T1 magnetic resonance. Extra-axial fluid collection adjacent to right frontal lobe with enhancement along the dural margin, consistent with a subdural empyema.

T1-weighted MR, the fluid will be hyperintense to CSF because of proteinaceous material—pus—within it (Fig. 29.25). Often, prominent enhancement is present along the margins of the collection. Signal changes in adjacent brain parenchyma are also commonly seen secondary to cerebritis. An empyema can develop as a complication of meningitis in younger patients. In older individuals, contiguous spread from a paranasal sinus or ear infection is the most common etiology. Occasionally, it can be difficult to determine if an epidural fluid collection is an abscess or a hematoma, in which case follow-up CT exam may be useful.

Subdural empyema, in its most basic form, is disruption of the arachnoid layer with a combination of both CSF and purulent material beneath the dura. The fluid collection can cover the convexities and tract within the interhemispheric fissure. A subdural empyema may present either acutely or chronically, and 10% of patients will go on to develop a brain abscess or venous thrombosis. MR is more sensitive than CT for its detection. The signal is low on T1-weighted images, and high on T2 and FLAIR images. A key imaging feature is that subdural empyemas demonstrate restricted diffusion and a subdural effusion does not. In the chronic setting, there is rim enhancement of the surrounding granulation tissue. An imaging pitfall is in differentiating a chronic subdural hematoma from a subdural empyema. Both look similar but should have a different clinical history.

SPINE

The spine consists of both osseous and ligamentous components that transmit forces to allow movement while protecting the spinal cord and vertebral arteries. In terms of mechanical forces, the spine is divided into three columns. The anterior column includes the anterior longitudinal ligament and the anterior two thirds of the vertebral body and the annulus fibrosis. The middle column consists of the posterior third of the vertebral body, the posterior annulus, and the posterior longitudinal ligament. The facet joints, laminae, spinous processes, and interspinous ligaments comprise the posterior column. Interruption of two contiguous columns, including both osseous and ligamentous components, creates instability.

Following trauma, plain films or CT is initially obtained and evaluated for fracture and ligamentous injury. An initial assessment must be made of appropriate alignment in both coronal and sagittal planes. Spinal alignment is assessed in the sagittal plane with the use of the anterior vertebral body line, posterior vertebral body line, spinolaminar line, and dorsal surface articular pillar lines (Fig. 29.26). The atlantoaxial and craniocervical relationship are evaluated with various measurements, including the basion–dens interval of 12 mm or less, the Power's ratio, and the atlantoaxial distance of less than 2 mm in an adult. Abnormal alignment or a widened facet joint or intervertebral disc space raises suspicion for ligamentous injury, and should prompt additional imaging. Dynamic flexion and extension plain films or MR with STIR (short tau inversion recovery) sequences are helpful. Abnormal motion during flexion and extension or increased signal within the ligaments on STIR images is consistent with ligamentous injury (Fig. 29.27).

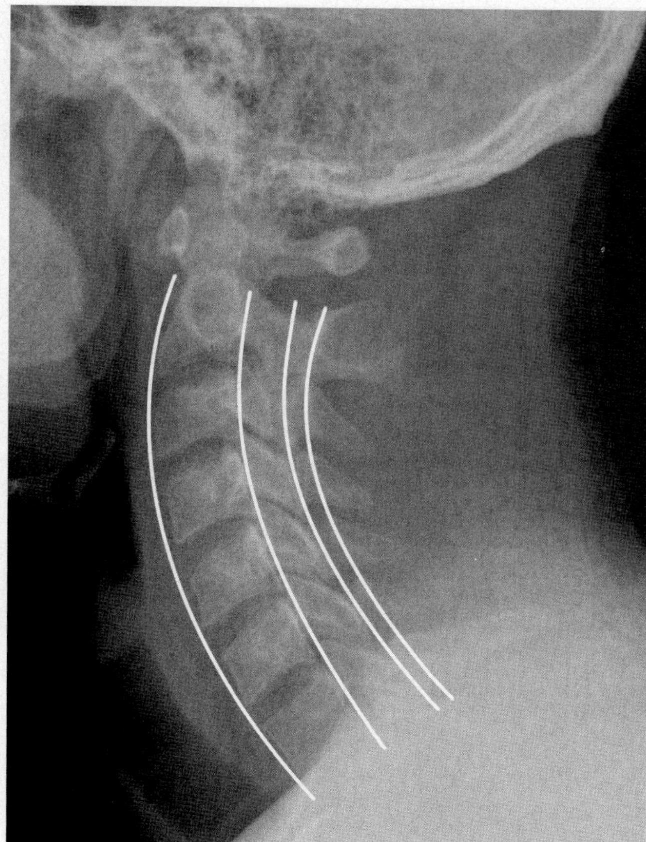

FIGURE 29.26. Normal lateral view of the cervical spine with normal smooth curvature of the anterior vertebral body line, posterior vertebral body line, dorsal surface articular pillar line, and spinal laminar line.

Spine fractures are classified according to the mechanism of injury as axial load, hyperflexion, hyperextension, lateral flexion, or rotational injuries. Variations of spine fractures are numerous and complex, and only the more common injuries are discussed in this section.

Axial load forces can produce a Jefferson fracture of C1 or a burst-type fracture. A Jefferson fracture is a C1 ring fracture where fractures are present in both the anterior and posterior rings and the lateral masses are dislocated laterally. Burst fractures are caused by severe axial compression leading to fractures of the anterior and posterior margins of the vertebral body with anterior and middle column involvement—an unstable injury, often with retropulsion of bony fragments into the canal.

Flexion injuries result in compression fractures, facet dislocations (unilateral or bilateral), or a flexion teardrop fracture. In contrast to a burst fracture, compression fractures only involve the anterior vertebral body (anterior column) and are stable as long as there is only anterior column involvement. A flexion teardrop injury is the most severe cervical spine injury. The "teardrop" is composed of a sheared fragment from the anteroinferior vertebral body, which is associated with bilateral facet subluxations, posterior subluxation of the vertebral body, and disruption of all major stabilizing ligaments. This

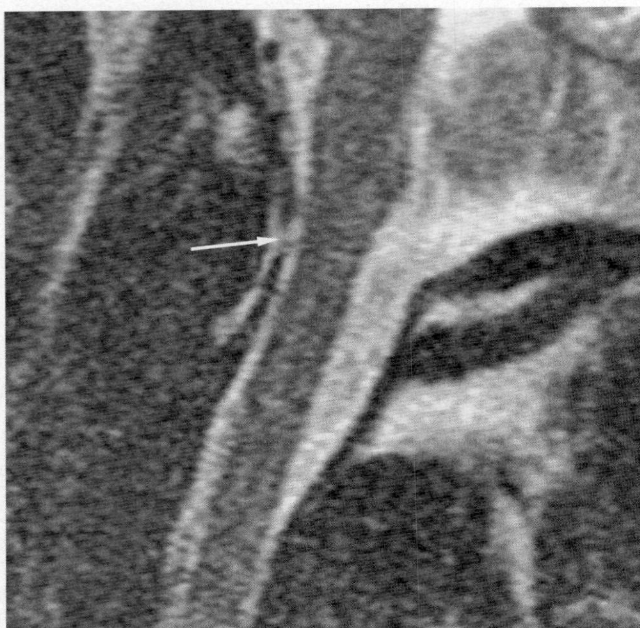

FIGURE 29.27. Sagittal short tau inversion recovery magnetic resonance. Focal disruption of the posterior longitudinal ligament at the C2 level (*arrow*).

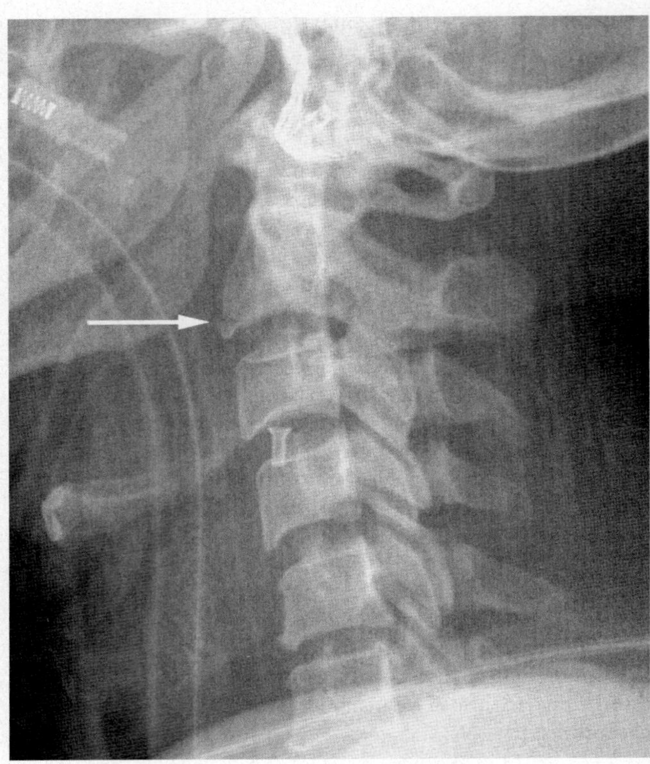

FIGURE 29.29. Lateral plain film of the cervical spine. Extension teardrop fracture (*arrow*) with an avulsed bony fragment from the anteroinferior corner of C2.

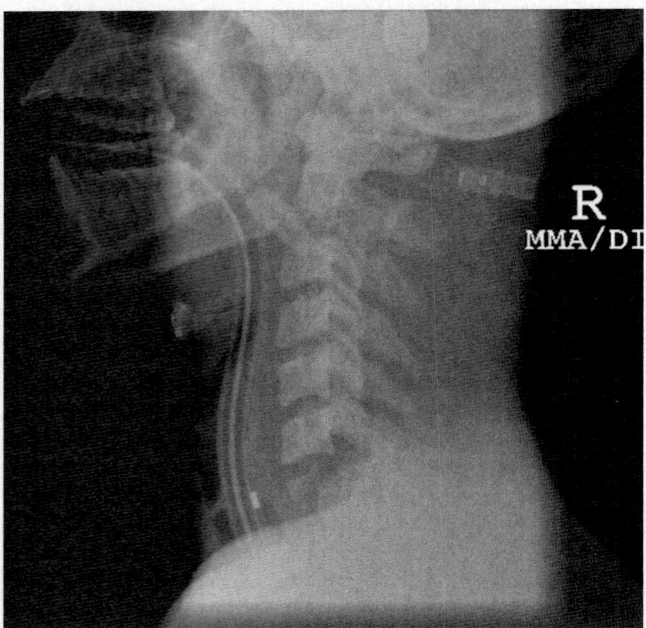

FIGURE 29.28. Lateral plain film. Flexion teardrop fracture involving C7 with posterior subluxation of the C7 vertebral body. In this case, the teardrop was avulsed from the anterosuperior corner of the vertebral body, whereas an anteroinferior corner avulsion is more commonly seen.

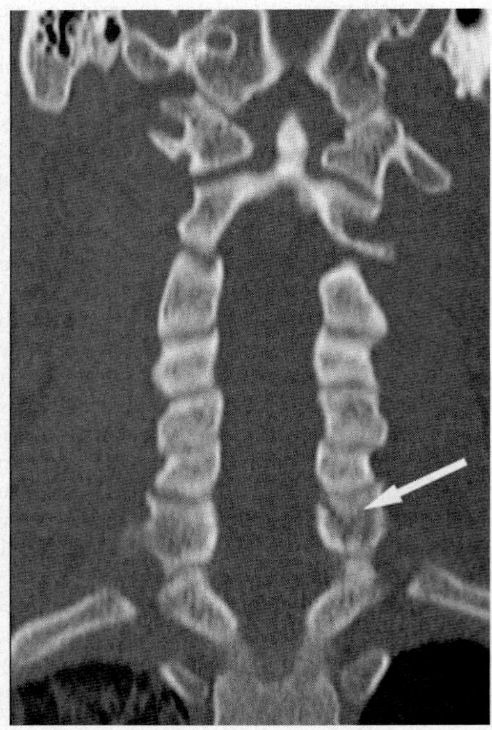

FIGURE 29.30. Coronal cervical spine computed tomography reconstruction. Lateral flexion injury resulting in fracture of the left articular pillar of C7 (*arrow*).

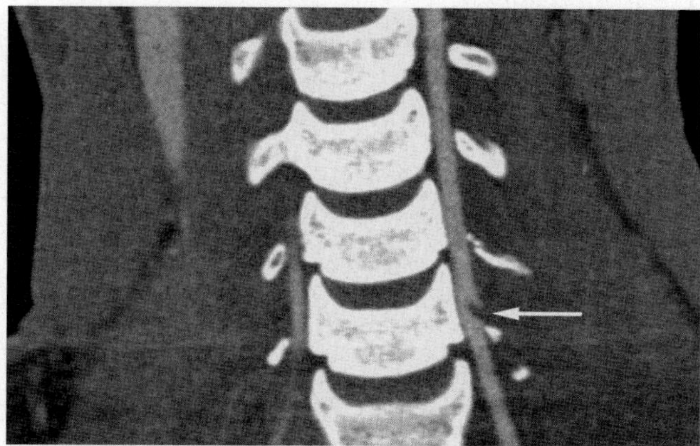

FIGURE 29.31. Coronal reformation of computed tomography angiography. A focal defect is present in the left vertebral artery (*arrow*) immediately adjacent to transverse process fracture consistent with traumatic dissection.

injury often results in severe compromise of the spinal canal, cord compression, and neurologic impairment (Fig. 29.28).

Extension injuries can result in a hangman's fracture, a pillar fracture, an extension teardrop fracture, or a hyperextension fracture–dislocation. A hangman's fracture is composed of bilateral pars or pedicle fractures of C2. This often results in widening of the canal, and there is usually no initial neurologic deficit; however, the injury is very unstable. Extension teardrop fractures commonly involve the upper cervical spine, most commonly at C2 where the anteroinferior corner avulses from the axis, tearing the anterior longitudinal ligament (Fig. 29.29). The unstable hyperextension fracture dislocation results from a severe hyperextension force. This causes a comminuted articular mass fracture with contralateral facet subluxation, mild anterior subluxation, and potential rupture of both the posterior and anterior longitudinal ligaments.

Injuries resulting in a lateral flexion force lead to transverse process fractures, lateral flexion dislocation of the dens, and lateral wedgelike compression fractures of a vertebral body (Fig. 29.30). Additionally, nerve root avulsions and damage to the brachial plexus are associated with a severe lateral flexion force.

Finally, rotational forces cause rotatory atlantoaxial subluxation, as well as injuries to the anterior and posterior longitudinal ligaments. Rotatory atlantoaxial subluxation can result in the patient holding the head in a persistently cocked orientation. In severe cases, rotatory atlantoaxial subluxation or fixation can compromise flow in the vertebral arteries. Radiographically, this presents as a persistent rotational abnormality in the alignment of C1 with C2.

Often, the direction of forces involved in a spinal injury is complex, and variations and combinations of the above-described injuries are seen. For example, dens fractures require a combination of flexion and extension as well as a shearing lateral force vector.

The vertebral arteries arise from the subclavian arteries and usually enter the cervical spine at C6. Should a fracture line cross the transverse foramen through which the vertebral artery runs, a CTA should be obtained to evaluate for traumatic injury. An intimal flap, focal narrowing, or even occlusion may be seen with vessel dissection (Fig. 29.31). Fractures that cross the carotid canal at the skull base may require similar evaluation with CTA.

When acute spinal cord compression symptoms present, an MR should be obtained to evaluate for a spinal epidural hematoma, acute disc herniation, or cord injury. Other than trauma, spinal epidural hematomas can be the result of anticoagulant therapy, vascular malformation, or systemic disease such as systemic lupus erythematosus. Even minor trauma can

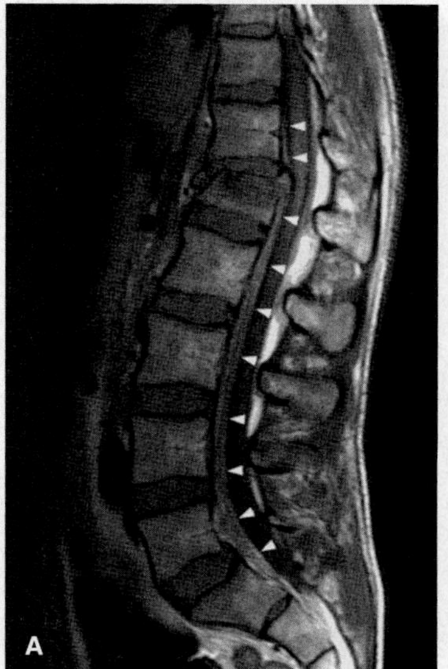

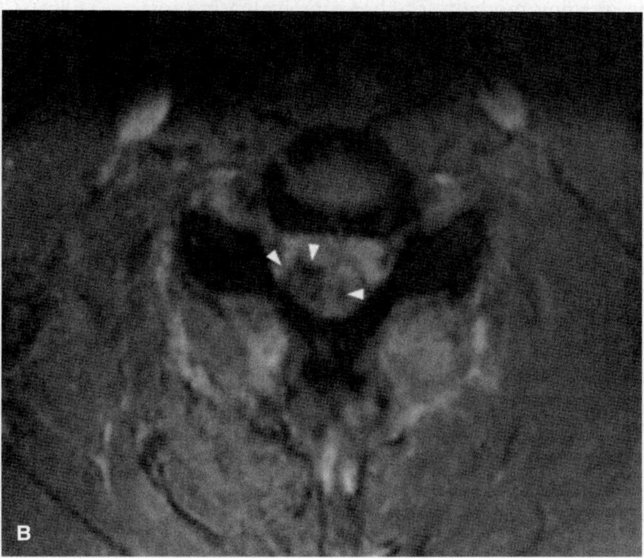

FIGURE 29.32. Sagittal (**A**) and axial (**B**) T1 magnetic resonance of the lumbar spine in a patient with an L1 burst fracture. There is heterogeneous high signal intensity within the anterior epidural space extending from L1 through the upper sacrum representing epidural blood products (*arrowheads*).

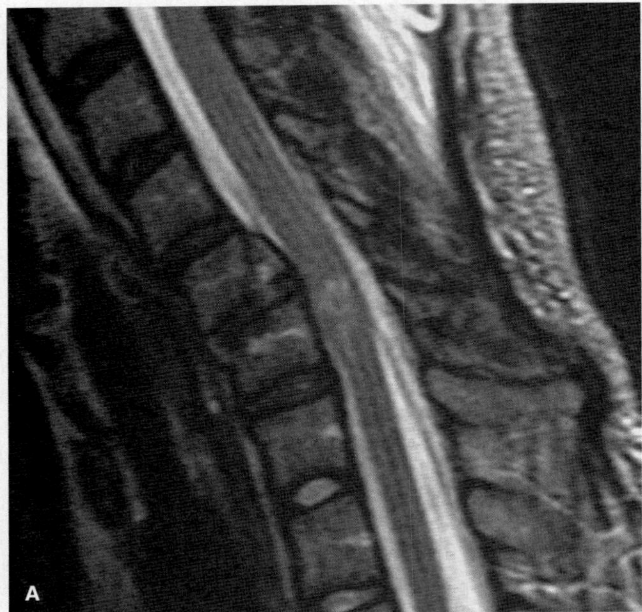

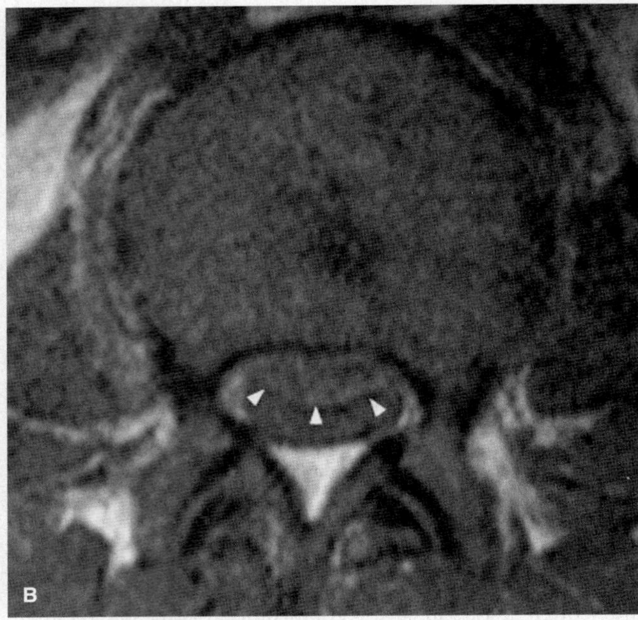

FIGURE 29.33. **A:** Sagittal T2 magnetic resonance (MR). A two-level fracture in the midcervical spine narrows the canal diameter and results in cord contusion manifested by high T2 signal in the cord. **B:** Axial gradient MR. Areas of dark signal representing blood products are seen within the area of cord contusion (*arrowheads*).

cause an epidural hematoma as the valveless venous plexus in the epidural space is prone to injury. MRI best demonstrates blood products in the epidural space (Fig. 29.32).

Spinal cord injury results in neurologic impairment. It can be caused by spinal cord compression from bony fragments, stretching injury, or impairment of the vascular supply (anterior spinal artery in the overwhelming majority of cases). Symptoms are related to the level and severity of injury. MR is the imaging modality of choice in evaluating for cord and nerve root injury. Increased T2 signal and enhancement are the hallmarks of injury (Fig. 29.33A). Cord contusions are often best visualized on gradient echo sequences, where the blood creates loss of signal and so appears black (Fig. 29.33B).

Suggested Readings

Gomori JM, Grossman RI. Mechanisms responsible for the MR appearance and evolution of intracranial hemorrhage. *Radiographics.* 1988;8:427.

Grossman RI, Yousem DM. *Neuroradiology: The Requisites.* 2nd ed. Philadelphia: Mosby; 2003.

Leach JL, Fortuna RB, Jones BV, et al. Imaging of cerebral venous thrombosis: current techniques, spectrum of findings, and diagnostic pitfalls. *Radiographics.* 2006;26:S19–S41.

Lell MM, Anders K, Uder M, et al. New techniques in CT angiography. *Radiographics.* 2006;26:S45–S62.

Lustrin ES, Karakas SP, Ortiz AO, et al. Pediatric cervical spine: normal anatomy, variants, and trauma. *Radiographics.* 2003;23:539.

Offiah CE, Turnbull IW. The imaging appearances of intracranial CNS infections in adult HIV and AIDS patients. *Clin Radiol.* 2006;61(5):393–401.

Srinivasan A, Goyal M, Azri FA, et al. State-of-the-art imaging of acute stroke. *Radiographics.* 2006;26:S75–S95.

CHAPTER 30 ■ INTENSIVE CARE UNIT POINT-OF-CARE TESTING

WILLIAM E. WINTER

INTRODUCTION

This chapter will focus on three aspects of laboratory testing in the intensive care unit (ICU) setting: (a) choice of point-of-care (POC) tests, (b) quality assurance in POC testing (POCT), and (c) regulatory issues germane to POCT.

DEFINITION OF POINT-OF-CARE TESTING

Point-of-care testing is the performance of laboratory tests in the immediate physical vicinity of the patient (1). A synonym for POCT is "near-patient testing." By definition, samples for POCT are not sent by courier or tube system to another geographically distant site.

POCT can be performed in the patient's home, business, or school; in a physician's office (e.g., a physician office laboratory [POL]); in a clinic; or near the patient's bedside in the hospital or emergency room. POC tests can essentially be performed anywhere where trained personel are present to provide patient care such as ICUs, operating rooms, ambulances, helicopters, ships, and airplanes. The most common POCT performed by patients is outpatient self-monitoring of blood glucose (SMBG) (2). In the outpatient setting, another commonly performed test—but far less common than SMBG—is self-testing for the prothrombin time-international normalized ratio (PT-INR) that is used to monitor and adjust warfarin doses in chronically anticoagulated patients (3).

Concerning inpatients, testing that is performed by medical technologists using central laboratory-type instruments near the patient's bedside can—geographically—qualify as POCT. However, such testing is outside the scope of this chapter, as such testing is really central laboratory testing in a noncentral laboratory location.

There are several strengths to POCT:

- Better sample stability between the time of sample drawing and analysis—often seconds in duration
- Shorter turnaround time (TAT); some results are available within a minute or less of sample acquisition
- Reduced sample volume requirements
- Immediate result availability to the respiratory therapist, nurse, or physician caring for the patient
- Opportunity for instantaneous notification of staff in cases of critical (e.g., "panic") values

CHOOSING WHICH TESTS TO RUN AT THE POINT OF CARE

POCT is most valuable when such test results immediately influence acute patient management (Tables 30.1 and 30.2) (1). An alternative way to provide similar rapid TATs is the placement of a satellite laboratory adjacent to the ICU or a tube system with direct sample delivery to a rapid response laboratory. Nevertheless, in resuscitations, it is difficult to argue against POCT being immediately adjacent to the patient.

If the test result will not immediately affect patient care, the higher cost of POCT compared with central laboratory testing is usually not justified. Also, POCT is usually not as accurate or precise as central laboratory testing, making central laboratory testing advantageous. In addition, if a nurse or respiratory therapist is performing POCT, this takes time away from his or her direct patient care activities. Other experts argue that the time to perform POCT is no longer than the time it takes to draw and label a sample for transit to a central or satellite laboratory.

A list of tests appropriate for POCT in the ICU include arterial blood gas (ABG) analysis, potassium, ionized calcium, glucose, and lactate. In addition to pH, pO_2, pCO_2, and calculated bicarbonate and hemoglobin saturation—either estimated from the pO_2 or measured directly via co-oximetry—ABG analysis provides a measurement of hemoglobin (g/dL) that can be of critical importance in postoperative patients or other patients who develop acute hypotension or manifest external evidence of bleeding, such as melena. If carbon monoxide poisoning or methemoglobinemia is present, pulse oximetry will not reflect the true hemoglobin saturation. In such instances, hemoglobin saturation must be directly determined by co-oximetry.

Sodium measurements are frequently performed concurrent with potassium measurements. However, unless a patient is suffering a seizure and hyponatremia must be excluded on an emergency basis, sodium measurements from a central laboratory are usually adequate to meet the clinical urgency of (nonseizure) circumstances. However, many POCT devices that measure potassium will concurrently and automatically measure sodium using ion-selective electrodes.

It can be argued that POCT for coagulation studies is not justified in the ICU setting because no immediate anticoagulation or procoagulation decisions need be made that cannot wait until coagulation studies are available from the central laboratory. This assumes a TAT for prothrombin time (PT), activated partial thromboplastic time (aPTT), and fibrinogen of less than 60 minutes. However, if cardiovascular intervention

TABLE 30.1

POINT-OF-CARE TESTING RECOMMENDATIONS FOR INTENSIVE CARE UNITS (ICUs)

Testing available at the point of care (POC), in a satellite laboratory adjacent to the ICU, or via rapid tube transport to a central laboratory
Arterial blood gases (includes hemoglobin concentration)
Lactate
Potassium (with or without sodium)
Glucose
Ionized calcium
Testing at a POC/satellite laboratory that is useful in special circumstances
Activated clotting time
Ionized magnesium
Examples of tests not justified at the POC or satellite laboratory
B-type natriuretic peptide/N-terminal-pro B-type natriuretic peptide (BNP/NT-proBNP)
Cardiac markers
Endocrine testing
Iron studies (serum iron, total iron binding capacity, ferritin)
Lipid testing
Liver function testing
Prothrombin time, activated partial thromboplastin time
Renal function testing
Total magnesium
Toxicology testing

procedures are carried out in the ICU, as opposed to the radiology suite, where heparin is administered in moderate to large doses, activated clotting times (ACTs) must be available within the unit to monitor heparin's effects. The ACT is monitored in such settings because such high doses of heparin will prolong the aPTT to infinity, as no clot forms. ACT is then monitored in place of the aPTT to determine when the arterial sheath can be removed. If an intravascular sheath is in place, the ACT is monitored to confirm that excessive anticoagulation is not present prior to sheath removal. The intensivist must be aware that while the term *ACT* is generic, ACT measurements performed on devices produced by different manufacturers are most often not equivalent. Thus, clotting time guidelines from one device are not necessarily transferable to another device, and such clotting guidelines must be determined for each manufacturer's ACT instrument.

While POC measurements of cardiac markers [myoglobin, MB isoenzyme of creatine kinase (CK-MB), troponine I, or troponin-T], markers of cardiac failure [BE type natriuretic peptide (BNP) or NT-proBNP (N-terminal-pro-B-type natriuretic peptide)], and emergency toxicology testing (ethanol, opiates, cocaine, PCP, and so forth) may be justified in the emergency room where patients require immediate triage (4), the performance of these tests at the POC in the ICU is not justified. The advantages of superior accuracy and reproducibility available through the central laboratory outweigh any TAT advantage of POCT. It is unlikely in the ICU that a cardiac marker result TAT of less than 30 to 60 minutes will improve patient care. Likewise, there are no emergency decisions concerning renal function assessment, such as creatinine, blood urea nitrogen, and urinalysis, or liver function assessment, such as total protein, albumin, total and direct bilirubin, alanine aminotransferase (ALT), aspartate aminotransferase (AST), and alkaline phosphatase, that warrant routine POCT for these analytes in the ICU.

PEARLS

- Every hospital and ICU is distinctive and has unique laboratory needs.
- The nursing staff, intensivists, POCT coordinators, and clinical pathologists should work together to define the appropriate testing mix for their institution.

TABLE 30.2

EXAMPLES OF LABORATORY TESTS AND THE DECISIONS BASED ON THEIR RESULTS

Test	Possible clinical impacts
Arterial blood gases	Administration of oxygen or ventilator support
Lactate	If elevated: Need for more aggressive acute intervention with intravenous fluids, pressors, and/or improved ventilation
Na^+, K^+, Cl^-, total serum CO_2, Cr, blood urea nitrogen, serum and urine osmolality	Rates and type of fluid resuscitation or fluid restriction, need for fluid boluses, des-amino-d-arginine vasopressin (DDAVP) administration, fluid restriction for renal failure
Glucose	Attainment and maintenance of tight glycemic control
Ionized calcium	Need for intravenous calcium administration
Hemoglobin/hematocrit	Assessment of need for transfusion of red blood cells
Platelet count	Assessment of need for platelet transfusions
Activated clotting time	Management of heparin anticoagulation and reversal of anticoagulation (e.g., protamine sulfate administration)
Prothrombin time, activated partial thromboplastin time, thrombin time, fibrinogen	Assessment of possible coagulopathy

QUALITY ASSURANCE IN POINT-OF-CARE TESTING

Because so many ICU decisions are based upon the results of laboratory analyses (Table 30.1), the intensivist must understand the strengths and the limitations of laboratory testing, whether performed in a central lab, in a satellite lab, or at the POC (1).

In order to provide quality results, an overview of quality assurance (QA) concepts in laboratory testing follows. The National Committee for Clinical Laboratory Standards (now the Clinical Laboratory Standards Committee [CLSC]) defined quality assurance as "the practice which encompasses all endeavors, procedures, formats and activities directed towards ensuring that a specified quality or product is achieved and maintained." QA programs encompass assessments of analytical quality control; monitoring of turnaround times, regulatory compliance, and success of proficiency testing; and supervision of personnel training and competency.

To provide quality results:

1. Standard operating procedures (SOPs) must be developed and followed
2. Systems must be in place to recognize and solve random and systematic problems
3. Result reliability must be defined in terms of suitable precision and accuracy

A QA program assesses all aspects of testing: Preanalytical, analytical, and postanalytical events. Preanalytical issues concern proper patient identification and tube labeling, proper sample acquisition, appropriate transport to the central lab or to the POCT device (e.g., cooling of ABG samples), and timing of the test (e.g., proper timing for therapeutic drug monitoring). Analytical matters concern the instrument performance, and postanalytical issues concern proper result reporting (e.g., the correct result is reported on the correct patient).

Theoretically, the goal of laboratory testing is to produce timely and reliable (e.g., quality) measurements of analytes that assist in the diagnosis, management, and prevention of human diseases. Analyte is a generic term for any substance that is measured in any fluid. Testing is most commonly carried out on blood or urine samples, but other fluids can be examined, such as cerebrospinal fluid (CSF), stool, semen, vitreous fluid, saliva, cyst fluids, exudates, and transudates. Blood tests can be performed on whole blood, serum, or plasma. The source of blood can be arterial, capillary, or venous. Essentially all capillary tests are performed on whole blood.

When whole blood is drawn into a tube containing an anticoagulant (e.g., heparin, potassium oxalate, or sodium citrate) and the tube is centrifuged, plasma results and floats above the level of the red blood cells. Platelet-poor plasma results when the anticoagulated blood is spun hard enough to sediment the platelets. For example, platelet-poor citrated plasma is used in the PT, aPTT, thrombin time (TT), and fibrinogen assays. On the other hand, when plasma is not spun vigorously (i.e., a "soft" spin), platelet-rich plasma results (i.e., plasma in which the platelet count is greater than 10,000 platelets/μL), which is used when certain types of specialized platelet function tests are carried out, such as platelet aggregation studies in response to agents such as thrombin, epinephrine, adenosine diphosphate (ADP), thromboxane A_2, or ristocetin.

When whole blood is placed into a tube containing no anticoagulant (e.g., a red top tube) and the blood is allowed to clot, serum results after centrifugation. Plasma contains clotting factors, whereas these are absent from serum. Plasma is what is present in living people; serum results when blood clots and serum is present in the bloodstream postmortem as blood clots following death.

In the ICU setting, the sample of choice is usually whole blood drawn from an artery when measuring blood gases, or arterial or venous whole blood when, for example, measuring sodium, potassium, glucose, lactate, or ionized calcium. If patients are not in shock and display satisfactory peripheral perfusion, a warmed finger or toe can be lanceted to obtain a capillary whole-blood sample for glucose measurement. In the ICU setting, besides hematocrit and glucose measurements, there are no other common reasons to obtain capillary blood.

The Value of Laboratory Test Results

The value of a test result can be conceptualized as the quality of the result divided by the TAT (Equation 1). This assumes that the laboratory data can be acted upon as soon as the data become available. Certainly, physiologic parameters that change the most rapidly attract and demand our attention, such as pH, pCO_2, pO_2, glucose, and potassium.

Quality results are accurate, and repeated measurements of the same sample demonstrate reproducibility (e.g., high precision; Equation 2). The central laboratory's ability to provide both quality results and a short TAT are often at odds with one another; more accurate and precise complex assays are usually more time-consuming, and such tests may not be available on POCT devices. Figure 30.1 depicts a theoretical curve for the relationship of result quality (y axis) and TAT (x axis). If assay time is reduced below a certain limit, the quality of the assay will be reduced. On the other hand, significant delays in making critical clinical decisions can adversely affect patient outcome. We must also acknowledge that POC tests rarely, if ever, will be as accurate or precise as tests accomplished in the central laboratory.

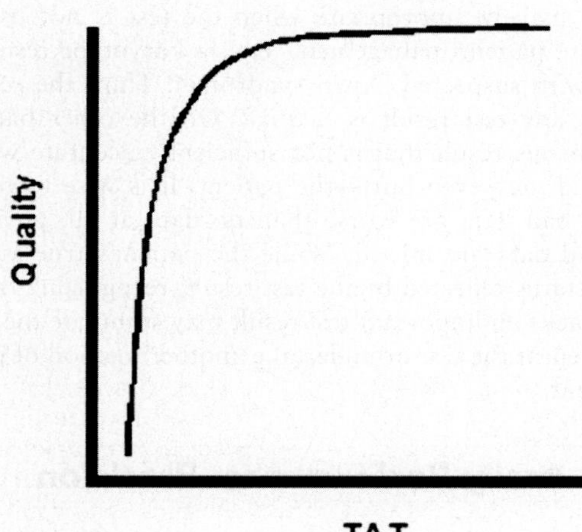

FIGURE 30.1. Relationship of quality to TAT. TAT, turnaround time.

Equation 1:

$$\text{Value of a test} \approx \text{Quality of the result} \times \text{Turnaround time}^{-1}$$

Note: Higher-quality results and lower turnaround times can provide higher-value tests.

Equation 2:

$$\text{Quality of the result} \approx \text{Bias}^{-1} \times \text{Coefficient of variation}^{-1}$$

Note: Reduced bias (e.g., higher accuracy) and reduced coefficients of variation (e.g., higher precision) improve the quality of the test result.

Desirable intrinsic characteristics of the assay for the diagnosis, management, or prediction of disease are a high sensitivity and specificity. In epidemiologic terms, *sensitivity* is the number of true positive results divided by the number of observations in a diseased population.

$$\text{Sensitivity} = \text{True Positives} \div (\text{True Positives} + \text{False Negatives})$$

Specificity is the number of true negative results divided by the number of observations undertaken in a nondiseased population.

$$\text{Specificity} = \text{True Negatives} \div (\text{True Negatives} + \text{False Positives})$$

In its broadest sense, TAT is the "vein to brain" time: The time it takes between sample acquisition (e.g., venipuncture: the *vein* time) to result recognition by the treating physician (e.g., the *brain* time). Usually TAT is defined as the duration of time between sample acquisition and result reporting. Unfortunately, the laboratory often has little control over factors that determine when a sample is delivered to the central laboratory after acquisition. Similarly, preanalytical problems frequently develop because the sample is not properly drawn, labeled, or preserved prior to delivery to the lab. To be of value, the correct sample must be drawn from the correct patient at the correct time in the correct volume and placed in the correct tube.

If the analysis produces the most accurate result possible, but the TAT is unacceptably long, the value of the result in patient management is significantly degraded. TAT is most important in the ICU setting when the test results are used to immediately alter the patient's care. Examples of such tests include arterial blood gases for ventilator patients and glucose measurements in tight glycemic control protocols. There are many instances, however, where a TAT of several hours or more may be appropriate when the test is not used for immediate patient management (e.g., a karyotype result in a patient with suspected Down syndrome). Thus, the *required* TAT for any test result is *relative*. On the other hand, an instantaneous result that is not sufficiently accurate will not help—and may even hurt—the patient. It is wise to remember that bad data are worse than no data at all; physicians using bad data are misled. While the patient's true status is not the status reflected by the test result, recognizing that the patient lacks an important test result may stimulate the physician to repeat the test or undertake another method of patient assessment.

Assay Performance: Precision

Precision is synonymous with reproducibility; for example, if aliquots of the original sample are retested, will the same result as the original result be observed (5)? Precision can be defined in terms of the assay's standard deviation (SD) and coefficient of variation (CV). When aliquots of a single sample are measured repeatedly, the histographic distribution of results will represent a bell-shaped curve. Other descriptions for such a distribution include a Gaussian distribution or parametric distribution.

The SD for an assay is the square root of the variance. The variance is calculated as follows: The difference between each individual value and the mean is squared, these values are summed, and the sum of the squares is then divided by the number of repeats minus one. Sixty-eight percent of the repeats will fall within ± 1 SD of the mean. Approximately 95% of the repeats will fall within ± 2 SD of the mean, and approximately 99% of the repeats will fall within ± 3 SD of the mean. This concept will be used in developing rules that will help us determine when an analysis and analyzer are or are not working properly.

CV is expressed as a percent: The SD is divided by the mean multiplied by 100. While SDs have values with units—mg/dL for glucose or mm Hg for pO_2—and are difficult to remember, CVs are unitless and allow easy comparisons among various analyses without needing to recall the specific SD or units. For example, electrolyte measurements using ion-selective electrodes usually display CVs of 1% to 2%. In comparison, analyses that use chemical reactions with spectrophotometric or electrical detection typically have CVs of 4% to 5%. As a consequence of their complex nature involving antigen–antibody interactions, immunoassays can show even greater variability, with CVs of 5% to 10%.

Precision can be further described as intra-assay or interassay reproducibility. Intra-assay precision is assessed when the same sample is run 10, 20, or more times in a single run. A "run" is the series of same analyses that are accomplished in a single day, shift, or other period of time during which the analyzer is believed to be analytically stable (e.g., does not require recalibration; many modern analyses are so stable that calibration may not be required for many days or longer). Intra-assay comparisons would not exceed 1 day.

Intra-assay precision is almost always superior to interassay precision. Interassay precision is determined by measuring the same sample serially on different days (e.g., measuring the same sample once per day for 20 or more workdays in a row). For a typical chemical analysis, the intra-assay CV might be 5% and the interassay CV might be 7%. Clinicians do need to know the total imprecision—the combined intra-assay (e.g., same-day or same-shift reproducibility) and interassay (e.g., reproducibility over several days) imprecision—because some patients may be, for example, on ventilatory support for days or weeks with various degrees of pulmonary failure. While CVs and SDs cannot be added together to determine total imprecision, the intra-assay and interassay variances can be added together. The square root of the *total* variance then provides the SD, and the SD divided by the sample mean (multiplied by 100) provides the percent CV.

Assay Performance: Accuracy

Accuracy is a measure of bias. *Bias* is the difference between the "real" (or "true") result and the measured result; bias can be positive or negative. A positive bias is present when the measured result exceeds the true result. A negative bias is found when the measured result is less than the true result. Bias must not be excessive; the bias that does exist must not lead to incorrect diagnosis, management, or disease prediction.

The true result of an assay may be difficult to define or determine. This is especially true when there is only one basic method available for the measurement of an analyte. For many measurements, the only method of analysis is the field method (i.e., the analytical procedure that is used in the central laboratories or at POC). For example, PO_2 can only be measured using an oxygen-sensitive electrode. Reference methods, by definition, are more specific for the measurement of the analyte in question than the field method. Definitive methods are the best available methods of measurement with the highest specificity. Ideally, reference and definitive methods also have better precision than field methods. A review of cholesterol measurements can be instructive in comparing field, reference, and definitive methods.

The field method for cholesterol measurements is a spectrophotometric enzymatic assessment using cholesterol esterase and cholesterol oxidase. The definitive cholesterol measurement involves direct acidic oxidation of cholesterol with spectroscopic assessment of the oxidation products. The definitive measurement is isotopic dilution mass spectroscopy. Certainly, isotopic dilution mass spectroscopy will never be carried out in central laboratories or at the POC. Even acid oxidation of cholesterol will not be carried out in central laboratories or at the POC because concentrated acids are highly toxic and dangerous to work with, and such methods are not automated. However, the definitive method can be used to create standards that can be used as calibrators for reference methods. The reference methods are then employed to develop calibrators for the field methods.

Because reference intervals (i.e., the "normal" ranges) are based on such calibrators, if there is a significant bias in calibration between the method used to establish the reference interval and the method in real-time use in the care of the patient, errors may be made in the interpretation of the result as to whether or not it falls within the reference interval, and to what degree the result may exceed or fall below the reference interval. On the other hand, relative change (i.e., the present result compared to a previous result) will not be affected by bias if instrument calibration is stable and the assay is precise. However, a lack of precision can have a major misleading effect on the interpretation of serial results. A lack of precision (i.e., imprecision) requires that larger absolute differences occur between serial measurements to ensure that any difference occurring is an actual difference in the patient, rather than a variation (e.g., imprecision) in the assay. With a highly precise assay, small serial differences are more likely to represent a true difference in the patient's condition. With a highly imprecise assay, larger serial differences are required to indicate a true difference in the patient's condition. To further complicate the consideration of a normal versus an abnormal result, we must consider biologic variation: The normal variation in a biologic measurement that can represent minute-to-minute or hour-to-hour fluctuations: Ultradian rhythms (e.g., luteinizing hormone [LH] or follicle-stimulating hormone [FSH] secretion); daily variations: Circadian rhythms (e.g., a.m. vs. p.m. levels of cortisol); or variations greater than a day: Infradian rhythm (e.g., the menstrual period).

Analytical Sensitivity and Specificity

In analytical terms, sensitivity is the lowest concentration of an analyte that can reliably be measured. As measurements approach zero concentration of the analyte, the uncertainty of the measurement increases. At a certain point with a progressive decline in analyte concentration, the uncertainty of the measurement is so great that to report a lower number becomes meaningless. Analyzer manufacturers should define their lower limit of detection (LLD) to inform the user of the analyzer's expected analytical sensitivity. In addition, it is routine policy for laboratories to define their own LLD or, at a minimum, to confirm the manufacturer's stated LLD. In the ICU setting, LLD is most probably important in the measurement of glucose: "How low a glucose concentration can our POCT analyzer reliably report?" This must be carefully defined.

Analytical specificity is the certainty that the assay only measures the analyte of interest and does not measure other unintended substances in solution (e.g., "What is the assay's cross-reactivity to other analytes?"). Cross-reactivity is not usually an issue for POCT in ICUs based on the types of assays run in such situations. However, in the central laboratory, cross-reactivity can be a significant issue. For example, cardiac troponin-T or troponin-I measurements should not cross-react with skeletal muscle troponin-T or troponin-I. On the other hand, assay cross-reactivity is desirable if one wishes to test for a class of drugs (e.g., drug abuse testing for benzodiazepines, opiates, sympathomimetics, or barbiturates).

Quality Control Testing

For all inpatient testing, whether waived-regulated testing, moderate complexity testing, or high-complexity testing (see below), quality control must be assessed at least daily for all analytes measured on the device. For certain types of testing, such as radioimmunoassays or enzyme-linked immunosorbent assays (ELISAs), control testing may need to be performed with each run of patient samples.

To perform quality control testing, a sample of known concentration is measured with the device in question (5). This is the "control material" or, simply, the "control." The control material is usually available in a large volume and is prepared in many aliquots (e.g., greater than 100) in a stable (e.g., frozen) form, so that the control material can be used over the course of many months to even longer than 1 year.

If the control result for a run of samples falls within previously defined limits, the device is said to be "in control," and patient results can be reported. If the control result is outside defined limits, the device is said to be "out of control," meaning an analytical error has occurred and patient results cannot be reported. Another way to express an out-of-control run is to state that the run was rejected. Thus, before any patient results can be reported, the operator must ensure that the analyzer is functioning correctly. Clearly, the control material must be measured prior to the release of any patient results. Many times, the control is placed at the beginning and at the end of the run. For moderate- and high-complexity testing, at least two levels of control are usually assessed. For example, the mean value of one control can be near a clinical decision point, while the mean value of the other control value can be considerably above the clinical decision point.

If the assay is out of control, the operator must troubleshoot the problem. Possible causes of out-of-control runs include:

- Machine mechanical errors (e.g., pipetting too little or too much liquid)
- Outdated reagents
- Reagents that have lost potency due to heating or lack of refrigeration
- Degraded control materials
- Operator error (e.g., mislabeled or switched controls, as in reversing the low-level and high-level controls)
- Spectrophotometric error (e.g., bulb loss or degraded function)
- Detector error

Fortunately, most POCT devices, even if moderately complex, are self-contained, are fairly robust, and can be simply "fixed" by replacing the reagent cartridge.

James Westgard created a series of rules that can be used to determine if a run or device is in control or is out of control (5). These "Westgard rules," or their variations, are used essentially universally throughout the laboratory community. For each control material, the performance of the material is initially established by running this sample daily over the course of 20 to 30 days when the assay is otherwise known to be in control by using previously characterized control materials. From these data, the mean and the SD for the sample's measurement—the performance—on the device in question can be calculated.

Once the performance of the control material is known (i.e., its mean value and SD are established), this material can then be used to determine if subsequent runs are in control. If a single control value is 3 or fewer SDs away from the mean, the assay is in control and the results can be released. While, strictly speaking, being in control—a control result of more than +2 to +3 SDs above or less than −2 to −3 SDs below the mean—is a warning, the operator should review previous control data and confirm that other instrument parameters are functioning normally.

If the control result exceeds the mean value ± 3 SDs, this is such an unlikely event (e.g., this should occur at random no more than ~1% of the time) as to suggest that the run is out of control. A single out-of-control run represents the consequence of a random error. On the other hand, if in two sequential runs a control displays a warning result each time, the second run is out of control. This is the 2_{2S} rule[1] and demonstrates a probable systemic (i.e., nonrandom) error. The Westgard quality control errors are summarized in Table 30.3. Systematic errors reflect recurrent errors such as short sampling and a degraded reagent, a constant interference, or loss of calibration.

For many POCT assays, the mechanics of the measuring device (e.g., electrodes) are designed into a single-use, disposable cartridge. In such cases, individual cartridges cannot be quality controlled, as measurement of a control material in the cartridge expends the cartridge. However, when such cartridges are manufactured using highly automated and monitored systems, the reproducibility of the manufacturing process can be so highly regulated that minimal variation exists among cartridges within a single manufacturing run, batch, or lot. While individual cartridges cannot be tested for quality control, the batch of cartridges can be assessed upon receipt by the health care institution by measuring a control material in one or more cartridges chosen at random from the batch received. Devices that use disposable cartridges can have their electronics or optics checked daily or more often via electronic quality control. In electronic quality control, a cartridge simulator is placed into the instrument to test if the instrument reports the proper result as defined for the simulator.

[1]Two sequential results that are between >2 and 3 SDs away from the mean constitute a quality control violation.

TABLE 30.3

WESTGARD QUALITY CONTROL RULES FOR A SINGLE LEVEL OF CONTROL

Rule name	Rule definition
1_{2s}	One control result greater than 2 to 3 standard deviations (SDs) above or below the mean (warning only; all other rules are rejection rules)
1_{3s}	One control result greater than 3 SDs above or below the mean (random error)
2_{2s}	Two sequential control results greater than 2 to 3 SDs above or below the mean (systematic error)
R_{4s}	Two sequential control results with a total range of greater than 4 SDs (random error)
4_{1s}	Four sequential control results greater than 1 SD above or below the mean (systematic error)
10_m	Ten sequential control results above or below the mean (systematic error)

PEARLS

- The take-home message for the intensivist and patient care staff is that POCT must be quality controlled to ensure a high reliability of test results.

REGULATORY ISSUES IN POINT-OF-CARE TESTING

Laboratory testing, both at the POC and in satellite or central laboratories, is highly regulated by the Clinical Laboratory Improvement Amendments (CLIA) passed by the U.S. Congress in 1988. The shorthand term for the subsequent regulations is "CLIA 88" or, more simply, "CLIA." Laboratories that perform ex vivo tests on any human tissue or body fluid must be certified by the Secretary of Health and Human Services (HHS).

Analyses where a biologic sample is not intentionally removed from the body does not fall under CLIA regulations. These types of analyses reflect *monitoring* and not *testing* according to CLIA. Examples of such analyses include measurement of the partial pressure of exhaled carbon dioxide, alcohol breathalyzers, exhalation of $^{13}CO_2$ after oral administration of ^{13}C-urea in search of *Helicobacter pylori* infection, transcutaneous bilirubinometers, pulse oximetry, and intermittent arterial sampling via indwelling canula for blood gases when the blood is returned to the patient's body. Incidentally, workplace drug abuse testing does not fall under the CLIA regulations.

The CLIA laboratory certification program is operated by the Centers for Medicare and Medicaid Services (CMS) (formerly the Health Care Financing Administration [HCFA]), the Food and Drug Administration (FDA), and the Centers for Disease Control and Prevention (CDC). Specific information on CLIA can be found at http://www.fda.gov/cdrh/clia (the FDA CLIA website that addresses complexity test categorizations and waivers); http://www.cms.hhs.gov/clia (the CMS CLIA website concerning program information, statistics, etc.); and http://www.phppo.cdc.gov/clia/ (the CDC CLIA website regarding regulations).

Currently the FDA determines whether an in vitro diagnostic test (including the test system) is waived or not waived (e.g., nonwaived test). Nonwaived tests are further classified as moderate complexity or high complexity. Therefore, there are three major CLIA regulatory categories: Waived testing, moderate-complexity testing, and high-complexity testing. Strictly speaking, the location of testing—POC versus satellite or central laboratory—does not define the complexity of the testing. Moderate-complexity testing can be performed immediately adjacent to the POC in a satellite laboratory, while, alternatively, a waived test (e.g., BNP, BioSite Incorporated, San Diego, CA) can be performed in a central laboratory.

Waived Testing

Waived tests are defined as determinations that can be performed at any site by any operator (including the patients themselves) following the manufacturer's recommendations. Theoretically, a waived test is a test that is so simple to perform that it is believed to carry little risk of error. CLIA describes waived tests as "simple procedures with little chance of negative outcomes if performed inaccurately." However in the real world, experience teaches us that even waived tests can be performed improperly. Furthermore, erroneous results from certain waived tests in various situations can undoubtedly lead to potentially serious or fatal adverse outcomes (e.g., underestimation or overestimation of the PT-INR in patients being treated with warfarin for anticoagulation).

Waived testing that a person performs on him- or herself is not directly regulated by CLIA. However, whenever a health care provider performs a waived test on a patient, the testing is regulated. This is a common situation in ICUs when, for example, blood glucose testing is carried out by nursing personnel. Thus, CLIA has implications for waived testing in inpatient settings.

According to CLIA, hospitals must develop procedures and policies that specify the circumstances in which waived-test results are employed in patient management, services, and treatment. To achieve this, waived-test results must be placed in the clinical record, along with the appropriate reference interval (i.e., the normal range). The need for confirmatory testing must be defined; for example, if the POCT blood glucose is less than 60 mg/dL or greater than 500 mg/dL, a blood sample is sent to the central laboratory for confirmation. Finally, the test usage must be consistent with other hospital policies and the manufacturer's recommendations.

For inpatient waived testing to be performed properly, CLIA mandates that the staff executing the test must be identified, supervised, and qualified to perform the test. This requires adequate specific training and orientation to test performance and documentation of a satisfactory level of competence. This applies to all health care providers, including physicians. Competency must be demonstrated at the time of orientation training and yearly thereafter. Determination of competency must include at least two of the following four assessments:

1. Performing a test on an unknown specimen
2. Observation by a supervisor or qualified delegate
3. Monitoring the user's quality control performance
4. Written testing relevant to the waived-test method

Other CLIA standards for inpatient waived testing include that written policies and procedures are readily available and kept up to date; quality control checks are defined and conducted on each procedure; and the quality control results are recorded and maintained for review.

Blood glucose testing at the POC is an example of a waived and regulated test. Other examples of waived tests are given in Table 30.4. Presently, there are at least 40 waived tests;

TABLE 30.4

EXAMPLES OF WAIVED TESTS

- B-type natriuretic peptide
- Bladder tumor–associated antigen
- Blood lead
- Estrone 3-glucuronide
- Fecal occult blood
- Gastric occult blood, gastric pH
- Hematocrit, spun
- Hemoglobin (whole blood)
- Hemoglobin A_{1c}
- Ketones in blood
- Lipids: Cholesterol, triglycerides, high-density lipoprotein cholesterol
- Lithium
- Nasal swab for influenza A/B
- Platelet aggregation studies
- Prothrombin time-international normalized ratio
- Saliva fern test
- Thyroid-stimulating hormone
- Urine creatinine
- Urine dipstick test strips (e.g., pH, specific gravity, protein, glucose, blood, ketones, urobilinogen, bilirubin, leukocytes, nitrites)
- Urine human chorionic gonadotropin, luteinizing hormone (an LH ovulation test), follicle-stimulating hormone (FSH for menopause testing)
- Urine microalbumin
- Urine toxicology testing (e.g., cocaine, tetrahydrocannabinol [THC], amphetamines, methamphetamine, phencyclidine [PCP], barbiturates, tricyclic antidepressants, methylenedioxymethamphetamine (MDMA), opiates, oxycodone, morphine, propoxyphene, etc.)
- Various chemistry tests (e.g., total protein, total bilirubin, alanine aminotransferase, alkaline phosphatase, amylase, γ-glutamyl transpeptidase, blood urea nitrogen)
- Various tests for infection (e.g., monospot, *Helicobacter pylori* antibodies, group A *Streptococcus*, vaginal aerobic/anaerobic organisms, adenovirus, respiratory syncytial virus)

Note: Approval of a test as being waived is device specific; listing a test in this table does not imply that all versions of the test are waived.

the current list of waived tests and devices can be found at http://www.accessdata.fda.gov/scripts/cdrh/cfdocs/cfClia/testswaived.cfm.

It is important to recognize that CLIA approval of a test as being waived is device-specific: The test and the device are together approved as being waived for a specific analysis. For example, just because one manufacturer's test for blood glucose is waived does not mean that all single-use strip measurements of glucose by all manufacturers are waived. In the outpatient setting, the most commonly performed waived tests include urine pregnancy tests, blood glucose measurements, urine dipstick/tablet chemistries, ovulation tests, and fecal occult blood tests.

A laboratory or health care unit performing only waived tests must obtain a certificate of waiver (COW). COW laboratories are required to follow manufacturers' test instructions, participate in the CLIA program, and pay applicable biennial certificate fees. This is relevant outside the formal boundaries of the hospital and ICU setting.

Moderate- and High-Complexity Testing

CLIA defines moderate-complexity tests as being more intricate than waived tests. Moderate-complexity testing is typically carried out on automated analyzers. Examples of such tests include blood counts and routine chemistries. High-complexity tests are still more complicated, usually involving nonautomated or complicated analyses requiring considerable technologist or laboratory professional judgment, such as cross-matching of blood or microbiology testing.

Seven categories are considered when classifying the complexity of a nonwaived test:

1. Required operator knowledge
2. Operator training and experience
3. Preparation of reagents and materials
4. Characteristics of the operational steps
5. Calibration, quality control, and proficiency testing
6. Test system troubleshooting and equipment maintenance
7. Test result interpretation and judgment

For each category, the complexity of the test is scored: A score of 1 indicates the lowest level of complexity, and a score of 3 indicates the highest level. A score of 2 indicates complexity intermediate between 1 and 3. If the total score for the seven criteria is 12 or less, the test/device system is categorized as moderate complexity, whereas those test/device systems receiving scores above 12 are codified as high complexity.

Moderate- and high-complexity tests require quality control, proficiency testing, a quality assurance program, and so forth. There are also specific and detailed requirements regarding personnel qualifications and, as an aside, we point out that the experienced laboratorian recognizes that their most important resource is a highly skilled staff. Excluding provider-performed microscopy (PPM), which is a subset of moderate-complexity testing, all nonwaived tests are generally the purview of the pathologist and the clinical laboratory, or supervised by the pathologist and the clinical laboratory. Similar to waived, but regulated, POC tests, all moderate-complexity tests performed at the POC are regulated and, at a minimum, require similar training, supervision, quality control, and proficiency testing as waived inpatient tests.

Many POC testing devices applicable to ICUs are of moderate complexity. Some POCT devices applicable to ICUs perform only blood gas measurements (pH, pO_2, pCO_2), while the option to perform co-oximetry may also be available. Other devices will measure Na^+, K^+, glucose, ionized Ca^{2+}, and/or lactate, in addition to blood gases. At least one device on the market has the capacity to measure cardiac markers and PT-INR in addition to the above parameters. Some devices can perform a wide battery of non–blood gas analyses and may not even be of moderate complexity (e.g., the Abraxis Piccolo POC Chemistry Analyzer [Abraxis North America, Union City, CA] is CLIA waived and regulated).

While not attempting to provide an exhaustive list of all available blood gas analyzers, robust blood gas analyzers are available from a variety of manufacturers, including the following:

Abbott Point of Care Inc., East Windsor, NJ: iStat
Bayer Diagnostics, MA: Rapidpoint 400
ITC, Edison, NJ: IRMA TRUpoint Blood Gas Analysis System
Nova Biomedical, Waltham, MA: Stat Profile CCX, pHOx and pHOx Plus
Radiometer America Inc., Westlake, OH: Radiometer ABL80 FLEX, ABL77, and NPT7

Some of these devices are completely mobile and hand-held (e.g., iStat), while other analyzers can be pole-mounted (Radiometer ABL80 FLEX) or only require a small amount of bench space (e.g., they have a small "footprint") (Radiometer NPT7).

PEARLS

- The "take-home" message here is that intensivists and patient care staff must ensure that all regulatory rules are followed and enforced. This provides the best environment possible for the provision of accurate and precise laboratory test results.

FURTHER CONSIDERATIONS IN POINT-OF-CARE TESTING IN THE INTENSIVE CARE UNIT

Intensivists should work closely with their hospital's clinical pathologists and POCT coordinators in determining what type of acute testing should be available in their ICU. With the emergence of tight glycemic control, blood glucose testing must be available at the POC in ICUs. Such testing should be robust, accurate, and precise, and suffer from few, if any, critical interferences. These characteristics must also be sought in any POCT device that is brought into the ICU.

The need for POCT for blood gases and other tests depends on the ease of sample delivery to a satellite or central hospital laboratory and result TAT. In our satellite "STAT" laboratory located immediately outside the operating room complex and adjacent to many of the ICUs, 90% of blood gas results are reported in 7 minutes or less.

If blood gas analyses are performed in the ICU, unless personnel are added to the ICU staff, the work load is transferred, to some extent, to the ICU nursing or respiratory care staffs from the laboratory staff. However, there may be time savings in the ICU if a sample does not need to be prepared for transit to the satellite or central laboratory, and it is this immediacy of the test result that *may* improve patient care. Nevertheless, it is very difficult to find evidence-based medicine studies that clearly demonstrate better patient outcomes that result from reduced laboratory turnaround times. Even if patient care is not markedly improved, reduced TATs may aid in transferring patients to the floor or home more quickly. Patients may be more rapidly weaned from ventilation, which may decrease the use of resources. After improving patient outcomes, the next most important outcome variable for most hospital administrators is the expense of care and the need to reduce those costs (6).

If the decision has been made to proceed with POCT in the ICU, the analyzer and the support system must be carefully chosen. Ideally, the POCT device should have the ability to easily interface with the laboratory information system (LIS) to enable laboratory data transfer, billing, quality control data management, and tracking of operator competency (7). The nursing staff or respiratory care staff that will perform the testing should have a voice in the analyzer choice. The device's reproducibility must be examined (i.e., the precision of the device) (5), and the device results should be correlated with those of the central laboratory in search of biases (i.e., the accuracy of the device) (5).

Just as important as the analyzer is the quality of the blood sample that will be used for testing. For example, blood for a glucose measurement that is drawn through a line though which glucose has been infused may give falsely elevated values unless a sufficient "blank" sample is drawn through the line—in other words, "clearing the line" beforehand. Recall that D5 has a glucose concentration of 500 mg/dL (five times greater than normal) and D10 has a glucose concentration of 1,000 mg/dL (ten times greater than normal). Another example of such a preanalytical error is the exposure of blood to room air when blood gas testing is warranted. Blood samples exposed to room air can exhibit an increased PO_2, decreased PCO_2, and increased pH. When POCT devices that require cartridges are used, proper filling of the cartridge is essential to obtain a valid result. Wasting cartridges is expensive; in some systems, individual cartridges may cost several dollars, as opposed to pennies per test in a central laboratory.

Analytical interferences must be considered in the choice of ICU POCT instruments. An interference is a characteristic of a patient sample that may bias the result. Examples of interferences affecting certain central laboratory tests include hyperlipidemia, hyperbilirubinemia, and hemolysis. At the POC, blood glucose testing devices that use glucose dehydrogenase and the PQQ reagent (pyrroloquinolinequinone) display positive interferences when maltose is present in the patient's bloodstream. Maltose is used as a stabilizer in drugs such as intravenous immunoglobulin, and icodextrin used in dialysis is metabolized to maltose. This positive interference can lead to an overestimate of the blood glucose and subsequent overtreatment of "hyperglycemia," with severe or even fatal hypoglycemia as the consequence. Glucose oxidase devices that use the patient's blood as a source of oxygen exhibit negative biases in the glucose measurement in cases of hypoxia or where the elevation is over approximately 5,000 feet. On the other hand, glucose oxidase devices that use ferricine or ferricyanide display positive biases in blood glucose when the patient is hypoxic and negative biases when the patient is hyperoxic, such as a ventilated patient receiving supplemental oxygen.

Quality control for the POCT must be carried out and monitored as part of an overall quality assurance program. All device operators will require initial training and competency testing. Cost per test must also be a consideration. POCT can be ten or more times as expensive as central laboratory testing. In considering any POCT in the ICU, the pathologist and POCT coordinator must be involved in this process from the start, as this fosters a collegial relationship. In the end, the ultimate goal is to provide excellent patient care. New laboratory tests will continue to appear that will influence ICU care such as test panels for stroke and sepsis and improved cardiac risk panels. Prudent review of the medical literature and cooperation between the ICU staff and the laboratory staff will help determine where such testing is best carried out.

References

1. Nichols JH. Point-of-care testing. In: Nichols JH, ed. *Point-of-Care Testing, Performance Improvement and Evidence-Based Outcomes.* New York: Marcel Dekker, Inc.; 2003:1.
2. Winter WE. Point-of-care testing in the management of diabetes mellitus. In: Nichols JH, ed. *Point-of-Care Testing, Performance Improvement and Evidence-Based Outcomes.* New York: Marcel Dekker, Inc.; 2003:235.
3. Nuttall GA, Santrach P. Hemoglobin and coagulation. In: Nichols JH, ed. *Point-of-Care Testing, Performance Improvement and Evidence-Based Outcomes.* New York: Marcel Dekker, Inc.; 2003:353.
4. Christenson RH, Azzazy El-Badaway HME. Point-of-care testing for biochemical markers of acute coronary syndromes. In: Nichols JH, ed. *Point-of-Care Testing, Performance Improvement and Evidence-Based Outcomes.* New York: Marcel Dekker, Inc.; 2003:379.
5. Westgard JO, Klee GG. Quality management. In: Burtis CA, Ashwood ER, Bruns DE, eds. *Tietz Textbook of Clinical Chemistry and Molecular Diagnostics.* St. Louis: Elsevier Saunders; 2006:485.
6. Schallom L. Point of care testing in critical care. *Crit Care Nurs Clin North Am.* 1999;11:99.
7. Halpern NA. Point of care diagnostics and networks. *Crit Care Clin.* 2000;16:623.

SECTION III ■ TECHNIQUES, PROCEDURES, AND TREATMENTS

CHAPTER 31 ■ CLEAN AND ASEPTIC TECHNIQUES AT THE BEDSIDE

RABIH O. DAROUICHE

IMPORTANCE OF NOSOCOMIAL BLOODSTREAM INFECTION

The success in using better technology and more effective medicinal agents to prolong the survival of critically ill, immunocompromised, and an older population of patients has, unfortunately, been associated with a surge in the incidence and complications of nosocomial infections. At the present time, more than 2 million cases of hospital-acquired infection occur each year in the United States, resulting in the death of about 90,000 patients.

Although bloodstream infection generally accounts for less than 15% of all cases of nosocomial infections, critically ill patients and persons with cancer have disproportionately higher rates of nosocomial bloodstream infections. This phenomenon can be explained, at least in part, by the fact that the critically ill patient is more dependent on vascular access, and the vascular catheter is the most important culprit for nosocomial bloodstream infections. For instance, not only do bloodstream infections account for 20% of all cases of nosocomial infections among ICU patients, but 87% of bacteremias originate from an infected central vascular catheter (1). Similarly, most cases of bloodstream infection among cancer patients are associated with an indwelling vascular catheter, including 70% of patients with solid tumors and 56% of those who suffer from hematologic malignancy (2).

The vast majority of the 175 million vascular catheters inserted each year in the United States are peripherally placed, and are very unlikely—less than 0.1% to 0.2%—to cause bloodstream infection (3). Most cases of catheter-related bloodstream infection (CRBSI) arise from the almost 6 million central vascular catheters inserted annually. These data include about 4.5 million short-term catheters, with a mean duration of placement of 7 to 10 days, and 1.5 million long-term catheters, over one million of which are mainly peripherally inserted central catheters (PICCs), and the rest are tunneled catheters (4).

We have witnessed over the last several years an escalating drive to prevent CRBSIs, with the intention of achieving four goals:

1. Reduce the unacceptably high incidence of catheter-related bloodstream infection. Since, on average, about 5% of the 6 million annually placed central vascular catheters result in bloodstream infection, about 300,000 cases of CRBSI occur each year in the United States, including at least 80,000 cases among ICU patients (5). The rates of CRBSI tend to be lower in the surgical care units than in medical and pediatric intensive care units; that difference is attributed, at least in part, to a relatively shorter mean duration of catheter placement in the surgical intensive care unit.
2. Avoid the serious complications of CRBSI, which can result in irreversible multiorgan damage and has an attributable mortality that can be as high as 23% (6) to 25% in critically ill patients (7–9).
3. Limit the economic sequelae, as the treatment of CRBSIs in a critically ill patient increases cost as much as $29,000 (7–9) to $56,000 (10) per case, and surviving patients are hospitalized for a mean of 6.5 (7–9) to 22 (10) days longer than those who do not develop such an infection. The overall annual cost of management approaches $2.3 billion.
4. Control the presence of organisms within the biofilm surrounding indwelling vascular catheters since this environment constitutes an optimal reservoir for emergence of antibiotic resistance, including vancomycin-intermediate or -resistant staphylococci (11,12).

To offer the increasingly time-constrained intensivists a scientifically based and clinically applicable assessment, this chapter will review only approaches that have been evaluated in prospective randomized clinical trials or meta-analyses that have already been reported in peer-reviewed journals. Clinical trials with less desirable designs, including nonrandomized, retrospective, and crossover studies, will not be considered because confounding variables may lead to scientifically invalid conclusions. Likewise, results of studies that have been reported in an abstract form but have not yet been subjected to the peer review process will not be addressed.

EPIDEMIOLOGY OF NOSOCOMIAL BLOODSTREAM INFECTIONS

In the largest and most informative assessment of the epidemiology and microbiology of nosocomial bloodstream infections, the study of Surveillance and Control of Pathogens of Epidemiologic Importance (SCOPE) identified a total of 24,179 episodes of bloodstream infection in 49 U.S. hospitals from 1995 to 2002, for a rate of 60 cases per 10,000 hospital admissions (13). This study revealed that 87% of bloodstream infections were caused by a single organism, and 13% were polymicrobial. The monomicrobial episodes of nosocomial bloodstream infection were primarily caused by Gram-positive bacteria (65%, including coagulase-negative staphylococci in

31%, *Staphylococcus aureus* in 20%, and *Enterococcus* spp. in 9%), followed by Gram-negative bacteria (25%) and *Candida* spp. (9%). The overall crude mortality rate among patients with nosocomial bloodstream infection was 27% and was organism-specific as patients infected with *Candida* spp. and coagulase-negative staphylococci were the most (40%) and least (21%) likely to die, respectively. Very importantly, the percentage of hospital isolates of methicillin-resistant *S. aureus* (MRSA) significantly ($p < 0.001$) increased from 22% in 1995 to 57% in 2002.

DIAGNOSIS OF CATHETER-RELATED INFECTION

Since bloodstream infection is the most common serious complication of indwelling vascular catheters, early and accurate diagnosis of this infectious complication is essential. According to the Centers for Disease Control and Prevention (CDC) (14), CRBSI is defined as the isolation of the same organism (i.e., the same species with identical antimicrobial susceptibility) from the colonized catheter and from peripheral blood in a patient with clinical manifestations of sepsis and no other apparent source of bloodstream infection. Until recently, catheter colonization was almost always defined as the growth in cultures from either the tip or subcutaneous segment of the catheter of greater than or equal to 15 colony-forming units/mL by the semiquantitative roll-plate method (15), or greater than or equal to 1,000 colony-forming units/mL by the quantitative sonication method (16).

This standard manner of diagnosing CRBSI, however, is retrospective, as it requires removal and culture of the vascular catheter. Regrettably, only 15% to 25% of central venous catheters removed because of suspected catheter-related infection yield growth from cultures of the catheter tips (17). This explains the escalating interest in assessing and implementing procedures that are intended to prospectively diagnose catheter-related infection without removal of the catheter (18). The potential roles of two such microbiologic methods that could indicate whether the catheter is the source of bloodstream infection have been recently assessed. Both methods require concurrent collection of peripheral and central (i.e., through the lumen of the catheter) blood cultures. The first qualitative method—differential time to positivity (DTP)—which relies on the understanding that the culture of a blood sample that contains higher bacterial concentration would become positive, as detected by production of carbon dioxide by multiplying organisms, at least 2 hours before this would occur in a culture from peripheral blood (2). In the setting of a CRBSI, in which the catheter itself was the source of infection, the supposition is that the bacterial load of the infected catheter is higher than that seen in peripheral blood. The other quantitative method—paired quantitative blood cultures (PQBC)—is based on the anticipation that the number of colony-forming units (CFU) retrieved from a central blood culture would be greater than or equal to fivefold higher than that grown from cultured peripheral blood (19). Although a meta-analysis of 51 studies of both short- and long-term catheters published from 1996 to 2004 demonstrated that the PQBC method is the more accurate method in diagnosing intravascular device-related bloodstream infection (20), the PQBC method is less accurate than the DTP method for diagnosing bloodstream infection associated with short-term catheters (2,19). Furthermore, the PQBC method is more laborious and less implemented in hospital microbiology laboratories than the DTP method. In addition to considering the sensitivity, specificity, and the positive and negative predictive values of different diagnostic methods that do not require catheter removal, other factors—such as availability, ease of performance, cost, and clinical scenarios of individual patients—often affect the frequency of implementing various diagnostic methods in different medical facilities.

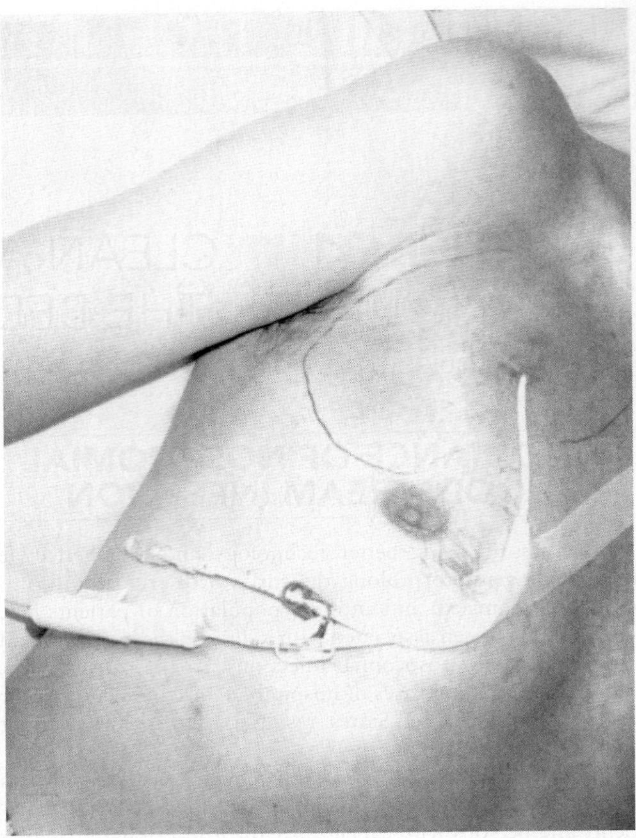

FIGURE 31.1. Exit-site infection around an indwelling double-lumen left subclavian central venous catheter that clinically manifested with pain, tenderness, erythema, and swelling.

Infections associated with vascular catheters can also present as an exit-site infection (Fig. 31.1), which manifest as erythema, tenderness, swelling, and drainage. Since inflammatory skin changes can be detected in only about one fourth of patients with bloodstream infection associated with central venous catheters, the absence of exit-site infection does not negate the existence of CRBSI. Patients with a tunneled vascular catheter can also develop tunnel infection which, like bloodstream infection but unlike exit-site infection, usually requires the removal of the infected catheter to establish cure.

PATHOGENESIS AND IMPACT ON PREVENTION

Source of Pathogens

The four potential sources of pathogens are the patient's skin around the site of catheter insertion, a contaminated catheter

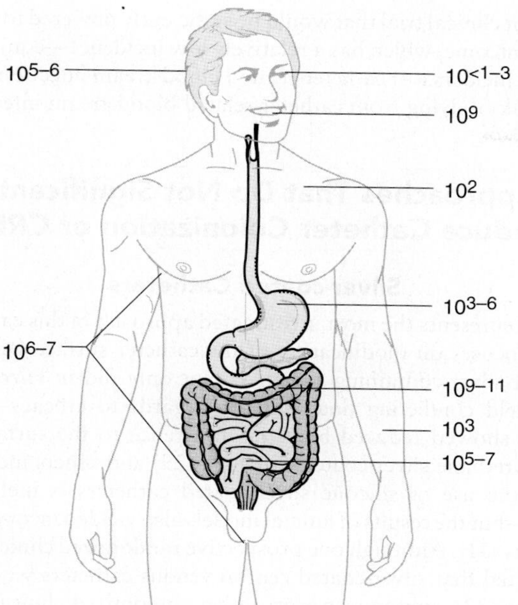

FIGURE 31.2. Colony-forming units of bacteria residing per square centimeter (cfu/cm^2) of skin surface in different body sites.

hub, hematogenous seeding from a distant site of infection, and infected infusate. The source of infecting organisms is not determined in about 25% of patients with CRBSI. Not only do both of the first two sources listed above originate from the skin—of the patient and health care providers—but they collectively are responsible for the vast majority of catheter-associated infections. The patient's skin around the catheter insertion site is the most common source of organisms that colonize central venous catheters with a short-term (mean duration, less than 7 to 10 days) indwelling time (21). As shown in Figure 31.2, the concentration of bacteria on the skin differs between various body sites, with the highest concentration generally present in the femoral area, which is greater than the jugular area, which itself is greater than the subclavian area. Factors that favor higher bacterial concentration on the skin where catheters are inserted include soiling by bacteria-containing bodily fluids and secretions, presence of hair follicles, high temperature, and moist environment. After colonizing the external surface of the catheter, skin-derived flora migrate along the subcutaneous segment into the distal intravascular segment to potentially result in bloodstream infection. In this clinical scenario of infection associated with long-term vascular catheters that are subjected to more extensive manipulation at the catheter hub, the catheter hub becomes contaminated by organisms that originate from the hands of medical personnel, then migrate along the internal surface of the catheter into the intravascular segment before causing bloodstream infection (22). The difference in the pathogenesis of infections associated with short-term versus long-term catheters helps explain why a surface-modified vascular catheter with antimicrobial activity only along the external surface is likely to protect against infection associated with short-term but not long-term catheters.

Type of Pathogens

The pathogenesis of infections associated with vascular catheters dictates the microbiology of this infection. Because the patient's skin around the catheter insertion site and the hands of medical personnel provide the two most common sources of pathogens, at least two thirds of cases of catheter-related infection are caused by staphylococcal organisms (coagulase-negative staphylococci and *Staphylococcus aureus*) (23). Less common pathogens, including Gram-negative bacteria and *Candida* spp., collectively cause about 25% of infection cases and are particularly prominent in infections from vascular catheters placed for long periods of time. Because of this wide array of potential pathogens, potentially preventive approaches that are active only against Gram-positive bacteria may not significantly reduce the overall rate of infection and, in some instances, may even predispose to superinfection by less common pathogens.

Milieu of Pathogens

Like other medical devices, infection of vascular catheters centers around the universal formation of a layer of biofilm surrounding the indwelling catheter (Fig. 31.3). The biofilm is composed of both bacterial products (fibroglycocalyx in the case of coagulase-negative staphylococci) and host factors—platelets and tissue ligands such as fibronectin, fibrinogen, and fibrin that variably adhere to well-described receptors on the surface of certain organisms, including staphylococcal and *Candida* organisms (24). Not only does the biofilm act as a protective barrier for embedded organisms against host immune defenses, including phagocytosis and opsonization (25,26), but it also can impair the activity (27) and, possibly, the penetration (28) of antibiotics against the slowly growing sessile organisms that inhabit the biofilm. This unique biofilm environment may explain why surface-modified vascular catheters containing antimicrobial agents that retain activity within the biofilm, and leach from the catheter surface to produce a zone of inhibition

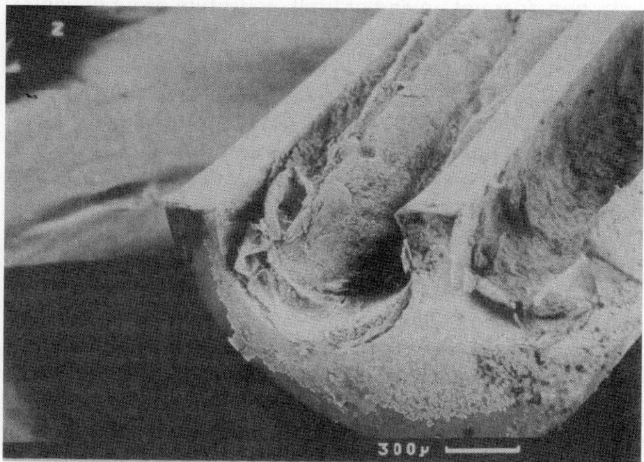

FIGURE 31.3. A cross-sectional image of a multilumen central venous catheter delineating the presence of a layer of biofilm around the luminal surface of the catheter.

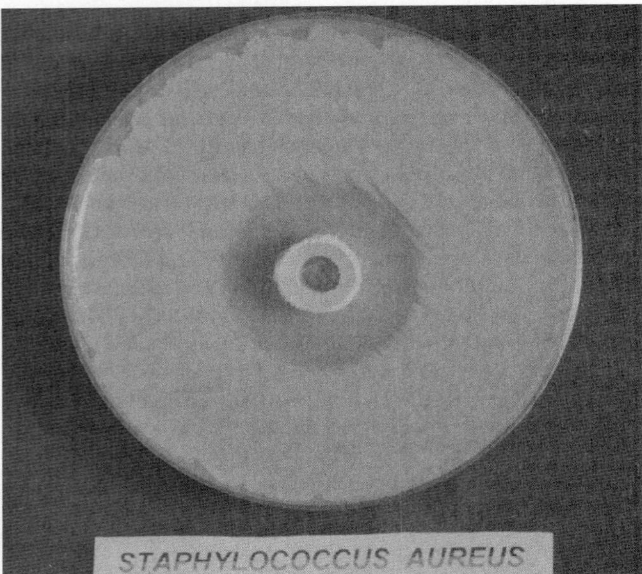

FIGURE 31.4. Zone of inhibition around an antimicrobial-coated device placed on the surface of an agar plate that had been freshly inoculated with a biofilm-producing clinical strain of *Staphylococcus aureus*. This zone of inhibition was assessed 24 hours after incubating the agar plate at 37°C and resulted from the leaching of the antimicrobial agent off the coated device surface into the surrounding agar to result in killing of bacteria.

against deeply embedded organisms within the biofilm, tend to be clinically protective (Fig. 31.4).

PREVENTION OF VASCULAR CATHETER-ASSOCIATED INFECTIONS

Bloodstream infection is the most common serious complication of indwelling vascular catheters. Although catheter colonization is a prelude to catheter-associated infection, most colonized catheters do not become clinically infected (24). Therefore, a significant reduction in the rate of catheter colonization does not, in and of itself, constitute proof of clinical efficacy. The ultimate proof of clinical efficacy is a significant reduction in the rate of CRBSI in a sufficiently powered, prospective, randomized clinical trial. As a corollary, if an inadequately powered clinical trial that fails to demonstrate a significant reduction in the rate of CRBSI despite a significantly lower rate of catheter colonization in the experimental versus control group, it is implied that the experimental strategy is either not clinically protective or needs to be examined in a larger clinical trial. In that regard, a properly conducted meta-analysis that adjusts well to confounding variables may help address the benefit of a potentially preventive approach. A critical analysis of the peer-reviewed literature allows the categorization of potentially preventive measures into three groups: (i) approaches that do not significantly reduce catheter colonization or CRBSI, (ii) approaches that significantly reduce catheter colonization but not CRBSI, and (iii) approaches that significantly reduce CRBSI. Although the most desirable impact of potentially preventive measures is a reduction in mortality associated with CRBSI, it would be impractical to conduct a several-thousand-patient clinical trial that would be sufficiently powered to assess this outcome, which has a relatively low incidence—equivalent to the incidence of catheter-related bloodstream infection times the risk of dying from catheter-related bloodstream infection.

Approaches That Do Not Significantly Reduce Catheter Colonization or CRBSI

Silver-coated Catheters

This represents the most investigated approach in this category and focuses on modification of the catheter surface with different silver-containing moieties. Not only did *in vitro* studies yield conflicting findings with regards to efficacy—since some showed reduced bacterial adherence to the surfaces of polyurethane silver-coated catheters (29) and others indicated that the use of silicone silver-coated catheters is ineffective (30)—but the results of animal models also yielded inconclusive results (31). Although one prospective randomized clinical trial reported that silver-coated central venous catheters were protective (32), subsequent prospective randomized clinical trials found no evidence of clinical efficacy (33,34). The most recent assessment showed that short-term, central venous catheters impregnated with silver ions bonded to an inert ceramic zeolite reduce neither catheter colonization nor CRBSI (35). Not only is the silver application to the surface of short-term catheters mostly ineffective, but its incorporation onto the surface of long-term catheters can negatively impact the incidence of infection and cause adverse events. For instance, a prospective randomized clinical trial of tunneled long-term (mean dwell time, 92 days) hemodialysis catheters demonstrated a statistically insignificant trend for higher rates of catheter colonization (2.8 versus 1.3 cases per 1,000 catheter-days) and catheter-related infection (1.8 versus 1.1 cases per 1,000 catheter-days) in patients with silver-coated versus uncoated catheters, respectively (36). In addition to being clinically ineffective, the silver-coated hemodialysis catheters were removed in 2 of 47 (4%) patients because of the chronic development of hyperpigmented skin lesions at the site of catheter insertion, thereby contributing to the decision to abandon the clinical use of that particular silver-coated catheter (36). Several factors are responsible for the poor clinical efficacy of silver-coated catheters: (a) Since incorporated silver molecules do not effectively leach off the surface of most coated catheters, they do not produce effective zones of inhibition around the catheter surface that would ensure access of the coating agents to biofilm-embedded organisms; (b) silver tends to bind to host proteins, thereby resulting in lower concentration of free active silver molecules; and (c) the antimicrobial activity of silver can be impaired in the presence of bodily fluids (37).

Catheters Coated with Benzalkonium Chloride

In vitro studies showed that heparin-coated catheters possess some antimicrobial activity, possibly attributable to the weak antiseptic benzalkonium chloride, which is applied to the catheter surface primarily for its surfactant activity to allow bonding with heparin (38). However, small prospective randomized clinical trials failed to show a decrease in the rate of CRBSI associated with the benzalkonium chloride–coated catheters (39,40).

Approaches That Significantly Reduce Catheter Colonization But Not CRBSI

Dipping Catheters in Antibiotic Solutions

This bedside approach relies on dipping positively charged surfactant (usually tridodecyl methyl ammonium chloride, TDMAC)-pretreated catheters in a solution of negatively charged antibiotics such as cephalosporins and glycopeptides just prior to catheter insertion. Although a prospective randomized clinical trial showed that short-term central venous and arterial catheters that were pretreated with TDMAC and dipped at the bedside in cefazolin were sevenfold less likely to be colonized than undipped catheters, there was no demonstrated impact on the occurrence of CRBSI (41). A not-so-well-designed prospective randomized clinical trial also reported that immersion of short-term central venous catheters in vancomycin just prior to insertion was associated with a 22% reduction in the rate of catheter colonization (defined in that study as any level of bacterial growth by roll-plate culture of the catheter tip) as compared with nonimmersed catheters (42). The drawbacks of dipping catheters in vancomycin are the absence of impact on the incidence of catheter-related bloodstream infection and the occurrence of *Candida* overgrowth.

Catheters Coated with Silver-Platinum-Carbon

A prospective randomized clinical trial showed that short-term central venous catheters coated with silver-platinum-carbon (so-called oligon) were significantly less likely to become colonized than conventional uncoated catheters (18.6% versus 29.6%, $p = 0.003$) (43). However, there was no significant reduction in the rate of bloodstream infection associated with coated versus uncoated catheters (3.3% versus 4.3%).

Approaches That Significantly Reduce CRBSIs

Quite understandably, the most recent CDC guidelines included new recommendations for using all of the following clinically protective measures, including cutaneous antisepsis with chlorhexidine (category IA), maximal sterile barriers (category IA), and catheters coated with the combinations of chlorhexidine plus silver sulfadiazine, or minocycline plus rifampin (category IB) (14).

Cutaneous Antisepsis with Chlorhexidine

The objective of antiseptic cleansing of the skin is to achieve a major reduction—preferably a greater than or equal to 3 log reduction—in bacterial concentration on the skin surface at the catheter insertion site. Prompted by an expanding body of supporting evidence, almost a dozen clinical guidelines issued by various scientific and regulatory organizations, both individually and in collaboration, have recommended the use of chlorhexidine-containing preparations rather than povidone-iodine or alcohol for cleansing the skin around the vascular catheter insertion site (14). A prospective randomized clinical trial showed that vascular catheters inserted when using 2% aqueous chlorhexidine were significantly less likely to become colonized than catheters placed by using either 10% povidone-iodine or 70% alcohol (3). More important, CRBSI was fourfold to fivefold less likely in the former group than in the latter two groups (0.55% versus 2.6% and 2.3%, respectively). In a meta-analysis of eight prospective randomized clinical trials that included a total of 4,143 vascular catheters, the relative risk of CRBSI was twice as high among patients who receive povidone-iodine versus chlorhexidine (44). The superiority of chlorhexdiine over iodophor and alcohol could be predicted by comparing their characteristics, as shown in Table 31.1. Unlike iodophor and alcohol, chlorhexidine provides a residual and persistent antimicrobial activity that is not impaired by exposure to organic matter such as blood, does not irritate the skin, and has minimal absorption through the skin. Although 2% chlorhexidine compounds appear to be optimal in terms of both efficacy and safety, only recently has aqueous chlorhexidine become available in the United States, where the most frequently used form of chlorhexidine is in combination with an alcohol, usually isopropyl alcohol. As Table 31.2 delineates, the combination of chlorhexidine and alcohol has many more favorable properties than the combination of iodophor and alcohol. These recognizable differences have contributed to the escalating application of antiseptic solution that contains the combination of chlorhexidine and alcohol on the skin surrounding the insertion site of vascular catheters.

TABLE 31.1

COMPARISON OF INDIVIDUAL ANTISEPTIC AGENTS

Characteristic of antimicrobial agent	Iodophor	Alcohol	Chlorhexidine
Broad-spectrum activity	Yes	Yes	Yes
Rapid activity	No	Yes	No
Residual activity	No	No	Yes
Preserved activity in contact with bodily fluids	No	No	Yes
Nonirritating	No	No	Yes
Minimal absorption	No	No	Yes

Maximal Sterile Barriers

In contrast to traditional sterile precautions that include the use of gloves and a small drape, maximal sterile precautions

TABLE 31.2

COMPARISON OF SOLUTIONS THAT CONTAIN COMBINATIONS OF ANTIMICROBIAL AGENTS

Characteristic of combination	Iodophor/ Alcohol	Chlorhexidione/ Alcohol
Broad-spectrum activity	Yes	Yes
Rapid activity	Yes	Yes
Residual activity	No	Yes
Preserved activity in contact with bodily fluids	No	Yes
Nonirritating	No	Yes
Minimal absorption	No	Yes

comprise the use of gloves, a large drape, a cap, a mask, and a gown. When compared in a prospective randomized fashion, the use of maximal sterile barriers versus traditional sterile precautions when inserting long-term (mean duration of placement, 70 days), noncuffed silicone vascular catheters was associated with a significantly lower incidence of catheter colonization (0.3 versus 1 per 1,000 catheter-days; $p = 0.007$) and CRBSI (0.08 versus 0.5 per 1,000 catheter-days, $p = 0.02$) (45,46). Although this protective measure is intended to be used for insertion of all central venous catheters, it is currently used less frequently outside the intensive care units and specialty care areas in which reside patients with a high risk of infection, including those with bone marrow transplant or leukemia.

Catheters Coated with Chlorhexidine and Silver Sulfadiazine

There exist two catheters coated with the combination of chlorhexidine and silver sulfadiazine. The first-generation, and most studied, catheter (47–56) has antimicrobial agent incorporated only along the external surface of the catheter. The second-generation catheter differs in two ways from the first-generation catheter: Both antimicrobial agents are incorporated onto the external and internal surfaces, and it contains three times the amount of chlorhexidine (57).

The largest prospective randomized clinical trial of the first-generation devices coated with chlorhexidine/silver sulfadiazine in 403 short-term (mean duration of placement, 6 days), polyurethane central venous catheters demonstrated a significant reduction in the rate of catheter colonization (13.5% versus 24.1%; $p = 0.005$) and CRBSI (1.0% versus 4.6%; $p = 0.03$) as compared with uncoated catheters (50). Although most other clinical trials (47,51–56) showed that chlorhexidine/silver sulfadiazine–coated catheters were significantly less likely to be colonized than uncoated catheters, they could not demonstrate a significant reduction in the rate of CRBSI; these studies were not sufficiently powered to detect significant differences in the rates of CRBSI. Additionally, however, a meta-analysis of 12 clinical trials showed that these antimicrobial-coated catheters resulted in a significant reduction in the rates of both catheter colonization (odds ratio = 0.44; $p < 0.001$) and CRBSI (odds ratio = 0.56; $p = 0.005$) (58).

Since this first-generation chlorhexidine/silver sulfadiazine–coated catheter provided only short-lived (about 1 week) antimicrobial activity, and only along the external surface of the catheter (53), it was not likely to protect against infection of long-term catheters that frequently become contaminated with bacteria migrating from the contaminated hub along the internal surface of the catheter. Not unexpectedly, a large (680 catheters) prospective randomized clinical trial showed that placement of chlorhexidine/silver sulfadiazine–coated central venous catheters for a mean of 20 days in patients with hematologic malignancy did not reduce the rate of CRBSI as compared with uncoated catheters (5% versus 4.4%) (59).

The second-generation chlorhexidine/silver sulfadiazine–coated catheters have a longer durability of antimicrobial activity than the first-generation catheters (60). A recent report of a large (842 catheters) prospective randomized clinical trial demonstrated that second-generation chlorhexidine/silver sulfadiazine–coated polyurethane short-term central venous catheters are less likely to become colonized than uncoated catheters (9% versus 16%, $p < 0.01$) but had a statistically insignificant trend for a lower rate of CRBSIs (0.3% versus 0.8%) (57). Since the incidence of CRBSI in the uncoated catheter group was lower than usual, this study may not have had sufficient power to assess the desired outcome. Because both the first-generation and second-generation chlorhexidine/silver sulfadiazine–coated catheters generally reduce catheter colonization to a similar degree, it is reasonable to regard these two catheters as being equally protective against infection.

Catheters Coated with Minocycline and Rifampin

This unique combination of antibiotics was selected for the following reasons: (a) Both agents are active against the vast majority of staphylococcal isolates, including MRSA and MRSE (61); (b) the combination of agents provides broad-spectrum antimicrobial activity against most pathogens that can cause CRBSI, thereby reducing the likelihood of developing superinfection by Gram-negative bacteria or *Candida* spp. (62,63); (c) since minocycline and rifampin have different mechanisms of activity, with minocycline retarding protein synthesis and rifampin inhibiting DNA-dependent RNA polymerase, it is unlikely that a bacterial strain will become concomitantly resistant to both agents; and (d) unlike many antibiotics–including vancomycin, ciprofloxacin, and the aminoglycosides–that are much less active against biofilm bacteria than planktonic bacteria, rifampin (64) and minocycline (65) are particularly active against biofilm-embedded bacteria.

The clinical efficacy of this catheter surface modification was initially confirmed in a prospective randomized clinical trial that showed that polyurethane short-term (mean duration of placement, 6 days) central venous catheters coated with minocycline and rifampin were significantly less likely than uncoated catheters to become colonized (8% versus 26%; $p < 0.001$) and cause bloodstream infection (0% versus 5%; $p < 0.01$) (66). In a large (738 catheters) prospective randomized clinical trial, polyurethane short-term (mean duration of placement, 8 days) central venous catheters coated with minocycline and rifampin were more protective than the first-generation chlorhexidine/silver sulfadiazine–coated catheters, with a threefold lower rate of catheter colonization (7.9% versus 22.8%; $p < 0.001$) and a 12-fold lower rate of CRBSI (0.3% versus 3.4%; $p < 0.002$) (67).

The superior clinical protection afforded by minocycline/rifampin–coated catheters was predictable, since these catheters were shown in an animal study to prevent *S. aureus* infection of percutaneously placed catheter segments better than first-generation chlorhexidine/silver sulfadiazine-coated catheters (63); and since they have a longer *in vivo* durability of antimicrobial activity than first-generation chlorhexidine/silver sulfadiazine–coated catheters, as determined by the residual zones of inhibition generated by catheters removed from patients (68). The production of an effective zone of inhibition by an antimicrobial-coated catheter surface may serve to inhibit adherence of organisms not only to the catheter surface, but also to various host-derived adhesins such as fibronectin, fibrinogen, fibrin, and laminin that exist within the biofilm layer surrounding the indwelling prosthesis (69,70). The size of the *in vitro* zone of inhibition against *S. aureus* around a coated vascular catheter is likely to predict the clinical efficacy, or lack thereof, in preventing catheter colonization and CRBSI (71). The optimal characteristics of antimicrobial-coated vascular catheters are listed in Table 31.3.

TABLE 31.3

COMPARISON OF ANTIBIOTIC DIPPED VERSUS ANTIMICROBIAL COATING OF VASCULAR CATHETERS

Characteristic	Antibiotic dipping	Antimicrobial coating
Practical	No	Yes
Determined amount of drugs bound to catheter	No	Yes
Known amount of drugs that leach off catheter	No	Yes
Determined durability of antimicrobial activity	No	Yes
Uses therapeutic drugs of choice	Yes	No
Clinical protection against infection	No	Yes/No[a]

[a]Clinical protection against catheter-related bloodstream infection is afforded by some but not all antimicrobial-coated vascular catheters.

The clinical benefit achieved by incorporating the combination of minocycline and rifampin onto the surfaces of short-term polyurethane central venous catheters prompted the assessment of this approach in long-term silicone catheters. Indeed, a prospective randomized clinical trial demonstrated that similarly coated long-term silicone central venous catheters were fourfold less likely than uncoated catheters to result in bloodstream infection (2% versus 8%, $p = 0.002$) (72). Even more important, in a prospective randomized multicenter clinical trial conducted to determine whether antimicrobial coating can obviate the need for the not-so-practical, time-consuming, and expensive practice of tunneling long-term central venous catheters, nontunneled minocycline/rifampin–coated catheters were significantly less likely than tunneled uncoated catheters to result in bloodstream infection (73). In general, clinical trials have shown no evidence of developing antimicrobial resistance when using either short-term (67,68) or long-term (74) central venous catheters coated with minocycline and rifampin and short-term chlorhexidine/silver sulfadiazine-coated catheters (50).

Table 31.4 summarizes the advantages of using antimicrobial-coated versus antibiotic-dipped catheters. Both patient-specific and institution-based factors should guide the use of antimicrobial-coated catheters. In general, the clinical protection afforded by antimicrobial-coated catheters has been documented only in populations of patients at high risk for infection—including critically ill patients, immunocompromised subjects, recipients of total parenteral nutrition, and so forth—and are not intended to be used in patients at low risk of infection, such as persons embarking on an elective surgical procedure and expected to have the central venous catheter in place for only 1 to 2 days. An institutional incidence of catheter-related bloodstream infection of more than 3.3 per 1,000 catheter-days (equivalent to about 2%) is felt by some authorities high enough to consider the use of antimicrobial-coated vascular catheters (50,75,76). Although clinically protective antimicrobial-coated catheters generally cost about 20% more than uncoated prototypes, tremendous savings can be incurred when using chlorhexidine/silver sulfadiazine (77) and, even more so, the more clinically protective minocycline/rifampin-coated catheters (78).

TABLE 31.4

OPTIMAL CHARACTERISTICS OF ANTIMICROBIAL-COATED VASCULAR CATHETERS THAT WOULD PREDICT CLINICAL EFFICACY

1. Broad-spectrum antimicrobial activity against most potential pathogens and not just against Gram-positive bacteria. This property helps augment the degree of clinical protection and circumvent the likelihood of superinfection by organisms other than staphylococci.
2. Presence of antimicrobial activity along both the external and internal catheter surfaces. This specification enhances the likelihood of protection against bacteria originating from both the patient's skin and catheter hub.
3. Durable antimicrobial activity. This characteristic provides the opportunity for procuring clinical efficacy for both short-term and long-term vascular catheters.
4. Production of zones of inhibition. It is essential that the coating antimicrobial agents have access to organisms that either adhere directly to the catheter surface or become embedded deep within the biofilm.
5. Preserved antimicrobial activity against biofilm-embedded organisms. This property augments the likelihood of clinical protection.

Controversial Practices

Unlike the above described measures that have attracted almost unanimous evidence-based agreement regarding their efficacy or lack thereof, the following practices continue to stir some controversy.

Guidewire Exchange of Vascular Catheters

The clinical practice of exchanging central venous catheters over a guidewire has been plagued by two controversies. The first one focuses on routine guidewire exchange of noninfected catheters, and the other controversy centers around guidewire exchange of infected catheters. Although suboptimally designed studies initially encouraged routine guidewire exchange of central venous catheters, well-designed prospective randomized clinical trials yielded different results (79–81). For instance, a prospective randomized clinical trial found that scheduled catheter replacement over a guidewire every 3 days is associated with a higher rate of infection but a lower incidence of mechanical complications, primarily pneumothorax, than replacement of catheters when clinically indicated (mean duration of catheter placement of 7 days) (79). Since the risk of catheter-related infection increases as the duration of catheter placement extends, the results of this study (79) may not necessarily apply to clinical scenarios where catheters are clinically used for much longer periods.

The prevailing (82,83), but not universal (84–86), clinical practice dictates that if catheters are removed because of suspicion of infection in patients who require another vascular access, a new catheter is placed at a different site. In such patients, there is a concern that guidewire-assisted exchange of the infected catheter may result in contamination of the newly placed catheter by organisms present in the subcutaneous tract and/or the lumen of the removed catheter that may transfer onto the guidewire. The potential drawback of catheter replacement at a different site is vascular thrombosis and, hence, compromise of future intravenous access, particularly in children with cancer and patients dependent on hemodialysis (84). In hemodynamically stable patients with limited vascular access and in whom catheter-related infection is possible but not very likely, it is reasonable to insert the new catheter over a guidewire as long as the removed catheter is cultured; should culture of the removed catheter yield growth, it is recommended to remove the catheter that was newly inserted over a guidewire and place yet another catheter at a different site. Although it is theoretically plausible that insertion at the same site of a vascular catheter with effective antimicrobial coating along both the external and internal catheter surfaces may obviate the need to manipulate another vascular site, this approach requires clinical investigation.

Antimicrobial Catheter Hub

It is important to mention that the definitions of outcomes used in clinical trials examining this approach were less rigorous than those adopted in most studies of other types of potentially preventive measures. A prospective randomized clinical trial initially showed that attachment of an antimicrobial hub containing iodinated alcohol to central venous catheters, with a mean duration of placement of 2 weeks, significantly reduced the rate of colonization of the catheter hub (1% versus 11%; $p < 0.01$) and CRBSI (4% versus 16%; $p < 0.01$) (87). However, a subsequent prospective randomized clinical trial of 130 central venous catheters with this antimicrobial hub versus standard catheters in critically ill patients showed no differences between the two groups in the rates of colonization of the catheter tip and hub and, more important, revealed a trend for a higher rate of catheter-related sepsis in association with the use of this technology (24% versus 15%) (88). Because this antimicrobial catheter hub protects only against organisms that migrate through the hub along the internal surface of the catheter, but not against skin organisms that advance along the external surface of the catheter, the potential clinical benefit of using this preventive approach in the context of vascular catheters that remain in place for less than or equal to 7 to 10 days is doubtful.

Flushing or Locking the Catheter Lumen with Antibiotic-Anticoagulant Solutions

The relationship between infection and thrombosis of vascular catheters prompted numerous investigations of the clinical efficacy of flushing or locking the catheter lumen with various antibiotic-anticoagulant combinations that do not result in systemic levels of the antibiotic. Because this approach provides antimicrobial activity against only organisms that exist in the catheter lumen, clinical investigations have generally focused on long-term vascular catheters that are frequently infected by such a route. Prospective randomized clinical trials in immunocompromised children (89) and adults (90) revealed that flushing the lumen of long-term central venous catheters with a solution that contains vancomycin and heparin significantly reduces the rate of CRBSI due to luminal colonization by vancomycin-susceptible organisms, as compared with flushing catheters with heparin alone (0% versus 21%, $p = 0.04$; and 0% versus 7%, $p = 0.05$, respectively). One of these two studies (89) also showed that the use of vancomycin-heparin catheter flush was associated with a statistically insignificant fourfold reduction (5% versus 21%) in the rate of CRBSI due to luminal colonization by vancomycin-resistant organisms. Another prospective randomized clinical trial in children with long-term central venous catheters showed significantly lower rates of CRBSI when catheters were flushed with either vancomycin-ciprofloxacin-heparin (0.55/1,000 versus 1.72/1,000 catheter-days, $p = 0.005$) or vancomycin-heparin solutions (0.37/1,000 versus 1.72/1,000 catheter-days, $p = 0.004$) than when flushed with heparin alone (91). Other clinical trials, however, yielded discrepant results. For instance, a prospective randomized clinical trial in pediatric patients who had cancer and/or were receiving total parenteral nutrition revealed that flushing the lumen of long-term central venous catheters with a solution that also consisted of vancomycin and heparin did not reduce the rate of CRBSI due to luminal colonization by vancomycin-susceptible organisms, as compared with flushing catheters with heparin alone (1.4/1,000 versus 0.6/1,000 catheter-days, $p = 0.25$) (92). Moreover, catheters flushed with the combination of vancomycin and heparin were associated with a significant fourfold increase in the rate of CRBSI due to luminal colonization by vancomycin-resistant organisms (2.3/1,000 versus 0.53/1,000 catheter-days, $p = 0.03$) (92). In a recent meta-analysis of four prospective randomized clinical trials in high-risk children or adults, the risk ratio of developing CRBSI was 0.34 ($p = 0.04$) among patients who receive vancomycin-containing catheter lock solution versus those who receive only heparin (93). Although there were no observed cases of infection of vancomycin-locked catheters by vancomycin-resistant organisms (93), the potential emergence of resistance to vancomycin, a drug that is still used to treat most cases of catheter infections, continues to underscore the equivocal role of this strategy.

PERSPECTIVE ON FUTURE WORK

Although institutional implementation of quality improvement programs to educate health care providers and improve their compliance with hand hygiene and basic infection control measures when inserting or maintaining a vascular catheter are generally beneficial, the level of adherence and duration of benefit are not optimal (94,95). Moreover, some preventive measures have probably reached a point of limited return as they have reduced but did not eliminate the occurrence of CRBSI (96). That is why it is essential that we strive to explore the potential benefit of either new innovative approaches or the application of already established technology in other clinical scenarios, which will be discussed.

Instilling a Catheter Lock Solution That Contains an Antibiofilm Plus an Antimicrobial Agent

This inclusion of an antibiofilm agent in a catheter lock combination solution would help enhance the access and activity of the antimicrobial agent against biofilm-embedded organisms.

Although numerous antibiofilm agents could theoretically be used, the use of N-acetyl cysteine is quite intriguing because of its well-established safety—FDA approved for both systemic and inhalational administration in doses that far exceed the amount that would be included in a catheter lock solution—and recent preliminary reports of in vitro efficacy (97,98).

Assessing the Clinical Value of Quorum-Sensing Inhibitors

This intriguing approach, which disrupts bacterial cell-to-cell communication, can impair the formation of biofilm in vitro and in animal models (99). However, there are no peer-reviewed clinical reports that have assessed this potentially protective approach, and the activity of different quorum-sensing inhibitors tends to be largely genus-specific; for example, the RNAIII-inhibiting peptide is active against only *S. aureus* and *S. epidermidis* (99), and yet another quorum-sensing inhibitor attenuates the virulence of *Pseudomonas aeruginosa* (100). It is prudent to clinically assess the safety, efficacy, and practicality of this approach.

Inserting Clinically Protective Antimicrobial-Coated Catheters to Safely Prolong the Duration of Catheter Placement

Since there is a direct relationship between the duration of catheter placement and risk of catheter-related infection (101), most clinical practitioners leave short-term central venous catheters in place for less than 10 days. Although not comprehensively investigated as of yet, it is likely that clinically protective antimicrobial-coated catheters with durable antimicrobial activity could be safely left in place for a longer period of time, perhaps for 2 to 3 weeks, without sacrificing anti-infective efficacy (102).

Applying Clinically Protective Antimicrobial Coating on Hemodialysis Catheters

Not only are hemodialysis catheters more likely to become infected than regular central venous catheters, but they are also associated with more serious clinical (including paucity of other body sites that would be amenable to placing a new hemodialysis access) and economic consequences once infection evolves (103).

Assessing the True Value of Bundled Preventive Interventions

A recent prospective cohort study of a bundle of five evidence-based measures—including hand washing, maximal sterile barriers, cleansing skin with chlorhexidine, avoiding femoral sites if possible, and removing catheters when no longer needed—reported a significant reduction in the rate of CRBSI in critically ill patients: The risk of infection compared to preintervention was 0.62 at 0 to 3 months and 0.36 at 18 months (104). These promising findings, however, were limited by the fact that the study was not randomized, potential underreporting of infection could have occurred after initiating the study, and the effect of the bundled interventions on different microbial pathogens was not investigated. Therefore, it is imperative that bundled interventions be assessed in a prospective randomized fashion.

PEARLS

- The infection-prone vascular catheter, an indispensable component of modern health care, is a vice in disguise.
- Although catheter colonization is a prelude to infection, most colonized catheters do not result in catheter-related infection.
- Proof of clinical protection against infection afforded by a potentially preventative approach is defined as significant reduction in catheter-related bloodstream infection.
- Adherence to optimal infection control measures is the mainstay for preventing infection, but consistent adherence to guidelines usually drops within months of institutional implementation of educational programs.
- Although optimal infection control measures save lives, more lives can be saved by combining infection control measures and clinically protective technology.
- Antimicrobial modification of the surface of vascular catheters is not necessarily indicative of clinical protection against catheter-related infection.
- A clinically protective anti-infective approach can also incur cost savings and reduce the reservoir of antimicrobial-resistant pathogens that exist within the biofilm surrounding indwelling catheters.

References

1. Richards MJ, Edwards JR, Culver DH, et al. Nosocomial infections in medical intensive care units in the United States. National Nosocomial Infections Surveillance System. *Crit Care Med.* 1999;27:887–892.
2. Raad I, Hanna HA, Alakech B, et al. Differential time to positivity: a useful method for diagnosing catheter-related bloodstream infections. *Ann Intern Med.* 2004;140:18.
3. Maki DG, Ringer M, Alvarado CJ. Prospective randomized trial of povidone-iodine, alcohol, and chlorhexidine for prevention of infection associated with central venous and arterial catheters. *Lancet.* 1991;338:339.
4. Darouiche RO, Berger DH, Khardori N, et al. Comparison of antimicrobial impregnation with tunneling of long-term central venous catheters: a randomized, controlled trial. *Ann Surg.* 2005;242:193.
5. Mermel LA. Prevention of intravascular catheter-related infections. *Ann Intern Med.* 2000;132:391–402.
6. Warren DK, Quadir WW, Hollenbeak CS, et al. attributable cost of catheter-associated bloodstream infections among intensive care patients in a nonteaching hospital. *Crit Care Med.* 2006;34:2084.
7. Pittet D, Tarara D, Wenzel RP. Nosocomial bloodstream infection in critically ill patients: excess length of stay, extra costs, and attributable mortality. *JAMA.* 1994;271:1598.
8. Heiselman D. Nosocomial bloodstream infections in the critically ill [Letter]. *JAMA.* 1994;272:1819.
9. Pittet D, Wenzel RP. Nosocomial bloodstream infections in the critically ill [Letter]. *JAMA.* 1994;272:1819.
10. Dimick JB, Pelz RK, Consunji, et al. Increased resource use associated with catheter-related bloodstream infection in the surgical intensive care unit. *Arch Surg.* 2001;136:229.
11. Sieradzki K, Roberts RB, Haber SW, et al. The development of vancomycin resistance in a patient with methicillin-resistant *Staphylococcus aureus* infection. *N Engl J Med.* 1999;340:517.
12. Smith TL, Pearson ML, Wilcox KR, et al. Emergence of vancomycin resistance in *Staphylococcus aureus. N Engl J Med.* 1999;340:493.
13. Wisplinghoff H, Wisplinghoff T, Tallent SM, et al. Nosocomial bloodstream infections in US hospitals: analysis of 24,179 cases from a prospective nationwide surveillance study. *Clin Infect Dis.* 2004;39:309.
14. O'Grady NP, Alexander M, Dellinger EP, et al. Guidelines for the prevention of intravascular catheter-related infections. Centers for Disease Control and Prevention. *MMWR Morb Mortal Wkly Rep* 2002;51(RR-10):1.
15. Maki DG, Weise CE, Sarafin HW. A semiquantitative culture method for identifying intravenous-catheter-related infection. *N Engl J Med.* 1977;296:1305.
16. Sherertz RJ, Raad II, Balani A, et al. Three-year experience with sonicated vascular catheter cultures in a clinical microbiology laboratory. *J Clin Microbiol.* 1990;28:76.

17. Bouza E, Alvarado N, Alcala L, et al. A randomized and prospective study of 3 procedures for the diagnosis of catheter-related bloodstream infection without catheter withdrawal. *Clin Infect Dis.* 2007;44:820.
18. Linares J. Diagnosis of catheter-related bloodstream infection: conservative techniques. *Clin Infect Dis.* 2007;44:827.
19. Chatzinikolaou I, Hanna H, Hachem R, et al. Differential quantitative blood cultures for the diagnosis of catheter-related bloodstream infections associated with short- and long-term catheters: a prospective study. *Diagn Microbiol Infect Dis.* 2004;50:167.
20. Safdar N, Fine JP, Maki DG. Meta-analysis: methods for diagnosis of intravascular device-related bloodstream infection. *Ann Intern Med.* 2005;142:451.
21. Maki DG, Cobb L, Garman JK, et al. An attachable silver-impregnated cuff for prevention of infection with central venous catheters: a prospective randomized multicenter trial. *Am J Med.* 1988;85:307.
22. Salzman MB, Isenberg HD, Shapiro JF, et al. A prospective study of the catheter hub as the portal of entry for organisms causing catheter-related sepsis in neonates. *J Infect Dis.* 1993;167:487.
23. Raad II, Bodey GP. Infectious complications of indwelling vascular catheters. *Clin Infect Dis.* 1992;15:197.
24. Darouiche RO. Device-associated infections: a macroproblem that starts with microadherence. *Clin Infect Dis.* 2001;33:1567.
25. Jensen ET, Kharazmi A, Lam K, et al. Human polymorphonuclear leukocyte response to *Pseudomonas aeruginosa* grown in biofilms. *Infect Immun.* 1990;58:2383–2385.
26. Costerton JW, Stewart PS, Greenberg EP. Bacterial biofilms: a common cause of persistent infections. *Science.* 1999;284:1318.
27. Darouiche RO, Dhir A, Miller AJ, et al. Vancomycin penetration into biofilm covering infected prostheses and effect on bacteria. *J Infect Dis.* 1994;170:720.
28. Kumon H, Tomochika K, Matunaga T, et al. A sandwich cup method for the penetration assay of antimicrobial agents through *Pseudomonas* exopolysaccharides. *Microbiol Immunol,* 1994;38:615.
29. Jansen B, Rinck M, Wolbring P, et al. In vitro evaluation of the antimicrobial efficacy and biocompatibility of a silver-coated central venous catheter. *J Biomat App.* 1994;9:55.
30. Kampf G, Dietze B, Grobe-Siestrup C, et al. Microbicidal activity of a new silver-containing polymer, SPI-ARGENT II. *Antimicrob Agents Chemother.* 1998;42:2440.
31. Gilbert JA, Cooper RC, Puryear HA, et al. A swine model for the evaluation of efficacy of anti-microbial catheter coatings. *J Biomater Sci Polym Ed.* 1998;9:931.
32. Goldschmidt H, Hahn U, Satwender HJ, et al. Prevention of catheter-related infections by silver-coated central venous catheters in oncological patients. *Zentralbl Bakteriol.* 1995;283:215.
33. Bach A, Eberhardt H, Frick A, et al. Efficacy of silver-coating central venous catheters in reducing bacterial colonization. *Crit Care Med.* 1999;27: 515.
34. Dunser MW, Mayr AJ, Hinterberger G, et al. Central venous catheter colonization in critically ill patients: a prospective, randomized, controlled study comparing standard with two antiseptic-impregnated catheters. *Anesth Analg.* 2005;101:1778.
35. Kalfon P, de Vaumus C, Samba D, et al. Comparison of silver-impregnated with standard multi-lumen central venous catheters in critically ill patients. *Crit Care Med.* 2007;35:1032.
36. Trerotola S, Johnson M, Shah H, et al. Tunneled hemodialysis catheters: use of a silver-coated catheter for prevention of infection-a randomized study. *Radiology.* 1998;207:491–496.
37. Darouiche RO. Anti-infective efficacy of silver-coated medical prostheses. *Clin Infect Dis.* 1999;29:1371–1377.
38. Mermel LA, Stolz SM, Maki DG. Surface antimicrobial activity of heparin-bonded and antiseptic-impregnated vascular catheters. *J Infect Dis.* 1993;167:920.
39. Moss HA, Tebbs Se, Faroqui MH, et al. A central venous catheter coated with benzalkonium chloride for the prevention of catheter-related microbial colonization. *Eur J Anesthesiol.* 2000;17:680–687.
40. Jaeger K, Osthaus A, Heine J, et al. Efficacy of a benzalkonium chloride-impregnated central venous catheter to prevent catheter-associated infection in cancer patients. *Eur J Chemother.* 2001;47:50–55.
41. Kamal GD, Pfaller MA, Rempe LE, et al. Reduced intravascular catheter infection by antibiotic bonding. *JAMA.* 1991;265:2364.
42. Thornton J, Todd NJ, Webster NR. Central venous line sepsis in the intensive care unit: a study comparing antibiotic coated catheters with plain catheters. *Anesthesia.* 1996;51:1018.
43. Ranucci M, Isgro G, Giomarelli PP, et al. Impact of oligon central venous catheters on catheter colonization and catheter-related bloodstream infection. *Crit Care Med.* 2003;31:52.
44. Chaivakunapruk N, Veenstra N, Lipsky BA, et al. Chlorhexidine compared with povidone-iodine solution for vascular catheter-site care: a meta-analysis. *Ann Intern Med.* 2002;136:792.
45. Raad II, Hohn DC, Gilbreath BJ, et al. Prevention of central venous catheter-related infections by using maximal sterile barrier precautions during insertion. *Infect Control Hosp Epidemiol.* 1994;15:231.
46. Maki DG. Yes, Virginia, aseptic technique is very important: maximal barrier precautions during insertion reduces the risk of central venous catheter-related bacteremia. *Infect Contr Hosp Epidemiol.* 1994;15:227.
47. Van heerden PV, Webb SA, Fong S, et al. Central venous catheters revisited–infection rates and an assessment of the new Fibrin Analyzing System brush. *Anesthes Intens Care.* 1996;24:330.
48. Ciresi D, Albrecht RM, Volkers PA, Scholten DJ. Failure of an antiseptic bonding to prevent central venous catheter-related infection and sepsis. *Am Surg.* 1996;62:641–646.
49. Pemberton LB, Ross V, Cuddy P, et al. No difference in catheter sepsis between standard and antiseptic central venous catheters. A prospective randomized trial. *Arch Surg.* 1996;131:986–989.
50. Maki DG, Stolz SM, Wheeler S, et al. Prevention of central venous catheter-related bloodstream infection by use of an antiseptic-impregnated catheter: a randomized, controlled study. *Ann Intern Med.* 1997;127;257.
51. Tennenberg S, Lieser M, Mccurdy B, et al. A prospective randomized clinical trial of an antibiotic- and antiseptic-coated central venous catheter in the prevention of catheter-related infections. *Arch Surg.* 1997;132:1348.
52. George SJ, Vuddamalay P, Boscoe MJ. Antiseptic-impregnated central venous catheters reduce the incidence of bacterial colonization and associated infection in immunocompromised transplant patients. *Eur J Anesthesiol.* 1997;14:428.
53. Heard SO, Wagle M, Vijayakumar E, et al. The influence of triple-lumen central venous catheters coated with chlorhexidine/silversulfadiazine on the incidence of catheter-related bacteremia: a randomized, controlled clinical trial. *Arch Intern Med.* 1998;158;81.
54. Collin GR. Decreasing catheter colonization through the use of an antiseptic-impregnated catheter: a continuous quality improvement project. *Chest.* 1999;115:1632.
55. Hannan M, Juste RN, Umasanker S, et al. Antiseptic-bonded central venous catheters and bacterial colonization. *Anesthesia.* 1999;54:868.
56. Sheng WH, Ko WJ, Wang JT, et al. Evaluation of antiseptic-impregnated central venous catheters for prevention of catheter-related infection in intensive care unit patients. *Diagn Microbiol Infect Dis.* 2000;38:1.
57. Rupp ME, Lisco SJ, Lipsett PA, et al. Effect of a second-generation venous catheter impregnated with chlorhexidine and silver sulfadiazine on central catheter-related infections: a randomized, controlled trial. *Ann intern Med.* 2005;143:570.
58. Veenstra DL, Saint S, Saha S, et al. Efficacy of antiseptic-impregnated central venous catheters in preventing catheter-related bloodstream infection. *JAMA.* 1999;281:261.
59. Logghe C, Van Ossel C, D'Hoore W, et al. Evaluation of chlorhexidine and silver-sulfadiazine impregnated central venous catheters for the prevention of bloodstream infection in leukemic patients: a randomized controlled trial. *J Hosp Infect.* 1997;37:145.
60. Bassetti S, Hu J, D'Agastino Jr, et al. Prolonged antimicrobial activity of a catheter containing chlorhexidine-silver sulfadiazine extends protection against catheter infection. *Antimicrob Agents Chemother.* 2001;45:1535.
61. Darouiche RO, Raad II, Bodey GP, et al. Antibiotic susceptibility of staphylococcal isolates from patients with vascular catheter-related bacteremia: potential role of the combination of minocycline and rifampin. *Int J Antimicrob Agents.* 1995;6:31.
62. Raad I, Darouiche R, Hachem R, et al. Antibiotics and prevention of microbial colonization of catheters. *Antimicrob Agents Chemother.* 1995; 39:2397.
63. Raad I, Darouiche R, Hachem R, et al. The broad spectrum activity and efficacy of catheters coated with minocycline and rifampin. *J Infect Dis.* 1996;173:418.
64. Widmer AF, Frei R, Rajacic Z, et al. Correlation between in vivo and in vitro efficacy of antimicrobial agents against foreign body infections. *J Infect Dis.* 1990;162:96.
65. Raad I, Hanna H, Jiang Y, et al. Comparative activities of daptomycin, linezolid, and tigecycline against catheter-related methicillin-resistant *Staphylococcus* bacteremic isolates embedded in biofilm. *Antimicrob Agents Chemother.* 2007;51:1656.
66. Raad I, Darouiche R, Dupuis J, et al. Central venous catheters coated with minocycline and rifampin for the prevention of catheter-related colonization and bloodstream infections: a randomized, double-blind trial. *Ann Intern Med.* 1997;127:267.
67. Darouiche RO, Raad II, Heard SO, et al. A comparison of two antimicrobial-impregnated central venous catheters. *N Engl J Med.* 1999; 340:1.
68. Marick PE, Abraham G, Carean P, et al. The ex vivo antibacterial activity and colonization rate of two antimicrobial-coated central venous catheters. *Crit Care Med.* 1999;27:1128.
69. Vaudaux P, Pittet D, Haeberli A, et al. Host factors selectively increase staphylococcal adherence on inserted catheters: a role for fibronectin and fibrinogen or fibrin. *J Infect Dis.* 1989;160:865.
70. Hermann M, Vaudaux PE, Pittet D, et al. Fibronectin, fibrinogen, and laminin act as mediators of adherence of clinical staphylococcal isolates to foreign material. *J Infect Dis.* 1988;158:693.
71. Bassetti S, Hu J, D'Agastiono, et al. In vitro zones of inhibition of coated vascular catheters predict efficacy in preventing catheter infection with *Staphylococcus aureus* in vivo. *Eur J Clin Microbiol Infect Dis.* 2000;19:612.
72. Hanna H, Benjamin R, Chatzinikolau I, et al. Long-term silicone central

venous catheters impregnated with minocycline and rifampin decrease rates of catheter-related bloodstream infection in cancer patients: a prospective, randomized clinical trial. *J Clin Oncol.* 2004;22:3163.

73. Darouiche RO, Berger DH, Khardori N, et al. Comparison of antimicrobial impregnation with tunneling of long-term central venous catheters: a randomized, controlled trial. *Ann Surg.* 2005;242:193.
74. Chatzinikolaou I, Hanna H, Graviss L, et al. Clinical experience with minocycline and rifampin-impregnated central venous catheters in bone marrow transplantation recipients: efficacy and low risk of developing staphylococcal resistance. *Infect Control Hosp Epidemiol.* 2003;24:961.
75. Crnich CJ, Maki DG. The promise of novel technology for the prevention of intravascular device-related bloodstream infection, I: pathogenesis and short-term devices. *Clin Infect Dis.* 2002;34:1232.
76. Crnich CJ, Maki DG. The promise of novel technology for the prevention of intravascular device-related bloodstream infection, II: long-term devices. *Clin Infect Dis.* 2002;340:1362.
77. Veenstra DL, Saint S, Sullivan SD. Cost-effectiveness of antiseptic-impregnated central venous catheters for the prevention of catheter-related bloodstream infection. *JAMA.* 1999;282:554.
78. Shorr AF, Humphreys CW, Helman DL. New choices for central venous catheters: potential financial implications. *Chest.* 2003;124:275.
79. Cobb DK, High KP, Sawyer RG, et al. A controlled trial of scheduled replacement of central venous and pulmonary-artery catheters. *N Engl J Med.* 1992;327:1062.
80. Eyer S, Brummit C, Crossley K, et al. Catheter-related sepsis: a prospective, randomized, study of three different methods of long-term catheter maintenance. *Crit Care Med.* 1990;18:1073.
81. Timsit JF. Scheduled replacement of central venous catheters is not necessary. *Infect Control Hosp Epidemiol.* 2000;21:371.
82. Reed CR, Sessler CN, Glauser FL, et al. Central venous catheter infections: concepts and controversies. *Intensive Care Med.* 1995;21:177.
83. Cook D, Randolph, Kernerman P, et al. Central venous catheter replacement strategies: a systematic review of the literature. *Crit Care Med.* 1997; 25:1417.
84. Robinson D, Suhocki P, Schwab SJ. Treatment of infected tunneled venous access hemodialysis catheters with guidewire exchange. *Kidney Int.* 1998;53:1792.
85. Bach A, Bohrer H, Geiss HK. Safety of a guidewire technique for replacement of pulmonary artery catheters. *J Cardiothorac Vasc Anesth.* 1992; 6:711.
86. Martinez E, Mensa J, Roviera M, et al. Central venous catheter exchange by guidewire for treatment of catheter-related bacteremia in patients undergoing BMT or intensive chemotherapy. *Bone Marrow Transplant.* 1999;23:41.
87. Segura M, Alvarez-Lerma F, Tellado JM, et al. Advances in surgical technique: a clinical trial on the prevention of catheter-related sepsis using a new hub model. *Ann Surg.* 1996;223:363.
88. Luna J, Masdeu G, Perez M, et al. Clinical trial evaluating a new hub device designed to prevent catheter-related sepsis. *Eur J Clin Microbiol Infect Dis.* 2000;19:655.
89. Schwartz C, Henrickson KJ, Roghmann K, et al. Prevention of bacteremia attributed to luminal colonization of tunneled central venous catheters with vancomycin-susceptible organisms. *J Clin Oncol.* 1990;8:591.
90. Carratala J, Njubo J, Fernandez-Sevilla A, et al. Randomized, double-blind trial of an antibiotic-lock technique for prevention of Gram-positive central venous catheter-related infection in neutropenic patients with cancer. *Antimicrob Agents Chemother.* 1999;43:2200.
91. Henrickson KJ, Axtell RA, Hoover SM, et al. Prevention of central venous catheter-related infections and thrombotic events in immunocompromised children by the use of vancomycin/ciprofloxacin/heparin flush solution: a randomized, multicenter, double-blind trial. *J Clin Oncol.* 2000;18:1269.
92. Rackoff WR, Weiman M, Jakobowski D, et al. A randomized, controlled trial of the efficacy of a heparin and vancomycin solution in preventing central venous catheter infections in children. *J Pediatr.* 1995;127:147.
93. Safdar N, Maki DG. Use of vancomycin-containing lock or flush solutions for prevention of bloodstream infection associated with central venous access devices: a meta-analysis of prospective, randomized trials. *Clin Infect Dis.* 2006;43:474.
94. Sherertz RJ, Ely EW, Westbrook DM, et al. Education of physicians-in-training can decrease the risk for vascular catheter infection. *Ann Intern Med.* 2000;132:641–648.
95. Warren DK, Zack JE, Mayfield JL, et al. The efect of an education program on the incidence of central venous catheter-associated bloodstream infection in amedical ICU. *Chest.* 2004;126:1612.
96. Bijma R, Girbes AR, Klejer DJ, et al. Preventing central venous catheter-related infection in a surgical intensive-care unit. *Infect Control Hosp Epidemiol.* 1999;20:618–620.
97. Aslam S, Trautner BW, Ramanathan V, et al. Combination of tigecycline and N-acetylcysteine reduces biofilm-embedded bacteria on vascular catheters. *Antimicrob Agents Chemother.* 2007;51:1556–1558.
98. Mansouri MD, Darouiche RO. In vitro antimicrobial activity of N-acetylcysteine against bacteria colonizing central venous catheters. *Int J Antimicrob Agents.* 2007;29:474–476.
99. Dell'Acqua G, Giacometti A, Cirioni O, et al. Suppression of drug-resistant staphylococcal infections by the quorum sensing inhibitor RNA-inhibiting peptide. *J Infect Dis.* 2004;190:318.
100. Hentzer M, Wu H, Anderson JB, et al. Attenuation of *Pseudomonas aeruginosa* virulence by quorum sensing inhibitors. *EMBO J.* 2003;22:3803–3805.
101. Ullman RF, Gurevich I, Schoch PE, et al. Colonization and bacteremia related to duration of triple-lumen intravascular catheter replacement. *Am J Infect Control.* 1990;18:201.
102. Norwood S, Wilkins HE, III, Vallina VL, et al. The safety of prolonging the use of central venous catheters: a prospective analysis of the effects of using antiseptic-bonded catheters with daily site care. *Crit Care Med.* 2000;28:1376.
103. Ramanathan V, Chiu EJ, Thomas JT, et al. Healthcare costs associated with hemodialysis catheter-related infections: a single-center experience. *Infect Control Hosp Epidemiol.* 2007;28:606–609.
104. Pronovost P, Needham D, Bernholtz S, et al. An intervention to decrease catheter-related bloodstream infections in the ICU. *N Engl J Med.* 2006;355:2725.

CHAPTER 32 ■ VASCULAR CANNULATION

INDERMEET S. BHULLAR • ERNEST F. J. BLOCK

DEFINITION

A central venous catheter (CVC) by definition has its tip in the superior vena cava.

HISTORY

The ancient Greek physician Galen (129–200 AD) first proposed the existence of blood in the human body. Born in Greece, he immigrated to Rome and became the principal doctor for the gladiators. With legal constraints limiting dissections on humans, he used animal dissections to provide some of the earliest anatomy charts. His work, *On the Element According to Hippocrates*, describes the philosopher's system of four bodily humors—blood, yellow bile, black bile, and phlegm—which were modeled after the four classic elements of Hippocrates: air, water, fire, and earth. In 1616, William Harvey proposed that contrary to Galen's writings, the heart did not constantly produce blood, but rather, there was a finite amount of blood that circulated in one direction throughout the body. His ideas raised doubts about the benefit of bloodletting, a popular medical practice at the time.

In 1727, an English naturalist and clergyman, Stephen Hales, was the first to determine arterial blood pressure. Inserting a brass pipe into a horse's central artery and connecting it to a glass tube, he observed the blood rise in the pipe and concluded that this must be due to a pressure in the blood. He published this work in 1733 in his second-volume *Haemastaticks*, which contained experiments on the "force of the blood" in various animals, its rate of flow, and the capacity of the different vessels. In this work Hales also described the first catheterization of the heart of a living animal. In an effort to measure the precise capacity of the heart he bled a sheep to death and then led a gun-barrel from the neck vessels into the still-beating heart. Through this, he filled the hollow chambers with molten wax and then measured from the resultant cast the volume of the heartbeat and the minute volume of the heart, which he calculated from the pulse beat.

In 1844, Claude Bernard inserted a mercury thermometer into the carotid artery of a horse and advanced it through the aortic valve into the left ventricle to measure the blood temperature. He adapted this experiment over the next 40 years for measuring intracardiac pressures in a variety of animals. Based on his work, the use of catheters became the standard method for physiologists to study the hemodynamics of the cardiovascular system. Another major step in the development of cardiac catheterization was taken by Adolph Fick in 1870. His famous but brief note on the calculation of blood flow is the basis for today's procedures.

In 1929, a German surgical trainee, Werner Forssmann, experimented on a human cadaver and realized how easy it was to guide a urologic catheter from an arm vein into the right atrium. He went so far as to dissect the veins of his own forearm and guide a urologic catheter into his right atrium using fluoroscopic control and a mirror. With the catheter in place, he walked to the x-ray room, and had his own chest x-rayed to prove the safety and feasibility of human right heart catheterization. This made Forssmann the first to document right heart catheterization in humans using radiographic techniques. In return, he was fired from his position at the hospital but subsequently won the Nobel Prize in 1956. In 1949, Duff presented the first series of 43 patients that underwent transfemoral catheterization of the inferior vena cava (IVC) for fluid and electrolyte management (1).

The clinical use of CVCs was first described by Aubaniac in a 1952 publication summarizing a 10-year experience with subclavian vein catheters for rapid infusion of fluids during resuscitation of wounded soldiers on the battlefield (2). Since then, several other access routes have been described. In 1969, Dudrick and Wilmore reported the use of long-term polyvinyl catheters placed in central veins for the administration of total parenteral nutrition (TPN) (3). In 1973, Broviac introduced the silicone rubber catheter for long-term home TPN, followed closely by the introduction of the peripherally inserted central catheter (PICC) line by Hoshell in 1975 (4,5). Hickman introduced a larger-bore Broviac catheter for bone marrow transplant patients to give and withdraw blood in 1979 (6). In 1982, Neidehuber implanted the first chest ports used clinically (7).

Approximately 5 million CVC insertions are done every year in the United States, of which 200,000 are ports and 400,000 are tunneled catheters. The utilization of CVC in the intensive care unit (ICU) is similar in adult and pediatric patients.

INDICATIONS

The decision to place a central venous access device should be made after considering the risks and benefits to each patient. Therapeutic indications include the following: Administration of chemotherapy, administration of TPN, administration of blood products, performance of plasmapheresis, and performance of hemodialysis. Patients who have difficult peripheral IV access, such as obese patients or drug abusers, should also be considered for CVCs. Many drugs are caustic, causing irritation of the venous intima leading to inflammation and thrombosis. Patients being administered these drugs also need central venous access. Some of these caustic drugs include amphotericin B, Bactrim, ciprofloxacin, dobutamine, doxycycline, erythromycin, ganciclovir, lidocaine, penicillins, pentamidine, Phenergan, phenytoin, potassium (depending on dilution), Rocephin, vancomycin, and tobramycin. Infusates with an osmolality >280 to 300 mOsm also require central dilution.

CONTRAINDICATIONS

There are no absolute contraindications to central line placement. However, relative contraindications include:

1. Infected sites
2. Anatomic abnormalities
3. Burns
4. Coagulopathy

Although caution is recommended in patients with an elevated international normalized ratio (INR), combined coagulopathy, thrombocytopenia, or liver disease, there is little evidence that transfusion of fresh frozen plasma (FFP) is required before insertion. Fisher and Mutimer evaluated 658 patients with liver disease and coagulopathy (INR >1.5 and/or platelet counts $<150 \times 10^9$/L) that underwent CVC insertion for complications. The subclavian vein approach was utilized in 352 patients (median INR 2.7) and the internal jugular (IJ) route in 302 patients (median INR 2.7). Only one patient developed a hemothorax after accidental subclavian artery puncture. There were no other major vascular complications. A significantly higher incidence of minor complications, such as superficial hematoma, was noted for patents that had multiple needle puncture attempts and failed guidewire cannulation of vein. Interestingly, patients with the IJ approach had a significantly higher rate of superficial hematoma formation compared to the subclavian route (11% vs. 3%). A significantly higher oozing rate was noted for patients with low platelets as compared to normal levels, indicating a possible role for platelet transfusion in select patients. We recommend that the presence of liver failure with elevated INR should not be considered an absolute contraindication to CVC placement. There is little evidence that FFP should be transfused beforehand or that the IJ route is better than the subclavian. Consideration should be given to platelet transfusion in patients with liver disease, elevated INR, and low platelets (8). Ultrasound guidance may play an important role in patients with coagulopathy (see below).

IMMEDIATE CONCERNS

More than 15% of all patients who receive CVCs have complications (9–11). At least 52% of the reported complications are related to practitioner technique. The level of experience of the physician reduces the risk of the complications (10,12). Physicians who have placed 50 or more CVCs are half as likely to have a mechanical complication as those who have performed less than 50 (10). The number of insertion attempts is also significant since the incidence of mechanical complications after three or more insertion attempts is six times that after one attempt (13). The complication rate is decreased with certification programs that provide formal education and practice simulators as well as placement under supervision (10,12). An increasingly important tool for improving safe learning curves for CVC placement is the two-dimensional ultrasound imaging and guidance.

PREPARATION

Informed Consent

The judgment by the war crimes tribunal at Nuremberg laid down ten standards to which physicians must conform when carrying out experiments on human subjects in a new code (the Nuremberg Code) that is now accepted worldwide. Among other requirements, this document enunciates the requirement of *voluntary informed consent* of the human subject. The principle of voluntary informed consent protects the right of the individual to control his or her own body.

Informed consent is a process of communication between a patient and physician that results in the patient's authorization or agreement to undergo a specific medical intervention. It originates from the legal and ethical right the patient has to direct what happens to his or her body and from the ethical duty of the physician to involve the patient in his or her health care. This communication process is both an ethical obligation and a legal requirement spelled out in statutes and case law in all 50 states.

The following criteria must be met in the process of securing an informed consent:

1. Establish that the patient is competent and capable of making rational decisions regarding his or her health. If the patient is determined to be too incapacitated/incompetent to make health care decisions, a surrogate decision maker must be identified. There is a specific hierarchy of appropriate decision makers defined by state law:
   a. *Surrogate hierarchy:*
      (1) Patient's agent as defined in the advanced care directive
      (2) Guardian
      (3) Spouse
      (4) Adult son or daughter
      (5) Custodial parent
      (6) Adult grandchild
      (7) Available adult relative with closest degree of kinship
2. Using words and language that the patient can understand (use an interpreter if necessary), the physician must convey the details of the planned procedure, its potential benefits, serious risks, and any feasible alternatives.
3. Review the risks and benefits of the alternative procedure.
4. Review the risks and benefits of not receiving the procedure.
5. Address all the patient's questions and concerns. The physician must verify that the patient has understood what has been said, accepted the risks involved, and agreed to proceed with the procedure.
6. Finally, the individual must sign the consent form, which documents in generic format the major points of consideration.
7. The only exception to this is securing informed consent during extreme emergencies. The patient's consent should only be "presumed," rather than obtained, in emergency situations when the patient is unconscious or incompetent and no surrogate decision maker is available.

Appropriate documentation must be made in the patient's chart defining the circumstances of the informed consent.

Obtain History

A procedure-directed history and physical exam are essential. Investigate the following:

1. Location and number of previous CVCs and ports
2. Location of known venous thrombi
3. History of infected ports and their sites
4. History of clavicle fracture
5. History of bleeding associated with CVC placement
6. History of pneumothorax or other complications from previous CVCs
7. History of IVC filter placement
8. Current or recent use of warfarin, aspirin, clopidogrel bisulfate, heparin, low-molecular-weight heparin, or other anticoagulants
9. History of pacemaker insertion

Potential access sites should be evaluated to determine if there are any anatomic or cutaneous abnormalities (such as scarring from trauma, previous radiation, surgery, infections, or burns) that would preclude placement of a central venous access device. A previous history of venous thrombi as documented by ultrasound would be crucial in selection of the insertion site and would help avoid unnecessary complications. In patients with a history of IVC filter, care must be exercised when using the femoral route to avoid entrapment of the guidewire in the filter. Placement of a pulmonary artery catheter using the femoral route is also contraindicated in these patients for the same reason. Previous fractures of the clavicle may make access difficult secondary to distortion of the anatomy and landmarks.

Sterile Preparation of Operator and Skin

Prior to starting the procedure, obtain all necessary items listed below and, using an aseptic technique, open them onto a working table in close proximity to the patient:

1. Sterile gown and gloves
2. Hat and mask
3. Central line kit with a large enough drape to cover the insertion area and to prevent contamination of long wires
4. 2% chlorhexidine or 10% povidone iodine
5. Sterile saline flush

Prepare the skin with 2% chlorhexidine or 10% povidone iodine. Ten percent povidone iodine has no immediate effect. It allows a slow release of iodine and takes about 2 minutes to be fully effective. Therefore, after application allow appropriate time for drying prior to draping. This gap can be filled as the time to obtain a "maximum sterile barrier." This includes the placement of a sterile cap, mask, gown, and gloves for every single procedure. The use of all four elements consistently along with appropriately prepped skin reduces catheter-related septicemia by sixfold (14).

The patient's scrub should include a generous area and extend 10 cm outward in a circular manner from the planned insertion point. If the line is placed in an area with hair, the hair need not be removed. Bacterial counts are the same after prepping with or without hair. Razors for hair removal can cause micro-abrasions and increase the risk of infection. A mechanical or frictional scrub is best in that it reduces both the microbial burden and the epithelial cellular debris.

Next, place the large sterile drape over the insertion site. Do not occlude the air supply or field of vision when draping neck areas of conscious patients. An assistant, electronic devices, or both must monitor relevant parameters of the patient's well-being continually through the procedure, because the operator may lose valuable clues while concentrating on the procedure and because much of the patient is obscured by drapes.

Prepare the CVC kit prior to starting the line placement as follows:

1. Load the 1% lidocaine.
2. Bring the wire onto the sterile field close to the insertion point to minimize movements after cannulation of the vein with the finder needle.
3. Adjust the wire by pulling the J-curve of the tip into the hub of the guidewire holder so that it is straightened out and ready for insertion.
4. Remove the distal port cap off the catheter for easier placement over the wire.
5. Flush the ports of the catheter with sterile saline to remove air.

Position Patient

Now you are ready for catheter insertion. At this point place the patient in a 10- to 25-degree Trendelenburg position. This significantly increases the diameter of the IJ as compared to the supine position and further helps to increase venous cannulation and decrease the risk for air embolism (15–17). However, special consideration must be taken prior to placing patients with traumatic brain injury in the Trendelenburg position since this position may exacerbate intracranial pressure elevation and secondary brain injury. Caution should also be used in patients with high aspiration risk, gastric distention, orthopnea, or hypoxia.

Analgesia

Analgesia and sedation to reduce pain and anxiety during any invasive procedure are often helpful. Local analgesia may be obtained by injecting 1 to 5 mL of 1% lidocaine without epinephrine subcutaneously so that a 1-cm wheal is raised. Use the smallest needle available and inject slowly to minimize discomfort of tissue distention. Attention should be paid to the track of local anesthetic instilled so that subsequent larger needles are not inserted into an area where there is minimum anesthetic. Some operators use the smallest needle to create a skin wheal, leave that needle in the skin after removing the syringe, and then replace the small needle with a longer 21- to 22-gauge needle into the same site to further infiltrate the deeper tissues. This longer needle is then left in the tissues after removing the syringe and serves as a guide to insert the final large needle precisely into the tissue that has been well anesthetized. Conscious sedation must be used with great caution in nonintubated patients. The operator should be aware of his or her institutional policy regarding conscious sedation. At minimum, a review of the patient's chart and history should be routinely performed to assess for underlying cardiac and other medical problems that may interfere with sedation and verify allergies. The patient should be appropriately monitored. Monitors for blood pressure measurements, electrocardiography, and pulse oximetry should be attached before the patient receives any sedatives, and these parameters should be checked every 5 to 10 minutes. Personnel certified in basic and advanced cardiac life support procedures must be present in the room to monitor the patient at all times during the administration of intravenous sedation. Reversal agents such as naloxone and flumazenil should be readily available and the operator should be familiar with their dosage and administration. The operator should be cautious with the use of flumazenil as a reversal agent in patients on chronic benzodiazepines to avoid the complication of seizures. Patients should be monitored postprocedure until their vital signs are stable and they are alert and back to their baseline.

CENTRAL VENOUS CANNULATION

Seldinger Technique

The Seldinger technique is a procedure to obtain safe access to blood vessels and other hollow organs. It is named after Dr. Sven-Ivar Seldinger (1921–1998), a Swedish radiologist from Mora, Dalarna County, who introduced the procedure in 1953 (18). In the procedure the desired vessel or cavity is punctured with a sharp hollow needle called a trocar. A round-tipped (J-tipped) guidewire is then advanced through the lumen of the trocar, and the trocar is withdrawn. Any hollow catheter or cannula can now be passed over the guidewire into the cavity or vessel. The guidewire is then withdrawn.

FEMORAL VEIN CANNULATION (FIGS. 32.1 TO 32.3)

Introduction

The femoral route for central venous catheterization was first described by Duffy in 1948 (1). He reported on 72 patients with polyethylene catheters inserted over extended periods of time into central veins with 28 of these utilizing the femoral route. However, subsequent independent reports by Moncrief (1958) and Bansmer et al. (1958) identified an unacceptably high rate of venous thrombosis and catheter-related sepsis associated with this technique (19,20). This led to the femoral route falling out of favor. Resurgence in interest came toward the end of 1960, when Dr. Stanley Shaldon et al., working at the Royal Free Hospital in London, developed a technique for hemodialysis by percutaneous catheterization of the femoral artery and vein. They developed single-lumen catheters having tapered tips for entry over a Seldinger wire to be used in hemodialysis. The technique was described in a 1961 publication of *The Lancet* and subsequently re-established the femoral route as a safe and effective means to obtain central venous access (21).

The femoral route is popular as it avoids many of the following complications associated with subclavian and IJ routes (22):

1. Pneumothorax
2. Hemothorax

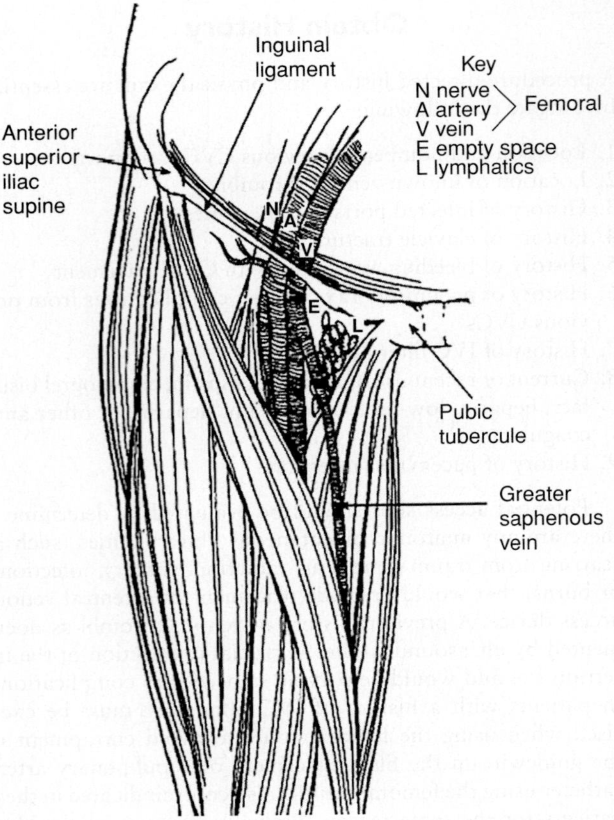

FIGURE 32.1. Anatomy of the femoral artery and vein. Use the pneumonic NAVEL (Nerve, Artery, Vein, Empty space, Lymphatics) to recall structures as you move in a lateral to medial direction toward the navel.

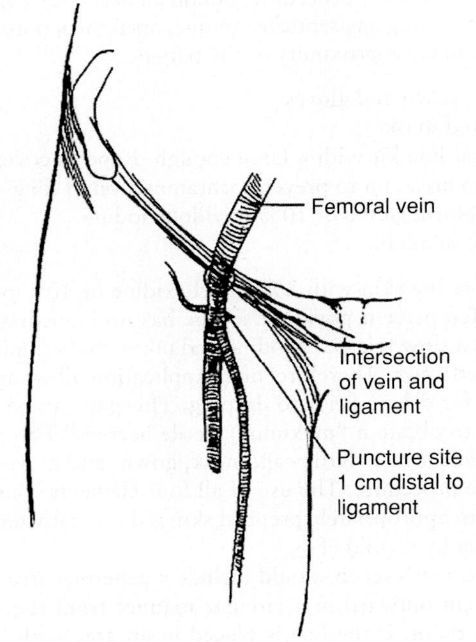

FIGURE 32.2. Choose a puncture site 1 to 2 cm inferior to the inguinal ligament to avoid intra-abdominal injury and retroperitoneal hematomas.

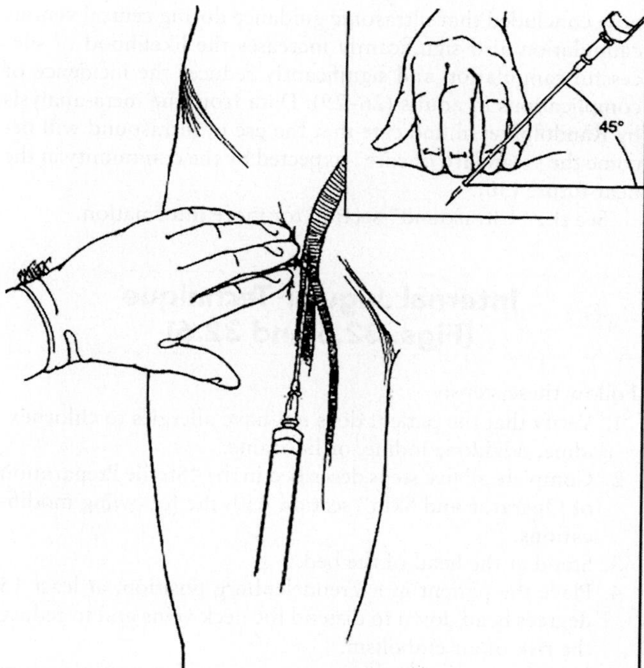

FIGURE 32.3. Locate the femoral artery, keep a finger on the artery, and introduce the finder needle attached to a 10-mL syringe at an angle of 45 degrees to the skin, about 1 cm medial to the femoral artery pulsation, 2 cm below the inguinal ligament.

3. Arrhythmias
4. Thoracic duct laceration
5. Damage to phrenic, vagus, and recurrent laryngeal nerves

Another benefit of the femoral route is that a radiograph is not necessary to verify proper position.

Bleeding from inadvertent arterial puncture (the main mechanical complication of femoral venous cannulation) is more easily controlled by manual pressure in the groin than in other sites (23). The femoral route is also felt to be the easiest site for rapid access and the best site for inexperienced operators to learn the basic techniques of central venous access using the Seldinger technique (24).

Anatomy and Patient Positioning

The femoral vein is punctured in the femoral triangle (inferior to the inguinal ligament, lateral to the adductor longus, and medial to the sartorius muscles), where it lies medial to the femoral artery.

Technique

Follow these steps:

1. Verify that the patient does not have allergies to chlorhexidine, povidone iodine, or lidocaine.
2. Complete all five steps described in the "Sterile Preparation of Operator and Skin" section.
3. Extend the patient's leg and abduct slightly at the hip.
4. Locate the femoral artery, keep a finger on the artery, and introduce the finder needle attached to a 10-mL syringe at an angle 45 degrees to the skin, about 1 cm medial to the femoral artery pulsation, 2 cm below the inguinal ligament.
5. Slowly advance the needle cephalad and posteriorly while continuously withdrawing the plunger. Too much suction applied to the plunger in a hypovolemic patient may lead to vein collapse with minimum blood return. This may mislead the operator into assuming the needle is not in the vessel lumen.
6. Once venous blood is obtained, use the Seldinger technique to complete the procedure.
7. Verify that all ports allow aspiration of venous blood and can be flushed with saline without resistance.
8. Secure the catheter, cover with a nonocclusive sterile dressing, and document the procedure appropriately in the chart.

STEPS TO PREVENT COMPLICATIONS

1. Do not force the wire through the finder needle; resistance of any type is an indication to stop, remove the needle and guidewire, and hold pressure on the vein. Verify that the patient does not have an IVC filter.
2. One hand should be on the guidewire at all times during the procedure to avoid losing the wire into the femoral vein.
3. Avoid overzealous dilation of the femoral vein with the dilator. Excessive dilation extending beyond the subcutaneous tissue and fat into the vein increases the risk of postprocedure complications (oozing, hematoma formation, arteriovenous fistula formation, and pseudoaneurysm formation).
4. Stay below the inguinal ligament. The distal tip of the finder needle should not traverse cephalad to the inguinal ligament to avoid retroperitoneal hematoma and/or intra-abdominal injuries.
5. Inadvertent arterial puncture and subsequent hematoma or pseudoaneurysm formation can be prevented by providing direct pressure manually or with a standard device for at least 30 minutes.

INTERNAL JUGULAR VEIN CANNULATION

Anatomy and Patient Positioning (Fig. 32.4)

The IJ vein exits the jugular foramen at the skull base and courses inferiorly in the carotid sheath along with the carotid artery and vagus nerve. It courses along a straight line from the mastoid process to the medial side of the insertion point of the clavicular head of the sternocleidomastoid (SCM) muscle. Although it sits posterior to the carotid artery at the skull base, as it courses down the neck, it spirals around the artery and ends up anteriorly at the level of the clavicle. For purposes of internal jugular vein access, an important anatomic triangle is formed by the two heads of the SCM and the medial one third of the clavicle. It is within this triangle that the right IJ is most safely and readily cannulated. Within this triangle, the carotid artery lies medial and slightly posterior to the internal jugular vein,

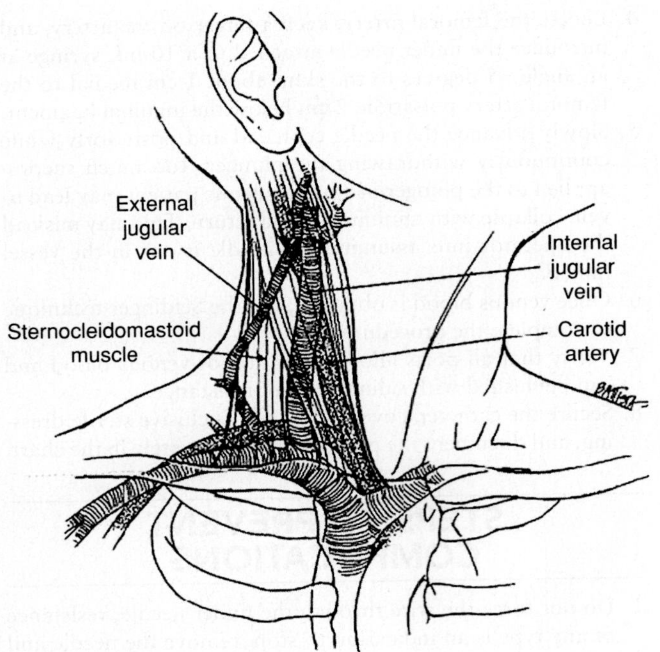

FIGURE 32.4. Anatomy of the internal jugular vein.

decreasing its chances of accidentally being punctured during catheter insertion. It joins with the subclavian vein to become the brachiocephalic vein. The Valsalva maneuver or Trendelenburg position can increase the size of the IJ. If these maneuvers do not increase the size, distal stenosis or obstruction should be considered. Also, avoid overextending the patient's neck since this may actually flatten and decrease the size of the IJ vein. The advantages to using the right IJ for CVC insertion include:

1. More superficial position than the subclavian vein
2. Apical pleura does not rise as high on the right as the left and the right side avoids the thoracic duct
3. Straighter course to the superior vena cava as compared to the left IJ or either subclavian route
4. Lower stenosis or occlusion rate as opposed to the subclavian vein

Role of Ultrasound

The anatomic relationship of the internal jugular vein to the carotid artery varies. Sonography lessens the complications of inadvertent puncture and/or cannulation of the carotid artery. Denys and Uretsky evaluated 200 consecutive patients with sonography and found that the IJ was normal size and position in 92%, nonvisualized in 2.5%, and exceedingly small in 3%. Other studies suggest that IJ variations from normal can occur in up to 28%. The variability among authors may relate to the level and degree of neck rotation when examined with ultrasound. As the neck is turned away from 30 to 90 degrees, the IJ assumes a more anterior position in relation to the carotid artery (25). Doppler-guided approaches to the IJ have been reported to reduce both the number of needle passes required to locate the vein and the incidence of inadvertent carotid puncture (26–29). Furthermore, two recent systematic reviews have now concluded that ultrasonic guidance during central venous cannulation also significantly increases the likelihood of successful cannulation and significantly reduces the incidence of complications in adults (26–29). Data from the meta-analysis by Randolph et al. indicate that the use of ultrasound will become the "standard of care" expected by the community in the near future (30).

See the "Ultrasound" section for more information.

Internal Jugular Technique (Figs. 32.5 and 32.6)

Follow these steps:

1. Verify that the patient does not have allergies to chlorhexidine, povidone iodine, or lidocaine.
2. Complete all five steps described in the "Sterile Preparation of Operator and Skin" section with the following modifications.
3. Stand at the head of the bed.
4. Place the patient in a Trendelenburg position, at least 15 degrees head down to distend the neck veins and to reduce the risk of air embolism.
5. Slightly turn the head (no more than 20 degrees) away from the puncture site. Turning it too far increases the risk of arterial puncture.
6. Obtain a "maximum sterile barrier," which includes the placement of a sterile cap, mask, gown, and gloves.
7. Cleanse the skin and drape the area with the large drape.
8. Identify the apex of the triangle formed by the two heads of the SCM and clavicle.
9. Use local anesthetic (1% lidocaine provided in the kit) and the smallest needle available to anesthetize the puncture site at the apex of the triangle.
10. SMALL NEEDLE LOCATOR: Use a 10-mL syringe attached to a small finder needle (usually 22 gauge 1 inch) to find the internal jugular vein. This helps to decrease inadvertent carotid artery injury.

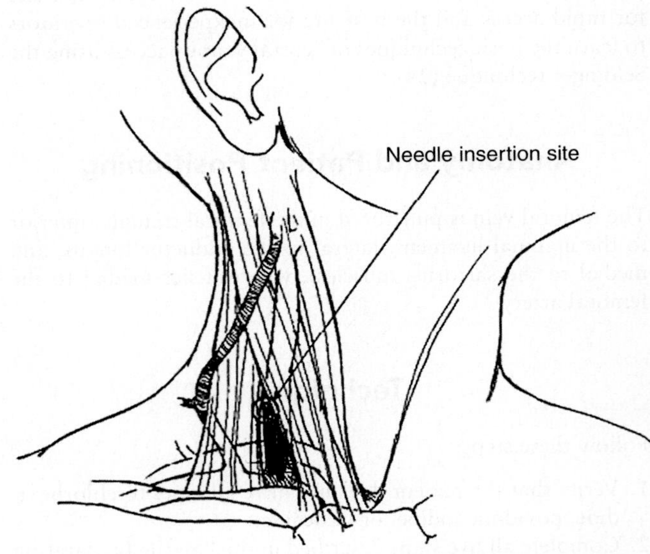

FIGURE 32.5. Identify the apex of the triangle formed by the two heads of the sternocleidomastoid (SCM) and clavicle.

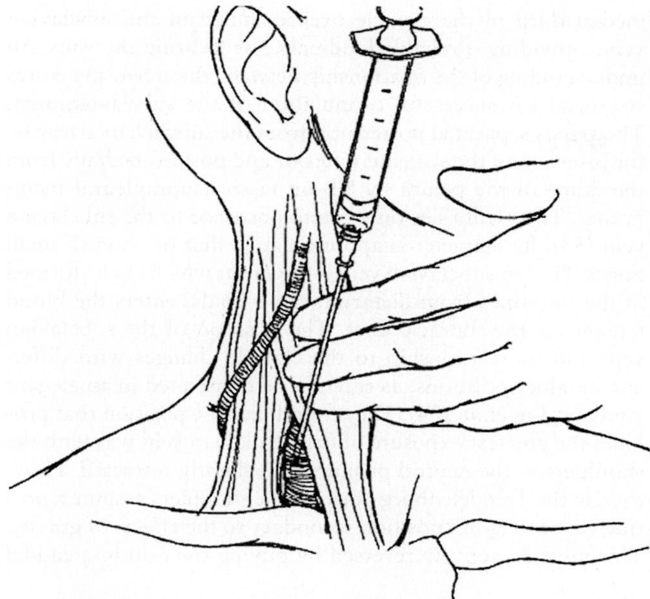

FIGURE 32.6. Attach a fresh 10-mL syringe to the large 18-gauge 2-inch finder needle and, using the previously placed 22-gauge needle as a guide, find the internal jugular vein.

11. Insert the 22-gauge needle at an angle of 30 to 40 degrees to the skin and advance it downward toward the ipsilateral nipple.
12. The syringe and needle should be stabilized by resting the hand on the mandible of the patient at its midpoint.
13. The vein is usually within 2 to 3 cm of the skin. If the vein is not found, redirect the needle more laterally.
14. More so than the subclavian vein, the jugular vein is easily compressed. As a result, a blood flashback is quite frequently not encountered until the needle is being withdrawn; therefore, withdraw slowly.
15. Once the IJ is identified, leave the 22-gauge needle in place and remove the 10-mL syringe. Some operators bypass the step of using a smaller finder needle.
16. BIG NEEDLE: Attach a fresh 10-mL syringe to the large 18-gauge 2-inch finder needle, and using the previously placed 22-gauge needle as a guide, find the IJ vein.
17. The practice of priming the aspirating syringe with saline is unwarranted and makes the differentiation of venous and arterial blood more difficult (31).
18. If the blood from the finder needle is pulsatile, remove the needle and hold pressure for a full 10 minutes prior to proceeding. Consider ultrasound-guided placement if not already being utilized.
19. Once venous blood is obtained, use the Seldinger technique to complete the procedure.
20. Verify that all ports allow aspiration of venous blood and can be flushed with saline without resistance.
21. Secure the catheter, cover with a nonocclusive sterile dressing, and document the procedure appropriately in the chart.
22. Obtain a stat chest radiograph to verify the position and exclude pneumothorax or other injuries.
23. Andrews et al. have recently measured the distance from skin puncture site to atria-caval junction in 100 patients undergoing central venous cannulation by various routes (32). Their findings are presented in Table 32.1.

TABLE 32.1

DISTANCE FROM SKIN PUNCTURE SITE TO ATRIA-CAVAL JUNCTION

Insertion site	Distance
Right internal jugular vein to atria-caval junction	16.0 cm
Right subclavian vein to atria-caval junction	18.4 cm
Left internal jugular vein to atria-caval junction	19.1 cm
Left subclavian vein to atria-caval junction	21.2 cm

From Tan BK, Hong SW, Huang MH, et al. Anatomic basis of safe percutaneous subclavian venous catheterization. *J Trauma.* 2000;48(1):82–86.

Steps to Prevent Complications

1. Do not force the wire through the finder needle; resistance of any type is an indication to stop, remove the needle and guidewire, and hold pressure on the vein.
2. One hand should be on the guidewire at all times during the procedure to avoid losing the wire into the IJ vein.
3. Avoid overzealous dilation of the IJ vein with the dilator. Excessive dilation extending beyond the subcutaneous tissue and fat into the vein increases the risk of postprocedure complications (oozing, hematoma formation, arteriovenous fistula formation, and pseudoaneurysm formation).
4. Verify that the guidewire moves easily back and forth through the dilator as the dilator is advanced toward the vein to avoid puncturing through the back wall of the vein due to bending of the wire at the dilator tip.
5. Inadvertent arterial puncture and subsequent hematoma or pseudoaneurysm formation can be prevented by providing direct pressure manually or with a standard device for at least 30 minutes.
6. If the patient is intubated and on high positive end-expiratory pressure (PEEP) settings, holding the inspiratory effort for a few seconds while cannulating the IJ vein may decrease the overinflation of the lung apex and decrease the chances of obtaining a pneumothorax. (This should only be performed if no deleterious effects occur toward the patient's oxygenation, ventilation, alveolar recruitment, or overall status.)

SUBCLAVIAN VEIN CANNULATION

Anatomy and Patient Positioning (Figs. 32.7 and 32.8)

The subclavian vein is a continuation of the axillary vein and runs from the outer border of the first rib to the medial border of anterior scalene muscle where it joins with the IJ vein to form the innominate vein (brachiocephalic vein). The position of the vein is defined by its name, *sub* meaning below, and *clavian* meaning pertaining to the clavicle. Anteriorly, the

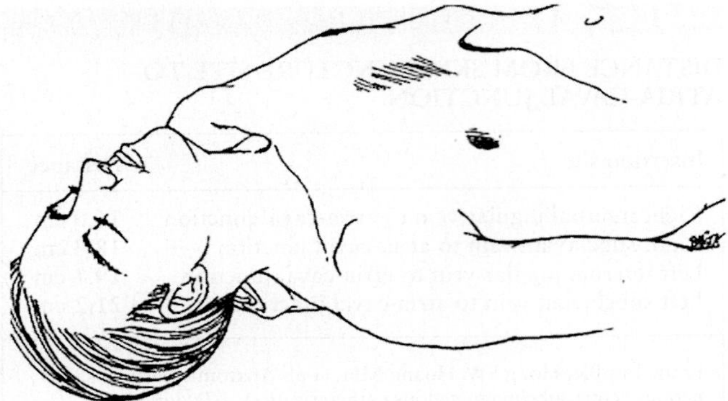

FIGURE 32.7. Patient positioning for subclavian vein cannulation.

medial third of the clavicle overlies much of the subclavian vein, providing a reliable landmark for locating the vein. An understanding of the relationship between these two structures is crucial for successful cannulation of the subclavian vein. The vein is separated posteriorly from the subclavian artery by the insertion of the scalenus anterior and posteromedially from the dome of the pleura by Sibson fascia (suprapleural membrane). The pleura lies only 5 mm posterior to the subclavian vein (33). Its diameter is approximately that of a man's small finger. The left subclavian vein is the site at which chyle, formed in the intestines from dietary fat and lipids, enters the blood stream via the thoracic duct. The position of the subclavian vein and its relationship to the clavicle changes with different shoulder positions, as recently demonstrated in an elegant study by Tan et al. (34). They found that the position that provides the greatest exposure of the subclavian vein was with the shoulders in the neutral position and slightly retracted. However, in the Trendelenburg position the shoulders assume a protracted (shrugging) position secondary to the effects of gravity. This must be actively reversed by pulling the arm in a caudal

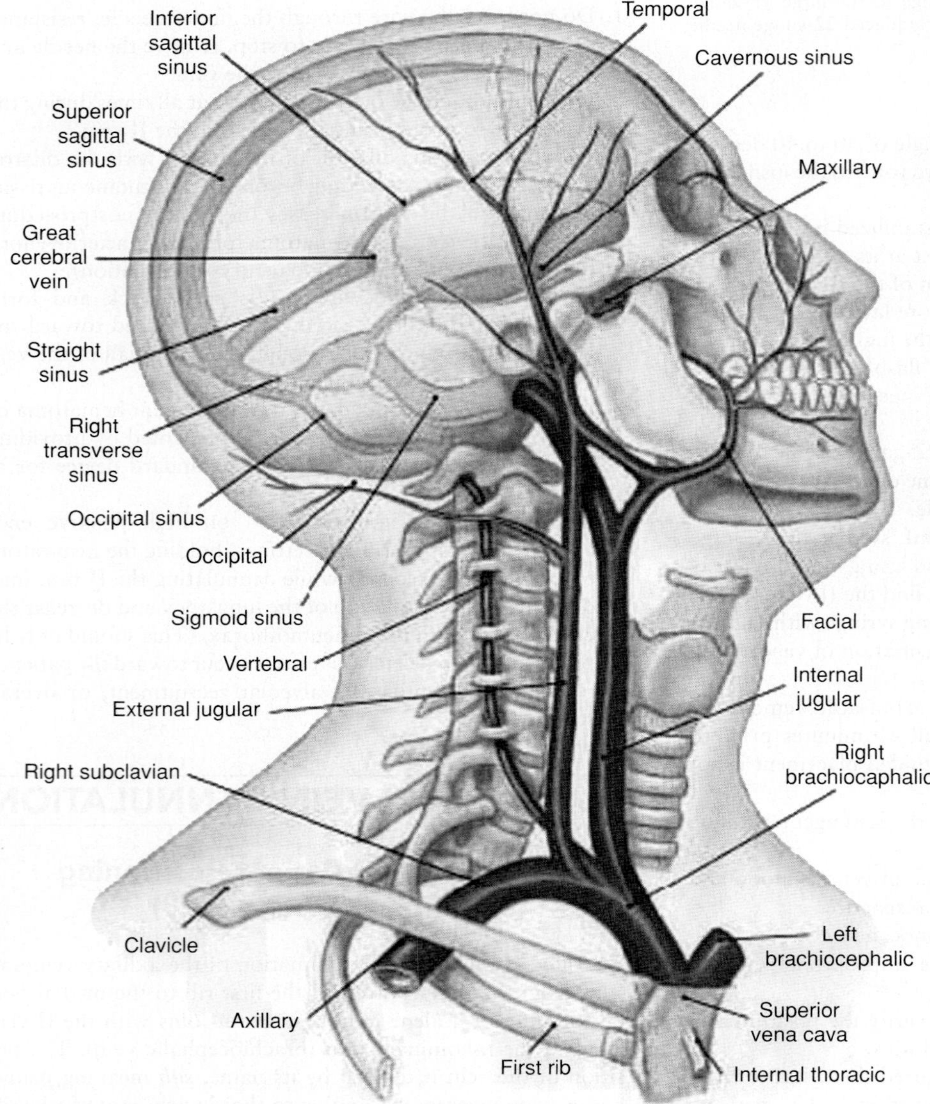

FIGURE 32.8. Anatomy of subclavian vein.

direction while performing the venipuncture to return the shoulder to a neutral position and maximize vein exposure from under the clavicle. This maneuver is extremely helpful even in patients who cannot be in the Trendelenburg position or who are unable to have a roll inserted between the scapulae. Secondly, a retracted position of the shoulder, as obtained by placing a rolled towel beneath the vertebral column between the scapulae to allow the shoulders to fall back, was shown to serve two very important purposes: (a) it prevents the interference between the path of the needle insertion and the humeral head of the shoulder, ensuring that the needle and syringe are always parallel to the coronal plane; and (b) it brings the subclavian vein into close contact with the undersurface of the clavicle, which is desirable for accurate identification of the vein (34). More, however, is not better. Jesseph et al. showed, using magnetic resonance imaging, that excessive shoulder retraction resulted in compression of the vein in the groove between the first rib and the clavicle (35). Understanding these relationships will improve the chances for successful cannulation of the vein.

Keeping the shoulder neutral and retracted was further emphasized by the radiologic studies by Land et al. They demonstrated using single-view venograms in 70 adult patients that the subclavian vein, which was in the path of the needle when the shoulder was in neutral position, moved out of its path when the shoulder was abducted or elevated. The left subclavian vein also ran more medial in relation to the clavicle as compared to the right (36,37).

Infraclavicular Technique (Figs. 32.9 through 32.12)

Follow these steps:

1. Verify that the patient does not have allergies to chlorhexidine, povidone iodine, or lidocaine.

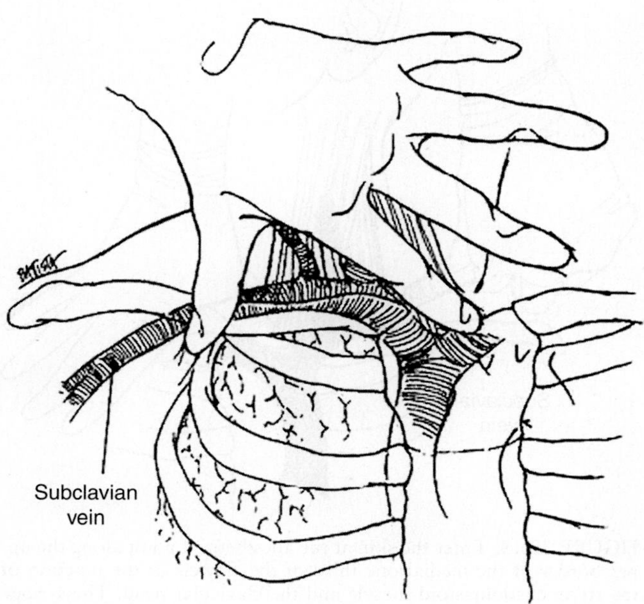

FIGURE 32.9. Identify the middle one third of the clavicle as it follows a gentle curve up toward the shoulder.

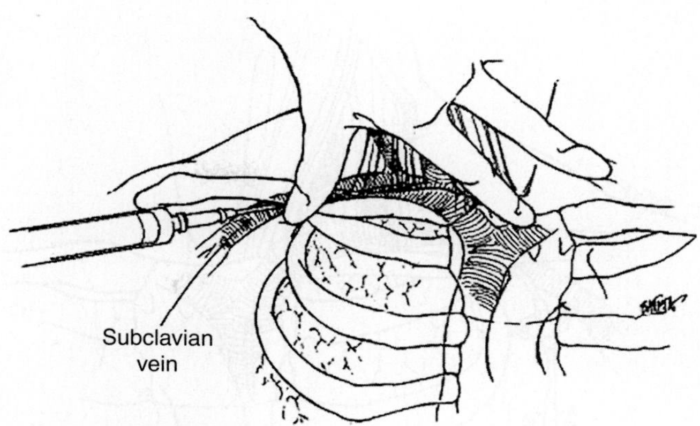

FIGURE 32.10. Enter the skin at the anesthetized point and point the needle tip toward the suprasternal notch. While maintaining constant suction on the syringe and a parallel line to the coronal plane and the floor, gently advance the needle tip cephalad until it passes under the clavicle and into the vein.

2. Complete all five steps described in the "Sterile Preparation of Operator and Skin" section with the following modifications.
3. Place a rolled towel beneath the vertebral column between the scapulae to allow the shoulders to fall back into a slight neutral-retracted position (CONTRAINDICATED in patients with cervical spine injuries since elevation of the shoulders may lead to neck flexion, and should not be done on trauma victims without spine clearance) (4). Place the patient in a Trendelenburg position, at least 15 degrees head down to distend the subclavian veins and to reduce the risk of air embolism.
4. Obtain a "maximum sterile barrier," which includes the placement of a sterile cap, mask, gown, and gloves.
5. Cleanse the skin and drape the area with the large drape provided in the kit.
6. Identify the middle one third of the clavicle as it follows a gentle curve up toward the shoulder.
7. Use local anesthetic (1% lidocaine provided in the kit) and use the smallest needle available to anesthetize the puncture site 2 cm inferior and lateral to the curving middle one third portion of the clavicle.
8. A common mistake, especially in overweight patients or patients with large stature, is to use a puncture site that is

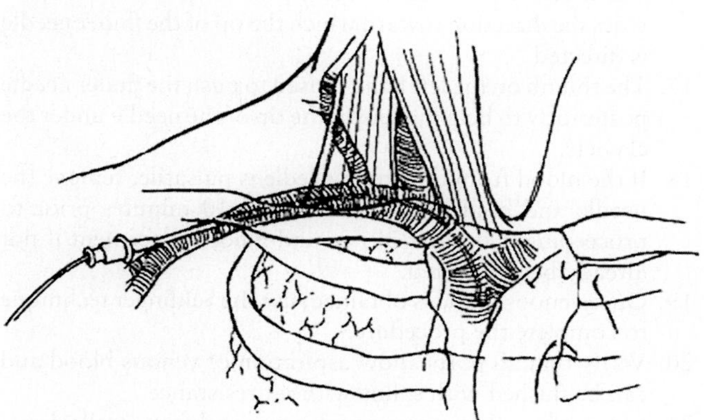

FIGURE 32.11. Once venous blood is obtained, use the Seldinger technique to complete the procedure.

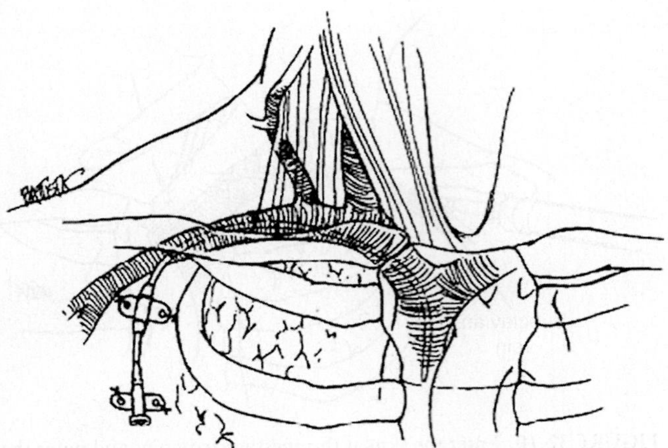

FIGURE 32.12. Secure the central line and flush all ports with sterile saline after aspirating back venous blood to eliminate trapped residual air bubbles.

too close to the clavicle. This makes it extremely difficult to pass the finder needle under the clavicle while maintaining the needle and syringe parallel to the coronal plane and the floor. As the angle of entry between the patient's chest and the syringe increase in an effort to get under the clavicle, the chances of producing a pneumothorax also increase proportionally. A distance more than 2 cm from the edge of the clavicle may be necessary in larger patients.

9. **Therefore, at all times maintain the needle and syringe parallel to the coronal plane and floor. Have an assistant pull the arm caudad at the initiation of venipuncture.**
10. Attach a fresh 10-mL syringe to the large needle.
11. Enter the skin at the anesthetized point and point the needle tip toward the suprasternal notch.
12. While maintaining constant suction on the syringe and a parallel line to the coronal plane and the floor, gently advance the needle tip cephalad until it hits the clavicle.
13. Withdraw the needle and syringe back 2 cm from the clavicle prior to making an effort to pass under the leading edge.
14. Not withdrawing the needle 2 to 4 cm is a common mistake and makes the maneuvering of the needle tip around the convex leading edge of the clavicle difficult.
15. The left hand acts as the guide for the finder needle.
16. The index finger rests on the suprasternal notch and provides the direction toward which the tip of the finder needle is directed.
17. The thumb on the left hand is used to push the finder needle posteriorly to help maneuver the tip of the needle under the clavicle.
18. If the blood from the finder needle is pulsatile, remove the needle and hold pressure for a full 10 minutes prior to proceeding. Consider ultrasound-guided placement if not already being utilized.
19. Once venous blood is obtained, use the Seldinger technique to complete the procedure.
20. Verify that all ports allow aspiration of venous blood and can be flushed with saline without resistance
21. Secure the catheter, cover with a nonocclusive sterile dressing, and document the procedure appropriately in the chart.
22. Obtain a stat chest radiograph to verify the position and exclude pneumothorax or other injuries.
23. Check the distance of the catheter inserted from skin entry site (Table 32.1).

Supraclavicular Technique (Fig. 32.13)

Follow these steps:

1. Verify that the patient does not have allergies to chlorhexidine, povidone iodine, or lidocaine.
2. Complete all five steps described in the "Sterile Preparation of Operator and Skin" section with the following modifications.
3. Place the patient in a Trendelenburg position, at least 15 degrees head down to distend the subclavian veins and to reduce the risk of air embolism.
4. Obtain a "maximum sterile barrier," which includes the placement of a sterile cap, mask, gown, and gloves.
5. Cleanse the skin and drape the area with the large drape provided in the kit.
6. Use local anesthetic (1% lidocaine provided in the kit) and the smallest needle available to anesthetize the puncture site at the junction of the sternocleidomastoid and the clavicular head.
7. Attach a fresh 10-mL syringe to the large needle.
8. Enter the skin at the anesthetized point along the upper border of the medial one third of the clavicle at the junction of the sternocleidomastoid muscle and the clavicular head.
9. The syringe is depressed 15 degrees below the coronal plane and the needle is directed at an angle 45 degrees to the sagittal plane.
10. The vein is met at an average depth of 1 to 1.5 cm from the skin.

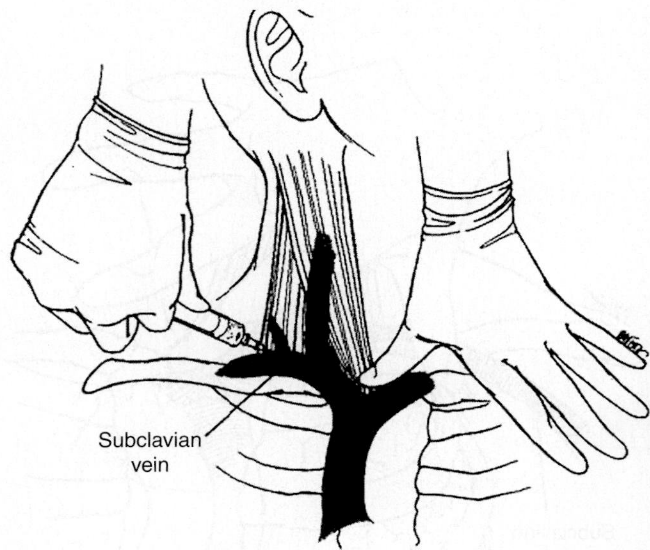

FIGURE 32.13. Enter the skin at the anesthetized point along the upper border of the medial one third of the clavicle at the junction of the sternocleidomastoid muscle and the clavicular head. The syringe is depressed 15 degrees below the coronal plane and the needle is directed at an angle 45 degrees to the sagittal plane. The vein is met at an average depth of 1 to 1.5 cm from the skin.

11. Once venous blood is obtained, use the Seldinger technique to complete the procedure.
12. Verify that all ports allow aspiration of venous blood and can be flushed with saline without resistance
13. Secure the catheter, cover with a nonocclusive sterile dressing, and document the procedure appropriately in the chart.
14. Obtain a stat chest radiograph to verify the position and exclude pneumothorax or other injuries.

Steps to Prevent Complications

1. Do not force the wire through the finder needle; resistance of any type is an indication to stop, remove the needle and guidewire, and hold pressure on the vein.
2. One hand should be on the guidewire at all times during the procedure to avoid losing the wire into the subclavian vein.
3. Avoid overzealous dilation of the subclavian vein with the dilator. Excessive dilation extending beyond the subcutaneous tissue and fat into the vein increases the risk of post-procedure complications (oozing, hematoma formation, arteriovenous fistula formation, and pseudoaneurysm formation).
4. Verify that the guidewire moves easily back and forth through the dilator as the dilator is advanced toward the vein to avoid puncturing through the back wall of the vein due to bending of the wire at the dilator tip.
5. Inadvertent arterial puncture and subsequent hematoma or pseudoaneurysm formation can be prevented by providing direct pressure manually or with a standard device for at least 30 minutes.
6. If the patient is intubated and on high PEEP settings, holding the inspiratory effort for a few seconds while cannulating the subclavian vein may decrease the overinflation of the lung apex and decrease the chances of obtaining a pneumothorax. (This should only be performed if no deleterious effects occur toward the patient's oxygenation, ventilation, alveolar recruitment, or overall status.)

ULTRASOUND-GUIDED VEIN CANNULATION

Review of Literature

Over 5 million CVCs are placed each year in the United States, with an associated overall complication rate of 10% to 15% (38,39). The traditional method of using surface anatomic landmarks for the placement of CVCs is fraught with complication risks, especially in patients with obesity, neck deformity or rigidity, previous surgery at the cannulation site, IJ vein thrombosis, hypovolemia, coagulopathy, or the inability to lie flat. There may also be variation in the normal anatomy of the IJ vein. Using ultrasound, Denys and Uretsky found that 8.5% of 200 patients had abnormal IJ vein anatomy with a small fixed IJ vein in 3%, no right IJ vein at all in 2.5%, an IJ vein medial to the carotid in 2%, and an IJ vein lateral to the carotid with no overlap in 1% (40). These common anatomic variants may explain the complication rate and need for multiple attempts to achieve success using the landmark technique alone. Mechanical complications, such as arterial puncture and pneumothorax, have been reported to occur in up to 12% of landmark-guided placements, and the risk increases sixfold after three needle passes (41). This risk can be reduced significantly with the use of ultrasound (US) guidance. The first description of audio-guided Doppler localization and cannulation of IJ vein was provided by Legler and Nugent in 1984 (42).

There are two types of real-time US guidance described in the literature for facilitating CVC placement:

1. Audio-guided Doppler US, which generates an audible sound from flowing venous blood, which helps the operator localize the vein and differentiate it from its companion artery
2. Two-dimensional (2-D) imaging US guidance, which is the more commonly used method, and provides real-time gray-scale imaging of the anatomy

Two-dimensional imaging involves the use of a 7.5-MHz linear array transducer to visualize the relevant anatomy and can be performed by two techniques. In the first technique, the US is used to mark the location of the vein relative to anatomic surface landmarks followed by sterile percutaneous cannulation. The second technique involves one or two operators and involves continuous real-time imaging of the great vessels during cannulation. This provides the operator with the advantage of continuous visualization of the desired vein and the surrounding anatomic structures before and during the insertion. The second technique requires the operators to have a "maximum sterile barrier" with sterile cap, mask, gown, and gloves; a sterile sheath to cover the ultrasound probe; gel to maintain acoustic coupling; and an assistant to place the probe into the sterile sheath.

There have been seven randomized trials comparing real-time 2-D US guidance to the landmark technique for IJ vein cannulation (40,43–48). These studies have found significant differences between the ultrasound and landmark techniques in the following parameters:

1. Higher success rate (100%) of cannulation of the IJ vein using US as compared to 76% to 95% using the landmark technique
2. Higher cannulation rate of the IJ vein on the first attempt using the US technique
3. Lower access time with the US technique (there is, however, a wide variation in the total access times from one study to the next due to inconsistent definitions of starting and stopping points while using the US technique)
4. Lower incidence of carotid artery puncture and hematoma complications with the US technique
5. Reduction in the number of passes necessary to achieve cannulation using the US technique as compared to the landmark technique

Cannulation failures in the landmark technique group were consistently salvaged with a single attempt using the US-guided cannulation technique.

A meta-analysis of eight randomized controlled trials comparing US-guided cannulation to the standard landmark technique was recently performed by Randolph et al. (30). Of the eight randomized studies, seven evaluated the IJ vein and one evaluated the subclavian vein (43,44,49–54). They concluded that the use of Doppler US or real-time 2-D US guidance for vessel location and CVC placement significantly improved success rates, decreased the complication rates, and decreased the need for multiple catheter placement attempts associated with IJ and subclavian vein cannulation.

On the basis of these data, the Agency for Healthcare Research and Quality listed the use of real-time ultrasound guidance for central venous catheterization as one of the 11 practices to improve patient care (55).

The National Institute for Health and Clinical Excellence (NICE) is located in the United Kingdom and provides the National Health Service (a publicly funded health care system of the United Kingdom) with guidelines based on the literature regarding the use of new technologies and procedures to improve health care treatment. They have also independently reviewed the literature and published guidelines, available on the Internet, that strongly recommend 2-D US imaging as the preferred method of insertion of CVCs into the IJ vein in adults and children in elective situations (56).

Recommendations

There is overwhelming evidence that all physicians involved in placing CVCs should complete appropriate training to achieve competence in the use of real-time 2-D US for venous cannulation. Furthermore, all elective IJ vein CVC placements should be performed under the guidance of real-time 2-D US. The newer portable ultrasound machines provide the additional advantage of being easily transported and available in the operating room, intensive care unit, and emergency department, as well as at the bedside on the hospital ward.

PULMONARY ARTERY CATHETER

Indications

1. Diagnosis of shock states
2. Management of fluid resuscitation and inotropic support in shock states
3. Management of severe burns
4. Monitoring and management of complicated acute myocardial infarction
5. Diagnosis of primary pulmonary hypertension
6. Diagnosis of valvular disease, intracardiac shunts, cardiac tamponade, and pulmonary embolus
7. Therapeutic: Aspiration of air emboli

Contraindications

1. Tricuspid or pulmonary valve mechanical prosthesis
2. Right heart mass (thrombus and/or tumor)
3. Tricuspid or pulmonary valve endocarditis

Technique

Follow these steps:

1. First, place a central venous introducer following the steps outlined above.
2. Verify placement of the introducer with a chest radiograph. Some operators will obtain a chest radiograph at the end of procedure when the pulmonary artery catheter (PAC) is in position unless a complication during venous cannulation is suspected.
3. Cleanse the skin and introducer thoroughly with chlorhexidine, after verifying patient's allergies.
4. Obtain a "maximum sterile barrier," which includes the placement of a sterile cap, mask, gown, and gloves.
5. Have your assistant open the PAC kit in a sterile fashion, being careful not to contaminate any of the contents.
6. Remove the PAC from the kit and have your assistant hook up the ports to the transducer and make sure that the readings are accurate as the catheter is being manipulated.
7. Take great care in maintaining sterile technique at all times while working closely with the nonsterile assistant. Protect the sterile portion of the catheter by resting it on the large sterile field while the transducers are attached.
8. Have the assistant check the proximal and distal ports for patency by flushing them with sterile saline. Also have the assistant check the patency of the balloon using the syringe provided in the kit.
9. On the surface of the catheter are line markings, which indicate distance from the tip of the catheter in centimeters. Familiarize yourself with these markings prior to placing the catheter. Single thin lines are used to indicate a distance of 10 cm, while a single wide line indicates a distance of 50 cm from the tip. These lines are used in combination to indicate the distance from the tip (Fig. 32.14).
10. Therefore, as the catheter is inserted you will see one thin line at 10 cm, two thin lines at 20 cm, three thin lines at 30 cm, four thin lines at 40 cm, and a single wide thick line at 50 cm. At 60 cm there is a wide thick line and a single thin line in combination. The wedge position is achieved in most patients 45 to 55 cm from the tip.
11. Place the sterile plastic sleeve over the catheter after flushing all ports to further protect the catheter in a sterile cover during manipulation (Fig. 32.15).
12. The distal end of the PAC is then inserted into the central venous introducer hub, and is threaded down the central vein into the superior vena cava.
13. The PAC must be placed at least 30 cm (three thin lines) into the introducer in order for the balloon to clear the distal end of the introducer sheath prior to inflation.

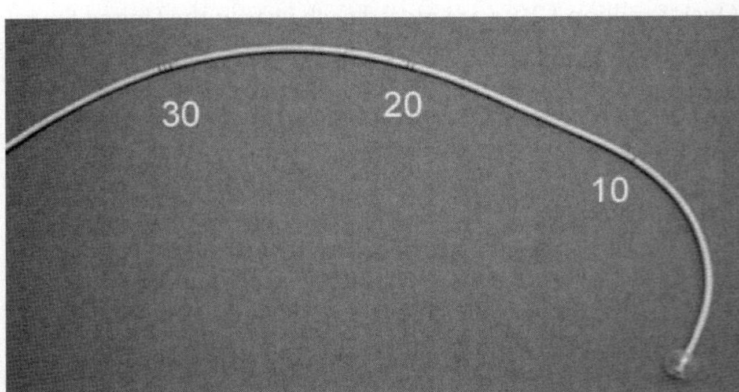

FIGURE 32.14. Each thin black line mark indicates 10-cm distance from the tip of the catheter.

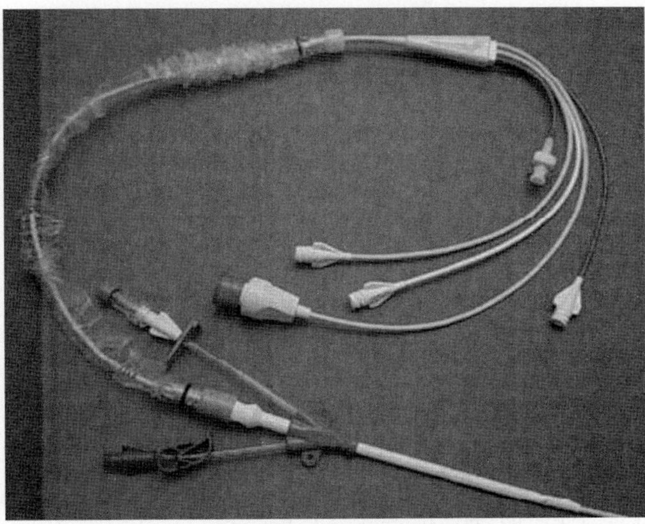

FIGURE 32.15. Place the plastic sleeve cover over the catheter to maintain sterility during placement and to help secure and lock its final position onto the introducer.

14. Once at 30 cm in the central vein, the balloon is inflated and the catheter is advanced through the right atrium, past the tricuspid valve into the right ventricle, quickly through the right ventricle (to minimize occurrence of arrhythmias), and past the pulmonary valve into the pulmonary artery. The waveforms and pressure readings on the monitor provide the information on the position of the catheter in the vasculature (Fig. 32.16).
15. Once in the pulmonary artery, the catheter should be carefully advanced until it wedges. At this point the balloon can be deflated, and pulmonary artery tracings should reappear. If the balloon wedges before maximal reinflation, then the catheter is "overwedged" and should be pulled back slightly until it wedges only with maximal inflation (this helps prevent pulmonary artery rupture).
16. General guidelines for the distance necessary to travel to reach the various structures of the heart are as follows:

    The right atrium: 20 to 25 cm
    The right ventricle: 30 to 35 cm
    The pulmonary artery: 40 to 45 cm
    The catheter usually wedges at 50 to 55 cm

17. Once the PAC is in the correct position, the balloon should be deflated and the catheter secured in place by locking the plastic sleeve tip onto the hub of the introducer.
18. Correct catheter placement is confirmed with a chest radiograph.

WARNING: AT NO POINT SHOULD THE PAC EVER BE WITHDRAWN WHILE THE BALLOON IS INFLATED! Always verify that the assistant has deflated the balloon prior to withdrawing the PAC. Only advance forward with the balloon inflated and never withdraw. This avoids the complication of rupture of the pulmonary artery, which can lead to massive life-threatening hemorrhage and death.

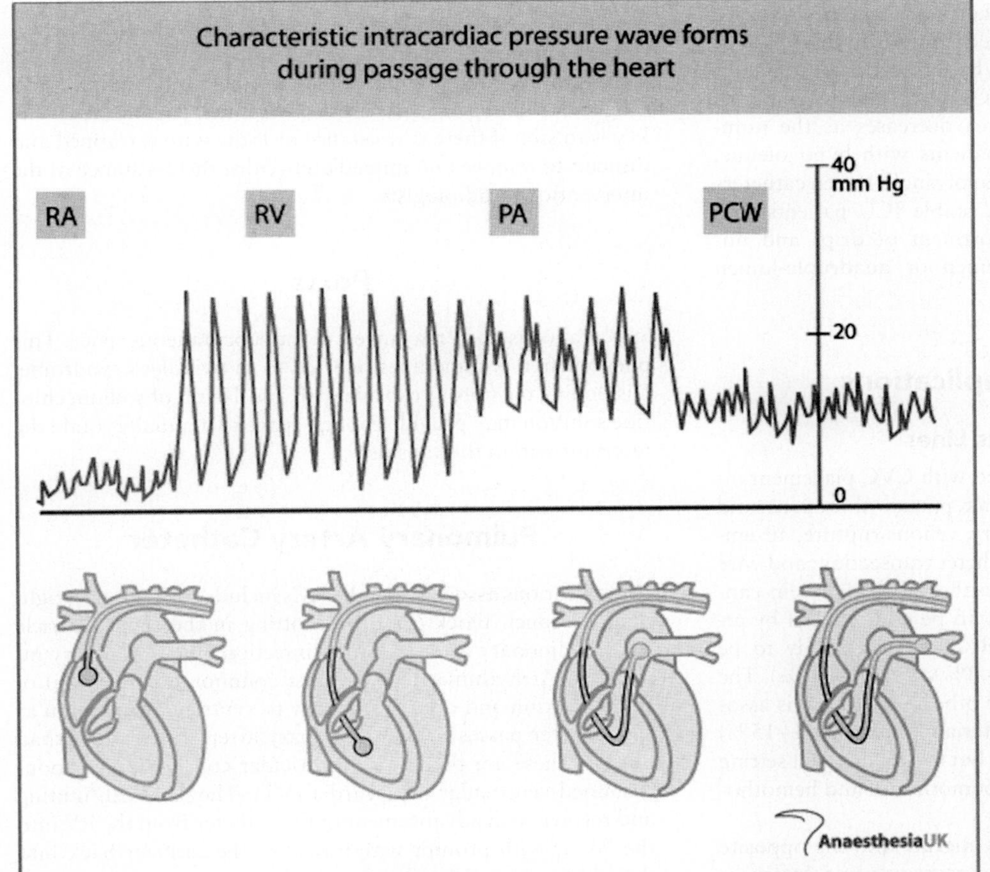

FIGURE 32.16. Use the waveforms to guide the placement of the pulmonary artery catheter from the right atrium, through the right ventricle, to the pulmonary artery, and finally into the wedge position. RA = right atrium, RV = right ventricle, PA = pulmonary artery, PCW = pulmonary capillary wedge.

Complications

The complication rate in patients with CVCs is as follows:

1. Overall complication rate of 15% (57–59)
2. Mechanical complication rate of 5% to 19% (57,58,60)
3. Infectious complication rate of 5% to 26% (14,57,59)
4. Thrombotic complication rate of 2% to 26% (57)

ANTIMICROBIAL-IMPREGNATED CATHETERS

The use of catheters impregnated with chlorhexidine and silver sulfadiazine as well as those impregnated with minocycline and rifampin have been shown in randomized trials to lower the rate of catheter-related bloodstream infections (14,61). The randomized trial by Maki et al. demonstrated that the use of chlorhexidine- and silver sulfadiazine–impregnated catheters significantly lowered bloodstream infections from 7.6 infections per 1,000 catheters to 1.6 infections per 1,000 catheters (61). Therefore, the use of antimicrobial-impregnated catheters should be considered in all circumstances, especially when the institution rate of catheter-related bloodstream infections is higher than 2% (61).

SINGLE-LUMEN AND MULTILUMEN CATHETERS

The number of lumens in the catheter has not been shown to affect the rate of catheter-related complications (62–64). Therefore, catheter choice should be based on the patient's needs and the indications for the CVC placement. Since the radius of the catheter of the lumen decreases as the number of ports increase, in trauma patients with hypovolemic, hemorrhagic shock, large dual-lumen or single-lumen catheters are preferred. On the other hand, stable ICU patients that require multiple ports for an assortment of drips and nutrition may benefit from triple-lumen or quadruple-lumen catheters.

Mechanical Complications

Central Venous Lines

Mechanical complications associated with CVC placement include cardiac tamponade, hemothorax, pneumothorax, carotid artery injury, subclavian artery injury, venous rupture, air embolism, catheter malpositioning, catheter transection, and wire or catheter embolism. Compared to the subclavian vein cannulation, the IJ route is more likely to be complicated by arterial puncture (3%–4% vs. 6%–9%) and less likely to be complicated by pneumothorax (1%–3% vs. 0.1%–0.2%). The femoral route, in comparison to the other two routes, is associated with a much higher rate of arterial puncture (9%–15%) and hematoma formation (3%–5%) but in the emergent setting offers the advantage of avoiding pneumothorax and hemothorax (57,58,60,65–67).

The tip of an intact catheter can migrate into the opposite brachiocephalic vein, jugular vein, or azygous veins. Interventional radiology can play an important role in repositioning misplaced catheters. If a catheter was placed without imaging guidance, it may be placed into an artery. Appropriate consultation of the vascular or cardiothoracic service should be obtained prior to removing misplaced catheters from the subclavian artery and especially the carotid artery. Malposition of the catheter tip into the lumbar venous plexus resulting in paraplegia has also been described as a rare complication of CVC placement.

Perforation of the great vessels occurs less than 1% of the time but carries nearly a 40% mortality rate. More commonly seen with the right subclavian vein approach, it usually is the result of guidewire kinking during advancement of the dilator (68).

Pinch-off syndrome has been described with the subclavian route when the catheter is crushed between a narrow path between the clavicle and the first rib. The catheter can become occluded, and with repeated trauma, it can fracture and embolize distally. The fragment can become lodged in the heart, resulting in cardiac arrhythmias or perforation, or it can be embolized further into the pulmonary artery. If recognized early, the interventional radiologist can usually capture the catheter fragments and successfully remove them. If the fragments remain unrecognized, thrombus formation and fibrosis around the catheter can result in catheter attachment to the vessel wall.

Guidewires used for venous access can become trapped in indwelling vena cava filters or electrodes from pacemakers and other implantable devices. Fluoroscopy often demonstrates that the J-wire has become trapped around the tip of an IVC filter.

Pulling back on the wire in the hope of dislodging it can have catastrophic results, with migration of the filter, tears in the IVC, hemorrhage, and death.

Several techniques are available to the interventional radiologist to remove broken wires or wires trapped in filters. The key is to **stop** if there is resistance or if the wire is trapped and difficult to remove and immediately enlist the assistance of the interventional radiologists.

Ports

Subcutaneous ports may invert in the subcutaneous space. This phenomenon is sometimes referred to as twiddler's syndrome. Distending the fibrous capsule with 5 to 10 mL of sodium chloride solution may provide enough space to manually rotate the reservoir within the capsule.

Pulmonary Artery Catheter

Complications associated with PACs include arrhythmias, right bundle branch block (RBBB), knotting in the right ventricle (RV), pulmonary artery rupture, infection, and pulmonary infarction. Arrhythmias are the most common complication of PAC insertion and occur secondary to ventricular irritation as the catheter passes to the pulmonary artery (PA). More than 80% of these are premature ventricular contractions or nonsustained ventricular tachycardia (VT). They are self-limiting and resolve with advancement of the catheter from the RV into the PA or with prompt withdrawal of the catheter back into the right atrium. Significant arrhythmias requiring treatment occur in less than 1% of patients, usually those with concurrent cardiac ischemia.

RBBB occurs in 5% of PAC insertions and usually is transient after positioning the catheter into the PA. The presence of a pre-existing left bundle branch block (LBBB) puts the patient at risk for complete heart block should RBBB occur. In these patients, temporary pacing equipment should be kept nearby on standby.

The incidence of knotting of the PAC on itself, on intracardiac structures, or on pacing wires is less than 1%. This risk is increased in patients with dilated cardiac chambers. A persistent RV tracing despite advancement of the PAC further than 20 cm into the patient should alert the physician to this possibility.

Pulmonary artery rupture is the most catastrophic complication of PAC insertion. Although it occurs in less than 1% of cases, it carries a mortality rate of 50%. Age over 60 years, anticoagulation therapy, and the presence of pulmonary hypertension increase the risk of rupture. The presence of sudden and large quantities of hemoptysis, especially immediately after PAC balloon inflation, greatly indicates this possibility. Management includes lateral decubitus positioning (bleeding side down), intubation with a double-lumen endotracheal tube (ET), and increasing PEEP. Embolization via bronchoscopy or angiography or lobectomy may be necessary if bleeding continues or is massive.

PAC-related infection is a fairly common complication. The incidence of positive catheter tip culture result is 45% in some series. Fortunately, the risk for clinical sepsis is less than 0.5% per day of catheter use.

The incidence of pulmonary infarction is less than 7%. Unintentional distal migration of the PAC tip is the usual cause. Some evidence indicates that catheter-related thrombi also may be a significant cause. While postmortem studies have shown that the rate of endocardial lesions (e.g., thrombi, hemorrhage, vegetations) related to PAC use is significant, correlation with clinical events has not been established.

Peripherally Inserted Central Catheter

Ignoring resistance during the placement of a CVC can lead to significant complications. This was illustrated best in a recent case report where surgical removal of a nonfunctional peripherally inserted central catheter (PICC) revealed an extensive extraluminal knot. Review of the placement procedure revealed multiple attempts at advancing and withdrawing the PICC against resistance. Aggressive approaches to the removal of difficult PICC lines may result in damage to the vein, or catheter fracture with subsequent embolization (69).

Air Embolism

Air embolism may also occur as a rare complication during CVC placement. It is more common in conditions that diminish the central venous pressure, such as decreased intravascular volume and upright sitting position. Rapid introduction of air into the venous circulation of greater than 300 to 400 mL at a rate of 100 mL/second is considered to be fatal. Clinically, the patient will have immediate hypoxemia and/or cardiovascular collapse. The hypoxemia is a result of V/Q mismatch (ventilation without perfusion) due to mechanical obstruction of vessels by the air bubbles. The air further has a chemical activation of the pulmonary endothelium resulting in activation of complement, free radicals, and inflammatory mediators, which results in bronchoconstriction and/or noncardiogenic pulmonary edema. The physical exam reveals the wheezing and crackles of heart failure. The classic finding of "mill wheel murmur," a churning sound heard throughout the entire cardiac cycle from air bubbles in the RV, is a relatively specific sign of air embolism, but is insensitive and occurs late in the course. Management includes securing the airway and placing the patient in the left lateral decubitus position with right side up, making it more difficult for the air to enter the right ventricular outflow tract (pulmonary artery) because it is in a dependent position. The best intervention is prevention; placing the patient in 15 degrees of Trendelenburg position prior to placing the CVC increases the central venous pressure and decreases the chance for air embolism to occur.

Infectious Complications

The subclavian vein cannulation is associated with a significantly lower rate of total infectious complications when compared to the femoral venous cannulation route (57,70). Although there are no randomized trials comparing the subclavian and IJ routes, there is evidence suggesting that subclavian catheterization is less likely to result in catheter-related infection (14,71,72).

Thrombotic Complications

Catheter-related venous thrombosis, diagnosed with US, occurs in approximately 15% of patients in the medical intensive care units (73). The risk of catheter-related thrombosis is directly proportional to the site of insertion; it occurred in 22% of patients with femoral venous catheters, and only 2% of patients with subclavian venous catheters (57). In a nonrandomized observational study the IJ vein was associated with four times the risk of thrombosis as compared to the subclavian vein (74). Therefore, subclavian vein cannulation carries the lowest risk of catheter-related thrombosis.

Maximal Sterile Barrier

We strongly recommend the use of all components of the maximal sterile barrier with ***each*** central line placement, which includes mask, cap, sterile gown, sterile gloves, and a large sterile drape. This strict practice has been shown to reduce the rate of catheter-related bloodstream infections and save an estimated $167 per catheter insertion (14). Chlorhexidine-based solutions are preferred for skin preparation over the povidone iodine solutions since the former have been shown to reduce the risk of catheter colonization in a number of studies (75,76).

PHYSICIAN EXPERIENCE

Increased complication rates have been associated with inexperienced physicians and with multiple failed attempts of

CVC insertion. Physicians who have performed more than 50 CVC insertions are *half* as likely to have a mechanical complication as those who have performed less than 50 (58). Furthermore, the incidence of mechanical complications after *three* or more insertion attempts is *six* times the rate after one attempt (60).

ULTRASOUND GUIDANCE

As summarized in the section on US guidance, there is clear evidence indicating that during IJ cannulation US guidance should be *routinely* used, since it significantly reduces the number of mechanical complications, the number of catheter placement failures, the number of attempts needed for insertion, and the time required for insertion (40,43–49). However, its use during subclavian vein cannulation has had mixed results in clinical trials and cannot be as strongly recommended, but should be considered in difficult cases where the landmark technique has failed (49,77,78).

OINTMENTS AND DRESSINGS

Antibiotic ointments (bacitracin, neomycin, and polymyxin) should not be used since they increase the rate of catheter colonization by fungi, promote the emergence of antibiotic-resistant bacteria, and do not lower the rate of catheter-related bacteremia (79–82). Similarly, silver-impregnated subcutaneous cuffs should not be used since they have not been shown to reduce the incidence of catheter-related bacteremia (79,83,84).

SCHEDULED CATHETER CHANGES

The risk of catheter-related bacteremia increases after the fifth to seventh day after insertion (14,61,85). Multiple trials have failed to demonstrate a decrease in catheter-related bacteremia with strategies for scheduled guidewire exchanges and scheduled replacement at a new site. In fact, scheduled exchanges over a guidewire have been associated with a trend toward an increased rate of catheter-related infections, and scheduled new site replacement has been associated with higher mechanical complications during insertion (86–88). Therefore, catheter exchange should not be performed on a scheduled basis at new sites or over the wire; rather, it should be based on the clinical status of the patient, the presence or absence of fever, and the appearance of the insertion site on the skin.

ALTERNATIVE ACCESS ROUTES

External Jugular Vein

The external jugular vein (EJV) may be used as an alternative route to gain central venous access. Although its superficial location makes it a preferred route in the presence of substantial coagulopathy, its valves and anatomic angles limit the ability to cannulate the superior vena cava to only 50% of the time. The EJV begins just anterior to the ear at the angle of the mandible. It courses obliquely across the anterior surface of the sternocleidomastoid muscle and joins the subclavian vein (SV) behind the medial third of the clavicle.

For cannulation, place the patient in a 15- to 30-degree modified Trendelenburg position with the head turned away from the site of venipuncture. The right side is preferred. The EJV is identified as it crosses the posterior margin of the sternocleidomastoid muscle. If the vein is not visible or palpable, a Valsalva maneuver or inflation hold applied to mechanically ventilated patients may help to distend the vein. If it cannot be visualized or palpated, another approach is preferred.

After introduction of local analgesia, a needle is advanced at an angle approximately 15 to 20 degrees above the skin. While slight negative pressure is maintained in the syringe lumen, the vein is sought. Once it is entered, advance the needle an additional 1 to 2 mm and then advance either the catheter or a guidewire through the needle, according to the selected technique.

If obstruction to guidewire passage is encountered, several maneuvers can be tried, including medial and lateral flexion of the neck as well as sequential or concomitant ipsilateral arm movements (abduction, adduction, and internal and external rotation). Another maneuver that is occasionally helpful is withdrawal of the J-wire for approximately 1 cm, followed by rotation and advancement of the wire.

Complications with significant morbidity are rare from this approach. Most complications are associated with catheter placement and catheter maintenance.

LONG-TERM ACCESS

Tunneled Catheters

Since the risk of catheter-related bacteremia increases after the fifth to seventh day after insertion of routine central lines, patients who require long-term venous access for chemotherapy or antibiotic treatment need more durable options (14,61,85). Tunneled catheters, such as the Hickman, Broviac, and Groshong, are composed of medical-grade silicone tubing, and are placed in a similar fashion to routine central lines except that a portion of the catheter is "tunneled" under the subcuticular tissue of the anterior chest wall or neck prior to exiting the skin. This technique was first described by Broviac et al. in 1973 and subsequently modified by Hickman et al. in 1979 (88,89). These catheters may be used for 6 to 12 months after placement if they are cared for diligently by the patient. The tunneled portion contains a fibrous cuff that induces an inflammatory reaction with the subcuticular tissue resulting in tissue ingrowth and attachment. The cuff-tissue ingrowth secures the catheter in place long term. Placement is routinely performed in the operating room or interventional radiology suite under fluoroscopic guidance since *exact* positioning of the catheter tip at the superior vena cava–right atrial junction is critical in preventing postoperative complications and in ensuring proper long-term functioning. Removal of infected catheters can be performed at the patient's bedside with local anesthetic and requires freeing the cuff from its fibrous subcuticular attachments either via the exit site or through a separate incision over the cuffed portion.

Ports

An alternative choice for long-term venous access is the completely implanted Port-a-Cath. The term "Port-a-Cath" is derived from the fusion of "portal" and "catheter." The "portal" is the reservoir compartment that has a silicone bubble cover for needle insertion (the septum) and is surgically inserted into a pocket created under the skin in the upper chest and appears as a bump under the epidermis. It is attached to the tunneled "catheter" that is placed under fluoroscopic guidance using routine technique for central line placement. The great advantage offered with the device is that it requires no special maintenance and is completely internal, so swimming and bathing are not a problem. The septum of the "portal" is made of a special self-sealing silicone rubber that can be punctured through the skin up to 1,000 times before it needs to be replaced. To administer treatment or to withdraw blood, the silicone cover of the portal is palpated under the skin of the anterior chest, sterilized, and then punctured with a special Huber point needle. Since the breach of skin integrity is very small and never larger than the caliber of the needle, there is a very low infection risk. This is another advantage over tunneled catheters such as the Hickman. However, unlike tunneled catheters that can be removed at the bedside, infected ports usually require the operating room setting for extraction of the device from the subcuticular pocket.

Peripherally Inserted Central Catheter Line

A PICC line provides long-term (1–6 months) intravenous access for chemotherapy regimens, extended antibiotic therapy, or total parenteral nutrition. First described in 1975, it is an alternative route of central access through a peripheral vein (brachial, basilic, or cephalic) with little risk of pneumothorax, air embolization, and cardiac arrhythmias (90). PICC lines are usually inserted under the guidance of fluoroscopy, US, or radiographs by radiologists or certified registered nurses. In a recent trial with over 200 pediatric patients undergoing US-guided PICC line placement, a 98% success rate and a 5% complication rate were reported (91). Complications may include phlebitis, hemorrhage, thrombosis, infection, and breakage/leakage. When compared to central lines, PICCs are associated with higher rates of phlebitis and more difficult insertion attempts (92,93). The rate of complications significantly increases as the number of PICC line days exceeds 30. More than 70% of complications occur after 30 days of placement (94). The infection rate for PICC lines is similar to conventionally placed CVCs; however, they have the added disadvantages of being more vulnerable to thrombosis and dislodgement and less useful for drawing blood specimens (95–98). Another concern is over usage that potentially exhausts upper extremity venous access sites. This may have serious implications in chronically ill patients, especially those with renal failure who may eventually require arteriovenous fistulas for dialysis access. Complication rates (infection, sepsis, and thrombosis requiring removal) as high as 40% to 50% have been reported with the use of PICC lines in chemotherapy patients (99). Based on the above evidence, we recommend strong caution against the routine use of PICC lines.

PERIPHERAL ARTERIAL CANNULATION

Introduction

Continuous blood pressure monitoring is essential for the management of critically ill patients. Significant differences may occur between arterial pressures measured by direct versus indirect invasive methods (100,101).

The indications for peripheral arterial cannulation include:

1. Continuous blood pressure (BP) monitoring in postoperative and critically ill patients
2. Hypotension or hypertension requiring continuous infusion
3. Mechanically ventilated patients that require repeated blood gases

Use caution in the following circumstances:

1. Extremities with burns or trauma
2. Extremities with carpal tunnel syndrome
3. Broken or infected skin
4. Coagulopathy
5. Raynaud disease

Also, locations near AV fistulas and insertion into synthetic grafts should be avoided.

The most frequently used site for direct arterial cannulation and BP measurement is the radial artery (102–108). Use of the femoral artery, axillary artery, dorsalis pedis artery, and temporal artery has also been described (109–112). Utilization of the brachial artery is not recommended due to poor collateral circulation and secondary ischemia to the radial and ulnar artery in the setting of obstruction, due to the potential for loss of the hand (113).

With regard to radial artery cannulation, the value of the Allen test in predicting potential ischemic damage after cannulation is at best unreliable. The original test described in 1929 was for the purpose of evaluating palmar collateral circulation in thromboangiitis obliterans (114). In critically ill patients the test has poor predictive power. Situations (such as shock, jaundice, or vasoconstriction) commonly found in the critically ill patient can significantly confound the test. A normal or negative test result does not rule out the possibility of digital ischemia after insertion of a radial arterial catheter. Furthermore, arterial catheterization has been performed in patients with a positive test result without ischemic consequences (115–117). Therefore, we do not advocate routine use of the visual modified Allen test. If an abnormality of the collateral circulation in an extremity is suspected, a Doppler Allen test or Doppler evaluation of the palmar arch, ulnar artery, or posterior dorsalis pedis can be performed before cannulation. The operator should document the impression of collateral circulation in the procedure note.

INSERTION TECHNIQUES

General Approach

Use an 18-gauge or 20-gauge Angiocath for cannulation of the artery. First palpate the artery at two points 2 cm apart. Using an 18-gauge needle, make a small superficial break through the skin over the artery. This penetrates the tough skin barrier and prevents shearing and damage of the tip of the Angiocath during subsequent arterial penetration. The Angiocath cannula is advanced through the puncture site along the course of the artery at a 30- to 45-degree angle to the skin. Once the anterior wall of the artery is penetrated, the needle is withdrawn and the plastic cannula is gently advanced into the arterial vessel at a lower angle (15–30 degrees) to facilitate smooth passage. The Angiocath may pass though the anterior and posterior walls of the artery. In this case, after removing the inner needle, gently withdraw the plastic cannula until pulsatile blood flows freely from the open end. Then advance the plastic cannula at a lower angle into the arterial lumen. The use of a guidewire and the Seldinger technique may be employed to assist with the threading of the cannula into the artery after penetration. Never try to thread the guidewire against even slight resistance.

If complications occur, such as distal ischemia, local infection, inability to withdraw blood effectively, or poor waveform, the arterial catheters should be changed to another site. Before removal, pressure should be applied proximally and distally to the insertion site. Attaching a syringe to the catheter and applying suction during extraction (for removal of developed clots) decreases the incidence of arterial thrombotic occlusion. After catheter removal, fingertip pressure should be applied for 10 minutes or as long as necessary to achieve hemostasis and prevent hematoma or aneurysm formation.

Specific Consideration: Radial Artery

The radial artery is one of the best cannulation sites due to its accessibility and the safety of extensive collateralization. The nondominant hand of the patient should be cannulated first. Placing a small rolled towel under the wrist and securing it with tape onto a backboard in a hyperextended position (about 20 degrees) diminishes the arterial tortuosity and dramatically increases the cannulation success rate. The artery should be cannulated 1 to 2 cm proximal to the wrist flexion point where there is a lower risk for digital ischemia because of better collateral circulation.

Specific Consideration: Femoral Artery

See the section above for identification and cannulation techniques for the femoral vein. The artery can be easily palpated in most patients. It should be punctured below the inguinal ligament to prevent intra-abdominal injury and retroperitoneal hematomas. The artery is usually reached 3 to 5 cm from the skin. The modified Seldinger technique is usually required for femoral cannulation. Consider using a Doppler US to guide cannulation in high-risk patients who are anticoagulated or obese.

Specific Consideration: Axillary Artery

The axillary artery should be cannulated as high as possible in the axilla, close to the thoracic apex, because of a rich anastomotic network surrounding the artery in this region (112). The axillary artery is fraught with a number of complications. Care must be taken with needle punctures high in the apex of the thoracic cavity to avoid pneumothorax or hemothorax. Thromboembolism can also occur from the axillary artery down to the radial or ulnar artery. Hematoma from a puncture leak of the artery can fill the axillary sheath around the neurovascular bundle and compress the brachial plexus, resulting in nerve damage and peripheral neuropathy. Since the risk of cerebral air embolism from accidental air injection into the axillary artery is higher with right-sided catheterization, placement should be performed preferentially on the left side first.

Specific Consideration: Dorsalis Pedis Artery

This small artery is congenitally absent in 3% to 12% of the population and is often difficult or impossible to cannulate. Furthermore, blood pressure measured in the dorsalis pedis artery may differ significantly from that measured in more central arteries, especially in the presence of vasopressor infusion (110,111).

Specific Consideration: Temporal Artery

Rich collateral circulation and easy accessibility makes the temporal artery an attractive site for cannulation. Tortuosity and its location, however, make cannulation and maintenance extremely difficult.

Complications

The most common complications include local ischemia, infection, hematoma, bleeding, thrombosis, distal embolism, ischemic necrosis, arteriovenous fistula formation, air embolism, and neuropathy (118–122). Of these, ischemic necrosis and thrombosis are two of the most concerning complications occurring 1% to 2.5% of the time (123,124). The incidence of local infection at the catheter insertion site is reported to be as high as 10% to 15%, while the incidence rate of catheter-related sepsis is 0.2% to 5% (121,125).

References

1. Duffy BJ. The clinical use of polyethylene tubing for intravenous therapy. *Ann Surg*. 1949;130:929–936.
2. Aubaniac RL. L'injection intraveninеuse sous-claviculaire; advantages et technique. *Presse Med*. 1952;60:1456.
3. Wilmore DW, Dudrick SJ. Safe long-term venous catheterization. *Arch Surg*. 1969;98:256–258.
4. Broviac JW, Cole JJ, Scribner BH. A silicone rubber atrial catheter for prolonged parenteral alimentation. *Surg Gynecol Obstet*. 1973;136(4):602–606.
5. Hoshal VL. Total intravenous nutrition with peripherally inserted silicone elastomer central venous catheters. *Arch Surg*. 1975;43:1937–1943.
6. Hickman RO, Buckner CD, Clift RA, et al. A modified right atrial catheter for access to the venous system in marrow transplant recipients. *Surg Gynecol Obstet*. 1979;148:871–875.
7. Niederhuber JE, Ensminger W, Gyves JW, et al. Totally implanted venous and arterial access system to replace external catheters in cancer treatment. *Surgery*. 1982;92:706–712.
8. Fisher NC, Mutimer DJ. Central venous cannulation in patients with liver disease and coagulopathy—a prospective audit. *Intensive Care Med*. 1999;25:481–485.

9. Merrer J, De Jonghe B, Golliot F, et al. Complications of femoral and subclavian venous catheterization in critically ill patients: a randomized controlled trial. *JAMA*. 2001;286:700–707.
10. Sznajder JI, Zveibil FR, Bitterman H, et al. Central vein catheterization: failure and complication rates by three percutaneous approaches. *Arch Intern Med*. 1986;146:259–261.
11. Veenstra DL, Saint S, Saha S, et al. Efficacy of antiseptic-impregnated central venous catheters in preventing catheter-related bloodstream infection: a meta-analysis. *JAMA*. 1999;281:261–267.
12. Fares LG II, Block PH, Feldman SD. Improved house staff results with subclavian cannulation. *Am Surg*. 1986;52:108–111.
13. Mansfield PF, Hohn DC, Fornage BD, et al. Complications and failures of subclavian-vein catheterization. *N Engl J Med*. 1994;331:1735–1738.
14. Raad I, Darouiche R, Dupuis J, et al. Central venous catheters coated with minocycline and rifampin for the prevention of catheter-related colonization and bloodstream infections: a randomized, double-blind trial. *Ann Intern Med*. 1997;127:267–274.
15. Parry G. Trendelenburg position, head elevation and a midline position optimize right IJ vein diameter. *Can J Anaesth*. 2004;51(4):379–381.
16. Schreiber SJ, Lambert UK, Doepp F, et al. Effects of prolonged head-down tilt on IJ vein cross-sectional area. *Br J Anaesth*. 2002;89(5):769–771.
17. Clenaghan S, McLaughlin RE, Martyn C, et al. Relationship between Trendelenburg tilt and IJ vein diameter. *Emerg Med J*. 2005;22(12):867–868.
18. Seldinger SI. Catheter replacement of the needle in percutaneous arteriography; a new technique. *Acta Radiol*. 1953;39:368–376.
19. Moncrief JA. Femoral catheters. *Ann Surg*. 1958;147:166–172.
20. Bansmer G, Keith D, Tesluk H. Complications following use of indwelling catheters of inferior vena cava. *JAMA*. 1958;1606–1611.
21. Shaldon S, Chiandussi L, Higgs B. Hemodialysis by percutaneous catheterization of the femoral artery an vein with regional heparinization. *Lancet*. 1961;II:857–859.
22. Polderman KH, Girbes AR. Central venous catheter use. Part I: mechanical complications. *Intensive Care Med*. 2002;28:1–17.
23. Smynrios NA. The jury on femoral vein catheterization is still out. *Crit Care Med*. 1997;25:1943–1946.
24. Swanson RS, Uhlig PN, Gross PL, et al. Emergency intravenous access through the femoral vein. *Ann Emerg Med*. 1984;13:244–247.
25. Armstrong PJ, Sutherland R, Scott DH. The effect of position and different manoeuvres on internal jugular vein diameter size. *Acta Anaesthesiol Scand*. 1994;38:229–231.
26. Gratz I, Afshar M, Kidwell P, et al. Doppler-guided cannulation of the internal jugular vein: a prospective, randomized trial. *J Clin Monit*. 1994;10(3): 185–188.
27. Gilbert TB, Seneff MG, Becker RB. Facilitation of internal jugular venous cannulation using an audio-guided Doppler ultrasound vascular access device: results from a prospective, dual-center, randomized, crossover clinical study. *Crit Care Med*. 1995;123:60–65.
28. Caridi JG, Hawkins IF Jr, Wiechmann BN, et al. Sonographic guidance when using the right internal jugular vein for central vein access. *Am J Roentgenol*. 1998;171(5):1259–1263.
29. Keenan SP. Use of ultrasound to place central lines. *J Crit Care*. 2002; 17(2):126–137.
30. Randolph AG, Cook DJ, Gonzales CA, et al. Ultrasound guidance for placement of central venous catheters: a meta-analysis of the literature. *Crit Care Med*. 1996;24(12):2053–2058.
31. Ho AM, Chung DC, Tay BA, et al. Diluted venous blood appears arterial: implications for central venous cannulation. *Anesth Analg*. 2000;91(6): 1356–1357.
32. Andrews RT, Bova DA, Venbrux AC. How much guidewire is too much? Direct measurement of the distance from subclavian and internal jugular vein access sites to the superior vena cava-atrial junction during central venous catheter placement. *Crit Care Med*. 2000;28(1):138–142.
33. Smith BE, Modell JH, Gaub M, et al. Complications of subclavian vein catheterization. *Arch Surg*. 1965;90:228–229.
34. Tan BK, Hong SW, Huang MH, et al. Anatomic basis of safe percutaneous subclavian venous catheterization. *J Trauma*. 2000;48(1):82–86.
35. Jesseph JM, Conces DJ, Augustyn GT. Patient positioning for subclavian vein catheterization. *Arch Surg*. 1987;122:1207–1209.
36. Land RE. Anatomic relationships of the right subclavian vein. *Arch Surg*. 1971;102:178–180.
37. Land RE. The relationship of the left subclavian vein to the clavicle: practical considerations pertinent to the percutaneous catheterization of the subclavian vein. *J Thorac Cardiovasc Surg*. 1972;63(4):564–568.
38. McGee DC, Gould MK. Preventing complications of central venous catheterization. *N Engl J Med*. 2003;348:1123–1133.
39. Mermel LA, Farr BM, Sherertz RJ, et al. Guidelines for the management of intravascular catheter-related infections. *Clin Infect Dis*. 2001;32:1249–1272.
40. Denys BG, Uretsky BF, Reddy PS. Ultrasound-assisted cannulation of the internal jugular vein: a prospective comparison to the external landmark-guided technique. *Circulation*. 1993;87:1557–1562.
41. Mansfield PF, Hohn DC, Fornage BD, et al. Complications and failures of subclavian-vein catheterization. *N Engl J Med*. 1994;331:1735–1738.
42. Legler D, Nugent M. Doppler localization of the internal jugular vein facilitates central venous cannulation. *Anesthesiology*. 1984;60:481–482.
43. Mallory DL, McGee WT, Shawker TH, et al. Ultrasound guidance improves the success rate of internal jugular vein cannulation: a prospective, randomized trial. *Chest*. 1990;98:157–160.
44. Troianos CA, Jobes DR, Ellison N. Ultrasound-guided cannulation of the internal jugular vein: a prospective, randomized study. *Anesth Analg*. 1991;72:823–826.
45. Slama M, Novara A, Safavian A, et al. Improvement of internal jugular vein cannulation using an ultrasound-guided technique. *Intensive Care Med*. 1997;23:916–919.
46. Teichgraber UK, Benter T, Gebel M, et al. A sonographically guided technique for central venous access. *AJR Am J Roentgenol*. 1997;169:731–733.
47. Nadig C, Leidig M, Schmiedeke T, et al. The use of ultrasound for the placement of dialysis catheters. *Nephrol Dial Transplant*. 1998;13:978–981.
48. Hayashi H, Amano M. Does ultrasound imaging before puncture facilitate internal jugular vein cannulation? Prospective randomized comparison with landmark-guided puncture in ventilated patients. *J Cardiothorac Vasc Anesth*. 2002;16:572–575.
49. Gilbert TB, Seneff MG, Becker RB. Facilitation of internal jugular venous cannulation using an audio-guided Doppler ultrasound vascular access device: results from a prospective, dual-center, randomized, crossover clinical study. *Crit Care Med*. 1995;23:60–65.
50. Branger B, Zabadani B, Vecina F, et al. Continuous guidance for venous punctures using a new pulsed Doppler probe: efficiency, safety. *Nephrologie*. 1994;15:137–140.
51. Scherhag A, Klein A, Jantzen JP. Cannulation of the internal jugular vein using 2 ultrasonic techniques: a comparative controlled study. *Anaesthesist*. 1989;38:633–638.
52. Vucevic M, Tehan B, Gamlin F, et al. The SMART needle. A new Doppler ultrasound-guided vascular access needle. *Anaesthesia*. 1994;49:889–891.
53. Gualtieri E, Deppe SA, Sipperly ME, et al. Subclavian venous catheterization: greater success rate for less experienced operators using ultrasound guidance. *Crit Care Med*. 1995;23:692–697.
54. Gratz I, Afshar M, Kidwell P, et al. Doppler-guided cannulation of the internal jugular vein: a prospective, randomized trial. *J Clin Monit*. 1994;10:185–188.
55. *Making Health Care Safer: A Critical Analysis of Patient Safety Practices*. Rockville, MD: Agency for Healthcare Research and Quality; 2001.
56. Calvert N, Hind D, McWilliams RG, et al. The effectiveness and cost-effectiveness of ultrasound locating devices for central venous access: a systematic review and economic evaluation. *Health Technol Assess*. 2003;7:1–84.
57. Merrer J, De Jonghe B, Golliot F, et al. Complications of femoral and subclavian venous catheterization in critically ill patients: a randomized controlled trial. *JAMA*. 2001;286:700–707.
58. Sznajder JI, Zveibil FR, Bitterman H, et al. Central vein catheterization: failure and complication rates by three percutaneous approaches. *Arch Intern Med*. 1986;146:259–261.
59. Veenstra DL, Saint S, Saha S, et al. Efficacy of antiseptic-impregnated central venous catheters in preventing catheter-related bloodstream infection: a meta-analysis. *JAMA*. 1999;281:261–267.
60. Mansfield PF, Hohn DC, Fornage BD, et al. Complications and failures of subclavian-vein catheterization. *N Engl J Med*. 1994;331:1735–1738.
61. Maki DG, Stolz SM, Wheeler S, et al. Prevention of central venous catheter-related bloodstream infection by use of an antiseptic-impregnated catheter: a randomized, controlled trial. *Ann Intern Med*. 1997;127:257–266.
62. Ma TY, Yoshinaka R, Banaag A, et al. Total parenteral nutrition via multilumen catheters does not increase the risk of catheter-related sepsis: a randomized, prospective study. *Clin Infect Dis*. 1998;27:500–503.
63. Farkas JC, Liu N, Bleriot JP, et al. Single- versus triple-lumen central catheter-related sepsis: a prospective randomized study in a critically ill population. *Am J Med*. 1992;93:277–282.
64. Clark-Christoff N, Watters VA, Sparks W, et al. Use of triple-lumen subclavian catheters for administration of total parenteral nutrition. *J Parenter Enteral Nutr*. 1992;16:403–407.
65. Martin C, Eon B, Auffray JP, et al. Axillary or internal jugular central venous catheterization. *Crit Care Med*. 1990;18:400–402.
66. Durbec O, Viviand X, Potie F, et al. A prospective evaluation of the use of femoral venous catheters in critically ill adults. *Crit Care Med*. 1997;25: 1986–1989.
67. Timsit JF, Bruneel F, Cheval C, et al. Use of tunneled femoral catheters to prevent catheter-related infection: a randomized, controlled trial. *Ann Intern Med*. 1999;130:729–735.
68. Robinson JF, Robinson WA, Cohn A, et al. *Arch Intern Med*. 1995;155: 1225–1228.
69. Marx M. The management of the difficult peripherally inserted central venous catheter line removal. *J Intraven Nurs*. 1995;18:246–249.
70. Henrickson KJ, Axtell RA, Hoover SM, et al. Prevention of central venous catheter-related infections and thrombotic events in immunocompromised children by the use of vancomycin/ciprofloxacin/heparin flush solution: a randomized, multicenter, double-blind trial. *J Clin Oncol*. 2000;18:1269–1278.
71. Heard SO, Wagle M, Vijayakumar E, et al. Influence of triple-lumen central venous catheters coated with chlorhexidine and silver sulfadiazine on the

incidence of catheter-related bacteremia. *Arch Intern Med.* 1998;158:81–87.

72. McKinley S, Mackenzie A, Finfer S, et al. Incidence and predictors of central venous catheter related infection in intensive care patients. *Anaesth Intensive Care.* 1999;27:164–169.
73. Hirsch DR, Ingenito EP, Goldhaber SZ. Prevalence of deep venous thrombosis among patients in medical intensive care. *JAMA.* 1995;274:335–337.
74. Timsit JF, Farkas JC, Boyer JM, et al. Central vein catheter-related thrombosis in intensive care patients: incidence, risk factors, and relationship with catheter-related sepsis. *Chest.* 1998;114:207–213.
75. Maki DG, Ringer M, Alvarado CJ. Prospective randomised trial of povidone-iodine, alcohol, and chlorhexidine for prevention of infection associated with central venous and arterial catheters. *Lancet.* 1991;338:339–343.
76. Mimoz O, Pieroni L, Lawrence C, et al. Prospective, randomized trial of two antiseptic solutions for prevention of central venous or arterial catheter colonization and infection in intensive care unit patients. *Crit Care Med.* 1996;24:1818–1823.
77. Lefrant JY, Cuvillon P, Benezet JF, et al. Pulsed Doppler ultrasonography guidance for catheterization of the subclavian vein: a randomized study. *Anesthesiology.* 1998;88:1195–1201.
78. Bold RJ, Winchester DJ, Madary AR, et al. Prospective, randomized trial of Doppler-assisted subclavian vein catheterization. *Arch Surg.* 1998; 133:1089–1093.
79. Flowers RH III, Schwenzer KJ, Kopel RF, et al. Efficacy of an attachable subcutaneous cuff for the prevention of intravascular catheter-related infection: a randomized, controlled trial. *JAMA.* 1989;261:878–883.
80. Zakrzewska-Bode A, Muytjens HL, Liem KD, et al. Mupirocin resistance in coagulase-negative staphylococci, after topical prophylaxis for the reduction of colonization of central venous catheters. *J Hosp Infect.* 1995;31:189–193.
81. Maki DG, Band JD. A comparative study of polyantibiotic and iodophor ointments in prevention of vascular catheter-related infection. *Am J Med.* 1981;70:739–744.
82. Pearson ML. Guideline for prevention of intravascular device-related infections. *Infect Control Hosp Epidemiol.* 1996;17:438–473.
83. Maki DG, Cobb L, Garman JK, et al. An attachable silver-impregnated cuff for prevention of infection with central venous catheters: a prospective randomized multicenter trial. *Am J Med.* 1988;85:307–314.
84. Smith HO, DeVictoria CL, Garfinkel D, et al. A prospective randomized comparison of an attached silver-impregnated cuff to prevent central venous catheter-associated infection. *Gynecol Oncol.* 1995;58:92–100.
85. Collin GR. Decreasing catheter colonization through the use of an antiseptic-impregnated catheter: a continuous quality improvement project. *Chest.* 1999;115:1632–1640.
86. Cook D, Randolph A, Kernerman P, et al. Central venous catheter replacement strategies: a systematic review of the literature. *Crit Care Med.* 1997; 25:1417–1424.
87. Cobb DK, High KP, Sawyer RG, et al. A controlled trial of scheduled replacement of central venous and pulmonary-artery catheters. *N Engl J Med.* 1992;327:1062–1068.
88. Broviac JW, Cole JJ, Scribner BH. A silicone rubber atrial catheter for prolonged parenteral administration. *Surg Gynecol Obstet.* 1973;136:602–606.
89. Hickman RO, Buckner CD, Clift RA, et al. A modified right atrial catheter for access to the venous system in marrow transplant recipients. *Surg Gynecol Obstet.* 1979;148:871–875.
90. Hoshal VL. Total intravenous nutrition with peripherally inserted silicone elastomer central venous catheters. *Arch Surg.* 1975;43:1937–1943.
91. Donaldson JS, Morello FP, Junewick JJ, et al. Peripherally inserted central venous catheters: US-guided vascular access in pediatric patients. *Radiology.* 1995;197(2):542–544.
92. Smith JR, Friedell ML, Cheatham ML, et al. Peripherally inserted central catheters revisited. *Am J Surg.* 1998;176:208–211.
93. Cowl CT, Weinstock JV, Al-Jurf A, et al. Complications and cost associated with parenteral nutrition delivered to hospitalized patients through either subclavian or peripherally inserted central catheters. *Clin Nutr.* 2000;19:237–243.
94. Matsuzaki A, Suminoe A, Koga Y, et al. Long-term use of peripherally inserted central venous catheters for cancer chemotherapy in children. *Support Care Cancer.* 2006;14(2):153–160.
95. Safdar N, Maki DG. Risk of catheter-related bloodstream infection with peripherally inserted central venous catheters used in hospitalized patients. *Chest.* 2005;128(2):489–495.
96. Allen AW, Megargell JL, Brown DB, et al. Venous thrombosis associated with the placement of peripherally inserted central catheters. *J Vasc Interv Radiol.* 2000;11:1309–1314.
97. Grove JR, Pevec WC. Venous thrombosis related to peripherally inserted central catheters. *J Vasc Interv Radiol.* 2000;11:837–840.
98. Duerksen DR, Papineau N, Siemens J, et al. Peripherally inserted central catheters for parenteral nutrition: a comparison with centrally inserted catheters. *J Parenter Enteral Nutr.* 1999;23:85–89.
99. Cheong K, Perry D, Karapetis C, et al. High rate of complications associated with peripherally inserted central venous catheters in patients with solid tumors. *Internal Med J.* 2004;34(5):234–238.
100. Venus B, Mathru M, Smith RA, et al. Direct versus indirect blood pressure measurements in critically ill patients. *Heart Lung.* 1985;14:228.
101. Brunner JMR, Krenis LJ, Kunsman JM. Comparison of direct and indirect methods of measuring arterial blood pressure. *Med Instrum.* 1981;15:11.
102. Slogoff S, Keats A, Arlund C. On the safety of radial artery cannulation. *Anesthesiology.* 1983;59:42–47.
103. Mandel M, Dauchot P. Radial artery cannulation in 1000 patients: precautions and complications. *J Hand Surg.* 1977;2:482–485.
104. Clarke W, Freund PR, Wasse L. Assessment of adequacy of ulnar arterial flow prior to radial artery catheterization. *Anesthesiology.* 1982;55:A38.
105. Wilkins RG. Radial artery cannulation and ischaemic damage: a review. *Anaesthesia.* 1985;40:896.
106. Jones RM, Hill AB, Nahrwold ML, et al. The effect of method of radial artery cannulation on postcannulation blood flow and thrombus formation. *Anesthesiology.* 1981;55:76.
107. Kondo K. Percutaneous radial artery cannulation using a pressure-curve-directed technique. *Anesthesiology.* 1984;61:639.
108. Stirt TA. "Liquid stylet" for percutaneous radial artery cannulation. *Can Anaesth Soc J* 1982;29:492.
109. Abou-Madi M, Lenis S, Archer D, et al. Comparison of direct blood pressure measurements at the radial and dorsalis pedis arteries. *Anesthesiology.* 1986;65:692–695.
110. Husum B, Eriksen T. Percutaneous cannulation of the dorsalis pedis artery. *Br J Anaesth.* 1979;51:1055.
111. Youngberg J, Miller E. Evaluation of percutaneous cannulations of the dorsalis pedis artery. *Anesthesiology.* 1976;44:80.
112. Bryan-Brown CW, Kwun KB, Lumb PD, et al. The axillary artery catheter. *Heart Lung.* 1983;12:492.
113. Barnes RW, Foster EJ, Janssen GA, et al. Safety of brachial arterial catheters as monitors in the intensive care unit: prospective evaluation with the Doppler ultrasonic velocity detector. *Anesthesiology.* 1976;44:260.
114. Allen EV. Thromboangiitis obliterans: methods of diagnosis of chronic occlusive arterial lesions distal to the wrist with illustrative cases. *Am J Med.* 1929;178:237–244.
115. Ejrup B, Fischer B, Wright, IS. Clinical evaluation of blood flow to the hand: the false-positive Allen test. *Circulation.* 1966;33:778–782.
116. Kamienski RW, Barnes RW. Critique of the Allen test for continuity of the palmar arch assessed by Doppler ultrasound. *Surg Gynecol Obstet.* 1976;142:861.
117. Slogoff S, Keats AS, Arlund C. On the safety of radial artery cannulation. *Anesthesiology.* 1983;59:42–47.
118. Puri VK, Carlson RW, Bander JJ, et al. Complications of vascular catheterization in the critically ill. *Crit Care Med.* 1980;8:495.
119. Gardner RM, Schwartz R, Wong HC, et al. Percutaneous indwelling radial-artery catheters for monitoring cardiovascular function. *N Engl J Med.* 1974;290:1227.
120. Bedford RF. Radial artery function following percutaneous cannulation with 18 and 20 gauge catheters. *Anesthesiology.* 1977;47:37.
121. Weinstein RA, Stamm WE, Kramer L. Pressure monitoring devices: overlooked sources of nosocomial infection. *JAMA.* 1976;236:936.
122. Shinozaki T, Deane R, Mazuzan JE, et al. Bacterial combination of arterial lines: a prospective study. *JAMA.* 1983;249:223.
123. Weiss BM, Gattiker RI. Complications during and following radial artery cannulation: a prospective study. *Intensive Care Med.* 1986;12:424.
124. Sladen A. Complications of invasive hemodynamic monitoring in the intensive care unit. *Curr Probl Surg.* 1988;17:69.
125. Band JD, Maki DG. Infections caused by arterial catheters used for pressure monitoring. *Am J Med.* 1970;67:735.

CHAPTER 33 ■ TEMPORARY CARDIAC PACEMAKERS

JAMIE B. CONTI • GREGORY W. WOO

Temporary pacing is an essential tool in the critical care setting for providing emergent cardiac pacing. This chapter will discuss (a) indications for temporary pacing, (b) types of temporary pacemakers available, (c) techniques for placement, (d) basic troubleshooting, and (e) potential complications.

INDICATIONS

The most common indication for temporary pacing is hemodynamically unstable bradycardia. Bradycardia may be the result of primary degenerative conduction system disease or secondary causes such as medications, metabolic abnormalities, or acute myocardial infarction (AMI) (1). Medications that may cause bradycardia include antiarrhythmic drugs and β- or calcium channel blockers, in particular diltiazem or verapamil. Hyperkalemia and other electrolyte disturbances can not only cause bradycardia, but also may contribute to high pacing thresholds. Therefore, secondary causes of bradycardia must be corrected for pacing to be successful. Table 33.1 lists some indications for temporary cardiac pacing.

Not all bradycardia in the setting of AMI requires temporary pacing (Tables 33.2A and B). For example, an atrioventricular (AV) block that occurs during an inferior wall MI from a right coronary artery occlusion may be secondary to ischemia of the region supplied by the AV nodal artery. In this setting, AV block rarely progresses to high-degree AV block, typically resolves within 2 weeks, and probably will not require temporary pacing. On the other hand, AV block in the setting of an anterior wall MI carries a worse prognosis. Anterior wall MIs can be more extensive, and AV block seen in this situation is usually from infarct involvement of the interventricular septum and infranodal conduction system. AV block from an anterior wall MI may rapidly deteriorate to asystole. Temporary pacing in the setting of an anterior wall MI and complete heart block (CHB) is strongly suggested.

Other indications for temporary pacemakers are considered prophylactic. There are some procedures performed in the cardiac catheterization or electrophysiology lab in which temporary pacing is strongly considered. These patients should be evaluated carefully preoperatively, and pacing initiated as necessary. For example, a patient undergoing alcohol septal ablation has a high risk of developing acute CHB. The incidence of acute CHB has been reported to be as high as 55% to 70%, but a much smaller percentage requires permanent cardiac pacing—11% to 17% (2,3). Other examples include percutaneous coronary rotational atherectomy (Rotoblation), rheolytic thrombectomy (AngioJet), or a generator replacement in a patient who is pacemaker dependent.

Temporary pacing is also commonly used after cardiac surgery. The incidence of hemodynamically unstable bradycardia after cardiac surgery has been reported to be as high as 4% (4). Specifically, AV block is not uncommon after valvular heart surgery and is likely a result of either direct injury to the surrounding conduction system or edema. Sinus bradycardia occurs in 64% of postcardiac transplant patients (5). Though this bradycardia often resolves, temporary pacing may be required to maintain adequate heart rates for optimal cardiac output in the immediate posttransplant recovery period. In addition, temporary atrial pacing may reduce the incidence of postoperative atrial fibrillation, which is quite common after cardiac surgery (6).

Temporary pacemakers may also be used for other reasons besides bradycardia and heart block. Pause or bradycardia-dependent polymorphic ventricular tachycardia, such as that occurring in the long QT syndrome, can be treated with temporary pacing, which will shorten the QT interval. Overdrive or rapid ventricular pacing may also prevent ventricular tachycardias triggered by premature ventricular contractions. In addition, some ventricular tachycardias may be terminated by ventricular pacing. Likewise, certain atrial tachycardias, such as atrial flutter, can be terminated with rapid atrial pacing.

TEMPORARY PACING CATHETERS

Deciding on Atrial, Ventricular, or Dual-chamber Pacing

Although most intensive care unit (ICU) pacing needs can be met with single-chamber, right ventricular pacing, there are some clinical situations in which dual-chamber pacing is necessary. Some patients rely on AV synchrony and atrial contraction to maintain optimal physiologic cardiac contraction for adequate cardiac output. Such patients include those with congestive heart failure, significant diastolic dysfunction, and right ventricular infarction with AV block. Dual-chamber pacing is most readily available in postcardiac surgical patients, as temporary epicardial wires are routinely placed at the time of surgery. However, if not available, insertion of two separate pacing catheters or a specialized dual-chamber pacing catheter will be necessary. Single-chamber atrial pacing can also be used in many of the aforementioned situations, as long as the only conduction system abnormality is from sinus node dysfunction and not AV block. Also, single-chamber atrial pacing may be preferred if the patient has a mechanical

TABLE 33.1

INDICATIONS FOR TEMPORARY CARDIAC PACING

BRADYARRHYTHMIAS
Asystole
Any symptomatic or hemodynamically unstable bradycardia
Second-degree Mobitz type II or third-degree heart block
Other conduction abnormalities at high risk for progression to complete heart block such as alternating bundle branch block or new bifascicular block

TACHYARRHYTHMIAS
Bradycardia or pause-dependent polymorphic ventricular tachycardia
Ventricular tachycardia that is treatable with overdrive pacing
Atrial tachycardias or atrial flutters that are treatable with overdrive pacing

PREVENTATIVE
Patient undergoing right heart catheterization with a left bundle branch block
Cardiac interventions with high risk of bradyarrhythmia such as rheolytic thrombectomy (AngioJet), rotational atherectomy (Rotoblation), or alcohol septal ablation
Pacemaker generator change in a patient who is pacemaker dependent

TABLE 33.2A

STANDARD AMERICAN COLLEGE OF CARDIOLOGY/AMERICAN HEART ASSOCIATION CLASSIFICATION FOR RECOMMENDATIONS AND INDICATIONS

Class I	Conditions for which there is evidence and/or general agreement that a given procedure or treatment is beneficial, useful, and effective
Class II	Conditions for which there is conflicting evidence and/or a divergence of opinion about the usefulness/efficacy of a procedure or treatment.
Class IIa	Weight of evidence/opinion is in favor of usefulness/efficacy.
Class IIb	Usefulness/efficacy is less well established by evidence/opinion.
Class III	Conditions for which there is evidence and/or general agreement that a procedure/treatment is not useful/effective and in some cases may be harmful

Gregoratos G, et al. ACC/AHA/NASPE 2002 guideline update for implantation of cardiac pacemakers and antiarrhythmia devices-summary article: a report of the American College of Cadiology/American Heart Association Task Force on Practice Guidelines (ACC/AHA/NASPE Committee to Update the 1998 Pacemaker Guidelines). *J Am Coll Cardiol.* 2002;40:1703–1719.

TABLE 33.2B

INDICATIONS FOR PACING IN ACUTE MYOCARDIAL INFARCTION

Class I	Class IIb	Class III
Asystole	Persistent second- or third-degree atrioventricular (AV) block at the AV node level	Transient AV block in the absence of intraventricular conduction defects
Persistent second-degree AV block in the His-Purkinje system with bilateral bundle branch block or third-degree AV block within or below the His-Purkinje system after acute myocardial infarction		Transient AV block in the presence of isolated left anterior fascicular block
Transient advanced (second- or third-degree) infranodal AV block and associated bundle branch block. If the site of block is uncertain, an electrophysiologic study may be necessary.		Acquired left anterior fascicular block in the absence of AV block
Persistent and symptomatic second- or third-degree AV block		Persistent first-degree AV block in the presence of bundle branch block that is old or age indeterminate

Gregoratos G, et al. ACC/AHA/NASPE 2002 guideline update for implantation of cardiac pacemakers and antiarrhythmia devices-summary article: a report of the American College of Cadiology/American Heart Association Task Force on Practice Guidelines (ACC/AHA/NASPE Committee to Update the 1998 Pacemaker Guidelines). *J Am Coll Cardiol.* 2002;40:1703–1719.

TABLE 33.3

COMMON PACING MODES AVAILABLE FOR TEMPORARY PACING

Mode	Chamber paced	Chamber sensed	Synchronous or asynchronous	Advantages	Disadvantages
VVI	Ventricle	Ventricle	Synchronous	Technically simple	Nonphysiologic; may exacerbate CHF
AAI	Atrium	Atrium	Synchronous	Physiologic (AV node intact)	Technically more difficult; requires intact AV nodal conduction
DDD	Atrium and ventricle	Atrium and ventricle	Synchronous	Physiologic	Technically more difficult; may require two pacing catheters
VOO	Ventricle	n/a	Asynchronous	Same as VVI	Same as VVI
AOO	Atrium	n/a	Asynchronous	Same as AAI	Same as AAI
DOO	Atrium and ventricle	n/a	Asynchronous	Same as DDD	Same as DDD

CHF, congestive heart failure; AV, atrioventricular.

tricuspid valve to avoid catheter entrapment or tricuspid valve endocarditis to avoid dislodgement of the vegetation. Table 33.3 summarizes the available pacing modes for temporary pacing.

Ventricular

Most temporary transvenous pacing catheters are designed for placement in the right ventricle. These pacing catheters are constructed of a wire insulated with a polymer such as polyethylene or polyvinyl chloride, and are available in various sizes (Fig. 33.1A). Firmer materials add to the maneuverability of torque-controlled catheters, allowing for more control during placement and more stability once positioned. However, because of their relative stiffness, added caution must be taken during placement to avoid perforation of the great vessels or heart. In general, these catheters should be placed with fluoroscopic guidance. Balloon-tipped catheters are available to allow for flow-assisted placement, which is critical if fluoroscopy is not available (Fig. 33.1B). There are also specialized pulmonary artery catheters that have dedicated pacing ports for the placement of a pacing wire electrode while still allowing for routine hemodynamic monitoring (Fig. 33.2). However, inflation of the balloon to obtain pulmonary artery wedge pressure may cause the electrode to migrate and can result in loss of pacing capabilities.

Atrial

There are also multiple catheter designs for atrial pacing. Some pacing catheters are preformed to facilitate placement into the right atrial appendage or coronary sinus, thus allowing atrial pacing (Fig. 33.3). Other atrial pacing catheters use a delivery system consisting of a guiding catheter to position the pacing

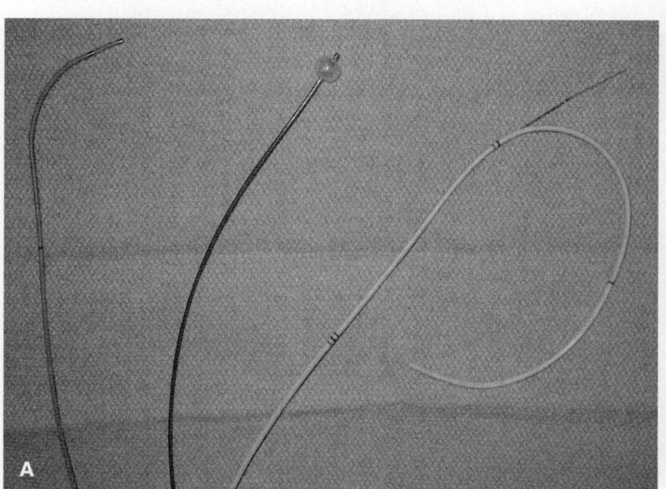

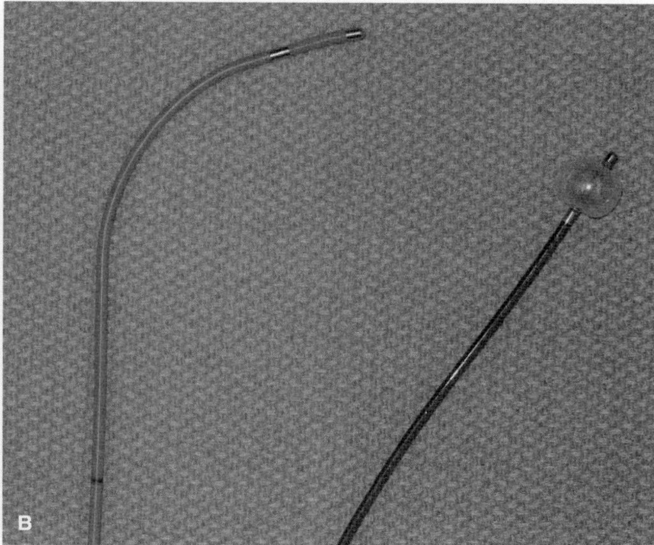

FIGURE 33.1. **A:** Transvenous pacing catheters. From left to right: 6F torque-guided bipolar pacing catheter, 5F balloon-tipped pacing catheter, and 7.5F pacing Swan-Ganz pulmonary artery catheter. **B:** Close-up view of the tips of the torque-guided and balloon-tipped pacing catheter.

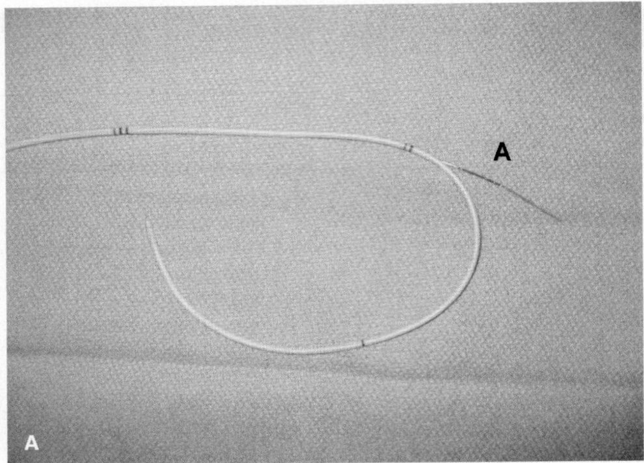

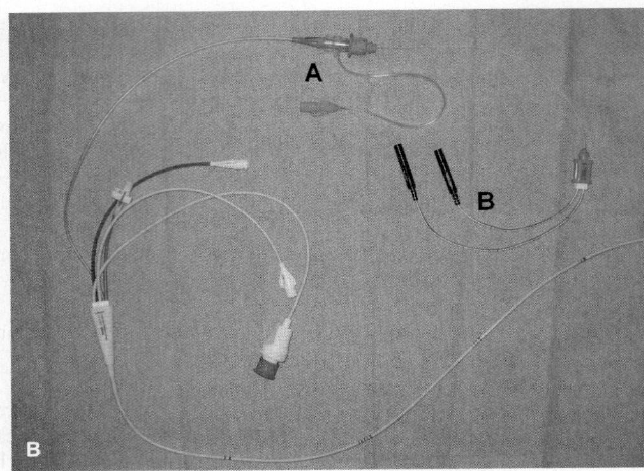

FIGURE 33.2. **A:** Swan-Ganz catheter with the pacing electrode extended out at the 20-cm mark (marked *A*). **B:** Pacing wire (marked *B*) inserted into a dedicated pacing port (marked *A*).

electrode catheter within the right atrium. A variety of new electrode catheters consist of several electrodes positioned 10 to 20 cm proximal to the distal-tip electrodes. These electrodes are positioned to lie along the lateral right atrial wall, allowing atrial sensing and pacing. An innovative modification of this technique allows for a small atrial J-wire to be placed through a dedicated lumen in the catheter into the right atrium, with distal electrodes already positioned in the right ventricular apex (Fig. 33.4). Both of these types of catheter adaptations have been developed to allow a "one venous stick" approach to AV pacing. However, the atrial electrodes provided by these catheters often do not reliably pace the atrium.

The vast majority of temporary pacing catheters are designed to lie against the ventricular myocardium once positioned (passive fix). However, newer catheter designs, especially those for right atrial pacing, have a deployable screw that is embedded in the myocardium (active fix) (Fig. 33.5). All leads placed in the heart carry a risk of migration and perforation (7), but active fix leads may reduce the risk of dislodgement (8).

Temporary pacing catheters can be bipolar or unipolar. Bipolar catheters have both the negative (anode) and positive (cathode) electrodes in contact with the heart (Fig. 33.6A). In a unipolar catheter, the anode is in contact with the heart, but the cathode is elsewhere on the body (Fig. 33.6B). Bipolar electrodes are preferred because they are less susceptible to external electrical interference.

EXTERNAL PACEMAKER UNIT

The external temporary pacemaker unit controls the pacing mode, stimulus output, stimulus frequency, and threshold for sensing intrinsic activity (Fig. 33.7). Pacing modes can be synchronous (demand/inhibited) or asynchronous to pace the atrium, ventricle, or both. The range of output varies from 0 to 20 mA. The frequency can be adjusted from 30 to 180 beats

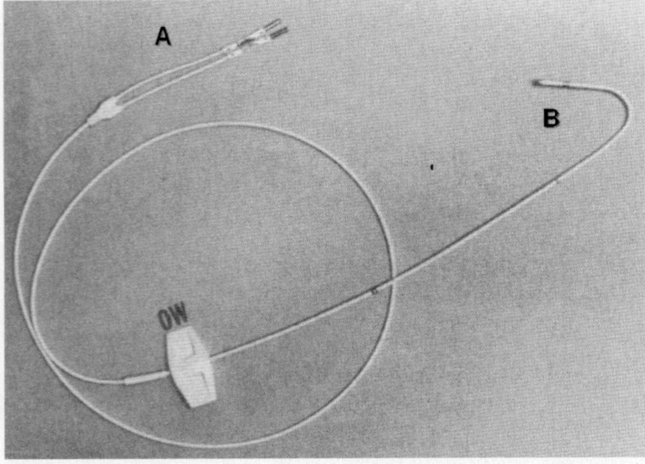

FIGURE 33.3. Atrial pacing catheter with a preformed "J" to facilitate placement in the right atrial appendage. *OW* marks the "orientation wing" to assist in the placement. *A* marks the proximal connectors that connect to the generator. *B* marks the distal preformed "J" tip.

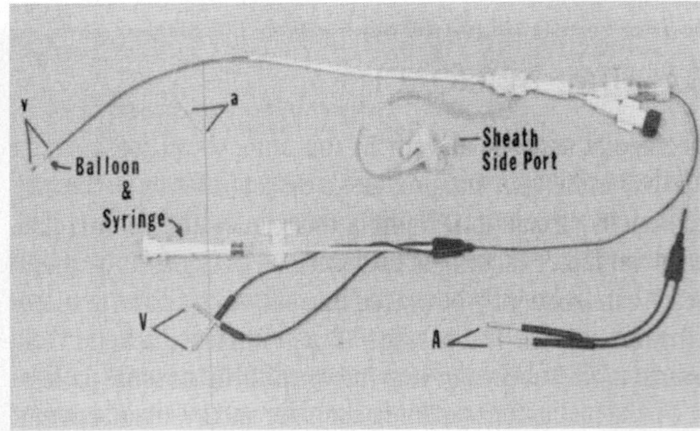

FIGURE 33.4. A balloon-tipped catheter designed for placement into the right ventricular apex. A small atrial "J" electrode (designated *a* on the picture) can be positioned through a lumen into the right atrium. *A* marks the connectors for pacing the atrium. *V* marks the connectors for pacing the ventricle, and *v* is the distal electrode that is positioned in the right ventricle.

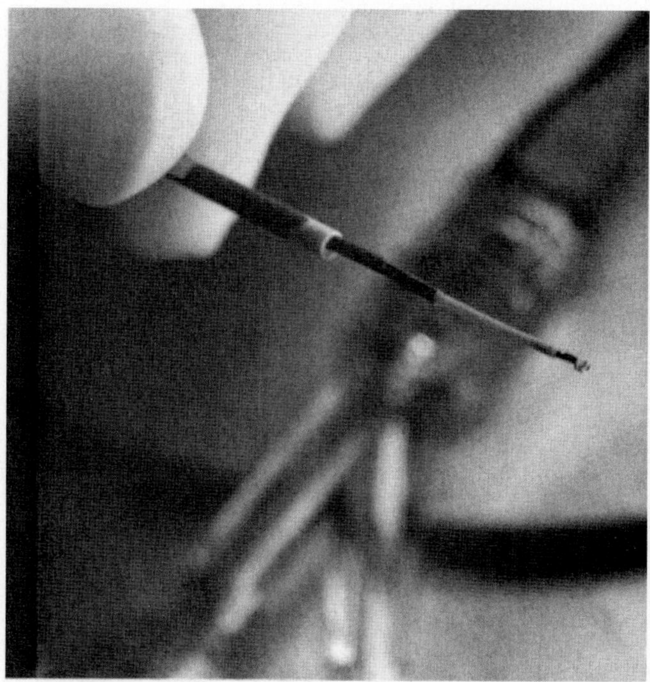

FIGURE 33.5. An example of an active fixation lead with a screw helix. (Compliments of Medtronic, Inc., Minneapolis, MN.)

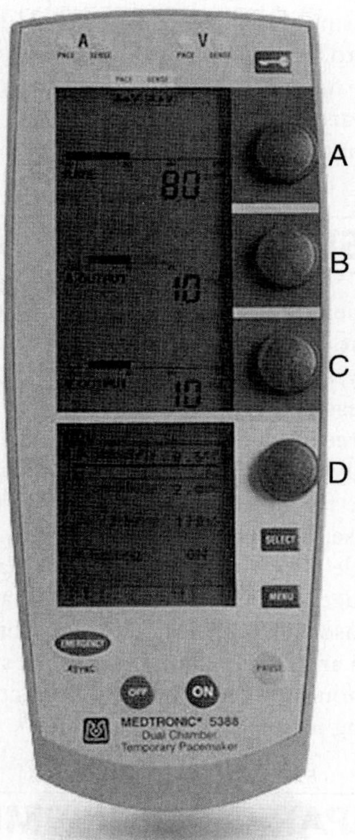

FIGURE 33.7. Temporary pacing unit. This unit has separate controls for atrial and ventricular programming. Controls *A*, *B*, and *C* adjust pacing rate, atrial pacing output, and ventricular pacing output, respectively. Control *D* selects pacing mode, atrioventricular (AV) interval, and sensitivities.

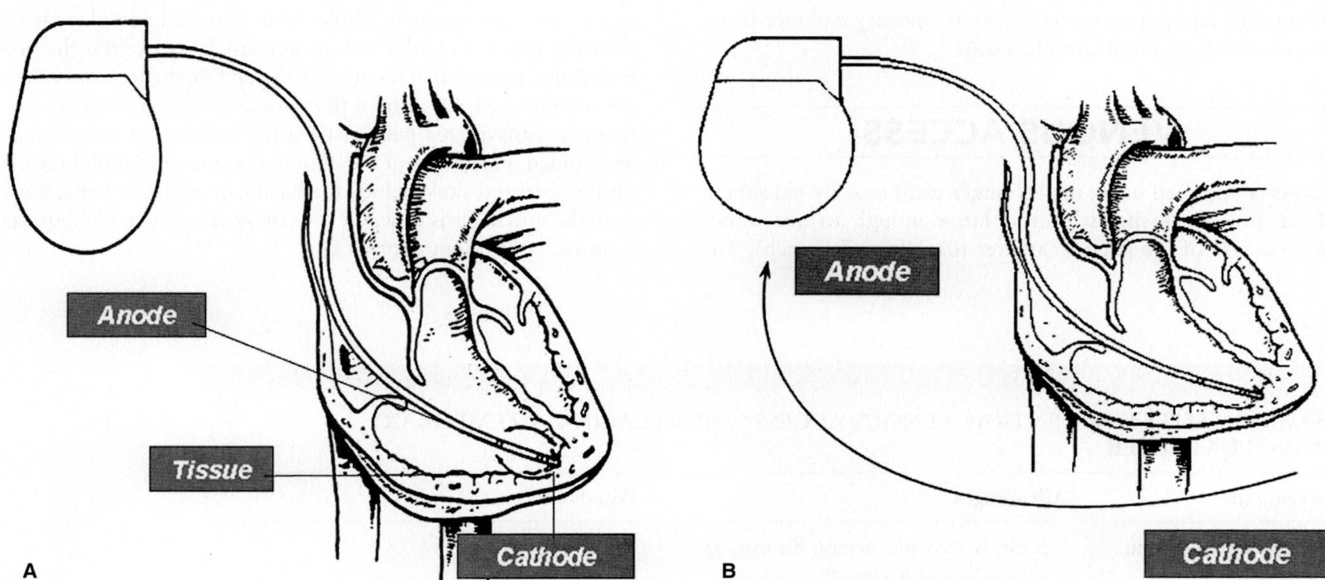

FIGURE 33.6. Diagrams representing bipolar and unipolar pacing configurations. **A:** In the bipolar configuration, both the positive (cathode) and negative (anode) electrodes are in contact with the myocardium. **B:** In the unipolar configuration, one electrode is in contact with the myocardium. The other electrode may be a patch on the skin, or in this example the generator.

per minute. Sensing threshold can be varied from no sensing (asynchronous) to less than 1.5 mV. The function of these units varies widely by manufacturer, making it imperative that staff and physicians are familiar with the routine function of the particular unit in their hospital.

ASSESSMENT OF THE PATIENT

A complete patient assessment must be made prior to pacemaker placement. Bradycardia alone is not sufficient. Hemodynamic instability, symptoms, or evidence of significant conduction system disease on the electrocardiogram (bundle branch block, high-degree heart block) favors therapy. Also, reversible causes, especially medications, should be sought. Glucagon may be effective for β-blocker overdose, calcium for calcium channel overdose, and digoxin immune Fab (Digibind®) for digitalis glycoside overdose. Some bradycardias can be treated medically with agents such as isoproterenol, a β_1-receptor agonist that increases heart rate. Electrolyte abnormalities such as hyperkalemia and other adverse metabolic states, such as severe acidosis, should be corrected, and in fact, if uncorrected, may make pacing ineffective.

PREPARING EQUIPMENT

All the necessary equipment should be available and inspected. The external pacing unit should be programmed to the desired settings and turned to the "On" position. A new battery should be installed. The lead should be examined for any defects. The connector cables should be inserted into the pacing generator to make sure that they are compatible (Fig. 33.8).

Continuous electrocardiographic monitoring and a defibrillator at the bedside are required. Fluoroscopy is preferred, but is not mandatory, if a balloon-tipped electrode catheter is being placed through the internal jugular or subclavian vein. Having the equipment ready before temporary catheter insertion is critical to avoid complications.

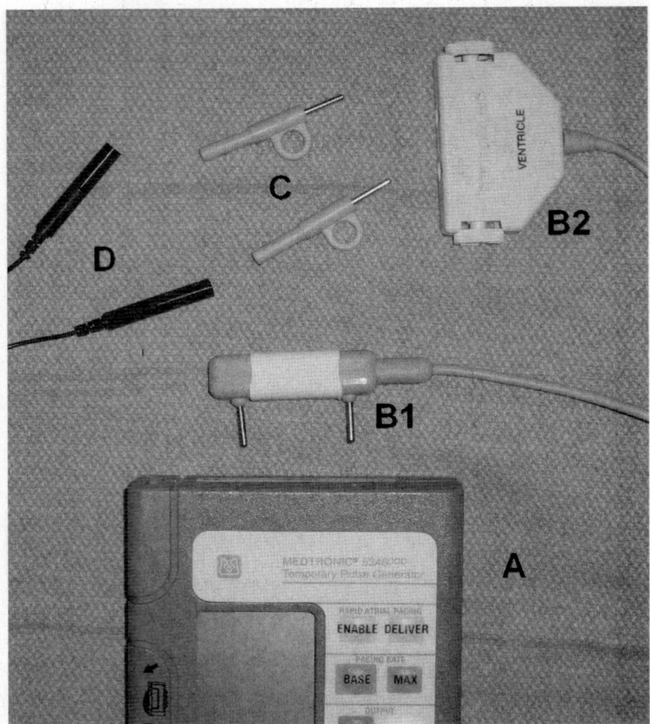

FIGURE 33.8. An example of a temporary pacing system setup. An inspection of the appropriate connectors, pins, and other accessories should be performed before placement. *A* is the generator unit. *B1* and *B2* are the proximal and distal ends of an extension adaptor. *C* shows connector pins. *D* shows the proximal connectors of the pacing catheter.

VENOUS ACCESS

Access is obtained using the Seldinger technique by placement of an introducer sheath that is large enough to accommodate the size of the pacing catheter (usually 4–7 French). The most common sites used are the internal jugular, subclavian, or femoral veins. The advantages and disadvantages of various access sites are given in Table 33.4. For bedside placement, the right internal jugular vein or left subclavian vein is the preferred site. In the cardiac catheterization lab, the femoral vein is commonly used. Of note, if the patient is likely to require permanent transvenous pacing, then the subclavian vein should be avoided on the side of the planned permanent implantation. Other potential sites include the basilic or cephalic veins; however, the downside is that access of these vessels usually requires a surgical cut-down approach.

TABLE 33.4

COMMON SITES FOR CENTRAL VENOUS ACCESS WHEN PLACING A TEMPORARY PACING CATHETER

Access site	Advantages	Disadvantages
Internal jugular vein	Relatively easy placement; fluoroscopy generally not necessary	Pneumothorax
Subclavian vein	Relatively easy placement; fluoroscopy generally not necessary	Pneumothorax; site commonly used for permanent pacing
Femoral vein	Relatively easy access	Leg immobilization; high risk of infection; fluoroscopy needed for placement

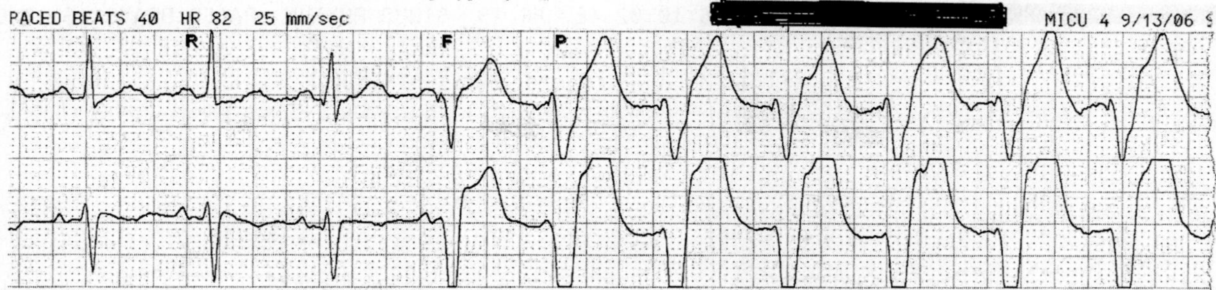

FIGURE 33.9. Evidence of ventricular capture during temporary pacing catheter placement. *R* denotes intrinsic ventricular conduction. *F* is a fusion beat. *P* is a paced ventricular beat.

PLACEMENT OF THE TRANSVENOUS PACING CATHETER

Once the sheath is in place, the pacing catheter is advanced through the sheath into the venous system. The lead is attached to the connector cables, which have been inserted into the pacing unit. The lead is gradually advanced under continuous electrocardiographic monitoring, with care not to use excessive force, as this may lead to perforation. If performed under fluoroscopic guidance, an inferior or septal position in the distal third of the apex is preferred. Apical right ventricular capture is noted by a left bundle branch, superior axis pattern. Once ventricular capture is obtained, threshold testing is performed. If no fluoroscopy is available, a balloon-tipped catheter must be used. Placement into the right ventricle is confirmed by ventricular capture on the electrocardiogram (ECG) with a left bundle branch block, superior axis pattern (Fig. 33.9). Once in place, the balloon is deflated to avoid advancement into the pulmonary artery.

Placement of a temporary atrial pacemaker should be performed by clinicians who implant permanent pacemakers, as the implant techniques are similar. Fluoroscopy is essential for this procedure.

Dual-chamber temporary pacing most commonly occurs after cardiac surgery when the patient has epicardial wires that were placed at the time of the surgery. Rarely is temporary endocardial dual-chamber pacing necessary. An example would be a patient with complete heart block and congestive heart failure who requires the hemodynamic benefit of atrioventricular synchrony and atrial contraction. In such a rare situation, separate catheters are placed, or if single access is preferred, a specialized dual-chamber pacing catheter is appropriate (Fig. 33.4).

PACE SENSING AND THRESHOLD DETERMINANTS

After obtaining good anatomic positioning of the pacing catheter, a stimulation threshold should be determined. With continuous electrocardiographic monitoring, pacing should begin at a rate at least 10 beats per minute faster than the patient's intrinsic heart rate, with the output set at 5 mA. The output of the pacemaker is gradually decreased until the stimuli fail to produce ventricular (or atrial) capture (Fig. 33.10). The current setting at which capture fails to occur is called the *pacing threshold* and should be less than 1 mA. The pacemaker output should be set at three to five times the pacing threshold.

If the pacemaker is to be used in a demand mode, it is also important that there is adequate sensing of the endocardial electrogram. To ensure good sensing, the pacing rate is set lower than the patient's intrinsic rate. The sensitivity of the pacing unit is set at its most sensitive level (lowest value), and is then decreased (higher values) gradually. The setting at which the pacemaker fails to sense and begins pacing competitively with the patient's intrinsic rhythm is called the *sensing threshold* (Fig. 33.11). For demand pacing, the sensitivity should be set at a more sensitive level than the sensing threshold.

POSTINSERTION CARE

The electrode catheter and its introducer should be secured to the skin under sterile conditions. Coiling the proximal electrode catheter around the insertion site and firmly taping to the skin prevents dislodgement of the distal catheter. An extension cable should be used to connect the catheter electrode pins to the pulse generator. The pulse generator should be secured to a

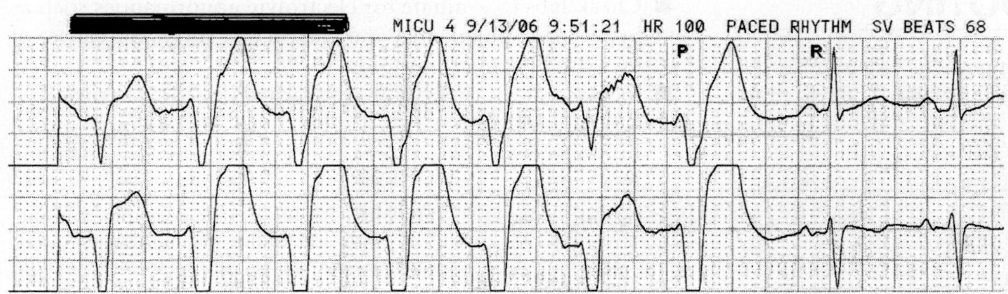

FIGURE 33.10. Loss of capture during threshold testing. Temporary pacing rate was set at 100 bpm. Loss of capture is obvious with change in QRS morphology. *P* is the last paced ventricular beat. The patient's own rhythm comes through with loss of ventricular pacing. *R* denotes an intrinsic ventricular beat.

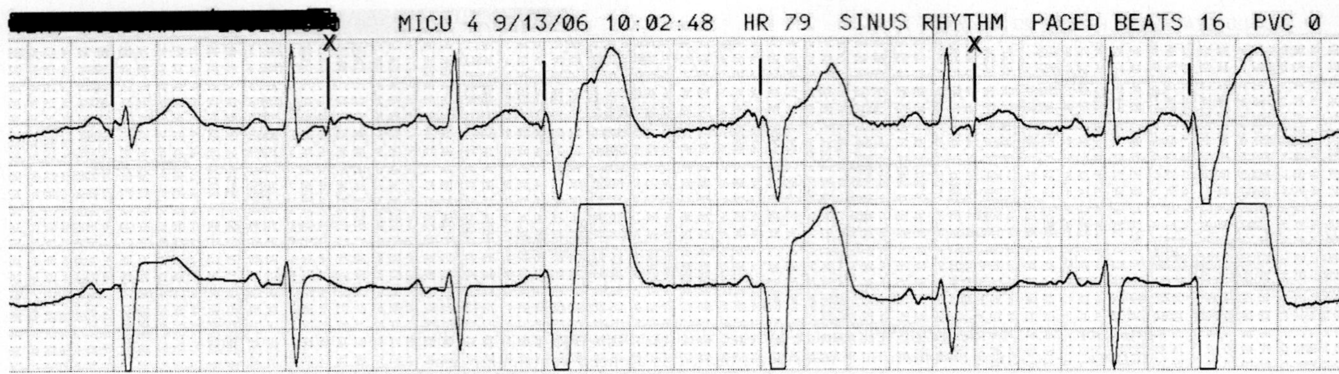

FIGURE 33.11. Sensitivity testing. Temporary pacing rate was set at 60 bpm. Sensitivity level was gradually set to lowest sensitivity (highest value). Ventricular pacing occurs at intervals when pacing should have been inhibited. Pacing artifacts (indicated by vertical marks) are appreciated and are "marching through" at 60 bpm. *X* denotes functional noncapture that occurs because a pacing stimulus was delivered at a time when the ventricle was refractory.

location where it will unlikely be moved or disconnected inadvertently. The plastic shield provided with the pulse generator should be slipped over its controls to prevent accidental control movement. Covering of the entire pacemaker unit (including shield) with a plastic see-through glove prevents exposure of the generator to liquids.

A portable chest radiograph should be obtained to ensure proper positioning of the pacing catheter and to assess for complications, particularly pneumothorax. A baseline 12-lead ECG should be obtained to document the QRS morphologic features, with the pacing catheter in proper position. A right bundle branch block morphology in lead V_1 with ventricular pacing may indicate pacing of the left ventricle (via an atrial septal defect [ASD], ventral septal defect [VSD], etc.) and increases the patient's risk of a thromboembolic stroke. A change in the morphology of the paced QRS may be the first sign of electrode displacement. Continuous electrocardiographic monitoring of the patient is imperative.

Daily evaluation should include inspection of the entry site, cardiac auscultation, threshold determinations, and evaluation of intrinsic rhythm. Complications of the pacemaker often can be determined by auscultation. For example, a pericardial friction rub may indicate ventricular penetration, and a clicking sound may imply intercostal muscle stimulation. Marked changes in thresholds may occur with catheter movement or perforation, requiring catheter repositioning. Any significant changes should be evaluated with an ECG and chest radiograph. The intrinsic rhythm can be evaluated by reducing the rate of the pacemaker until the underlying rhythm emerges.

TROUBLESHOOTING

Problems will arise, and a stepwise approach to determine the problem should be taken to determine the cause. The two most common problems are failure to capture (pacing artifact without a conducted QRS) and failure to pace (no pacing artifact).

Common reasons for noncapture usually include lead dislodgement, change in pacing threshold, or *undersensing*. Noncapture from lead dislodgment may simply be from lack of apposition of the catheter against tissue. However, a more concerning cause is cardiac perforation. Changes in the patient's clinical status or introduction of new medications can lead to increased pacing thresholds. Electrolyte abnormalities and acidosis may prevent pacing. Antiarrhythmic medications, especially sodium channel blockers such as flecainide or propafenone, may also increase pacing thresholds. Undersensing is failure of the pacemaker to sense intrinsic conduction (Fig. 33.12), and can appear as noncapture when a pacing stimulus is delivered during the refractory period (Figs. 33.11 and 33.12).

Failure to pace may occur due to loss of output from the pacemaker generator, break in the circuit, or *oversensing*. Potential causes of loss of output from the generator include loss of power (low batteries) or disconnection of the pacing catheter from the generator. Also, a break in the insulation or wiring anywhere between the connectors to the pacing catheter may result in failure to pace. Oversensing is the inhibition of the pacemaker by events that the pacemaker should ignore (Fig. 33.13), and may be caused by electromagnetic interference (EMI), T waves, and myopotentials. It is important to note that EMI is prevalent in most ICU settings.

Troubleshooting begins with a thorough review of the patient's clinical status and medications. It also includes the following steps:

- Check labs to evaluate for electrolyte abnormalities such as hyper- or hypokalemia, and correct any reversible causes of increased pacing thresholds.
- Increase the output of the generator to restore capture.

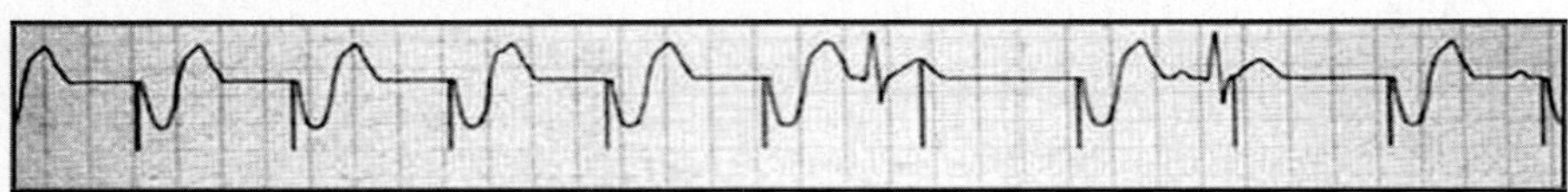

FIGURE 33.12. Ventricular undersensing. The sixth and eighth pacing artifacts occur at times when pacing should have been inhibited.

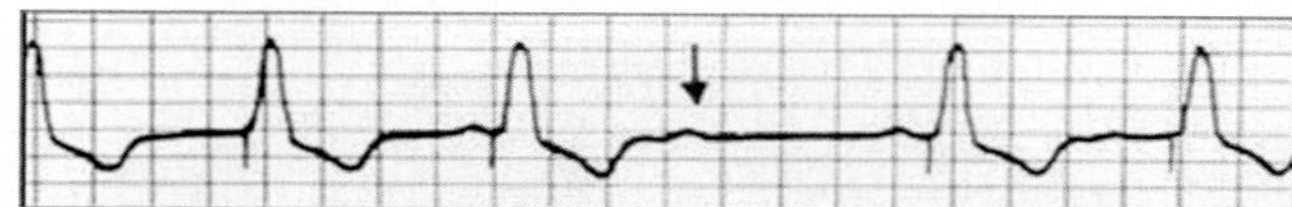

FIGURE 33.13. Ventricular oversensing. The *arrow* points to a time when a ventricular paced event should have occurred.

- Review the settings on the generator box for appropriate programming and to see if the device has been turned on.
- Replace the batteries if they are suspected to be depleted.
- Inspect the box for any obvious abnormalities and examine the connectors from the generator to the pacing catheter for any loose connections, fractures, or insulation breaks.
- A chest radiograph should be part of any workup for pacing problems; it is useful to evaluate for not only lead dislodgment, but also pneumothorax.
- An echocardiogram may help in determining if there is a new effusion, which may be seen if a perforation has occurred.

A specific problem that may be encountered with dual-chamber pacing is pacemaker-mediated tachycardia (PMT). For dual-chamber pacing, the postventricular atrial refractory period (PVARP) and the AV delay must also be programmed (Fig. 33.14A). The PVARP is the time after a ventricular-sensed or paced beat when atrial activity is ignored. The PVARP prevents tracking of retrograde atrial contractions, which could lead to PMT (Fig. 33.14B). However, too long of a PVARP setting may result in loss of AV synchrony, as the intrinsic P wave will not be sensed. The AV delay is the time from an atrial-sensed or paced beat to a ventricular-paced beat. This is analogous to the PR interval on a standard electrocardiogram.

COMPLICATIONS

Although the insertion of a temporary transvenous pacing catheter is generally a safe and well-tolerated procedure, there are potential complications that can occur as with any invasive intervention. The potential for a complication can occur at any point during the procedure from the time of initial catheter insertion to the time that the catheter is finally removed. Complications include:

- Vascular injury
- Inadvertent arterial puncture
- Bleeding
- Infection
- Cardiac tamponade
- Tricuspid valve injury
- Pneumothorax
- Hemothorax
- Air embolism
- Phrenic nerve injury
- Thoracic duct injury
- Guidewire fracture
- Thromboembolism
- Atrial or ventricular arrhythmia

Insertion of a temporary pacemaker in the setting of an acute MI may increase the risk of certain complications. Bleeding risk is increased because the patient is usually anticoagulated. The infarcted myocardium may be soft and necrotic, increasing the risk of cardiac perforation. Additionally, infarcted tissue may result in high pacing thresholds or inability to capture. The myocardium may be irritable, increasing the risk of arrhythmia. Metabolic and electrolyte abnormalities may also result in high pacing thresholds or myocardial irritability, and must be corrected.

If a complication is suspected, physical exam, chest radiography, and an echocardiogram should be performed immediately. The physical exam may reveal a new pericardial friction rub, suggesting cardiac perforation. The radiograph will help to evaluate the lead location and potential cardiopulmonary complications, such as a pneumothorax or pericardial or pleural effusion. Limited echocardiogram images can quickly assess the presence of an effusion.

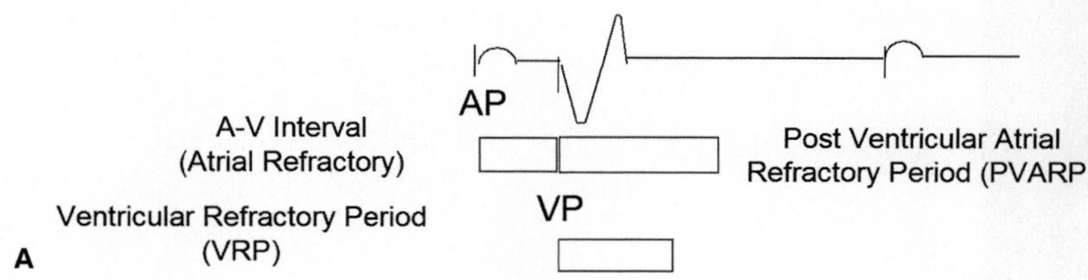

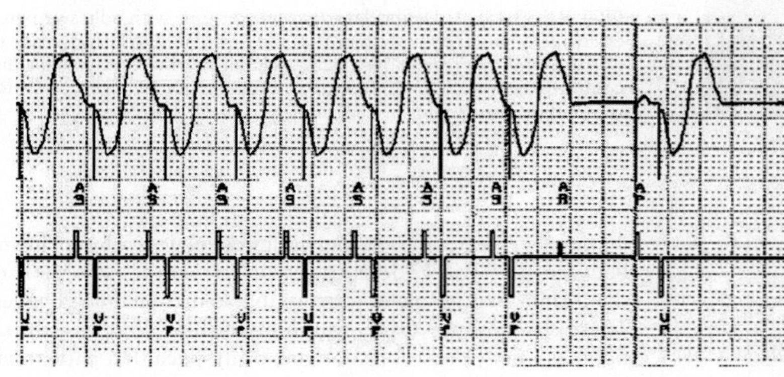

FIGURE 33.14. A, B: Schematic of postventricular atrial refractory period (PVARP) and an example of pacemaker-mediated tachycardia (PMT). *AP* is atrial paced; *VP* is ventricular paced. PVARP is the period after a ventricular event during which no atrial event will be ignored. Example of PMT that occurred in a patient with a permanent dual-chamber pacemaker. The top recording is an electrocardiogram lead; the bottom recording is a marker channel. Atrial-sensed (AS) activity occurs because of retrograde conduction after a ventricular-paced (VP) event. The pacemaker, therefore, tracks the atrial event, leading to the pacing rate at the upper tracking limit. PMT was terminated by placement of a magnet. Lengthening of the PVARP would have prevented sensing of the retrograde atrial activity. (Diagrams are compliments of Medtronic, Inc., Minneapolis, MN.)

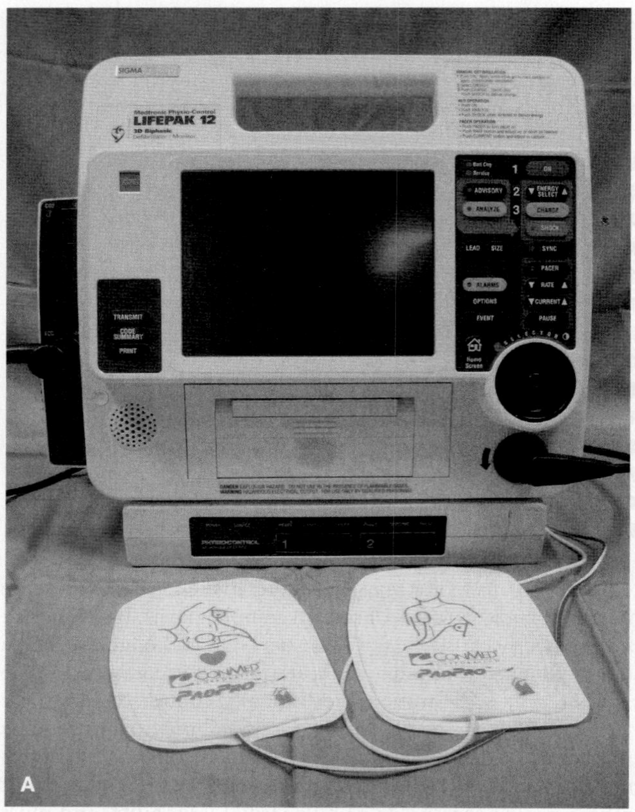

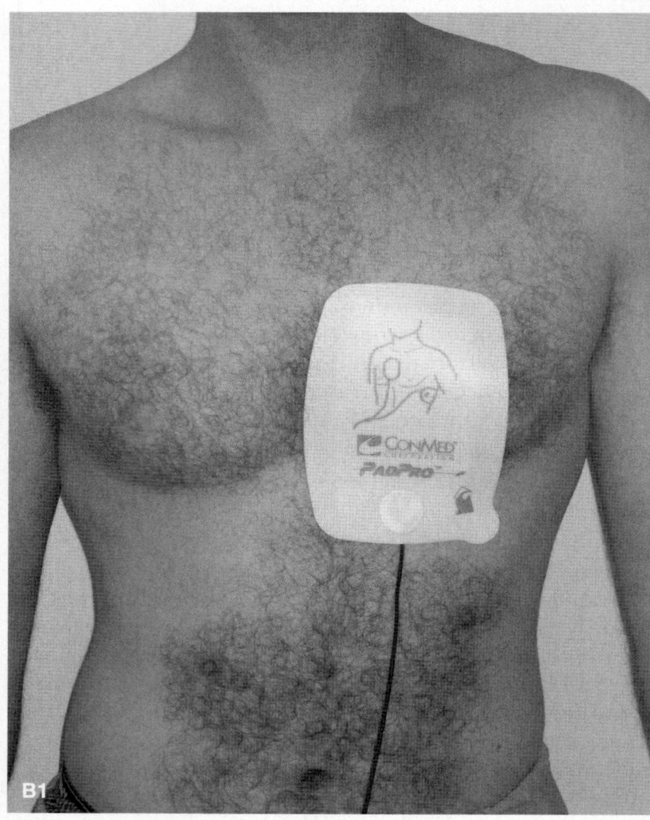

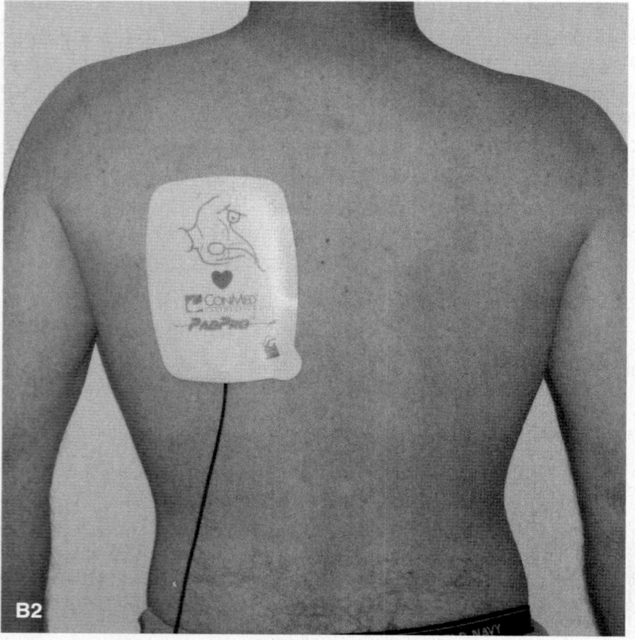

FIGURE 33.15. **A:** Defibrillator/pacemaker unit with adhesive patch electrodes. This type of system is readily available, relatively easy to operate, and has reasonable pacing reliability. However, patient discomfort limits its use. **B:** Typical anteroposterior patch location for transcutaneous pacing.

Pacemaker Syndrome

One significant problem that the practitioner should be cognizant of is that of "pacemaker syndrome." Occasionally, when temporary ventricular pacing is initiated, loss of synchrony between the atria and ventricles or retrograde activation of the atrium may result in unfavorable hemodynamic changes. These changes may cause symptoms such as dizziness, throat tightness, neck pulsations, fatigue, or dyspnea. If a patient has symptoms suggestive of "pacemaker syndrome" during temporary ventricular pacing, a dual-chamber system is strongly advised if permanent pacing is necessary.

ALTERNATIVE TEMPORARY PACING METHODS

External Noninvasive (Transcutaneous) Pacing

External transcutaneous pacing was introduced by Zoll in 1952, before other pacing techniques were developed (9). Pacing is achieved through two large, self-adhesive electrode pads, usually placed in an anteroposterior position, which are connected to an external pulse generator (Fig. 33.15A, B). Since its introduction, improvements have been made that have resulted in better stimulation thresholds and pacing reliability. Successful pacing with this method has been reported to be as high as 94% (10). However, pectoral muscle stimulation is common and may require sedation of the patient (10), and reliable capture is still not as consistent as with other pacing methods. Because external pacing does not require central venous access and is relatively easy to perform, this method is still frequently utilized as a bridge to a more reliable pacing method.

Transesophageal Pacing

Transesophageal pacing is possible because of the posterior position of the esophagus to the left atrium. The advantages of this technique are that its placement is relatively noninvasive and has minimum complications; the major disadvantage is that ventricular capture is unreliable. Therefore, transesophageal pacing is most useful for patients that need atrial pacing only. This technique requires a special transesophageal pacing electrode and generator, which provides higher outputs necessary for transesophageal pacing—usually between 2 and 530 mA (Fig. 33.16). The electrode is introduced orally or nasally, and is advanced to the proximity of the left atrium. Optimal electrode position occurs at a location with the largest atrial electrograms.

Transthoracic Pacing

A transthoracic approach has been used successfully on many occasions, but less invasive temporary pacing techniques have made this procedure quite uncommon. This highly invasive technique is performed by direct percutaneous placement of pacing catheters or wires into the right ventricle through a transthoracic needle, utilizing an approach from the precordium or from the subxiphoid region. A needle and stylet are introduced into the right ventricle. As the needle and stylet are being advanced, they are connected to the V_1 lead of a standard ECG. A current of injury pattern is seen upon penetration of the right ventricular wall, providing that there is not complete ventricular asystole. Removal of the stylet and aspiration of blood verifies intracardiac positioning. The pacing catheter is then passed through the needle, the needle is removed, and the electrodes are connected to a standard pacing box. There are several complications that are potentially severe, including pneumothorax, coronary artery perforation, mediastinal bleeding, and cardiac tamponade. This approach should thus be used only when other pacing options are not available.

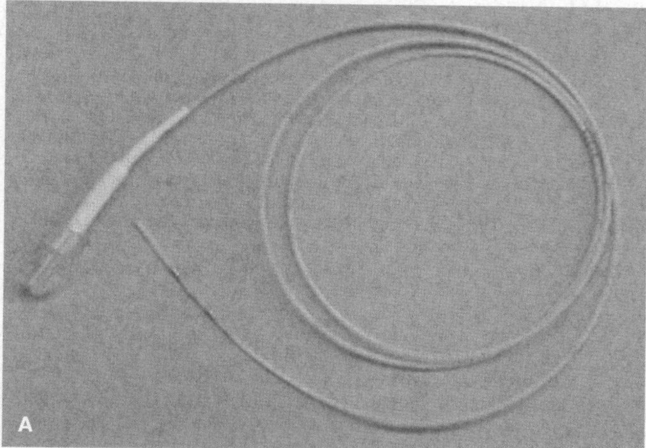

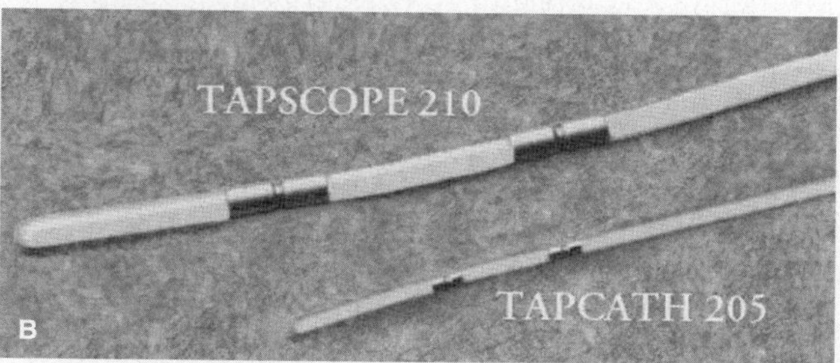

FIGURE 33.16. **A:** Temporary transesophageal pacing catheter. **B:** 10F (*top*) and 5F (*bottom*) catheters. (Compliments of CardioCommand, Inc., Tampa, FL.)

SUMMARY

Temporary pacing is an invaluable tool for the management of cardiac rhythm disturbances, including not only bradyarrhythmias, but also some tachyarrhythmias. There are multiple transvenous pacing catheters available, in addition to other modalities if temporary transvenous pacing is not possible. Basic familiarity with its indications, placement, and management is essential for all of those who work in the critical care setting.

References

1. Atkins J, Leshin S, Blomqvist C. Ventricular conduction blocks and sudden death in acute myocardial infarction. Potential indications to pacing. *N Engl J Med.* 1973;288(6):281–284.
2. Geitzen F, Leuner C, Raute-Kreinsen U, et al. Acute and long-term

results after transcoronary ablation of septal hypertrophy (TASH). Catheter interventional treatment for hypertrophic obstructive cardiomyopathy. *Eur Heart J.* 1999;20(18):1342–1354.

3. Faber L, Seggewiss H, Gleichmann U. Percutaneous transluminal septal myocardial ablation in hypertrophic obstructive cardiomyopathy: results with respect to intraprocedural myocardial contrast echocardiography. *Circulation.* 1998;98(22):2415–2421.
4. Baerman J, Kirsh M, de Buitleir M, et al. Natural history and determinants of conduction defects following coronary artery bypass surgery. *Ann Thorac Surg.* 1987;44(2):150–153.
5. Miyamoto Y, Curtiss E, Kormos R, et al. Bradyarrhythmia after heart transplantation. Incidence, time course, and outcome. *Circulation.* 1990;82(5 Suppl.):IV313–317.
6. Daoud E, Snow R, Hummel J, et al. Temporary atrial epicardial pacing as prophylaxis against atrial fibrillation after heart surgery: a meta-analysis. *J Cardiovasc Electrophysiol.* 2003;14(2):127–132.
7. Cooper JP, Swanton RH. Complications of transvenous temporary pacemaker insertion. *Br J Hosp Med.* 1995;53(14):155–161.
8. Pinto N, Jones T, Dyamenahalli U, et al. Temporary transvenous pacing with an active fixation bipolar lead in children: a preliminary report. *PACE.* 2003;26(7 Pt 1):1519–1522.
9. Zoll PM. Resuscitation of the heart in ventricular standstill by external electric stimulation. *N Engl J Med.* 1952;247(20):768–771.
10. Madsen J, Meibom J, Videbak R, et al. Transcutaneous pacing: experience with the Zoll noninvasive temporary pacemaker. *Am Heart J.* 1988(1 Pt 1); 116:7–10.

CHAPTER 34 ■ IMPORTANT INTENSIVE CARE PROCEDURES

GEORGE C. VELMAHOS

Invasive procedures are performed at the bedside of critically ill patients with increasing frequency to avoid the risks, resources, and inconvenience of transportation to other areas of the hospital (1,2). With the development of safety systems and new techniques, the morbidity of these bedside procedures is not higher than the morbidity of similar procedures performed in the operating room, emergency department, or angiography suite (3,4). Knowledge of anatomy, attention to detail, and understanding of potential pitfalls need to be mastered by the specialists involved in bedside procedures. Collaboration across specialties is crucial, as boundaries are continuously crossed and traditional turfs make little sense in the age of technology.

Below I will describe the following procedures, which can safely be performed at the bedside: open and percutaneous thoracostomy, thoracentesis, pericardiocentesis, diagnostic peritoneal aspiration and lavage, percutaneous tracheostomy, open and percutaneous cricothyroidotomy, percutaneous gastrostomy, abdominal pressure monitoring, and percutaneous vena cava filter placement (5). Routine procedures such as central venous and arterial catheterization will be described in other chapters. The described procedures are selected from a myriad of possible bedside procedures (spanning from urologic, neurosurgical, gynecologic, and general surgical to orthopedic, pediatric, or radiographic) on the basis of two criteria: they can potentially be performed not only by surgeons but also by any adequately trained physician functioning within appropriate patient safety systems, and on occasions several of these procedures must be performed emergently and without the luxury of waiting for a subspecialty expert. Therefore, critical care physicians from different tracks should familiarize themselves with the technique, indications, and complications associated with these procedures.

TUBE THORACOSTOMY

Indications

Fluid or air that remains undrained into the pleural cavity may cause infection, lung collapse, or entrapment, and therefore needs to be drained. A pneumothorax is usually drained if it exceeds 15% to 20% of the hemithoracic volume or causes hemodynamic instability (6). Smaller pneumothoraces can be observed. There is no universally-accepted volume threshold for the drainage of a hemothorax. Usually, all hemothoraces of penetrating traumatic cause are drained. Hemothorax after blunt trauma is drained if more than 200 mL of blood is in the thoracic cavity, as found by blunting of the costodiaphragmatic angle on erect chest radiograph or estimated on computed tomographic imaging. Fluids of other cause (hydrothorax, chylothorax, etc.) are drained according to volume and patient symptomatology.

Following trauma, the chest tube output is used as an indication to operation. A thoracotomy is offered if the output is more than 1,500 mL shortly after placement or if output of more than 200 mL per hour persists over 4 to 6 hours after placement (7). However, these are not absolute criteria. One must remember that chest tubes are not reliable drains of intrathoracic blood because they often clog, kink, or are misplaced. A hemodynamically unstable patient who is bleeding in the chest should be taken to the operating room even with lower than the above chest tube outputs.

Technique

Percutaneous Thoracostomy

The percutaneous technique is safe for patients who do not have risk factors for intrathoracic adhesions (e.g., previous thoracic operation, empyema, clotted hemothorax, etc.). A 28 Fr or 32 Fr chest tube is adequate according to the size of the patient and does not cause excessive pain. For the drainage of simple pneumothorax, smaller tubes (18 Fr or 22 Fr) may be used.

The site of placement is chosen and prepared. The most common site is at the intercostal space above the nipple (usually the fourth intercostal space) and at the midaxillary line. The diaphragm can elevate up to the nipple in expiration, and for this reason, lower placement of chest tubes is not safe and may risk injury to the diaphragm and intra-abdominal organs. Adequate local analgesia is key because tube thoracostomy is a painful procedure (Fig. 34.1). The entire track should be infiltrated and not just the subcutaneous tissue.

A needle, covered by a plastic sheath and connected to a fluid-filled syringe, is inserted through the skin with the intent to hit the underlying rib. Once the rib is felt, the needle is slightly withdrawn and then redirected immediately over the rib to avoid injury to the neurovascular intercostals bundle that travels under each rib. Under continuous suction the syringe and needle are slowly advanced until bubbles of air are aspirated. This indicates that the needle has entered into the pleural space. The needle and syringe are withdrawn, and the plastic sheath left in place. A guidewire is inserted into the sheath (Fig. 34.2). If there is any resistance during advancement of the guidewire, the procedure should be repeated from the beginning. With the guidewire in place, the plastic sheath is removed. A 2-cm skin incision is made, and

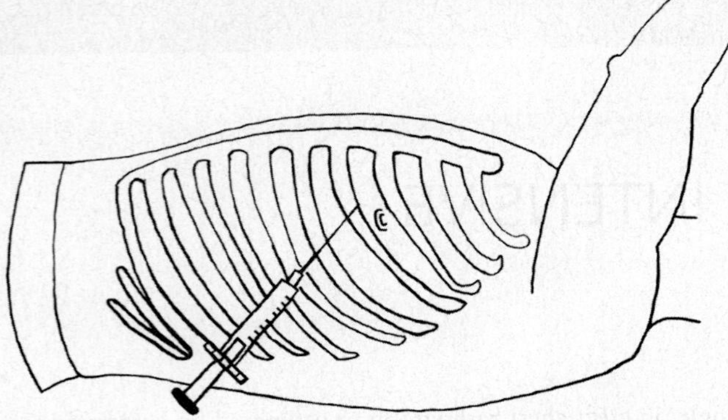

FIGURE 34.1. Site for generous injection of local anesthetic prior to chest tube insertion, usually at the fourth intercostal space, above the rib margin, at midaxillary line.

sequential dilatation with three consecutive dilators is done over the guidewire. Following this, the chest tube, loaded on a plastic guide, is placed over the guidewire into the chest. The plastic guide and guidewire are withdrawn, and the chest tube is left in place.

Securing the chest tube is a very important part of the procedure. The tube is tied to the skin with a 0 nonabsorbable suture. A separate suture should be placed as a purse-string around the tube and left untied. This suture will serve to close the incision once the chest tube is removed. The tube should also be taped to the skin. Extra precautions should be taken to have the chest tube and its connection to the drainage bottles secured to avoid inadvertent partial or complete removal. Usually, 20 cm H_2O negative suction is applied at least for the first 48 hours although there is no evidence that this shortens the period of placement or decreases the rate of residual pneumothorax compared to water seal.

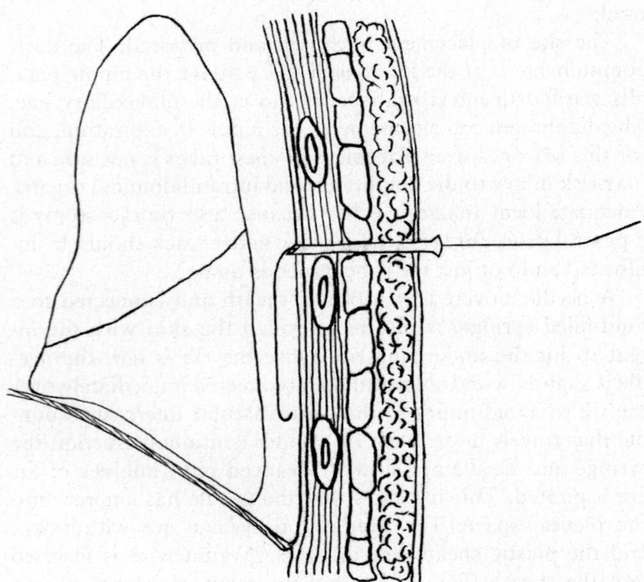

FIGURE 34.2. A guidewire is inserted through the sheath into the pleural space, guiding sequential enlargement of the tract by tapered dilators.

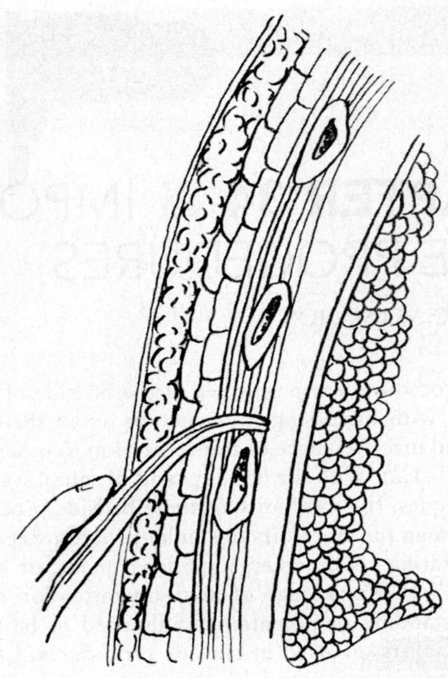

FIGURE 34.3. A sturdy clamp is necessary to spread the muscles wide to allow easy insertion of the chest tube.

Open Thoracostomy

The site of placement is marked as above. A 4-cm incision is made parallel to the ribs. Blunt dissection follows through the subcutaneous tissue and muscle. The clamp is finally inserted into the pleural space in a controlled way over the rib underlying the skin incision (Fig. 34.3). It is then opened wide to spread the muscles and enlarge the tract. This is an important step since the novice tends to make the skin incision large but the intermuscular tract too small, resulting in difficulty with tube insertion. There is no reason to "tunnel" the track to the rib above the skin incision. Tunneling causes more pain, makes the procedure more difficult, and offers no benefit.

A finger is inserted to explore for the presence of adhesions at the site of insertion (Fig. 34.4). Then, the chest tube is guided by a clamp into the opening and toward the superior and posterior hemithorax (Fig. 34.5). The clamp is removed, and the tube is secured as discussed above.

Removal of Chest Tubes

Removal takes place when there is no air leak and fluid output is less than 2 mL/kg per 24 hours. The patient is asked to inspire maximally and hold the breath. With one hand against the chest wall, the physician pulls abruptly the chest tube with the other hand and immediately ties the purse string to seal the insertion site. The site is dressed. If a purse-string suture is absent, it is important to apply occlusive dressing to prevent air entry into the chest.

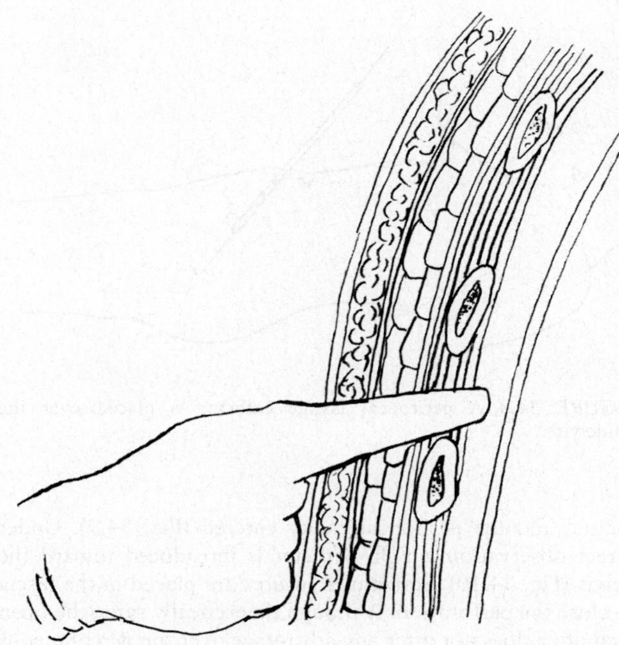

FIGURE 34.4. A finger is inserted into the track prior to tube insertion to ensure a clear pleural space and absence of adhesions.

Pitfalls and Complications

A misplaced chest tube may not drain adequately. Do not assume that air or fluid will be drained because a chest tube is in place (8). Confirm correct placement with a chest radiograph, and have a low threshold to replace or add a chest tube, if the symptoms are not relieved, hemodynamic instability persists, or drain seizes abruptly. A chest tube may cause more harm than benefit if the technique is wrong. Injury to the intercostals vessels or lung may cause significant bleeding. The chest tube should then be removed and on rare occasions the bleeding site explored if the hemorrhage continues. Intraparenchymal placement may cause a persistent air leak. It is usually diagnosed by computed tomography. The tube should be removed, and the leak usually seals. The chest tubes should be securely tied and taped to the skin and checked daily. Accidental removal of a tube equals a sloppy technique. Infection is the most common related complication. Poor aseptic technique, long duration of the tube in the chest, and no antibiotic prophylaxis (one dose before tube placement) are associated with this complication (9). Significant undrained hemothorax (estimated at more than 400 mL) should be managed by thoracoscopic evacuation or intrathoracic thrombolysis (10,11).

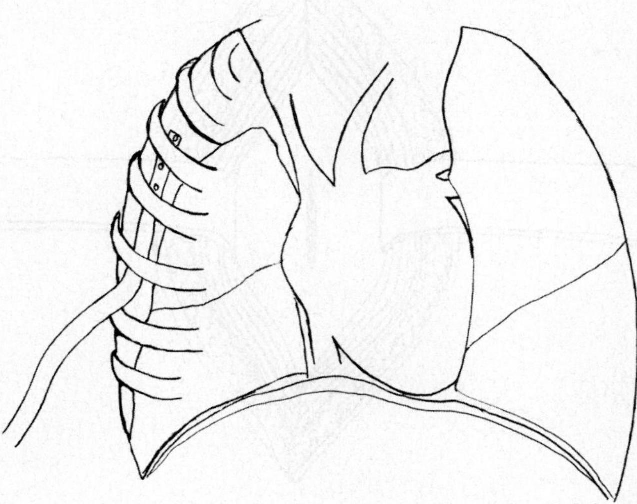

FIGURE 34.5. The final position of the chest tube.

DIAGNOSTIC PERITONEAL ASPIRATION (DPA) AND LAVAGE (DPL)

Indications

The most common reason for a diagnostic peritoneal aspiration and lavage (DPA/DPL) is the diagnosis of intra-abdominal injury. A count of more than 100,000 red blood cells/mm^3 or 500 white blood cells/mm^3 or the presence of bile, enteric content, or high-amylase fluid in the effluent of the lavage are considered indications for an operation following abdominal trauma (12). However, these criteria are oversensitive and frequently lead to unnecessary operations. Furthermore, these cell counts are valid for blunt but not for penetrating trauma. Portable ultrasonography and the liberal use of helical computed tomography have limited the usefulness of DPL. Currently, DPA/DPL is used only on rare occasions due to lack of appropriate technologic resources or due to major physiologic instability that precludes patient transport to computed tomography (13). Another indication for DPL may be to detect bowel injury since CT scan may miss intestinal infarction and perforation. Aspiration or paracentesis of the abdomen is also performed to diagnose and treat ascites.

Technique

Percutaneous Insertion of Peritoneal Catheter

A 0.5-cm skin incision is placed under the umbilicus (or over it in the presence of pregnancy, pelvic hematoma, or a lower midline operative scar). A sheathed needle is introduced with direction toward the pelvis. The needle is connected to a fluid-filled syringe and advanced slowly. When the flow of fluid becomes unobstructed, the needle is in the peritoneal cavity (Fig. 34.6). Needle and syringe are withdrawn, and the plastic sheath is left in place. A guidewire is introduced through the sheath, which is then removed (Fig. 34.7). A dilator is placed over the guidewire and withdrawn. Then, the DPL catheter is introduced and the guidewire is removed (Fig. 34.8). Aspiration is performed first (DPA) and is considered positive if 10 mL of gross blood is aspirated. If the DPA is negative, 1 L of normal saline is infused (DPL). By lowering the normal saline bag below the level of the body, the lavage fluid returns into the bag; the fluid is sent for analysis.

A simpler DPL system includes only a catheter fed over a trocar. The trocar and catheter are introduced in a controlled and slow fashion into the abdomen. Two points of resistance

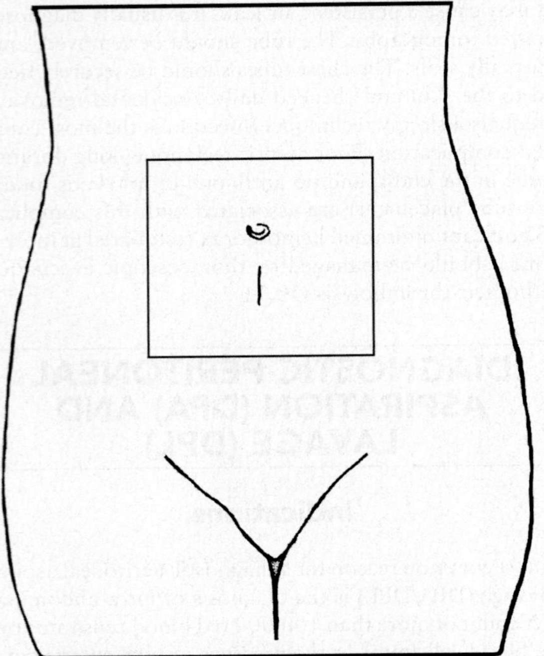

FIGURE 34.6. Site for peritoneal lavage catheter placement, just below the umbilicus.

are felt as the trocar passes through the anterior fascia and the peritoneum. As soon as the tip of the trocar passes the second point of resistance—and is presumably into the abdomen—the catheter is fed over it toward the pelvis and the trocar is removed. Experience is needed to perform this technique to prevent trocar injury of abdominal contents.

Open Technique for Peritoneal Catheter Insertion

A 2- to 4-cm skin incision is performed under or over the umbilicus. The fascia is visualized and retracted. The fascia is then

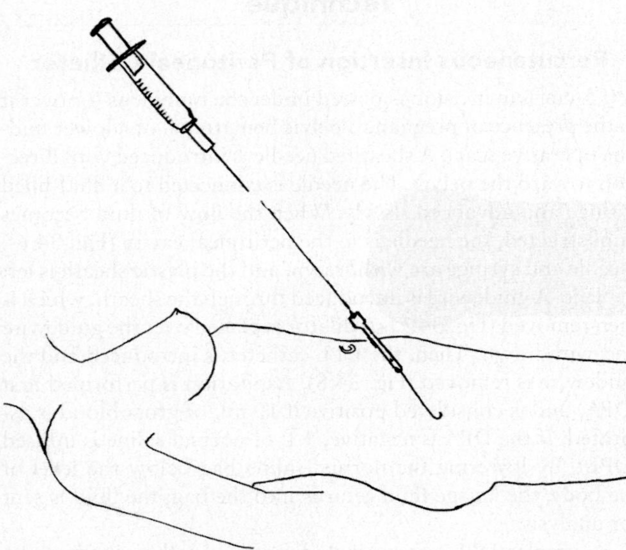

FIGURE 34.7. The needle is removed, and the remaining plastic sheath allows guidewire insertion.

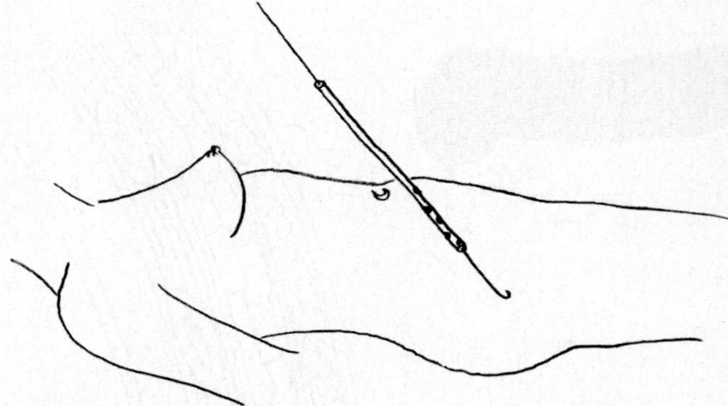

FIGURE 34.8. A peritoneal lavage catheter is placed over the guidewire.

incised and the peritoneal cavity entered (Fig. 34.9). Under direct observation a DPL catheter is introduced toward the pelvis (Fig. 34.10). Sometimes sutures are placed in the fascia to close the perforation. Although theoretically safer, the open technique does not offer any advantage over the percutaneous technique. It takes longer to perform and may potentially be complicated in obese patients. I recommend the percutaneous technique routinely although the choice of technique is based on operator preference.

Pitfalls and Complications

The introduction of needles and catheters in the abdominal cavity carries the (very low) risk of injuring the bowel or vessels. The procedure needs to be performed by physicians experienced with the procedure, which is becoming uncommon as

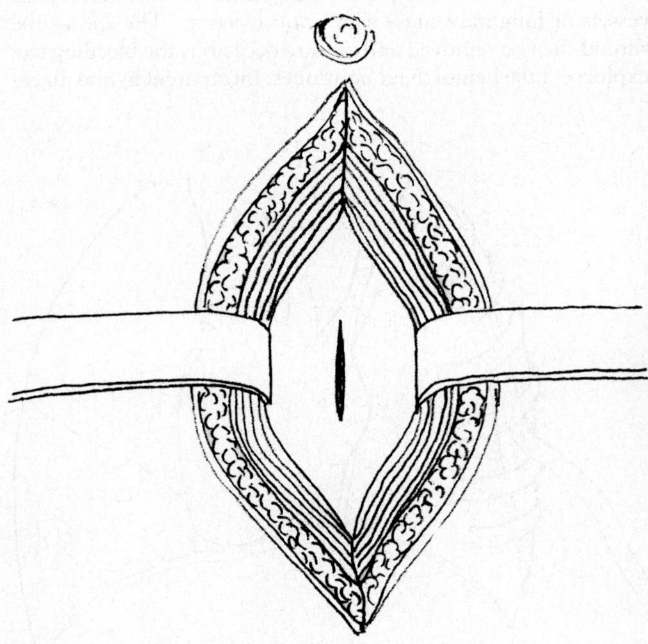

FIGURE 34.9. Open technique for peritoneal lavage catheter insertion with direct visualization and incision of the abdominal fascia.

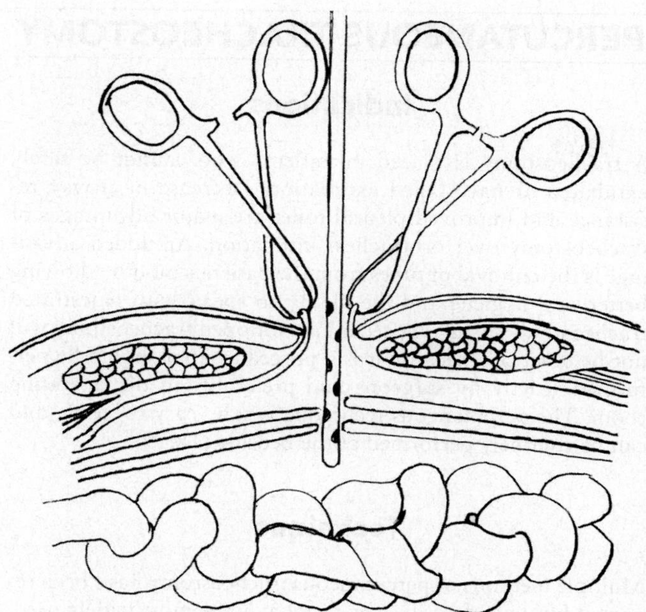

FIGURE 34.10. Insertion of the peritoneal lavage catheter under direct vision.

the procedure is not frequently performed (14). Once-useful cell counts need to be viewed with caution, as the indications for surgical exploration after abdominal trauma have changed and many injuries are managed nonoperatively. Infusing the lavage fluid but being unable to retrieve it is not uncommon. Slight reposition of the catheter may help.

CRICOTHYROIDOTOMY

Indications

Cricothyroidotomy is a real emergency and reserved for those patients who cannot be intubated orally or nasally or have lost a preexisting oral airway and are desaturating. It would be a mistake to attempt a tracheostomy in such patients, as this consumes considerably more time. Because the cricothyroid space is superficial in relationship to the skin, it should be selected as the easiest point—even if suboptimal—for insertion of a lifesaving airway.

Technique

Open Cricothyroidotomy

A vertical incision is placed above the cricothyroid space (Fig. 34.11). This incision is preferred over a horizontal or collar-type incision because it can be extended over the trachea and decreases the likelihood of bleeding from injury to the anterior jugular veins, which run close to the midline of the neck. After sharp incision of any soft tissue between the skin and cricoid cartilage, the cricothyroid space is identified by palpation (Fig. 34.12). Any bleeding at this point is ignored, as the sheer goal is to establish an airway as soon as possible. A pointed clamp is introduced through the cricothyroid membrane and opened

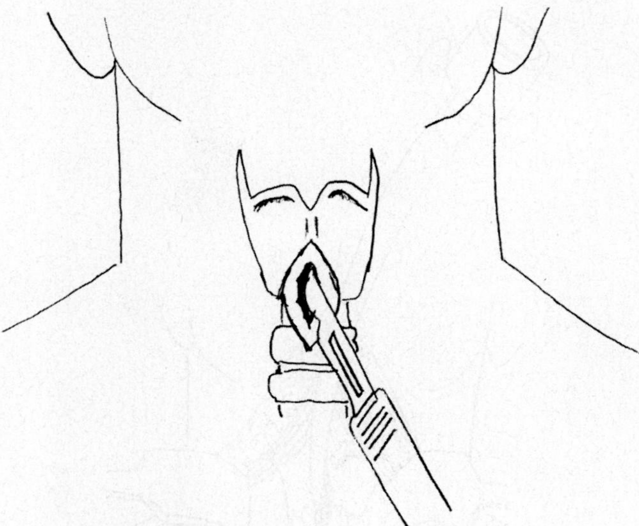

FIGURE 34.11. Vertical incision at the cricothyroid space.

to dilate the space (Fig. 34.13). Experienced surgeons can use the scalpel to incise the membrane, although the risk exists for injuring the cartilage or posterior wall. The thyroid cartilage is immobilized and pulled upward and anteriorly with a tracheostomy hook. The tracheostomy hook is essential for this procedure. A no. 4 tracheostomy tube is introduced. If the space is wide, a no. 6 tube is preferable. The bleeding is controlled by sutures, electrocoagulation, or pressure.

Percutaneous Cricothyroidotomy

A vertical incision is made. A hollow needle is introduced through the cricothyroid space (Fig. 34.14A, B) and a guidewire is introduced through the needle (Fig. 34.14C), which is then removed. Dilation of the trachea takes place over the guidewire by introducing a dilator (Fig. 34.15A). Finally, a no. 4 tracheostomy tube is placed over a guiding dilator and the guidewire (Fig. 34.15B). The dilator and guidewire are removed, and the tube is left in place and secured to the skin.

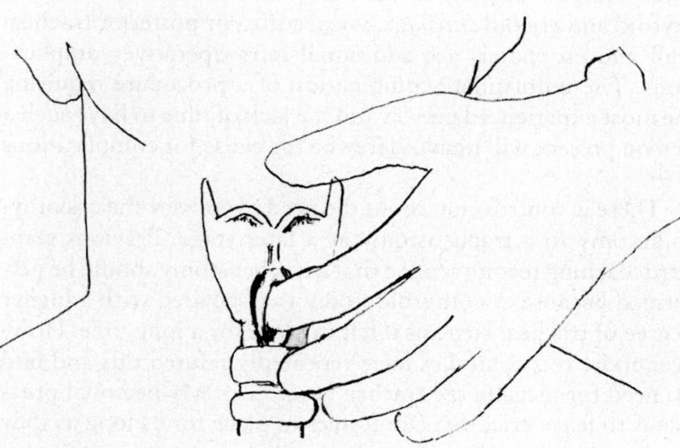

FIGURE 34.12. Digital identification of the cricothyroid space.

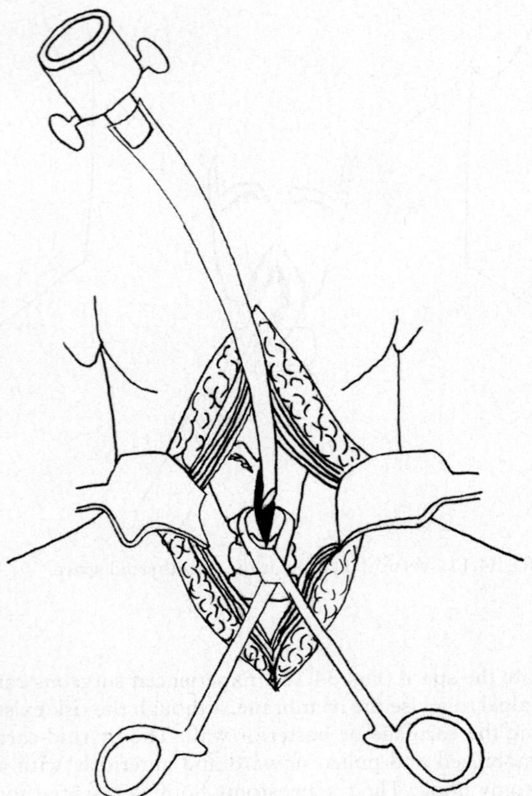

FIGURE 34.13. Dilatation of the cricothyroid membrane and insertion of the tracheostomy tube.

Pitfalls and Complications

Despite the apparent simplicity of the technique, a cricothyroidotomy can become a challenging procedure, as the pressure to establish an airway in a dying patient is great. Blood can obscure the field and create additional difficulty. Incorrect identification of the cricothyroid space and placement of the incision above the thyroid cartilage is possible (15). Inadequate opening of the cricothyroid membrane and loss of valuable minutes while trying to insert the tracheostomy tube through a very narrow opening is again not uncommon. Injury of the thyroid and cricoid cartilage, vocal cords, or posterior tracheal wall and esophagus are additional intra-operative complications. The unfortunate combination of a procedure requiring the most experienced person and the lack of time to have such a person present will unavoidably be the cause for complications (16).

There is controversy about the need to convert the cricothyroidotomy to a tracheostomy at a later stage. Previous standard teaching recommended that a tracheostomy should be performed because cricothyroidotomy is associated with a higher degree of tracheal stenosis if left in place for a long time. However, more recent studies have repeatedly refuted this and find no need for incising the trachea twice (17). My personal practice is to leave cricothyroidotomies in place for as long as they are needed to ventilate the patient without converting to a tracheostomy.

PERCUTANEOUS TRACHEOSTOMY

Indications

A tracheostomy is placed in patients who cannot be safely extubated or have failed extubation. Decrease in airway resistance and improved pleural toilet are major advantages of tracheostomy over orotracheal intubation. An added advantage is the removal of tubes from the patient's mouth, allowing better oral hygiene and the ability to speak with fenestrated tracheostomy tubes. The technique for open tracheostomy will not be described because it is a procedure that should be performed strictly by surgeons and preferably in the operating room. The percutaneous technique is safe, easy to teach, and can be routinely performed at the bedside (18,19).

Technique

Multiple methods of percutaneous tracheostomy have been reported but one, described by Ciaglia, is the most widely used, validated by multiple articles from different groups, and described below. Ideally, the neck is hyperextended by placing a pillow under the patient's shoulders but can be left in the neutral position if spinal precautions are maintained. After preparation of the neck, the site of incision is selected to be in the middle between the cricoid cartilage and sternal notch, which corresponds to the second or third tracheal cartilage. The procedure is performed under bronchoscopic guidance. The bronchoscope is introduced through the orotracheal tube, and the tube is pulled to the level immediately below the vocal cords. A 2- to 3-cm vertical incision is placed, and the subcutaneous tissue and pretracheal muscles are bluntly dissected until the trachea is palpated (Fig. 34.16). A sheathed needle connected to a fluid-filled syringe is introduced. Aspiration of bubbles into the syringe indicates entry into the trachea, also confirmed by the bronchoscope (Fig. 34.17). The needle is pushed in 2 mm farther since the sheath is shorter than the needle. The needle and syringe are removed, and the sheath remains in place. The syringe is placed back on the sheath and air aspirated to confirm that the sheath remains in the airway and has not dislodged during removal of the needle. A J-tipped guidewire is introduced through the sheath into the trachea, and the sheath is then removed (Fig. 34.18). The track is dilated by a short firm dilator, following which a large curved dilator (Fig. 34.19), fed over a guiding tube, is introduced over the guidewire. The large curved dilator has a mark to guide how deep it should be inserted into the airway. Now the trachea is adequately dilated to accommodate the tracheostomy tube. The curved dilator is removed, and the tracheostomy tube (usually a Shiley no. 8) is fed over a 28 Fr dilator, guided by the guidewire/guiding tube complex into the trachea (Fig. 34.20). Although I almost routinely use a no. 8 tracheostomy tube, on the rare occasions that a no. 6 is required, it will be fed over a 26 Fr dilator. The kit contains several sizes of dilators to accommodate different caliber tracheostomy tubes. A single cannula tracheostomy tube will have the same internal diameter as a double cannula tube but a smaller external diameter making it easier for insertion. All these steps are visualized through the bronchoscope although during insertion of the main dilator, the force required to push the dilator may temporarily collapse the trachea for

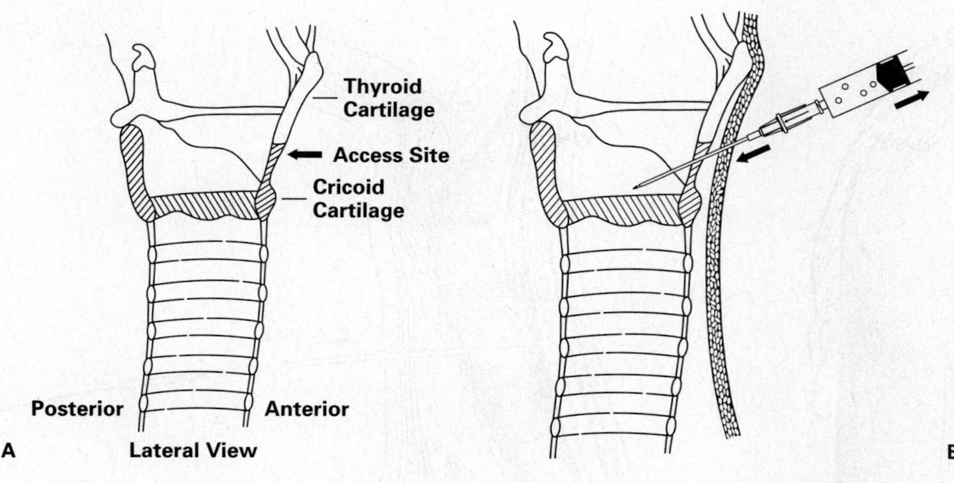

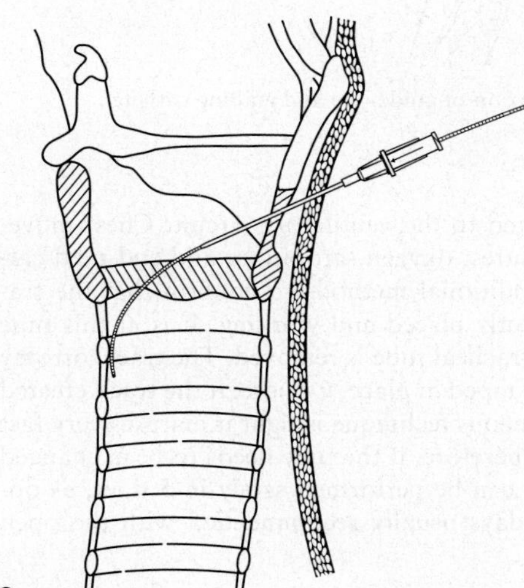

FIGURE 34.14. **A:** Access site for cricothyroidotomy (lateral view). (From Cook Medical, Inc., with permission.) **B:** Localization of the cricothyroid space and placement of catheter (lateral view). (From Cook Medical, Inc., with permission.) **C:** Insertion of guidewire through the hollow catheter (lateral view). (From Cook Medical, Inc., with permission.)

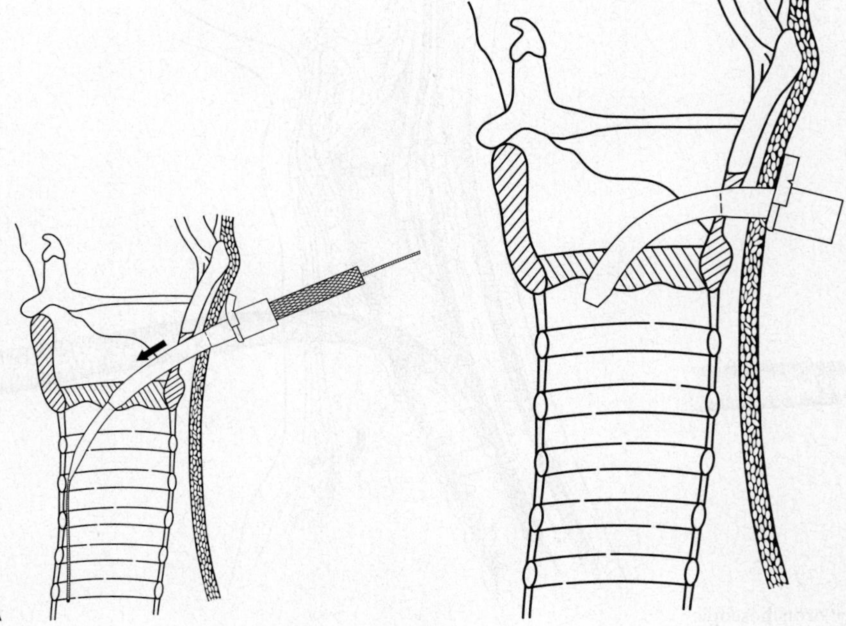

FIGURE 34.15. **A:** Dilatation of the tract (lateral view). (From Cook Medical, Inc., with permission.) **B:** Placement of the tracheostomy tube in the cricothyroid space (lateral view). (From Cook Medical, Inc., with permission.)

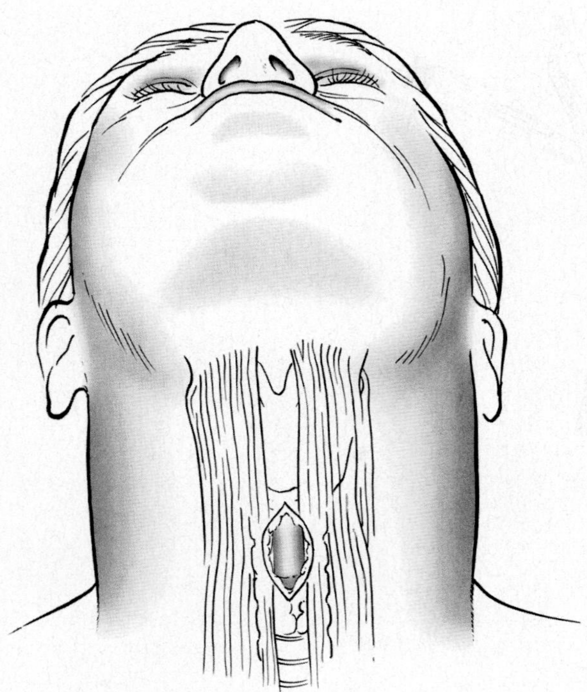

FIGURE 34.16. Placement of incision for percutaneous tracheostomy.

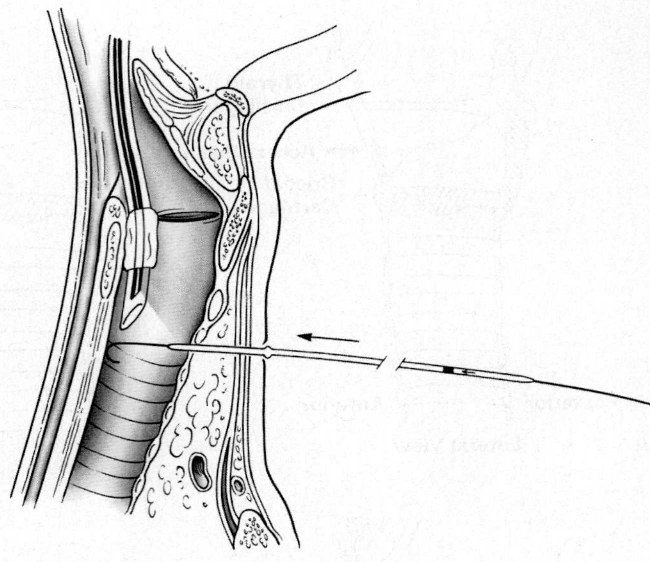

FIGURE 34.18. Insertion of guidewire and guiding catheter.

several seconds with poor visualization through the bronchoscope.

Finally, the guidewire, guiding tube, and curved dilator are removed and the tracheostomy tube is left in place. The bronchoscope is withdrawn from the endotracheal tube (which remains in place) and inserted into the newly placed tracheostomy tube to confirm correct placement by visualizing the carina. The cuff of the tracheostomy tube is inflated, and the tube is connected to the ventilatory circuit. Chest movement, airway pressures, oxygen saturation, and end-tidal carbon dioxide are additional methods to confirm that the tracheostomy is correctly placed and working. It is at this time only that the endotracheal tube is removed. The tracheostomy tube is sutured and taped in place. Of note, if the track created during the percutaneous technique is tight it matures very fast around the tube. Therefore, if the tube needs to be exchanged or downsized, this can be performed safely in 5 days, as opposed to 8 to 10 days usually recommended with the open technique.

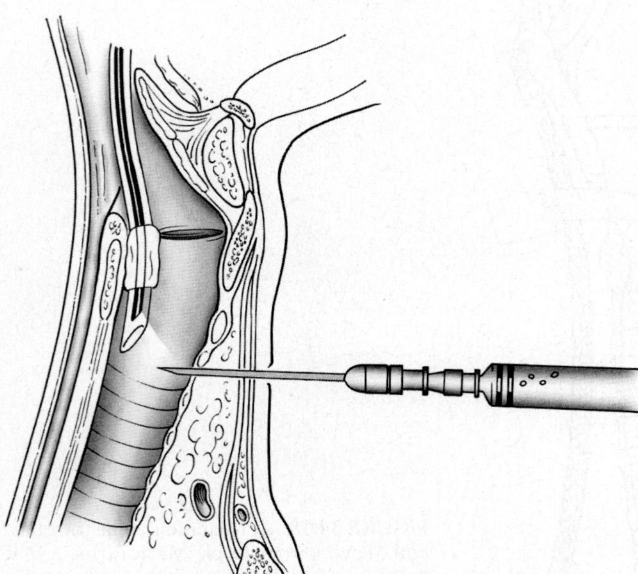

FIGURE 34.17. Insertion of fluid-filled syringe under bronchoscopic guidance and aspiration of bubbles.

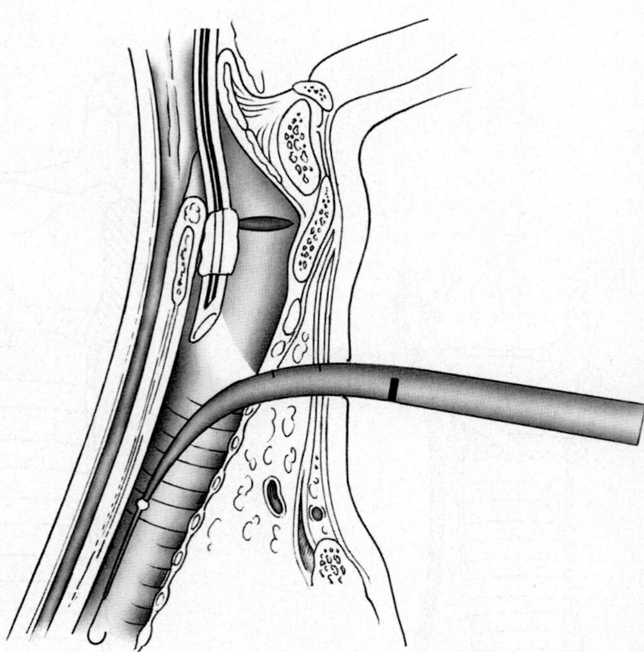

FIGURE 34.19. Dilation with the large progressive curved dilator.

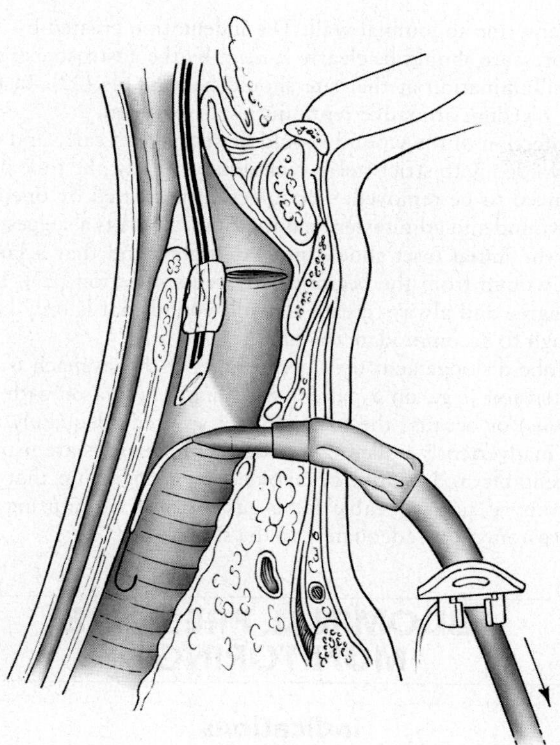

FIGURE 34.20. Insertion of the tracheostomy tube over a guiding dilator.

Pitfalls and Complications

Loss of airway is the most important concern (20). It can occur by unrecognized pretracheal or paratracheal placement of the dilators, which dilate the soft tissues instead of the trachea, leading to placement of the tracheostomy tube outside of the trachea. Bronchoscopic guidance is key to avoid this, and although I do not consider it necessary for experienced surgeons, I would encourage most physicians to use it. Also, the endotracheal tube should not be removed before the very end of the procedure and after correct placement of the tracheostomy tube is confirmed bronchoscopically and/or by unobstructed introduction of a suction catheter through the tube, normal chest movements, and expected ventilatory parameters. The bronchoscope may be used to suction blood clots, which can cause major airway occlusion, and also to obtain sputum cultures if indicated.

Bleeding is usually not a problem, and I routinely do not use electrocoagulation. On occasion, however, injury to an anterior vessel or the thyroid may cause bleeding through the wound. In most cases, one needs to complete the procedure fast to prevent blood from draining into the airway and achieve hemostasis by compression of the tracheostomy tube against the track. It is very rare that bleeding will persist, and under such circumstances the incision should be enlarged and the wound explored at the bedside or ideally in the operating room. Superficial bleeders may easily be suture ligated.

A common error is not withdrawing the endotracheal tube far enough, leading to impalement of the tube/balloon (or even the bronchoscope) with the finder needle.

Tube dislodgement may be a catastrophic complication, particularly if it occurs early after the operation (21). For this reason, the tube should be secured in place by sutures and a tape. Morbidly obese patients with particularly thick necks may need longer tracheostomy tubes.

PERCUTANEOUS GASTROSTOMY

Indications

A gastrostomy is required for patients who cannot be fed through the mouth because of inability to swallow, prolonged intubation, obstructing lesions of the pharynx or esophagus, or extensive neck operations. Although short-term nutrition can be offered through a nasogastric tube, a gastrostomy is preferred for longer needs.

Technique

The epigastrium and left upper quadrant are prepared. The procedure starts with an esophagogastroscopy and insufflation of the stomach, so that it apposes the anterior abdominal wall. An appropriate site of placement is selected by applying digital pressure on the skin, which is seen through the gastroscope as an indentation to the stomach. Transillumination should also be possible at the selected site of placement. A long needle covered by a plastic sheath is introduced through the skin and abdominal muscles into the stomach (Fig. 34.21). The needle is withdrawn and the plastic sheath left in place. A snare is introduced through the appropriate port of the gastroscope. A guidewire is placed in the stomach through the plastic sheath and grasped by the snare (Fig. 34.22). The gastroscope, snare, and guidewire are withdrawn out of the mouth. The guidewire is disengaged from the snare and tied to the tip of a percutaneous gastrostomy tube. A 2-cm incision is made on

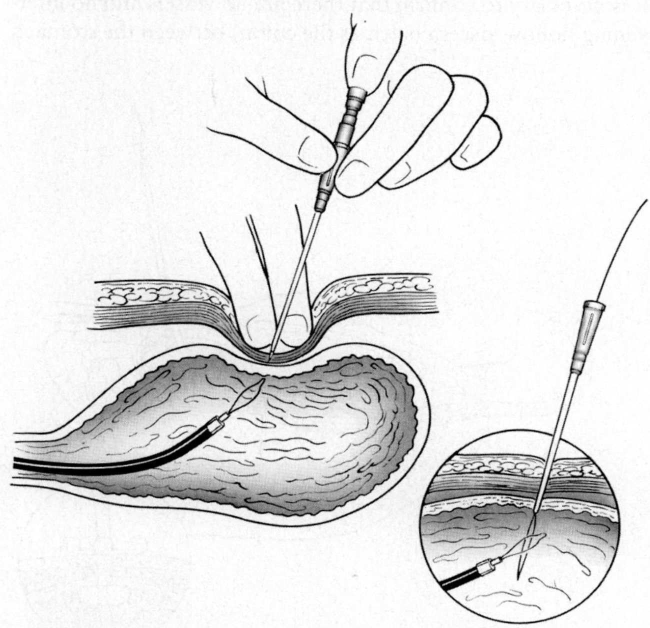

FIGURE 34.21. Insertion of needle into the stomach under endoscopic guidance.

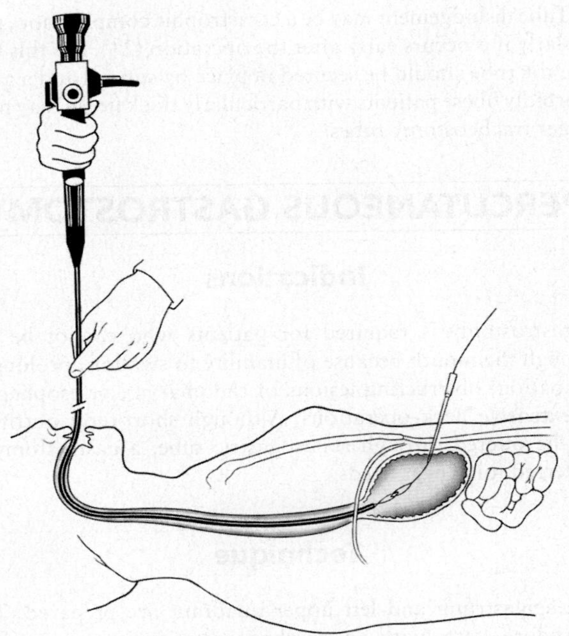

FIGURE 34.22. Guidewire snared and pulled with gastroscope through mouth.

the skin, and the guidewire is pulled. In this way, the gastrostomy tube is also pulled back into the mouth and, through the esophagus and stomach, out of the skin (Fig. 34.23). The gastroscope is reintroduced into the stomach and confirms correct placement of the tube. The tube is secured by placing a flange and suturing it to the skin. It can be used within 6 hours for medication and 12 hours for feeds.

Pitfalls and Complications

It is necessary to confirm that there are no vessels and no intervening hollow viscera (such as the colon) between the stomach and anterior abdominal wall. The indentation created by digital pressure should be clearly evident by the gastroscope, and transillumination at that site should be possible (22). In this way, bleeding or inadvertent injuries are avoided.

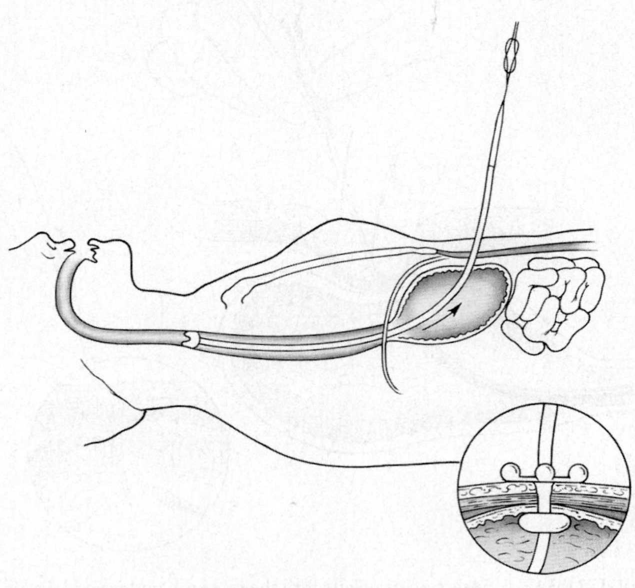

FIGURE 34.23. Gastrostomy tube pulled through stomach.

Infection of the wound should be recognized early and can be avoided with strict sterile technique. Usually, the tube does not need to be removed. The infection is treated by opening the wound and administering antibiotics. There is a suggestion that the initial tract should not be "tight" and that a larger skin wound from the beginning prevents infection (23). I do not agree and always create a small wound that is only large enough to accommodate the tube.

Tube dislodgement may occur either if the stomach is under tension (e.g., on a patient with hiatal hernia or with adhesions) or because the tube was not secured adequately and was inadvertently pulled (24). Both complications are usually preventable and should be avoided by recognizing that the anatomy is not favorable for a gastrostomy or suturing the gastrostomy tube adequately to the skin.

ABDOMINAL PRESSURE MONITORING

Indications

Patients at risk of or developing abdominal compartment syndrome should have the intra-abdominal pressures measured routinely. Abdominal hypertension, the elevation of pressure in the abdominal cavity due to bleeding or visceral swelling, leads to compromise of cardiac output, tissue perfusion, and ventilation, all eventually resulting in death if untreated (25). Clinical diagnosis is important, as the experienced physician will recognize a tense abdomen in the presence of hypotension, oliguria, and high airway pressures. Multiple methods have been described to monitor the intra-abdominal pressure. The most widely accepted method is the measurement of bladder pressure because of the logical assumption that the intraperitoneal pressure is transmitted on the bladder wall. Pressures below 10 cm H_2O are considered normal, 10 to 15 acceptable for postoperative patients, 15 to 20 worrisome and possibly in need of action, and over 20 as cause for decompression in most cases (26). This technique is described below.

Technique

Presumably the bladder is empty because such patients always have a Foley catheter. With the patient lying flat and under aseptic technique, a three-way stopcock is connected to a syringe and pressure monitor. Fifty to 100 mL of saline are injected into the bladder, and the stopcock is opened toward the pressure monitor. It is important to level the monitor in advance, so that the 0 mark corresponds to the level of the pubic symphysis (see Fig. 73.3 in Secondary and Tertiary Triage of the Trauma Patient). There is currently in the market a system that allows continuous measurement of pressures without interrupting the continuity of the Foley circuit and therefore decreasing the risk of urinary infection.

An easy and simple technique that does not require any instruments is the U-tube technique. According to it, the Foley

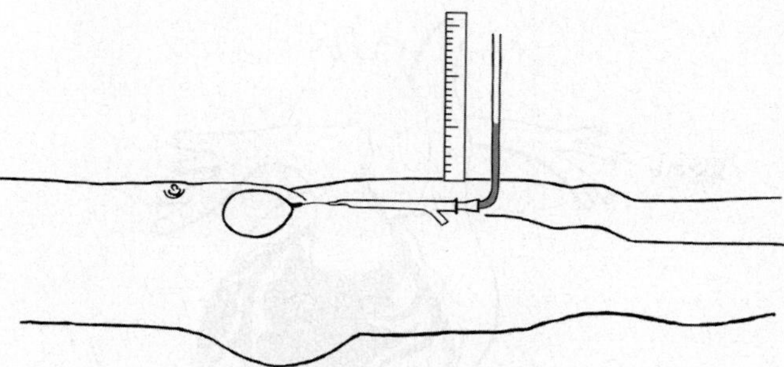

FIGURE 34.24. Measurement of intra-abdominal pressure using column of urine/water in the Foley catheter tubing.

is elevated while allowing a U-loop to form. If there is not enough urine in the tube, saline needs to be injected. The column of urine or injected fluid that forms is measured between the pubic symphysis and meniscus (Fig. 34.24). This measurement represents the abdominal pressure.

Pitfalls and Complications

The most dangerous pitfall is the exclusive reliance on bladder pressure measurements. Clinical examination should always be the principal reason for continued observation or immediate decompression. Bladder pressure measurements should only support the clinical diagnosis.

PERICARDIOCENTESIS

Indication

The pericardial space can accommodate large volumes of fluid if accumulation occurs over a long period of time, whereas cardiac tamponade develops with even small quantities of fluid; it thus happens abruptly. Pericardiocentesis is indicated to treat tamponade or diagnose the nature of chronic fluid (27). The latter is performed under ultrasonographic guidance. The former will be described below, although pericardiocentesis for traumatic tamponade is rarely useful. Unless the patient is in a remote area with difficult access to a trauma center, pericardiocentesis is not indicated; rapid sternotomy and control of the bleeding is.

Technique

With the patient supine, a standard pericardiocentesis kit or, in true emergencies, a central line kit can be used. A hollow needle is inserted approximately 1 cm below the costal margin and slightly to the left of the midline. The direction is toward the left shoulder. The needle is advanced slowly under the rib (Fig. 34.25). Electrocardiographic monitoring is possible by attaching an alligator clip to the needle. ST-segment elevations indicate contact of the needle with the epicardium. Aspiration of fluid or blood obviously indicates that the needle is in the pericardial sac. Aspiration of blood relieves the pericardial tamponade, and a guidewire is inserted through the needle. Using a

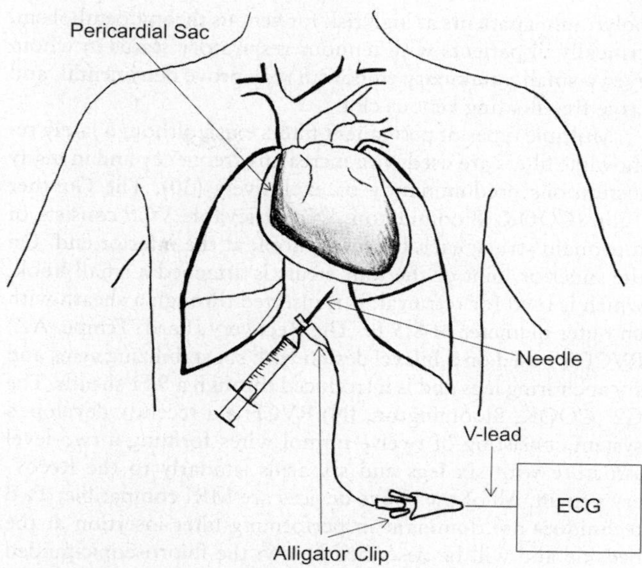

FIGURE 34.25. Technique of pericardiocentesis.

Seldinger technique, a catheter is inserted and used to withdraw further fluid or blood over time, if needed. With wide availability of portable ultrasound machines, emergent tapping of pericardial space may be safer than the previously used "blind" technique as described above.

Pitfalls and Complications

Pericardiocentesis is a potentially dangerous technique, if performed blindly (28). When done by radiologic guidance for stable conditions, little risk if involved. When performed under emergency situations for presumed cardiac tamponade, there is risk of injuring the heart, particularly if the clinical diagnosis of tamponade is not correct and the space between the pericardium and epicardium is very narrow. Additionally, misplacement of the needle—most typically under the heart—is not unusual. As mentioned previously, blind pericardiocentesis for traumatic injury purposes has been nearly abandoned in urban hospital settings.

PERCUTANEOUS INFERIOR VENA CAVA FILTER PLACEMENT

Indications

Inferior vena cava filter (VCF) use has met an explosive growth for the treatment and prophylaxis of pulmonary embolism (29). The evidence about its effectiveness is contradictory, another interesting medical example of how standard of care is formed in the absence of solid evidence. Absolute indications for filter placement are as follows: recurrent pulmonary embolism despite anticoagulation, contraindications to anticoagulation in the presence of pulmonary embolism or proximal deep venous thrombosis, and complications of anticoagulation prompting its cessation. Relative indications include polytrauma patients at high risk for venous thromboembolism, critically ill patients with tenuous respiratory status in whom even a small pulmonary embolism may prove detrimental, and large free-floating venous clot.

Multiple types of permanent filters exist, although lately removable filters are used with increasing frequency and in many institutions predominantly or exclusively (30). The Gunther Tulip (COOK, Bloomington, IN) retrievable VCF consists of four main struts, each bearing a hook at the inferior end. On the superior joint of the four struts is attached a small hook, which is used for retrieval. It is inserted through a sheath with an outer diameter of 8.5 Fr. The Recovery (Bard, Tempe, AZ) RVCF is based on a bilevel design with six stabilizing arms and six anchoring legs and is introduced through a 9 Fr sheath. The G2 (COOK, Bloomington, IN) RVCF is a recently developed system consisting of twelve nitinol wires forming a two-level structure with six legs and six arms similarly to the Recovery system. All of the above devices are MRI compatible. Two techniques are dominant in performing filter insertion at the bedside and will be described below: the fluoroscopic-guided and the endovascular ultrasound-guided techniques.

Technique

Fluoroscopy Guided

After a screening duplex ultrasound is performed to examine for femoral venous clots, portable fluoroscopy is used to define the L2-4 lumbar region. The site of venous access is selected—typically the left or right femoral vein—and venous cannulation is performed using a Seldinger technique. A 4 or 5 Fr angiographic catheter is advanced over a guidewire into the inferior vena cava and up to the second lumbar vertebra. Contrast material is injected, and the cava is imaged to delineate its anatomy and size. In particular, the renal veins are defined as the landmark below which the filter should be placed. After venography is completed, the pigtail catheter is exchanged for the sheath, which is inserted over a dilator. The sheath is positioned under the renal veins, and the filter carrier system is advanced into the sheath. The filter is then deployed, completion venography is performed, and the sheath is withdrawn. The filter sits caudad to the renal veins (Fig. 34.26).

Intravascular Ultrasonographic (IVUS) Guided (31)

Insertion is usually performed through a right femoral vein approach. A micropuncture is made in the vein using a 4 Fr catheter, and a 0.035 wire is introduced. An 8 Fr sheath is inserted into the inferior vena cava, and the IVUS (In-Vision Gold, Volcano Corp, Rancho Cordova, CA) is advanced over the wire through the iliac venous system up to the level of the right atrium. Then, it is slowly withdrawn to evaluate the inferior vena cava in a retrograde fashion. The right renal artery and bilateral veins are visualized, and the maximum diameter of the vena cava is measured. After a second puncture in the right common femoral vein, the delivery sheath for a VCF is introduced over a 0.035 guidewire. The sheath and then the VCF are advanced to the level of the renal veins. Deployment is performed under direct IVUS visualization. Confirmation of correct placement below the renal and above the iliac veins is established ultrasonographically. The catheters and sheaths are removed and direct pressure held over the femoral puncture sites. A postinsertion plain radiograph is routinely performed to verify correct placement at the L2-4 level. This technique is valuable in patients at risk for renal failure due to avoidance of radiocontrast dye.

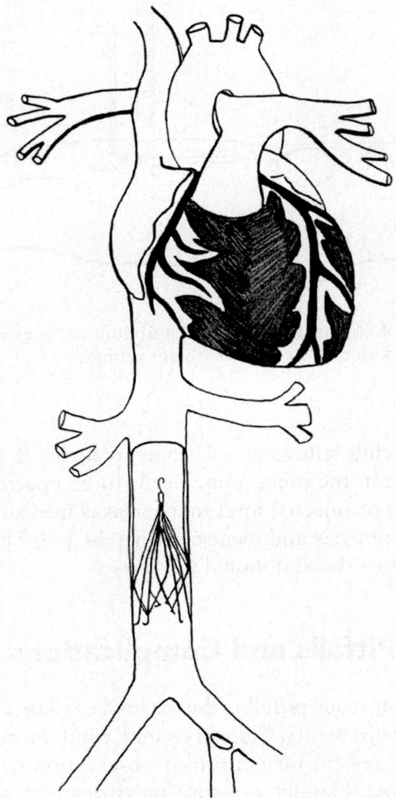

FIGURE 34.26. Position of vena cavae filters, caudad to the renal veins.

Pitfalls and Complications

The potential for complications starts with the venous access. Access complications (the same as any central venous access) include bleeding, hematoma, arteriovenous fistula, hemopneumothorax, and cardiac dysrhythmias. Misplacement outside the IVC or at an incorrect location is a common complication of insertion and has been reported to be as high as 4.6% (32). Locations for filter misplacement include renal veins, gonadal veins, or unintended suprarenal placement. Insertion site venous thrombosis and vena cava occlusion are potential complications of filters. Access via the internal jugular or subclavian vein results in a lower incidence of thrombosis when compared to femoral access. Caval thrombosis rates do not appear to vary significantly among the available filters. Some reports show very high rates of caval thrombosis (up to 25%) while others for the same filter are much lower (33). Two explanations for this disparity are: different patient populations (i.e., trauma versus malignancy) and provider related. It is expected that with the increasing use of retrievable VCFs, the rate of caval thrombosis will decrease. Pulmonary embolism in the presence of an IVC filter has been reported in 3% to 7% of patients after filter placement in series >50 patients (34). Guidewire entrapment occurs during placement of central venous and pulmonary artery catheters as well as during catheter exchanges. Attempts at removal of an entrapped item can lead to filter displacement and vessel damage when excessive force is applied. Straight guidewires should be used for all new central venous catheters in patients with indwelling IVC filters.

References

1. Gillman L, Leslie G, Williams T, et al. Adverse events experienced while transferring the critically ill patient from the emergency department to the intensive care unit. *Emerg Med J.* 2006;23:858–861.
2. Venkataraman ST, Orr RA. Intrahospital transport of critically ill patients. *Crit Care Clin N Am.* 1992;8:525–531.
3. Warren J, Fromm RE Jr, Orr RA, et al. American College of Critical Care Medicine. Guidelines for the inter- and intrahospital transport of critically ill patients. *Crit Care Med.* 2004;32:256–262.
4. Barba C. The intensive care unit as an operating room. *Surg Clin N Am.* 2000;80:957–973.
5. Van Natta TL, Morris JA, Eddy VA, et al. Elective bedside surgery in critically injured patients is safe and cost-effective. *Ann Surg.* 1998;227:618–624.
6. Dalbec DL, Krome RL. Thoracostomy. *Em Med Clin N Am.* 1986;4:441–457.
7. *Advanced Trauma Life Support Manual: Thoracic Trauma.* Chicago, IL: American College of Surgeons; 1993.
8. Demetriades D. Tube thoracotomy. In: Shoemaker WC, Demetriades D, Velmahos G, eds. *Procedures and Monitoring for the Critically Ill.* Philadelphia, PA: WB Saunders; 2002:47–53.
9. Demetriades D, Breekon V, Breckon C, et al. Antibiotic prophylaxis in penetrating injuries of the chest. *Ann R Coll Surg Engl.* 1991;73:348–351.
10. Vassiliu P, Velmahos GC, Toutouzas KG. Timing, safety, and efficacy of thoracoscopic evacuation of undrained post-traumatic hemothorax. *Am Surg.* 2001;67:1165–1169.
11. Kimbrell JB, Yamzon J, Petorne P, et al. Intrapleural thrombolysis for the management of undrained traumatic hemothorax: a prospective observational study. *J Trauma.* 2007;62:1175–1180.
12. Root HD, Hauser CW, McKinley CR, et al. Diagnostic peritoneal lavage. *Surgery.* 1965;5:633–636.
13. Kuncir E, Velmahos GC. Diagnostic peritoneal aspiration: the foster child of DPL. *Intern J Surg.* 2007;5:167–171.
14. Velmahos GC, Demetriades D, Stewart M, et al. Open versus closed diagnostic peritoneal lavage: a comparison on safety, rapidity, efficacy. *J R Coll Surg Edinb.* 1998;43:235–238.
15. Goumas P, Kokkinis K, Petrocheilos J, et al. Cricothyroidotomy and the anatomy of the cricothyroid space. An autopsy study. *J Laryngol Otol.* 1997;111:354–356.
16. Cornwell EE, III. Cricothyroidotomy. In: Shoemaker WC, Demetriades D, Velmahos GV, eds. *Procedures and Monitoring for the Critically Ill.* Philadelphia, PA: WB Saunders, 2002:43–45.
17. Wright MJ, Greenberg DE, Hunt JP, et al. Surgical cricothyroidotomy in trauma patients. *South Med J.* 2003;96:465–467.
18. Friedman Y, Fildes J, Mizock B, et al. Comparison of percutaneous and surgical tracheostomies. *Chest.* 1996;110:480–485.
19. Velmahos GC, Gomez H, Boicey CM, et al. Bedside percutaneous tracheostomy is safe and easy to teach: prospective evaluation of a modification of the current techniques on 100 patients. *World J Sur.* 2000;24:1109–1115.
20. Dulguerov P, Gysin C, Perneger TV, et al. Percutaneous or surgical tracheostomy: a meta-analysis. *Crit Care Med.* 1999;27:1617–1625.
21. Velmahos GC, Demetriades D. Common bedside procedures in the intensive care unit. In: Shoemaker WC, Ayres SM, Grenvik A, et al., eds. *Textbook of Critical Care.* 4th ed. Philadelphia, PA: WB Saunders; 2000:114–119.
22. Miller RE, Castlemain B, Lacqua FJ, et al. Percutaneous endoscopic gastrostomy. Results in 316 patients and review of literature. *Surg Endosc.* 1989; 3:186–190.
23. Sharma VK, Howden CW. Meta-analysis of randomized, controlled trials of antibiotic prophylaxis before percutaneous endoscopic gastrostomy. *Am J Gastroenterol.* 2001;96:1951–1952.
24. Shallman RW, Norfleet RG, Hardache JM. Percutaneous endoscopic gastrostomy feeding tube migration and impaction in the abdominal wall. *Gastrointest Endosc.* 1988;34:367–368.
25. Diebel LN, Wilson RF, Dulchavsky SA, et al. Effect of increased intra-abdominal pressure on hepatic, arterial, portal, venous microcirculatory blood flow. *J Trauma.* 1992;33:279–283.
26. World Society of the Abdominal Compartment Syndrome. www.wsacs.org.
27. Allen KB, Faber LP, Warren WH, et al. Pericardial effusion: subxiphoid pericardiostomy versus percutaneous catheter drainage. *Ann Thor Surg.* 1999;67:437–440.
28. Focht G, Becker RC. Pericardiocentesis. In: Rippe JM, Irwin RS, Fink MP, et al., eds. *Procedures and Techniques in Intensive Care Medicine.* Boston, MA: Little & Brown; 1995:111–116.
29. Sing RF, Smith CH, Miles WS, et al. Preliminary results of bedside inferior vena cava filter placement: safe and cost-effective. *Chest.* 1998;114:315–316.
30. Karmy-Jones R, Jurkovich G, Velmahos GC, et al. Practice patterns and outcomes after retrievable vena cava filters in trauma patients: an AAST multicenter study. *J Trauma.* 2007;62:17–25.
31. Garrett JV, Passman MA, Guzman RJ, et al. Expanding options for bedside placement of inferior vena cava filters with intravascular ultrasound when transabdominal duplex ultrasound imaging is inadequate. *Ann Vasc Surg.* 2004;18:329–334.
32. Kazmers A, Ramnauth S, Williams M. Intraoperative insertion of Greenfield filters: lessons learned in a personal series of 152 cases. *Am Surg.* 2002;68(10):877–882.
33. AbuRahma AF, Robinson PA, Boland JP, et al. Therapeutic and prophylactic vena caval interruption for pulmonary embolism: caval and venous insertion site patency. *Ann Vasc Surg.* 1993;7:561–568.
34. Geisinger MA, Zelch MG, Risius B. Recurrent pulmonary embolism after Greenfield filter placement. *Radiology.* 1987;165:383–384.

CHAPTER 35 ■ INTERVENTIONAL RADIOLOGY IN THE CRITICAL CARE UNIT

KEITH R. PETERS • SCOTT W. PETERSON

Image-guided procedures have increasingly become the standard care due to their minimally invasive nature and comparable or improved outcomes relative to similar procedures without image guidance. Many of these procedures, such as drain placement, can be performed at the bedside allowing unstable patients to remain in the intensive care unit. Procedures that require transport to the radiology department can often be performed with mild sedation or monitored anesthesia care (MAC), without the need for general anesthesia.

Some of the procedures that will be discussed require advanced techniques acquired during fellowship training. For these procedures, the indications, patient preparation, expected outcomes, and potential complications will be discussed. Other procedures, however, may simply represent the use of image guidance to improve outcome and safety of standard clinical procedures, as in the case of ultrasound guided thoracentesis. In discussing these procedures, a more detailed technical description will be provided to assist the clinician performing procedures following appropriate training and supervision. The primary skill to be acquired in the performance of image-guided procedures is the ability to translate the 2-D images that are obtained to the 3-D space in which the procedure is performed. So, as this chapter is read, please consider how some existing procedures could be modified and improved with the use of image guidance and which procedures could be referred to radiology rather than requiring a more open procedure.

Imaging devices that may be used include ultrasound (US), computed tomography (CT), fluoroscopy, and digital subtraction imaging (DSI). All use ionizing radiation, with the exception of ultrasound, and therefore must be performed in areas with appropriate radiation shielding, usually in the radiology department. In some cases, a portable fluoroscopic device in the shape of a "C"—typically described as a portable C-arm—can be brought to the intensive care area provided sufficient radiation shielding is provided the other patients and health care workers, and provided a fluoroscopic-compatible bed/table is available. Federal law requires the use of devices producing ionizing radiation to be supervised by a physician; however, hospital credentialing bodies may have specific training requirements that must also be met. Such is not usually the case with ultrasound. The options for ultrasound devices range from small highly portable handheld units that may be adequate for vascular access and for some drainage procedures, to highly advanced systems with the ability to perform measurements, evaluate vascular flow, and perform 3-D reconstructions. Most ultrasound devices are supplied with multiple probes that vary in frequency of sound wave emitted and device shape, allowing for evaluation of various viewing windows and depths of view.

As each of these procedures is discussed, the more standard imaging methods used at our institution will be described, followed by a brief notation of other possible modalities, for completeness.

PERCUTANEOUS FLUID AND ABSCESS DRAINAGE

Percutaneous drainage is an accepted technique for removal of fluid from most locations in the body. The need for exploratory surgery has decreased with improved imaging techniques such as CT, magnetic resonance imaging (MRI), and ultrasound, which can precisely localize a fluid collection. These imaging modalities can then be used to guide the drainage procedure. Combination of percutaneous drainage and antibiotic administration can frequently resolve the infection without the need for surgical intervention. And in cases where subsequent surgery is required, the drains placed under image guidance can be used as a guide to the abscess and potentially decrease the area and extent of surgical dissection.

Evaluation

CT, MRI, and ultrasound can be used in the detection and localization of fluid collections. Ultrasound has the advantage of portability and is very good in the evaluation of fluid in the thorax and in the evaluation of subdiaphragmatic and paracolic collections in the abdomen. However, it is limited by collections of air and is therefore often not able to evaluate mediastinal or central abdominal regions. MRI can localize areas of pathology and fluid collections but is often a less optimal examination due to scan time, exam degradation due to patient motion, and limited availability of interventionally oriented MR scanners and MR-compatible devices for subsequent fluid drainage. Therefore, CT is usually the modality of choice for both localization and drainage.

Image Guidance

As previously stated, most abdominal and central thoracic drainage procedures are performed with CT guidance. Ultrasound can be used for pleural, subpleural, subdiaphragmatic, and paracolic collections. The decision is not only based on location and size but also on operator preference. Imaging must be adequate to define a pathway to the fluid collection. A critical concept is to ensure that the bowel and significant vasculature structures are not entered, and this is best ensured by CT visualization.

Patient Preparation

Review of the patient's medications and coagulation profile is necessary to evaluate potential bleeding risk; we require normalization of prothrombin time (PT) and partial thromboplastin time (PTT). The international normalized ratio (INR) must be less than 1.5, and platelets should be in excess of 75,000 to 100,000 cells/μL. With the potential exception of a thoracentesis or pleural catheter placement, most of these procedures require conscious sedation with an intravenous (IV) narcotic such as fentanyl or hydromorphone, in combination with a short-acting hypnotic sedative such as midazolam. Constant physiologic monitoring is required. Antibiotic coverage should be instituted prior to abscess manipulation due to the concern for precipitation of a septic episode. Previous concerns regarding alterations of culture results have not been sufficiently documented and are outweighed by the potential for life-threatening sepsis. However, if there is low suspicion of infection, such as the case with a large pleural fluid collection, and the patient's white count is within normal limits, antibiotic coverage may not be necessary.

Equipment

Initial access to a fluid collection is usually with an 18-, 20-, or 22-gauge needle. This guide needle can then be used to allow for parallel placement of a drainage catheter with direct stick trocar technique or a wire can be inserted through the guide needle to allow for placement of a drainage catheter using the over-the-wire Seldinger technique.

For drainage catheters, various catheter shapes and sizes are available. Dual-lumen sump catheters, accordion catheters, and locking loop catheters can be used. The French size of the tube is determined by the type and viscosity of the fluid being drained. An 8 to 12 French catheter can be used to drain a sterile pleural effusion; however, a 16 to 20 French catheter may be required for an abdominal abscess.

Also available for very-short-term use is a Safe-T-Centesis catheter (Cardinal Health, McGraw Park, IL). This is an all-inclusive kit that can be used for draining presumed sterile fluid collections in the chest or abdomen, and in which a drain will not need to be kept in place. This kit also has the advantage of sharps protection in all of the devices (Fig. 35.1A–C).

Drainage Technique

Once localized, an access pathway is identified on CT or ultrasound. The pathway needs to be clear of adjacent solid organs and bowel. A skin entry site is selected and sterilely prepped; in our institution, the prep of choice is 2% chlorhexidine solution in 70% isopropyl alcohol.

Under ultrasound guidance, the needle can be visualized as it is advanced. With CT guidance, small incremental advancements of the needle are made and the position evaluated with repeat imaging. If a Hawkins blunt needle system is used, a sharp inner cannula is used to penetrate the skin and muscle with the blunt cannula used along the remainder of the pathway to displace small vessels. Once at the margin of the collection, the sharp inner cannula is used for final entry. When the fluid collection is entered, a small amount of the material can be aspirated and evaluated by Gram stain to determine if it is infected. This can often be determined by the gross

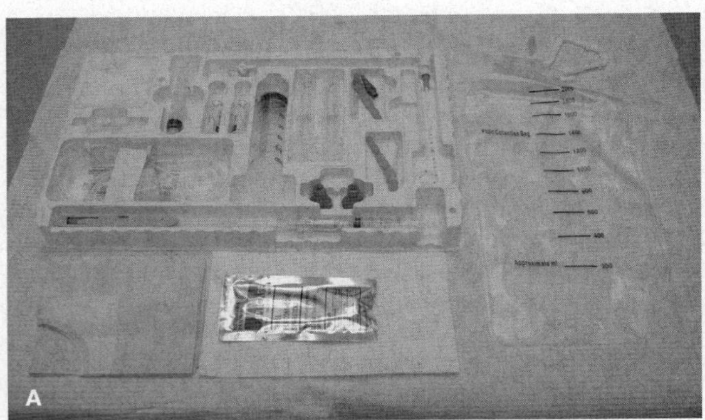

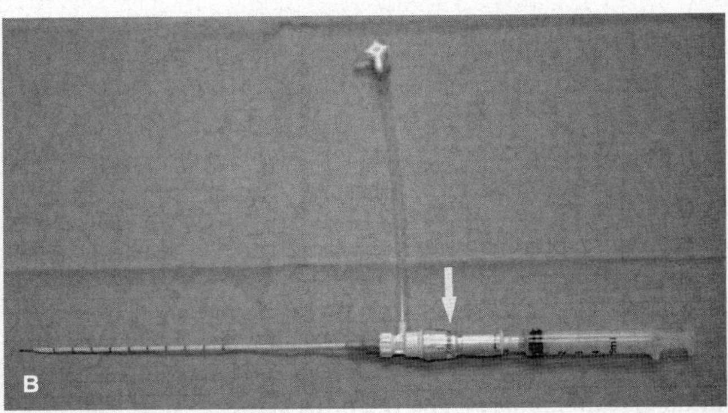

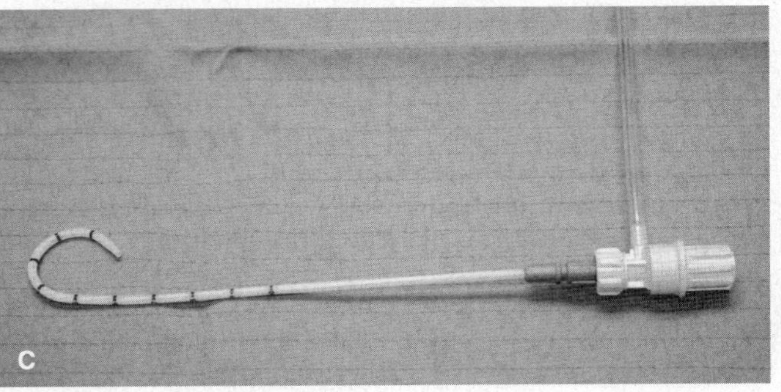

FIGURE 35.1. Typical drainage tray. **A:** Layout and contents of the Safe-T-Centesis Catheter Drainage Tray. The kit includes patient prep supplies, a 6 Fr temporary pigtail drainage catheter, and a fluid collection system. **B:** Safe-T-Centesis device. At the juncture of the syringe and the drainage catheter is an indicator (*arrow*) that signals the operator when the needle tip enters a free cavity with a color change and an audible click. **C:** Pigtail catheter unrestrained in the shape it will assume in free cavity.

examination of the material. A guidewire is advanced through the needle and coiled in the collection. Fascial dilators are then used to dilate the tract to at least the size of the planned drainage catheter. Finally the catheter is advanced over the wire into the collection, making sure that all side holes are in the collection. This process is monitored by serial CT imaging. When performed under ultrasound guidance for abscess entry, the guidewire and catheter placements are often monitored fluoroscopically if the procedure is performed in radiology. When the catheter is in the fluid collection and imaging has confirmed the position, the contents are completely aspirated. For sterile collections, such as a simple pleural effusion, the catheter can then be removed. For infected or recurrent collections, the drainage catheter is left in place and a drainage collection device attached. The catheter is also secured in place externally by suturing it to the skin with nonabsorbable suture; some institutions use commercially available adhesive devices (Figs. 35.2A–C and 35.3A, B).

An alternative method for catheter placement that can be used for larger and more superficial collections, where there is a larger access window, is the trocar technique. After placement of the guide/reference needle, a selected drainage catheter with its sharp stylet is advanced through a dermatotomy immediately adjacent to and in parallel with the reference needle. There is usually a decrease in resistance to the advancement of the drain when the collection is entered. The sharp stylet is removed, fluid aspirated to confirm position, and the catheter is advanced into the collection off of its internal stiffener and then coiled within the collection. Once drained, the collection is reimaged to ensure complete evacuation. This will also demonstrate the possible presence of loculated areas that must be drained by placement of additional catheters.

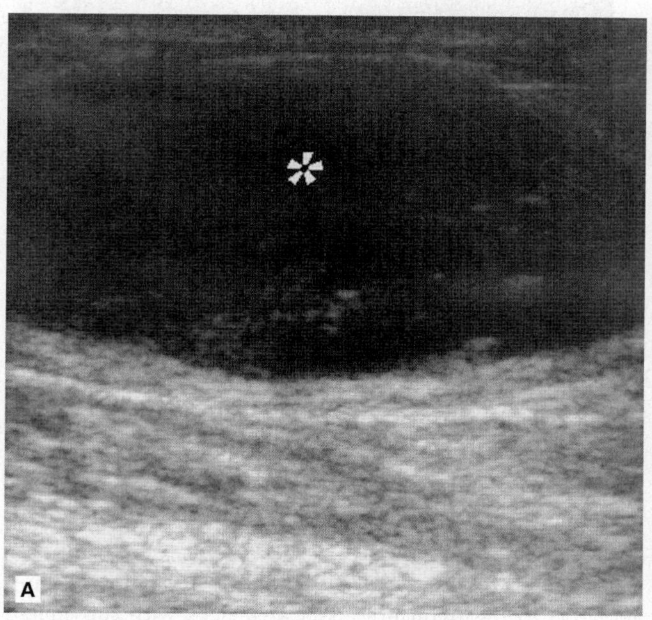

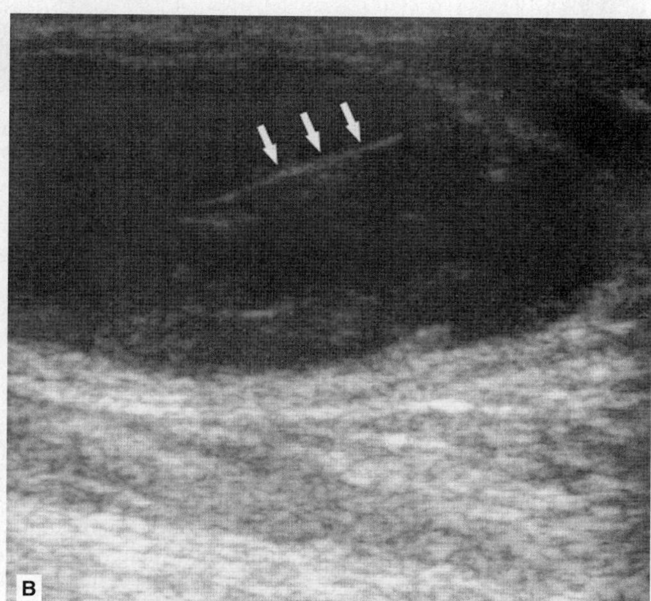

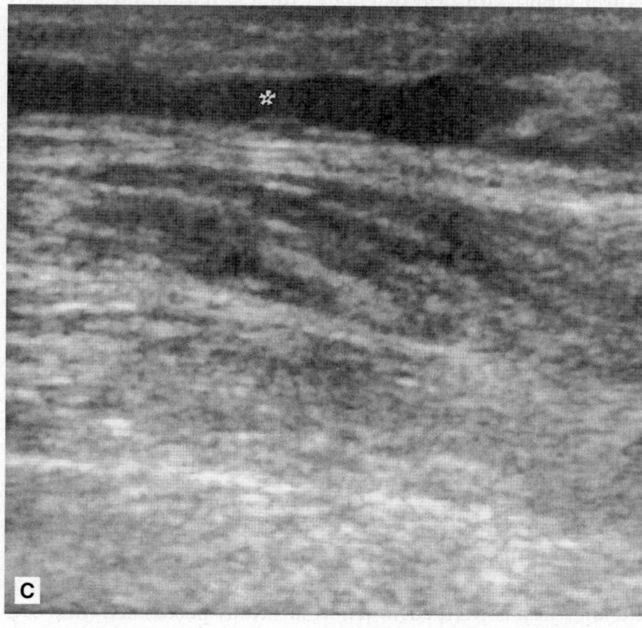

FIGURE 35.2. A 74-year-old patient on Coumadin developed a focal lower extremity area of swelling, erythema, and progressive pain adjacent to the knee following trauma. **A:** Ultrasound (US) examination demonstrates a 5.5-mL hypoechoic superficial fluid collection (*asterisk*). **B:** Hyperechoic needle (*arrows*) seen entering the fluid collection. **C:** Postevacuation US demonstration near complete drainage of the fluid collection (*asterisk*). The fluid was sterile and consistent with liquefied hematoma.

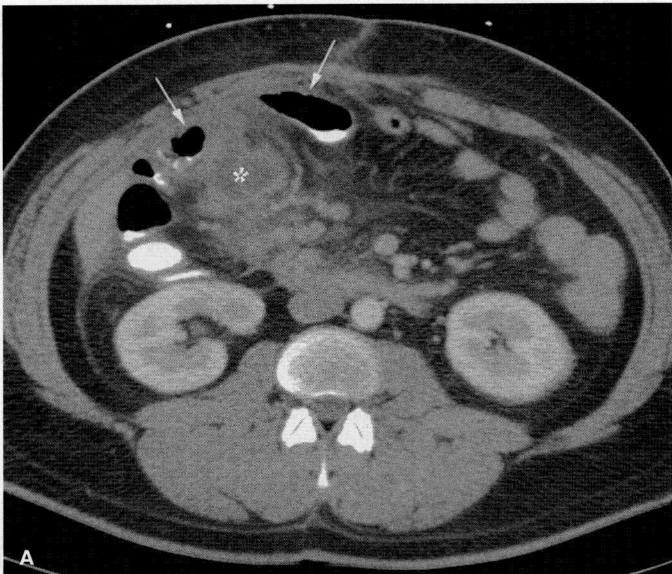

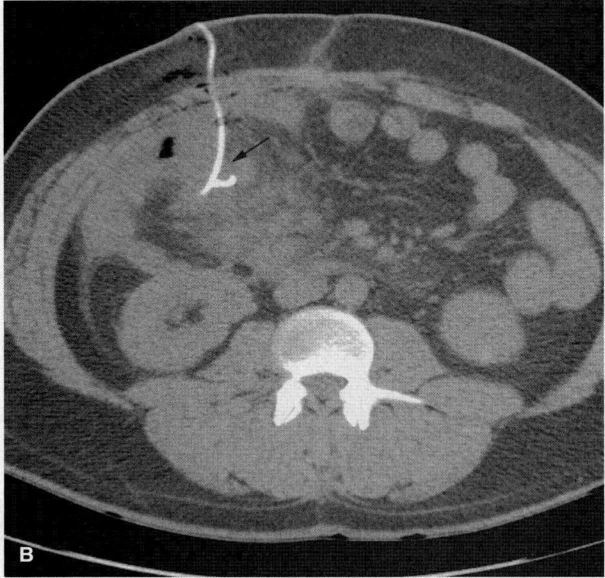

FIGURE 35.3. Patient with diverticular disease and mesenteric abscess. **A:** Close proximity of bowel loops (*arrows*) to the 4-mL fluid collection (*asterisk*). **B:** Required CT guidance for drain placement (*arrow*).

Postplacement Catheter Care

The catheter is connected to either a gravity drain or a suction device such as a Jackson-Pratt bulb. Output should be recorded by the nursing staff, and the catheter should be irrigated three times a day with sterile saline to maintain patency. The catheter needs to be evaluated daily to confirm patency, evaluate output, evaluate the skin entry site, and to monitor patient clinical status including temperature trend and white count.

End points to determine the time for catheter removal are as follows: decrease in the catheter output to less than 20 mL per day, normalization of temperature and white count, and overall clinical improvement of the patient. When these end points are achieved, the patient is usually reimaged and the tube withdrawn if the collection is no longer present. However, if after 2 to 3 days these end points are not achieved, repeat imaging should also be performed to determine the need for further intervention. Reported success rates for percutaneous abscess drainage are 90% to 100% (1–3) with a recurrence rate of 8% to 20%, most commonly related to early catheter removal (4).

Special Considerations

Abscess–Fistula Complex

This is a type of enteric abscess that should be suspected when high fluid output greater than 100 mL per day persists. In this scenario, follow-up evaluation may include injection of iodinated nonionic contrast under fluoroscopic guidance. Results of this study will help determine the need for catheter placement directly into the fistula or surgical intervention. This subgroup often requires 3 to 6 weeks of drainage in association with medical management and nutritional support.

Solid Organ Abscess Drainage

Hepatic, splenic, and renal abscesses can be drained percutaneously, although this sometimes requires an intercostal approach. The lowest possible intercostal level should be used if this approach is necessary to decrease the risk of pneumothorax or the potential spread of infection into the thorax, resulting in empyema. Also, due to the higher risk of bleeding with access into these organs, it is necessary to select the shortest pathway possible through normal tissue, to use a blunt needle system when traversing normal tissue, and to use smaller drainage catheters, usually 8 French. Simple needle aspiration of these collections is preferred over catheter drainage, especially when the collections are small (Fig. 35.4A–C).

Pancreatic Collections

Drainage of pancreatic fluid collections often require CT guidance due to the frequently associated ileus with subsequent overlying bowel loops. Therefore excellent opacification of bowel loops with oral or enteral tube administration of contrast is necessary. Pancreatic abscesses usually contain highly viscous material, which necessitates use of larger-bore catheters (greater than 16 French). Pancreatic pseudocysts usually require only an 8 to 10 French drainage catheter. Additionally, not all pseudocysts require drainage, as most spontaneously resolve. Factors influencing the decision to drain the collection include suspected infection, pain, or obstruction of adjacent bowel or bile duct. Successful pseudocyst drainage can be as high as 90%. However, the results of pancreatic abscess drainage are more variable, with reports of a success rate between 32% and 80%. This wide range is possibly due to difficulty in differentiation of infected pancreatic necrosis, which is difficult to treat, from a focal abscess (5).

Empyema

Drainage of an empyema can frequently be performed at the bedside under ultrasound guidance, with the patient's position dependent on his or her ability to assist and the exact location of the collection; a sitting position is often preferred. The collection is localized, entry site marked, site prepped, local anesthesia obtained, and dermatotomy performed followed

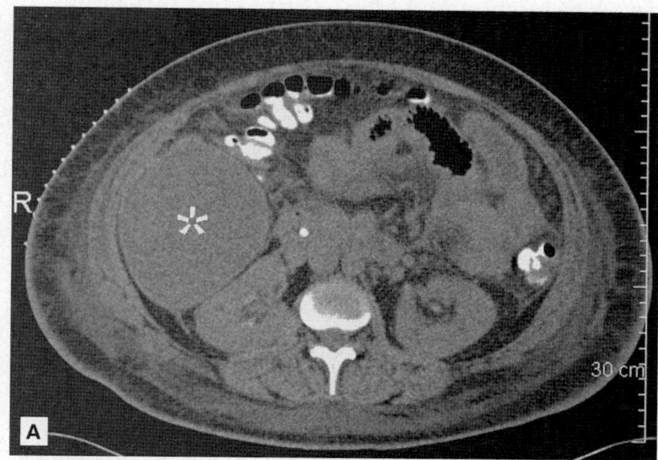

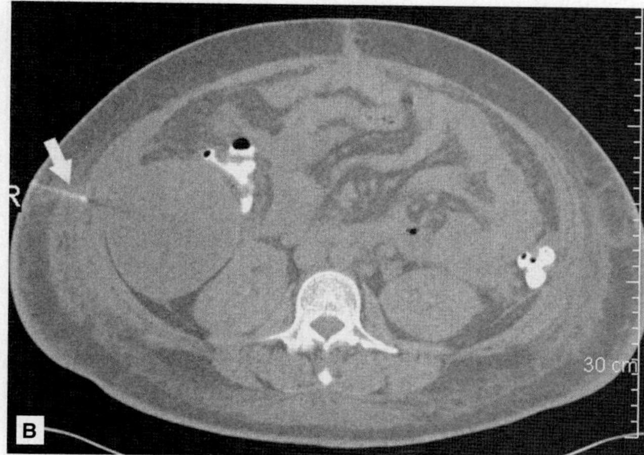

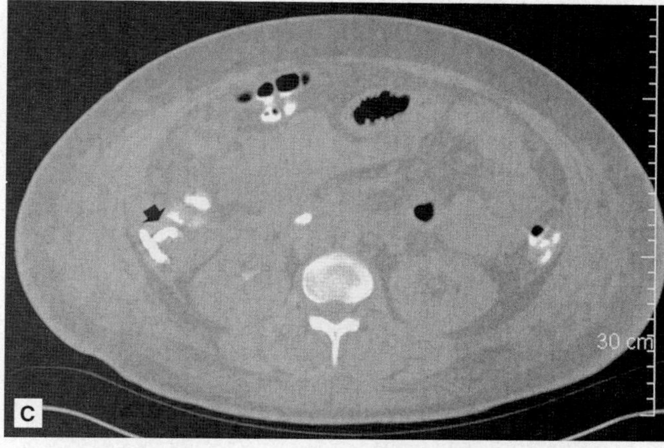

FIGURE 35.4. CT-guided drainage of infrahepatic abscess. **A:** CT scan through the fluid collection (*asterisk*) with localizer grid applied on the skin over the target. **B:** Following determination of pathway, entry site marking, sterile skin prep and drape, and local anesthesia the access needle is advanced under CT guidance into the fluid collection. Repeat CT is performed to evaluate needle path and depth (*arrow*). **C:** Postdrainage obtained at the same level as **A** shows loop of drainage catheter (*short arrow*) in markedly decompressed abscess cavity. (Case courtesy of Lauren Alexander, MD, Gainesville, FL.)

by deep blunt dissection. A 14 to 20 French catheter is then inserted, often with the trocar technique. The empyema is aspirated and the catheter connected to Pleur-Evac water seal pleural drainage system. The overall success rate for percutaneous drainage of empyema is 77% (6) (Fig. 35.5A–D).

Thick fluid collections may require the use of intrapleural thrombolytic injection such as t-PA, to disrupt fibrin septae. This can be accomplished with an infusion of rt-PA solution containing 2 to 6 mg of rt-PA in 50 to 250 mL of normal saline. This is infused daily for 1 to 3 days. There does not appear to be any significant systemic effect associated with this intralesional infusion of the thrombolytic medication, and there is an approximate 94% clinical improvement rate (7).

Diagnostic and Therapeutic Thoracentesis

Image-guided thoracentesis can easily be performed at the bedside with ultrasound. This is most frequently performed with the patient sitting on the side of the bed facing away from the operator. In some cases, due to severity of the patient's condition, this procedure may need to be performed with the patient supine. This can significantly increase the difficulty of the procedure, especially with smaller collections. This situation can be improved by placing the patient on a cardiopulmonary resuscitation (CPR) backboard to slightly elevate him or her off the bed, and by raising the head of bed as tolerated to drain more of the fluid into a focal dependent position near the diaphragm. Sedation is usually not required as sufficient pain control can be obtained with local anesthesia. Of note, CT may be required in some cases due to the small size and/or location of the fluid.

Diagnostic thoracentesis is often used to differentiate a transudate from an exudate, and in the case of an exudate, to evaluate for malignancy or infection. This diagnostic procedure can be performed with a 20 to 22 gauge needle. Ultrasound is used to localize the collection, and the site of entry is marked. This area is prepped and local anesthesia obtained. The needle is then advanced close to the superior rib margin at the selected intercostal space to avoid the neurovascular bundle that courses along the inferior margin of the rib. Once entered, sufficient pleural fluid is aspirated for laboratory analysis consisting of pH, Gram stain and culture, total protein, lactate dehydrogenase (LDH), glucose, and cytology. At completion of the procedure, the needle is removed and an air-occlusive dressing applied.

Therapeutic thoracentesis is usually requested due to dyspnea or in association with catheter placement for a chemical pleurodesis. A posterolateral approach is used to decrease patient discomfort when lying down and potentially pressing on the tube rather than a direct posterior approach, which is used in standard diagnostic thoracentesis. When a catheter will be necessary only during the short drainage procedure, we use the 6 French catheter that comes in the Safe-T-Centesis kit, with its three-way stopcock and internal valves to decrease the risk of pneumothorax. The fluid is then removed with syringe

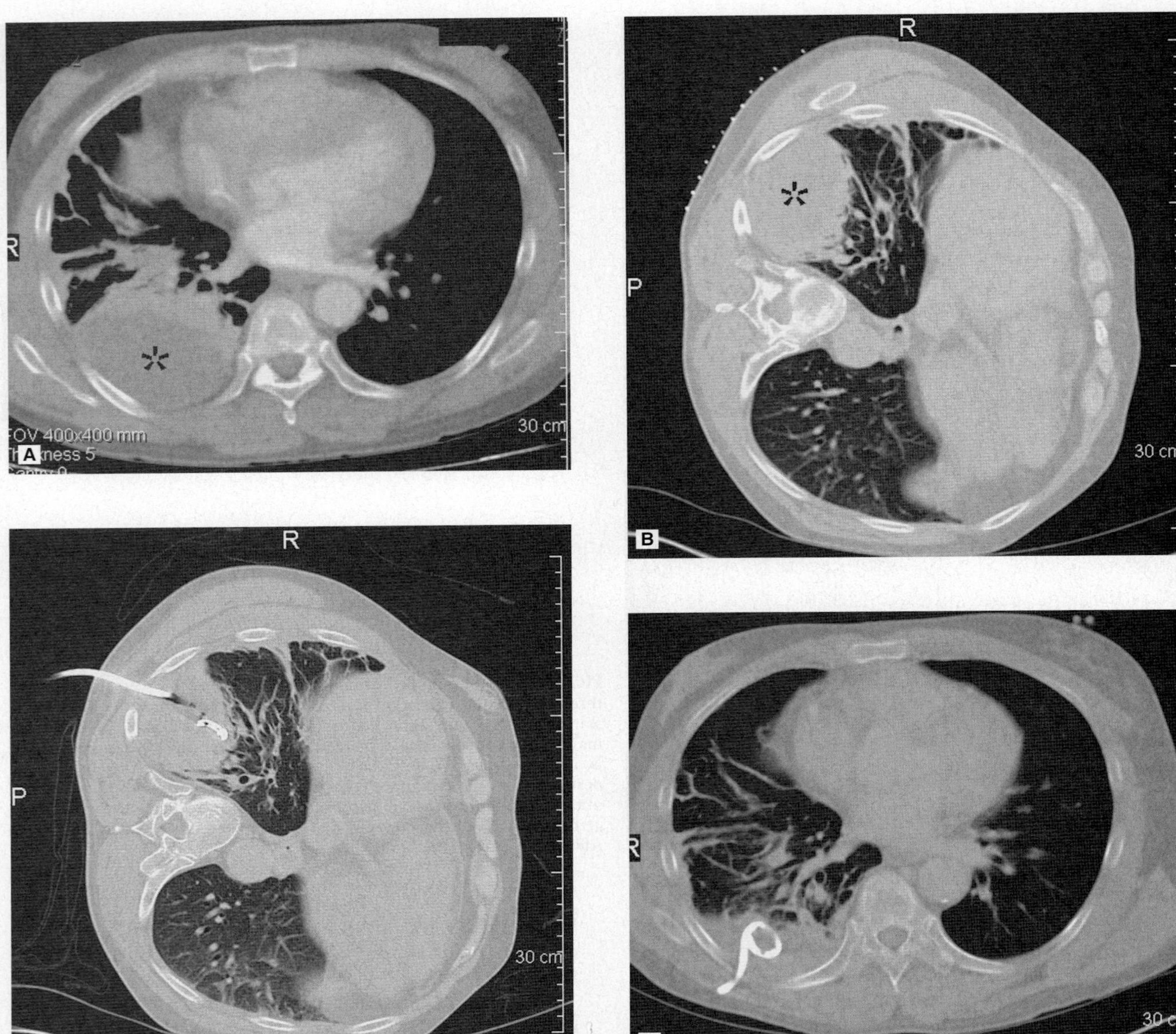

FIGURE 35.5. A 19-year-old patient with sepsis and cough. **A:** Axial CT at the level of the midchest demonstrates an 8.5-cm fluid collection in the right posterior hemithorax (*asterisk*) with compression atelectasis of the adjacent lung. Direct percutaneous access is blocked due to inferior margin of the scapula, overlying ribs, and aerated lung. **B:** Patient was placed in a left-side-down decubitus position. Change in position provides direct posterior access to the fluid collection. A localizer grid has been placed to mark site of access. **C:** Access gained with micropuncture needle system and then a 14 Fr drain placed over a wire. Fluid aspirated with syringe and then drain was secured in place and connected to suction bulb. **D:** Postdrain placement CT. (Case courtesy of Lauren Alexander, MD, Gainesville, FL.)

aspiration or by connection to a vacuum bottle that can be changed when full. Chest pain can occur with rapid fluid removal; however, this usually resolves with temporary cessation of the drainage and with subsequent resumption of the drainage procedure at a slower rate. Coughing often occurs toward the end of the procedure as the pleural surfaces become reapposed. When longer-term access is required, a 10 to 14 French tube is placed by either trocar or Seldinger technique and connected to Pleur-Evac water seal drainage system. The overall incidence of pneumothorax with ultrasound-guided procedures approximates 3% (Fig. 35.6).

If a pneumothorax occurs in association with thoracic intervention, or secondary to underlying lung disease, a chest tube/pleural catheter may be required. The indications for tube placement include size of pneumothorax greater than 25%, pain, shortness of breath, or progressive enlargement on serial radiography. These tubes are easily placed in the second or third intercostal space anteriorly. Our preference is to place an 8 French catheter under fluoroscopic guidance using the Seldinger technique to avoid injury to the adjacent lung. We gain access with a 4 French micropuncture system (Angio Dynamics, Queensbury, NY) followed by insertion of a 0.035

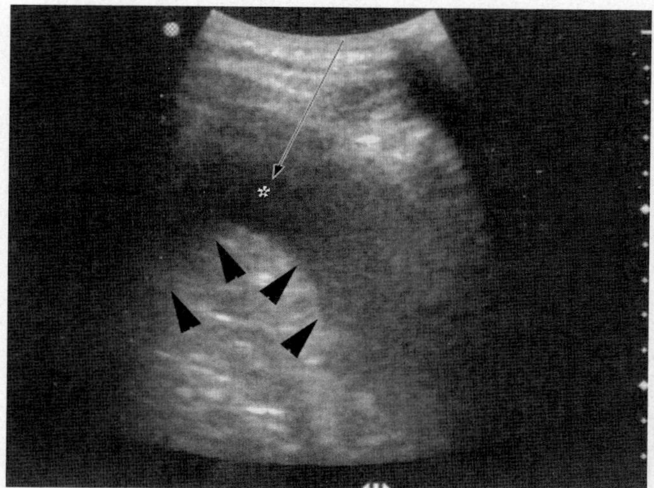

FIGURE 35.6. Ultrasound image showing typical appearance for thoracentesis guidance. The central target (pleural effusion) is identified by an *asterisk*, lung margin by *arrowheads*, and drainage catheter pathway with an *arrow*.

guidewire over which the chest tube is advanced. This is secured in place with nonabsorbable suture and covered with petroleum jelly gauze to decrease the risk of air leak. Most of the pneumothorax is aspirated using a 60-mL syringe with the aid of a three-way stopcock. Then the tube is connected to a Pleur-Evac drainage system as is done with surgically placed chest tubes. The pleural catheter remains in place until there is no significant residual pneumothorax and there is no evidence of air leak when the tube is connected to water seal (Fig. 35.7A–C).

Abdominal Paracentesis

Ultrasound or CT guidance can be used to drain diffuse or loculated fluid collections in the abdomen. In most cases, ultrasound is sufficient and can be performed at the bedside. The site of maximal fluid collection is localized without evidence of intervening loops of bowel, and this area is marked and prepped. The procedure can usually be performed with local anesthesia without sedation. The preference at our institution is to use the 6 French Safe-T-Centesis catheter kit. This drainage procedure can be performed for diagnostic and/or therapeutic purposes. When performed as a therapeutic procedure, the catheter and

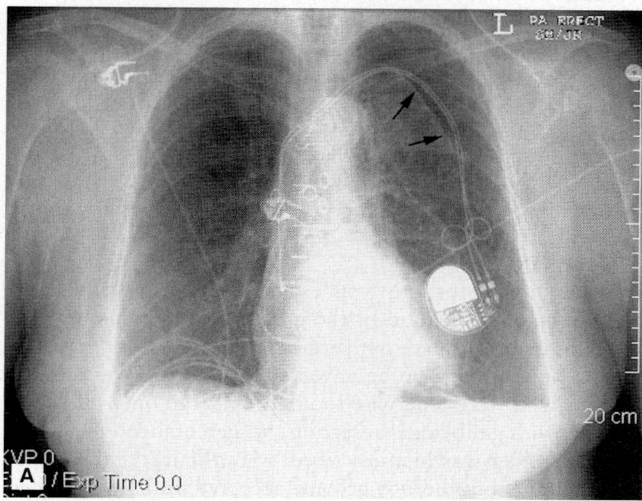

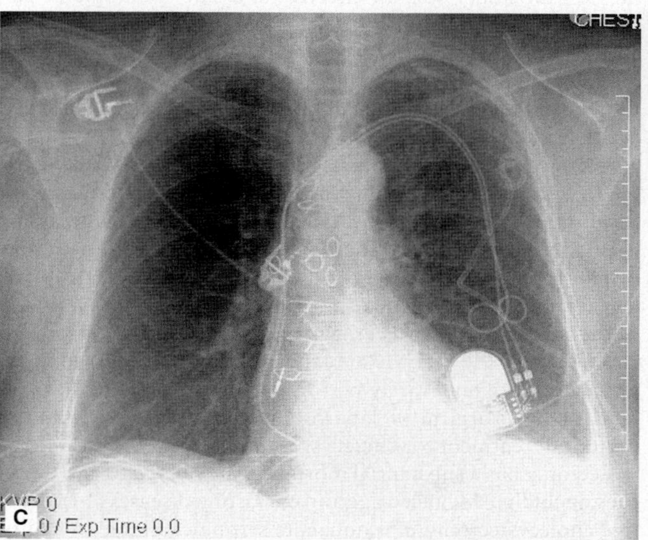

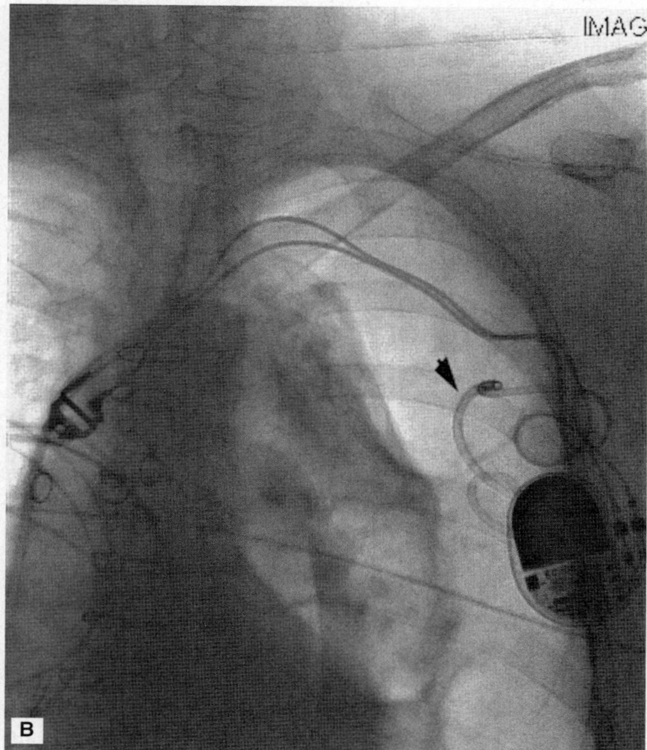

FIGURE 35.7. A 70-year-old female with progressive pneumothorax following placement of transvenous cardiac pacing device. **A:** *Arrows* indicate the partially collapsed left lung following pacing device placement. **B:** Fluoroscopic image obtained at time of 8 Fr chest tube insertion. The tube was placed slightly lower than the usual apical position to avoid potential damage to the pacing device or wires. **C:** Following chest tube insertion, the pneumothorax was evacuated with syringe aspiration of the air. Follow-up chest radiograph demonstrates near-completed resolution. The chest tube was connected to Pleur-Evac drainage system.

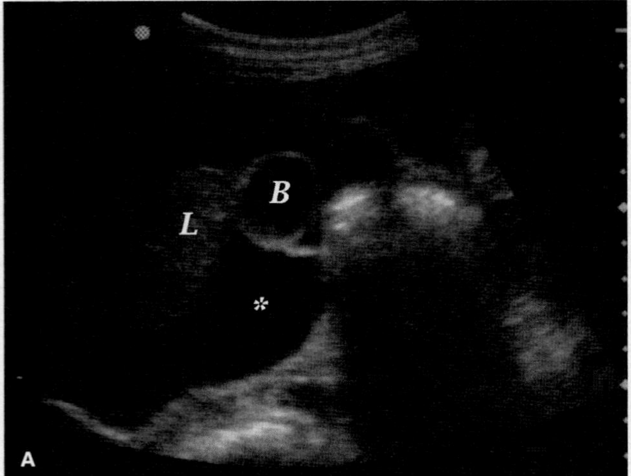

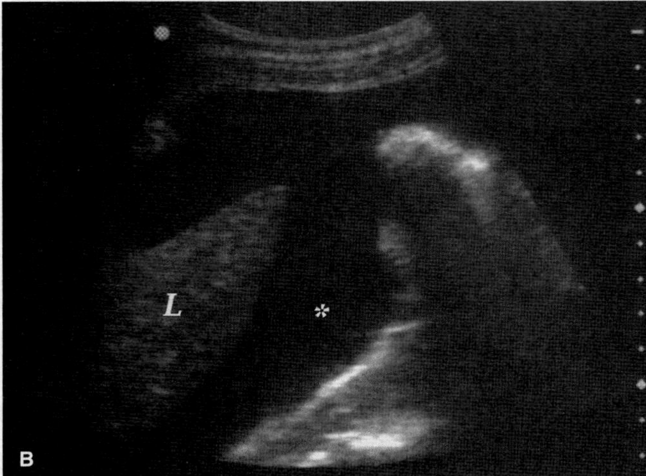

FIGURE 35.8. Abdominal paracentesis. **A:** Initial position shows a segment of bowel blocking access to the perihepatic fluid. *B*, segment of bowel; *L*, liver; *asterisk*, fluid. **B:** Slight change in transducer position yields a safe pathway for drainage.

tubing can be connected to either a three-way stopcock and drainage bag or to a 1-L vacuum bottle system. Removal of volumes greater than 5 L can lead to volume redistribution and may require IV albumin infusion (Fig. 35.8A, B).

Suprapubic Drain Placement

The patients in whom placement of a suprapubic cystostomy tube are performed are those with bladder neck obstruction from prostatic hypertrophy or prostate cancer, and with a neurogenic bladder. However, there is an increasing population of ICU patients following pelvic trauma who may also require this procedure.

The procedure is performed under local anesthesia and with conscious sedation. The procedure is usually performed with both ultrasound and fluoroscopic guidance, although in some cases this may be performed at the bedside with ultrasound guidance alone. The bladder must be distended to displace loops of small bowel out of the pelvis. This can be accomplished by the normal filling of the bladder, in the case of outflow obstruction, by filling of the bladder through an indwelling Foley, or by insertion of a 20-gauge needle into the bladder and subsequent filling of the bladder with normal saline. After preparation of the site, if direct access with a needle is used, ultrasound guidance is used to localize the bladder and avoid adjacent loops of small bowel. Once distended, a point 2 to 3 cm above the pubic symphysis is localized in a paramedian location. An 18-gauge needle is advanced under ultrasound guidance, again to avoid any loops of small bowel. The position is confirmed by return of urine, or if saline has been used to distend the bladder, iodinated contrast material can be injected. On confirmation of position, a 0.035-inch stiff guidewire is coiled in the bladder and the tract serially dilated. The degree of dilatation is dependent on type of catheter to be used. For short-term drainage, a soft, 10 to 12 French locking loop catheter can be used. However, for longer-term use, a 16 to 20 French Foley catheter should be used, which can be inserted through a peel-away sheath. Either the locking loop catheter or the peel-away sheath is advanced over the indwelling stiff guidewire under fluoroscopic guidance after sufficient tract dilatation.

Catheter maintenance primarily centers around risk of infection. Some authors recommend use of long-term trimethoprim/sulfamethoxazole. Additionally, the catheter should be exchanged every 2 to 3 months or whenever it becomes clogged with debris. The overall success rate for the procedure approaches 100% (8).

CHOLECYSTOSTOMY

Surgical cholecystostomy was established as a definite technique for decompression of the gallbladder by Sims in 1878 (9). Sims demonstrated that surgical cholecystostomy with insertion of a drainage tube gave rapid relief of symptoms in patients who were otherwise too ill to undergo open cholecystectomy with gallbladder resection (9). Percutaneous access to the gallbladder was first described by Burkhardt and Mueller (10) in 1921, but did not become accepted until 1980, when Shaver et al. (11) demonstrated that percutaneous drainage of the gallbladder was an effective and safe technique in patients with acute cholecystitis who were unfit for surgery (9–11). This technique consists of a minimally invasive method of removing gallbladder contents by placing a drainage catheter into the gallbladder lumen using some form of image guidance (9,12,13).

Aside from safe decompression of the gallbladder, percutaneous access to the gallbladder lumen allows additional interventional procedures to be carried out on the gallbladder and biliary tree. Some of these procedures include dissolution of gallstones using methyl-*tert*-butyl ether (MTBE), gallbladder ablation, percutaneous cholecystolithotomy, and drainage of the biliary tree. However, due to the advent of laparoscopic techniques in the early 1980s, these additional interventional procedures are now rarely performed.

Although surgical or laparoscopic cholecystectomy is the preferred treatment for cholecystitis in the acute setting, cholecystectomy has a substantial mortality rate related to patient issues, including advanced age and coexisting diseases (14). Elective cholecystectomy in a nonacute setting carries a mortality

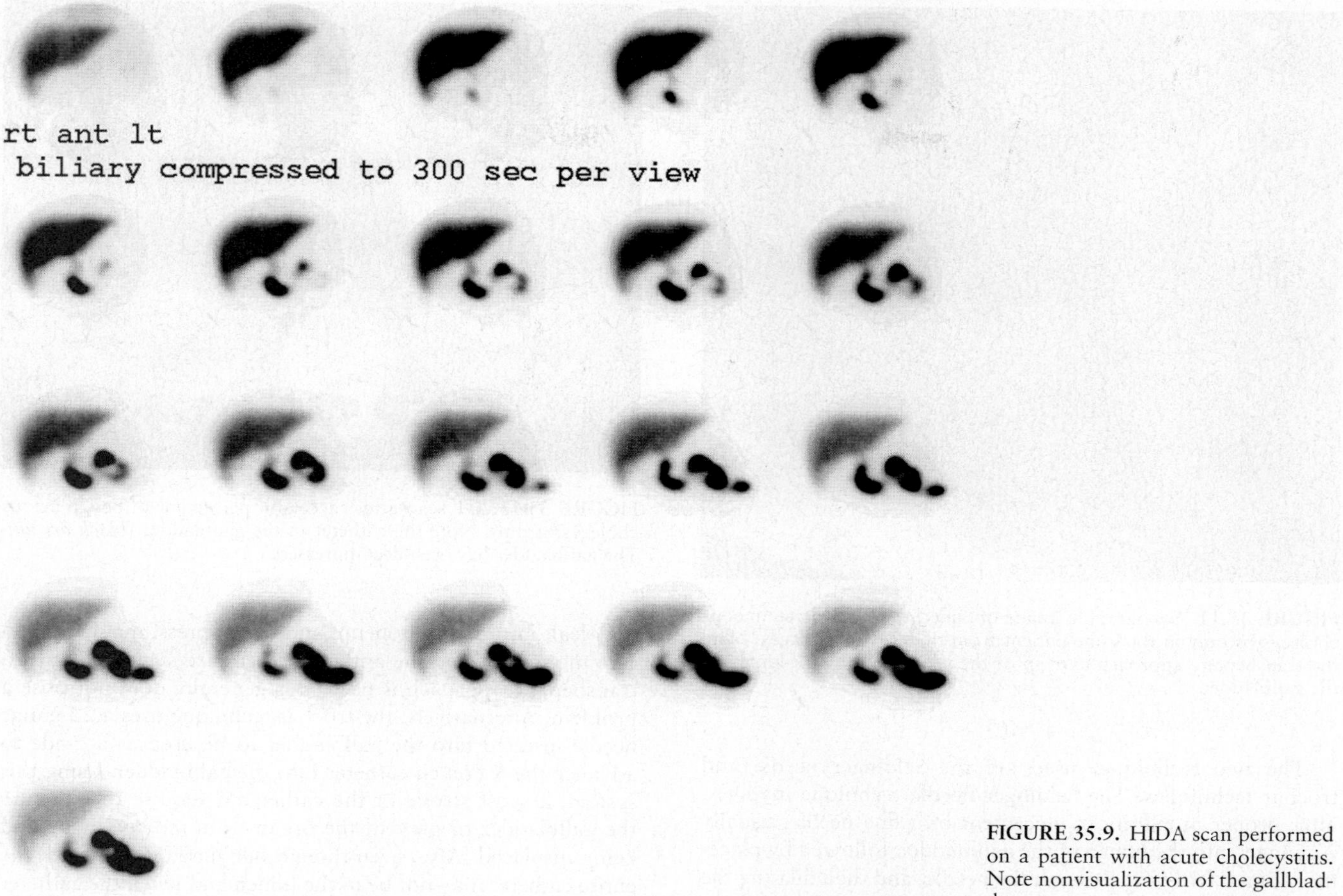

FIGURE 35.9. HIDA scan performed on a patient with acute cholecystitis. Note nonvisualization of the gallbladder.

as low as 0.7% to 2%. However, cholecystectomy in the acute patient may have a mortality rate as high as 14% to 19% (14). Percutaneous cholecystostomy can be performed in the acute setting with low mortality rates as a temporizing measure. When the patient has improved and is better able to tolerate an operative intervention, cholecystectomy can be performed electively. In addition, in patients with acalculous cholecystitis, percutaneous cholecystostomy will decompress the gallbladder and may eliminate the need for later cholecystectomy (9).

Acalculous cholecystitis typically occurs in patients admitted for shock, major surgery, and thermal injury, as well as in patients receiving total parenteral nutrition. It is believed to be caused by inflammation and ischemia of the gallbladder, not related to the presence of stones, but rather to intravesicular hemorrhage or inspisated bile causing obstruction, leading to inflammation and infection (14,15). The diagnosis of acalculous cholecystitis can be elusive, as ultrasound and scintigraphy are diagnostically unreliable (9). Percutaneous cholecystostomy has been advocated as a therapeutic trial in these patients provided other sources of sepsis have been excluded (16).

Other indications for percutaneous cholecystostomy include hydrops, empyema of the gallbladder, and complications of cholecystitis including perforation and pericholecystic abscess (17) (Fig. 35.9).

Percutaneous cholecystostomy is usually performed in the angiography suite using ultrasound and fluoroscopy. Computed tomography (CT) scan is another modality that may be of benefit in certain patients (Fig. 35.10). The procedure may also be performed at the patient's bedside using only ultrasound (Fig. 35.11). Although conscious sedation is usually administered, occasionally, if the patient is unable to tolerate conscious sedation, the procedure can be safely performed using only local anesthesia (Figs. 35.12 and 35.13).

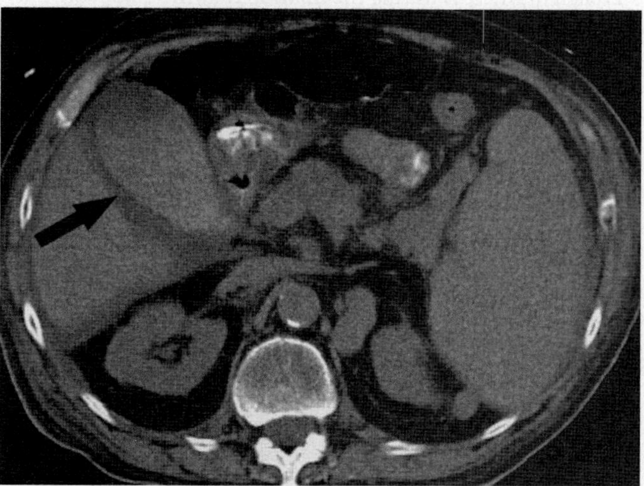

FIGURE 35.10. CT scan of the same patient as in previous image. Note the thickened gallbladder wall and fluid surrounding the gallbladder.

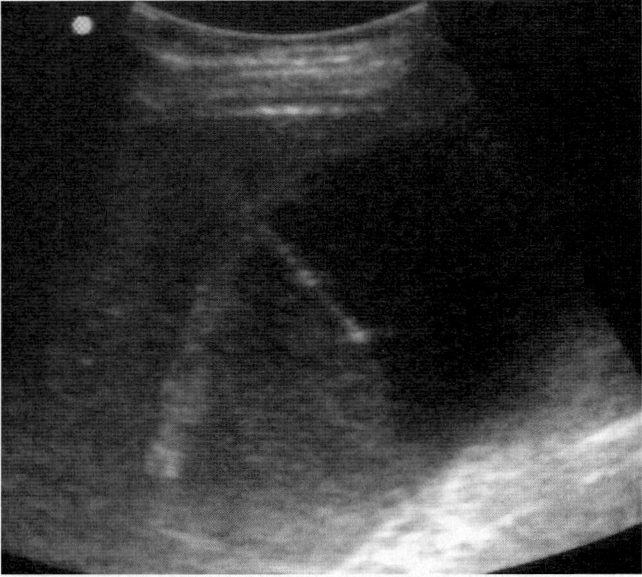

FIGURE 35.11. Sonographic image obtained during a percutaneous cholecystostomy in the same patient from the previous images. Note the transhepatic approach and tip of the needle within the lumen of the gallbladder.

The two techniques used are the Seldinger needle and trochar techniques. The Seldinger needle technique involves, after proper preparation, placement of a fine needle, usually 22 gauge, into the lumen of the gallbladder, followed by placement of a 0.018-wire through the needle, and then dilating the site over the wire to accommodate larger wires, if needed, or placement of a drainage catheter. The trochar technique involves placement of a catheter, usually 8 French, which is held on a rigid needle with sharp stylet. This system is advanced as a unit under image guidance into the lumen of the gallbladder. Each needle technique has its own merits and is usually chosen based on operator comfort.

The Seldinger technique allows for a single puncture of the gallbladder, which is then sequentially dilated to accommodate a 0.035 wire. Fascial dilators are then used to accommodate the 8 French drain. It is during the dilation that the guidewire may buckle and access may be lost. If this occurs, the gallbladder may leak into the peritoneum and decompress, making puncture more difficult. The author's experience suggests that if a transhepatic approach is used, this generally does not pose a problem. Alternatively, the trochar technique uses a 22-gauge needle inserted into the gallbladder to be used as a guide to advance the 8 French catheter into the gallbladder. Using this system, a swift stroke of the catheter is require to puncture the gallbladder to prevent the organ from moving away and being displaced. Also, even though bile may be aspirated, the entire catheter may not be in the lumen and when the catheter is advanced, dislodgement may occur. Again, both techniques are widely used and accepted and depend on the operator's comfort level.

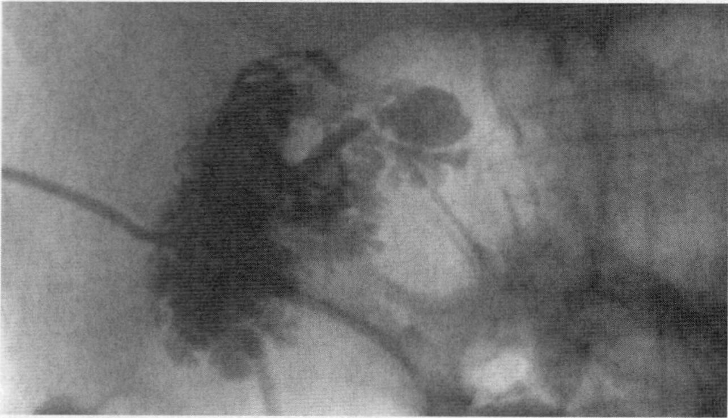

FIGURE 35.12. Contrast injection through the cholecystostomy tube. Note the irregular filling defects consistent with sludge or pus in the gallbladder.

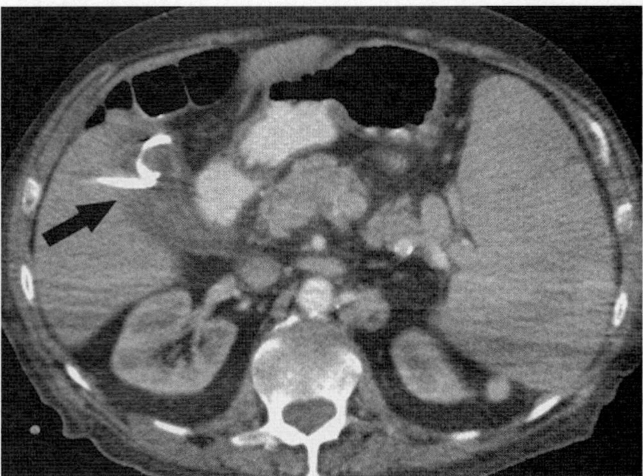

FIGURE 35.13. CT scan after successful placement of percutaneous cholecystostomy. Note the catheter in the gallbladder (*black arrow*). The gallbladder has been decompressed.

The gallbladder can be approached either via the transhepatic route (Fig. 35.11), attempting to enter through the anatomic bare area, or using a transperitoneal approach. The bare area is formed embryologically when the mesentery that surrounds the gallbladder fuses with the undersurface of the liver. The transhepatic approach tends to minimize bile leak in the presence of ascites. This approach also minimizes gallbladder motion by puncturing near the bare area. This is of significance as it is gallbladder motion that will lead to tube dislodgement. Puncture of the gallbladder by this approach minimizes leakage of bile as the liver will act to tamponade the tract. However, puncture through the bare area has proven difficult in all cases (18). The transperitoneal approach is more direct in some cases and allows better access than the transhepatic approach if percutaneous cholecystolithotomy is planned using a large scope because of the large tract that would have to be formed through the parenchyma of the liver to accommodate the endoscopic device. The main drawback of the transperitoneal approach is when the Seldinger technique is planned, as the gallbladder mobility allows for easy buckling of the catheters due to a lack of parenchymal support, leading to misplaced or dislodged catheters. This problem is largely eliminated if the trochar system is used in combination with the transperitoneal approach.

Cholecystostomy has been well studied and has a 100% technical success rate (11,13,14,16,19) (Fig. 35.13). Procedure-related mortality rates are well documented in the range of 0%

to 2%, well below the published rate of complications for surgical cholecystostomy in the acute setting (14,20–22). Procedure-related complications include bleeding, vagal response, and biliary peritonitis related to bile leak. Clinical improvement has been shown to occur in 1 to 2 days, and response rates of 87% have been shown at 3 days (9,23). Browning et al. (24) reported that patients with pericholecystic fluid or gallstones were the most likely to have a positive response to the procedure. Ninety-two percent of patients with gallstones showed clinical improvement after percutaneous cholecystostomy. In the ICU, where acute acalculous cholecystitis is most likely to occur, it has been shown that in patients with unexplained sepsis, percutaneous cholecystostomy has shown dramatic clinical improvement, defined as decreased white blood cell count, normalization of body temperature, and reduction in the use of vasopressors, in up to 59% of patients (9,16,19).

HEPATOBILIARY DRAINAGE

Although the technique of percutaneous cholangiography was first described by Burkhardt and Muller in 1921 (25), it was not until 1966 that percutaneous transhepatic biliary drainage was described by Seldinger (26), using a simple sheathed needle technique. In 1974, Molnar and Stockum (27) described percutaneous biliary drainage using a transhepatic catheter. Subsequent to this description, numerous technical advances were made in the area of guidewires and catheters, which allowed an increased ability to negotiate areas of stricture and stenosis within the biliary tree using a percutaneous approach (25). At present, there is a wide array of devices and instrumentation that allow for increased percutaneous biliary interventions, including management of biliary strictures, biliary leaks, biliary fistulae, stone extraction, biopsies, and radiation therapy.

Whereas percutaneous biliary interventions gained popularity in the 1970s and 1980s, the development of endoscopic retrograde cholangiopancreatography (ERCP) has largely replaced the percutaneous approach for many disease states. However, the technique of choice will mainly depend on the skills available by physicians at the local institution (28). Additionally, there are instances where a percutaneous approach is preferred over an ERCP, mainly instances where ERCP fails, or ERCP is not an option due to prior intestinal surgery that does not allow the endoscope to reach the biliary tree (Figs. 35.14 and 35.15).

Prior to the initiation of the procedure, any coagulopathy should be corrected and prophylactic antibiotics administered. Preprocedure imaging includes either a CT scan, ultrasound, or magnetic resonance imaging (MRI) to look for the location of dilated bile ducts and also to evaluate the anatomy of the liver. The right upper quadrant of the abdomen in the midaxillary line is prepped, using sterile technique, for an intercostal approach. Although the right-sided approach is commonly used, many interventional radiologists prefer to access the biliary tree via a left-sided ductal approach.

After conscious sedation is administered, a 22-gauge needle is advanced into the liver using fluoroscopic guidance. Diluted contrast is injected as the needle is slowly withdrawn; alternatively, the needle can be advanced and contrast injected. This technique works well for the nondilated system. After identifying the biliary system, further contrast is injected slowly to opacify the biliary tree and identify a suitable access site in the bile ducts. Next, with the contrast-filled duct as a target, the system is entered using a 22-gauge needle with fluoroscopic guidance. Thereafter, there are two options. First, an external drain can be placed to decompress the system, with the patient being brought back to the interventional radiology (IR) suite 24 hours later; this reduces the risk of introducing infected bile into the bloodstream. The second option is to attempt internal/external drainage. Although this may save the patient one step in a staged procedure and allow for physiologic drainage of bile, there is a risk of introducing infection as previously described. It is the authors' preference to achieve external drainage first and allow the ducts to drain overnight

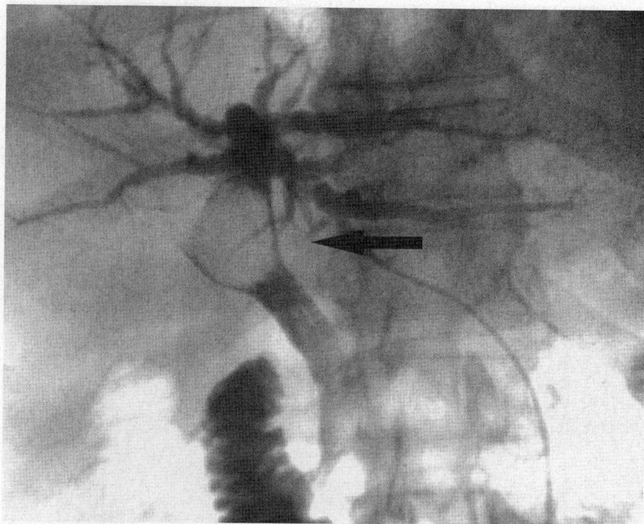

FIGURE 35.14. Failed endoscopic placement of common bile duct (CBD) stent due to the presence of a large mass (*black arrow*) within the CBD. (Image courtesy of James Caridi, MD.)

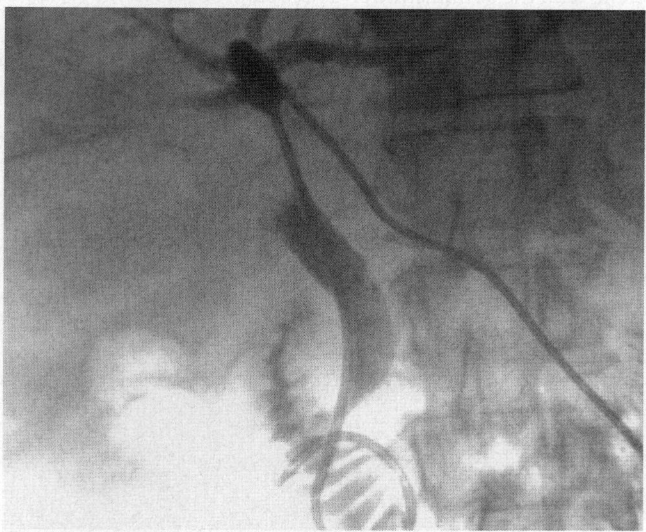

FIGURE 35.15. Successful percutaneous drainage using a left-sided biliary duct. Note that the drainage catheter has been advanced past the obstruction and into the small intestine. (Image courtesy of James Caridi, MD.)

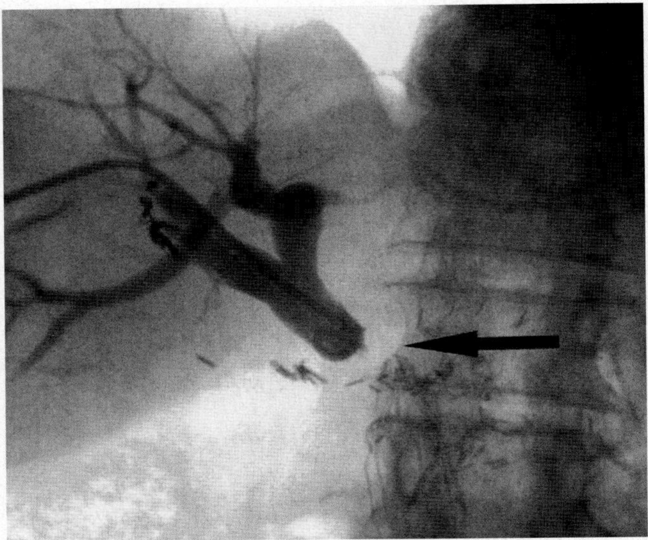

FIGURE 35.16. Patient presents with biliary obstruction. On hospital day 1, external drainage has been achieved using a right-sided bile duct approach. Cholangiogram shows complete obstruction in the mid common bile duct (CBD) (*black arrow*).

before attempting any lengthy intervention (Figs. 35.16 and 35.17).

The indications for percutaneous biliary drainage include palliation of an unresectable primary or secondary malignancy of the liver causing biliary obstruction, benign strictures including biliary-enteric anastomosis as seen in liver transplant patients, sepsis secondary to biliary obstruction, preoperative decompression, stone removal, bile leak after laparoscopic cholecystectomy, biopsies, permanent internalization of drainage by placement of internal stent, and radiation therapy (29) (Figs. 35.18 and 35.19).

The only true contraindication to percutaneous biliary drainage is a bleeding diathesis. Usually this problem is overcome with the administration of blood products in the form of

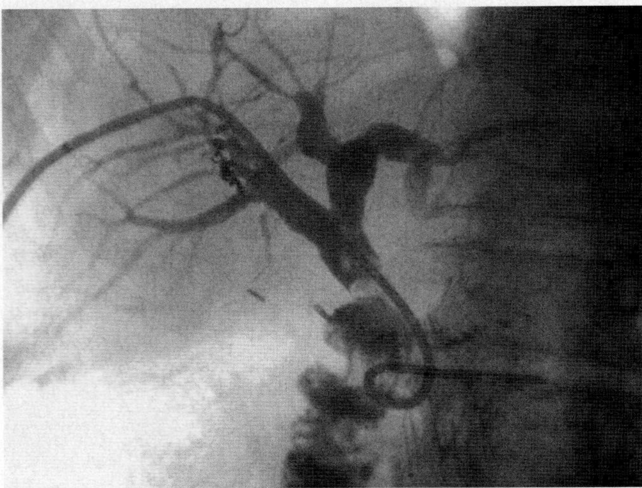

FIGURE 35.17. On hospital day 2, internal/external drainage has been achieved by gaining access to the small intestine across the area of obstruction.

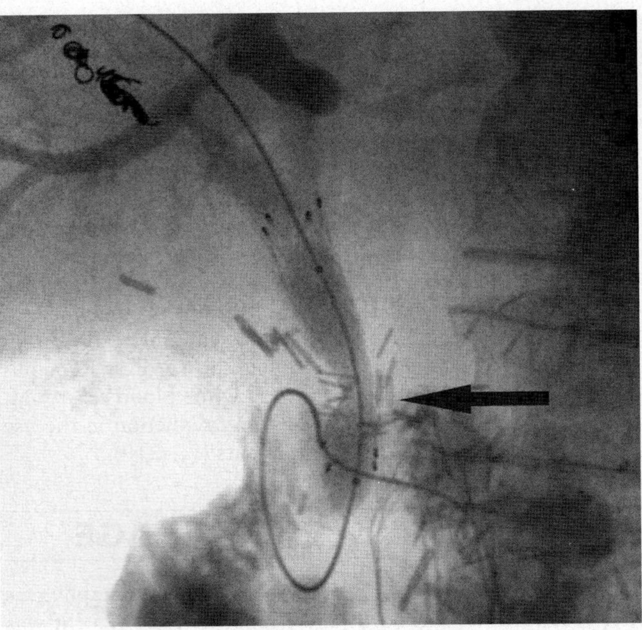

FIGURE 35.18. This is the same patient as in Figures 35.16 and 35.17. A metallic self-expanding stent has been placed across the area of obstruction in the distal common bile duct. Note the waist in the stent (*black arrow*) due to the surrounding mass.

fresh frozen plasma, platelets, and vitamin K. Relative contraindications include the presence of sepsis, unless it is of biliary origin. The presence of ascites increases the risk of bleeding, and catheter misplacement, as well as making the procedure technically more difficult; hence ascitic fluid should be drained prior to performing the procedure. The presence of

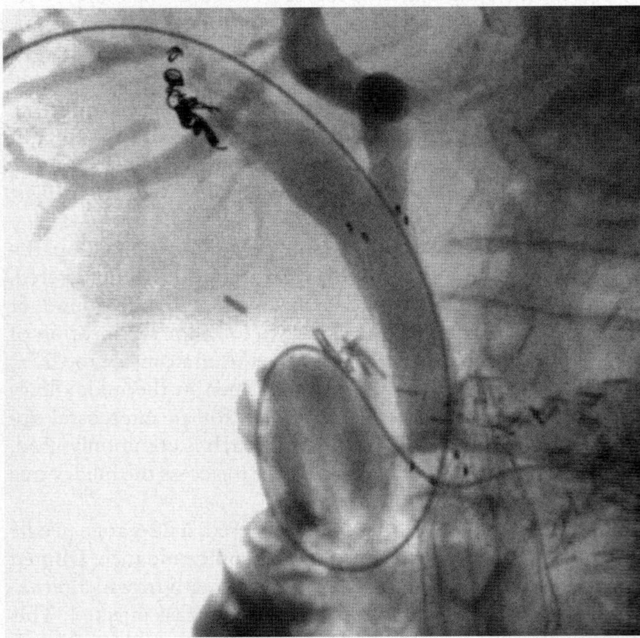

FIGURE 35.19. Post–stent placement and balloon angioplasty. No residual stenosis is noted, and the stent is fully expanded.

multiple intrahepatic obstructions also raises the risk of introducing bacteria to a bile duct that is not drained and that can rapidly become infected.

The catheter should be anchored to the skin. This is usually performed with a suture from the skin to the tube. Approximately 2 cm of slack should be available to prevent tube dislodgement from hepatic motion with respiration. The tube should be flushed with 5 mL of saline every 6 hours for the first 48 hours the tube is in place and then as needed thereafter. The drainage from the tube should be monitored daily to identify any signs of obstruction of the catheter or evidence of bleeding. If brisk bleeding occurs, this may be the result of erosion of the tube through an adjacent hepatic blood vessel that is in continuity with one of the many side holes of the drainage catheter; this usually occurs in the setting of a tube that has migrated out of position with patient motion or inadequate tube anchorage.

The tube site should be cleaned routinely to discourage bacterial colonization. Patients with an external biliary drain in place should receive IV fluids if there is marked choleresis, as this may precipitate hepatorenal failure. If any problem is identified with the tube, IR should be contacted if the problem cannot be resolved immediately on the unit (28).

Burke et al. (30) have reviewed the published success rates of the technique in the literature. Canalization is easier when the intrahepatic ducts are dilated, and success rates approach 95% for the dilated system, whereas it is 70% for the nondilated biliary tree. Internal drainage is achieved in 90% of patients with successful biliary canalization. Stone removal is successful in 90% of cases. Stents placed as palliation for malignant disease are patent 50% of the time at 6 months after placement.

Percutaneous transhepatic biliary drainage carries a significant risk, approximately 10% for all patients (30), and this risk may increase or decrease based on the patient's overall medical condition. Patients presenting with coagulopathy, cholangitis, biliary stones, malignant obstruction, or proximal obstruction will have higher complication rates (30). Complications related to insufficient bile drainage and tube dislodgement is usually relieved with placement of a tube 10 French in size. Sepsis, reported in 2.5% of cases, may be considerable unless prophylactic antibiotics are used prior to the procedure; bleeding is reported with 2.5% of cases as well. Abscess formation or peritonitis is noted in 1.2% of patients; pleura entry is noted in 0.5% of cases. Death is reported in 1.7% of patients.

Although this procedure has several associated complications, it is difficult to compare rates from one institution to another, as patient selection and the presence of other comorbidities may influence complication rates. It is, therefore, important that each institution monitor its own complication rates to ensure quality.

TRANSJUGULAR INTRAHEPATIC PORTOSYSTEMIC SHUNT

Portal hypertension refers to a pathologic increase in pressure in the portal vein. Although it is defined as an increase in portal venous pressure above 12 mm Hg, the standard is to report the portal pressure as a gradient between the portal vein and the inferior vena cava (31). The gradient becomes important because there are several conditions, including pregnancy and ascites, that may elevate the absolute portal pressure or the pressure in the inferior vena cava (IVC).

The liver is the main source of resistance to blood flow in the portal vein (32). Certain disease states, including cirrhosis, disrupt the normal architecture of the liver and lead to formation of fibrosis around the hepatic venules and sinusoids. This fibrosis reduces the diameter of the sinusoids, thus acting to increase resistance. As the pressure in the portal vein increases, one of the ways the body responds is by finding alternate pathways for blood to return to the heart, so called portosystemic collaterals. This is seen as an increase in size of normally small veins within the body, which, as the veins increase to a pathologic size, are called *varices*. Certain patterns of varices are commonly seen, with the classic distribution in the lower esophagus and stomach. Other common patterns include mesenteric varices and connections between the spleen and kidney. Generally, varices begin to form with a portal pressure greater than 12 mm Hg. Risk of variceal hemorrhage increases as the portal pressure rises to 18 mm Hg.

There have been several methodologies used in treating the complications associated with chronic portal hypertension. Nicolai Eck was the first to achieve surgical portal flow diversion in 1877 (33). In 1945, Whipple et al. (34) and others (35) began using portacaval and conventional splenorenal shunts in clinical practice. Since that time, other shunt procedures have been developed, including end-to-side portacaval shunt, side-to-side portacaval shunt, distal splenorenal shunt, as well as various interposition shunts, all aimed at reducing the pressure in the portal vein and treating variceal hemorrhage (32). Surgery remained the standard until the 1980s when endoscopic techniques were popularized, including direct injection of the bleeding varix with a sclerosing agent. Additional therapies offered through use of an endoscope include banding and ligation of the bleeding varices. Other forms of medical management include administration of vasopressin or vasopressin combined with nitroglycerin using an intravenous route. Vasopressin and its derivatives act by constricting the vascular smooth muscle altering the body's arterial beds including the splanchnic arteries, and thereby reducing the portal pressure by reducing the portal inflow (32). Sclerotherapy has also been performed by direct injection of sclerosing agents into the varices.

The main complication of a successful surgical shunt is the development of encephalopathy, whereas the main drawback to endoscopic and other forms of medical management is that the offending process, portal hypertension, is not addressed, which leads to high rates of rebleeding. These two reasons pressed physicians to develop new treatments.

Transjugular intrahepatic portacaval shunting (TIPS) was first conceived of and performed in dogs in 1969 by Josef Rosch et al. (36). The first human case of percutaneous TIPS was reported in 1988 (37). It is an effective nonsurgical and nonendoscopic means to control variceal bleeding by decompressing the portal venous system (38). A CT scan, ultrasound, or MRI is recommended to evaluate for patency of the portal vein as well as exclude hepatic neoplasm and evaluate for other anatomic considerations. The usual laboratory studies to check for hematocrit and coagulopathy should also be performed. IV antibiotics should be administered prior to the procedure. The technique consists of a percutaneous approach, usually ultrasound-guided canalization of the right internal jugular vein. From this approach, access is gained to the hepatic veins

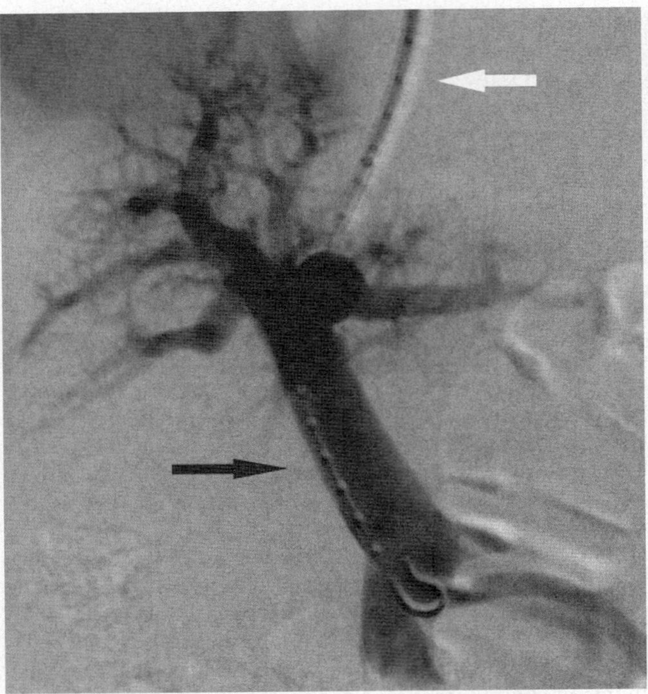

FIGURE 35.20. Patient with cirrhosis undergoing a transjugular intrahepatic, portacaval shunting (TIPS) procedure. Catheter (*white arrow*) is positioned from a hepatic venous approach, through the hepatic parenchyma into the portal vein (*black arrow*). (Image courtesy of Harry K. Meisenbach, MD.)

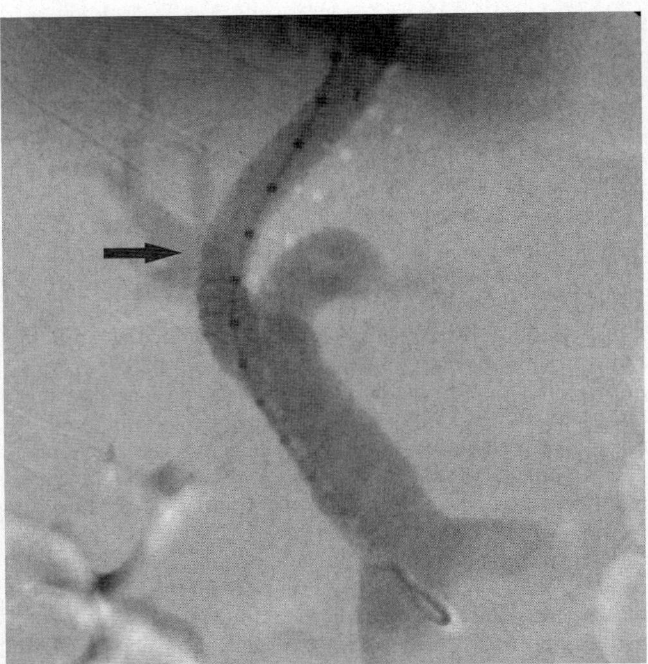

FIGURE 35.21. Post–transjugular intrahepatic, portacaval shunting (TIPS) angiogram shows a patent TIPS shunt with a covered stent (*black arrow*). (Image courtesy of Harry K. Meisenbach, MD.)

and pressure measurements are made from the portal vein using a wedged technique to the right atrium. A hepatic venogram is performed, followed by angiogram of the portal vein, using carbon dioxide and either a wedged technique or puncture of the hepatic parenchyma through the jugular access. Passage of a long curved needle is then performed from a satisfactory location in the hepatic vein, usually the right hepatic vein, into the identified location in the intrahepatic portion of the portal vein or its branches. Direct pressure measurements are made using the transjugular pathway (Fig. 35.20). If acceptable, balloon angioplasty of the intrahepatic tract between the hepatic vein and the portal vein is then performed. A stent, usually covered, is deployed from the portal vein to the hepatic vein through the tract to keep it patent and prevent hepatic recoil and restenosis (Fig. 35.21). Repeat pressure measurements are performed to confirm satisfactory pressures have been reached. Any additional adjustments that need to be made to the stent can be performed at this time, as well as embolization of varices if indicated.

When TIPS was first described, it was indicated for uncontrollable esophageal variceal hemorrhage; other indications included gastric or intestinal variceal hemorrhage. The indications have since expanded and now include recurrent variceal hemorrhage despite repeated endoscopic treatment, refractory ascites, hepatic hydrothorax, Budd-Chiari syndrome, and as a bridge to liver transplantation.

TIPS produces profound hemodynamic effects secondary to portosystemic diversion, including decreasing flow to the liver and increasing that to the heart. There are several situations where TIPS is absolutely contraindicated. These include severe or rapidly progressive liver failure, severe encephalopathy, and congestive heart failure. Relative contraindications include biliary obstruction, hepatic malignancy, portal vein thrombosis, and polycystic liver disease; additional considerations include the patient's coagulation status. The most frequent complication is bleeding related to perforation of the hepatic capsule by the needle during attempted canalization of the portal vein. Other considerations include the patient's overall medical condition.

The patient's ability to tolerate a TIPS procedure, as well as being a predictor of early mortality, has been calculated in the past using the Child-Pugh classification and the acute physiology and chronic health evaluation II (APACHE II) scores. Today the model for end-stage liver disease (MELD) score has largely replaced other calculations as the best predictor of early mortality. The MELD score is based on the patient's INR, total bilirubin, and creatinine (Cr). The formula is as follows:

$$\text{MELD score} = 10\{0.957\text{Ln(Cr)} + 0.378\text{Ln(Total bili)} + 1.12\text{Ln(INR)} + 0.643\}$$

where Ln is.

There are a few additional rules when using this formula. For any of the three variables, 1 is the minimum acceptable value. The maximum acceptable value for serum creatinine is 4. The maximum value for the MELD score is 40. It is recognized that a patient's MELD score may change with time and therefore recertification is necessary. How often the score is calculated increases with an increasing MELD score. A MELD score of 18 has generally been shown to be the cutoff for performing a TIPS procedure.

A TIPS procedure is one of the most difficult procedures performed in the IR suite. It involves many steps and as such carries

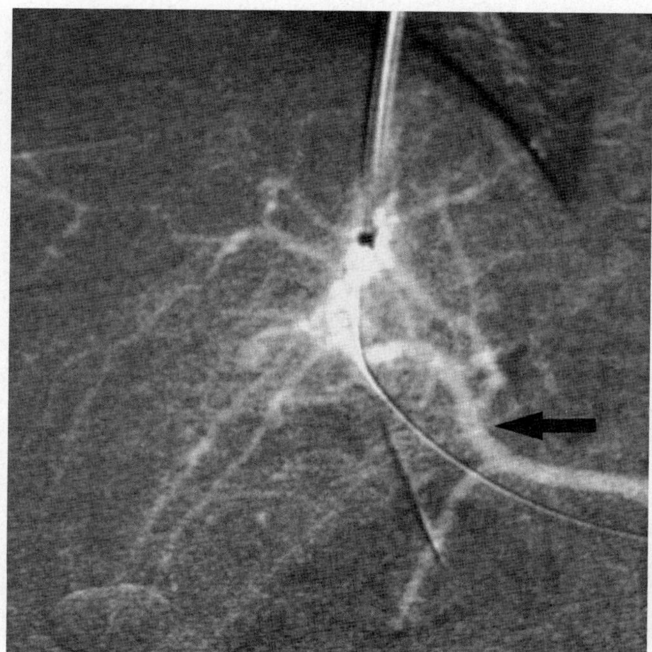

FIGURE 35.22. Attempted canalization of the portal vein during a transjugular intrahepatic, portacaval shunting (TIPS) procedure. This CO_2 injection identifies canalization of the hepatic artery (*black arrow*).

with it a large number of potential complications ranging from bleeding at the puncture site to death. However, many studies have been performed and there are a few likely complications (39,40). It should be noted, too, that there is a learning curve for performing the procedure, which may alter the number and severity of complications.

Puncturing the portal vein has proved to be difficult in some cases. Thrusting a large needle blindly through the liver parenchyma can cause a host of complications including bleeding from the liver capsule if the needle perforates the capsule of the liver. Hemobilia can be seen if the needle perforates a bile duct in close proximity to a vascular structure. The needle may leave the capsule of the liver and puncture adjacent organs including the intestine, gallbladder, kidney, and aorta, among others (Figs. 35.22–35.24).

Dilation and stenting of the tract through the liver may also produce numerous complications. If the puncture of the portal vein is extrahepatic, as it has been shown to be in 50% of patients (41), and the tract dilated, fatal hemoperitoneum may result. Stent migration and misplacement have been described. Stents have migrated to the heart, pulmonary arteries, and into the portal vein. Manipulation of wire and catheters within the portal and splenic veins during TIPS may lead to thrombosis of these vessels. Additionally, stents may develop immediate thrombosis after placement, particularly if the angle of the stent is acute or it forms a tight angle with the portal or hepatic vein. There is also a possibility of pulmonary embolism should the thrombus migrate.

Delayed complications occur as well, and a few should be noted. These include contrast-induced nephropathy, hematoma, encephalopathy, stent migration, thrombosis, and elevated right atrial pressures. Often, the procedure may take

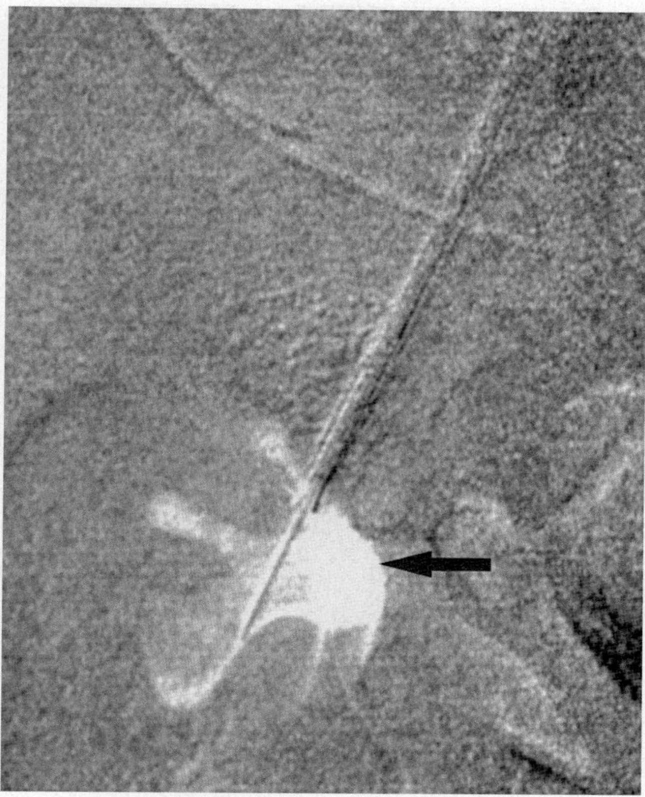

FIGURE 35.23. Attempted canalization of the portal vein during a transjugular intrahepatic, portacaval shunting (TIPS) procedure. The tip of the cannula is in the renal pelvis (*black arrow*).

additional time or a procedural complication may occur, requiring additional contrast that may lead to nephropathy. Rarely a hematoma may occur at the puncture site. Often, TIPS patients are coagulopathic. Although the risk of bleeding is usually recognized at the time of the procedure, as with any angiogram, delayed bleeding may occur. Encephalopathy is not uncommon post-TIPS and ranges from 12% to 34% (38). Treatment consists of lactulose, given orally to help reduce ammonia. If this fails, a flow-reducing stent could be placed to decrease flow through the stent and increase flow back to the liver. Finally, the shunt could be occluded to return the patient to the pre-TIPS state. Although rare, fever may occur postprocedure and may be related to infection or the trauma of the procedure itself. In either case, infection should be ruled out.

Shunt malfunction can also be considered a complication. Acute thrombosis has already been discussed, but delayed thrombosis is also noted, as well as restenosis and stent shortening. Stenoses within the TIPS may form anywhere along the shunt from the portal vein to the IVC. Stenosis near the end of the stent is usually caused by a stent that is too short and leaves an area of the liver exposed. This leads to narrowing and, ultimately, stent occlusion. Restenosis within the stent itself has been seen, particularly with uncovered stents, and is thought to be related to bile being exposed to the shunt and the development of intimal hyperplasia; this has largely been resolved by the use of covered stents. Finally, the postprocedure right atrial pressures are going to be higher than preprocedure values. If the absolute value is greater than 10 mm Hg, diuresis is recommended.

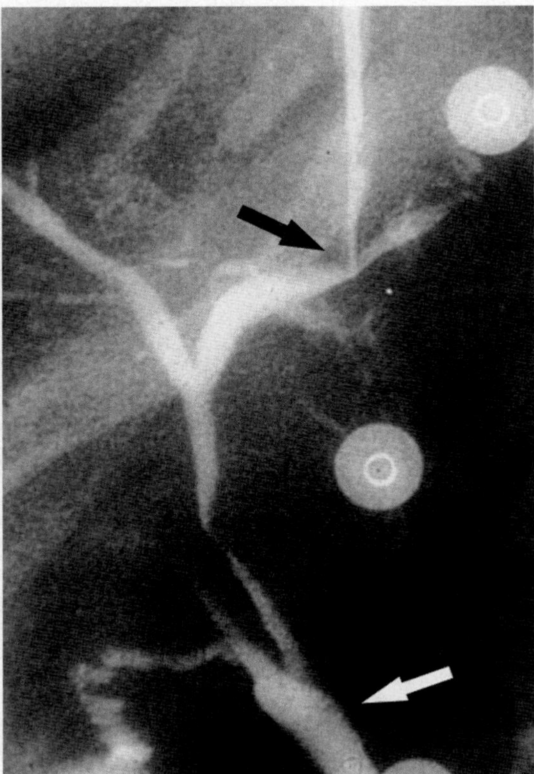

FIGURE 35.24. Attempted canalization of the portal vein during a transjugular intrahepatic, portacaval shunting (TIPS) procedure. The tip of the cannula is in the left hepatic duct (*black arrow*). Contrast is noted throughout the biliary system and into the common bile duct (*white arrow*).

Follow-up care for TIPS patients is relatively uncomplicated. In addition to evaluating for and treating the delayed complications noted above, one must follow the patient routinely with ultrasound to confirm patency and exclude restenosis or thrombosis of the stent. If this is noted, it is a relatively simple procedure to perform angioplasty of the stenosed segment and return the shunt to its normal function. Ultrasound is usually performed within 1 to 2 weeks after placement of the TIPS; it is repeated at 3 months, 6 months, and then every 6 months and as needed for early identification of any problems with the shunt. It is much easier to maintain a working shunt than to place a new TIPS.

TIPS can be performed with extremely high rates of success, approximating 92% to 99%. Reasons for a failed TIPS procedure include portal vein thrombosis, atrophic hepatic veins, small hard livers, and massive ascites. For patients in whom TIPS was performed for hemorrhage, the procedure was successful in stopping the bleeding acutely in 91.1%, although the risk of rebleeding increases with time up to 20.7% at 2 years. Fatal complications decrease proportionately with the number of procedures that are performed, consistent with a learning curve. Even so, the fatality rate ranges from 0.6% to 4.3%. Published less than 30-day mortality rates range from 4% to 36%. The reason for the variation is multifactorial, based on patient selection and the center performing the procedure. The 5-year mortality rate averages 31.7%, with the most common cause of death being progressive hepatic failure (38).

CENTRAL VENOUS ACCESS

Central venous access and maintenance is one of the most commonly performed procedures in IR (42). The demand for stable, secure, and dependable central venous access has increased dramatically over the past several years as medical therapies have become more complex, and patients present with multiple comorbidities. Additionally, outpatient services have increased sharply as providers have come under increased pressure to reduce hospital costs (43). Today, over 5 million central venous catheters (CVCs) are placed each year in the United States (44,45). CVCs are used in the ICU for infusion of a wide array of medications, blood products, total parenteral nutrition, and can be used for blood draws, hemodialysis, and plasmapheresis as well as many other reasons including contrast administration for diagnostic imaging.

Traditionally, CVCs have been placed by the surgical service, with the radiologist's role limited to confirming satisfactory placement and identifying complications on the postprocedure radiographs. The advent of image-guided procedures allows the IR service to be more involved with vascular access, predominantly in difficult access patients (Fig. 35.25). With time, studies have shown that image-guided vascular access is generally superior to blind insertion, with fewer immediate complications and improved long-term function (1–3). Generally, response time for vascular access placement is decreased with IR. Additionally, there are much lower hospital costs in radiology compared to the operating room (46). Certainly, imaging is critical during any complex vascular access procedure including translumbar and revascularization techniques, but the role for image guidance is gaining importance even in routine vascular access procedures as the need for rapid and safe central venous access increases.

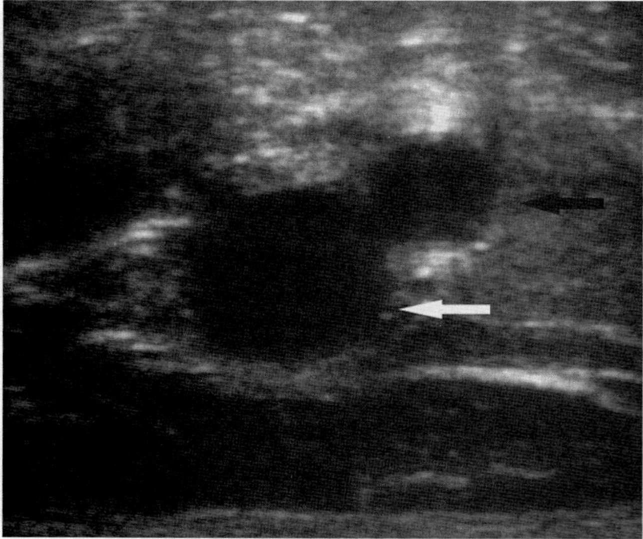

FIGURE 35.25. Grayscale sonographic image of the neck demonstrates clear visualization of the left internal jugular vein (*white arrow*). The left internal carotid artery is seen as well (*black arrow*). Additional features used to differentiate the two structures are the increase in vein caliber with Valsalva maneuver compared with the typical arterial pulsation of the carotid artery.

The field of central venous access has blossomed into a very large industry, with a plethora of devices on the market and virtually every manufacturer of medical equipment supplying their own line of CVCs. It would be difficult to review every manufacturer's devices in this section, but the general categories and catheters will be reviewed.

Peripherally Inserted Central Catheters

In peripherally inserted central catheters (PICC), a peripheral vein in the upper extremity (usually the antecubital, basilica, or cephalic) is cannulated, usually with ultrasound guidance, and a long flexible catheter, essentially a long IV line, is advanced from this puncture site to position its tip in the superior vena cava (SVC) near the right atrium. PICCs come in various sizes and styles, either single- or double-lumen versions, and range from 3 to 7 French. They may have internal valves near the hub, or even on the tip of the catheter, which are important for patients with an allergy to heparin. These valved PICCs are able to be flushed with normal saline, as heparin is not needed to maintain patency. There may also be external clamps that occlude the catheter when it is not in use. The advantage of PICCs include the fact that they are well tolerated by patients, they look and function like a peripheral IV, which allows for ease of use by the nursing staff, and additionally, PICCs carry a lower procedural risk than central lines because they are placed in a peripheral vein, usually avoiding the vital structures in the chest. The single- and double-lumen varieties usually provide sufficient access for most patients. A new "power" PICC configuration has been developed that allows for higher pressures during high-flow contrast injections as seen in CT scans for diagnostic purposes. Many hospitals have entire PICC line teams which are composed of nurses who specialize in placing these at the bedside. If the team is unsuccessful, then the PICC line can usually be placed by an IR clinician or another caregiver specializing in these procedures. Although PICCs are widely used with rapidly increasing acceptance by patients and clinicians alike, there are some associated complications with this type of catheter. One should be aware of the potential complications and long-term ramifications so that the appropriate access can be chosen for each patient.

Venous thrombosis rates, in veins where PICCs are placed, may be as high as 38% (47). It should be noted that Grove and Pevec (48) showed a lower thrombosis rate, up to 9.8% with 6 French catheters, but also demonstrated a positive correlation with catheter size; 3 French catheters had a lower rate of thrombosis than did the 6 French devices. This becomes especially important in planning for dialysis access. If the veins of the upper extremity, commonly used for dialysis fistula, are occluded, fistula creation is more difficult and longevity is reduced. Therefore, in patients with diabetes, chronic renal insufficiency, overt renal failure, or other medical conditions that may lead to renal failure in the future, the preservation of upper extremity and central venous access takes on significant importance (47). Indeed, guideline 7 of the National Kidney Foundation's initiative states that arm veins, which may potentially be used in the creation of a dialysis fistula, should be preserved (49). Any procedure that may increase the risk of venous thrombosis should be avoided.

Bloodstream infections have also been studied with respect to PICCs. Safdar and Maki (50) have noted that PICCs used in the hospital setting have a much higher rate of infection than those used in outpatients. Additionally, they have the same rate of infection as nontunneled central lines and a higher rate of infection than those that are tunneled and cuffed.

Clotting of PICCs has decreased somewhat with the development of valved catheters, although, due to their small size, occluded lumens remain common and require a change of catheter over the wire.

Nontunneled Central Venous Catheters

Nontunneled central venous catheters are generally placed in either the right or left internal jugular veins, or they may be placed in either the right or left subclavian veins, although this location is discouraged due to the potential for venous stenosis. These catheters have either a single-, double-, or triple-lumen configuration. The triple lumen is primarily used for inpatients, especially in the ICU. The triple-lumen catheter is used for relatively short periods of time, up to 14 days, and can accommodate fluids, antibiotics, blood, dialysis, plasmapheresis, and other acute care needs (51). These catheters come in predetermined lengths depending on the site of placement, with left-sided catheters being longer than right-sided catheters, and range in size from 5 to 13 French. They have tapered tips, and some are impregnated with an antibiotic compound to reduce the risk of infection. Although these catheters are usually placed by the clinical team, image guidance is frequently necessary in patients who are obese, coagulopathic, or who have venous abnormalities such as thrombosis or stenosis (51). Complications are still relatively rare with these catheters but are more common and severe than with the PICCs. Again, complications are fewer with image-guided placement than with blind placement (52). Complications include, but are not limited to, hematomata, air embolism, pneumothorax, and nerve injury (53); longer-term complications include mechanical, thrombotic, and infectious causes.

Hematomata are usually treated by applying pressure and correcting any coagulopathy. Air emboli are noted immediately and are usually self-limiting as the air will be dissipated in a few minutes. In extreme cases, additional measures are required, including turning the patient so the left side is down, attempting to aspirate some of the air through the catheter, and administration of oxygen through nasal cannula or mask. Pneumothorax is rare with image guidance, less than 1%, but if this occurs, usually a Heimlich valve chest tube can be placed in the midclavicular line in the second intercostal space. Nerve injury is usually avoided by choosing an appropriate puncture site away from the usual location of nerve pathways. Mechanical complications include fragmentation and migration of the catheter. Fragmentation is more common with subclavian catheters than with internal jugular catheters, due to the pinch-off mechanism between the subclavius muscle, costoclavicular ligament, clavicle, and first rib. Thrombotic complications include thrombus in the catheter, around the catheter, or in the vein near the tip of the catheter. Inability to aspirate blood is usually the first indication of thrombus, and various measures are used to treat this problem. Thrombolytic agents can be placed in the lumen of the catheter in an attempt to lyse the clot. If there is a fibrin sheath around the tip, this can be stripped away using radiologic techniques, such as endovascular balloon disruption of the fibrin sheath or endovascular migration of a snare around the catheter, which is then tightened and pulled down along the catheter to remove the fibrin deposits. If the vein is thrombosed, thrombolysis can be performed if there are no contraindications. Finally, the catheter can be replaced over the wire in certain instances, if one is unable to clear the obstruction from the catheter and other causes have been excluded.

Tunneled Catheters

Tunneled chest wall catheters range in size from 6 to 14 French. They typically have a small Dacron cuff attached circumferentially to the shaft of the catheter, which is placed in a subcutaneous location within the tunnel and allows in-growth of fibrous tissue that secures the catheter in place and reduces the risk of infection. Some cuffs are impregnated with antimicrobial compounds (51). These catheters are generally used long term, on the order of months to years. The typical use for a tunneled catheter includes antibiotics, chemotherapy, fluids, total parenteral nutrition (TPN), blood administration, dialysis, and plasmapheresis. The risks with these catheters are essentially the same as for nontunneled central venous catheters, although fragmentation and thrombosis are seen more commonly in the tunneled devices because they are usually placed for longer periods of time.

Port Catheters

Subcutaneous ports are the final category of central venous catheters to be discussed. Implanted ports are completely contained within the body, with no portion of the device exposed (54). They are either single or double lumen and are constructed of stainless steel, titanium, or plastic and come in various sizes, which helps in choosing a specific port for a patient. These devices are used for chemotherapy, blood administration, fluids, TPN, and antibiotics and require the use of a special noncoring needle. Typically a small subcutaneous pocket is made on the chest wall to accommodate the port. Alternatively, a pocket can be created in the upper extremity and the port placed from this location. However, there is an increased risk of venous thrombosis using ports from the extremity location, and it is generally discouraged (55). Access is obtained into one of the central veins, with the right internal jugular (IJ) vein preferred, as this access carries the lowest immediate and long-term risk to the central veins. The catheter is then advanced through the tunnel and puncture site into the vein. The catheter is cut after measuring the appropriate length from the port to the SVC/atrial junction. The skin overlying the port is closed and, ultimately, heals completely. These devices are used when long-term access is needed, usually on the order of months to years. Advantages of this type of device are its long-term capacity to provide safe, dependable central access, and it allows for a more normal quality of life as there are no exposed portions of the access device; the patient is able to swim and bathe in the usual fashion. The port is easily accessible and is low maintenance. Disadvantages include a more involved initial placement as a subcutaneous pocket is needed. A needle stick is required every time the port is used. Additionally, if a port becomes infected, it requires a more involved procedure to remove it than devices that are not implanted.

Catheter and Site Selection

Choosing the appropriate access site and type of catheter is a complex decision and cannot be standardized, given the complexities of patient care. However there are several basic principles that will help guide one to the most appropriate choice. If the access is to be used for dialysis or plasmapheresis, obviously, high flow rates are needed and larger-sized catheters are needed. A central vein puncture is more appropriate than an extremity vein and, depending on the length of time the catheter is needed, will sway the physician to either a nontunneled or tunneled variety. If the patient is coagulopathic or has other significant comorbidities and access is needed for fluids and routine medications, a PICC could be considered, although caution is recommended if there is a chance the patient may need dialysis in the future. Additionally, a central vein nontunneled device could be considered. If the device is needed infrequently on the order of once per month, an implanted port would be most appropriate.

In general, the safest device that will still meet the needs of the patient should be used. However we realize that supplies and standards vary from hospital to hospital, and that patient and physician preference plays a role as well.

The previously identified and discussed locations and catheters represent the usual and standard approach to central venous access. However, it is not uncommon to have patients with complex histories in whom central venous access is not easily obtained (Figs. 35.26–35.31). For instance, if the subclavian and jugular veins and superior vena cava are occluded and are unable to be revascularized by endovascular techniques, alternate routes must be used. One should be familiar with these alternate pathways for central venous access.

The femoral veins represent a simple approach to the inferior vena cava (Fig. 35.32). These are generally large, relatively superficial veins, the puncture of which is routine using image guidance. Once accessed, a catheter can be placed to the IVC/right atrial junction without difficulty. The main drawback to using this access route is an increased risk of infection. Additionally, it is uncomfortable for patients who are ambulatory.

If the femoral routes are unable to be used, the next appropriate site would be a translumbar access. This involves puncturing the inferior vena cava directly from a posterior approach over the right iliac crest below the level of the renal veins. Once accessed, the tract is dilated to accommodate the catheter, which is directed into the superior portion of the inferior vena cava. This procedure definitely requires fluoroscopic guidance and carries increased risk of procedure-related complications.

One additional site that should be mentioned is the transhepatic approach. When the IVC is occluded and all other sites have been exhausted, vascular access can be achieved by puncturing the intrahepatic portion of the hepatic vein from a right upper quadrant approach, much as if performing a biliary drainage catheter placement. However, instead of aiming for the bile ducts, the hepatic vein is cannulated and the tract dilated to accommodate the appropriate catheter, which is positioned with its tip in the right atrium (Figs. 35.33 and 35.34).

Finally, direct surgical placement of a catheter into the right atrium has been described but is rarely used as access can

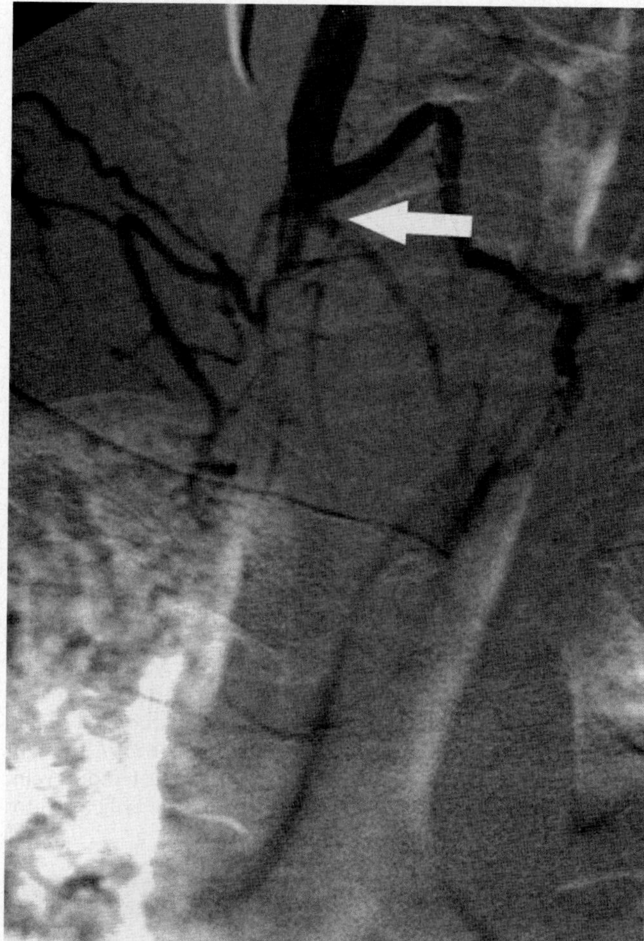

FIGURE 35.26. Contrast injection of the right internal jugular vein shows complete occlusion at the level of the base of the neck (*white arrow*).

generally be placed using revascularization techniques from alternate routes (56).

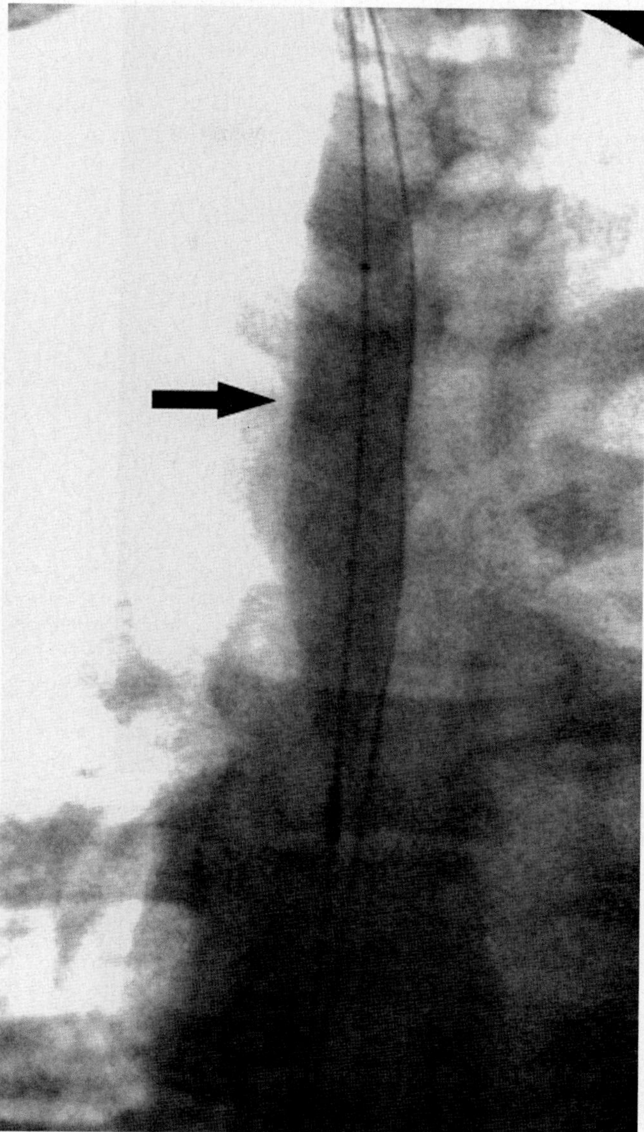

FIGURE 35.27. Same patient as in Figure 35.26. Access has been obtained across the area of obstruction, and balloon angioplasty is being performed with a 14-mm balloon (*black arrow*).

VENA CAVA FILTERS

Vena cava filters are small intravascular devices designed to prevent pulmonary embolism by trapping venous emboli. Filters do not prevent formation of new thrombus, nor do they promote lysis of a pre-existing thrombus or embolus. Pulmonary embolism (PE) occurs when thrombus that has formed in peripheral veins breaks free and is carried by the normal venous return to the heart and lungs (57) (Fig. 35.35).

PE is one of the principle causes of hospital mortality, accounting for approximately 200,000 deaths annually in the United States (58). The annual incidence of PE is estimated to be approximately 630,000 (59). The most common source of PE is from deep vein thrombus (DVT) within the lower extremities, although veins in the pelvis and upper extremities can also give rise to PE (57,60). It has been shown that 11% of patients with acute PE die within 1 hour and do not receive therapy. Of those surviving the first hour, the diagnosis is established and treatment initiated in only 29%. The vast majority of patients die because of *failure to diagnose*. Less than 10% of PE deaths occur in patients in whom treatment is initiated. However, due to advances in diagnostic technology and improvements in treatment, the percentage of patients who die after treatment has been initiated has been decreasing (59).

The mainstay of treatment of PE has consisted of anticoagulation, primarily through the use of heparin acutely followed by long-term anticoagulation with warfarin for at least 6 months (57). There are certain situations where patients either fail anticoagulation therapy or in whom anticoagulation therapy is contraindicated. Examples include those patients at high risk for falling, hemorrhagic stroke, trauma, or neoplasm. In these cases, interruption of the vena cava is indicated.

Surgical interruption of the venous system began in the 1930s with the performance of ligation of the common femoral and superficial femoral veins (60). Additional techniques

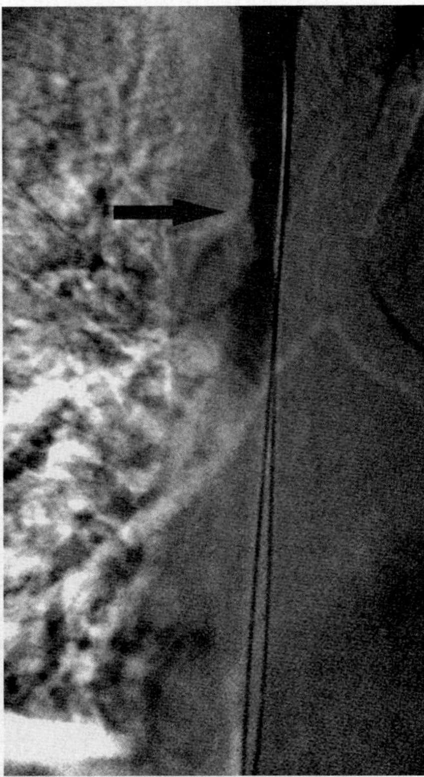

FIGURE 35.28. Postangioplasty contrast injection demonstrates improved flow in the superior vena cava (*black arrow*).

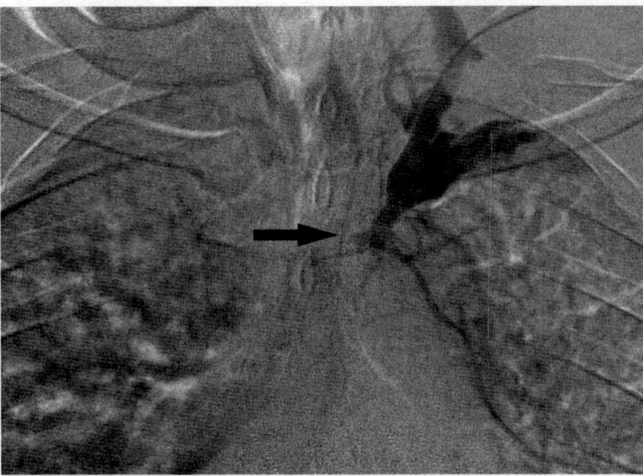

FIGURE 35.30. Contrast injection of the left internal jugular vein shows complete occlusion of the innominate vein (*black arrow*).

included phlebotomy with thrombectomy. There was a significant incidence of limb edema with vein ligation. Clips that occlude a portion of the inferior vena cava (IVC) were developed throughout the 1960s in an attempt to reduce the amount of limb edema (61). Ligation of the IVC just below the level of the renal veins was described by Oschner in 1970 (62). Although this technique had the same operative mortality as femoral vein ligation, it had a lower incidence of recurrent PE. Still, 10% to

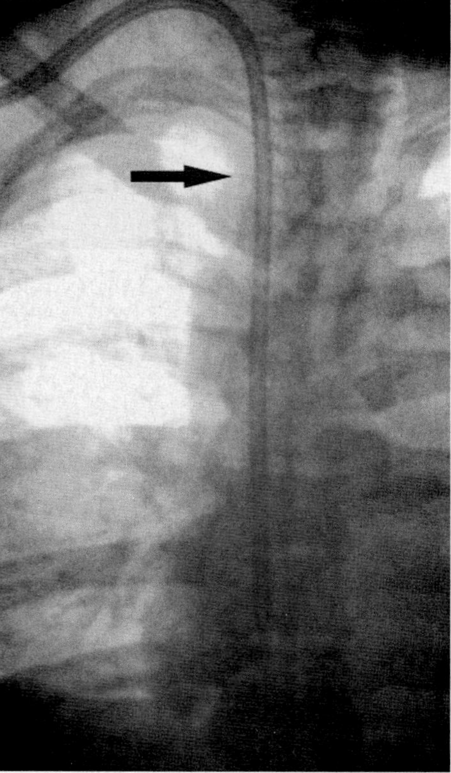

FIGURE 35.29. Successful placement of a tunneled dialysis catheter (*black arrow*) in a previously occluded right internal jugular vein. This is the same patient as in Figures 35.26–35.28.

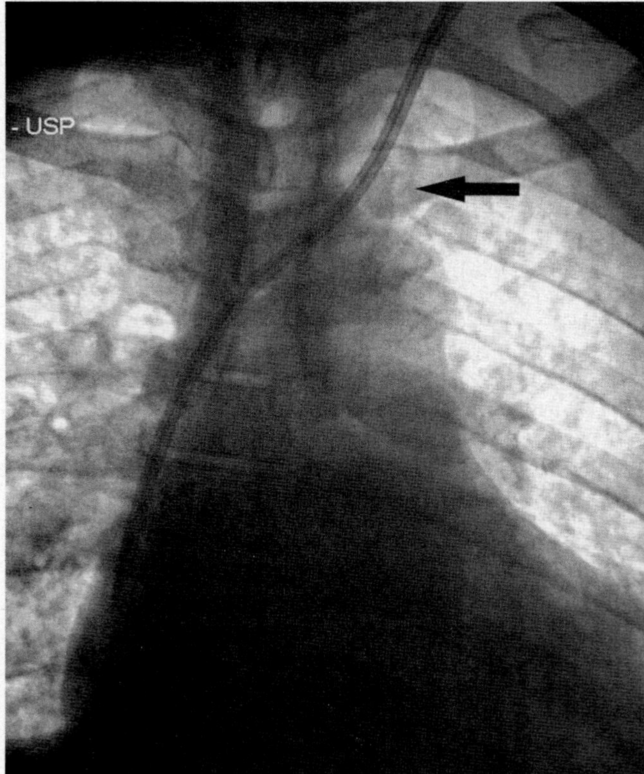

FIGURE 35.31. Successful revascularization of the previously occluded innominate vein with placement of a tunneled dialysis catheter by this left internal jugular venous approach.

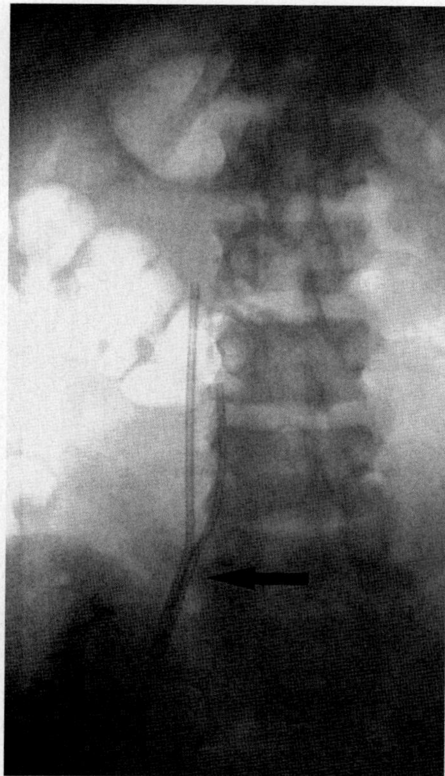

FIGURE 35.32. Dialysis catheter is noted with its tip (*black arrow*) in the inferior vena cava, from a right common femoral venous approach.

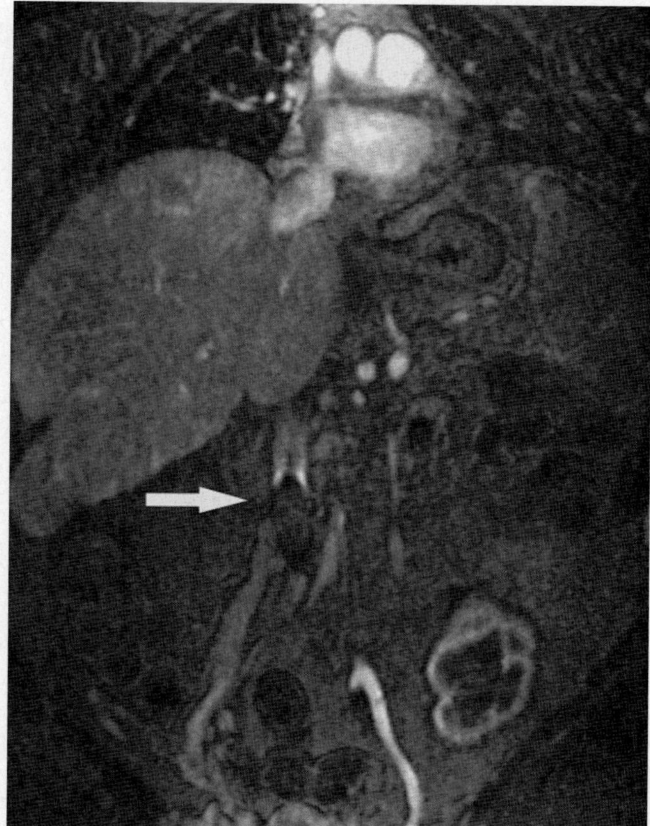

FIGURE 35.33. Magnetic resonance venogram of the inferior vena cava was performed in this patient with difficult venous access. *White arrow* shows a filter in the inferior vena cava. There is occlusion of the iliac veins.

16% of patients had immediate lower extremity edema. New techniques for caval interruption were pursued, and in 1967, the first umbrella filter was developed as a replacement for surgical ligation of the femoral veins and caval clips. Currently, filters represent the standard of care when partial interruption of the vena cava is indicated to prevent PE (60). Most filters have been placed in the inferior vena cava as 75% to 90% of PEs originate in the legs and pelvis (63).

It is of significant interest that therapy for upper extremity DVT has been controversial. Some centers elect not to use anticoagulation due to a low incidence of thromboembolism (60). However, more recent studies with larger patient populations have shown an incidence of PE from upper extremity DVT of between 4% and 28%, similar to that for DVT in the lower extremities. In addition, there have been several documented reports of fatal PE due to upper extremity DVT (64). Studies have shown that filters may also be placed safely and effectively in the superior vena cava (64,65) (Figs. 35.36 and 35.37).

The primary indication for filter placement in the vena cava is in a patient with DVT or PE when a contraindication for anticoagulation exists. Contraindications to anticoagulation include hemorrhagic stroke, major trauma, recent neurosurgery, active gastrointestinal (GI) bleeding, intracranial neoplasm, pregnancy, high risk for falling, and poor patient compliance. Additional indications include free-floating thrombus in the vena cava or iliofemoral veins and recurrent PE while undergoing anticoagulation therapy. The indications for filter placement have continued to expand, particularly with the development of retrievable filters (Figs. 35.38–35.41). Placement of a vena cava filter as prophylaxis in patients with high risk for developing PE has also been advocated. These patients include those with marginal pulmonary reserve, those with known DVT about to undergo major surgery, hypercoagulable states like neoplastic processes, and patients with severe trauma who will be in bed for long periods of time (60).

There are only a few relative contraindications to placement of a filter in the vena cava. These include those patients with thrombus between the access site and the deployment site. This has largely been overcome due to the new advances in technology that allow for placement of filters from various locations, including the femoral, jugular, subclavian, and brachial veins. Although MRI was a contraindication in the past, new filters that are MRI compatible have been developed and are now widely used. Infection has long posed a problem in patients needing an IVC filter because the filter could become infected and necessitate surgical removal. However, with the advent of retrievable filters, this has become less of an issue.

The IVC is usually the largest vein in the body. It is responsible for drainage of blood from the legs, pelvis, and abdomen back to the right atrium of the heart. It is formed by the confluence of the common iliac veins at or about the level of L5. It should be noted that at this location, the left common iliac vein crosses under the right common iliac artery and is compressed between the artery and the vertebral body at this location. This often leads to thickening of the vein and leads to thrombosis

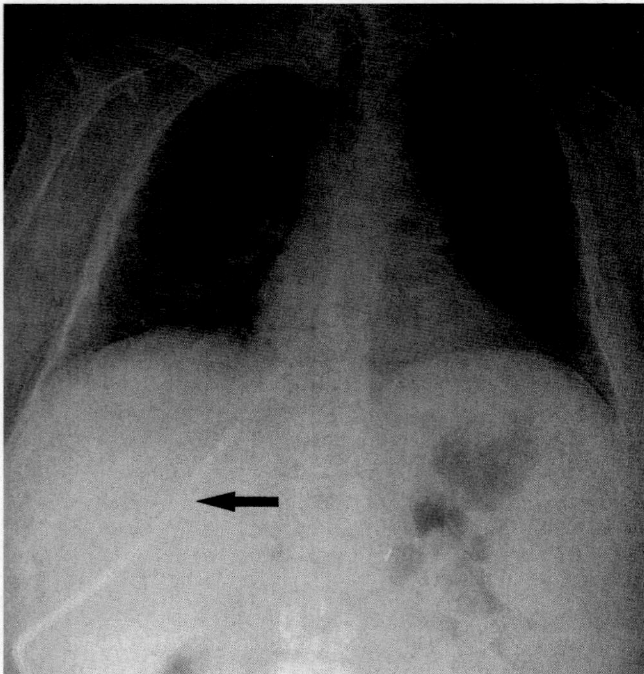

FIGURE 35.34. Same patient as in Figure 35.33. The patient has undergone placement of a dialysis catheter into the hepatic vein (*black arrow*) with its tip in the inferior vena cava at the level of the right atrium. (Image courtesy of James Caridi, MD.)

in the left common iliac vein, the so-called May-Thurner syndrome. Treatment usually consists of stent placement, and the results are best if the stent is placed prior to thrombosis.

As the IVC runs superiorly, it is joined by the lumbar veins. It is positioned anterior to the right side of the spine and psoas muscle. The right gonadal vein also joins the IVC. The left gonadal vein usually joins the left renal vein. Both renal veins

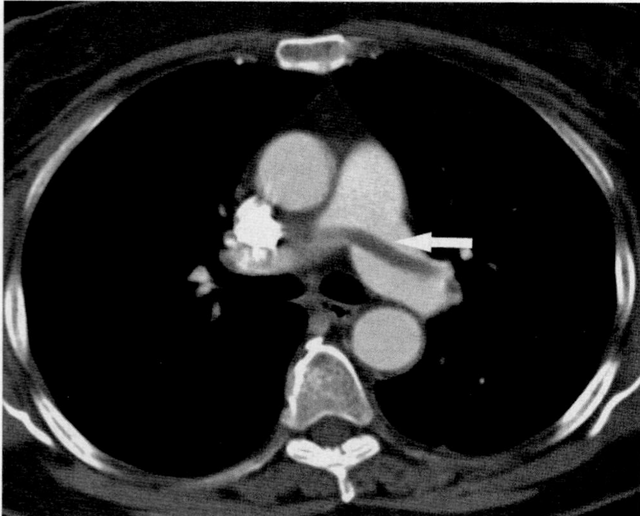

FIGURE 35.35. CT scan of the pulmonary arteries demonstrates a saddle pulmonary embolism (*white arrow*) extending into both the right and left pulmonary arteries.

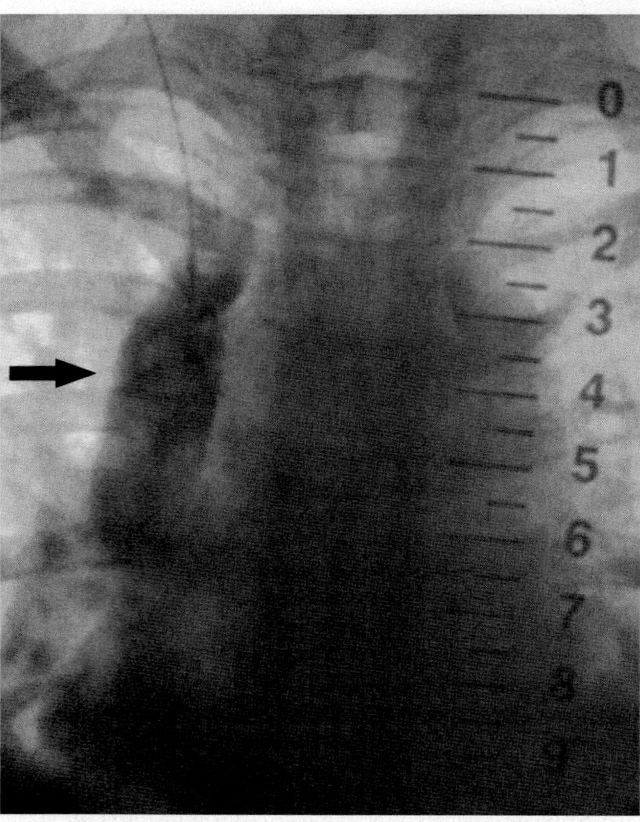

FIGURE 35.36. Venogram of the superior vena cava (*black arrow*) prior to placement of a vena cava filter.

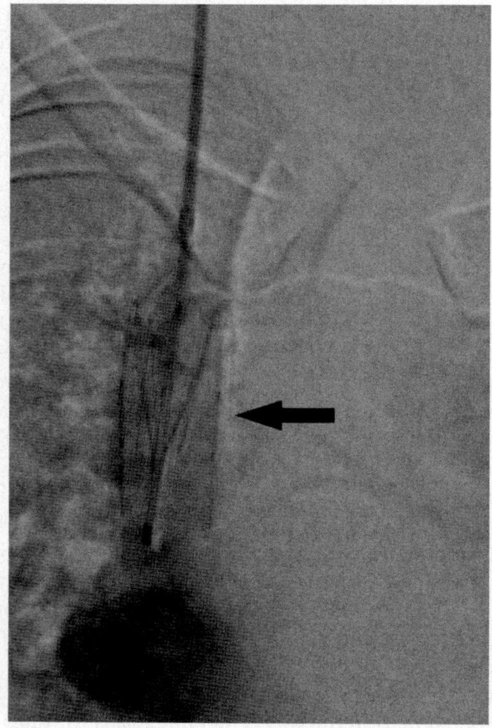

FIGURE 35.37. Vena cava filter has been placed in the superior vena cava (*black arrow*).

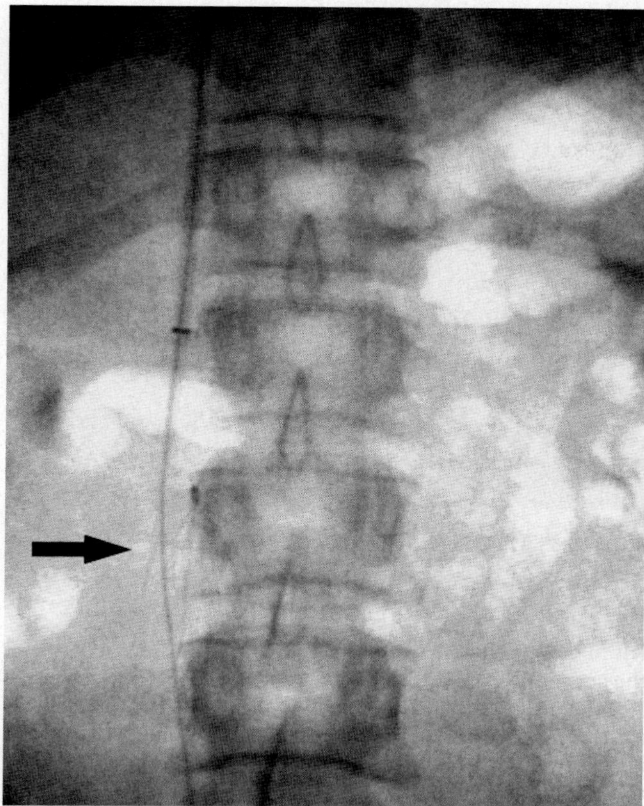

FIGURE 35.38. Access has been obtained from a jugular venous approach with its wire past the filter, Bard G2, to be retrieved (*black arrow*).

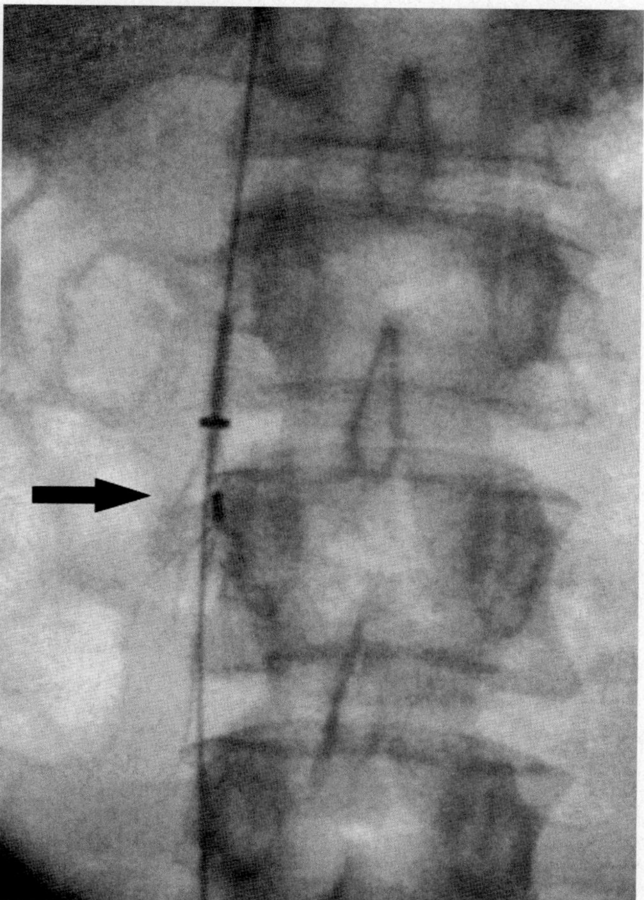

FIGURE 35.39. Recovery cone (*black arrow*) is positioned over the tip of the vena cava filter.

join the IVC at or about L1. Above the right renal vein, the right adrenal veins join the IVC. More superiorly, the three hepatic veins join the IVC just before it empties into the right atrium of the heart at or about T9 (66). The vast majority of IVC's measure between 19 and 20 mm in diameter. There are occasional IVCs with a much greater diameter, the so-called megacavas. This becomes important because many of the filters available at present are indicated for IVCs with a diameter of 2.8 cm or less.

Common variant anatomy seen in the IVC includes the double inferior vena cava. This anomaly is seen in 0.2% to 3.0% of patients (67). The embryologic cause is secondary to the persistence of the right and left cardinal veins (63). The left-sided IVC runs superiorly to join the left renal vein, which then crosses anterior to the aorta and joins the IVC. This is important because a filter placed in the right IVC may not fully protect against PE as thrombus may migrate superiorly through the left-sided IVC (Figs. 35.42–35.45). A circumaortic left renal vein is seen in 8.7% of the population. In this scenario, there are two left renal veins. One passes anterior to the aorta to join the IVC in the usual manner while the second runs posterior to the aorta and joins the IVC, frequently at a lower level than the anterior left renal vein. This is important because if a filter is placed between the renal veins, thrombus may travel retrograde in the left posterior renal vein and anterograde through the left anterior renal vein, making the filter ineffective. The retroaortic left renal vein has an incidence of 1.8% to 2.4% and usually enters the IVC at a lower location than the usual left renal vein. This necessitates a lower placement of the IVC filter (63). The left-sided IVC, also called transposition of the IVC, has an incidence of 0.2% to 0.5% (Figs. 35.46–35.48). Interrupted IVC with azygous or hemiazygous continuation occurs in 0.6% of the population. When this is the case, placement of the filter is recommended in the azygous or hemiazygous veins (67). The megacava is seen in approximately 3% of the population and is important as the diameter exceeds the ability of many filters. If an inappropriate filter is chosen, there is a high likelihood of migration centrally. In this case, filters are usually placed in the iliac veins, which will usually accommodate the filters.

The superior vena cava (SVC) is formed by the confluence of the two brachiocephalic veins at the lower margin of the first right costal cartilage. It is generally 7 cm in length and measures 2 cm in diameter. As it courses inferiorly, it enters the superior and posterior portion of the right atrium at the level of the third costal cartilage. It is important to note that the inferior half of the SVC lies within the pericardium. The main tributaries include the azygous vein and other small veins from the mediastinum and pericardium. The double SVC is seen as a result of failure of the left brachiocephalic vein to form and persistence of the left anterior cardinal vein. The left SVC drains into the right atrium via the coronary sinus; this variant is seen in 0.35% of the population. A single left SVC occurs if the right anterior cardinal vein regresses instead of the

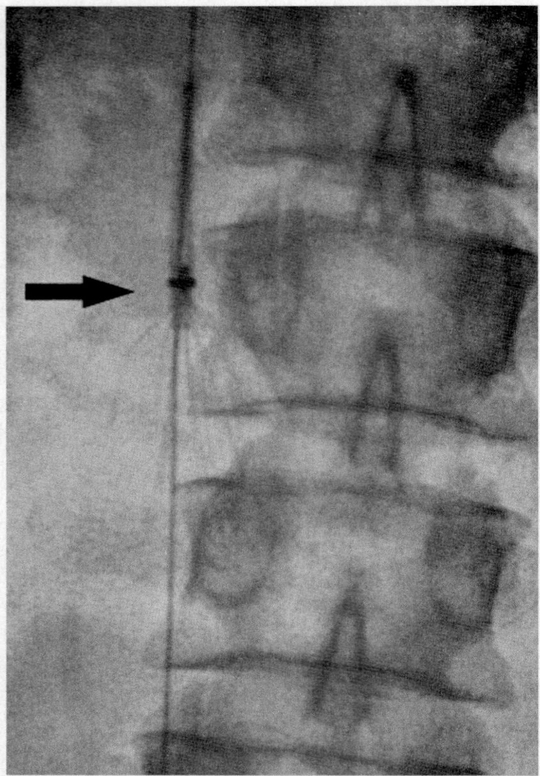

FIGURE 35.40. The tip of the vena cava filter is contained by the recovery cone and is now in the distal portion of the sheath (*black arrow*).

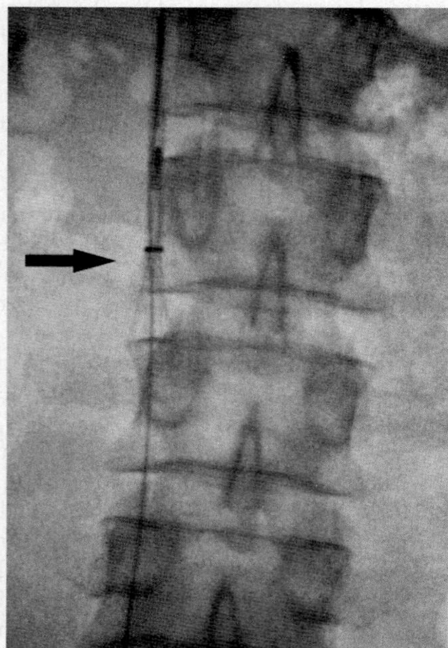

FIGURE 35.41. Vena cava filter has been completely recovered and is now contained within the sheath (*black arrow*).

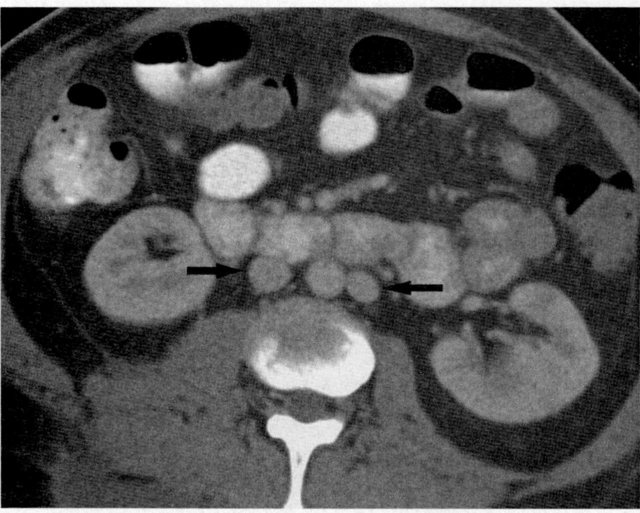

FIGURE 35.42. Duplicated inferior vena cava (*black arrows*) as seen on CT scan.

left. This left-sided SVC also drains into the right atrium via the coronary sinus (68).

Imaging of the vena cava is imperative prior to placement of a filter. The cavagram is performed by injecting contrast directly into the vena cava while obtaining a film sequence. The injection should be forceful enough to reflux into the left common iliac vein to exclude a duplicated IVC. The injection should also identify the location of the renal veins and diameter of the

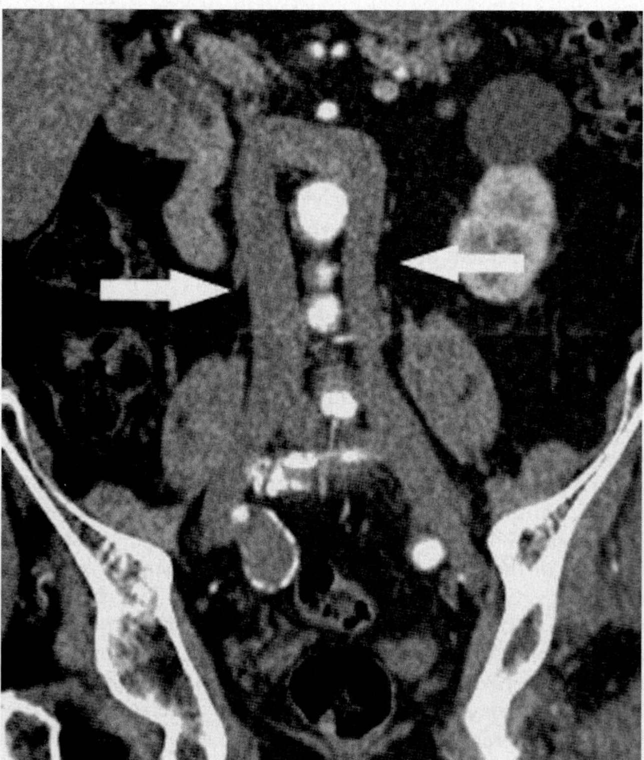

FIGURE 35.43. Coronal reconstruction of the CT in the previous image shows the duplicated inferior vena cava (*white arrows*).

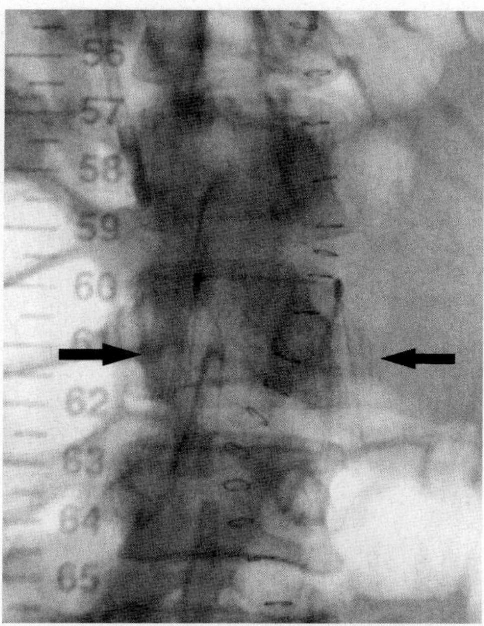

FIGURE 35.44. Radiograph of the abdomen demonstrates two separate filters (*black arrows*) corresponding to filters in each limb of the duplicated inferior vena cava.

IVC. This is the gold standard and is usually performed immediately prior to placement of a filter. However, it is often helpful in planning the access site to have additional studies prior to filter placement. CT scan is perhaps the most widely available modality. Additionally, MRI is very helpful. Ultrasound can be used but is limited by operator dependence and is often limited due to bowel gas.

The first filter used was the Mobin-Uddin umbrella filter in 1967. Since the initial success of this filter, numerous other devices have been developed. Currently, there are 11 different filters available for placement, which are approved by the Food and Drug Administration (FDA) and include the following:

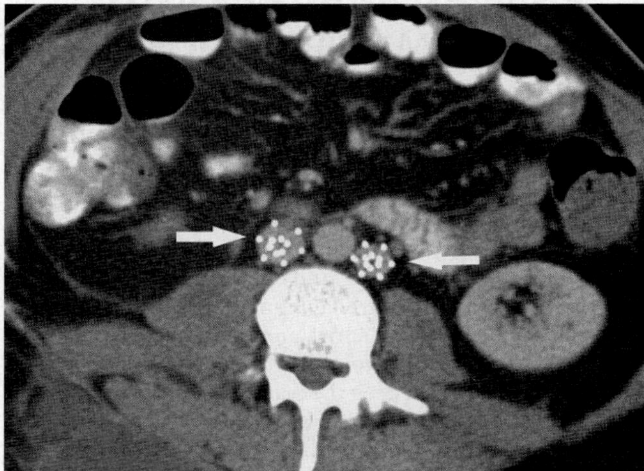

FIGURE 35.45. CT scan of the abdomen demonstrates filters (*white arrows*) in each limb of the duplicated inferior vena cava.

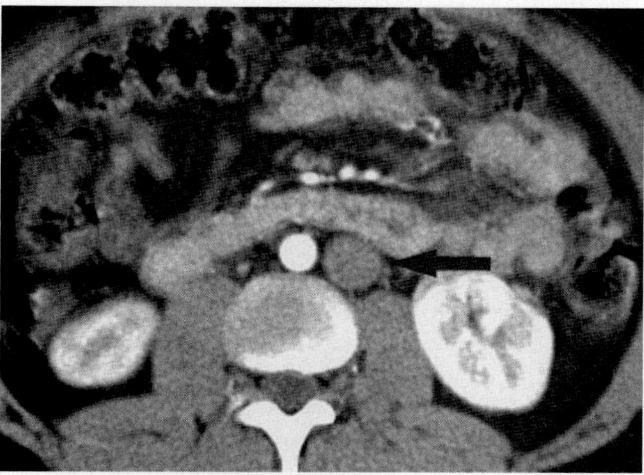

FIGURE 35.46. CT scan of the abdomen demonstrates the inferior vena cava (*black arrow*) to be positioned on the left side of the aorta.

1. Stainless steel Greenfield filter (SGF)
2. Titanium Greenfield filter (TGF)
3. Stainless steel Greenfield filter (12F SGF)
4. Vena Tech-LGM filter
5. Vena Tech-LP filter
6. Simon nitinol filter
7. Bird's nest filter (BNF)
8. TrapEase filter
9. Günther Tulip filter
10. Recovery filter
11. OptEase filter

These are made of different materials and all have a slightly different shape and architectural modifications. There are

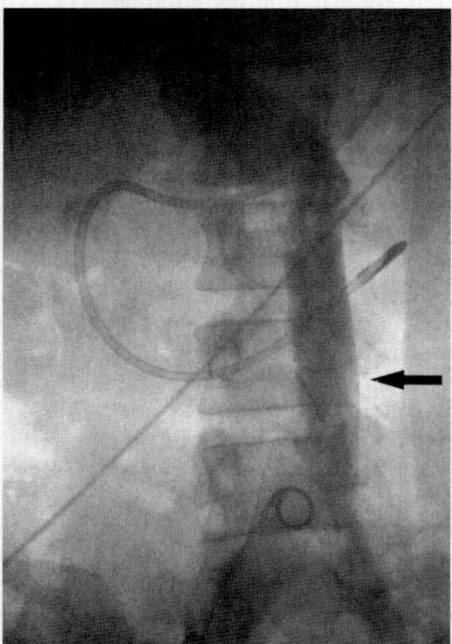

FIGURE 35.47. Venogram of the inferior vena cava in the same patient as in Figure 35.46. Note that the inferior vena cava (IVC) is to the left of midline (*black arrow*).

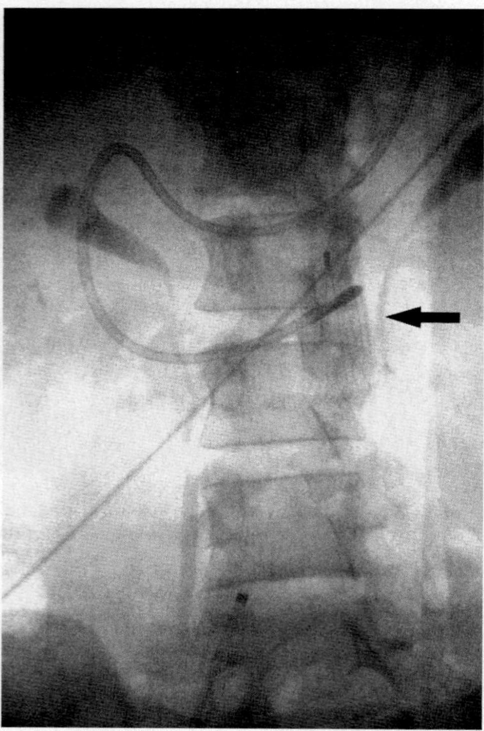

FIGURE 35.48. Plain radiograph of the abdomen demonstrates a filter (*black arrow*) in the left-sided inferior vena cava (IVC).

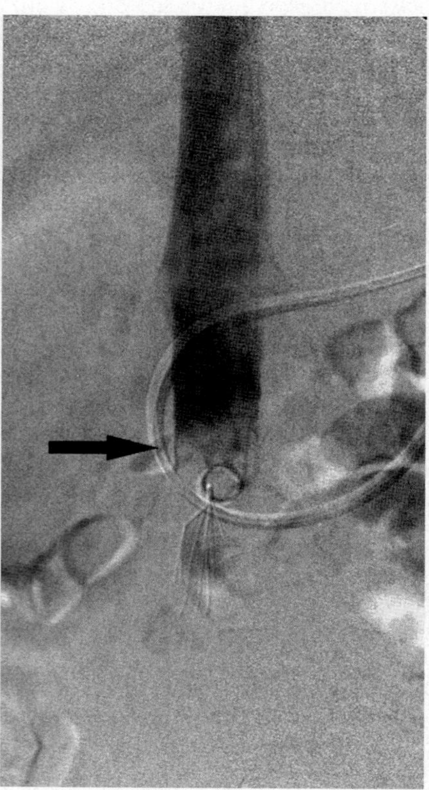

FIGURE 35.49. Venogram of the inferior vena cava (IVC) shows occlusion of the IVC at the level of the filter. There is some clot (*black arrow*) extending superior to the filter.

currently three types of filters approved in North America for retrieval. These include the Günther Tulip, Recovery, and the OptEase filters. It should be noted that although some filters are designated as retrievable, this is not possible in all patients. Some limiting factors include trapped clot in the filter, filter tilt, and ingrowth of the filter into the wall of the vena cava.

Most filters are placed in the infrarenal IVC. The filter is usually placed as closely as possible to the inferior extent of the renal veins. This reduces the potential dead space between the filter and the renal veins, which is a potential space for clots to form above the filter if the IVC were to occlude secondary to the filter (Figs. 35.49 and 35.50). Placement of the filter above the renal veins is not recommended due to the potential thrombosis of the renal veins. However, it is acceptable to place the filter above the renal veins in certain conditions including renal vein thrombosis, IVC thrombosis extending above the renal veins, recurrent PE in spite of having an infrarenal filter in place, pregnancy, and ovarian vein thrombosis.

Filters have been shown to be safe and effective at preventing PE from an upper extremity venous source. However, there are a few technical considerations. The SVC is shorter than the IVC, and therefore, there is less room to place the filter. Additionally, the filter needs to be inverted, compared to the IVC location. Therefore, it is appropriate to use a filter designed for the IVC from a jugular access and place this in the SVC from a femoral access.

There are many complications reported in the literature, from the initial placement of the filter to long-term complications. Some of the reported complications are unique to each filter based on design and materials used in the construction of the filter. Some of the commonly identified complications include wound hematomas from the access site (2%), sepsis (less than 1%), recurrent PE (5%), filter migration (less than 1%), acute and delayed caval thrombosis (5%), limb edema, retroperitoneal hemorrhage, perforation of the IVC as well as adjacent organs including the aorta, tilting of the filter, and wire prolapse specific to the bird's nest type of filter, failure of the filter to open, fractured filter (1%), and misplacement of the filter in the vena cava (57).

FOREIGN BODY RETRIEVAL AND MANIPULATION

Foreign bodies have been identified within the vasculature since invasive procedures were first instituted as medical therapy. Foreign bodies pose a particular health risk of infection and hemorrhage. In addition, they can migrate within the body to unsafe locations including the heart and pulmonary vasculature, causing dysrhythmia and shortness of breath. They can migrate to small blood vessels and cause thrombosis. When a foreign body is lost uncontrollably in the vasculature, it puts the patient's life potentially at risk and is intensely anxiety provoking for all caregivers involved.

Surgical removal has been the mainstay for retrieval of foreign bodies until 1964, when the first percutaneous retrieval of a foreign body was described by Thomas et al. (69). At that time, Thomas and Sinclair retrieved a broken segment of steel spring from the right atrium and IVC. Since that time, the number and complexity of percutaneous procedures has

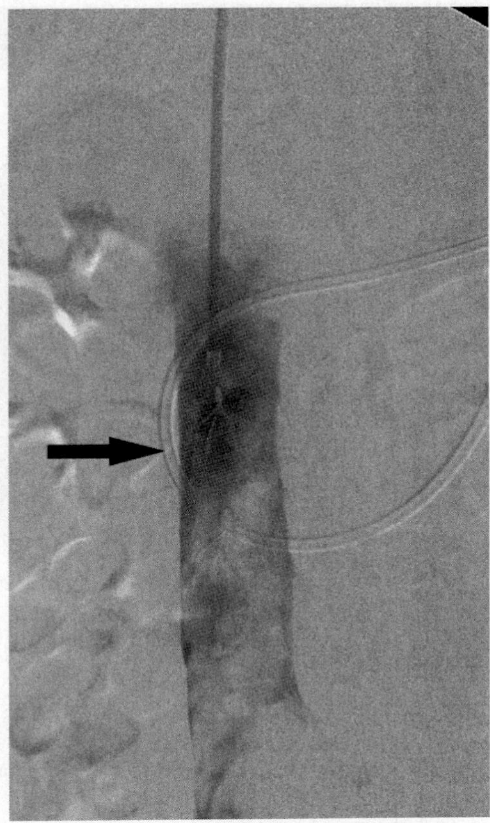

FIGURE 35.50. Venogram of the inferior vena cava (IVC) shows deployment of a filter (*black arrow*) above the clot in the IVC.

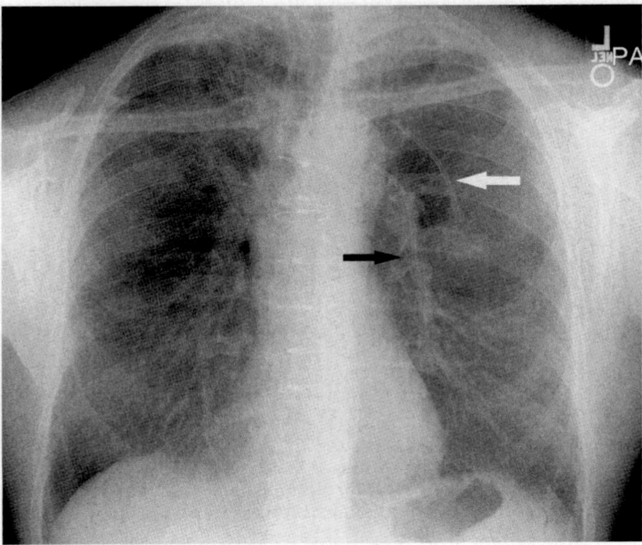

FIGURE 35.51. A chest radiograph was obtained in this patient with a nonfunctioning portacath in the left subclavian vein. Note the implanted port (*white arrow*) in the left chest wall. There is disruption of the catheter at the thoracic inlet. The distal fragment is noted in the left pulmonary artery (*black arrow*). (Image courtesy of Harry K. Meisenbach, MD.)

increased dramatically. As technology has advanced, producing more therapeutic devices, which are made continually smaller and more technical, the potential for treating numerous diseases with minimal invasion increases. With this tremendous growth of percutaneous procedures come increasing numbers of foreign bodies that are found within the vasculature and body. Percutaneous retrieval of foreign objects has become a mainstay of interventional radiology (70). Egglin et al. (71) have published success rates of 97% for percutaneous foreign body retrieval, and it is now the initial choice of retrieval treatment options (72).

The initial foreign bodies identified were related to procedures in which had been lost wires, fragments of diagnostic angiography catheters, portions of balloons, and misplaced or migrating endovascular stents. Increasing numbers and types of procedures have resulted in an increase in foreign bodies, including migrating IVC filters, fragmented catheters—including PICCs—implanted portacaths, dialysis catheters, and CVCs (Figs. 35.51 and 35.52). More recently with the development of embolization techniques using coils, there have been increasing numbers of nontarget embolizations that have prompted additional foreign bodies to be retrieved (73). It is important to note that any device placed within the vascular system is prone to breaking or fragmenting, including fractured pacemaker wires, portions of intra-aortic balloon pumps, biopsy needles, and fragmented deployment catheters, to name but a few (73–75). Foreign bodies are not unique to the vascular system. Many examples are discussed in the literature including broken nasogastric tubes, gastrostomy tubes, nephrostomy and ureteral catheters as well as broken drains and others. All of these foreign bodies, while still relatively uncommon, pose a significant threat and usually need to be addressed emergently.

Initial retrieval techniques consisted of using homemade snares, which were essentially a diagnostic catheter with an angiographic wire looped through the end to create a loop that was used to encircle the free end of the foreign body and ultimately remove the fragment. Additional devices that were

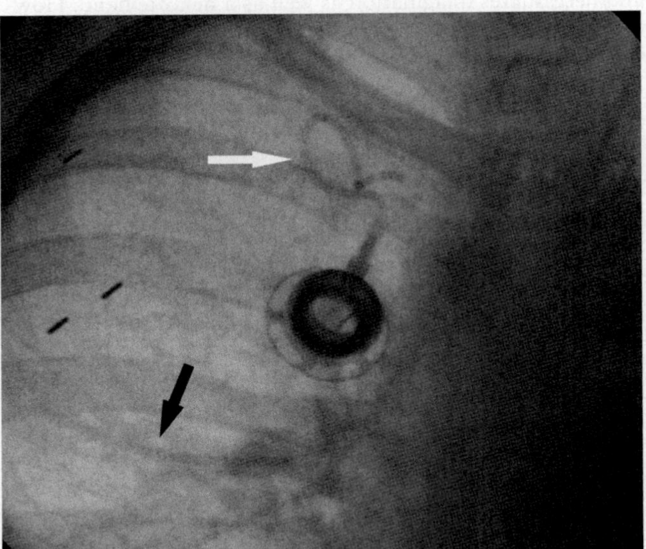

FIGURE 35.52. A second patient with a nonfunctioning portacath in the right chest wall. The implanted port is noted (*white arrow*). The free fragment of catheter has migrated into the right pulmonary artery (*black arrow*). (Image courtesy of Harry K. Meisenbach, MD.)

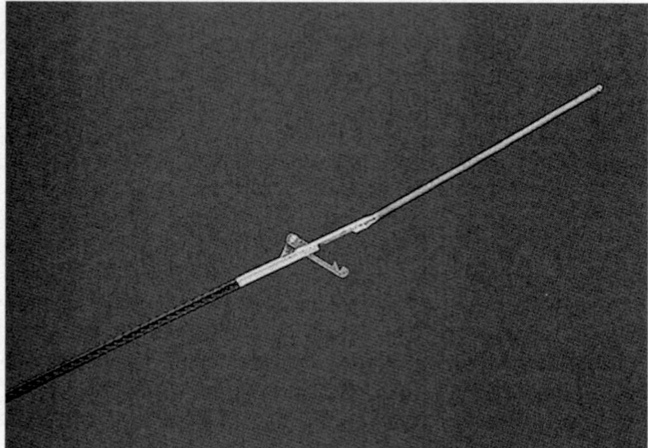

FIGURE 35.53. Endovascular forceps allow for grasping foreign bodies. (Image reproduced with permission from Cook Corporation.)

developed were metallic forceps or graspers (70) (Fig. 35.53). It was learned that using fluoroscopic guidance, these biopsy forceps could be guided to the foreign body and used to gain control of the object and pull it out of the body. Other devices include metallic baskets, balloons, and wires with magnetic tips to adhere to the object (73) (Fig. 35.54). Perhaps the greatest single advance was the development of the gooseneck snare originally described by Casteneda in 1991 (76) (Fig. 35.55). This was the first snare device that exits the catheter at a right angle and comes in different sizes, making retrieval of foreign bodies much easier in different-sized vessels. Today, there are many variations of the gooseneck snare; perhaps the most popular is the Ensnare device, which has three loops or snares in one (Fig. 35.56). Additional devices used are deflecting wires, baskets, and suction devices.

Unlike other routine angiographic procedures, which are essentially standardized and do not vary significantly from one institution to the next, each foreign body retrieval is unique and necessitates imagination as well as a delicate hand. However, there are some basic principles that should be adhered to when attempting foreign body retrieval. First, does the re-

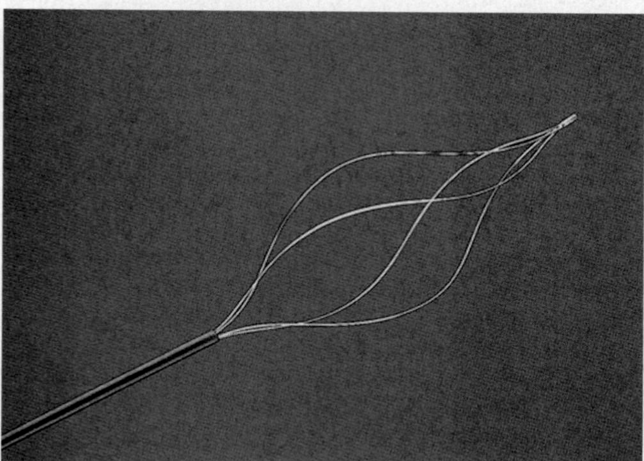

FIGURE 35.54. Endovascular basket also allows for retrieval of foreign bodies. (Image reproduced with permission from Cook Corporation.)

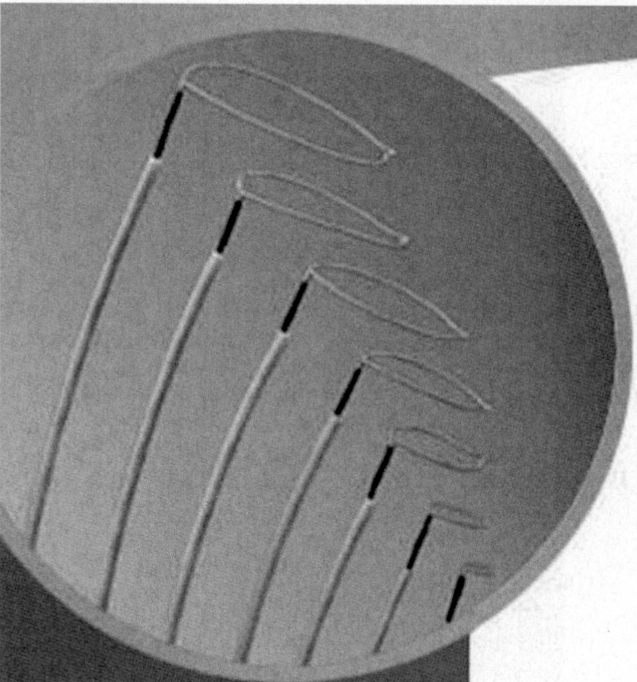

FIGURE 35.55. The gooseneck snare has the snare loop at a 90-degree angle from the wire. This allows for endovascular retrieval of foreign bodies. (Image reproduced with permission from EV3 Corporation.)

trieval procedure pose more risk to the patient than simply leaving the foreign body in its current location? An example of this scenario is an embolized coil to a peripheral branch of the hepatic artery during embolization of a hepatic artery pseudoaneurysm. Although the coil may occlude a small distal branch of the hepatic artery, the dual blood supply to the liver will likely prevent any infarction or ill outcome.

Second, is the foreign body likely to migrate to an unstable position where it poses more of a risk to the patient? An example of this is a fragment of a dialysis catheter that is lodged in the superior vena cava. While at present, the patient may be

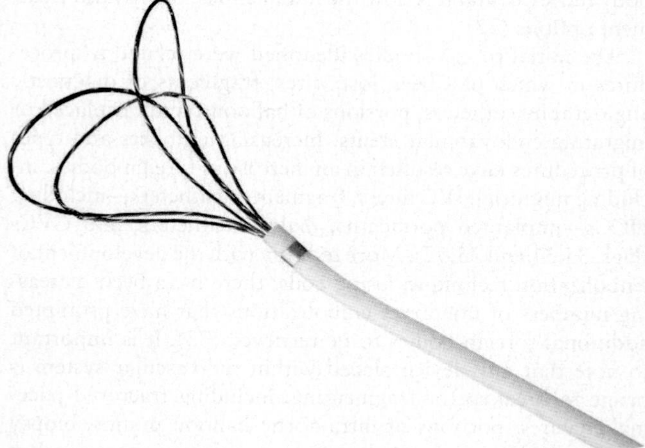

FIGURE 35.56. The Ensnare device has three loops to increase the ability of the snare to trap foreign bodies. (Image reproduced with permission from Angiotech Corporation.)

asymptomatic, the fragment could easily move to the right atrium, right ventricle, or pulmonary vasculature where it could lead to increased risk of pulmonary embolism or dysrhythmia.

Third, it is important to know the exact location of the foreign body. If it has migrated outside the vascular system, then an endovascular approach will be futile and another approach will be necessary. An example of this has been described in the literature with IVC filters that have migrated from their normal infrarenal location to the heart and have a strut extending outside the myocardium (77). Obviously an endovascular approach would not be advised for filter removal in this case.

Finally, can the object be physically removed from the body without causing harm? Some endovascular stents or stent grafts are difficult to remove given their large size. Therefore, in these instances, it is usually in the patient's best interest to move the stent to a location that poses less risk. One example is stents that have migrated from their normal location. These have been successfully repositioned into vessels and locations to minimize any threat of complication.

In general, endovascular retrieval is accepted as a safer, faster, and cheaper method than the surgical alternative. Several examples follow of common retrieval scenarios seen in the ICU.

1. Vascular access catheter fragment in the pulmonary artery. The concept is that most fragments occur at the confluence of the subclavian vein, clavicle, and first rib. When a catheter is present in this location, motion of the arm creates a pinch-type event on the catheter. Over time, the catheter weakens in this location and is susceptible to fragmenting. The approach to the removal of a catheter is to identify the free end of the fragment and attempt snaring, usually from a femoral vein access. This vein is chosen given its size and ability to accommodate larger sheaths and catheters, if needed, for removal. If a free end of the fragment is not readily snared, the catheter can often be moved, using a pigtail catheter, to a more practical location. Alternatively, a wire can be snared around the central portion of the catheter, and the snare and catheter are both pulled out through the same sheath, in effect creating a snare from a regular angiographic guidewire and affecting removal of the foreign body.
2. Migrating, unopened filter in the inferior vena cava. IVC filters are commonly used to prevent fatal pulmonary embolism in patients who have a contraindication to anticoagulation. These devices are made from various metals and come in various shapes and sizes. They are generally sized to the diameter of the IVC. Occasionally, these devices fail to open on release from the deployment sheath. Generally, it is the opening of the filter that anchors it into its location, usually in the infrarenal IVC. When the filter does not open fully on its release, it is prone to cephalad migration and may end up in the heart. With the development of retrievable filters, there are several devices available to grab the tip of the filter and remove it safely, in its entirety.
3. Embolic coils are sometimes challenging to place and may reach a nontarget location if the coil is not sized appropriately to the vessel being embolized. When this happens, the coil should be retrieved if possible, assuming retrieval does not pose additional risk to the patient.

There are a few special scenarios that deserve mention. The following examples are not uncommon to patients in the ICU, and knowledge of their cause and appropriate treatment is important.

1. The "stuck wire" has been described in the literature and is not uncommon (78,79). This usually occurs when the health care provider is placing a central line in the right internal jugular vein. After gaining access to the vein using a needle, a wire is advanced to maintain access while dilating the puncture site to accommodate the central line. After placement of the catheter, the provider meets resistance when pulling on the wire and is unable to withdraw the wire. When a radiograph is obtained, it is noted that the wire is fouled on the struts of an IVC filter. Do not pull the wire as this will result in either dislodging the filter or further tightening the attachment of the wire to the filter. The appropriate next step is to secure the wire on the patient's neck and notify IR. The technique for freeing the wire is the "monorail technique" and has been described in the literature (80). This entails making a small hole in an angiographic catheter approximately 1 cm from its tip and advancing this catheter over the existing wire with the wire exiting the catheter at the newly placed side hole. The stiff end of a wire is then advanced into the catheter from the hub, and the unit is advanced to the level of the filter. This will allow enough torque to free the wire and allow safe removal. This technique should only be performed using direct fluoroscopic visualization.
2. The "knotted catheter" is well known and is usually related to placement of a Swan-Ganz catheter. The balloon tip fails to float freely into the pulmonary artery and as a result, the provider retracts the catheter and then readvances it in an attempt to make it reach the appropriate location. In the process, the catheter becomes entangled on itself and forms a knot. Again, once this is discovered, do not pull the catheter in an attempt to undo the knot as this will only tighten it further making removal more difficult. The appropriate treatment is to notify IR who can then use a series of wires and catheters to undo the free end of the catheter and ultimately remove the knot under direct fluoroscopic guidance.
3. The "migrated PICC" is common to the ICU. Briefly, the patient has had a PICC placed with its tip in the SVC and confirmed by x-ray film. On a subsequent film, the tip of the PICC line is in a suboptimal location in the internal jugular vein. Depending on the medications and fluids going through the PICC, this could pose some risk to the patient. Again, IR is ideally suited for correcting this problem, using fluoroscopic guidance and either a guidewire or other deflecting device, including rapid injection of 5 mL of saline to move the tip into a satisfactory location.

As long as procedures are being performed on patients, we are likely to see various foreign bodies within the vasculature and other organ systems. Increasing technology allows physicians to develop new treatments and increase the number of procedures available. This will certainly lead to an increased variety of foreign bodies identified and with it, place new demands for imaginative techniques to safely remove these objects. Although a loose foreign body inside a patient can be anxiety provoking and may have a potentially hazardous outcome, it is likely that others have encountered the same complication. By understanding the devices used and the techniques available, retrieval should be a relatively mundane experience.

VASCULAR MESENTERIC PATHOLOGY

Frequent mesenteric pathologies encountered in the ICU are mesenteric ischemia, gastrointestinal bleeding, and solid organ trauma with hemorrhage. A brief review of the vascular anatomy is essential to the understanding of these pathologies and their treatment. The three major aortic branches supplying the abdominal organs are the celiac artery, the superior mesenteric artery, and the inferior mesenteric artery. The *celiac artery* arises from the abdominal aorta at approximately the T12/L1 disc space and provides the arterial supply to the liver, spleen, stomach, and pancreas. There are three primary branches—the left gastric artery, which supplies the fundus of the stomach, the common hepatic artery, and the splenic artery. The *superior mesenteric artery* (SMA) arises from the anterior abdominal aorta approximately 1 to 2 cm distal to the celiac artery and supplies the pancreas, most of the small bowel, and the right colon. The *inferior mesenteric artery* (IMA) arises from the anterior distal abdominal aorta at the level of L3 and supplies the left colon, the sigmoid colon, and the superior rectum.

Numerous collateral pathways exist between the mesenteric vessels such as the pancreaticoduodenal artery connection between the celiac axis and the SMA, or the middle colic connection between the SMA and IMA. Collateral pathways also exist within these vessel territories such as the communication of the splenic and left gastric branches of the celiac axis through the short gastric arteries. These communications are important in providing collateral circulation in chronic states where atherosclerotic disease is present but may also aid in tissue perfusion when transarterial embolization is required in the treatment of an acute gastrointestinal hemorrhage.

Imaging

Imaging of the mesenteric vessels can be performed with digital subtraction angiography (DSA), CT angiography (CTA), MR angiography, and, to some extent, with ultrasound and nuclear medicine. DSA remains the gold standard in the evaluation of the mesenteric vessels. This study requires performance in the angiography suite, and, depending on the patient's condition, conscious sedation administration or anesthesia may be required. Most of the bowel must be free of significant amounts of residual barium or Gastrografin contrast agents from prior studies. The procedure includes abdominal aortography and selective catheterizations of at least the celiac trunk, SMA, and IMA. However selective catheterizations of additional vessels such as the splenic artery, the left gastric artery, or hepatic artery are often required. Therefore proper renal function or support is critical due to potential total iodinated contrast dose.

CTA can also be used in the initial evaluation of suspected abdominal pathology. This is performed with a baseline noncontrast CT of the abdomen and pelvis followed by rapid IV bolus administration of 100 to 150 mL of iodinated contrast material with associated thin-section imaging followed by postadministration contrast-enhanced CT. Multiplanar reformations and CT angiography can be performed off line of the thin-section CT data to create arterial images. CT has advantages of not only being able to evaluate the proximal vessels but also the ability to evaluate the perfusion of the visceral organs and status of the bowel wall. MR and magnetic resonance angiography (MRA) can provide similar data as with CT; however, the study is often degraded by patient motion or the presence of metallic implants such as IVC filters or surgical clips. The lack of significant nephrotoxicity of the gadolinium contrast agents may allow for a more focused DSA examination in patients with compromised renal function. Ultrasound can be used in the initial evaluation of abdominal pathology but is limited in its ability to evaluate the vasculature. The aorta can be well demonstrated as can the celiac trunk and SMA. However, distal branches of these vessels and the IMA are usually not imaged due to their small caliber (Fig. 35.57A–F).

Nuclear medicine imaging is of importance in evaluation of patients with gastrointestinal bleeding. Evaluation with a ^{99m}technetium-tagged red blood cell study can detect bleeding at a rate of 0.1 mL per minute compared with the 0.5 to 1 mL per minute required for DSA.

Mesenteric Ischemia

This process resulting from inadequate blood supply to the intestine is usually seen in elderly patients and results in bowel inflammation and injury. The most common form is acute mesenteric ischemia, a result of emboli or hypotension. The less common chronic form is most often secondary to atherosclerotic disease producing hemodynamically significant stenoses in at least two of the three mesenteric arteries (81). Our discussion will focus on acute mesenteric ischemia, as it is not only a cause of admission to the intensive care unit, but can also be present as a comorbidity in the ICU patient population.

Acute mesenteric ischemia can be a true emergency with mortality exceeding 80% without rapid intervention in most reports. Many cases—approximately 50%—are secondary to an embolic event, usually cardiac or aortic in origin. However, approximately 20% are due to thrombosis of an existing atherosclerotic lesion, 20% due to prolonged hypotension, and 10% due to mesenteric venous thrombosis (82,83).

Findings on plain abdominal film are nonspecific early in the course of ischemia, with air in the bowel wall or in the portal vein seen only as a late finding. CT is an excellent screening examination, especially when combined with CT angiography. However, if intestinal ischemia is suspected, oral contrast should not be administered as this will degrade any subsequent DSA study. CT examination with IV contrast administration will allow visualization of the bowel wall and the arterial and venous structures. DSA remains the gold standard in the imaging evaluation of suspected acute mesenteric ischemia. The most common finding is that of an embolus within the SMA, particularly at its origin. Many of these emboli will fragment and migrate distally in the SMA and result in more significant ischemia as the collateral pathways are occluded. Emboli to other sites may also occur. The primary role of interventional radiology in these cases is diagnostic (84). In those patients without peritoneal signs or evidence of bowel infarction, intra-arterial thrombolysis or suction thrombectomy may be attempted and has been shown to be beneficial in select case reports. However, surgical thrombectomy and resection of infarcted bowel remains the standard of care (85).

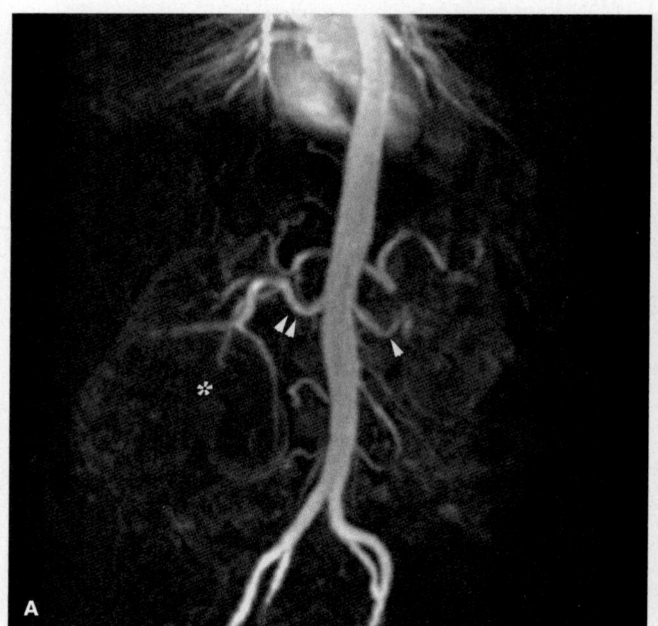

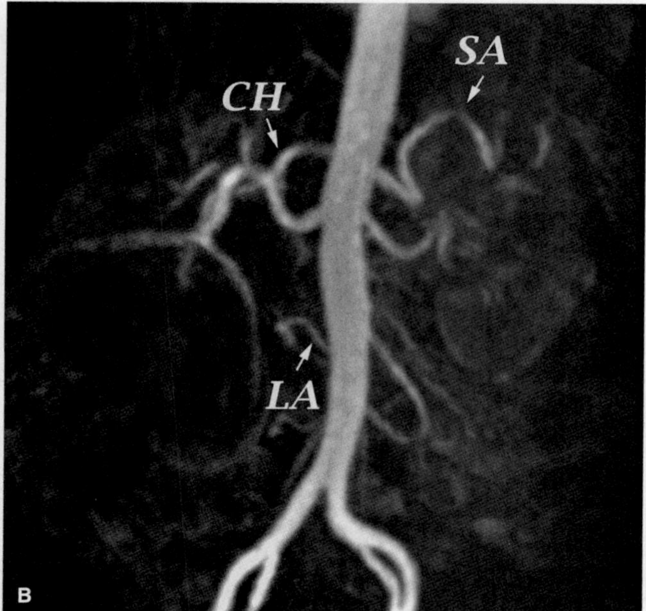

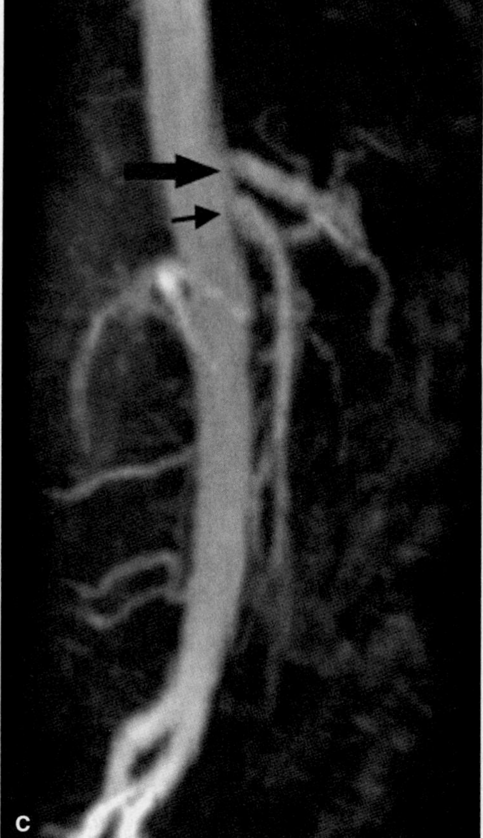

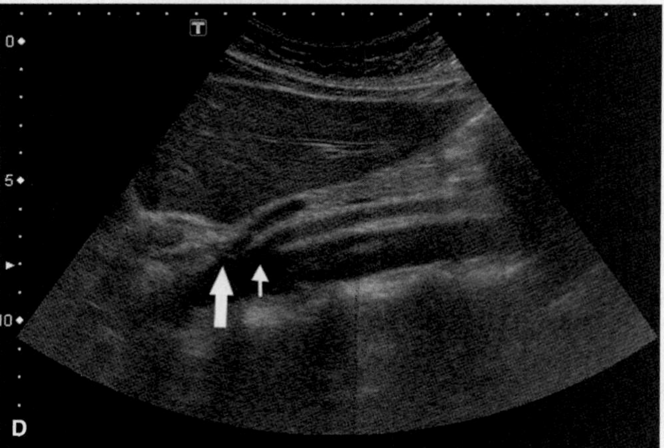

FIGURE 35.57. Rotational views from a magnetic resonance (MR) abdominal aortogram in a patient with right-sided renal hypernephroma. **A:** Frontal view with full field of view demonstrates normal caliber left renal artery (*arrowhead*) compared with dilated right renal artery (*double arrowheads*). The branches of the right renal artery are splayed around a large mass extending from the lower pole of the kidney (*asterisk*). **B:** Magnified view of **A.** Also note the appearance of the normal splenic artery (*SA*), common hepatic artery (*CH*), and lumbar arteries (*LA*). **C:** Further rotation of B to the lateral projection allows visualization of the celiac trunk (*thick arrow*) and the superior mesenteric artery (*arrow*). **D–F:** Three other patients demonstrating imaging modalities of the aorta. **D:** Long axis of the abdominal aorta with ultrasound origins of the celiac axis (*thick arrow*) and superior mesenteric artery (*arrow*) are well seen. The distal aspects of the vessels cannot be visualized due to bowel gas interference. (Image courtesy of Patricia Mergo, MD, Gainesville, FL.)

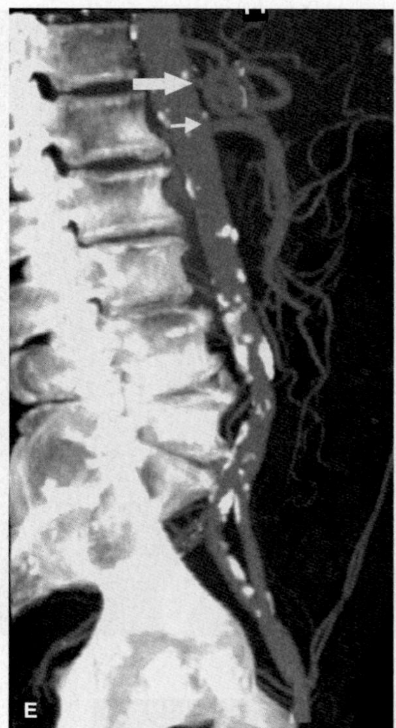

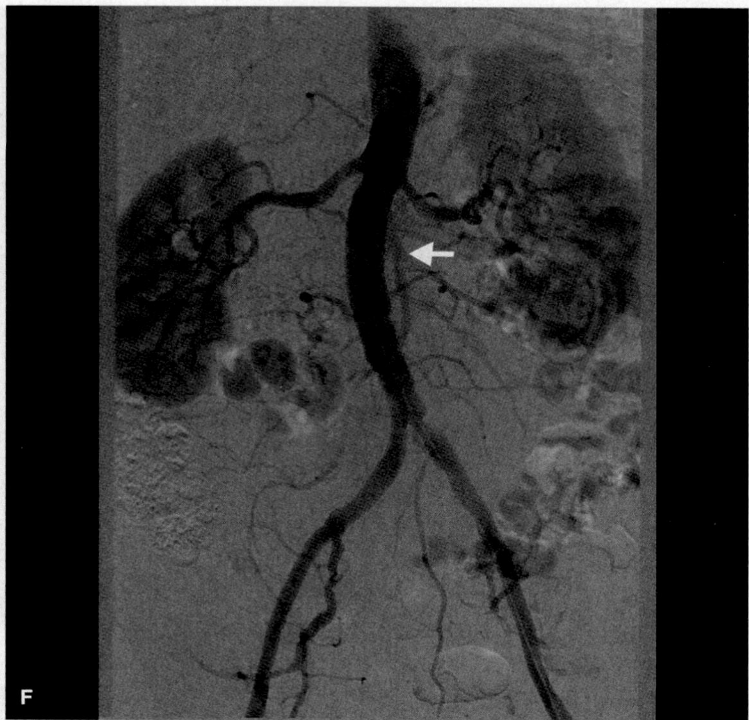

FIGURE 35.57. **E:** Sagittal CT angiogram reconstruction of the abdominal aorta. Again origins of the celiac axis (*thick arrow*) and the superior mesenteric artery (*arrow*) are well seen. Additionally, the more distal aspects of the vessels can also be visualized. The image can be rotated as was done with the MR angiogram (**A–C**) to allow better visualization of specific areas. **F:** Frontal view of an abdominal aortogram. In this early-phase image, the superior mesenteric artery and its proximal branches can be seen (*arrow*). (Image courtesy of Chris Spinosa, RT, Gainesville, FL.)

In those patients with low flow in the SMA without evidence of a focal stenosis, endovascular treatment of so-called nonocclusive mesenteric ischemia (NOMI) may be attempted with intra-arterial infusion of papaverine. This agent is infused at a rate of 30 to 60 mg per hour for 12 to 24 hours, with repeat angiographic evaluation every 12 to 24 hours (86). The infusion can be continued for several days but is discontinued if peritoneal signs are persistent or worsen, if the patient's cardiac status does not permit continuation of the infusion, or on resolution of symptoms (Fig. 58A–C).

Acute Arterial Gastrointestinal Bleeding

Three primary phases exist in the treatment plan of patients with acute gastrointestinal bleeding: stabilization, diagnosis of bleeding source, and definitive treatment of underlying cause. The mainstay of patient management in acute arterial gastrointestinal bleeding is supportive care and stabilization in the ICU, including placement of large-bore IV lines, fluid resuscitation, blood product transfusion, correction of clotting factor abnormalities, and nasogastric (NG) tube placement. Between 75% and 85% of patients experience spontaneous resolution of the bleeding episode.

After stabilization, the next step is localization of the bleeding source. The GI tract is divided into upper and lower tracts by the ligament of Treitz. Upper gastrointestinal bleeding is much more frequent and usually manifests with hematemesis, and may have a positive aspirate for blood from the NG tube. The most common causes of an upper GI bleed are gastritis or ulcers involving the esophagus, stomach, or duodenum. Other key diagnoses to consider are portal hypertension with varices, a Mallory-Weiss tear, tumor, or an aortoenteric fistula. Lower gastrointestinal bleeding is less frequent and presents with melena or hematochezia. This is usually secondary to a colonic lesion. The most common causes of a lower GI bleed are diverticulosis or angiodysplasia in patients older than 40 years of age, and a Meckel diverticulum or inflammatory bowel disease in younger patients. Most cases (95%) of upper gastrointestinal bleeding are successfully evaluated and treated endoscopically with electrocautery, sclerotherapy, or banding. However, in some cases of persistent bleeding ulcers, treatment with intra-arterial vasopressin infusion or embolization may be required.

Endoscopic evaluation of lower GI bleeding is also limited secondary to residual fecal material and clot. Therefore radiographic evaluation and treatment are frequently necessary. If the patient is actively bleeding at a brisk rate—with bright red blood per rectum—he or she may go directly to angiography; however, with slower bleed rates, initial evaluation is usually with a ^{99m}technetium-tagged red blood cell scan. This nuclear medicine imaging study can detect bleed rates of 0.1 mL per minute and has increased sensitivity when cine scintigraphic methods are used.

Arteriography requires the patient be stable both for transport and the procedure. Selective arteriography is focused at the most likely site based on endoscopic and nuclear imaging. Arterial, capillary, and venous phases are acquired to detect acute extravasation, tumoral blush, or variceal development. The key to diagnosis of an arterial source is the extravasation and pooling of contrast (87). This finding is present in approximately 50% of patients undergoing arteriography for a GI bleed.

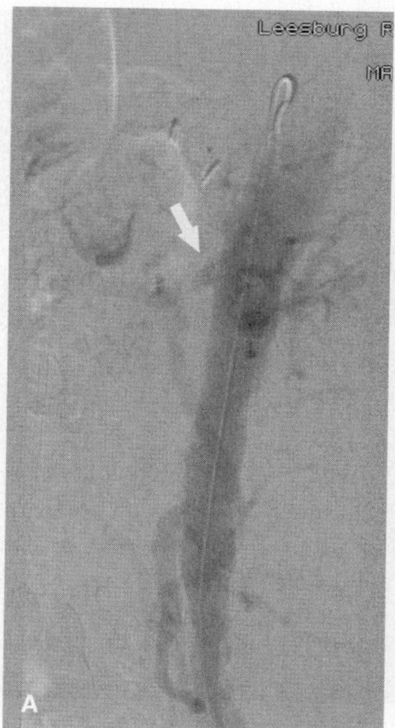

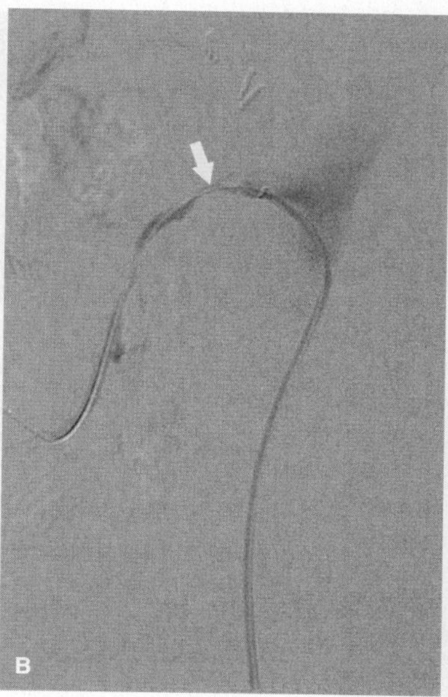

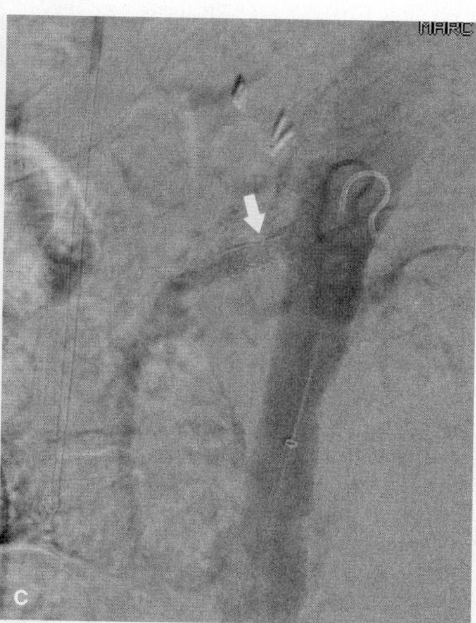

FIGURE 35.58. Elderly female with weight loss and abdominal pain exacerbated with eating. **A:** Lateral aortogram demonstrating a high-grade stenosis of the superior mesenteric artery (SMA) (*arrow*). **B:** Lateral image demonstrating selective catheterization of the SMA with migration of a catheter and guidewire across the area of stenosis. **C:** Following balloon angioplasty and stenting, there is wide patency at the origin of the SMA (*arrow*). (Case courtesy of Marc Schwartzberg, MD, Leesburg, FL.)

If a bleeding site is identified, two primary endovascular treatment options are available—vasopressin infusion or embolization therapy. Vasopressin constricts smooth muscle and can effectively treat focal small vessel or mucosal source bleeding with 90% efficacy. Therefore, it is of primary utility in treatment of diverticular bleeding or diffuse gastritis. The infusion is used to stabilize the patient so as to allow medical management of the gastric or diverticular inflammation, as up to 50% may rebleed following cessation of the infusion. The vasopressin infusion requires selective catheter placement and is performed at a rate of 0.2 to 0.4 units per minute for 24 hours. This treatment is contraindicated in the presence of severe cardiac disease, peripheral vascular disease, or bowel ischemia. Embolization is reserved for larger vessel bleeding sites, especially ulcers in the upper gastrointestinal tract and in areas of angiodysplasia in the lower gastrointestinal tract (88,89). The risk of GI tract ischemia or infarction is less in the upper gastrointestinal system due to extensive collaterals. This increased risk of postembolization infarction in the lower gastrointestinal tract can be minimized with superselective catheter placement and by proper selection of embolic agents. In those cases in which the lesion to be treated can be reached with a catheter, embolization with microparticles, such as 700- to 900-μm polyvinyl alcohols (PVA) or Gelfoam, may be used. When only the arterial pedicle supplying the lesion can be catheterized or if the lesion is a high-flow bleeding site, microcoils may be deployed. Embolization is successful in 90% of cases and has an approximately 20% rebleed rate (90) (Fig. 35.59A–E).

Post–traumatic Abdominal and Pelvic Hemorrhage

Penetrating and high-impact blunt trauma can result in major vascular injury to the abdominal solid organs or pelvis. The presence of significant vascular injury can usually be identified by routine trauma CT protocols, which include noncontrast CT, CT angiography, and post–contrast-enhanced CT studies. Diagnostic angiography is rarely indicated in evaluation of these patients. Key findings that can be demonstrated include free fluid/hemorrhage in the abdomen, subcapsular areas of hemorrhage, parenchymal hematomas, active extravasation of contrast, and pseudoaneurysm formation. Presence of these findings in association with a decreasing hematocrit is an indication for angiography with the intent to embolize, especially in the unstable or difficult to stabilize patient.

The CT examination will have previously identified the areas to be treated, so a complete abdominal diagnostic angiogram is usually not necessary; rather, selective studies are usually appropriate. For hepatic injuries, the examination can focus on the celiac trunk, proper hepatic artery, and SMA. For splenic injuries, the exam focuses on the celiac trunk and splenic artery. For pelvic injuries, the examination includes a pelvic arteriogram with a pigtail catheter in the distal abdominal aorta followed by selective catheterization and angiography of the internal and external iliac arteries bilaterally.

For hepatic trauma, the area of vascular injury is localized and particulate embolization performed, usually followed by coil occlusion. Distal embolization is required due to the extensive network of intrahepatic collaterals. Hepatic infarction secondary to therapeutic embolization is rare due to the portal venous supply to the liver. Transarterial embolization has been shown to decrease the volume required for fluid resuscitation and the volume of blood transfusion required but presents similar complications as compared with open repair. Complications of both procedures include hepatic necrosis, hepatic abscess, and bile leaks with an overall morbidity rate of 58% (91). However, studies have also suggested that hepatic injury patients with grade 4 or 5 liver injury, greater than 25% parenchymal disruption, based on the American

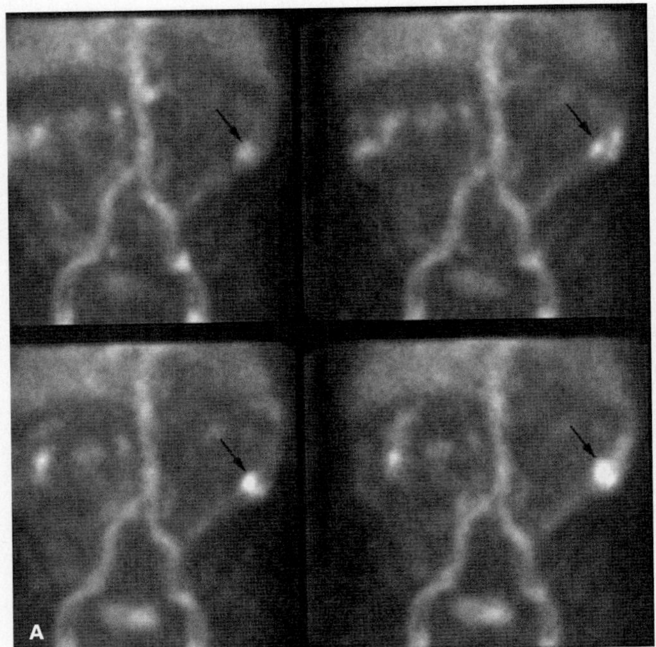

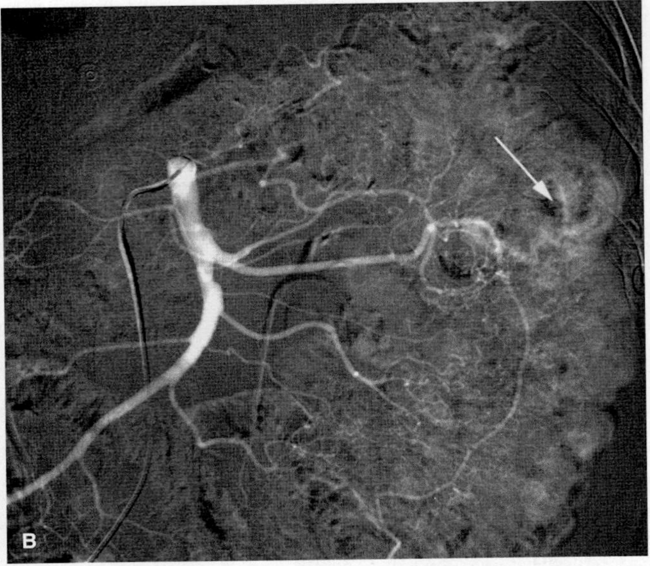

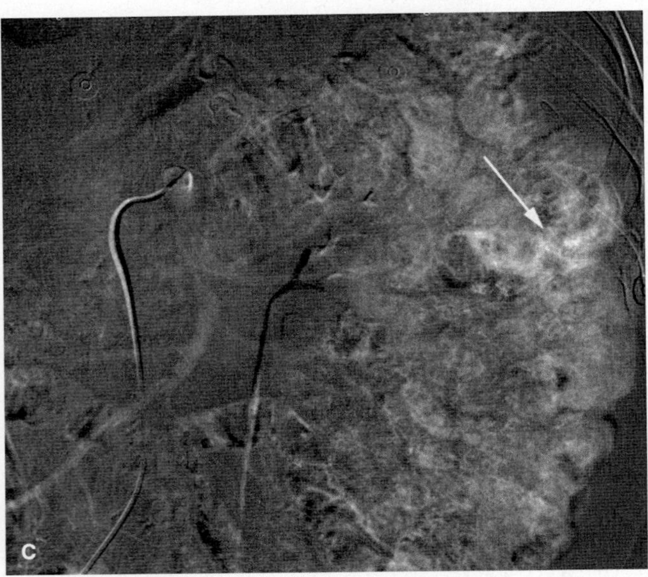

FIGURE 35.59. Elderly patient with acute onset of intermittent lower gastrointestinal hemorrhage with associated anemia and hypotension. **A:** Nuclear medicine tagged red blood cell (RBC) bleeding study demonstrating an abnormal collection of radioisotope in the left midabdomen laterally with shape and movement consistent with localization within the bowel (*arrow*). **B:** Selective superior mesenteric angiogram. **C:** Demonstrates an abnormal area of contrast enhancement and blush in the proximal ileum (noted in both B and C [*arrow*]).

Association for the Surgery of Trauma classification (Mirvis classification) and requiring greater than 2,000 mL per hour fluid resuscitation to maintain normotensive state undergo open repair (92) (Fig. 35.60A–C).

Splenic embolization can be performed at the site of injury if the lesion is small and focal. However, diffuse or major injuries require embolization of the main splenic artery. Embolization of the splenic artery is thought to decrease the risk of rebleed while complete infarction is avoided due to the collateral supply provided from the short gastric arteries. Although embolization decreases the risk of further bleeding, these patients may have significant pain due to splenic infarction and should also be monitored for subsequent splenic abscess development (93,94) (Fig. 35.61A, B).

Pelvic trauma is associated with major bleeding, especially in the setting of a pelvic fracture. Although much of the bleeding can be controlled with pelvic fixation, many of these patients are too unstable and require embolization to stabilize the patient prior to definitive surgical intervention. Due to the acuity of the patient, selective proximal internal iliac embolization is usually performed with 1 to 2 mm Gelfoam pledgets and coils in an attempt to decrease the local arterial pressure and flow. The primary complication of concern is possible embolic material reflux into the external iliac artery leading to lower limb ischemia. Superselective distal catheterization is frequently too time consuming for these critically ill patients, and small particle embolization has the added risk of pelvic ischemia or infarction (95).

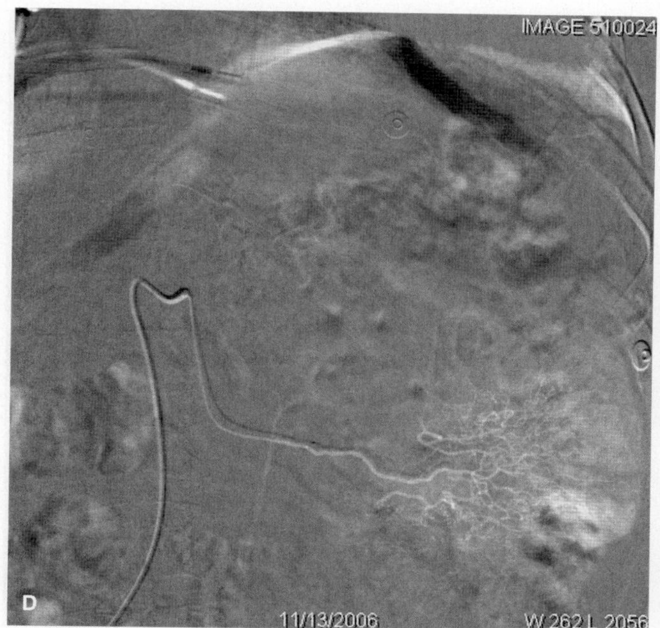

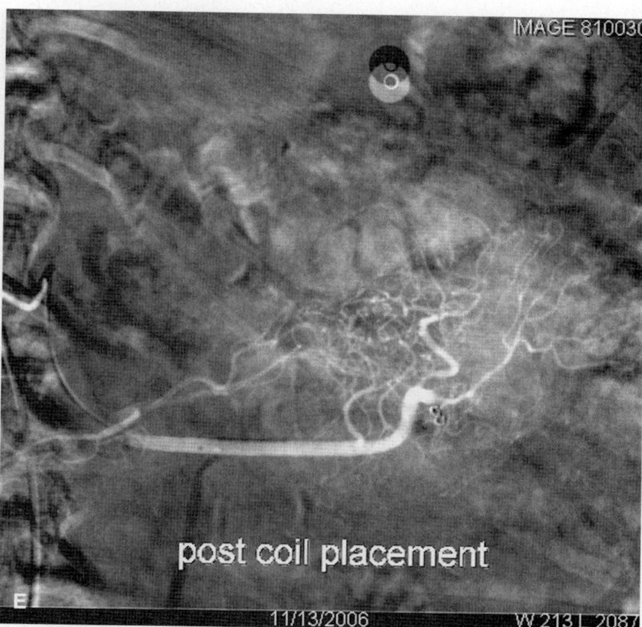

FIGURE 35.59. **D:** Selective catheterization of the abnormal vessel with a 4 Fr catheter. **E:** Post–coil embolization angiogram of the superior mesenteric artery shows nonfilling of the abnormal branch. The patient recovered without further episodes of bleeding.

PERIPHERAL LIMB ISCHEMIA

Patients with acute limb ischemia will often require admission to the ICU. These patients have approximately 25% mortality related to associated vascular disease, which can lead to myocardial ischemia, stroke, renal insufficiency, or limb loss as complicating factors. Additionally these patients may require intensive monitoring secondary to intra-arterial infusion of thrombolytic medications.

The initial presentation of these patients is usually a pale, pulseless extremity. This is associated with pain, paresthesias, and paralysis due to the sensitivity of neural tissue to ischemia. Acute ischemia is a surgical emergency, as irreversible tissue loss can occur with 4 to 6 hours of complete ischemia.

Following diagnosis of limb ischemia, the patient is evaluated to determine whether the event is related to an embolic or thrombotic event. Thrombosis is usually seen in the setting of a pre-existing stenosis and therefore may be better tolerated due to prior development of collateral circulation pathways. The patient will usually have contralateral peripheral vascular disease clinically and on imaging studies, including Doppler, CT angiography, and MR angiography. Embolic occlusions usually present with profound ischemia as collateral pathways have not had time to develop. In these patients, the more proximal pulses may be normal; evaluation must include a search for the source of embolus.

Patients with critical ischemia may be taken directly to surgery for intraoperative angiography and exploration, with subsequent embolectomy and bypass grafting. Patients who develop compartment syndrome may require fasciotomies. These procedures result in limb salvage rates of 75% to 90%.

More stable patients may be candidates for angiography and percutaneous intervention. Angiography is performed to determine the sites of occlusion, possible treatment options, cause of ischemia, and any secondary sites of disease. In the case of an embolic event, this may include evaluation of the aorta for aneurysm or other sources of emboli, along with evaluation of the mesenteric vasculature, renal arteries, and contralateral limb for asymptomatic areas of emboli. Endovascular techniques for recanalization include mechanical thrombectomy, aspiration thrombectomy, balloon angioplasty, and pharmacologic thrombolysis. Success rate and patency rates are similar to surgery. However, patients undergoing pharmacologic thrombolysis deserve special attention.

Pharmacologic thrombolysis is currently performed with agents such as tissue plasminogen activator (t-PA). Prior agents have included streptokinase and urokinase (96). When an intra-arterial infusion is performed, a catheter is advanced under fluoroscopic guidance to the site of the thrombus. Mechanical disruption of the clot is attempted and followed by thrombolytic infusion. The infusion can be rapid and performed in the angiography suite with the so-called pulse spray technique for acute thrombi, or performed with an extended slow infusion in the treatment of more chronic/organized thrombi. In the case of the slow infusion, patients will return to the ICU with a catheter in place. The catheter is positioned with its tip at the level of the clot and a constant infusion of thrombolytic agent via a mechanical pump. The infusion of t-PA can vary but will be approximately 0.5 to 1.0 mg per hour. The patient will need to undergo follow-up angiography every 6 to 12 hours to monitor progress. It is important to note that, in up to 20% of cases, distal emboli will lead to an increase in symptoms following the fragmentation/lysis of the primary clot. However, this usually resolves within 1 to 2 hours with continued thrombolytic infusion and lysis (Fig. 35.62A–C).

As expected, the primary complication with thrombolytic infusion is hemorrhage at the site of catheter insertion. To decrease this risk, an access sheath is used and the access limb is immobilized. Any bleeding will require decrease in the drug infusion rate and decrease in degree of anticoagulation.

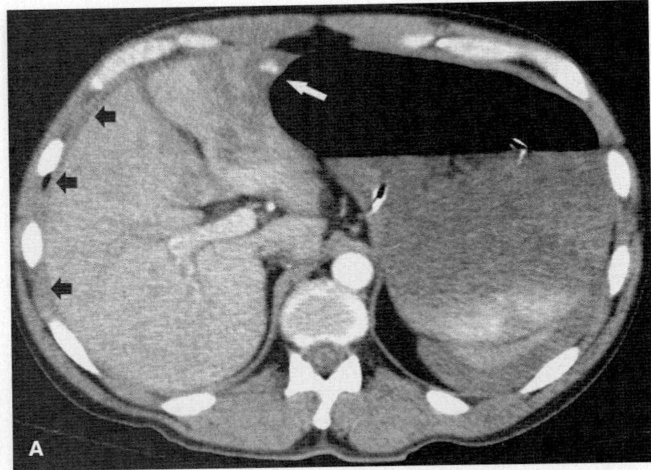

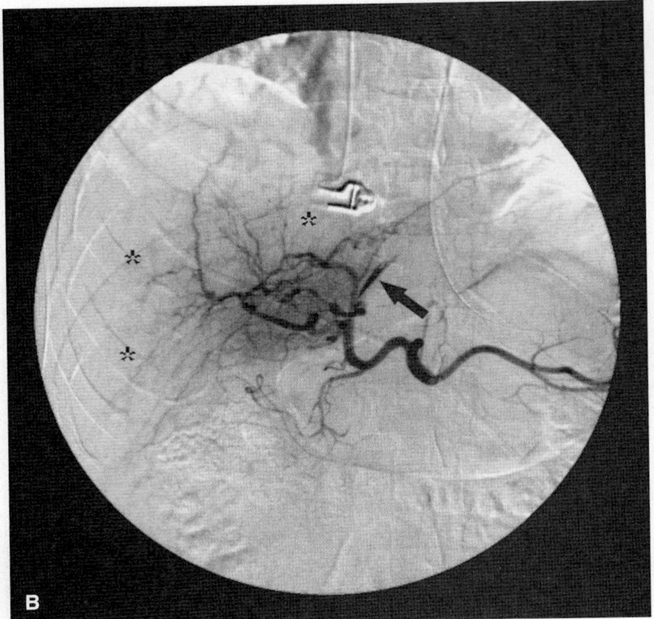

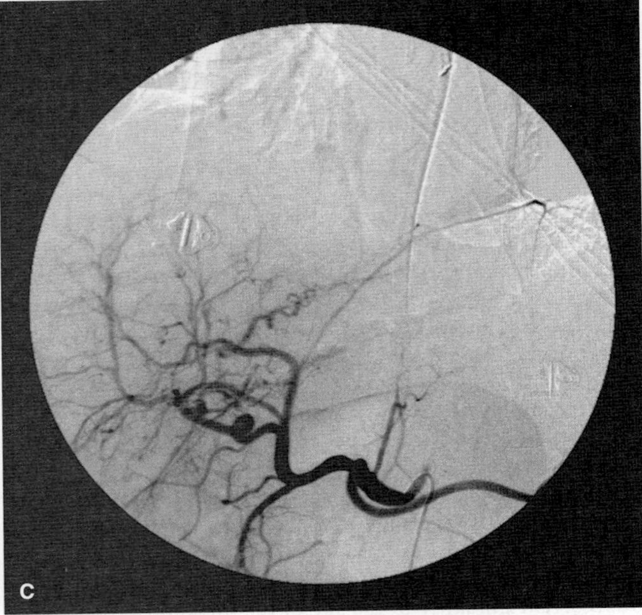

FIGURE 35.60. Patient with grade 3 liver laceration and grade 1 splenic trauma following motor vehicle crash. Patient was stabilized and taken to radiology for embolization. **A:** Axial CT demonstrating liver laceration with subcapsular hematoma (*arrow*) and perihepatic hematoma (*short arrows*). **B:** Selective right hepatic angiogram demonstrating hypovascular areas of hepatic contusion (*asterisks*), and contrast extravasation indicative of active bleeding (*arrow*). **C:** Patient underwent embolization with Gelfoam. Follow-up angiogram demonstrates no evidence of persistent bleed.

There are numerous contraindications to intra-arterial infusion of thrombolytic agents. Absolute contraindications include active or recent—within 10 days—internal bleeding, stroke within 2 months, intracranial neoplasm, or mobile left heart thrombus (97). Preprocedure laboratory evaluation should include hemoglobin/hematocrit, platelet count, PTT, PT, INR, and activated clotting time (ACT).

During the infusion, the patient is most often monitored in the ICU. The arterial entry site should be closely watched and evaluated at least every 30 minutes, and peripheral pulses should be checked every 2 to 4 hours. Repeat analysis of the laboratory parameters should be performed on a 2-hour basis. The hemoglobin and hematocrit should be maintained at or about 10 mg/dL and about 30%, respectively. The patient will most often be re-evaluated angiographically every 6 to 12 hours. Endovascular thrombolysis has a reported success rate of 85% to 95% for acute lower limb ischemia. Success appears to be related to the acuity of the thrombus and a rapid early response to the thrombolytic agent (98–100). Long-term patency is improved if underlying lesions can be treated contemporaneously with either endovascular or surgical methods (101–103).

A major complication of thrombolytic infusion is severe bleeding. If this occurs, the infusion will need to be discontinued. The patient may need transfusion of blood products. Evaluation of the source of hemorrhage may be required for bleeding that persists. Of note, a review of the literature by Kandarpa and Aruny (104) demonstrated an incidence of 6.6% for intracranial hemorrhage. Other complications that may occur include peripheral embolization seen in 5% to 20%, usually secondary to lysis of the thrombus being treated, compartment syndrome seen in approximately 2%, and pseudoaneurysm formation at the arterial access site seen in less than 1% (105,106).

NUTRITION

The importance of adequate nutritional support for the hospitalized patient has become increasingly clear over the past decades. Malnutrition is associated with altered immune

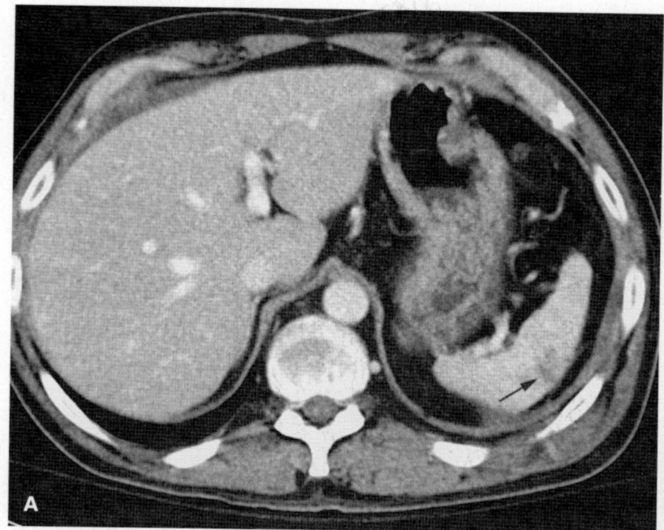

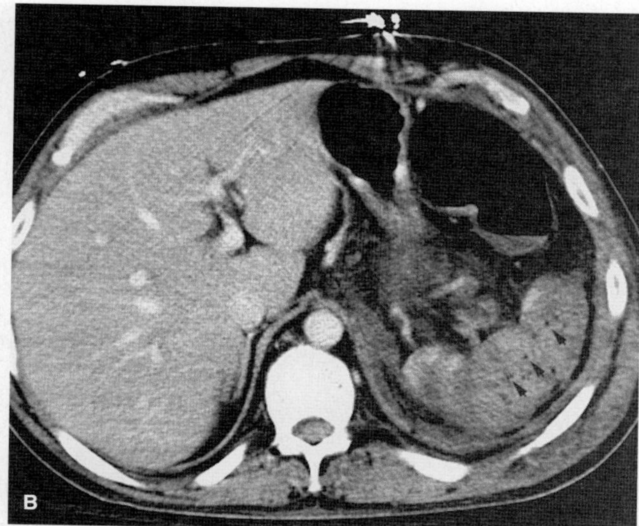

FIGURE 35.61. Patient with blunt abdominal trauma following motor vehicle crash with splenic laceration. Patient was treated with transarterial splenic embolization with subsequent development of splenic abscess. **A:** Preembolization contrast-enhanced CT scan of the abdomen at the level of the splenic hilum demonstrating the grade 2 splenic laceration (*arrow*). **B:** Postembolization day 3 contrast-enhanced CT scan demonstrating an enlarged, edematous, minimally enhancing spleen with small foci of air consistent with necrosis (*arrowheads*).

function, delayed wound healing, susceptibility to infection, reduced quality of life, increased caregiver burden, and mortality. Up to 60% of older adults in hospitals and long-term facilities are malnourished and require supplemental nutrition. The decision to initiate tube feedings is made by the health care provider, usually after a nutritional assessment has been performed and a detailed discussion with the patient or surrogate, outlining the risks and benefits, has taken place (107).

The oral pathway is the preferred route for nutrient delivery. However, when patients are no longer able to independently maintain an acceptable caloric intake, nutritional supplementation should then be considered. As long as the gastrointestinal tract is functional, the enteral route is preferable to the parenteral route and is accomplished through the use of feeding tubes, which may include nasogastric (NG), nasojejunal, gastrostomy, gastrojejunostomy, and jejunostomy tubes (107).

Surgical gastrostomy was initially proposed in 1837 but first successfully performed in 1876 (108,109); the endoscopic technique for gastrostomy was originally published in 1980 (113). The first nonendoscopic percutaneous technique using fluoroscopic guidance and a trochar was described and performed by Preshaw in 1981 (110). Subsequently, Wills and Oglesby, and Tao and Gillies, independently developed gastrostomy procedures using the Seldinger technique in 1983 (109,110).

Nutritional support should be considered in any patient who is going to be without adequate caloric intake for a period of time. There are many feeding tubes available, and choosing one is sometimes difficult. In choosing the correct tube, one considers the length of time the additional support will be needed, the overall medical condition of the patient, as well as the risk of reflux and aspiration. Occasionally, these tubes will also be placed for bowel decompression secondary to prolonged ileus or intestinal obstruction.

In patients who will need short-term support, on the order of 2 to 3 weeks, an NG tube should be the first tube considered as this is the least invasive and the simplest to place. NG tubes are not intended for long-term nutritional use as they may lead to mucosal erosions and sinusitis (107). Additionally, these should not be used in patients with recent esophageal surgery.

For longer periods of time or more chronic conditions, one should consider a gastrostomy tube, which is more invasive than the NG tube but is better tolerated for long periods of time. In patients at risk for aspiration or esophageal reflux, a gastrojejunostomy or jejunostomy tube is more appropriate. Placing the tip of the feeding tube in the jejunum reduces the risk of reflux and aspiration.

There are several relative, and a few absolute, contraindications to percutaneous feeding tube placement. Gastric varices, colonic interposition, infiltrating gastric carcinoma, and uncorrectable coagulopathy are absolute contraindications. The presence of ascites, inability to place a nasogastric tube, partial gastrectomy, enlarged spleen, and hepatomegaly are considered relative contraindications.

Although gastrostomy tubes can be placed both in an open manner and endoscopically, a few situations preclude these services from placing gastrostomy tubes. In many of these instances, interventional radiology can still achieve satisfactory placement. One example includes patients with esophageal stricture. Endoscopic placement is dependent on the ability to pass the endoscope from the oral cavity to the stomach. This may not always be possible due to narrowing of the esophageal lumen. However, a 4 French hydrophilic catheter can usually be advanced over a glide wire even through the tightest of strictures. Additionally, not every patient is able to undergo general anesthesia, and in the IR suite placement of a gastrostomy tube percutaneously often requires only local anesthesia. Finally, there are patients with deformed stomachs secondary to gastric surgery including Billroth I and II. Although tube placement is difficult, the stomach can be safely punctured using CT guidance, and then the tract dilated in the usual fashion. Other anatomic considerations that would persuade one to use CT guidance include patients with a narrow window between the

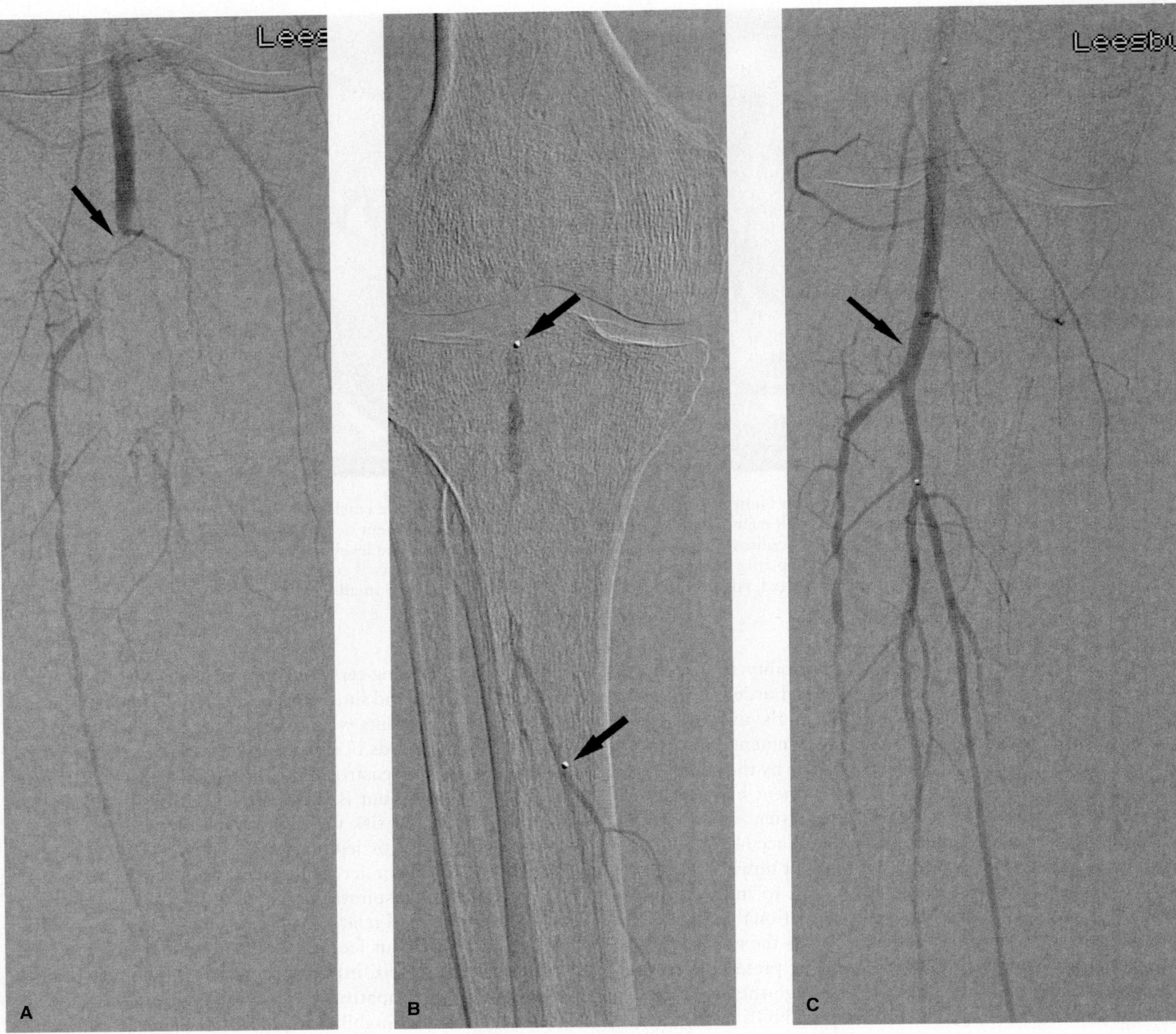

FIGURE 35.62. A 70-year-old male with acute left and right leg pain and ischemia. **A:** Catheter for angiogram at the level of the left knee demonstrates thrombosis of the popliteal artery (*arrow*). **B:** Selective microcatheter placement in the popliteal artery. Distal catheter segment with infusion side holes is marked. **C:** Follow-up angiogram obtained after 24 hours of selective intra-arterial thrombolytic infusion demonstrates patency of the popliteal artery and its runoff. (Case courtesy of Marc Schwartzberg, MD, Leesburg, FL.)

liver, spleen, and colon. The scaphoid abdomen, in which the stomach is tucked underneath the costal margin, is often difficult using only fluoroscopy.

One of the main complications of a gastrostomy tube is the relatively high rate of esophageal reflux, with its associated risk of pulmonary aspiration. One study used scintigraphy to evaluate for gastroesophageal reflux and to determine if gastrostomy tubes caused reflux (107). Patients were evaluated immediately before and 1 week after placement of percutaneous gastrostomy tubes. Almost half of these patients showed evidence for reflux. Although gastrojejunostomy is technically slightly more difficult than placing a gastrostomy tube, it should be considered in all patients with known aspiration.

It is important to be aware of three additional sites that are rarely used but have been described in the literature (108). Translumbar duodenostomy is used in patients being dialyzed peritoneally, in whom any leakage from a feeding tube may lead to peritonitis. To eliminate this risk, the patient is placed prone in the CT scanner and a safe approach to the retroperitoneal portion of the duodenum is identified. Using sterile technique, the duodenum is punctured using the Seldinger technique. The tract is then dilated in the usual fashion. If leak of contents occurs, it is retroperitoneal and is unlikely to lead to peritonitis.

Transhepatic enteral feeding has been described in patients with pancreatic carcinoma that is obstructing the duodenum. Access is obtained into the biliary tree using a transhepatic approach. Two wires are placed, one in the biliary tree while the other is advanced into the small intestine distal to the site of obstruction. An external biliary drain is placed in the biliary tree while a feeding tube is advanced over the second wire into the small intestine for feeding purposes.

Jejunostomy in liver transplant patients could also be considered using the afferent limb of the jejunum. This route has traditionally been used as access to the biliary tree in transplant patients but could also be used for enteral feeding. Briefly, access is obtained into the biliary tree using a transhepatic approach. From this location, a snare-type catheter is advanced into an anterior loop of small intestine. From a percutaneous approach, the snare is used as a target and canalization of the snare is performed. The wire is then pulled through the biliary tree for a through and through access, and a feeding tube can then be advanced into the small intestine.

References

1. Stabile B, Puccio E, vanSonnenberg E, Neff CC. Preoperative percutaneous drainage of diverticular abscess. *Am J Surg.* 1990;159(1):99–104.
2. Nunez D Jr, Huber JS, Yuzarry JM, et al. Nonsurgical drainage of appendiceal abscess. *Am J Roentgenology.* 1986;146(3):587–589.
3. Lambiase RE, Cronan JJ, Dorfman GS, et al. Percutaneous drainage of abscesses in patients with Crohn's disease. *Am J Roentgenology.* 1988;150(5): 1043–1045.
4. Lang EK, Springer RM, Glorioso LW 3rd, et al. Abdominal abscess drainage under radiologic guidance; cause of failure. *Radiology.* 1986;159(2):329–336.
5. Balthazar EJ, Freeny PC, vanSonnenberg E. Imaging and intervention in acute pancreatitis. *Radiology.* 1994;193(2):297–306.
6. Lee MJ, Saini S, Brink JS, et al. Interventional radiology of the pleural space: management of thoracic empyema with image guided catheter drainage. *Semin Interv Radiol.* 1991;8:29–35.
7. Kandarpa K, Aruny J. *Handbook of Interventional Radiologic Procedures.* 3rd ed. Philadelphia, PA: Lippincott Williams & Wilkins; 2001:157–158.
8. Pender SM, Lee MJ. Percutaneous suprapubic cystostomy for long-term bladder drainage. *Semin Interv Radiol.* 1996;13(2):93.
9. Farrell MA, Lee MJ. Interventional radiology of the gallbladder. In: Gazell G. *Hepatobiliary and Pancreatic Radiology.* New York, NY: Thieme Medical Publishers; 1998.
10. Burkhardt H, Meuller W. Versuche uber die Punktion der Gallensblsg und ihre Roentgendarsteeung. *Dtsch Zschr Chir.* 1921;161:168–170.
11. Shaver RW, Hawkins IF, Soong J. Percutaneous cholecystostomy. *AJR Am J Roentgenol.* 1982;138:1133–1136.
12. Pearse DM, Hawkins IF, Shaver R, et al. Percutaneous cholecystostomy in acute cholecystitis and common duct obstruction. *Radiology.* 1984;152: 365–367.
13. Vogelzang RL, Nemcek AA. Percutaneous cholecystostomy: diagnostic and therapeutic efficacy. *Radiology.* 1988;168:29–34.
14. Sosna J, Kruskal JB, Copel L, et al. US-guided percutaneous cholecystostomy: features predicting culture-positive bile and clinical outcome. *Radiology.* 2004;230:785–791.
15. Nahrwold DL. Acute cholecystitis. In: Sabiston D Jr, ed. *Textbook of Surgery.* 15th ed. Philadelphia, PA: WB Saunders; 1997:1126–1131.
16. Lee MJ, Saini S, Brink J, et al. Treatment of critically ill patients with sepsis of unknown cause: value of percutaneous cholecystostomy. *AJR Am J Roentgenol.* 1991;156:1163–1166.
17. Ramakrishnan KG, et al. Percutaneous cholecystostomy—an alternative to surgery in a high-risk patient with acalculous cholecystitis. *Indian J Radiol Imaging.* -year;13:3:307–310.
18. Nemcek AA, Bernstein JE, Vogelzang RL. Percutaneous cholecystostomy: does transhepatic puncture preclude a transperitoneal catheter route? *J Vasc Interv Radiol.* 1991;2:543–547.
19. Boland GW, Lee MJ, Leung J, et al. Percutaneous cholecystostomy in critically ill patients: early response and final outcome in 82 patients. *AJR Am J Roentgenol.* 1994;163(2):339–342.
20. Ghahreman A, McCall JL, Windsor JA. Cholecystostomy: a review of recent experience. *Aust N Z J Surg.* 1999;69:837–840.
21. England RE, McDermott VG, Smith TP, et al., Percutaneous cholecystostomy: who responds? *AJR Am J Roentgenol.* 1997;168:1247–1251.
22. Lee MJ. Gallbladder intervention. In: *The Requisites, Vascular and Interventional Radiology.* Philadelphia, PA: Mosby, 2004:589–597.
23. Hatzidakis AA, Prassopoulos P, Petinarakis I, et al. Acute cholecystitis in high-risk patients: percutaneous cholecystostomy vs conservative treatment. *Eur Radiol.* 2002;12:1778–1784.
24. Browning P, McGahan J, Gerscovich E. Percutaneous cholecystostomy for the suspected acute cholecystitis in the hospitalized patient. *J Vasc Interv Radiol.* 1993;4:531–538.
25. Yedlicka JW, et al. Biliary tract intervention, 1: interventional techniques in the hepatobiliary system. In: *Casteneda's, Interventional Radiology.* Philadelphia, PA: Williams & Wilkins, 1997:1439–1574.
26. Seldinger SI. Percutaneous transhepatic cholangiography. *Acta Radiol.* 1966;253(Suppl):1.
27. Molnar W, Stockum AE. Relief of obstructive jaundice through percutaneous transhepatic catheter—a new therapeutic method. *AJR Am J Roentgenol.* 1974;122:356.
28. Lee MJ. Biliary intervention. In: *Kaufman and Lee's Vascular and Interventional Radiology.* Philadelphia, PA: Mosby; 2004:558–587.
29. Trambert JJ. The biliary tree and pancreas. In: *Bakal's Vascular and Interventional Radiology.* New York, NY: Thieme Medical Publishers; 2002:391–410.
30. Burke DR, et al. Quality improvement guidelines for percutaneous transhepatic cholangiography and biliary drainage. *J Vasc Interv Radiol.* 2003;14:S243–S246.
31. Bosch J, Navasa M, Garcia-Pagan JC, et al. Portal hypertension. *Med Clin North Am.* 1989;73:931.
32. Tadavarthy SM. Transjugular intrahepatic portosystemic shunting. In: *Castaneda's Interventional Radiology.* Philadelphia, PA: Williams & Wilkins; 1997:253–297.
33. Hahn M, Massen O, Nencki M, et al. Die eck sche fistel zwischen der unteren hohevene and der pfortaden und ihre folgen fur den organismus. *Arch Exp Pathol Phramokol.* 1893;32:162–210.
34. Whipple AO. The problem of portal hypertension in relation to the hepatosplenopathies. *Ann Surg.* 1945;122:440–475.
35. Blakemore AH, Lord JW Jr. The technique of using Vitallium tubes in establishing portocaval shunts for portal hypertension. *Ann Surg.* 1945; 122:476–489.
36. Rosch J, Hanafee WN, Snow H. Transjugular portal venography and radiologic portal caval shunt: an experimental study. *Radiology.* 1969;91:1112–1114.
37. Richter GM, Noeldge G, Palmaz JC, et al. Transjugular intrahepatic portocaval stent shunt: preliminary clinical results. *Radiology.* 1990;174;1027–1030.
38. Keller FS, et al. TIPS. In: *Gazelle's Hepatobiliary and Pancreatic Radiology.* New York, NY: Thieme Medical Publishers; 1998:417–447.
39. Freedman A, Sanyal A. Complications of transjugular intrahepatic portosystemic shunts. *Semin Intervent Radiol.* 1994;11:161–177.
40. Freedman A, Sanyal A, et al. Complications of transjugular intrahepatic portosystemic shunts: a comprehensive review. *Radiographics.* 1993;13: 1185–1210.
41. Shultz SR, LaBerge JM. Location of the portal vein bifurcation with relation to the liver capsule: an anatomic study. *Radiology.* 1993;189(P):253.
42. Valji. Vascular access placement and foreign body retrieval. In: Valji *Vascular and Interventional Radiology.* Philadelphia, PA: WB Saunders; 1999:337–355.
43. Cole D. Selection and management of central venous access devices in the home setting. *J Intravenous Nurs.* 1999;22:315–319.
44. Silberzweig JE, Sacks D, Khorsandi AS, et al. Reporting standards for central venous access. *J Vasc Interv Radiol.* 2000;11:391–400.
45. Scott W. Central venous catheters: an overview of Food and Drug Administration activities. *Surg Oncol Clin North Am.* 1995;4:377–393.
46. Foley MJ: Radiology Placement of long-term central venous peripheral access system ports (PAS port): results in 150 patients. *J Vasc Interv Radiol.* 1995;6:255.
47. Allen AW, Megargell JL, Brown DB, et al. Venous thrombosis associated with the placement of peripherally inserted central catheters. *J Vasc Interv Radiol.* 2000;11:1309–1314.
48. Grove JR, Pevec WC. Venous thrombosis related to peripherally inserted central catheters. *J Vasc Interv Radiol.* 2000;11:837–840.
49. Schwab S, Besarab A, Beathard G, et al. *Dialysis Outcomes Quality Initiative Clinical Practice Guidelines for Vascular Access.* New York, NY: National Kidney Foundation; 1997.
50. Safdar N, Maki D. Risk of catheter-related bloodstream infection with peripherally inserted central venous catheters used in hospitalized patients. *Chest.* 2005;128:489–495.
51. Mauro M, Black S. Central venous access. In: Bakal , et al. *Vascular and Interventional Radiology.* New York, NY: Thieme Medical Publishers; 2002:441–457.
52. Lameris JS, Post PJM, Zonderland HM, et al. Percutaneous placement of Hickman catheters: comparison of sonographically guided and blind techniques. *AJR Am J Roentgenol.* 1990;155:1097–1099.
53. Lund GB. Complications from long term tunneled venous access catheters: a review. *Semin Intervent Radiol.* 1994;2:340–348.
54. Morris SL, Jaques PF, Mauro MA. Radiology-assisted placement of implantable subcutaneous infusion ports for long-term venous access. *Radiology.* 1992;184:149–151.
55. Kuriakose P, Colon-Otero G, Paz-Fumagalli R. Risk of deep venous thrombosis associated with chest versus arm central venous subcutaneous port catheters: a 5-year single institution retrospective study. *J Vasc Interv Radiol.* 2002;13:179–184.

56. Kaufman JA. Upper extremity, neck, and central thoracic veins. In: *Kaufman's Vascular and Interventional Radiology.* Philadelphia, PA: Mosby; 2004:163–193.
57. Kaufman JA. Vena caval filters. In: *Kandarpa's Handbook of Interventional Radiologic Procedures.* 3rd ed. Philadelphia, PA: Lipincott Williams & Wilkins; 2002:245–264.
58. Kaufman JA. Pulmonary circulation. In: *Kaufman and Lee's Vascular and Interventional Radiology.* Philadelphia, PA: Mosby, 2004:194–218.
59. Dalen JE, Albert JS. Natural history of pulmonary embolism. *Progr Cardiovasc Dis.* 1975;17:259–270.
60. Dalen JE. Pulmonary embolism: what have we learned since Virchow?: Natural history, pathophysiology, and diagnosis. *Chest.* 2002;122:1440–1456.
61. Oschner A, Oschner JL, Sanders HS. Prevention of pulmonary embolism by caval ligation. *Ann Surg.* 1970;171:923–938.
62. Qian Z, Tadavarthy SM, Casteneda-Zuniga WR. Inferior vena cava filters. In: *Casteneda's Interventional Radiology.* Philadelphia, PA: Williams & Wilkins; 1997:854–896.
63. Siskin GP. Inferior vena cava filters. *eMedicine* 2006;1:28.
64. Miles RM, Chappell F, Renner O. A partially occluding vena cava clip for prevention of pulmonary embolism. *Am Surg.* 1964;30:40–47.
65. Spence LD, et al. Acute upper extremity deep venous thrombosis: safety and effectiveness of superior vena caval filters. *Radiology.* 1999;210:53–58.
66. Ascher E, et al. Clinical experience with superior vena caval Greenfield filters. *J Endovasc Ther.* 1999;6(4):365–369.
67. Lundell C, Kadir S. Inferior vena cava and spinal veins. In: *Kadir's Atlas of Normal and Variant Angiographic Anatomy.* Philadelphia, PA: WB Saunders; 1991:187–202.
68. Mejia EA, Saroyan M, Balkin PW, et al. Analysis of inferior venacavography before Greenfield filter placement. *Ann Vasc Surg.* 1989;3:232.
69. Thomas J, Sinclair-Smith B, Bloomfield D, et al. Nonsurgical retrieval of a broken segment of steel spring guide from right atrium and inferior vena cava. *Circulation.* 1964;30:106–108.
70. Selby JB, Tegtmeyer CJ, Bittner GM. Experience with new retrieval forceps for foreign body removal in the vascular, urinary and biliary systems. *Radiology.* 1990;176:535–538.
71. Egglin TKP, Dickey KW, Rosenblatt M, et al. Retrieval of intravascular foreign bodies: experience in 32 cases. *AJR Am J Roentgenol.* 1995;164:1259–1264.
72. Gustavo Andrade, Romero Margues, et al. Intravenous catheter fragments: endovascular retrieval. *Radiol Brasileira* 2006;39:no. 3.
73. Gabelmann A, Kramer S, Gorich J. Percutaneous retrieval of lost or misplaced intravascular objects. *AJR Am J Roentgenol* 2001;176:1509–1513.
74. Zoarski GH, Bear HM, Clouston JC, et al. Endovascular extraction of malpositioned fibered platinum microcoils from the aneurysm sac during endovascular therapy. *AJNR Am J Neuroradiol.* 1997;18:691–695.
75. Morse SS, Strauss EB, Hashim SW, et al. Percutaneous retrieval of an unusually large, nonopaque intravascular foreign body. *AJR Am J Roentgenol.* 1986;146:863–864.
76. Yedlicka JW Jr, Carlson JE, Hunter DW, et al. Nitinol gooseneck snare for removal of foreign bodies: experimental study and clinical evaluation. *Radiology.* 1991;178:691–693.
77. Urena R, Greenwood L. Bird's nest filter migration to the right atrium. *AJR Am J Roentgenol.* 2004;183:1037–1039.
78. Marelich G, Tharrat R. Greenfield inferior vena cava filter dislodged during central venous catheter placement. *Chest.* 1994;106:957–959.
79. Loesberg A, Taylor F. Dislodgement of inferior vena caval filters during "blind" insertion of central venous catheters. *AJR Am J Roentgenol.* 1993; 161:637–638.
80. Morgan J, Sussman S. "Monorail technique" for removal of entrapped exchange wire in a Greenfield filter. *J Vasc Interv Radiol.* 1998;9(3):469–470.
81. Kaufman JA, Lee MJ. *Vascular and Interventional Radiology, the Requisites.* Philadelphia, PA: Mosby; 2004:294–296.
82. Nemcek AA, Vogelzang RL. Interventional management of acute mesenteric ischemia. In: Strandness DE, van Breda A, eds. *Vascular Disease: Surgical and Interventional Therapy.* New York, NY: Churchill Livingston; 1994:785–793.
83. Bakal CW, Sprayregen S, Wolf EL. Radiology of intestinal ischemia. Angiographic diagnosis and management. *Surg Clin North Am.* 1992;72(1):125–141.
84. Edwards MS, Cherr, GS, Craven TE, et al. Acute occlusive mesenteric ischemia: surgical management and outcomes. *Ann Vasc Surg.* 2003;17:72–79.
85. Lock G. Acute mesenteric ischemia: classification, evaluation and therapy. *Acta Gastroenterol Belg.* 2002;65(4):220–225.
86. Kandarpa K. Acute mesenteric ischemia. In: Kandarpa K, Aruny J, eds. *Handbook of Interventional Radiologic Procedures.* 3rd ed. Philadelphia, PA: Lippincott Williams & Wilkins; 2002:214.
87. Hastings GS. Angiographic localization and transcatheter treatment of gastrointestinal bleeding. *Radiographics.* 2000;20:1160–1168.
88. Guy GE, Shetty PC, Sharma RP, et al. Acute lower gastrointestinal hemorrhage: treatment by superselective embolization with polyvinyl alcohol particles. *AJR Am J Roentgenology* 1992;159(3):521–526.
89. Okazaki M, Furui S, Higashihara H, et al. Emergent embolotherapy of small intestine hemorrhage. *Gastrointest Radiol.* 1992;17:223–228.
90. Gomes AS, Lois JF, McCoy RD. Angiographic treatment of gastrointestinal hemorrhage: comparison of vasopressin infusion and embolization. *AJR Am J Roentgenol.* 1986;146(5):1031–1037.
91. Mohr AM. Angiographic embolization for liver injuries: low mortality, high morbidity. *J Trauma.* 2003;55(6):1077–1082.
92. Hagiwara A, Yukioka T, Ohta S, et al. Nonsurgical management of patients with blunt hepatic injury: efficacy of transcatheter arterial embolization. *AJR Am J Roentgenol.* 1997;169:1151–1156.
93. Hagiwara A, Yukioka T, Ohta S, et al. Nonsurgical management of patients with blunt splenic injury: efficacy of transcatheter arterial embolization. *AJR Am J Roentgenol/* 1996;167(1):159–166.
94. Pachter HL, Guth AA, Hofstetter SR, et al. Changing patterns in management of splenic trauma: the impact of non operative management. *Ann Surg.* 1998;227(5):708–717; discussion 717–719.
95. Velmahos G. A prospective study on the safety and efficacy of angiographic embolization for pelvic and visceral injuries. *J Trauma.* 2002;53(2):303–308.
96. McNamara TO, Fischer JR. Thrombolysis of peripheral arterial and graft occlusions: improved results using high dose urokinase. *AJR Am J Roentgenol.* 1985;144(4):764–775.
97. Kandarpa K, Aruny J. *Handbook of Interventional Radiologic Procedures.* 3rd ed. Philadelphia, PA: Lippincott Williams & Wilkins; 2002:406.
98. Thrombolysis in the management of lower limb peripheral arterial occlusion–a consensus document. Working Party on Thrombolysis in the Management of Limb Ischemia. *Am J Cardiol.* 1998;81(2):207–218.
99. McNamara TO. Thrombolysis as an alternative initial therapy for the acutely ischemic limb. *Semin Vasc Surg.* 1991;5:89–98.
100. Graor RA, Olin J, Bartholomew JR, et al. Efficacy and safety of intra-arterial local infusion of streptokinase, urokinase, or tissue plasminogen activator for peripheral arterial occlusion: a retrospective review. *J Vasc Med Biol.* 1990;2:310–315.
101. Sullivan KL, Gardinar GA Jr, Kandarpa K, et al. Efficacy of thrombolysis in infrainguinal bypass grafts. *Circulation.* 1991;83(2 Suppl):I-99–I-105.
102. McNamara TO, Bomberger RA. Factors affecting initial and 6 month patency rates after intra-arterial thrombolysis with high dose urokinase. *Am J Surg.* 1986;152(6):709–712.
103. Durham JD, Rutherford RB. Assessment of long-term efficacy of fibrinolytic therapy in the ischemic extremity. *Semin Interv Radiol.* 1992;9:166–173.
104. Kandarpa K, Aruny J. *Handbook of Interventional Radiologic Procedures.* 3rd ed. Philadelphia, PA: Lippincott Williams & Wilkins; 2002:413.
105. Gardiner GA, Sullivan KL. Complication of regional thrombolytic therapy. In: Kadir S, ed. *Current Practice of Interventional Radiology.* Philadelphia, PA: BC Decker; 1991:87–91.
106. McNamara TO, Goodwin SC, Kandarpa K. Complications associated with thrombolysis. *Semin Interv Radiol.* 1994;2:134–144.
107. Dharmarajan TS, Unnikrishnan D. Tube feeding in the elderly: the technique, complications, and outcome. *Postgrad Med.* 2004;115(2):51–61.
108. Llerena J, Gorriz E, et al. Gastrointestinal tract intervention. In: *Casteneda's Interventional Radiology.* 3rd ed. Philadelphia, PA: Williams & Wilkins; 1997:1609–1619.
109. Lee MJ. GI tract intervention. In: *Kaufman and Lee's Vascular and Interventional Radiology, the Requisites.* Philadelphia, PA: Mosby; 2004:521–557.
110. Giuliano AW, Yoon HC, Lomis NN, et al. Fluoroscopically guided percutaneous placement of large-bore gastrostomy and gastrojejunostomy tubes: review of 109 cases. *J Vasc Interv Radiol.* 2000;11:239–246.

CHAPTER 36 ■ FEEDING TUBE PLACEMENT

LAWRENCE J. CARUSO • LARRY C. MARTIN

IMMEDIATE CONCERNS

Major Problems

For critically ill patients, enteral nutrition is preferable to parenteral whenever feasible. However, enteral feeding can be accompanied by multiple challenges. In addition to feeding intolerance and metabolic alterations, enteral support may be hindered by difficulties inserting and maintaining the feeding tube itself. Problems include inability to place a feeding tube into the stomach or small intestine, occlusion of the tube by inspissated feeds or medications, and tube dislodgment.

Mechanical complications of feeding tube placement can be life-threatening. In deeply sedated or comatose patients, inadvertent placement of a nasoenteral tube into the bronchial tree is not uncommon. Percutaneous tube placement can be complicated by bowel perforation or insertion site infection. Thoughtful consideration of the appropriate tube placement method as well as careful technique will minimize complications.

Stress Points

1. The initial consideration for determining the choice of an enteral access system is the anticipated duration of enteral feeding.
   - *Short term:* Patients predicted to need enteral feeding for 2 weeks or less are said to have short-term requirements. These patients are best served with bedside placement of a nasoenteric tube.
   - *Long term:* Patients thought to need enteral feeding for greater than 6 to 8 weeks are described as having long-term requirements. Percutaneous or surgically placed tubes are most appropriate for this subgroup of patients.
   - *Intermediate:* Patients with the anticipated need for enteral feeding for greater than 2 weeks but less than 6 to 8 weeks are said to have an intermediate requirement. These patients are well served by nasally, percutaneously, or surgically placed feeding tubes.
2. Roughly half of critically ill patients have gastric emptying dysfunction. For these patients, enteral tubes may need to be placed beyond the pylorus.
3. Several bedside techniques have been described to aid in achieving postpyloric placement of tubes inserted through the nose. These techniques are highly successful in experienced hands.
4. Fluoroscopic or endoscopic support may be necessary for passing the tip of the nasoenteric tube beyond the pylorus. Even with the assistance of these modalities, success is not guaranteed.
5. Percutaneous gastrostomy has been shown to be less costly and less time consuming, and has fewer complications than surgical gastrostomy.
6. While bolus gastric feeding may occasionally be used, continuous infusion of enteral feeds is better tolerated than bolus feeding (1).
7. Surgically placed jejunostomy tubes are excellent for long-term infusion feeding, but expose the critically ill patient to the risks and complications of an operative procedure.

ESSENTIAL DIAGNOSTIC TESTS AND PROCEDURES

1. Auscultation of air instilled into the nasogastric or nasoenteric tube is useful for determining proper tube placement. It is important to confirm that the tube was not inadvertently placed into the bronchial tree.
2. After placement of a nasogastric or nasoenteric feeding tube, an abdominal radiograph should be obtained to confirm proper tube location before infusing the enteral formula.
3. If there is concern that a nasoenteric tube has migrated back into the stomach, its position must be clarified with a radiograph.
4. Dislodged percutaneous tubes should be replaced as soon as possible to prevent closure of the tube tract.

Initial Therapy

1. Determine whether the patient can tolerate enteral nutrition.
2. Based on the patient's overall condition, associated medical conditions, the functional status of the gastrointestinal tract, and available hospital resources, the most appropriate type of feeding tube and placement technique can be chosen.
3. If the attempted placement technique is unsuccessful, reconsider the above and choose another enteral access option.

OVERVIEW

Critically ill patients will almost invariably require nutritional intervention. Current guidelines support the preferential use of enteral nutrition over parenteral nutrition (1). While parenteral nutrition can effectively deliver protein and calories, it does not prevent intestinal mucosal atrophy (2,3). It is now well recognized that the healthy gut mucosal layer provides a barrier to pathogen invasion (4,5). Microbial invasion through the gut into the systemic circulation is thought to represent a major cause of the nosocomial sepsis, and possibly the multiple organ dysfunction, seen with critical illness (6–9).

Enteral nutrition is preferable to parenteral in terms of cost, complications, gut mucosal maintenance, and metabolic and immune function (10–13). However, feeding the patient via the gastrointestinal tract is more difficult than through a central vein. Enteral feeding is commonly frustrated by gastric dysmotility, aspiration, diarrhea, and occasionally intestinal ileus (14). Feeding intolerance, fluid restrictions, and metabolic derangements further limit attempts to establish total enteral support. Appropriate gastrointestinal access can also be challenging to obtain and maintain, and may require surgical placement. Often, after successful access placement, feeding tubes occlude, dislodge, or are inadvertently removed. Despite the obvious obstacles listed in the first paragraph, it is clear that the benefits of enteral nutrition far outweigh the concerns.

Fortunately, there are a multitude of commercially available tube designs and a variety of placement techniques to meet most needs. The choice of tube type, access site, and placement technique will depend on a number of considerations including each patient's unique requirements, clinician preference, and even available resources. This chapter will review the assortment of tube types, the differences between gastrointestinal placement sites, and the variety of access options available. In addition, it will describe the decision-making process required for choosing the best combination of tube, site, and method of placement.

DETERMINING THE MOST APPROPRIATE TUBE TYPE, SITE, AND PLACEMENT TECHNIQUE

When considering the initiation of enteral feeding, the clinician must first decide on the most appropriate type of tube to employ, the region in the gastrointestinal tract in which to place the tube, and the technique to access the lumen. Several factors influence the ultimate decision (15):

1. Duration of enteral feeding
2. Current status of the patient
3. Coexisting medical conditions
4. Functional status of the gastrointestinal tract
5. Previous abdominal surgeries
6. Tube brands in stock
7. Availability of radiologic, gastroenterologic, and surgical support

Duration of Enteral Feeding

The initial consideration is the anticipated duration of enteral feeding. Based on the patient's current status and comorbidity, it must be estimated whether the access requirement is to be short, intermediate, or long term. The distinction between the three classifications is somewhat artificial and there are no absolute time separations.

Short Term

Short term usually implies the need for enteral feeding for up to 2 weeks in duration. Short-term enteral feeding is commonly used for patients who tend to be free of significant underlying medical conditions, such as trauma victims and younger patients who undergo uncomplicated major surgery. In most of these patients, access requirements can be satisfied by placing the tube into the gastrointestinal tract using the nasal approach. These tubes are considered to be temporary in that they can be easily removed when they are no longer required. Placement techniques tend to be relatively inexpensive and minimally invasive, and carry a low complication rate. Although these tubes easily dislodge, replacement is usually straightforward.

Long Term

Long-term enteral access can be defined as the need to administer enteral nutritional support for an extended period of time or even permanently. Some authors describe long-term support as that requiring access for more than 4 to 6 weeks (16,17). Regardless of the time, the important consideration for these patients is that the tube needs to be more permanently secured. In most cases, nasally placed tubes are not adequate. For this subgroup of patients, tube placement tends to be more invasive and more expensive and has greater potential for complications. It also usually requires surgical or percutaneous procedures. Patients requiring long-term enteral nutrition are those whose illness is such that recovery will be delayed or permanently incomplete. These patients typically are older, have significant comorbid conditions or end-stage organ dysfunction, and have had a serious acute event.

Intermediate Duration

Intermediate duration is also a relative term but encompasses all patients with requirements for enteral feeding access for greater than 2 weeks but less than 6 to 8 weeks. These patients can be served by any of the available access routes. Though nasally placed tubes are less secure, the ease of replacement can often extend their use for the duration of their necessity. Tubes placed percutaneously or surgically tend to be considered permanent but can be removed without much difficulty should feeding access no longer be necessary. In most cases, the decision can be based on factors such as previous abdominal surgery and the availability of resources.

Site of Tube Placement and Technique

Although the patient's current medical status and comorbid conditions indirectly influence the choice of tube by their effects on the duration of tube utilization, these factors also directly impact the choice of placement site and technique. The more critically ill patients are less likely to tolerate a surgical or endoscopic procedure. In these patients, if enteral feeding is desired, less invasive techniques such as nasal access can be used temporarily until conditions are more conducive to long-term access placement. Patients with complications such as intestinal fistulae, laparotomy wound infections, open abdomens, or sepsis from other sources also may be inappropriate for surgically or percutaneously placed tubes. Other groups at increased risk for complications with surgically or percutaneously placed tubes include obese patients and those with diabetes, cancer, malnutrition, immunocompromised conditions, end-stage liver disease, cirrhosis, ascites, renal failure, uremia, thrombocytopenia, coagulopathy states, and significant heart disease.

Inadequate gastric emptying is common in critically ill patients, occurring in roughly half of general intensive care unit (ICU) patients and up to 80% of patients with traumatic brain injury (18–20). Interleukin-1, a cytokine released during stressed states, has been shown to delay gastric emptying when administered to rats (21). Many underlying conditions such as diabetes mellitus, medication use, gastritis, sepsis, and electrolyte abnormalities also affect gastric emptying (22). Due to concerns about inadequate gastric emptying and potential aspiration, many physicians feel compelled to place the tip of the feeding tube in the small bowel. However, while postpyloric feeding has a lower incidence of gastroesophageal regurgitation and a trend toward less aspiration compared to gastric feeding (23), evidence that postpyloric feeding improves outcomes is somewhat lacking.

The Canadian Critical Care Nutrition Guidelines recommended feeding in the small bowel whenever feasible (1). This recommendation is based largely on a meta-analysis of a number of prospective, randomized studies. However, the analysis relied heavily on one particular study (24). Unfortunately, the majority of patients in the postpyloric group were fed into the stomach, calling into question whether the study should be included in the meta-analysis. Two other meta-analyses found no significant differences in the incidence of pneumonia or mortality between patients fed into the stomach or postpyloric (25,26). It should be noted that all of the studies analyzed were fairly small, with the largest study including 101 patients. As a result, the individual studies were underpowered to detect a small but clinically meaningful difference in outcomes. For example, in order to detect a 20% reduction in the incidence of aspiration pneumonia with a baseline rate of 22%, over 2,600 patients would be required (26). Given that the studies were underpowered to show small but meaningful differences in the rates of pneumonia, along with the documented increases in gastroesophageal reflux and microaspiration with gastric compared to postpyloric feeding, it seems appropriate to place the feeding tube postpyloric whenever feasible. However, attempts at postpyloric placement should not unduly delay the start of enteral nutrition, as gastric feedings are often well tolerated.

The extra workload and cost to place the feeding beyond the pylorus is not trivial. While nasogastric tubes can typically be placed fairly easily, placement of postpyloric tubes often involves multiple attempts with as many radiographs. If the tube cannot be properly positioned with a blind technique, endoscopy or fluoroscopy may be required, the latter requiring a trip out of the unit with the associated costs and personnel requirements. Bedside techniques to improve the success of tube placement are discussed below.

BEDSIDE TECHNIQUES

Motility Agents

If gastric feeding is used, the addition of a promotility agent may be helpful. Metoclopramide increases upper gastrointestinal motility by blocking dopamine receptors. It has been shown to improve gastric emptying and decrease gastric residual volumes in ICU patients (27–29). Erythromycin, a macrolide antibiotic that is also a motilin agonist, increases gastric emptying and tolerance to gastric feeding (29–31). The commonly used dose is 200 mg, but 70 mg may be just as effective (32). Unfortunately, patients often develop tachyphylaxis to the drugs after several days, requiring close monitoring of gastric volumes and feeding tolerance (29). Safety concerns should be taken into account when using motility agents. Metoclopramide is associated with movement disorders, which may be irreversible. Erythromycin can prolong the Q-T interval and has many drug interactions. In addition, the long-term use of any antibiotic raises concerns about the development of resistance.

Functional Status of Gastrointestinal Tract

The functional status of the gastrointestinal tract also may influence the technique of tube placement in other ways. Gastroesophageal disease or obstruction may preclude the ability to pass tubes nasally and may also make percutaneous tube placement using the endoscopic approach difficult or impossible. Adhesions from previous upper abdominal surgeries or the anatomic alterations seen after procedures such as gastrectomy or pancreaticoduodenectomy diminish the likelihood of endoscopic and radiologic placement and may make a surgical placement more complicated.

Hospital Resources

Hospital resources—both supplies and personnel—also influence the decision-making process. Hospitals may have a limited selection of tube products, as the cost has become a significant determinant of hospital purchasing. Because many tube designs are similar, substitutions can be successful, and the inability to obtain a specific tube should not preclude the use of enteral nutrition. Human resources also vary from facility to facility. Not all hospitals offer equal expertise in each of the support services required. The choice between radiologic, gastroenterologic, or surgical support may be based to some degree on the strength and weaknesses of these departments within the hospital.

Summary

The selection of the most appropriate tube type, access site, and placement technique for the critically ill is based on the consideration of these interrelated factors. Therefore, the final decision varies from patient to patient. Success is never ensured but occurs most often when all of the dependent variables are considered and the approach is flexible to allow for change when the situation warrants creativity. To aid in the decision-making process, a useful algorithm is provided (Fig. 36.1).

TUBE OPTIONS AND DESIGNS

Currently, a large variety of tube designs are commercially available. For nasal placement, tubes tend to be thin, soft, and flexible. Most are polyvinyl chloride, silicone, or polyurethane. Many are weighted at the tip with mercury, whereas others are

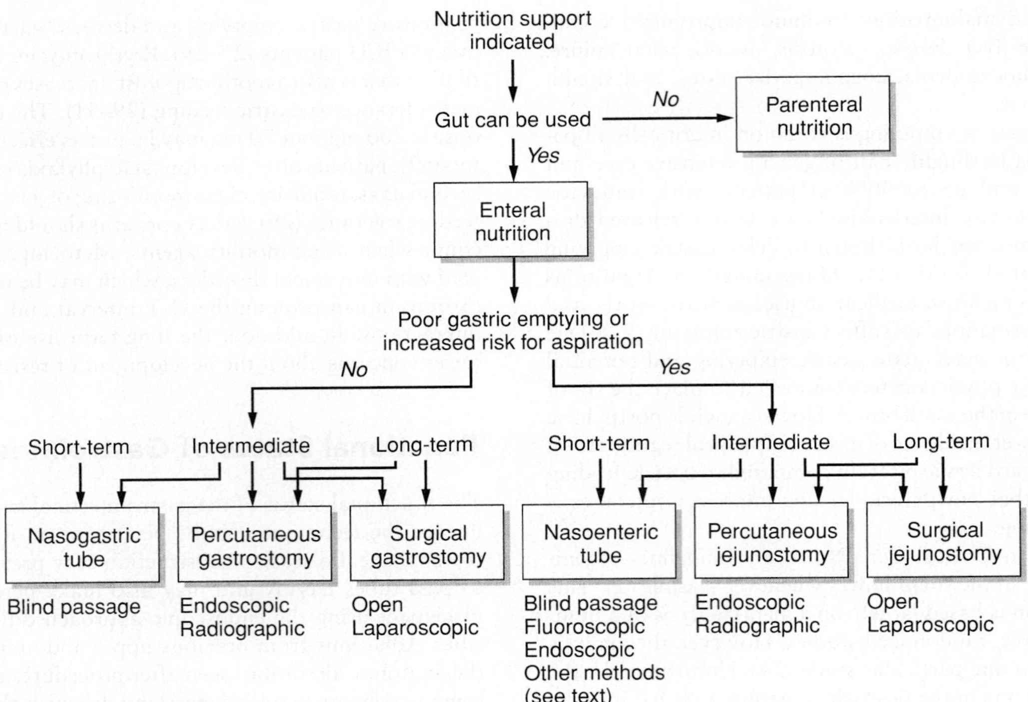

FIGURE 36.1. Algorithm for determining appropriate enteral access for the critically ill.

unweighted. Most contain a thin metal stylet to assist in placement. All are radiopaque to enable confirmation of position by radiographic study. Their soft, flexible construction and narrow diameter enables these tubes to be well tolerated by the patient. However, these tubes are prone to occlusion, particularly if feeding is interrupted without irrigating the tube free of formula and when the tube is used for the delivery of crushed or dissolved medications.

Percutaneous

Percutaneously placed tubes also come in a variety of commercially prepared designs. These tubes tend to be wider in diameter than those used for nasal placement, which decreases but does not completely prevent the likelihood of occlusion. Placement requires fluoroscopic or endoscopic assistance to direct the tube into the appropriate lumen after skin puncture. These tubes are less likely to dislodge but can leak, cause pain at the insertion site, and induce a local soft tissue infection. With long-term use, they also may begin to deteriorate. Some models have separate ports for simultaneous jejunal feeding and gastric decompression. Most are secured from within the lumen of the viscus by a small flange or balloon contained within the tip; removal may require endoscopy.

Surgical

The choices for surgical access are also extensive. Balloon- and mushroom-tipped soft rubber tubes are commonly used for gastrostomy tubes. These have a wide bore and are flexible. Like their percutaneously placed counterparts, they may leak, cause pain at the insertion site, and induce a local soft tissue infection. The rubber tubes also have been known to deteriorate with time. Some models on the market have multiple lumens and ports to allow for gastric decompression and jejunal nutrient infusion.

Jejunostomy Tubes

Feeding tubes used for jejunal access tend to be smaller in diameter than surgically placed gastrostomy tubes but wider than the nasally inserted models. In the early 1970s, the needle catheter jejunostomy was introduced (33). This consisted of a tube similar in design to those used for nasal insertion in that it was extremely narrow in diameter. Although easy to insert, the needle catheter jejunostomy has fallen from favor because it is a poor conduit for most enteral formulas. The small tube size employed was prone to kinking and frequently was too narrow to allow rapid flow of the more viscous feeding solutions (15,34), and the small diameter did not allow for medication administration through the tube. Other acceptable options for jejunostomy placement include soft rubber tubes and biliary T tubes. Their wider internal diameter improves infusion and decreases the likelihood of occlusion. Red rubber or Robinson catheters are excellent choices. Unfortunately, these tubes are prone to dislodgement and need to be secured diligently. Balloon- and mushroom-tipped tubes are less susceptible to inadvertent removal because their tips are wider than their shafts and anchor them in place. Although popular with some, these tubes are disdained by many. The widened tip can potentially obstruct the narrow lumen or erode the wall of the jejunum. The biliary T tube provides some of the security of the balloon- and mushroom-tipped tubes with less risk of intestinal obstruction or erosion, but must be fashioned for easy removal. As with the gastric tubes, tube deterioration, leakage, and site infection may occur.

PLACEMENT TECHNIQUE OPTIONS

The myriad techniques available for feeding tube placement ensure the potential for obtaining enteral access in nearly all critically ill patients. As stated earlier, the many factors involved in choosing the most appropriate tube type and access site also determine the technique for placement.

Nasogastric

The least complicated and quickest feeding access is the nasogastric tube. Although the stiffer, wider tubes used for gastric decompression also can be used for feeding, it may be preferable to replace these tubes with the thin, softer, more flexible tubes. Placement is similar to that of the drainage sump tubes. The tube is lubricated and then passed blindly through a nostril. It travels down the posterior pharynx into the esophagus and then into the stomach. Placement is aided by wire stylets or weighted tips. Complications are similar to those of the sump tube, such as epistaxis, rhinitis, esophageal perforation or hemorrhage, pneumothorax, and inadvertent placement into the trachea or bronchus.

Nasoduodenal and Nasojejunal

Zaloga (35) found that only 5% of weighted small-bore feeding tubes pass spontaneously through the pylorus. Manually passing the soft, thin, flexible tube across the length of the stomach and beyond the pylorus is often challenging. Often, the tube coils back into the fundus or cannot easily be negotiated through the antrum and pylorus. In most cases, the difficulty in tube advancement into the duodenum is related to the blind nature of the passage and to the inability to steer or guide the tube (Fig. 36.2). Success varies from 49% to 92% (35,36).

Several techniques have been described to aid in passage. Some authors have reported improved success with simple maneuvers such as placing the patient in the right lateral decubitus position, giving the tube a gentle clockwise twist as it is being passed, or bending the tip of the stylet (35,37). Using a dedicated feeding tube placement service, Zaloga reported a success rate of 92% with such a technique. House officers who learned the technique were able to achieve placement rates of 70% to 80%.

The use of ultrasound (38), electrocardiogram (39), or an electromagnetic transmitter (40) for location of the tip of the tube during insertion have all been described and may decrease the time of insertion and the number of confirmatory radiographs. However, these techniques do not actually guide the tube in its course. A technique using an industrial magnet to guide a magnet-tipped tube into the duodenum has also been described (41). All these techniques have reported success rates above 75%, but large trials comparing them to other techniques are lacking.

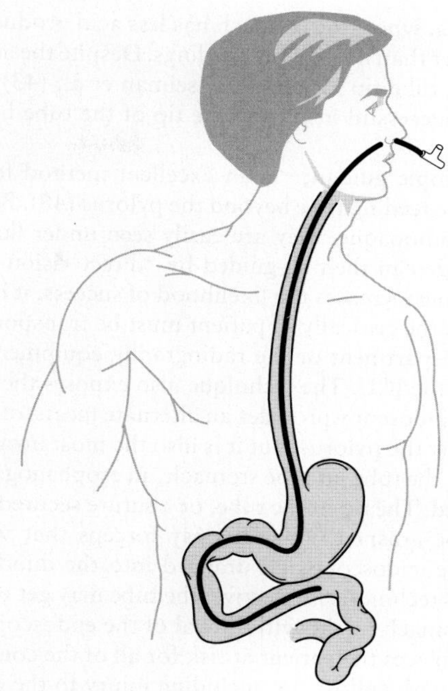

FIGURE 36.2. Nasoenteric feeding tube.

Another approach to postpyloric feeding tube placement involves the administration of a promotility agent just prior to tube insertion. Metoclopramide and erythromycin have been commonly used to increase upper gastrointestinal motility. In one study of 10 patients, metoclopramide, 20 mg IV, given 10 minutes before insertion increased the success rate of transpyloric feeding tube placement compared to placebo (42). However, a larger study using 10 mg of metoclopramide showed no benefit (43). Kittinger et al. (44) found that when metoclopramide was given after tube insertion into the stomach, it improved tube passage only in diabetic patients. The data for erythromycin are limited but more consistent. Administration of erythromycin 200 mg or 500 mg IV prior to feeding tube insertion has been shown to increse the success of postpyloric placement and to decrease the time needed for insertion (45,46).

Continuous pH monitoring using a specially designed tube that has a built-in pH sensor in the tip has been described to facilitate passage by enabling recognition of the tube tip location (43,47). Generally, lower pH values are found in the stomach compared with the duodenum, even in patients receiving H_2-receptor antagonists (35). This device may obviate the need for radiographic confirmation of tube location. Of course, where the need for fewer radiographs may save money, the requirement for specialized tubes and a pH monitor may offset the savings. These tubes are generally two to three times more expensive than traditional tubes, and most pH monitors cost a few hundred dollars.

Serial or continuous pH monitoring also can be used to indicate if the tube has migrated back into the stomach. Strong et al. (47) reported a 100% correlation between the radiographic documentation of tube location with the measured pH in eight patients. In that study, all changes in tube tip location as interpreted by pH were confirmed by radiography. However, the ability to use pH values to determine location may be less accurate in the setting of H_2-blocker administration or with achlorhydria, where the stomach has less acid production and, hence, higher than normal pH readings. Despite the advantages of knowing tube tip location, Heiselman et al. (43) were still only 79% successful in getting the tip of the tube beyond the pylorus.

Fluoroscopic guidance is an excellent method for placing the tip of the feeding tube beyond the pylorus (48). Because the tubes are radiopaque, they are easily seen under fluoroscopy. Tube passage can then be guided by "direct vision." Though this technique increases the likelihood of success, it has several drawbacks: the critically ill patient must be transported to the radiology department or the radiography equipment must be brought to the ICU. The technique also exposes the patient to radiation. Endoscopy provides an alternate means of delivering the tube past the pylorus, but it is also the most invasive. After positioning the tube into the stomach, an esophagogastroscopy is performed. The tip of the tube, or a suture secured to the tip, can then be grasped with a biopsy forceps that was passed through the endoscope and dragged into the duodenum. Although this technique is effective, the tube may get pulled back into the stomach by the withdrawal of the endoscope, and the procedure places the patient at risk for all of the complications associated with endoscopy, including injury to the esophagus, stomach, or duodenum; perforation; bleeding; and aspiration. Nasoenteric tubes also can be placed at the time of laparotomy for patients requiring temporary jejunal access.

There is no consensus in the literature as to whether weighted or unweighted tubes pass into the duodenum more often. Levenson et al. (49) demonstrated that there was no apparent difference in the likelihood of tube passage between weighted and unweighted tubes. Lord et al. (50) found that with the addition of preinsertion metoclopramide, unweighted tubes were significantly more likely to pass than weighted (84% vs. 36%, respectively). In contrast, Whatley et al. (42) found that 80% of weighted tubes passed when metoclopramide was given before insertion.

Even after the successful nasoenteric placement, tubes easily can be inadvertently removed or pulled back into the stomach. No method for tube immobilization (i.e., sutures, bridles, or taping) is completely secure. Occasionally, replacement requires considerable effort.

Percutaneous Gastrostomy

Although surgically placed gastrostomy tubes have long been heralded as the gold standard for obtaining stable, long-term gastric luminal access, numerous published reports demonstrate that percutaneous placement offers all of the same advantages but with a significantly lower complication rate. This technique involves the placement of an access tube into the gastric lumen using a direct puncture of the skin and abdominal and gastric walls. Endoscopic or radiographic assistance is essential. Percutaneous endoscopic gastrostomy (PEG) tube placement generally requires one of two techniques, termed "push" and "pull." There are numerous commercially available insertion kits that contain the tube and the equipment necessary for placement. A formal esophagogastroduodenoscopy is performed first to rule out upper gastrointestinal disease that precludes tube placement. The endoscope is then steered against the anterior gastric wall to transilluminate the stomach's position through the abdominal wall and skin. If successful, a small needle is then passed through a skin puncture into the gastric lumen. With the pull technique, a long nylon guidewire is inserted through the needle and grabbed with a snare that was fed through the endoscope. The guidewire is then dragged out of the patient's mouth and used to guide the tube down the esophagus, into the stomach, and out through the skin. With the push method, the catheter is passed directly over the guidewire with a peel-away sheath.

Complication Rates

The incidence of major complications with this technique is generally described as between 1% and 3%, and the reported mortality rate is about 0.5% (51,52). Complications include colonic injury, gastric perforation, hemorrhage, leakage with peritonitis, necrotizing fasciitis, and skin infection (53,54). In addition to having a lower complication rate than the open technique, the PEG procedure has been shown to require less time (10–30 minutes) to perform and has a lower cost overall (52,55,56). It also can usually be performed under local or intravenous sedation. Conditions that preclude the ability to perform upper endoscopy such as obstruction, varices, and severe *Candida* esophagitis are contraindications to this procedure. Relative contraindications include ascites—with its attendant risk of peristomal leakage as well as peritonitis from gastric leakage—and previous upper abdominal surgery, because the adhesions that form after surgery may prevent the stomach from being manipulated up to the abdominal wall. If transillumination cannot be achieved, the procedure should be aborted.

An alternative method for percutaneous gastrostomy is the radiographic approach. The stomach is distended with air using a nasogastric tube. Radiopaque contrast is then instilled in the stomach to enable it to be seen with fluoroscopy. The abdominal wall then can be pressed down onto the stomach. A needle is passed into the lumen and a guidewire inserted through the needle. The tract is dilated to the appropriate diameter and the tube is pushed into the lumen. This technique eliminates the need for endoscopy; however, many of the same contraindications and complications apply. In addition, this method does not allow inspection of the mucosa before tube placement or direct visualization of tube position after it is in place.

Percutaneous Jejunostomy

With the success of the percutaneous gastrostomy, an interest arose in applying the same technology to jejunal access for patients with a significant risk of aspiration or abnormal gastric motility. Specialized two-lumen tubes are available, with a gastric port for decompression and an extended jejunal limb for feeding. These tubes can be inserted either by the endoscopic technique or with radiographic assistance (57).

Complication Rates

Despite the similarity of the percutaneous endoscopic jejunostomy (PEJ) technique with percutaneous gastrostomy placement, the procedure has been found to have a much higher complication rate. The published rate of tube dysfunction ranges from 30% to 85% (58–60). Ironically, there seemed to be no decrease in aspiration rate with these jejunal tubes for patients with an increased aspiration risk. This may not be indicative of a failure of the tube in preventing the reflux of feeding formula. In fact, formula is rarely recovered from the tracheal aspirate. In all likelihood, the lack of improvement in aspiration suggests that the aspiration is mainly oral and pharyngeal secretions. In addition, like nasojejunal access, passage of these tubes through the pylorus is not always successful, and they have been known to migrate back into the stomach.

In one study of PEJ tubes, DiSario et al. (59) described a 95% serious complication rate, a 50% mortality rate, and a 70% incidence rate of tube failure. The alarmingly high mortality rate resulted predominantly from aspiration. However, the investigators did not make the distinction as to whether patients aspirated feeds or oropharyngeal secretions. In addition, they did not radiographically check tube position after aspiration to see if the tip had migrated back into the stomach. Tube failure was also a significant problem in this study. Occlusion represented greater than half of the tube complications. This was attributed to using the tube to deliver crushed tablets and inspissated feeding solutions. Proper use of the catheters should minimize these problems. Wolfsen et al. (58) also reported a higher incidence of complications with PEJ catheters compared with PEG tubes. However, in contrast to the DiSario study, they reported a 36% incidence of tube dysfunction and a 17% incidence of aspiration. Although complications were more likely to occur in patients with PEJ versus PEG tubes, the study was not randomized, and the differences may be related more to the underlying diseases of the patients than to the tubes themselves. The significant complication and tube failure rates reported in the literature suggest that, currently, the percutaneous endoscopically placed jejunostomy tube may not be the best option for long-term feeding (60).

Surgical Gastrostomy

Before the development of safe and effective methods for percutaneous tube placement, surgical techniques were the most commonly employed. After entering the abdominal cavity, a large-bore tube is placed directly into the gastric lumen and then pulled through the abdominal wall and out through the skin. The tubes used are usually balloon or mushroom tipped to prevent dislodgement. To minimize the risk of leakage and peritonitis, the tube is secured with two or three concentric pursestring sutures, and the anterior wall of the stomach is tacked to the undersurface of the abdominal wall to obliterate any potential space around the tube. This technique is generally referred to as the *Stamm gastrostomy*.

Complication Rates

The overall complication rate varies from 2.5% to 24% in the literature, with a major complication rate of about 10% (51,52). However, the wide range may be more indicative of the severity of illness of the patient populations than from the procedure itself. In addition to the complications associated with any gastric tube, surgical placement adds the increased risks associated with surgery and anesthesia. For patients requiring laparotomy for other reasons, the gastrostomy tube can be inserted at that time with minimal additional time or morbidity. However, for patients not requiring abdominal surgery, this technique requires a laparotomy and an anesthetic. In patients without previous abdominal surgery, the procedure can be brief and limited. The incision type can be either limited vertical midline or small left upper quadrant transverse one. Some surgeons can perform this procedure with local anesthesia, which avoids the risk associated with general anesthetics. Patients who have had previous abdominal surgery may pose a greater risk for complications because the procedure may be more involved. Adhesions—scar tissue that forms in the abdominal cavity as a result of surgery—may extend the incision size and the length of time necessary for tube placement. In addition, it increases the likelihood of injury to the stomach or intestines.

Recently, new minimally invasive techniques have been described using laparoscopy (61). These procedures have a decreased morbidity compared with the traditional open techniques because they do not require the laparotomy incision. However, they require a surgeon with experience in laparoscopic surgery and may be impossible in patients with previous abdominal surgery.

Surgical Jejunostomy

Like the surgically placed gastrostomy, the technique for open jejunostomy tube placement is generally safe; however, it can be more risky in patients who have had abdominal surgery, and typically requires general anesthesia. The most commonly employed techniques minimize the risks of leak from the bowel around the tube by either placing a pursestring suture around the tube (Stamm) or creating a serosal tunnel from the bowel wall overlying a portion of the tube (Witzel). After tube insertion into the jejunal lumen, the bowel is plicated to the undersurface of the anterior abdominal wall with three to four silk sutures placed circumferentially around the tube to further minimize the risk of leak and peritonitis (Fig. 36.3). The bowel is also carefully positioned for plication to prevent kinking or tube erosion.

To facilitate tube placement and minimize the risk of leak, the needle catheter jejunostomy technique was developed. It was first described by Delaney et al. (33) in 1973 as a safe and simple alternative to standard jejunostomy tube placement.

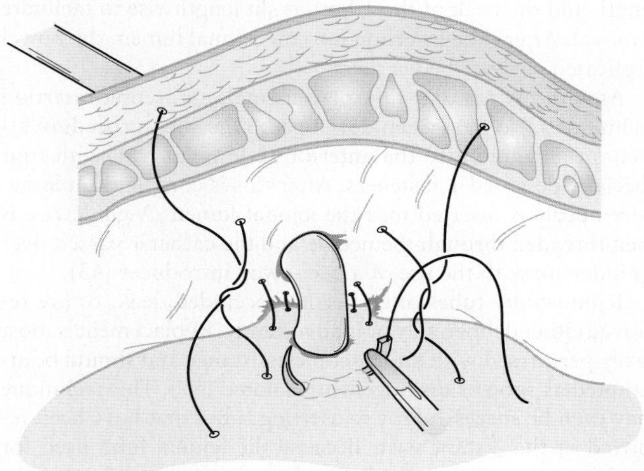

FIGURE 36.3. Plication of the jejunum to the anterior abdominal wall. By suturing the jejunum to the abdominal wall circumferentially around the tube, the risk of leakage is decreased.

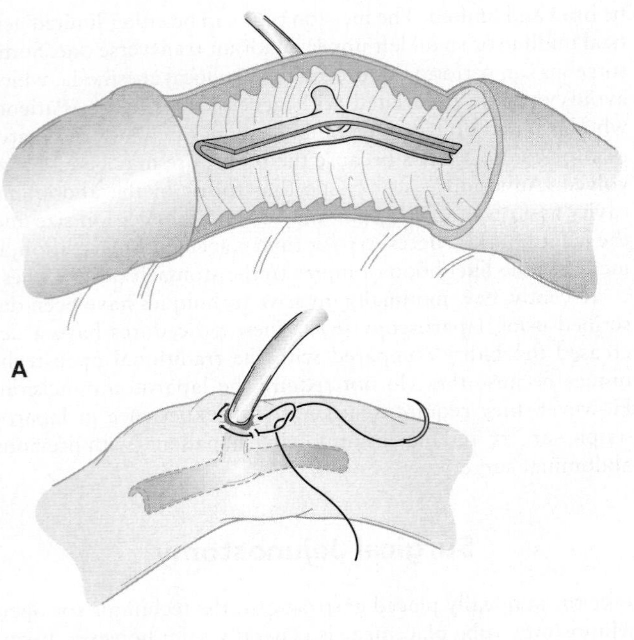

FIGURE 36.4. A surgically placed jejunostomy tube using a biliary T tube.

This method employs a narrow tube that is inserted by needle puncture through the antimesenteric border of the jejunal wall obliquely to create a subserosal tunnel. The tube is secured with a pursestring suture and then passed through the abdominal wall and skin. Few major complications were reported with this technique. Page et al. (62) had a 1% major and 1.5% minor complication rate in 199 patients. As stated earlier, these tubes tend to be unreliable and therefore are unpopular with many surgeons.

More commonly used is a large-bore, soft flexible catheter with additional holes placed into the jejunal lumen with a single pursestring suture. A biliary T tube can also be used for jejunal feeding, and is less likely to dislodge than the straight tube (Fig. 36.4). The limbs are each cut to approximately 3 cm in length and the back of the T limb is slit lengthwise to facilitate removal. After tube insertion into the jejunal lumen, the bowel is plicated as described earlier.

As with gastrostomy tube placement, laparoscopic insertion techniques also have been developed. One such procedure attaches the jejunum to the anterior abdominal wall with four specially designed T fasteners. After this is completed, a large-bore needle is inserted into the jejunal lumen. A guidewire is then threaded through the needle and the catheter passed over a guidewire with the use of a peel-away introducer (63).

Jejunostomy tubes often become occluded, leak, or are removed either deliberately or inadvertently. Replacement is most easily performed with fluoroscopic assistance and should be attempted as soon as dislodgement is noted (57). This technique may even be successful for reinserting tubes that have been removed in the distant past. Because the jejunal limb used for the jejunostomy is routinely fixed to the undersurface of the abdominal wall, luminal access can be achieved by passing a needle catheter through the skin site or scar. Once the tip of the needle is in the lumen, a long guidewire is then directed into the lumen and used to direct the tube.

NOVEL APPROACHES TO ENTERAL ACCESS

A few novel approaches to enteral access are included for completeness. These techniques were performed in patients unable to have access established with more conventional methods. In two case reports, the duodenal lumen was safely cannulated by fluoroscopy- or computed tomography–guided puncture using a lumbar approach (64,65).

SUMMARY

Enteral nutrition is fully recognized as an important addition to the comprehensive care of the critically ill and the preferred means of nutritional support. However, the successful establishment of secure and dependable enteral feeding access may be challenging. Several factors, including the patient's current condition, past medical and surgical history, status of the gastrointestinal tract, and hospital resources available to the clinician determine the best tube type, access choice, and placement method. Fortunately, several options are currently available so that there should be few reasons—short of gastrointestinal tract dysfunction—that preclude the use of enteral nutrition.

No single enteral access combination is superior to the others. None guarantees success in all instances. Using a flexible strategy based on the unique characteristics of the patient and the patient care environment will maximize the likelihood of success. Persistence also pays dividends. Failure of one attempt should not be a cause to abandon enteral feeding. A fresh new approach, possibly using another access option, may ultimately succeed. Only with patience, determination, and an understanding of the available access options will the greatest number of critically ill patients reap the benefits of enteral nutrition.

References

1. Clinical Practice Guideline for Nutrition Support in the Mechanically Ventilated, Critically Ill Adult Patient. http://www.criticalcarenutrition.com/index.php?option=com_content&task=view&id=34&Itemid=59. Accessed February 20, 2008.
2. Moore FA, Moore EE, Jones TN, et al. TEN versus TPN following major abdominal trauma-reduced septic morbidity. *J Trauma.* 1989;29:916.
3. Kudsk KA, Croce MA, Fabian TC, et al. Enteral versus parenteral feeding: effects on septic morbidity after blunt and penetrating abdominal trauma. *Ann Surg.* 1992;215:503.
4. Gianotti L, Alexander JW, Nelson JL, et al. Role of early enteral feeding and acute starvation on postburn bacterial translocation and host defense: prospective, randomized trials. *Crit Care Med.* 1994;22:265.
5. Heyland DK, Cook DJ, Guyatt GH. Enteral nutrition in the critically ill patient: a critical review of the literature. *Intensive Care Med.* 1993;19:435.
6. Babineau TJ, Blackburn GL. Time to consider early gut feeding. *Crit Care Med.* 1994;22:191.
7. Grant JP, Snyder BA. Use of L-glutamine in total parenteral nutrition. *J Surg Res.* 1988;44:506.
8. Johnson LR, Copeland EM, Dudrick JT, et al. Structural and hormonal alterations in the gastrointestinal tract of parenterally fed rats. *Gastroenterology.* 1975;68:1170.
9. Wilmore DW, Smith RJ, O'Dwyer ST, et al. The gut: a central organ after surgical stress. *Surgery.* 1988;104:917.
10. Page CP. The surgeon and gut maintenance. *Am J Surg.* 1989;158:485.
11. Deitch EA. Multiple organ failure: pathophysiology and potential future therapy. *Ann Surg.* 1992;216:117.
12. Carrico J, Meakin JL. Multiple organ failure syndrome. *Arch Surg.* 1986;121:196.

13. Border JR, Hassett J, LaDuca J, et al. The gut origin septic states in blunt multiple trauma (ISS = 40) in the ICU. *Ann Surg.* 1987;206:427.
14. Marshall JC, Christou NV, Meakins JL. The gastrointestinal tract: the "undrained abscess" of multiple organ failure. *Ann Surg.* 1993;218:111.
15. Thibault A: Care of feeding tubes. In: Borlase BC, Bell SJ, Blackburn GL, et al., eds. *Enteral Nutrition.* New York: Chapman & Hall; 1994:197.
16. Koruda MJ, Guenter P, Rombeau JL. Enteral nutrition in the critically ill. *Crit Care Clin.* 1987;3:133.
17. Minard G. Enteral access. *Nutr Clin Pract.* 1994;9:172.
18. Ritz MA, Fraser R, Edwards N, et al. Delayed gastric emptying in ventilated critically ill patients: Measurement by ^{13}C-octanoic acid breath test. *Crit Care Med.* 2001;29(9):1744.
19. Tarling MM, Toner CC, Withington PS. A model of gastric emptying using paracetamol absorption in intensive care patients. *Intensive Care Med.* 1997;23:256.
20. Kao CH, ChangLai SP, Chieng PU, et al. Gastric emptying in head-injured patients. *Am J Gastroenterol.* 1998;93(7):1108.
21. Suto G, Kiraly A, Tache Y. Interleukin 1 beta inhibits gastric emptying in rats: mediation through prostaglandin and corticotrophin-releasing factor. *Gastroenterology.* 1994;106(6):1568.
22. McClave SA, Snider HL, Lowen CC, et al. Use of residual volume as a marker for enteral feeding intolerance: prospective blinded comparison with physical examination and radiographic findings. *JPEN J Parenter Enter Nutr.* 1992;16:99.
23. Heyland DK, Drover JW, MacDonald S, et al. Effect of postpyloric feeding on gastroesophageal regurgitation and pulmonary microaspiration: results of a randomized controlled trial. *Crit Care Med.* 2001;29:1495.
24. Taylor SJ, Fettes SB, Jewkes C, et al. Prospective, randomized, controlled trial to determine the effect of early enhanced enteral nutrition on clinical outcome in mechanically ventilated patients suffering head injury. *Crit Care Med.* 1999;27(11):2525.
25. Marik PE, Zaloga GP. Gastric versus post-pyloric feeding: a systematic review. *Crit Care.* 2003;7(3):R46.
26. Ho KM, Dobb GJ, Webb SAR. A comparison of early gastric and post-pyloric feeding in critically ill patients: a meta-analysis. *Intensive Care Med.* 2006;32:639.
27. Jooste CA, Mustoe J, Collee G. Metoclopramide improves gastric motility in critically ill patients. *Intensive Care Med.* 1999;25:464.
28. Calcroft RM, Joynt G, Hung V. Gastric emptying in critically ill patients: a randomized, blinded, prospective comparison of metoclopramide with placebo. *Intensive Care Med.* 1997;23(Suppl):S138.
29. Nguyen NQ, Chapman MJ, Fraser RJ, et al. Erythromycin is more effective than metoclopramide in the treatment of feed intolerance in critical illness. *Crit Care Med.* 2007;35:483.
30. Dive A, Miesse C, Galanti L, et al. Effect of erythromycin on gastric motility in mechanically ventilated critically ill patients: a double-blind, randomized, placebo-controlled study. *Crit Care Med.* 1995;23:1356.
31. Chapman MJ, Fraser RJ, Kluger MT, et al. Erythromycin improves gastric emptying in critically ill patients intolerant of nasogastric feeding. *Crit Care Med.* 2000;28:2334.
32. Ritz MA, Chapman MJ, Fraser RJ, et al. Erythromycin dose of 70 mg accelerates gastric emptying as effectively as 200 mg in the critically ill. *Intensive Care Med.* 2005;31:949.
33. Delaney HM, Carnevale NH, Garvey JW. Jejunostomy by a needle catheter technique. *Surgery.* 1973;73:786.
34. Jones TN, Moore EE, Moore FA. Early postoperative feeding. In: Borlase BC, Bell SJ, Blackburn GL, et al. eds. *Enteral Nutrition.* New York: Chapman & Hall; 1994:78.
35. Zaloga GP. Bedside method for placing small bowel feeding tubes in critically ill patients: a prospective study. *Chest.* 1991;100:1643.
36. Welch SK, Hanlon MD, Waits M, et al. Comparison of four bedside indicators used to predict duodenal feeding tube placement with radiography. *JPEN J Parenter Enter Nutr.* 1994;18:525.
37. Thurlow PM. Bedside enteral feeding tube placement into duodenum and jejunum. *JPEN J Parenter Enter Nutr.* 1986;10:104.
38. Hernandez-Socorro CR, Marin J, Ruiz-Santana S, et al. Bedside sonographic-guided versus blind nasoenteric feeding tube placement in critically ill patients. *Crit Care Med.* 1996;24(10):1690.
39. Keidan I, Gallagher TJ. Electrocardiogram-guided placement of enteral feeding tubes. *Crit Care Med.* 2000;28:2631.
40. Gray R, Tynan C, Reed L, et al. Bedside electromagnetic-guided feeding tube placement: an improvement over traditional placement technique? *Nutr Clin Pract.* 2007;22(4):436.
41. Gabriel SA, Ackermann RJ, Castresana M. A new technique for placement of nasoenteral feeding tubes using external magnetic guidance. *Crit Care Med.* 1997;25(4):641.
42. Whatley K, Turner WW, Dey M, et al. When does metoclopramide facilitate transpyloric intubation? *JPEN J Parenter Enter Nutr.* 1984;8:679.
43. Heiselman DE, Vidovich RR, Milkovich G, et al. Nasointestinal tube placement with a pH sensor feeding tube. *JPEN J Parenter Enter Nutr.* 1993;17:562.
44. Kittinger JW, Sandler RS, Heizer WD. Efficacy of metoclopramide as an adjunct to duodenal placement of small-bore feeding tubes: a randomized, placebo-controlled, double-blind study. *JPEN J Parenter Enter Nutr.* 1987;11:33.
45. Kalliafas S, Choban PS, Ziegler D, et al. Erythromycin facilitates postpyloric placement of nasoduodenal feeding tubes in intensive care unit patients: randomized, double-blinded, placebo-controlled trial. *JPEN J Parenter Enteral Nutr.* 1996;20(6):385.
46. Griffith DP, McNally T, Battey CH, et al. Intravenous erythromycin facilitates bedside placement of postpyloric feeding tubes in critically ill adults: a double-blind, randomized, placebo-controlled study. *Crit Care Med.* 2003;31:39.
47. Strong RM, Gribbon R, Durling S, et al. Enteral tube feedings utilizing a pH sensor enteral feeding tube. *Nutr Suppl Sero.* 1988;8:11.
48. Grant JP, Curtas MS, Kelvin FM. Fluoroscopic placement of nasojejunal feeding tubes with immediate feeding using a nonelemental diet. *JPEN J Parenter Enter Nutr.* 1983;7:299.
49. Levenson R, Turner WW, Dyson A, et al. Do weighted nasogastric feeding tubes facilitate duodenal intubations? *JPEN J Parenter Enter Nutr.* 1988;12:135.
50. Lord LM, Weser-Maimone A, Pulhamus M, et al. Comparison of weighted vs unweighted enteral feeding tubes for efficacy of transpyloric intubation. *JPEN J Parenter Enter Nutr.* 1993;17:271.
51. Larson DE, Burton DD, Schroeder KW, et al. Percutaneous endoscopic gastrostomy: indications, success, complications, and mortality in 314 consecutive patients. *Gastroenterology.* 1987;93:48.
52. Grant JP. Comparison of percutaneous endoscopic gastrostomy with Stamm gastrostomy. *Ann Surg.* 1988;270:598.
53. Peasarini AC, Dittler HJ. Feeding tube perforation as a complication of percutaneous endoscopic gastrostomy. *Endoscopy.* 1992;24:235.
54. Saltzberg DM, Anand K, Juvan P, et al. Colocutaneous fistula: an unusual complication of percutaneous endoscopic gastrostomy. *JPEN J Parenter Enter Nutr.* 1987;11:86.
55. Dwyer KM, Watts DD, Thurber JS, et al. Percutaneous endoscopic gastrostomy: the preferred method of elective feeding tube placement in trauma patients. *J Trauma.* 2002;52:26.
56. Kirby DF, Craig RM, Tsang T-K, et al. Percutaneous endoscopic gastrostomies: a prospective evaluation and review of the literature. *JPEN J Parenter Enter Nutr.* 1986;10:155.
57. Lambiase RE, Dorfman GS, Cronan JJ, et al. Percutaneous alternatives in nutritional support: a radiologic perspective. *JPEN J Parenter Enter Nutr.* 1988;12:513.
58. Wolfsen HC, Kozarek RA, Ball TJ, et al. Tube dysfunction following percutaneous gastrostomy and jejunostomy. *Gastrointest Endosc.* 1990;36:261.
59. DiSario JA, Foutch PG, Sanowski RA. Poor results with percutaneous endoscopic jejunostomy. *Gastrointest Endosc.* 1990;36:257.
60. Henderson JM, Strudel WE, Gilinsky NH. Limitations of percutaneous endoscopic jejunostomy. *JPEN J Parenter Enter Nutr.* 1993;17:546.
61. Reiner DS, Leitman IM, Ward RJ. Laparoscopic Stamm gastrostomy with gastropexy. *Surg Laparosc Endosc.* 1991;1:189.
62. Page CP, Carlton PK, Andrassy RJ, et al. Safe, cost-effective postoperative nutrition: defined formula diet via needle catheter jejunostomy. *Am J Surg.* 1979;138:939.
63. Duh Q-Y, Way LW. Laparoscopic jejunostomy using T-fasteners as retractors and anchors. *Arch Surg.* 1993;128:105.
64. Cwikiel W. Percutaneous duodenostomy-alternative route for enteral nutrition. *Acta Radiol.* 1991;32:153.
65. Koolpe HA, Dorfman D, Kramer M. Translumbar duodenostomy for enteral feeding. *AJR Am J Roentgenol.* 1989;153:299.

CHAPTER 37 ■ FLEXIBLE BRONCHOSCOPY

MICHAEL A. JANTZ

Flexible bronchoscopy is an essential diagnostic and therapeutic tool in the intensive care unit (ICU). Potential indications for flexible bronchoscopy in the ICU include airway management (intubation, changing of endotracheal tubes, and extubation); diagnosis of respiratory infections, parenchymal lung disease, acute inhalational injury, or airway injury from intubation or chest trauma; and treatment of hemoptysis, atelectasis, foreign bodies, obstructing airway lesions, and bronchopleural fistulae. From a diagnostic standpoint, flexible bronchoscopy can identify the etiology of hemoptysis and the cause of pulmonary infection.

Compared with rigid bronchoscopy, flexible bronchoscopy offers enhanced visualization of the proximal and distal airways, is associated with fewer complications, and can be performed at the bedside, averting the need for general anesthesia and operating room resources. However, for management of massive hemoptysis, difficult-to-extract foreign bodies, bronchoscopic laser resection, and benign or malignant obstruction of the trachea or bilateral mainstem bronchi, rigid bronchoscopy may be the procedure of choice.

Both fiberoptic and video bronchoscopes are utilized for flexible bronchoscopy in the ICU. Video bronchoscopy allows for better resolution of the image because of the greater number of pixels on the charge-coupled device for image acquisition. In contrast, the resolution of the traditional fiberoptic bronchoscope is determined by the diameter of the optical fibers and seems to have reached its technological limit. With the video bronchoscope, as well as with attachment of a camera head to the fiberoptic bronchoscope, observation by multiple parties is possible, which decreases the possibility of missed findings and facilitates teaching and education. Compared with video bronchoscopes, the fiberoptic bronchoscope is less expensive, although improper use and care can result in broken optical fibers and thus higher repair costs over time.

PROCEDURE

General Considerations

In nonintubated patients, flexible bronchoscopy can be performed by the transnasal or transoral route with a bite block. In the mechanically ventilated patient, gas exchange abnormalities may occur due to the bronchoscope occupying a significant portion of the internal diameter of the endotracheal tube (ET) (1). This reduction in the cross-sectional area of the ET may lead to hypoventilation, hypoxemia, and air trapping with intrinsic positive end-expiratory pressure (auto-PEEP). The outer diameter of the bronchoscope should be at least 2 mm smaller than the lumen of the ET to minimize these effects. As most adult bronchoscopes have an outer diameter of 5 to 6 mm, an 8-mm ET is generally recommended for performing bronchoscopy safely in the intubated patient. A pediatric bronchoscope with an outer diameter of 3 to 4 mm should be used if the ET is smaller.

Informed consent for the procedure should be obtained prior to starting bronchoscopy. Enteral feeding or oral intake should be discontinued for 4 hours before and 2 hours after the procedure. Patients with asthma should receive bronchodilators prior to bronchoscopy. Platelet counts and coagulation studies should be obtained in those patients with risk factors for bleeding if the bronchoscopic procedure will include biopsies. In the ICU setting, most patients will be monitored with a continuous electrocardiogram, pulse oximetry, and intra-arterial blood pressure or intermittent cuff blood pressure every 3 to 5 minutes. Monitoring intracranial pressure (ICP) and end-tidal CO_2 has been suggested for patients with a serious head injury (2).

Equipment for reintubation and bag-valve-mask ventilation should be readily available, and suctioning equipment, including Yankauer and endotracheal catheters, should be accessible at the bedside. In addition to sedatives and analgesics, resuscitation medications should also be on hand. It is prudent to have materials for chest tube thoracostomy located in the ICU.

Premedication

Topical anesthesia is typically used to suppress the gag reflex and coughing. Nonintubated patients will undergo topical anesthesia of the nares and oropharynx with lidocaine jelly and nebulized or sprayed lidocaine. The tracheal and bronchial mucosa is anesthetized with 1% lidocaine solution. In intubated patients, the 1% lidocaine can be administered through the endotracheal tube or through the working channel of the bronchoscope after insertion into the ET. Lidocaine is absorbed through the mucous membranes and achieves peak serum concentrations that are similar to that of intravenous administration. The total dose of lidocaine should not exceed 3 to 4 mg/kg. Patients with cardiac or hepatic insufficiency have reduced clearance of lidocaine, and thus the dose should not exceed 2 to 3 mg/kg. The use of lidocaine should be kept to a minimum if samples for culture are to be obtained, as bacteriostatic lidocaine preparations may decrease culture yields. The administration of antisialagogues, such as atropine or glycopyrrolate, has been recommended in the past to reduce secretions and prevent bradycardia, although recent studies suggest no benefit from use of these drugs (3).

Sedation and analgesic agents are often used during bronchoscopy to provide anxiolysis, antegrade amnesia, analgesia, and cough suppression. A combination of opiates and benzodiazepines is typically used. The most commonly used benzodiazepine is midazolam, given its short elimination half-life and rapid onset of action. Fentanyl is the most commonly used opiate, again due to a short elimination half-life. Meperidine has also been used for bronchoscopy, although clearance is decreased with hepatic and renal failure, and accumulation of a toxic metabolite, normeperidine, may cause seizures. Propofol may also be used in intubated patients and patients with adjunctive airway support (4); advantages include rapid onset and offset of action, with the potential disadvantage of drug-induced hypotension. The type and level of sedation required depend on the clinical status. Nonintubated patients, particularly with borderline oxygenation and ventilation or with central airway obstruction, should likely receive light or moderate sedation. Unstable hypoxic patients with acute respiratory distress syndrome (ARDS) and patients with brain injury may require deep sedation, or even neuromuscular blockade, to safely perform the procedure (5).

Mechanical Ventilation

In mechanically ventilated patients, a special swivel adapter, with a perforated diaphragm through which the bronchoscope is passed, is used to prevent loss of delivered tidal volumes (6).

As previously noted, bronchoscopy in the mechanically ventilated patient may cause hypoxemia, hypoventilation, generation of auto-PEEP, and potential barotrauma. The lumen of the ET should be 2 mm larger than the external diameter of the bronchoscope. Decreases in delivered tidal volumes will occur during pressure-limited, time-cycled ventilator modes, as well as when flow-limited, volume-cycled breaths become pressure limited. To reliably ensure tidal volume delivery, volume-cycled breaths should be used during bronchoscopy. Because the increase in peak pressure is dissipated along the endotracheal tube and does not represent an increased risk for barotrauma, the peak pressure limit on the ventilator can be significantly elevated to ensure delivery of tidal volume. The high peak pressures seen during bronchoscopy are not reflective of pressures distal to the endotracheal tube. The problem with high peak pressures is ventilator pressure limiting, resulting in decreased effective tidal volume. Decreasing inspiratory flow rate decreases peak pressures and pressure limiting, but may paradoxically increase predisposition to auto-PEEP by decreasing the expiratory time. Set tidal volumes may need to be increased by 40% to 50% in some patients to achieve adequate tidal volumes. Barotrauma and hypotension may occur if the bronchoscope-added expiratory resistance leads to auto-PEEP. Some authors advocate reducing set PEEP or discontinuing PEEP prior to bronchoscopy (1). The fraction of inspired oxygen (FiO_2) should be increased to 1.0 prior to and during the procedure to ensure adequate oxygenation. Exhaled tidal volumes should be monitored during the procedure. The bronchoscope should be withdrawn periodically to allow for adequate ventilation; prolonged suctioning through the bronchoscope can decrease delivered tidal volumes and oxygenation.

Bronchoalveolar Lavage

Bronchoalveolar lavage (BAL) allows for sampling of cellular and noncellular components from the lower respiratory tract. The tip of the bronchoscope is wedged into a distal airway, and sterile saline solution is instilled through the bronchoscope and then aspirated with the syringe or suctioned into a sterile trap. Aliquots of 20 mL to 60 mL are generally used. Infusions of 120 mL to 240 mL are needed to ensure adequate sampling of secretions in the distal respiratory bronchioles and alveoli (7–9). Aspiration of aliquots by syringes in a serial fashion allows for detection of progressively bloodier aliquots, which strongly suggests the presence of alveolar hemorrhage. The first aliquot of aspirated fluid is likely to contain a significant amount of material from the proximal airways. As such, some authors recommend discarding this aliquot or analyzing the aliquot separately from the remainder of the fluid (7). In patients with emphysema, collapse of the airways with negative pressure during aspiration or suctioning may limit the amount of fluid obtained. The very small fluid return in these patients may contain only diluted material from the proximal bronchi rather than the alveoli, and thus may give rise to false-negative results (10). Suctioning prior to having the bronchoscope in the appropriate wedged position should be minimized to avoid contamination with upper airway secretions and potential false-positive results.

In addition to quantitative bacterial cultures for the diagnosis of ventilator-associated pneumonia, BAL samples may also be sent for cytology, antigen tests, and polymerase chain reaction tests, which provide additional information for the diagnosis of noninfectious and infectious etiologies of pulmonary disease as compared to the protected specimen brush.

Protected Specimen Brush

The protected specimen brush (PSB) is used to obtain a lower respiratory tract specimen for microbiology that is not contaminated by organisms in the proximal airways. The PSB consists of a retractable brush within a double-sheathed catheter that has a distal dissolvable plug occluding the outer catheter (11,12). After the tip of the bronchoscope is positioned in the desired area, the catheter is advanced through the working channel and situated 1 to 3 cm beyond the distal end of the bronchoscope to prevent collection of secretions pooled around the distal end of the bronchoscope. The inner cannula containing the brush is advanced to eject the distal plug, and the brush is then advanced into the desired subsegment under direct visualization. Once the sample is obtained, the brush is retracted into the inner cannula, the inner cannula is then withdrawn into the outer sheath, and the entire catheter is removed from the bronchoscope. The distal ends of the outer and inner cannula are wiped with alcohol, cut with sterile scissors, and discarded. The brush is advanced beyond the remaining portion of the inner cannula, cut with sterile scissors, and placed in 1 mL of nonbacteriostatic sterile saline or transport media.

Quantitative Bronchoalveolar Lavage and Protected Specimen Brush Cultures

Specimens for culture should be rapidly processed to prevent a decrease in pathogen viability or contaminant overgrowth. The BAL sample should be transported in a sterile, leakproof container. The initial aliquot, which is thought to be representative of proximal airway secretions, should be discarded or analyzed separately from the remaining pooled fractions. It is recommended that specimens for microbiologic analysis be processed within 30 minutes, although refrigeration can be used when the specimens cannot be immediately processed (7,13). The specimens should be processed according to clearly defined protocols (14). Pathogens are present in lower respiratory tract secretions, at concentrations of at least 10^5 to 10^6 colony forming units (CFU)/mL, in patients with pneumonia, while contaminant bacteria are present at concentrations of less than 10^4 CFU/mL (15,16). The diagnostic thresholds proposed for BAL and PSB are based on these concentrations with 10^4 CFU/mL for BAL, which collects 1 mL of secretions in 10 to 100 mL of saline and represents 10^5 to 10^6 CFU/mL, which is considered supportive of the diagnosis of ventilator-associated pneumonia. Similarly, the concentration of 10^3 CFU/mL for PSB, which collects 0.001 to 0.01 mL of secretions in 1 mL of saline, is considered supportive of the diagnosis of ventilator-associated pneumonia.

Transbronchial and Endobronchial Biopsies

Histologic samples of lung parenchyma may be obtained with transbronchial lung biopsies. In patients with diffuse or localized parenchymal diseases, transbronchial lung biopsies may be useful and offer a less invasive option to open lung biopsy. It should be noted, however, that for some interstitial lung diseases and pulmonary vasculitides, transbronchial biopsy specimens are inadequate to make a definitive diagnosis. The major risks of transbronchial biopsies are bleeding and pneumothorax. The risk of pneumothorax is higher when performing transbronchial biopsies in the mechanically ventilated patient (17). Fluoroscopy may not be required to perform transbronchial biopsies in mechanically ventilated patients with diffuse parenchymal disease; however, I would recommend the use of fluoroscopy, if available, to minimize the risk of a life-threatening pneumothorax. A chest radiograph should be obtained in all critically ill or mechanically ventilated patients after transbronchial lung biopsy.

Samples of bronchial mucosa and endobronchial abnormalities may be obtained with endobronchial biopsies. Transbronchial and endobronchial biopsies may be sent for bacterial, mycobacterial, and fungal cultures as indicated, in addition to histology.

CONTRAINDICATIONS

Only a few absolute contraindications to flexible bronchoscopy exist in critically ill patients. Flexible bronchoscopy should not be performed in the absence of informed consent, if trained personnel are not available, if adequate oxygenation cannot be maintained during the procedure, if unstable cardiac conditions are present, or if uncontrolled bronchospasm is present (18,19). The inability to normalize the platelet count and coagulation parameters if biopsy or PSB is planned is a relative contraindication. Airway inspection and BAL may likely be done safely despite thrombocytopenia or coagulopathy unless the abnormalities are profound. The general recommendation is that the platelet count should be at least 50,000 cells/μL if biopsies are going to be performed. Performing biopsies or PSB in patients on antiplatelet agents is controversial. Patients with uremia, which causes a functional platelet defect, are at increased risk for hemorrhage with biopsy procedures (20). Patients with pulmonary hypertension have also been noted to be at risk for greater bleeding with transbronchial biopsies.

Patients with stable COPD may safely undergo flexible bronchoscopy. Sedation during the procedure should be used cautiously, and the possibility of supplemental oxygen-induced hypoventilation should be considered.

Patients with increased ICP should be carefully monitored during flexible bronchoscopy. Bronchoscopy has been noted to increase ICP by at least 50% in 88% of patients with head trauma, despite the use of deep sedation and paralysis (5). Cerebral perfusion pressure may not change, however, due to concurrent increases in mean arterial pressure during bronchoscopy. Despite an increase in ICP, no significant neurologic complications were noted in studies of patients with severe head trauma or space-occupying lesions who were undergoing flexible bronchoscopy (2,5,21). In spite of these observations, caution is warranted in performing bronchoscopy in patients with markedly elevated ICP.

COMPLICATIONS

With appropriate care, flexible bronchoscopy is an extremely safe procedure. The incidence rate of major complications ranges from 0.08% to 0.15%, and the mortality rate ranges from 0.01% to 0.04%. Minor complications (e.g., vasovagal reaction, fever, bleeding, nausea, and vomiting) occur in as many as 6.5% of these patients (22–24). Flexible bronchoscopy in mechanically ventilated patients has the potential for life-threatening complications including hypoxemia, hypercapnia, barotrauma, cardiac arrhythmias, myocardial ischemia, intracranial hypertension, local anesthetic toxicity, and pulmonary hemorrhage. Careful patient selection, meticulous preparation before the procedure, and vigilant physiologic monitoring during the procedure limit complications and mortality. The characteristics of high-risk patients are summarized in Table 37.1.

A prospective clinical trial in critically ill, mechanically ventilated patients with ARDS provides important information with regard to the safety of BAL in this patient population. Careful attention was directed toward maintenance of minute ventilation and the limitation of auto-PEEP during the procedure. Severe hypoxemia and hypotension were seen in 4.5% and 3.6% of patients, respectively. No significant reduction occurred in postprocedure pulmonary function, such as static compliance or PaO_2/FiO_2 ratio. No deaths were attributed to the procedure. The incidence of pneumothorax was 0.9% (1 of 110 patients) (25).

These results are in contrast to other investigators who have shown the potential for significant decline in oxygenation, which can persist for up to 2 hours after the procedure (26). In healthy patients, the arterial partial pressure of oxygen (PaO_2) may decline by 20 to 30 mm Hg during flexible bronchoscopy (26). In critically ill patients, the decrement in PaO_2 can exceed 30 to 60 mm Hg (27,28). In a more recent study of bronchoscopy in critically ill patients, hypoxemia was observed in 29 of 147 procedures (19.7%) (29). The greater the amount of normal saline instilled for lavage during bronchoscopy, the more frequent the hypoxemia—seen in as many as 23% of patients—and the longer its duration, up to 8 hours (30,31). Hypoxemia- and hypercapnia-induced increased

TABLE 37.1

CHARACTERISTICS OF INCREASED-RISK PATIENTS FOR BRONCHOSCOPY ON MECHANICAL VENTILATION

PULMONARY
PaO_2 <70 mm Hg with FiO_2 >0.70
PEEP >10 cm H_2O
Auto-PEEP >15 cm H_2O
Active bronchospasm
CARDIAC
Recent myocardial infarction (<48 h)
Unstable dysrhythmia
Mean arterial pressure <65 mm Hg on vasopressor therapy
COAGULOPATHY
Platelet count <20,000 cells/μL
Increase of prothrombin time or partial thromboplastin time 2.0 times control
CENTRAL NERVOUS SYSTEM
Increased intracranial pressure

FiO_2, fraction of inspired oxygen; PEEP, positive end-expiratory pressure.

sympathetic tone can result in dysrhythmias, myocardial ischemia, hypotension, and cardiac arrest.

Bronchoscopy-associated hypoxemia may be minimized by providing 100% oxygen during the procedure, shortening bronchoscopy time, and frequently withdrawing the bronchoscope from the airway to allow adequate ventilation. Adequate tidal volume delivery should be monitored by observing chest excursions and exhaled tidal volumes in patients undergoing mechanical ventilation. Tidal volume and flow rates must be adjusted to provide adequate ventilation (1,26,32).

Complications associated with the administration of sedation, analgesia, and topical anesthesia include hypotension and allergic reactions, as well as hypoventilation, and hypoxemia from oversedation and respiratory depression. The overzealous use of local anesthetic agents within the airways has potential for toxicity with the rapid uptake of these agents into the systemic circulation from the bronchial mucosa (33). Lidocaine is the most commonly used airway anesthetic. The risks of toxicity are decreased with total doses of less than 4 mg/kg of body weight. The duration of airway anesthesia induced by lidocaine is approximately 20 to 40 minutes. Lidocaine in excessive doses can cause sinus arrest and atrial ventricular block, especially in patients with underlying heart disease. Other potential adverse reactions include respiratory arrest, seizures, laryngospasm, and, rarely, hypersensitivity reactions. Although not as commonly used for topical anesthesia, benzocaine has been associated with the development of methemoglobinemia (34).

Although rarely associated with bronchoscopy, dysrhythmias are more likely to occur in critically ill patients (35). Major cardiac dysrhythmias occur in 3% to 11% of all patients undergoing bronchoscopy. Hypoxemia is the major risk factor for the development of dysrhythmias (36,37).

Laryngospasm (in the nonintubated patient) or bronchospasm can occur in any patient undergoing flexible bronchoscopy, but are more common in patients with pre-existing reactive airway disease. Preoperative bronchodilator therapy significantly reduces the risk of bronchoscopy-induced bronchospasm in most patients with reactive airway disease (38).

Although transbronchial biopsy is a relatively safe procedure in patients with normal hemostasis and pulmonary vascular pressures, it is associated with a 2.7% and 0.12% risk of morbidity and mortality, respectively (39). Hemorrhage (more than 50 mL of blood) is more likely to occur in patients who undergo transbronchial biopsy. Risk factors for hemorrhage include thrombocytopenia, coagulopathy, uremia, and pulmonary hypertension. Transbronchial biopsy should be restricted to nonuremic patients with platelet counts greater than 50,000 cells/μL and prothrombin times and activated partial thromboplastin times less than twice that of controls (22, 39, 40). The incidence rate of bronchoscopy-related hemorrhage in normal hosts approaches 1.4%. In immunocompromised hosts, the rate of hemorrhage ranges from 25% to 29%, while hemorrhage occurs in as many as 45% of uremic patients (22,41,42). Administration of desmopressin, 0.3 μg/kg, can reverse the uremic effect on platelet function, although no controlled study evaluating the safety of performing transbronchial biopsies after treatment with desmopressin exists (43). Pneumothorax occurs in fewer than 5% of nonventilated patients undergoing transbronchial biopsy. Tube thoracostomy is required in approximately half of these patients (22). A major risk factor for pneumothorax is positive pressure ventilation, especially if PEEP is used. Rates of pneumothorax after transbronchial lung biopsy in mechanically ventilated patients have been reported up to 7% and 23% (44–46). Fluoroscopic guidance may diminish the risk of pneumothorax. No patient should undergo bilateral transbronchial biopsy procedures during the same bronchoscopic episode because of the small risk of bilateral pneumothorax.

Postbronchoscopy fever occurs in as many as 16% of patients. Bronchoscopy-related pneumonia is rare, occurring in fewer than 5%, and bacteremia is exceedingly rare (47,48). In general, endocarditis prophylaxis is not required with flexible bronchoscopy (49).

Neurosurgical patients are at risk for intracranial hypertension as a result of bronchoscopy-induced elevation of intrathoracic pressure, arterial hypertension, and hypercapnia. Bronchoscopy-associated cough or retching must therefore be avoided. Deep sedation with or without neuromuscular blockade may be utilized if bronchoscopy is deemed necessary.

DIAGNOSTIC AND THERAPEUTIC BRONCHOSCOPY

Airway Management

Flexible bronchoscopy can provide an efficient and effective means to secure a difficult airway, change an endotracheal tube, and inspect an airway during extubation (50,51). Endotracheal intubation can be technically difficult in select patient groups (Table 37.2). Intubation using flexible bronchoscopy under topical anesthesia, with or without conscious sedation, is an important technique in these patients with compromised airways, particularly if the airway is obstructed or if the trachea is extrinsically compressed by a mediastinal mass. Spontaneous ventilation keeps the airway open and assists the

TABLE 37.2

FACTORS ASSOCIATED WITH DIFFICULT ENDOTRACHEAL INTUBATIONS

ANATOMIC	**NEOPLASIA**
Short muscular neck	Laryngeal papillomatosis
Receding mandible	Stylohyoid ligament calcification
Prominent upper incisors	Laryngeal carcinoma
Microglossia	Mediastinal carcinoma
Limited mandible movement	**TRAUMA**
Large breasts	Mandibular fracture
Cervical rigidity	Maxillary fracture
CONGENITAL ABNORMALITIES	Laryngeal and tracheal trauma
Absence of nose	Mediastinal carcinoma
Choanal atresia	**ENDOCRINE**
Macroglossia	Obesity
INFECTIOUS	Acromegaly
Bacterial retropharyngeal abscess	Thyromegaly
Epiglotitis	
Diphtheria	
Infectious mononucleosis	
Croup	
Leprosy	
NONINFECTIVE INFLAMMATION	
Rheumatoid arthritis	
Instability of cervical spine	
Cervical fixation	
Temporomandibular disease	
Cricoarytenoid disorders	
Hypoplastic mandible	
Ankylosing spondylitis	

bronchoscopist in locating the glottis when airway anatomy is distorted (50,52). Bronchoscopic examination of the airway also identifies the nature of the obstructed airway and helps to plan for additional therapeutic maneuvers to relieve the airway obstruction.

Bronchoscopic endotracheal intubation can be performed using either a nasal or oral approach. With the nasal approach, after preparation of the nasal mucosa with a local anesthetic such as lidocaine and a mucosal vasoconstrictor such as 1% phenylephrine, the bronchoscope is passed through the nares and situated directly above the glottic opening. It is then passed into the trachea and the ET is passed over the bronchoscope into the trachea. The major limitation of this approach in many ICU patients with concomitant abnormalities of coagulation is epistaxis and the potential for sinusitis with prolonged nasal intubation. The development of epistaxis can significantly impair the bronchoscopic examination and can seriously hamper subsequent nasal or laryngoscopic attempts at intubation. Other difficulties associated with nasal intubation include adenoid dislocation and difficulty passing the ET in patients with a limited diameter of the nares.

Oral flexible bronchoscopic intubation effectively avoids these difficulties associated with nasal intubation. Topical anesthesia of the oropharynx is achieved with spraying of 4% lidocaine. Translaryngeal injection of 3 mL of 4% lidocaine through the cricothyroid membrane to provide topical anesthesia to the larynx and trachea, in addition to lidocaine sprays to the oropharynx, is favored by some practitioners. Others favor a "spray as you go" technique, with injection of lidocaine through the working channel of the bronchoscope to provide laryngeal and tracheal topical anesthesia. Alternatively, nebulization of 6 to 8 mL of 4% lidocaine is used for topical anesthesia in some institutions (50). A bite block should be in place to prevent scope damage from the patient biting. In some patients, the use of an oral intubating airway, such as the Williams Airway Intubator, the Ovassapian Airway, or the Berman Airway, may be helpful in successfully intubating the patient with a difficult airway (53). The oral intubating airway directs the flexible bronchoscopy past the tongue and directly over the larynx, facilitating endotracheal intubation. Use of these airways in the completely awake patient with inadequate topical anesthesia may be problematic due to gagging and vomiting. This is less of a problem in the sedated or unconscious patient. After exposure of the vocal cords, the bronchoscope is passed into the trachea and the ET is then passed over the bronchoscope into the airway. In some patients, the endotracheal tube impinges on laryngeal structures despite the smooth entrance of the bronchoscope into the trachea. In this situation, the ET may be withdrawn back over the bronchoscope, rotated 90 degrees clockwise or counterclockwise to change the position of the tube bevel relative to the larynx, and readvanced during inspiration (50). Mild to moderate conscious sedation may be used in some patients to improve patient comfort and tolerance of nasal or oral bronchoscopic intubation. Great caution should be taken in patients with highly compromised airways, however, and sedatives may need to be completely avoided.

In addition to the oral intubating airway, other airway adjuncts have been used in combination with the flexible bronchoscope for intubation of patients with a difficult airway. A special facial mask with a diaphragm for the bronchoscope has been developed for the critically ill and for use in the operating room (54). The mask is useful for bronchoscopic intubation in sedated or comatose patients with limited respiratory reserve, providing a tight seal for assisted ventilation during the procedure. The intubating laryngeal mask airway (LMA) has also been used successfully in combination with the flexible bronchoscope (55).

Flexible bronchoscopy allows for ET changes in patients with endotracheal tube cuff leaks, inadequate ET internal diameters, and nasotracheal tube–associated sinusitis. Before bronchoscopy, the oropharynx should be suctioned thoroughly. For oral tracheal intubation, the endotracheal tube should be shortened 2 to 3 cm at its proximal end and advanced over the bronchoscope before its placement in the pharynx. The bronchoscope tip is advanced to the level of the cuff of the existing endotracheal tube, and secretions are aspirated through the suction channel. If necessary, the cuff is deflated and the bronchoscope advanced into the tracheal lumen. The endotracheal tube is then withdrawn with the cuff fully deflated, the bronchoscope tip advanced to the carina, and the new endotracheal tube advanced over the bronchoscope into the trachea. Adequate positioning of the tube 3 to 4 cm proximal to the carina is confirmed by visual inspection, and the cuff is inflated. After intubation, a chest radiograph is not required to confirm adequate placement of the endotracheal tube (56). Tube changes by the oral or nasal routes are possible. Contralateral nasal reintubation, however, may be difficult because of the lateral displacement of the septum by the existing nasotracheal tube.

Percutaneous dilatational tracheostomy (PDT) has become a well-accepted method for performing bedside tracheostomy in the ICU. While not universally utilized, flexible bronchoscopy is routinely used in performing PDT (57). Bronchoscopy facilitates proximal positioning of the ET prior to introducing the guidewire needle into the trachea, reducing the risk of ET impalement by the needle, and facilitates reintubation if the ET is dislodged out of the airway. Bronchoscopic visualization ensures that the guidewire needle is introduced in the appropriate interspace in a midline position and that the needle does not penetrate the membranous posterior tracheal wall, thereby decreasing the risk of misplacement of the tracheostomy tube and creation of a false paratracheal passage. Bronchoscopy also provides feedback to the operator during dilator passage so that pressure on the posterior wall is minimized and the potential for posterior wall tears is reduced.

Flexible bronchoscopy can be extremely useful in the placement of a double-lumen ET. If a right-sided tube is used, adequate positioning of the tube with the tracheal port proximal to the carina and bronchial port proximal to the right upper lobe orifice can be confirmed by using a small-diameter (3.5-mm outer diameter) flexible bronchoscope to inspect the airway through each lumen (58,59). Positioning of left-sided tubes is not as problematic given the longer length of the left mainstem bronchus relative to the right mainstem bronchus and less likelihood of obstructing the left upper or left lower lobe. In general, bronchoscopic confirmation of proper bronchial port positioning should be performed after all double-lumen ET intubations, given the significant rate of malpositioning with a blind technique (60).

Flexible bronchoscopy provides an excellent opportunity to inspect the airways at the time of extubation in patients at risk for airway compromise, including those intubated for inhalation injury, trauma, subglottic stenosis, and laryngeal edema. The bronchoscope is advanced through the ET to its most distal aspect, and the ET and bronchoscope are withdrawn slowly together to allow inspection of the airway. If bronchoscopy confirms persistent mucosal edema or airway obstruction, the endotracheal tube can be readvanced over the bronchoscope into the tracheal lumen and secured, with extubation postponed until a later time.

Atelectasis

Segmental or lobar atelectasis presents radiographically as a parenchymal density associated with a combination of shift of an interlobar fissure, crowding of vessels or bronchi, ipsilateral mediastinal shift, or elevation of the diaphragm. Complete lung atelectasis will produce opacification of the hemithorax and usually ipsilateral mediastinal shift. Atelectasis is most commonly due to mucous plugging; however, in patients who do not improve after chest physiotherapy, endobronchial obstruction due to endobronchial tumor, foreign body, or blood clot should be excluded by bronchoscopy. Predisposing conditions for mucous plugging and atelectasis include inadequate inspiratory effort (pain, sedation, and muscle weakness), immobility, obesity, excessive airway secretions, pre-existing airway disease, and endobronchial obstructing lesions. Lobar or whole lung atelectasis produces hypoxemia by right-to-left vascular shunting and ventilation/perfusion mismatching. The clinical significance of atelectasis is directly related to its extent and to the pre-existing pulmonary reserve of the patient.

Much of the evidence supporting the role of flexible bronchoscopy in the treatment of atelectasis is anecdotal. Success rates for bronchoscopy range from 19% to 89% (61). One randomized trial comparing bronchoscopy to aggressive chest physiotherapy and nebulizer therapy found no advantage for bronchoscopy, although the study methodology has been criticized (62–64). Patients with whole lung or lobar atelectasis tend to respond better than those with segmental atelectasis. With the exception of large, obstructing central airway mucous plugs, the radiographic response to successful removal of secretions is delayed from 6 to 24 hours. Therapeutic bronchoscopy is, in general, indicated for patients with life-threatening whole lung or lobar atelectasis and for patients who have not responded to chest physiotherapy measures. Chest physiotherapy should be continued after successful bronchoscopy to prevent new airway obstructions. Instillation of saline or a dilute 10% solution of acetylcysteine through the working channel may help to clear thick, tenacious secretions. Acetylcysteine is a bronchial irritant, however, and may exacerbate bronchospasm in patients with reactive airway disease. Typically 10- to 20-mL aliquots of saline are used as the irrigant to facilitate clearing of mucous plugs. If saline irrigation fails, then instillation of acetylcysteine or rhDNase (Pulmozyme) may be considered (65–67). In some patients, holding continuous suction while withdrawing the bronchoscope through the ET allows removal of large mucous plugs that cannot be suctioned directly through the working channel. Extremely tenacious mucous plugs may require the use of biopsy forceps or a foreign body basket to be successfully extracted. Blood clots may similarly be removed with saline irrigation. Instillation of acetylcysteine may be helpful in more difficult to remove blood clots. The use of biopsy forceps or a foreign body basket may be needed to remove blood clots that cannot be removed with irrigation and suction extraction.

Selective intrabronchial insufflation by the flexible bronchoscope, preceded by suctioning of mucus from large airways, has been used in patients with refractory atelectasis (61). One study in a surgical ICU study using air insufflation for lobar collapse reported an overall effectiveness of 82%, with 92% effectiveness when collapse was less than 72 hours' duration (68). Although only minor clinically insignificant complications have been described, selective positive pressure insufflation does carry the potential risk of barotrauma (69–71).

Hemoptysis

Flexible bronchoscopy plays a central role in the evaluation of hemoptysis. Bronchoscopy should be considered in all critically ill patients with hemoptysis, regardless of the degree of hemoptysis, to localize the site of bleeding and attempt to determine the underlying etiology. Localization of the site of bleeding is important to guide temporizing therapy such as angiographic embolization and definitive therapy such as surgical resection. Early rather than delayed bronchoscopy should be performed to increase the likelihood of localizing the source of bleeding. Bronchoscopy performed within 48 hours of bleeding onset successfully localized bleeding in 34% to 91% of patients, depending on the case series, as compared to successful localization in 11% to 52% of patients if bronchoscopy was delayed (72). Bronchoscopy performed within 12 to 24 hours may provide an even higher yield.

Massive hemoptysis is defined as expectoration of blood exceeding 200 to 1,000 mL over a 24-hour period, with expectoration of greater than 600 mL in 24 hours as the most commonly used definition (73). In practice, the rapidity of bleeding and ability to maintain a patent airway are critical factors, and life-threatening hemoptysis can alternatively be defined as the amount of bleeding that compromises ventilation. Only 3% to 5% of patients with hemoptysis have massive hemoptysis, with the mortality rates approaching 80% in various case series. Most patients who die from massive hemoptysis do so from asphyxiation secondary to airway occlusion by clot and blood, not exsanguination. The causes of massive hemoptysis are listed in Table 37.3. Infections associated with bronchiectasis, tuberculosis, lung abscess, and necrotizing pneumonia are commonly responsible for the massive bleeding. Other common causes include bronchogenic carcinoma, mycetoma, invasive fungal diseases, chest trauma, cystic fibrosis, pulmonary infarction, coagulopathy, and alveolar hemorrhage due to Wegener granulomatosis and Goodpasture syndrome.

Airway patency must be ensured in patients with massive hemoptysis. While preparing for intubation and bronchoscopy, the patient may be positioned in the lateral decubitus position with the bleeding side down. Most patients with massive hemoptysis will require intubation and mechanical ventilation. While intubation generally preserves oxygenation and facilitates blood removal from the lower respiratory tract, the ET may become obstructed by blood clots with inability to oxygenate and ventilate the patient. The largest possible ET should be inserted to allow for use of bronchoscopes with a 2.8- to 3.0-mm working channel for more effective suctioning and to allow for better ventilation with the bronchoscope in the airway for prolonged periods of time. In severe cases, the mainstem bronchus of the nonbleeding lung can be selectively intubated under bronchoscopic guidance to preserve oxygenation and ventilation from the normal lung.

Some authors have recommended the use of a double-lumen ET to isolate the normal lung and permit selective intubation. While double-lumen endotracheal tubes have been used successfully in the airway management of massive hemoptysis, there are a number of potential pitfalls. First, placement of

TABLE 37.3

POTENTIAL CAUSES OF MASSIVE HEMOPTYSIS

NEOPLASM
Bronchogenic cancer
Metastasis (parenchymal or endobronchial)
Carcinoid
Leukemia
INFECTIOUS
Lung abscess
Bronchiectasis
Tuberculosis
Necrotizing pneumonia
Fungal pneumonia
Septic pulmonary emboli
Mycetoma (aspergilloma)
PULMONARY
Bronchiectasis
Cystic fibrosis
Sarcoidosis (fibrocavitary)
Diffuse alveolar hemorrhage
Airway foreign body
CARDIAC/VASCULAR
Mitral stenosis
Pulmonary embolism/infarction
Arteriovenous malformation
Bronchoarterial fistula
Ruptured aortic aneurysm
Congestive heart failure
Pulmonary arteriovenous fistula
IATROGENIC/TRAUMATIC
Blunt or penetrating chest trauma
Tracheal/bronchial tear or rupture
Tracheoinnominate artery fistula
Bronchoscopy
Pulmonary artery rupture from Swan-Ganz catheter
Endotracheal tube suctioning trauma
HEMATOLOGIC
Coagulopathy
Disseminated intravascular coagulation
Thrombocytopenia
DRUGS/TOXINS
Anticoagulants
Antiplatelet agents
Thrombolytic agents
Crack cocaine

a double-lumen ET is difficult for less experienced operators, particularly with a large amount of blood in the larynx and oropharynx. Second, the individual lumens of the ET are significantly smaller than a standard ET and are at significant risk of being occluded by blood and blood clots. Lastly, positioning of the double-lumen ET and subsequent bronchoscopic suctioning of the distal airways require a small pediatric bronchoscope with working channels of 1.2 to 1.4 mm. Adequate suctioning of large amounts of blood and blood clots through such bronchoscopes is extremely problematic. In one series of 62 patients with massive hemoptysis, death occurred in four of seven patients managed with a double-lumen ET due to loss of tube positioning and aspiration (74). I do not recommend the use of double-lumen ETs for airway management in massive hemoptysis. As an alternative to selective mainstem bronchial intubation or intubation with a double-lumen ET, an ET that incorporates a bronchial blocker, such as the Univent tube, may be used.

Endobronchial tamponade with flexible bronchoscopy can prevent aspiration of blood into the contralateral lung and preserve gas exchange in patients with massive hemoptysis. Endobronchial tamponade can be achieved with a 4-French Fogarty balloon-tipped catheter. The catheter may be passed directly through the working channel of the bronchoscope or the catheter can be grasped by biopsy forceps placed though the working channel of the bronchoscope prior to introduction into the airway. The bronchoscope and catheter—with the latter held in place adjacent to the bronchoscope by the biopsy forceps—are then inserted as a unit into the airway. Care must be taken not to perforate the catheter or balloon by the forceps. The catheter tip is inserted into the bleeding segmental orifice, and the balloon is inflated. If passed through the suction channel, the proximal end of the catheter is clamped with a hemostat, the hub cut off, and a straight pin inserted into the catheter channel proximal to the hemostat to maintain inflation of the balloon catheter. The clamp is removed, and the bronchoscope is carefully withdrawn from the bronchus with the Fogarty catheter remaining in position, to provide endobronchial hemostasis (75–77). The catheter can safely remain in position until hemostasis is ensured by surgical resection of the bleeding segment or bronchial artery embolization. Right heart balloon catheters have been used in a similar fashion (78). A modified technique for placement of a balloon catheter has been described using a guidewire for insertion. A 0.035-inch soft-tipped guidewire is inserted through the working channel of the bronchoscope into the bleeding segment. The bronchoscope is withdrawn, leaving the guidewire in place. A balloon catheter is then inserted over the guidewire and placed under direct visualization after reintroduction of the bronchoscope (79). The use of endobronchial blockers developed for unilateral lung ventilation during surgery may hold promise for management of massive hemoptysis in tamponading bleeding and preventing contralateral aspiration of blood (80). The Arndt endobronchial blocker is placed through a standard ET and directly positioned with a pediatric bronchoscope. Suctioning and injection of medications can be performed through the lumen of the catheter after placement. The Cohen tip-deflecting endobronchial blocker is also placed through a standard ET and directed into place with a self-contained steering mechanism under bronchoscopic visualization. At this time, there is limited published experience with these blockers in the setting of massive hemoptysis, although the author has successfully used them for this application. The prolonged use of endobronchial blockers may cause mucosal ischemic injury and postobstructive pneumonia.

Additional bronchoscopic techniques may be useful as a temporizing measure in patients with massive hemoptysis. Bronchoscopically administered topical therapies such as iced sterile saline lavage or topical 1:10,000 or 1:20,000 epinephrine solution may be helpful (81). Direct application of a solution of thrombin or a fibrinogen–thrombin combination solution has been used (82). The use of bronchoscopy-guided topical hemostatic tamponade therapy using oxidized regenerated cellulose mesh has recently been described (83). Although anecdotal, the author has had success with topical application of 5 to 10 mL of a 1 mEq/mL (8.4%) sodium bicarbonate solution.

For patients who have hemoptysis due to endobronchial lesions, particularly endobronchial tumors, hemostasis may be achieved with the use of neodymium-yttrium-aluminum-garnet (Nd:YAG) laser phototherapy, electrocautery, or cryotherapy via the bronchoscope.

Diagnosis of Ventilator-associated Pneumonia

For the diagnosis of ventilator-associated pneumonia (VAP), the use of bronchoscopic modalities remains controversial and is often institution dependent. Although commonly attributed to pneumonia, the chest radiographic finding of alveolar infiltrates in the ICU patient can represent a broad differential diagnosis, requiring a wide range of therapies. The use of standard clinical criteria for the diagnosis of pneumonia such as new pulmonary infiltrates, hypoxemia, leukocytosis or leukopenia, fever, and pathogenic bacteria in respiratory secretions has been associated with a significant rate of misdiagnosis (84). Bacterial colonization of the upper airways and endotracheal tube can confound the reliability of the Gram stain and cultures from tracheal aspirates obtained in the intubated patient. Concern about the inaccuracy of clinical approaches to the diagnosis of VAP and the possibility of antibiotic overprescribing with a clinical strategy has led some investigators to postulate that bronchoscopic methods such as PSB and BAL would improve the diagnosis of VAP and treatment outcomes (15,16).

The methodology for performing PSB and BAL quantitative cultures is outlined in a previous section of this chapter. PSB and BAL should be performed in the most abnormal segment as determined by radiographic studies or where endobronchial abnormalities are most pronounced. Alternatively, samples may be obtained from the right lower lobe, as this is the most commonly affected area on autopsy studies. A quantitative culture result of more than 10^4 CFU/mL is considered diagnostic for pneumonia with BAL, while more than 10^3 CFU/mL is considered diagnostic for pneumonia with PSB. An evidence-based review of 23 prospective studies of BAL in suspected VAP showed a sensitivity of 42% to 93% with a mean of 73% ± 18%, and a specificity of 45% to 100% with a mean of 82% ± 19% (85). In 12 studies, the detection of intracellular organisms in 2% to 5% of recovered cells was used to diagnose pneumonia, with a mean sensitivity of 69% ± 20% and a specificity of 75% ± 28% (85). An advantage of looking for intracellular organisms is the ability to obtain information of high predictive value in a rapid time frame without waiting for the results of cultures to define the presence of pneumonia, although not the specific identity of the etiologic pathogen (84).

In a review of studies evaluating PSB, the sensitivity ranged from 33% to 100% with a median sensitivity of 67%, while the specificity ranged from 50% to 100% with a median specificity of 95% (86). It is unclear if BAL is superior to PSB or vice versa in the diagnosis of VAP. In a meta-analysis of 18 studies on PSB (795 patients) and 11 studies on BAL (435 patients), there was no difference in the accuracy of the two tests (87). BAL does offer an advantage in that additional microbiologic tests beyond routine bacterial cultures, as well as cytologic analysis, can be performed on the sample if an infectious process is suspected other than typical bacterial pneumonia. PSB may potentially have a greater complication rate compared with BAL, but this has not been formally compared.

Despite studies of BAL and PSB showing a greater accuracy than tracheal aspirates, the routine use of bronchoscopy for establishing the diagnosis of VAP remains controversial (84,88). This controversy is in part due to critiques in study methodologies and in part due to some studies showing a benefit in patient outcomes while others have not. One prospective, nonrandomized study noted a difference in mortality between patients managed with an invasive bacteriologic strategy (19%) versus those managed with a clinical strategy (35%) (89). One large, prospective randomized trial did show an advantage to the quantitative bronchoscopic approach when compared with a clinical approach in a multicenter study of 413 patients suspected of having VAP. Compared with patients managed clinically, those receiving invasive management had a lower mortality rate on day 14 (16% vs. 25%; $p < 0.02$), but not on day 28, and lower mean sepsis-related organ failure assessment scores on days 3 and 7. At 28 days, the quantitative culture group had significantly more antibiotic-free days (11 ± 9 vs. 7 ± 7 days; $p < 0.001$), but only a multivariate analysis showed a significant difference in mortality (hazard ratio 1.54; 95% confidence interval [CI] 1.10–2.16) (90). No differences in mortality were observed in three randomized single-center studies when invasive techniques (PSB and/or BAL) were compared with either quantitative or semiquantitative endotracheal aspirate culture techniques (91–93). However, these studies included few patients (51, 76, and 88, respectively), and antibiotics were continued in all patients, even those with negative cultures, thereby negating one of the potential advantages of the bacteriologic strategy. A meta-analysis of these randomized controlled trials noted that an invasive approach did not alter mortality (odds ratio 0.89, 95% CI 0.56–1.41), although invasive testing affected antibiotic utilization (odds ratio for change in antibiotic management after invasive sampling 2.85, 95% CI 1.45–5.59) (94).

Performing microbiologic cultures of pulmonary secretions for diagnostic purposes after initiating new antibiotic therapy can lead to false-negative results and is likely of little value regardless of the manner in which the secretions are sampled. Studies have demonstrated that culture positivity at 24 and 48 hours after the onset of antimicrobial treatment is markedly diminished (95,96). The decrease in positive cultures after initiation of antibiotic therapy appears to affect PSB more so than BAL. If patients have been treated with antibiotics but did not have a change in antibiotic class prior to bronchoscopy for a suspected new episode of VAP, the yield of BAL and PSB appears to be similar to that in patients who have not received antibiotics (97). If an invasive bronchoscopy strategy is used to establish a diagnosis of VAP, BAL and/or PSB should be performed prior to administration of antibiotics or administration of new antibiotics if the patient was previously on antimicrobial therapy.

Diagnosis of Other Respiratory Infections

Flexible bronchoscopy is an essential modality in evaluating the critically ill, immunocompromised patient with pulmonary infiltrates. These patients are at risk for fungal, viral, protozoal, mycobacterial, and atypical bacterial pulmonary infections. Critically ill patients who have no underlying immunocompromised condition, such as acquired immunodeficiency syndrome (AIDS), leukemia, neutropenia, hematopoietic stem cell/bone marrow transplant, or solid organ transplant, may also develop respiratory infections other than bacterial pneumonias, such as fungal and viral infections. In addition to these patients, those who present with acute respiratory failure and apparent community-acquired pneumonia, but fail to respond appropriately to antibiotic therapy, may benefit from bronchoscopy to evaluate for more unusual infections and noninfectious causes of acute respiratory failure with infiltrates. Bronchoscopy is not recommended for routine community-acquired pneumonia.

BAL, as compared to PSB, provides the opportunity for more extended microbiologic studies and for cytology. It is unclear if the addition of transbronchial biopsy to BAL improves diagnostic accuracy in immunocompromised patients with pulmonary infiltrates. Transbronchial biopsy may increase the yield for the diagnosis of infectious etiologies, but more commonly establishes an alternate noninfectious cause of infiltrates in these patients (98). The benefits versus risks, including life-threatening pneumothorax and bleeding, need to be individualized in the critically ill immunocompromised patient.

In immunocompromised and critically ill patients who are suspected to have an atypical infection, BAL fluid should be sent for cytopathology to evaluate for viral cytologic changes, as well as Gomori methenamine silver staining (GMS) to evaluate for fungal organisms and *Pneumocystis jiroveci*. Alternatively, Papanicolaou, Giemsa, toluidine blue O, or direct fluorescent antibody staining may be used for detection of *Pneumocystis*.

For *Pneumocystis* in AIDS patients, BAL has a sensitivity rate in diagnosing *Pneumocystis* pneumonia of approximately 85% to 90%, and for transbronchial biopsy, the diagnostic yield approaches 87% to 95%. When BAL and transbronchial biopsy are performed in AIDS patients with *Pneumocystis* pneumonia, the diagnostic yield is 95% to 98% (99–102). Given the high yield of BAL and the potential risk of transbronchial biopsy in critically ill patients, transbronchial biopsy is not recommended in AIDS patients for diagnosing *Pneumocystis*. In immunocompromised patients without HIV, the yield of BAL is lower, and transbronchial biopsies to establish a diagnosis may be required. Although not used routinely in clinical practice, polymerase chain reaction (PCR) for *Pneumocystis* on BAL specimens may increase diagnostic rates (103).

For the diagnosis of pulmonary fungal infections in immunocompromised patients, BAL fluid should be sent for fungal stains and cultures in addition to cytology stains. It is unclear if the addition of transbronchial biopsy to BAL increases the diagnostic yield for fungal infections. If transbronchial biopsies are obtained, the samples should be sent for culture in addition to histology. Some fungi, such as *Mucor* and *Rhizopus,* are difficult to grow on culture, and diagnosis relies on BAL cytology or biopsy specimens. *Aspergillus* is the most commonly encountered pulmonary fungal infection. BAL cytology and culture are diagnostic in approximately 50% to 60% of cases of invasive pulmonary aspergillosis. The diagnostic yield from BAL appears to be increased with the use of galactomannan antigen and PCR testing, although galactomannan antigen testing is more readily available (104–106). Antigen testing for histoplasmosis and blastomycosis on BAL samples is now available (107).

To evaluate for viral infections, respiratory viral cultures and a respiratory syncytial virus antigen assay should be obtained. BAL cytology may demonstrate characteristic intracytoplasmic inclusions, but sensitivity is lacking. Immunofluorescence and PCR for cytomegalovirus (CMV) may be performed on BAL specimens (108).

If there is suspicion for tuberculosis or nontuberculous mycobacteria, BAL samples should be sent for acid-fast bacillus stains and mycobacterial culture. BAL samples of sputum smear–negative patients with tuberculosis are smear positive in 12% to 42% of patients and culture positive in 66% to 95% (109). In one third to one half of initially sputum smear–negative patients, bronchoscopy specimens yield the only positive source of mycobacterial tuberculosis (110–112). Although not routinely used, PCR for tuberculosis may be obtained on BAL to provide a more rapid diagnosis (113,114).

For atypical bacterial infections, additional stains and cultures may be required. *Legionella* requires specific culture media. A direct fluorescence antibody stain is also available for *Legionella.* Some laboratories utilize specific media if *Nocardia* is suspected. *Nocardia* can often be identified with a combination of Gram stain and modified Ziehl-Neelsen stains, and are observed as delicately branched, weakly Gram-positive, variably acid-fast bacilli. Methenamine-silver stains may demonstrate the organisms in tissue specimens.

Diagnosis of Noninfectious Pulmonary Infiltrates

Although most helpful in excluding infectious etiologies for pulmonary infiltrates in ICU patients, bronchoscopy with BAL and/or transbronchial biopsy may be able to establish the etiology of noninfectious infiltrates in some patients (115,116). In some cases, surgical lung biopsy will be required to make a definitive diagnosis. The appearance of the BAL and a cell count and differential on the BAL fluid can be helpful in suggesting a diagnosis. A bloody BAL that does not decrease, or increases in the degree of blood return with serial fluid aliquots, is diagnostic of alveolar hemorrhage. This can be confirmed with iron staining that demonstrates hemosiderin-laden alveolar macrophages. BAL fluid that has a milky or whitish, cloudy appearance with flocculent debris that settles to the bottom of the container is suggestive of pulmonary alveolar proteinosis. Additional support for this diagnosis is provided with a positive periodic acid–Schiff (PAS) stain. The diagnosis of pulmonary alveolar proteinosis can be confirmed with transbronchial or surgical lung biopsy. A BAL with a differential count greater than 25% eosinophils is virtually diagnostic of eosinophilic lung disease. In the patient with acute respiratory failure, this finding will most commonly be due to acute eosinophilic pneumonia, although parasitic lung infections such as strongyloidiasis rarely have a similar presentation. A finding of greater than 25% lymphocytes on BAL differential is suggestive of sarcoidosis, hypersensitivity pneumonitis, drug reaction, or viral infection.

Transbronchial biopsy can confirm the above diagnoses in most cases. In addition, transbronchial biopsy may be able to establish other noninfectious diagnoses of pulmonary infiltrates in the ICU including idiopathic interstitial pneumonia and graft versus host disease in stem cell or bone marrow transplant patients, leukemic infiltrates, drug-induced pneumonitis, bronchiolitis obliterans organizing pneumonia/cryptogenic organizing pneumonia (BOOP/COP), bronchoalveolar carcinoma, lymphangitic carcinomatosis, and acute rejection after lung transplantation.

Traumatic Airway Injury

The classic signs of tracheobronchial disruption include shortness of breath, massive subcutaneous emphysema, persistent pneumothorax despite chest tube insertion, and a large air leak after tube thoracoscopy. On occasion, however, only subtle signs exist, even in the presence of significant injury. Flexible bronchoscopy should be performed early in any patient with chest trauma in whom airway injury may have occurred (117). Signs and symptoms of tracheobronchial injury are listed in Table 37.4. Tracheobronchial disruption rarely occurs as an isolated injury (118). A history of a rapid deceleration injury, such as a motor vehicle accident with the patient's chest striking the steering wheel or dashboard, is typical. The pathogenesis of tracheobronchial rupture in blunt chest trauma is caused by shearing, wrenching, or compressive forces, acting alone or in concert. Rapid deceleration results in shearing forces, acting predominantly at the distal trachea near the carina where the relatively fixed trachea joins the more mobile distal airways (119,120). If the trachea and mainstem bronchi are crushed

TABLE 37.4

SIGNS AND SYMPTOMS OF TRACHEOBRONCHIAL INJURY

- Fracture of upper ribs
- Fracture of clavicle or sternum
- Chest wall contusions
- Chest radiograph showing:
  - Subcutaneous emphysema
  - Pneumothorax
  - "Sagging" lung
  - Pneumomediastinum
  - Atelectasis
  - Pulmonary contusion
- Hemoptysis
- Bronchopleural fistula
- Dyspnea
- Cough

between the chest wall and vertebral column and the glottis closed, airway pressure suddenly increases, and resultant rupture of the airway may occur (118).

In patients with tracheal or bronchial disruption, early bronchoscopy can reliably detect the site of airway injury (121–126). Prompt diagnosis and surgical correction or tracheobronchial disruption produce a better outcome, and delay in diagnosis is usually detrimental to the patient (118). Patients with partial tracheal or bronchial disruption may be relatively asymptomatic and present with a paucity of physical findings. Delays in diagnosis unfortunately are common and have been associated with decreased frequency of successful repair. Failure to diagnose disruption may result in a delayed stricture formation at the site of injury, resulting in dyspnea, distal atelectasis, and chronic recurrent infections.

If an airway injury is suspected, flexible bronchoscopy should be performed through an endotracheal tube prepositioned on the bronchoscope to assess tracheal or bronchial disruption. If a persistent bronchopleural fistula exists because of proximal airway trauma, the cuff of the endotracheal tube sometimes can be positioned just distal to the rupture site and inflated, and adequate ventilation can be established before surgical repair. Cervical tracheal rupture is less common than rupture of the intrathoracic trachea. Cervical tracheal rupture, however, may be more difficult to diagnose once the patient is intubated because of the proximal location of the tear, and may itself be an impediment to intubation (127).

Bronchopleural Fistula

In patients who are not candidates for surgical management of a bronchopleural fistula (BPF), flexible bronchoscopic techniques may offer alternative methods for closure of the BPF. Detection of a proximal BPF due to stump breakdown after lobectomy or pneumonectomy or a BPF due to bronchial dehiscence is usually relatively straightforward, as these abnormalities can be directly visualized. In the setting of a BPF due to a rent or tear on the lung periphery, locating the bronchial segment that provides ventilation to that area of the lung can be more difficult. Several techniques can be employed by bronchoscopy to localize the proximal endobronchial site of the fistulous tract. Occasionally, air bubbles can be seen emanating from the segmental bronchus. Washing the suspected segment with normal saline and coughing may accentuate the bubbling. A balloon-tipped catheter, such as a Fogarty catheter or a single-lumen right heart catheter, can be passed through the working channel of the bronchoscope and selectively positioned in suspect segmental bronchial orifices that lead to the peripheral fistula. After positioning the catheter in the suspect segment, the balloon is inflated to occlude the orifice, and the bronchoscopist then looks for cessation of bubbling in the water seal chamber of the pleural drainage unit (121). The lack of bubbling after balloon inflation confirms that the bronchial segment has been occluded and allows the BPF to heal.

Successful endobronchial occlusion of BPFs has been reported with cyanoacrylate-based tissue adhesives (Histoacryl, Bucrylate), fibrin sealants (Tisseal, Hemaseal, thrombin plus fibrinogen or cryoprecipitate), absorbable gelatin sponge (Gelfoam), vascular occlusion coils, doxycycline and blood, Nd:YAG laser, silver nitrate, and lead shot (128–130). The agent initially seals the leak by acting as a plug and subsequently induces an inflammatory process with fibrosis and mucosal proliferation permanently sealing the area. Of these techniques, the uses of cyanoacrylate tissue adhesives and fibrin sealants have been most widely reported.

Airway stents may be used to cover and seal the fistula in selected patients, depending on the location of the fistula. BPFs due to breakdown of a stump after lobectomy or pneumonectomy or bronchial dehiscence after lung transplantation or bronchoplastic procedures are the most amenable to successful closure with airway stenting. More recently, the successful closure of BPFs using bronchoscopic placement of endobronchial valves designed for emphysema has been described (131–133).

Foreign Body Removal

Risk factors for foreign body aspiration include age younger than 3 years, altered consciousness, trauma, and disordered swallowing mechanisms. Although occurring less frequently in adults than in children, tracheobronchial foreign bodies are problematic in adults (134,135). Patients may present with dyspnea, coughing, wheezing, or stridor. Foreign body aspiration may be relatively occult, with no obvious history for aspiration. Radiographically, there may be evidence of atelectasis, bronchiectasis, or recurrent pneumonitis.

Bronchoscopy to remove an aspirated foreign body should be performed by an experienced bronchoscopist. For pediatric patients, the foreign body may be successfully extracted via flexible bronchoscopy. For most situations, however, the rigid bronchoscope remains the instrument of choice in young children and infants (135). In adults, flexible bronchoscopy has clearly been shown to be an effective diagnostic and therapeutic tool in cases of suspected foreign body aspiration (134,136,137). Several extraction devices are available for use through the flexible bronchoscope (138). Biopsy forceps, graspers, and foreign body baskets are most commonly employed. Large foreign bodies may be extracted by applying continuous suction and withdrawing the bronchoscope with the foreign body adhered to the tip of the scope. Compared with rigid bronchoscopy, flexible bronchoscopy offers an enhanced visualization of the more peripheral airways, can be performed at the bedside, and averts the need for general anesthesia and operating room facilities. Occasionally, combined flexible and rigid bronchoscopy are required to enhance retrieval of the foreign body.

Inhalation Injury

Exposure to fire or smoke in an enclosed environment puts the patient at risk for thermal airway injury. Patients with singed nasal hairs, facial burns around the nose or mouth, oral/nasopharyngeal burns, carbonaceous sputum, or hoarseness should be suspected of having an upper airway injury. Stridor, wheezing, or other manifestations of upper airway symptomatology may imply impending ventilatory failure. In patients with suspected inhalation injury, flexible bronchoscopy should be performed early by an experienced bronchoscopist to identify evidence of thermal airway injury. Flexible bronchoscopy allows direct examination of the supraglottic and infraglottic areas. The need for intubation should be anticipated and an endotracheal tube placed over the bronchoscope before examining the airways. If intubation is deemed necessary, the bronchoscope can function as a guide for endotracheal tube placement. Serial examinations may be necessary in patients with apparent minimal thermal airway injury on initial evaluation (139). Signs indicating impending airway obstruction include inflammation, edema, ulceration, or hemorrhage of the upper airway mucosa (140–143).

By using flexible bronchoscopy, inhalation injury can be classified into acute, subacute, and chronic phases. In the acute stage, upper airway obstruction from mucosal edema and respiratory failure from pulmonary edema and hemorrhage are the main characteristics. Soot deposition in the airways and carbon monoxide poisoning also may be found. The subacute stage, which lasts from hours to several days, is manifested by necrosis of the tracheobronchial mucosa, hemorrhagic tracheal bronchitis, persistent pulmonary edema with or without hemorrhage, and secondary infection. Scarring and stenosis of the tracheobronchial tree with formation of granulation tissue, as well as bronchiectasis due to bronchiolitis obliterans, are the hallmarks of the chronic stage. Flexible bronchoscopy may offer significant utility in identifying these three stages of significant injury (144).

In the intubated patient, repeat airway examination by bronchoscopy may be necessary before extubation to ensure airway patency and resolution of the supraglottic or laryngeal edema. The endotracheal tube can be withdrawn over the bronchoscope while inspecting the airway mucosa and replaced if the airway is compromised (145).

Acute Upper Airway Obstruction

Causes of upper airway obstruction include epiglottitis, bilateral vocal cord paralysis, laryngeal edema, and foreign body. In the pediatric patient, subglottic stenosis secondary to croup should also be considered. Flexible bronchoscopy can be helpful to make a diagnosis in these circumstances. Flexible bronchoscopy may be particularly helpful for diagnosis and therapeutic intubation in upper airway obstruction after burn and smoke inhalation injury and trauma to the face and neck. The flexible bronchoscope affords immediate direct visualization of the upper airway and, if performed with an ET placed over the bronchoscope, affords visualization and guidance for endotracheal intubation. If epiglottitis is suspected, it may be prudent to perform bronchoscopy in the surgical suite, with the surgical team available for emergency tracheostomy in case of failure. When performing bronchoscopic intubation in suspected upper airway obstruction, the nasotracheal approach may be preferable because the turbinates offer stabilization and a more controlled approach to the area of acute airway obstruction (146). Flexible bronchoscopic intubation in upper airway obstruction may be performed in the sitting position with decreased posterior displacement of the epiglottis over the compromised upper airway as compared with laryngoscopic examination in the supine position. If foreign body obstruction is known or suspected as the cause of the upper airway obstruction, rigid bronchoscopy may be the bronchoscopy method of choice.

Central Airway Obstruction

Patients may develop impending or acute respiratory failure due to central airway obstruction from primary lung cancer or metastatic malignancies. Treatment for malignant airway obstruction from endoluminal tumor has typically consisted of Nd:YAG laser photoresection and metal or silicone stent placement, although endobronchial electrocautery or argon plasma coagulation has more recently been used in lieu of the Nd:YAG laser (147–149). Other modalities such as cryotherapy, photodynamic therapy, and brachytherapy have been used to treat malignant airway obstruction; however, there is a delay in airway patency after treatment with these therapies and, as such, they may be less satisfactory in treating the patient with acute respiratory failure who would benefit from immediate airway patency. Airway obstruction from extrinsic tumor compression is typically treated with placement of metal or silicone stents.

Patients may also develop respiratory failure from benign causes, most commonly previous intubation or tracheostomy tube placement, causing a cicatricial stenosis with or without granulation tissue. Patients who have an indwelling tracheostomy tube may also develop a fibrous stenosis or granulation tissue just beyond the tip of the tracheostomy tube, thereby causing airway obstruction. The granulation tissue may be resected with laser electrocautery therapy. The stenosis may be dilated with a rigid bronchoscope or balloon dilatation catheters. In selected patients, silicone stents may be placed after dilatation. In general, metal stents should not be used for tracheal stenosis due to a higher complication rate and difficulty in removing the stent should problems develop.

Status Asthmaticus

The usefulness of bronchoscopy in patients with status asthmaticus is the subject of controversy (32,150). Success has been reported with bronchial lavage in patients with obstructive airway disease who could not be weaned from ventilatory support (151,152). Bronchial lavage may benefit selected mechanically ventilated patients with thick, tenacious secretions who are unresponsive to aggressive bronchodilator therapy (65,153). Mucous plugs impacted in airways may be extracted using the flexible bronchoscope for lavage, thus improving ventilation and oxygenation (65,154). Critically ill, mechanically ventilated asthmatic patients are, however, poor candidates for bronchial lavage; the procedure is likely to produce a significant increase in auto-PEEP and worsening of hypoxemia. The extolled benefits of lung lavage are limited to case reports (155–157). Normal saline lavage solution has been traditionally used, but diluted acetylcysteine may enhance mucous clearance from the airways by a mucolytic effect (65,155). Acetylcysteine should be used with caution because it may provoke bronchospasm in patients with reactive airway disease. Asthmatics should receive aggressive bronchodilator therapy before bronchoscopy.

References

1. Lindholm CE, Oilman B, Snyder JV, et al. Cardiorespiratory effects of flexible fiberoptic bronchoscopy in critically ill patients. *Chest.* 1978;74:363.

2. Peerless J, Snow N, Likavec M, et al. The effect of fiberoptic bronchoscopy on intracranial pressure in patients with brain injury. *Chest.* 1995;108:962.
3. Cowl CT, Prakash UB, Kruger BR. The role of anticholinergics in bronchoscopy: a randomized clinical trial. *Chest.* 2000;118:188.
4. Clarkson K, Power CK, O'Connell F, et al. A comparative evaluation of propofol and midazolam as sedative agents in fiberoptic bronchoscopy. *Chest.* 1993;104:1029.
5. Kerwin AJ, Croce MA, Timmons SD, et al. Effects of fiberoptic bronchoscopy on intracranial pressure in patients with brain injury: a prospective clinical study. *J Trauma.* 2000;48:878.
6. Reichert WW, Hall WJ, Hyde RW. A simple disposable device for performing fiberoptic bronchoscopy on patients requiring continuous artificial ventilation. *Am Rev Respir Dis.* 1974;109:394.
7. Meduri GU, Chastre J. The standardization of bronchoscopic techniques for ventilator-associated pneumonia. *Chest.* 1992;102(Suppl 1):557S.
8. American Thoracic Society. Clinical role of bronchoalveolar lavage in adults with pulmonary disease. *Am Rev Respir Dis.* 1990;142:481.
9. Klech H, Pohl W. Technical recommendations and guidelines for bronchoalveolar lavage (BAL). *Eur Respir J.* 1989;2:561.
10. Rennard SI, Aalbers R, Bleecker E, et al. Bronchoalveolar lavage: performance, sampling procedure, processing and assessment. *Eur Respir J.* 1998;26(Suppl):13S.
11. Wimberley N, Faling LJ, Bartlett JG. A fiberoptic bronchoscopy technique to obtain uncontaminated lower airway secretions for bacterial culture. *Am Rev Respir Dis.* 1979;119:337.
12. Wimberley NW, Bass JB Jr, Boyd BW, et al. Use of a bronchoscopic protected catheter brush for the diagnosis of pulmonary infections. *Chest.* 1982;81:556.
13. de Lassence A, Joly-Guillou ML, Martin-Lefevre L, et al. Accuracy of delayed cultures of plugged telescoping catheter samples for diagnosing bacterial pneumonia. *Crit Care Med.* 2001;29:1311.
14. Baselski VS, Wunderink RG. Bronchoscopic diagnosis of pneumonia. *Clin Microbiol Rev.* 1994;7:533.
15. Chastre J, Combes A, Luyt CE. The invasive (quantitative) diagnosis of ventilator-associated pneumonia. *Respir Care.* 2005;50:797.
16. Fagon JY. Diagnosis and treatment of ventilator-associated pneumonia: fiberoptic bronchoscopy with bronchoalveolar lavage is essential. *Semin Respir Crit Care Med.* 2006;27:35.
17. O'Brien JD, Ettinger NA, Shevlin D, et al. Safety and yield of transbronchial biopsy in mechanically ventilated patients. *Crit Care Med.* 1997;25:440.
18. British Thoracic Society Bronchoscopy Guidelines Committee, a Subcommittee of Standards of Care Committee of British Thoracic Society. British Thoracic Society guidelines on diagnostic flexible bronchoscopy. *Thorax.* 2001;56(Suppl 1):i1.
19. Guidelines for fiberoptic bronchoscopy in adults. American Thoracic Society. *Am Rev Respir Dis.* 1987;136:1066.
20. Hanson RR, Zavala DC, Rhodes ML, et al. Transbronchial biopsy via flexible fiberoptic bronchoscope; results in 164 patients. *Am Rev Respir Dis.* 1976;114:67.
21. Bajwa MK, Henein S, Kamholz SL. Fiberoptic bronchoscopy in the presence of space-occupying intracranial lesions. *Chest.* 1993;104:101.
22. Credle WF, Smiddy JF, Elliott RC. Complications of fiberoptic bronchoscopy. *Am Rev Respir Dis.* 1974;109:67.
23. Udaya BS, Prakash MD, Stubbs SE. Bronchoscopy: indications and technique. *Semin Respir Med.* 1981;3:17.
24. Pereira W, Kovnat DM, Snider GL. A prospective cooperative study of complications following flexible fiberoptic bronchoscopy. *Chest.* 1978;73:813.
25. Steinberg KP, Mitchell DR, Maunder RJ, et al. Safety of bronchoalveolar lavage in patients with adult respiratory distress syndrome. *Am Rev Respir Dis.* 1993;148:556.
26. Albertini RE, Harrell JH, Kurihara N. Arterial hypoxemia induced by fiberoptic bronchoscopy. *JAMA.* 1974;230:1666.
27. Albertini R, Harrell JH, Moser KM. Hypoxemia during fiberoptic bronchoscopy. *Chest.* 1974;65:117.
28. Ghows MB, Rosen MJ, Chuang MT, et al. Transcutaneous oxygen monitoring during fiberoptic bronchoscopy. *Chest.* 1986;89:543.
29. Turner JS, Willcox PA, Hayhurst MD, et al. Fiberoptic bronchoscopy in the intensive care unit—a prospective study of 147 procedures in 107 patients. *Crit Care Med.* 1994;22:259.
30. Trouillet JL, Guiguet M, Gibert C, et al. Fiberoptic bronchoscopy in ventilated patients. Evaluation of cardiopulmonary risk under midazolam sedation. *Chest.* 1990;97:927.
31. Weinstein HJ, Bone RC, Ruth WE. Pulmonary lavage in patients treated with mechanical ventilation. *Chest.* 1977;72:583.
32. Dubrawsky C, Awe RJ, Jenkins DE. The effect of bronchofiberscopic examination on oxygenation status. *Chest.* 1976;67:137.
33. Wu FL, Razzaghi A, Souney PF. Seizure after lidocaine for bronchoscopy: case report and review of the use of lidocaine in airway anesthesia. *Pharmacotherapy.* 1993;13:72.
34. Khan NA, Kruse JA. Methemoglobinemia induced by topical anesthesia: a case report and review. *Am J Med Sci.* 1999;318:415.
35. Barrett CR. Flexible fiberoptic bronchoscopy in the critically ill patient. *Chest.* 1978;73:746.
36. Shrader DL. The effect of fiberoptic bronchoscopy on cardiac rhythm. *Chest.* 1978;73:821.
37. Katz AS, Michelson EL, Stawick J, et al. Cardiac arrhythmias: frequency during fiberoptic bronchoscopy and correlation with hypoxemia. *Arch Intern Med.* 1981;141:603.
38. Belen J, Neuhaus A, Markowitz D, at al. Modification of the effect of fiberoptic bronchoscopy on pulmonary mechanics. *Chest.* 1981;79:516.
39. Zavala DC. Pulmonary hemorrhage in fiberoptic transbronchial biopsy. *Chest.* 1976;70:584.
40. Fulkerson WJ. Current concepts: fiberoptic bronchoscopy. *N Engl J Med.* 1984;311:511.
41. Landa JF. Indications for bronchoscopy. *Chest.* 1978;73:687.
42. Johnston H, Reisz G. Changing spectrum of hemoptysis: underlying causes in 148 patients undergoing diagnostic flexible fiberoptic bronchoscopy. *Arch Intern Med.* 1989;149:1666.
43. Kobrinsky NL, Israels ED, Gerrard JM, et al. Shortening of bleeding time by 1-deamino-8-D-arginine vasopressin in various bleeding disorders. *Lancet.* 1984;1:1145.
44. Pincus PS, Kallenbach JM, Hurwitz MD, et al. Transbronchial biopsy during mechanical ventilation. *Crit Care Med.* 1987;15:1136.
45. O'Brien JD, Ettinger NA, Shevlin D, et al. Safety and yield of transbronchial biopsy in mechanically ventilated patients. *Crit Care Med.* 1997;25:440.
46. Bulpa PA, Dive AM, Mertens L, et al. Combined bronchoalveolar lavage and transbronchial lung biopsy: safety and yield in ventilated patients. *Eur Respir J.* 2003;21:489.
47. Pereira W, Kovnat DM, Khan MA, et al. Fever and pneumonia after flexible fiberoptic bronchoscopy. *Am Rev Respir Dis.* 1975;112:59.
48. Kane RC, Cohen MH, Fossieck BE, et al. Absence of bacteremia after fiberoptic bronchoscopy. *Am Rev Respir Dis.* 1975;111:102.
49. Dajani AS, Bisno AL, Chung KJ, et al. Antimicrobial prophylaxis for the prevention of bacterial endocarditis in patients with underlying cardiac conditions. *JAMA.* 1990;264:2919.
50. Ovassapian A. The flexible bronchoscope: a tool for anesthesiologists. *Clin Chest Med.* 2001;22:281.
51. Weiss YG, Deutschman CS. The role of fiberoptic bronchoscopy in airway management of the critically ill patient. *Crit Care Clin.* 2000;16:445.
52. Ovassapian A. Flexible bronchoscopic intubation of awake patients. *J Bronchol.* 1994;1:240.
53. Greenland KB, Irwin MG. The Williams Airway Intubator, the Ovassapian Airway and the Berman Airway as upper airway conduits for fiberoptic bronchoscopy in patients with difficult airways. *Curr Opin Anaesthesiol.* 2004;17:505.
54. Ovassapian A, Randel GI. The role of the fiberscope in the critically ill patient. *Crit Care Clin.* 1995;11:29.
55. Caponas G. Intubating laryngeal mask airway. *Anaesth Intensive Care.* 2002;30:551.
56. O'Brien D, Registrar S, Curran J, et al. Fiberoptic assessment of tracheal tube position: a comparison of tracheal tube position as estimated by fiberoptic bronchoscopy and by chest x-ray. *Anaesthesia.* 1985;40:73.
57. deBloisblanc BP. Percutaneous dilational tracheostomy techniques. *Clin Chest Med.* 2003;24:399.
58. Shinnick JP, Freedman AP. Bronchofiberscopic placement of a double-lumen endotracheal tube. *Crit Care Med.* 1981;10:544.
59. Ovassapian A. Fiberoptic bronchoscope and double-lumen tracheal tubes. *Anesthesia.* 1983;38:1104.
60. Klein U, Karzai W, Bloos F, et al. Role of fiberoptic bronchoscopy in conjunction with the use of double-lumen tubes for thoracic anesthesia: a prospective study. *Anesthesiology.* 1998;88:346.
61. Kreider ME, Lipson DA. Bronchoscopy for atelectasis in the ICU: a case report and review of the literature. *Chest.* 2003;124:344.
62. Marini JJ, Pierson DJ, Hudson LD. Acute lobar atelectasis: a prospective comparison of fiberoptic bronchoscopy and respiratory therapy. *Am Rev Respir Dis.* 1979;119:971.
63. Mehrishi S. Is bronchoscopy indicated in the management of atelectasis? Pro bronchoscopy. *J Bronchol.* 2002;9:46.
64. Raoof S. Is bronchoscopy indicated in the management of atelectasis? Con bronchoscopy. *J Bronchol.* 2002;9:52.
65. Millman M, Goodman AH, Goldstein IM, et al. Status asthmaticus: use of acetylcysteine during bronchoscopy and lavage to remove mucous plugs. *Ann Allergy.* 1983;50:85.
66. Perruchoud A, Ehrsam R, Heitz M, et al. Atelectasis of the lung: bronchoscopic lavage with acetylcysteine: experience in 51 patients. *Eur J Respir Dis Suppl.* 1980;111:163.
67. Slattery DM, Waltz DA, Denham B, et al. Bronchoscopically administered recombinant human DNase for lobar atelectasis in cystic fibrosis. *Pediatr Pulmonol.* 2001;31:38.
68. Haenel JB, Moore FA, Moore EE, et al. Efficacy of selective intrabronchial air insufflation in acute lobar collapse. *Am J Surg.* 1992;164:501.
69. Harada K, Mutsuda T, Saoyama N, et al. Re-expansion of refractory atelectasis using a bronchofiberscope with a balloon cuff. *Chest.* 1983;84:725.
70. Millen JE, Vandree J, Glauser FL. Fiberoptic bronchoscopic balloon occlusion and re-expansion of refractory unilateral atelectasis. *Crit Care Med.* 1978;6:50.

71. Tsao TC, Tsai YH, Lan RS, et al. Treatment for collapsed lung in critically ill patients. *Chest.* 1990;97:435.
72. Dweik RA, Stoller JK. Role of bronchoscopy in massive hemoptysis. *Clin Chest Med.* 1999;20:89.
73. Jean-Baptiste E. Clinical assessment and management of massive hemoptysis. *Crit Care Med.* 2000;28:1642.
74. Gourin A, Garzon AA. Operative treatment of massive hemoptysis. *Ann Thorac Surg.* 1974;18:52.
75. Gottlieb LS, Hillberg R. Endobronchial tamponade therapy for intractable hemoptysis. *Chest.* 1975;67:482.
76. Saw EC, Gottlieb LS, Yokoyama T, et al. Flexible fiberoptic bronchoscopy and endobronchial tamponade in the management of massive hemoptysis. *Chest.* 1976;70:589.
77. Lee SM, Kim HY, Ahn Y. Parallel technique of endobronchial balloon catheter tamponade for transient alleviation of massive hemoptysis. *J Korean Med Sci.* 2002;17:823.
78. Jolliet P, Soccal P, Chevrolet JC. Control of massive hemoptysis by endobronchial tamponade with a pulmonary artery balloon catheter. *Crit Care Med.* 1992;20:1730.
79. Kato R, Sawafuji M, Kawamura M, et al. Massive hemoptysis successfully treated by modified bronchoscopic balloon tamponade technique. *Chest.* 1996;109:842.
80. Kabon B, Waltl B, Leitgeb J, et al. First experience with fiberoptically directed wire-guided endobronchial blockade in severe pulmonary bleeding in an emergency setting. *Chest.* 2001;120:1399.
81. Conlan AA, Hurwitz SS. Management of massive haemoptysis with the rigid bronchoscope and cold saline lavage. *Thorax.* 1980;35:901.
82. Tsukamoto T, Sasaki H, Nakamura H. Treatment of hemoptysis patients by thrombin and fibrinogen-thrombin infusion therapy using a fiberoptic bronchoscope. *Chest.* 1989;96:473.
83. Valipour A, Kreuzer A, Koller H, et al. Bronchoscopy-guided topical hemostatic tamponade therapy for the management of life-threatening hemoptysis. *Chest.* 2005;127:2113.
84. American Thoracic Society; Infectious Diseases Society of America. Guidelines for the management of adults with hospital-acquired, ventilator-associated, and healthcare-associated pneumonia. *Am J Respir Crit Care Med.* 2005;171:388.
85. Torres A, El-Ebiary M. Bronchoscopic BAL in the diagnosis of ventilator-associated pneumonia. *Chest.* 2000;117(Suppl 2):198S.
86. Baughman RP. Protected-specimen brush technique in the diagnosis of ventilator-associated pneumonia. *Chest.* 2000;117(Suppl 2):203.
87. de Jaeger A, Litalien C, Lacroix J, et al. Protected specimen brush or bronchoalveolar lavage to diagnose bacterial nosocomial pneumonia in ventilated adults: a meta-analysis. *Crit Care Med.* 1999;27:2548.
88. Fujitani S, Yu VL. Quantitative cultures for diagnosing ventilator-associated pneumonia: a critique. *Clin Infect Dis.* 2006;43(Suppl 2):S106.
89. Heyland DK, Cook DJ, Marshall J, et al. The clinical utility of invasive diagnostic techniques in the setting of ventilator-associated pneumonia. Canadian Critical Care Trials Group. *Chest.* 1999;115:1076.
90. Fagon JY, Chastre J, Wolff M, et al. Invasive and noninvasive strategies for management of suspected ventilator-associated pneumonia: a randomized trial. *Ann Intern Med.* 2000;132:621.
91. Sanchez-Nieto JM, Torres A, Garcia-Cordoba F, et al. Impact of invasive and noninvasive quantitative culture sampling on outcome of ventilator-associated pneumonia: a pilot study. *Am J Respir Crit Care Med.* 1998;157:371.
92. Ruiz M, Torres A, Ewig S, et al. Noninvasive versus invasive microbial investigation in ventilator-associated pneumonia: evaluation of outcome. *Am J Respir Crit Care Med.* 2000;162:119.
93. Sole Violan J, Fernandez JA, Benitez AB, et al. Impact of quantitative invasive diagnostic techniques in the management and outcome of mechanically ventilated patients with suspected pneumonia. *Crit Care Med.* 2000;28:2737.
94. Shorr AF, Sherner JH, Jackson WL, et al. Invasive approaches to the diagnosis of ventilator-associated pneumonia: a meta-analysis. *Crit Care Med.* 2005;33:46.
95. Prats E, Dorca J, Pujol M, et al. Effects of antibiotics on protected specimen brush sampling in ventilator-associated pneumonia. *Eur Respir J.* 2002;19:944.
96. Montravers P, Fagon JY, Chastre J, et al. Follow-up protected specimen brushes to assess treatment in nosocomial pneumonia. *Am Rev Respir Dis.* 1993;147:38.
97. Souweine B, Veber B, Bedos JP, et al. Diagnostic accuracy of protected specimen brush and bronchoalveolar lavage in nosocomial pneumonia: impact of previous antimicrobial treatments. *Crit Care Med.* 1998;26:236.
98. Jain P, Sandur S, Meli Y, et al. Role of flexible bronchoscopy in immunocompromised patients with lung infiltrates. *Chest.* 2004;125:712.
99. Ognibene FP, Shelhamer J, Gill V, et al. The diagnosis of Pneumocystis carinii pneumonia in patients with the acquired immunodeficiency syndrome using subsegmental bronchoalveolar lavage. *Am Rev Respir Dis.* 1984;129:929.
100. Stover DE, White DA, Romano PA, et al. Diagnosis of pulmonary disease in acquired immune deficiency syndrome (AIDS). *Am Rev Respir Dis.* 1984;130:659.
101. Wollschlager C, Khan F. Diagnostic value of fiberoptic bronchoscopy in acquired immunodeficiency syndrome. *Cleve Clin Q.* 1985;52:489.
102. Broaddus C, Dake MD, Stulbarg MS, et al. Bronchoalveolar lavage and transbronchial biopsy for the diagnosis of pulmonary infections in the acquired immunodeficiency syndrome. *Ann Intern Med.* 1985;102:747.
103. Flori P, Bellete B, Durand F, et al. Comparison between real-time PCR, conventional PCR and different staining techniques for diagnosing Pneumocystis jiroveci pneumonia from bronchoalveolar lavage specimens. *J Med Microbiol.* 2004;53:603.
104. Musher B, Fredricks D, Leisenring W, et al. Aspergillus galactomannan enzyme immunoassay and quantitative PCR for diagnosis of invasive aspergillosis with bronchoalveolar lavage fluid. *J Clin Microbiol.* 2004;42:5517.
105. Klont RR, Mennink-Kersten MA, Verweij PE. Utility of Aspergillus antigen detection in specimens other than serum specimens. *Clin Infect Dis.* 2004;39:1467.
106. Sanguinetti M, Posteraro B, Pagano L, et al. Comparison of real-time PCR, conventional PCR, and galactomannan antigen detection by enzyme-linked immunosorbent assay using bronchoalveolar lavage fluid samples from hematology patients for diagnosis of invasive pulmonary aspergillosis. *J Clin Microbiol.* 2003;41:3922.
107. Hage CA, Davis TE, Egan L, et al. Diagnosis of pulmonary histoplasmosis and blastomycosis by detection of antigen in bronchoalveolar lavage fluid using an improved second-generation enzyme-linked immunoassay. *Respir Med.* 2007;101:43.
108. Ison MG, Fishman JA. Cytomegalovirus pneumonia in transplant recipients. *Clin Chest Med.* 2005;26:691.
109. Danek JJ, Bower JS. Diagnosis of pulmonary tuberculosis by fiberoptic bronchoscopy. *Am Rev Respir Dis.* 1979;119:677.
110. Jett JR, Cortese DA, Dines DE. The value of bronchoscopy in the diagnosis of mycobacterial disease. *Chest.* 1981;80:575.
111. Pant K, Chawla R, Mann PS, et al. Fiberbronchoscopy in smear-negative miliary tuberculosis. *Chest.* 1989;95:1151.
112. de Gracia J, Curull V, Vidal R, et al. Diagnostic value of bronchoalveolar lavage in suspected pulmonary tuberculosis. *Chest.* 1988;93:329.
113. Tueller C, Chhajed PN, Buitrago-Tellez C, et al. Value of smear and PCR in bronchoalveolar lavage fluid in culture positive pulmonary tuberculosis. *Eur Respir J.* 2005;26:767.
114. Chen NH, Liu YC, Tsao TC, et al. Combined bronchoalveolar lavage and polymerase chain reaction in the diagnosis of pulmonary tuberculosis in smear-negative patients. *Int J Tuberc Lung Dis.* 2002;6:350.
115. Meyer KC. Bronchoalveolar lavage as a diagnostic tool. *Semin Respir Crit Care Med.* 2007;28:546.
116. Meyer KC. Bronchoalveolar lavage in the diagnosis and management of interstitial lung diseases. *Clin Pulm Med.* 2007;14:148.
117. Barmada H, Gibbons JR. Tracheobronchial injury in blunt and penetrating chest trauma. *Chest.* 1994;106:74.
118. Baumgartner F, Sheppard B, de Virgilio C, et al. Tracheal and main bronchial disruptions after blunt chest trauma: presentation and management. *Ann Thorac Surg.* 1990;50:569.
119. Caster R, Wareham EE, Brewer LA. Rupture of the bronchus following closed chest trauma. *Am J Surg.* 1962;104:212.
120. Kirsh MM, Orringer MB, Douglas MB, et al. Management of tracheobronchial disruption secondary to nonpenetrating trauma. Current review: tracheobronchial disruption from blunt trauma. *Ann Thorac Surg.* 1976;22:93.
121. Hara KS, Prakash UBS. Fiberoptic bronchoscopy in the evaluation of acute chest and upper airway trauma. *Chest.* 1989;96:627.
122. Ecker RR, Libertini RV, Rea WJ, et al. Injuries of the trachea and bronchi. *Ann Thorac Surg.* 1971;11:280.
123. Grover FL, Ellestad C, Arom KV, et al. Diagnosis and management of major tracheobronchial injuries. *Ann Thorac Surg.* 1979;28:384.
124. Kelly JP, Webb WR, Moulder PV, et al. Management of airway trauma: combined injuries of the trachea and esophagus. *Ann Thorac Surg.* 1987;43:160.
125. Jones WS, Mavroudis C, Richardson JD, et al. Management of tracheobronchial disruption resulting from blunt trauma. *Surgery.* 1984;95:319.
126. Roxburgh JC. Rupture of the tracheobronchial tree. *Thorax.* 1987;42:681.
127. Major CP, Floresguerra CA, Messerschmidt WH, et al. Traumatic disruption of the cervical trachea. *J Tenn Med Assoc.* 1992;85:517.
128. Sippel JM, Chesnutt MS. Bronchoscopic therapy for bronchopleural fistulas. *J Bronchol.* 1998;5:61.
129. McManigle JE, Fletcher GL, Tenholder MF. Bronchoscopy in the management of bronchopleural fistula. *Chest.* 1990;97:1235.
130. Lois M, Noppen M. Bronchopleural fistulas: an overview of the problem with special focus on endoscopic management. *Chest.* 2005;128:395.
131. Toma TP, Kon OM, Oldfield W, et al. Reduction of persistent air leak with endoscopic valve implants. *Thorax.* 2007;62:830.
132. Feller-Kopman D, Bechara R, Garland R, et al. Use of a removable endobronchial valve for the treatment of bronchopleural fistula. *Chest.* 2006;130:273.
133. Ferguson JS, Sprenger K, Van Natta T. Closure of a bronchopleural fistula using bronchoscopic placement of an endobronchial valve designed for the treatment of emphysema. *Chest.* 2006;129:479.

134. Limper AH, Prakash UBS. Tracheobronchial foreign bodies in adults. *Ann Intern Med.* 1990;112:604.
135. Swanson KL, Edell ES. Tracheobronchial foreign bodies. *Chest Surg Clin N Am.* 2001;11:861.
136. Cunanan OS. The flexible fiberoptic bronchoscope in foreign body removal. *Chest.* 1978;73:725.
137. Lan RS, Lee CH, Chiang YC, et al. Use of fiberoptic bronchoscopy to retrieve bronchial foreign bodies in adults. *Am Rev Respir Dis.* 1989;140:1734.
138. Atul MC, Rafanan AL. Extraction of airway foreign body in adults. *J Bronchol.* 2001;8:123.
139. Hunt JL, Agee RN, Pruitt BA Jr. Fiberoptic bronchoscopy in acute inhalation injury. *J Trauma.* 1975;15:641.
140. Wald PH, Balmes JR. Respiratory effects of short-term, high-intensity toxic inhalations: smoke, gases, and fumes. *J Intensive Care Med.* 1987;2:260.
141. Crapo RO. Smoke-inhalation injuries. *JAMA.* 1981;246:1694.
142. Hunt JL, Agec RN, Pruitt BA Jr. Fiberoptic bronchoscopy in acute inhalation injury. *J Trauma.* 1975;15:641.
143. Williams DO, Vanecko RM, Glassroth J. Endobronchial polyposis following smoke inhalation. *Chest.* 1983;84:774.
144. Sueoka N, Kato O, Aoki Y, et al. Fiberoptic bronchoscopy in inhalation injury. *J Jpn Soc Bronchol.* 1994;16:454.
145. Dellinger RP. Fiberoptic bronchoscopy in adult airway management. *Crit Care Med.* 1990;18:882.
146. Giudice JC, Komansky H, Gordon R, et al. Acute upper airway obstruction: fiberoptic bronchoscopy in diagnosis and therapy. *Crit Care Med.* 1981;9:878.
147. Seijo LM, Sterman DH. Interventional pulmonology. *N Engl J Med.* 2001; 344:740.
148. Beamis J. Interventional pulmonology techniques for treating malignant large airway obstruction: an update. *Curr Opin Pulm Med.* 2005;11: 292.
149. Wahidi MM, Herth FJ, Ernst A. State of the art: interventional pulmonology. *Chest.* 2007;131:261.
150. Satin SA, Scoggin C. Fiberoptic bronchoscopy in bronchial asthma: a word of caution. *Chest.* 1976;69:39.
151. Lang DM, Simon RA, Mathison DA, et al. Safety and possible efficacy of fiberoptic bronchoscopy with lavage in the management of refractory asthma with mucous impaction. *Ann Allergy.* 1991;67:324.
152. Henke CA, Hertz M, Gustafson P. Combined bronchoscopy and mucolytic therapy for patients with severe refractory status asthmaticus on mechanical ventilation: a case report and review of the literature. *Crit Care Med.* 1994;22:1880.
153. Shridharani M, Maxson TR. Pulmonary lavage in a patient in status asthmaticus receiving mechanical ventilation: a case report. *Ann Allergy.* 1982;49:157.
154. Weinstein HJ, Bone RC, Ruth WE. Pulmonary lavage in patients treated with mechanical ventilation. *Chest.* 1977;72:583.
155. Niederman MS, Gambino A, Lichter J, et al. Tension ball valve mucus plug in asthma. *Am J Med.* 1985;79:131.
156. Millman M, Goodman AH, Goldstein IM, et al. Bronchoscopy and lavage for chronic bronchial asthma. *Immunol Allerg Pract.* 1981;3:10.
157. Brashear RE, Meyer SC, Manion MW. Unilateral atelectasis in asthma. *Chest.* 1973;63:847.

CHAPTER 38 ■ AIRWAY MANAGEMENT

THOMAS C. MORT • ANDREA GABRIELLI • TIMOTHY J. COONS • ELIZABETH CORDES BEHRINGER • A. JOSEPH LAYON

IMMEDIATE CONCERNS

Major Problems

Maintenance of the airway must be one of the most essential goals of critical care. Critical care personnel apply their expertise in resuscitating the critically ill patient by volume infusion, invasive line placement, titration of vasoactive medications, analysis of laboratory studies, and performing radiographic examinations, but may neglect the "A" of the ABCs until further clinical deterioration turns the need for airway management into an emergency. Airway functions are numerous and, though it primarily supports the exchange of oxygen and carbon dioxide, the airway assists in the regulation of temperature, contributes to the warming and humidification of inspired gas, traps and expels foreign particles, and protects against foreign body entry into the lungs through a complex array of reflex responses.

Many of these functions are altered or lost in critically ill patients. Airway obstruction can result from infection, trauma, laryngospasm, soft tissue edema, and aspiration of gastric or other noxious materials. Protective reflexes may be lost as a result of disease and depression with narcotics, sedatives, or paralytic agents. Humidification can also be lost as various appliances that bypass the nose, pharynx, and upper airway are inserted to maintain airway patency. Clinicians must then employ methods to maintain airway hydration, including humidifiers, nebulizers, and heat–moisture exchangers. These devices introduce additional problems such as nosocomial infections and increased work of breathing.

GENERAL PRINCIPLES

Primum non nocere (first do no harm) applies most fittingly to the airways of critically ill patients. The intensivist must not only be knowledgeable of respiratory pathophysiology, but also must possess technical skill and sound judgment in airway management. Various options are available, including bag-valve-mask ventilation, translaryngeal intubation (oral or nasal), tracheotomy, and cricothyroidotomy. Adjunctive drugs such as local anesthetics, narcotics, benzodiazepines, barbiturates, muscle relaxants, ketamine, and propofol play an important role. Their use facilitates airway control and improves respiratory support.

In most instances, bag-valve-mask (Fig. 38.1) ventilation precedes tracheal intubation. Immediate correction of hypoxemia should be attempted by application of a mask and initiation of bag ventilation with an increased FiO_2 while equipment for intubation is prepared. An appropriate mask provides a tight seal around the nose and mouth, and the colorless plastic with soft and pliable edges allows visualization of the

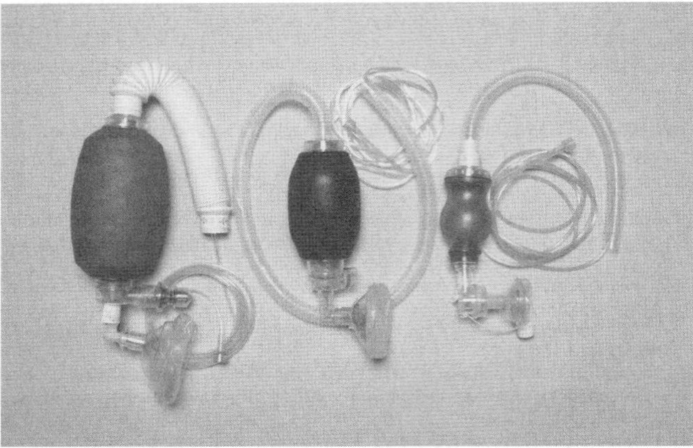

FIGURE 38.1. Standard bag-valve-mask setup. Note that the bag is self-inflating, so it can be used with (usual) or without (in emergencies) an external gas supply. The "tail" of the bag serves as an oxygen reservoir.

mouth and secretions. The mask is attached to the resuscitation (self-inflating or collapsible) bag with a high-flow oxygen source. Various systems will supply an FiO_2 between 0.60 and 1.0, depending upon the mask fit, the manufacturer, the oxygen flow rate, and the style of bag design based on the Mapleson (Fig. 38.2) designation (1–3). Proper inflation requires two hands: One to hold the mask firmly in place against the patient's face, and the other to compress the bag (4). The mandible must be lifted to create a seal without airway occlusion. An oropharyngeal or nasal airway facilitates oxygen delivery by bypassing or retracting the tongue (5,6). Forceful bag compression should be avoided to prevent gastric distention and possible pulmonary aspiration. Gentle insufflation allows clinical assessment of lung compliance and minimizes complications. Contraindications to bag-valve-mask ventilation include airway obstruction, pooling of blood or secretions in the pharynx, and severe facial trauma (7,8).

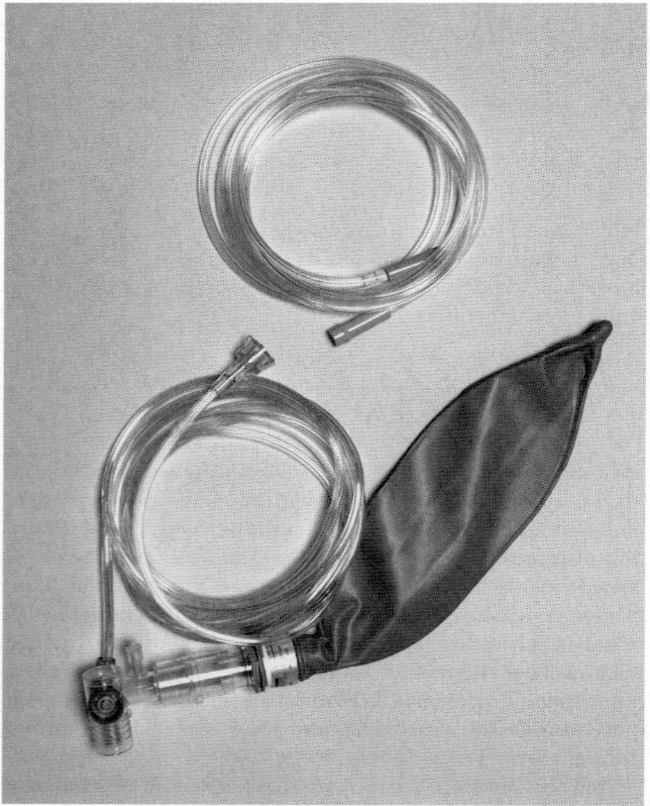

FIGURE 38.2. A Mapleson D bag. Note that this is not a self-inflating bag, and hence must be used with an external gas source. The positioning of the fresh gas inlet—designating the Mapleson bag class—and the fresh gas flow impact the amount of rebreathing. It is possible, in an inadvertent situation, if the fresh gas runs out and the pressure regulating ("pop off") valve is closed, to continuously rebreathe exhaled gas. This would ultimately result in injury or death.

TABLE 38.1

INDICATIONS FOR TRACHEAL INTUBATION

Open an obstructed airway
Provide airway pressure support to treat hypoxemia
PaO_2 less than 60 mm Hg with an FiO_2 greater than 0.5
Alveolar-to-arterial oxygen gradient 300 mm Hg
Intrapulmonary shunt more than 15%–20%
Provide mechanical ventilation
Respiratory acidosis
Inadequate respiratory mechanics
Respiratory rate more than 30 breaths/min
FVC less than 10 mL/kg
NIF more than –20 cm H_2O
V_D/V_T more than 0.6
Facilitate suctioning, instillation of medications, and bronchoscopy
Prevent aspiration
Gag and swallow reflexes absent

FiO_2, fraction of inspired oxygen; FVC, forced vital capacity; NIF, negative inspiratory force; V_D/V_T, dead space/tidal volume ratio.

Critically ill patients require tracheal intubation (Table 38.1) for several reasons (7). When inadequate ventilation is observed, tracheal intubation becomes necessary. It provides airway patency, facilitates tracheobronchial suctioning, and minimizes aspiration of blood, gastric contents, or secretions into the pulmonary tree. Oxygen administration and mechanical ventilation correct hypoxemia and hypercapnia, improve the alveolar-to-arterial oxygen partial pressure gradient, and reduce intrapulmonary shunting. In emergency situations in which intravascular access is absent, drug administration into the endotracheal tube can be life saving. Epinephrine, atropine, lidocaine, and naloxone exert their pharmacologic effects after tracheal administration (9–12).

Relative or absolute contraindications to conventional tracheal intubation exist in patients with traumatic or severe degenerative disorders of the cervical spine; in those with acute infectious processes such as acute supraglottitis or intrapharyngeal abscess; and in patients with extensive facial injury and basal skull fracture (13–15). Blind nasal intubation may be contraindicated in upper airway foreign body obstruction because the tube may push the foreign body distally and exacerbate airway compromise (13–16).

ANATOMIC CONSIDERATIONS

Adult

Specific anatomic characteristics may determine the ease or difficulty of intubation. The intensivist sometimes does not have

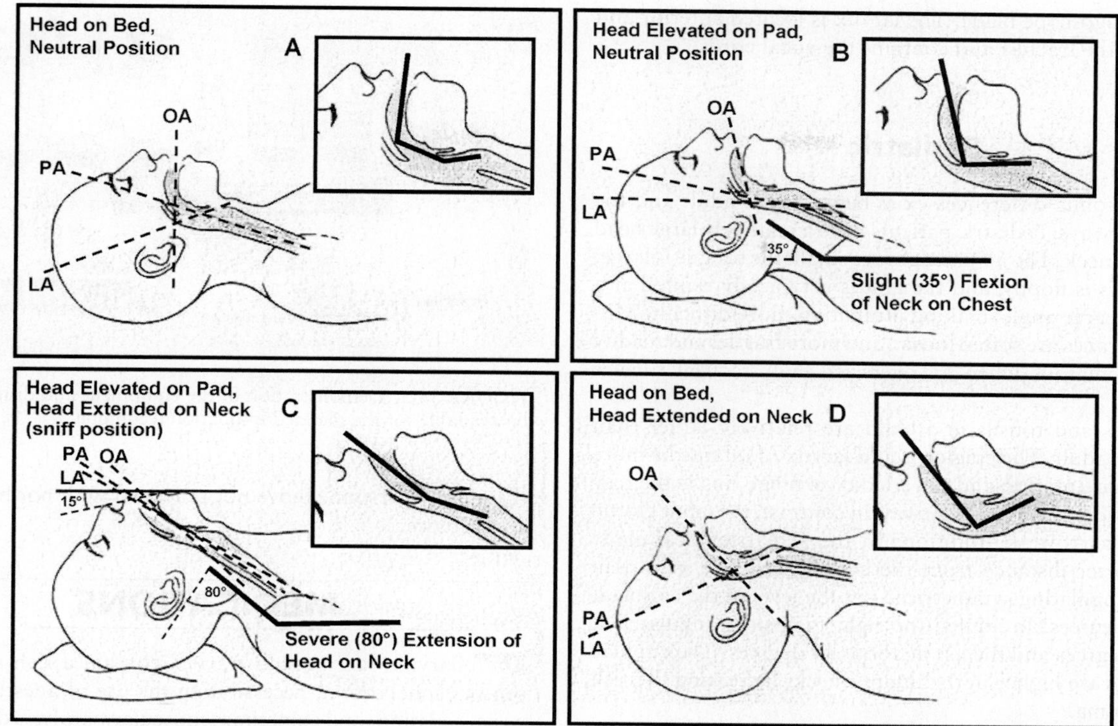

FIGURE 38.3. Demonstration of the "sniffing position" for optimal visualization of the glottic opening.

the flexibility to examine and assess the airway at leisure but must act quickly with skill and confidence. A good working knowledge of the anatomy of the mouth, neck, cervical spine, and pulmonary tree is mandatory for a successful and safe intubation. Examination of cervical spine mobility includes flexion and extension. Neck flexion aligns the pharyngeal and tracheal axes, whereas head extension on the neck and opening of the mouth align the oral passage with the pharyngeal and tracheal axes. This maneuver places the patient in a "sniffing position" (17) (Fig. 38.3). Incorrect positioning of the head and neck accounts for one of the common errors in orotracheal intubation. Flexion and extension of the head decreases 20% by 75 years of age. Degenerative arthritis limits cervical spine motion, more so with extension than flexion. Movement of the spine is contraindicated in the presence of potential cervical spine injury; hence, patients are maintained in a neutral position with in-line stabilization. Barring the edentulous patient, the front component of the hard cervical collar is commonly removed to allow full mandibular movement and optimize mouth opening. This maneuver removes the standard flexion and extension movements used to optimize the line of sight and therefore reduces one's ability to see "around the corner" in many cases (18–22). Each technique, maneuver, or accessory airway device available may alter the alignment of the cervical spine to a small degree based on the device itself, combined with the force and maneuvering performed by the operator, despite in-line stabilization (18,23–25). The available data and accumulated clinical experience do not dictate one method over another, especially when many practitioners who suggest an awake fiberoptic intubation is the "best" approach may themselves have reservations and concerns regarding their own comfort and competency at performing such a technique (18,26,27). The most appropriate technique is debatable but it would be prudent that the practitioner do his or her best with familiar equipment and approaches. This would not be the time to attempt to use a newly purchased item (e.g., rigid fiberscope), since one has not become competent and familiar with its use on a manikin and elective "easy" patients. Other diseases may place the patient at risk for atlantoaxial and cervical spine instability, and reduced mouth opening beyond those with known or suspected neck pathology (28).

Important anatomic landmarks may help the physician during direct laryngoscopy (Fig. 38.4). The cricoid, a circle of cartilage above the first tracheal ring, can be compressed to occlude the esophagus (Sellick maneuver), thereby preventing passive gastric regurgitation into the trachea during intubation (29). The epiglottis, a large cartilaginous structure, lies in the anterior pharynx. The vallecula, a furrow between the epiglottis and base of the tongue, is the placement site for the tip of a

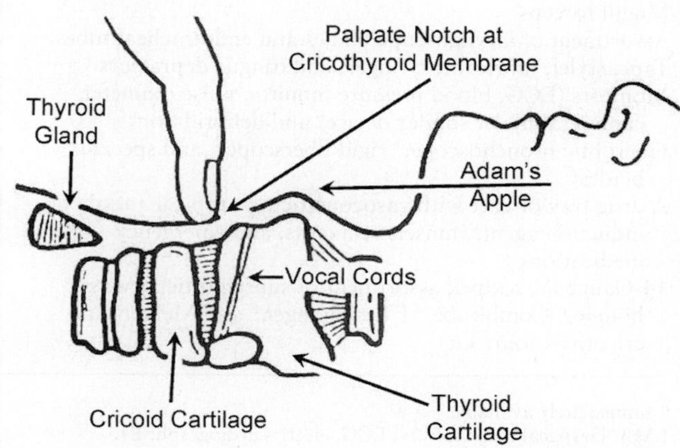

FIGURE 38.4. Laryngoscopic landmarks. Panel shows the cricoid cartilage.

curved laryngoscope blade. The larynx is located anterior and superior to the trachea and contains the vocal cords.

Pediatric

Several anatomic differences exist between the adult and the pediatric airways. Pediatric patients have a relatively large head and flexible neck. The air passages are small, the tongue is large, the epiglottis is floppy, and the glottis is typically slanted at a 40- to 50-degree angle, making intubation more difficult. Mucous membranes are softer, looser, and more fragile, and readily become edematous when an oversized endotracheal tube is used.

Adenoids and tonsils in a child are relatively larger than those in the adult. The epiglottis and larynx of infants lie more cephalad and anterior, and the cricoid cartilage ring is the narrowest portion of the upper airway. In contrast, the adult glottic opening is narrowest. Additionally, the pediatric vocal cords have a shorter distance from the carina, with the mainstem bronchus angulating symmetrically at the level of the carina at about 55 degrees. In adults, the right mainstem angulates at about 25 degrees and the left at about 45 degrees. The cupulae of the lungs are higher in the infant's neck, increasing the risk of lung trauma.

To avoid delay and minimize complications, all anticipated equipment and drugs must be available for the planned intubation technique (Table 38.2, Fig. 38.5). Additionally, a difficult airway cart or bag with a variety of airway rescue devices—as well as a bronchoscope and/or fiberoptic laryngoscope—should be readily available (30,31). It is far better to have a limited assortment of airway devices with which personnel are familiar and competent to handle than to have an expensive, well-stocked cart containing a plethora of devices that the airway personnel have not practiced with nor have gained competence.

TABLE 38.2

STANDARD EQUIPMENT AND DRUGS FOR TRANSLARYNGEAL INTUBATION

Bag-valve-mask resuscitation bag
LMA-type device
Oxygen source
Suction apparatus
Selection of oral and nasal airways
Magill forceps
Assortment of laryngoscope blades and endotracheal tubes
Tape, stylet, lubricant, syringes, and tongue depressors
Monitors (ECG, blood pressure monitor, pulse oximeter, capnography, or similar device) and defibrillator[a]
Fiberoptic bronchoscope,[a] rigid fiberscope,[a] and specialty blades[a]
A drug tray or cart with vasoconstrictors, topical anesthetics, induction agents, muscle relaxants, and emergency medications
14-Gauge IV, scalpel, assortment of supraglottic airways,[a] bougie,[a] Combitube,[a] ET exchanger,[a] and Melker-type cricothyrotomy kit

[a] Immediately available.
LMA, laryngeal mask airway; ECG, electrocardiograph; ET, endotracheal tube.

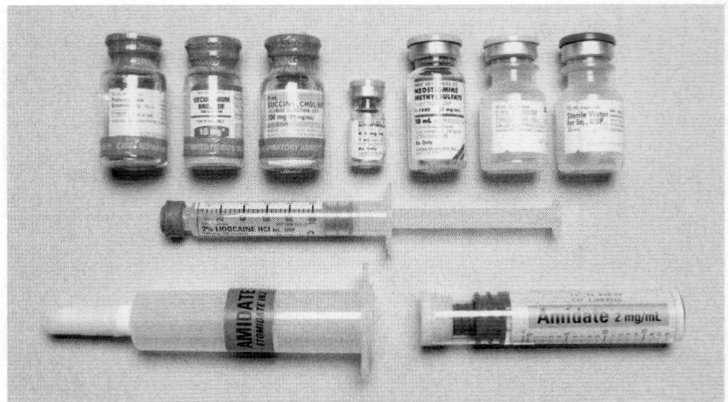

FIGURE 38.5. Demonstration of the equipment and drugs that must be available for the planned intubation technique.

MEDICATIONS

The pharynx, larynx, and trachea contain a rich network of sensory innervation, necessitating the use of anesthesia, analgesia, sedation, and sometimes muscular paralysis during intubation of a spontaneously breathing, awake, or semiconscious patient. Drugs commonly used are local anesthetics, sedative-hypnotics (sodium thiopental, propofol, etomidate), narcotics (fentanyl, morphine sulfate, hydromorphone, remifentanil), sedative-anxiolytics (benzodiazepine class—midazolam), muscle relaxants (depolarizing and nondepolarizing agents), and miscellaneous agents such as ketamine and dexmedetomidine.

Local Anesthetics

The use of local anesthetics is often overlooked in the intensive care unit (ICU) setting for a number of reasons: (a) it is far easier to administer an intravenous agent than to take the time to prepare the patient with topical anesthetics or local nerve blocks; (b) the urgency of the situation may preclude their timely use; (c) the patient's anatomic/physical characteristics may limit their effective application (poor or nonexistent landmarks, coagulopathy, excessively dry mucosa, excessive secretions, patient uncooperation); and (d) the underappreciation of their value in managing the airway and the underestimation of airway difficulty in the ICU setting. Moreover, access to the proper local anesthetic agents and the accessories for their accurate delivery (nebulizer, atomizer, Krause forceps, cotton balls, Abraham laryngeal cannula, etc.) may be limited in the ICU setting unless they have been prepared and gathered in advance (difficult airway cart).

Aerosolized or nebulized 1% to 4% lidocaine can readily achieve nasopharyngeal and oropharyngeal anesthesia if the patient is cooperative and capable of deep inhalation, thus limiting its usefulness in the ICU. The author has found this method less desirable due to its time-consuming application process and its limited effectiveness when compared to topically applied local anesthetics or local blocks. Transtracheal (cricothyroid membrane) instillation of 2 to 4 mL of 1% to 4% lidocaine with a 22- to 25-gauge needle causes sufficient coughing-induced reflex to afford ample distribution to anesthetize the subglottic and supraglottic regions plus the posterior pharynx in 90% of patients (32–34). Cocaine provides excellent conditions for facilitating intubation through the nasopharynx due to its outstanding topical anesthetic and mucosal and vascular shrinkage capabilities (33). However, in-hospital availability may limit its use in favor of phenylephrine or oxymetazoline combined with readily available local anesthetics. Lidocaine ointment applied to the base of the tongue with a tongue blade or similar device allows performance of direct laryngoscopy in many patients. If time permits, nasal spraying with a vasoconstrictor followed by passing a progressively larger nasal airway trumpet from 24 French to 32 French that is coated/lubricated with lidocaine gel/ointment provides exceptional coverage of the nasocavity in preparing for a nasal intubation. Instillation of liquid lidocaine via the *in situ* nasal trumpet offers an excellent conduit to distribute additional topical anesthetic to the orohypopharynx. It is best performed in the sitting-up position to enhance coverage of the airway structures.

Barbiturates

Sodium thiopental, an ultra-short-acting barbiturate, decreases the level of consciousness and provides amnesia without analgesia after an intubation dose of 4 to 7 mg/kg ideal body weight (IBW) dose over 20 to 50 seconds (administered via a peripheral IV) in the otherwise healthy patient. Its short duration of action (5–10 minutes) makes it ideal for short procedures such as intubation. Thiopental has an excellent cerebral metabolic profile in regards to lowering cerebral metabolic rate while maintaining cerebral blood flow as long as systemic blood pressure is maintained within an adequate range. However, thiopental may lead to hypotension in critically ill patients due to its vasodilatation properties, especially in the face of hypovolemia (34). Though inexpensive, its use in the operating room has declined in favor of propofol. Unfortunately, many upcoming personnel do not develop a working knowledge of the barbiturates. In the ICU setting, reducing the dose of thiopental to 1 to 2 mg/kg IBW is very useful for preparing the patient for tracheal intubation with or without a muscle relaxant.

Narcotics

Narcotics such as morphine, hydromorphone, fentanyl, and remifentanil reduce pain perception and allay anxiety, making intubation less stressful. In addition, they have some sedative effect, suppress cough, and relieve dyspnea (35,36). Fentanyl and the ultra-short-acting remifentanil have a more rapid onset and shorter duration of action than the conventional narcotics used in the ICU setting for analgesia (37–39). Morphine may lead to histamine release and its potential sequelae. Though all narcotics cause respiratory depression, the newer synthetic narcotics may lead to muscular chest wall rigidity that may hamper ventilation and may contribute to episodes of bradycardia. Narcotics, titrated to effect, are quite effective in settling the patient undergoing an awake intubation. Their analgesic, antitussive, and antihypertensive qualities are extremely valuable especially in light of the ability to rapidly reverse excessive narcotization.

Benzodiazepines

Benzodiazepines such as lorazepam and midazolam have excellent amnestic and sedative properties (40). Diazepam has seen its use decline markedly due to its less favorable distribution and clearance characteristics. This drug class does not provide analgesia and may be combined with an analgesic agent during intubation, especially if an awake or semiconscious state with maintenance of spontaneous ventilation is the goal. Midazolam largely has replaced diazepam for intubation because of its more rapid onset and shorter duration of action. Lorazepam use for intubation is possible, but it is hampered by a slower pharmacodynamic onset (2–6 minutes) as compared to midazolam. Hypotension may occur in hypovolemic patients, and benzodiazepines potentiate narcotic-induced respiratory depression.

Muscle Relaxants

The clinician may desire or need to administer a muscle relaxant to optimize intubation conditions, but the vast majority of ICU intubations may be accomplished without such agents. There are basically two perspectives regarding the use of muscle relaxants in the critically ill patient:

1. The administration of a sedative-hypnotic agent with a rapid-acting muscle relaxant, typically succinylcholine, as the standard technique for tracheal intubation is often cited as improving intubation conditions and leading to fewer complications (41). Though this recommendation has much merit, the ubiquitous acceptance of this approach has fallen into the hands of practitioners who frequently do not fully contemplate the patient's risk for airway management difficulties and may not have access or a good working knowledge of airway rescue devices to bail them out if conventional laryngoscopy techniques fail (42–46). Many who use this approach may do so regardless of their patient assessment. This is akin to a "shoot first, ask questions later" approach. One may expect outcomes with this approach akin to those noted when it is used in social situations.
2. The alternative approach is to assess the patient's airway-related risk factors, the patent's potential needs, and the patient's ability to tolerate methods of preparation (e.g., topical, light sedation, and then proceed with induction) followed by customization of the preparation of the patient rather than a "one size fits all" mentality. Though the decision for their use is the clinician's to make, one must be a patient advocate since he or she rarely ever has any say in the matter. It is our opinion that any clinician who administers drugs such as induction agents, including paralytics, thus rendering the patient entirely dependent on the airway management team, must have developed a rescue strategy coupled with the equipment to deploy such a strategy (43,45,46).

The indications for muscle relaxants include agitation or lack of cooperation not related to inadequate or no sedation, increased muscle tone (seizures, tetanus, and neurologic diseases), avoidance of intracranial hypertension, limiting patient movement (potential cervical spine injury), and the need for shortening the time frame from an awake state with protective reflexes to an asleep state with the goal of rapid tracheal intubation (upper gastrointestinal bleed).

Neuromuscular blocking agents may cause depolarization of the motor end-plate (succinylcholine, a depolarizing agent) or prevent depolarization (nondepolarizer: pancuronium, vecuronium, rocuronium). Succinylcholine has a rapid onset and short duration of effect, making it useful in the critical care setting; however, it may raise serum potassium levels by 0.5 to 1.0 mEq/L. It is contraindicated in bedridden patients and in those with pre-existing hyperkalemia, burns, or recent or long-term neurologic deficits (47–49). Other side effects are elevation of intragastric and intraocular pressures, muscle fasciculation, myalgia, malignant hyperthermia, cardiac bradyarrhythmias, and myoglobinuria. Depending on the initial dose—our recommendation is 0.25 mg/kg IBW—and systemic conditions, succinylcholine has a relatively short duration of 3 to 10 minutes. However, if airway management difficulties exist, one should never presume the muscle relaxant will wear off in time to "save" the patient and allow spontaneous patient-initiated ventilation. Emergency rescue techniques should be deployed as early as possible when conventional intubation methods prove unsuccessful.

Nondepolarizing muscle relaxants have a longer time to onset and duration of action as compared to succinylcholine. Rocuronium (typical operating room dose, 0.6 mg/kg) can approach succinylcholine in rapid time of onset if dosed accordingly (1.2 mg/kg), but the increased dosage requirements to meet this objective come with some cost: extended duration of drug action and increased cost.

One controversy to consider when faced with a known or suspected difficult airway: If the practitioner is contemplating the use of a muscle relaxant, which agent is most advantageous? Standard dosing of succinylcholine potentially offers the awake option earlier than a nondepolarizing agent, but if it wears off too soon, then a period of poor or marginal ventilation may hamper patient care and require a transition to a rescue option. Conversely, a short-acting nondepolarizer offers good transition to a rescue plan if mask ventilation is adequate, but does not allow an early-awaken option (46).

Ketamine

Ketamine, a phencyclidine derivative, provides profound analgesia, amnesia, and dissociative anesthesia (50,51). The patient may appear awake but is uncommunicative. Airway reflexes are often, but not always, preserved. Ketamine has a rapid onset and relatively short duration of action. Its profile is unique: it is a myocardial depressant, but this is often countered by its sympathomimetic properties, thus leading to hypertension and tachycardia in many patients. Its use in the critically ill patient with ongoing activation of his or her sympathetic outflow could lead to profound hemodynamic instability since the underlying myocardial depression may not be successfully countered. Though it offers favorable bronchodilatory properties, it promotes bronchorrhea, salivation, and a high incidence of dreams, hallucinations, and emergence delirium (50,51).

Propofol

Propofol also is useful during intubation, especially if titrated to the desired effect rather than simply administering a one-time bolus (52–55). After intravenous administration via a peripheral IV (1–3 mg/kg IBW), unconsciousness occurs within 30 to 60 seconds. Awakening is observed in 4 to 6 minutes with a lower lingering level of sedation compared to other induction agents (52,53,55). Side effects include pain on injection, involuntary muscle movement, coughing, and hiccups. Hypotension, cardiovascular collapse, and, rarely, bradycardia may complicate its use, especially if administered in rapid single-bolus dosing in the critically ill patient with relative or absolute hypovolemia, a systemic capillary leak syndrome, or pre-existing vasodilatation (e.g., sepsis, systemic inflammatory response syndrome [SIRS]). It, however, is an excellent agent that may be titrated to a desired effect while maintaining spontaneous ventilation.

Etomidate

Etomidate is considered by many to be the preferred induction agent in the critically ill patient due to its favorable hemodynamic profile, as compared to the other available induction agents. The hemodynamic stabilization offered by etomidate, however, should not be considered a panacea since it too may lead to hemodynamic deterioration (56,57). Currently, its role as a single-dose induction agent is in question due to its transient depression of the adrenal axis. Once regarded as a minor concern, this adrenal suppression may be much more influential in the outcome of the critically ill. Some have expressed caution with etomidate's use as a single-dose induction agent, especially in the septic or trauma populations. A variety of opinions exist, ranging from an opinion that etomidate should be avoided completely, to its avoidance in select populations such as the septic population, to its use—if at all—with empiric steroid replacement therapy for at least 24 hours (58–60). Perhaps well-designed clinical trials should be performed to determine the relevance of these published precautions. Until more information is available, the practitioner who chooses to use etomidate would be wise and prudent to consider communicating with the ICU care team so they are aware of its use and may act accordingly if hemodynamic instability occurs within 24 hours of administration.

Dexmedetomidine

Dexmedetomidine is an ultra-short-acting α_2 agonist that, when administered intravenously, provides analgesia and mild to moderate sedation with relatively minimal respiratory depression while affording tolerance of "awake" fiberoptic and conventional tracheal intubation (61,62). While a most useful drug, its cost prevents its use in many centers.

EQUIPMENT FOR ACCESSING THE AIRWAY

Esophageal Tracheal Combitube

The esophagotracheal airway (Combitube, ETC) (Fig. 38.6), recommended by the American Heart Association (AHA) Advanced Cardiovascular Life Support (ACLS) course and other national guidelines (30,63,64), is an advanced variant of the

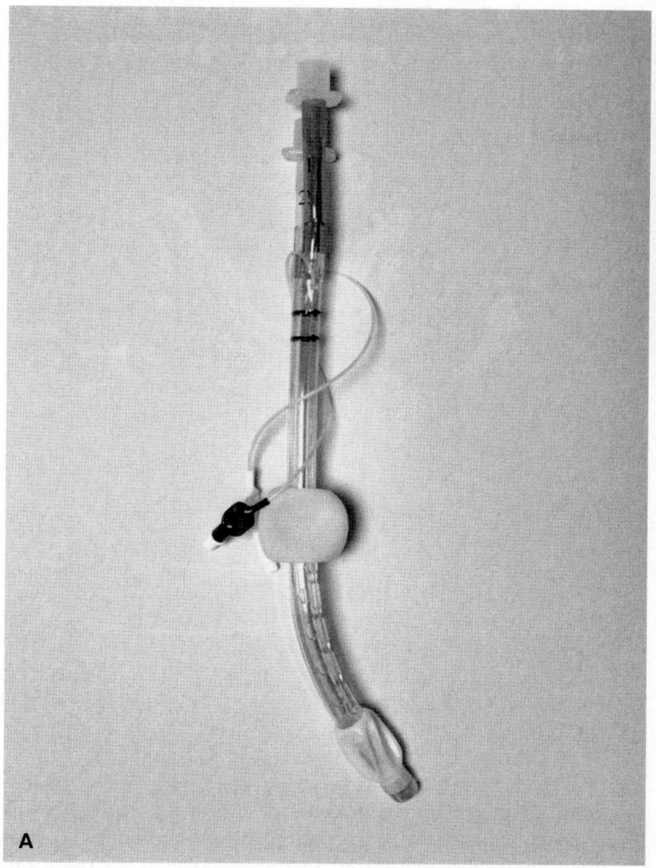

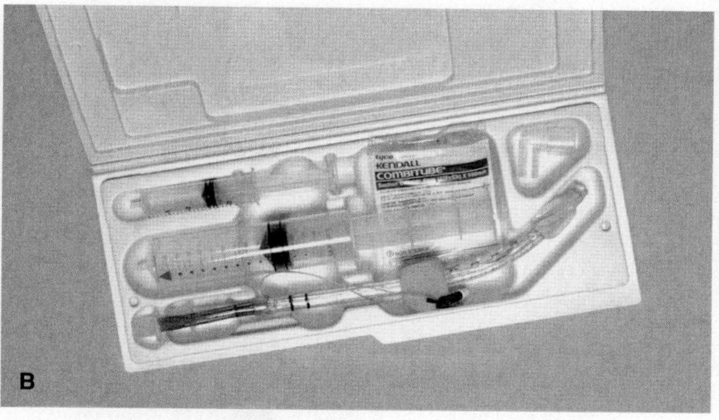

FIGURE 38.6. The esophagotracheal double-lumen airway, the Combitube.

older esophageal obturator airway and the pharyngeal tracheal lumen airway (PTLA). The double lumens with proximal and distal cuffs allow ventilation and oxygenation in a majority of nonawake patients whether placed in the esophagus (95% of all insertions) or the trachea (65,66). Its proximal cuff is placed between the base of the tongue and the hard palate and the distal cuff within the trachea or upper esophagus (67,68). The ETC is inserted blindly, assisted by a jaw thrust or laryngoscopic assistance. Its role in emergency airway management is well recognized and though less popular than the laryngeal mask airway (LMA) or fiberoptic bronchoscope, it may serve a vital role in offering airway rescue when laryngoscopy, bougie insertion, or LMA-assisted ventilation/intubation fails (69). A recent latex-free modification of the Combitube, the Easytuber (Teleflex Ruesch; www.teleflexmedical.com) has a shorter and thinner pharyngeal section, which allows the passage of a fiberscope via an opening of the pharyngeal lumen to inspect the trachea while ventilating.

Tracheal Intubation

When the decision has been made to provide mechanical ventilatory support or airway control, the second question to answer is the route of tracheal intubation: oral versus nasal (unless a surgical airway is clinically indicated). Most commonly, orotracheal intubation is the preferred procedure to establish an airway because it usually can be performed more rapidly, offers a direct view of the glottis, has fewer bleeding complications, avoids nasal necrosis and sinus infection, and allows a larger tracheal tube to be placed as compared to the nasal approach. Finally, the blind nasal approach is particularly benefited by spontaneous ventilation. Airway vigilance should be a goal of the critical care practitioner; thus, conventional and advanced airway rescue equipment must be immediately available during any attempts at airway management. Before attempting to intubate, all anticipated equipment and drugs must be prepared. This may best be provided by an organized "intubation box" containing conventional intubation equipment, with a selection of lubricants, local/topical anesthetics, intravenous induction agents, and medications to assist in treating peri-intubation hemodynamic alterations (heart rate, blood pressure). The box should have a visible lock with hand-breakable deterrent devices to reduce the problem of "missing" equipment. The wide spectrum of patient preparation for tracheal intubation ranges from an unconscious and paralyzed patient, to preparation with mild to moderate dosing of sedatives and analgesics, to the other extreme of topical anesthetics or no medication at all.

Critically ill patients often require only a fraction of the drug doses provided to their elective operating room counterparts. Careful intravenous titration may attenuate hemodynamic alterations, loss of consciousness, apnea, and aspiration. Controversy lies in whether or not to preserve spontaneous ventilation: In essence, should one administer pharmacologic paralyzing agents to the critically ill patient, thus placing the patient in a state in which the practitioner is solely responsible for ventilation, oxygenation, and tracheal intubation? Advocates for paralysis, the majority of which practice in the emergency department locale, cite a low rate of complications and

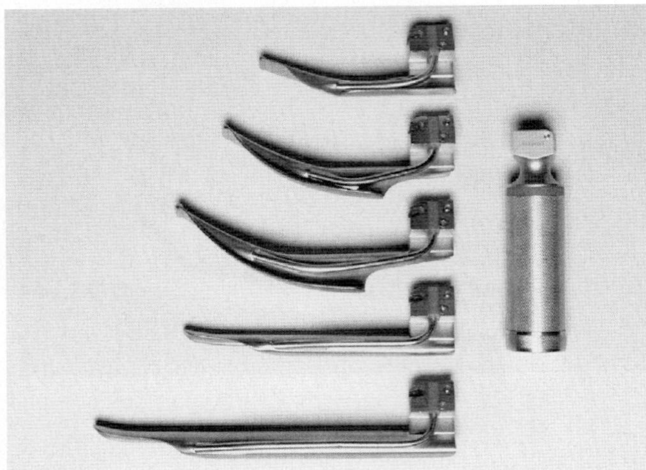

FIGURE 38.7. Examples of fiberoptic laryngoscope handle and blades, in which the bulb is in the handle and the light is transmitted through fiberoptic bundles.

ease of intubation. Conversely, critical care databases suggest that emergency tracheal intubation is far from "safe" and devoid of complications whether or not paralyzing agents are administered (41,43–45,70). From a patient advocate standpoint, any practitioner who ablates the patient's ability to spontaneously ventilate via neuromuscular blocking agents must be properly trained and experienced in basic and advanced airway management so that the depth of his or her ability to provide airway control lies well beyond simply conventional laryngoscopy and intubation (45).

Equipment

Laryngoscopes. A laryngoscope (Fig. 38.7) (fiberoptic vs. conventional) is used to expose the glottis to facilitate passage of the tracheal tube. Unfortunately, proper skill and experience using this standard airway management technique varies widely among critical care practitioners. The utility of the laryngoscope under elective circumstances, with otherwise healthy surgical patients, is essentially limited to individuals with a grade I or II view that can be easily intubated (22). Though a difficult view is mentioned by many as being uncommon (22), Kaplan et al. (71) documented a 14% incidence of grade III or IV views despite optimizing maneuvers such as the optimal external laryngeal manipulation (OELM) and the backward upward right pressure (BURP) technique (Fig. 38.8). This is further complicated, as up to 33% of critically ill patients have a limited view with laryngoscopy (epiglottis only or no view at all) (44,45,72). This is why the critical care practitioner responsible for airway management must be prepared to embark on a Plan B or Plan C immediately if conventional direct laryngoscopy fails to offer a reasonable glottic view that allows timely and accurate intubation.

Blades. Laryngoscope blades are of two principal kinds, curved and straight, varying in size for use in infants, children, or adults (Fig. 38.9). Many varieties of both the curved and straight blades have been redesigned in the hopes of augmenting visualization to facilitate passage of an endotracheal tube. Innovations to improve laryngeal exposure include a hinged blade tip to augment epiglottic lifting during laryngoscopy (73),

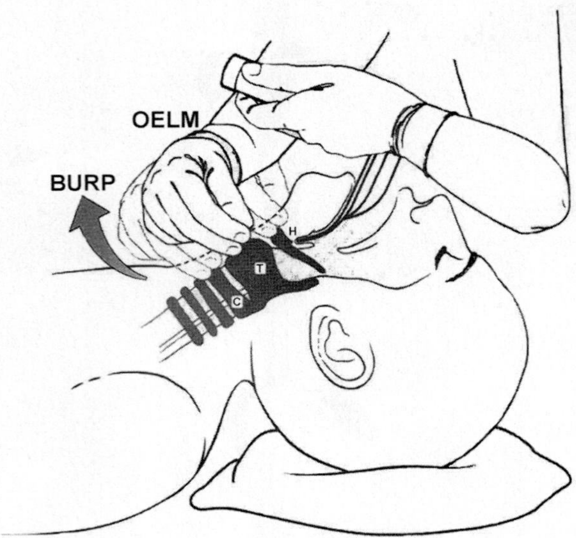

FIGURE 38.8. Diagrammatic representation of the optimal external laryngeal movement (OELM) and backward upward rightward pressure (BURP) maneuvers for optimal visualization of the glottis.

rigid fiberscopes, and video-assisted laryngoscopy (74–80). These innovations may, depending on the individual patient airway characteristics, offer an improved view of the glottis to improve the first-pass success rate, reduce intubation attempts, potentially reduce the time to intubation in the difficult airway, and potentially result in a reduction in esophageal intubation and other airway-related complications that are relatively commonplace with standard techniques. The future lies with visualizing "around the corner" in the hopes of improving patient airway safety (74–80).

Endotracheal Tubes. Most endotracheal tubes (ETs) are disposable and are made of clear, pliable polyvinylchloride, with

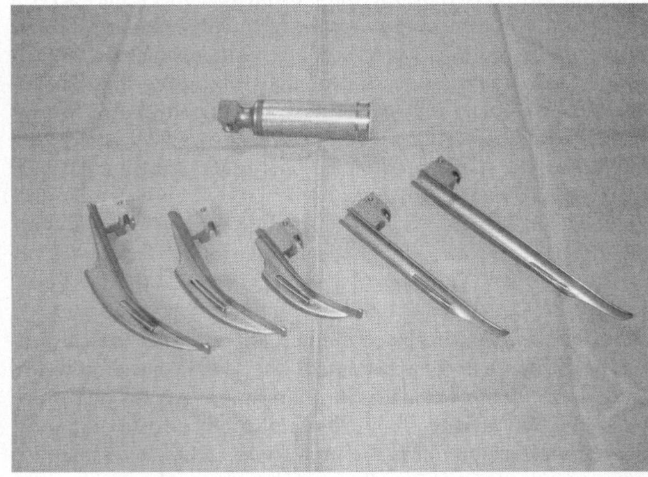

FIGURE 38.9. Various types of laryngoscope blades in common use.

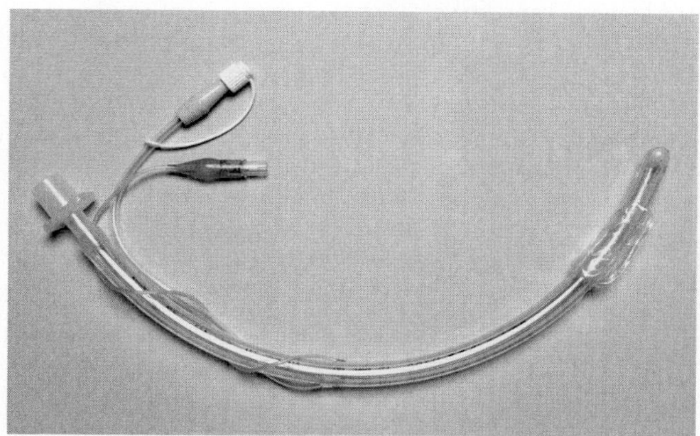

FIGURE 38.10. The Malinkrodt Hi-Lo Evacuation tube. While it comes in various sizes, it is not optimal for all patients. There is level 1 evidence that, with proper use, it decreases risk of ventilator-associated pneumonia. (From American Thoracic Society. Guidelines for the management of adults with hospital-acquired, ventilator-associated and healthcare-associated pneumonia. *Am J Respir Crit Care Med.* 2005;171:388–416.)

little tendency to kink until they attain body temperature. Though the ETs mold to the contour of the upper airway and present a smooth interior, affording easy passage of suction catheters or a flexible bronchoscope, they may become encrusted with secretions, biofilm, and concretions that may decrease luminal patency and endanger patient care.

In adults, all commonly used ETs are of the cuffed variety, and many now used are types that allow suctioning of subglottic secretions—the Hi-Lo Evacuation ET (Fig. 38.10). The ET cuff ensures a closed system, permitting control of ventilation and reducing the possibility of silent or active aspiration of oronasal secretions, vomitus, or blood, although microaspiration is well recognized. Commonly, ET cuffs are the high volume–low pressure models that offer a broad contact with the tracheal wall and potentially limit ischemic damage to the mucosa. The tube size used depends upon the size of the patient (Table 38.3).

TABLE 38.3

RECOMMENDED SIZES FOR ENDOTRACHEAL TUBES

Patient age	Internal diameter of tube (mm)[a]
Newborn	3.0
6 mo	3.5
18 mo	4.0
3 y	4.5
5 y	5.0
6 y	5.5
8 y	6.0
12 y	6.5
16 y	7.0
Adult female	7.0–7.5
Adult male	8.0–9.0

[a] One size larger and one size smaller should be allowed for individual intra-age variations and shorter-stature individuals. Where possible, the subglottic suction endotracheal tube should be used.

The primary reasons for tracheal intubation will vary from patient to patient and by practitioner, related to not only the patient's pathophysiology, but also the physician's judgment and experience in caring for the critically ill. The main goals of tracheal intubation include protecting the airway from contamination, providing positive-pressure ventilation, providing a patent airway, and permitting access to the tracheobronchial tree for suctioning, instillation of medications, or diagnostic/therapeutic bronchoscopy. While the vast majority of tracheal intubations are via the oral route, the choice between the oral and the nasal—or the transcricoid/transtracheal route—will again be primarily determined by the patient's physical and airway conditions, the expected duration of mechanical support, and the judgment and skills of the practitioner.

Malleable Stylet. A well-lubricated malleable stylet (Fig. 38.11) is preferred by many to preform the ET into a shape that may expedite passing through the glottis. The stylet should be viewed as a guide, not a "spear," and its tip should be safely inside the ET, never distal to the ET tip (81,82). It should not be used to force the ET into the airway or ram its way through the vocal cords when they are closed or otherwise inaccessible. Also, the popular "hockey stick"–shaped tip used by many is useful, yet its angle must be appreciated by the operator. The angle often will impede advancement into the airway since the ET tip may impinge on the anterior tracheal wall and the sharp angulations of the stylet may impede its own removal from the ET (81–83). Ideally, the styleted ET tip should be placed at the entrance of the glottis, and then, with stylet removal, the ET will advance into the trachea less traumatically. Unfortunately, many practitioners unknowingly advance the styleted ET deep into the trachea without appreciating the potential damage the stylet-stiffened ET tip may cause to the tracheal wall.

HOW MIGHT THE AIRWAY BE ACCESSED?

General Indications and Contraindications

The oral approach is the standard method for tracheal intubation today. The indications are numerous and it may be best to focus on the contraindications. The oral route would not be a reasonable choice when there is limited access to the oral cavity due to trauma, edema, or anatomic difficulties. These contraindications for the oral route would presume that the nasal approach is feasible from both the patient's and clinician's standpoint. If not, a surgical approach via the cricothyroid membrane or a formal tracheostomy would be clinically indicated. Though nasal intubations were a mainstay in earlier decades, the oral approach has displaced it due to the popularity of the "rapid sequence intubation" and the better appreciation of the potential detriments of long-term nasal intubation.

Orotracheal Intubation

The airway care team members should expediently prepare both the patient and the equipment for the airway management procedure. While bag ventilation (preoxygenation) is being provided, obtaining appropriate towels for optimizing head

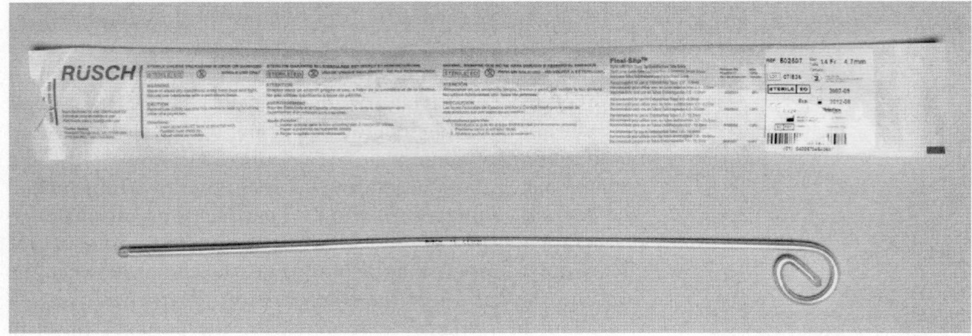

FIGURE 38.11. Malleable stylet for use with insertion of an endotracheal tube.

and neck position or blankets for ramping the obese patient and adjusting the bed height and angulation should be carried out (Fig. 38.12, left panel); how *not* to position is noted in the right panel of Figure 38.12. Assembling the necessary equipment, such as the ET, syringes, suction equipment, lubricant, CO_2 detector, and a stylet if desired, should be quickly carried out for the primary airway manager. During this time, a rapid medical-surgical history is obtained, the review of previous intubation procedures sought, and an airway examination completed (30,42). Intravenous access is ensured and a primary plan for induction developed. Access to airway rescue devices should be addressed and, of course, it is best if they are at the bedside. Clear communication among team members is imperative as well as discussion of the plan with the patient, if appropriate. Chaos is to be avoided and, in this context, the individual managing the procedure must insist that unnecessary talking and agitation be limited.

A tube of appropriate diameter and length should be selected and, though gender is an important factor in size selection, patient height is equally important as there is a linear relationship between the latter and glottic size. Typically, the choice in a woman would be a 7.0 to 8.0 mm ET, and in males an 8 to 9 mm ET would be used. Nonetheless, smaller-diameter ETs should be readily available for any eventuality. A team member should examine the ET for patency and cuff integrity. The 15-mm proximal adapter should fit snugly and the ET kept in its sterile wrapper and not handled until insertion. It may be placed in warm water to soften the PVC tubing, which may assist with passing the ET over a stylet, a tracheal introducing catheter (bougie), or a fiberscope, or during an ET exchange.

Based on the patient history and physical examination, combined with the practitioner's judgment, past experience, available equipment, and the needs of the patient, a determination is made as to what induction method is best. Patient preparation for tracheal intubation may range from little to no medication to the other extreme of unconsciousness with muscle relaxation (41,84,85). Considering the earlier discussion involving airway risk assessment, the practitioner will need to determine if preservation of spontaneous ventilation is in the patient's best interest, as well as the depths of amnesia, hypnosis, and analgesia the patient may require so that airway manipulation is tolerated (30,63,64). Titration of a sedative-hypnotic or analgesic to render the patient tolerant of airway manipulation is often based on the practitioner's knowledge and experience of the available induction agents, combined with the perceived needs of the patient plus the predicted tolerance of their administration. The pharmacodynamic effects following administration via an IV site will depend on the IV location (central vs. peripheral, hand vs. antecubital fossa), vein patency, catheter diameter and length, IV flow rate, and the patient's cardiac output.

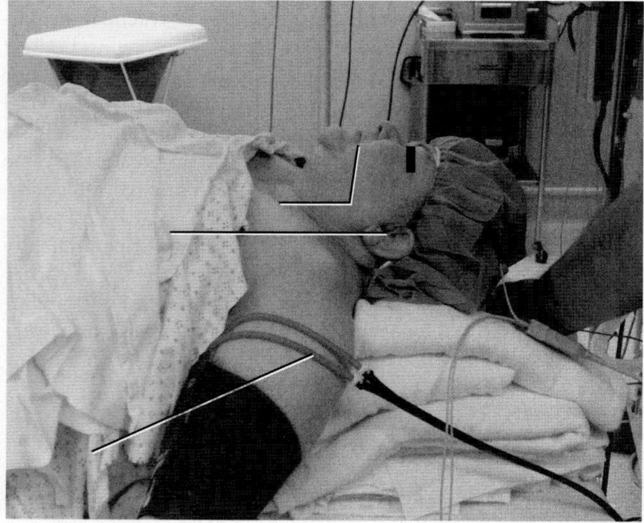

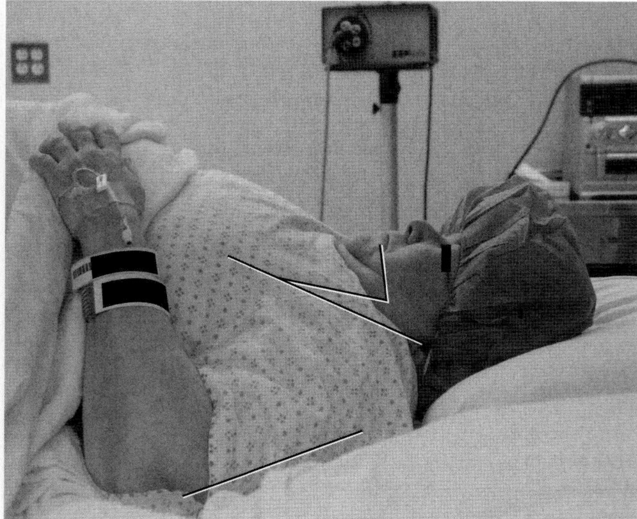

FIGURE 38.12. Ramping of an obese patient's torso to improve glottic visualization is noted on the left panel. The right panel shows the patient position *without* proper ramping.

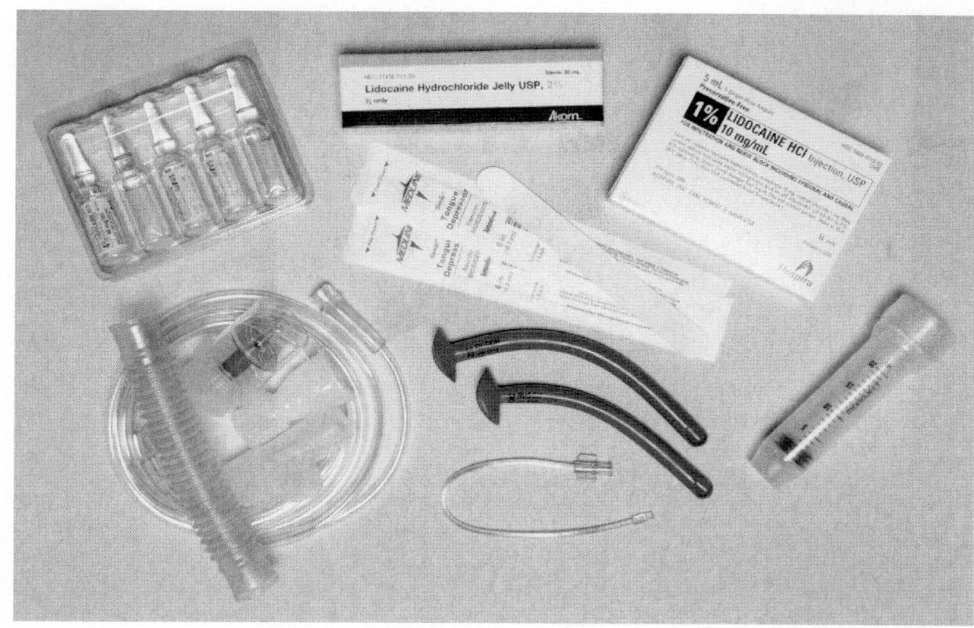

FIGURE 38.13. Equipment used to topicalize the airway prior to instrumentation: Tongue blade with lidocaine jelly, nebulizer with 4% lidocaine, and nasal dilators of various sizes.

Central IV access may speed administration and time to onset plus potentially deliver a more concentrated medication bolus as compared to an equal dose administered through an IV on the dorsum of the hand.

The practitioner has several choices for patient preparation: (a) awake with no medication; (b) awake with topical anesthesia or local nerve blocks, and with or without light sedation; (c) sedation/analgesia only with the option of neuromuscular blocker use; and (d) a set induction regimen for a rapid sequence intubation (e.g., etomidate and succinylcholine) (41,77,84,85). Faced with a variety of preparation choices and a wide breadth of patient circumstances, the critical care physician will need to decide what approach to pursue based on the medical, surgical, and airway situation; the patient's needs and level of tolerance, balanced by the practitioner's judgment; and access to and experience with airway equipment (41,44,45,84,85).

Awake Intubation

Awake intubation techniques comprise both nasal and oral routes and, most often, involve topically applied local anesthetics (Fig. 38.13) or local nerve blocks. Conversely, if the patient's mental status and response to oropharyngeal stimulation are depressed, no medication may be needed to accomplish intubation. The application of topical anesthesia and a local nerve block requires more time and effort, expanded access to such agents and equipment, more patience, and finesse combined with a broader familiarity of head and neck anatomy (24,86). If done properly, the patient's airway may be managed with nearly all conventional and accessory devices with the exception of the Combitube. Practitioners may prefer to maintain spontaneous ventilation during emergency airway management by avoiding excessive sedative-hypnotic agents and/or muscle relaxants (87). Light sedation and analgesics, however, are typically administered despite the label of being "awake." Awake intubation techniques have been largely supplanted by induction of unconsciousness or deep sedation with or without muscle relaxation (87,88). Though the "awake intubation" is an extremely useful approach, its reduced utilization means that practitioners and their students will be less comfortable with this method through lack of experience and confidence. Its subsequent use by less experienced practitioners may complicate patient care due to poorly administered topical anesthesia, ineffective local nerve block techniques, and the lack of judicious and creative sedative/analgesic measures.

Awake intubation may benefit from the addition of a narcotic agent by providing analgesia, antitussive action, and better hemodynamic control. Many reserve an awake approach for the known or suspected difficult airway to avoid "burning any bridges" and for those with severe cardiopulmonary compromise, pre-existing unconsciousness, or marked mental or neurologic depression. However, if the patient is a poor candidate for an awake approach, or preparation for an awake approach is suboptimal, patient injury and difficult management may still ensue since an awake approach does not guarantee successful intubation nor is it devoid of morbidity or mortality (89–91).

Following proper preparation, unless the patient is unconscious or has markedly depressed mental status, the "awake look" technique incorporates conventional laryngoscopy to evaluate the patient's airway to gauge the feasibility and ease of intubation (46); explanation to the patient (if applicable) is imperative for cooperation. If viewing the airway structures during an "awake look" proves fruitful, intubation should be performed during the same laryngoscopic attempt either directly—grade I or II view—or by bougie assistance—grade I, II, or III—or by other means (92,93). Many "awake look" procedures that yield a reasonable view, but in which intubation is not performed, are followed by anesthetic induction with the potential for a worse view due to airway tissue collapse and obstruction by redundant tissue due to loss of pharyngeal tone. Too often, patient comfort is placed well above patient safety. The critically ill patient is often tolerant of bougie-assisted intubation (Fig. 38.14), supraglottic airway placement (e.g., LMA) (Fig. 38.15), or the placement of specialty airway devices such

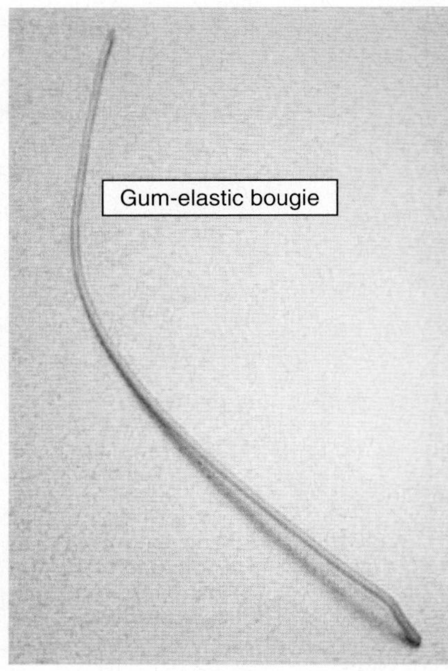

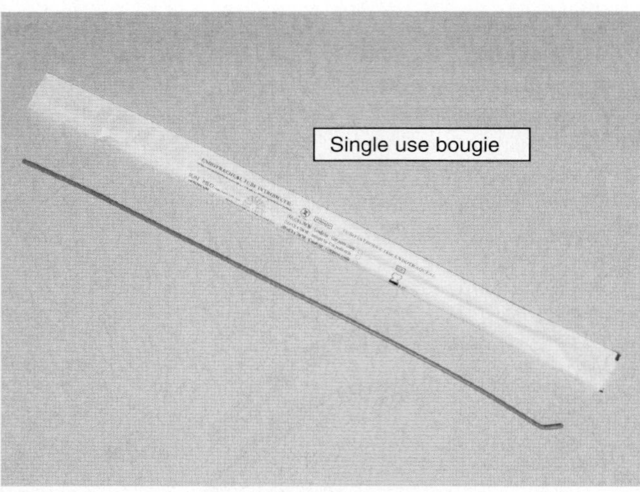

FIGURE 38.14. Array of tracheal "bougies" used to access the airway in difficult situations.

as the rigid fiberscopes following topical anesthetic application, local nerve blocks, or even light sedation (24,93–96).

Sedated to Asleep Techniques

Titration of medication to provide amnesia, analgesia, anxiolysis, sedation, or a combination of these desirable effects with the goal of providing comfort while preserving spontaneous ventilation is possible (44,97). Muscle relaxants may be added as an option if pharmacologic attempts to render the patient accepting of airway manipulation prove suboptimal or unsatisfactory. Sedation and amnesia are mandatory when paralysis is induced (43,44,87,88). The variety of agents available to render the patient accepting of airway manipulation and ultimately tracheal intubation have been outlined previously. Though more physical effort is required when spontaneous ventilation is maintained, allowing continued respiratory efforts may assist the practitioner in navigating the ET successfully into the trachea by the appreciation of audible breaths via the ET, coughing after intubation, ventilation bag expansion/contraction, vocalization with esophageal intubation, following the pathway of bubbles percolating around the otherwise hidden glottis, or the "up and down" movement of secretions that may offer direction in the difficult-to-visualize airway (43,44,76,87,88). Breath-holding, glottic closure, laryngospasm, swallowing, biting, jaw clenching, and gagging may contribute adversely to the intubation process, but most of these are overcome with patience and the acceptance that these are "signs of life." In difficult situations, titration techniques that provide sedation/analgesia offer the opportunity to abort such "signs of life" with the hope of returning the patient to his or her previous state at a later time (30,63,64). The "awake" approach is accomplished by the application of topical local anesthetics and/or local nerve blocks or simply proceeding without medication based on the concurrent suppression of mental status and gag reflexes.

Rapid Sequence Intubation

Rapid sequence intubation (RSI) refers to the administration of an induction agent followed by a neuromuscular blocking agent, with the goal of hastening the time needed to induce unconsciousness and muscle paralysis based on a concern for aspiration of orogastric secretions. By minimizing the

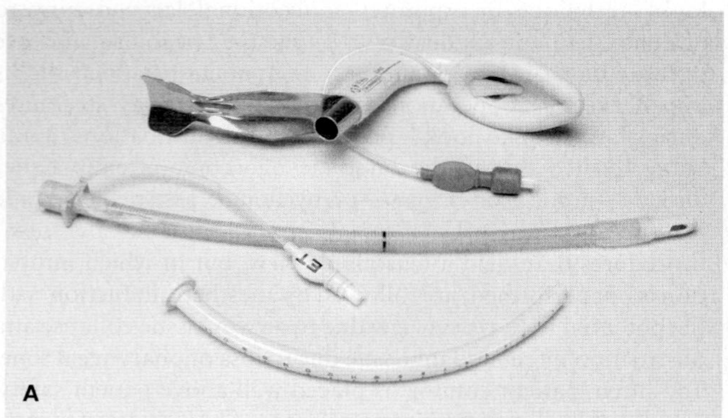

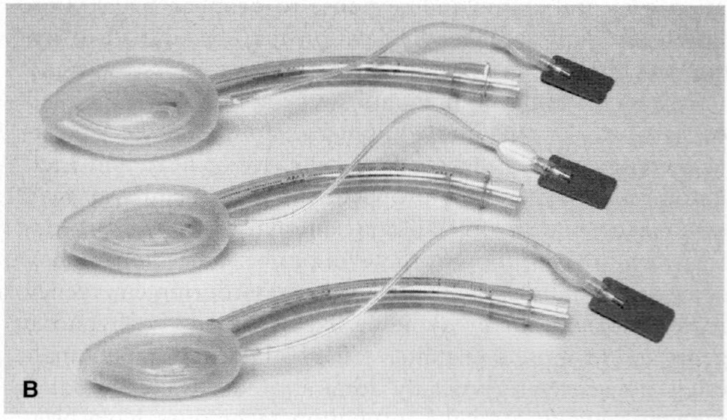

FIGURE 38.15. Laryngeal mask airways for emergent/difficult intubation. **A:** The intubating laryngeal mask airway (LMA). **B:** Various sized LMAs for patients of different sizes and ages.

time the airway is unprotected, the risk of aspiration theoretically should be reduced. Preoxygenation is paramount since oxygenation/ventilation efforts via a bag-mask during the induction process are not typically carried out, thus hypothetically avoiding esophagogastric insufflation (41,98,99). Cricoid pressure is applied, in theory, to reduce the risk of passive regurgitation of any stomach contents (29). These practices during an RSI may not always be practical nor able to be carried out, since patients do desaturate during the apneic phase of the RSI, particularly in obesity, pregnancy, poor or suboptimal preoxygenation efforts or the presence of cardiopulmonary pathology.

If needed, bag-mask support should be delivered despite the concern about esophagogastric insufflation and subsequent regurgitation/aspiration. Additionally, the application of cricoid pressure—both quantitative and qualitative—is so variable that concerns with its ubiquitous use and overall effectiveness have been raised (100–104). Cricoid pressure may actually improve or worsen the laryngoscopic view, plus impede mask ventilation; hence, adjustment or release of cricoid pressure should be considered in these circumstances. Further, cricoid pressure may alter the ability to place accessory devices, such as the LMA, and impede fiberoptic viewing (105–108). Despite these potential limitations of cricoid pressure, no desaturating patient—high risk for aspiration or not—should have bag-mask ventilation support withheld because of the fear of aspiration.

When performing an RSI or, for that matter, any induction method involving a neuromuscular blocking agent, an understanding of ventilation, and intubation options in the event conventional methods fail, and a preplanned strategy to assist the patient must be in place *prior* to induction. The development of such strategies during a crisis is difficult, often short-sighted and incomplete, and may be counterproductive and destructive to patient care. Education, training, and immediate access to airway rescue equipment that the practitioner can competently incorporate in an airway crisis is a goal worthy of expanded effort, time, and finances (30,41,43,45,46,63,64).

The proponents of rapidly controlling the airway using RSI cite a reduction in the risk of aspiration as a main thrust for this technique. Moreover, an RSI is said to be associated with a lower incidence of complications and higher first-pass intubation success rate as compared to the "sedation only" method (41,43,98,99). A predetermined induction regimen, such as etomidate and succinylcholine, is popular, easy to teach and replicate, easy to administer (e.g., 0.25 mg/kg IBW etomidate and 0.25 mg/kg IBW of succinylcholine), requires little planning or forethought, can be standardized, and, most importantly, generally works well for most critically ill patients. Though the standard dosing regimen of succinylcholine is 1 to 1.5 mg/kg, the authors find that a variety of doses may fit the needs of the operator. One should consider that the higher the dose administered, the longer the duration to recover (patient-initiated spontaneous ventilation).

Nevertheless, it appears that this approach is so commonly practiced by some individuals that it becomes the chosen induction regimen, with little regard for the patient's individual clinical condition and airway status. Several authors tout near-perfect success rates with RSI coupled with a minimum number of complications (41,43,98,99). This "slam-dunk" approach may not be the best for a significant number of the critically ill patients, namely the obese, the known or suspected difficult airway patient, the hemodynamically unstable patient, or those with significant cardiopulmonary compromise, such as pulmonary embolism, cardiac tamponade, and/or myocardial ischemia. Though there is little argument that many intubations may be made easier by the administration of a muscle relaxant, selective use based on the patient evaluation and clinical circumstances is the best option (30,44–46,63,64,70,72,87,88).

Positioning the Patient

One of the most important factors in improving the success rate of orotracheal intubation is positioning the patient properly (Fig. 38.3). Classically, the sniffing position, namely cervical flexion combined with atlanto-occipital extension, will assist in improving the line of sight of the intubator. Bringing the three axes into alignment (oral, pharyngeal, and laryngeal) is commonly optimized by placing a firm towel or pillow beneath the head (providing mild cervical flexion) combined with physical backward movement of the head at the atlanto-occipital joint via manual extension. This, when combined with oral laryngoscopy, will improve the "line of sight" for the intubator to better visualize the laryngeal structures in most patients (46). Optimizing bed position is imperative, as is the angle at which the patient lies on the bed. The variety of mattress material (air, water, foam, gel) provides a challenge to the practitioner since these mattresses may worsen positioning characteristics in an emergency setting. Optimizing the position of the obese (Fig. 38.12, left panel) patient is an absolute requirement to assist with (a) spontaneous ventilation and mask ventilation; (b) opening the mouth; (c) gaining access to the neck for cricoid application, manipulation of laryngeal structures, or invasive procedures; (d) improving the "line of sight" with laryngoscopy; and (e) prolonging oxygen saturation after induction (109–113). A ramp is constructed with blankets, a preformed wedge, or angulation of the mechanical bed to bring the ear and the sternal notch into alignment by ramping the patient's head, shoulders, and upper torso, thus facilitating spontaneous ventilation, mask ventilation, and laryngoscopy. The extra time spent to properly position the patient will reap great benefits (77,110,113).

Blade Use

The Curved Blade. Following opening of the mouth, either by the extraoral technique (finger pressing downward on chin) or the intraoral method (the finger scissor technique to spread the dentition), the laryngoscope blade is introduced at the right side of the mouth and advanced to the midline, displacing the tongue to the left. The epiglottis is seen at the base of the tongue and the tip of the blade inserted into the vallecula. If the oropharynx is dry, lubricating the blade is helpful; otherwise, suctioning out excessive secretions may assist greatly in visualizing airway structures. The laryngoscope blade should be lifted toward an imaginary point in the corner of the wall opposite the patient to avoid using the upper teeth as a fulcrum for the laryngoscope blade. Moreover, a forward and upward lift of the laryngoscope and blade stretches the hyoepiglottic ligament, thus folding the epiglottis upward and further exposing the glottis. As a result, the larynx is suspended on the tip of the blade by the hyoid bone. The practitioner's right hand, prior to picking up the ET, should be used to apply external pressure on the laryngeal cartilage (thyroid cartilage) to potentially afford better visualization of the glottis. OELM (Fig. 38.8), as this maneuver is called, is optimized and turned over to an assistant who attempts to replicate the optimal position for the operator's viewing. This description, while obviously optimal, is not always feasible.

With visualization of the glottic structures, the ET is passed to the right of the laryngoscope through the glottis into the trachea until the cuff passes 2 to 3 cm beyond the vocal cords. As described earlier, a Lehane-Cormack grade II or III airway may preclude easy placement of the tracheal tube. Thus, a blind guide underneath the epiglottis (tracheal tube introducer, bougie) or a rigid fiberoptic stylet may be incorporated to improve the insertion success rate.

The Straight Blade. Intubation with a straight blade involves the same maneuvers but with one major difference. The blade is slipped *beneath* the epiglottis, and exposure of the larynx is accomplished by an upward and forward lift at a 45-degree angle toward the corner of the wall opposite the patient. Again, leverage must not be applied against the upper teeth.

With either technique, the common causes of failure to intubate include inadequate position of the head, misplacement of the laryngoscope blade, inadequate muscle relaxation, insufficient depth of sedation/analgesia or general anesthesia, obscuring of the glottis by the tongue, and lack of familiarity with the anatomy, especially where pathologic changes are present. Inserting a laryngoscope blade too deeply, usually past the larynx and into the cricopharyngeal area, results in lifting of the entire larynx. If familiar landmarks are not appreciated, stop advancing the scope, withdraw the blade, and start over. If more than 30 seconds have passed or there is evidence that the oxygen saturation has dropped from the prelaryngoscopy level, bag-mask support to reoxygenate the patient is imperative. There is now evidence that repetitive laryngoscopies are not in the best interest of patient care and may place the patient at extreme risk for potentially life-threatening airway-related complications (44,45). Unless the first one to two laryngoscopy attempts were performed by less experienced members of the team, attempts at conventional laryngoscopy alone to intubate the trachea should be abandoned in favor of incorporating an airway adjunct to assist the clinician in hastening the process of gaining airway control (30,44,45,63,64,114,115).

Nasotracheal Intubation

Nasotracheal intubation, once the mainstay approach in the emergency setting, is still commonly used in oral and maxillofacial operative interventions, but less commonly in emergency situations outside the operating room. Nasotracheal intubation is an alternative to the oral route for patients with trismus, mandibular fracture, a large tongue, or edema of the oral cavity or oropharynx, and is a useful approach for the spontaneously breathing patient who refuses to lie supine or in the presence of excessive secretions. The presence of midfacial or posterior fossa trauma and coagulopathy are absolute contraindications to this technique. Thus, it is best avoided in patients with a basilar skull fracture, a fractured nose, or nasal obstruction. It is also contraindicated in the presence of acute sinusitis or mastoiditis. Additionally, as the nasal portal dictates a smaller-diameter tracheal tube, it must be remembered that as downsizing takes place, the length of the tracheal tube is shortened; hence, the length must be considered when placing a small-caliber tube (e.g., a 6.0-mm diameter in an individual taller than about 69 inches), as the nasal tracheal tube may end up as an elongated nasal trumpet, without entrance into the trachea (116–118).

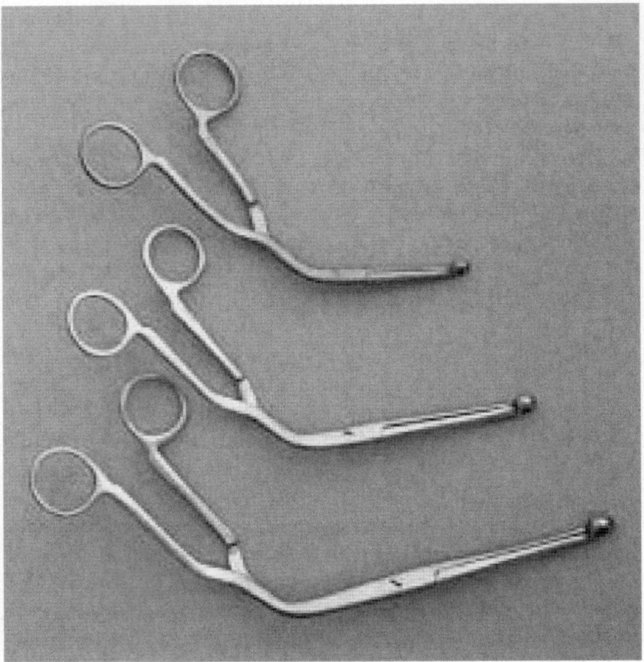

FIGURE 38.16. Magill forceps for manipulating the endotracheal tube into the glottis. These come in several sizes.

The method of intubation via the nasal approach is variable. It may be placed blindly during spontaneous ventilation, combined with oral laryngoscopic assistance to aid with ET advancement utilizing Magill forceps (Fig. 38.16); utilize indirect visualization through the nares via an optical stylet (Fig. 38.17) or a flexible (Fig. 38.18) or rigid fiberscope (Fig. 38.19); or incorporate a lighted stylet (Fig. 38.20) for transillumination of the laryngeal structures (78,119,120).

Technique

The patient may be prepared for the nasal approach by pretreatment of the mucosa of both nostrils with a solution of 0.1% phenylephrine and a decongestant spray such as

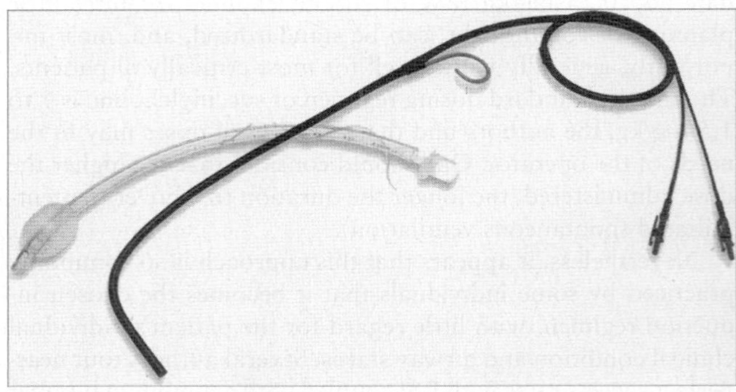

FIGURE 38.17. An optical stylet, allowing visualization of the glottis as the endotracheal tube is advanced.

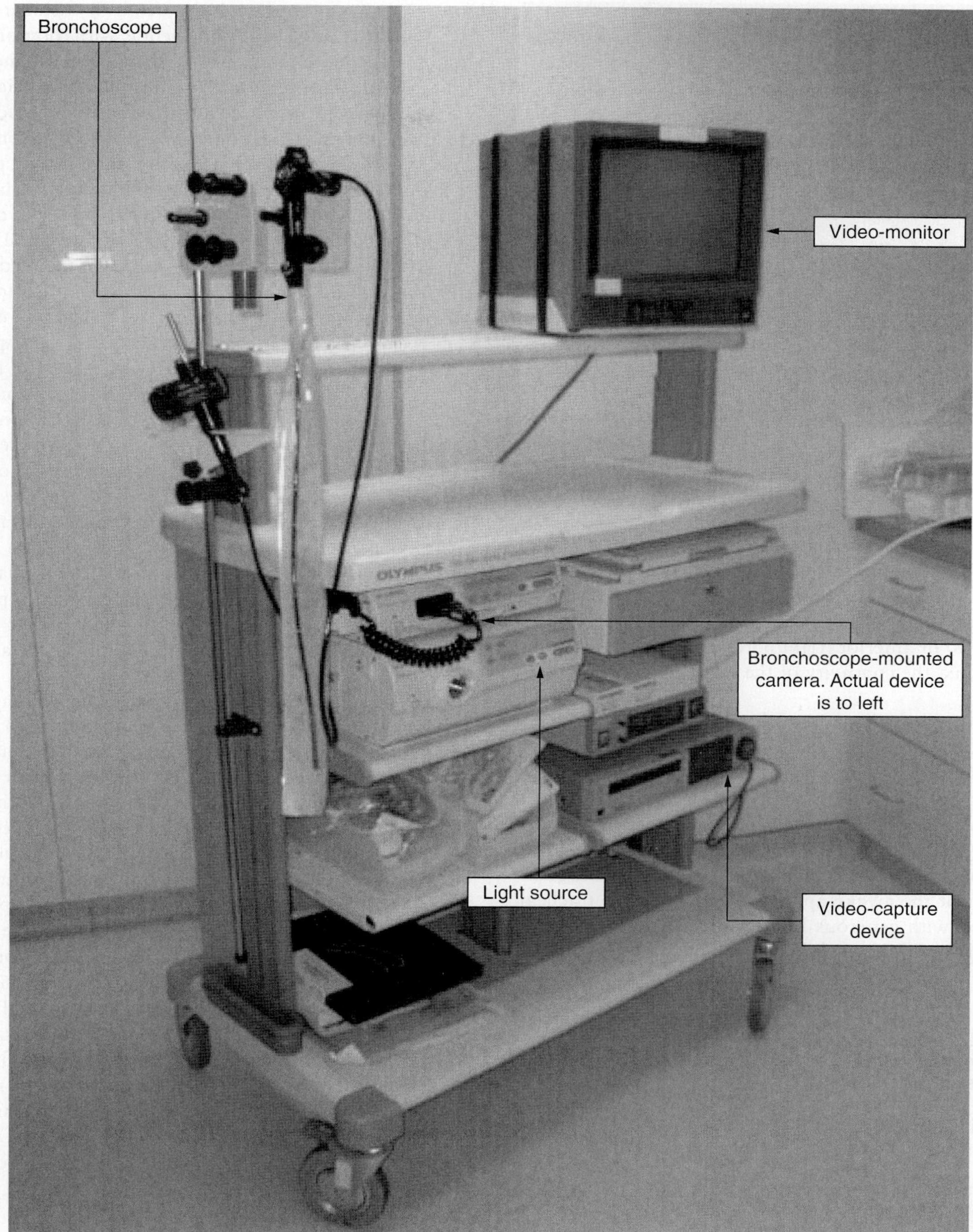

FIGURE 38.18. A fiberoptic bronchoscope with associated cart as used at Shands Hospital at the University of Florida.

oxymetazoline for 3 to 10 minutes. This is followed by progressive dilation, starting with either a 26 French or 28 French nasal trumpet, and progressing to a 30 French to 32 French trumpet lubricated with 2% lidocaine jelly (Fig. 38.13). The method is relatively expedient. Conversely, placement of cotton pledgets soaked in a mixture of vasoconstrictor agent and local anesthetic is equally effective if one is experienced with the nasal anatomy and the proper equipment is available. Supplemental oxygen may be provided by nasal cannulae placed between the lips or via a face mask. The patient is best intubated with spontaneous ventilation maintained, yet incremental sedation/analgesia may be provided to optimize patient comfort and cooperation. Sitting upright has the advantage of maximizing the oropharyngeal diameter (116,121).

Orientation of the tracheal tube bevel is important for patient comfort and to reduce the risk of epistaxis and tearing or

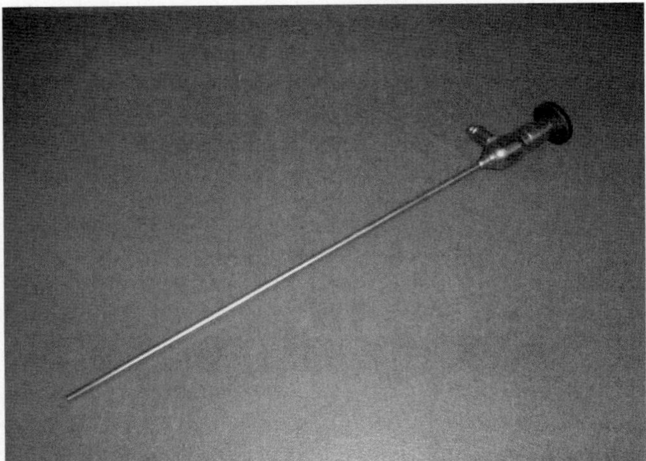

FIGURE 38.19. A rigid bronchoscope.

dislocation of the nasal turbinates. On either side of the nose, the bevel should face the turbinate (away from the septum). Due to bevel orientation, the tracheal tube's manufactured curve (concavity) may be facing posterior "toward the patient's face" (left nares) or anterior (right nares); once the ET reaches the nasopharynx, the concavity of the tube should face posteriorly.

In the ICU setting, this approach may be helpful in those with restricted cervical spine motion, trismus, and oral cavity swelling/obstruction, to name but a few conditions of interest. Awake, sitting upright with spontaneous ventilation is an ideal setting for nasal intubation. The blind approach is best accomplished with ventilation preserved. Topically applied local anesthetics, local nerve blocks, and judicious sedation and analgesia supplement the awake approach. Warming the tracheal tube combined with generous lubrication will assist rotation and advancement while providing a soft and pliable airway to reduce injury to the nasal mucosa or turbinates. Tube advancement should be slow and gentle, with rotation when resistance is encountered. Excessive force, rough maneuvers, poor lubrication, and use of force against an obstruction should be discouraged. If advancement is met with resistance from glottic/anterior tissues, helpful maneuvers to overcome these obstacles include sitting the patient upright, flexing the head forward on the neck, and manually pulling the larynx anteriorly. Conversely, if advancement is met with posterior displacement into the esophagus, sitting the patient upright, extending the head on the neck, and applying posterior-directed pressure on the thyrocricoid complex may assist in intubation. Rotation of the tube and manual depression or elevation of the larynx may be required to succeed. Voluntary or hypercapnic-induced hyperpnea helps if the patient is awake because maximal abduction of the cords is present during inspiration. Entry into the trachea is signified by consistent breath sounds transmitted by the tube and inability to speak if the patient is breathing, as well as by lack of resistance, often accompanied by cough. Often one can then feel the inflation of the tracheal cuff below the larynx and above the manubrium sterni, followed by connecting the tube to the rebreathing system and expanding the lungs (122). Confirmation with end-tidal CO_2 measurement or fiberoptic viewing is imperative. Application of a specially designed airway "whistle" that assists the clinician with spontaneous ventilation intubation may be advantageous (123).

Nasotracheal intubation may also be accomplished with *fiberoptic assistance*. When the blind approach is met with difficulty, the fiberoptic adjunct may expedite intubation, but may be of limited assistance if secretion control is poor or if relied upon as a salvage method following nasal trauma. However, use of a fiberoptic bronchoscope is an excellent choice for the primary nasal approach with the patient sitting upright and the intubator preferentially standing in front or to the side of the patient as opposed to "over the top" (124,125). Advancement of the ET into the glottis may be impeded by hang-up on the laryngeal structures: The vocal cord, the posterior glottis, or, typically, the right arytenoid (126,127). When resistance is met, a helpful tip is as follows: withdrawing the tube 1 to 2 cm, rotate the tube counterclockwise 90 degrees, then readvance with the bevel facing posteriorly (126,127). Matching the tracheal tube to the fiberscope to minimize the gap between the internal diameter of the tube and the scope may also improve advancement (126). Tracheal confirmation and tip positioning are added advantages to fiberoptic-assisted intubation.

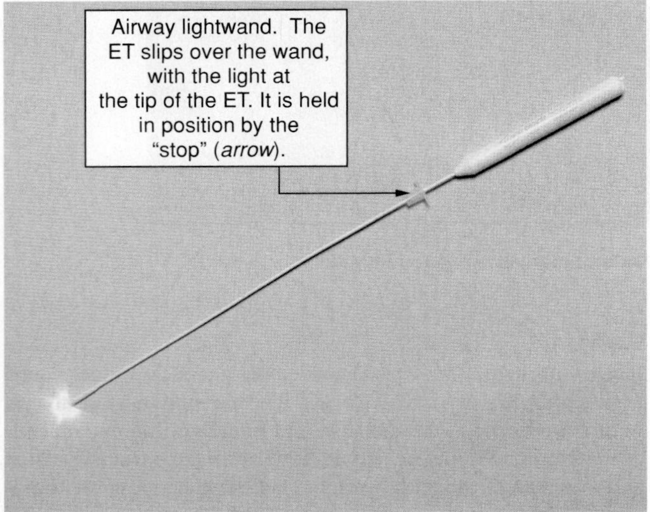

Airway lightwand. The ET slips over the wand, with the light at the tip of the ET. It is held in position by the "stop" (*arrow*).

FIGURE 38.20. A lighted stylet (Lightwand) for blind insertion of an endotracheal tube. Utilization of this technique requires significant practice.

Complications of Nasal Intubation

Though the nasally placed ET has the advantage of overall stability, the nasal approach has decreased in popularity due to a restriction of tube size, the potential to add epistaxis to an already tenuous airway situation, the potential for sinus obstruction and infection beyond 48 hours, nasal tissue damage, and perceived discomfort during insertion. Nasotracheal intubation can cause avulsion of the turbinate bone when the tube engages the anterior end of the middle turbinate's lateral attachment in the nose and forces the avulsed turbinate into the nasopharynx (116–118,128,129). Additionally, prolonged nasotracheal intubation may contribute to sinusitis, ulceration, and tissue breakdown (117,130,131).

INTUBATION ADJUNCTS

Indirect Visualization of the Airway

Fiberoptic Bronchoscopy

There is an immense amount of interest in advancing airway management well beyond simply placing a laryngoscope blade into the oropharynx in the hopes that tracheal intubation can be quickly and easily accomplished. It is the critically ill ICU patient who precisely would benefit from improving the "line of sight," a straight line from the operator's eyes to the level of the glottic opening (71,72,80,132). Being able to see "around the corner" is immensely important when one's goal is to minimize intubation attempts and hasten the time to securing the airway (74,77–79,83). Flexible bronchoscopy is the gold standard in indirect visualization of the airway. Its role in the critically ill ICU patient is as broad as it is adaptable to various clinical scenarios, and serves many life-saving roles, both diagnostic and therapeutic. Flexible bronchoscopy does require expertise and patience and may be limited by secretions and edema (124). Its role in tracheal intubation in the critically ill patient probably best lies in its use as a first-line technique (124), rather than as a rescue technique (26,115,132,133) (Table 38.4). Edema, secretions, and bleeding often complicate visualization of the airway following multiple failed conventional laryngoscopies, thus leaving fiberoptic capabilities limited.

Incorporating a portable TV monitor to broadcast the fiberoptic view (Fig. 38.18) to the airway team is an excellent teaching modality, plus it allows input by other team members to optimize communication, positioning, and other maneuvers to hasten the intubation process (124,134). Fiberoptic intubation effectiveness is reduced by inadequate patient preparation (e.g., topical local anesthesia application when mucosal desiccation or excessive secretions are present, or excessive sedation in an attempt to counter poorly functioning topical anesthesia coverage or inadequate local anesthesia blocks). An inexperienced practitioner, one of the prime reasons for failure or suboptimal or no assistance (hence the inability to provide adequate jaw thrust or lingual retraction); improper choice of equipment (using a pediatric-sized bronchoscope to place a 9.0 ET); and improper positioning (utilizing the supine approach in a morbidly obese patient) all will impact negatively on success. An awake technique chosen in an uncooperative patient, the lack of bronchoscope defogging, inadequate lubrication, and poor judgment in the approach (e.g., a nasal fiberoptic approach in the face of a coagulopathy or nasofacial abnormalities, or a fiberoptic approach when patient has excessive, uncontrollable secretions or bleeding) further contribute to failure and frustration. Inadequate patient preparation with medication (e.g., too light sedation leading to discomfort or an uncooperative patient, or excessive sedation leading to hypoventilation, airway obstruction, or excessive coughing or procedural pain due to lack of narcotic administration) will place an undue and likely uncorrectable burden on the fiberoptic technique.

Successful fiberoptic intubation is dependent on a wide range of factors, each being performed in a timely manner (Table 38.5). Any single factor that is neglected or improperly executed may hamper the fiberoptic effort; hence, the practitioner's inexperience is a primary factor in both failures and difficulty encountered. A properly prepared and positioned patient undergoing fiberoptic nasal intubation may become a challenge—or the procedure may even fail—if too large an ET is chosen to pass through the nasal cavity or when arytenoid hang-up is encountered upon advancing the ET without counterclockwise rotation (124).

TABLE 38.4

CLINICAL USES OF FIBEROPTIC BRONCHOSCOPY IN THE INTENSIVE CARE UNIT

Primary tracheal intubation
Intubation adjunct for LMA-type airway device
Confirmation of intubation
Airway evaluation for extubation
ET/tracheostomy evaluation of position and patency
Diagnostic/therapeutic interventions for a cuff leak
Bronchial lavage for diagnostic/therapeutic reasons
ET exchange

LMA, laryngeal mask airway; ET, endotracheal tube.

TABLE 38.5

KEYS TO FIBEROPTIC INTUBATION SUCCESS

Patient preparation
Sedatives, narcotics, topical, local blocks, secretion control. Is patient cooperative?
Is fiberoptic approach a reasonable choice for intubation?
Choice of approach
Oral *vs.* nasal
Position
Supine, upright, elevated head of bed
Choice of fiberoptic equipment
Diameter, pediatric *vs.* adult
Other
Adequacy of light source, lubrication, assistance, ET warming capabilities, proper ET size

ET, endotracheal tube.

Video-laryngoscopy and Rigid Fiberscopes

In an effort to overcome the difficulty of "seeing around the corner," various advancements have been made to the standard laryngoscope. Though a difficult-to-visualize glottis is reported to be uncommon (22), Kaplan et al. reported that direct laryngoscopy in a large cohort of elective general anesthesia patients had a Lehane-Cormack view of III or IV in 14% despite maneuvers to optimize viewing with a curved laryngoscope blade (71). The incidence of a grade III/IV view in the emergency intubation population is more than double this rate; hence the need to improve visualization capabilities "around the corner" (44,135).

The addition of optical fibers or mirrors plus design alterations have improved one's line of sight over conventional blades. Devices such as the Bullard (20,22,76) (Fig. 38.21) and the Wu scopes (25,136–138) and the Upsher-Scope rigid fiberscopes (138) provide unparalleled visualization of the airway in most instances and may be particularly

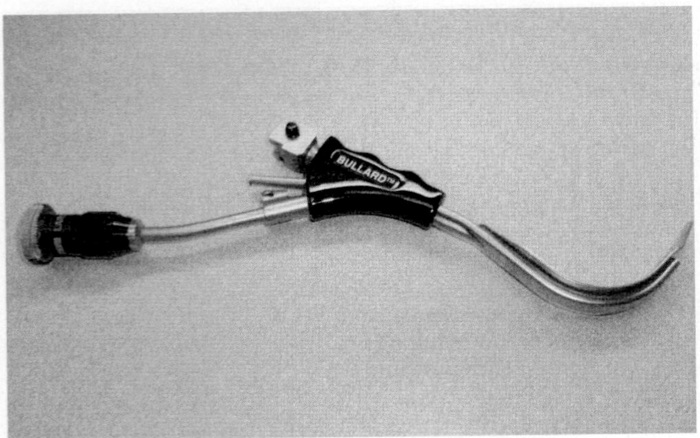

FIGURE 38.21. Bullard intubating laryngoscope.

useful in the presence of restricted cervical mobility (18,74,75). Each has an eyepiece for viewing via fiberoptic bundles for a single operator but may be attached to a teaching video head for team viewing and instruction (124,134). Video capabilities allow viewing on a television monitor, pushing video-laryngoscopy to a new and higher level of sophistication. The Macintosh (curved) video-laryngoscope (Karl Storz Endoscopy) was developed and produced by modifying a standard laryngoscope to contain a small video camera (71,139). Currently, improvements in video screen resolution, portable power sources, and the refinement in optics have afforded a new class of airway devices to assist in management of the difficult airway in the operating room, the ICU, and even remote floor locations (78,135,137,140). Alterations of the curved blade with an approximate 60-degree tip deflection separate the GlideScope and McGrath scope from the others. Though visualization is excellent, a principal observation to appreciate is that these instruments allow visualization, but they do not perform intubation of the trachea. Visualization of structures with failure to intubate is uncommon (less than 4%) (140,141), though various ET maneuvers and the use of a bougie may overcome many of these failures (142). The effectiveness and efficiency of these advanced devices require an

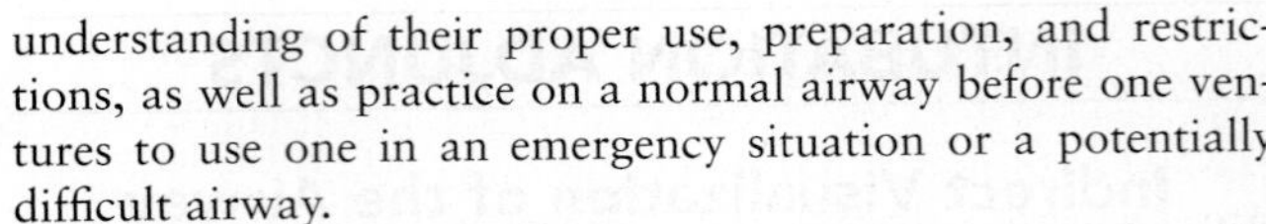
understanding of their proper use, preparation, and restrictions, as well as practice on a normal airway before one ventures to use one in an emergency situation or a potentially difficult airway.

A recent addition to advanced airway management is a disposable, low cost, J-shaped rigid optical laryngoscope utilizing mirrors and lenses, and which offers a clear and panoramic view of the glottic structures when placed midline in the lower airway (143). The Airtraq laryngoscope (Fig. 38.22) is an excellent adjunct for tracheal intubation, for evaluating the difficult airway for extubation, and for providing impressive indirect viewing of the glottic structures of the difficult airway during ET exchange (144). For advancement into the airway, a minimum amount of mouth opening must exist; its bulky dimensions may limit its use in the presence of a Halovest and restricted mouth opening.

Optical Stylets

Another class of intubation adjuncts that are very useful in improving success in the difficult-to-visualize airway (Lehane-Cormack grade III/IV) is the fiberoptic tracheal tube introducer or stylet. Typically fashioned like a stylet, the ET is loaded onto the fiberoptic shaft and then the stylet is maneuvered into the trachea. Visualization via an eyepiece on the scope or from a video screen affords a view of the airway structures that would otherwise remain restricted or blind (18,19,77,78,135). The ability to navigate the ET-loaded stylet past airway structures and visually confirm entrance into the trachea may hasten intubation in the difficult airway that otherwise would be considered difficult or impossible with conventional laryngoscopy (77,135,145). Again, edema, secretions, mucosal swelling, and limited mouth opening, as well as operator inexperience, may limit visualization capabilities (135). Several manufacturers produce relatively inexpensive hand-held rigid fiberoptic stylets that facilitate "seeing around the corner"; hence, they can be transported to the bedside in the ICU or to remote locations throughout the hospital (77,78,135). The use of these devices is improved by optimal positioning, lubrication, defogging, warming the ET/scope, secretion control, and, above all, practice under controlled conditions prior to deployment in the emergency setting (77,78,80,135).

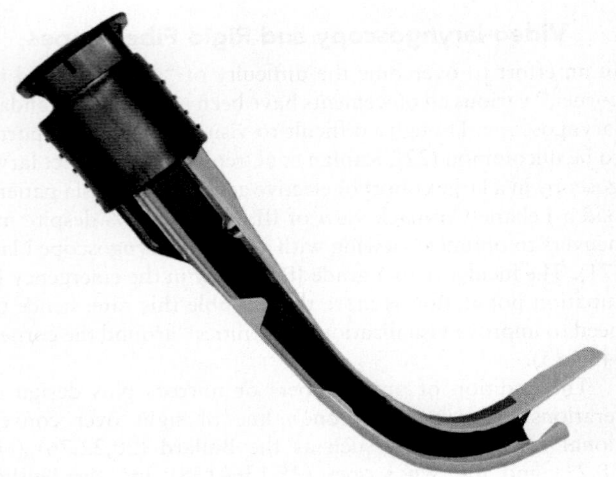

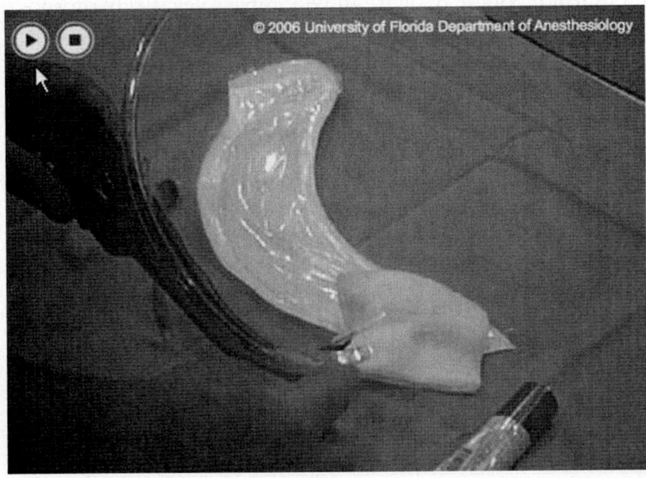

FIGURE 38.22. The Airtraq laryngoscope.

Tracheal Tube Introducer/Bougie

The tracheal tube introducer (TTI, or bougie) (Fig. 38.14) has earned a position in anesthesia care as an effective airway adjunct by assisting navigation of the ET into the trachea when anatomic constraints and/or an overhanging epiglottis limit the view of the glottic opening. A grade II (arytenoids and posterior cords only) or grade III laryngeal view (epiglottis only) is ideal for bougie-assisted intubation (93,146). The TTI is listed as a rescue option in national guidelines and should be included in a difficult airway cart or portable bag (30,31,63,64). The advantages of the bougie include low cost, no power supply, portability, a rapid learning curve, minimal set-up time, and a relatively high success rate and its immediate use reduces intubation-related complications (93,146). Placement involves passing it underneath the epiglottis with further navigation through the glottis to a depth of 20 to 24 cm, with potential tactile feedback as the curved tip bounces over the cartilaginous trachea rings. The tracheal ring "clicks" may not be appreciated in all cases. Further gentle advancement to 28 to 34 cm leads to the "hang-up test" or Cheney test. This maneuver is useful not only for bougie-assisted intubation itself, but also when ET verification maneuvers and devices are imprecise or confusing. Passing the ET is assisted by laryngoscopy to clear the airway of obstacles, lubricating the ET, and counterclockwise rotation to limit arytenoid hang-up of the ET tip. The bougie's role in difficult airway management is underappreciated and, given its potentially prominent role as a simple "no frills" airway tool, more attention to its position in an airway management strategy is warranted (114,115,147).

CONFIRMATION OF TRACHEAL INTUBATION

Physical Examination

Confirmation of ET location following intubation is imperative to optimize patient safety (30,46,63,64,89,91,92,148,149). Indirect clinical indicators of intubation such as chest excursions, breath sounds, tactile ET placement test, ET condensation, observing abdominal distension or auscultating the epigastrium, and oxygen saturation monitoring are considered nonfail-safe methods since each may be lacking, misinterpreted, or falsely negative or positive in the elective setting, and this fallibility is exaggerated in the emergency setting (149). Clinician interpretation of these and many other clinical findings in an acutely ill patient in a noisy environment under adverse conditions is marginal at best (149). Even experienced personnel are plagued by inadequacies of their interpretation and understanding (89,91,92). Nonetheless, and notwithstanding these limitations, our practice for **initial** confirmation of ET placement is as follows:

1. Observation of the ET passing through the vocal cords
2. Chest rise with bagging
3. Presence of condensation upon exhalation
4. Absence of gurgling over the stomach
5. Presence of breath sounds over the **lateral** midhemithoraces
6. Presence of CO_2 (Fig. 38.23)

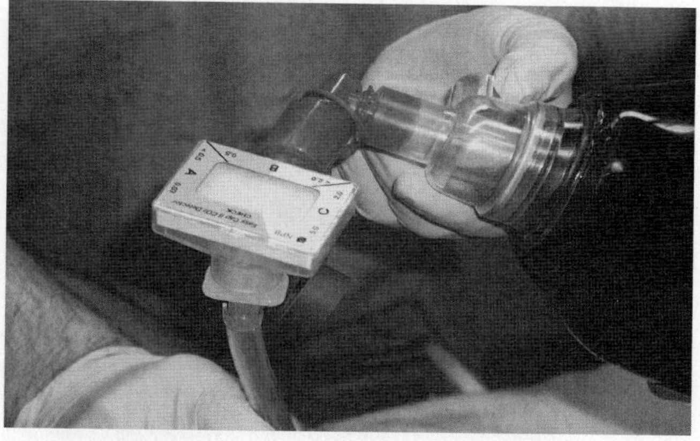

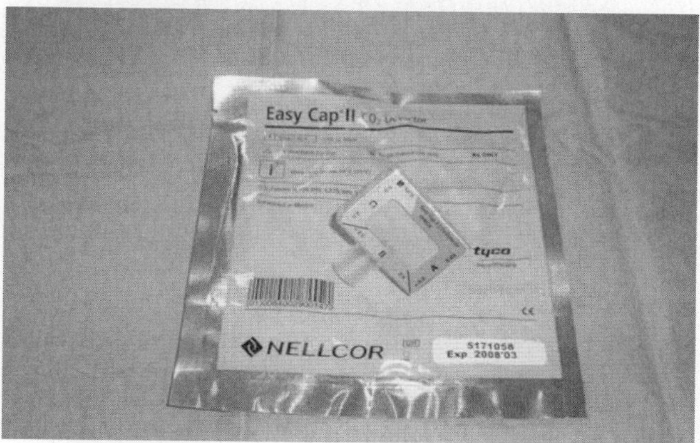

FIGURE 38.23. Disposable colorimetric CO_2 detector. Yellow signifies the presence of CO_2, violet its absence.

Capnography

To supplement the clinician's skill of accurately assessing ET location, the identification of exhaled CO_2 via disposable colorimetric devices or capnography should be considered an accepted standard of practice for elective as well as out-of-the-operating-room intubation (30,46,148). Considered "almost fail-safe," these methods may fail due to a variety of causes, namely the disposable colorimetric devices may fail in low-flow or no-flow cardiac states (no pulmonary blood flow as a source of exhaled carbon dioxide), or the color change may fail or confuse the clinician due to simple misinterpretation or more commonly by soilage from secretions, pulmonary edema fluid, or blood. Conversely, capnography may fail due to temperature alterations (outside, helicopter rescue), soilage of the detector, battery or electrical failure, or equipment failure due to age, missing accessories, or lack of maintenance.

Other Devices

Esophageal detector devices, either the syringe or the self-inflating bulb (Fig. 38.24) models, assist in the detection of ET location based on the anatomic difference between the trachea (an air-filled column) and the esophagus (a closed and collapsible column) (150). Applying a 60-mL syringe to the

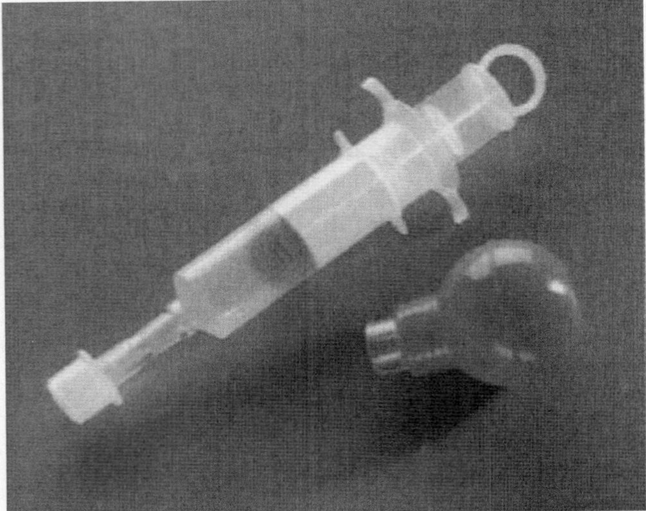

FIGURE 38.24. Esophageal detector devices, either the syringe or the self-inflating bulb models, assist in the detection of endotracheal tube location based on the anatomic difference between the trachea (an air-filled column) and the esophagus (a closed and collapsible column). Note that a 15 mm adaptor inserts onto the tip of the bulb syringe so that the connection may be made.

ET and withdrawing air should collapse the esophagus, while the trachea should remain patent. This concept was simplified by replacing the syringe with a self-inflating bulb that can be attached to the ET following placement. Either compression of the bulb prior to attachment to the ET or following attachment may still lead to false-negative results (no reinflation even though the ET is in the trachea) in less than 4% of cases (150). Failures of this technique include ET soilage, carinal or bronchial intubation in the obese, and those with severe pulmonary disease (chronic obstructive pulmonary disease [COPD], bronchospasm, thick secretions, or aspiration), and gastric insufflation. This technique is not affected by a low-flow or arrest state and, hence, it may be useful when capnography or colorimetric devices fail (150–152).

Two techniques considered infallible or fail-safe when used under optimal conditions are extremely accurate in detecting and confirming ET position: (a) visualizing the ET within the glottis and (b) fiberoptic visualization of tracheal/carinal anatomy (46). However, the critically ill population may have limited glottic visualization on laryngoscopy in up to 33% of cases (44,135). Following intubation, visualization of laryngeal structures may be obscured due to the presence of the ET. Likewise, fiberoptic visualization may be hampered by secretions and blood, as well as access to and the expertise to use such equipment.

Cheney Test

A clinically useful adjunct for assisting in the verification of the ET location includes the hang-up test, consisting of passing a bougie or similar catheterlike device for the purpose of detecting tip impingement on the carinal or bronchial lumen. Typically, gently advancing a bougie to 27 to 35 cm depth may allow the practitioner to appreciate hang-up on distal structures as compared to unrestricted advancement if the ET is in the esophagus (153).

DEPTH OF ENDOTRACHEAL TUBE INSERTION

Classic depth of insertion is height and gender based, as well as impacted by the route of ET placement (i.e., oral vs. nasal) and the patient's intrinsic anatomy. The depth will vary with head extension/flexion and lateral movement. Final tip position is best at about 2 to 4 cm above the carina to limit irritation with head movement and patient repositioning. Typically, the height of the patient is most specific in determining ET tip depth. ET depth in the adult patient less than or equal to 62 inches (157 cm) in height should be approximately 18 to 20 cm; otherwise, 22 to 26 cm may be the appropriate depth. Chest radiography only determines the tip depth at the time of film exposure. Fiberoptic depth assessment is the real-time method that garners the most clinical data for diagnostic and therapeutic purposes (123,154).

AMERICAN SOCIETY OF ANESTHESIOLOGISTS PRACTICE GUIDELINES

These guidelines and others specifically suggest that airway management procedures should be accompanied by capnography or similar technology to reduce the incidence of unrecognized esophageal intubation, hypoxia, brain injury, and death (30,63,64). We can think of no reason, in the economically advanced countries, why these recommendations would not be followed.

AMERICAN SOCIETY OF ANESTHESIOLOGISTS DIFFICULT AIRWAY PRACTICE GUIDELINES

Though reviewed earlier in this chapter, the salient points of the algorithm (Table 38.6) as they relate to the critically ill patient requiring emergency airway management are well worth repeating. Preintubation evaluation in the hopes of recognizing the difficult airway is paramount, yet is meshed with the understanding that the unrecognized or underappreciated difficult airway (mask ventilation, intubation, or both) occurs frequently. Examination of the patient, however, may be restricted due to emergent conditions, and the medical record may provide little to no useful data, especially when the patient previously had an easily managed airway but the airway status has changed substantially. When difficulty is known or predicted, patient preparation and access to airway equipment become primary focal points. This is not the case with the unrecognized or underestimated difficult airway. The induction technique is obviously not customized to the known difficulty; hence, the practitioner must counter this "surprise" by a preplanned rescue strategy, immediate access to advanced airway equipment, and personnel assistance combined with the expertise and competence to initiate and accomplish such a rescue strategy (30,63,64).

TABLE 38.6

AMERICAN SOCIETY OF ANESTHESIOLOGISTS DIFFICULT AIRWAY ALGORITHM

ASA AMERICAN SOCIETY OF ANESTHESIOLOGISTS

DIFFICULT AIRWAY ALGORITHM

1. Assess the likelihood and clinical impact of basic management problems:
   - A. Difficult Ventilation
   - B. Difficult Intubation
   - C. Difficulty with Patient Cooperation or Consent
   - D. Difficult Tracheostomy
2. Actively pursue opportunities to deliver supplemental oxygen throughout the process of difficult airway management
3. Consider the relative merits and feasibility of basic management choices:

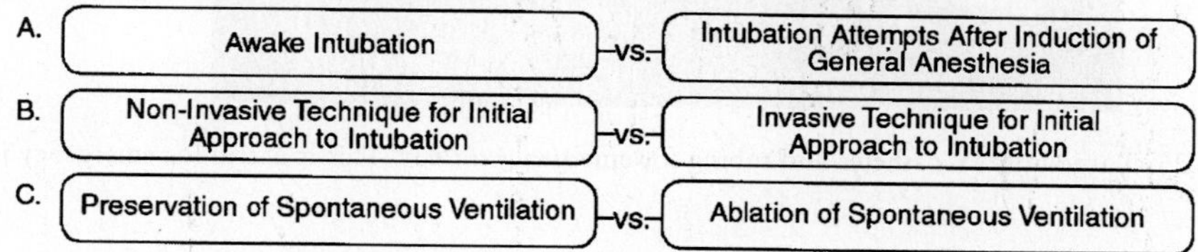

4. Develop primary and alternative strategies:

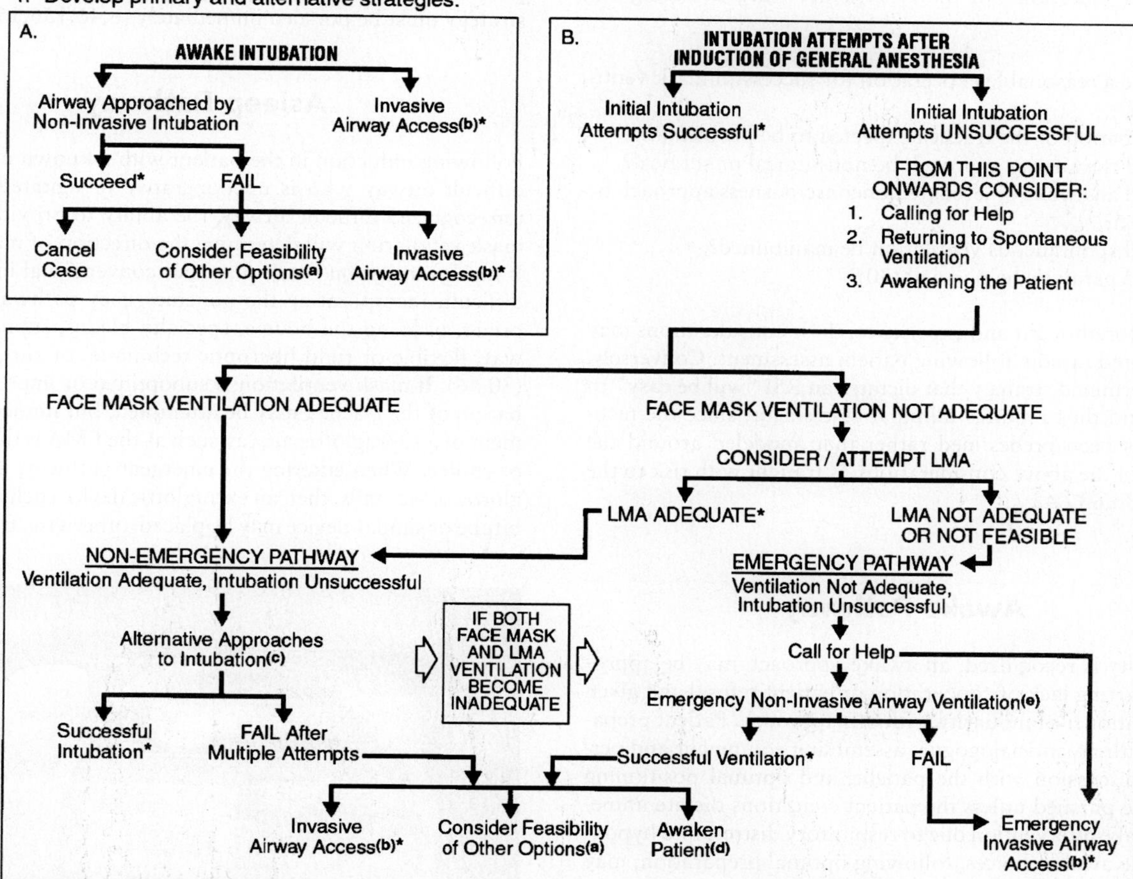

*** Confirm ventilation, tracheal intubation, or LMA placement with exhaled CO_2**

a. Other options include (but are not limited to): surgery utilizing face mask or LMA anesthesia, local anesthesia infiltration or regional nerve blockade. Pursuit of these options usually implies that mask ventilation will not be problematic. Therefore, these options may be of limited value if this step in the algorithm has been reached via the Emergency Pathway.

b. Invasive airway access includes surgical or percutaneous tracheostomy or cricothyrotomy.

c. Alternative non-invasive approaches to difficult intubation include (but are not limited to): use of different laryngoscope blades, LMA as an intubation conduit (with or without fiberoptic guidance), fiberoptic intubation, intubating stylet or tube changer, light wand, retrograde intubation, and blind oral or nasal intubation.

d. Consider re-preparation of the patient for awake intubation or canceling surgery.

e. Options for emergency non-invasive airway ventilation include (but are not limited to): rigid bronchoscope, esophageal-tracheal combitube ventilation, or transtracheal jet ventilation.

Source: http://www.asahq.org/publicationsAndServices/Difficult%20Airway.pdf.

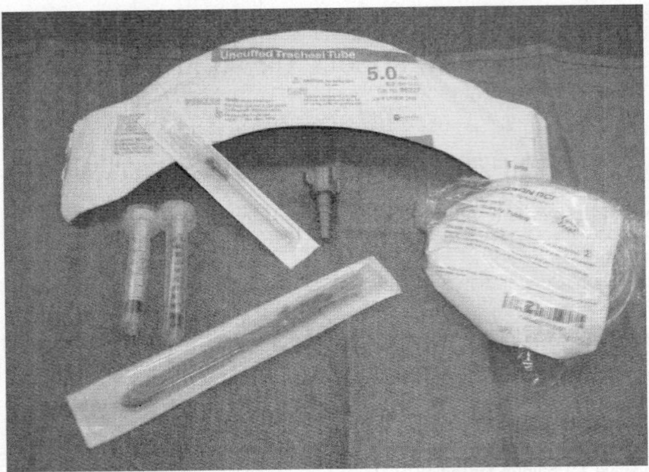

FIGURE 38.25. Large-bore IV catheter and tubing for emergency airway. This is useful for emergency jet ventilation.

Primary questions for the practitioner when accessing the patient are:

1. Is there a reasonable expectation for successful mask ventilation?
2. Is intubation of the trachea expected to be problematic?
3. Should the airway approach be nonsurgical or surgical?
4. Should an awake or a sedated/unconsciousness approach be pursued?
5. Should spontaneous ventilation be maintained?
6. Should paralysis be pursued (30)?

With forethought and experience, these considerations may be answered rapidly following patient assessment. Conversely, a predetermined strategy that dictates an RSI "will be easy" to pursue and thus requires minimal assessment, since the technique has been predestined rather than modeled around the findings of the above considerations, is fraught with risk to the patient (30,63,64).

Awake Pathway

If difficulty is recognized, an awake approach may be appropriate, barring lack of cooperation or patient refusal and given the practitioner's familiarity with this approach. Patient preparation with an antisialogogue, assembling equipment and personnel, discussion with the patient, and optimal positioning should be pursued unless the patient conditions dictate immediate awake intervention due to respiratory distress and hypoxemia. The awake choices, following optimal preparation, may allow the practitioner to take an "awake look" with conventional laryngoscopy; utilize bougie-assisted intubation, LMA insertion, or indirect fiberoptic techniques (rigid and flexible); or proceed with a surgical airway. The Combitube would not be indicated in the awake state. Access to the airway via cricothyroid membrane puncture via large-bore catheter insertion (Fig. 38.25A) with either modified tubing or a jet device (Fig.38.25B) to ventilate, or Melker cricothyrotomy kit (Fig. 38.26) is an option prior to other awake or asleep methods, but is often forgotten and rarely executed. If the awake approach fails or the patient deteriorates, prompting rapid intervention, the rescue strategy must be pursued immediately (6,46,155,156).

Asleep Pathway

Following induction in the patient with a known or suspected difficult airway who is uncooperative or agitated, or in the unrecognized difficult airway, the ability to provide adequate mask ventilation will determine the direction of management. If mask ventilation is adequate but conventional intubation is difficult, incorporating the nonemergency pathway is appropriate, utilizing the bougie, specialty blades, supraglottic airway, flexible or rigid fiberoptic technique, or surgical airway (30,46). If mask ventilation is suboptimal or impossible, intubation of the trachea may be attempted, but immediate placement of a supraglottic airway such as the LMA is the treatment of choice. When entering the emergent pathway, if the supraglottic device fails, then an extraglottic device such as the Combitube or similar device may be placed; otherwise, transtracheal

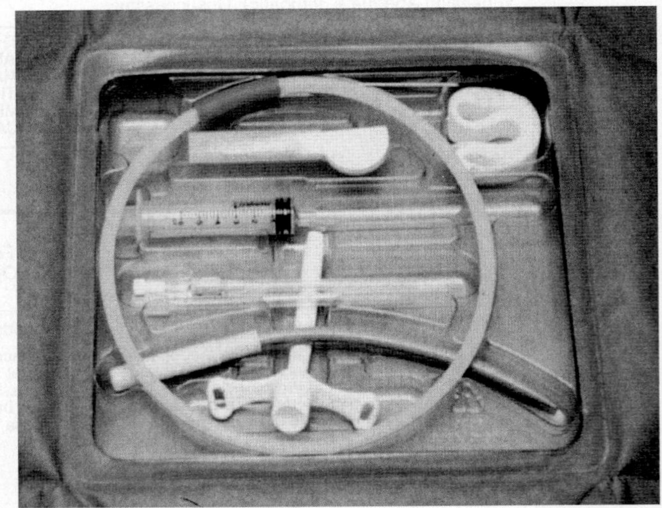

FIGURE 38.26. The Melker cricothyrotomy kit for emergency subglottic access to the airway.

TABLE 38.7

STRATEGY FOR EMERGENCY AIRWAY MANAGEMENT OF THE CRITICALLY ILL PATIENT

1. Conventional intubation—grade I or II view
2. Bougie—grade III view
   a. May use for grade I and II if needed
3. LMA/supraglottic device—grade III or IV view
   a. LMA/supraglottic rescue for bougie failure
   b. Or use the LMA/supraglottic device as a primary device (i.e., known difficult airway, cervical spine limitations, Halo-vest)
4. Combitube—rescue device for any failure or as a primary device if clinically appropriate
5. Fiberscope (optical/video-assisted rigid or flexible models)—primary mode of intubation, an adjunct for intubation via the LMA

LMA, laryngeal mask airway.

jet ventilation may be pursued by personnel knowledgeable in its application and execution, or a surgical airway placed (30,46).

A recently suggested strategy for emergency airway management of the critically ill patient outside the operating room is shown in Table 38.7 (114,115). Patient care was compared before (no immediate access to rescue equipment or $ETCO_2$ monitoring) and after (immediate access to rescue equipment and $ETCO_2$ monitoring) the management strategy was in place. A substantial improvement in patient care was realized with the following strategy: Hypoxemia, defined as SpO_2 <90%, was reduced from 28% to 12%; severe hypoxemia, defined as SpO_2 <70%, was reduced by 50%; esophageal intubation was reduced by 66%; multiple esophageal intubations were reduced by 50%; regurgitation and aspiration were reduced by 87%; and the rate of bradycardia fell by 60%. Any rescue strategy, however, should be customized to the practitioner's skill level, his or her access to rescue equipment, and his or her knowledge and competence of using such equipment (113, 114). Similar strategies have been used in the operating room with an improved margin of safety for airway management (84,85,147).

COMPLICATIONS RELATED TO ACCESSING THE AIRWAY

Tracheal intubation is an important source of morbidity and, occasionally, of mortality (30,43–46,89,91,92,148). Complications occur in four time periods: during intubation, after placement, during extubation, and after extubation (Table 38.8). Patients with smaller airways, especially infants and children, have a higher incidence of complications, combined with an increased risk of upper airway obstruction secondary to glottic edema and subglottic stenosis.

Cuffed tube usage for prolonged intubation and artificial ventilation substantially increases the rate of tracheal and laryngeal injury. The extent of injury is dependent on duration of exposure, the presence of infected secretions, and severity of respiratory failure. Cuff pressures above 25 to 35 mm Hg further add to risk by compressing tracheal capillaries, which predisposes to ischemic mucosal damage despite the high-volume, low-pressure cuffs that are standard today (157–160). Other factors of importance include the duration of intubation, reintubation, and route of intubation, with nasal intubation producing more complications than oral; patient-initiated self-extubation; excessive tracheal tube movement; trauma during procedures; and poor tube care. As one might expect, clinicians unskilled in intubation techniques increase the complication rate.

TABLE 38.8

RISKS OF TRACHEAL INTUBATION

Time	Tissue injury	Mechanical problems	Other
Tube placement	Corneal abrasion; nasal polyp dislodgement; bruise/laceration of lips/tongue; tooth extraction; retropharyngeal perforation; vocal cord tear; cervical spine subluxation or fracture; hemorrhage; turbinate bone avulsion	Esophageal/endobronchial intubation; delay in cardiopulmonary resuscitation; ET obstruction; accidental extubation	Dysrhythmia; pulmonary aspiration; hypertension; hypotension; cardiac arrest
Tube in place	Tear/abrasion of larynx, trachea, bronchi	Airway obstruction; proximal or distal migration of ET; complete or partial extubation; cuff leak	Bacterial infection (secondary); gastric aspiration; paranasal sinusitis; problems related to mechanical ventilation (e.g., pulmonary barotrauma)
Extubation	Tear/abrasion of larynx, trachea, bronchi	Difficult extubation; airway obstruction from blood, foreign bodies, dentures, or throat packs	Pulmonary aspiration; laryngeal edema; laryngospasm; tracheomalacia; intolerance of extubated state

ET, endotracheal tube.

During Intubation

Trauma

Tracheal intubation dangers begin at the time of initial tube insertion. Direct airway trauma depends on operator skill and the degree of difficulty encountered during intubation (27). Injuries include bruised or lacerated lips and tongue, inadvertent tooth extraction, upper airway hemorrhage, vocal cord tears, and nasal polyp dislodgement. Inadvertent contact of the cornea by the operator's hand may cause a corneal abrasion. Nasopharyngeal mucosa perforation can create a false passage, whereas a tear in the pyriform fossa mucosal lining may lead to mediastinal emphysema, tension pneumothorax, and infectious complications (27,89,91,92). Fracture or subluxation of the cervical spine, though rare, may result from careless movement of the head or forceful hyperextension during attempts to improve laryngeal exposure (18). Laryngoscopy may lead to swelling, edema, and bleeding of the oropharyngolaryngeal complex. Pre-existing edema or a coagulopathy will only exaggerate further swelling and bleeding. Continued efforts to control the airway with conventional laryngoscopic attempts may prove detrimental if supraglottic-glottic edema/swelling/closure results from repetitive trauma. Accessory devices such as the LMA and Combitube are dependent on a patent glottic opening; thus, exacerbating tissue damage with repetitive attempts may reduce rescue success with these devices (46).

Delay

Excessive delay in cardiopulmonary resuscitation may occur while an inexperienced practitioner tries to visualize the vocal cords. If intubation cannot be accomplished within 30 seconds, a more experienced person should make the attempt whenever possible. Multiple intubation attempts by any practitioner, unskilled or skilled, may make subsequent attempts more problematic and markedly increase the risk of hypoxemia, esophageal intubation, regurgitation, aspiration, bradycardia, cardiovascular collapse, and arrest (44–46). If effective mask ventilation and oxygen delivery are not possible during cardiopulmonary resuscitation (CPR), then prompt placement of an accessory device (LMA, Combitube) to support ventilation and oxygenation should be pursued (30,46,63,64). The LMA may assist with tracheal intubation itself and/or support ventilation and oxygenation in lieu of intubation.

Airway-related Complications

Airway-related complications in the emergency setting are similar in variety but outflank their elective counterpart in magnitude, occurrence, and consequence. Excessive secretions, edema, and bleeding, especially from repetitive instrumentation, may plague these interventions. The incidences of laryngospasm, bronchospasm, bleeding, tissue trauma, aspiration, inadequate ventilation, and difficult intubation remain relatively poorly documented.

Hypoxemia. Hypoxemia during emergency intubation has a variable incidence, ranging from 2% to 28% (12,44,89,90, 140,161–163). Currently, there is little specific literature reporting the influence of age, comorbid conditions, and pathologic states on the incidence of hypoxemia during emergency airway management, yet the risk increases as the patient's clinical situation worsens (Table 38.9) (70,163). Moreover, the patient's oxygenation reserves, obesity-related pulmonary limitations, and difficulty with airway management will influence the incidence of hypoxemia (112,164–167).

Hypoxemia-related concerns for emergency airway management include:

1. The limits of preoxygenation in the critically ill
2. The increased incidence of multiple intubation attempts
3. The increased incidence of encountering a "difficult airway" in the emergency setting (30,44,45,72,85,90)

Esophageal Intubation. Delayed recognition of esophageal intubation (EI) is a leading adverse event contributing to hypoxemia, aspiration, central neurologic system damage, and death (27,30,89–92,148,149). Failure to recognize EI is not limited to inexperienced trainees and, despite the use of verification devices, EI-related catastrophes persist (88,90,91). Indirect clinical signs of detecting tracheal tube location are imprecise and their interpretation is further restricted under emergent circumstances (Fig. 38.27) (46,89,91,149). Curbing the ill effects of EI by vigilant monitoring and rapid detection is warranted (148,149). Viewing the tube between the vocal cords, considered fail-safe, is impractical in 10% to 30% of patients due to anatomic limitations (44,168). Fiberoptic verification is fail-safe, yet is limited by blood and secretions, the operator's skill, and equipment access (124).

Regurgitation and Aspiration. Perioperative pulmonary aspiration is uncommon, occurring in approximately 1 in every 2,600 cases, but is magnified in the emergency surgical

TABLE 38.9

AIRWAY COMPLICATIONS CONTRIBUTING TO HYPOXEMIA

Esophageal intubation	Regurgitation/aspiration
Mainstem bronchial intubation	Multiple attempts
Inadequate or no preoxygenation	Duration of laryngoscopy attempt
Failure to "reoxygenate" between attempts	Airway obstruction, unable to ventilate
Tracheal tube occlusion: Biting, angulation	Accidental extubation after intubation
Tracheal tube obstruction after intubation	Bronchospasm, coughing, bucking
Due to:	
Particulate matter	
Blood clots	
Thick, tenacious secretions	

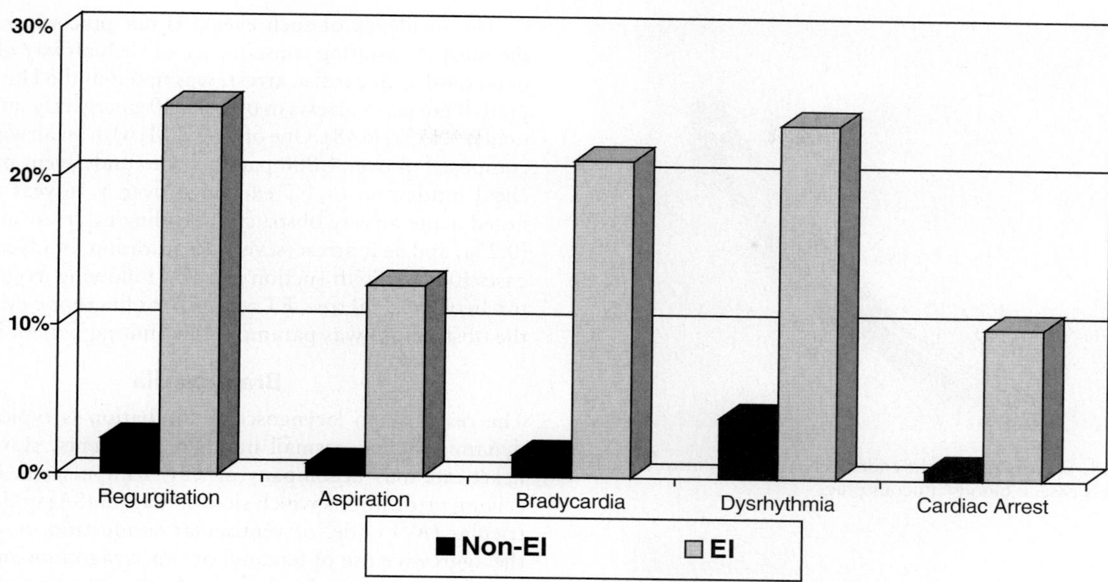

FIGURE 38.27. Incidence of complications with (EI) and without (non-EI, i.e., tracheal intubation) esophageal intubation detected by indirect clinical signs. (From Mort TC. Esophageal intubation with indirect clinical tests during emergency tracheal intubation: a report on patient morbidity. *J Clin Anesth.* 2005;17[4]:255.)

setting (169). Regurgitation during emergency intubation varies widely, ranging between 1.6% and 8.5%, with aspiration of the regurgitated material ranging between 0.4% and 5% (44,45,90,170). Emergently, there is little control over NPO status, ileus, upper gastrointestinal bleeding, or altered airway reflexes. Hypoxemia, bradycardia, and arrest may be magnified during regurgitation/aspiration (44,45,84,170). Immediate access to, and use of, accessory devices and ET-placement verifying equipment has reduced regurgitation and aspiration by 43% and 75%, respectively (148,149). Upper gastrointestinal bleeding is particularly risky, as it increases regurgitation by a factor of 4 and aspiration by a factor of 7 when compared to nonbleeding patients undergoing emergency intubation (95,171).

Airway Injury. The "airway" may sustain minor, nondisabling to catastrophic, life-threatening degrees of trauma during emergency intubation unbeknown to the practitioner. Difficult intubation is a factor in many, but not all, cases; for example, in several series, 50% of intubations resulting in esophageal perforations were believed to have been atraumatic intubations (27,89,91,92). Injury, shrouded by generalized nonspecific signs and symptoms combined with sedated, intubated patients unable to communicate, may limit the consideration of any injury (27,92). Pneumothorax, subcutaneous emphysema, pneumomediastinum, dysphasia, chest pain, coughing, or deep cervical pain advancing to a febrile state should be investigated (27,92).

Bronchial Intubation. Undetected bronchial intubation discovered by a postintubation chest radiograph is common, being seen in between 3.5% and 15.5% of cases. This undetected event increases substantially following difficult intubation, often leading to hypoxemia, atelectasis, bronchospasm, lobar collapse, and barotrauma if left uncorrected (44,45,172–176). Lung auscultation and palpation of the inflated cuff above the sternal notch may decrease bronchial intubation or carinal impingement, but are not fail-safe (122). Fiberoptic evaluation is definitive; thus, access to this modality in the ICU is important to allow for investigation of any unexplained oxygen desaturation, coughing, bronchospasm, or changes in peak inspiratory pressures, or an abrupt or gradual reduction in tidal volume (174–178).

Multiple Intubation Attempts. National guidelines define a difficult intubation as the inability to intubate within three attempts, at which point alternative airway techniques should be incorporated (30). Repeated interventions increase tissue trauma, bleeding, and edema, and may transform a "ventilatable" airway to one that is not (44–46). The number of laryngoscopic attempts directly increases complications, increasing with the second laryngoscopic attempt and accelerating rapidly with three or more attempts (44,45). All critically ill patients who require emergency airway management likely should be regarded as a potentially unanticipated difficult airway. Hence, observing the one or two attempts "rule" under "optimal conditions" before rapidly moving to an alternative strategy is prudent (27,43–46,85).

Though the literature has recommended a rapid sequence intubation technique as the definitive method of patient preparation, airways are as individual as their owners, and practitioner skills are variable. Thus, patients may benefit from an individualized approach (41,97,98). Incorporating a strategy that is adaptable to the practitioner and the patient (and his or her airway) may lead to a lower incidence of complications (27,44,45,85–88,114,115).

After Intubation

Acute Endotracheal Tube Obstruction Following Intubation

Acute ET obstruction has a differential diagnostic list that is long but, in most cases, can be discerned rapidly. Biting may be from an awake, agitated, or delirious patient or, on the other

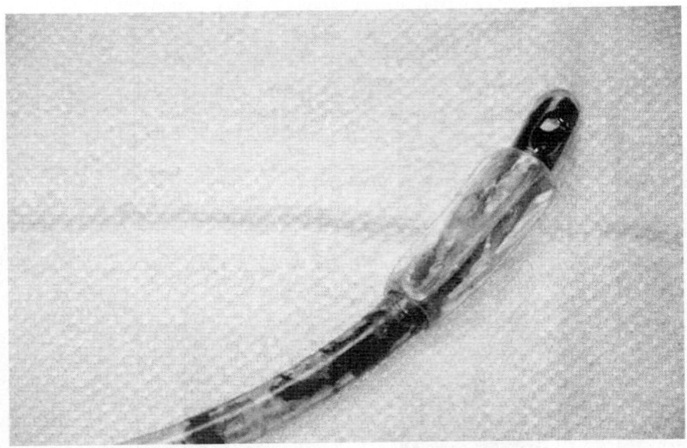

FIGURE 38.28. Obstruction of the endotracheal tube by intraluminal material, in this case, a bloody mucous plug.

hand, the ET tip may abut the tracheal wall. A bite block in the patient's mouth, additional sedation/analgesic agents, or slight rotation of the tube may correct the obstruction. Kinking of the tube or herniation of the cuff can occlude the airway and compromise ventilation, as can blood clots, tissue, dried secretions, tube lubricants, and foreign bodies. Partial or complete obstruction (Fig. 38.28) of a newly placed ET or tracheostomy tube by intraluminal or extraluminal sources may present as a life-threatening emergency requiring immediate corrective measures to reduce the risk of hypoxia-related morbidity and mortality (155,179).

Signs of ET or tracheobronchial obstruction are high inflation pressures, absent or impaired chest excursion, marked respiratory effort with paradoxical movement, cyanosis, hypoxemia, and venous congestion. Acute severe bronchospasm following primary tracheal intubation or during a tube exchange may mimic acute obstruction.

The rescue therapy differs between the *in situ* ET obstruction—depending upon its degree—and obstruction distal to the ET tip. Rapid removal of a completely obstructed ET may be life saving and, conversely, partial obstruction of the ET or tracheobronchial tree by inspissated mucus, blood, or tissue may require rapid irrigation and suctioning, either blindly via a suction catheter or utilizing a fiberoptic bronchoscope.

The etiology of the airway obstruction following intubation in the emergency setting in the ICU is often related to thick secretions. The patient undergoing emergency tracheal intubation may require mechanical support based on respiratory insufficiency due to poor secretion-clearing capabilities, poor cough, retained secretions, and shallow respirations. Once the trachea is intubated and positive pressure is delivered, the retained and dormant secretions mobilize more proximally toward the upper tracheobronchial tree, potentially contributing to airway obstruction. Conversely, during an ET exchange in a patient maintained on positive end-expiratory pressure (PEEP), especially when the level is approximately 8 cm H_2O or above, the sudden loss of expiratory pressure during the exchange appears to allow proximal movement of retained secretions, previously undetected or unreachable by standard ET suction techniques, to rapidly migrate toward the tracheocarinal region, potentially leading to very difficult or impossible ventilation.

The incidence of such events is not precisely known, but the most devastating consequence of such airway obstruction, hypoxia-driven cardiac arrest, was noted in the Hartford Hospital database (5 arrests in over 3,000 emergently intubated patients, 0.17%) (148). One of us (TCM) with an airway database composed of over 1,800 patients who underwent primary tracheal intubation or ET exchange over a 16-year period has noted acute airway obstruction leading to arrest in four cases (0.2%) and near arrest (severe desaturation, bradycardia) in 16 cases (0.9%). Swift suction removal following irrigation of the tracheobronchial tree, ET removal, or fiberoptic evacuation of the obstruction was paramount in limiting patient injury.

Bradycardia

The response to laryngoscopy intubation is typically hyperdynamic, but in a small number of patients, slowing of the heart rate may accompany airway manipulation. Patients receiving medications which slow sinoatrial (SA) node, atrioventricular (AV) node, or ventricular conduction, in addition to the aggressive use of fentanyl or other vagotonic medications, may be at increased risk for a further slowing of the heart rate. Preintubation bradycardia due to medication, an intrinsically slow heart rate in hypertensive disease of the elderly and the physically fit, and occasionally severe hypoxemia or the Cushing reflex in elevated intracranial pressure (ICP) may place the patient at a lower threshold to experience bradycardia. Vigorous laryngoscopy and tracheal intubation, inadvertent EI, and airway-related complications with severe or prolonged hypoxemia have led to bradycardia and cardiac arrest (44,45,148,149). Moreover, progressive bradycardia has been noted to precede intraoperative cardiac arrests in the majority of cases (146,148,180–182). Propofol's role in bradycardia remains ill-defined, but may be more relevant in the ICU patient on a continuous intravenous infusion rather than when using the agent in a single dose for intubation.

Vagotonic influences related to airway manipulation and hypoxemia appear to be primary factors. While an uncomplicated laryngoscopy may reduce the heart rate, airway-associated complications during difficult laryngoscopy and intubation with concurrent hypoxemia increase the incidence of bradycardia dramatically (148,170). The sympathetic outflow stimulated by a moderate reduction in oxygen tension may be overwhelmed by the parasympathetic influence with ongoing or worsening hypoxemia, thus leading to medullary ischemia. In addition, the drop in heart rate is typically associated with a significant reduction in blood pressure, often requiring aggressive therapy. When confronted with bradycardia, it behooves the practitioner to optimize oxygen delivery via the rapid deployment of accessory devices, call for the code cart, and provide pharmacologic intervention as well as interventions for potentially catastrophic pathology such as a tension pneumothorax, unrecognized esophageal intubation, or mainstem bronchus intubation.

Dysrhythmias

The acute onset of a new dysrhythmia during the manipulation of the airway or immediately after completion of securing the airway is infrequently reported. Pre-existing rhythm disturbances may be exaggerated by even rapid, straightforward airway manipulation, but may pale in comparison to the response initiated by a vigorous laryngoscopy, especially if it is associated with multiple attempts, inadequate sedation, or additional myocardial compromise. Bradycardia (see above), supraventricular tachycardia, atrial fibrillation or flutter with a rapid ventricular response, and ventricular disturbances are usually poorly tolerated by the critically ill patient, often complicated by varying degrees of hypotension. Further, succinylcholine—often used in RSI—is a well-known causative factor in contributing to a multitude of atrial and ventricular rhythm disturbances. Ongoing myocardial injury or a prolonged, vigorous, or traumatic manipulation of the airway can potentiate life-threatening dysrhythmias (44,183).

Cardiac Arrest

Anesthesia-related cardiac arrest in the operating room is relatively infrequent (0.01%), with the majority related to airway mishaps/difficulties (146,180–182). The risk of cardiac arrest in the ICU patient during emergency airway management may be as high as 2% (44,45,148,170). Specific risk factors contributing to cardiac arrest during airway manipulation included three or more intubation attempts, hypoxemia, regurgitation with aspiration, bradycardia, and esophageal intubation, often with one or more of these complications cascading from one to another (148,149). Nonairway-related cardiac arrests may result from ET obstruction, tension pneumothoraces, massive pulmonary thromboembolism, induction medication, and deterioration in patients suffering from acute myocardial infarction with cardiogenic shock (148). The varied list of etiologic factors that may contribute, singly or in combination, to the risk of cardiopulmonary arrest and cardiovascular collapse related to tracheal intubation is noted in Table 38.10 (170). Immediate access and use of advanced airway equipment and airway-placement verifying devices appear to have a significant impact on the incidence of hypoxemia-driven cardiac arrest (148).

TABLE 38.10

FACTORS CONTRIBUTING TO POSTINTUBATION HEMODYNAMIC INSTABILITY

- Anesthetic medications
- Sympathetic surge, vasovagal response
- Excessive parasympathetic tone
- Loss of spontaneous respirations
- Positive pressure ventilation
- Positive end-expiratory pressure (PEEP)
- Auto- or intrinsic PEEP
- Hyperventilation with pre-existing hypercarbia
- Decrease in patient work
- Underlying disease process (i.e., myocardial insufficiency)
- Volume imbalances (sepsis, diuretics, hypovolemia, hemorrhage)
- Preload dependent physiology
  - Valvular heart disease, congestive heart failure, pulmonary embolus, right ventricular failure, restrictive pericarditis, cardiac tamponade
  - Hypoxia-related hemodynamic deterioration
- Hyperkalemia-induced deterioration (succinylcholine)

Modified from Schwab TM, Greaves TH. Cardiac arrest as a possible sequela of critical airway management and intubation. *Am J Emerg Med.* 1998;16:609.

The Hyperdynamic Response to Airway Management

A brief or prolonged hyperdynamic response frequently accompanies direct laryngoscopy and intubation, and may reflect a number of physiologic factors, including wakefulness; the magnitude, vigor, and extent of the airway manipulation; underlying hypertension and cardiovascular disease; intravascular volume status; underlying sympathetic outflow; any related renal and cerebral pathology; induction medication; and the functional reserve of the patient among other clinical causes. Patients with central nervous system (CNS) pathology (stroke, intracerebral hemorrhage, seizure disorder) will have a higher likelihood of hypertension and/or tachycardia with airway manipulation (184–186). A persistent hyperdynamic response post intubation may reflect ongoing pain, anxiety, and/or wakefulness that may respond to additional anesthetic induction agents, or may reflect an exaggerated response seen in the high-risk individual with diabetes mellitus, renal or cardiovascular disease, or a CNS insult, and may also be seen in the intoxicated and the traumatized patient (184,185,187,188). Treatment with additional induction agents or vasodilators, diltiazem, or β antagonists may suffice, but overly aggressive treatment may quickly introduce further hemodynamic compromise when the therapy outlasts the self-limited phase of postintubation hypertension (186,187). Pathologic conditions which dictate aggressive therapy include head injury, intracerebral bleed, cerebral vascular accident, or seizure disorder.

Recognizable causes of an exaggerated hyperdynamic response may include balloon inflation, ET suctioning, mainstem bronchial/carinal impingement, coughing, bucking, or "fighting" the ventilator. The aggressive administration of anesthesia induction agents is literally a double-edged sword: capable of limiting the hyperdynamic response during airway manipulation but the quiescent, stimulation-free period that usually follows securing the airway may lead to a sharp reduction in the blood pressure (184,186).

Hypotension

The incidence of postintubation hypotension in the emergency setting is the most common of the hemodynamic alterations stemming from a variety of single and multiple etiologies (44,45,148,189,190). Being mindful of the pre-existing comorbidities and the current clinical deterioration prompting intubation, the airway manager's judgment and experience will influence the medication choices and techniques to prepare the patient for airway instrumentation. The major challenge is to select the agents that will achieve the goal of blunting, attenuating, or blocking the postlaryngoscopy hyperdynamic response, typically lasting for only a brief amount of time, with minimal subsequent influence or contribution to postintubation hypotension. Strategies are best tailored to the individual patient's needs based on the experience and judgment of the airway manager rather than, as we have commented several times previously, a standard intubation protocol such as etomidate and succinylcholine being administered to each and every patient (43,45). The addition of a neuromuscular blocking agent may impact the dosing of induction agents and the subsequent need for vasoactive medications, especially when blood pressure is maintained by agitation, struggling, straining, and muscle contraction of the critically ill patient.

The aggressive use of induction agents may potentiate the reduction in blood pressure following airway manipulation, particularly if no additional stimulation is provided post intubation. The institution of positive-pressure ventilation with PEEP plus any vasodilatation and myocardial depression from anesthetic agents may contribute to postintubation hypotension (189,190). This response is accentuated in incidence and magnitude in the critically ill patient who is struggling with underlying cardiopulmonary deterioration, acid-base imbalance, sepsis, hemorrhage, hypovolemia, and other maladies (44,148,189,190). Postintubation hypotension may require crystalloid resuscitation and/or a vasoactive agent such as ephedrine, Neo-Synephrine, vasopressin, or norepinephrine. Postintubation hypotension, *per se*, has not been studied in detail, though brief hypotension, in general, has been suggested as a significant contributing factor to patient morbidity and poor outcomes, especially in the traumatized and the neurologically injured patient (191).

Published reports that mention postintubation hypotension suggest that it is a rare occurrence despite the disposition of the critically ill patient. For example, two emergency department studies of nearly 1,200 patients reported less than 0.3% (four patients) developed hypotension (systolic less than 90 mm Hg) (98,99). Conversely, emergency intubation outside the operating room—including the emergency department—by anesthesiologists reported that four of every ten patients suffered hypotension requiring vasoactive medications to supplement crystalloid administration in one half of the victims (44,45,148). Nonetheless, the extent and degree of hypotension will be influenced by the induction agent, volume status, pre-existing comorbidities, and reason for the clinical deterioration, plus numerous other factors. Sepsis and cardiovascular injury such as myocardial infarction, congestive cardiomyopathy, pulmonary embolism, or cardiac tamponade appear to place the patient at greater risk for postintubation hypotension and the subsequent need for vasoactive medications.[1]

Age appears to play a prominent role in the incidence of postintubation hypotension: The octogenarian (52%) and nonagenarian (61%) are at higher risk as compared to those younger than 30 years old (22%) and the group between 30 and 60 years (35%). The need for vasoactive agents to counter the hypotension is twice as likely in the octogenarian and older groups when compared to those younger than 50 years old (62% vs. 30%) (192).

Endotracheal Tube Displacement/Extubation

Tube displacement out of the trachea or migration of the tube tip into a bronchus may compromise the airway (177,178). Appropriate securing and notation of tube markings in relation to the lip may minimize this complication, but the location of the markings at the dentition level has little bearing on the position of the ET tip (178,193). A chest radiograph may assist in confirming tip location, but only at the time of the filming. Fiberoptic evaluation of the tracheal tube positions offer real-time information that a chest radiograph taken 4 hours earlier cannot offer (154). Hyperextension of the head may cause migration of the tracheal tube tip away from the carina toward the pharynx; conversely, head flexion may advance the tube tip, with an average 1.9 cm movement of the tube (158).

Lateral rotation of the head may move the tube to 0.7 to 1 cm away from the carina. If tube tip position is in question and there is any clinical sign or symptom suggesting a problem (e.g., desaturation, tachypnea, and so forth), then one should consider aggressively pursuing a fiberoptically assisted determination of the tube placement rather than awaiting the call for a chest radiograph or waiting until an emergent situation has developed.

Accidental Extubation

Accidental extubation is a well-known clinical problem with the potential of significant patient morbidity and mortality (193). Accidental extubation, either patient-initiated self-extubation or resultant from external forces (nurse/physician moving patient, radiology team, transport, etc.), is another potential complication after intubation, occurring in 8% to 13% of intubated, critically ill patients (194). To prevent unplanned extubation, secure the tube by taping circumferentially around the upper neck. A variety of manufactured ET securing devices are available for purchase in lieu of the taping option. Tincture of benzoin improves adhesiveness of the tape to the skin and the tube. Restraining the patient's hands, care in turning and moving the patient, and good nursing practices minimize—but do not eliminate—this complication. Proper sedation regimens, close observation, and hastening extubation in those who meet criteria may reduce patient-initiated self-extubations (195,196).

Complete extubation of the trachea is most obvious when the patient self-extubates. However, the trachea may only be partially extubated when the ET cuff-tip complex is displaced proximally between or above the cords (193). An audible cuff leak is common, regardless of whether the final position of the ET cuff is just below, between, or proximal to the vocal cords. Moreover, complete extubation of the trachea—the cuff and ET tip lying in the hypopharynx—may present with a continuous or intermittent leak, or none at all (193). An ET secured at the lips/dentition at a level of 21 to 26 cm does not always equate to a correct tip position within the trachea (193). ET thermolability at body temperature may result in a coiled, kinked, or spirally misshaped (S-shaped) tube. If a cuff leak is heard, an attempt at remediation on a repetitive basis by adding air to the cuff may lead to further cuff-tip displacement (herniation). The hypopharynx may accommodate an ET with an overinflated cuff containing as much as 30 to 150 mL of air. Repetitive "fixing" of a cuff leak with small increments of air over several hours to days may lead to a stretched, highly compliant cuff positioned in the hypopharynx with continued ventilation and oxygenation. Cuff pressure measurements may be misleading due to altered cuff compliance and its position in the upper airway (193).

If a cuff leak—either intermittent or continuous—is noted, the pilot balloon should be checked for integrity. If inflated, the cuff-tip complex may be displaced at or above the glottic opening. Cuff deflation with blind advancement toward the airway should be discouraged by personnel not fully capable of managing the airway in the event of ET displacement, kinking, esophageal intubation, or loss of the airway. Evaluating the airway with direct laryngoscopy (DL) may be very helpful in assessing the location and status of the ET, but ET thermolability reduces one's ability to advance the softened, floppy, or deformed ET (193).

[1]Data from the Hartford Hospital emergency intubation database.

Conversely, a more proximal displaced ET (visible cuff in the hypopharynx) should not be advanced by hand unless the view of the airway is clear. Diagnostic/therapeutic bronchoscopy is the optimal choice. Diagnosing the location and deformity of the ET is possible coupled with its unparalleled utility for advancing the ET into the trachea. Secretions, operator skill, lack of immediate access to such equipment, and an ET tip abutting on the glottic, supraglottic, or hypopharyngeal structures may present reintubation challenges (193). If cuff hyperinflation is noted, complete deflation must be done prior to advancement over the fiberoptic bronchoscope (FOB). Once the airway is resecured, changing the deformed ET to a new one (via an airway exchanger cannula) may be considered (193). This clinical problem is common and life threatening; therefore, equipping the ICU with advanced airway devices is imperative (27,31,44,46).

The Failed Intubation

In the clinical situation in which the patient has been positioned to the best of the practitioner's abilities, the operator is experienced at performing the airway management intervention, and optimal efforts at conventional mask ventilation and tracheal intubation have been attempted but are unsuccessful (a CVCI [can't ventilate, can't intubate] situation), the practitioner will need to rapidly deploy his or her rescue plan in an attempt to salvage the airway and to save the patient's life. Following *failure* of conventional mask ventilation (no ventilation or oxygen delivery) or when mask ventilation is *failing (inadequate gas exchange, SpO_2 less than 90%, or a falling SpO_2)*, a supraglottic airway (LMA) should be placed (30,46,63,64). In some instances in which mask ventilation and oxygen delivery fail, or are failing—yet prior to any intubation attempt—intubation could be attempted if it is reasonably assumed to be straightforward and can likely be rapidly completed, as in the case of a patient with a slender habitus, who is edentulous, with no obvious difficult airway risk factors. If unsuccessful, placement of the LMA or a Combitube should proceed immediately (30,46). Conversely, the Combitube may serve as a backup for LMA failure (69). Both devices have a high rate of success for ventilation, are placed rapidly and blindly, and require a relatively simple skill set. However, in the situation described, most practitioners would choose the LMA due to its wider familiarity and because it readily serves as an intubation conduit, whereas the Combitube does not (46).

Limiting intubation attempts is a key to successful management, since repeated attempts that are probably futile (e.g., a grade IV view with conventional methods) waste time; increase trauma, edema, and bleeding; and markedly increase the risk of hypoxemia and other potentially devastating complications (27,30,44,45,63,64). It must be stressed that conventional intubation failure should be supplemented by an airway adjunct such as the bougie, specialty blades, or fiberscopes if immediately available. A key point is: **Use them early, and use them often.**

The American Society of Anesthesiologists (ASA) guidelines list both the LMA and the Combitube as ventilatory devices in the CVCI situation as less invasive options (30,46). More invasively, transtracheal jet ventilation (TTJV) via a large-gauge (12 or 14 gauge) IV catheter through the cricothyroid membrane may be an appropriate alternative, but advanced planning with ready access to the proper equipment and a sound understanding of "jetting" principles (lowest PSI setting to maintain SpO_2 in the 80%–90% range, prolonged inspiration-to-expiration ratio [i.e., 1:5], 6–12 quick breaths per minute, allowing a path for exhalation, constant catheter stabilization, and barotrauma vigilance) must be followed; otherwise, the consequences may be very serious, indeed (46,197).

It is imperative to appreciate the difference between an upper airway CVCI and a lower airway CVCI. A lower airway CVCI due to glottic abnormalities such as spasm, tumor, abscess, massive swelling, or subglottic pathology cannot be solved with a device dependent on glottic patency such as the LMA or Combitube (46). Only a subglottic approach, such as TTJV or a surgical airway, will suffice. Likewise, repetitive intubation attempts leading to airway trauma, bleeding, and edema not only markedly reduce the effectiveness of many intubation adjuncts, but also the once ventilatable airway may deteriorate into one that cannot be managed effectively, thus transforming the airway to a CVCI situation. If, however, management of an upper airway CVCI with noninvasive techniques fails, then rapid transition to TTJV or a surgical approach must be rendered (30,46,63,64). Conversely, successful ventilation and oxygen delivery via a supraglottic device does allow time to gain surgical access if intubation via the supraglottic device is difficult or fails.

All these life-saving maneuvers cannot be accomplished by carrying a laryngoscope in our back pocket or by grabbing the bare essential airway management equipment from a plastic storage bin in the ICU. Advanced planning to acquire and properly deploy conventional and advanced airway equipment, coupled with the education to execute a rescue strategy, is warranted given the precarious airway status of many critically ill patients who require airway management (30,31,46,63,64). Availability of personnel is imperative, as intubation is a team activity. The CVCI situation is very terrifying—indeed, bloodcurdling—so planning ahead to reduce the risks of airway management is both a justifiable and sound endeavor.

Laryngeal/Tracheal Damage

Prolonged intubation may cause laryngeal or tracheal injury (110,112–115,164). Excessive cuff pressure and prolonged intubation can initiate mucosal erosion, cartilage necrosis, and eventually tracheal stenosis. Movement of the tube during assisted ventilation may erode the trachea, usually in the posterior membranous portion. Blood-tinged sputum or any degree of new-onset hemoptysis should prompt evaluation of the ET or tracheostomy tube position. Erosions, granulation tissue growth, mucosal tears, and suction catheter–related trauma may contribute to bloody secretions, as may an undiagnosed lung tumor or necrotizing infectious process. Tracheal or bronchial rupture occurs more frequently in infants, the elderly, or patients with chronic obstructive lung disease. Because signs and symptoms may be delayed, chest radiographs and prompt endoscopy may confirm the diagnosis.

Miscellaneous

Other problems encountered during intubation are aspiration of gastric contents secondary to passive (silent) regurgitation, and leakage of orogastric secretions past the cuff. Regimens to cleanse the nasal and oropharyngeal cavity suggest a potential reduction in nosocomial pneumonia in the ICU setting. Paranasal sinusitis develops in 2% to 5% of nasally intubated patients and commonly involves the maxillary sinus (119–121). Signs and symptoms include fever and purulent nasal discharge, often appearing 2 to 4 days after nasal intubation. Infrequently, a middle ear infection results from bacterial reflux into the eustachian tube, followed by contiguous spread into the middle ear (122,123).

During Extubation

Problems during extubation arise secondary to mechanical damage, which develops while the tube is in place or in response to tissue injury. Failure to deflate the cuff, adhesion of the tube to the tracheal wall, or transfixation of the tube by a suture to a nearby structure may result in a difficult or impossible extubation. Laryngospasm and acute airway obstruction represent the most serious complications during the immediate postextubation period. Positive-pressure ventilation via a bag-mask assembly may assist in oxygen exchange, but prompt relief may require reintubation or rapid administration of a quick-onset muscle relaxant for laryngospasm. Collapse of redundant supraglottic tissue postextubation combined with rapid accumulation of laryngeal edema may occur immediately upon extubation of the trachea. Moreover, edema formation occurs in two other phases of the postextubation period: Acutely during the first 5 to 20 minutes post extubation or on a delayed basis, within 30 minutes to 8 hours of extubation. Laryngeal edema may involve the supraglottic, retroarytenoidal, and subglottic areas. Severe respiratory obstruction may occur after extubation, and frequently requires urgent reintubation or tracheotomy. Steroid use in the treatment of laryngeal edema is controversial, but may reduce postextubation stridor, reduce the need for reintubation in select patients, and hasten the resolution of existing traumatic edema. Utilization of bilevel positive airway pressure (BiPAP) or heliox (helium–oxygen mixture) may also be of use in the postextubation patient with stridor.

Other causes of airway obstruction after extubation are blood clots, foreign bodies, dentures, traumatized dentition, and throat packs inadvertently left in the airway. Passive regurgitation or active vomiting at extubation may result in gastric content aspiration; stridor may be the presenting clinical sign if air movement is possible. Rapid deployment of therapy is imperative; nebulized racemic epinephrine, heliox, judicious use of anxiolytics, noninvasive positive pressure modalities, or tracheal intubation may be in order.

After Extubation

Complications after extubation are divided into early (up to 72 hours) and late (more than 72 hours).

Early Complications

Early complications are listed in Table 38.11. Mechanical irritation to the pharyngeal mucosa causes sore throat. Short-lived or prolonged aphonia—a weakened voice—is common, especially following prolonged intubation. Laryngeal incompetence following extubation is the rule; hence, resumption of an oral diet must be timed appropriately to the patient's ability to cough, control secretions, and competently and safely swallow liquids and solids.

TABLE 38.11

TRACHEAL INTUBATION COMPLICATIONS SEEN AFTER EXTUBATION

Time of occurrence	Complications
Early (0–72 h)	Numbness of tongue Sore throat Laryngitis Glottic edema Vocal cord paralysis
Late (>72 h)	Nostril stricture Laryngeal ulcer, granuloma, or polyp Laryngotracheal webs Laryngeal or tracheal stenosis Vocal cord synechiae

Vocal cord paralysis and arytenoid dislocation and dysfunction may be appreciated following extubation (198–204). Paralysis may be unilateral or bilateral, with the left cord twice as frequently affected as the right, and males predominating with this complication. Damage to the external laryngeal nerve may cause lasting voice change, with unilateral nerve injury usually causing hoarseness. Paralysis can result and, if the injury is bilateral, may lead to airway obstruction.

Late Complications

Late postextubation complications include laryngeal ulcer, granuloma, polyp, synechiae (fusion) of the vocal cords, laryngotracheal membrane webs, laryngeal or tracheal fibrosis, and nostril stricture from damage to the alae (202,203,205). Laryngeal ulcerations or granulomata are more commonly located at the posterior region of the vocal cords where the endotracheal tube tends to have more continual contact. The patient may complain of foreign body sensation, fullness or discomfort at the back of the throat, and persistent hoarseness. Any patient complaining of airway-related pain, discomfort, fever, or systemic signs of infection following difficult airway management should be evaluated for tissue injury in the upper and lower airway and pharyngoesophageal region (27,92).

EXTUBATION OF THE DIFFICULT AIRWAY IN THE INTENSIVE CARE UNIT

Airway management also constitutes maintaining control of the airway into the postextubation period. The known or suspected difficult airway patient should be evaluated in regard to factors that may contribute to his or her inability to tolerate extubation. A comprehensive review of medical and surgical conditions and previous airway interventions, an evaluation of the airway, and formulation of a primary plan for extubation as well as a rescue plan for intolerance are essential for optimizing safety (206–208). Reintubation, immediately or within 24 hours, may be required in up to 25% of ICU patients (209–211). Measures to avert reintubation such as noninvasive ventilation for those at highest risk for extubation failure are effective in preventing reintubation and may reduce mortality rate if done so upon extubation (212). However, a delay in the

TABLE 38.12

RISK FACTORS FOR DIFFICULT EXTUBATION

Known difficult airway
Suspected difficult airway based on the following factors:
Restricted access to airway
Cervical collar, Halo-vest
Head and neck trauma, procedures, or surgery
ET size, duration of intubation
Head and neck positioning (i.e., prone *vs.* supine)
Traumatic intubation, self-extubation
Patient bucking or coughing
Drug or systemic reactions
Angioedema
Anaphylaxis
Sepsis-related syndromes
Excessive volume resuscitation

ET, endotracheal tube.

application of noninvasive ventilation when the patient displays signs of early or late postextubation respiratory distress or failure results in a less effective application in most patients, except those with COPD (213–216). Factors beyond routine extubation criteria that may be helpful in predicting failure include neurologic impairment, previous extubation failure, secretion control, and alterations in metabolic, renal, systemic, or cardiopulmonary issues (209–211).

"Difficult extubation" is defined as the clinical situation when a patient presents with known or presumed risk factors that may contribute to difficulty re-establishing access to the airway (Table 38.12). The extubation of the patient with a known or presumed difficult airway and the potential for subsequent intolerance of the extubated state poses an increased risk to patient safety. An extubation strategy should be developed that allows the airway manager to (a) replace the ET in a timely manner and (b) ventilate and oxygenate the patient while he or she is being prepared for reintubation, as well as during the reintubation itself (30).

The practitioner should assess the patient's risk on two levels: The patient's predicted ability to tolerate the extubated state and the ability (or inability) to re-establish the airway if reintubation becomes necessary (206–208). Weaning criteria and extubation parameters will not be discussed as they vary by locale, practitioner, and the patient's clinical situation. Table 38.13 outlines two categories for pre-extubation evaluation (208).

NPO Status

The NPO status of the patient to be extubated and the subsequent need for reintubation has not been thoroughly studied, but it makes clinical sense to consider 2 to 4 hours off of distal enteral feeds prior to extubation while maintaining the NPO status post extubation until the patient appears at low risk for failing the extubation "trial." Unfortunately, the ICU patient may succumb to reintubation based on a multitude of factors; hence, predictability of failure and when it will occur is difficult to discern.

TABLE 38.13

THE DIFFICULT EXTUBATION: TWO CATEGORIES FOR EVALUATION

1. Evaluate the patient's inability to tolerate extubation
a. Airway obstruction (partial or complete)
b. Hypoventilation syndromes
c. Hypoxemic respiratory failure
d. Failure of pulmonary toilet
e. Inability to protect airway
2. Evaluate for potential difficulty re-establishing the airway
a. Difficult airway
b. Limited access to the airway
c. Inexperienced personnel pertaining to airway skills
d. Airway injury, edema formation

Modified from Cooper RM. Extubation and changing endotracheal tube. In Benumof J, ed. *Airway Management.* St. Louis: Mosby; 1995.

The Cuff Leak

Hypopharyngeal narrowing from edema or redundant tissues, supraglottic edema, vocal cord swelling, and narrowing in the subglottic region of any etiology may contribute to the lack of a cuff leak (217–222). Too large of a tracheal tube in a small airway should, of course, be considered. A higher risk of post extubation stridor or the need for reintubation is prevalent in those without a cuff leak, in women, and in patients with a low Glasgow coma score (217–222). Attempting to determine the etiology for the lack of a cuff leak may impact patient care, as individuals may remain intubated longer than is required or receive an unneeded tracheostomy. If airway edema is the culprit, steps to decrease airway edema include elevation of the head, diuresis, steroid administration, minimizing further airway manipulation, and "time" (223–225). The cuff leak test as an indicator for predicting postextubation stridor is helpful, but the performance of a cuff leak test varies by institution and protocol, as does its interpretation by the individual physician. Testing to predict successful extubation is inconclusive (223–225). A relatively crude yet effective method of cuff leak test involves auscultation for cuff leak with or without a stethoscope. A more precise method is to take an indirect measurement of the *volume of gas escaping* around the ET following cuff deflation, determined by calculating the average difference between inspiratory and expiratory volume while on assisted ventilation (218,225). Cuff leak volume (CLV) may be measured as the difference of tidal volume delivered with and without cuff deflation and stated as a percentage of leak, or as an absolute volume. The percentage CLV will vary with the tidal volume administered during the test (8 mL/kg vs. 10–12 mL/kg), but several authors have found an absolute CLV less than 110 to 130 mL (218,219) or 10% to 24% of delivered tidal volume as helpful in predicting postextubation stridor (219–221,225). Stridor increases the risk of reintubation. Single- or multiple-dose steroids may reduce postextubation airway obstruction in pediatric patients, depending on dosing protocols, patient age, and duration of intubation (223). Steroid use in adults administered 6 hours prior to extubation—rather than 1 hour prior—may reduce postextubation stridor and decrease the need for reintubation in critically ill patients (210,223–225).

Risk Assessment: Direct Inspection of the Airway

Garnering useful information about the airway status may need to go well beyond the cuff leak test since it is relatively crude, provides little direct data regarding one's ability to access the airway in the event of a need for reintubation, and is relatively uninformative as to the actual status of the glottis. While it is mandatory that the records of the known difficult airway patient be reviewed, it is also the case that a record of previous airway interventions in a patient who may have undergone a marked alteration in their airway status could be less than informative. Practitioners should weigh the pros and cons of evaluating such an airway to determine ease or difficulty in the ability to gain access via conventional or advanced techniques. Additionally, some patients may need evaluation of their hypopharyngeal structures and supraglottic airway to assess airway patency and resolution of edema, swelling, and tissue injury. Conventional laryngoscopy is a standard choice for evaluation, but often fails due to a poor "line of sight." Additionally, the relationship of grading and comparing the laryngeal view of a nonintubated to an intubated glottis is inconsistent (226). Flexible fiberoptic evaluation is useful but may be limited by secretions and edema (124). Video-laryngoscopy and other indirect visualization techniques that allow one to see "around the corner" are especially helpful. The Airtraq, as may other optical or video-laryngoscopy devices, has been found to be particularly useful by offering outstanding wide-angle visualization of the periglottic structures in the critically ill patient with a known difficult airway (144).

American Society of Anesthesiologists Practice Guidelines Statement Regarding Extubation of the Difficult Airway

The ASA guidelines (30) have suggested that a preformulated extubation strategy should include:

1. A consideration of the relative merits of awake extubation versus extubation before the return of consciousness; this is clearly more applicable to the operating room setting than to the ICU
2. An evaluation for general clinical factors that may produce an adverse impact on ventilation after the patient has been extubated
3. The formulation of an airway management plan that can be implemented if the patient is not able to maintain adequate ventilation after tracheal decannulation
4. Consideration of the short-term use of a device that can serve as a guide to facilitate intubation and/or provide a conduit for ventilation/oxygenation

Clinical Decision Plan for the Difficult Extubation

A variety of methods are available to assist the practitioner's ability to maintain continuous access to the airway following extubation, each with limitations and restrictions. Though no method guarantees control and the ability to re-secure the airway at all times, the LMA offers the ability for fiberoptic-assisted visualization of the supraglottic structures while serving as a ventilating and reintubating conduit; it is hampered by a limited time frame in which it may be left in place. The bronchoscope is useful for periglottic assessment following extubation, but requires advanced skills and minimal secretions. Moreover, it offers only a brief moment for airway assessment and access to the airway following extubation (124). Conversely, the airway exchange catheter (AEC, Fig. 38.14) allows continuous control of the airway after extubation, is well tolerated in most patients, and serves as an adjunct for reintubation and oxygen administration (206,227–229). Patient intolerance, accidental dislodgment, and mucosal and tracheobronchial wall injury have been reported, but are rare (230–234). Carinal irritation may be treated with proximal repositioning, the instillation of topical agents to anesthetize the airway, and explanation and reassurance. Dislodgment may occur, resultant from an uncooperative patient or a poorly secured catheter. Observation in a monitored environment with experienced personnel should be given top priority, as should the immediate availability of difficult airway equipment in the event of intolerance to tracheal decannulation (206–208). Tips for success with the use of this device are shown in Table 38.14.

TABLE 38.14

AIRWAY EXCHANGE CATHETER (AEC)-ASSISTED EXTUBATION: TIPS FOR SUCCESS

1. Access to advanced airway equipment
2. Personnel
   a. Respiratory therapist
   b. Individual competent with surgical airway?
3. Prepare circumferential tape to secure the airway catheter after extubation
4. Sit patient upright; discuss with patient
5. Suction ET, nasopharynx, and oropharynx
6. Pass lubricated AEC to 23–26 cm depth
7. Remove the ET while maintaining the AEC in its original position
8. Secure the AEC with the tape (circumferential); mark AEC "airway only"
9. Administer oxygen:
   a. Nasal cannula
   b. Face mask
   c. Humidified O_2 via AEC (1–2 L/min)
10. Maintain NPO
11. Aggressive pulmonary toilet

ET, endotracheal tube.

Clinical judgment and the patient's cardiopulmonary and other systemic conditions, combined with the airway status, should guide the clinician in establishing a reasonable time period for maintaining a state of "reversible extubation" with the indwelling AEC (Table 38.15) (206).

EXCHANGING AN ENDOTRACHEAL TUBE

Exchanging an ET due to cuff rupture, occlusion, damage, kinking, a change in surgical or postoperative plans, or self-extubation masquerading as a cuff leak, or when the

TABLE 38.15

SUGGESTED GUIDELINES FOR MAINTAINING PRESENCE OF AIRWAY EXCHANGE CATHETER

Difficult airway only, no respiratory issues, no anticipated airway swelling	1–2 h
Difficult airway, no direct respiratory issues, **potential** for airway swelling	>2 h
Difficult airway, respiratory issues, multiple extubation failures	>4 h

requesting team prefers a different size or alteration in location, is a common procedure. Preparation for the possible failure of the exchange technique and appreciation of the potential complications is imperative (30).

Four methods typify the airway manager's armamentarium of exchanging an ET: Direct laryngoscopy, a flexible or rigid fiberscope, the airway exchange catheter, or a combination of these techniques (2). Proper preparation is imperative and patients should undergo a comprehensive airway exam. Access to a variety of airway rescue devices is of paramount importance in the event of difficulty with ET exchange (208).

Direct Laryngoscopy

DL is the most common and easiest technique for exchanging an ET, but has several pitfalls and limitations. Airway collapse following removal of the ET may impede visualization and, thus, reintubation. This method leaves the patient without continuous access to the airway and should be restricted to the uncomplicated "easy" airway (94).

Fiberscopic Bronchoscope–assisted Exchange

Fiberscopic bronchoscope–assisted exchange (FBAE) is useful for nasal to oral or vice versa exchanges and oral-to-oral exchanges, as well as for immediate confirmation of ET placement within the trachea and positioning precision (3–5). Though difficult in the edematous or secretion-filled airway, FBAE allows continuous airway access in skilled hands. Passing the flexible fiberscope through the glottis along the side of the existing ET, although not without significant difficulty, the old ET can be backed out, followed by advancing the ET—preloaded onto the fiberoptic bronchoscope—into the trachea. Conversely, the preloaded flexible fiberscope may be placed immediately adjacent to the glottis. The old ET is then backed out over an AEC and the glottis is intubated with the FOB-ET complex. A larger flexible model is better maneuvered than a pediatric-sized scope. Passing a lubricated, warmed ET that is rotated 90 degrees will reduce arytenoid-glottic impingement. Rigid fiberscopes such as the Bullard, the Wu scope, the Upsher, and the Airtraq are very useful for visualizing the otherwise difficult airway during the exchange by offering the ability to "see around the corner" (124,235–238). The fiberscope may be rendered useless by unrecognizable airway landmarks, edema, and secretions as well as operator inexperience.

Airway Exchange Catheter

The AEC incorporates the Seldinger technique for maintaining continuous access to the airway. Strategy and preparation are the keys to successful and safe exchange (Table 38.16). Proper sizing of the AEC to best approximate the inner diameter of the ET will allow a smoother replacement. A chin lift–jaw thrust maneuver and/or laryngoscopy will assist the passing of a well-lubricated *warmed* ET that may need to be rotated counterclockwise by 90 degrees to reduce glottic impingement. A larger-diameter (19 French is the size we most often use) AEC is best in passing an adult-sized ET. Exchanging a tracheostomy tube over an AEC is especially valuable when the peristomal tissues are immature. The use of a tracheal hook to elevate the tracheal cartilage and proper head/neck positioning (shoulder roll) will optimize the exchange. The exchange is often performed "blindly" since laryngoscopy in the ICU patient often reveals little to no view of the supraglottic airway. Thus, incorporation of any of the advanced laryngoscopes that assist in "seeing around the corner" (Bullard, Wu, Glidescope, McGrath, Airtraq, etc.) offer certain advantages to the operator and the patient: (a) assessment of the airway is improved; (b) there is better estimation of what size ET the glottis will accept; (c) visualization during the exchange offers the ability to direct the new ET into the trachea and reduce arytenoid hang-up or impingement; (d) it confirms that the AEC remains in the trachea during the exchange; and (e) it allows visual confirmation that the ET is placed in the trachea and the ET cuff is lowered below the glottis. Finally, the advanced airway device would be in position to assist in reintubation if any unforeseen difficulties arise during the exchange.

TABLE 38.16

STRATEGY AND PREPARATION FOR ENDOTRACHEAL TUBE (ET) EXCHANGE

1. Place on 100% oxygen
2. Review patient history, problem list, medications, and level of ventilatory support
3. Assemble conventional and rescue airway equipment including capnography
4. Assemble personnel (nursing, respiratory therapy, surgeon, airway colleagues)
5. Prepare sedation/analgesia ± neuromuscular blocking agents
6. Optimal positioning; consider DL of airway
7. Discuss primary/rescue strategies and role of team members; choose new ET (soften in warm water)
8. Suction airway; advance lubricated large AEC via ET to 22–26 cm depth
9. Elevate airway tissues with laryngoscope/hand, remove old ET, and pass new ET
10. Remove AEC and check ET with capnography/bronchoscope or use a closed system and place small bronchoscope through swivel adapter while at the same time ventilating, checking for CO_2, with the AEC still in place

DL, direct laryngoscopy; AEC, airway exchange catheter.

Minimizing the gap between the ET and the AEC is important for ease of exchange. If, due to luminal size restrictions, the smaller-sized AEC (4 mm, 11 French) is used when going from, for example, a double-lumen to a single-lumen ET in a high-risk ICU patient, then temporary reintubation with a smaller warmed (6.5 mm) ET as opposed to a larger (8–9 mm) ET may ease passage into the trachea. Once secured, a larger AEC may be passed via the indwelling ET with subsequent exchange to a larger ET. Various AEC exchange techniques are practiced, and customized variations of the standard methods assist the practitioner to tackle individual patient characteristics (94,235–238).

ET exchange, while simple conceptually, is not a simple procedure as hypoxemia, esophageal intubation, and loss of the airway may occur. The decision on the method of exchange is based on known or suspected airway difficulty, edema and secretions, and most significantly, the experience and judgment of the clinician. It is recommended that continuous airway access be maintained in all but the simplest and most straightforward airway situations (94).

Follow-up Care

Following a life-threatening airway encounter with a patient, dissemination of such information is often overlooked and there is currently no standard method of relaying information from one caregiver to another (30,89). Notes written in the chart are a start, as is a discernible or highly visible label on the outside of the medical chart, but these may be inadequate. Informative and accurate medical records of airway interventions should be promoted as a potentially life-saving exercise; hence, detailed accounting of an intubation with more information written in the chart—not less—is best for patient care. However, a caveat to note is as follows:

> If the chart states difficulty was encountered, assume it will again be difficult; if the notes states it was "easy" or no details are provided, assume and plan on the potential for difficulty.

Discussing difficulties with the patient in this setting is certainly different from the elective surgical case in the operating room. For the future care of the patient, opening a Medic Alert file has many advantages for improved dissemination of patient care information, especially in our mobile society. Obtaining medical records in a timely fashion is a constant deterrent. However, the Medic Alert file will not assist the care for the current hospitalization, only in future ones (27,30,89). Hence, steps for the current hospitalization can be taken to improve communication for efficient transfer of needed information to the airway team. Initially identifying the patient by a colorful wrist bracelet, analogous to a medication or latex allergy bracelet, is a simple but effective trigger for the airway team to investigate the patient's airway status. A computerized medical record may allow a "Difficult Airway Alert" to be readily and prominently displayed, thus allowing identification of the patient on the current and possibly future hospitalizations—although only at the current hospital. Future airway interventions in the unrecognizable or unanticipated difficult airway are particularly benefited by "flagging" the patient. The Medic Alert system is dependent on patient compliance and payment.

References

1. Campbell TP, Stewart RD. Oxygen enrichment of bag valve mask units during positive pressure ventilation: a comparison of various techniques. *Ann Emerg Med.* 1988;17:232.
2. Dorges V, Wenzel V, Knacke P, et al. Comparison of different airway management strategies to ventilate apneic, nonpreoxygenated patients. *Crit Care Med.* 2003;31:800.
3. Mazzolini DG, Marshall NA. Evaluation of 16 adult disposable manual resuscitators. *Respir Care.* 2004;49:1509.
4. Hayes H. Cardiopulmonary resuscitation. In: Wilkens EW, ed. *Emergency Medicine.* Baltimore: Williams & Wilkins; 1989:10.
5. Hocbaum SR. Emergency airway management. *Emerg Clin North Am.* 1986;4:411.
6. Jorden RC. Airway management. *Emerg Clin North Am.* 1988;6:671.
7. Florete OG. Airway management. In: Civetta JM, Taylor RW, Kirby RR, eds.. *Critical Care.* 2nd ed. Philadelphia: JB Lippincott; 1992:1419.
8. Yokoyama T, Yamashita K, Manabe M. Airway obstruction caused by nasal airway. *Anesth Analg.* 2006;103(2):508.
9. Hasegawa EA. The endotracheal use of emergency drugs. *Heart Lung.* 1986;15:66.
10. Greenberg MI. Endotracheal drugs: state of the art. *Ann Emerg Med.* 1984;13:789.
11. Greenberg MI, Mayeda DV, Chrzanowski R, et al. Endotracheal administration of atropine sulfate. *Ann Emerg Med.* 1982;10:546.
12. Powers RD, Donowitz LG. Endotracheal administration of emergency medications. *South Med J.* 1983;77:340.
13. Dauphine K. Nasotracheal intubation. *Emerg Clin North Am.* 1988;6:715.
14. Moore EE, Eiseman B, Vanuy CW. *Critical Decisions in Trauma.* St. Louis: CV Mosby; 1984:30.
15. Donlon JV. Anesthetic management of patients with compromised airways. *Anesth Rev.* 1980;VII:22.
16. Linscott MS, Horton WC. Management of upper airway obstruction. *Otolaryngol Clin North Am.* 1979;12:351.
17. Stone DJ, Gal TJ. Airway management. In: Miller RD, ed. *Anesthesia.* 4th ed, Vol. 2. New York: Churchill Livingstone; 1994.
18. Crosby ET. Airway management in adults after cervical spine trauma. *Anesthesiology.* 2006;104(6):1293.
19. Rudolph C, Schneider JP, Wallenborn J, et al. Movement of the upper cervical spine during laryngoscopy: a comparison of the Bonfils intubation fiberscope and the Macintosh laryngoscope. *Anaesthesia.* 2005;60:668.
20. Agro F, Barzoi G, Montechia F. Tracheal intubation using a Macintosh laryngoscope or a Glidescope in 15 patients with cervical spine immobilization. *Br J Anaesth.* 2003;90:705.
21. Turkstra TP, Craen RA, Pelz DM, et al. Cervical spine motion: A fluoroscopic comparison during intubation with lighted stylet, Glidescope, and Macintosh laryngoscope. *Anesth Analg.* 2005;101:910.
22. Rose DK, Cohen MM. The airway: problems and predictions in 18,500 patients. *Can J Anaesth.* 1994;41:372.
23. McGuire G, El-Beheiry H. Complete upper airway obstruction during awake fiberoptic intubation in patients with unstable cervical spine fractures. *Can J Anesth.* 1999;46:176.
24. Cohn AI, Zornow MH. Awake endotracheal intubation in patients with cervical spine disease: a comparison of the Bullard laryngoscope and the fiberoptic bronchoscope. *Anesth Analg.* 1995;81:1283.
25. Smith CE, DeJoy SJ. New equipment and techniques for airway management in trauma. *Curr Opin Anaesth.* 2001;14(2):197.
26. Fuchs G, Schwarz G, Baumgartner A, et al. Fiberoptic intubation in 327 patients with lesions of the cervical spine. *J Neurosurg Anesth.* 1999;11:11.
27. Peterson GN, Domino KB, Caplan RA, et al. Management of the difficult airway: a closed claims analysis. *Anesthesiology.* 2005;103:33.
28. Tokunaga D. Atlantoaxial subluxation in different intraoperative head positions in patients with rheumatoid arthritis. *Anesthesiology.* 2006;104(4):675.
29. Sellick BA. Cricoid pressure to control regurgitation of stomach contents during induction of anesthesia. *Lancet.* 1961:404.
30. Practice guidelines for management of the difficult airway: an updated report by the American Society of Anesthesiologists Task Force on Management of the Difficult Airway. *Anesthesiology.* 2003;98:1269.
31. Kane BG, Bond WF, Worrilow CC, et al. Airway carts: a systems-based approach to airway safety. *J Patient Saf.* 2006;2(3):154.
32. Stoelting RK. Local anesthetics. In: *Pharmacology and Physiology in Anesthetic Practice.* 2nd ed. Philadelphia: JB Lippincott; 1991:148.
33. Gross JB, Hartigan ML. A suitable substitute for 4% cocaine before blind nasotracheal intubation: 3% lidocaine-0.25% phenylephrine nasal spray. *Anesth Analg.* 1984;63:915.
34. Marshall BE, Wollman H. General anesthetics. In: Gilman AG, Goodman RS, Rall RW, eds. *The Pharmacologic Basis of Therapeutics.* New York: Macmillan; 1985:276.
35. Flacke JW, Bloor BC, Kripke E-A, et al. Comparison of morphine, meperidine, fentanyl and sufentanil in balanced anesthesia: a double blind study. *Anesth Analg.* 1985;64:897.

36. Stanski DR, Hug CC. Alfentanil: aldnetically predictable narcotic analgesic. *Anesthesiology.* 1982;87:435.
37. Drover DR. Determination of the pharmacodynamic interaction of propofol and remifentanil during esophagogastroduodenoscopy in children. *Anesthesiology.* 2004;100(6):1382.
38. Bouillon TW. Pharmacodynamic interaction between propofol and remifentanil regarding hypnosis, tolerance of laryngoscopy, bispectral index, and electroencephalographic approximate entropy. *Anesthesiology.* 2004;100(6):1353.
39. Warner OJ, Rai MR, Parry TM. Is remifentanil better than propofol at providing optimal conditions for an awake intubation? *Anesthesiology.* 2006;105:A824.
40. Reves JG, Fragen RJ, Vinik HR, et al. Midazolam: pharmacology and uses. *Anesthesiology.* 1981;54:66.
41. Reynolds SF. Airway management of the critically ill patient: rapid-sequence intubation. *Chest.* 2005;127(4):1397.
42. Levitan RM. Limitations of difficult airway prediction in patients intubated in the emergency department. *Ann Emerg Med.* 2004;44(4):307.
43. Levitan R. The importance of a laryngoscopy strategy and optimal conditions in emergency intubation. *Anesth Analg.* 2005;100(3):899.
44. Mort TC. Emergency tracheal intubation: complications associated with repeated laryngoscopic attempts. *Anesth Analg.* 2004;99:607.
45. Mort TC. The importance of a laryngoscopy strategy and optimal conditions in emergency intubation. *Anesth Analg.* 2005;100(3):900.
46. Benumof JL. The ASA management of the difficult airway algorithm and explanation. In: Benumof JL, ed. *Airway Management Principles and Practice.* St. Louis: Mosby-Year Book; 1996:151.
47. Cooperman LH, Strobel GE, Kennel EM. Massive hyperkalemia after administration of succinylcholine. *Anesthesiology.* 1970;32:161.
48. Gronert GA, Theye RA. Pathophysiology of hyperkalemia induced by succinylcholine. *Anesthesiology.* 1975;65:89.
49. Levitan R. Safety of succinylcholine in myasthenia gravis. *Ann Emerg Med.* 2005;45(2):225.
50. Green SM. Incidence and severity of recovery agitation after ketamine sedation in young adults. *Am J Emerg Med.* 2005;23(2):142.
51. Berkenbosch JW. Safety and efficacy of ketamine sedation for infant flexible fiberoptic bronchoscopy. *Chest.* 2004;125(3):1132.
52. Sebel PS, Lowdon JD. Propofol: a new intravenous anesthetic. *Anesthesiology.* 1989;71:260.
53. Taylor MB, Grounds RM, Dulrooney PD, et al. Ventilatory effects of propofol during induction of anaesthesia: comparison with thiopentone. *Anaesthesia.* 1986;41:816.
54. Eastwood PR. Collapsibility of the upper airway at different concentrations of propofol anesthesia. *Anesthesiology.* 2005;103(3):470.
55. Doufas AG. Induction speed is not a determinant of propofol pharmacodynamics. *Anesthesiology.* 2004;101(5):1112.
56. Jacoby J. Etomidate versus midazolam for out-of-hospital intubation: a prospective, randomized trial. *Ann Emerg Med.* 2006;47(6):525.
57. Cone D. Etomidate as a sole agent for endotracheal intubation in the prehospital air medical setting. *Ann Emerg Med.* 2004;43(1):147.
58. Jackson WL. Should we use etomidate as an induction agent for endotracheal intubation in patients with septic shock? — a critical appraisal. *Chest.* 2005;127(3):1031.
59. Murray H. Etomidate for endotracheal intubation in sepsis: acknowledging the good while accepting the bad. *Chest.* 2005;127(3):707.
60. Bloomfield R. Exploring the role of etomidate in septic shock and acute respiratory distress syndrome. *Crit Care Med.* 2006;34(6):1858.
61. Cortinez LI. Dexmedetomidine pharmacodynamics: part II: crossover comparison of the analgesic effect of dexmedetomidine and remifentanil in healthy volunteers. *Anesthesiology.* 2004;101(5):1077.
62. Jooste EH, Ohkawa S, Sun LS. Fiberoptic intubation with dexmedetomidine in two children with spinal cord impingements. *Anesth Analg.* 2005;101(4):1248.
63. Henderson JJ, Popat MT, Latto IP, et al. Difficult Airway Society Guidelines for management of the unanticipated difficult intubation. *Anaesthesia.* 2004;59(7):675.
64. Crosby ET, Cooper RM, Douglas MJ, et al. The unanticipated difficult airway with recommendations for management. *Can J Anaesth.* 1998;45(8):757.
65. Frass M, Frenzer R, Zdrahl F, et al. The esophageal tracheal Combitube: preliminary results with a new airway for CPR. *Ann Emerg Med.* 1987;16:768.
66. Cady CE. The effect of Combitube use on paramedic experience in endotracheal intubation. *Am J Emerg Med.* 2005;23(7):868.
67. Gaitini LA. The esophageal-tracheal Combitube resistance and ventilatory pressures. *J Clin Anesth.* 2005;17(1):26.
68. McGlinch B. Recommendation of the minimal volume technique to avoid tongue engorgement with prolonged use of the esophageal-tracheal Combitube. *Ann Emerg Med.* 2005;45(5):566.
69. Mort TC. Laryngeal mask airway and bougie intubation failures: the Combitube as a secondary rescue device for in-hospital emergency airway management. *Anesth Analg.* 2006;103(5):1264.
70. Leibowitz AB. Tracheal intubation in the intensive care unit: extremely hazardous even in the best of hands. *Crit Care Med.* 2006;34(9):2497.
71. Kaplan MB, Hagberg CA, Ward D, et al. Comparison of direct and video-assisted views of the larynx during routine intubation. *J Clin Anesth* 2006;18(5):357–362.
72. Ali AK, Trottier SJ, Christopher V, et al. Prevalence of difficult/failed airway: medical-surgical intensive care unit. *Crit Care Med.* 2006;34(12)S:A135.
73. Sugiyama K, Yokoyama K. Head extension angle required for direct laryngoscopy with the mccoy laryngoscope blade. *Anesthesiology.* 2001;94(5):939.
74. Smith CE, Pinchak AB, Sidhu TS, et al. Evaluation of tracheal intubation difficulty in patients with cervical spine immobilization: fiberoptic (WuScope) versus conventional laryngoscopy. *Anesthesiology.* 1999;91(5):1253.
75. Hastings RH, Vigil AC, Hanna R, et al. Cervical spine movement during laryngoscopy with the Bullard, Macintosh and Miller laryngoscopes. *Anesthesiology.* 1995;82:859.
76. Cooper SD, Benumof JL, Ozaki GT. Evaluation of the Bullard laryngoscope using the new intubating stylet: comparison with conventional laryngoscopy. *Anesth Analg.* 1994;79:965.
77. Levitan RM. Emergency airway management in a morbidly obese, noncooperative, rapidly deteriorating patient. *Am J Emerg Med.* 2006;24(7):894.
78. Levitan RM. Design rationale and intended use of a short optical stylet for routine fiberoptic augmentation of emergency laryngoscopy. *Am J Emerg Med.* 2006;24(4):490.
79. Rudolph C, Schneider JP, Wallenborn J, et al. Movement of the upper cervical spine during laryngoscopy: a comparison of the Bonfils intubation fiberscope and the Macintosh laryngoscope. *Anaesthesia.* 2005;60:668.
80. Bein B, Caliebe D, Romer T, et al. Using the Bonfils intubation fiberscope with a double-lumen tracheal tube. *Anesthesia.* 2005;102(6):1290.
81. Borasio P, Ardissone F, Chiampo G. Post-intubation tracheal rupture. A report on ten cases. *Eur J Cardiothoracic Surg.* 1997;12:98–100.
82. Massard G, Rougé C, Dabbagh A, et al. Tracheobronchial lacerations after intubation and tracheostomy. *Ann Thorac Surg.* 1996;61:1483.
83. Agro FE, Antonelli S, Cataldo R. Use of Shikani flexible seeing stylet for intubation via the intubating laryngeal mask airway. *Can J Anaesth.* 2005;52(6):657.
84. Rosenblatt, William HMD. Preoperative planning of airway management in critical care patients. *Crit Care Med.* 2004;32:186.
85. Rosenblatt WH. The Airway Approach Algorithm: a decision tree for organizing preoperative airway information. *J Clin Anesth.* 2004;16(4):312.
86. Sanchez A, Trivedi NS, Morrison DE. Preparation of the patient for awake intubation. In: Benumof JL, ed. *Airway Management: Principles and Practice.* St. Louis: Mosby-YearBook; 1996:159.
87. Atlas GM, Mort TC. Attempts at emergent tracheal intubation of inpatients: a retrospective practice analysis comparing adjunct sedation with or without neuromuscular blockade. *Internet J Anesth.* 2003;7(2).
88. Vijayakumar E, Bosscher H, Renzi FP, et al. The use of neuromuscular blocking agents in the emergency department to facilitate tracheal intubation in the trauma patient: help or hindrance? *J Crit Care.* 1998;13:1.
89. Caplan RA, Posner KL, Ward RJ et al. Adverse respiratory events in anesthesia: a closed claim analysis. *Anesthesiology.* 1990;72:828.
90. Schwartz DE, Matthay MA, Cohen N. Death and other complications of emergency airway management in critically ill adults: a prospective investigation of 297 tracheal intubations. *Anesthesiology.* 1995;82:367.
91. Cheney RW, Posner KL, Caplan RA. Adverse respiratory events infrequently leading to malpractice suits: a closed claim analysis. *Anesthesiology.* 1991;75:932.
92. Domino KB, Posner KL, Caplan RA, et al. Airway injury during anesthesia: a closed claims analysis. *Anesthesiology.* 1999;91(6):1703–1711.
93. Orelup CM, Mort TC. Airway rescue with the bougie in the difficult emergent airway. *Crit Care Med.* 2004;32(12)S:A118.
94. Sugarman J, Mort TC. Exchange of the endotracheal tube in the "normal" airway: strategies & complications. *Crit Care Med.* 2004;32(12)S:A80.
95. Oliwa N, Mort TC. Is a rapid sequence intubation always indicated for emergency airway management of the upper GI bleeding patient? *Crit Care Med.* 2005;33(12)S:A97.
96. Donahue S, Mort TC. LMA placement with light sedation/topical anesthesia in the critically ill. *Crit Care Med.* 2005;33(12)S:A86.
97. Ikeda H. The effects of head and body positioning on upper airway collapsibility in normal subjects who received midazolam sedation. *J Clin Anesth.* 2006;18(3):185.
98. Sakles JC, Laurin EG, Rantapaa AA, et al. Airway management in the emergency department: a one year study of 610 intubations. *Ann Em Med.* 1998;31(3):325.
99. Tayal VS, Riggs RW, Marx JA, et al. Rapid-sequence intubation at an emergency medicine residency: success rate and adverse events during a two-year period. *Acad Emerg Med.* 1999;6:31.
100. Shorten GD, Alfille PH, Gliklich RE. Airway obstruction following application of cricoid pressure. *J Clin Anesth.* 1991;3:403.
101. Georgescu A, Miller JN, Lecklitner ML. The Sellick maneuver causing complete airway obstruction. *Anesth Analg.* 1992;74:457.
102. Ho AMH, Wong W, Ling E, et al. Airway difficulties caused by improperly applied cricoid pressure. *J Emerg Med.* 2001;20:29.
103. Vanner RG, Clarke P, Moore WJ, et al. The effect of cricoid pressure and neck support on the view at laryngoscopy. *Anaesthesia.* 1997;52:896.

104. Palmer JH, Ball DR. The effect of cricoid pressure on the cricoid cartilage and vocal cords: an endoscopic study in anaesthetised patients. *Anaesthesia.* 2000;55:263.
105. Aoyama K, Takenaka I, Sata T, et al. Cricoid pressure impedes positioning and ventilation through the laryngeal mask airway. *Can J Anaesth.* 1996;43:1035.
106. Harry RM, Nolan JP. The use of cricoid pressure with the intubating laryngeal mask. *Anaesthesia.* 1999;54:656.
107. Asai T, Murao K, Shingu K. Cricoid pressure applied after placement of laryngeal mask impedes subsequent fibreoptic tracheal intubation through mask. *Br J Anaesth.* 2000;85:256.
108. Brimacombe J, White A, Berry A. Effect of cricoid pressure on the ease of insertion of the laryngeal mask airway. *Br J Anaesth.* 1993;71:800.
109. Collins JS, Lemmens HJ, Brodsky JB, et al. Laryngoscopy and morbid obesity: a comparison of the "sniff" and "ramped" positions. *Obes Surg.* 2004;14:1171.
110. Brodsky JB, Lemmens HJ, Brock-Utne JG, et al. Morbid obesity and tracheal intubation. *Anesth Analg.* 2002;94:732.
111. Neill AM, Angus SM, Sajkov D, et al. Effects of sleep posture on upper airway stability in patients with obstructive sleep apnea. *Am J Respir Crit Care Med.* 1997;155:199.
112. Berthoud MC, Peacock JE, Reilly CS. Effectiveness of preoxygenation in morbidly obese patients. *Br J Anaesth.* 1991;67:464.
113. Boyce JR, Ness T, Castroman P, et al. A preliminary study of the optimal anesthesia positioning for the morbidly obese patient. *Obes Surg.* 2003;13:4.
114. Mort TC. Emergency airway management: a strategy to improve the first pass success rate and improve patient safety. *Crit Care Med.* 2004;32(12)S:A80.
115. Sugarman J, Mort TC. Efficacy of an emergency airway management algorithm toward improving resident intubation success. *Crit Care Med.* 2004;32(12)S:A76.
116. Elwood T, Stillions DM, Woo D, et al. Nasotracheal intubation: a randomized trial of two methods. *Anesthesiology.* 2002;96(1):51.
117. Scamman FL, Babin RW. An unusual complication of nasotracheal intubation. *Anesthesiology.* 1983;59:352.
118. Sherry KM. Ulceration of the inferior turbinate: a complication of prolonged nasotracheal intubation. *Anesthesiology.* 1983;59:148.
119. Xue F, Zhang G, Liu J, Li X, et al. A clinical assessment of the Glidescope videolaryngoscope in Nasotracheal intubation with general anesthesia. *J Clin Anesth.* 2006;18(8):611.
120. Agro F, Hung OR, Cataldo R. Lightwand intubation using the Trachlight: a brief review of current knowledge. *Can J Anaesth.* 2001;48(6):592.
121. Xue FS, Li CW, Sun HT. The circulatory responses to fiberoptic intubation: a comparison of oral and nasal routes. *Anaesthesia.* 2006;61(7):639–645.
122. Pollard RJ, Lobato EB. Endotracheal tube location verified reliably by cuff palpation. *Anesth Analg.* 1995;81(1):135.
123. Rich JM. Recognition and management of the difficult airway with special emphasis on the intubating LMA-Fastrach/whistle technique: a brief review with case reports. *Proc (Bayl Univ Med Cent).* 2005;18(3):220.
124. Ovassapian A. *Fiberoptic Endoscopy and the Difficult Airway.* Philadelphia: Lippincott-Raven; 1996.
125. Randell T, Yli-Hankala A, Valli H, et al. Topical anesthesia of the nasal mucosa for fiberoptic airway endoscopy. *Br J Anaesth.* 1991;66:164.
126. Johnson DM. Endoscopic study of mechanisms of failure of endotracheal tube advancement into the trachea during awake fiberoptic orotracheal intubation. *Anesthesiology.* 2005;102(5):910.
127. Katsnelson T, Frost EAM, Farcon E, et al. When the endotracheal tube will not pass over the flexible fiberoptic bronchoscope. *Anesthesiology.* 1992;76:152
128. Patiar S, Ho EC, Herdman RC. Partial middle turbinectomy by nasotracheal intubation *Ear Nose Throat J.* 2006;85(6):380–382.
129. Prior S. Foreign body obstruction preventing blind nasal intubation. *Anesth Prog.* 2006;53(2):49.
130. Gallagher TJ, Civetta JM. Acute maxillary sinusitis complicating nasotracheal intubation: a case report. *Anesth Analg.* 1976;55:885.
131. Grindlinger GA, Niehoff J, Hughes SL, et al. Acute paranasal sinusitis related to nasotracheal intubation of head-injured patients. *Crit Care Med.* 1987;15:214.
132. Kerwin AJ, Croce MA, Timmons SD, et al. Effects of fiberoptic bronchoscopy on intracranial pressure in patients with brain injury: a prospective clinical study. *J Trauma.* 2000;48:878.
133. Tinnesz P, Mort TC. Emergency airway rescue by the 2nd airway team after failed attempts. *Crit Care Med.* 2004;32(12)S:A118.
134. Shulman GB, Nordin NG, Connelly NR. Teaching with a video system improves the training period but not subsequent success of tracheal intubation with the Bullard laryngoscope. *Anesthesiology.* 2003;98(3):615.
135. Jacobson D, Mort TC. Comparison of direct laryngoscopy and a fiberoptic stylet for emergency intubation. *Anesthesiology.* 2006;105(3):A816.
136. Sprung J, Weingarten T, Dilger J. The use of WuScope fiberoptic laryngoscopy for tracheal intubation in complex clinical situations. *Anesthesiology.* 2003;98(1):263.
137. Smith CE, DeJoy SJ. New equipment and techniques for airway management in trauma. *Curr Opin Anaesth.* 2001;14(2):197.
138. Connelly NR, Ghandour K, Robbins L, et al. Management of unexpected difficult airway at a teaching institution over a 7-year period. *J Clin Anesth.* 2006;18(3):198.
139. Kaplan M, Ward D, Berci G. A new video laryngoscope: an aid to intubation and teaching. *J Clin Anesth.* 2002;14:620.
140. Cooper R, Pacey JA, Bishop MJ, et al. Early clinical experience with a new video laryngoscope (Glidescope) in 728 patients. *Can J Anesth.* 2005;52:191.
141. Watts ADJ, Gelb AW, Bach DB, et al. Comparison of Bullard and Macintosh laryngoscopes for endotracheal intubation of patients with a potential cervical spine injury. *Anesthesiology.* 1997;87:1335–1342.
142. Heitz JW. The use of a gum elastic bougie in combination with a videolaryngoscope. *J Clin Anesth.* 2005;17(5):408.
143. Maharaj CH, Chonghaile MN, Higgins BD, et al. Tracheal intubation by inexperienced medical residents using the Airtraq and Macintosh laryngoscopes—a manikin study. *Am J Em Med.* 2006;24(7):769.
144. Mort TC. Laryngoscopy vs. optical stylet vs. optical laryngoscope (Airtraq) for extubation evaluation. *Anesthesiology.* 2006;105(3):A823.
145. Turkstra T, Pelz D, Shaikh A. Comparison of Shikani optical stylet to macintosh laryngoscope for intubation of patients with potential cervical spine injury: a randomized controlled fluoroscopic trial. *J Neurosurg Anesthesiol.* 2006;18(4):327.
146. Jabre P. Use of gum elastic bougie for prehospital difficult intubation. *Am J Emerg Med.* 2005;23(4):552.
147. Combes X, Le Roux B, Suen P, et al. Unanticipated difficult airway in anesthetized patients: prospective validation of a management algorithm. *Anesthesiology.* 2004;100(5):1146.
148. Mort TC. The incidence and risk factors for cardiac arrest during emergency tracheal intubation: a justification for incorporating the ASA Guidelines in the remote location. *J Clin Anesth.* 2004;16(7):508.
149. Mort TC. Esophageal intubation with indirect clinical tests during emergency tracheal intubation: a report on patient morbidity. *J Clin Anesth.* 2005;17(4):255.
150. Salem MR. Verification of endotracheal tube position. *Anesth Clin NA.* 2001;19(4):813.
151. Andres AH, Langenstein H. The esophageal detector device is unreliable when the stomach has been ventilated. *Anesthesiology.* 1999;91(2):566–568.
152. Wright RS, Burdumy TJ. Acute endotracheal tube occlusion caused by use of an esophageal detector device: report of a case and a discussion of its utility. *Ann Emerg Med.* 2004;43(5):626–629.
153. Bair AE, Laurin EG, Schmitt BJ. An assessment of a tracheal tube introducer as an endotracheal tube placement confirmation device. *Am J Emerg Med.* 2005;23(6):754.
154. Ezri T, Khazin V, Szmuk P, et al. Use of the Rapiscope vs. chest auscultation for detection of accidental bronchial intubation in non-obese patients undergoing laparoscopic cholecystectomy. *J Clin Anesth.* 2006;18(2):118.
155. Kemmots O. Six cases of endotracheal tube obstruction. *Jpn J Anesthesiol.* 1971;21:259.
156. Keenan RL, Boyan CP. Decreasing frequency of anesthetic cardiac arrests. *J Clin Anesth.* 1991;3:354–357.
157. Hedden M, Erosoz CEJ, Donnelly WH, et al. Laryngotracheal damage after prolonged use of orotracheal tubes in adults. *JAMA.* 1969;207:703.
158. Dubick MN, Wright BD. Comparison of laryngeal pathology following long term oral and nasal endotracheal intubation. *Anesth Analg.* 1978;57:663.
159. Kastanos N, Miro RE, Perez AM, et al. Laryngotracheal injury due to endotracheal intubation incidence, evolution and predisposing factors: a prospective long term study. *Crit Care Med.* 1983;11:362.
160. Esteller-More E, Ibanez J, Matino E, et al. Prognostic factors in laryngotracheal injury following intubation and/or tracheotomy in ICU patients. *Eur Arch Otorhinolaryngol.* 2005;262(11):880.
161. Mort TC. When failure to intubate is failure to oxygenate. *Crit Care Med.* 2006;34:2030.
162. Mort TC. Preoxygenation remains essential before emergency tracheal intubation. *Crit Care Med.* 2006;34:1860.
163. Mort TC. Preoxygenation in critically ill patients requiring emergency tracheal intubation. *Crit Care Med.* 2005;33(11):2672–2675.
164. Mort TC. Morbid obesity—risky airway business. *Crit Care Med.* 2005;33(12)S:A81.
165. Benumof JL. Preoxygenation: best method for both efficacy and efficiency? *Anesthesiology.* 1999;91:603.
166. Baraka AS, Taha SK, Aouad MT, et al. Preoxygenation: comparison of maximal breathing and tidal volume breathing techniques. *Anesthesiology.* 1999;91:612.
167. Salem MR, Joseph NJ, Crystal GJ, et al. Preoxygenation: comparison of maximal breathing and tidal volume techniques. *Anesthesiology.* 2000;92:1845.
168. Bair AE, Filbin MR, Kulkarni RG, et al. The failed intubation attempt in the emergency department: analysis of prevalence, rescue techniques, and personnel. *J Emerg Med.* 2002;23:131.
169. Warner MA. Is pulmonary aspiration still an important problem in anesthesia. *Curr Opin Anaesth.* 2000;13(2):215.
170. Schwab TM, Greaves TH. Cardiac arrest as a possible sequela of

critical airway management and intubation. *Am J Emerg Med.* 1998;16:609.

171. Oliwa N, Mort TC. Airway management of the upper GI bleeding patient: are extra measures warranted? *Crit Care Med.* 2006;33(12)S:A98.
172. McCoy EP, Russell WJ, Webb RK. Accidental bronchial intubation. An analysis of AIMS incident reports from 1988 to 1994 inclusive. *Anaesthesia.* 1997;52(1):24.
173. Schwartz DE, Liberman JA, Cohen NH. Confirmation of endotracheal tube position. *Crit Care Med.* 1995;23(7):1307–1308.
174. Seto K, Goto H, Hacker DC, et al. Right upper lobe atelectasis after inadvertent right main bronchial intubation. *Anesth Analg.* 1983;62:851.
175. Gandhi SK, Munshi CA, Kampine JP. Early warning sign of an accidental endobronchial intubation: A sudden drop or sudden rise in $PaCO_2$? *Anesthesiology.* 1986;65:114.
176. Owen RL, Cheney FW. Endobronchial intubation: a preventable complication. *Anesthesiology.* 1987;67:255.
177. Greene ER Jr, Gutierez FA. Tip of polyvinyl chloride double-lumen endotracheal inadvertently wedged in left lower lobe bronchus. *Anesthesiology.* 1986;64:406.
178. Brodsky JB, Shulman MS, Mark JBD. Malposition of left-sided double-lumen endotracheal tubes. *Anesthesiology.* 1985;62:667.
179. Glinsman D, Pavlin EG. Airway obstruction after nasal-tracheal intubation. *Anesthesiology.* 1982;56:229.
180. Keenan RL, Boyan CP. Cardiac arrest due to anesthesia. *JAMA.* 1985;253:2373–2377.
181. Chopra V, Bovill JG, Spierdijk H. Accidents, near accidents and complications during anaethesia. *Anaethesia.* 1990;45:3.
182. Kubota Y, Toyoda Y, Kubota H, et al. Frequency of anesthetic cardiac arrest and death in the operating room at a single general hospital over a 30-year period. *J Clin Anesth.* 1994;6:227.
183. Kane DM, Mort TC. Emergency intubation in the cardiac catheterization suite: hemodynamic consequences. *Crit Care Med.* 2004;32(12)S:A46.
184. Wintermark M, Chioléro R, van Melle G, et al. Relationship between brain perfusion computed tomography variables and cerebral perfusion pressure in severe head trauma patients. *Crit Care Med.* 2004;32(7):1579.
185. Jellish WS. Anesthetic issues and perioperative blood pressure management in patients who have cerebrovascular diseases undergoing surgical procedures. *Neurol Clin.* 2006;24(4):647.
186. Yastrebov K. Intraoperative management: carotid endarterectomies. *Anesthesiol Clin NA.* 2004;22(2):265.
187. Nicholls TP, Shoemaker WC, Wo CCJ. Survival, hemodynamics, and tissue oxygenation after head trauma. *J Am Coll Surg.* 2006;202(1):120.
188. Rose DK, Cohen MM. The incidence of airway problems depends on the definition used. *Can J Anaesth.* 1996;43(1):30–34.
189. Franklin C, Samuel J, Hu TC. Life-threatening hypotension associated with emergency intubation and the initiation of mechanical ventilation. *Am J Emerg Med.* 1994;12(4):425.
190. Klinger JR. Hemodynamics and positive end-expiratory pressure in critically ill patients. *Crit Care Clin.* 1996;12:841.
191. Demetriades D, Martin M, Ali Salim A, et al. Relationship between American College of Surgeons trauma center designation and mortality in patients with severe trauma. *J Am Coll Surg.* 2006;202(2):212–215.
192. Mort TC. Emergency intubation: octogenarians and beyond. *Crit Care Med.* 2005;33(12)S:A85.
193. Mort TC. ETT cuff leak: a safety strategy. *Crit Care Med.* 2005; 33(12)S:A85.
194. Mort TC. Unplanned tracheal extubation outside the operating room: a quality improvement audit of hemodynamic and tracheal airway complications associated with emergency tracheal reintubation. *Anesth Analg.* 1998;86:1171.
195. Jaber S, Chanques G, Altairac C, et al. A prospective study of agitation in a medical-surgical ICU incidence, risk factors, and outcomes. *Chest.* 2005;128(4):2749.
196. Krinsley JS, Barone JE. The drive to survive unplanned extubation in the ICU. *Chest.* 2005;128(2):560.
197. Benumof JL, Scheller MD. The importance of transtracheal jet ventilation in the management of the difficult airway. *Anesthesiology.* 1989;71: 769.
198. Cinar SO. Isolated bilateral paralysis of the hypoglossal and recurrent laryngeal nerves (Bilateral Tapia's syndrome) after transoral intubation for general anesthesia. *Acta Anaesthesiol Scand.* 2005;49(1):98.
199. Rubin AD. Arytenoid cartilage dislocation: a 20-year experience. *J Voice.* 2005;19(4):687.
200. Sagawa M. Bilateral vocal cord paralysis after lung cancer surgery with a double-lumen endotracheal tube: a life-threatening complication. *J Cardiothorac Vasc Anesth.* 2006;20(2):225.
201. Dimarakis I. Vocal cord palsy as a complication of adult cardiac surgery: surgical correlations and analysis. *Eur J Cardiothorac Surg.* 2004;26(4):773.
202. Ulrich-Pur H. Comparison of mucosal pressures induced by cuffs of different airway devices. *Anesthesiology.* 2006;104(5):933.
203. Gomes Cordeiro AM. Possible risk factors associated with moderate or severe airway injuries in children who underwent endotracheal intubation. *Pediatr Crit Care Med.* 2004;5(4):364.
204. Gaylor EB, Greenberg SB. Untoward sequelae of prolonged intubation. *Laryngoscope.* 1985;95:1461.
205. Fan CM. Tracheal rupture complicating emergent endotracheal intubation. *Am J Emerg Med.* 2004;22(4):289.
206. Cooper RM. The use of an endotracheal ventilation catheter in the management of difficult extubations. *Can J Anaesth.* 1996;43:90.
207. Benumof JL. Airway exchange catheters: simple concept, potentially great danger. *Anesthesiology.* 1999;91(2):342–344.
208. Cooper RM. Extubation and changing endotracheal tube. In: Benumof J, ed. *Airway Management.* St. Louis: Mosby; 1995.
209. Frutos-Vivar F, Ferguson ND, Esteban, A, et al. Risk factors for extubation failure in patients following a successful spontaneous breathing trial. *Chest.* 2006;130(6):1664.
210. Epstein SK. Preventing postextubation respiratory failure. *Crit Care Med.* 2006;34(5):1547.
211. Epstein SK, Ciubotaru RL. Independent effects of etiology of failure and time to reintubation on outcome for patients failing extubation. *Am J Respir Crit Care Med.* 1998;158(2):489–493.
212. Ferrer M, Valencia M, Nicolas JM, et al. Early non-invasive ventilation averts extubation failure in patients at risk. A randomized trial. *Am J Respir Crit Care Med.* 2006;173(2):164.
213. Esteban A, Frutos-Vivar F, Ferguson ND, et al. Noninvasive positive-pressure ventilation for respiratory failure after extubation. *N Engl J Med.* 2004;350:2452.
214. Keenan SP, Powers C, McCormack DG, et al. Noninvasive positive-pressure ventilation for postextubation respiratory distress: a randomized controlled trial. *JAMA.* 2002;287:3238.
215. Nava SGC, Fanfulla F, Squadrone E, et al. Noninvasive ventilation to prevent respiratory failure after extubation in high-risk patients. *Crit Care Med.* 2005;33:2456.
216. Salam A, Tilluckdharry L, Amoateng-Adjepong Y, et al. Neurologic status, cough, secretions and extubation outcomes. *Intensive Care Med.* 2004;30:1334.
217. Chung YH, Chao TY, Chiu CT, et al. The cuff-leak test is a simple tool to verify severe laryngeal edema in patients undergoing long-term mechanical ventilation. *Crit Care Med.* 2006;34(2):409.
218. Miller RL, Cole RP. Association between reduced cuff leak volume and postextubation stridor. *Chest.* 1996;110:1035.
219. Jaber S, Chanques G, Matecki S, et al. Post-extubation stridor in intensive care unit patients. Risk factors evaluation and importance of the cuff-leak test. *Intensive Care Med.* 2003;29:6.
220. De Bast Y, De Backer D, Moraine JJ, et al. The cuff leak test to predict failure of tracheal extubation for laryngeal edema. *Intensive Care Med.* 2002;28:1267–1272.
221. Sandhu RS, Pasquale MD, Miller K, et al. Measurement of endotracheal tube cuff leak to predict postextubation stridor and need for reintubation. *J Am Coll Surg.* 2000;190:682.
222. Kwon B, Yoo JU, Furey CG, et al. Risk factors for delayed extubation after single-stage, multi-level anterior cervical decompression and posterior fusion. *J Spinal Disord Tech* 2006;19(6):389.
223. Markovitz BP, Randolph AG. Corticosteroids for the prevention of reintubation and postextubation stridor in pediatric patients: a meta-analysis. *Pediatr Crit Care Med.* 2002;3:223.
224. Meade MO, Guyatt GH, Cook DJ, et al. Trials of corticosteroids to prevent postextubation airway complications. *Chest.* 2001;120:464S.
225. Cheng K-C, Hou C-C, Huang H-C, et al. Intravenous injection of methylprednisolone reduces the incidence of postextubation stridor in intensive care unit patients. *Crit Care Med.* 2006;34:1345.
226. Dower AM, George RB, Law JA, et al. Comparison of pre & postintubation Cormack-Lehane and POGO scores using the AirwayCam(r) video system. *Anesthesiology.* 2006;105:A527.
227. Dosemeci L, Yilmaz M, Yegin A, et al. The routine use of pediatric airway exchange catheter after extubation of adult patients who have undergone maxillofacial or major neck surgery: a clinical observational study. *Crit Care.* 2004;8:385.
228. Loudermilk EP, Hartmanngruber M, Stoltfus DP, et al. A prospective study of the safety of tracheal extubation using a pediatric airway exchange catheter for patients with a known difficult airway. *Chest.* 1997;111: 1660.
229. Mort TC. Continuous airway access for the difficult extubation: the efficacy of the airway exchange catheter. *Anesth Analg.* 2007;105(5):1357–1362.
230. Baraka AS. Tension pneumothorax complicating jet ventilation via Cook airway exchange catheter. *Anesthesiology.* 1999;91:557–558.
231. DeLima L, Bishop M. Lung laceration after tracheal extubation over a plastic tube changer. *Anesth Analg.* 1991;73:350–351.
232. Seitz PA, Gravenstein N. Endobronchial rupture from endotracheal reintubation with an endotracheal tube guide. *J Clin Anesth.* 1989;1:214–217.
233. Benumof JL, Gaughan SD. Concerns regarding barotrauma during jet ventilation. *Anesthesiology.* 1992;76:1072–1073.
234. Fetterman D, Dubovoy A, Reay M. Unforeseen esophageal misplacement of airway exchange catheter leading to gastric perforation. *Anesthesiology.* 2006;104:1111–1112.

235. Mort TC. Exchange of a nasal ETT to the oral position: patient safety vs method. *Crit Care Med.* 2005;33(12)S:A114.
236. Smith CE. Exchange of a double-lumen endobronchial tube using fiber-optic laryngoscopy (WuScope) in a difficult intubation patient. *J Clin Anesth.* 2006;18(5):398.
237. Muto T, Akizuki K, Wolford LM. Simplified technique to change the endotracheal tube from nasal to oral to facilitate orthognathic and nasal surgery. *J Oral Max Surg.* 2006;64(8):1310–1312.
238. Wolpert A, Goto H. Exchanging an endotracheal tube from oral to nasal intubation during continuous ventilation. *Anesth Analg.* 2006;103(5):1335.

CHAPTER 39 ■ HYPERBARIC OXYGEN THERAPY

RICHARD E. MOON • JOHN PAUL M. LONGPHRE

The first recorded attempt to use hyperbaric therapy was in 1662, when Henshaw in Britain used an organ bellows to manipulate the pressure within an enclosed chamber designed to seat a patient. He recommended high pressure for acute diseases and low pressure for chronic diseases (1). The pressure fluctuations in either direction were probably quite small. Widespread use of hyperbaric therapy began in the 19th century. At that time, powerful pneumatic pumps were designed, which could be used to compress chambers with air. Physicians in France and Britain used compressed air treatment for miscellaneous conditions. Junod used pressures of 1.5 atmospheres absolute (ATA) to treat patients, but did experiments up to 4 ATA (2). Simpson, using pressures in the range of 1.3 to 1.5 ATA, reported treating a variety of complaints, including dysphonia, asthma, tuberculosis, menorrhagia, and deafness (1), although without any physiologic basis.

Compressed air construction work was also developed in the 1800s, in which men were exposed to elevated ambient pressure within compartments for the purpose of excavating tunnels or bridge piers in muddy soil that was otherwise subject to flooding. Upon decompression at the end of a work shift, workers often developed joint pains or neurologic manifestations (*caisson disease*, *the bends*, or *decompression sickness*). Although the pathophysiology (nitrogen bubble formation in tissues; see below) was not understood, it was observed that recompression of these individuals could relieve the symptoms. Administration of recompression therapy became routine during construction of the Hudson River tunnel in the 1890s (3). All of these treatments used compressed air. Although oxygen breathing under pressure had been suggested for the treatment of decompression sickness as early as 1897 (4) and was used intermittently over the next 30 years, systematic study and use of hyperbaric oxygen would not occur until much later.

Oxygen administration during recompression therapy for decompression sickness increased the efficacy of the treatment (5,6) and is now routinely used for both decompression sickness and gas embolism. The administration of oxygen at increased ambient pressure became known as hyperbaric oxygen (HBO) therapy. In the 1950s, pilot investigations were performed of HBO as a therapy for diseases other than those related to gas bubbles, including carbon monoxide poisoning, clostridial myonecrosis (gas gangrene), and later, selected chronic wounds.

For many years, the Undersea and Hyperbaric Medical Society has regularly reviewed and published information regarding the use of HBO in selected diseases (7), and its recommendations have been widely accepted. The list of accepted indications (7) contains a heterogeneous group of conditions (Table 39.1), suggesting that more than one mechanism mediates the clinical effects of HBO, including the increase in ambient pressure (partly responsible for its efficacy in conditions caused by gas bubble disease) and pharmacologic effects of supraphysiologic increases in blood and tissue PO_2 as discussed below.

EFFECTS OF HYPEROXIA

Blood Gas Values

Under normal clinical HBO therapy conditions (2–3 ATA), breathing 100% oxygen can lead to arterial PO_2 (PaO_2) values that are 10 to 17 times higher than normal (8,9). PaO_2 levels can rise from the normal of 90 to 100 mm Hg (breathing air at sea level, i.e., 1 ATA or normobaria) to 1,000 to 1,700 mm Hg in healthy subjects breathing 100% oxygen at 2 to 3 ATA (see Table 39.2).

One effect is an increase in blood oxygen content:

$$\text{Blood } O_2 \text{ content (mL/dL)} = 1.34 \cdot \text{Hb} \cdot SaO_2/100 + 0.003 \cdot PaO_2 \quad [1]$$

where Hb is hemoglobin concentration (g/dL), SaO_2 is arterial Hb-O_2 saturation, and PaO_2 is arterial oxygen tension.

The second term of Eq. 1 represents the dissolved oxygen proportion, which under normal circumstances represents a small fraction of total arterial oxygen content, and is therefore often disregarded. However, during HBO, this dissolved fraction is substantially increased (see Table 39.2). In fact, mixed venous Hb-O_2 saturation is 100% under resting conditions while breathing 100% oxygen at 3 ATA. Thus, oxygen delivery can be maintained under these circumstances without hemoglobin. This was shown by Boerema et al. in a swine model (10).

$PaCO_2$ is not significantly affected by the increased pressure (8,9,11), although the venoarterial PCO_2 difference is slightly increased, mostly because of a reduction in cardiac output.

TABLE 39.1

CONDITIONS AMENABLE TO TREATMENT WITH HYPERBARIC OXYGEN THERAPY

Gas bubble disease
- Air or gas embolism[a] (236–238)
- Decompression sickness[a] (237,238)

Poisonings
- Carbon monoxide poisoning[a] (151–153,239)
- Cyanide (154,165)
- Carbon tetrachloride (176,240)
- Hydrogen sulfide (154,168,169)

Necrotizing soft tissue infections
- Clostridial myositis and myonecrosis[a] (181,241–243)
- Mixed aerobic/anaerobic necrotizing soft tissue infections[a] (182,184,243,244)
- Mucormycosis (187,245)

Aerobic infections
- Refractory osteomyelitis[a] (7)
- Intracranial abscess[a] (7)
- Streptococcal myositis (48)

Acute ischemia
- Crush injury, compartment syndrome, and other acute traumatic ischemic conditions[a] (246)
- Compromised skin grafts and flaps[a] (31,33,247,248)

Acute hypoxia
- Acute exceptional anemia[a] (191)
- Support of oxygenation during therapeutic lung lavage (219,249)

Thermal burns[a] (197,198,200,250)

Delayed radiation injury (soft tissue and osteoradionecrosis)[a] (7,251–254)

Enhancement of healing in selected problem wounds[a] (7,255)

Envenomation
- Brown recluse spider bite (256,257)

[a]Approved by the Undersea and Hyperbaric Medical Society (Gesell LB, ed. *Hyperbaric Oxygen Therapy: A Committee Report.* Durham, NC. Undersea and Hyperbaric Medical Society; 2008; see also: http://www.uhms.org).

Vasoconstriction

Hyperoxia causes peripheral vasoconstriction (8,9,12), regardless of atmospheric pressure (13). At a mere 2 ATA, systemic vascular resistance can increase by 30% in dogs (14). The mechanisms for this include scavenging of nitric oxide (NO) by superoxide anion (O_2^-) (15) and increased binding of NO at high PO_2 to hemoglobin, forming S-nitrosohemoglobin (9). Vasoconstriction has the positive effect of reducing edema in injured tissues and surgical flaps (discussed later). During HBO, the arterial blood O_2 content is sufficiently high that despite vasoconstriction and reduced blood flow, oxygen delivery is increased (16) (see also Table 39.2). Although peripheral vasoconstriction occurs in normal skin during hyperbaric oxygen exposure, repetitive intermittent HBO appears to increase the microvascular blood flow of healing wounds (17).

Hemodynamics

Heart rate and cardiac output both decrease by 13% to 35% under hyperbaric conditions (Table 39.2) (8,9,14,18,19). Small changes may occur in systemic and pulmonary artery pressure, with an increase in systemic vascular resistance (SVR) and a decrease in pulmonary vascular resistance (PVR) (9). Despite the reduced cardiac output, oxygen delivery is increased (Fig. 39.1).

Organ Blood Flow

Studies in large animals indicate that the decrease in peripheral blood flow is limited primarily to the cerebral and peripheral vascular beds, with other organs unaffected (14). In rats, HBO has been shown to decrease organ blood flow, including the myocardium, kidney, brain, ocular globe, and gut (15,20–22). In autonomically blocked conscious dogs at 3 ATA, coronary blood flow is decreased (23). Another dog study at 2 ATA revealed no change in coronary, hepatic, renal, or mesenteric blood flow (14).

Cellular and Tissue Effects

In a myocutaneous flap model during reperfusion following 4 hours of ischemia, Zamboni et al. described a delayed decrease in blood flow (24). This flow reduction appears to be associated with adherence of leukocytes to the endothelium of the small vessels, an effect that is significantly inhibited by HBO. A delayed reduction in cerebral blood flow has also been observed after arterial gas embolism in the brain (25), which has similarly been attributed to leukocyte accumulation in the capillaries (26). HBO reduces cerebral infarct volume and myeloperoxidase activity, a marker of neutrophil recruitment (27). In other studies using animal models, it has been observed that HBO pretreatment reduces ischemia/reperfusion injury to the liver (28). HBO reduces ischemia/reperfusion injury to the intestine (29,30) and muscle (31), as well as reducing ischemia-induced necrosis in muscle (32–37), brain (38,39), and kidney (40). One mechanism for this effect of HBO appears to be the inhibition of leukocyte β_2-integrin function (41–43). Part of the beneficial effect of HBO in these settings is speculated to be due to the prevention of endothelial leukocyte adherence. After focal ischemia, HBO also reduces postischemic blood–brain barrier damage and edema (44) and has an anti-apoptotic effect (45).

Antibacterial Effects

The increase in PO_2 during HBO can be toxic to anaerobic bacteria, which lack antioxidant defense mechanisms. In addition, HBO has effects on aerobic organisms via neutrophil mechanisms. Killing of aerobic bacteria by leukocytes is related to the O_2-dependent generation of reactive oxygen species within the lysosomes. *In vitro* studies have demonstrated that phagocytic killing of *Staphylococcus aureus* by polymorphonuclear leukocytes becomes less effective as ambient PO_2 is decreased. This mechanism appears to be important *in vivo* when tissue

TABLE 39.2

BLOOD GAS AND HEMODYNAMIC VALUES IN 14 HEALTHY ADULTS BREATHING SPONTANEOUSLY (MEAN ± STANDARD DEVIATION)

Condition	PaO_2 (mm Hg)	SaO_2 (%)	$P\bar{v}O_2$ (mm Hg)	$S\bar{v}O_2$ (%)	$PaCO_2$ (mm Hg)	$P\bar{v}CO_2$ (mm Hg)	Hb (g/dL)	Arterial O_2 content (mL/dL)	Dissolved O_2 (%)
1 ATA, air	93 ± 9	96 ± 2	42 ± 2	76 ± 3	38 ± 3	42 ± 3	12.7 ± 0.8	16.6 ± 1.1	1.7 ± 0.2
3 ATA, 100% O_2	1,493 ± 224	98 ± 3	378 ± 164	98 ± 2	35 ± 2	43 ± 3	12.7 ± 0.8	21.1 ± 1.3	21.2 ± 3.0

Condition	HR (bpm)	Cardiac output (L min^{-1})	Mean arterial pressure (mm Hg)	Mean pulmonary artery pressure (mm Hg)	PA wedge pressure (mm Hg)	SVR (dynes sec cm^{-5})	PVR (dynes sec cm^{-5})
1 ATA, air	66.6 ± 8.2	6.5 ± 1.1	92.5 ± 10.5	13.6 ± 3.4	8.2 ± 3.9	1,118 ± 235	67 ± 24
3 ATA, 100% O_2	62.7 ± 12.5	5.9 ± 1.0	94.9 ± 9.4	12.4 ± 2.1	9.3 ± 2.5	1,286 ± 309	41 ± 11

ATA, atmospheres absolute; HR, heart rate; SVR, systemic vascular resistance; PVR, pulmonary vascular resistance. These data obtained in part from McMahon TJ, Moon RE, Luschinger BP, et al. Nitric oxide in the human respiratory cycle. *Nat Med.* 2002;8:711–717.

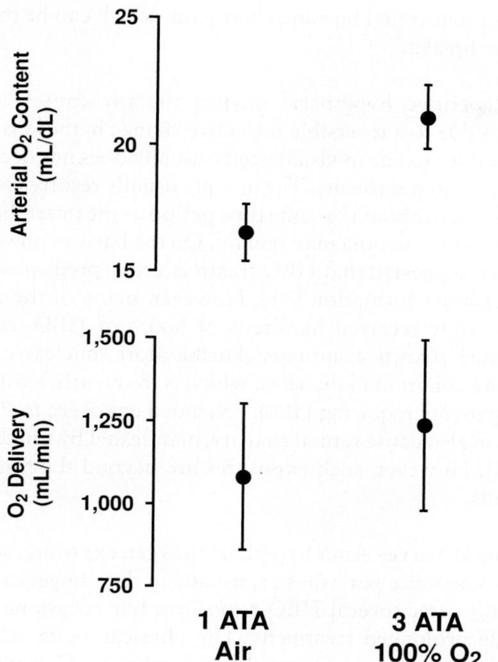

FIGURE 39.1. Arterial O_2 content and delivery while breathing air at 1 atmosphere absolute (ATA) or 100% oxygen at 3 ATA. Measurements are shown in a group of normal volunteers. (Data from McMahon TJ, Moon RE, Luschinger BP, et al. Nitric oxide in the human respiratory cycle. *Nat Med.* 2002;8:711–717.)

PO_2 is low (e.g., in osteomyelitis) (46). In an animal model of osteomyelitis, the cidal effect of tobramycin against *Pseudomonas* was increased when tissue PO_2 was raised by the administration of 100% O_2 at increased ambient pressure (47). Published evidence also supports an augmentation of penicillin by HBO in the treatment of soft tissue streptococcal infections (48).

Oxygen Toxicity

Pharmacology

Exposure of an animal to increased partial pressure of oxygen results in higher rates of endogenous production of reactive oxygen species, including superoxide anion (O_2^-), hydroxyl radical ($OH^\bullet$), hydrogen peroxide (H_2O_2), and singlet oxygen, which are responsible for tissue oxygen toxicity (49–51). Tissue O_2 toxicity includes the following: Lipid peroxidation, sulfhydryl group inactivation, oxidation of pyridine nucleotides, inactivation of Na^+–K^+–ATPase and inhibition of DNA, and protein synthesis. Toxic effects of these species depend upon both dose and duration of O_2 exposure. In the central nervous system, HBO initially reduces NO availability and causes vasoconstriction. HBO stimulates neuronal nitric oxide production and causes the accumulation of peroxynitrite. Prior to onset of a seizure, NO levels and blood flow both increase above control levels (52,53). This, in turn, decreases brain γ-aminobutyric acid (GABA) levels, creating an imbalance between glutamatergic and GABAergic synaptic function, which is believed to be partly responsible for central nervous system (CNS) O_2 toxicity (54).

Clinical Effects

At sufficiently high PO_2, any organ can be susceptible to oxygen toxicity. However, within the clinical range of inspired PO_2 (1–3 ATA), the most susceptible tissues are the lung, brain, retina, lens, and peripheral nerve.

Brain. Oxygen toxicity of the central nervous system produces a wide variety of manifestations (55). The most common mild symptom is nausea; the most dramatic is generalized nonfocal convulsions. These are usually self-limited, even without pharmacologic treatment, and have no long-term effects. The occurrence of a hyperoxic seizure does not imply the development of a convulsive disorder. Factors that increase the risk of CNS oxygen toxicity include hypercapnia and probably fever.

CNS O_2 toxicity is uncommon when inspired PO_2 is less than 3 ATA. While in-water convulsions in divers have been recorded at an inspired PO_2 of 1.3 ATA, convulsions during clinical hyperbaric oxygen therapy occur in only a small fraction of treatments. Approximately 0.02% of treatments at an inspired PO_2 of 2 ATA and 4% at 3 ATA. At an inspired PO_2 less than 3 ATA, the risk of convulsions increases markedly, particularly in patients with sepsis. While anecdotal reports suggest that HBO may precipitate seizures in patients who have an underlying predisposition (56), there are no epidemiologic data to confirm this. When indicated, HBO should not be withheld on the basis of an underlying seizure disorder.

Both CNS and pulmonary toxicity can be delayed by the use of air breaks (a period of a few minutes where air is administered in lieu of 100% oxygen) (57–60). Oftentimes, the aura of a hyperoxic convulsion occurs in the form of nausea or facial paresthesias. The patient can be given an air break to avert such a convulsion. Once the symptoms have resolved (usually within a few minutes), the oxygen can be restarted without recurrence. During the tonic-clonic phase of a seizure, the airway may be obstructed. Therefore, it is imperative that chamber pressure not be reduced during this time in order to avoid pulmonary barotrauma and the possibility of arterial gas embolism. After a convulsion, some practitioners recommend administering prophylactic medication for the duration of HBO.

Prophylactic anticonvulsants such as phenytoin, phenobarbital, or benzodiazepines can reduce the chance of convulsions when utilizing clinical treatment schedules with a significant risk of CNS O_2 toxicity (e.g., treatment pressure >3 ATA). The authors' practice is to load septic patients intravenously with phenobarbital as tolerated, up to 12 mg/kg, prior to hyperbaric oxygen treatment at 3 ATA, with doses every 8 hours to maintain a serum concentration in the therapeutic anticonvulsant range. When using inspired $PO_2 \leq 2.8$ ATA, the risk of CNS toxicity is sufficiently low that prophylactic anticonvulsant therapy is not required.

Hyperoxic seizures and other CNS manifestations in diabetics can be caused by HBO-induced reduction in blood glucose. Therefore, the occurrence of CNS O_2 toxicity in a patient with diabetes during HBO treatment should prompt the immediate measurement of plasma glucose. When blood PO_2 is extremely high, bedside glucose measurement devices, particularly those dependent upon a glucose oxidase reaction, can be inaccurate, producing measurements that significantly underestimate the true value (61). Laboratory-based glucose measurement is usually accurate.

Lungs. Pulmonary oxygen toxicity during hyperbaric oxygen therapy is also PO_2 and time dependent. Clinical HBO protocols have been empirically developed to minimize the risk of pulmonary O_2 toxicity, which almost never occurs during routine daily or twice-daily clinical treatments. However, it can occur during extended treatments that are used for treating gas embolism or decompression sickness, in which inspired PO_2 is as high as 2.8 ATA. The initial manifestation is usually a burning substernal chest pain and cough (62), which is most likely due to tracheobronchitis. Continued exposure to oxygen can produce more severe manifestations such as dyspnea and acute respiratory distress syndrome (ARDS). Measurable abnormalities include reduced forced vital capacity and carbon monoxide transfer factor (DLCO). Pulmonary oxygen toxicity symptoms may not be evident in patients who are sedated and mechanically ventilated. Moreover, such patients often have pulmonary infiltrates for a variety of reasons and it may be impossible to distinguish the possible additive effects of pulmonary O_2 toxicity.

While the maximum safe inspired PO_2 during clinical hyperbaric oxygen therapy is based mainly upon CNS O_2 toxicity limits, the safe exposure *duration* is determined by pulmonary limits. Prediction formulas have been developed that approximate the average reduction in vital capacity after continuous oxygen exposure (63–65). However, the usefulness of these algorithms for individual patients is severely limited due to individual variability and comorbid factors that may affect O_2 susceptibility, such as prior exposure, intermittent exposure, and endotoxemia. HBO treatment schedules that include periods of air breathing ("air breaks") interspersed between O_2 periods reduce the rate of onset of both pulmonary and CNS toxic manifestations and can increase the overall dose of oxygen that is tolerated. In the awake patient, the occurrence of burning, retrosternal chest pain is a more useful indicator of incipient pulmonary toxicity.

If standard HBO treatment schedules are used (e.g., 2 ATA/2 hours, 2.5 ATA/90 minutes one to two times daily, or U.S. Navy treatment tables), pulmonary O_2 toxicity is almost never clinically evident. It is seen only with the most extreme levels of hyperbaric exposure such as may be required for severe neurologic decompression illness. Furthermore, most minor pulmonary oxygen toxicity resolves within 12 to 24 hours of air breathing. Complete reversal of vital capacity (VC) decrements, as large as 40% of control, has been observed after extended O_2 exposure at 2 ATA (66). Therefore, in clinical situations requiring aggressive HBO therapy such as spinal cord decompression sickness or arterial gas embolism, some degree of pulmonary O_2 toxicity is acceptable.

Supplemental O_2 administration at 1 ATA between HBO treatments can accelerate the onset of symptoms of pulmonary O_2 toxicity during subsequent HBO. Thus, if O_2 is absolutely required between HBO treatments, it is prudent to use the lowest concentration.

Some antineoplastic agents, such as bleomycin (67,68) and mitomycin C (69), can predispose to fatal pulmonary O_2 toxicity, probably due to drug-induced reduction in antioxidant defenses. The risk of pulmonary O_2 toxicity due to HBO therapy in patients with previous exposure to either of these agents is unknown, although 6 months after the agent has been discontinued, HBO seems to be safe. Even after this point, in some patients, HBO induces mild pulmonary O_2 toxicity symptoms such as retrosternal burning chest pain, which can be managed with air breaks.

Eye. Repetitive hyperbaric oxygen therapy causes myopia, which is due to a reversible refractive change in the lens (70). A measurable change in visual acuity usually does not occur until after 20 or so treatments. The myopia usually resolves over several weeks, in about the same time period as the onset; however, some residual myopia may remain. On the basis of one study, it has been suggested that HBO treatment may predispose to nuclear cataract formation (71). However, many of the patients in this study received hundreds of hours of HBO, considerably more than is customary. Furthermore, nuclear cataracts are more common in diabetes, which is frequently a comorbidity in patients requiring HBO. Extended exposure to PO_2 of 3 ATA can also cause retinal toxicity, manifested by tunnel vision (72,73). However, such exposures are beyond the range used clinically.

Peripheral Nerve. After hyperbaric oxygen exposure, some patients experience paresthesias, usually in their fingers and toes, generally after several HBO exposures but occasionally after a single prolonged treatment. The physical exam is normal, and the symptoms resolve within a few hours. This manifestation has no known clinical significance and is not a reason to discontinue hyperbaric therapy.

PHYSICAL EFFECTS OF COMPRESSION/DECOMPRESSION

Boyle's Law

Clinically, the complications of HBO therapy that most frequently occur are those related to the body's gas-containing spaces (74). Dealing with volume changes in these gas-containing spaces is unique to HBO therapy. For a gas, absolute pressure and volume are inversely related. The increase in pressure during HBO treatment will therefore decrease the volume of closed gas-containing spaces within the body, such as the gastrointestinal tract or middle ear and, in the event of gas embolism or decompression sickness, bubbles.

EFFECTS OF GASES OTHER THAN OXYGEN

Nitrogen

The narcotic properties of compressed air were first reported by Junod in 1835 as described by Bennett and Rostain (75). Hyperbaric nitrogen causes narcosis or pleasant intoxication at pressures greater than about 4 ATA in most individuals and near unconsciousness at greater than 10 ATA (76). Since patients breathe oxygen, nitrogen narcosis is only a problem for tenders in multiplace hyperbaric chambers. However, most hyperbaric treatments occur between 2 and 3 ATA, where symptoms of nitrogen narcosis are exceedingly mild.

Nitrogen (and other inert breathing gases such as helium) is the major causative agent of decompression sickness. During decompression, excess tissue nitrogen can become supersaturated, come out of solution, and form bubbles. This can lead to decompression sickness, with manifestations depending on their location and secondary effects.

Trace Gases

The pharmacologic effects of gases are proportional to their partial pressures. Although a trace gas may only be present in minute quantities, as the chamber pressure rises, so does the partial pressure of a gas. Therefore, gases such as carbon monoxide or carbon dioxide in concentrations that have no pharmacologic or toxic effects at 1 ATA may exert measurable effects in a hyperbaric environment.

USE OF HYPERBARIC OXYGEN FOR SPECIFIC DISEASES

Gas Embolism and Decompression Sickness

Gas bubbles in the body can be due to direct gas entry via veins or arteries (arterial or venous gas embolism) or via *in situ* formation due to gas supersaturation in divers, compressed air workers, or aviators (decompression sickness). Since the two conditions often both occur in the same patient (particularly in divers), the principles of treatment of the two are the same. The syndrome of either or both condition is commonly referred to as *decompression illness* (DCI).

Arterial and Venous Gas Embolism

Entry of gas into the circulation can occur via several mechanisms. Gas embolism has recently been reviewed (77,78). In divers breathing compressed gas, arterial gas embolism (AGE) can ensue if decompression (ascent) occurs while the diver holds his or her breath or due to gas trapping caused by focal or generalized airways obstruction. AGE due to this mechanism can result after an ascent to the surface of as little as 1 meter. AGE can also occur during diagnostic or therapeutic procedures such as angiography.

Venous gas embolism (VGE) can result due to direct injection or entry via an open vein in which ambient pressure exceeds venous pressure. This can exist during laparoscopic surgical procedures due to the elevated intra-abdominal pressure, or open procedures in which venous pressure in the surgical wound is subatmospheric. The classic scenario for this is an intracranial procedure in the sitting position. However, it has also been described in procedures such as liver resection, cesarean section, and spine surgery. VGE can also occur due to oral hydrogen peroxide (H_2O_2) ingestion. H_2O_2 absorbed into the circulation is broken down by catalase into water and oxygen bubbles. VGE can result if a central venous catheter is opened to air, particularly if the patient is breathing spontaneously. It has also been reported in patients with ARDS being ventilated with positive end-expiratory pressure (79). VGE has been described during orogenital sex after blowing air intravaginally (80). Intravenous injection is better tolerated than intra-arterial injection because of the pulmonary filter. However, if the rate of entry of gas into the veins is sufficiently high, bubbles can traverse the pulmonary capillary network and become arterial emboli. Large volumes can obstruct the right heart or pulmonary artery and cause cardiac arrest.

Large volumes of arterial gas can cause acute obstruction of large vessels. Small quantities tend to remain in the circulation only transiently; however, they can precipitate a sustained reduction in local blood flow (25). The mechanism appears to be endothelial damage (81) and adherence of leukocytes (26,82–84). Endothelial barrier function is also impaired in both the brain and lung, resulting in edema (85,86) and impaired endothelial-dependent vasoactivity (87). Animal models of AGE have revealed a significant elevation of intracranial pressure (ICP) and depression of cerebral PO_2 (88,89). In a pig model, hyperventilation failed to correct these parameters (90); however, HBO at 2.8 ATA (U.S. Navy Table 6, Fig. 39.4) restored both ICP and brain PO_2 toward normal (Fig. 39.3).

Clinical manifestations of AGE include acute loss of consciousness, confusion, focal neurologic abnormalities, and cerebral edema. VGE causes acute dyspnea, tachypnea, hypotension, cardiac ischemia or arrest, and pulmonary edema (86). In monitored patients, VGE is often heralded by a decrease in end-tidal PCO_2 (91), although sometimes, with small volumes of CO_2 embolism such as during laparoscopy, it may be increased. A mill-wheel murmur can be heard in some patients, although this sign is neither sensitive nor specific. Venous gas bubbles in sufficient quantities can cross into the arterial circulation (producing AGE) either through the pulmonary capillary network or via an intracardiac shunt, such as a patent foramen ovale.

Imaging is not useful for diagnosing either VGE or AGE. Gas bubbles are rarely visible on radiographic images (92). Except in cases where associated conditions such as pneumothorax are suspected or neurologic conditions such as hemorrhage require exclusion, imaging studies are not necessary and tend to delay definitive treatment.

Decompression Sickness

During diving or exposure to a compressed gas environment such as a hyperbaric chamber, inert gas (usually nitrogen) is taken up by tissues. During decompression, inert gas can become supersaturated and form bubbles *in situ* in tissues. Certain tissues are more susceptible to *in situ* bubble formation.

Manifestations of decompression sickness (DCS) can range from mild to severe (Fig. 39.2). The most common

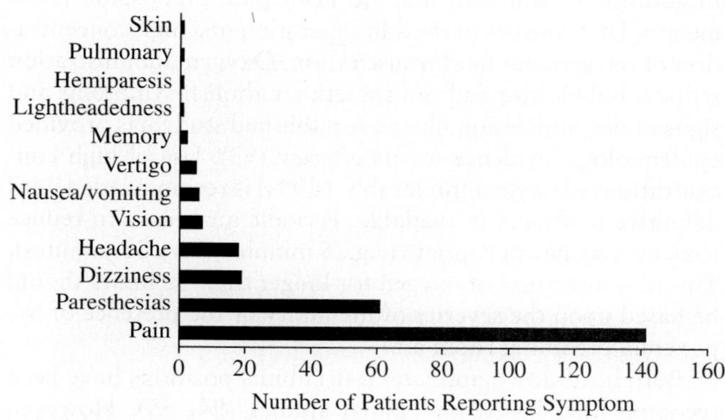

FIGURE 39.2. Symptoms of decompression illness in a series of recreational divers. (Redrawn from Divers Alert Network. *Annual Diving Report.* Durham, NC: Divers Alert Network; 2006.)

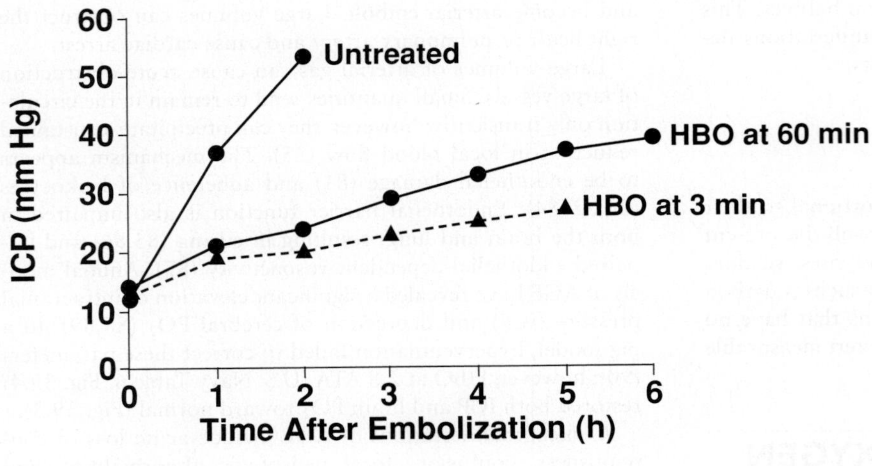

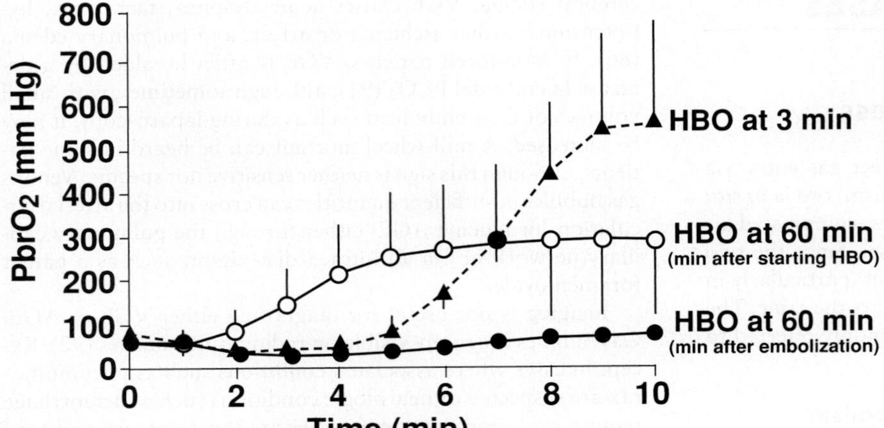

FIGURE 39.3. Effect of hyperbaric oxygen (HBO) on intracranial pressure (ICP) and brain PO_2 in pigs after air embolism. **Top panel:** HBO initially at 2.8 atmospheres absolute (ATA) (U.S. Navy Table 6) reduces ICP compared with no treatment, whether it is started 3 minutes or 60 minutes after embolization. **Bottom panel:** Brain tissue PO_2 in the two groups of animals. For the 60-minute group, the closed circles represent $PbrO_2$ in the first 10 minutes after embolization; the open circles represent $PbrO_2$ in the first 10 minutes after the start of HBO. Values in lower panel are mean ± standard deviation. (Redrawn from van Hulst RA, Drenthen J, Haitsma JJ, et al. Effects of hyperbaric treatment in cerebral air embolism on intracranial pressure, brain oxygenation, and brain glucose metabolism in the pig. *Crit Care Med.* 2005;33:841–846.)

manifestations are joint pain and paresthesias. Although mild cases can progress to severe, severe manifestations almost always occur within 12 hours after surfacing.

Treatment of Decompression Sickness and Arterial Gas Embolism

Prehospital Treatment

In addition to standard first aid principles, prehospital treatment of DCI consists of the administration of a high concentration of oxygen and fluid resuscitation. Oxygen administration reduces bubble size and can sometimes abolish symptoms and signs of decompression illness. A published study has provided epidemiologic evidence for its efficacy (93). Use of high concentrations of oxygen (preferably 100%) is recommended until definitive treatment is available. Periodic air breaks to reduce toxicity may be appropriate (e.g., 5 minutes every 30 minutes). The administration of oxygen for longer than 12 hours should be based upon the severity of the injury or the presence of hypoxemia breathing room air.

Both head-down and lateral decubitus positions have been recommended based on animal studies (94, 95). However, the hemodynamic response to venous gas embolism is unaffected by body position (96,97), and prolonged head-down position may exacerbate cerebral edema (98). Supine position is therefore recommended, also because patient access and supportive therapies can be more easily administered in this position.

Hospital Treatment

Standard treatment of gas embolism includes airway and ventilatory management, maintaining a high PaO_2 and normal $PaCO_2$ (99) (Fig. 39.3), and support of arterial pressure. Like other forms of neurologic injury, it is recommended that when managing neurologic DCI, both hyperthermia and hyperglycemia (>140–185 mg/dL, 7.8–10.3 mM/L) should be avoided or treated (100).

Physical Removal of Gas

Physical removal of gas after massive arterial gas embolism has been described in cardiopulmonary bypass (101,102). Venous gas embolism has been successfully treated with chest compression (103) and aspiration through catheters in the right atrium (104,105) or pulmonary artery (106).

Recompression

Although symptomatic improvement can be obtained with oxygen at 1 ATA, the definitive treatment of both forms of decompression illness is hyperbaric oxygen. The safety and efficacy of HBO for the treatment of divers was initially shown 70 years ago (6). Since then, treatment protocols have been

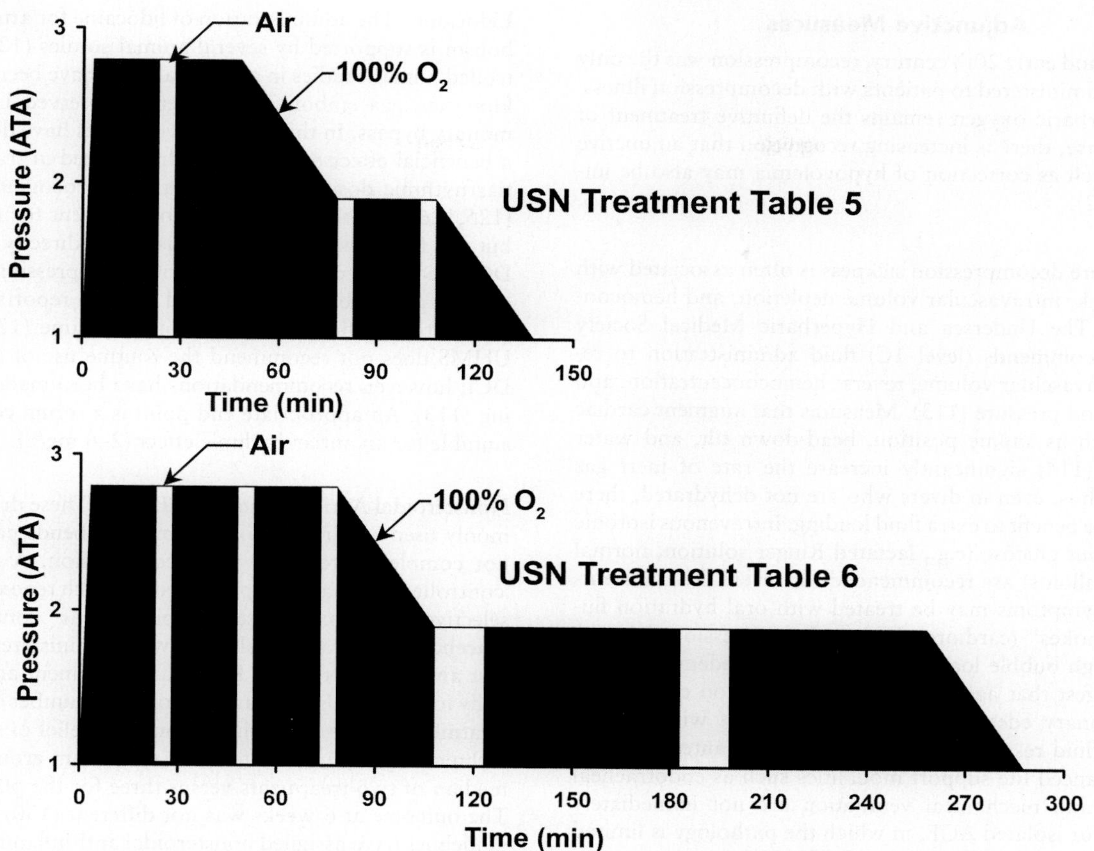

FIGURE 39.4. **Top:** U.S. Navy (USN) Treatment Table 5. According to USN guidelines, this table may be used for symptoms involving skin (except for cutis marmorata), the lymphatic system, muscles and joints, with a normal neurologic exam, and when all symptoms have completely resolved within 10 minutes of reaching 2.8 atmospheres absolute (ATA). **Bottom:** USN Treatment Table 6. This table may be used for all types of decompression illness. Extensions (additional oxygen breathing cycles) can be administered at either treatment pressure (2.8 and 1.9 ATA). (Data from Navy Department. *US Navy Diving Manual.* Revision 4. Vol. 5: Diving Medicine and Recompression Chamber Operations. NAVSEA 0910-LP-103-8009. Washington, DC: Naval Sea Systems Command; 2005.)

empirically developed that have been shown to have a high degree of success with a low probability of oxygen toxicity (107). The most widely used treatment protocols ("tables") were developed by the U.S. Navy and promulgated via the *Diving Manual* (108) (Fig. 39.4). Both U.S. Navy Treatment Tables 5 and 6 use 100% oxygen breathing periods ("O_2 cycles") interspersed with air breathing periods ("air breaks") at 2.8 and 1.9 ATA in a two-step pattern (see Fig. 39.4). Guidelines are available to administer additional O_2 cycles ("extensions") at both pressures (108). The vast majority, if not all cases, of DCI can be adequately treated using U.S. Navy treatment tables.

The U.S. Navy tables were designed for use in multiplace chambers, where air breaks can easily be administered by discontinuing O_2. Since monoplace chambers were designed to be compressed with 100% O_2, shorter alternate treatment tables were designed for their use (109,110) (Fig. 39.5). Although direct comparisons with U.S. Navy tables have never been performed, case series suggest that these tables are efficacious for DCI (110). Monoplace chambers fitted with an air supply and delivery system can be used to administer treatment according to traditional Navy tables (111).

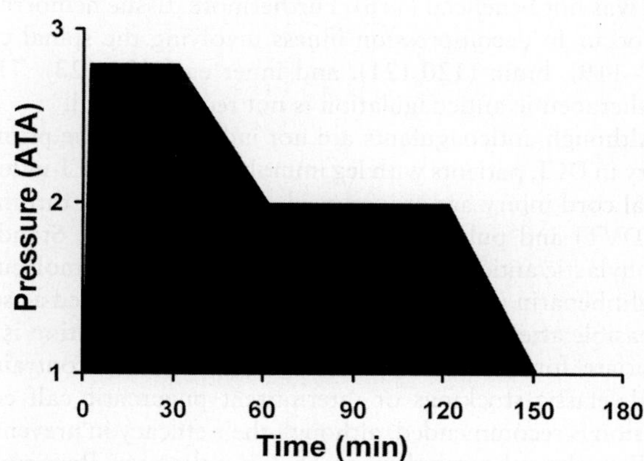

FIGURE 39.5. Hart-Kindwall monoplace treatment table. This table was designed for use in monoplace chambers without the capability of administering air breaks. Except for the lack of air breaks and limited ability for extension, it is similar to U.S. Navy Table 5, with a shorter time at 2.8 atmospheres absolute (ATA) and longer time at 1.9 ATA. (Data from Boerema I, Meyne NG, Brummelkamp WH, et al. Life without blood. *J Cardiovasc Surg [Torino]*. 1960;1:133–146.)

Adjunctive Measures

In the 19th and early 20th century, recompression was the only treatment administered to patients with decompression illness. While hyperbaric oxygen remains the definitive treatment of bubble disease, there is increasing recognition that adjunctive therapies such as correction of hypovolemia may also be important (112).

Fluids. Severe decompression sickness is often associated with capillary leak, intravascular volume depletion, and hemoconcentration. The Undersea and Hyperbaric Medical Society (UHMS) recommends (level 1C) fluid administration to replenish intravascular volume, reverse hemoconcentration, and support blood pressure (113). Measures that augment cardiac preload such as supine position, head-down tilt, and water immersion (114) significantly increase the rate of inert gas washout. Thus, even in divers who are not dehydrated, there may be some benefit to extra fluid loading. Intravenous isotonic fluids without glucose (e.g., lactated Ringer solution, normal saline, or colloids) are recommended for severe DCI. Patients with mild symptoms may be treated with oral hydration fluids. For "chokes" (cardiorespiratory decompression sickness, in which high bubble loads cause pulmonary edema), animal studies suggest that aggressive fluid resuscitation can exacerbate pulmonary edema. Thus, for the patient with chokes, aggressive fluid resuscitation may not be warranted, particularly if advanced life support modalities such as endotracheal intubation and mechanical ventilation are not immediately available. For isolated AGE, in which the pathology is limited to cerebral infarction, aggressive fluid administration is also unwarranted.

Anticoagulants. Intravascular bubbles can induce platelet accumulation, adherence, and thrombus formation. Indeed, in a canine model of arterial gas embolism, therapeutic anticoagulation promoted a return in a short-term outcome: evoked potential amplitude, but only when heparin was combined with prostaglandin I_2 (PGI_2) and indomethacin (115). In this model, heparin alone was ineffective. In other experiments, heparin given either prophylactically or therapeutically to dogs with DCI was not beneficial (116). Furthermore, tissue hemorrhage can occur in decompression illness involving the spinal cord (117–119), brain (120,121), and inner ear (122,123). Thus, full therapeutic anticoagulation is not recommended.

Although anticoagulants are not indicated for the primary injury in DCI, patients with leg immobility due to DCI-induced spinal cord injury are at increased risk of deep vein thrombosis (DVT) and pulmonary thromboembolism (PE). Standard prophylactic anticoagulant measures, typically low-molecular-weight heparin (LMWH), are therefore recommended as soon as feasible after the onset of injury. Full anticoagulation is appropriate for established DVT/PE. If LMWH is contraindicated, elastic stockings or intermittent pneumatic calf compression is recommended, although their efficacy in preventing DVT or thromboembolism in DCI is unknown. Recommendations have been extrapolated from guidelines for traumatic spinal cord injury; neither their efficacy nor safety in neurologic DCI has been specifically confirmed. Thus, when facilities exist, a screening test for DVT a few days after injury is appropriate (113).

Lidocaine. The administration of lidocaine for arterial gas embolism is supported by several animal studies (124). No controlled human studies in accidental AGE have been performed. However, gas emboli are frequently observed in cardiopulmonary bypass. In this setting, two studies have demonstrated a beneficial effect of lidocaine administered in traditional antiarrhythmic doses on postoperative neurocognitive function (125,126). Another study has shown benefit for nondiabetics but not for diabetics (127). Human data directly pertinent to DCI are confined to three cases of decompression sickness or arterial gas embolism, published as case reports, which appeared to benefit from intravenous lidocaine (128,129). The UHMS does not recommend the routine use of lidocaine for DCI; however, recommendations have been made for its dosing (113). An appropriate end point is a serum concentration suitable for an antiarrhythmic effect (2–6 mg/L).

Nonsteroidal Anti-inflammatory Drugs. These drugs are commonly used empirically for treatment of bends pain that does not completely resolve with recompression. A randomized, controlled trial has been published in which tenoxicam, a nonselective cyclo-oxygenase inhibitor, was compared with placebo. Tenoxicam or placebo was administered during the first air break of the first hyperbaric treatment and continued daily for 7 days. Using as an end point the number of hyperbaric treatments required to achieve complete relief of symptoms or a clinical "plateau" of effect, the tenoxicam group required a median of two treatments versus three for the placebo group. The outcome at 6 weeks was not different (130). The UHMS guidelines have assigned nonsteroidal anti-inflammatory drugs a level 2B recommendation (113).

Corticosteroids. Unless given prophylactically, corticosteroids have not been shown to be of benefit in animal models of DCI (131–133). In a pig study, methylprednisolone treatment did not protect against severe DCS, and the treated animals had a greater mortality (134). In the absence of human trials of corticosteroids in DCI and the lack of benefit in animal studies, corticosteroids are not recommended.

Perfluorocarbons. Perfluorocarbons (PFCs) are a family of chemically inert, water-insoluble, synthetic compounds with a high solubility for both inert gases and oxygen, which may eventually become available for human use as blood substitutes. Intravenous injection of PFC emulsions could augment oxygen delivery to ischemic tissues with impaired circulation and facilitate inert gas washout from tissues (135). Indeed, beneficial effects have been observed in animal studies of both decompression sickness and gas embolism (136–140). There may also be a benefit from the surfactant properties in the treatment of intravascular gas bubbles (141).

Arterial Gas Embolism and Decompression Sickness Treatment Summary

Immediate treatment of AGE or DCS includes standard principles of first aid, including the administration of oxygen and fluids during transport to a hyperbaric chamber. If the patient is in an extremely remote location from which transport is not feasible and the manifestations are minor, if the patient's condition does not progress for 24 hours, and if the neurologic exam is normal, the risk of emergent transport may exceed the risk of conservative treatment (142).

Carbon Monoxide

Carbon monoxide (CO) is an important cause of unintentional poisoning fatalities in the United States each year (143). CO binds to hemoproteins, including hemoglobin and myoglobin, interfering with oxygen transport. It also binds to the mitochondrial cytochrome C oxidase in the electron transport chain (similar to cyanide), impairing oxidative phosphorylation, stopping the cell's energy production, and resulting in cellular hypoxia (144–146) and oxidative stress (147). In addition, CO exposure induces intravascular platelet–neutrophil activation (148). CO-related oxidative stress can cause chemical alterations in myelin basic protein (149), triggering immune-mediated neurologic deficits.

The symptoms and signs of CO poisoning include headache (or tightness across forehead), weakness, nausea and vomiting, syncope, tachycardia, tachypnea, and encephalopathy. Myocardial ischemia is also a common finding.

For survivors of this poisoning, the most debilitating results can be the late neurologic sequelae. These are often cognitive problems such as a decrement in short-term memory (150–152). Some patients improve clinically and then deteriorate several days after the event.

HBO therapy is known to accelerate the elimination of CO (153,154). Pace et al. found that the half-life of CO was longest when breathing air (214 minutes). Half-life decreased to 42 minutes breathing 100% O_2 at 1 ATA and further to 18 minutes with 100% O_2 at 2.5 ATA (153). The reduction in half-life may be important in preventing cell death by allowing mitochondrial adenosine triphosphate (ATP) production to resume before the cell would have otherwise died (144,155). In animal studies, HBO administration after acute CO exposure appears to minimize the lipid peroxidation in the brain, which occurs during or after removal of CO (147), and results in more rapid repletion of brain energy stores (155).

A double-blind randomized control trial carried out by Weaver et al. indicates that HBO therapy can prevent the occurrence of the late neurologic sequelae of CO poisoning if the patients are treated within 24 hours of the exposure (152).

All patients should be initially treated with 100% normobaric oxygen. HBO therapy is usually reserved for patients who have more severe poisoning, as determined by high HbCO level (e.g. $\geq$25%), loss of consciousness, or other neurologic manifestations, or myocardial ischemia, arrhythmias, or other cardiac abnormalities (152,154,156–158). A systematic analysis of 163 patients with CO poisoning who did not receive HBO revealed the following two risk factors for sequelae: older age and longer CO exposure (159). However, some patients without these risk factors also developed sequelae. The authors concluded that, in addition to other indications, regardless of HbCO level or loss of consciousness, anyone older than 36 years with symptoms should receive HBO.

Pregnant women should be treated according to maternal indications. Pregnant women may therefore have an HbCO level that is 10% to 15% less than that of the fetus. There is evidence that short periods of HBO therapy are not dangerous to the fetus or mother (160).

Cyanide

Cyanide leads to hypoxia on a cellular level by rapidly binding to mitochondrial cytochrome oxidase. Inhalation of high concentrations of cyanide (270 ppm) is rapidly fatal in humans (with blood levels reaching 3 μg/mL), whereas ingestion of cyanide is less rapidly fatal (161). When very low doses of cyanide are absorbed (whole blood levels of 0.5–2.53 μg/mL), tachycardia and decreased level of consciousness are possible (161,162).

There are very few studies and case reports of the use of HBO therapy in the treatment of cyanide poisoning (163–167). This is likely due partly to the effectiveness of chemical treatments (with sodium nitrite and thiosulfate) but also possibly related to the fact that the bonding of cyanide to the mitochondria's cytochrome C oxidase is not an oxygen-dependent mechanism. Chemical treatment of cyanide poisoning leads to the formation of methemoglobin. Utilizing HBO therapy to increase the amount of circulating dissolved oxygen has been shown to have both prophylactic and antagonistic effects on cyanide poisoning in rabbits (166). Human case reports also hint that HBO therapy may be useful when the response to chemical antidotes has been incomplete (165).

Hydrogen Sulfide

Like CO and cyanide, hydrogen sulfide (H_2S) reacts with mitochondrial cytochrome C oxidase, impairing electron transport. This is not an oxygen-dependent mechanism. The rationale for using HBO therapy is the same as for cyanide poisoning, in that HBO therapy can increase the dissolved fraction of oxygen. Use of HBO therapy for H_2S poisoning is based on two case reports suggesting a positive benefit (168,169).

Carbon Tetrachloride

Carbon tetrachloride (CCl_4) is a CNS depressant, hepatotoxin, and nephrotoxin, with renal failure being the most common cause of death from very high-level exposures (170). In the setting of CCl_4 poisoning of the rat, HBO has been shown to improve survival (171), decrease liver necrosis (172), decrease conversion of CCl_4 to toxic free-radical metabolites (173,174), and decrease CCl_4 metabolite-induced lipid peroxidation (175). One case report describes an obtunded patient treated with HBO for presumed CO poisoning. There was no historical evidence for CO exposure; the patient improved, regained consciousness, and admitted to ingestion of a normally lethal dose of 250 mL of CCl_4 (176).

NECROTIZING INFECTIONS

Clostridial Infections

This soil-based anaerobic organism causes a type of rapidly progressive disease known as gas gangrene, which, if left untreated, is almost uniformly fatal. In most cases, it is introduced to the human via accidental trauma. The most common species that cause the disease are *Clostridium perfringens* (80%–90%),

Clostridium oedematiens, and *Clostridium septicum.* These organisms release α-toxin, which is a lecithinase related to the form found in snake, bee, and scorpion venoms, causing a liquefaction necrosis (177).

These organisms lack antioxidant defenses and therefore are susceptible to HBO therapy. The first to report this finding was Brummelkamp et al. in 1961 (178,179). Around the same time, it was discovered that at 3 ATA, α-toxin production quickly ceases (180); since then, animal studies (181) and meta-analyses of human case series support the use of HBO (182). If treatment is initiated within 24 hours of diagnosis, disease-specific mortality can be as low as 5% (177).

The typical HBO treatment schedule varies between 2.5 and 3 ATA for 90 minutes, with three treatments in the first 24 hours, followed by two treatments per day at 2 to 3 ATA until clinical stability. Aggressive surgical debridement and antibiotic therapy are also essential.

Nonclostridial Bacterial Infections

These are often necrotizing infections, usually polymicrobial, including at least one anaerobic species. These infections often follow local trauma and are enhanced by both local ischemia and reduced host defenses (many patients are diabetic with atherosclerosis) (183). The mainstays of therapy are surgical debridement and antibiotics. Individual case series and meta-analyses support the use of HBO as an adjunct (182,184,185). The HBO treatment schedule is similar to that of clostridial disease.

Mucormycosis

Rhinocerebral mucormycosis is a rare but devastating invasive disease of the head and neck with 30% to 50% or greater mortality when treated, often found in immunocompromised patients such as diabetics in ketoacidosis, or patients receiving antineoplastic agents and/or steroids (186). It is primarily treated with wide debridement and amphotericin B. Due to the rarity of this disease, randomized trials have not been performed. Several case reports have suggested that HBO therapy may be an effective adjunct (187–189). Recommended treatment protocol is 2 to 2.5 ATA for 2 hours, twice daily, for 40 to 80 treatments (190).

Severe Anemia

Hyperbaric oxygen increases dissolved oxygen in the plasma and thus enhances arterial oxygen content. Tissue oxygen delivery can therefore be supported acutely, even in the absence of hemoglobin. Therefore, HBO at 2 to 3 ATA can be used for temporary support of severely anemic patients if definitive therapy in the form of cross-matched blood is not immediately available (191). Evidence that intermittent repetitive HBO is effective therapy for patients who refuse blood has no basis in controlled outcome studies (192).

Head Injury

Evidence in animal studies suggests that HBO can prevent secondary injury after head trauma (193). HBO does reduce intracranial pressure after head injury (194), presumably due to cerebral vasoconstriction, but it is logistically very difficult to transport and monitor such patients for HBO. Although randomized studies have demonstrated a reduction in mortality with HBO treatment, the proportion of patients with good long-term results is not increased (194,195).

Thermal Injury

In a series of patients with carbon monoxide poisoning due to coal mine explosions and fire, those treated for CO poisoning with HBO who also had burns showed more rapid healing and less infection than others who did not receive HBO (196). Since then, some studies have supported its use (197,198), but others have failed to demonstrate a significant beneficial effect of HBO (199–202). In the randomized prospective study by Brannen et al. (202), twice-daily HBO at 2 ATA for 90 minutes had no effect on mortality or length of stay, although one of the authors reported in the discussion that HBO reduced the fluid loss, and the patients appeared to heal earlier. HBO appeared to reduce the volume of fluid required for initial resuscitation. A systematic review of the published evidence did not support the routine use of HBO in thermal burns (203). It should be noted that thermal burns are often accompanied by acute carbon monoxide poisoning for which HBO is indicated.

Myocardial Infarction

Increasing the blood O_2 content using HBO causes bradycardia, as well as a reduction in cardiac output (204) and myocardial O_2 consumption (23). HBO has been shown to improve wall motion abnormalities in patients with resting myocardial ischemia (205). In a rabbit model after 30 minutes of left coronary occlusion, HBO at 2.5 ATA reduced infarct size when administered either during or immediately after occlusion (206). A pilot randomized prospective study revealed lower peak creatine phosphokinase (CPK) levels and shorter time to pain relief with tissue plasminogen activator (tPA) with a single 2 ATA HBO treatment versus tPA and O_2 at 1 ATA delivered via face mask (207). The complete study revealed small, statistically insignificant differences in favor of HBO, but was underpowered to detect differences in mortality (208).

Stroke

A series of 13 patients with stroke treated with HBO at 2 to 3 ATA within 5 hours of onset was published by Heyman et al. (209). At that time, no imaging was available to exclude hemorrhage. Nevertheless, of 13 patients treated within 5 hours of symptom onset, nine improved during HBO treatment, and two stuporous patients with hemiparesis or hemiplegia improved dramatically immediately upon exposure to HBO and maintained their improvement permanently. The use of HBO in stroke is supported by animal studies demonstrating smaller infarct volume, reduced edema, and attenuation of hemorrhagic transformation (38,39,44,210–214). Human studies have not been encouraging (215–217), possibly because few if any patients since Heyman's study have been treated within the same short time frame. Routine use of HBO in this context will have to await further human outcome studies.

Support of Arterial Oxygenation

HBO has been reported as a method of attempting to support arterial blood oxygenation in respiratory distress syndrome (RDS) of the newborn, with disastrous results because of pulmonary oxygen toxicity (218). HBO is occasionally used for short periods to support oxygenation during therapeutic lung lavage (219–221).

Sedation and General Anesthesia during Hyperbaric Treatment

Anesthetic agents may be required for surgery while in a saturation diving system (e.g., offshore), for therapeutic lung lavage, or for sedation during mechanical ventilation. Inhaled agents can be used with conventional anesthetic vaporizers, which deliver a constant partial pressure of agent, irrespective of chamber pressure. Nitrous oxide can be used as a sole agent at increased pressure, although it induces several disagreeable side effects, including tachypnea, tachycardia, hypertension, diaphoresis, muscle rigidity, catatonic jerking of the extremities, eye opening, and opisthotonus. It is also associated with severe nausea and vomiting after recovery (222). Nitrous oxide must be avoided entirely in helium atmospheres because its administration induces intravascular bubble formation due to isobaric counterdiffusion through the skin (223). Nitrous oxide should also be avoided even at 1 ATA in patients who have recently scuba dived or experienced decompression illness. In such patients, tissue bubbles may be present, which could enlarge due to nitrous oxide diffusion and cause symptoms (224).

Inside hyperbaric chambers, intravenous agents such as propofol, ketamine, midazolam, and narcotics are preferred because their use avoids atmospheric pollution. Pressure-induced reversal of anesthesia is not significant up to 10 ATA, and if it occurs at higher pressures, it can be offset by appropriate titration.

HYPERBARIC CHAMBER OPERATION

Types of Hyperbaric Chambers

Monoplace

As implied by the name, these chambers have space for only one average-sized adult. Generally speaking, modern chambers of this type are cylindrical in shape and made of a large (approximately 0.6–1 m internal diameter and 2.1–2.3 m long) clear acrylic tube with a cap on one end and entry/exit hatch on the other. Patients slide into the chamber through the hatch to rest supine while they receive HBO therapy (Fig. 39.6).

Other than their small size, these chambers differ from their multiplace counterparts (described below) in that they are pressurized with 100% oxygen (in most cases) and are generally limited to no more than approximately 3 ATA operating pressure. This limitation makes them unsuitable for some high-

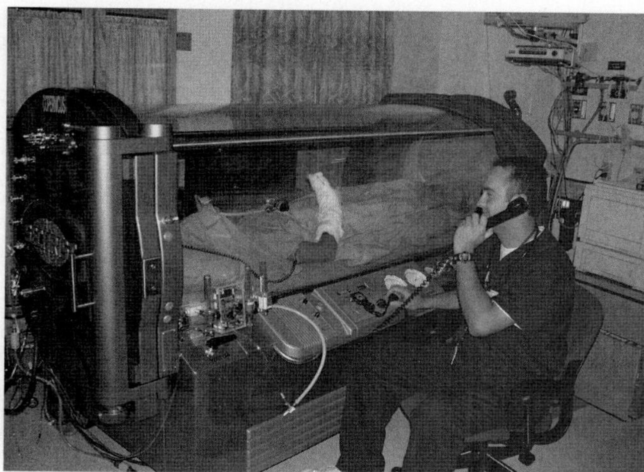

FIGURE 39.6. Monoplace chamber. This type of chamber has room for one patient or a tender with a small child. Chamber atmosphere is 100% O_2. The chamber is constructed of transparent Plexiglas to allow observation. Through-hull penetrators in the door on the left can be seen and allow monitoring, intravenous fluid administration, and control of a ventilator inside the chamber. (Photograph courtesy of Dr. Lindell Weaver.)

pressure treatment tables occasionally used for some types of decompression illness. Monoplace chambers can be fitted such that air breaks can be administered using a tight-fitting mask.

A challenge with the use of these chambers is lack of direct access to the patient. However, almost all monitoring and ventilatory care (invasive blood pressure monitoring, mechanical ventilation, chest tube management, etc.) previously only available to patients in multiplace chambers can now be delivered in monoplace chambers (111,225).

Multiplace

These chambers can hold two or more patients/tenders. They exist in many shapes and sizes, usually large cylindrical or spherical shapes made of high-quality steel. Most of these chambers have a personnel lock as well, which allows patients or medical staff to exit or enter the chamber while it is at pressure. Transfer locks allow medicines, materials, and food to be moved into or out of the chamber. Patients are generally accompanied in the chamber by a tender or nurse, who can attend to the needs of the patient during the treatment. Administration of all critical care modalities is relatively easy inside a multiplace chamber (Fig. 39.7).

Due to their sturdier construction, multiplace chambers are generally able to withstand much higher pressures than their acrylic monoplace counterparts, and thus can be used for a wider range of treatment pressures.

Minimization of Fire Hazards and Atmosphere Control

Hyperbaric chambers are unique among medical equipment in that the nurse, tender, or physician is frequently also inside the treatment vessel (chamber) with the patient (in the case of multiplace chambers) and not easily accessible in the event of an emergency. The environment must be carefully managed to ensure atmosphere quality, with specified limits for oxygen

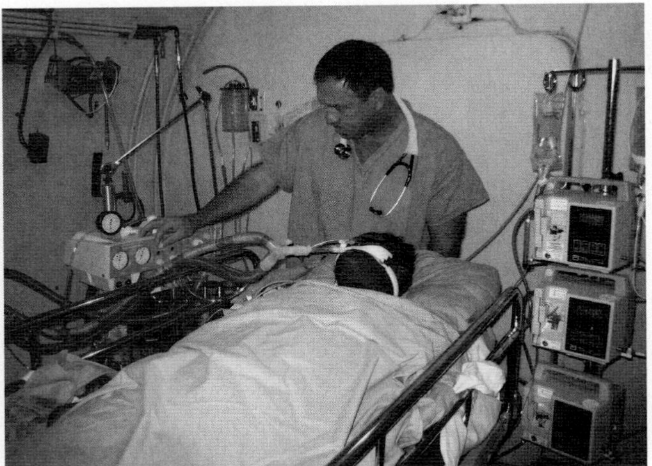

FIGURE 39.7. Patient treatment in a multiplace chamber.

and carbon dioxide, and to eliminate sources of ignition such as matches and cigarette lighters. Cotton suits are worn by patients and staff. Oil-based cosmetics and/or wigs (frequently made of synthetic materials) are prohibited (226).

Additionally, stretchers and equipment must have the petroleum-based lubricants removed from their wheels and other lubricated parts. Any other objects with petroleum-based lubricants must be cleaned of these lubricants prior to chamber treatment. At the time of this writing, there has not been a reported fire in a hyperbaric chamber that has resulted in a loss of life in the United States, although several such incidents have occurred overseas.

Ventilatory Care

Mechanical Ventilation

Certain precautions must be taken when diving a mechanically ventilated patient in a hyperbaric chamber. First of all, the ventilator must be approved for hyperbaric use. They should be fluidically or pneumatically controlled. Electrically driven ventilators are arguably less safe than ones using pneumatic or fluidic control. Although not commonly used at very high chamber pressures (6 ATA), ventilators powered by compressed oxygen have an inlet PO_2 of up to 4,560 mm Hg (227), which can present a significant fire hazard.

As pressure rises, so does the gas density, which leads to a corresponding increase in airway resistance. Unless the ventilator is volume cycled, the tidal volumes may drop as pressure rises (227). Therefore, tidal volumes should be monitored closely (228).

Prior to chamber pressurization, inflating the endotracheal cuff with water or saline will prevent leakage due to cuff volume compression.

Suction

Since the chamber is at pressure, suction can be created simply by venting a hose to the outside world attaching a regulator to a through-hull penetrator. Normal hospital equipment can be modified for this use (229). In patients with copious secretions or ventilated patients, it is preferable to perform deep suctioning immediately prior to both compression and decompression of the chamber. This removes any mucous plugs that could contribute to air trapping.

Chest Tube Management

Conventional water seal or one-way valve pleural drainage systems operate satisfactorily inside hyperbaric chambers, with or without applied suction. During chamber decompression, expansion of gas volume within the tubing connecting the chest tube with the drainage system is automatically vented via the water seal or one-way valve. On the other hand, during chamber compression, the same gas volume is compressed and the connecting tubing and gas-containing space on the patient side of the water seal will tend to collapse, therefore producing high negative intrapleural pressures. Standard commercially available pleural evacuation systems have a manually activated pressure relief valve, which should be activated during the compression phase to relieve this excessive negative pressure.

Intravenous Infusion Devices

Several different IV infusion devices have been tested inside multiplace hyperbaric chambers and found to deliver fluid accurately. While it is the policy of some facilities not to use electrical equipment inside a chamber, others minimize a fire hazard by purging the device with 100% nitrogen. For monoplace use, the IV infusion device must be outside the chamber. Glass IV bottles should be avoided in order to prevent explosion during decompression due to expansion of any contained air bubble.

Arterial Blood Gas Measurement

Arterial blood gas analysis can be performed inside a multiplace hyperbaric chamber using an analyzer adapted for hyperbaric use. Alternatively, blood samples can be decompressed and analyzed at 1 ATA. The latter procedure is simpler, but subject to error. While pH and PCO_2 are relatively stable during decompression, PO_2 usually exceeds ambient pressure outside the chamber, and thus it tends to decline rapidly as oxygen is released from solution. Reasonably accurate values can be obtained if the sample is analyzed immediately after decompression (230).

Alternatively, it is possible to predict arterial PO_2 during HBO therapy from a 1 ATA arterial blood gas measurement using the following equations. All that is needed is a 1 ATA blood gas measurement (at known FiO_2), the HBO treatment pressure in ATA (P_{ATA}, usually between 2 and 3 ATA), barometric pressure (P_b, in mm Hg, usually near 760 mm Hg), the vapor pressure of water at body temperature (P_{H2O}, at or near 47 mm Hg), the respiratory exchange ratio (usually 0.8), and $PaCO_2$ and the following formulas:

$$PaO_2(1\ ATA) = (P_b - PH_2O) \cdot FiO_2 - PaCO_2 \cdot \left[FiO_2 + \frac{1 - FiO_2}{R}\right] \quad [2]$$

$$PaO_2\ (\text{predicted during HBO}) = PaO_2\ (1\ ATA)/PaO_2\ (1\ ATA) \cdot [(760 \bullet P_{ATA} - 47) - PCO_2] \quad [3]$$

where Pb is the barometric pressure outside the chamber; PaO_2 (1 ATA) is the arterial PO_2 at 1 ATA; PaO_2 (1 ATA) is the alveolar PO_2 at 1 ATA; FiO_2 is the inspired O_2 fraction; R is the respiratory exchange ratio (usually 0.8); P_{ATA} is the ambient pressure in the chamber in ATA; and PCO_2 is the arterial PCO_2 measured at 1 ATA, assumed to be unchanged during HBO.

Patient Monitoring

Most monitoring modalities used in hyperbaric chambers are identical to those used in normobaric situations, with few exceptions. Whenever inflatable pressure bags are used, such as for invasive blood pressure measurement, as the chamber pressurizes, the volume of air and the pressure in the pressure bag decreases, and thus one must periodically pump it up during compression; when decompressing the chamber, the air in the pressure bag expands, which must be released periodically to avoid rupture. For the same reason, pulmonary artery catheter balloons should be left open to the atmosphere during chamber compression and decompression.

Invasive pressure monitoring (or any monitoring where an electrical signal is transmitted via cable/wire) can be performed using through-hull penetrators to connect the transducer inside the chamber with the preamplifier outside.

Standard stethoscopes and sphygmomanometers can be used without difficulty in a multiplace chamber. Mercury pressure gauges should be avoided to prevent chamber contamination in the event of breakage.

Cardiac Arrest and Defibrillation

If a patient requires cardioversion or defibrillation while receiving HBO treatment, it is necessary to have through-hull penetrators for the high-voltage cables connecting an outside defibrillator with the paddles inside. Use of a low-impedance gel will prevent sparks or heat buildup at the site of paddle contact. Careful design and testing are necessary to confirm adequacy of energy delivery. The only alternative is to decompress the chamber and cardiovert or defibrillate at 1 ATA.

Tenders, Nurses, and Other Chamber Staff Considerations

Inside tenders in a multiplace chamber will take up nitrogen. While there is no requirement for a decompression stop for typical 2 ATA/2 hour or 2.5 ATA/90 minute treatments, many facilities require their staff to breathe 100% oxygen during decompression to reduce the very small risk of DCS. Additionally, repetitive exposures within a short time to even these low pressures may incur some risk of DCS. Minimum time intervals between hyperbaric exposures for staff are routine. Longer treatments or higher treatment pressures generally mandate specific decompression or oxygen breathing requirements for the inside staff. Emergency decompression from such exposures due to patient instability may therefore place the accompanying tender at risk. In the event of such an emergency, the tender should be immediately recompressed. The most widely accepted management schedule is described on p. 9–13 of the U.S. Navy *Diving Manual* (108).

Critical Care in a Hyperbaric Chamber in the Field

Field chambers are used in the offshore oil industry and at some remote inland dive sites. Divers injured due to decompression illness or trauma may require critical care in this setting. This is particularly the case for divers decompressing from saturation dives, in which an injured diver may require many days of decompression before he or she can be transferred to a hospital. Tracheal intubation, chest tube insertion, mechanical ventilation, hemodynamic and CNS monitoring, and treatment of convulsions may all be necessary (231). Portable radiographs can be obtained by passing an x-ray beam through a Plexiglas port, with the x-ray plate inside the chamber (232).

HYPERBARIC TREATMENT COMPLICATIONS

Barotrauma

Otic

As many as 17% of all HBO therapy patients report ear pain with compression, making otic barotraumas the most common complication of HBO therapy (74). This is the result of difficulty with middle ear pressure equalization (i.e., eustachian tube opening). As the chamber is compressed, the increased pressure on the tympanic membrane can cause it to stretch medially just as when one dives in a swimming pool. Only rarely does this result in perforation of the tympanic membrane in awake patients, as they are able to notify the chamber operator of their progressive discomfort. Most often, there is unilateral otic discomfort associated with an erythematous tympanic membrane that heals over the following 5 to 7 days. In patients who are unable to adequately perform a Valsalva maneuver required to equalize pressure (i.e., sedated, intubated, with eustachian tube/sinus dysfunction, or with tracheostomy tube), bilateral myringotomies with or without tube placement are performed. Because myringotomies heal in 2 to 3 days, for patients unable to equalize, bilateral tympanostomy tubes are normally placed in patients who are expected to receive repetitive treatments for longer.

Sinus

Sinus barotrauma ("sinus squeeze") is a relatively infrequent occurrence, which occurs in patients with active sinus infection, allergic rhinitis, or nasal polyps. During pressure change, the patient will feel discomfort in the region of the affected sinus, particularly if it is the frontal sinus (233). Sinus squeeze can usually be prevented using topical decongestants such as oxymetazoline and slow compression of the chamber (233).

Pulmonary

Although this is far more frequent with scuba diving, it can also occur rarely in dry hyperbaric chambers, causing AGE (234), pneumomediastinum, or pneumothorax. Patients with cystic or bullous disease are presumably at risk; however, many such patients have received HBO without complication. In patients with a pre-existing pneumothorax, tube decompression is recommended, especially if the patient is to be treated in a monoplace chamber.

Pulmonary Edema

Peripheral vasoconstriction induced by HBO and the resulting increase in afterload can precipitate pulmonary edema in patients with impaired ventricular function (235).

Evaluation of a Patient for Hyperbaric Oxygen Therapy

In assessing a patient for hyperbaric therapy, two aspects need to be evaluated: Potential efficacy of treatment and risk of adverse effects. Indications for hyperbaric oxygen therapy as determined by the Undersea and Hyperbaric Medical Society (7) are listed in Table 39.1. A second factor is the predicted arterial PO_2, which must be within a therapeutic range during HBO therapy (>1,000 mm Hg). If a patient has pulmonary gas exchange impairment that precludes attainment of an arterial PO_2 that is sufficiently high, then HBO is unlikely to be effective. A method for predicting arterial oxygenation during HBO makes use of the relative constancy of the ratio of arterial to alveolar PO_2 (PaO_2/PAO_2 ratio) as described above (Eq. 2 and 3). Finally, the assessment must include evaluating for the risk of pulmonary barotrauma. During decompression, pulmonary cysts or bullae can rupture (234), although such complications are extremely rare. Patients with untreated pneumothorax usually require a tube thoracostomy, unless immediate chest decompression can be performed. Patients with a pneumothorax for whom monoplace treatment is planned require prophylactic chest tube insertion irrespective of the size of the pneumothorax. Patients in heart failure in whom left ventricular function may not be able to tolerate an increase in afterload are also at risk (235).

Susceptibility to otic barotrauma and occasionally to sinus barotrauma also plays a role in determining fitness for HBO therapy. Obtunded patients are especially at risk of otic barotrauma, and many practitioners advocate prophylactic myringotomy.

SUMMARY

Although hyperbaric oxygen therapy has limited indications, it represents definitive therapy for some critically ill patients, especially those with gas bubble disease (decompression sickness or gas embolism) and carbon monoxide poisoning. The available evidence also strongly suggests that it is an effective adjunct in necrotizing soft tissue infections. HBO can be safely administered to the critically ill patient using an appropriately equipped hyperbaric chamber and implementing standard monitoring and supportive measures.

References

1. Simpson A. *Compressed Air, as a Therapeutic Agent, in the Treatment of Consumption, Asthma, Chronic Bronchitis, and Other Diseases.* Edinburgh: Sutherland & Knox; 1857.
2. Junod VT. Recherches physiologiques et thérapeutiques sur les effets de la compression et de la raréfaction de l'air, tant sur le corps que sur les membres isolés. *Rev Med Fr Étrange.* 1834;3:350–368.
3. Phillips JL. *The Bends.* New Haven, CT: Yale University; 1998.
4. Zuntz N. Zur Pathogenese und Therapie der durch rasche Luftdruckänderungen erzeugten Krankheiten. *Fortschr Med.* 1897;15:632–639.
5. Behnke AR, Shaw LA. The use of oxygen in the treatment of compressed air illness. *Navy Med Bull.* 1937;35:1–12.
6. Yarbrough OD, Behnke AR. The treatment of compressed air illness using oxygen. *J Ind Hyg Toxicol.* 1939;21:213–218.
7. Gesell LB, ed. *Hyperbaric Oxygen Therapy: A Committee Report.* Durham, NC: Undersea and Hyperbaric Medical Society; 2008.
8. Whalen RE, Saltzman HA, Holloway DH Jr, et al. Cardiovascular and blood gas responses to hyperbaric oxygenation. *Am J Cardiol.* 1965;15:638–646.
9. McMahon TJ, Moon RE, Luschinger BP, et al. Nitric oxide in the human respiratory cycle. *Nat Med.* 2002;8:711–717.
10. Boerema I, Meyne NG, Brummelkamp WH, et al. Life without blood. *J Cardiovasc Surg (Torino).* 1960;1:133–146.
11. Bergofsky EH, Wang MC, Yamaki T, et al. Tissue oxygen and carbon dioxide tensions during hyperbaric oxygenation. *JAMA.* 1964;189:841–844.
12. Bergofsky EH, Bertun P. Response of regional circulations to hyperoxia. *J Appl Physiol.* 1966;21:567–572.
13. Bird AD, Telfer AB. Effect of hyperbaric oxygen on limb circulation. *Lancet.* 1965;13:355–356.
14. Berry JM, Doursout MF, Butler BD. Effects of hyperbaric hyperoxia on cardiac and regional hemodynamics in conscious dogs. *Aviat Space Environ Med.* 1998;69:761–765.
15. Demchenko IT, Boso AE, Bennett PB, et al. Hyperbaric oxygen reduces cerebral blood flow by inactivating nitric oxide. *Nitric Oxide.* 2000;4:597–608.
16. Dooley JW, Mehm WJ. Noninvasive assessment of the vasoconstrictive effects of hyperoxygenation. *J Hyperbar Med.* 1990;4:177–187.
17. Sheikh AY, Rollins MD, Hopf HW, et al. Hyperoxia improves microvascular perfusion in a murine wound model. *Wound Repair Regen.* 2005;13:303–308.
18. Hahnloser PB, Domanig E, Lamphier E, et al. Hyperbaric oxygenation: alterations in cardiac output and regional blood flow. *J Thorac Cardiovasc Surg.* 1966;52:223–231.
19. Villanucci S, Di Marzio GE, Scholl M, et al. Cardiovascular changes induced by hyperbaric oxygen therapy. *Undersea Biomed Res (Suppl).* 1990;17:117.
20. Demchenko IT, Boso AE, Natoli MJ, et al. Nitric oxide is involved in the mechanism of HBO-induced cerebral vasoconstriction. *Undersea Hyperb Med.* 1998;25(Suppl):54.
21. Demchenko IT, Oury TD, Crapo JD, et al. Regulation of the brain's vascular responses to oxygen. *Circ Res.* 2002;91:1031–1037.
22. Hordnes C, Tyssebotn I. Effect of high ambient pressure and oxygen tension on organ blood flow in conscious trained rats. *Undersea Biomed Res.* 1985;12:115–128.
23. Savitt MA, Rankin JS, Elberry JR, et al. Influence of hyperbaric oxygen on left ventricular contractility, total coronary blood flow, and myocardial oxygen consumption in the conscious dog. *Undersea Hyperb Med.* 1994;21:169–183.
24. Zamboni WA, Roth AC, Russell RC, et al. Morphological analysis of the microcirculation during reperfusion of ischemic skeletal muscle and the effect of hyperbaric oxygen. *Plast Reconstr Surg.* 1993;91:1110–1123.
25. Helps SC, Meyer-Witting M, Rilley PL, et al. Increasing doses of intracarotid air and cerebral blood flow in rabbits. *Stroke.* 1990;21:1340–1345.
26. Helps SC, Gorman DF. Air embolism of the brain in rabbits pre-treated with mechlorethamine. *Stroke.* 1991;22:351–354.
27. Miljkovic-Lolic M, Silbergleit R, Fiskum G, et al. Neuroprotective effects of hyperbaric oxygen treatment in experimental focal cerebral ischemia are associated with reduced brain leukocyte myeloperoxidase activity. *Brain Res.* 2003;971:90–94.
28. Chen MF, Chen HM, Ueng SW, et al. Hyperbaric oxygen pretreatment attenuates hepatic reperfusion injury. *Liver.* 1998;18:110–116.
29. Tjarnstrom J, Wikstrom T, Bagge U, et al. Effects of hyperbaric oxygen treatment on neutrophil activation and pulmonary sequestration in intestinal ischemia-reperfusion in rats. *Eur Surg Res.* 1999;31:147–154.
30. Yamada T, Taguchi T, Hirata Y, et al. The protective effect of hyperbaric oxygenation on the small intestine in ischemia-reperfusion injury. *J Pediatr Surg.* 1995;30:786–790.
31. Zamboni WA, Wong HP, Stephenson LL. Effect of hyperbaric oxygen on neutrophil concentration and pulmonary sequestration in reperfusion injury. *Arch Surg.* 1996;131:756–760.
32. Haapaniemi T, Nylander G, Sirsjo A, et al. Hyperbaric oxygen reduces ischemia-induced skeletal muscle injury. *Plast Reconstr Surg.* 1996;97:602–607; discussion 8–9.
33. Zamboni WA, Roth AC, Russell RC, et al. The effect of acute hyperbaric oxygen therapy on axial pattern skin flap survival when administered during and after total ischemia. *J Reconstr Microsurg.* 1989;5:343–347.
34. Hong JP, Kwon H, Chung YK, et al. The effect of hyperbaric oxygen on ischemia-reperfusion injury: an experimental study in a rat musculocutaneous flap. *Ann Plast Surg.* 2003;51:478–487.

35. Bosco G, Yang ZJ, Nandi J, et al. Effects of hyperbaric oxygen on glucose, lactate, glycerol and anti-oxidant enzymes in the skeletal muscle of rats during ischaemia and reperfusion. *Clin Exp Pharmacol Physiol.* 2007;34:70–76.
36. Buras JA, Reenstra WR. Endothelial-neutrophil interactions during ischemia and reperfusion injury: basic mechanisms of hyperbaric oxygen. *Neurol Res.* 2007;29:127–131.
37. Riccio M, Pangrazi PP, Campodonico A, et al. Combined use of WEB2170 and HBO therapy can reduce ischemia and reperfusion injury to the skeletal muscle in a rabbit model. *Microsurgery.* 2007;27:43–47.
38. Henninger N, Kuppers-Tiedt L, Sicard KM, et al. Neuroprotective effect of hyperbaric oxygen therapy monitored by MR-imaging after embolic stroke in rats. *Exp Neurol.* 2006;201:316–323.
39. Schabitz WR, Schade H, Heiland S, et al. Neuroprotection by hyperbaric oxygenation after experimental focal cerebral ischemia monitored by MRI. *Stroke.* 2004;35:1175–1179.
40. Gurer A, Ozdogan M, Gomceli I, et al. Hyperbaric oxygenation attenuates renal ischemia-reperfusion injury in rats. *Transplant Proc.* 2006;38:3337–3340.
41. Kalns J, Lane J, Delgado A, et al. Hyperbaric oxygen exposure temporarily reduces Mac-1 mediated functions of human neutrophils. *Immunol Lett.* 2002;83:125–131.
42. Thom SR. Effects of hyperoxia on neutrophil adhesion. *Undersea Hyperb Med.* 2004;31:123–131.
43. Thom SR, Mendiguren I, Hardy K, et al. Inhibition of human neutrophil beta2-integrin-dependent adherence by hyperbaric O_2. *Am J Physiol.* 1997;272:C770–C777.
44. Veltkamp R, Siebing DA, Sun L, et al. Hyperbaric oxygen reduces blood-brain barrier damage and edema after transient focal cerebral ischemia. *Stroke.* 2005;36:1679–1683.
45. Lou M, Chen Y, Ding M, et al. Involvement of the mitochondrial ATP-sensitive potassium channel in the neuroprotective effect of hyperbaric oxygenation after cerebral ischemia. *Brain Res Bull.* 2006;69:109–116.
46. Mader JT, Brown GL, Guckian JC, et al. A mechanism for the amelioration by hyperbaric oxygen of experimental staphylococcal osteomyelitis in rabbits. *J Infect Dis.* 1980;142:915–922.
47. Mader JT, Adams KR, Sutton TE. Infectious diseases: pathophysiology and mechanisms of hyperbaric oxygen. *J Hyperbar Med.* 1987;2:133–140.
48. Zamboni WA, Mazolewski PJ, Erdmann D, et al. Evaluation of penicillin and hyperbaric oxygen in the treatment of streptococcal myositis. *Ann Plast Surg.* 1997;39:131–136.
49. Carraway MS, Piantadosi CA. Oxygen toxicity. *Respir Care Clin N Am.* 1999;5:265–295.
50. Freeman BA, Crapo JD. Biology of disease: Free radicals and tissue injury. *Lab Invest.* 1982;47:412–426.
51. Gerschman R, Gilbert DL, Nye SW, et al. Oxygen poisoning and x-irradiation: a mechanism in common. *Science.* 1954;119:623–626.
52. Demchenko IT, Atochin DN, Boso AE, et al. Oxygen seizure latency and peroxynitrite formation in mice lacking neuronal or endothelial nitric oxide synthases. *Neurosci Lett.* 2003;344:53–56.
53. Demchenko IT, Boso AE, Whorton AR, et al. Nitric oxide production is enhanced in rat brain before oxygen-induced convulsions. *Brain Res.* 2001;917:253–261.
54. Demchenko IT, Piantadosi CA. Nitric oxide amplifies the excitatory to inhibitory neurotransmitter imbalance accelerating oxygen seizures. *Undersea Hyperb Med.* 2006;33:169–174.
55. Donald KW. Oxygen poisoning in man, I & II. *BMJ.* 1947;1:667–672, 712–717.
56. Doherty MJ, Hampson NB. Partial seizure provoked by hyperbaric oxygen therapy: possible mechanisms and implications. *Epilepsia.* 2005;46:974–976.
57. Bleiberg B, Kerem D. Central nervous system oxygen toxicity in the resting rat: postponement by intermittent oxygen exposure. *Undersea Biomed Res.* 1988;15:337–352.
58. Chavko M, McCarron RM. Extension of brain tolerance to hyperbaric O2 by intermittent air breaks is related to the time of CBF increase. *Brain Res.* 2006;1084:196–201.
59. Harabin AL, Survanshi SS, Weathersby PK, et al. The modulation of oxygen toxicity by intermittent exposure. *Toxicol Appl Pharmacol.* 1988;93:298–311.
60. Lambertsen CJ. Extension of oxygen tolerance in man: philosophy and significance. *Exp Lung Res.* 1988;14(Suppl):1035–1058.
61. Vote DA, Doar O, Moon RE, et al. Blood glucose meter performance under hyperbaric oxygen conditions. *Clin Chim Acta.* 2001;305:81–87.
62. Clark JM, Lambertsen CJ. Pulmonary oxygen toxicity: a review. *Pharmacol Rev.* 1971;23:37–133.
63. Bardin H, Lambertsen CJ. *A Quantitative Method for Calculating Cumulative Pulmonary Oxygen Toxicity. Use of the Unit Pulmonary Toxicity Dose (UPTD).* Philadelphia: Institute of Environmental Medicine, University of Pennsylvania; 1970.
64. Clark JM. Oxygen toxicity. In: Bennett PB, Elliott DH, eds. *The Physiology and Medicine of Diving.* Philadelphia: WB Saunders; 1993:121–169.
65. Harabin AL, Homer LD, Weathersby PK, et al. An analysis of decrements in vital capacity as an index of pulmonary oxygen toxicity. *J Appl Physiol.* 1987;63:1130–1135.
66. Clark JM, Lambertsen CJ. Rate of development of pulmonary O_2 toxicity in man during O_2 breathing at 2.0 Ata. *J Appl Physiol.* 1971;30:739–752.
67. Goldiner PL, Carlon GC, Cvitkovic E, et al. Factors influencing postoperative morbidity and mortality in patients treated with bleomycin. *BMJ.* 1978;1:1664–1667.
68. Nygaard K, Smith-Erichsen N, Hatlevoll R, et al. Pulmonary complications after bleomycin, irradiation and surgery for esophageal cancer. *Cancer.* 1978;41:17–22.
69. Thompson CC, Bailey MK, Conroy JM, et al. Postoperative pulmonary toxicity associated with mitomycin C therapy. *South Med J.* 1992;85:1257–1259.
70. Anderson B Jr, Shelton DL. Axial length in hyperoxic myopia. In: Bove AA, Bachrach AJ, Greenbaum LJ Jr, eds. *Underwater and Hyperbaric Physiology IX Proceedings of the Ninth International Symposium on Underwater and Hyperbaric Physiology.* Bethesda, MD: Undersea and Hyperbaric Medical Society; 1987:607–611.
71. Palmquist BM, Philipson B, Barr PO. Nuclear cataract and myopia during hyperbaric oxygen therapy. *Br J Ophthalmol.* 1984;68:113–117.
72. Behnke AR, Forbes HS, Motley EP. Circulatory and visual effects of oxygen at 3 atmospheres pressure. *Am J Physiol.* 1936;114:436–442.
73. Clark JM, Thom SR. Oxygen under pressure. In: Brubakk AO, Neuman TS, eds. *Physiology and Medicine of Diving.* London: Saunders; 2003:376.
74. Plafki C, Peters P, Almeling M, et al. Complications and side effects of hyperbaric oxygen therapy. *Aviat Space Environ Med.* 2000;71:119–124.
75. Junod T. Recherches sur les effets physiologiques et thérapeutiques de la compression et de raréfaction de l'air, tant sur le corps que les membres isolés. *Ann Gén Med sér 2,* 1835;9:157–172.
76. Behnke AR, Thomas RM, Motley EP. The psychologic effects from breathing air at 4 atmospheres pressure. *Am J Physiol.* 1935;112:554–558.
77. Muth CM, Shank ES. Gas embolism. *N Engl J Med.* 2000;342:476–482.
78. Fukaya E, Hopf HW. HBO and gas embolism. *Neurol Res.* 2007;29:142–145.
79. Morris WP, Butler BD, Tonnesen AS, et al. Continuous venous air embolism in patients receiving positive end-expiratory pressure. *Am Rev Respir Dis.* 1993;147:1034–1037.
80. Kaufman BS, Kaminsky SJ, Rackow EC, et al. Adult respiratory distress syndrome following orogenital sex during pregnancy. *Crit Care Med.* 1987;15:703–704.
81. Nossum V, Koteng S, Brubakk AO. Endothelial damage by bubbles in the pulmonary artery of the pig. *Undersea Hyperb Med.* 1999;26:1–8.
82. Dutka AJ, Kochanek PM, Hallenbeck JM. Influence of granulocytopenia on canine cerebral ischemia induced by air embolism. *Stroke.* 1989;20:390–395.
83. Hallenbeck JM, Dutka AJ, Tanishima T, et al. Polymorphonuclear leukocyte accumulation in brain regions with low blood flow during the early postischemic period. *Stroke.* 1986;17:246–253.
84. Levin LL, Stewart GJ, Lynch PR, et al. Blood and blood vessel wall changes induced by decompression sickness in dogs. *J Appl Physiol.* 1981;50:944–949.
85. Chryssanthou C, Springer M, Lipschitz S. Blood-brain and blood-lung barrier alteration by dysbaric exposure. *Undersea Biomed Res.* 1977;4:117–129.
86. Zwirewich CV, Müller NL, Abboud RT, et al. Noncardiogenic pulmonary edema caused by decompression sickness: rapid resolution following hyperbaric therapy. *Radiology.* 1987;163:81–82.
87. Nossum V, Hjelde A, Brubakk AO. Small amounts of venous gas embolism cause delayed impairment of endothelial function and increase polymorphonuclear neutrophil infiltration. *Eur J Appl Physiol.* 2002;86:209–214.
88. van Hulst RA, Lameris TW, Haitsma JJ, et al. Brain glucose and lactate levels during ventilator-induced hypo- and hypercapnia. *Clin Physiol Funct Imaging.* 2004;24:243–248.
89. van Hulst RA, Lameris TW, Hasan D, et al. Effects of cerebral air embolism on brain metabolism in pigs. *Acta Neurol Scand.* 2003;108:118–124.
90. van Hulst RA, Haitsma JJ, Lameris TW, et al. Hyperventilation impairs brain function in acute cerebral air embolism in pigs. *Intensive Care Med.* 2004;30:944–950.
91. Mann C, Boccara G, Fabre JM, et al. The detection of carbon dioxide embolism during laparoscopy in pigs: a comparison of transesophageal Doppler and end-tidal carbon dioxide monitoring. *Acta Anaesthesiol Scand.* 1997;41:281–286.
92. Benson J, Adkinson C, Collier R. Hyperbaric oxygen therapy of iatrogenic cerebral arterial gas embolism. *Undersea Hyperb Med.* 2003;30:117–126.
93. Longphre JM, Denoble PJ, Moon RE, et al. First aid normobaric oxygen for the treatment of recreational diving injuries. *Undersea Hyperb Med.* 2007;34:43–49.
94. Atkinson JR. Experimental air embolism. *Northwest Med.* 1963;62:699–703.
95. Van Allen CM, Hrdina LS, Clark J. Air embolism from the pulmonary vein. *Arch Surg.* 1929;19:567–599.
96. Mehlhorn U, Burke EJ, Butler BD, et al. Body position does not affect the hemodynamic response to venous air embolism in dogs. *Anesth Analg.* 1994;79:734–739.
97. Geissler HJ, Allen SJ, Mehlhorn U, et al. Effect of body repositioning

after venous air embolism. An echocardiographic study. *Anesthesiology.* 1997;86:710–717.

98. Dutka AJ. Therapy for dysbaric central nervous system ischemia: adjuncts to recompression. In: Bennett PB, Moon RE, eds. *Diving Accident Management.* Bethesda, MD: Undersea and Hyperbaric Medical Society; 1990:222–234.
99. van Hulst RA, Klein J, Lachmann B. Gas embolism: pathophysiology and treatment. *Clin Physiol Funct Imaging.* 2003;23:237–246.
100. Adams HP Jr, del Zoppo G, Alberts MJ, et al. Guidelines for the early management of adults with ischemic stroke: a guideline from the American Heart Association/American Stroke Association Stroke Council, Clinical Cardiology Council, Cardiovascular Radiology and Intervention Council, and the Atherosclerotic Peripheral Vascular Disease and Quality of Care Outcomes in Research Interdisciplinary Working Groups: the American Academy of Neurology affirms the value of this guideline as an educational tool for neurologists. *Stroke.* 2007;38:1655–1711.
101. Brown JW, Dierdorf SF, Moorthy SS, et al. Venoarterial cerebral perfusion for treatment of massive arterial air embolism. *Anesth Analg.* 1987;66:673–674.
102. Stark J, Hough J. Air in the aorta: treatment by reversed perfusion. *Ann Thorac Surg.* 1986;41:337–338.
103. Ericsson JA, Gottlieb JD, Sweet RB. Closed-chest cardiac massage in the treatment of venous air embolism. *N Engl J Med.* 1964;270:1353–1354.
104. Michenfelder JD, Martin JT, Altenburg BM, et al. Air embolism during neurosurgery. An evaluation of right-atrial catheters for diagnosis and treatment. *JAMA.* 1969;208:1353–1358.
105. Bowdle TA, Artru AA. Treatment of air embolism with a special pulmonary artery catheter introducer sheath in sitting dogs. *Anesthesiology.* 1988;68:107–110.
106. Marshall WK, Bedford RF. Use of a pulmonary-artery catheter for detection and treatment of venous air embolism: a prospective study in man. *Anesthesiology.* 1980;52:131–134.
107. Thalmann ED. Principles of US Navy recompression treatments for decompression sickness. In: Moon RE, Sheffield PJ, eds. *Treatment of Decompression Illness.* Kensington, MD: Undersea and Hyperbaric Medical Society; 1996:75–95.
108. Navy Department. *US Navy Diving Manual.* Revision 4. Vol. 5: Diving Medicine and Recompression Chamber Operations. NAVSEA 0910-LP-103-8009. Washington, DC: Naval Sea Systems Command; 2005.
109. Hart GB, Strauss MB, Lennon PA. The treatment of decompression sickness and air embolism in a monoplace chamber. *J Hyperbar Med.* 1986;1:1–7.
110. Cianci P, Slade JB Jr. Delayed treatment of decompression sickness with short, no-air-break tables: review of 140 cases. *Aviat Space Environ Med.* 2006;77:1003–1008.
111. Weaver LK. Monoplace hyperbaric chamber use of U.S. Navy Table 6: a 20-year experience. *Undersea Hyperb Med.* 2006;33:85–88.
112. Moon RE, ed. *Adjunctive Therapy for Decompression Illness.* Kensington, MD: Undersea and Hyperbaric Medical Society; 2003.
113. Undersea and Hyperbaric Medical Society. UHMS Guidelines for Adjunctive Therapy of DCI. In: Moon RE, ed. *Adjunctive Therapy for Decompression Illness.* Kensington, MD: Undersea and Hyperbaric Medical Society; 2003:184–189.
114. Balldin UI. Effects of ambient temperature and body position on tissue nitrogen elimination in man. *Aerosp Med.* 1973;44:365–3670.
115. Hallenbeck JM, Leitch DR, Dutka AJ, et al. Prostaglandin I_2, indomethacin and heparin promote postischemic neuronal recovery in dogs. *Ann Neurol.* 1982;12:145–156.
116. Reeves E, Workman RD. Use of heparin for the therapeutic/prophylactic treatment of decompression sickness. *Aerosp Med.* 1971;42:20–23.
117. Broome JR. Association of CNS hemorrhage with failure to respond to recompression treatment—implications for management of refractory cases of decompression illness. In: Moon RE, Sheffield PJ, eds. *Treatment of Decompression Illness.* Kensington, MD: Undersea and Hyperbaric Medical Society; 1996:364–373.
118. Elliott DH, Hallenbeck JM, Bove AA. Venous infarction of the spinal cord in decompression sickness. *J Roy Nav Med Serv.* 1974;60:66–71.
119. Palmer AC, Blakemore WF, Payne JE, et al. Decompression sickness in the goat: nature of brain and spinal cord lesions at 48 hours. *Undersea Biomed Res.* 1978;5:275–286.
120. Gorman DF, Browning DN. Cerebral vaso-reactivity and arterial gas embolism. *Undersea Biomed Res.* 1986;13:317–335.
121. Waite CL, Mazzone WF, Greenwood ME, et al. Cerebral air embolism I. Basic studies. US Naval Submarine Medical Center Report No. 493. Panama City, FL: US Navy Submarine Research Laboratory; 1967. Report No.: 493.
122. Landolt JP, Money KE, Topliff ED, et al. Pathophysiology of inner ear dysfunction in the squirrel monkey in rapid decompression. *J Appl Physiol.* 1980;49:1070–1082.
123. McCormick JG, Holland WB, Brauer RW, et al. Sudden hearing loss due to diving and its prevention with heparin. *Otolaryngol Clin North Am.* 1975;8:417–430.
124. Mitchell SJ. Lidocaine in the treatment of decompression illness: a review of the literature. *Undersea Hyperb Med.* 2001;28:165–174.
125. Mitchell SJ, Pellett O, Gorman DF. Cerebral protection by lidocaine during cardiac operations. *Ann Thorac Surg.* 1999;67:1117–1124.
126. Wang D, Wu X, Li J, et al. The effect of lidocaine on early postoperative cognitive dysfunction after coronary artery bypass surgery [comment]. *Anesth Analg.* 2002;95:1134–1141, table of contents.
127. Mathew J, Grocott H, Phillips-Bute B, et al. Lidocaine does not prevent cognitive dysfunction after cardiac surgery. *Anesth Analg.* 2004;98(Suppl): SCA13.
128. Cogar WB. Intravenous lidocaine as adjunctive therapy in the treatment of decompression illness. *Ann Emerg Med.* 1997;29:284–286.
129. Mitchell SJ, Benson M, Vadlamudi L, et al. Cerebral arterial gas embolism by helium: an unusual case successfully treated with hyperbaric oxygen and lidocaine. *Ann Emerg Med.* 2000;35:300–303.
130. Bennett M, Mitchell S, Dominguez A. Adjunctive treatment of decompression illness with a non-steroidal anti-inflammatory drug (tenoxicam) reduces compression requirement. *Undersea Hyperb Med.* 2003;30:195–205.
131. Francis TJR, Dutka AJ, Clark JB. An evaluation of dexamethasone in the treatment of acute experimental spinal decompression sickness. In: Bove AA, Bachrach AJ, Greenbaum LJ, Jr, eds. *Underwater and Hyperbaric Physiology IX Proceedings of the Ninth International Symposium on Underwater and Hyperbaric Physiology.* Bethesda, MD: Undersea and Hyperbaric Medical Society; 1987:999–1013.
132. Dutka AJ, Mink RB, Pearson RR, et al. Effects of treatment with dexamethasone on recovery from experimental cerebral arterial gas embolism. *Undersea Biomed Res.* 1992;19:131–141.
133. Francis TJR, Dutka AJ. Methylprednisolone in the treatment of acute spinal cord decompression sickness. *Undersea Biomed Res.* 1989;16:165–174.
134. Dromsky DM, Toner CB, Fahlman A, et al. Prophylactic treatment of severe decompression sickness with methylprednisolone. *Undersea Hyperb Med.* 1999;26(Suppl):15.
135. Novotny JA, Bridgewater BJ, Himm JF, et al. Quantifying the effect of intravascular perfluorocarbon on xenon elimination from canine muscle. *J Appl Physiol.* 1993;74:1356–1360.
136. Mahon RT, Dainer HM, Nelson JW. Decompression sickness in a swine model: isobaric denitrogenation and perfluorocarbon at depth. *Aviat Space Environ Med.* 2006;77:8–12.
137. Dainer H, Nelson J, Brass K, et al. Short oxygen prebreathing and intravenous perfluorocarbon emulsion reduces morbidity and mortality in a swine saturation model of decompression sickness. *J Appl Physiol.* 2007; 102:1099–1104.
138. Dromsky DM, Spiess BD, Fahlman A. Treatment of decompression sickness in swine with intravenous perfluorocarbon emulsion. *Aviat Space Environ Med.* 2004;75:301–305.
139. Yoshitani K, de Lange F, Ma Q, et al. Reduction in air bubble size using perfluorocarbons during cardiopulmonary bypass in the rat. *Anesth Analg.* 2006;103:1089–1093.
140. Zhu J, Hullett JB, Somera L, et al. Intravenous perfluorocarbon emulsion increases nitrogen washout after venous gas emboli in rabbits. *Undersea Hyperb Med.* 2007;34:7–20.
141. Eckmann DM, Armstead SC, Mardini F. Surfactants reduce platelet-bubble and platelet-platelet binding induced by in vitro air embolism. *Anesthesiology.* 2005;103:1204–1210.
142. Mitchell SJ, Doolette DJ, Wachholz CJ, et al., eds. *Management of Mild or Marginal Decompression Illness in Remote Locations.* Durham, NC: Divers Alert Network; 2005.
143. Centers for Disease Control and Prevention (CDC). Unintentional poisoning deaths—United States, 1999–2004. *MMWR Morb Mortal Wkly Rep.*2007;56:93–96.
144. Brown SD, Piantadosi CA. Reversal of carbon monoxide-cytochrome c oxidase binding by hyperbaric oxygen *in vivo*. *Adv Exp Med Biol.* 1989;248: 747–754.
145. Brown SD, Piantadosi CA. *In vivo* binding of carbon monoxide to cytochrome c oxidase in rat brain. *J Appl Physiol.* 1990;68:604–610.
146. Chance B, Erecinska M, Wagner M. Mitochondrial responses to carbon monoxide toxicity. *Ann N Y Acad Sci.* 1970;174:193–204.
147. Thom S. Antagonism of carbon monoxide-mediated brain lipid peroxidation by hyperbaric oxygen. *Toxicol Appl Pharmacol.* 1990;105:340–344.
148. Thom SR, Bhopale VM, Han ST, et al. Intravascular neutrophil activation due to carbon monoxide poisoning. *Am J Respir Crit Care Med.* 2006;174: 1239–1248.
149. Thom SR, Bhopale VM, Fisher D. Hyperbaric oxygen reduces delayed immune-mediated neuropathology in experimental carbon monoxide toxicity. *Toxicol Appl Pharmacol.* 2006;213:152–159.
150. Werner B, Back W, Akerblom H, et al. Two cases of acute carbon monoxide poisoning with delayed neurological sequelae after a "free" interval. *J Toxicol Clin Toxicol.* 1985;23:249–265.
151. Thom S, Taber R, Mendiguren I, et al. Delayed neuropsychologic sequelae after carbon monoxide poisoning: prevention by treatment with hyperbaric oxygen. *Ann Emerg Med.* 1995;25:474–480.
152. Weaver LK, Hopkins RO, Chan KJ, et al. Hyperbaric oxygen for acute carbon monoxide poisoning. *N Engl J Med.* 2002;347:1057–1067.
153. Pace N, Strajman E, Walker EL. Acceleration of carbon monoxide elimination in man by high pressure oxygen. *Science.* 1950;111:652–654.
154. Piantadosi CA. Diagnosis and treatment of carbon monoxide poisoning. *Respir Care Clin N Am.* 1999;5:183–202.
155. Brown SD, Piantadosi CA. Recovery of energy metabolism in rat brain after carbon monoxide hypoxia. *J Clin Invest.* 1992;89:666–672.

156. Ernst A, Zibrak JD. Carbon monoxide poisoning. *N Engl J Med.* 1998;339:1603–1608.
157. Tibbles PM, Edelsberg JS. Hyperbaric-oxygen therapy. *N Engl J Med.* 1996;334:1642–1648.
158. Thom SR. Hyperbaric-oxygen therapy for acute carbon monoxide poisoning. *N Engl J Med.* 2002;347:1105–1106.
159. Weaver LK, Valentine KJ, Hopkins RO. Carbon monoxide poisoning: risk factors for cognitive sequelae and the role of hyperbaric oxygen. *Am J Respir Crit Care Med.* 2007;176:491–497.
160. Van Hoesen KB, Camporesi EM, Moon RE, et al. Should hyperbaric oxygen be used to treat the pregnant patient for acute carbon monoxide poisoning? A case report and literature review. *JAMA.* 1989;261:1039–1043.
161. Meyers RA, Thom SR. Carbon monoxide and cyanide poisoning. In: Kindwall EP, ed. *Hyperbaric Medicine Practice.* Flagstaff, AZ: Best Publishing; 1994:344–366.
162. Cope C, Abramowitz S. Respiratory responses to intravenous sodium cyanide, a function of the oxygen-cyanide relationship. *Am Rev Respir Dis.* 1960;81:321–328.
163. Carden E. Hyperbaric oxygen in cyanide poisoning. *Anaesthesia.* 1970;25:442–443.
164. Goodhart GL. Patient treated with antidote kit and hyperbaric oxygen survives cyanide poisoning. *South Med J.* 1994;87:814–816.
165. Litovitz TL, Larkin RF, Myers RA. Cyanide poisoning treated with hyperbaric oxygen. *Am J Emerg Med.* 1983;1:94–101.
166. Takano T, Miyazaki Y, Nashimoto I, et al. Effect of hyperbaric oxygen on cyanide intoxication: in situ changes in intracellular oxidation reduction. *Undersea Biomed Res.* 1980;7:191–197.
167. Way JL, End E, Sheehy MH, et al. Effect of oxygen on cyanide intoxication. IV. Hyperbaric oxygen. *Toxicol Appl Pharmacol.* 1972;22:415–421.
168. Smilkstein MJ, Bronstein AC, Pickett HM, et al. Hyperbaric oxygen therapy for severe hydrogen sulfide poisoning. *J Emerg Med.* 1985;3:27–30.
169. Whitcraft DD 3rd, Bailey TD, Hart GB. Hydrogen sulfide poisoning treated with hyperbaric oxygen. *J Emerg Med.* 1985;3:23–25.
170. ATSDR. Toxicological Profile for Carbon Tetrachloride. U.S. Dept. of Health and Human Services PHS, Agency for Toxic Substances and Disease Registry; 2005.
171. Burkhart KK, Hall AH, Gerace R, et al. Hyperbaric oxygen treatment for carbon tetrachloride poisoning. *Drug Saf.* 1991;6:332–338.
172. Marzella L, Muhvich K, Myers RA. Effect of hyperoxia on liver necrosis induced by hepatotoxins. *Virchows Arch B Cell Pathol Incl Mol Pathol.* 1986;51:497–507.
173. Burk RF, Lane JM, Patel K. Relationship of oxygen and glutathione in protection against carbon tetrachloride-induced hepatic microsomal lipid peroxidation and covalent binding in the rat. Rationale for the use of hyperbaric oxygen to treat carbon tetrachloride ingestion. *J Clin Invest.* 1984;74:1996–2001.
174. Burk RF, Reiter R, Lane JM. Hyperbaric oxygen protection against carbon tetrachloride hepatotoxicity in the rat. Association with altered metabolism. *Gastroenterology.* 1986;90:812–818.
175. Bernacchi A, Myers R, Trump BF, et al. Protection of hepatocytes with hyperoxia against carbon tetrachloride-induced injury. *Toxicol Pathol.* 1984;12:315–323.
176. Truss CD, Killenberg PG. Treatment of carbon tetrachloride poisoning with hyperbaric oxygen. *Gastroenterology.* 1982;82:767–769.
177. Heimbach RD. Gas gangrene. In: Kindwall EP, ed. *Hyperbaric Medicine Practice.* Flagstaff, AZ: Best Publishing; 1994:374–388.
178. Brummelkamp WH, Boerema I, Hoogendyk L. Treatment of clostridial infections with hyperbaric oxygen drenching. A report on 26 cases. *Lancet.* 1963;1:235–238.
179. Brummelkamp WH, Hogendijk J, Boerema I. Treatment of anaerobic infections (clostridial myositis) by drenching tissues with oxygen under high atmospheric pressure. *Surgery.* 1961;49:299–302.
180. Van Unnik AJM. Inhibition of toxin production in Clostridium perfringens in vitro by hyperbaric oxygen. *Antoine von Leeuwenhoek.* 1965;31:181–186.
181. Demello FJ, Haglin JJ, Hitchcock CR. Comparative study of experimental *Clostridium perfringens* infection in dogs treated with antibiotics, surgery and hyperbaric oxygen. *Surgery.* 1973;73:936–941.
182. Clarke LA, Moon RE. Hyperbaric oxygen in the treatment of life threatening soft tissue infections. *Respir Care Clin N Am.* 1999;5:203–219.
183. Bakker DJ. Selected aerobic and anaerobic soft tissue infections diagnosis and the use of hyperbaric oxygen as an adjunct. In: Kindwall EP, ed. *Hyperbaric Medicine Practice.* Flagstaff, AZ: Best Publishing; 1994:396–415.
184. Riseman JA, Zamboni WA, Curtis A, et al. Hyperbaric oxygen therapy for necrotizing fasciitis reduces mortality and the need for debridements. *Surgery.* 1990;108:847–850.
185. Dahm P, Roland FH, Vaslef SN, et al. Outcome analysis in patients with primary necrotizing fasciitis of the male genitalia. *Urology.* 2000;56:31–35; discussion 5–6.
186. Blitzer A, Lawson W, Meyers BR, et al. Patient survival factors in paranasal sinus mucormycosis. *Laryngoscope.* 1980;90:635–648.
187. Price JC, Stevens DL. Hyperbaric oxygen in the treatment of rhinocerebral mucormycosis. *Laryngoscope.* 1980;90:737–747.
188. Couch L, Theilen F, Mader JT. Rhinocerebral mucormycosis with cerebral extension successfully treated with adjunctive hyperbaric oxygen therapy. *Arch Otolaryngol Head Neck Surg.* 1988;114:791–794.
189. Ferguson BJ, Mitchell TG, Moon R, et al. Adjunctive hyperbaric oxygen for treatment of rhinocerebral mucormycosis. *Rev Infect Dis.* 1988;10:551–559.
190. Farmer JC, Kindwall EP. Use of adjunctive hyperbaric oxygen in the management of fungal disease. In: Kindwall EP, ed. *Hyperbaric Medicine Practice.* Flagstaff, AZ: Best Publishing; 1994:582–586.
191. Hart GB, Lennon PA, Strauss MD. Hyperbaric oxygen in exceptional acute blood-loss anemia. *J Hyperbar Med.* 1987;2:205–210.
192. Van Meter KW. A systematic review of the application of hyperbaric oxygen in the treatment of severe anemia: an evidence-based approach. *Undersea Hyperb Med.* 2005;32:61–83.
193. Palzur E, Vlodavsky E, Mulla H, et al. Hyperbaric oxygen therapy for reduction of secondary brain damage in head injury: an animal model of brain contusion. *J Neurotrauma.* 2004;21:41–48.
194. Rockswold SB, Rockswold GL, Vargo JM, et al. Effects of hyperbaric oxygenation therapy on cerebral metabolism and intracranial pressure in severely brain injured patients. *J Neurosurg.* 2001;94:403–411.
195. Rockswold GL, Ford SE, Anderson DC, et al. Results of a prospective randomized trial for treatment of severely brain-injured patients with hyperbaric oxygen. *J Neurosurg.* 1992;76:929–934.
196. Ikeda K, Ajiki H, Nagao H, et al. Experimental and clinical use of hyperbaric oxygen in burns. In: Wada J, Iwa T, eds. *Proceedings of the 4th International Congress on Hyperbaric Medicine.* Baltimore, MD: Williams & Wilkins; 1970:377–380.
197. Hart GB, O'Reilly RR, Broussard ND, et al. Treatment of burns with hyperbaric oxygen. *Surg Gynecol Obstet.* 1974;139:693–696.
198. Niezgoda JA, Cianci P, Folden BW, et al. The effect of hyperbaric oxygen therapy on a burn wound model in human volunteers. *Plast Reconstr Surg.* 1997;99:1620–1625.
199. Perrins DJD. A failed attempt to limit tissue destruction in scalds of pig skins with hyperbaric oxygen. In: Wada J, Iwa T, eds. *Proceedings of the 4th International Congress on Hyperbaric Medicine.* Baltimore, MD: Williams & Wilkins; 1970:381–387.
200. Cianci P, Lueders HW, Lee H, et al. Adjunctive hyperbaric oxygen therapy reduces length of hospitalization in thermal burns. *J Burn Care Rehabil.* 1989;10:432–435.
201. Cianci P, Williams C, Lueders H, et al. Adjunctive hyperbaric oxygen in the treatment of thermal burns. An economic analysis. *J Burn Care Rehabil.* 1990;11:140–143.
202. Brannen AL, Still J, Haynes M, et al. A randomized prospective trial of hyperbaric oxygen in a referral burn center population. *Am Surg.* 1997;63:205–208.
203. Villanueva E, Bennett MH, Wasiak J, et al. Hyperbaric oxygen therapy for thermal burns. *Cochrane Database Syst Rev.* 2004:CD004727.
204. Whalen R, Saltzman H, Holloway D, et al. Cardiovascular and blood gas responses to hyperbaric oxygenation. *Am J Cardiol.* 1965;15:638–646.
205. Swift PC, Turner JH, Oxer HF, et al. Myocardial hibernation identified by hyperbaric oxygen treatment and echocardiography in postinfarction patients: comparison with exercise thallium scintigraphy. *Am Heart J.* 1992;124:1151–1158.
206. Sterling DL. Hyperbaric oxygen limits infarct size in ischemic rabbit myocardium in vivo. *Circulation.* 1993;88:1931–1936.
207. Shandling AH, Ellestad MH, Hart GB, et al. Hyperbaric oxygen and thrombolysis in myocardial infarction: the "HOT MI" pilot study. *Am Heart J.* 1997;134:544–550.
208. Stavitsky Y, Shandling AH, Ellestad MH, et al. Hyperbaric oxygen and thrombolysis in myocardial infarction: the "HOT MI" randomized multicenter study. *Cardiology.* 1998;90:131–136.
209. Heyman A, Saltzman HA, Whalen RE. The use of hyperbaric oxygenation in the treatment of cerebral ischemia and infarction. *Circulation.* 1966;33 (Suppl II):20–27.
210. Veltkamp R, Warner DS, Domoki F, et al. Hyperbaric oxygen decreases infarct size and behavioral deficit after transient focal cerebral ischemia in rats. *Brain Res.* 2000;853:68–73.
211. Gunther A, Kuppers-Tiedt L, Schneider PM, et al. Reduced infarct volume and differential effects on glial cell activation after hyperbaric oxygen treatment in rat permanent focal cerebral ischaemia. *Eur J Neurosci.* 2005;21:3189–3194.
212. Veltkamp R, Siebing DA, Heiland S, et al. Hyperbaric oxygen induces rapid protection against focal cerebral ischemia. *Brain Res.* 2005;1037:134–138.
213. Qin Z, Karabiyikoglu M, Hua Y, et al. Hyperbaric oxygen-induced attenuation of hemorrhagic transformation after experimental focal transient cerebral ischemia. *Stroke.* 2007;38:1362–1367.
214. Veltkamp R, Bieber K, Wagner S, et al. Hyperbaric oxygen reduces basal lamina degradation after transient focal cerebral ischemia in rats. *Brain Res.* 2006;1076:231–237.
215. Anderson DC, Bottini AG, Jagiella WM, et al. A pilot study of hyperbaric oxygen in the treatment of human stroke. *Stroke.* 1991;22:1137–1142.
216. Nighoghossian N, Trouillas P, Adeleine P, et al. Hyperbaric oxygen in the treatment of acute ischemic stroke. A double-blind pilot study. *Stroke.* 1995;26:1369–1372.

217. Rusyniak DE, Kirk MA, May JD, et al. Hyperbaric oxygen therapy in acute ischemic stroke: results of the Hyperbaric Oxygen in Acute Ischemic Stroke Trial Pilot Study. *Stroke.* 2003;34:571–574.
218. Cochran WD, Levison H, Muirhead DM Jr, et al. A clinical trial of high oxygen pressure for the respiratory-distress syndrome. *N Engl J Med.* 1965;272:347.
219. Camporesi EM, Moon RE. Hyperbaric oxygen as an adjunct to therapeutic lung lavage in pulmonary alveolar proteinosis. In: Bove AA, Bachrach AJ, Greenbaum LJ Jr, eds. *Underwater and Hyperbaric Physiology IX Proceedings of the Ninth International Symposium on Underwater and Hyperbaric Physiology.* Bethesda, MD: Undersea and Hyperbaric Medical Society; 1987:955–960.
220. Biervliet JD, Peper JA, Roos CM, et al. Whole lung lavage under hyperbaric conditions: 1. The monitoring. *Adv Exp Med Biol.* 1992;317:115–120.
221. van der Kleij AJ, Peper JA, Biervliet JD, et al. Whole lung lavage under hyperbaric conditions: 2. Monitoring tissue oxygenation. *Adv Exp Med Biol.* 1992;317:121–124.
222. Russell JB, Snider MT, Richard RB, et al. Hyperbaric nitrous oxide as a sole anesthetic agent in humans. *Anesth Analg.* 1990;70:289–295.
223. Lambertsen CJ, Idicula J. A new gas lesion syndrome in man, induced by "isobaric gas counterdiffusion." *J Appl Physiol.* 1975;39:434–443.
224. Acott CJ, Gorman DF. Decompression illness and nitrous oxide anaesthesia in a sports diver. *Anaesth Intensive Care.* 1992;20:249–250.
225. Weaver LK, Howe S. Noninvasive Doppler blood pressure monitoring in the monoplace hyperbaric chamber. *J Clin Monit.* 1991;7:304–308.
226. NFPA. National Fire Protection Association, Standards for Healthcare Facilities. Document 99, Chapter 20; 2005.
227. Moon RE, Bergquist LV, Conklin B, et al. Monaghan 225 ventilator use under hyperbaric conditions. *Chest.* 1986;89:846–851.
228. Weaver LK, Greenway L, Elliott CG. Performance of the Sechrist 500A hyperbaric ventilator in a monoplace hyperbaric chamber. *J Hyperbar Med.* 1988;3:215–225.
229. Weaver LK. Operational use and patient care in the monoplace hyperbaric chamber. *Respir Care Clin N Am.* 1999;5:51–92.
230. Weaver LK, Howe S. Normobaric measurement of arterial oxygen tension in subjects exposed to hyperbaric oxygen. *Chest.* 1992;102:1175–1181.
231. Van Meter K. Medical field management of the injured diver. *Respir Care Clin N Am.* 1999;5:137–177.
232. Booth L. Details of an X-ray system for use in diving medicine. In: Smith G, ed. *Proceedings of the Sixth International Congress on Hyperbaric Medicine.* Aberdeen: Aberdeen University Press; 1979:443–444.
233. Kindwall EP. Contraindications and side effects to hyperbaric oxygen treatment. In: Kindwall EP, ed. *Hyperbaric Medicine Practice.* Flagstaff, AZ: Best Publishing; 1994:46–54.
234. Wolf HK, Moon RE, Mitchell PR, et al. Barotrauma and air embolism in hyperbaric oxygen therapy. *Am J Forensic Med Pathol.* 1990;11: 149–153.
235. Weaver LK, Churchill S. Pulmonary edema associated with hyperbaric oxygen therapy. *Chest.* 2001;120:1407–1409.
236. Leitch DR, Green RD. Pulmonary barotrauma in divers and the treatment of cerebral arterial gas embolism. *Aviat Space Environ Med.* 1986;57:931–938.
237. Moon RE, Gorman DF. Treatment of the decompression disorders. In: Neuman TS, Brubakk AO, eds. *The Physiology and Medicine of Diving.* New York, NY: Elsevier Science; 2003:600–650.
238. Moon RE, Sheffield PJ. Guidelines for treatment of decompression illness. *Aviat Space Environ Med.* 1997;68:234–243.
239. Piantadosi CA. The role of hyperbaric oxygen in carbon monoxide, cyanide and sulfide intoxication. *Prob Resp Care.* 1991;4:215–231.
240. Berk RF, Lane JM, Patel K. Relationship of oxygen and glutathione in protection against carbon tetrachloride-induced hepatic microsomal lipid peroxidation and covalent binding in the rat. Rationale for the use of hyperbaric oxygen to treat carbon tetrachloride ingestion. *J Clin Invest.* 1984; 74:1996–2001.
241. Bakker DJ, van der Kleij AJ. Soft tissue infections including clostridial myonecrosis: diagnosis and treatment. In: Oriani G, Marroni A, Wattel F, eds. *Handbook on Hyperbaric Medicine.* New York: Springer-Verlag; 1996: 343–361.
242. Bakker DJ, van der Kleij AJ. Clostridial myonecrosis. In: Oriani G, Marroni A, Wattel F, eds. *Handbook on Hyperbaric Medicine.* New York: Springer-Verlag; 1996:362–385.
243. Escobar SJ, Slade JB, Jr., Hunt TK, et al. Adjuvant hyperbaric oxygen therapy (HBO_2) for treatment of necrotizing fasciitis reduces mortality and amputation rate. *Undersea Hyperb Med* 2005;32:437–443.
244. Zamboni WA, Kindwall EP. Author's reply to: still unproved in necrotising fasciitis. *BMJ.* 1993;307:936.
245. Yohai RA, Bullock JD, Aziz AA, et al. Survival factors in rhino-orbital-cerebral mucormycosis. *Surv Ophthalmol.* 1994;39:3–22.
246. Bouachour G, Cronier P, Gouello JP, et al. Hyperbaric oxygen therapy in the management of crush injuries: a randomized double-blind placebo-controlled clinical trial. *J Trauma.* 1996;41:333–339.
247. Nemiroff PM. Synergistic effects of pentoxifylline and hyperbaric oxygen on skin flaps. *Arch Otolaryngol Head Neck Surg.* 1988;114:977.
248. Zamboni WA, Roth AC, Russell RC, et al. The effect of hyperbaric oxygen on reperfusion of ischemic axial skin flaps: a laser Doppler analysis. *Ann Plast Surg.* 1992;28:339–341.
249. Jansen HM, Zuurmond WW, Roos CM, et al. Whole-lung lavage under hyperbaric oxygen conditions for alveolar proteinosis with respiratory failure. *Chest.* 1987;91:829–832.
250. Niu AKC, Yang C, Lee HC, et al. Burns treated with adjunctive hyperbaric oxygen therapy—a comparative study in humans. *J Hyperbar Med.* 1987; 2:75–85.
251. Bevers RF, Bakker DJ, Kurth KH. Hyperbaric oxygen treatment for haemorrhagic radiation cystitis. *Lancet.* 1995;346:803–805.
252. Farmer JC Jr, Shelton DL, Angelillo JD, et al. Treatment of radiation-induced tissue injury by hyperbaric oxygen. *Ann Otol Rhinol Laryngol.* 1978;87:707–715.
253. Ferguson BJ, Hudson WR, Farmer JC, Jr. Hyperbaric oxygen therapy for laryngeal radionecrosis. *Ann Otol Rhinol Laryngol.* 1987;96:1–6.
254. Norkool DM, Hampson NB, Gibbons RP, et al. Hyperbaric oxygen therapy for radiation-induced hemorrhagic cystitis. *J Urol.* 1993;150:332–334.
255. Fife CE, Buyukcakir C, Otto GH, et al. The predictive value of transcutaneous oxygen tension measurement in diabetic lower extremity ulcers treated with hyperbaric oxygen therapy: a retrospective analysis of 1,144 patients. *Wound Repair Regen.* 2002;10:198–207.
256. Broughton G 2nd. Management of the brown recluse spider bite to the glans penis. *Mil Med.* 1996;161:627–629.
257. Maynor ML, Moon RE, Klitzman B, et al. Brown recluse spider envenomation: a prospective trial of hyperbaric oxygen therapy. *Acad Emerg Med.* 1997;4:184–192.
258. Divers Alert Network. *Annual Diving Report.* Durham, NC: Divers Alert Network; 2006.
259. van Hulst RA, Drenthen J, Haitsma JJ, et al. Effects of hyperbaric treatment in cerebral air embolism on intracranial pressure, brain oxygenation, and brain glucose metabolism in the pig. *Crit Care Med.* 2005;33:841–846.

CHAPTER 40 ■ ANESTHESIA IN THE ICU

AVNER SIDI • YAKOV YUSIM

THE NEED

The intensive care unit (ICU) provides services for patients with life-threatening disorders. Most require analgesia and sedation for pain and anxiety management as well as mechanical ventilation, or as adjuvant therapy for bedside procedures done in the ICU (i.e., tracheostomy, venous and arterial catheterization, etc.). These patients may undergo surgical interventions outside the traditional operating room (OR) and/or "off-department" procedures such as magnetic resonance imaging (MRI) and computed tomography (CT) scan, or other radiographic examinations (1).

The roots of critical care medicine (CCM) are founded in anesthesiology, in our predecessors' efforts to extend the OR care delivered to the critically ill to the postanesthetic care unit (PACU). ICUs were developed to deal with real-time problems: Respiratory failure caused by polio epidemics in the early 1950s (2) and, later, that seen after cardiothoracic surgery (3). The needs of these high-acuity patients led to the development of better OR monitoring and more aggressive management. These devices and this approach were used not only in the OR, but also in the high-acuity areas that evolved into today's ICUs. In that regard, anesthesiology and intensive care medicine influenced and fertilized one another. This symbiosis was mostly, although not completely, positive.

ANESTHESIOLOGY IN CRITICAL CARE MEDICINE: A CONTINUATION OR SYMBIOSIS?

As it is difficult to safely sedate the critically ill, it is not surprising that anesthetic agents moved from the OR for use in the ICU. Of course, problems may occur with long-term ICU use of drugs initially conceived for short-term OR anesthetic use (4).

Long- and Short-term Use of Anesthetic Drugs and Techniques

Pharmacotherapy

Nitrous oxide has been a key component of general anesthesia for several decades. It has also been used to provide sedation for patients in the ICU. As a result of long-term administration of nitrous oxide, a previously unseen complication developed: severe bone marrow depression due to interference with vitamin B_{12} metabolism (5). Similarly, when etomidate, with its excellent safety profile in the OR, was used for continuous sedation in the ICU, acute adrenal insufficiency due to impaired 11-β-hydroxylase activity was noted (6).

More recently, the difficulties with moving drugs from the OR into the ICU continue to surface. Some patients with acute respiratory distress syndrome (ARDS) require the prolonged use of neuromuscular blockers to facilitate mechanical ventilation. Ventilatory modes such as pressure control–inverse inspiration/expiration (I:E) ratio and partial liquid ventilation with perfluorocarbons all require profound sedation and, often, paralysis. When the neuromuscular blocking drugs are discontinued, patients may be profoundly weak for extended periods of time. This condition has become known as the neuromyopathy of critical illness and, while commonly reported with pancuronium, vecuronium, and other steroid-ring–based agents, it may be seen with other agents as well (7). This syndrome is prevalent in patients having received glucocorticoids during their ICU admission.

Propofol, which has many advantages over other sedative drugs in the ICU, has been associated with sepsis, which is attributed to failure to use appropriate sterile techniques with a lipid-based solution. In the pediatric and adult populations, there have been reports of fatal lactic acidosis—the *propofol infusion syndrome*—in association with high doses for an extended period (8,9).

Other problems can occur with the long-term use of drugs initially conceived for short-term anesthetic use. Metabolites of agents such as diazepam, midazolam, and morphine can accumulate in patients, especially the elderly or those with major organ dysfunction, resulting in prolonged sedation.

Technique: Monitoring Devices

It is not just drugs from the OR that are of interest to intensivists. The pulmonary artery catheter, initially used by cardiologists in coronary care units and coronary angiography suites in the early 1970s, was met with enthusiasm by OR anesthesiologists, especially those caring for patients during cardiac procedures. Another device developed for the OR, but of great interest in the ICU, is the bispectral index (BIS) monitor. Especially when neuromuscular blockers are used in the ICU patient for an extended period, how does one ensure that the patient is adequately sedated? Although there are few good studies documenting the utility of BIS in the ICU, increasing recognition and a possible role for such a device are evolving. Neither of these devices is without risk and controversy, although both, in our opinion, have their utility (10,11); this is discussed further in other chapters herein.

NEWER THERAPIES IN ANESTHESIA AND THE INTENSIVE CARE UNIT

As clinical medicine has advanced, new syndromes have emerged. ARDS was first reported in 1967 (12), probably because before that time, patients rarely survived long enough for the full-blown syndrome to develop. Today, we have multiple organ failure/dysfunction syndrome (MODS), and it is the unusual death that results from acute hypoxia or acute hypotension.

A similar pattern is found in the OR analogues of the critically ill patient: The American Society of Anesthesiologists (ASA) physical status (PS) V patient. Although the perioperative mortality in these patients has decreased to less than 60%—both intraoperatively and in the 24 hours postoperatively—mortality occurring at greater than two weeks postoperatively during hospitalization has increased from 0% to more than 15% (13), suggesting not an actual decrease in mortality rate, but a shift in time when mortality occurs. This may also be seen in posttrauma deaths, where immediate death is related to neurologic or cardiovascular injury, or hemorrhage, and late death is due to infection, multiorgan failure, or both (14).

To a great extent, perioperative mortality is a product of the severity of illness and the advances in life support that constitute the body of the practice of anesthesiology (15). Thus, our interventions can affect the rate of acute mortality. But is mortality being decreased overall, or just postponed? In any case, to determine our priorities while practicing anesthesia in the ICU environment, we need to learn and assess patient risk and safety in the ICU.

RISK ASSESSMENT

American Society of Anesthesiologists Classification and Intensive Care Unit Patients

Assessing patient risk in the perioperative period is traditionally and routinely done using the ASA classification system. The ASA PS classification was developed in 1941 (16) and revised in 1963 (17,18) to include five categories, and modified "unofficially" and expanded in 1994 to include a sixth category for organ donors (19). Category V indicates that the "patient is moribund and not expected to survive for 24 hours with or without operation" (17–19). Although the ASA PS V category is associated with a high mortality, it is less clear that it is a valid predictor of death shortly *after* operation (13). While studies regarding morbidity and mortality in this group were published in the 1960s and 1970s (18,20–23) and in the late 1980s and 1990s (13,24–37), the original purpose of the system was only to describe the preoperative condition in order to facilitate tabulation of statistical data in anesthesiology (16). Even though the ASA PS V category predicts that a patient is *at risk* for death, it was never intended to be a multifactorial index or predictor of outcome (22). We have shown (12), as have others (38), that the ASA PS V category is likely not a sensitive predictor of intraoperative mortality, even though an ASA PS V status may correlate with overall perioperative mortality (18,20,21). Interestingly enough, the ASA PS score may correlate with perioperative mortality similar to or better than other systems devised to predict mortality or morbidity, such as the Goldman index in noncardiac surgery patients (39), the Reiss index in the elderly (29,30), the Hachinski Ischemic Score (HIS) in ICU patients (31), various perioperative variables (blood loss, ventilation, ICU stay) (32) or age (28,33), and in cancer patients (34). We found that the ASA PS V classification is associated with a higher incidence of untoward respiratory and cardiac events during emergency surgery (13). This finding is similar to that reported elsewhere (25,40,41). An ASA PS classification greater than 3 was found to be one of the independent predictors of severe adverse outcome associated with general anesthesia (27). Univariate analysis showed a significant correlation between ASA class and perioperative variables (intraoperative blood loss, duration of postoperative ventilation, and duration of intensive care stay), postoperative complications, and mortality rate (32) (Table 40.1).

Univariate analysis demonstrated the importance of the ASA PS classification in the development of postoperative complications in the related organ systems. Estimating the increased risk odds ratio for single variables, it was found that the risk of a complication was influenced mainly by ASA class, with ASA PS class IV having a risk odds ratio = 4.2 and ASA class III a risk odds ratio = 2.2. Thus, it is obvious that ASA physical status classification is a predictor of postoperative outcome (32).

Among ASA PS V patients, there is a high incidence of death after diagnostic procedures (13). This is probably related to the new era in both diagnostic testing and anesthetic care, such as CT and/or MRI scans of critically ill patients that involve general anesthesia or anesthesia care and monitoring during transport and the procedure. The ASA score subjectively categorizes patients into five subgroups by preoperative physical fitness. Since inception, it has been revised on several occasions and now also includes an "E" suffix denoting an emergency case (42). ASA classification makes no adjustment for age, gender, weight, or pregnancy, nor does it reflect the nature of the planned surgery, the skill of the anesthetist or surgeon, or the degree of pretheater preparation or facilities for postoperative care. While the ASA PS score does not predict risk for a particular patient or intervention—since underlying fitness is an important predictor of survival from surgery—the ASA PS score does have *some* correlation with outcome. As it is simple and widely understood, it is commonly used as a part of the preoperative assessment, and is an easy tool for audit.

In the United Kingdom, patients are coded according to their ASA and CEPOD (confidential enquiry into perioperative deaths) (43) scores. These describe the patient from the perspectives of basic risk banding and urgency of surgery. The scores allow anesthesiologists and surgeons to describe their workload and outcomes, which may be helpful for audit purposes and outcomes research.

Acute Physiology and Chronic Health Evaluation Score, American Society of Anesthesiologists Classification, and Other Scoring Systems

Interestingly, prediction of morbidity and mortality by the Acute Physiology and Chronic Health Evaluation (APACHE)

TABLE 40.1

PERIOPERATIVE VARIABLES IN RELATION TO AMERICAN SOCIETY OF ANESTHESIOLOGISTS (ASA) CLASSIFICATION

Perioperative variable	ASA I	ASA II	ASA III	ASA IV
Duration of operation (h)	1.25	1.3	2.1	1.9
Blood loss, intraoperative (L)	0.08	0.1	0.3	1.5
Postoperative ventilation (h)	1	4	8	47
ICU stay (d)	0.2	1	2	5
Postoperative stay (d)	9	16	21	18
Pulmonary infection (%)	0.5	2	5	12
Pulmonary complication—other (%)	0.6	2	4	10
Cardiac complications (%)	0.1	2	5	18
Urinary infection (%)	2	5	6	5
Wound infection (%)	2	4	6	11
Mortality (%)	0.1	1	4	18

Each variable has a significant difference of $p < 0.05$ according to Fisher's exact test or Student's test between the ASA I and the ASA II, ASA III, or ASA IV classification. Data from Sidi A, Lobato EB, Cohen JA. The American Society of Anesthesiologists Physical Status: category V revisited. *J Clin Anesth.* 2000;12:328–334.

II system, which has only up to an 85% success rate in predicting mortality (44,45), has been compared to the ASA PS score several times in the last decade. APACHE II was found to be similar to the ASA PS system in its ability to predict outcome in nonelderly patients undergoing major surgery (35); APACHE II may, however, be better in certain groups of ICU patients (31) and in elderly patients with gastrointestinal bleeding (36). Comparison of the APACHE II system to other severity classification scoring systems has been performed (44,46), and is discussed elsewhere in this textbook.

Cardiac surgery remains a difficult area for outcome prediction in the ICU (45). A combination of intraoperative and postoperative variables, including the Parsonnet scoring system and the APACHE II and III scores, can improve predictive ability. The Parsonnet study (47) demonstrated that it is possible to design a simple method of risk stratification of open-heart surgery patients that makes it feasible to analyze operative results by risk groups and to compare results in similar groups between institutions.

Cardiac Risk and Anesthetic Risk in Intensive Care Unit Patients

Little information is available regarding the interaction of perioperative management (including ICU) and clinical outcome in patients undergoing major surgery such as cardiovascular and cardiothoracic interventions. Most data are derived from patients with ischemia undergoing aortocoronary bypass, and are extrapolated to other groups. Thirty years ago, Goldman et al. analyzed more than 1,000 patients having undergone major noncardiac surgery (48). Using multivariate analysis, they identified nine preoperative variables that independently correlated with postoperative cardiac complications. Although the patient population was "noncardiac," the Goldman Cardiac Risk Index became popular because of the relative weight and value assigned to each factor, which facilitated calculation of "overall cardiac risk." Eventually, this index was used to quantitate preoperative cardiac recommendations.

The scientific validity of this index has been questioned (49), as was its prediction for adverse cardiac outcome in comparison to the ASA PS classification for noncardiac surgery (50). The latter work showed that patients undergoing abdominal aortic aneurysm surgery were at higher risk for cardiac complication than suggested by the Goldman index. Another study investigated the utility of the Goldman index in vascular surgery (51), and found that more cardiac events occurred than it predicted. Thus, as a tool to plan postoperative management, the original Goldman index failed in cardiovascular patient populations.

Another prospective assessment of risk was the one conducted by Detsky et al. in patients undergoing noncardiac surgery (52,53). Changes in the index were proposed to improve its accuracy. The modified index added risk factors such as angina, pulmonary edema, and old myocardial infarction (MI), and deleted the risk factor of major surgery. Detsky et al. presented a statistical approach to assessing cardiac risk by converting average risk for patients undergoing particular surgical procedures (pretest probabilities) to average risks for patients with each index score (posttest probabilities). The likelihood ratios, presented in Table 40.2, convert a given pretest probability of complications into the posttest probability or change in risk, based on points assigned by the Detsky index. A likelihood ratio of more than 1 denotes an incremental risk over the pretest probability in a given procedure (52).

A more recent evaluation score—the Cardiac Anesthesia Risk Evaluation (CARE) score—is a simple risk classification system for cardiac surgical patients (54). It is based on clinical judgment and three clinical variables: comorbid conditions categorized as controlled or uncontrolled, surgical complexity, and urgency of the procedure (Table 40.3). This scoring system can rapidly stratify a patient for the probability of morbidity and mortality. The multifactorial risk scores of CARE were also compared to the risk indexes developed for general cardiac surgical populations in ICU patients by Parsonnet et al. (47), Tuman et al. (55), and Tu et al. (56). When the CARE score was compared to these other three multifactorial risk indexes for prediction of mortality and morbidity after cardiac surgery,

TABLE 40.2

PERIOPERATIVE CARDIAC COMPLICATION RATIO ACCORDING TO THE DETSKY CARDIAC RISK INDEX[a]

		Ratio		
Class	Points	Minor surgery	Major surgery	All surgery
I	0–15	0.4	0.4	0.4
II	15–30	2.8	3.6	3.4
III	>30	12.2	14.9	10.6

[a] Perioperative cardiac complication ratio, in minor, major, and all surgery cases, according to the Detsky Cardiac Risk Index. Detsky presented a statistical approach to assessing cardiac risks by converting average risks for patients undergoing particular surgical procedures (pretest probabilities) to average risks for patients with each index score (posttest probabilities). Data from Detsky AS, Abrams HB, McLaughlin JR, et al. Predicting cardiac complications in patients undergoing non-cardiac surgery. *J Gen Intern Med.* 1986;1(4):211–219; and Detsky AS, Abrams HB, Forbath N, et al. Cardiac assessment for patients undergoing noncardiac surgery. A multifactorial clinical risk index. *Arch Intern Med.* 1986;146(11): 2131–2134.

the CARE score performs as well as multifactorial risk indexes for outcome prediction in cardiac surgery. Cardiac anesthesiologists use those scores in their practice and can predict patient outcome with acceptable accuracy.

These classifications contain variables available in most of our patients and, like the CARE score, they apply to all cardiac surgical patients, and not only to those undergoing coronary artery surgery. Another system was developed in Europe by Peter and Lutz as an instrument for grading the level of anesthetic risk for a patient (57). Twenty parameters are involved in that scoring system: patient status, nature of the operation, age, weight, fasting status, consciousness, blood pressure, heart rate, pulse rate, respirations, renal function, liver function, blood glucose, electrolytes, hydration, hemoglobin, allergies, other major diseases, expected operative time, and burns (Table 40.4). Patients with a previous myocardial infarction were compared to those with no prior infarction to determine the influence of previous infarction on perioperative cardiac complications. Patients with a previous myocardial infarction had a higher perioperative myocardial infarction rate (3.8%) than did those patients with no prior history of myocardial infarction (0.4%) (57).

Although good predictive accuracy was found, there are problems. Measured ejection fraction was not included as an independent component in multifactorial risk indexes, even though evidence suggests that the degree of left ventricular (LV) dysfunction predicts outcome in noncardiac surgery (58). Thus, the cardiac risk indexes remain imperfect but useful tools for determining perioperative risk for cardiac events. Additional cardiac tests should be routinely employed in determining the individual patient's current risk status. Indeed, in an editorial, Goldman recognized that the new techniques and information changed the methods for prospective evaluation (59). The first technical breakthrough was the use of biostatistical analysis; the second used sophisticated evaluation such as echocardiography and scintigraphy to deal with the less well-defined middle-risk group. The next breakthrough may be utilization of randomized control trials—a methodologic rather than a technologic change. Work is ongoing by different investigators (60) to continuously update the cardiac risk indexes, which remain important tools in the current era.

In estimating an updated probability, it is quite possible that the risk indexes derived from a general patient population may not be accurate or perfectly applicable to more selected patient samples—such as those patients undergoing cardiac or aortic surgery, or who are in the ICU. By integrating the patient's score on a risk index with the prior probability of major complications in a large population of similar patients, the resulting "risk estimate" may be superior to the prior probability or the old risk index alone (Table 40.5).

INTENSIVE CARE UNIT PROCEDURES: COST SAVINGS AND PATIENT SAFETY

ICU management of critically ill patients often includes anesthesia for minor procedures such as tracheostomy and percutaneous endoscopic gastrostomy (PEG) tube. Although advances in ICU airway management include percutaneous tracheostomy, semi-open tracheostomy, and conventional tracheostomy, many critically ill, surgical and injured patients still receive open tracheostomy in the OR (61). While percutaneous tracheostomy is performed routinely in many medical ICU settings, in high-risk surgical and trauma patients, often with unstable cervical spine injury and tissue edema, direct visualization of the cervical structures and trachea is imperative during tracheostomy. Open tracheostomy and PEG in the ICU can be undertaken in selected patients as part of a collaborative, multidisciplinary ICU patient management strategy (61). This is done to address the risk of patient transport, the inappropriate use of OR time, and the cost to the patient as part of an effort to standardize and improve patient care. The OR costs included basic room fee and charge per minute for general surgery and anesthesia and the anesthesia professional fee; the ICU costs included supplies. The surgical professional fee, tracheostomy tube cost, and gastroscope maintenance were not included in the analysis. For purposes of analysis, OR tracheostomy and OR PEG times were defined as 120 minutes and 60 minutes, respectively, although analysis through the fiscal year yielded widely divergent average OR times for these procedures. A cost comparison for individual procedure, total to date, and associated cost savings was shown by Knudsen et al. (61). By that comparison tracheostomy versus PEG had OR costs of $37,000 versus $17,000, ICU costs of $1,300 versus $1,700, and cost savings of $35,700 versus $15,300, respectively. Although the study is very small, tracheostomy and PEG placement in the ICU in selected patients were noted to be safe, avoided patient travel, improved OR utilization, and yielded a significant reduction in cost; in this study, there were no complications (61).

ANALGESIA AND SEDATION IN THE INTENSIVE CARE UNIT

Principles

Sedation is an essential component in the management of intensive care patients. It is required to relieve the discomfort

TABLE 40.3

CARDIAC ANESTHESIA RISK EVALUATION SCALE (CARE SCORE)

Part A

Parameter	Status	Group
Cardiac disease	Stable	A1
	Uncontrolled	A2
	Advanced (end stage)	A3
Other medical diseases	None	B1
	One or more controlled	B2
	One or more uncontrolled	B3
Cardiac surgery complexity	Noncomplex	C1
	Complex	C2
	Undertaken as last hope to save or improve life	C3
Urgency of surgery	Nonemergency	D1
	Emergency (surgery performed as soon as diagnosis is made and an operating room is available)	D2

Part B

Situation	Score	Risk category
A1 and B1 and C1	1	1
A1 and B2 and C1	2	2
(A2 or B3 or C2) and D1	3	3
(A2 or B3 or C2) and D2	3E	4
(A2 or A3 or B3) and C2 and D1	4	5
(A2 or A3 or B3) and C2 and D2	4E	6
A3 and C3 and D1	5	7
A3 and C3 and D2	5E	8

Part C

Risk category	Morbidity (%)	Prolonged length of stay (%)	Mortality (%)
1	5.4	2.9	0.5
2	10.3	5.1	1.1
3	19.0	8.8	2.2
4	32.1	14.7	4.5
5	48.8	23.5	8.8
6	65.8	35.4	16.7
7	79.6	49.4	29.3
8	88.7	63.6	46.2

Controlled medical problems include:

- Controlled hypertension
- Controlled diabetes mellitus
- Controlled peripheral vascular disease
- Controlled chronic obstructive pulmonary disease
- Controlled systemic disease

Uncontrolled cardiac or medical problems include:

- Unstable angina pectoris treated with intravenous heparin or nitroglycerin
- Preoperative intra-aortic balloon pump
- Heart failure with pulmonary or peripheral edema
- Uncontrolled hypertension
- Renal insufficiency (serum creatinine >140 mol/L)
- Other debilitating systemic disease

(continued)

TABLE 40.3

(CONTINUED)

Part C			
Risk category	Morbidity (%)	Prolonged length of stay (%)	Mortality (%)
Complex surgery includes: ■ Reoperation ■ Combined valve and coronary artery surgery ■ Multiple valve surgery ■ Left ventricular aneurysmectomy ■ Repair of ventricular septal defect after myocardial infarction ■ Coronary artery bypass of diffuse or heavily calcified vessels			

The Cardiac Anesthesia Risk Evaluation scale (CARE score) is a risk classification system for patients undergoing cardiac surgery. Assessing disease and surgery status (part A) and risk category according to the combined situation (part B), this scale can be used to assess patients for the probability of morbidity and mortality (part C).
Data from Dupuis JY, Wang F, Nathan H, et al. The cardiac anesthesia risk evaluation score: a clinically useful predictor of mortality and morbidity after cardiac surgery. *Anesthesiology.* 2001;94(2):194–204; and http://www.medal.org/visitor/www/Active/ch31/ch31.01/ch31.01.02.aspx.

and anxiety caused by procedures such as tracheal intubation, ventilation, suction, and physiotherapy. It can also minimize agitation and maximize rest and appropriate sleep. Analgesia is an almost universal requirement for the intensive care patient. Adequate sedation and analgesia ameliorates the metabolic response to surgery and trauma. Too much or too little sedation and analgesia can increase morbidity.

Sedation in the ICU varies widely, from producing complete unconsciousness and paralysis to being nursed awake, yet in comfort. There are many components to the ideal regimen, but key elements include recognition of pain, anxiolysis, amnesia, sleep, and muscle relaxation. The following are indications for sedation:

- Fear and/or anxiety
- Difficult sleeping
- Control of agitation
- Facilitation of mechanical ventilation/airway management
- Protection against myocardial ischemia
- Amnesia during neuromuscular blockade

Although the mainstay of therapy is pharmacologic, other patient needs are equally important:

- Good communication with regular reassurance from nursing staff
- Environmental control such as humidity, lighting, temperature, and noise
- Explanation prior to procedures
- Management of thirst, hunger, constipation, and full bladder
- Variety for the patient (e.g., radio, visits from relatives, washing/shaving)
- Appropriate diurnal variation—gives pattern to days

An essential goal of all critical care physicians should be to maintain an optimal level of pain control and sedation for their patients. This has become increasingly important because of evidence showing that the combined use of sedatives and analgesics may ameliorate the detrimental stress response in critically ill patients. Unfortunately, both pain and anxiety are subjective and difficult to measure, thereby limiting our ability to analyze these states and making management more challenging.

Although there is still a lack of high-quality, randomized, prospective, controlled trials that compare agents, monitoring techniques, and scoring systems, several societies have come together to publish clinical practice guidelines for sedation and analgesia. Recommended opioids are fentanyl or hydromorphone for short-term use, and morphine or hydromorphone for longer-term therapy. Midazolam or diazepam is recommended for sedation of the acutely agitated patient, while lorazepam is recommended for longer infusions. Propofol is preferred when rapid awakening is desired. The challenge for critical care physicians is to use these medications to provide comfort and safety without increasing morbidity or mortality. Most studies support the use of protocols in order to help achieve these goals. The bottom line is that most protocols end up stressing some common issues. These include, when consistent with patient safety, daily cessation of drugs to evaluate the patient and frequent reassessment of the level of sedation required by each specific patient. Much is unknown about the long-term effects of sedative and analgesic drugs used as infusions from weeks to months.

Complications from Pain and Anxiety

Undertreated pain results in many physiologic responses associated with poor outcomes (62). Stimulation of the autonomic nervous system and release of humoral factors—catecholamines, cortisol, glucagons, leukotrienes, prostaglandins, vasopressin, and β endorphins—following injury, sepsis, or surgery represent the "stress response." This activation of the sympathetic nervous system increases heart rate, blood pressure, and myocardial oxygen consumption, which can lead to myocardial ischemia or infarction (63). An altered humoral response can lead to hypercoagulability as a result of increased level of factor VIII, fibrinogen platelet activity, and inhibition of fibrinolysis (64). Stress hormones also produce insulin resistance, increased metabolic rate, and protein catabolism. Immunosuppression is common with a noted reduction in number and function of lymphocytes and granulocytes (65). The stress response has been considered a

TABLE 40.4

MODIFICATION OF THE ANESTHETIC RISK ASSESSMENT, ACCORDING TO OPERATION TYPE AND SYSTEM FUNCTIONS (PART A) AND ASSESSING RISK CATEGORIES (PART B)

Part A: Modification of the Anesthetic Risk Assessment, according to general, system involvement, diseases, and metabolic parameters

Parameter	Finding	Points
GENERAL		
Status	"Status" (in good shape)	0
	Ambulant (? walking wounded)	1
	Emergency	2
Type of operation	Planned, scheduled	0
	Urgent	1
	Immediate	2
Anticipated operation time	≤120 min	0
	121–180 min	1
	>180 min	2
Age	0–1 y	1
	1–39 y	0
	40–69 y	1
	70–79 y	2
	>80 y	4
Weight	>50% over	4
	30%–50% over	2
	10%–30% over	1
	Normal (10% over or under)	0
	10%–15% under	1
	15%–25% under	2
	>25% under	4
Fasting	>6 h	0
	1–6 h	1
Allergies	None	0
	Allergies	1
	≤1 h	2
CENTRAL NERVOUS SYSTEM		
Consciousness	Conscious	0
	Drowsy	1
	Comatose	2
CARDIOVASCULAR SYSTEM		
Blood pressure	Stable	0
	Hypotension	1
	Labile hypertension	2
	Fixed hypertension	4
	Compensated shock	8
	Uncompensated shock	16
Heart	Healthy	0
	Compensated heart failure	1
	Decreased cardiac function	2
	Myocardial infarction <2 mo	4
	Heart failure	8
	Decompensated heart failure	16
Pulse	Normal	0
	Irregular rhythm	1
	Tachycardia	2
	Arrhythmias	2
	Preventricular contractions	4
	Complete atrioventricular block	16

(*continued*)

TABLE 40.4

(CONTINUED)

Part A: Modification of the Anesthetic Risk Assessment, according to general, system involvement, diseases, and metabolic parameters

Parameter	Finding	Points
PULMONARY SYSTEM		
Respirations	Normal	0
	Dyspnea	1
	Bronchitis	2
	Pneumonia	4
	Respiratory failure	8
OTHER SYSTEMS/DISEASES		
Renal function	Normal	0
	Renal failure	1
	Anuria or uremia	2
Liver function	Normal	0
	Liver failure	1
	Hepatic coma	2
Other diseases	None	0
	Other severe disease	2
Burns	None	0
	<15% body surface area (BSA) with no pulmonary	1
	15%–50% BSA with no pulmonary	4
	>50% BSA or pulmonary	8
	>50% BSA and pulmonary	16
METABOLIC FUNCTIONS		
Blood sugar	Normal	0
	Controlled diabetes	1
	Uncontrolled diabetes	2
Electrolytes	Normal (3 to 5 mmol/L)	0
	Hyperkalemia >5 mmol/L	1
	Hypokalemia 2.5–2.99 mmol/L	2
	Hypokalemia <2.5 mmol/L	4
Hydration	Normal	0
	Dehydrated	4
Hemoglobin	>12.5 g/dL	0
	7.5–12.5 g/dL	1
	<7.5 g/dL	2

Part B: Assessing risk categories

Risk score	Risk group
0 or 1	I
2 or 3	II
4–7	III
8–15	IV
>15	V

Risk score = SUM (points for all 20 parameters). Interpretation: minimum score: 0; maximum score: 109. The higher the score is, the greater the anesthetic risk.
Data modified from Peter K, Lutz H. [Proceedings: preoperative exploration (author's trans.)]. *Langenbecks Arch Chir.* 1973;334:681–687.

beneficial hemostatic mechanism, but more recent data have shown that this response may be, in part, detrimental. There are data to suggest that the adequate treatment of pain can decrease the magnitude of the changes occurring following surgery, and thereby may decrease postoperative complications (66–69).

The ICU environment can lead to psychological difficulties. Memories of vivid nightmares, hallucinations, and paranoid delusions were prominent in studies of ICU patients after discharge (70). Patients who have been sedated and paralyzed during ventilation have reported experiencing hallucinations,

TABLE 40.5

POTENTIAL USE OF THE ORIGINAL MULTIFACTORIAL CARDIAC RISK INDEX TO ESTIMATE THE PROBABILITY OF CARDIAC COMPLICATIONS IN DIFFERENT TYPES OF PATIENTS

Type of patient surgery	Baseline risk (%)	Adjusted risk using multifactorial index (%)			
		Class I	Class II	Class III	Class IV
Minor surgery	1	0.3	1	3	19
Major noncardiac surgery	3	1	3.5	10	45
High-risk cardiac surgery	10	3	10	30	75

Baseline or adjusted risk of major cardiac complications.
Class I: 0–5 points; class II: 6–12 points; class III: 13–25 points; and class IV: ≥26 points. Adjusted risk was calculated with multifactorial index using data from Goldman L, Caldera DL, Nussbaum SR, et al. Multifactorial index of cardiac risk in noncardiac surgical procedures. *N Engl J Med.* 1977;297(16):845–850; Jeffrey CC, Kunsman J, Cullen DJ, et al. A prospective evaluation of cardiac risk index. *Anesthesiology.* 1983;58(5):462–464; and Detsky AS, Abrams HB, McLaughlin JR, et al. Predicting cardiac complications in patients undergoing non-cardiac surgery. *J Gen Intern Med.* 1986;1(4):211–219.

delusions, and an altered sense of reality (71). Although some procedures can be explained to patients in order to relieve anxiety, not all patients requiring interventions during the acute stage of illness are in a state receptive to reasoning. These experiences result in some patients developing posttraumatic stress syndromes after their ICU stay (72). Effective therapy for anxiety and pain can reduce some of the adverse emotional experiences and decrease the incidence of postoperative neurosis (73).

ASSESSMENT OF PAIN AND ANXIETY

Sedative/analgesic dosage of commonly used agents varies between patients. A valid method for monitoring sedation would allow sedation to be tailored to the individual. Any scoring system should be simple, easily performed, noninvasive, and, most importantly, reproducible. Physiologic variables, serum concentrations of drugs, and neurophysiologic tools such as electroencephalography (EEG), cerebral function analyzing monitor (CFAM), and lower esophageal contractility have all been used but are both expensive and unreliable. The best systems are clinically based; six levels of sedation are used:

1. Anxious and agitated
2. Cooperative, orientated, and tranquil
3. Responds to verbal commands only
4. Asleep but brisk response to loud auditory stimulus/light glabellar tap
5. Asleep but sluggish response to loud auditory stimulus/light glabellar tap
6. Asleep, no response

Evaluation of the sedation level should be completed hourly by the ICU nurse, with reduction in frequency as the patient stabilizes. It is suggested that levels 2 to 4 be considered suitable for patients in the ICU. An increase in the sedation score must prompt the physician to consider the differential diagnoses of oversedation, decreased consciousness level due to neurologic/biochemical disorder, or ICU-associated depression. It is preferable to allow the patient to breathe as soon as possible on synchronized intermittent mandatory ventilation (SIMV) or triggered ventilation, such as pressure support. Deep sedation, with or without paralysis, is reserved for severe head injury, inadequate oxygen delivery, and diseases such as tetanus.

Pain and anxiety are subject to interpretation, and are difficult to objectify and monitor from one care provider to another unless a standard is developed for assessing and monitoring these states. This is what makes management of sedation in critically ill patients one of the more challenging areas in ICU care. For pain, the most widely used scale is the visual analog scale (VAS). Patients point to a number on a horizontal line that is a representation of the spectrum of pain—from "no pain" to "the worse pain I have ever had." The scale is simplistic and has a high degree of reliability and validity (74), but ignores other dimensions such as quantitative aspects of pain. Not all critically ill patients can use the scale because of the severity of their illnesses. Sometimes bedside nurses have to use behavioral signs such as facial expressions, movements, or posturing, or physiologic signs such as tachycardia, hypertension, or tachypnea. Unfortunately, none of these methods is exact. They depend on cultural interpretation of pain, type of illness, and use of other drugs that can alter the hemodynamic or movement parameters.

Monitoring sedation is also inexact, and a true gold standard has not been established. The Glasgow coma scale (GCS) is widely used for the assessment of level of consciousness, but validity is established only in patients with neurologic deficits. The sedation scale used most commonly worldwide is the 6-point Ramsay scale (75). The Ramsay scale is a numerical scale of motor responsiveness based on increasing depth of sedation (Table 40.6). Most comparative studies have used the Ramsay scale, but it has drawbacks. Based as it is on motor response, the scale must be modified for patients receiving muscle relaxants and, similar to pain assessment, there is no consensus as to what represents an adequate level of sedation in an individual patient. Other scales include the Sedation-Agitation Scale (SAS) (Appendix 40.1), Pain Intensity Scale (Appendix 40.2), and Motor Activity Assessment Scale (MAAS) (Table 40.7), but all have similar drawbacks.

The BIS of the EEG is known to provide information about the cortical and subcortical regions (76). The BIS scale, based on a score between 0 and 100, is an index of level of consciousness (77). It is more often used in the OR as an index of depth of anesthesia. Recently, attempts have been made to extend the use of BIS into the ICU, but preliminary reports have been

TABLE 40.6

RAMSAY'S SEDATION SCALE

Level	Description
Awake	
1	Anxious and/or agitated
2	Cooperative, oriented, and tranquil
3	Responds to commands
Asleep	
4	Quiescent with brisk response to light glabellar tap or loud auditory stimulus
5	Sluggish response to light glabellar tap or loud auditory stimulus
6	No response

Data from Ramsay MA, Savege TM, Simpson BR, et al. Controlled sedation with alphaxalone-alphadolone. *BMJ.* 1974;2(920):656–659.

conflicting because of muscle-based electrical activity or metabolic or structural abnormalities of the brain in ICU patients (78,79). More work is required to validate this technique in the ICU patient, but the theoretical benefits of a noninvasive monitor of cerebral function are self-evident. However, to date, no data have shown that BIS monitoring, when used to assess depth of sedation, significantly alters patient outcomes in the ICU (80). Because of the lack of evidence, routine use of this device was not recommended in the latest clinical practice guidelines (81).

Comparisons of Sedation Scoring Systems

As discussed above, for the assessment of sedation, several scoring systems have been introduced into clinical practice, but the differentiation of deeper sedation levels in particular remains poor. Auditory-evoked potentials (AEPs), as an objective method, were compared in assessing level of sedation to five different sedation scoring systems (Ramsay, Cohen, O'Sullivan, Armstrong, and Cook systems) (75,82–85) and studied in a prospective clinical study (86). Previous studies have shown that AEPs, especially latencies of the midlatency component N_b, could serve as an indicator of depth of anesthesia (87). Using electrophysiologic methods to evaluate sedation during ICU therapy, changes in latency of peak N_b were compared with various levels of sedation assessed by the five sedation scoring systems. As in anesthesia, latencies of N_b increased with increasing depth of sedation. Among the scoring systems, the one developed by Ramsay correlated best with changes in N_b latency ($r^2 = 0.68$). The coefficient of determination, r^2, of the other scores ranged from 0.56 to 0.61. Objective electrophysiologic monitoring is desirable during long-term sedation.

TABLE 40.7

MOTOR ACTIVITY ASSESSMENT SCALE

Motor activity description	Motor score
Minimal or no response to noxious stimuli (suctioning or 5 s of vigorous orbital, sternal, or nail bed pressure)	0
Responds to physical stimuli, but does not follow commands	1
Responds to verbal or physical stimuli, but drifts off again	2
Calm, easily arousable, cooperative, follows commands	3
Anxious, but calms down on verbal instructions	4
Requires physical restraints, biting endotracheal tube (ET), does not calm down on verbal instructions	5
Dangerously agitated and uncooperative, tries to remove ET/catheters, striking, thrashing	6

Data modified from Dahaba AA, Grabner T, Rehak P, et al. Remifentanil versus morphine analgesia and sedation for mechanically ventilated critically ill patients: a randomized double blind study. *Anesthesiology.* 2004;101(2):640–646.

Sedatives Used in the Intensive Care Unit

The "ideal" sedative agent should possess the following qualities:

- Both sedative *and* analgesic properties
- Minimal cardiovascular side effects
- Controllable respiratory side effects
- Rapid onset/offset of action
- No accumulation in renal/hepatic dysfunction
- Inactive metabolites
- Inexpensive
- No interactions with other ICU drugs

Such a drug does not exist, and therefore, drug combinations are usually required. Sedative drugs may be given as boluses or infusions, although as a rule, infusions are preferable, with boluses utilized for procedures. Anxiety in the critically ill is best treated with a benzodiazepine, after adequate treatment of pain and correction of any reversible causes such as hypoxia, metabolic abnormalities, treatable neurologic abnormalities, infections, renal or hepatic failure, or nonclinical seizure activity (88). In recent clinical guidelines (81), the recommended choices have been narrowed to diazepam, lorazepam, midazolam, and propofol. Other drugs are haloperidol—useful for delirium—and dexmedetomidine, a new α_2-receptor agonist, which is being used for ICU sedation (Table 40.8).

Benzodiazepines

These are anxiolytic, anticonvulsant, and amnesic drugs, and provide some muscle relaxation in addition to their hypnotic effect. Their effects are mediated by depressing the excitability of the limbic system via reversible binding at the γ-aminobutyric acid (GABA)–benzodiazepine receptor complex. They have minimal cardiorespiratory depressant effects, but these are synergistic with opioids. Rapid bolus doses can cause both hypotension and respiratory arrest. All benzodiazepines are metabolized in the liver. The common drugs in this class are diazepam, midazolam, and lorazepam. Overdose or accumulation can be reversed by flumazenil, the benzodiazepine receptor antagonist. It should be given in small aliquots—1 mg in 0.2-mg increments—which may be repeated once in 30 minutes, as large doses can precipitate seizures. Because of the short half-life, an infusion may be required.

TABLE 40.8

SEDATIVES RECOMMENDED FOR PATIENTS IN THE INTENSIVE CARE UNIT

Drug	Elimination half-life	Peak effect	Minimal suggested dosage	Recommended infusion dosage
Diazepam	20–40 h	3–5 min	5- to 10-mg bolus	Infusion not recommended
Midazolam	3–5 h	2–5 min	1- to 2-mg bolus	0.5–10 mg/h
Lorazepam	10–20 h	2–20 min	1- to 2-mg bolus	0.5–10 mg/h
Propofol	20–30 h	90 s	Bolus dose not recommended	25–100 μg/kg/min
Haloperidol	10–24 h	3–20 min	2- to 10-mg bolus	2–10 mg/h
Dexmedetomidine (α_2-adrenoceptor agonist)	2 h	1–2 min	Bolus dose not recommended	0.2–1 μg/kg/h

There is wide interpatient variability in the potency, efficacy, and pharmacokinetics of benzodiazepines, and thus, the dose must be titrated to the level of sedation. After long-term administration, the dose should be reduced gradually, or a lower dose reinstated if there are withdrawal symptoms (insomnia, anxiety, dysphoria, and sweating).

Benzodiazepines are administered intermittently (intravenous diazepam) or continuously (intravenous midazolam). The potential advantages of midazolam are its water solubility, short distribution and elimination half-lives (20 minute and 90 minute, respectively) (89), and lack of long-acting active metabolites. In contrast, diazepam has an elimination half-life of 44 hours (90) and its major active metabolite, desmethyldiazepam, has a half-life of 93 hours (91). These data are derived from a single-dose administration in normal subjects; much of midazolam's pharmacokinetic advantage is lost when administered by infusion to critically ill patients (90,92,93). In ICU patients, midazolam's elimination half-life may be greatly prolonged (91), and clinically important accumulation may occur (94). By using intermittent diazepam, there is a clinical disincentive to overdosage, as administration of each dose is a deliberate action by the bedside nurse. Continuous infusions of sedatives are more convenient, but risk oversedation if the infusion rate is not regularly reduced to test the lower limit of acceptable sedation. In terms of cost, diazepam has a clear advantage, being one-tenth the price. Although some may argue that, because of cost and the prolonged elimination half-life of midazolam in the critically ill, the standard sedative regimen should be intermittent intravenous diazepam, midazolam is more commonly used in our experience. Both regimens produced a rapid onset of acceptable sedation, but undersedation appeared more common with the less expensive diazepam regimen. Additionally, used alone, a sedation score may be an inappropriate outcome measure for a sedation trial (95).

Propofol (2, 6-Diisopropylphenol)

The mode of action of propofol is thought to be via the GABA receptor, but at a different site than the benzodiazepines. First developed as an intravenous anesthetic agent and with a rapid onset of action, it is metabolized rapidly—both hepatically and extrahepatically—and is thus ideal for continuous infusion. Recovery usually occurs within 10 minutes of discontinuation, but the agent can accumulate with prolonged use, particularly in the obese patient. It is solubilized as an emulsion, and the formulation can cause thrombophlebitis and pain, so it is ideally infused via a large or central vein. Prolonged infusions can lead to increased triglyceride and cholesterol levels and, indeed, its use is not licensed in children because of associated deaths attributable to this drug. A theoretical maximum recommended dose is thus 4 mg/kg/hour. Disadvantages also include cardiorespiratory depression, particularly in the elderly, septic, or hypovolemic patient. Infusions may color the urine green.

Ketamine

Ketamine acts at the *N*-methyl-D-aspartate (NMDA) receptor. In subanesthetic doses, ketamine is both a sedative and analgesic. However, it is generally not used because of the increase in blood pressure, intracranial pressure (ICP), and pulse rate that may result. It may also cause hallucinations, but these can be avoided if administered concomitantly with a benzodiazepine. It appears not to accumulate and, given its bronchodilatory properties, sometimes has a role in severe asthma. Its use in the ICU is often in conjunction with a narcotic for synergistic effect.

Etomidate

Etomidate was historically used in the ICU as an infusion, but is now no longer used in this manner. For maintenance of hypnosis, target concentration of 300 to 500 ng/mL may be achieved by administration of a two- or three-stage infusion (e.g., 100 μg/kg/minute for 10 minutes followed by 20 μg/kg/minute for 30 minutes, and then 10 μg/kg/minute), since its pharmacokinetics are described by a three-compartment model (96). It is used as a single dose (0.2–0.4 mg/kg) for induction when cardiovascular stability is desired. Some have ceased using the agent, even as a single dose, as it has been shown to cause adrenal suppression, even when used in this manner (97).

Barbiturates

Barbiturates such as Pentothal have been used in the ICU, especially in the management of patients with head injuries and seizure disorders. They cause significant cardiovascular depression and accumulate during infusions, leading to prolonged recovery times. Pentothal is still used occasionally in critically high levels of ICP to induce a "barbiturate coma" and in intractable seizure activity.

Butyrophenones and Phenothiazine

Although classified as major tranquilizers, these agents remain useful in the ICU, particularly in delirious patients. An aggressive dosing regimen of haloperidol may be particularly useful in a patient with delirium to promote calm, 2 to 10 mg IV every

10 to 15 minutes until the desired response is achieved (81). Haloperidol, in particular, causes minimal respiratory depression and has less α-blocking tendency than chlorpromazine, and hence, less hypotension. Significant side effects include prolongation of the QT interval, extrapyramidal effects, or neuroleptic malignant syndrome—and hence, haloperidol must be used with caution. Special care must be taken when using this agent with erythromycin, which may, in itself, prolong the QT interval.

Clonidine

This is the most well known of the α_2 agonists, but also has α_1-agonistic properties. A more specific agonist is dexmedetomidine; however, it is expensive and uncommonly available at present. It is particularly useful in patients with sympathetic overactivity such as alcohol withdrawal and tetanus, as it inhibits catecholamine release. Clonidine also is synergistic with opioids and acts at the spinal cord to inhibit nociceptive inputs, thus imparting analgesia. It is contraindicated in hypovolemia and can cause hypotension, bradycardia, and dry mouth.

Volatile Agents

Isoflurane has been used in concentrations of up to 0.6% and produces good long-term sedation, with minimal cardiorespiratory side effects and rapid awakening. Scavenging and pollution are a problem, as is incorporating the vaporizer into the ventilator. Although rarely used anymore, free fluoride ions from metabolized methoxyflurane can cause renal failure. More recently, desflurane has been shown to be effective in sedation, with rapid offset of effects.

Analgesics

Pain in the critically ill is best treated with a pure opioid agonist. The commonly available opiates all work at the μ receptors, so that the selection of the agent used should be based on pharmacokinetic characteristics. In a recent clinical guideline (81), the recommended choices have been narrowed to morphine, fentanyl, and hydromorphone. As the use of meperidine (pethidine), nonsteroidal anti-inflammatory drugs (NSAIDs), and mixed opioid agonist-antagonist agents are discouraged due to potential adverse effects, their use is not discussed. However, drugs such as morphine, a long-acting opioid that can be given parenterally or enterally, and ketamine, a sedative drug with analgesic qualities, are discussed at the end of this section because they do have specific advantages in the ICU patient, and can be used for the difficult to sedate patient. Table 40.9 lists some of the recommended drugs and their minimal suggested dosages for the treatment of pain.

Morphine, a long-acting opioid recommended by the consensus conference as the preferred analgesic agent for the critically ill, is the most frequently used intravenous analgesic agent in the ICU (98). Remifentanil hydrochloride is a potent μ-receptor agonist with unique features of rapid onset and rapid predictable offset of action (99), which makes it quickly adjustable to the required level of sedation. This agent may be a useful tool for sedation and analgesia in postsurgical ICU patients.

Drugs Used for Analgesia/Sedation in the Intensive Care Unit

Remifentanil. Remifentanil, an ultra-short-acting opioid metabolized by nonspecific tissue and blood esterases, has a rapid onset of action and does not accumulate after infusions even in organ dysfunction. It is, however, very expensive and can cause significant bradycardia. The efficacy and safety of a remifentanil–midazolam regimen versus a standard morphine–midazolam combination in short- and medium-term mechanically ventilated ICU subjects was recently compared (100). Remifentanil dosing was based on recommendations from a previous study evaluating remifentanil analgesia and sedation in mechanically ventilated ICU patients (101), whereas doses of morphine and midazolam were based on guidelines issued by the Society of Critical Care Medicine (98). The primary end point of the study (100) was to compare the efficacy of the two regimens, defined as the mean percentage of hours of the Sedation Agitation Scale (SAS) score (102) of 4 (Appendix 40.1). A remifentanil-based regimen was found to be more effective in providing optimal analgesia/sedation than a standard, morphine-based regimen. The remifentanil-based regimen allowed a more rapid emergence from sedation and facilitated earlier extubation. The agent is relatively expensive.

Morphine. Morphine is very commonly used and is the drug against which all other opioids are measured. The analgesic dose is highly variable, and may be delivered as an intermittent bolus—although there are problems with peak and trough effects but less accumulation—or as a continuous infusion. Morphine is primarily hepatically metabolized to two products: Morphine-3-glucuronide and morphine-6-glucuronide; both are excreted renally and may accumulate in renal dysfunction. The latter metabolite has independent, long-lasting sedative activity.

Morphine has minimal cardiovascular side effects unless given as a large bolus to hypovolemic patients or resultant from histamine release. It is relatively contraindicated in asthma and

TABLE 40.9

ANALGESICS RECOMMENDED FOR PATIENTS IN THE INTENSIVE CARE UNIT

Drug	Elimination half-life	Peak effect: intravenous	Minimal suggested dosage	Recommended infusion dosage
Morphine	2–4 h	30 min	1- to 4-mg bolus	1–10 mg/h
Fentanyl	2–5 h	4 min	25- to 100-μg bolus	25–200 μg/h
Hydromorphone	2–4 h	20 min	0.2- to 1-mg bolus	0.2–2 mg/h
Ketamine	2–3 h	30–60 s	100- to 200-μg/kg bolus	1–2 μg/kg/min

renal failure, and should be given in small increments in uncorrected hypovolemia. However, its use in renal failure is acceptable as long as the dosing interval is increased or the infusion rate reduced. Normal duration of action after a single dose is about 2 hours. As with all opioids, care should be taken in patients with hepatic failure.

Fentanyl. Fentanyl is a potent synthetic opioid derived from meperidine (pethidine). While it is considered a short-acting opioid with a rapid onset, after prolonged infusion the duration of action approaches that of morphine, although it does not accumulate in renal failure. It does not cause histamine release and is suitable for analgesia in the hemodynamically unstable patient.

Alfentanil. Alfentanil is a relatively expensive synthetic opioid with an onset of action about five times faster than fentanyl, due to the small volume of distribution, but is not as prone to accumulation as it is less lipid soluble. The duration of action is about one-third that of fentanyl and it, too, is safe in renal failure. Alfentanil has minimal cardiovascular effects and is a potent antitussive agent. Although not particularly sedating, alfentanil does possess many of the qualities desired of the ideal ICU analgesic.

Other agents include meperidine, which is not suitable for use in infusions, as the metabolite, normeperidine, may accumulate and cause convulsions. Naloxone is a specific receptor antagonist working at the OP3 (old μ) receptor; it completely abolishes the effects of all opioids at this site. The dose should be titrated slowly at the risk of unmasking arrhythmias or seizures in certain patients.

α_2-Adrenoceptor Agonists. Clonidine and dexmedetomidine cause sedation, anxiolysis, and amnesia by their action at the central α_2 adrenoceptors, and also have the advantages of not causing respiratory depression, in addition to their significant anesthetic-sparing effect (103). Dexmedetomidine is the newer agent, and has a greater specificity for the α_2 adrenoceptor than clonidine. It has an elimination half-life of 2 hours, and is metabolized in the liver to methyl and glucuronide metabolites. Its clearance is reduced in liver failure, and it inhibits the CYP2D6 component of the enzyme cytochrome P450 (CYP) (104). Clonidine has been investigated in head-injured patients for its role in reducing catecholamine release and causing cerebral vasoconstriction, rather than as a sedative. There are conflicting studies regarding its effect on ICP, cerebral blood flow (CBF), or cerebral metabolism in head-injured patients (105).

Other Agents

Neuromuscular Blocking Agents

In some patients, muscle relaxation may be needed in addition to sedation and analgesia. It is vital to remember that neuromuscular blocking agents (NMBAs) have no effect on consciousness or comfort, and should be avoided if possible. There are no standard clinical techniques to monitor the level of consciousness in the patient receiving NMBAs, so it is necessary to give generous doses of sedative drugs. Use of NMBAs has fallen from about 90% of patients in the 1980s to 10% of patients in the 1990s in Europe and the United Kingdom (106–108).

Some NMBAs used in anesthesia have limited ICU use. For example, succinylcholine (suxamethonium) is used predominantly during emergency tracheal intubation, but a resultant rise in serum potassium must be expected, which makes it particularly inappropriate for use in cases of renal failure. Excessive potassium release also occurs after 48 hours in extensive burns and spinal cord injury. Pancuronium, on the other hand, is long acting, but may cause undesirable tachycardia; it may also accumulate in renal failure. Vecuronium is an analogue of the aminosteroid pancuronium, but causes minimal cardiovascular side effects. It is suitable for intubation and infusion. The dosage for intubation is 0.1 mg/kg as a bolus, while the continuous infusion is 1 to 2 μg/kg/minute as an infusion; the drug may accumulate in renal failure.

Atracurium is a benzylisoquinolinium agent metabolized by ester hydrolysis and Hoffman (spontaneous) elimination. Its metabolites are inactive and do not accumulate in renal or hepatic dysfunction. Histamine release occasionally occurs with boluses, but recovery occurs predictably within 1 hour, regardless of the duration of infusion. The intubating dose is 0.5 mg/kg, and the infusion dose is 4 to 12 μg/kg/minute.

Monitoring of NMBAs is performed using an ulnar nerve stimulator to follow the train-of-four count at the thenar eminence. Clinical monitoring such as cardiovascular reflexes to noxious stimuli should also be observed. Full "surgical" relaxation may not be necessary.

Problems with Relaxants

- The patient may be aware as a result of inadequate sedation. This can be evaluated by withdrawing muscle relaxants for a time period to allow recovery of muscular function.
- Accumulation may occur, especially with aminosteroids in acute renal failure (ARF), with prolonged paralysis after discontinuation.
- Severe myopathy and/or critical illness polyneuropathy occasionally occurs (especially with use of corticosteroids).
- There is a loss of protective reflexes.
- There is a tendency to oversedate.
- There is enhanced paralysis from other common ICU situations such as hypokalemia, aminoglycoside antibiotics, and hypophosphatemia.

THE PRACTICE: GLOBAL PRACTICES AND PRACTICE GUIDELINES

As noted above, a variety of pharmacologic agents can be used for the treatment of pain and anxiety. Although recommendations have been made for sedation and analgesic regimens in the ICU, practice continues to vary widely between different ICUs. Several studies have attempted to characterize international practices by sending out surveys and questionnaires. In Europe, 63% of participants used midazolam often or always for patients requiring sedation, followed by 35% who used propofol and 9% who used haloperidol often or always for ICU patients (106). Use of narcotics was more evenly divided, with one third using morphine often or always, one third using fentanyl, and one fourth using sufentanil. Only 43% of the European ICUs used a sedation scale. When a scale was used, the Ramsay scale was used 74% of the time (106).

In Denmark, midazolam and propofol were used more frequently than diazepam (100%, 92%, and 24%, respectively) (107). For analgesia, the preferred drugs were morphine (94%), fentanyl (76%), and sufentanil (43%). Only 16% of the ICUs used a sedation scale, but they all used the Ramsay scale if one was used (107). In England, propofol was slightly more popular than midazolam, while almost no ICUs used lorazepam (108); after 72 hours of sedation, midazolam infusions are more popular. Analgesic usage included morphine, alfentanil, and fentanyl, in that order. A sedation scale was used in 67% of ICUs but, while the Ramsay scale was still the most popular, almost one third of the ICUs used another scoring system (108). Overall, although differences do exist between countries (98,109), most ICUs around the world are using similar drugs for pain and sedation. Almost all recognized the importance of adequate analgesia and anxiolysis, and very few used neuromuscular blocking agents, unless required for specific indications.

TABLE 40.10

CLINICAL PRACTICE GUIDELINES FOR SEDATION AND ANALGESIA FROM THE SOCIETY OF CRITICAL CARE MEDICINE AND AMERICAN COLLEGE OF CRITICAL CARE MEDICINE

PAIN
1. An assessment of pain and the response to therapy should be regularly assessed using an appropriate pain scale.
2. Therapeutic plans and goals should be developed for all patients.
3. Recommended intravenous opioids are fentanyl for acute distress, fentanyl or hydromorphone for patients with hemodynamic instability or renal insufficiency, and morphine and hydromorphone for longer-term therapy.
4. Scheduled doses or continuous infusions are preferred over intermittent boluses.
5. Nonsteroidal anti-inflammatory drugs and acetaminophen can be useful adjuncts, but beware of renal insufficiency or gastrointestinal bleeding.

SEDATION
1. Treatment of pain and other reversible causes should be conducted before sedating an agitated patient.
2. A treatment plan/goal should be established for each patient; therapy should be assessed with a sedation scale.
3. Midazolam or diazepam is useful for the acutely agitated patient.
4. Propofol is preferred when rapid awakening is crucial; triglyceride levels should be monitored for >2 d of continuous infusions.
5. Lorazepam is recommended for longer infusions.
6. Doses should be tapered daily to assess underlying mental status, and sedation protocols can be helpful and beneficial.
7. Haloperidol is the preferred agent for the treatment of delirium.

Data from De Deyne C, Struys M, Decruyenaere J, et al. Use of continuous bispectral EEG monitoring to assess depth of sedation in ICU patients. *Intensive Care Med.* 1998;24(12):1294–1298; and Jacobi J, Fraser GL, Coursin DB, et al. Task Force of the American College of Critical Care Medicine (ACCM) of the Society of Critical Care Medicine (SCCM), American Society of Health-System Pharmacists (ASHP), American College of Chest Physicians clinical practice guidelines for the sustained use of sedatives and analgesics in the critically ill adult. *Crit Care Med.* 2002;30(1):119–141.

The use of a sedation score seems to be gaining popularity, but a consensus as to the optimal level of sedation is lacking. Further work will be needed to see if the use of these scores can improve ICU morbidity and mortality.

The Society of Critical Care Medicine (SCCM) and the American College of Critical Care Medicine (ACCM), in 1995, published clinical practice guidelines for sedation and analgesia for the critically ill patient (109). These two societies have joined with the American Society of Health System Pharmacists (ASHP), and they have recently published revised clinical practice guidelines (82) (Table 40.10).

SEDATION PROTOCOLS

The challenge for critical care physicians who use analgesics and sedatives is to provide patient comfort and safety without increasing morbidity and mortality. Because of the variety in practice styles, pathways to standardize patient care have attracted attention. From a mechanical ventilation standpoint, weaning protocols have been shown to improve efficiency, reduce resource utilization, improve patient outcomes, reduce overall ICU expenditures, and decrease the frequency of tracheostomies (110).

For sedation, there have been two prospective, randomized, controlled trials examining the effects of sedation protocols in the intubated patient. Brook et al. randomized 321 medical ICU patients to a nurse-implemented sedation protocol or to standard care (111). They showed that the protocol group had shorter mechanical ventilation time, length of stay, and tracheostomy rates. Kress et al. also studied medical ICU patients, but their protocol group had sedation infusions interrupted daily for a "wake-up test," and the sedation was restarted at half the previous dose (112). The control group did not have scheduled daily decreases in the infusion rate, and care was left to the discretion of the ICU team. This group of investigators also found a statistically significant shorter duration of mechanical ventilation and length of ICU stay in the intervention group.

On the basis, in part, of the above data, recent clinical guidelines recommend that a sedation protocol be instituted and that it include daily cessation, and patient-specific targeted goals, of sedation and analgesia administration (81).

To provide the highest quality of patient care, the intensivist must constantly review treatment of sedation regimens in search of "'best practice." While randomized controlled trials (RCTs) are considered the gold standard for the evaluation of competing treatments, these have nevertheless been criticized, as strict inclusion and exclusion criteria may exclude the very patients who clinicians are obliged to treat (113). The conduct of trials in the ICU is further complicated by the varying case mix between different units so that the results of even perfectly conducted studies may not be relevant to a unit with a different case mix. As a result, it becomes necessary to develop protocols and systems for examining practice in one's own unit (95).

Daily Interruption of Sedation Protocols

Continuous sedation for patients undergoing mechanical ventilation is a double-edged sword. On the one hand, it may promote comfort and reduce agitation; on the other hand, it may prolong the duration of mechanical ventilation and interfere with assessment of neurologic status. The administration of sedative drugs by continuous infusion offers a more consistent level of sedation than intermittent bolus administration, and thus may improve patient comfort (114). Adequate sedation is often difficult to achieve with intermittent administration, and such regimens can be taxing on nurses and can hamper other aspects of patient care (115–117). However, a potential drawback to continuous infusions is the accumulation of the drug and the accompanying delays in the improvement of mental status. It is hypothesized that daily interruption of the sedative infusion will decrease these problems (112).

Care of critically ill patients is costly. In the United States in 1997, approximately $80.8 billion was spent on intensive care (118), and about 10% of this amount was spent on drugs (119). Ten to fifteen percent of the drug costs resulted from the purchase of sedative agents (120). Thus, a conservative estimate of the yearly cost of sedative drugs administered in intensive care units in the United States in 1997 (121) is between $0.8 billion and $1.2 billion; the cost may be higher if the use of sedative drugs increases the duration of mechanical ventilation and the length of stay in the intensive care unit.

Daily interruption of the infusion of sedative drugs shortened the duration of mechanical ventilation by more than 2 days and the length of stay in the intensive care unit by 3.5 days (112). Compared with the control group, the group assigned to daily interruption of sedation had a significantly shorter median duration of mechanical ventilation (7.3 vs. 4.9 days) and a significantly shorter median length of ICU stay (9.9 vs. 6.4 days) (112). Reducing the duration of mechanical ventilation will probably cut costs—both direct costs and those related to complications of mechanical ventilation, such as ventilator-associated pneumonia and barotrauma. Daily interruption of the sedative infusion is a practical, cost-effective intervention that can be readily performed by the nurses caring for patients in the ICU. The results of neurologic assessments can then be relayed to physicians, and infusions of sedative drugs can be restarted and adjusted as needed by the nurses. These results suggest that daily interruption of the sedative infusion provides acceptable sedation while minimizing adverse effects.

In addition, daily interruption of the sedative infusion reduced the total dose of midazolam administered by almost half (112). A trend toward using lower doses of benzodiazepines has previously been reported (122,123) and is at least partly related to the concomitant administration of opiates such as morphine. Benzodiazepines may enhance the analgesic effects of morphine (124), and this synergism may decrease the doses of benzodiazepines needed to achieve adequate sedation. In the above-mentioned study, daily interruption of the sedative infusion did not alter the doses of propofol administered (112). The concentration of propofol in plasma declines rapidly after administration is discontinued (125), which is probably why the daily period of drug stoppage in the intervention group was shorter among patients assigned to propofol than among those assigned to midazolam. Despite this difference, the patients were awake on more than 80% of days in both the intervention subgroups; this percentage did not differ according to the sedative agent used. In addition, there were no differences in the duration of mechanical ventilation or the length of stay in the intensive care unit when patients were grouped according to the sedative they received. However, the percentage of patients successfully discharged to their homes was greater in the group assigned to daily interruption of infusions than in the control group (112).

One drawback to continuous intravenous sedation is impaired mental status (126), which may prevent the early detection of neurologic dysfunction resulting from new insults. Stopping the sedative infusion for a period during each day is a simple way to improve the clinician's ability to perform daily neurologic examinations. Avoiding unnecessary diagnostic studies may reduce the rate of complications related to the transport of patients (127,128), in addition to reducing costs.

In conclusion, daily interruption of the infusion of sedative drugs is a safe and practical approach to treating patients who are mechanically ventilated. This practice decreases the duration of mechanical ventilation, ICU length of stay, and doses of benzodiazepines required. It also improves the ability of clinicians to perform daily neurologic examinations and reduces the need for diagnostic studies to evaluate unexplained alterations in mental status.

The guidelines for mechanically ventilated adults can be incorporated in three pathways: according to the level of pain, anxiety, or refractory sedation/delirium (129) (Fig. 40.1). Essential to the guidelines is the method of assessing sedation—that is, the Ramsay scale. The goal of the sedation algorithm is to maintain patients at a Ramsay score of 2 to 3. Achieving the appropriate level of sedation in a patient may be as simple as administering a midazolam bolus and a scheduled lorazepam dose, or may require the use of multiple agents. Once a patient is adequately sedated, therapy can be converted to a scheduled longer-acting lorazepam dose within 24 hours if he or she requires a midazolam or propofol infusion (Table 40.11). These guidelines use pathways that address pain and delirium, both reasons why patients often continue to be agitated and unresponsive to sedation. Midazolam and propofol are restricted to use in short-term sedation (less than 24 hours). Lorazepam can be the preferred agent for long-term sedation in critically ill patients. All patients are converted to lorazepam after 24 hours. Midazolam can still be used for loading doses in unresponsive patients receiving lorazepam or other sedatives.

Doses of Sedation Drugs

Dosing Algorithm

As mentioned above, the variety in practice styles and the pathways used to attempt to standardize patient care, choose drugs, and titrate doses can be very complicated and confusing. An example for choosing a dosing algorithm is outlined in the flow chart (Fig. 40.2) (100).

Doses of Sedation and Analgesic Drugs

The loading dose, boluses, maintenance dose, and onset and duration of common sedating and analgesic drugs are outlined in Tables 40.12 and 40.13. One can see that those doses are very similar and comparable to conscious-sedation drugs. The loading dose, maintenance dose, and plasma level of common drugs used for conscious sedation are presented in Table 40.14. The doses used in various procedures are also comparable to those used in ICU patients, and are presented in Table 40.15.

TABLE 40.11

LORAZEPAM CONVERSION GUIDE

		Lorazepam IV starting dose	
Drug (infusion rate)	**Infusion rate**	**Infusion rate (mg/h)**	**Bolus (mg q2h)**
Propofol (mg/kg/h)	>30	4	8
	15–30	2	4
	<15	—	2
Midazolam (mg/h)	>8	4	8
	4–8	2	4
	<4	—	2

Data modified from Shah S. *ICU Analgesia/Sedation Guidelines Created*. Current Topics from the Drug Information Center, College of Pharmacy, University of Kentucky; 2000;30(1):1–4.

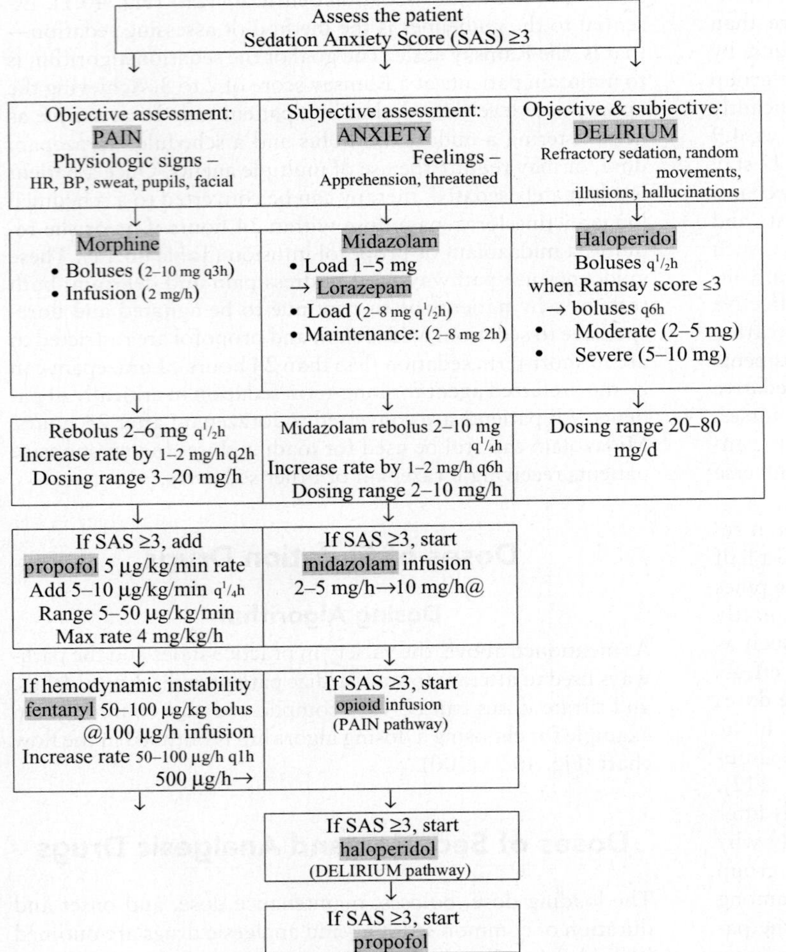

FIGURE 40.1. Guidelines for sedation and analgesia in the intensive care unit.

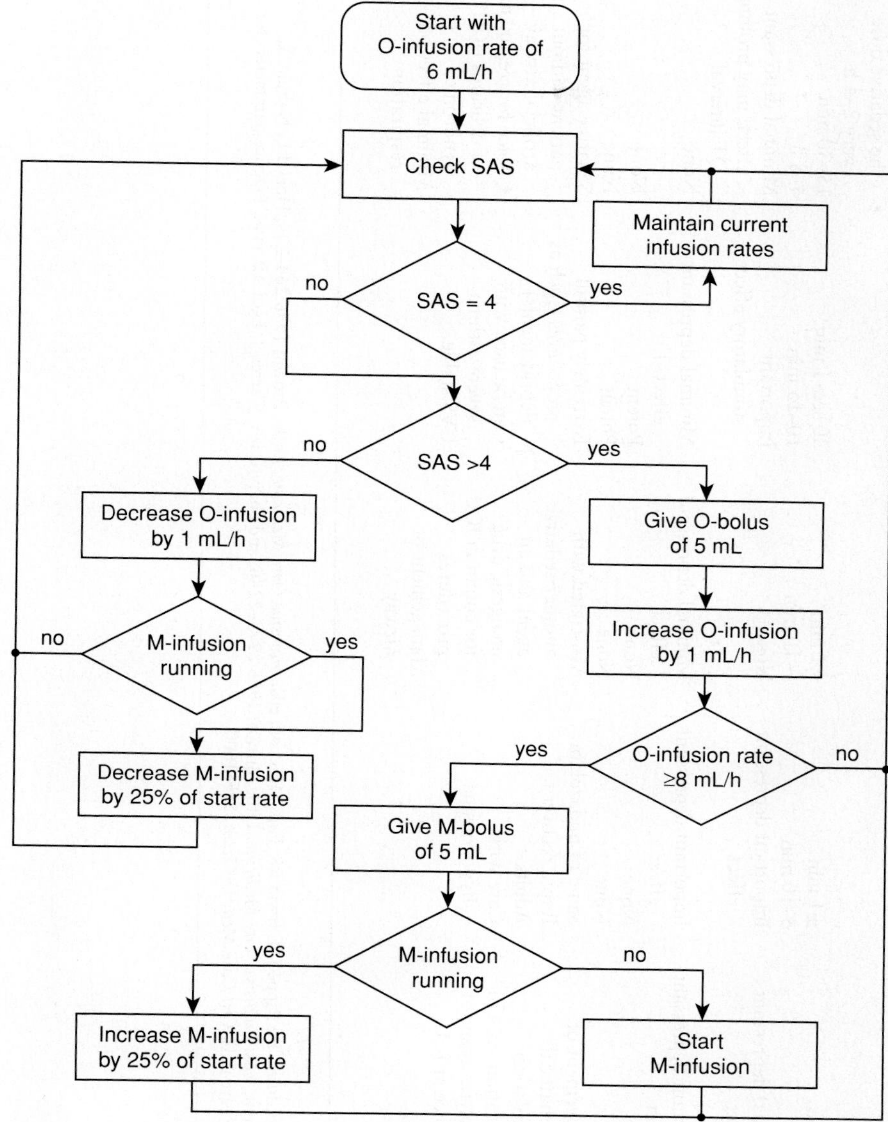

O-infusion: Opioid infusion (morphine or remifentanil)
O-bolus: Morphine bolus or placebo bolus (remifentanil group)
M-infusion: Midazolam infusion
M-bolus: Midazolam bolus

Whenever Pain Intensity Score exceeded 2, an O-bolus of 5 mL was given and O-infusion was increased by 1 mL/h irrespective of the SAS at that time.

FIGURE 40.2. Flow chart of the study of opioid (remifentanil or morphine) and midazolam dosing algorithms. SAS, Sedation Anxiety Score. (From Dahaba AA, Grabner T, Rehak P, et al. Remifentanil *versus* morphine analgesia and sedation for mechanically ventilated critically ill patients: a randomized double blind study. *Anesthesiology.* 2004;101[3]:640–646.)

SPECIAL PROBLEMS IN INTENSIVE CARE UNIT SEDATION

Sedation for the Neurosurgical Patient in the Neurointensive Care Unit

Context for Use of Sedation in Head Injury

Following head injury, sedation may be instituted in emergency situations in the prehospital phase. More commonly, it is instituted in the emergency department, usually to allow for airway control. Continued use may be required in the short term (e.g., to allow an agitated patient to undergo radiologic imaging). It may also be required over the longer term in the neurointensive care unit (NICU). Sedation in the NICU is required to provide the amnesia, anxiolysis, and compliance with treatment that is required in any ICU. Additionally, it may represent an intrinsic part of the management of the head-injured patient by reduction of cerebral metabolism, with coupled reductions in cerebral blood volume (CBV) and, hence, ICP. Such agents may also be required for the control of refractory acute, posttraumatic epilepsy.

TABLE 40.12

ONSET, DURATION, EFFECTS, AND INDICATIONS OF COMMON SEDATING DRUGS

	Midazolam	Lorazepam	Propofol	Etomidate	Ketamine	Haloperidol
Loading doses	0.1–0.3 mg/kg *or* 2- to 4-mg bolus	0.03–0.07 mg/kg	0.5–2.0 mg/kg *or* 5- to 50-mg bolus	0.2–0.5 mg/kg	0.5–1.0 mg/kg *or* 1- to 2-mg/kg bolus	5–10 mg
Maintenance dose	0.03–0.25 mg/kg/h *or* 0.5–10 mg/h	0.03–0.07 mg/kg at 4- to 6-h intervals	1.0–6.0 mg/kg/h	Not recommended	1.2–6.0 mg/kg/h *or* 10–45 μg/kg/min	Increase 5 mg every 15–20 min until sedative effect is achieved; repeat the sedative dose every 2–4 h
Onset	±2 min	≥3 min	±1 min	±1 min	30 sec–1 min	15–30 min
Duration	15–30 min	6–8 h	5–10 min	5–10 min	10–15 min	4–8 h
Cardiac effects	Minimal depressant effect	Minimal depressant effect	Important depressant effect	None	Important stimulatory effect	Minimal depressant effect; may prolong QT interval
Respiratory effects	Important depressant effect	Important depressant effect	Important depressant effect	Minimal depressant effect	Minimal depressant effect	None
Analgesia	None	None	None	None	Potent	None
Amnesia	Potent	None	None	None	Potent	None
Indications	Management of airway Improvement of mechanical ventilation (duration <24 h) Associated with another sedative agent and an analgesic drug for common ICU procedures	Improvement of mechanical ventilation (duration <24 h) Anxiolytic agent of choice at ICU	Same of midazolam Rapid recovery Adults Care with hypovolemia	Associated with another sedative agent and an analgesic drug for common ICU procedures Management of airway	Extremely painful procedures (such as debridements) Can be used with severe asthma CVS stable	Sedative agent for patient without an artificial airway Choice for treatment of delirious (ICU syndrome) Minimal effect on respiration

ICU, intensive care unit; CVS, cardiovascular system.
Data from Landow L, Joshi-Ryzewics W. Anesthesia for bedside procedures. In: Rippe JM, Irwin RS, Fink MP, et al., eds. *Intensive Care Medicine*. Little, Brown; 1996:264–274; Hoey LL, Nahum A, Vance-Bryan K. Sedative agents. In: Rippe JM, Irwin RS, Fink MP, et al., eds. *Intensive Care Medicine*. Little, Brown; 1996:2273–2286; and Shapiro BA, Warren J, Egol AB, et al. Practice parameters for intravenous analgesia and sedation for adult patients in the intensive care unit. *Crit Care Med*. 1995;23:1596–1600.

TABLE 40.13

THE LOADING DOSE, BOLUSES, MAINTENANCE DOSE, ONSET, AND DURATION OF COMMON ANALGESIC DRUGS

	Dose			
Drug	**Infusion**	**Bolus**	**Pediatric use**	**Comments/indications**
Morphine	1 mg/h	2–5 mg	0.5 mg/kg in 50 mL normal saline (N/S) Infuse 1–4 mL/h	Histamine release Accumulates especially in renal failure
Fentanyl	1–3 μg/kg/h	50–100 μg	50 μg/kg in 50 mL N/S Infuse 1–4 mL/h	Less histamine release Less accumulation in renal failure
Alfentanil	1–5 mg/h	0.5–1 mg	NA	Expensive Short acting and little accumulation
Pentothal	50–250 mg/h	1–2 mg/kg	NA	Use in epilepsy/raised intracranial pressure Very prolonged wakeup

Properties of the Ideal Sedative Agent

The concept of the "ideal" sedative agent must be modified for use in the NICU. Traditional properties of the ideal sedative and the additional demands made by neurointensive care are specified in Table 40.16 and Figures 40.3 and 40.4. Perhaps more so than in any other critical care setting, there is a need for ease of ability to titrate agents for sedation in head injury. Such patients may require rapid increases in sedation levels to cover clinical procedures or other stimuli that could result in dangerous ICP elevations if left untreated. Other patients may require high doses of sedatives to achieve metabolic suppression.

On the other hand, there may be a clinical need to achieve a rapid reversal of sedation to enable neurologic evaluation. These considerations underline the need for drugs that have not only a rapid onset, but also a rapid offset. Commonly used agents, such as sodium thiopental (thiopentone) and fentanyl, have short-lasting effects when used as a single bolus. However, cessation of drug action in these settings is achieved by rapid redistribution of the drug to a large volume of distribution (Vd), rather than by rapid drug metabolism or elimination. Repeated doses, or prolonged infusions, of such agents may saturate the Vd, and the drug effects—which are now critically dependent upon clearance rather than redistribution—may be significantly prolonged. The dependence of offset of drug effects on the duration of therapy has led to the concept of context-sensitive half-time, which takes account of the cumulative effects of drugs with prolonged administration (Fig. 40.5) (130). Thus, the most desirable agents are those with a short duration of action as a consequence of rapid excretion or metabolism—with no active metabolites—and show little or no prolongation of their duration of effect with increases in duration of administration. Even short-acting agents, such as propofol and alfentanil, may show some prolongation of effect with long-term use (Fig. 40.6). Perhaps the only current agent that seems substantially immune to this phenomenon is remifentanil (Fig. 40.6, Table 40.17) (131).

TABLE 40.14

DOSAGES OF DRUGS FOR CONSCIOUS SEDATION

Drug	**Loading dose (μg/kg)**	**Maintenance infusion rate (μg/kg/min)**	**Plasma drug level**
Thiopental	1,000–3,000	100–300	8–4 μg/mL
Methohexital	250–1,000	10–50	2–5 mg/mL
Diazepam	50–150		
Midazolam	25–100	0.25–1	40–100 ng/mL
Droperidol	5–17		
Propofol	250–1,000	10–50	1–2 μg/mL
Ketamine	500–1,000	10–20	0.1–1 μg/mL
Etomidate	100–200	7–14	100–300 ng/mL
Fentanyl	1–3	0.01–0.03	1–2 ng/mL
Alfentanil	10–25	0.25–1	25–75 ng/mL
Sufentanil	0.1–0.5	0.005–0.01	0.02–0.2 ng/mL

Reproduced from Greenberg CP, DeSoto H. Sedation techniques. In: Twersky RS, ed. *The Ambulatory Anesthesia Handbook*. St. Louis: Mosby Yearbook; 1995.

TABLE 40.15

INTRAVENOUS BOLUS SEDATION TECHNIQUE

PROCEDURE	DRUG
Dental	Alphaprodine 30 mg, Atropine 0.6 mg, Hydroxyzine 50 mg, Methohexital 30–60 mg
Dental/ear–nose–throat	Diazepam 10–20 mg, Fentanyl 50-μg increments, Scopolamine 0.25 mg
Oral surgery	Midazolam 0.12 mg/kg, Fentanyl 100 μg
Neuroradiology	Midazolam 2.5–20 mg, Fentanyl 50–300 μg or Propofol 100–150 mg, Fentanyl 50–125 μg
Endoscopy	Diazepam 10 mg, Meperidine 50–75 mg Midazolam 0.05 mg/kg, Alfentanil 5 mcg/kg
Multiple ambulatory surgery procedures	Midazolam 2–3 mg Alfentanil 250–500 μg or Fentanyl 50–100 μg, Methohexital 20–30 mg or Propofol 10–20 mg

Reproduced from Greenberg CP, DeSoto H. Sedation techniques. In: Twersky RS, ed. *The Ambulatory Anesthesia Handbook*. St. Louis: Mosby Yearbook; 1995.

TABLE 40.16

CHARACTERISTICS OF AN IDEAL SEDATIVE USED ON THE NEUROINTENSIVE CARE UNIT

GENERAL REQUIREMENTS
- Good-quality sedation
- Rapid onset and offset of action
- Noncumulative
- No systemic adverse effects
- Inexpensive

NEUROINTENSIVE CARE REQUIREMENTS
- Maintain cerebral autoregulation and cerebrovascular response to $PaCO_2$
- Reduce $CMRO_2$, to an extent that provides an isoelectric or burst-suppressed EEG
- Reduce CBV and hence ICP
- Reduce seizure activity
- Have rapid offset of action to enable neurologic assessment
- Result in rapid changes in CNS depression in response to changes in dose

$PaCO_2$, partial carbon dioxide pressure; $CMRO_2$, cerebral metabolic rate; EEG, electroencephalogram; CBV, cerebral blood volume; ICP, intracranial pressure; CNS, central nervous system.

Pattern of Sedative Use

Many different sedatives have been used over the years in the NICU. A survey of sedative use in the United Kingdom and Ireland in 1995 showed the frequency of use of different sedative and analgesic agents in neurointensive care units (132,133). Most centers used a combination of a hypnotic and an opioid, the usual agents being propofol (65%), midazolam (80%), morphine (60%), fentanyl (46%), and alfentanil (26%). None of these agents is ideal, and there are few published studies that compare sedative drugs either within or between the different pharmacologic subclasses. See Table 40.17 for a summary of the main classes of sedatives.

To conclude, there is no ideal sedative for use in head injury, and few studies directly compare the effectiveness and adverse effects of different agents in this group of patients. Among the existing drugs, propofol appears to have most of the properties required but, as with all commonly used agents, it is at the expense of systemic blood pressure. The other frequently used agents, such as opioids and benzodiazepines, also have features to recommend them. In the absence of new, improved drugs, sedation of head-injured patients will likely continue to involve a number of agents. The introduction of remifentanil is promising, with its unique metabolic pathway allowing intense narcosis with a rapid and reliable offset of action, and the potential neuroprotective action of dexmedetomidine is worthy of further study.

Sedation in the Thermally Injured Patient

The quality and intensity of pain in severely burned patients during ICU treatment frequently changes due to repeated operations and dressing changes. Adequate analgesia is crucial in the critical care of burn victims, and not only to increase patient comfort, although this is of obvious concern. Either administration of too much or too little analgesia can worsen outcome: Pain decreases wound healing and immunologic competence, while overdosage of analgesics decreases intestinal motility and increases the length of stay in the ICU. The optimal concept of analgesia, following the World Health Organization (WHO) guidelines for pain management, should therefore consist of sufficient basic pain relief combined with a fast-onset "rescue" medication that provides on-top (additive) analgesia if needed (134). The combination of a NSAID and a long-acting opioid (morphine hydrochloride) with the short-acting esterase-metabolized opioid remifentanil on top seemed to be a promising concept for burn patients. The experience with this new concept of analgesia in severely burned ICU patients, with burn wounds of 20% to 80% total body surface area (TBSA), has been detailed (134). These patients received 75 mg diclofenac twice daily with a continuous IV infusion of morphine; a remifentanil infusion was added on demand if necessary. Morphine was administered in a mean dosage of 4 mg/hour. Remifentanil was administered at a median dosage of 0.7 mg/hour. This method of treatment allowed adequate individual analgesia according to actual demand, without serious side effects in severely burned patients. It can be used in both intubated and spontaneously breathing, nonintubated patients. Additionally, a cost analysis showed benefits compared to a conventional regimen (134).

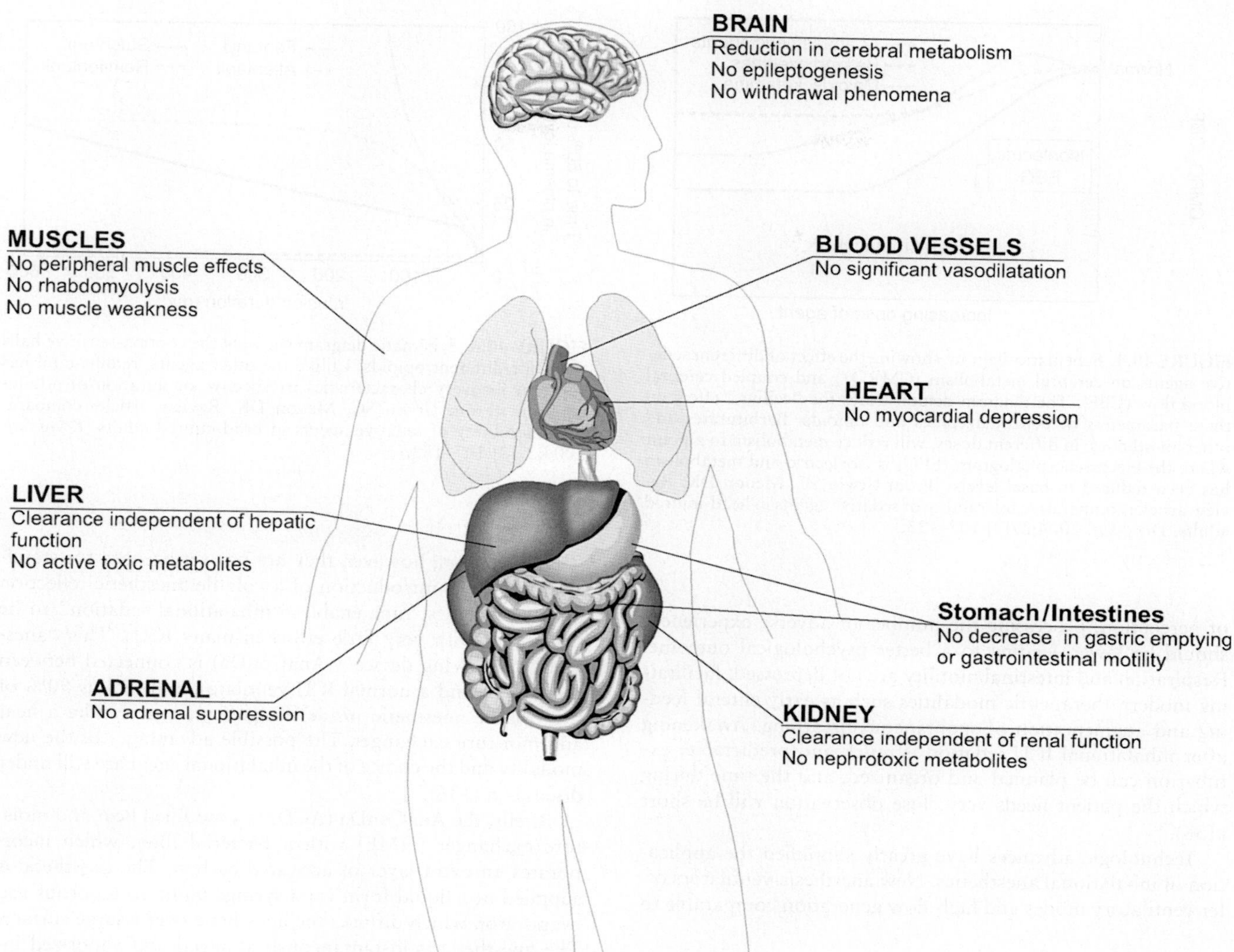

FIGURE 40.3. Desirable organ-specific effects, of the ideal sedative agent, used in intensive care unit patients with brain injury. Several organ systems may be compromised by extracranial injury, making the patient more susceptible to unwanted effects of sedative agents.

Analgesia and Sedation following Cardiac Surgery

Maintaining homeostasis after heart surgery is central to the patient's outcome. Pain and anxiety are factors contributing to postoperative morbidity, since they correlate with elevated heart rate and blood pressure, increased peripheral O_2 consumption, and elevated serum adrenergic neurohormone levels.

Multiple drug combinations can be administered in the cardiac ICU. In a trial to identify the most adequate drug for the postoperative ICU setting, a prospective, randomized, open-label study was performed (135). This study's aim was a comparative analysis of a central adrenergic α_2 blocker, dexmedetomidine, versus a short-acting opioid, remifentanil, with regard to analgesia, sedation, and side effects. Both drugs proved effective for controlling pain and anxiety. Remifentanil was more efficient in this study, especially when time was not considered, based on the better results in the first 4 hours of the postoperative period.

Short-acting Drugs for Long-term Intensive Care Unit Sedation

Inhalational Intensive Care Unit Sedation

ICU sedation poses many problems. The action and side effects of intravenous drugs in the severely ill patient population of an ICU are difficult to control. The incidence of posttraumatic stress disorder (PTSD) after long-term sedation is high. The recent focus on propofol infusion syndrome entails restrictions in the use of this drug. On the other hand, volatile anesthetics very selectively suppress consciousness but leave many autonomic functions intact. In the absence

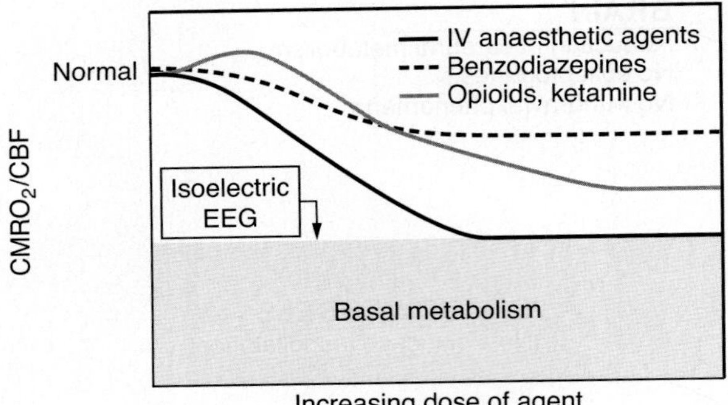

FIGURE 40.4. Schematic diagram showing the effect of different sedative agents on cerebral metabolism ($CMRO_2$) and coupled cerebral blood flow (CBF). The diagram demonstrates the "ceiling" effect on these parameters of benzodiazepines and opioids. Barbiturates and other anesthetics, in different doses, will reduce metabolism to a point where the electroencephalogram (EEG) is isoelectric and metabolism has been reduced to basal levels. (From Urwin SC, Menon DK. Review article: comparative tolerability of sedative agents in head-injured adults. *Drug Saf.* 2004;27[2]:107–133.)

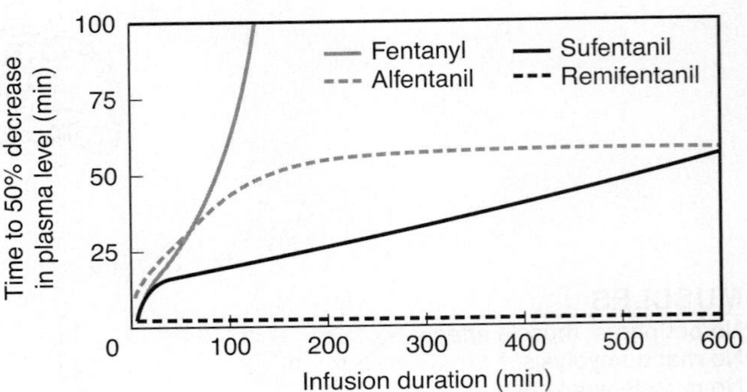

FIGURE 40.6. Schematic diagram showing the context-sensitive half-times for different opioids. Unlike the other agents, remifentanil has constant recovery characteristics irrespective of duration of administration. (From Urwin SC, Menon DK. Review article: comparative tolerability of sedative agents in head-injured adults. *Drug Saf.* 2004;27[2]:107–133.)

of perception, processing the number of adverse experiences should be lower, leading to a better psychological outcome. Respiration and intestinal motility are not depressed, facilitating modern therapeutic modalities such as early enteral feeding and augmentation of spontaneous breathing. Awakening after inhalational ICU sedation is quick and predictable; extubation can be planned and organized, and the time during which the patient needs very close observation will be short (136).

Technologic advances have greatly simplified the application of inhalational anesthetics. New anesthesia ventilators offer ventilatory modes and high-flow generation comparable to

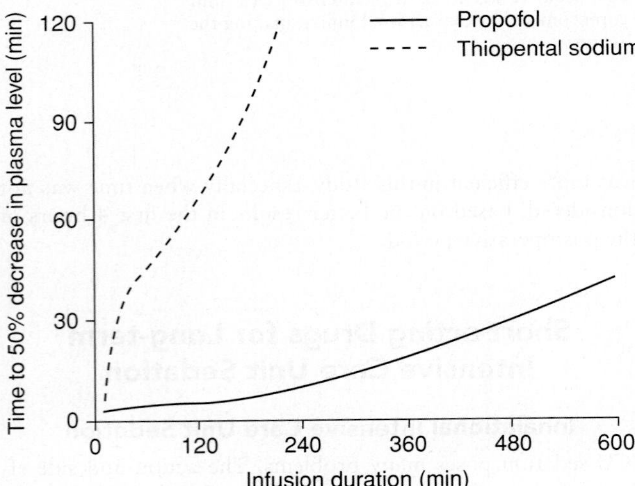

FIGURE 40.5. Schematic diagram showing the context-sensitive half-times for thiopental sodium and propofol. Note that the recovery characteristics of both drugs worsen with increasing duration of administration, but that this effect is much more prominent for thiopental sodium. (From Urwin SC, Menon DK. Review article: comparative tolerability of sedative agents in head-injured adults. *Drug Saf.* 2004;27[2]:107–133.)

ICU ventilators; however, they are not yet licensed for stand-alone use. The introduction of a volatile anesthetic reflection filter for the first time enables "inhalational sedation" to be performed with very little effort in many ICUs. This "anesthetic conserving device" (AnaConDa) is connected between the patient and a normal ICU ventilator, and retains 90% of the volatile anesthetic inside the patient, exactly like a heat and moisture exchanger. The possible advantages of the new modality and the choice of the inhalational agent are still under discussion (136).

Briefly, the AnaConDa (ACD) is a modified heat and moisture exchanger (HME) with a bacterial filter, which incorporates an extra layer of activated carbon. The anesthetic is supplied in a liquid form via a syringe pump to a porous rod evaporator, which diffuses the anesthetic over a large surface. The anesthetic is instantaneously dragged and vaporized inside the ACD by the inspiratory gas flow and delivered to the lungs. The activated carbon layer absorbs some of the expired anesthetic vapor and desorbs some of it in the next inspiration (137). In this way, it can be used as a vaporizer device with a standard critical care ventilator, saving anesthetic loss like a low-flow circle anesthetic system. In fact, it has proved to reduce anesthetic consumption to a level equivalent to that produced in a circle system using a fresh gas flow of 1.5 L (138). Figure 40.7 shows the main components of ACD (139).

BEDSIDE ANESTHESIA IN THE INTENSIVE CARE UNIT

Principles of Procedural Anesthesia at the Bedside

Prospective planning requires knowledge of the patient's condition and an assessment of the anesthetic requirements of the proposed procedure. The spectrum of anesthetic options ranges from sedation and analgesia and monitored anesthesia care (MAC) to total intravenous anesthesia (TIVA) (138).

Procedural anesthesia at the bedside offers patients relief from anxiety, discomfort, and pain, and may expedite the

TABLE 40.17

MAIN SEDATIVE AGENTS USED IN THE TREATMENT OF HEAD-INJURED PATIENTS IN THE NEUROINTENSIVE CARE UNIT

Drug	$t_{1/2}$ (h)	Metabolite accumulation	CBF	$CMRO_2$	ICP	MAP	Seizure threshold	Other effects
Midazolam	2–2.5	+	↓	↓	(↓)	↓	↑	Interaction with peripheral benzodiazepine leukocyte receptors (clinical relevance?)
Lorazepam	0–20	++	↓	↓	(↓)	↓	↑	
Diazepam	20–40	+++	↓	↓	(↓)	↓	↑	
Morphine	1.7–4.5	++	(↓)^{a}	(↓)^{a}	(↑)^{a,b}	(↓)^{a}	(↓)^{c}	↓ Reticuloendothelial cell function, macrophage migration, and microbial killing in vitro
Fentanyl	3.7	+	(↓)^{a}	(↓)^{a}	(↑)^{a,b}	(↓)^{a}	(↓)^{c}	
Alfentanil	1.5	+	(↓)^{a}	(↓)^{a}	(↑)^{a,b}	(↓)^{a}	(↓)^{c}	
Remifentanil	0.15	–	(↓)^{a}	(↓)^{a}	(↑)^{a,b}	(↓)^{a}	(↓)^{c}	Remifentanil pharmacokinetics unique, with excellent titratability and wake-up characteristics
Thiopental sodium (thiopentone)	11.5	+++	↓	↓	↓	↓	↑	Marrow suppression, and leukocyte respiratory burst suppression with high doses
Pentobarbital (pentobarbitone)	11.7–19.5	++	↓	↓	↓	↓	↑	
Methohexital (methohexitone)	4	–	↓	↓	↓	↓	↑	
Propofol	7.2	–^{d}	↓	↓	↓	↓	↑	Lipid load, propofol infusion syndrome Antioxidant (clinical relevance?)
Ketamine	2.6	+	↑	↑	↑	↑^{e}	↓	No adrenal suppression NMDA antagonist (clinical relevance?)
Etomidate	4.8	–	↓	↓	↓	↓	↑	Adrenal suppression, renal failure with propylene glycol (vehicle for infusion)
Haloperidol	(24)^{f}	–	↓			↓	↑	Extrapyramidal effects
Dexmedetomidine	2	–	↓	↔	↓	↓	?	
Clonidine	20	–	↓	↔	↓	↓	?	Part of Lund protocol

↓ = decrease; ↑= increase; ↔ = no change; ? = inadequate data.

[a] While opioids and benzodiazepines reduce CBF and $CMRO_2$, there is a ceiling to these effects and they do not produce burst-suppression or an isoelectric EEG.

[b] Rapid infusions or large doses of potent opioids may reduce MAP and CPP, and the resulting autoregulation-induced cerebral vasodilatation may increase CBV and ICP.

[c] Several studies suggest that high-dose opioids may increase epileptiform activity.

[d] Consider context-sensitive half-time.

[e] High doses of ketamine may result in MAP drops, especially in hypovolemic patients, but MAP is generally elevated or maintained.

[f] Figure shows duration of maximum.

$t_{1/2}$, elimination half-life; CBF, cerebral blood flow; $CMRO_2$, cerebral metabolic rate; ICP, intracranial pressure; MAP, mean arterial pressure; NDMA, *N*-methyl-D-aspartate; EEG, electroencephalogram; CPP, cerebral perfusion pressure; CBV, cerebral blood volume.

Data from Rhoney DH, Parker D. Use of sedative and analgesic agents in neurotrauma patients: effects on cerebral physiology. *Neurol Res.* 2001;23:237–259; and Urwin SC, Menon DK. Review article: comparative tolerability of sedative agents in head-injured adults. *Drug Saf.* 2004;27(2):107–133.

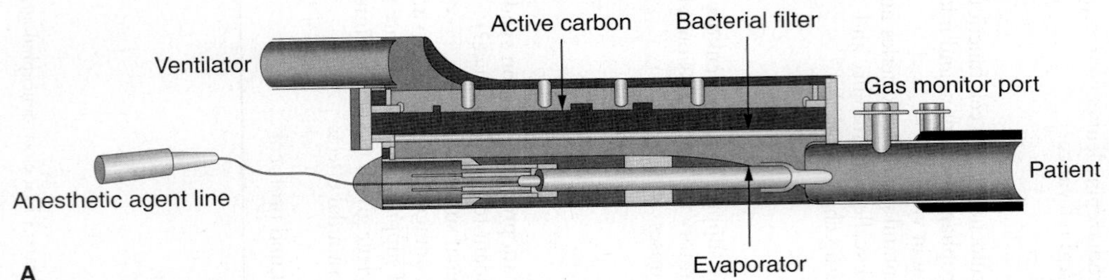

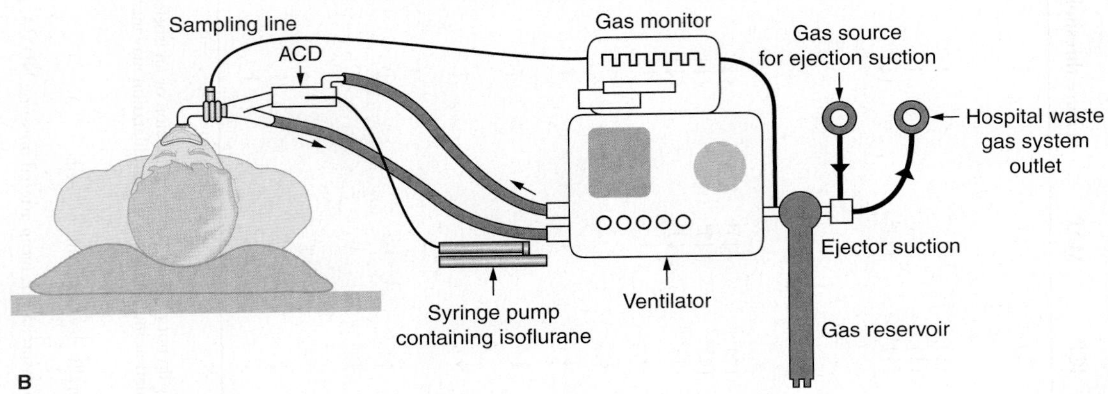

FIGURE 40.7. **A:** Anesthetic converting device, AnaConDa. **B:** Breathing circuit with anesthetic converting device (AnaConDa) at the inspiratory limb of the breathing circuit. (From Sackey PV, Martling CR, Radell PJ. Three cases of PICU sedation with isoflurane delivered by AnaConDa. *Paediatr Anaesth.* 2005;15[10]:879–885.)

procedure by increasing patient cooperation. Identification of the at-risk patient and modifying the anesthetic should reduce complications (see Risk Assessment section). The choice of pharmaceuticals (see above) depends upon the level of anticipated required anesthesia. Personnel requirements also vary. Although an anesthesiologist is not required to administer medications and monitor the patient for sedation and analgesia or monitored anesthesia care, TIVA does require the services of an anesthesiologist. Costs are influenced by the personnel requirements and length of the procedure, which sets the drug requirements and drug costs. In the end, personal experience combined with knowledge should guide the provider to offer efficacious and cost-effective procedural anesthesia in the ICU.

Inhalational Anesthetic Agents: The Nonresponding Patient

Halothane, isoflurane, and sevoflurane are potent bronchodilators in asthmatic patients receiving mechanical ventilation who have failed to respond to conventional β-adrenergic agents (140). Experimental evidence indicates a direct effect on bronchial smooth muscle mediated via calcium-dependent channels, as well as by modulating vagal-, histamine-, allergen-, and hypoxia-induced bronchoconstrictor mechanisms (141,142). Furthermore, these agents reduce pulmonary vascular tone, resulting in lower pulmonary artery pressures in acute asthma (143). Bronchodilator responses are seen in the form of reduced peak airway pressures within minutes, associated with improved ventilation—resulting in a lower $PaCO_2$—and reduced air trapping (144). Although the bronchodilator effects are seen at subanesthetic concentrations, these agents also offer a relatively expensive method of sedation. A few ICU ventilators, such as the Seimens Servo 900 series, can be fitted with a vaporizer, allowing anesthetic gases to be administered. Effective exhaled gas scavenging systems are required when using inhalational anesthetics in the ICU. If this system is not available, a Cardiff canister can be added to the expiratory port of the ventilator to remove effluent anesthetic gases. Significant side effects such as hypotension and myocardial irritability exist, and prolonged administration of some agents may result in bromide or fluoride toxicity (145). Sevoflurane, a halogenated ether, is largely devoid of cardiorespiratory side effects, and may be the preferred agent. The administration of subanesthetic concentrations of these agents via a face mask may relieve bronchospasm refractory to conventional treatment (146).

One of the difficult aspects of mechanical ventilation of the acute asthmatic patient is the weaning and extubation process. The presence of the endotracheal tube within the larynx and trachea induces bronchoconstriction, which becomes troublesome as the sedation is withdrawn in preparation for extubation (147,148). Use of an inhalational anesthetic agent allows the endotracheal tube to be removed under anesthesia, with the confident expectation of rapid recovery once the anesthetic is discontinued (149).

SPECIAL PROCEDURES

Bedside Procedures and Monitoring

The long list of bedside ICU procedures includes special monitoring of critically ill patients, and provides guidance on all aspects of treatment, from the emergency room to the ICU. On that list, most are the commonly performed procedures used by critical care specialists, surgeons, emergency room physicians, and certified registered nurse anesthetists (Table 40.18) (150).

TABLE 40.18

LIST OF ALL ASPECTS OF *PROCEDURES AND MONITORING* IN THE INTENSIVE CARE UNIT FOR WHICH SEDATION OR ANESTHESIA IS PROVIDED

PROCEDURES
- Central venous catheterization/arterial catheterization
- Pulmonary artery catheterization
- Intraosseous infusion at the bedside
- Tracheostomy/cricothyroidotomy
- Tube thoracostomy
- Pericardiocentesis
- Pericardial window
- Percutaneous feeding catheter
- Placement of diagnostic abdominal paracentesis
- Peritoneal lavage
- Assisted ventilation and intubation
- Flexible bronchoscopy
- Intra-abdominal pressure monitoring
- Intracranial pressure monitoring
- Jugular bulb oximetry
- Cardiac pacemaker placement
- Inferior vena caval filter
- Placement of epidural analgesia
- Suprapubic urinary tube placement
- Bedside spinal immobilization

MONITORING
- Routine clinical monitoring in acute illnesses
- Invasive hemodynamic monitoring
- Noninvasive cardiac output monitoring: Bioimpedance and partial CO_2, rebreathing methods
- Transesophageal Doppler monitoring
- Gastric tonometry
- Renal function
- Support noninvasive autonomic nervous system monitoring in critical care physiology of shock and acute circulatory failure
- Hemodynamic therapy for circulatory dysfunction

Mini-surgery

Bedside Diagnostic Minilaparoscopy and Minilaparotomy

The use of bedside minilaparoscopy as a diagnostic aid in the ICU patient with a possible intra-abdominal process is a rescue operation in a potential catastrophic condition. Although the workup of potential abdominal pathology in critically ill ICU patients uses conventional methods, including physical examination, CT, ultrasonography, and diagnostic peritoneal lavage, a delay in the diagnosis of intra-abdominal pathology is a major contributor to morbidity and mortality. The reasons for delay are multifactorial, including failure to consider the diagnosis, lack of sensitivity of noninvasive diagnostic modalities, and difficulty in safely transporting a critically ill patient. Bedside diagnostic laparoscopy is a modality that is safe, accurate, time efficient, and potentially therapeutic.

Recent laparotomy is no longer a contraindication to bedside laparoscopy. A recent study by Bauer et al. described the use of laparoscopy in patients with acute abdominal findings after urologic surgery (151). It is in the group of patients with recent previous laparotomy that diagnostic laparoscopy may have its greatest advantage over CT scanning. Postoperative changes may be difficult to differentiate from acute abdominal pathology on CT (e.g., free air, fluid, inflammation). Diagnostic laparoscopy, though, allows direct examination of the abdominal cavity. By avoiding negative laparotomies and limiting the reopening of recent abdominal incisions, it is possible to decrease wound complications and ultimately reduce the length of the hospital stay. Although not a new revelation, it is of significance to note that intubation is not a requirement for laparoscopy. Fabian et al. (152) showed that laparoscopy can be used safely in trauma patients. Diagnostic laparoscopy is often used as an operating room procedure under general anesthesia (152). Iberti et al. found it useful for identifying intestinal ischemia following aortobifemoral bypass (153). Others have described it as a tool that can be used outside the operating room, but exclusively to evaluate trauma by both blunt (154) and penetrating (155) mechanisms. Still others describe the use of diagnostic laparoscopy in the ICU; however, in this setting, the patient is required to be intubated and under general anesthesia (156,157); patients who have had a recent laparotomy are specifically excluded (157). The diagnosis of acute abdominal conditions in the critically ill patient remains difficult. ICU patients with abdominal pain, unexplained acidosis or sepsis, or suspected mesenteric ischemia are eligible for bedside diagnostic minilaparoscopy (158). Bedside minilaparoscopy can be a safe and accurate method to evaluate critically ill patients in whom the possibility of mesenteric ischemia or other intra-abdominal process is entertained. Bedside diagnostic laparoscopy can be a useful replacement for diagnostic laparotomy in the operating room. It should be included in the diagnostic algorithm when evaluating the unstable ICU patient with a suspected acute intra-abdominal process.

The procedure can be performed at the bedside in the ICU with the patient under local anesthesia and intravenous (conscious or asleep) sedation. In some reports (158,159) most of the patients did not require general anesthesia, although local anesthetics and sedation with midazolam or propofol were used. Most of the patients in these studies were intubated prior to laparoscopy. They required mechanical ventilation because of their disease process; none of them was intubated solely to perform the procedure. Local anesthesia with lidocaine and sedation with midazolam or propofol was used in all cases.

Pneumoperitoneum can be established with nitrous oxide (NO) to a relatively low pressure of 8 to 10 mm Hg.

Hemodynamics and ventilatory parameters should be monitored before, during, and after the procedure. Such procedures typically last a relatively short time (mean 21 minutes [158]). Laparoscopy performed at the bedside in the ICU may be used as a routine diagnostic tool in the evaluation of critically ill patients, similar to the use of CT, ultrasonography, and radiography (159), as there are minimal complications directly related to the procedure. Thus, bedside laparoscopy in the ICU under local or general anesthesia is a diagnostic and potentially therapeutic tool that can be used safely in the workup of potential abdominal pathology in critically ill patients. The application of diagnostic laparoscopy could become a routine procedure in the ICU to evaluate critically ill patients. No limitations, such as need for intubation or general anesthesia, should compromise the performance of the procedure. Additionally, patients with recent abdominal surgery were not excluded from consideration (159).

Laparoscopic Procedures

Laparoscopic procedures can reveal findings such as turbid fluid consistent with viscus perforation, sterile hemorrhagic fluid, a retroperitoneal mass, and an abdominal abscess (160). Thus, bedside laparoscopy in the ICU is feasible, informative, and accurate. It has a role in diagnosing abdominal pathologies and planning further treatment. It may avert a nontherapeutic laparotomy. Unfortunately, the prognosis in these patients is poor. Earlier use of this diagnostic modality may improve patient outcome.

Tracheostomy

Tracheostomy is one of the most frequent procedures carried out in critically ill patients, with major advantages compared to translaryngeal endotracheal intubation such as reduced laryngeal anatomic alterations, reduced inspiratory load, better patient tolerance, and improved nursing care. Thus, tracheostomy can enhance care in patients who need prolonged mechanical ventilation and/or airway control. The right timing for a tracheostomy remains controversial; however, it appears that early tracheostomy in selected severe trauma, burn, and neurologic patients could be effective to reduce the duration of mechanical ventilation, intensive care stay, and costs. ICU growth and improvements in technology have led to an increasing number of critically ill patients who require prolonged mechanical ventilation; these can be managed most appropriately with tracheostomies (161). Until recently, surgical tracheostomy performed in the OR was the only option available. However, morbidity from surgical tracheostomy ranges from 6% to 66%, and mortality ranges from 0% to 5% (162,163). Complications resulting from surgical tracheostomy performed in the ICU are comparable to those performed in the OR (162,163). The "classical" technique of percutaneous dilatational tracheostomy using progressive dilators was introduced by Ciaglia et al. in 1985 and, today, has become the procedure of choice in the majority of the cases, as it is safe, easy, and quick, with minor complications (164).

Percutaneous dilatational tracheostomy (PDT) has been recognized as a reliable alternative to the surgical placement of an artificial airway in patients with persistent respiratory failure due to various medical conditions (164,165). PDT may offer several advantages over conventional surgical tracheostomy placement, as PDT is associated with lower periprocedural and postprocedural complication rates (163); moreover, PDT can be performed at the bedside, thus avoiding the scheduling, time commitments, and costs associated with surgical operating facilities (Table 40.19A).

TABLE 40.19A

ADVANTAGES OF TRACHEOSTOMY COMPARED WITH ORO-/NASOTRACHEAL INTUBATION

- Secure airway
- Avoid laryngeal and vocal cord injury
- Reduced airway resistance and dead space
- Ease of airway suction and mouth care
- Oral feeding possible
- Improved patient comfort

All PDT procedures are performed at the ICU bedside with continuous monitoring of blood pressure, heart rate, respiratory rate, oxygen saturation, and cardiac rhythm. Mechanical ventilatory support should be maintained throughout the procedure, the fraction of inspired oxygen increased to 1.0, and all patients placed on mandatory mechanical ventilation mode. Most procedures are attended by an anesthesiologist to assist in the management of the airway in the event of complications.

PDT has gained widespread acceptance in the ICU setting and presents a valid alternative to operative tracheostomy. In fact, recent data suggest several potential advantages compared to surgical tracheostomy, including ease of performance and a lower incidence of both peristomal bleeding and postoperative infection (166).

Among the relative contraindications for PDT are patients with altered neck anatomy due to severe neck burns and scarring from a previous tracheostomy (167). In addition, obese patients with large and thick necks are considered poor candidates for PDT, and are commonly referred for surgical tracheostomy placement (Table 40.19B).

Thrombocytopenia is another relative contraindication, and a higher incidence of bleeding, a prolonged stay in the ICU, and increased mortality are often associated with this finding (168). Many physicians consider thrombocytopenia a contraindication for performing the procedure (169,170); hence, thrombocytopenic patients often are excluded from comparative trials (166,171,172). PDT procedures take place under bronchoscopic control and are either performed or supervised by at least one pulmonologist or critical care medicine physician. Informed consent for these procedures is obtained from an appropriately designated surrogate. The procedure is performed in all patients following a standardized protocol, as previously described by Cantais et al. (171) using a commercially available kit (SIMS; Portex; Hythe, Kent, United Kingdom). The

TABLE 40.19B

ABSOLUTE AND RELATIVE CONTRAINDICATIONS FOR PERCUTANEOUS DILATATIONAL TRACHEOSTOMY

- Age <15 y
- Intubation difficulty
- Documented or suspected tracheomalacia
- Anatomic problems in the neck
- Fat and/or short neck, thyroid enlargement
- Uncorrectable bleeding problems
- Previous neck and/or thorax surgery

only modification consisted of the local administration of a 2% solution of lidocaine with epinephrine (1:200,000) before proceeding with tracheal puncture.

Immediately after the tracheostomy insertion, a bronchoscopic examination is performed through the tracheostomy to confirm the correct position of the tracheostomy tube and to identify injuries or bleeding. Subsequently, the trachea proximal to the percutaneously placed tracheostomy is inspected bronchoscopically via the remaining orotracheal tube to identify fractures of tracheal rings or blood. After the procedure, a chest radiograph was performed to rule out the presence of a pneumothorax.

Percutaneous Endoscopic Gastrostomy

Aspiration pneumonia due to gastroesophageal reflux is a frequent complication in ICU. The most commonly chosen method for long-term enteral access—gastrostomy—also reduces the risk of aspiration and shortens the hospital stay. A decrease in positive tracheal aspirate cultures was seen after PEG insertion—3.14 ± 1.95 times before PEG and 1.52 ± 1.47 times after PEG (173). Nasogastric tubes, used in the past, have been inadequate for long-term therapy due to patient discomfort, among other risks (174). The advantages of enteral versus parenteral feeding, in patients with a normal functioning gastrointestinal tract, are well known and include better patient compliance, maintenance of gastrointestinal tube integrity, and decreased costs, as well as minimizing villous atrophy and, at least theoretically, minimizing translocation of bacteria/fungi (174–176).

PEG placement seems to be a safe and cost-effective alternative to operative gastrostomy, especially as the latter requires general anesthesia and it is not without significant morbidity and mortality. Additionally, a failed PEG does not preclude subsequent operative gastrostomy. Surgical gastrostomy and jejunostomy are always performed in the operating theater with general anesthesia, and are associated with measurable morbidity and mortality (177). Ferraro et al. (178) performed PEG at the bedside in the ICU, using TIVA for patients with spontaneous ventilation and local anesthesia for sedated patients on mechanical ventilation. Enteral feeding through PEG usually started 24 hours after the end of the procedure. Early PEG in critically injured patients is a safe and effective method of providing access to the gastrointestinal tract for nutritional support. In patients with significant brain injuries, adequate sedation and the presence of an ICP monitor help to minimize secondary insults to the brain (179).

The indications for PEG placement are as follows: neurologic diseases with swallowing incapacity, pharyngeal and esophageal neoplasms, and long-term hospitalized patients after major surgical procedures who are unable to swallow. Absolute PEG contraindications are massive ascites, gastric varices, hepatomegaly, coagulopathy, and total esophageal stenosis. Previous abdominal surgery may not represent a problem if there is good adhesion between the abdominal and the gastric wall.

Burns and Wound Debridement

The main aim of care in a burn center is to control hypovolemia and obtain maximal tissue perfusion and oxygen delivery to damaged but viable tissues, as well as to healthy organs. To manage the burn shock, catecholamines are often indicated when appropriate fluid loading is inadequate to maintain perfusion. Mechanical ventilation is indicated in several cases: A deep burn over more than 60% of TBSA, facial and cervical burns, severe pulmonary burn injury from smoke inhalation, carbon monoxide intoxication, tracheobronchial thermal injury, and blast injury, among other reasons. Because of the severity of burn-related pain, continuous sedation is usually required. Early surgical treatment such as escharotomies, excision and grafting—which cause significant pain as well as blood loss—and hydrotherapy often require general anesthesia (180,181). Burn injury can modify the volume of distribution and the pharmacokinetics of anesthetic agents and muscle relaxants (181). Finally, chemical or electrical burns, radiation, associated CO intoxication, multiple trauma, and burn injury in infants raise specific problems.

The care of critically ill burn patients can be challenging because of the rapidly escalating tolerance for opioids. A recent study evaluated the safety and efficacy of anesthesiologist-administered anesthesia in the burn intensive care unit treatment room. The review suggested that these procedures can be performed safely with appropriate supervision and monitoring without detrimental effects on patient activity level or nutritional status (180).

Adequate analgesia is crucial in the critical care of burn victims. The quality and intensity of pain in severely burned patients during the ICU treatment changes frequently due to repeated operations and dressing changes. The administration of too much or too little analgesia can worsen outcome: Pain prolongs wound healing and immunologic incompetence, while overdosage of analgesics decreases intestinal motility and increases the length of stay at the ICU.

Greher et al. reported their first experiences with a new concept of analgesia—NSAIDs and narcotics—in severely burned ICU patients. This concept allowed adequate individual analgesia according to the actual demand without serious side effects. Analysis showed a reduction in cost by one third compared to a conventional analgesic regimen with sufentanil. This manner of analgesia provision in severely burned patients is safe, highly effective, and flexible enough to meet the actual analgesic demands of the patient. It can be used in both intubated and spontaneously breathing, nonintubated patients (134).

Ketamine is traditionally used for short- and long-term sedation and analgesia of a burn patient (181). Edrich et al. used ketamine for long-term sedation and analgesia of burn patients. Under escalating opiate dosages—even without adequate analgesia—the patient had developed persistent ileus as well as abdominal distension that caused respiratory compromise. The opiate-sparing effect of the continuous ketamine infusion allowed a decrement in dosage of more than 90%; the ileus resolved within 24 hours. The quality of sedation also changed for the better. There were no obvious adverse effects of ketamine (182).

Disease Treatment (Asthma, Epilepsy)

Status Epilepticus

Refractory status epilepticus (SE) is a major neurologic emergency, each year affecting 10 to 50 per 100,000 persons; in adults, its mortality rate ranges from 7% to 20% (183,184). Prompt initiation of treatment is essential, because SE becomes more refractory to treatment with time (183–185). SE that fails to respond to first-line therapy of benzodiazepines followed by second-line therapy (phenytoin, valproate, or phenobarbital) is defined as refractory SE (183,185). Refractory SE occurs in about 30% of patients with SE and is associated with a mortality rate of greater than 20% (183).

Management of refractory SE requires induction of coma with potent anesthetics under continuous EEG monitoring, requiring mechanical ventilation in an ICU setting. The aim of treatment is to terminate SE and prevent late SE-associated complications, including hyperthermia, hypotension, hypoglycemia, rhabdomyolysis, pulmonary edema, cerebral edema, and failure of cerebral autoregulation (185). Barbiturates are the anesthetics most commonly used to induce coma in this setting, especially in Europe (186,187). Propofol, the widely used intravenous anesthetic, has been shown to control SE in animals (188) and humans (189–194), and to shorten the duration of electroconvulsive therapy (195). It is still debated whether propofol should be used as an alternative to barbiturates or as first-choice treatment in refractory SE (196). A recent study showed that propofol was effective in the management of most refractory SE episodes in adults (196). Despite relatively high total doses of propofol, the incidence of treatment-related adverse events was quite low. In particular, no patient experienced life-threatening adverse effects or the so-called propofol infusion syndrome. The deaths were attributable to refractory SE itself or its etiology.

Propofol works possibly through modulation of GABA-α receptors at a site different from that targeted by benzodiazepines and barbiturates (188). Although propofol is currently considered as an alternative to barbiturates or midazolam for the management of patients with refractory SE (185), only limited clinical data are available. In a retrospective review of patients receiving propofol for refractory SE, it was found to be ineffective in only 14% (190). Another refractory SE series found no difference in terms of duration of ICU stay or the incidence of arterial hypotension between patients receiving propofol and those receiving barbiturates, whereas time to seizure control was significantly shorter in the propofol group (2.6 vs. 123 minute) (191). A retrospective comparison of propofol and midazolam in refractory SE did not find any difference in terms of seizure control (clinical or EEG), infectious complications, hemodynamic compromise, duration of mechanical ventilation, and mortality (193), and a recently published systematic review of 28 series—including 193 refractory SE patients (54 receiving midazolam, 33 propofol, and 106 barbiturates) (194)—showed that barbiturates were most effective for controlling seizures, followed by propofol and then midazolam; however, more patients receiving barbiturates had continuous EEG monitoring, introducing a possible bias. Furthermore, this study showed less hypotension with propofol, suggesting possible subtherapeutic dosage of propofol. Finally, propofol was recently reported to control complex-partial refractory SE (192). In the study of Rossetti et al. (196), 77% of refractory SE episodes were successfully treated, allowing permanent seizure control in 67% of patients with propofol alone, and 10% with propofol and subsequent barbiturate therapy. Propofol was administered at relatively high doses (mean, 4.8 mg/kg/hour) for several days (mean, 3 days). The overall mortality rate was 23%, which is identical to that found in another retrospective refractory SE study (183). The large variation in previously reported mortality rates, ranging from 17% to 80%, can be explained by discrepancies in the definition, management, and etiology of refractory SE (183,191,197,198). The median duration of mechanical ventilation and ICU stay in the Mayer study (183) were shorter than previously reported in series of refractory SE treated with barbiturates (197,198). However, discrepancies in patient selection between series may account for these differences. The relatively short duration of mechanical ventilation may be related to the pharmacokinetic properties of propofol, especially its short elimination half-life (190,191).

To our knowledge, no fatal case of propofol infusion syndrome has been described in patients with refractory SE. Although some of the patients had high propofol infusion rates for a prolonged time (i.e., $\geq$9 days), isolated hyperlipidemia was rarely seen (196).

Some patients with long propofol treatment had transient movement disorders, showing tremor on emergence from general anesthesia and transient focal dystonia of a limb. Whereas some case reports underlined the efficacy of propofol in the management of refractory SE (189), others described abnormal movements, posturing, and seizurelike activity related to its use (199,200). Other studies—prospectively investigating motor phenomena related to propofol by using EEG monitoring—concluded that these were nearly always nonepileptic (201). It is thus likely that the aforementioned "seizures" might have been confused with abnormal movements, including opisthotonus, increased tone with twitching, and rhythmic movements (202,203), which are probably caused by subcortical dopaminergic excitatory activity induced by a low dose of propofol. These movements disappear as cortical GABA inhibition occurs at higher doses (201). Propofol might also act as a glycine antagonist in subcortical and spinal structures (203), explaining the occurrence of opisthotonus. Similar abnormal movements can be encountered with many other anesthetics (204).

Status Asthmaticus

Status asthmaticus is defined as an attack of bronchial asthma that resists conventional treatment and continues for more than 24 hours. Most deaths from acute asthma occur outside the hospital, but the at-risk patient may be recognized on the basis of prior ICU admission and asthma medication history. Patients who fail to improve significantly in the emergency department should be admitted to an ICU for observation, monitoring, and treatment. Hypoxia, dehydration, acidosis, and hypokalemia render the severe acute asthmatic patient vulnerable to cardiac dysrhythmia and cardiorespiratory arrest. Mechanical ventilation may be required for a small proportion of patients for whom it may be life saving. Aggressive bronchodilator (e.g., continuous nebulized β-agonist treatment) and anti-inflammatory therapy must continue throughout the period of mechanical ventilation. Recognized complications of mechanical ventilation include hypotension, barotrauma, and nosocomial pneumonia. Low ventilator respiratory rates, long expiratory times, and small tidal volumes help to prevent hyperinflation. Volatile anesthetic agents may produce bronchodilation in patients resistant to β agonists. Fatalities in acute asthmatics admitted to the ICU are relatively uncommon (205).

Drug Therapy for Intubation and Mechanical Ventilation in Status Asthmaticus

Anesthetic Agents and Sedatives

Etomidate and thiopentone are short-acting imidazole and barbiturate drugs, respectively, that are commonly used for intubation, although there are rare reports of bronchospasm and anaphylactoid reactions with these agents. Longer-term sedation may be obtained by infusion of midazolam (2–10 mg/hour), although metabolites may accumulate in renal and hepatic impairment. Ketamine is a general anesthetic agent that has been used before, during, and after intubation in patients with acute severe asthma. It has sympathomimetic and bronchodilating properties. The usual dose for intubation is 1 to 2 mg/kg given intravenously over 2 to 4 minutes. It may increase blood pressure and heart rate, lower seizure threshold, alter mood, and cause delirium. Inhalational anesthetics used as induction agents have the advantage of bronchodilation and may make muscle relaxation unnecessary; however, specialized anesthetic equipment is required for this approach.

Opioids are a useful addition to sedatives and provide analgesia during intubation and mechanical ventilation. Morphine as a bolus may cause histamine release, which can worsen bronchoconstriction and hypotension. Some intravenous preparations also contain metabisulphite, to which some asthmatics are sensitive. Fentanyl is a better choice of opioid for intubation as it inhibits airway reflexes and is short acting. It causes less histamine release than morphine, but large boluses may cause bronchospasm and chest wall rigidity.

Neuromuscular Blocking Drugs

Rocuronium, a nondepolarizing muscle relaxant with an acceptably rapid onset, offers an alternative to succinylcholine. Allergic sensitivity may occur to any neuromuscular blocking agent, and many may also cause histamine release with the potential for bronchospasm, particularly in bolus doses. Atracurium boluses should be avoided because of the bronchospastic potential, and vecuronium or pancuronium infusions should be used for longer-term maintenance of muscle relaxation.

Myopathy and muscle weakness are well-recognized complications of the long-term administration of nondepolarizing neuromuscular blocking agents in asthmatic patients, with an incidence of about 30%. In most cases, the myopathy is reversible, but may take weeks to resolve. There is an association between neuromyopathy and the duration of muscle relaxant drug use that is independent of corticosteroid therapy. The use of neuromuscular blocking agents should, therefore, as possible be kept to a minimum.

Inhalational Anesthetic Agents: The Nonresponding Patient

Status asthmaticus can be successfully treated with volatile anesthetics such as isoflurane. The tidal volume, pH, and $PaCO_2$ can be improved within 6 hours after anesthesia (205). When patients who were not treated with isoflurane were compared to patients treated with the agent in an attempt to assess the usefulness of isoflurane inhalation therapy, isoflurane inhalation therapy seemed useful for intractable status asthmaticus, and earlier introduction of this agent was expected to achieve a greater therapeutic effect (205). The patients treated with isoflurane stayed in the ICU and underwent mechanical ventilation for a shorter period. These patients had hypotension and liver dysfunctionafter the inhalation anesthesia, but these symptoms were improved by decreasing the concentration of isoflurane.

Halothane, isoflurane, and sevoflurane are potent bronchodilators in asthmatic patients receiving mechanical ventilation who have failed to respond to conventional ß-adrenergic agents. Experimental evidence indicates a direct effect on bronchial smooth muscle mediated via calcium-dependent channels as well as by modulating vagal-, histamine-, allergen-, and hypoxia-induced bronchoconstrictor mechanisms. Furthermore, these agents reduce pulmonary vascular tone, resulting in lower pulmonary artery pressures in acute asthmatic episodes. Bronchodilator responses are seen in the form of reduced peak airway pressures within minutes, associated with improved distribution of ventilation—resulting in a lower $PaCO_2$—and reduced air trapping. Although bronchodilator effects are seen at subanesthetic concentrations, these agents also offer a relatively expensive method of sedation. Several ICU ventilators, such as the Seimens Servo 900 series, can be fitted with a vaporizer, which allows anesthetic gases to be administered. Effective exhaled gas scavenging systems are required when using inhalational anesthetics in the ICU. Significant side effects such as hypotension and myocardial irritability exist, and prolonged administration of some agents may result in bromide or fluoride toxicity. The halogenated ether sevoflurane is largely devoid of cardiorespiratory side effects and may be the preferred agent. Administration of subanesthetic concentrations of one of these agents via face mask may relieve bronchospasm refractory to conventional treatment.

Imaging and Interventional Radiology

Among the long list of bedside procedures in the ICU that require special monitoring and care of the critically ill patient are MRI and CT scan, umbrella insertion, and angiographic manipulation (150). Among the critically ill, there is a significant incidence of death after diagnostic procedures (Fig. 40.8) (13), probably related to the aggressive use of diagnostic techniques (CT, MRI) in seriously ill patients, which mandates the use of general anesthesia or anesthesia care and monitoring during transport and the procedure.

Umbrella Insertion or Inferior Vena Cava Filter

For some ICU patients—at high risk for development of deep vein thrombosis and pulmonary embolism but with contraindications for anticoagulation therapy—the inferior vena cava filters are very useful and safe. Inferior vena cava filters are traditionally placed in the angio suite or operating room under fluoroscopy. Performing the procedure under such circumstances, in spite of being very efficient, presents two inconveniences: The need to transport the patient to the site where the fluoroscopy equipment is located and the use of iodinated contrast for proper location, and release of the devices. For patients with normal renal function and for those with conditions that require them being taken to the procedure room, such facts do not seem relevant. However, for patients with compromised renal function—mainly those on the edge of acute

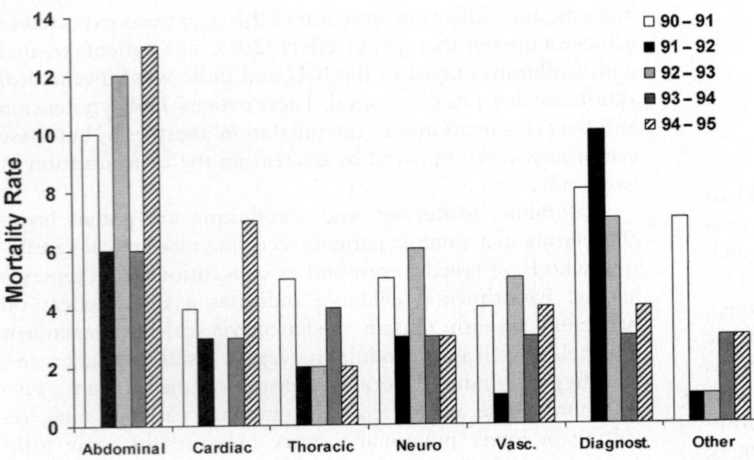

FIGURE 40.8. The rate of mortality by type of surgery for patients in the American Society of Anesthesiologists Physical Status (ASA PS) V category. Mortality rate was the highest in the abdominal surgery and the diagnostic procedures groups. (From Sidi A, Lobato EB, Cohen JA. The American Society of Anesthesiologists Physical Status: category V revisited. *J Clin Anesth.* 2000;12:328–334.)

kidney failure—the use of iodinated contrast, even in small quantities, may cause worsening of the nephrologic prognosis. On the other hand, critically ill patients who are hemodynamically unstable, are dependent on mechanical ventilation, and require high fractions of O_2 often present a high risk and are not candidates for transportation to environments with fluoroscopy to insert inferior vena cava filters. There are reports indicating an increased risk for complications—from 5.9% to 15.5%—during the intrahospital transportation of critically ill patients (206–208). For patients in these circumstances, it may be more appropriate to perform bedside procedures if possible. Some authors described the use of ultrasound for inferior vena cava filter placement, with a 97% success rate (209). Moreover, the vena cava filter placement guided by ultrasound seems to be effective, safe, and economically advantageous in relation to the conventional method (210,211).

SUMMARY

Most ICU patients require analgesia and sedation for pain and anxiety management and mechanical ventilation, or as adjuvant therapy for bedside procedures done in the ICU. These patients may undergo surgical interventions outside the traditional OR procedures. The roots of CCM are to be found in anesthesiology, extending the OR care delivered to the critically ill to the PACU. The needs of these high-acuity patients led to the development of better OR monitoring and more aggressive management. In that regard, anesthesiology and intensive care medicine influenced and fertilized one another, and this symbiosis was mostly positive. Of course, problems may occur with long-term ICU use of drugs initially conceived for short-term OR anesthetic use. It is not just drugs from the OR, but also monitoring devices that are of interest to intensivists, such as the pulmonary artery catheter and the BIS monitor.

Perioperative mortality is a product of the severity of illness, the advances in life support, and our interventions that affect the rate of acute mortality. To determine our priorities while practicing anesthesia in the ICU environment, we need to learn and assess patient risk and safety in the ICU.

Sedation is an essential component in the management of intensive care patients. It is required to relieve the discomfort and anxiety caused by procedures such as tracheal intubation, ventilation, suction, and physiotherapy. It can also minimize agitation and maximize rest and appropriate sleep. Analgesia is an almost universal requirement for the intensive care patient. Adequate sedation and analgesia ameliorates the metabolic response to surgery and trauma. Too much or too little sedation and analgesia can increase morbidity. Sedative/analgesic dosage of commonly used agents varies between patients. A valid method for monitoring sedation would allow sedation to be tailored to the individual. Any scoring system should be simple, easily performed, noninvasive, and, most importantly, reproducible. Physiologic variables, serum concentrations of drugs, and neurophysiologic tools such as EEG have all been used but proven to be expensive and unreliable. The challenge for critical care physicians who use analgesics and sedatives is to provide patient comfort and safety without increasing morbidity and mortality. Because of the variety in practice styles, pathways to standardize patient care have attracted attention. From a mechanical ventilation standpoint, weaning protocols have been shown to improve efficiency, reduce resource utilization, improve patient outcomes, reduce overall ICU expenditures, and decrease the frequency of tracheostomies.

ICU sedation poses many problems. The action and side effects of intravenous drugs in the severely ill patient population of an ICU are difficult to control. The incidence of posttraumatic stress disorder after long-term sedation is high. The recent focus on propofol infusion syndrome entails restrictions in the use of this drug. On the other hand, volatile anesthetics very selectively suppress consciousness but leave many autonomic functions intact. In the absence of perception, processing the number of adverse experiences should be lower, leading to a better psychological outcome. Respiration and intestinal motility are not depressed, facilitating modern therapeutic modalities such as early enteral feeding and augmentation of spontaneous breathing. Awakening after inhalational ICU sedation is quick and predictable; extubation can be planned and organized, and the time during which the patient needs very close observation will be short.

ICU management of critically ill patients often includes anesthesia for minor procedures such as tracheostomy and percutaneous endoscopic gastrostomy tube. Prospective planning requires knowledge of the patient's condition and an assessment of the anesthetic requirements of the proposed procedure. The spectrum of anesthetic options ranges from sedation and analgesia and monitored anesthesia care, tototal intravenous anesthesia.

References

1. Maccioli GA, Cohen NH. General anesthesia in the intensive care unit? Is it ready for "prime time"? *Criti Care Med.* 2005;33(3):687–688.
2. Lassen HCA. A preliminary report on the 1952 epidemic of poliomyelitis in Copenhagen with special reference to the treatment of acute respiratory insufficiency. *Lancet.* 1953;1:37–40.
3. Bjork VO, Engstrom CG. The treatment of ventilatory insufficiency after pulmonary resection by tracheostomy and artificial ventilation. *J Thorac Surg.* 1957;34:228–241.
4. Ramsay JG. Anesthesiology in critical care medicine: a symbiosis? *ASA Newslett.* 2000;64(3).
5. Lassen HCA, Hinriksen E, Neukirch F, et al. Treatment of tetanus: Severe bone marrow suppression after prolonged nitrous oxide anesthesia. *Lancet.* 1956;1:527–530.
6. Ledingham IM, Finlay WEI, Watt I, et al. Etomidate and adrenocortical function (letter). *Lancet.* 1983;1:1434.
7. Watling SM, Dasta JF. Prolonged paralysis in intensive care unit patients after the use of neuromuscular blocking agents: a review of the literature. *Crit Care Med.* 1994;22:884–893.
8. Cray SH, Robinson BH, Cox PN. Lactic acidemia and bradyarrhythmia in a child sedated with propofol. *Crit Care Med.* 1998;26:2087–2092.
9. Kang TM. Propofol infusion syndrome in critically ill patients. *Ann Pharmacother.* 2002;36:1453–1456.
10. Connors AF, Speroff T, Dawson NV, et al. The effectiveness of right heart catheterization in the initial care of critically ill patients. *JAMA.* 1996;276:889–897.
11. De Deyne C, Struys M, Decruyenaere J, et al. Use of continuous bispectral EEG monitoring to assess depth of sedation in ICU patients. *Intens Care Med.* 1998;24:1294–1298.
12. Ashbaugh DG, Bigelow DB, Petty TL, et al. Acute respiratory distress syndrome in adults. *Lancet.* 1967;2:319–323.
13. Sidi A, Lobato EB, Cohen JA. The American Society of Anesthesiologists Physical Status: category V revisited. *J Clin Anesth.* 2000;12:328–334.
14. Trunkey DD. Trauma. *Sci Am.* 1983;249:28.
15. Keats AS. The ASA classification of physical status—a recapitulation. *Anesthesiology.* 1978;49:233–236.
16. Saklad M. Grading of patients for surgical procedures. *Anesthesiology.* 1941;2:281–284.
17. New Classification of Physical Status. American Society of Anesthesiologists, Inc. *Anesthesiology.* 1963;24:111.
18. Dripps RD, Lamont A, Eckenhoff JE. The role of anesthesia in surgical mortality. *JAMA.* 1961;178:261–266.
19. Preoperative evaluation and the choice of anesthetic techniques. In: Stoelting RK, Miller RD, eds. *Basics of Anesthesia.* 3rd ed. New York: Churchill Livingstone; 1994:108.
20. Vacanti CJ, vanHouten RJ, Hill RC. A statistical analysis of the relationship of physical status to postoperative mortality in 68,388 cases. *Anesth Analg.* 1970;49:564–566.
21. Marx GF, Mateo CV, Orkin LR. Computer analysis of postanesthetic deaths. *Anesthesiology.* 1973;39:54–58.
22. Keats AS. The ASA classification of physical status—a recapitulation. *Anesthesiology.* 1978;49:233–236.
23. Owens WD, Felts JA, Spitznagel EL. ASA physical status classifications. *Anesthesiology.* 1978;49:239–243.
24. Warden JC, Horan BF. Deaths attributed to anaesthesia in New South Wales, 1984–1990. *Anaesth Intensive Care.* 1996;24:66–73.
25. Cullen DJ, Nemeskal AR, Cooper JB, et al. Effect of pulse oximetry, age, and ASA physical status on the frequency of patients admitted unexpectedly to a postoperative intensive care unit and the severity of their anesthesia-related complications. *Anesth Analg.* 1992;74:181–188.
26. Ruiz K, Aitkenhead AR. Was CEPOD right? *Anaesthesia.* 1990;45:978–980.
27. Forrest JB, Rehder K, Cahalan MK, et al. Multicenter study of general anesthesia. III. Predictors of severe perioperative adverse outcomes. *Anesthesiology.* 1992;76:3–15.
28. Tiret L, Hatton F, Desmonts JM, et al. Prediction of outcome of anaesthesia in patients over 40 years: a multifactorial risk index. *Stat Med.* 1988;7:947–954.
29. Leardi S, De Santis C, Ciccarelli O, et al. Risk of surgery in the geriatric age: prospective evaluation of risk factors. *Ann Ital Chir.* 1998;69:575–579.
30. Leardi S, De Santis C, Ciuca B, et al. Risk indices in geriatric surgery: ASA index versus Reiss index. *Minerva Chir.* 1997;52:255–260.
31. Wahl W, Pelletier K, Schmidtmann S, et al. Experience with various scores in evaluating the prognosis of postoperative intensive care patients. *Chirurg.* 1996;67:710–717.
32. Wolters U, Wolf T, Stutzer H, et al. ASA classification and perioperative variables as predictors of postoperative outcome. *Br J Anaesth.* 1996;77:217–222.
33. Hall JC, Hall JL. ASA status and age predict adverse events after abdominal surgery. *J Qual Clin Pract.* 1996;16:103–108.
34. Hessman O, Bergkvist L, Strom S. Colorectal cancer in patients over 75 years of age—determinants of outcome. *Eur J Surg Oncol.* 1997;23:13–19.
35. Goffi L, Saba V, Ghiselli R, et al. Perioperative APACHE II and ASA scores in patients having major general surgical operations: prognostic value and potential clinical applications. *Eur J Surg.* 1999;165:730–735.
36. Di Paolo S, Giangreco L, Staudacher C. Operative risk in elderly patients with gastrointestinal hemorrhage. *Minerva Chir.* 1996;51:953–957.
37. Groenendijk RP, Croiset van Uchelen FA, Mol SJ, et al. Factors related to outcome after pneumonectomy: retrospective study of 62 patients. *Eur J Surg.* 1999;165:193–197.
38. Goldstein A Jr, Keats AS. The risk of anesthesia. *Anesthesiology.* 1970;33:130–143.
39. Waters J, Wilkinson C, Golmon M, et al. Evaluation of cardiac risk in noncardiac surgical patients [Abstract]. *Anesthesiology.* 1981;55:A343.
40. Schwilk B, Muche R, Bothner U, et al. Quality control in anesthesiology. Results of a prospective study following the recommendations of the German Society of Anesthesiology and Intensive Care. *Anaesthetist.* 1995;44:242–249.
41. Del Guercio LRM, Cohn JD. Monitoring operative risk in the elderly. *JAMA.* 1980;243:1350–1355.
42. Anon. New classification of physical status. *Anesthesiology.* 1963;24:111.
43. Buck N, Devlin HB, Lunn JN. *The Report of a Confidential Enquiry into Perioperative Deaths.* London: The Nuffield Provincial Hospitals Trust and Kings Fund; 1987.
44. Bein R, Fröhlich D, Pömsl J, et al. The predictive value of four scoring systems in liver transplant recipients. *Intens Care Med.* 1995;21:32–37.
45. Turner JS, Morgan CJ, Thakrar B, et al. Difficulties in predicting outcome in cardiac surgery patients. *Crit Care Med.* 1995;23:1843–1850.
46. Le Gall J-R, Lemeshow S, Saulnier F. A new Simplified Acute Physiology Score (SAPS II) based on a European/North American multicenter study. *JAMA.* 1993;270:2957–2963.
47. Parsonnet V, Dean D, Bernstein AD. A method of uniform stratification of risk for evaluating the results of surgery in acquired adult heart disease. *Circulation.* 1989;79(suppl I):3–12.
48. Goldman L, Caldera DL, Nussbaum SR, et al. Multifactorial index of cardiac risk in noncardiac surgical procedures. *N Engl J Med.* 1977;297(16):845–850.
49. Ross AF, Tinker JH. Cardiovascular disease. In: Brown DL, ed. *Risk and Outcome in Anesthesia.* Philadelphia: JB Lippincott Co; 1988:39.
50. Schoeppel SL, Wilkinson C, Waters J, et al. Effects of myocardial infarction on perioperative cardiac complications. *Anesth Analg.* 1983;62(5):493–498.
51. Jeffrey CC, Kunsman J, Cullen DJ, et al. A prospective evaluation of cardiac risk index. *Anesthesiology.* 1983;58(5):462–464.
52. Detsky AS, Abrams HB, McLaughlin JR, et al. Predicting cardiac complications in patients undergoing non-cardiac surgery. *J Gen Intern Med.* 1986;1(4):211–219.
53. Detsky AS, Abrams HB, Forbath N, et al. Cardiac assessment for patients undergoing noncardiac surgery. A multifactorial clinical risk index. *Arch Intern Med.* 1986;146(11):2131–2134.
54. Dupuis JY, Wang F, Nathan H, et al. The cardiac anesthesia risk evaluation score: a clinically useful predictor of mortality and morbidity after cardiac surgery. *Anesthesiology.* 2001;94(2):194–204.
55. Tuman KJ, McCarthy RJ, March RJ, et al. Morbidity and duration of ICU stay after cardiac surgery. A model for preoperative risk assessment. *Chest.* 1992;102:36–44.
56. Tu JV, Jaglal SB, Naylor D, the Steering Committee of the Provincial Adult Care Network of Ontario. Multicenter validation of a risk index for mortality, intensive care unit stay, and overall hospital length of stay after cardiac surgery. *Circulation.* 1995;91:677–684.
57. Peter K, Lutz H. [Proceedings: Preoperative exploration (author's trans.)]. *Langenbecks Arch Chir.* 1973;334:681–687.
58. Goldman L. Perioperative myocardial ischemia. To everything there is a season. *Anesthesiology.* 1992;76(3):331–333.
59. Goldman L. Cardiac risk in noncardiac surgery: an update [Review]. *Anesth Analg.* 1995;80(4):810–820.
60. Foster ED, Davis KB, Carpenter JA, et al. Risk of noncardiac operation in patients with defined coronary disease: the Coronary Artery Surgery Study (CASS) registry experience. *Ann Thorac Surg.* 1986;41(1):42–50.
61. Knudsen NW, Sebastian MW, Perez-Tamayo RA, et al. Intensive care unit procedures: cost savings and patient safety. *Crit Care.* 1999;3(suppl 1):P2.
62. Lewis KS, Whipple JK, Michael KA, et al. Effect of analgesic treatment on the physiological consequences of acute pain. *Am J Hosp Pharm.* 1994;51(12):1539–1554.
63. Mangano DT, Siliciano D, Hollenberg M, et al. Postoperative myocardial ischemia. Therapeutic trials using intensive analgesia following surgery. The Study of Perioperative Ischemia (SPI) Research Group. *Anesthesiology.* 1992;76(3):342–353.
64. Britton BJ, Hawkey C, Wood WG, et al. Stress—a significant factor in venous thrombosis? *Br J Surg.* 1974;61(10):814–820.
65. Slade MS, Greenberg LJ, Yunis EJ, et al. Integrated immune response to standard major surgical trauma in normal patients. *Surg Forum.* 1974;25(0):425–427.

66. Swinamer DL, Phang PT, Jones RL, et al. Effect of routine administration of analgesia on energy expenditure in critically ill patients. *Chest.* 1988;93(1):4–10.
67. Moller IW, Dinesen K, Sondergard S, et al. Effect of patient-controlled analgesia on plasma catecholamine, cortisol and glucose concentrations after cholecystectomy. *Br J Anaesth.* 1988;61(2):160–164.
68. Modig J, Borg T, Bagge L, et al. Role of extradural and of general anaesthesia in fibrinolysis and coagulation after total hip replacement. *Br J Anaesth.* 1983;55(7):625–629.
69. Salomaki TE, Leppaluoto J, Laitinen JO, et al. Epidural versus intravenous fentanyl for reducing hormonal, metabolic, and physiologic responses after thoracotomy. *Anesthesiology.* 1993;79(4):672–679.
70. Jones C, Griffiths RD, Macmillan RR, et al. Psychological problems occurring after intensive care. *Br J Int Care.* 1994;2:46–53.
71. Parker MM, Schubert W, Shelhamer JH, et al. Perceptions of a critically ill patient experiencing therapeutic paralysis in an ICU. *Crit Care Med.* 1984;12(1):69–71.
72. Schelling G, Stoll C, Haller M, et al. Health-related quality of life and posttraumatic stress disorder in survivors of the acute respiratory distress syndrome. *Crit Care Med.* 1998;26(4):651–659.
73. Bond M. Psychological and psychiatric aspects of pain. *Anaesthesia.* 1978;33(4):355–361.
74. Chapman CR, Casey KL, Dubner R, et al. Pain measurement: an overview. *Pain.* 1985;22(1):1–31.
75. Ramsay MA, Savege TM, Simpson BR, et al. Controlled sedation with alphaxalone-alphadolone. *BMJ.* 1974;2(920):656–659.
76. Shapiro BA. Bispectral Index: better information for sedation in the intensive care unit? *Crit Care Med.* 1999;27(8):1663–1664.
77. Liu J, Singh H, White PF. Electroencephalographic bispectral index correlates with intraoperative recall and depth of propofol-induced sedation. *Anesth Analg.* 1997;84(1):185–189.
78. Shah N, Clack S, Chea F, et al. Does bispectral index of EEG correlate with Ramsay sedation score in ICU patients [Abstract]? *Anesthesiology.* 1996;85:A469.
79. Frenzel D, Greim CA, Sommer C, et al. Is the bispectral index appropriate for monitoring the sedation level of mechanically ventilated surgical ICU patients? *Intensive Care Med.* 2002;28(2):178–183.
80. De Deyne C, Struys M, Decruyenaere J, et al. Use of continuous bispectral EEG monitoring to assess depth of sedation in ICU patients. *Intensive Care Med.* 1998;24(12):1294–1298.
81. Jacobi J, Fraser GL, Coursin DB, et al. Task Force of the American College of Critical Care Medicine (ACCM) of the Society of Critical Care Medicine (SCCM), American Society of Health-System Pharmacists (ASHP), American College of Chest Physicians Clinical practice guidelines for the sustained use of sedatives and analgesics in the critically ill adult. *Crit Care Med.* 2002;30(1):119–141.
82. Cohen AT, Kelly DR. Assessment of alfentanil by intravenous infusion as long term sedation in intensive care. *Anaesthesia.* 1987;42:545–548.
83. O'Sullivan G, Park GR. The assessment of sedation in critically ill patients. *Clin Intensive Care.* 1991;2:116–122.
84. Armstrong RF, Bullen C, Cohen SL, et al. Intermittent positive pressure ventilation. *Clin Intensive Care.* 1992;3:284–287.
85. Cook S. *Technical Problems in Intensive Care. Intensive Care Rounds.* Abingdon, UK: The Medicine Group Ltd.; 1991:19–22.
86. Schulte-Tamburen AM, Scheier J, Briegel J, et al. Comparison of five sedation scoring systems by means of auditory evoked potentials. *Intensive Care Med.* 1999;25:377–382.
87. Thornton C, Barrowcliffe MP, Konieczko KM, et al. The auditory evoked response as an indicator of awareness. *Br J Anaesth.* 1989;63:113–115.
88. Cohen IL. The management of the agitated ICU patient. *Crit Care Med.* 2002;30(Suppl. 1):S97–123.
89. Bell DM, Richards G, Dhillon S, et al. A comparative pharmacokinetic study of intravenous and intramuscular midazolam in patients with epilepsy. *Epilepsy Res.* 1991;10:183–190.
90. Shelly MP, Mendel L, Park GR. Failure of critically ill patients to metabolise midazolam. *Anaesthesia.* 1987;42:619–626.
91. Greenblatt DJ, Divoll MK, Soong MH, et al. Desmethyldiazepam pharmacokinetics: studies following intravenous and oral desmethyldiazepam, oral clorazepate, and intravenous diazepam. *J Clin Pharmacol.* 1988;28:853–859.
92. Barrientos-Vega R, Sanchez-Soria M, Morales-Garcia C, et al. Prolonged sedation of critically ill patients with midazolam or propofol: impact on weaning and costs. *Crit Care Med.* 1997;25:33–40.
93. Dirksen MS, Vree TB, Driessen JJ. Clinical pharmacokinetics of long-term infusion of midazolam in critically ill patients—preliminary results. *Anaesth Intensive Care.* 1987;15:440–444.
94. Shelly MP, Sultan MA, Bodenham A, et al. Midazolam infusions in critically ill patients. *Eur J Anaesthesiol.* 1991;8:21–27.
95. Finfer SR, O'Connor AM, Fisher MM. A prospective randomised pilot study of sedation regimens in a general ICU population: a reality-based medicine study. *Crit Care.* 1999;3(3):79–83.
96. Van Hamme MJ, Ghoneim MM, Ambre JJ. Pharmacokinetics of etomidate, a new intravenous anesthetic. *Anesthesiology.* 1978;49(4):274–277.
97. Wagner RL, White PF, Kan PB, et al. Inhibition of adrenal steroidogenesis by the anesthetic etomidate. *N Engl J Med.* 1984;310(22):1415–1421.
98. Shapiro BA, Warren J, Egol AB, et al. Practice parameters for intravenous analgesia and sedation for adult patients in the intensive care unit: An executive summary. Society of Critical Care Medicine. *Crit Care Med.* 1995;23:1596–1600.
99. Glass PSA, Hardman D, Kamiyama Y, et al. Preliminary pharmacokinetics and pharmacodynamics of an ultra-short-acting opioid: remifentanil (GI87084B). *Anesth Analg.* 1993;77:1031–1040.
100. Dahaba AA, Grabner T, Rehak P, et al. Remifentanil versus morphine analgesia and sedation for mechanically ventilated critically ill patients: a randomized double blind study. *Anesthesiology.* 2004;101(3):640–646.
101. Cavaliere F, Antonelli M, Arcangeli A, et al. A low-dose remifentanil infusion is well tolerated for sedation in mechanically ventilated, critically-ill patients. *Can J Anesth.* 2002;49:1088–1094.
102. Riker RR, Picard JT, Fraser GL. Prospective evaluation of the Sedation-Agitation Scale for adult critically ill patients. *Crit Care Med.* 1999;27:1325–1329.
103. Segal IS, Vickery RG, Walton JK, et al. Dexmedetomidine diminishes halothane anesthetic requirements in rats through postsynaptic alpha-2 adrenergic receptor. *Anesthesiology.* 1988;69:818–823.
104. Urwin1 SC, Menon DK. Review article: comparative tolerability of sedative agents in head-injured adults. *Drug Saf.* 2004;27(2):107–133.
105. Asgeirsson B, Grande PO, Nordstrom CH, et al. Effects of hypotensive treatment with β2-agonist and β1-agonist on cerebral haemodynamics in severely head injured patients. *Acta Anaesthesiol Scand.* 1995;39:347–351.
106. Soliman H, Melot C, Vincent J. Sedative and analgesic practice in the intensive care unit: the results of a European survey. *Br J Anaesth.* 2001;87(2):186–192.
107. Christensen BV, Thunedborg LP. Use of sedatives, analgesics and neuromuscular blocking agents in Danish ICUs 1996/97: a national survey. *Intensive Care Med.* 1999;25(2):186–191.
108. Murdoch S, Cohen A. Intensive care sedation: a review of current British practice. *Intensive Care Med.* 2000;26(7):922–928.
109. Liu LL, Gropper MA. Review: postoperative analgesia and sedation in the adult intensive care unit. A guide to drug selection. *Drugs.* 2003;63(8):755–767.
110. Ely EW, Baker AM, Dunagan DP, et al. Effect on the duration of mechanical ventilation of identifying patients capable of breathing spontaneously. *N Engl J Med.* 1996;335(25):1864–1869.
111. Brook AD, Ahrens TS, Schaiff R, et al. Effect of a nursing-implemented sedation protocol on the duration of mechanical ventilation. *Crit Care Med.* 1999;27(12):2609–2615.
112. Kress JP, Pohlman AS, O'Connor MF, et al. Daily interruption of sedative infusions in critically ill patients undergoing mechanical ventilation. *N Engl J Med.* 2000;342(20):1471–1477.
113. Proctor S. Is this the end of research as we know it? *BMJ.* 1997;315(7105):388.
114. Jacobs JR, Reves JG, Glass PSA. Rationale and technique for continuous infusions in anesthesia. *Int Anesthesiol Clin.* 1991;29:23–38.
115. Shelly MP. Sedation, where are we now? *Intensive Care Med.* 1999;25:137–139.
116. Olsson GL, Leddo CC, Wild L. Nursing management of patients receiving epidural narcotics. *Heart Lung.* 1989;18:130–138.
117. Covington H. Use of propofol for sedation in the ICU. *Crit Care Nurse.* 1998;18(4):34–39.
118. Halpern NA, Bettes L, Greenstein R. Federal and nationwide intensive care units and healthcare costs: 1986–1992. *Crit Care Med.* 1994;22:2001–2007.
119. Gundlach CA, Faulkner TP, Souney PF. Drug usage patterns in the ICU: profile of a major metropolitan hospital and comparison with other ICUs. *Hosp Formul.* 1991;26:132–136.
120. Cheng EY. The cost of sedating and paralyzing the critically ill patient. *Crit Care Clin.* 1995;11:1005–1019.
121. *1999 New York Times Almanac.* New York: Penguin Reference Books; 1998:316.
122. Kress JP, O'Connor MF, Pohlman AS, et al. Sedation of critically ill patients during mechanical ventilation: a comparison of propofol and midazolam. *Am J Respir Crit Care Med.* 1996;153:1012–1018.
123. Swart EL, van Schijndel RJM, van Loenen AC, et al. Continuous infusion of lorazepam versus midazolam in patients in the intensive care unit: sedation with lorazepam is easier to manage and is more cost-effective. *Crit Care Med.* 1999;27:1461–1465.
124. Sivam SP, Ho IK. GABA in morphine analgesia and tolerance. *Life Sci.* 1985;37:199–208.
125. Ronan KP, Gallagher TJ, George B, et al. Comparison of propofol and midazolam for sedation in intensive care unit patients. *Crit Care Med.* 1995;23:286–293.
126. Mirski MA, Muffelman B, Ulatowski JA, et al. Sedation for the critically ill neurologic patient. *Crit Care Med.* 1995;23:2038–2053.
127. Braman SS, Dunn SM, Amico CA, et al. Complications of intrahospital transport in critically ill patients. *Ann Intern Med.* 1987;107:469–473.
128. Indeck M, Peterson S, Smith J, et al. Risk, cost, and benefit of transporting ICU patients for special studies. *J Trauma.* 1988;28:1020–1025.

129. Shah S. *ICU Analgesia/Sedation Guidelines Created.* Current Topics from the Drug Information Center, College of Pharmacy, University of Kentucky; 2000;30(1):1–4.
130. Shafer SL. Advances in propofol pharmacokinetics and pharmacodynamics. *J Clin Anesth.* 5;(6 Suppl 1):15S.
131. Westmoreland CL, Hoke JF, Sebel PS, et al. Pharmacokinetics of remifentanil (GI87084B) and its major metabolite (GI90291) in patients undergoing elective inpatient surgery. *Anesthesiology.* 1993;79(5):893–903.
132. Matta B, Menon D. Severe head injury in the United Kingdom and Ireland: a survey of practice and implications for management. *Crit Care Med.* 1996;24:1743–1748.
133. Rhoney DH, Parker D. Use of sedative and analgesic agents in neurotrauma patients: effects on cerebral physiology. *Neurol Res.* 2001;23:237–259.
134. Greher M, Sitzwohl C, Andel D, et al. A new concept of analgesia in severely burned patients based on the who guidelines for pain management. *Anesthesiology.* 2001;95:A384.
135. Campos LA, Soares LG, Fernandes MA, et al. Immediate postoperative analgesia and sedation following heart surgery: a comparative analysis of dexmedetomidine chlorohydrate versus remifentanyl hydrochloride. *Crit Care.* 5;(Suppl 3):70.
136. Meiser A, Laubenthal H. Inhalational anaesthetics in the ICU: theory and practice of inhalational sedation in the ICU, economics, risk-benefit. *Best Pract Res Clin Anaesthesiol.* 2005;19(3):523–538.
137. Enlund M, Wiklund L, Lambert H. A new device to reduce the consumption of a halogenated anesthetic agent. *Anaesthesia.* 2001;56(5):429–423.
138. Tempia A, et al. The anesthetic conserving device compared with conventional circle system used under different flow conditions for inhaled anesthesia. *Anesth Analg.* 2003;96:1056–1061.
139. Sackey PV, Martling CR, Radell PJ. Three cases of PICU sedation with isoflurane delivered by the 'AnaConDa'. *Paediatr Anaesth.* 2005;15(10): 879–885.
140. Eger EI. The pharmacology of isoflurane. *Br J Anaesth.* 1984;56:71–99S.
141. Hirshman CA, Edelstein G, Peetz S, et al. Mechanism of action of inhalational anesthesia on airways. *Anesthesiology.* 1982;56:107–111.
142. Korenaga S, Takeda K, Ito Y. Differential effects of halothane on airway nerves and muscle. *Anesthesiology.* 1984;60:309–318.
143. Saulnier FF, Durocher AV, Deturck RA, et al. Respiratory and hemodynamic effects of halothane in status asthmaticus. *Intensive Care Med.* 1990;16:104–107.
144. Maltais F, Reissmann H, Navalesi P, et al. Comparison of static and dynamic measurements of intrinsic PEEP in mechanically ventilated patients. *Am J Respir Crit Care Med.* 1994;150:1318–1324.
145. Echeverria M, Gelb AW, Wexler HR, et al. Enflurane and halothane in status asthmaticus. *Chest.* 1986;89:152–154.
146. Padkin AJ, Baigel G, Morgan GA. Halothane treatment of severe asthma to avoid mechanical ventilation. *Anaesthesia.* 1997;52:994–997.
147. Gal TJ. Pulmonary mechanics in normal subjects following endotracheal intubation. *Anesthesiology.* 1980;52:27–35.
148. Habre W, Scalfaro P, Sims C, et al. Respiratory mechanics during sevoflurane anesthesia in children with and without asthma. *Anesth Analg.* 1999;89:1177–1181.
149. Phipps P, Garrard CS. The pulmonary physician in critical care • 12: acute severe asthma in the intensive care unit. *Thorax.* 2003;58:81–88.
150. Shoemaker WC, Belzberg H, Wo CC, et al. Multicenter study of noninvasive monitoring systems as alternatives to invasive monitoring of acutely ill emergency patients. *Chest.* 1998;114(6):1643–1652.
151. Bauer JJ, Schulam PG, Kaufman HS, et al. Laparoscopy for the acute abdomen in the postoperative urologic patient. *Urology.* 1998;51:917–919.
152. Fabian TC, Croce MA, Stewart RM, et al. A prospective analysis of diagnostic laparoscopy in trauma. *Ann Surg.* 1993;217:557–564.
153. Iberti TJ, Salky BA, Onofrey D. Use of bedside laparoscopy to identify intestinal ischemia in postoperative cases of aortic reconstruction. *Surgery.* 1989;105:686–689.
154. Berci G, Sachier JM, Paz Parlow M. Emergency laparoscopy. *Am J Surg.* 1991;161:332–335.
155. Ivatury RR, Simon RJ, Stahl WM. A critical evaluation of laparoscopy in penetrating abdominal trauma. *J Trauma.* 1993;34:822–827.
156. Forde KA, Treat MR. The role of peritoneoscopy (laparoscopy) in the evaluation of the acute abdomen in critically ill patients. *Surg Endosc.* 1992;6:219–221.
157. Walsh RM, Popovich MJ, Hoadley J. Bedside diagnostic laparoscopy and peritoneal lavage in the intensive care unit. *Surg Endosc.* 1998;12:1405–1409.
158. Gagne DJ, Malay MB, Hogle NJ, et al. Bedside diagnostic minilaparoscopy in the intensive care patient. *Surgery.* 2002;131(5):491–496.
159. Pecoraro AP, Cacchione RN, Sayad P, et al. The routine use of diagnostic laparoscopy in the intensive care unit. *Surg Endosc.* 2001;15:638–641.
160. Rosin D, Haviv Y, Kuriansky J, et al. Bedside laparoscopy in the ICU: report of four cases. *J Laparoendosc Adv Surg Tech.* 2001;11(5):305–309.
161. Plummer AL, Gracey DR. Consensus conference on artificial airways in patients receiving mechanical ventilation. *Chest.* 1989;96(1):178–180.
162. Stock MC, Woodward CG, Shapiro BA, et al. Perioperative complications of elective tracheostomy in critically ill patients. *Crit Care Med.* 1986;14(10):861–863.
163. Friedman Y, Fildes J, Mizock B, et al. Comparison of percutaneous and surgical tracheostomies. *Chest.* 1996;110(2):480–485.
164. Ciaglia P, Firsching R, Syniec C. Elective percutaneous dilatational tracheostomy. A new simple bedside procedure; preliminary report. *Chest.* 1985;87(6):715–719.
165. Mansharamani NG, Koziel H, Garland R, et al. Safety of bedside percutaneous dilatational tracheostomy in obese patients in the ICU. *Chest.* 2000;117(5):1426–1429.
166. Freeman BD, Isabella K, Lin N, et al. A metaanalysis of prospective trials comparing percutaneous and surgical tracheostomy in critically ill patients. *Chest.* 2000;118:1412–1418.
167. Ernst A, Garland R, Zibrak J. Percutaneous tracheostomy. *J Bronchol.* 1998;5:247–250.
168. Kluge S, Meyer A, Kuhnelt P, et al. Percutaneous tracheostomy is safe in patients with severe thrombocytopenia. *Chest.* 2004;126(2):547–551.
169. Hubner N, Rees W, Seufert K, et al. Percutaneous dilatational tracheostomy done early after cardiac surgery: outcome and incidence of mediastinitis. *Thorac Cardiovasc Surg.* 1998;46:89–92.
170. Westphal K, Byhahn C, Lischke V. Tracheostomy in intensive care. *Anaesthesist.* 1999;48:142–156.
171. Cantais E, Kaiser E, Le-Goff Y, et al. Percutaneous tracheostomy: prospective comparison of the translaryngeal technique versus the forceps-dilational technique in 100 critically ill adults. *Crit Care Med.* 2002;30:815–819.
172. Van Natta TL, Morris JA, Eddy VA, et al. Elective bedside surgery in critically injured patients is safe and cost-effective. *Ann Surg.* 1998;227:618–626.
173. Akinci IO, Ozcan P, Tugrul S, et al. Percutaneous endoscopic gastrostomy in the ICU. *Ulus Travma Derg.* 2000;6(4):281–283.
174. Russel RR, Brotman M, Norris F. Percutaneous gastrostomy—a new simplified and cost-effective technique. *Am J Surg.* 1984;148:132–137.
175. Campos AC, Marchesini JB. Recent advances in the placement of tubes for enteral nutrition. *Curr Opin Clin Nutr Metab Care.* 1999;2:265–269.
176. Jeffrey L, Ponsky MD, Michael WL, et al. Percutaneous endoscopic gastrostomy: indications, limitations, techniques, and results. *World J Surg.* 1989;13:165–170.
177. Wasljew BK, Ujlkl GT, Beal JM. Feeding gastrostomy; complications and mortality. *Am J Surg.* 1982;143:194–195.
178. Ferraro F, Capasso A, Troise E. Enteral nutrition in the ICU: clinical experience of percutaneous endoscopic gastrostomy. *Riv Ital Nutr Parenter Enter Anno.* 2004;22(2):86–90.
179. Carrillo E, Heniford B, Osborne D, et al. Bedside percutaneous endoscopic gastrostomy: a safe alternative for early nutritional support in critically ill trauma patients. *Surg Endosc.* 1997;11(11):1068–1071.
180. Dimick P, Helvig E, Heimbach D, et al. Anesthesia-assisted procedures in a burn intensive care unit procedure room: benefits and complications. *J Burn Care Rehabil.* 1993;14(4):446–449.
181. Gueugniaud PY. [Management of severe burns during the 1st 72 hours] [article in French]. *Ann Fr Anesth Reanim.* 1997;16(4):354–369.
182. Edrich T, Friedrich AD, Holger K. International Anesthesia Research Society critical care and trauma; ketamine for long-term sedation and analgesia of a burn patient. *Anesth Analg.* 2004;99:893–895.
183. Mayer SA, Claassen J, Lokin J, et al. Refractory status epilepticus frequency, risk factors, and impact on outcome. *Arch Neurol.* 2002;59:205–210.
184. Lothman E. The biochemical basis and pathophysiology of status epilepticus. *Neurology.* 1990;40(suppl 2):13–23.
185. Shorvon S. The management of status epilepticus. *J Neurol Neurosurg Psychiatry.* 2001;70(suppl II):ii22–ii27.
186. Coeytaux A, Jallon P, Galobardes B, et al. Incidence of status epilepticus in French-speaking Switzerland (EPISTAR). *Neurology.* 2000;55:693–697.
187. Holtkamp M, Masuhr F, Harms L, et al. The management of refractory generalised convulsive and complex partial status epilepticus in three European countries: a survey among epileptologists and critical care neurologists. *J Neurol Neurosurg Psychiatry.* 2003;74:1095–1099.
188. Rasmussen PA, Yang Y, Rutecki PA. Propofol inhibits epileptiform activity in rat hippocampal slices. *Epilepsy Res.* 1996;25:169–175.
189. Wood PR, Browne GPR, Pugh S. Propofol infusion for the treatment of status epilepticus. *Lancet.* 1988;I:480–481.
190. Brown LA, Levin GM. Role of propofol in refractory status epilepticus. *Ann Pharmacother.* 1998;32:1053–1059.
191. Stecker MM, Kramer TH, Raps EC, et al. Treatment of refractory status epilepticus with propofol: clinical and pharmacokinetic findings. *Epilepsia.* 1998;39:18–26.
192. Begemann M, Rowan AJ, Tuhrim S. Treatment of refractory complex-partial status epilepticus with propofol: case report. *Epilepsia.* 2000;41:105–109.
193. Prasad A, Worral BB, Bertram EH, et al. Propofol and midazolam in the treatment of refractory status epilepticus. *Epilepsia.* 2001;42:380–386.
194. Claassen J, Hirsch LJ, Emerson RG, et al. Treatment of refractory status epilepticus with pentobarbital, propofol, or midazolam: a systematic review. *Epilepsia.* 2002;43:146–153.
195. Rampton AJ, Griffin RM, Durcan JJ, et al. Propofol and electroconvulsive therapy. *Lancet.* 1988;I:196–197.

196. Rossetti AO, Reichhart MD, Schaller MD, et al. Propofol treatment of refractory status epilepticus: a study of 31 episodes. *Epilepsia.* 2004;45(7):757–763.
197. Parviainen I, Uusaro A, Kälviäinen R, et al. High-dose thiopental in the treatment of refractory status epilepticus in intensive care unit. *Neurology.* 2002;59:1249–1251.
198. Krishnamurthy KB, Drislane FW. Depth of EEG suppression and outcome in barbiturate anesthetic treatment for refractory status epilepticus. *Epilepsia.* 1999;40:759–762.
199. Sutherland MJ, Burt P. Propofol and seizures. *Anaesth Intens Care.* 1994;22:733–737.
200. Iwasaki F, Mimura M, Yamazaki Y, et al. Generalized tonic-clonic seizure induced by propofol in a patient with epilepsy. *Masui.* 2001;50:168–170.
201. Borgeat A, Dessibourg C, Popovic V, et al. Propofol and spontaneous movements: an EEG study. *Anesthesiology.* 1991;74:24–27.
202. Walder B, Tramèr MR, Seeck M. Seizure-like phenomena and propofol: a systematic review. *Neurology.* 2002;58:1327–1332.
203. Borgeat A. Propofol: pro- or anticonvulsant? *Eur J Anaesth.* 1997;14(suppl 15):17–20.
204. Modica PA, Tempelhoff R, White PF. Pro- and anticonvulsant effects of anesthetics (part II). *Anaesth Analg.* 1990;70:433–444.
205. Iwaku F, Otsuka H, Kuraishi H, et al. [The investigation of isoflurane therapy for status asthmaticus patients] [article in Japanese] *Arerugi.* 2005;54(1):18–23.
206. Allen J, Shirk MB. Sedation and paralysis in the MICU. *Intensive Care Med.* 1999;25:377–382.
207. Szem JW, Hydo LJ, Fischer E, et al. High-risk intrahospital transport of critically ill patients: safety and outcome of the necessary "road trip." *Crit Care Med.* 1995;23:1660–1666.
208. Stearley HE. Patients' outcomes: intrahospital transportation and monitoring of critically ill patients by a specially trained ICU nursing staff. *Am J Crit Care.* 1998;7:282–287.
209. Corriere MA, Passman MA, Guzman RJ, et al. Comparison of bedside transabdominal duplex ultrasound versus contrast venography for inferior vena cava filter placement: what is the best imaging modality? *Ann Vasc Surg.* 2005;19:229–234.
210. Conners MS 3rd, Becker S, Guzman RJ, et al. Duplex scan-directed placement of inferior vena cava filters: a five-year institutional experience. *J Vasc Surg.* 2002;35:286–291.
211. Neser RA, Filho MC, de Oliveira Homa CM. Placement of inferior vena cava filter guided by ultrasound: report of two cases. *J Vasc Br.* 2006;5(1):71–73.

APPENDICES ■ SEDATION AND PAIN SCALES

APPENDIX 40.1

SEDATION/AGITATION SCALE

Sedation description	Sedation category	Sedation score
Minimal or no response to noxious stimuli	Unarousable	1
Responds to physical stimuli, but does not follow commands	Very sedated	2
Difficult to arouse, responds to verbal or physical stimuli, but drifts off again	Sedated	3
Calm, easily arousable, cooperative, follows commands	Calm & cooperative	4
Anxious, but calms down on verbal instructions	Agitated	5
Requires physical restraints, biting endotracheal tube (ET), does not calm down on verbal instructions	Very agitated	6
Tries to remove ET or catheters, striking, thrashing	Dangerously agitated	7

Data modified from Dahaba AA, Grabner T, Rehak P, et al. Remifentanil versus morphine analgesia and sedation for mechanically ventilated critically ill patients: a randomized double blind study. *Anesthesiology*. 2004;101(2):640–646.

APPENDIX 40.2

PAIN INTENSITY SCALE

Pain category	Pain score
None	1
Mild	2
Moderate	3
Severe	4
Very severe	5
Worst probable	6

Data modified from Dahaba AA, Grabner T, Rehak P, et al. Remifentanil versus morphine analgesia and sedation for mechanically ventilated critically ill patients: a randomized double blind study. *Anesthesiology*. 2004;101(2):640–646.

SECTION IV ■ ESSENTIAL PHYSIOLOGIC CONCERNS

CHAPTER 41 ■ FLUIDS AND ELECTROLYTES

STEVEN G. ACHINGER • JUAN CARLOS AYUS

Fluid and electrolyte disorders are very common in critically ill patients. There are some circumstances in which a patient is placed in intensive care for the management of a specific electrolyte disturbance such as hyponatremia or hyperkalemia. The development of electrolyte disturbances among critically ill patients is also common due to breakdown of homeostatic mechanisms that prevent the development of electrolyte disturbances. These impairments in homeostatic function are numerous such as renal failure, use of diuretics, and nonosmotic release of antidiuretic hormone (ADH) due to nausea, pain, or other stimuli. In this chapter the pathophysiology of electrolyte disturbances will be addressed with a focus on presentations common among intensive care unit (ICU) patients. Disorders of water balance (hyponatremia and hypernatremia) will be addressed in more detail due to the importance of these disorders as a cause of morbidity and mortality and the prevalence of impaired water balance in ICU patients.

GENERAL COMMENTS

In an average person without extremes of weight, approximately 60% of total body weight is water. Of this total body water, two thirds (40% of total body weight) is in the intracellular (ICF) space, and one third (20% of total body weight) is outside the cells, i.e., extracellular (ECF) space. Extracellular volume is divided into intravascular space and interstitial fluid (5% and 15% of total body weight, respectively). The intravascular space containing plasma is the most mobile fluid compartment and the first to be released to areas of injury and the first to be repleted through intravenous infusion. In the intravascular space are red cells in addition to plasma. Red cell volume plus plasma volume compose the blood volume (BV), which is estimated to be 7% of the total body weight. In a 70-kg person, total body water is 42 L (60% × 70 kg), circulating BV is 4.9 L (7% × 70 kg), ICF is 28 L (40% × 70 kg), and ECF is 14 L (20% × 70 kg). The percentage of weight used will vary depending on deviation from ideal body weight and sex (see Blood Volume chapter).

Water is freely permeable between body compartments and migrates to areas of higher solutes, but this takes time. Therefore, chronic hypotonic losses with ability to "borrow" from ICF (28 L) is better tolerated than acute isotonic losses, which has only the ECF (14 L) to borrow from. Osmolality (tonicity) defined as number of particles in solution is normally 280 to 300 mOsm/L in the serum.

The ICF concentration of solutes is vastly different from that of the ECF, and approximately 80% of adenosine triphosphate (ATP) generated is used to maintain this gradient. Some of the ECF cations (in mEq/L) are as follows: sodium (Na^+), 142; potassium (K^+), 4; calcium (Ca), 5; and magnesium (Mg), 3. The ICF cations (in mEq/L) are: K^+, 150; Mg, 40; and Na^+, 10. Some of the ECF anions (in mEq/L) are chloride (Cl^-), 103; and bicarbonate, 27. The major ICF anions (in mEq/L) are phosphates, 107; proteins, 40; and sulfates, 43. This difference in ICF and ECF electrolyte composition explains the clinical observations that large amounts of certain electrolytes are needed to replete small deficiencies in the serum (ECF) if the ICF stores are depleted. One of our limitations is the inability to assess ICF electrolyte composition easily at the bedside.

Due to water being freely permeable, the osmolality of all body compartments should be the same, but in reality, the protein concentration in the plasma to interstitial fluid is 16:1, generating an oncotic pressure difference between the two compartments. Starling forces describe net fluid flux between intravascular space and the interstitium:

$$Q = Kf\{(Pc - Pi) - \sigma(\pi c - \pi i)\}$$

where Q is the net fluid flux (mL/minute), (Pc − Pt) is hydrostatic pressure difference between capillary (c) and interstitium (i), and ($\pi c - \pi i$) is the oncotic pressure difference between the capillary and interstitium. Kf is the filtration coefficient for that membrane (mL/minute per mm Hg), and is the product of capillary surface area and capillary hydraulic conductance, and σ is the permeability factor (i.e. reflection coefficient) with one being impermeable, and zero being completely permeable.

The permeability factor explains why, in times of capillary leak as in shock states, colloids cannot maintain an oncotic pressure difference and tend to leak out into the interstitium. The general principle of fluid resuscitation is that intravascular hypovolemia should be replaced with isotonic fluid, which tends to distribute in the ECF (3:1) intravascular:interstitium. Hypotonic fluid will distribute between all body compartments with only a small amount remaining in the intravascular space (since water is freely permeable). Maintaining intravascular blood volume is of primary importance to deliver nutrition (via plasma) and oxygen (via red cells) to the tissues. Frequently used isotonic solutions are 0.9% normal saline (154 mEq/L of Na^+ and Cl each) and lactated Ringer solution (130 mEq/L Na^+, 109 mEq/L Cl^-, 4 mEq/L K^+, 3 mEq/L Ca^{2+}, 28 mEq/L lactate).

The end point of fluid resuscitation continues to be an area of great debate since routine measurement of intravascular (plasma) volume is not the norm. Surrogate markers are used to assess adequate fluid resuscitation: blood pressure, heart rate, urine output, and parameters of perfusion and cardiac function. Although every clinician wants to treat patients to "euvolemia," there are only a few centers measuring intravascular volume using radioisotope studies (see Blood Volume chapter). Debate will continue on how much fluid to give until an easy method of measuring intravascular volume is available.

DISORDERS OF WATER METABOLISM

Overview of Water Balance

Dysnatremias (hyponatremia or hypernatremia) are among the most common electrolyte disturbances and usually are associated with poor outcomes. This problem persists due to failure to promptly recognize a life-threatening condition and initiate appropriate treatment. This chapter will focus on the pathogenesis, diagnosis, treatment, and prevention of dysnatremias.

Regulation of Water Balance

Extracellular fluid (ECF) tonicity is generally reflected in the concentration of sodium in the serum. The serum sodium is proportional to the total body exchangeable sodium (Na_e) plus the total body exchangeable potassium (K_e). This critical relationship is shown mathematically in Equation 41.1. Equation 41.1 is not used clinically; rather, it illustrates the relationship between total body solutes and total body water. Decreases in potassium often accompany hyponatremia, and replacement of intracelllular solute losses can also be an important part of treating hyponatremia. As water intake and excretion are tightly regulated to maintain near-constant plasma osmolality (Fig. 41.1), disturbances in serum sodium indicate disorders in water balance, not gains or loss of sodium. This is a crucial point in understanding dysnatremias. The actions of antidiuretic hormone (ADH), also called arginine vasopressin (AVP) (1) on the kidney tightly regulates water excretion. To maintain water balance, an intact thirst mechanism and the ability of the kidneys to vary urinary concentration are required.

$$\frac{Na_e + K_e}{\text{Total body water}} \alpha \; Na_{pl} \qquad [1]$$

Renal Water Handling

The kidney can vary urinary concentration significantly and either excrete a large water load in very dilute urine or conserve water significantly such that the daily solute load is excreted in a small volume of urine. When the urinary filtrate passes into the cortical collecting duct, it is very dilute (as low as 50 mOsm/kg). As the urine moves through the cortical collecting duct into the collecting tubule, water reabsorption occurs in the presence of ADH. In the absence of ADH activity (as in diabetes insipidus), urine concentration will remain very low (50–80 mOsm/kg). When ADH activity is maximal, urinary concentration can be as high as 1,200 mOsm/kg. This ability to excrete very dilute or a very concentrated urine allows the body to achieve water balance across a very wide range of water intake (between approximately 0.8 L per day and 15 L per day). Impairments of this hormonal system that links perturbations in serum osmolality as detected by osmoreceptors in the hypothalamus to variations in urinary concentration can lead to impairments in water balance. Administration of water to a patient with impaired water excretion (Table 41.1) can lead to hyponatremia.

Electrolyte Free Water

Electrolyte free water is a useful concept in the approach to the patient with a disturbance in water balance. Electrolyte free water is a conceptual volume of a body fluid (usually urine) that represents the volume of that fluid that would be required to dilute the electrolytes contained within total volume of the fluid to the same tonicity as plasma electrolytes (Fig. 41.2). The remainder of the volume (total volume minus electrolyte free water) can be thought of as containing the nonelectrolyte osmoles. This nonelectrolyte water excretion is the amount of

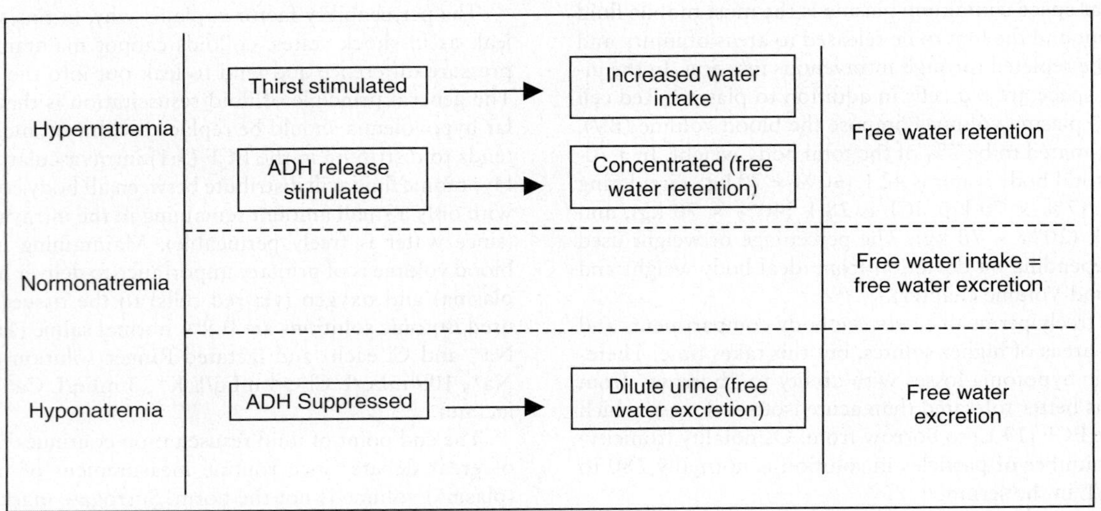

FIGURE 41.1. Water intake and excretion regulation. ADH, antidiuretic hormone.

TABLE 41.1

STATES OF IMPAIRED WATER EXCRETION IN THE ICU RESULTING IN HYPONATREMIA

Volume-depleted states
Volume depletion
Diuretics
Normal-volume states
SIADH
Pain
Postoperative state
Nausea
Hypothyroidism
Volume-expanded states
Congestive heart failure
Renal failure
Cirrhosis

SIADH, syndrome of inappropriate antidiuretic hormone.

water excreted above the excretion of electrolyte solutes, and thus if it is not replaced, will have an effect on the plasma sodium concentration. In other words, the osmolality of a solution is not important in determining if it contains "free water"; rather, it is the concentration of electrolytes that is important. An example of this is that the administration of dextrose solutions provides the same amount of free water as an equal volume of deionized water, whereas 0.45% normal saline contains approximately 50% less. Electrolyte free water clearance can be calculated as a convenient clinical tool in assessing water need in a patient. The amount of electrolyte free water in a body fluid (e.g., urine, sweat, nasogastric [NG] aspirate) is calculated by the following formula:

$$[1 - ([Na^+]fl + [K^+]fl)/([Na^+]pl + [K^+]pl)] \times \text{volume of fluid (mL)} = \text{electrolyte free water clearance} \quad [2]$$

where fl is body fluid and pl is plasma.

Clinical Application of Electrolyte Free Water Clearance

The most important conceptual point to understand is that the urine electrolytes and *not* the urine osmolality determine the degree of free water excretion in the urine. It is not always necessary to calculate an exact value for the electrolyte free water clearance if the relationship between the plasma electrolytes and the urine electrolytes is understood. If the concentration of electrolytes in the urine is greater than the concentration of electrolytes in the plasma, then free water is not being excreted in the urine. If the concentration of electrolytes in the urine is less than that in the plasma, then the patient is excreting free water in the urine. This relationship is illustrated in Figure 41.3. This is a simple test that can allow for a quick assessment of the ongoing losses of water in the urine.

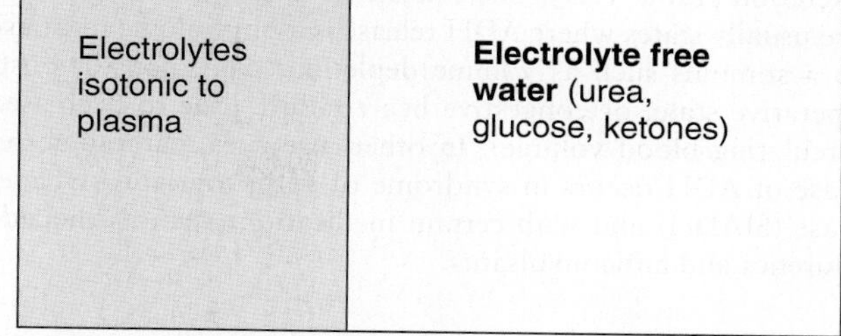

FIGURE 41.2. Electrolyte free water.

HYPONATREMIA

Hyponatremia commonly occurs in hospital settings and especially in the ICU setting. Often the condition is asymptomatic, but hyponatremic encephalopathy (brain dysfunction due to cerebral edema in turn due to hyponatremia) can result (2–4). Hyponatremic encephalopathy is a life-threatening medical emergency, and it must be recognized and promptly treated as it can often lead to death or devastating neurologic complications (5,6). Differentiating between these two spectrums of the disease presentation is critical. Among risk factors for life-threatening hyponatremia are female gender of premenopausal age (7), children (5), and hypoxia (7). Research over the last decade has elucidated the pathogenetic mechanisms that underlie these risk factors, and this has prompted new thinking and mandated shifts in the clinical approach to hyponatremia.

Pathogenesis of Hyponatremia

Hyponatremia is defined as a serum sodium of <135 mEq/L. The ability of the kidney to dilute the urine and thus excrete free water is the body's primary defense against the development of hyponatremia. Excess ingestion of water as the sole cause of hyponatremia is rare since the typical adult with normal renal function can excrete a massive free water load (15 L of free water per day). The combination of factors necessary for the development of hyponatremia are free water intake in the setting of an underlying condition that impairs free water

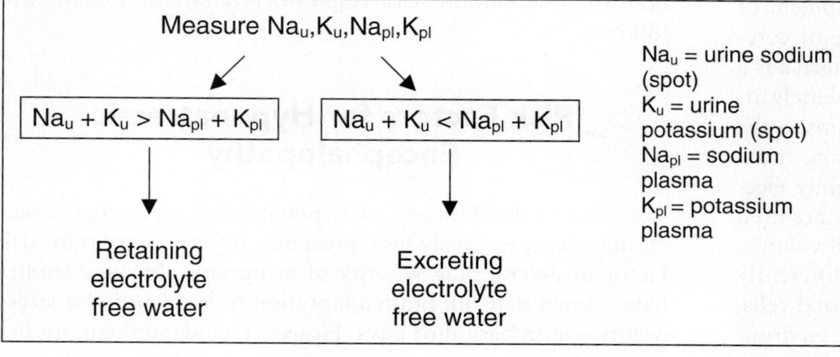

FIGURE 41.3. Relationship of electrolyte concentration in urine and plasma to the amount of free water excreted.

excretion (Table 41.1). The states that impair water excretion are usually states where ADH release is a physiologic response to a stimulus such as volume depletion, pain, nausea, postoperative state, or congestive heart failure (due to decreased circulating blood volume). In other instances, pathologic release of ADH occurs in syndrome of inappropriate ADH release (SIADH) and with certain medications such as thiazide diuretics and anticonvulsants.

Brain Defenses against Cerebral Edema

Hyponatremia induces an osmotic gradient that favors water movement into the brain leading to cerebral edema and neurologic injury. However, the brain is contained within a specialized compartment separated from the systemic circulation by the blood–brain barrier that impedes entry of water and has specialized mechanisms for handling water fluxes (8–10). The blood–brain barrier is a specialized structure with tight junctions between vascular endothelial cells (11–13) that interface with glial cells (astrocytes) on the brain side of the blood–brain barrier. Astrocytes form an important part of the microvascular compartment in the brain and project foot processes that abut the endothelial cells of the brain capillaries (14). This highly specialized cell performs many supporting functions in maintaining the fluid environment and the electrolyte milieu of the extracellular space of the brain (15,16). Among these functions is shunting of potassium from the microenvironment by uptake and release of potassium with water accompanying, in the perivascular space away from neurons. This function is accomplished through a concentration of aquaporin 4 (AQ4) water channels and Kir4.1 potassium channel located at the end-feet around the perivascular space (8). There is increasing evidence that glial cells also have an important role in brain water handling. The observation that glial cells (but not neurons) selectively swell following hypotonic stress presaged the existence of a glial-specific water pore, which has now been shown to be aquaporin 4 (AQ4). Mice lacking AQ4 do not develop cerebral edema in response to hyponatremia, suggesting that these channels may have an important role not only in normal water regulation in the brain, but also in the pathogenesis of hyponatremia-induced cerebral edema (17). During states of cytotoxic brain edema, water is shunted through the astrocyte, which swells, and the neuron is protected from this influx of water. Therefore, astrocytes are the principal regulator of the brain water content as they comprise the bulk of the intracellular space, and the response of these cells following osmolar stress is an important determinant of the changes in brain volume during hyponatremia.

The brain has several defenses against the development of cerebral edema. The first response is the shunting of cerebrospinal fluid from within the brain, but this mechanism has a limited capacity to buffer volume changes (18). Immediately after a volume stress, cell volume regulatory mechanisms in the cerebral astrocytes play an important role in reducing brain volume through reduction in cellular osmolyte (mainly electrolyte) content. These are adaptive mechanisms that are used by multiple cell types to counteract an increase in cell volume; however, the astrocyte responds to cellular swelling differently than many other cells (19). In erythrocytes, white blood cells, and epithelial cells, swelling occurs due to a hypotonic environment and calcium influx that begins a series of events termed the *regulatory volume decrease* (RVD) mediated by activation of K^+ and Cl^- channels that allow these ions to be released into the extracellular environment. In glial cells this is not the predominant response. The glial cell uses ATP-dependent mechanisms (19) that require the Na^+/K^+ ATPase during which ions are extruded from the glial cell and water obligatorily follows the extruded ions, reducing brain volume and protecting from the development of cerebral edema. This response is ongoing, and in animal models of acute hyponatremia, brain water content is close to the baseline value 6 hours after induction of acute hyponatremia (20). The Na^+/K^+ ATPase is ubiquitous and plays an essential role in cellular ion homeostasis. In the brain, this enzyme is very important in the response of the cell to volume stress and hypotonic insult (19). The enzyme has binding domains for sodium, potassium, and cardiac glycosides and requires the hydrolysis of ATP to ADP to provide energy for moving these ions against concentration gradients (21). Therefore, *in vitro* evidence suggests that the actions of the sodium potassium ATPase are the important immediate responses in determining the brain's response to hypo-osmolar stress (Fig. 41.4).

In summary, during times of systemic hypo-osmolality, water enters the brain through aquaporin 4 channels located in the glial cell end-feet surrounding brain capillaries. This osmotic swelling may also allow sodium into the glial cell, and expansion of the glial cell quickly ensues. Immediate shunting of cerebrospinal fluid (CSF) accommodates some of this expansion, but this is a limited mechanism. The glial cell reduces the intracellular volume by energy-dependent extrusion of solutes via the Na^+/K^+ ATPase pump. Several clinical factors have been shown to impair these glial cell adaptive responses, resulting in poor patient outcomes.

Clinical Manifestations

Symptoms of hyponatremia are due to osmotic swelling of the brain that accompanies the decrease in plasma osmolality. Manifestations are varied, and they depend on the degree of central nervous system adaptation to hypo-osmolality. Significant degrees of hyponatremia can be asymptomatic, such as chronic hyponatremia secondary to cirrhosis or heart failure. Conversely, hyponatremic encephalopathy is the clinical term for symptomatic cerebral edema secondary to hyponatremia, and this condition can have a fulminant presentation. Early signs are usually nonspecific—nausea, vomiting, headaches (22)—and often go unrecognized and are thought to be due to cerebral edema. When pressure is exerted on the skull by the brain, seizures may occur and if uncorrected, brainstem herniation with respiratory failure and death will follow (23).

Risk Factors for Hyponatremic Encephalopathy

The time to development of hyponatremia, i.e., acute versus chronic, has previously been presumed to be an important risk factor in determining severity of symptoms. *In vitro* studies have shown that full brain adaptation to hypo-osmolar stress occurs over a period of days. However, epidemiologic studies

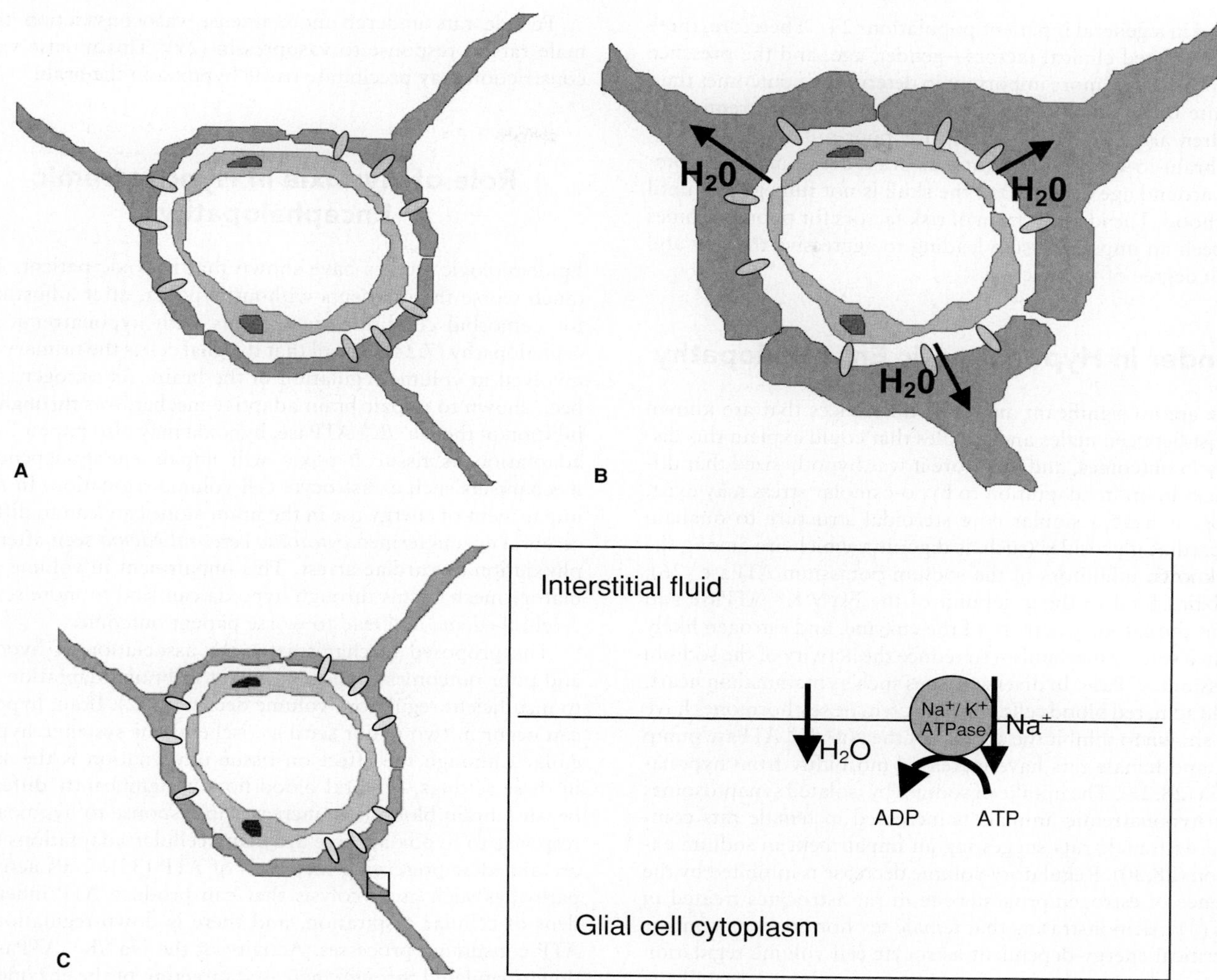

FIGURE 41.4. The brain's response to hypo-osmolar stress based on action of the sodium potassium ATPase. A: Normal glial cell. B: Glial cell swelling following water influx under hyponatremic conditions. C: Restoration of glial cell volume through extrusion of solutes via sodium-potassium ATPase. ADP, adenosine diphosphate; ATP, adenosine triphosphate.

have not demonstrated time to development of hyponatremia to be predictive of death (7,24). There is disparity in patient outcomes even when the time to development of hyponatremia is similar. For an example of the perplexing problem presented by hyponatremia, consider that an elderly male following transurethral resection of the prostate may acutely develop a serum sodium of 110 or a mentally ill patient may ingest large volumes of water to develop hyponatremia of similar degree, and encephalopathy does not result. However, young female patients following surgery may develop respiratory arrest and die due to brainstem herniation with serum sodium as high as 128 mEq/L (7). Although a component of acuity of the insult is important in affecting the outcomes, other factors appear to affect outcomes independent of the time course. A predilection for hyponatremic encephalopathy to affect females is a clue that patient-specific factors may be important in determining patient outcomes (7,25).

Neurologic symptoms of hyponatremic encephalopathy are due to pressure of the brain on the rigid skill. Brain size is determined by the incremental change in cell size due to osmotic influx of water, minus the regulatory volume decrease in response to hypo-osmolality. There are three major risk factors for poor outcomes following hyponatremic encephalopathy, which are discussed below. Patient factors play an important role in outcome.

In an epidemiologic study, being female of premenopausal age was shown to be the most important factor in predicting poor outcomes among postsurgical patients developing hyponatremia (7). Although male and female patients were equally likely to develop hyponatremia and hyponatremic encephalopathy postoperatively, permanent brain damage or death was 25 times more likely to occur in female patients (7). The degree of reduction in serum sodium and time to development of hyponatremia did not influence outcome. Comorbid conditions (coronary artery disease, chronic obstructive pulmonary disease, and peripheral vascular disease) were all more prevalent in male survivors than in female nonsurvivors with hyponatremic encephalopathy. Hypoxia at disease presentation was also identified as an important risk factor for hyponatremic encephalopathy. These findings have subsequently been verified in a general inpatient population (24). Therefore, three patient-related clinical factors—gender, age, and the presence of hypoxia—are more important in determining outcomes than the rate of development or the severity of hyponatremia (7). Children are another risk group for poor outcomes due to a high brain-to–cranial vault ratio as brain development is complete around age 6 years, but the skull is not fully grown until adulthood. The identification of risk factors for poor outcomes has been an important step leading to aggressive therapy and a high degree of vigilance.

Gender in Hyponatremic Encephalopathy

There are no significant anatomic differences that are known to exist between males and females that could explain this disparity in outcomes, and therefore it was hypothesized that differences in brain adaptation to hypo-osmolar stress may exist. Estrogens have a similar core steroidal structure to ouabain and cardiac glycosides (such as digoxin), which are among the best known inhibitors of the sodium potassium ATPase (26). Ouabains bind to the α subunit of the Na^+/K^+ ATPase and inhibit the catalytic activity of the enzyme, and estrogen likely acts in a similar mechanism to reduce the activity of the sodium potassium ATPase. In diverse tissues such as mammalian heart, diaphragm, red blood cells, and liver, female sex hormones have been shown to inhibit the activity of the Na^+/K^+ ATPase pump (27), and female rats have increased morbidity from hyponatremia (28,29). The uptake of sodium by isolated synaptosomes from hyponatremic animals is increased in female rats compared with male rats suggesting an impairment in sodium extrusion (28,30). Regulatory volume decrease is inhibited by the presence of estrogen/progesterone in rat astrocytes treated *in vitro* (31), demonstrating that female sex hormones can impair the critical energy-dependent astrocyte cell volume regulation that actively extrudes ions from the intracellular space of the edematous astrocytes.

Female rats undergo more intense vasoconstriction than male rats in response to vasopressin (29). This intense vasoconstriction may precipitate tissue hypoxia in the brain.

Role of Hypoxia in Hyponatremic Encephalopathy

Epidemiologic studies have shown that hypoxic patients fare much worse than patients without hypoxia, after adjustment for comorbid conditions in patients with hyponatremic encephalopathy (7,24). Recall that the glial cell is the primary cell involved in volume regulation in the brain. As estrogens had been shown to impair brain adaptive mechanisms through inhibition of the Na^+/K^+ ATPase, hypoxia may also impair brain adaptation as tissue hypoxia will impair energy-dependent mechanisms such as astrocyte cell volume regulation. In fact, impairment of energy use in the brain alone can lead to diffuse cerebral edema termed *cytotoxic cerebral edema* seen after asphyxiation or cardiac arrest. This impairment in volume regulatory mechanisms through hypoxia can lead to more severe cerebral edema and lead to worse patient outcomes.

The proposed mechanism for the association of hypoxia and poor outcomes is an impairment in brain adaptation due to insufficient regulatory volume decrease (32). Brain hypoxia can occur in two major settings: ischemia or systemic hypoxemia. Although the effect on tissue oxygenation is the same in these settings, cerebral blood flow is significantly different because brain blood flow increases in response to hypoxia. In response to hypoxia, there are many cellular adaptations that are aimed at preserving the levels of ATP (33). Cells activate pathways such as glycolysis that can produce ATP independent of cellular respiration, and there is down-regulation of ATP-consuming processes. Activity of the Na^+/K^+ ATPase is down-regulated through increased targeting of the enzyme for endocytosis; thus the cell favors maintenance of intracellular

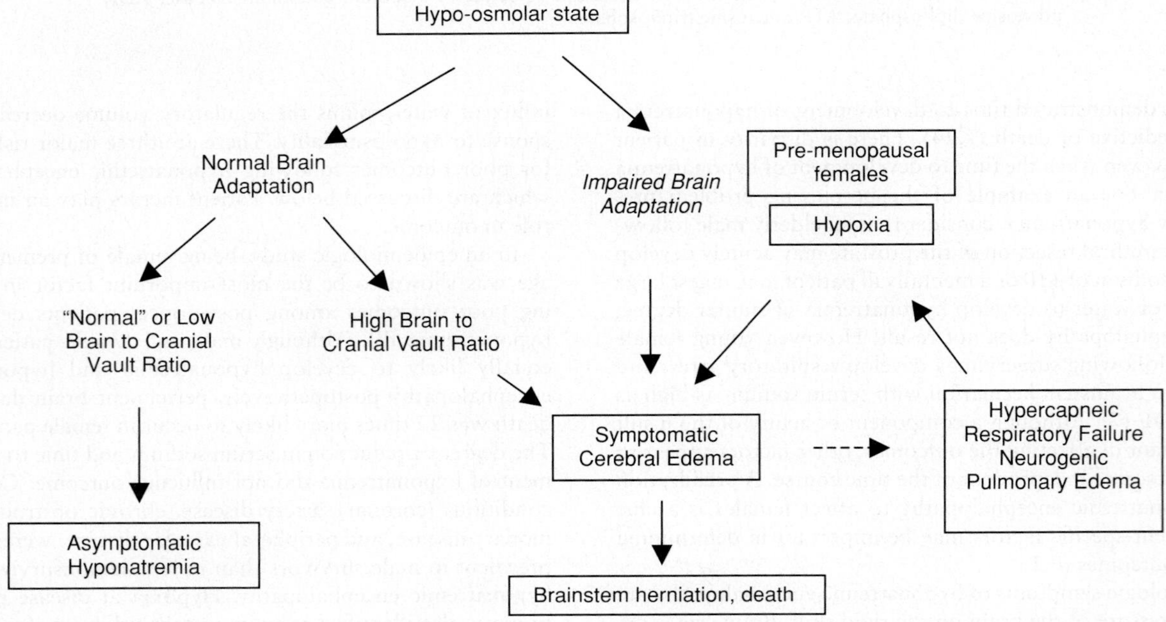

FIGURE 41.5. The role of hypoxia.

ATP levels over cell volume regulatory mechanisms. This may contribute to the glial cell impairment in volume regulation. Subsequent animal studies have shown that in brain hypoxia induced by either tissue ischemia or by systemic hypoxia, brain adaptation and survival are significantly impaired (32,34).

Hypoxia has been shown to develop in patients with hyponatremic encephalopathy through two mechanisms: hypercapnic respiratory failure and neurogenic pulmonary edema (35,36). Hypercapnic respiratory failure usually develops as a consequence of central respiratory depression and is a first sign of impending brain herniation. Neurogenic pulmonary edema is a well-described complication of cerebral edema from other causes as well as in hyponatremic encephalopathy (35,36). Neurogenic pulmonary edema is a complex disorder characterized by increased vascular permeability and increased catecholamine release (37) that occurs secondary to elevated intracranial pressure. Hypoxemia plays the role of both a risk factor and pathogenetic mechanism in severe cerebral edema. Whether hypoxia is present initially or develops as a consequence of hyponatremia through hypercapnic respiratory failure and/or neurogenic pulmonary edema (35,36), poor outcomes ensue (Fig. 41.5).

Approach to Hyponatremic Patient

The first step in working up the hyponatremic patient is to exclude hyperosmolar hyponatremia (Fig. 41.6). An osmotically active substance that is confined to the extracellular fluid (usually glucose or mannitol) will remove water from the intracellular space and will dilute the serum sodium concentration (translocational hyponatremia). To assess for a sodium disturbance in the setting of hyperglycemia, one must correct the serum sodium by adding 1.6 mEq/L for every 100 mg/dL increase of the serum glucose above 100 mg/dL. Significant hyperosmolality can exist in the setting of a normal or low serum sodium in cases of hyperglycemia. For example, a patient has a serum glucose of 650 mg/dL and a serum sodium of 130 mEq/L. Correct the serum sodium as follows:

$$\frac{(650\,\text{mg/dL} - 100\,\text{mg/dL})}{(100\,\text{mg/dL})} \times 1.6\,\text{mEq/L}$$
$$= 5.5 \times 1.6\,\text{mEq/L} = 8.8\,\text{mEq/L}$$

Thus the corrected serum sodium in this patient is 139 mEq/L.

The entity of pseudohyponatremia should also be kept in mind. Hyperproteinemia and hyperlipidemia can lead to spuriously low serum sodium measurements when *samples are diluted* prior to measurement of the serum sodium. If a potentiometric method is used, then this is not a concern. In pseudohyponatremia, the measured serum osmolality will be normal.

The remainder of the diagnostic approach is based on the history, urinary electrolytes, and clinical assessment of the patient's intravascular volume status. Physical examination can be unreliable in the clinical assessment of volume status and thus should be interpreted with caution (Fig. 41.6). A difficult group of patients not emphasized in Figure 41.6 are those with total body fluid overload (with edema, weight gain) due to shock and loss of fluid into the interstitial space, but who are intravascular volume depleted. Despite edema, they would be categorized as the "volume depletion" group, and the intravascular volume may best be assessed by blood volume measurements.

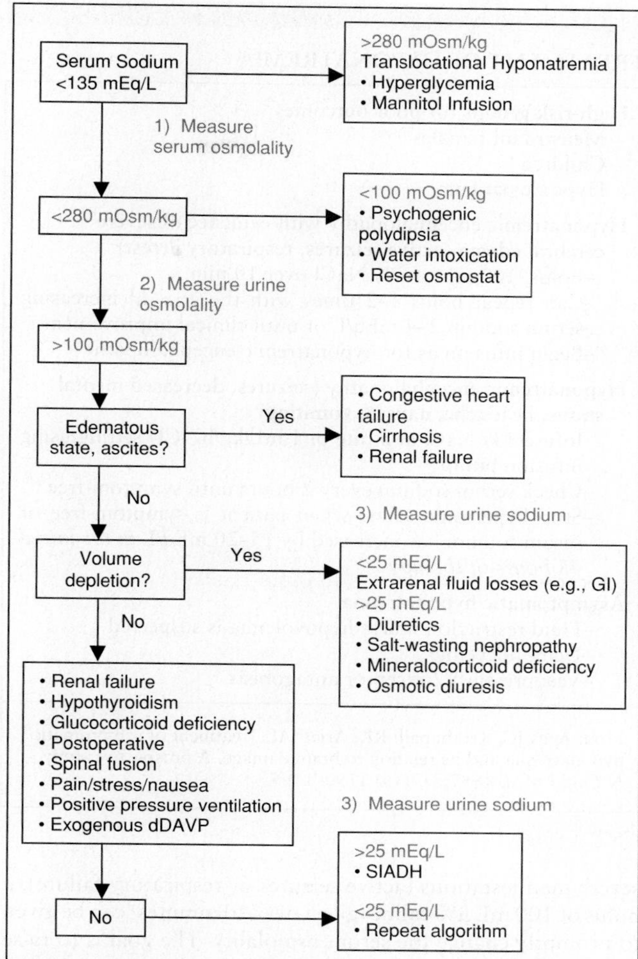

FIGURE 41.6. Diagnostic approach to hyponatremia. DDAVP, desmopressin; GI, gastrointestinal; SIADH, syndrome of inappropriate antidiuretic hormone.

Treatment of Hyponatremic Encephalopathy

Use of hypertonic saline to correct hyponatremia is reserved for patients with signs of hyponatremic encephalopathy and is not appropriate in asymptomatic patients regardless of serum sodium (6). Also, the serum osmolality should be measured prior to beginning therapy with hypertonic saline to verify that a hypotonic state exists (22). Fluid restriction alone is never appropriate to manage a patient with hyponatremic encephalopathy, especially in intravascular hypovolemic states. Early recognition of the problem and prompt therapy are the most important factors associated with successful intervention and good neurologic outcomes (22).

The rationale for treatment with hypertonic saline can be summarized as follows: (i) Remove patients with severe manifestations of cerebral edema from immediate danger, (ii) correct serum sodium to a mildly hyponatremic level, and (iii) maintain this level of serum sodium to allow for the brain to adapt to the change in serum osmolality. Table 41.2 gives an overview of the approach to therapy. Prompt therapy should be instituted in all patients with hyponatremic encephalopathy. In patients with

TABLE 41.2

TREATMENT OF HYPONATREMIA

High-risk groups for poor outcomes
Menstruant females
Children
Hypoxic patients

Hyponatremic encephalopathy with evidence of severe cerebral edema (active seizures, respiratory arrest)
–Bolus, 100 mL of 3% NaCl over 10 min
–Can repeat bolus 1–2 times with the goal of increasing serum sodium 2–4 mEq/L or until clinical improvement
–Begin infusion as for hyponatremic encephalopathy

Hyponatremic encephalopathy (seizures, decreased mental status, headache, nausea, vomiting)
–Infuse 3% NaCl at a rate of 1 mL/kg/h. ICU setting using infusion pump
–Check serum sodium every 2 hours until symptom-free
–Stop hypertonic saline when patient is symptom-free or serum sodium has increased by 15–20 mEq/L *in the initial 48 hours of therapy*

Asymptomatic hyponatremia
–Fluid restriction unless hypovolemia is suspected
–Demeclocycline
–Vasopressin V2 receptor antagonists

From Ayus JC, Krothapalli RK, Arieff AI. Treatment of symptomatic hyponatremia and its relation to brain damage. A prospective study. *N Engl J Med.* 1987;317(19):1190–1195.

severe manifestations (active seizures or respiratory failure), a bolus of 100 mL 3% saline (given over 10 minutes) can be given to promptly change the serum osmolality. The goal is to raise the serum sodium by about 2 to 4 mEq/L. If seizures or respiratory failure persist, the bolus may be repeated. Following the bolus, an infusion of hypertonic saline should be given with the goal of raising the serum sodium to mildly hyponatremic levels. However, the total change in serum sodium should not exceed 15 to 20 mEq/L over 48 hours (6). For patients with hyponatremic encephalopathy without active seizures or respiratory arrest, an infusion of 3% saline without a bolus is appropriate. Again, the goal is also to raise the serum sodium to mildly hyponatremic levels; the total change in serum sodium should not exceed 15 to 20 mEq/L over 48 hours (6).

Additional precautionary steps are necessary to prevent therapy-induced brain injury. The serum sodium should never be corrected to normonatremic or hypernatremic levels for a few days following hyponatremic encephalopathy. This maintenance period will allow the patient to adjust to the new plasma tonicity. In patients with impaired cardiac output in whom pulmonary edema may develop with vigorous volume expansion, intravenous furosemide should be given in addition to hypertonic saline to prevent volume overload.

There are formulas that have been advocated to calculate the infusion rate when giving hypertonic saline; however, we do not endorse their use. This practice can lead to patient injury when a calculated rate is used as a substitute for proper patient monitoring. Any patient receiving 3% saline should have the serum sodium checked at least every 2 hours until the patient and the serum sodium values are stable. All patients with severe manifestations must be placed in an intensive care setting. The rationale for close monitoring is that ongoing water losses cannot be predicted, and equations that calculate infusion rates assume a closed system (i.e., no ongoing water losses) and significant overcorrection can occur. To guide initial therapy, an infusion of 3% saline of 1 mL/kg will estimate an increase in serum sodium by approximately 1 mEq/L. Initial infusion rates should be adjusted based on repeated serum sodium values and the patient's clinical response.

During the treatment of hyponatremia, the clinician needs to be vigilant to be sure that a free water diuresis does not occur. Clinical scenarios where this is more of concern are interruption of desmopressin (DDAVP) therapy, psychogenic polydipsia, and drug-induced hyponatremia when the offending agent is stopped. To prevent ongoing water losses in the urine and "autocorrection" of the serum sodium, DDAVP can be given to increase urinary concentration and reduce free water losses. This must be done carefully with the patient strictly fluid restricted or kept with no enteral intake in an intensive care unit setting. If unrestricted fluid intake occurs during DDAVP administration, significant hyponatremia can develop. Consultation with an expert experienced in treating sodium disorders is mandatory in such cases. An increase in urine output is the first sign that a water diuresis is ensuing, and therefore hourly urine output needs to be followed in all patients with hyponatremic encephalopathy. The difficulty in treating cases where autocorrection can occur is illustrated in the special case studies below.

Risk Factors for the Development of Cerebral Demyelination

Cerebral demyelination is a rare, serious complication associated with the correction of severe hyponatremia. When symptoms manifest, it is usually a delayed phenomenon occurring days to weeks following correction of hyponatremia and can manifest as a pseudocoma with a locked-in stare. This condition can also be asymptomatic and therefore magnetic resonance imaging (MRI) (which is sensitive for the detection of demyelinating lesions) is necessary for the diagnosis. It is important to understand that the rate of correction of serum sodium alone does not predict the development of cerebral demyelination; rather, the absolute change in serum sodium over 48 hours is predictive (6). Other clinical factors such as liver disease and hypoxia increase the risk of demyelination, and care must be exercised in these groups (6). As noted above, the serum sodium can be quickly be corrected in an acutely symptomatic patient without increasing the risk of demyelination as long as the absolute change over 48 hours does not exceed 15 to 20 mEq/L and the patient is not corrected to normonatremic levels. *Patients with liver disease are particularly susceptible to cerebral demyelination, and caution should be exercised in this setting; the safe degree of correction over 48 hours in this group is not known (6).*

Management of Asymptomatic Hyponatremia

Regardless of the cause and regardless of the absolute level of the serum sodium, asymptomatic hyponatremia does not require aggressive therapy, but the diagnostic approach to hyponatremia is similar (Fig. 41.6), and treatment should be based on the cause. Fluid restriction can be used alone if hypovolemia is not suspected, but this will typically not result in resolution of the hyponatremia, especially in cases of SIADH where electrolyte free water excretion is negative. Precipitating medications such as thiazide diuretics and anticonvulsants should be stopped. If hyponatremia persists despite fluid restriction, demeclocycline can be used to lower osmolality and increase free water excretion. Vasopressin receptor (V2) blockers are new agents that show promise for the treatment of hyponatremia (38). There is currently limited experience with these medications. However, they may become the mainstay of therapy for asymptomatic hyponatremia in the future as demeclocycline has potential side effects.

Approach to Fluid Therapy and Prevention of Hospital-Acquired Hyponatremia

Until proven otherwise, a patient in a critical care setting should be assumed to have an impairment in free water excretion. In patients with intact kidney function, ADH levels are likely to be high. In patients with renal failure, free water excretion is also impaired. Common situations where water balance is impaired include the following: cases of effective circulating volume depletion (cirrhosis, heart failure, and third spacing of fluid), gastrointestinal fluid losses, diuretic use (especially thiazides), renal failure (acute and chronic), SIADH, cortisol deficiency, and hypothyroidism (Table 41.1). As noted above, hypotonic intravenous fluids should not be used except in the setting of replacement of a water deficit (i.e., hypernatremia). Isotonic solution normal saline (0.9% NaCl) containing 154 mEq/L of Na^+ and Cl^- is the most appropriate parenteral fluid when intravenous fluids are indicated for the maintenance of intravascular volume in the postoperative period (39). Also, any patient receiving fluid therapy should have the serum sodium measured at least daily.

Hospital-acquired hyponatremic encephalopathy occurs most commonly when hypotonic fluids are administered to a patient with an impairment of free water excretion. A clinical setting that merits specific discussion is the postoperative state. Approximately 1% of patients develop a serum sodium of <130 mEq/L following surgery, and clinically important hyponatremia complicates 20% of these cases (7). The postoperative state commonly includes multiple stimuli for ADH release including pain, stress, nausea, vomiting, narcotic medications, and volume depletion (7). Administration of a hypotonic intravenous fluid in the postoperative state or in other clinical settings characterized by impaired free water excretion can have disastrous consequences.. The use of hypotonic fluids is reserved for treatment of a free water deficit, such as exists in the setting of hypernatremia.

Special Case Studies

Postoperative Hyponatremia

A 32-year-old female with no significant past medical history undergoes elective laparoscopic bilateral tubal ligation at 8:00 a.m.; 5% dextrose, 1/4 normal saline is started by the anesthesiologist and maintained at 125 mL per hour. The patient remains in recovery until late in the afternoon and is kept because she is too sedated to leave. Intravenous meperidine is given, with adequate pain relief. She does not tolerate oral intake, and the IV fluids are continued at the current rate. At 2:45 a.m. the following day, the patient complains of headache and she is given Vicodin by the on-call physician. At 9:00 a.m., a nurse notifies the surgeon of a sodium of 129 mEq/L; no new orders are received, and intravenous fluids are continued. Later that morning the patient is noted to be lethargic, and the surgeon is notified by the nursing staff; an order is received to hold pain medications. At 3:30 p.m., the patient has a generalized seizure and goes into respiratory failure. She is intubated and mechanical ventilation is initiated. Serum sodium at this time is 124 mEq/L.

Key Points:

- This patient has multiple stimuli for ADH release and thus impaired free water excretion. Administration of a hypotonic fluid was not appropriate and placed the patient at risk for hyponatremia.
- The most important measure to prevent postoperative hyponatremia is to avoid the use of a hypotonic fluid in a postsurgical patient and administer 0.9% sodium chloride when parenteral fluids are indicated.
- In this case the clinicians failed to recognize the early signs of hyponatremic encephalopathy (headache, nausea, and vomiting), which occurred when the patient's sodium was 129 mEq/L. *The presence or absence of symptoms of hyponatremic encephalopathy and not the absolute level of the serum sodium determines whether or not a life-threatening condition exists.*

Exercise-induced Hyponatremia

A 21-year-old woman collapses 30 minutes after completing a marathon and is brought to the emergency room. She is disoriented and significantly short of breath on arrival. Physical exam reveals a normal cardiac exam, crackles in all lung fields, and a nonfocal neurologic exam with depressed mental status. Chest radiograph reveals pulmonary edema. Serum electrolytes include sodium of 126 mEq/L and potassium of 3.1 mEq/L.

Key Points:

- Exercise-associated hyponatremia has been described in marathon runners. Those who develop this problem consume large amounts of water throughout the race, in excess of the water lost through sweating (36,40). The proposed mechanism is that significant portions of consumed water remains sequestered in the gut as there is divergence of blood flow from the splanchnic circulation during the race. Additionally, ADH is released secondary to the extreme physical exertion of the race. Following completion of the marathon, the ingested water is absorbed and acute hyponatremia ensues, which can be fatal.
- Noncardiogenic pulmonary edema induced by cerebral edema has been described in association with exercise-induced hyponatremia. Paradoxically, treatment with 3% saline leads to resolution of the pulmonary edema by treating the underlying cerebral edema (41).
- Limiting fluid intake is necessary as hypotonic electrolyte sports drinks or salt consumption during the race do not appear to be effective in prevention of this condition (40).

DDAVP Withdrawal

A 76-year-old nursing home patient with a history of urinary incontinence, following transurethral resection of the prostate, is treated with intranasal DDAVP, 10 μg each night. On a routine chemistry panel 1 week prior to admission, his sodium was 138 mEq/L and the patient was doing quite well. Two days prior to presentation he was started on DDAVP, 10 μg in the late morning. On the day of admission, the patient is found to be lethargic and unresponsive and is transported to an emergency room. His serum sodium is 104 mEq/L and serum potassium is 4.0 mEq/L. Urine sodium is 95 mEq/L and urine potassium is 45 mEq/L. He is treated with a 75-mL bolus, then infusion of 3% saline, and his neurologic status improves. Infusion of 3% saline is held when the serum sodium is 120 mEq/L. DDAVP has also been withheld because it is noted to have caused the hyponatremia. Urine output increases significantly over the ensuing night and on the following morning his serum sodium is 139 mEq/L, urine sodium is 17 mEq/L, and urine potassium is 11 mEq/L.

Key Points:

- DDAVP alone will not induce hyponatremia. DDAVP will cause retention of free water, and thus the dosing needs to be titrated in conjunction with the patient's fluid intake. Proper patient instruction and close monitoring are essential during dose changes.
- If DDAVP is withheld, which is commonly done in cases of DDAVP-associated hyponatremia, a free water diuresis will

ensue and dangerous overcorrection of the serum sodium hypernatremia may occur.

- The best approach to a patient with hyponatremic encephalopathy due to DDAVP-associated hyponatremia is to continue DDAVP and restrict all enteral fluid intake. Three percent NaCl should be used to correct the patient to the desired serum sodium level, then should be discontinued. A slow infusion of 0.9% can be continued if necessary to support volume status, and absolutely no hypotonic fluids should be administered. This will prevent overcorrection of the serum sodium secondary to a water diuresis. Consultation with a specialist is recommended in these complex cases.

HYPERNATREMIA

Hypernatremia, a serum sodium greater than 145 mEq/L, is commonly encountered in the intensive care unit. Thirst is a powerful protective mechanism, and therefore, restricted access to water is nearly always necessary for the development of hypernatremia. Restricted access to water occurs in various settings, often at the extremes of age: patients who are debilitated by an acute or chronic illness, in neurologic impairment such as dementia, in infants, in moribund patients, or in those on mechanical ventilation with inability to drink water, or in any situation without free access to water. Hypernatremia can develop in essentially any critically ill patient with altered mental status or intubated for mechanical ventilation, because these patients have restricted access to fluids. In most patients in the ICU with hypernatremia, there is a combination of impaired access to water and ongoing free water losses. Renal water losses may occur secondary to solute diuresis (typically urea or glucose), renal concentrating defects (such as loop diuretics), excess hypertonic sodium bicarbonate administration and gastrointestinal fluid losses (especially nasogastric suction and lactulose administration).

Pathogenesis of Hypernatremia

The thirst mechanism and the kidney's urinary concentrating ability that minimize water losses in the urine are the body's defenses against the development of hypernatremia. The common causes of hypernatremia in the ICU usually involve states of impaired water access in conjunction with excessive free water losses (Fig. 41.7). Hypernatremia is a relatively uncommon diagnosis on admission to the intensive care unit but frequently develops during critical illness, and the cause is nearly always iatrogenic. Failure to recognize significant electrolyte free water losses in the urine and to provide adequate replacement in either parenteral or enteral solutions is a common cause of hypernatremia in the intensive care setting.

During hypernatremic states, the brain is subject to osmolar stress that favors the movement of water out of the brain and can lead to significant brain damage. *In vivo* studies have shown that the brain adapts to hypernatremia through increases in osmotically active ions and *de novo* generation of osmotically active idiogenic osmoles. The osmotically active cations that are increased in the brain during hypernatremia are sodium and potassium. Idiogenic osmoles refer to a heterogeneous group of osmotically active substances such as myoinositol, glycerophosphocholine, choline, and sorbitol (42,43). This response is seen in the acute setting, and no further changes in brain osmolality are observed after 1 week of hypernatremia (44). These defenses preserve brain volume during elevations in the plasma osmolality and prevent significant decrease in brain size due to osmotic water losses in the brain. In correction of chronic hypernatremia, idiogenic osmoles do not dissipate quickly, and rapid correction of chronic hypernatremia over 24 hours can lead to cerebral edema (44).

Approach to the Hypernatremic Patient

A detailed history focusing on fluid intake and losses is the first step in the evaluation of the hypernatremic patient. Various sources of water losses in the critically ill patient are (Fig. 41.8) water losses in the urine, from the gastrointestinal tract (diarrhea and nasogastric suction), and insensible losses (fever, sepsis, massive diaphoresis, burns). These amounts should be calculated (when accurate counts are available) or estimated. In assessing urinary water losses, both the urine osmolality and electrolytes should be measured in evaluation of urinary concentrating ability and to assess urinary water losses. Caution should be exercised in the interpretation of the urine osmolality as this is an area where error is frequently made. The urine osmolality alone cannot be used to determine whether or not there is free water loss in the urine. This is because water is excreted with nonelectrolyte osmoles (which under physiologic conditions is typically urea) and with electrolyte osmoles. Both contribute to the osmolality of the urine but have differential effects on water balance. Water that is excreted with nonelectrolyte osmoles is water that is lost in excess of electrolyte loss. Recall that the serum sodium is proportional to total body electrolytes relative to total body water (Equation 41.1). Therefore loss of water with the nonelectrolyte osmoles will raise the serum sodium. By contrast, water that is excreted with electrolyte osmoles will not affect the serum sodium (as long as the concentration of electrolytes in the urine and serum are similar). This is because both the numerator and denominator of Equation 41.1 is decreasing and therefore the proportion is unchanged. In cases where there is a high urea or glucose load, significant amounts of water can be lost in the urine

Lack of water intake	Increased water losses
Decreased thirst (dementia, neurologic impairment) Mechanical ventilation Bowel rest/nasogastric suction	Solute diuresis (hyperlgycemia, urea loading from tube feeds or hyperalimentation) Loop diuretics Gastrointestinal water losses Diabetes insipidus

FIGURE 41.7. Common causes of hypernatremia in the ICU.

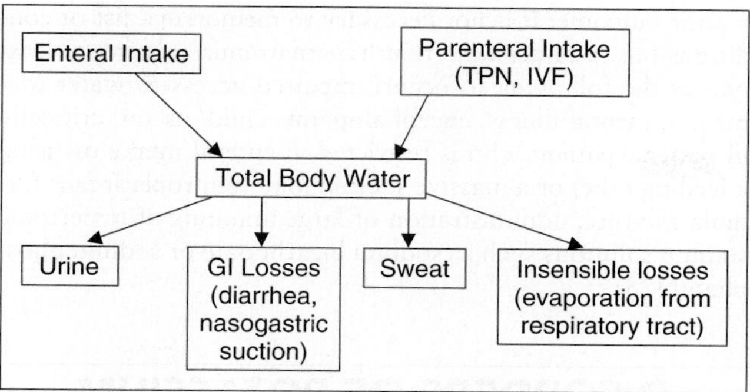

FIGURE 41.8. Sources of water intake and loss in the ICU. GI, gastrointestinal; IVF, intravenous fluid; TPN, total parenteral nutrition.

despite maximal urinary concentration. Failure to concentrate the urine in the face of hypernatremia should raise suspicion of a urinary concentrating defect. Renal failure, loop diuretics, tubulointerstitial renal disease, and diabetes insipidus are the main causes of urinary concentrating defects. In summary, all sources of water intake and water loss should be considered in assessing the water needs of a critically ill patient (Fig. 41.8) as an imbalance favoring water loss over water intake will lead to hypernatremia.

Clinical Manifestations of Hypernatremia

Hypernatremia leads to an efflux of fluid from the intracellular space to the extracellular space to maintain osmotic equilibrium across the cell membranes. The primary clinical manifestations are due to central nervous system depression as cerebral dehydration and cell shrinkage occurs. Hypernatremia carries an overall mortality between 40% and 70% in children (45). The elderly and patients with end-stage liver disease are at particular risk for complications from hypernatremia. Treatment of hepatic encephalopathy with lactulose frequently causes an osmotic diarrhea that leads to water losses in the stool. As a result, hypernatremia can quickly develop and lead to severe morbidity. Patients with liver disease are at high risk for cerebral demyelination in the setting of changes in serum sodium (6).

Central Diabetes Insipidus

Central diabetes insipidus (CDI) is a unique cause of hypernatremia that can be seen in the ICU and is most commonly in the setting of head injury, pituitary surgery, and cerebral hemorrhages. Specific therapy is indicated for this condition and therefore it needs to be recognized early. With polyuria secondary to water diuresis, severe hypernatremia can rapidly develop in an individual who has restricted access to fluids such as an ICU patient. Sodium-retentive mechanisms are intact in patients with CDI, and therefore clinical volume depletion is not a characteristic feature. The diagnosis of CDI should be suspected if the urine is not concentrated in the setting of hypernatremia (46). In general, the plasma osmolality typically exceeds the urine osmolality in CDI. Formal diagnostic testing for diabetes insipidus is beyond the scope of this text and is usually undertaken in consultation with a nephrologist. A simple and reliable clinical test that can be used to distinguish CDI from nephrogenic diabetes insipidus is to administer a V2 receptor agonist, such as DDAVP. A 50% increase in urine osmolality following DDAVP administration strongly suggests CDI. Once the diagnosis is established, DDAVP can be given either subcutaneously or intranasally. When DDAVP is administered, water intake should be adjusted appropriately to avoid precipitation of significant hyponatremia, and serial serum electrolytes should be monitored during dose titration (23).

Treatment of Hypernatremia

The goal of treatment of hypernatremia is to achieve normal circulatory volume as patients typically have circulatory volume depletion and then to correct the serum sodium with free water replacement (Table 41.3). The first step is to assess the ongoing water losses in the urine to determine if the water losses are renal in origin, or if the kidneys are appropriately conserving water. A simple method for assessing free water loss in the urine is displayed in Equation 41.3, which is Equation 41.2 but looking specifically at the urine:

$$\left(1 - \frac{[\text{Na}^+]_\text{U} + [\text{K}^+]_\text{U}}{[\text{Na}^+]_\text{P} + [\text{K}^+]_\text{P}}\right) \times \text{urine output rate} \quad [3]$$
$$= \text{rate of urinary water loss}$$

The degree of ongoing water losses in the urine will assist in determining the rate of fluid administration. In cases of extrarenal fluid losses, the fluid loss will need to be estimated. Fluid resuscitation with normal saline or colloid to replenish the circulating volume should precede correction of the water deficit (Table 41.3). In hypernatremic states, insulin resistance has also been observed (47). This can lead to severe hyperglycemia and potential worsening of hyperosmolality during therapy with glucose-containing solutions. For this reason, glucose-containing solutions are potentially harmful and should be avoided if possible. If intravenous glucose solutions must be used (for example, 5% dextrose in water), hourly measurement of the plasma glucose should be made and an insulin drip considered if plasma glucose becomes elevated.

TABLE 41.3

TREATMENT OF HYPERNATREMIA

1. Replete intravascular volume with colloid solution, isotonic saline, or plasma.
2. Estimate water deficit. Deficit should be replaced over 48–72 hours, aiming for a correction of 1 mOsm/L/hour. In severe hypernatremia (>170 mEq/L), serum sodium should not be corrected to below 150 mEq/L in the first 48–72 hours. Replacement of ongoing water losses are given in addition to the deficit.
3. Hypotonic fluid should be used. Usual replacement fluid is 77 mEq/L (0.45 N saline). A lower sodium concentration may be needed if there is a renal concentrating defect or sodium overload. Glucose-containing solutions should be avoided, and an oral route of administration should be used.
4. Monitor plasma; electrolytes should be monitored every 2 hours until patient is neurologically stable.

Reproduced from Medical Knowledge Self-assessment Program (MKSAP) 2006.

Oral hydration is preferable to parenteral and should be used when possible. Serial measurement of electrolytes every 2 hours is necessary until the patient is neurologically stable. In patients without evidence of hypernatremic encephalopathy, the serum sodium should not be corrected more quickly than 1 mEq/hour or 15 mEq/24 hours. In severe cases (>170 mEq/L), sodium should not be corrected to below 150 mEq/L in the first 48 to 72 hours (36).

Case Scenario: Solute Diuresis from Excess Urea Load

A 46-year-old man is admitted with severe necrotizing pancreatitis. He has a history of alcohol abuse, hepatitis C, and chronic liver disease. The patient weighs 76 kg. Admission labs are listed below. The patient is kept without enteral intake overnight and volume expanded with 6 L of normal saline. Twenty-four hours after admission, abdominal pain worsens and he is continued without enteral intake. Serum sodium is 145. Over the next 24 hours, urine output increases and isotonic saline is continued at 100 mL per hour. Total parenteral nutrition is initiated with a total volume of 2 L, 120 mEq of sodium, and high amino acid content. The chemistry and urine studies 48 hours after admission are listed.

	Admission	48 hours after admission
Sodium (mEq/L)	137	155
Potassium (mEq/L)	3.5	3.1
Chloride (mEq/L)	103	112
Bicarbonate (mmol/L)	21	24
Blood urea nitrogen (mg/dL)	23	53
Creatinine (mg/dL)	1.3	1.1
Urine output (mL per hour)	40	200
Urine sodium (mEq/L)	—	45
Urine potassium (mEq/L)	—	22
Urine osmolality (mOsm/kg)	—	610

What is the cause of the polyuria in this patient? Answer: Solute diuresis.

Learning Point:

- Solute diuresis secondary to a high urea load is a common cause of hypernatremia in the critical care setting.

This patient presents a typical example of a solute diuresis leading to hypernatremia in the critical care setting. By taking the ratio of the sodium plus potassium in the urine over the sodium plus potassium in the serum, urinary water losses can be assessed. The sodium plus potassium in the urine is lower than that in the blood. In this case, the ratio is 70/156 = 0.45. This means that 45% of his urine is electrolyte containing and conversely that 55% of the urine is electrolyte free water. At his current urine output, he is losing (0.55 × 200 mL/hour) = 110 mL of water per hour in the urine. Water replacement must be at least equal to this to replace his ongoing water losses in the urine. The urine osmolality is high due to ADH secretion, and this is increasing the urine concentration. The low urine sodium and potassium, at a time when the urine osmolality is high, signifies that there is a nonelectrolyte osmole in the urine that is obligating water loss. This is a classic presentation of an osmotic diuresis secondary to urea. The high urea load in this case is probably multifactorial, being secondary to the hypercatabolic state with muscle breakdown in addition to the necessarily high protein in the total parenteral nutrition.

Prevention of Hypernatremia in the ICU

The prevention of hypernatremia is best accomplished by recognition of patients at risk for this disorder and at risk of a poor outcome. It is not necessary to memorize a list of conditions but to understand that hypernatremia requires at least one of the following to occur: impaired access to water (dementia, mental illness, encephalopathy, child/ infant, critically ill patient, patient who is restricted in enteral intake or using a feeding tube) or a massive sodium load (improper infant formula mixture, administration of large amounts of hypertonic sodium solutions such as sodium bicarbonate or sodium phosphate) (23).

DISORDERS OF POTASSIUM BALANCE

Physiology of Potassium Homeostasis

Potassium is present mainly in the intracellular space (approximately 4,000 mEq of total body stores) and is sequestered in the intracellular space through the action of the Na^+/K^+ ATPase pump. The serum potassium level is tightly regulated so that the potential differences across membranes, especially cardiac, are not affected by alterations in potassium level. As the extracellular space contains very little of the total body potassium, shifting of potassium from one space to another is a major cause of both hyperkalemia and hypokalemia. The major influences that favor potassium movement into cells are insulin and β_2-adrenergic stimulation. Metabolic acidosis favors potassium movement out of cells as H^+ is exchanged for K^+ when H^+ moves intracellularly. However, this may have less importance in settings where an organic anion is generated as a result of the acidosis (such as lactic acidosis) as the organic ions may also move intracellularly and thus negate the electrogenic stimulus for potassium to move out of the cell.

Potassium excretion is tightly regulated, and the excretion of potassium can be varied such that potassium balance is maintained across a wide range of potassium intake. There are two main determinants of potassium excretion of clinical significance: flow of tubular filtrate into the distal nephron and secretion of potassium into the electronegative filtrate through epithelial potassium channels. The electronegativity of the tubular filtrate is determined by reabsorption of sodium from the filtrate at a faster rate than reabsorption of Cl^-. This reabsorption occurs through the epithelial sodium channel ENaC (47,48). The effect of aldosterone with sodium retention is the most important influence increasing the action of ENaC and therefore stimulates potassium excretion. Medications such as amiloride, triamterene, and trimethoprim (49) block ENaC and lead to decreased K^+ secretion and can lead to clinically important hyperkalemia. Decrease in the rate of tubular flow into the distal nephron stimulates the renin angiotensin system, which in turn stimulates release of aldosterone. The renin angiotensin axis, in addition to stimulating the release of aldosterone, also affects hemodynamic changes at the glomerular level, which act to maintain glomerular filtration rate and therefore maintain distal flow into the nephron with the ability to excrete potassium. In summary, the renal excretion of potassium is enhanced during states of high tubular flow and also under the actions of aldosterone. Therefore, inhibition of either of these through a decrease in glomerular filtration rate (of any cause) or inhibition of the action of aldosterone (e.g., adrenal insufficiency or pharmacologic blockade) can lead to potassium retention.

Hyperkalemia

Pathophysiology

Hyperkalemia occurs through two major mechanisms: shifting of potassium from intracellular compartment to the extracellular fluid compartment or through total body excess (Table 41.4). Total body potassium excess nearly always implies a deficiency in renal potassium excretion as the kidney. It is difficult to overcome a normal kidney's ability to increase potassium excretion by increasing potassium intake except in cases of a massive potassium load (rhabdomyolysis, tumor lysis syndrome). Chronic renal failure alone typically does not lead to hyperkalemia until the glomerular filtration rate (GFR) falls below approximately 15 mL/minute. Other mitigating factors will exacerbate hyperkalemia in the setting of chronic renal failure such as medications (Table 41.5). Hyperkalemia commonly complicates acute renal failure and is less tolerated in the acute setting. Hyperkalemia is most often encountered in unexpected development of acute renal failure such as in postsurgery (especially after cardiac or vascular surgery), post–intravenous contrast study, administration of nephrotoxic antibiotics (especially aminoglycosides), post–cardiac catheterization. Other settings include end-stage renal disease, adrenal insufficiency, type IV renal tubular acidosis (RTA) (usually seen in diabetics), crush injury, diabetes, and massive blood transfusion. Medications are a very important risk factor for the development of hyperkalemia (Table 41.5).

Management of Hyperkalemia

The first step in the management of hyperkalemia is to differentiate life-threatening hyperkalemia from less urgent cases and then to identify the diagnosis. The absolute levels of the potassium cannot be reliably used to determine if a life-threatening condition exists, and the effect of elevated potassium on the cardiac membrane must be determined through an electrocardiogram. The management of emergent hyperkalemia is detailed in Table 41.6. As a temporizing measure, shifting of potassium intracellularly with insulin or beta-agonists can be used until definitive removal therapy is instituted. If normal renal function is present, diuretics and intravenous saline can be used to remove potassium. Cation exchange resins can be used as an adjunctive therapy. In patients with renal failure, especially with oliguria, emergency dialysis is often necessary. Hyperkalemia not associated with electrocardiographic changes can sometimes be managed with discontinuation of the offending agent. Some medications causing hyperkalemia such as spironolactone can have a long half-life, and the effect can last for up to 1 to 2 weeks. Close follow-up is mandatory with serial measurements of serum potassium and renal function (50). If managed properly, hyperkalemia is usually associated with good long-term prognosis.

TABLE 41.4

CAUSES OF HYPERKALEMIA

Assess for increased potassium intake
Low-sodium salt substitutes and potassium supplements
Assess for shift of potassium intracellular fluid to extracellular fluid
Metabolic acidosis
Tissue necrosis (rhabdomyolysis, bowel infarction, tumor lysis) or depolarization
Insulin deficiency
β_2-Blockade
Assess for reduced potassium excretion in urine
Renal failure
Low aldosterone action (Think drugs: especially heparin, cyclosporine, tacrolimus, ARB, ACE-I)
Decreased distal nephron flow rate

ACE-I, angiotensin-converting enzyme inhibitor; ARB, angiotensin receptor blockers.
From {MKSAP 2006}.

TABLE 41.5

MEDICATIONS THAT CAUSE HYPERKALEMIA

Drugs that interfere with potassium excretion
Interfere with renin–angiotensin–aldosterone axis:
ACE-I, ARB, aldosterone blockers, heparin (decrease aldosterone synthesis), beta-blockers (decrease renin release)
Interfere with tubular potassium handling:
Potassium-sparing diuretics (amiloride, triamterene), trimethoprim, calcineurin inhibitors (cyclosporine, tacrolimus)
Drugs that shift potassium from intracellular fluid to extracellular
β_2-blockers, depolarizing paralytics (e.g., succinylcholine), digitalis

ACE-I, angiotensin-converting enzyme inhibitor; ARB, angiotensin receptor blockers.
From {MKSAP 2006}.

Case Scenario: Heparin-induced Hyperkalemia

A 60-year-old female patient is 5 days post–total hip replacement for osteoarthritis. She has a history of diabetes, hypertension, and a seizure disorder and no known kidney disease. Her outpatient medications include insulin, metformin, atenolol, hydrochlorothiazide, and Dilantin. The surgery was uneventful, but on postsurgical day 2, she develops severe shortness of breath and chest pain. A pulmonary embolism is diagnosed, and she is placed on unfractionated heparin and transferred to the intensive care unit. Following the surgery, she has additionally been receiving promethazine, 12.5 mg as needed (prn) for nausea and vomiting, and meperidine, 25 mg prn for pain. Her preoperative labs were all normal; today's chemistry panel (on postoperative day 4) is listed below:

Sodium (mEq/L)	138
Potassium (mEq/L)	5.9
Chloride (mEq/L)	102
Bicarbonate (mEq/L)	27
Blood urea nitrogen (BUN) (mg/dL)	18
Creatinine (mg/dL)	1.1
Glucose (mg/dL)	153

Which of the following best explains the development of hyperkalemia? Answer: Use of heparin.

Key Point:

- Heparin can lead to hyperkalemia by decreasing aldosterone levels (51).

Heparin is a frequent cause of hyperkalemia in the hospital setting in both patients with normal renal function and in those

TABLE 41.6

TREATMENT OF HYPERKALEMIA

Immediate actions
Electrocardiogram. Look for peaked T waves, loss of p waves, widened QRS. Loss of p wave and widened QRS suggest impending ventricular fibrillation.
Send repeat serum potassium to confirm diagnosis (do not wait for confirmatory test to initiate emergency therapy).
Hyperkalemia with electrocardiographic (ECG) changes
Stabilize cardiac membrane
–Intravenous (IV) calcium gluconate or chloride to stabilize cardiac membrane, may repeat in 5 min if ECG changes persist
–Place patient on cardiac monitoring
Shift potassium into cells
–IV insulin (with IV dextrose if necessary to prevent hypoglycemia)
–Albuterol, 10–20 mg by nebulization (caution in heart disease)
–IV $NaHCO_3$ may be of benefit
Potassium removal
–Dialysis
–Diuretics (with IV saline if patient is not volume overloaded) if renal function is normal
–Cation exchange resins (caution with decreased GI motility as bowel necrosis can occur)
Hyperkalemia without electrocardiographic changes
–Remove offending agents
–Otherwise follow same therapy as above with dialysis, diuretics, and/or cation exchange resins.

GI, gastrointestinal.

with renal insufficiency. In this case, renal function appears to be normal. Heparin inhibits the synthesis of aldosterone and leads to impairment of renal potassium secretion in the distal tubule. Two major factors are necessary for potassium excretion to occur: distal flow of urine to the distal nephron (this is impaired in acute renal failure) and aldosterone action. The necessity for distal secretion of potassium to maintain potassium balance is because of the very low filtered load of potassium due to the low concentration of potassium in the blood. Aldosterone acts by promoting the exchange of potassium for sodium in the distal tubule. The glomerular filtration rate is normal in this case, but due to decreased distal secretion of potassium, potassium excretion is impaired.

HYPOKALEMIA

Pathophysiology

Hypokalemia can occur either through shifting from ECF to ICF or through total body potassium depletion via gastrointestinal losses (distal to the stomach) or urinary losses (Table 41.7). Gastric secretion contains only 10 mEq/L of K^+, but hypovolemia associated with vomiting/NG suction stimulates aldosterone with sodium retention and potassium excretion. Shifting of potassium into the intracellular compartment is a physiologic process that normally occurs in response to insulin secretion. Without this process, a meal could lead to a dangerously high potassium level since the total amount of potassium contained within the extracellular space is quite low. β_2-adrenergic stimulation is another avenue for cellular uptake of potassium. This is clinically significant as β_2 agonists can be used to transiently treat hyperkalemia and possibly lead to hypokalemia in certain clinical settings.

TABLE 41.7

COMMON CAUSES OF HYPOKALEMIA

Potassium shift into cells
Alkalosis, recovery from diabetic ketoacidosis, β_2-agonists, insulin
Gastrointestinal potassium losses
Vomiting, nasogastric suction, diarrhea
Renal potassium losses
Diuretics, hypomagnesemia, hyperaldosteronism, drugs (amphotericin B, cisplatin), proximal (type II) and distal (type I) renal tubular acidosis (RTA), Bartter and Gitelman syndromes.
Decreased potassium intake

Intestinal secretion contains 30–60 mEq/L of potassium.
Gastric secretion contains only 10 mEq/L of potassium, and hypokalemia may be a result of hypovolemia with stimulation of aldosterone. Aldosterone will lead to sodium retention and potassium excretion in the kidneys.
From {MKSAP 2006}.

Clinical Manifestations

The effects of hypokalemia are related to the effect of low potassium on neuromuscular transmission and conduction in the heart. A decrease in extracellular potassium makes the membrane less excitable and muscle weakness results. Hypokalemia can lead to arrhythmias (especially in patients on digitalis or with heart disease). Other effects include ileus, muscular cramps, augmented ammonia production in the kidney (which can potentiate hepatic encephalopathy), and rhabdomyolysis. Hypokalemia is often associated with hypomagnesemia, and serum magnesium status should be assessed in all patients with hypokalemia.

Management of Hypokalemia

Potassium can be replaced with potassium chloride (KCl). For severe hypokalemia, potassium chloride should be given intravenously (IV) at a rate of 10 to 20 mEq per hour. Hypomagnesemia should also be corrected if present. Total body potassium deficits are typically large (200–300 mmol for serum potassium of 3.0 mEq/L, i.e., for each 1 mEq below normal), and repeated replacements may be needed with serial measurements (50).

Since K^+ is a major intracellular cation, serum levels may not reflect the severity of deficiency.

Case Scenario: Hypokalemia Associated with Metabolic Acidosis
A 21-year-old woman is admitted for a 1-week history of muscular weakness and shortness of breath. Her past medical history is insignificant except for a history of dental caries and dry eyes. Her admission laboratories are listed below:

Sodium (mEq/L)	137
Potassium (mEq/L)	1.8
Chloride (mEq/L)	115
Bicarbonate (mEq/L)	9
BUN (mg/dL)	16
Creatinine (mg/dL)	0.9
Glucose (mg/dL)	110
Arterial pH	7.09
PCO_2	14
PO_2	115

The patient is placed in the intensive care unit on a cardiac monitor.

What is the most likely diagnosis? This is a dramatic presentation of distal renal tubular acidosis with profound hypokalemia. Her history is suggestive of Sjögren syndrome, which can be complicated by distal renal tubular acidosis (52).

What is the next appropriate step in electrolyte and acid-base management? Replete potassium with intravenous potassium chloride. It is important not to treat this patient initially with alkali therapy; this can lead to shifting of potassium intracellularly and fatal hypokalemia. Once her potassium has been corrected, she can be treated with intravenous sodium bicarbonate.

DISORDERS OF DIVALENT IONS

The divalent ions phosphorus, calcium, and magnesium play important roles in cellular function such as regulation of enzymes and energy metabolism. In critical illness, the homeostasis of these ions is often altered, and abnormal levels are commonly encountered. The best treatment of these conditions requires knowledge of the pathophysiology of the alterations in the levels in these ions.

Phosphate Homeostasis

Phosphate is important for many basic processes of cellular metabolism and bone metabolism. Clinically in the intensive care setting, the need for phosphate for proper cellular energy metabolism through high-energy phosphate compounds (e.g., adenosine triphosphate) is among the most important. Phosphate is obtained in the diet primarily through protein intake. The typical Western diet contains sufficient phosphate to meet metabolic demands; however, in patients with poor nutritional status, often seen in alcoholics, hypophosphatemia may develop. The phosphate excretion in the kidney is regulated by several factors that favor tubular phosphate reabsorption (such as insulin, prostaglandin E_2, and thyroid hormone) and factors that inhibit phosphate reabsorption (such as parathyroid hormone and the newly characterized phosphaturic hormone FGF-23 that plays a role in hereditary and acquired phosphate-wasting disorders). Phosphate reabsorption is handled principally in the proximal tubule through the NPT2 sodium phosphate cotransporter. Therefore, disorders of the proximal tubule, such as Fanconi syndrome, may lead to renal phosphate wasting.

Hypophosphatemia

Pathophysiology

There are three major mechanisms of hypophosphatemia (Table 41.8): shifting of phosphate from the extracellular to the intracellular space, renal phosphate losses, and gastrointestinal losses. Very often the disorder occurs as a multifactorial disease with acid-base disturbances, decreased intake, and renal losses all contributing. Phosphate, like potassium and magnesium, is mainly an intracellular ion. Therefore, low serum phosphate usually represents significant total body phosphate depletion. Hypophosphatemia commonly occurs in alcoholics and in hospitalized patients. The diagnosis is usually evident from the history; however, if the cause is in doubt, renal phosphate losses can be assessed by calculating the fractional excretion of phosphorus.

$$\frac{[\text{P}]\text{u} \times [\text{Cr}]\text{pl}}{[\text{P}]\text{pl} \times [\text{Cr}]\text{u}} = \text{fractional excretion of phosphorus}$$

where P is phosphorus level, u is urine, pl is plasma, and Cr is creatinine level.

This will help discern if the phosphate losses are gastrointestinal (GI) in origin or if the losses are in the urine. The fractional excretion of phosphorus should be measured at a time when serum phosphorus is low, and if the fractional excretion of phosphorus is below 5%, the kidney is appropriately conserving phosphate and therefore the losses are extrarenal. In critically ill patients, there are many common conditions and

TABLE 41.8

CAUSES OF HYPOPHOSPHATEMIA

Decreased phosphate absorption, GI phosphate losses
- Alcoholism/poor nutrition
- Diarrhea
- GI tract surgery
- Ingestion of phosphate-binding medications or antacids
- TPN preparations with inadequate phosphorus
- Vitamin D deficiency
- Use of corticosteroids

Shifting of phosphate from extracellular space
- Refeeding syndrome
- Respiratory alkalosis
- Hungry bone syndrome
- High-grade lymphoma, acute leukemia
- Administration of glucagon, epinephrine

Increased renal losses of phosphate
- Hyperparathyroidism
- Fanconi syndrome (proximal tubular dysfunction seen in several diseases especially multiple myeloma)
- Diuretics, especially carbonic anhydrase inhibitors
- Acute volume expansion
- Amphotericin B
- Oncogenic osteomalacia
- Hypophosphatemic rickets (X-linked and AD)

AD, autosomal dominant; GI, gastrointestinal; TPN, total parenteral nutrition.
From {MKSAP 2006}.

circumstances that set the patient up to be at risk for hypophosphatemia. Alcoholism, nasogastric suction, malnutrition, extensive bowel resection, malignancy, low sun exposure, and diuretic use are among the conditions seen in ICU patients that are associated with hypophosphatemia.

Clinical Manifestations

Symptoms are often absent in mild cases. In severe depletion, muscular weakness (especially large muscle groups, proximal extremity weakness), arrhythmias, rhabdomyolysis, hypotension, hypoventilation, seizures, coma, and hemolytic anemia may occur. The most life threatening is cardiac and ventilatory failure. Other undesirable effects of hypophosphatemia are the following: shift of oxygen dissociation curve to the left from deficiency of 2,3,DPG; depressed immune function (chemotaxis, phagocytosis, bacteriocidal activity); platelet dysfunction (adhesion and aggregation); metabolic acidosis (impaired bicarbonate resorption and ammonia production); and abnormal glucose metabolism from decreased entry into the cell to make high-energy phosphates.

Treatment

Phosphorus replacement in asymptomatic patients should be oral and can be given as a potassium or sodium salt. Parenteral phosphorus administration should be undertaken in symptomatic patients or in patients with severe depletion (<1.0 mg/dL) or when the oral route is not appropriate. Parenteral phosphate preparations are generally ordered in millimoles. One millimole (mmol) of phosphate equals 31 mg of phosphorus. Since phosphate is administered as either a sodium salt or a potassium salt, intolerance to either of these should be considered in settings such as renal failure or congestive heart failure. Phosphate replacement should be judicious in patients with renal failure as significant hyperphosphatemia can occur.

Case Scenario: Refeeding Syndrome

A 37-year-old man with a long history of alcoholism is admitted to the intensive care unit with severe pancreatitis. His friends state that for the last several weeks he has been drinking beer all day and has been eating very little except for salty snacks. Over the course of the next 3 days, his ICU course is complicated by development of sepsis and a pancreatic abscess that has required drainage. Five days into his hospital course he remains on mechanical ventilation and vasopressor support. On this day, his chemistry panel is given below:

Serum	
Sodium (mEq/L)	136
Potassium (mEq/L)	4.3
Chloride (mEq/L)	105
Bicarbonate (mEq/L)	22
BUN (mg/dL)	6
Creatinine (mg/dL)	0.6
Calcium (mg/dL)	7.0
Albumin (g/dL)	2.7
Phosphorus (mg/dL)	2.1
Magnesium (mg/dL)	2.0
Glucose (mg/dL)	98

He is started on total parenteral nutrition with 2,000 total calories, 20% from fat. There is 120 mEq of sodium and 80 mEq of potassium, and the total volume is 2 L a day.

This patient is at high risk for which complications following the institution of total parenteral nutrition? Answer: Refeeding syndrome and rhabdomyolysis.

Learning Points:

- Refeeding syndrome is a potential complication in patients who are malnourished and suddenly given a large calorie load.
- Rhabdomyolysis is a potentially severe complication of the refeeding syndrome.

This patient is at high risk for the refeeding syndrome, and therefore the potential for rhabdomyolysis is a concern (53). His history and laboratory values (low BUN and albumin) suggest malnutrition, and thus phosphate depletion is likely present despite the close-to-normal value for serum phosphate. The phosphate is sequestered in the intracellular compartment, and it is the intracellular depletion of phosphate that is critical. Once this patient is supplied with calories, especially carbohydrates, oxidative phosphorylation and generation of ATP will quickly deplete the intracellular phosphate and lead to rhabdomyolysis. The best means of preventing this complication from occurring is recognizing patients who are at high risk and monitoring serum phosphate closely.

Hyperphosphatemia

Pathophysiology

Hyperphosphatemia occurs primarily in the setting of impaired renal function and is not typically seen outside of iatrogenic causes in patients with normal kidney function. Significant phosphate loading can occur due to exogenous phosphate administration or as part of the tumor lysis syndrome (however, renal insufficiency also commonly complicates this condition). Occult sources of phosphate loading include sodium phosphate solutions (either orally or as an enema), which can produce significant and, in some rare cases, fatal outcomes. In renal failure, elevated serum phosphorus is associated with cardiovascular disease and cardiovascular mortality and should be avoided.

Clinical Manifestations

There are few overt symptoms of hyperphosphatemia, and the syndrome may be insidious. Nephrocalcinosis can complicate hyperphosphatemia and manifest as renal insufficiency. On rare occasions, acute dialysis may be indicated to treat hyperphosphatemia. Extended dialysis session (>4 hours) may be necessary as phosphorus mobilization is time dependent and phosphorus removal in short dialysis sessions is limited (54).

Case Scenario: Hyperphosphatemia as a Complication of Sodium Phosphate Administration

An 85-year-old man with a history of hypertension is admitted to the intensive care unit with refractory hypotension. His wife states that he had been complaining of constipation and had used several enemas at home over the past 48 hours. His wife then stated that he has become progressively lethargic throughout the day, and she called an ambulance because he fell after trying to get up from a chair and was severely confused. He takes only hydrochlorothiazide for hypertension and is otherwise without significant medical history. The physical exam is significant for blood pressure of 85/45 and pulse of 58; respirations are 8 breaths per minute, and he is afebrile. The physical exam is otherwise significant only for Chvostek sign.

The chemistry panel on admission is given below:

Serum	
Sodium (mEq/L)	149
Potassium (mEq/L)	4.5
Chloride (mEq/L)	109
Bicarbonate (mEq/L)	20
BUN (mg/dL)	23
Creatinine (mg/dL)	1.7
Calcium (mg/dL)	4.8
Albumin (g/dL)	3.8
Phosphorus (mg/dL)	8.2
Magnesium (mg/dL)	2.0
Glucose (mg/dL)	98

What risk factor for hyperphosphatemia did this patient have? Answer: Renal insufficiency put this patient at risk. The creatinine level of 1.7 in a patient of his age is indicative of significant decrease in GFR (estimated at 41 mL/minute). The use of hyperosmolar phosphate enemas is a risk in this population. The time that the solution is allowed to dwell determines the amount of phosphate absorbed. Fatal cases have been reported even in patients without renal failure (55). This patient is exhibiting signs of hypocalcemia, hypotension, and impending cardiovascular collapse that can occur with acute hyperphosphatemia.

Overview of Calcium Balance

Calcium concentration in plasma is tightly regulated. Intracellular calcium levels are very low whereas the total body calcium stores in the bone are plentiful. Calcium balance and the calcium concentration in the blood are maintained by regulatory processes that promote calcium influx into the extracellular fluid (mainly intestinal calcium absorption and release of calcium from bone demineralization) and remove calcium from the extracellular fluid (urinary calcium excretion and bone formation). Disturbances in serum calcium occur when there is an imbalance between these processes regulating calcium movement. The hormonal influences that regulate these processes are complex but involve the actions of two principal hormones: parathyroid hormone and calcitriol. Calcium exists in the plasma as protein-bound calcium and ionized calcium, usually measured in mmol/L. Measurement of the total serum calcium reflects the aggregate amount of these two pools of plasma calcium. Ionized calcium is the active component and the more important physiologically.

The total measured serum calcium needs to take into account changes in the amount of albumin, which is the predominant calcium-binding protein in the circulation. A simple correction for the total calcium based on perturbations of the serum albumin is the following: a reduction in plasma albumin of a 1 g/L will decrease the serum total calcium by 0.8 mg/dL (56). If the decrease in total serum calcium is within the range as would be expected based on the decrease in albumin, then it can be surmised that the ionized serum calcium is probably normal. The validity of this correction in critical illness has been questioned, possibly due to factors that affect binding of calcium to albumin. Measurement of ionized calcium levels in critically ill patients is a good practice, and results may be available within minutes of using point-of-care testing.

Hypocalcemia

Pathophysiology

The causes of hypocalcemia can be divided into either efflux of calcium out of the extracellular space or by decreased entry of calcium into the extracellular space (Table 41.9) (57). Under normal circumstances, homeostatic mechanisms can maintain serum calcium levels despite low intake by increasing mobilization from the bone. Hypocalcemia can result from decreased calcium absorption and decreased calcium mobilization from bone stores in hypoparathyroidism and vitamin D deficiency. Increased calcium removal from the serum occurs in severe pancreatitis through saponification of fats and in osteoblastic metastatic disease (Table 41.9). The ionized calcium is the important factor for determining severity, and conditions that alter protein binding of calcium in the blood may precipitate symptomatic hypocalcemia. Alkalemia will increase the affinity of albumin for calcium (through altering the net charge of the protein) and will lower the ionized calcium. Acute increases in total albumin may lower ionized calcium. Risk factors for hypocalcemia include the following: neck irradiation, parathyroid surgery, renal transplantation in patients with tertiary hyperparathyroidism, malignancy, alcoholism, low sun exposure, and malnutrition.

Clinical Manifestations

The clinical manifestations include altered mental status and tetany (Chvostek and Trousseau signs). The association between hypocalcemia and sepsis is not well understood although it is now recognized that elevated intracellular calcium levels are a common mechanism for cell death. Possible mechanisms for the association of sepsis and hypocalcemia are parathyroid hormone (PTH) insufficiency, altered vitamin D metabolism, hypomagnesemia, chelation of calcium by lactate and also calcitonin precursors (58–62). Hypocalcemia in critical illness is a common finding and is often asymptomatic.

TABLE 41.9

CAUSES OF HYPOCALCEMIA

Hypoparathyroidism/pseudohypoparathyroidism
Hyperphosphatemia
Hypomagnesemia
Vitamin D deficiency
- Dietary deficit
- Reduced sun exposure
- Decreased 25-hydroxylation of vitamin D (liver disease, alcoholism)
- Decreased vitamin D–sensitive rickets type 1 (1-α hydroxylase deficiency) and type 2 (receptor deficiency)

Renal failure (reduced 1-hydroxylation of vitamin D)
Osteoblastic metastases (prostate, breast)
Saponification in severe pancreatitis
Citrate load (blood transfusion)

From {MKSAP 2006}.

Management of Hypocalcemia

One of the first questions to be addressed in approaching a patient with altered levels of serum calcium is to what degree is the ionized calcium altered and why? If the ionized calcium is decreased due to chelation from hyperphosphatemia, treatment of the hypocalcemia can be dangerous as it can precipitate vascular calcification. In sepsis, hypocalcemia is common and treatment is not usually necessary unless cardiovascular collapse with ionized calcium levels of less than 0.8 mmol/L is present. Data from animal models suggest that it may be harmful to treat hypocalcemia in the setting of sepsis (63,64). There are no randomized clinical studies to guide treatment of hypocalcemia in sepsis, and treatment should be reserved for those with symptomatic hypocalcemia and/or severe hypocalcemia. Reflex treatment of hypocalcemia without consideration of the underlying cause (especially in the setting of hyperphosphatemia) can be detrimental: therefore, it is important to determine the cause and degree of symptoms before deciding to initiate therapy.

For acute symptomatic hypocalcemia, administer intravenous calcium chloride or calcium gluconate (56). Calcium gluconate is advantageous because it is less caustic to veins. Calcium should not be infused more rapidly than 2.5 to 5 mmol in 20 minutes because of the risk of cardiac abnormalities and asystole. Intravenous calcium will transiently normalize the calcium level, and an infusion should be started following the bolus, especially in settings where there is an ongoing process such as the hungry bone syndrome following parathyroidectomy. Magnesium deficiency, by inducing resistance to the actions of parathyroid hormone, can be an important cause of hypocalcemia in the critical care setting. If magnesium deficiency is the cause, calcium levels should return to normal once magnesium is replaced.

Case Scenario: Hypocalcemia Associated with Sepsis

A 43-year-old man with end-stage liver disease secondary to chronic hepatitis C infection presents with shortness of breath and abdominal pain. He has significant ascites and has decreased urine output for the last week. His appetite has been very poor over the last week although he has no other complaints. His blood pressure is 71/50, pulse is 86, and temperature 98.4°F. Admission labs are given below:

Sodium (mEq/L)	131
Potassium (mEq/L)	4.9
Chloride (mEq/L)	108
Bicarbonate (mEq/L)	20
BUN (mg/dL)	24
Creatinine (mg/dL)	1.6
Albumin (mg/dL)	2.4
Calcium (mg/dL)	6.8
Phosphorus (mg/dL)	2.8
Glucose (mg/dL)	78

He is admitted to the intensive care unit and treated with broad-spectrum antibiotics and vasopressor for presumed septic shock.

What considerations should be taken in determining if this hypocalcemia should be treated? Answer: The cause is an important factor. This is likely a case of mild hypocalcemia due to sepsis. Check the ionized calcium level, serum magnesium level, and assess the degree of symptoms including electrocardiogram. If the serum magnesium level is decreased, this should be treated. If the ionized calcium is <0.8 mmol/L or if the patient appears to be symptomatic, the patient may benefit from treatment with intravenous calcium.

Key Point:

- Sepsis is a common cause of hypocalcemia. Check the level of ionized calcium and magnesium in critically ill patients with hypocalcemia.

Hypercalcemia

Pathophysiology

Hypercalcemia is caused by entrance of calcium into the intravascular space in excess of renal excretion and calcium incorporation into bone. Two sources of calcium influx into the intravascular space are intestinal absorption and bone reabsorption. The most common causes are primary hyperparathyroidism, malignancy, and granulomatous diseases. Other causes are listed in Table 41.10. Additionally, hypercalcemia can be caused by decreased renal excretion as occurs in primary hyperparathyroidism and thiazide diuretics. Total calcium must be corrected for serum albumin because of protein binding, and ionized calcium should be measured in hypercalcemic patients.

Clinical Manifestations

Hypercalcemia produces a decrease in neuromuscular excitability and decreased muscular tone. Clinical manifestations of hypercalcemia include: lethargy, confusion, coma, nausea, constipation, polyuria, and hypertension. Hypercalcemia can lead to volume depletion, nephrolithiasis, and nephrogenic diabetes insipidus.

Approach to Diagnosis

The causes of hypercalcemia are listed in Table 41.10. The first step is to measure PTH level. The normal response of the parathyroid gland in the presence of elevated ionized calcium levels is to decrease secretion of parathyroid hormone. Failure to suppress parathyroid hormone secretion in the face of

TABLE 41.10

CAUSES OF HYPERCALCEMIA

Excess calcium influx into vascular space
- –Primary hyperparathyroidism (usually adenoma, gland hyperplasia; parathyroid malignancy is rare)
- –Malignancy (multiple myeloma, carcinomas through production of PTH-related peptide, osteosarcomas)
- –Immobilization
- –Granulomatous disease (increased vitamin D production?)
  - –Sarcoidosis
  - –Tuberculosis
- –Paget disease
- –Milk-alkali syndrome
- –Vitamin D intoxication
- –Hyperparathyroidism (stimulation of osteoclasts)

Decreased calcium excretion
- –Primary hyperparathyroidism
- –Thiazide diuretics
- –Familial hypocalciuric hypercalcemia

PTH, parathyroid hormone.
From {MKSAP 2006}.

hypercalcemia denotes hyperparathyroidism. Primary hyperparathyroidism is among the most common causes of hypercalcemia in the general population but typically does not result in severe, symptomatic hypercalcemia. In hypercalcemia of malignancy, parathyroid hormone is usually suppressed (this is the normal response of the parathyroid gland). PTH-related peptide (PTHrp) should also be ordered if malignancy is suspected as many cancers express this protein product that stimulates PTH receptors (65). Additionally, 1,25-hydroxyvitamin D and 25-hydroxyvitamin D levels can be helpful if abnormal vitamin D metabolism is suspected. Certain granulomatous conditions lead to increased 1,25 vitamin D (66), and in cases of vitamin D intoxication, high levels of 25-OH vitamin D reflective of total body vitamin D stores may be seen (67).

Management of Hypercalcemia

In most patients with symptomatic hypercalcemia, volume depletion occurs and one of the first steps is volume repletion with intravenous saline (0.9% saline is the treatment of choice). This replacement of the extracellular volume will increase calcium excretion in the urine. Caution is advised in infusing large amounts of saline to an oliguric patient. After fluid resuscitation, normal saline should be continued and furosemide can also be given to increase urinary calcium excretion. A common mistake is to administer furosemide at the same time as starting fluid resuscitation. Diuretics should not be given until the patient is completely volume resuscitated. The action of loop diuretics is distinct from that of thiazide diuretics. Loop diuretics act in the ascending limb of Henle and will promote calcium excretion in the urine. Thiazide diuretics act more distally in the nephron and will decrease calcium excretion. Bisphosphonates are good long-term treatment for hypercalcemia of malignancy by impairing bone reabsorption, but these agents must be used with caution in patients with renal insufficiency (Table 41.11). Calcitonin is usually effective in the short term, but tachyphylaxis develops. It is best used early in the management while waiting for diuresis to remove calcium from the body. In patients with renal failure, dialysis is usually necessary to treat symptomatic hypercalcemia.

Case Scenario: Hypercalcemia of Malignancy

A 46-year-old man with a 1-year history of pain in his legs and back is brought to the emergency room for decreased mental status. His wife states that he is very active and works as an attorney, but he has been easily fatigable over the last several months. Over the last 12 hours, he has gotten progressively more lethargic and is difficult to arouse.

Sodium (mEq/L)	136
Potassium (mEq/L)	4.8
Chloride (mEq/L)	108
Bicarbonate (mEq/L)	16
BUN (mg/dL)	51
Creatinine (mg/dL)	5.8
Albumin (mg/dL)	3.8
Calcium (mg/dL)	16.8
Magnesium (mg/dl)	2.8
Phosphorus (mg/dL)	4.6
Glucose (mg/dL)	98

A Foley catheter is inserted, and the urine output is 50 mL. In the emergency room, he is administered 2 L of 0.9% NaCl intravenously, and over the next 2 hours there is no urine output.

What is the next appropriate step in management of hypercalcemia in this patient? Answer: This patient should undergo emergency hemodialysis, which can be used in cases of renal failure and severe hypercalcemia (68). From history, this patient likely has multiple myeloma with complications of this disorder: hypercalcemia and renal failure. It is appropriate to give a volume challenge with normal saline to treat prerenal azotemia. However, with no urine output after 2 L of saline, acute renal failure is likely, and hemodialysis offers the best treatment for severe hypercalcemia. The patient should be dialyzed on a hypocalcemic bath in an intensive care setting, with cardiac monitoring and very close monitoring of the ionized calcium.

TABLE 41.11

TREATMENT OF SEVERE HYPERCALCEMIA

1. Replete intravascular volume with normal saline.
2. Use intravenous furosemide to increase calcium excretion (after volume repletion).
3. In hypercalcemia of malignancy, use bisphosphonates to decrease calcium reabsorption from the bone.
4. Adjunctive therapy includes calcitonin (effect is usually short term; tachyphylaxis develops).
5. Start hemodialysis.

Hypomagnesemia

Pathophysiology

Magnesium depletion occurs in many conditions (Table 41.12) and is common in critical illness (69). Hypomagnesemia, because of its effect on the myocardial membrane, is important to identify, especially in those with known (or at risk for) cardiac arrhythmias. Sources of magnesium loss can be through urinary losses or also in the GI tract. Often, inadequate intake in malnourished patients is the principal cause of the magnesium deficiency. High-risk patients at particular risk for hypomagnesemia include hospitalized patients, alcoholics, and intensive

TABLE 41.12

CAUSES OF HYPOMAGNESEMIA

Gastrointestinal losses
- Diarrhea
- Nasogastric suction
- Malabsorption
- Steatorrhea
- Extensive bowel resection
- Acute pancreatitis
- Intestinal fistula

Urinary losses
- Diuretics, aminoglycosides, cisplatin, alcohol
- Pentamidine, foscarnet, cyclosporine, amphotericin B
- Phosphorus depletion
- Metabolic acidosis

From {MKSAP 2006}.

care unit patients. Magnesium depletion has effects on the homeostasis of other ions, and therefore, magnesium depletion often occurs in the presence of hypokalemia and hypocalcemia. Magnesium depletion causes a potassium-wasting state, and patients with hypokalemia should be assessed for magnesium depletion. Hypomagnesemia induces a state of reduced parathyroid hormone secretion and PTH resistance. Tissue magnesium depletion can be present in the absence of decreased serum magnesium levels (since most magnesium is in the intracellular space), and that tissue depletion can lead to adverse outcomes (70).

Decreased total serum magnesium levels are common in critically ill patients. This is often due to a decrease in serum albumin, which is the principal binding protein of magnesium, and many of these patients do not have decreased ionized magnesium levels (69). The correlation of ionized hypomagnesemia and mortality in ICU patients is controversial (69). Magnesium is not actively mobilized from a body pool (unlike calcium), and therefore, serum levels are very dependent on intake. If magnesium intake is exceeded by magnesium loss (e.g., urinary losses), then the serum magnesium levels will be decreased.

Clinical Manifestations

The most serious consequences of hypomagnesemia are its cardiovascular effects. Hypomagnesemia is associated with poor outcomes in acute myocardial infarction and may predispose to arrhythmias (71). Magnesium treatment may decrease arrhythmias after myocardial infarction, but studies conflict on whether outcomes are improved with magnesium treatment (72–74). Magnesium depletion increases the risk of torsades des pointes, a form of polymorphic ventricular tachycardia. Intravenous magnesium is regarded as treatment for torsades des pointes and refractory ventricular tachycardia even in the absence of documented hypomagnesemia. Additionally, hypomagnesemia may contribute to atrial arrhythmias following cardiopulmonary bypass (75) Other manifestations include altered mental status, seizures, and muscular weakness. Magnesium is an important cofactor for multiple enzyme function (including ATPase) and an essential electrolyte.

Treatment of Hypomagnesemia

For acutely symptomatic patients, parenteral administration should be undertaken. In asymptomatic patients, the oral route should be used although absorption is variable. Parenterally administered magnesium inhibits magnesium reabsorption in the ascending limb of Henle, and much of a parenterally administered dose may be wasted in the urine. For patients with severe manifestations, 8 to 16 mEq should be administered intravenously in 5 to 10 minutes followed by 48 mEq over the next 24 hours.

Case Scenario: Hypomagnesemia and Associated Electrolyte Disturbances

A 56-year-old man is admitted to the surgical intensive care unit after an emergency coronary artery bypass performed following the dissection of his left anterior descending artery during an attempted percutaneous coronary intervention. He has a history of hypertension, smoking, and alcohol abuse. His medications are atenolol and aspirin. His surgery was uncomplicated, and his urine output was 70 mL per hour. His chemistry panel on admission to the intensive care unit is given:

Sodium (mEq/L)	138
Potassium (mEq/L)	3.1
Chloride (mEq/L)	106
Bicarbonate (mEq/L)	24
BUN (mg/dL)	22
Creatinine (mg/dL)	1.4
Albumin (mg/dL)	3.7
Calcium (mg/dL)	7.3
Magnesium (mg/dL)	1.3
Phosphorus (mg/dL)	2.4
Ionized calcium (mmol/L)	0.8
Glucose (mg/dL)	98

Treatment of hypomagnesemia in this patient is likely to improve which other electrolyte disorders in this patient? Answer: magnesium deficiency due to poor dietary intake is the most likely cause of both the hypokalemia and hypocalcemia. Treatment of the hypomagnesemia will likely lead to resolution of the hypocalcemia. Potassium replacement should be given as well, as hypomagnesemia has lead to renal potassium wasting.

Hypermagnesemia

Pathophysiology

Hypermagnesemia is not a common condition, and it is often iatrogenic. Magnesium is readily excreted by the kidney in patients with normal renal function, and this disorder is uncommon except in cases of large ingestions (Epsom salt and magnesium-containing cathartics). In the presence of gastrointestinal disease such as peptic ulcer disease, magnesium absorption can be enhanced, and magnesium-containing antacids in this setting can lead to toxic hypermagnesemia (76). Patients with renal failure are at highest risk for developing hypermagnesemia, and the administration of magnesium-containing cathartics to these patients can be fatal (77). Clinical manifestations of hypermagnesemia include hypotension, bradycardia, respiratory depression, decreased mental status, and ECG abnormalities.

Management

Removal of the offending agent may be sufficient in mild cases with normal renal function. In symptomatic hypermagnesemia, the neuromuscular membrane can be stabilized by administration of 1 g of calcium chloride intravenously over 5 to 10 minutes. Dialysis is usually necessary in the setting of renal insufficiency or severe toxicity.

Case Scenario: Hypermagnesemia and Risk Factors for Development

An 84-year-old man is brought in from a nursing home with decreased level of consciousness. He has a past medical history significant for hypertension and peptic ulcer disease. He was recently diagnosed with a gastric ulcer and erosive esophagitis by esophagogastroduodenoscopy, and he has been taking lansoprazole. He has had continuous heartburn and symptoms, and he has been taking antacids frequently according to his wife. His physical exam is significant for blood pressure of 85/40 and pulse of 72. Respiratory rate is 8 breaths per minute.

Sodium (mEq/L)	138
Potassium (mEq/L)	4.0
Chloride (mEq/L)	106
Bicarbonate (mEq/L)	22
BUN (mg/dL)	23
Creatinine (mg/dL)	1.5
Albumin (mg/dL)	3.9
Calcium (mg/dL)	7.3
Magnesium (mg/dL)	6.8
Phosphorus (mg/dL)	2.2
Glucose (mg/dL)	91

Why did this patient develop severe hypermagnesemia? Answer: this patient has two risk factors that predisposed to the development of hypermagnesemia. He has chronic renal dysfunction, which was not appreciated by the treating physicians. He also has gastrointestinal disease, which can increase the absorption of magnesium from the gut, especially in magnesium-containing antacids.

References

1. Dunn FL, Brennan TJ, Nelson AE, et al. The role of blood osmolality and volume in regulating vasopressin secretion in the rat. *J Clin Invest.* 1973;52(12):3212–3219.
2. Arieff AI, Ayus JC. Endometrial ablation complicated by fatal hyponatremic encephalopathy. *JAMA.* 1993;270(10):1230–1232.
3. Arieff AI, Ayus JC. Pathogenesis of hyponatremic encephalopathy. Current concepts. *Chest.* 1993;103(2):607–610.
4. Ayus JC, Levine R, Arieff AI. Fatal dysnatraemia caused by elective colonoscopy. *BMJ.* 2003;326(7385):382–384.
5. Arieff AI, Ayus JC, Fraser CL. Hyponatraemia and death or permanent brain damage in healthy children. *BMJ.* 1992;304(6836):1218–1222.
6. Ayus JC, Krothapalli RK, Arieff AI. Treatment of symptomatic hyponatremia and its relation to brain damage. A prospective study. *N Engl J Med.* 1987;317(19):1190–1195.
7. Ayus JC, Wheeler JM, Arieff AI. Postoperative hyponatremic encephalopathy in menstruant women. *Ann Intern Med.* 1992;117(11):891–897.
8. Nielsen S, Nagelhus EA, Amiry-Moghaddam M, et al. Specialized membrane domains for water transport in glial cells: high-resolution immunogold cytochemistry of aquaporin-4 in rat brain. *J Neurosci.* 1997;17(1):171–180.
9. Agre P, Preston GM, Smith BL, et al. Aquaporin CHIP: the archetypal molecular water channel. *Am J Physiol.* 1993;265(4 Pt 2):F463–476.
10. Nielsen S, Smith BL, Christensen EI, et al. Distribution of the aquaporin CHIP in secretory and resorptive epithelia and capillary endothelia. *Proc Natl Acad Sci U S A.* 1993;90(15):7275–7279.
11. Simard M, Arcuino G, Takano T, et al. Signaling at the gliovascular interface. *J Neurosci.* 2003;23(27):9254–9262.
12. Amiry-Moghaddam M, Ottersen OP. The molecular basis of water transport in the brain. *Nat Rev Neurosci.* 2003;4(12):991–1001.
13. Dolman D, Drndarski S, Abbott NJ, et al. Induction of aquaporin 1 but not aquaporin 4 messenger RNA in rat primary brain microvessel endothelial cells in culture. *J Neurochem.* 2005;93(4):825–833.
14. Abbott NJ, Ronnback L, Hansson E. Astrocyte-endothelial interactions at the blood-brain barrier. *Nat Rev Neurosci.* 2006;7(1):41–53.
15. Simard M, Nedergaard M. The neurobiology of glia in the context of water and ion homeostasis. *Neuroscience.* 2004;129(4):877–896.
16. Paulson OB, Newman EA. Does the release of potassium from astrocyte endfeet regulate cerebral blood flow? *Science.* 1987;237(4817):896–898.
17. Manley GT, Fujimura M, Ma T, et al. Aquaporin-4 deletion in mice reduces brain edema after acute water intoxication and ischemic stroke. *Nat Med.* 2000;6(2):159–163.
18. Reulen HJ, Tsuyumu M, Tack A, et al. Clearance of edema fluid into cerebrospinal fluid. A mechanism for resolution of vasogenic brain edema. *J Neurosurg.* 1978;48(5):754–764.
19. Olson JE, Sankar R, Holtzman D, et al. Energy-dependent volume regulation in primary cultured cerebral astrocytes. *J Cell Physiol.* 1986;128(2):209–215.
20. Melton JE, Patlak CS, Pettigrew KD, et al. Volume regulatory loss of Na, Cl, and K from rat brain during acute hyponatremia. *Am J Physiol.* 1987;252(4 Pt 2):F661–669.
21. Blanco G, Mercer RW. Isozymes of the Na-K-ATPase: heterogeneity in structure, diversity in function. *Am J Physiol.* 1998;275(5 Pt 2):F633–650.
22. Moritz ML, Ayus JC. The pathophysiology and treatment of hyponatraemic encephalopathy: an update. *Nephrol Dial Transplant.* 2003;18(12):2486–2491.
23. Achinger SG, Moritz ML, Ayus JC, et al. Why are patients still dying? *South Med J.* 2006;99(4):1–12.
24. Nzerue CM, Baffoe-Bonnie H, You W, et al. Predictors of outcome in hospitalized patients with severe hyponatremia. *J Natl Med Assoc.* 2003;95(5):335–343.
25. Arieff AI. Hyponatremia, convulsions, respiratory arrest, and permanent brain damage after elective surgery in healthy women. *N Engl J Med.* 1986;314(24):1529–1535.
26. Chen JQ, Contreras RG, Wang R, et al. Sodium/potassium ATPase (Na(+), K (+)-ATPase) and ouabain/related cardiac glycosides: a new paradigm for development of anti-breast cancer drugs? *Breast Cancer Res Treat.* 2006;96(1):1–15.
27. Davis RA, Kern F Jr, Showalter R, et al. Alterations of hepatic Na+,K+-atpase and bile flow by estrogen: effects on liver surface membrane lipid structure and function. *Proc Natl Acad Sci U S A.* 1978;75(9):4130–4134.
28. Fraser CL, Kucharczyk J, Arieff AI, et al. Sex differences result in increased morbidity from hyponatremia in female rats. *Am J Physiol.* 1989;256(4 Pt 2):R880–885.
29. Arieff AI, Kozniewska E, Roberts TP, et al. Age, gender, and vasopressin affect survival and brain adaptation in rats with metabolic encephalopathy. *Am J Physiol.* 1995;268(5 Pt 2):R1143–1152.
30. Fraser CL, Sarnacki P. Na+-K+-ATPase pump function in rat brain synaptosomes is different in males and females. *Am J Physiol.* 1989;257(2 Pt 1):E284–289.
31. Fraser CL, Swanson RA. Female sex hormones inhibit volume regulation in rat brain astrocyte culture. *Am J Physiol.* 1994;267(4 Pt 1):C909–914.
32. Vexler ZS, Ayus JC, Roberts TP, et al. Hypoxic and ischemic hypoxia exacerbate brain injury associated with metabolic encephalopathy in laboratory animals. *J Clin Invest.* 1994;93(1):256–264.
33. Hochachka PW, Buck LT, Doll CJ, et al. Unifying theory of hypoxia tolerance: molecular/metabolic defense and rescue mechanisms for surviving oxygen lack. *Proc Natl Acad Sci U S A.* 1996;93(18):9493–9498.
34. Ayus JC, Armstrong D, Arieff A. Hyponatremia with hypoxia: effects on brain adaptation, perfusion and histology in rodents. *Kidney Int* 2006;69(8):1318–1325.
35. Ayus JC, Arieff AI. Pulmonary complications of hyponatremic encephalopathy. Noncardiogenic pulmonary edema and hypercapnic respiratory failure. *Chest.* 1995;107(2):517–521.
36. Ayus JC, Varon J, Arieff AI. Hyponatremia, cerebral edema, and noncardiogenic pulmonary edema in marathon runners. *Ann Intern Med.* 2000;132(9):711–714.
37. McClellan MD, Dauber IM, Weil JV. Elevated intracranial pressure increases pulmonary vascular permeability to protein. *J Appl Physiol.* 1989;67(3):1185–1191.
38. Schrier RW, Gross P, Gheorghiade M, et al. Tolvaptan, a selective oral vasopressin V2-receptor antagonist, for hyponatremia. *N Engl J Med.* 2006;355(20):2099–2112.
39. Moritz ML, Ayus JC. Prevention of hospital-acquired hyponatremia: a case for using isotonic saline. *Pediatrics.* 2003;111(2):227–230.
40. Hew-Butler T, Almond C, Ayus JC, et al. Consensus statement of the 1st International Exercise-Associated Hyponatremia Consensus Development Conference, Cape Town, South Africa 2005. *Clin J Sport Med.* 2005;15(4):208–213.
41. Ayus JC, Arieff AI. Noncardiogenic pulmonary edema in marathon runners. *Ann Intern Med.* 2000;133(12):1011.
42. Heilig CW, Stromski ME, Blumenfeld JD, et al. Characterization of the major brain osmolytes that accumulate in salt-loaded rats. *Am J Physiol.* 1989;257(6 Pt 2):F1108–1116.
43. Lien YH, Shapiro JI, Chan L. Effects of hypernatremia on organic brain osmoles. *J Clin Invest.* 1990;85(5):1427–1435.
44. Ayus JC, Armstrong DL, Arieff AI. Effects of hypernatraemia in the central nervous system and its therapy in rats and rabbits. *J Physiol.* 1996;492 (Pt 1):243–255.
45. Moritz ML, Ayus JC. The changing pattern of hypernatremia in hospitalized children. *Pediatrics.* 1999;104(3 Pt 1):435–439.
46. Moritz ML, Ayus JC. Dysnatremias in the critical care setting. *Contrib Nephrol.* 2004;144:132–157.
47. Ayus JC, Krothapalli RK. Hyperglycemia (HG) associated with non-diabetic hypernatremia (NDH) patients. *J Am Soc Nephrol.* 1990;1:317A.
48. Halperin ML, Kamel KS. Potassium. *Lancet.* 1998;352(9122):135–140.
49. Schlanger LE, Kleyman TR, Ling BN. K(+)-sparing diuretic actions of trimethoprim: inhibition of Na+ channels in A6 distal nephron cells. *Kidney Int.* 1994;45(4):1070–1076.
50. Gennari FJ. Disorders of potassium homeostasis. Hypokalemia and hyperkalemia. *Crit Care Clin.* 2002;18(2):273–288, vi.
51. Leehey D, Gantt C, Lim V. Heparin-induced hypoaldosteronism. Report of a case. *JAMA.* 1981;246(19):2189–2190.
52. al-Jubouri MA, Jones S, Macmillan R, et al. Hypokalaemic paralysis revealing Sjögren syndrome in an elderly man. *J Clin Pathol.* 1999;52(2):157–158.
53. Marinella MA. Refeeding syndrome and hypophosphatemia. *J Intensive Care Med.* 2005;20(3):155–159.
54. Achinger SG, Ayus JC. The role of daily dialysis in the control of hyperphosphatemia. *Kidney Int Suppl.* 2005(95):s28–32.

55. Pitcher DE, Ford RS, Nelson MT, et al. Fatal hypocalcemic, hyperphosphatemic, metabolic acidosis following sequential sodium phosphate-based enema administration. *Gastrointest Endosc.* 1997;46(3):266–268.
56. Body JJ, Bouillon R. Emergencies of calcium homeostasis. *Rev Endocr Metab Disord.* 2003;4(2):167–175.
57. Tohme JF, Bilezikian JP. Hypocalcemic emergencies. *Endocrinol Metab Clin North Am.* 1993;22(2):363–375.
58. Zaloga GP, Chernow B. The multifactorial basis for hypocalcemia during sepsis. Studies of the parathyroid hormone-vitamin D axis. *Ann Intern Med.* 1987;107(1):36–41.
59. Robertson GM Jr., Moore EW, Switz DM, et al. Inadequate parathyroid response in acute pancreatitis. *N Engl J Med.* 1976;294(10):512–516.
60. Weir GC, Lesser PB, Drop LJ, et al. The hypocalcemia of acute pancreatitis. *Ann Intern Med.* 1975;83(2):185–189.
61. Hersh T, Siddiqui DA. Magnesium and the pancreas. *Am J Clin Nutr.* 1973;26(3):362–366.
62. Cooper DJ, Walley KR, Dodek PM, et al. Plasma ionized calcium and blood lactate concentrations are inversely associated in human lactic acidosis. *Intensive Care Med.* 1992;18(5):286–289.
63. Zaloga GP, Sager A, Black KW, et al. Low dose calcium administration increases mortality during septic peritonitis in rats. *Circ Shock.* 1992;37(3): 226–229.
64. Malcolm DS, Zaloga GP, Holaday JW. Calcium administration increases the mortality of endotoxic shock in rats. *Crit Care Med.* 1989;17(9):900–903.
65. Moseley JM, Kubota M, Diefenbach-Jagger H, et al. Parathyroid hormone-related protein purified from a human lung cancer cell line. *Proc Natl Acad Sci U S A.* 1987;84(14):5048–5052.
66. Adams JS, Singer FR, Gacad MA, et al. Isolation and structural identification of 1,25-dihydroxyvitamin D3 produced by cultured alveolar macrophages in sarcoidosis. *J Clin Endocrinol Metab.* 1985;60(5):960–966.
67. Dusso AS, Brown AJ, Slatopolsky E. Vitamin D. *Am J Physiol Renal Physiol.* 2005;289(1):F8–28.
68. Camus C, Charasse C, Jouannic-Montier I, et al. Calcium free hemodialysis: experience in the treatment of 33 patients with severe hypercalcemia. *Intensive Care Med.* 1996;22(2):116–121.
69. Soliman HM, Mercan D, Lobo SS, et al. Development of ionized hypomagnesemia is associated with higher mortality rates. *Crit Care Med.* 2003;31(4):1082–1087.
70. Ryzen E, Elkayam U, Rude RK. Low blood mononuclear cell magnesium in intensive cardiac care unit patients. *Am Heart J.* 1986;111(3):475–480.
71. Dyckner T. Serum magnesium in acute myocardial infarction. Relation to arrhythmias. *Acta Med Scand.* 1980;207(1–2):59–66.
72. Woods KL, Fletcher S, Roffe C, et al. Intravenous magnesium sulphate in suspected acute myocardial infarction: results of the second Leicester Intravenous Magnesium Intervention Trial (LIMIT-2). *Lancet.* 1992;339(8809):1553–1558.
73. ISIS-4: a randomised factorial trial assessing early oral captopril, oral mononitrate, and intravenous magnesium sulphate in 58,050 patients with suspected acute myocardial infarction. ISIS-4 (Fourth International Study of Infarct Survival) Collaborative Group. *Lancet.* 1995;345(8951):669–685.
74. Early administration of intravenous magnesium to high-risk patients with acute myocardial infarction in the Magnesium in Coronaries (MAGIC) Trial: a randomised controlled trial. *Lancet.* 2002;360(9341):1189–1196.
75. Maslow AD, Regan MM, Heindle S, et al. Postoperative atrial tachyarrhythmias in patients undergoing coronary artery bypass graft surgery without cardiopulmonary bypass: a role for intraoperative magnesium supplementation. *J Cardiothorac Vasc Anesth.* 2000;14(5):524–530.
76. Clark BA, Brown RS. Unsuspected morbid hypermagnesemia in elderly patients. *Am J Nephrol.* 1992;12(5):336–343.
77. Onishi S, Yoshino S. Cathartic-induced fatal hypermagnesemia in the elderly. *Intern Med.* 2006;45(4):207–210.

CHAPTER 42 ■ BLOOD GAS ANALYSIS AND ACID-BASE DISORDERS

STEVEN G. ACHINGER • JUAN CARLOS AYUS

Acid-base physiology is among the most complex topics in clinical medicine. Disturbances of this system are common in the critically ill, and important clinical decisions based on measured acid-base parameters occur on a daily, even hourly basis. Therefore, a sound understanding of acid-base physiology is mandatory for the intensivist.

The field is full of complicated concepts and equations that, at times, have only limited applicability to the practicing clinician due to the failure of any current model to faithfully and completely recapitulate the complex buffering process *in vivo*. The purpose of this chapter is to provide a conceptual introduction to the current approach to acid-base physiology, while de-emphasizing calculations and formulas. The goal is not to know how to derive the commonly used formulas, but rather to understand the meaning of measured and derived acid-base parameters that are used clinically, and how they may—or may not—help in answering three essential questions in the critically ill patient with an acid-base disturbance:

- What acid-base disorder(s) is (are) present?
- How severe is the disturbance?
- What is the etiology underlying the derangements?

MAINTENANCE OF THE ARTERIAL pH AND ACID-BASE BALANCE: BUFFERING AND ACID EXCRETION

Buffering of acids is the first line of defense against perturbations in systemic pH. Recall that the pH is a logarithmic scale that is a function of the concentration of H_3O^+ species in solution (H^+ will be used interchangeably with H_3O^+ in this chapter). In neutral solution, $[H^+]$ is $\times\ 10^{-7}$ M and $[OH^-]$ is 10^{-7} M; this satisfies the dissociation constant for water:

$$[H_2O] \leftrightarrow [H^+] + [OH^-]\,Ksp = 10^{-14} \qquad [1]$$

The pH, defined by Sorenson, is the negative log of the concentration of H^+. Therefore, in neutral solution, the pH is 7. This is a very small concentration of $[H^+]$, and therefore, addition of small amounts of $[H^+]$ to water will lead to significant fluctuations in pH. For example, we will consider an experiment performed by Jorgensen and Astrup (1) in which 1.25 mEq/L of HCl is added to hemolyzed human blood. Assuming that the blood contained no buffers (i.e., if the blood was imagined to be a container of water that starts at a neutral pH), the expected pH following such an infusion would be calculated by the following:

1.25×10^{-2} moles (number of moles of H^+ added)
$+\,1 \times 10^{-7}$ moles (number of moles of H^+ in neutral water)
$= 1.25 \times 10^{-2}$ moles/L.

Taking the negative log yields a pH of 1.9; this would be the expected pH if there were not buffers available. However, following the infusion, the pH of the blood changed approximately 0.2 pH points. This means that less than 1/10,000th of the H^+ added remains unbound in the blood. This illustrates the tremendous buffering capacity of the blood. A buffer can be thought of as a substance that, when present in solution, takes up $[H^+]$ and therefore resists change in pH when $[H^+]$ is added. The overall buffering system of the body is complex and includes several components. These are listed in Table 42.1. The most important system is the carbon dioxide–bicarbonate system, which is the principal buffer in the extracellular fluid. This buffering system is also very important clinically since it is the only buffering system where the two components (acid and conjugate base) are readily measurable in the extracellular fluid (ECF). Buffers work by binding the free H^+ as the conjugate base, which is a weak acid.

Buffers allow the body to resist acute changes in pH; however, buffering capacity will eventually be depleted if acid is continually added. For example, in humans, the net fixed acid production is approximately 70 to 100 mmol/day. It is the excretion of the daily acid load that ultimately allows the body to maintain acid-base balance. The excretion of the daily acid load occurs through two distinct mechanisms: (a) the renal excretion of fixed acid and (b) the respiratory excretion of volatile acid (i.e., carbon dioxide). Through the interconversion of bicarbonate, carbonic acid, and carbon dioxide, fixed and volatile acids can be buffered until they can be excreted through the urine or respiration (Fig. 42.1). In the lung, CO_2 is released, which ultimately leads to more H^+ reacting with HCO_3^- to generate water and more CO_2. In the kidneys, the entire filtered load of bicarbonate is—in order to avoid losing base—reabsorbed. When the kidney excretes one H^+ in the urine, one "new" HCO_3^- is generated. These two processes are both important in the excretion of the acid load, and modulation of these processes is also important in compensating for acid-base disturbances.

Urinary Excretion of Fixed Acids

In the reabsorption of bicarbonate, the corresponding H^+ produced in the process must be excreted in the urine. As most bicarbonate reabsorption occurs in the proximal tubule, the renal

TABLE 42.1

BLOOD AND EXTRACELLULAR FLUID BUFFERS

Acid	Conjugate base
H_2CO_3	HCO_3^-
Albumin-H	$Albumin^-$
H_2PO_4	HPO_4^-
Hgb-H	Hgb^-

secretion of H^+ is ten times greater in the proximal tubule—approximately 4,000 mmol/day—as compared with the distal tubule—approximately 400 mmol/day. However, in the distal tubule, there is a much higher luminal–intracellular H^+ gradient than that seen in the proximal tubule—a ratio of approximately 500:1. This high gradient is due to active secretion of H^+ into the tubule. If the excretion of acid occurred in the absence of buffers, the ability to excrete acid in the urine would be limited. In much the same way that the body can absorb large amounts of acid without much change in pH, the kidney accomplishes a similar task in the excretion of large amounts of fixed acid through the use of buffers in the urine with modestly acidic pH (approximately 5.5 under maximal conditions). The excretion of H^+ in the urine occurs with different conjugate bases, which are grouped as titratable acids—mostly phosphates—and nontitratable acids—ammonium. The excretion of titratable acid has a limit that is, for the most part, dependent on the filtered load of phosphate, as this is the main buffer for nontitratable acids. However, the kidney can generate its own buffer—ammonia; moreover, the renal capacity to generate ammonia and to excrete acid as ammonium under normal conditions is substantial. This capacity may be significantly up-regulated in the face of systemic acidosis. Ammonia is produced in the kidney, traverses the plasma membrane, and is "trapped" in the tubular lumen because the low pH drives the following reaction to the right, as the plasma membrane is much less permeable to the charged species ammonium.

$$NH_3 + H^+ \leftrightarrow NH_4^+ \quad [2]$$

Therefore, ammonia–ammonium acts as a urinary buffer system, allowing the elimination of one H^+ for nearly every ammonia produced. The buffering of acid in the urine, especially via ammonium, allows for substantial amounts of acid to be excreted without generating excessively acidic urine.

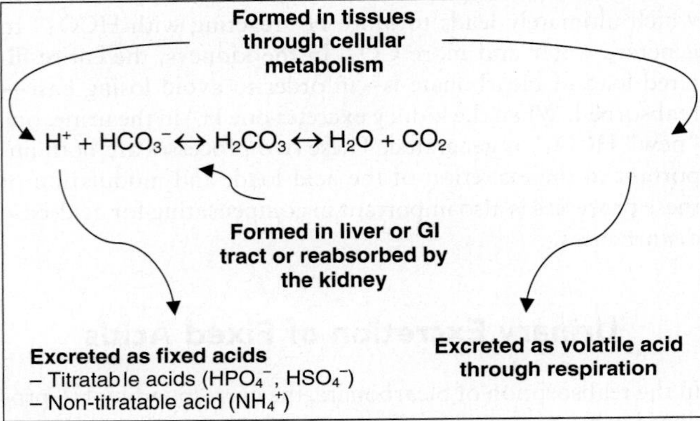

FIGURE 42.1. Normal acid-base homeostasis.

Titratable acids make up a relatively small proportion of the acid excreted and do not increase to near the degree that nontitratable acidity (ammonium) increases in the face of systemic acidosis.

The kidney, through active secretion of H^+ in the distal tubule, is able to achieve an H^+ concentration gradient of approximately 100:1 between the urine and the intracellular space of the tubular epithelial cells. This corresponds to the maximally acidic urine of approximately pH 5. Without any buffers, it would require 7,000 liters of urine to excrete a daily load of 70 mEq of acid in buffer-free urine of pH 5.0! Therefore, urinary buffers are very important in allowing the body to excrete the daily fixed acid load. Chronic metabolic acidosis stimulates the renal production of ammonia as a physiologic response; this response reaches its maximum production after several days.

Assessing Urinary Acid Excretion

In the presence of systemic acidosis, the kidney will compensate by increasing the excretion of fixed acids, mainly in the nontitratable form (i.e., ammonium). The increase in ammonium—which is a cation; recall that ammonia is predominantly in the form of NH_4^+ at a pH of 7 or below—excretion results in a perturbation in the electrolytes present in the urine. This manifests as a change in the urine anion gap where ammonium is the unmeasured anion. The urinary anion gap is a useful clinical test that can be used to gauge the amount of ammonium excreted in the urine without directly measuring it (2). It may be used to indirectly estimate the amount of ammonium in the urine and is calculated using the following formula:

$$[Na^+] + [K^+] - [Cl^+] = \text{urinary anion gap} \quad [3]$$

The urine anion gap is assessed in patients with metabolic acidosis and is used to determine if the renal response to the systemic acidosis is appropriate. In other words, the urine anion gap answers the question, Are the kidneys excreting the acid load appropriately or are the kidneys part of the acid-base problem? If the kidneys are excreting the acid load appropriately, there must be a nonrenal source of the acidosis—for example, diarrhea. Because ammonium is not a measured cation in this equation, the presence of significant amounts of ammonium causes an abundance of chloride relative to the measured cationic constituents of the urine (sodium and potassium). Therefore, if there is a high level of ammonium in the urine, the urine anion gap will be negative. The relationship between the amount of ammonium in the urine and the urine anion gap is illustrated in Figure 42.2. As a general rule, a negative urinary anion gap suggests that the kidney is excreting ammonium in the urine. This is a continuous variable, and the more negative the value, the greater the renal response. In the face of systemic acidosis, if the renal response is appropriate, there will be a high amount of ammonium in the urine, and the urine anion gap will be highly negative. This is sometimes referred to as a *negative net urinary charge*; however, this is a bit misleading because the urine is, of course, electroneutral; it is simply because we are not considering the contribution of ammonium that the net urinary charge seems negative. A

Scenario 1. *Small amount of NH_4+ in the urine.*
Urine anion gap close to zero or positive

$$[Na^+] + [K^+] + [NH_4^+] \sim [Cl^-] \longrightarrow [Na^+] + [K^+] \sim [Cl^-]$$

Scenario 2. *Large amount of NH_4+ in the urine.*
Urine anion gap very negative

$$[Na^+] + [K^+] + [NH_4^+] \sim [Cl^-] \longrightarrow [Na^+] + [K^+] < [Cl^-]$$

FIGURE 42.2. Effect of urine ammonium concentration on the urine anion gap.

highly negative urine anion gap is strong evidence that the renal response to metabolic acidosis is normal. Conversely, an anion gap that is near zero or positive suggests that there is little or no ammonium in the urine, which is reflected by a paucity of chloride in the urine relative to the concentration of measured cations. This is evidence that the kidney is not appropriately excreting ammonium in the urine and suggests a renal contribution to the acidosis. A caveat that is often clinically important is that the presence of unmeasured anions in the urine (such as β-hydroxybutyrate) may falsely depress the urinary anion gap, and therefore this test does have some limitations, such as during ketonuria.

RELATIONSHIP BETWEEN SYSTEMIC pH AND BUFFER CONCENTRATIONS: AN EVOLVING CONCEPT

We have previously noted that, because of the presence of buffers, addition of—or conversely, removal of—$[H^+]$ to the body does not produce the expected change in pH that would occur in unbuffered solutions. In this section, we will address the question of the relationship between pH and the concentrations of buffers.

Traditional Paradigm

One of the earliest observations in this field, and still very important clinically today, was the observation by Hendersen that the concentration of H^+ in the blood was dependent upon the concentration of CO_2, H_2CO_3, and HCO_3^-. The Henderson-Hasselbalch equation was later derived by using the Sorenson convention of expressing $[H^+]$ as pH. This relationship is usually expressed as:

$$pH = 6.1 + \log[HCO_3^-]/[H_2CO_3]$$

As the $[H_2CO_3]$ in plasma is related to the partial pressure of CO_2, this relationship can be rewritten as:

$$pH = 6.1 + \log([HCO_3^-]/0.03 \times PCO_2) \quad [4]$$

This relationship became very meaningful clinically as the methodologies to measure the key variables pH, HCO_3^-, and PCO_2 were developed. Now the concentration of the constituents of the principal buffering system could be related to the systemic pH. This allowed, among other things, a framework around which to understand how much alkali must be added in order to affect systemic pH in an acidemic patient. However, it became apparent that the relationship between pH, HCO_3^-, and PCO_2 failed to completely describe the relative contributions of fixed acids and volatile acids (the respiratory component) to acidosis. This is because PCO_2 and HCO_3^- are not truly independent of each other, as changes in one will lead to changes in the other, as will be seen later, according to the relationship given in Eq. 11. Additionally, it was noted that no single value accurately quantifies the degree of fixed acids present during metabolic acidosis or alkalosis. The degree of acidemia could be considered as simply the pH, as the pH is ultimately a composite of the net respiratory and metabolic components of the acid-base disturbance. However, because of the buffering capacity of the body, a quantification of the fixed acid derangement is not explained by this relationship alone.

Historically, several theoretical frameworks have been developed in an attempt to overcome this lack of exactitude in the concepts of quantification and etiology. The first obstacle to accurate quantification is the reality that the HCO_3^- system was not the only quantitatively important buffering system to be considered. The erythrocyte membrane is permeable to H^+, and therefore H^+ can diffuse inside the cell and hemoglobin can act as an intracellular buffer. Other buffering systems, such as phosphate and circulating proteins, can act as clinically relevant buffers as well (Table 42.1). By quantitative chemistry, the pH of a system is dependent on the relative concentrations of the acids and conjugate bases of all of the buffering systems present. Clinically, we measure accurately the concentration of the acid (CO_2) and conjugate base (HCO_3^-) of only one buffering system. Therefore, perturbations in the other buffering systems are not accounted for in the framework that only considers carbonate species.

Another major complicating factor is the fact that the human body is not a closed system. CO_2 is both continually being generated in the tissues and continually excreted through the respiratory system. Therefore, changes in CO_2 can, and frequently do, occur very rapidly in humans as the respiratory rate increases or decreases. Additionally, the kidney can modulate the production of HCO_3^- to adjust the HCO_3^- concentration and, albeit at a much slower pace than respiratory effects, change the pH. If the rate of HCO_3^- production exceeds consumption of HCO_3^-, the serum bicarbonate increases; conversely, if it is below the rate of production, HCO_3^- will decrease. What this means is that the concentration of the measured parameters—HCO_3^- and PCO_2—are not just dependent on the inciting insult—the disease process—that caused them to change, but also on the body's response to that change (i.e., compensation).

Base Excess and Standard Base Excess

The change in pH of a system is dependent on both the amount of acid (or base) added and that present on the buffering capacity. As acid is added to a buffered solution, for every H^+ that is buffered, one molecule of conjugate base of the buffer is consumed. Therefore, assessing changes in concentrations of the conjugate base is more helpful than the degree of change in the pH in quantifying the degree of fixed acids present. The difficulty in describing the buffering system of a patient is the inaccessibility for measurement of a fair proportion of the buffers (Table 42.1), especially intracellular buffers. Several expressions have been proposed to quantify the degree of acid loading based on the change in body buffers. The most commonly used concept in this regard is the *base excess*. Siggaard-Andersen defined the base excess of blood as the number of mEq of acid (or base) needed to titrate 1 L of blood to a pH of 7.4 at 37° C with a PCO_2 of 40 mm Hg; note that this is an experimentally arrived upon value. The standard base excess is the base excess corrected for changes in hemoglobin, recalling that hemoglobin is an important intracellular buffer. The base excess can be considered as a measurement of the "metabolic" portion of an acid-base disturbance since the concentration of CO_2 is being held constant at a normal level. The base excess has become a widely used parameter to characterize acid-base disturbances. One major drawback of the base excess is that it is a measured parameter of whole blood. However, *in vivo*, the blood is circulating and comes into contact with other tissues that can serve to provide buffering capacity. In clinical practice, however, the base excess is not measured by titration; rather, it is calculated from a nomogram that assumes normal nonbicarbonate buffers. This simplification, while allowing the widespread application of the base excess, has, in one sense, the drawback of losing the actual measurement of nonbicarbonate buffers that occurs when blood is directly titrated. Despite potential drawbacks, the base excess is very useful in describing the magnitude of a metabolic disturbance on the concentration of buffers and has become a widely used parameter to assess the degree of a metabolic disturbance.

The Anion Gap

The anion gap is calculated by taking the difference between the concentrations of the measured cations and the measured anion; it takes on a value of approximately 8 to 12 mEq/L in healthy individuals (3–5). The anion gap is an indirect estimation of the amount of "extra anions" in the circulation. The anion gap normally reflects the serum albumin (negatively charged at physiologic pH) (6), phosphate, and other minor anions (7). The unmeasured anions that may, under pathologic situations, lead to an increased anion gap can be either endogenous substances normally found in lower levels such as lactate or β-hydroxybutyrate or exogenous substances such as salicylates. The anion gap is calculated using the following formula:

$$[Na^+] - ([Cl^-] + [HCO_3^-]) \quad [5]$$

Metabolic acidosis is subdivided into anion gap and non-anion gap metabolic acidosis based on the value of the anion gap. In general, metabolic acidosis is caused either by the loss of bicarbonate—as in gastrointestinal losses or impaired renal acid excretion—or by a gain of acid associated with an unmeasured anion. The gain of acid is usually associated with the presence of an unmeasured anion (e.g., lactic acid); an exception might be intake of HCl. The extra base present—again, using the example of lactate—leads to a greater difference between the measured anions and cations, and therefore a greater anion gap. There is a wide range for the normal anion gap (4) and, in our experience, a normal anion gap is approximately 8 to 10 mEq/L—slightly lower than the value referenced above—but this may vary with methodologies in various labs; thus, checking with the local laboratory is imperative (4,8). When interpreting the anion gap, caution must be exercised, as there is significant variation in the anion gap and it can be influenced by many conditions other than metabolic acidosis.

Hypoalbuminemia is the most common condition that affects the normal anion gap since albumin normally contributes to the net negative charge of the blood (9). For every 1 mg/dL fall in the plasma albumin concentration, the anion gap should decrease by approximately 3 mEq/L (3). In plasma cell dyscrasias, such as multiple myeloma, the presence of cationic proteins in the serum is a cause for falsely depressing the anion gap (10), which has been attributed to an increased net positive charge due to the presence of net cationic immunoglobulins (11). Conditions that have been noted to increase the anion gap in the absence of metabolic acidosis are renal failure, volume depletion, metabolic alkalosis (12), and some penicillins. The anion gap can be lowered by hypoalbuminemia, hypercalcemia, and hyponatremia (13). Because of the wide variation in the anion gap and the variety of conditions that can affect it, it is best to directly measure "unmeasured anions" such as lactate whenever feasible.

Case Scenario #1: Use of Henderson-Hasselbalch Equation to Guide Ventilation

A 48-year-old morbidly obese patient is admitted to the hospital with shortness of breath and fever. In the emergency room, he is started on intravenous antibiotics. Over the next 3 hours, he becomes severely short of breath and develops a diminished level of consciousness. He is intubated and placed on mechanical ventilation. His past medical history is significant for diabetes mellitus and hypertension. Social history is significant for one pack per day tobacco abuse for 20 years. Current medications include amlodipine 5 mg PO daily, enalapril 5 mg PO bid, and hydrochlorothiazide 12.5 mg PO bid. Physical exam shows blood pressure of 156/88 mm Hg, pulse 76 beats/minute, and temperature 96°F. The patient is morbidly obese. Cardiovascular exam is normal. Lung exam reveals bilateral breath sounds with diffuse crackles on the right and egophony. The initial ventilator settings are synchronous intermittent mandatory ventilation (SIMV) with a rate of 20, tidal volume of 800 mL, and positive end-expiratory pressure (PEEP) of 5 cm H_2O, with an FiO_2 of 1.0. Thirty minutes after mechanical ventilation is initiated, the following labs are drawn:

Serum	
Sodium (mEq/L)	141
Potassium (mEq/L)	4.2
Chloride (mEq/L)	100
Bicarbonate (mEq/L)	34
Blood urea nitrogen (BUN) (mg/dL)	13
Phosphorus (mg/dL)	3.8
Creatinine (mg/dL)	0.8
Albumin (g/dL)	3.8
Glucose (mg/dL)	152

Arterial blood gas	
pH	7.65
PO_2 (mm Hg)	340
PCO_2 (mm Hg)	32

- **What acid-base disorder is present in this patient?**
This patient has an underlying respiratory acidosis with compensation (note elevated HCO_3^-). When a patient with chronic respiratory acidosis and appropriate renal compensation is placed on mechanical ventilation, he or she is at risk of developing severe alkalemia. This occurs because mechanical ventilation can remove PCO_2 from the blood quickly, hence increasing the pH precipitously. However, it takes time for the kidney to adapt to the change in blood pH. In time, the kidney can adapt by decreasing bicarbonate reabsorption, leading to loss of bicarbonate in the urine if the patient is not chloride depleted, but this does not happen in the acute setting. Following the start of mechanical ventilation in this patient, he has developed an iatrogenic respiratory alkalosis and a dangerously high arterial pH.
- **In order to correct the pH to 7.35, what goal CO_2 should be maintained?**
The appropriate measure is to decrease the minute ventilation to allow the PCO_2 to rise to a level that would lead to a normal or slightly acidic pH. To determine the PCO_2 that corresponds to a pH of 7.35, use the Henderson-Hasselbalch relationship. In the acute setting, the HCO_3^- will not change since renal adjustments take several days to have full effect, and therefore the best way to change the pH is to adjust PCO_2.

$$7.35 = 6.1 + \log(34/0.03 * PCO_2)$$
$$PCO_2 = 64\,\text{mm Hg}$$

Therefore, the ventilation rate should be decreased to maintain a PCO_2 of approximately 64 to achieve a pH of 7.35.

Newer Models of Acid-base Quantification: Stewart Approach

The assumptions made in the traditional model are that acids behave as Brønsted/Lowry acids—that is, proton donors—and that the degree of a metabolic disturbance causes a decrease in buffers, which is best approximated by the decrease in serum bicarbonate. Therefore, every mole of H^+ added results in a reciprocal decrease in the concentration of buffers. This decrease in buffers occurs principally as a decrease in serum bicarbonate, but other unmeasured buffers, such as Hgb-H, are also decreased during acidosis. An approach that is gaining popularity, especially among critical care physicians, is the Stewart model, a deviation from the traditional approach to acid-base quantification, which makes different assumptions about the definition of acids and bases. In essence, in the Stewart model, an acid is defined as any substance that raises the $[H^+]$ of a solution, not necessarily limited to an H^+-donating species. Many excellent reviews have been written on this topic (14–17); discussion in this chapter will be limited to an introduction to the key derived parameters of the Stewart model so that they can be contrasted with the standard approach. The most strikingly different concept of the Stewart model is that the serum bicarbonate is not used as the measure of buffering capacity present. This model uses the strong ion difference as a fundamental measure of the presence of buffers.

The Strong Ion Difference

Strong ions are the ions in the blood that can be considered as completely dissociated in solution (18). *The strong ion difference (SID) is analogous to the buffer base of a solution.* The SID is calculated as:

$$[SID] = \{[Na^+] + [K^+]\} - \{[Cl^-] - [lactate]\} \qquad [6]$$

The remaining anions in solution are the buffers, which can be thought of as the bicarbonate plus the nonbicarbonate buffers, denoted $[A^-]$. $[A^-]$ is the sum of negative charge (buffering capacity) of albumin and phosphate.

$$[SID] = [HCO_3^-] + [A^-] \qquad [7]$$

SID in the Stewart model is considered more reflective of the concentrations of buffers and not the serum bicarbonate. In fact, the Stewart equation describes the pH in terms of three independent variables: The strong ion difference [SID], $[A_{tot}]$, and PCO_2, where A_{tot} is the concentration of weak acids. This is in contrast to the Henderson-Hasselbalch equation, which relates pH to $[HCO_3^-]$ and PCO_2 (Eq. 4). In the Stewart model, bicarbonate concentration varies dependently on these other more fundamental parameters. The arguments for and against this claim are many, and are beyond the scope of this text. It can be stated, however, that the traditional approach to acid-base disturbances is still practiced most frequently, and the Stewart model has gained widest acceptance in the critical care field. This makes sense in that the Stewart model may have advantages in description of extreme acid-base conditions, especially when the assumption that noncarbonate buffers are constant may not be true, such as in critical illness. A high SID denotes metabolic alkalosis, and a low SID denotes metabolic acidosis. There are modifications of the standard model that attempt to take into account perturbations in noncarbonate species such as the correction of the anion gap for disturbances in serum albumin; this will be illustrated later in examples.

Expected and Apparent Strong Ion Difference. The SID under normal conditions can be thought as the sum of the buffer anions (bicarbonate and nonbicarbonate buffer anions) and should be about 40 mEq/L. As noted above, when the SID deviates from this value, a metabolic acid-base disturbance should be suspected. As noted above, the SID is one of three independent variables that determines $[H^+]$, and therefore, conversely, the SID can be related to the three fundamental values: pH, PCO_2, and $[A_{tot}]$. The expected SID (SIDe) is the SID that would be predicted based on the pH, PCO_2, and A_{tot} (in this case A_{tot} is approximated based on the albumin and phosphate). This relationship is given below:

$$\begin{aligned}[SIDe] = {} & (1{,}000 \times 2.46 \times 10^{-11} \times PCO_2/10^{-pH}) + [albumin] \\ & \times (0.123 \times pH - 0.631) + [phosphate] \\ & \times (0.309 \times pH - 0.469)\end{aligned} \qquad [8]$$

The apparent SID (SIDa) is the strong ion difference considering the concentrations of the strong ions that are normally present in the serum: Na^+, K^+, and Cl^-. This definition is given below:

$$[SIDa] = \{[Na^+] + [K^+]\} - [Cl^-] \qquad [9]$$

When the SIDa and SID differ, there is a strong anion gap, which is described below.

Strong Ion Gap

The strong ion gap (SIG) should be considered as an evaluation of unmeasured anions, analogous to the traditional anion gap. The strong anion gap is normally zero and is defined as:

$$SIG = \text{anion gap} - [A^-]$$

where A^- is the composite of nonbicarbonate buffers in the blood. $[A^-] = 2.8$ (albumin in g/dL) $+ 0.6$ (phosphate in mg/dL) at a pH of 7.4.

$$SIG = [SID_e] - [SID_a] \quad [10]$$

When the strong ion gap exceeds zero, there is an unmeasured anion present. This is analogous to the traditional anion gap, with a correction factor for the presence of hypoalbuminemia (19). The traditional anion gap is rarely corrected for disturbances in phosphate, although, as can be seen in the above formula for A^-, the contribution of deviations in phosphate is much smaller than that of albumin, reflecting that, quantitatively, albumin has much greater buffering capacity than phosphate.

The Stewart model has also been used to classify metabolic acid-base disorders based on the SID. An elevated SID is consistent with metabolic alkalosis, and a low SID is consistent with metabolic acidosis. The metabolic acidoses are further subdivided based on a high SIG (analogous in many ways to a high anion gap) and a low SIG (analogous to a low or normal anion gap). In this regard, the two approaches approximate each other. The use of the SIG may be advantageous over the use of the standard anion gap, given that the anion gap can have a wide range of values and is thus somewhat imprecise. This is especially true in settings where nonbicarbonate buffers deviate from normal—for example, the patient with acidosis, sepsis, and acute renal failure with serum albumin of 1.9, phosphorus of 7.0, and hemoglobin of 7.2 mg/dL. Clearly in this extreme, the assumption that only changes in serum bicarbonate species reflect the metabolic component of the acidosis may not hold true.

Stewart versus Traditional Approach

Despite the differences in these two approaches to acid-base quantification presented, it should be noted that they are quite similar. The advantage of the Stewart approach is that nonbicarbonate buffers are considered in quantifying acid-base disturbances and, as noted before, this is most likely to be pivotal in critical illness. However, accurate quantification of acid-base status is only part of managing acid-base disturbances. Correctly diagnosing acid-base disorders and treating them appropriately is the ultimate goal; in this regard, we do not find considerable advantage of the Stewart approach over more traditional methodologies. It is important that the clinician understand the limitation of any of the acid-base models, such as understanding when perturbations in the anion gap are significant and when they are not. In the cases presented in this chapter, we have used a traditional approach to acid-base analysis, and we continue use this approach in our own practice.

Key Points

1. The buffering of acids allows the body to "absorb" large amounts of acid without significant disturbance in pH. It is through the excretion of the daily acid load, however, that the body is allowed to maintain acid-base balance. A highly negative urinary anion gap suggests that there is significant ammonium in the urine; in response to metabolic acidosis, this would indicate that the renal compensation is intact. A urinary anion gap that is near zero or positive suggests that there is little or no ammonium in the urine and, in the face of systemic acidosis, would indicate renal acid wasting.
2. Bicarbonate is the principal buffer in the body; however, other buffers play an important role in maintaining systemic pH, and disturbances in nonbicarbonate buffers may be more important in critical illness than in other settings.

Volatile Acidity

Up until now, we have dealt exclusively with fixed acids. Disturbances in fixed acids cause a change in available buffers and change in systemic pH. It is critical to note that volatile acidity plays a very important role in determining the systemic pH both in primary respiratory disturbances and in compensation to metabolic disturbances as will be discussed.

Carbon dioxide is soluble in water, and in solution, reacts with water molecules to form carbonic acid, which can then further react as the following:

$$CO_2 + H_2O \leftrightarrow H_2CO_3 \leftrightarrow H^+ + HCO_3^- \quad [11]$$

H_2CO_3 is the acid portion of the bicarbonate buffer; however, its concentration is proportional to the partial pressure of CO_2, and therefore its direct measurement is not necessary. By the equilibrium expressions above, it can be seen that primary changes in PCO_2 will alter the amount of H_2CO_3. A high PCO_2 will increase the concentration of H_2CO_3, and a low PCO_2 will decrease the concentration of H_2CO_3. By quantitative chemistry, as you increase the concentration of the conjugate acid, the pH of a buffered solution will increase, and as you decrease concentration of conjugate acid, the opposite occurs. The PCO_2 in the circulation is the sum of its production and excretion. The production of CO_2 is not frequently altered; however, the excretion of CO_2—occurring only through respiration—is variable based upon the minute ventilation.

Mechanisms of Compensation

The previous sections have detailed how buffering allows the body to absorb significant amounts of H^+ without large fluctuations in pH. These buffering systems allow pH to remain constant during physiologic changes in endogenous acid production, and they also form the first defense against an acid-base insult (Table 42.1). The buffering systems and respiratory compensation are very rapid, whereas renal compensation may take days to become fully effective (20). The capacity of the body's buffering system is substantial, and therefore significant amounts of acid can be absorbed before a relatively small change in systemic pH occurs. Buffers act immediately and are thus the first line of defense.

In response to systemic changes in pH, compensatory mechanisms act to counteract the primary disturbance. Figure 42.3 gives an overview of the compensatory responses to the primary acid-base disturbances. In response to metabolic acidosis, there is increased ventilation to decrease PCO_2; the kidney responds by increasing the excretion of H^+, thereby generating more HCO_3^- (Fig. 42.3A). The opposite response occurs during metabolic alkalosis, except that the kidneys are usually not able to respond to the increase in HCO_3^- appropriately, as failure of the kidney to respond to elevated HCO_3^- is necessary for the development of metabolic alkalosis (this is

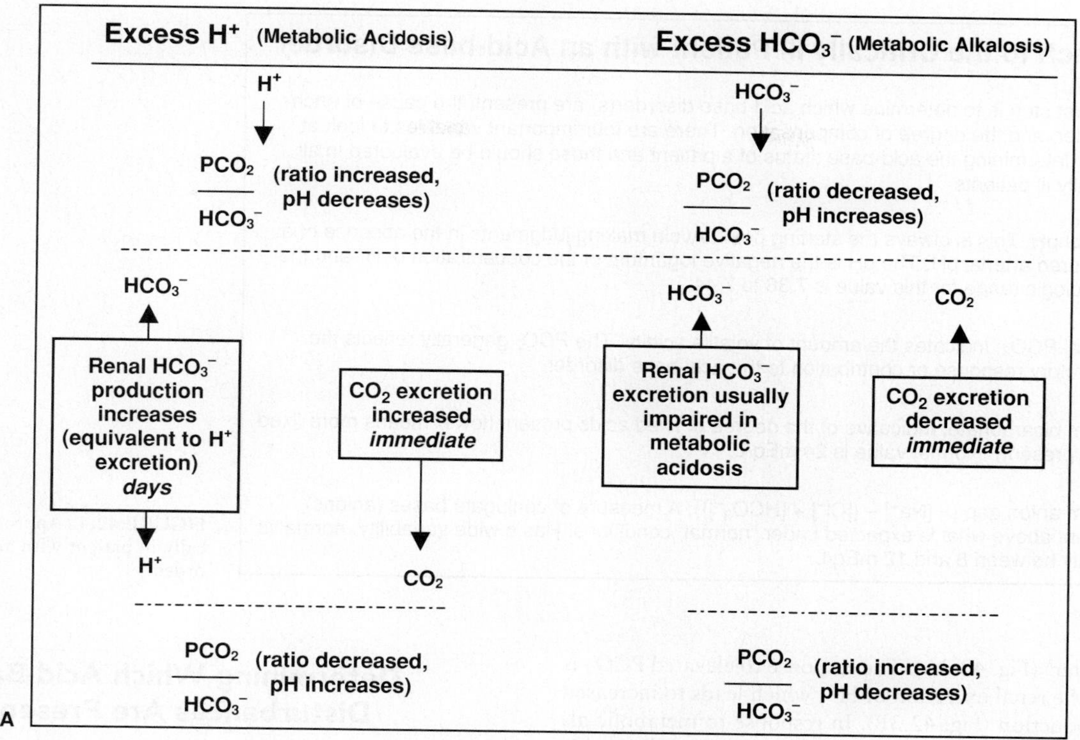

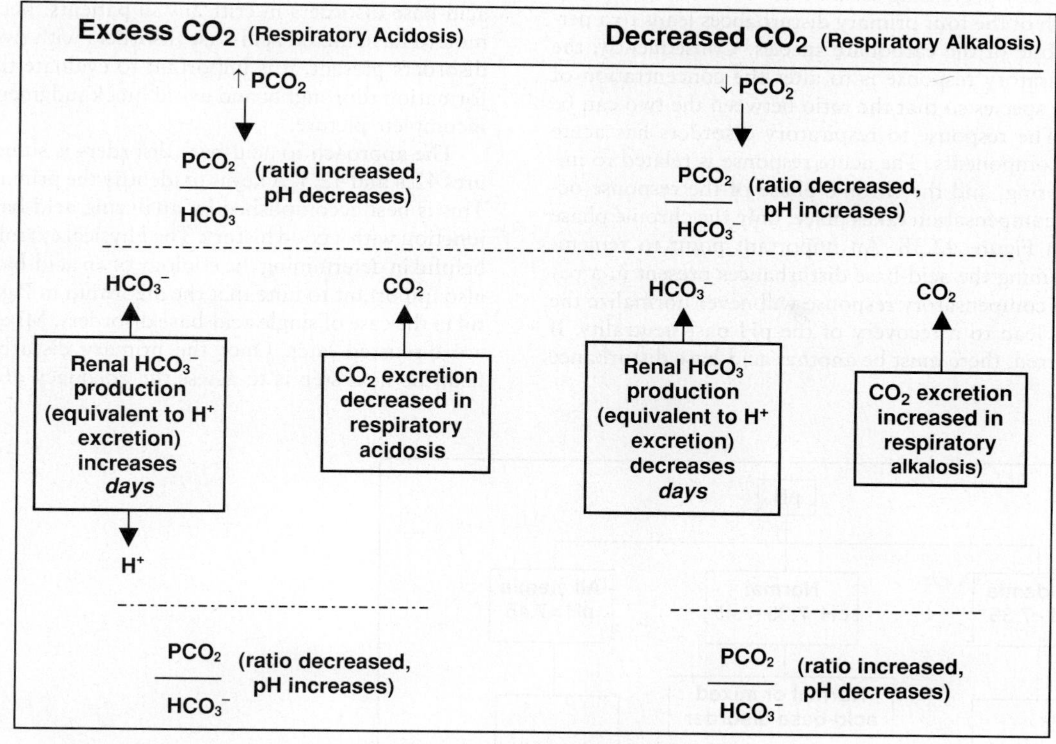

FIGURE 42.3. **A:** Primary metabolic acid-base disturbances and compensatory mechanisms. **B:** Primary respiratory acid-base disturbances and compensatory mechanisms.

Approach to the Critically Ill Patient with an Acid-base Disorder

The first step is to determine which acid-base disorder(s) are present, the cause of each disorder, and the degree of compensation. There are four important variables to look at when determining the acid-base status of a patient and these should be evaluated in all critically ill patients:

- Arterial pH: This is always the starting point. Avoid making judgments in the absence of a measured arterial pH. The pH is the negative logarithm of the concentration of H^+ and the physiologic range for this value is 7.38 to 7.44
- Arterial PCO_2: Indicates the amount of volatile acidity. The PCO_2 generally reflects the respiratory response or contribution to the acid-base disorder.
- Serum bicarbonate: Indicative of the degree of fixed acids present (lower means more fixed acids present). Normal value is 24 mEq/L.
- Serum anion gap (= $[Na^+] - \{[Cl^-] + [HCO_3^-]\}$): A measure of conjugate bases (anions) present above what is expected under "normal" conditions. Has a wide variability, normal is usually between 8 and 12 mEq/L.

FIGURE 42.4. Approach to the critically ill patient with an acid-base disorder.

described later) (Fig. 42.3A). The response to elevated PCO_2 is to increase the renal excretion of H^+, which leads to increased HCO_3^- production (Fig. 42.3B). In response to metabolic alkalosis, the excretion of H^+ decreases and less bicarbonate is produced, thereby decreasing serum bicarbonate (Fig. 42.3B). Note that each of the four primary disturbances leads to a perturbation of one of the carbonate species. Consequently, the main compensatory response is to alter the concentration of the conjugate species so that the ratio between the two can be maintained. The response to respiratory disorders has acute and chronic components. The acute response is related to immediate buffering, and the chronic phase of the response occurs as renal compensation takes place; only the chronic phase is depicted in Figure 42.3B. An important point to remember in determining the acid-base disturbances present in a patient is that a compensatory response will never normalize the serum pH or lead to a recovery of the pH past neutrality. If this has occurred, there must be another acid-base disturbance present.

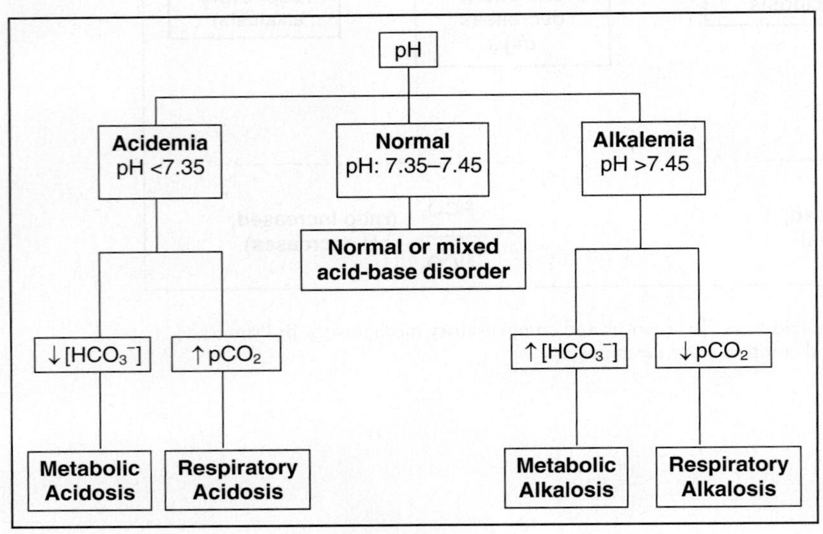

FIGURE 42.5. General approach to acid-base disorders. (From Ayus JC. MKSAP 14, 2006, Nephrology Section. Medical Knowledge Self Assessment Program. American College of Physicians; 2006. Copyrighted by the American College of Physicians.)

Determining Which Acid-Base Disturbances Are Present

A systematic approach is important in correctly diagnosing acid-base disorders in critically ill patients. Because it is common to have mixed acid-base disorders with two or even three disorders present, it is important to evaluate the available information thoroughly and avoid quick judgments based on an incomplete picture.

The approach to acid-base disorders is summarized in Figures 42.4 and 42.5. A key is to identify the primary disturbance. This is best accomplished by analyzing acid-base data in conjunction with a good history. The physical examination is rarely helpful in determining the etiology of an acid-base disorder. It is also important to note that the algorithm in Figure 42.5 is useful in the case of single acid-base disorders. Mixed disturbances are discussed later. Once the primary disturbance is identified, the next step is to assess the adequacy of compensation.

TABLE 42.2

COMPENSATIONS FOR ACID-BASE DISORDERS

Metabolic acidosis	■ For every 1 mmol/L decrease in HCO_3^- → 1 mm Hg decrease in PCO_2 ■ Expected PCO_2 = 1.5 (HCO_3^-) + 8 ± 2 ■ PCO_2 should approach last two digits of pH
Metabolic alkalosis	■ For every 1 mmol/L increase in HCO_3^- → 0.7 mm Hg increase in PCO_2
Respiratory acidosis	■ **Acute:** For 10 mm Hg increase in PCO_2 → 1 mmol/L increase in HCO_3^- ■ **Chronic:** For 10 mm Hg increase in PCO_2 → 4 mmol/L increase in HCO_3^-
Respiratory alkalosis	■ **Acute:** For every 10 mm Hg decrease in PCO_2 → 2 mmol/L decrease in HCO_3^- ■ **Chronic:** For every 10 mm Hg decrease in PCO_2 → 4 mmol/L decrease in HCO_3^-

Table 42.2 gives the expected values of PCO_2 and HCO_3^- following compensations for primary disturbances. In the setting of respiratory disorders, acute compensation occurs over hours, while the chronic compensation occurs over days. If there is only one disturbance, and the compensation is adequate, there is nothing more to do. On the other hand, if the compensation is inappropriate, then a second disorder is present. Recall that a compensation will never normalize the pH or "compensate" past the point of neutrality (e.g., a primary metabolic acidosis as a single disorder cannot lead to a neutral or alkaline pH). In these cases, a mixed acid-base disorder is present. An additional clue that a mixed acid-base disorder is present is an elevated anion gap when a metabolic acidosis is not suspected. For this reason, it is good practice to calculate the anion gap in all critically ill patients.

CAUSES OF ACID-BASE DISORDERS

In determining the etiology, the clinician usually must rely on the history, clinical presentation, and, most importantly, laboratory data in order to determine the inciting disease state (Fig. 42.6).

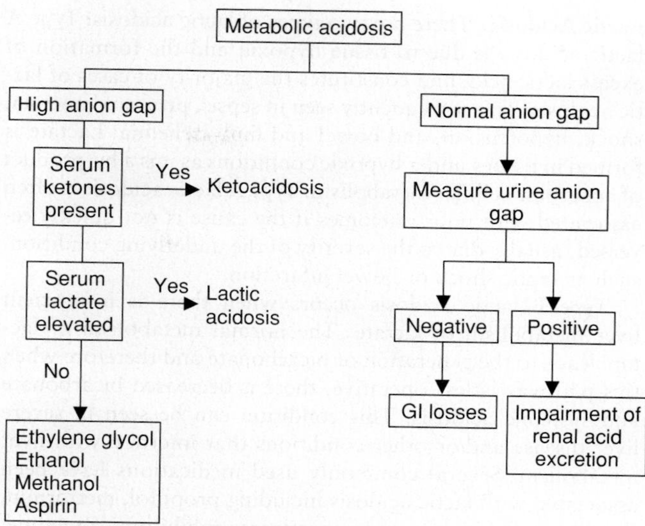

FIGURE 42.6. Diagnostic approach to metabolic acidosis. (From Ayus JC. MKSAP 14, 2006, Nephrology Section. Medical Knowledge Self Assessment Program. American College of Physicians; 2006. Copyrighted by the American College of Physicians.)

Metabolic Acidosis

Causes of Anion Gap Acidosis

The common etiologies of elevated anion gap metabolic acidosis are listed in Table 42.3.

Diabetic Ketoacidosis. Insulin is secreted and mediates the metabolism of carbohydrates and the storage of fat during times of normal enteral intake. Under fasting conditions, insulin secretion decreases. Diabetic ketoacidosis occurs when a deficit of insulin activity leads to altered cellular metabolism and glucose utilization is impaired. The deficiency of insulin causes the liberation of fatty acids and pathophysiologic keto acid production. The degree of increase in the anion gap is related to the amount of retained ketones, and therefore diabetic ketoacidosis can be present with varying degrees of hyperchloremia (21). In addition to abnormal ketoacid production, diabetic ketoacidosis is typically also associated with hyperglycemia, a decrease in circulatory volume, and, oftentimes, free water deficits as well, in addition to hypokalemia and hypophosphatemia. Even though total body potassium stores are decreased, the serum potassium concentration is frequently elevated on presentation due to the effects of insulin deficiency, hyperglycemia, and acidosis on potassium distribution. The treatment of diabetic ketoacidosis includes re-expansion of the extracellular fluid volume, administration of insulin to halt acid production, and correction of potassium and phosphorus deficits, with close monitoring of plasma electrolytes.

TABLE 42.3

COMMON CAUSES OF ELEVATED ANION GAP METABOLIC ACIDOSIS

Lactic acidosis
Diabetic ketoacidosis
Renal failure
Ingestions
■ Methanol
■ Ethylene glycol
■ Paraldehydes
■ Salicylates

Lactic Acidosis. There are two types of lactic acidosis: Type A lactic acidosis is due to tissue hypoxia and the formation of excess lactic acid, and constitutes the majority of cases of lactic acidosis. This is frequently seen in sepsis, profound anemia, shock, hypotension, and bowel and limb ischemia. Lactate is formed in tissues under hypoxic conditions as it is a by-product of anaerobic cellular metabolism. Type A lactic acidosis is often associated with poor outcomes if the cause is not quickly reversed, usually due to the severity of the underlying condition, such as septic shock or bowel infarction.

Type B lactic acidosis occurs when there is insufficient liver metabolism of lactate. The normal metabolism of lactate leads to the generation of bicarbonate and therefore when this pathway is less operative, there is decreased bicarbonate and systemic acidosis. This condition can be seen in severe liver disease and/or other conditions that interfere with liver metabolism. Several commonly used medications have been associated with lactic acidosis including propofol, metformin, the nonnucleotide reverse transcriptase inhibitors, stavudine, didanosine, and zidovudine. Carbon monoxide poisoning can present with nonspecific symptoms and lead to lactic acidosis by inhibiting oxygen utilization in the tissues.

Toxic Ingestions Associated with Elevated Anion Gap Acidosis. Ingestions are important causes of acidosis in the critical care setting (22). Common ingestions that often lead to elevated anion gap metabolic acidosis are listed in Table 42.3. The presence of ingested alcohols or other solvents can be inferred by measurement of the osmolal gap when an ingestion is suspected.

The osmolal gap can be calculated using the following formula:

(Measured serum osmolality) − (Calculated serum osmolality)

where the calculated serum osmolality is obtained as follows:

$$2 \times [Na^+]\,(mEq/L) + \text{Urea nitrogen}\,(mg/dL)/2.8 + \text{Glucose}\,(mg/dL)/18 \quad [12]$$

The osmolal gap is normally approximately 10 mOsm/kg H_2O. The normal osmolal gap is a reflection of substances normally present in the serum that exert oncotic forces. These are plasma proteins and ions found in smaller quantities, such as calcium and magnesium. An elevated osmolal gap is an indication that an unmeasured osmole is present in the serum; in the intensive care setting, this is commonly due to ethanol. The osmolal gap can also be used to quantify the level of ethylene glycol or methanol, although direct measurement of these toxins is indicated if their presence is suspected; however, therapy should not be delayed while waiting for confirmation.

Case Scenario #2: Salicylate Toxicity

A 68-year-old man presents to the emergency room following an intentional toxic ingestion. He was brought in by his son, who found him confused when he stopped by his (the patient's) house. One month prior to admission, he suffered the loss of his wife and has felt hopeless since that time. Upon presentation, he is lethargic and weak. His past medical history is significant for hypertension and gout. Past surgical history is significant for an appendectomy 20 years ago and coronary artery bypass graft (CABG) 2 years ago. He smokes one and a half packs of cigarettes a day and he denies the use of alcohol or illicit drugs. Physical exam is significant for blood pressure of 156/80 mm Hg, pulse of 79 beats/minute, respirations of 32 breaths/minute, and temperature of 98°F. He is lethargic, in moderate respiratory distress, and oriented only to place and person. Cardiovascular exam is normal, and there is no wheezing on chest exam. Laboratory data are given below:

Serum	
Sodium (mEq/L)	141
Potassium (mEq/L)	3.9
Chloride (mEq/L)	105
Bicarbonate (mEq/L)	9
BUN (mg/dL)	21
Creatinine (mg/dL)	1.2
Glucose (mg/dL)	128
Arterial blood gas	
pH	7.40
PO_2	67
PCO_2	15

Salicylate toxicity is typically associated with an anion gap metabolic acidosis and respiratory alkalosis; this is the acid-base disorder present in this patient. In diagnosing the acid-base disturbance in this patient, the first step is to look at the serum pH. The pH is normal with low serum bicarbonate. This is the first clue that a complex disorder is present since a compensatory response to metabolic acidosis would not normalize the serum pH. We can determine that there is a metabolic acidosis present because of the elevated anion gap (anion gap = 27). Given the presence of a metabolic acidosis, we can then predict what the PCO_2 should be. Using the Winter formula, the expected PCO_2 is approximately 21 mm Hg (Table 42.2), and thus a respiratory alkalosis is present. This pattern is strongly suggestive of salicylate toxicity (23).

Case Scenario #3: Lactic Acidosis in the Setting of Abnormal Levels of Nonbicarbonate Buffers

A 44-year-old female with cirrhosis secondary to autoimmune hepatitis is admitted to the hospital for fever and abdominal pain. The patient is listed for an orthotopic liver transplantation and has been clinically stable for the past month. She noted abdominal pain and fever that have gotten progressively worse over the last 2 days. Her past medical history is otherwise nonsignificant. Current medications include spironolactone 100 mg PO bid, furosemide 80 mg PO bid, and lactulose 30 mL PO bid. Previous surgeries include the placement of a transjugular intrahepatic portosystemic shunt (TIPS) and a cholecystectomy. Physical exam is significant for blood pressure of 74/55 mm Hg, pulse of 72 beats/minute, temperature 100.8°F, and respiratory rate of 24 breaths/minute. She appears cachectic. Cardiovascular and chest exams are normal. Her abdomen is distended and there is diffuse tenderness. She has 1+ pitting edema in the lower extremities. Spontaneous bacterial peritonitis is suspected, and the patient is admitted to the hospital. Admission labs are given below:

Serum	
Sodium (mEq/L)	128
Potassium (mEq/L)	5.1
Chloride (mEq/L)	106
Bicarbonate (mEq/L)	11
BUN (mg/dL)	20
Creatinine (mg/dL)	1.3
Phosphorus (mg/dL)	2.1
Albumin (g/dL)	1.4
Glucose (mg/dL)	84
Arterial blood gas	
pH	7.23
PO_2 (mm Hg)	78
PCO_2 (mm Hg)	28

■ **What is the best characterization of the acid-base disturbance in this patient?**

The acid-base disorder is an anion gap metabolic acidosis, likely lactic acidosis. While the anion gap appears normal, the degree of hypoalbuminemia needs to be considered because the negative charge on albumin is a significant component of the "normal"

TABLE 42.4

ETIOLOGIES OF NON–ANION GAP METABOLIC ACIDOSIS

Extrarenal source	Renal source
Gastrointestinal disorders	
■ Diarrhea	■ Renal tubular acidosis
■ Pancreatic and biliary fistulas	■ Renal failure
■ Laxatives, cholestyramine	■ Hypoaldosteronism
■ Ureterointestinal diversions (ileal conduit)	

unmeasured anions. For every 1 g/dL decrease in the serum albumin, the expected anion gap decreases by 2.5 mEq/L. Thus, in this patient, to consider her anion gap at a normal level, it should not exceed approximately 5 to 6 mEq/L. Again, caution should be used in interpreting the anion gap in these settings; if any suspicion exists for lactic acidosis, the serum lactate should be measured directly.

Non–Anion Gap Acidosis

In a non–anion gap/hyperchloremic acidosis, there is a primary decrease in the serum bicarbonate and an associated increase in the serum chloride. The serum bicarbonate decreases because of renal or extrarenal, gastrointestinal losses (Table 42.4). One of the key etiologic questions to be answered in the approach to a patient with a non–anion gap acidosis is whether or not the kidney is appropriately responding to the acidosis by excreting the acid load or if the cause of the acidosis is improper acid excretion by the kidney. This allows one to differentiate renal from nonrenal causes of the acidosis. The urine anion gap, which is calculated using Eq. 3, is a convenient methodology to assess urinary acid excretion. If the urine anion gap is positive or close to zero, this suggests that (a) there is very little ammonium in the urine (Fig. 42.2) and (b) the kidney is not appropriately excreting acids. If the urine anion gap is highly negative, this suggests that (a) there is a large amount of ammonium in the urine and (b) the kidney is excreting acids appropriately (Fig. 42.2).

Causes of Non–Anion Gap Metabolic Acidosis

Diarrhea. Severe diarrhea leads to non–anion gap metabolic acidosis through loss of bicarbonate, and is typically associated with volume depletion and hypokalemia. In very severe cases, circulatory collapse can occur, and an anion gap (lactic) acidosis may supervene upon the non–anion gap acidosis. Patients who chronically abuse laxatives may develop metabolic acidosis and hypokalemia. However, frequently, these patients also abuse diuretics and therefore can have an associated metabolic alkalosis. In order to determine if the renal response to the acidosis is normal, the urine anion gap should be measured.

Ureterointestinal Diversions. In a ureterointestinal diversion, urine in the intestine leads to reabsorption of chloride and water. Consequently, the absorption of chloride can induce secretion of bicarbonate into the intestine. Additionally, urease-positive bacteria in the intestine metabolizes the urea in the urine to form ammonium, which, when absorbed, liberates excess acid after it is metabolized in the liver. Also, chronic pyelonephritis is common in the diverted kidney, and a superimposed distal renal tubular acidosis (RTA) may occur.

Renal Tubular Acidosis. Renal tubular acidosis is a heterogeneous mix of disorders that is characterized by defects in urinary acid excretion in the setting of intact renal function. Proximal (type 2) RTA is caused by a decrease in proximal bicarbonate reabsorption, whereas in distal (type 1) RTA, the primary defect is impairment of distal acidification (24,25). The net result is that the urine pH is not maximally acidified. The lack of acidification—in other words, secretion of H^+—leads to less ammonium trapping in the urine and therefore to an anion gap that is either positive or near zero. In the intensive care unit, renal tubular acidosis often presents with profound acidosis and hypokalemia. It is important to treat the hypokalemia first with potassium chloride before correcting the acidosis, as administration of bicarbonate in the setting of severe potassium depletion can lead to fatal hypokalemia as potassium is taken up by cells when H^+ exits the cells. Type 4 RTA is a clinical syndrome of hyperkalemia and hyperchloremic metabolic acidosis (26) caused by a lack of aldosterone effect on the kidney and is seen most commonly in the following settings: diabetes, advanced age, acquired immunodeficiency syndrome (AIDS), interstitial nephritis, obstructive uropathy, postrenal transplant status, use of angiotensin-converting enzyme inhibitors and heparin (both of which impair aldosterone production), and use of cyclosporine.

RTA should be suspected if the renal response to systemic acidemia is impaired as evidenced by a positive urine anion gap. The next step is to determine the type. The most practical starting point is to differentiate a proximal from a distal RTA. To understand this, some physiology must be discussed. Recall that bicarbonate is reabsorbed predominantly in the proximal tubule. Proximal RTA develops because of impaired reabsorption of bicarbonate. The lack of bicarbonate reabsorption in patients with normal serum bicarbonate leads to wasting of bicarbonate in the urine until a steady state is reached in which the serum bicarbonate drops to a level at which the reabsorptive capacity of the proximal tubule is no longer overwhelmed. At this point, there is no longer any bicarbonate in the urine. For this reason, in a patient with proximal RTA, the serum bicarbonate will be low; however, the urine pH will be low—this is because the distal acidification mechanisms are functional. If such a patient is given an alkali load, serum bicarbonate is temporarily increased, and bicarbonate "spills" into the urine because the filtered load of bicarbonate exceeds the reabsorptive threshold, which leads to an increase in the urine pH. Once the alkali load is stopped, serum bicarbonate drops, bicarbonate no longer appears in the urine, and the urine pH can now drop to its maximally acidic level of approximately 5.5. This is the basis for the provocative testing to demonstrate a proximal RTA, and also explains why these patients often have to take a tremendous amount of alkali in order to achieve normal serum pH.

Renal Failure. The kidneys have the capacity to excrete acids to such a degree that acid-base balance is maintained until kidney function deteriorates to below a glomerular filtration rate of approximately 20 mL/minute. The resulting acidosis is of a mixed type and it is generally, but not universally, associated with an elevated anion gap. Chronic metabolic acidosis should be treated to prevent bone demineralization, which may occur with time. The goal of treatment is to maintain normal acid-base status.

Pancreatic or Biliary Fistula. These disorders can lead to the loss of bicarbonate-rich solutions through the gastrointestinal tract and result in systemic acidosis. If correction of the underlying fistula is not possible, treatment with alkali salts can be helpful.

Hypoaldosteronism. Similar to type 4 RTA acidosis, hypoaldosteronism can lead to an impairment in renal acid excretion. Aldosterone activity in the kidney leads to hypokalemia and metabolic alkalosis; conversely, lack of this activity decreases aldosterone secretion and leads to hyperkalemia and metabolic acidosis.

Case Scenario #4: Non–Anion Gap Metabolic Acidosis: Assessing Urinary Acid Excretion

A 66-year-old man is seen in the emergency room. He has had 8 days of severe diarrhea, abdominal pain, and decreased food intake, but adequate intake of liquids. He believes that he became sick after babysitting his grandson who had similar symptoms. His medical history is significant for diabetes and hypertension. Surgical history only consists of coronary artery bypass grafting 3 years ago. His medications include enalapril 20 mg PO bid, aspirin 81 mg PO daily, atenolol 50 mg PO daily, hydrochlorothiazide 25 mg PO daily, and metformin 1 g PO bid. He has a family history of diabetes and premature coronary artery disease. He does not smoke or use drugs, and drinks alcohol occasionally. Physical exam is significant for blood pressure of 105/70 mm Hg and a pulse of 72 beats/minute; blood pressure drops to 90/50 mm Hg when the patient stands. Temperature is 98.8°F, and respiratory rate is 32 breaths/minute. There is a small amount of occult blood in the stool. Labs are given below:

Serum	
Sodium (mEq/L)	136
Potassium (mEq/L)	3.9
Chloride (mEq/L)	114
Bicarbonate (mEq/L)	13
BUN (mg/dL)	21
Creatinine (mg/dL)	1.2
Albumin (g/dL)	4.0
Glucose (mg/dL)	128
Urine	
pH	6
Sodium (mEq/L)	32
Potassium (mEq/L)	21
Chloride (mEq/L)	80
Arterial blood gas	
pH	7.27
PO_2	90
PCO_2	30

■ **Which acid-base disorder is present and what is the likely etiology?**

This patient has a non–anion gap metabolic acidosis from a nonrenal origin. The low pH and decreased serum bicarbonate indicate the presence of metabolic acidosis. Respiratory compensation is adequate, and therefore there is no complex acid-base disorder present. The serum anion gap is not elevated. The urine electrolytes and the calculation of the urine anion gap are useful to distinguish between a renal source and a gastrointestinal (GI) source of the acidosis. If gastrointestinal losses are the cause of the acidosis and the renal response to the acidosis is normal, a significant amount of ammonium will be present in the urine. The presence (or absence) of ammonium can be inferred by calculating the urine anion gap. The formula for the urine anion gap is as follows: $[K^+] + [Na^+] - [Cl^-]$. If there is an unmeasured anion present, then $[Cl^-]$ exceeds $[K^+] + [Na^+]$ and the urine anion gap is significantly negative. When there is little or no unmeasured anion present, the urine anion gap will take on a positive value. In this case, the urine anion gap = 32 mEq/L + 21 mEq/L – 80 mEq/L = –27 mEq/L, and therefore there is a significant amount of ammonium (NH_4^+) in the urine, which implies a normal renal response to the systemic acidosis—thereby designating an extrarenal cause of the acidosis.

Treatment of Metabolic Acidosis

Treatment of Anion Gap Metabolic Acidosis. The treatment of an anion gap metabolic acidosis is focused on reversing the pathogenesis of the endogenous acid production and eliminating excess acid. By far the most important aspect of treatment is to identify the source of the acidosis if it is not already apparent, such as in diabetic ketoacidosis or septic shock. Treatment of an anion gap acidosis with bicarbonate replacement therapy remains controversial, especially in lactic acidosis. It has been argued that bicarbonate may be used as a bridge until homeostatic mechanisms reverse the condition through the metabolism of endogenous bases, such as lactate and ketone bodies, and therefore bicarbonate regeneration. This approach of using alkali therapy assumes that there is a detriment to a low pH (or serum bicarbonate) above and beyond the harm caused by the underlying condition. However, evidence from animal models argues that bicarbonate therapy may have deleterious effects on pH, serum lactate levels, and cardiac function (27–29). Bicarbonate leads to the generation of CO_2 during buffering and, as CO_2 readily diffuses across cell membranes, intracellular acidosis has been shown to worsen during bicarbonate therapy. Worsening of cardiac function, which has been associated with intracellular acidosis, is the proposed mechanism for worsening of lactic acidosis following the administration of bicarbonate during lactic acidosis (30). Hemodialysis rapidly corrects acidosis and is typically necessary to treat acidosis in the setting of renal failure.

Treatment of Non–Anion Gap Metabolic Acidosis. Bicarbonate therapy is generally indicated in non–anion gap acidosis since the primary disturbance is a decrease in bicarbonate. This is contrasted to anion gap acidosis where correction of the underlying cause is the primary concern. Oral bicarbonate or oral citrate solutions are agents for chronic therapy for non–anion gap acidosis. For acute presentations, especially in patients who may not be able to tolerate prolonged hyperventilation, intravenous bicarbonate therapy may be used.

Medications and Metabolic Acidosis

Medications are an increasingly important cause of severe acidosis and can be life threatening in many cases. Lactic acidosis has been reported with all nonnucleoside reverse transcriptase inhibitors used to treat human immunodeficiency virus (HIV); this effect is related to the drug's inhibition of mitochondrial function, with resultant anaerobic metabolism (31–34). The newer-generation anticonvulsant topiramate has also been associated with lactic acidosis (34). Metformin is also well known to lead to lactic acidosis, which can be treated with hemodialysis (35). The propofol infusion syndrome is a dangerous complication sometimes seen with the use of this drug; it is associated with head injury, use of propofol for more than 48 hours, use in children, and concomitant use of catecholamines and steroids (36–38).

Case Scenario #5: Propofol Infusion Syndrome

A 25-year-old male is in the intensive care unit following a craniotomy for a traumatic head injury. He had suffered a depressed skull fracture to the left frontal bone from blunt trauma during an altercation. He has no known medical problems and takes no medications. Family members state that he occasionally uses intravenous cocaine and smokes cigarettes. Intraoperatively, he is given intravenous cefazolin and phenytoin. It is now postoperative day 2, and he is currently receiving propofol infusion at 8 μg/kg/minute. Blood pressure is 155/90 mm Hg, pulse 80 beats/minute, temperature 97.4°F, and respiratory rate 12 breaths/minute. He is currently mechanically ventilated on SIMV mode with bilateral breath sounds. He has a normal cardiac exam, and there is no peripheral edema. Laboratory data are as follows:

	Day 3	Day 6
Sodium (mEq/L)	136	137
Potassium (mEq/L)	3.9	4
Chloride (mEq/L)	104	103
Bicarbonate (mEq/L)	20	12
BUN (mg/dL)	18	19
Creatinine (mg/dL)	1.1	1.0
Albumin (g/dL)	4.0	4.0
Glucose (mg/dL)	128	112
Lactate (mmol/L)		7
pH	7.37	7.21
PCO_2	38	32

- **What is the likely cause of the acidosis in this patient?** Propofol infusion syndrome is an important entity in the intensive care unit (37,39,40). The patients who appear to be at the greatest risk for the condition are those receiving prolonged infusions after suffering brain injury. Treatment for the condition appears to be discontinuation of propofol; hemofiltration has been used successfully (41,42). It is important to note that many fatalities have occurred when the condition is not recognized promptly, and thus early recognition is critical.

Key Points

1. Bicarbonate therapy is indicated for non–anion gap acidosis.
2. The primary concern in anion gap acidosis is correction of the underlying cause.

Metabolic Alkalosis

Metabolic alkalosis occurs when there is an excess of buffers present, raising the systemic pH. In metabolic alkalosis, there is a primary elevation in the serum bicarbonate. This condition is common in the intensive care setting and can have severe complications. As the primary problem is an increase in bicarbonate, metabolic alkalosis can be readily corrected by renal bicarbonate excretion. Under normal circumstances the potential for bicarbonate excretion is tremendous, and thus, alterations in the renal handling of bicarbonate must occur to maintain the alkalosis. Without an impairment of the renal capacity to excrete bicarbonate, the kidneys would simply excrete the bicarbonate load. The most common reason for impairment of renal excretion of bicarbonate is chloride deficiency and renal failure. In general, metabolic alkaloses are generated by either bicarbonate intake in excess of loss or by the primary loss of H^+ (Table 42.5).

TABLE 42.5

CAUSES OF ALKALOSIS GENERATION

Excessive alkaline load	Loss of hydrogen ions
Bicarbonate infusion, hemodialysis $CaCO_3$ supplements Oral citrate solutions Parenteral nutrition (acetate, glutamate)	**Gastrointestinal losses:** Vomiting, nasogastric suction **Renal losses:** Diuretics, excessive mineralocorticoid

Chloride-sensitive Metabolic Alkalosis

Nasogastric suction, vomiting, and diuretics are very frequent causes of metabolic alkalosis. Hypokalemia develops in the setting of vomiting or nasogastric suction not due to gastrointestinal losses, as the stomach contents are not rich in potassium; rather, the losses of potassium are renal losses due to potassium bicarbonate excretion and secondary hyperaldosteronism. In these settings, renal losses of sodium and potassium are obligatory in order to excrete bicarbonate. In this situation, the urinary chloride (not the urinary sodium) better reflects the effective blood volume of the patient. Similar to the loss of gastric secretions, diuretic-induced extracellular fluid volume depletion stimulates aldosterone secretion. The action of aldosterone stimulates sodium reabsorption in the distal tubule, which is coupled with secretion of potassium and H^+. Therefore, a urine that is paradoxically acidic is generated. Other causes of metabolic alkalosis that are sensitive to the administration of chloride include those occurring after hypercapnic and after diuretic use.

As noted above, in order to maintain the alkalosis, renal bicarbonate excretion must be impaired in some way. In the setting of chloride depletion, the kidney is unable to excrete the excess bicarbonate, and therefore the alkalosis is maintained (43,44) (Table 42.6). Among patients with normal renal

TABLE 42.6

CLASSIFICATION OF METABOLIC ALKALOSIS BY CHLORIDE HANDLING

Chloride sensitive (urine Cl^- less than 20 mEq/L)	Chloride resistant (urine Cl^- greater than 40 mEq/L)
Gastrointestinal acid losses ■ Nasogastric suction, vomiting ■ Congenital Cl^- losses in stool? ■ Rectal adenoma	**Hypertensive** ■ Renovascular hypertension ■ Hyperaldosteronism ■ Liddle syndrome ■ Glycyrrhizic acid
Renal acid losses ■ Penicillins, citrate ■ Postdiuretic ■ Posthypercapnic	**Normotensive** ■ Diuretics ■ Bartter and Gitelman syndromes ■ Administration of alkali

function and normal chloride status, attempting to raise the serum bicarbonate concentration 2 to 3 mEq/L above the normal value is virtually impossible because the kidneys can easily excrete the excess bicarbonate.

Chloride-insensitive Metabolic Alkalosis

The chloride-insensitive metabolic alkalosis commonly encountered in the critical care setting is that occurring after the use of loop diuretics. The loss of large amounts of bicarbonate-free fluid in a patient with expanded ECF space—such as during therapy with a loop diuretic—is thought to lead to a reduction in the ECF space, with relative conservation of bicarbonate concentration. This has been termed *contraction alkalosis*. Other causes of chloride-insensitive metabolic alkalosis are hyperaldosteronism—both primary and secondary—such as might be seen with renovascular disease (Table 42.6). Rare causes of chloride-insensitive metabolic alkalosis are Bartter and Gitelman syndromes.

Renal and Extrarenal Compensation

Immediately following the generation of metabolic alkalosis, buffering systems begin to decrease the effects of the alkaline load. Respiratory compensation for a metabolic alkalosis involves respiratory suppression and an increase in the PCO_2 (Fig. 42.3A, Table 42.2). Respiratory compensation for severe metabolic alkalosis has practical limits, as respirations can be suppressed only to a certain degree. Without the effect of mitigating factors such as volume depletion, the kidney will respond to metabolic alkalosis through increasing the renal excretion of bicarbonate. Severe chloride depletion can theoretically inhibit this exchange and therefore inhibit bicarbonate secretion. Finally, hyperaldosteronism secondary to diuretic use stimulates the tubular secretion of potassium and H^+. The net effect is an acidic urine that also helps to maintain the alkalosis. In patients with low urinary chloride, chloride replacement is indicated to allow bicarbonate excretion.

Treatment of Metabolic Alkalosis

The metabolic alkalosis seen in the intensive care unit often develops as a complication rather than a presenting disorder. H_2 blockers and proton pump inhibitors can be used as a measure to decrease losses of H^+ in patients with prolonged gastric aspiration or chronic vomiting, which may help prevent the development of metabolic alkalosis. In patients with chloride-sensitive metabolic alkalosis, treatment usually consists of replacement of the chloride deficit—usually with normal saline since volume depletion is also often present. Potassium chloride is almost always indicated when hypokalemia is also present, although potassium concentrations may increase as the alkalosis is corrected. In severe, symptomatic metabolic alkalosis—a pH greater than 7.6—hemodialysis may be indicated and can be used to correct alkalemia, especially when associated with renal failure (45). The use of acidic solutions is rarely indicated (Table 42.7).

Case Scenario #6: Diabetic Ketoacidosis with Concomitant Metabolic Alkalosis

A 21-year-old male presents to the emergency room with severely diminished mental status. He states that he has felt nauseated for the last few days and has been unable to eat well. This morning, he vomited several times and was brought to the emergency room by his girlfriend. His past medical history is negative for any chronic medical problems. He had a tonsillectomy as a child but no other surgeries. Physical exam is significant for blood pressure of 122/57 mm Hg, pulse of 105 beats/minute, respiratory rate of 28 breaths/minute, and temperature of 99.3°F. He is thin and in moderate distress. Chest exam is normal. His abdomen is soft and nontender. Stool is negative for occult blood. In the emergency room, the patient begins to vomit large amounts, and he aspirates a significant amount of stomach contents and develops respiratory failure. He is intubated and started on mechanical ventilation. After 1 hour of mechanical ventilation, the following laboratory values are received:

Serum	
Sodium (mEq/L)	138
Potassium (mEq/L)	3.7
Chloride (mEq/L)	91
Bicarbonate (mEq/L)	16
BUN (mg/dL)	11
Phosphorus (mg/dL)	2.2
Albumin (g/dL)	3.6
Creatinine (mg/dL)	1.7
Glucose (mg/dL)	980
Arterial blood gas	
pH	7.41
pO_2	67
PCO_2	27

- **What is the acid-base disturbance present in this patient?** This patient has a mixed acid-base disorder, metabolic acidosis/metabolic alkalosis. The patient presents with diabetic ketoacidosis. The anion gap is 31, which signifies a large degree of ketoacid production. Because of the nausea and vomiting, he also has developed a metabolic alkalosis, and thus the bicarbonate level is higher than one would expect with this degree of acid production. This can be formalized by calculating the delta–delta anion gap. Another method of conceptualizing what is occurring is to take the difference of the anion gap and a normal anion gap. To illustrate how this works, we define the normal anion gap as 12 mEq/L. In this case, the difference between the patient's anion gap and the normal anion gap is: 31 – 12 = 19 mEq/L. This difference is often referred to as the delta–delta anion gap. If this number is added to the patient's bicarbonate, the result is 35. This significantly exceeds the normal bicarbonate of 24, which indicates that a metabolic alkalosis is present. What this tells us is that if all of the unmeasured anions—which are potentially bicarbonate—are converted back to bicarbonate, the patient would be considered to have a metabolic alkalosis.

TABLE 42.7

TREATMENT OF METABOLIC ALKALOSIS

Chloride sensitive	■ IV normal saline volume expansion ■ Discontinue diuretics if possible ■ H_2 blockers or proton pump inhibitors in cases of nasogastric suction and vomiting
Chloride resistant	■ Remove offending agent ■ Replace potassium if deficient
Extreme alkalosis	■ Hemodialysis ■ NH_4Cl or HCl can also be used

Key Points

1. Metabolic alkalosis is often accompanied by a decrease in chloride such that the decrease offsets the incremental increase in bicarbonate.
2. Metabolic alkalosis is caused by excessive bicarbonate intake or loss of H^+.

3. Vomiting, nasogastric suction, and diuretics are the most frequent causes of metabolic alkalosis in the intensive care unit setting.
4. In patients with metabolic alkalosis and low urinary chloride, normal saline is indicated to expand the extracellular space.

Respiratory Acid-base Disorders

Under normal conditions, through endogenous metabolism, approximately 15,000 mmol/day of CO_2 is produced. Carbon dioxide enters the plasma and forms carbonic acid, which subsequently dissociates to bicarbonate and H^+. The majority of this CO_2 generated is transported to the lungs in the form of bicarbonate. The H^+ produced in the process is exchanged across the erythrocyte cell membrane and is buffered intracellularly. In the alveoli, this process is reversed and the bicarbonate combines with H^+, liberating CO_2, which is then excreted through respiration. Carbon dioxide is the main stimulus for respiration, which is activated by small elevations in the PCO_2. Hypoxia is a minor stimulus for respiration and is typically effective when the PO_2 is in the range of 50 to 55 mm Hg. Derangements in respiratory CO_2 excretion lead to alterations in the ratio of PCO_2 to bicarbonate in the serum and therefore alter systemic pH (recall the Henderson-Hasselbalch relationship, Eq. 4).

Respiratory Acidosis

Respiratory acidosis results from the primary retention of carbon dioxide; a variety of disorders that reduce ventilation can lead to respiratory acidosis. The common etiologies of respiratory acidosis seen in intensive care unit patients are listed in Table 42.8.

The increase in the plasma PCO_2 decreases the pH by formation of carbonic acid (Eq. 11). The principal compensatory defense mechanisms against respiratory acidosis are buffering and renal compensation. Recalling the Henderson-Hasselbalch relationship (Eq. 4), the pH of the blood is dependent on the relative concentrations of CO_2 and bicarbonate. Therefore, when there is an increase in PCO_2, the renal response to increase HCO_3^- is an action to normalize this relationship (Fig. 42.3B). In respiratory acidosis, the extracellular buffering capacity is severely limited because bicarbonate cannot buffer carbonic acid. Intracellular buffers—hemoglobin and other intracellular proteins—serve as the protection against acute rises in PCO_2. In circulating erythrocytes, the H^+ that is produced as carbonic acid is formed from CO_2 that is buffered by hemoglobin; bicarbonate then leaves the cell in exchange for chloride. The buffering response to an elevation of CO_2 occurs within 10 to 15 minutes.

Renal compensation occurs in response to chronic respiratory acidosis. Hypercapnia stimulates secretion of protons in the distal nephron. Additionally, the urinary pH decreases and urinary ammonium excretion is increased, as is titratable acid excretion and excretion of chloride. The net effect is enhanced reabsorption of bicarbonate. The kidney's response to an acute increase in PCO_2 through compensation takes 3 to 4 days to reach completion (Table 42.2).

Aside from the compensatory mechanisms mentioned above, an increase in alveolar ventilation is ultimately required in order to eliminate excess CO_2 and therefore to re-establish equilibrium. If ventilation increases quickly during the acute period, the decrease in PCO_2 re-establishes equilibrium. However, following sustained hypercapnia that has elicited an appropriate renal response (i.e., a compensatory increase in serum bicarbonate), bicarbonaturia accompanies the return of the PCO_2 to normal. However, in order for this to occur, the chloride intake must be sufficient to replenish the deficit that developed during the renal compensation to the chronic respiratory acidosis, which induces a negative chloride balance. If chloride is deficient, the serum bicarbonate will remain persistently elevated, a phenomenon termed posthypercapnic metabolic alkalosis.

TABLE 42.8

CAUSES OF RESPIRATORY ACIDOSIS

Airway obstruction	■ Foreign body, aspiration ■ Obstructive sleep apnea ■ Laryngospasm or bronchospasm
Neuromuscular disorders of respiration	
Acute:	■ Myasthenia gravis ■ Guillain-Barré syndrome ■ Botulism, tetanus, drugs ■ Hypokalemia, hypophosphatemia (respiratory muscle impairment) ■ Cervical spinal injury
Chronic:	■ Morbid obesity (aka Pickwickian syndrome) ■ Central sleep apnea
Central respiratory depression	■ Drugs (opiates, sedatives), anesthetics ■ Oxygen administration in acute hypercapnia ■ Brain trauma or stroke
Respirator disorders	
Acute:	■ Severe pulmonary edema ■ Asthma or pneumonia ■ Acute respiratory distress syndrome ■ Chronic obstructive pulmonary disorder ■ Pulmonary fibrosis
Chronic:	■ Chronic pneumonitis

Clinical Presentation. Acute respiratory acidosis can produce headaches, confusion, irritability, anxiety, and insomnia, although the symptoms are difficult to separate from concomitant hypoxemia. Symptoms may progress to asterixis, delirium, and somnolence. The severity of the clinical presentation correlates more closely with the rapidity of the development of the disturbance rather than the absolute PCO_2 level.

Treatment. The treatment of respiratory acidosis is focused on alleviating the underlying disorder. In patients with acute respiratory acidosis and hypoxemia, supplemental oxygen is appropriate. However, to treat the hypercapnia, an increase in effective alveolar ventilation is necessary through either reversal of the underlying cause or, if necessary, mechanical ventilation. The administration of bicarbonate in respiratory acidosis when a coexisting metabolic acidosis is not present is potentially harmful. Bicarbonate in the setting of acute respiratory acidosis may precipitate acute pulmonary edema, metabolic alkalosis, and augmented carbon dioxide production, leading to increased PCO_2 in patients with inadequate respiratory reserve (45).

During chronic respiratory acidosis, renal compensation leads to a near-normalization of the arterial pH. In treating chronic respiratory acidosis, the objective is to ensure adequate oxygenation and, if possible, to increase alveolar ventilation. The administration of excessive oxygen and use of sedatives should be avoided because these treatments can depress the respiratory drive. Mechanical ventilation may be indicated when there is an acute exacerbation of chronic hypercapnia. If mechanical ventilation is used, the PCO_2 should be decreased gradually, avoiding precipitous drops, as rapid correction may cause severe alkalemia. Also, this may increase the cerebrospinal fluid pH, because carbon dioxide rapidly equilibrates across the blood–cerebrospinal fluid barrier. This complication can lead to serious neurologic problems, including seizures and death.

Special Scenario: Permissive Hypercapnia. It has been shown that ventilator strategies to reduce ventilator-associated lung injury (VALI) improve intensive care unit outcomes (46–49). This strategy is referred to as permissive hypercapnia and may reduce VALI through several mechanisms: by reducing stretch trauma and associated release of cytokines, and by preventing translocation of endotoxin and bacteria across the alveolar capillary barrier (50–54). It is not known for certain if respiratory acidosis per se has a beneficial effect, though there are recent data to suggest such an effect (55). Primary elevation of PCO_2 is also suggested to be deleterious on cardiac function (27,28), though this may be outweighed by protective effects of hypercapnia on lung injury (56). Further studies will be needed to delineate the specific roles of low tidal volume and respiratory acidosis with or without buffering in the management of acute lung injury.

Case Scenario #7: Respiratory Acidosis

A 56-year-old morbidly obese patient is admitted to the hospital with severe cellulitis of the right lower extremity that fails to respond to intravenous antibiotics. On hospital day 3, he undergoes a right below-knee amputation and, although recovering well, complains of severe pain postoperatively. His blood cultures drawn at admission are negative. His past medical history is significant for diabetes mellitus and chronic lower extremity ulceration that is felt to be secondary to venous stasis. Current medications include hydrochlorothiazide 25 mg PO daily, amlodipine 10 mg PO daily, enalapril 10 mg PO bid, metformin 1,000 mg PO bid, and a fentanyl patch 25 μg/hour. Two days following the operation he is found to have diminished mental status and the following laboratory data are obtained:

Serum	
Sodium (mEq/L)	140
Potassium (mEq/L)	4.4
Chloride (mEq/L)	98
Bicarbonate (mEq/L)	34
BUN (mg/dL)	19
Creatinine (mg/dL)	1.2
Phosphorus (mg/dL)	4.3
Albumin (g/dL)	3.7
Glucose (mg/dL)	180
Arterial blood gas	
pH	7.09
PO_2 (mm Hg)	55
PCO_2 (mm Hg)	110

■ **Which medication contributed most to the acid-base disorder prior to initiation of mechanical ventilation?**

The laboratory values are consistent with acute respiratory acidosis, secondary to fentanyl, likely in the setting of a chronic respiratory acidosis, itself probably secondary to restrictive lung disease from obesity. The chronic respiratory acidosis is evidenced by the increased serum bicarbonate with a decreased pH. This is consistent with a history of obesity, which can lead to a restrictive pattern of lung disease characterized by chronic respiratory insufficiency. An acute respiratory acidosis is present because the expected degree of renal compensation is not present as it would be if the patient had a chronic elevation of the PCO_2 to levels of 110 mm Hg. The acute respiratory failure is most likely secondary to narcotic overdose, and thus fentanyl is the most likely causative agent.

Respiratory Alkalosis

Pathophysiology. Respiratory alkalosis is due to a primary increase in ventilation, which leads to a decrease in the PCO_2 and occurs commonly in the intensive care unit either as a treatment (e.g., for elevated intracranial pressure), as an iatrogenic complication of mechanical ventilation, or as part of a disease presentation (Table 42.9) (57). The lowered PCO_2 in turn reduces carbonic acid levels, which decreases systemic pH. The buffering system and, ultimately, renal compensation are the counterregulatory measures that are directed at maintaining plasma pH in this setting. In the setting of acute respiratory alkalosis, proteins, phosphates, and hemoglobin liberate H^+. These liberated protons subsequently react with bicarbonate to form carbonic acid. At the level of the erythrocyte, a shift of chloride to the extracellular compartment ensues, as bicarbonate and cations enter in exchange for protons. The net effect of this buffering system reduces plasma pH and accounts for a 2 mEq/L decrease in the serum bicarbonate for every 10 mm Hg decrease in the PCO_2 that occurs in the acute setting (Table 42.2). Persistent respiratory alkalemia elicits the renal response, which leads to a net decrease in the secretion of H^+. This renal compensation causes a decrease in the proximal reabsorption of bicarbonate and a decrease in the excretion of titratable acids and of ammonium. Recall that the excretion of one H^+ in the kidney leads to the regeneration of a HCO_3^- molecule; therefore, these renal changes decrease renal

TABLE 42.9

CAUSES OF RESPIRATORY ALKALOSIS

Cause	Examples
Hypoxia	■ High altitude ■ Congestive heart failure ■ Severe V/Q mismatch
Lung diseases	■ Pulmonary fibrosis ■ Pulmonary edema ■ Pneumonia ■ Pulmonary embolism
Drugs	■ Salicylates ■ Progesterone ■ Nicotine
Direct stimulation of respiratory drive	■ Psychogenic hyperventilation ■ Cirrhosis ■ Gram-negative sepsis ■ Pregnancy (progesterone) ■ Excessive mechanical ventilation ■ Neurologic disorders (e.g., pontine tumors)

production of HCO_3^-. This compensatory response is maximal 3 to 4 days following the onset of alkalemia and leads to further decrease in serum HCO_3^-.

Clinical Presentation. Respiratory alkalosis may lead to a wide range of clinical manifestations ranging from alteration in consciousness, perioral paresthesias, and muscle spasms to cardiac arrhythmias. In addition, alkalemia also can affect metabolism of divalent ions. By stimulating glycolysis, alkalemia causes phosphate to shift from the extracellular space into the intracellular compartment as glucose-6-phosphate is formed. Additionally, the level of ionized calcium in the blood may also decrease due to increased binding of calcium to albumin.

Treatment. The underlying cause for respiratory alkalosis should be sought (Table 42.9). Cirrhosis can lead to respiratory alkalosis through impaired clearance from the circulation of progesterones and estrogens, similar to pregnancy (58). This is a commonly seen acid-base disorder in the intensive care unit. In psychogenic hyperventilation, rebreathing air using a bag increases the systemic PCO_2 and can treat alkalemia. Specific therapy, other than treatment of the underlying cause, is typically not necessary.

Case Scenario #8: Severe Acute Respiratory Alkalosis: A Potential Complication of Mechanical Ventilation

A 42-year-old patient with morbid obesity is admitted to the hospital with shortness of breath and fever. In the emergency room, he is started on intravenous antibiotics. Over the next 3 hours, he becomes severely short of breath and develops a diminished level of consciousness. He is intubated and placed on mechanical ventilation. His past medical history is significant for diabetes mellitus and hypertension. The social history is significant for one pack per day of smoking for 20 years. Current medications include amlodipine 5 mg PO daily, enalapril 5 mg PO bid, and hydrochlorothiazide 12.5 mg PO bid. Physical exam shows blood pressure of 156/80 mm Hg, pulse of 70 beats/minute, and temperature of 100.8°F. The patient is morbidly obese. The cardiovascular exam is normal. Lung exam reveals bilateral breath sounds with diffuse crackles on the right and egophony. Thirty minutes after mechanical ventilation laboratory studies are sent, with the following results:

Serum	
Sodium (mEq/L)	140
Potassium (mEq/L)	4.4
Chloride (mEq/L)	97
Bicarbonate (mEq/L)	35
BUN (mg/dL)	15
Creatinine (mg/dL)	0.9
Phosphorus (mg/dL)	4.0
Albumin (g/dL)	3.9
Glucose (mg/dL)	146
Arterial blood gas	
pH	7.66
PO_2 (mm Hg)	340
PCO_2 (mm Hg)	31

■ **What PCO_2 goal should be targeted in order to correct the acid-base disorder and attain a normal pH?**

The respiratory rate should be decreased to maintain the pH at a level of about 55 mm Hg, as this will lead to a pH of approximately 7.4. When a patient with chronic respiratory acidosis and appropriate renal compensation is placed on mechanical ventilation, he or she is at risk of developing a posthypercapnic metabolic alkalosis, as occurred in this case. Quickly lowering the PCO_2 in a patient with an elevated bicarbonate can lead to a dangerous degree of alkalemia. This occurs because mechanical ventilation can remove PCO_2 from the blood quickly, thus increasing the pH precipitously. However, it takes time for the kidney to adapt to the change in blood pH. In time, the kidney can adapt by decreasing bicarbonate reabsorption, leading to loss of bicarbonate in the urine; but this does not happen quickly, usually requiring a minimum of 24 to 36 hours. The appropriate measure is to decrease the minute ventilation to allow the PCO_2 to rise to a level that would lead to a normal or slightly acidic pH. The target PCO_2 can be calculated by using the Henderson-Hasselbalch equation; however, this degree of precision is not always necessary. The minute ventilation can simply be decreased and titrated to achieve the desired pH.

MIXED ACID-BASE DISORDERS

Mixed acid-base disorders are more difficult to diagnose than simple acid-base disorders. A good general rule is to keep in mind that in patients with a known primary acid-base disorder, a mixed disorder needs to be suspected if the pH is normal or if the apparent "compensation" has led to a pH that is beyond the normal. For example, if a patient with metabolic acidosis has a pH of 7.47, this indicates an accompanying respiratory alkalosis since a compensation would not lead to an alkaline pH if the primary disorder is an acidosis.

Metabolic and Respiratory Acidosis

In this mixed disorder, respiratory compensation is insufficient for the degree of decrease in bicarbonate. The most extreme example of this mixed-condition disorder occurs following cardiopulmonary arrest. In this setting, there is a decrease in bicarbonate levels—a metabolic acidosis secondary to lactic acidosis—and retention of carbon dioxide secondary to respiratory arrest. The pH in this setting is very low. Mixed metabolic and respiratory acidosis is also commonly seen in patients with a primary metabolic acidosis and concomitant lung disease. The lung disease impairs the ability of the patient to increase the ventilatory rate to appropriately decrease the PCO_2. Furthermore, this combination of disorders can manifest as a patient with a chronically elevated PCO_2 and an inability to increase the serum bicarbonate. This would indicate a chronic respiratory acidosis and possibly a metabolic acidosis due to a "normalized" serum bicarbonate in a setting in which the bicarbonate would be expected to be elevated. Finally, the presence of an anion gap, despite a normal serum bicarbonate level, should raise the index of suspicion for this combination of conditions.

Metabolic and Respiratory Alkalosis

Acidemia is better tolerated than is alkalemia. For example, a pH of 7.2 is well tolerated, whereas a pH of greater than 7.6 is associated with significant mortality. Mixed metabolic and respiratory alkalosis can lead to a significant elevation in the pH and is therefore very serious. This condition typically occurs in patients on mechanical ventilation. Often, mechanical ventilation, by mandating a minimum minute ventilation, will not allow the patient to elevate the PCO_2 significantly in response to alkalemia. Frequently, the metabolic alkalosis in this setting is due to diuretic use, administration of bicarbonate solutions, or massive transfusions with a citrate load.

Respiratory Alkalosis and Metabolic Acidosis

Most commonly, this combination is seen in Gram-negative sepsis, which can stimulate the respiratory drive—resulting in respiratory alkalosis—and also cause circulatory collapse with subsequent lactic acidosis. In the medical intensive care unit, salicylate intoxication classically leads to a mixed metabolic acidosis and respiratory alkalosis (23). Salicylates directly lead to an anion gap metabolic acidosis, and they also directly stimulate respiration.

Approach to Mixed Acid-base Disorders

There is no simple algorithm to use in the approach to a mixed acid-base disorder. The approach outlined in Figure 42.5 assumes that only a single disorder is present. Complex acid-base problems should be suspected when the values cannot be explained by a single disorder and its compensation. An example of this might be a patient with lactic acidosis and an alkaline pH.

Key Points

1. In patients with a known primary acid-base disturbance, a mixed acid-base disorder should always be suspected if the pH is normal or the "compensation" has surpassed the normal pH.
2. Mixed metabolic and respiratory acidosis occurs when the respiratory compensation is insufficient for the degree of decrease in bicarbonate.
3. The presence of an increased anion gap despite normal serum bicarbonate levels should raise suspicion for mixed metabolic acidosis and metabolic alkalosis.
4. Non–anion gap metabolic acidosis and anion gap metabolic acidosis can coexist.
5. Gram-negative sepsis is a common cause of respiratory alkalosis and metabolic acidosis.
6. Mixed metabolic acidosis and metabolic alkalosis occurs commonly in diabetic ketoacidosis.

Case Scenario #9: Mixed Acid-base Disorder: Metabolic Acidosis and Respiratory Acidosis

A 64-year-old is admitted to the intensive care unit with pneumonia and septic shock. The patient states that he has had increasing shortness of breath and fever over the past 4 days. His past medical history is significant for hypertension. Surgical history is significant for a previous cholecystectomy. Medications include amlodipine and hydrochlorothiazide. Physical exam shows a blood pressure of 85/50 mm Hg, pulse of 110 beats/minute, respiratory rate of 22 breaths/minute, and temperature of 101.8°F. The cardiovascular examination is significant for a 2/6 systolic murmur and there are crackles over his entire right lung field. There is trace pedal edema. Chemistry values on admission are given below:

Serum	
Sodium (mEq/L)	135
Potassium (mEq/L)	4.8
Chloride (mEq/L)	103
Bicarbonate (mEq/L)	10
BUN (mg/dL)	22
Creatinine (mg/dL)	1.4
Phosphorus (mg/dL)	2.8
Albumin (g/dL)	3.8
Glucose (mg/dL)	115
Arterial blood gas	
pH	6.95
PO_2 (mm Hg)	51
PCO_2 (mm Hg)	48

■ **What acid-base disorder(s) is (are) present in this patient?**
The acid-base disorder is a mixed anion gap metabolic acidosis with a respiratory acidosis. The decrease in bicarbonate accompanied by an elevated anion gap is consistent with a primary metabolic acidosis. The expected PCO_2 using the Winter formula $= 10(1.5) + 4 = 19$. The PCO_2 is significantly elevated above this level, and thus a respiratory acidosis is present. The PCO_2 is much higher than would be expected based on the degree of acidemia, and thus a respiratory acidosis, secondary to inadequate ventilation from pneumonia, is present.

References

1. Jorgensen K, Astrup P. Standard bicarbonate, its clinical significance, and a new method for its determination. *Scand J Clin Lab Invest.* 1957;9(2):122–132.
2. Batlle DC, Hizon M, Cohen E, et al. The use of the urinary anion gap in the diagnosis of hyperchloremic metabolic acidosis. *N Engl J Med.* 1988; 318(10):594–599.
3. Gabow PA. Disorders associated with an altered anion gap. *Kidney Int.* 1985;27(2):472–483.
4. Winter SD, Pearson JR, Gabow PA, et al. The fall of the serum anion gap. *Arch Intern Med.* 1990;150(2):311–313.
5. Sadjadi SA. A new range for the anion gap. *Ann Intern Med.* 1995;123 (10):807.
6. Figge J, Rossing TH, Fencl V. The role of serum proteins in acid-base equilibria. *J Lab Clin Med.* 1991;117(6):453–467.
7. Fencl V, Jabor A, Kazda A, et al. Diagnosis of metabolic acid-base disturbances in critically ill patients. *Am J Respir Crit Care Med.* 2000;162 (6):2246–2251.
8. Moe OW, Fuster D. Clinical acid-base pathophysiology: disorders of plasma anion gap. *Best Pract Res Clin Endocrinol Metab.* 2003;17(4):559–574.
9. Hassan H, Joh JH, Bacon BR, et al. Evaluation of serum anion gap in patients with liver cirrhosis of diverse etiologies. *Mt Sinai J Med.* 2004;71(4):281–284.
10. Schnur MJ, Appel GB, Karp G, et al. The anion gap in asymptomatic plasma cell dyscrasias. *Ann Intern Med.* 1977;86(3):304–305.
11. Murray T, Long W, Narins RG. Multiple myeloma and the anion gap. *N Engl J Med.* 1975;292(11):574–575.
12. Madias NE, Ayus JC, Adrogue HJ. Increased anion gap in metabolic alkalosis: the role of plasma-protein equivalency. *N Engl J Med.* 1979;300(25): 1421–1423.
13. Salem MM, Mujais SK. Gaps in the anion gap. *Arch Intern Med.* 1992; 152(8):1625–1629.
14. Story DA, Kellum JA. New aspects of acid-base balance in intensive care. *Curr Opin Anaesthesiol.* 2004;17(2):119–123.
15. Corey HE. Stewart and beyond: new models of acid-base balance. *Kidney Int.* 2003;64(3):777–787.
16. Wooten EW. Science review: quantitative acid-base physiology using the Stewart model. *Crit Care.* 2004;8(6):448–452.
17. Story DA. Bench-to-bedside review: a brief history of clinical acid-base. *Crit Care.* 2004;8(4):253–258.
18. Kellum JA, Kramer DJ, Pinsky MR. Strong ion gap: a methodology for exploring unexplained anions. *J Crit Care.* 1995;10(2):51–55.
19. Feldman M, Soni N, Dickson B. Influence of hypoalbuminemia or hyperalbuminemia on the serum anion gap. *J Lab Clin Med.* 2005;146(6):317–320.

20. Pierce NF, Fedson DS, Brigham KL, et al. The ventilatory response to acute base deficit in humans. Time course during development and correction of metabolic acidosis. *Ann Intern Med.* 1970;72(5):633–640.
21. Adrogue HJ, Wilson H, Boyd AE 3rd, et al. Plasma acid-base patterns in diabetic ketoacidosis. *N Engl J Med.* 1982;307(26):1603–1610.
22. Judge BS. Differentiating the causes of metabolic acidosis in the poisoned patient. *Clin Lab Med.* 2006;26(1):31–48, vii.
23. Krause DS, Wolf BA, Shaw LM. Acute aspirin overdose: mechanisms of toxicity. *Ther Drug Monit.* 1992;14(6):441–451.
24. Kurtzman NA. Disorders of distal acidification. *Kidney Int.* 1990;38(4):720–727.
25. Narins RG, Goldberg M. Renal tubular acidosis: pathophysiology, diagnosis and treatment. *Dis Mon.* 1977;23(6):1–66.
26. DeFronzo RA. Hyperkalemia and hyporeninemic hypoaldosteronism. *Kidney Int.* 1980;17(1):118–134.
27. Arieff AI, Leach W, Park R, et al. Systemic effects of NaHCO3 in experimental lactic acidosis in dogs. *Am J Physiol.* 1982;242(6):F586–591.
28. Graf H, Leach W, Arieff AI. Evidence for a detrimental effect of bicarbonate therapy in hypoxic lactic acidosis. *Science.* 1985;227(4688):754–756.
29. Jeffrey FM, Malloy CR, Radda GK. Influence of intracellular acidosis on contractile function in the working rat heart. *Am J Physiol.* 1987;253(6 Pt 2): H1499–1505.
30. Ayus JC, Krothapalli RK. Effect of bicarbonate administration on cardiac function. *Am J Med.* 1989;87(1):5–6.
31. Kalkut G. Antiretroviral therapy: an update for the non-AIDS specialist. *Curr Opin Oncol.* 2005;17(5):479–484.
32. Wohl DA, McComsey G, Tebas P, et al. Current concepts in the diagnosis and management of metabolic complications of HIV infection and its therapy. *Clin Infect Dis.* 2006;43(5):645–653.
33. Moyle GJ, Datta D, Mandalia S, et al. Hyperlactataemia and lactic acidosis during antiretroviral therapy: relevance, reproducibility and possible risk factors. *Aids.* 2002;16(10):1341–1349.
34. Tebb Z, Tobias JD. New anticonvulsants–new adverse effects. *South Med J.* 2006;99(4):375–379.
35. Guo PY, Storsley LJ, Finkle SN. Severe lactic acidosis treated with prolonged hemodialysis: recovery after massive overdoses of metformin. *Semin Dial.* 2006;19(1):80–83.
36. Parke TJ, Stevens JE, Rice AS, et al. Metabolic acidosis and fatal myocardial failure after propofol infusion in children: five case reports. *BMJ.* 1992;305(6854):613–616.
37. Cremer OL, Moons KG, Bouman EA, et al. Long-term propofol infusion and cardiac failure in adult head-injured patients. *Lancet.* 2001;357(9250):117–118.
38. Perrier ND, Baerga-Varela Y, Murray MJ. Death related to propofol use in an adult patient. *Crit Care Med.* 2000;28(8):3071–3074.
39. Vasile B, Rasulo F, Candiani A, et al. The pathophysiology of propofol infusion syndrome: a simple name for a complex syndrome. *Intensive Care Med.* 2003;29(9):1417–1425.
40. Corbett SM, Moore J, Rebuck JA, et al. Survival of propofol infusion syndrome in a head-injured patient. *Crit Care Med.* 2006;34(9):2479–2483.
41. Wolf A, Weir P, Segar P, et al. Impaired fatty acid oxidation in propofol infusion syndrome. *Lancet.* 2001;357(9256):606–607.
42. Cray SH, Robinson BH, Cox PN. Lactic acidemia and bradyarrhythmia in a child sedated with propofol. *Crit Care Med.* 1998;26(12):2087–2092.
43. Luke RG, Galla JH. Chloride-depletion alkalosis with a normal extracellular fluid volume. *Am J Physiol.* 1983;245(4):F419–424.
44. Galla JH, Bonduris DN, Luke RG. Effects of chloride and extracellular fluid volume on bicarbonate reabsorption along the nephron in metabolic alkalosis in the rat. Reassessment of the classical hypothesis of the pathogenesis of metabolic alkalosis. *J Clin Invest.* 1987;80(1):41–50.
45. Ayus JC, Olivero JJ, Adrogue HJ. Alkalemia associated with renal failure. Correction by hemodialysis with low-bicarbonate dialysate. *Arch Intern Med.* 1980;140(4):513–515.
46. Amato MB, Barbas CS, Medeiros DM, et al. Effect of a protective-ventilation strategy on mortality in the acute respiratory distress syndrome. *N Engl J Med.* 1998;338(6):347–354.
47. Hickling KG, Walsh J, Henderson S, et al. Low mortality rate in adult respiratory distress syndrome using low-volume, pressure-limited ventilation with permissive hypercapnia: a prospective study. *Crit Care Med.* 1994;22(10):1568–1578.
48. Brower RG, Rubenfeld GD. Lung-protective ventilation strategies in acute lung injury. *Crit Care Med.* 2003;31(4 Suppl):S312–316.
49. Laffey JG, O'Croinin D, McLoughlin P, et al. Permissive hypercapnia–role in protective lung ventilatory strategies. *Intensive Care Med.* 2004;30(3):347–356.
50. Maggiore SM, Jonson B, Richard JC, et al. Alveolar derecruitment at decremental positive end-expiratory pressure levels in acute lung injury: comparison with the lower inflection point, oxygenation, and compliance. *Am J Respir Crit Care Med.* 2001;164(5):795–801.
51. Boussarsar M, Thierry G, Jaber S, et al. Relationship between ventilatory settings and barotrauma in the acute respiratory distress syndrome. *Intensive Care Med.* 2002;28(4):406–413.
52. Slutsky AS, Tremblay LN. Multiple system organ failure. Is mechanical ventilation a contributing factor? *Am J Respir Crit Care Med.* 1998;157(6 Pt 1): 1721–1725.
53. Tremblay L, Valenza F, Ribeiro SP, et al. Injurious ventilatory strategies increase cytokines and c-fos m-RNA expression in an isolated rat lung model. *J Clin Invest.* 1997;99(5):944–952.
54. Murphy DB, Cregg N, Tremblay L, et al. Adverse ventilatory strategy causes pulmonary-to-systemic translocation of endotoxin. *Am J Respir Crit Care Med.* 2000;162(1):27–33.
55. Kregenow DA, Rubenfeld GD, Hudson LD, et al. Hypercapnic acidosis and mortality in acute lung injury. *Crit Care Med.* 2006;34(1):1–7.
56. Sinclair SE, Kregenow DA, Lamm WJ, et al. Hypercapnic acidosis is protective in an in vivo model of ventilator-induced lung injury. *Am J Respir Crit Care Med.* 2002;166(3):403–408.
57. Laffey JG, Kavanagh BP. Hypocapnia. *N Engl J Med.* 2002;347(1):43–53.
58. Lustik SJ, Chhibber AK, Kolano JW, et al. The hyperventilation of cirrhosis: progesterone and estradiol effects. *Hepatology.* 1997;25(1):55–58.

CHAPTER 43 ■ CENTRAL NERVOUS SYSTEM

EDWARD M. MANNO • ALEJANDRO A. RABINSTEIN

The last few decades have yielded significant insights into the mechanisms of acute cerebral injury. The most important finding has been that a significant proportion of neurologic damage after injury occurs secondarily and, thus, is potentially preventable or treatable. This discovery has altered the approach to acute neurologic injury and, coupled with improved diagnostic techniques, has reversed the therapeutic nihilism that had previously marked the field. In this chapter, we will attempt to provide a foundation in the basics of cerebrovascular physiology. Based on these foundations, we will attempt to outline a rational approach to the treatment of both general and specific neurologic emergencies.

CEREBRAL METABOLISM AND HYPOXIC ISCHEMIC BRAIN INJURY

Approximately 20% of the cardiac output and oxygen consumption is utilized by the human brain, which accounts for only 2% of the total body mass (1). The majority of cerebral oxygen consumption occurs at the highly metabolically active gray matter structures of the brain. The relatively high metabolic activity of these cells is needed to sustain the electrical gradients of neurons needed to transmit electrical signals, synthesize transmitters, and maintain the infrastructure of the cell (2).

The central nervous system utilizes intracellular stores of phosphocreatine and adenosine triphosphate (ATP) as its energy source. These stores are constantly replenished through the aerobic oxidative phosphorylation of glucose at the inner membrane of the neuronal mitochondria. Glucose is the main substrate for brain metabolism, with specific glucose transferases in the capillary endothelium providing entry into the neuronal cytoplasm. Brain energy reserves are limited. Electrical activity is inhibited within seconds, and cellular breakdown occurs within minutes of lack of oxygen delivery to the neurons. Anaerobic metabolism provides only a small amount of the energy needed to maintain neuronal cellular activity (2).

Under normal conditions, cerebral blood flow (CBF) and regional distribution of oxygen are tightly coupled. Increases in cerebral metabolism lead to an increase in the delivery of oxygen and glucose to metabolically active tissue. Cerebral blood flow is, by convention, measured in milliliters of flow per 100 g of tissue per minute. Normal CBF ranges between 30 and 70 mL/100 g/minute. The cerebral metabolic rate of oxygen consumption ($CMRO_2$) is the rate of oxygen utilized by cerebral tissue. It is calculated by the Fick method of measuring the product of CBF and the cerebral oxygen arterial–venous difference of an inert nondiffusible substance. Direct and indirect methods exist to estimate both CBF and $CMRO_2$. Cerebral oxygen delivery (CDO_2) is the product of CBF and the oxygen-carrying capacity of hemoglobin. The normal mean capillary partial pressure of oxygen (PO_2) is approximately 65 mm Hg, representing a difference between normal arterial PO_2 (90–95 mm Hg) and venous PO_2 (35–40 mm Hg). Normal values for standard measures of CBF, $CMRO_2$, and CDO_2 are detailed in Table 43.1.

Cerebral ischemia develops if cerebral oxygen utilization cannot meet metabolic demands. This can result from problems with cerebral oxygen delivery, increased metabolic demands, or impaired oxygen utilization. Decreases in CDO_2 can occur with decreases in cerebral blood flow due to stroke, increased intracranial pressure (ICP), decreased cardiac output, or hypotension. The cerebral metabolic rate increases with increased cerebral activity, seizures, or hyperthermia. Blood loss or carbon monoxide poisoning can decrease the oxygen-carrying capacity (3).

Inadequate oxygen delivery due to decreased CBF is the most common cause of cerebral ischemia. Synaptic transmission, and hence electrical activity, discontinues at CBF below 15 to 20 mL/100 g/minute. Further decreases in CBF lead to ionic pump failure and membrane destabilization (3). Cerebral oxygen delivery can also be affected by changes in the concentration of oxygen bound to hemoglobin. Hemoglobin has a high affinity for binding oxygen, with greater than 90% of the hemoglobin binding sites for oxygen saturated at arterial partial pressures of oxygen (PaO_2) greater than 70 mm Hg. Increasing PaO_2 with increases in inspired oxygen above this level, therefore, has little effect on oxygen delivery. However, a large oxygen gradient is needed at the cellular level to provide an adequate pressure gradient for the oxygen molecule to diffuse to the mitochondrial inner membrane. The critical required PO_2 at the level of the mitochondria is estimated at 5 mm Hg; hence, at low oxygen gradients (venous PO_2 levels below 30 mm Hg), cerebral insufficiency will develop (2).

TABLE 43.1

NORMAL VALUES FOR CEREBRAL BLOOD FLOW AND METABOLISM

Cerebral blood flow (CBF)	50 mL/100 g/min
Systemic arterial oxygen content (CaO_2)	14–20 mL/100 mL
Jugular venous oxygen content ($CjvO_2$)	8–13 mL/100 mL
Jugular venous oxygen saturation ($SjvO_2$)	65%
Cerebral arterial–venous oxygen content difference [$C(a\text{-}v)O_2 = CaO_2 - CjvO_2$]	6.3 mL/100 mL
Cerebral oxygen delivery ($CDO_2 =$ CBF $\times$ CaO_2)	10 mL/100 g/min
Cerebral metabolic rate of oxygen consumption $CMRO_2 -$ CBF $\times$ $C(a\text{-}v)O_2$	3.5 mL/100 g/min

Several mechanisms exist to maintain oxygen delivery to the brain. Cerebral hypoperfusion will lead to the depolarization of medullary neurons mediating sympathetic output, which consequently results in a compensatory increase in blood pressure and heart rate. Decreased cerebral perfusion leading to decreased arterial oxygen delivery to the cerebral capillary bed will lead to venodilation lowering of the postcapillary pressure and increasing flow across the capillary bed. Oxygen extraction bound to hemoglobin is increased across the capillary bed as CBF continues to decrease. This increase in oxygen extraction can be detected by measuring jugular venous blood and comparing it to arterial oxygen content. Finally, increases in local hydrogen ion concentration will occur as ischemia develops, presumably due to lactate production from anaerobic metabolism. The resultant shift in the oxygen displacement curve of hemoglobin to the right will result in increased oxygen released from hemoglobin to the local cerebral tissue.

Cerebral ischemia can be categorized into focal and global causes. *Focal ischemia* occurs when there is severe or complete reduction of blood flow to one of the major arteries of the brain. Neurologic impairment develops in functional patterns attributable to the particular arterial distribution that is involved. This most commonly is seen secondary to embolic or atherosclerotic large vessel occlusion. *Global ischemia* refers to severe reductions or cessation of blood flow to the entire brain. This most commonly occurs after cardiac arrest but can be seen in any condition that leads to global cerebral hypoperfusion or hypoxia (2,3).

Cerebral tissues exhibit selective vulnerability to ischemia. Neurons are the least resistant to cerebral ischemia, followed by oligodendroglia, astrocytes, and endothelial cells in order of susceptibility. Specific neuronal populations also exhibit selective vulnerability to ischemia and hypoxia. The most susceptible neurons to anoxia are the CA_1 and CA_3 cell populations located in the medial hippocampus. These cells are the most widely connected and have the highest resting metabolic rate of all neurons. Similarly, highly metabolically active cells with high susceptibility to ischemia include the cerebellar Purkinje cells, cortical cell levels 3 and 5, and the medium-size neurons of the striatum (2,4).

Vascular patterns of neuronal injury encountered with cerebral anoxia can be attributed to the selective ischemic vulnerability of varying cerebral cell types, coupled with the different mechanisms by which ischemia or hypoxia can occur. Watershed or border zone infarctions occur at the boundary between the perfusion territories of the large cerebral arteries. Hypotension after cardiac, septic, or hemorrhagic shock is the most common etiology for this phenomenon. Selective loss of neurons in the hippocampus, basal ganglia, cortex, and cerebellum can lead to laminar necrosis of these tissues, and may occur after ischemia leads to cell death in these cells, but circulation is restored prior to involvement of other neuronal cell populations. Dysmyelination of the central white matter can develop in the setting of hypotension where hypoxia does not occur. Cerebral white matter is believed to be selectively vulnerable to this condition due to its decreased resting regional CBF compared to the more metabolically active gray matter (2).

Neuronal cell death is a product of both the severity and time of ischemia; thus, incomplete degrees of ischemia can be tolerated for longer periods of time. However, there is some critical threshold of ischemia that will ultimately lead to necrosis. The duration and severity of ischemia needed to reach a critical threshold can be modified by metabolic factors such as hyperglycemia, temperature, and metabolic activity. Critical reductions of oxygen, therefore, produce significant but nonfatal degrees of ischemia and neuronal function. Lethal reductions of oxygen imply that some threshold has been crossed that will lead to a series of events, and ultimately to cell death (2).

Oxygen deprivation leading to neuronal cell death proceeds through several distinctive steps. The high metabolic activity of neurons rapidly depletes oxygen-derived ATP and phosphocreatine stores, resulting in failure of synaptic transmission. The electroencephalogram (EEG) at this point becomes flat, and consciousness is lost. Electrical failure occurs as CBF falls below 16 to 20 mL/100 g tissue/minute and cerebral oxygen consumption falls below one third of its normal resting metabolism, but restoration of CBF after electrical failure will allow functional recovery of the cell. Further decreases in CBF to less than 10 mL/100 g tissue/minute will lead to failure of the energy needed to maintain the activity of the membrane sodium potassium pump. As flow continues to decrease, membrane depolarizations occur, and ionic gradients are lost as potassium effluxes from the cell and sodium and water enters the cells, leading to the development of cytotoxic edema (Fig. 43.1).

Release of excessive amounts of glutamate is believed to mediate the process of excitatory cell death after ischemia. Normally, glutamate, an excitatory neurotransmitter, is released into the synaptic cleft and rapidly cleared by energy-dependent cellular uptake mechanisms. In the setting of energy failure, extracellular glutamate levels increase. Most glutamate neurotoxicity is mediated through *N*-methyl D-aspartate (NMDA) receptors. Stimulation of these receptors activates calcium channel–mediated entry into the cell. Intracellular calcium subsequently activates a number of destructive enzymatic processes, including protease destruction of structural proteins and phospholipase destruction of plasma membranes, with release of arachidonic acid and endonucleases capable of fragmenting DNA repair mechanisms. Mitochondrial uptake of calcium leads to the interruption of electron transport and the development of oxygen-free radicals (1,3,5,6).

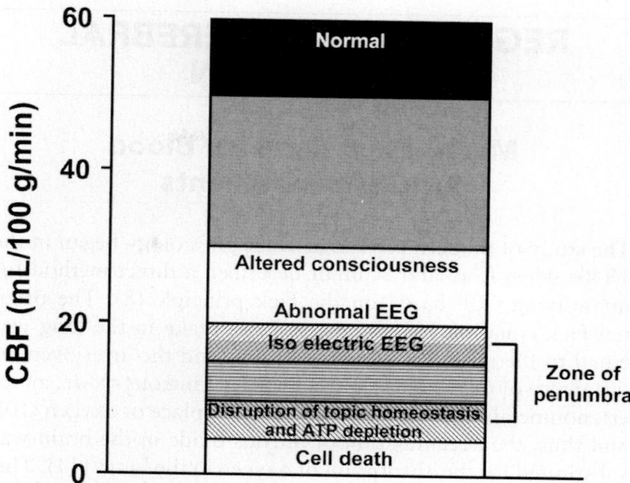

FIGURE 43.1. Blood flow thresholds for cerebral function and metabolism. As blood flow decreases, synaptic transmission and electrical activity ceases (electroencephalographic silence). Further decreases in flow lead to loss of ionic homeostasis and cell death. The ischemic penumbra describes brain tissue with blood flows below electrical failure but above membrane failure. CBF, cerebral blood flow; EEG, electroencephalogram; ATP, adenosine triphosphate. (From Veremakis CV, Lindner DH. Central nervous system injury: essential physiologic and therapeutic concerns. In: Civetta JM, Taylor RW, Kirby RR, eds. *Critical Care.* Philadelphia: Lippincott–Raven Publishers; 1997:273–289.)

The above process leads to necrosis of brain tissue with distinctive neuropathologic features. Necrosis is characterized by cellular swelling, membrane wall lysis, and a resultant inflammatory reaction to clear the necrotic tissue. Cells die in groups, leaving large areas of necrotic tissue (7). Apoptosis, or programmed cell death, also occurs in cerebral ischemia. Apoptosis is an organized and regulated form of cell death where intra- and extracellular signals lead to a programmed process of cell death with preservation of the mitochondria. Pathologically, apoptosis leads to cell shrinkage, chromatin condensation, and dissolution of the cell membrane. Inflammation is not commonly seen. These two distinctive forms of cell death probably represent a spectrum of the biochemical and morphologic changes that can occur in cerebral ischemia (1).

In focal ischemia and infarction, a central region of necrosis can be surrounded by a potentially viable area of tissue described as the *ischemic penumbra*. The ischemic penumbra can be defined through CBF measurements and electrophysiology, or biochemical and genetic methods. The penumbra, by definition, is tissue that is potentially salvageable if circulation is restored. Neurocritical care focuses on methods to restore flow to the ischemic penumbra and potentially limit the extent of neuronal cell death.

REGULATION OF CEREBRAL CIRCULATION

Methods of Cerebral Blood Flow Measurements

The study of modern cerebrovascular physiology began in the 1940s when Kety and Schmidt described a direct method for quantifying CBF based on the Fick principle (8). The original Fick equation stated that oxygen uptake in the lung was equal to the product of cardiac output and the arteriovenous difference of oxygen (9). Kety substituted nitrous oxide, an inert, nonmetabolizable, diffusible tracer in place of oxygen (10), and thus, the accumulation of nitrous oxide in the brain was substituted for the absorption of oxygen in the lungs (11). This technique is still considered the gold standard for quantifying CBF, but is invasive and limits measurements only to global CBF (12).

The development of external detection systems allowed for the use of radioactive tracers to measure regional areas of CBF. Focal perfusion and washout of substances could be used to determine flow into local brain regions. Xenon^{133}, a diffusible γ-emitting substance, was used initially as an injection and later through inhalation. Perfusion and washout were calculated using a rotating γ-counter. Later, the application of computed tomographic techniques (Xenon CT) allowed for improved resolution of regional areas of cerebral blood flow (rCBF) (13). Single photon emission computed tomography (SPECT) uses technetium^{99} as a ligand to measure rCBF, and is the most commonly used technique to measure CBF. Technetium^{99} crosses the blood–brain barrier and is trapped within cells. The tracer accumulates in varying brain regions according to the rate of delivery, and thus is a marker for rCBF. Multidetector systems are used to quantify the accumulation of tracer (14). Positron emission tomography (PET) is similar to SPECT in that an external detecter is used to measure an accumulated radioactive substance. The generation and use of positrons, however, significantly improve resolution. A positron is an electron with a positive charge formed by the decay of radionuclides. It requires a cyclotron or linear accelerator for its production. The collision of a positron with an electron produces two photons that are sent off at 180 degrees. The simultaneous detection of these photons allows for improved resolution and three-dimensional reconstruction of rCBF. In addition to measuring CBF, different radiolabeled ligands can be used to measure cerebral blood volume (CBV), glucose metabolism, or cerebral oxygen extraction. PET provides the highest quantifiable measure of rCBF and can be used for a variety of physiologic experiments (15). However, it is expensive, requires a cyclotron, and is limited to a few academic centers (Fig. 43.2).

New techniques of bolus tracking with magnetic resonance imaging (MRI) and computed tomography (CT) have allowed for acute assessments of cerebral perfusion. In these techniques, a bolus of a contrast agent is detected either through changes in the T_2 signal or Hounsfield units. Estimations of CBF can be made by measuring the transit time required for these boluses to pass through cerebral tissue. These techniques are being used widely for the acute assessments of cerebral infarctions (16,17).

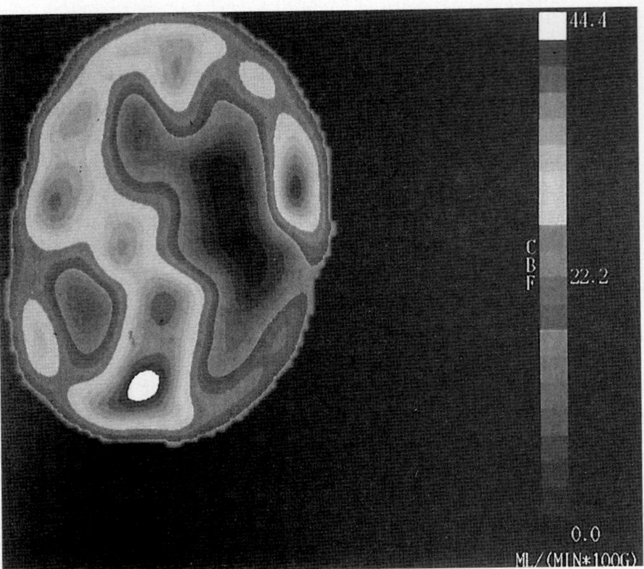

FIGURE 43.2. Positron emission tomography image of an intracerebral hemorrhage. Note central area of necrosis surrounded by area of decreased perfusion. (Courtesy of Michael Diringer, Washington University School of Medicine.)

Factors that Regulate Cerebral Blood Flow

Cerebral Autoregulation

Cerebral autoregulation refers to the capacity of CBF to remain constant despite changes in cerebral perfusion pressure. It is a pressure phenomenon that needs to be differentiated from the effect of carbon dioxide and arterial oxygen tension on CBF. This control, and thus the shape of the autoregulatory curve, can be modified by a number of extrinsic factors. Hypertension, hypocarbia, and increased sympathetic nervous activity will increase both the upper and lower ranges of autoregulation. Chronic hypotension, hypercarbia, and parasympathetic activity will lower the set points of autoregulation. The autoregulatory curve will shift upward with advancing age. In the healthy, normotensive individual, CBF is a pressure-passive phenomenon below perfusion pressures of 50 to 60 mm Hg and above perfusion pressures of 150 to 160 mm Hg. Between these broad parameters, CBF increases only slightly (18,19) (Fig. 43.3).

In most vascular beds, autoregulation occurs at the level of the arterioles. A significant proportion of vascular resistance in the cerebral circulation, however, is modulated at the level of the cerebral arteries. In cats, dogs, and monkeys, approximately 40% of the cerebral vascular resistance is mediated by changes in the baseline pial artery diameter of vessels greater than 400 μm in diameter (20).

In response to hypotension, both cerebral arteries and arterioles will dilate to maintain constant CBF. Vessel dilation progresses from the largest vessels to the smallest with decreases in cerebral perfusion pressure (21). Cerebral arterioles will also continue to dilate below the lower limit of autoregulation (19). Further drops in pressure flow slowly across the capillary bed and lead to an increase in the oxygen extraction coefficient

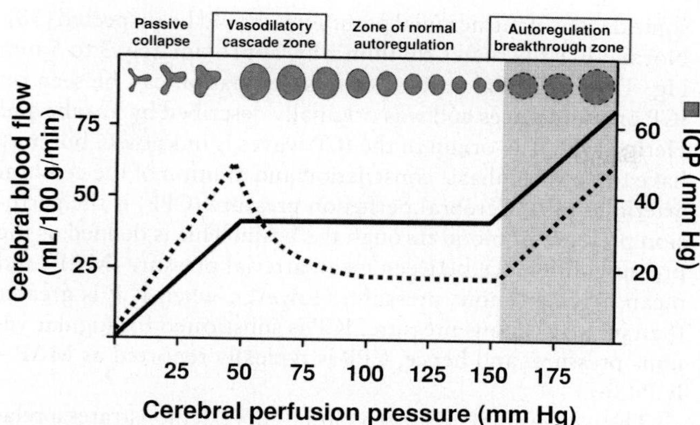

FIGURE 43.3. Cerebral autoregulatory curve with cerebral blood flow remaining constant between cerebral perfusion pressures (CPP) of 50 and 150 mm Hg (*solid line*). Superimposed curve of cerebral blood volume (CBV) at variable CPP (*dotted line*). The top portion of the figure illustrates the cerebral arteriolar caliber. Note that at CPP below the level of cerebral autoregulation, arteries and arterioles begin to collapse (passive collapse). CBV decreases from a point of maximal dilation seen near the lower end of CA (vasodilatory cascade zone) to a constant blood volume (zone of normal autoregulation). Higher CPP leads to autoregulatory breakthrough and parallel increases in both CBF and CBV (autoregulatory breakthrough zone). ICP, intracranial pressure. (From Rose JC, Mayer SA. Optimizing blood pressure in neurological emergencies. *Neurocrit Care.* 2004;1:287–299.)

from hemoglobin (18). Continued hypotension progresses to cerebral hypoperfusion and ischemia as previously discussed.

In a similar fashion, cerebral pial arteries and arterioles will constrict as perfusion pressure increases. Maximal vasoconstriction occurs at cerebral perfusion pressures of 160 to 170 mm Hg. Above these pressures, there is a forced vasodilation of the cerebral vessels with a large increase in CBF. The ensuing hypertensive encephalopathy is due to blood–brain barrier disruption and the development of cerebral edema (21). The initial distribution of this edema commonly is located in the occipital lobes. This is speculated to occur due to the limited sympathetic innervation of the posterior circulation.

Mechanisms of Cerebral Autoregulation

There are several theories that have been proposed to explain the mechanisms of cerebral autoregulation. These can be broadly categorized into the myogenic, metabolic, and neurogenic hypotheses of autoregulatory control (18).

Myogenic Theory. The myogenic theory postulates that the smooth muscle cells of the cerebral arteries and arterioles constrict or dilate in response to the transmural pressure generated across the vessel wall (22). This may be mediated by alterations in the position of the actin myosin filament in the vessel wall (23). Another theory is that changes in vessel wall shear stress induced by alterations in blood flow induce the release of vasoactive substances from the vascular endothelium that subsequently leads to vessel wall constriction or dilation (24). The myogenic theory is supported by the rapidity with which cerebral autoregulation occurs, although the myogenic theory by itself cannot account for all of the regulation that occurs. In jugular venous hypertension, cerebral arterial pressure is increased. While this condition should lead to arterial vasoconstriction, vasodilation is most commonly found under these circumstances (25). It is thus postulated that myogenic factors may play a significant role only when metabolic factors are not significant. Alternately, myogenic factors may work synergistically with metabolic factors, providing changes in vascular tone that may optimize the metabolic response (26).

Metabolic Theory. The metabolic theory of pressure autoregulation postulates that the local changes in cerebral blood flow found with changes in cerebral metabolic activity are mediated through the release of local neurochemical substances from the nonvascular cells of the central nervous system (18). The tight coupling of flow to metabolism and the timing of autoregulation support this postulated mechanism. Several substances have been suggested including hydrogen ion concentrations, carbon dioxide, nitric oxide, adenosine, potassium, and calcium (27). Experimental evidence exists in favor of and against all of the postulated mediators (18,28–30). Varying combinations have also been suggested. Most recently, changes in potassium levels mediated through alterations in calcitonin gene-related peptides have been suggested as a mechanism of arteriolar dilation (31). Changes in cerebral perfusion pressure have been observed that alter the degree of endothelial oxygen tension, and have been suggested as an important mechanism for autoregulation (32).

Neurogenic Influences. The role of direct neurogenic influences on cerebral autoregulation is limited. As mentioned, the sympathetic and parasympathetic nervous system plays a role in modulating the cerebral autoregulatory curve. However, direct neural control over small arteries or arterioles that regulate focal changes in CBF does not occur, and other intrinsic nerve fibers may be in a position to regulate vascular tone (33). The localization or central control of these nerves has so far proved elusive (18,34).

Regulation of Cerebral Blood Flow by Carbon Dioxide and Oxygen

Changes in the partial pressure of carbon dioxide ($PaCO_2$) have significant effects on CBF. A 1-mm Hg change in $PaCO_2$ results in an approximately 2.5% to 4% change in CBF. This effect is more pronounced in the gray matter than white matter. The response curve of $PaCO_2$ is sigmoidal, with the CBF response flattening below 15 to 20 mm Hg and above 100 mm Hg. The vasodilation occurs in all vessel sizes but is most pronounced on the smaller arterioles (11) (Fig. 43.4).

Changes in vessel diameter are mediated through alterations in cerebrospinal hydrogen ion concentrations (CSF pH). The direct application of CO_2 or bicarbonate to pial arterioles does not affect vessel diameters. Since CO_2 is freely diffusible across the blood–brain barrier, changes in $PaCO_2$ will affect both cerebrospinal fluid hydrogen ion and bicarbonate concentrations (35). The response of changes in hydrogen ion concentration is relatively short-lived, lasting only a few hours, as the choroid plexus of the brain will compensate for changes in hydrogen ion concentration by adjusting the production of cerebrospinal fluid bicarbonate (36).

At partial pressures of oxygen below 50 mm Hg, there is a rapid increase in CBF. Again, this is more significant in gray, as opposed to white, matter. There is a linear relationship between

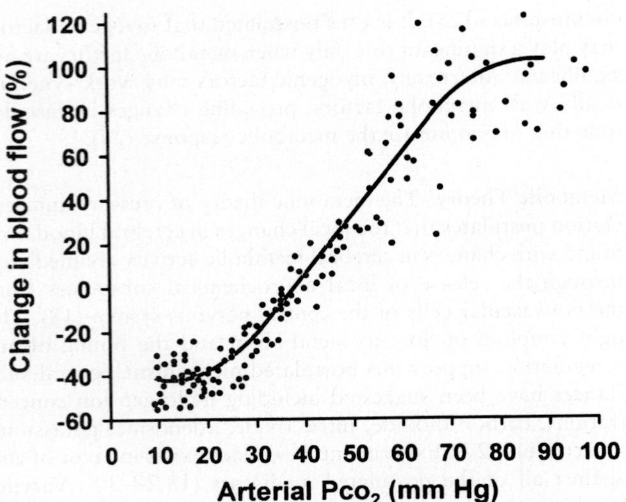

FIGURE 43.4. Alterations in cerebral blood flow with changes in the partial pressure of carbon dioxide. Note the S-shaped curve, with flat portions at the extremes of the curve. Data obtained from normotensive dogs. (From Harper AM, Glass HI. Effect of alterations in the arterial carbon dioxide tension on the blood flow through the cerebral cortex at normal and low arterial pressures. *J Neurol Neurosurg Psychiatry.* 1965;28:449–452.)

the arterial oxygen content and CBF in hypoxia (Fig. 43.5) (21,37). Vasoactive effects may be mediated directly through oxygen or adenosine A_2 receptors (11).

Cerebral Blood Volume and Intracranial Hemodynamics

Normal ICP measures between 5 and 8 mm Hg, with statistical variations ranging as high as 15 mm Hg. Beyond this level,

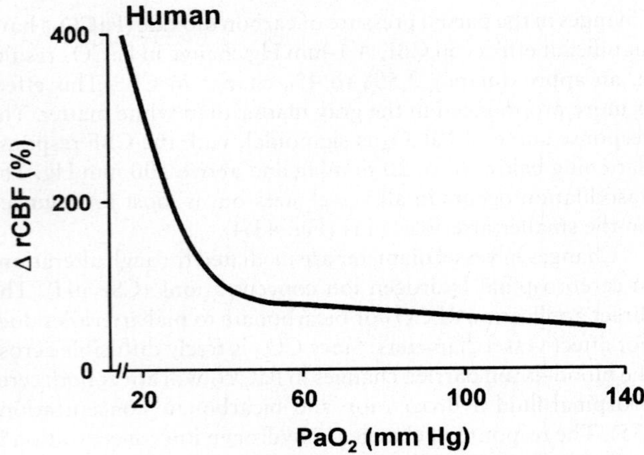

FIGURE 43.5. Alterations of regional cerebral blood flow to changes in arterial oxygen tension. Note oxygen tensions below approximately 50 lead to a sharp increase in regional cerebral blood flow. rCBF, regional areas of cerebral blood flow. (From Golanov EV, Reisw DJ. Oxygen and cerebral blood flow. In: Welch KMA, Caplan LR, Reis DJ, et al., eds. *Primer on Cerebrovascular Disease*. San Diego: Academic Press; 1997:58–60.)

some degree of intracranial pathology should be suspected (38). Normal ICP fluctuates rhythmically, approximately 3 to 5 mm Hg. The sinusoidal pattern of this fluctuation can be seen on ICP pressure traces and was originally described by Traube and Hering (39). The origin of the ICP waves is unknown, but may have to do with phasic constriction and dilation of the cerebral arterioles (40). Cerebral perfusion pressure (CPP) is the perfusion pressure of blood through the brain. This is defined as the pressure difference between mean arterial pressure (MAP) and mean jugular venous pressure. However, when ICP is greater than jugular venous pressure, ICP is substituted for jugular venous pressure, and hence, CPP is typically reported as MAP – ICP (36).

The intracranial pressure volume curve demonstrates a relatively flat portion where increases in volume are accommodated with little change in pressure. At some inflection point, these processes are exhausted, and small changes in volume lead to larger increases in ICP (Fig. 43.6). This pressure volume curve may, thus, represent the displacement of various fluids from the intracranial space.

The approximate contents of the intracranial cavity consist of the brain parenchyma (75%), blood (20%), and CSF (5%). Most of the intracranial blood resides on the venous side of the circulation (38). According to the Monroe doctrine, the overall volume of the contents of the intracranial cavity must remain constant. Accordingly, any increase in the intracranial contents from venous engorgement, intracerebral hemorrhage, tumors, edema, etc., must be compensated by an equal displacement of fluids or tissue. Monroe postulates that the flat portion of the ICP volume curve represents displacement of CSF into the more compliant spinal subarachnoid space. Progressive increases in volume lead to further displacement of venous and arterial blood. Finally, brain tissue is displaced and herniation will occur (Fig. 43.6) (41).

The ICP volume curve can be affected by the speed and duration of changes that occur in the intracranial cavity. Tumors, for example, can grow to large volumes before becoming problematic. The slow-growing process allows for a gradual increase in intracranial compliance. Similarly, an acute hemorrhage of the same size will not be tolerated.

Intracranial compliance can be determined by measuring the change in ICP to a given volume. A volume pressure response (VPR) is estimated by measuring the ICP response to an infusion of 1 mL of sterile saline into an intraventricular catheter (42). Small changes in response to this increased volume suggest that the patient was on the flat portion of the volume pressure curve. Increases in ICP greater than 4 mm Hg in response to 1 mL of fluid would suggest that intracranial reserve was limited. A more widely used index to measure intracranial compliance has been the pressure volume index (PVI). This index estimates the volume needed to increase ICP by a factor of 10 (43).

Spontaneous and sustained elevations in ICP were noted by Lunberg early in the study of cerebral hemodynamics (44). The origin of these "plateau waves" had been speculative until the 1980s when Rosner et al. provided a potential rationale as to how these could develop. Rosner accounted for these waves through the observation of subtle changes in MAP and ICP, and their effect on CBV and ICP. Rosner observed that plateau waves were always preceded by subtle drops in CPP. As previously noted, decreases in CPP will lead to cerebral vasodilation of the cerebral arterioles and arteries, which consequently

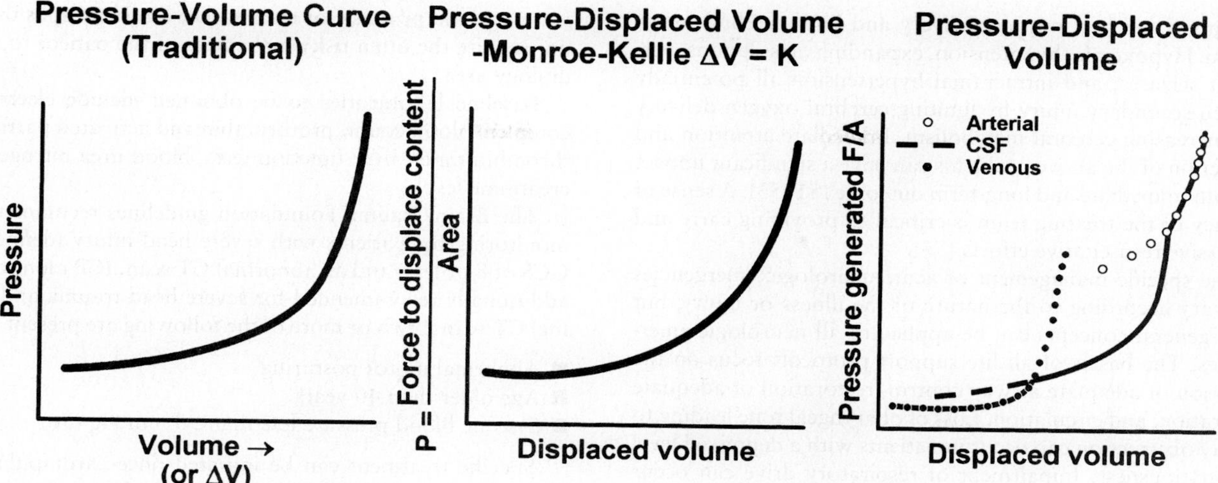

FIGURE 43.6. Three forms of the intracranial pressure volumes curves. The curve on the left represents the traditional teaching that compensatory mechanisms allow for small changes in pressure as intracranial volume increases. The middle section suggests that pressure may be better defined as the force per unit area needed to displace a certain volume of the intracranial contents. The last section suggests that the traditional pressure volume curve actually represents superimposed displacement curves of varying substances in the cranial cavity. At low pressures (flat portion), cerebral spinal fluid is displaced downward into the compliant spinal subarachnoid space. As pressure increases, venous and arterial blood are displaced before brain parenchyma is displaced at very high pressures (cerebral herniation). CSF, cerebrospinal fluid. (From Rosner MJ. Pathophysiology and management of increased intracranial pressure. In: Andrews BT, ed. *Neurosurgical Intensive Care*. New York: McGraw-Hill; 1993:57–112.)

result in an increase in total CBV through an increase of blood in the cerebral venous system. At some point, however, continued decreases in CBF will lead to a decrease in CBV (Fig. 43.3) (45). The cerebral engorgement of blood that occurs with the initial decrease in MAP increases ICP and decreases CPP, thus initiating a cycle of decreasing CPP, increasing CBV, and increasing ICP. The process is spontaneously reversed by an acute elevation of blood pressure from a Cushing response. This sympathetic response occurs in the setting of decreased CPP as the brainstem center's modulating sympathetic activity becomes oligemic (46). Rosner has used these observations as the basis for management of cerebral perfusion pressure due to head trauma (41).

Cerebral Edema

Intracranial hypertension can be caused by expanding masses, cerebral engorgement, or the development of cerebral edema. Cerebral edema may compress brain structures, leading to herniation, or reduce cerebral perfusion with subsequent infarction (47). Cerebral edema is roughly defined as an increase in the brain tissue water and sodium content of the extravascular space (48). Cerebral edema is, therefore, different from brain engorgement, which represents an increase in the blood volume of the intravascular space (49).

Cerebral edema can be defined according to its location or mechanism of production. According to location, edema can occur either inside the brain cells (intracellular) or outside the cells and the intravascular space in the interstitium (interstitial). While certain forms of cerebral edema may predominate, pure forms of either type of edema rarely exist. *Cytotoxic edema* is the term employed to describe the intracellular edema that develops after the loss of cell wall integrity (50). The terminology implies a toxic etiology, but it is most often seen in cellular energy failure due to ischemia or hypoxia. Vasogenic edema represents an expansion of the interstitium due to disruption of the capillary blood–brain barrier, which allows the extravasation of fluid from the intravascular space. Interstitial edema develops secondary to increases in the hydrostatic pressures of the ventricular system draining the CSF. Osmotic edema refers to the intracellular swelling that occurs due to rapid changes in brain sodium concentrations or the osmotic disequilibrium syndromes (48).

MECHANISMS OF BRAIN INJURY AND THERAPEUTIC CONCERNS

Immediate Concerns

The most important features in managing acute neurologic injury are rapid transport to a trauma center or stroke center; management of airway, oxygenation, and circulation issues; careful and repeated monitoring; and prompt head imaging, with immediate medical or surgical management of expanding mass lesions (51). The mechanisms of neurologic injury will, of course, vary depending upon the nature of the injury, but all will include—to some degree—secondary injury caused by cerebral ischemia. In head trauma, shearing injury develops due to different deceleration rates of gray and white matter. The resultant disruption of neurologic tracts is followed by a period of ischemia and secondary injury. Prolonged seizure activity in status epilepticus leads to hippocampal ischemia, cell death, and atrophy (52). A zone of ischemia surrounds all areas of cerebral infarction and cerebral hemorrhage (53).

The primary goal of acute neurologic management is to prevent secondary injury. This is attained by initiating measures to support cerebral oxygen delivery and limit cerebral metabolism. Hypoxemia, hypotension, expanding mass lesions, persistent seizures, and intracranial hypertension all potentially worsen secondary injury by limiting cerebral oxygen delivery and increasing cerebral metabolism. Immediate attention and correction of the above problems can have a significant impact on both immediate and long-term outcome (51–53). A sense of urgency of the treating team is critical to providing early and aggressive resuscitative efforts (53).

The specific management of acute neurologic emergencies will vary according to the nature of the illness or injury, but some general concepts can be applied to all neurologic emergencies. The basics of all life support protocols focus on the initiation of adequate airway control, restoration of adequate respiration, and circulation. Loss of pharyngeal tone leading to airway obstruction can occur in patients with a depressed level of consciousness. Impairment of respiratory drive can occur after seizures, head trauma, anoxic injury, stroke, or metabolic disturbances. Decreases in cerebral perfusion are common after head or multisystem injury, shock, sepsis, and hemorrhage.

The acute management of neurologic injury must focus on the maintenance of cerebral oxygen delivery. To accomplish this goal, adequate oxygenation, respiration, and blood pressure must be ensured. Airway control via endotracheal intubation for the neurologic patient should be performed immediately in all patients with a Glasgow coma score (GCS) of 8 or less. Supplemental oxygenation and red blood cell transfusions should be given to provide adequate oxygenation.

Once the basics of life support have been secured, a rapid history should be obtained from supporting personnel or family since, in many circumstances, the patient will be unable to provide an adequate history. The immediate details surrounding the incident are crucial to understanding the nature or type of injury. A general physical exam prior to the neurologic assessment should focus on possible trauma or other medical conditions. Raccoon eyes or a Battle sign (bruising of the orbits and mastoid region respectively) is evidence for a basilar skull fracture. In head trauma with loss of consciousness, neck injury should be assumed and cervical stabilization provided. A funduscopic exam may reveal papilledema or subhyaloid hemorrhages. Underlying body or breath odors may suggest intoxication. New onset atrial fibrillation may be the only clue to the mechanism of a cerebral infarct. Subtle eye, finger, or limb movements may be the only indication for subclinical seizure activity. A rapid neurologic assessment focusing on the level of consciousness, the cranial nerve exam, and any localizing features can be obtained within minutes. The GCS is commonly used as a quantitative assessment of neurologic function (54). More recently, a new coma score has been developed that has been validated in the neurointensive care unit (55) (Fig. 43.7). Further validations of this scale are under way in nonneurologic staff and intensive care units.

Emergent head imaging is obtained as soon as the patient is considered hemodynamically stable to leave the emergency room or intensive care unit. CT is the usual initial choice due to accessibility. A head CT without contrast is the best test to assess for skull or bone fractures and the possibility of acute intracranial blood. Large intracerebral, epidural, or subdural hematomas may need emergent evacuation. New imaging techniques such as CT perfusion and MRI for perfusion diffusion imaging may be able to identify specific salvageable ischemic brain regions that are at risk for infarction. New portable CT scanners hold promise for even earlier assessment, as these do not require the often risky movement of the patient to the radiology area.

Baseline laboratories to be obtained include electrolytes, complete blood count, prothrombin and activated partial prothrombin times, liver function tests, blood urea nitrogen, and creatinine levels.

The Brain Trauma Foundation guidelines recommend ICP monitoring for patients with severe head injury (defined as a GCS of 8 or less) and an abnormal CT scan. ICP monitoring is additionally recommended for severe head trauma and a normal CT scan if two or more of the following are present (56):

- Abnormal motor posturing
- Age older than 40 years
- Systolic blood pressure less than 90 mm Hg (56)

Specific treatment can be initiated once cardiopulmonary status has been stabilized and general and neurologic assessments have been completed. Guidelines and protocols currently exist for prehospital management of head trauma, intravenous and intra-arterial lysis of cerebral thrombosis, intracerebral hemorrhage, and status epilepticus (52,57–60).

General Therapeutic Considerations

In addition to the above measures designed to maintain adequate cerebral oxygen delivery, there has been a growing interest in the role of temperature, glucose, and blood pressure modulation in the management of neurologic injury. There is a large body of evidence in standardized laboratory animal models of cerebral ischemia that elevations in brain temperature both increase the amount of neuropathologic damage to injured tissue and induce damage to brain areas not usually involved (61). Excitotoxicity is believed to be the most likely mechanism for induction of these changes.

Hyperthermia

Hyperthermia increases both glutamate release and extracellular concentration. Free radical production is accelerated, and the sensitivity of neurons to excitotoxic injury is increased (62, 63). The role for excitotoxicity is corroborated by a noted increase in cellular acidosis and depolarization in the ischemic penumbra. Other postulated mechanisms for neurologic damage with hyperthermia include inhibition of protein kinases responsible for synaptic transmission and cellular repair, and the release of neuronal proteases. The latter is believed to be the mechanism for worsening cerebral edema at higher brain temperatures (64–67). Hyperthermia worsens outcomes in ischemic stroke patients (68), with a 2.2-fold increase in morbidity and mortality for every 1° increase in temperature above 37.5°C (69). Similarly, these results have been extended to the neurologic intensive care unit population. Hyperthermia in this population both worsened outcome and increased length of stay (70).

Hypothermia

Hypothermia may have a neuroprotective role in preventing many of the neuropathologic changes described with hyperthermia. Early applications of hypothermia protocols were problematic, with significant cardiac complications occurring below temperatures of 30°C. Most protocols were used during

Eye response

4 Eyelids open or opened, tracking, or blinking to command

3 Eyelids open but not tracking

2 Eyelids closed but open to loud voice

1 Eyelids closed but open to pain

0 Eyelids remain closed with pain

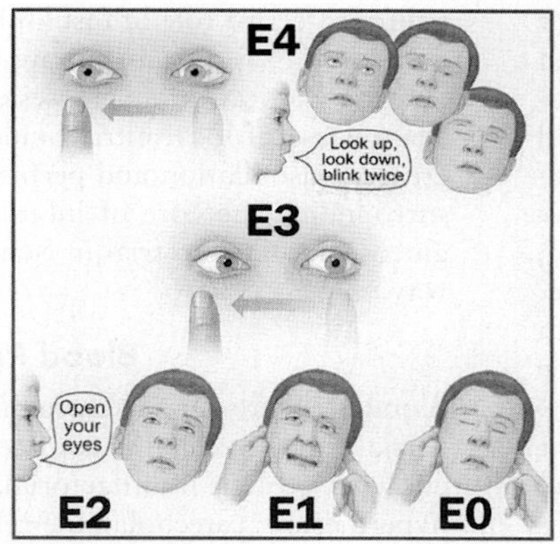

Eye response (E)
Grade the best possible response after at least 3 trials in an attempt to elicit the best level of alertness. A score of **E4** indicates at least 3 voluntary excursions. If eyes are closed, the examiner should open them and examine tracking of a finger or object. Tracking with the opening of 1 eyelid will suffice in cases of eyelid edema or facial trauma. If tracking is absent horizontally, examine vertical tracking. Alternatively, 2 blinks on command should be documented. This will recognize a locked-in syndrome (patient is fully aware). A score of **E3** indicates the absence of voluntary tracking with open eyes. A score of **E2** indicates eyelids opening to loud voice. A score of **E1** indicates eyelids open to pain stimulus. A score of **E0** indicates no eyelids opening to pain.

Motor response

4 Thumbs-up, fist, or peace sign to command

3 Localizing to pain

2 Flexion response to pain

1 Extensor posturing

0 No response to pain or generalized myoclonus status epilepticus

Motor response (M)
Grade the best possible response of the arms. A score of **M4** indicates that the patient demonstrated at least 1 of 3 hand positions (thumbs-up, fist, or peace sign) with either hand. A score of **M3** indicates that the patient touched the examiner's hand after a painful stimulus compressing the temporomandibular joint or supraorbital nerve (localization). A score of **M2** indicates any flexion movement of the upper limbs. A score of **M1** indicates extensor posturing. A score of **M0** indicates no motor response or myoclonus status epilepticus.

Brainstem reflexes

4 Pupil and corneal reflexes present

3 One pupil wide and fixed

2 Pupil *or* corneal reflexes absent

1 Pupil *and* corneal reflexes absent

0 Absent pupil, corneal, and cough reflex

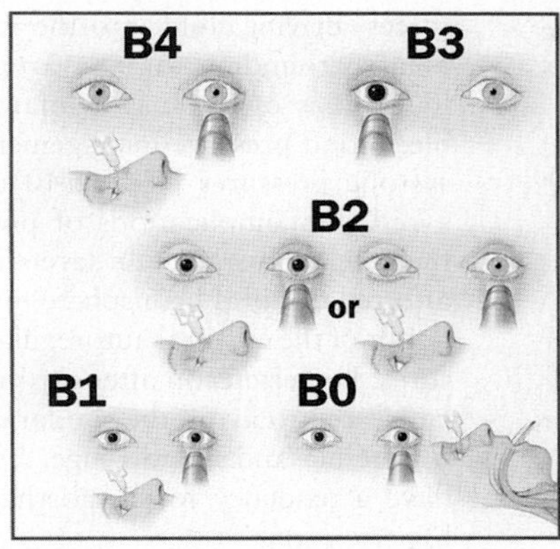

Brainstem reflexes (B)
Grade the best possible response. Examine pupillary and corneal reflexes. Preferably, corneal reflexes are tested by instilling 2–3 drops of sterile saline on the cornea from a distance of 4–6 inches (this minimizes corneal trauma from repeated examinations). Cotton swabs can also be used. The cough reflex to tracheal suctioning is tested only when both of these reflexes are absent. A score of **B4** indicates pupil and cornea reflexes are present. A score of **B3** indicates one pupil wide and fixed. A score of **B2** indicates either pupil or cornea reflexes are absent, **B1** indicates both pupil and cornea reflexes are absent, and a score of **B0** indicates pupil, cornea, and cough reflex (using tracheal suctioning) are absent.

Respiration

4 Not intubated, regular breathing pattern

3 Not intubated, Cheyne-Stokes breathing pattern

2 Not intubated, irregular breathing pattern

1 Breathes above ventilator rate

0 Breathes at ventilator rate or apnea

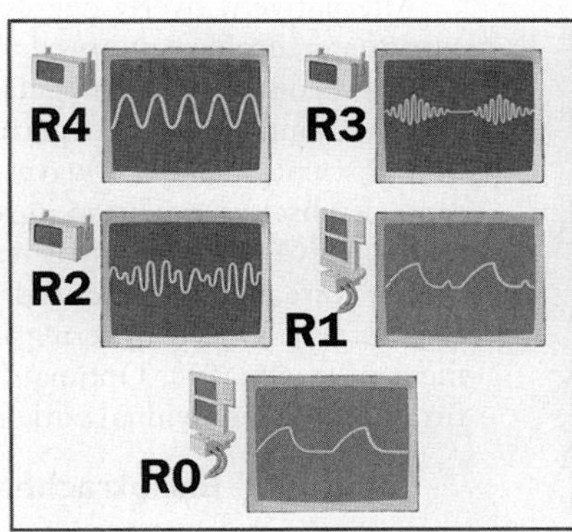

Respiration (R)
Determine spontaneous breathing pattern in a nonintubated patient and grade simply as regular **R4**, irregular **R2**, or Cheyne-Stokes **R3** breathing. In mechanically ventilated patients, assess the pressure waveform of spontaneous respiratory pattern or the patient triggering of the ventilator **R1**. The ventilator monitor displaying respiratory patterns is used to identify the patient-generated breaths on the ventilator. No adjustments are made to the ventilator while the patient is graded, but grading is done preferably with $Paco_2$ within normal limits. A standard apnea (oxygen-diffusion) test may be needed when patient breathes at ventilator rate **R0**.

FIGURE 43.7. Instructions for the assessment of the individual categories of the FOUR score. (From Wijdicks EFM, Bamlet WR, Maramattom BV, et al. Validation of a new coma scale: the FOUR score. *Ann Neurol.* 2005;58:585–593. © 2007. Mayo Foundation for Medical Education and Research.)

cardiac arrest with cardiac and neurosurgical procedures with varying results (71). Moderate hypothermia (33°C) has been employed successfully, with significant improvements in neurologic outcome in two randomized trials for global cerebral ischemia after cardiac arrest (72,73). In both of these protocols, hypothermia was induced early—within 2 to 8 hours—and maintained for 12 to 24 hours before passive rewarming. Sedation and pharmacologic paralysis were instituted to prevent the hypermetabolism and hyperthermia that occurs with shivering. Hypothermia, however, failed to improve outcome in a randomized trial of patients with severe head trauma (74). Subgroup analysis revealed worse outcomes in patients older than 45 years and in spontaneous hypothermic patients who were actively rewarmed. It is speculated that the lack of efficacy was due to the delay in the initiation of treatment (71). Hypothermia has been applied to patients with ischemic stroke in a small case series with promising results (75). A multicenter trial using a randomized application of hypothermia for large hemispheric infarcts is currently under way.

Hyperglycemia

Glucose control in patients with neurologic injury has recently received a considerable amount of attention. Hyperglycemia has been well documented to increase infarct size and worsen outcome in ischemic stroke (76,77). More recent studies in patients treated with thrombolytics have supported these observations (78–81). The negative effects of hyperglycemia may be limited to large-vessel ischemia or occlusions (82). Hyperglycemia has also been associated with a worsened outcome in subarachnoid hemorrhage (83), and results in head trauma have been inconsistent (84,85).

Hyperglycemia in acute neurologic injury may be attributed to several different mechanisms. The most common proposed mechanism for the development of hyperglycemia is a hormonally induced stress response that occurs with neurologic injury, thus leading to an increase in catecholamine and cortisol release. Other proposed means by which hyperglycemia can occur in neurologic injury include pituitary ischemia, direct irritation of glucose regulatory centers, and the discovery of latent diabetes (76).

Hyperglycemia may increase neurologic injury through a number of mechanisms, which include:

- Expansion of infarct size, due to an associated reduction in perfusion (86)
- Increases in cerebral metabolism (87) and cerebral edema (88)
- Potentiated calcium entry directly into neurons (89)
- The production of free radical–induced oxidative stress and inflammation (90,91) (the most widely supported mechanism of hyperglycemia-induced neuronal injury)

Intensive insulin therapy to maintain blood glucose below 110 mg/dL reduced morbidity and mortality in a prospective, randomized, single-center, surgical intensive care unit (92). A subgroup analysis of 63 patients with isolated head injury revealed improved ICP control, fewer vasopressor requirements, and a decreased incidence of diabetes insipidus and seizures. A reduction in ventilator dependency and improvement in long-term rehabilitation was attributed to prevention of or reduction in the development of a critical illness polyneuropathy (93). Insulin reduces ischemic brain damage in animal models during acute ischemia (94). However, there may be a direct neuroprotective role of insulin beyond the modulation of glucose levels (95). Insulin suppresses mediators of inflammation and coagulation, and increases endothelial nitric oxide release. The release of local nitric oxide could potentially lead to increased vasodilation and perfusion of the ischemic penumbra surrounding the core of infarcted tissue (96). A multicenter glucose and insulin trial in ischemic stroke is currently under way.

Blood Pressure

Blood pressure management in neurologic injury is controversial. Hypertension is common after neurologic injury. The etiology is often multifactorial, and may include underlying hypertension, catecholamine release to pain and stress, direct hypothalamic damage, or a physiologic response to volume depletion. The center of the controversy, thus, is determining whether the hypertension encountered during neurologic injury is pathologic or a normal compensatory and protective physiologic response. In addition, cerebral autoregulation is disturbed to varying degrees after brain injury; after the complete loss of autoregulation, CBF directly correlates with MAP. Disturbances in cerebral autoregulation can be global or focal, involving only areas adjacent to the damaged brain.

The controversy surrounding the optimal blood pressure after neurologic injury is based on competing processes. In areas surrounding neurologic injury, the blood–brain barrier is often damaged. In these areas, hypertension can lead to the development of cerebral edema by increasing the intravascular Starling forces, driving fluid into the interstitium of the brain. Brain area surrounding tumors, arteriovascular malformations, or local areas of trauma or infarction are particularly susceptible. Blood pressure management is often titrated to maintain systolic pressures below 140 mm Hg after neurosurgery to avoid the complications of postoperative edema and breakthrough hemorrhage. In severe carotid stenosis, the CPP to the affected cerebral hemisphere may be compromised, leading to a shift of the cerebral autoregulatory curve to lower blood pressures. Hypertension after carotid endarterectomy may need to be treated to avoid the similar complications of breakthrough hyperemia and hemorrhage. Large cerebral infarcts similarly have a tendency for hemorrhagic conversion with sustained hypertension.

Alternatively, overly aggressive management of hypertension after neurologic injury can be potentially deleterious. Brain areas with disturbed autoregulation may require a specific pressure to maintain adequate perfusion. An example of this is the development of plateau waves after head trauma that represents cerebral vasodilation in response to inadequate cerebral perfusion. Cerebral vasospasm after subarachnoid hemorrhage (SAH) is treated with induced hypertension. In selected small case series, induced hypertension has been used in the treatment of stroke (97). Optimal blood pressure may need to be titrated to the individual patient and disease process.

Endotracheal Intubation

Medical complications are common after neurologic injury and worsen outcome (98,99). The risk of aspiration pneumonia is increased in patients with a depressed level of consciousness. Early recognition and treatment of this complication are needed. Endotracheal intubation is required for neurologic patients who are unable to maintain airway patency or protect their airway from secretions. Endotracheal intubation portends a poor outcome for patients with ischemic and hemorrhagic stroke (100). The timing of extubation in the neurologic patient is controversial, since many patients remain intubated solely for airway protection. Dogma mandates that patients remain intubated until their GCS improves to greater than 8. However, a more recent prospective study has suggested that prolonged intubation in neurologic patients increases the rate of ventilator-acquired pneumonias, increases length of stay, and worsens outcomes. The authors recommend early extubation based on the patient's ability to control secretions (101). Alternatively, early tracheostomy may be considered.

Cardiac Stunning and Neurogenic Pulmonary Edema

Cardiac stunning and neurogenic pulmonary edema can occur after acute neurologic catastrophes. This is most commonly seen after severe head trauma, subarachnoid hemorrhage, status epilepticus, or intracerebral hemorrhage. The mechanism of cardiopulmonary damage is believed to occur through massive catecholamine release mediated through the sympathetic nervous system (102). In neurogenic pulmonary edema, sympathetic-mediated pulmonary venoconstriction is believed to create the Starling forces necessary to develop pulmonary edema (103). The sympathetic nervous system also innervates the contractile elements of the pulmonary endothelial cells. Catecholamine-mediated contraction of these cells can lead to opening of the tight junctions of the capillaries, allowing protein to flux into the pulmonary parenchyma (104). The process is self-limited, and aggressive diuresis and high levels of positive end-expiratory pressure (PEEP) are usually adequate to improve oxygenation.

Sympathetically-induced cardiac changes may be more severe. The sympathetic innervation of the heart parallels the cardiac conductive system, which probably accounts for the noted electrocardiogram (ECG) changes that can occur with severe neurologic injury. Deep T-wave inversions are usually reported as "cerebral T waves"; however, the spectrum of sympathetically induced ECG changes is broad, and includes ST elevations and depressions (102). Pathologically, cardiac contraction bands are seen surrounding the entry zone of the sympathetic endplates into the myocardium. These bands represent reperfusion injury from ischemic cardiac muscle. The muscle dies in a hypercontracted state and ultimately becomes calcified (105). Cardiac enzymes are elevated, but this finding does not necessarily implicate coronary artery disease. Clinically, myocardial contraction is impaired, and cardiac output and ejection fraction are decreased. Pulmonary edema is common, complicating an oftentimes concurrent process of neurogenic pulmonary edema. More recently, apical ballooning has been described with catecholamine excess, the so-called "Tako-Tsubo" cardiomyopathy (106). Serial echocardiography suggests that cardiac function usually improves over the course of a week, although it is important to note that the diagnosis of catecholamine-induced cardiac stunning implies a more severe neurologic injury, complicates medical management, and may portend a worse outcome (99).

Sodium Metabolism and Homeostasis

Disturbances in sodium metabolism and homeostasis are found in a variety of neurologic diseases. The syndrome of inappropriate antidiuretic hormone (SIADH) may be seen early in head trauma. Circulating levels of antidiuretic hormone (ADH) are elevated in a number of acute neurologic emergencies secondary to a catecholamine-induced stress response. This raises the question of whether the hyponatremia encountered is itself due to inappropriate ADH release or simply represents an appropriate but significant release of the hormone. In either case, the release of ADH has significant implication for the management of the neurologic patient. Acute hyponatremia leads to the development of intracellular edema, with expansion of the size of the neuronal cell body. Unlike other cells in the body, the neuron needs to maintain its cell size and integrity in order to transmit electrical signals. The cellular response of the neuron to intracellular edema is to extrude intracellular osmoles to reduce the intracellular osmolality and return the cell size to normal (107). Thus, chronic hyponatremia can be tolerated well. However, cellular swelling in response to acute hyponatremia will lead to mental obtundation and seizures. Due to these considerations, normal saline is the preferred intravenous solution in the neurologic intensive care unit.

Salt-wasting Nephropathy

A self-limited, salt-wasting nephropathy can develop after SAH. This process will lead to hyponatremia and volume depletion if not recognized and treated (108). The etiology remains somewhat difficult to identify. In dogs and guinea pigs, the process is mediated through the renal sympathetic nerve. Transection of this nerve will prevent salt wasting. This response is species specific, and is not true for rats; the human response is unknown (109). A variety of circulating hormones or substances have been proposed to initiate this response. The leading candidate is the B isoform of atrial natriuretic peptide (ANP), which has been found in some series to be elevated prior to the development of hyponatremia and cerebral vasospasm (110).

Diabetes insipidus (DI) leading to hypernatremia is expected after pituitary surgery, and is seen in any process that affects the hypothalamus or pituitary stalk. Head trauma leading to shearing injury of the pituitary stalk is a common cause for delayed DI. The diagnosis is made by the development of hypernatremia in the setting of hypotonic diuresis that is not induced by diuretics. This process must be differentiated from a postoperative diuresis. Normal postoperative diuresis will not spontaneously develop hypernatremia. Correction of the hypernatremia must be achieved slowly if hypernatremia has been present for more than a few hours (107).

SPECIFIC THERAPEUTIC CONCERNS AND TREATMENT OPTIONS

Head Trauma and Intracranial Hypertension

Severe head trauma remains a significant source of morbidity and mortality in the United States, accounting for approximately 50,000 deaths a year. It is the leading source of death for people younger than 44 years of age (51). Historically, treatment has focused on the management of sustained intracranial hypertension, and was based largely on retrospective data obtained from the National Traumatic Coma data bank. Survival was greater than 80% in patients who were able to have their ICP maintained at less than 20 mm Hg compared with more than 90% mortality for patients who had uncontrollable sustained intracranial hypertension (53,111). Therefore, treatment was focused on measures to decrease ICP, which might include diuresis, aggressive treatment of hypertension, keeping the patient relatively hypovolemic, and elevation of the head of bed.

The work by the Richmond group in the 1970s and 1980s largely changed the focus on head trauma treatment from using measures designed to lower ICP to those designed to maintain adequate CPP. As previously described, in some circumstances, elevations in ICP may be related to inadequate perfusion (41). Treatment thus shifted to include maintaining adequate blood volume and cerebral perfusion, as well as treating sustained elevations in ICP. What constitutes an adequate CPP has been debatable and may vary under different conditions; however, the most recent Brain Trauma Foundation guidelines have recommended a minimum CPP of 60 mm Hg (112).

In addition to maintaining adequate cerebral perfusion, a treatment strategy has been proposed that tailors hyperventilation based on the results of jugular venous O_2 ($SjvO_2$) monitoring (113). In some circumstances, elevated ICP can be attributed to cerebral hyperemia. In this condition, a narrow arterial venous gradient can be normalized by inducing cerebral vasoconstriction through hyperventilation. Similarly, widened arterial venous gradients would suggest a high risk of cerebral ischemia and prompt efforts to increase cerebral perfusion. Both methods have their proponents, but most agree that attention to details and standardization of care in the severely injured neurologic patient are crucial (114,115).

More recently, brain tissue oxygen monitoring has been used in head trauma to guide therapy. Brain tissue oxygen tension is measured by placement of a small flexible probe, usually through a cranial bolt directly into the brain parenchyma. CBF and PET studies have reported that low oxygen tensions correlate with low CBF measures and high oxygen extraction ratios (116,117). Two small observational studies have suggested an improved neurologic outcome with therapies designed to maintain brain tissue oxygen tensions greater than 10 mm Hg (118); however, to date, no randomized trials have been completed (119).

Intracranial hypertension is treated through the removal of space-occupying lesions, decreasing cerebral edema or venous engorgement, or expanding the cranial vault. Expanding brain masses—tumors, subdural or epidural hematomas—need to be evacuated as soon as possible to avoid cerebral herniation and damage to important brain structures. Removal of CSF through an external ventricular drain is a means to reduce the volume of the intracranial contents. Placement of an external ventricular drain also allows for the direct measurement of ICP.

Hyperventilation is useful for the acute management of intracranial hypertension. Intracranial hypertension is treated through decreases in CBV that are mediated through arteriolar vasoconstriction. Chronic hyperventilation is generally avoided due to concerns that prolonged vasoconstriction may worsen cerebral ischemia (120). The effect of hyperventilation on ICP is also self-limited, generally lasting only 3 to 6 hours; thus, hyperventilation is usually used for ICP control in the acute setting until a longer-acting strategy can be employed.

Osmotic agents are typically employed to lower ICP. Mannitol, given in boluses of 0.25 to 1.0 g/kg, is the most commonly used agent in the United States. Mannitol lowers ICP through a number of mechanisms. The intravascular osmotic gradient

$$F = \frac{8dPr^4}{\pi nl}$$

$$\begin{aligned} \text{where } F &= \text{flow} \\ dP &= \text{pressure gradient (CPP)} \\ r &= \text{vessel diameter} \\ n &= \text{viscosity} \\ l &= \text{vessel length} \end{aligned}$$

FIGURE 43.8. Rearrangement of the Pouisselle equation. Flow is directly related to the fourth power of the radius of the cerebral vessel and inversely related to serum viscosity. If flow remains constant and viscosity is reduced, then vessel diameter must decrease. CPP, cerebral perfusion pressure. (From Rosner MJ. Pathophysiology and management of increased intracranial pressure. In: Andrews BT, ed. *Neurosurgical Intensive Care*. New York: McGraw-Hill; 1993:57–112.)

created by mannitol can lead to extracellular fluid being drawn into the intravascular space and removed through osmotic diuresis. Paczynski et al. were able to demonstrate a decrease in hemispheric brain water in a rat stroke model with large boluses of mannitol, although the effect was small and delayed for several hours (121). More likely, mannitol exerts its effect on ICP by decreasing CBV. According to this theory, the osmotic gradient initiated by an infusion of mannitol causes an influx of extravascular water into the intravascular space. This leads to a decrease in blood viscosity due to a hemodilution of red blood cell mass and fibrinogen. The decrease in ICP can be explained through the use of the Hagen-Pouisselle equation. In this equation, flow is indirectly related to serum viscosity and a constant—a product of π (pi) times the length of the vessel (Fig. 43.8). Assuming constant cerebral blood flow and cerebral vessel reactivity, according to this equation, the radius of this vessel must decrease in response to both an increase in CPP and a decrease in viscosity (48). Rosner describes this as passive vasoconstriction (41).

Hypertonic saline in place of mannitol has been recently advocated. Hypertonic saline may have an advantage of less nephrotoxicity, although this has not been studied. Theoretically, its mechanism of action should be the same as mannitol. Widespread use of hypertonic saline, however, has been limited by a lack of a standardized dosing regimen (122,123).

An overall strategy for treating intracranial hypertension is to attempt to maintain the most optimal CPP at the lowest possible ICP. To attain this goal, other maneuvers may be necessary. Sedation and paralysis can be helpful to decrease ICP if chest wall compliance is high or if the patient is exhibiting respiratory dyssynchrony with the ventilator. Since the spinal venous plexus lacks valves, there is a theoretical concern that elevations in PEEP could be transmitted directly to the brain, thus increasing ICP. This is rarely problematic in noncompliant pulmonary states, but can occur if PEEP is elevated—some would say at a value of greater than 20 cm H_2O—under conditions of increased pulmonary and decreased intracranial compliance (125).

Corticosteroids are useful in treating the vasogenic edema from tumors and meningitis. The use of glucocorticoids in head trauma, though, is not recommended as several randomized trials have found no therapeutic benefit (125–127).

Barbiturates are effective in lowering ICP by decreasing cerebral metabolism. Their use is generally reserved for cases of refractory intracranial hypertension, and dosing is often titrated to a burst suppression pattern monitored on the EEG. One randomized trial reported improved mortality (128) with barbiturate use, although in head trauma, this remains debatable due to the limited quality of life of survivors (129).

Early hemicraniectomy—defined as occurring within 48 hours—with duraplasty is gaining recognition as a possible alternative for treatment of recalcitrant traumatic cerebral edema (130). Future randomized trials will need to be performed for further research.

Seizure Control and Status Epilepticus

Seizures are common after neurologic injury and can worsen outcome by increasing metabolic demands beyond oxygen delivery capabilities. Anticonvulsant prophylaxis may be employed for patients with subarachnoid hemorrhage, or intracerebral hemorrhages that abut the cortical surface of the brain. Anticonvulsants are recommended during the first week after severe head trauma to prevent posttraumatic epilepsy (131). Immediate treatment of seizures should utilize generous dosing of benzodiazepines.

Status epilepticus (SE) is a neurologic emergency that is associated with significant morbidity and mortality. Traditional definitions of SE that require 30 minutes of sustained seizure activity or nonarousal between sequential seizures have proved impractical to initiating timely treatment. A new operational definition suggests the immediate treatment of all seizures that last more than 5 minutes (52). Protocols have been developed for the sequential application of anticonvulsants (52). Aggressive early initiation of treatment is important, *as SE becomes more difficult to control as seizures continue.* It is important to note that SE is often underrecognized. Generalized tonic-clonic movements during electrical seizure activity evolve through a progression of clinical stages where a form of electrical mechanical disassociation can occur. Over time, physical movements become progressively more subtle and are manifested only by slight movements of the lips, fingers, or eyelids. A common mistake is to assume that seizures have discontinued after loading with anticonvulsants and initiating pharmacologic paralysis. This underscores the importance of EEG monitoring to ensure that seizures have been adequately treated. Attention to airway management and hemodynamics is important, as many of the anticonvulsants will have respiratory and cardiovascular depressant effects.

Refractory SE is defined as SE that has not responded to the usual first-line medications. Propofol, midazolam, and thiopental—or pentobarbital infusions under EEG monitoring—are required for treatment. However, propofol use has fallen into relative disfavor due to several case reports of deaths during infusions (132,133). It is not used in children with SE due to concerns over the development of a propofol infusion syndrome (134).

Subarachnoid Hemorrhage

Mortality from aneurysmal SAH remains high, with 15% of patients dying before getting medical attention (135). The care of patients with SAH can be divided into management before and after a cerebral aneurysm is secured. Management prior to aneurysmal treatment is designed to prevent rebleeding. Rebleeding occurs in approximately one third of all patients with aneurysmal SAH, and is highest within a few days after SAH. Neurosurgical repair or endovascular coil embolization of the aneurysm is therefore instituted as soon as possible.

Most patients will have acute elevations in blood pressure due to the stress of significant pain and the catecholamine surge that occurs after SAH. Management of blood pressure after SAH is controversial, although most neurosurgeons and neurointensivists will treat acute hypertension in patients with unsecured aneurysms. The rationale for treatment is based on the International Cooperative Aneurysmal trial (136) and, more recently, on a large Japanese observational study that noted a higher incidence of rebleeding in patients with sustained systolic elevations in blood pressure of more than 160 mm Hg (137). Blood pressure is preferentially treated with β-blockers, which do not significantly affect CBF and can narrow the pulse pressure. Hydralazine and angiotensin-converting enzyme (ACE) inhibitors have minimal effects on CBF. In general, nitroprusside is avoided due to concerns that it may induce cerebral venodilation and increase ICP. Intravenous nicardipine is the drug of choice if intravenous infusion is needed to control blood pressure (135).

The use of antifibrinolytic agents to prevent rebleeding is controversial. Previously a mainstay of treatment, the use of antifibrinolytic agents was largely abandoned after studies revealed increased mortality from the development of cerebral vasospasm. More recently, however, a randomized nonblinded study suggested that rebleeding rates could be decreased without increasing the rate of cerebral vasospasm (138). This study awaits further confirmation. Acute hydrocephalus is common after SAH and requires the placement of an external ventricular drain.

Once the aneurysm is secured, care focuses on the evaluation and treatment of cerebral vasospasm. Cerebral vasospasm is a pathologic narrowing of the basal cerebral arteries that occurs after SAH. Pathologically, the cerebral vessels display intimal hyperplasia, collagen remodeling, and a diffuse cellular infiltrate (139). The process takes approximately 4 days to develop and resolves after approximately 2 weeks. This process is initiated by a breakdown product of hemoglobin found in the subarachnoid space. The likelihood of developing cerebral vasospasm is predicted by the amount of subarachnoid blood visualized on a 24-hour CT scan (140). Larger amounts of blood predict a higher likelihood of vasospasm, and the location of the clot usually correlates with the site of most severe vasospasm (141).

Cerebral vessel narrowing can be monitored by the use of transcranial Doppler ultrasonography (TCD). Rising flow velocities may precede the development of neurologic deficits but, oftentimes, will ideally need to be verified by CBF measures to verify the significance of TCD findings (139). The onset of vasospasm is treated with intravascular fluid expansion and hemodynamic augmentation. Cerebral salt wasting can occur, and is best treated with hypertonic solutions and fludrocortisone. Cerebral autoregulation is impaired in cases of cerebral vasospasm and may require induced hypertension to treat neurologic deficits. There is a theoretical advantage to the use of phenylephrine since there are decreased α-receptors in the cerebral vasculature, although this has not been verified with CBF studies (139,142). Some studies had advocated the use of dobutamine to increase cardiac index in patients with vasospasm (143). Nonrandomized studies have shown reversal of nearly 75% of ischemic lesions from cerebral vasospasm with the above measures (144). Recalcitrant deficits may require interventional angioplasty to open the narrowed vessels. Nimodipine, a calcium channel blocker, is used as a neuroprotectant in patients with SAH.

Intracerebral Hemorrhage

Intracerebral hemorrhage (ICH) is bleeding that occurs directly into the brain parenchyma. ICH is classified as primary, secondary to underlying lesions, or spontaneous. The most common etiology of ICH is hypertension, which weakens and ruptures the small perforating vessels of the basal cerebral arteries. A growing source of ICH is secondary to long-term anticoagulant use (145).

Clinically, ICH presents with severe headaches and focal neurologic deficits, usually prompting an immediate transfer to an emergency room. Serial head CT studies have revealed that hematoma expansion occurs in approximately 40% of patients with ICH within the first 6 hours (146). A double-blinded randomized trial suggested that recombinant factor VII used within the first 4 hours of ictus decreased the hematoma expansion and improved outcome (147), but questions still remain, since an increase in thrombotic complications was noted in the treatment group. Acute hypertension is, again, common after ICH, and blood pressure control is controversial since aggressive management may extend the ischemic penumbra surrounding the hematoma. Conversely, PET studies suggest that modest control of hypertension is safe (148). A large randomized study evaluating the surgical evacuation of supratentorial ICH did not report a benefit over medical management. However, subgroup analysis did suggest a benefit to evacuation of primarily cortical hemorrhages (149). A subsequent study is currently ongoing. Corticosteroids have not shown any benefit in the treatment of ICH (150).

Ischemic Stroke

The use of thrombolytics has dramatically changed the management of acute ischemic stroke. The National Institute of Neurological Disorders and Stroke (NINDS) trial demonstrated improved 3-month outcomes in patients treated within 3 hours of onset with intravenous tissue plasminogen activator (tPA) (59). Intra-arterial lysis of clots has been successfully used in small trials and has extended the treatment windows up to 6 hours for the anterior circulation and 12 hours for the posterior circulation (58). Most recently, devices used for direct mechanical disruption and removal of intra-arterial clots have been approved (151).

Hypertension is common in the setting of an acute stroke, but usually resolves within a few hours of ictus, and treatment is controversial. Hemorrhagic conversion of ischemic infarctions is increased with sustained systolic pressures greater than 180 mm Hg; blood pressure must be below this limit prior to tPA administration (59). However, overly aggressive treatment of blood pressure is commonplace and may actually result in extension of the primary ischemic insult.

Large hemispheric infarctions—defined as strokes involving more than 50% of the middle cerebral artery (MCA) territory—are at risk for the subsequent development of cerebral edema and herniation (152). Close neurologic monitoring is required to identify any signs of deterioration. Treatments designed to lower ICP can be effective but act only as temporizing measures, since cerebral tissue shifts and not increased ICP are most likely to be the source of neurologic deterioration (153). Hemicraniectomy has been successfully used in a small case series and one pilot trial (154–156). The application and timing of this procedure, however, remain debatable.

SUMMARY

This chapter has attempted to provide an overview of cerebral vascular physiology and cerebral ischemia. A grasp of these principles is vital to understanding the nature of treatments designed to maintain adequate CBF and prevent secondary neurologic injury. Future treatments that focus on the details of critical care and maintaining tissue oxygenation show promise in improving outcome after neurologic injury.

PEARLS

Physiology

- Cerebral ischemia develops if oxygen utilization cannot meet the metabolic requirements of the tissue. This most commonly occurs due to a decrease in oxygen delivery to the cell.
- Ischemia is categorized into focal and global etiologies, with varying brain cell subtypes and neurons displaying selective vulnerability to ischemia.
- Neuronal cell death is a product of the degree and time of ischemia modulated by several metabolic factors.
- Cell death proceeds through several distinctive steps, leading to either necrosis or apoptosis.
- In focal ischemia, a core of central necrotic tissue is surrounded by ischemic but potentially viable tissue.

Cerebral Circulation

- Various methods to measure CBF and $CMRO_2$ have been developed and utilized to study cerebrovascular physiology. Newer perfusion techniques involving magnetic resonance and computed tomography perfusion may expand clinical applications.
- Cerebral autoregulation refers to the ability of the cerebral vasculature to maintain constant CBF over a range of CPP.
- Cerebral autoregulation is maintained through a variety of proposed mechanisms that lead to vasoconstriction and dilation of both the cerebral arteries and arterioles.
- Cerebral autoregulation is disturbed in most neuropathologic processes and increases the risk of secondary ischemic insult.
- Carbon dioxide and oxygen tensions have distinctive effects on CBF. The effects of carbon dioxide are mediated through changes in CSF hydrogen ion concentration.
- Intracranial pressure volume curves may reflect the pressure needed to displace various cerebral contents from the intracranial cavity.

- Acute elevations in ICP, known as plateau waves, can be explained by cerebral vasodilation induced by decreases in CPP.
- Cerebral edema is described by its location and mechanism of production.

Treatment Issues

- Secondary injury accounts for a significant proportion of the neurologic injury that occurs after stroke, trauma, or seizures.
- Secondary injury can be reduced by:
  - Prompt transport to a trauma or stroke center
  - Initiation of brain resuscitative measures designed to improve cerebral oxygen delivery
  - Emergent brain imaging with available neurosurgical procedures as needed
  - Serial neurologic assessment and monitoring
- Specific protocols exist for treatment of specific neurologic emergencies.

General Therapeutic Considerations

- Hyperthermia and hyperglycemia extend neurologic damage in animal models of ischemia and are associated with worse neurologic outcomes.
- Moderate hypothermia improved neurologic outcomes in patients with cerebral anoxia after cardiac arrest and may be helpful for other types of neurologic injury.
- Control of hyperglycemia may lead to improved outcomes in neurologic injury.
- Blood pressure management after acute neurologic injury needs to be titrated to maintain adequate cerebral perfusion, but not worsen the development of cerebral edema.
- Medical complications are frequent after acute neurologic injuries and need to be treated aggressively.

Specific Treatment Options

- Management of head trauma has expanded from the primary focus on lowering ICP to maintaining adequate CPP. Attention to oxygen extraction ratios and brain tissue oxygenation may also improve outcome.
- Status epilepticus is an emergency that can be successfully treated if recognized and treated early.
- Treatment of aneurysmal SAH focuses on methods to prevent rebleeding prior to aneurysmal repair and methods to increase CBF during cerebral vasospasm after aneurysm repair.
- Early strategies to lyse clots in ischemic stroke and prevent hematoma expansion after ICH have changed the acute management of stroke.

References

1. Wieloch T. Molecular mechanisms of ischemic brain damage. In: Edvinsson L, Krause DN, eds. *Cerebral Blood Flow and Metabolism*. 2nd ed. Philadelphia: Lippincott Williams & Wilkins; 2002:423–451.
2. Plum F, Pulsinelli WA. Cerebral metabolism and hypoxic-ischemic brain injury. In: Asbury AK, McKhann GM, McDonald WI, eds. *Diseases of the Nervous System. Clinical Neurobiology.* 2nd ed. Philadelphia: Saunders; 1992:1002–1015.
3. Bhardwaj A, Alkayed NJ, Kirsch JR, et al. Mechanisms of ischemic brain damage. *Curr Cardiol Rep.* 2003;5:160–167.
4. Auer RN, Sutherland GR. Hypoxia and other related conditions. In: Graham DI, Lantos PL, eds. *Greenfields Neuropathology.* 7th ed. London: Arnold Publisher; 2002:233–280.
5. Choi DW. The excitotoxic concept. In: Welch KMA, Caplan LR, Reis DJ, et al., eds. *Primer on Cerebrovascular Disease.* San Diego: Academic Press; 1997:187–190.
6. Astrup J, Symon L, Branston N, et al. Cortical evoked potentials and extracellular potassium and hydrogen ions at critical levels of brain ischemia. *Stroke.* 1977;8:51.
7. Kerr JF, Wyllie AH, Currie AR. Apoptosis: a basic biological phenomenon with wide ranging implications in tissue kinetics. *Br J Cancer.* 1972;26:239.
8. Kety SS, Schmidt CF. The determination of cerebral blood flow in man by the use of nitrous oxide in low concentrations. *Am J Physiol.* 1945;143:53.
9. Fick A. Ueber die Messung des Blutquantums in den Herzventrikeln. *Sitz ber Physik-Med Ges Wurzburg.* 1870;2:16–28.
10. Marino P. Oxygen transport. In: Marino P, ed. *The ICU Book.* Philadelphia: Lea and Febiger; 1991:14–24.
11. Ginsberg MD. Cerebral circulation: its regulation, pharmacology, and pathophysiology. In: Asbury AK, McKhann GM, McDonald WI, eds. *Diseases of the Nervous System. Clinical Neurobiology.* Philadelphia: Saunders; 1992:989.
12. Manno EM, Koroshetz WJ. Cerebral blood flow. In: Babikian VL, Weschler LR, eds. *Transcranial Doppler Ultrasonography.* 2nd ed. Boston: Butterworth-Heinemann; 1999:67–86.
13. Gur D, Good WF, Wolfson SK Jr, et al. In vivo mapping of local cerebral blood flow by xenon-enhanced computed tomography. *Science.* 1982;5:1267.
14. Masdeu JC, Brass LM, Holman BL, et al. Brain single-photon emission tomography. *Neurology.* 1994;44:1970.
15. Powers WJ, Raichle ME. Positron emission tomography and its application to the study of cerebrovascular disease in man. *Stroke.* 1985;16:361.
16. Villringer A, Rosen BR, Belliveau J, et al. Dynamic imaging with lanthanide chelates in normal brain: contrast due to magnetic susceptibility effects. *Magn Reson Med.* 1988;6:164.
17. Hunter GJ, Hamberg LM, Ponzo JA, et al. Assessment of cerebral perfusion and arterial anatomy in hyperacute stroke with three-dimensional functional CT: early clinical results. *AJNR Am J Neuroradiol.* 1998;19:29.
18. Chillon JM, Baumbach GL. Autoregulation: arterial and intracranial pressure. In: Edvinsson L, Krause DN, eds. *Cerebral Blood Flow and Metabolism.* 2nd ed. Philadelphia: Lippincott Williams & Wilkins; 2002:395–412.
19. Chillon JM, Baumbach GL. Autoregulation of cerebral blood flow. In: Welch KMA, Caplan LR, Reis DJ, et al., eds. *Primer on Cerebrovascular Disease.* San Diego: Academic Press; 1997:51–54.
20. Shapiro HM, Stromberg DD, Lee DR, et al. Dynamic pressures in the pial arterial microcirculation. *Am J Physiol.* 1971;221:279.
21. Kontos HA, Wei EP, Navari RM, et al. Responses of cerebral arteries and arterioles to acute hypotension and hypertension. *Am J Physiol Heart Circ Physiol.* 1978;234:H371.
22. Folkow B. Description of the myogenic hypothesis. *Circ Research* 1964;15:279–287.
23. Bayliss WM. On the local reaction of the arterial wall to changes of internal pressure. *J Physiol.* 1902;28:220.
24. Rubanyi GM, Freay A, Kauser K, et al. Mechanoreception by the endothelium: mediators and mechanisms of pressure- and flow-induced vascular responses. *Blood Vessels.* 1990;27:246–257.
25. Wei EP, Kontos HA. Responses of cerebral arterioles to increased venous pressure. *Am J Physiol Heart Cir Physiol.* 1982;243:H442.
26. Osol G, Halpern W. Myogenic properties of cerebral blood vessels from normotensive and hypertensive rats. *Am J Physiol Heart Circ Physiol.* 1985;249:H914.
27. Kuschinsky W, Wahl M. Local chemical and neurogenic regulation of cerebral vascular resistance. *Physiol Rev.* 1978;58:656.
28. Magistretti PJ. Coupling of cerebral blood flow and metabolism. In: Welch KMA, Caplan LR, Reis DJ, et al., eds. *Primer on Cerebrovascular Disease.* San Diego: Academic Press; 1997:70–75.
29. Dirnagl U, Dreier J. Regulation of cerebral blood flow by ions. In: Welch KMA, Caplan LR, Reis DJ, et al., eds. *Primer on Cerebrovascular Disease.* San Diego: Academic Press; 1997:75–77.
30. Winn RH. Adenosine and its receptors: influence on cerebral blood flow. In: Welch KMA, Caplan LR, Reis DJ, et al., eds. *Primer on Cerebrovascular Disease.* San Diego: Academic Press; 1997:77–79.
31. Kitazano T, Heistad DD, Farachi FM. Role of ATP-sensitive potassium channels in CGRP-induced dilation of the basilar artery in vivo. *Am J Physiol Heart Circ Physiol.* 1994;266:H11.
32. Wei EP, Kontos HA. Increased venous pressure causes myogenic constriction of cerebral arterioles during focal hypoxia. *Circ Res.* 1984;55:249–252.

33. Edvisson L. Neurogenic mechanisms in the cerebrovascular bed. Autonomic nerves, amine receptors and their effects on cerebral blood flow. *Acta Physiol Scand Suppl.* 1975;427:1.
34. Lou HC, Edvisson L, MacKenzie ET. The concept of coupling blood flow to brain function: revision required? *Ann Neurol.* 1987;22:289.
35. Traystman RJ. Regulation of cerebral blood flow by carbon dioxide. In: Welch KMA, Caplan LR, Reis DJ, et al., eds. *Primer on Cerebrovascular Disease.* San Diego: Academic Press; 1997:55–58.
36. Ropper AH. Treatment of intracranial hypertension. In: Ropper AH, ed. *Neurological and Neurosurgical Intensive Care.* 3rd ed. New York: Raven Press; 1993:29–52.
37. Heistad DD, Kontos HA. Cerebral circulation. In: Shepard JT, Abboud FM, eds. *Handbook of Physiology. Section 2. The Cardiovascular System. Vol III. Peripheral Circulation and Organ Blood Flow.* Bethesda: American Physiological Society; 1983:137–182.
38. Lindsey KW, Bone I, Callander R. *Neurology and Neurosurgery Illustrated.* 4th ed. Edinburgh: Churchill Livingstone; 2004:52.
39. Szidon JP, Cherniack NS, Fishman AP. Traube-Hering waves in the pulmonary circulation of the dog. *Science.* 1969;164:75.
40. Newell DW, Aaslid R, Stoos R, et al. The relationship of blood flow velocity fluctuations to intracranial pressure B waves. *J Neurosurg.* 1992;76:415.
41. Rosner MJ. Pathophysiology and management of increased intracranial pressure. In: Andrews BT, ed. *Neurosurgical Intensive Care.* New York: McGraw-Hill; 1993:57–112.
42. Miller JD, Garibi J, Pickard JD. Induced changes of cerebrospinal fluid volume. Effects during continuous monitoring of ventricular fluid pressure. *Arch Neurol.* 1973;28:265.
43. Marmarou A, Shulman K, Rosende RM. A nonlinear analysis of the cerebrospinal fluid system and intracranial pressure dynamics. *J Neurosurg.* 1978;48:332.
44. Lunberg N. Continuous recording and control of ventricular fluid pressure in neurosurgical practice. *Acta Psychiatr Scand.* 1960;36(Suppl 149):1.
45. Rose JC, Mayer SA. Optimizing blood pressure in neurological emergencies. *Neurocrit Care.* 2004;1:287.
46. Schrader H, Zwentnow NM, Mokrid L. Regional cerebral blood flow and CSF pressures during Cushing response induced by a supratentorial expanding mass. *Acta Neurol Scand.* 1985;71:453.
47. Rapoport SI. Brain edema and the blood-brain barrier. In: Welch KMA, Caplan LR, Reis DJ, et al., eds. *Primer on Cerebrovascular Disease.* San Diego: Academic Press; 1997:25–28.
48. Manno EM. When to use hyperventilation, mannitol, or corticosteroid to reduce increased intracranial pressure from cerebral edema. In: Rabinstein AA, Wijdicks EFM, eds. *Tough Calls in Acute Neurology.* Amsterdam: Elsevier; 2004:107–124.
49. Fishman RA. Brain edema and disorders of intracranial pressure. In: Rowland LP, ed. *Merritt's Neurology.* 10th ed. Philadelphia: Lippincott Williams & Wilkins; 2000:284–290.
50. Klatzo I. Neuropathological aspects of brain oedema. *J Neuropathol Exp Neurol.* 1967;26:1–14.
51. Stone JL, Ghaly RF, Di Gianfilippo AD, et al. Acute head trauma management and pathophysiological principles. In: Stone JL, ed. *Head Injury and Its Complications.* Costa Mesa, CA: PMA Publishing; 1993:1–22.
52. Manno EM. New treatment strategies in the management of status epilepticus. *Mayo Clin Proc.* 2003;78:508.
53. Veremakis CV, Lindner DH. Central nervous system injury: essential physiologic and therapeutic concerns. In: Civetta JM, Taylor RW, Kirby RR, eds. *Critical Care.* 3rd ed. Philadelphia: Lippincott-Raven Publishers; 1997:273–289.
54. Teasdale G, Jennett B. Assessment of coma and impaired consciousness. A practical scale. *Lancet.* 1974;2:81.
55. Wijdicks EFM, Bamlet WR, Maramattom BV, et al. Validation of a new coma scale: the FOUR score. *Ann Neurol.* 2005;58:585.
56. Guidelines for the treatment of severe head injury. Brain Trauma Foundation, American Association of Neurological Surgeons, Joint Section of Neurotrauma and Critical Care. *J Neurotrauma.* 1996;13:641.
57. Gabriel EJ, Ghajar J, Jagoda A, et al. , Brain Trauma Foundation. Guidelines for prehospital management of traumatic brain injury. *J Neurotrauma.* 2002;1:111.
58. Furlan A, Higashida R, Weschler L, et al. Intra-arterial prourokinase for acute ischemic stroke. The PROACT II study: a randomized controlled trial. Prolyse in Acute Cerebral Thromboembolism. *JAMA.* 1999;282:2003.
59. The National Institute of Neurological Disorders and Stroke rt-PA Stroke Study Group. Tissue plasminogen activator for acute ischaemic stroke. *N Engl J Med.* 1995;333:1581.
60. Manno EM, Atkinson JA, Fulgham JR, et al. Emerging medical and surgical management strategies in the evaluation and treatment of intracerebral hemorrhage. *Mayo Clin Proc.* 2005;80(3):420.
61. Ginsberg G, Busto R. Combating hyperthermia in acute stroke. A significant clinical concern. *Stroke.* 1998;29:529.
62. Dietrich WD, Busto R. Hyperthermia and brain ischemia. In: Welch KMA, Caplan LR, Reis DJ, et al., eds. *Primer on Cerebrovascular Disease.* San Diego: Academic Press; 1997.
63. Manno EM, Farmer CJ. Acute brain injury: if hypothermia is good, then is hyperthermia bad? *Crit Care Med.* 2004;32:1611.
64. Chen H, Chopp M, Welch KMA. Effect of mild hyperthermia on the ischemic infarct volume after middle cerebral artery occlusion in the rat. *Neurology.* 1991;41:1133.
65. Chen Q, Chopp M, Bodzin G, et al. Temperature modulation of cerebral depolarization during focal cerebral ischemia in rats: correlation with ischemic injury. *J Cereb Blood Flow Metab.* 1993;13:389.
66. Chopp M, Welch KMA, Tidwell CD, et al. Effect of mild hyperthermia on the recovery of metabolic function after global cerebral ischemia in cats. *Stroke.* 1988;19:1521.
67. Morimato T, Ginsberg MD, Dietrich WD, et al. Hyperthermia enhances spectrin breakdown in transient focal cerebral ischemia. *Brain Res.* 1997;746:43.
68. Azzimondi G, Bassein L, Nonino F, et al. Fever in acute stroke worsens prognosis: a prospective study. *Stroke.* 1995;26:2040.
69. Reith J, Jorgensen HS, Pedersen PM, et al. Body temperature in acute stroke: relation to stroke severity, infarct size, mortality, and outcome. *Lancet.* 1996;347:422.
70. Diringer MN, Reaven NL, Funk SE. Elevated body temperature independently contributes to increased length of stay in neuro ICU patients. *Crit Care Med.* 2004;32:1489.
71. Clifton GL. Is keeping cool still hot? An update on hypothermia in brain injury. *Curr Opin Crit Care.* 2004;10:116.
72. Bernard SA, Gray TW, Buist MD, et al. Treatment of comatose survivors of out-of-hospital cardiac arrest with induced hypothermia. *N Engl J Med.* 2002;346:557.
73. Holzer M. The Hypothermia After Cardiac Arrest Study Group. Mild therapeutic hypothermia to improve the neurologic outcome after cardiac arrest. *N Engl J Med.* 2002;346:549.
74. Clifton GL, Miller E, Choi SC, et al. Lack of effect of induction of hypothermia after acute brain injury. *N Engl J Med.* 2001;344:556.
75. Schwab S, Schwartz S, Spranger M, et al. Moderate hypothermia in the treatment of patients with severe middle cerebral artery infarctions. *Stroke.* 1998;29:1437.
76. Garg R, Chauduri A, Munschauer F, et al. Hyperglycemia, insulin, and acute stroke. A mechanistic justification for a trial of insulin infusion therapy. *Stroke.* 2006;37:267.
77. Capes SE, Hunt D, Malmberg K, et al. Stress hyperglycemia and prognosis of stroke in nondiabetic and diabetic patients: a systematic overview. *Stroke.* 2001;32:2426.
78. Leigh R, Zaidat OO, Suri MF, et al. Predictors of hyperacute clinical worsening in ischemic stroke patients receiving thrombolytic therapy. *Stroke.* 2004;35:1903.
79. Alvarez-Sabin J, Molina CA, Montaner J, et al. Effects of admission hyperglycemia on stroke outcome in reperfused tissue plasminogen activator–treated patients. *Stroke.* 2003;34:1235.
80. Baird TA, Parsons MW, Phanh T, et al. Persistent poststroke hyperglycemia is independently associated with infarct expansion and worse clinical outcome. *Stroke.* 2003;34:2208.
81. Williams LS, Rotich J, Qi R, et al. Effects of admission hyperglycemia on mortality and costs in acute ischemic stroke. *Neurology.* 2002;59:67.
82. Bruno A, Biller J, Adams HP Jr, et al. Acute blood glucose level and outcome from ischemic stroke. Trial of org 10172 in acute stroke treatment (TOAST) investigators. *Neurology.* 1999;52:280.
83. Wartenberg KE, Mayer SA. Medical complications after subarachnoid hemorrhage: new strategies for prevention and management. *Curr Opin Crit Care.* 2006;12:78.
84. Cochran A, Scaife ER, Hansen KW, et al. Hyperglycemia and outcomes from pediatric traumatic brain injury. *J Trauma.* 2003;55:1035.
85. Parish RA, Webb KS. Hyperglycemia is not a poor prognostic sign in head injured children. *J Trauma.* 1988;28:517.
86. Duckrow RB, Beard DC, Brennan RW. Regional cerebral blood flow decreases during hyperglycemia. *Ann Neurol.* 1985;17:267.
87. Folbergrova J, Memezawa H, Smith ML, et al. Focal and perifocal changes in tissue energy state during middle cerebral artery occlusion in normo- and hyperglycemic rats. *J Cereb Blood Flow Metab.* 1992;12:25.
88. Li PA, Shuaib A, Miyashita H, et al. Hyperglycemia enhances extracellular glutamate accumulation in rats subjected to forebrain ischemia. *Stroke.* 2000;31:183.
89. Berger L, Hakim AM. The association of hyperglycemia with cerebral edema in stroke. *Stroke.* 1986;17:865.
90. Mohanty P, Hamouda W, Garg R, et al. Glucose challenge stimulates reactive oxygen species (ROS) generation by leucocytes. *J Clin Endocrinol Metab.* 2000;85:2970.
91. Dhindsa S, Tripathy D, Mohanty P, et al. Differential effects of glucose and alcohol on reactive oxygen species generation and intranuclear nuclear factor-kappab in mononuclear cells. *Metabolism.* 2004;53:330.
92. Van den Berghe G, Wouters P, Weekers F, et al. Intensive insulin therapy in critically ill patients. *N Engl J Med.* 2001;345:1359.
93. Van den Berghe G, Schoonheydt K, Becx P, et al. Insulin therapy protects the central nervous system of intensive care patients. *Neurology.* 2005;64:1348.
94. Fukuoka S, Yeh H, Mandybur TI, et al. Effect of insulin on acute experimental cerebral ischemia in gerbils. *Stroke.* 1989;20:396.
95. Voll CL, Auer RN. Insulin attenuates ischemic brain damage independent of its hypoglycemic effect. *J Cereb Blood Flow Metab.* 1991;11:1006.

96. Aljada A, Saadeh R, Assian E, et al. Insulin inhibits the expression of intercellular adhesion molecule-1 by human aortic endothelial cells through stimulation of nitric oxide. *J Clin Endo and Metab.* 2000;85: 2572–2575.
97. Rordorf G, Koroshetz WJ, Ezzaddine MA, et al. A pilot study of drug-induced hypertension for treatment of acute stroke. *Neurology.* 2001; 56:1210.
98. Bae HJ, Yoon DS, Lee J, et al. In hospital medical complications and long term mortality after ischemic stroke. *Stroke.* 2005;36:2441.
99. Wartenberg KE, Schmidt JM, Classen J, et al. Impact of medical complications on outcome after subarachnoid hemorrhage. *Crit Care Med.* 2006;34:617.
100. Gujjar AR, Deibert E, Manno EM, et al. Mechanical ventilation for ischemic stroke and intracerebral hemorrhage: indications, timing, and outcome. *Neurology.* 1998;51:447.
101. Coplin WM, Pierson DJ, Cooley KD, et al. Implications of extubation delay in brain-injured patients meeting standard weaning criteria. *Am J Respir Crit Care Med.* 2000;161:1530.
102. Samuels MA. Cardiopulmonary aspects of acute neurologic diseases. In: Ropper AH, ed. *Neurological and Neurosurgical Intensive Care.* 3rd ed. New York: Raven Press; 1993:103–119.
103. Smith WS, Matthay MA. Evidence for a hydrostatic mechanism in neurogenic pulmonary edema. *Chest.* 1997;111:1326.
104. Simon RP, Bayne LL. Pulmonary lymphatic flow alterations during intracranial hypertension in sheep. *Ann Neurol.* 1984;15:188.
105. Karch SB, Billingham ME. Myocardial contraction bands revisited. *Hum Pathol.* 1986;17:9.
106. Connelly KA, MacIsaac AI, Jelinek VM. Stress, myocardial infarction, and the "tako-tsubo" phenomenon. *Heart.* 2004;90:52.
107. Young GB, DeRubeis DA. Metabolic encephalopathies. In: Young GB, Ropper AH, Bolton CF, eds. *Coma and Impaired Consciousness. A Clinical Perspective.* New York: McGraw-Hill; 1998:307–392.
108. Maroon JC, Nelson PB. Hypovolemia in patients with subarachnoid hemorrhage: therapeutic implications. *Neurosurgery.* 1979;4:223.
109. Dibona GF, Kopp UC. Neural control of renal function. *Physiol Rev.* 1997; 77:75.
110. Sviri GE, Feinsod M, Soustiel JF. Brain natriuretic peptide and cerebral vasospasm after subarachnoid hemorrhage: clinical and TCD correlations. *Stroke.* 2000;31:118.
111. Narayan RK, Kishore PR, Becker DP, Intracranial pressure: to monitor or not to monitor? *J Neurosurg.* 1982;56:650.
112. Guidelines for the management of severe traumatic brain injury: cerebral perfusion pressure. Update notice on reference 56. Available at: www.braintrauma.org/site/PageServer?program=Guidelines. Accessed March 19, 2008.
113. Cruz J, Miner ME, Allen SJ, Continuous monitoring of cerebral oxygenation in acute brain injury: injection of mannitol during hyperventilation. *J Neurosurg.* 1990;73:725.
114. Chestnut RM. Hyperventilation versus cerebral perfusion pressure management: time to change the question. *Crit Care Med.* 1998;26:210.
115. Bulger EM, Nathens AB, Rivara FP, et al. Management of sever head injury: institutional variations in care and effect on outcome. *Crit Care Med.* 2002;30:1870.
116. Hemphill JC 3rd, Smith WS, Sonne DC, et al. Relationship between brain tissue oxygen tension and CT perfusion: feasibility and initial results. *AJNR Am J Neuroradiol.* 2005;26:1095.
117. Johnston AJ, Steiner LA, Coles JP, et al. Effect of cerebral perfusion pressure augmentation on regional oxygenation and metabolism after head injury. *Crit Care Med.* 2005;33:189.
118. Meixensberger J, Jaeger M, Vath A, et al. Brain tissue oxygen guided treatment supplementing ICP/CPP therapy after traumatic brain injury. *J Neurol Neurosurg Psychiatry.* 2003;74:760.
119. Rose JC, Neill TA, Hemphill JC. Continuous monitoring of the microcirculation in neurocritical care: an update on brain tissue oxygenation. *Curr Opin Crit Care.* 2006;12:97.
120. Chesnut RM. Medical management of sever head injury: present and future. *New Horizons.* 1995;3:581.
121. Paczynski RP, He YY, Diringer MN, et al. Multiple-dose mannitol reduces brain water content in a rat model of cortical infarction. *Stroke.* 1997;28:437.
122. Shackford SR, Bourguignon PR, Wald SL, et al. Hypertonic saline resuscitation of patients with head injury: a prospective randomized clinical trial. *J Trauma.* 1998;44:50.
123. Quershi AI, Suarez JI. Use of hypertonic saline solutions in treatment of cerebral edema and intracranial hypertension. *Crit Care Med.* 2000;28:3301.
124. Cooper KR, Boswell PA, Choi SC. Safe use of PEEP in patients with severe head injury. *J Neurosurgery.* 1985;63:552.
125. Deardon NM, Gibson JS, McDowell DG, et al. Effect of high-dose dexamethasone on outcome after severe head injury. *J Neurosurg.* 1986;64: 81.
126. Cooper PR, Moody S, Clark WK, et al. Dexamethasone and severe head injury. A prospective double-blinded study. *J Neurosurg.* 1979;51:307.
127. Giannotta SL, Weiss MH, Apuzzo MLJ, et al. High dose glucocorticoids in the management of severe head injury. *Neurosurgery.* 1984;15:497.
128. Eisenberg HM, Frankowski RF, Constant CF. High-dose barbiturate control of elevated intracranial pressure in patients with severe head injury. *J Neurosurg.* 1988;69:15.
129. Schalen W, Sonesson B, Messeter K, et al. Clinical outcome and cognitive impairment in patients with severe head injury treated with barbiturate coma. *Acta Neurchir.* 1992;17:153.
130. Bullock MR, Chesnut R, Ghajar J, et al. Surgical Management of Traumatic Brain Injury Author Group. Surgical management of traumatic parenchymal lesions. *Neurosurgery.* 2006;58(3 Suppl):S25.
131. Temkin NR, Dikmen SS, Wilensky AJ, et al. A randomized double-blind study of phenytoin for the prevention of post traumatic seizures. *N Engl J Med.* 1990;323:497.
132. Kumar MA, Urrutia VC, Thomas CE, et al. The syndrome of irreversible acidosis after prolonged propofol infusion. *Neurocritical Care.* 2005;3: 257.
133. Friedman JA, Manno EM, Fulgham JR. Propofol use in the neuro ICU. *J Neurosurg.* 2002;96:1161.
134. Propofol-infusion syndrome in children. *Lancet.* 1999;353:2074.
135. Manno EM. Subarachnoid hemorrhage. *Neurol Clin N Am.* 2004;22:347.
136. Adams HP Jr, Kassell NF, Torner JC, et al. Early management of aneurysmal subarachnoid hemorrhage: a report of the cooperative aneurysm study. *J Neurosurg.* 1981;54:141.
137. Ohkuma H, Tsurutani H, Suzuki S. Incidence and significance of early aneurysmal rebleeding before neurosurgical or neurological management. *Stroke.* 2001;32:1176.
138. Hillman J, Fridrikson S, Nilsson O, et al. Immediate administration of tranexamic acid and reduced incidence of early rebleeding after aneurysmal subarachnoid hemorrhage: a prospective randomized study. *J Neurosurg.* 2002;97:771.
139. Manno EM, Gress DR, Schwamm LH, et al. Effects of induced hypertension on transcranial Doppler ultrasound velocities in patients after subarachnoid hemorrhage. *Stroke.* 1998;29:422.
140. Fisher CM, Kistler JP, Davis JM. Relation of cerebral vasospasm to subarachnoid hemorrhage visualized on computed tomographic scanning. *Neurosurgery.* 1980;6:1.
141. Kistler JP, Crowell RM, Davis KR. The relation of cerebral vasospasm to the extent and location of subarachnoid blood visualized by CT scanning: a prospective study. *Neurology.* 1983;33:424.
142. Bevan JA, Duckworth J, Laher I, et al. Sympathetic control of cerebral arteries: specialization in receptor type, reserve, affinity, and distribution. *FASEB J.* 1987;1:193.
143. Levy ML, Rabb CH, Zelman V, et al. Cardiac performance enhancement from dobutamine in patients refractory to hypervolemic therapy for cerebral vasospasm. *J Neurosurg.* 1993;79:494.
144. Kassell NF, Peerless SJ, Durwaed QJ, et al. Treatment of ischemic deficits from vasospasm with intravascular volume expansion and induced arterial hypertension. *Neurosurgery.* 1982;11:337.
145. Manno EM, Atkinson JLD, Fulgham JR, et al. Emerging medical and surgical management strategies in the evaluation and treatment of intracerebral hemorrhage. *Mayo Clin Proc.* 2005;80:420.
146. Brott T, Broderick J, Kothari R, et al. Early hemorrhagic growth in patients with intracerebral hemorrhage. *Stroke.* 1997;28:1.
147. Mayer SA, Brun NC, Begtrup K, et al. Recombinant Activated Factor VII Intracerebral Hemorrhage Trial Investigators. Recombinant activated factor VII for acute intracerebral hemorrhage. *N Engl J Med.* 2005;352: 777.
148. Powers WJ, Zazulia AR, Videen TO, et al. Autoregulation of cerebral blood flow surrounding acute (6 to 22 hours) intracerebral hemorrhage. *Neurology.* 2001;57:18.
149. Mendelow AD, Gregson BA, Fernandes HM, et al., STICH investigators. Early surgery versus initial conservative treatment in patients with spontaneous supratentorial intracerebral haematomas in the International Surgical Trial in Intracerebral Haemorrhage (STICH): a randomised trial. *Lancet.* 2005;365(9457):387.
150. Poungvarin N, Bhoopat W, Virijavwjakul A, et al. Effects of dexamethasone in primary supratentorial intracerebral hemorrhage. *N Engl J Med.* 1987;315:1229.
151. Gobin YP, Starkman S, Duckwiler GR, et al. MERCI 1: a phase 1 study of Mechanical Embolus Removal in Cerebral Ischemia. *Stroke.* 2004;35:2848.
152. Manno EM. The management of large hemispheric cerebral infarcts. *Compr Ther.* 2005;31:124.
153. Frank JI. Large hemispheric infarction, clinical deterioration, and intracranial pressure. *Neurology.* 1995;45:1286.
154. Delashaw JB, Broaddus WC, Kassall WF, et al. Treatment of right hemispheric cerebral infarctions by hemicraniectomy. *Stroke.* 1990;21:874.
155. Rieke K, Schwab S, Krieger D, et al. Decompressive surgery in space occupying hemispheric infarctions by hemicraniectomy. *Crit Care Med.* 1995;23:1576.
156. Frank JI. Preliminary results of the HeADDFIRST trial. Paper presentation at the Neurocritical Care Society Meeting. Neurocritical Care Society, Baltimore, MD, November 2006.

CHAPTER 44 ■ THE LUNG STRUCTURE AND FUNCTION

JOHN J. MARINI • DAVID J. DRIES • JOHN F. PERRY, JR.

Many aspects of cardiopulmonary life support are rooted in understanding the anatomy and physiology of the respiratory system. The purpose of this chapter is to review those aspects of normal structure and function of the lungs and chest wall that impact most directly on daily practice. Intentionally, we have only dipped tentatively into the physiology of pathologic conditions, as to attempt to do so would clearly exceed our page allocation and scope of this assignment. Nonetheless, we hope that this overview serves as a starting point by underlining the principles of undeniable clinical relevance.

ANATOMIC CONSIDERATIONS

Tracheobronchial Tree

A useful approach to understanding the tracheobronchial tree (Fig. 44.1) is that of Weibel (1), who numbered successive generations of air passages from the trachea to the alveolar sacs. In some sectors, there may be as few as eight generations, while in others, the air pathway may divide 23 times from the trachea (generation 0) to the alveoli (generation 23). It may be assumed that the number of passages in each generation is double that in the previous generation, and the number of passages in each generation is 2 raised to the power of the generation number.

The trachea has a mean diameter of 1.8 cm and a length of 11 cm. It is supported by U-shaped cartilage, which is joined posteriorly by smooth muscle bands. Despite the presence of cartilage, the posterior wall is deformable so that the trachea can be occluded by a pressure on the order of 50 to 70 cm H_2O. Within the chest, the trachea can be compressed by elevated intrathoracic pressure, as may occur during cough when the decreased diameter increases the efficiency of secretion removal. The tracheal mucosa is a columnar ciliated epithelium containing mucus-secreting goblet cells. Cilia beat in a coordinated manner, creating an upward stream of mucus and foreign material. Anesthetics render the cilial beat ineffective. Cilial movement of mucus and respiratory debris is also compromised by drying, which occurs in patients breathing dry gas through a tracheostomy.

The trachea bifurcates asymmetrically, with the right bronchus wider and better aligned with the long axis of the trachea. It is more likely, therefore, to receive aspirated material. Main, lobar, and segmental bronchi have firm cartilaginous support, which is horseshoe shaped. Cartilage is arranged in irregular plates more distally. Where cartilage is irregular and discontinuous, bronchial smooth muscle in helical bands forms a network (1,2). The bronchial epithelium is similar to that in the trachea, although the height of cells diminishes in more peripheral passages until it becomes cuboidal in bronchioles. Bronchi down to generation 4 are sufficiently regular to be individually named. By the third generation, total cross-sectional area of the respiratory tract is still minimal.

When bronchi in generations 1 through 4 are subjected to large changes in intrathoracic pressure, collapse occurs when intrathoracic pressure exceeds intraluminal pressure by about 50 cm H_2O. Collapse occurs in larger bronchi during a forced expiration since the greater part of the alveolar-to-mouth pressure difference is taken up in the segmental bronchi. Intraluminal pressure, particularly within larger bronchi, is well below intrathoracic pressure, particularly with emphysema. Collapse of larger bronchi limits peak expiratory flow in the normal subject (3).

Small bronchi extend through about seven generations, with diameter progressively falling from 3.5 to 1 mm. Since their number approximately doubles with each generation, the total cross-sectional area increases rapidly with each generation to a value at generation 11, which is about seven times the total cross-sectional area at the level of the lobar bronchi. Down to the level of true bronchi, air passages lie in close proximity to branches of the pulmonary artery in a sheath also containing pulmonary lymphatics. Distension of these lymphatics gives rise to classic cuffing seen with pulmonary edema. Small bronchi are not directly attached to pulmonary parenchyma and are not subject to direct traction. They rely on cartilage within their walls for patency and on transmural pressure, which is normally a positive gradient from the lumen to the intrathoracic space. Intraluminal pressure in small bronchi rapidly rises to more than 80% of alveolar pressure during forced expiration.

At the 11th generation, where diameter usually approximates 1 mm, cartilage disappears from the wall of airways, and structural rigidity ceases to be the factor maintaining patency. Beyond this level, air passages are embedded in pulmonary parenchyma, and elastic recoil of the lung holds the air passages open. The caliber of the airways below the 11th generation is strongly influenced by lung volume, as forces holding the lumen open are greater at higher lung volumes. Airway closure may occur at reduced lung volumes.

In succeeding generations, the number of bronchioles increases more rapidly than caliber diminishes. The total cross-sectional area increases until, in terminal bronchioles, it is about 30 times the area at the level of the large bronchi. The flow resistance of the smaller air passages (<2 mm) approximates one tenth of the total. Contraction of helical muscle bands wrinkles the cuboidal epithelium into longitudinal folds, which increases flow resistance and, in some cases, results in airway obstruction. Down to the terminal bronchiole level, air

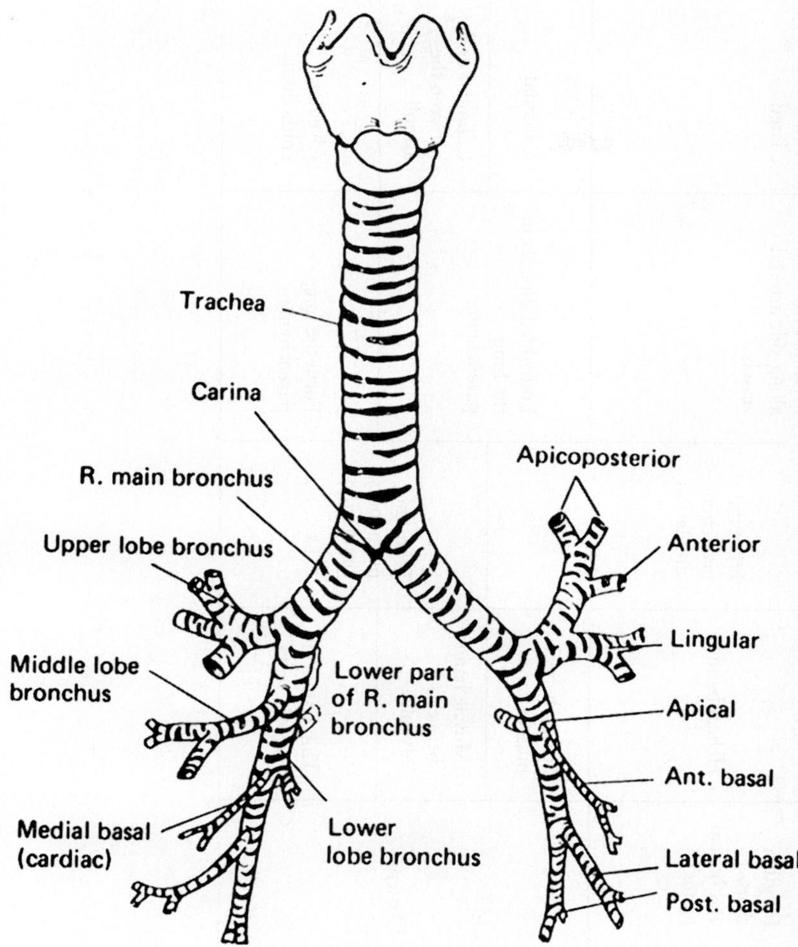

FIGURE 44.1. Named branches of the tracheobronchial tree, viewed from the front. (Reused with permission from Nunn JF. *Applied Respiratory Physiology.* 3rd ed. London: Butterworths; 1987.)

passages derive nutrition from bronchial circulation, and are influenced by systemic arterial blood gas levels. Beyond this point, air passages rely on pulmonary circulation for nutrition (Table 44.1).

From the trachea to the smallest bronchioles, the functions of air passages are conduction and humidification. Beyond this point, there is a transition from conduction to gas exchange. In the three generations of respiratory bronchioles, there is a gradual increase in the number of alveoli in the walls. The epithelium is cuboidal between the mouths of the mural alveoli in the earlier generations of respiratory bronchioles but becomes progressively flatter until it is entirely alveolar epithelium in the alveolar ducts. Like the conductive bronchioles, the respiratory bronchioles are embedded in the pulmonary parenchyma. The respiratory bronchioles have well-marked muscle layers, with bands looping over the opening alveolar ducts and the openings of mural alveoli. The total cross-sectional area at this level is in the order of hundreds of square centimeters.

The primary lobular terminal respiratory unit is the likely equivalent of the alveolus when considered from the standpoint of function. The primary lobule is defined as the zone supplied by a first-order respiratory lobule. There are approximately 130,000 primary lobules with a diameter of about 3.5 mm containing approximately 2,000 alveoli each.

Alveolar ducts (generations 20–22) arise from terminal respiratory bronchioles and differ from terminal respiratory bronchioles by having no walls other than the mouths of mural alveoli (approximately 20 in number). Approximately half of alveoli arise from ducts. The last generation of air passages differs from the alveolar ducts solely in the fact that they are blind pouches. Approximately 17 alveoli arise from these alveolar sacs and account for half of the total number of alveoli.

Alveoli

The total number of alveoli is approximately 300 million but ranges from 200 to 600 million, corresponding to the height of the subject. The size of the alveoli is proportional to the lung volume. The alveoli are larger in the upper part of the lung, except at maximal inflation when the vertical size gradient disappears. The reduction in the size of alveoli and the corresponding reduction in the caliber of smaller airways in the dependent parts of the lung comprise the most important implications in gas exchange. At functional residual capacity, the mean diameter is 0.2 mm (4).

Alveolar walls, which separate adjacent alveoli, consist of two layers of alveolar epithelium on a separate basement membrane enclosing the interstitial space. These layers contain pulmonary capillaries, elastin and collagen, nerve endings, and occasional neutrophils and macrophages. On one side of the interstitium, the capillary endothelium and alveolar epithelium

TABLE 44.1

	Generation (mean)	Number	Mean diameter (mm)	Area supplied	Cartilage	Muscle	Nutrition	Emplacement	Epithelium
Trachea	0	1	18	Both lungs	U-shaped	Links open end of cartilage			Columnar cilated
Main bronchi	1	2	13	Individual lungs			From the bronchial circulation	Within connective tissue sheath along-side arterial vessels	
Lobar bronchi	2 ↓ 3	4 ↓ 8	7 ↓ 5	Lobes	Irregular shaped and helical plates	Helical bands			
Segmental bronchi	4	16	4	Segments					
Small bronchi	5 ↓ 11	32 ↓ 2,000	3 ↓ 1	Secondary lobules					
Bronchioles Terminal bronchioles	12 ↓ 16	4,000 ↓ 65,000	1 ↓ 0.5		Absent	Strong helical muscle bands		Embedded directly in the lung parenchyma	Cuboidal
Respiratory bronchioles	17 ↓ 19	130,000 ↓ 500,000	0.5	Primary lobules		Muscle bands between alveoli	From the pulmonary circulation		Cuboidal to flat between the alveoli
Alveolar ducts	20 ↓ 22	1,000,000 ↓ 4,000,000	0.3	Alveoli		Thin bands in alveolar septa		Form the lung parenchyma	Alveolar epithelium
Alveolar sacs	23	8,000,000	0.3						

are closely opposed, and the total thickness from gas to blood is usually less than 0.4 μm. This is the active side of the capillary, and gas exchange is more efficient at this site. The opposite side of the capillary is usually more than 1 to 2 μm thick and contains collagen and elastin fibers in an expanded tissue space. Herein is situated the connective tissue framework, which maintains pulmonary geometry. Alveolar septa are generally flat due to the tension generated by elastic fibers and surface tension at the air–fluid interface. The surface tension of the alveolar lining fluid is modified in the presence of surfactant. Septa are perforated by fenestrations known as pores of Kohn. These pores provide collateral ventilation, which can be demonstrated between the air spaces supplied by large bronchi (2).

Alveolar Cellular Morphology

The alveoli are divided by septa lined by flattened, continuous epithelial cells covering the thin interstitium (5). This epithelium, in humans, consists primarily of two distinct cells—type I and type II—with occasional neuroendocrine cells. In addition, although not frequently a part of the alveolar wall, the alveolar macrophage is, in fact, normally present on the alveolar epithelial surface.

Type I Epithelium

The type I alveolar cell (squamous lining cell), although comprising only 8% of parenchymal lung cells and inconspicuous by light microscopy, covers approximately 95% of the alveolar surface area, and has a total volume twice that of the histologically more prominent type II cell. Its nucleus is small and flattened. The nucleus is covered by a thin rim of cytoplasm containing few organelles. The remainder of the cytoplasm is aligned in broad sheets measuring 0.3 to 0.4 μm in thickness and extending in all directions for 50 μm or more over the alveolar surface. Sheets of adjacent type I cells interdigitate, and individual plates may reach into neighboring alveoli by winding the septal tip or by extending through the alveolar pores. Localized gap junctions have been identified between adjacent type I cells and between type I and type II alveolar cells frequently in association with an occluding junction (6).

The cytoplasm of type I epithelium contains few organelles but numerous pinocytotic vesicles, which are thought to transport fluid or proteins across the air–blood barrier. Type I cells have shown the ability to take up intra-alveolar particulate material. This particle clearance may be small in comparison with alveolar macrophages and the mucociliary apparatus. However, movement of materials across type I epithelium may allow particles to be deposited in regional lymph nodes.

Type II Epithelium

The type II epithelial cell (granular pneumocyte) is cuboidal in shape and protrudes into the alveolar lumen. Thus, it is easily identified on light microscopy. These cells may occur in groups of two or three. Type II epithelium is often located near corners where adjacent alveoli meet. The cytoplasm of type II epithelium is rich in organelles, including endoplasmic reticulum with ribosomes, Golgi complexes, mitochondria, and membrane-bound osmiophilic granules. There is evidence from ultrastructural, biochemical tissue culture and immunologic studies that type II cells and their osmophilic granules supply alveolar surfactant. These granules appear to function in a storage capacity, although some aspects of surfactant synthesis may also occur. Release of granule contents into the alveolar lumen occurs by exocytosis.

A second major function of type II epithelium is repopulation of normal and damaged alveolar epithelium. The type I cell is thought to be incapable of replication. On the other hand, the type II population is mitotically active and repopulates the alveolar surface. In addition, cytoplasmic simplicity and the large surface area of type I cells make them susceptible to damage from a variety of stimuli. In such circumstances, type II cells proliferate and temporarily repopulate alveolar walls, providing epithelial integrity. In time, they transform into type I cells. This sequence has been demonstrated with pulmonary injury from a variety of agents including oxygen, nitrous oxide, and other chemicals. Microvilli cover the surface of type II cells, suggesting that these cells may function in resorption of fluid or other materials from the alveolar air space.

Alveolar Macrophage

Pulmonary macrophages can be divided into three groups based on anatomic locations: (a) airway macrophage situated within the lumen or beneath the epithelial lining of conducting airways, (b) interstitial macrophage found isolated or in relation to lymphoid tissue in the interstitial connective tissue space, and (c) alveolar macrophage located on the alveolar surface. The alveolar macrophage has been the most extensively studied due to its accessibility by bronchoalveolar lavage (7,8).

The alveolar macrophage ranges from 15 to 50 μm in diameter and is round in shape with a foamy granular cytoplasm. The nuclei are eccentric and may be multiple within the cell. Ultrastructurally, macrophages show prominent cytoplasmic projections that appear as microvilluslike structures. The cytoplasm contains a well-developed Golgi apparatus, scattered mitochondria, endoplasmic reticulum, ribosomes, microtubules and microfilaments, and membrane-bound granules of varying appearance. These granules contain primary and secondary lysosomes.

Pulmonary alveolar macrophages differ from other macrophages by having aerobic energy production, increased mitochondria and mitochondrial enzymes, and more numerous and larger lysosomes. Alveolar macrophages are ultimately derived from bone marrow precursors, presumably by way of the peripheral blood monocyte. In addition, there is evidence for a population of alveolar interstitial macrophages capable of division and replenishment or augmentation of the alveolar macrophage population in the absence of a functioning bone marrow or in times of increased stress. The average lifespan of a pulmonary macrophage in the air space is estimated at 80 days. Various inhaled toxins, including cigarette smoke, have a negative effect on macrophage viability and activity.

The functions of the alveolar macrophage are numerous. They can be considered within the context of phagocytosis and clearance of unwanted intra-alveolar debris, immunologic interactions, and production of inflammatory and other chemical mediators. Subpopulations of macrophages may have capacities for one or more of these functions. Macrophage surface receptors include IgG, IgE, and C3. In association with these and other opsonins such as fibronectin, phagocytosis of foreign material occurs. Ingested microorganisms are subjected to lysosomal enzymes and, in many cases, are destroyed. Alveolar macrophages also ingest and eliminate endogenous pulmonary material, including dying type I and type II epithelial cells, alveolar surfactant, and inflammatory exudates, as may be produced during pneumonitis. Macrophages ingesting foreign material typically die within the alveoli or enter the mucociliary elevator, allowing their clearance. Alveolar macrophages present antigens to T lymphocytes for specific immunity and, ultimately, T- and B-cell activation. The production of a variety of mediators has been attributed to the alveolar macrophage population. Among substances identified are fibronectin, prostaglandins, leukotrienes, interferons, and α_1 antitrypsin.

Pulmonary Vasculature

Pulmonary Arterial and Venous Circulation

The pulmonary circulation carries the same flow as the systemic circulation, but arterial pressure and vascular resistance are normally one-sixth as great (2). The media of the pulmonary arteries are half as thick as in the systemic arteries of the corresponding size. In larger vessels, the media consist mainly of elastic tissue, but in smaller vessels, they are mainly muscular, with a transition being in vessels of 1 mm in diameter. Pulmonary arteries lie close to corresponding air passages in connective tissue sheaths.

The transition to arterioles occurs at an internal diameter of 100 μm. These vessels differ radically from the systemic circulation, as they are virtually devoid of muscular tissue. There is a thin medium of elastic tissue separated from blood by the endothelium. There is little structural difference between the pulmonary arterioles and venules.

Pulmonary capillaries arise from larger vessels—the pulmonary metarterioles—and form a dense network over the walls of the alveoli; the spaces between them are similar in size to the capillaries themselves. About 75% of the capillary bed is filled in the resting state, but the percentage is higher in the dependent parts of the lung. This gravity-dependent effect is the basis of the vertical gradient of ventilation/perfusion ratios. Inflation of alveoli reduces the cross-sectional area of the capillary bed and increases the resistance to blood flow. Pulmonary capillary blood is collected into venules, which are structurally similar to arterioles. Unlike pulmonary arteries, pulmonary veins run close to the septa, which separate segments of the lung.

Bronchial Circulation

At the level of terminal bronchioles, air passages and accompanying blood vessels receive nutrition from bronchial vessels, which arise from systemic circulation. Part of this bronchial circulation returns to the systemic venous beds but mingles with pulmonary venous drainage, contributing to shunt. It has been established that when pulmonary arterial pressure in animals is raised as by massive pulmonary emboli, pulmonary arterial blood is able to reach pulmonary veins without traversing the capillary bed. This physiologic arteriovenous communication may offer an explanation for abnormalities of gas exchange during anesthesia.

Pulmonary Lymphatics

There are no lymphatics visible in the interalveolar septa, but small lymph vessels commence at the junction between the alveolar and extra-alveolar spaces. A well-developed lymphatic system courses around the bronchi and pulmonary vessels, capable of containing up to 500 mL of lymph, and draining toward the hilum (9). Down to airway generation 11, lymphatics lie in a potential space around air passages and vessels, separating them from lung parenchyma. This space becomes distended with lymph and pulmonary edema and accounts for the characteristic "butterfly shadow" seen on a chest radiograph. In the hilum, lymphatic drainage passes through groups of tracheobronchial lymph nodes, where tributaries from superficial subpleural lymphatics contribute. Most of the lymph from the left lung enters the thoracic duct. Lymph from the right lung drains into the right lymphatic duct. Pulmonary lymphatics often cross the midline.

RESPIRATORY PHYSIOLOGY AND MECHANICAL VENTILATION

Positive pressure ventilation as a life-sustaining measure first proved its merit during the polio epidemics of the 1950s. Since that time, the use of mechanical ventilatory support has been synonymous with the growth of critical care medicine. Early ventilation used neuromuscular blocking agents to provide control of patient respiratory efforts. Today, patient–ventilator interaction is critical, and there is a growing awareness of complications associated with neuromuscular blockade. Finally, there is increasing recognition that ventilators can induce various forms of lung injury, which has led to reappraisal of the goals of ventilatory support (10). While it seems that each manufacturer has introduced differing modes of mechanical ventilation, the fundamental principles of ventilatory management of critically ill patients remain unchanged.

Positive pressure ventilation can be life saving in patients with hypoxemia or respiratory acidosis refractory to simpler measures. In patients with severe cardiopulmonary distress with excessive work of breathing, mechanical ventilation substitutes or supplements the action of respiratory muscles (11). In the setting of respiratory distress, respiratory muscles may account for as much as 40% of total oxygen consumption. In these circumstances, mechanical ventilation allows diversion of oxygen to other tissue beds that may be vulnerable. In addition, reversal of respiratory muscle fatigue, which may contribute to respiratory failure, depends on respiratory muscle rest. Positive pressure ventilation can reverse or prevent atelectasis by allowing inspiration at a more favorable region of the pressure–volume curve describing pulmonary function (Fig. 44.2). With improved gas exchange and relief from excessive respiratory muscle work, an opportunity is provided for the lungs and airways to heal. Mechanical ventilation is not therapeutic in and of itself, and positive pressure ventilation may aggravate or initiate alveolar damage. These dangers of ventilator-induced lung injury have led to a reappraisal of the objectives of mechanical ventilation. Rather than seeking normal arterial blood gas values, it is often better to accept a degree of respiratory acidosis and possibly relative hypoxemia to avoid large tidal volumes and high inflation pressures.

Mechanical ventilation may have hemodynamic effects as well. When applied to a passively breathing individual, positive pressure ventilation frequently lowers cardiac output, primarily as a result of decreased venous return. (This is especially true when gas trapping occurs during passive inflation [12]). In other circumstances, this form of ventilation may increase

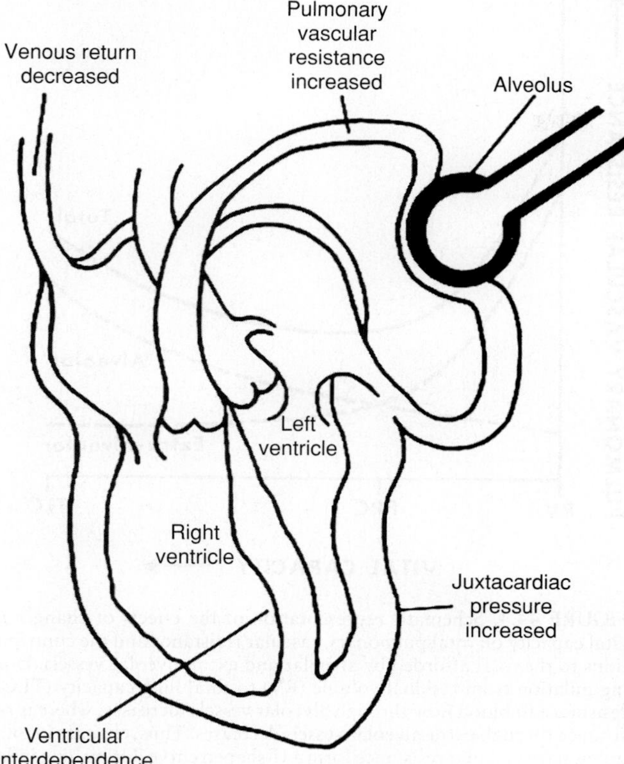

FIGURE 44.2. Factors responsible for the hemodynamic effects seen with positive pressure ventilation. An increase in intrathoracic pressure compresses the vena cava and thus decreases venous return. Alveolar distension compresses the alveolar vessels, and the resulting increases in pulmonary vascular resistance and right ventricular afterload produce a leftward shift in the interventricular septum. Left ventricular compliance is decreased by both the bulging septum and the increased juxtacardiac pressure resulting from distended lungs. (Reused with permission from Tobin MJ. Mechanical ventilation. *N Engl J Med.* 1994;330:1056–1061.)

cardiac output in the setting of impaired myocardial contractility because left ventricular afterload decreases with an increase in intrathoracic pressure. Alveolar distension compresses alveolar vessels, and the resulting increase in pulmonary vascular resistance and right ventricular afterload produces a leftward shift in the interventricular septum. Left ventricular compliance is decreased both by the bulging interventricular septum and increased juxtacardiac pressure from the distended lungs. There seems little doubt that adding mechanical ventilation or removing this support from critically ill patients can be a significant imposed stress.

Mechanical ventilation strategies are clearly affected by underlying pulmonary disease. For example, in patients with acute respiratory failure, chronic obstructive pulmonary disease (COPD), asthma, or other conditions associated with a high minute ventilation, gas trapping develops in alveoli because patients have inadequate expiratory time available for exhalation before the next breath begins. Patients experiencing this "breath stacking" have a residual, peripheral positive end-expiratory pressure (PEEP). Also termed auto-PEEP, this retained peripheral gas makes triggering the ventilator more difficult, since the patient needs to generate a negative pressure equal in magnitude to the level of auto-PEEP in addition to the trigger threshold of the machine. This is one factor that may contribute to the patient's inability to trigger the ventilator despite the obvious respiratory effort. Auto-PEEP may be undetected because it is not registered routinely on the pressure manometer of the ventilator. Newer machines have software to detect auto-PEEP. In older machines, occluding the expiratory port of the circuit at the end of expiration in a relaxed patient causes pressure in the lungs and the ventilator circuit to equilibrate, and the level of auto-PEEP is displayed on the manometer (13). Fortunately, in most patients, auto-PEEP does not become a problem until the respiratory rate reaches 30 breaths/minute. If auto-PEEP or breath stacking is detected, the respiratory rate and tidal volume should be reduced to permit this (breath stacking) process to resolve.

LUNG MECHANICS

Respiratory Muscles

Air flows to and from the alveoli, driven by differences in pressure between the airway opening and the alveolus. During spontaneous breathing, mouth (atmospheric) pressure remains constant, while alveolar pressure fluctuates under the influence of changing pleural pressure and tissue recoil forces (14–16). The diaphragm powers inspiration both by displacing the abdominal contents caudally and by raising the lower ribs, expanding them outward by a bucket handle effect (17,18). This latter action is aided by the external intercostal muscles. Normal exhalation is passive. When faced with a large ventilatory requirement or with impeded gas flow due to airway obstruction or parenchymal restriction, the accessory muscles of respiration are recruited to aid inhalation. Forceful exhalation is assisted by the internal intercostal muscles. The phrenic nerves (C3–C5) innervate the diaphragm, while the spinal nerves (T2–L4) innervate the intercostal and abdominal muscles.

The primary disorders of respiratory muscle function are usefully considered as problems of the diaphragm or problems of the accessory respiratory muscles (18,19). When upright, patients with isolated paralysis of both hemidiaphragms can often sustain adequate ventilation by the coordinated use of the intercostal and abdominal muscles. First, the diaphragm is forced upward as the muscles contract to raise the abdominal pressure. The diaphragm then descends, aided by gravity, as muscle relaxation allows abdominal pressure to fall. This mechanism cannot work effectively in the supine position, a circumstance that explains why orthopnea is a prominent symptom of this disorder. Patients with spinal cord injury (quadriplegia) have the converse anatomic problem: The intact diaphragm provides adequate ventilation to meet the normal requirement, but paralysis of the expiratory musculature severely limits ventilatory reserve and coughing efficiency.

Pressure–Volume Relationships

The lung and its thoracic shell occupy identical volumes, except when air or fluid separates them (20–22). At any specified volume, the pressure acting to distend the lung is alveolar pressure minus pleural pressure, while the pressure across the chest wall is pleural pressure minus atmospheric pressure. The volume of the lung is determined uniquely by lung compliance (distensibility) and the pressure difference acting to distend it (transpulmonary pressure). Thus, lung volume is the same whether the alveolar pressure is 0 and pleural pressure is –5, or if alveolar pressure is 25 and pleural pressure is 20. A similar relationship between the distending pressure, compliance, and volume also applies to the chest wall. When the chest wall muscles are relaxed at functional residual capacity (FRC), the tendency of the chest wall to spring outward balances the tendency of the lung to recoil to a smaller volume. Should either the lung or the chest wall become less compliant (as in interstitial fibrosis or obesity), the pressure–volume curve shifts rightward and flattens, causing FRC to decrease (20). Conversely, an increased lung compliance (as in emphysema) allows a higher resting volume.

Pleural Pressure

The fraction of change in alveolar pressure sensed in the pleural space depends on the relative compliances of the lung (C_L) and chest wall (C_W). For a given change in alveolar pressure (ΔPa), the amount transmitted to the pleural space (ΔPpl) will be:

$$\Delta Ppl = \Delta Pa(C_L/(C_L + C_W))$$

An inherently stiff chest wall would allow no volume change of the lung and complete transmission of a given increment in alveolar pressure to the pleural space. Conversely, an infinitely stiff lung would transmit none of it. Under normal circumstances, the lung and chest wall are almost equally compliant throughout the tidal range, so that approximately half of any change in alveolar pressure (as when PEEP is applied) is recorded in the pleural space. In clinical practice, average pleural pressure is estimated for clinical purposes as esophageal pressure (23).

Although clinicians speak fondly of pleural pressure as if it were a unique number, pleural pressure varies considerably throughout the chest because of hydrostatic gradients (which at FRC averages 0.37 cm water per centimeter vertical height), and because the pleural space and mediastinum have irregular contours caused by bony and vascular structures. At FRC, the average pleural pressure at midlung level is negative because the lungs are held open at greater than their relaxed volume. Pleural pressure surrounds the heart, the great vessels, and large airways, therefore affecting the vascular pressures measured at intrathoracic sites.

Effects of Changes in Lung Volume

Airway Resistance

Lung volume exerts a strong influence on airway resistance because resistance is inversely proportional to the fourth power of the radius. Pleural pressure surrounds the largest airways, while airways deeper within the lung are tethered open by the wall tension forces of the alveoli. Hence, as lung volume increases, the diameter of all airways increases, and resistance falls. Conversely, if a normal lung is held at a low resting lung volume, as in obesity, airway resistance will be high. In most restrictive diseases of lung tissue (e.g., interstitial fibrosis), the effects of heightened recoil on the airway diameter and driving force are usually more than sufficient to offset the effect of reduced volume, and flow rates are high relative to volume.

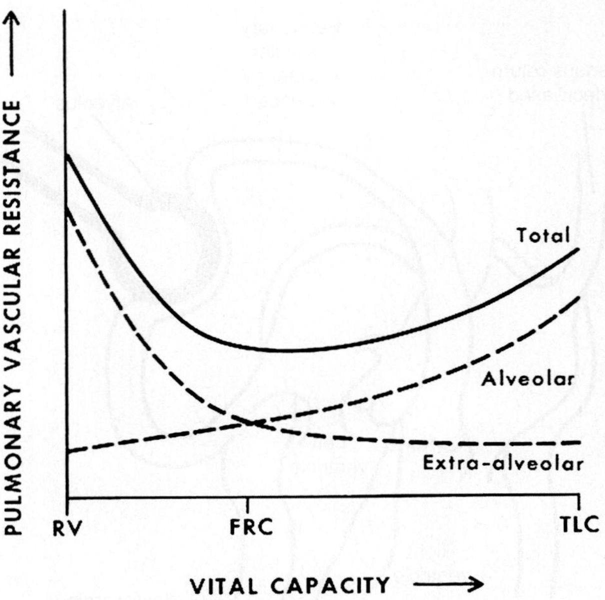

FIGURE 44.3. Schematic representation of the effects of changes in vital capacity on total pulmonary vascular resistance and the contributions to the total afforded by alveolar and extra-alveolar vessels. During inflation from residual volume (RV) to total lung capacity (TLC), resistance to blood flow through alveolar vessels increases, whereas resistance through extra-alveolar vessels decreases. Thus, changes in total pulmonary vascular resistance form a U-shaped curve during lung inflation. FRC, functional residual capacity. (Reused with permission from Murray JF. Circulation. In: *The Normal Lung: The Basis for Diagnosis and Treatment of Pulmonary Disease*. Philadelphia: WB Saunders; 1976:131.)

Pulmonary Vascular Resistance

Raising the lung volume has a different effect on the resistance of pulmonary vessels. Although the extra-alveolar vessels expand for reasons similar to those outlined for the airways, the capillaries are compressed as vascular pressures fall relative to alveolar pressure, and net pulmonary vascular resistance increases with each increment of lung volume above FRC (Fig. 44.3).

Muscular Force

The lung volume has an important effect on the maximal inspiratory and expiratory muscular forces that can be generated. The magnitude of these forces can be quantified by measuring the pressure recorded against the occluded airway. At total lung capacity (TLC), the lung and chest wall exert their highest recoil pressures. More importantly, the muscles of expiration are stretched maximally and are able to generate their highest contractile forces. If the occluded airway port is suddenly released, as during coughing, intraluminal airway pressure falls. The flexible posterior walls of the central airways invaginate, and the lumen narrows markedly to a slit. As gas accelerates to a high velocity through this narrow region, it shears mucus from the airway walls and delivers it to the oropharynx. To be maximally effective, a coughing effort must be forceful and start from a high lung volume. Gas flows should not be obstructed in small airways, and the glottis must be sealed to allow pressure within the airway to build. In critically ill patients, all of these conditions may be violated simultaneously. For intubated patients, a vital capacity greater than 20 mL/kg

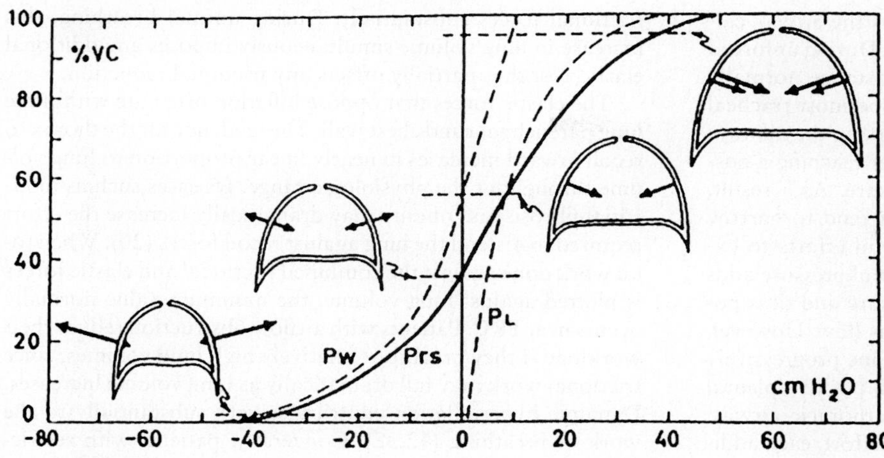

FIGURE 44.4. Static volume–pressure curves of the lung (P_L), chest wall (P_W), and total respiratory system (P_{rs}) during relaxation in the sitting posture. The static forces of the lung and the chest wall are pictured by the arrows in the side drawings. The dimensions of the arrows are not to scale; the volume corresponding to each drawing is indicated by the horizontal broken lines. (Reused with permission from Vassilakopoulos T, Zakynthinios S, Roussos C. Muscle function: basic concepts. In: Marini JJ, Slutsky AS, eds. *Physiological Basics of Ventilatory Support.* New York: Marcel Dekker, Inc.; 1998:114.)

and a maximal expiratory pressure of 60 mm Hg against an occluded airway at TLC are good predictors of an effective cough post extubation. The greatest negative end-inspiratory pressure can be generated at a residual volume where the muscle fibers of the diaphragm are stretched maximally to a position of favorable mechanical advantage. This encourages some patients to unintentionally misuse incentive spirometers that place emphasis on achieving a high flow rate rather than a high inhaled volume; they often exhale below FRC in order to take advantage of higher inspiratory muscle efficiency (and the relatively minor tendency of the chest wall to spring outward) at lower volumes. Conversely, hyperinflation causes the diaphragm to work less effectively, adding to the sense of dyspnea experienced by patients with COPD (Fig. 44.4).

Position and Lung Volume

Position has an important influence on lung volume. In assuming a recumbent supine position, FRC falls approximately 25% to 30% (approximately 1,000 mL) in the adult, with most of the decrease occurring before the Fowler (30-degree) position (24). This reduction in lung volume occurs because the abdominal contents push the diaphragm upward. In either lateral recumbent position, the lung volume at FRC is only about 15% to 20% less than the upright sitting value because the nondependent (uppermost) lung maintains its sitting lung volume, or actually distends, partially offsetting the loss of volume from the lower lung. These observations have relevance for the nursing care of postoperative and critically ill patients.

Normal Pattern of Breathing

To provide fresh gas at 5 to 7 L/minute to the lungs, the thoracic pump moves a stroke volume of 5 to 7 mL/kg at a frequency of 10 to 16 per minute. Once every 8 to 10 minutes, a sigh of two to four times the normal tidal volume occurs, which apparently serves to reverse the natural tendency for the individual alveoli to collapse when ventilated at a normal but monotonous volume. Breath-to-breath FRC changes continuously, at about a constant average value (25).

Dead Space

The bronchial, nasal, and pharyngeal passages do not participate in gas exchange. This anatomic dead space varies with airway caliber and lung volume, averaging roughly 2.2 mL/kg of lean body weight at FRC. Because approximately 50% of this dead space resides in the upper airways, orotracheal intubation and tracheostomy decrease anatomic dead space significantly (26). On the other hand, face masks and ventilator tubing unflushed by fresh gas can become an extension of the anatomic dead space, increasing the work of breathing. In addition to anatomic dead space, some volume of fresh gas (the alveolar dead space) reaches alveoli but does not participate in gas exchange because of inadequate perfusion. A portion of the increased ventilation requirement observed after a large pulmonary embolus results from this mechanism. Taken together, anatomic and alveolar dead space constitute the physiologic dead space (i.e., the volume of gas moved during each tidal breath that does not participate in gas exchange). The fraction of each tidal breath wasted in this fashion, the dead space volume–to–tidal volume (V_D/V_T) ratio, can be accurately approximated by the formula:

$$V_D/V_T = (PaCO_2 - PECO_2)/PaCO_2$$

where $PaCO_2$ and $PECO_2$ are the partial pressures of CO_2 in arterial blood and mixed expired gas, respectively. At a normal tidal volume, V_D/V_T increases with age; expressed as a percentage:

$$V_D/V_T = 24.6 + 0.17\,(\text{age in years})$$

At very low tidal volumes, V_D/V_T rises to a high value because anatomic dead space does not decrease proportionately. (Nonetheless, even at tidal volumes theoretically below the anatomic dead space value, some alveolar gas exchange does occur.). During exercise, the V_D/V_T may fall to 20% or less, owing both to large tidal breaths and better perfusion throughout the lung.

Flow Limitation

The rate of airflow depends on the pressure difference driving the flow and the resistance: flow = driving pressure/resistance. Flow rates during exhalation are volume dependent because the recoil pressure that drives gas flow, as well as the airway caliber, increases progressively with lung volume. During unforced tidal breathing, the major site of airway resistance normally resides in the nasal passages, larynx, and uppermost tracheal airway. The average pleural pressure surrounding the airways varies from –2 cm H_2O to –10 cm H_2O, never reaching a positive value relative to the intraluminal pressure. As a result, there are no compressive pleural forces that tend to narrow the airway during passive exhalation. Forceful efforts to exhale raise the pleural pressure. Increased pleural pressure adds to the recoil pressure to boost alveolar pressure and thus potentially improves the driving pressure for gas flow. However, because pressure within the airway must decline progressively to zero as the airway opening is approached, positive pleural pressure also narrows the compressible intrathoracic airway. Above approximately two thirds of maximal effort, each additional increment in pressure narrows the airway sufficiently to offset the increment in alveolar pressure. The maximal flow rate is then said to be effort-independent at that lung volume, and remains so at smaller lung volumes, so long as the forceful effort is sustained. According to classic teaching, the point within the airway where pleural pressure and intraluminal pressure are equal (the *equal pressure point*) determines where "critical narrowing" occurs (27). Normally, it resides in the trachea or main bronchi at high lung volumes and migrates toward the alveolus as forceful expiration proceeds. A less well-known theory of flow limitation is the *wave speed theory*. Although scientifically more defensible than the equal pressure point theory, it is less intuitive and less widely known. Both theories predict that once flow limitation occurs, flow rate is determined only by the recoil pressure of the lung and resistance of the airway segment upstream of the critical pressure point.

Reproducibility stemming from effort independence is the main reason why effort-independent, forced spirometry values (such as FEV_1) enjoy popularity as indices for evaluating airflow obstruction. Peak flow rate, which occurs before 25% of the vital capacity has been exhaled and all inspiratory flow rates are effort dependent, is therefore less reproducible. There are some disadvantages in using maximal flow rates, however. Some patients with emphysema have such collapsible airways that flow rates demonstrate negative effort dependence (i.e., flow rates worsen with increasing effort). Presumably, this helps account for the practice of pursed lip breathing among patients who are so severely limited by their disease that they must utilize optimal rates of exhalation during tidal breathing.

Work of Breathing

Energy must be expended in moving gas to and from the alveoli, primarily against frictional and elastic forces (28–31). Under extreme ventilatory burdens, such exertion may contribute substantially to total oxygen consumption. The main portion of fractional resistance arises from collisions of gas molecules with the surfaces of the airway. Work done against friction depends strongly upon airway size, increasing rapidly as airway caliber narrows. For this reason, frictional work varies inversely with lung volume, which influences luminal diameter. When airways are narrowed by obstructive disease, a relatively small increase in resting lung volume can reduce the work dissipated against frictional forces substantially. During normal breathing, this increase in lung volume simultaneously imposes an additional elastic cost that partially offsets any frictional reduction.

The elastic forces that oppose inflation originate within the lung parenchyma and chest wall. The tendency for the thorax to recoil inward increases in nearly linear proportion to lung volume throughout the physiologic range. Diseases such as interstitial fibrosis and obesity may dramatically increase the effort required to distend the lung against recoil forces (20). When total work done against the combined frictional and elastic forces is plotted against lung volume, the minimum value normally occurs near FRC. Patients with airflow obstruction reduce their workload if they breathe at relatively high lung volumes, since frictional work may fall dramatically as lung volume increases. Dynamic hyperinflation contributes very substantially to the work of breathing (12,32). Conversely, patients with restrictive parenchymal disease may perform less total work at lower lung volumes as the reduction in elastic work more than compensates for the increase in frictional work. Under normal circumstances, FRC is set near the volume at which total work of breathing is minimized. In cases of advanced airflow obstruction, maintenance of acceptable ventilation may require that the patient sustain a higher lung volume in order to take advantage of the higher flow rates achievable at that level. (At a lower FRC, expiratory flow is too slow to allow adequate alveolar ventilation.) Positive alveolar pressure generated during this process is termed *dynamic hyperinflation,* and is quantified by stopping flow at end expiration. This allows auto-PEEP (intrinsic PEEP) to be approximated (12,33).

VENTILATION/PERFUSION RELATIONSHIPS

Distribution of Ventilation and Perfusion

Ventilation

Alveoli contiguous to the pleura are kept open by a positive distending pressure (alveolar minus pleural). At the same horizontal level, a net pressure—very nearly equal to pleural pressure—surrounds the alveoli deep within the lung parenchyma due to the phenomenon of interdependence (which links each alveolar wall to its immediate and distant neighbors). Although the alveolar distending pressures across a given horizontal slice of the lung are similar, the vertical gradient of pleural pressure (approximately 0.3 cm water/vertical centimeter at FRC) causes a more negative pleural pressure at the apex of the upright lung than at the base (34,35). Consequently, the apical alveoli and airways are larger at FRC than their basal counterparts. However, as pleural pressure falls during inhalation, it does so unevenly; pressure falls most in the dependent regions closer to the diaphragm. This larger pressure swing, together with the fact that smaller alveoli are more compliant than larger ones, causes the bases to ventilate better than the apices. The same principles hold in the supine, prone, and lateral positions; uppermost lung regions are held open at higher volumes, but the dependent lung regions are better ventilated—a good rationale for periodically turning bedridden patients from side to side. These principles, which apply to spontaneous breathing, do not necessarily hold for patients receiving positive pressure ventilation in a passive mode.

Perfusion

The relationship of ventilation to dependency is fortunate, considering that the distribution of pulmonary blood flow follows a similar rule. Because of its low resistance, the normal pulmonary vascular bed is a low-pressure circuit, with resting pressures in the central arteries averaging approximately 25/10 mm Hg (mean 15 mm Hg). Pulmonary venous pressure is similar to that of the left atrium, oscillating between 3 and 10 mm Hg with the cardiac cycle. Because the apices are positioned at least 10 cm above the hila in the upright position, many capillaries therein must wink open and closed at different phases of the breathing cycle during the tidal breathing cycle. Hydrostatic pressure adds to luminal pressure so that vessels in the dependent regions are relatively dilated and the driving pressure for flow is relatively high. Hence, perfusion improves markedly, proceeding from apex to base (36). This helps explain why emboli localize to the lower lobes and why collapse of the air spaces at the base can cause profound hypoxemia, while upper lobe atelectasis seldom does. Given the patient with unilateral parenchymal disease and a choice of placing the patient in either lateral position to improve gas exchange, the good lung should be placed dependent for two reasons: The good lung will receive a higher percentage of total ventilation and perfusion, and the bad lung will be subjected to higher distending pressures. One should be concerned, however, that mucus and other noxious liquids produced in the "bad" lung could flood the dependent "good" lung, unless precautions are taken. Although dependency causes both ventilation and perfusion per unit volume to increase, the effect on perfusion is more striking, and therefore the regional ventilation-to-perfusion ratio is highest at the apex and lowest at the base (35,36).

Regulation of Regional Perfusion

Blood flow through a lung region depends on the relationship between the alveolar pressure and pulmonary arterial and venous pressures. According to what is presently believed, if alveolar pressure exceeds arterial pressure, alveolar capillaries will pinch closed, and no blood will flow except through "corner" vessels that are subjected to different distending forces (37). If alveolar pressure is less than arterial pressure but exceeds venous pressure, flow through the region will be driven by the difference between arterial and alveolar (not venous) pressures. If venous pressure is higher than alveolar pressure, flow will be dependent on the arterial minus venous pressure difference, independent of alveolar pressure. Zones reflecting each of these conditions can be identified during tidal breathing (36,38–40). The influence of alveolar pressure on capillary patency is particularly important to consider when high levels of positive end-expiratory pressure are applied to the airway. If alveolar pressure exceeds pulmonary venous pressure, balloon occlusion pulmonary (wedge) pressure will reflect alveolar—not pulmonary venous—pressure through at least a portion of the respiratory cycle.

Capillary Recruitment

At a given lung volume, pulmonary vascular resistance falls as flow increases. Rising pulmonary arterial pressure recruits previously unperfused capillaries so that a fivefold increase in cardiac output during exercise results in a smaller than twofold increase in mean pulmonary arterial pressure. (The ventilation-to-perfusion match-up also becomes more uniform under these conditions.) In a patient with a partially obliterated pulmonary vascular bed (e.g., emphysema or interstitial fibrosis), no capillaries may remain to be recruited at rest. In this condition, even modest increments in cardiac output or pulmonary vascular resistance cause pulmonary artery pressure to increase dramatically.

Active Vasoconstriction

Apart from the effect of capillary recruitment, pulmonary blood flow can be regionally controlled by active constriction of vascular smooth muscle. If vascular smooth muscle hypertrophy is due to chronic hypertension, the response to vasoconstricting stimuli may be exaggerated. Alveolar hypoxia exerts by far the most important influence on variations of local vascular tone (39). Normally, this property serves a useful purpose, diverting blood away from alveoli that are poorly ventilated. However, acting against a background of a restricted capillary bed, widespread hypoxic vasoconstriction may cause excessive pulmonary artery pressure and precipitate acute right ventricular failure, as in exacerbated COPD. Acidemia is a weaker stimulus to pulmonary artery vasoconstriction that adds to the effect of alveolar hypoxia.

Other stimuli can influence vasomotor tone. Hypertonic fluids, such as angiographic contrast media, can cause a striking vasoconstrictor response. (This is believed to be a major mechanism causing sudden death in angiographic studies of patients with pulmonary hypertension [40].) Vasoactive substances such as serotonin, histamine, and prostaglandin F_2-α also produce notable vasoconstriction. α-Adrenergic vasopressors (e.g., levarterenol) cause little response. Unfortunately, relatively few available drugs produce potent vasodilation. Prostacyclin (intravenous or aerosolized) and inhaled nitric oxide, however, are exceptions (41). Aminophylline, isoproterenol, and calcium channel blockers (e.g., nifedipine) also act as pulmonary vasodilators. In the outpatient setting, bosentan and sildenafil have an undeniable vasodilating effect, but over a longer term.

Regulation of Regional Ventilation

Ventilation to a given lung region depends not only on the stress (pressure difference) applied, but also on the regional compliance of that unit and the resistance to air entry (42,43). The product of resistance and compliance is known as the *time constant*, RC, by analogy to electrical capacitors. A region with a low time constant (e.g., a stiff lung unit with open conducting airway) will fill and empty rapidly, and be relatively well ventilated for the amount of stress applied, compared to immediate neighbors having higher time constants. Healthy lungs depend upon contraction and relaxation of the bronchial smooth muscle to change the resistance and compliance of local units. Both β sympathetic and parasympathetic nerves innervate the bronchial smooth muscle. Vagal fibers are distributed throughout the tracheobronchial tree, while sympathetic fibers appear to concentrate in small airways. Under normal resting conditions, there is tonic vagal tone. Irritating stimuli, such as smoke, can trigger mild generalized bronchoconstriction, even among normal subjects. Localized bronchoconstriction occurs in an inflamed bronchus. Although found in some animal species, α receptors on bronchial smooth muscle are difficult to demonstrate in man. Carbon dioxide bronchodilates while hypocarbia bronchoconstricts. Diminished CO_2 delivery and resulting bronchoconstriction may partially explain the ventilation defects occasionally seen in the region of a pulmonary embolus. Hypoxemia and acidosis may also cause some degree of bronchoconstriction. Many circulating agents affect bronchial tone. Epinephrine and other catecholamines that stimulate β_2 receptors bronchodilate, as do cholinergic blockers, certain prostaglandins, nitric oxide, and theophylline derivatives. Histamine, prostaglandin F_2-α, and perhaps α-adrenergic stimulators bronchoconstrict.

GAS EXCHANGE AND TRANSPORT

The Respiratory Quotient

The primary function of ventilation is to allow the exchange of CO_2 generated in body tissues for the oxygen available in the inspired gas mixture. In the adult of average size at rest, approximately 250 mL of oxygen are consumed by the tissues per minute, whereas 200 mL of CO_2 are generated—a respiratory quotient ($CO_2/O_2 = RQ$) of 0.8. Over a long period of time, the ratio of gases exchanged with the atmosphere, R, must equal the RQ. Transiently, however, this atmospheric exchange ratio may exceed or be less than RQ, as during hyper- or hypoventilation. Important increases in the CO_2 production relative to the oxygen consumption ratio can occur with the shift to a high-carbohydrate diet. Starvation and the development of certain metabolically stressful conditions (e.g., sepsis) reduce CO_2 generation.

Alveolar Gas Equation

Gases move between the blood and alveolar spaces by diffusing from areas of higher partial pressure to those with lower partial pressure (44). As fresh gas is inspired at local barometric pressure, it is warmed to body temperature and humidified before it reaches the main carina. At saturation, the partial pressure exerted by water vapor at 37°C is 47 mm Hg, independent of barometric pressure. Thus:

$$PiO_2 = FiO_2 \cdot (P_B - 47)$$

where PiO_2 is the partial pressure of oxygen in the central airways, FiO_2 is the fraction of oxygen in the inspired gas mixture, and P_B is barometric pressure in millimeters of mercury. Barometric pressure falls with ascending altitude (45). Although 750 mm Hg at sea level, P_B is 520 mm Hg at 10,000 feet.

In the steady state, the partial pressure of oxygen at the alveolar level (PaO_2) can be estimated from the simplified alveolar gas equation, which is based on the principle of conservation of mass:

$$PaO_2 = PiO_2 - (PaCO_2)/RQ$$

$PaCO_2$, the partial pressures of CO_2 in arterial blood, and the alveolar PCO_2 of well-perfused units remain nearly equivalent, even in disease, so that $PaCO_2$ is usually measured and substituted. Transient episodes of hyperventilation and breath-holding can result in oxygen tensions that are considerably higher or lower than the values predicted.

Alveolar-Arterial Oxygen Tension Difference

The alveolar gas equation is worth remembering because the difference between calculated PAO_2 and measured PaO_2 (known variously as the A-a PO_2 difference, A-a DO_2, or the A-a gradient) provides a measure of the efficiency of gas exchange between the alveolus and the arterial blood. The normal A-a gradient increases with FiO_2 and with age. When supine, A-a DO_2 is approximately 10 mm Hg for a healthy young person at sea level when breathing air and 100 mm Hg while breathing 100% oxygen. Hyper- and hypoventilation do not noticeably affect it. The A-a DO_2 is a particularly useful index when monitoring patients who require supplemental oxygen.

Causes of Arterial Hypoxemia

Arterial oxygen content may fall due to one of six mechanisms: (a) inhalation of a hypoxic gas mixture, (b) hypoventilation, (c) impaired diffusion of oxygen from alveolar space to pulmonary capillary, (d) ventilation/perfusion mismatching, (e) shunting of venous blood past alveolar capillaries, and (f) admixture of abnormally desaturated systemic venous blood (34). A decrease in the inspired fraction of oxygen, as at high altitude, will cause hypoxemia for obvious reasons. In the steady state and in accordance with the alveolar gas equation, hypoventilation will cause alveolar PO_2 to fall as oxygen is consumed, but not replenished, at a sufficient rate. The impaired diffusion of oxygen can result in incomplete equilibration of alveolar and pulmonary capillary blood, but this appears to be of limited clinical importance except when the lung parenchyma is seriously abnormal and cardiac output is high. The increased distance for diffusion between the alveolus and erythrocyte, the decreased gradient for O_2 diffusion, and the shortened transit time of the red cell through the capillary all adversely influence diffusion (44). Under ordinary circumstances, however, none of these factors acting in isolation slows the equilibration sufficiently to prevent the saturation of end-capillary blood. Nonetheless, a combination of adverse influences may cause enough impairment of diffusion to contribute to hypoxemia (e.g., diffusion impairment probably contributes to the hypoxemia of a person with interstitial fibrosis during exercise).

Ventilation/Perfusion Mismatch

Regional mismatching of ventilation and perfusion is perhaps the most frequent cause of clinically important desaturation (e.g., COPD). *Regional* is the key word when the entire lung is considered. It is not the ratio of minute ventilation relative to total pulmonary blood flow that determines whether hypoxemia occurs, but rather whether ventilation and perfusion distribute appropriately (e.g., one lung could receive all ventilation and the other lung all perfusion, for an overall ventilation/perfusion [V/Q] ratio of 1.0). Units that are relatively poorly ventilated in relation to the perfusion they receive cause desaturation; high V/Q units contribute to alveolar and physiologic dead space, but not to hypoxemia. Unfortunately, overventilating some units to compensate for others that are underventilated may keep $PaCO_2$—but not PaO_2—at the proper level. Aliquots of blood exiting from different lung units mix gas *contents*, not partial pressures. For CO_2 content, which relates linearly to alveolar ventilation in the physiologic range, a unit with good ventilation can compensate for an underventilated unit. However, at normal barometric pressure, a little more oxygen can be loaded onto blood with already saturated hemoglobin, no matter how high the oxygen tension in the overventilated units may rise. Hence, when equal amounts of blood from well and poorly ventilated units blend their contents, the result is blood with O_2 content halfway between them and a PaO_2 only slightly higher than that of the lower V/Q unit. Supplementing the inspired fraction of oxygen will cause arterial hypoxemia to reverse impressively as the alveolar oxygen partial pressure of even poorly ventilated units climbs high enough to achieve saturation. After breathing 100% oxygen for a sufficient period of time, only those units that are totally—or almost totally—unventilated will contribute to hypoxemia.

Shunt

Hypoventilation, impaired diffusion, and V/Q mismatching all respond to supplemental oxygen. Units that are totally unventilated are unresponsive to oxygen therapy and contribute to intrapulmonary shunt. Shunt can also be intracardiac, as in cyanotic (right-to-left) congenital heart disease, or can result from the passage of blood between abnormal vascular communications within the lung, as occurs with pulmonary arteriovenous communications. If given oxygen for 15 minutes, the percentage of blood flow being shunted can be calculated from the formula:

$$[(CcO_2 - CaO_2)/(CcO_2 - CvO_2)] \times 100$$

where C denotes content, and c, a, and v denote end-capillary, arterial, and mixed venous, respectively (46). End-capillary PO_2 is assumed to equal alveolar oxygen tension, which in turn is calculated from the simplified alveolar gas equation. (Although it is best to measure mixed venous oxygen content directly, stable patients with presumed normal cardiac output and hemoglobin and oxygen consumption can reasonably be estimated to have a normal CvO_2, so long as arterial blood is near full saturation.) For a patient breathing pure oxygen, a shunt fraction less than 25% can be estimated rapidly by dividing the A-a difference ($670-PaO_2$) by 20, again with the proviso that the mixed venous oxygen content is normal. At lower inspired oxygen fractions, true shunt cannot be reliably estimated by an analysis of oxygen contents, but venous admixture or physiologic shunt can. Although V/Q mismatch as well as true shunt may contribute to a lower than normal PaO_2, any desaturation can be considered as if it originated from true shunt units. To calculate venous admixture, CcO_2 in the shunt formula is calculated from the ideal PAO_2 existing at that particular inspired oxygen fraction. At the bedside, a very imprecise but commonly used indicator of gas exchange is the PaO_2/FiO_2 ratio (the "P-to-F" ratio). In healthy adults, this ratio exceeds 400, independently of the FiO_2.

As the percentage of true shunt rises, supplemental oxygen becomes progressively less effective in raising PaO_2. When true shunt fraction is higher than 25%, little benefit accrues from raising the inspired oxygen fraction above 0.5. As a shunt increases, the P-to-F ratio becomes increasingly insensitive. These considerations have practical significance, because concentrations of oxygen higher than 0.5 markedly increase the risk of oxygen toxicity, but may have only marginal benefit in high shunt lungs (47). Hence, in patients with true shunt, FiO_2 can frequently be lowered out of a dangerous range without changing PaO_2 noticeably. Conversely, at low shunt percentages, even small changes in shunt fraction or at FiO_2 can cause major changes in oxygen tension. If the venous admixture is due primarily to V/Q mismatching, the response to raising FiO_2 will depend on whether most admixture arises from units with nearly normal, moderately low, or very low V/Q ratios (48). If hypoxemia is caused by very low V/Q (but not shunt) units, little improvement may accrue until the oxygen fraction approaches 1.0, at which level PaO_2 rises abruptly.

Admixture of Abnormally Desaturated Venous Blood

Admixture of abnormally desaturated venous blood is a potentially important mechanism acting to lower PaO_2 in patients with impaired pulmonary gas exchange and reduced cardiac output. The oxygen content of venous blood is determined by the interplay between oxygen consumption and oxygen delivery. O_2 consumption equals cardiac output times CaO_2 minus CvO_2. Oxygen delivery will be impaired if arterial saturation falls without a compensatory increase in tissue perfusion, or if tissue perfusion falls. In the first instance, the peripheral tissues will strip the usual amount of oxygen from an already desaturated hemoglobin molecule, and the resulting venous O_2 content will drop, provided that O_2 consumption remains normal. In the second instance, venous content will fall as an abnormal amount of oxygen is removed from each unit volume of sluggishly passing blood.

If all returning venous blood goes to well-ventilated units, abnormally desaturated venous blood presents no problem, as blood exiting from the lung will be fully saturated. However, to the extent that venous admixture exists, reduced venous saturation translates into arterial desaturation. When lung parenchymal disease develops, patients with limited cardiac reserves are those at greatest jeopardy for serious desaturation by this mechanism. In such patients, there is a "positive feedback loop"—arterial desaturation leads to venous desaturation, which adds to venous admixture and impairs arterial oxygenation further. Even with stable lung parenchymal disease, serious arterial desaturation can occur if cardiac output falls disproportionately to oxygen consumption. Thus, in many intensive care patients, PaO_2 fluctuates considerably, independent of changes in the lungs.

GAS TRANSPORT AND STORAGE

Oxygen Carriage

In blood, hemoglobin binds the vast majority of oxygen, and plasma dissolves the remaining small fraction. The oxyhemoglobin dissociation relationship is curvilinear, with the knee of the curve at approximately 60 mm Hg at normal pH (49). Acidosis, increased temperature, raised $PaCO_2$, and increased erythrocyte 2,3-diphosphoglycerate (DPG) shift the curve rightward, mildly hampering loading at the alveolus but facilitating unloading of oxygen at the low PO_2 of tissue. At sea level, normal PaO_2 is age dependent, varying from approximately 100 mm Hg at age 20 to 80 mm Hg at age 80. Because hemoglobin binding is 90% complete at a partial pressure of 60 mm Hg and falls rapidly below that level, a PaO_2 of $\geq$60 mm Hg and SaO_2 of $\geq$90% are commonly agreed to represent adequate oxygen loading, and are used as benchmark values for clinical purposes. Raising the PaO_2 10-fold raises the oxygen-carrying capacity a scant 12.5%. The volume of oxygen carried in 100 mL of blood can be calculated from the following formula:

$$CaO_2 = 1.39\,[Hgb]\ \%\ Sat + 0.0034\,[PaO_2]$$

where Hgb is hemoglobin, expressed in grams per 100 mL of blood, and % Sat equals percentage of hemoglobin saturation. At normal rates of oxygen consumption and delivery, mixed venous blood has a PO_2 of 40 mm Hg, a saturation of 75%, and an oxygen content of 15 mL oxygen per 100 mL of blood. The content difference between simultaneous arterial and mixed venous samples—the a-v O_2 difference—averages 5 mL of oxygen per 100 mL of blood under normal circumstances. However, this difference widens when O_2 consumption is disproportionate to the rate of O_2 delivery to the tissues, as commonly occurs in states of low cardiac output. Conversely, the difference will be narrow in sites of abnormally high blood flow or if there are functional arteriovenous shunts in peripheral tissues.

CO_2 Carriage

Carbon dioxide is carried in the blood in three forms. The small proportion physically dissolved in plasma contributes little to CO_2 exchange between venous blood and the alveolus (about 10% of the total). CO_2 is also bound to blood proteins (mainly hemoglobin) more avidly by venous than by arterial blood. Approximately 30% of the CO_2 delivered to the alveolus is released from these "carbamino" compounds (50). Quantitatively, the majority of CO_2 carried in the blood takes the form of bicarbonate ion. With the help of erythrocyte carbonic anhydrase to speed its conversion to CO_2 as it reaches the alveolus, bicarbonate delivers approximately 60% of the total CO_2 offered for exchange.

Stores of O_2 and CO_2

Exclusive of the gas volume of the lungs, total body tissue stores of oxygen are small, scarcely more than 1 L. In addition, a considerable proportion of that stored volume is not available to the tissues without unacceptable reductions in PO_2 and the gradient for diffusion of oxygen at the tissue level. Following sudden cessation of the circulation, supplies are rapidly exhausted, and irreversible damage to certain vital organs occurs within minutes. The lungs act as a reservoir of approximately 500 mL of oxygen when breathing air; hence, PaO_2 falls more slowly during apnea than it does during circulatory arrest. (For this reason, attempts to maintain adequate forward blood flow must not be interrupted during management of circulatory arrest.) When filled with pure oxygen rather than air, the capacity of the lung reservoir is increased fivefold, and the duration of apnea before hypoxemia occurs is prolonged threefold or longer. Breathing oxygen does little to increase storage in blood and other body tissues, and PAO_2 falls precipitously upon returning to room air breathing. Thus, "preoxygenating" a patient before tracheal suctioning is ineffective if more than a few seconds elapse after oxygen is removed from the face, and is maximally effective when oxygen is continued up to the time that suction is applied. Similar considerations apply during endotracheal intubation; if the tube cannot be placed quickly and the patient continues to breathe spontaneously, the attempt to intubate should not be prolonged.

By comparison with oxygen stores, body stores of carbon dioxide are enormous—on the order of 100 times as great. As a result, it takes much longer for CO_2 to find a steady-state level after a step change in ventilation (51). Interestingly, $PaCO_2$ more rapidly achieves the steady-state value following a step *increase* in ventilation than following a step decrease. The $PaCO_2$ will have achieved its final value within 10 to 15 minutes after a ventilatory increase, although not for almost an hour or more following a decrease. These rules of thumb are helpful when deciding the time for arterial blood gas sampling during weaning efforts or when adjusting ventilator settings.

Consequences of Altered PaO_2, $PaCO_2$, and pH

Hypoxemia

Whether hypoxemia is tolerated well or poorly depends not only on the degree of desaturation, but also on compensatory mechanisms and the sensitivity of the vital organs to hypoxic stress. The major mechanisms of compensation are an increased cardiac output to improve perfusion of vital tissues (due to capillary recruitment and changes in distribution of resistance) and increases in hemoglobin concentration. Other adaptations, such as improved downloading of oxygen by tissue acidosis and increased anaerobic metabolism, assume less importance until failure of the primary methods calls them into action (as during circulatory arrest).

If a conscious individual without cardiac limitation or anemia is made mildly hypoxic over a short period of time, no important effect will be noted until PaO_2 falls below 50 to 60 mm Hg. At that level malaise, lightheadedness, mild nausea, vertigo, impaired judgment, and discoordination are the first symptoms, reflecting the extreme sensitivity of cerebral tissue to hypoxia (52). Although minute ventilation increases, little dyspnea develops unless hypercapnia uncovers underlying mechanical lung problems, as in COPD. Marked confusion resembling alcohol intoxication appears as PaO_2 falls into the 35- to 50-mm Hg range, especially in older individuals with ischemic cerebrovascular disease. Heart rhythm disturbances also develop. Between 25 and 35 mm Hg, renal blood flow decreases and urine output slows. Lactic acidosis appears at this level, even with normal cardiac function. The patient becomes lethargic or obtunded, and minute ventilation is maximal. At approximately 25 mm Hg, the normal individual loses consciousness; and below that tension, minute ventilation falls due to depression of the respiratory drive center.

The sequence of events will be shifted to occur at progressively higher levels of oxygen tension if any of the major compensatory mechanisms for hypoxemia is defective. Even mild decreases in oxygen tension are poorly tolerated by an anemic patient with impaired cardiac output. In addition, critically ill patients may have impaired autonomic control of perfusion distribution due either to endogenous pathology (e.g., sepsis) or to vasopressor therapy.

Hyperoxia

At normal barometric pressure, venous and mean tissue oxygen tensions rise less than 10 mm Hg above normal when pure oxygen is administered to healthy subjects; hence, nonpulmonary tissues are little altered. However, high concentrations of oxygen in the lung eventually replace nitrogen even in poorly ventilated regions, causing collapse of low V/Q units as oxygen is absorbed by venous blood faster than it is replenished. Diminished lung compliance results. More importantly, high oxygen tensions injure bronchial and parenchymal tissues. The toxic effects of oxygen are both time-and concentration-dependent (47). Several hours of pure oxygen breathing is sufficient to cause some sternal discomfort due to irritation of bronchial epithelium. Within 12 hours, histologic evidence of alveolar injury begins to develop. At high concentrations, parenchymal infiltration and fibrosis occur eventually, a process usually requiring days to weeks. However, many patients subjected to similar conditions undergo no detectable adverse changes. There is general agreement that very high oxygen concentrations are well tolerated for up to 48 hours. At concentrations of inspired oxygen less than 50%, clinically detectable oxygen toxicity is unusual; however long, such therapy is required.

Carbon Dioxide

Hypercapnia

The major waste product of oxidative metabolism, CO_2 is a relatively innocuous gas. Apart from its key role in regulation of ventilation, the clinically important effects of CO_2 relate to changes in cerebral blood flow, pH, and adrenergic tone. Hypercapnia dilates cerebral vessels and hypocapnia constricts them, a point of importance for patients with raised intracranial pressure. Acute increases in CO_2 depress consciousness, probably a result of neuronal acidosis. Similar but slowly developing increases in CO_2 are well tolerated. Nonetheless, a higher $PaCO_2$ signifies alveolar hypoventilation, which causes a decrease in alveolar and arterial PO_2. With hypoxemia averted by supplemental oxygen, some outpatients with severe airflow obstruction and $PaCO_2$ carry levels that chronically exceed 90 mm Hg and continue to lead active lives. The adrenergic stimulation that accompanies acute hypercapnia causes cardiac output to rise and peripheral vascular resistance to increase. Diaphoresis and plethora are accompanying clinical signs. During acute respiratory acidosis, these effects may partially offset those of the hydrogen ion on cardiovascular function, allowing better tolerance of low pH than with metabolic acidosis of a similar degree. During acute respiratory acidosis, constriction of glomerular arterioles also occurs by adrenergic stimulation, sometimes producing oliguria. Muscular twitching, asterixis, and seizures may be observed at extreme levels of hypercapnia in patients made susceptible by electrolyte or neural disorders.

Hypocapnia

The major effects of acute hypocapnia relate to alkalosis and diminished cerebral blood flow. Abrupt lowering of $PaCO_2$ reduces cerebral blood flow and raises neuronal pH, causing altered cortical and peripheral nerve function. Sudden major reduction of $PaCO_2$ (e.g., shortly after initiating mechanical ventilation) can produce life-threatening seizures. Cardiac arrhythmias are also an important consequence of abruptly lowering $PaCO_2$.

Hydrogen Ion Concentration

For mammalian cells to function optimally, hydrogen ion concentration must be rigidly controlled. The widest pH range that can be sustained for more than a few hours and is compatible with life is approximately 6.8 to 7.8 units. Although all organs malfunction to some extent during acidosis, cardiovascular function is perhaps the most impaired. Myocardial fibers contract less efficiently, systemic vessels react sluggishly to vasoconstrictive stimuli, vasomotor control deteriorates, blood pressure falls, arrhythmias develop, and pulmonary hypertension is accentuated (53). As a result, defibrillation and cardiopulmonary resuscitation are especially difficult in an acidotic patient. In addition, acidosis profoundly affects neuronal performance, acts synergistically with alveolar hypoxia to cause pulmonary vasoconstriction, and blunts the action of adrenergic bronchodilators on the conducting airways. Each of these effects accelerates dramatically in severity as pH falls below 7.20. Above 7.20, pH is not a major concern of itself, and should not prompt therapy aimed solely at pH correction. (In fact, the rightward shift of the oxyhemoglobin dissociation curve may improve tissue oxygen delivery if cardiovascular performance remains adequate.) In this higher pH range, acutely developing acidosis is more alarming for what it signifies: Seriously compromised ventilatory, metabolic, or cardiovascular systems in need of urgent attention.

Alkalosis causes less apprehension among physicians than acidosis of a similar degree because the etiology is usually less life threatening. However, alkalosis is detrimental with regard to the release of oxygen to the tissues, shifting the oxyhemoglobin dissociation curve leftward. Raised pH does not exert the dangerously depressing influence on myocardium and blood vessels seen with a similar degree of acidosis. Furthermore, unless very abrupt and severe, the effects of raised pH on the brain are limited to confusion and encephalopathy. The major risk of extreme alkalosis appears to relate to cardiac arrhythmias, which are caused in part by electrolyte shifts (decreased calcium, increased potassium) and diminished oxygen delivery.

To keep hydrogen ion concentration within narrow limits, its generation rate must equal the elimination rate. The hydrogen ion is generated in two ways: One by hydration of CO_2 from "volatile" acid (according to the reaction complex formula) and another by the production of fixed acid from the by-products of metabolism such as sulfates and phosphates (49,53). Ventilation eliminates the volatile acid load after reversal of the CO_2 hydration reaction in the lung capillaries, while the kidney excretes the bulk of the fixed acid load. Quantitatively, the lungs are much more important, as they eliminate a much greater acid load (53). If the excretion of CO_2

speeds or slows inappropriately, the result is respiratory derangement of the acid-base balance. If the excretion rate of fixed acid speeds or slows in relation to production, or if abnormal metabolic loads of acid or alkali develop that cannot be handled, metabolic acidosis or alkalosis occurs. A complete discussion of acid-base physiology is beyond the scope of this chapter.

Control of Ventilation

The respiratory center of the medulla modifies its own cyclic rhythm by integrating signals from many sources (54). These inputs, which may be of cortical, chemical, or reflex origin, cause changes in the timing frequency in the depth of tidal breathing. In general, each potential modifier of medullary activity is much more potent as a stimulus to increase breathing than as a depressant to retard the endogenous level of breathing set by the respiratory center. Efferent flow descends via the phrenic nerves to the diaphragm and via the spinal nerves to the intercostal and abdominal muscles. Control of output from the medullary respiratory center is an interactive process. For example, the precise effect of a given rise in $PaCO_2$ will depend on the levels of cortical arousal, PaO_2, and pH. The result of that neural output will depend on the ability of the ventilatory muscles to contract in a coordinated fashion and on the lungs to ventilate upon command.

Chemical Stimuli

Under normal resting conditions, intracerebral hydrogen ion concentration is the predominant influence over ventilation. As in the periphery, the ratio of bicarbonate concentration to PCO_2 determines pH. Unlike CO_2, which transports passively across the blood–brain barrier, the bicarbonate concentration of the cerebrospinal fluid is maintained somewhat lower than in blood by an active process (the "brain kidney"). This mechanism is capable of making relatively rapid compensatory adjustments in bicarbonate so that cerebrospinal fluid (CSF) pH is restored almost completely to its normal resting value of 7.3 within 12 hours following a derangement (54,55). By comparison, the CO_2 crosses the juxtamedullary area quickly and passively. Thus, an abrupt rise in $PaCO_2$ precipitates intracerebral acidosis, prompting increased ventilation to restore pH balance. The potency of an increase in $PaCO_2$ wanes with time, as CSF bicarbonate rises to compensate. Conversely, the ventilatory compensation for sustained metabolic acidosis is maximized 12 or more hours following its onset, since initially peripheral pH receptors drive $PaCO_2$ to low levels and create CSF alkalosis, which temporarily limits the ventilatory increase.

$PaCO_2$ drives ventilation mainly through its effect on intracerebral hydrogen ion concentration. However, a rise in $PaCO_2$ also stimulates receptors at the carotid bifurcation (perhaps to the peripheral pH receptors located there). The level of PaO_2 modifies the ventilatory response to CO_2, increasing it when hypoxemia occurs. Thus, when hypoxemia is relieved (as during treatment of the compensated COPD), $PaCO_2$ is expected to rise somewhat, even if the respiratory center is otherwise normally responsive to CO_2. The rise in CO_2 will be exaggerated if CO_2 sensitivity is reduced. Cortical depression, whether caused by sleep or sedative drugs, limits the response to CO_2, especially in patients with a previously blunted drive to breathe. Prolonged mechanical stress may also alter the sensitivity to chemical stimuli. Although the most common example occurs in chronic airflow obstruction, even normal individuals increase the CO_2 set point if made to breathe against resistance for an extended period of time. Teleologically, this occurs because total work of breathing lessens when $PaCO_2$ rises to make each tidal exchange more efficient.

Although an effect can be demonstrated up to 150 mm Hg, PaO_2 is an important stimulus for ventilation only when the blood is significantly desaturated (54). Oxygen receptors located mainly in the carotid body send neural signals to the medulla. Extreme hypoxia depresses rather than stimulates ventilation by direct depression of the respiratory center. With advancing age, the ventilatory response to hypoxemia (into low blood pH) diminishes, perhaps a consequence of carotid artery sclerosis. Starvation and sedatives also attenuate the hypoxic ventilatory drive. Systemic acidosis is a very potent drive to ventilation, with its effect at least additive to that of hypoxemia when the two occur together, as they often do clinically. The receptors for peripheral blood pH are located in the carotid body.

Nonchemical Stimuli

Neural reflexes originating from receptors located within the lung or chest wall may drive ventilation. Thus, the hyperventilation that occurs during the early phases of asthma and pulmonary edema, as well as the chronic hyperventilation of interstitial fibrosis, may result from stimulation of normally quiescent receptors. Central neurogenic hyperventilation and Cheyne-Stokes breathing (on average, also a hyperventilatory pattern) usually result from intracerebral pathology and may be modified by neuromuscular input.

Clinical Disorders of Ventilatory Control

For therapeutic purposes, it is important when evaluating hypercapnia to distinguish patients with depressed drives ("won't" breathers) from those whose condition, such as COPD or neuromuscular disease, will not allow them to achieve normal alveolar ventilation ("can't" breathers). Many patients present with combined problems of drive and mechanics. For example, because advanced age and starvation may blunt ventilatory drives, an elderly patient within acutely elevated ventilation requirements and mechanical stress (e.g., pneumonia) often presents with a component of respiratory acidosis as well as hypoxemia. Clues to primary respiratory center dysfunction include no evidence of obstruction or neuromuscular disease, normal A-a DO_2, and the preserved ability to drive $PaCO_2$ considerably below normal with voluntary hyperventilation. Because a wide spectrum of response to PCO_2 and PaO_2 exist even among healthy normal subjects, it is not surprising that two otherwise indistinguishable patients with the same pulmonary pathology may set very different levels of alveolar ventilation.

Sleep routinely blunts the chemical drives to breathe (56–58). Many chronic disorders can depress the respiratory center function. Among these, hypothyroidism, narcotic overdose, and the obesity hypoventilation syndrome are perhaps the most reversible. The utility of respiratory center stimulants is limited. Stimulants are contraindicated for patients with problems confined to disordered mechanics, such as COPD, since dyspnea may worsen with little beneficial effect. Progesterone increases CO_2 drive in pregnant women and has been used therapeutically as a ventilatory stimulant for primary hypoventilation (59). Its maximal effect is delayed several days. Conversely, testosterone blunts CO_2 responsiveness (60). Newer drugs touted to selectively improve alertness (e.g., modafinil, atomoxetine) may prove useful when somnolence contributes to hypoventilation.

References

1. Weibel ER. *Morphometry of the Human Lung.* Berlin: Springer; 1963.
2. Nunn JF. *Applied Respiratory Physiology.* 3rd ed. London: Butterworths; 1987.
3. Macklem PT, Wilson NJ. Measurement of intrabronchial pressure in man. *J Appl Physiol.* 1965;20:653–663.
4. Glazier JB, Hughes JM, Maloney JE, et al. Vertical gradient of alveolar size in lungs of dogs frozen intact. *J Appl Physiol.* 1967;23:694–705.
5. Fraser RG, Paré JA, Paré PD, et al. *Diagnosis of Diseases of the Chest.* 3rd ed. Philadelphia: Saunders; 1988.
6. Crapo JD, Barry BE, Gehr P, et al. Cell number and cell characteristics of the normal human lung. *Am Rev Respir Dis.* 1982;126:332–337.
7. Hocking WG, Golde DW. The pulmonary-alveolar macrophage (first of two parts). *N Engl J Med.* 1979;301:580–587.
8. Hocking WG, Golde DW. The pulmonary-alveolar macrophage (second of two parts). *N Engl J Med.* 1979;301:639–645.
9. Staub NC. J Pulmonary edema. *Physiol Rev.* 1974;54:678–811.
10. Dreyfuss D, Saumon G. Ventilator-induced lung injury: lessons from experimental studies. *Am J Respir Crit Care Med.* 1998;157:294–323.
11. Tobin MJ. Mechanical ventilation. *N Engl J Med.* 1994;330:1056–1061.
12. Pepe PE, Marini JJ. Occult positive end-expiratory pressure in mechanically ventilated patients with airflow obstruction. The auto-PEEP effect. *Am Rev Respir Dis.* 1982;126:166–170.
13. Chatburn RL, Primiano FP Jr. A new system for understanding modes of mechanical ventilation. *Respir Care.* 2001;46:604–621.
14. Loring SH. Mechanics of lungs and chest wall. In: Marini JJ, Slutsky AS, eds. *Physiological Basis of Ventilatory Support.* New York: Marcel Dekker Inc.; 1998:177–208.
15. Agostoni E, Mead J. Statics of the respiratory system. In: Fenn WO, Rahn H, eds. *Handbook of Physiology, Section 3: Respiration.* Vol. 1. Washington, D.C.: American Physiology Society; 1964:387–409.
16. Rodarte JH. Lung and chest wall mechanics: basic concepts. In: Scharf SM, Cassidy SS, eds. *Heart-Lung Interactions in Health and Disease.* New York: Marcel Dekker; 1989:221–242.
17. DeTroyer A, Loring SH. Actions of the respiratory muscles. In: Roussos C, Macklem PT, eds. *The Thorax.* 2nd ed. New York: Marcel Dekker Inc; 1994:535–563.
18. Vassilakopoulos T, Zakynthinos S, Roussos C. Muscle function: basic concepts. In: Marini JJ, Slutsky AS, eds. *Physiological Basis of Ventilatory Support.* New York: Marcel Dekker Inc.; 1998:103–152.
19. Roussos C, Macklem PT. The respiratory muscles. *N Engl J Med.* 1982; 307:786–797.
20. Sharp JT, Barrocas M, Chokroverty S. The cardiorespiratory effects of obesity. *Clin Chest Med.* 1980;1:103–118.
21. Otis AB, Fenn WO, Rahn H. Mechanics of breathing in man. *J Appl Physiol.* 1950;2:592–607.
22. Mead J. Mechanical properties of lungs. *Physiol Rev.* 1961;41:281–330.
23. Baydur A, Behrakis PK, Zin WA, et al. A simple method for assessing the validity of the esophageal balloon technique. *Am Rev Respir Dis.* 1982;126: 788–791.
24. Marini JJ, Tyler ML, Hudson LD, et al. Influence of head-dependent positions on lung volume and oxygen saturation in chronic air-flow obstruction. *Am Rev Resp Dis.* 1984;129(1):101–105.
25. Tobin MJ. Breathing pattern analysis. *Intensive Care Med.* 1992;18:193–201.
26. Fowler WS. The respiratory dead space. *Am J Physiol.* 1948;154:405–416.
27. Hyatt RE. Expiratory flow limitation. *J Appl Physiol.* 1983;55(1 Pt 1):1–7.
28. Sassoon CSH, Mahutte CK. Work of breathing during mechanical ventilation. In: Marini JJ, Slutsky AS, eds. *Physiological Basis of Ventilatory Support.* New York: Marcel Dekker Inc.; 1998:261–310.
29. Tobin MJ. Respiratory monitoring in the intensive care unit. *Am Rev Respir Dis.* 1988;138:1625–1642.
30. Otis AB. The work of breathing. In: Fenn WO, Rahn H, eds. *Handbook of Physiology, Section 3: Respiration.* Vol. 1. Washington, D.C.: American Physiology Society; 1964:463–476.
31. Aubier M, Viires N, Syllie G, et al. Respiratory muscle contribution to lactic acidosis in low cardiac output. *Am Rev Respir Dis.* 1982;126:648–652.
32. Kimball WR, Leith DE, Robins AG. Dynamic hyperinflation and ventilator dependence in chronic obstructive pulmonary diseases. *Am Rev Respir Dis.* 1982;126:991–995.
33. Hoffman RA, Ershowsky P, Krieger BP. Determination of auto-PEEP during spontaneous and controlled ventilation by monitoring changes in end-expiratory thoracic gas volume. *Chest.* 1989;96:613–616.
34. Otis AB, McKerrow CB, Bartlett RA, et al. Mechanical factors in distribution of pulmonary ventilation. *J Appl Physiol.* 1956;8:427–443.
35. Permutt S, Howell JB, Proctor DF, et al. Effect of lung inflation on static pressure-volume characteristics of pulmonary vessels. *J Appl Physiol.* 1961;16:64–70.
36. West JB, Dollery CT, Naimark A. Distribution of blood flow in isolated lung: Relation to vascular and alveolar pressures. *J Appl Physiol.* 1964;19:713–724.
37. Albert RK, Lakshminarayan S, Charan NB, et al. Extra-alveolar vessel contribution to hydrostatic pulmonary edema in in situ dog lungs. *J Appl Physiol.* 1983;54(4):1010–1017.
38. Riley RL, Cournand A. Analysis of factors affecting partial pressures of oxygen and carbon dioxide in gas and blood of lungs: theory. *J Appl Physiol.* 1951;4:77–101.
39. Peake MD, Harabin AL, Brennan NJ, et al. Steady-state vascular responses to graded hypoxia in isolated lungs of five species. *J Appl Physiol.* 1981;51(5):1214–1219.
40. Peck WW, Slutsky RA, Hackney DB, et al. Effects of contrast media on pulmonary hemodynamics: comparison of ionic and nonionic agents. *Radiology.* 1983;149:371–374.
41. Sastry BK. Pharmacologic treatment for pulmonary arterial hypertension. *Curr Opin Cardiol.* 2006;21(6):561–568.
42. Mead J, Whittenberger JL. Physical properties of human lungs measured during spontaneous respiration. *J Appl Physiol.* 1953;5:779–796.
43. Grassino AE, Roussos C, Macklem PT. Static properties of the chest wall. In: Crystal RG, West JB, et al., eds. *The Lung: Scientific Foundations.* New York: Raven Press; 1991:855–867.
44. Forster RE. Diffusion of gases across the alveolar membrane. In: *Handbook of Physiology.* Section 3. Washington, DC: American Physiological Society; 1987.
45. West JB. The physiologic basis of high-altitude diseases. *Ann Int Med.* 2004; 141(10):789–800.
46. Pontoppidan H, Geffin B, Lowenstein E. Acute respiratory failure in the adult. Parts 1-3. *N Engl J Med.* 1972;287(14):690–698,743–752, 799–806.
47. Deneke SM, Fanburg BL. Normobaric oxygen toxicity of the lung. *N Engl J Med.* 1980;303(2):76–86.
48. Dantzker DR, Brook CJ, Dehart P, et al. Ventilation-perfusion distributions in the adult respiratory distress syndrome. *Am Rev Resp Dis.* 1979;120(5):1039–1052.
49. Corey HE. Stewart and beyond: new models of acid-base balance. *Kidney Int.* 2003;64(3):777–787.
50. Severinghaus JW. Simple, accurate equations for human blood O2 dissociation components. *J Appl Physiol.* 1979;46:599–602.
51. Ivanov SD, Nunn JF. Influence of duration of hyperventilation on rise time of P-CO2 after step reduction of ventilation. *Respir Physiol.* 1968;5(2):243–249.
52. Kafer ER, Sugioka K. Respiratory and cardiovascular responses to hypoxemia and the effects of anesthesia. *Intl Anesthesiol Clin.* 1981;19(3):85–122.
53. Kellum JA. Clinical review: reunification of acid-base physiology. *Crit Care.* 2005;9(5):500–507.
54. Younes M, Georgopoulos D. Control of breathing relevant to mechanical ventilation. In: Marini JJ, Slutsky AS, eds. *Physiological Basis of Ventilatory Support.* New York: Marcel Dekker Inc.; 1998:1–74.
55. Bisgard GE, Busch MA, Forster HV. Ventilatory acclimatization to hypoxia is not dependent on cerebral hypocapnic alkalosis. *J Appl Physiol.* 1986; 60(3):1011–1015.
56. Weinhouse GL, Schwab RJ. Sleep in the critically ill patient. *Sleep.* 2006; 29(5):707–716.
57. Phillips B. Sleep, sleep loss, and breathing. *Southern Med J.* 1985;78(12): 1483–1486.
58. Skatrud JB, Dempsey JA. Interaction of sleep state and chemical stimuli in sustaining rhythmic ventilation. *J Appl Physiol.* 1983;55:813–822.
59. Sutton FD Jr, Zwillich CW, Creagh CE, et al. Progesterone for outpatient treatment of Pickwickian syndrome. *Ann Int Med.* 1975;83(4):476–479.
60. Matsumoto AM, Sandblom RE, Schoene RB, et al. Testosterone replacement in hypogonadal men: effects on obstructive sleep apnoea, respiratory drives, and sleep. *Clin Endocrinol.* 1985;22(6):713–721.

CHAPTER 45 ■ CARDIOVASCULAR SYSTEM

MICHAEL SCHLAME • THOMAS J. J. BLANCK

STRUCTURE OF THE HEART

Structure of Cardiac Myocytes

Cardiac myocytes are the main cell type of cardiac tissue (1). They have two important functions: (a) to contract in response to an electrical stimulus and (b) to pass the electrical stimulus on to neighboring cells. The simultaneous performance of these two activities requires a highly specialized array of intracellular membranes and contractile elements. Cardiac myocytes are distinct in many ways from skeletal muscle cells. For instance, cardiac myocytes are approximately 10 to 15 μm in diameter and about 50 μm long, which is only a fraction of the size of skeletal myocytes, which may extend up to several centimeters.

Cardiac myocytes are surrounded by the sarcolemma, a specialized plasma membrane that harbors the pumps responsible for ion exchange between the intracellular and the extracellular space (see section 2). The sarcolemma not only lines the surface of the cardiac myocyte, but it also forms a series of tubular invaginations, so-called *T tubules* (transverse tubules). These tubules effectively increase the surface area of the cell and bring the extracellular environment into close proximity of intracellular structures. T tubules are rich in L-type calcium channels, so that extracellular calcium gets delivered rapidly into the core of the cell.

Cardiac myocytes contain a number of organelles in specific spatial arrangement. These organelles include sarcomers, mitochondria, the sarcoplasmic reticulum, the nucleus, and the Golgi apparatus. Sarcomeres (about 50% of cell volume) and mitochondria (30% to 40% of cell volume) are the dominant components of cardiac myocytes (Fig. 45.1). These two organelles are responsible for contraction and supply of energy, respectively. It is therefore not surprising that the majority of inborn cardiomyopathies are caused by defects in either of these structures. The cardiac sarcomere consists of (a) actin filaments, built from actin monomers with associated troponin and tropomyosin; and (b) myosin filaments (see section 3). The sarcomere structure of the heart is similar to that of the skeletal muscle. Between the sarcomere bundles, mitochondria form elongated sacs, which are oriented parallel to the sarcomeres, reflecting a close spatial relationship between intracellular energy supply and energy consumption.

The sarcoplasmic reticulum is a network of tubes and cysts, spreading throughout the cell. Together with the T tubules, the sarcoplasmic reticulum accounts for about 2% of the cellular volume. The cisternal parts of the sarcoplasmic reticulum lie in close apposition to the T tubules. The two structures interact closely in order to generate cyclic changes in the calcium concentration. These signaling events are triggered by the depolarization-induced influx of calcium through the T tubules, which causes a second wave of massive release of calcium from the sarcoplasmic reticulum (see section 2).

Finally, cardiac myocytes contain a nucleus that accounts for about 5% of the cell volume. The nucleus is localized in the center of the cell and is associated with the rough endoplasmic reticulum, where the synthesis of proteins takes place. Some of the proteins are then processed in the Golgi apparatus, which is also associated with the endoplasmic reticulum.

Cardiac myocytes form a functional syncytium in which cells act in concert, both mechanically and electrically. This aspect requires sophisticated communication between cardiac myocytes at the intercalated discs, a specialized portion of the sarcolemma where individual cells make contact with each other. Intercalated discs send processes deep into the neighboring cell, which creates an interdigitating junction with a large surface area. Mechanical cooperation between cells is provided by specific anchor sites for actin filaments and by spot desmosomes that allow actin filaments to run from one cell to another. Electrical cooperation between cells is provided by gap junctions that contain microchannels. Gap junctions allow the passage of ions and small molecules between adjacent myocytes.

The above discussion applies mostly to the prototype of cardiac myocytes located in the ventricular myocardium. However, the heart contains three modifications of this prototype: (a) atrial cardiomyocytes located in the right and left atrium, (b) pacemaker cells located in the sinoatrial and atrioventricular nodes, and (c) Purkinje cells located in the Tawara branches. *Atrial cardiomyocytes* are smaller than ventricular cardiomyocytes (about 20 μm long and 5 μm in diameter) and they are elliptical in shape. They have a lesser concentration of T tubules than ventricular cells, but many more intercellular connections, both end to end and side to side, in order to spread the electrical impulse rapidly. Pacemaker cells have the ability to generate an action potential, and Purkinje cells have the ability to transmit this action potential with high speed. Both pacemaker and Purkinje cells are myocytes in principle, but they have specialized electrical properties. On the other hand, atrial and ventricular myocytes have specialized mechanical properties, but they also have the ability to generate and propagate action potentials.

Gross Anatomy of the Heart

The human heart is a four-chamber pump that ejects blood by rhythmic contractions (Fig. 45.2). Two thick-walled chambers, the left and the right ventricles, drive the systemic and pulmonary circulation. Two thin-walled chambers, the left and the right atria, eject blood into the respective ventricles at the end of their relaxation phase. Thus, atrial systole occurs during ventricular diastole and vice versa. Although atrial contractions

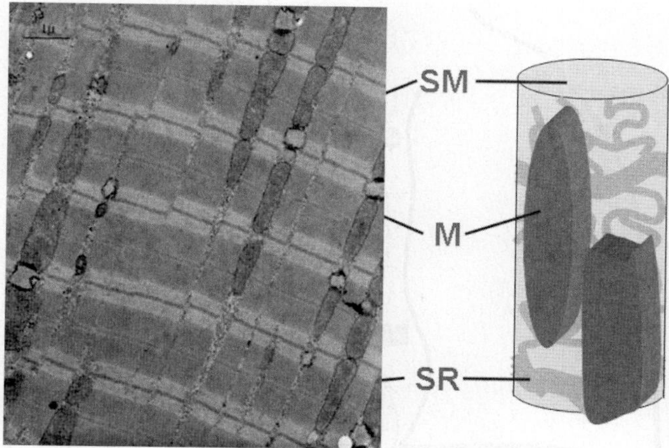

FIGURE 45.1. Internal structure of cardiomyocytes. The electron micrograph shows sarcomers (SMs) and mitochondria (M), the dominant intracellular organelles. Sarcomers form rods, which are surrounded by a web of sarcoplasmic reticulum (SR). Sarcomers and mitochondria are oriented in parallel.

may contribute up to 20% of the cardiac output by increasing ventricular filling, it is, in principle, dispensable, and the heart may function as a two-chamber pump in patients with atrial fibrillation or atrial asystole. In order to generate unidirectional blood flow, valves are positioned at the outflow orifices of each chamber. The atrioventricular valves (tricuspid and mitral) are located between atria and ventricles, whereas the semilunar valves (aortic and pulmonic) are located between ventricles and main arteries. As a result, the ventricles may close alternatively their inflow and outflow tract, but atria close their outflow tract only. For this reason, partial reversal of blood flow may occur in patients with atrioventricular (AV) valve regurgitation or in patients with untimely atrial contraction (atrial flutter, junctional rhythm).

The left ventricle has the shape of a conic cylinder that contracts by shortening both its long axis and its diameter (Fig. 45.3). As it connects the left atrium with the aortic root, it has to pump blood against a large pressure gradient. The left ventricle is the actual generator of blood pressure and is

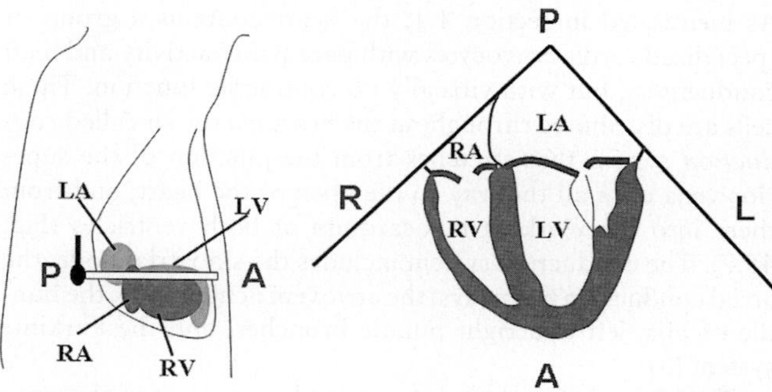

FIGURE 45.2. Four-chamber view of the heart by transesophageal echocardiography. The left drawing shows the orientation of the echo beam relative to the four heart chambers. The right drawing shows the four chambers in the echocardiographic image. LA, left atrium; RA, right atrium; LV, left ventricle; RV, right ventricle; A, anterior; P, posterior; R, right; L, left.

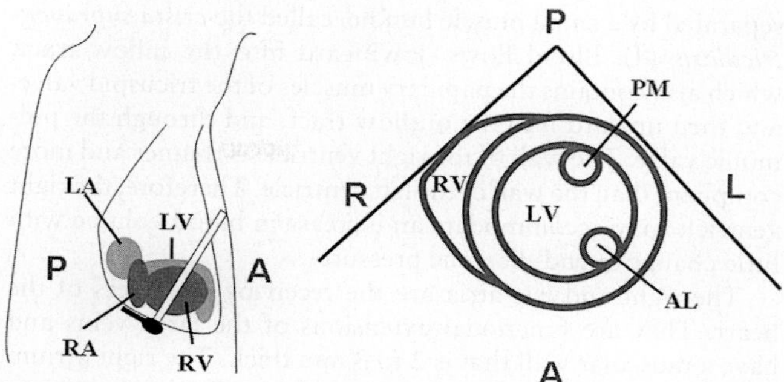

FIGURE 45.3. Transgastric view of the left ventricle. The left drawing shows the orientation of the echo beam relative to the heart chambers. The right drawing shows the two ventricles in the echocardiographic image. LV, left ventricle; RV, right ventricle; AL, anterolateral papillary muscle; PM, posteromedial papillary muscle; A, anterior; P, posterior; R, right; L, left.

the main engine of blood flow. In extreme cases, such as in patients with Fontan correction of congenital defects, the entire circulation may be driven by a single left-type ventricle (2). The ventricular wall consists of three distinct layers of tissue: the endocardium, the myocardium, and the epicardium (3). The endocardium is endothelial tissue that lines the ventricular cavity. It covers the inside of the myocardium, including the beamlike projections of the myocardium in the ventricle called *trabeculae*. The myocardium is the middle layer that contains the contractile cardiac myocytes. The myocardium makes up most of the ventricular wall, which is about 1 cm thick. The outside of the myocardium is covered by epicardium. The space between epicardium and myocardium contains coronary blood vessels and some fat tissue.

The right ventricle has a more complex geometry than the left ventricle (Fig. 45.4). It consists of a trabeculated inflow tract and a nontrabeculated outflow tract, both of which are

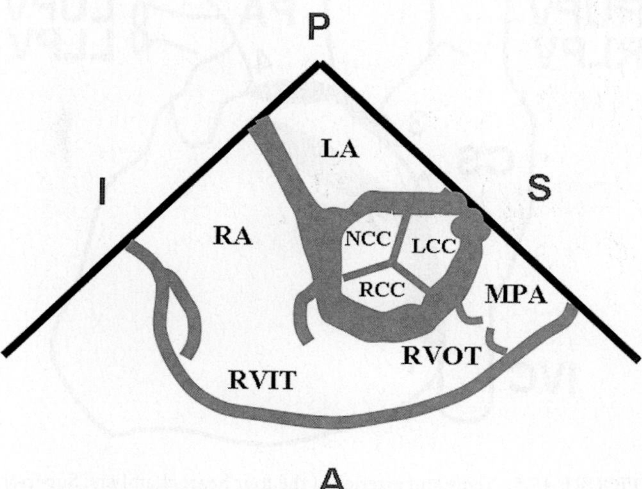

FIGURE 45.4. Echocardiographic view of the right ventricle. It is divided into a right ventricular inflow tract (RVIT) and a right ventricular outflow tract (RVOT). In this view, the right ventricle wraps around the aortic valve, of which all three cusps are seen in cross section. LCC, left coronary cusp; RCC, right coronary cusp; NCC, noncoronary cusp; LA, left atrium; RA, right atrium; MPA, main pulmonary artery; A, anterior; P, posterior; I, inferior; S, superior.

separated by a small muscle bundle, called the *crista supraventricularis* (4). Blood flows downward into the inflow tract, which also contains the papillary muscles of the tricuspid valve, and then upward into the outflow tract, and through the pulmonic valve. The wall of the right ventricle is thinner and more compliant than the wall of the left ventricle. Therefore, the right ventricle may accommodate an increase in blood volume with little change in end-diastolic pressure.

The right and left atria are the receiving chambers of the heart. They are functional extensions of the large veins and have a muscular wall that is 2 to 3 mm thick. The right atrium is located superior and medial to the right ventricle. It receives blood from the superior vena cava, the inferior vena cava, and the coronary sinus. The left atrium is located superior and posterior to the left ventricle. It receives blood from four pulmonary veins that enter the posterior wall of the left atrium in the left inferior, left superior, right inferior, and right superior position (Fig. 45.5). Atria have trabeculated auricular appendages of variable size. These appendages may become the site of blood clot formation.

The atrioventricular valves originate from connective tissue rings located at the atrioventricular junction. The valves are formed from endocardial tissue flaps that grow into the lumen of the junction. The free edges of the flaps are anchored to papillary muscles of the ventricular myocardium via chordae tendineae. The right-sided tricuspid valve has three flaps (anterior, posterior, and septal), whereas the left-sided mitral valve has only two (anterior and posterior). The semilunar valves are

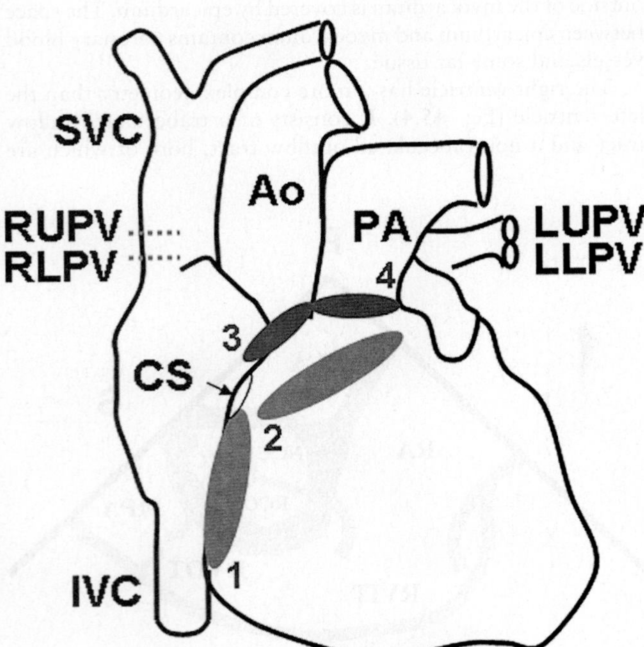

FIGURE 45.5. Veins and arteries of the four heart chambers. Superior vena cava (SVC), inferior vena cava (IVC), and coronary sinus (CS) empty into the right atrium. Left upper (LU), left lower (LL), right upper (RU), and right lower (RL) pulmonary veins (PVs) empty into the left atrium. The aorta (Ao) receives blood from the left ventricle and the pulmonary artery (PA) receives blood from the right ventricle. The positions of the four heart valves are shown in anteroposterior projection: 1, tricuspid valve; 2, mitral valve; 3, aortic valve; 4, pulmonic valve.

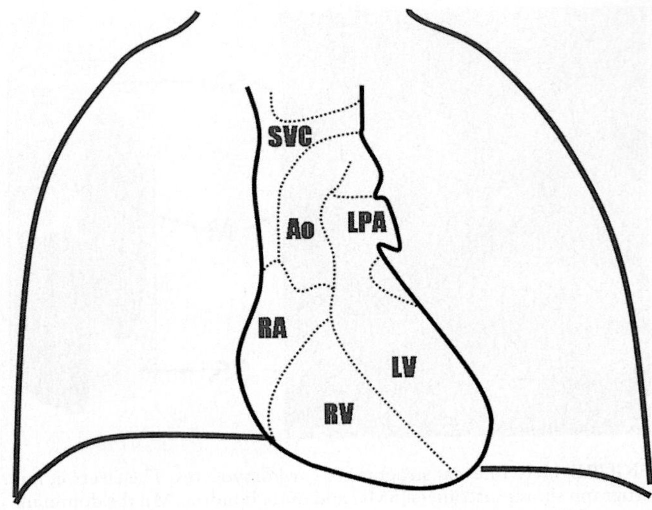

FIGURE 45.6. Anteroposterior projection of the cardiac silhouette on x-ray film of the chest. SVC, superior vena cava; RA, right atrium; Ao, aorta; LPA, left pulmonary artery; RV, right ventricle; LV, left ventricle.

derived from the same connective tissue ring as the atrioventricular valves. However, they have a smaller orifice and smaller, semi-lunar cusps that grow into the lumen of the main arteries. These cusps close the valvular orifice if there is sufficient back pressure from the arterial side. The three cusps of the pulmonic valve are positioned anterior, left, and right. The three cusps of the aortic valve are referred to as left coronary, right coronary, and noncoronary. The aortic valve is tilted about 40 degrees to the horizontal plane. The pulmonic valve is oriented near perpendicularly to the aortic valve.

Critically ill patients are routinely followed by serial radiographic studies of the chest. The anteroposterior projection of the cardiac silhouette on radiographs may yield specific information about the structures that contribute to the silhouette borders (Fig. 45.6). The right border of the silhouette is formed by the superior vena cava and the right atrium. The left border is formed by the aortic arch, the left pulmonary artery, and the left ventricle.

Pacemakers and Conduction System

As mentioned in section 1.1, the heart contains a group of specialized cardiac myocytes with pacemaker activity and high conductivity, but with virtually no contractile function. These cells are distributed throughout the heart *via* the so-called *conduction system* that stretches from the junction of the superior vena cava all the way to the apex of the heart, and from there into the working myocardium of both ventricles (Fig. 45.7). The conduction system includes the sinoatrial node, the atrial conduction pathways, the atrioventricular node, the bundle of His, left and right bundle brunches, and the Purkinje system (3).

The sinoatrial node is located at the junction of the right atrium and the superior vena cava. The node is 4 × 20 mm in size, and contains a collection of specialized cardiac myocytes with very dependable automaticity. The ability of these cells to depolarize spontaneously in short constant time intervals makes them the physiologic pacemaker, silencing all other

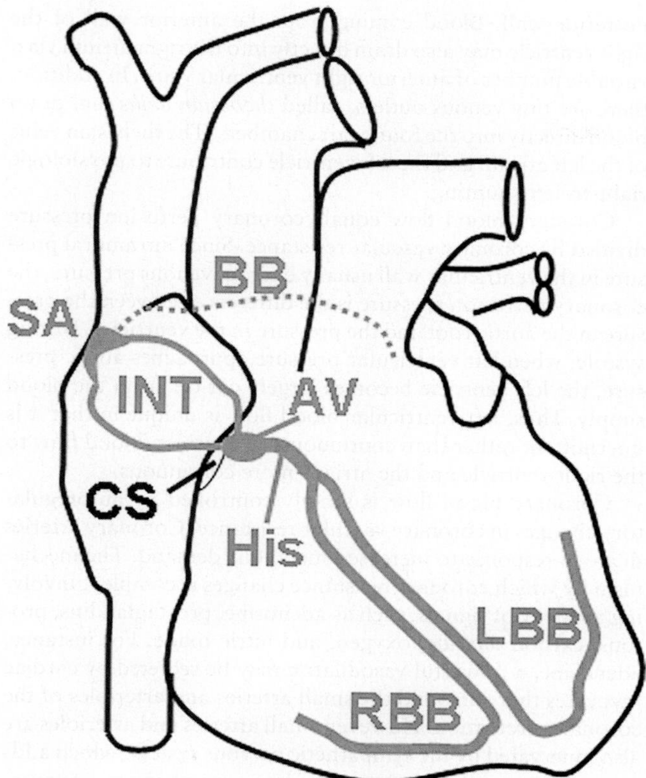

FIGURE 45.7. Major pathways of the cardiac conduction system. SA, sinoatrial node; INT, internodal tracts; BB, Bachmann bundle (connection between left and right atria); AV, atrioventricular node; His, bundle of His; RBB, right bundle branch; LBB, left bundle branch; CS, coronary sinus.

potential centers of automaticity in the heart. The rate of depolarization of the sinoatrial node is under control of the autonomic nervous system (see section 2). Parasympathetic impulses from the vagus nerve (cranial nerve X) decrease the rate of depolarization, whereas sympathetic impulses from accelerator fibers (originating from ventral roots T1-T4) increase the rate of depolarization.

Because of its anatomic location, the sinoatrial node directly depolarizes the right atrium. In addition, the sinoatrial activity is conducted to the left atrium via the Bachmann bundle. Additionally, internodal conduction pathways exist to facilitate the transmission of electrical impulses from the sinoatrial node to the atrioventricular node. The atrioventricular node is only 2 × 4 mm in size. It is located near the ostium of the coronary sinus on the right side of the central fibrous body that provides the scaffold of the four heart valves at the atrioventricular junction. The atrioventricular node is the main conduction pathway that links atrial and ventricular depolarization. However, additional strands of conducting muscle tissue are sometimes present in normal human hearts and may become functionally active under pathologic conditions (e.g., pre-excitation syndromes). Like the sinoatrial node, the atrioventricular node has the ability to depolarize spontaneously, but its activity is normally suppressed by the sinoatrial node because the latter fires at a much higher rate. Nevertheless, the atrioventricular node may become the dominant pacemaker in patients with sinus node dysfunction (junctional heart rhythm).

The atrioventricular node transmits the depolarization wave to the bundle of His, a 20-mm-long array of fibers that extends from the node posteriorly and inferiorly into the interventricular septum. The conduction of impulses through the atrioventricular node is delayed in order to allow enough time between atrial and ventricular systole. This delay also limits the number of impulses that can be transmitted to the ventricles, so that patients with atrial fibrillation do not develop life-threatening ventricular fibrillation. The bundle of His penetrates the central fibrous body between the tricuspid, mitral, and aortic valves. It divides at the top of the interventricular septum into the right and left bundle branches. The bundle branches travel downward in the interventricular septum toward the papillary muscles. They connect to the Purkinje system, which activates the ventricular myocardium.

Coronary Perfusion

Blood is supplied to the heart through the right and left main coronary arteries, which arise from ostia located near the top of the sinus of Valsalva (Fig. 45.8). The left coronary artery divides after a 2- to 10-mm course into the left anterior descending artery and the circumflex artery. The left anterior descending artery gives off two diagonal branches, and supplies primarily the left ventricle and the interventricular septum as well as a small portion of the anterior wall of the right ventricle next to the septum (Table 45.1). The circumflex artery travels posteriorly around the heart and supplies the left atrium and the left ventricle. In 10% to 15% of patients, the circumflex artery continues as the posterior descending artery (left dominant

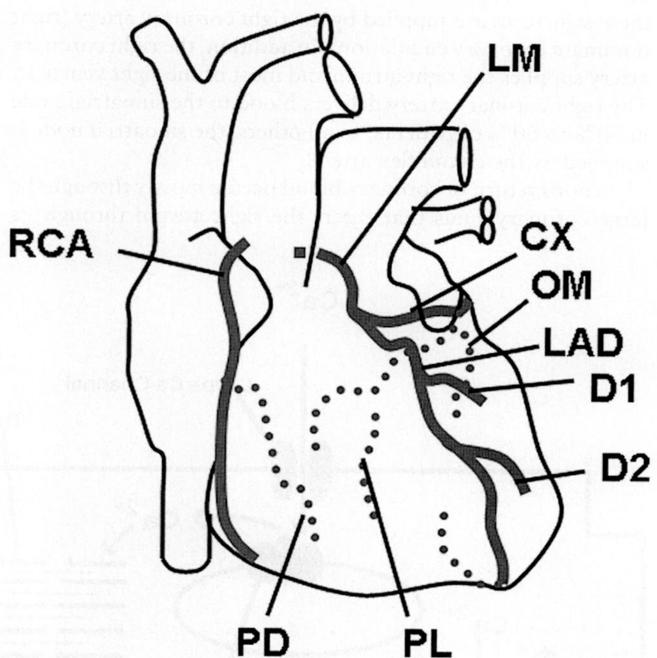

FIGURE 45.8. Coronary arteries. *Dotted lines* are on the posterior aspect of the heart. LM, left main coronary artery; CX, circumflex artery; OM, obtuse marginal artery; LAD, left anterior descending artery; D1, first diagonal artery; D2, second diagonal artery; PL, posterolateral artery; RCA, right coronary artery; PD, posterior descending artery.

TABLE 45.1

CORONARY BLOOD SUPPLY

Artery	Supplied structure
LAD	LV (anterior, lateral, and apical walls; anterolateral papillary muscle) RV (portion of anterior wall) IVS (anterior two thirds, most of bundle branches)
CX	LA LV (lateral, posterior, and inferior[a] walls; anterolateral and posteromedial[a] papillary muscles) IVS[a] (posterior third, proximal bundle branches) SA node[a] AV node[a]
RCA	RA RV LV[a] (inferior wall, posteromedial papillary muscle) IVS[a] (posterior third, proximal bundle branches) SA node[a] AV node[a]

[a]Variable blood supply coming either from RCA or from CX.
LAD, left anterior descending artery; CX, circumflex artery; RCA, right coronary artery; LV, left ventricle; RV, right ventricle; IVS, interventricular septum; LA, left atrium; SA, sinoatrial; AV, atrioventricular; RA, right atrium; RV, right ventricle.

coronary circulation). In these cases, the circumflex artery is the main blood supply to the inferior wall of the left ventricle, the posterior third of the interventricular septum, and the atrioventricular node. However, in 85% to 90% of patients, these structures are supplied by the right coronary artery (right dominant coronary circulation). In addition, the right coronary artery supplies the right atrium and most of the right ventricle. The right coronary artery delivers blood to the sinoatrial node in 50% to 60% of patients. In all others, the sinoatrial node is supplied by the circumflex artery.

Venous return of coronary blood occurs mostly through the large coronary sinus that enters the right atrium through its posterior wall. Blood coming from the anterior wall of the right ventricle may also drain directly into the right atrium via a variable number of anterior right ventricular veins. In addition, there are tiny venous outlets, called *thebesian veins* that drain blood directly into the four heart chambers. The thebesian veins of the left atrium and the left ventricle contribute to physiologic right-to-left shunting.

Coronary blood flow equals coronary perfusion pressure divided by coronary vascular resistance. Since intramural pressure in the ventricular wall usually exceeds venous pressure, the coronary perfusion pressure is the difference between the pressure in the aortic root and the pressure in the ventricles. During systole, when left ventricular pressure approaches aortic pressure, the left ventricle becomes largely cut off from the blood supply. Thus, left ventricular blood flow is unique in that it is intermittent rather than continuous. In contrast, blood flow to the right ventricle and the atria is more continuous.

Coronary blood flow is strictly controlled by autoregulatory changes in coronary vascular resistance. Coronary arteries dilate in response to increased metabolic demand. The mechanism by which coronary resistance changes is complex, involving an array of signals, such as adenosine, prostaglandins, protons, carbon dioxide, oxygen, and nitric oxide. For instance, adenosine, a powerful vasodilator, may be secreted by cardiac myocytes that surround the small arteries and arterioles of the coronary circulation. However, small arteries and arterioles are also innervated by the sympathetic nervous system, which adds extrinsic control to the autoregulatory mechanisms. Sympathetic control may involve both constriction of blood vessels via α_1 receptors and dilation of blood vessels via β_2 receptors. Coronary constriction appears to be important in equalizing blood flow through the layers of the heart (1).

ELECTRICAL CYCLE OF THE HEART

The electrical cycle of the heart derives from the excitable nature of each cardiac myocyte. These are typical cells that have become specialized in two major ways: (a) to transmit electrical signals and (b) to transduce that electrical signal into a mechanical function, contraction (Fig. 45.9). We will first examine the excitable characteristics of the individual cardiac myocyte.

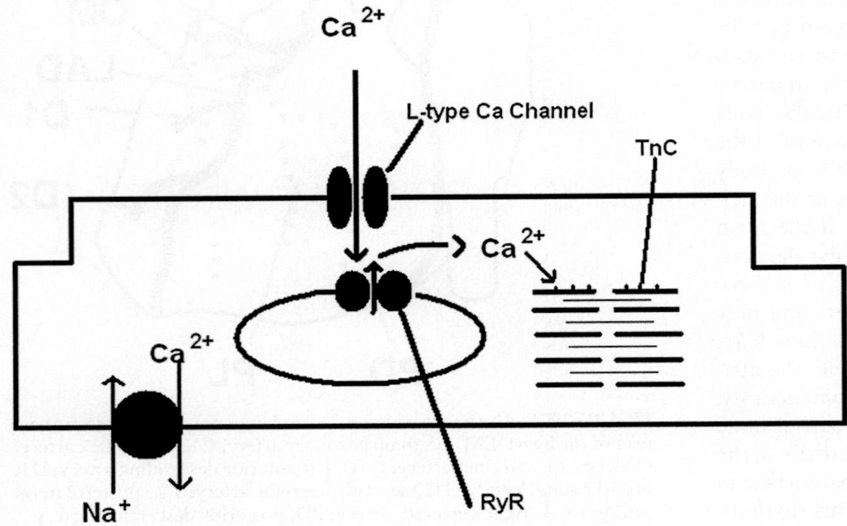

FIGURE 45.9. A schematic representing a cardiac myocyte demonstrating a few of the important Ca^{2+} regulatory sites. TnC represents troponin C and RyR represents the ryanodine receptor.

Resting Membrane Potential

As already discussed above, the cardiac myocyte is engulfed by a plasma membrane called the *sarcolemma*, which ensures the separation of the intracellular from the extracellular environment. The sarcolemma is a lipid bilayer with many voltage- and ligand-gated ion channels and other pumps, transporters, and receptors that allow the cell to fulfill its excitable function. The most significant elements of the sarcolemma that allow the electrical signals to be both generated and transmitted are the voltage-gated ion channels, the Na^+–Ca^{2+} exchanger and the Na^+-K^+-ATPase electrogenic pump. While every cell has a membrane potential, the factor that makes cardiac cells, and other excitable cells such as neurons, unique is the high density of voltage-gated ion channels. However, unlike other excitable cells, intercalated discs and their imbedded gap junctions allow the conduction of an electrical impulse between adjacent cardiac myocytes.

The cardiac myocyte has an electrical cycle that lasts from 500 to 800 msec, while the action potential (AP) is 300 msec or less (5). Therefore, there is a significant period of time when the cardiac myocyte is at "rest." At rest, the myocyte is relaxed and is maintained at its resting membrane potential, E_m. The resting membrane potential results from the open K^+ channels in the sarcolemma and the small "leak" of Na^+ through the sarcolemma. The resting membrane potential is described by the Nernst equation, which takes into account the permeability of the sarcolemma and its ion gradients. Since K^+ channels are the only open channels at rest, the resting membrane potential is strongly dependent on the intra- and extracellular K^+ gradient.

$$E_K = 61.54 \log_{10} ([K^+]_o / [K^+]_i$$

E_K is the potential due to the K^+ gradient, $[K^+]_o$ is the extracellular K^+ concentration, $[K^+]_i$ is the intracellular K^+ concentration, and 61.54 is a conversion factor (2.303 × RT/zF), which includes z, the valence of K^+; F, the Faraday constant; R, the gas constant; the body temperature in Kelvin; and 2.303, the factor to transform a natural log into a logarithm to the base 10. Depending on the values used for extra- and intracellular K^+, the resting membrane potential is calculated to be between –80 and –90 mV. Since the sarcolemma is not completely impermeable to all ions, ion gradients and the resulting membrane potential would ultimately dissipate if the Na^+-K^+-ATPase pump were not able to maintain the K^+ gradient. The Na^+-K^+-ATPase pump hydrolyzes adenosine triphosphate (ATP) to adenosine diphosphate (ADP) in order to eliminate three Na^+ from the cell for every two K^+ that are pumped into the cell until electrical and chemical energy is balanced, resulting in a resting membrane potential of approximately –85 mV for cardiac myocytes.

Action Potential

Within the sinoatrial (SA) node are pacemaker cells that contain few contractile elements, but have the important characteristics of *spontaneous diastolic depolarization*. The pacemaker cells undergo a gradual depolarization from their "resting" membrane potential of –65 mV to approximately –40 mV, which is the *threshold* at which an *action potential* is initiated.

The action potential is a regenerative all-or-none event that occurs when the membrane potential depolarizes to a level where a sufficient number of ion channels open, leading to an inward current that can begin a positive feedback loop (6). The predominant ion channels responsible for the action potential in the SA node pacemaker cells are T- and L-type Ca^{2+} channels. The T- and the L-type channels activate and inactivate ten times more slowly than Na^+ channels and provide the broader profile of the SA and AV nodal AP, as well as the long plateau, which is evident in the AP of both the atrial and ventricular cardiac myocyte (Fig. 45.10). The dependence on Ca^{2+} as the depolarizing current makes the SA and AV nodes particularly sensitive to pharmacologic manipulation with Ca^{2+} channel blockers.

The configuration of the SA node AP is markedly different from that in the atrial and ventricular cardiac myocytes, where voltage-gated Na^+ channels predominate and provide the major fast inward current responsible for depolarization. Figure 45.10 provides examples of the action potentials from the SA node through the atria and the AV node down the bundle of His

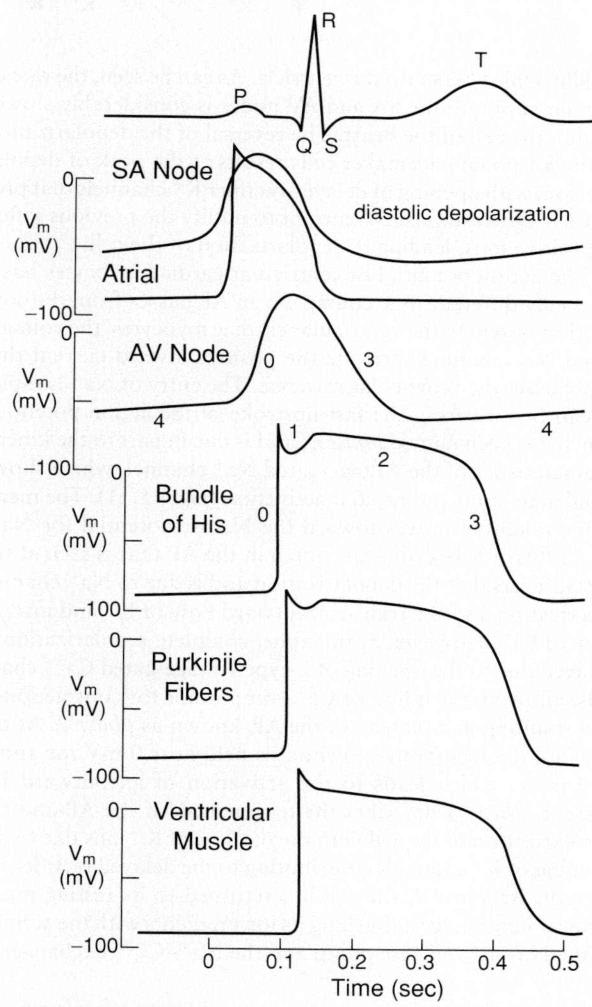

FIGURE 45.10. The surface electrocardiogram at the top of the figure and the action potential profiles throughout the heart and their temporal relationships to each other. SA, sinoatrial; AV, atrioventricular. (Reused with permission from Lynch C. Cellular electrophysiology of the heart. In: Lynch C, ed. *Clinical Cardiac Electrophysiology: Perioperative Considerations*. Philadelphia: JB Lippincott; 1994:1.)

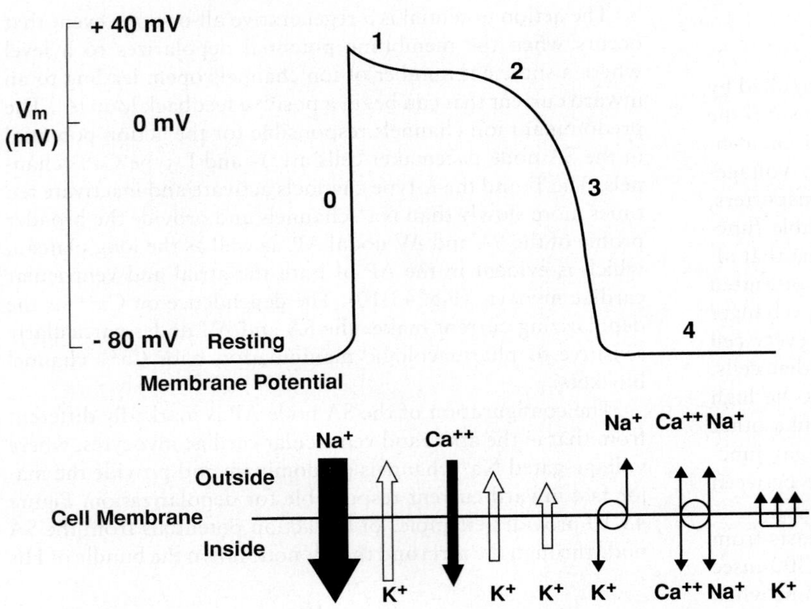

FIGURE 45.11. Proposed model of sarcoplasmic reticulum (SR) Ca^{2+} transport as a cardiac pacemaker. After a normal Ca^{2+} release, the SR Ca^{2+} uptake refills the SR with Ca^{2+} and triggers, via the ryanodine receptor, a local SR Ca^{2+} release, which triggers a Na^+–Ca^{2+} exchange current leading to the depolarization of the sinoatrial nodal cell. SL, sarcolemma. (Reused with permission from Bers DM. The beat goes on. *Circ Res.* 2006;99:921.)

and Purkinje fibers into the ventricle. As can be seen, the rate of depolarization in the SA and AV nodes is considerably slower than in the rest of the heart. The reversal of the depolarization of the SA nodal pacemaker cells results at the peak of depolarization, with opening of delayed rectifier K^+ channels that provide the outward positive current to nullify the previous influx of positive ions, leading to repolarization of the cell.

The action potential in ventricular cardiac myocytes has a markedly different time course. As an AP passes from the conduction system to the ventricular cardiac myocytes, the voltage-gated Na^+ channels provide the positive inward current that depolarizes the ventricular myocyte. The entry of Na^+ is rapid, as can be seen from the fast upstroke of the action potential, which has been named *phase 0*, and is due in part to the kinetic characteristics of the voltage-gated Na^+ channel, which shows rapid activation and rapid inactivation (Fig. 45.11). The membrane potential moves toward the Nernst potential for Na^+, $E_{Na}{}^+$. *Phase 1* describes the notch in the AP that is seen at the initial reversal of the depolarization and is due to Na^+ channel inactivation and the transient outward flow of K^+ and inward flow of Cl^-. However, at this time, complete repolarization is delayed due to the opening of L-type voltage-gated Ca^{2+} channels, allowing the influx of Ca^+—important for contraction—and resulting in a plateau of the AP, known as *phase 2*. At the plateau, the membrane potential is held near 0 mV for about 100 msec, which leads to the activation of an outward K^+ current. *Phase 3* describes the termination of the AP and the repolarization of the cell with the outflow of K^+ ions due to the opening of K^+ channels contributing to the delayed rectifier K^+ current. At *phase 4*, the cell has returned to its resting membrane potential, reestablishing its ion gradients with the activity of the Na^+-K^+-ATPase pump and the Na^+–Ca^{2+} exchanger.

Autonomic Control of the Cardiac Electrical Activity

The autonomic nervous system plays a major role in controlling the initiation of the heart beat and the rate of pacemaker firing. Both parasympathetic and sympathetic nervous inputs converge on the SA and AV nodal cells, exerting opposite influences on heart rate (7).

Parasympathetic

The parasympathetic nervous system contributes nerve fibers from its cranial outflow through the cervical ganglia where preganglionic fibers course down to the cardiac plexus, and from there send postganglionic unmyelinated axons that impinge on the SA and AV nodal cells. The cardiac plexus is divided into a superficial and deep plexus. The superficial plexus is found at the base of the heart at the arch of the aorta, while the deep plexus is found on the anterior aspect of the trachea near its bifurcation. The parasympathetic fibers carried by the vagus nerve are cholinergic and release acetylcholine (ACh) when activated. ACh has three principal actions that result in the slowing of heart rate and a decrease in contractility. ACh activates an outward K^+ current, which leads to hyperpolarization and reduction of the slope of the spontaneous diastolic depolarization of SA and AV nodal cells. In atrial cells, the duration of the AP is decreased, leading to a decrease in the atrial filling phase and a consequent decrease in contractility. A third mechanism of inhibition that occurs through ACh synaptic release and muscarinic activation is a decrease in I_{Ca} (the entry of calcium into atrial myocytes upon initiation of the action potential), which leads directly to a decrease in atrial contractility (7).

Sympathetic

Sympathetic nervous input to the heart derives from preganglionic neurons in the upper four or five thoracic spinal segments. Axons pass to postganglionic neurons in thoracic and cervical ganglia. The cervical ganglia supply the superior, middle, and inferior cardiac nerves to the cardiac plexus where they meet the thoracic cardiac nerves from the thoracic ganglia. Sympathetic nervous outflow then supplies the pacemaker cells in the SA and AV nodes, the conduction system, and both the atrial and ventricular myocytes. β-Adrenergic activation through the sympathetic input to the heart leads to cardiac acceleration and increased contractility. Norepinephrine is the major adrenergic synaptic mediator in the heart. The action of adrenergic stimulation is relatively simple: To increase the heart rate. The mechanism of this effect, however, is complex. β-Adrenergic stimulation leads to increased activation of I_f, the inward current that accelerates diastolic depolarization, so that a threshold is reached earlier in the AP, leading to earlier opening of L-type Ca^{2+} channels, since their threshold is reached sooner. The L-type Ca^{2+} channel is also activated by β-adrenergic stimulation. The channel is phosphorylated, which results in faster channel opening and more frequent channel openings. Depolarization is thus faster, leading to faster activation of I_K and repolarization. The net result is more frequent firing of the AP and a faster heart rate (7).

Recent work has focused on the primacy of Ca^{2+} in regulating the pacemaker function of the SA node (8,9). Bogdanov et al. (8) have proposed that the ryanodine receptor (RyR) in SA nodal cells is important in regulating the firing rate of the SA node. They have demonstrated that the interaction of the sarcoplasmic reticulum (SR) Ca^{2+} pump, intraluminal Ca^{2+}, the RyR receptor, and the Na^+–Ca^+ exchanger can work in concert toward diastolic depolarization and activation of a regenerative AP. Blocking of RyR Ca^{2+} release limits depolarization, while β-adrenergic stimulation activates the SR Ca^{2+} pump and RyR gating, resulting in more Ca^{2+} sparks and faster refiring of APs (Fig. 45.11). While this proposal is new, it certainly broadens the previous view of pacemaker generation and unifies aspects of pacemaker activity and arrhythmia generation.

If both parasympathetic and sympathetic inputs to the heart are totally blocked pharmacologically, the heart rate actually increases, as manifested by the overriding parasympathetic inhibition seen in most individuals (7).

CONTRACTION–RELAXATION CYCLE OF THE HEART

Initiating Events

The concerted and synchronous activity of the heart for the approximately 2.5 billion heart beats over a lifetime depends on tight physiologic control; that is, the spontaneous and rhythmic electrical activity of the pacemaker cells must be transformed into regular and synchronized contraction and relaxation. The atrial and ventricular myocytes are designed to provide this contractile function. Each cardiac myocyte transforms electrical activity into a synchronized contraction. The electrical signal is uniformly passed through gap junctions from cardiac myocyte to cardiac myocyte, producing the AP previously described. The unique characteristic of the AP essential for the initiation of the contractile process is the *plateau phase* (10). The plateau phase, as seen in Figure 45.12, is due to the prolonged opening of the L-type Ca^{2+} channel, which provides an inward positive current of Ca^{2+}, thus maintaining the depolarization for a prolonged period. The entry of Ca^{2+} through the L-type channel initiates the sequence of events leading to contraction.

Role of Calcium

As already explained in section 1, the ventricular myocyte has an extensive membranous system called the T tubules that allow the extracellular fluid to invaginate into the central recesses of the cell (Fig. 45.13). Depolarization that occurs with the action potential leads to the opening of L-type Ca^{2+} channels. The L-type channels are present in the T-tubular structure and are in close apposition to the calcium release channels, known as RyRs, which are located in the SR. Upon depolarization, Ca^{2+} (I_{Ca}) courses through the voltage-gated L-type Ca^{2+} channels into the cleft that separates the sarcolemma (T tubule) from the SR. The cleft is approximately 10 nm wide. This area of the SR is densely populated with RyRs. The Ca^{2+} that enters through the L-type channel diffuses through the cleft to activate RyRs, initiating the opening of the RyR and the release of large amounts of Ca^{2+} from the SR. Although it has yet to be measured, it is estimated that the concentration of Ca^{2+} reaches several millimolars and subsequently leads to the activation of the myofibrils. This process of depolarization, Ca^{2+} entry, and subsequent Ca^{2+} release has been termed *Ca^{2+} sparks*. These sparks cause the concerted activation of clusters of RyRs. Since the T tubules and the SR are spread throughout the myocyte (Fig. 45.13), the Ca^{2+} that is released floods the cell and interacts with the Ca^{2+}-sensitive protein in the myofibrils, troponin C.

The activation of contraction is similar in atrial and ventricular myocytes in that depolarization initiates the opening of Ca^{2+} channels and the entry of Ca^{2+}, but quite different in extent because of the differing architecture of the two types of myocytes (11) (Fig. 45.13). The major difference is that a T-tubular network does not exist in the atrial myocyte, resulting in a markedly different Ca^{2+} distribution during depolarization between the atrial and ventricular myocyte. In the ventricular myocyte, a T tubule occurs at every Z line and penetrates perpendicularly into the myocyte. In addition, the T tubule has extensive branching but always maintains its intimate relationship to the SR. Furthermore, the SR in the ventricular myocyte

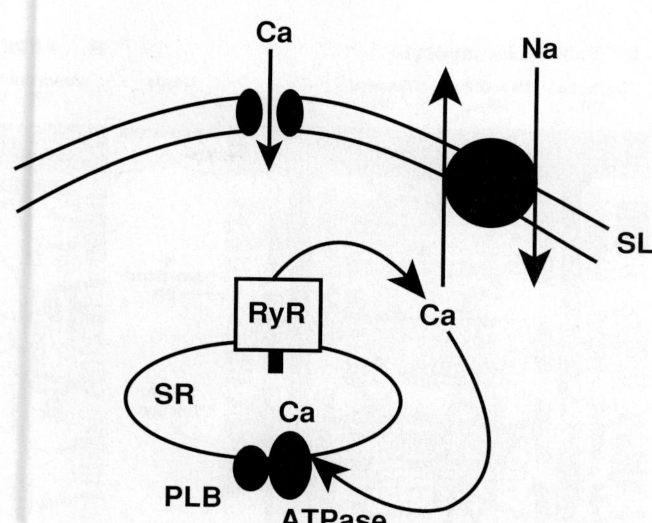

FIGURE 45.12. The ventricular cardiac myocyte action potential (AP). The numbers along the AP indicate the phases of the AP. The lower panel schematically represents the relative quantity and temporal relationship of the ionic movements involved in the AP. SL, sarcolemma; RyR, ryanodine receptor; SR, sarcoplasmic reticulum; PLB, phospholamban. (Reused with permission from Barber MJ. Class I antiarrhythmic agents. In: Lynch C, ed. *Clinical Cardiac Electrophysiology: Perioperative Considerations*. Philadelphia: JB Lippincott; 1994:85.)

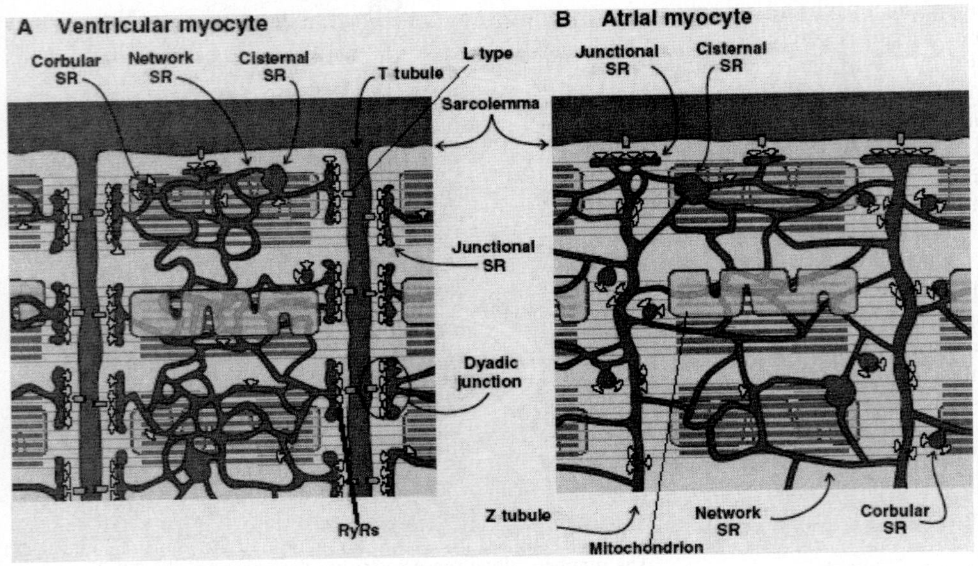

FIGURE 45.13. Comparison of the ventricular and atrial sarcoplasmic reticulum (SR). Note the T-tubular structure in the ventricular myocyte and the marked absence of T tubules in the atrial myocyte. (Reused with permission from Bootman M, Higazi DR, Coombes S, et al. Calcium signaling during excitation-contraction coupling in mammalian atrial myocytes. *J Cell Sci.* 2006;119:3915.)

forms an intricate network that surrounds the myofibrils, while the SR in the atrial myocyte forms a much simpler and less elaborate network. Hence, in the ventricular myocyte, a depolarization results in Ca^{2+} entry and release throughout the cell. The Ca^{2+} profile within the ventricular myocyte is thus homogeneous due to the synchronous recruitment of Ca^{2+} sparks throughout the cell. The profile in the atrial myocytes is quite different due to the absence of a T-tubular system and the presence of a "Z-tubular" system. The Z tubule is an SR element rather than a sarcolemmal element. The Z tubules are tubular extensions of the SR that are perpendicular to the long axis of the cell and contain RyRs. There are two main RyR populations in the atrial myocyte: one population at the periphery and a second, more extensive population deeper in the atrial myocyte. A depolarization therefore results in a markedly different Ca^{2+} profile. One observes mainly a rise in Ca^{2+} around the periphery of the cell and not the homogeneous Ca^{2+} profile seen throughout the ventricular myocyte.

Depolarization initiates Ca^{2+} entry. Ca^{2+} entry initiates large amounts of Ca^{2+} release from the RyR to initiate contraction. Prior to discussing the elements of contraction, it is important to consider the process of Ca^{2+} sequestration that completes the excitation–contraction–relaxation process. The SR is an extensive network of tubules and cysts and contains multiple imbedded proteins, but the two most significant are the RyR and the Ca^{2+} pump, known as the *SERCA* (sarcoendoplasmic reticulum calcium pump). The SERCA is essential for re-establishing the low concentration of Ca^{2+} in the cytosol, allowing relaxation to occur. It achieves this by using energy from the hydrolysis of ATP to pump Ca^{2+} from the cytosol back into the SR. However, one must remember that excess Ca^{2+} from the extracellular space enters the myocyte upon depolarization, and therefore a second mechanism for Ca^{2+} removal must exist to re-establish the initial cytosolic Ca^{2+} concentration. The additional mechanism is the Na^+–Ca^{2+} exchanger, a sarcolemmal protein that exchanges three Na^+ ions for one Ca^{2+} ion. Recall that excess sodium is pumped out of the cell by the Na^+-K^+-ATPase pump.

The SERCA is a pump that is regulated by adrenergic stimulation. The SERCA increases its activity (i.e., its ability to utilize ATP to accumulate Ca^{2+} within the SR) when exposed to β-adrenergic stimulation (12). Activation of the SERCA occurs through a series of kinases, such as protein kinase C, protein kinase A, and calmodulin-dependent protein kinase, which phosphorylate a protein called phospholamban (PLB). PLB is bound to the SERCA in its unphosphorylated form and inhibits pump activity. β-Adrenergic stimulation of the heart has three major effects: (a) to enhance tension development, (b) to increase the rate of tension development, and (c) to increase the rate of relaxation. The increased rate of relaxation has been shown to be mainly related to the phosphorylation of PLB. PLB functions as a brake on the SERCA. In knockout mice deficient in PLB, heart rate, contractility, and the rate of relaxation are all markedly enhanced. The SERCA works at a higher frequency in the absence of PLB, resulting in a greater Ca^{2+} load in the SR, which translates into a positive inotropic effect since there is more Ca^{2+} available for release from the SR during depolarization. Mutations of PLB have recently been shown in humans to be associated with heart failure, and PLB and its phosphorylation are now considered important potential pharmacologic targets for the treatment of heart failure (13).

Ca^{2+} availability is tightly regulated in the myocardial cell because Ca^{2+} ions are the switch that finally initiates the contractile process. The final step in the Ca^{2+} cascade is the binding of the Ca^{2+} that floods the myoplasm to troponin C.

Molecular Interactions

Ca^{2+} triggers the contractile process by interacting with the Ca^{2+}-binding protein, troponin C, which is an integral part of the sarcomere. The sarcomere is the smallest contractile unit and is defined from Z line to Z line (Fig. 45.14). The myofibrillar structure is made up of interacting filaments, termed thick and thin filaments. The light area adjacent to the Z line consists of thin filaments, which are polymers of actin monomers that are anchored to the Z line. The A band consists of overlapping thick and thin filaments, and the H band in stretched muscle is due to thick filaments alone. The thick filament consists of myosin, a large protein made up of six subunits. Each

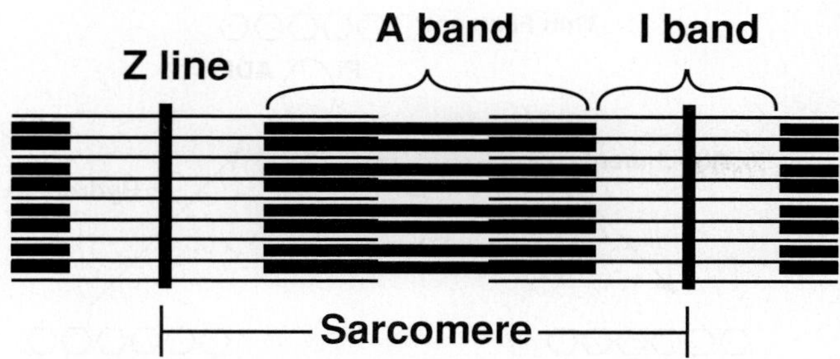

FIGURE 45.14. The sarcomere, the minimal unit of contraction in the cardiac myocyte. The A band demonstrates the overlap of thick and thin filaments. The I band represents the thin filaments anchored to the Z line.

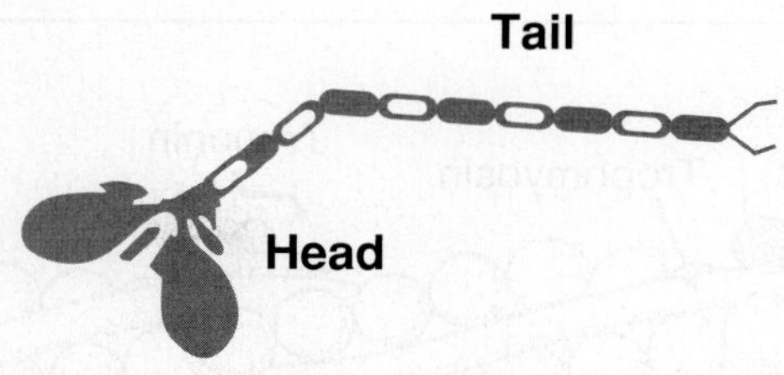

FIGURE 45.15. A schematic of the myosin molecule. A two-headed molecule with a flexible neck and an α-helical tail. The head contains a binding site for adenosine triphosphate. The head and neck have attached essential and regulatory light chains that are referred to in the text.

myosin molecule contains two heavy chains, each of 220 kDa; two essential light chains (MLC1) of about 17 kDa; and two regulatory light chains (MLC2), each more than 20 kDa. The myosin molecule has a unique structure (Fig. 45.15) consisting of a tail area of two long α-helical segments due to the intertwining of heavy chains, a hinge area, and two globular head segments. The heads have a site for actin binding, an ATP binding pocket, and enzymatic ATPase activity. The MLC1 chains are bound to the rodlike neck of the heavy chains, and are believed to mechanically stabilize the myosin heads during force generation. The MLC2 chains are involved in the beat-to-beat tuning of force development. Phosphorylation of MLC2 leads to increased force development and an increased rate of force development, but a slowing of the kinetics of relaxation (14). Beside the thin and thick filament made up of actin and myosin, respectively, a third filament exists, which has been identified and characterized over the last 35 years. That third filament consists of the titin molecule. Titin is a giant endosarcomeric protein that extends from Z line to Z line (15,16) (Fig. 45.16). It has elastic properties that convey passive force to the cardiac myocyte. If a myocyte is stretched beyond overlap of the thick and thin filaments, the restoring force to resting length is provided by titin. In the cardiac myocyte, two isoforms of titin exist (N2B and N2BA), which differ in their extensibility. The N2BA isoform endows the cell with greater compliance. In patients with diastolic dysfunction and diastolic heart failure, the less compliant isoform, N2B, dominates. On the other hand, in patients with systolic heart failure, the more compliant isoform of titin, N2BA, dominates (17). Besides conferring passive tension to the cell, titin also aligns T tubules and the SR within the sarcomere and localizes the myosin thick filaments to a central location within the sarcomere.

The thin filament consists of individual actin molecules of 43 kDa that combine to form long polymer chains in a double helical array. Interposed at regular spacing along the actin double helix are complexes of tropomyosin (Tm) and troponin (Tn) (Fig. 45.17). Tropomyosin is a linear molecule of approximately 70 kDa that lies in the groove of the actin double helix. Tn is found at the amino terminal end of the Tm molecule. Tn consists of a complex of three protein components: TnT, TnI, and TnC. Each of these components has a unique function essential for the orderly contractile process. **TnT** contains the binding site for tropomyosin and thus allows the Tn complex to be bound to Tm. **TnI** is an inhibitory subunit, blocking the interaction of actin with the myosin head and preventing force development. Finally, **TnC**, the molecular switch that activates contraction, has four Ca^{2+} binding sites, two of which are always occupied, even at a resting cytosolic Ca^{2+} concentration of 100 to 150 nM. The other two sites are of lower affinity and only bind Ca^{2+} when the concentration of Ca^{2+} is raised following release of Ca^{2+} from the RyR during the AP. Once the two low-affinity sites are filled with two Ca^{2+} ions, a conformational change occurs, resulting in a movement of the Tn complex and Tm and activation of the actin–myosin interaction (18).

Cardiac Contraction Cycle

At the molecular level, contraction and force generation occur because of the interaction of the myosin head with actin.

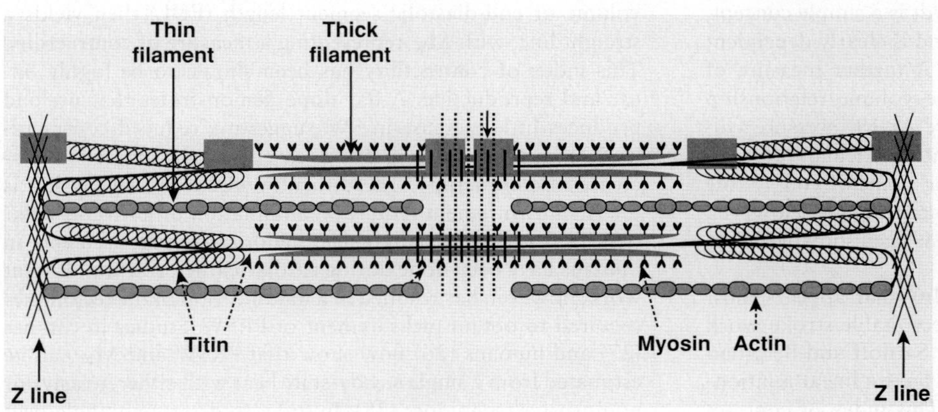

FIGURE 45.16. A representation of the sarcomere, demonstrating the essential role of the titin molecule in anchoring the thick filament to the Z line. (Reused with permission from Katz AM, Zile MR. New molecular mechanism in diastolic heart failure. *Circulation.* 2006;113:1922.)

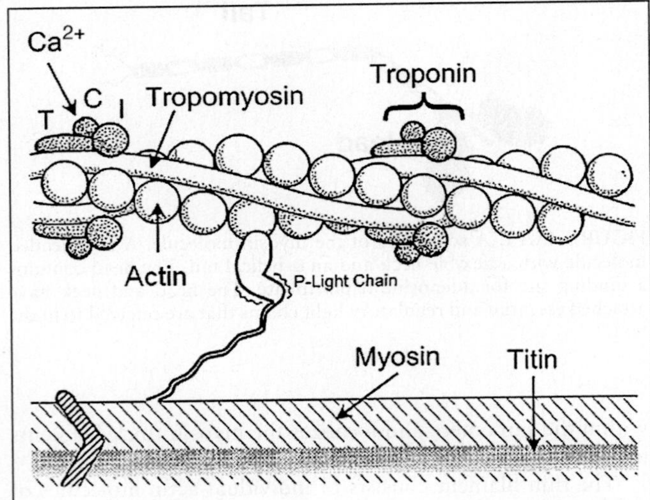

FIGURE 45.17. Schematic representation of protein interactions comprising the contractile apparatus in the cardiac myocyte. (Reused with permission from Ruegg JC. Cardiac contractility: how calcium activates the myofilaments. *Naturwissenschaften.* 1998;85:575.)

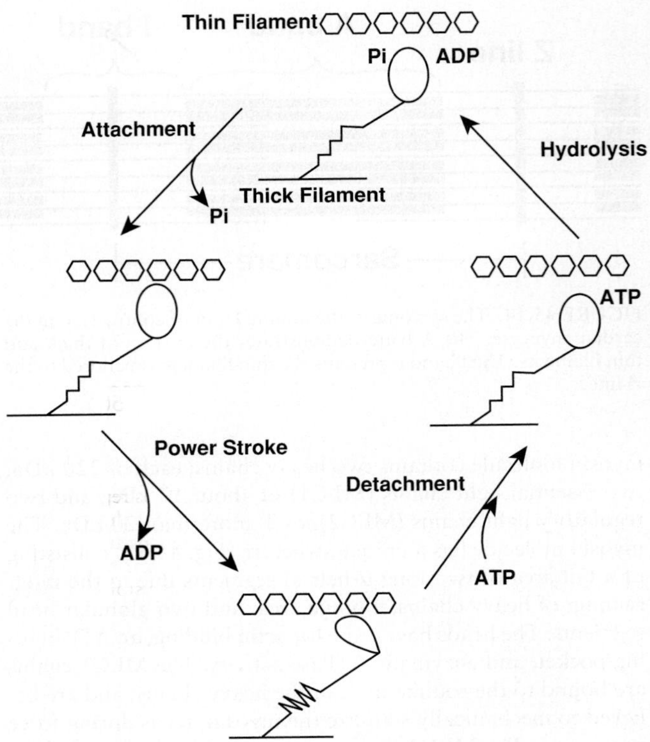

FIGURE 45.18. Schematic of the contractile cycle of the actin–myosin interaction. Energy for contraction is provided by adenosine triphosphate (ATP). The myosin head contains enzymatic ATPase activity. When ATP is hydrolyzed, a high-energy phosphate intermediate (P_i) is formed on the myosin head. The dissociation of P_i leads to attachment of actin to myosin, and adenosine diphosphate (ADP) dissociation is associated with the actin–myosin power stroke.

That interaction involves ATP binding and hydrolysis to form ADP, and the formation of a high-energy P_i intermediate at the myosin head (Fig. 45.18). Upon attachment of the head to actin, P_i is released, followed by release of ADP; the "power stroke" occurs wherein the myosin head changes conformation, pulling the thin filament toward the Z line. ATP then binds to a myosin head, leading to detachment of actin and myosin. ATP is hydrolyzed, forming the P_i intermediate and the ADP myosin complex, allowing reattachment to another site on the actin filament, since the relative position of myosin to actin has changed (19).

Two processes control contractility in the cardiac myocyte: (a) the length of the sarcomere and (b) the intrinsic contractility of the contractile elements. It was not until after 1950 that this latter phenomenon was first appreciated (20). The measurement of contractility *in vivo* has neither been easy nor satisfactory to accomplish. Several indices of contractility have been developed, but they usually require a great deal of technical expertise and invasive monitoring. Positive peak dP/dt, the time differential of ventricular pressure, has been employed as a simple index of contractile function. In order to appropriately measure it, a high fidelity micromanometer needs to be inserted into the left or right ventricle. While dP/dt is a simple concept, it is technically challenging to obtain, and is clearly dependent on preload, afterload, and heart rate. A further measure of contractility is the end-systolic pressure–volume relationship (ESPVR) (21). As can be seen in Figure 45.19, pressure volume loops may be generated at different ventricular volumes, and the slope of the line connecting the point of end systole on a family of loops gives a measure of contractility. However, even this measurement of contractility has been shown to yield inconsistent results (22).

Currently, the measure of contractility that appears most reliable and consistent is the preload recruitable stroke work (PRSW) relationship. First proposed by Sarnoff and Berglund in 1954 (23), PRSW has been proven to have a linear relationship to the end-diastolic volume (24). This index of contractility has survived two decades of investigation and appears to reliably measure contractility despite changes in preload and afterload. The PRSW is obtained from the integrals of a family of pressure–volume loops, the measure of stroke work (SW), at varying end-diastolic volumes (EDVs) (25) (Fig. 45.20). The relationship is quantified by the following equation:

$$SW = M_W \times (EDV - V_W)$$

where M_W is the slope and V_W is the volume axis intercept (26).

A plot of the stroke work as a function of end-diastolic volume or end-diastolic segment length (EDL) then yields a straight line, with M_W representing a measure of contractility. This index of contractility has been shown to be highly linear and reproducible. A flat slope demonstrates that preload produces little increase in SW, suggesting reduced contractility. On the other hand, an increase in slope suggests an increase in contractility. The difficulty with this relationship is that its measurement requires manipulation of left ventricular (LV) pressure and volume. The majority of measurements in humans have been done during cardiac catheterization. Recent work, however, has resulted in a modification of the techniques required to obtain measurement of PRSW. Studies in canines (27) and humans (26) now show that PRSW and M_W can be estimated from a single steady-state beat with either invasive or noninvasive techniques (28). In order to determine single-beat

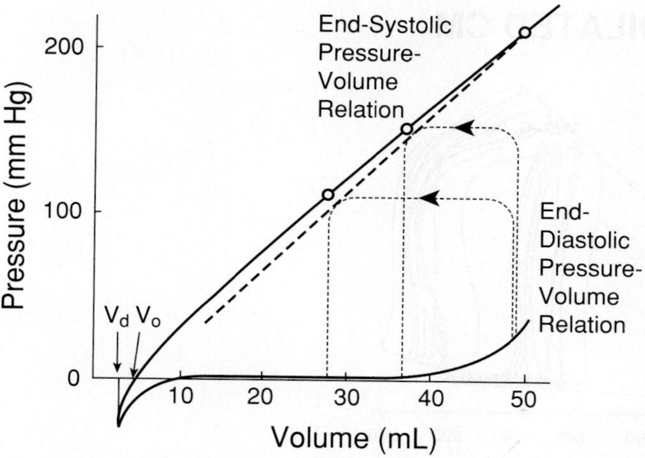

FIGURE 45.19. The pressure volume loops. The *y* axis represents the pressure in the left ventricle, while the *x* axis represents the volume in the ventricle. The line connecting pressure–volume loops at end systole is a straight line called the end-systolic pressure–volume relationship. (Reused with permission from Sagawa K. The end-systolic pressure-volume relation of the ventricle: definition, modification, and clinical use. *Circulation.* 1981;63:1223.)

PRSW, the following formula has been derived:

$$SB\,M_W = SW_B/[EDV_B - k \times EDV_B + (1 - k) \times LV_{Wall}$$

where SW_B is stroke work for a single beat, EDV_B is the end-diastolic volume, LV_{Wall} is the LV wall volume estimated from an echocardiographic LV mass determination, and k is a constant that varies little in healthy and diseased hearts. SW_B can be estimated noninvasively from Doppler-derived SV and an oscillometric blood pressure measurement.

The pressure–volume loop provides a graphic representation of the active and passive properties of the heart as a pump. The shape and position of the pressure–volume loop can be of great value in characterizing the clinical picture. As shown in Figures 45.21 and 45.22, a particular pathologic state can be identified by the pressure–volume loop (29). The pressure–volume loop for patients with dilated cardiomyopathy and restrictive cardiomyopathy are markedly shifted to the right, while in hypertrophic cardiomyopathy, they are shifted to the left compared to normal individuals. Acute coronary ischemia also markedly alters the pressure–volume loops. SW can be calculated from the integration of the loop and gives a good idea of the energy expenditure involved with each heart beat. Fortunately, noninvasive techniques are now available to assess ventricular function in a quantitative way.

BLOOD FLOW AND BLOOD PRESSURE

Basic Hemodynamic Model

The function of the cardiovascular system is to circulate blood, which is essential for the maintenance of the internal environment of the human body. Blood flows only if a pressure gradient exists. Although blood flow is the purpose of the circulation, it is blood pressure that is commonly used as a surrogate to determine its operational performance. Pressure and flow are related by Ohm's law:

$$Q = \Delta P/R$$

where Q is the flow (volume per time), ΔP is the pressure gradient, and R is the resistance to flow. Although this law, in a strict sense, only holds true for a rigid tube, it has been successfully applied to cardiovascular physiology. For instance, Ohm's law can be used to calculate the vascular resistance in patients in whom blood flow (by means of a balloon-tipped pulmonary artery catheter) and blood pressure (by means of an arterial catheter) are measured simultaneously. Such measurements have shown that the systemic vascular resistance is normally about ten times higher than the pulmonary vascular resistance (Table 45.2). In clinical practice, the systemic vascular resistance (SVR) is calculated from the cardiac output (Q), the mean arterial blood pressure (MAP), and the central venous pressure (CVP):

$$SVR = (MAP - CVP)/Q$$

Likewise, the pulmonary vascular resistance (PVR) is calculated from the cardiac output, the mean pulmonary artery

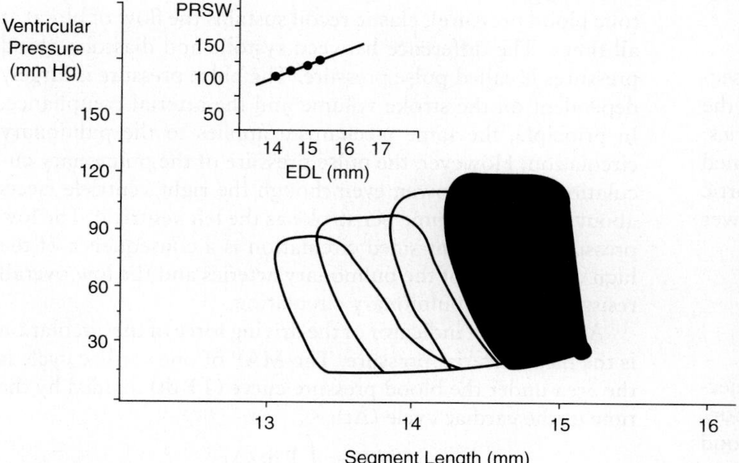

FIGURE 45.20. Pressure–segment length loop. In the inset, integrals of a family of pressure–segment length loops are plotted against end-diastolic segment length (EDL). The slope of this relationship, M_W, is a measure of contractility. (Adapted from Pagel PS, Kampine JP, Schmeling WT, et al. Comparison of end-systolic pressure-length relations and preload recruitable stroke work as indices of myocardial contractility in the conscious and anesthetized chronically instrumented dog. *Anesthesiology.* 1990;73:278.)

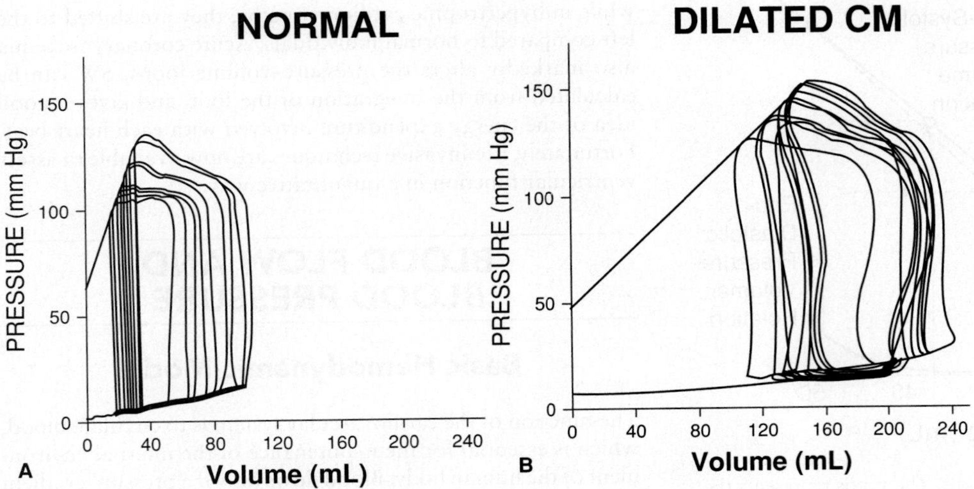

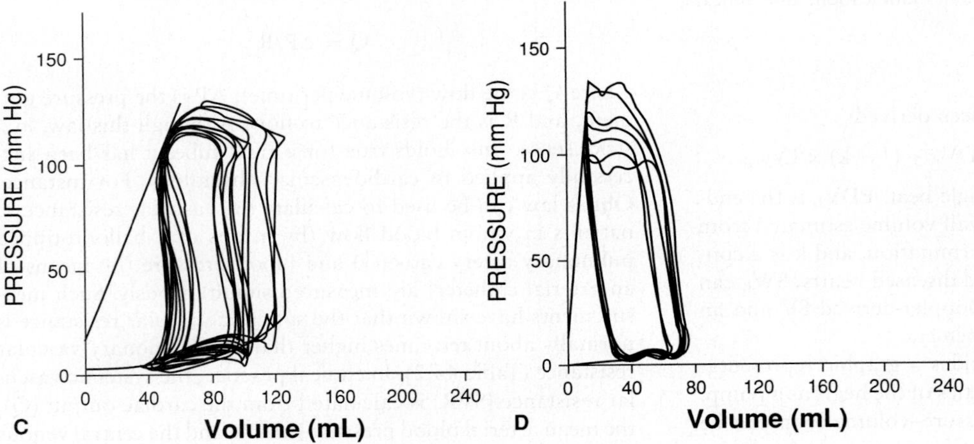

FIGURE 45.21. A comparison of pressure–volume loops of patients with distinct types of cardiomyopathy (CM) in comparison to a normal patient. (Reused with permission from Kass DA. Clinical ventricular pathophysiology: a pressure-volume view. In: Waltier D, ed. *Ventricular Function*. Baltimore: Williams & Wilkins; 1995:131.)

pressure (PAP_m), and the capillary wedge pressure (CWP). The latter is measured after balloon occlusion of a branch of the pulmonary artery and is normally in equilibrium with the pulmonary venous pressure:

$$PVR = (PAP_m - CWP)/Q$$

These values may be indexed to body surface area.

In a steady state, the blood flow is equal at any two cross sections in series along the circulation. Thus, the flow through the aorta equals the flow through all of the systemic capillaries. Although the aorta is the largest blood vessel, the combined cross-sectional area of the capillaries far exceeds the aortic cross section. As a result, the velocity of flow is much lower in the capillaries than in the aorta.

Generation of Blood Pressure

The pressure of the systemic circulation is produced by ejection of blood from the left ventricle. As a result of this ejection, blood is accelerated, and the elastic walls of the central blood vessels are slightly distended. The distension is crucial for normal circulatory function because it stores potential energy in vascular structures, resulting in a continuous flow of blood, even after the actual ejection period is completed. Although the pressure during the ejection period (systolic blood pressure) is higher than the pressure after the ejection period (diastolic blood pressure), elastic recoil sustains the flow of blood at all times. The difference between systolic and diastolic blood pressures is called pulse pressure. The pulse pressure is largely dependent on the stroke volume and the arterial compliance. In principle, the same mechanism applies to the pulmonary circulation. However, the pulse pressure of the pulmonary circulation is much lower, even though the right ventricle ejects about the same volume per stroke as the left ventricle. The low pressure in the right-sided circulation is a consequence of the high compliance of the pulmonary arteries and the low overall resistance of the pulmonary circulation.

An important indicator of the driving force of the circulation is the mean arterial pressure. The MAP of one cardiac cycle is the area under the blood pressure curve ($\int P\,dt$) divided by the time of the cardiac cycle (Δt):

$$MAP = \int P\,dt/\Delta t$$

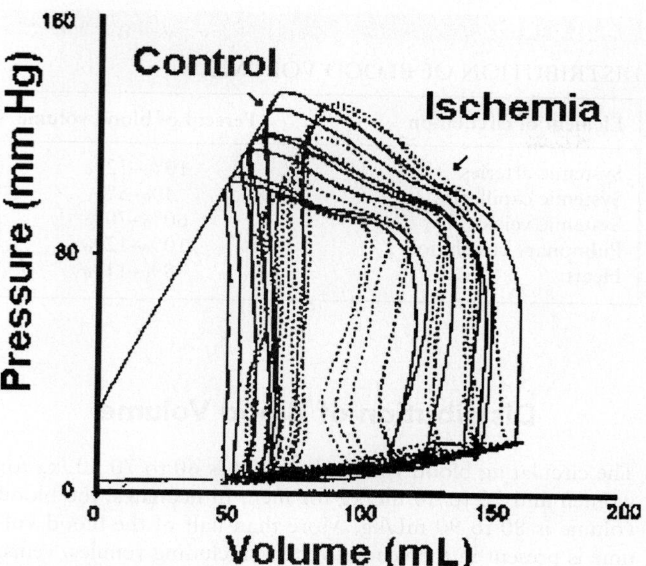

FIGURE 45.22. Pressure–volume loops from a patient prior to and during acute coronary occlusion. Note the marked shift to the right of the family of loops during the ischemic period. (Reused with permission from Kass DA. Clinical ventricular pathophysiology: a pressure-volume view. In: Warltier D, ed. *Ventricular Function.* Baltimore: Williams & Wilkins; 1995:131.)

Determination of MAP by this equation requires invasive monitoring of a continuous blood pressure trace. When blood pressure is measured by noninvasive techniques, MAP can be approximated from diastolic (DBP) and systolic (SBP) blood pressures by the following equation:

$$\text{MAP} = (2\text{DBP} + \text{SBP})/3$$

The mean arterial pressure changes very little between the aorta and the small arteries. However, in arterioles and capillaries, a large pressure gradient exists, which eventually dissipates the mean pressure to a value near zero (venous pressure). Despite the constant mean pressure in all small and large arteries, there are noticeable changes in systolic and diastolic blood pressure.

TABLE 45.2

HEMODYNAMIC VARIABLES

Variable	Normal value
Mean arterial pressure	70–105 mm Hg
Systolic blood pressure	90–140 mm Hg
Diastolic blood pressure	60–90 mm Hg
Central venous pressure	0–5 mm Hg
Mean pulmonary artery pressure	10–20 mm Hg
Systolic pulmonary pressure	15–25 mm Hg
Diastolic pulmonary pressure	5–10 mm Hg
Capillary wedge pressure	5–12 mm Hg
Cardiac index (CI)	2.5–3.5 L/min/m^2
Stroke volume index (CI/heart rate)	36–48 mL/m^2
Systemic vascular resistance index	1,200–1,500 dyne-sec cm^{-5}/m^2
Pulmonary vascular resistance index	80–240 dyne-sec cm^{-5}/m^2

The systolic blood pressure increases from proximal to distal arteries, whereas the diastolic blood pressure decreases in the same direction. This phenomenon (i.e., increase in pulse pressure from central to distal) is caused by reflections of the pulse wave in the vascular tree.

Vascular Resistance and Compliance

The resistance to blood flow is one of the most important physiologic variables, one that constantly changes in response to external and internal factors. The resistance (R) to laminar flow through a rigid tube can be expressed by Poiseuille's law, which states that:

$$R = 8\eta L/\pi r^4$$

where η is the viscosity, L is the length of the tube, and r is its radius (1). Thus, the resistance depends on both the composition of blood and the properties of blood vessels. Specifically, the viscosity increases with hematocrit and with the plasma protein concentration (Fig. 45.23), whereas the radius of blood vessels is under tight control of the autonomic nervous system (see below). Poiseuille's law gives only an approximation of the true hemodynamic resistance because the human circulation deviates in many ways from the conditions under which the law applies. Blood vessels are not rigid, but they form branching and tapering elastic tubes; blood flow is not steady but pulsatile, and it is not necessarily laminar, but has turbulent flow components at certain locations.

Among the three independent variables of Poiseuille's law, it is the radius of blood vessels that undergoes the most significant changes. Total vessel radius, adjusted by a fine balance between vasodilation and vasoconstriction, is the main

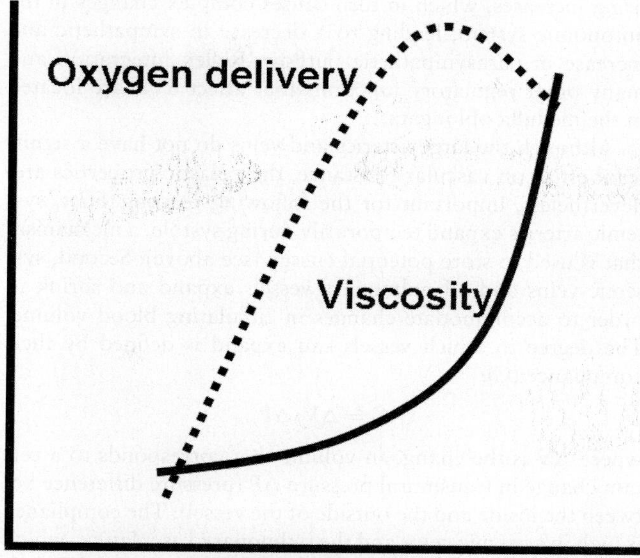

FIGURE 45.23. Effect of hematocrit on blood viscosity and oxygen delivery. Abnormally high hematocrits produce a sharp increase in viscosity, which raises vascular resistance to a point that oxygen delivery decreases. The decrease in oxygen delivery results from a decrease in cardiac output, which more than offsets the increase in oxygen-carrying capacity.

regulator of vascular resistance. SVR is the net result of the resistance offered by many vessels arranged both in series and in parallel. In analogy to electrical circuits, resistances in series are summed as (1):

$$SVR = R_{arteries} + R_{arterioles} + R_{capillaries} + R_{venules} + R_{veins}$$

In contrast, resistances in parallel are related to total SVR by the following equation (1):

$$1/SVR = 1/R_{coronary} + 1/R_{cerebral} + 1/R_{muscle} + 1/R_{splanchnic} + 1/R_{renal} + 1/R_{skin} + \cdots$$

Individual components of the systemic circulation make very different contributions to total SVR. In particular, it holds that:

$$R_{arterioles} + R_{capillaries} >> R_{arteries} + R_{venules} + R_{veins}$$

Arterioles in particular are the main targets of the various regulatory mechanisms that lead to vasodilation or vasoconstriction. Since the resistances of the coronary, cerebral, and renal circulations are primarily controlled by local demand, the main factor that regulates total SVR is the net radius of arterioles in muscles, skin, and the gut. This net radius is under hormonal and autonomic nervous control and it can be affected by a number of drugs.

Hormones that are powerful vasoconstrictors include epinephrine, norepinephrine, angiotensin II, and arginine vasopressin (1). Nitric oxide is a vasodilator, with a very short half-life and an action that is mainly local. The autonomic nervous system exerts control over the SVR by an array of sympathetic fibers that innervate arterioles and capillaries at multiple sites, which is why sympathetic tone has such a profound effect on blood pressure. All these mechanisms act in concert and are linked by reflex pathways, such as the baroreceptor reflex. The baroreceptor reflex responds to mechanoreceptors located in the aorta, carotid sinuses, atria, ventricles, and pulmonary vessels. When the wall of these structures is stretched, receptor firing increases, which in turn causes complex changes in the autonomic system, leading to a decrease in sympathetic and increase in parasympathetic outflow. Reflex integration and many other regulatory functions that affect SVR are located in the medulla oblongata.

Although the large arteries and veins do not have a significant effect on vascular resistance, their elastic properties are, nevertheless, important for the following reasons. First, systemic arteries expand temporarily during systole, a mechanism that is used to store potential energy (see above). Second, systemic veins and all pulmonary vessels expand and shrink in order to accommodate changes in circulating blood volume. The degree to which vessels can expand is defined by their compliance (C):

$$C = \Delta V/\Delta P$$

where ΔV is the change in volume that corresponds to a certain change in transmural pressure ΔP (pressure difference between the inside and the outside of the vessel). The compliance is high in systemic veins and the pulmonary vasculature, which is why changes in blood volume will primarily affect the volume of these structures. In contrast, the compliance is low in the systemic arteries; as a result, their total volume is relatively stable, and they distend only minimally when the arterial pressure rises during systole. Compliance is inversely related to resistance.

TABLE 45.3

DISTRIBUTION OF BLOOD VOLUME

Element of circulation	Percent of blood volume
Systemic arteries	10%–12%
Systemic capillaries	4%–5%
Systemic veins	60%–70%
Pulmonary circulation	10%–12%
Heart	8%–11%

Distribution of Blood Volume

The circulating blood volume in adults is 60 to 70 mL/kg for women and 70 to 80 mL/kg for men. In neonates, the blood volume is 80 to 90 mL/kg. More than half of the blood volume is present in the venous system, including venules, veins, and the cava (Table 45.3). As discussed above, the compliance of veins is about 20 times higher than that of systemic arteries. Thus, small changes in venous pressure are associated with large changes in venous volume, and the venous system serves as a reservoir to accommodate shifts in total blood volume.

Stroke volume and cardiac output are highly sensitive to the degree of filling of the cardiac ventricles. Cardiac filling in turn depends on the central blood volume, which is defined as intrathoracic blood present in the heart, cava, pulmonary circulation, and intrathoracic arteries. The distribution of blood between the central (intrathoracic) compartment and the peripheral (extrathoracic) compartment can change with body position and with sympathetic tone. Redistribution of blood occurs mainly between compliant structures, such as the heart, the veins, and the pulmonary vasculature. The variable portion of the peripheral blood volume is located in the veins of the extremities and the abdominal cavity. In contrast, the blood volume in systemic arteries changes very little because of their low compliance. Changes in central venous pressure can be used as an indicator of changes in central blood volume. Although this technique is widely employed in the practice of critical care, it is not very sensitive, and it is only accurate if a number of preconditions apply, such as normal cardiac function, normal intrathoracic pressures, and accurate positioning of the pressure transducer.

Just like the vascular resistance, blood volume and blood distribution are under endocrine and autonomic nervous control. Angiotensin II and aldosterone decrease renal excretion of sodium, which leads to an increase in total plasma volume. Atrial natriuretic peptide is released into the bloodstream when atria are stretched, causing increased renal sodium excretion, which therefore leads to a decrease in plasma volume. Erythropoietin is a hormone released by the kidneys that causes bone marrow to increase the production of red blood cells, which also increases total blood volume. The distribution of blood volume is sensitive to the sympathetic tone. High sympathetic outflow causes venoconstriction in addition to the constriction of arterioles. The main effect of venoconstriction is an increase of the central blood volume at the expense of the peripheral blood volume.

References

1. Rhoades RA, Tanner GA, eds. *Medical Physiology.* 2nd ed. Philadelphia: Lippincott Williams & Wilkins; 2003.
2. Davies LK, Knauf DG. Anesthetic management for patients with congenital heart disease. In: Hensley FA, Martin DE, Gravlee GP, eds. *Cardiac Anesthesia.* 3rd ed. Philadelphia: Lippincott Williams & Wilkins; 2003.
3. Thibodeau GA, Patton KT. *Anatomy and Physiology.* 6th ed. St. Louis: Mosby Elsevier; 2007.
4. Sidebotham D, Merry A, Legget M, eds. *Practical Perioperative Transesophageal Echocardiography.* Edinburgh, Scotland: Butterworth Heinemann; 2003.
5. Lynch C. Cellular electrophysiology of the heart. In: Lynch C, ed. *Clinical Cardiac Electrophysiology: Perioperative Considerations.* Philadelphia: JB Lippincott; 1994:1.
6. Study R. The structure and function of neurons. In: Hemmings H, Hopkins P, eds. *Foundations of Anesthesia Basic and Clinical Sciences.* London: Mosby; 2000:179.
7. Opie LH. *The Heart Physiology from Cell to Circulation.* 3rd ed. Philadelphia: Lippincott-Raven; 1998.
8. Bogdanov KY, Maltsev VA, Vinogradova TM, et al. Membrane potential fluctuations resulting from submembrane Ca^{2+} releases in rabbit sinoatrial nodal cells impart an exponential phase to the late diastolic depolarization that controls their chronotropic state. *Circ Res.* 2006;99:979.
9. Bers DM. The beat goes on. *Circ Res.* 2006;99:921.
10. Barber MJ. Class I antiarrhythmic agents. In: Lynch C, ed. *Clinical Cardiac Electrophysiology: Perioperative Considerations.* Philadelphia: JB Lippincott; 1994:85.
11. Bootman M, Higazi DR, Coombes S, et al. Calcium signaling during excitation-contraction coupling in mammalian atrial myocytes. *J Cell Sci.* 2006;119:3915.
12. Tada M, Kirchberger M, Repke DI, et al. The stimulation of calcium transport in cardiac sarcoplasmic reticulum by adenosine 3 prime:5 prime–monophosphate-dependent protein kinase. *J Biol Chem.* 1974;249:6174.
13. Koss KL, Kranias EG. Phospholamban: a prominent regulator of myocardial contractility. *Circ Res.* 1996;79:1059.
14. Moss RL, Fitzsimons DP. Myosin light chain 2 into the mainstream of cardiac development and contractility. *Circ Res.* 2006;99:225.
15. Granzier H, Wu Y, Siegfried L, et al. Titin: physiological function and role in cardiomyopathy and failure. *Heart Failure Rev.* 2005;10:211.
16. Katz AM, Zile MR. New molecular mechanism in diastolic heart failure. *Circulation.* 2006;113:1922.
17. van Heerebeck L, Borbely A, Niessen WM, et al. Myocardial structure and function differ in systolic and diastolic heart failure. *Circulation.* 2006;113:1966.
18. Ruegg JC. Cardiac contractility: how calcium activates the myofilaments. *Naturwissenschaften.* 1998;85:575.
19. Blanck TJJ, Lee DL. Cardiac physiology. In: Miller RD, ed. *Anesthesia.* Vol. 1. Philadelphia: Churchill Livingstone; 2000:619.
20. Katz AM, Lorell BH. Regulation of cardiac contraction and relaxation. *Circulation.* 2000;102(S IV):69.
21. Sagawa K. The end-systolic pressure-volume relation of the ventricle: definition, modification, and clinical use. *Circulation.* 1981;63:1223.
22. Blanck TJJ, Lee DL. Cardiac physiology. In: Miller RD, ed. *Anesthesia.* Vol. 1. Philadelphia: Churchill Livingstone; 2000:619.
23. Sarnoff SJ, Berglund EI. Starling's law of the heart studied by means of simultaneous right and left ventricular function curves in the dog. *Circulation.* 1954;9(5):706–718.
24. Glower DD, Spratt JA, Snow ND, et al. Linearity of the Frank-Starling relationship in the intact heart: the concept of pre-load recruitable stroke work. *Circulation.* 1985;71:994.
25. Pagel PS, Kampine JP, Schmeling WT, et al. Comparison of end-systolic pressure-length relations and preload recruitable stroke work as indices of myocardial contractility in the conscious and anesthetized chronically instrumented dog. *Anesthesiology.* 1990;73:278.
26. Lee W, Huang W, Yu W, et al. Estimation of preload recruitable stroke work relationship by a single-beat technique in humans. *Am J Physiol.* 2003;284:744.
27. Karunanithi MK, Feneley MP. Single-beat determination of preload recruitable stroke work relationship: derivation and evaluation in conscious dogs. *J Am Coll Cardiol.* 2000;35:502.
28. Baicu CF, Zile MR, Aurigemma GP, et al. Left ventricular systolic performance, function, and contractility in patients with diastolic heart failure. *Circulation.* 2005;111:2306.
29. Kass DA. Clinical ventricular pathophysiology: a pressure-volume view. In: Warltier D, ed. *Ventricular Function.* Baltimore: Williams & Wilkins; 1995:131.

CHAPTER 46 ■ FUNDAMENTALS OF CARDIOPULMONARY RESUSCITATION

IKRAM U. HAQUE • ANDREA GABRIELLI • ARNO L. ZARITSKY

Cardiopulmonary resuscitation (CPR) is described as a series of assessments and interventions performed during a variety of acute medical and surgical events where death is likely without immediate intervention. Among these events, sudden cardiac arrest (SCA) is a leading cause of death in the United States (1) and Canada (2) in adults. Cardiac arrest (CA) is defined as "cessation of cardiac mechanical activity as confirmed by the absence of signs of circulation." As its name implies, in the prehospital arena, adult SCA is most commonly due to ventricular fibrillation (VF) (3) secondary to ischemic heart disease; asystole and pulseless electrical activity (PEA) are less common initial rhythms with SCA, although these rhythms may represent the initial identified rhythm in adults who actually experienced an acute VF or ventricular tachycardia (VT) event. Although VF and VT are considered to be the most common out-of-hospital (OOH) arrest rhythms, only 20% to 38% of in-hospital arrest patients have VF or VT as their initial rhythm. In contrast, children and young adults require CPR most commonly for respiratory arrest, airway obstruction, or drug toxicity. VF/VT is identified as the initial rhythm in 5% to 15% of OOH arrests in children (4). Other conditions such as trauma, external or internal hemorrhage, and drowning may call for resuscitation at any age.

Regardless of the cause, immediate and effective CPR can save lives. In patients with witnessed VF CA, CPR doubles (3) or triples (5) the rate of survival. Unfortunately, only ~27% of OOH arrest victims receive bystander CPR.

The primary goal of CPR is to generate sufficient oxygen delivery to the coronary and cerebral circulations in order to maintain cellular viability while attempting to restore a perfusing cardiac rhythm by defibrillation, pharmacologic intervention, or both.

IMMEDIATE CONCERNS

Effective CPR can be performed by following a few basic rules:

- Immediately assess the environment for danger and move the patient if necessary. Never assume that an environment is safe.
- Minimize the time from cardiac arrest recognition to starting effective CPR. For every minute without CPR during witnessed VF CA, survival decreased by 7% to 10% in contrast to a decrease in survival by 3% to 4% per minute when bystander CPR preceded attempted defibrillation (6).
- Defibrillate immediately if a defibrillator is rapidly available (<3–5 minutes) in patients with VF. This should be the primary treatment focus within the first few minutes of SCA due to ventricular fibrillation. For each minute delay in defibrillation, chances of eventual hospital discharge decreased by 8% to 10% (7). Note that if the time from arrest to emergency medical service (EMS) arrival and initiation of CPR is more than 5 minutes, provision of 2 minutes of CPR before attempted defibrillation was associated with improved outcome (8,9).
- "Push hard and fast" during chest compressions and minimize the duration of interruptions to reassess the patient's rhythm. It is recommended to interrupt chest compressions only briefly and about every 2 minutes to assess the rhythm and switch rescuer if feasible.
- While CPR is in progress, attempt to identify the cause of arrest. Although the steps of CPR are uniform, other resuscitation interventions may be indicated based on the cause of CA. If the patient fails to respond to standard CPR interventions, think about delayed recognition and recall the H's and T's (Table 46.1) to help identify a potentially correctable cause for ongoing cardiac arrest.
- Good teamwork increases the effectiveness of resuscitation when more than one rescuer is available.
- Attention to postresuscitation care is an important element of neurologic outcome. Focus on restoring and supporting adequate cardiac output and tissue perfusion, monitor and maintain normal blood glucose concentrations, treat the underlying cause of the arrest, maintain normothermia, and consider therapeutic hypothermia to maximize survival and cerebral recovery.
- If the patient fails to respond to effective CPR, appropriate judgment is needed in determining when to stop resuscitative efforts.

TABLE 46.1

POTENTIAL CORRECTABLE PROBLEMS DURING CARDIAC ARREST: "6 H'S AND 5 T'S"

Hypovolemia
Hypoxia
Hydrogen ion (acidosis)
Hypo-/hyperkalemia
Hypoglycemia
Hypothermia
Toxins
Tamponade, cardiac
Tension pneumothorax
Thrombosis, coronary or pulmonary
Trauma

Adapted from 2005 American Heart Association Guidelines for Cardiopulmonary Resuscitation and Emergency Cardiovascular Care. *Circulation.* 2005;112[24]SIV-1–IV-211.

Guidelines for CPR and advanced adult and pediatric advanced life support are published every 5 years by the American Heart Association (AHA) (10). These guidelines are based on an extensive evidence-based review by national and international experts leading to the publication of a consensus on science and treatment recommendations prepared by the International Liaison Committee on Resuscitation (ILCOR) (11,12). ILCOR is a collaborative organization of American, European, Australian, Canadian, South African, and Latin American resuscitation councils with the goal of identifying the best resuscitation evidence (13).

OUTCOME OF CARDIOPULMONARY RESUSCITATION

Measuring Outcome after Cardiac Arrest

Retrospective and prospective observational outcome reports have been published about the success rates of both in-hospital and out-of-hospital cardiac arrest, but most of these are single-center reports with relatively few subjects. More recently, cardiac arrest events and outcomes have been systematically monitored in large multicenter settings. To facilitate data comparison across communities, international guidelines were published for data collection using standard definitions of events and outcome for both adults and children (the Utstein Guidelines) (14–16). In 2000, the AHA established a National Registry of Cardiopulmonary Resuscitation (NRCPR) to systematically collect data on the epidemiology, processes of care, and outcome of in-hospital CPR (4,17). This comprehensive database has, at the time of this writing, an excess of 100,000 cardiac arrest events and provides important insights into the mechanism, logistics, and outcomes of cardiac arrest and helps evaluate the impact of interventions such as a rapid response team. The standard consensus terms used to describe outcome of CA are as follows (13):

1. **Successful defibrillation:** Termination of fibrillation to an organized electrical rhythm (including PEA for at least 5 seconds after shock delivery).
2. **Return of spontaneous circulation (ROSC):** Restoration of a spontaneous perfusing heart rhythm in the absence of external chest compressions for approximately >30 seconds. This term is not applicable when extracorporeal support is used, such as extracorporeal membrane oxygenation or a biventricular assist device.
3. **Survived event:**
   a. **Out-of-hospital setting:** Sustained ROSC with spontaneous circulation until admission and transfer of care to medical staff at the receiving hospital.
   b. **In-hospital setting:** Sustained ROSC for >20 minutes (or support of circulation if extracorporeal circulatory support is applied).

4. **End of event:** A resuscitation event is deemed to have ended when either death is declared or spontaneous circulation is restored and sustained for 20 minutes or longer. If extracorporeal life support is being provided, the end of event is 20 minutes after the establishment of extracorporeal circulation.
5. **Survival to hospital discharge:** Survival to hospital discharge is the point at which the patient is discharged from the hospital acute care unit regardless of neurologic status, outcome, or destination.
6. **Neurologic outcome at discharge:** Assessment of neurologic recovery is measured at discharge in terms of recovery of consciousness and achievement of precardiac arrest level of functioning.

Out-of-hospital Cardiac Arrest

Despite improvement in the scientific basis for resuscitation practices and extensive efforts at CPR training of lay and professional rescuers over the years, the outcome of most adult victims of out-of-hospital cardiac arrest remains poor, with a median reported survival to hospital discharge of 6.4% (7,18). A recent study suggested that adults who had a cardiac arrest in a public location (i.e., witnessed) were more likely to arrive to the hospital alive (39% vs. 31%, $p = 0.049$) and were more likely to have a good neurologic outcome after 6 months (35% vs. 25%, $p = 0.023$) compared with patients who had a cardiac arrest in a nonpublic location (19).

In children, the epidemiology and physiology of OOH cardiac arrest is different. In this group of patients, a recent systematic review of 41 studies of out-of-hospital cardiac arrest, including trauma, revealed an ROSC of 30%, with survival to admission of 24% but survival to discharge of 12% and neurologically intact survival of only 4% (20). The initial cardiac rhythms observed in these children were asystole, 78%; PEA, 12.8%; VF/pulseless VT, 8.1%; and bradycardia with a pulse, 1%.

In-hospital Cardiac Arrest

Despite efforts to train professional in-hospital rescuers to deliver effective CPR and use various devices and therapeutic drugs during resuscitation, the objective survival rates over the years have hardly changed (21,22). Currently, in-hospital cardiac arrest in adults has an overall survival of about 18% (17,23–25). Analysis of data from the NRCPR found that the prevalence of VF or pulseless VT as the first documented pulseless rhythm during in-hospital cardiac arrest was only 23% in adults and 14% in children (4). The prevalence of asystole as the initial rhythm was 35% in adults and 40% in children, whereas the prevalence of PEA was 32% versus 24% in adults and children, respectively. The rate of survival to hospital discharge following pulseless cardiac arrest was higher in children than adults, 27% versus 18%, respectively. Of these survivors, 65% of children and 73% of adults had good neurologic outcome. After adjusting for known predictors, such as arrest location and monitoring at time of arrest, outcome was surprisingly worse when the rhythm was VF/VT in children compared with asystole and PEA (4). Further analysis of these data showed that VF/VT occurred during CPR in children more commonly than it occurred as the initial rhythm (26). Survival to discharge is highest (35%) when VF/VT is the initial rhythm compared with much worse survival (11%) if this rhythm develops during resuscitation (26).

Neurologic Outcome

Neurologic outcome is determined by the cause of arrest (e.g., degree of shock or hypoxemia prior to arrest), the duration of no flow, adequacy of flow during CPR, restoration of adequate flow following ROSC, and subsequent injury secondary to postarrest management such as the occurrence of hyperthermia or hypoglycemia. Survivors who ultimately have a good outcome generally awaken within 3 days after CA. Most patients who remain neurologically unresponsive due to anoxic-ischemic encephalopathy for more than 7 days will fail to survive, and those who do survive often have poor neurologic recovery (27–29). Neurocognitive impairment ranges from dependency on others for care to remaining in a minimally conscious or vegetative state. Achieving good functional outcome is the ultimate goal for successful CPR because survival with severe neurologic injury is a terrible cost to patients, their family members and friends, and society at large. The financial implications of caring for these patients with disordered consciousness are substantial (30).

Unfortunately, most studies reporting outcome data lack these difficult-to-obtain elements or have used crude methods to describe neurologic outcome, such as the composite scores from the Glasgow outcome scale (GOS) (31) and Cerebral Performance Category (CPC) (32,33). One important limitation of these scales is the possibility of wide variation of neurologic function for the same score. In children, other scales such as the Pediatric Cerebral Performance Category (PCPC) and Pediatric Overall Performance Category (POPC) have been used (34–36). Currently, 11% to 48% of CA patients admitted to the hospital will be discharged with good neurologic outcome (21,37,38). Recent data from the NRCPR show that neurologic outcome in discharged adult survivors is generally good with 73% of patients with Cerebral Performance Category 1 (17).

INITIAL CONSIDERATIONS

CPR is primarily based on two principles:

1. Providing artificial ventilation and oxygenation through an unobstructed airway to maintain gas exchange. Since cardiac output is limited, the rescuer needs to avoid ventilation in excess of that required for adequate ventilation/perfusion matching.
2. Delivering chest compressions to maintain threshold blood flow, especially to the heart and brain, while minimizing interruption of compressions.

Basic Life Support

Basic life support (BLS) is the initial phase of CPR recognized as the "ABCs" of CPR: A, airway; B, breathing; C, circulation. Effective BLS can provide almost 30% of normal cardiac output with adequate arterial oxygen content; this is sufficient to protect the brain for minutes until effective defibrillation or other definitive therapeutic maneuvers are provided (39). With the 2000 guidelines for CPR, a new evidence-based approach to ventilation during CPR was introduced that continued with the 2005 edition. New evidence from laboratory and clinical science led to a de-emphasis on the role of ventilation following a dysrhythmic cardiac arrest (arrest primarily resulting from an acute cardiovascular event, such as ventricular fibrillation or tachycardia) (40). However, after asphyxial cardiac arrest (cardiac arrest primarily resulting from respiratory arrest and less commonly from shock), the traditional emphasis on ensuring airway patency, effective ventilation, and circulation remains fundamental to achieving survival and the intact neurologic outcome of patients. The following section summarizes BLS in adults; differences in BLS for infants and children compared with adults are seen in Table 46.2.

Airway

After establishing unresponsiveness and calling for help, opening the airway and maintenance of airway patency are the next steps of CPR. Provision and maintenance of a patent upper airway should be provided with the maneuvers listed below. These maneuvers are described in detail in basic airway management chapters.

1. Head tilt/chin lift
2. Jaw-thrust maneuver
3. Triple airway maneuver
4. Mandibular forward displacement

If airway obstruction is felt to be present and foreign body is suspected, immediate removal should be done using basic airway management guidelines.

Breathing

Determination of Apnea. There are several recommended methods of determining the absence of spontaneous breathing in an unconscious patient when no pulse oximetry is present. Spontaneous respiration may be difficult to observe unless the airway is opened (41). Once airway patency is established, the rescuer should place his or her ear over the victim's mouth and nose. The rise and fall of the chest should be noted while

TABLE 46.2

SUMMARY OF BASIC LIFE SUPPORT ABCD MANEUVERS FOR INFANTS, CHILDREN, AND ADULTS FOR LAY RESCUERS AND HEALTH CARE PROVIDERS (NEWBORN INFORMATION NOT INCLUDED)

Maneuver	Adult Lay rescuer: ≥8 y HCPs: Adolescent and older	Child Lay rescuers: 1–8 y HCPs: 1 y to adolescent	Infant ≤1 y of age
Airway	Head tilt–chin lift (HCPs: Suspected trauma, use jaw thrust)		
Breathing: Initial	Two breaths at 1 sec/breath	Two breaths at 1 sec/breath	
HCPs: Rescue breathing without chest compressions	10–12 breaths/min (approximate)	12–20 breaths/min (approximate)	
HCPs: Rescue breaths for CPR with advanced airway	←8–10 breaths/min (approximately)→		
Foreign body airway obstruction	Abdominal thrusts		Back slaps and chest thrust
Circulation **HCPs:** Pulse check (≤10 s)	Carotid		Brachial or femoral
Compression landmarks	Lower half of sternum, between nipples		Just below nipple line (lower half of sternum)
Compression method ■ Push hard and fast ■ Allow complete recoil	Heel of one hand, other hand on top	Heel of one hand or as for adults	Two or three fingers HCPs (two rescuers): Two thumb–encircling hands
Compression depth	1½ to 2 inches	Approximately one-third to one-half the depth of the chest	
Compression rate	←Approximately 100/min→		
Compression:ventilation ratio	30:2 (one or two rescuers)	30:2 (single rescuer) HCPs: 15:2 (two rescuers)	
Defibrillation AED	Use adult pads Do not use child pads	Use AED after five cycles of CPR (out of hospital) Use pediatric system for child 1–8 y if available HCPs: For sudden collapse (out of hospital) or in-hospital arrest use AED as soon as available	No recommendation for infants <1 y of age

Note: Maneuvers used by only health care providers are indicated by HCPs. AED, automated external defibrillator; CPR, cardiopulmonary resuscitation. Adapted from 2005 American Heart Association Guidelines for Cardiopulmonary Resuscitation and Emergency Cardiovascular Care. *Circulation.* 2005;112[24]SIV-1–IV-211.

listening for breath sounds and feeling for expired air. The absence of these signs is indicative of apnea. Frequently, gasping, gurgling, snoring sounds or agonal respiratory efforts may be observed during sudden cardiac arrest, especially within the first few minutes of collapse. This is typically not sustained, and should not be mistaken for adequate spontaneous respiration. In some instances, the victim may exhibit respiratory efforts but no air exchange is observed. This indicates severe upper airway obstruction; opening the airway will facilitate the resumption of air movement. Despite the widespread diffusion of these recommendations, studies showed that lay rescuers as well as professional rescuers are unable to accurately determine adequate breathing in unresponsive patients (42,43). Currently, it is recommended that if breathing cannot be confirmed within 10 seconds, two rescue breaths should be given.

Initiation of Rescue Breathing. If the patient is not breathing, immediate rescue breaths are delivered using the maneuver appropriate for the situation. Most first-responder personnel and medical professional staff in hospitals are trained to use adjunct devices during BLS. When a bag-mask ventilation (BMV) is not immediately available, mouth-to-mouth rescue breathing can still be life saving.

Intuitively, the presence of vomitus and fear of infectious contamination can affect the willingness of rescuers to perform mouth-to-mouth resuscitation. Lawrence and Sivaneswaran showed that only 13% of 70 hospital staff members surveyed would use mouth-to-mouth ventilation during CPR and 59% would prefer to do mouth-to-mask ventilation (44). Specialized breathing masks with a one-way valve can be utilized during CPR. The valve prevents the exhaled air from entering the rescuer's mouth.

During both one and two-rescuer CPR, two mouth-to-mouth breaths are given during a pause after every 30th chest compression. This ratio is the same for adults, children, and infants when there is only one rescuer. If two or more professional rescuers are present, a 15:2 ratio is used in children (defined as child if there are no signs of puberty such as facial hair or breast development) and infants.

Once an advance airway (i.e., endotracheal tube, laryngeal mask airway [LMA], or pharyngotracheal Combitube) is obtained, chest compressions are given continuously at a rate of 100 compressions per minute without interruption for ventilation. A ventilation rate of eight to ten can sufficiently match the perfusion achieved by chest compression (20%–30% of normal at best) (45). Rescue breathing when there is a pulse should not exceed 12 breaths/minute (45).

Manual Resuscitators (Bag-valve Devices). Bag-valve devices (BVDs) of various designs and sizes are available for adults and children to deliver manual breaths. A self-inflating, manually operated bag with a nonrebreathing valve is preferred because it allows ventilation even if there is no connection to an oxygen source. This device may be used in conjunction with a face mask, endotracheal tube, or other invasive airway device.

The standard parts of a BVD include (a) a delivery port with a 15-mm/22-mm adapter coupling that can be connected to the mask or tracheal tube; (b) a one-way, non jam valve that allows a minimum of 15 L/minute oxygen flow rate for spontaneous and controlled ventilation; and (c) a system for ensuring delivery of a high oxygen concentration through an auxiliary oxygen inlet at the back of the bag or by an oxygen reservoir. The bag holds a volume up to 1,600 mL. Some pediatric resuscitator bags are provided with a 25- to 30-cm H_2O pop-off valve to avoid excessive positive airway pressure, thereby reducing the risk of gastric insufflation and hyperinflation of the lungs and subsequent pulmonary barotrauma, but a pop-off valve is not recommended during CPR in adults since higher airway pressures may be needed to achieve adequate ventilation. A malfunctioning valve may lead to improper venting and inadequate ventilation. This can be recognized by the sound of air escaping through the relief valve while squeezing the bag. Adjusting or partially occluding a malfunctioning valve may be life saving.

The operator should be positioned at the top of the victim's head. Appropriate face mask size should be selected, the airway opened, and a tight seal created covering the mouth and the nose as described previously. After proper head positioning, the bag is squeezed to deliver the breath over 1 second. Tidal volume is sufficient if visible chest rise is present. An oropharyngeal airway or nasopharyngeal airway may be used to facilitate bag-mask ventilation in case of upper airway obstruction. Proper bag-mask ventilation requires training, practice, and familiarity with the equipment.

A single rescuer may have difficulty maintaining a correct head position and delivering adequate tidal volume at the same time (46–48). Thus, two rescuers may be more effective where one rescuer seals the mask to the mouth, performs a jaw thrust, and maintains head extension while the other rescuer squeezes the bag with both hands (49). Oxygen supplementation during bag-mask ventilation delivers 40% to 60% O_2 without an oxygen reservoir and over 90% with an oxygen reservoir (50,51).

Complications associated with the use of a bag-mask device are primarily due to excessive ventilating pressures causing pneumothorax, pneumomediastinum, and gastric distention that can lead to decreased total lung compliance, regurgitation, and gastric rupture (52). Unless the rescuer is proficient in the use of flow-inflating devices (e.g., Mapleson D system, typically used by anesthesia personnel) during CPR, it is preferable to use a self-inflating handheld resuscitator bag.

Special consideration should be applied for pediatric patients. In fact, the pediatric airway may be flattened by excessive extension of the cervical spine during the head tilt–chin lift maneuver. Smaller breaths must be used to avoid abdominal distention, regurgitation, and pulmonary barotrauma. As with adults, appropriate tidal volume is characterized by visible chest rise.

Oxygen-powered, Manually Triggered Ventilation Devices. Oxygen-powered breathing devices may be used when available during CPR. These simple ventilatory devices require high oxygen flow rates to overcome air leak (44). Although they may be able to deliver adequate tidal volumes, high-flow-rate time-cycled oxygen-powered devices carry a risk of severe gastric distention when used with a face mask.

Inspiratory Impedance Valve. A small inspiratory impedance valve device was recently introduced to occlude the airway selectively during the decompression phase of chest compressions without interfering with exhalation or resuscitation bag ventilation. This device, as shown in Figure 46.1, is placed between the end of an endotracheal tube or face mask and the resuscitation bag, which then limits air entry into the lungs during chest recoil or when the patient spontaneously breathes. In the

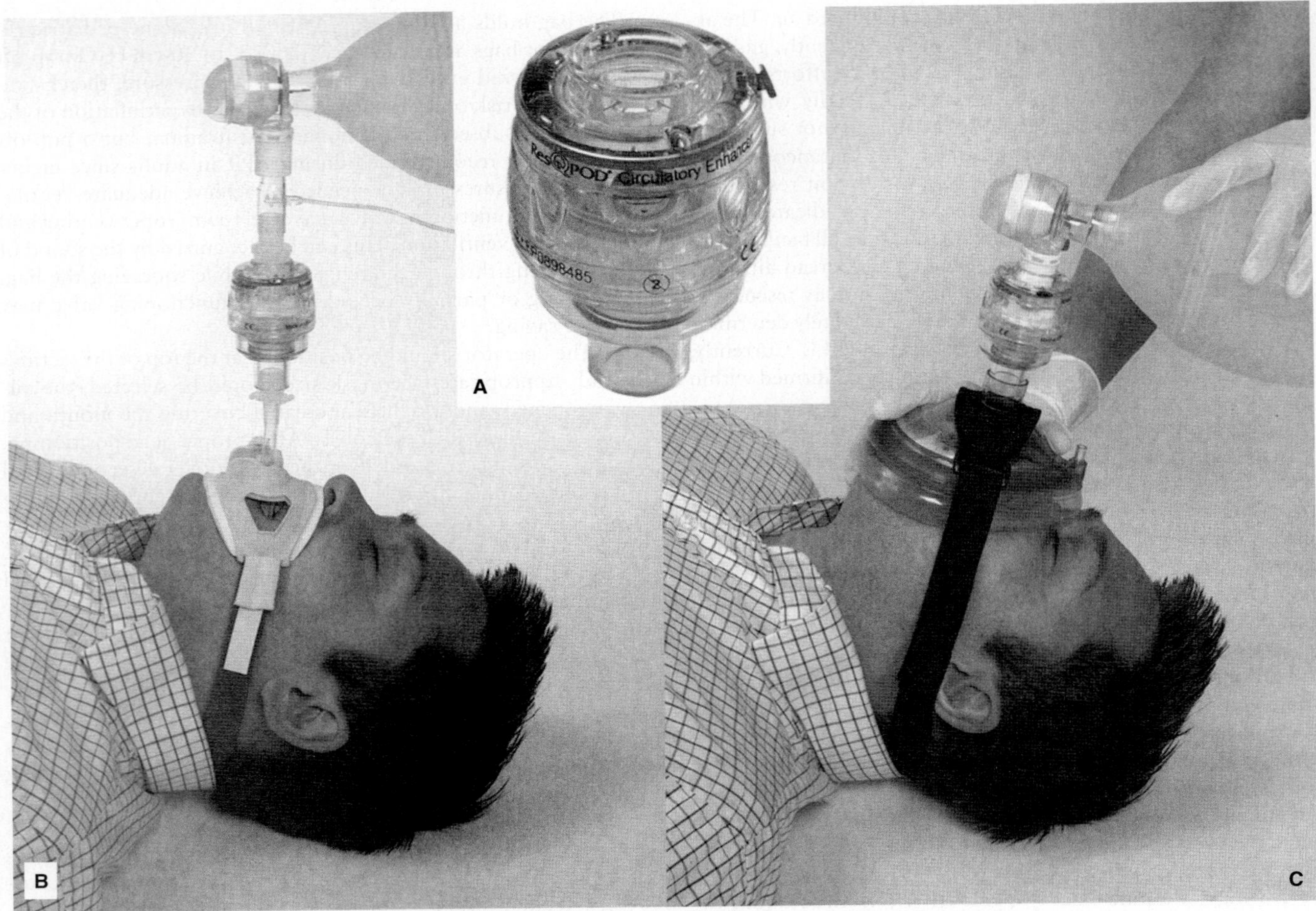

FIGURE 46.1. Top center (A) showing an inspiratory impedance valve device (ResQPOD, Advanced Circulatory Systems, Inc., Minneapolis, MN). The device is applied between the resuscitation bag and endotracheal tube as shown in bottom left (B) or between the resuscitation bag and face mask as shown in bottom right (C). (Pictures courtesy of ResQPOD, Advanced Circulatory Systems, Inc., Minneapolis, MN.)

latter circumstance, the patient needs to overcome the inspiratory threshold pressure for air flow to occur. The resulting modest reduction in intrathoracic pressure enhances venous return to the heart between chest compressions and thus cardiac output. This device has no deleterious effect on ventilation, and can enhance coronary and cerebral blood flow during CPR in animals and humans along with a higher rate of ROSC after defibrillation (53,54). An enhancement of cardiac output during spontaneous ventilation has also been observed in hypovolemic shock states (55). In spite of the favorable hemodynamic effect, the use of this device so far has not demonstrated a definitive long-term neurological improvement after ROSC. At the time of this writing, a large multicenter clinical trial is under way.

Circulation

Determination of Circulation. In the absence of a continuous arterial line monitoring, palpation for carotid or femoral pulses has been traditionally the gold standard for a diagnosis of cardiac arrest. Recent studies, however, showed that both lay rescuers (56) and health professionals are unable to accurately determine the presence or absence of a pulse; most required more than the recommended 10 seconds to feel confident about whether a pulse was present (42,57). Based on this observation that can significantly delay chest compression, the pulse check was eliminated for lay rescuers and de-emphasized for health professionals in the 2000 and 2005 guidelines (45,58), where verification of "no pulse" is not recommended beyond 10 seconds.

Mechanism of Blood Flow during Chest Compression. In the early 19th century, open cardiac massage was used successfully by Kristian et al. in the emergency treatment of cardiac arrest (59). In a short time, this became the method of choice for CPR (60,61), with variable outcomes reported. Open cardiac massage requires a thoracotomy and the heart is squeezed directly by the hands of the rescuer (61,62). The basic idea was to produce an effective perfusion pressure gradient for blood flow from the heart to vital organs. Open cardiac massage has been utilized in a variety of special situations where the access to the chest is immediately feasible (63–66). For example, in the cardiac intensive care unit (ICU), open cardiac compression is used both in adult and pediatric patients in the immediate postoperative setting (67). Outside of the operating room (OR), the use of open cardiac massage, although it improved coronary perfusion pressure and increased ROSC, was not followed by improved survival (68).

In 1960, Kouwenhoven et al. reported successful resuscitation of dogs and subsequently humans with ventricular fibrillation cardiac arrest using the combination of closed chest compression, artificial respiration, and electrical defibrillation (69,70). They hypothesized that the heart was physically squeezed between the sternum and vertebral column, whereby the blood flow generated is similar to the mechanism of spontaneous contraction of the heart; hence, this is called the "cardiac pump" model. This model, however, does not explain several clinical observations in contrast with the cardiac pump theory such as the ineffectiveness of CPR during flail chest, although theoretically it should be easier to compress the heart in this condition, or the effectiveness of closed chest CPR in patients with hyperinflated chest due to severe emphysema.

The cardiac pump model was challenged in the 1970s when Criley et al. reported ROSC with cough during ventricular fibrillation (71,72). In 1980, Rudikoff et al. reported that fluctuations of intrathoracic pressures were primarily responsible for blood flow during CPR (73,74). These findings supported a noncardiac or "thoracic pump" mechanism for blood flow during CPR. This model proposes that increased intrathoracic pressure during chest compression elevates the pressure of blood located in structures within the thorax, creating the gradient for forward blood flow from the intrathoracic to lower pressure extrathoracic arteries. During relaxation, intrathoracic pressure drops, resulting in refilling of the heart with blood. In this model, the heart acts as a passive conduit. Echocardiographic studies to elucidate the pumping mechanism during cardiac arrest have failed to resolve the controversy (75–77). It appears that in adults with thin chest walls, direct cardiac compression does occur, whereas in prolonged resuscitation and in patients with thick chest walls or hyperinflated lungs, the thoracic pump mechanism becomes the predominant flow mechanism. It is also likely that both mechanisms are involved in some cases.

In infants and children, a mechanism of direct cardiac compression is well supported by the observation of CPR performed in young animal models (78). Currently, closed chest compression is the standard method of producing blood flow during CPR for both adult and pediatric victims.

Closed Chest Compression. Closed chest compressions consist of the rhythmic application of pressure over the lower half of the sternum. Even if properly performed, in adults, chest compressions can only produce systolic arterial pressures of 60 to 80 mm Hg; diastolic pressure is usually low and mean arterial pressure in the carotid artery seldom exceeds 40 mm Hg (79). These values are low compared to normal but still can provide critical blood flow to the heart and brain while attempts to restore definitive cardiac activity are implemented. To achieve maximum benefit from chest compressions during CPR, attention should be given to the following components:

1. **Positioning the patient:** The victim should lie supine on a hard surface. If the patient is on a soft bed, then place a backboard beneath the patient (80). The rescuer should kneel beside the victim's thorax if the victim is on the floor (81), or adjust the bed to the level of the rescuer's hip if the victim is on a bed. Other positions like over-the-head CPR and two-person straddle CPR are described, but the efficacy of these techniques has not been established (82).
2. **Positioning of rescuer hands:** In adults, the rescuer ideally should compress the lower half of the victim's sternum. Locating proper hand position, however, has been confusing in lay rescuer education, so it is easier to teach that the rescuer should place the heel of the hand on the sternum in the center (middle) of the chest between the nipples and then place the heel of the second hand on top of the first so that the hands are overlapped and parallel (83,84). Compressions are delivered while keeping the arms straight at elbow. This is best achieved by leaning over the victim, which allows the rescuer's weight to be used in producing effective chest compression, but the rescuer should avoid maintaining compression on the chest during the relaxation phase, since this impairs venous return (85,86).

   In children, the rescuer again should ideally compress the lower half of the sternum, avoiding the xiphoid process and the ribs, but the lay rescuer is taught to position the heel of one hand at the midnipple line. Either one or two hands can be used in children, depending on the strength of the rescuer. In a child, the use of two hands generates higher compression pressures compared with one hand and is less fatiguing in a manikin study (87), but no outcome study has shown superiority of one method over the other.

   In infants, two different techniques are used: The two-finger technique and the two-thumb encircling technique. With the two-finger technique, the rescuer compresses the lower half of the sternum just below the intermammary line with the second and third or third and fourth fingers (78,88–90). This is the only technique to be used by lay rescuers. The two-thumb encircling hands technique is recommended when there are two health care provider rescuers. The infant's chest is encircled with both hands with the thumbs placed on the lower half of the sternum and the fingers spread around the thorax. Compression is delivered with both thumbs while the lateral chest is squeezed simultaneously with the fingers. The two-thumb encircling technique produces more consistent compression depth and higher coronary perfusion pressures (91–93).
3. **Depth of compression:** The sternum is depressed approximately $1\frac{1}{2}$ to 2 inches (approximately 4 to 5 cm) in adults. In children and infants, the chest should be compressed to achieve one-half to one-third the depth of the anterior-posterior diameter of the chest. The higher proportional depth of compression is appropriate in infants, whereas one-third the depth of compression is appropriate in children. Data in manikin models show that rescuers often do not sustain an adequate depth of compression during CPR for more than 2 minutes. In studies of adults undergoing CPR in both the out-of-hospital (94) and in-hospital (95) setting, inadequate compression depth is commonly observed. Since adequate depth of compression is important in achieving optimal forward flow, emphasis should be placed on compressing "hard" as well as fast enough, and the rescuer performing chest compressions should change approximately every 2 minutes during the time when the patient's rhythm is being reassessed.
4. **Compression rate:** Recent studies in animals (96) and in humans (97,98) support that a rate of at least 80 per minute should be achieved to provide optimal forward blood flow during CPR, with some experts suggesting higher cardiac

output with compression rates up to 150 per minute. Higher compression rates, however, are more difficult to sustain. It is important to remember that the compression rate refers to the speed of compressions, not the actual number of compressions delivered per minute. The actual number of chest compressions delivered per minute is determined by the rate of chest compressions and the number and duration of interruptions to open the airway, deliver rescue breaths, and time for analysis of cardiac rhythm and delivery of shock. To maximize the beneficial effects of chest compressions producing blood flow, the 2005 guidelines recommend compressions at a rate of approximately 100 per minute with interruptions in chest compressions kept to a minimum.

5. **Decompression:** After achieving the maximum depth of compression, the chest should be released to recoil on its own. It is crucial to let the chest recoil completely before the next compression is started. Incomplete chest recoil leaves residual positive (relative to atmospheric) intrathoracic pressure that decreases both coronary and cerebral perfusion (86).
6. **Duty cycle:** Duty cycle refers to the sum of the time interval from the start of compression until maximum compression is achieved (i.e., "compression cycle") plus the time interval from the maximum compression to complete decompression (i.e., "decompression cycle") prior to the next compression. Studies in animals and in manikin models showed that coronary and cerebral perfusion directly increased with increasing compression rate up to 130 to 150 per minute using a compression cycle between 20% and 50% of the duty cycle (99,100). Current guidelines recommend a 50% compression cycle (101).

Compression-to-Ventilation Ratio during Basic Life Support

Different compression-to-ventilation (C:V) cycles were recommended when one or two rescuers are present. In children, additional ratios were used to provide more ventilation. Recent studies show that both lay and health care rescuers provide poor chest compressions (94,95), and there is often a prolonged hands-off period during CPR while breaths are being given or the rhythm is being assessed, resulting in no cardiac output. Both animal data and theoretic models suggest that higher cardiac output will be achieved using a higher ratio of chest compressions and fewer interruptions for ventilation. The latter is acceptable since the overall cardiac output is only 25% to 30% of normal at best, which means that ventilation only needs to be 25% to 30% of normal to achieve adequate matching of ventilation to cardiac output during CPR. Therefore, the new guidelines recommend one universal ratio of 30 compressions to two ventilations in adults, children, and infants with one rescuer. If two health professionals are present, they should use a 15:2 ratio in children and infants. This approach maximizes chest compressions and minimizes time for ventilation, rhythm analysis, and shock, and improves ROSC and outcome (9,102).

In addition to being easy to teach and recall, the 30:2 compression:ventilation rate is designed to reduce the likelihood of hyperventilation, which impairs venous return as shown in a well-done animal study (103). Additionally, other data suggest that no ventilation is needed for the first few minutes of sudden cardiac arrest and need for initial ventilations has remained a matter of debate (9).

As previously noted, when the airway is secured, continuous chest compressions should be delivered continuously in an asynchronous mode with the ventilation. Unfortunately, the by-product of increasing the speed of chest compression is fatigue, detected by both animal (104) and human studies (105).

Acceptable Variations of Closed Chest Compressions

1. **Interposed abdominal compression.** The interposed abdominal compression (IAC) CPR technique uses a dedicated second rescuer to provide manual compression of the abdomen (midway between the xiphoid and the umbilicus) during the relaxation phase of chest compression. The purpose is to enhance venous return during CPR (106,107). When IAC CPR performed by trained providers was compared with standard CPR for in-hospital cardiac arrest, IAC CPR improved ROSC and short-term survival in two randomized trials and improved survival to hospital discharge in one study (108,109). The implementation of this technique is limited by the extensive complex training needed and the need for at least three rescuers to provide coordinated compressions and ventilation.
2. **Active Compression-decompression.** Active compression-decompression CPR (ACD CPR) is performed with a handheld device equipped with a suction cup to actively lift the anterior chest during decompression. It is thought that decreasing intrathoracic pressure during the decompression phase enhances venous return to the heart. Although substantial animal data demonstrated that the device improves cardiac output during CPR, clinical trials reported mixed results, with some showing improved survival (110–112) and others finding no effect when compared to standard CPR (113–116). The reason for the disparate results is not clear, but some data suggest that extensive training is required to use this device effectively, and there is a higher rate of rescuer fatigue from the increased effort required during both compression and relaxation. At the time of this writing, no ACD CPR device is approved by the Food and Drug Administration (FDA) for sale in the United States.
3. **Phased thoracic-abdominal compression-decompression.** This technique is essentially a combination of the IAC CPR and ACD CPR techniques described above. A handheld device is used to alternate chest compression and abdominal decompression with chest decompression and abdominal compression. The utility of this technique is also limited by the need for a dedicated rescuer and the complexity of training (117).

Mechanical Adjuncts for Circulation

1. **Mechanical piston device.** This device is composed of a plunger mounted on a backboard, which is driven by compressed gas to depress the sternum. The rate and depth of compressions is adjustable with a 50% compression cycle. Use of this device resulted in improved end-tidal CO_2 in both in-hospital and out-of-hospital settings (118–120). The expense and bulkiness of the device has limited its widespread distribution and use.
2. **Vest device (load distributing band).** The load-distributing band (LDB) is a circumferential chest compression device composed of a pneumatically or electrically actuated constricting band and backboard. The band is wrapped around the patient and compresses the entire chest, producing

thoracic pump CPR. Use of this device improved survival to emergency department arrival in one study (121); an FDA-approved device (AutoPulse) is available. A cohort study conducted before and after introduction of the load-distributing band found an improved rate of ROSC and survival to hospital discharge (122), whereas a randomized multicenter trial reported at the same time found no survival benefit 4 hours after the arrest and a lower rate of survival to hospital discharge (123).

Advanced Life Support

Advanced life support (ALS) entails advanced airway management including use of ancillary equipment to support ventilation and oxygenation, prompt recognition, and, when appropriate, treatment of life-threatening arrhythmias using electrical therapy including defibrillation, cardioversion, pacemaker insertion, and pharmacologic therapy. ALS includes the use of pharmacologic therapy and advanced procedures extending into the postarrest setting such as the use of therapeutic hypothermia.

Advanced Airway Management

Tracheal Intubation. Endotracheal intubation is indicated when the rescuer is unable to adequately ventilate or oxygenate the arrested or unconscious patient with bag-mask ventilation, or if prolonged ventilation is required and airway protective reflexes are absent in the patient with a perfusing rhythm. A properly placed endotracheal tube (ET) is the gold standard method for securing the airway. It maintains a patent airway to deliver effective positive pressure ventilation and use of positive end-expiratory pressure when indicated. It possibly reduces the risk from aspiration, especially if a cuffed tube is used, and it provides a means to suction airway secretions and provides an alternate route for resuscitation drugs delivery (124). No randomized adult studies have compared the outcome from endotracheal intubation to bag-mask ventilation, but one prospective randomized controlled trial in children showed no survival benefit of endotracheal intubation over bag-mask ventilation by trained EMS personnel (125).

Attempted endotracheal intubation by less skilled rescuers results in complications. Retrospective studies reported a 6% to 14% incidence of misplaced or displaced ETs (126–128). To minimize the risk of esophageal intubation, it is important to use an end-tidal CO_2 ($ETCO_2$) detector or esophageal detector device in addition to careful auscultation and observing symmetric chest rise. In patients requiring movement, exhaled CO_2 monitoring (capnography) is helpful to detect tube displacement. Proper tube position should be confirmed by chest radiography when feasible. The intensivist is expected to master endotracheal intubation. However, expert personnel may not be immediately available in the ICU. Due to the technical difficulty and skill level needed for endotracheal intubation, there is increased emphasis on learning bag-mask ventilation, which could be used primarily for ventilation and can serve as rescue backup if attempted endotracheal intubation fails.

Confirmation of Correct Endotracheal Tube Placement. Clinical signs used to confirm correct ET placement are (a) visualization of bilateral chest rise, (b) bilateral breath sounds over the lateral lung fields, (c) absent breath sounds over the epigastrium, and (d) presence of water vapor/mist in the tube. None of these signs is confirmatory, however, and an $ETCO_2$ detector or esophageal detector is indicated to confirm correct tube placement.

$ETCO_2$ detector device. A disposable colorimetric device that detects $ETCO_2$ has been investigated as a guide to correct endotracheal tube placement (129–131). The device fits on the end of the ET and is normally purple in color; exhaled CO_2 turns the color to bright yellow indicating that the ET is in the trachea. The positive predictive value of this device for correct tube placement is close to 100%, but the negative predictive value ranges from 20% to 100% depending on whether the patient has a perfusing rhythm (132). False-negative results are seen if there is no or very low pulmonary blood flow, such as during cardiac arrest or with a large pulmonary embolus. Conversely, false-positive (i.e., the detector remains yellow) results are seen when it is contaminated with an acidic drug (e.g., epinephrine) or gastric contents. Currently, it is recommended to confirm each endotracheal intubation with an $ETCO_2$ capnograph or an esophageal detector device. If doubt exists about whether the tube is correctly placed, direct visualization of the larynx is advised.

Esophageal detector device. There are two versions: The bulb and the syringe esophageal detector devices (EDD). The bulb EDD consists of a bulb that is compressed and attached to the endotracheal tube. When the squeezed bulb is released, if the tube is in the esophagus, the suction collapses the lumen of the esophagus or pulls the esophageal tissue against the tip of the tube, and the bulb will not re-expand (positive result for esophageal placement). The syringe EDD consists of a syringe attached to the ET; the rescuer attempts to pull the plunger of the syringe. If the tube is in the esophagus, it will not be possible to pull out the plunger (i.e., aspirate air) with the syringe. This device has high sensitivity for esophageal placement of ETs in both cardiac arrest and patients with a perfusing rhythm (133–135), but poor specificity for tracheal placement. The device may suggest esophageal placement when the tube is in the trachea in patients who are morbidly obese, in late pregnancy, and with pulmonary edema or severe airway obstructive disease (e.g., asthma). These false-positive events occur because either the trachea collapses (obesity and late pregnancy) or air is not easily recruitable from the lung (pulmonary edema and severe airway obstruction). Sensitivity and specificity of EDDs are poor in children younger than 1 year old, and they are not recommended in children weighing less than 20 kg (136).

Advanced Airway Adjuncts. Multiple airway adjuncts are available in cases of failed endotracheal intubation and difficult bag-mask ventilation. Two of these devices, the laryngeal mask airway and esophageal tracheal Combitube, are widely used and discussed in depth in Chapter 38 (Airway Management). These adjuncts are "rescue airways," a bridge rather than alternate to endotracheal intubation that is readily mastered with appropriate training. Although they facilitate effective ventilation, they do not allow tracheal suctioning or provide reliable airway protection.

Electrical Therapy

Electrical therapy is one of the mainstays of ALS, especially in adults. Electrical energy is used to treat life-threatening cardiac dysrhythmias, which constitutes 16% to 85% (137–140) of out-of-hospital and 14% to 56% (17,141–144) of in-hospital cardiac arrests. Recent data suggest that ventricular fibrillation and ventricular tachycardia are decreasing, with only 24% of the initial rhythms in over 36,000 adult arrests being VF- or VT-based on a recent analysis from the National Registry for Cardiopulmonary Resuscitation (NRCPR) (4). In hospitalized children with cardiac arrest, VF is the initial rhythm in approximately 10% of cases and subsequently occurs during 15% of the cases (26). Despite the fall in prevalence, early recognition of a shockable rhythm is critical since the outcome following effective treatment is much better than after asystole or PEA (4). Several different modes of electrical therapies are available for treatment of different rhythm problems. These include defibrillation, cardioversion, and cardiac pacing.

Defibrillation. Defibrillation is defined as delivery of electrical energy resulting in termination of VF for at least 5 seconds following the shock (145,146). The goal is to quickly depolarize the whole myocardium, terminating the rhythm and hoping that a sinus rhythm will start. Defibrillation should not be confused with ROSC or survival. In most adults, the initial postshock rhythm is asystole or an organized slow rhythm without a pulse (i.e., PEA). This observation is the basis for the current guideline recommendation to immediately begin chest compressions after shock delivery.

Defibrillator device. There are two types of defibrillator devices available: (a) manual defibrillator devices require the rescuer to analyze the rhythm and then manually set and determine the electrical energy dose; (b) automatic defibrillator devices analyze the rhythm, determine if a shock is required, and deliver the shock if needed automatically. There are two types of automatic defibrillators: internal implantable cardioverter defibrillator (ICD) and automated external defibrillator (AED). Defibrillators are also characterized by the mode and waveform of electrical current delivered into monophasic and biphasic defibrillators. Animal and human data show that biphasic defibrillators have a higher first shock success in terminating VF compared with monophasic devices; the latter are no longer produced. Manufacturers use various methods of delivering the biphasic energy, and more recently, triphasic and quadriphasic defibrillators are being developed and appear to be potentially more effective than biphasic defibrillators (147,148).

Monophasic defibrillators deliver current in one direction or polarity so current flows from one paddle (or electrode) to the other throughout the duration of shock. As noted, these defibrillators are being replaced by biphasic defibrillators.

Biphasic defibrillators deliver current sequentially in both directions or polarity during one shock. In the first phase, the current moves from one paddle to the other as with monophasic defibrillators, and during the second phase, the current flow reverses direction. Biphasic defibrillators can also be further classified based on the waveform changes into (a) biphasic truncated exponential waveform and (b) rectilinear biphasic waveform. Several randomized trials (149–151) showed that defibrillation with biphasic waveforms of relatively low energy (200 J) is safe and has equivalent or higher efficacy for termination of VF than monophasic waveform shocks of equivalent or higher energy, which decreases the risk of myocardial injury and increases shock efficacy.

Defibrillation dose. The optimal energy dose for the first of subsequent shocks required for effective defibrillation remains unknown despite multiple studies (151,152). The ideal shock dose for a biphasic device is one that falls within the range documented as effective using that specific device. It is reasonable to use selected energies of 150 J to 200 J with a biphasic truncated exponential waveform or 120 J with a rectilinear biphasic waveform for the initial shock. For second and subsequent biphasic shocks, the same or higher energy can be given. The rescuer should have knowledge of the type of defibrillator being used and select the energy dose accordingly. Most manual defibrillators are set to an initial default of 200 J of energy. This is not necessarily the optimal dose in all cases, but was selected because it falls within the reported range of doses effective for first and subsequent biphasic shocks. If only a monophasic defibrillator is available, then an energy dose of 360 J is recommended for all shocks.

During shock, the average current delivered is the key determinant of successful defibrillation (153–155). Current delivery is determined by the energy level selected and by the patient's transthoracic impedance. The average adult human transthoracic impedance is 70 to 80 Ω (156–158). While mean current determines the success of defibrillation, high peak currents during the shock are associated with myocardial injury. Biphasic waveforms deliver lower peak current values compared to monophasic waveforms. If transthoracic impedance is high, a low-energy shock will not generate sufficient current to achieve defibrillation. To improve current delivery, conductive gels are recommended in place of manual paddles. Adhesive pads have the added advantage of reducing the risk of inadvertent rescuer shock. Regardless of the device used, the rescuer needs to press the paddles or pads firmly on the chest wall to ensure a good electrical contact.

The optimal dose for effective defibrillation in infants and children is not known. The upper limit for safe defibrillation is also not known, but doses more than 4 J/kg (as high as 9 J/kg) have effectively defibrillated children (159,160) and pediatric animal models (161) with no significant reported adverse effects. Recommended manual defibrillation (monophasic or biphasic) doses for children are 2 J/kg for the first attempt and 4 J/kg for subsequent attempts.

Electrode position. Either handheld paddles or self-adhesive pads are used for shocks. Electrodes are applied to the bare chest in the conventional sternal-apical (anterolateral) position. The right (sternal) chest pad is placed on the victim's right superior-anterior (infraclavicular) chest and the apical (left) pad is placed on the victim's inferior-lateral left chest, lateral to the left breast. Other acceptable pad positions are placement on the lateral chest wall on the right and left sides (biaxillary) or the left pad in the standard apical position and the other pad on the right or left upper back (avoiding the scapular bone). Similar positions are recommended for children, particularly the anterior-posterior position since many defibrillators have only a single size electrode pad and there should be at least 1 inch between the pads. The rescuer should make sure that electrodes are not overlapping and are not on top of implanted devices or transdermal medicine patches if present. If the patient is wet, the chest should be wiped dry before placement. Another caution is to avoid placing the oxygen source near the electrodes, particularly in children where the distance from the face to the chest is short.

Electrode size. In general, the largest pad or paddle that can be placed on the chest while avoiding contact between the pads or paddles should be used. There should be at least 1 inch between the pads. Paddles that are too small increase the risk of skin burn injury.

Automatic rhythm analysis and automatic external defibrillators. AEDs are computerized compact devices that use voice and visual prompts to guide lay rescuers and health care providers to safely defibrillate VF or pulseless VT (139,162–164). In a large prospective randomized trial (165) funded by the AHA, the National Heart, Lung, and Blood Institute (NHLBI), and several AED manufacturers, lay rescuer CPR AED programs in targeted public settings doubled the number of survivors from out-of-hospital VF SCA when compared with programs that provided early EMS call and early CPR.

Despite limited evidence, AEDs should be considered within the hospital as a way to facilitate early defibrillation (a goal of <3 minutes from collapse), especially in areas where staff have limited to no rhythm recognition skills or defibrillators are used infrequently.

For children 1 to 8 years of age, the rescuer should use a pediatric dose-attenuator system with the AED if one is available (160). If the rescuer provides CPR to a child in cardiac arrest and does not have an AED with a pediatric attenuator system, the rescuer should use a standard AED.

Electrical Cardioversion. Electrical cardioversion is used for some life-threatening arrhythmias causing rapid cardiovascular deterioration. These include VT and supraventricular tachycardias (SVTs), such as paroxysmal atrial tachycardia (PAT), atrial flutter, or atrial fibrillation with a rapid ventricular response. The electrode size and positioning is the same as that used in defibrillation; the difference between cardioversion and defibrillation is described below.

Technique. Unlike defibrillation, cardioversion must be synchronized with the patient's electrocardiogram (ECG). The ideal discharge point is during the upstroke of the R wave of the QRS complex. Delivery of the energy during the T wave of the QRS may result in ventricular fibrillation. Most commercially available defibrillators automatically coordinate the discharge to the patient's ECG if the machine is placed in the synchronized mode and the QRS complex is of adequate size for consistent detection. If the defibrillator does not "sense" the QRS complex, increasing the ECG gain improves sensing. Cardioversion should never be attempted with quick-look paddles, because ECG artifact may make synchronization impossible. Unsynchronized cardioversion should only be used when the available equipment does not allow synchronization.

Energy level. The amount of energy recommended for emergency cardioversion varies with the rhythm (166,167); 100 J is recommended for atrial fibrillation and 50 J for atrial flutter (168). Monomorphic ventricular tachycardia responds well to cardioversion, and 100 J should be attempted first. Pulseless ventricular tachycardia behaves like ventricular fibrillation, and 200 J should be used initially. For cardioversion in conscious patients, sedation with intravenous diazepam, midazolam, or methohexital is indicated, and the cardioversion accomplished with the lowest energy possible (50–200 J). In children, the recommended initial cardioversion dose is 0.5 to 1 J/kg.

External Cardiac Pacing. While, in general, external (transcutaneous) pacing is not recommended for patients in asystolic cardiac arrest, it is our opinion that it should be always considered in the ICU or other critical care areas of the hospital where the device and adequate skill are promptly available. However, three randomized controlled trials (169,170) of fair quality indicated no improvement in the rate of admission to hospital or survival to hospital discharge when paramedics or physicians attempted to provide pacing in asystolic patients in the prehospital or hospital (emergency department) setting. Pacing can be considered in patients with symptomatic bradycardia when a pulse is present.

Pharmacologic Therapy

Pharmacologic therapy in CA is used to increase the rate of ROSC and terminate or limit the risk of recurrent arrhythmias. It is recognized that there are no placebo-controlled studies showing that any vasopressor during human CA increases survival to discharge; indeed, some studies questioned the benefit of their use (171). For obvious reasons, it is unlikely that a large prospective randomized study on this issue will ever be available. However, drug administration is now a secondary priority during CPR with primary emphasis placed on high-quality chest compressions with minimal hands-off time. Since there is little evidence for their use, the number of pharmacologic agents recommended during CPR decreased.

Route of Administration for Resuscitation Medications. It is important to remember that a central venous line may not be available at the time of the arrest, nor is its immediate placement necessary to ensure survival. Peripheral intravenous access can be used effectively with the advantage of not interrupting CPR. When only a peripheral vascular access is available, it is crucial to rapidly follow the medication bolus with a 10- to 20-mL fluid bolus to ensure central delivery. If obtaining any venous access is difficult despite numerous attempts, intraosseous (IO) cannulation is an effective alternate for drug delivery. Studies in both children (172,173) and adults (174) suggest the effectiveness of this route in all age groups. Commercially available kits are available for easy use.

If IV or IO access cannot be achieved, then some resuscitation medications can be administered via instillation through an ET, if available. Lipid-soluble medications that can be delivered via ET are lidocaine, epinephrine, atropine, naloxone, and vasopressin. This route, however, results in much lower blood concentrations compared with IV administration. Optimal doses of the medications delivered via the ET route are not known, but it is recommended to administer at least 2 to $2\frac{1}{2}$ times the IV recommended doses. In fact, animal data suggest that using standard intravenous epinephrine doses via the ET route may not achieve high enough plasma concentrations to be effective (175,176).

Once vascular access is achieved, resuscitation drugs should be immediately readministered if cardiac arrest is still present.

Epinephrine. Epinephrine is the most commonly used medication during CPR. Epinephrine's primary action in CA is to increase the coronary perfusion pressure through systemic vasoconstriction mediated by its α-adrenergic effects. The

β-adrenergic effects are relatively unimportant. Indeed, even when complete β-adrenergic blockade is used in an animal cardiac arrest model, epinephrine is effective, whereas α-adrenergic blockade completely eliminates epinephrine's effects (177).

Epinephrine is used primarily during CA due to asystole and PEA. It is a second-line agent used for shock-refractory VF or pulseless VT. Although there are no clinical trials demonstrating that epinephrine is effective in CA, there is substantial animal data and anecdotal clinical experience that epinephrine elevates the coronary perfusion pressure and thus myocardial blood flow. There are little pharmacologic data supporting the currently recommended dose of 1 mg of epinephrine in adult cardiac arrest and 0.01 mg/kg in children. Epinephrine should be given intravascularly whenever possible since intratracheal doses are erratically absorbed as noted above. If only the endotracheal route is available, the dose should be increased to 2 to 2.5 mg in adults and 0.1 mg/kg in children.

Since epinephrine's beneficial effect is through systemic vasoconstriction, it seems reasonable to speculate that higher doses would produce a greater increase in coronary and cerebral perfusion pressure. This hypothesis was supported by initial animal data (178), but subsequent animal studies (179,180) and clinical trials in adults (181,182) and children (183) failed to show a beneficial effect. Indeed, clinical experience suggests that high-dose epinephrine is harmful rather than beneficial and is only indicated in clinical conditions characterized by poor adrenergic responsiveness, such as severe septic shock and β blocker, neuraxial anesthesia, or systemic bupivacaine overdose.

Vasopressin. Vasopressin is an endogenous antidiuretic hormone that, when given at high doses, causes vasoconstriction by directly stimulating vascular smooth muscle V1 receptors (184). Vasopressin improves coronary perfusion pressure, but unlike epinephrine, offers theoretical advantages of cerebral vasodilation, possibly improving cerebral perfusion. Its lack of β_1-adrenergic activity potentially avoids unnecessary increases of myocardial oxygen consumption, resulting in postresuscitation arrhythmias. Vasopressin has a longer half-life of 10 to 20 minutes compared to the 3 to 5 minutes observed with epinephrine.

Several human studies suggested that vasopressin achieved a comparable ROSC in CA, although no additional benefit was seen compared with epinephrine (185,186). A recent meta-analysis showed a trend favoring vasopressin (187) compared to epinephrine. Recent guidelines continue to recommend epinephrine as the agent of choice, but one dose of vasopressin 40 units IV/IO is now indicated as an alternative to replace the first or second dose of epinephrine in all CA including asystole and PEA.

Vasopressin is not currently recommended for pediatric use since in an animal model of pediatric asphyxial CA, ROSC was higher in the epinephrine group (188). Vasopressin is contraindicated in conscious patients with ischemic heart disease as it may provoke angina. Other adverse effects include increased mesenteric and renal vascular resistance, bronchial constriction, and uterine contractions in women.

Sodium bicarbonate. Metabolic and respiratory acidosis develops during CA resulting from anaerobic metabolism, leading to lactic acid generation and inadequate ventilation along with reduced blood flow during CPR, which leads to inadequate pulmonary delivery of carbon dioxide for elimination. Untreated acidosis suppresses spontaneous cardiac activity, decreases the electrical threshold required for the onset of ventricular fibrillation, decreases ventricular contractile force, and decreases cardiac responsiveness to catecholamine such as epinephrine. An elevated PCO_2 tension probably is more detrimental to myocardial function and catecholamine responsiveness than metabolic acidosis. CO_2 readily diffuses across myocardial cell membranes, causing intracellular acidosis and resulting in life-threatening derangements of myocardial function. Likewise, cerebrospinal fluid acidosis may occur secondary to the diffusion of CO_2 across the blood–brain barrier, producing postarrest cerebral acidosis. Since sodium bicarbonate buffering of excess protons transiently increases the PCO_2 tension, sodium bicarbonate administration without sufficient ventilation and circulation to remove the CO_2 that it produces seems to be more detrimental than helpful (189,190). Sodium bicarbonate therapy may be useful after interventions such as defibrillation, cardiac compression, intubation, ventilation, and more than one trial of epinephrine have been used. Some evidence suggests that any benefit from bicarbonate therapy may be related more to volume expansion from its high sodium content rather than its buffering effects (191).

If arterial blood gas and pH measurements are not available, the recommended initial dose of sodium bicarbonate is 1 mEq/kg intravenously; half of this dose may be repeated at 10-minute intervals. For pediatric patients, the 1 mEq/kg dose should be diluted 1:1 with sterile water to reduce the osmolality.

Administration of excessive amounts of sodium bicarbonate can result in metabolic alkalosis, leftward shift of the oxyhemoglobin dissociation curve, interference with tissue oxygenation, hypernatremia, hypokalemia, and worsening of respiratory and myocardial acidosis if adequate ventilation and perfusion cannot be achieved and maintained.

Atropine. Atropine is used during CPR for its vagolytic actions. A reduced vagal influence on the heart improves both the rate of sinoatrial node discharge and impulse conduction through the atrioventricular (AV) conduction system, with a resulting increase in heart rate.

Atropine is used in sinus bradycardia when accompanied by hypotension or frequent premature ventricular contractions (PVCs) secondary to unsuppressed ectopic electrical activity arising in the area of injured tissue during the prolonged period after repolarization. Sinus bradycardia after myocardial infarction may predispose the heart to the onset of ventricular fibrillation (192). When profound bradycardia is present, acceleration of the heart rate above 60 beats per minute (bpm) may improve cardiac output and reduce the incidence of ventricular fibrillation. Atropine also may be useful for treating high-degree AV block with a slow ventricular rate and asystole occurring after increased parasympathetic tone that results in suppression of the electrical activity to the heart (193).

The dosage of atropine for severe symptomatic bradycardia is 0.5 to 1.0 mg intravenously repeated every 3 to 5 minutes until the desired pulse rate is obtained or a maximum of 0.04 mg/kg has been given. A larger dose has little therapeutic value, and a smaller dose may actually slow the heart rate. Endotracheal dose is 2 to 2.5 mg. Although not routinely recommended in the treatment of asystole, when used, incremental doses of

1 mg are preferred, using up to three doses given every 3 to 5 minutes of CA.

Ventricular tachycardia and fibrillation after intravenous administration of atropine have been reported. In second-degree type II heart block, a paradoxical decrease in ventricular response may result (189).

Lidocaine. Lidocaine decreases ectopic electrical myocardial activity by raising the electrical stimulation threshold of the ventricle during diastole. In ischemic myocardial tissue after infarction, it may suppress re-entrant arrhythmias such as ventricular tachycardia or fibrillation. There is now good evidence, however, that other agents are superior to lidocaine in terminating VT (194,195); hence, it is not considered a first-line agent. The 2005 guidelines recommend lidocaine only when amiodarone is not available.

Lidocaine may be used in stable monomorphic VT and polymorphic VT with normal or prolonged QT interval if ventricular function is not decreased.

The loading dose of lidocaine is approximately 1 to 1.5 mg/kg given as an intravenous bolus. If needed, repeat 0.5 to 0.75 mg/kg every 5 to 10 minutes, up to a total of 3 mg/kg, followed by a continuous infusion of 30 to 50 μg/kg/minute (1–4 mg/minute in a 70-kg patient) (192).

Excessive doses may induce heart block or depression of sinus node discharge, especially in patients with pre-existing conduction disturbances. Toxicity may occur in oliguric or anuric patients because renally excreted lidocaine degradation products also have pharmacologic effects and toxic potential. Early signs of lidocaine toxicity are due to central nervous system (CNS) effects and include anxiety, loquacity, tremors, metallic taste, and tinnitus. These may be followed by somnolence, respiratory depression, apnea, and, in severe cases, cardiovascular collapse. If CNS irritability occurs, lidocaine therapy should be withdrawn and a barbiturate or a benzodiazepine may be administered if deemed necessary and if the patient's circulatory status is sufficiently stabilized.

Procainamide. Procainamide suppresses both atrial and ventricular arrhythmias with similar mechanisms of action to those of lidocaine. It may suppress an ectopic irritable focus and blocks re-entrant arrhythmias by slowing electrical conduction. Procainamide may be superior to lidocaine in terminating VT (196).

Procainamide is used in the management of PVCs, ventricular tachycardia, and persistent ventricular fibrillation, but amiodarone is usually preferred.

Incremental bolus injections of procainamide are slowly infused at 20 mg/minute until (a) the arrhythmia is controlled, (b) hypotension occurs, (c) the QRS complex is widened 50% from baseline, or (d) a total dose of 17 mg/kg (1.2 g in a 70-kg adult) is given followed by a continuous infusion of 1 to 4 mg/minute to prevent recurrent arrhythmias. Other effective administration schedules have been tested and approved; all are designed to maintain a therapeutic plasma level of 4 to 8 μg/mL.

Procainamide can have profound myocardial depressant effects, especially after myocardial infarction; therefore, continuous ECG and arterial blood pressure monitoring are mandatory. End points of therapy include hypotension and a greater than 50% widening of the QRS complex.

Amiodarone. IV amiodarone is a complex drug with effects on sodium, potassium, and calcium channels on myocardial cells as well as α- and β-adrenergic blocking properties. The 2005 guidelines denote that it is the preferred agent for both atrial and ventricular arrhythmias, especially in the presence of impaired cardiac function.

Amiodarone is recommended for narrow-complex tachycardias that originate from a re-entry mechanism (re-entry SVT); ectopic atrial focus; control of hemodynamically stable VT, polymorphic VT with a normal QT interval, or wide-complex tachycardia of uncertain origin (195,197); and control of rapid ventricular rate due to accessory pathway conduction in pre-excited atrial arrhythmias with AV nodal blockade in patients with preserved or impaired ventricular function (198).

In the treatment of arrhythmias with a pulse, 150 mg amiodarone is given IV over 10 minutes, followed by a 1 mg/minute infusion for 6 hours and then a 0.5 mg/minute maintenance infusion over 18 hours. Supplementary infusions of 150 mg can be repeated every 10 minutes as necessary for recurrent or resistant arrhythmias to a maximum manufacturer-recommended total daily IV dose of 2.2 g. One study found amiodarone to be effective in patients with atrial fibrillation when administered at relatively high doses of 125 mg/hour for 24 hours (total dose 3 g) (199).

When used in the treatment of VF or pulseless VT, a bolus dose of 300 mg is recommended diluted in 20 to 30 mL of D5W. A single second dose may be given (150 mg) in 3 to 5 minutes for shock-refractory VF or VT. In children, 5 mg/kg is given as a rapid bolus and may be repeated up to 15 mg/kg.

The major adverse effects of amiodarone are hypotension and bradycardia, which can be prevented by slowing the rate of drug infusion. In addition, amiodarone can increase the QT interval, and therefore its use should be carefully considered when other drugs that can prolong the QT interval are administered.

Calcium. Calcium ion plays a critical role in myocardial contractility and action potential generation, but studies have shown no benefit of calcium in CA (200,201), and therefore calcium probably should not be considered during CA only when acute hyperkalemia or hypocalcemia is suspected or calcium channel blockers were administered. The use of calcium during CA is controversial because of the fear that it may produce a tetanic contraction of an irritable myocardium or depression of the sinus node, resulting in asystole. Since maintenance of the 10,000-fold higher extracellular calcium concentration compared with the intracellular concentration is energy dependent, exposing hypoxic-ischemic cells to high plasma calcium concentrations may result in calcium overload, which activates a number of toxic mechanisms. This effect is particularly worrisome in the brain because it is so sensitive to hypoxia.

When indicated, the recommended dose is 5 to 10 mL of a 10% solution of calcium chloride (8–16 mg/kg). A bolus may be repeated at 10-minute intervals, if necessary. Calcium salts cannot be mixed directly with sodium bicarbonate because it precipitates as calcium carbonate. Several calcium preparations are available for intravenous use: Calcium chloride and calcium gluconate are the most popular. Calcium gluconate is given in a dose of 6 to 8 mL if peripheral IV access is available. Undiluted calcium chloride given through a peripheral vein may cause sclerosis and tissue injury; therefore, if a central site is not available and the patient is not in cardiac arrest, it should either be diluted or calcium administered in a less irritating form (e.g., calcium gluconate). In children, a dose of 10 to 20 mg/kg of calcium chloride is recommended.

Rapid administration of a large bolus of calcium chloride, especially through a central venous catheter, may produce severe sinus bradycardia or sinus arrest. Calcium must also be used cautiously in patients receiving digitalis, because it can produce or accentuate digitalis toxicity.

Magnesium. Magnesium is recommended for the treatment of torsades de pointes VT with or without cardiac arrest. It has not been shown to be helpful during non–torsades de pointes VT (202,203). Although magnesium is a calcium channel blocker and theoretically may protect ischemic cells from overload, there are no data supporting its routine use in cardiac arrest. If needed, magnesium is given at a dose of 1 to 2 g diluted in D5W over 10 to 60 minutes. In children, a dose of 25 to 50 mg/kg is used.

Rapid administration may result in hypotension and bradycardia. Magnesium also should be used cautiously in patients with renal failure.

Algorithms for Advanced Life Support

The treatment algorithms of pulseless cardiac arrest and tachycardia with pulse are summarized in Figures 46.2 and 46.3, respectively.

Monitoring during Cardiopulmonary Resuscitation

Clinical

There are no reliable clinical indicators of the effectiveness of CPR provided. Although feeling for a pulse during chest compressions is used clinically to assess the effectiveness of chest compressions, no study has validated this technique. Moreover, data show that a palpated femoral pulse may be from retrograde venous pulsation rather than antegrade arterial flow (204).

Hemodynamics

When invasive arterial and central venous pressure monitoring are present, coronary perfusion pressure (CoPP) monitoring is possible. It is calculated as CoPP = aortic diastolic pressure minus the right atrial pressure (CoPP = DBP – RAP). A CoPP >15 mm Hg is predictive of ROSC (193,205) and increased CoPP correlates with improved 24-hour survival in animal studies (206).

Arterial Blood Gas

The acidosis gradient between arterial and central venous blood (largely determined by PCO_2) reflects the effectiveness of blood flow during low-flow states such as CPR (207). Similarly, animal studies and case reports report similar arteriovenous differences in PCO_2 between arterial and venous blood at the organ level (e.g., heart) and the entire organism (208–210). These studies suggest that measurement and comparison of a venous and arterial blood gas may be predictive during cardiac arrest. Furthermore, it suggests that the arterial blood gas does not accurately reflect the severity of tissue acidosis, hypoxia, or hypercarbia during both in-hospital and out-of-hospital cardiac arrest. Instead, the arterial blood gas often reflects the effectiveness of ventilation during cardiac arrest. Similarly, both animal and human data show a significant worsening of the arterial blood gas values for acidosis and oxygenation with ROSC, representing the washout of built-up tissue acids.

End-tidal Carbon Dioxide

Aerobic and anaerobic cellular metabolism generates CO_2, which rapidly diffuses out of the cell and into tissue capillaries, is transported to the lungs, is exhaled, and can be measured as end-tidal CO_2 (211,212). Under normal conditions, end-tidal PCO_2 is 2 to 5 mm Hg less than the $PaCO_2$. Although ischemic hypoxia can alter the respiratory quotient, systemic metabolism changes little during CPR, which is relatively brief, so that changes in end-tidal PCO_2 during CPR typically reflects changes in the effective pulmonary blood flow (211,212). Under conditions of constant minute ventilation, end-tidal CO_2 is linearly related to cardiac output, even during extremely low blood flow rates (213), and is therefore useful clinically as a monitor of perfusion during shock and CPR. Indeed, a number of studies showed that end-tidal CO_2 varies directly with cardiac output during cardiac arrest (214–216) and provides a useful indicator of the efficacy of resuscitation efforts. Not surprisingly, $ETCO_2$ also predicts outcome in adults (217–220) and children (221). Additionally, capnography is used in resuscitation research as an indication of pulmonary blood flow, which serves as a proxy for the direct measurement of cardiac output (120,222,223).

Following the administration of epinephrine, end-tidal CO_2 typically falls, suggesting that the relationship of end-tidal CO_2 to cardiac output is altered, but in fact it is maintained and reflects a global fall in cardiac output due to changes in pulmonary and peripheral vascular resistance and preferential redirection of blood flow (219). When used in cardiac arrest, epinephrine decreases pulmonary blood flow (i.e., overall cardiac output) and end-tidal CO_2 while increasing coronary perfusion pressure and myocardial blood flow because of increased peripheral vascular resistance (224).

Coronary artery perfusion pressure also correlates closely with end-tidal CO_2 (218,225). Several studies of end-tidal carbon dioxide during low blood flow states found that levels changed significantly with changes in minute ventilation (226). When minute ventilation doubled, end-tidal carbon dioxide decreased by 50%, and when minute ventilation decreased by 50%, end-tidal carbon dioxide doubled. Thus, end-tidal carbon dioxide varies inversely with minute ventilation and can be used to monitor ventilation during low-flow conditions. If both perfusion and ventilation are changed, end-tidal carbon dioxide levels can be difficult to interpret.

Postresuscitation Care

After ROSC, the risk of mortality remains high for cardiac arrest patients as most deaths happen during the first 24 hours following successful resuscitation (227,228). Postresuscitation care is one of the most important elements of CPR that can potentially result in improved outcome (229). The goals of postresuscitation care are to (a) optimize cardiovascular and neurologic support, (b) identify the possible cause of arrest

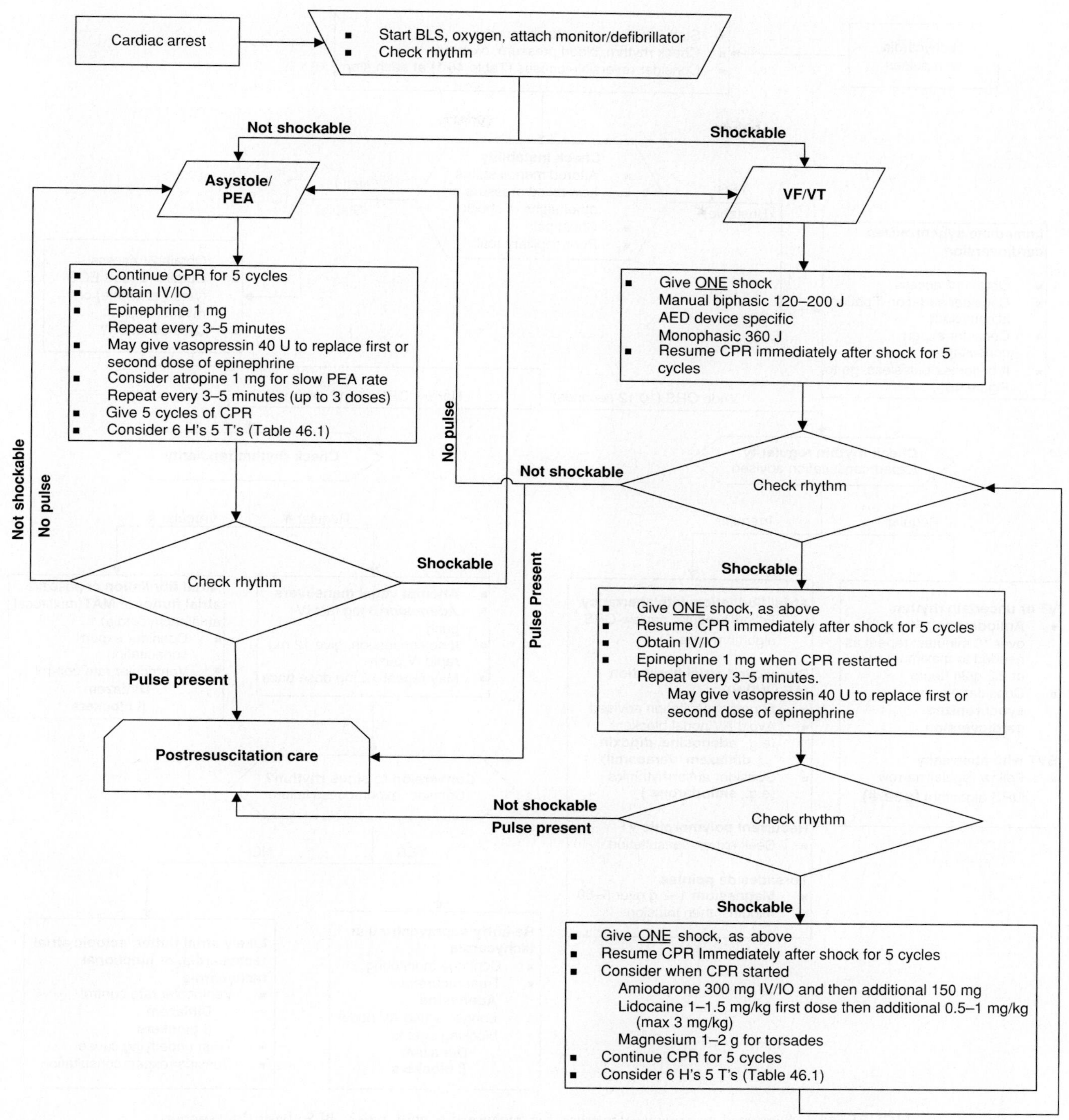

FIGURE 46.2. Suggested treatment algorithm for pulseless cardiac arrest. It is important that resuscitation drugs should be given during the cardiopulmonary resuscitation (CPR) cycles to minimize "no CPR" time. BLS, basic life support; PEA, pulseless electrical activity; VF, ventricular fibrillation; VT, ventricular tachycardia; AED, automated external defibrillator; IO, intraosseous. (Adapted and modified from 2005 American Heart Association Guidelines for Cardiopulmonary Resuscitation and Emergency Cardiovascular Care. *Circulation.* 2005;112[24]SIV-1–IV-211.)

and prevent recurrence, and (c) use measures that may improve long-term neurologic outcome.

After ROSC, vital signs, clinical and laboratory signs of tissue perfusion, the occurrence of cardiac arrhythmias, and neurologic status should be frequently monitored. Obtain appropriate intravenous and intra-arterial vascular access as needed to monitor the patient and obtain frequent laboratory studies. Obtain an arterial or central venous blood gas (preferably both) to assess for the presence of acid-base abnormalities, and obtain electrolytes including magnesium, phosphorus, ionized

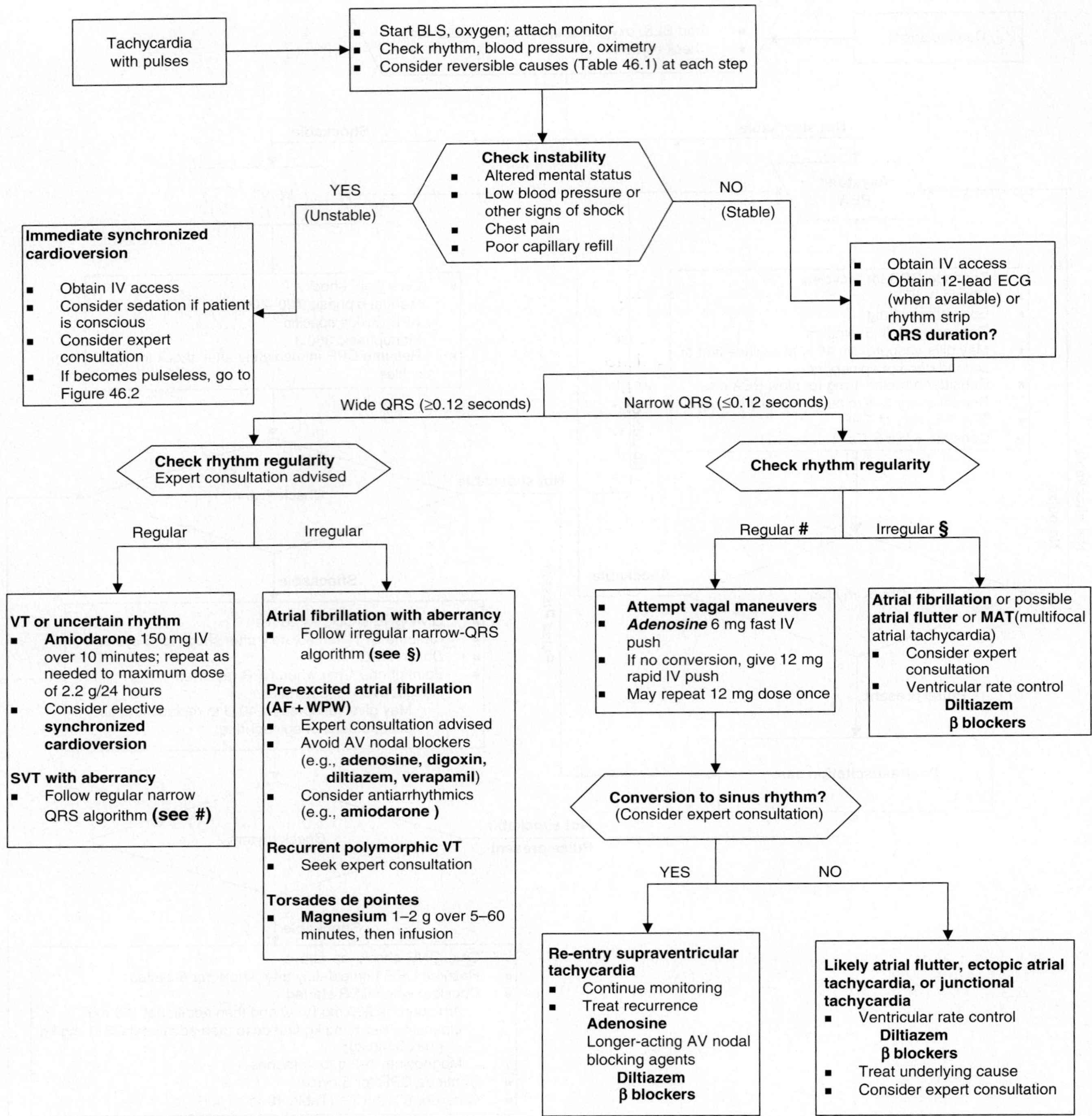

FIGURE 46.3. Suggested treatment algorithm for tachycardia with pulse. BLS, basic life support; ECG, electrocardiogram; VT, ventricular tachycardia; SVT, supraventricular tachycardia; WPW, Wolff-Parkinson-White syndrome. (Adapted and modified from 2005 American Heart Association Guidelines for Cardiopulmonary Resuscitation and Emergency Cardiovascular Care. *Circulation.* 2005;112[24]SIV-1–IV-211.)

calcium, and blood urea nitrogen (BUN) to ensure that there are no electrolyte abnormalities and to help assess renal function. The gradient between arterial and venous oxygen saturation can help evaluate the adequacy of tissue perfusion. Trained personnel with resuscitation equipment must accompany the patient during transport to an appropriate monitoring unit.

It is increasingly recognized that postresuscitation care has an important effect on ultimate survival following cardiac arrest. Studies are currently evaluating optimal treatments for postresuscitation care (230). The following are generally accepted as part of postresuscitation care.

Glucose Control

Many studies showed a strong association between hyperglycemia after cardiac arrest and poor neurologic outcome (28,231–233). Hyperglycemia developing after cardiac arrest likely reflects the effects of epinephrine and endogenous stress hormones as well as reduced glucose metabolism by the injured brain. What is not clear, however, is whether control of the glucose concentration following cardiac arrest results in an improved outcome. Data from studies in adult surgical and medical critical care patients showed reduced mortality with tight glucose control (234,235). Based on these data in critically ill patients, it seems reasonable to normalize the glucose concentration in patients after cardiac arrest, but the evidence for this approach is lacking. Furthermore, it is not clear if glucose should be restricted or if insulin should be used to normalize the glucose concentration, but the general approach is to frequently monitor the glucose concentration and use an insulin infusion to normalize the glucose concentration if it is elevated. The target range for glucose concentration in this situation is not known, but a range of 80 to 110 mg/dL is commonly used. The risk of this approach is that hypoglycemia may occur, resulting in further injury to at-risk brain cells.

Respiratory System

Some respiratory dysfunction can be present after ROSC, and patients require ongoing mechanical ventilation and oxygen administration. ET position should be assessed upon arrival to the critical care unit. Ventilator support should be adjusted to help normalize the patient's acid-base status and work of breathing, while recognizing that high respiratory rates and airway pressure may impair venous return and thus cardiac output. If an end-tidal CO_2 monitor is available, ventilation rate should be adjusted to maintain end-tidal CO_2 within a range of about 35 mm Hg to 45 mm Hg. In patients with obstructive pulmonary disease and increased resistance to exhalation, a lower ventilation rate should be used (e.g., six to eight breaths per minute) to prevent air trapping and to allow enough time for complete exhalation (132).

If more severe injury is present, it is usually due to pulmonary edema, gastric content aspiration, or acute respiratory distress syndrome (ARDS). While generally in these cases oxygenation may be improved by the application of positive end-expiratory pressure, more detailed treatment guidelines are reviewed in other sections of this textbook.

Cardiovascular System

Cardiac function and rhythm can be altered after cardiac arrest. This results from both global ischemia and reperfusion injury post ROSC or by the effect of defibrillation itself, which can cause myocardial stunning (236,237). Hemodynamic instability is common after cardiac arrest and may be multifactorial including a combination of cardiac dysfunction, altered capillary permeability, variations in venous and arterial vascular tone, and the elaboration of cytokines that may mimic sepsis (238). Invasive hemodynamic monitoring and judicious use of inotropes with vasopressor or vasodilators properties may be needed (227).

Although post–cardiac arrest arrhythmias may be detrimental, prophylactic treatment may also produce adverse effects, so prophylactic antiarrhythmics are not recommended. If an antiarrhythmic was used to achieve ROSC, then it should be continued, although the selection of antiarrhythmic agents for longer-term use is best made in consultation with a cardiologist.

Central Nervous System

After ROSC, the brain often experiences an initial brief increased blood flow ("hyperemia") phase, which is followed by a significantly reduced ("no-reflow phenomenon") phase due to microvascular dysfunction and thrombosis (239,240). In addition, excitatory neurotransmitters are released, increasing metabolic demand in vulnerable areas of the brain such as the hippocampus. In general, efforts are focused on optimizing cerebral perfusion pressure by treating hypotension and maintaining, when feasible, a 20% to 30% higher than normal mean arterial pressure, especially in cases at risk for increased intracranial pressure. Fever and seizures can be seriously detrimental to the brain and should be aggressively treated. There are insufficient data to recommend for or against the use of prophylactic anticonvulsants in postcardiac arrest.

Temperature Control

Avoiding Hyperthermia. Temperature dysregulation may be present after ROSC, which may result from brain injury as shown in animal models of cardiac arrest (241–244). Fever is associated with worse neurologic outcome in humans after cardiac arrest or ischemic brain injury (245,246). Antipyretics and surface cooling techniques should be used to achieve normothermia. Some experts recommend routine administration of antipyretics, and the 2005 guidelines recommend frequent or continuous temperature monitoring and aggressive treatment of fever in the postarrest setting.

Hypothermia after Cardiac Arrest. In 2002, two prospective randomized controlled clinical trials of therapeutic hypothermia were conducted in comatose survivors after cardiac arrest in adults. In the Australian study (247), survivors of out-of-hospital VF cardiac arrest with coma were randomized in the field by EMS providers to hypothermia or normothermia, with cooling beginning in the prehospital setting. Cooling was maintained for 12 hours followed by passive rewarming. Good outcome (survival and good functional recovery) was observed in 21 of 43 (49%) hypothermic patients versus 9 of 34 (26%) normothermic patients ($p = 0.046$; number needed to treat [NNT] = 5; 95% confidence interval [CI], 2.3–81). A larger European trial in a similar patient population (248) showed favorable neurologic outcome at 6 months with the use of 24 hours of therapeutic hypothermia begun after hospital arrival following out-of-hospital ventricular fibrillation cardiac arrest (75 of 136 [55%]) compared with the normothermic group (54 of 137 [39%]). The risk ratio for this study was 1.40 (95% CI, 1.08–1.81) and the NNT was 7 (95% CI, 3.6–25). Subsequently, the ILCOR recommended the use of therapeutic hypothermia for adult patients who were comatose following ventricular fibrillation cardiac arrest and suggested that hypothermia should be considered in comatose patients with other rhythms after out-of-hospital cardiac arrest (249).

Several neonatal trials also showed a beneficial effect of 72 hours of therapeutic hypothermia following perinatal asphyxia (250,251), but there are no clinical data in children to recommend for or against the routine use of hypothermia in the postarrest setting.

Hypothermia can be applied in two ways after cardiac arrest: (a) permissive hypothermia, maintaining the mild hypothermia >33°C that is often present in postarrest patients; or (b) induced hypothermia, where patients are actively cooled to the 32°C to 34°C range. Currently, consensus guidelines for induction, maintenance, and weaning of therapeutic hypothermia do not exist. Some recent studies have explored methods of internal cooling using cold saline boluses or endovascular catheters (252). We recently surveyed a sample from the pediatric critical care community and found that despite awareness of this technique, it is not widely applied. There is variation in methods, temperature goal, and duration of cooling, with most clinicians using external cooling techniques with target temperature ranging from 33°C to 35°C for 12 to 24 hours (253).

Prolonged or deeper hypothermia increases the risk of infection, coagulopathy, thrombocytopenia, renal impairment, and pancreatitis (254,255). It is likely that induced hypothermia will affect drug metabolism, but there are little objective data to guide clinical therapy. Further studies are needed to develop standard protocols for this brain-protective therapy.

Extracorporeal Life Support and Cardiopulmonary Resuscitation

Rapid use of extracorporeal membrane oxygenation (ECMO) in the context of CPR is termed extracorporeal cardiopulmonary resuscitation (ECPR). This technique is invasive and requires emergent cannulation of a large central vein and artery. Venous blood is passed through a membrane oxygenator for oxygenation and removal of CO_2 and returned in an artery to augment blood circulation. The setup and personnel required for this procedure are available in few large tertiary care centers with an in-house multidisciplinary team available to rapidly prepare the ECMO circuit. ECPR has been used in both pediatric and adult patients with primarily cardiac disease with a reported survival of 64% in neonates, 50% in children, and 51% in adults (256,257). In a large single-center report (258), 64 children who failed initial advanced life support were placed on ECMO during active CPR with the median duration of chest compressions of 50 minutes (range 5–105 minutes); remarkably, 33 (50%) survived for 24 hours and 21 (33%) survived to hospital discharge. Five of the survivors were noted to have significant neurologic impairment at hospital discharge. Use of extraordinary measures like ECPR and ECMO seems reasonable if the patient's condition is reversible and ECMO can be established before irreversible brain damage happens during the cardiac arrest. One advantage of extracorporeal circulatory support is that it is relatively easy to rapidly cool the patient and maintain the target temperature for brain protection.

ETHICAL CONSIDERATIONS

Termination of Cardiopulmonary Resuscitation Efforts

CPR is inappropriate when survival is not expected. Even in the ICU, CPR can be administered by rescuers who may not know the patient or the advanced directive status of the patient. There are few criteria that can reliably predict the futility of CPR. Therefore, it is recommended that all patients with cardiopulmonary arrest receive CPR with the following exceptions:

1. There is a valid Do Not Attempt Resuscitation (DNAR) order, which can be verified.
2. Signs of irreversible death are already present (e.g., rigor mortis, decapitation, decomposition, dependent lividity).
3. No physiologic benefit can be expected with further CPR.
4. In newborns, gestational age or congenital abnormality is related to almost certain early death.

In the ICU, CPR is started without a physician's order, which is based on implied consent for emergency treatment. As a minimal standard, it is expected that all nursing staff in the unit are able to immediately start BLS and be knowledgeable on the use of an automatic external defibrillator. However, the decision to stop CPR should be made by a physician treating the patient, ideally familiar with the patient's pre-existing conditions. Although many factors have been studied as a guide to determine the futility of CPR, such as the presence of comorbidities, time to CPR, time to defibrillate, and initial rhythm, none of these either alone or in combination reliably predicts chances of neurologically intact survival (259,260). On rare occasions, good outcome with prolonged CPR has been reported (261–263). It is acceptable to prolong resuscitative efforts in children with recurrent VF or VT, drug toxicity, or a primary hypothermic insult.

Family Presence during Cardiopulmonary Resuscitation

It has been a common practice to exclude family of the arrest victim during CPR efforts. Helping the family of a dying patient is an important part of CPR and should be done in a compassionate manner considering the family's cultural and religious beliefs and practices. Although there is concern that allowing family presence may become disruptive, interfere with resuscitation, cause them to experience syncope, and increase the risk of legal liability (264–266), these concerns were not substantiated by good evidence, and in the authors' experience these factors are not a major issue. Family surveys following CPR suggested that the majority of family members want to be present during CPR (267,268). It is also suggested that being present at the time of death was comforting and helped with adjustment later (269). In pediatric arrest, most parents surveyed wanted an option to be present during CPR (270). The resuscitation team should be sensitive to the family's presence and a team member should be assigned to comfort the family, answer questions, and clarify the procedures.

Future Considerations

Current Performance during Cardiopulmonary Resuscitation

Although U.S. and international guidelines continue to recommend high-quality CPR to improve survival from cardiac arrest (271), disturbing evidence seems to indicate that this is not happening in most cases. Studies suggest that bystander CPR in witnessed cardiac arrest is performed in only about one third of the cases (272,273). There are several suggested reasons for this finding: CPR algorithms are complicated, training is inadequate, retention of skills is difficult, and both lay rescuer and professionals are afraid of transmission of diseases (274–276).

An out-of hospital cardiac arrest observational study in 176 adults showed that chest compressions were given only half of the available time during the resuscitation event. When CPR was performed by professional rescuers, compression time increased but still averaged 80% of the total resuscitation time (94). In the same setting (277), it was reported that police and firefighters performed CPR correctly only 45% of the time while waiting for ambulance personnel. Prehospital data indicate that most of the time "wasted" without CPR could be explained by programmed interruptions from automated defibrillators or pulse check. The quality of in-hospital CPR is also discouraging. Even highly trained hospital personnel such as ICU physicians often fall short of CPR guidelines during resuscitation efforts (95).

One other issue is the inability to completely relax the chest during the decompression phase (85). Recent laboratory data suggest that rescuer fatigue is an important cause of poor BLS CPR. Reduced performance due to fatigue was noted after just 1 minute and the magnitude was proportional to the compression speed. In a manikin model, an increased compression-to-ventilation ratio of 15:2 provided only 14.5% more compressions than a C:V ratio of 5:1, but nearly 81% of the rescuers perceived that a C:V ratio of 15:2 was more tiring than a 5:1 ratio (104). The quality of compressions seems to decrease significantly after 1 minute and then again between 4 and 5 minutes of CPR, suggesting the need for frequent rescuer rotations, between 1 and 5 minutes, to optimize the effectiveness of chest compression. Interestingly, subjective awareness of fatigue is usually present only after 5 minutes, despite the substantial decrease of chest compression depth at 1 minute (278). Decay of chest compression quality always includes rate and depth.

Studies have shown that the decay of skill mastery is almost immediate after a CPR class with a trend toward too shallow compressions by lay rescuers (279) and too deep compressions by health professionals (280). In general, repeated manikin training is more successful in correcting too shallow compressions than too deep (280).

Another study revealed that most trained personnel provided too much ventilation, $\sim$30 breaths/minute, during out-of-hospital cardiac arrest. Hyperventilation increases mean airway pressure, resulting in decreased venous return and cardiac output, which worsens survival (40).

Training Needs for Quality Improvement

Involvement of Lay Rescuers

Few advanced life support interventions improve survival of SCA patients. It is recognized that early and effective CPR and defibrillation are effective. Therefore, there is a need to increase access to CPR education and improve CPR training quality and retention of skills.

Feedback Devices

Use of devices that can help rescuers by prompting or giving voice feedback or tone may increase the effectiveness of CPR. These devices improve $ETCO_2$ and quality of CPR in both in-hospital and out-of-hospital settings (98,281–283).

Medical Emergency Teams

Recently, there is increased emphasis on the use of a dedicated in-hospital rapid response system (RRS) for early intervention in at-risk patients. There are two components of this system: (a) case recognition and team activation, and (b) the emergent medical response. Medical emergency teams (METs) are the response component of an RRS that has the capability of prescribing therapy, providing advance airway management, securing central venous access, and beginning ICU-level care at the bedside (284). These teams are often composed of experienced nurses and doctors with skills in critical care who are available 24 hours a day to seek out, assess, and manage patients who clinically pose a threat to develop cardiac arrest. Several small studies documented reduction in cardiac arrest rates with the use of METs (285,286), but a recent large clustered randomized study was not able to show any difference in cardiac arrest, unexpected death, and unplanned ICU admissions with the use of METs (287). Further studies are needed to evaluate the effectiveness and feasibility of METs.

Research Considerations

Research in patients with CA is extremely challenging. Most of the interventions need to be applied very quickly to be beneficial, which makes it hard for researchers to obtain institutional review board approval.

Ethical Considerations and Informed Consent

Obtaining consent from family is not always possible or practical at the time of cardiac arrest. Some researchers argue that presuming consent in these patients serves a benefit to the living and others argue that since the patient is clinically dead, consent is unnecessary since a dead patient is without autonomy. This argument does not account for the potential emotional harm to the family, who may oppose use of a deceased loved one for research, and also does not account for their cultural and religious beliefs.

Recently the importance of CPR research was recognized and the FDA adopted regulations that allow exception for consent in certain circumstances. Obtaining an exception requires the researcher to consult with experts in the field and representative lay persons, along with open and full public disclosure of the study, including the methodologic details of, need for, and benefit of the research.

References

1. Chugh SS, Jui J, Gunson K, et al. Current burden of sudden cardiac death: multiple source surveillance versus retrospective death certificate-based review in a large U.S. community. *J Am Coll Cardiol.* 2004;44(6):1268–1275.
2. Vaillancourt C, Stiell IG. Cardiac arrest care and emergency medical services in Canada. *Can J Cardiol.* 2004;20(11):1081–1090.
3. Valenzuela TD, Roe DJ, Cretin S, et al. Estimating effectiveness of cardiac arrest interventions: a logistic regression survival model. *Circulation.* 1997;96(10):3308–3313.
4. Nadkarni VM, Larkin GL, Peberdy MA, et al. First documented rhythm and clinical outcome from in-hospital cardiac arrest among children and adults. *JAMA.* 2006;295(1):50–57.
5. Holmberg M, Holmberg S, Herlitz J. Effect of bystander cardiopulmonary resuscitation in out-of-hospital cardiac arrest patients in Sweden. *Resuscitation.* 2000;47(1):59–70.

6. Larsen MP, Eisenberg MS, Cummins RO, et al. Predicting survival from out-of-hospital cardiac arrest: a graphic model. *Ann Emerg Med.* 1993; 22(11):1652–1658.
7. Callans DJ. Out-of-hospital cardiac arrest—the solution is shocking. *N Engl J Med.* 2004;351(7):632–634.
8. Wik L, Hansen TB, Fylling F, et al. Delaying defibrillation to give basic cardiopulmonary resuscitation to patients with out-of-hospital ventricular fibrillation: a randomized trial. *JAMA.* 2003;289(11):1389–1395.
9. Kellum MJ, Kennedy KW, Ewy GA. Cardiocerebral resuscitation improves survival of patients with out-of-hospital cardiac arrest. *Am J Med.* 2006;119(4):335–340.
10. 2005 American Heart Association (AHA) guidelines for cardiopulmonary resuscitation (CPR) and emergency cardiovascular care (ECC) of pediatric and neonatal patients: pediatric basic life support. *Pediatrics.* 2006; 117(5):e989–1004.
11. Gasco Garcia MC, Rabanal Llevot JM. [New directives for basic and advanced cardiopulmonary resuscitation from the International Liaison Committee on Resuscitation (ILCOR). Directives of the European Resuscitation Council (ERC) for 2005.] *Rev Esp Anestesiol Reanim.* 2006;53(5):273–274.
12. The International Liaison Committee on Resuscitation (ILCOR) consensus on science with treatment recommendations for pediatric and neonatal patients: neonatal resuscitation. *Pediatrics.* 2006;117(5):e978–988.
13. Jacobs I, Nadkarni V, Bahr J, et al. Cardiac arrest and cardiopulmonary resuscitation outcome reports: update and simplification of the Utstein templates for resuscitation registries. A statement for healthcare professionals from a task force of the international liaison committee on resuscitation (American Heart Association, European Resuscitation Council, Australian Resuscitation Council, New Zealand Resuscitation Council, Heart and Stroke Foundation of Canada, InterAmerican Heart Foundation, Resuscitation Council of Southern Africa). *Resuscitation.* 2004;63(3):233–249.
14. Cummins RO. The Utstein style for uniform reporting of data from out-of-hospital cardiac arrest. *Ann Emerg Med.* 1993;22(1):37–40.
15. Cummins RO, Chamberlain D, Hazinski MF, et al. Recommended guidelines for reviewing, reporting, and conducting research on in-hospital resuscitation: the in-hospital 'Utstein style'. A statement for healthcare professionals from the American Heart Association, the European Resuscitation Council, the Heart and Stroke Foundation of Canada, the Australian Resuscitation Council, and the Resuscitation Councils of Southern Africa. *Resuscitation.* 1997;34(2):151–183.
16. Zaritsky A, Nadkarni V, Hazinski MF, et al. Recommended guidelines for uniform reporting of pediatric advanced life support: the pediatric Utstein Style. A statement for healthcare professionals from a task force of the American Academy of Pediatrics, the American Heart Association, and the European Resuscitation Council. Writing Group. *Circulation.* 1995;92(7):2006–2020.
17. Peberdy MA, Kaye W, Ornato JP, et al. Cardiopulmonary resuscitation of adults in the hospital: a report of 14720 cardiac arrests from the National Registry of Cardiopulmonary Resuscitation. *Resuscitation.* 2003; 58(3):297–308.
18. Myerburg RJ, Fenster J, Velez M, et al. Impact of community-wide police car deployment of automated external defibrillators on survival from out-of-hospital cardiac arrest. *Circulation.* 2002;106(9):1058–1064.
19. Eisenburger P, Sterz F, Haugk M, et al. Cardiac arrest in public locations—an independent predictor for better outcome? *Resuscitation.* 2006;70(3):395–403.
20. Donoghue AJ, Nadkarni V, Berg RA, et al. Out-of-hospital pediatric cardiac arrest: an epidemiologic review and assessment of current knowledge. *Ann Emerg Med.* 2005;46(6):512–522.
21. Herlitz J, Bahr J, Fischer M, et al. Resuscitation in Europe: a tale of five European regions. *Resuscitation.* 1999;41(2):121–131.
22. Berger R, Kelley M. Survival after in-hospital cardiopulmonary arrest of noncritically ill patients. A prospective study. *Chest.* 1994;106(3):872–879.
23. Brindley PG, Markland DM, Mayers I, et al. Predictors of survival following in-hospital adult cardiopulmonary resuscitation. *CMAJ.* 2002;167(4):343–348.
24. Cohn AC, Wilson WM, Yan B, et al. Analysis of clinical outcomes following in-hospital adult cardiac arrest. *Intern Med J.* 2004;34(7):398–402.
25. Sandroni C, Ferro G, Santangelo S, et al. In-hospital cardiac arrest: survival depends mainly on the effectiveness of the emergency response. *Resuscitation.* 2004;62(3):291–297.
26. Samson RA, Nadkarni VM, Meaney PA, et al. Outcomes of in-hospital ventricular fibrillation in children. *N Engl J Med.* 2006;354(22):2328–2339.
27. Levy DE, Caronna JJ, Singer BH, et al. Predicting outcome from hypoxic-ischemic coma. *JAMA.* 1985;253(10):1420–1426.
28. Longstreth WT Jr, Diehr P, Inui TS. Prediction of awakening after out-of-hospital cardiac arrest. *N Engl J Med.* 1983;308(23):1378–1382.
29. Longstreth WT Jr, Inui TS, Cobb LA, et al. Neurologic recovery after out-of-hospital cardiac arrest. *Ann Intern Med.* 1983;98(5 Pt 1):588–592.
30. Gray WA, Capone RJ, Most AS. Unsuccessful emergency medical resuscitation—are continued efforts in the emergency department justified? *N Engl J Med.* 1991;325(20):1393–1398.
31. Jennett B, Bond M. Assessment of outcome after severe brain damage. *Lancet.* 1975;1(7905):480–484.
32. A randomized clinical study of a calcium-entry blocker (lidoflazine) in the treatment of comatose survivors of cardiac arrest. Brain Resuscitation Clinical Trial II Study Group. *N Engl J Med.* 1991;324(18):1225–1231.
33. Safar PB, Bircher NG. *Cardiopulmonary Cerebral Resuscitation: Basic and Advanced Cardiac and Trauma Life Support: An Introduction to Resuscitation Medicine.* 3rd ed. London: W.B. Saunders; 1988.
34. Fiser DH. Assessing the outcome of pediatric intensive care. *J Pediatr.* 1992; 121(1):68–74.
35. Fiser DH, Long N, Roberson PK, et al. Relationship of pediatric overall performance category and pediatric cerebral performance category scores at pediatric intensive care unit discharge with outcome measures collected at hospital discharge and 1- and 6-month follow-up assessments. *Crit Care Med.* 2000;28(7):2616–2620.
36. Fiser DH, Tilford JM, Roberson PK. Relationship of illness severity and length of stay to functional outcomes in the pediatric intensive care unit: a multi-institutional study. *Crit Care Med.* 2000;28(4):1173–1179.
37. Bottiger BW, Grabner C, Bauer H, et al. Long term outcome after out-of-hospital cardiac arrest with physician staffed emergency medical services: the Utstein style applied to a midsized urban/suburban area. *Heart.* 1999; 82(6):674–679.
38. Westal RE, Reissman S, Doering G. Out-of-hospital cardiac arrests: an 8-year New York City experience. *Am J Emerg Med.* 1996;14(4):364–368.
39. Waalewijn RA, Nijpels MA, Tijssen JG, et al. Prevention of deterioration of ventricular fibrillation by basic life support during out-of-hospital cardiac arrest. *Resuscitation.* 2002;54(1):31–36.
40. Aufderheide TP, Lurie KG. Death by hyperventilation: a common and life-threatening problem during cardiopulmonary resuscitation. *Crit Care Med.* 2004;32(9 Suppl):S345–351.
41. Safar P, Escarraga LA, Chang F. Upper airway obstruction in the unconscious patient. *J Appl Physiol.* 1959;14:760–764.
42. Eberle B, Dick WF, Schneider T, et al. Checking the carotid pulse check: diagnostic accuracy of first responders in patients with and without a pulse. *Resuscitation.* 1996;33(2):107–116.
43. Ruppert M, Reith MW, Widmann JH, et al. Checking for breathing: evaluation of the diagnostic capability of emergency medical services personnel, physicians, medical students, and medical laypersons. *Ann Emerg Med.* 1999;34(6):720–729.
44. Lawrence PJ, Sivaneswaran N. Ventilation during cardiopulmonary resuscitation: which method? *Med J Aust.* 1985;143(10):443–446.
45. 2005 International Consensus on Cardiopulmonary Resuscitation and Emergency Cardiovascular Care Science with Treatment Recommendations. Part 2: Adult basic life support. *Resuscitation.* 2005;67(2-3):187–201.
46. Johannigman JA, Branson RD, Davis K Jr, et al. Techniques of emergency ventilation: a model to evaluate tidal volume, airway pressure, and gastric insufflation. *J Trauma.* 1991;31(1):93–98.
47. McSwain GR, Garrison WB, Artz CP. Evaluation of resuscitation from cardiopulmonary arrest by paramedics. *Ann Emerg Med.* 1980;9(7):341–345.
48. Hess D, Baran C. Ventilatory volumes using mouth-to-mouth, mouth-to-mask, and bag-valve-mask techniques. *Am J Emerg Med.* 1985;3(4):292–296.
49. Jesudian MC, Harrison RR, Keenan RL, et al. Bag-valve-mask ventilation; two rescuers are better than one: preliminary report. *Crit Care Med.* 1985;13(2):122–123.
50. Campbell TP, Stewart RD, Kaplan RM, et al. Oxygen enrichment of bag-valve-mask units during positive-pressure ventilation: a comparison of various techniques. *Ann Emerg Med.* 1988;17(3):232–235.
51. Nam SH, Kim KJ, Nam YT, et al. The changes in delivered oxygen fractions using laerdal resuscitator bag with different types of reservoir. *Yonsei Med J.* 2001;42(2):242–246.
52. Hirschman AM, Kravath RE. Venting vs ventilating. A danger of manual resuscitation bags. *Chest.* 1982;82(3):369–370.
53. Lurie K, Zielinski T, McKnite S, et al. Improving the efficiency of cardiopulmonary resuscitation with an inspiratory impedance threshold valve. *Crit Care Med.* 2000;28(11 Suppl):N207–209.
54. Lurie KG, Mulligan KA, McKnite S, et al. Optimizing standard cardiopulmonary resuscitation with an inspiratory impedance threshold valve. *Chest.* 1998;113(4):1084–1090.
55. Sigurdsson G, Yannopoulos D, McKnite SH, et al. Effects of an inspiratory impedance threshold device on blood pressure and short term survival in spontaneously breathing hypovolemic pigs. *Resuscitation.* 2006;68(3): 399–404.
56. Bahr J, Klingler H, Panzer W, et al. Skills of lay people in checking the carotid pulse. *Resuscitation.* 1997;35(1):23–26.
57. Moule P. Checking the carotid pulse: diagnostic accuracy in students of the healthcare professions. *Resuscitation.* 2000;44(3):195–201.
58. Guidelines 2000 for Cardiopulmonary Resuscitation and Emergency Cardiovascular Care. Part 3: adult basic life support. The American Heart Association in collaboration with the International Liaison Committee on Resuscitation. *Circulation.* 2000;102(8 Suppl):I22–59.
59. Keen WW. Case of total laryngectomy (unsuccessful) and a case of abdomen hysterectomy (successful) in both which massage of the heart for chloroform collapse was employed, with notes of 25 other cases of cardiac massage. *Ther Gaz.* 1904;28:217–220.

60. Lee WE, Downs TM. Resuscitation by direct massage of the heart in the cardiac arrest. *Ann Surg.* 1924;80:555–561.
61. Bircher N, Safar P. Manual open-chest cardiopulmonary resuscitation. *Ann Emerg Med.* 1984;13(9 Pt 2):770–773.
62. Ewer MS, Ali MK, Frazier OH. Open chest resuscitation for cardiopulmonary arrest related to mechanical impairment of circulation: a report of two cases. *Crit Care Med.* 1982;10(3):198–199.
63. Alifimoff JK. Open versus closed chest cardiac massage in non-traumatic cardiac arrest. *Resuscitation.* 1987;15(1):13–21.
64. Robertson C. Open-chest cardiac massage for non-traumatic cardiac arrest. *Arch Emerg Med.* 1987;4(4):207–210.
65. Boczar ME, Howard MA, Rivers EP, et al. A technique revisited: hemodynamic comparison of closed- and open-chest cardiac massage during human cardiopulmonary resuscitation. *Crit Care Med.* 1995;23(3):498–503.
66. Pottle A, Bullock I, Thomas J, et al. Survival to discharge following open chest cardiac compression (OCCC). A 4-year retrospective audit in a cardiothoracic specialist centre–Royal Brompton and Harefield NHS Trust, United Kingdom. *Resuscitation.* 2002;52(3):269–272.
67. Raman J, Saldanha RF, Branch JM, et al. Open cardiac compression in the postoperative cardiac intensive care unit. *Anaesth Intensive Care.* 1989; 17(2):129–135.
68. Geehr EC, Lewis FR, Auerbach PS. Failure of open-heart massage to improve survival after prehospital nontraumatic cardiac arrest. *N Engl J Med.* 1986;314(18):1189–1190.
69. Kouwenhoven WB, Jude JR, Knickerbocker GG. Closed-chest cardiac massage. *JAMA.* 1960;173:1064–1067.
70. Jude JR, Kouwenhoven WB, Knickerbocker GG. Cardiac arrest. Report of application of external cardiac massage on 118 patients. *JAMA.* 1961; 178:1063–1070.
71. Criley JM, Blaufuss AH, Kissel GL. Cough-induced cardiac compression. Self-administered from of cardiopulmonary resuscitation. *JAMA.* 1976;236(11):1246–1250.
72. Criley JM, Blaufuss AH, Kissel GL. Self-administered cardiopulmonary resuscitation by cough-induced cardiac compression. *Trans Am Clin Climatol Assoc.* 1976;87:138–146.
73. Chandra N, Rudikoff M, Weisfeldt ML. Simultaneous chest compression and ventilation at high airway pressure during cardiopulmonary resuscitation. *Lancet.* 1980;1(8161):175–178.
74. Rudikoff MT, Maughan WL, Effron M, et al. Mechanisms of blood flow during cardiopulmonary resuscitation. *Circulation.* 1980;61(2):345–352.
75. Rich S, Wix HL, Shapiro EP. Clinical assessment of heart chamber size and valve motion during cardiopulmonary resuscitation by two-dimensional echocardiography. *Am Heart J.* 1981;102(3 Pt 1):368–373.
76. Werner JA, Greene HL, Janko CL, et al. Two-dimensional echocardiography during CPR in man: implications regarding the mechanism of blood flow. *Crit Care Med.* 1981;9(5):375–376.
77. Deshmukh HG, Weil MH, Gudipati CV, et al. Mechanism of blood flow generated by precordial compression during CPR. I. Studies on closed chest precordial compression. *Chest.* 1989;95(5):1092–1099.
78. Orlowski JP. Optimum position for external cardiac compression in infants and young children. *Ann Emerg Med.* 1986;15(6):667–673.
79. Paradis NA, Martin GB, Goetting MG, et al. Simultaneous aortic, jugular bulb, and right atrial pressures during cardiopulmonary resuscitation in humans. Insights into mechanisms. *Circulation.* 1989;80(2):361–368.
80. Tweed M, Tweed C, Perkins GD. The effect of differing support surfaces on the efficacy of chest compressions using a resuscitation manikin model. *Resuscitation.* 2001;51(2):179–183.
81. Handley AJ, Handley JA. Performing chest compressions in a confined space. *Resuscitation.* 2004;61(1):55–61.
82. Perkins GD, Stephenson BT, Smith CM, et al. A comparison between over-the-head and standard cardiopulmonary resuscitation. *Resuscitation.* 2004;61(2):155–161.
83. Handley AJ. Teaching hand placement for chest compression—a simpler technique. *Resuscitation.* 2002;53(1):29–36.
84. Kundra P, Dey S, Ravishankar M. Role of dominant hand position during external cardiac compression. *Br J Anaesth.* 2000;84(4):491–493.
85. Aufderheide TP, Pirrallo RG, Yannopoulos D, et al. Incomplete chest wall decompression: a clinical evaluation of CPR performance by EMS personnel and assessment of alternative manual chest compression-decompression techniques. *Resuscitation.* 2005;64(3):353–362.
86. Yannopoulos D, McKnite S, Aufderheide TP, et al. Effects of incomplete chest wall decompression during cardiopulmonary resuscitation on coronary and cerebral perfusion pressures in a porcine model of cardiac arrest. *Resuscitation.* 2005;64(3):363–372.
87. Stevenson AG, McGowan J, Evans AL, et al. CPR for children: one hand or two? *Resuscitation.* 2005;64(2):205–208.
88. Clements F, McGowan J. Finger position for chest compressions in cardiac arrest in infants. *Resuscitation.* 2000;44(1):43–46.
89. Finholt DA, Kettrick RG, Wagner HR, et al. The heart is under the lower third of the sternum. Implications for external cardiac massage. *Am J Dis Child.* 1986;140(7):646–649.
90. Shah NM, Gaur HK. Position of heart in relation to sternum and nipple line at various ages. *Indian Pediatr.* 1992;29(1):49–53.
91. Houri PK, Frank LR, Menegazzi JJ, et al. A randomized, controlled trial of two-thumb vs two-finger chest compression in a swine infant model of cardiac arrest [see comment]. *Prehosp Emerg Care.* 1997;1(2):65–67.
92. Dorfsman ML, Menegazzi JJ, Wadas RJ, et al. Two-thumb vs. two-finger chest compression in an infant model of prolonged cardiopulmonary resuscitation. *Acad Emerg Med.* 2000;7(10):1077–1082.
93. Whitelaw CC, Slywka B, Goldsmith LJ. Comparison of a two-finger versus two-thumb method for chest compressions by healthcare providers in an infant mechanical model. *Resuscitation.* 2000;43(3):213–216.
94. Wik L, Kramer-Johansen J, Myklebust H, et al. Quality of cardiopulmonary resuscitation during out-of-hospital cardiac arrest. *JAMA.* 2005; 293(3):299–304.
95. Abella BS, Alvarado JP, Myklebust H, et al. Quality of cardiopulmonary resuscitation during in-hospital cardiac arrest. *JAMA.* 2005;293(3):305–310.
96. Yu T, Weil MH, Tang W, et al. Adverse outcomes of interrupted precordial compression during automated defibrillation. *Circulation.* 2002;106(3): 368–372.
97. Swenson RD, Weaver WD, Niskanen RA, et al. Hemodynamics in humans during conventional and experimental methods of cardiopulmonary resuscitation. *Circulation.* 1988;78(3):630–639.
98. Kern KB, Sanders AB, Raife J, et al. A study of chest compression rates during cardiopulmonary resuscitation in humans. The importance of rate-directed chest compressions. *Arch Intern Med.* 1992;152(1):145–149.
99. Halperin HR, Tsitlik JE, Guerci AD, et al. Determinants of blood flow to vital organs during cardiopulmonary resuscitation in dogs. *Circulation.* 1986;73(3):539–550.
100. Feneley MP, Maier GW, Kern KB, et al. Influence of compression rate on initial success of resuscitation and 24 hour survival after prolonged manual cardiopulmonary resuscitation in dogs. *Circulation.* 1988;77(1):240–250.
101. Handley AJ, Handley JA. The relationship between rate of chest compression and compression:relaxation ratio. *Resuscitation.* 1995;30(3):237–241.
102. Rea TD, Helbock M, Perry S, et al. Increasing use of cardiopulmonary resuscitation during out-of-hospital ventricular fibrillation arrest: survival implications of guideline changes. *Circulation.* 2006;114(25):2760–2765.
103. Aufderheide TP, Sigurdsson G, Pirrallo RG, et al. Hyperventilation-induced hypotension during cardiopulmonary resuscitation. *Circulation.* 2004;109(16):1960–1965.
104. Greingor JL. Quality of cardiac massage with ratio compression-ventilation 5/1 and 15/2. *Resuscitation.* 2002;55(3):263–267.
105. Odegaard S, Saether E, Steen AS, et al. Quality of lay person CPR performance with compression:ventilation ratios 15:2, 30:2 or continuous chest compressions without ventilations on maikins. *Resuscitation.* 2006;doi10.1016/j.resuscitation.2006.05.012.
106. Beyar R, Kishon Y, Kimmel E, et al. Intrathoracic and abdominal pressure variations as an efficient method for cardiopulmonary resuscitation: studies in dogs compared with computer model results. *Cardiovasc Res.* 1985;19(6):335–342.
107. Voorhees WD, Niebauer MJ, Babbs CF. Improved oxygen delivery during cardiopulmonary resuscitation with interposed abdominal compressions. *Ann Emerg Med.* 1983;12(3):128–135.
108. Sack JB, Kesselbrenner MB, Jarrad A. Interposed abdominal compression-cardiopulmonary resuscitation and resuscitation outcome during asystole and electromechanical dissociation. *Circulation.* 1992;86(6):1692–1700.
109. Sack JB, Kesselbrenner MB, Bregman D. Survival from in-hospital cardiac arrest with interposed abdominal counterpulsation during cardiopulmonary resuscitation. *JAMA.* 1992;267(3):379–385.
110. Lurie KG, Shultz JJ, Callaham ML, et al. Evaluation of active compression-decompression CPR in victims of out-of-hospital cardiac arrest. *JAMA* 1994;271(18):1405–1411.
111. Plaisance P, Lurie KG, Vicaut E, et al. A comparison of standard cardiopulmonary resuscitation and active compression-decompression resuscitation for out-of-hospital cardiac arrest. French Active Compression-Decompression Cardiopulmonary Resuscitation Study Group. *N Engl J Med.* 1999;341(8):569–575.
112. Tucker KJ, Galli F, Savitt MA, et al. Active compression-decompression resuscitation: effect on resuscitation success after in-hospital cardiac arrest. *J Am Coll Cardiol.* 1994;24(1):201–209.
113. Schwab TM, Callaham ML, Madsen CD, et al. A randomized clinical trial of active compression-decompression CPR vs standard CPR in out-of-hospital cardiac arrest in two cities. *JAMA.* 1995;273(16):1261–1268.
114. Stiell IG, Hebert PC, Wells GA, et al. The Ontario trial of active compression-decompression cardiopulmonary resuscitation for in-hospital and prehospital cardiac arrest. *JAMA.* 1996;275(18):1417–1423.
115. Mauer D, Schneider T, Dick W, et al. Active compression-decompression resuscitation: a prospective, randomized study in a two-tiered EMS system with physicians in the field. *Resuscitation.* 1996;33(2):125–134.
116. Luiz T, Ellinger K, Denz C. Active compression-decompression cardiopulmonary resuscitation does not improve survival in patients with prehospital cardiac arrest in a physician-manned emergency medical system. *J Cardiothorac Vasc Anesth.* 1996;10(2):178–186.
117. Arntz HR, Agrawal R, Richter H, et al. Phased chest and abdominal compression-decompression versus conventional cardiopulmonary resuscitation in out-of-hospital cardiac arrest. *Circulation.* 2001;104(7):768–772.
118. Dickinson ET, Verdile VP, Schneider RM, et al. Effectiveness of mechanical

versus manual chest compressions in out-of-hospital cardiac arrest resuscitation: a pilot study. *Am J Emerg Med.* 1998;16(3):289–292.
119. McDonald JL. Systolic and mean arterial pressures during manual and mechanical CPR in humans. *Ann Emerg Med.* 1982;11(6):292–295.
120. Ward KR, Menegazzi JJ, Zelenak RR, et al. A comparison of chest compressions between mechanical and manual CPR by monitoring end-tidal PCO2 during human cardiac arrest. *Ann Emerg Med.* 1993;22(4):669–674.
121. Casner M, Andersen D, Isaacs SM. The impact of a new CPR assist device on rate of return of spontaneous circulation in out-of-hospital cardiac arrest. *Prehosp Emerg Care.* 2005;9(1):61–67.
122. Ong ME, Ornato JP, Edwards DP, et al. Use of an automated, load-distributing band chest compression device for out-of-hospital cardiac arrest resuscitation. *JAMA.* 2006;295(22):2629–2637.
123. Hallstrom A, Rea TD, Sayre MR, et al. Manual chest compression vs use of an automated chest compression device during resuscitation following out-of-hospital cardiac arrest: a randomized trial. *JAMA.* 2006;295(22):2620–2628.
124. Pepe PE, Copass MK, Joyce TH. Prehospital endotracheal intubation: rationale for training emergency medical personnel. *Ann Emerg Med.* 1985; 14(11):1085–1092.
125. Gausche M, Lewis RJ, Stratton SJ, et al. Effect of out-of-hospital pediatric endotracheal intubation on survival and neurological outcome: a controlled clinical trial. *JAMA.* 2000;283(6):783–790.
126. Jones JH, Murphy MP, Dickson RL, et al. Emergency physician-verified out-of-hospital intubation: miss rates by paramedics. *Acad Emerg Med.* 2004;11(6):707–709.
127. Sayre MR, Sakles JC, Mistler AF, et al. Field trial of endotracheal intubation by basic EMTs. *Ann Emerg Med.* 1998;31(2):228–233.
128. Katz SH, Falk JL. Misplaced endotracheal tubes by paramedics in an urban emergency medical services system. *Ann Emerg Med.* 2001;37(1):32–37.
129. Bhende MS, Thompson AE, Cook DR, et al. Validity of a disposable end-tidal CO2 detector in verifying endotracheal tube placement in infants and children. *Ann Emerg Med.* 1992;21(2):142–145.
130. Ornato JP, Shipley JB, Racht EM, et al. Multicenter study of a portable, hand-size, colorimetric end-tidal carbon dioxide detection device. *Ann Emerg Med.* 1992;21(5):518–523.
131. Vukmir RB, Heller MB, Stein KL. Confirmation of endotracheal tube placement: a miniaturized infrared qualitative CO2 detector. *Ann Emerg Med.* 1991;20(7):726–729.
132. 2005 American Heart Association Guidelines for Cardiopulmonary Resuscitation and Emergency Cardiovascular Care. *Circulation.* 2005;112 (24 Suppl):IV1–203.
133. Bozeman WP, Hexter D, Liang HK, et al. Esophageal detector device versus detection of end-tidal carbon dioxide level in emergency intubation. *Ann Emerg Med.* 1996;27(5):595–599.
134. Sharieff GQ, Rodarte A, Wilton N, et al. The self-inflating bulb as an airway adjunct: is it reliable in children weighing less than 20 kilograms? *Acad Emerg Med.* 2003;10(4):303–308.
135. Williams KN, Nunn JF. The oesophageal detector device. A prospective trial on 100 patients. *Anaesthesia.* 1989;44(5):412–414.
136. Haynes SR, Morton NS. Use of the oesophageal detector device in children under one year of age. *Anaesthesia.* 1990;45(12):1067–1069.
137. Capucci A, Aschieri D, Piepoli MF, et al. Tripling survival from sudden cardiac arrest via early defibrillation without traditional education in cardiopulmonary resuscitation. *Circulation.* 2002;106(9):1065–1070.
138. Holmberg M, Holmberg S, Herlitz J. Incidence, duration and survival of ventricular fibrillation in out-of-hospital cardiac arrest patients in Sweden. *Resuscitation.* 2000;44(1):7–17.
139. White RD, Hankins DG, Bugliosi TF. Seven years' experience with early defibrillation by police and paramedics in an emergency medical services system. *Resuscitation.* 1998;39(3):145–151.
140. Culley LL, Rea TD, Murray JA, et al. Public access defibrillation in out-of-hospital cardiac arrest: a community-based study. *Circulation.* 2004; 109(15):1859–1863.
141. Skogvoll E, Isern E, Sangolt GK, et al. In-hospital cardiopulmonary resuscitation. 5 years' incidence and survival according to the Utstein template. *Acta Anaesthesiol Scand.* 1999;43(2):177–184.
142. Parish DC, Dane FC, Montgomery M, et al. Resuscitation in the hospital: relationship of year and rhythm to outcome. *Resuscitation.* 2000;47(3):219–229.
143. Cooper S, Cade J. Predicting survival, in-hospital cardiac arrests: resuscitation survival variables and training effectiveness. *Resuscitation.* 1997;35(1):17–22.
144. Andreasson AC, Herlitz J, Bang A, et al. Characteristics and outcome among patients with a suspected in-hospital cardiac arrest. *Resuscitation.* 1998;39(1–2):23–31.
145. White RD. External defibrillation: the need for uniformity in analyzing and reporting results. *Ann Emerg Med.* 1998;32(2):234–236.
146. Gliner BE, White RD. Electrocardiographic evaluation of defibrillation shocks delivered to out-of-hospital sudden cardiac arrest patients. *Resuscitation.* 1999;41(2):133–144.
147. Zhang Y, Rhee B, Davies LR, et al. Quadriphasic waveforms are superior to triphasic waveforms for transthoracic defibrillation in a cardiac arrest swine model with high impedance. *Resuscitation.* 2006;68(2):251–258.
148. Zhang Y, Ramabadran RS, Boddicker KA, et al. Triphasic waveforms are superior to biphasic waveforms for transthoracic defibrillation: experimental studies. *J Am Coll Cardiol.* 2003;42(3):568–575.
149. van Alem AP, Chapman FW, Lank P, et al. A prospective, randomised and blinded comparison of first shock success of monophasic and biphasic waveforms in out-of-hospital cardiac arrest. *Resuscitation.* 2003;58(1):17–24.
150. Schneider T, Martens PR, Paschen H, et al. Multicenter, randomized, controlled trial of 150-J biphasic shocks compared with 200- to 360-J monophasic shocks in the resuscitation of out-of-hospital cardiac arrest victims. Optimized Response to Cardiac Arrest (ORCA) Investigators. *Circulation.* 2000;102(15):1780–1787.
151. Morrison LJ, Dorian P, Long J, et al. Out-of-hospital cardiac arrest rectilinear biphasic to monophasic damped sine defibrillation waveforms with advanced life support intervention trial (ORBIT). *Resuscitation.* 2005; 66(2):149–157.
152. Walsh SJ, McClelland AJ, Owens CG, et al. Efficacy of distinct energy delivery protocols comparing two biphasic defibrillators for cardiac arrest. *Am J Cardiol.* 2004;94(3):378–380.
153. Higgins SL, O'Grady SG, Banville I, et al. Efficacy of lower-energy biphasic shocks for transthoracic defibrillation: a follow-up clinical study. *Prehosp Emerg Care.* 2004;8(3):262–267.
154. Bourland JD, Tacker WA Jr, Geddes LA. Strength-duration curves for trapezoidal waveforms of various tilts for transchest defibrillation in animals. *Med Instrum.* 1978;12(1):38–41.
155. Bourland JD, Tacker WA Jr, Geddes LA, et al. Comparative efficacy of damped sine wave and square wave current for transchest ventricular defibrillation in animals. *Med Instrum.* 1978;12(1):42–45.
156. Kerber RE, Grayzel J, Hoyt R, et al. Transthoracic resistance in human defibrillation. Influence of body weight, chest size, serial shocks, paddle size and paddle contact pressure. *Circulation.* 1981;63(3):676–682.
157. Kerber RE, Kouba C, Martins J, et al. Advance prediction of transthoracic impedance in human defibrillation and cardioversion: importance of impedance in determining the success of low-energy shocks. *Circulation.* 1984;70(2):303–308.
158. Lerman BB, DiMarco JP, Haines DE. Current-based versus energy-based ventricular defibrillation: a prospective study. *J Am Coll Cardiol.* 1988; 12(5):1259–1264.
159. Gurnett CA, Atkins DL. Successful use of a biphasic waveform automated external defibrillator in a high-risk child. *Am J Cardiol.* 2000;86(9):1051–1053.
160. Atkins DL, Jorgenson DB. Attenuated pediatric electrode pads for automated external defibrillator use in children. *Resuscitation.* 2005;66(1):31–37.
161. Berg RA, Chapman FW, Berg MD, et al. Attenuated adult biphasic shocks compared with weight-based monophasic shocks in a swine model of prolonged pediatric ventricular fibrillation. *Resuscitation.* 2004;61(2):189–197.
162. Cummins RO, Eisenberg M, Bergner L, et al. Sensitivity, accuracy, and safety of an automatic external defibrillator. *Lancet.* 1984;2(8398):318–320.
163. White RD, Vukov LF, Bugliosi TF. Early defibrillation by police: initial experience with measurement of critical time intervals and patient outcome. *Ann Emerg Med.* 1994;23(5):1009–1013.
164. Davis EA, Mosesso VN Jr. Performance of police first responders in utilizing automated external defibrillation on victims of sudden cardiac arrest. *Prehosp Emerg Care.* 1998;2(2):101–107.
165. Hallstrom AP, Ornato JP, Weisfeldt M, et al. Public-access defibrillation and survival after out-of-hospital cardiac arrest. *N Engl J Med.* 2004;351 (7):637–646.
166. Sirna SJ, Ferguson DW, Charbonnier F, et al. Factors affecting transthoracic impedance during electrical cardioversion. *Am J Cardiol.* 1988; 62(16):1048–1052.
167. Kerber RE, Martins JB, Kienzle MG, et al. Energy, current, and success in defibrillation and cardioversion: clinical studies using an automated impedance-based method of energy adjustment. *Circulation.* 1988;77(5): 1038–1046.
168. Kerber RE, Kienzle MG, Olshansky B, et al. Ventricular tachycardia rate and morphology determine energy and current requirements for transthoracic cardioversion. *Circulation.* 1992;85(1):158–163.
169. Barthell E, Troiano P, Olson D, et al. Prehospital external cardiac pacing: a prospective, controlled clinical trial. *Ann Emerg Med.* 1988;17(11):1221–1226.
170. Cummins RO, Graves JR, Larsen MP, et al. Out-of-hospital transcutaneous pacing by emergency medical technicians in patients with asystolic cardiac arrest. *N Engl J Med.* 1993;328(19):1377–1382.
171. van Walraven C, Stiell IG, Wells GA, et al. Do advanced cardiac life support drugs increase resuscitation rates from in-hospital cardiac arrest? The OTAC Study Group. *Ann Emerg Med.* 1998;32(5):544–553.
172. Guy J, Haley K, Zuspan SJ. Use of intraosseous infusion in the pediatric trauma patient. *J Pediatr Surg.* 1993;28(2):158–161.
173. Banerjee S, Singhi SC, Singh S, et al. The intraosseous route is a suitable alternative to intravenous route for fluid resuscitation in severely dehydrated children. *Indian Pediatr.* 1994;31(12):1511–1520.

174. Glaeser PW, Hellmich TR, Szewczuga D, et al. Five-year experience in prehospital intraosseous infusions in children and adults. *Ann Emerg Med.* 1993;22(7):1119–1124.
175. Efrati O, Ben-Abraham R, Barak A, et al. Endobronchial adrenaline: should it be reconsidered? Dose response and haemodynamic effect in dogs. *Resuscitation.* 2003;59(1):117–122.
176. Manisterski Y, Vaknin Z, Ben-Abraham R, et al. Endotracheal epinephrine: a call for larger doses. *Anesth Analg.* 2002;95(4):1037–1041, table of contents.
177. Hilwig RW, Kern KB, Berg RA, et al. Catecholamines in cardiac arrest: role of alpha agonists, beta-adrenergic blockers and high-dose epinephrine. *Resuscitation.* 2000;47(2):203–208.
178. Chase PB, Kern KB, Sanders AB, et al. Effects of graded doses of epinephrine on both noninvasive and invasive measures of myocardial perfusion and blood flow during cardiopulmonary resuscitation. *Crit Care Med.* 1993; 21(3):413–419.
179. Berg RA, Otto CW, Kern KB, et al. A randomized, blinded trial of high-dose epinephrine versus standard-dose epinephrine in a swine model of pediatric asphyxial cardiac arrest. *Crit Care Med.* 1996;24(10):1695–1700.
180. Berg RA, Otto CW, Kern KB, et al. High-dose epinephrine results in greater early mortality after resuscitation from prolonged cardiac arrest in pigs: a prospective, randomized study. *Crit Care Med.* 1994;22(2):282–290.
181. Gueugniaud PY, Mols P, Goldstein P, et al. A comparison of repeated high doses and repeated standard doses of epinephrine for cardiac arrest outside the hospital. European Epinephrine Study Group. *N Engl J Med.* 1998;339(22):1595–1601.
182. Vandycke C, Martens P. High dose versus standard dose epinephrine in cardiac arrest - a meta-analysis. *Resuscitation.* 2000;45(3):161–166.
183. Perondi MB, Reis AG, Paiva EF, et al. A comparison of high-dose and standard-dose epinephrine in children with cardiac arrest. *N Engl J Med.* 2004;350(17):1722–1730.
184. Krismer AC, Lindner KH, Wenzel V, et al. The effects of endogenous and exogenous vasopressin during experimental cardiopulmonary resuscitation. *Anesth Analg.* 2001;92(6):1499–1504.
185. Stiell IG, Hebert PC, Wells GA, et al. Vasopressin versus epinephrine for inhospital cardiac arrest: a randomised controlled trial. *Lancet.* 2001; 358(9276):105–109.
186. Wenzel V, Krismer AC, Arntz HR, et al. A comparison of vasopressin and epinephrine for out-of-hospital cardiopulmonary resuscitation. *N Engl J Med.* 2004;350(2):105–113.
187. Aung K, Htay T. Vasopressin for cardiac arrest: a systematic review and meta-analysis. *Arch Intern Med.* 2005;165(1):17–24.
188. Voelckel WG, Lurie KG, McKnite S, et al. Comparison of epinephrine and vasopressin in a pediatric porcine model of asphyxial cardiac arrest. *Crit Care Med.* 2000;28(12):3777–3783.
189. Kette F, Weil MH, Gazmuri RJ. Buffer solutions may compromise cardiac resuscitation by reducing coronary perfusion pressure. *JAMA.* 1991; 266(15):2121–2126.
190. Graf H, Leach W, Arieff AI. Evidence for a detrimental effect of bicarbonate therapy in hypoxic lactic acidosis. *Science.* 1985;227(4688):754–756.
191. Benjamin E, Oropello JM, Abalos AM, et al. Effects of acid-base correction on hemodynamics, oxygen dynamics, and resuscitability in severe canine hemorrhagic shock. *Crit Care Med.* 1994;22(10):1616–1623.
192. Gunnar RM, Passamani ER, Bourdillon PD, et al. Guidelines for the early management of patients with acute myocardial infarction. A report of the American College of Cardiology/American Heart Association Task Force on Assessment of Diagnostic and Therapeutic Cardiovascular Procedures (Subcommittee to Develop Guidelines for the Early Management of Patients with Acute Myocardial Infarction). *J Am Coll Cardiol.* 1990;16(2):249–292.
193. Paradis NA, Martin GB, Rivers EP, et al. Coronary perfusion pressure and the return of spontaneous circulation in human cardiopulmonary resuscitation. *JAMA.* 1990;263(8):1106–1113.
194. Marill KA, Greenberg GM, Kay D, et al. Analysis of the treatment of spontaneous sustained stable ventricular tachycardia. *Acad Emerg Med.* 1997;4(12):1122–1128.
195. Somberg JC, Bailin SJ, Haffajee CI, et al. Intravenous lidocaine versus intravenous amiodarone (in a new aqueous formulation) for incessant ventricular tachycardia. *Am J Cardiol.* 2002;90(8):853–859.
196. Gorgels AP, van den Dool A, Hofs A, et al. Comparison of procainamide and lidocaine in terminating sustained monomorphic ventricular tachycardia. *Am J Cardiol.* 1996;78(1):43–46.
197. Schutzenberger W, Leisch F, Kerschner K, et al. Clinical efficacy of intravenous amiodarone in the short term treatment of recurrent sustained ventricular tachycardia and ventricular fibrillation. *Br Heart J.* 1989;62(5): 367–371.
198. Cybulski J, Kulakowski P, Makowska E, et al. Intravenous amiodarone is safe and seems to be effective in termination of paroxysmal supraventricular tachyarrhythmias. *Clin Cardiol.* 1996;19(7):563–566.
199. Cotter G, Blatt A, Kaluski E, et al. Conversion of recent onset paroxysmal atrial fibrillation to normal sinus rhythm: the effect of no treatment and high-dose amiodarone. A randomized, placebo-controlled study. *Eur Heart J.* 1999;20(24):1833–1842.
200. Stueven HA, Thompson B, Aprahamian C, et al. The effectiveness of calcium chloride in refractory electromechanical dissociation. *Ann Emerg Med.* 1985;14(7):626–629.
201. Stueven HA, Thompson B, Aprahamian C, et al. Lack of effectiveness of calcium chloride in refractory asystole. *Ann Emerg Med.* 1985;14(7):630–632.
202. Fatovich DM, Prentice DA, Dobb GJ. Magnesium in cardiac arrest (the magic trial). *Resuscitation.* 1997;35(3):237–241.
203. Miller B, Craddock L, Hoffenberg S, et al. Pilot study of intravenous magnesium sulfate in refractory cardiac arrest: safety data and recommendations for future studies. *Resuscitation.* 1995;30(1):3–14.
204. Connick M, Berg RA. Femoral venous pulsations during open-chest cardiac massage. *Ann Emerg Med.* 1994;24(6):1176–1179.
205. Halperin HR, Tsitlik JE, Gelfand M, et al. A preliminary study of cardiopulmonary resuscitation by circumferential compression of the chest with use of a pneumatic vest. *N Engl J Med.* 1993;329(11):762–768.
206. Kern KB, Ewy GA, Voorhees WD, et al. Myocardial perfusion pressure: a predictor of 24-hour survival during prolonged cardiac arrest in dogs. *Resuscitation.* 1988;16(4):241–250.
207. Weil MH, Rackow EC, Trevino R, et al. Difference in acid-base state between venous and arterial blood during cardiopulmonary resuscitation. *N Engl J Med.* 1986;315(3):153–156.
208. Kette F, Weil MH, Gazmuri RJ, et al. Intramyocardial hypercarbic acidosis during cardiac arrest and resuscitation. *Crit Care Med.* 1993;21(6):901–906.
209. Tucker KJ, Idris AH, Wenzel V, et al. Changes in arterial and mixed venous blood gases during untreated ventricular fibrillation and cardiopulmonary resuscitation. *Resuscitation.* 1994;28(2):137–141.
210. Gudipati CV, Weil MH, Gazmuri RJ, et al. Increases in coronary vein CO2 during cardiac resuscitation. *J Appl Physiol.* 1990;68(4):1405–1408.
211. Bircher NG. Acidosis of cardiopulmonary resuscitation: carbon dioxide transport and anaerobiosis. *Crit Care Med.* 1992;20(9):1203–1205.
212. Gravenstein JS, Paulus DA, Hayes TJ, et al. *Capnography in Clinical Practice.* Boston: Butterworths; 1989.
213. Idris AH, Staples ED, O'Brien DJ, et al. End-tidal carbon dioxide during extremely low cardiac output. *Ann Emerg Med.* 1994;23(3):568–572.
214. Gazmuri RJ, Weil MH, Bisera J, et al. End-tidal carbon dioxide tension as a monitor of native blood flow during resuscitation by extracorporeal circulation. *J Thorac Cardiovasc Surg.* 1991;101(6):984–988.
215. Gudipati CV, Weil MH, Bisera J, et al. Expired carbon dioxide: a noninvasive monitor of cardiopulmonary resuscitation. *Circulation.* 1988;77(1): 234–239.
216. Sanders AB, Atlas M, Ewy GA, et al. Expired PCO2 as an index of coronary perfusion pressure. *Am J Emerg Med.* 1985;3(2):147–149.
217. Falk JL, Rackow EC, Weil MH. End-tidal carbon dioxide concentration during cardiopulmonary resuscitation. *N Engl J Med.* 1988;318(10):607–611.
218. Sanders AB, Kern KB, Otto CW, et al. End-tidal carbon dioxide monitoring during cardiopulmonary resuscitation. A prognostic indicator for survival. *JAMA.* 1989;262(10):1347–1351.
219. Wiklund L, Soderberg D, Henneberg S, et al. Kinetics of carbon dioxide during cardiopulmonary resuscitation. *Crit Care Med.* 1986;14(12):1015–1022.
220. Callaham M, Barton C. Prediction of outcome of cardiopulmonary resuscitation from end-tidal carbon dioxide concentration. *Crit Care Med.* 1990;18(4):358–362.
221. Bhende MS, Thompson AE. Evaluation of an end-tidal CO2 detector during pediatric cardiopulmonary resuscitation. *Pediatrics.* 1995;95(3):395–399.
222. Ornato JP, Gonzalez ER, Garnett AR, et al. Effect of cardiopulmonary resuscitation compression rate on end-tidal carbon dioxide concentration and arterial pressure in man. *Crit Care Med.* 1988;16(3):241–245.
223. Ornato JP, Levine RL, Young DS, et al. The effect of applied chest compression force on systemic arterial pressure and end-tidal carbon dioxide concentration during CPR in human beings. *Ann Emerg Med.* 1989;18(7):732–737.
224. Martin GB, Gentile NT, Paradis NA, et al. Effect of epinephrine on end-tidal carbon dioxide monitoring during CPR. *Ann Emerg Med.* 1990;19(4):396–398.
225. Sanders AB, Ewy GA, Bragg S, et al. Expired PCO2 as a prognostic indicator of successful resuscitation from cardiac arrest. *Ann Emerg Med.* 1985; 14(10):948–952.
226. Idris AH, Staples ED, O'Brien DJ, et al. Effect of ventilation on acid-base balance and oxygenation in low blood-flow states. *Crit Care Med.* 1994;22(11):1827–1834.
227. Laurent I, Monchi M, Chiche JD, et al. Reversible myocardial dysfunction in survivors of out-of-hospital cardiac arrest. *J Am Coll Cardiol.* 2002; 40(12):2110–2116.
228. Negovsky VA. The second step in resuscitation—the treatment of the 'post-resuscitation disease'. *Resuscitation.* 1972;1(1):1–7.
229. Safar P. Resuscitation from clinical death: pathophysiologic limits and therapeutic potentials. *Crit Care Med.* 1988;16(10):923–941.
230. Skrifvars MB, Pettila V, Rosenberg PH, et al. A multiple logistic regression analysis of in-hospital factors related to survival at six months in patients resuscitated from out-of-hospital ventricular fibrillation. *Resuscitation.* 2003;59(3):319–328.

231. Longstreth WT Jr, Inui TS. High blood glucose level on hospital admission and poor neurological recovery after cardiac arrest. *Ann Neurol.* 1984; 15(1):59–63.
232. Calle PA, Buylaert WA, Vanhaute OA. Glycemia in the post-resuscitation period. The Cerebral Resuscitation Study Group. *Resuscitation.* 1989; 17(Suppl):S181–188; discussion S199–206.
233. Longstreth WT Jr, Copass MK, Dennis LK, et al. Intravenous glucose after out-of-hospital cardiopulmonary arrest: a community-based randomized trial. *Neurology.* 1993;43(12):2534–2541.
234. van den Berghe G, Wouters P, Weekers F, et al. Intensive insulin therapy in the critically ill patients. *N Engl J Med.* 2001;345(19):1359–1367.
235. Van den Berghe G, Wilmer A, Hermans G, et al. Intensive insulin therapy in the medical ICU. *N Engl J Med.* 2006;354(5):449–461.
236. Weaver WD, Cobb LA, Copass MK, et al. Ventricular defibrillation—a comparative trial using 175-J and 320-J shocks. *N Engl J Med.* 1982; 307(18):1101–1106.
237. Kern KB, Hilwig RW, Rhee KH, et al. Myocardial dysfunction after resuscitation from cardiac arrest: an example of global myocardial stunning. *J Am Coll Cardiol.* 1996;28(1):232–240.
238. Adrie C, Adib-Conquy M, Laurent I, et al. Successful cardiopulmonary resuscitation after cardiac arrest as a "sepsis-like" syndrome. *Circulation.* 2002;106(5):562–568.
239. Gisvold SE, Sterz F, Abramson NS, et al. Cerebral resuscitation from cardiac arrest: treatment potentials. *Crit Care Med.* 1996;24(2 Suppl):S69–80.
240. del Zoppo GJ, Mabuchi T. Cerebral microvessel responses to focal ischemia. *J Cereb Blood Flow Metab.* 2003;23(8):879–894.
241. Hickey RW, Kochanek PM, Ferimer H, et al. Induced hyperthermia exacerbates neurologic neuronal histologic damage after asphyxial cardiac arrest in rats. *Crit Care Med.* 2003;31(2):531–535.
242. Dietrich WD, Busto R, Halley M, et al. The importance of brain temperature in alterations of the blood-brain barrier following cerebral ischemia. *J Neuropathol Exp Neurol.* 1990;49(5):486–497.
243. Dietrich WD, Busto R, Valdes I, et al. Effects of normothermic versus mild hyperthermic forebrain ischemia in rats. *Stroke.* 1990;21(9):1318–1325.
244. Kim Y, Busto R, Dietrich WD, et al. Delayed postischemic hyperthermia in awake rats worsens the histopathological outcome of transient focal cerebral ischemia. *Stroke.* 1996;27(12):2274–2280; discussion 2281.
245. Zeiner A, Holzer M, Sterz F, et al. Hyperthermia after cardiac arrest is associated with an unfavorable neurologic outcome. *Arch Intern Med.* 2001;161(16):2007–2012.
246. Soukup J, Zauner A, Doppenberg EM, et al. The importance of brain temperature in patients after severe head injury: relationship to intracranial pressure, cerebral perfusion pressure, cerebral blood flow, and outcome. *J Neurotrauma.* 2002;19(5):559–571.
247. Bernard SA, Gray TW, Buist MD, et al. Treatment of comatose survivors of out-of-hospital cardiac arrest with induced hypothermia. *N Engl J Med.* 2002;346(8):557–563.
248. Mild therapeutic hypothermia to improve the neurologic outcome after cardiac arrest. *N Engl J Med.* 2002;346(8):549–556.
249. Nolan JP, Morley PT, Hoek TL, et al. Therapeutic hypothermia after cardiac arrest. An advisory statement by the Advancement Life support Task Force of the International Liaison committee on Resuscitation. *Resuscitation.* 2003;57(3):231–235.
250. Shankaran S, Laptook AR, Ehrenkranz RA, et al. Whole-body hypothermia for neonates with hypoxic-ischemic encephalopathy. *N Engl J Med.* 2005;353(15):1574–1584.
251. Gluckman PD, Wyatt JS, Azzopardi D, et al. Selective head cooling with mild systemic hypothermia after neonatal encephalopathy: multicentre randomised trial. *Lancet.* 2005;365(9460):663–670.
252. Bernard S, Buist M, Monteiro O, et al. Induced hypothermia using large volume, ice-cold intravenous fluid in comatose survivors of out-of-hospital cardiac arrest: a preliminary report. *Resuscitation.* 2003;56(1):9–13.
253. Haque IU, Latour MC, Zaritsky AL. Pediatric critical care community survey of knowledge and attitudes toward therapeutic hypothermia in comatose children after cardiac arrest. *Pediatr Crit Care Med.* 2006;7(1):7–14.
254. Schubert A. Side effects of mild hypothermia. *J Neurosurg Anesthesiol.* 1995;7(2):139–147.
255. Metz C, Holzschuh M, Bein T, et al. Moderate hypothermia in patients with severe head injury: cerebral and extracerebral effects. *J Neurosurg.* 1996;85(4):533–541.
256. National Registry of CPR (NRCPR). *National Registry of CPR SAB Participant Report.* American Heart Association, Dallas, TX; 2002.
257. Younger JG, Schreiner RJ, Swaniker F, et al. Extracorporeal resuscitation of cardiac arrest. *Acad Emerg Med.* 1999;6(7):700–707.
258. Morris MC, Wernovsky G, Nadkarni VM. Survival outcomes after extracorporeal cardiopulmonary resuscitation instituted during active chest compressions following refractory in-hospital pediatric cardiac arrest. *Pediatr Crit Care Med.* 2004;5(5):440–446.
259. Ronco R, King W, Donley DK, et al. Outcome and cost at a children's hospital following resuscitation for out-of-hospital cardiopulmonary arrest. *Arch Pediatr Adolesc Med.* 1995;149(2):210–214.
260. Schindler MB, Bohn D, Cox PN, et al. Outcome of out-of-hospital cardiac or respiratory arrest in children. *N Engl J Med.* 1996;335(20):1473–1479.
261. Reis AG, Nadkarni V, Perondi MB, et al. A prospective investigation into the epidemiology of in-hospital pediatric cardiopulmonary resuscitation using the international Utstein reporting style. *Pediatrics.* 2002;109(2):200–209.
262. Lopez-Herce J, Garcia C, Rodriguez-Nunez A, et al. Long-term outcome of paediatric cardiorespiratory arrest in Spain. *Resuscitation.* 2005;64(1):79–85.
263. Parra DA, Totapally BR, Zahn E, et al. Outcome of cardiopulmonary resuscitation in a pediatric cardiac intensive care unit. *Crit Care Med.* 2000;28(9):3296–3300.
264. Adams S, Whitlock M, Higgs R, et al. Should relatives be allowed to watch resuscitation? *BMJ.* 1994;308(6945):1687–1692.
265. Meyers TA, Eichhorn DJ, Guzzetta CE. Do families want to be present during CPR? A retrospective survey. *J Emerg Nurs.* 1998;24(5):400–405.
266. Robinson SM, Mackenzie-Ross S, Campbell Hewson GL, et al. Psychological effect of witnessed resuscitation on bereaved relatives. *Lancet.* 1998;352(9128):614–617.
267. Eichhorn DJ, Meyers TA, Mitchell TG, et al. Opening the doors: family presence during resuscitation. *J Cardiovasc Nurs.* 1996;10(4):59–70.
268. Offord RJ. Should relatives of patients with cardiac arrest be invited to be present during cardiopulmonary resuscitation? *Intensive Crit Care Nurs.* 1998;14(6):288–293.
269. Doyle CJ, Post H, Burney RE, et al. Family participation during resuscitation: an option. *Ann Emerg Med.* 1987;16(6):673–675.
270. Beckman AW, Sloan BK, Moore GP, et al. Should parents be present during emergency department procedures on children, and who should make that decision? A survey of emergency physician and nurse attitudes. *Acad Emerg Med.* 2002;9(2):154–158.
271. Cummins RO, Ornato JP, Thies WH, et al. Improving survival from sudden cardiac arrest: the "chain of survival" concept. A statement for health professionals from the Advanced Cardiac Life Support Subcommittee and the Emergency Cardiac Care Committee, American Heart Association. *Circulation.* 1991;83(5):1832–1847.
272. Herlitz J, Ekstrom L, Wennerblom B, et al. Effect of bystander initiated cardiopulmonary resuscitation on ventricular fibrillation and survival after witnessed cardiac arrest outside hospital. *Br Heart J.* 1994;72(5):408–412.
273. Stiell I, Nichol G, Wells G, et al. Health-related quality of life is better for cardiac arrest survivors who received citizen cardiopulmonary resuscitation. *Circulation.* 2003;108(16):1939–1944.
274. Locke CJ, Berg RA, Sanders AB, et al. Bystander cardiopulmonary resuscitation. Concerns about mouth-to-mouth contact. *Arch Intern Med.* 1995; 155(9):938–943.
275. Brenner BE, Kauffman J. Reluctance of internists and medical nurses to perform mouth-to-mouth resuscitation. *Arch Intern Med.* 1993;153(15): 1763–1769.
276. Brenner B, Stark B, Kauffman J. The reluctance of house staff to perform mouth-to-mouth resuscitation in the inpatient setting: what are the considerations? *Resuscitation.* 1994;28(3):185–193.
277. van Alem AP, Sanou BT, Koster RW. Interruption of cardiopulmonary resuscitation with the use of the automated external defibrillator in out-of-hospital cardiac arrest. *Ann Emerg Med.* 2003;42(4):449–457.
278. Hightower D, Thomas SH, Stone CK, et al. Decay in quality of closed-chest compressions over time. *Ann Emerg Med.* 1995;26(3):300–303.
279. Brennan RT, Braslow A. Skill mastery in public CPR classes. *Am J Emerg Med.* 1998;16(7):653–657.
280. Thoren AB, Axelsson A, Holmberg S, et al. Measurement of skills in cardiopulmonary resuscitation—do professionals follow given guidelines? *Eur J Emerg Med.* 2001;8(3):169–176.
281. Berg RA, Sanders AB, Milander M, et al. Efficacy of audio-prompted rate guidance in improving resuscitator performance of cardiopulmonary resuscitation on children. *Acad Emerg Med.* 1994;1(1):35–40.
282. Wik L, Thowsen J, Steen PA. An automated voice advisory manikin system for training in basic life support without an instructor. A novel approach to CPR training. *Resuscitation.* 2001;50(2):167–172.
283. Handley AJ, Handley SA. Improving CPR performance using an audible feedback system suitable for incorporation into an automated external defibrillator. *Resuscitation.* 2003;57(1):57–62.
284. Devita MA, Bellomo R, Hillman K, et al. Findings of the first consensus conference on medical emergency teams. *Crit Care Med.* 2006;34(9):2463–2478.
285. Bellomo R, Goldsmith D, Uchino S, et al. A prospective before-and-after trial of a medical emergency team. *Med J Aust.* 2003;179(6):283–287.
286. Buist MD, Moore GE, Bernard SA, et al. Effects of a medical emergency team on reduction of incidence of and mortality from unexpected cardiac arrests in hospital: preliminary study. *BMJ.* 2002;324(7334):387–390.
287. Hillman K, Chen J, Cretikos M, et al. Introduction of the medical emergency team (MET) system: a cluster-randomised controlled trial. *Lancet.* 2005;365(9477):2091–2097.

CHAPTER 47 ■ RENAL PHYSIOLOGY AND ITS SYSTEMIC IMPACT

MARCELO E. HEINIG • A. AHSAN EJAZ

MAIN POINTS

- The prevalence of acute renal failure continues to increase.
- Mortality of acute renal failure, despite improvements, remains high.
- Loss of autoregulation of renal blood flow, vasoconstriction, and subsequent downstream effects potentiate the inflammatory cascade in acute renal failure.
- Pre-existing organ dysfunction affects the prognosis of critically ill patients.
- The decrease in physiologic reserve in acute renal failure influences drug dosing, treatment modality, and response to interventions in patients in the intensive care unit.
- The treatment of acute renal failure is based on the principle that the preservation of renal blood flow and optimal perfusion pressure improves outcomes.

Acute renal failure (ARF) is a common finding in hospitalized patients. The accurate incidence of acute renal failure is undetermined due to the differences in definitions used in databases at different time points. However, data from hospitalized Medicare beneficiaries—using an acute renal failure definition from ICD-9-CM as "the sudden, severe onset of inadequate kidney function"—yields an overall incidence rate of 23.8 cases per 1,000 discharges (1). Others have reported incidences of hospital-acquired acute renal failure of 4.9% to 7%. Patients who develop ARF have an in-hospital mortality of 15.2%, which increases to 32.9% if dialysis is also required. In the intensive care unit (ICU), the incidence of ARF—again, depending on the definitional criteria used—has been reported to range between 5% and 17%. Nonetheless, the mortality rates of ICU patients with ARF were high in every study, ranging between 24% and 53%; when renal replacement therapy was required, the mortality was even higher, ranging between 45% and 79% (2,3).

Knowledge of risk factors for ARF in the ICU can be helpful in the determination of clinical outcome and contribute to more defined risk assessment and management in this cohort (Table 47.1). This chapter reviews pertinent renal physiology, the mechanisms and outcomes of ischemic acute renal failure, the progression of chronic kidney disease and its impact on acute critical illness, and the principles of management of acute renal failure. Specifics on the treatment of ARF and a detailed description of the various treatment modalities are to be found in later chapters of this textbook.

PHYSIOLOGY OF THE KIDNEY

General Anatomy

The ability of the kidney to maintain the equilibrium of the corporal fluids and electrolytes depends on three essential processes: (i) filtration of the circulating blood by the glomerulus to form an ultrafiltrate, (ii) reabsorption of specific solutes from the tubular fluid to the blood, and (iii) secretion from the peritubular capillary blood system to the tubular space. The functions of the kidney are dependent on the unique anatomic arrangement of its structures.

The afferent arteriole divides into several branches after entering the glomerular tuft and forms the capillary network present in the glomerulus (Fig. 47.1). The confluence of several capillaries forms the efferent arteriole, which drains the blood from the glomerulus. During the ultrafiltration process, water and solutes pass through the endothelium, the glomerular basement membrane, and the slit-diaphragm between the podocytes. The determinant of the filtration of a substance is its size and charge. Substances with molecular radius of less than 2 nm are filtered freely, whereas ionic charges of substances measuring between 2 and 4 nm determine the amount of their filtration. Substances with molecular radius greater than 4 nm are not filtered.

The medullary region of the kidneys is characterized by low oxygen tension (10 to 15 mm Hg) under normal conditions. The tubular segments located in this region—pars recta or S3 segment of proximal tubule and medullary thick ascending limb—are characterized by active transport of Na^+, which is dependent on oxidative phosphorylation for energy. The high rates of oxygen consumption associated with the precarious blood flow in the medullary region are responsible for the vulnerability of this area to ischemia.

General Renal Physiology

Glomerular Filtration Rate and Renal Plasma Flow

The glomerular filtration rate (GFR) and the renal plasma flow (RPF) are rate measurements that help to characterize the status of renal function. The total rate at which fluid is filtered into all the glomeruli constitutes the *glomerular filtration rate* (GFR). The normal GFR varies between 100 and 120 mL/min/1.73 m^2, depending on various factors including gender, age, and body weight. Changes in the GFR can result from changes in the

TABLE 47.1

PREDICTORS OF ACUTE RENAL FAILURE IN THE INTENSIVE CARE UNIT

Risks	All patients OR $N = 194^a$	Sepsis OR $N = 2{,}442^b$	CV Surgery OR $N = 43{,}642^c$	Trauma OR $N = 153^d$
Demographics				
Age	0.93	1.1		2.82
Acute Clinical Setting				
High-risk surgery	1.51		1.98	
Sepsis	3.11			
High injury severity score				5.75–13.7
Emergency procedure			7.61*	
Cardiopulmonary bypass			2.64*	
Pre-Existing Condition				
Chronic kidney disease	1.77	1.02	1.31–5.80[b]	
Cardiac failure	1.85		1.55	
Cancer	3.75		—	
Prior cardiac surgery			1.93	
COPD			1.26	
Hypertension (SBP >160 mm Hg)			1.03–1.98[c]	
Peripheral vascular disease			1.51	
Clinical Findings				
Elevated A-a gradient	1.04			
Elevated serum bilirubin	3.6	9.7		
Hypotension				3.04
Hemoperitoneum				6.80
Long bone fractures				2.36
Morbid obesity	2.1		1.11*	
APACHE II quartile	1.57			
Elevated CVP		1.5		

CV, cardiovascular; OR, odds ratio; COPD, chronic obstructive pulmonary disease; SBP, systolic blood pressure; CVP, central venous pressure.
[a]Source: Chawla LS, Abell L, Mazhari R, et al. Identifying critically ill patients at high risk for developing acute renal failure: a pilot study. *Kidney Int.* 2005;68:2274–2280.
[b]Source: Yegenaga I, Hoste E, Van Biesen W, et al. Clinical characteristics of patients developing ARF due to sepsis/systemic inflammatory response. *Am J Kidney Dis.* 2004;43:817–824.
[c]Source: Chertow GM, Lazarus JM, Christiansen CL, et al. Preoperative renal risk stratification. *Circulation.* 1997;95:878–884.
[d]Source: Vivino G, Antonelli M, Moro ML, et al. Risk factors for acute renal failure in trauma patients. *Intensive Care Med.* 1998;24:808–814.

glomerular permeability or capillary surface area or from changes in the net ultrafiltration. In a single glomerulus, the driving pressure for the glomerular filtration is determined by the difference of the gradient of the hydrostatic and oncotic pressures between the capillaries and the Bowman space.

The rate at which plasma flows through the kidney is called *renal plasma flow. Renal blood flow* (RBF) is the volume of blood delivered to the kidney per unit time (1 to 1.2 L/min). Renal blood flow calculations are based on renal plasma flow and hematocrit:

$$\text{RBF} = \text{RPF}/1 - \text{hematocrit}$$

It is possible to measure the RPF using para-aminohippurate as a tracer in humans, with a normal value about 625 mL/min, but the test is not commonly used in clinical practice due to labor intensity and cost.

Autoregulatory Control of Renal Blood Flow

Despite the significant variations in mean arterial pressure, renal blood flow and GFR remain constant, a phenomenon known as *autoregulation.* Autoregulation is affected via changes in diameter of the afferent arterioles in response to a combination of two mechanisms:

1. *The myogenic reflex:* When the renal perfusion pressure increases, the afferent arteriole constricts automatically.
2. *Tubuloglomerular feedback:* Situations associated with an increased delivery of NaCl to the macula densa result in vasoconstrictive response of the afferent arteriole. The increased uptake of chloride ions by the macula densa cells leads to ATP release into the surrounding extracellular space. ATP is then converted to adenosine which binds to adenosine A_1 receptors causing afferent arteriolar vasoconstriction.

Basic Principles of Tubular Transport

The kidneys filter about 180 L of plasma, and all but 2 L are reabsorbed. This massive reabsorption is accomplished through several modifications of the glomerular ultrafiltrate, consisting of absorption and secretion of water and solutes before becoming the final urine. In general, three different tubular segments

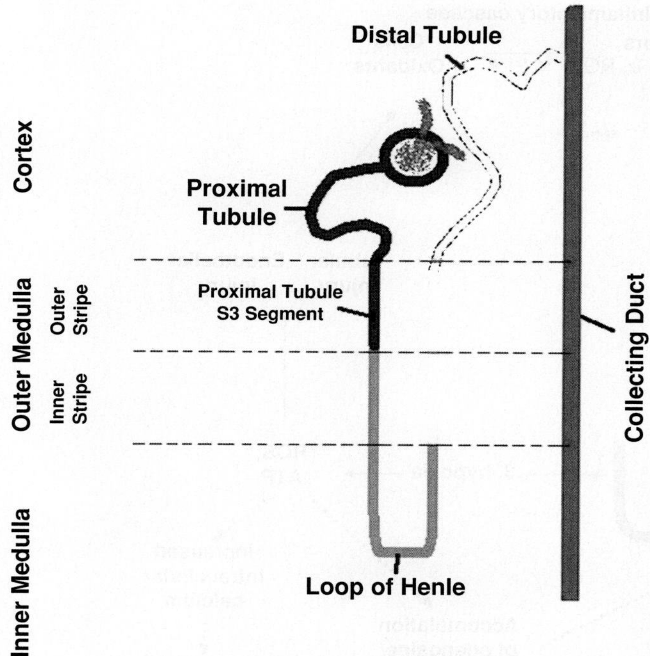

FIGURE 47.1. Nephron—the functional unit of the kidney.

are involved in this process and can be recognized based on the differences in the function of their cells.

1. The *proximal tubule* reabsorbs most of the filtered glucose, amino acids, low-molecular-weight proteins, and water (approximately 65%). Other solutes, such as Na^+, K^+, Cl^-, HCO_3^-, Ca^{2+}, phosphate, and urea are also absorbed in this nephron segment. The terminal segment of the proximal tubule—the pars recta or S3—is responsible for the secretion of numerous drugs and toxins.
2. The straight portion of the proximal tubule, the thin ascending and descending limbs, and the thick ascending limb constitute the region known as the *loop of Henle*. This region is responsible for the continuing reabsorption of the solutes that escaped the proximal tubules (Na^+, Cl^-, K^+, Ca^{2+}, Mg^{2+}). It is the major area responsible for the ability of the kidneys to concentrate or dilute the final urine. The principal luminal transporter expressed in the thick ascending limb is the Na-K_2Cl cotransporter, which is the target of diuretics such as furosemide.
3. The *distal nephron* is responsible for the final adjustments in the urine. Critical regulatory hormones such as vasopressin and aldosterone regulate the acid and potassium excretion and the urinary concentration at this segment. Thiazide diuretics act at the distal convoluted tubule through an apical cotransporter of Na^+.

The Glomerulotubular Balance

The fact that the tubules tend to reabsorb a constant proportion of a glomerular filtrate rather than a constant amount is called *glomerular balance*. As an example, if the filtered load of Na^+ was increased by 10%, total Na^+ reabsorption in the tubules would also increase by 10%, keeping the final amount of Na^+ in the urine—100 to 250 mEq/day—stable. In the absence of this mechanism, even small changes in the GFR would cause major changes in the final amount excreted of any solute. The mechanisms responsible for this balance are not fully understood, but changes in the oncotic pressure in the peritubular capillaries and in the delivery of certain solutes (glucose and amino acids) to the proximal tubule are probably involved.

Control of Effective Circulating Volume via Integrated Mechanisms

Most volume-regulatory mechanisms in the kidney use the *effective circulating volume*, or the degree of fullness of the vasculature, as the final target. Under normal conditions, the effective circulating volume varies in direct proportion to the extracellular fluid volume. As Na^+ is the most abundant extracellular solute, the kidney excretion or retention of Na^+ is a crucial step to control of effective circulatory fluid volume. Osmoregulation is under the control of a single hormonal system, the antidiuretic hormone (ADH), but volume regulation requires a complex set of redundant and overlapping mechanisms.

The kidneys are able to conserve water by excreting the solute load in concentrated urine in conditions of excess water loss. Similarly, in high water intake states, the urinary volume may increase to as high as 14 L/day, with an osmolality significantly lower than that of the plasma. Vasopressin or ADH regulates the water permeability in the distal nephron and is the principal hormone responsible for the determination of the urinary concentration and volume. Normally, the major stimulus to secretion of ADH is the plasma osmolality, but in situations of extracellular volume depletion, the set point to release ADH is shifted, and higher levels of this hormone are common even in hypotonic states.

The renin-angiotensin system plays a central role in the control of effective circulatory fluid volume. The afferent arteriolar cells that form part of the juxtaglomerular apparatus release renin in response to increased sympathetic nervous stimulation, reduced arterial blood pressure, or reduced delivery of NaCl to the macula densa region. Renin cleaves angiotensinogen into angiotensin I and is then converted to angiotensin II by the angiotensin-converting enzyme. Angiotensin plays important roles in the control of blood pressure and the effective circulatory fluid volume:

- Angiotensin II has the direct effect of increasing the sodium reabsorption in the proximal tubule (stimulation of Na^+/H^+ exchange).
- The aldosterone secreted by the adrenal glands in response to the angiotensin II stimulates sodium reabsorption in the distal nephron.
- Angiotensin II causes general arteriolar vasoconstriction, thereby increasing arterial pressure.

Increased renal sympathetic tone enhances renal salt reabsorption and can decrease renal blood flow at higher frequencies. In addition to its direct effects on renal function, increased sympathetic outflow promotes the activation of the renin-angiotensin system.

PATHOPHYSIOLOGY OF ACUTE RENAL FAILURE

Ischemic acute renal failure is a syndrome that develops following a sudden transient drop in total or regional blood flow to the kidney. Classically, a decrease in mean arterial pressure has

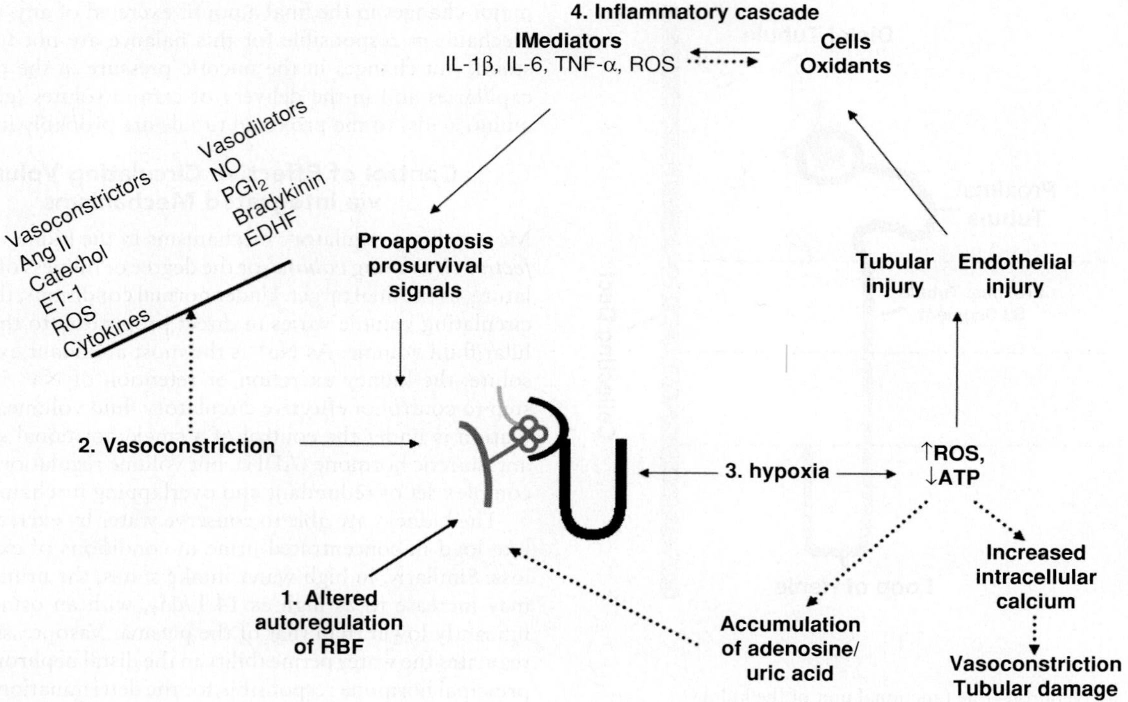

FIGURE 47.2. Theories of the mechanism of acute renal failure.

been associated with a reduction in renal blood flow with subsequent tissue hypoxia, tubular and vascular injury, and loss of renal structure and function. However, renal blood flow and glomerular filtration rate can decrease by as much as 50% despite the maintenance of mean arterial pressure (4), suggesting the presence of renal vasoconstriction. Mechanisms for these observations in ischemic acute renal failure are discussed below (Fig. 47.2).

Theories of the Mechanism of Acute Renal Failure

Loss of Autoregulation of Renal Blood Flow

Renal blood flow is dependent on systemic blood pressure and intrarenal vascular resistance. The autoregulatory mechanisms, through changes in vascular resistance, ensure that over a wide range of perfusion pressures, renal blood flow remains stable and glomerular filtration can be maintained. However, in ischemic acute renal failure, autoregulation of renal blood flow is lost. Consequently, renal blood flow diminishes with decreased mean arterial pressure over the autoregulatory range (5). The loss of autoregulation of renal blood flow is related to an increase in renovascular resistance.

Imbalance of Mediators of Vascular Tone

The paradoxical rise in renovascular resistance seen with decreasing renal perfusion in ischemic acute renal failure is due to the loss of the usual balance of vasoconstrictors and the vasodilators required to maintain the normal tone of the renal vasculature. The aberrant responses to neurohormonal stimuli and the persistent vasoconstriction worsen renal perfusion and impair oxygen and nutrient delivery to the areas supplied by the postglomerular vessels.

Tissue Hypoxia

The partial pressure of oxygen in the outer medulla is about 10 to 15 mm Hg. Even a mild decrease in renal perfusion can lead to a hypoxic insult (oxidative stress) to the vulnerable medullary nephron segments. Tissue hypoxia can result in depletion of cellular ATP stores, increased intracellular calcium, and subsequent disruption of actin cytoskeleton in the endothelial and vascular smooth muscle cells, with resultant hemodynamic impairment and tubular injury. Adenosine nucleotide metabolic products are not reused for the regeneration of ATP and are, instead, diverted through the degradatory pathways to generate xanthine and uric acid. Accumulation of adenosine and uric acid worsens vasoconstriction and renal perfusion via their effects on adenosine receptors and afferent arterioles, respectively. Cellular activation also leads to reactive oxygen species generation, phospholipase activation, and membrane lipid alterations.

The Inflammatory Cascade

Hypoxia, with subsequent reperfusion, leads to acute inflammatory changes. Inflammation is one of the major pathophysiologic pathways contributing to ischemic acute renal failure. Ischemic injury to the vasa recta results in enhanced adherence of leukocytes to the vascular endothelial cells, sequestration of leukocytes, vascular congestion—that is, a no-flow phenomenon—cellular infiltration, production of inflammatory mediators, and generation of reactive oxygen species. Cytokines and chemokines, released from the injured cells, attract and activate inflammatory cells to the site of injury and potentiate the inflammatory cascade. A similar inflammatory response is also seen with tubular cell injury, which is also capable of producing inflammatory mediators. The inflammatory changes are most pronounced in the outer medullary stripe, the region that is most susceptible to hypoxic insult.

Prosurvival and Proapoptotic Signaling Pathways

Numerous stress response mechanisms are rapidly activated in response to oxidative insults. Some of the pathways are preferentially linked to cell survival whereas others are proapoptotic. These pathways intersect and modulate each other's activities. Whether a particular insult leads to cell repair and survival—or death—depends on the nature and severity of the insult, the balance between the proapoptotic and antiapoptotic signals, and the basal state of the cells. Ongoing efforts to elucidate factors that play a role in microvascular endothelial injury and dysfunction, expression of adhesion molecules that facilitate leukocyte-endothelial interactions, the cytokine network, the cellular response to oxidative stress, and the gene activation patterns that regulate tissue injury and repair will result in a better understanding of the complex mechanisms involved in the pathogenesis of ischemic acute renal failure.

Role of Uric Acid in Acute Renal Failure

Serum uric acid is frequently elevated during cardiovascular surgery and has been shown to correlate with the risk of developing acute renal failure (6). Hyperuricemia worsens cisplatin-induced acute renal failure via a crystal-independent mechanism. Uric acid decreases the bioavailability of nitric oxide, increases afferent arteriolar vasoconstriction, and decreases the glomerular filtration rate. Uric acid causes preglomerular arteriolar smooth muscle proliferation and may interfere with autoregulation of the renal blood flow. The proinflammatory and prooxidative properties of uric acid can potentiate the inflammatory cascade, mediating acute renal failure.

OUTCOME OF ACUTE RENAL FAILURE OF CRITICAL ILLNESS

The outcome of acute renal failure of critical illness is of immense importance. The mean duration of in-hospital acute renal failure is 14 days. Most episodes resolve in the first month of evolution (7), and only 11% of the patients require renal replacement therapy (2). However, the requirement for renal replacement therapy increases to over 70% when acute renal failure is severe, that is, in the presence of oliguria or severe azotemia (3,8). The usual ICU mortality approximates 5% without acute renal failure, 23% with acute renal failure, and over 60% with acute renal failure requiring renal replacement therapy (Fig. 47.3). Of the patients with acute renal failure who expire, 78% do so within 2 weeks after the renal insult. The 90-day and 1-year survival of those who are discharged from the hospital are 64% and 50%, respectively (8). Interestingly, the ICU mortality of patients with end-stage renal disease is 11%, much lower than for acute renal failure patients who do not need dialysis support (2). The increased mortality associated with the acute decline in renal function is not explained simply by loss of organ function.

The recovery of renal function is influenced by many factors, including pre-existing chronic illness. In one review, only 41% of the patients were reported to be in good health 3 months before entry into the intensive care unit (9); chronic kidney disease has been reported in 30% of all patients admitted to the intensive care unit (3,8,9). Most of the survivors of acute renal failure recover their renal function within 2 weeks, and 65% to 94% of them have independent renal function at discharge from the hospital (3,8,10).

PATHOPHYSIOLOGY OF CHRONIC KIDNEY DISEASE

Epidemiology

An increasingly elderly population with pre-existing renal dysfunction is treated in our intensive care units. The presence of chronic renal disease on admission to the intensive care unit is associated with an incremental increase in long-term mortality in survivors of acute renal failure (Fig. 47.4). Furthermore, recovery from acute renal failure is often accompanied by

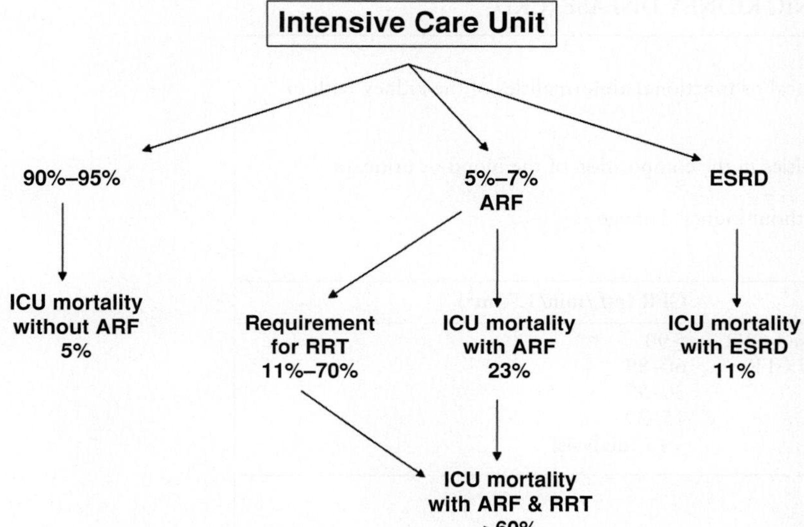

FIGURE 47.3. Outcome of acute renal failure of critical illness.

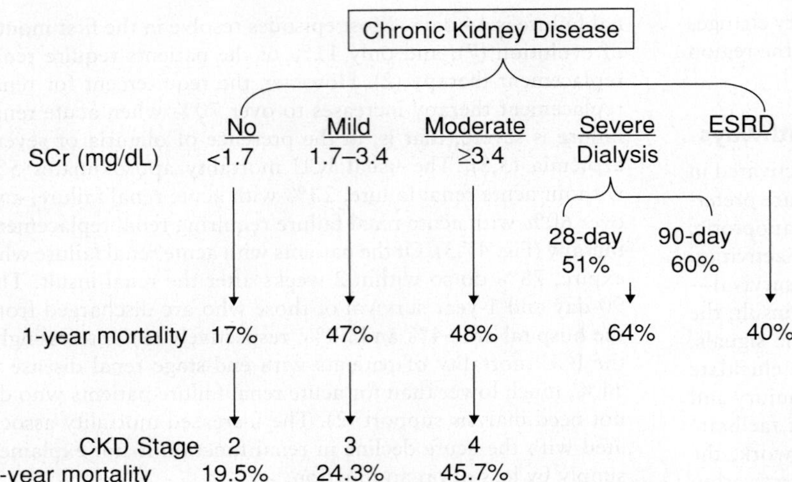

FIGURE 47.4. Effect of the stage of chronic kidney disease on ICU mortality.

residual renal dysfunction and the perils associated with chronic kidney disease. Chronic kidney disease affects 12% of the U.S. population (11). The prevalence of chronic kidney disease is relatively stable, but the number of end-stage renal disease patients who require maintenance dialysis treatments continues to grow. It is estimated that the number of end-stage renal disease treatments will increase 60% by the year 2010. One reason for the discrepancy between the size of the chronic kidney disease pool and the incidence of end-stage renal disease may be the premature cardiovascular death in many patients before progression to end-stage renal disease. In fact, chronic kidney disease has a five to ten times higher risk of death than end-stage renal disease (12). The 5-year mortality of patients with chronic kidney disease stages 2, 3, and 4 are 19.5%, 24.3%, and 45.7%, respectively; 1.1%, 1.3%, and 19.9% progress to renal replacement therapy, respectively (13). The above data underscore the impact of pre-existing organ dysfunction on the prognosis of critically ill patients.

Theories of Chronic Kidney Disease

The U.S. National Kidney Foundation's Kidney Disease Outcomes Quality Initiative classification of chronic kidney disease (Table 47.2) facilitates the development of appropriate management plans but does not provide information on the future risk of decline in renal function. Once renal damage reaches a certain threshold, the progression of renal damage is consistent, irreversible, and independent of initial insult. The characteristic histologic findings of tubular atrophy, interstitial fibrosis, and glomerulosclerosis in chronic kidney disease of diverse causes suggest that multifactorial and complex interactions between numerous pathways of cellular damage by both cellular and humoral pathways contribute to their progression to a common final pathway. Brief overviews of the proposed mechanisms that are involved in the progression of chronic kidney disease are provided below.

TABLE 47.2

DEFINITION AND CLASSIFICATION OF CHRONIC KIDNEY DISEASE (CKD)

DEFINITION

1. Kidney damage for ≥3 months, as defined by structural or functional abnormalities of the kidney with or without decreased GFR, manifested by either:
   - Pathologic abnormalities, or
   - Markers of kidney damage, including abnormalities in the composition of the blood or urine, or abnormalities in imaging tests
2. GFR <60 mL/min/1.73 m^2 for 3 months, with or without kidney damage

CLASSIFICATION

CKD stage	Description	GFR (mL/min/1.73m^2)
I	Kidney damage with normal/increased GFR	≥90
II	Kidney damage with mild decreased GFR	60–89
III	Moderate decreased GFR	30–59
IV	Severe decreased GFR	15–29
V	Kidney failure	<15 (dialysis)

GFR, glomerular filtration rate.

The Hyperfiltration Theory

The hyperfiltration theory (14) emphasizes glomerular hemodynamic changes as the final common pathway in progressive chronic kidney disease. Accordingly, renal injury from diverse causes results in hyperfunction of the remaining glomeruli. The sustained elevations in glomerular pressures and flows favor hyperfiltration and the loss of selectivity of the permeability of the glomerulus. The ensuing proteinuria causes tubule cell injury by "misdirected filtration"—the accumulation of glomerular filtrate outside of the Bowman space and into periglomerular space, creation of a cellular cover around the focus of misdirected filtration by interstitial fibroblasts, extension over the entire glomerulus leading to global sclerosis (15), luminal obstruction, and overwhelming the tubular mechanism by excessive uptake and degradation of filtered protein by the proximal tubule cells. The subsequent extravasation of the accumulated filtered plasma protein into the interstitium causes inflammatory reaction and tubulointerstitial fibrosis (16).

The Complement Activation Theory

The complement activation theory maintains that the proteinuria-induced intraluminal activation of the terminal complement cascade, leading to the formation of C5b-9 membrane attack complex, is the principal mediator of chronic progressive interstitial damage and progressive renal failure in proteinuric renal disease, irrespective of primary glomerular injury. This is supported by the demonstration of increased urinary excretion of C5b-9 in nonimmunologic glomerular injury, correlation of tubulointerstitial deposition of the C5b-9 with interstitial myofibroblast accumulation and proteinuria, and the observation that, in experimental models, progressive interstitial injury was maintained only in hypocomplementemic animals.

The Chronic Hypoxia Theory

The chronic hypoxia theory emphasizes chronic ischemic damage in the tubulointerstitium as a final common pathway in end-stage renal injury. The extent of tubulointerstitial damage is better correlated with impaired renal function than the degree of glomerular injury. The countercurrent arrangement of the descending postglomerular vessels and ascending vasa recta vessels, elevated vasa recta permeability to oxygen, and high metabolic requirement results in a graded fall in oxygen tension from the outer cortex to the inner medulla. In extensive tubulointerstitial injury, the loss and distortion of peritubular capillaries, increased transposition of extracellular matrix, vasoconstriction, glomerular damage, anemia, and oxidative stress impair oxygen supply to the corresponding regions. Hypoxia leads to apoptosis or epithelial-mesenchymal transdifferentiation and exacerbates fibrosis of the kidney and subsequent hypoxia, setting in motion the vicious cycle to end-stage renal disease (17).

Elevated Asymmetric Dimethylarginine

The endothelium plays a crucial role in the maintenance of vascular tone and structure. Endothelium produces nitric oxide, a crucial mediator of vasodilation, inhibition of vasoconstrictor influences, antithrombosis, anti-inflammation, and antiproliferation. The generation of nitric oxide by nitric oxide synthase is inhibited by asymmetric dimethylarginine (ADMA). Elevated plasma ADMA levels are inversely related to GFR and significantly associated with progression of chronic kidney disease (18,19). Elevated ADMA in chronic kidney disease is not due to impaired urinary clearance, but to increased ADMA generation (synthesized by protein methyltransferase) and decreased degradation (mainly by dimethylarginine dimethylaminohydrolase). It is speculated that uremic oxidative stress is involved in the dysregulation of protein methyltransferase and dimethylarginine dimethylaminohydrolase (20).

Anemia

Erythrocytes represent a major antioxidant component of blood. The generation of oxidants is amplified in anemia; it is also enhanced in chronic kidney disease due to increased oxygen consumption by the remnant hyperfunctioning nephrons. Hypoxia of the tubular cells due to decreased delivery of oxygen may be the main link between interstitial fibrosis and tubular destruction. Hypoxia stimulates the production of extracellular matrix by tubular cells and renal interstitial fibroblasts and the release of profibrotic cytokines. Treatment with erythropoetin increases red blood cell mass, improves red blood cell survival by antiapoptotic effects, and decreases oxidative stress. Whether the correction of anemia can decrease the progression of chronic kidney disease remains to be seen (21).

Microvascular Endothelium

Renal microvasculature is maintained by the balance of angiogenic growth factors, alteration of which impairs capillary repair, causes loss of microvasculature, and leads to a decrease in glomerular filtration rate, and oxygen and nutrient supply to the tubules and interstitial cells. The progressive loss of the endothelium results in capillary collapse and development of glomerulosclerosis, impaired blood flow, and tubulointerstitial fibrosis. Increased expression of thrombospondin-1 and other antiangiogenic factors, and decreased expression of vascular endothelial growth factor (VEGF) and other proangiogenic factors, influence the renal microvasculature in progressive chronic kidney disease. VEGF expression correlates with the severity of peritubular capillary loss and inversely correlates with the degree of tubulointerstitial inflammation; it is inhibited by macrophage-derived inflammatory cytokines (IL-10, IL-6, TNF-α) and angiotensin II, and modulated by nitric oxide—factors involved in the pathogenesis of renal injury (22).

IMPACT OF CHRONIC KIDNEY DISEASE ON CRITICAL ILLNESS

Chronic kidney disease is associated with a decrease in structural and functional reserve. The renal capacity to autoregulate renal blood flow; maintain normal systemic blood pressure; excrete solutes, fluids, electrolytes, and the daily acid load; and metabolize drugs is diminished (Table 47.3). The reduction in physiologic reserves influence drug dosing, treatment modality, and response to interventions in patients in the intensive care unit.

Blood Pressure

Some degree of autonomic dysfunction occurs in most patients with moderate to severe chronic kidney disease. The presence

TABLE 47.3

IMPACT OF CHRONIC KIDNEY DISEASE ON OTHER ORGAN SYSTEMS

Cardiovascular System
- Blood pressure control
  - Inadequate sympathetic response due to autonomic dysfunction
  - Elevated frequency of cardiac tamponade leading to low blood pressure during dialysis
- Coronary disease
  - High prevalence of severe coronary heart disease
  - Atypical presentation
  - False positive elevations in creatine kinase and troponin T
  - Appropriate medical therapy is significantly underused
- Arrhythmias
  - High frequency caused by anatomic and biochemical abnormalities
  - Especially common during hemodialysis

Respiratory Failure
- Pulmonary edema and/or pleural effusion
  - Restrictive effects of fluid retention contribute to the development of acute ventilatory failure
- Metabolic acidosis
  - High demand for ventilation caused by acidosis makes the weaning a challenge
- Auto-PEEP
  - Airway mucosal edema predisposes to air trapping and endogenous positive end-expiratory pressure

Central Nervous System
- Uremic encephalopathy
  - Usually present when creatinine clearance level falls below 15 mL/min
- Disequilibrium syndrome
  - Neurologic dysfunction caused by rapid correction of uremia

PEEP, positive end-expiratory pressure.

of autonomic dysfunction impairs the patient's ability to maintain the systemic blood pressure, which may complicate dialysis treatment of patients in the ICU who require removal of large quantities of fluid. Despite the significant down-regulation of alpha and beta adrenergic receptors, plasma catecholamine levels are often elevated in these patients and may increase the risk of cardiac complications. Uremic pericardial effusion may also cause vasopressor-resistant hypotension that, if unrecognized, may have dire consequences for the patient, as the onset of cardiac tamponade can be rapid without premonitory signs.

Cardiac Dysrhythmias

Cardiac dysrhythmias are common in patients with chronic renal failure due to underlying left ventricular hypertrophy, calcific cardiomyopathy that involves the conducting tissues, a "disturbed" metabolic milieu, and chronic tissue hypoxia. An increased incidence of cardiac dysrhythmias is seen in patients with postoperative acute renal failure that may be exacerbated with rapid fluctuations in hemodynamics and electrolyte concentrations in those requiring dialysis support.

Chest Pain

The presence of renal dysfunction can influence the symptoms, manifestations, and progression of coronary syndromes. Chronic kidney disease affects outcome in patients with acute coronary syndrome and is an independent risk factor for the development of coronary artery disease and for more severe coronary heart disease. Chronic kidney disease is also associated with an adverse effect on prognosis from cardiovascular disease. Many dialysis patients with angina often have a fairly typical history of exercise-induced chest discomfort that is similar to those with normal renal function. However, silent myocardial ischemia is also common among patients with severe kidney disease. It has been speculated that the extremely poor prognosis among dialysis patients with an acute myocardial infarction may be due in part to a relatively increased number of atypical clinical presentations, resulting in both underdiagnosis and undertreatment. The presence of dyspnea alone due to an acute myocardial infarction in an individual scheduled to undergo a regular chronic dialysis procedure may be mistakenly attributed to volume overload. In addition, baseline abnormalities on the electrocardiogram, such as left ventricular hypertrophy, may mask characteristic changes with ischemia.

Respiratory Failure

Most patients with acute respiratory failure on mechanical ventilation require some form of renal replacement therapy. Conversely, alterations in respiratory drive, mechanics, muscle function, and gas exchange are frequent consequences of uremia. The development of acute renal failure predisposes patients to overall fluid overload, decreased plasma oncotic pressure, and leakage of fluid from pulmonary capillaries. The restrictive effects of pulmonary interstitial and alveolar edema, pleural effusion, and chest wall edema increase the work of spontaneous breathing and may contribute to the development of acute ventilatory failure. In addition, the metabolic acidosis present in most instances of acute renal failure increases the demand for ventilation through compensatory respiratory alkalosis, further disrupting the relationship between the patient's ventilatory needs and capabilities. Pulmonary edema and ventilation at low lung volumes can cause or worsen hypoxemia.

Acute renal failure can necessitate several modifications in the management of mechanical ventilation. Higher airway pressure is required to maintain the same level of ventilation in the presence of pulmonary edema, pleural effusion, or total-body fluid overload. Airway mucosal edema can reduce effective airway diameter, predisposing to air trapping and intrinsic positive end-expiratory pressure, which can reduce venous return, further compromising cardiac function and increasing the risk of alveolar rupture. The management of acute lung injury and acute respiratory distress syndrome using lung-protective ventilation is made more difficult in the presence of metabolic acidosis, which increases ventilatory drive and worsens acidemia related to permissive hypercapnia.

Disordered Consciousness

Uremic encephalopathy is an organic brain disorder that develops in patients with acute or chronic renal failure, usually when creatinine clearance falls, and remains, below 15 mL/min. Accumulation of toxins, increases in intracellular concentration of calcium in brain cells, and imbalances of neurotransmitter amino acids within the brain are thought to be responsible, although urea itself is not thought to be causative. Clinical manifestations vary with worsening uremia, but prompt identification and initiation of dialysis treatment can readily reverse the symptoms. Initiation of dialysis treatment can also lead to disordered consciousness, especially when advanced states of uremia are dialyzed for excessive lengths of time during their first treatment sessions—the *dialysis disequilibrium syndrome.*

Decreased Metabolism of Drugs

The pharmacokinetics of most drugs are altered in renal dysfunction; their clearances are impaired or they accumulate in tissues and continue to exert their effects long after their administration. Some are broken down into their metabolites with deleterious consequences. Most of the drugs are not removable by dialysis due to their high protein binding. Many effective drug therapies cannot be used because of the risk of accumulation and toxicity. Some drugs are removed by dialysis and require postdialysis supplementation. The varying clearances of the different continuous renal replacement therapies mandate the knowledge of the clearance of the particular modality used to effectively dose a particular drug.

GENERAL PRINCIPLES OF MANAGEMENT

Despite the remarkable progress achieved in understanding the pathophysiology of acute renal failure, no specific pharmacologic agent has yet been approved for its treatment and prevention remains the principle element in its management.

The treatment of established acute renal failure is based on the following principles:

- The preservation of renal blood flow and optimal perfusion pressure favorably influences the deterioration of renal function.
- Correction of uremia, electrolyte, acid-base, endocrine, hematologic and nutritional disorders, and hypervolemia can favorably affect outcome
- The pharmacokinetics and clearance of drugs are altered in renal failure, and the appropriate dosage adjustment requires knowledge of the pharmacokinetic parameters of the drugs and clearance characteristics of the different renal replacement techniques.
- The treatment and complications of secondary causes of acute renal failure may determine its outcome.
- The appropriate integration of care provided by intensivists and organ specialists can favorably affect outcome.

In certain clinical situations, such as in cardiovascular surgery, ischemic acute renal failure is strongly associated with occult renal ischemia—associated with poor cardiac performance, fixed atherosclerotic disease of the renal arteries and/or prolonged hypoxemia, and reduced renal functional reserve. Due to the silent nature of renal ischemia, prognostic stratification using reliable surrogates can guide clinical decision making (23–26). Recently, the use of atrial natriuretic peptides has been shown to improve dialysis-free survival in thoracic aortic aneurysm surgery patients with impaired renal function. However, the use of atrial peptides in acute renal failure remains controversial—two major clinical trials have reported unfavorable outcomes whereas two smaller clinical trials have shown favorable outcomes.

The prevalence of acute renal failure continues to rise; however, there are indications that the mortality of patients with acute renal failure may be declining. This decline in mortality is not due to the effects of newer drugs in the treatment of acute renal failure, but rather, it is due to the increased cooperation between the intensivists and subspecialists, which has led to a concerted approach to treatment. This has resulted in increased awareness of disease states, early initiation and higher doses of dialysis treatments, maintenance of euglycemia, and other interventions that play important roles in reversing mortality.

References

1. Xue JL, Daniels F, Star RA, et al. Incidence and mortality of acute renal failure in Medicare beneficiaries, 1992 to 2001. *J Am Soc Nephrol.* 2006;17:1135–1142.
2. Clermont G, Acker CG, Angus DC, et al. Renal failure in the ICU: comparison of the impact of acute renal failure and end-stage renal disease on ICU outcomes. *Kidney Int.* 2002;62:986–996.
3. Uchino S, Kellum JA, Bellomo R, et al; Beginning and Ending Supportive Therapy for the Kidney (BEST Kidney) Investigators. Acute renal failure in critically ill patients: a multinational, multicenter study. *JAMA.* 2005;294:813–818.
4. Lundberg S. Renal function during anaesthesia and open-heart surgery in man. *Acta Anaesthesiol Scand Suppl.* 1967;27:1–81.
5. Kelleher SP, Robinette JB, Conger JD. Sympathetic nervous system in the loss of autoregulation in acute renal failure. *Am J Physiol.* 1984;246:F379–386.
6. Ejaz AA, Mu W, Kang DH, et al. Could uric acid have a role in acute renal failure? *Clin J Am Soc Nephrol.* 2007;2(1):16–21.
7. Liano I, Liaño F, Pascual J; the Madrid ARF Study Group. Epidemiology of acute renal failure: a prospective, multicenter, community-based study. *Kidney Int.* 1996;50:811–818.
8. Hegarty J, Middleton RJ, Krebs M, et al. Severe acute renal failure in adults: place of care, incidence and outcomes. *QJM.* 2005;98:661–666.
9. Silvester W, Bellomo R, Cole L. Epidemiology, management, and outcome of severe acute renal failure of critical illness in Australia. *Crit Care Med.* 2001;29:1910–1915.
10. Bagshaw SM, Laupland KB, Doig CJ, et al. Prognosis for long-term survival and renal recovery in critically ill patients with severe acute renal failure: a population-based study. *Crit Care.* 2005;9:R700–709.
11. Coresh J, Byrd-Holt D, Astor BC, et al. Chronic kidney disease awareness, prevalence, and trends among U.S. adults, 1999 to 2000. *J Am Soc Nephrol.* 2005;16:180–188.
12. Go AS, Chertow GM, Fan D, et al. Chronic kidney disease and the risks of death, cardiovascular events, and hospitalization. *N Engl J Med.* 2004;351:1296–1305.
13. Keith DS, Nichols GA, Gullion CM, et al. Longitudinal follow-up and outcomes among a population with chronic kidney disease in a large managed care organization. *Arch Intern Med.* 2004;164:659–663.
14. Brenner BM, Meyer TW, Hostetter TH. Dietary protein intake and the progressive nature of kidney disease: the role of hemodynamically mediated glomerular injury in the pathogenesis of progressive glomerular sclerosis in aging, renal ablation, and intrinsic renal disease. *N Engl J Med.* 1982;307:652–659.
15. Kriz W, Elger M, Hosser H, et al. How does podocyte damage result in tubular damage? *Kidney Blood Press Res.* 1999;22:26–36.
16. Zandi-Nejad K, Eddy AA, Glassock RJ, et al. Why is proteinuria an ominous biomarker of progressive kidney disease? *Kidney Int.* 2004;92:S76–89.
17. Nangaku M. Chronic hypoxia and tubulointerstitial injury: a final common pathway to end-stage renal failure. *J Am Soc Nephrol.* 2006;17:17–25.
18. Fliser D, Kronenberg F, Kielstein JT, et al. Asymmetric dimethylarginine and progression of chronic kidney disease: the mild to moderate kidney disease study. *J Am Soc Nephrol.* 2005;16:2456–2461.
19. Ravani P, Tripepi G, Malberti F, et al. Asymmetrical dimethylarginine predicts progression to dialysis and death in patients with chronic kidney disease: a competing risks modeling approach. *J Am Soc Nephrol.* 2005;16:2449–2455.
20. Matsuguma K, Ueda S, Yamagishi S, et al. Molecular mechanism for

elevation of asymmetric dimethylarginine and its role for hypertension in chronic kidney disease. *J Am Soc Nephrol.* 2006;17:2176–2183.
21. Rossert J, Fouqueray B, Boffa JJ. Anemia management and the delay of chronic renal failure progression. *J Am Soc Nephrol.* 2003;14:S173–177.
22. Kang DH, Kanellis J, Hugo C, et al. Role of the microvascular endothelium in progressive renal disease. *J Am Soc Nephrol.* 2002;13:806–816.
23. Chertow GM, Lazarus JM, Christiansen CL, et al. Preoperative renal risk stratification. *Circulation.* 1997;95:878–884.
24. Chawla LS, Abell L, Mazhari R, et al. Identifying critically ill patients at high risk for developing acute renal failure: a pilot study. *Kidney Int.* 2005;68:2274–2280.
25. Yegenaga I, Hoste E, Van Biesen W, et al. Clinical characteristics of patients developing ARF due to sepsis/systemic inflammatory response. *Am J Kidney Dis.* 2004;43:817–824.
26. Vivino G, Antonelli M, Moro ML, et al. Risk factors for acute renal failure in trauma patients. *Intensive Care Med.* 1998;24:808–814.

CHAPTER 48 ■ GASTROINTESTINAL PHYSIOLOGY

JORGE H. CASTRO • JUAN B. OCHOA

The splanchnic organs, composed of liver, pancreas, the large and small bowel, and the gut-associated lymphoid tissue (GALT), can be a source of critical illness. These splanchnic organs also play central roles in perpetuating the multiorgan dysfunction syndrome (MODS) and failure (MOSF). As such, the critical care physician must have a significant understanding of the illnesses that arise in and relate to these organs, particularly regarding their identification and contribution to the systemic inflammatory response, to ultimately design an appropriate treatment plan and minimize the potential complications.

The complexity of the splanchnic organs is such that entire books have been dedicated to the subject. Because of its complexity, an isolated chapter will, by necessity, be only an introduction to the topic. We will describe some of the concepts that are considered most important in the relationship between gut and systemic inflammatory response syndrome (SIRS)/MODS, including the preservation of a functional intestinal barrier and the function of the GALT. The goal of this chapter, therefore, is to stimulate and prepare the reader for a more in-depth study of this area.

BASIC GASTROINTESTINAL PHYSIOLOGY

The gastrointestinal (GI) tract is a dual-functioning organ system that works actively in the selective absorption process; it also plays an important role in providing continuous immune surveillance and protection. The absorption of nutrients—the best-studied function of the GI tract—is essential for the processing, presentation, and delivery of all nutrients into the body. Nutrient processing is also important for maintaining a healthy gut mucosa. In addition, the gut harbors approximately 70% of all the body's immune tissue and function (1). The GALT is actively exposed to multiple antigens, and it processes these antigens and develops immunity against several environmental antigens (2–4).

Working in concert, the GI tract, including its mucosa and the GALT, create a sophisticated organ whose function and complexity we only partially understand. The mucosa of the GI tract is, in fact, a semipermeable membrane that acts as an *intestinal barrier* and is maintained by adequate blood perfusion, the secretion of mucin, and other substances such as IgA (2,5,6). Normal GI motility avoids bacterial overgrowth, and the presence of commensal organisms prevents the growth of pathogenic bacteria. Not surprisingly, alterations in all of these factors can result in disease and the development or perpetuation of SIRS or MODS (1,6–8).

DISEASE PROCESSES THAT AFFECT THE SPLANCHNIC ORGANS

In critical illness, two main disease processes can lead to, or contribute to, critical illness: An inflammatory process in which an infectious agent is not initially involved, and an inflammatory process in which infection, particularly of bacterial origin, is an essential component of the disease process. However, it is important to state that in many cases, soon after the initiation of the process, which was originally without infection, bacterial contamination and invasion may play an essential role in the pathophysiology of the disease.

Inflammatory Processes Not Caused by an Infectious Agent

These include processes such as shock and ischemia–reperfusion, toxic hepatitis, or acute pancreatitis. In such disorders, the inflammatory response and activation of the immune system may proceed in the absence of infection. The clinical presentation of severe inflammation in these cases may be indistinguishable from those of diseases in which an infectious process predominates.

Inflammatory Processes in Which Infection Plays a Major Role

Disorders such as perforated appendicitis or diverticulitis with peritonitis are typical examples of this situation. In such cases, bacterial invasion of the peritoneum plays a key role in triggering the inflammatory process. The clinical presentation is classically observed as sepsis, with an acute surgical abdomen. In general, the hollow viscus is a preferred portal of entry for infection. There are, however, other forms of splanchnic organ infection not conforming to the presentation of an acute abdomen that may also be the source of a severe inflammatory response. For example, infectious pancreatitis and acute viral hepatitis can initiate the inflammatory process. A thorough review of each of these disease states is impossible in the context of this chapter; however, much is covered elsewhere in this textbook. In this chapter, we provide an outline of some of the most important and frequent processes below.

Representative Diseases of the Splanchnic Organs

Acute Pancreatitis

Acute pancreatitis is a disease process with a wide spectrum of clinical presentations and causes that can challenge any critical care physician. Only 10% to 15% of cases are severe enough to threaten patient survival, and therefore, the critical care physician tends to be involved in only the most severe cases. The most frequent causes of acute pancreatitis are gallstones and alcohol intake, constituting more than 85% of the cases (9). Other causes include hyperlipidemia, viral infections, and certain drugs such as propofol (10,11) (Tables 48.1 and 48.2).

In the intensive care unit, we should take into special consideration the association between using sedation with propofol and the presence of hypertriglyceridemia and acute pancreatitis. Devlin et al. (10) retrospectively studied 159 patients in the intensive care unit (ICU) with propofol sedation. They found that 29 (18%) patients developed hypertriglyceridemia, and among these 29 patients, 3 presented a clinical picture of acute pancreatitis. Their final recommendation was to monitor the serum triglycerides levels and pancreas enzymes after 48 hours on propofol.

Acute pancreatitis triggers the activation of endogenous enzymes such as trypsin, causing autolysis and activation of the inflammatory response. Inflammatory responses to pancreatitis can be severe enough to lead to organ failure. Bacterial seeding of the necrotic pancreas can occur, most probably through bacterial translocation from the gut, sometimes leading to the development of sepsis—one of the main causes of delayed death. It may be difficult to differentiate a severe aseptic inflammatory response to pancreatitis from a septic response due to bacterial contamination (9,12–15).

The usual initial workup for acute pancreatitis is to obtain serum amylase and lipase values and determine the severity of the disease by either APACHE II score or Ramson criteria (10) (Tables 48.3 and 48.4).

Ideally, the extension of necrosis should be determined in all cases of severe acute pancreatitis; the gold standard to make such determinations is contrast-enhanced computed tomography (CT). The CT is important for other reasons as well. For example, at times, the severity of SIRS and the early presence of shock indicates that the patient may be suffering from life-threatening complications such as major bleeding and/or hollow viscus erosion/perforation; the abdominal CT scan is useful to assess such possibilities.

After the first 2 weeks of the disorder, the incidence of infection is increased. The patient may show a persistent inflammatory state, and can deteriorate with SIRS, sepsis, or septic shock. Although the presence of pancreatic air bubbles on abdominal CT scan suggests infection, the gold standard to rule out this possibility is CT-guided needle aspiration of the necrotic pancreatic bed (9,12–15).

TABLE 48.1

CLASSIFICATION SYSTEM OF DRUG-INDUCED ACUTE PANCREATITIS

Class Ia Drugs: At least one case report with positive rechallenge, excluding all other causes, such as alcohol, hypertriglyceridemia, gallstones, and other drugs

Class Ib Drugs: At least one case report with positive rechallenge; however, other causes, such as alcohol, hypertriglyceridemia, gallstones, and other drugs were not ruled out

Class II Drugs:

- At least four cases in the literature.
- Consistent latency (≥75% of cases)

Class III Drugs:

- At least two cases in the literature
- No consistent latency among cases
- No rechallenge

Class IV Drugs: Drugs not fitting into the earlier-described classes; single case report published in medical literature, without rechallenge.

From Badalov N, Baradarian R, Iswara K, et al. Drug-induced acute pancreatitis: an evidence-based review. *Clin Gastroenterol Hepatol.* 2007;5:648–661, with permission.

Acute Mesenteric Ischemia

The splanchnic organs are perfused by three major vessels: the celiac axis, which perfuses the liver, stomach, and spleen; the superior mesenteric artery, which supplies most of the small bowel and the right side of the colon; and the inferior mesenteric artery, which supplies the left side of the colon, sigmoid, and superior portion of the rectum. Acute mesenteric ischemia is caused by several conditions including classic arterial occlusion due to atherosclerosis or embolism (frequently from the left atrium or left ventricle); low flow states due to shock, including cardiogenic shock; or mesenteric venous occlusion. Acute mesenteric ischemia frequently manifests as a devastating disease process. However, mesenteric ischemia can also present in a more subtle manner—for instance, mild abdominal distention and/or mild pain. Reperfusion of the splanchnic organs, which occurs with treatment, may also be associated with a significant and occasionally dramatic systemic inflammatory response (16,17).

TABLE 48.2

SUMMARY OF DRUG-INDUCED ACUTE PANCREATITIS BASED ON DRUG CLASS

Class Ia	Class Ib	Class II	Class III	Class IV
α-Methyldopa	All-trans-retinoic acid	Acetaminophen	Alendronate	Adrenocorticotrophic hormone
Azodisalicylate	Amiodarone	Chlorthiazide	Atorvastatin	Ampicillin
Bezafibrate	Azathioprine	Clozapine	Carbamazepine	Bendroflumethiazide
Cannabis	Clomiphene	DDI	Captopril	Benzapril
Carbimazole	Dexamethasone	Erythromycin	Ceftriaxone	Betamethazone
Codeine	Ifosfamide	Estrogen	Chlorthalidone	Capecytabine
Cytosine Arabinoside	Lamivudine	L-asparaginase	Cimetidine	Cisplatin
Dapsone	Losartan	Pegasparagase	Clarithromycin	Colchicine
Enalapril	Linesterol/methoxy ethinylestradiol	Propofol	Cyclosporin	Cyclophosphamide
Furosemide	6-MP	Tamoxifen	Gold	Cyproheptidine
Isoniazid	Meglumine		Hydrochlorothiazide	Danazol
Mesalamine	Methimazole		Indomethacin	Diazoxide
Metronidazole	Nelfinavir		Interferon/ribavirin	Diclofenac
Pentamidine	Norethindrone/mestranol		Irbesartan	Difenoxylate
Pravastatin	Omeprazole		Isotretinoin	Doxorubicin
Procainamide	Premarin		Ketorolac	Ethacrinic acid
Pyritonol	Sulfamethazole		Lisinopril	Famciclovir
Simvastatin	Trimethoprim–sulfamethazole		Metalozone	Finasteride
Stibogluconate			Metformin	5-Fluorouracil
Sulfamethoxazole			Minocycline	Fluvastatin
Sulindac			Mirtazapine	Gemfibrozil
Tetracycline			Naproxen	Interleukin-2
Valproic acid			Paclitaxel	Ketoprofen
			Prednisone	Lovastatin
			Prednisolone	Mefanamic acid
				Nitrofurantoin
				Octreotide
				Oxyphenbutazone
				Penicillin
				Phenophthalein
				Propoxyphene
				Ramipril
				Ranitidine
				Rifampin
				Risperidone
				Ritonovir
				Roxithromycin
				Rosuvostatin
				Sertraline
				Strychnine
				Tacrolimus
				Vigabatrin/lamotrigine
				Vincristine

From Badalov N, Baradarian R, Iswara K, et al. Drug-induced acute pancreatitis: an evidence-based review. *Clin Gastroenterol Hepatol.* 2007; 5:648–661, with permission.

The presence of severe abdominal pain with few abdominal findings on physical exam, in any patient with risk factors, obliges the clinician to rule out this entity. Performing the examination can be made quite difficult in a sedated and ventilated patient. Hemoconcentration and/or an unexplained metabolic acidosis are indications of this disorder; occasionally, lower GI tract bleeding can be noted, or a positive stool guaiac study is obtained. Plain abdominal films are less specific, showing everything from normal findings to the demonstration of ileus, portal vein air, air in the colonic wall, or free intraperitoneal air (Figs. 48.1 and 48.2). A contrast-enhanced abdominal CT scan is useful, as it may identify the precise location of the compromised vessel (artery or vein) and extension of the damage, and signs such as portal vein air, air in the bowel wall, and complications such as free intraperitoneal air. When the patient is too unstable to be moved for a CT scan, bedside diagnostic laparotomy/laparoscopy is an option (16,17).

Extrahepatic Biliary Disease

Benign extrahepatic biliary disease (EBD) is frequently associated with varying degrees of sepsis and inflammatory response and is a common reason for admission to the ICU. Extrahepatic

TABLE 48.3

RAMSON'S PROGNOSTIC SIGNS OF PANCREATITIS CRITERIA FOR ACUTE PANCREATITIS NOT DUE TO GALLSTONES

At admission	During the initial 48 h
Age >55 y	Hematocrit fall >10 points
WBC >16,000/mm^3	BUN elevation >5 mg/dL
Blood glucose >200 mg/dL	Serum calcium <8 mg/dL
Serum LDH >300 IU/L	Arterial PO_2 <60 mm Hg
Serum AST >250 U/dL	Base deficit >4 mEq/L
	Estimated fluid sequestration >6 L

WBC, white blood cells; LDH, lactate dehydrogenase; AST, aspartate aminotransferase; BUN, blood urea nitrogen.
From Ramson JHC. Etiological and prognostic factors in human acute pancreatitis: a review. *Am J Gastroenterol.* 1982;77:633–638, with permission.

biliary disease includes cholecystitis and/or cholangitis. The severity of EBD increases with extremes of age and neglect related to delayed time to surgical consultation, and in patients with chronic diseases such as diabetes mellitus or those who are immunosuppressed for any reason. The main cause of EBD is the presence of gallbladder calculi.

Cholecystitis in the absence of calculi is also observed in the ICU, particularly in those patients who are in shock, kept without oral intake, or who received total parenteral nutrition (TPN). Acute acalculous cholecystitis may be an occult cause of sepsis and is difficult to diagnose, particularly because studies such as ultrasound lose their accuracy in the critically ill (18–20). Thus, the diagnosis of acalculous cholecystitis is sometimes difficult, and the intensivist must have a high index of suspicion. Usual findings are fever, hyperbilirubinemia, and right upper quadrant pain; sometimes, however, there are only signs of SIRS.

The initial study is bedside ultrasound of the right upper quadrant. Specific signs of inflammation are thickening of the gallbladder wall to greater than 3.5 mm or pericholecystic fluid. The abdominal CT scan may also be helpful in demonstrating pericholecystic fluid and pericholecystic tissue inflammation (one can obtain similar findings with ultrasound [US]), with a main disadvantage of having to transport the patient outside the ICU. On the other hand, other studies such as nuclear medicine have almost no role in the workup of the ICU patient because of the lack of specificity (18–20) and the need to transport the patient for this study.

Perforation of a Hollow Viscus

Perforation of a hollow viscus with resultant intra-abdominal sepsis is a common cause for admission to the ICU. As such, the critical care physician will frequently manage these patients who present a picture of bacterial sepsis. Patients with colonic perforations may demonstrate varying degrees of septic shock. Patients with perforated peptic ulcer disease most often present initially with chemical peritonitis, which will progress to bacterial peritonitis if left untreated. Surgical management of patients with a perforated hollow viscus is an essential aspect of their care, and thus coordination between the anesthesia, surgery, and critical care teams is of great importance (21–23).

The combination of an acute abdomen with rapid deterioration of the patient's condition should trigger the possibility of a perforated hollow viscus. The emergent nature of the presentation will dictate the next step. Bedside plain abdomen films may, on occasion, demonstrate pneumoperitoneum; ultrasound usually does not show specific signs. The CT scan has the ability to demonstrate very small degrees of pneumoperitoneum, free fluid, duodenal wall inflammatory changes, and inflammation of surrounding organs (21).

TABLE 48.4

CRITERIA FOR ACUTE GALLSTONE PANCREATITIS

At admission	During the initial 48 h
Age >70 y	Hematocrit fall >10 points
WBC >18,000/mm^3	BUN elevation >2 mg/dL
Blood glucose >220 mg/dL	Serum calcium <8 mg/dL
Serum LDH >400 IU/L	Arterial PO_2 <60 mm Hg
Serum AST >250 U/dL	Base deficit >5 mEq/L
	Estimated fluid sequestration >4 L

WBC, white blood cells; LDH, lactate dehydrogenase; AST, aspartate aminotransferase; BUN, blood urea nitrogen.
From Ramson JHC. Etiological and prognostic factors in human acute pancreatitis: a review. *Am J Gastroenterol.* 1982;77:633–638, with permission.

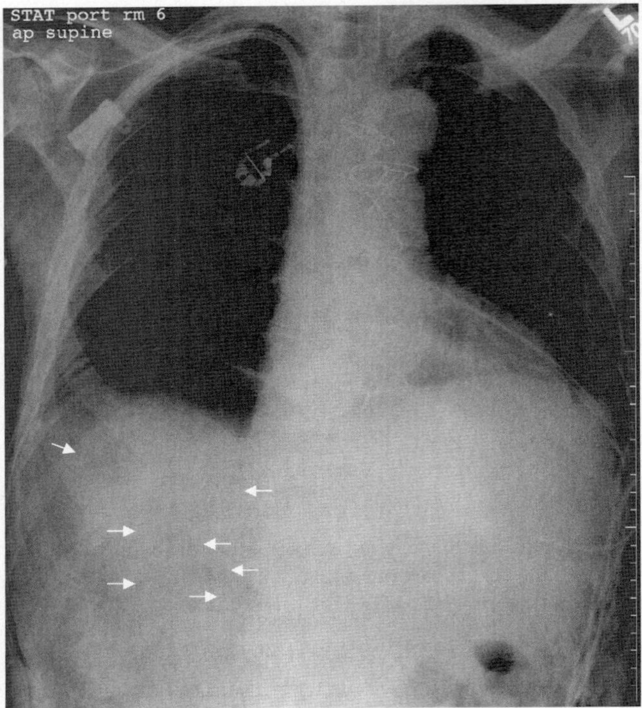

FIGURE 48.1. This abdominal plain film shows the presence of air inside the portal vein—a classic sign for mesenteric ischemia (*arrows*).

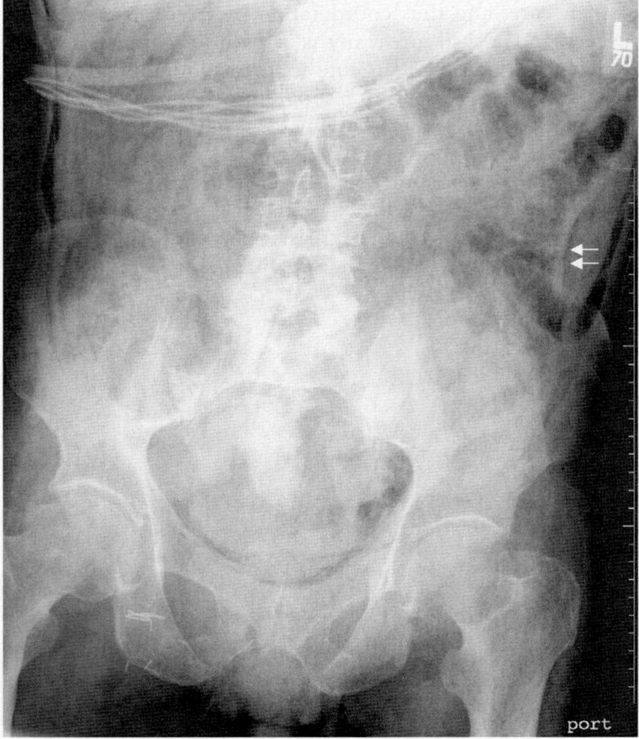

FIGURE 48.2. Note the colonic wall thickening and air bubbles in colonic wall—nonspecific signs for mesenteric ischemia (*arrows*).

Clostridium difficile Colitis

The selective pressure of antibiotic use may lead to the disruption of normal fecal flora, with the emergence of resistant organisms, which can, in turn, cause disease. Best known of these organisms is *Clostridium difficile*, which can cause diarrheal outbreaks in health care institutions. The emergence of a hypervirulent strain of *C. difficile*, which produces both toxins A and B (24)—and is frequently fluoroquinolone-resistant—has been a problem of particular importance in ICUs in many countries (25). *Clostridium difficile* colitis can be a lethal disease, particularly if not adequately treated. There is an increased risk of developing severe *C. difficile* colitis in patients who are chronically ill, as well as in the elderly and immunosuppressed. Early identification and treatment are critical, and the presence of significant leukocytosis should trigger the possibility of such a diagnosis (26). The current mainstay of treatment is oral vancomycin and/or metronidazole—the latter given either intravenously or orally. Aggressive fluid resuscitation and careful monitoring of the clinical condition, along with timely surgical intervention, is important to decrease mortality. Morbidity from this disease and a significant incidence of recurrence continue to be a problem. Other adjunct treatments, including dietary manipulations, the use of probiotics and toxin-binding agents, and restoration of the colonic flora through the use of probiotics are all treatments that are being tested, though their exact role in the treatment of this disease is unclear (27). An interesting, though not appealing, idea is that of transplantation of the fecal flora, which refers to the administration of fecal flora directly to the lumen of the colon or via a nasogastric (NG) tube; preliminary results of this procedure has had promising results in small studies.

The diagnosis of *C. difficile* colitis may be a challenge. However, laboratory data most frequently show a leukemoid reaction on the complete blood count, and hypoalbuminemia; the most commonly used study is the toxin A and B enzyme immunoassay. If there is suspicion of megacolon, an initial abdominal radiograph—a KUB (kidney, ureters, and bladder) study—may reveal significant colonic dilatation with pneumatosis in the colonic wall. The abdominal CT scan is useful to assess colon integrity and rule out other pathologies (24).

THE ABDOMEN AS AN "UNKNOWN SOURCE OF SEPSIS"

Evaluation of the abdomen as the source of sepsis in the ICU patient is difficult. Clinical examination in a neurologically intact patient remains the gold standard used to rule out an acute surgical abdomen and the identification of the abdomen as a source of sepsis. This is not the case in many critically ill patients in whom neurologic impairment due to the primary disease, or resultant from sedation, abrogates good communication with the patient and a dependable clinical examination. In fact, performing a good clinical examination was not possible in 43% to 69% of patients in the ICU (28). Particularly difficult are those who have had recent previous abdominal surgery, and in whom an intra-abdominal septic complication could be a potential cause of critical illness.

How is one to open the "black box" of the abdomen and identify an occult source of sepsis? Several conditions such as

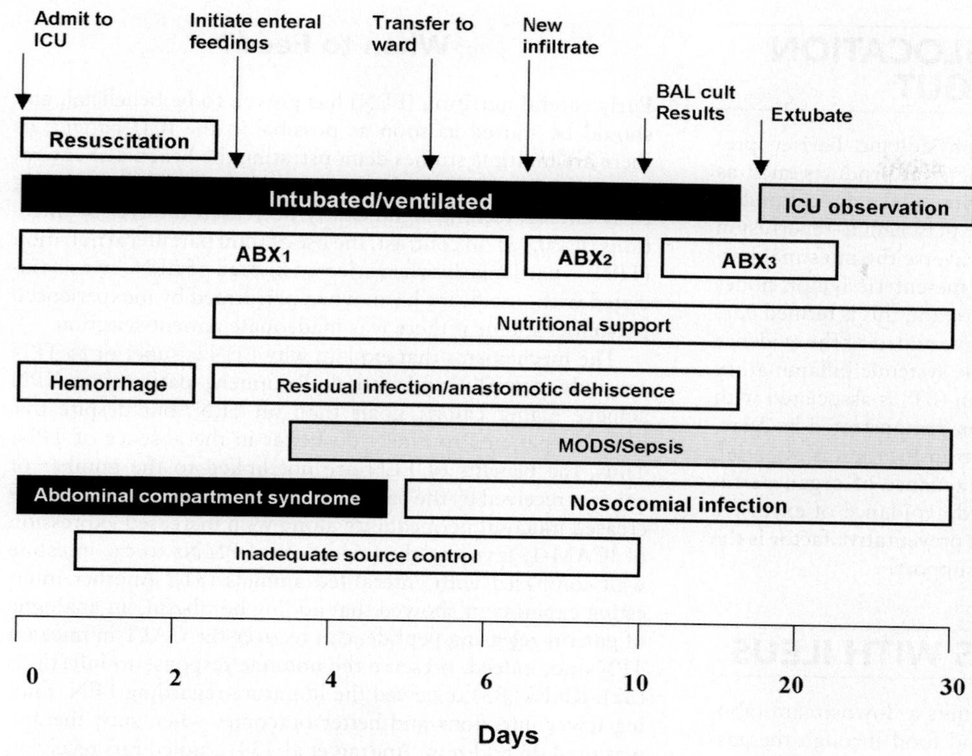

FIGURE 48.3. Scheme showing when, during the course of an intensive care unit admission, intra-abdominal problems are more likely to be seen, especially after abdominal or interventional procedures. ABX, antibiotics; BAL cult, bronchoalveolar lavage culture; ICU, intensive care unit; MODS, multiorgan dysfunction syndrome. (From Crandakk M, West MA. Evaluation of the abdomen in the critically ill patient: opening the black box. *Curr Opin Crit Care.* 2006;12:333–339, with permission.)

pancreatitis and mesenteric ischemia could develop during the intensive care unit admission or may be the primary reason for admission. The diagnostic approach in these patients is dictated by several factors, including the severity of the critical illness, the availability of different diagnostic tools, and the availability of specialized consultants (Fig. 48.3). In patients with severe hemodynamic instability and/or marginal ventilatory status, transport to radiologic suites or other diagnostic facilities may not be possible; also, portable CT scanners are often not available. Therefore, it is important for the critical care physician to identify the available tools that can assist him or her in the timely diagnosis and management of occult abdominal sepsis.

The use of radiologic studies such as CT scan, ultrasound, and nuclear medicine imaging require careful evaluation of the risks associated with the specific study versus the benefit from the information obtained. It is important to emphasize that none of the imaging studies used to diagnose an acute intra-abdominal process is risk-free. For example, studies such as abdominal CT scanning require transport outside of the ICU, and the use of contrast material can produce serious toxicity, such as acute renal failure with intravenous (IV) contrast media administration, as well as discomfort and pain. The information yielded by any of the studies may be poor or lead to misinterpretation, thereby increasing morbidity; thus, the authors discourage the use of diagnostic tests in a "fishing expedition" mode. The studies requested must be done to answer a specific question or questions and the results provided by the study. Furthermore, the risks must be offset by the benefits accruing to the patient, which is not always a simple calculation.

Occasionally, the intensivist appeals to the surgeon to perform an exploratory laparotomy as a means to diagnose and treat intra-abdominal illness. Blind exploratory laparotomies, however, have yielded uniformly poor results, generally not identifying the source of infection, while significantly increasing morbidity or mortality (28). Other less aggressive modes of surgical diagnostic interventions have, therefore, been designed, including diagnostic peritoneal lavage (DPL), paracentesis, and bedside laparoscopy.

ABDOMINAL COMPARTMENT SYNDROME

Increased intra-abdominal pressures compromising blood flow to splanchnic organs have been described in an increased percentage of patients in the ICU. In a recent article, for example, Malbrain et al., from the European Community (29), analyzed 265 consecutive patients in the ICU, measuring intra-abdominal pressures via transduction of the urinary bladder. This work demonstrated that nonsurvivors tended to have higher intra-abdominal pressures. Furthermore, patients with prior elevated intra-abdominal pressures exhibited increased sepsis-related organ failure assessment (SOFA) scores.

Determining when abdominal decompression should be done remains controversial and is partially subjective. For some, intra-abdominal hypertension (IAH) is defined as a pressure greater than 20 mm Hg in the presence of at least one organ failure. In these cases, opening the abdomen should be considered and should be viewed as a therapeutic maneuver to improve splanchnic organ perfusion. Demonstrating that surgical therapy improves outcome is, however, difficult. Nonetheless, it is logical that increasing organ perfusion should improve physiologic function, or at least not worsen the outcome.

BACTERIAL TRANSLOCATION FROM THE GUT

Maintenance of the gut mucosal physiologic barrier prevents the passage of bacteria—or bacterial products such as endotoxin—into the systemic circulation. Once the gut undergoes a predisposing condition, such as an ischemia–reperfusion insult, bacteria and endotoxins can traverse the intestinal barrier and seed distant organs such as mesenteric lymph nodes (MLNs), solid organs, and the bloodstream; this is termed *bacterial translocation*. Several studies have added to the evidence linking bacterial translocation and the systemic inflammatory response (1–4). Bacterial translocation (BT) is associated with postoperative sepsis in up to 14%, as demonstrated by MacFie et al. (3). Prevention of bacterial translocation is essential, and is accomplished by careful maintenance of organ perfusion, judicious use of antibiotics, and avoidance of excessive IV fluids. Perhaps the most important preventative factor is the early institution of enteral nutrition support.

SPECIAL CONCERNS WITH ILEUS

Normal gastrointestinal motility permits a downstream (aboral) progression of secreted fluids and food through the gastrointestinal tract. It also prevents bacterial overgrowth and provides the adequate contact of nutrients with the gut mucosa, thereby allowing digestion and absorption. Loss of coordinated propulsive motor impulses may result in decreased digestion and absorption of food and liquids, gastrointestinal intolerance, and the lack of passage of flatus or stool; this is called *ileus*. Ileus is therefore a *functional intestinal obstruction* in the absence of mechanical evidence of obstruction.

Ileus, in its worse clinical presentation, is a manifestation of organ (gastrointestinal) dysfunction or failure. Ileus can result in abdominal compartment syndrome, severe electrolytic disturbances, and bacterial overgrowth. Furthermore, the presence of ileus precludes successful enteral nutritional interventions. For these reasons, adequate identification of ileus is an essential aspect of care of the critical care physician.

The diagnosis of ileus is often inaccurate and is based on significant preconceptions that are frequently erroneous. For example, it is often believed that surgical intervention on the gastrointestinal tract results in ileus, and that, postoperatively, this patient population should be kept without oral or enteral intake. Similar misconceptions are often observed with artificially established amounts of gastric residuals or nasogastric outputs. Paradoxically, multiple patients are often kept without enteral intake, which only exacerbates gastrointestinal dysfunction and provides an inadequate and/or inappropriate diagnosis of ileus.

Ileus has to be carefully identified by radiographs and a thorough clinical assessment. Careful hydration and restoration of splanchnic blood flow through adequate resuscitation are essential. The judicious use of enteral nutritional support and avoiding prolonged time periods without enteral intake are essential to the prevention and treatment of ileus. Furthermore, the careful treatment of the cause of an ileus, such as sepsis, will often result in the spontaneous resolution of the gastrointestinal process. Maintenance of fluid and electrolyte balance are also important.

When to Feed?

Early enteral nutrition (EEN) has proven to be beneficial, and should be started as soon as possible in the ICU patient, as there are multiple studies demonstrating the benefits of enteral nutrition. For example, Moore et al. (30) found that starting early enteral feeding significantly decreased the risk of infections ($p < 0.05$). In contrast, the use of total parenteral nutrition (TPN)—particularly when selected instead of EEN—was associated with significant harm when performed by inexperienced personnel and/or if there was inadequate patient selection.

The mechanisms that explain why EEN is superior to TPN are only partially understood. Routinely, patients on TPN achieve higher caloric goals than on EEN, but despite this practice, patients routinely do better in the absence of TPN. Thus, the benefits of EEN are not linked to the number of calories received by the patient. Starvation is associated with increased mucosal permeability along with increased expression of ICAM-1, favoring the migration of PMNs to the intestine wall compared with enteral-fed animals (31). Another interesting experiment showed that adding bombesin, an analogue of gastrin-releasing peptide, can recover the GALT in mice on TPN and, indeed, preserve the immune response to infections (32). Kudsk (33) reviewed the literature regarding EEN, finding fewer infections and better outcomes when such therapy was used. In addition, Andrad et al. (34) studied rats receiving either standard TPN or glutamine-enriched TPN. They found less bacterial translocation in the group on glutamine-enriched TPN, suggesting that glutamine, an amino acid, improves the response to antigens and increases the IgA levels, as reported previously (35). Other authors have reported that EEN prevents GALT atrophy and the development of SIRS/MOD (36–38).

SUMMARY

Splanchnic organs continue to be a challenge for intensivists. Splanchnic organs can both be a source of disease and perpetuate existing problems. Maintenance of normal splanchnic organ function is essential for the survival of the patient. Gut trophism and immune function is better preserved by enteral/oral nutrition. Therefore, EEN should be the standard of care in trauma services.

References

1. Schmidt H, Martindale R. The gastrointestinal tract in critical illness. *Curr Opin Clin Nutr Metab Care.* 2001;4:547–551.
2. Achenson DWK. Mucosal immune responses. *Best Pract Res Clin Gastroenterol.* 2004;18:387–404.
3. MacFie J, Reddy BS, Gatt M, et al. Bacterial translocation studied in 927 patients over 13 years. *Br J Surg.* 2006;93:87–93.
4. Moore F. The role of the gastrointestinal tract in postinjury multiple organ failure. *Am J Surg.* 1999;178:449–453.
5. Moore E, Moore FA, Franciose RJ, et al. The postischemic gut serves as a priming bed for circulating neutrophils that provoke multiple organ failure. *J Trauma.* 1994;37:881–887.
6. Leaphart CL, Tepas III JJ. The gut is a motor of organ dysfunction. *Surgery.* 2007;141:563–569.
7. Laughlin RS, Musch MW, Hollbrook CJ, et al. The key role of Pseudomonas aeruginosa PA-I lectin on experimental gut-derived sepsis. *Ann Surg.* 2000;232:133–142.

8. Reinhart K, Bloos F, Brunkhorst. Pathophysiology of sepsis and multiple organ dysfunction. In: Fink M, Abraham E, Vincent JL, et al., eds. *Textbook of Critical Care.* 5th ed. Philadelphia, PA: Elsevier Saunders; 2005: 1257.
9. Badalov, N, Baradarian, R, Iswara, K, et al. Drug-induced acute pancreatitis: an evidence-based review. *Clin Gastroenterol Hepatol.* 2007;5:648–661.
10. Devlin JW, Lau AK, Tanios MA. Propofol-associated hypertriglyceridemia and pancreatitis in the intensive care unit: an analysis of frequency and risk factors. *Pharmacotherapy.* 2005;10:1348–1352.
11. Beger HG, Rau B, Mayer J, et al: Natural course of acute pancreatitis. *World J Surg.* 1997;21:130–135.
12. Zhao X, Anderson R, Wang X, et al. Acute pancreatitis-associated lung injury: pathophysiological mechanisms and potential future therapies. *Scand J Gastroenterol.* 2002;37:1351–1358.
13. Mann DV, Hershman MJ, Hittinger R, et al. Multicenter audit of death from acute pancreatitis. *Br J Surg.* 1994;81:890–893.
14. Hartwig W, Werner J, Uhl W, et al. Management of infection in acute pancreatitis. *J Hepatobiliary Pancreat Surg.* 2002;9:423–428.
15. Ramson JHC. Etiological and prognostic factors in human acute pancreatitis: a review. *Am J Gastroenterol.* 1982;77:633–638.
16. Haglund U. Gut ischaemia. *Gut.* 1994;35:S73–76.
17. Brandt LJ, Boley SJ. AGA technical review on intestinal ischemia. American Gastrointestinal Association. *Gastroenterology.* 2000;118:954–968.
18. Glenn F, Becker CG. Acute acalculous cholecystitis: an increasing entity. *Ann Surg.* 1982;195:131–136.
19. Boland G, Lee MJ, Mueller PR. Acute cholecystitis in the intensive care unit. *New Horiz.* 1993;1:246–260.
20. Ryu JK, Ryu KH, Kim KH. Clinical features of acute acalculous cholecystitis. *J Clin Gastroenterol.* 2003;36:166–169.
21. Solomkin JS, Wittman DW, West MA, et al. Intraabdominal infections. In Schwartz SI, Shires GT, Spencer FC, et al., eds. *Principles of Surgery,* 7th ed. New York, NY: McGraw-Hill; 1999:1515–1550.
22. Anaya DA, Nathens AB. Risk factors for severe sepsis in secondary peritonitis. *Surg Infect (Larchmt).* 2003;4:355–362.
23. Fry DE, Pearlstein DE, Fulton RL, et al. Multiple system organ failure: the role of uncontrolled infection. *Arch Surg.* 1980;115:136–140.
24. Fekety R, Shah AB: Diagnosis and treatment of *Clostridium difficile* colitis. *JAMA.* 1993;269:71.
25. Razavi B, Apisarnthanarak A, Mondy LM. *Clostridium difficile*: emergence of hypervirulence and fluoroquinolone resistance. *Infection.* 2007;5:300–307.
26. Wanahita A, Goldsmith EA, Musher DM. Conditions associated with leukocytosis in a tertiary care hospital with particular attention to the role of infection caused by *Clostridium difficile. Clin Infect Dis.* 2002;34:1585–1592.
27. Miller MA. Clinical management of *Clostridium difficile*-associated disease. *Clin Infect Dis.* 2007;45:S122–S128.
28. Crandall M, West MA. Evaluation of the abdomen in the critically ill patient: opening the black box. *Curr Opin Crit Care.* 2006;12:333–339.
29. Malbrain M, Chiumello D, Pelosi P, et al. Incidence and prognosis of intraabdominal hypertension in a mixed population of critically ill patients: a multiple-center epidemiological study. *Crit Care Med.* 2005;33:315–322.
30. Moore FA, Feliciano DV, Andrassy RJ, et al. Early enteral feeding, compared with parenteral, reduces postoperative septic complications. The results of a meta-analysis. *Ann Surg.* 1992;216:172–183.
31. Fukatsu K, Zarzaur BL, Johnson CD, et al. Enteral nutrition prevents remote organ injury and death after a gut ischemic insult. *Ann Surg.* 2001;233:660–668.
32. DeWitt RC, Wu Y, Renegar KB, et al. Bombesin recovers gut-associated lymphoid tissue and preserves immunity to bacterial pneumonia in mice receiving total parenteral nutrition. *Ann Surg.* 2000;231:1–8.
33. Kudsk KA. Early enteral nutrition in surgical patients. *Nutrition.* 1998;14: 541–544.
34. Andrade M, Santos D, Fernandez S, et al. Prevention of bacterial translocation using glutamine: a new strategy of investigation. *Nutrition.* 2006;22: 419–424.
35. Sawai T, Goldstone N, Drongowski RA, et al. Effect of secretory immunoglobulin A on bacterial translocation in an enterocyte-lymphocyte coculture model. *Pediatr Surg Int.* 2001;17:275–279.
36. Avenell A. Glutamine in critical care: current evidence from systematic reviews. *Proc Nutr Soc.* 2006;65:236–241.
37. Wildhaber B, Yang H, Spencer A, et al. Lack of enteral nutrition. Effects on the immune system. *J Surg Res.* 2005;123:8–16.
38. MacFie J. Enteral versus parenteral nutrition: the significance of bacterial translocation and gut-barrier function. *Nutrition.* 2000;16:606–611.

CHAPTER 49 ■ COAGULATION

MAUREANE HOFFMAN

Normal coagulation represents a balance between intact local hemostatic mechanisms in response to injury and the regulatory mechanisms that prevent systemic extension of coagulation. Plasma proteins and cellular components are both necessary for appropriate hemostasis. The coagulation reactions are normally localized on cell surfaces by specific receptors on the cells and protease inhibitors in the fluid phase. The process of hemostasis can be divided into primary hemostasis (formation of an initial platelet plug), secondary hemostasis (stabilization of the platelet plug in a fibrin polymer), and fibrinolysis (dissolution of the clot to allow healing or remove a thrombus) (Table 49.1). Disorders of coagulation result when local coagulation pathways are impaired, the protective mechanisms to prevent intravascular coagulation (thrombosis) are inadequate, or these protective measures overrespond and interfere with local hemostasis. Hemostasis can also be impaired by alterations in the local environment, such as acidosis or hypothermia. The components of the coagulation system can be assessed in clinical laboratory tests. However, no test is currently available that reflects the overall adequacy of the hemostatic process.

POINTS OF EMPHASIS

- Primary hemostasis refers to the adhesion of circulating platelets at the site of injury. In many instances the initial platelet plug, assisted by local vasoconstriction, is sufficient to stop bleeding from small-caliber vessels.
- Secondary hemostasis involves the activation of plasma coagulation proteins leading to generation of thrombin on the activated platelet surface. This process culminates in stabilization of the initial platelet plug in a crosslinked fibrin meshwork.
- The hemostatic process is prevented from extending inappropriately through the vasculature by antithrombotic regulatory mechanisms.
- The role of fibrinolysis is to remove clots that are formed within the vasculature and to degrade hemostatic clots to allow normal progression of wound healing.
- The events in the coagulation process are regulated by the cell surfaces on which they take place.
- Laboratory tests can evaluate aspects of hemostatic function, but no laboratory tests provide a global assessment of the risk of bleeding or hemostatic adequacy.
- Local tissue conditions, such as hypothermia and acidosis, can strongly influence the effectiveness of the hemostatic process, even in the presence of adequate levels of coagulation factors and platelets.

PRIMARY HEMOSTASIS

Components

Primary hemostasis is composed of several important activities: reflex vasoconstriction after vascular injury, platelet adhesion to extracellular matrix components, platelet activation, and degranulation. These are modulated by biochemical and physiologic stimuli. Therefore, when any agents interfere with any of these steps, increased bleeding can result.

Vasculature

Constituents of the vessel wall are important components of primary hemostasis. In the baseline state vascular endothelial cells provide a nonthrombogenic interface with the circulating blood. An injury, however, exposes extracellular matrix proteins in the subendothelial and perivascular tissues (such as collagen, fibronectin, von Willebrand factor [vWF], thrombospondin, and laminin) that mediate platelet adhesion. The perivascular tissues also express significant levels of tissue factor (TF) activity, which initiates the process of thrombin generation on the adjacent platelet surfaces and leads to formation of a fibrin clot. Vascular injury typically also triggers reflex vasoconstriction, which assists the coagulation process in staunching bleeding.

Platelets

Platelets adhere at a site of injury and, in concert with local vasoconstriction, provide initial hemostasis. Once hemostasis is achieved by these mechanisms, the subsequent stabilization of the platelet plug in a fibrin meshwork can proceed more effectively than if bleeding continues. Initial hemostasis may be established even if a defect in the coagulation protein cascade is present. However, the platelet plug is insufficient to provide long-term hemostasis, and delayed rebleeding will occur if it is not reinforced by a stable fibrin clot during secondary hemostasis.

Platelets not only plug the vascular defects at a site of injury, but also provide the specialized cell surface on which activation of many of the coagulation proteins takes place. As they circulate in an unactivated state, platelets do not support activity of the coagulation proteases. However, when activated, they rapidly undergo a variety of alterations that allow them to support and regulate procoagulant activity.

Unactivated platelets express a very low level of phosphatidylserine, the primary procoagulant phospholipid, on their surfaces. Upon activation, phosphatidylserine is rapidly translocated from the inner to the outer leaflet of the platelet

TABLE 49.1

OVERVIEW OF THE COMPONENTS INVOLVED IN NORMAL HEMOSTASIS

PRIMARY HEMOSTASIS
Vessel wall
Platelets
Fibrinogen
von Willebrand factor
SECONDARY HEMOSTASIS
Coagulation proteins
Protease inhibitors
Cell membrane phospholipid
FIBRINOLYSIS
Plasminogen
Tissue-type plasminogen activator (tPA)
Plasminogen activator inhibitors (PAIs)

plasma membrane. It is then available to support binding and activity of the coagulation complexes (1).

The platelet plasma membrane also provides a ready source of substrate (arachidonic acid) for the synthesis of prostaglandins and thromboxanes—compounds that modulate many of the functions of platelets (2). Platelet aggregation, granule release, and reflex vasoconstriction all are influenced by prostaglandins and thromboxanes.

Membrane receptors for collagen and other subendothelial and adhesive proteins are present on the platelet membrane (3,4) and can mediate binding of unactivated platelets at sites of injury. These binding events can transmit an activation signal to the platelet. However, full platelet activation probably also requires stimulation by thrombin that is produced as the coagulation reactions are initiated. Other platelet surface receptors, such as glycoprotein (GP) IIb/IIIa, the receptor for fibrinogen, rapidly change conformation from an inactive to an active form upon platelet activation (5). This allows the activated platelets to aggregate with fibrinogen serving as a bridge between platelets.

Platelet degranulation occurs somewhat more slowly after activation than do membrane surface changes. Dense and α-granules within the platelet cytoplasm contain numerous components that play a role in the coagulation process, such as factors V, VIII, and XIII; fibrinogen; von Willebrand factor; protease inhibitors; and platelet agonists (adenosine diphosphate [ADP], epinephrine, and serotonin). Secretion of these platelet agonists further enhances platelet activation and hemostasis. Platelet granules also contain chemotactic factors, growth factors, and other cytokines that play a role in the inflammatory response and wound healing.

Function in Normal Coagulation

When the integrity of a blood vessel is disrupted, the subendothelial tissues are exposed. Within seconds, platelets begin to adhere to the subendothelial binding sites both directly and indirectly via fibrinogen and von Willebrand factor. Exposure of extravascular tissue factor simultaneously initiates secondary hemostasis as discussed below.

Platelets are "activated" both by collagen and by small amounts of thrombin generated on nearby TF-bearing cells, resulting in release of the α-granule and dense granule contents and the production of thromboxane. These events occur within seconds after platelet adhesion and have a positive feedback effect on the procoagulant response. Vasoconstriction and formation of a platelet plug establish initial hemostasis within minutes if the injured vessel is not of very large caliber.

Laboratory Evaluation

A careful history should be taken before beginning a laboratory evaluation of any bleeding disorder. This should include an assessment of the duration, pattern, and severity of bleeding problems, including whether the bleeding is spontaneous or associated with trauma or surgery. A lifelong bleeding tendency may suggest a congenital disorder, but an onset in adulthood does not necessarily exclude a congenital problem. In obtaining a history of bleeding pattern, it is necessary to determine whether a true hemorrhagic disorder exists. In this regard, it is often helpful to assess if the bleeding is out of proportion to the degree of trauma, or whether blood transfusions were required for relatively minor surgical procedures. Since many drugs and foods can affect platelet function, a complete drug history is also important. Platelet-mediated bleeding disorders usually result in a mucocutaneous bleeding pattern, with ecchymosis, petechiae, purpura, epistaxis, and gingival bleeding commonly observed (6), in contrast to coagulation protein disorders, in which deep tissue bleeding and hemarthroses are more common.

Abnormalities of primary hemostasis can be due to either quantitative or qualitative platelet defects. The microscopic review of a peripheral blood smear allows one to estimate circulating numbers of platelets if a blood count is not available. Each platelet visualized per high-power oil-immersion field approximates 15,000 platelets per microliter of whole blood. A normal count is roughly 150,000 to 400,000/μL. However, 50,000 to 100,000/μL is usually sufficient for hemostasis if platelet function is normal. The cause of reduced circulating platelet numbers cannot be ascertained from a smear review, and bone marrow aspiration and biopsy are typically required to distinguish decreased platelet production from increased destruction.

Bleeding Time

Qualitative abnormalities of platelet function can be assessed by several different techniques, and algorithms for the evaluation of such disorders have been developed (7). The template bleeding time can provide an assessment of primary hemostasis in patients with a suspected platelet abnormality (8). However, the bleeding time has sometimes been used as a preoperative screening test of overall hemostasis. In the absence of a history of a bleeding disorder, the bleeding time is not a useful predictor of the risk of hemorrhage associated with surgical procedures, nor does a normal bleeding time exclude the possibility of excessive hemorrhage associated with invasive procedures (9).

In the several modern variations of the bleeding time test, a disposable template is used to make a standardized incision on the forearm after inflating a blood pressure cuff to 40 mm Hg on the upper arm. The time required for bleeding to stop is measured in a standardized fashion. Simple as it sounds, the bleeding time test requires a significant degree of skill and experience to perform reproducibly. Qualitative defects in platelet function, von Willebrand factor deficiency, afibrinogenemia, marked thrombocytopenia, and abnormalities in vascular collagen all can result in a prolonged bleeding time (normal is less than 10 minutes). The bleeding time result also depends on orientation and size of the incision, site of the incision, skin quality, skin temperature, operator technique, and patient cooperation. Disorders of coagulation (secondary hemostasis) do *not* generally affect the bleeding time.

Platelet Aggregation Tests

Platelet function can be assessed in the laboratory by aggregation studies. This approach is considered the gold standard in assessing qualitative platelet defects. Platelet-rich plasma is incubated with a platelet agonist, such as ADP, collagen, epinephrine, or thrombin, resulting in platelet activation and consequent aggregation. Aggregation is measured as an increase in light transmission through the platelet suspension. An analysis of the aggregation curves with different agonists often provides information on the nature of the platelet defect. Platelet aggregation studies also require an extremely skilled and experienced operator. In addition, preanalytic variables such as the blood collection technique and transport conditions can significantly impair platelet function. Aggregation studies cannot be done reliably if the platelet count is less than 100,000/μL. A "false normal" on platelet aggregation testing is very unlikely, but abnormal platelet aggregation results should be confirmed by repeat testing, if possible.

PFA-100

Semi-automated techniques have made platelet function testing much more readily available by removing the requirement for an extremely experienced operator. The oldest and most well-established of these is the PFA-100 (10). This instrument uses a disposable test cartridge to simulate primary hemostasis. Inside the cartridge is a membrane coated with collagen and epinephrine and/or ADP. An anticoagulated blood sample is aspirated through an aperture in the membrane and the time required for occlusion of the aperture is measured. While the PFA-100 test appears to be a useful screen for platelet dysfunction, there is no consensus that it is *the* replacement test for the bleeding time. Neither the bleeding time nor the PFA-100 is able to predict the likelihood that a patient will bleed excessively during an invasive procedure.

There are many other commercial tests that measure particular aspects of platelet aggregation or clot formation. Some are still only being used for research, while others are being used in selected clinical settings. The VerifyNow Aspirin Assay (formerly Ultegra RPFA-ASA), for instance, is a test that detects platelet dysfunction due to aspirin effects (11). A VerifyNow P2Y12 test is now available to monitor the effects of the antiplatelet agent clopidogrel (12), and VerifyNow IIb/IIIa Assay to monitor the effects of abciximab and other anti-IIb/IIIa agents (11). Plateletworks is a testing method used to monitor changes in platelet function by measuring aggregation ability (13). This is not a comprehensive list, and new tests are appearing regularly. However, none of them has emerged as being useful for the global assessment of platelet function at this time.

TABLE 49.2

PROCOAGULANTS OF SECONDARY HEMOSTASIS

VITAMIN K–DEPENDENT FACTORS
Factor II (prothrombin)
Factor VII (proconvertin)
Factor IX (Christmas factor)
Factor X (Stuart-Prower factor)
CONTACT FACTORS
Factor XI
THROMBIN-SENSITIVE FACTORS
Fibrinogen
Factor V (proaccelerin)
Factor VIII (antihemophilic factor)
Factor XIII (Laki-Lorand factor)

SECONDARY HEMOSTASIS

Components

From a biochemical standpoint, the individual components of secondary hemostasis can be classified by their structural features into three groups: the contact factors, the vitamin K–dependent factors, and the thrombin-sensitive factors. Table 49.2 lists each of these groups and their respective factors that are involved in hemostasis. Proteins C and S are vitamin K–dependent; however, they function as anticoagulant rather than procoagulant proteins. Protein Z is a procoagulant; its precise role in hemostasis remains to be clarified.

Contact Factors

Factor XI (FXI), FXII, high-molecular-weight kininogen (HK), and prekallikrein (PK) are referred to as the "contact factors." Patients who are deficient in FXII, HK, or PK do not have a clinical bleeding tendency, although their activated partial thromboplastin time (aPTT; see below) is prolonged.

When factor XII contacts a negatively charged surface, such as the "activator" in the aPTT or subendothelial collagen, its activation from a zymogen form begins. It undergoes a conformational change that provides partial activation and, more importantly, renders it susceptible to further activation by PK. HK, a precursor of bradykinin, is also involved in the factor XII activation process. In a reciprocal action, activated FXII (FXIIa) in turn cleaves and activates PK to kallikrein, which activates still more FXII. Kallikrein and FXIIa are now thought to primarily have a role in the activation of plasminogen (discussed in the section on fibrinolysis) and in inflammatory responses rather than in normal hemostasis. However, there is evidence that the contact factors can play a role in promoting thrombosis under some circumstances.

By contrast, FXI is clearly involved in normal hemostasis, since its deficiency is associated with a clinical bleeding tendency. It is a zymogen precursor of a serine protease that circulates in complex with the nonenzymatic cofactor HK. While FXI is activated by FXIIa in the aPTT assay, it is activated by thrombin during hemostasis in vivo. Both thrombin and FXI bind to sites on the platelet surface glycoprotein Ib, and this interaction facilitates FXI activation.

Vitamin K–dependent Factors

The vitamin K–dependent coagulation factors include prothrombin (factor II) and factors VII, IX, and X. In addition, three other vitamin K–dependent plasma proteins that are involved in normal coagulation have been identified: Proteins C, S, and Z. With the exception of protein S, the vitamin K–dependent factors are zymogens, which are inert precursors of serine proteases that must be proteolytically activated to express their enzymatic activity. Their activity is dramatically enhanced by binding to a specific cofactor that does not have enzymatic activity of its own. Thus, TF is the cofactor for FVIIa, FVIIIa for FIXa, FVa for FXa, and protein S for activated protein C. Thrombin is fully active to clot fibrinogen and activate platelets in the absence of any cofactor. However, binding to a cofactor on the surface of endothelial cells, thrombomodulin, changes its activity so that it is no longer procoagulant, but rather activates protein C, which has anticoagulant/antithrombotic effects. The complex of activated protein C/protein S cleaves and inactivates the cofactors FVa and FVIIIa. This means that any thrombin that escapes from the vicinity of an injury and reaches healthy endothelium initiates antithrombotic responses, so that clotting is not propagated throughout the vascular tree.

The vitamin K–dependent factors all have a homologous protein structure (14). Each of them has an amino-terminal γ-carboxy glutamic acid (Gla) domain with 9 to 12 Gla residues. The negatively charged Gla residues bind calcium ions and maintain the Gla domain in an appropriate conformation to mediate binding of the protein to lipid membranes. Thus, calcium chelators such as ethylenediaminetetraacetic acid (EDTA) and citrate exert their anticoagulant effects by preventing the binding of Gla-containing factors to membranes.

Each vitamin K–dependent factor is posttranslationally modified by a γ-glutamyl carboxylase that catalyzes carboxylation of glutamic acid to form the Gla residues. This carboxylase requires oxygen, carbon dioxide, and the reduced form of vitamin K for its action. For each glutamyl residue that is carboxylated, one molecule of reduced vitamin K is converted to the epoxide form. A separate enzyme complex, the vitamin K epoxide reductase (15), converts the epoxide form of vitamin K back to the reduced form. Warfarin (Coumadin) blocks the activity of the reductase and prevents recycling of vitamin K back to the reduced form. Warfarin thus blocks γ-glutamyl carboxylation, with the result that a heterogeneous population of undercarboxylated forms of the vitamin K–dependent factors appears in circulation. These undercarboxylated forms have reduced coagulant activity. Since warfarin blocks recycling of vitamin K rather than blocking the carboxylase itself, the effects of warfarin can be reversed by administration of vitamin K.

Protein Z functions as a cofactor for a protein Z–dependent serine protease inhibitor (ZPI) (16). Protein Z actually binds to FXa and facilitates its inhibition by ZPI, and thus protein Z/ZPI appear to have an anticoagulant function. This is supported by the finding that deficiency of protein Z is associated with a thrombotic tendency in a mouse model (17). The full physiologic and pathophysiologic roles of protein Z/ZPI are not yet understood, but their levels appear to contribute to the risk of thrombosis in humans.

Thrombin-sensitive Factors

The thrombin-sensitive factors are so named because of their susceptibility to proteolysis by thrombin, which in most cases leads to their enzymatically active forms. These include fibrinogen and factors V, VIII, and XIII. The central importance of thrombin formation to normal coagulation and its regulation is again emphasized by these interactions, along with others discussed previously. Factors V and VIII have homologous structures, but factor XIII and fibrinogen are structurally very different.

Conversion of fibrinogen to fibrin, and its subsequent polymerization and incorporation into the matrix of a platelet plug, represents the end point for secondary hemostasis. Fibrinogen is a comparatively large, complex coagulation protein. Conversion to fibrin occurs when thrombin symmetrically cleaves two pairs of short polypeptides, fibrinopeptides A and B, from its amino terminal ends. This exposes cryptic binding sites, allowing spontaneous polymerization of fibrin. As fibrin is polymerized and becomes insoluble, it is also stabilized by the action of activated factor XIII, which forms covalent crosslinks between fibrin monomers. FXIII is activated by the action of thrombin as well. In the absence of FXIII, the fibrin polymers that are formed are unstable and cannot provide sufficient matrix rigidity to the primary platelet plug. Deficiency of this factor results in delayed bleeding as a consequence of early clot breakdown.

FV is also proteolytically activated by thrombin. Recall, too, that FV is also present in platelet α-granules and is secreted and expressed on the platelet membrane surface, where many of the coagulation reactions occur. In fact, the platelet as a source of FVa for initial *in vivo* coagulation is probably more important than the FVa provided by plasma.

FVIII circulates in complex with very-high-molecular-weight multimers of the adhesive protein vWF. Von Willebrand factor stabilizes the inherently unstable FVIII as well as mediating platelet adhesion to extracellular matrix components under high shear conditions. By binding vWF to the platelet surface, GPIb also localizes FVIII to the platelet surface, where it is activated and released from vWF by thrombin. It then complexes with its partner protease, FIXa, to form the complex that will activate FX on the platelet surface.

Function in Normal Coagulation

The Coagulation Cascade

In the 1960s two groups proposed a similar model of the interactions of the coagulation factors. Each clotting factor was thought to exist as a proenzyme that was converted to an active enzyme by proteolysis. In these "cascade" or "waterfall" models, sequential activation of the plasma clotting factors served to progressively amplify a procoagulant signal and ultimately lead to a burst of thrombin generation (18,19). The original model was subsequently modified to include the observation that some of the procoagulants were cofactors that did not have enzymatic activity.

Initially, the scheme of coagulation only included what we now call the "intrinsic" pathway—so named because all of its components are present in the blood. While it had long been known that tissue extracts (thromboplastin) could trigger blood clotting, the intrinsic pathway was thought to be

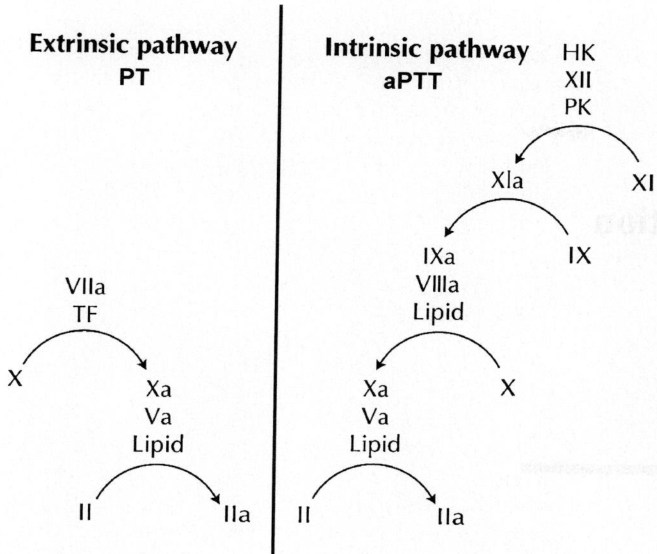

FIGURE 49.1. The cascade model of coagulation. PT, prothrombin time; TF, tissue factor; aPTT, activated partial thromboplastin time; HK, high-molecular-weight kininogen; PK, prekallikrein.

of primary physiologic importance because deficiency of FVIII or FIX was known to result in a severe bleeding condition (hemophilia). Later the tissue factor or "extrinsic" pathway was added to the model to produce the familiar coagulation cascade as shown in Figure 49.1.

In the modern cascade model the intrinsic pathway is initiated by activation of the contact factors. FXIa can then activate FIX, which then acts with its cofactor, FVIII, on a phospholipid surface to activate FX. The extrinsic pathway consists of FVIIa and TF. Both pathways can activate FX, which, in complex with its cofactor FVa on a phospholipid surface, converted prothrombin to thrombin. Our current screening coagulation tests follow the outline of this model: The prothrombin time (PT) test is initiated by adding TF, calcium, and phospholipid to plasma and measuring the time required for clotting. The aPTT is initiated by adding a charged surface and phospholipid to plasma to allow activation of the contact factors (the "activation" phase). The plasma is then recalcified and the time to clotting is measured. Thus, the cascade model of coagulation is useful as a guide to interpreting the PT and aPTT.

However, the cascade model has severe limitations as a model of physiology. The key observation that the FVIIa/TF complex activated not only FX but also FIX (20) suggested that the intrinsic and extrinsic pathways were in fact linked. Several groups demonstrated points of interaction between the pathways and suggested that they could not operate as independent and redundant systems, as the cascade model implied. Furthermore, this model fails to provide insight into why patients with coagulation abnormalities bleed. For example, patients with deficiencies of the contact factors have a prolonged aPTT only and no clinical bleeding tendency. Patients with FXI deficiency have a similarly prolonged aPTT and variable bleeding. Patients with classic hemophilia A (FVIII deficiency) and hemophilia B (FIX deficiency) have a less prolonged aPTT but a significant bleeding tendency.

A Cell-based Model of Coagulation

It was recognized from the earliest studies of coagulation that cells were important participants in the coagulation process. Of course, it is clear that normal hemostasis is not possible in the absence of platelets. In addition, TF is an integral membrane protein and thus its activity is normally associated with cells. Since different cells express different levels of pro- and anticoagulant proteins as well as having different complements of receptors for components of hemostasis, simply representing the cells involved in coagulation as phospholipid vesicles overlooks the important contributions of cells in directing hemostasis in vivo. Thus, a model that gives insight into the physiology and pathophysiology of hemostasis requires due consideration to the role of living cells in the process. A cell-based model of coagulation has been proposed (21), which views the coagulation process as occurring in a series of steps that take place on two different cell surfaces: the TF-bearing cells and platelets. This model is illustrated in Figure 49.2.

Initiation. The *initiation* step takes place on the TF-bearing cell surface, which is exposed to blood when an injury occurs (Fig. 49.2A). Functioning as a receptor for FVII, the transmembrane protein TF promotes conversion of the FVII to its proteolytically active form, FVIIa. The FVIIa/TF complex catalyzes conversion of FIX and FX to their active forms, FIXa and FXa, respectively. On the TF-bearing cell, the FXa formed during this step combines with its cofactor FVa and forms a prothrombinase complex sufficient to generate a small amount of thrombin in the milieu of the TF-bearing cell. This small quantity of thrombin is not sufficient to clot fibrinogen. It does, however, promote platelet activation and the conversion of FV, FVIII, and FXI to their active forms in the next step.

Amplification. The *amplification* step (Fig. 49.2B) takes place on the platelet surface, where the small amount of thrombin formed during initiation can bind to specific receptors. Protease-activated receptors (PAR-1 and PAR-4) mediate platelet activation. Thrombin also binds to GPIb, which facilitates the activation of FVIII and its release from vWF, as well as activation of FXI. Platelet activation leads to secretion of partially activated FV from platelet α-granules, with thrombin acting to complete its conversion to FVa. Cofactors Va and VIIIa are quickly bound to specific sites on the platelet surface once they are activated. Factor IXa activated by the FVIIa/TF complex is capable of diffusing from the TF-bearing cell to adjacent activated platelet surfaces, where it binds to its cofactor to form FVIIIa/FIXa complexes. At the end of the amplification step, activated platelets have bound activated factors in preparation to produce large amounts of thrombin.

Propagation. During the *propagation* step (Fig. 49.2C), plasma FX is converted to FXa on the activated platelet surface, where it can move into direct association with its cofactor FVa while remaining surface bound. The platelet surface FXa/FVa acts on plasma prothrombin to produce a thrombin burst of sufficient magnitude to clot fibrinogen.

The role of FXI in hemostasis has been a point of some controversy, since even severe FXI deficiency does not result in a hemorrhagic tendency as severe as that seen in severe

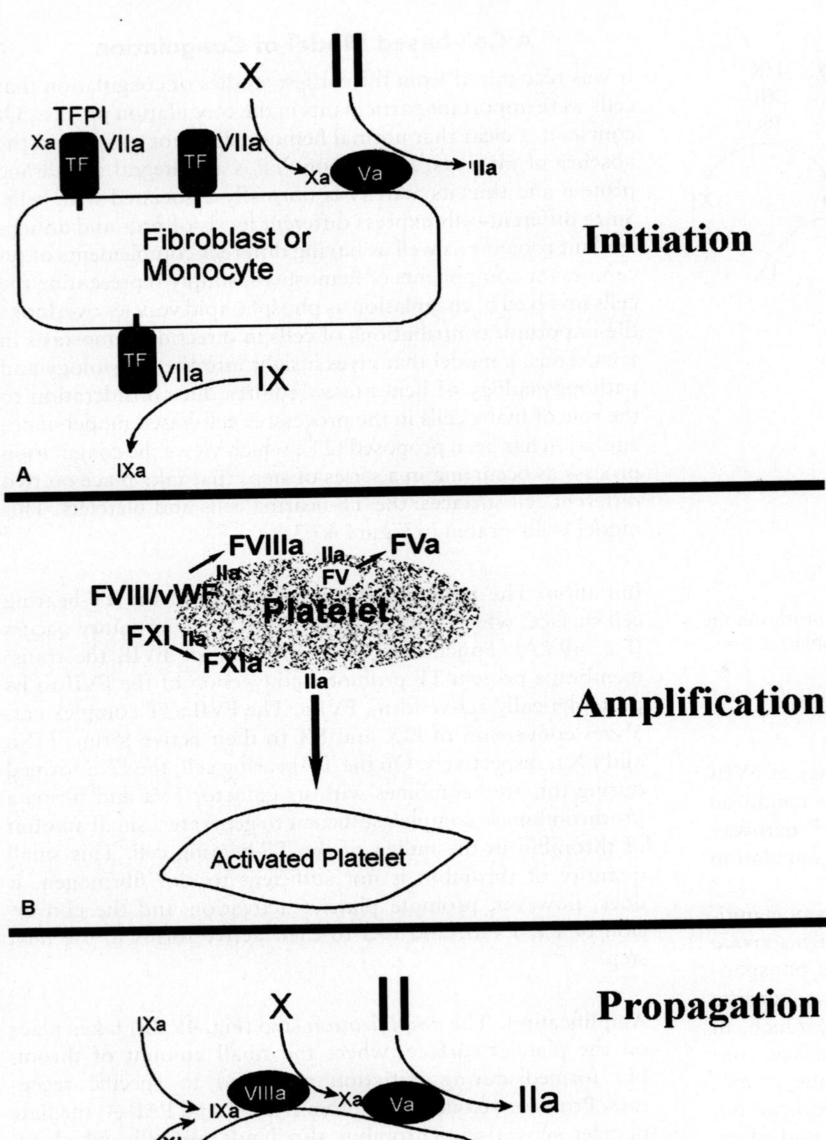

FIGURE 49.2. A cell-based model of coagulation. TFPI, tissue factor pathway inhibitor; vWF, von Willebrand factor.

FVIII or IX deficiency. This can be explained if FXI is viewed as an "enhancer" or "booster" of thrombin generation during the propagation phase. FXIa activates additional FIXa on the platelet surface to supplement FIXa/FVIIIa complex formation and enhance platelet surface FXa and thrombin generation. Thus, FXI is not essential for platelet-surface thrombin generation, as are FIX and FVIII, and its deficiency does not compromise hemostasis to the degree seen in FIX and FVIII deficiency.

Fibrin Polymerization. Thrombin now cleaves two pairs of short polypeptides from fibrinogen, and the resulting fibrin monomer rapidly and spontaneously polymerizes. Thrombin also activates FXIII, and FXIIIa in turn catalyzes covalent linkages between fibrin monomers, vastly increasing the tensile strength of the fibrin mesh that now stabilizes the initial platelet plug.

Laboratory Evaluation

The cell-based model of coagulation shows us why the "extrinsic" and "intrinsic" pathways are not redundant. Let us consider the "extrinsic" pathway to consist of the FVIIa/TF complex working with the FXa/Va complex, and the "intrinsic" pathway to consist of FXIa working with the complexes of factors VIIIa/IXa and factors Xa/Va. As illustrated in the right hand panel of Figure 49.3, the "extrinsic" pathway operates on the TF-bearing cell to initiate the coagulation process. By contrast, as shown in Figure 49.4, the "intrinsic" pathway operates on the activated platelet surface to produce the burst of thrombin that causes formation of the fibrin clot. Thus, these two pathways are specialized to carry out functions on different cell surfaces. The PT can be considered to be a test of the adequacy of the components of the initiating pathway, while the aPTT is a test of the components needed for platelet

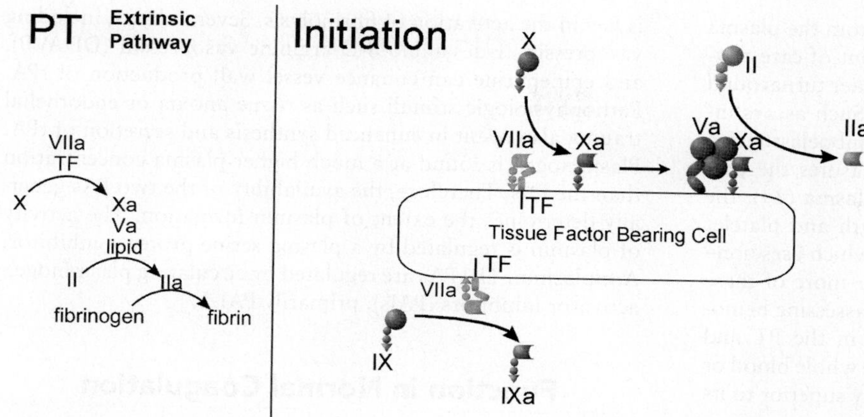

FIGURE 49.3. The prothrombin time (PT) tests the extrinsic/initiation pathway. TF, tissue factor.

surface thrombin generation. Each can provide useful information about the cause of abnormal bleeding, but either can be expected to give us an overall view of hemostatic function or accurately predict the risk of bleeding.

Prothrombin Time

Although the first step in identifying and classifying disorders of secondary hemostasis is *always* a careful history and physical examination, the focus here is on the laboratory evaluation of clotting disorders. The most commonly ordered screening test of clotting is PT. In this test, plasma is incubated with a thromboplastin reagent that contains TF and phospholipid vesicles to bind FVII from the plasma and activate the extrinsic pathway (Fig. 49.3). Acquired or congenital deficiencies of factors VII, X, V, prothrombin or fibrinogen can prolong the PT. The PT is also commonly used to monitor oral anticoagulant therapy, that is, warfarin. Any acquired or congenital deficiencies of factors VII, X, or V; thrombin; or fibrinogen can also prolong the PT.

Activated Partial Thromboplastin Time

The aPTT is another commonly measured parameter of coagulation. Plasma is incubated with a reagent that provides a negatively charged surface for activation of the contact factors of coagulation. The reagent also contains phospholipid vesicles and calcium, which are required for activity of the distal portion of the intrinsic pathway. As shown in the left-hand panel of Figure 49.4, the aPTT is sensitive to a deficiency of any of the factors in the intrinsic and common pathways.

Thrombin Time

The thrombin time assesses both the quantitative and qualitative aspects of the conversion of fibrinogen to fibrin. Thrombin is added to plasma, and the time until appearance of a fibrin clot is measured. The myriad disorders associated with either availability or function of fibrinogen are assessed with this test. It is exquisitely sensitive to the presence of heparin and inhibitors of fibrin monomer polymerization (i.e., fibrin degradation products, dysfibrinogens). The reptilase time also provides an assessment of fibrinogen and its function. Like thrombin, the reptilase enzyme (derived from snake venom) cleaves polypeptides from fibrinogen, leading to activation and fibrin monomer formation. Unlike the thrombin time, however, the reptilase time is not affected by heparin.

Specific Factor Assays

Factor assays are also available for most of the important coagulation proteins involved in the clotting of blood. The general concept behind these assays involves providing the specific substrate for the factor that is suspected to be deficient. Subsequent time to clotting is then measured and clotting factor activity is reported as a percentage of normal activity.

"Global" Tests of Coagulation

As the critical role of cells in coagulation has become more clear, a number of coagulation tests have become available that can be run on whole blood or platelet-rich plasma.

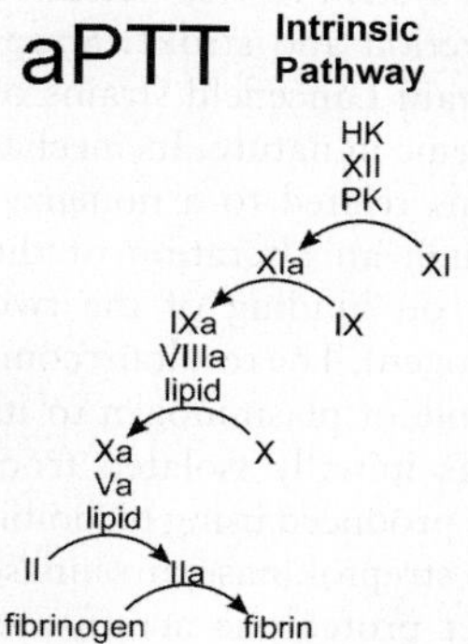

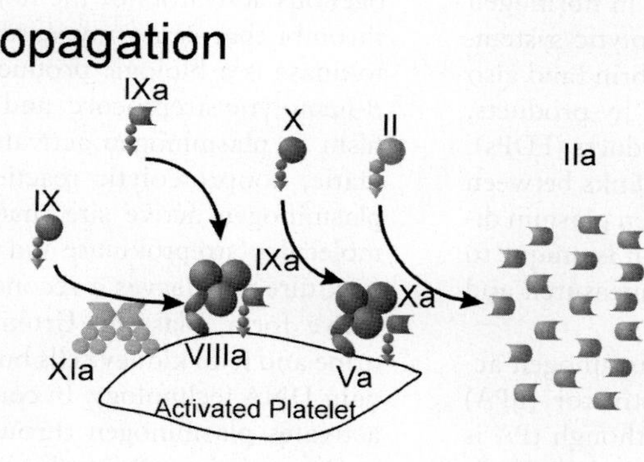

FIGURE 49.4. The activated partial thromboplastin time (aPTT) tests the intrinsic/platelet surface pathway. HK, high-molecular-weight kininogen; PK, prekallikrein.

Because the cells do not have to be separated from the plasma for these assays and some are suitable for point-of-care testing, some of these assays also have a much quicker turnaround time than tests run in the clinical laboratory. Such assays include several variations on the venerable thromboelastogram (TEG) (22,23); the Thrombogram, which measures the pattern of thrombin generation in platelet-rich plasma (24); the Hemodyne, which measures fibrin clot strength and platelet contraction (25); the Clot Signature Analyzer, which uses non–anticoagulated blood (26); and others. One or more of these assays seem likely to play an important role in assessing hemostatic parameters that are not well reflected in the PT and aPTT. However, none of the currently available whole blood or platelet-rich plasma tests has emerged as clearly superior to its competitors.

An additional test that deserves mention is the activated clotting time (ACT). It is not considered a test of "global" hemostasis, but does use whole blood and is performed as point-of-care testing (27). It is similar to a whole blood aPTT because clotting is initiated with charged materials that activate the contact pathway, such as celite, kaolin, or a combination of celite, kaolin, and glass. The ACT is commonly used for monitoring blood anticoagulant response to heparin during cardiopulmonary bypass and cardiac catheterization. However, some other anticoagulants and other agents, such as aprotinin, can affect the ACT. Furthermore, the test does not reflect the anticoagulant effect of some agents, such as low-molecular-weight heparins. Since the test has not been standardized, different reagent/instrument systems may give different results under the same clinical conditions. In spite of these caveats, the ACT has proven to be useful in the cardiac cath lab and during cardiac surgery when a single system is used consistently and local "cutoff" levels have been determined for assessing adequate anticoagulation and adequate reversal by protamine.

PHYSIOLOGY AND BIOCHEMISTRY OF FIBRINOLYSIS

Components

The major enzyme component of the fibrinolytic system is plasminogen, the zymogen form of plasmin. It is primarily synthesized in the liver and circulates in the plasma at 10- to 20-mg/dL concentrations under basal conditions. Plasminogen concentrations, however, can greatly increase in response to inflammatory states, paralleling changes seen in fibrinogen levels. Plasmin is the final effector of the fibrinolytic system, which degrades the fibrin clot. Plasmin cleaves fibrin (and also fibrinogen) at multiple sites, resulting in several by-products, known clinically as fibrin(ogen) degradation products (FDPs). After polymerization of fibrin, factor XIIIa crosslinks between the D-domains of adjacent fibrin monomers. When plasmin digests crosslinked fibrin, a product is produced that is unique to fibrin cleavage, called the *d-dimer*. This can be measured and quantitated (discussed later).

Plasmin is produced by the action of two plasminogen activators (PAs): Urokinase-type plasminogen activator (uPA) and tissue-type plasminogen activator (tPA). Although tPA is present in many tissues, its release by vascular endothelial cells is key in the activation of fibrinolysis. Several drugs, including vasopressin, 1-desamino-8-D-arginine vasopressin (DDAVP), and epinephrine can enhance vessel wall production of tPA. Pathophysiologic stimuli such as tissue anoxia or endothelial trauma also result in enhanced synthesis and secretion of tPA. Plasminogen is found at a much higher plasma concentration than the PAs. Therefore, the availability of the two PAs generally determines the extent of plasmin formation. The activity of plasmin is regulated by a plasma serine protease inhibitor: Antiplasmin. The PAs are regulated by circulating plasminogen activator inhibitors (PAIs), primarily PAI-1.

Function in Normal Coagulation

Even as the fibrin clot is being formed in the body, the fibrinolytic system is being initiated to disrupt it. If a clot is formed in the vicinity of an intact endothelial layer, fibrinolysis is activated as a protective mechanism. tPA release from endothelial cells is provoked by thrombin as well as venous occlusion (28). Both the secreted tPA and plasma plasminogen bind to the evolving fibrin polymer, which dramatically enhances the activation of plasminogen by tPA. Plasmin is formed in the vicinity of the thrombus and acts to degrade it.

When a hemostatic clot is formed at a site of tissue injury, fibrinolysis must still take place to remove the clot during wound healing. PAs released from leukocytes, probably primarily uPA, begin the fibrinolytic process in this case.

Thrombin activatable fibrinolysis inhibitor (TAFI) is a zymogen that can be activated (TAFIa) by thrombin or plasmin (29). As fibrin is degraded by plasmin, C-terminal lysines are exposed that enhance activation of additional plasminogen to plasmin. TAFIa removes the C-terminal lysines from fibrin and thereby inhibits the cofactor activity of fibrin for plasminogen activation.

Fibrinolysis is essential for removal of clots during the process of wound healing as well as for removing intravascular clots that might otherwise be manifest as thrombosis. Intravascular deposition of fibrin is also associated with the development of atherosclerosis. Therefore, an effective fibrinolytic system tends to protect against the chronic process of atherosclerotic vascular disease as well as the acute process of thrombosis. Conversely, defects of fibrinolysis increase the risk of atherothrombotic disease. For example, elevated levels of PAI-1, an inhibitor of fibrinolysis, are associated with an increased risk of atherosclerosis and thrombosis (30), as are decreased levels of plasminogen (31).

Streptokinase and urokinase have been used clinically as exogenous activators of the fibrinolytic system to lyse occlusive thrombi that cause myocardial infarction and stroke. Streptokinase is a biologic product of certain Lancefield strains of β-hemolytic streptococci and is antigenic in nature. Its mechanism of plasminogen activation seems related to a nonenzymatic, nonproteolytic reaction through an alteration of the plasminogen active site that occurs on binding of the two molecules (streptokinase and plasminogen). The resultant complex directly cleaves a second molecule of plasminogen to its active form, plasmin. Urokinase was initially isolated from urine and fetal kidney cells but is now produced using recombinant DNA technology. In contrast to streptokinase, urokinase activates plasminogen through direct proteolytic action and is not antigenic. Recombinant human tPA (rh-tPA) also can be infused intravenously to activate fibrinolysis. Exogenously administered rh-tPA has identical actions as endogenously produced tPA.

After activation by any of the above described methods, excess fibrinolysis has the potential to interfere with normal hemostatic mechanisms. Since tPA normally activates plasminogen in the vicinity of fibrin, fibrinolytic activity is confined to the site of clot formation. However, plasmin can digest both fibrinogen and fibrin. When excess plasmin activity is produced or it is not inhibited appropriately, plasmin can degrade and deplete circulating fibrinogen. Thus, therapeutic activation of fibrinolysis produces a systemic lytic state with dose-dependent depletion of plasma fibrinogen.

Laboratory Evaluation

Tests that directly measure fibrinolytic function or activity are not as readily available as those that measure secondary hemostasis. In general, the PT, aPTT, and thrombin time are relatively insensitive to changes in fibrinolytic activity (including those induced by streptokinase or urokinase). Therefore, these tests are not useful in the diagnosis of increased fibrinolysis. An assay of plasma fibrinogen and fibrin degradation product levels provides some useful information concerning fibrin(ogen)olysis, if basal levels are known. These assays are not the tests of choice for either diagnosing or monitoring hyperfibrinolysis.

The test that has historically been most used to evaluate the possibility of hyperfibrinolysis is the euglobulin clot lysis time. However, it is not quantitative and is at best only a gross indicator of increased fibrinolytic activity. The test involves the precipitation of fibrinogen, plasminogen, and plasminogen activators by mixing a plasma sample with an acidic solution of low ionic strength. These precipitated proteins are then redissolved and allowed to clot, and the time to clot lysis is measured. A shortened time to clot lysis (less than 3 hours) indicates a state of increased fibrinolysis. Unfortunately, the degree of shortening of the euglobulin clot lysis time does not correlate with the extent of increased fibrinolysis. Further, difficulties in test interpretation can occur if the level of fibrinogen is low or if amounts of fibrin degradation products sufficient to impede clot formation are present. Because this test is very labor intensive and its interpretation can be problematic, it is now rarely performed.

The one assay that is commonly performed to monitor an aspect of fibrinolysis is the D-dimer assay. D-dimer is a specific proteolysis product of the action of plasmin on crosslinked fibrin. The presence of increased amounts of D-dimer in plasma or serum indicates that thrombin has been generated, fibrin has formed, and some degree of fibrinolysis has occurred. The D-dimer level is increased any time the coagulation response has been activated—whether appropriate or inappropriate. Thus, D-dimer levels are elevated following surgery or trauma, as well as in the setting of intravascular coagulation (thrombosis) and disseminated intravascular coagulation (DIC). This test is theoretically negative in instances of primary fibrinolysis, where fibrinogen—not crosslinked fibrin—is being degraded. The D-dimer assay can be extremely useful as part of an algorithm for the evaluation of pulmonary embolism—primarily when a normal D-dimer level can rule out thrombosis/embolism.

COAGULATION FUNCTION IN THE TISSUE ENVIRONMENT

The compartmentalization of the various aspects of coagulation, as presented here, is intended to ease the burden of conceptualization for the reader. *In vivo* coagulation, however, occurs in a tissue environment. While we have discussed, to some extent, the important role of the vessel wall and vascular endothelial cells in controlling the coagulation process, there are additional local attributes that can have a very significant impact on the effectiveness of hemostasis. First and foremost, hemostasis is unlikely to be effective when a very large vessel has been transected and primary hemostasis is unable to stop or slow the hemorrhage. This type of problem requires a surgical rather than a biochemical approach. In addition, two of the most important variables that can impair the effectiveness of the coagulation process are low temperature and pH.

Hypothermia

Hypothermia is defined as a body temperature of less than 35°C. Hypothermia occurs in a number of clinical settings, including both deliberate and accidental circumstances. In some instances, such as during cardiopulmonary bypass surgery, hypothermia is desired for its neuroprotective effects. However, hypothermia that accompanies severe trauma is associated with a significantly worse prognosis than either trauma or hypothermia alone. The primary risk of hypothermia in both regulated and nonregulated environments is that of abnormal bleeding. Mild hypothermia increases transfusion requirements, even during elective surgery (32). Several mechanisms have been proposed to contribute to impaired hemostasis associated with hypothermia, including reduced activity of clotting factors and platelets, activation of fibrinolysis, and endothelial injury (33). It appears that the defect in hemostasis observed in mild hypothermia (37°C–33°C) results primarily from impaired platelet adhesion/aggregation, but that reduced coagulant enzyme activity becomes a compounding factor of profound hypothermia (34). Of course, local hypothermia will not be reflected in the results of laboratory coagulation testing. Therefore, it is important for the clinician to consider the possibility that hypothermia may be contributing to bleeding in certain patients.

Metabolic Derangements

Like hypothermia, acidosis is also associated with worse survival in trauma and surgery patients. It can result from metabolic derangements that develop in the sickest patients. Excess lactic acid production associated with tissue hypoxia is the best recognized cause. Lactic acid is the end product of anaerobic metabolism and its level is related to oxygen availability. Acidosis can impair coagulation and worsen the risk of serious hemorrhage (35). Massive transfusion can exacerbate acidosis, since stored blood has a reduced pH.

Small changes in pH have a much greater impact on the effectiveness of the coagulation system than do small changes in temperature. Most of the coagulation proteases have a structure analogous to trypsin, a digestive enzyme. Trypsin has a pH optimum in the alkaline range (8.0–8.5), which suits it well to functioning in the alkaline environment of the small intestine. The coagulation proteases similarly have a pH optimum in the alkaline range, which does not equip them to work well in acidotic tissues. A drop in pH from 7.4 to 7.0 reduces the activity of the enzyme complex that activates thrombin by more than 70% (36). Acidosis is also not reflected in the results of laboratory coagulation testing and the clinician must be aware of the profound effect that modest changes in the pH can have on hemostasis.

SUMMARY

The process of hemostasis is intricately intertwined with other aspects of the host response to injury. Laboratory testing is critical to the evaluation of a patient with a disorder of coagulation. However, laboratory testing must be coupled with a careful clinical evaluation and interpretation, including recognition of other conditions such as hypothermia and acidosis that can impact hemostasis.

References

1. Rosing J, van Rijn JL, Bevers EM, et al. The role of activated human platelets in prothrombin and factor X activation. *Blood.* 1985;65:319.
2. FitzGerald GA. Mechanisms of platelet activation: thromboxane A2 as an amplifying signal for other agonists. *Am J Cardiol.* 1991;68:11B.
3. Canobbio I, Balduini C, Torti M. Signaling through the platelet glycoprotein Ib-V-IX complex. *Cell Signal.* 2004;16:1329.
4. Moroi M, Jung SM. Platelet glycoprotein VI: its structure and function. *Thromb Res.* 2004;114:221.
5. Bennett JS. Structure and function of the platelet integrin alphaIIbbeta3. *J Clin Invest.* 2005;115:3363.
6. Marcus A. Platelets and their disorders. In: Ratnoff O, Forbes C, eds. *Disorders of Hemostasis.* Philadelphia: WB Saunders; 1996:79.
7. Kottke-Marchant K, Corcoran G. The laboratory diagnosis of platelet disorders. *Arch Pathol Lab Med.* 2002;126:133.
8. Sramek R, Sramek A, Koster T, et al. A randomized and blinded comparison of three bleeding time techniques: the Ivy method, and the Simplate II method in two directions. *Thromb Haemost.* 1992;67:514.
9. Peterson P, Hayes TE, Arkin CF, et al. The preoperative bleeding time test lacks clinical benefit: College of American Pathologists' and American Society of Clinical Pathologists' position article. *Arch Surg.* 1998;133:134.
10. Mammen EF, Comp PC, Gosselin R, et al. PFA-100 system: a new method for assessment of platelet dysfunction. *Semin Thromb Hemost.* 1998;24:195.
11. Wheeler GL, Braden GA, Steinhubl SR, et al. The Ultegra rapid platelet-function assay: comparison to standard platelet function assays in patients undergoing percutaneous coronary intervention with abciximab therapy. *Am Heart J.* 2002;143:602.
12. Malinin A, Pokov A, Spergling M, et al. Monitoring platelet inhibition after clopidogrel with the VerifyNow-P2Y12(R) rapid analyzer: the VERIfy Thrombosis risk ASsessment (VERITAS) study. *Thromb Res.* 2006;119:277.
13. White MM, Krishnan R, Kueter TJ, et al. The use of the point of care Helena ICHOR/Plateletworks and the Accumetrics Ultegra RPFA for assessment of platelet function with GPIIB-IIIa antagonists. *J Thromb Thrombolysis.* 2004;18:163.
14. Roberts H, Monroe D, Hoffman M. Molecular biology and biochemistry of the coagulation factors, and pathways of blood coagulation. In: Beutler E, Lichtman M, Coller B, et al., eds. *William's Hematology.* New York: McGraw-Hill Publishing; 2000.
15. Li T, Chang CY, Jin DY, et al. Identification of the gene for vitamin K epoxide reductase. *Nature.* 2004;427:541.
16. Han X, Fiehler R, Broze GJ Jr. Isolation of a protein Z-dependent plasma protease inhibitor. *Proc Natl Acad Sci U S A.* 1998;95:9250.
17. Yin ZF, Huang ZF, Cui J, et al. Prothrombotic phenotype of protein Z deficiency. *Proc Natl Acad Sci U S A.* 2000;97:6734.
18. Macfarlane RG. An enzyme cascade in the blood clotting mechanism, and its function as a biological amplifier. *Nature.* 1964;202:498.
19. Davie EW, Ratnoff OD. Waterfall sequence for intrinsic blood clotting. *Science.* 1964;145:1310.
20. Østerud B, Rapaport SI. Activation of factor IX by the reaction product of tissue factor and factor VII: additional pathway for initiating blood coagulation. *Proc Natl Acad Sci U S A.* 1977;74:5260.
21. Hoffman M, Monroe DM 3rd. A cell-based model of hemostasis. *Thromb Haemost.* 2001;85:958.
22. De Nicola P, Mazzetti GM. How to interpret a thromboelastogram. *Minerva Med.* 1956;47:2043.
23. Robert Valeri C, Ragno G. In vitro testing of platelets using the thromboelastogram, platelet function analyzer, and the clot signature analyzer to predict the bleeding time. *Transfus Apher Sci.* 2006;35:33.
24. Al Dieri R, Peyvandi F, Santagostino E, et al. The thrombogram in rare inherited coagulation disorders: its relation to clinical bleeding. *Thromb Haemost.* 2002;88:576.
25. Reid TJ, Snider R, Hartman K, et al. A method for the quantitative assessment of platelet-induced clot retraction and clot strength in fresh and stored platelets. *Vox Sang.* 1998;75:270.
26. Fricke W, Kouides P, Kessler C, et al. A multicenter clinical evaluation of the Clot Signature Analyzer. *J Thromb Haemost.* 2004;2:763.
27. Doherty TM, Shavelle RM, French WJ. Reproducibility and variability of activated clotting time measurements in the cardiac catheterization laboratory. *Catheter Cardiovasc Interv.* 2005;65:330.
28. Szymanski LM, Pate RR, Durstine JL. Effects of maximal exercise and venous occlusion on fibrinolytic activity in physically active and inactive men. *J Appl Physiol.* 1994;77:2305.
29. Bajzar L, Manuel R, Nesheim ME. Purification and characterization of TAFI, a thrombin-activable fibrinolysis inhibitor. *J Biol Chem.* 1995;270:14477.
30. Huber K, Christ G, Wojta J, et al. Plasminogen activator inhibitor type-1 in cardiovascular disease. Status report 2001. *Thromb Res.* 2001;103(Suppl 1):S7.
31. Xiao Q, Danton MJ, Witte DP, et al. Plasminogen deficiency accelerates vessel wall disease in mice predisposed to atherosclerosis. *Proc Natl Acad Sci U S A.* 1997;94:10335.
32. Schmied H, Kurz A, Sessler DI, et al. Mild hypothermia increases blood loss and transfusion requirements during total hip arthroplasty. *Lancet.* 1996;347:289.
33. Kirkpatrick AW, Chun R, Brown R, et al. Hypothermia and the trauma patient. *Can J Surg.* 1999;42:333.
34. Wolberg AS, Meng ZH, Monroe DM 3rd, et al. A systematic evaluation of the effect of temperature on coagulation enzyme activity and platelet function. *J Trauma.* 2004;56:1221.
35. Cosgriff N, Moore EE, Sauaia A, et al. Predicting life-threatening coagulopathy in the massively transfused trauma patient: hypothermia and acidoses revisited. *J Trauma.* 1997;42:857.
36. Meng ZH, Wolberg AS, Monroe DM 3rd, et al. The effect of temperature and pH on the activity of factor VIIa: implications for the efficacy of high-dose factor VIIa in hypothermic and acidotic patients. *J Trauma.* 2003;55:886.

CHAPTER 50 ■ ALLERGY AND IMMUNOLOGY

PETAR J. POPOVIC • BENJAMIN M. MATTA • JUAN B. OCHOA

OVERVIEW

The modern word *immunity* is derived from the Latin word *immunis,* which referred to exemption from military services, tax payments, or other public services. Throughout the medical history literature, the term *immunity* referred to those who were disease free or protected from getting disease. Immunity as a medical term defines a state of having sufficient biologic defenses to avoid infectious disease or other unwanted biologic invasion. The collection of tissues, cells, and molecules responsible for immunity constitute the *immune system,* and their coordinated response to the potentially harmful (mostly foreign) substances is called the *immune response*.

The main physiologic function of the immune system—protection of the host from infection—for many years characterized the immune response in its ability to distinguish between "foreign" and "self"—the key issue being that foreign was to be attacked and eradicated, while self was not to be attacked. In recent years, however, from the wide range of diseases that are consequent to inappropriate immune functions, we have learned that the ability of the immune system to distinguish between harmful and harmless molecules or cells—rather than characterizing the dichotomy as foreign and self—is essential for mounting protective immune responses and preventing the induction of pathology (Table 50.1). For example, in addition to infectious diseases that develop when immune cells fail to recognize and quickly eradicate microorganisms (foreign and harmful), failure to recognize and eliminate transformed "self" cells (self, but harmful) might result in tumor growth and produce an even more serious clinical condition. On the other hand, the unwanted response to harmless self-proteins produces a variety of autoimmune (*auto* meaning directed at the self) diseases, some of which are severe and life threatening. Autoimmune diseases are classified as systemic or organ specific, although there is often a significant overlap between the two because some diseases that start as organ specific later affect other organs. Finally, immune response toward foreign but harmless substances produces a wide variety of clinical syndromes, defined as allergic diseases or *allergies*. The word *allergy* is derived from the Greek words *allos*, meaning different or changed, and *ergos,* meaning work or action, and roughly refers to an "altered or unusual reaction." Allergy-producing substances are called *allergens*. Examples of allergens include the dust mite, pollens, molds, and foods. It is estimated that more than 50 million North Americans are affected by allergic conditions, with a cost of more than $10 billion dollars yearly. Fortunately, in the majority of cases, allergic diseases are mild in onset and development, and annoying rather than serious medical conditions. However, sometimes serious and life-threatening clinical conditions that require immediate medical intervention develop as a result of allergic reactions. Some of those adverse allergic reactions, such as anaphylactic shock and severe asthma exacerbation, are elaborated in more detail in Chapters 60 and 142, respectively. Besides the previously mentioned, naturally occurring pathology associated with inappropriate immune response, additional problems arise with the development of transplantation medicine. Transplantation is the process of taking cells, tissues, or organs, termed *graft*, from one individual (graft donor) and placing them into a different individual (graft recipient). Although, from our point of view, transplantation is not only harmless but also beneficial and therapeutic, recipient immune cells recognize graft as foreign and potentially harmful. Unless suppressed, recipient immune cells respond to foreign molecules within the graft and induce graft rejection. In clinical practice, it is important to distinguish immune-mediated graft rejection from graft failure induced by other causes. On the other hand, transplanted cells sometimes contain a significant number of donor immune cells that can respond to recipient tissue and produce a serious and life-threatening condition, termed *graft-versus-host disease* (GVHD).

Immunology as a discipline is the study of immunity at the level of cellular and molecular events that control homeostasis and activation of the immune system. Immunology is helping us to better understand the complex processes involved in the immune reactions and to find a way to more appropriately modulate those processes once their malfunction (function) becomes harmful to the host.

CELLS AND TISSUES OF THE IMMUNE SYSTEM

There are two basic types of immune reactions: innate and adaptive (Table 50.2). Innate immunity (also called natural or native immunity) consists of cellular and biochemical defense mechanisms that are in place even before encounter with microbes, and are poised to respond rapidly to infection before the development of the adaptive immune response. The principal components of the innate immunity are (a) physical and chemical barriers, (b) phagocytes (neutrophils, macrophages) and NK (natural killer) cells, (c) the complement system and acute-phase proteins, and (d) cytokines. In contrast to innate immunity, the adaptive immune response needs to be stimulated by exposure to infectious agents or molecules, and it increases in magnitude and defensive capabilities with each successive exposure to a particular molecule. The defining characteristics of adaptive immunity are exquisite specificity for distinct molecules and an ability to "memorize" and respond more vigorously to repeated exposure. Because of its specificity for a particular antigen, adaptive immunity is also

TABLE 50.1

CHARACTERISTICS OF ANTIGEN AND IMMUNOPATHOLOGY

	Antigen	Pathology	Immune response	Treatment
Foreign	Harmful	Infections	Wanted	Stimulation
	Harmless	Allergies	Unwanted	Suppression
	Harmless	Graft rejection or GVHD	Unwanted	Suppression
Self	Harmful	Cancer	Wanted	Stimulation
	Harmless	Autoimmunity	Unwanted	Suppression

GVHD, graft versus host disease.

referred to as *specific immunity*. The main components of adaptive immunity are lymphocytes and their products. Substances and molecules that induce specific immune responses, or are the targets of such responses, are termed *antigens*. There are two types of adaptive response: *Humoral immunity* mediated by antibodies and B lymphocytes and *cell-mediated immunity,* which involves T lymphocytes. The cardinal features of adaptive immune responses, besides specificity and memory, are (a) diversity, the ability to respond to a large variety of antigens; (b) specialization, the optimal response for a particular antigen; (c) self-limitation, allows immune homeostasis; and (d) self-tolerance, nonreactivity to self. Both innate and adaptive immune responses can be divided into distinct phases: recognition of antigen, activation, and the effector phase of antigen elimination, followed by the return to homeostasis; and in the case of adaptive response, the maintenance of memory (1).

Lymphoid tissues are classified as generative or primary lymphoid organs and as peripheral or secondary lymphoid organs. Primary lymphoid organs are *bone marrow,* where all lymphocytes arise and also where B lymphocytes mature, and the *thymus*, where T lymphocytes mature and reach a stage of functional competence. The peripheral lymphoid organs and tissues include *lymph nodes, spleen,* and the *cutaneous and mucosal immune system*. Specialized microenvironments within primary immune organs support immune cell growth and maturation, while secondary lymphoid organs are sites in which optimal adaptive immune responses are initiated and developed. Lymph nodes are sites of immune response to lymph-borne antigens, and the spleen is the major site of immune response to bloodborne antigens. Similarly, cutaneous and mucosal immune systems are specialized for the best response to potential antigens coming through skin and mucosal surfaces, respectively. It is important to mention that, although some cells are permanently resident in one tissue, lymphocytes continuously move through the bloodstream and lymphatic system, from one peripheral (secondary) lymphoid tissue to another. Lymphocyte recirculation and migration to particular tissues are tightly regulated and mediated by adhesion molecules, chemokines, and their receptors, and depend on the cell maturation and activation stage. The main cells of the immune system involved in the adaptive immune response are antigen-specific lymphocytes, specialized antigen-presenting cells (APCs) that display antigens and activate lymphocytes, and effector cells that function to eliminate antigens (microbes). Lymphocytes are the only cells in the body capable of specifically recognizing and distinguishing different antigens. Lymphocytes consist of subsets that are different in their function, but are morphologically indistinguishable. Two main subpopulations of lymphocytes are designated as *B* and *T lymphocytes,* which refer to the organs in which those cells are found to mature, *bursa of Fabricius* in birds (equivalent to *bone marrow* in mammals) and *thymus*, respectively.

TABLE 50.2

TYPES OF IMMUNE RESPONSE

	Innate	Adaptive
Characteristics		
Specificity	Pathogen-associated molecular patterns	Antigenic determinants of protein, microbial and nonmicrobial
Diversity	Limited; germline encoded	Very large; somatic hypermutations of gene segments
Memory	None	Yes
Self-tolerance	Yes (innately)	Yes (acquired)
Components		
Physical barriers	Skin; mucosal epithelia	None
Chemical barriers	Antimicrobial substances	None
Blood proteins	Complement	Antibodies
Cells	Phagocytes (macrophages, neutrophils) and natural killer cells	Lymphocytes (B and T cells)

B lymphocytes are the only cells capable of producing antibodies. They recognize extracellular (soluble or cell surface) antigens and differentiate into antibody-secreting cells, thus functioning as the mediators of humoral immunity. T lymphocytes, the mediators of cellular immunity, consist of functionally distinct populations, the best defined of which are *helper* T cells, cytolytic or *cytotoxic* T cells (CTLs), and *regulatory* T cells. NK cells are the third population of lymphocytes with receptors different from those of B and T cells and with major function involving innate immunity (2).

In modern times, the use of monoclonal antibodies has allowed us to define unique surface proteins, which are present only in that particular cell population and have been used as their characteristic identification marker. The standard nomenclature for these proteins is the *CD* (cluster of differentiation) numerical designation that currently consists of 350 different molecules. The majority of characterized molecules, however, are present on more than one cell population, where their presence defines maturation stage or particular effector function. The classification of lymphocytes by CD antigen expression is now widely used in clinical medicine and experimental immunology. According to the CD classification, helper T cells are defined as $CD3^+$ and $CD4^+$; most CTLs are $CD3^+$ and $CD8^+$, while regulatory T cells are a subgroup of helper cells with an additional low expression of the CD25 activation marker—the α-chain of the surface receptor for interleukin-2 (IL-2Rα)—and are defined as $CD3^+$, $CD4^+$, and $CD25^+$. B cells are characterized with the expression of CD19, while NK cells express the CD56 molecule.

APCs are a cell population that are specialized to capture microbial and other antigens, display them to lymphocytes, and provide signals that stimulate the proliferation and differentiation of lymphocytes. The major type of APCs is the dendritic cell, which is found under epithelia and in most organs, where it is poised to capture antigens and transport them to peripheral lymphoid organs. There are two major subtypes of dendritic cells: myeloid and plasmacytoid. Dendritic cells are the most potent APCs capable of stimulating "naive" T cells as they encounter antigens for the first time. Mature mononuclear phagocytes, tissue macrophages, also function as APCs in a T cell–mediated, adaptive immune response. Macrophages that have ingested microbes may activate "naive" T cells, while, in turn, effector T cells may stimulate the macrophages to more efficiently kill ingested pathogens. Follicular dendritic cells (FDCs) are cells present in the lymphoid tissue that trap antigens in the complex with antibodies or complement products and display those antigens for recognition by B lymphocytes.

After being stimulated by APCs, lymphocytes differentiate into effector cells. Differentiated effector helper T cells secrete cytokines and interact with and activate macrophages and B lymphocytes. Effector CTLs develop granules containing proteins that kill virus-infected and transformed host (tumor) cells. B-cells differentiate into plasma cells that actively synthesize and secrete antibodies. Some antigen-stimulated B and T lymphocytes differentiate into memory cells whose function is to mediate rapid and enhanced responses to second and subsequent exposures to antigens (1,2).

Cytokines are proteins secreted by the cells of innate and adaptive immunity that mediate many of the functions of those cells. Cytokines are produced in response to microbes and other antigens, and different cytokines stimulate diverse responses of cells involved in immunity and inflammation. In the activation phase of the adaptive immune response, cytokines stimulate growth and differentiation of lymphocytes; in the effector phase, they activate different cells to eliminate microbes and other antigens. Based on their principal biologic action, cytokines might be classified into three main functional categories: those that mediate innate immunity (IL-1, IL-6, and tumor necrosis factor [TNF]-α), those that regulate adaptive immunity (IL-2, IL-4, IL-5, and interferon [IFN]-γ), and those that stimulate hematopoiesis (IL-3, IL-7, and some growth factors). Although different cells produce cytokines of innate and adaptive immunity, and those cytokines act on different target cells, this distinction is not absolute because cytokines produced during such reactions often have overlapping action (IL-10 and IL-12). Additionally, cytokine signals from multiple immune cells tightly regulate antigen-processing and clearance responses (3).

ANTIGEN RECOGNITION AND PROCESSING

Antigen recognition is the first phase of the adaptive immune response. Antibodies, major histocompatibility complex (MHC), and T-cell antigen receptors (TCRs) are the three classes of molecules used in adaptive immunity to recognize antigens. Antibodies produced in a membrane-attached form function as B-cell receptors for antigen recognition. The interaction of antigen with membrane antibodies initiates B-cell activation and, thus, constitutes the recognition phase of the humoral immune response. B-lymphocyte differentiation, upon activation, proceeds along two pathways: one that requires stimulation by helper T lymphocytes, the T cell–dependent pathway, or the T cell–independent pathway. The antigens recognized by B cells may be in their native, nondegraded form and not require prior processing of the antigen by other immune system cells. In order to get help from T cells, however, B cells need to internalize the membrane antibody–antigen complex, degrade protein, and display it back on the cell surface membrane in complex with the class II MHC molecule. As explained below, T cells can recognize antigens only if they are processed and presented on the membrane surface of APCs in complex with the MHC molecules. Antibodies are also produced in a secreted form by activated B cells. In the effector phase of the humoral immune response, secreted antibody binds to antigens and triggers several effector mechanisms that eliminate the antigens. Although of the same antigen specificity, membrane-bound antibodies are involved in antigen recognition and B-cell activation, while secreted antibodies are responsible for triggering the effector phase of the humoral immune response and antigen clearance. It is essential to know that specificity and effector functions of antibodies depend on their basic structure. An antibody molecule has a symmetric core structure composed of two identical light chains and two identical heavy chains. Both heavy chains and light chains consist of amino terminal variable (V) regions and carboxyl terminal constant (C) regions. While light- and heavy-chain amino terminal variable regions together participate in antigen recognition, only the constant regions of the heavy chains are involved in antibody effector functions (1,2).

In contrast to B cells and their secreted antibodies that can recognize soluble as well as cell-associated antigens in their native form, T cells can only recognize antigens that are displayed on other cell surfaces and are degraded into fragments by the body's various APCs. The task of displaying cell-associated antigens for recognition by T cells is performed by specialized proteins that are encoded by genes in a locus called the *major histocompatibility complex*. MHC molecules are integral components of the ligands that most T cells recognize, because the antigen receptors of T cells are actually specific for the complex of (foreign) peptide antigens and (self) MHC molecules. MHC molecules are found on immune and nonimmune cells. There are two main types of MHC gene products: class I and class II MHC molecules, which sample different pools of protein antigens, cytosolic or intracellular antigens and extracellular antigens that have been endocytosed, respectively. MHC class I molecules are present on virtually all nucleated cells where they display antigens to be recognized by $CD8^+$ cytotoxic T lymphocytes. MHC class II molecules are found primarily on APCs and primarily activate $CD4^+$ helper T cells. Once an antigen enters an APC, it is degraded to its peptide fragments. These antigen fragments are then integrated with the MHC molecule and transported to the cell membrane, where they are exposed to neighboring cells within a complex that includes either class I or class II MHC molecules. T lymphocytes subsequently recognize the MHC–antigen (MHC–Ag) complex and initiate antigenic response (1,2).

All T lymphocytes recognize an antigen by specific T-cell receptor (TCR) molecules expressed on their cell membrane. These TCR molecules function similarly to a lock and key with the MHC–Ag complex. It is important to understand that only a few T lymphocytes constituting one T-cell clone are specific for one particular antigen. In addition to T-cell receptor binding to the MHC–Ag complex, multiple membrane receptors are used in APC–T-cell interaction. During the infection-free time, however, cells still express MHC–Ag complexes containing self-antigens that should not provoke an immune response under normal conditions because potentially harmful lymphocytes that might be activated by regular self-antigens are eliminated during their maturation process within the thymus or bone marrow. Unfortunately, not all self-antigens are presented during lymphocyte maturation, and some might be exposed later during their lifespan. Exposure of those "hidden" self-antigens could initiate an unwanted immune response toward self-molecules, resulting in the development of an autoimmune disease (1).

In contrast to appropriately processed antigens that stimulate a limited number of T cells (one clone) bearing the same TCR (approximately one in a million circulating T cells), some bacterial proteins and toxins are able to stimulate T cells without first undergoing endocytosis and degradation. Those molecules, characterized as *superantigens*, can simultaneously stimulate T cells with different antigen specificity, and subsequently induce *polyclonal activation* with the extensive systemic release of cytokines. The stimulatory effect of superantigens is a consequence of direct binding to the class II MHC on APCs and the non–antigen-specific part of TCR on T cells, thus being able to activate 2% to 20% of all T cells. The massive T-cell activation results in the release of large amounts of inflammatory cytokines that induce T-cell anergy or death (apoptosis), which severely disturbs the ability of the immune system to respond appropriately to infection. As a consequence of the systemic effects of released cytokines, infected patients may develop toxic shock syndrome. Systemic effects include fever, endothelial damage, profound hypertension, disseminated intravascular coagulation, and multiorgan failure (4).

ANTIGEN CLEARANCE AND INFLAMMATION: IMMUNE EFFECTOR FUNCTIONS

Once the immune system recognizes an antigen, inflammation and clearance processes are initiated. Activation and the effector phase of the adaptive immune response are intended to eliminate antigen in the most appropriate and efficient way. For example, one set of components of the immune system is activated in response to the extracellular antigen (antibodies and helper T cells), while others are more effective in the elimination of the intracellular antigen (CTLs and NK cells). Regardless of the type of antigen, processes involved in the activation and effector phase of immune response induce changes in the surrounding tissue, defined as *inflammation*. The antigen clearance process is enhanced within inflamed tissues by increased vascular flow, altered vascular permeability, and the recruitment of immune cells. Those changes also produce four cardinal clinical signs of inflammation or ongoing immune response: (a) warmness (*calor*), (b) redness (*rubor*), (c) swelling (*tumor*), and (d) pain (*dolor*), often accompanied by malfunction of the involved organ (*functio laesa*).

Several physiologic mechanisms are involved in circulating inflammatory cell adhesion to vascular endothelium and subsequent diapedesis. Multiple adhesion molecules are present on both circulating inflammatory cells (L-selectin, LFA-1, and MAC-1) and endothelial cells (P-selectin, E-selectin, ICAM-1, and ICAM-2 molecules) after stimulation. Expression and function of these molecules is modulated by "early response" cytokines (TNF-α and IL-1) secreted by activated tissue macrophages and other APCs. Additionally, IL-8 production by endothelial cells and tissue fibroblasts is a major component of the chemotactic gradient facilitating neutrophil migration across the endothelial surface. Neutrophils are capable of direct recognition and phagocytosis of circulating antigens. After neutrophil phagocytosis, enzyme-laden lysosomes fuse with the antigen-containing phagosome, digesting and destroying the antigen. Neutrophils possess receptors for the Fc portion of immunoglobulins as well as receptors for complement components. Thus, opsonization or coating of antigens by immunoglobulins and complement markedly enhances phagocytic capability and antigen elimination (5).

The predominant mechanism for adequate reaction to, and rapid clearance of, extracellular antigen involves antibodies or immunoglobulins. Antibodies possess unique antigen specificity, thereby narrowing the inflammatory response to the specific antigenic target. Antibodies circulating in the bloodstream or interstitial fluid promptly recognize, and bind to, an antigen; but because antibodies do not directly perform any effector function, the elimination of antigen requires interaction of antibody with the components of innate immunity such as complement proteins or phagocytes and eosinophils. Antibody-mediated effector functions include neutralization of microbes or toxic microbial products, activation of the complement system, opsonization (coating) of antigens for enhanced phagocytosis, antibody-dependent cell-mediated cytotoxicity

(ADCC), and immediate hypersensitivity in which antibodies trigger mast cell activation.

Antibody molecules or immunoglobulins (Ig) can be divided into distinct classes and subclasses on the basis of differences in the structure (heavy chain), tissue and biologic fluid distribution, and functional capability. In order from the highest to the lowest serum concentration, those classes of antibody molecules (also referred to as isotypes) are designated as IgG, IgA, IgM, IgD, and IgE. It is important to note that different classes of antibodies perform different effector functions. Among the most notable functions of immunoglobulins are opsonization and the capacity to activate complement. IgG, IgM, and IgA are crucial to normal opsonization functions. Opsonization by IgG and IgM expedites the clearance of circulating antigens, whereas the secretion of IgA onto mucosal surfaces facilitates the clearance of invaders by mucosal surface macrophages and neutrophils. Because of its larger size, the function of IgM is confined primarily to the intravascular clearance of antigens, whereas IgG readily diffuses into the extravascular space. After being coupled with an antigen, antigen–antibody complexes—also termed immune complexes—are normally cleared by phagocytic and red blood cells. The clearance of immune complexes from the circulation is dependent on effective opsonization, binding of the immune complex–bound C3b fragment to CR1 on erythrocytes, and subsequent transport to the liver and spleen (6). IgD is primarily found on the surface of naive B cells where it functions as the receptor for antigen recognition. Although a little amount of IgD is also secreted, it is believed that IgD does not perform any physiologic immune function. In contrast to other immunoglobulin classes, once secreted, IgE is present free in the serum for a very short time, since it binds rapidly to the specific receptor on basophils, eosinophils, and mast cells. Antigen activation of cell-bound IgE results in the immediate release of various mediators, including histamine, serotonin, and leukotrienes. Although IgE is commonly connected to the allergic reactions, the physiologic function of IgE seems to be an immediate response to antigen and the induction of vascular dilation, increased vascular permeability, and the recruitment of immune cells. An important immune function of IgE is also to protect the host against parasites.

The complement system is capable of generating a broad series of inflammatory actions associated with antigen clearance. These actions include lysis of cells bearing antigen–antibody complexes, opsonization of antigens, chemotaxis of inflammatory cells, and generation of anaphylactic reactions. Complement activation may be accomplished by either the classic pathway, initiated by antigen–antibody complexes, or the alternate route initiated by antigenic protein aggregates, endotoxin, or insoluble compounds with certain surface characteristics. With sequential proteolysis of complement substrates, various complement fragments with neutrophil and eosinophil chemotactic properties, as well as vasodilatory effects, are generated that produce the previously mentioned cardinal signs of inflammation (7).

The major cells involved in antigen clearance include APCs and lymphocytes, neutrophils, and various organ-specific structural cells or tissue macrophages. Although many antigens may be destroyed within mononuclear phagocytic cells by intracellular enzymes, some antigens may become sheltered within the cells. Elimination of these antigens requires additional activation from helper T cells, which predominates in the case of bacterial infection. In general, the helper population of T lymphocytes ($CD4^+$) supports the function of mononuclear phagocytic cells and enhances antibody production by the B-lymphocyte population, thus supporting the clearance of extracellular antigens. Activated T cells increase the secretion of cytokines that are crucial for regulation of the immune response. On the basis of the pattern of cytokines secreted, $CD4^+$ lymphocytes are subdivided into two major classes: Th1 or Th2. The Th2 group of $CD4^+$ cells secretes cytokines, such as IL-4 and IL-10, that stimulate secretion of antibodies but partially suppress the cellular immune response and initiate the healing process. The cytokines secreted by the Th1 group of $CD4^+$ cells, including IL-2 and IFN-γ, are potent stimulants of the cell-mediated immune response. The systemic predominance of $CD4^+$ cell stimulation with either the Th1 or Th2 cytokine pattern has been associated with altered resistance to certain infections (8).

The $CD8^+$ population of T lymphocytes (CTLs) functions to destroy cells sheltering an antigen presented within a class I MHC complex, and is involved in the clearance of intracellular antigens. Lysis of the infected cell by CTLs, however, dominates during viral infections. Besides the important role of the T lymphocyte in clearing microbial pathogens, those cells are crucial for the recognition and elimination of self-transformed tumor cells. As a part of tumor cell growth, new antigens arise, which are presented on the cell surface in the complex with class I MHC molecules. As those antigens are new or changed self-antigens, CTLs cells might recognize them and induce tumor cell lysis. The CTL response refers primarily to cell killing by cytotoxic $CD8^+$ lymphocytes. After exposure to processed antigen, and under the influence of the lymphokines IL-2 and IFN-γ, activated $CD8^+$ cells proliferate, synthesize, and secrete membrane attack molecules, which results in lysis of the antigen-bearing cell. Similar to the cell lysis by CTLs, natural killer cells lyse neighboring cells by secreting membrane attack molecules (perforin and granzymes). Unlike the CTL response, the natural killer cell lysis of antigen-bearing cells does not seem to be antigen specific. Killer lymphocytes, the third major cytolytic cell population, are coated with surface receptors for antibodies. Killer lymphocytes may localize to antigen–antibody-coated cells, where they release their cytotoxic granules. Antibody recognition is crucial to this system, and killer lymphocyte function seems to be a component of antibody-dependent cytotoxicity. Natural killer cells and killer lymphocytes can be activated and made to proliferate in vitro under the influence of cytokines. These lymphokine-activated killer (LAK) cells may be reinfused into the body and have been investigated as cancer immunotherapy (8,9).

In addition to the primary immune APCs or professional APCs, structural cells, such as those of the endothelium, epithelium, and connective tissue, are also important to an effective immune response. Not only are these cells capable of secreting cytokines and inflammatory mediators, but after stimulation, they also express class II MHC molecules and may function in antigen presentation to T lymphocytes. Those cells are termed *nonprofessional APCs*, and their activation by particular cytokines (IFN-γ) may underlie the organ dysfunction associated with chronic immune stimulation and inflammation (1).

The release of multiple inflammatory mediators from migrating leukocytes—proteases, oxygen radicals, leukotrienes, platelet-activating factor—expands the local inflammatory process. Conversely, several cytokines and soluble cytokine receptors are normally present to down-regulate or limit the inflammatory response. Among these "anti-inflammatory" factors are IL-4, IL-10, IL-13, transforming growth factor (TGF)-β, and IL-1 receptor antagonist. Cytokines released into the systemic circulation as a consequence of either localized or systemic inflammation have been directly implicated in the pathophysiologic mechanisms of the organ dysfunction associated with major trauma, sepsis, and burns. If high plasma concentrations are achieved, IL-1, TNF-α, and IL-6 have been shown to have profound effects on body metabolism and are capable of inducing hypotension, fever, and cachexia. Their functions have been implicated in the manifestations of septic shock, and their concentration correlates with mortality. In response to TNF-α, nitric oxide is produced by endothelial cells and, along with the other mediators, promotes smooth muscle relaxation and vasodilation. Whether these cytokines and mediators are the primary pathogenetic mediators for the shock syndrome or are markers for systemic inflammation is unclear (10).

Adequate response to the antigen, and successful and fast antigen elimination, results in the development of signs and symptoms defined as *acute* inflammation. In contrast, failure of immune cells to appropriately respond and eliminate antigen might result in the long-term stimulation of immune reaction and the development of *chronic* inflammation. Chronic inflammation is characteristic of most autoimmune diseases in which unwanted, rather than inappropriate, response toward self-antigens induces pathology.

HYPERSENSITIVITY REACTIONS

Adaptive immunity serves the important function of host defense against microbial infections, but immune responses are also capable of causing tissue injury and disease. Disorders caused by immune responses are termed *hypersensitivity diseases* (Table 50.3). This term arose from the clinical definition of immunity as "sensitivity," which is based on observations that an individual who has been exposed to an antigen exhibits a detectable reaction or is "sensitive" to subsequent encounters with the antigen. A common cause of hypersensitivity diseases is failure of self-tolerance, which, under physiologic conditions, ensures that the individual's immune system does not respond to his or her own antigens. Hypersensitivity diseases also result from uncontrolled or excessive responses against foreign antigens, such as microbes and noninfectious environmental antigens (11).

Hypersensitivity diseases represent a clinically heterogeneous group of disorders. The two principal factors that determine the clinical and pathologic manifestations of such diseases are the type of immune response that causes tissue injury, and the nature and location of antigen that is the target of this response. According to the nature of the immune response and the effector mechanisms responsible for cell and tissue injury, hypersensitivity diseases are commonly classified into four main types.

Type I

Type I hypersensitivity reaction, also called *immediate* hypersensitivity, is the most prevalent type of hypersensitivity diseases. IgE antibodies that are bound to mast cells, basophils, and eosinophils cause immediate hypersensitivity. When cell-associated IgE antibodies are cross-linked by the antigen, the cells are activated to rapidly release a variety of mediators. These mediators collectively cause increased vascular permeability, vasodilation, bronchial and visceral smooth muscle contraction, and local inflammation. Under normal conditions, this type of response is first triggered by antigen, but is short lived and beneficial for antigen clearance. In clinical medicine, these reactions are commonly referred to as allergy or atopy, and are the most common disorders of immunity that affect 20% of all individuals in the United States. The most common forms of atopic disease are allergic rhinitis (hay fever), bronchial asthma, atopic dermatitis (eczema), and food allergies. Immediate systemic hypersensitivity, characterized by edema in many tissues and fall in blood pressure secondary to vasodilation, is termed *anaphylaxis*, and may be fatal.

TABLE 50.3

TYPES OF PATHOLOGIC IMMUNE REACTIONS

Type	Effectors	Mechanism injury	Diseases
Type I, immediate hypersensitivity	IgE antibodies, Mast cells	Cell degranulation and mediator release	Hay fever, asthma, anaphylaxis
Type II, antibody mediated	Antibodies to single cell's antigens	Complement-dependent lysis and phagocytosis of cells	Anemia, thrombocytopenia, agranulocytosis
	Antibodies to tissue antigens	Enzyme release from activated leukocytes	Goodpasture disease, blistering skin diseases
	Antibodies to hormones or receptors	Function inhibition or activation	Diabetes, hyperthyroidism, myasthenia gravis
Type III, immune complex mediated	Antibody–antigen complexes	Immune complex–mediated leukocyte activation	Glomerulonephritis, vasculitis, SLE, serum sickness
Type IV, T-cell mediated	$CD4^+$ helper T cells	Macrophage activation and inflammation	Diabetes, multiple sclerosis, RA
	$CD8^+$ cytotoxic T cells	Target cell lysis	Acute hepatitis, graft rejection

SLE, systemic lupus erythematosus; RA, rheumatoid arthritis.

Type II

Antibodies other than IgE can cause tissue injury by recruiting and activating inflammatory cells. Diseases induced by such antibodies are identified as type II *hypersensitivity reactions.* Those antibodies are specific for antigens of particular cells or the extracellular matrix, and are found attached to these cells or tissue. Antibodies against tissue antigens cause disease by three main mechanisms:

1. First, antibodies against antigens on circulating cells promote complement activation and cell lysis or phagocytosis. Those antibodies might promote development of anemia, thrombocytopenia, and/or agranulocytosis.
2. Second, antibodies deposited in the tissue recruit neutrophils and macrophages. As phagocytosis is not possible, those cells release their products and induce tissue injury. This is the case with blistering skin diseases, vasculitis, and some forms of glomerulonephritis.
3. Third, some antibodies to a hormone, hormone receptors, blood-clotting factors, growth factors, an enzyme, or a drug might cause disease or treatment failure by inactivating or activating vital biologic function of these molecules without inducing any inflammation and tissue damage. Diseases mediated by this mechanism are myasthenia gravis, hyperthyroidism (Graves disease), diabetes, and myeloblastic anemia.

Type III

Immune complex disease or type III hypersensitivity is caused by antibody–antigen complexes formed in tissues. In certain disease states, immune complexes may freely circulate or be deposited within tissues, stimulating inflammatory reactions throughout the body. Immune complexes easily activate and complement neutrophils that cause tissue injury. In contrast to the type II diseases, type III hypersensitivity diseases are often systemic, such as serum sickness and systemic lupus erythematosus (SLE).

Type IV

Finally, tissue injury may be due to T lymphocytes that activate the effector mechanisms of delayed-type hypersensitivity (DTH) or directly kill target cells. Such conditions are type IV hypersensitivity *disorders.* In those diseases, tissue injury results from the products of activated macrophages, such as hydrolytic enzymes, reactive oxygen species, nitric oxide, and proinflammatory cytokines. Many organ-specific autoimmune diseases are caused by hypersensitivity reactions induced by T cells, such as insulin-dependent diabetes mellitus, multiple sclerosis, rheumatoid arthritis, contact sensitivity, and inflammatory bowel diseases (IBDs) (11).

IMMUNE DEFECTS AND CRITICAL ILLNESS

In contrast to the hypersensitivity reactions, many life-threatening diseases represent the consequences of immune system defects or deficiencies. Recurrent or unusual infections, increased susceptibility to tumors, and delayed healing characterize patients with immune system disorders. Although many immune system diseases overlap in immunopathogenesis, most may be classified on the basis of the predominant immune defect, be that defect congenital or acquired (Tables 50.4A and B). Additionally, many other chronic illnesses might be associated with subtle immunologic abnormalities, potentially contributing to clinical disease. Immune system disorders may be grouped into disorders of humoral immunity (Table 50.4A), cell-mediated immunity (Table 50.4B), and phagocytic cell function.

TABLE 50.4A

IMMUNODEFICIENCY SYNDROMES: ANTIBODY AND COMPLEMENT

Defect	Etiology	Consequence
IgG deficiency	Acquired, common variable hypogammaglobulinemia; congenital, X-linked or associated with ataxia telangiectasia	Recurrent infections, especially with *Streptococcus pneumoniae* and *Haemophilus* sp.
IgA deficiency	Thought to occur primarily as a congenital abnormality	Recurrent sinopulmonary infections, especially with *S. pneumoniae*
Early complement component (C2–C4) deficiencies	Congenital	Predisposition to autoimmune disease (e.g., SLE), increased risk for infections
Late complement component (C5–C8) deficiencies	Congenital	Increased risk for infections, especially with *Neisseria*
C1 inhibitor deficiency	Primarily congenital, rarely acquired	Angioedema, abdominal distress, upper airway obstruction
Complement receptor deficiency	Congenital or acquired	Predisposition to autoimmune disease
Alternate complement pathway defects	Associated with sickle cell disease	Increased risk for infections, especially with *S. pneumoniae*

SLE, systemic lupus erythematosus

TABLE 50.4B

IMMUNODEFICIENCY SYNDROMES: CELL MEDIATED

Defect	Etiology	Consequence
T-lymphocyte defects	AIDS, lymphoma, iatrogenic (especially glucocorticoid therapy and immunosuppressants used in solid organ transplantation)	Infection with opportunistic pathogens, *Pneumocystis jirovecii,* CMV, herpes simplex, *Cryptococcus neoformans,* and *Legionella*
Chronic granulomatous disease	Abnormal neutrophil oxidative metabolism, ineffective microbicidal activity, congenital	Recurrent bacterial and fungal infections; pyogenic infection of the skin, lymph nodes, liver, and lungs
Neutropenia	Most commonly iatrogenic (cytotoxic chemotherapy)	Bacterial and fungal infections
Leukocyte adhesion deficiency	Congenital absence of leukocyte adhesion molecules (LFA, MAC-1, selectins)	Recurrent skin, soft tissue, and lung infections; persistently elevated peripheral leukocyte counts
Chediak-Higashi syndrome	Congenitally abnormal neutrophil chemotaxis and degranulation, decreased microbicidal capacity	Associated with albinism and photophobia; recurrent infections
Job syndrome	Congenitally abnormal neutrophil chemotaxis, delayed catabolism of IgE	Elevated serum IgE; sinusitis; otitis media; eczema; recurrent skin and soft tissue infections, with *Staphylococcus aureus*

AIDS, acquired immunodeficiency syndrome; CMV, cytomegalovirus.

Defects of the complement system include deficiencies of individual complement component proteins, regulatory proteins, or complement receptors. Complement component deficiencies may be broadly grouped into early (C1–C4) or late component (C5–C8) deficiencies. A predisposition to *Streptococcus pneumoniae* and *Haemophilus influenzae* infections has been observed in patients deficient in early complement components. *Neisseria meningitidis* infections have been recognized as sequelae of late-component deficiencies. In contrast to patients with late-component deficiencies, patients with early-component deficiencies possess a uniquely higher incidence of autoimmune disease, especially SLE. In these patients, it has been suggested that the complement deficiency impairs effective clearance of circulating immune complexes, predisposing to autoimmune diseases. The consumption of complement in sepsis and septic shock has been clearly demonstrated. Whether complement activation is pathogenic or physiologic in septic shock remains unclear. Both the alternate and classic pathways of complement activation have been shown to be activated in septic shock, potentially related to a sepsis-induced inactivation of C1 inhibitors (12).

The most clinically significant complement regulatory protein deficiency is loss of C1 inhibitor activity. This nonspecific esterase inhibitor is strategic in controlling the classic complement cascade and inhibiting the action of several clotting factors. Although acquired forms of C1 inhibitor deficiency have been described, the autosomally dominant genetic defect is the most common. In patients with hereditary angioedema, trauma or stress may precipitate uncontrolled activation of the complement system, culminating in a systemic angioedema–nonpruritic limb edema, gastrointestinal disturbances, and upper airway obstruction. Unlike the angioedema associated with anaphylaxis, the angioedema associated with C1 inhibitor deficiency is much less responsive to epinephrine and glucocorticoids. In addition to subcutaneous or inhaled epinephrine, the management of acute angioedema may include the use of fresh frozen plasma or, when available, purified C1 inhibitor replacement. As maintenance therapy, androgens such as danazol or stanozolol offer effective therapy and are usually effective in increasing the levels of serum C1 inhibitor. C1 inhibitor deficiency is characterized by deficient C1 functional activity in serum, along with low levels of C2 and C4, especially during acute episodes. Notably, the serum level of C3 or total hemolytic complement activity is commonly normal. Few patients deficient in complement receptors have been described. The lack of cell surface complement receptors results in poor clearance of immune complexes. The elevated level of circulating immune complexes is thought to underlie the high prevalence of SLE in these patients (12).

Abnormalities of immunoglobulin production manifest most commonly as deficiencies, although the excessive production of immunoglobulins occasionally results in severe sequelae, as may occur in Waldenstrom macroglobulinemia. Infectious consequences of immunoglobulin deficiency result from most forms of immunoglobulin deficiency. The most common adult type of primary immunoglobulin deficiency is a selective deficiency of IgA. Although IgA deficiency has been associated with recurrent sinopulmonary infections and with *Giardia* intestinal infections, many of these patients remain asymptomatic. The clinical consequences of hypogammaglobulinemia are more frequent in patients with the heterogeneous disorders that compose common variable hypogammaglobulinemia. Common variable hypogammaglobulinemia includes a group of disorders characterized by low or absent serum immunoglobulin levels and an enhanced risk for bacterial infections, especially sinopulmonary infections. Because the infections are usually recurrent and generally responsive to treatment, these patients may present in adulthood with bronchiectasis and lung destruction. Infections with encapsulated bacteria, such as *Haemophilus* and *Streptococcus,* are especially prevalent. The most frequently diagnosed immunoglobulin deficiency pattern in these patients is a decrease in all classes of immunoglobulins. Prophylactic therapy with γ-globulin has proven to be effective in preventing infections (7,13).

Among the many disorders associated with elevated serum concentrations of immunoglobulins, diseases associated with excessive IgM production are especially notable for acute clinical sequelae. Because of their size and structure, IgM globulins possess unique properties, including cold insolubility (cryoglobulins) and the potential to greatly increase blood viscosity. Excessive IgM production may result from a clearly benign response to mycoplasma and viral infections, or a neoplastic-like B-lymphocyte response (Waldenstrom macroglobulinemia). The cold agglutinin response to infections rarely results in more than a mild hemolytic anemia, but the IgM levels associated with Waldenstrom macroglobulinemia may produce life-threatening consequences. Viscosity-related sequelae include confusion, coma, visual impairment, and congestive heart failure. Plasmapheresis to lower the serum IgM level is effective therapy for these acute complications (7,13).

A normal antibody immune response to foreign material may occasionally result in dramatic clinical symptomatology. Especially notable examples are serum sickness and leukoagglutinin reactions. Serum sickness is characterized by the formation of circulating antigen–antibody complexes 7 to 10 days after injection of an antigenic protein into the body. With systemic deposition of the immune complexes, complement is activated and edema, rash, arthralgia, and fever result. The most common cases of serum sickness follow treatment with antithymocyte globulin (equine or rabbit origin) or snake antivenom (equine origin). Glucocorticoid therapy is usually indicated for severe serum sickness symptoms. The leukoagglutinin reaction results from the incidental transfusion of antibodies with red blood cells or plasma. Leukoagglutinin reactions result from the interaction of transfused antibodies with recipient neutrophils, prompting neutrophil sequestration in the lungs. Cough, dyspnea, and respiratory failure may follow the transfusion. Treatment is supportive, as there is no specific therapy for the reactions (14).

Acquired defects in lymphocyte- and macrophage-regulated immunity are the most common immunodeficiencies encountered in adults. Three major groups of disorders account for most of these disorders: the acquired immunodeficiency syndrome (AIDS), various lymphohematologic malignancies, and iatrogenic immunosuppression. These diseases are associated with enhanced susceptibility to infections with common pathogens, as well as a unique predisposition to infections with opportunistic microorganisms. The pathogenesis of one of the most devastating immune disorders, AIDS, involves selective depletion of the $CD4^+$ subset of T lymphocytes by retroviral infection. In these patients, lymphocyte depletion, combined with abnormal macrophage function and certain B-lymphocyte malfunctions, culminates in a plethora of potentially life-threatening infections. As with other patients with profound defects in lymphocyte-regulated immunity, patients with AIDS may commonly present with acute and severe respiratory failure in association with diffuse pulmonary infiltrates. Notable opportunistic respiratory pathogens in patients with defects in lymphocyte-regulated immunity include *Pneumocystis jirovecii, Listeria monocytogenes, Nocardia* sp., *Mycobacteria* sp., *Cryptococcus neoformans,* and cytomegalovirus. Before the AIDS epidemic, most cases of *Pneumocystis* pneumonia in adults occurred among iatrogenically immunosuppressed patients or patients with lymphoma, especially Hodgkin lymphoma. Immunosuppressants primarily affecting lymphocyte function include those used in organ transplantation: glucocorticoids, antithymocyte globulin, OKT3 antilymphocyte globulin, azathioprine, and cyclosporine.

The most common abnormalities of phagocytic function are related to either an abnormal number or function of circulating neutrophils. The consequence of almost all neutrophil defects is infection, primarily bacterial and fungal, and, less commonly, viral. The incidence of infection among neutropenic patients correlates with the depression of the circulating neutrophil count and the duration of neutropenia. Neutropenia is graded based on absolute neutrophil count as mild (1,000 to 1,500 cells/μL), moderate (500 to 1,000 cells/μL), or severe (less than 500 cells/μL) (15). The risk of infection increases proportionally as the circulating neutrophil count falls and is greater when the neutropenia persists over several days. Universally, patients with an absolute neutrophil count below 1,000 cells/μL have a substantially increased risk of infection over time, while serious infections are uncommon until more severe neutropenia develops with counts less than 500 cells/μL. With neutrophil counts below 100 cells/μL, the incidence of severe infection increases dramatically (15, 16). This risk forms the basis for empiric antimicrobial therapy in neutropenic patients before pathogen identification. The pathogenesis of neutrophil functional abnormalities has been most extensively studied among patients with congenital neutrophil defects. A history of recurrent lymphocutaneous or pulmonary infections with staphylococci or Gram-negative bacilli, especially *Pseudomonas* sp. or *Serratia* sp., provides a clue to a potential underlying neutrophil function disorder. Notably, infections with obligate anaerobic bacilli are exceedingly rare among patients with neutrophil defects. Multiple congenital functional defects of neutrophils have been identified and are outlined in Table 50.4B. Specific therapy exists for only one of these congenital disorders. Among certain patients with chronic granulomatous disease, the administration of IFN-γ has been shown to partially correct the neutrophil abnormality and dramatically lessen the incidence of infections (17).

IMMUNOTHERAPY

A broad spectrum of immunotherapies has evolved over the last several years (Table 50.5A). Immunotherapies may be broadly classified as either immune system stimulants or suppressants, but there is much mechanistic overlap. For example, the therapeutic effect of intravenous immune globulin (IVIG) administration in the treatment of idiopathic thrombocytopenia purpura has been partially attributed to the immunosuppressive properties of the transfused immunoglobulin complexes. Likewise, the actions of most immunosuppressive drugs are relatively global, with alterations in both cell-mediated immunity and humoral immunity (18).

Immunotherapies and Critical Illness

Although the complications of immunosuppression commonly result in serious illnesses, only a few specific immunotherapies are used in caring for critically ill patients. These immunotherapies include the use of certain antibodies, antibody fragments,

TABLE 50.5A

IMMUNOTHERAPY

Agents	Indications	Major side effects
Immunosuppressive drugs		
Corticosteroids	Multiple diseases associated with inflammation, graft rejection	Adrenal suppression, infection, altered glucose metabolism, cataracts, osteoporosis
Cytotoxic chemotherapies	Cancer therapy	Neutropenia, infection, mucosal ulceration
Methotrexate	Multiple diseases associated with inflammation, cancer therapy	Pneumonitis, hepatitis, neutropenia, infection
Cyclosporine	Graft rejection	Nephrotoxicity, hypertension
Azathioprine	Graft rejection, rheumatoid arthritis	Leukopenia, thrombocytopenia, infection
Immunomodulatory drugs		
Levamisole	Cancer therapy	Diarrhea, nausea, stomatitis, neurotoxicity, leukopenia, rash

and plasmapheresis (Table 50.5B). Multiple other forms of immunotherapy for critically ill patients have been used less consistently or with no success. The use of immunosuppressives and antibodies in the management of septic shock has failed to demonstrate any clinical benefit. The administration of antibodies, either as pooled γ-globulin fractions or antigen-specific immunoglobulins, has demonstrable efficacy in many chronic medical illnesses. Certain antibodies and antibody fragments occupy a novel therapeutic role in the management of the critically ill patient (19).

A unique detoxifying mechanism for digoxin intoxication involves the use of the Fab fragment of an anti-digoxin antibody. These fragments, produced in sheep, facilitate digoxin clearance with minimal side effects. Within minutes of infusion, serum-free digoxin levels are usually undetectable, whereas immunoreactive digoxin levels (detecting the inactive digoxin–Fab complexes) are usually elevated. Digoxin–Fab complexes are excreted by the kidneys without the latent release of digoxin. In general, anti-digoxin Fab therapy is indicated for digoxin-intoxicated patients presenting with life-threatening arrhythmias or digoxin intoxication accompanied by hyperkalemia. In addition to correcting the cardiac toxicity, the occasional hyperkalemia induced by digoxin poisoning commonly resolves with the Fab therapy. The commercially available anti-digoxin Fab product contains 40 mg of the Fab fragment, which is capable of binding 0.6 mg digoxin. The amount of Fab to be administered may be calculated either from knowledge of the amount ingested or by the formula (assuming that the drug has reached equilibrium levels):

$$\text{Body burden of digoxin (mg)} = [\text{Serum digoxin level (ng/mL)} \times 5.6(\text{L/kg, distribution volume}) \times \text{Weight (kg)}]/1{,}000$$

The body burden of digoxin should be calculated and the appropriate number of anti-digoxin Fab vials administered. Clinical experience suggests that it is better to deliver the correct number or a slight excess of Fab vials rather than underdose the patient. Side effects, even in the presence of moderate renal

TABLE 50.5B

IMMUNOTHERAPY: ANTIBODIES

Agents	Indications	Major side effects
Immunoglobulin (pooled human)	Ig deficiency diseases, ITP, myasthenia gravis, Guillain-Barré syndrome, CMV pneumonia in immunosuppressed patients	Myalgia, arthralgia, fever, aseptic meningitis, reactions in IgA-deficient patients, rarely anaphylaxis
Hyperimmune human Ig (hepatitis B, rabies, tetanus, Rho globulin, hepatitis A, measles)	Passive prophylaxis for specific diseases	Myalgia and injection site inflammation when administered intramuscularly
Hyperimmune sera	Antidotes for envenomization	Anaphylaxis, serum sickness
Antithymocyte globulin	Graft rejection, aplastic anemia	Fever, chills, thrombocytopenia, serum sickness, anaphylaxis
OKT3 (monoclonal antibody to T cells)	Graft rejection	Cytokine syndrome (especially with first injection, infection)
Anti-digoxin Fab fragment	Digoxin intoxication with arrhythmias	Hypokalemia, heart failure
Antiplatelet integrin receptor (ReoPro)	Prevention of acute reocclusion after coronary angioplasty	Hemorrhage

ITP, idiopathic thrombocytic purpura; CMV, cytomegalovirus.

TABLE 50.5C

IMMUNOTHERAPY: CYTOKINES AND GROWTH FACTORS

Agents	Indications	Major side effects
Interleukin-2 (IL-2)	Cancer therapy	Capillary leak syndrome, hypotension, pulmonary edema
Interferon-α (IFN-α)	Cancer therapy, certain forms of hepatitis	Flu-like syndrome: fever, headache, chills, myalgia
Interferon-γ (IFN-γ)	Chronic granulomatous disease with recurrent infections	Flu-like syndrome
Interferon-β (IFN-β)	Multiple sclerosis	Flu-like syndrome: injection site inflammation
Granulocyte colony stimulating factor (GCSF)	Prevention of infections and episodes of febrile neutropenia after chemotherapy	Bone pain
Granulocyte–macrophage colony stimulating factor (GM-CSF)	Myeloid reconstitution after bone marrow transplantation	Capillary leak syndrome; pulmonary edema; pericardial effusion; flulike syndrome

insufficiency, have been mild. Rarely is there a need to readminister a Fab dose. After the Fab administration, serum potassium levels should be monitored because the most common side effect is hypokalemia, and cautious potassium supplementation may be necessary. Once the anti-digoxin Fab has been administered, serum digoxin levels are uninterpretable. With normal renal function, the digoxin–Fab complex is excreted with a half-life of 10 to 20 hours (20).

Multiple immunomodulatory agents, including cytokines (Table 50.5C), antibodies to cytokines, and soluble cytokine receptors, are under active investigation in the management of critical illnesses and their complications. Whereas initial clinical trials suggested some efficacy of certain anti-endotoxin antibodies, studies in larger patient populations clearly demonstrated no benefit and perhaps a harmful effect. Considering the complexity of the immune system regulatory mechanisms in critical illnesses, the interpretation of preliminary immunomodulatory studies should be done with caution (21).

Plasmapheresis, the removal of plasma from blood with the reinfusion of cells and replacement fluids, has been used in many illnesses with variable success. Plasmapheresis has been shown to be effective in several illnesses that commonly require management in the intensive care unit, including idiopathic thrombocytopenia purpura (ITP), Guillain-Barré syndrome, myasthenia gravis, Waldenstrom macroglobulinemia, and Goodpasture syndrome. In general, plasmapheresis requires placement of either large-bore peripheral venous catheters or a temporary hemodialysis catheter. Most of the severe complications associated with plasmapheresis have been related to placement and maintenance of the venous access catheter. Hemorrhagic and septic complications are major concerns with respect to the choice of vascular access because of catheter manipulation during the pheresis sessions, the predisposition to hemorrhage associated with plasma extraction, and underlying renal and hemostatic derangements. Peripheral venous catheters or femoral catheters are probably preferable to subclavian or internal jugular sites for patients with hemostatic derangements. Similarly, the appropriate replacement fluid varies with the clinical condition and disease. In general, fresh frozen plasma is the most appropriate replacement fluid in treating ITP, whereas 5% albumin with isotonic saline is usually used for most neurologic indications. The volume of replacement fluid is estimated by approximating the amount of plasma removed. Considering that one plasma volume is commonly removed with each session, the replacement volume can be estimated from the following equation:

$$\text{Blood volume} = \text{Weight (kg)} \times 70\text{ mL}$$
$$\text{Replacement volume} = \text{Blood volume} \times (1 - \text{hematocrit, as a decimal})$$

Hence, for a 70-kg adult with a hematocrit of 40%, the replacement volume would be 2,940 mL. The plasma volume to be removed, replacement volume, and type of replacement fluid must be individualized based on the patient's clinical condition. Almost 50% of patients undergoing plasmapheresis experience some complication. Most of the complications, such as muscle cramps, are mild and have been related to the citrate used in the circuit. Less commonly, hypofibrinogenemia, electrolyte deficiencies, and total protein deficiencies may develop. Patients undergoing frequent sessions should be monitored regularly for electrolyte levels, blood counts, and fibrinogen levels. Fibrinogen depletion, especially in patients with clinical conditions predisposing to hemorrhage, may be treated with cryoprecipitate (22).

Complications of Immunotherapy

The side effects of many immunotherapies include several severe illnesses. Infectious complications of immunosuppressive therapy account for the most common severe consequences of immunotherapies. However, several other severe, noninfectious clinical syndromes have been attributed to certain immunotherapies. These systemic reactions have been described most commonly with certain immunoglobulin or cytokine therapies. The infusion of γ-globulin (IVIG) may result in myalgia, low-grade fever, and back pain. These relatively minor symptoms have been partially attributed to complement activation by immunoglobulin complexes, and are usually effectively managed by slowing the rate of infusion or prophylaxis with antihistamines (23). Occasionally, IVIG infusions may result in systemic hypotension or anaphylaxis. These severe reactions, although rare, have been described most commonly among patients with IgA deficiencies who have pre-existing antibodies to IgA. The IgA in the IVIG infusate is thought to initiate the subsequent antigen–antibody reaction. Immunoglobulins produced in animals, such as antithymocyte globulin and the antivenins, are among the most common causes of anaphylaxis or serum sickness. The immunosuppressive monoclonal antibody OKT3 is occasionally associated with a "cytokine release syndrome" shortly after infusion. OKT3 is a murine monoclonal antibody that selectively depletes T lymphocytes and has proven useful in solid organ transplantation. The cytokine release syndrome manifests as fever, myalgia, dyspnea, and hypotension. This reaction is most common after the initial OKT3 infusion and has been attributed to the systemic release of IFN-γ and TNF-α. This syndrome may be prevented by prophylaxis with corticosteroids. Another cytokine-mediated syndrome is the capillary leak syndrome associated with IL-2 administration and used in certain cancer therapies and multiple other investigational studies. The capillary leak syndrome, although apparently dose related, is common, and in certain patient populations, the incidence rate approaches 50%. The sepsis-like syndrome consists of hypotension, extravascular fluid sequestration, and, occasionally, pulmonary edema. Treatment includes vasopressor cardiovascular support and corticosteroids. Development of the syndrome may require a decrease in the interleukin dose or cessation of therapy (24).

SUMMARY

It is important to keep in mind that all aspects of immunity are tightly integrated, such that cell-mediated immune responses and humoral responses do not function as independently of each other as was once thought. Similarly, almost all non-immune cellular and organ functions, such as those responsible for hemodynamic stability and body metabolism, have been shown to be partially modulated by networking cytokine messages from the multiple immune system cells. Appropriate immunologic responses are crucial to recovery from most critical illnesses. The complex intercommunication among immune and non-immune system cells manifests itself as many of the systemic symptoms commonly associated with acute illness, such as fever, hypotension, and protein depletion. Perturbation of the immune defense systems, whether on a congenital or acquired basis, complicates the recovery process and commonly prolongs otherwise curable illnesses. The expanding use of immunotherapies has been accompanied by the recognition of several severe systemic side effects and infectious consequences that, in themselves, result in serious illnesses.

References

1. Sakaguchi S. Regulation of immune response. In: Rich RR, ed. *Clinical Immunology: Principles and Practice.* 2nd ed. St. Louis: Mosby-Year Book; 1995:15.1.
2. Nossal GJ. The basic components of the immune system. *N Engl J Med.* 1987;316:1320.
3. Romagnani S. Lymphokine production by human T cells in disease states. *Annu Rev Immunol.* 1994;12:227.
4. Marrack P. The staphylococcal enterotoxins and their relatives. *Science.* 1990;248:705.
5. Abbas KA, Lichtman HA. Innate immunity. In: Abbas KA, Lichtman HA, eds. *Cellular and Molecular Immunology.* 5th ed. Philadelphia: Saunders; 2003:275.
6. Schifferli JA, Ng YC, Peters DK. The role of complement and its receptor in the elimination of immune complexes. *N Engl J Med.* 1986;315:488.
7. Popovic P, Dubois D, Rabin SB, et al. Immunoglobulin titers and immunoglobulin subtypes. In: Lotze MT, Thomson AW. *Measuring Immunity.* San Diego, CA: Elsevier Academic Press; 2005:159.
8. Abbas AK, Lichtman AH. Effector mechanisms of cell-mediated immunity. In: Abbas AK, Lichtman AH, eds. *Cellular and Molecular Immunology.* 5th ed. Philadelphia: Saunders; 2003:298.
9. Rosenberg SA. Adoptive immunotherapy for cancer. *Sci Am.* 1990;262:62.
10. Casey LC, Balk RA, Bone RC. Plasma cytokine and endotoxin levels correlate with survival in patients with the sepsis syndrome. *Ann Intern Med.* 1993;119:771.
11. Sell S. Immunopathology. In: Rich RR, Fleisher TA, eds. *Clinical Immunology: Principles and Practice.* St. Louis: Mosby-Year Book; 1995:449.
12. Frank MM. Complement in the pathophysiology of human disease. *N Engl J Med.* 1987;316:1525.
13. Rosen FS, Cooper MD, Wedgwood RJP. The primary immunodeficiencies. *N Engl J Med.* 1984;311:300.
14. Welborn JL, Hersch J. Blood transfusion reactions. *Postgrad Med.* 1991;90:125.
15. Schwartzberg LS. Neutropenia: etiology and pathogenesis. *Clin Cornerstone.* 2006;8(Suppl 5):S5.
16. Bodey G, Buckley M, Sathe Y, et al. Quantitative relationships between circulating leukocytes and infection in patients with leukemia. *Ann Intern Med.* 1966;64:328.
17. Ezekowitz RAB, Dinauer MC, Jaffe HS, et al. Partial correction of the phagocytic defect in patients with X-linked chronic granulomatous disease by subcutaneous interferon gamma. *N Engl J Med.* 1988;319:146.
18. Abe Y, Horiuchi A, Miyake M, et al. Anti-cytokine nature of natural human immunoglobulin: one possible mechanism of the clinical effect of intravenous immunoglobulin therapy. *Immunol Rev.* 1994;139:5.
19. Suffredini AF. Current prospects for the treatment of clinical sepsis. *Clin Exp Immunol.* 1994;22:(Suppl):12.
20. Taboulet P, Baud FJ, Bismuth C. Clinical features and management of digitalis poisoning: rationale for immunotherapy. *Clin Toxicol.* 1993;31:247.
21. Luce JM. Introduction of new technology into critical care practice: a history of HA-1A human monoclonal antibody against endotoxin. *Crit Care Med.* 1993;21:1233.
22. Strauss RG, Ciavarella D, Gilcher RO, et al. An overview of current management. *J Clin Apheresis.* 1993;8:189.
23. Duhem C, Dicato MA, Ries F. Side-effects of intravenous immune globulins. *Clin Exp Immunol.* 1994;97(Suppl 1):79.
24. Rieves DR, Levine SJ, Shelhamer SH. Allergy and immunology. In: Civetta MJ, Taylor RW, Kirby RR, eds. *Critical Care.* 3rd ed. Philadelphia: Lippincott-Raven; 1997:303.

SECTION V ■ MODULATING THE RESPONSE TO INJURY

CHAPTER 51 ■ MOLECULAR BIOLOGY: GENOMICS AND PROTEONOMICS

BRYCE A. HEESE • ROBERTO T. ZORI

The Human Genome Project (HGP), initiated in 1990 and completed in 2001, promised to revolutionize the practice of medicine with cheap and efficient technology. Traditionally, genetic testing has consisted of broad genome screening studies (e.g. chromosome karyotype, comparative genomics hybridization) or DNA-based techniques for a select number of single gene disorders. However, the HGP has provided a wealth of information for scientific discovery and has led to development of new and more efficient methods for genetic analysis. Both the number of disease-causing genes being discovered and the number of applicable gene tests being developed are increasing exponentially. The future of genomics promises personalized health management, such as selection of specific therapies and drugs based on individualized genetic information from whole genome screening. However, for many nongenetic clinicians, the promised revolution is not yet obvious, and the use of genetic information in daily clinical practice can be confusing and difficult to manage.

The complexity of the human genome is highlighted by the knowledge that the set of human proteins (several million) is significantly greater than the relatively small number of genes (estimated to be only about 25,000). This underscores the importance of epigenetics, such as alternate splicing (alternate coding sequence) within the same gene, or posttranslational modification of the coded protein to create innumerable gene products. Proteomics is the study of the physiologic composition of proteins (or the proteome) as affected by different biologic processes. Of note, the use of certain protein biomarkers, such as C-reactive protein and creatine kinase isoforms, have been commonly used in clinical practice for decades in disease profiling. More recently, the FDA has emphasized the role of protein biomarkers in drug development and clinical analysis, which is also helping to spur research in the field. Proteomics shows great promise in critical care, since drugs typically target proteins and not genes. However, the complexity and massive expanse of human proteins and gene expression are added barriers to proteomic research, often causing difficulty in producing reliable results. The future promise of proteomics, similar to genomics, is to provide revolutionary information for the managing clinician. Like genomics, however, its clinical applicability is presently limited.

Population screening for genetic disease is another current topic in clinical genetics that proposes to change clinical medicine. The purpose of population screening is to reduce morbidity and mortality by detecting an individual's risk prior to manifesting clinical disease. The original principles for population screening by the World Health Organization have been adapted to fit the construct of a new genomics era (1). The key feature of any population screen is to weigh relative costs, ethics, and other considered risks compared to the benefits, particularly the ability to treat based on early detection (2). Prenatal screening for genetic diseases is steadily increasing, as is the promise of population genetic screening in adults and children for common genetic diseases. In reality, population genetic screening has been implemented for decades. A particular example is the mass newborn screening primarily used to detect inherited metabolic diseases, as well as genetic disorders such as sickle cell anemia. The early detection and management of genetic disorders has increased survival of these previously unrecognized and devastating diseases. Such detection and management also provides a significant clinical problem for the future, as there will be a deficiency in metabolic specialists, typically pediatric trained, to care for long-term surviving children who achieve adulthood with inherited metabolic disorders. This will place a burden on intensivists due to the added risk of surgery and illness for these individuals.

This chapter will concentrate primarily on genetic conditions that may present in a catastrophic fashion and frequently require attendance in a critical care unit. The purpose is to alert the critical care physician to the presence of genetic or inherited metabolic diseases, as well as to provide some guidance for emergency therapy in unique situations, in particular, those involving patients in acute metabolic crises. This section is not intended to be a comprehensive list of genetic diseases encountered, as such information is far too detailed for this chapter and, additionally, will likely be outdated shortly after publication. Instead, the reader is encouraged to use the information summarized herein as a starting point to find up-to-date, peer-reviewed, Web-based information for the proper management of genetic conditions.

FUNDAMENTALS OF GENOMICS/GENETICS

The term *genome* refers to the complete set of DNA (deoxyribonucleic acid) within an organism. In humans, the nuclear genome consists of 46 chromosomes (or 23 pairs of chromosomes), half of which are maternally inherited (from the egg) and half inherited paternally (from sperm). The nucleus of most cells within the body contain a single copy of the human genome. A distinction should be made between the 46 chromosomes found within the cell's nucleus and the mitochondrial genome, which is found within each mitochondria of the cell.

Mitochondria, and thus, mitochondrial DNA, is inherited only maternally (the sperm does not contribute mitochondria to the zygote). Mitochondrial disorders will be discussed again in the following mitochondrial disease section.

A single nuclear chromosome consists of a continuous chain of double-stranded DNA, which if stretched from end to end would measure about 1 yard in length. Each strand contains a sequence of nucleotides (adenine, thymine, cytosine, or guanine) in various combinations. The order of the nucleotides contributes to the genetic information and is, essentially, the organism's blueprint. When two complementary strands of DNA are in a dormant stage, they are bonded together as a double strand, forming the chromosome. During replication or gene expression (transcription and translation; see below), parts of the double strand must be separated by a complex molecular process to expose the genes.

Genes are regions of DNA that contain a sequence of nucleotides coding for a single strand of RNA (ribonucleic acid), a process called *transcription*. RNA, in turn, exits the nucleus and serves as the template from which amino acids are combined to form a protein, a process referred to as *translation*. Depending on its structure, shape, and a complex process of posttranslational modifications, a protein may have any number of functions, such as a structural component (the cell membrane or extracellular matrix), cellular receptors, plasma transporters, enzymes, or numerous other functions within the body. Each gene is about 10,000 base pairs in length, but can range from a few hundred to several thousands of base pairs, and they are located on various sites throughout the genome. Genes also contain promoter regions, introns, and other nontranscribed sequences that are important regulatory factors for efficient and timely gene expression. The Human Genome Project described about 25,000 genes, accounting for only about 10% of the full genome. Much of the remainder of the genome consists of vast expansions of highly conserved repeat sequences, the function of which is not presently understood.

Individual humans share over 99.9% of this sequence with one another. However, given the size of the human genome, about 3 billion base pairs, this allows for significant differences between individuals. An individual's genotype refers to the structural makeup of DNA. Genotype is typically used in reference to a single gene of interest; however, it may also be used in the context of a set of genes and gene modifiers, or even the entire genome. An individual's *phenotype* is a term used to describe the physical manifestations, which are typically determined by both gene expression and environmental influences. Genetic variations, or mutations, can be in the form of a single nucleotide substitution, or small insertions or deletions of nucleotides within a DNA sequence. If a mutation occurs within the translational region of a gene, it may potentially change the transcription or translation of that gene, causing an alteration in the gene product, and therefore changing an individual's phenotype. A mutation may also occur within a regulatory region of a gene, which may alter the expression of a gene, causing decreased or increased translation. Alternatively, mutations may occur within the translated segment of a gene but have little or no affect on the gene product or clinical phenotype. In many cases, mutations occur outside of the gene sequence or within untranslated regions of a gene (e.g., introns) where there would not be an affect on gene expression.

Traditionally, genetics has focused on monogenetic and/or Mendelian disorders in which an identifiable change in DNA material, such as a mutation in a gene or chromosomal anomaly, results in an identifiable genetic disorder. More and more, genetics research is involving polygenic diseases such as cardiovascular disease, hyperlipidemia, or asthma, where genetics likely plays a role in disease susceptibility; in most cases, there is not an identifiable single gene defect, but rather multiple genetic variations. Single-nucleotide polymorphisms (SNPs) are a method of looking at DNA sequence variation. SNPs may occur within or outside of a coding region, and may or may not cause a change in an amino acid and/or protein structure. The HapMap project is an offshoot of the Human Genome Project that is working on cataloging haplotypes, or variations of SNPs, within the population. This information can then be used in research and eventually medicine to identify genetic variants that lead to increased susceptibility to complex (or polygenic) diseases.

Genetic Testing

The promise of genomics is to provide a cheap and efficient personalized genomic profile for every person. Today's reality, however, is sporadic testing for several well-characterized genetic disorders. However, the number of genetic tests available has increased tenfold within the past decade, and technology and discovery are rapidly evolving. The breadth of genetic testing will likely continue to grow exponentially (3). For the nongeneticist, deciding on how to proceed with genetic testing can be cumbersome and confusing. Because of scientific discovery and the continued expansion of genetic testing, it would be overwhelming to list all of the genetic testing available, particularly as the information quickly becomes outdated. The clinician, thus, must be able to use updated, often Web-based, materials to aid in this decision process.

Genetic testing may consist of whole chromosome screening (e.g., chromosomal karyotype or comparative genomic hybridization arrays) and FISH (fluorescence *in situ* hybridization). These tests look for large deletions or duplications, often associated with specific syndromes, within the genome. This section will primarily discuss DNA-based gene tests that typically identify single gene disorders.

Common gene testing includes sequence analysis, targeted mutation analysis, and mutation scanning. *DNA sequence analysis* identifies a given nucleotide sequence in an individual and compares it to the known normal sequence to look for alterations. This method of testing has traditionally been time-consuming and costly. It can be particularly burdensome for large gene regions. However, as technology becomes more efficient, more gene tests will likely turn to sequencing, as it has a slightly higher rate of detection. *Targeted mutation analysis* is used as a diagnostic tool when a small number of mutations within a single gene are known to cause a disease. Often, when a mutation is not detected by this method, gene sequencing is performed to look for a possible mutation not included in the targeted analysis. Finally, *mutation scanning*, a screening tool using various methods to detect variations in DNA segments, is used when other methods are too time consuming or costly because several mutations are distributed along large segments of DNA. Each method has benefits and deficiencies for detecting mutations, depending on the specific situation. It is, therefore, important to keep in mind that there are multiple detection techniques available when making the decision to proceed with genetic testing.

Several factors must be taken into account when considering genetic testing:

1. The clinician should, first, establish a clinical basis for suspecting a particular genetic disease. Today, genetic testing is relatively expensive and can be time-intensive, depending on the study. A personal and family history, physical exam, screening laboratory and radiographic tests, as well as any supporting studies can provide evidence pointing to a specific diagnosis and should be used when deciding whether to proceed with genetic testing. In the circumstance of inherited metabolic diseases, screening metabolic laboratory tests and enzyme assays may also be used to eliminate the need for specific genetic studies (discussed in inherited metabolic diseases section below).
2. The clinician must weigh the necessity of genetic testing, particularly taking into account whether management or treatment options will change as a result of testing. Although in some cases, test results may not alter the management of a patient, the genetic results may be useful for screening family members who are at risk of inheriting the condition.
3. No genetic test is perfect. False-positive and -negative results, test sensitivity, and other measures must be evaluated when deciding the utility of testing. This information can often be found in sources such as GeneTests (discussed below), or should be available from the testing laboratory itself.
4. Both the clinician and the patient should understand the purpose and utility of genetic testing. A common pitfall is for a clinician to evaluate genetic results as strictly positive or negative when, in fact, there is a certain level of uncertainty in almost every test. Genetic testing is rarely 100% sensitive. False-negative results are possible when a mutation occurs in a region of the gene that is not evaluated, such as a regulatory sequence or intron. Additionally, many diseases exhibit locus heterogeneity (more than one gene may be responsible); therefore, a genetic test may miss a significant portion of affected individuals. At the same time, it is not uncommon to find an abnormality in a gene that is predicted (or known) to be completely benign. A common pitfall is to interpret these benign variant results as a positive test. Furthermore, genetic testing is commonly performed without discussing options with the patient or patient's family. As genetic testing may have consequences (e.g., ethical, insurance, or familial inheritance factors) beyond the patient's acute setting, many—but not all—genetic centers require consent prior to testing, but it is always appropriate to keep the patient informed regardless of the laboratory's procedures. Careful consideration of each component is essential, and assistance from a genetic counselor or geneticist can be useful in the decision process and interpretation of genetic tests.

Clinical genetic testing is constantly evolving. Along with current journal articles and reviews, Web-based information is becoming essential for the proper evaluation and management of genetic diseases. A commonly used site for comprehensive literature review of DNA-based diseases is the Online Mendelian Inheritance in Man. OMIM* also provides links to MEDLINE and many related databases. Another helpful resource for updated genetic testing is GeneTests† (4). GeneTests encompasses several hundred current, peer-reviewed articles of common genetic disorders. The site includes information on specific tests offered from both clinical and strictly research laboratories as well as estimates of mutation detection rates, alternate genes, and differential diagnostic considerations. GeneTests provides suggestions for management and counseling, as well as links to educational resources for many of these diseases.

*OMIM; http://www.ncbi.nlm.nih.gov/entrez/query.fcgi?db=OMIM; from the National Center for Biotechnology Information provided by the National Library of Medicine and National Institutes of Health.

INHERITED DISORDERS OF METABOLISM

Inherited disorders of metabolism comprise a heterogeneous group of genetic diseases, several of which present in acute metabolic distress, which require emergency management and critical care monitoring. Each disorder involves a defective enzyme or transport protein that normally contributes to proper biochemical process within the body. As a group, the clinical manifestations of metabolic disorders can be extremely variable depending on the affected biochemical pathway, severity of the molecular defect (e.g., the amount of residual enzyme activity), and environmental factors (e.g., illness, fasting, or dietary intake). Although there are approximately 1,000 metabolic disorders described, each disorder is relatively rare; collectively, however, there is an estimated incidence of about 1:4,000.

Increased awareness and detection in all ages, as well as advances in our understanding and management of metabolic diseases, has decreased morbidity and increased survival in children with metabolic disorders, even into adulthood (5,6). For example, expanded newborn screening identifies more infants with metabolic disorders. In addition to improved early detection of presymptomatic infants with metabolic disorders, newborn screening has secondarily identified affected siblings and family members of all ages. Furthermore, case reports of adult-onset metabolic disease are not uncommon, typically described in the setting of an acute metabolic stressor such as a prolonged presurgical fast or an illness with vomiting and dehydration (7,8). It is essential for the intensivist to be knowledgeable about the possible presentation, initial evaluation, and emergency management for patients of all ages with this group of disorders.

Metabolism refers to the sum of the process of biochemical synthesis (anabolism) and breakdown (catabolism) of compounds, such as proteins, carbohydrates, and lipids from the diet or stored within the body. Inherited metabolic disorders are genetic defects that affect an enzyme or a transport protein important to normal metabolism. Clinically, inherited metabolic disorders manifest with a wide range of symptoms, from chronic progressive disease to acute metabolic crises, following an apparently asymptomatic interval. Depending on the severity and type of disorder, any number of organ systems may be involved. Hepatic failure may present in tyrosinemia type I, Wilson disease, and Gaucher disease. Cardiomyopathy may be a feature in infantile and juvenile Pompe disease, very-long-chain acyl-CoA dehydrogenase deficiency, and various lysosomal storage diseases. Muscle disease, either myopathy and/or rhabdomyolysis, may occur in mitochondrial encephalomyopathy, lactic acidosis, and stroke-like episodes

†http://www.genetests.org

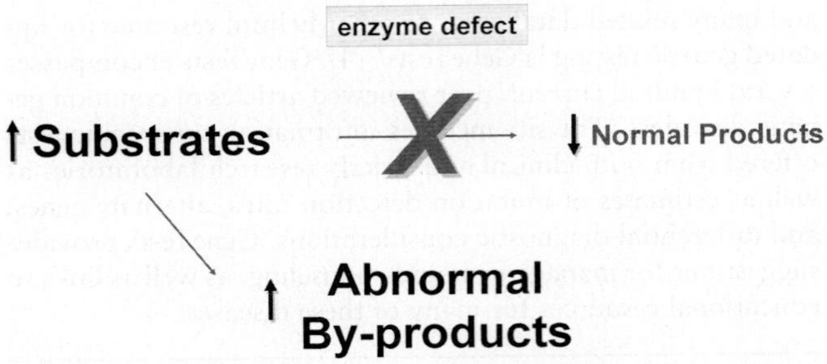

FIGURE 51.1. Most inborn errors of metabolism are due to an enzyme defect within a metabolic pathway. The defect may lead to toxic accumulation of substrate, or metabolic by-products, or to deficiency of an essential product within that pathway.

(MELAS), very-long-chain acyl-CoA dehydrogenase deficiency, and McArdle disease. Acute encephalopathy is a concern in many organic acidurias, urea cycle defects, and fatty acid oxidation defects.

Often, the acute presentation of an inherited metabolic disorder may mimic a more common, systemic disease such as sepsis or intoxication; however, swift recognition and management of a metabolic disorder is important for improving the overall morbidity and mortality. Saudubray et al. (9) loosely classified these disorders into three groups:

1. *Metabolic disorders of intermediary metabolism that cause toxic accumulation of metabolites.* This may be conceptualized as a road block in the normal metabolic pathway causing a traffic jam and the buildup of potentially toxic intermediary metabolites. Some of these metabolites will be directed to alternative pathways, which may lead to the accumulation of toxic byproducts (Fig. 51.1). Examples of this group include organic acidurias, aminoacidopathies, fatty acid oxidation defects, urea cycle defects, disorders of metal transport (e.g., Wilson disease), and carbohydrate defects. In critical care, many of these diseases present in acute metabolic crises with some combination of encephalopathy, liver disease, multisystem failure, metabolic acidosis, ketoacidosis, lactic acidosis, or hyperammonemia.
2. *Metabolic defects that affect cellular respiration or mitochondrial energy production.* This group includes enzyme defects of the mitochondrial respiratory chain itself. It also includes enzymes in glycolysis (the breakdown of glucose, for energy), glycogenosis (utilization of glycogen stores for energy), gluconeogenesis (glucose synthesis for transport to other organs), and the tricarboxylic acid (TCA or Kreb) cycles. Fatty acid oxidation disorders, which cause toxic accumulation of fatty acids and other byproducts (group 1), are also considered here, as the products of these reactions are an essential energy source for the TCA cycle and mitochondrial respiratory chain, particularly during fasting stress.
3. *Disorders involving the synthesis or breakdown of complex (large) molecules.* This group includes lysosomal storage disorders, peroxisomal disorders (e.g., X-linked adrenoleukodystrophy), disorders of glycosylation, and cholesterol synthesis defects. In general, these disorders are chronic progressive disease, and though they may rapidly worsen during illness or stress, they rarely present in acute metabolic crises.

For an exhaustive discussion of all known metabolic disorders, the reader is referred to comprehensive reviews (10,11). Herein, we focus on metabolic disorders and associated scenarios that may present to the critical care unit.

FATTY ACID OXIDATION DISORDERS

Fatty acid oxidation disorders encompass a group of metabolic defects of mitochondrial beta-oxidation. Beta-oxidation is the process of breaking down fatty acids to aid in energy production, as adenosine triphosphate (ATP), via the respiratory chain complex. Several 2-carbon molecules (acetyl-CoA) are also produced by beta-oxidation of each fatty acid. Acetyl-CoA can be utilized in the tricarboxylic acid cycle for aerobic respiration or as a precursor for the production of ketone bodies. Therefore, the beta-oxidation cycle is essential for the normal physiologic response to fasting after typical energy sources, such as glucose and glycogen, are depleted. In the fasting state, vital organs, in particular the brain, require an alternate source of energy in the form of ketone bodies.

Several enzymes are essential in the beta-oxidation of fatty acids. Carnitine palmitoyltransferase 1 (CPT1), carnitine palmitoyltransferase 2 (CPT2), and carnitine acylcarnitine carrier protein are important for the transfer of fatty acids into the mitochondria. Long-chain fatty acids (12–18 carbon-length molecules) are acted on by the enzyme's very long-chain acyl-CoA dehydrogenase (VLCAD), mitochondrial trifunctional protein, and long-chain 3-hydroxyacyl-CoA dehydrogenase (LCHAD). Medium-chain fatty acids (6–12 carbon-length molecules) are broken down by the enzyme medium-chain acyl-CoA dehydrogenase (MCAD) (Fig. 51.2).

Disease manifestation, age of onset, and severity vary greatly, depending on the enzyme defect. The most common of these conditions, MCAD deficiency, with an estimated incidence of 1 in 15,000, can present at any age, with fasting intolerance, metabolic encephalopathy, and hypoketotic hypoglycemia. Often, the acute presentation is a result of an illness with vomiting and dehydration. This condition may also cause liver disease with significant hyperammonemia, referred to as *Reye-like syndrome.* Of note, myopathy and cardiomyopathy are rare in MCAD deficiency. Individuals with MCAD deficiency are essentially completely asymptomatic between acute episodes. Long-chain fatty acid defects (VLCADD, LCHADD, or TFP [trifunctional protein] deficiency) and CPT2 deficiency may also present early in childhood with similar fasting intolerance and hypoketotic hypoglycemia, along with cardiomyopathy. However, milder forms of these diseases may not present until adolescence or early adulthood, typically with only muscle disease associated with rhabdomyolysis and/or cardiomyopathy.

ORGANIC ACIDURIAS AND AMINOACIDOPATHIES

Organic acidurias are caused by defects in the normal cellular breakdown of amino acids or odd-chain fatty acids. Examples include propionic aciduria and methylmalonic aciduria, which are disorders of the breakdown of the amino acids isoleucine and valine. Other disorders include isovaleric aciduria, 3-methylglutaconic aciduria, glutaric aciduria type I, multiple carboxylase deficiency, and biotinidase deficiency.

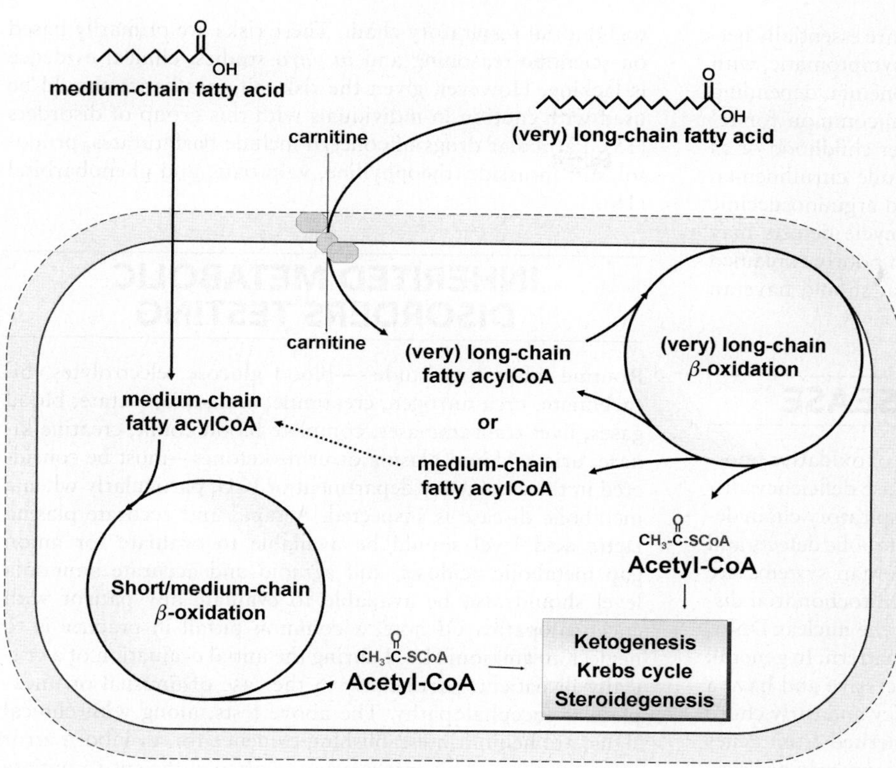

FIGURE 51.2. Fatty acid oxidation occurs primarily in the mitochondria. Carnitine plays an important role in transport of long-chain fatty acids into the mitochondria. Each fatty acid molecule is broken down by several enzymatic cycles (beta-oxidation) in which each cycle produces a 2 carbon molecule (acetyl-CoA). Beta-oxidation enzymes are fatty acid chain-length specific (i.e. medium-chain acyl-CoA dehydrogenase breaks down fatty acids that are of medium chain length, 6–10 carbons). Acetyl-CoA is important for ketogenesis, energy production, and other essential biochemical roles.

Aminoacidopathies, disorders marked by the abnormal accumulation of specific amino acids, can be included within this group, as there is clinical overlap in many of these conditions. Amino acids are organic acids (which include a carboxylic group) that are unique in that they have an amino group (containing nitrogen). As a group, aminoacidopathies can have much more variability in clinical presentation. Examples may include maple syrup urine disease (MSUD), a defect involving the catabolism of the branched chain amino acids leucine, isoleucine, and valine, or tyrosinemia type I, which can cause accumulation of the by-product succinylacetone, a metabolite toxic to liver cells.

In the ICU, it is important to be aware of this group of disorders, many of which present with acute metabolic crises that may mimic or accompany more typical scenarios such as sepsis or drug overdose.

UREA CYCLE DISORDERS

Defects of the urea cycle affect the normal detoxification of ammonia (Fig. 51.3). Ammonia primarily results from nitrogen waste accumulated from excess intake of protein or the endogenous catabolism of protein. The most common urea cycle disorder, X-linked ornithine transcarbamylase (OTC) deficiency, severely affects neonatal males shortly after birth. This often presents as significant encephalopathy and respiratory alkalosis at a few days of life, after significant protein intake.

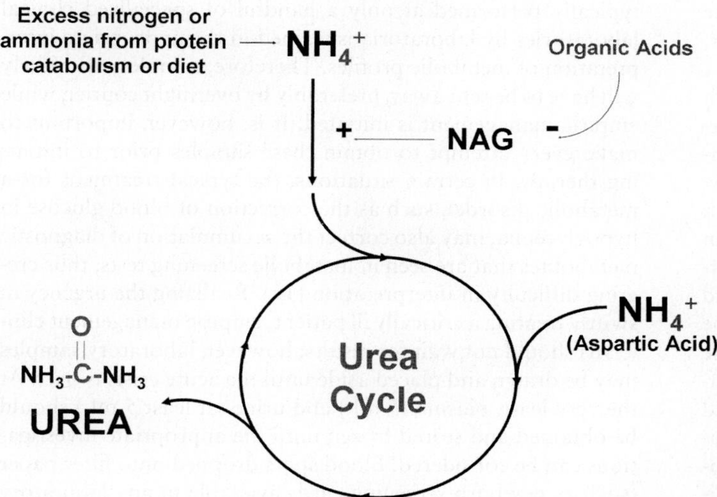

FIGURE 51.3. Removal of excess nitrogen (ammonium, NH_4^+) waste from dietary intake and catabolism of protein is facilitated by several enzyme steps in the urea cycle. The end product is a water soluble compound, urea, which is readily excreted by the kidneys. N-acetylglutamate (NAG) is an important positive activator of carbamyl phosphate synthetase, the first enzyme in the urea cycle. The formation of NAG is inhibited by accumulation of organic acid metabolites from the breakdown of organic acids, amino acids, fatty acids and other organic compounds, thus potentially leading to secondary hyperammonemia.

Females who are carriers for OTC deficiency are essentially heterozygous for the condition but may also be symptomatic, with significant recurrent episodes of hyperammonemia, depending on the extent of X-inactivation. It is not uncommon for females with OTC deficiency to present in later childhood or as adults. Additional urea cycle disorders include citrullinemia, carbamylphospate synthase-1 deficiency, and argininosuccinic aciduria. Acute hyperammonemia in urea cycle defects may manifest at any age. Thus, an individual with poorly explained encephalopathy, including lethargy or coma, should have an ammonia level evaluated.

MITOCHONDRIAL DISEASE

Mitochondrial disorders consist of disorders of oxidative phosphorylation, including pyruvate dehydrogenase deficiency, disorders of the tricarboxylic acid cycle, and respiratory chain defects. These are a heterogeneous group of metabolic defects and should be considered whenever unrelated organ systems are affected without a reasonable explanation. Mitochondrial disorders can be caused by gene defects within the nuclear DNA, which have a typical Mendelian inheritance pattern. In general, these conditions are inherited autosomal recessive and have a clinically more severe onset, usually in infancy and early childhood. Mitochondrial disorders that are inherited from genes within mitochondrial DNA itself are more commonly progressive and present later in life (12).

Defects involving mitochondrial DNA are only maternally inherited, because only the egg—not the sperm—donates mitochondria to the zygote. Another consideration in mitochondrial (maternal) inherited disorders is that each cell in the body contains multiple sets of mitochondria; therefore, the same cell—and thus an individual—may have a mixture of both mutated and normal mitochondrial DNA. This is referred to as *heteroplasmy* and contributes to the phenotypic heterogeneity observed in patients with maternally inherited mitochondrial disorders. The clinician should be aware of mitochondrial disorders, such as the more common mitochondrial encephalomyopathy, lactic acidosis, and stroke-like episodes (MELAS), which may present to the ICU with multisystem disease. Of particular concern in these disorders is metabolic stroke and lactic acidosis (see respective sections below).

Although understanding and awareness of mitochondrial disorders is improving, treatment remains limited. In the acute setting, supportive management including ventilatory support, treatment of lactic acidosis, fluid and nutritional support (i.e., limiting glucose intake to 3–5 g/kg/min and supplementing with lipids), and management of seizures is important. Specific therapies, such as a "mitochondrial cocktail" of vitamins and cofactors, are predicted to aid in ATP production, and are used by most specialists who treat mitochondrial disorders. Although considered safe, the efficacy of these vitamins and cofactors in treating these conditions is not well established. This generally includes CoQ10, L-carnitine, vitamin B_1 (thiamine), and vitamin B_2 (riboflavin) (13,14). Particular attention should be given to mitochondrial patients requiring anesthetics. These individuals are inherently at risk due to the mitochondria's inability to deal with added oxidative stress from surgery and anesthesia. Additionally, most anesthetic agents affect mitochondrial function in some fashion, such as depressing carbohydrate metabolism or inhibiting certain components of the mitochondrial respiratory chain. These risks are primarily based on scientific reasoning and *in vitro* studies; clinical evidence is lacking. However, given the risk, all anesthetics should be used with caution in individuals with this group of disorders (15). Particular drugs of concern include barbiturates, propofol, nitroprusside, theophylline, valproate, and phenobarbital (16).

INHERITED METABOLIC DISORDERS TESTING

Routine laboratory studies—blood glucose, electrolytes, bicarbonate, urea nitrogen, creatinine, ammonia, lactate, blood gases, liver transaminases, complete blood count, creatine kinase, uric acid and plasma or urine ketones—must be considered in the emergency department or ICU, particularly when a metabolic disease is suspected. A rapid and accurate plasma lactic acid level should be available to evaluate for anion gap metabolic acidosis, and a rapid and accurate ammonia level should also be available to evaluate any patient with encephalopathy. Of note, a common pitfall in practice is to neglect an ammonia level during the initial evaluation of a critically ill patient, particularly in the case of unusual or unexplained encephalopathy. The above tests, along with clinical signs, are helpful in establishing evidence for an inborn error of metabolism. This information is often sufficient to initiate appropriate empiric therapy for metabolic diseases while diagnostic and confirmatory studies are performed. Please refer to Table 51.1 for a list of routine laboratory studies which can aid in the workup of a suspected metabolic disorder.

Specialized Metabolic Laboratories

The basic laboratory studies, as noted above, are important in the initial evaluation of any critically ill patient, particularly if an etiologic explanation for the observed symptom complex is not readily apparent. When a metabolic disease is suspected, special laboratory investigations are warranted (Table 51.2). These include plasma amino acids, plasma acylcarnitines, and urine organic acids. The relative pattern of accumulated and deficient metabolites is useful in suggesting, or even diagnosing, specific inherited metabolic disorders. These studies are typically performed at only a handful of specialized clinical laboratories by laboratorians trained in the appropriate interpretation of metabolic profiles. Therefore, samples most likely will have to be sent away, preferably by overnight courier, while empiric management is initiated. It is, however, important to make every attempt to obtain these samples prior to initiating therapy. In certain situations, the typical treatment for a metabolic disorder, such as the correction of blood glucose in hypoglycemia, may also correct the accumulation of diagnostic metabolites that are seen in metabolic screening tests, thus creating difficulty in interpretation (12). Realizing the urgency in swiftly treating a critically ill patient, empiric management clinicians should not wait for results; however, laboratory samples may be drawn and placed aside until the acute crisis is over. At the very least, plasma (5 mL) and urine (at least 5 mL) should be obtained and stored frozen until the appropriate investigations can be considered. Blood spots dropped onto filter paper (such as newborn screening cards available in any laboratory

TABLE 51.1

ROUTINE LABORATORY STUDIES IN KNOWN/SUSPECTED METABOLIC DISORDERS

Test	Findings	Considerations
Electrolytes, blood gas	Metabolic acidosis, metabolic alkalosis	OA, LA, UCD
Glucose	Hypoglycemia	FAO, OA, glycogenosis disorders
Complete blood count	Neutropenia, pancytopenia	OA, LA, glycogenosis disorders
Liver transaminases	Liver dysfunction	AA, OA, FAO, LA, carbohydrate disorders, α_1-antitrypsin, Wilson disease
Ammonia	Hyperammonemia	UCD, OA
Lactic acid	Lactic acidosis	LA, glycogenosis disorders, HFI
CPK		Muscular dystrophies, glycogenosis disorders, FAO
Ketones (serum/urine)	Ketoacidosis	AA, OA, glycogenosis disorders, LA
	Abnormally low in response to fasting	FAO
Uric Acid	Hyperuricemia	Glycogenosis disorders, purine defects (e.g., Lesch-Nyhan)

OA, organic aciduria; LA, lactic acidemia (e.g., primary lactic acidemia, mitochondrial respiratory chain disorder); UCD, urea cycle defect; FAO, fatty acid oxidation defect; AA, disorder of amino acid metabolism; HFI, hereditary fructose intolerance; CPK, creatine phosphokinase.

affiliated with a nursery), completely dried and stored with a desiccant, may also be saved for further analysis such as an acylcarnitine profile and, in some cases, molecular gene testing (17).

Plasma Acylcarnitines

Plasma acylcarnitines aid in diagnoses of fatty acid oxidation disorders and certain organic acidurias. This is the same technology used in expanded newborn screening programs due to the ability to screen for several metabolites—and, thus, several different disorders—by a single technique. A common pitfall in the hospital setting is to mistakenly order total and free carnitine levels in place of a plasma acylcarnitine profile. Although carnitine levels are useful in the workup of primary carnitine deficiency, caused by a defective carnitine uptake transporter protein, which is manifested by muscle myopathy and cardiomyopathy, carnitine levels also evaluate specifically for carnitine deficiency, which may accompany several metabolic disorders. Although the carnitine levels are of significance in the management of a suspected metabolic disorder, plasma acylcarnitines will likely be more useful when the diagnosis of a metabolic disease is in question.

TABLE 51.2

SPECIALIZED METABOLIC LABORATORY STUDIES FOR SUSPECTED METABOLIC DISORDERS

Test	Considerations
Plasma amino acids (quantitative)	Urea cycle defects, amino acidopathies
Plasma acylcarnitine analysis	Fatty acid oxidation defect, organic acidurias
Urine organic acids	Organic acidurias, fatty acid oxidation defect

Quantitative Plasma Amino Acids

Quantitative plasma amino acids aid in the diagnoses of urea cycle disorders, certain organic acidurias, and primary lactic acidoses (i.e., an elevated alanine is indirect evidence of chronic lactic acidosis). This test is also essential for the safe monitoring of patients who are on a protein-restricted diet or specific amino acid–restricted diet. Another common pitfall in the hospital is to mistakenly order a urine amino acid profile. Aside from evaluating for renal tubular disease and a handful of inherited disorders of amino acid transport (e.g., cystinuria), urine amino acids have little value in the workup of metabolic disorders, particularly in the setting of an acute metabolic crisis.

Urine Organic Acids

Urine organic acids aid in the diagnoses of organic acidurias, primary lactic acidemias (e.g., respiratory chain disorders and pyruvate dehydrogenase deficiency), as well as certain fatty acid oxidation disorders. This test is also essential in establishing a specific diagnosis in devastating disorders such as tyrosinemia type I (by the presence of the metabolite succinylacetone) and glutaric aciduria type I (by the presence of 3-hydroxyglutaric acid).

Endocrine studies, such as an insulin level, a random cortisol level, C-peptide, thyroid function studies, or growth hormone levels, are also important in the workup of individuals with atypical acute presentations, particularly in unusual fasting hypoglycemia, but will not be described in detail within the realm of genetic diseases. Additionally, there are several other metabolic screening studies, such as a very long-chain fatty acid panel (to identify peroxisomal disorders such as X-linked adrenoleukodystrophy), urine glycosaminoglycans and oligosaccharides (to identify various lysosomal storage disorders), or plasma sterols (to identify cholesterol biosynthesis disorders). These studies may be helpful in the workup of certain, often chronic, progressive disorders. However, they are not typically useful in evaluating a patient in acute metabolic crises.

Confirmatory Studies

When a specific metabolic disorder is suggested by the screening laboratory studies discussed above, confirmatory studies are typically performed to ensure proper diagnosis and management. This may include specific enzyme studies performed on leukocytes or biopsied samples, such as hepatocytes, myocytes, or other tissues, depending on the disorder in question. Increasingly, specific DNA-based gene studies are being used for diagnostic testing in metabolic disorders. This level of testing is typically performed only in selected laboratories with an interest in the specific disorder. Such studies can be time-consuming and often costly, and are generally not useful for management of a patient in the emergency department or ICU.

POSTMORTEM EVALUATION FOR METABOLIC DISORDERS

When a metabolic disease is suspected in a patient who has died, several key samples must be taken for follow-up testing. Plasma (5 mL, stored frozen) and urine (any amount, stored frozen) should be drawn, preferably prior to death. Additionally, when a metabolic disease is in question, the ICU should be prepared to obtain proper consent for retrieving and storing tissue for future metabolic studies. Fresh tissues from biopsied liver, muscle, and skin (fibroblasts) should be obtained as quickly and efficiently as possible after death. Obviously, this can be a very stressful situation for medical staff and for family members; therefore, the hospital and ICU should establish a postmortem metabolic protocol in anticipation of such an event to help the process flow as smoothly as possible. When it is not feasible to retrieve the above samples, a blood spot, dried on filter paper as described above, should be obtained for possible metabolic or genetic testing. Ideally, this would also include dried bile spots on filter paper for a more thorough analysis. However, this, too, requires a postmortem examination (18).

GENETIC SCENARIOS IN CRITICAL CARE

Emergency Protocol

Patients with a previously diagnosed metabolic disorder, prone to acute metabolic crisis, often possess an emergency protocol letter that has been drafted by a treating genetic or metabolic specialist. The protocol should contain general information about the condition and how it affects the particular patient. It should also provide important recommendations for management during an acute metabolic episode. Depending on the disorder, emergency therapies may include one or more of the following components:

1. Management of the acute insult (e.g., dehydration, infection, and trauma) with supportive care
2. Detoxification of accumulated metabolites (e.g., with hydration, bicarbonate, scavenger therapy, or hemodialysis)
3. Reversing the catabolic process (typically by increasing caloric intake).

HYPOGLYCEMIA IN METABOLIC DISEASE

Hypoglycemia is a serious concern in critical care. It is typically defined by a blood glucose level less than 40 mg/dL in all ages. However, the American Diabetes Association describes hypoglycemia in nondiabetic individuals as a blood glucose less than 70 mg/dL due to normal physiologic triggers that occur below this level (19). In any event, tight control of blood sugars—in most centers to a level between 80 and 110 mg/dL—is ideal in the management of critically ill patients (20). In the critical care setting, hypoglycemia can be a normal physiologic response to severe systemic illness, multiple organ failure, or liver damage. More commonly, it is the result of drugs such as insulin or alcohol, although rare causes of hypoglycemia include endocrine and metabolic disorders.

Postprandial hypoglycemia—that occurring within four to six hours of a meal—may indicate an endocrine disorder such as hyperinsulinism. Hyperinsulinism also presents with low or no ketone production, which is contrary to a normal physiologic response to low blood sugar. Postprandial hypoglycemia may also be observed in glycogen storage disease type I, which typically presents in the neonatal or infant stage, and is often accompanied by hepatomegaly.

Atypical hypoglycemic response to prolonged fasting, defined as six to 24 hours, may indicate a metabolic defect of fatty acid oxidation. Fatty acid oxidation is the normal physiologic response to fasting in which fatty acids are broken down into ketone bodies for energy. Due to the inability to produce ketones from fatty acids, these disorders may present as hypoketotic hypoglycemia, as well as acute encephalopathy from accumulation of toxic metabolites combined with low ketones and glucose. For example, medium-chain acyl-CoA dehydrogenase (MCAD) deficiency is believed to have an incidence of 1 in 15,000. Acute metabolic attacks in MCAD deficiency can be severe, often presenting in infancy or childhood after an inciting illness or fast. However, between attacks, individuals with this disorder may be completely asymptomatic, and some individuals potentially reach adulthood undiagnosed and without symptoms. In critical care, it is important to be aware of these conditions when working up patients with an atypical response to illness, stress, or prolonged fasting, such as a routine surgical procedure (8).

Other metabolic disorders may include hypoglycemia in their presentation. Elevated ketones with low blood sugar may be observed as secondary effects of acute decompensation in individuals with an organic aciduria, such as propionic aciduria. In this case, accumulated toxic metabolites may also manifest with encephalopathy and metabolic acidosis. Hypoglycemia that accompanies lactic acidosis can be a sign of a respiratory chain disorder or a defect in mitochondrial energy metabolism. Depending on the severity and cause of the respiratory chain dysfunction, other signs and symptoms may accompany a respiratory chain defect, such as encephalopathy, myopathy, stroke-like episodes, and various other organ diseases.

Laboratory Investigations for Metabolic Causes of Hypoglycemia

When suspecting a metabolic disorder, the basic metabolic laboratory studies, including accurate blood glucose, electrolytes, bicarbonate, blood urea nitrogen, creatinine, ammonia, blood gas analysis, lactic acid, liver transaminases, complete blood count, creatine kinase, and uric acid, should be obtained. Blood for insulin, cortisol, and C-peptide levels should be obtained while an individual is hypoglycemic to evaluate for a potential endocrine disorder. The normal physiologic response to fasting hypoglycemia is to produce ketone bodies. Thus, abnormally low plasma and/or urine ketone levels may indicate either inappropriate insulin production or a disorder of fatty acid oxidation. Elevated plasma-free fatty acids may also be indicative of a fatty acid oxidation defect. Plasma acylcarnitines, urine organic acids, and plasma amino acids are important screening studies when suspecting a metabolic disorder. It is essential that these studies—including the above-cited endocrine laboratories—be obtained prior to initiating management for hypoglycemia. Correction of the blood glucose will cause difficulty in the interpretation of many laboratory results—for example, a normal or elevated insulin level in the setting of a corrected blood glucose level would not be useful. In certain cases, correction of hypoglycemia may also correct the accumulation of diagnostic metabolites that are seen in metabolic screening tests (12).

Management of Hypoglycemia

When oral correction of hypoglycemia is not possible, an initial intravenous bolus of 25 g of dextrose—50 mL of a 50% solution (for children: 1 mg/kg glucose of a 20% solution)—may be used, followed by continuous infusion of a 10% dextrose solution with appropriate electrolytes. Management of a suspected metabolic disorder may require 7 to 10 mg/kg/min to maintain appropriate glucose levels, or even greater in certain cases of hyperinsulinism. Although glucagon may be administered for transient correction of hypoglycemia, it will be ineffective in conditions where glycogen reserves are not available, as in certain glycogen storage diseases or where glycogen reserves are depleted as in a fatty acid oxidation defect, organic aciduria, as well as alcohol ingestion.

Glucose, lactic acid, and acid-base status must be closely monitored due to the high glucose concentration administered. In many cases, hypoglycemia is accompanied by significant dehydration requiring fluid correction. With high fluids and glucose administration, electrolytes—particularly sodium—must be carefully monitored, and sodium levels should be maintained above 135 mMol/L to avoid complications of cerebral edema (21). If a fatty acid oxidation defect or organic aciduria is suspected, carnitine (100 mg/kg per day; maximum 5 g per day may be given IV or orally) should be initiated empirically until a more definitive diagnosis is made. Carnitine will aid by conjugating and facilitating the excretion of accumulated toxic fatty acid and organic acid metabolites.

KETOACIDOSIS IN METABOLIC DISEASE

Ketone bodies, including 3-hydroxybutyrate, acetoacetate, and acetate, are derived from excess acetyl-CoA and generally formed in the mitochondria of liver cells from fatty acid breakdown. Ketogenesis is a physiologic response to the depletion of carbohydrates, such as glucose and glycogen, as seen in prolonged fasting. Vital tissues, particularly the brain, can convert ketone bodies back into acetyl-CoA for use in the tricarboxylic cycle and use acetyl-CoA as an alternate energy source when glucose is not available.

Ketoacidosis is the abnormal accumulation of these acidic ketone bodies, causing significantly low pH. Exhaled acetone, the "fruity" breath odor can be a sign of ketoacidosis. Diabetic ketoacidosis (discussed elsewhere in this textbook) is a common problem in critical care due to absence of insulin, which normally suppresses fatty acid breakdown into ketone bodies. Ketoacidosis is also observed in individuals on a ketogenic diet, a possible treatment for certain refractory seizure disorders. Alcoholic ketoacidosis may occur in chronic alcoholics following abrupt withdrawal of ethanol along with depletion of carbohydrates. Several metabolic disorders, including organic acidurias (e.g., propionic aciduria, methylmalonic aciduria), aminoacidopathies (e.g., maple syrup urine disease) and respiratory chain defects, may be associated with profound ketoacidosis as a secondary effect during acute metabolic decompensation. A neonate, child, or adult presenting with any combination of ketoacidosis, metabolic acidosis, lactic acidosis, hypoglycemia, hyperammonemia, systemic disease, liver disease, lethargy, encephalopathy, or coma should be evaluated for a metabolic disease, particularly if a reasonable explanation for the presentation cannot be found.

Laboratory Investigation for Metabolic Ketoacidosis

Evaluation for ketoacidosis, particularly when a metabolic disorder is suspected, should include initial basic laboratory studies including blood glucose, electrolytes, bicarbonate, blood urea nitrogen, creatinine, ammonia, blood gas analysis, lactic acid, liver transaminases, complete blood count, creatine kinase, and uric acid. An ammonia level should be obtained, as secondary hyperammonemia may be suggestive of a metabolic disease such as an organic aciduria. A complete blood count may show neutropenia or pancytopenia in certain organic acidurias, respiratory chain abnormalities, or glycogen storage diseases. Specialized laboratory tests to screen for a suspected metabolic disorder include plasma acylcarnitines, plasma amino acids, and urine organic acids.

Management of Metabolic Ketoacidosis

Management strategies for ketoacidosis, in the context of a known or suspected metabolic disease, begins with treatment of the underlying stress, such as infection or fever, followed by careful improvement of metabolic acidosis and prevention of further protein catabolism. Intake of protein and fatty acids should be discontinued, and administration of fluids up to 1.5 times maintenance and dextrose as a 10% solution, up to 10 mg/kg/min with appropriate electrolytes will also help to reverse the catabolic state, which, if left unchecked, will worsen the acute metabolic crisis (17,21). High volumes of fluid may be important, as metabolic decompensation often follows an inciting stressor such as vomiting and dehydration. Intravenous sodium bicarbonate can be used, but the goal should be to raise and maintain arterial blood pH to 7.2 and keep plasma bicarbonate levels greater than 10 mMol/L—and not to correct the acidosis to normal. Electrolyte, fluid, and acid-base status and frequent neurologic assessment must be monitored closely. Serum sodium levels should be maintained above 135 mMol/L to prevent cerebral edema. However, the administration of sodium bicarbonate can also lead to hypernatremia. Hypokalemia may occur as a response to rising pH and should be closely monitored throughout therapy.

A specific example of a disease that may present with profound ketoacidosis during metabolic crises is maple syrup urine disease (MSUD). These individuals, particularly older children and adults who are no longer growing, can be very difficult to manage. In cases of severe ketoacidosis with MSUD, the administration of IV insulin in combination with a steady supply of high glucose has been shown to enhance anabolism in addition to preventing hyperglycemia from excess carbohydrate infusion (17,22). Obviously, careful and frequent monitoring of blood glucose is necessary when using high concentrations of glucose, particularly with the use of insulin. Another important factor in managing metabolic defects with profound ketoacidosis is that prolonged (greater than 48 hours) restriction of protein will cause the body to become deficient in certain essential amino acids and therefore resume breakdown of endogenous protein stores, thus worsening the ketoacidosis (23). Consultation with a metabolic specialist and/or metabolic nutritionist familiar with these disorders is essential in both short- and long-term management.

HYPERAMMONEMIA IN METABOLIC DISEASE

An ammonia level should be standard in any critical care situation involving an obtunded patient, particularly if the cause is not readily apparent. A normal ammonia level in a healthy adult is typically less than 50 μM/L and slightly higher in healthy neonates, up to 80 μM/L. Elevated ammonia is toxic to brain cells and can result in lethargy with plasma ammonia levels as low as 100 to 200 μM/L; severe encephalopathy and coma may result from higher levels (24). Respiratory alkalosis from hyperventilation is caused by ammonia's effect on the brain's respiratory drive. Regardless of the cause, hyperammonemia should be managed quickly and efficiently to reduce significant morbidity.

Plasma ammonia may be artificially elevated as a result of sample handling and/or difficult blood draw—for example, with the use of a tourniquet during phlebotomy. Severe liver disease and overproduction of ammonia by colonized urease-producing bacteria are possible causes of hyperammonemia (25). Several inherited metabolic disorders should be considered in patients of all ages presenting with hyperammonemia. Severe urea cycle disorders may present in the neonatal period shortly after birth, with ammonia levels well above 1,000 μM/L; however, milder cases may not present until adolescence or adulthood (7,26). The urea cycle is essential in the disposal of excess nitrogen wastes, including ammonia, by forming soluble urea which is more readily excreted by the kidneys. Thus, the physiologic process of protein catabolism (e.g., in the case of fasting or illness) leads to toxic accumulation of ammonia in patients with urea cycle defects. Other metabolic disorders that cause the accumulation of toxic organic acid, amino acid, or fatty acid metabolites may also cause a prominent elevation in ammonia by secondarily inhibiting the enzyme N-acetylglutamate synthase, a component in the urea cycle (Fig. 51.3). Therefore, a thorough investigation into metabolic causes of hyperammonemia may be warranted.

Laboratory Investigations for Metabolic Causes of Hyperammonemia

When suspecting a metabolic cause of hyperammonemia, the clinician should obtain basic metabolic laboratory investigations, as described above. Of note, an abnormally low blood urea nitrogen in the context of elevated ammonia may be further evidence of an underlying urea cycle defect (25). Further laboratory investigation for a suspected urea cycle defect includes plasma quantitative amino acids to measure levels of the urea cycle intermediates, particularly citrulline and arginine. These compounds, in addition to urine orotic acid measurement, will be useful in differentiating the specific defect within the urea cycle. As mentioned above, certain organic acidurias and fatty acid oxidation disorders may present with hyperammonemia. Therefore, plasma acylcarnitines and urine organic acids should also be obtained.

Management of Hyperammonemia

Hyperammonemia should be aggressively managed, as it can be toxic to the brain. Excess nitrogen must be reduced by halting the protein intake. If a diagnosis is not immediately known, fat must also be restricted until a disorder of fatty acid oxidation has been formally ruled out. In addition, administration of high glucose, 10 mg/kg/min, will provide extra calories and prevent further protein catabolism, and thus the accumulation of excess nitrogen. It will be difficult to achieve this level of glucose infusion in adult patients. Typically, a safe place to start is a 10% dextrose solution with appropriate electrolytes to run at 1.5 times maintenance. Glucose, lactate, and acid-base levels must be closely monitored while the patient is receiving high glucose concentrations. The increased fluid intake—again, up to 1.5 times maintenance—will assist in the excretion of ammonium. Electrolytes, particularly sodium, must be carefully monitored and kept above 135 mMol/L. Additional diuresis may be necessary to avoid complications of fluid overload and cerebral edema (21). The nitrogen scavenging drugs—sodium benzoate, 5.5 g/m^2 (250 mg/kg in children) and sodium phenylacetate, also 5.5 g/m^2 (250 mg/kg in children)—should be readily available to aid in the removal of excess ammonia by allowing an alternate pathway for nitrogen excretion (17). These medications can be diluted in 10% dextrose and administered intravenously as a loading dose over 90 minutes, and then this same dose given continuously over 24 hours. Sodium benzoate and sodium phenylacetate are now FDA-approved for the management of hyperammonemia, and dosage and administration should comply with the manufacturer's recommendations. Additionally, the essential amino acid, arginine, is an intermediate in the urea cycle found downstream from most of the common defects, and it is often deficient in urea cycle defects. Intravenous infusion of L-arginine, 4 g/m^2 (300 mg/kg in children), may be administered with sodium benzoate and sodium phenylacetate as a loading dose over 90 minutes, followed by a continuous infusion over 24 hours (27). Alternatively, arginine may be given orally if the patient is able to take it. If the diagnosis is uncertain, carnitine, 100 mg/kg/day, IV or orally, should be given for empiric treatment of a potential organic aciduria or fatty acid oxidation defect (21). Dialysis should be readily available for refractory cases or for severe hyperammonemia—that is, with levels greater than 400 μM/L. This can be in the form of hemodialysis, hemofiltration, or peritoneal dialysis, although obviously the former are more efficient in the removal of toxic metabolites.

LACTIC ACIDOSIS IN METABOLIC DISEASE

Lactic acidosis is a common problem in intensive care and is typically a secondary effect from inadequate oxygen supply or tissue hypoperfusion as seen in respiratory failure, systemic shock, or tissue infarction. Signs and symptoms indicative of lactic acidosis include metabolic acidosis (pH <7.3, bicarbonate <15 mEq/L) with hyperventilation, and an abnormal anion gap (>15 mEq/L). Drugs such as ethanol, ethylene glycol, and salicylates may cause secondary lactic acidosis (28). A related isoform, D-lactate, is produced by bacteria colonized primarily in the gut and may contribute to significant metabolic acidosis. D-lactic acidosis should be considered in a patient who presents with encephalopathy, metabolic acidosis with a high serum anion gap, and symptoms of short bowel syndrome or gastric malabsorption (29,30). Plasma and/or urine D-lactate levels must be determined separately, as the regular assay for plasma lactic acid may be normal and miss the isoform.

Any metabolic disorder that presents with acute decompensation, such as certain organic acidurias, urea cycle defects, and fatty acid oxidation defects, may also develop significant lactic acidosis secondary to systemic disease. Because acute metabolic attacks are often triggered by an inciting stressor, such as illness with vomiting and dehydration, the clinician should consider metabolic disorders in patients with atypical presentations of lactic acidosis or unusual response to therapy.

Defects that affect glycogen metabolism (e.g., certain glycogen storage disorders), gluconeogenesis (e.g., fructose diphosphatase deficiency), and disorders of cellular aerobic respiration (e.g., pyruvate carboxylase deficiency, pyruvate dehydrogenase deficiency, and disorders of the respiratory chain complex) constitute a group of metabolic disorders referred to as *primary lactic acidoses*. In these cases, lactic acid is the accumulated byproduct from the metabolic defect itself rather than a secondary effect from systemic disease. Timing in relation to a carbohydrate load may be useful in the evaluation of lactic acidosis. For example, the lactic acid level in disorders of gluconeogenesis generally improves after the fed state with normal glucose levels, and lactic acidosis worsens with fasting hypoglycemia. In contrast, certain glycogen storage disorders and disorders of cellular aerobic respiration respond with a paradoxical elevation of lactic acid following a carbohydrate load due to the inherent block in carbohydrate utilization (31). Mitochondrial disorders will also be discussed in this section, as well as metabolic stroke.

Laboratory Investigations for Metabolic Causes of Lactic Acidosis

When the presentation of lactic acidosis suggests a possible metabolic disorder, basic metabolic laboratory investigations, as noted above, should be obtained immediately. As with serum ammonia levels, lactic acid levels may be artificially elevated as a result of sample handling and/or difficult blood draw—for example, with use of a tourniquet during phlebotomy. Additional screening laboratory tests for a suspected metabolic disease should include a plasma acylcarnitine profile, urine organic acids, and plasma amino acids. An abnormal elevated alanine seen in plasma amino acids may be an indirect measurement of pyruvate and lactate but is not affected by a tourniquet lab draw (12). Abnormal ketosis, particularly paradoxical postprandial ketosis, may be indicative of a primary lactic acidosis defect. An elevated cerebrospinal fluid (CSF) lactate may be helpful in the evaluation of a suspected primary lactic acidosis. As noted above, a d-lactic acid level should be considered in a patient who presents with encephalopathy, metabolic acidosis with a high serum anion gap, and symptoms of short bowel syndrome or gastric malabsorption.

A pyruvate level and differential measurements of the two serum ketones—3-hydroxybutyrate and acetoacetate—can be helpful in distinguishing between the different primary lactic acidoses. For example, an elevated lactate-to-pyruvate ratio with an elevated 3-hydroxybutyrate-to-acetoacetate ratio, in the setting of paradoxical postprandial ketosis and lactic acidosis, would highly suggest a respiratory chain disorder. These ratios act as an indirect method of measuring cellular oxidation/reduction status (31). However, due to the difficulty in collection, handling, and interpretation of these studies, this level of analysis is generally not feasible nor necessary for the acute management of patients with a primary lactic acidosis.

Management of Lactic Acidosis

Managing the underlying cause of lactic acidosis is the mainstay of treatment in most cases. For example, adequate ventilation and oxygenation, tissue perfusion, antimicrobial coverage, and other strategies common to the critical care setting should be continually monitored and adjusted. Intravenous sodium bicarbonate to correct anion gap acidosis caused by excess lactic acid can be used, but the goal should be to raise and maintain arterial blood pH to 7.2 and keep plasma bicarbonate levels greater than 10 mMol/L rather than correct the acidosis to normal. Large amounts of sodium bicarbonate may be necessary to achieve this goal. Therefore, sodium should be closely monitored for the risk of developing hypernatremia from large amounts of sodium bicarbonate. Potassium should also be monitored for the risk of hypokalemic response to rising pH. Diuretics such as furosemide, with adequate potassium supplementation, can be considered in this case. Other considerations might include the use of tris-hydroxymethyl aminomethane (THAM) or dialysis for cases refractory to typical treatment (17).

If a primary lactic acidosis is confirmed or highly suspected, glucose should be limited to between 3 and 5 mg/kg/min, as carbohydrates may worsen the accumulation of lactic acid (21).

Alternative calories—for example, lipids—should be sought. Before restricting glucose, however, note that disorders of fatty acid oxidation cannot handle excess lipids efficiently, and organic acidurias require high caloric loads to prevent acute protein catabolism. Both of these conditions should be reasonably ruled out. The diagnosis of a primary versus secondary causes of lactic acidosis is tricky, and consultation with a metabolic specialist familiar with the diagnosis and management of these disorders is recommended.

GENETIC CONSIDERATIONS IN RHABDOMYOLYSIS

Rhabdomyolysis, or myonecrosis, refers to skeletal muscle destruction and release of toxic substances in the circulatory system. Laboratory markers for rhabdomyolysis include elevated serum creatine kinase (CK) and the presence of myoglobinuria, or red-brown, cola-colored urine. Rapid identification and management is important to decrease morbidity, particularly the development of acute renal failure.

Rhabdomyolysis most commonly results from direct muscle trauma, particularly crush injury. Excessive muscle exertion such as in status epilepticus may cause a significant elevation of CK. It has also been described in an unconditioned otherwise healthy individual, although this would be a rare circumstance (32). Drug exposure may be the most common cause of rhabdomyolysis, particularly in critical care. Common medications that have been associated include diuretics, statins, clofibrate, narcotics, theophylline, corticosteroids, benzodiazepines, phenothiazines, and tricyclic antidepressants, as well as recreational drugs of abuse including alcohol, cocaine, amphetamines, heroin, phencyclidine, and lysergic acid diethylamide (33). Late-onset muscular dystrophies—for example, X-linked Becker muscular dystrophy—may present with exertional rhabdomyolysis; however, these individuals are often limited by weakness (31).

Recurrent rhabdomyolysis, or severe disease for which there is not a reasonable cause, may indicate an underlying metabolic disorder. These disorders may present at any age, and it is not uncommon for onset to occur in early adulthood despite a typical active childhood. Active muscle has a high energy demand for adenosine triphosphate (ATP), generated primarily from stored glycogen during the initial part of exercise and free fatty acids during prolonged exercise. Defects in these metabolic processes may lead to exercise intolerance and potentially rhabdomyolysis. McArdle disease (myophosphorylase deficiency, or glycogen storage disease type V) is a defect in glycolysis and often presents in late childhood to early adulthood with muscle fatigue and cramps. Certain long-chain fatty acid oxidation defects—such as long-chain 3-hydroxy acyl-CoA dehydrogenase deficiency (LCHAD), very long-chain acyl-CoA dehydrogenase deficiency (VLCAD), carnitine palmitoyltransferase deficiency type II (CPT2), and primary carnitine deficiency—can present with exercise intolerance and rhabdomyolysis in older children and adults. In addition, myoadenylate deaminase deficiency, a defect in the recycling of purines—and hence ATP—can have a similar presentation. Finally, respiratory chain disorders (see mitochondrial diseases, below) should be considered in recurrent myoglobinuria when accompanied by multisystemic involvement and lactic acidosis (31).

Laboratory Investigation for Metabolic Causes of Rhabdomyolysis

Laboratory investigations important in the management and workup of rhabdomyolysis include basic laboratory investigations, as noted above. Lactic acidosis can acutely accompany muscle damage or hypoperfusion, but a history of chronic lactic acidosis may be an indicator of an underlying mitochondrial respiratory chain disorder. A plasma acylcarnitine analysis should be drawn to evaluate for a possible fatty acid oxidation defect (e.g., LCHAD, VLCAD, CPT2). Further diagnostic workup for metabolic causes of rhabdomyolysis may require an open muscle biopsy for muscle enzyme studies, such as CPT2, myophosphorylase, and myoadenylate deaminase. This is important to consider; however, time-intensive specialized enzyme studies are not likely helpful in the acute management of rhabdomyolysis.

Management of Rhabdomyolysis

Management of rhabdomyolysis involves preventing further muscle damage and providing supportive care to prevent significant morbidity from acute renal failure, hypovolemia, metabolic acidosis, hyperkalemia, disseminated intravascular coagulation, and respiratory and hepatic insufficiency. Early and aggressive fluid management with normal saline, at the rate of 1.5 L per hour, is the only therapy that has been proven beneficial. However, many centers also use the administration of bicarbonate to alkalinize urine, as well as mannitol for theoretical benefit in minimizing kidney damage (34,35). In disorders of fatty acid oxidation, rhabdomyolysis is caused by muscle tissue damage due to lack of energy from fatty acid metabolism. Consider the administration of dextrose (up to a 10% solution) for known or highly suspected metabolic disorders to minimize continued muscle breakdown in these conditions.

GENETIC CONSIDERATIONS IN STROKE

Stroke is a heterogeneous neurologic condition that refers to the presentation of focal cerebral damage. A strong familial predilection suggests a genetic component (36,37). However, with rare exception (e.g., CADISIL, see below), single genes have a relatively low impact on the overall stroke risk (38). Therefore, it is well established that stroke is multifactorial, or influenced by environmental factors with a certain genetic predisposition. Well-known modifiable risk factors, including smoking, hypertension, hyperlipidemia, and diabetes mellitus, have a significant environmental component. However, these risk factors, particularly hypertension, hyperlipidemia, and diabetes, also have a familial predisposition and thus contribute to the genetic susceptibility of stroke as well.

Single gene disorders that cause isolated stroke, such as cerebral autosomal dominant arteriopathy with subcortical infarcts and leukoencephalopathy or (CADISIL), are rare. Alternatively, most genes (and/or genetic disorders) associated with stroke are part of a multisystem disease in which stroke is a secondary manifestation of the disorder. This includes multifactorial disorders such as hyperlipidemia, hypertension, and diabetes mellitus, as noted above, as well as single-gene disorders that affect cerebral vascular structure (e.g., connective tissue disorders) or hematologic conditions that increase the risk for thromboembolism (e.g., antithrombin III deficiency). Certain inherited metabolic disorders are also associated with a secondary risk of stroke. We will present several defined genetic disorders that either cause or predispose to stroke. The reader is referred to more comprehensive reviews on stroke (37,39); nonetheless, caution should be used, as there is ever-increasing knowledge and discovery of new genes in stroke, as is the case in any multigenic disorder.

Causative Gene Disorders in Stroke

Single-gene disorders that cause familial, isolated stroke are rare. An example is CADISIL, which typically presents in mid-adult life with clinical manifestations of migraines, transient ischemic attacks, lacunar infarcts, and multi-infarct dementia. The condition is diagnosed by clinical findings, distinct MRI studies showing subcortical white matter lesions, and traditionally by skin biopsy showing electron dense granules within smooth muscle cells. The gene for CADISIL (Notch3) has been identified and is clinically available for diagnostic testing (40). Clinical genetic testing should be considered in any unusual presentation of isolated stroke, particularly in adults younger than 50 years of age with clinical and radiographic evidence of CADISIL (37). Although the specific pathophysiology of CADISIL is still unknown, it is believed to be due to the increased fragility of cerebral microvessels. An autosomal recessive counterpart, CARASIL (cerebral autosomal recessive arteriopathy with subcortical infarcts and leukoencephalopathy), and other candidate genes causing isolated stroke are under investigation. However, currently, only CADISIL gene testing appears to have clinical applicability.

Genetic Susceptibility to Stroke

Connective tissue disorders that affect cervical and intracranial arteries can cause the formation of aneurysms and/or arterial dissection and lead to ischemic stroke. Disorders such as vascular type (or type IV) Ehlers-Danlos syndrome (EDS) and Marfan syndrome are well-known connective disorders affecting large vessels; both are inherited autosomal dominant. This underscores the importance of obtaining a personal or family history, particularly when there is a presentation of recurrent arterial dissection or aneurysm. Individuals with Marfan syndrome and vascular type EDS typically have an identifiable physical phenotype, and clinical diagnostic criteria exist for these conditions. Genetic and molecular testing is available for these disorders and can be helpful, not only to confirm the diagnosis, but also for family screening. Of note, vascular involvement in Marfan syndrome typically affects the larger arteries, particularly the aortic root; however, several related connective tissue diseases, such as the Marfanlike Loeys-Dietz syndrome, have recently been described with a possible predisposition to arterial involvement (41). Genetic and molecular testing is available for some of these disorders. Furthermore, there are likely several, yet undiscovered, connective tissue genes that predispose to abnormalities in the vascular wall. Additionally, many of these conditions are likely multifactorial, and many investigators are looking for candidate susceptibility genes (42,43). Finally, autosomal dominant polycystic kidney disease has also been described with intracranial aneurysms and should be considered in the workup for stroke (44).

Vascular disease may predispose to vessel occlusion and ischemic disease, and thus stroke. Genetic disorders that can lead to cerebrovascular disease include fibromuscular dysplasia (more commonly affecting renal arteries) and Moyamoya disease (cerebrovascular disease of arteries near basal ganglia, typically seen in children). Another vascular defect, Fabry disease, is an X-linked lysosomal storage disorder affecting the breakdown of specific glycosphingolipids. The disorder typically manifests in male adolescents or adults with recurrent pain crises, and leads to renal failure and cardiovascular disease if left untreated. Accumulated deposition of glycosphingolipids in small arteries, particularly vertebrobasilar arteries, leads to occlusion and infarcts (45).

Thromboembolism contributes to about 30% of ischemic stroke. Therefore, coagulation studies should be obtained to rule out common causes of thrombotic disease. Genetic predisposition to coagulopathy leading to thrombosis may include protein C deficiency, protein S deficiency, factor V Leiden mutation, antiphospholipid antibody syndromes, homocystinemia, and sickle cell anemia.

Inherited Metabolic Disorders and Susceptibility to Stroke

Homocystinuria is a metabolic disorder associated with a significant risk for thromboembolism. Clinical features of homocystinuria can be quite variable; many individuals have low IQ, psychiatric problems, and extrapyramidal signs. A tall, marfanoid body habitus has also been described. Similarly, mild to moderate homocystinemia can be caused by acquired nutritional deficiency of folic acid, vitamin B_{12} or vitamin B_6, or by a congenital defect in the gene coding for 5, 10-methylenetetrahydrofolate reductase (MTHFR). In any case of thromboembolic stroke, a plasma homocystine level should be obtained (39).

Methylmalonic aciduria (MMA) is a metabolic defect in the breakdown of certain amino acids. MMA also has been described with MRI and/or CT findings involving bilateral lesions of the globus pallidus and cortical atrophy, along with clinical findings of dystonia and choreoathetosis. The rare onset of stroke in these patients is generally not isolated. Rather, it is typically observed in the setting of acute metabolic decompensation, such as profound anion gap metabolic acidosis and ketoacidosis (46) (See the section on ketoacidosis, above).

Metabolic Stroke in Mitochondrial Disorders

Metabolic stroke, or stroke-like episodes observed in patients with mitochondrial encephalomyopathy, lactic acidosis, and stroke-like episodes (MELAS), as well as other inherited mitochondrial disorders, can be devastating. However, the etiology of these strokes is not well understood (14,47). Of note, stroke-like episodes have also been described in children with certain congenital disorders of glycosylation, a diverse group of disorders often presenting with dysmorphic features and multisystem involvement (48). Stroke-like episodes typically present with infarcts within the posterior temporal, parietal, and occipital lobes on imaging. The infarcts are atypical in that they are localized in regions near large vessels as opposed to watershed regions (49,50). Aside from supportive care, no definitive therapy has been established for treating metabolic stroke. Koga et al. (51) administered L-arginine, 0.5 g/kg per dose, intravenously during acute metabolic stroke in a few patients with MELAS with positive results. The rationale behind using arginine in mitochondrial patients is that stroke-like episodes may, in part, be due to poor vasodilatation of cerebral arteries, and arginine, a precursor to nitric oxide, may improve vascular tone. Caution must be observed with use of intravenous L-arginine. Hypotension may be a side effect of IV infusion, and acid-base status should be monitored carefully due to the common preparation of IV arginine hydrochloride. Arginine is not considered standard therapy in this situation, and therefore consultation with a metabolic specialist is recommended for determining the appropriate therapy for metabolic stroke (14).

GENETIC CONSIDERATIONS IN CARDIOMYOPATHY AND SUDDEN CARDIAC DEATH

Cardiomyopathies encompass a heterogeneous group of disorders with multiple clinical, molecular, and histiologic presentations. Traditionally, these have been categorized according to various pathophysiologic manifestations, such as hypertrophic (increased myocardial tissue thickness; e.g., increased myocyte size, fibrosis, or storage material), dilated (enlarged cardiac chamber volume), restrictive (inhibited ventricular filling), and mixed disorders (52). Definitions and classification schemes can be confusing due to the marked variability of causes and presentation. In particular, many traditional schemes do not account for the increasingly updated genetic and molecular discoveries. Furthermore, ion channelopathies, or dysrhythmic disorders, such as long QT syndrome (LQTS), present with a structurally normal heart, distinct from cardiomyopathies. It is well known that most forms of familial hypertrophic cardiomyopathy and long QT syndrome are inherited autosomal dominant. Both conditions predispose the affected individual to sudden cardiac death, often with little or no warning. This underscores the importance of not only properly diagnosing and managing the affected individual, but also screening and monitoring family members at risk for inheriting the condition (53–55). DNA-based genetic testing is available for several genes responsible for both hypertrophic cardiomyopathy and LQTS. Genetic testing should be considered in any patient presenting with a significant clinical picture suspicious for either condition, in particular young individuals presenting with sudden cardiac death. Finally, several metabolic disorders are at risk for developing cardiomyopathy—for example, fatty acid oxidation defects affecting mitochondrial energy (ATP) production or lysosomal storage diseases leading to cardiac tissue infiltration of storage material. This section is an overview of the genetic considerations in cardiomyopathies and causes of sudden cardiac death.

Ion Channelopathies

The most common congenital arrhythmia, long QT syndrome (LQTS), is inherited either autosomal dominant (Romano-Ward syndrome) or autosomal recessive (Jervell, Lange-Nielsen). About half of the individuals with these conditions are symptomatic, commonly with tachydysrhythmias resulting in syncopal events. However, some individuals remain asymptomatic (56). The autosomal dominant conditions, Andersen-Tawil syndrome and Timothy syndrome, are also associated with dysmorphic findings. The autosomal recessive forms of LQTS are typically associated with sensorineural deafness. Traditionally, these disorders are diagnosed clinically by history and rate-corrected QT interval. However, today, several genes responsible for this condition have been found, and genetic testing for many of these genes is clinically available. This is an example that genetic testing is not only beneficial for confirming the diagnosis but also for potential screening of first-degree relatives who may be asymptomatic and at risk for inheriting the condition. Family members who inherit the condition can have early and appropriate management to prevent complications, particularly death. All individuals who have a known mutation causing LQTS, and all first-degree relatives at risk for LQTS in whom a causative mutation is not found, are recommended to have at least a 12-lead ECG performed, followed by an exercise ECG, the latter particularly to evaluate a borderline resting ECG (57). Other less common ion channelopathies include Brugada syndrome (autosomal dominant sodium channelopathy causing a distinctive ECG pattern), catecholaminergic polymorphic ventricular tachycardia (autosomal dominant with normal resting ECG), and short QT syndrome (linked to mutations seen in ion channel genes of LQTS) (55).

Hypertrophic Cardiomyopathy

Familial hypertrophic cardiomyopathy (HCM), commonly autosomal dominant, is the most common cause of sudden cardiac death in young individuals. This condition is inherited as autosomal dominant, and therefore, a thorough family history is important in the workup. As with LQTS, many individuals with HCM may be completely asymptomatic. Clinically, HCM may be diagnosed by standard imaging, such as an echocardiogram showing left ventricular wall thickening. Several causative genes, typically coding for contractile proteins within the muscle cell, have been identified. Many of these genes are clinically available for genetic testing. As with LQTS, genetic testing for HCM may be useful not only for confirmatory diagnosis, but also for screening first-degree relatives at risk to inherit the condition. Recommendations for asymptomatic individuals at risk for HCM due to either a known mutation or a first-degree relative with HCM include a yearly physical exam, 12-lead ECG, and echocardiogram until the age of 18 years (58). Beyond 18 years of age, it is generally recommended to continue screening at least every 5 years, although management strategies may differ (58–60).

Dysrhythmogenic right ventricular cardiomyopathy/dysplasia (ARVC/D), caused by abnormal fibrofatty infiltration and tissue replacement within the right ventricle, is another cause of sudden cardiac death in young individuals. It has an autosomal dominant inheritance and is clinically difficult to diagnose. Several genes have been determined to have a role in this condition (55).

Several storage diseases lead to the infiltration of large molecules within the cardiac tissue. Although the pathophysiology is significantly different, clinically, these disorders may mimic hypertrophic cardiomyopathy. Dominant mutations in the gene PRKAG2 have been shown to cause glycogen accumulation in vacuoles within myocytes, clinically manifesting as HCM (61). Another condition, Danon disease, is an X-linked glycogen storage disease that presents with cardiomyopathy and typically skeletal myopathy, primarily in adolescent males. Mental retardation has also been seen in Danon disease. Glycogen storage disease type II has been shown to cause significant hypertrophic cardiomyopathy, with severe hypotonia in the infantile-onset form. However, adolescents and adults with milder forms of Pompe disease present later with proximal muscle weakness and do not typically have the cardiac manifestations. Other inherited metabolic disorders causing infiltrative hypertrophic cardiomyopathy typically accompany other significant clinical manifestations. Examples include Hunter syndrome (X-linked), Hurler (autosomal recessive), and Fabry disease (X-linked).

Dilated Cardiomyopathy

Dilated cardiomyopathy (DCM), or ventricular enlargement with systolic dysfunction, leads to progressive failure and is a common reason for heart transplant. The causes of DCM are variable, typically from acquired disorders such as infection, toxic exposures, and nutritional deficiencies (such as carnitine deficiency). Duchenne and Becker muscular dystrophy, as well as other diseases of the heart muscle, may lead to progressive cardiac failure and a dilated cardiomyopathy presentation. In addition, inherited metabolic disorders, such as organic acidurias, fatty acid oxidation defects, and respiratory chain disorders, may manifest with cardiomyopathy. Although potential carnitine deficiency or defects in mitochondrial aerobic respiration have been implicated as a cause of cardiomyopathy in metabolic acute metabolic disease, the specific pathophysiologic mechanism is not readily known. A cardiac evaluation is generally recommended in individuals with metabolic defects presenting in acute metabolic crises.

Familial DCM has been suggested in about 20% to 35% of cases by autosomal dominant, autosomal recessive or X-linked inheritance patterns. Several genes have been implicated in these conditions; however, clinical testing is not yet feasible for most cases of DCM. A particular exception is tafazzin, a mitochondrial protein responsible for the X-linked Barth syndrome typically seen in young males. As with HCM, family screening and monitoring is recommended, particularly in at-risk first-degree relatives (62).

ANESTHESIA RISKS IN GENETIC AND METABOLIC DISORDERS

Certain genetic, and particularly metabolic, diseases have an increased anesthesia risk. This not only includes an increased risk via the anesthetics themselves but also increased risks due to specific structural abnormalities that accompany some genetic disorders.

Individuals with metabolic disorders, such as fatty acid oxidation defects, organic acidurias, and urea cycle disorders, are predisposed to metabolic decompensation from physical and catabolic tissue breakdown from the stress of surgery and anesthetics. Preventative measures, such as high glucose infusion (typically 10% dextrose solution) and hydration (generally 1.5 times maintenance fluids with appropriate electrolyte) before, during, and after surgery are necessary to avoid a catabolic state (17). Consultation with a specialist familiar with metabolic disorders will aid in determining the appropriate management of these patients.

Particular attention should be given to mitochondrial patients requiring anesthetics. These individuals are inherently at risk due to the mitochondria's inability to deal with added oxidative stress from surgery and anesthesia. Additionally, most anesthetics affect mitochondrial function in some fashion, such as depressing carbohydrate metabolism or inhibiting certain components of the mitochondrial respiratory chain. These risks are primarily based on scientific reasoning and *in vitro* studies, resulting in inadequate or nonexistent clinical evidence. However, given the inherent risk, all anesthetics should be used with caution in this group of disorders (15). Drugs that should be used with particular caution in mitochondrial disorders include barbiturates, propofol, nitroprusside, theophylline, valproate, and phenobarbital (16).

Presedation evaluations should include an assessment for the presence of a genetic condition that carries a heightened risk of anesthesia. Well-described risks in genetic conditions include airway difficulty from structural and functional defects, abnormal respiratory mechanics, gastric reflux, cardiovascular disease, neuromuscular problems, liver disease, and renal disease, as well as risk for hyperthermia. Butler et al. (63) recently published an extensive review encompassing 163 single-gene, chromosomal, and multifactorial genetic conditions with anesthesia risks. Examples of airway management problems in genetic conditions include Down syndrome and certain skeletal dysplasias in which there is a risk of cervical cord compression due to atlantoaxial instability or kyphoscoliosis, respectively (17,64). In these patients, recent cervical spine radiographs should be reviewed prior to intubation and head positioning.

PHARMACOGENETICS AND PHARMACOGENOMICS

Personalized medicine is not a new concept. Many drugs and therapies are adjusted according to age, weight, body mass, and even gender and ethnicity. In many cases, treatment is modified depending on individual drug response. The preoperative evaluation includes personal and family history, including medications and drug use, and history of drug reactions, and anesthetic and bleeding complications, all of which may affect the management of a patient. The era of genomics has promised to personalize medicine according to an individual's specific genotype. The Human Genome Project has accelerated academic and pharmaceutical research in this field; however, in practical terms, the use of genetic- or genomic-based drug therapy is currently used only in specific situations. *Pharmacogenetics* refers to a drug's response according to differences in a single gene (e.g., CYP2D6, which codes for a specific enzyme responsible for metabolizing several drugs). *Pharmacogenomics* refers to a drug's response according to the effects of multiple genes and environmental factors. Although these terms have slightly different meanings, they are often used synonymously. Currently, there are few examples of clinically applicable genetic tests that influence drug therapy. Current pharmacogenetic testing relies on single-gene mutation studies, even though it is clear that most drug response is influenced by multigenic (multiple genes affecting the metabolism of a drug) and multifactorial (combination of genetic and environmental) factors.

Drugs—and other foreign chemicals (e.g., pollutants, carcinogens, or food additives)—are typically subject to extensive metabolism by cellular enzymes and transporters. This is the body's natural mechanism for detoxifying and eliminating potentially harmful compounds. Pharmaceutical drugs are formulated and dosed accordingly with this process in mind. Many drugs are administered as an inactive compound (prodrug) that relies on cellular metabolism to convert it to an active metabolite (65).

Early observations relevant to pharmacogenetics occurred over 50 years ago. For example, during World War II, African American soldiers given the antimalarial drug, primaquine, were noted to develop hemolytic anemia much more commonly than Caucasians (66). It is now recognized that the susceptibility to hemolytic anemia is related to an inherited defect in the enzyme, glucose-6-phosphate dehydrogenase, which is more common in certain ethnicities. Similarly, in the 1950s, Kalow and Gunn (67) noted an atypical response to the muscle relaxant, succinylcholine, in a small subset of Caucasians, which is now known to be caused by differences in the enzyme pseudocholinesterase, responsible for the metabolism of this drug.

A handful of examples of genetic testing are relevant to individualized drug therapy. 6-Mercaptopurine (6-MP) and its prodrug, azathioprine, are commonly used in treating certain forms of leukemia or rheumatologic disorders, respectively. This drug is metabolized, in part, by an enzyme called thiopurine methyltransferase (TPMT). It is recognized that about 1 in 300 individuals have a deficiency in TPMT and are unable to effectively metabolize these drugs, thus leading to toxic accumulation of thiopurine metabolites, which can be fatal (68). Many centers typically screen for TPMT genotype and dose these drugs accordingly to avoid adverse effects, while at the same time optimizing therapeutic response. A second example of pharmacogenetics entering the field of medicine is testing for polymorphisms (or genetic variants) in the CYP2D6 gene. CYP2D6 is a member of a superfamily of genes that code for cytochrome P450 enzymes responsible for metabolizing many commonly used drugs. CYP2D6 is one of the most studied enzymes within this group and is responsible for metabolizing a diverse group of drugs such as codeine, dextromethorphan, metoprolol, and nortriptyline (69). Polymorphisms within this gene or gene deletions are believed to be responsible for 'slow metabolism' of some commonly used drugs. An example is codeine, which has little or no affect in about 10% of the population due to poor metabolism of this prodrug to active metabolites, such as morphine. It is conceivable that genetic testing, comprising a panel of susceptible genes and their related polymorphisms such as in CYP2D6, could be invaluable in optimizing drug doses in patients; indeed, clinical genotyping has recently become clinically available (70). The efficacy, as well as practical clinical application, particularly in a critical scenario, of this type of testing (pharmacogenomic) has yet to be realized. For more information about pharmacogenomics and its potential application in clinical practice, the reader is referred to more in-depth reviews on this subject (71–74).

References

1. Wilson JM, Jungner YG. Principles and practice of mass screening for disease. Public Health Papers 34. Geneva, Switzerland: World Health Organization; 1968.
2. Burke W, Coughlin SS, Lee NC, et al. Application of population screening principles to genetic screening for adult-onset conditions. *Genet Test.* 2001;5(3):201–211.
3. Glabman M. Genetic testing, major opportunity, major problems. *Manag Care.* 2006;15(11):20–32.
4. GeneTests: Medical information resource (database online). Copyright, University of Washington, Seattle. 1993–2006. Available at http://www.genetests.org. Accessed December 15, 2006.
5. Lee PJ. Growing older: the adult metabolic clinic. *J Inherit Metab Dis.* 2002; 25:252–260.
6. Brenton DP. The adult and adolescent clinic for inborn errors of metabolism. *J Inherit Metab Dis.* 2000;23:215–228.
7. Smith W, Kishnani PS, Lee B, et al. Urea cycle disorders: clinical presentation outside the newborn period. *Crit Care Clin.* 2005;4(Suppl):S9–17.
8. Raymond K, Bale AE, Barnes CA, et al. Medium-chain acyl-CoA dehydrogenase deficiency: sudden and unexpected death of a 45-year-old woman. *Genet Med.* 1999;1(6):293–294.
9. Saudubray JM, Sedel F, Walter JH. Clinical approach to treatable inborn metabolic diseases: an introduction. *J Inherit Metab Dis* 2006;29:261–274.
10. Scriver CR, Beaudet AL, Sly WS, et al., eds. *The Metabolic and Molecular Bases of Inherited Disease.* New York, NY: McGraw-Hill; 2001.
11. Nyhan WL, Ozand PT. *Atlas of Metabolic Diseases.* London, England: Chapman & Hall; 1998.
12. Zschocke J, Hoffmann GF. Vademecum metabolicum. In: *Manual of Metabolic Paediatrics.* 2nd Ed. Stuttgart, Germany: Schattauer; 2004.
13. Shoffner J. Oxidative phosphorylation diseases. In: Scriver C, Beaudet S, Valle D, et al., eds. *The Metabolic & Molecular Bases of Inherited Disease.* New York, NY: McGraw-Hill; 2001.
14. Scaglia F, Northrop J. The mitochondrial encephalopathy, lactic acidosis with stroke-like episodes (MELAS) syndrome: a review of treatment options. *CNS Drugs.* 2006;20(6):443–464.
15. Muravchick S, Levy R. Clinical implications of mitochondrial dysfunction. *Anesthesiology.* 2006;105:819–837.
16. Boelen C, Smeitink J. Mitochondrial energy metabolism. In: Blau N, Hoffman GF, Leonard J, et al., eds. *Physician's Guide to the Treatment and Follow-Up of Metabolic Diseases.* Berlin, Germany: Springer-Verlag; 2004.
17. Hoffmann GF, Clarke J, Leonard JV. Emergency management of metabolic diseases. In: Blau N, Hoffmann GF, Leonard J, Clarke J, eds. *Physician's Guide to the Treatment and Follow-Up of Metabolic Diseases.* Berlin, Germany: Springer-Verlag; 2005.
18. Rinaldo P, Matern D. Contemporary diagnostic techniques: biochemical diagnosis of inborn errors of metabolism. In: Colin D, Rudolph AM, Rudolph MK, et al. *Rudolph's Pediatrics.* 21st ed. New York: McGraw-Hill; 2003.
19. American Diabetes Association Workgroup on Hypoglycemia. Defining and reporting hypoglycemia in diabetes. *Diabetes Care.* 2005;28:1245–1249.
20. Van Den Berghe G, Wouters P, Weekers F. Intensive insulin therapy in critically ill patients. *N Engl J Med.* 2001;345:1359–1367.
21. Prietsch V, Linder M, Zschocke J, et al. Emergency management of inherited metabolic diseases. *J Inherit Metab Dis.* 2002;25:531–546.
22. Biggemann B, Zass R, Wendel U. Postoperative metabolic decompensation in maple syrup urine disease is completely prevented by insulin. *J Inherit Metab Dis.* 1993;16:912–913.
23. Strauss K, Puffenberger E, Morton DH. Maple syrup urine disease (updated January 6, 2006). In: GeneTests: Medical information resource (database online). Copyright, University of Washington, Seattle. 1993–2006. Available at http://www.genetists.org. Accessed December 15, 2006.
24. Summar M, Tuchman M. Proceedings of a consensus conference for the management of patients with urea cycle disorders. *J Pediatr.* 2001;138:S6–10.
25. Bachmann C. Inherited hyperammonemias. In: Blau N, Duran M, Blaskovics ME, et al., eds. *Physician's Guide to the Laboratory Diagnosis of Metabolic Diseases.* Berlin, Germany: Springer-Verlag; 1996.
26. Felig DM, Brusilow SW, Boyer JL. Hyperammonemic coma due to parenteral nutrition in a woman with heterozygous ornithine transcarbamylase deficiency. *Gastroenterology.* 1995;109(1):282–284.
27. Leonard JV. Inherited hyperammonemias. In: Blau N, Hoffman GF, Leonard J, et al., eds. *Physician's Guide to the Treatment and Follow-Up of Metabolic Diseases.* Berlin, Germany: Springer-Verlag; 2004.
28. Clarke JA. Metabolic acidosis. In: Clarke J, ed. *A Clinical Guide to Inherited Metabolic Diseases.* 2nd ed. United Kingdom: Cambridge University Press; 2002.
29. DuBose T. Metabolic acidosis. In: Kasper DL, Braunwald E, Fauci A, et al.

Harrison's Principles of Internal Medicine. 16th ed. New York, NY: McGraw-Hill; 2005.
30. Uribarri J, Oh MS, Carroll HJ. D-lactic acidosis: a review of clinical presentation, biochemical features, and pathophysiologic mechanisms. *Medicine.* 1998;77(2):73–82.
31. Saudubray JM, Charpentier C. Clinical phenotypes: diagnosis/algorithms. In: Scriver C, Beaudet S, Valle D, et al., eds. *The Metabolic & Molecular Bases of Inherited Disease.* New York, NY: McGraw-Hill; 2001.
32. Sinert R, Kohl L, Rainone T. Exercise-induced rhabdomyolysis. *Ann Emerg Med.* 1994;23:1301–1306.
33. Counselman F. Rhabdomyolysis. In: Tintinalli J, Kelen G, Stapczynski S, et al., eds. *Tintinalli's Emergency Medicine.* 6th ed. New York, NY: McGraw-Hill; 2004.
34. Allison R, Bedsole L. The other medical causes of rhabdomyolysis. *Am J Med Sci.* 2003;326(2):79–88.
35. Huerta-Alardin A, Varon J, Marik P. Bench-to-bedside review: rhabdomyolysis—an overview for clinicians. *Crit Care.* 2005;9(2):159–169.
36. Liao D, Myers R, Hunt S. Familial history of stroke and stroke risk. The Family Heart Study. *Stroke.* 1997;28:1908–1912.
37. Wang MM. Genetics of ischemic stroke: future clinical applications. *Semin Neurol.* 2006;26(5):523–530.
38. Flossmann E, Schulz UG, Rothwell PM. Systematic review of methods and results of studies of the genetic epidemiology of ischemic stroke. *Stroke.* 2004;35:212–227.
39. Hademenos GJ, Alberts MJ, Awad MD, et al. Advances in the genetics of cerebrovascular disease and stroke. *Neurology.* 2001;56:997–1008.
40. Joutel A, Corpechot C, Ducros A. Notch3 mutations in CADISIL, a hereditary adult-onset condition causing stroke and dementia. *Nature.* 1996;383: 707–710.
41. Loeys BL, Chen ER, Neptune ER, et al. A syndrome of altered cardiovascular craniofacial, neurocognitive and skeletal development caused by mutations in TGFBR1 or TGFBR2. *Nat Genet.* 2005;37:275–81.
42. Rubenstein SM, Peerdemann SM, van Tulder MW, et al. A systematic review of the risk factors for cervical artery dissection. *Stroke.* 2005;36:1575–1580.
43. Krischek B, Inoue I. The genetics of intracranial aneurysms. *J Hum Genet.* 2006;51(7):587–594.
44. Pirson Y, Chauveau D, Torres V. Management of cerebral aneurysms in autosomal dominant polycystic kidney disease. *J Am Soc Nephrol.* 2002;13:269–276.
45. Desnick RJ, Astrin KH. Fabry disease (updated August 2004). In: GeneTests: medical information resource (database online). Copyright, University of Washington, Seattle. 1993–2006. Available at http://www.genetists.org. Accessed December 15, 2006.
46. Fenton WA, Gravel RA, Rosenblatt DS. Disorders of propionate and methylmalonate metabolism. In: Scriver C, Beaudet S, Valle D, et al. *The Metabolic & Molecular Bases of Inherited Disease.* New York, NY: McGraw-Hill; 2001.
47. Hirano M, Pavlakis SG. Mitochondrial encephalomyopathy, lactic acidosis, and stroke-like episodes (MELAS): current concepts. *J Child Neurol.* 1994;9(1):4–13.
48. Patterson MC. Metabolic mimics: the disorders of N-linked glycosylation. *Semin Pediatr Neurol.* 2005;12:144–151.
49. Shoffner J. Oxidative phosphorylation diseases. In: Scriver C, Beaudet S, Valle D, et al., eds. *The Metabolic & Molecular Bases of Inherited Disease.* New York, NY: McGraw-Hill; 2001.
50. Koga Y, Akita Y, Junko N, et al. Endothelial dysfunction in MELAS improved by L-arginine supplementation. *Neurology.* 2006;66:1766–1769.
51. Koga Y, Akita Y, Nishioka J, et al. L-Arginine improves the symptoms of strokelike episodes in MELAS. *Neurology.* 2005;64(4):710–712.
52. Richarson P, McKenna W, Bristow M, et al. Report of the 1995 World Health Organization/International Society and Federation of Cardiology Task Force on the Definition and Classification of Cardiomyopathies. *Circulation.* 1996;93:841–842.
53. Ackerman MJ. Genetic testing for risk stratification in hypertrophic cardiomyopathy and long QT syndrome: fact or fiction? *Curr Opin Cardiol.* 2005;20:175–181.
54. Corrado D, Basso C, Thiene G. Is it time to include ion channel diseases among cardiomyopathies? *J Electrocardiology.* 2005;38:81–87.
55. Maron BJ, Towbin JA, Thiere G, et al. Contemporary definitions and classifications of the cardiomyopathies: an American Heart Association scientific statement from the Council on Clinical Cardiology, Heart Failure and Transplantation Committee; Quality of Care and Outcomes Research and Functional Genomics and Translational Biology Interdisciplinary Working Groups; and Council on Epidemiology and Prevention. *Circulation.* 2006;113:1807–1816.
56. Schwartz PJ, Priori SG, Bloise R, et al. Molecular diagnosis in a child with sudden infant death syndrome. *Lancet.* 358:1342–1343.
57. Swan H, Toivonen L, Viitasalo M. Rate adaptation of QT intervals during and after exercise in children with congenital long QT syndrome. *Eur Heart J.* 1998;19:508–513.
58. Maron BJ, McKenna WJ, Danielson GK, et al. American College of Cardiology/European Society of Cardiology clinical expert consensus document on hypertrophic cardiomyopathy: a report of the American College of Cardiology Foundation Task Force on Clinical Expert Consensus Documents and the European Society of Cardiology Committee for Practice Guidelines. *Eur Heart J.* 2003;24:1965–1991.
59. Sen-Chowdhry S, McKenna WJ. Sudden cardiac death in the young: a strategy for prevention by targeted evaluation. *Cardiology.* 2006;105: 196–206.
60. Crispell KA, Hanson EL, Coats K, et al. Periodic rescreening is indicated for family members at risk of developing familial dilated cardiomyopathy. *J Am Coll Cardiol.* 2002;39(9):1503–1537.
61. Arad M, Benson DW, Perez-Atayde AR, et al. Constitutively active AMP kinase mutations cause glycogen storage disease mimicking hypertrophic cardiomyopathy. *J Clin Invest.* 2002;109:357–362.
62. Burkett EL, Hershberger RE. Clinical and genetic issues in familial dilated cardiomyopathy. *J Am Coll Cardiol.* 2005;45(7):969–981.
63. Butler MG, Hayes BG, Hathaway MM, et al. Specific genetic diseases at risk for sedation/anesthesia complications. *Anesth Analg.* 2000;91:838–855.
64. Ali FE, Al-Bustan MA, Al-Busairi WA, et al. Cervical spine abnormalities associated with Down syndrome. *Int Orthop.* 2006;30(4):284–289.
65. Gonzalez FJ, Tukey RH. Drug metabolism. In: Brunton LL, ed. *Goodman & Gilman's Pharmacology.* 11th ed. New York, NY: McGraw-Hill; 2006.
66. Carsen PE, Flanagan CL, Iokes CE. Enzymatic deficiency in primaquine-sensitive erythrocytes. *Science.* 1956;124:484–485.
67. Kalow W, Gunn DR. Some statistical data on atypical cholinesterase of human serum. *Ann Hum Genet.* 1959;23:239.
68. McLeod HL, Krynetski EY, Relling MV, et al. Genetic polymorphism of thiopurine methyltransferase and its clinical relevance for childhood acute lymphoblastic leukemia. *Leukemia.* 2000;14(4):567–572.
69. Kroemer HK, Eichelbaum M. "It's the genes, stupid." Molecular bases and clinical consequences of genetic cytochrome P450 2D6 polymorphism. *Life Sci.* 1995;56:2285–2298.
70. Jain KK. Applications of Amplichip CYP450. *Mol Diagn.* 2005;9(3):119–127.
71. Evans WE, McLeod HL. Pharmacogenomics—drug disposition, drug targets, and side effects. *N Engl J Med.* 2003;348(6):538–549.
72. Weinshilboum R. Inheritance and drug response. *New Engl J Med.* 2003; 348(6):329–337.
73. Goldstein DB, Tate SK, Sisodiya SM. Pharmacogenetics goes genomic. *Nat Rev Genet.* 2004;4:937–947.
74. Sweeny BP. Watson and Crick 50 years on. From double helix to pharmacogenomics. *Anaesthesia.* 2004;59:150–165.

CHAPTER 52 ■ GENE THERAPY IN CRITICAL ILLNESS: PAST APPLICATIONS AND FUTURE POTENTIAL

ROBERT D. WINFIELD • LYLE L. MOLDAWER

INTRODUCTION

Gene therapy refers to the transfer or delivery of nucleic acids to somatic cells, resulting in a therapeutic effect through the correction of a genetic defect, the production of a therapeutically useful protein, or the attenuation of endogenous mRNA (1). While traditional medical and surgical treatment modalities are often effective in the treatment of disease processes, most small-molecule approaches are nonspecific, carrying with them the risks of adverse side effects and the possibility of harm to the patient (2). Even protein-based therapies, such as monoclonal antibodies or receptor antagonists, frequently have associated untoward side effects related to antigen recognition and activation of acquired immunity. Additionally, in disease processes such as inborn errors of metabolism, or chronic inflammatory or autoimmune diseases such as diabetes mellitus or rheumatoid arthritis, medication is frequently temporizing, and not curative, and must be taken indefinitely. In theory, gene therapy is a more tailored approach to disease, with results that are not only therapeutically successful, but also specific to a disease process, often lacking in significant side effects, and potentially curative in chronic disease states.

Unfortunately, while gene therapy offers these potential opportunities, in most cases, they remain only theoretical and unrealized, and have not yet been applied to practice. A number of significant practical hurdles exist to the use of gene therapy in the clinical arena, and, despite some 20 years of experimental work, few clinical successes have resulted. However, the prognosis for gene therapy is, in general, quite bright, and there have been a number of impressive results demonstrating the power and potential utility of this approach. This chapter will briefly review these research areas and summarize the essential aspects of human gene therapy, including the mechanism, possible risks, disease states amenable to gene therapy, and clinical use now and in the future. Our emphasis in the latter sections of this review will focus on the clinical application of gene therapy to acute inflammatory conditions in critical illness, such as sepsis, traumatic injury, and adult respiratory distress syndromes.

OVERVIEW

While the concept of gene therapy is a relatively simple one, the practice is complex and requires the following:

- The identification of a gene target in a disease of interest
- Creation of a DNA sequence that will generate a therapeutically active product
- Selection and incorporation of the sequence into an appropriately selected vector with an appropriate promoter sequence
- Delivery of the vector into the cells of interest
- The successful incorporation of the sequence into the host's cellular machinery for expression

A good deal of groundwork has been laid for the identification of gene targets and the creation of DNA sequences through efforts such as the recently completed Human Genome Project. Utilizing the information obtained through this and other undertakings, the number of areas for potential intervention has continued to multiply.

VECTORS

With targets identified, the first step toward the integration of the gene sequence into the cells of interest is the selection of a vector. In this context, we use the term *vector* to refer to the delivery system for exogenous genetic material, and it can be as simple as a bacterial plasmid (Fig. 52.1) or as complicated as a recombinant virus. In general, we are not referring to the direct administration of nucleic acids with catalytic or other activities, such as ribozymes or small inhibitory RNA (siRNA) sequences. Rather, we are discussing expression systems where the host synthetic machinery is required to express either the induced protein or RNA sequences. Immediate goals for the creation and use of a vector are the delivery of genetic material to the correct site and expression of that material at a meaningful (therapeutic) level, all in a controlled fashion (3). No vector currently in use is completely successful at achieving this end. What follows is a discussion of a few of the more commonly considered vectors utilized at present, with a brief summary evaluation of some of their positive and negative features in critical illness.

Viral Vectors

Viral vectors represented the first vehicle utilized in gene therapy, and their use is still commonplace today. In general, viral vectors offer the advantages of intrinsic delivery methods combined with an inherent means for incorporating genetic material into the host cells (either episomal or with integration into the host genome). This takes advantage of the evolutionary

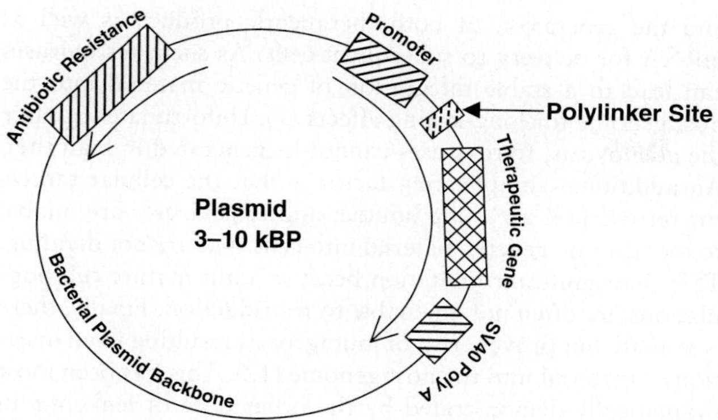

FIGURE 52.1. Prototypical expression plasmid used for nonviral gene therapy. Circular DNA generally based on a traditional bacterial plasmid (e.g., pBR), usually 3 to 10 kBP in size containing a promoter sequence (in this case, cytomegalovirus [CMV] early enhancer/promoter), the expressed transgene, an SV40 polyadenylation sequence, and one or more polylinker sites for splicing in and out DNA. In many cases, the plasmid may also contain a promoter and gene that conveys antibiotic resistance, which aids in the production of the plasmid in the bacterial host.

success that viruses have attained in inserting their genetic material into eukaryotic cells and manipulating their expression machinery. Their overall disadvantages include generation of an immune response to varying degrees, as well as variable assimilation of genetic material into the host and its expression.

In fact, the major challenge today with the use of viral vectors is controlling the host immune and other cellular processes that have evolved to control and ultimately eliminate viral infections.

Viral vectors can also be divided based on whether they integrate their genetic information into the host genome (such as retroviruses and adeno-associated viruses (AAVs) or remain primarily episomal (such as adenovirus). While the former generally results in prolonged expression, often in excess of several months, the latter generally results in transient expression, lasting several days to a few weeks. While multiple different viruses have been proposed and are occasionally used as vectors, three primary viral vectors are in common use today, and will be presently discussed: adenoviruses, retroviruses, and AAVs.

Adenoviruses

Adenoviruses are the most commonly utilized vector in human gene therapy, accounting for 26% of all vectors currently being utilized in gene therapy clinical trials (4). Adenoviruses have a number of characteristics that account for their popularity in this field (Table 52.1):

1. They are easily grown in high viral titers.
2. They have a large capacity for transgene insertion.
3. They are efficiently transduced into both dividing and nondividing cells.
4. Only under very rare conditions do they incorporate into the host genome.

TABLE 52.1

ADVANTAGES AND DISADVANTAGES OF DIFFERENT GENE THERAPY VECTORS

Viral vector	Advantages	Disadvantages
Adenovirus	1. Generation of high viral titers 2. Rapidly transfects dividing and nondividing cells 3. Rapid onset of expression (within hours) 4. Transient high-level expression 5. Large genome available for expressed transgene 6. Incorporation into host genome is rare 7. Many existing methods for manipulating genome	1. Significant inflammatory response and activation of innate immunity 2. Pre-existing exposure to and humoral immunity in human population 3. Transient expression precludes use in chronic conditions
AAV	1. Nonpathogenic 2. Mild immunogenicity 3. Stable integration into host with long-term expression 4. Many variants 5. Many existing methods for manipulating genome 6. Many existing production and purification methods	1. Small size of vector limits ability to package larger genes 2. Long lag time between administration and maximal expression 3. Stable integration precludes use in acute inflammation
Retro- or lentivirus	1. Membrane coat protects genetic material 2. Target receptors allow uptake by specific cells 3. "Self-contained" mechanisms for incorporation of genetic material into host genome 4. Generates both gene product and mRNA for stable integration into genome	1. Low titer 2. Limited cellular targets 3. Targets dividing cells only 4. Stable integration precludes use in acute inflammation

5. There are a variety of different serotypes with varying affinities for different cell types.
6. Many methods have been developed for manipulation of the adenoviral genome, allowing for tailored approaches to individual clinical scenarios and the potential for overcoming obstacles associated with immune responses and the duration of therapeutic activity (5).

The primary disadvantage of using adenovirus as a therapeutic vector is its intense activation of innate and both humoral and cellular immune responses. We and others have previously shown that administration of adenovirus into an immunocompetent host produces an often unwanted and dose-dependent induction of a number of proinflammatory cytokines, including tumor necrosis factor (TNF)-α (6,7). This activation of innate immunity and inflammation was most dramatically presented in the case of a subject who died from a "cytokine storm" and multisystem organ failure following the intravenous injection of adenovirus (8). In less dramatic but more frequent cases, adenovirus may activate inflammatory and immune processes, with the potential to prove harmful to the patient and undoubtedly limit expression of the therapeutic gene, and can prevent the effectiveness with repeated administration of the vector (9). Because of the ubiquitous nature of adenoviruses and because most patients have some existing acquired immunity to adenovirus infections, adenoviral vectors are often neutralized quickly in the setting of previous exposure. Furthermore, adenovirus receptors are present on many different types of cells, making targeting of specific cell types difficult, although this latter concern can be remedied to some degree with tissue-specific promoters (5,9). As a result, there are considerable ongoing research efforts to modify the adenoviral delivery system, in some cases by removing the adenoviral genes that, when expressed, are recognized by the host immune system. These "gutless" adenoviral recombinants reduce, but do not eliminate, their recognition by host immune tissues (10). Even with all of these limitations well known, the advantages of adenovirus still make it the most popular vector, in large part because of the high degree of, but transient, expression that is achieved. For the critically ill patient, adenovirus remains a potentially effective tool for the short-term delivery and expression of therapeutic proteins. As we will see, many of the hurdles associated with its inflammatory and immune processes can still be managed, even in the setting of acute inflammation.

Retroviruses

Retroviruses are second among the commonly utilized vectors (4) and are attractive for use in gene therapy, owing to the presence of three features:

- Membrane-coated viral particles are taken up through a receptor-mediated mechanism into target cells.
- A plus-stranded RNA genome is then incorporated into a double-stranded DNA within cellular chromosomes via reverse transcriptase.
- Particles are assembled in the cytoplasm with incorporation of the full-length retroviral mRNA as the mobile form of genetic information (11).

Clearly, these features could be beneficial, as the retrovirus offers a protective environment for delivery, an inherent mechanism for incorporation of genetic material into the host genome and the generation of both therapeutic product as well as mRNA for delivery to subsequent cells. As such, retroviruses can lead to a stable integration of genetic material into the host genome for long-lasting effects (1). Unfortunately, unlike the adenovirus, retroviruses cannot be generated in high titer. An additional complicating factor is that the cellular targets for retroviruses are quite limited, and retroviruses are unable to incorporate genetic material into cells that are not dividing. This is a significant limitation because adult mature cell populations are often not amenable to transduction. Finally, there is a small, but proven, risk of mutagenesis resulting from insertion of material into the host genome (12). This has been most dramatically demonstrated by the occurrence of leukemia in two patients with primary combined immunodeficiency treated with retrovirus-based gene therapy (13).

Adeno-associated Vectors

Adeno-associated viral vectors are less commonly employed in clinical trials than adenoviruses or retroviruses; however, their promise as a delivery method that can produce prolonged expression in the absence of a host inflammatory response has led to a recent increase in enthusiasm for their use. Adeno-associated virus is a replication-deficient parvovirus found in humans as well as nonhuman primates, and exists in over 100 distinct variants (14). The advantageous features of AAV are many, including its nonpathogenicity, long duration of infection, large number of variants, generally mild immunogenicity, ease of genomic modification, and the fact that a number of recombinant production and purification methods have been developed for it (15). A number of experimental studies have demonstrated long-term expression of a variety of genetic materials following transfection of recombinant AAV vectors into a number of tissues, including muscle, lung, liver, gut, the central nervous system, and eye (16). The primary limitation to the use of AAV is its small size, which limits the amount of material that may be packaged into the vector. A second potential drawback is the presence of a significant lag time between the administration of the AAV and maximal gene expression, which may limit its efficacy in conditions where a rapid response is desirable, as in the acute inflammatory conditions to be discussed later. Additionally, since the expression of genetic material is so durable when AAV is utilized, improved regulatory mechanisms are necessary to control expression in disease states where constitutive expression would be deleterious (16). Again, this is potentially problematic in acute inflammation, where long-term immune suppression or enhancement could be undesirable.

Nonviral Vectors

With the intrinsic problems associated with the use of viral vectors, it is not surprising that significant research has been directed toward the development of synthetic vectors that do not rely on viral delivery systems. Interestingly, the exploration of nonviral delivery systems goes back to the early 1970s when it was first shown that exogenous nucleic acids could be readily taken up into cells (17). Initially, it was believed in the mid-1990s that these nonviral vectors would have the potential to overcome the previously discussed issues of generated immune responses, nonspecificity, and potential mutagenesis associated with viral delivery systems. Additionally, the perfect nonviral vector would be incorporated efficiently into dividing and nondividing cells, and have a large DNA capacity (18). As with viral vectors, these ideals have not been fully realized. In fact, a number of significant hurdles remain that have limited the usefulness of current nonviral approaches. The primary difficulties with nonviral approaches are the recognition of plasmid DNA by components of the innate immune system and generation of an inflammatory response; at the same time, the incorporation of DNA tends to be poor, and their expression is limited. At present, the most commonly utilized nonviral vector is plasmid DNA, administered either as naked DNA or incorporated into liposomal delivery systems. An overview of these vectors follows.

Naked DNA

Naked DNA is appealing for use in human gene therapy because its introduction into a patient generally does not stimulate an acquired immune response. Unfortunately, plasmid DNA, generally composed of bacterial sequences, is often recognized by the innate immune system, and can generate a potentially limiting inflammatory response. Bacterial DNA generally has a methylation pattern distinct from eukaryotic DNA and, as such, is recognized by toll-like receptors, specifically TLR9. Activation of TLR9 by CpG sequences in plasmid DNA can induce a proinflammatory cytokine response via nuclear factor (NF)-κB–dependent signaling pathways (19). We have shown that the administration of plasmid DNA can exacerbate existing inflammation and increase mortality during acute inflammatory processes (20).

In addition, the administration of naked DNA is not target specific, nor does it have defenses against host nucleases. Under normal conditions, greater than 99% of administered DNA is destroyed by circulating, lysosomal, and cytosolic endonucleases (21); thus, the use of naked DNA generally relies upon the administration of relatively large amounts of DNA and novel approaches that can circumvent these limitations. A variety of methods have been introduced in an attempt to present naked DNA into host cells, as well as to prevent it from being destroyed. High-pressure delivery systems have been among the most studied and utilized (18). The process is a conceptually simple one, placing DNA onto a metallic microparticle and then using a "gene gun" to deliver the particles into target cells utilizing electromotive force (22). There is some evidence to suggest that uptake and incorporation of DNA is increased in injured or damaged cells, and these high-pressure delivery systems may inadvertently injure cell populations and induce cell recovery mechanisms. Unfortunately, though, while these mechanical delivery systems such as the gene gun deliver the DNA to cells of interest, they do so over a very limited area and have primarily been demonstrated to be effective only in superficial tissues; thus, different high-pressure methods, such as hydroporation (intravenous injection of a large volume of DNA in solution) and jet injection (intravenous injection of a small volume of DNA in solution), have been proposed to overcome these obstacles for the systemic delivery of DNA, and have each shown success in different animal and human models (23,24).

Electroporation is a technique that uses electrodes implanted in the tissue of interest to generate an electric field, with a resultant increase in permeability for the subsequently introduced DNA. While gene transfer is increased substantially through this technique, it is limited by the need for surgery to place electrodes and the tissue damage generated by the electric field (18); additionally, the exact mechanism for the success of electroporation has been called into question (25). More recently described techniques include laser beam gene transduction, ultrasonic gene delivery, magnetofaction (using magnetic nanoparticles to carry DNA to target tissues via direction by a magnetic field), and photochemical internalization (using light-sensitive endosomal vesicles to deliver DNA, and then lysing these vesicles with wavelength-appropriate light). Each of these methods has been shown to either increase the efficiency of gene transfer or increase expression in target tissues (reviewed in reference 18).

Liposomal Delivery

Liposomal delivery methods are the most common traditional approaches to nonviral DNA delivery, and have been utilized extensively since their introduction as one of the initial gene delivery methods (26). The concept is that the cationic lipid forms an electrostatic association with the DNA, leading to collapse of the anionic polymer, forming what is known as a lipoplex (18). These lipoplexes may be modified by the addition of ligands, antibodies, or other lipids in an attempt to improve target specificity, improve their stability, or decrease their toxicity. The lipoplexes fuse with the cellular membrane and are incorporated into endosomes. While liposomes do not trigger cellular immunity per se, they can activate the innate immune system, and their toxicity is the major limitation to their widespread use as a vector. Recent efforts have focused on diminishing the toxicity of these vectors, and two recent efforts have proven effective at lessening the immune response. The first, a simple staged procedure involving injection of liposome followed by injection of DNA—rather than injection of a formed lipoplex—led to a decrease in cytokine production as well as a reduced inflammatory response denoted by diminished neutropenia, lymphopenia, thrombocytopenia, and complement depletion with an increased transgene expression in the lung (27). The second method involves the creation of a "safeplex" containing anti-inflammatory entities such as glucocorticoids, nonsteroidal anti-inflammatory drugs (NSAIDs), or NF-κB inhibitors (28). The authors demonstrated significant suppression of inflammatory cytokine production via this method to go along with efficient gene delivery and expression.

SEPSIS AND ACUTE INFLAMMATION

Inflammation is, in a general sense, a principal component of innate immunity and is the body's first reaction to an infectious or injurious agent (29). Under normal circumstances, this response is a well-orchestrated series of events designed to promote the isolation or destruction of a bacterial or viral invader, or healing from a traumatic insult. However, when unchecked, the activation of the innate immune system may trigger additional inflammatory responses in distant organ systems in what has been termed the *systemic inflammatory response syndrome* (SIRS) (29). When SIRS occurs in the setting of a microbial infection, it is defined as sepsis. Patients who develop SIRS may recover from this condition or progress to multiple organ dysfunction syndrome (MODS), in which they develop signs and symptoms of failure in multiple organ systems. These conditions take a heavy toll on affected patients, with significant morbidity and, in the case of sepsis, a mortality rate ranging from 25% to 80% (reviewed in reference 30).

Despite significant advances in both our understanding of the mechanisms underlying inflammation and in the resuscitation of critically ill patients with SIRS and sepsis, mortality rates from these conditions have not changed significantly over the past three decades. Current modalities utilized in the treatment of patients suffering from these disease states remain largely supportive or carry with them potentially dangerous side effects. Immune modulation through gene therapy carries a great deal of promise and would appear to be well suited for treatment of patients with these conditions; however, barriers still exist to the use of gene therapy clinically.

The Perfect Gene Therapy Vector

What would the perfect gene therapy vector look like for a critically ill patient, if technically possible? The vector would, when administered to a critically ill patient or organism, be rapidly taken up by the target cells and the transgene expressed quickly, within minutes to hours. Administration of the vector would not require any invasive procedure other than current critical care management, and the vector itself would be silent in terms of eliciting or exacerbating an inflammatory or immune response. Expression would be transient and could be turned off or silenced once the patient or animal was in a recovery mode. Finally, there would be no long-term consequences associated with the vector administration or expression of the transgene.

Clearly, the perfect vector does not presently exist, and one could argue that no single vector will be optimal for all critically ill patients. What is clearly obvious, however, is that all of the research to date has used vectors and delivery systems that were not optimal. Progress in gene therapy for the treatment of critically ill patients will remain dependent upon advances in the technology and science of gene therapy, as well as in defining the optimal therapeutic gene to be administered.

Over the past 15 years, significant efforts have been made to define the role of gene therapy in acute inflammatory conditions. In the following discussion, recent developments in gene therapy for acute endotoxemia and sepsis will be summarized.

ENDOTOXICOSIS

Most studies involving gene therapy for acute endotoxemia have focused on the immunomodulatory roles of interleukin-10 (IL-10). Our laboratory was the first to explore the possibilities of gene therapy in endotoxemia, demonstrating the beneficial effect of expressing either a soluble TNF receptor or the human IL-10 gene on mortality (31). In a subsequent study by Drazan et al., the authors also achieved inhibition of TNF-α and IL-1β by using an adenoviral vector to express viral IL-10 in the livers of neonatal mice; interestingly, though, they did not note significant modulation of IL-6 production (32). Xing et al. likewise used an adenoviral vector given intramuscularly to express murine IL-10, finding that they achieved expression not only at the site, but also in distant tissues; further, they showed a decrease in the levels of TNF-α as well as IL-6 (33). IL-10 gene transfer has also been shown to decrease endotoxin-induced pulmonary inflammation when given intratracheally (34). Finally, it has been demonstrated that pretreatment with an AAV expressing IL-10 also confers a survival advantage in mice undergoing an endotoxemic challenge, suggesting that it may be possible to pretreat susceptible individuals (35).

While IL-10 has received the most attention with gene therapy for the treatment of endotoxicosis, other targets have been explored. Among the first to utilize a different approach, Baumhofer et al. performed gene transfer of other anti-inflammatory cytokines, IL-4 and IL-13, using cationic liposomes, finding a decreased TNF-α response to a lethal endotoxin challenge and showing a survival advantage in experimental mice when compared with controls (36). Alexander et al. showed similar results utilizing an adenoviral vector expressing *bacterial permeability increasing protein* prior to lethal endotoxicosis (37).

Given the beneficial effects of IL-10–based gene therapy, there has been increasing interest in therapeutic approaches aimed at interfering directly with inflammation signaling pathways. One such approach has been to target nuclear factor-κB (NF-κB) activation during inflammation. For example, Matsuda et al. evaluated the effect of transfecting an NF-κB decoy into lung tissue and demonstrated decreased expression of inflammatory mediators in lung tissue, decreased pulmonary vascular permeability, and improved blood gas parameters when compared to control (38). A similar approach has been to overexpress another group of targeted proteins, the suppressor of cytokine signaling (SOCS) family, which has been determined to be a group of feedback inhibitors of cytokine receptor signaling. Fang et al. used a liposomal delivery system to transfer SOCS3 and IL-10 into mice that were subsequently given an endotoxic challenge. The authors reported that delivery of SOCS3 in addition to IL-10 led to the greatest improvement in survival, but that administration of either independently improved the survival of mice at 48 hours (39). Finally, Nakamura et al. found that they could diminish the degree of renal dysfunction typically seen in endotoxemia by using adenoviral-mediated delivery of β_2-adrenoceptor to rat kidneys (40).

While these approaches have yielded generally positive results in animal models, concerns have been raised regarding the safety of administering a potentially immunogenic vector in the setting of acute inflammation. Our laboratory evaluated this possibility, showing that there is TNF-α–mediated hepatic injury when first-generation adenoviral vectors were administered in the setting of endotoxicosis (7); however, we also demonstrated that utilizing lower doses and incorporating an IL-10 construct into the vector abrogated this injury. These data were later supported by findings by Fejer et al., who demonstrated dramatic increases in TNF-α and nitric oxide levels in the kidney, liver, lung, and spleen. They further showed that these findings correlated with a diminished survival in animals treated with adenovirus and lipopolysaccharide (LPS) (41).

SEPSIS

Sepsis is a particularly challenging disorder for treatment by gene therapy because sepsis is a systemic disease (29), and targeting therapy to a single tissue or organ is generally ineffective. In addition, the failure of most monotherapies for the treatment of sepsis has convincingly shown that the pathologic basis for sepsis is multifactorial, and treatment against a single component of sepsis is unlikely to be dramatically successful.

With that said, however, the primary effort of using gene therapy in sepsis has been directed against the exuberant inflammatory response; as in endotoxicosis, by far the most commonly used approach has been the forced expression of the anti-inflammatory protein, IL-10. IL-10 is a particularly attractive transgene in sepsis for a number of reasons (42,43). IL-10 is a profoundly anti-inflammatory cytokine and is known to suppress the expression of early proinflammatory genes like TNF-α and IL-1 by preventing NF-κB translocation. As previously discussed, IL-10 gene therapy has been frequently successful in lethal endotoxicosis. Importantly, IL-10 works through what is known as a "bystander effect," meaning that transfection does not need to occur in every cell, since expression and secretion of IL-10 by a few transfected cells can produce biologic effects in adjacent, but not transfected, cells or tissues. Unfortunately, treatment of septic animals with the systemic administration of IL-10 protein has produced variable results, with most investigators unable to show any therapeutic benefit (44).

Because of the need for rapid but transient expression of the transgene, most transfection schemes have used either adenovirus or plasmid-based nonviral approaches for sepsis and acute inflammatory injury. Although it is difficult to compare results from different investigators with different vectors and delivery systems, the results have generally been positive with IL-10–based gene therapies in severe sepsis. Probably the most convincing data with systemic IL-10–based gene therapy has come from the recent studies of Kabay et al. in Turkey (45,46). These investigators used a plasmid-based approach with cationic liposomes, and demonstrated that the prior intraperitoneal injection of plasmids expressing human IL-10 could improve survival and reduce end-organ injury in a cecal ligation and puncture model of sepsis. The authors were able to demonstrate—using immunohistochemistry—human IL-10 expression in the liver, kidney, and lung following gene therapy.

We used plasmid-based IL-10 gene therapy for the treatment of experimental pancreatitis and were also able to show transient expression and improved outcomes (20,47,48). However, the data were complicated by the fact that the administration of cationic liposomes and the plasmid DNA without the transgene alone actually exacerbated the inflammatory response to pancreatitis and worsened outcome (20). In this case, expression of the IL-10 was required to dampen the inflammatory response not only to the experimental pancreatitis, but also to the administered plasmid and cationic liposomes.

During the initial studies with nonviral approaches and IL-10, we were disappointed by the low level of expression and its very transient nature (47,48). As a result, we switched early to the use of adenovirus to express the human IL-10 gene, with the idea that we could achieve therapeutic levels with the protein, with sufficiently low infection titers that would not exacerbate the already activated innate immunity. We were well aware of the studies of Doerschug et al., who had shown that administration of first-generation adenoviral recombinants during polymicrobial sepsis (cecal ligation and puncture) actually worsened survival (49). In fact, we demonstrated that the clearance of adenovirus from the lungs of mice was due to the TNF-mediated activation of innate and acquired immune processes (6). Importantly, expression of IL-10 reduced the inflammatory response to the adenovirus and prolonged expression (6,50).

In our initial studies, we administered first-generation adenoviral recombinants to mice intravenously prior to the induction of sepsis by either a cecal ligation and puncture or zymosan administration (51,52). In both cases, transfection occurred primarily in the liver and resulted in high circulating levels of human IL-10 (ng/mL). Although we did not see a worsening in outcome as was reported by Doerschug et al. (49), we did not see any improvements in outcome either, despite good expression of the transgene. The studies suggested to us that the systemic expression of IL-10 following the intravenous administration of the viral vector would be ineffective, similar to the systemic administration of the protein, as reported by Remick et al. (44).

We were surprised, however, when we saw that the compartmentalized expression of the IL-10 adenoviral vector was beneficial in both experimental models. Interestingly, the intratracheal administration of adenovirus expressing human or viral IL-10 improved outcome in the zymosan model of acute lung injury and multiorgan failure (51). Interestingly, better effects were seen with viral IL-10 expression, which appeared to be more tissue-associated than in the systemic circulation (50), and the beneficial effects of human IL-10 expression were strongly dose dependent (51,53). Actually, higher doses of adenovirus administered intratracheally and producing systemic concentrations of protein were frequently less effective than lower doses producing only local expression (53). Interestingly, the adenovirus also had to be administered prior to the inflammatory stimulus; once the process was ongoing, gene therapy was ineffective (51).

Also exciting was the observation that when very small quantities of adenovirus expressing human IL-10 were injected either subcutaneously into the footpad of mice or directly into the thymus, outcome from a cecal ligation and puncture-induced sepsis was markedly improved (52,54). Subsequent studies revealed that this compartmentalized administration of the adenoviral vector resulted in the transfection and expression of IL-10 by primarily dendritic cells (54,55). In the case of footpad injections, these IL-10 expressing dendritic cells then migrated to the draining lymph nodes where they expressed the protein in the context of class II expression and antigen presentation (Fig. 52.2). In these studies, we learned that autocrine production of IL-10 created a novel dendritic cell that had a phenotype consistent with an immature, tolerant, regulatory dendritic cell (56). Surprisingly, we subsequently showed that we could *ex vivo* transfect myeloid dendritic cells with this adenoviral recombinant expressing IL-10, and when they were reintroduced into a mouse prior to sepsis, could also improve outcome (56). Although the mechanism of protection is still unknown, it is speculated that this novel dendritic cell population expressing IL-10 may have fostered the expansion of regulatory T cells with the capacity of reducing the magnitude of the inflammatory response.

Although IL-10 has been the primary transgene used in models of sepsis as an anti-inflammatory agent, other approaches have been considered. As previously discussed, blocking NF-κB activation in endotoxicosis is an alternate approach aimed at preventing an exuberant inflammatory response (38); however, other approaches targeting more specific components of the injury response have been considered. For example, Weiss et al. used an adenoviral vector to delivery HSP70 into the lungs of mice following a cecal ligation and puncture (57). These investigators observed a

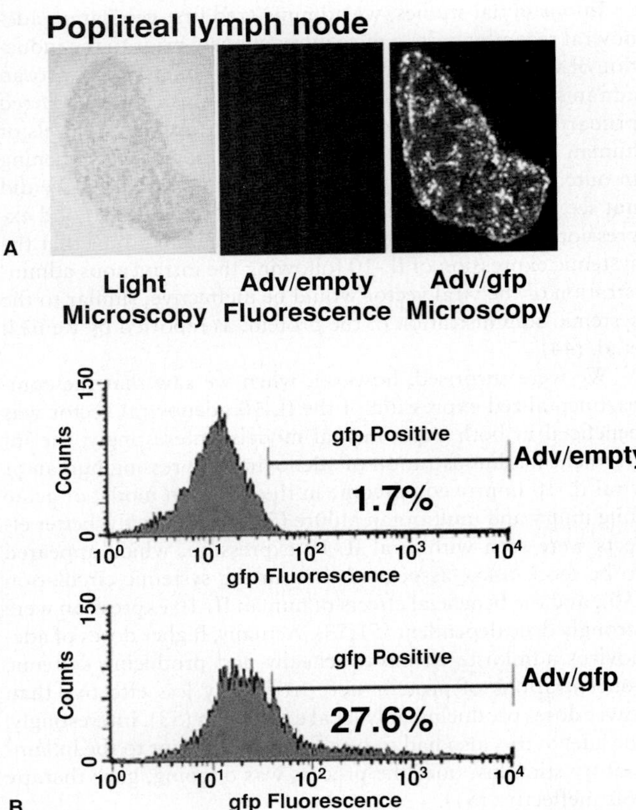

Tymus after Intrathymic Injection

C CLP + Adv/empty Fluorescence

CLP + Adv/gfp Microscopy

Light Microscopy

FIGURE 52.2. Transfection efficiency following adenoviral gene transfer. A: An empty adenoviral vector or one expressing green fluorescent protein (gfp) was injected directly into the footpad of mice. Twenty-four hours later the popliteal lymph node was removed and green fluorescence determined by microscopy. Cells transfected with the adenovirus expressing gfp could be detected in accessory cells, predominantly dendritic cells. (Reprinted from Oberholzer A, Oberholzer C, Moldawer LL. Sepsis syndromes: understanding the role of innate and acquired immunity. *Shock*. 2001;16:83, with permission.) B: The same adenoviral vectors were injected into the thymus of mice, and 24 hours later, the thymi were removed, and gfp fluorescence determined in CD11c$^+$ dendritic cells. Approximately 27% of the CD11c$^+$ dendritic cells were expressing the gfp. C: Fluorescent microscopy confirms the gfp expression in the accessory cells of thymi injected with recombinant adenovirus expressing gfp. (Reprinted with permission from Oberholzer A, Oberholzer C, Moldawer LL. Sepsis syndromes: understanding the role of innate and acquired immunity. *Shock*. 2001;16:83.)

significantly improved survival and reduced pulmonary inflammation.

Targeting the lung with adenovirus has been frequently used to deliver other therapeutic genes. Zhou et al. used adenovirus to deliver a mutant surfactant enzyme (CTP; phosphocholine cytidylyltransferase) to the lungs of mice prior to *Pseudomonas* infection and showed improved lung function and delayed mortality (58). Similar improvements in mortality and reduced lung injury were seen by Shu et al. when adenoviral expression of β-defensin-2 was also induced prior to *Pseudomonas* pneumonia (59). In both cases, the inflammatory potential of adenovirus did not appear to exacerbate the pneumonia response. Along these same lines, Chen et al. actually used an adenovirus to deliver TNF-α to the lungs of mice after a cecal ligation and puncture, but *prior* to a secondary *Pseudomonas* pneumonia (60). They hypothesized that the bacterial peritonitis might produce a defect in the pulmonary TNF response to the *Pseudomonas*, and adenoviral expression of TNF-α would improve host responses and outcome.

THE FUTURE OF GENE THERAPY FOR CRITICAL ILLNESS

Gene therapy for critical illness remains an elusive target in the future. There has been considerable progress made using gene therapy for the correction of inherited genetic disorders, and the possibility of cures for primary combined immunodeficiency, cystic fibrosis, α_1-antitrypsin deficiency, Pompe disease, and other genetic diseases are on the horizon (Table 52.2). In contrast, progress as a drug (protein) delivery system for acute illnesses remains a considerable challenge. Limitations are primarily centered on optimizing the vector and promoter, which must still undergo further refinements to yield a delivery system that is rapid, transient, tissue specific, and safe, and one that does not exacerbate activated inflammatory and innate immune systems. Although adenovirus and plasmid-based delivery systems are most frequently used today, both have significant limitations in their current iterations.

In addition, there is little consensus about the optimal gene target to express, as critical illness, sepsis, trauma, and shock simultaneously affect a large number of immune and somatic cell systems, including innate and acquired immunity, thrombosis, fibrinolysis, acute phase, and neuron–endocrine, endocrine, and renal systems. Most approaches to date have been focused on either the global inflammatory response, the interaction between innate and acquired immunity, or specific lung functions. Whether a global approach will be superior to targeting specific components of the response in critical illness is still unproven.

FUTURE GOALS

Gene therapy remains an exciting and potentially important approach for the treatment of critically ill patients. It is unlikely that gene therapy will ever replace protein or small-molecule therapeutics, but because of its potential specificity and the ability to manipulate expression over extended periods of time, gene therapy remains an attractive but elusive goal for the treatment of the critically ill patient.

TABLE 52.2

ANNOTATED SUMMARY OF STUDIES USING GENE THERAPY IN MODELS OF CRITICAL ILLNESS

Investigators	Vector and mode of delivery	Experimental model	General results
Rogy et al., 1995[a]	Plasmid-based human IL-10, IP injection	Endotoxicosis	Improved survival, reduced TNF-α
Drazan et al. 1996[b]	Adenoviral viral IL-10, IP injection	Endotoxicosis	Reduced TNF-α and IL-1β; no impact on IL-6
Xing et al., 1996[c]	Adenoviral murine IL-10, IM injection	Endotoxicosis	Reduced TNF-α and IL-6
Baumhofer et al., 1998[d]	Plasmid-based human IL-4 and IL-13, IP injection	Endotoxicosis	Improved survival, reduced TNF-α, decreased peritoneal macrophage function
Denham et al., 1998[e]	Plasmid-based human IL-10, IP injection	Pancreatitis	Improved histologic findings
Chen et al., 2000[f]	Adenoviral TNF-α, IT injection	Cecal ligation and puncture, Pseudomonal acute lung injury	Improvement in pulmonary function, improved survival
Dokka et al., 2000[g]	Cytomegaloviral murine IL-10, IT injection	Endotoxicosis	Reduced lung inflammation
Minter et al., 2000[h]	Adenoviral human IL-10, IT, IV injection	Multisystem organ failure and pancreatitis	Attenuated inflammatory response, improved survival in multisystem organ failure when given IV
Norman et al., 2000[i]	Cationic liposomal plasmid DNA, IP injection	Pancreatitis	Increased severity and mortality in pancreatitis
Oberholzer et al., 2001[j]	Adenoviral human IL-10, intrathymic and IV injection	Cecal ligation and puncture	Decreased inflammation, improved survival with intrathymic injection
Doerschug et al., 2002[k]	First- and second-generation adenoviral vectors, IV injection	Cecal ligation and puncture	Decreased survival when first-generation vectors used
Oberholzer et al., 2002[l]	Adenoviral human IL-10, SQ injection	Cecal ligation and puncture	Dose-dependent improvement in survival
Weiss et al., 2002[m]	Adenoviral heat shock protein, IT injection	Cecal ligation and puncture	Improvement in survival, improvement in pulmonary function
Chen et al., 1999[n]	Plasmid-based TFPI–CD4–P-selectin and hirudin–CD4–P-selectin, IV injection	Endotoxicosis	Reduced intravascular thrombosis and consumptive coagulopathy
Alexander et al., 2004[o]	Cytomegaloviral murine BPI, IP injection	Endotoxicosis	Reduced TNF-α and MIP-2, improved survival
Matsuda et al., 2004[p]	NF-κB decoy oligonucleotide, IV injection	Endotoxicosis	Reduced lung inflammation, blood gas improvement
Fang et al., 2005[q]	Cationic liposomal SOCS3, IP injection	Endotoxicosis	Reduced TNF-α, improved survival
Fejer et al., 2005[r]	Adenoviral deletion mutants and UV inactivated adenovirus, IP and IV injection	Endotoxicosis	Synergistic increase in TNF-α and NO production, decreased survival
Nakamura et al., 2005[s]	Adenoviral β_2-adrenoceptor, SQ injection	Endotoxicosis	Diminished reduction in renal function
Kabay et al., 2006[t]	Plasmid-based human IL-10, IP injection	Cecal ligation and puncture	Improved survival
McAuliffe et al., 2006[u]	Adenoviral human and viral IL-10, inhalation	Acute lung injury, multisystem organ failure	Dose-dependent worsening of inflammation and survival

(*Continued*)

TABLE 52.2

(*Continued*)

Investigators	Vector and mode of delivery	Experimental model	General results
Shu et al., 2006[v]	Adenoviral β-defensin-2, intranasal	Pseudomonal acute lung injury	Improvement in pulmonary function, delayed mortality
Zhou et al., 2006[w]	Adenoviral CTP: phosphocholine cytidylyltransferase, IT injection	Pseudomonal acute lung injury	Improvement in pulmonary function, delayed mortality

IL, interleukin; IP, intraperitoneal; TNF, tumor necrosis factor; IM, intramuscular; IT, intratracheal; IV, intravenous; SQ, subcutaneous; TFPI, tissue factor pathway inhibitor; BPI, bactericidal/permeability-increasing protein; MIP, macrophage inflammatory protein; NF, nuclear factor; SOCS, suppressor of cytokine signaling; NO, nitric oxide.

Data from:

[a] *J Exp Med.* 1995;181(6):2289–2293.
[b] *J Pediatr Surg.* 1996;31(3):411–414.
[c] *J Leukoc Biol.* 1996;59(4):481–488.
[d] *Eur J Immunol.* 1998;28(2):610–615.
[e] *J Gastrointest Surg.* 1998;2(1):95–101.
[f] *J Immunol.* 2000;165(11):6496–6503.
[g] *Am J Physiol Lung Cell Mol Physiol.* 2000;279(5):L872–877.
[h] *J Immunol.* 2000;164(1):443–451.
[i] *Gene Ther.* 2000;7(16):1425–1430.
[j] *Proc Natl Acad Sci U S A.* 2001;98(20):11503–11508.
[k] *J Immunol.* 2002;169(11):6539–6545.
[l] *J Immunol.* 2002;168(7):3412–3418.
[m] *J Clin Invest.* 2002;110(6):801–806.
[n] *Transplantation.* 1999;68(6):832–839.
[o] *Blood.* 2004;103(1):93–99.
[p] *Mol Pharmacol.* 2005;67(4):1018–1025.
[q] *Cell Mol Immunol.* 2005;2(5):373–377.
[r] *J Immunol.* 2005;175(3):1498–1506.
[s] *Clin Sci (Lond).* 2005;109(6):503–511.
[t] *World J Surg.* 2007;31(1):105–115.
[u] *Gene Ther.* 2006;13(3):276–282.
[v] *Shock.* 2006;26(4):365–371.
[w] *Gene Ther.* 2006;13(12):974–985.

References

1. Rubanyi GM. The future of human gene therapy. *Mol Aspects Med.* 2001; 22:113.
2. Riedl MA, Casillas AM. Adverse drug reactions: types and treatment options. *Am Fam Physician.* 2003;68:1781.
3. Anderson WF. Human gene therapy. *Nature.* 1998;392:25.
4. *Vectors Used in Gene Therapy Clinical Trials.* Vol. 2006.
5. McConnell MJ, Imperiale MJ. Biology of adenovirus and its use as a vector for gene therapy. *Hum Gene Ther.* 2004;15:1022.
6. Minter RM, Rectenwald JE, Fukuzuka K, et al. TNF-alpha receptor signaling and IL-10 gene therapy regulate the innate and humoral immune responses to recombinant adenovirus in the lung. *J Immunol.* 2000;164:443.
7. Oberholzer C, Oberholzer A, Tschoeke SK, et al. Influence of recombinant adenovirus on liver injury in endotoxicosis and its modulation by IL-10 expression. *J Endotoxin Res.* 2004;10:393.
8. Marshall E. Gene therapy death prompts review of adenovirus vector. *Science.* 1999;286:2244.
9. Ritter T, Lehmann M, Volk HD. Improvements in gene therapy: averting the immune response to adenoviral vectors. *Biodrugs.* 2002;16:3.
10. Kochanek S, Schiedner G, Volpers C. High-capacity 'gutless' adenoviral vectors. *Curr Opin Mol Ther.* 2001;3:454.
11. Baum C, Schambach A, Bohne J, et al. Retrovirus vectors: toward the plentivirus? *Mol Ther.* 2006;13:1050.
12. Nabel EG, Nabel GJ. Complex models for the study of gene function in cardiovascular biology. *Annu Rev Physiol.* 1994;56:741.
13. Marshall E. Gene therapy. Second child in French trial is found to have leukemia. *Science.* 2003;299:320.
14. Flotte TR. AAV-based gene therapy for inherited disorders. *Pediatr Res.* 2005;58:1143.
15. Monahan PE, Samulski RJ. AAV vectors: is clinical success on the horizon? *Gene Ther.* 2000;7:24.
16. Le Bec C, Douar AM. Gene therapy progress and prospects–vectorology: design and production of expression cassettes in AAV vectors. *Gene Ther.* 2006; 13:805.
17. Bhargava PM, Shanmugam G. Uptake of nonviral nucleic acids by mammalian cells. *Prog Nucleic Acid Res Mol Biol.* 1971;11:103.
18. Conwell CC, Huang L. Recent advances in non-viral gene delivery. *Adv Genet.* 2005;53:3.
19. Zhao H, Hemmi H, Akira S, et al. Contribution of toll-like receptor 9 signaling to the acute inflammatory response to nonviral vectors. *Mol Ther.* 2004;9:241.
20. Norman J, Denham W, Denham D, et al. Liposome-mediated, nonviral gene transfer induces a systemic inflammatory response which can exacerbate preexisting inflammation. *Gene Ther.* 2000;7:1425.
21. Wolff JA, Budker V. The mechanism of naked DNA uptake and expression. *Adv Genet.* 2005;54:3.
22. Yang NS, Burkholder J, Roberts B, et al. In vivo and in vitro gene transfer to mammalian somatic cells by particle bombardment. *Proc Natl Acad Sci U S A.* 1990;87:9568.
23. Zhang G, Gao X, Song YK, et al. Hydroporation as the mechanism of hydrodynamic delivery. *Gene Ther.* 2004;11:675.
24. Walther W, Stein U, Fichtner I, et al. Low-volume jet injection for efficient nonviral in vivo gene transfer. *Mol Biotechnol.* 2004;28:121.
25. Liu F, Heston S, Shollenberger LM, et al. Mechanism of in vivo DNA transport into cells by electroporation: electrophoresis across the plasma membrane may not be involved. *J Gene Med.* 2006;8:353.
26. Felgner PL, Gadek TR, Holm M, et al. Lipofection: a highly efficient, lipid-mediated DNA-transfection procedure. *Proc Natl Acad Sci U S A.* 1987;84: 7413.
27. Tan Y, Liu F, Li Z, et al. Sequential injection of cationic liposome and plasmid DNA effectively transfects the lung with minimal inflammatory toxicity. *Mol Ther.* 2001;3:673.
28. Liu F, Shollenberger LM, Huang L. Non-immunostimulatory nonviral vectors. *Faseb J.* 2004;18:1779.
29. Oberholzer A, Oberholzer C, Moldawer LL. Sepsis syndromes: understanding the role of innate and acquired immunity. *Shock.* 2001;16:83.
30. Efron P, Moldawer LL. Sepsis and the dendritic cell. *Shock.* 2003;20:386.

31. Rogy MA, Auffenberg T, Espat NJ, et al. Human tumor necrosis factor receptor (p55) and interleukin 10 gene transfer in the mouse reduces mortality to lethal endotoxemia and also attenuates local inflammatory responses. *J Exp Med.* 1995;181:2289.
32. Drazan KE, Wu L, Bullington D, et al. Viral IL-10 gene therapy inhibits TNF-alpha and IL-1 beta, not IL-6, in the newborn endotoxemic mouse. *J Pediatr Surg.* 1996;31:411.
33. Xing Z, Ohkawara Y, Jordana M, et al. Adenoviral vector-mediated interleukin-10 expression in vivo: intramuscular gene transfer inhibits cytokine responses in endotoxemia. *Gene Ther.* 1997;4:140.
34. Dokka S, Malanga CJ, Shi X, et al. Inhibition of endotoxin-induced lung inflammation by interleukin-10 gene transfer in mice. *Am J Physiol Lung Cell Mol Physiol.* 2000;279:L872.
35. Yamano S, Scott DE, Huang LY, et al. Protection from experimental endotoxemia by a recombinant AAV encoding interleukin 10. *J Gene Med.* 2001;3:450.
36. Baumhofer JM, Beinhauer BG, Wang JE, et al. Gene transfer with IL-4 and IL-13 improves survival in lethal endotoxemia in the mouse and ameliorates peritoneal macrophages immune competence. *Eur J Immunol.* 1998;28:610.
37. Alexander S, Bramson J, Foley R, et al. Protection from endotoxemia by adenoviral-mediated gene transfer of human bactericidal/permeability-increasing protein. *Blood.* 2004;103:93.
38. Matsuda N, Hattori Y, Takahashi Y, et al. Therapeutic effect of in vivo transfection of transcription factor decoy to NF-kappaB on septic lung in mice. *Am J Physiol Lung Cell Mol Physiol.* 2004;287:L1248.
39. Fang M, Dai H, Yu G, et al. Gene delivery of SOCS3 protects mice from lethal endotoxic shock. *Cell Mol Immunol.* 2005;2:373.
40. Nakamura A, Imaizumi A, Niimi R, et al. Adenoviral delivery of the beta2-adrenoceptor gene in sepsis: a subcutaneous approach in rat for kidney protection. *Clin Sci (Lond).* 2005;109:503.
41. Fejer G, Szalay K, Gyory I, et al. Adenovirus infection dramatically augments lipopolysaccharide-induced TNF production and sensitizes to lethal shock. *J Immunol.* 2005;175:1498.
42. Scumpia PO, Moldawer LL. Biology of interleukin-10 and its regulatory roles in sepsis syndromes. *Crit Care Med.* 2005;33:S468.
43. Oberholzer A, Oberholzer C, Moldawer LL. Interleukin-10: a complex role in the pathogenesis of sepsis syndromes and its potential as an anti-inflammatory drug. *Crit Care Med.* 2002;30:S58.
44. Remick DG, Garg SJ, Newcomb DE, et al. Exogenous interleukin-10 fails to decrease the mortality or morbidity of sepsis. *Crit Care Med.* 1998;26:895.
45. Kabay B, Kocaefe C, Baykal A, et al. 2006. Interleukin-10 gene transfer: prevention of multiple organ injury in a murine cecal ligation and puncture model of sepsis. *World J Surg.* 2007;31(1):200–209.
46. Kabay B, Kocaefe YC, Baykal A, et al. Liposome-mediated intraperitoneal interleukin 10 gene transfer increases survival in cecal litigation and puncture model of sepsis. *Shock.* 2006;26:37.
47. Denham W, Denham D, Yang J, et al. Transient human gene therapy: a novel cytokine regulatory strategy for experimental pancreatitis. *Ann Surg.* 1998;227:812.
48. Denham W, Yang J, MacKay S, et al. Cationic liposome-mediated gene transfer during acute pancreatitis: tissue specificity, duration, and effects of acute inflammation. *J Gastrointest Surg.* 1998;2:95.
49. Doerschug K, Sanlioglu S, Flaherty DM, et al. First-generation adenovirus vectors shorten survival time in a murine model of sepsis. *J Immunol.* 2002;169:6539.
50. Minter RM, Ferry MA, Rectenwald JE, et al. Extended lung expression and increased tissue localization of viral IL-10 with adenoviral gene therapy. *Proc Natl Acad Sci U S A.* 2001;98:277.
51. Minter RM, Ferry MA, Murday ME, et al. Adenoviral delivery of human and viral IL-10 in murine sepsis. *J Immunol.* 2001;167:1053.
52. Oberholzer C, Oberholzer A, Bahjat FR, et al. Targeted adenovirus-induced expression of IL-10 decreases thymic apoptosis and improves survival in murine sepsis. *Proc Natl Acad Sci U S A.* 2001;98:11503.
53. McAuliffe PF, Murday ME, Efron PA, et al. Dose-dependent improvements in outcome with adenoviral expression of interleukin-10 in a murine model of multisystem organ failure. *Gene Ther.* 2006;13:276.
54. Oberholzer A, Oberholzer C, Bahjat KS, et al. Increased survival in sepsis by in vivo adenovirus-induced expression of IL-10 in dendritic cells. *J Immunol.* 2002;168:3412.
55. Oberholzer C, Tschoeke SK, Bahjat K, et al. In vivo transduction of thymic dendritic cells with adenovirus and its potential use in acute inflammatory diseases. *Scand J Immunol.* 2005;61:309.
56. Oberholzer A, Oberholzer C, Efron PA, et al. Functional modification of dendritic cells with recombinant adenovirus encoding interleukin 10 for the treatment of sepsis. *Shock.* 2005;23:507.
57. Weiss YG, Maloyan A, Tazelaar J, et al. Adenoviral transfer of HSP-70 into pulmonary epithelium ameliorates experimental acute respiratory distress syndrome. *J Clin Invest.* 2002;110:801.
58. Zhou J, Wu Y, Henderson F, et al. Adenoviral gene transfer of a mutant surfactant enzyme ameliorates pseudomonas-induced lung injury. *Gene Ther.* 2006;13:974.
59. Shu Q, Shi Z, Zhao Z, et al. Protection against Pseudomonas aeruginosa pneumonia and sepsis-induced lung injury by overexpression of beta-defensin-2 in rats. *Shock.* 2006;26:365.
60. Chen GH, Reddy RC, Newstead MW, et al. Intrapulmonary TNF gene therapy reverses sepsis-induced suppression of lung antibacterial host defense. *J Immunol.* 2000;165:6496.

CHAPTER 53 ■ THE HOST RESPONSE TO INJURY AND CRITICAL ILLNESS

JAMIE TAYLOR • CLIFFORD S. DEUTSCHMAN

In 1794 John Hunter wrote, "There is a circumstance attending accidental injury which does not belong to disease—namely, that the injury has in all cases a tendency to produce both the disposition and the means of a cure." This first described the stress response, a biphasic physiologic response that, when uninterrupted by complications, has predictable characteristics and lasts 7 to 10 days (Fig. 53.1). When not altered by intervention or complications, the stress response is initiated by a global depression of energy expenditure and metabolism. This 24-hour phase that occurs immediately following injury is followed by a period of hypermetabolism that characteristically persists for 5 to 7 days. The driving force for this second phase appears to lie with the need to mount an immune or inflammatory response to combat infection and facilitate repair of damaged tissues. Most markers for ongoing inflammation and metabolism peak on postinjury day 2 and return to baseline around day 7. Although the intensity of the response may change or the time course may be altered by intervention, these events must take place or the organism will not survive.

It is possible for the normal stress response to be altered by coexisting disease or interrupted by adverse events such as recurrent bleeding, systemic inflammatory response syndrome (SIRS), or progression of SIRS into sepsis. The organism then may enter a state of persistent hypermetabolism. This continued inflammation has been postulated to lead to organ dysfunction and immune incompetence (Fig. 53.2). The onset of

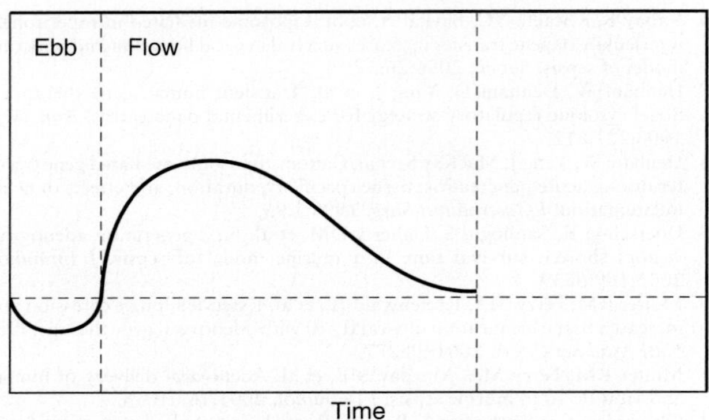

FIGURE 53.1. The stress response. (Reprinted with permission from Kohl BA, Deutschman CS. The inflammatory response to surgery and trauma. *Curr Opin Crit Care.* 2006;12(4):325–332.)

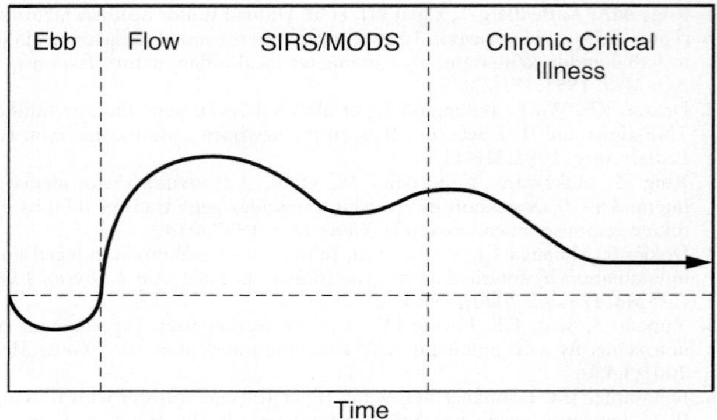

FIGURE 53.3. The onset of immune incompetence marks a transition from a hyperfunctional to a hypofunctional state in which patients are at higher risks for nosocomial infections and demonstrate a pervasive endocrinopathy. SIRS, systemic inflammatory response syndrome; MODS, multiple organ dysfunction syndrome.

immune incompetence marks a transition from a hyperfunctional to a hypofunctional state in which patients are at higher risks for nosocomial infections and demonstrate a pervasive endocrinopathy (Fig. 53.3). It is from this state that most intensive care unit (ICU) deaths occur (1).

THE NORMAL STRESS RESPONSE

David P. Cuthbertson was perhaps the first to study the host response to injury. In 1929, while working at Glasgow University, Cuthbertson was charged with the duty of investigating why fractures of the distal femur were slow to heal. He discovered that if prolonged immobilization occurred postinjury, the urinary excretion of sulphur, nitrogen, phosphorus, and calcium was elevated. As an aside to these studies, Cuthbertson noted that body temperature followed a characteristic pattern (Fig. 53.1). In the first 24 hours following the fracture, temperature decreased. Following this period, temperature rose, peaking on postinjury day 3 and returning to baseline by postinjury day 7. He correlated this change in temperature with alterations in oxygen consumption and carbon dioxide production. Further, he noted that the sulphur : nitrogen ratio closely matched that of muscle. This led to Cuthbertson's proposal of a paradigm by which the body responded to injury. If the damage to the patient is not immediately fatal, there is a compensatory reaction in which vasoconstriction shunts blood away from the periphery and to the central organs, most notably the heart and brain. This promotes short-term survival. Hypothermia and oliguria are associated with a global decrease in oxygen consumption and energy expenditure. In an effort to expand plasma volume and avoid failed oxygen delivery, the body conserves salt and water by increasing aldosterone secretion (2). These effects are seen throughout the body in the first 24 hours after injury. Cuthbertson termed this sequence of events the "ebb" phase or traumatic shock. When it becomes clear that death is not imminent, a second aspect of the response emerges. The key to these reactions is an attempt to repair tissue damage, a process that is accomplished via the activity of white blood cells (WBCs). Slowed circulation in the ebb phase allows WBCs to move toward the periphery and adhere to the endothelium. Neutrophils react first, with macrophages following. With restoration of the circulation, the process becomes active. It is characterized by phagocytosis and lysis of bacterial, viral, or fungal invaders and removal of cellular debris. In addition, macrophages, lymphocytes, and antigen-presenting cells (APCs) secrete proteins called cytokines. To a great extent, these are growth factors that facilitate repair of damaged tissue. This process requires enormous amounts of energy, with a 2- to 20-fold increase in oxygen consumption and resting energy expenditure (REE). Body temperature rises and oxygen consumption and carbon dioxide production increase (2,3). Monk et al. showed an increase in REE of up to 55% above predicted in trauma patients (4). Some studies suggest that survival is dependent on this ability to maintain hypermetabolism and adequate oxygen utilization (3,5–8). Because WBCs are more or less obligate glucose users, there is an associated increase in glucose requirements (9). After the first 24 hours, hepatic glycogen stores are depleted and a source of *de novo* glucose is required. This is generated by hepatic gluconeogenesis. Cuthbertson proposed that the body was able to provide its own source of nutrients by breaking down protein, a theory that has since been validated. This provides substrate for gluconeogenesis and constituent amino acids for synthesis of hepatic proteins and repair in the area of injury. However, adequate mobilization is not enough to ensure substrate delivery. Therefore, the response includes

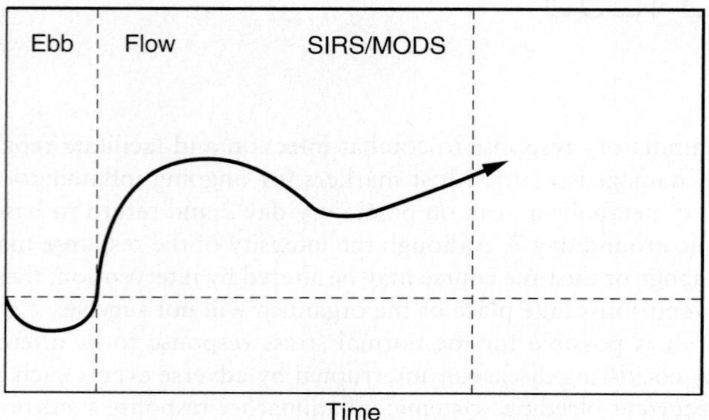

FIGURE 53.2. Continued inflammation, which has been postulated to lead to organ dysfunction and immune incompetence. SIRS, systemic inflammatory response syndrome; MODS, multiple organ dysfunction syndrome.

capillary dilatation to increase flow and improve delivery. Unfortunately, due to thrombosis in damaged tissue, most injured areas are avascular. To allow substrate delivery to these regions, capillary tight junctions separate, allowing fluid and substrate to "leak" from the vasculature. Increased vascular permeability results in redistribution of extracellular fluid and plasma proteins to form edema and exudate (10). Glucose and other nutrients move down their concentration gradients across the extracellular matrix to areas of damage. Removal of waste requires an increase in renal blood flow and glomerular filtration to enable excretion of amino acid degradation products. The liver detoxifies nitrogenous wastes by the production of urea; metabolizes alanine, lactate, and glycerol through gluconeogenesis; and produces acute-phase proteins that bind metabolic by-products and limit the activity of proteolytic enzymes secreted by activated WBCs (1). Because this process increases delivery to nearly every part of the body, Cuthbertson termed this part of the response the "flow" phase.

Work by Cuthbertson and Francis C. Moore demonstrated that initiation of the flow phase is in part hormonally modulated. An initial dramatic release of endogenous catecholamines (11) is supplemented by alterations in the somatotropic system (growth hormone and insulinlike growth factor) such that anabolism is postponed and energy substrates are redirected to vital organs. Both the thyroid and the gonadal axes are suppressed. Adrenocorticotropin hormone (ACTH) secretion is heightened by increased corticotropin-releasing hormone (CRH), arginine vasopressin (AVP), catecholamines, angiotensin II, serotonin, and some inflammatory cytokines (interleukin [IL]-1, IL-2, IL-6, and tumor necrosis factor [TNF]). ACTH stimulates the adrenal glands to produce glucocorticoids and mineralocorticoids. Glucocorticoids and glucagon promote glucogenesis and glycogenolysis and induce peripheral insulin resistance, leading to increased glucose production (12). This in turn increases insulin secretion, producing an "insulin-resistant" state.

Tissue repair is initiated by these activities. Traumatized tissue and hemorrhage initiate platelet accumulation and activation. The coagulation cascade is triggered by both the intrinsic and extrinsic pathways. This serves to sustain and enhance immune cell migration and activation. In addition, fibroblasts at the edge of the wound divide, migrate toward the center, and produce collagen. Surviving capillaries bud, and these new capillaries also migrate toward the center. Eventually the wound edges will fuse and consist of vascularized granulation tissue (13). This process is thought to be mediated by an increase in fibroblast growth factors, epidermal growth factor, platelet-derived growth factor, and vascular endothelial growth factor (14).

This massive mobilization of defense mechanisms may also affect normal tissue. Therefore, one of the most important characteristics of the normal stress response is that it is a balance between the inflammatory and the anti-inflammatory systems. This involves the proinflammatory cytokine TNF, released by the activated macrophage. When TNF "spills over" from the interstitium into the bloodstream, it stimulates the medullary reticular formation and the hypothalamus in the brain. This activation of the hypothalamic-pituitary-adrenal axis ultimately causes increased anti-inflammatory activity. For example, glucocorticoids released as a result of this process limit the negative biologic consequences caused by inflammation (15). TNF also stimulates the dorsal vagal complex and alters the efferent vagal output. This is in part responsible for "sickness" behavior (i.e., anorexia and fever) (16–18). More importantly, however, is neuromodulation of the immune response. The "inflammatory reflex" or the cholinergic anti-inflammatory pathway occurs when proinflammatory cytokines such as IL-1 and TNF stimulate the parasympathetic nervous system through receptors on the vagus nerve. The afferent input travels to the nucleus solitarius and is relayed to the dorsal motor nucleus, resulting in an increase in acetylcholine release at cholinergic nerve terminals in the areas of inflammation. Activated macrophages have acetylcholine receptors that, when stimulated, decrease the release of proinflammatory cytokines (19,20). This balance of the systems is crucial in limiting the stress response.

Moore et al. also observed changes in the size of body fluid compartments. In a normal stress response, catabolism is accompanied by an increase in the vascular space (recruitment); expansion of the extravascular, extracellular space; and a decrease in the intracellular compartment. This process ends 4 to 5 days after injury with a shift to anabolism (11). The vasculature contracts, fluid is removed from the extracellular space and either moves back into cells or is excreted by the kidneys, and the intracellular shift is accompanied by an influx of protein and electrolytes. While the physiologic "signal" that initiates this transition is still unknown, it is telling that the transition occurs at the completion of the first wave of angiogenesis. The generation of a new vascular highway obviates the need for nutrient concentration gradients, increased vascular permeability, and water and electrolyte conservation. Conservation of salt and water is no longer a priority and a brisk diuresis results. In addition, as the intracellular space expands, increases in intracellular anions and cations are required. These must come from the vascular space. Therefore, resolution of catabolism is accompanied by decreases in serum levels of potassium, magnesium, and phosphate ions and, therefore, diuresis and decreases in serum electrolytes are the hallmarks of resolution of the stress response.

The cellular immune response to normal inflammatory stimuli involves neutrophils, monocytes (macrophages), lymphocytes, and APCs. Neutrophils are recruited to areas of injury early in the process. This is stimulated in part by protein antigens and chemoattractant molecules (chemokines) released by endothelial cells and fixed tissue macrophages. Their function is removal of cellular debris by phagocytosis and secretion of lytic molecules such as digestive enzymes and free radicals. While the influx of neutrophils is self-limited, lasting about 48 hours, the rest of the response, which starts within hours of neutrophil influx, may be more persistent. It consists of infiltration by macrophages, APCs, and lymphocytes. Macrophages are of key importance in innate immunity, a process that is nonspecific and involves natural barriers such as skin, natural killer cells, and chemicals in the blood that act immediately upon antigen introduction. Macrophages respond to stimulation with phagocytosis of foreign or damaged material and secretion of cytokines that stimulate inflammation and also function as growth factors. In addition, they contribute to adaptive immunity by presenting antigens, a function that also is served by APCs. Antigen-presenting cells such as dendritic cells capture antigens, transport them to lymph nodes, and present them to T cells, initiating cell-mediated immunity. Follicular dendritic cells have a similar function except that they present antigens to B cells and therefore initiate humoral immunity. Lymphocytes are the prime components of the adaptive immune response. They have specific receptors for antigens. B cells produce antibodies and are mediators of humoral immunity. T cells recognize peptide fragments of protein antigens bound to APCs and are involved in cell-mediated immunity. T cells can be further divided into CD4 cells, which enhance or inhibit the immune response; CD8 cells, which lyse other cells with intracellular pathogens; and natural killer (NK) cells, which do not express antigen receptors and contribute to innate immunity.

Adaptive immunity is antigen specific and can be divided into five phases. The first phase is presentation of the antigen to a B or T cell by an APC. In the second phase, B and T cells are activated, undergoing clonal expansion, differentiation, and antibody production. Antigens are eliminated in the third or effector phase. Decline is the fourth phase: The stimulus has been removed and there is apoptosis of immune cells and phagocytosis of cellular debris. The last phase involves the surviving immune cells acquiring memory (21). As the process proceeds, there is a change in the phenotype of CD4 T cells that is profoundly important. The catabolic phase of inflammation is characterized by an abundance of CD4 cells of the type 1 helper T cell (Th1) phenotype. This results in secretion of proinflammatory cytokines such as IL-2, TNF-α, and interferon-γ. The switch to anabolism is accompanied by a predominance of type 2 helper T cells (Th2), which secrete anti-inflammatory cytokines such as IL-4 and IL-10. In a normal stress response, immune function declines and the transition from Th1 to Th2 occurs by the fourth or fifth day. The switch from Th1 to Th2 may be hormonally mediated. It is known that cortisol and androgens, which are secreted in great quantities in catabolism, stimulate Th2 cell production.

One clinical manifestation of this is in the blood. That is, early in the response there is a mixed leukocytosis with neutrophil predominance. This gives way to a macrophage/lymphocyte-rich pattern and is followed by an overall decline in the white blood cell count.

DEVIATION FROM THE NORMAL STRESS RESPONSE

The stress response is considered to be adaptive and vital in order to survive an injury. However, many aspects of the process may become excessive or unbalanced. This converts an adaptive response into a pathologic one. Risk factors that predispose to the development of an abnormal response include inadequate or delayed resuscitation, persistent inflammatory or infectious sources, baseline organ dysfunction, age older than 65 years, immunosuppression, alcohol abuse, malnutrition, and invasive instrumentation (22). There are two such common occurrences in the surgical or trauma population. The first is hemorrhage, uncorrected fluid loss, or underresuscitation. These result in a recurrence of shock, with vasoconstriction, decreased perfusion and cardiac output, and impaired tissue substrate delivery. The treatment is identification and treatment of the underlying cause accompanied by correction of the fluid imbalance.

The second common abnormality is prolonged hypermetabolism. Persistence of a hyperdynamic circulation and secretion of immunologic markers; elevations of serum potassium, magnesium, and phosphate; and/or marginal urine output indicate a prolonged or renewed stress response and warn of a new or recurrent abnormality. This state commonly is referred to as systemic inflammatory response syndrome. If SIRS is suspected to be from an infectious cause, then the condition is referred to as sepsis or the sepsis syndrome. Initially, the normal stress response, SIRS, and sepsis may mimic each other. Differentiation lies in the time course and in the etiology of the metabolic perturbations. The definitions of SIRS, sepsis, and severe sepsis, as formulated in 2001, are detailed in Table 53.1.

Sepsis is the most common cause of death in noncardiac intensive care units. The increasing use of broad-spectrum antibiotics, immunosuppression therapy, and invasive technology may be responsible (23). Recent studies estimate the incidence of sepsis in the United States as 240 to 300 cases of severe sepsis per 100,000 people, an increase from 74 cases per 100,000 people in 1979. The mortality rate ranges from 17.9% for sepsis, 28.6% for severe sepsis, and up to 50% in those with septic

TABLE 53.1

DIAGNOSTIC CRITERIA FOR SEPSIS IN ADULTS

SUSPECTED OR DOCUMENTED INFECTION
General variables
Fever (T >38.3°C)
Hypothermia (T <36°C)
Heart rate (>90 bpm or >2 SDs above normal for age)
Tachypnea
Altered mental status
Edema or positive fluid balance (>20 mL/kg over 24 h)
Hyperglycemia (plasma glucose >120 mg/dL or 7.7 mmol/L) without DM
Inflammatory variables
Leukocytosis (WBC >12,000/μL)
Leukopenia (WBC <4,000/μL)
Normal WBC count with >10% immature forms
Plasma C-reactive protein >2 SDs above the normal value
Plasma procalcitonin >2 SDs above the normal value
Hemodynamic variables
Arterial hypotension (SBP <90 mm Hg, MAP <70 or SBP ↓ >40 mm Hg or <2 SDs below normal)
SvO_2 >70%
Cardiac index >3.5 L/min/m^2
Organ dysfunction variables
Arterial hypoxemia (PaO_2/FiO_2 <300)
Acute oliguria (urine output <0.5 mL/kg/h for at least 2 h)
Creatinine increase >0.5 mg/dL
Coagulation abnormalities (INR >1.5 or aPTT >60 s)
Ileus
Thrombocytopenia (platelets <100,000/μL)
Hyperbilirubinemia (plasma total bilirubin >4 mg/dL or 70 mmol/L)
Tissue perfusion variables
Hyperlactatemia (>1 mmol/L)
Decreased capillary refill or mottling

T, temperature; SDs, standard deviations; DM, diabetes mellitus; WBC, white blood cell; SBP, systolic blood pressure; MAP, mean arterial pressure; SvO_2, mixed venous saturation; PaO_2, arterial partial pressure of oxygen; FiO_2, fraction of inspired oxygen; INR, international normalized ratio; aPTT, activated partial thromboplastin time.
From Levy MM, et al. 2001 SCCM/ESICM/ACCP/ATS/SIS international sepsis definitions conference. *Crit Care Med.* 2003;31(4): 1250–1256.

shock and comorbid conditions. The etiology of sepsis has also changed over time. In the 1970s and 1980s, Gram-negative bacteria were the predominant cause of sepsis. Gram-positive organisms are now the leading pathogens, with fungal organisms on the rise (24).

Sepsis likely predisposes to organ dysfunction. When this dysfunction is overt, the process is referred to as multiple organ dysfunction syndrome (MODS). However, abnormalities in MODS seem to be confined to cellular and organ dysfunction as histology and infrastructure are preserved. The most proximal defect that has been identified to date in SIRS/sepsis/MODS is an abnormality of oxygen utilization at the subcellular level. Two theories to explain this have been advanced. The first is that there is an impairment of microcirculatory autoregulation. Vasodilation of some vascular beds coexists with vasoconstriction of others, causing a maldistribution of flow and, therefore, oxygen (25). The second theory assumes adequate perfusion but an alteration in cellular metabolism with an inability to extract and use oxygen (26). This is supported by recent studies demonstrating a defect in mitochondrial function (27–29). In either case, the result is a block in cellular metabolism. As a result, the ability of cells and organs to respond to external stimuli may be lost. For example, there is a progressive loss of hormonal responsiveness. The liver becomes unresponsive to insulin and glucagons and the cardiovascular system to catecholamines (30–32). As such, the hyperfunctional state cannot be maintained. It has been proposed that cells enter a "preservation mode" in which viability is maintained but the capacity to communicate with each other is lost. Cellular interaction is lost and thus organ function is compromised (33–35). Acute lung injury (ALI) progresses to acute respiratory distress syndrome (ARDS) and hypotension from vasoplegia is compounded by cardiac dysfunction that requires vasopressors and inotropic and chronotropic support. Renal function decreases to a point that renal replacement therapy must be considered and hepatic dysfunction results in severe ascites and coagulopathy, both having the potential to lead to a profound encephalopathy. The immune system is one of the most important systems to be affected. The development of immune incompetence coupled with a pervasive endocrinopathy places the patient at a higher risk for nosocomial infections, and it is in this state that most deaths from sepsis occur.

The issue of immune incompetence requires further discussion. Historically, sepsis has been viewed as a condition ruled by uncontrolled inflammation. However, an increasing number of studies indicate that sepsis is in fact a state of inflammatory failure (36–39). More specifically, sepsis is associated with an alteration in the adaptive immune response (40). The early phase of sepsis resembles normal stress in that there is a hormonal milieu that stimulates Th2 responses and these responses are observed. Indeed, studies have shown that patients with sepsis have increased Th2 cells and IL-10 and that these levels predict mortality (41,42). However, as sepsis progresses, there is a profound endocrinopathy and progressive anergy (12). That is, chronic critical illness is associated with a loss of T-cell responsiveness on any level (43). This may reflect enhanced lymphocyte apoptosis (44–46). Hotchkiss et al. also demonstrated that there were decreased levels of follicular dendritic cells, B cells, and CD4 T cells at the time of death of septic patients, resulting in impaired antigen presentation, antibody production, and B-cell and macrophage stimulation (44–46). The ultimate result of immunosuppression is the development of sequential infections, often invoking the decision to withdraw therapy.

One major contributor to the development of complications from inflammation is the presence of comorbidities. Chronic comorbid conditions are present in over 50% of patients with sepsis and are associated with an increase in mortality (47–49). Diseases reported to increase the risk of the normal stress response developing into sepsis are diabetes mellitus (DM), human immunodeficiency virus (HIV), chronic liver disease, and cancer (47). Esper et al. conducted a historical cohort study that reviewed patients with the diagnosis of sepsis in U.S. acute care hospitals from 1979 to 2003, characterizing the type and source of infections and comorbid diseases. They found that men were more likely than women and African Americans were more likely than Caucasians to develop sepsis. Non-Caucasian patients who were septic were more likely to have concomitant DM, HIV, chronic renal failure, and alcohol abuse. Caucasians had higher incidences of cancer and chronic obstructive pulmonary disease (COPD). The presence of one comorbidity increased the risk of developing at least one organ system failure by 30%. Those with two comorbidities had a 39% chance and those with three or more had a 45% chance of developing acute organ failure (50).

It is not difficult to imagine how baseline insufficiencies affect the stress response. For example, the ability to maintain a circulatory system capable of providing oxygen and nutrients to areas of injury is paramount to survival. In the setting of underlying coronary artery disease (CAD), this ability may be impaired. Kern et al. (51) found that patients with CAD have a significantly decreased cardiac index and oxygen delivery and, not surprisingly, an increased oxygen extraction ratio during sepsis. They also showed that these patients had increased endothelial adhesion molecule expression, which may correlate with the severity of sepsis, shock, and organ failure and predict poor outcome (52,53). Chronic pulmonary disease, regardless of the etiology, increases the chance of intubation and the requirement for prolonged ventilatory support. Intubation places the patient at risk for ventilator-associated pneumonia, aspiration, and respiratory muscle atrophy. A patient with chronic renal or liver failure is at risk for anemia, coagulopathies, and immunosuppression prior to being injured. With an impaired functional reserve in vital organs and responses, the stress response to injury has a high likelihood of progressing to a state of prolonged critical illness.

TREATMENT OR PREVENTION

It is logical that treatment of pre-existing disorders and comorbidities will alter the stress response. Indeed, a number of studies have examined the role of perioperative β-blockade and concluded that, in appropriate patients, outcome is improved. More problematic are attempts to alter the course of the prolonged state that constitutes SIRS, sepsis, MODS, and chronic critical illness. Despite promising animal data, most approaches have failed in patients. The successes are notable. Herndon et al. showed that in the pediatric burn population, resting energy expenditure decreased and net muscle protein balance increased with administration of propranolol. However, there have been several experiments conducted with mice in septic or hemorrhagic shock showing an increase in mortality from immunosuppression after β-blockade (54,55).

Adequate analgesia via epidural and intravenous use of agents such as opiates, α-blockers, nonsteroidal anti-inflammatory drugs, and local anesthetics have been shown to both decrease inflammation and improve immune function (56–59). Early goal-directed resuscitation has been shown to improve outcome in a single-center trial (60). A multicenter trial in the United States is beginning. Similarly, a protocol using insulin infusions to maintain serum glucose levels between 80 and 110 mg/dL has been shown to reduce mortality and complications in a surgical ICU in a single institution (61). However, similar results were not observed in the medical ICU in the same institution (62) or in an as yet unpublished multicenter European trial (GLUCONTROL, confirmed by personal communication). The benefit of insulin appeared to be confined to patients in the ICU for more than 3 to 5 days. This would suggest that insulin is one of many hormones that become ineffective in chronic critical illness.

SUMMARY

Injury is present in the form of elective surgery, trauma, infection, and medical illnesses such as pancreatitis. It is crucial for the clinician to understand the underlying course of events that comprise the stress response. This enables the detection of deviations from normal physiology. Although intervention may be useful in reducing the extremes of the stress response and limiting the untoward impact of comorbidities, balance is the hallmark of a normal response. Pre-existing disease and persistent hypermetabolism offset this balance and pathologic conditions prevail. Both anti-inflammatory and inflammatory strategies may offer therapeutic benefit to attenuating the abnormalities, but most therapy has proved disappointing.

References

1. Kohl BA, Deutschman CS. The inflammatory response to surgery and trauma. *Curr Opin Crit Care.* 2006;12(4):325–332.
2. Clowes G, et al. Energy metabolism and proteolysis in traumatized and septic man. *Surg Clin North Am.* 1976;56:1169–1184.
3. Cerra FB, et al. Correlations between metabolic and cardiopulmonary measurements in patients after trauma, general surgery, and sepsis. *J Trauma.* 1979;19(8):621–629.
4. Monk DN, et al. Sequential changes in the metabolic response in critically injured patients during the first 25 days after blunt trauma. *Ann Surg.* 1996;223(4):395–405.
5. Russell JA, et al. Oxygen delivery and consumption and ventricular preload are greater in survivors than in nonsurvivors of the adult respiratory distress syndrome. *Am Rev Respir Dis.* 1990;141(3):659–665.
6. Shoemaker WC, et al. Physiologic patterns in surviving and nonsurviving shock patients. Use of sequential cardiorespiratory variables in defining criteria for therapeutic goals and early warning of death. *Arch Surg.* 1973; 106(5):630–636.
7. Hayes MA, et al. Oxygen transport patterns in patients with sepsis syndrome or septic shock: influence of treatment and relationship to outcome. *Crit Care Med.* 1997;25(6):926–936.
8. Hayes MA, et al. Response of critically ill patients to treatment aimed at achieving supranormal oxygen delivery and consumption. Relationship to outcome. *Chest.* 1993;103(3):886–895.
9. Woolf N. *Pathology: Basic and Systemic.* Philadelphia: WB Saunders; 1998: 41–62.
10. Cuthbertson DP. Post-traumatic metabolism: a multidisciplinary challenge. *Surg Clin North Am.* 1978;58(5):1045–1054.
11. Moore F, Olsen K, McMurrey J. *The Body Cell Mass and Its Supporting Environment.* Philadelphia: WB Saunders; 1978.
12. Van den Berghe G, de Zegher F, Bouillon R. Clinical review 95: acute and prolonged critical illness as different neuroendocrine paradigms. *J Clin Endocrinol Metab.* 1998;83(6):1827–1834.
13. Hunt TK, et al. Studies on inflammation and wound healing: angiogenesis and collagen synthesis stimulated in vivo by resident and activated wound macrophages. *Surgery.* 1984;96(1):48–54.
14. Frank S, et al. Regulation of vascular endothelial growth factor expression in cultured keratinocytes. Implications for normal and impaired wound healing. *J Biol Chem.* 1995;270(21):12607–12613.
15. Landry DW, Oliver JA. The pathogenesis of vasodilatory shock. *N Engl J Med.* 2001;345(8):588–595.
16. Goehler LE, et al. Vagal immune-to-brain communication: a visceral chemosensory pathway. *Auton Neurosci.* 2000;85(1-3):49–59.
17. Hermann GE, et al. c-Fos generation in the dorsal vagal complex after systemic endotoxin is not dependent on the vagus nerve. *Am J Physiol Regul Integr Comp Physiol.* 2001;280(1):R289–299.
18. Emch GS, Hermann GE, Rogers RC. TNF-alpha activates solitary nucleus neurons responsive to gastric distension. *Am J Physiol Gastrointest Liver Physiol.* 2000;279(3):G582–586.
19. Borovikova LV, et al. Vagus nerve stimulation attenuates the systemic inflammatory response to endotoxin. *Nature.* 2000;405(6785):458–462.
20. Bernik TR, et al. Pharmacological stimulation of the cholinergic antiinflammatory pathway. *J Exp Med.* 2002;195(6):781–788.
21. Abbas AK, Lichtman AH. *Immunology: Function and Disorders of the Immune System.* 2nd ed. Philadelphia: Saunders; 2004:6–11.
22. Orbach S, Weiss Y, Deutschman CS. Care of the patient with sepsis or the systemic inflammatory response syndrome. In: Murray M, et al., eds. *Critical Care Medicine: Perioperative Management.* Philadelphia: Lippincott-Raven Publishers; 2002.
23. Levy MM, et al. 2001 SCCM/ESICM/ACCP/ATS/SIS international sepsis definitions conference. *Crit Care Med.* 2003;31(4):1250–1256.
24. Angus DC, Pereira CA, Silva E. Epidemiology of severe sepsis around the world. *Endocr Metab Immune Disord Drug Targets.* 2006;6(2):207–212.
25. Ince C, Sinaasappel M. Microcirculatory oxygenation and shunting in sepsis and shock. *Crit Care Med.* 1999;27(7):1369–1377.
26. Cerra FB. The systemic septic response: concepts of pathogenesis. *J Trauma.* 1990;30(12 Suppl):S169–174.
27. Levy RJ, et al. Competitive and noncompetitive inhibition of myocardial cytochrome C oxidase in sepsis. *Shock.* 2004;21(2):110–114.
28. Deutschman CS, Levy RJ, Weiss YG. Glutamine and heat shock proteins: one more approach to lung injury. *Crit Care Med.* 2005;33(6):1422–1424.
29. Singer M, Brealey D. Mitochondrial dysfunction in sepsis. *Biochem Soc Symp.* 1999;66:149–166.
30. Clemens MG, et al. Insulin resistance and depressed gluconeogenic capability during early hyperglycemic sepsis. *J Trauma.* 1984;24(8):701–708.
31. Deutschman CS, De Maio A, Clemens MG. Sepsis-induced attenuation of glucagon and 8-BrcAMP modulation of the phosphoenolpyruvate carboxykinase gene. *Am J Physiol.* 1995;269(3 Pt 2):R584–591.
32. Breslow MJ, et al. Effect of vasopressors on organ blood flow during endotoxin shock in pigs. *Am J Physiol.* 1987;252(2 Pt 2):H291–300.
33. Godin PJ, Buchman TG. Uncoupling of biological oscillators: a complementary hypothesis concerning the pathogenesis of multiple organ dysfunction syndrome. *Crit Care Med.* 1996;24(7):1107–1116.
34. Buchman TG. The community of the self. *Nature.* 2002;420(6912):246–251.
35. Buchman TG, et al. Complex systems analysis: a tool for shock research. *Shock.* 2001;16(4):248–251.
36. Lederer JA, Rodrick ML, Mannick JA. The effects of injury on the adaptive immune response. *Shock.* 1999;11(3):153–159.
37. Oberholzer A, Oberholzer C, Moldawer LL. Sepsis syndromes: understanding the role of innate and acquired immunity. *Shock.* 2001;16(2):83–96.
38. Ertel W, et al. Downregulation of proinflammatory cytokine release in whole blood from septic patients. *Blood.* 1995;85(5):1341–1347.
39. Venet F, et al. Both percentage of gammadelta T lymphocytes and CD3 expression are reduced during septic shock. *Crit Care Med.* 2005;33(12):2836–2840.
40. Shelley O, et al. Interaction between the innate and adaptive immune systems is required to survive sepsis and control inflammation after injury. *Shock.* 2003;20(2):123–129.
41. Opal SM, DePalo VA. Anti-inflammatory cytokines. *Chest.* 2000;117(4): 1162–1172.
42. Gogos CA, et al. Pro- versus anti-inflammatory cytokine profile in patients with severe sepsis: a marker for prognosis and future therapeutic options. *J Infect Dis.* 2000;181(1):176–180.
43. Meakins JL, et al. Delayed hypersensitivity: indicator of acquired failure of host defenses in sepsis and trauma. *Ann Surg.* 1977;186(3):241–250.
44. Hotchkiss RS, et al. Apoptotic cell death in patients with sepsis, shock, and multiple organ dysfunction. *Crit Care Med.* 1999;27(7):1230–1251.
45. Hotchkiss RS, et al. Depletion of dendritic cells, but not macrophages, in patients with sepsis. *J Immunol.* 2002;168(5):2493–2500.
46. Hotchkiss RS, et al. Sepsis-induced apoptosis causes progressive profound depletion of B and CD4+ T lymphocytes in humans. *J Immunol.* 2001;166(11):6952–6963.
47. Angus DC, et al. Epidemiology of severe sepsis in the United States: analysis of incidence, outcome, and associated costs of care. *Crit Care Med.* 2001;29(7):1303–1310.

48. Alberti C, et al. Epidemiology of sepsis and infection in ICU patients from an international multicentre cohort study. *Intensive Care Med.* 2002;28(2):108–121.
49. Martin GS, et al. The epidemiology of sepsis in the United States from 1979 through 2000. *N Engl J Med.* 2003;348(16):1546–1554.
50. Esper AM, et al. The role of infection and comorbidity: factors that influence disparities in sepsis. *Crit Care Med.* 2006;34(10):2576–2582.
51. Kern H, et al. Increased endothelial injury in septic patients with coronary artery disease. *Chest.* 2001;119(3):874–883.
52. Sessler CN, et al. Circulating ICAM-1 is increased in septic shock. *Am J Respir Crit Care Med.* 1995;151(5):1420–1427.
53. Boldt J, et al. Circulating adhesion molecules in the critically ill: a comparison between trauma and sepsis patients. *Intensive Care Med.* 1996;22(2):122–128.
54. Schmitz D, et al. beta-Adrenergic blockade during systemic inflammation: impact on cellular immune functions and survival in a murine model of sepsis. *Resuscitation.* 2007;72(2):286–294.
55. Oberbeck R, et al. Influence of beta-adrenoceptor antagonists on hemorrhage-induced cellular immune suppression. *Shock.* 2002;18(4):331–335.
56. Akural EI, et al. The effects of pre-emptive epidural sufentanil on human immune function. *Acta Anaesthesiol Scand.* 2004;48(6):750–755.
57. Wu CT, et al. The effect of epidural clonidine on perioperative cytokine response, postoperative pain, and bowel function in patients undergoing colorectal surgery. *Anesth Analg.* 2004;99(2):502–509.
58. Volk T, et al. Postoperative epidural anesthesia preserves lymphocyte, but not monocyte, immune function after major spine surgery. *Anesth Analg.* 2004;98(4):1086–1092.
59. Molina PE. Opioids and opiates: analgesia with cardiovascular, haemodynamic and immune implications in critical illness. *J Intern Med.* 2006;259(2):138–154.
60. Rivers E, et al. Early goal-directed therapy in the treatment of severe sepsis and septic shock. *N Engl J Med.* 2001;345(19):1368–1377.
61. van den Berghe G, et al. Intensive insulin therapy in the critically ill patients. *N Engl J Med.* 2001;345(19):1359–1367.
62. Van den Berghe G, et al. Intensive insulin therapy in the medical ICU. *N Engl J Med.* 2006;354(5):449–461.
63. Curi R, et al. Molecular mechanisms of glutamine action. *J Cell Physiol.* 2005;204(2):392–401.

CHAPTER 54 ■ MULTIPLE ORGAN DYSFUNCTION SYNDROME

J. MATTHIAS WALZ • STEPHEN O. HEARD

IMMEDIATE CONCERNS

Major Problems

Progressive dysfunction of multiple organ systems, culminating in the syndrome of multiple organ dysfunction syndrome (MODS), has become a leading cause of death in critically ill and injured patients. MODS is a disease of medical progress. Broader use of intensive care unit (ICU) resources, combined with improvements in single organ–directed therapy, such as mechanical ventilation and renal replacement therapy, has reduced early mortality after major physiologic insults. The result is a longer ICU stay for an increasing number of patients after severe sepsis and trauma, during which inflammation and tissue injury may result in MODS.

MODS represents a systemic disorder of immunoregulation, endothelial dysfunction, and hypermetabolism, with varying manifestations in individual organs. The mortality of MODS will increase as the number of failing organs increases, suggesting that changes in the function of all organs have equal significance in outcome. However, organs differ in their host defense functions and sensitivity to host-derived inflammatory mediators or reductions in oxygen delivery ($\dot{D}O_2$). Therefore, diagnosis and therapy focus, whenever possible, on preventive measures. Changes in the cellular oxygen (O_2) supply and metabolism may cause and complicate MODS. Consequences can include direct hypoxic organ damage, secondary ischemia/reperfusion (I/R) injury mediated by neutrophils and reactive O_2 species (ROS), and enhanced injury by activation of cytokines, including tumor necrosis factor-α (TNF-α). Initial and subsequent therapy follows a two-tiered approach, targeting systemic factors that contribute to ongoing inflammation and single organ–related problems. Efforts are first directed at stabilizing $\dot{D}O_2$ while addressing life-threatening derangements in acid-base balance and gas exchange. Prompt correction of hemodynamic instability to defined end points that correlate with resolution of tissue O_2 debt minimizes ischemia-related organ damage. The element of time is a critical factor. Delays in completing initial resuscitation, eliminating foci of infection or devitalized tissue, or treating de novo organ-specific problems such as oliguria all worsen outcome. Late-phase (e.g., over 72 hours) problems involve acquired immunosuppression, predisposition to secondary infection, and hypermetabolism, which impairs wound healing and host defense.

Initial Essential Diagnostic Tests and Procedures

Hemodynamic and Metabolic Monitoring

1. Begin assessing the adequacy of initial resuscitation efforts by noninvasive measures including skin color and temperature, arterial blood pressure, pulse rate, respiratory rate, mental status, and urine output; determine if metabolic acidosis is present from arterial blood gas and plasma bicarbonate ($NaHCO_3$) determinations. If acidosis is present, establish whether the anion gap and plasma lactate concentrations are increased.

2. Consider invasive hemodynamic monitoring by arterial and central vascular catheterization. Central venous pressure estimates right heart filling but may not accurately gauge left ventricular preload with tricuspid insufficiency, pre-existing heart disease, pulmonary hypertension, or acute respiratory distress syndrome (ARDS). Exclude myocardial infarction as a cause of hemodynamic instability by electrocardiography, creatine kinase isoenzyme, and troponin I levels.
3. Targeted hemodynamic management can be accomplished by invasive or noninvasive means (e.g., pulmonary artery catheterization, pulse contour analysis, or esophageal Doppler monitoring). Mixed or central venous O_2 saturation and lactate concentrations—if the latter are initially elevated—should be monitored to determine the adequacy of resuscitation and assist in the titration of therapy.
4. Hemodynamic instability despite adequate fluid resuscitation in patients with severe sepsis should be treated with inotropes as indicated, and the hemoglobin level should be raised to 10 mg/dL in the early stages of resuscitation according to the principles of early goal-directed therapy (EGDT).

Evaluation for Infection

1. For suspected sepsis upon ICU admission, blood cultures—including fungal cultures where appropriate—should be immediately obtained, as should Gram stains and cultures of urine, an adequate sputum specimen (where "adequate is defined by 25 or more leukocytes per low-power field") or tracheobronchial washings, and wound discharges before antimicrobial therapy. Suspicious skin lesions should undergo culture by aspiration and biopsy. On discovery of fluid collections, perform thoracentesis and paracentesis within 12 hours or less; determine pH; and perform a Gram stain, culture, cell count, cytologic studies, glucose level, and other chemistries.
2. Evaluate the patient thoroughly for all infectious and potential noninfectious etiologies of MODS.
3. For suspected nosocomial sepsis, reculture blood, urine, and sputum; evaluate all sites of vascular cannulation and remove catheters, if possible; and consider fiberoptic bronchoscopy to obtain protected brush specimen or bronchoalveolar lavage (BAL) samples in patients with pneumonia. Exclude infective endocarditis or endovascular infection by echocardiography and scintigraphic scanning for high-grade or recurrent bacteremia.
4. Serially monitor renal, pancreatic, and hepatic function; exclude acalculous cholecystitis or pancreatitis by abdominal ultrasound. Perform computed tomography of the sinuses, chest, abdomen, and pelvis when appropriate to define fluid collections.
5. Maintain a high index of suspicion for opportunistic fungal infection with *Candida* sp. despite negative results on blood culture.

Initial Therapy

1. Resuscitation of hemodynamic instability should be rapidly initiated with crystalloid or colloid infusions, followed by replenishment of the red cell mass.
2. Vasopressors—dopamine, norepinephrine, vasopressin—are titrated to a systolic pressure of 90 to 100 mm Hg or a mean arterial pressure of 70 mm Hg or higher.
3. In patients with septic shock and hypotension despite adequate fluid resuscitation, evaluate the patient for evidence of adrenal insufficiency and initiate therapy with low-dose corticosteroids if indicated.
4. Evaluate and treat ionized hypocalcemia and severe metabolic acidosis if the response to catecholamine therapy is inadequate.
5. If shock persists despite rapid and aggressive fluid resuscitation, consider endotracheal intubation and mechanical ventilation, irrespective of arterial blood gas values. Proper titration of ventilatory therapy averts respiratory muscle fatigue and arrest by reducing shock-related increases in the O_2 cost of breathing.
6. Evaluate and treat oliguria. Differentiate prerenal causes by obtaining serum and urine Na^+, creatinine, and urea nitrogen to calculate the fractional excretion of sodium (FeNa) or urea nitrogen.
7. Stabilize long bone fractures early.
8. Initiate broad-spectrum antimicrobial therapy, including coverage against methicillin-resistant *Staphylococcus aureus*, *Staphylococcus epidermidis,* and *Pseudomonas aeruginosa.* Add coverage for suspected anaerobic intra-abdominal sepsis.
9. Begin antifungal therapy in patients at high risk for fungal sepsis despite negative results on blood culture when clinical findings are suggestive (e.g., extensive colonization by *Candida,* nonintertriginous skin rash, myositis, or retinitis).
10. Perform prompt re-exploration for suspected intra-abdominal sepsis and abscess formation.

EPIDEMIOLOGY OF MULTIPLE ORGAN DYSFUNCTION SYNDROME

Significant advances have been made in critical care medicine over the last 30 years, particularly in the last decade. Nonetheless, many critically ill patients often suffer the progressive deterioration in the function of one or more organs, a phenomenon that has been termed *multiple organ dysfunction syndrome* (1). MODS is the leading cause of death for patients in the intensive care unit. Furthermore, the death rate remains high for patients who survive their ICU admission. In addition, the financial costs are significant, with more than 60% of ICU resources consumed by these patients (2).

Individual organ dysfunction may result from a direct insult, such as pulmonary aspiration of gastric contents (primary MODS), or it can be associated with a systemic process such as shock or pancreatitis (secondary MODS) (1). Alterations in organ function seen during MODS are a continuum rather than a discrete, dichotomous event indicating the failure of an organ. A number of organ dysfunction scores have been developed to predict the clinical outcome of these patients (Table 54.1). These scores not only serve to establish the baseline degree of organ dysfunction, but also enable the clinician to evaluate the progression or resolution of organ dysfunction over time. In general, an increase in the number of dysfunctional organs increases the risk of death. Examples of early scores of organ failure include those published by Goris et al. (3) and Knaus et al. (4). Refinement of these scores led to the development

TABLE 54.1

COMPARISON OF THE PHYSIOLOGIC AND BIOCHEMICAL PARAMETERS USED BY FOUR SCORING SYSTEMS FOR ORGAN DYSFUNCTION AND FAILURE

Organ system	Sequential organ failure assessment (SOFA) (6)	Multiple organ dysfunction score (MOD) (5)	Logistic organ dysfunction (LOD) (184)	Brussels (185)
Cardiovascular	Blood pressure and vasopressor use	Blood pressure and adjusted heart rate	Blood pressure and heart rate	Blood pressure, fluid responsiveness, and acidosis
Pulmonary	PaO_2/FiO_2 and mechanical ventilation	PaO_2/FiO_2	PaO_2/FiO_2 and mechanical ventilation	PaO_2/FiO_2
Hepatic	Bilirubin	Bilirubin	Bilirubin and prothrombin time	Bilirubin
Hematologic	Platelets	Platelets	Platelets and white blood cell count	Platelets
Renal	Creatinine and urine output	Creatinine	Creatinine, blood urea nitrogen, or urine output	Creatinine
Central nervous system	Glasgow coma score (GCS)	GCS	GCS	GCS

Reprinted from Bernard GR. Quantification of organ dysfunction: seeking standardization. *Crit Care Med.* 1998;26:1767–1768, with permission.

of the multiple organ dysfunction (MOD) score (5) and the sequential organ failure assessment (SOFA) score (6). In principle, these scores are based on parameters for six organ systems: Cardiovascular, respiratory, hematologic, renal, central nervous system (CNS), and hepatic (7). The difference in these scores lies in the parameter to describe cardiovascular dysfunction. The MOD score describes the degree of cardiovascular dysfunction as a composite of heart rate, central venous pressure, and mean arterial pressure (pressure-adjusted heart rate), whereas the SOFA score describes cardiovascular dysfunction by the dose of vasoactive agents administered.

Several trials have evaluated the performance of these scores as descriptors of multiple organ dysfunction and failure, and to assess the incidence of MODS in the intensive care unit. Moreno et al., in a prospective, international multicenter trial composed of 1,449 patients, were able to demonstrate that total maximum SOFA score and change in SOFA score over time (δ) can be used to quantify the degree of organ dysfunction present on ICU admission, the degree of dysfunction or failure that appears during the ICU stay, and the cumulative insult suffered by the patient (7). These findings were subsequently confirmed by Ferreira et al. (8), who demonstrated that changes in the SOFA score were a good indicator of prognosis. In their study of 352 consecutive patients, an increase in SOFA score during the first 48 hours of intensive care predicted a mortality rate of at least 50% (8). In a group of patients with ARDS, the Toronto ARDS Outcomes Group found a significant relationship between the change in MOD score over time of the ICU stay and the distance walked in 6 minutes up to 1 year following discharge from the ICU (9). The recent European Sepsis Occurrence in Acutely Ill Patients (SOAP) multicenter trial analyzed data from 3,147 adult ICU admissions to determine the incidence of MODS and its associated mortality in mixed medical and surgical ICU populations (10). The overall rate of MODS, defined as severe acquired dysfunction in two or more organ systems, was 43% for patients without a diagnosis of sepsis and 73% of those with a diagnosis of severe sepsis, which represents a substantially higher incidence than in some previously published reports (4). Like other investigators, they found a direct relationship between the number of organs failing and the ICU mortality (Fig. 54.1). Single organ failure carried an ICU mortality rate of 6%, whereas patients with four or more failing organs had mortality rates of 65%. While earlier reports have suggested that the increase in mortality associated with an increased number of failed organs is independent of the identity of dysfunctional organ systems

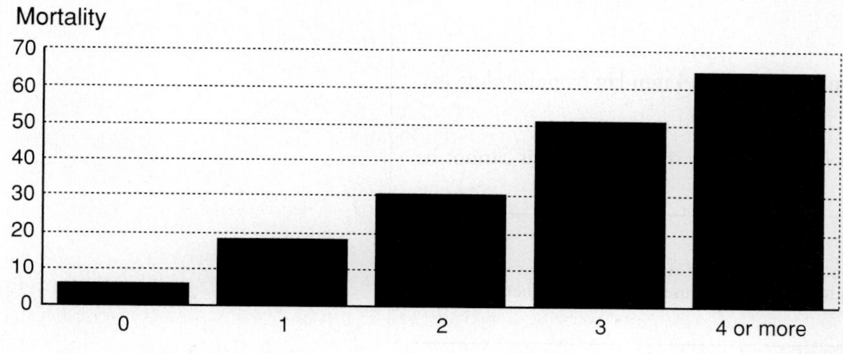

FIGURE 54.1. Relationship between the number of failed organs on admission and intensive care unit mortality. (Reproduced from Vincent J-L, Sakr Y, Sprung CL, et al. Sepsis in European intensive care units: results of the SOAP study. *Crit Care Med.* 2006;34:344–353, with permission.)

(11–13), the SOAP investigators found different results. Organ failure in patients with severe sepsis generally carried a higher mortality than in those patients without a diagnosis of severe sepsis. As for individual organ systems in the group of patients with severe sepsis, failure of the coagulation system carried the highest mortality (52.9%), followed by the hepatic (45.1%), CNS (43.9%), cardiovascular (42.3%), and renal system (41.2%). Respiratory failure in this analysis was associated with a mortality risk of 34.5%. Certain subsets of patients admitted to the ICU appear to be at greater risk of MODS: patients older than 65 years (older than 55 years in trauma patients [13]), increased severity of illness as assessed by APACHE II scores (20 or more), and diagnosis of sepsis or acute lung injury (ALI) on admission. Among the patients with severe sepsis, the SOAP investigators found as independent predictors of mortality the following: "Medical" admissions, *Pseudomonas* species infection, SAPS II score on admission, SOFA score at the onset of sepsis, bloodstream infection, cirrhosis, and cumulative fluid balance within the first 72 hours of the onset of sepsis. The latter variable has not previously been identified as an independent predictor of mortality; further investigations will be necessary to distinguish whether a positive fluid balance in the ICU is simply a marker of severity of illness or is harmful, *per se*.

PATHOPHYSIOLOGY

MODS usually occurs in patients who exhibit signs of a generalized inflammatory response (systemic inflammatory response syndrome [SIRS], Table 54.2) (1). Although SIRS is often the result of infection, other conditions such as necrotizing pancreatitis or trauma can also lead to systemic manifestations of inflammation; SIRS due to infection has been defined as sepsis. Recent guidelines (14) have broadened the diagnostic criteria for sepsis that were originally proposed in 1992. For those patients who present with SIRS only, a significant number will progress to sepsis, septic shock, and, ultimately, MODS (15). Although suspected or documented infection is not required for the development of MODS, the syndromes of SIRS, sepsis, and MODS are closely related. Consequently, the review of the pathophysiology of MODS will also include discussions of SIRS and MODS.

Derangements in Oxygen Delivery and Consumption

In most tissues, oxygen consumption (VO_2) is determined by metabolic demand and is independent of $\dot{D}O_2$. When $\dot{D}O_2$ is

TABLE 54.2

AMERICAN COLLEGE OF CHEST PHYSICIANS/SOCIETY OF CRITICAL CARE MEDICINE DEFINITIONS OF SEPSIS AND ORGAN FAILURE

A. **Infection**
Microbial phenomenon characterized by an inflammatory response to the presence of the micro-organism or the invasion of normally sterile host tissue by those organisms

B. **Bacteremia**
The presence of viable bacteria in the blood

C. **Systemic inflammatory response syndrome (SIRS)**
The systemic inflammatory response to a variety of severe clinical insults, manifested by two or more of the following conditions:
(1) Temperature greater than 38°C or less than 36°C
(2) Heart rate greater than 90 beats/min
(3) Respiratory rate more than 20 breaths/min or $PaCO_2$ less than 32 mm Hg
(4) WBC more than 12,000 cells /μL, less than 4,000 cells/μL, or more than 10% immature (band) forms

D. **Sepsis**
The systemic response to infection. The manifestations are the same as those enumerated for SIRS.

E. **Severe sepsis**
Sepsis associated with organ dysfunction, hypoperfusion, or hypotension

F. **Septic shock**
Sepsis with hypotension, despite adequate fluid resuscitation, and perfusion abnormalities, including but not limited to the following:
(1) Lactic acidosis
(2) Oliguria
(3) Acute alteration in mental status

G. **Hypotension**
A systolic BP less than 90 mm Hg or a reduction of more than 4 mm Hg from baseline in the absence of other causes for hypotension

H. **Multiple organ dysfunction syndrome**
Presence of altered organ function in an acutely ill patient such that homeostasis cannot be maintained without intervention

WBC, white blood cell; BP, blood pressure.
Condensed from American College of Chest Physicians/Society of Critical Care Medicine Consensus Conference. Definitions for sepsis and organ failure and guidelines for the use of innovative therapies in sepsis. *Crit Care Med.* 1992;20:864–874.

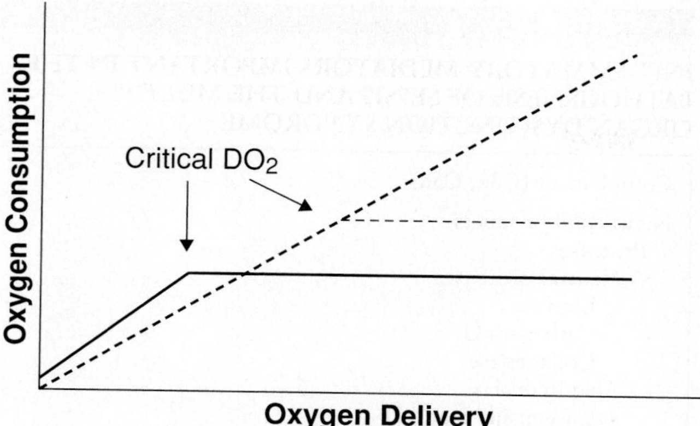

FIGURE 54.2. The relationship between oxygen delivery and consumption. The solid line represents the normal relationship. The dashed line shows pathologic supply dependency. (Reproduced from Heard SO, Fink MP. Multiple-organ dysfunction syndrome. In: Murray MJ, Coursin DB, Pearl RG, et al., eds. *Critical Care Medicine. Perioperative Management.* Philadelphia: Lippincott Williams & Wilkins; 2002.)

reduced, VO_2 is maintained by increased oxygen extraction by the tissues. If $\dot{D}O_2$ is reduced to the point where the metabolic need cannot be met, then VO_2 becomes "supply dependent" (Fig. 54.2). The point at which VO_2 decreases is called the critical $\dot{D}O_2$. Although one study (16) suggested that the critical $\dot{D}O_2$ in anesthetized humans is 330 mL/minute/m^2, another investigation where life support was withdrawn in critically ill patients demonstrated that the value is substantially lower (17).

A number of studies from the 1970s, 1980s, and early 1990s seemed to suggest that systemic VO_2 was supply dependent over a wide range of $\dot{D}O_2$ in patients with sepsis or ARDS. Since VO_2 and $\dot{D}O_2$ are independent of each other, the linking of these two variables in patients with ARDS or sepsis was coined pathologic supply dependency. This concept is important, as it implies that inadequate oxygen is being delivered to the tissues and anaerobic metabolism is occurring despite "normal" global perfusion. As a consequence, inadequate production of adenosine triphosphate (ATP) and other high-energy phosphates may contribute to the development of MODS in these patients.

The validity of the concept of pathologic supply dependency was subsequently challenged. Mathematical coupling of data (e.g., VO_2 and $\dot{D}O_2$ both determined by use of a pulmonary artery catheter), pooling of data, and spontaneous changes in metabolic demand (which would increase $\dot{D}O_2$) can explain many of the results of the studies purporting to show pathologic supply dependency. Clinical investigations that utilized independent means to measure both $\dot{D}O_2$ and VO_2 failed to demonstrate pathologic supply dependency in patients with ARDS or sepsis. Furthermore, critical $\dot{D}O_2$ in these patients was no higher than in other critically ill patients.

More recently, there has been a recognition that supply dependency may be occurring in patients, but not at the global level. There is an increasing appreciation that the regional circulation and microcirculation—arterioles, capillary bed, and postcapillary venules—play a crucial role in the pathogenesis of organ dysfunction in shock. Heterogeneous microcirculatory abnormalities occur due to changes in the activation state and shape of endothelial cells, alterations in vascular smooth muscle tone, activation of the clotting system, and changes in red and white blood cell deformability (discussed later). The surface receptors and mediators associated with these changes are now being identified, and include oxidants, lectins, proteases, vasoactive products of inducible nitric oxide synthase (iNOS), and altered adrenergic receptor sensitivity. Alterations in microvascular circulation have been demonstrated in congestive heart failure, cardiogenic shock, hemorrhage, and sepsis. Microcirculatory changes of congestive heart failure include reduced conjunctival microvascular density and attenuated nailfold capillary recruitment during postocclusive reactive hyperemia (18). Animal models of hemorrhagic shock demonstrate attenuated functional capillary perfusion—a measure of the number of capillaries that are actively moving blood—of skeletal muscle and the intestinal villi (19,20). Renal and intestinal regional blood flow are reduced despite resuscitation and return of global hemodynamics back to baseline values (21). In patients with severe sepsis, forearm reactive hyperemia measured by air plethysmography is diminished following arterial occlusion, and red blood cell deformability is reduced compared to controls (22). Tissue (skeletal muscle) oxygen saturation in septic patients is no different than that observed in healthy controls or postsurgical patients (23); however, microvascular compliance and skeletal muscle oxygen consumption is reduced, and postischemic reperfusion time is increased compared to controls. Orthogonal polarization spectral (OPS) imaging is a technique by which perfusion of small and large vessels in the microcirculation of mucosal surfaces can be seen and quantified. Clinical studies (24, 25) where OPS imaging has been utilized have shown that the fraction of perfused small vessels in patients with severe heart failure, cardiogenic shock, or sepsis is significantly lower than in those critically ill patients without those conditions (Fig. 54.3).

Functional cellular hypoxia—"cytopathic hypoxia"—or metabolic failure is a condition where the cell is incapable of utilizing oxygen to produce ATP despite adequate oxygen delivery. Indeed, in patients with sepsis and in animal models of sepsis, oxygen tension in the intestine, bladder, and skeletal muscle is elevated, suggesting that the problem is not one of inadequate $\dot{D}O_2$ but one of oxygen utilization (26–28). The defect in oxygen utilization likely resides in the mitochondrion. Muscle biopsies from septic patients reveal that skeletal muscle ATP concentrations and respiratory chain activity are lower compared to samples obtained from control patients (29). Furthermore, patients dying from sepsis have even lower ATP concentrations and respiratory chain activity (complex 1) compared to sepsis survivors (29,30). The mechanism by which cytopathic hypoxia or metabolic failure occurs has not been fully elucidated. However, nitric oxide and its metabolite, peroxynitrite, are mediators that are released during sepsis and are inhibitors of the mitochondrial electron transport chain (31). Single-strand breaks in nuclear DNA can occur in sepsis by a variety of endogenously formed oxidants, including peroxynitrite. Poly (ADP-ribose) polymerase (PARP) is an enzyme that is activated by the formation of these DNA breaks. Since the substrate for PARP is NAD$^+$, the activation of PARP can result in a profound reduction in the cellular levels of NAD$^+$, thereby causing cellular energy depletion (32, 33).

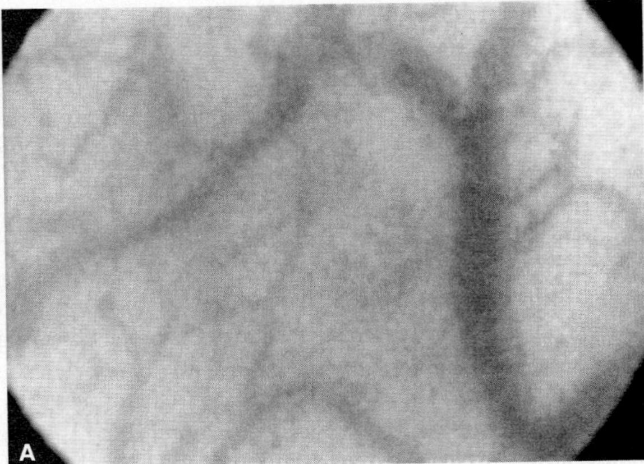

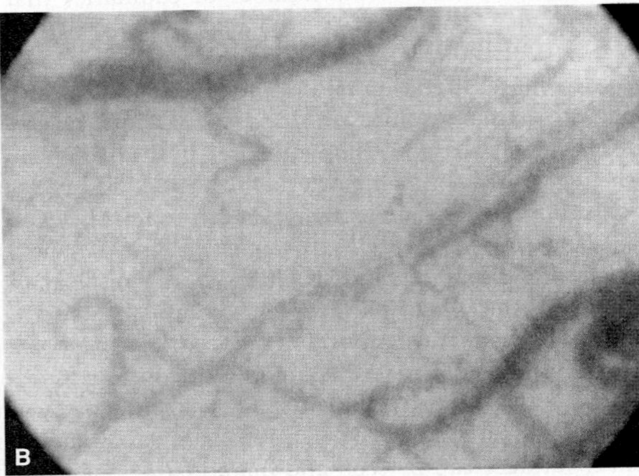

FIGURE 54.3. Sublingual microcirculation as assessed by orthogonal polarization spectral imaging in a healthy volunteer (**A**) and in a patient with early septic shock (**B**). Normal capillary density is observed in panel A whereas low capillary density is observed in panel B. Real time images may be viewed at http://www.cooperhealthorg/content/gme_fellowship_shock.htm. (Reproduced from De Backer D, Creteur J, Preiser J-C, et al. Microvascular blood flow is altered in patients with sepsis. *Am J Respir Crit Care Med.* 2002;166:98–104, with permission.)

TABLE 54.3

INFLAMMATORY MEDIATORS IMPORTANT IN THE PATHOGENESIS OF SEPSIS AND THE MULTIPLE ORGAN DYSFUNCTION SYNDROME

Complement (C3a, C5a)
Neutrophil products
Proteases
Neutral proteases
Elastase
Cathepsin G
Collagenase
Acid hydrolase
Cathepsins B and D
β-glucuronidase
Glucosaminase
Oxygen radicals
Superoxide anion
Hydroxyl radical
Hydrogen peroxide
Peroxynitrite
Bradykinin
Lipid mediators
Prostaglandins
Thromboxane A_2
Prostaglandin I_2
Prostaglandin E_2
Leukotrienes (LTB_4, LTC_4, LTD_4, LTE_4)
Platelet-activating factor (PAF)
Cytokines
Tumor necrosis factor-α (TNF-α)
Interleukins (IL-1, IL-6, IL-8)
High-mobility group 1 (HMG-1)
Macrophage migration inhibition factor (MIF)
Nitric oxide

Reprinted from Heard SO, Fink MP. Multiple-organ dysfunction syndrome. In: Murray MJ, Coursin DB, Pearl RG, et al., eds. *Critical Care Medicine. Perioperative Management.* Philadelphia: Lippincott Williams & Wilkins; 2002, with permission.

ROLE OF INFLAMMATORY AND VASOACTIVE MEDIATORS

Although early clinical series emphasized the implication of uncontrolled infection in the development of MODS, it is clear that MODS can occur with either extensive tissue injury such as that seen with trauma, pancreatitis, or sepsis. A large amount of evidence is available that implicates the release of inflammatory mediators in the pathogenesis of MODS (Table 54.3).

Complement, Neutrophils, and Reactive Oxygen Metabolites

The complement cascade is activated via three pathways (Fig. 54.4). The **classical pathway** is triggered by antibody-coated targets or antigen–antibody complexes. The **alternative pathway** is activated by aggregated immunoglobulins, products of tissue trauma, lipopolysaccharide (LPS), and other complex polysaccharides. The **lectin-ficolin pathway** is initiated by the binding of organisms to mannose binding-lectin (MBL), a protein important in innate immunity (34). Once MBL is bound to a pathogen, an MBL-associated serine protease is produced, which forms a C3 convertase by cleavage of C4 and C2. Products of the complement pathway activate neutrophils, which can obstruct capillaries and release oxygen radicals and lysosomal enzymes—among other mediators, thereby damaging the endothelium. Furthermore, adhesion molecules, which are expressed on both polymorphonuclear leukocytes (PMNs) and vascular endothelium in response to LPS and other inflammatory mediators, facilitate the adherence and diapedesis of PMNs through the endothelium.

A significant amount of evidence exists, suggesting that complement activation is important in the pathophysiology of MODS. In an animal model of generalized inflammation (e.g., with zymosan treatment), C5-deficient mice had a lower mortality compared to wild-type mice; however, late organ

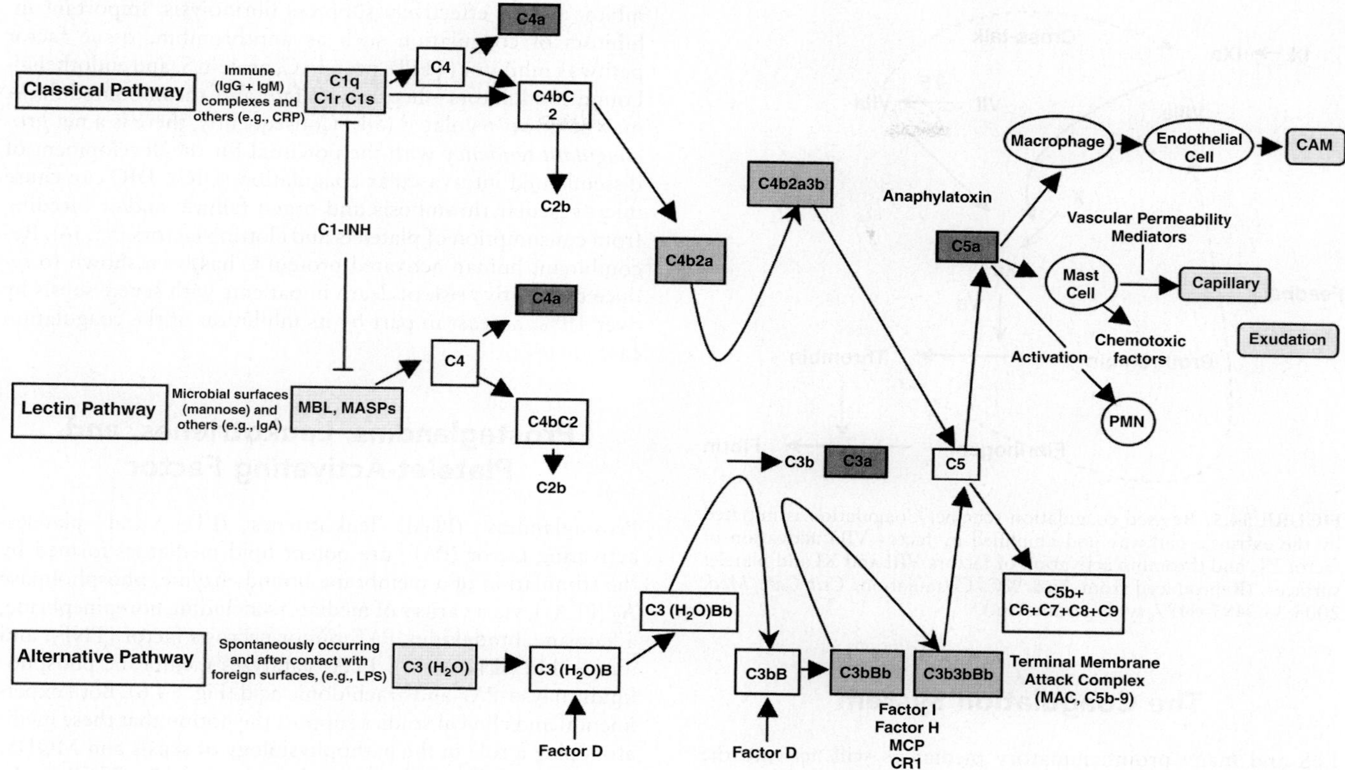

FIGURE 54.4. The three complement activation pathways (classic, alternative, and lectin). IgG, immunoglobulin G; IgM, immunoglobulin M; IgA, immunoglobulin A; CRP, C-reactive protein; MBL, mannose-binding lectin protein; MASP, MBL-associated proteases; C1-INH, C1-inhibitor; LPS, lipopolysaccharide; CAM, cell adhesion molecules; MAC, membrane attack complex; PMN, polymorphonuclear leukocytes; MCP, monocyte chemoattractant protein; CR1, complement component receptor 1. (Reproduced from Goldfarb RD, Parrillo JE. Complement. *Crit Care Med.* 2005;33:S482–S484, with permission.)

failure was not different between the groups (35). An inhibitor of complement, bisbenzylisoquinoline alkaloid, will decrease mortality and the percentage of animals with organ injury in zymosan-treated mice (36). In a rodent model of abdominal aortic aneurysm rupture, a complement C5a receptor antagonist attenuated lung and intestinal permeability indices and lung myeloperoxidase activity compared to controls (37). Clinically, activation of both complement and neutrophils occurs in patients with ARDS or burns (38,39), and circulating plasma levels of C3a correlate with severity of injury and outcome in patients with multiple trauma (40). Evidence of complement and neutrophil activation has also been found in bronchoalveolar lavage (BAL) from patients with ARDS (41). Administration of a C1-inhibitor in patients with severe sepsis and septic shock reduces neutrophil activation (42) and improves renal function and SOFA scores compared to untreated control patients (43).

Reactive oxygen species—superoxide anion, hydrogen peroxide, and the hydroxyl radical—are released by activated PMNs and can injure tissues by damaging DNA, cross-linking cellular proteins, and causing peroxidation of membrane lipids (44,45). Lipid peroxidation diminishes membrane fluidity and increases membrane permeability, thereby impairing cellular function. The conclusion that toxic oxygen radicals are important in the pathophysiology of respiratory dysfunction comes from clinical studies of patients with ARDS where plasma levels of lipid peroxides are elevated, levels of hydrogen peroxide are increased in the expiratory condensate (46), and oxidative damage to proteins in BAL fluid is found (47). In addition, patients with ARDS have reduced levels of oxygen radical scavengers (e.g., α-tocopherol, ubiquinone, and glutathione), a sign of "oxidant stress" (48,49). Despite these data, antioxidant therapies have not translated into improved outcome for patients with ARDS or MODS, although such interventions may increase the number of days "free" of acute lung injury (50) or mechanical ventilation (51), decrease the incidence of new organ failures (51), and reduce the oxidative stress during septic shock (52).

The Kallikrein-Kinin System

The kallikrein-kinin system is part of the contact system, and is composed of complement, coagulation, and kallikrein-kinins. Bradykinin, the end product of this cascade, is a potent vasodilator and increases vascular permeability. Some of these effects are mediated by the release of secondary mediators, such as nitric oxide and eicosinoids. Although some experimental and clinical data suggest that the kallikrein-kinin system is important in the pathogenesis of sepsis and MODS, a clinical trial of a bradykinin receptor antagonist (CP-0127) for the adjuvant therapy of sepsis failed to alter the 28-day mortality (53).

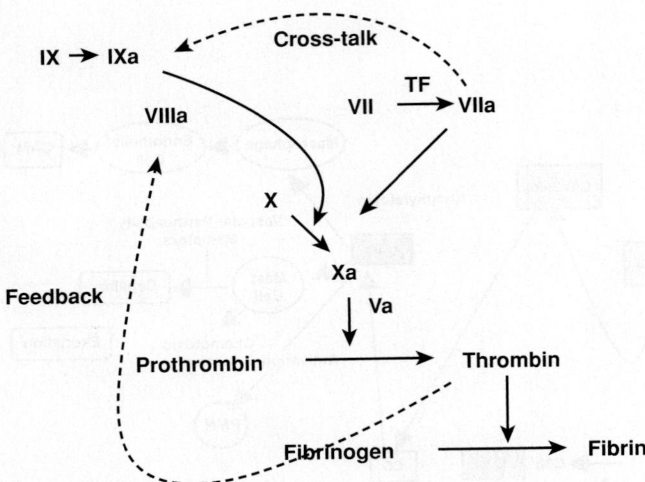

FIGURE 54.5. Revised coagulation scheme. Coagulation is initiated by the extrinsic pathway and amplified by factor VIIa activation of factor IX, and thrombin activation of factors VIII and XI and platelet surfaces. (Reproduced from Aird WC. Coagulation. *Crit Care Med.* 2005;33:S485–S487, with permission.)

The Coagulation System

LPS and many proinflammatory mediators will activate the coagulation system (Fig. 54.5). Coagulation in sepsis or inflammatory states is initiated primarily by the extrinsic tissue factor–dependent pathway, as these mediators induce the expression of tissue factor (TF) on monocytes and endothelial cells (54). Although these same mediators activate the fibrinolytic system, subsequent increases in plasminogen activator inhibitor-1 (PAI-1) and thrombin-activatable fibrinolysis inhibitor (TAFI) effectively suppress fibrinolysis. Important inhibitors of coagulation such as antithrombin, tissue factor pathway inhibitor (TFPI), protein C, protein S, and endothelial-bound modulators—heparan sulfate and thrombomodulin—may be down-regulated (54). Consequently, there is a net *procoagulant tendency* with the potential for the development of disseminated intravascular coagulation (DIC). DIC can cause microvascular thrombosis and organ failure, and/or bleeding from consumption of platelets and clotting factors (55,56). Recombinant human activated protein C has been shown to reduce the relative risk of death in patients with severe sepsis by over 19%, at least in part by its inhibition of the coagulation cascade (57).

Prostaglandins, Leukotrienes, and Platelet-Activating Factor

Prostaglandins (PGs), leukotrienes (LTs), and platelet-activating factor (PAF) are potent lipid mediators formed by the stimulation of a membrane-bound enzyme, phospholipase A_2 (PLA_2), via a variety of mediators including norepinephrine, adenosine, bradykinin, PAF, tumor necrosis factor (TNF), and interleukin (IL)-1β (58). PLA_2 catalyzes membrane phospholipids to lyso-PAF and arachidonic acid (Fig. 54.6). Both experimental and clinical studies support the notion that these mediators play a role in the pathophysiology of sepsis and MODS.

Elevated plasma levels of thromboxane B_2 (TXB_2), the metabolite of the prostaglandin thromboxane A_2 (TXA_2), are observed in animal models of sepsis and are correlated with organ injury and outcome. Inhibitors of cyclo-oxygenase and thromboxane synthase abrogate the organ injury and improve survival. Clinically, elevated plasma levels of TXB_2 and PGI_2 have been measured in patients with Gram-negative septic

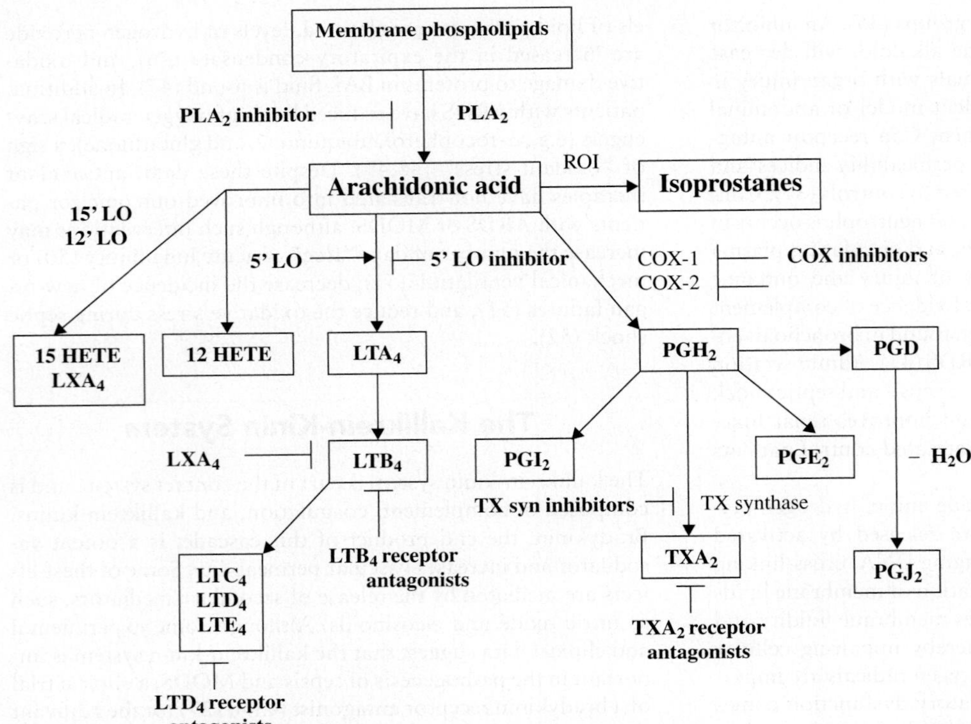

FIGURE 54.6. The eicosanoid pathway. PLA_2, phospholipase A_2; ROI, reactive oxygen intermediates; COX, cyclo-oxygenase; LO, lipo-oxygenase; HETE, hydroxyeicosatetraenoic acid; LT, leukotriene; TX, thromboxane; LX, lipoxin; PG, prostaglandin. (Reproduced from Cook JA. Eicosanoids. *Crit Care Med.* 2005;33:S488–S491, with permission.)

shock and correlate with the severity of organ failure and survival. However, clinical trials of nonselective inhibitors of cyclo-oxygenase (ibuprofen) have failed to show any effect on survival (59), and a recent trial evaluating the effectiveness of a selective inhibitor of a group IIA secretory phospholipase in patients with suspected sepsis and organ failure showed no survival benefit nor effect on organ dysfunction (60). The antifungal agent, ketoconazole, is an imidazole derivative that inhibits thromboxane synthase. Use of ketoconazole in patients at risk for ARDS prevents the development of ARDS (61,62); however, once ARDS is established, this agent is ineffective at reversing the syndrome or improving survival (63). Other clinical trials evaluating inhibitors of prostaglandin production have been underpowered to show any effect.

A significant role of leukotrienes in the pathophysiology of the cardiovascular dysfunction observed in sepsis is unlikely, since the administration of leukotrienes (LTC_4 and LTD_4) to primates and sheep results in increased systemic vascular resistance and depressed cardiac output. However, intratracheal administration of these leukotrienes in animals results in a significant increase in capillary permeability, leading to a pattern of pulmonary edema not inconsistent with ARDS. Furthermore, elevated concentrations of LTB_4, LTC_4, and LTD_4 have been measured in the BAL fluid recovered from patients with ARDS. Although leukotriene receptor antagonists have improved pulmonary hemodynamics and oxygenation in experimental sepsis studies, no clinical trials using these agents for sepsis or ARDS have been performed.

A large amount of data exists supporting the role of PAF in the pathogenesis of sepsis and MODS. *In vitro*, incubation of macrophages with PAF will lead to an exaggerated release of TNF and tissue factor by these cells following exposure to LPS. Conversely, LPS-induced release of TNF by macrophages is inhibited by PAF receptor antagonists. PAF expression on the surface of endothelial cells will result in PMN adherence and activation. In addition, stimulation of PAF receptors on the endothelium results in changes in cell shape and cytoskeletal structure. In animal models of endotoxicosis, elevated plasma levels of PAF have been measured and are associated with many of the physiologic abnormalities seen in sepsis: myocardial dysfunction, vasodilatation, and microvascular permeability. Infusion of PAF into animals reproduces many of the findings observed in endotoxicosis or sepsis. In animal models of sepsis, PAF receptor antagonists have had variable effects on outcome; however, most studies have demonstrated an improvement in organ function (58). Clinically, depressed plasma levels of PAF acetylhydrolase (PAF-AH), the enzyme responsible for metabolizing PAF, have been observed in critically ill patients and correlate inversely with organ dysfunction. However, a phase III trial of recombinant PAF-AH failed to improve outcome or prevent organ dysfunction (64). A subsequent study of critically ill patients revealed that plasma levels of PAF-AH were variable over time and with severity of illness (65). Such a finding provides a partial explanation for the lack of efficacy of recombinant PAF-AH.

Cytokines

Cytokines are small proteins that are secreted by nearly all nucleated cells and exhibit autocrine, paracrine, or endocrine activity (66,67); they are generally classified as proinflammatory or anti-inflammatory molecules. This classification, however, is somewhat arbitrary as an individual cytokine may act in either a proinflammatory or anti-inflammatory fashion, depending on the underlying biologic process. Proinflammatory cytokines such as TNF and IL-1 can stimulate the release of other mediators: PAF, nitric oxide, LTs, and PGs.

TNF assumes an important role in the pathogenesis of human sepsis, septic shock, and MODS. TNF is directly cytotoxic to some cell types and will induce the expression of adhesion molecules on neutrophils and endothelial cells to promote the recruitment of these white cells to the site of injury or infection. Furthermore, endothelial permeability is increased. Metabolic effects attributable to TNF include activation of the acute-phase response, fever (along with IL-1), skeletal muscle catabolism, and increased peripheral lipolysis and hepatic lipogenesis (67). When injected into normal volunteers, small doses of LPS or recombinant TNF will reproduce many of the metabolic and hemodynamic changes observed in sepsis (68,69). Similar findings are observed in animal studies, and treatment with anti-TNF antibodies will prevent many of the adverse consequences of endotoxic or live Gram-negative bacterial shock (70). However, in studies of critically ill patients, the correlation of plasma TNF levels and outcome is variable (71,72). Such disparate results may be due to timing and method of the TNF assay, as well as to the acuity, etiology, or treatment of the patient's illness, or genetic differences in patients. Results from multicenter studies of adjuvant therapy with either anti-TNF antibodies or soluble TNF receptors have demonstrated that neither passive immunization nor the soluble receptors reduce mortality from sepsis. However, in one recent trial where patients were stratified according to initial plasma levels of IL-6 (as a marker of severity of illness), outcome was improved, and organ dysfunction was ameliorated with the administration of a monoclonal antibody to TNF (73).

Like TNF, IL-1 has a wide variety of biologic actions and has been implicated in the pathogenesis of sepsis and MODS (74). In addition, TNF and IL-1 often act in a synergistic fashion. IL-1 induces the expression of cyclo-oxygenase (COX)-2 and iNOS expression (75). Furthermore, IL-1 increases the expression of other cytokines—most notably TNF and IL-6—chemokines, adhesion molecules, and a number of tissue proteases and matrix metalloproteases (75). IL-1 also stimulates the release of myeloid progenitor cells, resulting in neutrophilia (75). Animal models suggest a role for IL-1 in sepsis and MODS, and the use of IL-1 receptor antagonist (IL-1RA) is beneficial in several human inflammatory diseases (e.g., rheumatoid arthritis). However, use of IL-1RA in patients with sepsis does not reduce mortality nor reverse organ failure (76–78).

Interleukin 6 (IL-6) is another cytokine that has been identified to be important in the response to infection and development of MODS. Small doses of endotoxin administered to normal volunteers will stimulate the release of IL-6 (79). IL-6 will persist for longer periods of time in the blood than other cytokines and may serve as an important marker for the outcome of patients with sepsis or septic shock. Both the IL-6 receptor and the signaling receptor gp130 are required for the biologic activity of IL-6 to be realized (79). Murine models of hemorrhagic shock indicate that IL-6 is important in the development of gut barrier dysfunction (see below) (79). In addition, IL-6 may be important in promoting thrombosis during sepsis. Passive immunization with an anti–IL-6 antibody reduces activation of the coagulation cascade in a primate model of endotoxicosis but has no effect on the coagulation abnormalities associated with low-dose LPS in humans (80).

IL-8 is a chemotactic cytokine (chemokine) and is expressed principally by monocytes and macrophages by stimulation with LPS, bacteria, TNF, and IL-1 (81). IL-8 induces chemotaxis of inflammatory cells, and its presence at sites of inflammation may persist for long periods of time (81). That IL-8 is important in the development of MODS is demonstrated by the observation of high IL-8 levels in BAL fluid from patients with ARDS or pneumonia (82). Although neutralizing IL-8 may reduce cardiac ischemia/reperfusion injury in dogs, a reduction in chemokines increases mortality in animal models of pneumonia (81).

High-mobility group box 1 (HMGB1) is a cytokine that was discovered over 30 years ago, but its importance as an inflammatory mediator was appreciated only recently (Fig. 54.7) (83). HMGB1 is released from a variety of cells in response to LPS or bacteria, and the response is delayed (84). Exposure of the lung to HMGB1 increases neutrophil accumulation, edema, and other proinflammatory cytokines, whereas gastrointestinal exposure results in increased gut permeability and translocation of bacteria to mesenteric lymph nodes (84). Administration of this cytokine to animals causes death as a result of epithelial barrier disruption. Treatment of experimental endotoxicosis or sepsis with antibodies to HMGB1 or HMGB1 antagonists improves survival (83,85). There have been no clinical studies to evaluate the efficacy of anti-HMGB1 therapies in sepsis or other inflammatory conditions.

Macrophage migration inhibitory factor (MIF) is a cytokine that is found in macrophages in preformed cytoplasmic pools (86). It is released rapidly in response to bacterial products and works to up-regulate and sustain the activation of a variety of cell types to produce TNF, IL-1, IL-6, and IL-8. The major action of MIF may be the regulation of p53-dependent apoptosis. Anti-MIF therapy in animal models of sepsis is protective (86). Although MIF appears to be an important mediator of sepsis and sepsis-induced MODS (87), it does not appear to play a prominent role in tissue injury resulting from trauma (88).

Nitric Oxide

Nitric oxide (NO) is an inorganic free-radical gas, produced by catalysis of one of the terminal guanidine nitrogens of L-arginine by the NO synthase (NOS) group of enzymes (89). Two general classes of NOS have been described: Constitutive (calcium-dependent) NOS (neuronal and endothelial) and inducible (calcium-independent) NOS (90). The production of the latter enzyme is induced by LPS, TNF, and a variety of other inflammatory mediators. A variety of cells and tissues release NO, including endothelium, vascular smooth muscle, neutrophils, and mononuclear, glial, mast, hepatic, and adrenal medullary cells (90). Vasorelaxation, neurotransmission, and microbicidal activity are some of the important functions that NO possesses. The role that NO plays in the host is a function of the rate and timing of its production and the surrounding

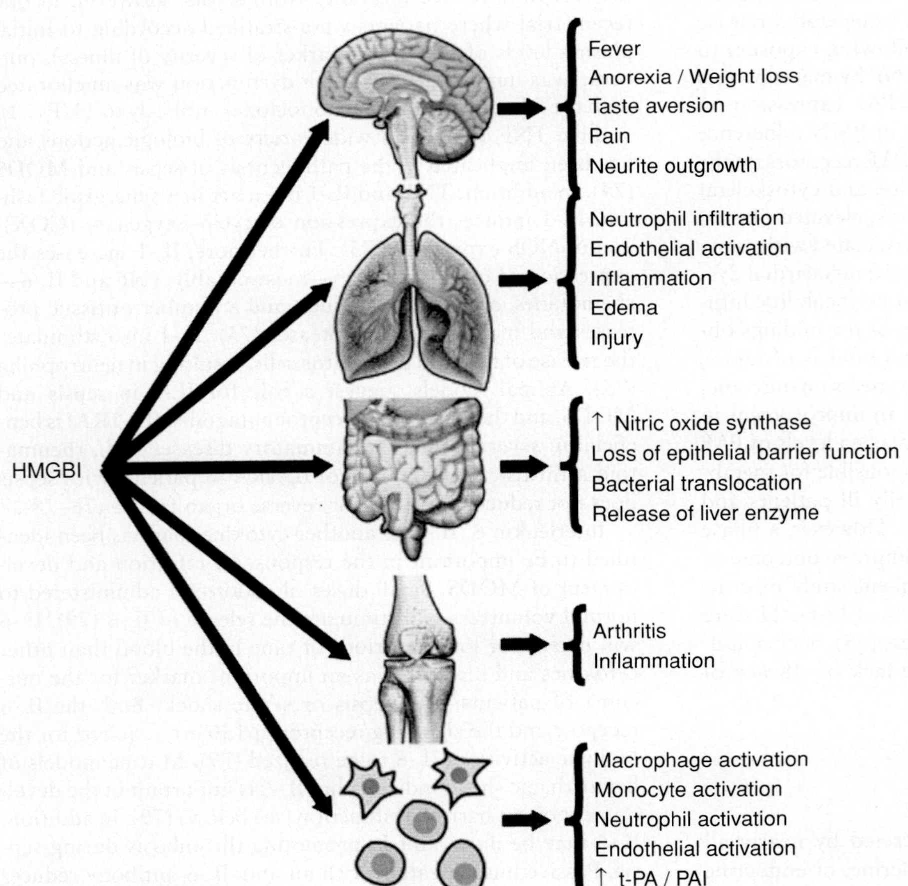

FIGURE 54.7. Inflammatory responses in various areas of the host that are medicated by high-mobility group box 1 (HMGB1). tPA, tissue plasminogen activator; PAI, plasminogen activator inhibitor. (Reproduced from Wang H, Yang H, Tracey KJ. Extracellular role of HMGB1 in inflammation and sepsis. *J Intern Med.* 2004;255:320–331, with permission.)

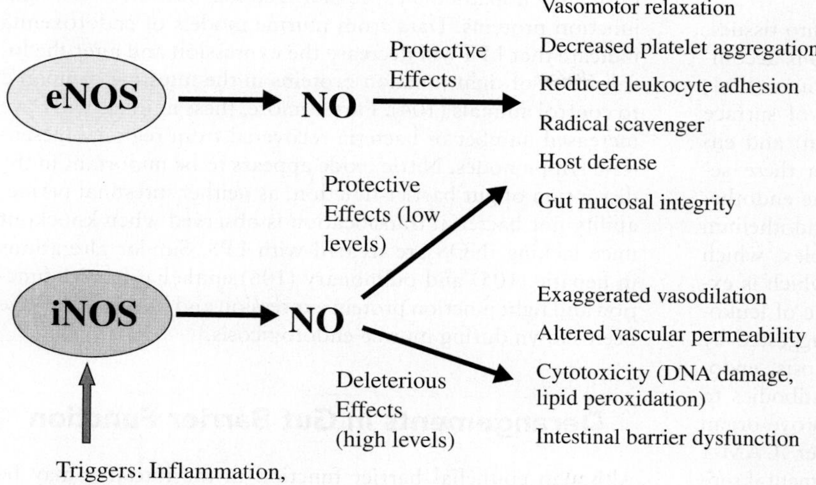

FIGURE 54.8. The divergent effects of nitric oxide (NO) derived from the endothelium (eNOS, endothelial nitric oxide synthase) or as a consequence of inflammation (iNOS, inducible or inflammatory NOS). (Reproduced from Levy RM, Prince JM, Billiar TR. Nitric oxide: a clinical primer. *Crit Care Med.* 2005;33:S492–S495, with permission.)

environment. Normally, NO acts as a direct signaling molecule (e.g., vasorelaxation and neurotransmission), and low levels of NO (produced by constitutive NOS and at times by inducible NOS) have protective effects (Fig. 54.8) (90). Alternatively, it may function as an indirect cytotoxic agent and induce intestinal barrier dysfunction.

A significant amount of experimental and clinical evidence suggests that NO plays an important role in the pathophysiology of sepsis and MODS. Inducible NOS and NO production increase in animals during both endotoxic and hemorrhagic shock. iNOS-deficient mice are protected from LPS-induced hypotension, and have a higher survival following endotoxicosis (91). NO contributes to TNF-induced cardiac dysfunction in a concentration-dependent fashion (92). Increased urinary excretion of NO metabolites (nitrite and nitrate) has been reported in septic patients and correlates inversely with systemic vascular resistance (SVR) (91).

Excess NO in the presence of superoxide anion results in the formation of peroxynitrite ($ONOO^-$), a reactive oxidant that causes lipid peroxidation, inhibits mitochondrial respiration, inactivates glyceraldehyde-3-phosphate dehydrogenase, inhibits membrane sodium/potassium ATP activity, and triggers DNA single-strand breakage. As mentioned previously, DNA damage activates the nuclear enzyme, PARP, which can lead to cellular energy depletion and death (93). Furthermore, excessive amounts of NO and peroxynitrite can activate the transcription factor, NFκB, and amplify the inflammatory response (94).

The efficacy of inhibitors of NOS in the treatment of sepsis and MODS is unclear, and the use of some inhibitors may actually be detrimental. Although hypotension, vascular leak, and vasopressor requirements can be reduced with the use of nonspecific NOS inhibitors, microcirculatory blood flow can be altered, resulting in organ injury. Indeed, a large randomized, prospective trial evaluating the efficacy of the nonspecific NOS inhibitor, L-N^G-monomethylarginine, in patients with septic shock was stopped early because the death rate was higher in the intervention group (95).

THE ENDOTHELIUM

The role of the vascular endothelium is to control the flow of nutrients, blood cells, and a broad array of biologically active molecules to the tissues; this is achieved via membrane-bound receptors for a plethora of molecules and through tight junction proteins and receptors that regulate cell–cell and cell–matrix relationships (96). Endothelial cell injury may well impair the delivery of nutrients to tissues and allow the extravasation of proinflammatory mediators into the interstitial space.

There is a large amount of data supporting the role of an impaired endothelium in the development of MODS. Endothelial cell exposure to LPS will cause anatomic changes including nuclear vacuolization, cytoplasmic swelling and fragmentation, and detachment from the internal elastic lamina (97). In humans with septic shock, elevated levels of circulating endothelial cells can be detected and correlate with outcome. High plasma levels of molecules that are expressed on the surface of endothelial cells (i.e., thrombomodulin [TM], intercellular adhesion molecule [ICAM]-1, and E-selectin) are observed during sepsis and acute lung injury, and are an indirect indication of endothelial damage (98). Furthermore, this injury appears to be sustained, as injection of small doses of LPS into human volunteers will result in high plasma levels of TM that peak at 24 hours and of TF that are still increasing at 48 hours (96).

In the uninjured state, the endothelial cell has important anticoagulant properties. Several heparin-like molecules are expressed on the surface of the cells to accelerate the inactivation of serine proteases of coagulation by antithrombin (96). Thrombomodulin binds thrombin and forms a complex that activates protein C. However, exposure of the endothelial cells to inflammatory or septic mediators will shift the endothelial cells to a procoagulant state by increasing expression of TF and internalization of TM. Furthermore, the endothelial cell will have impaired release of tissue plasminogen activator and an increased release of PAI-1. This procoagulant/antifibrinolytic state is associated with fibrin deposition, platelet consumption, microthrombi, tissue ischemia and necrosis, and an increased risk of death (99).

Before leukocytes and monocytes can migrate into tissues, they must adhere to the endothelium. This process is accomplished by the local synthesis of PAF and cytokines (IL-1, IL-8, and TNF), which stimulates the expression of surface molecules called selectins on leukocytes (L-selectin) and endothelial cells (E-selectin). The interplay between these selectins allows loose binding of the leukocyte to the endothelium. Leukocytes are bound more strongly to the endothelium by the interaction between the CD11/CD18 complex, which is expressed on the leukocyte, and the ICAM-1, which is expressed on the endothelial cell membrane. The role of leukocyte adhesion in the development of MODS is suggested by several lines of evidence. In animal models of sepsis, endotoxicosis, or ischemia/reperfusion, monoclonal antibodies to the CD11/CD18 integrin or to L-selectin will improve organ dysfunction (100). Knockout animals lacking either ICAM-1 or E-selectin have improved survival during experimental sepsis (101). Clinically, plasma ICAM-1 levels are higher in patients with septic shock than in healthy controls or patients with SIRS (98), and the levels correlate with the severity of shock.

Endothelium-derived relaxation is also impaired in sepsis, and such alteration may contribute to MODS. Acetylcholine-induced relaxation of aortic rings obtained from septic animals is attenuated. In animals with chronically overexpressed endothelial cell nitric oxide synthase (ecNOS), resistance to LPS-induced hypotension, lung injury, and death are observed (96). In normal volunteers, small doses of LPS will also impair endothelium-dependent relaxation for days (102). These data help explain the observations that reactive forearm hyperemia is attenuated in patients with sepsis. In addition, the importance of intact ecNOS in these patients is supported by the observation that treatment of patients with septic shock by nonselective NOS inhibitors is associated with no change or an increase in mortality compared to untreated patients (95).

EPITHELIAL BARRIER DYSFUNCTION

Epithelial cells help maintain normal function of organs by the maintenance of distinct compartments. The tight junctions between adjacent epithelial cells serve several important functions: (a) differentiation (103) of the cell into apical and basolateral domains, (b) preservation of cellular polarity, (c) generation of distinct internal environments formed by the epithelial layer, and (d) providing a semipermeable barrier that regulates the passive diffusion of solutes between the paracellular pathway and prevents entry of microbes and toxins (e.g., intestine and lung) (103).

Data from studies using cultured epithelial monolayers show that nitric oxide and peroxynitrate, as well as other proinflammatory mediators, increase the permeability of the monolayer. The mechanism for this increase in permeability is incompletely understood; however, some data suggest that there is a decrease in the expression and improper localization of some of the tight junction proteins. Other investigations have determined that inhibition of the epithelial cell membrane Na^+-K^+-ATPase pump by these mediators results in cellular swelling and an increase in intracellular sodium concentration, which ultimately impairs the expression and localization of the tight junction proteins. Data from murine models of endotoxemia indicate that LPS will decrease the expression and alter the localization of tight junction proteins in the intestine compared to control animals (104). Furthermore, these animals will have increased number of bacteria recovered from regional mesenteric lymph nodes. Nitric oxide appears to be important in the disruption of gut barrier function, as neither intestinal permeability nor bacterial translocation is observed when knockout mice lacking iNOS are treated with LPS. Similar alterations in hepatic (105) and pulmonary (106) epithelial barrier function and tight junction protein expression and localization have been shown during murine endotoxicosis.

Derangements in Gut Barrier Function

Although epithelial barrier function in the intestine may be altered during sepsis and other inflammatory states, thereby allowing bacterial translocation to occur, there are other components of the gut barrier that will prevent the bacteria or bacterial products from gaining access to systemic organs (107). In addition to alterations in the epithelial barrier described previously, other clinical conditions that can contribute to altered gut barrier function include antibiotics, stress ulcer prevention, hypoalbuminemia, vasoactive agents, and use of hyperosmolar feeding preparations. The clinical importance of the disrupted gut barrier function in the pathogenesis of MODS remains ill defined at this point.

APOPTOSIS

Apoptosis (programmed cell death) is the term used to describe a specific method by which cells die. The event is a well-defined, active, and energy-dependent process. There are two primary pathways involved in apoptosis: The intrinsic (mitochondrial and endoplasmic reticulum) pathway and the extrinsic ("death receptor") pathway (108). The latter pathway is activated by receptors such as Fas, with the subsequent activation of two enzymes, caspase-8 or -10. The intrinsic pathway stimulates caspase-9 by loss of the mitochondrial membrane potential and movement of cytochrome c into the cytosol. These initiator caspases cleave effector caspases (e.g., caspase-3 and -7), which results in the cleavage of cellular proteins and DNA and, ultimately, apoptosis (109).

The exact role of apoptosis in the development of MODS is unclear. In animal models of infection, lymphocyte, endothelial cell, kidney, lung, and skeletal muscle, apoptosis is increased (110). Data from clinical studies show that upregulation of apoptotic pathways is increased in patients with ARDS (111). Furthermore, widespread apoptosis occurs in splenic and colonic lymphoid populations in patients who die from sepsis and MODS (112,113). The effect of apoptosis on the immune function includes loss of various immune cells and impairment of immunity by apoptosis-induced immunosuppression of the remaining immune cells (114). Therapies directed against these programmed pathways are under intense investigation and include inhibition of cytochrome c release, use of RNA interference for gene silencing, and caspase inhibitors (114).

COMPLEX NONLINEAR SYSTEMS

The body may be considered a biologic network that is complex, highly coupled, and nonlinear (115). The host response to trauma, shock, or sepsis—involving metabolic, neural, endocrine, inflammatory, and immune components—is such an example (116). The behavior of such a system cannot be predicted with great reliability; however, the system is "attracted" to specific states or stable configurations: "organized variability" (116,117). A large enough perturbation to an organ or mediator network may have unexpected and significant results elsewhere in the host and ultimately lead to MODS (118). In the healthy individual, there is a high degree of heart rate (beat-to-beat) variability. Several studies have shown a relationship between loss of heart rate variability and increased mortality in critically ill patients (119). In fact, normal volunteers injected with small doses of LPS exhibit loss of heart rate variability (120). Other examples of increased regularity of rhythms associated with disease include Cheyne-Stokes respiration, parkinsonian gait, neutrophil count in chronic myelogenous leukemia, and fever in Hodgkin disease (117). However, several diseases—acromegaly and Cushing disease—are associated with increased complexity (117). These data suggest that health is determined by "distance" from thermodynamic equilibrium: too much or too little variation (low or high entropy) represents pathologic conditions (117). A causal link between perturbations in complex systems and outcome remains elusive. However, following variability over time might allow greater accuracy in patient prognostication or may suggest a medical intervention (121). For example, a low level of complexity in the temperature curve of critically ill patients with MODS portends a poor prognosis (122). More research is needed into nonlinear dynamics to determine its importance and role in the development of MODS.

GENETIC SUSCEPTIBILITY

Single base variations in DNA—single nucleotide polymorphisms (SNPs)—are commonly used to discern genetic differences among patient populations (123). Approximately 1 in every 1,000 bases in the human genome is different between two unrelated individuals (123). Although more than 10 million SNPs have been mapped, only 4% of these occur in genes. By comparing healthy individuals to patients, SNPs involved in disease can be identified. Indeed, some—but not—all clinical studies have documented an increased risk of death and organ dysfunction in patients suffering from sepsis or ARDS and who are homozygotes for SNPs (124–128). In the future, patients may be identified in advance as to who should be monitored more closely or who might be benefit from certain interventions (e.g., anticytokine therapies) (123).

PREVENTION AND TREATMENT OF MULTIPLE ORGAN DYSFUNCTION SYNDROME

Although much progress has been made in our understanding in the pathogenesis of MODS, our knowledge remains incomplete. Consequently, the prevention and treatment of MODS are nonspecific and include the goals of maintaining adequate tissue oxygenation, finding and treating infection, providing adequate nutrition support, minimizing iatrogenic complications, and when necessary, providing artificial support (e.g., dialysis or mechanical ventilation) for individual dysfunctional organs.

Resuscitation

An episode of circulatory shock is probably the most common event that occurs before the development of MODS. As a result, timely restoration of intravascular volume and oxygen delivery is important in preventing or abrogating MODS in high-risk patients.

Controversy continues regarding the correct fluid for resuscitation and the optimal circulating hemoglobin concentration. Crystalloid solutions are efficacious and cheaper than colloid solutions. In a prospective study of a diverse population of critically ill patients comparing the efficacy of normal saline to albumin for fluid resuscitation, there was no overall difference in outcome—death, length of stay, or organ dysfunction—between the two groups (129). Subgroup analysis demonstrated an increased relative risk of death for trauma patients who received albumin, whereas the relative risk of death for severe sepsis patients was higher if saline was used (129). Colloids or hypertonic crystalloid solutions—or colloid/hypertonic crystalloid mixtures—may have beneficial effects on the inflammatory response or the development of edema, and may allow for faster resuscitation (130), but these effects have not been proven to be of overall value when these solutions are used clinically.

Assessing the adequacy of tissue oxygenation can often be difficult. The clinical parameters used most often, including arterial blood pressure, skin color, temperature, urine flow, mixed venous oxygen saturation, and blood-lactate concentrations, may be unreliable. Since observational studies have shown that "supranormal" levels of $\dot{D}O_2$ (660 mL/minute/m^2), VO_2 (170 mL/minute/m^2), and cardiac index (4.5 L/minute/m^2) are associated with higher survival rates, some clinicians have advocated resuscitation to such end points in critically ill patients. Although some studies of patients undergoing high-risk surgery or suffering from trauma suggest that such an approach may be of benefit, the majority of studies over the past 15 years clearly show that resuscitation to these end points in critically ill patients is of no benefit, or actually worsens outcome. Likewise, the use of the pulmonary artery catheter to guide therapy has not been shown to be of benefit in a large number of studies (131–133) and pulmonary capillary wedge pressure does not accurately reflect ventricular volume, even in normal volunteers (134). Less invasive and probably safer monitors have been developed for monitoring cardiac output that compare favorably with the accuracy of the thermodilution method. Use of systolic blood pressure variation, pulse pressure variation, stroke volume variation, or left ventricular end-diastolic area (as assessed by transesophageal echocardiography) may be of greater benefit to guide volume resuscitation than the use of pulmonary capillary wedge pressure. More recent data suggest that such aggressive resuscitation in the ICU may be too late. Early (i.e., in the emergency department before hospital admission), goal-directed therapy can reduce mortality and organ dysfunction in patients with severe sepsis and septic shock (135). Practice parameters for the hemodynamic support of the patient with sepsis and septic shock have been recently revised and provide useful guidelines for the practitioner (136).

Other largely experimental approaches that may be of value for assessing the adequacy of resuscitation include tonometric determination of subcutaneous tissue PCO_2; monitoring of conjunctival PO_2; use of near-infrared spectroscopy to assess the oxidation state of cytochrome a, a_3; sublingual PCO_2 measurements; and tonometric estimation of gastric intramucosal pH (pHi) or PCO_2. The latter two techniques are simple and "minimally invasive." Tonometric evidence of gastric mucosal acidosis (or hypercarbia) has been shown to correlate with both short-term and long-term mortality in critically ill patients, complications after cardiac surgery, and organ dysfunction in patients with pancreatitis (137,138). Sublingual hypercarbia has also been shown to be associated with increased mortality in critically ill patients (139). In addition, prevention of gastric intramucosal acidosis by timely fluid resuscitation and inotropic therapy may reduce mortality (140). However, more recent data have failed to demonstrate the usefulness of using gastric intramural pH as a therapeutic end point for resuscitation (141). Furthermore, the notion that gastric intramucosal acidosis or hypercarbia reflects the hemodynamics of the entire splanchnic bed has been cast into doubt (142).

Mechanical Ventilation

The method by which patients are mechanically ventilated can contribute to organ dysfunction. A plethora of experimental and clinical data indicate that overdistension of the lung through the use of large tidal volumes will cause lung injury, stimulate the release of inflammatory mediators, and effect derangements in organs other than the lung (143–145). Use of small tidal volumes (6 mL/kg) in the care of patients with ALI and ARDS will decrease mortality and increase ventilator-free and organ failure–free days (146). It is crucial to note that oxygenation cannot be used as a proxy for efficacy of therapy since patients who are ventilated with small tidal volumes require a longer period of time before PaO_2 improves.

Cyclic "opening" and "closing" of collapsed airways during tidal ventilation is also thought to cause lung injury (147). A recent small study of patients with ARDS suggests that the use of positive end-expiratory pressure (PEEP) above the lower inflection point of the respiratory system compliance curve reduces mortality and the number of failed organs compared to control patients (148). However, this concept has been called into question by data demonstrating that efforts to improve recruitment of collapsed lung units with high levels of PEEP do not reduce mortality or duration of mechanical ventilation (149) and a computed tomography (CT) scan investigation of patients with ARDS showing that ventilator-induced hyperinflation rather than cyclic recruitment/derecruitment is associated with a greater release of pulmonary inflammatory mediators (150).

Other methods of improving oxygenation in the patient with ARDS or ALI, such as the recruitment maneuver and the prone position, have been attempted. However, prospective randomized studies (151,152) have failed to demonstrate an outcome benefit to these approaches.

Fluid management is also an important component in the care of the patient with ARDS or ALI. Recent data show that a restrictive fluid strategy where cumulative fluid balance is kept close to zero in these patients improves the oxygenation index and increases the number of ventilator-free days without increasing the number of other organ failures (153).

Acute Renal Failure

Acute tubular necrosis (ATN) accounts for over 75% of the cases of acute renal failure (ARF) in the ICU (154), with a mortality rate ranging from 40% to 80%. The most common insult that predisposes ICU patients to ATN is persistent prerenal azotemia (154). Furthermore, in the critically ill patient, there is often more than one insult to the kidney: sepsis; exposure to aminoglycosides, amphotericin B, or radiocontrast agents; and the administration of nonsteroidal anti-inflammatory agents. Efforts to minimize these insults to the kidneys should be maximized. Timely resuscitation as mentioned previously is very important to prevent renal ischemia (135,155). If aminoglycosides must be used to treat infection, once-daily dosing (156) or the use of drug levels to discern pharmacokinetics (157) appears to reduce the risk of nephrotoxicity. Use of liposomal preparations of amphotericin B reduces the risk of renal damage (156). If patients are to receive contrast agents, hydration with sodium bicarbonate solutions have been shown to reduce the risk of subsequent renal dysfunction (158). Although N-acetylcysteine has been purported to reduce the risk of contrast-induced ARF (159), the observed results may be a reflection of the activation of creatinine kinase or an increase in the tubular secretion of creatinine (156). Medications such as "low-dose" dopamine or fenoldopam, which increase renal blood flow or loop diuretics, have no impact on preserving renal function in high-risk patients and should be avoided (156). The various methods of renal replacement therapy for patients with established renal failure are beyond the scope of this chapter; the reader is referred to Chapter 161.

Debridement of Necrotic Tissue and Fracture Stabilization

The presence of dead or devitalized tissue appears to predispose patients to the development of MODS; timely debridement of dead tissue is an important component in the prevention of the syndrome. Early surgical fixation of major lower extremity fractures will result in a lower incidence of ARDS and pneumonia. However, "damage control" orthopedics has recently gained popularity and is a concept whereby fractures are initially treated with external fixation. Definitive therapy occurs later when the patient is more stable. The inflammatory response appears to be attenuated in these patients, and the incidence of organ dysfunction is no higher compared to patients undergoing definitive therapy (160).

Infection

Sepsis is an important cause (or correlate) of MODS. It is important that the presence of infection is excluded in critically ill patients with signs of deteriorating organ function.

Empiric administration of broad-spectrum antibiotics is often necessary in the patient with suspected infection. Failure to administer the correct antibiotic(s) (161) in a timely fashion (162) can increase the risk of death for the patient.

Intra-abdominal Sepsis

Early and adequate drainage of intra-abdominal sepsis is important to prevent the development of MODS. Some surgeons have advocated multiple planned reoperations or open packing for severe cases of intra-abdominal sepsis or necrotizing pancreatitis. However, recent retrospective studies have questioned the utility of the open abdomen for intra-abdominal sepsis therapy because ICU and hospital length of stay and fistula rates appear higher than in matched controls (163). Randomized, prospective trials will be needed to determine when the open approach is optimal; one such trial is under way for patients with pancreatitis (164). Without clinical or radiologic evidence of intra-abdominal infection, "blind" laparotomy in the patient with worsening MODS is unlikely to be fruitful.

Pulmonary Sepsis

Ventilator-associated pneumonia (VAP) can play a role in the development and course of MODS; this is discussed in more detail in Chapter 111. Proven preventive measures include noninvasive positive pressure ventilation, elevation of the head of the bed (165), continuous subglottic suctioning, weaning protocols, optimization of sedation with daily "wake-ups" for the patient (166), and chlorhexidine oral rinse.

Selective digestive decontamination (SDD) is a technique by which topical nonabsorbable antibacterial and antifungal agents (usually with a concomitant 3- to 5-day course of systemic antibiotic therapy) are applied to the oropharynx and proximal bowel in mechanically ventilated patients to reduce the incidence of nosocomial infections, organ dysfunction, and mortality. A meta-analysis of 57 randomized controlled trials demonstrated a favorable effect on bloodstream infections and mortality (167). Fears concerning the emergence of resistance organisms do not appear to be well founded. SDD may very well reduce the incidence and prevalence of colonization with resistant Gram-negative aerobic bacteria (168). However, the use of SDD in the United States does not enjoy widespread popularity for reasons that are unclear.

Catheter-related Sepsis

Catheter-related bloodstream infections (CRBSIs) may contribute to the development and propagation of MODS. Proven strategies to reduce the risk of CRBSIs include handwashing prior to catheter insertion, use of maximum barrier precautions (cap, mask, sterile gloves and gown, and a large sterile drape that covers the patient), use of an aqueous chlorhexidine skin preparation solution, avoiding the femoral site for catheter insertion, and removing catheters when no longer needed (169). If these measures are ineffective in reducing the risk of infection, catheters with antiseptic surfaces (170,171) or impregnated with antibiotics (172) or the use of chlorhexidine dressing sponges can reduce the risk of infection.

Other Sources of Sepsis

Many other sources of infection in critically ill patients may contribute to the development of MODS. These infections are not always readily apparent, and the practitioner caring for the patient should remain alert to their presence. Some of these sources of infection include purulent sinusitis, suppurative thrombophlebitis, otitis media, perirectal abscess, epididymitis, prostatitis, calculous or acalculous cholecystitis (173), meningitis or brain abscess (particularly after instrumentation of the central nervous system), prosthetic intravascular graft infection, lower or upper urinary tract infection, and endocarditis. Physical examination and appropriate laboratory and radiographic studies should exclude these conditions.

Nutrition Support

Malnutrition can contribute to the morbidity and mortality of sepsis and MODS (see Chapter 64). Proteolysis is a prominent finding in sepsis and, although it cannot be suppressed by infusing amino acids, protein anabolism can be achieved by appropriate nutritional support. Furthermore, catabolism is mediated by endogenous catecholamines, and administration of β-adrenergic blocking agents can reverse the hypermetabolic response and protein catabolism (174). Early nutritional support may be beneficial in patients at risk for developing MODS (175). The consensus among experts is that if nutritional support is started, enteral feeding is preferable to the parenteral route in a variety of critically ill patients (176).

Regardless of the route of feeding, overfeeding should be avoided. The excessive administration of carbohydrates can alter the respiratory quotient with adverse effects on weaning from mechanical ventilation and affect hepatic metabolic function, thereby altering drug clearance and inducing hyperglycemia. Current guidelines for support of hypermetabolic patients with sepsis or MODS include a total caloric intake (exclusive of protein) of 20 to 25 kcal/kg/day—2 to 5 g/kg/day of glucose, plus 0.5 to 1.0 g/kg/day of fat, and 1.2 to 1.5 g/kg/day of protein. The number of calories needed for a given patient can be estimated using the Harris-Benedict equation or refined using indirect calorimetry.

Hyperglycemia can be a difficult problem, even when patients are not being fed. A strategy using a continuous infusion of insulin to maintain a range of serum glucose of 80 to 110 mg/dL in surgical patients can reduce mortality and organ dysfunction (e.g., renal failure and critical-illness polyneuropathy) (177). In medical ICU patients, morbidity, but not mortality, is reduced with such an intensive insulin regimen (178). Such a strategy is cost effective, with average savings of over $1,500 per patient (179). Maintenance of normal serum glucose levels appears to be the factor associated with the favorable outcome rather than the insulin dose (180).

Specialty Formulas

A number of enteral nutritional formulas are available that provide specific nutrients: glutamine, peptides, arginine, omega-3 fatty acids, nucleic acids, and antioxidants (e.g., vitamins E and C, β-carotene). Arginine is the substrate for NO synthase and is important in lymphocyte proliferation and wound healing (181). Omega-3 fatty acids change membrane lipid composition and can alter the inflammatory response (182). Nucleic acids assist in the proliferation of lymphocytes and intestinal crypt cells, as well as DNA and RNA synthesis (181). Several enteral nutrition formulas are available that include combinations of these additives. The Canadian Critical Care Clinical Practice Guideline Committee (183) recommends that arginine

TABLE 54.4

SUGGESTED STRATEGIES FOR THE PREVENTION OF MULTIPLE ORGAN DYSFUNCTION SYNDROME

1. **Prevention of hospital-acquired infection**
    a. Prevention of catheter-related bloodstream infections
        – Implementation of educational initiatives
        – Use of chlorhexidine solution for skin preparation
        – Use of maximum barrier precautions
        – Avoidance of the femoral insertion site
        – Removing catheter as soon as possible when no longer needed
    b. Strict infection control measures and hand hygiene
2. **Metabolic control and support**
    a. Strict glucose control
    b. Early enteral nutrition
3. **Early and appropriate treatment of infection and trauma**
    a. Early goal-directed therapy for severe sepsis
    b. Early and aggressive resuscitation of trauma victims
    c. Prompt eradication of documented sources/foci of infection
    d. Early fracture stabilization in multiple trauma
    e. Appropriate empiric antibiotic therapy according to consensus guidelines where available with earliest possible de-escalation of therapy according to culture results
4. **Prevention of acute lung injury (ALI), acute respiratory distress syndrome (ARDS), and ventilator-associated and aspiration pneumonia**
    a. Elevation of the head of bed to 30 degrees in all patients without spine precautions
    b. Stress gastritis prophylaxis according to consensus guidelines
    c. Lung protective ventilation strategies in patients with ALI/ARDS
    d. Implementation of weaning protocols
    e. Daily sedation holidays
    f. Chlorhexidine oral rinse
    g. Selective decontamination of the digestive tract
5. **Prevention of acute renal failure**
    a. Normal saline administration to prevent contrast-induced nephropathy with the addition of sodium bicarbonate or N-acetylcysteine as indicated
    b. Discontinuation of nephrotoxic drugs whenever possible; consider once-daily dosing regimens for aminoglycoside antibiotics

and other "select" nutrients not be used for enteral nutrition. However, in patients with ARDS, a formula supplemented with fish oil, borage oil, and antioxidants should be used (183). Although routine use of glutamine is discouraged, in patients with trauma and burns, enteral glutamine should be considered (183).

SUMMARY

Standard therapy for patients with MODS includes adequate cardiovascular resuscitation, identification and timely treatment of infection, early enteral nutrition, "tight" glucose control, individualized support for dysfunctional organs, and minimizing iatrogenic complications by following clinical practice guidelines based on evidence-based medicine for mechanical ventilation and prevention of ventilator-associated pneumonia and catheter-related bloodstream infections (Table 54.4) (184,185). Development of well-functioning ICU teams helps facilitate these paradigms of care. Improved outcome may be realized if patients at high risk for developing the syndrome can be identified earlier so that preventive measures can be instituted when appropriate. Because the pathogenesis of MODS involves numerous mediators, it is doubtful that all patients can be treated with a single agent or mode of therapy.

PEARLS

- MODS develops in up to 40% of critically ill patients without a diagnosis of sepsis and up to 70% of those with a diagnosis of severe sepsis. Mortality attributable to MODS rises as the number of failing organ systems increases; mortality rates in patients with one, two, or three failing organs average 30%, 50%, and greater than 70%, respectively, depending on the etiology of MODS and the organ systems involved.
- Population-based, but not individual, risks of mortality can be predicted with high degrees of precision by several severity-of-illness scoring systems and models.
- MODS may result from "single-hit" insults such as severe infection or trauma, or may evolve through several stages, each having characteristic clinical features.
- An uncontrolled focus of infection, ongoing perfusion deficits resulting in diminished tissue $\dot{D}O_2$, injured or devitalized tissue, and persistent inflammation commonly initiate and sustain MODS.
- Fever or hypothermia and leukocytosis are not always the manifestations of sepsis but may represent systemic inflammation.
- TNF-α, IL-1, IL-6, IL-8, platelet-activating factor, ROS, and NO are pivotal early mediators in the host response to

infection and have multiple pathophysiologic effects relevant to MODS.

- Inappropriate regulation of the production of cytokines, eicosanoids, ROS, and NO is thought to be of causal significance in MODS, as are pathologic neutrophil–endothelial interactions and cross-talk among elements of the coagulation, complement, and kinin cascades.
- Alterations in microvascular blood flow play an important role in the pathogenesis of organ dysfunction in shock. The surface receptors and mediators associated with these alterations include oxidants, lectins, proteases, vasoactive products of iNOS, and altered adrenergic receptor sensitivity.
- Clinically occult dysfunction of the gastrointestinal (GI) mucosal barrier in the ICU is common because of splanchnic ischemia from shock, and may result in endogenous endotoxemia and bacterial translocation.
- Neutrophil- and ROS-mediated intestinal I/R injury in the postresuscitation period is a potential mechanism of remote organ damage. This may lead to a domino-like sequence of organ failures.
- The liver plays a pivotal but clinically inapparent role in systemic host defense through four mechanisms. First, mononuclear phagocytic (Kupffer) cell uptake processes control the magnitude and circulating half-life of endotoxin, bacteria, and vasoactive by-products. Second, production and export of TNF-α with other mediators directly modulate lung function and cardiovascular stability. Third, hepatobiliary clearance is important in the metabolic inactivation and detoxification of such mediators. Fourth, the synthesis of acute-phase reactants regulates several key aspects of metabolism and inflammation.
- Reductions in total hepatic blood flow ($\dot{Q}L$) and $\dot{D}O_2$, or its partitioning between portal venous and hepatic arterial flows, may alter the aforementioned mechanisms, thereby influencing systemic immunoregulation.
- Signs of established MODS are manifested differently in each organ (e.g., ARDS, ARF), yet such changes often reflect generalized endothelial injury and inflammation.
- Diverse medical conditions may mimic sepsis-related MODS and should be excluded when appropriate. These include connective tissue diseases, intoxications, and neoplasms.
- Typical metabolic responses in MODS include hyperglycemia from insulin resistance, accelerated Cori cycle activity, and hepatic glucose release from gluconeogenesis and glycogenolysis. Hypertriglyceridemia results from TNF-α–related reductions in lipoprotein lipase activity. Hepatic lipogenesis is enhanced, increasing the respiratory quotient and minute ventilation. Marked protein catabolism from cytokine-mediated muscle proteolysis and urinary nitrogen wasting is typical.
- Early rapid resuscitation from shock, irrespective of its etiology, attenuates injury to regional organs and may decrease the incidence of MODS.
- Goal-oriented hemodynamic therapy should be initiated early (within 6 hours) after presentation and target values achieved within 12 to 24 hours.

ACKNOWLEDGMENTS

The authors thank Marguerite Eckhouse and Susan St. Martin for their editorial assistance. This chapter is a revision of the chapter authored by George M. Matuschak, MD, in the third edition of this textbook and relies on material previously coauthored by the senior author (Heard SO, Fink MP. Multiple-organ dysfunction syndrome. In: Murray MJ, Coursin DB, Pearl RG, et al., eds. *Critical Care Medicine. Perioperative Management.* Philadelphia: Lippincott Williams & Wilkins; 2002).

References

1. American College of Chest Physicians/Society of Critical Care Medicine Consensus Conference. Definitions for sepsis and organ failure and guidelines for the use of innovative therapies in sepsis. *Crit Care Med.* 1992; 20:864.
2. Garcia Lizana F, Manzano Alonso JL, Gonzalez Santana B, et al. [Survival and quality of life of patients with multiple organ failure one year after leaving an intensive care unit]. *Med Clin (Barc).* 2000;114(Suppl 3):99.
3. Goris RJ, te Boekhorst TP, Nuytinck JK, et al. Multiple-organ failure. Generalized autodestructive inflammation? *Arch Surg.* 1985;120:1109.
4. Knaus WA, Draper EA, Wagner DP, et al. Prognosis in acute organ-system failure. *Ann Surg.* 1985;202:685.
5. Marshall JC, Cook DJ, Christou NV, et al. Multiple organ dysfunction score: a reliable descriptor of a complex clinical outcome. *Crit Care Med.* 1995;23:1638.
6. Vincent JL, Moreno R, Takala J, et al. The SOFA (Sepsis-related Organ Failure Assessment) score to describe organ dysfunction/failure. On behalf of the Working Group on Sepsis- Related Problems of the European Society of Intensive Care Medicine. *Intensive Care Med.* 1996;22:707.
7. Moreno R, Vincent JL, Matos R, et al. The use of maximum SOFA score to quantify organ dysfunction/failure in intensive care. Results of a prospective, multicentre study. Working Group on Sepsis related Problems of the ESICM. *Intensive Care Med.* 1999;25:686.
8. Ferreira FL, Bota DP, Bross A, et al. Serial evaluation of the SOFA score to predict outcome in critically ill patients. *JAMA.* 2001;286:1754.
9. Herridge MS, Cheung AM, Tansey CM, et al. One-year outcomes in survivors of the acute respiratory distress syndrome. *N Engl J Med.* 2003; 348:683.
10. Vincent JL, Sakr Y, Sprung CL, et al. Sepsis in European intensive care units: results of the SOAP study. *Crit Care Med.* 2006;34:344.
11. Bell RC, Coalson JJ, Smith JD, et al. Multiple organ system failure and infection in adult respiratory distress syndrome. *Ann Intern Med.* 1983;99:293.
12. Knaus WA, Wagner DP, Draper EA, et al. The APACHE III prognostic system. Risk prediction of hospital mortality for critically ill hospitalized adults. *Chest.* 1991;100:1619.
13. Sauaia A, Moore FA, Moore EE, et al. Early predictors of postinjury multiple organ failure. *Arch Surg.* 1994;129:39.
14. Levy MM, Fink MP, Marshall JC, et al. 2001 SCCM/ESICM/ACCP/ATS/SIS International Sepsis Definitions Conference. *Crit Care Med.* 2003; 31:1250.
15. Rangel-Frausto MS, Pittet D, Costigan M, et al. The natural history of the systemic inflammatory response syndrome (SIRS). A prospective study. *JAMA.* 1995;273:117.
16. Komatsu T, Shibutani K, Okamoto K, et al. Critical level of oxygen delivery after cardiopulmonary bypass. *Crit Care Med.* 1987;15:194.
17. Ronco JJ, Fenwick JC, Tweeddale MG, et al. Identification of the critical oxygen delivery for anaerobic metabolism in critically ill septic and nonseptic humans. *JAMA.* 1993;270:1724.
18. Houben AJ, Beljaars JH, Hofstra L, et al. Microvascular abnormalities in chronic heart failure: a cross-sectional analysis. *Microcirculation.* 2003;10:471.
19. Vajda K, Szabo A, Boros M. Heterogeneous microcirculation in the rat small intestine during hemorrhagic shock: quantification of the effects of hypertonic-hyperoncotic resuscitation. *Eur Surg Res.* 2004;36:338.
20. Arslan E, Sierko E, Waters JH, et al. Microcirculatory hemodynamics after acute blood loss followed by fresh and banked blood transfusion. *Am J Surg.* 2005;190:456.
21. Cryer HM, Gosche J, Harbrecht J, et al. The effect of hypertonic saline resuscitation on responses to severe hemorrhagic shock by the skeletal muscle, intestinal, and renal microcirculation systems: seeing is believing. *Am J Surg.* 2005;190:305.
22. Astiz ME, DeGent GE, Lin RY, et al. Microvascular function and rheologic changes in hyperdynamic sepsis. *Crit Care Med.* 1995;23:265.
23. De Blasi RA, Palmisani S, Alampi D, et al. Microvascular dysfunction and skeletal muscle oxygenation assessed by phase-modulation near-infrared spectroscopy in patients with septic shock. *Intensive Care Med.* 2005;31: 1661.
24. De Backer D, Creteur J, Dubois MJ, et al. Microvascular alterations in patients with acute severe heart failure and cardiogenic shock. *Am Heart J.* 2004;147:91.

25. De Backer D, Creteur J, Preiser J-C, et al. Microvascular blood flow is altered in patients with sepsis. *Am J Respir Crit Care Med.* 2002;166:98.
26. VanderMeer TJ, Wang H, Fink MP. Endotoxemia causes ileal mucosal acidosis in the absence of mucosal hypoxia in a normodynamic porcine model of septic shock. *Crit Care Med.* 1995;23:1217.
27. Rosser DM, Stidwill RP, Jacobson D, et al. Oxygen tension in the bladder epithelium rises in both high and low cardiac output endotoxemic sepsis. *J Appl Physiol.* 1995;79:1878.
28. Boekstegers P, Weidenhofer S, Kapsner T, et al. Skeletal muscle partial pressure of oxygen in patients with sepsis. *Crit Care Med.* 1994;22:640.
29. Brealey D, Brand M, Hargreaves I, et al. Association between mitochondrial dysfunction and severity and outcome of septic shock. *Lancet.* 2002;360:219.
30. Svistunenko DA, Davies N, Brealey D, et al. Mitochondrial dysfunction in patients with severe sepsis: an EPR interrogation of individual respiratory chain components. *Biochim Biophys Acta.* 2006;1757:262.
31. Singer M. Metabolic failure. *Crit Care Med.* 2005;33(12 Suppl):S539.
32. Szabo C, Zingarelli B, O'Connor M, et al. DNA strand breakage, activation of poly (ADP-ribose) synthetase, and cellular energy depletion are involved in the cytotoxicity of macrophages and smooth muscle cells exposed to peroxynitrite. *Proc Natl Acad Sci U S A.* 1996;93:1753.
33. Szabo C, Zingarelli B, Salzman AL. Role of poly-ADP ribosyltransferase activation in the vascular contractile and energetic failure elicited by exogenous and endogenous nitric oxide and peroxynitrite. *Circ Res.* 1996;78:1051.
34. Dommett RM, Klein N, Turner MW. Mannose-binding lectin in innate immunity: past, present and future. *Tissue Antigens.* 2006;68:193.
35. Nieuwenhuijzen GA, Meyer MP, Hendriks T, et al. Deficiency of complement factor C5 reduces early mortality but does not prevent organ damage in an animal model of multiple organ dysfunction syndrome. *Crit Care Med.* 1995;23:1686.
36. Ivanovska N, Hristova M, Philipov S. Complement modulatory activity of bisbenzylisoquinoline alkaloids isolated from Isopyrum thalictroides–II. Influence on C3–9 reactions *in vitro* and antiinflammatory effect *in vivo*. *Int J Immunopharmacol.* 1999;21:337.
37. Harkin DW, Romaschin A, Taylor SM, et al. Complement C5a receptor antagonist attenuates multiple organ injury in a model of ruptured abdominal aortic aneurysm. *J Vasc Surg.* 2004;39:196.
38. Robbins RA, Russ WD, Rasmussen JK, et al. Activation of the complement system in the adult respiratory distress syndrome. *Am Rev Respir Dis.* 1987;135:651.
39. Fosse E, Pillgram-Larsen J, Svennevig JL, et al. Complement activation in injured patients occurs immediately and is dependent on the severity of the trauma. *Injury.* 1998;29:509.
40. Hecke F, Schmidt U, Kola A, et al. Circulating complement proteins in multiple trauma patients–correlation with injury severity, development of sepsis, and outcome. *Crit Care Med.* 1997;25:2015.
41. Fowler AA, Hyers TM, Fisher BJ, et al. The adult respiratory distress syndrome. Cell populations and soluble mediators in the air spaces of patients at high risk. *Am Rev Respir Dis.* 1987;136:1225.
42. Zeerleder S, Caliezi C, van Mierlo G, et al. Administration of C1 inhibitor reduces neutrophil activation in patients with sepsis. *Clin Diagn Lab Immunol.* 2003;10:529.
43. Caliezi C, Zeerleder S, Redondo M, et al. C1-inhibitor in patients with severe sepsis and septic shock: beneficial effect on renal dysfunction. *Crit Care Med.* 2002;30:1722.
44. Lindsay TF, Luo XP, Lehotay DC, et al. Ruptured abdominal aortic aneurysm, a "two-hit" ischemia/reperfusion injury: evidence from an analysis of oxidative products. *J Vasc Surg.* 1999;30:219.
45. Saikumar P, Dong Z, Weinberg JM, et al. Mechanisms of cell death in hypoxia/reoxygenation injury. *Oncogene.* 1998;17:3341.
46. Kietzmann D, Kahl R, Muller M, et al. Hydrogen peroxide in expired breath condensate of patients with acute respiratory failure and with ARDS. *Intensive Care Med.* 1993;19:78.
47. Lamb NJ, Gutteridge JM, Baker C, et al. Oxidative damage to proteins of bronchoalveolar lavage fluid in patients with acute respiratory distress syndrome: evidence for neutrophil-mediated hydroxylation, nitration, and chlorination. *Crit Care Med.* 1999;27:1738.
48. Richard C, Lemonnier F, Thibault M, et al. Vitamin E deficiency and lipoperoxidation during adult respiratory distress syndrome. *Crit Care Med.* 1990;18:4.
49. Lang JD, McArdle PJ, O'Reilly PJ, et al. Oxidant-antioxidant balance in acute lung injury. *Chest.* 2002;122(6 Suppl):314S.
50. Bernard GR, Wheeler AP, Arons MM, et al. A trial of antioxidants N-acetylcysteine and procysteine in ARDS. The Antioxidant in ARDS Study Group. *Chest.* 1997;112:164.
51. Gadek JE, DeMichele SJ, Karlstad MD, et al. Effect of enteral feeding with eicosapentaenoic acid, gamma-linolenic acid, and antioxidants in patients with acute respiratory distress syndrome. Enteral Nutrition in ARDS Study Group. *Crit Care Med.* 1999;27:1409.
52. Ortolani O, Conti A, De Gaudio AR, et al. Protective effects of N-acetylcysteine and rutin on the lipid peroxidation of the lung epithelium during the adult respiratory distress syndrome. *Shock.* 2000;13:14.
53. Fein AM, Bernard GR, Criner GJ, et al. Treatment of severe systemic inflammatory response syndrome and sepsis with a novel bradykinin antagonist, deltibant (CP-0127). Results of a randomized, double-blind, placebo-controlled trial. CP-0127 SIRS and Sepsis Study Group. *JAMA.* 1997;277:482.
54. Levi M. Disseminated intravascular coagulation: what's new? *Crit Care Clin.* 2005;21:449.
55. Gando S, Iba T, Eguchi Y, et al. A multicenter, prospective validation of disseminated intravascular coagulation diagnostic criteria for critically ill patients: comparing current criteria. *Crit Care Med.* 2006;34:625.
56. Ten Cate H. Trombocytopenia: one of the markers of disseminated intravascular coagulation. *Pathophysiol Haemost Thromb.* 2003;33:413.
57. Bernard GR, Vincent JL, Laterre PF, et al. Efficacy and safety of recombinant human activated protein C for severe sepsis. *N Engl J Med.* 2001; 344:699.
58. Bulger EM, Maier RV. Lipid mediators in the pathophysiology of critical illness. *Crit Care Med.* 2000;28(4 Suppl):N27.
59. Bernard GR, Wheeler AP, Russell JA, et al. The effects of ibuprofen on the physiology and survival of patients with sepsis. The Ibuprofen in Sepsis Study Group. *N Engl J Med.* 1997;336:912.
60. Abraham E, Naum C, Bandi V, et al. Efficacy and safety of LY315920Na/S-5920, a selective inhibitor of 14-kDa group IIA secretory phospholipase A2, in patients with suspected sepsis and organ failure. *Crit Care Med.* 2003;31:718.
61. Slotman GJ, Burchard KW, D'Arezzo A. Ketoconazole prevents acute respiratory failure in critically ill surgical patients. *J Trauma.* 1988;28:648.
62. Yu M, Tomasa G. A double-blind, prospective, randomized trial of ketoconazole, a thromboxane synthetase inhibitor, in the prophylaxis of the adult respiratory distress syndrome. *Crit Care Med.* 1993;21:1635.
63. Ketoconazole for early treatment of acute lung injury and acute respiratory distress syndrome: a randomized controlled trial. The ARDS Network. *JAMA.* 2000;283:1995.
64. Opal S, Laterre PF, Abraham E, et al. Recombinant human platelet-activating factor acetylhydrolase for treatment of severe sepsis: results of a phase III, multicenter, randomized, double-blind, placebo-controlled, clinical trial. *Crit Care Med.* 2004;32:332.
65. Claus RA, Russwurm S, Dohrn B, et al. Plasma platelet-activating factor acetylhydrolase activity in critically ill patients. *Crit Care Med.* 2005;33:1416.
66. Dinarello CA. Proinflammatory and anti-inflammatory cytokines as mediators in the pathogenesis of septic shock. *Chest.* 1997;112(6 Suppl):321S.
67. Gosain A, Gamelli RL. A primer in cytokines. *J Burn Care Rehabil.* 2005; 26:7.
68. Michie HR, Manogue KR, Spriggs DR, et al. Detection of circulating tumor necrosis factor after endotoxin administration. *N Engl J Med.* 1988;318:1481.
69. Michie HR, Spriggs DR, Manogue KR, et al. Tumor necrosis factor and endotoxin induce similar metabolic responses in human beings. *Surgery.* 1988;104:280.
70. Tracey KJ, Fong Y, Hesse DG, et al. Anti-cachectin/TNF monoclonal antibodies prevent septic shock during lethal bacteraemia. *Nature.* 1987; 330:662.
71. Martins GA, Da Gloria Da Costa Carvalho M, Rocha Gattass C. Sepsis: a follow-up of cytokine production in different phases of septic patients. *Int J Mol Med.* 2003;11(5):585–591.
72. Oberholzer A, Souza SM, Tschoeke SK, et al. Plasma cytokine measurements augment prognostic scores as indicators of outcome in patients with severe sepsis. *Shock.* 2005;23:488.
73. Panacek EA, Marshall JC, Albertson TE, et al. Efficacy and safety of the monoclonal anti-tumor necrosis factor antibody F(ab')2 fragment afelimomab in patients with severe sepsis and elevated interleukin-6 levels. *Crit Care Med.* 2004;32:2173.
74. Oberholzer A, Oberholzer C, Moldawer LL. Cytokine signaling–regulation of the immune response in normal and critically ill states. *Crit Care Med.* 2000;28(4 Suppl):N3.
75. Dinarello CA. Interleukin-1beta. *Crit Care Med.* 2005;33(12 Suppl):S460.
76. Vincent JL, Slotman G, Van Leeuwen PA, et al. IL-1ra administration does not improve cardiac function in patients with severe sepsis. *J Crit Care.* 1999;14:69.
77. Opal SM, Fisher CJ Jr, Dhainaut JF, et al. Confirmatory interleukin-1 receptor antagonist trial in severe sepsis: a phase III, randomized, double-blind, placebo-controlled, multicenter trial. The Interleukin-1 Receptor Antagonist Sepsis Investigator Group. *Crit Care Med.* 1997;25:1115.
78. Fisher CJ Jr, Dhainaut JF, Opal SM, et al. Recombinant human interleukin 1 receptor antagonist in the treatment of patients with sepsis syndrome. Results from a randomized, double-blind, placebo-controlled trial. Phase III rhIL-1ra Sepsis Syndrome Study Group. *JAMA.* 1994;271:1836.
79. Song M, Kellum JA. Interleukin-6. *Crit Care Med.* 2005;33(12 Suppl):S463.
80. Derhaschnig U, Bergmair D, Marsik C, et al. Effect of interleukin-6 blockade on tissue factor-induced coagulation in human endotoxemia. *Crit Care Med.* 2004;32:1136.
81. Remick DG. Interleukin-8. *Crit Care Med.* 2005;33(12 Suppl):S466.
82. Rodriguez JL, Miller CG, DeForge LE, et al. Local production of interleukin-8 is associated with nosocomial pneumonia. *J Trauma.* 1992;33:74.
83. Wang H, Bloom O, Zhang M, et al. HMG-1 as a late mediator of endotoxin lethality in mice. *Science.* 1999;285:248.

84. Yang H, Tracey KJ. High mobility group box 1 (HMGB1). *Crit Care Med.* 2005;33(12 Suppl):S472.
85. Yang H, Ochani M, Li J, et al. Reversing established sepsis with antagonists of endogenous high-mobility group box 1. *Proc Natl Acad Sci USA.* 2004;101:296.
86. Leng L, Bucala R. Macrophage migration inhibitory factor. *Crit Care Med.* 2005;33(12 Suppl):S475.
87. Calandra T, Echtenacher B, Roy DL, et al. Protection from septic shock by neutralization of macrophage migration inhibitory factor. *Nat Med.* 2000; 6:164.
88. Joshi PC, Poole GV, Sachdev V, et al. Trauma patients with positive cultures have higher levels of circulating macrophage migration inhibitory factor (MIF). *Res Commun Mol Pathol Pharmacol.* 2000;107:13.
89. Liaudet L, Soriano FG, Szabo C. Biology of nitric oxide signaling. *Crit Care Med.* 2000;28(4 Suppl):N37.
90. Levy RM, Prince JM, Billiar TR. Nitric oxide: a clinical primer. *Crit Care Med.* 2005;33(12 Suppl):S492.
91. Ochoa JB, Udekwu AO, Billiar TR, et al. Nitrogen oxide levels in patients after trauma and during sepsis. *Ann Surg.* 1991;214:621.
92. Horton JW, Maass D, White J, et al. Nitric oxide modulation of TNF-alpha-induced cardiac contractile dysfunction is concentration dependent. *Am J Physiol Heart Circ Physiol.* 2000;278:H1955.
93. Szabo C, Billiar TR. Novel roles of nitric oxide in hemorrhagic shock. *Shock.* 1999;12:1.
94. Zingarelli B. Nuclear factor-kappaB. *Crit Care Med.* 2005;33(12 Suppl): S414.
95. Lopez A, Lorente JA, Steingrub J, et al. Multiple-center, randomized, placebo-controlled, double-blind study of the nitric oxide synthase inhibitor 546C88: effect on survival in patients with septic shock. *Crit Care Med.* 2004;32:21.
96. Vallet B. Bench-to-bedside review: endothelial cell dysfunction in severe sepsis: a role in organ dysfunction? *Crit Care.* 2003;7:130.
97. Lee MM, Schuessler GB, Chien S. Time-dependent effects of endotoxin on the ultrastructure of aortic endothelium. *Artery.* 1988;15:71.
98. Sessler CN, Windsor AC, Schwartz M, et al. Circulating ICAM-1 is increased in septic shock. *Am J Respir Crit Care Med.* 1995;151:1420.
99. Vincent JL, De Backer D. Does disseminated intravascular coagulation lead to multiple organ failure? *Crit Care Clin.* 2005;21:469.
100. Gardinali M, Borrelli E, Chiara O, et al. Inhibition of CD11-CD18 complex prevents acute lung injury and reduces mortality after peritonitis in rabbits. *Am J Respir Crit Care Med.* 2000;161:1022.
101. Xu H, Gonzalo JA, St Pierre Y, et al. Leukocytosis and resistance to septic shock in intercellular adhesion molecule 1-deficient mice. *J Exp Med.* 1994;180:95.
102. Bhagat K, Moss R, Collier J, et al. Endothelial "stunning" following a brief exposure to endotoxin: a mechanism to link infection and infarction? *Cardiovasc Res.* 1996;32:822.
103. Fink MP. Intestinal epithelial hyperpermeability: update on the pathogenesis of gut mucosal barrier dysfunction in critical illness. *Curr Opin Crit Care.* 2003;9:143.
104. Han X, Fink MP, Yang R, et al. Increased iNOS activity is essential for intestinal epithelial tight junction dysfunction in endotoxemic mice. *Shock.* 2004;21:261.
105. Han X, Fink MP, Uchiyama T, et al. Increased iNOS activity is essential for hepatic epithelial tight junction dysfunction in endotoxemic mice. *Am J Physiol Gastrointest Liver Physiol.* 2004;286:G126.
106. Han X, Fink MP, Uchiyama T, et al. Increased iNOS activity is essential for pulmonary epithelial tight junction dysfunction in endotoxemic mice. *Am J Physiol Lung Cell Mol Physiol.* 2004;286:L259.
107. Magnotti LJ, Deitch EA. Burns, bacterial translocation, gut barrier function, and failure. *J Burn Care Rehabil.* 2005;26:383.
108. Perl M, Chung CS, Ayala A. Apoptosis. *Crit Care Med.* 2005;33(12 Suppl): S526.
109. Bredesen DE, Rao RV, Mehlen P. Cell death in the nervous system. *Nature.* 2006;443:796.
110. Mahidhara R, Billiar TR. Apoptosis in sepsis. *Crit Care Med.* 2000;28(4 Suppl):N105.
111. Hashimoto S, Kobayashi A, Kooguchi K, et al. Upregulation of two death pathways of perforin/granzyme and FasL/Fas in septic acute respiratory distress syndrome. *Am J Respir Crit Care Med.* 2000;161:237.
112. Hotchkiss RS, Schmieg RE Jr, Swanson PE, et al. Rapid onset of intestinal epithelial and lymphocyte apoptotic cell death in patients with trauma and shock. *Crit Care Med.* 2000;28:3207.
113. Hotchkiss RS, Swanson PE, Freeman BD, et al. Apoptotic cell death in patients with sepsis, shock, and multiple organ dysfunction. *Crit Care Med.* 1999;27:1230.
114. Hotchkiss RS, Nicholson DW. Apoptosis and caspases regulate death and inflammation in sepsis. *Nat Rev Immunol.* 2006;6:813.
115. Godin PJ, Buchman TG. Uncoupling of biological oscillators: a complementary hypothesis concerning the pathogenesis of multiple organ dysfunction syndrome. *Crit Care Med.* 1996;24:1107.
116. Seely AJ, Christou NV. Multiple organ dysfunction syndrome: exploring the paradigm of complex nonlinear systems. *Crit Care Med.* 2000;28:2193.
117. Seely AJ, Macklem PT. Complex systems and the technology of variability analysis. *Crit Care.* 2004;8(6):R367.
118. Aird WC. Endothelial cell dynamics and complexity theory. *Crit Care Med.* 2002;30(5 Suppl):S180.
119. Haji-Michael PG, Vincent JL, Degaute JP, et al. Power spectral analysis of cardiovascular variability in critically ill neurosurgical patients. *Crit Care Med.* 2000;28:2578.
120. Godin PJ, Fleisher LA, Eidsath A, et al. Experimental human endotoxemia increases cardiac regularity: results from a prospective, randomized, crossover trial. *Crit Care Med.* 1996;24:1117.
121. Papaioannou VE, Maglaveras N, Houvarda I, et al. Investigation of altered heart rate variability, nonlinear properties of heart rate signals, and organ dysfunction longitudinally over time in intensive care unit patients. *J Crit Care.* 2006;21:95.
122. Varela M, Churruca J, Gonzalez A, et al. Temperature curve complexity predicts survival in critically ill patients. *Am J Respir Crit Care Med.* 2006;174:290.
123. Villar J, Maca-Meyer N, Perez-Mendez L, et al. Bench-to-bedside review: understanding genetic predisposition to sepsis. *Crit Care.* 2004;8:180.
124. Stuber F, Petersen M, Bokelmann F, et al. A genomic polymorphism within the tumor necrosis factor locus influences plasma tumor necrosis factor-alpha concentrations and outcome of patients with severe sepsis. *Crit Care Med.* 1996;24:381.
125. Lorenz E, Mira JP, Frees KL, et al. Relevance of mutations in the TLR4 receptor in patients with gram-negative septic shock. *Arch Intern Med.* 2002;162:1028.
126. Gong MN, Zhou W, Williams PL, et al. Polymorphisms in the mannose binding lectin-2 gene and acute respiratory distress syndrome. *Crit Care Med.* 2007;35:48.
127. Walley KR, Russell JA. Protein C-1641 AA is associated with decreased survival and more organ dysfunction in severe sepsis. *Crit Care Med.* 2007;35:12.
128. Lin MT, Albertson TE. Genomic polymorphisms in sepsis. *Crit Care Med.* 2004;32:569.
129. Finfer S, Bellomo R, Boyce N, et al. A comparison of albumin and saline for fluid resuscitation in the intensive care unit. *N Engl J Med.* 2004;350:2247.
130. Wills BA, Nguyen MD, Ha TL, et al. Comparison of three fluid solutions for resuscitation in dengue shock syndrome. *N Engl J Med.* 2005;353:877.
131. Richard C, Warszawski J, Anguel N, et al. Early use of the pulmonary artery catheter and outcomes in patients with shock and acute respiratory distress syndrome: a randomized controlled trial. *JAMA.* 2003;290:2713.
132. Harvey S, Harrison DA, Singer M, et al. Assessment of the clinical effectiveness of pulmonary artery catheters in management of patients in intensive care (PAC-Man): a randomised controlled trial. *Lancet.* 2005;366:472.
133. Gattinoni L, Brazzi L, Pelosi P, et al. A trial of goal-oriented hemodynamic therapy in critically ill patients. SvO2 Collaborative Group. *N Engl J Med.* 1995;333:1025.
134. Kumar A, Anel R, Bunnell E, et al. Pulmonary artery occlusion pressure and central venous pressure fail to predict ventricular filling volume, cardiac performance, or the response to volume infusion in normal subjects. *Crit Care Med.* 2004;32:691.
135. Rivers E, Nguyen B, Havstad S, et al. Early goal-directed therapy in the treatment of severe sepsis and septic shock. *N Engl J Med.* 2001;345:1368.
136. Hollenberg SM, Ahrens TS, Annane D, et al. Practice parameters for hemodynamic support of sepsis in adult patients: 2004 update. *Crit Care Med.* 2004;32:1928.
137. Heard SO. Gastric tonometry: the hemodynamic monitor of choice (Pro). *Chest.* 2003;123(5 Suppl):469S.
138. Kovacs GC, Telek G, Hamar J, et al. Prolonged intestinal mucosal acidosis is associated with multiple organ failure in human acute pancreatitis: gastric tonometry revisited. *World J Gastroenterol.* 2006;12:4892.
139. Marik PE, Bankov A. Sublingual capnometry versus traditional markers of tissue oxygenation in critically ill patients. *Crit Care Med.* 2003;31:818.
140. Gutierrez G, Palizas F, Doglio G, et al. Gastric intramucosal pH as a therapeutic index of tissue oxygenation in critically ill patients. *Lancet.* 1992;339:195.
141. Splanchnic hypoperfusion-directed therapies in trauma: a prospective, randomized trial. *Am Surg.* 2005;71:252.
142. Creteur J, De Backer D, Vincent JL. Does gastric tonometry monitor splanchnic perfusion? *Crit Care Med.* 1999;27:2480.
143. Chiumello D, Pristine G, Slutsky AS. Mechanical ventilation affects local and systemic cytokines in an animal model of acute respiratory distress syndrome. *Am J Respir Crit Care Med.* 1999;160:109.
144. Ranieri VM, Suter PM, Tortorella C, et al. Effect of mechanical ventilation on inflammatory mediators in patients with acute respiratory distress syndrome: a randomized controlled trial. *JAMA.* 1999;282:54.
145. Ranieri VM, Giunta F, Suter PM, et al. Mechanical ventilation as a mediator of multisystem organ failure in acute respiratory distress syndrome. *JAMA.* 2000;284:43.
146. Ventilation with lower tidal volumes as compared with traditional tidal volumes for acute lung injury and the acute respiratory distress syndrome. The Acute Respiratory Distress Syndrome Network. *N Engl J Med.* 2000;342:1301.
147. Rouby JJ, Brochard L. Tidal recruitment and overinflation in acute respiratory distress syndrome: yin and yang. *Am J Respir Crit Care Med.* 2007; 175:104.
148. Villar J, Kacmarek RM, Perez-Mendez L, et al. A high positive

end-expiratory pressure, low tidal volume ventilatory strategy improves outcome in persistent acute respiratory distress syndrome: a randomized, controlled trial. *Crit Care Med.* 2006;34:1311.
149. Brower RG, Lanken PN, MacIntyre N, et al. Higher versus lower positive end-expiratory pressures in patients with the acute respiratory distress syndrome. *N Engl J Med.* 2004;351:327.
150. Terragni PP, Rosboch G, Tealdi A, et al. Tidal hyperinflation during low tidal volume ventilation in Acute Respiratory Distress Syndrome. *Am J Respir Crit Care Med.* 2007;175:160.
151. Oczenski W, Hormann C, Keller C, et al. Recruitment maneuvers after a positive end-expiratory pressure trial do not induce sustained effects in early adult respiratory distress syndrome. *Anesthesiology.* 2004;101:620.
152. Gattinoni L, Tognoni G, Pesenti A, et al. Effect of prone positioning on the survival of patients with acute respiratory failure. *N Engl J Med.* 2001; 345:568.
153. Wiedemann HP, Wheeler AP, Bernard GR, et al. Comparison of two fluid-management strategies in acute lung injury. *N Engl J Med.* 2006;354:2564.
154. Gill N, Nally JV Jr, Fatica RA. Renal failure secondary to acute tubular necrosis: epidemiology, diagnosis, and management. *Chest.* 2005;128: 2847.
155. Lin SM, Huang CD, Lin HC, et al. A modified goal-directed protocol improves clinical outcomes in intensive care unit patients with septic shock: a randomized controlled trial. *Shock.* 2006;26:551.
156. Venkataraman R, Kellum JA. Prevention of acute renal failure. *Chest.* 2007;131:300.
157. Rybak MJ, Abate BJ, Kang SL, et al. Prospective evaluation of the effect of an aminoglycoside dosing regimen on rates of observed nephrotoxicity and ototoxicity. *Antimicrob Agents Chemother.* 1999;43:1549.
158. Merten GJ, Burgess WP, Gray LV, et al. Prevention of contrast-induced nephropathy with sodium bicarbonate: a randomized controlled trial. *JAMA.* 2004;291:2328.
159. Duong MH, MacKenzie TA, Malenka DJ. N-acetylcysteine prophylaxis significantly reduces the risk of radiocontrast-induced nephropathy: comprehensive meta-analysis. *Catheter Cardiovasc Interv.* 2005;64:471.
160. Harwood PJ, Giannoudis PV, van Griensven M, et al. Alterations in the systemic inflammatory response after early total care and damage control procedures for femoral shaft fracture in severely injured patients. *J Trauma.* 2005;58:446.
161. Micek ST, Heuring TJ, Hollands JM, et al. Optimizing antibiotic treatment for ventilator-associated pneumonia. *Pharmacotherapy.* 2006;26:204.
162. Kumar A, Roberts D, Wood KE, et al. Duration of hypotension before initiation of effective antimicrobial therapy is the critical determinant of survival in human septic shock. *Crit Care Med.* 2006;34:1589.
163. Adkins AL, Robbins J, Villalba M, et al. Open abdomen management of intra-abdominal sepsis. *Am Surg.* 2004;70:137.
164. van Santvoort HC, Besselink MG, Cirkel GA, et al. A nationwide Dutch study into the optimal treatment of patients with infected necrotising pancreatitis: the PANTER trial. *Ned Tijdschr Geneeskd.* 2006;150:1844.
165. Drakulovic MB, Torres A, Bauer TT, et al. Supine body position as a risk factor for nosocomial pneumonia in mechanically ventilated patients: a randomised trial. *Lancet.* 1999;354:1851.
166. Schweickert WD, Gehlbach BK, Pohlman AS, et al. Daily interruption of sedative infusions and complications of critical illness in mechanically ventilated patients. *Crit Care Med.* 2004;32:1272.
167. Silvestri L, van Saene HK, Milanese M, et al. Selective decontamination of the digestive tract reduces bacterial bloodstream infection and mortality in critically ill patients. Systematic review of randomized, controlled trials. *J Hosp Infect.* 2007;65:187.
168. de Jonge E, Schultz MJ, Spanjaard L, et al. Effects of selective decontamination of digestive tract on mortality and acquisition of resistant bacteria in intensive care: a randomised controlled trial. *Lancet.* 2003;362:1011.
169. O'Grady NP, Alexander M, Dellinger EP, et al. Guidelines for the prevention of intravascular catheter-related infections. *Infect Control Hosp Epidemiol.* 2002;23:759.
170. Maki DG, Stolz SM, Wheeler S, et al. Prevention of central venous catheter-related bloodstream infection by use of an antiseptic-impregnated catheter. A randomized, controlled trial. *Ann Intern Med.* 1997;127:257.
171. Ranucci M, Isgro G, Giomarelli PP, et al. Impact of oligon central venous catheters on catheter colonization and catheter-related bloodstream infection. *Crit Care Med.* 2003;31:52.
172. Darouiche RO, Raad II, Heard SO, et al. A comparison of two antimicrobial-impregnated central venous catheters. Catheter Study Group. *N Engl J Med.* 1999;340:1.
173. Laurila J, Laurila PA, Saarnio J, et al. Organ system dysfunction following open cholecystectomy for acute acalculous cholecystitis in critically ill patients. *Acta Anaesthesiol Scand.* 2006;50:173.
174. Herndon DN, Hart DW, Wolf SE, et al. Reversal of catabolism by beta-blockade after severe burns. *N Engl J Med.* 2001;345:1223.
175. Perel P, Yanagawa T, Bunn F, et al. Nutritional support for head-injured patients. *Cochrane Database Syst Rev.* 2006;(4):CD001530.
176. McClave SA, Chang WK, Dhaliwal R, et al. Nutrition support in acute pancreatitis: a systematic review of the literature. *JPEN J Parenter Enteral Nutr.* 2006;30:143.
177. van den Berghe G, Wouters P, Weekers F, et al. Intensive insulin therapy in the critically ill patients. *N Engl J Med.* 2001;345:1359.
178. Van den Berghe G, Wilmer A, Hermans G, et al. Intensive insulin therapy in the medical ICU. *N Engl J Med.* 2006;354:449.
179. Krinsley JS, Jones RL. Cost analysis of intensive glycemic control in critically ill adult patients. *Chest.* 2006;129:644.
180. Van den Berghe G, Wouters PJ, Bouillon R, et al. Outcome benefit of intensive insulin therapy in the critically ill: insulin dose versus glycemic control. *Crit Care Med.* 2003;31:359.
181. Cerra FB, Benitez MR, Blackburn GL, et al. Applied nutrition in ICU patients. A consensus statement of the American College of Chest Physicians. *Chest.* 1997;111:769.
182. Endres S, Ghorbani R, Kelley VE, et al. The effect of dietary supplementation with n-3 polyunsaturated fatty acids on the synthesis of interleukin-1 and tumor necrosis factor by mononuclear cells. *N Engl J Med.* 1989;320:265.
183. Canadian Critical Care Clinical Practice Guidelines. Summary of Topics and Recommendations. 2007. http://www.criticalcarenutrition.com. Accessed January 30, 2007.
184. Le Gall JR, Klar J, Lemeshow S, et al. The Logistic Organ Dysfunction System. A new way to assess organ dysfunction in the intensive care unit. ICU Scoring Group. *JAMA.* 1996;276:802.
185. Russell JA, Singer J, Bernard GR, et al. Changing pattern of organ dysfunction in early human sepsis is related to mortality. *Crit Care Med.* 2000; 28:3405.

CHAPTER 55 ■ SHOCK: GENERAL

S. ROB TODD • KRISTA L. TURNER • FREDERICK A. MOORE

HISTORY

Despite significant technologic advances and the improved understanding of shock, it remains a diagnosis associated with significant morbidity and mortality. Hippocrates and Galen were the first to describe a "posttraumatic syndrome." Then in 1737, LeDran, a French surgeon, used the term *choc* to characterize a severe impact or jolt (1). However, it was not until 1867 that Edwin Morris popularized the term (2). He defined shock as "a peculiar effect on the animal system, produced by violent injuries from any cause, or from violent mental emotions."

In the late 1800s, Fischer and Maphoter further delineated the pathophysiology of shock (3,4). Fischer proposed a generalized "vasomotor paralysis" resulting in splanchnic blood pooling as the underlying mechanism of shock, while Maphoter suggested that the clinical manifestations appreciated in shock were the result of the extravascular leakage of fluids. A variation of Fischer's theory was supported by Crile in 1899 (5).

In the early 1900s, Walter B. Cannon proposed a toxin as the source of this altered capillary permeability and intravascular volume loss (6). Blalock challenged this theory in 1930 (7). He charged that significant hemorrhage alone could account for insufficient cardiac output in shock states and that it wasn't the result of circulating toxins. Then in the 1940s, Carl Wiggers demonstrated that following prolonged shock, irreversible circulatory failure could occur (8). At that time, hypotension was synonymous with shock, and blood pressure was the primary end point of resuscitation in shock. As such, volume resuscitation was the primary management strategy.

It wasn't until the turn of the 19th century that sources other than trauma were thought to cause shock. Sepsis was first depicted as causing shock during the Spanish American War (9). This was followed in 1906 with the description of anaphylactic shock. And subsequently in 1935, Tennant and Wiggers documented decreased myocardial contractility following coronary perfusion deprivation (10).

DEFINITION OF SHOCK

The definition of shock has historically been a moving target. Initially equated with hypotension, this is no longer the case (11,12). Shock is defined as an acute clinical syndrome resulting when cellular dysoxia occurs, ultimately leading to organ dysfunction and failure (13). Cellular dysoxia or inadequate tissue perfusion is critical in diagnosing shock, as there are many other causes of organ dysfunction and failure that are not resultant from shock.

Note the emphasis on shock as a syndrome, as this constellation of signs and symptoms predictably follows a well-described series of pathophysiologic events (14). Its clinical presentation varies widely based on the underlying etiology, the degree of organ perfusion, and prior organ dysfunction.

CLASSIFICATION OF SHOCK

The incidence and prevalence of shock are poorly characterized for a multitude of reasons. First and foremost, the definition of shock continues to lack consensus. As such, the screening for shock tends to be inadequate, and thus it is underreported. Additionally, patients presumably die in the prehospital setting. Taking these facts into account, one can readily appreciate why the reported incidence and mortality of shock varies widely.

In 1937, Blalock classified shock (15). He defined four categories: hematogenic or oligemic (hypovolemic), cardiogenic, neurogenic, and vasogenic. Subsequently, Weil and Shubin characterized shock based on cardiovascular parameters (16). The categories included hypovolemic, cardiogenic, extracardiac obstructive, and distributive. Table 55.1 represents an adaptation of this system (17). It is important to appreciate that most shock states incorporate different components of each of the aforementioned shock categories.

Hypovolemic Shock

Hypovolemic shock represents a state of decreased intravascular volume. Inciting events include internal or external hemorrhage, significant fluid losses from the gastrointestinal tract (emesis, high-output fistulae, or diarrhea) or urinary tract (hyperosmolar states), and "third spacing" ("capillary leakage" into the interstitial tissues or the corporeal cavities) (Table 55.1). Additional etiologies include malnutrition and large open wounds (burns and the open abdomen) (16,18).

The pathophysiology of shock is dependent upon its classification. Hypovolemic shock is characterized by a decrease in intravascular volume with resultant decreases in pulmonary capillary wedge pressure and cardiac output (Table 55.2). There is a subsequent increased sympathetic drive in an attempt to increase peripheral vasculature tone, cardiac contractility, and heart rate. These initially beneficial measures ultimately turn detrimental, as their resultant hypermetabolic state predisposes tissues to localized hypoxia (14). Furthermore, the aforementioned increased peripheral vascular tone may result in tissue ischemia via an inconsistent microcirculatory flow. In cases of

TABLE 55.1

SHOCK CLASSIFICATIONS

HYPOVOLEMIC
Hemorrhagic
–Trauma, gastrointestinal, retroperitoneal
Nonhemorrhagic
–Dehydration, emesis, diarrhea, fistulae, burns, polyuria, "third spacing," malnutrition, large open wounds

CARDIOGENIC
Myocardial
–Infarction, contusion, myocarditis, cardiomyopathies, pharmacologic
Mechanical
–Valvular failure, ventricular septal defect, ventricular wall defects
Arrhythmias

OBSTRUCTIVE
Impairment of diastolic filling
–Intrathoracic obstructive tumors, tension pneumothorax, positive-pressure mechanical ventilation, constrictive pericarditis, pericardial tamponade
Impairment of systolic contraction
–Pulmonary embolism, acute pulmonary hypertension, air embolism, tumors, aortic dissection, aortic coarctation

DISTRIBUTIVE
–Septic, anaphylactic, neurogenic, pharmacologic, endocrinologic

From Jimenez EJ. Shock. In: Civetta JM, Taylor RW, Kirby RR, eds. *Critical Care*. 3rd ed. Philadelphia: Lippincott–Raven Publishers; 1997:359; and Kumar A, Parrillo JE. Shock: classification, pathophysiology, and approach to management. In: Parrillo JE, Dellinger RP, eds. *Critical Care Medicine*. 2nd ed. St. Louis: Mosby, Inc.; 2002:371.

severe hypovolemic shock, a significant inflammatory component coexists.

Cardiogenic Shock

Cardiogenic shock is defined as inadequate tissue perfusion due to primary ventricular failure. Its incidence has remained fairly stable, and ranges from 6% to 8% (19–23). In the United States, it is the most common cause of mortality from coronary artery disease (19). Despite medical advances, it remains the number one cause of in-hospital mortality in patients experiencing a transmural myocardial infarction, with rates ranging between 70% and 90% (21,24). Other causes include myocarditis, cardiomyopathies, valvular diseases, and arrhythmias (Table 55.1).

The most common inciting event in cardiogenic shock is an acute myocardial infarction. Historically, once 40% of the myocardium has been irreversibly damaged, cardiogenic shock may result. From a mechanical perspective, decreased cardiac contractility diminishes both stroke volume and cardiac output (Table 55.2). These lead to increased ventricular filling pressures, cardiac chamber dilatation, and ultimately univentricular or biventricular failure with resultant systemic hypotension. This further reduces myocardial perfusion and exacerbates ongoing ischemia. The end result is a vicious cycle with severe cardiovascular decompensation. Similar to hypovolemic shock, a significant systemic inflammatory response has been implicated in the pathophysiology of cardiogenic shock.

Obstructive Shock

In obstructive shock, external forces compress the thin-walled chambers of the heart, the great vessels, or any combination thereof. These forces impair either the diastolic filling or the systolic contraction of the heart (Table 55.1). Large obstructive intrathoracic tumors, tension pneumothoraces, pericardial

TABLE 55.2

SHOCK HEMODYNAMIC PARAMETERS

	CVP	PCWP	CO	SVR	$S\bar{v}O_2$
Hypovolemic	↓↓	↓↓	↓↓	↑	↓
Cardiogenic					
Left ventricular myocardial infarction	Nl or ↑	↑	↓↓	↑	↓
Right ventricular myocardial infarction	↑↑	Nl or ↑	↓↓	↑	↓
Obstructive					
Pericardial tamponade	↑↑	↑↑	↓ or ↓↓	↑	↓
Massive pulmonary embolism	↑↑	Nl or ↓	↓↓	↑	↓
Distributive					
Early	Nl or ↑	Nl	↓ or Nl or ↑	↑ or Nl or ↓	Nl or ↓
Early after fluid administration	Nl or ↑	Nl or ↑	↑	↓	↑ or Nl or ↓
Late	Nl	Nl	↓	↑	↑ or ↓

CVP, central venous pressure; PCWP, pulmonary capillary wedge pressure; CO, cardiac output; SVR, systemic vascular resistance; $S\bar{v}O_2$, mixed venous oxygen saturation; Nl, normal.
From Jimenez EJ. Shock. In: Civetta JM, Taylor RW, Kirby RR, eds. *Critical Care*. 3rd ed. Philadelphia: Lippincott–Raven Publishers; 1997:359; and Kumar A, Parrillo JE. Shock: classification, pathophysiology, and approach to management. In: Parrillo JE, Dellinger RP, eds. *Critical Care Medicine*. 2nd ed. St. Louis: Mosby, Inc.; 2002:371.

tamponade, and constrictive pericarditis limit ventricular filling, while pulmonary emboli and aortic dissection impede cardiac contractility.

The hemodynamic parameters witnessed in obstructive shock include increases in central venous pressure and systemic vascular resistance and decreases in cardiac output and mixed venous oxygen saturation (Table 55.2). The pulmonary capillary wedge pressure and other hemodynamic indices are dependent on the obstructive cause. In pericardial tamponade, there is equalization of the right and left ventricular diastolic pressures, the central venous pressure, and the pulmonary capillary wedge pressure (increased). However, following a massive pulmonary embolus, right ventricular failure leads to increased right heart pressures and a normal or decreased pulmonary capillary wedge pressure.

Distributive Shock

Distributive shock is characterized by a decrease in peripheral vascular tone. Septic shock is the most common form. Additionally, distributive shock includes the other oft-quoted classes of shock including anaphylactic, neurogenic, and adrenal shock (Table 55.1).

Physiologically, all forms of distributive shock exhibit a decreased systemic vascular resistance (Table 55.2). Subsequently, these patients experience a relative hypovolemia as evidenced by a decreased (or normal) central venous pressure and pulmonary capillary wedge pressure. The cardiac output is initially diminished; however, following appropriate volume loading, the cardiac output is increased.

CELLULAR ALTERATIONS

All forms of shock, especially hemorrhagic and septic, induce a host response that is characterized by local and systemic release of proinflammatory cytokines, arachidonic acid metabolites, and activation of complement factors, kinins, and coagulation as well as hormonal mediators. Clinically, this is the systemic inflammatory response syndrome. Paralleling the systemic inflammatory response syndrome is an anti-inflammatory response referred to as the compensatory anti-inflammatory response syndrome. An imbalance between these responses appears to be responsible for increased susceptibility to infection and organ dysfunction (25–29).

Systemic Inflammatory Response Syndrome

In 1991, a consensus conference of the American College of Chest Physicians and the American Society of Critical Care Medicine defined systemic inflammatory response syndrome (SIRS) as a generalized inflammatory response triggered by a variety of infectious and noninfectious events (30). They arbitrarily established clinical parameters through a process of consensus. Table 55.3 summarizes the diagnostic criteria for systemic inflammatory response syndrome. At least two of the four criteria must be present to fulfill the diagnosis of systemic inflammatory response syndrome. Note, this definition emphasizes the inflammatory process regardless of its etiology. Subsequent studies have validated these criteria as predictive of increased intensive care unit mortality, and indicated that this risk increases concurrent with the number of criteria present.

TABLE 55.3

CLINICAL PARAMETERS OF THE SYSTEMIC INFLAMMATORY RESPONSE SYNDROME

1. Heart rate >90 beats/min
2. Respiratory rate >20 breaths/min, or $Paco_2$ <32 mm Hg
3. Temperature >38°C or <36°C
4. Leukocytes >12,000/mm^3 or <4,000/mm^3 or ≥10% juvenile neutrophil granulocytes

$Paco_2$, arterial co_2 partial pressure.

The systemic inflammatory response syndrome is characterized by the local and systemic production and release of multiple mediators, including proinflammatory cytokines, complement factors, proteins of the contact phase and coagulation system, acute phase proteins, neuroendocrine mediators, and an accumulation of immunocompetent cells at the local site of tissue damage (31).

Compensatory Anti-inflammatory Response Syndrome

Shock stimulates not only the release of proinflammatory mediators, but also the parallel release of anti-inflammatory mediators (26). This compensatory anti-inflammatory response is present concurrently with systemic inflammatory response syndrome (Fig. 55.1) (32). When these two opposing responses are appropriately balanced, the patient is able to effectively recover without incurring secondary injury from the autoimmune inflammatory response (25). However, overwhelming compensatory anti-inflammatory response syndrome appears responsible for postshock immunosuppression, which leads to increased susceptibility to infections and sepsis (26,31,33). With time, the systemic inflammatory response syndrome ceases to exist and the compensatory anti-inflammatory response syndrome is the predominant force.

Cytokine Response

Proinflammatory cytokines, tumor necrosis factor-α (TNF-α), and interleukin-1β (IL-1β) are key to the resultant inflammation (34,35). Secondary proinflammatory cytokines are released in a subacute fashion and include IL-2, IL-6, IL-8, platelet-activating factor (PAF), interferon-γ, endothelin-1, leukotrienes, thromboxanes, prostaglandins, and the complement cascade (34,36).

Interleukin-6 also acts as an immunoregulatory cytokine by stimulating the release of anti-inflammatory mediators such as IL-1 receptor antagonists and TNF receptors, which bind circulating proinflammatory cytokines (35). IL-6 also triggers the release of prostaglandin E_2 (PGE_2) from macrophages (35). Prostaglandin E_2 is potentially the most potent endogenous immunosuppressant (35). Not only does it suppress T-cell and macrophage responsiveness, but it also induces the release of

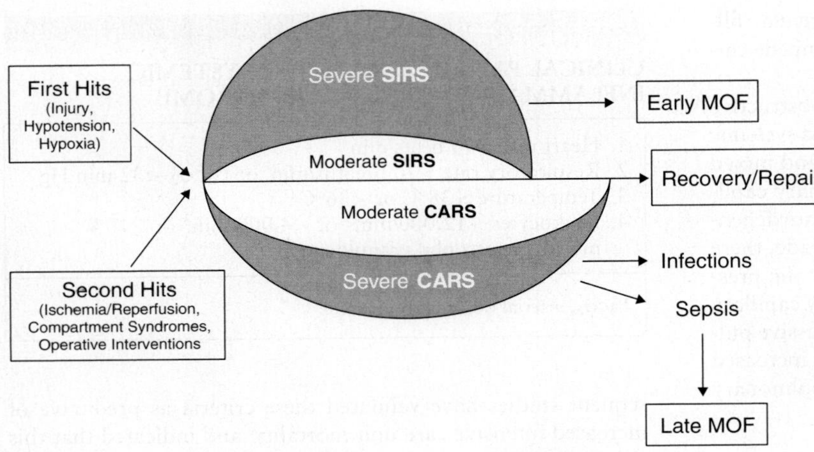

FIGURE 55.1. Postinjury multiple organ failure occurs as a result of a dysfunctional inflammatory response. SIRS, systemic inflammatory response syndrome; MOF, multiple organ failure; CARS, compensatory anti-inflammatory response syndrome.

IL-10, a potent anti-inflammatory cytokine that deactivates monocytes (35). A listing of pro- and anti-inflammatory mediators may be found in Tables 55.4 and 55.5.

Cell-mediated Response

Shock alters the ability of splenic, peritoneal, and alveolar macrophages to release IL-1, IL-6, and TNF-α, leading to

TABLE 55.4

PROINFLAMMATORY MEDIATORS

Mediator	Action
IL-1	IL-1 is pleiotropic. Locally, it stimulates cytokine and cytokine receptor production by T cells as well as stimulating B-cell proliferation. Systemically, IL-1 modulates endocrine responses and induces the acute phase response.
IL-6	IL-6 induces acute phase reactants in hepatocytes and plays an essential role in the final differentiation of B cells into Ig-secreting cells. Additionally, IL-6 has anti-inflammatory properties.
IL-8	IL-8 is one of the major mediators of the inflammatory response. It functions as a chemoattractant and is also a potent angiogenic factor.
IL-12	IL-12 regulates the differentiation of naive T cells into T_H1 cells. It stimulates the growth and function of T cells and alters the normal cycle of apoptotic cell death.
TNF-α	TNF-α is pleiotropic. TNF-α and IL-1 act alone or together to induce systemic inflammation as above. TNF-α is also chemotactic for neutrophils and monocytes, as well as increasing neutrophil activity.
MIF	MIF forms a crucial link between the immune and neuroendocrine systems. It acts systemically to enhance the secretion of IL-1 and TNF-α.

IL, interleukin; Ig, immunoglobulin; TNF, tumor necrosis factor; MIF, migration inhibitory factor.

TABLE 55.5

ANTI-INFLAMMATORY MEDIATORS

Mediator	Action
IL-4	IL-4, IL-3, IL-5, IL-13, and CSF2 form a cytokine gene cluster on chromosome 5q, with this gene particularly close to IL-13.
IL-10	IL-10 has pleiotropic effects in immunoregulation and inflammation. It down-regulates the expression of T_H1 cytokines, MHC class II antigens, and costimulatory molecules on macrophages. It also enhances B-cell survival, proliferation, and antibody production. In addition, it can block NF-κB activity, and is involved in the regulation of the JAK-STAT signaling pathway.
IL-11	IL-11 stimulates the T-cell–dependent development of immunoglobulin-producing B cells. It is also found to support the proliferation of hematopoietic stem cells and megakaryocyte progenitor cells.
IL-13	IL-13 is involved in several stages of B-cell maturation and differentiation. It up-regulates CD23 and MHC class II expression, and promotes IgE isotype switching of B cells. It down-regulates macrophage activity, thereby inhibiting the production of proinflammatory cytokines and chemokines.
IFN-α	IFN-α enhances and modifies the immune response.
TGF-β	TGF-β regulates the proliferation and differentiation of cells, wound healing, and angiogenesis.
α-MSH	α-MSH modulates inflammation by way of three mechanisms: direct action on peripheral inflammatory cells; actions on brain inflammatory cells to modulate local reactions; and indirect activation of descending neural anti-inflammatory pathways that control peripheral tissue inflammation.

IL, interleukin; CSF, colony-stimulating factor; T_H, T helper; MHC, major histocompatibility complex; Ig, immunoglobulin; IFN, interferon; TGF, transforming growth factor; MSH, melanocyte-stimulating hormone.

decreased levels of these proinflammatory cytokines (35). Kupffer cells, however, have an enhanced capacity for production of proinflammatory cytokines. Cell-mediated immunity requires not only functional macrophage and T cells, but also intact macrophage–T-cell interaction (35). Following injury, human leukocyte antigen (HLA-DR) receptor expression is decreased, leading to a loss of antigen-presenting capacity and decreased TNF-α production. Prostaglandin E_2, IL-10, and TGF-β all contribute to this "immunoparalysis" (25,35).

T helper cells differentiate into either T_H1 or T_H2 lymphocytes. T_H1 cells promote the proinflammatory cascade through the release of IL-2, interferon-γ (IFN-γ), and TNF-β, while T_H2 cells produce anti-inflammatory mediators (25,35). Monocytes/macrophages, through the release of IL-12, stimulate the differentiation of T-helper cells into T_H1 cells (35). Because IL-12 production is depressed following trauma, there is a shift toward T_H2, which has been associated with an adverse clinical outcome (25,35).

Adherence of the leukocyte to endothelial cells is mediated through the up-regulation of adhesion molecules. Selectins such as leukocyte adhesion molecule-1 (LAM-1), endothelial leukocyte adhesion molecule-1 (ELAM-1), and P-selectin are responsible for polymorphonuclear leukocytes (PMNLs) "rolling" (25,37). Up-regulation of integrins such as the CD11/18 complexes or intercellular adhesion molecule-1 (ICAM-1) is responsible for PMNL attachment to the endothelium (25). Migration, accumulation, and activation of the PMNLs are mediated by chemoattractants such as chemokines and complement anaphylotoxins (25). Colony-stimulating factors (CSFs) likewise stimulate monocyte- or granulocytopoiesis and reduce apoptosis of PMNLs during SIRS. Neutrophil apoptosis is further reduced by other proinflammatory mediators, thus resulting in PMNL accumulation at the site of local tissue destruction (25).

Leukocyte Recruitment

Proinflammatory cytokines enhance PMNL recruitment, phagocytic activity, and the release of proteases and oxygen-free radicals by PMNLs. This recruitment of leukocytes represents a key element for host defense following trauma, although it allows for the development of secondary tissue damage (38–41). It involves a complex cascade of events culminating in transmigration of the leukocyte, whereby the cell exerts its effects (42). The first step is capture and tethering, mediated via constitutively expressed leukocyte selectin denoted L selectin. L selectin functions by identifying glycoprotein ligands on leukocytes and those up-regulated on cytokine-activated endothelium (42).

Following capture and tethering, endothelial E selectin and P selectin assist in leukocyte rolling or slowing (37,43–48). P selectin is found in the membranes of endothelial storage granules (Weibel-Palade bodies) (45). Following granule secretion, P selectin binds to carbohydrates presented by P selectin glycoprotein ligand (PSGL-1) on the leukocytes (25). In contrast, E selectin is not stored, yet it is synthesized *de novo* in the presence of inflammatory cytokines (43,44). These selectins cause the leukocytes to roll along the activated endothelium, whereby secondary capturing of leukocytes occurs via homotypic interactions.

The third step in leukocyte recruitment is firm adhesion, which is mediated by membrane-expressed β_1- and β_2-integrins (49–51). The integrins bind to ICAM, resulting in cell–cell interactions and ultimately signal transduction. This step is critical to the formation of stable shear-resistant adhesion, which stabilizes the leukocyte for transmigration (49–51).

Transmigration is the final step in leukocyte recruitment following the formation of bonds between the aforementioned integrins and immunoglobulin (Ig)-superfamily members (42). The arrested leukocytes cross the endothelial layer via bicellular and tricellular endothelial junctions in a process coined diapedesis (52). This is mediated by platelet-endothelial cell adhesion molecules (PECAMs), proteins expressed on both the leukocytes and intercellular junctions of endothelial cells (42).

Proteases and Reactive Oxygen Species

Polymorphonuclear lymphocytes and macrophages are not only responsible for phagocytosis of micro-organisms and cellular debris, but can also cause secondary tissue and organ damage through degranulation and release of extracellular proteases and formation of reactive oxygen species or respiratory burst (25,39,40,41,53–55). Elastases and metalloproteinases, which degrade both structural and extracellular matrix proteins, are present in increased concentrations following trauma (25). Neutrophil elastases also induce the release of proinflammatory cytokines (25).

Reactive oxygen species are generated by membrane-associated nicotinamide adenine dinucleotide phosphate (NADPH)-oxidase, which is activated by proinflammatory cytokines, arachidonic acid metabolites, complement factors, and bacterial products (56,57). Superoxide anions are reduced in the Haber-Weiss reaction to hydrogen peroxide by superoxide dismutase located in the cytosol, mitochondria, and cell membrane (25). Hydrochloric acid is formed from H_2O_2 by myeloperoxidase, while the Fenton reaction transforms H_2O_2 into hydroxyl ions (25). These free reactive oxygen species cause lipid peroxidation, cell membrane disintegration, and DNA damage of endothelial and parenchymal cells (58–60). Oxygen radicals also induce PMNLs to release proteases and collagenase as well as inactivating protease inhibitors (61).

Reactive nitrogen species cause additional tissue damage following trauma (62). Nitric oxide (NO) is generated from L-arginine by inducible nitric oxide synthase (iNOS) in PMNLs or vascular muscle cells and by endothelial nitric oxide synthase in endothelial cells (62). Nitric oxide induces vasodilatation (25). Inducible nitric oxide synthase is stimulated by cytokines and toxins, whereas endothelial nitric oxide synthase (eNOS) is stimulated by mechanical shearing forces (62,63). Damage by reactive oxygen and nitrogen species leads to generalized edema and the capillary leak syndrome (62).

Complement, Kinins, and Coagulation

The complement cascade, kallikrein-kinin system, and coagulation cascade are intimately involved in the immune response to shock. They are activated through proinflammatory mediators, endogenous endotoxins, and tissue damage. The classic pathway of complement is normally activated by antigen–antibody complexes (Ig M or G) or activated coagulation factor XII (FXII), while the alternative pathway is activated by bacterial products such as lipopolysaccharide (64–66). Complement activation following trauma is most likely from the release of proteolytic enzymes, disruption of the endothelial lining, and tissue ischemia. The degree of complement activation correlates with the severity of injury. The cleavage of C3 and C5 by their respective convertases results in the formation of opsonins, anaphylotoxins, and the membrane attack complex (MAC) (64–66). The opsonins C3b and C4b enhance phagocytosis of cell debris and bacteria by means of opsonization (64,65). The anaphylotoxins C3a and C5a support inflammation via the recruitment and activation of phagocytic cells (i.e., monocytes, polymorphonuclear cells, and macrophages), enhancement of the hepatic acute phase reaction, and release of vasoactive mediators (i.e., histamine) (52,65). They also enhance the adhesion of leukocytes to endothelial cells, which results in increased vascular permeability and edema. C5a induces apoptosis and cell lysis through the interaction of its receptor and the MAC (52,65,66). Additionally, C3a and C5a activate reparative mechanisms (65). C1 inhibitor inactivates C1s and C1r, thereby regulating the classic complement pathway. However, during inflammation, serum levels of C1 inhibitor are decreased via its degradation by PMNL elastases (65).

The plasma kallikrein-kinin system is a contact system of plasma proteases related to the complement and coagulation cascades. It consists of the plasma proteins FXII, prekallikrein, kininogen, and factor XI (FXI) (67). The activation of FXII and prekallikrein is via contact activation when endothelial damage occurs exposing the basement membrane (67). Factor XII activation forms factor XIIa (FXIIa), which initiates the complement cascade through the classic pathway, whereas prekallikrein activation forms kallikrein, which stimulates fibrinolysis through the conversion of plasminogen to plasmin or the activation of urokinaselike plasminogen activator (uPA) (67). Tissue plasminogen activator (tPA) functions as a cofactor. Additionally, kallikrein supports the conversion of kininogen to bradykinin (67). The formation of bradykinin also occurs through the activation of the tissue kallikrein-kinin system, most likely through organ damage as the tissue kallikrein-kinin system is found in many organs and tissues including the pancreas, kidney, intestine, and salivary glands. The kinins are potent vasodilators. They also increase vascular permeability and inhibit the function of platelets (67).

The intrinsic coagulation cascade is linked to the contact activation system via the formation of factor IXa (FIXa) from factor XIa (FXIa). Its formation leads to the consumption of FXII, prekallikrein, and FXI while plasma levels of enzyme–inhibitor complexes are increased (25). These include FXIIa-C1 inhibitor and kallikrein-C1 inhibitor. C1 inhibitor and α1-protease inhibitor are both inhibitors of the intrinsic coagulation pathway (68,69).

Although the intrinsic pathway provides a stimulus for activation of the coagulation cascade, the major activation following trauma is via the extrinsic pathway. Increased expression of tissue factor (TF) on endothelial cells and monocytes is induced by the proinflammatory cytokines TNF-α and IL-1β (69–71). The factor VII (FVII)–TF complex stimulates the formation of factor Xa (FXa) and ultimately thrombin (FIIa) (25). Thrombin-activated factor V (FV), factor VIII (FVIII), and FXI result in enhanced thrombin formation (25). Following cleavage of fibrinogen by thrombin, the fibrin monomers polymerize to form stable fibrin clots. The consumption of coagulation factors is controlled by the hepatocytic formation of antithrombin (AT) III (25). The thrombin–antithrombin complex inhibits thrombin, FIXa, FXa, FXIa, and FXIIa (72). Other inhibitors include TF pathway inhibitor (TFPI) and activated protein C in combination with free protein S (72). Free protein S is decreased during inflammation due to its binding with the C4b binding protein (68,72).

Disseminated intravascular coagulation (DIC) may occur following shock. After the initial phase, intra- and extravascular fibrin clots are observed. Hypoxia-induced cellular damage is the ultimate result of intravascular fibrin clots. Likewise, there is an increase in the interactions between endothelial cells and leukocytes (68–70,73). Clinically, coagulation factor consumption and platelet dysfunction are responsible for the diffuse hemorrhage (68,71). Consumption of coagulation factors is further enhanced via the proteolysis of fibrin clots to fibrin fragments (68,71). The consumption of coagulation factors is further enhanced through the proteolysis of fibrin clots to fibrin fragments by the protease plasmin (25,69,74).

Acute Phase Reaction

The acute phase reaction describes the early systemic response following shock and other insult states. During this phase, the biosynthetic profile of the liver is significantly altered. Under normal circumstances, the liver synthesizes a range of plasma proteins at steady-state concentrations. However, during the acute phase reaction, hepatocytes increase the synthesis of positive acute phase proteins (i.e., C-reactive protein [CRP], serum amyloid A [SAA], complement proteins, coagulation proteins, proteinase inhibitors, metal-binding proteins, and other proteins) essential to the inflammatory process at the expense of the negative acute phase proteins. The list of acute phase proteins is in Table 55.6 (75,76).

The acute phase response is initiated by hepatic Kupffer cells and the systemic release of proinflammatory cytokines (76). IL-1, IL-6, IL-8, and TNF-α act as inciting cytokines (77,78). The acute phase reaction typically lasts for 24 to 48 hours prior to its down-regulation (35). IL-4, IL-10, glucocorticoids, and various other hormonal stimuli function to down-regulate the proinflammatory mediators of the acute phase response (35). This modulation is critical. In instances of chronic or recurring inflammation, an aberrant acute phase response may result in exacerbated tissue damage (35).

The major acute phase proteins include CRP and SAA, the activities of which are both poorly understood (79,80). C-reactive protein was so named secondary to its ability to bind the C-polysaccharide of *Pneumococcus*. During inflammation, CRP levels may increase by up to 1,000-fold over several hours depending on the insult and its severity (35). It acts as an opsonin for bacteria, parasites, and immune complexes; activates complement via the classic pathway; and binds chromatin (35). Binding chromatin may minimize autoimmune responses by disposing of nuclear antigens from sites of tissue debris (35). Clinically, CRP levels are relatively nonspecific and not predictive of posttraumatic complications. Despite this fact, serial measurements are helpful in trending a patient's clinical course (35).

Serum amyloid A interacts with the third fraction of high-density lipoprotein (HDL3), thus becoming the dominant

TABLE 55.6

ACUTE PHASE PROTEINS

Group	Individual proteins
POSITIVE ACUTE PHASE PROTEINS	
Major acute phase proteins	C-reactive protein, serum amyloid A
Complement proteins	C2, C3, C4, C5, C9, B, C1 inhibitor, C4 binding protein
Coagulation proteins	Fibrinogen, prothrombin, von Willebrand factor
Proteinase proteins	α_1-Antitrypsin, α_1-antichymotrypsin, α_2-antiplasmin, heparin cofactor II, plasminogen activator inhibitor I
Metal-binding proteins	Haptoglobin, hemopexin, ceruloplasmin, manganese superoxide dismutase
Other proteins	α_1-Acid glycoprotein, heme oxygenase, mannose-binding protein, leukocyte protein I, lipoprotein (a), lipopolysaccharide-binding protein
NEGATIVE ACUTE PHASE PROTEINS	Albumin, prealbumin, transferrin, apolipoprotein AI, apolipoprotein AII, α_2-Heremans-Schmid glycoprotein, inter-α-trypsin inhibitor, histidine-rich glycoprotein, protein C, protein S, antithrombin III, high-density lipoprotein

Positive acute phase proteins increase production during an acute phase response. Negative acute phase proteins are those that have decreased production during an acute phase response.

apolipoprotein during acute inflammation (81). This association enhances the binding of HDL3 to macrophages, which may engulf cholesterol and lipid debris. Excess cholesterol is then utilized in tissue repair or excreted (35). Additionally, SAA inhibits thrombin-induced platelet activation and the oxidative burst of neutrophils, potentially preventing oxidative tissue destruction (35).

DIAGNOSIS OF SHOCK

Early diagnosis of shock affords the patient the best possible outcome. The patient in overt shock with hypotension and tachycardia is relatively easy to diagnose. However, more often than not, shock presents in more insidious forms, whereby underrecognition and delay in treatment can lead to a poor outcome. Moreover, the concurrent presence of mixed shock states can confuse the picture. Diagnosis of shock relies on both basic history and physical examination skills, as well as more advanced technology available to the clinician.

Numerous clues in a patient's history may help alert the physician to the possibility of impending shock. Large fluid losses via traumatic or gastrointestinal hemorrhage, third spacing from intra-abdominal surgery or pancreatitis, prolonged dehydration from vomiting or diarrhea, or insensible losses from burns may very easily tip the patient into hypovolemic shock. A history of infection, presence of indwelling catheters, or recent surgery may be implicated in septic shock. Neurogenic shock occurs almost exclusively after trauma, although limited forms are seen with spinal anesthesia. History of prolonged steroid use, particularly in the elderly, may indicate adrenal shock in the patient with hypotension postoperatively. Exposures to drugs, transfusions, or other allergens should be sought to rule out anaphylactic shock. Recent myocardial infarction or cardiac intervention can lead to pump failure and cardiogenic shock. A detailed history is especially important for obstructive forms of shock, in which any intervention involving the chest can lead to either immediate or delayed compromise via cardiac tamponade or tension pneumothorax. Likewise, a history of deep venous thrombosis (DVT) or risk factors for thrombosis should alert the physician to the possibility of acute massive pulmonary embolism in the hypotensive patient.

Physical examination can provide more clues than just basic blood pressure measurements. As noted previously, hypotension alone is neither exclusive to shock nor absolute for a diagnosis, and therefore is only a small component of the physical examination. Certain findings may vary based on the type and timing of shock. The end result of any form of shock, however, is diminished end-organ perfusion. Therefore, any signs or symptoms of organ dysfunction should be considered as possible indicators of shock (Table 55.7). Often, the first sign of shock manifests as mental status changes, whether excitatory or somnolent in nature. The patient may appear diaphoretic and clammy in cardiogenic shock or warm and dry in early distributive shock. Heart rate may also be variable, with tachycardia compensating for diminished cardiac output in the patient with intact sympathetic drive. Vasoplegic shock such as neurogenic or adrenal (or in the β-blocked patient) may not have the compensatory increase in heart rate normally seen, and may itself provide a clue as to the type of shock. Tachypnea is almost universally seen, as the body tries to buffer the lactate produced in a state of tissue hypoxia. The kidneys provide a sensitive measure of adequate end-organ perfusion, as manifested by low urinary output. Cardiogenic shock has its own specific physical findings including increased venous jugular distension, acute pulmonary edema, and new murmurs or arrhythmias.

TABLE 55.7

CLINICAL RECOGNITION OF SHOCK

Organ system	Symptoms or signs	Causes
CNS	Mental status changes	↓ Cerebral perfusion
Circulatory		
Cardiac	Tachycardia	Adrenergic stimulation, depressed contractility
	Other dysrhythmias	Coronary ischemia
	Hypotension	Depressed contractility secondary to ischemia or MDFs, right ventricular failure
	New murmurs	Valvular dysfunction, VSD
Systemic	Hypotension	↓ SVR, ↓ venous return
	↓ JVPs	Hypovolemia, ↓ venous return
	↑ JVPs	Right heart failure
	Disparate peripheral pulses	Aortic dissection
Respiratory	Tachypnea	Pulmonary edema, respiratory muscle fatigue, sepsis, acidosis
	Cyanosis	Hypoxemia
Renal	Oliguria	↓ Perfusion, afferent arteriolar vasoconstriction
Skin	Cool, clammy	Vasoconstriction, sympathetic stimulation
Other	Lactic acidosis	Anaerobic metabolism, hepatic dysfunction
	Fever	Infection

CNS, central nervous system; MDFs, myocardial depressant factors; VSD, ventricular septal defect; SVR, systemic vascular resistance; JVPs, jugular venous pulsations.
From Jimenez EJ. Shock. In: Civetta JM, Taylor RW, Kirby RR, eds. *Critical Care.* 3rd ed. Philadelphia: Lippincott–Raven Publishers; 1997:359.

Various modalities for evaluating shock may be used either alone or in combination. Pooling data from multiple sources, however, is often required to get an adequate picture of shock resuscitation. Basic laboratory studies such as lactate level, base deficit, hemoglobin, creatinine, and cortisol may help provide evidence of or reason for shock. Likewise, a more advanced evaluation of shock may include echocardiogram, central venous pressure monitoring, tissue oxygenation and capnography, or advanced methods of determining cardiac output. Advantages and disadvantages of these more advanced modalities will be discussed later within the context of shock monitoring.

MANAGEMENT OF SHOCK

Optimal management of shock depends first and foremost on early recognition of the syndrome and correct determination of its etiology. Ongoing assessment of interventions is likewise paramount, as adjustments can be made in type and degree of specific therapies. The underlying goal of shock management is to improve tissue oxygen perfusion. This may be accomplished by manipulating one or multiple physiologic parameters involved in oxygen delivery and extraction.

Forms of obstructive shock require the most prompt diagnosis, as continued mechanical impairment can be rapidly fatal. Conversely, adequate treatment of these etiologies can be just as rapid. Performing needle decompression for a tension pneumothorax or pericardiocentesis for cardiac tamponade can be all that is required for these forms of shock. Pharmacologic and fluid support can be used as an adjunct while relief of mechanical obstruction is ongoing.

Management of distributive and hypovolemic forms of shock likewise involves attempted source control early in the diagnosis. This may be in the form of hemorrhage control, removal of infected tissue, or avoidance of sources of anaphylaxis. Once the inflammatory cascade has set in, vasoactive medications are often used in addition to fluid provision to increase perfusion.

Treatment of cardiogenic shock in particular warrants keen understanding of the physiologic process. Currently, initial therapy of cardiogenic shock consists of volume optimization, control of arrhythmias, use of the intra-aortic balloon pump, addition of vasopressors, and early revascularization in primary myocardial ischemia, with addition of inotropes only when these measures fail (82).

Classically, all forms of shock are treated in some capacity with a combination of fluids and vasoactive agents. Deliberation is ongoing regarding the dosing and selection of these modalities for resuscitation, and will be examined in greater detail.

Fluid Resuscitation

The initial treatment for all forms of shock is fluid administration. Provision of fluid helps restore perfusion and replace volume lost via hemorrhage, capillary leak, or redistribution. Historically, Blalock demonstrated reversal of shock state induced by tissue injury by using vigorous resuscitation of intravascular volume (83). As such, the use of fluids for shock management has become a cornerstone of therapy. Intravenous fluid is readily available, inexpensive, and easy to administer, and has low intrinsic morbidity. The etiology of shock and response to fluid will further dictate continued use of volume as primary therapy; however, all forms of shock potentially benefit from an initial fluid challenge (84). There are endless means of administering fluid given a particular clinical setting. General guidelines can be followed; however, considerable debate exists regarding the nuances of this most basic therapy. Deliberation should be given to the method of delivery, timing of administration, type of fluid, and volume of administration. Complications of fluid resuscitation, as well as emerging research in this area, should also be considered.

Route of Administration

The setting of shock dictates administration of fluid primarily via the intravenous route. Factors such as endotracheal intubation, mental status, adynamic or mechanical ileus, rapidity of response, and questionable absorption from the gastrointestinal tract preclude the enteric route as a primary vessel for fluid resuscitation in most cases. Intravenous access may be in the form of a peripheral or central venous catheter. Although the type of shock may guide the choice of catheter (i.e., an introducer catheter for a rapid infusion system or anticipated pulmonary artery catheter placement in cardiogenic shock, or a triple lumen for anticipated vasopressor therapy), the dictum of "two large-bore peripheral IVs" cannot be overstated (85). As per Poiseuille's Law, width and length of the catheter dictates flow; therefore, a long, narrow, peripherally inserted central catheter will be of little utility when infusing a large bolus of fluid quickly. In the severely volume depleted patient with collapsed veins, obtaining percutaneous venous access can prove difficult. Saphenous vein cut-downs or interosseus access, particularly in the trauma patient, can provide means of fluid administration until more permanent intravenous access can be obtained.

Timing of Administration

As stated previously, fluid is the initial therapy in all forms of shock. For forms of hypovolemic shock in particular, the concept of early restoration of intravascular volume to prevent circulatory collapse has long been recognized. In the hemorrhagic patient, aggressive volume resuscitation combined with source control may limit or prevent a state of irreversible shock, or the more currently described "lethal triad" of hypothermia, coagulopathy, and acidosis (86,87). The importance of the timing of volume loading is also being recognized in other forms of shock, particularly in sepsis (88). Amplification of the previously described immune response can potentially be avoided if perfusion is restored early in the pathophysiologic process (89). Often the resuscitation process begins in the prehospital phase, with ambulance personnel administering combinations of crystalloid and colloids en route. In this setting, timing of fluid resuscitation is given due attention. Delayed aggressive fluid resuscitation once the patient is already in the intensive care unit, and therefore later in the course of shock, as well as excessive doses of dobutamine (5–200 μg/kg/minute) can be detrimental (90).

Continued administration of fluid alone, however, should be based on the patient's underlying pathology. While vigorous fluid provision may be life sustaining in certain patients, an equal measure could prove counterproductive in others. Ongoing replacement of fluid should be based on both direct and insensible losses, keeping in mind the huge potential third-spacing loss into the interstitium. Again, the idea of pushing fluid beyond the initial phases of ischemia may propagate reperfusion injury, emphasizing early recognition and treatment of shock.

Volume of Resuscitation

Although there is general consensus regarding the timing of administration of fluids, there is little information to support the optimum volume to be given. Guidelines reference various quantities for crystalloid administration, including 500 mL, 1,000 mL, or the more universal 20 mL/kg bolus. The speed of the bolus likewise varies, although common sense dictates that rapid administration is preferred in the setting of hypotension.

Continued fluid administration beyond an initial bolus relies more on patient response than on arbitrary numbers. Physical examination characteristics such as jugular venous distension, skin turgor, and basic vital signs may give clues to volume state, but are notoriously subject to interpretation. The examiner is often misled by the appearance of gross edema, insomuch that it has no bearing on effective extracellular fluid volume in the patient with capillary leak. Efforts to measure intravascular volume status should be made, but these values should be interpreted in the context of cardiac output and ongoing therapy. Tools used to measure volume status include central venous pressure, pulmonary artery occlusion pressure, esophageal Doppler, and echocardiography, each with its own strengths and weaknesses (91–94). There is renewed interest in the actual measurement of blood volume rather than relying on surrogate markers (see Blood Volume chapter).

The amount of fluid required to achieve these goals will vary with patient size, cardiac status, type of fluid given, and timing and type of shock. Prominent guidelines direct the clinician to volume load to a central venous pressure of 8 to 10 mm Hg or a pulmonary capillary wedge pressure of >12 mm Hg prior to initiating vasopressor therapy for shock (95,96). Ideal volumes for shock resuscitation continue to be debated. In fact, restrictive fluid therapies for resuscitation have emerged in an effort to reduce the cardiac, wound healing, and pulmonary complications associated with large crystalloid infusions (97).

Fluid therapy in excess may lead to numerous complications. The coagulation profile may be altered secondary to dilution with excessive crystalloid infusion (98). Red blood cell mass is also diluted, and while this may not have a net effect on oxygen delivery, it may complicate interpretation of bleeding states. Tissue edema is also a consequence of volume resuscitation, and of these, the pulmonary component is most visible to the practitioner. Lung edema will manifest most readily with crystalloid therapy in the setting of hypoproteinemia—a common state in the shock patient (99). While some degree of pulmonary edema can be tolerated, critical hypoxia often threatens the recovery of patients who survive via massive volume resuscitation. The added mechanical impairment of ventilation induced by abdominal compartment syndrome, also seen with large volume resuscitation, further exacerbates the situation (100).

Types of Fluid

Considerable debate abounds regarding the types of fluid to be administered for shock resuscitation. The physiologic makeup of the human body allows for movement of fluids and solutes across compartments, specifically between the interstitium and intravascular space. Hydrostatic and oncotic forces dictate this movement at the capillary level, as explained by the Starling equation:

$$J_v = K_f\{(P_c - P_i) - \sigma(\pi_c - \pi_i)\}$$

where J_v is the net fluid flux (mL/minute). $(P_c - P_i)$ is hydrostatic pressure difference between capillary (c) and interstitium (i), and $(\pi_c - \pi_i)$ is the oncotic pressure difference between the capillary and interstitium, K_f is the filtration coefficient for that membrane (mL/minute per mm Hg), and is the product of capillary surface area and capillary hydraulic conductance. σ is the permeability factor (i.e. reflection coefficient) with one being impermeable, and zero being completely permeable. Imbalance in the forces—whether decreased oncotic pressure from hypoalbuminemia, increased hydrostatic pressure from heart failure, or decreased protein reflection coefficient with sepsis—occurs often with shock states. The choice of fluid type therefore requires appropriate knowledge of the characteristics of the fluid, as well as the pathophysiology of the shock state.

Crystalloids. Invariably, the workhorse of shock resuscitation is isotonic crystalloid. Composed of varying amounts of electrolytes and sugar, crystalloids are inexpensive, require no special tubing or preparation, and pose little to no allergy or transfusion risk. Almost every patient receives some form of intravenous crystalloid upon entering a hospital with little consequence as to the type given due to the low volumes given on average.

Crystalloids used in shock resuscitation are generally categorized as isotonic or hypertonic, describing the *in vivo* tonicity of the fluid. Typical isotonic crystalloids used are normal saline, lactated Ringer solution, or other commercially available combinations of electrolytes with sodium as the primary ion. Lacking protein components, the isotonic crystalloids readily distribute to the extracellular fluid compartment and will require larger volumes of infusion to maintain intravascular filling. Traditional philosophy dictates that a threefold volume of crystalloid to colloid is required for intravascular expansion. This ratio has recently been debated, however, and may actually be closer to a ratio of 1.5:1 when comparing crystalloid to 5% albumin (101).

Normal saline and lactated Ringer solution compromise the majority of isotonic crystalloid used for shock. Normal saline simply provides sodium with an equal amount of chloride for buffer. Hypernatremia and hyperchloremic metabolic acidosis are therefore potential consequences of continued normal saline administration (102). While the tonicity is essentially the same, the electrolyte composition of lactated Ringer is considered more physiologic, with inclusion of potassium and calcium, and reduction in chloride concentrations. Conversion of the lactate in lactated Ringer to bicarbonate in theory provides a buffer to metabolic acidosis in the patient with adequate liver function. Current compositions of lactated Ringer contain a racemic mixture of D- and L-lactate in solution. The presence of this D-isomer has been implicated as a potentiator of neutrophil activation in large volume infusions (103). Likewise, the presence of a large lactate load has been implicated in promoting respiratory acidosis in the spontaneously breathing patient (104).

Hypertonic Crystalloid. Combining the convenience of crystalloid with the tonicity of colloids, hypertonic saline has emerged as an important tool in shock resuscitation. Hypertonicity of the sodium concentration promotes influx of fluid from the interstitial space. As such, hypertonic saline is advantageous for rapid, low-volume resuscitation for hypovolemic shock, particularly in situations where resources may be scarce. Hypertonic solutions also favorably impact immune modulatory function. Studies particularly investigating hemorrhagic shock have found a decrease in neutrophil activation, and upregulation of anti-inflammatory cytokine production with use of hypertonic saline (105,106).

While relatively safe compared to colloid infusion, the administration of high concentrations of sodium for volume resuscitation carries the concern for hypernatremia and hyperosmolarity. The neurologic consequences of rapid sodium flux are well known; however, these have not been described in the hypertonic saline resuscitation population. Compromise of renal function is likewise feared with high sodium and osmolar loads. While some patient populations exhibit increases in creatinine without clinical renal dysfunction, studies in the burn population support this trepidation regarding hypertonic saline (107,108). Reports of hypokalemia, metabolic acidosis, and impaired platelet aggregation have also been documented with hypertonic saline use (109).

Colloids. Pertaining to volume resuscitation, colloids generally consist of fluids that have a higher molecular weight based on composition consisting of protein, starches, or cells. These components increase the cost of colloids, make them susceptible to shortage, and mandate specialized tubing for delivery. Possibility for transfusion reaction is increased as some of these compounds are derived from blood products. Likewise, allergic reactions can be noted with some of the synthetic formulations.

Conceptually, colloids more rapidly expand intravascular volume owing to their higher oncotic pressure. This effect may not necessarily persist beyond a few hours, especially in the critically ill patient in which capillary permeability is altered (110). In addition to more rapid volume expansion with less fluid infusion, this same increase in intravascular oncotic pressure has prompted the employment of colloids with the intent to reduce or prevent secondary edema. This mechanism does not hold in critical illness, particularly for lung edema in which dysfunction is unrelated to capillary oncotic pressure in shock (111).

Despite these findings, colloids are an important component of shock resuscitation. Integration of colloids into most protocols usually follows initial infusion of crystalloids or while awaiting blood product transfusion (112).

Albumin. First used for fluid resuscitation during World War II, albumin is a colloid derived from pooled human plasma and diluted with sodium. Preparations consist of 5% or 25% solution in quantities of 250 to 500 mL or 50 mL, respectively. As a blood product derivative, albumin is subject to disadvantages faced by other donated products—namely periodic shortages, high acquisition costs, and refusal based on religious grounds. While transmission of viruses or other blood-borne diseases is theoretically a risk, only a few cases have been reported. Like any resuscitation fluid, patients are subject to sequelae of volume overload if infusion amounts are not monitored.

While indications for albumin use are broad, proven benefit to particular therapies is increasingly narrow. Numerous studies detailing poor prognosis with low serum albumin levels in critically ill patients prompted attempts to improve survival with intravenous supplementation (113–115). Compared with other colloid administration, albumin itself has no benefit in this patient population (116,117).

Albumin as a resuscitation fluid likewise has come under scrutiny. Previously, studies investigating albumin as a volume expander have been underpowered, prompting meta-analysis as the primary statistical measure of its worth. An initial Cochrane review comparing albumin to crystalloid examined 24 studies and found a 6% increase in absolute risk of death with albumin infusion (118). To confuse matters, subsequent meta-analysis of 55 studies bore out no difference in mortality between albumin and crystalloid for resuscitation (119). In 2004, the Saline versus Albumin Fluid Evaluation (SAFE) trial prospectively compared albumin to isotonic crystalloid for fluid resuscitation in a mixed intensive care unit population (101). Results showed no difference in morbidity or mortality overall with albumin use. Advocates for albumin hail this study as an indicator that its use poses no harm as previously indicated. Opponents likewise cite the study, but as an indicator that there is no advantage to using albumin for volume resuscitation. A revised Cochrane analysis following the SAFE study again reported no advantage to albumin infusion for hypovolemic patients (120). Results must be interpreted in light of the heavy weight thus given to the SAFE trial in this review.

Starches. In an attempt to retain the oncotic properties of albumin while decreasing cost and transfusion risk, synthetic colloid polymers have been developed for use in volume resuscitation. As one of the primary synthetic colloids, starches, of which hydroxyethyl starch is most popular, consist of polymers of amylopectin. Like other colloids, hydroxyethyl starch owes its main advantage to providing appropriate volume expansion with less infusion than that of crystalloids. Initial formulations of hydroxyl ethyl starch (HES) included high-molecular-weight moieties, accounting for an increased risk of coagulation and renal disturbances associated with their use (121–123). Lower-molecular-weight HES solutions have since been developed, with resultant fewer negative effects on bleeding (124).

Of particular interest in colloid resuscitation, hydroxyethyl starch has favorable effects both on vascular permeability and inflammatory properties in animal models. Reduced pulmonary capillary leakage has been described with hydroxyethyl starch use in comparison to crystalloid and gelatin resuscitation (125,126). While numerous studies have illustrated downregulation of proinflammatory cytokines with hydroxyethyl starch use, some of these results may be an effect of the efficiency of volume resuscitation, and not necessarily the fluid itself (127–129). How this anti-inflammatory effect is translated into clinical outcomes is the subject of ongoing research.

Dextran. Among the lower-molecular-weight colloids, dextran consists of large glucose polymers of varying sizes. As a colloid, it does expand intravascular volume; however, the smaller-sized molecules redistribute quickly, giving it a short half-life. It improves microcirculation by decreasing blood viscosity and therefore primarily is used in situations where platelet adherence and red blood cell aggregation is discouraged, such as postcarotid endarterectomy. As such, the risk of bleeding limits their use as a primary resuscitation fluid. The combination of dextran with other fluids, most notably hypertonic saline, limits the adverse effects of dextran alone. Conceptually, the combination of the two would increase the amount and duration of oncotic pressure in the intravascular space compared with either alone. In animal models, the use of hypertonic saline plus dextran-70 is associated with improved hypovolemic resuscitation when compared to hypertonic saline alone. This effect has not translated well into human clinical studies, in which the combination shows no benefit over hypertonic saline alone in prehospital resuscitation (130,131). The administration of dextran plus hypertonic saline is considered safe, however, resulting in fewer complications than crystalloid in trauma resuscitation (132). Additional studies are needed to establish appropriate use of dextrans as they apply to shock resuscitation.

Gelatins. Gelatins consist of moderate-size molecular weight colloids derived from porcine sources. A perceived high level of antigenicity limits their use, particularly in the United States where they are not Food and Drug Administration (FDA) approved. The absolute incidence of anaphylaxis, however, is only 0.066% (133). Modified fluid gelatin is the most common colloid used worldwide, owing to its otherwise favorable side effect profile and inexpensive production costs. In comparison to crystalloids for shock resuscitation, gelatins provide superior volume expansion without additionally noted adverse effects of bleeding or pulmonary dysfunction (134–136). As gelatins gain approval throughout worldwide markets, further research is emerging to investigate their utility in shock resuscitation.

Blood Products. Provision of blood products as either a primary or adjunctive resuscitation fluid should be considered carefully. The risk of infection, immunosuppression, and transfusion reaction are well known (137,138). The cost of preparation, as well as short supply, also limits their use.

Blood products do provide an effective source of colloid for increasing oncotic pressure, but should only be used when secondary properties of the specific product are sought. Transfusing packed red blood cells, while increasing oxygen-carrying capacity, does not necessarily translate into improved survival in all situations. Targeting a specific hemoglobin concentration in critically ill patients may only benefit those with active coronary artery disease; otherwise, a restrictive transfusion policy to a hemoglobin level of 7.0 g/dL is safe (139). Specifically, in septic shock, the administration of red blood cells may benefit a subset of patients who have a low mixed venous oxygenation and low hemoglobin level after volume resuscitation with crystalloids (88). Measurement of red cell volume may be a better guide to blood transfusion rather than hemoglobin or hematocrit since the hemoglobin/hematocrit reflect red cell volume in relationship to plasma volume.

Fresh frozen plasma, cryoprecipitate, and platelets also have utility as colloids based on the coagulation profile. Each has the same adverse transfusion profile as administering red blood cells, however, and should only be used in combination with packed red blood cells for hemorrhagic shock, or in the setting of the coagulopathic patient requiring fluid resuscitation. Standard teaching of administering 1 unit of plasma for every 3 units of red blood cells has recently been challenged. More advanced hemorrhagic shock resuscitation requires a one-to-one ratio of plasma to red blood cell administration, with addition of platelets and cryoprecipitate based on laboratory evaluation (140).

Fluid Choices for Different Classifications of Shock

Debate abounds regarding appropriate use of crystalloids versus colloids in various shock states as illustrated by the numerous meta-analyses found in the literature. Differences in mortality are illustrated when subgroup analysis is performed; therefore, fluids for shock resuscitation can be examined based on underlying pathophysiology of the shock state. The two most studied categories are trauma-induced hemorrhagic shock and septic shock.

Hemorrhagic Shock Resuscitation. Current guidelines for hemorrhagic shock emphasize mixed crystalloid and colloid provision until blood products (either type specific or O negative) are available. Aggressive use of crystalloids during the Vietnam conflict resulted in improved mortality and reduction in renal failure, but also led to the emergence of acute lung injury and acute respiratory distress syndrome in the trauma population. Extensive use of crystalloids for trauma followed, with the popular concept of pushing fluids beyond supranormal resuscitation goals (141). Meta-analyses at the time provided further encouragement for this practice, with mortality favoring crystalloids over colloids in the trauma population (142). The advancement of damage control surgery led to improved outcomes while compensating for the accepted postoperative edema by leaving the abdomen open. Consequences of this large-volume approach are becoming more evident, with adverse cardiac, pulmonary, coagulation, and immunologic effects documented with massive crystalloid infusion (143).

The advent of synthetic colloids, as well as further research regarding hypertonic saline use, renewed interest in the concept of small-volume resuscitation, particularly on the battlefield. Hypertonic saline, dextran, and hydroxyethyl starch have the advantages of long shelf life, convenient preparation, and small aliquot volumes for equal resuscitation. This is particularly important in combat situations, where low-bolus 7.5% hypertonic saline is now the standard for initial resuscitation (144). Current battlefield practice has translated to civilian trauma, with the use of these compounds in the prehospital setting (132).

Hypotensive resuscitation in the hemorrhagic patient is an additional emerging concept. This strategy may be applied to the patient in whom mechanical control of bleeding has not been achieved—whether in traumatic injury, aortic aneurysm rupture, or gastrointestinal bleed (145–147). Measures to raise blood pressure, particularly with fluid administration, may be counterproductive. In the penetrating thoracic trauma patient, early administration of large volumes of crystalloid has been shown to increase bleeding and subsequent mortality (148). This is a very specific patient population, however, and further examination of fluid administration by a recent Cochrane review provided insufficient evidence for or against the use of early, large-volume resuscitation in hemorrhagic shock (149).

Septic Shock Resuscitation. Resuscitation for septic shock is currently a highly investigated topic, with numerous guidelines and protocols taking the forefront in hospital initiatives. While a large number of investigations seek the optimal pharmacologic therapy, fluid management is still a source of debate. The inflammatory process and resulting capillary leak inherent to sepsis creates an additional variable when considering which fluids to administer. The logical choice would therefore be a colloid with the idea of maintaining higher intravascular oncotic pressure. When comparing filling pressures and oxygen delivery, however, there is no appreciable difference between colloids and crystalloids, except in amount of fluid required. Despite delivering two to three times more fluid with crystalloid, patient outcomes are the same (150). With the exception of small subgroup analyses indicating a trend toward improved outcome with albumin resuscitation (SAFE), there are insufficient data to definitively support colloids over crystalloids for septic shock resuscitation. As such, large practice guidelines such as the Surviving Sepsis Campaign either incorporate a combination of fluids or simply leave this choice to the practitioner (95).

Pharmacotherapy in Shock

When incorporating pharmacotherapy for treatment of shock, catecholamines classically come to mind. Sympathomimetics are still the standard for raising the mean arterial pressure (MAP) in the hypotensive patient who is not responding to fluids. Shock is not hypotension alone, however, and other agents can be used to compensate for the diminished tissue perfusion defined by this syndrome. Drugs used for shock will be examined here by the classifications of vasopressor, inotrope, and miscellaneous, although these categories may overlap to a degree. An overview of the more common sympathomimetics is listed in Table 55.8.

Vasopressors

End-organ arterial autoregulation generally compensates for decreased MAP within a certain range. Local vasoconstriction and vasodilatation may be unable to overcome extremes of perfusion. Administering vasopressors may help improve MAP and therefore improve tissue perfusion by redistributing cardiac output. The venous compartment also benefits from vasopressor therapy by decreasing compliance and therefore improving effective volume.

Vasopressors are generally given after an initial fluid bolus has failed or had marginal effect. Within the context of avoiding the consequences of excessive fluid administration, vasopressors may help limit volumes of fluid given; however, peripheral and end-organ vasoconstriction have their own adverse effects. Striking the balance between volume and pressors in the context of timing and type of shock is therefore a key component to resuscitation. With early recognition of shock, vasopressors can often be avoided by restoration of volume.

Classifications of vasopressors consist of natural and synthetic versions of catecholamines (Table 55.8). Each pressor has its own advantage and disadvantage, although practitioners generally use only a few common agents in their armamentarium. The limited number of randomized controlled trials for *in vivo* use of pressors makes selection often one of familiarity, availability, and current trends (151). Often, surrogate end points serve as the basis for judging responsiveness to a drug agent, a strategy that may or may not manifest in improved patient outcome. There are some general recommendations, however, for certain drug regimens in particular types of shock.

Norepinephrine. A naturally occurring vasopressor, norepinephrine is released by the postganglionic adrenergic nerves in response to stress. It has potent α-adrenergic effects, with less potent β_1 stimulation. The α-adrenergic effects lead to increased systolic and diastolic pressure, with the addition of increased venous return via decreasing venous capacitance. This subsequently leads to increased cardiac filling pressure. Effect

TABLE 55.8

SYMPATHOMIMETIC DRUGS

Drug	Usual IV dose	Adrenergic effects α	β	Dopa	Arrhythmogenic potential	Setting
Dopamine	1–2 μg/kg/min[a]	1+	1+	3+	1+	Oliguria despite "normal" blood pressure
	2–10 μg/kg/min	2+	2+	3+	2+	Initial emergency treatment of hypotension (any cause)
	10–30 μg/kg/min	3+	2+	3+	3+	Alternative treatment for bradycardia
Dobutamine	2–30 μg/kg/min	1+	3+	0	2+	Cardiac shock Pulmonary edema with marginal blood pressure
Norepinephrine	0.5–80 μg/min	3+	2+	0	2+	Initial emergency treatment of hypotension (any cause, especially sepsis)
Epinephrine	0.5–1 **mg**[b] (1:10,000) 1–200 μg/min	1+	2+	0	3+	Cardiac arrest Severe hypotension and bradycardia
	0.3–0.5 **mg** SQ (1:1,000)[c]	2+	3+	0	3+	Anaphylaxis
Phenylephrine	20–200 μg/min	3+	0	0	0	Distributive shock when no cardiac effect is desired
Isoproterenol	2–10 μg/min	0	3+	0	3+	Refractory bradycardia Denervated hearts
Milrinone[d]	Load: 50 μg/kg over 10 min Then: 0.375–0.75 μg/kg/min	0	0	0	2+	Cardiogenic shock

Dopa, dopamine.
[a]Increases renal and splanchnic blood flow.
[b]Milligram doses are in bold to differentiate from micrograms.
[c]SQ: Subcutaneous dosing, may be repeated every 15–20 min.
[d]Phosphodiesterase inhibitors; require loading dose.
From Jimenez EJ. Shock. In: Civetta JM, Taylor RW, Kirby RR, eds. *Critical Care*. 3rd ed. Philadelphia: Lippincott–Raven Publishers; 1997:359.

on the coronary arterial flow is enhanced via the increase in diastolic blood pressure. The β-adrenergic effects lead to increased chronotropic function, although this is limited by the baroreflex of vasoconstriction, resulting in zero net change in heart rate. Enhanced inotrope stimulation and stroke volume are likewise negated by an increase in left ventricular afterload, leading to a limited increase in cardiac output.

Historically, the exaggerated peripheral vasoconstrictive properties of the drug have promoted a level of distrust leading to the often quoted "Leave 'em Dead." These fears are largely unfounded at indicated dosing ranges, and use of the drug may actually enhance renal function (152). The drug is safe and easily titratable, and lacks the tachyarrhythmic properties of other frequently used agents for shock. A resurgence in the use of norepinephrine has occurred with the recognition of its beneficial properties, and is now recommended as the first-line vasopressor in the treatment of septic shock (95). Norepinephrine is also useful for other forms of distributive shock and as a temporizing agent in cardiogenic shock.

Epinephrine. Epinephrine is the major physiologic adrenergic hormone of the adrenal medulla and represents the maximum in catecholamine stimulation. The agent potently stimulates α_1 receptors with resultant marked venous and arterial vasoconstriction. These changes may lead to detrimental effects on regional blood flow, particularly on mesenteric and renal vascular beds. β effects lead to increased heart rate and inotropism. Due to counter effects of β_2 vasodilation, the diastolic blood pressure is only slightly affected, with a lesser degree of increase in MAP than norepinephrine. Stimulation of β_2 receptors and blunting of mast cell response also makes epinephrine highly effective for anaphylaxis. Epinephrine has dose-dependent effects, with very low doses stimulating primarily β receptors. This property makes epinephrine attractive as a primary inotrope; however, the range of that particular low dose varies with each patient and titration may prove dangerous. In general, the use of epinephrine is considered a drug of last choice or in extreme situations such as cardiac arrest.

Dopamine. Dopamine has long been the workhorse in shock resuscitation, although the preponderance of its use has slowed with increasing evidence of deleterious effects (153). As the hormone precursor of norepinephrine and epinephrine, dopamine stimulates α, β, and dopaminergic receptors in a dose-dependent fashion. This results in mixed vasoconstrictive, inotropic, chronotropic, and vasodilatory effects.

Classically, "renal-dose" dopamine ranges from 0 to 5 μg/kg/minute and results in vasodilation of renal and mesenteric vascular beds via dopamine receptors. Although this stimulation results in diuresis, the overall effect on renal function and need for renal replacement therapy is unchanged and may actually be worsened (154). Conversely, at high doses of 10 to 20 μg/kg/minute, α effects predominate, resulting in almost pure vasoconstriction. β-Receptor stimulation at middle doses of 5 to 10 μg/kg/minute results in increased inotropic and chronotropic function leading to increased MAP similar to norepinephrine. However, without simultaneous activation of α receptors at this dose, vasodilatation by dopamine receptors is unopposed and reflex tachycardia may predominate. These dose-related effects are simply a guideline, as responsiveness to titration varies patient to patient, particularly in critical illness.

In the past, dopamine has been postulated as the first inotrope of choice in cardiogenic failure with hypotension (155). More recent recommendations, however, identify sympathetic inotropes such as dopamine as increasing mortality when used for primary left heart failure (156). Likewise, in septic shock, norepinephrine has a more reliable dosing profile and has demonstrated more beneficial outcomes compared to dopamine (157).

Phenylephrine. Phenylephrine is a rapidly acting vasopressor with a short duration of action and pure α_1 stimulation. As such, it increases MAP primarily by increasing systemic vascular resistance. Reflex bradycardia may develop; therefore, it is occasionally used for distributive shock in the face of tachyarrhythmias. This same unopposed increase in vascular resistance also impairs cardiac output in the patient with impaired pump function. The use of phenylephrine has since fallen out of favor, and is generally reserved for the pregnant patient with shock for whom other vasopressors may be detrimental.

Inotropes

As a group, inotropic agents augment cardiac output by increasing contractility. Sources of left ventricular failure are many, including exacerbation of congestive heart failure, acute infarction, or sepsis-related cardiomyopathy. Although improvement of pump function in these situations seems logical as a primary therapy, no literature supports any positive benefit on mortality when inotropes are used. This may be particularly true when the agents are used in a long-term fashion. As with other forms of pharmacotherapy for shock, inotropes should be used only in a short-term situation until underlying pathology can be corrected. Prolonged use can increase myocardial work and exacerbate ischemia.

The classic paradigm of cardiogenic shock with resulting reflexive increase in afterload has been recently challenged, with recognition of an inflammatory component to acute infarction. This inflammatory state results in vasodilation, making particular inotropes less useful for restoration of tissue perfusion (158). Likewise, the concept of pushing oxygen delivery to supranormal levels with excessive amounts of dobutamine (5–200 μg/kg/minute) to enhanced cardiac output has been largely abandoned, as it may worsen outcome (90).

Dobutamine. Dobutamine is a synthetic adrenergic agent derived from dopamine. Current formulation of the drug is as a racemic mixture, with the L-isomer stimulating α_1 and the D-isomer stimulating β_1 and β_2 receptors. This combined stimulation results in a net increase in inotropic and chronotropic parameters. In theory, vasodilatory (β_2) effects are limited, making dobutamine useful in increasing pump function without lowering blood pressure. In practice, some degree of vasodilation is encountered, resulting in decreased blood pressure and tachycardia acutely. With increase in cardiac output, however, the blood pressure generally corrects to normal. For this reason, adequate volume loading prior to initiation of dobutamine is emphasized. Likewise, the lack of increase in blood pressure makes dobutamine a poor selection as monotherapy in primary cardiogenic shock. Currently, dobutamine is the standard inotrope used in noncardiogenic shock (such as sepsis) when cardiac contractility is compromised (159).

Dopexamine. Another of the synthetic catecholamines, dopexamine uniquely stimulates β_2 and dopaminergic receptors with no α-adrenergic effects and minimal β_1 stimulation. Resultant effects therefore include vasodilation and positive inotropy via increased stroke volume. The agent may also exert indirect vasoactive changes via inhibition of norepinephrine reuptake at the postganglionic synapse (160). Dopexamine is often compared to dobutamine in trials, with the possible benefit of improved splanchnic perfusion (161).

Isoproterenol. With practically no α-adrenergic stimulation, isoproterenol functions as a pure β agonist. β_1 stimulation results in increased stroke volume and heart rate, while β_2 stimulation induces vasodilatation. The net result is that of enhanced cardiac output without the benefit of distribution of blood flow. Increased myocardial oxygen consumption exacerbated by lack of coronary perfusion due to decreased diastolic pressures may lead to cardiac ischemia. Use of isoproterenol is generally limited to β-blocker overdose or in the atropine-resistant transplanted heart.

Milrinone. A novel agent in vasoactive treatment, milrinone is a synthetic phosphodiesterase III inhibitor. Reduction in this enzyme results in an increase in cyclic adenosine monophosphate (cAMP), a modulator of myocardial contractility. Additional increase in cAMP results in vasodilation, with the net effect of increasing cardiac output and tachycardia at higher doses. This vasodilatory effect may decrease effective left ventricular preload, but may also benefit afterload reduction, reducing cardiac work. In the hypotensive patient, this vasodilation may not be tolerated acutely. While not recommended in vasodilatory shock for this reason, milrinone may be used in specific situations for cardiogenic shock. These include advanced heart failure in patients awaiting heart transplant, in acute decompensation of congestive heart failure (CHF) on standard medications, and in patients in cardiogenic shock with long-term β-blocker use (162).

Levosimendan. Levosimendan is the singular drug in a new class of inotropic agents. Primary mechanism of action is by increasing the sensitivity of troponin C for calcium without enhancing influx of calcium itself. The advantage of this physiology would be increased contractility without risk of arrhythmias. The drug shows promise as a new agent and is currently undergoing further investigation (163).

Miscellaneous Pharmacologic Therapy

Numerous other noncatecholamine agents have been used for various shock states. These may work by treating the symptoms, such as increasing vascular tone, or by treating the source depending on the type of shock. Examples of drug therapy for source treatment include antibiotics for septic shock, histamine blockers for anaphylactic shock, or somatostatin analogues for gastrointestinal hemorrhagic shock (164–166). Septic shock, in particular, is a syndrome for which the "magic bullet" is constantly sought. Numerous drugs under investigation seek to manipulate the inflammatory cascade at multiple levels. The agents reviewed here are more commonly incorporated into shock management.

Vasopressin. Vasopressin is an attractive hormone for use in shock states not only for its vasoconstrictive properties, but also for its antidiuretic effects. As a noncatecholamine vasopressor, it acts via V1 receptors to restore vascular tone. Catecholamine responsiveness may decrease over time during severe sepsis, possibly due to an increase in nitric oxide–induced vasodilatation. This alternate mode of action makes vasopressin a logical treatment for catecholamine-resistant shock. Studies of hemorrhagic and vasodilatory shock have demonstrated a relative deficiency of vasopressin. For this reason, vasopressin is often used at a low dose without titration, in the manner of hormone replacement. Potentiation of adrenergic agents makes vasopressin particularly useful in combination with norepinephrine, and has been recommended for the treatment of septic shock (167). Addition of vasopressin allows for reduced dosing of more harmful catecholamines in this situation. The ongoing Vasopressin and Septic Shock Trial (VASST) will help to define the role of vasopressin compared to norepinephrine in sepsis (168).

Terlipressin. Terlipressin is an analogue of vasopressin that is used in countries in which vasopressin is not available. It is employed in a similar fashion, usually for the treatment of catecholamine-resistant shock. Early studies are favorable, showing an increase in MAP and a decrease in the need for catecholamine vasopressors (169). Splanchnic circulation is spared excessive vasoconstrictive effects, as demonstrated by an increase in gastric mucosal perfusion (170). Terlipressin is used as a single bolus in these studies due to its long half-life (6 hours). This long duration of action may be disadvantageous as the effects are not easily discontinued if necessary, as with a vasopressin drip.

Steroids. The use of steroids in critical care has long been the topic of debate and refinement. For the purposes of shock, however, more definitive literature is emerging to help clarify their role. The role of "stress-dose steroids" perioperatively to prevent hypotension in the adrenal-insufficient patient has been supported for many years. The concept of relative adrenal insufficiency complicating shock states is now established as a recognizable and treatable entity. A recent meta-analysis reviewed the use of 200 to 300 mg of hydrocortisone daily for patients with septic shock. Administration for 5 days or more reduced duration of shock and mortality without increasing associated side effects of infection (171). Use of steroids should be limited to patients with shock refractory to fluids and vasopressors, and with a chemical diagnosis of adrenal insufficiency. Fludrocortisone at a dose of 50 mg/day orally may be added to the hydrocortisone regimen (172).

Drotrecogin Alfa. Among the newer immunomodulatory agents, drotrecogin alfa has received the most attention. The agent is a recombinant form of activated protein C, which acts to down-regulate the proinflammatory state, anticoagulate, and enhance fibrinolysis to enhance reopening of the microcirculation. As such, it is used for severe sepsis rather than shock per se. Due to its effect on the coagulation profile, the drug has limitations in patients with a risk of bleeding. When used as a drip (24 g/kg/hour for 96 hours), the drug provided a 6% reduction in 28-day mortality for patients with severe sepsis. The drug is expensive, and treatment should be limited to the patient with septic shock requiring renal or respiratory support, as outlined in the PROWESS trial (173).

END POINTS OF RESUSCITATION

The primary goal in the management of shock is a return to normal tissue perfusion. If shock is recognized promptly and timely appropriate treatment strategies are implemented, reversal of its clinical signs may be appreciated. These include improvement in mental status, normalization of vital signs, and restoration of urine output. However, despite these findings, many patients remain in a state of occult hypoperfusion and ongoing tissue acidosis with resultant multiple organ failure and death (12,174). This has been termed "compensated shock." Consequently, better end points of resuscitation are needed to guide resuscitation efforts.

The ideal end point should be operator independent, noninvasive, readily available, safe, and inexpensive. Unfortunately, no single parameter has proven superior in its ability to drive resuscitation efforts. This being said, numerous parameters have been proposed and/or utilized including basic hemodynamic monitoring, invasive hemodynamic monitoring, oxygen delivery, oxygen consumption, mixed venous oxygen saturation, lung water, arterial base deficit, arterial lactate, capnometry, tissue oxygen and carbon dioxide electrodes, and near infrared spectroscopy. We will discuss several of these in more depth in the following paragraphs.

Basic Hemodynamic Monitoring

Basic monitoring in patients with shock includes noninvasive vital sign measurements, cardiac rhythm, and urinary output. During this timeframe, an accurate blood pressure reading is essential. There are several states that underestimate blood pressure measurements including tachycardia in instances of a narrow pulse pressure, arrhythmias, and peripheral vascular disease, all of which are not uncommon in this population (175). The utilization of Doppler is helpful in such instances; however, it does not always rectify the problem (176). When more detailed information is desired, invasive hemodynamic monitoring is indicated.

Invasive Hemodynamic Monitoring

The hemodynamic profiles of shock are depicted in Table 55.2. It is these parameters that often guide the management of shock. As such, meticulous equipment calibration and documentation are essential (177,178). These measurements are subject to many potential artifacts as seen in Table 55.9 (14).

TABLE 55.9

COMMON ARTIFACTS IN HEMODYNAMIC MEASUREMENTS

Variable	Artifact	Causes	Comments/corrective action
Vascular pressures (including PCWP)	*Preload overestimation*	*Technical:*	
		Improper leveling of transducer	Avoid with rigid nursing protocols
		Improper calibration	
		Improper system frequency response	
		Respiratory:	
		Not recording pressures at end-expiration during mechanical ventilation	Avoid digital readouts Use analog tracings
		Active expiratory effort	Suspect with respiratory distress; consider muscle paralysis
		Positive end-expiratory pressure	Usually not significant with <10 cm H_2O PEEP
		Improper positioning of catheter tip	Suspect if tip in upper lobes on chest radiograph or PAD < PCWP
		Cardiac:	
		Mitral regurgitation	Read PCWP as post–A wave
		Mitral stenosis	Interpret with caution as preload estimate
		Acute changes in left ventricle compliance	Suspect in presence of myocardial ischemia
	Preload underestimation	*Technical: (as above)*	
		Respiratory:	
		Not recording pressures at end-expiration during spontaneous breathing	
Cardiac output	*Inaccuracies*	*Technical:*	
		Incorrect injectable volume; thermistor contact with vessel wall; incorrect computational constant	Inspect temperature curves; suspect if pulmonary artery waveform is dampened; follow rigid nursing protocol
		Cardiac:	
		Tricuspid regurgitation	Do not use in presence of significant tricuspid regurgitation
	Wide variation	*Technical: (as above)*	Delete measurements with >20% variation from the mean
		Respiratory:	
		Variable respiratory rate during mechanical ventilation	Average measurements throughout respiratory cycle
Mixed venous oxygen saturation	*Inaccuracies*	*Technical:*	
		Light reflecting against vessel wall, catheter kinking	Note computer error messages
		Presence of significant HgbCO	Measure HgbCO directly at least once
	Misinterpretation	Shifts in oxygen dissociation curve	Correlate with PvO_2 measurements
		Dependence on oxygen delivery	Correlate with oxygen delivery measurements
Extravascular lung water	*Inaccuracies*	Inaccurate measurement of cardiac output (as above)	Correlate cardiac output with regular thermodilution measurements
	Underestimation	Presence of significant areas of nonperfused lung	Measurements suspect in presence of significant regional disease (i.e., lobar pneumonia) or known vascular obstruction
Systemic vascular resistance	*Inaccuracies*	Inaccurate measurement of cardiac output (as above)	
		Inaccurate measurement of blood pressure	Measure directly (see above)

PCWP, pulmonary capillary wedge pressure; PEEP, positive end-expiratory pressure; PAD, pulmonary artery diastolic; HgbCO, carboxyhemoglobin; PvO_2, mixed venous oxygen partial pressure.
From Jimenez EJ. Shock. In: Civetta JM, Taylor RW, Kirby RR, eds. *Critical Care*. 3rd ed. Philadelphia: Lippincott–Raven Publishers; 1997:359.

Therefore, it is critical for the clinician to evaluate these variables in concert with the patient's clinical picture.

Central venous catheters are commonly used in this patient population. As such, central venous pressure measurements are readily available, and often serve as a rough guideline in the resuscitation of shock. The problem is the lack of a well-defined goal for central venous pressure. Similarly, with pulmonary artery catheters, numerous additional hemodynamic parameters become available; however, it is not clear that the appropriate end point is the normalization of these values, nor is it clear how these end points should be achieved (179–182).

In fact, observational studies have suggested that pulmonary artery catheters may actually increase mortality, intensive care unit length of stay, hospital costs, and resource utilization (183). In 2005, Shah et al. performed a meta-analysis of 13 randomized clinical trials evaluating the use of pulmonary artery catheters (184). They documented no improvement in overall mortality or hospital length of stay. An even more recent randomized controlled trial by the National Heart, Lung, and Blood Institute Acute Respiratory Distress Syndrome (ARDS) Clinical Trials Network found no survival benefit and increased catheter-associated complications when comparing pulmonary artery catheters to central venous catheters in the management of patients with acute lung injury when utilized relatively late (within 48 hours), which is the time when resuscitation should already be completed (185). The only positive trial involving pulmonary artery catheters was in older trauma patients who were in severe shock (186). In this subset, Friese et al. documented a survival benefit when patients were managed with a pulmonary artery catheter. This was, however, a retrospective review of the National Trauma Data Bank.

Oxygen Delivery

Oxygen delivery (DO_2) is a function of cardiac index (CI), hemoglobin (Hb), and oxygen saturation (SaO_2) as seen in the Fick equation:

$$DO_2\ (\text{mL/minute/m}^2) = (\text{CI}) \times (1.34\ \text{mL}\ O_2 \text{ carried by 1 g of Hb if 100\% saturated}) \times (\text{Hb})(SaO_2)$$

The use of oxygen delivery as a resuscitation end point has had varying results. In the 1970s, Shoemaker et al. reviewed the physiologic patterns in surviving and nonsurviving shock patients (187,188). They observed that survivors had significantly increased oxygen delivery, oxygen consumption, and cardiac index values (oxygen delivery $\geq$600 mL/minute/m^2, oxygen consumption $\geq$170 mL/minute/m^2, and cardiac index $\geq$4.5 L/minute/m^2). In a subsequent prospective study, they documented decreased complications, lengths of stay, and hospital costs when employing these parameters as goals of resuscitation in high-risk surgical patients (189). Further work by Shoemaker's group and others have shown that utilization of this "supranormal resuscitation" strategy decreases morbidity and mortality in critically ill patients (180,190–192).

Others have been unable to demonstrate any benefit to supranormal oxygen delivery (193–195). Moreover, supranormal resuscitation has been associated with significant morbidity (i.e., ongoing tissue ischemia, abdominal compartment syndrome, coagulopathy, and congestive heart failure) and mortality (196). In 2000, Velmahos et al. documented improved survival in patients who achieved supranormal oxygen delivery; however, they concluded that "this was not a function of the supranormal resuscitation, but rather the patient's own ability to achieve these parameters" (197,198). More recently, Kern and Shoemaker reviewed all randomized clinical trials of hemodynamic optimization (199). They determined that a survival benefit was only appreciable in those studies with interventions prior to the onset of organ failure and mortality of >20% in the control group (200). As demonstrated here, the utilization of oxygen delivery and more specifically "supranormal resuscitation" in the management of shock has had varying degrees of success.

Mixed Venous Oxygen Saturation

Another end point previously examined was mixed venous oxygen saturation. In critically ill patients, Gattinoni resuscitated patients to one of three hemodynamic goals (193). These included a cardiac index between 2.5 and 3.5 L/minute/m^2, cardiac index >4.5 L/minute/m^2, and $SvO_2 \geq 70\%$. There were no differences in multiple organ failure or mortality between the groups. This is in contrast to Rivers' study of severe sepsis/septic shock patients where reaching $SvO_2 \geq 70\%$ within 6 hours of resuscitation improved survival (88).

Base Deficit

Base deficit is defined as the amount of base in millimoles required to increase 1 liter of whole blood to the predicted pH based on the $PaCO_2$ (161). It may be calculated using the arterial blood gas as follows (201):

$$\text{Base Deficit} = -[(HCO_3) - 24.8 + (16.2)(\text{pH} - 7.4)]$$

In shock states, the base deficit may serve as a surrogate marker for anaerobic metabolism and subsequent lactic acidosis if metabolic acidosis is the primary disorder and not a compensatory response (202). In this sense, it is superior to pH secondary to the many compensatory mechanisms in place to normalize pH (203).

Secondary to its availability and rapidity, base deficit has been extensively studied as an end point of resuscitation. In a retrospective review, Davis et al. demonstrated that an increasing base deficit correlated directly with admission hypotension and increasing fluid requirements within the first 24 hours of admission (204). Furthermore, they determined that failure to normalize the base deficit was associated with increased mortality. Others have documented correlations between base deficit and blood product requirements, lengths of stay, acute lung injury, acute respiratory distress syndrome, renal failure, coagulopathy, multiple organ failure, and mortality (205–219).

In the clinical arena, base deficit levels have numerous confounders. These include alcohol intoxication, hyperchloremic metabolic acidosis secondary to aggressive normal saline or lactated Ringer resuscitation, and sodium bicarbonate administration (220,221). Base deficit may also be a normal compensatory response to respiratory alkalosis. As such, base deficit may be useful in trending resuscitation efforts; however, it is not a definitive stand-alone end point.

Lactate

Serum lactate levels are used extensively in monitoring shock resuscitation. In patients suffering from noncardiogenic shock, Vincent et al. documented a correlation between initial serum lactate levels and patient outcomes (222). However, in shock resuscitation it is the lactate trend that is most predictive of mortality. In trauma patients managed with "supranormal resuscitation," Abramson et al. determined that the time to lactate normalization was an important predictor of mortality (223). Patients whose lactate levels normalized (serum levels below 2 mmol/L) within 24 hours had a <10% mortality, those who normalized between 24 and 48 hours had a 25% mortality, while those who did not normalize by 48 hours had a >80% mortality. This trend was corroborated by McNelis et al. in postoperative surgical patients (224). In the trauma population, Manikas et al. further demonstrated that initial and peak lactate levels correlated with multiple organ failure (225). Although the serum lactate level signifies shock and ongoing tissue ischemia, its utilization as an end point in the resuscitation of shock has yet to be validated.

Bicarbonate

During anaerobic metabolism, bicarbonate serves as a buffer for released hydrogen ions. Serum bicarbonate levels decrease as the acidosis worsens, and in essence act as a surrogate for metabolic acidosis. In recent studies, serum bicarbonate levels have been determined to better predict metabolic acidosis and mortality than pH, anion gap, or lactate (226,227). Unfortunately, bicarbonate suffers from the same limitations as base deficit; therefore, its use as an end point of resuscitation is unclear at this time.

Capnometry

During periods of shock and ongoing tissue hypoperfusion, blood flow to the most vulnerable organs (brain and heart) is preserved at the expense of other organs (kidneys, intestinal tract, and musculoskeletal system) (200). In theory, the expended organs will manifest this state with an increase in tissue PCO_2 and a subsequent decrease in tissue pH. The splanchnic and oral mucosa are especially sensitive to such hypoxemic states; therefore, buccal, sublingual, and gastric capnometry would seem invaluable in monitoring shock resuscitation. Gastric capnometry is limited by gastric enteral nutrition, endogenous gastric acid secretion, and H_2 blockers (228,229).

Buccal and sublingual capnography have been shown to directly correspond with blood pressure, cardiac output, and tissue perfusion in animal models (230,231). Furthermore, they are more accurate in predicting mortality than blood pressure is. Povoas et al. documented a correlation between sublingual and duodenal PCO_2 and mesenteric blood flow during hemorrhagic shock in swine (232). In acutely ill humans, Weil et al. demonstrated a correlation between sublingual PCO_2 and lactate levels, the presence of shock, and survival (233,234). Additional studies have shown a correlation between sublingual PCO_2 and changes in regional microcirculatory blood flow and ongoing bleeding (235,236). Unfortunately, PCO_2 levels vary widely in the population, making standardization quite difficult (198). Monitoring device for sublingual capnography was recalled in 2004 for infectious complications and may be reinstated in the future.

Near-infrared Spectroscopy

Near-infrared spectroscopy is the measurement of the wavelength and intensity of the absorption of near-infrared light by a sample. In medicine, it uses chromophores such as hemoglobin to do so and allows for the measurement of tissue oxygenation, PO_2, PCO_2, and pH (237). Taylor et al. documented a close correlation between tissue oxygenation measurements and hemodynamic parameters in a hemorrhagic shock model (238). In this study, near-infrared spectroscopy was also better able to differentiate "responder" from "nonresponder" animals in comparison to lactate levels or global oxygen delivery. McKinley et al. studied near-infrared spectroscopy in critically injured trauma patients (239). They determined that the oxygen saturation of hemoglobin in tissue (StO_2) correlated well with systemic oxygen delivery, base deficit, and lactate. This modality is increasing in popularity with trials currently ongoing.

In shock resuscitation, the treatment strategy is to return normal tissue perfusion. Resuscitation end points are critical in this management. The ideal end point should be operator independent, noninvasive, readily available, safe, and inexpensive. Currently, no single parameter has proven superior in its ability to drive resuscitation efforts.

SUMMARY

Shock is likely the most common life-threatening diagnosis made in the intensive care unit. Despite technologic advances, it remains a significant source of morbidity and mortality. Its etiology is vast. As such, the diagnosis of shock and its inciting source can be difficult to identify if not elusive. Aggressive diagnostic testing is required to avoid irreversible cellular injury, multiple organ failure, and potentially death. The primary goal in the management of shock is a return to normal tissue perfusion. This is attained via various volume resuscitation modalities, pharmacologic agents, and resuscitation end points. Past and current research efforts continue in hopes of optimizing the diagnosis and management of shock with the ultimate goal of improving patient outcomes.

References

1. LeDran HF. *A Treatise, or Reflections Drawn from Practice on Gun-Shot Wounds*. London: England; 1737.
2. Morris EA. *A Practical Treatise on Shock after Operations and Injuries*. London: Hardwicke; 1867.
3. Fischer H. Ueber den Shock. *Samml Klin Vortr.* 1870:10.
4. Maphoter ED. Shock, its nature, duration, and mode of treatment. *BMJ*. 1879;2:1023.
5. Crile GW. *An Experimental Research into Surgical Shock*. Philadelphia: JB Lippincott; 1899.
6. Cannon WB. *Traumatic Shock*. New York: D. Appleton and Company; 1923.
7. Blalock A. Experimental shock: the cause of the low blood pressure produced by muscle injury. *Arch Surg*. 1930;20:959.
8. Wiggers CJ. *The Physiology of Shock*. Cambridge, MA: Harvard University Press; 1950.
9. Report of the Surgeon General of the Army. 1900:318.

10. Tennant R, Wiggers CJ. The effect of coronary occlusion on myocardial contraction. *Am J Physiol.* 1935;211:351.
11. Wo CJ, Shoemaker WC, Appel PL, et al. Unreliability of blood pressure and heart rate to evaluate cardiac output in emergency resuscitation and critical illness. *Crit Care Med.* 1993;21:218.
12. Scalea TM, Maltz S, Yelon J, et al. Resuscitation of multiple trauma and head injury: role of crystalloid fluids and inotropes. *Crit Care Med.* 1994;22:1610.
13. Viega C, Mello PM, Sharma VK, et al. Shock overview. *Semin Respir Crit Care Med.* 2004;25:619.
14. Jimenez EJ. Shock. In: Civetta JM, Taylor RW, Kirby RR, eds. *Critical Care.* 3rd ed. Philadelphia: Lippincott–Raven Publishers; 1997:359.
15. Blalock A. Shock: further studies with particular reference to the effects of hemorrhage. *Arch Surg.* 1937;29:837.
16. Weil MH, Shubin H. Proposed reclassification of shock states with special reference to distributive effects. In: Hinshaw LB, Cox BG, eds. *The Fundamental Mechanisms of Shock.* New York: Plenum Press; 1972:13.
17. Kumar A, Parrillo JE. Shock: classification, pathophysiology, and approach to management. In: Parrillo JE, Dellinger RP, eds. *Critical Care Medicine.* 2nd ed. St. Louis: Mosby, Inc.; 2002:371.
18. Warden GD. Burn shock resuscitation. *World J Surg.* 1992;16:16.
19. National Center for Health Statistics: Health, United States, 1986, DHHS Pub No (PHS) 87-1232, Washington, DC: US Government Printing Office; 1986.
20. Gruppo Italiano per lo Studio della Streptochinasi nell'Infarto Miocardico (GISSI). Effectiveness of intravenous thrombolytic treatment in acute myocardial infarction. *Lancet.* 1986;1:397.
21. Goldberg RJ, Gore JM, Alpert JS, et al. Cardiogenic shock after acute myocardial infarction: incidence and mortality from a community-wide perspective, 1975 to 1988. *N Engl J Med.* 1991;325:1117.
22. Collaborative Group. Third International Study of Infarct Survival. ISIS-3 a randomised comparison of streptokinase vs tissue plasminogen activator vs anistreplase and of aspirin plus heparin vs aspirin alone among 41, 299 cases of suspected acute myocardial infarction. *Lancet.* 1992;339:753.
23. The GUSTO Investigators. An international randomized trial comparing four thrombolytic strategies for acute myocardial infarction. *N Engl J Med.* 1993;329:673.
24. Hochman JS, Boland J, Sleeper LA. Current spectrum of cardiogenic shock and effect of early revascularization on mortality: results of an international registry. *Circulation.* 1995;91:873.
25. Keel M, Trentz O. Pathophysiology of trauma. *Injury Int J Care Injured.* 2005;36:691.
26. Bone R.C. Sir Isaac Newton, sepsis, SIRS, and CARS. *Crit Care Med.* 1996; 24:1125.
27. Lyons A, Kelly JL, Rodrick ML, et al. Major injury induces increased production of interleukin-10 by cells of the immune system with a negative impact on resistance to infection. *Ann Surg.* 1997;226:450.
28. Malone DL, Kuhls D, Napolitano LM, et al. Back to basics: validation of the admission systemic inflammatory response syndrome score in predicting outcome in trauma. *J Trauma.* 2001;51:458.
29. Rangel-Frausto MS, Pittet D, Costigan M, et al. The natural history of the systemic inflammatory response syndrome (SIRS). A prospective study. *JAMA.* 1995;273:117.
30. Definitions for sepsis and organ failure and guidelines for the use of innovative therapies in sepsis, American College of Chest Physicians/Society of Critical Care Medicine Consensus Conference. *Crit Care Med.* 1992;20: 864.
31. Van Griensen M, Krettek C, Pape HC. Immune reactions after trauma. *Eur J Trauma.* 2003;29:181.
32. Neidhardt R, Keel M, Steckholzer U, et al. Relationship of interleukin-10 plasma levels to severity of injury and clinical outcome in injured patients. *J Trauma.* 1997;42:863.
33. Schroder O, Laun RA, Held B, et al. Association of interleukin-10 promoter polymorphism with the incidence of multiple organ dysfunction following major trauma: results of a prospective pilot study. *Shock.* 2004;21:306.
34. Dinarello CA. Proinflammatory cytokines. *Chest.* 2000;118:503.
35. Cook MC. Immunology of trauma. *Trauma.* 2001;3:79.
36. Giannoudis PV, Hildebrand F, Pape HC. Inflammatory serum markers in patients with multiple trauma. *J Bone Joint Surg Br.* 2004;86:313.
37. Seekamp A, Jochum M, Ziegler M, et al. Cytokines and adhesion molecules in elective and accidental trauma-related ischemia/reperfusion. *J Trauma.* 1998;44:874.
38. Botha AJ, Moore FA, Moore EE, et al. Postinjury neutrophil priming and activation: an early vulnerable window. *Surgery.* 1995;118:358.
39. Cochrane CG. Immunologic tissue injury mediated by neutrophilic leukocytes. *Adv Immunol.* 1968;9:97.
40. Fujishima S, Aikawa N. Neutrophil-mediated tissue injury and its modulation. *Intensive Care Med.* 1995;21:277.
41. Smith JA. Neutrophils, host defense, and inflammation: a double-edged sword. *J Leuk Biol.* 1994;56:672.
42. Kubes P, Ward PA. Leukocyte recruitment and the acute inflammatory response. *Brain Pathol.* 2000;10:127.
43. Abbassi O, Kishimoto TK, McIntire LV, et al. E-selectin supports neutrophil rolling *in vitro* under conditions of flow. *J Clin Invest.* 1993;92:2719.
44. Bevilacqua MP, Pober JS, Mendrick DL, et al. Identification of an inducible endothelial-leukocyte adhesion molecule. *Proc Natl Acad Sci.* 1987;84:9238.
45. Geng J-G, Bevilacqua MP, Moore KL, et al. Rapid neutrophil adhesion to activated endothelium mediated by GMP-140. *Nature.* 1990;343:757.
46. Jones DA, Abbassi O, McIntire LV, et al. P-selectin mediates neutrophil rolling on histamine-stimulated endothelial cells. *Biophys J.* 1993;65:1560.
47. Kanwar S, Steeber DA, Tedder TF, et al. Overlapping roles for L-selectin and P-selectin in antigen-induced immune responses in the microvasculature. *J Immunol.* 1999;162:2709.
48. Robinson SD, Frenette PS, Rayburn H, et al. Multiple, targeted deficiencies in selectins reveal a predominant role for P-selectin in leukocyte recruitment. *Proc Natl Acad Sci.* 1999;96:11452.
49. Diamond MS, Springer TA. The dynamic regulation of integrin adhesiveness. *Curr Biol.* 1994;4:506.
50. Berlin C, Bargatze RF, Campbell JJ, et al. a4 integrins mediate lymphocyte attachment and rolling under physiologic flow. *Cell.* 1995;80:413.
51. Hemler ME. VLA proteins in the integrin family: structures, functions, and their role on leukocytes. *Ann Rev Immunol.* 1990;8:365.
52. Schmidt OI, Infanger M, Heyde CE, et al. The role of neuroinflammation in traumatic brain injury. *Eur J Trauma.* 2004;30:35.
53. Goris RJ, te Boekhorst TP, Neytinck JK, et al. Multiple organ failure—generalized autodestructive inflammation? *Arch Surg.* 1985;120:1109.
54. Martins PS, Kallas, EG, Neto MC, et al. Upregulation of reactive oxygen species generation and phagocytosis, and increased apoptosis in human neutrophils during severe sepsis and septic shock. *Shock.* 2003;20:208.
55. Powell WC, Fingleton B, Wilson CL, et al. The metalloproteinase matrilysin proteolytically generates active soluble Fas ligand and potentiates epithelial cell apoptosis. *Curr Biol.* 1999;9:1441.
56. Grote K, Flach I, Luchtefeld M, et al. Mechanical stretch enhances mRNA expression and proenzyme release of matrix metalloproteinase-2 (MMP-2) via NAD(P)H oxidase-derived reactive oxygen species. *Circ Res.* 2003;92:e80.
57. Winterbourn CC, Buss IH, Chan TP, et al. Protein carbonyl measurements show evidence of early oxidative stress in critically ill patients. *Crit Care Med.* 2000;28:143.
58. Kazzaz JA, Xu J, Palaia TA, et al. Cellular oxygen toxicity. Oxidant injury without apoptosis. *J Biol Chem.* 1996;271:15182.
59. Kretzschmar M, Pfeiffer L, Schmidt C, et al. Plasma levels of glutathione, alpha-tocopherol and lipid peroxides in polytraumatized patients; evidence for a stimulating effect of TNF alpha on glutathione synthesis. *Exp Toxicol Pathol.* 1998;50:477.
60. Shohami E, Beit-Yannai E, Horowitz M, et al. Oxidative stress in closed-head injury: brain antioxidant capacity as an indicator of functional outcome. *J Cereb Blood Flow Metab.* 1997;17:1007.
61. Lewen A, Matz P, Chan PH. Free radical pathways in CNS injury. *J Neurotrauma.* 2000;17:871.
62. Laroux FS, Pavlick KP, Hines IN, et al. Role of nitric oxide in inflammation. *Acta Physiol Scand.* 2001;173:113.
63. Skidgel RA, Gao XP, Brovkovych V, et al. Nitric oxide stimulates macrophage inflammatory protein-2 expression in sepsis. *J Immunol.* 2002; 169:2093.
64. Fosse E, Pillgram-Larsen J, Svennevig JL, et al. Complement activation in injured patients occurs immediately and is dependent on the severity of the trauma. *Injury.* 1998;29:509.
65. Mollnes TE, Fosse E. The complement system in trauma-related and ischemic tissue damage: a brief review. *Shock.* 1994;2:301.
66. Stahel PF, Morganti-Kossmann MC, Kossmann T. The role of the complement system in traumatic brain injury. *Brain Res Rev.* 1998;27:243.
67. Sugimoto K, Hirata M, Majima M, et al. Evidence for a role of kallikrein–kinin system in patients with shock after blunt trauma. *Am J Physiol.* 1998;274:1556.
68. Abraham E. Coagulation abnormalities in acute lung injury and sepsis. *Am J Respir Cell Mol Biol.* 2000;22:401.
69. Idell S. Coagulation, fibrinolysis, and fibrin deposition in acute lung injury. *Crit Care Med.* 2003;31:s213.
70. Fan J, Kapus A, Li YH, et al. Priming for enhanced alveolar fibrin deposition after haemorrhagic shock: role of tumor necrosis factor. *Am J Respir Cell Mol Biol.* 2000;22:412.
71. Gando S, Kameue T, Matsuda N, et al. Combined activation of coagulation and inflammation has an important role in multiple organ dysfunction and poor outcome after severe trauma. *Thromb Haemost.* 2002;88:943.
72. Rigby AC, Grant MA. Protein S: a conduit between anticoagulation and inflammation. *Crit Care Med.* 2004;32:s336.
73. Levi M, de Jonge E, van der Poll T. New treatment strategies for disseminated intravascular coagulation based on current understanding of the pathophysiology. *Ann Med.* 2004;36:41.
74. Lo EH, Wang X, Cuzner ML. Extracellular proteolysis in brain injury and inflammation: role for plasminogen activators and matrix metalloproteinases. *J Neurosci Res.* 2002;69:1.
75. Du Clos TW. Function of C-reactive protein. *Ann Med.* 2000;32:274.
76. Whicher JT, Evans SW. Acute phase proteins. *Hosp Update.* 1990:899.
77. Lennard AC. Interleukin-1 receptor antagonist. *Crit Rev Immunol.* 1995; 15:77.

78. Chikanza IC, Grossman AB. Neuroendocrine immune responses to inflammation: the concept of the neuroendocrine immune loop. *Bailliere's Clin Rheumatol.* 1996;10:199.
79. Emsley J, White HE, O'Hara BP, et al. Structure of pentameric human serum amyloid P component. *Nature.* 1994;367:338.
80. Gabay C, Kushner I. Acute-phase proteins and other systemic responses to inflammation. *N Engl J Med.* 1999;340:448.
81. Urieli-Shoval S, Linke RP, Matzner Y. Expression and function of serum amyloid A, a major acute-phase protein, in normal and disease states. *Curr Opin Hematol.* 2000;7:64.
82. Babaev A, Frederick PD, Pasta DJ, et al. Trends in management and outcomes of patients with acute myocardial infarction complicated by cardiogenic shock. *JAMA.* 2005;294:448.
83. Sabiston DC Jr. The fundamental contributions of Alfred Blalock to the pathogenesis of shock. *Arch Surg.* 1995;130:736.
84. Moore FA, McKinley BA, Moore EE, et al. Inflammation and the host response to injury, a large-scale collaborative project: patient-oriented research core—standard operating procedures for clinical care III. Guidelines for shock resuscitation. *J Trauma.* 2006;61:82.
85. American College of Surgeons. *Advanced Trauma Life Support for Doctors.* 7th ed. Chicago: American College of Surgeons; 2004.
86. Wiggers CJ. *Experimental Hemorrhagic Shock.* New York: Commonwealth Fund; 1950.
87. Bergstein JM, Slakey DP, Wallace JR, et al. Traumatic hypothermia is related to hypotension, not resuscitation. *Ann Emerg Med.* 1996;27:39.
88. Rivers E, Nguyen B, Havstad S, et al. Early goal-directed therapy in the treatment of severe sepsis and septic shock. *N Engl J Med.* 2001;345:1368.
89. O'Neill PJ, Cobb LM, Ayala A, et al. Aggressive fluid resuscitation following intestinal ischemia-reperfusion in immature rats prevents metabolic derangements and down regulates interleukin-6 release. *Shock.* 1994;1:381.
90. Hayes MA, Timmins AC, Yau EHS, et al. Elevation of systemic oxygen delivery in the treatment of critically ill patients. *N Engl J Med.* 1994; 330:1717.
91. Smith T, Grounds RM, Rhodes A. Central venous pressure: uses and limitations In: Pinsky MR, Payen D, eds. *Functional Hemodynamic Monitoring. Update in Intensive Care and Emergency Medicine.* No. 42. New York: Springer-Verlag; 2005:99.
92. Marini JJ, Leatherman JW. Pulmonary artery occlusion pressure: measurement, significance, and clinical uses In: Pinsky MR, Payen D, eds. *Functional Hemodynamic Monitoring. Update in Intensive Care and Emergency Medicine.* No. 42. New York: Springer-Verlag; 2005:111.
93. Singer M. Esophageal Doppler monitoring. In: Pinsky MR, Payen D, eds. *Functional Hemodynamic Monitoring. Update in Intensive Care and Emergency Medicine.* No. 42. New York: Springer-Verlag; 2005:193.
94. Vignon P. Hemodynamic assessment of critically ill patients using echocardiography Doppler. *Curr Opin Crit Care.* 2005;11:227.
95. Dellinger RP, Carlet JM, Masur H. Surviving Sepsis Campaign for management of severe sepsis and septic shock. *Crit Care Med.* 2004;32:858.
96. McKinley BA, Marvin RG, Cocanour CS, et al. Blunt trauma resuscitation: the old can respond. *J Trauma.* 2000;135:688.
97. Brandstrup B, Tonnesen H, Beier-Holgersen R, et al. Effects of intravenous fluid restriction on postoperative complications: comparison of two perioperative fluid regimens: a randomized assessor-blinded multicenter trial. *Ann Surg.* 2003;238:641.
98. Riddez L, Johnson L, Hahn RG. Central and regional hemodynamics during crystalloid fluid therapy after uncontrolled intra-abdominal bleeding. *J Trauma.* 1998;44:433.
99. Rackow EC, Weil MH, Macneil AR, et al. Effects of crystalloid and colloid fluids on extra vascular lung water in hypoproteinemic dogs. *J Appl Physiol.* 1987;62:2421.
100. Balogh Z, McKinley BA, Cocanour CS, et al. Secondary abdominal compartment syndrome is an elusive early complication of traumatic shock resuscitation. *Am J Surg.* 2002;184:538.
101. Finfer S, Bellomo R, Boyce N. A comparison of albumin and saline for fluid resuscitation in the intensive care unit. *N Engl J Med.* 2004;350:2247.
102. Williams EL, Hildebrand KL, McCormick SA, et al. The effect of intravenous lactated Ringer's solution versus 0.9% sodium chloride solution on serum osmolality in human volunteers. *Anesth Analg.* 1999;88:999.
103. Koustova E, Stanton K, Gushchin V, et al. Effects of lactated Ringer's solutions on human leukocytes. *J Trauma.* 2002;52:872.
104. Takil A, Eti Z, Irmak P, et al. Early postoperative respiratory acidosis after large intravascular volume infusion of lactated ringer's solution during major spine surgery. *Anesth Analg.* 2002;95:294.
105. Rhee P, Wang D, Ruff P, et al. Human neutrophil activation and increased adhesion by various resuscitation fluids. *Crit Care Med.* 2000;28:74.
106. Gushchin V, Stegalkina S, Alam HB, et al. Cytokine expression profiling in human leukocytes after exposure to hypertonic and isotonic fluids. *J Trauma.* 2002;52:867.
107. Khanna S, Davis D, Peterson B, et al. Use of hypertonic saline in the treatment of severe refractory posttraumatic intracranial hypertension in pediatric traumatic brain injury. *Crit Care Med.* 2000;28:1144.
108. Huang PP, Stucky FS, Dimick AR, et al. Hypertonic sodium resuscitation is associated with renal failure and death. *Ann Surg.* 1995;221:543.
109. Kreimeier U, Messmer K. Small-volume resuscitation: from experimental evidence to clinical routine: advantages and disadvantages of hypertonic solutions. *Acta Anaesthesiol Scand.* 2002;46:625.
110. Fleck A, Hawker F, Wallace PI, et al. Increased vascular permeability: a major cause of hypoalbuminaemia in disease and injury. *Lancet.* 1985;1:781.
111. Kohler JP, Rice CL, Zarins CK, et al. Does reduced colloid oncotic pressure increase pulmonary dysfunction in sepsis? *Crit Care Med.* 1981;9:90.
112. Vermeulen LC Jr, Ratko TA, Erstad BL, et al. A paradigm for consensus. The University Hospital Consortium guidelines for the use of albumin, nonprotein colloid, and crystalloid solutions. *Arch Intern Med.* 1995;155:373.
113. Blunt MC, Nicholson JP, Park GR. Serum albumin and colloid osmotic pressure in survivors and non-survivors of prolonged critical illness. *Anaesthesia.* 1998;53:755.
114. Golub R, Sorrento JJ, Cantu RJ, et al. Efficacy of albumin supplementation in the surgical intensive care unit: a prospective, randomized study. *Crit Care Med.* 1994;22:613.
115. McCluskey A, Thomas AN, Bowles BJM, et al. The prognostic value of serial measurements of serum albumin in patients admitted to an intensive care unit. *Anaesthesia.* 1996;51:724.
116. Stockwell MA, Soni N, Riley B. Colloid solutions in the critically ill. A randomized comparison of albumin and polygeline. I. Outcome and duration of stay in the intensive care unit. *Anaesthesia.* 1992;47:3.
117. Boldt J, Hessen M, Mueller M, et al. The effects of albumin versus hydroxyethyl starch solution on cardiorespiratory and circulatory variables in critically ill patients. *Anesth Analg.* 1996;83:245.
118. Cochrane Injuries Group Albumin Reviewers. Human albumin administration in critically ill patients: systematic review of randomised controlled trials. *BMJ.* 1998;317:235.
119. Wilkes MM, Navickis RJ. Patient survival after human albumin administration: a meta-analysis of randomized, controlled trials. *Ann Intern Med.* 2001;135:149.
120. Alderson, P, Bunn F, Li Wan Po A, et al. Human albumin solution for resuscitation and volume expansion in critically ill patients. *Cochrane Library.* 2006;3.
121. Treib J, Haass A, Pindur G. Coagulation disorders caused by hydroxyethyl starch. *Thromb Haemost.* 1997;78:974.
122. Cittanova ML, Leblanc I, Legendre C, et al. Effect of hydroxyethyl starch in brain-dead kidney donors on renal function in kidney-transplant recipients. *Lancet.* 1996;348:1620.
123. Schortgen F, Lacherade JC, Bruneel F, et al. Effects of hydroxyethylstarch and gelatin on renal function in severe sepsis: a multicentre randomised study. *Lancet.* 2001;357:911.
124. Treib J, Haass A, Pindur G, et al. All medium starches are not the same: influence of the degree of hydroxyethyl substitution of hydroxyethyl starch on plasma volume, hemorrheologic conditions, and coagulation. *Transfusion.* 1996;36:450.
125. Vincent JL. Plugging the leaks? New insights into synthetic colloids. *Crit Care Med.* 1991;19:316.
126. Feng X, Liu J, Yu M, et al. Hydroxyethyl starch, but not modified fluid gelatin, affects inflammatory response in a rat model of polymicrobial sepsis with capillary leakage. *Anesth Analg.* 2007;104:624.
127. Schmand JF, Ayala A, Morrison MH, et al. Effects of hydroxyethyl starch after trauma-hemorrhagic shock: restoration of macrophage integrity and prevention of increased circulating IL-6 levels. *Crit Care Med.* 1995;23:806.
128. Handrigan MT, Burns AR, Donnachie EM, et al. Hydroxyethyl starch inhibits neutrophil adhesion and transendothelial migration. *Shock.* 2005; 24:434.
129. Dieterich HJ, Weissmuller T, Rosenberger P, et al. Effect of hydroxyethyl starch on vascular leak syndrome and neutrophil accumulation during hypoxia. *Crit Care Med.* 2006;34:1775.
130. Vassar MJ, Perry CA, Holcroft JW. Prehospital resuscitation of hypotensive trauma patients with 7.5% NaCl versus 7.5% NaCl with added dextran: a controlled trial. *J Trauma.* 1993;34:622.
131. Vassar MJ, Fischer RP, O'Brien PE, et al. A multicenter trial for resuscitation of injured patients with 7.5% sodium chloride. The effect of added dextran 70. The Multicenter Group for the Study of Hypertonic Saline in Trauma Patients. *Arch Surg.* 1993;128:1003.
132. Mattox KL, Maningas PA, Moore EE, et al. Prehospital hypertonic saline/dextran infusion for post-traumatic hypotension. The U.S.A. Multicenter Trial. *Ann Surg.* 1991;213:482.
133. Ring J, Messmer K. Incidence and severity of anaphylactoid reactions to colloid volume substitutes. *Lancet.* 1977;1:466.
134. Wu J, Huang M, Tang G, et al. Hemodynamic response of modified fluid gelatin compared with lactated ringer's solution for volume expansion in emergency resuscitation of hypovolemic shock patients: preliminary report of a prospective, randomized trial. *World J Surg.* 2001;25:598.
135. Evans PA, Garnett M, Boffard K, et al. Evaluation of the effect of colloid (Haemaccel) on the bleeding time in the trauma patient. *J R Soc Med.* 1996;89:101.
136. Tollofsrud S, Svennevig JL, Breivik H, et al. Fluid balance and pulmonary functions during and after coronary artery bypass surgery: Ringer's acetate compared with dextran, polygeline, or albumin. *Acta Anaesthesiol Scand.* 1995;39:671.
137. Bordin JO, Heddle NM, Blajchman MA. Biologic effects of leukocytes present in transfused cellular blood products. *Blood.* 1994;84:1703.

138. van de Watering LMG, Hermans J, Houbiers JGA. Beneficial effects of leukocyte depletion of transfused blood on postoperative complications in patients undergoing cardiac surgery: a randomized clinical trial. *Circulation.* 1998;97:562.
139. Hébert PC, Wells GW, Blajchman MA. A multicenter, randomized, controlled clinical trial of transfusion requirements in critical care. *N Engl J Med.* 1999;340:409.
140. Gonzalez EA, Moore FA, Holcomb JB, et al. Fresh frozen plasma should be given earlier to patients requiring massive transfusion. *J Trauma.* 2007;62:112.
141. Shippy CR, Shoemaker WC. Hemodynamic and colloid osmotic pressure alterations in the surgical patient. *Crit Care Med.* 1983;11:191.
142. Velanovich V. Crystalloid versus colloid fluid resuscitation: a meta-analysis of mortality. *Surgery.* 1989;105:65.
143. Cotton BA, Guy JS, Morris JA, et al. The cellular, metabolic, and systemic consequences of aggressive fluid resuscitation strategies. *Shock.* 2006;26:115.
144. Committee on Fluid Resuscitation for Combat Casualties. Washington DC: Institute of Medicine, National Academy Press; 1999.
145. Dutton RP, MacKenzie CF, Scalea TM. Hypotensive resuscitation during active hemorrhage: impact on in-hospital mortality. *J Trauma.* 2002;52:1141.
146. Roberts K, Revell M, Youssef H, et al. Hypotensive resuscitation in patients with ruptured abdominal aortic aneurysm. *Eur J Vasc Endovasc Surg.* 2006;31:339.
147. Blair SD, Janvrin SB, McCollum CN, et al. Effect of early blood transfusion on gastrointestinal haemorrhage. *Brit J Surg.* 1986;73:783.
148. Bickell WH, Wall MJ, Pepe PE, et al. Immediate versus delayed fluid resuscitation for hypotensive patients with penetrating torso injuries. *N Engl J Med.* 1994;331:1105.
149. Kwan I, Bunn F, Roberts I. Timing and volume of fluid administration for patients with bleeding. *Cochrane Library.* 2006;3.
150. Rackow EC, Falk JL, Fein IA, et al. Fluid resuscitation in circulatory shock: a comparison of the cardiorespiratory effects of albumin, hetastarch, and saline solutions in patients with hypovolemic and septic shock. *Crit Care Med.* 1983;11:839.
151. Mullner M, Urbanek B, Havel C, et al. Vasopressors for shock. *Cochrane Database Syst Rev.* 2004;3:CD003709.
152. Albanese J, Leone M, Garnier F, et al. Renal effects of norepinephrine in septic and nonseptic patients. *Chest.* 2004;126:534.
153. Task Force of the American College of Critical Care Medicine, Society of Critical Care Medicine. Practice parameters for hemodynamic support of sepsis in adult patients in sepsis. *Crit Care Med.* 1999;27:639.
154. Bellomo R, Chapman M, Finfer S, et al. Low-dose dopamine in patients with early renal dysfunction: a placebo-controlled randomised trial. Australian and New Zealand Intensive Care Society (ANZICS) Clinical Trials Group. *Lancet.* 2000;356:2139.
155. Hollenberg SM, Kavinsky CJ, Parrillo JE. Cardiogenic shock. *Ann Intern Med.* 1999;131:47.
156. Sakr Y, Reinhart K, Vincent JL, et al. Does dopamine administration in shock influence outcome? Results of the Sepsis Occurrence in Acutely Ill Patients (SOAP) Study. *Crit Care Med.* 2006;34:589.
157. Martin C, Viviand X, Leone M, et al. Effect of norepinephrine on the outcome of septic shock. *Crit Care Med.* 2000;28:2758.
158. Kohsaka S, Menon V, Lowe AM, et al. Systemic inflammatory response syndrome after acute myocardial infarction complicated by cardiogenic shock. *Arch Intern Med.* 2005;165:1643.
159. Vallet B, Chopin C, Curtis SE, et al. Prognostic value of the dobutamine test in patients with sepsis syndrome and normal lactate values: a prospective, multicenter study. *Crit Care Med.* 1993;21:1868.
160. Hoffman BB, Lefkowitz RJ. Catecholamines, sympathomimetic drugs, and adrenergic receptor antagonists. In: Hardman JC, Limbird LE, eds. *Goodman and Gilman's The Pharmacological Basis of Therapeutics.* 9th ed. New York: McGraw-Hill; 1995.
161. Thoren A, Elam M, Ricksten SE. Differential effects of dopamine, dopexamine, and dobutamine on jejunal mucosal perfusion early after cardiac surgery. *Crit Care Med.* 2000;28:2338.
162. Cuffe MS, Califf RM, Adams KF, et al. Short-term intravenous milrinone for acute exacerbation of chronic heart failure: a randomized controlled trial. *JAMA.* 2002;287:1541.
163. Greenberg B, Borghi C, Perrone S. Pharmacotherapeutic approaches for decompensated heart failure: A role for the calcium sensitiser levosimendan? *Eur J Heart Fail.* 2003;5:13.
164. Garnacho-Montero J, Garcia-Garmendia JL, Barrero-Almodovar A, et al. Impact of adequate empirical antibiotic therapy on the outcome of patients admitted to the intensive care unit with sepsis. *Crit Care Med.* 2003;31:2742.
165. Sheikh A, Ten Broek V, Brown S, et al. H1-antihistamines for the treatment of anaphylaxis with and without shock. *Cochrane Database Syst Rev.* 2007;24:CD006160.
166. Gotzsche PC, Hrobjartsson A. Somatostatin analogues for acute bleeding oesophageal varices. *Cochrane Database Syst Rev.* 2005;25:CD000193.
167. Landry DW, Oliver JA. The pathogenesis of vasodilatory shock. *N Engl J Med.* 2001;345:588.
168. Cooper DJ, Russell JA, Walley KR, et al. Vasopressin and septic shock trial (VASST): innovative features and performance. *Am J Respir Crit Care Med.* 2003;167:A838.
169. Leone M, Albanese J, Delmas A, et al. Terlipressin in catecholamine-resistant septic shock patients. *Shock.* 2004;22:314.
170. Morelli A, Rocco M, Conti G, et al. Effects of terlipressin on systemic and regional haemodynamics in catecholamine-treated hyperkinetic septic shock. *Intensive Care Med.* 2004;30:597.
171. Annane D, Bellissant E, Bollaert P, et al. Corticosteroids for severe sepsis and septic shock: a systematic review and meta-analysis. *BMJ.* 2004;329:480.
172. Annane D, Sebille V, Charpentier C, et al. Effect of treatment with low doses of hydrocortisone and fludrocortisone on mortality in patients with septic shock. *JAMA.* 2002;288:862.
173. Bernard GR, Vincent JL, Laterre PF, et al. Recombinant Human Protein C Worldwide Evaluation in Severe Sepsis (PROWESS) study group. Efficacy and safety of recombinant human activated protein C for severe sepsis. *N Engl J Med.* 2001;344:699.
174. Abou-Khalil B, Scalea TM, Trooskin SZ, et al. Hemodynamic responses to shock in young trauma patients: need for invasive monitoring. *Crit Care Med.* 1994;22:633.
175. Bruner JMR, Krenis LJ, Krunsman JM, et al. Comparison of direct and indirect methods of measuring blood pressure. Parts I-III. *Med Instrum.* 1981;15:11, 97, 182.
176. Aaslid R, Brubakk AO. Accuracy of an ultrasound Doppler servo method for noninvasive determination of instantaneous and mean blood pressure. *Circulation.* 1981;64:753.
177. Eisenberg PR, Jaffe AS, Schuster DP. Clinical evaluation compared to pulmonary artery catheterization in the hemodynamic assessment of critically ill patients. *Crit Care Med.* 1984;12:349.
178. Connors AF Jr, McCafree DR, Gray BA. Evaluation of right heart catheterization in the critically ill patient without acute myocardial infarction. *N Engl J Med.* 1983;308:263.
179. Shoemaker WC, Bland RD, Appel PL. Therapy of critically ill postoperative patients based on outcome prediction and prospective clinical trials. *Surg Clin North Am.* 1985;65:811.
180. Bishop MH, Shoemaker WC, Appel PL, et al. Prospective, randomized trial of survivor values of cardiac index, oxygen delivery, and oxygen consumption as resuscitation endpoints in severe trauma. *J Trauma.* 1995;38:780.
181. Pinsky MR. Beyond global oxygen supply-demand relations: in search of measures of dysoxia. *Intensive Care Med.* 1994;20:1.
182. Shoemaker WC, Appel PL, Kram HB. Hemodynamic and oxygen transport responses in survivors and nonsurvivors of high-risk surgery. *Crit Care Med.* 1993;21:977.
183. Connors AF, Speroff T, Dawson NV, et al. The effectiveness of right heart catheterization in the initial care of critically ill patients. SUPPORT Investigators. *JAMA.* 1996;276:889.
184. Shah MR, Hasselblad V, Stevenson LW, et al. Impact of the pulmonary artery catheter in critically ill patients: meta-analysis of randomized clinical trials. *JAMA.* 2005;294:1664.
185. The National Heart, Lung, and Blood Institute Acute Respiratory Distress Syndrome (ARDS) Clinical Trials Network. Pulmonary-artery versus central venous catheter to guide treatment of acute lung injury. *N Engl J Med.* 2006;354:2213.
186. Friese R, Shafi S, Gentilello LM. Pulmonary artery catheter use is associated with reduced mortality in severely injured patients: a National Trauma Date Bank analysis of 53,312 patients. *Crit Care Med.* 2006;34:1597.
187. Shoemaker WC, Montgomery ES, Kaplan E, et al. Physiologic patterns in surviving and nonsurviving shock patients: use of sequential cardiorespiratory variables in defining criteria for therapeutic goals and early warning of death. *Arch Surg.* 1973;106:630.
188. Shoemaker WC, Appel P, Bland R. Use of physiologic monitoring to predict outcome and to assist in clinical decisions in critically ill postoperative patients. *Am J Surg.* 1983;146:43.
189. Shoemaker WC, Appel PL, Kram HB, et al. Prospective trial of supranormal values of survivors as therapeutic goals in high risk surgical patients. *Chest.* 1988;94:1176.
190. Boyd O, Grounds R, Bennett ED. A randomized clinical trial of the effect of deliberate perioperative increase of oxygen delivery on mortality in high-risk surgical patients. *JAMA.* 1993;270:2699.
191. Bishop MH, Shoemaker WC, Appel PL, et al. Relationship between supranormal circulatory values, time delays, and outcome in severely traumatized patients. *Crit Care Med.* 1993;21:56.
192. Fleming A, Bishop M, Shoemaker W, et al. Prospective trial of supranormal values as goals of resuscitation in severe trauma. *Arch Surg.* 1992;127:1175.
193. Gattinoni L, Brazzi L, Pelosi P, et al. A trial of goal-oriented hemodynamic therapy in critical ill patients. *N Engl J Med.* 1995;333:1025.
194. McKinley B, Kozar RA, Cocanour CS, et al. Normal versus supranormal oxygen delivery goals in shock resuscitation: the response is the same. *J Trauma.* 2002;53:825.
195. Heyland DK, Cook DJ, King D, et al. Maximizing oxygen delivery in critically ill patients: a methodological appraisal of the evidence. *Crit Care Med.* 1996;24:517.

196. Balogh Z, McKinley BA, Cocanour CS, et al. Supranormal trauma resuscitation causes more cases of abdominal compartment syndrome. *Arch Surg.* 2003;138:637.
197. Velmahos GC, Demetriades D, Shoemaker WC, et al. Endpoints of resuscitation of critically injured patients: normal or supranormal? A prospective randomized trial. *Ann Surg.* 2000;232:409.
198. Englehart MS, Schreiber MA. Measurement of acid-base resuscitation endpoints: lactate, base deficit, bicarbonate or what? *Curr Opin Crit Care.* 2006;12:569.
199. Kern JW, Shoemaker WC. Meta-analysis of hemodynamic optimization in high-risk patients. *Crit Care Med.* 2002;30:1686.
200. Tisherman SA, Barie P, Bokhari F, et al. Clinical practice guideline: endpoints of resuscitation [EAST Website]. 2003. http://www.east.org. Accessed November 2, 2006.
201. Martin MJ. Venous bicarbonate correlates linearly with arterial base deficit only if pH is constant—reply. *Arch Surg.* 2006;141:105.
202. Balasubramanyan N, Havens PL, Hoffman GM. Unmeasured anions identified by the Fenci-Stewart method predict mortality better than base excess, anion gap, and lactate in patients in the pediatric intensive care unit. *Crit Care Med.* 1999;27:1577.
203. Davis JW, Kaups KL, Parks SN. Base deficit is superior to pH in evaluating clearance of acidosis after traumatic shock. *J Trauma.* 1998;44:114.
204. Davis JW, Shackford SR, MacKersie RC, et al. Base deficit as a guide to volume resuscitation. *J Trauma.* 1988;28:1464.
205. Rutherford EJ, Morris JA, Reed GW, et al. Base deficit stratifies mortality and determines therapy. *J Trauma.* 1992;33:417.
206. Falcone RE, Santanello SA, Schultz MA, et al. Correlation of metabolic acidosis with outcome following injury and its value as a scoring tool. *World J Surg.* 1993;17:575.
207. Sauaia A, Moore FA, Moore EE, et al. Early predictors of postinjury multiple organ failure. *Arch Surg.* 1994;129:39.
208. Kincaid EH, Miller PR, Meredith JW, et al. Elevated arterial base deficit in trauma patients: a marker of impaired oxygen utilization. *J Am Coll Surg.* 1998;187:384.
209. Rixen D, Raum M, Bouillon B, et al. Base deficit development and its prognostic significance in posttrauma critical illness: an analysis by the trauma registry of the Deutsche Gesellschaft für unfallchirurgie. *Shock.* 2001;15:83.
210. Siegel JH, Rivkind AI, Dalal S, et al. Early physiologic predictors of injury severity and death in blunt multiple trauma. *Arch Surg.* 1990;125:498.
211. Eachempati SR, Robb T, Ivatury RR, et al. Factors affecting mortality in penetrating abdominal vascular trauma. *J Surg Res.* 2002;108:222.
212. Krishna G, Sleigh JW, Rahman H. Physiological predictors of death in exsanguinating trauma patients undergoing conventional trauma surgery. *Aust NZ J Surg.* 1998;68:826.
213. Davis JW, Parks SN, Kaups KL, et al. Admission base deficit predicts transfusion requirements and risk of complications. *J Trauma.* 1996;41:769.
214. Eberhard LW, Morabito DJ, Matthay MA, et al. Initial severity of metabolic acidosis predicts the development of acute lung injury in severely traumatized patients. *Crit Care Med.* 2000;28:125.
215. Rixen D, Siegel JH. Metabolic correlates of oxygen debt predict posttrauma early acute respiratory distress syndrome and the related cytokine response. *J Trauma.* 2000;49:392.
216. Botha AJ, Moore EA, Moore EE, et al. Base deficit after major trauma directly relates to neutrophil CD11b expression: a proposed mechanism of shock induced organ injury. *Int Care Med.* 1997;23:504.
217. Bannon MP, O'Neill CM, Martin M, et al. Central venous oxygen saturation, arterial base deficit, and lactate concentration in trauma patients. *Am Surg.* 1995;61:738.
218. Kincaid EH, Chang MC, Letton RW, et al. Admission base deficit in pediatric trauma: a study using the National Trauma Data Bank. *J Trauma.* 2001;51:332.
219. Randolph LC, Takacs M, Davis KA. Resuscitation in the pediatric trauma population: admission base deficit remains an important prognostic indicator. *J Trauma.* 2002;53:838.
220. Dunham CM, Watson LA, Cooper C. Base deficit level indicating major injury is increased with ethanol. *J Emerg Med.* 2000;18:165.
221. Brill SA, Schreiber MA, Stewart TR, et al. Base deficit does not predict mortality when secondary to hyperchloremic acidosis. *Shock.* 2002;17: 459.
222. Vincent J-L, Dufaye P, Berre J, et al. Serial lactate determinations during circulatory shock. *Crit Care Med.* 1983;11:449.
223. Abramson D, Scalea TM, Hitchcock R, et al. Lactate clearance and survival following injury. *J Trauma.* 1993;35:584.
224. McNelis J, Marini CP, Jurkiewicz, et al. Prolonged lactate clearance is associated with increased mortality in the surgical intensive care unit. *Am J Surg.* 2001;182:481.
225. Manikis P, Jankowski S, Zhang H, et al. Correlation of serial blood lactate levels to organ failure and mortality after trauma. *Am J Emerg Med.* 1995;13:619.
226. FitzSullivan E, Salim A, Demetriades D, et al. Serum bicarbonate may replace the arterial base deficit in the trauma intensive care unit. *Am J Surg.* 2005;190:961.
227. Martin MJ, FitzSullivan E, Salim A, et al. Use of serum bicarbonate measurement in place of arterial base deficit in the surgical intensive care unit. *Arch Surg.* 2005;140:745.
228. Calvet X, Baigorri F, Duarte M, et al. Effect of ranitidine on gastric intramucosal pH in critically ill patients. *Intensive Care Med.* 1998;24:12.
229. Marik PE, Lorenzaza A. Effect of tube feedings on the measurement of gastric intramucosal pH. *Crit Care Med.* 1996;24:1498.
230. Cammarata GA, Weil MH, Fries M, et al. Buccal capnometry to guide management of massive blood loss. *J Appl Physiol.* 2006;100:304.
231. Pellis T, Weil MH, Tang W, et al. Increases in both buccal and sublingual partial pressure of carbon dioxide reflect decreases of tissue blood flows in a porcine model during hemorrhagic shock. *J Trauma.* 2005;58:817.
232. Povoas HP, Weil MH, Tang W, et al. Decrease in mesenteric blood flow associated with increase in sublingual PCO_2 during hemorrhagic shock. *Shock.* 2001;15:398.
233. Weil MH, Nakagawa Y, Tang W, et al. Sublingual capnography: a new noninvasive measurement for diagnosis and quantitation of severity of circulatory shock. *Crit Care Med.* 1999;27:1225.
234. Baron BJ, Dutton RP, Zehtabchi S, et al. Sublingual capnometry for rapid determination of the severity of hemorrhagic shock. *J Trauma.* 2007;62: 120.
235. Creteur J, De Backer D, Sakr Y, et al. Sublingual capnometry tracks microcirculatory changes in septic patients. *Intensive Care Med.* 2006;32: 516.
236. Baron BJ, Sinert R, Zehtabchi S, et al. Diagnostic utility of sublingual PCO_2 for detecting hemorrhage in patients with penetrating trauma. *J Trauma.* 2004;57:69.
237. Horecker BL. The absorption spectra of hemoglobin and its derivatives in the visible and near infra-red regions. *J Biol Chem.* 1943;148:173.
238. Taylor JH, Mulier KE, Myers DE, et al. Use of near-infrared spectroscopy in early determination of irreversible hemorrhagic shock. *J Trauma.* 2005;58: 1119.
239. McKinley BA, Marvin RG, Cocanour CS, et al. Tissue hemoglobin O_2 saturation during resuscitation on traumatic shock monitored using near infrared spectrometry. *J Trauma.* 2000;48:637.

CHAPTER 56 ■ CARDIOGENIC SHOCK

MARC A. SIMON • MICHAEL R. PINSKY

IMMEDIATE CONCERNS

Definition

Cardiogenic shock is a major and frequently fatal complication of a variety of acute and chronic disorders that results in a primary impairment of the ability of the heart to maintain adequate tissue perfusion despite sufficient intravascular volume.

Essential Diagnostic Tests and Procedures

1. Bedside clinical criteria that provide evidence of reduced organ perfusion include oliguria, confusion, peripheral cyanosis, and evidence of peripheral vasoconstriction.
2. An accurate definition of cardiogenic shock also requires persistence of the shock state after correction of extracardiac conditions, such as hypovolemia or a variety of metabolic abnormalities including significant disturbances in acid-base metabolism, electrolyte abnormalities, or arrhythmias.
3. The pulmonary artery occlusion pressure (PAOP) is frequently in excess of 18 mm Hg, and the cardiac index (CI) is usually less than 2.2 L/minute/m^2.

Initial Therapy

1. Cardiogenic shock in the setting of acute myocardial infarction warrants pharmacologic intervention to limit infarct size and includes using heparin, aspirin, nitrates, β-blockers, calcium channel blockers, or a combination thereof. Primary coronary artery stenting is now recommended for patients with ST elevation or left bundle branch block who develop shock within 36 hours of acute myocardial infarction and are suitable for revascularization that can be performed within 18 hours of shock onset (1). Thrombolytic therapy may be used if early revascularization is not available (2).
2. Hemodynamic management includes optimization of preload and afterload and augmentation of contractility, when appropriate, with agents such as dobutamine, dopamine, norepinephrine, digitalis preparations, or phosphodiesterase inhibitors.
3. Surgical intervention in myocardial infarction has been used to limit infarct size by direct revascularization or correction of mechanical defects of an acute ischemic event such as ventricular septal defects (VSDs), acute mitral insufficiency, free wall rupture, or left ventricular aneurysm.
4. Mechanical assist devices such as the intra-aortic balloon pump (IABP) are used as temporizing measures to optimize blood pressure, cardiac output, and tissue perfusion in patients with cardiogenic shock while further diagnostic procedures and disease staging are performed. Newer percutaneous ventricular assist devices (VADs) providing 2 to 5 L/minute blood flow are now available and hold promise for rapid restoration of peripheral perfusion.

CLASSIFICATION

A variety of classification schemes have been proposed for the division of circulatory shock according to etiology and underlying hemodynamic mechanisms. Circulatory shock can be subdivided into four distinct classes on the basis of underlying mechanism plus hemodynamics; these classes should be considered and excluded before establishing a definite diagnosis of cardiogenic shock.

Hypovolemic Shock

Hypovolemic shock results from volume loss caused by conditions such as gastrointestinal bleeding or extravasation of plasma.

Obstructive Shock

Obstructive shock results from impedance of the circulatory channels by an intrinsic or extrinsic obstruction. Pulmonary embolism, dissecting aneurysm, and pericardial tamponade result in obstructive shock.

Distributive Shock

Distributive shock is caused by conditions such as direct arteriovenous shunting and is characterized by decreased resistance or increased venous capacity from the vasomotor dysfunction.

Cardiogenic Shock

Cardiogenic shock is characterized by primary myocardial dysfunction resulting in the inability of the heart to maintain an adequate cardiac output with subsequent compromising of metabolic requirements (Fig. 56.1). The most common

This work is supported in part by NIH grants HL007820, HL067181, and HL073198, and the NIH Roadmap Multidisciplinary Clinical Research Career Development Award Grant (K12 RR023267) from the National Institutes of Health.

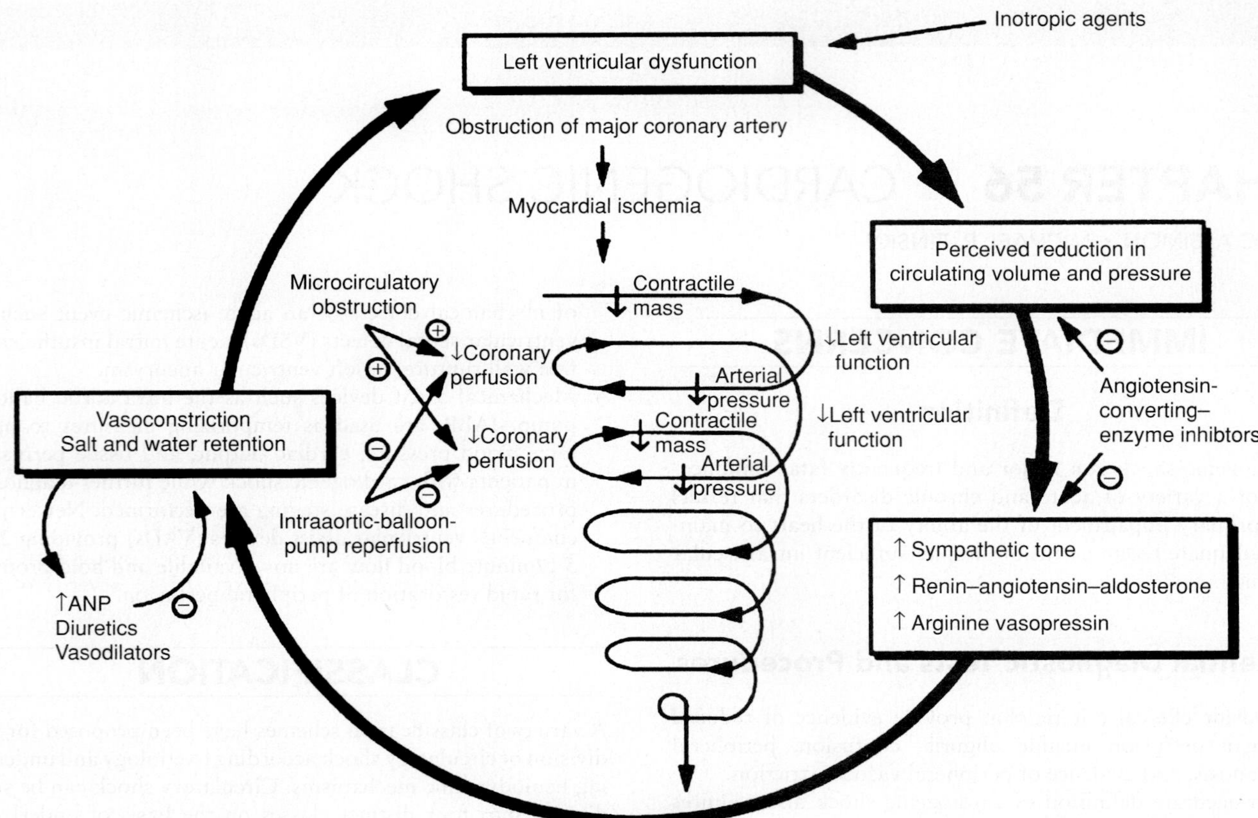

FIGURE 56.1. Neurohumoral and mechanical events that lead to death in patients with cardiogenic shock. ANP, atrial natriuretic peptide. (Used with permission from Pasternak RC, Braunwald E. Acute myocardial infarction. In: Wilson JD, Braunwald E, Isselbacher KJ, eds. *Harrison's Principles of Internal Medicine.* 12th ed. Vol. 1. New York: McGraw-Hill; 1991:953–964; and Francis GS. Neuroendocrine manifestations of congestive heart failure. *Am J Cardiol.* 1988;62[Suppl]:9A–13A.)

etiologies are myocardial infarction and cardiomyopathy with a superimposed hemodynamic stress.

ETIOLOGY

In order to understand the therapeutic approaches used to support left ventricular (LV) ejection and aid acutely decompensated hearts, it is important to understand the mechanisms underpinning LV systole. Systolic ventricular function is determined by preload, afterload, and contractility. Preload is the wall stress on the left ventricle prior to ejection. Operationally, we use LV end-diastolic volume to reflect this wall stress. Since measures of volumes can be difficult at the bedside, LV end-diastolic pressure, left atrial pressure, or pulmonary artery occlusion pressure are often used as surrogates for LV end-diastolic volume. Afterload is the maximal LV wall stress during ejection. By LaPlace's law, wall stress is proportional to the product of LV radius of curvature and transmural pressure. Under normal conditions, maximal LV afterload occurs at the instant of aortic value opening. Contractility is a more difficult term to define and quantify. A reasonable definition is the amount of force capable of being produced by the contracting myocardium (3). On a cellular level, contractility is related to the integrity of the actin–myocin coupling, intracellular calcium (Ca^{2+}) flux rate, and quantity. Functionally, one measures contractility by varying preload and afterload. Numerous measures have been attempted to quantify contractility with varying degrees of success depending upon the degree of true independence they have from preload or afterload. Measures of contractility include the maximal rate of isovolumic pressure development (dP/dt_{max}), the Frank-Starling law relating peak systolic activity (defined as either maximal developed pressure, volume ejected, or the product of the two) directly to end-diastolic volume (4), and left ventricular end-systolic pressure–volume relation (ESPVR) derived from pressure–volume loops. Systolic performance is the ability of the left ventricle to empty. This is a function of end-systolic volume; a commonly used calculation is the LV ejection fraction (effective ejection fraction in the case of valvular regurgitation).

The most common etiology of cardiogenic shock is acute myocardial infarction (MI) with a resultant loss of approximately 40% of functioning myocardium. Following myocardial infarction, the final infarct size has been shown to correlate with the degree of LV dysfunction (5). Loss of myocardial function may occur in one massive MI or may result in a cumulative loss of pump function caused by serial smaller infarcts. Cardiogenic shock more commonly results from infarction of the left ventricle, although recent clarification of the potential role of the right ventricle in the precipitation of the shock state

TABLE 56.1

CONTRIBUTING FACTORS TO THE DEVELOPMENT OF CARDIOGENIC SHOCK IN MYOCARDIAL INFARCTION

1. Loss of left ventricular function
   Cumulative loss of myocardial tissue exceeding 40% of ventricular mass, particularly anterior infarcts
   Myocardial infarction associated with bradyarrhythmias or tachyarrhythmias
   Hypovolemia or hypervolemia
2. Right ventricular infarction
3. Mechanical defects
   Papillary muscle dysfunction or rupture causing acute regurgitation
   Ventricular septal defect
   Ventricular pseudoaneurysm
   Free wall rupture and/or cardiac tamponade

has been recognized. Additionally, acute mechanical complications of myocardial infarction such as mitral insufficiency, free wall rupture, and acute VSD may result in cardiogenic shock during the peri-infarct period, as does the late development of left ventricular aneurysm (Table 56.1). Other causes of cardiogenic shock include end-stage or fulminant cardiomyopathy, myocarditis, acute chordal rupture causing valvular regurgitation, obstruction to left ventricular ejection (severe aortic stenosis or hypertrophic cardiomyopathy) or left ventricular filling (mitral stenosis or left atrial myxoma), or severe septic shock with myocardial depression.

Left Ventricular Acute Myocardial Infarction

Reduction in left ventricular performance is one of the major complications of ischemic heart disease. Several classifications that attempt to standardize the clinical and hemodynamic presentation of myocardial infarction have been proposed to aid in determining prognosis and the therapeutic approaches in patients with established cardiogenic shock or those who have the potential to progress to the shock state.

The Killip classification uses pure clinical bedside evaluation of the patient to establish prognostic indicators to predict the mortality associated with an acute myocardial infarction using the physical findings of congestive heart failure (6).

- *Class I* patients developed no overt signs of congestive heart failure, and these individuals had a low in-hospital mortality rate. This subgroup represented approximately 40% to 50% of all patients who presented with an acute MI. The in-hospital fatality rate was approximately 6%.
- *Class II* patients demonstrated evidence of impaired ventricular function as manifest by persistent bibasilar rales and an audible third heart sound. This subset of patients accounted for approximately 30% to 40% of patients with acute MI. The in-hospital mortality rate of 17% was triple relative to class I patients.
- *Class III* patients were characterized by the development of acute pulmonary edema, which was seen in approximately 10% to 15% of patients admitted to the hospital. A significant mortality rate of 38% was seen in this group treated conservatively before the thrombolytic era.
- *Class IV* patients had established cardiogenic shock with hypotension and signs of organ hypoperfusion. Cardiogenic shock occurred in 5% to 10% of infarct patients in this series but was associated with a high in-hospital mortality rate of 80%, which was a function of both severity of the underlying illness plus the limited availability of definitive treatment at the time this classification was proposed.

TABLE 56.2

HEMODYNAMIC SUBSETS AND MORTALITY IN MYOCARDIAL INFARCTION

Swan-Forrester class	Mortality rate (%)
I: CI >2.2; PAOP <18	<3
II: CI >2.2; PAOP >18	9
III: CI <2.2; PAOP <18	23
IV: CI <2.2; PAOP >18	51

PAOP, pulmonary artery occlusion pressure; CI, cardiac index in liters per minute per square meter.

The group at Cedars Sinai Medical Center, Los Angeles, also developed a clinical classification of heart failure associated with acute MI, which was subsequently refined by the availability of invasive hemodynamic monitoring using pulmonary artery catheters (PACs) (7) (Table 56.2). The Cedars Sinai classification also subdivided patients with acute myocardial into four subsets based on the measurement of the PAOP, CI, and clinical assessment.

Class I patients had no clinical evidence of pulmonary congestion or tissue hypoperfusion. Hemodynamic parameters measured in these subjects revealed the PAOP to be less than 18 mm Hg and the CI to be in excess of 2.2 L/minute/m^2. The advent and widespread use of pulmonary artery catheters clarified the concept of the ideal wedge that established the impact of diastolic dysfunction secondary to acute ischemia, with resultant impaired relaxation and elevated filling pressures being required to maintain adequate cardiac output.

Class I patients accounted for 25% of subjects admitted to the coronary care unit, and there was a low in-hospital mortality rate of 1%. Patients who on clinical grounds demonstrated no evidence of hypoperfusion or pulmonary congestion would not be expected to benefit from invasive cardiac monitoring. Frequent clinical reassessments and close attention paid to blood pressure and evidence of organ perfusion would represent adequate care.

Class II patients demonstrated pulmonary congestion as manifest by only an elevated PAOP greater than 18 mm Hg with an associated normal cardiac index. Class II patients accounted for approximately 25% of patients admitted to the coronary care unit, but an 11% mortality rate was associated with this group. Mild pulmonary congestion is transiently seen in a significant percentage of patients admitted to the coronary care unit and has a multifactorial etiology. Diastolic dysfunction induced by ischemia with retrograde transmission of elevated filling pressures into the pulmonary venous circuit results in extravasation of fluid into the pulmonary bed when hydrostatic pressure exceeds oncotic pressure. Ischemic papillary muscle dysfunction with mild degrees of mitral insufficiency is also a potential cause of pulmonary congestion in this subgroup. Physical examination of these patients reveals mild to moderate rales and potentially an audible third heart sound associated with radiographic evidence of pulmonary venous hypertension. Dyspnea and orthopnea are the main symptoms superimposed on the clinical presentation of myocardial ischemia. Treatment in this group is centered on reduction of filling pressures to a level that relieves pulmonary venous congestion but does not result in an overzealous reduction of filling pressures below the ideal wedge as the reduced cardiac contractility will require some increased filling volume and pressure to maintain adequate stroke volume and perfusion pressure (Starling mechanism). Excessive diuresis should be assiduously avoided, especially in patients who were euvolemic before the onset of their infarct. Despite signs of pulmonary congestion, patients presenting with acute pulmonary congestion frequently are not intravascularly volume overloaded, and diuretic therapy may reduce filling pressures to a level that would impair cardiac output. It is often difficult to ascertain at the bedside which patients are actually euvolemic and which are hypervolemic. Afterload reduction therapy will benefit both groups of patients and may allow time to assess total effective circulating blood volume by indirect measures, such as the existence of hyponatremia, peripheral edema, and S_4 gallop. Inotropic agents should be considered in such a situation so that pulmonary congestion can be relieved by diuresis if afterload reduction is not immediately effective since the increased inotropic state mitigates against a reduction in cardiac output induced by any reduction in cardiac filling pressures. Oxygenation should be maintained with adequate arterial saturation that may be monitored by oximetry. Vasodilator therapies in the form of nitroglycerin or inotropic agents with vasodilating capacity such as dobutamine are effective to return the hemodynamic parameters to normal. The usefulness and risk–benefit ratio of invasive hemodynamic monitoring in this subgroup of patients are controversial, although these patients frequently may be managed on clinical grounds.

Class III patients are characterized predominantly by clinical evidence of hypoperfusion. Hemodynamic monitoring reveals a PAOP less than 18 mm Hg and a cardiac index of less than 2.2 L/minute/m^2. The class III subgroup accounted for approximately 15% of patients with acute MI and was associated with a 23% mortality rate. Patients in this subgroup may be extremely difficult to manage on clinical grounds, and treatment can be facilitated by invasive hemodynamic monitoring to establish the volume status. Relative hypovolemia is determined by measuring the pulmonary artery occlusion pressure, which falls below that of the ideal wedge as predicted in ischemic states. Excessive diuresis is extremely problematic in this group of patients and may excessively decrease cardiac output because of the pre-existent relative hypovolemia. Class III patients require restoration of intravascular volume to increase filling pressures to a degree that ensures adequate cardiac output and organ perfusion.

Class IV patients demonstrated elevated PAOP in excess of 18 mm Hg and a depressed cardiac index of less than 2.2 L/minute/m^2 and frequently manifested signs of cardiogenic shock with clinical evidence of organ hypoperfusion and dysfunction. This subgroup accounted for approximately 35% of patients with MI and was associated with an in-hospital mortality rate of approximately 50%. Class IV patients may have a mechanical defect such as acute mitral insufficiency, free wall rupture, or VSD underlying the acute myocardial infarction; these are discussed separately. Oxygenation with the potential assisted ventilation in addition to inotropic and judicious use of vasodilator support is the recommended therapy in these subgroups.

Right Ventricular Infarction

Although isolated right ventricular (RV) infarction is rare, evidence of RV infarction and RV dysfunction is found in up to half of all infarcts and is clinically significant in nearly half of all inferior infarcts (8, 9). The clinical diagnosis of RV infarction should be considered when elevated jugular venous pressure is accompanied by hypotension while the lung fields are clear. But the diagnosis may be difficult to establish clinically unless hemodynamic measurements, special electrocardiographic leads, echocardiography, or nuclear imaging are performed (10). Right-sided precordial leads obtained by electrocardiography that demonstrates at least 1-mm ST elevation is approximately 70% sensitive in the diagnosis of RV infarction and confers a particularly poor prognosis (11). Echocardiography is an easily obtainable noninvasive study that demonstrates RV dilation and impairment of wall motion of the right ventricle. Radionuclide angiography currently is considered to be the most sensitive means to diagnose RV infarction, although more recent data suggest that magnetic resonance imaging is comparable (12,13). A decrease in RV ejection fraction that is associated with wall motion abnormalities is more than 90% sensitive in the diagnosis of an RV infarction. Hemodynamic studies that are supportive of significant ischemic involvement of the right ventricle are manifest by increases in right atrial pressures plus demonstration of resistance to diastolic filling, as shown by blunting of the y-descent that follows tricuspid valve opening. A "square root" sign or "dip and plateau" pattern in the diastolic pressure curve is commonly demonstrated in RV infarctions but is not specific and may be associated with pericardial tamponade or restrictive cardiomyopathy (14).

The Should We Emergently Revascularize Occluded Coronaries for Cardiogenic Shock (SHOCK) trial registry reported on the clinical characteristics of patients presenting with isolated RV shock (15). Patients with RV shock compared to LV shock were younger and had a lower prevalence of previous MI (25.5% vs. 40.1%), a lower prevalence of anterior MI (11% vs. 59%), and less multivessel disease (34.8% vs. 77.8%). As expected, the infarct-related vessel involved the right coronary artery more in RV shock (96% of cases) versus LV shock (27% of cases). These patients had a shorter median time between myocardial infarction and the diagnosis of shock (2.9 vs. 6.2 hours) compared to patients with left ventricular shock. Right atrial pressure was a highly significant distinguishing factor of right from left ventricular shock (mean pressure 23.0 $\pm$ 9.9 vs. 14.2 $\pm$ 7.4, $p = 0.0001$), while all other hemodynamic measures were similar. Interestingly, in-hospital mortality was not significantly different between RV and LV shock (53.1% vs. 60.8%). Improvement in survival due to revascularization was similar between groups and multivariate analysis revealed that RV shock was not an independent predictor of lower in-hospital mortality (odds ratio 1.07, 95% confidence interval 0.54–2.13). This similarity in survival was despite patients with RV shock being younger; thus, RV shock may carry a worse prognosis.

Cardiogenic shock in patients with RV infarction frequently represents a substantial loss of functioning myocardium and carries a poor prognosis. RV infarction accompanied by cardiogenic shock is frequently associated with a variety of conduction abnormalities, including a high-grade atrioventricular block or significant rhythm disturbances. The treatment of RV infarction complicated by cardiogenic shock centers around maintaining RV filling pressures and assurance of adequate volume. Hemodynamic measurements may facilitate the estimate of volume loading required. Nitrates, diuretics, and other predominantly vasodilating compounds should be avoided. Atrial fibrillation is frequently poorly tolerated by these patients and may require immediate electrical cardioversion. The use of digitalis in acute RV infarction, even in the presence of atrial fibrillation, is controversial. Adequate inotropic support with vasodilating inotropic agents such as dobutamine is used if cardiac output fails to optimize after adequate volume loading. Percutaneous revascularization should be considered as it has been shown to improve outcomes (16).

Mechanical Defects

A variety of mechanical defects may be associated with cardiogenic shock in the peri-infarction stage (Table 56.3). Myocardial infarction resulting in cardiogenic shock from the appearance of mechanical defects such as acute mitral insufficiency, VSD, or free wall rupture represents a major complication and requires aggressive diagnostic and therapeutic interventions if the patient is expected to survive. Despite improvements in imaging techniques plus mechanical assist devices and emergency surgery, the mortality from these complications remains extremely high.

Acute Mitral Insufficiency

The mitral valve is a complicated apparatus and consists of the valvular annulus, leaflets, chorda tendineae, and papillary muscles plus potential functional alterations from involvement of the adjacent myocardium. Abnormalities affecting any of the components of the mitral valve may result in acute or chronic mitral insufficiency. The mitral valve annulus may be dilated and contribute to mitral insufficiency, although this complication is primarily associated with cardiomyopathies or connective tissue diseases such as Marfan syndrome rather than an acute myocardial infarction. Calcification of the mitral valve annulus is common in the elderly and may alter coaptation of the mitral valve leaflets and result in mitral incompetence.

Acute mitral insufficiency caused by involvement of the valvular leaflets is associated with infective endocarditis from necrotizing organisms such as *Staphylococcus aureus* or *Enterococcus,* resulting in destruction of the valvular apparatus. Traumatic penetrating injuries that involve the valve itself are rare. Rupture of the chorda tendineae may also be seen in endocarditis or a variety of connective tissue diseases, including myxomatous degeneration or Marfan syndrome.

Chordal rupture that results in severe impairment of left ventricular function depends on the number of involved structures and the rapidity with which the rupture occurs. Mitral insufficiency in the peri-infarction state may result from involvement of the surrounding myocardium or papillary muscles. Papillary muscles located adjacent to the infarction zone may simply become dysfunctional because of alteration of synchrony of contraction related to ischemia or frank rupture from ischemic necrosis.

The degree of mitral insufficiency is a function of the degree of involvement and anatomic competence. The two papillary muscles (posteromedial and anterolateral papillary muscles) have different ischemic vulnerabilities because of the blood supply from the coronary arteries. The anatomic vascular supply represents end arteries that are solely supplied by terminal portions of the coronaries, thus rendering the papillary muscles vulnerable to ischemic involvement during an acute myocardial infarction. Papillary muscle dysfunction may result from intermittent ischemia during unstable angina or myocardial infarction with involvement of the adjacent myocardium (17). Papillary muscle dysfunction is characterized by mild flow murmurs, which may be grade I or grade II by auscultation. The anterolateral papillary muscle has a dual blood supply, which provides partial protection during ischemia. The diagonal branches of the left anterior descending and marginal branches from the circumflex supply blood to the anterolateral papillary muscle. The posteromedial papillary muscle is generally supplied solely from the posterior descending branch of the right coronary artery, increasing its vulnerability to ischemic-related dysfunction.

TABLE 56.3

COMPLICATIONS OF MYOCARDIAL INFARCTION

Characteristic	Ventricular septal rupture	Papillary muscle rupture	Papillary muscle dysfunction
Incidence	Unusual	Rare	Common
Murmur			
Type	Pansystolic	Early to pansystolic	Variable
Location	Left sternal border (95%)	Apex → axilla (50%)	Apex
Thrill	>50%	Rare	No
Clinical presentation	Left and right ventricular failure	Profound pulmonary edema	None to moderate left ventricular failure
Catheterization	O_2 step-up in right ventricle	Large left atrial V wave	Mild to moderate elevation of left atrial pressure

With permission from Crawford MH, O'Rourke RA. The bedside diagnosis of the complications of myocardial infarction. In: Eliot RS, ed. *Cardiac Emergencies.* Mount Kisco, NY: Futura; 1962.

Significant ischemia involving the papillary muscle that results in complete rupture with fulminant mitral insufficiency is generally fatal because of the marked volume load ejected retrograde into the left atria and pulmonary venous bed (18). However, if the major ischemic-related necrosis is distal and only involves rupture of the head of the papillary muscle, the resultant mitral insufficiency may be tolerated hemodynamically long enough to allow recognition, proper diagnosis, and surgical intervention. Mild ischemic involvement of the papillary muscle may be increased in hemodynamic significance in the presence of pre-existing left ventricular dilation, which alters the ability of the mitral leaflets to coapt. Severe ischemic-related mitral insufficiency is more frequently a result of posteromedial papillary muscle necrosis resulting from inferior or posterior myocardial infarctions, although one third of cases may result from anterior infarction (19,20). Less than half of cases present with electrocardiographic evidence of ST elevation or Q waves (20). Right ventricular papillary muscle rupture may occur but is uncommon. Involvement of papillary muscles in the right ventricle results in tricuspid insufficiency, which if severe may result in right ventricular failure.

Papillary muscle rupture is a relatively uncommon complication and occurs in approximately 1% of patients having an acute ischemic event. The incidence has decreased in the thrombolytic era (21). After acute MI with cardiogenic shock, the incidence of acute severe mitral regurgitation is 6.9% (22). The peak incidence of papillary muscle rupture is within the first week, with the majority occurring between days 3 and 5 after an acute MI. The diagnosis of papillary muscle rupture may be suspected on physical examination and has been facilitated with the advent of hemodynamic monitoring and echocardiography.

The physical examination in acute mitral insufficiency secondary to papillary muscle rupture differs from the findings associated with chronic valvular regurgitation. In the acute setting a palpable thrill is uncommon and the radiation of the murmur differs from chronic conditions. The systolic murmur is soft, is decrescendo, generally ends before the second heart sound, and is best audible at the base of the heart as opposed to the apex with radiation to the neck or the top of the head.

Echocardiography and Doppler ultrasound has been a major advance in the diagnosis of acute mitral insufficiency and its clinical separation from other mechanical lesions associated with a new murmur (23). The left atrium and left ventricle are generally of normal size, and the ejection fraction is increased and frequently hyperdynamic. The mitral leaflet flails and may prolapse into the left atrium. Doppler ultrasound with color flow study determines the presence and severity of mitral insufficiency and presence of an intracardiac shunt and quantifies the degree of mitral regurgitation. Data from the Should We Emergently Revascularize Occluded Coronaries for Cardiogenic Shock (SHOCK) trial, which randomized patients with cardiogenic shock within 36 hours of an acute myocardial infarction, has shown that the severity of mitral regurgitation quantified by Doppler echocardiography is an independent predictor of survival (24).

Pulmonary artery catheter placement with measurement of PAOP and cardiac output is useful in mitral insufficiency. The presence of a regurgitant wave in the PAOP tracing may be visible in acute mitral regurgitant lesions, especially when there is no evidence of a step-up in oxygen concentration in the right atria or right ventricle. Pulmonary artery catheterization is not necessary for diagnosis, but the use of invasive monitoring allows optimization of cardiac output, filling pressures, and adjustment of inotropic, vasodilator, and diuretic therapy on the basis of induced changes in pressures.

Ventricular Septal Defect

Rupture of the interventricular septum may present in a similar clinical manner as mitral insufficiency with the abrupt onset of congestive heart failure plus a new murmur, making the two conditions difficult to separate on clinical grounds. Rupture of the interventricular septum also occurs in the first week after the acute ischemic event with a peak incidence occurring between days 3 and 5. The prevalence rate of acute VSDs after an infarction is difficult to accurately determine but occurs within the range of 0.5% to 2.0% and is the cause of death in approximately 5% of all fatal MIs. Incidence of VSD as a cause of cardiogenic shock after acute myocardial infarction in the SHOCK trial registry was 3.9% (22). Blood supply to the septum is supplied by septal perforating branches of the left anterior descending vessel and acute VSD is more common in anterior myocardial infarctions. These patients frequently have multivessel disease and are older patients experiencing an initial myocardial infarction (25).

The diagnosis of acute VSD may be inferred on clinical grounds but frequently requires more sophisticated evaluation to accurately diagnose and quantify the defect, which is located in the muscular septum and may be multiple. The physical examination in acute VSD depends on the magnitude of the shunt, which is, in turn, a function of the size of the ventricular defect, right ventricular compliance, pulmonary artery pressures, and inotropic state. A significant VSD is associated with the characteristic findings of shock in addition to a new holosystolic murmur associated with a precordial thrill. A precordial thrill may be palpated in approximately 50% of patients with an acute VSD and is a function of the magnitude of pressure gradient between the two chambers.

The diagnosis of VSD and its separation from acute mitral insufficiency has been facilitated by the advent of noninvasive and invasive diagnostic procedures. Two-dimensional echocardiography combined with Doppler flow study generally identifies a significant defect (26). Contrast echocardiography using microbubble techniques also may aid in the diagnosis of acute VSD and establish the presence of an intracardiac shunt. Pulmonary artery catheterization demonstrates the absence of a V wave in the pulmonary wedge tracing and an increase in oxygen saturation by ~10% in the right ventricle compared with the right atrium. The mortality rate for septal defects is significant, with approximately 25% of patients dying within the first 24 hours and a 50% mortality rate at 1 week. Less than 10% survive 1 year when treated solely with medical therapy (27). When occurring in the setting of cardiogenic shock, in-hospital mortality has been reported as high as 87% (22).

Free Wall Rupture and Tamponade

Free wall rupture is a major complication of myocardial infarction and is difficult to diagnose premortem. The prevalence of this complication is unknown but may occur in up to 8% of all myocardial infarctions with approximately one third occurring in the first 24 hours after the onset of the ischemic event and the peak incidence between days 5 and 7 (28). The SHOCK trial registry reported a 1.4% incidence of free wall rupture as a cause of cardiogenic shock after acute MI (22).

Rupture of the free wall is a major cause of mortality in acute ischemic events and is associated with large transmural infarcts with inadequate collateral circulation. This serious complication occurs more commonly in elderly hypertensive patients. Involvement of the left ventricle is the rule, although free wall rupture involving the right ventricle has been reported. Rupture of the free wall is frequently associated with the ventricular remodeling process in which a segmental infarction results in elevated left ventricular and diastolic pressure with expansion of the infarcted area. Expansion involves thinning of the affected area with regional hypertrophy in the adjacent region surrounding the infarct. A disproportionate dilatation occurs in the infarcted area and the risk of free wall rupture is enhanced with high shearing forces and elevated pressures. Free wall rupture generally occurs in the border zone between the infarcted area and the normal surrounding myocardium. The advent of thrombolytic therapy has been postulated to potentially increase the risk of free wall rupture, although this has not been definitely confirmed. Thrombolytic therapy may actually minimize the extent of myocardial necrosis and decrease free wall rupture. The use of agents such as corticosteroids, previously used to blunt inflammatory response and infarct size, has been associated with increased risk of free wall rupture.

Cardiac rupture is a catastrophic event resulting in sudden cardiac death unless a pseudoaneurysm forms. Hemopericardium with cardiac tamponade is difficult to diagnose early enough to institute definitive therapy. Cardiac tamponade after acute myocardial infarction also may be secondary to hemorrhagic pericarditis, but massive hemopericardium is usually due to cardiac rupture with rapid development of electromechanical dissociation and death. The diagnosis of free wall rupture is difficult but should be suspected with sudden hypotension, elevated jugular venous pressures, muffled heart sounds, and a pulsus paradoxus. Echocardiography can document the presence of pericardial fluid and occasionally demonstrates the perforated free wall (29,30). The classic signs of tamponade are present on echocardiography and are caused by the rising intrapericardial pressure compressing the right atrium and right ventricle, resulting in equalization of pressures and right ventricular diastolic collapse. Definitive therapy involves pericardiocentesis plus volume and pressure support with early surgical intervention being necessary for salvage. Untreated free wall rupture is universally fatal, although isolated instances of successful aggressive intervention with surgical therapy have been reported (31).

Left Ventricular Aneurysm

Left ventricular aneurysm is a relatively common complication of MI and may occur in up to 15% of survivors (32). A true aneurysm has a wide base with the ventricular walls composed entirely of myocardium, compared with a pseudoaneurysm, which generally has a narrow base with the walls consisting of pericardium and thrombotic debris. True aneurysms have a relatively low risk of free wall rupture but are associated with increased mortality due to sudden death from ventricular arrhythmias, emboli from mural thrombus, and progressive loss of left ventricular function (33). Aneurysms may develop early in the postinfarction period and can be asymptomatic or present with significant deterioration of left ventricular function. The presence of left ventricular aneurysm may be inferred by persistent ST elevation in the absence of chest pain or enzyme leakage (34).

Echocardiography demonstrating dyskinesis is a valuable tool in diagnosing aneurysms, as is left ventricular angiography. Left ventricular angiography demonstrates paradoxic systolic distention during ventricular contraction. Successful treatment of the aneurysm may be achieved with resection of the involved myocardium, frequently in combination with saphenous vein or mammary artery bypass grafting because of the high associated prevalence of multivessel coronary artery disease. Surgical resection has been advocated in the presence of arrhythmias to eliminate the substrate for ventricular tachycardia, but electrophysiologic mapping techniques are necessary to demonstrate that the origin of the arrhythmia arises from the left ventricular aneurysm.

CLINICAL MANIFESTATIONS

The clinical manifestations of cardiogenic shock are a function of the underlying cause, and mechanical defects must be aggressively sought because of the need for definitive therapy. Clinical recognition of the shock syndrome frequently requires prompt and aggressive stabilization procedures to be instituted before the definitive diagnosis of the underlying etiology (Fig. 56.2). A history and physical examination should be obtained with special attention to mental status, jugular venous pulsations, quality and intensity of heart sounds, presence and localization of a murmur, and presence of oliguria. Diagnostic tests such as electrocardiogram, portable chest radiograph, arterial blood gases, and echocardiography frequently provide adequate clinical information to make a diagnosis and initiate stabilization therapy. A quarter of patients presenting with cardiogenic shock secondary to predominant left ventricular dysfunction do not have evidence of pulmonary congestion (35).

THERAPY

Percutaneous Revascularization

Prior to 1999, interventions for the management of cardiogenic shock complicating acute MI were not systematically studied. The landmark SHOCK trial demonstrated that a strategy of early revascularization by angioplasty or surgery reduced mortality from 63% to 50% at 6 months (36). This finding has resulted in a major paradigm shift in the management of cardiogenic shock. The first branch-point in the decision algorithm is whether or not shock is present in the setting of an acute MI. If shock is present, patients should undergo immediate coronary angiography with percutaneous intervention if feasible.

The SHOCK trial studied patients with onset of shock within 36 hours of an MI and randomized the patients to immediate revascularization versus initial medical stabilization. Almost all patients required inotropes or vasopressors. Treatment in the revascularization group (64% of patients) was angioplasty or stenting (stents were not available at the beginning of the trial in 1993, but were actively used by the end of the trial in 1998) and coronary artery bypass graft surgery in 36%. In a subgroup analysis, survival was similar between percutaneous and surgically revascularized patients (55.6% vs. 57.4% at 30 days and 51.9% vs. 46.8% at 1 year, respectively) despite a higher incidence of diabetes and multivessel disease in those patients surgically revascularized (37).

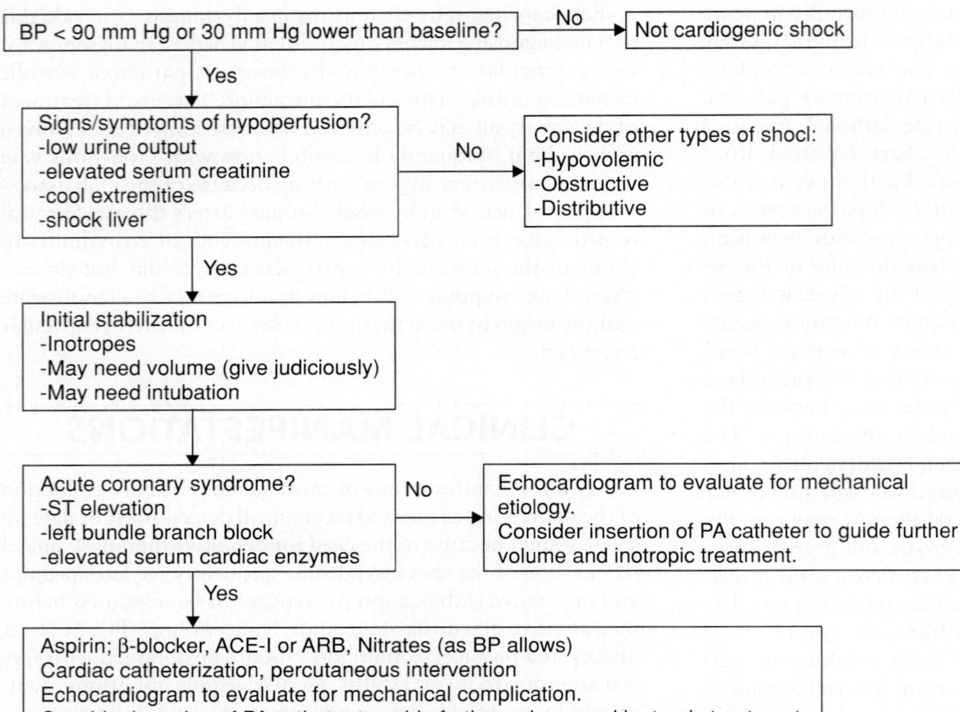

FIGURE 56.2. Management algorithm for cardiogenic shock. ACE-I, angiotensin-converting enzyme inhibitor; ARB, angiotensin II receptor blocker; PA, pulmonary artery.

Thrombolytic therapy was used in 49% of patients in the revascularization group and in 63% of the medical therapy group. There was no difference in survival at 30 days (53.3% in the revascularization group vs. 44.0% in the medical therapy group), likely a result of improved medical therapy. Age older than 75 years was associated with significantly higher 30-day mortality. Follow-up reports have shown persistent benefit to early revascularization with survival rates of 47% versus 34% at 1 year and 33% versus 20% at 6 years (38, 39). Of the patients surviving to hospital discharge (143/302), 6-year survival was 62% versus 44% (39).

An exciting aspect of the SHOCK trial was the registry that was created from patients screened for enrollment but not randomized, whose data was reported separately in a dedicated supplement to the *Journal of the American College of Cardiology* in September 2000. This registry described 1,190 patients and is the largest prospectively collected database for cardiogenic shock (22). Etiology of shock from the registry was left ventricular failure (78.5%), acute severe mitral regurgitation (6.9%), ventricular septal rupture (3.9%), isolated right ventricular shock (2.8%), and tamponade from free wall rupture (1.4%). Electrocardiographic site of infarction was anterior (55%), inferior (46%), posterior (19%), lateral (32%), and apical (11%), with multiple sites present in half of the cases. There was ST elevation, Q waves, or new left bundle branch block in 79% of cases. Systolic blood pressure averaged 88 mm Hg with a mean heart rate of 96 beats per minute. Of the subset of patients with invasive hemodynamics measured, PAOP was 23 mm Hg, cardiac index was 2.08 L/minute/m^2, and left ventricular ejection fraction was 33%. In-hospital mortality averaged 60% and ranged from 55% for acute severe mitral regurgitation, isolated right ventricular shock, and tamponade to 87% for ventricular septal rupture. Of the 717 patients who underwent coronary angiography, 15.5% had significant left main stenosis and 53.4% had three-vessel disease. Coronary artery disease severity also correlated with in-hospital mortality: No or single-vessel disease was associated with a 35% mortality rate as compared with three-vessel disease with a mortality rate of 50.8% (40).

Since the SHOCK trial, stenting has replaced angioplasty alone as the primary treatment for ischemic coronary artery disease due to its reduced incidence of restenosis. One recent case series has shown that stenting for cardiogenic shock decreased mortality compared to angioplasty alone (from 68% to 43%) (41). Primary coronary artery stenting is now recommended for patients with ST elevation or left bundle branch block who develop shock within 36 hours of acute myocardial infarction and are suitable for revascularization that can be performed within 18 hours of shock onset (1). Thrombolytic therapy may be used if early revascularization is not available (2).

While drug-eluting stents, which slowly elute a pharmacologic agent (currently either sirolimus or paclitaxel), are now widely used instead of bare metal stents due to their proven efficacy in reducing the incidence of restenosis, to date they have not been studied in the setting of cardiogenic shock (42,43).

Pharmacologic Limitation of Infarct Size

Several pharmacologic interventions have been used during acute myocardial infarction to minimize the extent of irreversible ischemic damage and decrease the likelihood of subsequent development of cardiogenic shock. Quantitative measurements of the extent of myocardial damage by electrocardiographic mapping and creatine kinase (CK) release are imprecise and frequently limit quantitative assessment of the potential therapeutic impact of pharmacologic interventions. Calcium channel blockers, β-blockers, and nitrates have been the main agents that have undergone clinical analysis to minimize myocardial damage, whereas a variety of experimental or uncommonly used therapies have been evaluated in small-scale clinical trials. Nitrates are complex pharmacologic agents with arterial and venodilating activity in addition to other potential beneficial effects, such as alteration of prostacyclin metabolism. Nitrates, when administered as topical, oral, or sublingual agents, are predominately venodilators with subsequent venous pooling, decreased venous return, and lowering of PAOP. Reduction in venous return and optimization of PAOP decrease left ventricular volume and improve subendocardial perfusion, thus reducing wall stress with the potential for minimizing infarct extent. Nitrates also have effects on systemic vascular resistance and epicardial coronary arteries, with resultant reduction of impedance to left ventricular ejection and increase in coronary blood flow.

Intravenously administered nitroglycerin has a more balanced arterial and venodilating effect. Clinical trials demonstrate that intravenous nitroglycerin administered at a level to decrease mean aortic pressure by 10% (44) results in a decrease in extension of MI and improves left ventricular ejection fraction and survival (45). Intravenous nitrates minimize the magnitude of infarct size as monitored by CK, and alter infarct expansion with reduction in the subsequent remodeling process and progression to congestive heart failure. Intravenous nitrates are potent vasodilators and require careful blood pressure monitoring to prevent significant hypotension and paradoxical bradycardia. Nitrates may result in a beneficial redistribution of coronary flow to the subendocardium without the coronary steal syndrome, a major detriment of other potent intravenous vasodilators such as nitroprusside.

Calcium channel blockers are important agents in managing patients with classic and vasospastic angina. The calcium channel blocking agents decrease systemic vascular resistance, decrease oxygen demand, and increase coronary flow, improving the balance between supply and demand. At pharmacologic doses, these agents also may have other potentially beneficial effects including antiplatelet activity.

Despite the documented beneficial effect of these agents in hypertension and angina, calcium channel blockers have not been proven to be beneficial in the treatment of MI and do not definitely limit infarct size. Studies using nifedipine have been unable to demonstrate benefit in patients with acute MI. Diltiazem has been advantageous in non–Q-wave infarction in the Diltiazem Reinfarction study (46). However, the Multicenter Diltiazem Postinfarction trial was not able to document a benefit to the administration of diltiazem in the postinfarction state when compared with placebo (47). Subgroup analysis demonstrated a mortality benefit with diltiazem therapy when no pulmonary congestion was present. However, mortality was increased when diltiazem was administered to subjects whose infarction was complicated by pulmonary congestion, implying that this agent should not be used in patients with cardiogenic shock. Studies performed in Denmark using intravenous verapamil followed by oral administration did not demonstrate a benefit. Later studies using only oral verapamil demonstrated a mortality reduction, although these trials have not been reconfirmed (48). Currently, the evidence for using calcium channel blockers for the treatment of acute MI to limit infarct size and progression to cardiogenic shock is limited.

β-Adrenergic blocking agents have been used in treating hypertension, atrial fibrillation, and a variety of ischemic conditions. β-Blockers act predominantly by decreasing myocardial oxygen demand caused by the negative chronotropic and inotropic activities of these agents. β-Blockers may have several other potentially beneficial effects including antiplatelet activity, regression of left ventricular hypertrophy, and reduction in sudden cardiac death. Clinical trials using β-blockade in acute MI have yielded conflicting results. The Goteborg trial administered metoprolol or placebo to subjects having an acute myocardial infarction and demonstrated a significant reduction in mortality at 90 days in the group randomly assigned to β-blocker therapy (49). Early administration of metoprolol was associated with a reduction in estimated infarct size, which presumably has an effect on early and long-term survival. Despite the fact that β-blockers are not commonly used as antiarrhythmic agents, there was a documented decrease in sudden cardiac death in the β-blocker group, which has been shown to be secondary to an increase in the ventricular fibrillatory threshold.

The Metoprolol in Acute Myocardial Infarction trial was able to demonstrate that the early administration of intravenous metoprolol followed by oral maintenance dose in acute MI was associated with a decrease in mortality in a high-risk subgroup of infarct patients (50). A subgroup study of the Goteborg Metoprolol trial found that early treatment with metoprolol in patients with suspected acute MI and signs of heart failure resulted in significantly reduced mortality at 3 months (10% vs. 19%), which persisted to 1 year (14% vs. 27%), compared to those who did not receive metoprolol (51). Propranolol, a noncardioselective β-blocker, has not uniformly been demonstrated to decrease mortality or limit infarct size when administered early in acute MI patients. However, the Beta-Blocker Heart Attack trial demonstrated reduced mortality when propranolol was administered after the acute phase of the infarction had subsided (52). Intravenous atenolol was studied in the First International Study of Infarct Survival Trial and demonstrated a 15% reduction in the early mortality of infarct patients who were given oral atenolol after the intravenous loading doses (53). β-Blockers also have been combined with thrombolytic therapy to limit infarct size. The Thrombolysis in Myocardial Infarction trial (TIMI II-B) studied the impact of three 5-mg boluses of metoprolol administered at 5-minute intervals followed by oral metoprolol compared with thrombolysis plus oral metoprolol. The TIMI II-B trial demonstrated a decrease in nonfatal reinfarctions and recurrent ischemic episodes in the group who received immediate intravenous metoprolol followed by oral therapy compared with the delayed subgroup. More recently, the CAPRICORN (Carvedilol Post Infarct Survival Control in Left Ventricular Dysfunction) trial studied carvedilol (6.25–25 twice per day in addition to standard therapy of aspirin, angiotensin converting enzyme [ACE] inhibition, and thrombolysis) versus placebo in a high-risk group of acute MI patients (n = 1,959) with an LV ejection fraction of ≤40%. Patients were treated for a mean of 1.3 years. All-cause mortality was lower in the carvedilol group than in the placebo group (54). Patients who had echocardiography demonstrated a significantly higher LV ejection fraction and decreased LV end-systolic volume in the carvedilol group at 6 months (55). Another post hoc analysis of the CAPRICORN study found that carvedilol suppressed atrial arrhythmias (2.3% vs. 5.4%) as well as ventricular arrhythmias (0.9% vs. 3.9%) compared to the control group (56). The beneficial effect on ventricular remodeling, in addition to the antiarrhythmic effect, may be one of the mechanisms by which carvedilol decreased mortality after acute MI in patients treated with ACE inhibitors. Use of β-blockers in acute myocardial infarction, while now standard of care, must be undertaken with caution because of the potential of precipitating atrioventricular block, reactive airways disease, and hypotension (57).

ACE inhibitors have been administered orally and intravenously in clinical trials to halt progression to congestive heart failure in the SAVE (Survival and Ventricular Enlargement) and Consensus-II (Cooperative New Scandinavian Enalapril Survival Study) trials. The SAVE study used captopril in over 2,000 patients who had an acute anterior MI when enrolled during the period from 3 to 16 days after the acute myocardial event (58). All patients with ejection fractions <40% were randomized to receive oral captopril or a placebo. Patients receiving captopril demonstrated less congestive heart failure, fewer recurrent MIs, fewer hospitalizations, and improved mortality over a 42-month period. The Consensus-II trial used intravenous enalapril in the early phase of infarction followed by oral enalapril, but there was no mortality benefit when compared with placebo (59). A review of the major post-MI heart failure trials such as SAVE, AIRE (Acute Infarction Ramipril Efficacy), and TRACE (Trandolapril Cardiac Evaluation), between 1992 and 1995, calculated that ACE inhibitors produced a relative risk reduction of 16% while β-blockade in addition to ACE inhibition in the CAPRICORN trial demonstrated an additional relative risk reduction of 23% (60). Oral ACE inhibitors are attractive agents because of their effects on hemodynamics, microcirculation, and angiotensin-mediated vasoconstriction and should be administered especially in anterior infarcts with significant reductions in ejection fraction unless there are contraindications (hyperkalemia, known drug sensitivity).

Selective aldosterone blockade with eplerenone for patients with LV ejection fraction of $\leq$40% after acute MI has been studied in one large, placebo-controlled trial, EPHESUS (Eplerenone Post-Acute Myocardial Infarction Heart Failure Efficacy and Survival Study). Eplerenone (in addition to treatment with β-blockers and ACE inhibitors) reduced all-cause mortality by 15%, cardiovascular mortality by 17%, heart failure hospitalizations by 23%, and sudden cardiac death by 21% (61). These outcomes were even more marked in the subgroup of patients with LV ejection fraction of $\leq$30%. In this group, all-cause mortality was reduced by 21%, cardiovascular mortality by 23%, sudden cardiac death by 33%, and heart failure mortality or hospitalization by 25% (62).

Angiotensin receptor blockade for LV ejection fraction of $\leq$40% after acute MI has been studied in the VALIANT (Valsartan in Acute Myocardial Infarction Trial) study (63). This was a multicenter, double-blind, randomized, active-controlled, parallel-group study comparing the efficacy and safety of long-term treatment with valsartan, captopril, and their combination in high-risk patients after MI. This compared three treatment groups consisting of patients receiving standard therapy plus valsartan (n = 4,909), valsartan plus captopril (n = 4,885), or captopril alone (n = 4,909). Valsartan treatment alone resulted in similar outcomes as captopril treatment alone and thus these agents can be used interchangeably. The combination of valsartan plus captopril increased the rate of adverse events (hypotension and renal dysfunction more commonly with valsartan; cough, rash, and taste disturbance more commonly with captopril) with no change in survival.

Adjunctive antiplatelet therapy with the glycoprotein IIb/IIIa inhibitor abciximab during emergent coronary artery stenting for cardiogenic shock has been shown to reduce mortality from 43% to 33% in one case series (41). The glycoprotein IIb/IIIa inhibitor eptifibatide used for non–ST-elevation myocardial infarction or unstable angina in the PURSUIT (Platelet Glycoprotein IIb/IIIa in Unstable Angina: Receptor Suppression in Using Integrelin Therapy) study has been shown to reduce 30-day mortality in the subset of patients developing cardiogenic shock (64). Clopidogrel in addition to aspirin is now standard of care after percutaneous coronary intervention and has been shown to decrease 1-year mortality in the setting of ST-elevation myocardial infarction (65). However, clopidogrel significantly increases the risk of postoperative bleeding in patients requiring surgical intervention.

Several agents have been used in small studies as adjunctive therapy in acute MI but have not reached widespread clinical use. Myocardial damage may be potentiated by the presence of reactive oxygen radicals, and free radical scavengers such as superoxide dismutase or catalase may provide potential benefit. Free radical scavengers have been shown to be effective when administered before the onset of experimental infarcts and definitive clinical studies are currently ongoing.

Glucose insulin potassium infusions (polarizing solution) have been used for several years to reduce infarct size by altering free fatty acid metabolism (66). Polarizing solution consists of 300 g of glucose, 50 units of regular insulin, and 80 mmol of potassium in 1 L of water delivered at 1.5 mL/kg/hour. Ejection fraction and wall motion abnormalities have been noted to improve after administering this solution, resulting in decreased mortality. Polarizing solution has not been studied extensively in double-blind, placebo-controlled trials and routine administration of this solution has not reached clinical acceptance.

Hyaluronidase may have anti-inflammatory activity and modulate the immune response postulated to play some role in the extent of infarct size. Hyaluronidase has been administered in small clinical studies and was associated with improved mortality and decreased development of Q waves implying myocardial salvage. There are no large-scale clinical trials available (67).

Thrombolysis

Thrombolysis induced by pharmacologic agents or direct angioplasty is an attractive treatment for re-establishing coronary perfusion to minimize the extent of myocardial infarction and progression to cardiogenic shock. The open artery hypothesis postulates that clinical outcome is dependent on maintaining adequate coronary perfusion to minimize ischemic damage mediated by vascular occlusion secondary to an intravascular thrombus. Recent trials of coronary thrombolysis, GISSI (Gruppo Italiano per lo Studio della Sopravvivenza nell'Infarto Miocardio), ISIS (International Study of Infarct Size), and GUSTO (Global Utilization of Strategies to Open Occluded Coronary Arteries), demonstrate the prevalence of cardiogenic shock in approximately 2% to 3% of acute MIs on arrival to the hospital with an additional 3% to 4% subsequently developing cardiogenic shock for a combined total of 7% (68,69). Early progression to cardiogenic shock is characterized demographically by elderly patients and the presence of anterior infarctions, low ejection fractions, diabetes, and previous MIs. Despite the theoretical attractiveness of administering recombinant tissue plasminogen activators or streptokinase in patients with established or impending cardiogenic shock, the mortality associated with cardiogenic shock remains high despite thrombolytic therapy, with the survival rate being only 35% as reported in the GISSI-I and GISSI-II trials (70). Prompt administration of thrombolytic agents within the first hour of acute MI may result in improved survival rates if reperfusion of the infarct-related artery can be sustained. Low coronary perfusion pressures in cardiogenic shock may play a potential role in the poor clinical outcome of these patients after thrombolytic therapy.

In vitro experimental infarct studies with reduced perfusion pressure have shown decreased diffusion of thrombolytic agents into clots with resultant impaired fibrinolysis (71). Enhanced pressure increases the rate of dissolution of an intravascular thrombus, implying that in cardiogenic shock with systemic hypotension, a reduced transcoronary pressure gradient may decrease efficacy of thrombolytic agents. The metabolic abnormalities associated with cardiogenic shock including lactic acidosis also may alter the conversion of plasminogen to plasmin and limit the efficacy of these drugs in clot lysis. Failure from lytic agents to sustain vascular patency in patients with cardiogenic shock is an indication for early cardiac catheterization and direct angioplasty if no contraindications exist. Persistent hypotension, nonevolving ST elevation, continuing clinical evidence of myocardial ischemia, CK elevations, and clinical instability are potential indications for rescue coronary angioplasty, which may result in increased survival (72). Rescue angioplasty has not been systematically studied in randomized controlled trials comparing it to thrombolytic therapy. If thrombolytic therapy does not result in establishment of coronary perfusion, angioplasty should be considered as a therapeutic option. The SHOCK trial reported that 49% of patients in the revascularization group received thrombolytic therapy and the early intervention group had a survival benefit (see section above) (36). Additionally, the SHOCK trial reported a survival benefit due to thrombolytic therapy (in-hospital mortality of 54% vs. 64%) (73). Cardiogenic shock secondary to mechanical defects such as papillary muscle dysfunction also has been treated successfully with percutaneous transluminal coronary angioplasty (PTCA), resulting in improved mitral regurgitation with resolution of cardiogenic shock (74).

Thrombolytic agents should be administered to all patients with acute MI who demonstrate evidence of the shock state if there are no contraindications and availability of a cardiac catheterization laboratory is >90 minutes. Failure of evidence of reperfusion is an indicator for rescue angioplasty.

Pharmacologic Agents

Inotropic Agents

The effectiveness of various inotropic agents in cardiogenic shock depends on the cause and underlying pathophysiologic mechanism of the shock state. With systemic hypotension, adequate perfusion of the coronary arteries must be maintained (Fig. 56.3).

Dopamine. Dopamine is an endogenous catecholamine with positive inotropic properties secondary to stimulation of α- and β-receptors plus dopamine receptors, which have been divided into two subtypes: DA_1 and DA_2 (75,76). DA_1 receptors are postsynaptic and induce dilation of the coronary, renal, and mesenteric vasculature. DA_2 receptors are located in autonomic ganglia and in the postganglionic sympathetic nervous system. Stimulation of DA_2 receptors blocks the release of endogenous catecholamines from intraneuronal storage sites. The effect of dopamine on α and β activity is dose related. Low infusion dosages of dopamine (2–5 μg/kg/minute) result in positive inotropic activity secondary to stimulation of the β_1 receptors. α-Receptor stimulation occurs at dosages above 10 μg/kg/minute and results in a secondary increase in systemic vascular resistance caused by peripheral vasoconstriction. In addition to the inotropic effect, dopamine results in increased atrioventricular conduction from adrenergic stimulation. The effects of dopamine are thus dose dependent, and pharmacologic activity is a function of the amount of dopamine infused corrected for body weight. The individual response may be variable and unless the clinical situation warrants large pressor doses to maintain blood pressure, dopamine infusion should begin at a low rate (1 μg/kg/minute) and gradually be increased to clinical responsiveness. Cardiogenic shock with low tissue perfusion accompanied by hypotension may be treated in a more aggressive manner with progressively increasing doses of dopamine at 5-minute intervals.

Low-dose dopamine infusion results in stimulation of DA_2 receptors and minimal or no changes in heart rate, cardiac output, or blood pressure. Stimulation of DA_2 receptors results in renal vasodilation and increases glomerular filtration rate, renal blood flow, and sodium excretion. Reduction in cardiac output in shock frequently results in shunting of blood away from the renal vasculature and induction of a prerenal state with elevated blood urea nitrogen–to–creatinine ratios and sodium retention. Dopamine reverses the redistribution of cardiac output and increases the amount of sodium presented to the loop of Henle, which allows increased efficacy of diuretics such as furosemide or bumetanide.

Medium dosing ranges of dopamine (5–10 μg/kg/minute) result in an increase in cardiac output, which may also improve volume status by increasing renal blood flow. The cardiac effects of dopamine in this dosing range are secondary to stimulation of the β_1-adrenergic receptors caused by a secondary release of norepinephrine. The effect of dopamine is indirect and depends on a pre-existent adequate storage level of endogenous catecholamines. Long-standing congestive heart failure is frequently associated with reduction in sympathetic receptors in the myocardium and the efficacy of dopamine may be limited if prolonged congestive heart failure was present before the shock syndrome. Dopamine infusion at this dose generally does not result in alterations of venous return secondary to venodilation, and right atrial and PAOP may not decrease. Dopamine may be combined with either direct vasodilating compounds or other inotropic agents such as dobutamine, which combine inotropism with vasodilation. Medium dosing range infusions of dopamine are generally safe and effective in maintaining blood pressure. Acid-base status and electrolyte levels should be optimized to avoid potential induction of arrhythmias with resultant malignant ventricular arrhythmias or marked sinus or supraventricular tachycardias, which would increase myocardial oxygen demand.

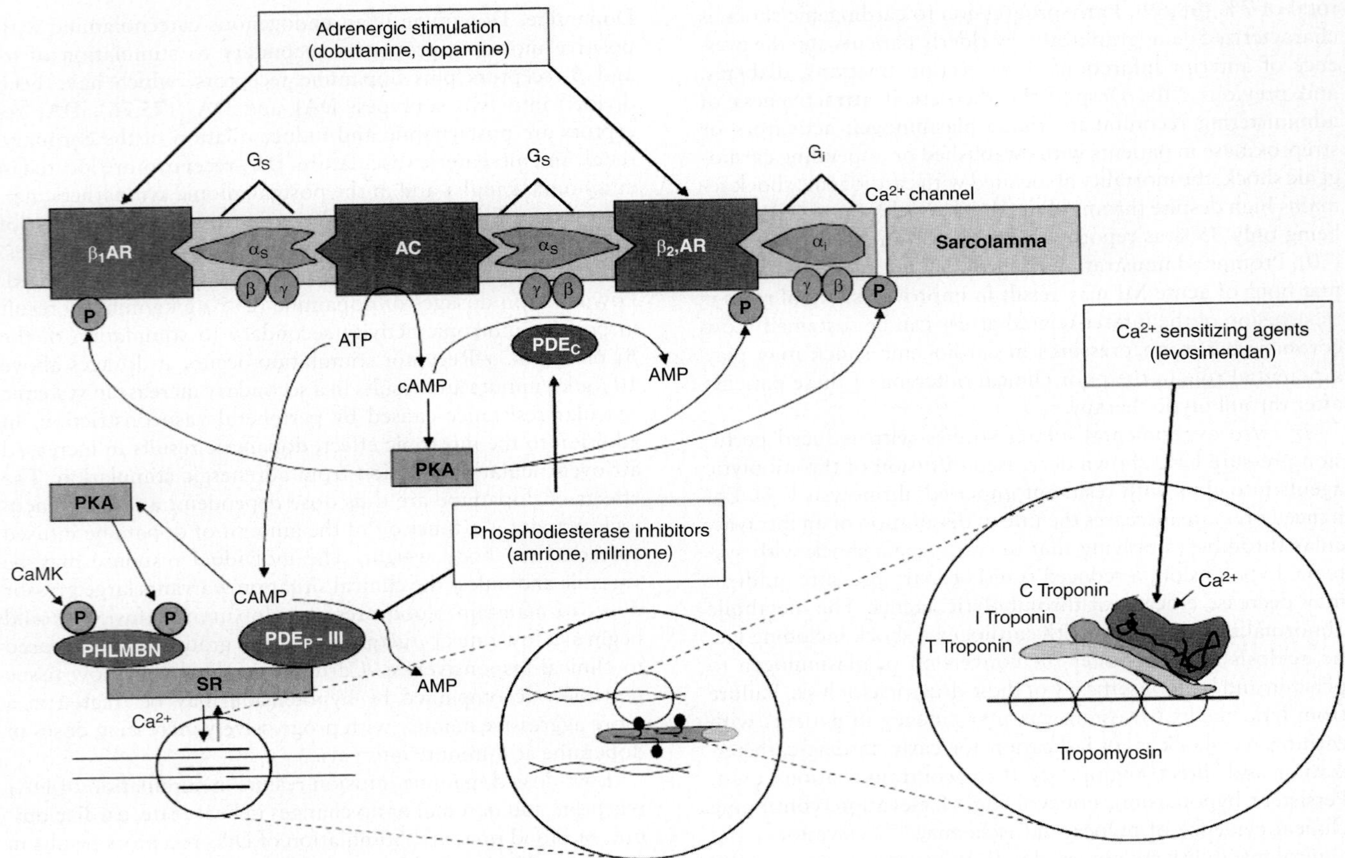

FIGURE 56.3. Mechanisms of action of inotropic drugs. (Used with permission from Garcia Gonzalez MJ, Dominguez Rodriguez A. Pharmacologic treatment of heart failure due to ventricular dysfunction by myocardial stunning: potential role of levosimendan. *Am J Cardiovasc Drugs*. 2006;6[2]:69–75.) β_1AR, β_1-adrenergic receptor; β_2AR, β_2-adrenergic receptor; AC, adenyl cyclase; AMP, adenosine monophosphate; ATP, adenosine triphosphate; Ca^{2+}, calcium; CaMK, calmodulin-activated kinase; cAMP, cyclic AMP; Gi, inhibitory G protein with α, β, and γ subunits; Gs, stimulatory G protein with α, β, and γ subunits; P, phosphorus; PDEc, cytosolic phosphodiesterases; PDEp-III, particulate, SR-associated PDE III; PHLMBN, phospholamban; PKA, cAMP-dependent protein kinase A; SR, sarcoplasmic reticulum.

High-range dopamine infusions (>10 μg/kg/minute) result in activation of α-adrenergic receptors and a secondary norepinephrine release with vasoconstriction and increased systemic vascular resistance. Patients in cardiogenic shock may need much higher doses of dopamine and ranges up to 50 μg/kg/minute have been used. Strict attention to volume status and repeated examinations for signs of excessive vasoconstriction are necessary. A central venous line is used for higher dopamine doses due to tissue necrosis should the solution extravasate. Dopamine may interact with certain coadministered drugs. Tricyclic antidepressants may increase the pressor response of direct-acting sympathomimetics and decrease the sensitivity to indirect-acting sympathomimetics. Because dopamine has direct and indirect effects on the vasculature, this agent should be used with caution, especially with overdoses of the tricyclic drugs (77). Although not commonly used, the rauwolfia alkaloids may potentiate the pressor response of direct-acting sympathomimetics resulting in hypertension. Monoamine oxidase inhibitors may increase pressor response of dopamine (78). Dopamine is an endogenous catecholamine that is degraded by catechol-o-methyltransferase and is not effective when administered in oral doses.

Dobutamine. As opposed to dopamine, which is an endogenous catechol and immediate precursor of norepinephrine and epinephrine, dobutamine is a synthetic agent that stimulates predominantly β_1-adrenoreceptors (79) (Table 56.4). Dobutamine is a direct-acting agent, unlike dopamine, and does not require the presence or release of intramyocardial norepinephrine to modulate its effects. Mild activation of β_2 and α receptors may be seen with this agent, but significantly less when compared with β_1 receptors. Administration of dobutamine results in a direct inotropic stimulation plus a secondary reflex vasodilation with reduction of systemic vascular resistance and an increase in cardiac output.

The pharmacologic mechanism of dobutamine is complicated because of its asymmetric structure and racemic mixture. The positive and negative isomers have been evaluated as to their relative activities in *in vitro* studies, and it seems that the positive isomer is predominantly responsible for the activation of the β receptors. The administration of dobutamine alters stimulation of β receptors in a differential manner with an increased binding affinity for the predominantly cardiac β_1-adrenergic receptors with a direct inotropic effect. The inotropic effects of this agent are not coupled with an increased

TABLE 56.4

DOBUTAMINE

Adrenergic receptor	Site	Action
β_1	Myocardium Sinoatrial node Atrioventricular conduction system	Increases atrial and ventricular contractility Increases heart rate Enhances atrioventricular conductions
β_2	Arterioles Lungs	Vasodilation Bronchodilation
α	Peripheral arterioles	Vasoconstriction
DA_1	Postsynaptic	Dilation of coronary, renal, and mesenteric vasculature
DA_2	Autonomic ganglia and postganglionic sympathetic nervous system	Decreased release of endogenous catechols

rate of arrhythmias when compared with epinephrine and norepinephrine and there seems to be fewer adverse electrophysiologic effects when compared with dopamine. Although a mild vasodilator, there are no major effects on arterial blood pressure due to an increase in cardiac output and stroke volume. The increase in cardiac output results in improved renal blood flow and enhanced ability to excrete sodium and water. Dobutamine is effective in cardiogenic shock, assuming that the underlying etiology is not caused by valvular or subvalvular stenosis and the pharmacologic infusion does not result in significant hypotension, and this agent may be combined with dopamine to maintain blood pressure.

Norepinephrine. Norepinephrine is a powerful α-adrenergic agonist that results in significant peripheral vasoconstriction when administered within the usual dosage range of 2 to 8 μg/minute. Norepinephrine is generally instituted in the treatment of cardiogenic shock after failure of volume correction and dopamine to maintain adequate cardiac output and blood pressure (80). Norepinephrine is a naturally occurring catecholamine that has both α- and β_1-adrenergic activity. Although generally associated with an increase in cardiac output, increases in systemic vascular resistance and mean aortic blood pressure may affect cardiac output adversely. The pressure work of the left ventricle and oxygen consumption are increased and blood may be shunted away from various organ beds because of volume redistribution secondary to catecholamine sensitivity. Oliguria and azotemia from impaired renal blood flow may be worsened secondary to the norepinephrine-mediated vasoconstriction. Norepinephrine has been associated with increased irritability of the ventricle with an increased electrical instability and potential adverse rhythm disorders. Clinical response will vary depending on the advantageous effects of increased perfusion pressure and cardiac output weighed against the detrimental effects of increased myocardial oxygen consumption and shunting from visceral organs.

Digitalis Preparations. The use of digitalis in general and cardiogenic shock specifically has been controversial because of theoretical objections involving the use of this agent and the lack of controlled clinical trials documenting a beneficial impact on mortality (81). Digitalis glycosides have complex mechanisms of action whose inotropic activity is modulated by increasing the availability of intracellular calcium secondary to inhibition of sodium–potassium ATPase. Inhibition of this ubiquitous enzyme, which is found not only in cardiac tissue but also in the central nervous system, gastrointestinal tract, and kidney, results in calcium influx by the activation of the sodium–calcium exchange mechanism. The level of free cytosolic calcium regulates the activity of tropomyosin with increased interactions between actin and myosin filaments and increased contractility. Alterations in contraction are caused by variations in levels of cytosolic calcium, which can be moved in and out of the sarcoplasmic reticulum.

The increase in cardiac output after administration of digitalis is modest when compared with the more powerful intravenous inotropes such as dobutamine, dopamine, and norepinephrine. Digitalis increases the refractory period at the atrioventricular node and decreases conduction velocity, resulting in a negative chronotropic effect in patients with atrial fibrillation. An advantage is that digitalis lacks the negative inotropic activity of other agents that have been used to slow the rate in atrial fibrillation, including β-blockers and calcium channel blockers such as diltiazem and verapamil (82). Digitalis increases vagal tone, decreases levels of norepinephrine in chronic heart failure possibly from decreased activity of the peripheral sympathetic nervous system, resets baroreceptor sensitivity, and may enhance natriuresis from increased cardiac output.

Digitalis withdrawal has been associated with worsening heart failure in a randomized, double-blind, placebo-controlled study of digitalis withdrawal in patients also treated with ACE inhibitors. However, the role of digitalis in cardiogenic shock is limited due to a modest increase in cardiac output, although the autonomic effects of this agent with decreases in the heart rate in atrial fibrillation are clinically beneficial.

Isoproterenol. Isoproterenol has both β_1- and β_2-adrenergic properties with increased myocardial contractility, heart rate, and cardiac output without vasoconstriction. The powerful chronotropic and inotropic activities of this agent increase myocardial work and oxygen. Isoproterenol is infrequently used in heart failure or cardiogenic shock unless the shock state is associated with bradyarrhythmias that do not respond to other therapies or with acute valvular insufficiency if blood pressure and volume status are maintained. Isoproterenol thus has a limited role in the acute management of cardiogenic shock.

Phosphodiesterase Inhibitors. Amrinone and milrinone are bipyridine derivatives that inhibit cellular levels of phosphodiesterase (83). Inhibition of this key enzyme results in increased levels of cyclic adenosine monophosphate (AMP) in cardiac muscle with resultant enhancement of protein phosphorylation by protein kinase with increased inotropic and chronotropic activities. The methylxanthines were known to nonspecifically inhibit phosphodiesterase activity and result in mild enhancement of the inotropic state. Both amrinone and milrinone have been shown in experimental and clinical studies to increase cardiac output in patients with severe congestive heart failure or cardiogenic shock (84).

Administering these agents results in reduction of central filling pressures and increases in stroke volume and cardiac output. The chronotropic effects of amrinone and milrinone are modest, but a mild increase in heart rate may be observed. Large doses may result in severe peripheral vasodilation, hypotension, and tachycardia. The phosphodiesterase inhibitors have been studied in patients with pump failure after myocardial infarctions, and at a dose of 200 μg/kg/hour, have been shown to improve cardiac function. Comparison in clinical trials of amrinone to other vasodilating inotropes such as dobutamine documented a greater decrease in systemic and pulmonary venous pressures in the group that received amrinone (85). The vasodilating activity of the phosphodiesterase inhibitors, while increasing cardiac output, may result in significant hypotension, requiring concomitant administration of sympathomimetic amines with at least partial α activity such as norepinephrine. The side effect profile of the phosphodiesterase inhibitors relates mainly to hematologic and gastrointestinal effects. Nausea, vomiting, and diarrhea occur in many patients. Thrombocytopenia is common with amrinone (approximately 15%), although the marked decreases in platelet counts to levels under 50,000 seems to be relatively rare and may require dose reduction. Milrinone is more potent on a milligram basis when compared with amrinone and also has effects on the inotropic state and ventricular relaxation. Incidence of thrombocytopenia seems less (<5%) than with amrinone. Enoximone is an imidazole derivative that also results in phosphodiesterase inhibition and increases levels of cyclic AMP and contractile force in isolated muscle preparations (86). Intravenous enoximone results in an increase in cardiac index with a decrease in right-sided filling pressures with minimal impacts on systemic vascular resistance and heart rate. Enoximone is currently undergoing a variety of controlled trials and seems to have a relatively mild side effect profile, and thrombocytopenia is uncommon with the use of this agent.

Glucagon. Glucagon is uncommonly used in cardiogenic shock but has a potential advantage in that it has a different mechanism of action from other sympathomimetic amines and does not require β-receptor stimulation to exert its inotropic effects (87,88). Glucagon is administered in a dosing range of 4 to 6 mg intravenously, which may be followed by a constant infusion of 4 to 12 mg/hour. Glucagon administration increases cardiac output by approximately 20%, which is associated with a decrease in peripheral vascular resistance with less myocardial oxygen demand when compared with norepinephrine. The indications for glucagon have not been delineated, although it seems justifiable to administer this agent to patients with cardiogenic shock who do not respond to conventional therapy or cannot tolerate other agents because of the development of significant arrhythmias or hematologic toxicity.

Levosimendan. Levosimendan is the first of a new class of inotropic agents called calcium sensitizers. Its mechanism of action involves increasing calcium sensitivity by binding to troponin C and stabilizing it in the calcium-induced conformation. This augments the effect of calcium binding to troponin C. Additionally, at high concentrations levosimendan inhibits phosphodiesterase 3, which also results in increased intracellular calcium concentration. These effects result in increased myocardial contraction associated with increased intracellular calcium transients (89). It improves myocardial contractility without increasing oxygen requirements and induces peripheral and coronary vasodilation with a potential antistunning, anti-ischemic effect (90). Given its vasodilatory properties, it is not primarily for cardiogenic shock but more for low-output heart failure. In addition to calcium sensitization, levosimendan also stimulates adenosine triphosphate (ATP)-sensitive potassium ion channels that are suppressed by intracellular ATP and acts synergistically with nucleotide diphosphates. This mechanism may contribute to the vasodilator action and may protect cardiomyocytes against ischemic damage (91). A loading dose of 6 to 24 mg/kg over 10 minutes followed by an infusion of 0.1 mg/kg/minute for 50 minutes, increased to 0.2 mg/kg/minute for an additional 23 hours, has been well tolerated (90). Initial clinical experience suggests that levosimendan causes dose-dependent increases in stroke volume and cardiac index, with minimum increase in heart rate (92). There are dose-dependent decreases in PAOP and right atrial, pulmonary arterial, and mean arterial pressures. The hemodynamic effects of levosimendan appear to be more pronounced than those seen with dobutamine (93) and sustained up to 24 hours after discontinuation of infusion due to an active metabolite (94). An initial clinical trial found no significant adverse events (92). Data from two published clinical trials indicate that levosimendan is associated with improved 6-month survival compared with dobutamine or placebo, although the studies were not powered to look at this outcome (93,95,96). There are several other trials not yet published but presented at national meetings that report a survival benefit of levosimendan compared with dobutamine or placebo. However, a 24-hour infusion of levosimendan had no effect on 6-month survival compared with dobutamine for patients with acutely decompensated heart failure in the Survival of Patients with Acute Heart Failure in need of Intravenous Inotropic Support (SURVIVE) trial reported at the American Heart Association Scientific Sessions in 2005 but not yet published (93). The European Society of Cardiology's 2005 guidelines on the diagnosis and treatment of acute heart failure include the use of levosimendan in patients with symptomatic low cardiac output secondary to systolic dysfunction without severe hypotension (97). This drug is not yet approved by the Food and Drug Administration (FDA), although it is available in some European countries.

Surgical Intervention

Surgical intervention in myocardial infarction has been used to limit infarct size by direct revascularization or to correct the mechanical defects of an acute ischemic event such as VSD, acute mitral insufficiency, free wall rupture, or left ventricular aneurysm. Surgical intervention for revascularization in acute myocardial infarction had been contraindicated on theoretic grounds because of the presumed high morbidity and mortality rates from cardiac catheterization and operative interventions during the unstable period of acute myocardial infarction. A variety of clinical studies determined that coronary bypass surgery could be performed in an expeditious manner with low mortality. Bypass surgery has been used as primary therapy in acute myocardial infarction with an overall operative rate of approximately 5% for transmural infarctions and a highly acceptable long-term mortality rate (98,99). Evidence is accumulating that early revascularization (<6 hours) by direct PTCA, intravenous or intracoronary thrombolytic agents, or bypass surgery in selected patients represents the treatment of choice. Congestive heart failure that occurs in the postmyocardial state may be amenable to revascularization by surgical interventions, although large-scale, controlled, randomized studies are lacking. However, several surgical series have reported on early and long-term survival of patients with an acute MI complicated by cardiogenic shock receiving coronary artery bypass surgery (98–102). Surgical intervention in cardiogenic shock is fraught with considerable clinical problems and requires the presence of surgically accessible and potentially viable myocardium. Surgical intervention has the advantage of re-establishing flow not only in the infarct-related artery, but also in vessels not involved in the acute ischemic process but significantly obstructed. Viability of the myocardium in the peri-infarction state may be difficult to determine secondary to problems with the acute delineation of stunned, hibernating, or irreversibly damaged myocardium. Nitroglycerin or dobutamine enhancement of ejection fraction is an indirect method of determining viability but is time consuming in a period where early revascularization is of prime importance.

Indications for surgical intervention in cardiogenic shock have not been completely delineated but should be considered in patients who fail to respond to volume correction and inotropic therapy. Failure of conventional medical interventions for cardiogenic shock should result in consideration of intra-aortic balloon counterpulsation, a temporizing measure before revascularization. Historically, emergent coronary artery bypass surgery preceded by placement of intra-aortic balloon pump has demonstrated improved survival rates in cardiogenic shock to approximately 75%. The SHOCK trial registry reported a 28% in-hospital mortality for the 290 patients undergoing coronary artery bypass surgery, which is comparable to other reported series (22,100). In a subgroup analysis of the SHOCK trial, survival was similar between percutaneous and surgically revascularized patients (55.6% vs. 57.4% at 30 days and 51.9% vs. 46.8%, respectively, at 1 year) despite a higher incidence of diabetes and multivessel disease in those patients surgically revascularized (37). Thus, surgical revascularization has an important role in patients with more extensive coronary artery disease.

Surgery for acute mitral insufficiency associated with cardiogenic shock in the postinfarction state is the only available definitive therapy. The impact of acute mitral insufficiency on left ventricular performance may be underestimated by studying the ejection fraction since the left ventricle ejects retrograde into the low-compliance left atrial and pulmonary venous system. Medical therapy with inotropic support and systemic peripheral vasodilation improves regurgitant flow as calculated by the regurgitant fraction. Severe mitral insufficiency is associated with a variety of adverse pathophysiologic changes that result in a poor survival after surgical intervention, but the results are significantly better than medical treatment that results in essentially 100% mortality if marked mitral insufficiency is associated with cardiogenic shock.

Surgical intervention is generally required for acute VSDs, which occur in the muscular portion of the interventricular septum and may be multiple. Two anatomic types of acute VSDs have been described. A VSD resulting from occlusion of a posterior descending coronary artery that arises from the right coronary is associated with a defect located in the inferobasilar region of the septum. Anteroseptal myocardial infarctions, which are associated with thrombotic occlusion of the left anterior descending, are associated with midapical to anterior defects in the septum. The physiologic impact of a left-to-right shunt is a function of the quantitative amount of involved myocardium plus associated left ventricular dysfunction, pulmonary artery pressures, and right ventricular compliance. A significant left-to-right shunt markedly decreases forward flow with poor peripheral perfusion and the clinical characteristics of cardiogenic shock. If the left ventricular end-diastolic pressure is markedly elevated, left-to-right shunting will also occur during diastole and is associated with an extremely high 24-hour mortality rate of approximately 25% (101,102). Medical treatment alone is associated with a 20% survival beyond 60 days and 1-year survival of less than 10%.

Surgical intervention in acute VSDs requires early and aggressive diagnostic and therapeutic interventions. Despite IABP and optimization with medical management, refinements in surgical technique have improved 1-year survival to 32% without coronary artery bypass. Evaluation of clinical trials that attempt to postpone therapy to improve the healing process have been questioned because this eliminates the most severely ill patients from definitive therapy and introduces a selection bias into the implications of therapy. Early surgical intervention with direct patch grafts plus coronary artery bypass may result in survival rates of up to 75%.

Free wall rupture of the left ventricle is a surgical disease even with a clotted hemopericardium tamponading further extravasation of blood into the pericardial space. The diagnosis of free wall rupture may be extraordinarily difficult on clinical grounds, and signs of pericardial tamponade should be actively sought. Pericardiocentesis with decompression of the pericardial space may be lifesaving in the short term but represents only a temporizing procedure. Cardiac rupture is essentially fatal, but surgical intervention may be successful with direct oversewing of the defect if recognized and managed in a timely fashion (103,104).

Left ventricular aneurysm as a cause of cardiogenic shock may require surgical intervention as a definitive therapy. The remodeling process, which begins after an acute ischemic event with regional thinning and expansion of the infarct zone, may result in progressive decrease in left ventricular performance and cardiogenic shock. If the aneurysmal dilation of the left ventricle involves more than 20% of the left ventricular mass, severe impairment of pumping ability ensues and potentially requires surgical intervention if there is a poor response to medical management including intra-aortic balloon pumping. Surgical intervention for aneurysms should be optimized in timing with adequate healing and fibrosis.

Mechanical Circulatory Support

The intra-aortic balloon pump has been in clinical use for over 20 years to increase diastolic coronary arterial perfusion and to decrease left ventricular afterload (105). The intra-aortic balloon pump is a temporizing measure that does not increase myocardial oxygen demand and results in reduction of ventricular diastolic volume and reduces pulmonary congestion with an increase in cardiac output. The intra-aortic balloon pump is the most widely used circulatory assist device in patients with cardiogenic shock because of the ease of insertion either percutaneously or surgically. Effective counterpulsation results in stabilization and potential reversal of the shock state with improvement in peripheral perfusion but does require an adequate systemic pressure and left ventricular performance to maximize its use. Profoundly hypotensive patients respond poorly to intra-aortic counterpulsation and the IABP has limited efficacy.

Balloon pumping in selected patients allows optimization of blood pressure, cardiac output, and tissue perfusion in patients with cardiogenic shock while further diagnostic procedures are performed. Hemodynamic effects of the IABP include the following (in percent change): Peak aortic systolic pressure (10%–15%), diastolic intra-aortic pressure (70%), arterial end-diastolic pressure (10%), peak ventricular pressure (10%), LV end-diastolic pressure (10%), dp/dt (10%), systemic vascular resistance (no change), mean arterial pressure (no change), cardiac index (10%–15%), and pulmonary capillary resistance (10%–15%). The intra-aortic balloon pump may be used prophylactically in patients with mechanical defects such as acute mitral insufficiency or VSD to increase coronary perfusion, allow time for healing, and restore cardiac output toward normal. The impact of intra-aortic balloon pumping on long-term survival is controversial and depends on the indications for insertion, hemodynamic status, and etiology of the cardiogenic shock. Patient selection is a key issue and early insertion of the intra-aortic balloon may result in increased clinical benefit rather than procrastination until overt low flow state has developed. The addition of the IABP to thrombolytic therapy for acute MI complicated by cardiogenic shock has been studied in a randomized clinical trial. There was no overall mortality benefit, but the subgroup of patients with Killip class III or IV benefitted with a 6-month mortality rate of 39% for combined therapy versus 80% for fibrinolysis alone (106). The SHOCK trial registry also reported a survival benefit with intra-aortic balloon pumping in addition to thrombolytic therapy (47% vs. 63% in-hospital mortality), but these results were heavily affected by higher revascularization rates in the group receiving the intra-aortic balloon pump (68% vs. 20%) (73).

Patients who are not expected to significantly benefit from an intra-aortic balloon pump are elderly patients, those with severe peripheral vascular disease, and those with large MIs exceeding 40% of the left ventricular myocardium. The overall survival rate of patients with cardiogenic shock treated with the intra-aortic balloon pump is approximately 40%. For subjects who required balloon insertion for large myocardial infarctions without a significant mechanical obstruction, the survival rate was only 27%. Complications may be documented in up to 30% of patients who undergo intra-aortic balloon pumping and relate mainly to local vascular problems, including surgical trauma, emboli, infection, and hemolysis.

Left ventricular assist devices (LVADs) function as prosthetic ventricles but require a sternotomy for insertion. Assist devices may be used to support left ventricular performance, right ventricular performance, or a combination, depending on the underlying condition. The indications for insertion of an LVAD are controversial, and traditionally have been reserved for medical and intra-aortic balloon pump failure and in the presence of the potentially salvageable myocardium and particularly as a bridge to cardiac transplantation. The Thoratec extracorporeal left ventricular assist device (Thoratec, Pleasanton, CA) has been used as a bridge to cardiac transplantation. Insertion of the Thoratec device in patients with severe left ventricular dysfunction allowed survival to transplant in approximately 75% of 29 patients (107). Similarly, in the Heartmate LVAD (Thoratec, Pleasanton, CA), survival to cardiac transplantation has been reported as 76% out of 97 patients (108). The REMATCH (Randomized Evaluation of Mechanical Assistance in the Treatment of Congestive Heart Failure) trial demonstrated improved outcomes in chronically ill patients too sick for cardiac transplantation as an alternative (destination therapy) to routine medical care (109). Hemodynamic unloading and myocardial rest after ventricular assist device (VAD) placement may lead to recovery of native cardiac function, allowing for removal of the device without cardiac transplantation (110–116). Ventricular assist device support is also associated with decreases in neurohormonal activation, alterations in myocyte calcium handling, and improvement in the proinflammatory cytokine milieu (117–125). Histologic analysis of the explanted heart at the time of transplantation demonstrated decreased fibrosis and myocyte size after VAD placement (121,126,127). Despite these salutatory changes as a result of VAD support, the frequency of bridge to recovery (BTR) in chronically supported subjects remains low, in the range of 3% to 10% in various series (111,114,115,128).

The Heartmate LVAD is approved for life-long support in patients deemed too ill for cardiac transplantation with several other devices undergoing clinical trials. There is retrospective data that early mechanical support as a bridge to transplantation after acute MI complicated by cardiogenic shock improves survival compared with a strategy of early revascularization (129). The technology has now advanced to include several other continuous flow pumps that offer the potential advantage of greater mechanical longevity, thus making them truly a lifelong option. Complications include hemolysis, thromboembolism, and infection, which have been decreased with increasing experience.

The Nimbus hemopump (Nimbus Medical, Inc., Rancho Cordova, CA) circumvented the problem associated with median sternotomy and allows a percutaneous placement of a cannula across the aortic valve, which is coupled to an extracorporeal power source. The Nimbus hemopump uses an Archimedes spiral screw valve that rotates at approximately 25,000 revolutions per minute without significant hemolysis (130). Although this pump is no longer available, there are several other percutaneous continuous rotary flow VADs, including the TandemHeart (Cardiac Assist, Pittsburgh, PA),

Cancion (Orqis Medical, Lake Forest, CA), and Impella (Abiomed, Danvers, MA). The TandemHeart is currently FDA approved, while the Impella is approved in Europe and in clinical trial in the United States. The Cancion system is also in clinical trial in the United States.

Future and Adjunctive Therapies

Autologous Stem Cells

Stem cells offer the hope of biologically rebuilding damaged myocardium due to their ability to differentiate into cardiomyocytes. There has been a substantial amount of research into the biology of various stem cells and now several clinical trials have been reported, with mixed results. Most trials have looked at stem cells' delivery percutaneously by intracoronary catheter after acute myocardial infarction in numbers ranging from 30 to 100 patients. The BOOST (Bone Marrow Transfer to Enhance ST-elevation Infarct Regeneration) trial found 6% improvement in ejection fraction compared to control but no significant difference at 18 months (131,132). The ASTAMI (Autologous Stem Cell Transplantation in Acute MI) trial found no difference in ejection fraction at 4 and 6 months, although Janssens et al. reported improved regional wall motion and decreased infarct size (133,134). The TOPCARE-CHD (Transcoronary Transplant of Progenitor Cells after MI with Chronic Ischemic Heart Disease) trial found 2.9% improvement in ejection fraction at 3 months, while the REPAIR-AMI (Intracoronary Administration of Bone Marrow-derived Progenitor Cells in Acute Myocardial Infarction) trial reported a 2.5% improvement in ejection fraction at 4 months (135,136). Multiple studies are currently under way including evaluating the safety and efficacy of stem cells implanted during surgery for VAD installation as well as coronary artery bypass surgery with depressed ventricular function and percutaneously for chronic angina. While this is a very promising therapy, considerable issues remain, including the risk of generating an arrhythmic focus, the best cell type, the amount of local myocardial blood flow necessary, the best method to deliver the cells to the myocardium, and the number of cells necessary.

Clenbuterol

Clenbuterol is a β_2-adrenergic receptor agonist that induces skeletal muscle hypertrophy and improves contraction. It also has been found to cause cardiomyocyte hypertrophy without apoptosis (137). In a recently reported single-center study, 15 patients requiring LVAD support were treated with clenbuterol in addition to lisinopril, carvedilol, spironolactone, and losartan (138). There was sufficient myocardial recovery to explant the LVAD in 11 of 15 patients, in whom 4-year survival was 89%, quality-of-life scores were almost normal, and mean left ventricular ejection fraction was 64%. These patients all had heart failure due to nonischemic cardiomyopathy without histologic evidence of active myocarditis. A multicenter trial in the United States is being planned.

Tissue-engineered Patches

Patches made from decellularized extracellular matrix may be another useful solution to biologic regeneration of myocardium. The patch retains biologically active substances such as growth factors providing paracrine as well as mechanical support for regrowth of cardiomyocytes. These devices are still in preclinical testing but have shown improvements in regional function in a myocardial infarction model (139).

CONCLUSIONS

Despite rapid advancement in pharmacologic thrombolytic therapy, mechanical revascularization techniques, and development of mechanical ventricular assist devices, cardiogenic shock remains a major clinical challenge with an associated high mortality. Improved survival in cardiogenic shock may be seen with an aggressive approach to diagnosis and management of the problem, with emphasis on early recognition and treatment of mechanical defects such as VSD, acute mitral insufficiency, and free wall rupture. Limitation of infarct size by minimizing the extent of infarcted tissue is the key component in all therapeutic strategies with the goal to maximize perfusion, limit irreversible cell death, and decrease potential for a secondary mechanical event.

PEARLS

- Clinical criteria used to establish the diagnosis of cardiogenic shock include absolute or relative hypotension, which is defined as a systolic blood pressure less than 90 mm Hg or a blood pressure that has fallen to at least 30 mm Hg less than the individual's baseline blood pressure.
- Cardiogenic shock thus may be a complication in patients with chronic hypertension who have an acute cardiac event that results in a decrease in blood pressure, but not to the 90 mm Hg systolic level.
- If signs of organ dysfunction and tissue hypoperfusion accompany this condition, the individual qualifies for the diagnosis of cardiogenic shock.
- The exact incidence of cardiogenic shock is difficult to ascertain because of variability in diagnostic criteria and survival rates in the early phase of acute MI. The Multicenter Investigation of Limitation of Infarct Size trial (140) documented an incidence rate of cardiogenic shock in 7.5% of subjects who were admitted to the hospital after having an acute myocardial infarction, a constant value from 1975 to 1997 (141). The Global Utilization of Streptokinase and Tissue Plasminogen Activator for Occluded Arteries (GUSTO-I) trial, the GUSTO-III trial, and other thrombolytic trials have reported incidences of 5% to 10% (68,142).
- The mortality rate for cardiogenic shock in the setting of acute MI is exceedingly high despite significant improvements due to a strategy of early revascularization as reported in the SHOCK (Should We Emergently Revascularize Occluded Coronaries for Cardiogenic Shock) trial. Historically, mortality rates were 81% as originally reported by Killip in 1967 (6). Early revascularization by angioplasty or surgery has been shown to reduce mortality from 63% to 50% at 6 months in the SHOCK trial (36).

References

1. Smith SC Jr, Feldman TE, Hirshfeld JW Jr, et al. ACC/AHA/SCAI 2005 Guideline Update for Percutaneous Coronary Intervention–summary

article: a report of the American College of Cardiology/American Heart Association Task Force on Practice Guidelines (ACC/AHA/SCAI Writing Committee to update the 2001 Guidelines for Percutaneous Coronary Intervention). *Circulation.* 2006;113(1):156.

2. Sanborn TA, Sleeper LA, Bates ER, et al. Impact of thrombolysis, intra-aortic balloon pump counterpulsation, and their combination in cardiogenic shock complicating acute myocardial infarction: a report from the SHOCK trial registry. Should we emergently revascularize occluded coronaries for cardiogenic shock? *J Am Coll Cardiol.* 2000;36(3 Suppl A): 1123.
3. Noble MI. Problems concerning the application of concepts of muscle mechanics to the determination of the contractile state of the heart. *Circulation.* 1972;45:252.
4. Sagawa K, Maughan WL, Sunagawa K, et al. *Cardiac Contraction and the Pressure-Volume Relationship.* New York: Oxford University Press, Inc.; 1988.
5. Mathey D, Biefield W, Hanrath P, et al. Attempt to quantitate relation between cardiac function and infarct size in acute myocardial infarction. *Br Heart J.* 1974;36(3):271.
6. Killip T, Kimball JT. Treatment of myocardial infarction in a coronary care unit. *Am J Cardiol.* 1967;20:457.
7. Forrester JS, Diamond GA, Chatterjee K. Medical therapy of acute myocardial infarction by application of hemodynamic subsets. *N Engl J Med.* 1976;295:1356.
8. Andersen HR, Falk E, Nielsen D. Right ventricular infarction: frequency, size and topography in coronary heart disease: a prospective study comprising 107 consecutive autopsies from a coronary care unit. *J Am Coll Cardiol.* 1987;10(6):1223.
9. Kinch JW, Ryan TJ. Right ventricular infarction. *N Engl J Med.* 1994;330(17):1211.
10. Andersen HR, Nielsen D, Falk E. Right ventricular infarction. *Am Heart J.* 1989;117:82.
11. Zehender M, Kasper W, Kauder E, et al. Right ventricular infarction as an independent predictor of prognosis after acute inferior myocardial infarction. *N Engl J Med.* 1993;328:981.
12. Dell'Italia LJ, Starling MR, Crawford MH. Right ventricular infarction. *J Am Coll Cardiol.* 1984;4:931.
13. Sato H, Murakami Y, Shimada T, et al. Detection of right ventricular infarction by gadolinium DTPA-enhanced magnetic resonance imaging. *Eur Heart J.* 1995;16(9):1195.
14. Goldstein JA, Barzilai, Rosamond TL. Determination of hemodynamic compromise with severe right ventricular infarction. *Circulation.* 1990;82:359.
15. Jacobs AK, Leopold JA, Bates E, et al. Cardiogenic shock caused by right ventricular infarction: a report from the SHOCK registry. *J Am Coll Cardiol.* 2003;41:1273.
16. Bowers TR, O'Neill WW, Grines C, et al. Effect of reperfusion on biventricular function and survival after right ventricular infarction. *N Engl J Med.* 1998;338(14):933.
17. Tcheng JE, Jackman JD, Nelson CL. Outcome of patients sustaining acute ischemic mitral regurgitation during myocardial infarction. *Ann Intern Med.* 1992;117:18.
18. Sharma SK, Seckler J, Israel DH. Clinical angiographic and anatomic findings in acute severe ischemic mitral regurgitation. *Am J Cardiol.* 1992;70:277.
19. Sharma SK, Seckler J, Israel DH, et al. Clinical, angiographic and anatomic findings in acute severe ischemic mitral regurgitation. *Am J Cardiol.* 1992;70(3):277.
20. Thompson CR, Buller CE, Sleeper LA, et al. Cardiogenic shock due to acute severe mitral regurgitation complicating acute myocardial infarction: a report from the SHOCK Trial Registry. Should we use emergently revascularize occluded coronaries in cardiogenic shock? *J Am Coll Cardiol.* 2000;36(3 Suppl A):1104.
21. Lear J, Feinberg MS, Vered Z. Effect of thrombolytic therapy on the evaluation of significant mitral regurgitation in patients with a first inferior myocardial infarction. *J Am Coll Cardiol.* 1993;21:1661.
22. Hochman JS, Buller CE, Sleeper LA, et al. Cardiogenic shock complicating acute myocardial infarction–etiologies, management and outcome: a report from the SHOCK trial registry. Should we emergently revascularize occluded coronaries for cardiogenic shock? *J Am Coll Cardiol.* 2000;36:1063.
23. Kisdnuke A, Otsuji Y, Kuroiwa R. Two dimensional echocardiographic assessment of papillary muscle contractility in patients with prior myocardial infarction. *J Am Coll Cardiol.* 1993;21:932.
24. Picard MH, Davidoff R, Sleeper LA, et al. Echocardiographic predictors of survival and response to early revascularization in cardiogenic shock. *Circulation.* 2003;107:279.
25. Menon V, Webb JG, Hillis LD, et al. Outcome and profile of ventricular septal rupture with cardiogenic shock after myocardial infarction: a report from the SHOCK trial registry. Should we emergently revascularize occluded coronaries in cardiogenic shock? *J Am Coll Cardiol.* 2000;36(3 Suppl A):1110.
26. Harrison MR, MacPhail B, Gurley JC. Usefulness of color flow Doppler imaging to distinguish ventricular septal defect from acute mitral regurgitation complicating acute myocardial infarction. *Am J Cardiol.* 1989;64:697.
27. Gray JM, Sethna D, Matloff JM. The role of cardiac surgery in acute myocardial infarction with mechanical complications. *Am Heart J.* 106:723.
28. Bates RJ, Beutler S, Resnekov L. Cardiac rupture: challenge in diagnosis and management. *Am J Cardiol.* 1977;40:1231.
29. Assmann PE, Roelandt JR. Two dimensional and Doppler echocardiography in acute myocardial infarction and its complications. *Ultrasound Med Biol.* 1987;13:507.
30. Buda AJ. The role of echocardiography in the evaluation of mechanical complications of acute myocardial infarction. *Circulation.* 1991;84(Suppl 3):109
31. Pappas PJ, Cerndianu AC, Baldino WA, et al. Ventricular free rupture after myocardial infarction: treatment and outcome. *Chest.* 1991;99:892.
32. Visser CA, Kan G, David CK, et al. Echocardiographic cineangiographic correlation in detecting left ventricular aneurysm. *Am J Cardiol.* 1982;50:337.
33. Heras M, Sany G, Etriu A, et al. Does left ventricular aneurysm influence survival after acute myocardial infarction. *Eur Heart J.* 1990;11:441.
34. Aryan S, Varat MA. Persistent ST elevation and ventricular wall abnormalities: a two-dimensional echocardiographic study. *Am J Cardiol.* 1984;53:1142.
35. Menon V, White H, LeJemtel T, et al. The clinical profile of patients with suspected cardiogenic shock due to predominant left ventricular failure: a report from the SHOCK trial registry. Should we emergently revascularize occluded coronaries in cardiogenic shock? *J Am Coll Cardiol.* 2000;36(3 Suppl A):1071.
36. Hochman JS, Sleeper LA, Webb JG, et al. Early revascularization in acute myocardial infarction complicated by cardiogenic shock. SHOCK investigators. Should we emergently revascularize occluded coronaries for cardiogenic shock. *N Engl J Med.* 1999;341(9):625.
37. White HD, Assmann SF, Sanborn TA, et al. Comparison of percutaneous coronary intervention and coronary artery bypass grafting after acute myocardial infarction complicated by cardiogenic shock: results from the should we emergently revascularize occluded coronaries for cardiogenic shock (SHOCK) trial. *Circulation.* 2005;112:1992.
38. Hochman JS, Sleeper LA, White HD, et al. One-year survival following early revascularization for cardiogenic shock. *JAMA.* 2001;285(2):190.
39. Hochman JS, Sleeper LA, Webb JG, et al. Early revascularization and long-term survival in cardiogenic shock complicating acute myocardial infarction. *JAMA.* 2006;295(21):2511.
40. Wong SC, Sanborn T, Sleeper LA, et al. Angiographic findings and clinical correlates in patients with cardiogenic shock complicating acute myocardial infarction: a report from the SHOCK trial registry. Should we emergently revascularize occluded coronaries for cardiogenic shock? *J Am Coll Cardiol.* 2000;36(3 Suppl A):1077.
41. Chan AW, Chew DP, Bhatt DL, et al. Long-term mortality benefit with the combination of stents and abciximab for cardiogenic shock complicating acute myocardial infarction. *Am J Cardiol.* 2002;89(2):132.
42. Moses JW, Leon MB, Popma JJ, et al. Sirolimus-eluting stents versus standard stents in patients with stenosis in a native coronary artery. *N Engl J Med.* 2003;349:1315.
43. Stone GW, Ellis SG, Cox DA, et al. A polymer-based, paclitaxel-eluting stent in patients with coronary artery disease. *N Engl J Med.* 2004;350(3):221.
44. Flaherty JT, Becker LC, Bulkley BH. Randomized prospective trial of intravenous nitroglycerin in patients with AMI. *Circulation.* 1983;68:576.
45. Jugoutt BI, Warnica JW. Intravenous nitroglycerin therapy to limit myocardial infarct size, expansion and complications. *Circulation.* 1988;78:906.
46. Gibson RS, Boden WE, Theroux P, et al. Diltiazem and reinfarction in patients with non–Q wave myocardial infarction. *N Engl J Med.* 1986;315:423.
47. The Multicenter Diltiazem Postinfarction Trial Group. The effect of diltiazem on mortality and reinfarction after myocardial infarction. *N Engl J Med.* 1988;319:385.
48. The Danish Study Group on Verapamil in Myocardial Infarction. Treatment with verapamil during and after an acute myocardial infarction: a review based on Danish Verapamil Infarction Trials I and II. *J Cardiovasc Pharmacol.* 1991;18(Suppl 6):520.
49. Herlity J, Hjalmarson A, Swedberg K, et al. The influence of early intervention in acute myocardial infarction on long term mortality and morbidity assessed in the Goteborg Metoprolol trial. *Int J Cardiol.* 1986;10:291.
50. Hjalmarson A, Elmfeldt D, Herlitz J, et al. Effect on mortality of metoprolol in acute myocardial infarction. A double-blind randomised trial. *Lancet.* 1981;2:823.
51. Herlitz J, Waagstein F, Lindqvist J, et al. Effect of metoprolol on the prognosis for patients with suspected acute myocardial infarction and indirect signs of congestive heart failure (a subgroup analysis of the Goteborg Metoprolol trial). *Am J Cardiol.* 1997;80:40J.
52. Viscoli CM, Horowitz RI, Singer BH. Beta blockers after myocardial infarction. *Ann Intern Med.* 1993;118:99.
53. ISIS-I Collaborative Group. Mechanisms for the early mortality reduction produced by beta blockade started early in myocardial infarction: ISIS-I. *Lancet.* 1988;i(8591):921.
54. Dargie HJ. Effect of carvedilol on outcome after myocardial infarction in patients with left-ventricular dysfunction: the CAPRICORN randomised trial. *Lancet.* 2001;357(9266):1385.

55. Doughty RN, Whalley GA, Walsh HA, et al. Effects of carvedilol on left ventricular remodeling after acute myocardial infarction: the CAPRICORN Echo Substudy. *Circulation.* 2004;109(2):201.
56. McMurray J, Kober L, Robertson M, et al. Antiarrhythmic effect of carvedilol after acute myocardial infarction: results of the Carvedilol Post-Infarct Survival Control in Left Ventricular Dysfunction (CAPRICORN) trial. *J Am Coll Cardiol.* 2005;45:525.
57. Roberts R, Rogers WJ, Mueller HS, et al. Immediate versus deferred beta blockade following thrombolytic therapy in patients with acute myocardial infarction (TIMI-IIB). *Circulation.* 1991;83:422.
58. The SAVE Investigators. Effect of captopril on mortality and morbidity in patients with left ventricular dysfunction after myocardial infarction. *N Engl J Med.* 1992;327:669.
59. Swedburg K, Held P, Kjekshus J. Effects of early administration of enalapril on mortality in patients with acute myocardial infarction: results of the Co-operative New Scandinavian Enalapril Survival Study (Consensus-II). *N Engl J Med.* 1992;327:678.
60. McMurray J, Pfeffer MA. New therapeutic options in congestive heart failure: part I. *Circulation.* 2002;105(17):2099.
61. Pitt B, Remme W, Zannad F, et al. Eplerenone, a selective aldosterone blocker, in patients with left ventricular dysfunction after myocardial infarction. *N Engl J Med.* 2003;348(14):1309.
62. Pitt B, Gheorghiade M, Zannad F, et al. Evaluation of eplerenone in the subgroup of EPHESUS patients with baseline left ventricular ejection fraction <or=30%. *Eur J Heart Fail.* 2006;8(3):295.
63. Pfeffer MA, McMurray JJ, Velazquez EJ, et al. Valsartan, captopril, or both in myocardial infarction complicated by heart failure, left ventricular dysfunction, or both. *N Engl J Med.* 2003;349(20):1893.
64. Hasdai D, Harrington RA, Hochman JS, et al. Platelet glycoprotein IIb/IIIa blockade and outcome of cardiogenic shock complicating acute coronary syndromes without persistent ST-segment elevation. *J Am Coll Cardiol.* 2000;36(3):685.
65. Zeymer U, Gitt AK, Junger C, et al. Effect of clopidogrel on 1-year mortality in hospital survivors of acute ST-segment elevation myocardial infarction in clinical practice. *Eur Heart J.* 2006;27(22):2661.
66. Rackley CE, Russel RO, Rogers WJ. Glucose-insulin-potassium infusion: review of clinical experience. *Postgrad Med.* 1979;65:93.
67. Henderson A, Campbell RWF, Julian DG. Effect of a highly purified hyaluronidase preparation on electrocardiographic changes in acute myocardial infarction. *Lancet.* 1982;i:874.
68. Holmes DR Jr, Bates ER, Kleiman NS, et al. Contemporary reperfusion therapy for cardiogenic shock: the GUSTO-I trial experience. The GUSTO-I investigators. Global Utilization of Streptokinase and Tissue Plasminogen Activator for Occluded Coronary Arteries. *J Am Coll Cardiol.* 1995;26:668.
69. Grella RD, Becker RC. Cardiogenic shock complicating coronary artery disease: diagnosis, treatment and management. *Curr Probl Cardiol.* 1994;12:693.
70. Gruppo Italiano Per lo Studio Della Streptochinase Mell Infarcto Miocardio (GISSI). Effectiveness of intravenous streptokinase treatment in acute myocardial infarction. *Lancet.* 1986;i:397.
71. Cox RH. Mechanical aspects of large coronary arteries. In: Santamore WP, Bove AA, eds. *Coronary Artery Disease.* Baltimore: Urban and Schwartzenberg; 1982:19.
72. Strack RS, Califf RM, Hinohara R, et al. Survival and cardiac event rates in the first year after emergent coronary angioplasty for acute myocardial infarction. *J Am Coll Cardiol.* 1988;11:1141.
73. Sanborn TA, Sleeper LA, Bates ER, et al. Impact of thrombolysis, intra-aortic balloon pump counterpulsation, and their combination in cardiogenic shock complicating acute myocardial infarction: a report from the SHOCK trial registry. Should we emergently revascularize occluded coronaries for cardiogenic shock? *J Am Coll Cardiol.* 2000;36:1123.
74. Shawl FA, Forman MB, Punja S, et al. Emergent coronary angioplasty in the treatment of acute ischemic mitral regurgitation. *J Am Coll Cardiol.* 1989;14:986.
75. Mueller HS, Evans R, Ayres SM. Effects of dopamine on hemodynamics and myocardial metabolism in shock following acute myocardial infarction in man. *Circulation.* 1978;57:361.
76. Goldberg LO. Cardiovascular and renal actions of dopamine: potential clinical applications. *Pharmacol Rev.* 1972;21:1.
77. Teba L, Schiebel F, Dedhia HV, et al. Beneficial effect of norepinephrine in the treatment of circulatory shock caused by tricyclic antidepressant overdose. *Am J Emerg Med.* 1988;6:566.
78. Horowitz D, Goldberg LI, Sjoerdsm A. Increased blood pressure response to dopamine and norepinephrine produced by MAO inhibitors. *J Lab Clin Med.* 1960;56:747.
79. Sonnenblick EH, Frishman WH, Lyeintel TH. Dobutamine: a new synthetic cardioactive sympathetic amine. *N Engl J Med.* 1979;300:17.
80. Mueller H, Ayres S, Giarinelli S, et al. Effect of isoproterenol, L-norepinephrine and intra-aortic balloon counterpulsation on hemodynamics and myocardial metabolism in shock following myocardial infarction. *Circulation.* 1972;55:325.
81. Kelly RA, Smith TW. Digoxin in heart failure: implications of recent trials. *J Am Coll Cardiol.* 1993;22(Suppl 4):107A.
82. Sarter BH, Marchinski FE. Redefining the role of digoxin in atrial fibrillation. *Am J Cardiol.* 1992;69:71.
83. Honerjager P. Pharmacology of bipyridine phosphodiesterase III inhibitors. *Am Heart J.* 1991;121:1939.
84. Benotti JR, Grossman W, Braunwald E, et al. Hemodynamic assessment of amrinone. *N Engl J Med.* 1978;299:1373.
85. Klein M, Siskind S, Frishman W. Hemodynamic comparison of intravenous amrinone and dobutamine in patients with chronic congestive heart failure. *Am J Cardiol.* 1981;48:160.
86. Dage RC, Kariya T, Hsiek CP, et al. Pharmacology of enoximone. *Am J Cardiol.* 1987;60:100.
87. Goldstein RE, Skelton CL, Levey GS. Effects of chronic heart failure on the capacity of glucagon to enhance contractility and adenyl cyclase. *Circulation.* 1971;44:638.
88. Scholtz H. Inotropic drugs and their mechanisms of action. *J Am Coll Cardiol.* 1984;4:389.
89. Hasenfuss G, Pieske B, Castell M, et al. Influence of the novel inotropic agent levosimendan on isometric tension and calcium cycling in failing human myocardium. *Circulation.* 1998;98(20):2141.
90. De Luca L, Colucci WS, Nieminen MS, et al. Evidence-based use of levosimendan in different clinical settings. *Eur Heart J.* 2006;27(16):1908.
91. Yokoshiki H, Katsube Y, Sunagawa M, et al. The novel calcium sensitizer levosimendan activates the ATP-sensitive K+ channel in rat ventricular cells. *J Pharmacol Exp Ther.* 1997;283(1):375.
92. Slawsky MT, Colucci WS, Gottlieb SS, et al. Acute hemodynamic and clinical effects of levosimendan in patients with severe heart failure. Study investigators. *Circulation.* 2000;102(18):2222.
93. Mebazaa A, Barraud D, Welschbillig S. Randomized clinical trials with levosimendan. *Am J Cardiol.* 2005;96(6A):74G.
94. Kivikko M, Lehtonen L, Colucci WS. Sustained hemodynamic effects of intravenous levosimendan. *Circulation.* 2003;107(1):81.
95. Moiseyev VS, Poder P, Andrejevs N, et al. Safety and efficacy of a novel calcium sensitizer, levosimendan, in patients with left ventricular failure due to an acute myocardial infarction. A randomized, placebo-controlled, double-blind study (RUSSLAN). *Eur Heart J.* 2002;23(18):1422.
96. Follath F, Cleland JG, Just H, et al. Efficacy and safety of intravenous levosimendan compared with dobutamine in severe low-output heart failure (the LIDO study): a randomised double-blind trial. *Lancet.* 2002;360(9328):196.
97. Nieminen MS, Bohm M, Cowie MR, et al. Executive summary of the guidelines on the diagnosis and treatment of acute heart failure. The Task Force on Acute Heart Failure of the European Society of Cardiology. *Eur Heart J.* 2005;26:384.
98. De Wood MA, Heit J, Spores J, et al. Anterior transmural myocardial infarction: effects of surgical coronary reperfusion on global and regional left ventricular function. *J Am Coll Cardiol.* 1983;1:1223.
99. De Wood MA, Notske RN, Berg R, et al. Medical and surgical management of early Q wave myocardial infarction. *J Am Coll Cardiol.* 1989;14:65.
100. Bolooki H. Emergency cardiac procedures in patients in cardiogenic shock due to complications of coronary artery disease. *Circulation.* 1989;79:I137.
101. Gray RJ, Sethna D, Matloff JM. The role of cardiac surgery in acute myocardial infarction with mechanical complications. *Am Heart J.* 1983;10:723.
102. Fox AC, Glassman E, Isom OW. Surgically remediable complications of myocardial infarction. *Prog Cardiovasc Dis.* 1979;21:461.
103. Bates RJ, Beutler S, Resnekov L, et al. Cardiac rupture: challenge in diagnosis and management. *Am J Cardiol.* 1977;40:1231.
104. Shapiro I, Isakov A, Burke M, et al. Cardiac rupture in patients with acute myocardial infarction. *Chest.* 1987;92:219.
105. Cohn LH. The role of mechanical devices. *J Cardiac Surg.* 1990;5:278.
106. Ohman EM, Nanas J, Stomel RJ, et al. Thrombolysis and counterpulsation to improve survival in myocardial infarction complicated by hypotension and suspected cardiogenic shock or heart failure: results of the TACTICS Trial. *J Thromb Thrombolysis.* 2005;19:33.
107. Farrar DJ, Hill JD, Gray LA, et al. Heterotopic prosthetic ventricles as a bridge to cardiac transplantation. *N Engl J Med.* 1988;318:333.
108. McCarthy PM, Smedira NO, Vargo RL, et al. One hundred patients with the HeartMate left ventricular assist device: evolving concepts and technology. *J Thorac Cardiovasc Surg.* 1998;115(4):904.
109. Rose EA, Gelijns AC, Moskowitz AJ, et al. Long-term use of a left ventricular assist device for end-stage heart failure. *N Engl J Med.* 2001;345:1435.
110. Gorcsan J 3rd, Severyn D, Murali S, et al. Non-invasive assessment of myocardial recovery on chronic left ventricular assist device: results associated with successful device removal. *J Heart Lung Transplant.* 2003;22:1304.
111. Farrar DJ, Holman WR, McBride LR, et al. Long-term follow-up of Thoratec ventricular assist device bridge-to-recovery patients successfully removed from support after recovery of ventricular function. *J Heart Lung Transplant.* 2002;21:516.
112. Maybaum S, Stockwell P, Naka Y, et al. Assessment of myocardial recovery in a patient with acute myocarditis supported with a left ventricular assist device: a case report. *J Heart Lung Transplant.* 2003;22:202.
113. Khan T, Delgado RM, Radovancevic B, et al. Dobutamine stress echocardiography predicts myocardial improvement in patients supported by left ventricular assist devices (LVADs): hemodynamic and histologic evidence

of improvement before LVAD explanation. *J Heart Lung Transplant.* 2003;22:137.

114. Mancini DM, Beniaminovitz A, Levin H, et al. Low incidence of myocardial recovery after left ventricular assist device implantation in patients with chronic heart failure. *Circulation.* 1998;98:2383.
115. Hetzer R, Muller JH, Weng Y, et al. Bridging-to-recovery. *Ann Thorac Surg.* 2001;71:S109.
116. Frazier OH, Delgado RM 3rd, Scroggins N, et al. Mechanical bridging to improvement in severe acute "nonischemic, nonmyocarditis" heart failure. *Congest Heart Fail.* 2004;10:109.
117. James KB, McCarthy PM, Thomas JD, et al. Effect of the implantable left ventricular assist device on neuroendocrine activation in heart failure. *Circulation.* 1995;92:II191.
118. Milting H, El Banayosy A, Kassner A, et al. The time course of natriuretic hormones as plasma markers of myocardial recovery in heart transplant candidates during ventricular assist device support reveals differences among device types. *J Heart Lung Transplant.* 2001;20:949.
119. Kucuker SA, Stetson SJ, Becker KA, et al. Evidence of improved right ventricular structure after LVAD support in patients with end-stage cardiomyopathy. *J Heart Lung Transplant.* 2004;23:28.
120. Terracciano CM, Hardy J, Birks EJ, et al. Clinical recovery from end-stage heart failure using left-ventricular assist device and pharmacological therapy correlates with increased sarcoplasmic reticulum calcium content but not with regression of cellular hypertrophy. *Circulation.* 2004;109:2263.
121. Barbone A, Holmes JW, Heerdt PM, et al. Comparison of right and left ventricular responses to left ventricular assist device support in patients with severe heart failure: a primary role of mechanical unloading underlying reverse remodeling. *Circulation.* 2001;104:670.
122. Bartling B, Milting H, Schumann H, et al. Myocardial gene expression of regulators of myocyte apoptosis and myocyte calcium homeostasis during hemodynamic unloading by ventricular assist devices in patients with end-stage heart failure. *Circulation.* 1999;100:II216.
123. Chaudhary KW, Rossman EI, Piacentino V 3rd, et al. Altered myocardial Ca2+ cycling after left ventricular assist device support in the failing human heart. *J Am Coll Cardiol.* 2004;44:837.
124. Torre-Amione G, Stetson SJ, Youker KA, et al. Decreased expression of tumor necrosis factor-alpha in failing human myocardium after mechanical circulatory support: a potential mechanism for cardiac recovery. *Circulation.* 1999;100:1189.
125. Goldstein DJ, Moazami N, Seldomridge JA, et al. Circulatory resuscitation with left ventricular assist device support reduces interleukins 6 and 8 levels. *Ann Thorac Surg.* 1997;63:971.
126. Bruckner BA, Stetson SJ, Perez-Verdia A, et al. Regression of fibrosis and hypertrophy in failing myocardium following mechanical circulatory support. *J Heart Lung Transplant.* 2001;20:457.
127. Zafeiridis A, Jeevanandam V, Houser SR, et al. Regression of cellular hypertrophy after left ventricular assist device support. *Circulation.* 1998;98:656.
128. Simon MA, Kormos RL, Murali S, et al. Myocardial recovery using ventricular assist devices: prevalence, clinical characteristics and outcomes. *Circulation.* 2005;112(Suppl I):I-32.
129. Tayara W, Starling RC, Yamani MH, et al. Improved survival after acute myocardial infarction complicated by cardiogenic shock with circulatory support and transplantation: comparing aggressive intervention with conservative treatment. *J Heart Lung Transplant.* 2006;25:504.
130. Merhige ME, Smalling RW, Cassidy D, et al. Effect of the hemopump left ventricular assist device on regional myocardial perfusion and function. *Circulation.* 1989;80(Suppl 3):158.
131. Wollert KC, Meyer GP, Lotz J, et al. Intracoronary autologous bone-marrow cell transfer after myocardial infarction: the BOOST randomised controlled clinical trial. *Lancet.* 2004;364:141.
132. Meyer GP, Wollert KC, Lotz J, et al. Intracoronary bone marrow cell transfer after myocardial infarction: eighteen months' follow-up data from the randomized, controlled BOOST (BOne marrOw transfer to enhance ST-elevation infarct regeneration) trial. *Circulation.* 2006;113:1287.
133. Janssens S, Dubois C, Bogaert J, et al. Autologous bone marrow-derived stem-cell transfer in patients with ST-segment elevation myocardial infarction: double-blind, randomised controlled trial. *Lancet.* 2006;367:113.
134. Lunde K, Solheim S, Aakhus S, et al. Intracoronary injection of mononuclear bone marrow cells in acute myocardial infarction. *N Engl J Med.* 2006;355:1199.
135. Assmus B, Honold J, Schächinger V, et al. Transcoronary transplantation of progenitor cells after myocardial infarction. *N Engl J Med.* 2006;355:1222.
136. Schächinger V, Erbs S, Elsässer A, et al. Intracoronary bone marrow-derived progenitor cells in acute myocardial infarction. *N Engl J Med.* 2006;355:1210.
137. Yacoub MH. A novel strategy to maximize the efficacy of left ventricular assist devices as a bridge to recovery. *Eur Heart J.* 2001;22:534.
138. Birks EJ, Tansley PD, Hardy J, et al. Left ventricular assist device and drug therapy for the reversal of heart failure. *N Engl J Med.* 2006;355:1873.
139. Kochupura PV, Azeloglu EU, Kelly DJ, et al. Tissue-engineered myocardial patch derived from extracellular matrix provides regional mechanical function. *Circulation.* 2005;112:I-144.
140. Hands ME, Rutherford JD, Muller JE, et al. The in-hospital development of cardiogenic shock after myocardial infarction: incidence, predictors of occurrence, outcome and prognostic factors. *J Am Coll Cardiol.* 1989; 14:40.
141. Goldberg RJ, Samad NA, Yarzebski J, et al. Temporal trends in cardiogenic shock complicating acute myocardial infarction. *N Engl J Med.* 1999;340(15):1162.
142. Hasdai D, Holmes DR Jr, Topol EJ, et al. Frequency and clinical outcome of cardiogenic shock during acute myocardial infarction among patients receiving reteplase or alteplase. Results from GUSTO-III. Global Use of Strategies to Open Occluded Coronary Arteries. *Eur Heart J.* 1999;20(2):128.

CHAPTER 57 ■ SEPSIS AND SEPTIC SHOCK

ANAND KUMAR • ASEEM KUMAR

Septic shock (shock due to infection) and sepsis-associated multiple organ failure are the dominant cause of death in intensive care units of the industrialized world. As many as 800,000 cases of sepsis are admitted every year to American hospitals (comparable to the incidence of first myocardial infarctions), with half of those developing septic shock (1). Historically, the mortality associated with sepsis and septic shock has been approximately 50% to 75% (2–4). The major advance in the therapy of septic shock was the development of antibiotic therapy 50 years ago, which resulted in a reduction in sepsis-associated mortality in the 30% to 50% range (2,3). However, the past 40 years have seen a gradual year-to-year increase in the incidence of sepsis (5). As a result, total deaths in the United States have increased even though the overall mortality rate has fallen from 27.8% to 17.9% during that period (5). At present, the total death toll from sepsis is comparable to that from myocardial infarction and far exceeds the impact of illnesses such as acquired immune deficiency syndrome (AIDS) or breast cancer (1,6).

The total number of cases continues to gradually increase due to a burgeoning population of patients with a chronic and high degree of susceptibility to infection (age, AIDS, organ failure with transplant, and other chronic illness); an increased use of invasive medical devices; and increased use of cytotoxic agents for autoimmune disease, transplants, and malignancy for patients at high risk for sepsis. Current estimates suggest a doubling of total United States cases by 2050 but with only a projected increase in population of 33% (1). Until recently, despite major advances in technology and constant refinement of our understanding of sepsis pathophysiology, numerous clinical trials have failed to produce any new drugs with consistent beneficial effects on this patient population. Nonetheless, the last 50 years have seen a gradual improvement in mortality, perhaps related to improvements in supportive care (5,7).

DEFINITIONS

Derived from the Greek word "sepo," meaning "I rot," the first introduction of the term *sepsis* occurs in the poems of Homer (circa eighth century B.C.) (8). Over the intervening 2,700 years, through Homer, Hippocrates, Aristotle, and Galen to current-day physicians, the term has continued to be used virtually unchanged in meaning. Hugo Schottmüller modernized the term with his 1914 definition, "Septicemia is a state of microbial invasion from a portal of entry into the blood stream which causes signs of illness" (9). From the time of Schottmüller's definition of septicemia until recent years, terms such as septicemia, sepsis, toxemia, and bacteremia were all used interchangeably to indicate patients exhibiting systemic responses to infection.

A significant problem with the term *septicemia* (as defined by Schottmüller) is that most patients with a septic response cannot be documented to have bacteremia/fungemia, and many with bacteremia/fungemia (e.g., endocarditis, catheter-related infection) do not exhibit overt sepsis. Recognizing that future large-scale clinical trials of novel sepsis therapies will require more consistent and precise definitions of the septic response, consensus definitions were developed in 1991 (10). These criteria were developed primarily as a tool to enhance the ability to perform clinical sepsis research. However, the terminology soon entered the clinical lexicon. These consensus definitions were revised in 2001 to accommodate the clinician's perspective (11). Current and previous definitions follow.

Infection: A microbial phenomenon characterized by an inflammatory response to the presence of micro-organisms or the invasion of normally sterile host tissue by these organisms.

Bacteremia: The presence of viable bacteria in the blood. The presence of other organisms in the blood should be described in like manner—viremia, fungemia, and so on. Bacteremia can either be transient, sustained, or intermittent.

Systemic Inflammatory Response Syndrome (SIRS): The systemic inflammatory response to various severe clinical insults, including but not limited to infection. Various other clinical insults include pancreatitis, ischemia, multiple trauma and tissue injury, hemorrhagic shock, immune-mediated organ injury, and exogenous administration of inflammatory mediators such as tumor necrosis factor or other cytokines. Previous criteria for SIRS are enumerated in Table 57.1. The more recent revision to sepsis definitions removed these SIRS criteria while retaining the concept. However, some understanding of these criteria remains crucial for the intensivist/clinical researcher, as most trials in the last 15 years have been predicated on patients having three or more of these criteria.

Sepsis: The systemic response to infection. This response is similar to SIRS, except that it is considered to result from an infection. The previously accepted definition required at least two of the four SIRS criteria in the presence of documented or suspected infection. The recent revision of the criteria enumerates multiple potential diagnostic criteria for sepsis (Table 57.2) and no longer specifically requires the discarded elements of the SIRS criteria.

Severe Sepsis: Sepsis associated with organ dysfunction, perfusion abnormalities, or hypotension. Organ system dysfunction can be described by organ failure scoring systems (12,13).

Septic Shock: Sepsis with hypotension despite adequate fluid resuscitation, in conjunction with perfusion abnormalities.

TABLE 57.1

DEFINITION OF SYSTEMIC INFLAMMATORY RESPONSE SYNDROME (SIRS)

Systemic inflammatory response syndrome (SIRS): The systemic inflammatory response to a wide variety of severe clinical insults manifests by two or more of the following conditions:

- Temperature greater than 38°C or less than 36°C
- Heart rate greater than 90 beats per minute (bpm)
- Respiratory rate greater than 20 breaths per minute or $PaCO_2$ less than 32 mm Hg
- White blood cell count greater than 12,000/μL, less than 4,000/μL, or 10% immature (band) forms

From Bone R. American College of Chest Physicians/Society of Critical Care Medicine Consensus Conference: definitions for sepsis and organ failure and guidelines for the use of innovative therapies in sepsis. *Crit Care Med.* 1992;20:864–874.

Standard abnormalities in an adult include mean arterial pressure (MAP) <60 mm Hg, systolic blood pressure <90 mm Hg, or a drop in systolic blood pressure >40 mm Hg from baseline.

Multiorgan Dysfunction Syndrome (MODS): The presence of altered organ function in an acutely ill patient, such that homeostasis cannot be maintained without intervention. Primary MODS is the direct result of a well-defined insult in which organ dysfunction occurs early and can be directly attributable to the insult itself. Secondary MODS develops as a consequence of a host response and is identified within the context of SIRS.

The relationship of many of these conditions to each other is demonstrated in Figure 57.1. An understanding of sepsis definitions has become increasingly important since most clinical trials in the last two decades have used the modified version of the 1991 sepsis definitions (usually requiring three rather than two SIRS criteria) in their entry criteria. The concept of a compensatory anti-inflammatory response has also been introduced after the demonstration that traditional anti-inflammatory mediators were also elevated during sepsis (14).

EPIDEMIOLOGY

Although the sepsis syndromes (from sepsis to septic shock) have been a major burden on human health in both the developed and undeveloped world, there has been a surprising dearth of epidemiologic information. In North America, this has been caused by the earlier lack of consensus definitions of these syndromes and, more recently, the absence of syndrome-specific diagnostic codes for sepsis within the International Classification of Disease (ICD) coding system. In the last 20 years, the development of consensus definitions and application of computerized hospital and government administrative databases has allowed substantial insight into the problem.

Martin et al. (5) have estimated 660,000 annual cases of sepsis in the United States during 2000 (adjusted rate 240/100,000 population) using an analysis of ICD-9 codes associated with National Hospital Discharge Survey data. With the exception of a single major study with much higher values (1), estimates for severe sepsis from sites across North America and Europe have been fairly consistent at 50 to 80/100,000 population (15–19). These cases account for approximately 10% to 15% of all intensive care unit (ICU) admissions (16,17,19–21). Approximately 25% of cases of sepsis (22) and 50% to 75% of cases of severe sepsis progress to septic shock (20). Septic

TABLE 57.2

REVISED DIAGNOSTIC CRITERIA FOR SEPSIS

Infection,[a] documented or suspected, and some of the following:

General variables
- Fever (core temerpature >38.3°C)
- Hypothermia (core temperature <36°C)
- Heart rate >90 min or >2 SD above the normal value for age
- Tachypnea
- Altered mental status
- Significant edema or positive fluid balance (>20 mL/kg over 24 h)
- Hyperglycemia (plasma glucose >120 mg/dL or 7.7 mmol/L) in the absence of diabetes

Inflammatory variables
- Leukocytosis (WBC count >12,000 μL)
- Leukopenia (WBC count <4,000 μL)
- Normal WBC count with >10% immature forms
- Plasma C-reactive protein >2 SD above the normal value
- Plasma procalcitonin >2 SD above the normal value

Hemodynamic variables
- Arterial hypotension[b] (SBP <90 mm Hg, MAP <70, or an SBP decrease >40 mm Hg in adults or <2 SD below normal for age)
- SvO_2 >70%[b]
- Cardiac index >3.5 L/min/m^2[b]

Organ dysfunction variables
- Arterial hypoxemia (PaO_2/FiO_2 <300)
- Acute oliguria (urine output <0.5 mL/kg/h or 45 mmol/L for ≥2 h)
- Creatinine increase >0.5 mg/dL
- Coagulation abnormalities (INR >1.5 or aPTT >60 s)
- Ileus (absent bowel sounds)
- Thrombocytopenia (platelet count <100,000 μL)
- Hyperbilirubinemia (plasma total bilirubin >4 mg/dL or 70 mmol/L)

Tissue perfusion variables
- Hyperlactatemia (>1 mmol/L)
- Decreased capillary refill or mottling

WBC, white blood cell; SBP, systolic blood pressure; MAP, mean arterial blood pressure; $S\bar{v}O_2$, mixed venous oxygen saturation; INR, international normalized ratio; aPTT, activated partial thromboplastin time.

[a]Infection defined as a pathologic process induced by a micro-organism.

[b]$S\bar{v}O_2$ sat >70% is normal in children (normally, 75%–80%), and CI 3.5–5.5 is normal in children; therefore, *neither* should be used as signs of sepsis in newborns or children.

From Levy MM, Fink MP, Marshall JC, et al. 2001 SCCM/ESICM/ACCP/ATS/SIS International Sepsis Definitions Conference. *Crit Care Med.* 2003;31(4):1250–1256.

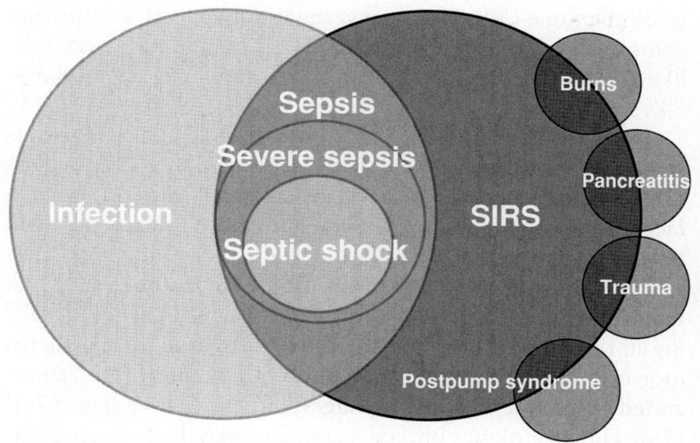

FIGURE 57.1. Venn diagram showing the relationship between infection and other sepsis-associated terms. The intersection of systemic inflammatory response syndrome (SIRS) and infection defines sepsis. Severe sepsis is a subset of sepsis defined by the presence of organ failure. Septic shock is a subset of severe sepsis in which the organ failure is cardiovascular (i.e., shock). Patients with certain inflammatory conditions (e.g., extensive burn injury, pancreatitis, major trauma, postpump syndrome, and so on) may demonstrate a "septic" appearance (i.e. SIRS) without the presence of infection required for a diagnosis of sepsis. (Adapted from Bone R. American College of Chest Physicians/Society of Critical Care Medicine Consensus Conference: definitions for sepsis and organ failure and guidelines for the use of innovative therapies in sepsis. *Crit Care Med.* 1992;20:864–874.)

shock represents between 5% and 8% of all ICU admissions (21,23). In the United States, the cost of sepsis and severe sepsis ranges from $22,000 to $60,000 per episode at a total cost of approximately $17 billion annually (1,24). Sepsis and related conditions are the tenth leading cause of death in the United States (6).

The incidence of sepsis appears to be increasing at a rate of about 9% per year in the United States (5) (Fig. 57.2). Reasons for this increase include the following: (a) An aging population with increased predisposition to illness; (b) increased proportion and longevity of the subpopulation with conditions that predispose to systemic infection including chronic organ failure (e.g., cirrhosis, renal failure, cardiomyopathy, chronic obstructive pulmonary disease [COPD]), and other conditions (e.g., diabetes, cancer, AIDS, etc.); (c) extensive use of invasive diagnostic and therapeutic modalities (indwelling catheters and devices), which lead to breakdown of native resistance to infection; and (d) widespread use of immunosuppressive chemotherapies for a wide range of diseases (asthma, inflammatory bowel disease, rheumatoid arthritis, systemic lupus erythematosus, and other autoimmune diseases).

Age is a substantial risk factor for sepsis, severe sepsis, and septic shock (1,5,25). Patients older than the age of 65 years are approximately 13-fold more likely to develop sepsis compared to others (5). Similarly, septic shock is 18 times more likely in the >80-year age group compared to those in the 20- to 29-year age group (23). Given that the average age of the North American population is increasing, and that the incidence of all the sepsis-related syndromes is markedly elevated in the elderly (23), the fact that the average age of patients with sepsis has climbed over the last few decades can be no surprise (1,5). That septic shock is substantially a geriatric illness is reflected in the median age of 67 years (25). The persistent 60:40 male:female preponderance in sepsis, severe sepsis, and septic shock may have its origins in men's increased predisposition to smoking-associated cases of pneumonia and peptic ulcer disease/gastrointestinal malignancy-associated gastric and bowel perforation (1,5,17,20,22,23). Nonwhite racial groups are also at substantially increased risk, particularly African Americans (5). However, low socioeconomic status is a substantial risk factor for septic shock (a fourfold increased risk in the lowest quintile of income compared to any other quintile) (23). In this context, it is unclear whether race may be relevant only as a marker of socioeconomic status. Comorbidities are common in patients with sepsis, as might be expected given an average age of 55 to 65 years for sepsis and perhaps higher for septic shock (5,19,25–29). Diabetes, COPD, renal failure, congestive heart failure, and malignancy can each be found in 10% to 20% of patients with sepsis or septic shock. At least 50% of patients with severe sepsis have at least one major medical comorbidity (5). Patients with septic shock have an even higher incidence (>90%) of major comorbidities. Alcoholism and substance abuse also substantially increases the risk of sepsis, as well as death from sepsis and septic shock (30).

As might be expected, mortality increases with the severity of the septic syndrome. Mortality is <15% for sepsis, 25% to 50% for severe sepsis, and >50% for septic shock (1,5,15–17,20–22,25,31). This mortality rate for septic shock, while staggering, nevertheless represents an improvement in survival

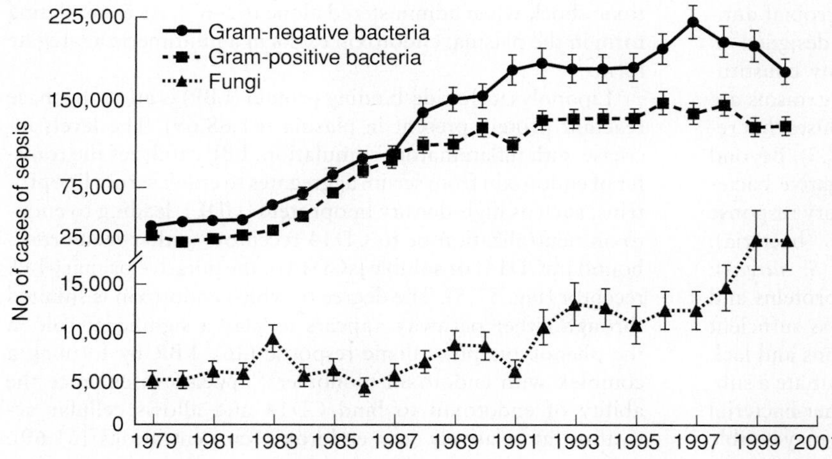

FIGURE 57.2. Incidence of sepsis in the United States stratified by organism group. The incidence of sepsis increased approximately 9% per year between 1979 and 2001 with the greatest relative increase in fungal infections. In addition, as of the late 1980s, Gram-positive pathogens became numerically dominant over Gram-negative organisms. (From Martin GS, Mannino DM, Eaton S, et al. The epidemiology of sepsis in the United States from 1979 through 2000. *N Engl J Med.* 2003;348(16):1546–1554.)

from 35 years ago when mortality rates frequently exceeded 80% (32,33). Early septic mortality (<3 days) appears to be associated most closely with shock with other deaths within the first week due to multiple organ failure. Later deaths tend to be most closely associated with pre-existing comorbidities (34). Of those succumbing to septic shock, approximately 75% are early deaths (within 1 week of shock), primarily due to hyperdynamic circulatory failure (35).

Throughout recorded history, there has been an evolution of the organisms that cause infectious diseases and the associated clinical syndromes. This phenomenon has become particularly pronounced since the advent of antibiotics in the last half of the previous century. By the 1960s and 70s, Gram-negative organisms had become the dominant pathogens over *Staphylococcus aureus* and streptococci. During the 1980s, resistant Gram-positive organisms (methicillin-resistant *S. aureus*, coagulase-negative staphylococci, penicillin-resistant *S. pneumoniae*, and enterococci) again re-emerged as major pathogens. Gram-positive cocci account for approximately 40% to 50% of single isolates (excluding fungi) in sepsis and septic shock (20,25,31,36–38).

Most recently, yeast and other fungi have demonstrated a remarkable increase in their contribution to sepsis (5% of total) and septic shock (8.2% of total), with an increase of about 10% per year (5,25,37,38). *Candida albicans* remains numerically dominant (about 60% of total fungal infections), but fluconazole-resistant yeasts are the most rapidly increasing species (39–41). Other major concerns in recent years include the emergence of vancomycin-resistant enterococci (42), extended spectrum β-lactamase (ESBL) resistance in Gram-negative organisms (reliably sensitive only to carbapenems) (43), and an endemic strain of virulent, methicillin-resistant *S. aureus* in the community (44). In addition, concerns regarding sporadic cases of vancomycin-resistant *S. aureus* (VRSA) are growing (45).

PATHOGENESIS OF SEPSIS, SEVERE SEPSIS, AND SEPTIC SHOCK

Sepsis and septic shock or sepsis-associated multiple organ failure typically begin with a nidus of infection within the body (e.g., pneumonia, peritonitis, urinary tract infection, abscess). Within that nidus, the organism replicates. Eventually, the infection at the inciting focus releases sufficient microbial antigens to elicit a systemic inflammatory response designed to eliminate the invading microbes (Fig. 57.3). Many constitutive and/or inducible elements of invasive microorganisms are capable of inciting the systemic inflammatory responses that result in sepsis and septic shock (Fig. 57.3, Table 57.3). Beyond endotoxin (lipopolysaccharide; LPS) of Gram-negative bacteria, other major triggers of the systemic inflammatory response characteristic of sepsis include various exotoxins (bacteria), peptidoglycans (streptococci), and teichoic acid (*S. aureus*); lipoarabinomannan of mycobacteria; and mannoproteins and β-glucan of fungi (46). Bacterial DNA may possess sufficient antigenic properties (based on unique CG repetitions and lack of deoxyribonucleic acid [DNA] methylation) to initiate a substantial inflammatory response independent of other bacterial elements (47–49). Bacterial ribonucleic acid (RNA) may be able to do the same (50). Recent investigations suggest a surprising commonality of signaling mechanisms in septic shock via Toll-like receptors from a broad range of etiologic agents (48,51–54).

Despite the large number of potential elements of pathogenic microorganisms that can drive the septic response, endotoxin of Gram-negative bacteria remains the prototype of such factors and the model for subsequent research. This antigen is thought to be central in initiating the powerful host response to infection with these organisms (55). LPS and other antigens interact with immune cells (particularly macrophages), resulting in the induction of proinflammatory cytokines such as tumor necrosis factor-α (TNF-α) and interleukin-1β (IL-1β) secreted by monocytes, macrophages, and other cells (Fig. 57.3) (56). These cytokines initiate a complex signaling sequence involving the release of secondary mediators (platelet-activating factor, leukotrienes, prostaglandins) and monocytes, as well as endothelial tissue factor expression, inducible nitric oxide synthetase induction, microvascular coagulation, cell-adhesion molecule up-regulation, and apoptosis (57–60). To maintain homeostasis (and likely as part of a feedback mechanism), several anti-inflammatory mediators are also released, including interleukin-10 (IL-10), transforming growth factor-β (TGFβ), and interleukin-1 receptor antagonist (IL-1ra). If homeostasis cannot be maintained, progressive and sequential dysfunction of various organ systems (i.e., MODS) may occur. If the inflammatory stimulus is particularly intense, or if there is limited cardiovascular reserve, effects on the cardiovascular system as manifested by septic shock may dominate the clinical presentation.

Microbial Antigen Signaling

As the prototypical and best-studied microbial antigen, an understanding of the signaling cascade of endotoxin is instructive. Endotoxin is an amphiphilic macromolecule located on the outer cell wall membrane of Gram-negative bacteria. It is composed of lipid A (a diglucosamine-based acylated phospholipid), and a polysaccharide side chain (61,62) (Fig. 57.4). The polysaccharide chain is composed of a short, highly conserved, proximal section (core polysaccharide) and a highly variable, longer distal oligosaccharide side chain. The core polysaccharide and lipid A are sometimes referred to as the *core glycolipid*. The highly conserved lipid A moiety is the toxic element of endotoxin and can reproduce the manifestations of endotoxic shock when administered alone (62–67). As a circulating form in the plasma, endotoxin exists in a multimeric aggregate form.

Lipopolysaccharide-binding protein (LBP) is an acute phase reactant protein present in plasma (61,68,69). The levels increase with inflammatory stimulation. LBP catalyzes the transfer of endotoxin from serum aggregates to either serum lipoproteins, such as high-density lipoprotein (HDL), leading to endotoxin neutralization or to CD14 receptors (either membrane-bound [mCD14] or soluble [sCD14]), the putative primary LPS receptor (Fig. 57.5). The degree to which endotoxin is shunted through either pathway appears to play a significant role in the phenotypic physiologic response (46). LBP, by forming a complex with endotoxin monomers, appears to enhance the ability of endotoxin to bind CD14 and allows cellular activation at relatively low endotoxin concentrations (61,69).

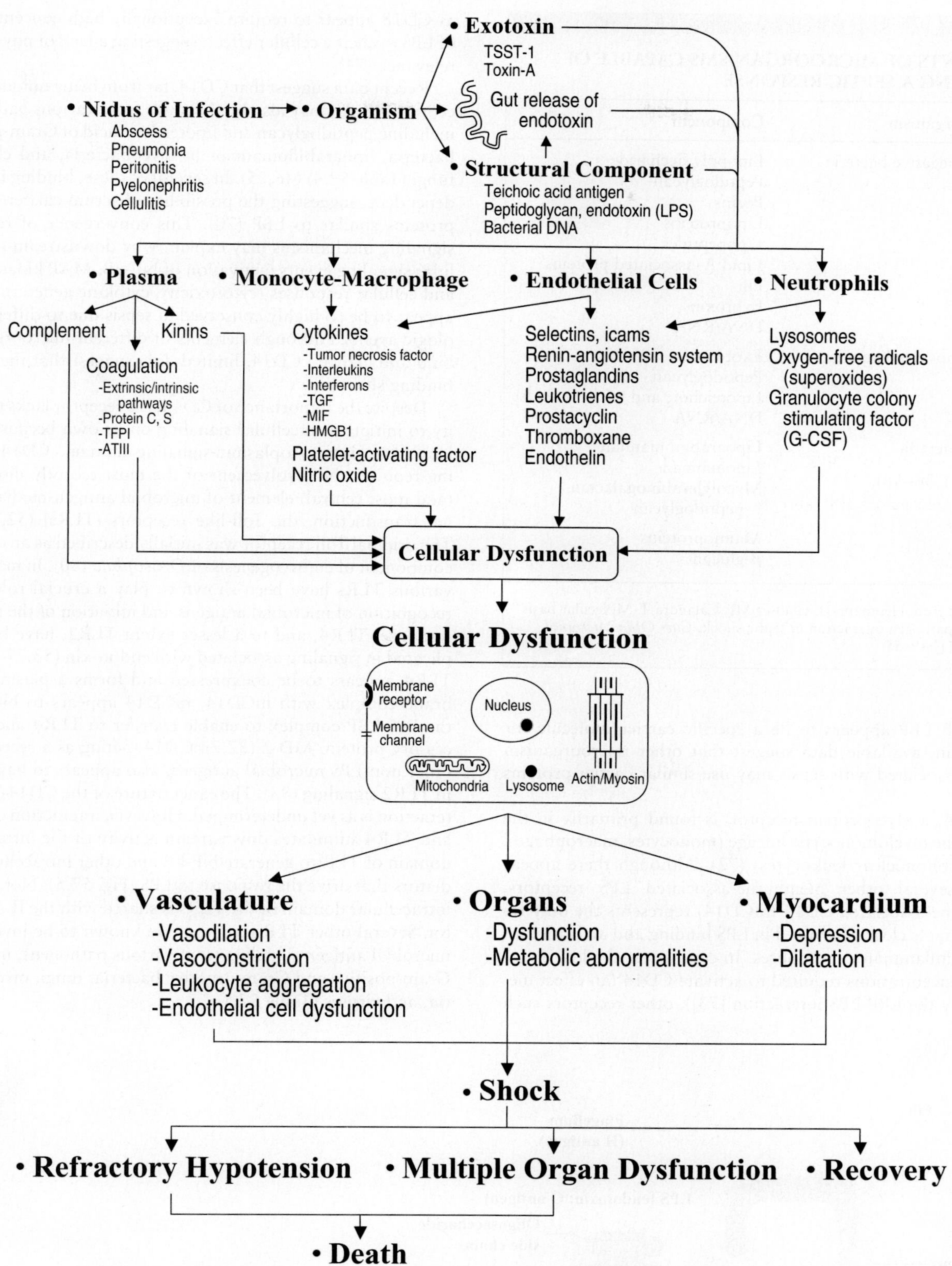

FIGURE 57.3. Pathogenesis of sepsis and septic shock. ATIII, antithrombin III; DNA, deoxyribonucleic acid; HMGB1, high mobility group box 1 protein; LPS, lipopolysaccharide; MIF, macrophage migration inhibitory factor; TFPI, tissue factor pathway inhibitor; TGF, transforming growth factor; Toxin A, *Pseudomonas* toxin A; TSST-1, toxic shock syndrome toxin 1. (Adapted from Parrillo JE. Pathogenic mechanisms of septic shock. *N Engl J Med.* 1993;328:1471–1477.)

TABLE 57.3

ELEMENTS OF MICROORGANISMS CAPABLE OF INDUCING A SEPTIC RESPONSE

Microorganism	Component
Gram-negative bacteria	Lipopolysaccharide Peptidoglycan Porins Lipoproteins Lipopeptides Lipid A–associated proteins Pili Exotoxins DNA/RNA
Gram-positive bacteria	Exotoxins Peptidoglycan Lipoteichoic and teichoic acids DNA/RNA
Mycobacteria	Lipoarabinomannan Lipomannan Mycolylarabinogalactan-peptidoglycan
Fungi	Mannoproteins β-glucan

Adapted from Heumann D, Glauser MP, Calandra T. Molecular basis of host-pathogen interaction in septic shock. *Curr Opin Microbiol.* 1998; 1(1):49–55.

Although LBP appears to be a specific carrier molecule for endotoxin, available data suggest that other microorganism toxins associated with sepsis may use similar carrier proteins (70,71).

CD14, a glycoprotein receptor, is found primarily in the cells of the myelomonocytic lineage (monocytes, macrophages, polymorphonuclear leukocytes) (72). Although there appear to be several other membrane-associated LPS receptors, membrane-associated CD14 (mCD14) represents the only receptor that is clearly involved in LPS binding and activation of cellular inflammatory responses. In contrast to the low endotoxin concentrations required to activate CD14 (an effect mediated by the LBP-LPS interaction [73]), other receptors such as CD18 appear to require exceptionally high concentrations of LPS to elicit a cellular effect, suggesting a lack of physiologic relevance (74).

Recent data suggest that CD14, far from being uniquely a receptor for LPS, may also bind ligands from various pathogens, including peptidoglycan and lipoteichoic acid of Gram-positive bacteria, lipoarabinomannan of mycobacteria, and chitin of fungi (Table 57.4) (46,75). In several of these, binding is serum dependent, suggesting the possibility of serum carrier/binding proteins similar to LBP (70). This convergence of receptor-signaling mechanisms may explain why downstream intracellular signaling events (activation of NF-κB, MAP kinases, etc.) and cellular responses (cytotoxicity, cytokine generation, etc.) appear to be so highly conserved in sepsis due to different etiologic agents. Although elements of different microorganisms bind and activate CD14, limited data suggest that the precise binding sites vary.

Despite the importance of CD14, the receptor lacks the ability to initiate intracellular signaling on its own because of the lack of an intracytoplasmic-signaling domain. CD14 signaling requires the involvement of the most recently discovered (and most central) element of microbial antigen-mediated signal transduction, the Toll-like receptors (TLRs) (52,76–79). The original Toll receptor was initially described as an essential component of embryogenesis of *Drosophila* (80). In mammals, various TLRs have been shown to play a crucial role in the recognition of microbial antigens and initiation of the immune response. TLR4, and to a lesser extent TLR2, have been implicated in signaling associated with endotoxin (53,77–79,81). TLR4 appears to be coexpressed and forms a plasma membrane complex with mCD14. mCD14 appears to bind with the LPS/LBP complex to enable transfer to TLR4 and an accessory protein, MD-2 (82). mCD14, acting as a receptor for other non-LPS microbial antigens, also appears to have a role in TLR2 signaling (83). The exact nature of the CD14-TLR interaction is as yet undetermined. However, interaction of CD14 and TLR4 stimulates downstream activity of the intracellular domain of TLR to generate NF-kB and other intracellular mediators that drive the response to LPS (Fig. 57.5). Notably, the intracellular domain of the TLRs is shared with the IL-1 receptor. Several other TLR receptors are known to be involved in microbial antigen signaling from various pathogens, including Gram-positive and Gram-negative bacteria, fungi, mycobacteria, and viruses (Table 57.5).

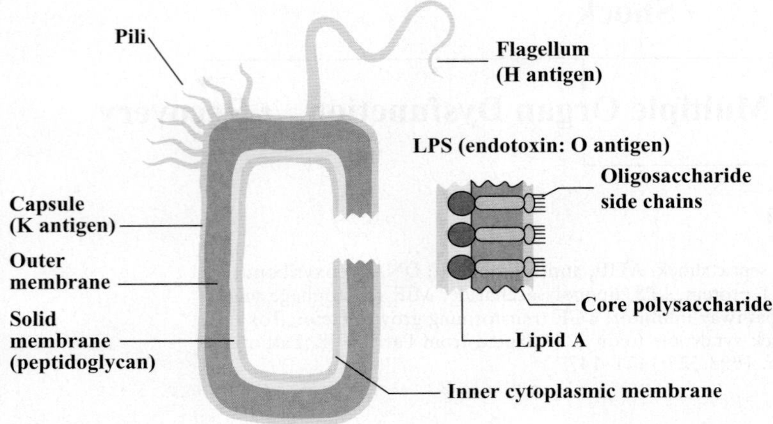

FIGURE 57.4. Endotoxin (lipopolysaccharide). Endotoxin is a component of the cell wall of Gram-negative bacilli. (From Young LS, Martin WJ, Meyer RD, et al. Gram-negative rod bacteremia: microbiologic, immunologic, and therapeutic considerations. *Ann Intern Med.* 1977;86:456–471, with permission.)

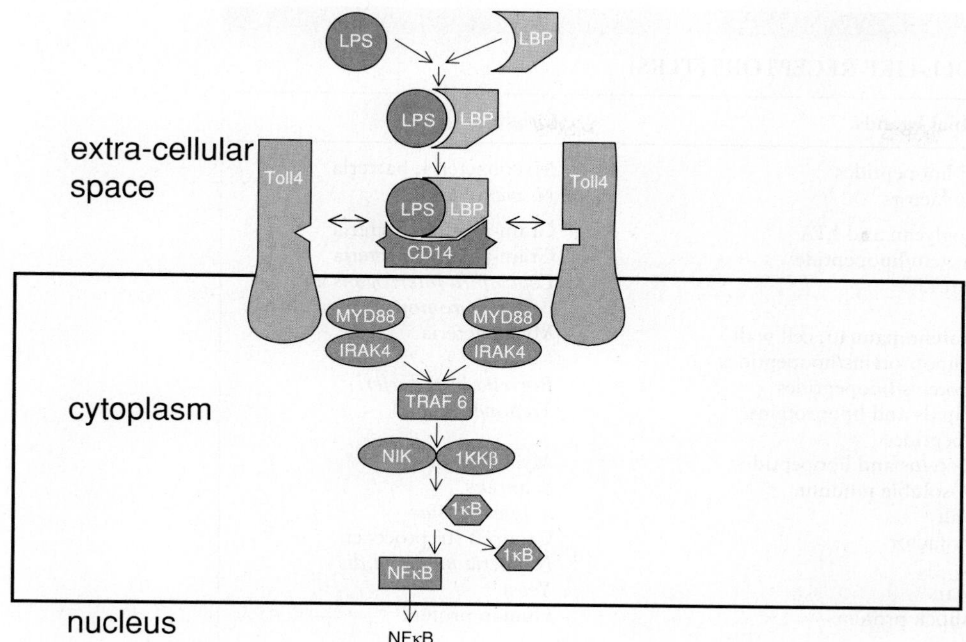

FIGURE 57.5. Endotoxin signaling pathway related to CD14 and TLR4 (Toll-like receptor 4). IκB, inhibitory κB; IKK, IκB kinase; IRAK, IL-1R–associated kinase; LBP, lipopolysaccharide-binding protein; LPS, lipopolysaccharide; MYD88, myeloid differentiation factor; NFκB, nuclear factor-κB; NIK, nuclear factor κB–inducing kinase; TRAF 6, tumor necrosis factor receptor associated factor.

Besides the Toll-like receptor pathways, other important routes of microbial antigen signaling exist. In particular, some Gram-positive organisms produce potent exotoxins that are implicated in the pathogenesis of toxic shock syndromes. These include the toxic shock syndrome toxin-1 associated with staphylococcal toxic shock and pyrogenic toxins predominantly associated with group A streptococci. These exotoxins appear to be superantigens in that they are able to activate broad polyclonal groups of lymphocytes, resulting in massive cytokine generation and toxic shock (84,85).

Cytokines

The concept of a systemic inflammatory response syndrome (SIRS) has already been discussed in the context of sepsis. The notion of an innate anti-inflammatory response, termed *compensatory anti-inflammatory response syndrome* (CARS), during sepsis also exists (14). This model suggests that a clinical insult (such as infection or injury) initiates a proinflammatory response that is countered by an endogenous anti-inflammatory reaction. The aggregate responses produce endogenous circulating mediators (cytokines, soluble receptors, adhesion molecules, growth factors, eicosanoids, etc.), generating systemic phenomena such as septic shock or immunosuppression. Clinical manifestations and patient outcome are dependent on the balance between proinflammatory and anti-inflammatory elements. The predominance of the inflammatory response corresponds to SIRS and may lead to cardiovascular compromise, shock, and organ dysfunction. However, a predominance of anti-inflammatory mediators produces a state of immune paralysis associated with a propensity to infection and inability to fight infection. Both may ultimately lead to death. In patients with sepsis, the duration of monocyte inactivation (a potential manifestation of CARS) correlates with mortality (86). If the counterinflammatory response is able to balance the inflammatory stimuli (while the infecting micro-organism is effectively cleared), homeostasis is achieved and clinical recovery will occur. In this model, sepsis has a dynamic nature based on the development and balance of the above-described responses (Fig. 57.6). This interplay is influenced by the nature of the inflammatory injury and the genetically determined variability of the host immune response (87,88).

Proinflammatory cytokines have multiple effects, including the stimulation of production and release of other proinflammatory mediators. TNF-α, interleukin-1β (IL-1β), and interleukin-6 (IL-6) are the best known proinflammatory cytokines and have overlapping and synergistic effects in stimulating the inflammatory cascade. The next phase in the cytokine response to infection is the endogenous counterinflammatory cascade in response to the systemic activity of proinflammatory cytokines. Cytokine inhibitors (e.g., IL-1 receptor antagonist [IL-1ra], soluble TNF receptor) and anti-inflammatory cytokines (e.g., TGFβ, IL-4, IL-10, and IL-13) are involved in this phase of the response. Other cytokines like HMGB1 may be involved even later in the syndrome. Thus, the cytokine network in sepsis involves proinflammatory cytokines,

TABLE 57.4

CD14 BINDING-CAPABLE MICROBIAL PRODUCTS

Ligands	Origin
Lipopolysaccharide	Gram-negative bacteria
Peptidoglycan	Gram-positive bacteria
Lipoteichoic acid	Gram-positive bacteria
Lipoarabinomannan	*Mycobacterium tuberculosis*
Rhamnose-glucose polymers	Streptococcus species
Polyuronic acids	Bacteria
Acylpolygalactoside	*Klebsiella pneumoniae*
Chitin	Yeast
Amphiphilic molecules	*Staphylococcus aureus*

TABLE 57.5

MICROBIAL LIGANDS OF THE TOLL-LIKE RECEPTORS (TLRS)

Receptor	Microbial ligands	Origin
TLR1	Triacyl lipopeptides	Mycobacteria, bacteria
	Soluble factors	*N. meningitidis*
TLR2	Peptidoglycan and LTA	Gram-positive bacteria
	Lipoprotein/lipopeptide	Gram-positive bacteria
	Atypical LPS	*Leptospira interrogans* and *Porphyromonas gingivalis*
	Lipoarabinomannan, cell wall and lipoproteins/lipopeptides	Mycobacteria
	Lipoproteins/lipopeptides	*Borrelia burgdorferi*
	Glycolipids and lipoproteins/ lipopeptides	*Treponema* spp.
	Lipoproteins and lipopeptides	*Mycoplasma* spp.
	Phenol-soluble modulin	*S. aureus*
	Cell wall	*S. pneumoniae*
	Soluble factor	Group B streptococci
	Porins	*Neisseria meningitidis*
	Zymosan	Yeast
	Heat shock protein	Human protein
TLR3	dsRNA	Virus
TLR4	LPS	Gram-negative bacteria
	LTA	Gram-positive bacteria
	Heat-sensitive compound	Mycobacteria
	Heat shock protein	*Chlamydia pneumoniae*
	Fusion protein	Respiratory syncytial virus
	Glycolipids	*Treponema brennaborense*
	Heat shock protein	Human protein
	Heat shock protein	Human protein
TLR5	Flagellin	Bacteria with flagella
TLR6	Diacyl lipopeptides	Mycoplasma
	Lipoteichoic acid	Gram-positive bacteria
	Zymosan	Fungi
TLR7	ssRNA	Virus
TLR8	ssRNA	Virus
TLR9	CpG DNA	Bacteria
TLR10	Unknown	Unknown
TLR11	Unknown	Unknown

LTA, lipoteichoic acid; LPS, lipopolysaccharide; dsRNA, double-stranded RNA; ssRNA, single-stranded RNA.
Adapted from Leaver SK, Finney SJ, Burke-Gaffney A, et al. Sepsis since the discovery of Toll-like receptors: disease concepts and therapeutic opportunities. *Crit Care Med.* 2007;35(5):1404–1410; and Van Amersfoort ES, Van Berkel TJ, Kuiper J, et al. Receptors, mediators, and mechanisms involved in bacterial sepsis and septic shock. *Clin Micro Rev.* 2003;16(3):379–414.

anti-inflammatory cytokines, and cytokine inhibitors (Table 57.6). It is the balance between these cytokines at different time points that determine the clinical manifestations and outcome of sepsis.

Nitric Oxide

Another important mediator, nitric oxide (NO), has a vital role in normal intracellular signal transduction (89). NO is synthesized by a family of enzymes called NO synthases (NOS) that incorporate nitrogen from one of the guanidine terminals of L-arginine with molecular oxygen to form NO and L-citrulline. Three distinct nitric oxide synthases have been purified, cloned, and characterized: (i) Neuronal NOS or nNOS, (ii) inducible NOS or iNOS, and (iii) endothelial NOS or eNOS, reflecting the cell types from which they were originally identified.

NO has several important roles in infection, sepsis, and septic shock. The iNOS gene is induced in immunoactivated cells. NO formed by these cells plays a role in host defense against bacterial, viral, and protozoan infections. Of particular importance in relation to septic shock, nitric oxide is the mediator through which endothelial cells normally cause relaxation of adjacent smooth muscle (89). Endothelial cells, through eNOS,

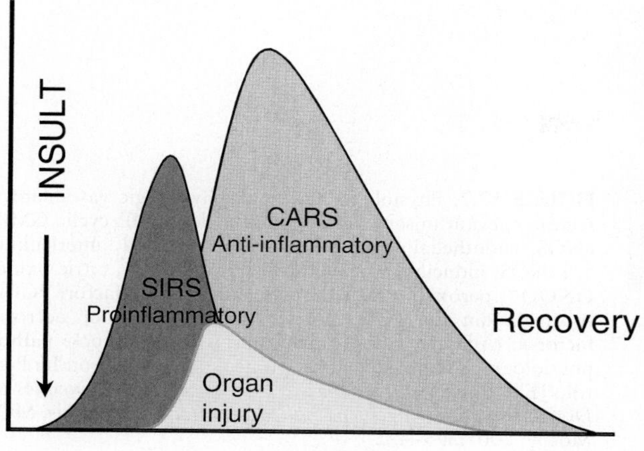

FIGURE 57.6. The dynamic cytokine inflammatory response. Sepsis is associated with an early transient dominance of proinflammatory cytokines corresponding to the systemic inflammatory response syndrome (SIRS) and the onset of organ damage. After this initial phase, the anti-inflammatory pathways of CARS (compensatory anti-inflammatory response syndrome) become active with the development of a refractory state characterized by a decreased capacity of mononuclear cells to produce proinflammatory cytokines. Recovery occurs if homeostasis is re-established. (Adapted from van der Poll T, van Deventer SJ. Cytokines and anticytokines in the pathogenesis of sepsis. *Infect Dis Clin North Am.* 1999;13(2):413–426.).

produce picomolar quantities of nitric oxide in response to several vasodilatory stimuli such as shear stress, acetylcholine, and bradykinin. This nitric oxide diffuses to adjacent smooth muscle and activates guanylate cyclase to produce cyclic GMP, which effects vascular relaxation. Activity of endothelial NOS is regulated and is calcium and calmodulin dependent.

During septic shock, an iNOS capable of producing nanomolar quantities of nitric oxide is generated in endothelium and vascular smooth muscle (89,90). Following this generation, the activity of this iNOS is unregulated and constant. Nitric oxide–mediated generation of cyclic guanosine monophosphate (cGMP) explains the profound loss of arterial vascular tone and venodilatation seen in septic shock (90,91) and may, in part, explain the irreversible vascular collapse seen late in hemorrhagic shock (92) (Fig. 57.7). A potential role for NO in inflammation-associated edema and third-spacing during shock has also been suggested (93). The *in vitro* myocardial depressant effects of TNF-α, IL-1β, and serum from septic humans may be mediated by a similar NO- and cGMP-dependent pathway (94,95). TNF-α, IL-1β, and IFN-γ have been identified as key mediators of iNOS activation. An alternative pathway by which NO may play a role in the cardiovascular pathophysiology of shock and sepsis involves the production of peroxynitrite ($ONOO^-$), a highly reactive oxidant, from the interaction of superoxide (OH^-) and nitric oxide (NO^-) (96).

HEMOSTASIS

The coagulation cascade represents a highly conserved antimicrobial defense mechanism common to even the most primitive complex organisms, such as the *Limulus* horseshoe crab. The hemolymph of the horseshoe crab, one of the oldest complex organisms still in existence, clots rapidly in response to minute quantities of endotoxin or beta-(1,3) glucan, a component of fungi. Pathogens are immobilized in the clot, allowing subsequent elimination (97,98). This commonality of purpose and function of the coagulation and inflammatory systems in eliminating invading microbes has persisted in evolution to present-day mammals including humans (99). These systems, in sharing common activation pathways, are inextricably linked.

Although both these systems are normally highly adaptive in nature, excessive activity of the coagulation and inflammation pathways can result in vascular injury, aberrant tissue blood flow, tissue damage, and, ultimately, organ dysfunction. Recent clinical and laboratory investigations have established that, in conjunction with the cytokine cascade, the coagulation system plays a key role in inflammatory states such as sepsis (100–102) (Fig. 57.8). A critical process in sepsis-induced coagulopathy is the activation of the extrinsic pathway (100).

During the normal hemostatic response, exposure of blood to nonvascular cell-bound tissue factor in the subendothelial layer initiates the extrinsic pathway through the binding of tissue factor to activated factor VII. The resulting enzyme complex, in turn, activates factor IX of the intrinsic pathway and factor X of the common pathway. With factor V as a cofactor,

TABLE 57.6

MAJOR PROINFLAMMATORY AND ANTI-INFLAMMATORY CYTOKINES AND RECEPTORS IN SEPSIS

Proinflammatory cytokines	Anti-inflammatory cytokines	Cytokine inhibitors
Tumor necrosis factor-α (TNF-α)	Transforming growth factor (TGF-β)	Soluble TNF receptors - Type I - Type II
Interleukin-1β (IL-1β)	Interleukin-4 (IL-4)	Interleukin-1 receptor antagonist (IL-1ra)
Interleukin-2 (IL-2)	Interleukin-6 (IL-6)	
Interleukin-6 (IL-6)	Interleukin-8 (IL-8)	
Interleukin-12 (IL-12)	Interleukin-9 (IL-9)	
Interferon-γ (IFN-γ)	Interleukin-10 (IL-10)	
Macrophage migration inhibitory factor (MIF)	Interleukin-11 (IL-11)	
High mobility group 1 protein (HMG-1)	Interleukin-13 (IL-13)	

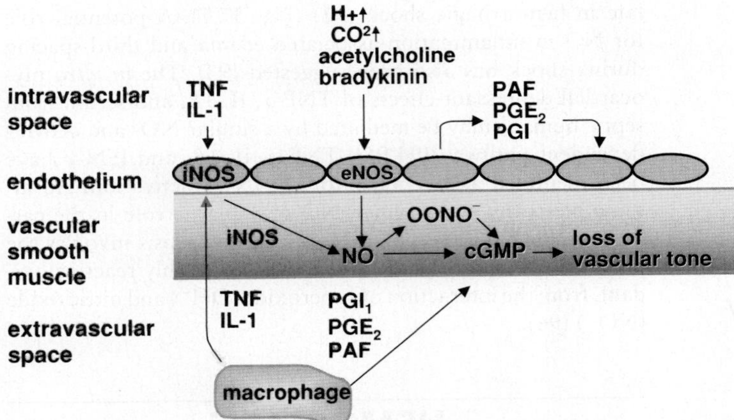

FIGURE 57.7. Physiologic and pathophysiologic vasodilatory factors relevant in sepsis and septic shock. cGMP, cyclic GMP; eNOS, endothelial nitric oxide synthetase; IL-1, interleukin-1β; iNOS, inducible nitric oxide synthetase; NO, nitric oxide; $ONOO^-$, peroxynitrite; PAF, platelet-activating factor; PGE_2, prostaglandin E_2; PGI_1, prostacyclin; TNF, tumor necrosis factor-α. (Adapted from Kumar A, Parrillo JE. Shock: pathophysiology, classification and approach to management. In: Parrillo JE, Dellinger RP, eds. *Critical Care Medicine: Principles of Diagnosis and Management in the Adult*. 3rd ed. St. Louis, MO: Mosby; 2007:379–422.)

activated factor X cleaves prothrombin to form thrombin. Thrombin then converts fibrinogen to fibrin, which results in clot formation (103).

In sepsis, however, the expression of tissue factor is either directly or indirectly induced by inflammatory cytokines. Overexpression of proinflammatory cytokines, such as TNF-α, IL-1β, and interleukin-8, are thought to upset the balance toward a procoagulant state (60,101,104) (Fig. 57.8). TNF-α and IL-1β, for example, can induce the expression of tissue factor in circulating monocytes and endothelial cells (101). The vascular endothelial injury resulting from inflammation can also further expose tissue factor in subendothelial tissue and perivascular cells. Endothelial injury also inhibits the production and activity of anticoagulants such as proteins C and S, the heparin–antithrombin complex, and thrombomodulin. Loss of native anticoagulant function is indicated by decreased activity and circulating levels of protein C (105,106), antithrombin III, (ATIII) (101,106), and tissue factor pathway inhibitor (TFPI) (107,108) in patients with severe sepsis and septic shock.

Current evidence suggests that the pathogenesis of sepsis is associated with (a) systemic activation of coagulation resulting in consumption of coagulant factors, (b) suppression of the anticoagulant system by the same proinflammatory mediators that activate coagulation, and (c) early activation followed by later suppression of fibrinolysis (60,101) (Fig. 57.8). Whereas the coagulation cascade is clearly activated in sepsis, the specific inciting events and the molecular linkages between inflammation and coagulation remain to be elucidated (60,101–103). Given observational studies demonstrating the depletion of anticoagulant factors (decreased activity levels of protein C [60,102], ATIII [101,103], and TFPI [28]) in patients with severe sepsis and septic shock, such markers may be useful to indicate the presence or severity of sepsis in the future.

HOST GENETIC FACTORS

Although the characteristics of the pathogen have much to do with the occurrence of clinical infection and progression to sepsis and septic shock, a growing body of data suggests that genomic variations between patients are equally important. These genomic variations in microbial and cell signaling, innate immunity, and coagulation and inflammatory stress cytokine responses appear to explain individual variations in susceptibility to infection, sepsis/septic shock, and septic death. They likely explain why identical organisms cause fulminant disease

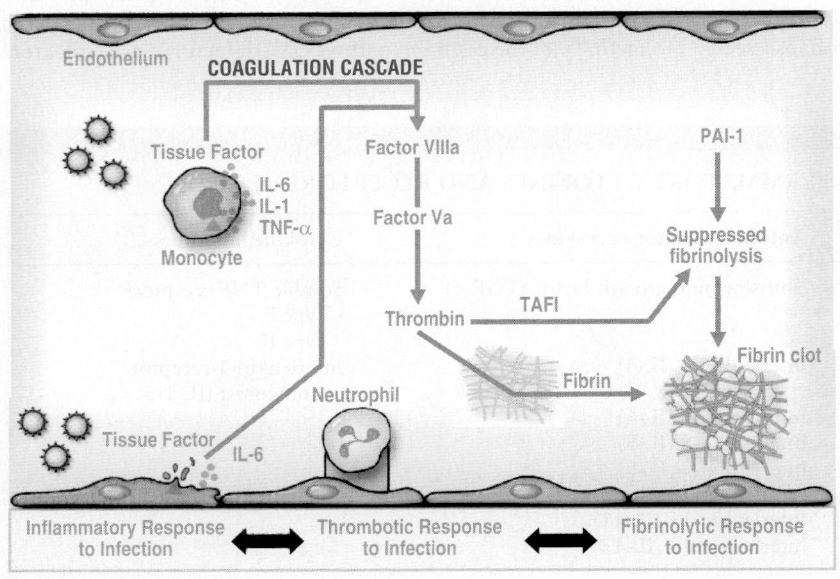

FIGURE 57.8. Cytokines induce the endothelial cell to shift from an antithrombotic to a prothrombotic phenotype. Expression of tissue factor by monocytes, and perhaps a subset of endothelial cells, initiates coagulation through the extrinsic system in patients with severe sepsis and septic shock. At the same time, fibrinolysis is inhibited through the release of thrombin-activatable fibrinolysis inhibitor (TAFI) and plasminogen activator inhibitor-1 (PAI-1). IL-1, interleukin-1β; IL-6, interleukin-6; TNF-α, tumor necrosis factor-α. (Copyright © 2002 Eli Lilly and Company. All rights reserved. Printed with permission. Permission to reproduce the copyrighted material must be obtained from Lilly prior to reproducing or using the image.)

TABLE 57.7

HUMAN GENETIC MARKERS ASSOCIATED WITH RISK OF INFECTION AND SEPSIS/SEPTIC SHOCK

Gene product group/ Gene product	Infection/sepsis association
Pattern Recognition Receptors	
TLR2	■ Tuberculosis
	■ Life-threatening bacterial infections
	■ *S. aureus* infections
TLR4	■ Gram-negative infection
	■ Septic shock
TLR5	■ *Legionella* infection
CD14	■ Septic shock and septic shock mortality
	■ Isolation of pathogenic bacteria in infection
Mannose-binding lectin	■ Bacterial infections
	■ Isolation of pathogenic bacteria in infection
Intracellular Proteins	
IRAK4	■ Recurrent Gram-positive infections
Cytokines	
TNF-α	■ Sepsis, septic shock, septic mortality
	■ Meningococcal mortality
TNF-β	■ Sepsis and septic mortality
IL-6	■ Septic mortality
IL-10	■ Sepsis and septic mortality
	■ CAP severity and mortality
	■ Pneumococcal septic shock
IFNγ	■ Infection
MIF	■ Sepsis and sepsis-induced acute lung injury
IL-1Ra	■ Sepsis and septic mortality
Coagulation Factors	
PAI-1	■ Meningococcal sepsis, septic shock, septic mortality, vascular complications
	■ Septic mortality
Protein C	■ Septic organ dysfunction and mortality
TAFI	■ Meningococcal and septic mortality
Fibrinogen-β	■ Septic mortality
Factor 5 (Leiden)	■ Septic mortality, pressor use, purpura fulminans

CD, cluster differentiation; IFN, interferon; IL, interleukin; IL-1Ra, IL-1 receptor antagonist; IRAK, interleukin-1 receptor-associated kinase; MIF, macrophage inhibitor factor; PAI, plasminogen activator inhibitor; TAFI, thrombin activatable fibrinolysis inhibitor; TLR, toll-like receptor; TNF, tumor necrosis factor.
Adapted from Arcaroli J, Fessler MB, Abraham E, et al. Genetic polymorphisms and sepsis. *Shock.* 2005;24(4):300–312; Lin MT, Albertson TE, Lin MT, et al. Genomic polymorphisms in sepsis. *Crit Care Med.* 2004;32(2):569–579; Texereau J, Pene F, Chiche JD, et al. Importance of hemostatic gene polymorphisms for susceptibility to and outcome of severe sepsis. *Crit Care Med.* 2004;32(5 Suppl):S313–S319; and Papathanassoglou ED, Giannakopoulou MD, Bozas E, et al. Genomic variations and susceptibility to sepsis. *AACN Adv Crit Care.* 2006;17(4):394–422.

with septic shock in some but only minimal clinical illness in others. The importance of inheritable elements in susceptibility and mortality risk of life-threatening infections is demonstrated by adopted twin studies which demonstrated remarkable convergence in the causes of death (including sepsis/infection) of such individuals (109).

The advent of complete gene mapping via high throughput analysis techniques (e.g., microarray gene chips, etc.) have resulted in a rapid expansion of the list of human genetic markers associated with risk of infection, sepsis/septic shock, and death. These markers fall into several broad groups, including those involved with microbial ligand binding, intracellular signaling, cytokine generation, and coagulation factor generation/activity as described in Table 57.7. It should be noted that some genetic polymorphisms may be linked to other genetic loci. An association between a given polymorphism and susceptibility to infection, sepsis, septic shock, or septic death does not always imply a direct causal relationship.

BIOENERGETIC FAILURE

The underlying metabolic defect in sepsis and septic shock has been the source of substantial controversy over the last 30 years. Most forms of shock are associated with low cardiac output (CO) and tissue hypoperfusion leading to overt tissue

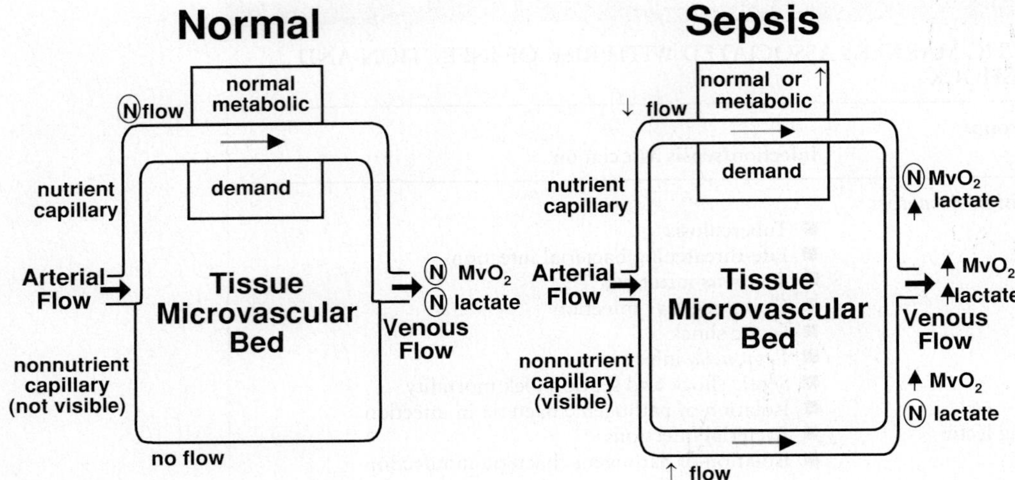

FIGURE 57.9. Microanatomic shunting in sepsis and septic shock. One explanation of the increased lactatic acidosis and MvO_2 found in septic shock is the potential presence of opening of nonnutrient blood vessels between the arterial and venous vascular beds. MvO_2, mixed venous oxygen saturation.

ischemia. This results in anaerobic glycolysis with intracellular acidosis, increased lactate, and high-energy phosphate depletion in the affected tissues. Blood oxygen extraction ratio (the ratio of oxygen consumed divided by the oxygen delivered) is increased as tissues maximize oxygen extraction in order to maintain oxygen consumption. During septic shock, the same tissue metabolic phenomenon of intracellular acidosis and increased lactate production is noted. However, cardiac output and total tissue perfusion is typically increased, and the oxygen extraction ratio falls. The explanation for tissue acidosis and lactate production in septic shock in the presence of tissue hyperperfusion is unknown.

Loss of vascular autoregulatory control may explain some of the typical metabolic findings of sepsis and septic shock. An early theory postulated the existence of microanatomic shunts between the arterial and venous circulations (110) (Fig. 57.9). During sepsis, these shunts were said to result in decreased systemic vascular resistance (SVR) and increased mixed venous oxygen saturation (MvO_2) (111). The resultant decrease in perfusion to tissue beds with normal or even increased metabolic demand could generate tissue ischemia and lactic acid. However, whereas microanatomic shunting has been noted in localized areas of inflammation, systemic evidence of this phenomenon in sepsis and septic shock is lacking (111–115). Another theory involving "functional" shunting due to defects of microcirculatory regulation in sepsis has also been proposed (Fig. 57.10) (116,117). Overperfusion of tissues with low metabolic requirements would result in increased MvO_2

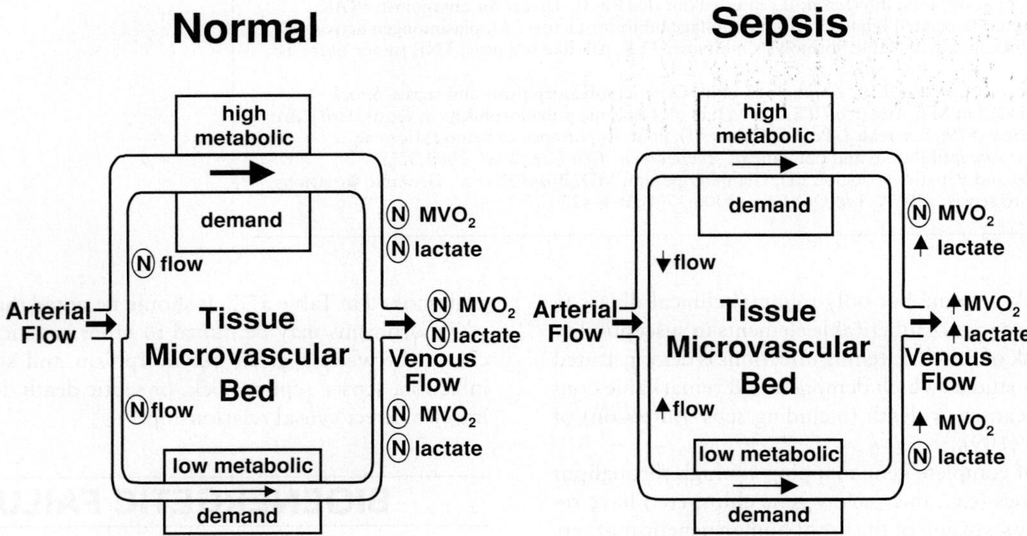

FIGURE 57.10. Functional shunting in sepsis and septic shock. Loss of ability to appropriately regulate microvascular flow according to tissue metabolic demand can lead to overperfusion of low-metabolic-demand tissue beds resulting in increased MvO_2 (mixed venous oxygen saturation). Underperfusion of high-metabolic-demand beds can result in tissue ischemia, anaerobic metabolism, and lactic acidosis.

and narrowing of the arteriovenous oxygen content difference. The relative vasoconstriction of vessels supplying more metabolically active tissues would result in tissue hypoxia and lactate production due to anaerobic metabolism. Observations that some capillary beds may be occluded by platelet microaggregates, leukocytes, fibrin deposits, and endothelial damage support this theory (112,116,118). Additional support comes from studies that demonstrate evidence of supply-dependent oxygen consumption in sepsis (119–123). Both of these theories of the metabolic defect of energy metabolism in sepsis and septic shock fall within the category of "stagnant" hypoxia as described by Barcroft in 1920 (124).

A third theory of the metabolic presentation of sepsis and septic shock suggests that circulating mediators cause an intracellular metabolic defect involving substrate use. This results in bioenergetic failure with high-energy phosphate (adenosine triphosphate [ATP] and phosphocreatine) depletion and lactate production (125–127). Increased mixed venous oxygen saturation could then be explained by perfusion, which is maintained in excess of tissue oxygen use capability. This phenomenon has been termed *histotoxic* (124) or *cytopathic* (127) hypoxia. Potential mechanisms to explain this form of hypoxia include impairment/ inactivation of pyruvate dehydrogenase; nitric oxide or peroxynitrite-mediated inhibition of mitochondrial respiration; uncoupling of oxidative phosphorylation or activation of poly-(ADP-ribosyl)-polymerase (PARP) (127). Observations demonstrating preservation of tissue PO_2 (128), absence of tissue hypoxia (129), and impairment of mitochondrial function (127,130–132) during sepsis and septic shock support this possibility.

In particular, near-infrared spectroscopy (NIRS) has been used to examine mitochondrial function in a primate model of septic shock using live *Escherichia coli* infusion. NIRS demonstrated the presence of mitochondrial dysfunction in skeletal muscle in animals with experimentally induced sepsis. This was manifested by the impairment of oxidation of cytochrome a,a3 with reperfusion after transient ischemia in septic animals compared to controls (131). Another primate study demonstrated early disturbance of mitochondrial redox state in skeletal muscle and brain in the presence of live *E. coli* bacteremia. Of note, these changes occurred before the onset of overt hemodynamic alterations (133). In a limited observational study, uncoupling of tissue oxyhemoglobin levels and mitochondrial oxygen consumption, as indicated by cytochrome a,a3 redox state (indicating mitochondrial oxidative stress), predicted the development of multiple organ failure in patients with major trauma (134). These data particularly support the possibility of a decreased ability of mitochondria to use oxygen as a potential cause of decreased tissue high-energy phosphate in sepsis.

All these theories of septic bioenergetic metabolism would be expected to result in a deficit of tissue high-energy phosphates during septic shock. A series of studies using biochemical analysis of harvested tissues and nuclear magnetic resonance (NMR) spectroscopy of septic animals have suggested that high-energy phosphate reserves are decreased in animal models of septic or endotoxic shock (125,135,136). It can be argued that in many of these studies, animals were inadequately fluid resuscitated, which resulted in tissue hypoperfusion. However, animals in at least one study (125) were clearly adequately resuscitated (cardiac output and tissue oxygen tension were maintained comparable to shams) and demonstrated similar evidence of high-energy phosphate depletion (skeletal muscle biopsy) along with an increased lactate/pyruvate ratio during rat peritonitis induced by cecal ligation and perforation (125). Little human data exist. In one study of critically ill patients (most of whom were septic), the acetoacetate/β-hydroxybutyrate ratio (a marker of mitochondrial redox state) rose significantly in nonsurvivors compared to survivors (137). Evidence of increased acetoacetate/β-hydroxybutyrate ratio, along with an increase in ATP degradation products in critically ill patients with sepsis, also exists (138,139). In addition, independent studies using skeletal muscle biopsies in patients with sepsis/septic shock observed decreased ATP and phosphocreatine but variable changes in lactate levels (140,141).

In contrast, other animal studies using NMR spectroscopy demonstrate that high-energy phosphates are not depleted in septic animals as would be expected in these theories of septic bioenergetic failure (142–144). According to these and other studies, cellular ischemia is not the dominant factor in metabolic dysfunction in sepsis (129,142–147). Rather, circulating mediators may result in cellular dysfunction, aerobic glycolysis, and lactate production in the absence of global ischemia (143). This position is weakened by data suggesting that increased lactate in septic shock is also associated with decreased pH (which would not be expected in aerobic glycolysis) (143). Nonetheless, ongoing controversy of this issue remains.

Cardiac and Vascular Responses

Prior to the introduction of the balloon-tipped pulmonary artery catheter (PAC) and echocardiography to assess cardiovascular performance, much of our understanding of septic hemodynamics was based on clinical findings. Two distinct clinical presentations of septic shock were proposed: Warm shock characterized with high CO, warm dry skin, bounding pulses and hypotension; and cold shock characterized with low CO, cold clammy skin, and diminished pulses (148). These two presentations were thought to represent a progressive continuum, starting with warm shock (in the initial hemodynamically well-compensated phase) and progressing to cold shock (indicating decompensation), culminating in death. This notion was supported by studies showing a correlation between survival and a high cardiac index (CI) (148,149). A major problem with this interpretation was that these studies used central venous pressure (CVP) as a reflection of left ventricular end-diastolic volume (LVEDV) and adequacy of fluid resuscitation. The central role of adequacy of intravascular volume status to CI and survival was suggested in a handful of studies at that time (150,151). Based on evidence collected over the past four decades, CVP is now accepted to be a poor measure of preload in critically ill patients, particularly those with sepsis and septic shock (152). Studies in recent years have clearly shown that adequately resuscitated septic shock patients typically exhibit a persistent hyperdynamic state, high CO, and low SVR (153,154). In nonsurvivors, this hyperdynamic state usually persists until death (Fig. 57.11) (35,155).

More than any other form of shock, distributive and, particularly, septic shock involves substantial elements of the hemodynamic characteristics of other shock categories. All forms of distributive shock involve decreased mean peripheral vascular resistance. Before fluid resuscitation, distributive shock also

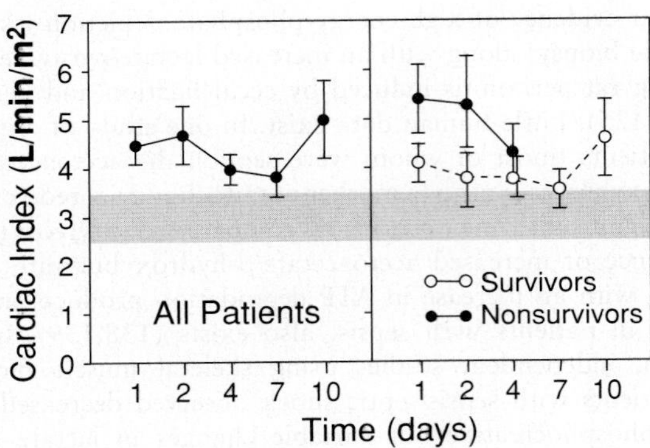

FIGURE 57.11. Cardiac index in resuscitated septic shock. The mean (standard error of the mean [SEM]) cardiac index plotted against time for all patients, survivors, and nonsurvivors. The *hatched areas* show the normal range. All groups maintained an elevated cardiac index throughout the study period. The difference between the survivors and nonsurvivors was not statistically significant. *Open circles*, survivors; *closed circles*, nonsurvivors. (Adapted from Parker MM, Shelhamer JH, Bacharach SL, et al. Profound but reversible myocardial depression in patients with septic shock. *Ann Intern Med*. 1984;100:483–490.)

involves a hypovolemic component with decreased central venous and pulmonary artery occlusion pressures. The primary cause of this relative hypovolemia is an increase of the vascular capacitance due to venodilatation. This phenomenon has been directly supported in animal models of sepsis (156–160) and is reinforced by the fact that clinical hypodynamic septic shock (low CO) can usually be converted to hyperdynamic shock (high CO) with adequate fluid resuscitation (35,148,161). Relaxation of vascular smooth muscle is attributed to several of the mediators known to circulate during sepsis. These same mediators also contribute to the second cause of hypovolemia in sepsis: Third-spacing of fluid to the interstitium due to loss of endothelial integrity. Further, decreased oral fluid and salt intake during the course of the illness may play a role. As a consequence, CO and central/mixed venous oxygen saturation in unresuscitated and poorly resuscitated septic shock patients is usually decreased (161,162). Septic shock also involves a cardiogenic element. Myocardial depression is common in human sepsis and septic shock (163,164). Circulating substances such as TNF-α, IL-1β, platelet-activating factor (PAF), leukotrienes, and most recently, IL-6 and macrophage migration inhibitory factor have been implicated in this process (95,165–172).

ORGAN SYSTEM DYSFUNCTION DUE TO SEPSIS AND SEPTIC SHOCK

Table 57.8 summarizes organ system dysfunction in sepsis and septic shock.

Central Nervous System

Septic encephalopathy is the most common neurologic manifestation of sepsis and septic shock, encompassing between 8% and 80% of patients with sepsis (173–176). The likely reason for the divergent frequencies of the syndrome in studies is the difficulty of identifying the condition in patients with superimposed hypotension, sedation, hypoxemia, acidosis, electrolyte disturbances, hypoglycemia/hyperglycemia, hypothermia/hyperthermia, and/or concurrent hepatic/renal failure/encephalopathy. The diagnosis, requiring the presence of altered mentation with an extracranial source of infection, is often one of exclusion. Although deficits can range from impairment of higher cognitive functions to delirium or coma, asterixis, myoclonus, and seizure activity are highly atypical (173,176). The diagnosis is best made by electroencephalography (EEG) (177). The occurrence and severity of septic encephalopathy (graded by EEG or Glasgow coma scale) appears to be associated with increased mortality (as high as 70%) (173,178).

Critical illness-associated neuromuscular syndromes (inclusive of critical illness polyneuropathy and myopathy) are the most common cause of neuromuscular problems in the ICU (179). The primary clinical manifestation of this condition is muscle weakness. Since many patients who are in the ICU with sepsis and septic shock require ventilatory support, the initial overt manifestation may be either respiratory failure or failure to wean from ventilation. Studies have suggested an incidence between 35% and 50% based on clinical criteria and 40% to 80% based on electromyography (EMG)/nerve conduction studies (180–182). Although the disorder is commonly

TABLE 57.8

ORGAN SYSTEM DYSFUNCTION IN SEPSIS AND SEPTIC SHOCK

CNS	Septic encephalopathy Critical illness polyneuropathy/ myopathy
Heart	Tachycardia Supraventricular tachycardia Ventricular ectopy Myocardial depression
Pulmonary	Acute respiratory failure Adult respiratory distress syndrome
Kidney	Prerenal failure Acute tubular necrosis
GI	Ileus Erosive gastritis Pancreatitis Acalculous cholecystitis Colonic submucosal hemorrhage Transluminal translocation of bacteria/antigens
Liver	Intrahepatic cholestasis
Hematologic	Disseminated intravascular coagulation Thrombocytopenia
Metabolic	Hyperglycemia Glycogenolysis Gluconeogenesis Hypertriglyceridemia
Immune System	Neutrophil dysfunction Cellular immune (T-cell/macrophage) depression Humoral immune depression

CNS, central nervous system; GI, gastrointestinal.

noted later in the recovery phase of sepsis and septic shock, EMG/nerve conduction data suggest that the onset is much earlier (concurrent or within days of the onset of septic shock) (183,184). The condition is a predominantly peripheral motor neuropathy in association with the presence of the systemic inflammatory response. Physical findings may include difficulty in weaning from the ventilator, symmetric paresis greater in the lower extremities, reduced deep tendon reflexes, and ataxia (180). A distal sensory neuropathy is also common. Approximately 25% of patients who are awake after a week on mechanical ventilation have significant weakness that lasts at least a week (185). The condition is considered to be an element of and is closely associated with the occurrence of MODS.

Cardiovascular System

The major clinically apparent manifestations of shock on the heart are due to sympathoadrenal stimulation. Heart rate is almost universally increased in the absence of disturbances of cardiac conduction; the degree of increase is predictive of outcome (35). In addition, catecholamine-driven supraventricular tachycardias and ventricular ectopy with ischemic electrocardiography (ECG) changes, particularly in patients predisposed to myocardial ischemia, may be found.

Like the brain, the blood supply to the heart is autoregulated, rendering it resistant to sympathetically driven vasoconstriction and shock-related hypoperfusion. Perfusion of the heart is unchanged or even increased during sepsis and septic shock (186,187). The occurrence of septic myocardial depression has already been addressed. Circulating myocardial depressant substances contribute to myocardial depression in sepsis and septic shock (188,189). This has been linked to decreased beta-adrenoreceptor affinity and density (190–192), as well as potential defects of intracellular signal transduction involving nitric oxide, G proteins, cyclic adenosine monophosphate (cAMP), and cGMP (95,193–197).

Although septic myocardial depression is a transient phenomenon in survivors, myocardial cell injury as evidenced by increased troponin levels does occur (198,199). Serum troponin is elevated in almost half of patients with septic shock (without myocardial creatine kinase [CK-MB] elevation or ischemic ECG changes) (200). A correlation between left ventricular (LV) dysfunction and troponin I (TnI) positivity has been shown (199). Serum TnI correlated with left ventricular dysfunction and was an independent predictor of the need for inotropic/vasopressor support, adverse outcome, and mortality in septic shock patients (200). Whether the clinically inapparent myocardial cell injury that is the source of elevated troponin contributes to, or is a consequence of, septic shock is yet to be determined. Although troponin is used as a marker of myocardial injury (particularly in the context of myocardial ischemia), it does not specifically suggest myocardial infarction in other contexts.

Respiratory System

Early respiratory responses to sepsis include tachypnea and hyperventilation. Gas exchange may be mildly abnormal. Later in the course of sepsis, patients may develop diffuse alveolar damage consistent with the acute lung injury (ALI) or adult respiratory distress syndrome (ARDS). Infections account for about one half of all cases of ARDS. These infections can involve local pneumonia or distant foci of infection associated with sepsis or septic shock. The risk of ARDS in association with sepsis increases with the severity of the syndrome (sepsis to septic shock) (201). From 40% to 60% of patients with Gram-negative septic shock develop ARDS. Sepsis is the single condition most closely associated with progression to acute lung injury or ARDS, with an incidence of 40% (202). Several comorbid factors increase the risk of ARDS, including chronic alcohol abuse, chronic lung disease, and severe acidemia (202). Most patients with septic ARDS also have other organ failure, i.e., MODS. Death is more commonly due to MODS or the underlying sepsis, although the impact of low tidal volume ventilation in ARDS studies suggest that the lung injury may still play a significant role (perhaps as a source of persistent inflammatory stimulation) (202–204). The mortality of ARDS/MODS is approximately 40%, although some recent reports suggest that it may be decreasing (202,205). Failure to improve in the first week is associated with progression of the syndrome and poor prognosis, as are MODS, chronic liver disease, and age; interestingly, indices of oxygenation and ventilation are not predictive (202).

Renal

Acute renal failure (ARF) is a major complication of sepsis and septic shock and occurs with increasing frequency in relation to the severity of the syndrome, from 16% to 19% with sepsis to 51% with septic shock (31,201,206). Sepsis has been the leading cause of acute tubular necrosis (ATN) in some ICU studies, accounting for almost 50% of cases (207–209). Sepsis-associated acute renal failure is associated with a substantially higher mortality risk (75%) than nonseptic ARF (45%); within this group, septic shock mortality is higher (80%) than in those with severe sepsis (70%) (201,208). Compared with nonsepsis-associated ARF, sepsis-related ARF patients are significantly older, sicker, require mechanical ventilation more often, and present later in the hospital course more frequently (208).

Gastrointestinal

The gut is relatively sensitive to circulatory failure due to the responsiveness of the splanchnic vasculature to vasoconstrictive stimulation by extrinsic factors. In addition, gut tissues may have increased sensitivity to proinflammatory cytokine-driven inflammatory injury. Typical clinical gut manifestations of hypoperfusion, sympathetic stimulation, and inflammatory injury associated with sepsis and septic shock include ileus, erosive gastritis, pancreatitis, acalculous cholecystitis, and colonic submucosal hemorrhage (210). In addition, enteric ischemia produced by circulatory shock and free radical injury with resuscitation may breach gut barrier integrity (211,212). Some theories propose that enteric bacteria and antigens (notably endotoxin) may translocate from the gut lumen to the systemic circulation during gut ischemia, resulting in irreversible shock (213) and MODS (214).

Hepatobiliary

Two major forms of organ injury can be seen in the liver with sepsis and septic shock (215,216). "Shock liver" (ischemic hepatitis) is associated with massive ischemic necrosis and major elevations of transaminases, which can occur with septic shock and is atypical in the absence of extensive hepatocellular disease (217). When it does occur, it can contribute substantially to lactic acidosis since the liver accounts for most serum lactate clearance. Hypoglycemia may also be seen. Centrilobular injury with mild increases of transaminases and lactate dehydrogenase is much more common. Transaminases usually peak within 1 to 3 days of the insult and resolve over 3 to 10 days. In both cases, there are only mild increases in bilirubin and alkaline phosphatase in the early phase. Despite the production of acute-phase reactants in early sepsis and septic shock, synthetic functions may be impaired, with decreased generation of prealbumin, albumin, and hepatic coagulation factors (increased prothrombin time [PT]). After, or independent of, the occurrence of septic shock, evidence of biliary stasis with increased bilirubin and alkaline phosphatase may be present (216). Increases in transaminases are modest.

Hematologic

Sepsis and septic shock are associated with a range of hematologic disorders including overt disseminated intravascular coagulation (DIC), thrombocytopenia, and coagulopathy. Thrombocytopenia and coagulopathy are multifactorial in nature. Bone marrow suppression, consumption, and medications can contribute to thrombocytopenia, whereas consumption and decreased liver production of coagulant factors, as well as malnutrition (leading to depleted vitamin K stores), contribute to coagulopathy. Nonetheless, whenever these findings are present, early disseminated intravascular coagulation (DIC) is possible.

Septic shock is the single most common cause of DIC, characterized by microangiopathic hemolysis, consumptive thrombocytopenia, consumptive coagulopathy, and microthrombi with tissue injury. Overt DIC occurs in one quarter to one half of cases of Gram-negative sepsis (218). Although Gram-positive sepsis has been thought to be less closely associated with DIC, the frequency of occurrence is quite similar (218,219). The occurrence of DIC in sepsis is associated with a doubling of projected mortality (218,220). DIC may also represent both a driver and manifestation of MODS. The deposition of microvascular thrombi can cause significant endothelial injury and inflammatory responses, leading to ischemic and inflammatory tissue injury, the basis of MODS.

A prolonged prothrombin time and partial thromboplastin time, hypofibrinogenemia, elevated level of fibrin split products, and the presence of the D-dimer herald the onset of disseminated intravascular coagulation. Since it is due to simultaneous systemic activation of coagulation and fibrinolysis cascades, it can be differentiated from the coagulopathy of liver failure by determination of endothelial cell-produced factor 8 (normal or increased with hepatic dysfunction). The pathogenesis of this disorder is linked to activation of tissue factor on endothelial cells and macrophages, probably by proinflammatory cytokines induced by exogenous bacterial toxins (220,221).

Metabolic

Specific, predictable, and overlapping metabolic alterations occur in both sepsis and shock. Foremost among these is hyperglycemia. There are two reasons for hyperglycemia in sepsis and states of shock. Early in sepsis, when hemodynamic stress initiates compensatory responses, endogenous catecholamines are released as a consequence of enhanced sympathoadrenal stimulation. In addition, increased release of adrenocorticotropic hormone (ACTH), glucocorticoids, and glucagon with a concomitant decreased release of insulin results in glycogenolysis and gluconeogenesis (222,223). Increased epinephrine also results in skeletal muscle insulin resistance, sparing glucose for use by glucose-dependent organs such as the heart and brain (224). In addition, proinflammatory, stress-related cytokines such as TNF-α, IL-1β, and IL-6 contribute to insulin resistance in peripheral tissues (225). Pharmacologic therapies of sepsis and shock, including catecholamine vasopressors/inotropes, steroids, and total parenteral nutrition, can add to these effects. It is notable that, despite insulin resistance, the increased metabolic demands of sepsis also result in increased overall glucose uptake and utilization (226).

With the evolution of sepsis to septic shock, metabolic responses progress. Late in shock, hypoglycemia may develop, possibly due to glycogen depletion or failure of hepatic glucose synthesis (227). Fatty acids are increased early in sepsis but fall later with hypoperfusion of adipose-containing peripheral tissue (226,228). Hypertriglyceridemia is often seen during shock as a consequence of catecholamine stimulation and reduced lipoprotein lipase expression induced by circulating TNF-α (223,226,229). Increased catecholamines, glucocorticoids, and glucagon also increase protein catabolism, resulting in a negative nitrogen balance (223,228).

Endocrine

Endocrine abnormalities are frequently underappreciated in sepsis and septic shock. Notable alterations in levels of pituitary, adrenal, thyroid, growth, and sex hormones are known to occur (225,230–236). In recent years, "relative" adrenal insufficiency in septic shock has received substantial attention. Few septic patients exhibit overt adrenal insufficiency. Relative bradycardia and a nontoxic appearance in a patient with septic shock is suggestive of this possibility. These are often elderly patients who have survived an initial episode of septic shock and either fail to fully recover or suffer a relapse. However, a considerable body of literature suggests that a suboptimal cortisol response (within the normal range) to sepsis and septic shock can have deleterious effects, including prolonged pressor dependence and increased mortality. Estimates of the frequency of adrenal insufficiency in septic shock vary wildly from 0% to 95% (237,238). In great part, this is due to the use of varying definitions based on baseline or cosyntropin-stimulated cortisol levels or changes in levels from baseline in response to cosyntropin. Common definitions in septic shock patients include random cortisol of $<$700 nmol/L (25 μg/dL), peak postcosyntropin level of $<$500 to 550 nmol/L (1–20 μg/dL), or postcosyntropin change in cortisol of $<$200 to 250 nmol/L (7–9 μg/dL) (230,237,239,240). Interestingly, pituitary dysfunction may play a role in many patients with adrenal insufficiency, as 85% of critically ill patients have decreased levels of adrenocorticotropic hormone (ACTH) (241).

Abnormalities of thyroid hormones are also present in sepsis and septic shock, although the clinical significance is less certain. In humans, serum T_4 and T_3 levels fall shortly after the onset of severe clinical infection. Euthyroid sick syndrome is manifested by low serum levels of thyroid hormones in clinically euthyroid patients with severe nonthyroidal systemic illness. Decreased T_3 levels are most common. Patients with more severe or prolonged illness also have decreased T_4 levels. Serum reverse T_3 (rT_3) is increased. Patients are clinically euthyroid and do not have clinically significant thyroid-stimulating hormone (TSH) elevations.

Sepsis and septic shock are clearly associated with perturbations of various hormones including insulin, growth hormone, TSH, thyroxin, ACTH, cortisol, growth hormone (242), and sex hormones. Perturbations of hormones of the posterior pituitary should be expected. In addition to abnormal prolactin levels (243), sepsis and septic shock are accompanied by relative deficiencies of vasopressin/antidiuretic hormone (ADH) levels. Vasopressin, produced in the hypothalamus and stored in the posterior pituitary gland, is released in response to hyperosmolarity. Hypotension as seen in shock states is an even more powerful stimulus for release. Recent human studies have suggested a relative deficit of circulating vasopressin in patients with septic shock (relative to those with cardiogenic or hypovolemic shock). This deficiency may be related to depletion of neurohypophyseal stores combined with NO-mediated inhibition of production (225,235). Clinically, vasopressin exerts powerful vasopressor effects in hypotensive patients, particularly those with septic shock. To some extent, this effect appears to be mediated through reestablishment of reduced sensitivity to catecholamine (244).

DIAGNOSIS OF SEPSIS

Under ideal circumstances, each patient with evidence of sepsis would undergo a thorough evaluation at presentation prior to the initiation of therapy. In the context of sepsis and septic shock, circumstances are rarely ideal, so an abbreviated initial assessment focusing on critical diagnostic and management planning elements is frequently necessary.

To ensure maximally rapid implementation of effective therapy, an initial presumptive diagnosis of severe sepsis and septic shock is mandated. The criteria for this presumptive diagnosis should be highly inclusive and based primarily on clinical criteria.

The initial presumptive diagnosis of sepsis with organ dysfunction (severe sepsis) may be made in the presence of the following elements:

- Suspected infection based on a minimal clinical constellation of localizing (e.g., dyspnea, cough, purulent sputum production, dysuria, pyuria, focal pain, local erythema, etc.) and systemic signs and/or symptoms of infection and sepsis (Table 57.9)
- Clinical evidence of organ dysfunction (e.g., hypotension with peripheral hypoperfusion, oliguria, hypoxemia, obtundation, etc.)

TABLE 57.9

CLINICAL SYMPTOMS/SIGNS FOR PRESUMPTIVE DIAGNOSIS OF SEVERE SEPSIS/SEPTIC SHOCK

Fever or hypothermia
Chills, rigors
Tachycardia
Widened pulse pressure
Tachypnea or hyperpnea
Confusion, decreased level of consciousness or delirium
Decreased urine output
Hypotension

Similarly, an initial diagnosis of septic shock is established in the presence of suspected infection with sustained hypotension without a definitive alternate explanation.

The initial presumptive diagnosis of severe sepsis or septic shock is based on clinical criteria and does not require microbiologic, radiographic, or other laboratory evidence of specific infection or organ injury. Only clinical evidence of infection and organ failure is necessary. For the most part, available laboratory tests or imaging studies represent supportive, not diagnostic, elements. This clinical approach allows a parallel, rapid initiation of empiric antimicrobials and supportive measures.

Although a suggestive clinical examination is sufficient for the presumptive diagnosis of severe sepsis and septic shock, more authoritative investigations (both laboratory and radiologic) are generally required for confirmation. For this reason, the definitive diagnosis of severe sepsis and septic shock involves a broader range of clinical and laboratory evidence of sepsis (Table 57.10) and organ dysfunction (arterial hypotension, lactic acidosis, or any organ dysfunction variables in Table 57.2). Establishment of a definitive diagnosis can help to more specifically target antimicrobial therapy and trigger specific therapies such as surgical source control and activated protein C.

TABLE 57.10

SUPPORTIVE/CONFIRMATORY FINDINGS FOR SEVERE SEPSIS/SEPTIC SHOCK

Leukocytosis, leukopenia, increased immature white blood cell (WBC) forms, toxic granulation, Dohle bodies
Thrombocytopenia ± increased INR or prothrombin time (PT)
Increased D-dimer or fibrin split products
Increased serum bilirubin, AST/ALT, C-reactive protein
Serum procalcitonin elevation
Metabolic acidosis with anion gap
Serum lactate elevation
Respiratory alkalosis or acidosis
Mixed venous saturation >70%
Diagnostic imaging findings
Positive microbiologic or pathologic samples for abnormal presence of microorganisms, leukocytes, or tissue necrosis

INR, international normalized ratio; AST/ALT, aspartate aminotransferase/alanine aminotransferase.

History

The initial history should focus on two major areas: The key symptoms with respect to diagnosis of sepsis and of the specific site of infection, and key factors that would modify initial empiric therapies such as antimicrobials, fluid resuscitation, and possibly, vasopressors/inotropes.

With respect to symptoms, constitutional complaints are entirely nonspecific. The classic pattern of fever, rigors, and chills is common but far from universal. Fatigue, malaise, anxiety, or confusion may be observed, particularly in the elderly. Occasionally, the elderly, the immunocompromised (nonspecific immune dysfunction due to chronic organ failure), and the immunosuppressed (specific immune defects) may present without classic signs and symptoms.

Fever is a common feature of infection and/or sepsis. Fever is caused by a direct effect of inflammatory mediators, such as IL-1β, on the hypothalamus. The fever response may be suppressed in septic shock and may be absent in the elderly, immunocompromised, or immunosuppressed patient. Hypothermia in septic shock is associated with reduced cardiac output and portends a poor prognosis (245). Septic encephalopathy manifested by disorientation or confusion is especially common in elderly individuals. Apprehension, anxiety, and agitation may all occur early in the course. With severe disease (i.e., septic shock) or progression of sepsis, overt encephalopathy with a decreased level of consciousness and coma can occur. Hyperventilation with respiratory alkalosis can manifest even before the onset of metabolic acidosis as a consequence of cytokine-mediated stimulation of the respiratory center in the medulla.

Localizing symptoms as described in Table 57.11 may be more helpful in determining the septic cause of the constitutional manifestations of sepsis. The key historical factors used to modify initial therapies include antimicrobial sensitivities/allergies, recent infections/antimicrobial use, the locale of infection acquisition (i.e., nosocomial vs. community), and major comorbidities. The existence of comorbidities (e.g., AIDS; chemotherapy; hematologic malignancy; neutropenia resulting in immunosuppression or chronic renal, heart, liver, or other organ failure; COPD; dementia; inflammatory bowel diseases; diabetes; or via invasive catheters/devices) resulting in immunocompromise mandate the use of extended-spectrum antimicrobial therapy. Chronic renal, liver, or heart failure may also influence the choice and volume/dose of antimicrobials, resuscitation fluids, and vasopressors. Recent antimicrobial use and nosocomial or institutional acquisition of infection may also mandate consideration of extended-spectrum antimicrobial therapy to adequately cover nosocomial pathogens.

Physical Examination

The physical examination should focus on ensuring that the patient is stable and on rapid localization of the site of infection. The physical examination should first ensure that the airway is patent, the patient is breathing satisfactorily, and vital signs and peripheral perfusion are acceptable.

Tachypnea and tachycardia are almost universal. Normothermia and fever are consistent with sepsis, but hypothermia should be of concern due to its association with shock/hypoperfusion. All patients with sepsis should be observed for signs of hypoperfusion (mottling, pallor, diaphoresis, impaired capillary refill in nail beds). An acutely ill, flushed, and toxic appearance is common in the septic patient, particularly early in the course. In the early stages of sepsis, CO is well maintained or even increased, skin and extremities are warm,

TABLE 57.11

LOCALIZING CLINICAL SYMPTOMS AND SIGNS IN SEVERE INFECTIONS

	History	Physical exam
Central nervous system	Headache, neck stiffness, photophobia	Meningismus (neck stiffness), focal neurologic signs (weakness, paralysis, paresthesia)
Head and neck	Earache, sore throat, sinus pain, or swollen lymph glands	Inflamed or swollen tympanic membranes or ear canal, sinus tenderness, pharyngeal erythema and exudates, inspiratory stridor, and cervical lymphadenopathy
Pulmonary	Cough (especially if productive), pleuritic chest pain, and dyspnea	Dullness on percussion, bronchial breath sounds, and localized crackles
Cardiovascular	Palpitations, syncope	New regurgitant valvular murmur
Intra-abdominal	Abdominal pain, nausea, vomiting, diarrhea, purulent discharge	Abdominal distention, localized tenderness, guarding or rebound tenderness, and rectal tenderness or swelling
Pelvic/genitourinary	Pelvic or flank pain, vaginal or urethral discharge, and urinary frequency and urgency	Costovertebral angle tenderness, pelvic tenderness, pain on cervical motion, and adnexal tenderness
Skin/soft tissue/joint	Localized limb pain or tenderness, focal erythema, edema, and swollen joint	Focal erythema or purple discoloration (subcutaneous necrosis), edema, tenderness, crepitus in necrotizing infections (*Clostridia* and Gram-negative infections), petechiae, purpura, erythema, ulceration, and bullous formation and joint effusion

Adapted from Sharma S, Mink S. Septic shock. http://www.emedicine.com/MED/topic2101.htm. 2007. Accessed Dec. 1, 2007.

and capillary refill is normal. As sepsis progresses, venodilation results in reduced central venous pressure and venous return. Hypovolemic manifestations with hypotension, reduced stroke volume, and CO with signs of tissue hypoperfusion develop. As patients are aggressively fluid resuscitated, a hyperdynamic circulatory state (albeit with distributive shock) again dominates the clinical picture and will usually persist until recovery or death.

The most common sites of infection causing sepsis and septic shock in order of frequency are respiratory, abdominal, urinary, and soft tissue. Abdominal infections are more closely associated with septic shock whereas urinary infections are more common in sepsis. Intravascular catheters are a frequently overlooked source of infection and sepsis. A recent study suggested that central venous catheters might account for as much as 3.7% of cases of septic shock (25). Similarly, cases of *Clostridium difficile*–related septic shock are often overlooked in the absence of overt toxic megacolon. Adding to the difficulty of managing the ICU patient with sepsis and/or septic shock is that many patients have simultaneous infection at more than one site.

Laboratory Studies

Patients with sepsis require urgent lab testing to help make a firm diagnosis and to evaluate the severity of the illness. Sepsis and septic shock typically present with somewhat different, though naturally overlapping, laboratory parameters (see Table 57.12). Lab tests usually start with a complete blood count (CBC). Hemoglobin is often decreased, although this is usually due to the presence of chronic disease. Hemoglobin can occasionally be increased in patients with substantial interstitial third-spacing and relative hypovolemia. The white cell count is increased in sepsis but may transiently normalize or even drop below normal range, with progression to septic shock. Although this phenomenon has been linked to Gram-negative septic shock, it can be seen in septic shock due to *any* pathogen. Leukopenia in this setting has been linked to poor outcome. Toxic granulation and the presence of Dohle bodies are also seen more frequently, with progression to more severe disease. Similarly, a marked left shift with increasing immature forms (bands) is more common in septic shock. Platelets often respond as an acute-phase reactant, with increases early in infection/sepsis. However, platelet counts drop, with septic shock reaching a nadir around day 5 in survivors.

In contrast, the international normalized ratio (INR) may be mildly abnormal at the onset of sepsis (due to malnourishment) and is usually most abnormal at onset of septic shock. Fibrinogen is an acute-phase reactant and is usually elevated with onset of infection/sepsis. However, levels will drop with septic shock, especially if DIC intervenes. Fibrin split products and D-dimers are very sensitive markers of progression of sepsis and are almost universally elevated with septic shock.

Serum creatinine and blood urea nitrogen (BUN) may actually be decreased due to increased renal blood flow in the early hyperdynamic phase of sepsis but will increase with the onset of septic shock. An increase in serum creatinine denotes an increased mortality risk even within a few hours of the onset of septic shock. Similarly, elevated serum lactate is closely correlated with increased mortality risk in septic shock.

TABLE 57.12

KEY LABORATORY VALUES IN INFECTION/SEPSIS VERSUS SEPTIC SHOCK

	Sepsis	Septic shock
Hb	N or ↓ (chronic disease)	↑ (hemoconcentration)
WBC	↑ + left shift	↑, N or ↓ -marked left shift with metamyelocytes, toxic granulation, and/or Dohle bodies
platelets	N or ↑	N or ↓
PT/INR	N or ↑ (malnutrition)	↑↑
fibrinogen	N or ↑	N or ↓
Fibrin split products/ D-dimer activity	↑	↑↑
Glucose	N or ↑	↑↑
Cr/BUN	N or ↑	↑↑
Bilirubin	N, late ↑	↑, late ↑↑
AST/ALT	N	↑-↑↑
Albumin	N or ↓ (malnutrition)	↓↓ (endothelial leakage/interstitial redistribution)
ABG	respiratory alkalosis	metabolic acidosis
HCO_3^-	N	↓
lactate	N	↑-↑↑
C-reactive protein	↑	↑↑
procalcitonin	↑	↑↑
Blood culture positivity	5%–10%	30%–40%

↑ increase, ↑↑ marked increase, ↓ decrease, ↓↓ marked decrease, N normal. Hb, hemoglobin; WBC, white blood cell count; PT, prothrombin time; INR, international normalized ratio; Cr/BUN, serum creatine and blood urea nitrogen; AST/ALT, serum aspartate transaminase and alanine transaminase; ABG, arterial blood gas; HCO_3^-, serum bicarbonate concentration.

Septic patients should have both site-specific and blood cultures drawn prior to initiation of antimicrobial therapy. In the case of septic shock, however, antimicrobial therapy should never be delayed to accommodate these cultures because of the antimicrobial delay-dependent increase in mortality risk (25). Gram stain should be performed on all site samples. Although there are some data to suggest that Gram stain is not useful in the initial management of certain infections (nosocomial pneumonia, peritonitis due to bowel perforation), a good specimen, appropriately interpreted, can provide invaluable information.

Imaging Studies

Although in most cases the clinical examination will localize the source of infection with a reasonable degree of confidence, basic radiographic imaging can be very useful in cases where an obvious site of infection is not apparent. Advanced imaging studies (computerized axial tomography [CAT], magnetic resonance imaging [MRI], ultrasound) rarely yield information regarding localization of the infection that has not been provided by the clinical examination and basic imaging studies. However, these techniques may be highly useful when definitive or precise localization and/or delineation of extent of disease are required.

A chest radiograph should be obtained in most patients admitted to the hospital with sepsis. Elderly, immunocompromised, and immunosuppressed patients with occult sepsis will often be found to have a pulmonary source on radiographic examination. Supine and upright or lateral decubitus abdominal films are useful if bowel perforation is of concern. In the appropriate clinical context of crepitus, bullae, hemorrhage, or foul-smelling exudate with intense local pain, evidence of gas in soft tissues on plain extremity radiographs is almost pathognomonic of necrotizing soft tissue infection with clostridia or facultatively anaerobic Gram-negative bacilli.

CT scan with contrast is the preferred imaging modality to rule out intra-abdominal, intracranial, epidural, perinephric, and soft tissue abscesses, as well as retroperitoneal abscess or mediastinal infection. They can also be useful for localizing bowel wall injury and assessing necrotizing soft tissue infections (although MRI is preferred for the latter). Ultrasound is the initial imaging modality of choice for biliary sepsis and obstructive uropathy, although CT scan is also sensitive and specific.

MANAGEMENT OF SEVERE SEPSIS AND SEPTIC SHOCK (I.E., THE SEPSIS SIX-PACK)

To optimize outcome in sepsis with organ dysfunction (severe sepsis), the initiating triggers, amplification cascade, and downstream organ dysfunction must be addressed; this requires monitoring and therapeutic elements. With respect to the initiating triggers, antimicrobials and, where possible, surgical and nonsurgical source control are mandated. With respect to the amplification cascade, one new agent (activated protein C) has been developed that directly dampens septic response by exerting both anti-inflammatory and antithrombotic effects, such that mortality is improved. Organ dysfunction is addressed through direct supportive measures. The most immediate of these—fluid and vasopressor/inotropic resuscitation—support the circulatory system. However, mechanical ventilation and dialysis have also been shown to improve outcome in severe sepsis and septic shock.

Six major areas in the evaluation and treatment of severe sepsis can be identified. These include the following:

1. Fluid resuscitation
2. Antimicrobial therapy
3. Vasopressors and inotropes
4. Invasive and noninvasive monitoring
5. Specific therapy
6. Miscellaneous supportive therapy

Fluid Resuscitation

The development of shock in patients with sepsis involves disturbances of global and regional perfusion. Initially, ventricular filling pressures as reflected by CVP and pulmonary wedge pressure (PWP) are decreased. As a consequence, venous return falls, resulting in limitation of CO. Although an increase in insensible losses and decreased fluid intake may contribute to this effect, nitric oxide–mediated venular dilatation and loss of endothelial barrier integrity (resulting in a drop in colloid oncotic pressure from loss of albumin into the interstitium) probably play a dominant role (246,247). A significant degree of hypovolemia is almost universal in early, untreated severe sepsis or septic shock. Available data suggest that initial isotonic fluid deficits can exceed 10 L (248).

Management of sepsis requires consideration of both global and regional perfusion defects, making the establishment of goals for therapy more complex than for other forms of shock. Support of global perfusion takes initial precedence. Since hypovolemia is a major factor in the hypotension and hypoperfusion of early septic shock, foremost among the appropriate initial therapeutic considerations is infusion of intravascular fluids. Fluid infusion should be implemented rapidly by large-bore peripheral intravenous catheters. Infusion of fluids can improve global perfusion indices (blood pressure, CO, and MvO_2/central venous oxygen saturation [$ScvO_2$]) and may reveal the presence of regional perfusion disturbances and/or myocardial depression that may require therapy with vasopressors/inotropes.

The three issues to consider in optimizing fluid resuscitation are the type of fluid used, the rapidity of infusion, and the amount of fluid administered.

Initial resuscitation of septic patients should be aimed at rapid intravascular volume expansion. The view that intravascular fluid depletion plays a central role in the pathogenesis of early septic shock has been recognized since the past midcentury. Several studies suggested that septic shock is associated with reduced total circulating blood volume (149,150). Since almost all untreated patients with severe sepsis or septic shock have a significant element of hypovolemia, a hypodynamic circulation with decreased cardiac output is typical prior to fluid resuscitation. This hypovolemia is probably the basis of early observations that death in sepsis is associated with decreased cardiac output. The patients in those studies were clearly inadequately resuscitated by current standards (149,150). Additional support for the central importance of functional hypovolemia in early septic shock comes from a more recent demonstration that the venous oxygen saturation is decreased in early preresuscitation septic shock (consistent with the findings in other forms of hypodynamic shock) (161).

Aggressive fluid loading is the standard early therapy of septic shock and results in the generation of a hyperdynamic circulatory state in over 90% of patients (249). Rapid fluid resuscitation may reveal severe sepsis without shock in a significant subset of patients with apparent septic shock (248). Increased total blood volume has been associated with higher cardiac output and increased survival in human septic shock (150). Intravascular volume dependence of the hyperdynamic circulatory state in sepsis has been confirmed in animal models (158). Although the demonstration that resuscitation from hypovolemia improves outcome in traumatic shock dates back to the early work of Cannon (250) and Cournand et al. (251), clear evidence that early aggressive fluid resuscitation improves outcome in septic shock is limited to a small series of pediatric septic shock (252) and a recent randomized study of goal-directed resuscitation (253).

Initial fluid resuscitation should be titrated to specific clinical end points. Aggressive fluid loading in patients with septic shock can increase total blood volume, cardiac output, oxygen delivery, and consumption while reducing lactic acidosis (119). Older studies have suggested that an increased blood volume associated with normalization of cardiac output is associated with improved survival (149,150).

In the absence of early invasive or echocardiographic monitoring, clinical end points can be used for titration of fluid resuscitation. Since both initial heart rate and blood pressure have been shown to be associated with outcome in septic shock as well as hypovolemic shock (35,254–256), standard goals may include the following:

- Heart rate ≤100 beats/minute
- Systolic blood pressure (≥90 mm Hg)
- Mean arterial pressure (≥60–65 mm Hg)
- Urine output (≥0.5 mL/kg/hour)

It should be noted that these clinical parameters can underestimate initial resuscitative requirements in critically ill subjects including those with septic shock (257–259).

Mortality in both septic and other forms of shock has also been associated with increased arterial lactate and base deficit levels (260). Normalization of these parameters can be used to augment clinical end points for titration of fluid resuscitation (261). However, both parameters represent relatively late responses to cellular stress, and resolution may similarly lag following the implementation of effective resuscitation (262).

Initial fluid resuscitation should be achieved using isotonic crystalloid solutions. Effective fluid resuscitation can be delivered with either isotonic crystalloid (e.g., normal saline, lactated Ringer solution) or colloid solutions (e.g., hydroxyethyl starch, human albumin). All of these solutions are equally effective if titrated to the same clinical end points. Given the difference in distribution of such compounds, it typically requires approximately four times more crystalloid to achieve the same hemodynamic effect as a given amount of colloid (263). Several animal and human studies have pointed out theoretical advantages to colloids in limiting interstitial fluid accumulation (which may benefit ARDS) in sepsis and septic shock (264–266). However, no clinical study has suggested improved clinical outcomes (morbidity or mortality) with colloid solutions (267,268). Although the severe sepsis subset of one recent randomized controlled trial (RCT) trended toward a more favorable outcome with albumin resuscitation (269), another (meta-analytic) study suggested an opposite trend toward increased mortality with albumin use (268,270). In addition, colloids are substantially more expensive than crystalloid solutions. For these reasons, isotonic crystalloids are recommended as the initial resuscitative solution for severe sepsis and septic shock. The development of a hyperchloremic acidosis can be anticipated with use of large volumes of normal saline. Use of lactated Ringer solution may limit this effect. Hypertonic saline is not recommended for the routine resuscitation of septic shock.

Rapid volume expansion (500 mL isotonic crystalloid every 10–30 minutes) should be continued until clinical and physiologic treatment targets are met. Vasopressor/inotropic support is required if fluid infusion alone fails to achieve physiologic response targets. Early aggressive resuscitation to achieve physiologically normal hemodynamic goals reduces subsequent morbidity and mortality in patients with septic shock. In a pediatric population with septic shock, rapid fluid resuscitation in the first hour of presentation to hospital improved survival (252). In an adult study, the effect of early goal-directed resuscitation to normal physiologic values in patients presenting to an emergency department with severe sepsis or septic shock was examined (253). All patients (both conventional and goal-directed therapy groups) were resuscitated in the emergency room for the first 6 hours to standard hemodynamic end points of CVP ≥8 mm Hg, MAP ≥65 mm Hg, and urine output ≥0.5 mL/kg per hour. The experimental early goal-directed therapy group, in addition, was managed using an experimental protocol to achieve both the standard goals and a central venous oxygen saturation ≥70% (as measured by an oximetric central venous catheter). During the 6 hours of their protocolized emergency room support, the experimental group received 1.5 L more fluid than the control group, and a substantially larger fraction of the patients in the experimental group achieved the physiologic resuscitative goals (99.2% vs. 86.1%). Overall mortality was significantly lower in the early goal-directed therapy group.

Antimicrobial Therapy and Source Control

Historically, critically ill patients with overwhelming infection have not been considered a unique subgroup comparable to neutropenic patients for purposes of selection of antimicrobial therapy. However, critically ill patients with severe sepsis and septic shock, similar to neutropenic patients, are characterized by distinct differences from the typical infected patient that impact on the optimal management strategy. These differences include the following:

- Marked alterations in antibiotic pharmacokinetics
- Increased frequency of hepatic and renal dysfunction
- High prevalence of unrecognized immune dysfunction
- Predisposition to infection with resistant organisms
- Marked increase in frequency of adverse outcome if there is a failure of rapid initiation of effective antibiotic therapy

Critical management decisions in this patient group must often be made emergently in the absence of definitive data regarding the infecting organism and its sensitivity pattern, patient immune status, and organ function. Since outcomes in severe sepsis and septic shock are strongly influenced by the rapidity of administration of an appropriate antimicrobial regimen at first presentation, a particularly thoughtful and judicious approach to initial empiric antimicrobial therapy is required (271–273).

Empiric antibiotic regimens should approach 100% coverage of pathogens for the suspected source of infection. Initial administration of inappropriate antimicrobials increases morbidity in a wide range of infections. The occurrence of initiation of inadequate antimicrobial therapy may occur as frequently as 17.1% in community-acquired and 34.3% in nosocomial bacteremia in patients admitted to the ICU (273). Similarly, 18.8% and 28.4% of septic shock cases were initially treated with inadequate antimicrobial therapy in another large study (274). Retrospective studies have shown that the risk of death increases from 30% to 60% in ICU bacteremia (4,272) to 70% to 100% in Gram-negative shock (4) when the initial empiric regimen fails to cover the inciting pathogen. More recent data suggest that the survival of septic shock with inappropriate initial antimicrobial therapy is reduced approximately 5-fold (range 2.5 to 10-fold in selected subgroups) to about 10% (274). These findings of a sharply increased mortality risk with initial inadequate antimicrobial therapy apply to serious infections caused by Gram-negative and Gram-positive bacteria as well as *Candida* species (4,274–278).

As a consequence, empiric regimens should err on the side of overinclusiveness. The most common cause of initiation of inappropriate antimicrobial therapy is a failure of the clinician to appreciate the risk of infection with antibiotic-resistant organisms (either uncommon organisms with increased native resistance or antibiotic-resistant isolates of common organisms). Selection of an optimal antimicrobial regimen requires knowledge of the probable anatomic site of infection; the patient's immune status, risk factors, and physical environment; and the local microbiologic flora and organism resistance patterns. Risk factors for infection with resistant organisms include a prolonged hospital stay, prior hospitalization, and prior colonization or infection with multiresistant organisms.

Superior empiric coverage can be obtained through the use of a local antibiogram or via consultation with an infectious disease specialist (279). Although not routinely required, extended-spectrum Gram-negative regimens, vancomycin, and/or antifungal therapy may be appropriate in specific high-risk cases with severe sepsis (Table 57.13). In addition, given that 90% to 95% of patients with septic shock have comorbidities or other factors that make them high risk for resistant organisms, it may be appropriate to initially treat all patients with septic shock using a combination of antimicrobials that result in a broadly expanded spectrum of coverage for the first few days. This approach should improve the adequacy of antimicrobial coverage initially, while ensuring that high-risk patients are not inappropriately categorized as low risk.

Intravenous administration of broad-spectrum antimicrobials should be initiated immediately (preferably <30 minutes) following the clinical diagnosis of septic shock. Appropriate intravenous, empiric broad-spectrum therapy should be initiated as rapidly as possible in response to clinical suspicion of infection in the presence of hypotension, i.e., presumptive septic shock. An assumption that hypotension is caused by anything other than sepsis in the setting of documented or suspected infection should be avoided, unless there is very strong data indicating a specific alternate cause. Retrospective studies of human bacteremia, pneumonia, and meningitis with sepsis suggest that mortality in sepsis increases with delays in antimicrobial administration (271,278,280–282). One major retrospective analysis of septic shock has suggested that a delay in the initial administration of effective antimicrobial therapy is the single strongest predictor of survival (25). Initiation of effective antimicrobial therapy within the first hour following the onset of septic shock-related hypotension was associated with 79.9% survival to hospital discharge. For every additional hour to effective antimicrobial initiation in the first 6 hours post onset of hypotension, survival dropped an average of 7.6%. With effective antimicrobial initiation between the first and second

TABLE 57.13

INDICATION FOR EXTENDED EMPIRIC ANTIBIOTIC THERAPY OF SEVERE SEPSIS/SEPTIC SHOCK

↑ Gram-negative coverage	■ Nosocomial infection ■ Neutropenic or immunosuppressed ■ Immunocompromised due to chronic organ failure (liver, renal, lung, heart, etc.)
↑ Gram-positive coverage (vancomycin)	■ High-level endemic MRSA (community or nosocomial) ■ Neutropenic patient ■ Intravascular catheter infection ■ Nosocomial pneumonia
Fungal/yeast coverage (triazole, echinocandin, amphotericin B)	■ Neutropenic fever or other immunosuppressed patient unresponsive to standard antibiotic therapy ■ Prolonged broad-spectrum antibiotic therapy ■ Positive relevant fungal cultures ■ Consider empiric therapy if high-risk patient with severe shock

MRSA, methicillin-resistant *Staphylococcus aureus*.

hour post hypotension onset, survival had already dropped to 70.5%. With effective antimicrobial therapy delay to 5 to 6 hours after hypotension onset, survival was just 42.0%, and by 9 to 12 hours, 25.4%. The adjusted odds ratio of death was already significantly increased by the second hour post hypotension onset, and the ratio continued to climb with longer delays.

Substantial delays before initiation of effective therapy have been shown in several studies of serious infections (271,282–284). In septic shock, the median time to delivery of effective antimicrobial therapy following initial onset of recurrent/persistent hypotension was 6 hours (25).

A potential survival advantage may exist if a pathogenic organism can be isolated in severe infections, including septic shock. Every effort should be made to obtain appropriate site-specific cultures to allow identification and susceptibility testing of the pathogenic organism; however, such efforts should not delay antimicrobial therapy.

Antimicrobial therapy should be initiated with dosing at the high end of the therapeutic range in all patients with life-threatening infection. Early optimization of antimicrobial pharmacokinetics can improve the outcome of patients with severe infection, including septic shock. This is most easily achieved by initiating antibiotic therapy with high-end dosing regimens.

Early in sepsis, before the onset of hepatic or renal dysfunction, cardiac output is increased in many patients. In association with increased free drug levels due to decreased albumin levels, drug clearance can be transiently increased (285). As the illness progresses, ICU patients with sepsis or septic shock exhibit substantially increased volumes of distribution and decreased clearance rates. Consequently, suboptimal dosing of antibiotics is common in these conditions (286–291). Data is most well developed in reference to aminoglycosides but also exists for fluoroquinolones, β-lactams, and carbapenems (286–291). Failure to achieve targets on initial dosing has been associated with clinical failure with aminoglycosides (292,293). Similarly, clinical success rate for treatment of serious infections tracks with higher peak blood levels of fluoroquinolones (nosocomial pneumonia and other serious infections) (294–296) and aminoglycosides (Gram-negative nosocomial pneumonia and other serious infections) (297,298). Although there are extensive data in experimental animals and less serious human infections, data for optimization of outcomes using β-lactams in critically ill, infected patients is relatively limited (299,300). A single recent paper has shown improved survival in patients with Pseudomonas bacteremia when treated with extended infusions rather than standard intermittent dosing of piperacillin/tazobactam (301).

Achievement of optimal serum concentrations of aminoglycosides (peak antibiotic serum concentration:pathogen minimal inhibitory concentration [MIC] ratio of $\geq$12) and longer periods of bactericidal β-lactam and carbapenem serum concentrations (minimum time above MIC in serum of 60% of dosing interval) are appropriate goals (294,302,303). This can most easily be attained with once-daily dosing of aminoglycosides (304). For β-lactams and related antibiotics, increased frequency of dosing (given identical total daily dose) is recommended. For example, piperacillin/tazobactam can be dosed at either 4.5 g every 8 hours or 3.375 g every 6 hours for serious infections; all things being equal, the latter would achieve a higher time above MIC and should be the preferred dosing option. A similar dosing approach should be used for other β-lactams in critically ill patients with life-threatening infections. Limited data suggest that continuous infusion of β-lactams and related drugs may be even more effective, particularly for relatively resistant organisms (305–309).

Multidrug antimicrobial therapy is preferred for the initial empiric therapy of septic shock. Probable pathogens should be covered by at least two antimicrobials with different bactericidal mechanisms. Given that highly resistant organisms are endemic in the critical care environment, multidrug antimicrobial therapy will reduce the probability of failure to cover these organisms. In addition, most patients with septic shock (even those without specific pre-existing immune defects) exhibit significant deficits of neutrophil and monocyte function during the course of their illness (310–316). Furthermore, malnutrition and organ dysfunction (e.g., renal or hepatic failure), which are common in ICU patients, suppress cell-mediated immunity. Based on these data, septic shock patients likely have a reduced ability to clear infection and may be best managed with multidrug therapy similar to that recommended for patients with neutropenic sepsis (317,318).

No prospective controlled study has specifically compared multiple versus single antimicrobial therapy in a broad range of severe sepsis or septic shock patients. Most infectious diseases physicians and other experts suggest no advantage to multidrug therapy in serious infections, including bacteremia (319,320). However, a subgroup analysis of the sickest subset of patients with Gram-negative bacteremia, with or without shock, has tended to suggest improved survival with the use of two or more antibiotics to which the causative organism is sensitive (321–324). Similarly, at least two retrospective and one prospective analyses of the most severe, critically ill patients with bacteremic pneumococcal pneumonia suggested improvement in outcome if two or more effective agents were used (325–327). This occurred even as patients with pneumococcal bacteremia with a lower severity of illness demonstrated no such benefit (325). A recent secondary analysis of a prospective study of community-acquired pneumonia has shown benefit with multidrug therapy compared to monotherapy but only in the subset of septic shock (328).

Empiric antimicrobial therapy should be adjusted to a narrower regimen within 48 to 72 hours if a plausible pathogen is identified or if the patient stabilizes clinically (i.e., resolution of shock). Although several retrospective studies have demonstrated that inappropriate therapy of bacteremic septic shock yields increased mortality (4,272,276–278), none have suggested that early narrowing of antibiotic therapy is detrimental if the organism is identified or if the patient is responding well clinically. This approach will maximize appropriate antibiotic coverage of inciting pathogens in septic shock while minimizing selection pressure toward resistant organisms. Although it is tempting to continue a broad-spectrum regimen in the 15% of improving patients who are culture-negative for a potential pathogen, intensivists must recognize that a strategy of broad-spectrum initial antimicrobial therapy will be sustainable only if overuse of these agents can be avoided. Aggressive de-escalation of antimicrobial therapy within 48 to 72 hours after initiation is required.

TABLE 57.14

COMMON SOURCES OF SEVERE SEPSIS/SEPTIC SHOCK REQUIRING URGENT SOURCE CONTROL

Toxic megacolon or *C. difficile* colitis with shock
Ischemic bowel
Perforated viscus
Intra-abdominal abscess
Ascending cholangitis
Gangrenous cholecystitis
Necrotizing pancreatitis with infection
Bacterial empyema
Mediastinitis
Purulent tunnel infections
Purulent foreign body infections
Obstructive uropathy
Complicated pyelonephritis/perinephric abscess
Necrotizing soft tissue infections (necrotizing fasciitis)
Clostridial myonecrosis

Where possible, early source control should be implemented in patients with severe sepsis, septic shock, and other life-threatening infections. Source control is a critical issue in the management of infection associated with severe sepsis. Infections found in ICU patients frequently require source control for optimal management. The need for such source control may initially be overlooked in many infections commonly found in the ICU (e.g., pneumonia-associated bacterial empyema, decubitus ulcers, *C. difficile* colitis). Causes of septic shock where source control may be required are noted in Table 57.14.

Source control may include removal of implanted or tunneled devices, open surgical/percutaneous drainage of infected fluids or abscesses, and surgical resection of infected tissues. In a broader sense, it is inclusive of elimination of inciting chemotherapies (e.g., antibiotics driving *C. difficile* colitis or chemotherapy causing gut injury). Efforts to identify infections requiring invasive forms of source control frequently require rapid (<2 hours) radiographic imaging (often CT scan) or, if clinical status and findings are supportive, direct and immediate surgical intervention without an imaging effort. With rare exceptions, surgical source control should follow aggressive resuscitative efforts to minimize intraoperative morbidity and mortality. In some cases (e.g., rapidly progressive necrotizing soft tissue infections, bowel infarction), optimal management mandates simultaneous aggressive resuscitation and surgical intervention. Subgroup analysis in at least one large prospective, severe sepsis study has suggested that failure to implement adequate source control is associated with increased mortality (329). Earlier surgical intervention has been shown to have a significant impact on outcome in certain rapidly progressive infections such as necrotizing fasciitis (330,331). In a large retrospective study of septic shock, time from hypotension to implementation of source control was found to be highly correlated with outcome (332).

The necessity for or efficacy of source control efforts should be reassessed within 12 to 36 hours following admission and/or source control efforts should be based on clinical response.

Vasopressors and Inotropes

Following fluid resuscitation, patients with severe sepsis or septic shock may demonstrate persistent vasomotor dysfunction characterized by regional perfusion deficits with or without systemic hypotension despite normal or increased CO. Clinical manifestations may include lactic acidosis and ongoing progression of organ failure.

Until recently, the only available approach to correction of regional perfusion defects was vasopressor therapy. Unfortunately, vasopressors do not represent a specific therapy for this problem. Their primary use is to increase systemic arterial pressure to a range that potentially sustains the ability of the vasculature to autoregulate flow on a tissue and organ level (333,334). This allows vital organ perfusion to be supported (potentially at the expense of peripheral perfusion) until definitive therapy (infection source control and antibiotics) can be implemented.

The aim of vasopressor/inotropic therapy in septic shock is simply the optimization of critical organ and tissue perfusion. However, the specific global and/or regional perfusion goals required to achieve this result are complex and controversial. Although specific targets can be suggested, therapy for each patient must be highly individualized and dynamic. Appropriate goals will change over time and should be re-evaluated on a continuing basis.

If hypotension and/or clinical evidence of tissue hypoperfusion persist after adequate fluid resuscitation of septic shock, vasopressor therapy is indicated. Norepinephrine and dopamine are both effective as initial therapy. Initiation of vasopressor support is dependent on the patient's clinical status following fluid resuscitation. If systemic hypotension in association with evidence of tissue/organ hypoperfusion (oliguria, obtundation, lactic acidosis) persists, vasopressor support is indicated. Selection of a vasopressor agent is based on an individualized assessment of the patient's needs. The patient's hemodynamic presentation, the anticipated cardiovascular effect of each vasoactive agent (based on the distribution of receptor activity), and the physician's experience and comfort with each drug should be considered. As a consequence of the variety of factors that may play a role in vasopressor selection, septic shock patients with a predominantly distributive hemodynamic pattern can be appropriately and effectively managed with one of several vasopressors including dopamine, norepinephrine, or phenylephrine.

Ideally, patients should have achieved the targeted intravascular volume status prior to initiation of vasopressors. Although vasopressors can be used to maintain blood pressure for brief periods while intravascular volume is repleted, the infusion of high-dose vasopressors to volume-depleted patients may substantially aggravate ischemic organ injury.

Studies suggesting that norepinephrine is superior to dopamine are less than definitive (335–340). No controlled study has directly assessed norepinephrine and dopamine in terms of survival, and few have compared the two agents with respect to markers of organ dysfunction. Studies assessing the effects of these agents on renal and splanchnic perfusion have been mixed, with neither agent demonstrating conclusive superiority (336,337,340–347). Norepinephrine may have more powerful vasopressor activity than dopamine (348). In addition, its inotropic effects are mediated by direct activity on myocardial β-adrenoreceptors. Dopamine pressor effects are weaker than those of norepinephrine, and inotropic effects are substantially indirect (through stimulation of release of myocardial catecholamine stores); excessive tachycardia may be more common. In addition, dopamine may exert significant immunosuppressive effects through suppression of prolactin production from the hypothalamus (349). Phenylephrine, a relatively pure β-adrenergic agonist, has minimal or absent inotropic effects and tends to cause reflex bradycardia. For that reason, it can be very useful in the context of excessive tachycardia or concurrent tachyarrhythmias. However, phenylephrine consistently decreases cardiac output and has an increased propensity to cause ischemic complications. Despite potent inotropic and vasopressor activity, epinephrine is not commonly used as the initial pressor therapy in septic shock because it can generate profound tachycardia, tissue ischemia, and metabolic disturbances.

Dobutamine is indicated for patients with low cardiac index or other evidence of hypoperfusion following achievement of adequate blood pressure. Milrinone can be used as an alternate agent if the response to dobutamine is suboptimal. In some cases of septic shock, clinical or laboratory evidence of hypoperfusion (e.g., oliguria, altered mentation, decreased mixed venous oxygen saturation, increased lactic acidosis) persists despite an adequate blood pressure. In this circumstance, the patient may require a higher blood pressure or assessment of cardiac output (via PAC or echocardiography) to determine the need for inotropic support. In the small proportion of septic shock patients who manifest overt myocardial depression following fluid resuscitation, dobutamine or milrinone may be indicated. Dobutamine can increase cardiac index in septic shock, although the inotropic response is frequently blunted relative to normal subjects (350,351). If catecholamine responsiveness is inadequate, low-dose milrinone may be effective since its inotropic activity is mediated through an alternate mechanism (352). When using either agent, patients must be adequately fluid resuscitated. Severe hypotension can result if intravascular volume is deficient when either dobutamine or milrinone is initiated (350,352).

Although the aim of inotropic therapy in severe sepsis/septic shock is to improve cardiac output and tissue perfusion, specific goals for cardiac index have been controversial; the currently recommended target is a CO within the normal range (approximately 2.5–4 L/minute per m^2). The utility of $MvO_2/ScvO_2$ as global indices of tissue perfusion adequacy in severe sepsis and septic shock is also uncertain. Limited studies suggest that an $MvO_2/ScvO_2$ below the normal range (65%–70%) may indicate inadequacy of resuscitation and/or total perfusion in early septic shock (161). If other hemodynamic targets have been achieved, an MvO_2 below 65% may represent an appropriate indication to increase oxygen delivery by starting inotropic agents. Recommendations to increase MvO_2 are based on mixed evidence. No benefit was noted in a randomized trial of goal-directed therapy using MvO_2 in critically ill patients after the onset of organ dysfunction (353,354). On the other hand, early goal-directed therapy targeting a $ScvO_2$ of $\geq$70% was associated with improved outcome in another study (253).

Supranormal hemodynamic goals are not indicated in the management of septic shock. Observational studies of medical and surgical critical care patients have demonstrated lower values of physiologic variables such as oxygen consumption (VO_2), oxygen delivery (DO_2), and CI in nonsurvivors relative to survivors of septic shock (355,356). These observations formed the basis of efforts to implement goal-directed therapy in septic shock to achieve supranormal physiologic parameters consistent with levels observed in survivors (i.e., CI $\geq$4.5 L/min/m^2, DO_2 $\geq$600 mL/minute per m^2, and VO_2 $\geq$170 mL/minute per m^2). Although a single clinical trial and at least one meta-analysis have suggested some promise with this approach (357,358), several large randomized trials have failed to demonstrate an overall significant benefit of supranormal oxygen delivery in patients with severe sepsis and septic shock (353,354,359–361). One has suggested increased mortality when supranormal oxygen delivery was generated with dobutamine (354). The absence of a beneficial effect with supranormal oxygen delivery in patients with severe sepsis and septic shock has been supported in recent meta-analytic reviews (362).

Continuous infusion of vasopressin (0.01–0.04 U/minute) exerts a strong pressor effect and may be beneficial in catecholamine-resistant septic shock following adequate volume resuscitation. Recently, vasopressin levels in septic shock patients have been shown to be decreased (363). Further studies have demonstrated that intravenous infusion of vasopressin in patients with septic shock results in a profound pressor response (236,364,365), an effect that is absent with even larger amounts of vasopressin in normotensive patients (235). A randomized, controlled, double-blind trial of 4-hour infusion of norepinephrine and vasopressin in high-dose, pressor-dependent shock has demonstrated significant improvement in urine output and creatinine clearance, along with a concomitant reduction in conventional vasopressor requirements in the vasopressin group (365). Another RCT has recently demonstrated that, while vasopressin can spare the need for high doses of sympathomimetic agents, outcome is not affected (366).

Because of the limited experience with this compound and the relatively prolonged pharmacologic effect of the drug, vasopressin should be used only after hemodynamic stabilization with standard agents (catecholamines) has been attempted.

At high dose (>0.04 U/minute), vasopressin may produce increased blood pressure, bradycardia, arrhythmias (premature atrial contractions, heart block), severe peripheral vasoconstriction, decreased cardiac output, myocardial ischemia, myocardial infarction, and cardiac arrest. In patients with vascular disease, even relatively modest doses can precipitate peripheral vascular insufficiency, mesenteric ischemia, or myocardial infarction. Given these potential side effects, the minimal amount of vasopressin required should be used to achieve the desired blood pressure goals. In addition, since vasopressin appears to be a pure vasopressor in the context of vasodilatory shock, cardiac output will usually decline. Consideration of placement of an intra-arterial and pulmonary artery catheter (PAC) should be given to all patients receiving vasopressin for shock.

Administration of low- or renal-dose dopamine (1–4 μg/kg per minute) to maintain renal or mesenteric blood flow in sepsis and septic shock is not recommended. Although concurrent infusion of low-dose dopamine during human septic shock does mitigate a decrease in renal perfusion that can occur as a consequence of norepinephrine infusion, the clinical benefit of this therapy is questionable (367,368). Low-dose dopamine infusions can cause a mild transient diuresis in the absence of other vasopressors in nonoliguric critically ill patients (369,370). However, low-dose dopamine does not prevent the development of renal dysfunction in these patients, including those with sepsis and septic shock (371,372).

Invasive and Noninvasive Monitoring

Controversy exists regarding the most appropriate monitoring methods for determining the adequacy of resuscitation in patients with severe sepsis and septic shock. The range of monitoring that must be considered in each patient begins with observation by specially trained nursing personnel, to routine noninvasive devices (e.g., continuous electrocardiographic monitors, intermittent mechanical sphygmomanometry, end-tidal carbon dioxide sensors, percutaneous oximetry), to commonly used invasive techniques (arterial, central venous, and pulmonary artery catheters). Prior to the advent of basic hemodynamic monitoring in the 1950s and early 1960s, clinical examination and manual sphygmomanometry were the only available methods for assessment of cardiovascular status. Clinical judgment correctly predicts the hemodynamic profile (including CO and central venous/pulmonary wedge pressures) of critically ill patients only about half of the time (373,374).

CVP has been considered a useful measure of intravascular volume since the early studies of hypovolemic shock in young men following battlefield trauma (250,251). However, CVP may be much less reliable as a reflection of left ventricular preload in older patients with various cardiopulmonary disorders as are typically found in a modern-day ICU (152,375). Although low filling pressures may reliably indicate hypovolemia in most patients, the presence of a normal or even elevated central venous pressure can be misleading in patients in whom right ventricular afterload is elevated or right ventricular contractility is impaired (376).

The PWP obtained by using a PAC has been considered to reflect intravascular volume more reliably than CVP. In addition, the device allows thermodilution-based derivation of CO (373,374,377). Although the PAC has gained widespread acceptance, significant questions about its use have been raised. Several studies have questioned the relationship of PAC-derived, pressure-based estimates of ventricular preload in specific groups of critically ill patients (375) and, more recently, even in normal subjects (378). In addition, the lack of randomized trials demonstrating benefit and the association of PAC with excess mortality in two observational cohort studies have led to concerns regarding the clinical utility and safety of PACs (379,380). Despite these concerns, the PAC remains the most commonly used modality for hemodynamic monitoring of unstable critically ill patients.

Patients with established septic shock should have continuous monitoring of blood pressure, oxygen saturation, electrocardiogram (ECG), and urine output in a closed ICU staffed with full-time dedicated intensivists and critical care–trained nurses. Several studies have demonstrated that a reduced mortality with decreased length of stay and overall cost for a wide range of individual conditions are obtained when critically ill patients are cared for in closed ICUs staffed with full-time dedicated intensivists and nurses (381–385). Similar improvements in outcome of sepsis and septic shock have been documented with the use of dedicated intensivists in closed ICUs (386). Among the practice differences associated with the use of full-time intensivists is a greater use of invasive monitoring (384).

Patients requiring vasopressor agents for a prolonged period or at high dose should be strongly considered for insertion of an arterial pressure catheter for continuous blood pressure monitoring, as well as to facilitate frequent measurements of arterial blood gases and chemistry. Accurate, continuous monitoring of blood pressure is required for optimal assessment of severity of shock, response to fluid resuscitation, and titration of vasopressors and inotropes. However, intense peripheral vasoconstriction may occur during shock as a consequence of the vascular compensatory response to hypotension or due to administration of vasopressors. Clinical ausculatory and noninvasive mechanical methods can be highly inaccurate in this setting (387,388). Patients with sustained shock, particularly those requiring vasopressor support, should be assessed for placement of an intra-arterial catheter for continuous blood pressure monitoring. However, such catheters should be preferentially placed in peripheral sites in non-end arteries (radial, dorsalis pedis), and should be used with caution in patients at high risk for vascular disease.

If volume resuscitation requirements exceed 2 L, placement of a central venous catheter for monitoring of CVP and for vasopressor/inotrope infusion should be considered. An initial target CVP of ≥8 mm Hg is recommended. Fluid deficits during septic shock in adults typically range from 5 to 10 L (248). In the absence of significant cardiopulmonary dysfunction, central venous pressure should accurately assess intravascular volume status. However, cardiopulmonary dysfunction is not uncommon in patients with septic shock either as an underlying predisposition to critical illness/sepsis or as a consequence of the injury (ARDS/acute lung injury [ALI], myocardial depression). Low central venous pressures remain indicative of hypovolemia; elevated or normal central venous pressures in this patient group may not necessarily indicate euvolemia. CVP monitoring should be entertained if substantial amounts of fluid resuscitation are required to ensure that overt hypovolemia is adequately addressed. The initial target CVP should be ≥8 mm Hg, with additional increases indicated by the effect of fluid boluses on cardiac output and clinical perfusion. The overall goal is to provide adequate cardiac output and tissue perfusion using the lowest necessary cardiac filling pressures.

Initiation of invasive cardiac monitoring using a pulmonary artery catheter should be considered if there has been an inadequate response to fluid resuscitation (3–5 L or CVP 8–12 mm Hg), if there is clinical suspicion of intravascular fluid volume overload, or if the patient has impaired cardiac function. An initial target of PWP of 12–15 mm Hg will ensure that hypovolemia is absent in most patients, but higher pressures may be required in certain subgroups. Although the maintenance of a blood pressure adequate for autoregulation of blood flow to vital organs and tissues is the first objective in the resuscitation of septic shock, support of global perfusion is also critical. Adequacy of global perfusion cannot always be reliably inferred from the clinical examination or CVP/arterial pressure monitoring (373,377,389). Patients who respond poorly to fluid resuscitation or are at high risk for fluid resuscitation–related complications may benefit from pulmonary artery catheterization. A substantial degree of variability in the relationship between PWP and end-diastolic volumes makes it difficult to specify target PWP goals that ensure adequate cardiac output and tissue perfusion (378,390,391). In general, a PWP titrated to at least 12 to 15 cm H_2O will optimize cardiac function (152). If hypotension persists, a higher PWP may be beneficial as assessed by measuring the effect of additional fluids on cardiac index. An elevated PWP may risk the development or aggravation of ALI and ARDS (392,393). Specific groups that may require higher PWP include those with congestive heart failure, left ventricular hypertrophy, restrictive or constrictive heart disease, or increased intrathoracic pressures, including those on high levels of positive end-expiratory pressure (PEEP).

In patients with vasopressor-requiring shock who develop progressive organ failure or hypoxemic respiratory failure, pulmonary artery catheterization may be a useful clinical management tool. The information available from a PAC can be used to help determine the cause of shock and provide a guide for interventions to maintain an appropriate cardiac output and intravascular volume to limit the risk of further progression of organ dysfunction/failure. If PACs are beneficial in patients with sepsis, the most likely candidates may be those in whom resuscitation by clinical assessment or CVP fails to reverse the progression of organ failure.

Invasive monitoring using a pulmonary artery catheter is not recommended for routine use in all patients with severe sepsis. At least one major prospective, nonrandomized multicenter study has suggested increased length of stay, costs, and mortality in a cohort of risk-matched patients receiving a PAC in the first 24 hours after ICU admission (394). A recent multicenter randomized controlled trial involving 676 subjects with shock (primarily septic), ARDS, or both has demonstrated no difference in organ failure–free days, renal support needs, vasopressor requirements, mechanical ventilation, ICU/hospital length of stay (14 and 90 day), or mortality between subjects randomized to pulmonary artery catheterization or controls (395). A second, smaller randomized trial of 200 patients (about 100 with sepsis) also demonstrated no mortality difference with or without the use of PAC (396). Other smaller studies, including one randomized trial in high-risk operative patients, failed to demonstrate any difference in mortality with PAC use (397,398). In contrast, one meta-analysis of RCTs demonstrated a reduced mortality risk in surgical ICU patients treated with PAC but no effect on mortality in medical or mixed ICU patients (399). On the basis of the total data available, routine use of PAC in patients with sepsis or other critical illness cannot be recommended.

Specific Therapy

As discussed, patients with severe sepsis and septic shock must first be treated using the following: (i) Appropriate resuscitation, (ii) broad spectrum antimicrobials, (iii) source control, and (iv) physiologic support of organ function in the intensive care unit. Immunomodulatory therapy has been evaluated only in association with adequate treatment based on these four elements.

In the last few decades, the dominant hypotheses regarding the pathogenesis of septic shock and septic organ dysfunction focused on inflammatory mediators including TNF α, IL-1β, interleukin-6, and platelet-activating factor. Several clinical trials have been performed evaluating both nonspecific inhibitors of inflammation such as nonsteroidal anti-inflammatory drugs and high-dose glucocorticoids and specific immunomodulatory agents such as monoclonal antibody against TNF α and IL-1 receptor antagonist (400,401). Despite an expenditure of over 1 billion dollars, these studies have failed to demonstrate a survival benefit. No primary immunomodulatory experimental agent has received regulatory approval.

Recently accepted models of the pathogenesis of sepsis have emphasized a central role for altered hemostatic/coagulant function. Three coagulation modulators have been assessed in large randomized controlled clinical trials: Tissue factor pathway inhibitor, antithrombin III, and drotrecogin alfa (activated) (recombinant human activated protein C). Drotrecogin alfa (activated) is the first and, to date, only specific therapy that has been shown to improve survival in patients with severe sepsis and septic shock.

Recombinant human-activated protein C should be administered in patients with suspected sepsis with organ dysfunction. Acceptable criteria include, but are not necessarily limited to, a minimum of one organ dysfunction with an Acute Physiology and Chronic Health Evaluation (APACHE) II score ≥25; or if an accurate APACHE II score is unavailable, the presence of two or more organ dysfunctions. Although clinical trials of modulation of the coagulation cascade for treatment of sepsis have been performed with several agents (e.g., antithrombin III [27], tissue factor pathway inhibitor [28]), only drotrecogin alfa (activated) has been shown to improve mortality (26). The pivotal study was an international multicenter RCT that compared drotrecogin alfa (activated) to placebo used in conjunction with standard treatment (antibiotics, physiologic support, and surgical source control) (26). Patients were entered into the study if they exhibited acute organ dysfunction due to a suspected infection (severe sepsis) within a 24-hour window. The study was stopped at a planned interim analysis because of definitive statistical evidence that supported a beneficial treatment effect. Using an intention-to-treat analysis, the study demonstrated an absolute mortality reduction of 6.5% from 31.3% in the placebo group to 24.8% in the drotrecogin alfa (activated) group, yielding a highly significant 21% relative risk reduction. Subsequent open-label studies of drotrecogin alfa (activated) using the same criteria as in the pivotal study have demonstrated a consistent mortality rate between 25.1% and 26.1% (402,403). A retrospective analysis of an open-label study suggests that earlier initiation of treatment (<24 hours after diagnosis of severe sepsis) yields superior outcomes (404).

The original study demonstrated a differential treatment effect based on either APACHE II scores or the number of acute organ dysfunctions present at the time of enrollment into the study. The absolute reduction in mortality was 1.7% among patients with a single dysfunctional organ and 7.4% among those with two or more dysfunctional organs (402,405). Similarly, there was no overall reduction in absolute mortality in the first 2 quartiles of APACHE score (score <25), whereas there was a 13% reduction in the last 2 quartiles (score ≥25) (405). A more recent RCT (prematurely terminated for futility) has underlined concerns regarding the utility of drotrecogin alfa (activated) in relatively low-risk (generally APACHE<25 or single organ failure) adult patients with a slight trend toward increased mortality risk in the treatment arm (29). Similarly, a study of drotrecogin alfa (activated) in pediatric septic shock with respiratory failure was also prematurely terminated due to its futility, along with evidence of an increased central nervous system (CNS) bleeding risk in neonates (406).

Drotrecogin alfa (activated) remains approved for management of high-risk patients with severe sepsis/septic shock, but new studies are ongoing to validate the continued use of this agent.

Intravenous immune globulin should be considered for patients suffering from streptococcal toxic shock syndrome. The potential utility of polyclonal immune globulin preparations for severe sepsis and septic shock in general is uncertain at present. One meta-analysis has suggested that sepsis-related mortality is significantly reduced when intravenous immunoglobulin (IVIG) is used in the management of such patients (407). A small randomized controlled trial of trauma patients has also demonstrated a reduced incidence of septic complications including pneumonia and other infections (other than catheter-related infections), although ICU length of stay and mortality were not reduced (408). Evidence favoring the use of polyclonal immunoglobulin for defined invasive streptococcal infections, including streptococcal septic shock, is more definitive. A case-matching study has demonstrated an improved 30-day survival in patients treated with intravenous polyclonal immune globulin, while a randomized controlled trial (aborted prematurely due to low enrollment) has shown decreased early sepsis-related organ failure with a trend toward improved survival (409).

Immunosuppressive doses of corticosteroids are contraindicated in the management of sepsis and septic shock. In the past, high-dose steroids had been advocated for sepsis with organ failure to dampen inflammatory responses and minimize organ dysfunction (410). Several large multicenter randomized controlled trials have definitively demonstrated that administration of high dose (15–30 mg/kg methylprednisolone equivalent) corticosteroids fail to improve outcome in adult septic shock (411–414). In some of these studies, mortality in specific subgroups appeared to be increased with steroid treatment (412).

Supportive Therapy

Although specific therapies for septic shock continue to be developed, general supportive care, in conjunction with antibiotics, remains the standard of care. Fluid and vasopressor/inotropic support have been addressed in this chapter. In addition, there has been an explosion of data in recent years regarding the efficacy of other elements of supportive care including ventilatory strategies, intensity of dialysis, endocrine support, and glycemic management. In other key areas (e.g., nutritional support), definitive data are lacking. Nonetheless, it is likely that an aggressive approach to optimization of supportive care, in combination with anti-infective therapy and resuscitative efforts, can improve morbidity and mortality. For that reason, application of appropriate support modalities in a timely manner should be the standard of care of septic patients in all ICUs.

Intensive renal replacement therapy (daily intermittent dialysis or continuous renal replacement therapy) is indicated for severe sepsis or septic shock with renal failure. Indications for acute dialysis in the ICU population are not dissimilar to those for other patients. These indications include volume overload, electrolyte imbalance, acid-base disturbances, elevated blood urea nitrogen, uremic pericarditis, or uremic encephalopathy. Unfortunately, ICU patients, especially those with acute renal failure, may have altered hemodialysis kinetics such that standard intermittent dialysis may offer suboptimal urea clearance kinetics despite apparently equivalent doses. Compared to standard intermittent dialysis, daily hemodialysis has been shown to yield higher urea clearance and improved mortality in ICU patients with acute renal failure (415). Similarly, another study has demonstrated that higher urea clearance with continuous venovenous hemodialysis yields reduced mortality (416). Whether these data can be extrapolated to include septic patients with a background of chronic renal failure is unknown. Peritoneal dialysis is not appropriate since even high-frequency exchanges yield relatively low urea clearance kinetics. A recent study of infection-related acute renal failure that included cases of sepsis demonstrated increased mortality among those treated with peritoneal dialysis compared to those treated with hemodialysis (417).

Intensive insulin therapy maintaining a blood glucose of 4.4 to 6.1 mmol/L (80–110 mg/dL) may be beneficial in critically ill ICU patients with severe sepsis. Hyperglycemia is a recognized risk factor for increased mortality in the critically ill independent of the APACHE II score (418). One single-center randomized, controlled, nonblinded trial has indicated that tight glycemic control in surgical ICU patients undergoing mechanical ventilation (mostly post–coronary artery bypass graft or other cardiovascular surgery) reduces the incidence of severe sepsis and decreases mortality, primarily because of a decreased incidence of multiple organ failure with septic foci (419). These data are consistent with other clinical and experimental studies suggesting the presence of granulocyte dysfunction and increased risk of infection in postoperative surgical patients with persistent hyperglycemia (420). However, another RCT by the same group has failed to demonstrate similar improvements in critically ill medical patients (421). A retrospective subgroup analysis, however, suggested mortality improvement in those patients admitted with an ICU length of stay of greater than 3 days. In addition, there was a decreased incidence of renal dysfunction and critical illness polyneuropathy, with fewer days on ventilator support and shorter ICU and hospital length of stay (421,422). No definitive data exist regarding the question of whether a tight control strategy is useful in patients who are already septic. In addition, these data should be interpreted with caution pending replication of these results in other centers.

Stress dose steroids may be administered at presentation to selected patients with septic shock pending the result of an ACTH stimulation test. Several previous large randomized, double-blind, multicenter trials have definitively demonstrated that administration of immunosuppressive (15–30 mg/kg methylprednisolone equivalent) corticosteroids fail to improve outcome in adult septic shock (411–414). However, some evidence suggests that low "stress-dose" corticosteroids may be beneficial. A relative adrenal insufficiency has been suggested to exist in a substantial subset of patients with septic shock (239,423). Among other deleterious effects, adrenal insufficiency can result in impairment of catecholamine sensitivity

(423–425). Administration of stress-dose steroids (150–300 mg hydrocortisone daily equivalent) to patients with septic shock can decrease pressor requirements while suppressing inflammatory markers (424,426,427). One recent RCT has demonstrated that 7 days of therapy with hydrocortisone, 50 mg IV every 6 hours, and fludrocortisone, 50 μg orally once daily, generates a significant reduction in mortality in patients with relative adrenal insufficiency (428). Subgroup analysis demonstrated that this improvement was restricted to those who fail to respond to an ACTH challenge (about 75% of septic shock patients), with an increase in serum cortisol of at least 250 nmol/L (9 μg/dL). In the recent past, these data were interpreted as suggesting that patients with pressor-dependent septic shock should undergo ACTH challenge on admission, followed immediately by initiation of stress-dose steroid therapy. If the ACTH stimulation test was within normal limits, corticosteroids were discontinued. If the test results indicated relative adrenal insufficiency, hydrocortisone and fludrocortisone were often continued for 7 days or as otherwise clinically indicated.

The major uncertainty with regard to stress-dose steroid therapy had been the appropriate test and value of serum cortisol to indicate adrenal insufficiency. Various studies supported using random cortisol levels between 275 and 950 nmol/L (10–35 μg/dL) during the acute stress, or increments of cortisol of 250 nmol/L (9 μg/dL) within the first hour following ACTH stimulation (239,423,428). Although no definitive data existed as to which cutoff value was best, many clinicians considered a random value of less than 400 nmol/L (15 μg/dL) to be sufficiently suggestive of relative adrenal insufficiency during the shock state to initiate and continue stress-dose therapy. Similarly, a value greater than 950 nmol/L (35 μg/dL) during shock has been thought to be sufficiently normal to discontinue stress-dose therapy without further assessment. Values between those two extremes were often interpreted to be an indication for ACTH challenge with a response of less than 250 nmol/L (9 μg/dL) supporting the need, for steroid therapy. Unfortunately, a recent study has challenged these accepted cutoffs in the critically ill by questioning the scientific validity of using total as opposed to free serum concentrations of serum cortisol in such patients (429).

Of most concern, a major multicenter, placebo-controlled, double-blind RCT of septic shock has failed to confirm an improvement in survival regardless of ACTH responsiveness (430). The steroid group did exhibit a reduction in pressor days but also had a higher incidence of superinfections and associated sepsis/septic shock events. Confounding these results, the steroid regimen (hydrocortisone alone) differed from the regimen used in the previous positive study and could also be implemented as late as 72 hours following onset of septic shock. Based on these data, stress-dose or low-dose steroid therapy should not be considered part of the routine management of septic shock pending further definitive trials.

Low-volume (6–8 mL/kg ideal body weight), pressure-limited ventilation is indicated in patients with sepsis-associated acute lung injury or acute respiratory distress syndrome. Animal and human studies have suggested that high levels of PEEP and large tidal volumes are associated with increased pulmonary generation of proinflammatory cytokines (431,432) and ventilation-induced lung injury (433). ALI and ARDS represent a manifestation of MODS that may occur in conjunction with severe sepsis and septic shock. Septic patients with bilateral persistent opacities, in association with an acute and persistent defect of oxygenation (PaO_2/FiO_2 ratio of $\leq$200 for ARDS and $\leq$300 for ALI) and no clinical evidence of left atrial hypertension or a pulmonary wedge pressure of $\geq$18 mm Hg, fit the criteria for this syndrome (434). Small randomized studies have supported the possibility that a lung-protective strategy using low tidal volumes and limited airway pressures may decrease pulmonary injury and decrease mortality (435). A single large multicenter, randomized controlled trial has demonstrated that ventilation of critically ill patients with ARDS with a low tidal volume (tidal volume of 6–8 mL/kg ideal body weight) reduces all-cause absolute mortality by 10% (from 40% to 30%; 25% relative risk reduction) (436). Patients with severe sepsis or septic shock who meet criteria for ALI or ARDS should be ventilated with a low-volume, pressure-limited strategy. Available evidence suggests that ventilation of patients at risk for ALI/ARDS with this strategy does not prevent the development of this pulmonary syndrome (437).

Endotracheal intubation and mechanical ventilation should be considered early in the management of all patients with sepsis and organ failure. Airway intubation is indicated for all patients with impaired airway protection reflexes (e.g., as a consequence of cerebral hypoperfusion or septic encephalopathy), refractory hypoxemia, respiratory acidosis, or respiratory distress associated with ongoing hypotension/hypoperfusion. Though not yet addressed by systematic studies, clinical experience suggests that respiratory arrest is a significant risk in such patients. These observations are consistent with observations of respiratory muscle compromise and respiratory failure in animal models of septic shock (438,439).

Enteral feeding should be considered within 24 hours of admission to the ICU for most patients with sepsis and septic shock. Parenteral feeding should be used only if enteral feeding is not possible despite best efforts. Recent meta-analyses suggest that early enteral feeding lowers the risk of infection and improves survival compared to delayed feeding in the critically ill (440). These findings are consistent with animal studies demonstrating that enteral nutrition maintains gut mucosal integrity, decreases bacterial translocation, and limits the systemic inflammatory response to bacterial toxins (441). Diminished bowel sounds should not prevent a trial of enteral feeding. Most patients will tolerate enteral feeding if a small bowel tube is used. Studies of parenteral feeding in the ICU have, in general, failed to demonstrate an improvement in mortality in critically ill patients (442). Other studies demonstrate the superiority of enteral over parenteral feeding in critically ill patients with respect to costs and complications, including risk of infection (441,443).

Intravenous administration of sodium bicarbonate is not indicated for sepsis-associated metabolic acidosis with a pH $\geq$7.15. Human investigations demonstrate that intravenous administration of sodium bicarbonate for lactic acidosis (pH $\geq$7.15) associated with septic shock does not improve cardiac performance or reduce vasopressor requirements compared to administration of an equimolar amount of normal saline (444,445). No human data exist in regard to the effect of intravenous bicarbonate administration for more severe degrees of metabolic acidosis.

TABLE 57.15

TIME LINE OF IMPLEMENTATION OF RECOMMENDED DIAGNOSTIC AND THERAPEUTIC INTERVENTIONS

	Resuscitation	Antimicrobials	Vasopressors/Inotropes	Monitoring	Specific Therapy	Supportive Therapy
First hour	■ Initiate crystalloid fluid resuscitation (500 mL every 10–15 min), titrating to HR <100, MAP ≥65 mm Hg, and urine output ≥0.5 mL/h	■ Initiate empiric, broad-spectrum, high-dose antimicrobial therapy with two or more cidal drugs where possible		■ Implement continuous monitoring of ECG, arterial saturation, blood pressure and UO		■ Supplemental oxygen ■ Consider intubation and mechanical ventilation prior to overt respiratory distress
1–8 hours	■ Titrate fluid resuscitation to elimination of base deficit and normalization of serum lactate	■ Initiate radiographic investigation for localization and delineation of infection ■ Implement source control if necessary	■ Initiate vasopressor therapy if circulatory shock persists following adequate fluid resuscitation ■ Initiate inotropes if CI or $S\bar{v}O_2$ are persistently decreased	■ ICU transfer with full monitoring support ■ Arterial catheter assessment ■ If shock persists with >2 L crystalloid resuscitation, venous catheter assessment ± placement (goal CVP ≥8 mm Hg)		■ Consider low-dose steroid therapy ± ACTH stimulation test
8–24 hours	■ Dynamic evaluation of resuscitative goals (based on clinical and invasive monitoring end points)		■ Consider vasopressin if shock refractory to first-line vasopressors persists	■ If persistently pressor dependent after 3–5 L crystalloid infusion, CVP ≥8 achieved, suspicion of intravascular volume depletion or limited cardiovascular reserve, PAC placement (initial goal PWP 12–15 mm Hg) ■ May be inserted earlier if clinically indicated	■ Consider initiation of drotrecogin-alfa (activated) if single organ failure with APACHE II ≥25, two or more organ failures in absence of APACHE score	■ Initiate enteral feeding ■ Consider intensive insulin therapy
>24 hours		■ Narrow antimicrobial regimen depending on isolation of pathogenic organisms and/or clinical improvement ■ Reassess necessity for or efficacy of source control		■ Consider PAC in vasopressor-dependent patients with progressive respiratory, renal, or multiple organ dysfunction		■ Intensive hemodialysis therapy for renal failure ■ Low-pressure, volume-limited ventilation for ARDS

HR, heart rate; MAP, mean arterial blood pressure; ECG, electroencephalograph; UO, urine output; Cl, chlorine; $S\bar{v}O_2$, mixed venous oxygen saturation; CVP, central venous pressure; ACTH, adrenocorticotropin hormone; PAC, pulmonary artery catheter; PWP, pulmonary wedge pressure; APACHE, Acute Physiology and Chronic Health Evaluation; ARDS, acute respiratory distress syndrome.

SUMMARY

Severe sepsis and septic shock continue to be a major cause of mortality and morbidity among patients requiring ICU support. In recent years, both basic and clinical research in the field have accelerated substantially. This has led to the publication of several studies with major implications regarding the appropriate management of patients with these conditions. Many of these new studies relate to optimization of supportive care. Although controversial, a single specific therapy, drotrecogin alfa (activated), has been shown to improve mortality in severe sepsis and septic shock. Few major studies in the areas of fluid resuscitation, vasopressors/inotropes, invasive and noninvasive monitoring, or antimicrobial therapy have been published in recent years. Nonetheless, outcome can most likely be improved by taking a systematic approach to therapy as described in Table 57.15. Although significant improvements in outcome have been made possible by new pharmacologic therapies, recent studies focusing on antimicrobial and supportive elements clearly demonstrate that close attention to established therapies can have a substantial impact on survival in severe sepsis and septic shock.

References

1. Angus DC, Linde-Zwirble WT, Lidicker J, et al. Epidemiology of severe sepsis in the United States: analysis of incidence, outcome, and associated costs of care. *Crit Care Med.* 2001;29(7):1303–1310.
2. Finland M, Jones WF, Barnes MW. Occurence of serious bacterial infections since the introduction of antibacterial agents. *JAMA.* 1959;84:2188–2197.
3. Hemminki E, Paakkulainen A. Effect of antibiotics on mortality from infectious diseases in Sweden and Finland. *Am J Public Health.* 1976;66:1180–1184.
4. Kreger BE, Craven DE, McCabe WR. Gram-negative bacteremia. IV. Re-evaluation of clinical features and treatment in 612 patients. *Am J Med.* 1980;68(3):344–355.
5. Martin GS, Mannino DM, Eaton S, et al. The epidemiology of sepsis in the United States from 1979 through 2000. *N Engl J Med.* 2003;348(16):1546–1554.
6. Minino AM, Heron MP, Smith BL. Deaths: preliminary data for 2004. *Natl Vital Stat Rep.* 2006;54(19):1–49.
7. Friedman G, Silva E, Vincent JL. Has the mortality of septic shock changed with time? *Crit Care Med.* 1998;26(12):2078–2086.
8. Geroulanos S, Douka ET. Historical perspective of the word "sepsis." *Intensive Care Med.* 2006;32:2077.
9. Budelmann G. Hugo Schottmuller, 1867–1936. The problem of sepsis [in German]. *Internist (Berl).* 1969;10(3):92–101.
10. Bone R. American College of Chest Physicians/Society of Critical Care Medicine Consensus Conference: definitions for sepsis and organ failure and guidelines for the use of innovative therapies in sepsis. *Crit Care Med.* 1992;20:864–874.
11. Levy MM, Fink MP, Marshall JC, et al. 2001 SCCM/ESICM/ACCP/ATS/SIS International Sepsis Definitions Conference. *Crit Care Med.* 2003;31(4):1250–1256.
12. Marshall JC, Cook DJ, Christou NV, et al. Multiple organ dysfunction score: a reliable descriptor of a complex clinical outcome. *Crit Care Med.* 1995;23(10):1638–1652.
13. Ferreira FL, Bota DP, Bross A, et al. Serial evaluation of the SOFA score to predict outcome in critically ill patients. *JAMA.* 2001;286(14):1754–1758.
14. Bone RC, Bone RC. Immunologic dissonance: a continuing evolution in our understanding of the systemic inflammatory response syndrome (SIRS) and the multiple organ dysfunction syndrome (MODS). *Ann Intern Med.* 1996;125(8):680–687.
15. Padkin A, Goldfrad C, Brady AR, et al. Epidemiology of severe sepsis occurring in the first 24 hrs in intensive care units in England, Wales, and Northern Ireland. *Crit Care Med.* 2003;31(9):2332–2338.
16. Finfer SBR, Bellomo R, Lipman J, et al. Adult-population incidence of severe sepsis in Australian and New Zealand intensive care units. *Intensive Care Med.* 2004;30:589–596.
17. Brun-Buisson C, Meshaka P, Pinton P, et al. EPISEPSIS: a reappraisal of the epidemiology and outcome of severe sepsis in French intensive care units. *Intensive Care Med.* 2004;30(4):580–588.
18. Sundararajan V, Macisaac CM, Presneill JJ, et al. Epidemiology of sepsis in Victoria, Australia. *Crit Care Med.* 2005;33(1):71–80.
19. Danai P, Martin GS. Epidemiology of sepsis: recent advances. *Curr Infect Dis Rep.* 2005;7:329–334.
20. Brun-Buisson C, Doyon F, Carlet J, et al. Incidence, risk factors, and outcome of severe sepsis and septic shock in adults. A multicenter prospective study in intensive care units. French ICU Group for Severe Sepsis. *JAMA.* 1995;274:968–974.
21. Annane D, Aegerter P, Jars-Guincestre MC, et al. Current epidemiology of septic shock: the CUB-Rea Network. *Am J Resp Crit Care Med.* 2003;168(2):165–172.
22. Sands KE, Bates DW, Lanken PN, et al. Epidemiology of sepsis syndrome in 8 academic medical centers. *JAMA.* 1997;278(3):234–240.
23. Pakhale S, Roberts D, Light B, et al. A geographically and temporally comprehensive analysis of septic shock: impact of age, sex and socioeconomic status. *Crit Care Med.* 2005;33:A79.
24. Zhan C, Miller MR. Excess length of stay, charges, and mortality attributable to medical injuries during hospitalization. *JAMA.* 2003; 290(14):1868–1874.
25. Kumar A, Roberts D, Wood KE, et al. Duration of hypotension before initiation of effective antimicrobial therapy is the critical determinant of survival in human septic shock. *Crit Care Med.* 2006;34(6):1589–1596.
26. Bernard GR, Vincent JL, Laterre PF. Efficacy and safety of recombinant human activated protein C for severe sepsis. *N Engl J Med.* 2001;344:699–709.
27. Warren BL, Eid A, Singer P, et al. High-dose antithrombin III in severe sepsis: a randomized controlled trial. *JAMA.* 2001;286(15):1869–1878.
28. Abraham E, Reinhart K, Opal S, et al. Efficacy and safety of tifacogin (recombinant tissue factor pathway inhibitor) in severe sepsis: a randomized controlled trial. *JAMA.* 2003;290(2):238–247.
29. Abraham E, Laterre PF, Garg R, et al. Drotrecogin alfa (activated) for adults with severe sepsis and a low risk of death. *N Engl J Med.* 2005; 353(13):1332–1341.
30. O'Brien JM Jr, Lu B, Ali NA, et al. Alcohol dependence is independently associated with sepsis, septic shock, and hospital mortality among adult intensive care unit patients. *Crit Care Med.* 2007;35(2):345–350.
31. Rangel-Frausto MS, Pittet D, Costigan M, et al. The natural history of the systemic inflammatory response syndrome (SIRS). A prospective study [comment]. *JAMA.* 1995;273(2):117–123.
32. Loeb HS, Cruz A, Teng CY, et al. Haemodynamic studies in shock associated with infection. *Br Heart J.* 1967;29(6):883–894.
33. Weil MH, Shubin H, Biddle M. Shock caused by gram-negative microorganisms. *Ann Intern Med.* 1964;60:384–400.
34. Kasal J, Jovanovic Z, Clermont G, et al. Comparison of Cox and Gray's survival models in severe sepsis. *Crit Care Med.* 2004;32(3):700–707.
35. Parker MM, Shelhamer JH, Natanson C, et al. Serial cardiovascular variables in survivors and nonsurvivors of human septic shock: heart rate as an early predictor of prognosis. *Crit Care Med.* 1987;15:923–929.
36. Alberti C, Brun-Buisson C, Burchardi H, et al. Epidemiology of sepsis and infection in ICU patients from an international multicentre cohort study. *Intensive Care Med.* 2002;28(2):108–121.
37. Richards MJ, Edwards JR, Culver DH, et al. Nosocomial infections in medical intensive care units in the United States. National Nosocomial Infections Surveillance System. *Crit Care Med.* 1999;27(5):887–892.
38. Wisplinghoff H, Bischoff T, Tallent SM, et al. Nosocomial bloodstream infections in US hospitals: analysis of. 24,179 cases from a prospective nationwide surveillance study. *Clin Infect Dis.* 2004;39(3):309–317.
39. Macphail GL, Taylor GD, Buchanan-Chell M, et al. Epidemiology, treatment and outcome of candidemia: a five-year review at three Canadian hospitals. *Mycoses.* 2002;45(5-6):141–145.
40. Berrouane YF, Herwaldt LA, Pfaller MA, et al. Trends in antifungal use and epidemiology of nosocomial yeast infections in a university hospital. *J Clin Microbiol.* 1999;37(3):531–537.
41. Abi-Said D, Anaissie E, Uzun O, et al. The epidemiology of hematogenous candidiasis caused by different Candida species. *Clin Infect Dis.* 1997; 24(6):1122–1128.
42. Murray BE, Murray BE. Vancomycin-resistant enterococcal infections. *N Engl J Med.* 2000;342(10):710–721.
43. Giamarellou H. Multidrug resistance in Gram-negative bacteria that produce extended-spectrum beta-lactamases (ESBLs). *Clin Microbiol Infect.* 2005;11(Suppl 4):1–16.
44. Miller LG, Perdreau-Remington F, Rieg G, et al. Necrotizing fasciitis caused by community-associated methicillin-resistant *Staphylococcus aureus* in Los Angeles. *N Engl J Med.* 2005;352(14):1445–1453.
45. From the Centers for Disease Control. *Staphylococcus aureus* resistant to vancomycin–United States, 2002. *JAMA.* 2002;288(7):824–825.
46. Heumann D, Glauser MP, Calandra T. Molecular basis of host-pathogen interaction in septic shock. *Curr Opin Microbiol.* 1998;1(1):49–55.
47. Hemmi H, Takeuchi O, Kawai T, et al. A Toll-like receptor recognizes bacterial DNA. *Nature.* 2000;408(6813):740–745.
48. Bauer S, Kirschning CJ, Hacker H, et al. Human TLR9 confers responsiveness to bacterial DNA via species-specific CpG motif recognition. *Proc Natl Acad Sci U S A.* 2001;98(16):9237–9242.

49. Sparwasser T, Miethke T, Lipford G, et al. Bacterial DNA causes septic shock. *Nature.* 1997;386(6623):336–337.
50. Alexopoulou L, Holt AC, Medzhitov R, et al. Recognition of double-stranded RNA and activation of NF-kappaB by Toll-like receptor 3. *Nature.* 2001;413(6857):732–738.
51. Dziarski R, Wang Q, Miyake K, et al. MD-2 enables Toll-like receptor 2 (TLR2)-mediated responses to lipopolysaccharide and enhances TLR2-mediated responses to Gram-positive and Gram-negative bacteria and their cell wall components. *J Immunol.* 2001;166(3):1938–1944.
52. Yang RB, Mark MR, Gray A, et al. Toll-like receptor-2 mediates lipopolysaccharide-induced cellular signalling. *Nature.* 1998;395(6699): 284–288.
53. Lien E, Sellati TJ, Yoshimura A, et al. Toll-like receptor 2 functions as a pattern recognition receptor for diverse bacterial products. *J Biol Chem.* 1999;274(47):33419–33425.
54. Schwandner R, Dziarski R, Wesche H, et al. Peptidoglycan- and lipoteichoic acid-induced cell activation is mediated by toll-like receptor 2. *J Biol Chem.* 1999;274(25):17406–17409.
55. Manocha S, Feinstein D, Kumar A, et al. Novel therapies for sepsis: antiendotoxin therapies. *Exp Opin Invest Drugs.* 2002;11(12):1795–1812.
56. Martich GD, Boujoukos AJ, Suffredini AF. Response of man to endotoxin. *Immunobiology.* 1993;187(3–5):403–416.
57. Ing DJ, Zang J, Dzau VJ, et al. Modulation of cytokine-induced cardiac myocyte apoptosis by nitric oxide, Bak, and Bcl-x. *Circ Res.* 1999;84:21–33.
58. Albelda SM, Smith CW, Ward PA. Adhesion molecules and inflammatory injury. *FASEB J.* 1994;8:504–512.
59. Balligand JL, Ungureanu-Longrois D, Simmons WW, et al. Cytokine-inducible nitric oxide synthase (iNOS) expression in cardiac myocytes. *J Biol Chem.* 1994;269:27580–27588.
60. Esmon CT. Role of coagulation inhibitors in inflammation. *Thromb Haemost.* 2001;86(1):51–56.
61. Heumann D. CD14 and LBP in endotoxemia and infections caused by Gram-negative bacteria. *J Endotoxin Res.* 2001;7(6):439–441.
62. Raetz CR, Ulevitch RJ, Wright SD, et al. Gram-negative endotoxin: an extraordinary lipid with profound effects on eukaryotic signal transduction. *FASEB J.* 1991;5(12):2652–2660.
63. Rietschel ET, Kirikae T, Schade FU, et al. Bacterial endotoxin: molecular relationships of structure to activity and function. *FASEB J.* 1994;8(2):217–225.
64. Hellman J, Warren HS. Antiendotoxin strategies. *Infect Dis Clin North Am.* 1999;13(2):371–386.
65. Kumar A, Zanotti S, Bunnell G, et al. Interleukin-10 blunts the human inflammatory response to lipopolysaccharide without affecting the cardiovascular response. *Crit Care Med.* 2005;33(2):331–340.
66. Kumar A, Bunnell E, Lynn M, et al. Experimental human endotoxemia is associated with depression of load-independent contractility indices: prevention by the lipid a analogue E5531. *Chest.* 2004;126(3):860–867.
67. Suffredini AF, Reda D, Banks SM, et al. Effects of recombinant dimeric TNF receptor on human inflammatory responses following intravenous endotoxin administration. *J Immunol.* 1995;155(10):5038–5045.
68. Le Roy D, Di Padova F, Tees R, et al. Monoclonal antibodies to murine lipopolysaccharide (LPS)-binding protein (LBP) protect mice from lethal endotoxemia by blocking either the binding of LPS to LBP or the presentation of LPS/LBP complexes to CD14. *J Immunol.* 1999;162(12):7454–7460.
69. Schumann RR, Leong SR, Flaggs GW, et al. Structure and function of lipopolysaccharide binding protein. *Science.* 1990;249(4975):1429–1431.
70. Heumann D, Barras C, Severin A, et al. Gram-positive cell walls stimulate synthesis of tumor necrosis factor alpha and interleukin-6 by human monocytes. *Infect Immun.* 1994;62(7):2715–2721.
71. Mattsson E, Rollof J, Verhoef J, et al. Serum-induced potentiation of tumor necrosis factor alpha production by human monocytes in response to staphylococcal peptidoglycan: involvement of different serum factors. *Infect Immun.* 1994;62(9):3837–3843.
72. Wright SD, Ramos RA, Tobias PS, et al. CD14, a receptor for complexes of lipopolysaccharide (LPS) and LPS binding protein. *Science.* 1990; 249(4975):1431–1433.
73. Hailman E, Lichenstein HS, Wurfel MM, et al. Lipopolysaccharide (LPS)-binding protein accelerates the binding of LPS to CD14. *J Exp Med.* 1994; 179(1):269–277.
74. Ingalls RR, Golenbock DT, Ingalls RR, et al. CD11c/CD18, a transmembrane signaling receptor for lipopolysaccharide. *J Exp Med.* 1995; 181(4):1473–1479.
75. Kusunoki T, Hailman E, Juan TS, et al. Molecules from *Staphylococcus aureus* that bind CD14 and stimulate innate immune responses. *J Exp Med.* 1995;182(6):1673–1682.
76. Kirschning CJ, Wesche H, Merrill AT, et al. Human toll-like receptor 2 confers responsiveness to bacterial lipopolysaccharide. *J Exp Med.* 1998;188(11):2091–2097.
77. Hoshino K, Takeuchi O, Kawai T, et al. Cutting edge: Toll-like receptor 4 (TLR4)-deficient mice are hyporesponsive to lipopolysaccharide: evidence for TLR4 as the Lps gene product. *J Immunol.* 1999;162(7):3749–3752.
78. Takeuchi O, Hoshino K, Kawai T, et al. Differential roles of TLR2 and TLR4 in recognition of gram-negative and gram-positive bacterial cell wall components. *Immunity.* 1999;11(4):443–451.
79. Chow JC, Young DW, Golenbock D, et al. Toll-like receptor-4 mediates lipopolysaccharide-induced signal transduction. *J Biol Chem.* 1999; 274(16):10689–10692.
80. Tauszig S, Jouanguy E, Hoffmann JA, et al. Toll-related receptors and the control of antimicrobial peptide expression in *Drosophila. Proc Natl Acad Sci U S A.* 2000;97(19):10520–10525.
81. Lien E, Means TK, Heine H, et al. Toll-like receptor 4 imparts ligand-specific recognition of bacterial lipopolysaccharide. *J Clin Invest.* 2000; 105(4):497–504.
82. Muroi M, Ohnishi T, Tanamoto K, et al. MD-2, a novel accessory molecule, is involved in species-specific actions of Salmonella lipid A. *Infect Immun.* 2002;70(7):3546–3550.
83. Muroi M, Ohnishi T, Tanamoto K, et al. Regions of the mouse CD14 molecule required for toll-like receptor. 2- and 4-mediated activation of NF-kappa B. *J Biol Chem.* 2002;277(44):42372–42379.
84. Muller-Alouf H, Alouf JE, Gerlach D, et al. Human pro- and anti-inflammatory cytokine patterns induced by *Streptococcus pyogenes* erythrogenic (pyrogenic) exotoxin A and C superantigens. *Infect Immun.* 1996;64(4):1450–1453.
85. Cohen J. The immunopathogenesis of sepsis. Review. *Nature.* 2002; 420(6917):885–891.
86. Docke WD, Randow F, Syrbe U, et al. Monocyte deactivation in septic patients: restoration by IFN-gamma treatment. *Nature Med.* 1997;3(6):678–681.
87. Mira JP, Cariou A, Grall F, et al. Association of TNF2, a TNF-alpha promoter polymorphism, with septic shock susceptibility and mortality: a multicenter study. *JAMA.* 1999;282(6):561–568.
88. Holmes CL, Russell JA, Walley KR. Genetic polymorphisms in sepsis and septic shock: role in prognosis and potential for therapy. *Chest.* 2003; 124:1103–1115.
89. Nathan C. Nitric oxide as a secretory product of mammalian cells. *FASEB J.* 1992;6:3051–3064.
90. Lorente JA, Landin L, Renes E, et al. Role of nitric oxide in the hemodynamic changes of sepsis. *Crit Care Med.* 1993;21:759–767.
91. Kilbourn RG, Gross SS, Jubran A, et al. N-methyl-L-arginine inhibits tumor necrosis factor-induced hypotension: implications for the involvement of nitric oxide. *Proc Natl Acad Sci U S A.* 1990;87:3629–3623.
92. Thiemermann C, Szabö C, Mitchell JA, et al. Vascular hyporeactivity to vasoconstrictor agents and hemodynamic decompensation in hemorrhagic shock is mediated by nitric oxide. *Proc Natl Acad Sci U S A.* 1993;90:267–271.
93. Kubes P. Nitric oxide modulates microvascular permeability. *Am J Physiol.* 1992;262(2):H611–H615.
94. Kumar A, Thota V, Dee L, et al. Tumor necrosis factor-alpha and interleukin-1 beta are responsible for depression of in vitro myocardial cell contractility induced by serum from humans with septic shock. *J Exp Med.* 1996;183:949–958.
95. Kumar A, Krieger A, Symeoneides S, et al. Myocardial dysfunction in septic shock, II: role of cytokines and nitric oxide. *J Cardiovasc Thorac Anesth.* 2001;15(4):485–511.
96. Beckman JS, Beckman TW, Chen J, et al. Apparent hydroxyl radical production by peroxynitrite: implications for endothelial injury from nitric oxide and superoxide. *Proc Natl Acad Sci U S A.* 1990;87(4):1620–1624.
97. Muta T, Iwanaga S, Muta T, et al. Clotting and immune defense in *Limulidae. Progr Molec Subcell Biol.* 1996;15:154–189.
98. Nachum R, Nachum R. Antimicrobial defense mechanisms in *Limulus polyphemus. Progr Clin Biol Res U S A.* 1979;29:513–524.
99. McGilvray ID, Rotstein OD, McGilvray ID, et al. Role of the coagulation system in the local and systemic inflammatory response. *World J Surg.* 1998;22(2):179–186.
100. Wheeler AP, Bernard GR. Treating patients with severe sepsis. *N Engl J Med.* 1999;340:207–214.
101. Gando S, Nanzaki S, Sasaki S. Activation of the extrinsic coagulation pathway in patients with severe sepsis and septic shock. *Crit Care Med.* 1998;26:2005–2009.
102. Mesters R, Helterbrand J, Utterback BG. Prognostic value of protein C concentrations in neutropenic patients at high risk of severe septic complications. *Crit Care Med.* 2000;28:2209–2216.
103. Rosenberg RD, Aird WC. Vascular-bed-specific hemostasis and hypercoagulable states. *N Engl J Med.* 1999;340:1555–1564.
104. van der Poll T, Bueller HR, ten Cate H, et al. Activation of coagulation after administration of tumor necrosis factor to normal subjects. *N Engl J Med.* 1990;322:1622–1627.
105. Esmon NL, Esmon CT. Protein C and the endothelium. *Semin Thromb Hemost.* 1988;14:210–215.
106. Mesters R, Mannucci PM, Coppola E. Factor VIIA and anti-thrombin III activity during severe sepsis and septic shock in neutropenic patients. *Blood.* 1996;88:881–886.
107. Abraham E. Tissue factor inhibition and clinical trial results of tissue factor pathway inhibitor in sepsis. *Crit Care Med.* 2000;28(9 Suppl):S31–S33.
108. Abraham E, Reinhart K, Svoboda P, et al. Assessment of the safety of recombinant tissue factor pathway inhibitor in patients with severe sepsis:

a multicenter, randomized, placebo-controlled, single-blind, dose escalation study. *Crit Care Med.* 2001;29(11):2081–2089.
109. Sorensen TI, Nielsen GG, Andersen PK, et al. Genetic and environmental influences on premature death in adult adoptees. *N Engl J Med.* 1988; 318(12):727–732.
110. Udhoji VN, Weil MH. Hemodynamic and metabolic studies on shock associated with bacteremia. *Ann Intern Med.* 1965;62:966–978.
111. Cohn JD, Greenspan M, Goldstein CR, et al. Arteriovenous shunting in high cardiac output shock syndromes. *Surg Gynecol Obstet.* 1968;127:282–288.
112. Thijs LG, Groenveld ABJ. Peripheral circulation in septic shock. *Appl Cardiopul, Pathol.* 1988;2:203–214.
113. Wright CJ, Duff JH, McLean APH, et al. Regional capillary blood flow and oxygen uptake in severe sepsis. *Surg Gynecol Obstet.* 1971;132:637–644.
114. Finley RJ, Duff JH, Holliday RL, et al. Capillary muscle blood flow in human sepsis. *Surgery.* 1975;78:87–94.
115. Cronenwett JL, Lindenauer SM. Direct measurement of arteriovenous anastomic blood flow in the septic canine hindlimb. *Surgery.* 1979;85:275–282.
116. Dantzker D. Oxygen delivery and utilization in sepsis. *Crit Care Clin.* 1989; 5:81–98.
117. Wolf YG, Cotev S, Perel A, et al. Dependence of oxygen consumption on cardiac output in sepsis. *Crit Care Med.* 1987;15:198–203.
118. Shoemaker WC, Chang P, Czer L, et al. Cardiorespiratory monitoring in postoperative patients, I: prediction of outcome and severity of illness. *Crit Care Med.* 1979;7:237–242.
119. Haupt MT, Gilbert EM, Carlson RW. Fluid loading increases oxygen consumption in septic patients with lactic acidosis. *Am Rev Respir Dis.* 1985;131:912–916.
120. Samsel RW, Nelson DP, Sanders WM, et al. Effect of endotoxin on systemic and skeletal muscle oxygen extraction. *J Appl Physiol.* 1988;65:1377–1382.
121. Vincent JL, Roman A, DeBacker D, et al. Oxygen uptake/supply dependency: effects of short-term dobutamine infusion. *Am Rev Respir Dis.* 1990;142:2–8.
122. Fenwick JC, Dodek PM, Ronco JJ, et al. Increased concentrations of plasma lactate predict pathological dependence of oxygen consumption on oxygen delivery in patients with adult respiratory distress syndrome. *J Crit Care.* 1990;5:81–87.
123. Gutierrez G, Pohil RJ. Oxygen consumption is linearly related to oxygen supply in critically ill patients. *J Crit Care.* 1986;1:45–53.
124. Barcroft J. On anoxaemia. *Lancet.* 1920;2:485–492.
125. Astiz M, Rackow EC, Weil MH, et al. Early impairment of oxidative metabolism and energy production in severe sepsis. *Circ Shock.* 1988;26: 311–320.
126. Mizock B. Septic shock: a metabolic perspective. *Arch Intern Med.* 1984; 144:579–585.
127. Fink MP. Cytopathic hypoxia. Mitochondrial dysfunction as mechanism contributing to organ dysfunction in sepsis. *Crit Care Clin.* 2001;17(1): 219–237.
128. VanderMeer TJ, Wang H, Fink MP. Endotoxemia causes ileal mucosal acidosis in the absence of mucosal hypoxia in a normodynamic porcine model of septic shock. *Crit Care Med.* 1995;23(7):1217–1226.
129. Hotchkiss RS, Rust RS, Dence CS, et al. Evaluation of the role of cellular hypoxia in sepsis by the hypoxic marker [18F] fluoromisonidazole. *Am J Physiol.* 1991;261:R965–R972.
130. King CJ, Tytgat S, Delude RL, et al. Ileal mucosal oxygen consumption is decreased in endotoxemic rats but is restored toward normal by treatment with aminoguanidine. *Crit Care Med.* 1999;27(11):2518–2524.
131. Simonson SG, Welty-Wolf K, Huang YT, et al. Altered mitochondrial redox responses in gram negative septic shock in primates. *Circ Shock.* 1994;43(1):34–43.
132. Brealey D, Brand M, Hargreaves I, et al. Association between mitochondrial dysfunction and severity and outcome of septic shock. *Lancet.* 2002;360(9328):219–223.
133. Griebel JA, Moore FA, Piantadosi CA. In-vivo responses of mitochondrial redox levels to *Escherichia coli* bacteremia in primates. *J Crit Care.* 1990;5:1–9.
134. Cairns CB, Moore FA, Haenel JB, et al. Evidence for early supply independent mitochondrial dysfunction in patients developing multiple organ failure after trauma. *J Trauma.* 1997;42(3):532–536.
135. Mori E, Hasebe M, Kobayashi K, et al. Alterations in metabolite levels in carbohydrate and energy metabolism of rat in hemorrhagic shock and sepsis. *Metabolism.* 1987;36:14–20.
136. Tanaka J, Sato T, Kamiyama Y, et al. Bacteremic shock: aspects of high-energy metabolism of rat liver following *Escherichia coli* injection. *J Surg Res.* 1982;33:49–57.
137. Yassen KA, Galley HF, Lee A, et al. Mitochondrial redox state in the critically ill. *Br J Anaesth.* 1999;83(2):325–327.
138. Grum CM, Simon RH, Dantzker D, et al. Evidence for adenosine triphosphate degradation in critically ill patients. *Chest.* 1985;88:763–767.
139. Ozawa K, Aoyama H, Yasuda K, et al. Metabolic abnormalities associated with postoperative organ failure. A redox theory. *Arch Surg.* 1983;118(11): 1245–1251.
140. Bergstrom J, Bostrom H, Furst P, et al. Preliminary studies of energy-rich phosphagens in muscle from severely ill patients. *Crit Care Med.* 1976; 4(4):197–204.
141. Liaw KY, Askanazi J, Michelson CB, et al. Effect of injury and sepsis on high-energy phosphates in muscle and red cells. *J Trauma.* 1980;20(9):755–759.
142. Song SK, Hotchkiss RS, Karl IE, et al. Concurrent quantification of tissue metabolism and blood flow via 2H/31P NMR in vivo, III: alterations of muscle blood flow and metabolism during sepsis. *Magn Reson Med.* 1992;25:67–77.
143. Hotchkiss RS, Karl IE. Reevaluation of the role of cellular hypoxia and bioenergetic failure in sepsis. *JAMA.* 1992;267:1503–1510.
144. Solomon MA, Correa R, Alexander HR, et al. Myocardial energy metabolism and morphology in a canine model of sepsis. *Am J Physiol.* 1994;266:H757–H768.
145. Hotchkiss RS, Song SK, Neil JJ, et al. Sepsis does not impair tricarboxylic acid cycle in the heart. *Am J Physiol.* 1991;260:C50–C57.
146. Chaudry IH, Wichterman KA, Baue AE. Effect of sepsis on tissue adenine nucleotide levels. *Surgery.* 1979;85:205–211.
147. Geller ER, Tankauskas S, Kirpatrick JR. Mitochondrial death in sepsis: a failed concept. *J Surg Res.* 1986;40:514–517.
148. MacLean LD, Mulligan WG, McLean APH, et al. Patterns of septic shock in man: a detailed study of 56 patients. *Ann Surg.* 1967;166:543–562.
149. Nishijima H, Weil MH, Shubin H, et al. Hemodynamic and metabolic studies on shock associated with gram-negative bacteremia. *Medicine (Baltimore).* 1973;52:287–294.
150. Weil MH, Nishijima H. Cardiac output in bacterial shock. *Am J Med.* 1978;64:920–922.
151. Blain CM, Anderson TO, Pietras RJ, et al. Immediate hemodynamic effects of gram-negative vs gram-positive bacteremia in man. *Arch Intern Med.* 1970;126:260–265.
152. Packman MI, Rackow EC. Optimum left heart filling pressure during fluid resuscitation of patients with hypovolemic and septic shock. *Crit Care Med.* 1983;11:165–169.
153. Winslow EJ, Loeb HS, Rahimtoola SH, et al. Hemodynamic studies and results of therapy in 50 patients with bacteremic shock. *Am J Med.* 1973; 54:421–432.
154. Krausz MM, Perel A, Eimerl D, et al. Cardiopulmonary effects of volume loading in patients with septic shock. *Ann Surg.* 1977;185:429–434.
155. Parker MM, Suffredini AF, Natanson C, et al. Responses of left ventricular function in surviviors and non-survivors of septic shock. *J Crit Care.* 1989;4:19–25.
156. Teule GJJ, Van Lingen A, Verweij-van Vught MA, et al. Role of peripheral pooling in porcine Escherichia coli sepsis. *Circ Shock.* 1984;12:115–123.
157. Natanson C, Fink MP, Ballantyne HK, et al. Gram-negative bacteremia produces both severe systolic and diastolic cardiac dysfunction in a canine model that simulates human septic shock. *J Clin Invest.* 1986;78:259–270.
158. Carroll GC, Snyder JV. Hyperdynamic severe intravascular sepsis depends on fluid administration in cynomolgus monkey. *Am J Physiol.* 1982; 243:131–141.
159. Teule GJJ, Den Hollander W, Bronsveld W, et al. Effect of volume loading and dopamine on hemodynamics and red cell distribution in canine endotoxic shock. *Circ Shock.* 1983;10:41–50.
160. Magder S, Vanelli G. Circuit factors in the high cardiac output of sepsis. *J Crit Care.* 1996;11(4):155–166.
161. Donnino M, Nguyen HB, Rivers EP. A hemodynamic comparison of early and late phase severe sepsis and septic shock. *Chest.* 2002;122:4S.
162. Kumar A, Haery C, Parrillo JE. Myocardial dysfunction in septic shock, I: clinical manifestation of cardiovascular dysfunction. *J Cardiothor Vasc Anesth.* 2001;15(3):364–376.
163. Ognibene FP, Parker MM, Natanson C, et al. Depressed left ventricular performance. Response to volume infusion in patients with sepsis and septic shock. *Chest.* 1988;93:903–910.
164. Parker MM, Shelhamer JH, Bacharach SL, et al. Profound but reversible myocardial depression in patients with septic shock. *Ann Intern Med.* 1984;100:483–490.
165. Garner LB, Willis MS, Carlson DL, et al. Macrophage migration inhibitory factor is a cardiac-derived myocardial depressant factor. *Am J Physiol.* 2003;285(6):H2500–H2509.
166. Eichenholz PW, Eichacker PQ, Hoffman WD, et al. Tumor necrosis factor challenges in canines: patterns of cardiovascular dysfunction. *Am J Physiol.* 1992;263:H668–H675.
167. Vincent JL, Bakker J, Marecaux G, et al. Administration of anti-TNF antibody improves left ventricular function in septic shock patients: results of a pilot study. *Chest.* 1992;101:810–815.
168. Hosenpud JD, Campbell SM, Mendelson DJ. Interleukin-1-induced myocardial depression in an isolated beating heart preparation. *J Heart Transplant.* 1989;8:460–464.
169. Massey CV, Kohout TR, Gaa ST, et al. Molecular and cellular actions of platelet-activating factor in rat heart cells. *J Clin Invest.* 1991;88:2106–2116.
170. Schutzer KM, Haglund U, Falk A. Cardiopulmonary dysfunction in a feline septic model: possible role of leukotrienes. *Circ Shock.* 1989;29:13–25.
171. Werdan K, Muller U, Reithmann C. "Negative inotropic cascades" in cardiomyocytes triggered by substances relevant to sepsis. In: Schlag G, Redl H, eds. *Pathophysiology of Shock, Sepsis and Organ Failure.* Berlin, Germany: Springer-Verlag; 1993:787–834.

172. Pathan N, Hemingway CA, Alizadeh AA, et al. Role of interleukin 6 in myocardial dysfunction of meningococcal septic shock. *Lancet.* 2004; 363(9404):203–209.
173. Papadopoulos MC, Davies DC, Moss R, et al. Pathophysiology of septic encephalopathy: a review. *Crit Care Med.* 2000;28(8):3019–3024.
174. Sprung CL, Peduzzi PN, Shatney CH, et al. Impact of encephalopathy on mortality in the sepsis syndrome. The Veterans Administration Systemic Sepsis Cooperative Study Group. *Crit Care Med.* 1990;18(8):801–806.
175. Pine RW, Wertz MJ, Lennard ES, et al. Determinants of organ malfunction or death in patients with intra-abdominal sepsis. A discriminant analysis. *Arch Surg.* 1983;118(2):242–249.
176. Young GB, Bolton CF, Austin TW, et al. The encephalopathy associated with septic illness. *Clin Invest Med.* 1990;13(6):297–304.
177. Young GB, Bolton CF, Archibald Y, et al. The electroencephalogram in sepsis-associated encephalopathy. *J Clin Neurophysiol.* 1992;9(1):145–152.
178. Kollef MH, Sherman G. Acquired organ system derangements and hospital mortality: are all organ systems created equally? *Am J Crit Care.* 1999;8(3):180–188.
179. De Jonghe B, Lacherade JC, Durand MC, et al. Critical illness neuromuscular syndromes. *Crit Care Clin.* 2006;22(4):805–818.
180. Leijten FS, Harinck-de Weerd JE, Poortvliet DC, et al. The role of polyneuropathy in motor convalescence after prolonged mechanical ventilation. *JAMA.* 1995;274(15):1221–1225.
181. Bercker S, Weber-Carstens S, Deja M, et al. Critical illness polyneuropathy and myopathy in patients with acute respiratory distress syndrome. *Crit Care Med.* 2005;33(4):711–715.
182. Lorin S, Sivak M, Nierman DM. Critical illness polyneuropathy: what to look for in at-risk patients. *J Crit Illness.* 1998;13(10):608–612.
183. Tennila A, Salmi T, Pettila V, et al. Early signs of critical illness polyneuropathy in ICU patients with systemic inflammatory response syndrome or sepsis [see comment]. *Intensive Care Med.* 2000;26(9):1360–1363.
184. Tepper M, Rakic S, Haas JA, et al. Incidence and onset of critical illness polyneuropathy in patients with septic shock. *Neth J Med.* 2000;56(6):211–214.
185. De Jonghe B, Sharshar T, Lefaucheur JP, et al. Paresis acquired in the intensive care unit: a prospective multicenter study. *JAMA.* 2002;288(22):2859–2867.
186. Cunnion RE, Schaer GL, Parker MM, et al. The coronary circulation in human septic shock. *Circulation.* 1986;73:637–644.
187. Dhainaut JF, Huyghebaert MF, Monsallier JF, et al. Coronary hemodynamics and myocardial metabolism of lactate, free fatty acids, glucose, and ketones in patients with septic shock. *Circulation.* 1987;75:533–541.
188. Reilly JM, Cunnion RE, Burch-Whitman C, et al. A circulating myocardial depressant substance is associated with cardiac dysfunction and peripheral hypoperfusion (lactic acidemia) in patients with septic shock. *Chest.* 1989;95:1072–1080.
189. Parrillo JE, Burch C, Shelhamer JH, et al. A circulating myocardial depressant substance in humans with septic shock. Septic shock patients with a reduced ejection fraction have a circulating factor that depresses in vitro myocardial cell performance. *J Clin Invest.* 1985;76:1539–1553.
190. Jones SB, Romano RD. Myocardial beta adrenergic receptor coupling to adenylate cyclase during developing septic shock. *Circ Shock.* 1990;30:51–61.
191. Bristow MR, Ginsburg R, Minobe W, et al. Decreased catecholamine sensitivity and beta adrenergic receptor density in failing human hearts. *N Engl J Med.* 1982;307:205–210.
192. Silverman HJ, Penaranda R, Orens JB, et al. Impaired beta-adrenergic receptor stimulation of cyclic adenosine monophosphate in human septic shock: association with myocardial hyporesponsiveness to catecholamines. *Crit Care Med.* 1993;21:31–39.
193. Kumar A, Brar R, Wang P, et al. The role of nitric oxide and cyclic GMP in human septic serum-induced depression of cardiac myocyte contractility. *Am J Physiol.* 1999;276:R265–R276.
194. Kumar A, Paladugu B, Mensing J, et al., Nitric oxide-dependent and -independent mechanisms are involved in TNFa-induced depression of cardiac myocyte contractility. *Am J Physiol.* 2007;292:R1900–R1906.
195. Anel R, Paladugu B, Makkena R, et al. TNFa induces a proximal defect of beta-adrenoreceptor signal transduction in cardiac myocytes. *Crit Care Med.* 1999;27:A95.
196. Gulick T, Chung MK, Pieper SJ, et al. Interleukin-1 and tumor necrosis factor inhibit cardiac myocyte adrenergic responsiveness. *Proc Natl Acad Sci.U S A.* 1989;86:6753–6757.
197. Chung MK, Gulick TS, Rotondo R, et al. Mechanism of cytokine inhibition of beta-adrenergic agonist stimulation of cyclic AMP in rat cardiac myoctyes: impairment of signal transduction. *Circ Res.* 1990;67:753–763.
198. Turner A, Tsamitros M, Bellomo R. Myocardial cell injury in septic shock. *Crit Care Med.* 1999;27(9):1775–1780.
199. ver Elst KM, Spapen HD, Nguyen DN, et al. Cardiac troponins I and T are biological markers of left ventricular dysfunction in septic shock. *Clin Chem.* 2000;46(5):650–657.
200. Mehta NJ, Khan IA, Gupta V, et al. Cardiac troponin I predicts myocardial dysfunction and adverse outcome in septic shock. *Intl J Cardiol.* 2004;95(1):13–17.
201. Schrier RW, Wang W. Acute renal failure and sepsis [see comment]. *N Engl J Med.* 2004;351(2):159–169.
202. Ware LB, Matthay MA, Ware LB, et al. The acute respiratory distress syndrome. *N Engl J Med.* 2000;342(18):1334–1349.
203. Sevransky JE, Levy MM, Marini JJ, et al. Mechanical ventilation in sepsis-induced acute lung injury/acute respiratory distress syndrome: an evidence-based review. *Crit Care Med.* 2004;32(11 Suppl):S548–S553.
204. The Acute Respiratory Distress Syndrome Network. Ventilation with lower tidal volumes as compared with traditional tidal volumes for acute lung injury and the acute respiratory distress syndrome. *N Engl J Med.* 2000; 342(18):1301–1308.
205. Piantadosi CA, Schwartz DA, Piantadosi CA, et al. The acute respiratory distress syndrome. *Ann Intern Med.* 2004;141(6):460–470.
206. Hoste EA, Lameire NH, Vanholder RC, et al. Acute renal failure in patients with sepsis in a surgical ICU: predictive factors, incidence, comorbidity, and outcome. *J Am Soc Nephrol.* 2003;14(4):1022–1030.
207. Rasmussen HH, Ibels LS. Acute renal failure. Multivariate analysis of causes and risk factors. *Am J Med.* 1982;73:211–218.
208. Neveu H, Kleinknecht D, Brivet F, et al. Prognostic factors in acute renal failure due to sepsis. Results of a prospective multicentre study. The French Study Group on Acute Renal Failure. *Nephrol Dial Transplant.* 1996;11(2):293–299.
209. Brivet FG, Kleinknecht DJ, Loirat P, et al. Acute renal failure in intensive care units–causes, outcome, and prognostic factors of hospital mortality; a prospective, multicenter study. French Study Group on Acute Renal Failure. *Crit Care Med.* 1996;24(2):192–198.
210. Astiz ME, Rackow EC, Weil MH. Pathophysiology and treatment of circulatory shock. *Crit Care Clin.* 1993;9:183–203.
211. Deitch E, Bridges W, Baker J, et al. Hemorrhagic shock-induced bacterial translocation is reduced by xanthine oxidase inhibition or inactivation. *Surgery.* 1988;104:191–198.
212. Mainous MR, Deitch EA. Bacterial translocation. In: Schlag G, Redl H, eds. *Pathophysiology of Shock, Sepsis and Organ Failure.* Berlin, Germany: Springer-Verlag; 1993:265–278.
213. Lillehei RC, MacLean LD. The intestinal factor in irreversible endotoxin shock. *Ann Surg.* 1958;148:513–519.
214. Meakins JL, Marshall JC. The gut as the motor of multiple organ failure. In: Marston A, Bulkley GB, Fiddian-Green RG, et al., eds. *Splanchnic Ischemia and Multiple Organ Failure.* London, England: Edward Arnold; 1989:339.
215. Marrero J, Martinez FJ, Hyzy R, et al. Advances in critical care hepatology. *Am J Resp Crit Care Med.* 2003;168(12):1421–1426.
216. Moseley RH. Sepsis and cholestasis. *Clin Liver Disease.* 1999;3:465–475.
217. Champion HR, Jones RT, Trump BF, et al. A clinicopathologic study of hepatic dysfunction following shock. *Surg Gynecol Obstet.* 1976;142:657–663.
218. Levi M, ten Cate H, Levi M, et al. Disseminated intravascular coagulation.[see comment]. *N Engl J Med.* 1999;341(8):586–592.
219. Bone RC. Gram positive organisms and sepsis. *Arch Intern Med.* 1994; 154:26–34.
220. Zeerleder S, Hack CE, Wuillemin WA, et al. Disseminated intravascular coagulation in sepsis. *Chest.* 2005;128(4):2864–2875.
221. ten Cate H. Pathophysiology of disseminated intravascular coagulation in sepsis. *Crit Care Med.* 2000;28(9 Suppl):S9–S11.
222. Woolf PD. Endocrinology of shock. *Ann Emerg Med.* 1986;15:1401–1405.
223. Arnold J, Leinhardt D, Little RA. Metabolic response to trauma. In: Schlag G, Redl H, eds. *Pathophysiology of Shock Sepsis and Organ Failure.* Berlin, Germany: Springer-Verlag; 1993:145–160.
224. Bessey PQ, Brooks DC, Black PR, et al. Epinephrine acutely mediates skeletal muscle insulin resistance. *Surgery.* 1983;94:172–179.
225. Brierre S, Kumari R, Deboisblanc BP, et al. The endocrine system during sepsis. *Am J Med Sci.* 2004;328(4):238–247.
226. Mizock B. Metabolic derangements in sepsis and septic shock. *Crit Care Clin.* 2000;16(2):319–336.
227. Naylor JM, Kronfeld DS. In-vivo studies of hypoglycemia and lactic acidosis in endotoxic shock. *Am J Physiol.* 1985;248:E309–E316.
228. Daniel AM, Pierce CH, Shizgal HM, et al. Protein and fat utilization in shock. *Surgery.* 1978;84:588–594.
229. Bagby GJ, Spitzer JA. Decreased myocardial extracellular and muscle lipoprotein lipase activities in endotoxin-treated rats. *Proc Soc Exp Biol Med.* 1981;168:395–398.
230. Ho HC, Chapital AD, Yu M, et al. Hypothyroidism and adrenal insufficiency in sepsis and hemorrhagic shock. *Arch Surg.* 2004;139(11):1199–1203.
231. Gardelis JG, Hatzis TD, Stamogiannou L, et al. Activity of the growth hormone/insulin-like growth factor-I axis in critically ill children. *J Pediatr Endocrinol.* 2005;18(4):363–372.
232. Beishuizen A, Thijs LG, Beishuizen A, et al. Endotoxin and the hypothalamo-pituitary-adrenal (HPA) axis. *J Endotoxin Res.* 2003;9(1):3–24.
233. Heemskerk VH, Daemen MA, Buurman WA, et al. Insulin-like growth factor-1 (IGF-1) and growth hormone (GH) in immunity and inflammation. *Cytokine Growth Factor Rev.* 1999;10(1):5–14.
234. Woods RJ, David J, Baigent S, et al. Elevated levels of corticotrophin-releasing factor binding protein in the blood of patients suffering from

arthritis and septicaemia and the presence of novel ligands in synovial fluid. *Br J Rheumatol.* 1996;35(2):120–124.
235. Holmes CL, Patel BM, Russell J, et al. Physiology of vasopressin relevant to management of septic shock. *Chest.* 2001;120(3):989–1002.
236. Landry DW, Levin HR, Gallant EM, et al. Vasopressin deficiency contributes to the vasodilatation of septic shock. *Circulation.* 1997;95:1122–1125.
237. Marik PE, Zaloga GP. Adrenal insufficiency during septic shock. *Crit Care Med.* 2003;31(1):141–145.
238. Zaloga GP, Marik P. Hypothalamic-pituitary-adrenal insufficiency. *Crit Care Clin.* 2001;17(1):25–42.
239. Annane D, Sebille V, Troche G, et al. A 3-level prognostic classification in septic shock based on cortisol levels and cortisol response to corticotropin. *JAMA.* 2000;283(8):1038–1045.
240. Manglik S, Flores E, Lubarsky L, et al. Glucocorticoid insufficiency in patients who present to the hospital with severe sepsis: a prospective clinical trial [see comment]. *Crit Care Med.* 2003;31(6):1668–1675.
241. Marik P, Rotello L, Zaloga G. Secondary adrenal insufficiency is common in critically ill patients. *Crit Care Med.* 2001;29:A163.
242. de Groof F, Joosten KF, Janssen JA, et al. Acute stress response in children with meningococcal sepsis: important differences in the growth hormone/insulin-like growth factor I axis between nonsurvivors and survivors. *J Clin Endocrinol Metab.* 2002;87(7):3118–3124.
243. Felmet KA, Hall MW, Clark RS, et al. Prolonged lymphopenia, lymphoid depletion, and hypoprolactinemia in children with nosocomial sepsis and multiple organ failure. *J Immunol.* 2005;174(6):3765–3772.
244. Medina P, Noguera I, Aldasoro M, et al. Enhancement by vasopressin of adrenergic responses in human mesenteric arteries. *Am J Physiol.* 1997; 272(3 Pt 2):H1087–H1093.
245. Peres BD, Lopes FF, Melot C, et al. Body temperature alterations in the critically ill. *Intensive Care Med.* 2004;30(5):811–816.
246. Gomez-Jimenez J, Salgado A, Mourelle M, et al. L-arginine: nitric oxide pathway in endotoxemia and human septic shock. *Crit Care Med.* 1995; 23:253–258.
247. Kubes P. Nitric oxide affects microvascular permeability in the intact inflamed vasculature. *Microcirculation.* 1995;2(3):235–244.
248. Rackow EC, Kaufman BS, Falk JL, et al. Hemodynamic response to fluid repletion in patients with septic shock: evidence for early depression of cardiac performance. *Circ Shock.* 1987;22:11–22.
249. Parrillo JE, Parker MM, Natanson C, et al. Septic shock in humans. Advances in the understanding of pathogenesis, cardiovascular dysfunction, and therapy. *Ann Intern Med.* 1990;113:227–242.
250. Cannon WB. *Traumatic Shock.* New York, NY: Appleton; 1923.
251. Cournand A, Riley RL, Bradley SE, et al. Studies of the circulation in clinical shock. *Surgery.* 1943;13:964–995.
252. Carcillo JA, Davis AL, Zaritsky A. Role of early fluid resuscitation in pediatric septic shock. *JAMA.* 1991;266(9):1242–1245.
253. Rivers E, Nguyen B, Havstad S, et al. Early goal-directed therapy in the treatment of severe sepsis and septic shock. *N Engl J Med.* 2001;345(19): 1368–1377.
254. Levraut J, Ichai C, Petit I, et al. Low exogenous lactate clearance as an early predictor of mortality in normolactatemic critically ill septic patients. *Crit Care Med.* 2003;31(3):705–710.
255. Abramson D, Scalea TM, Hitchcock R, et al. Lactate clearance and survival following injury. *J Trauma.* 1993;35(4):584–588.
256. Davis JW, Shackford SR, Mackersie RC, et al. Base deficit as a guide to volume resuscitation. *J Trauma.* 1988;28(10):1464–1467.
257. Oud L, Haupt MT. Persistent gastric intramucosal ischemia in patients with sepsis following resuscitation from shock. *Chest.* 1999;115(5):1390–1396.
258. Wo CC, Shoemaker WC, Appel PL, et al. Unreliability of blood pressure and heart rate to evaluate cardiac output in emergency resuscitation and critical illness. *Crit Care Med.* 1993;21(2):218–223.
259. Ward KR, Ivatury RR, Barbee WR. Endpoints of resuscitation for the victim of trauma. *Intensive Care Med.* 2001;16(2):55–75.
260. Bakker J, Coffemils M, Leon M, et al. Blood lactate levels are superior to oxygen-derived variables in predicting outcome in human septic shock. *Chest.* 1992;99:956–962.
261. Nguyen HB, Rivers EP, Knoblich BP, et al. Early lactate clearance is associated with improved outcome in severe sepsis and septic shock. *Crit Care Med.* 2004;32(8):1637–1642.
262. James JH, Luchette FA, McCarter FD, et al. Lactate is an unreliable indicator of tissue hypoxia in injury or sepsis. *Lancet.* 1999;354(9177):505–508.
263. Ernest D, Belzberg AS, Dodek PM. Distribution of normal saline and 5% albumin infusions in septic patients. *Crit Care Med.* 1999;27(1):46–50.
264. Rackow EC, Falk JL, Fein IA, et al. Fluid resuscitation in circulatory shock: a comparison of the cardiorespiratory effects of albumin, hetastarch, and saline solutions in patients with hypovolemic and septic shock. *Crit Care Med.* 1983;11:839–850.
265. Haupt MT, Teerapong P, Green D, et al. Increased pulmonary edema with crystalloid compared to colloid resuscitation of shock associated with increased vascular permeability. *Circ Shock.* 1984;12:213–224.
266. Haupt MT, Rackow EC. Colloid osmotic pressure and fluid resuscitation with hetastarch, albumin, and saline solutions. *Crit Care Med.* 1982; 10:159–162.
267. Wilkes MM, Navickis RJ. Patient survival after human albumin administration. A meta-analysis of randomized, controlled trials. *Ann Intern Med.* 2001;135(3):149–164.
268. Alderson P, Bunn F, Lefebvre C, et al. Human albumin solution for resuscitation and volume expansion in critically ill patients. *Cochrane Database Syst Rev.* 2002;(1):CD001208.
269. Finfer S, Bellomo R, Boyce N, et al. A comparison of albumin and saline for fluid resuscitation in the intensive care unit. *N Engl J Med.* 2004; 350(22):2247–2256.
270. Schierhout G, Roberts I. Fluid resuscitation with colloid or crystalloid solutions in critically ill patients: a systematic review of randomised trials [see comment]. *BMJ.* 1998;316(7136):961–964.
271. Meehan TP, Fine MJ, Krumholz HM, et al. Quality of care, process, and outcomes in elderly patients with pneumonia. *JAMA.* 1997;278(23):2080–2084.
272. Ibrahim EH, Sherman G, Ward S, et al. The influence of inadequate antimicrobial treatment of bloodstream infections on patient outcomes in the ICU setting [see comment]. *Chest.* 2000;118(1):146–155.
273. Kollef MH, Sherman G, Ward S, et al. Inadequate antimicrobial treatment of infections: a risk factor for hospital mortality among critically ill patients. *Chest.* 1999;115(2):462–474.
274. Kumar A, Suppes R, Gulati H, et al. The impact of initiation of inadequate antimicrobial therapy on survival in human septic shock. *Antimicrob Agents Chemother.* 2007;111:271.
275. Young LS, Martin WJ, Meyer RD, et al. Gram-negative rod bacteremia: Microbiologic, immunologic, and therapeutic considerations. *Ann Intern Med.* 1977;86:456–471.
276. Romero-Vivas J, Rubio M, Fernandez C, et al. Mortality associated with nosocomial bacteremia due to methicillin-resistant *Staphylococcus aureus.* *Clin Infect Dis.* 1995;21(6):1417–1423.
277. Nguyen MH, Peacock JE Jr, Tanner DC, et al. Therapeutic approaches in patients with candidemia. Evaluation in a multicenter, prospective, observational study. *Arch Intern Med.* 1995;155(22):2429–2435.
278. Vergis EN, Hayden MK, Chow JW, et al. Determinants of vancomycin resistance and mortality rates in enterococcal bacteremia. a prospective multicenter study. *Ann Intern Med.* 2001;135(7):484–492.
279. Byl B, Clevenbergh P, Jacobs F, et al. Impact of infectious diseases specialists and microbiological data on the appropriateness of antimicrobial therapy for bacteremia [see comment]. *Clin Infect Dis.* 1999;29(1):60–66.
280. Aronin SI, Peduzzi P, Quagliarello VJ. Community-acquired bacterial meningitis: risk stratification for adverse clinical outcome and effect of antibiotic timing. *Ann Intern Med.* 1998;129(11):862–869.
281. Miner JR, Heegaard W, Mapes A, et al. Presentation, time to antibiotics, and mortality of patients with bacterial meningitis at an urban county medical center. *J Emerg Med.* 2001;21(4):387–392.
282. Proulx N, Frechette D, Toye B, et al. Delays in the administration of antibiotics are associated with mortality from adult acute bacterial meningitis. *QJM.* 2005;98(4):291–298.
283. Houck PM, Bratzler DW, Nsa W, et al. Timing of antibiotic administration and outcomes for Medicare patients hospitalized with community-acquired pneumonia. *Arch Intern Med.* 2004;164(6):637–644.
284. Natsch S, Kullberg BJ, Van der Meer JW, et al. Delay in administering the first dose of antibiotics in patients admitted to hospital with serious infections. *Eur J Clin Microbiol Infect Dis.* 1998;17(10):681–684.
285. Pinder M, Bellomo R, Lipman, et al. Pharmacological principles of antibiotic prescription in the critically ill. *Anaesth Intensive Care.* 2002; 30(2):134–144.
286. Pimentel FL, Abelha F, Trigo MA, et al. Determination of plasma concentrations of amikacin in patients of an intensive care unit. *J Chemother.* 1995;7(1):45–49.
287. Whipple JK, Ausman RK, Franson T, et al. Effect of individualized pharmacokinetic dosing on patient outcome. *Crit Care Med.* 1991;19(12):1480–1485.
288. Joukhadar C, Frossard M, Mayer BX, et al. Impaired target site penetration of beta-lactams may account for therapeutic failure in patients with septic shock. *Crit Care Med.* 2001;29(2):385–391.
289. Franson TR, Quebbeman EJ, Whipple J, et al. Prospective comparison of traditional and pharmacokinetic aminoglycoside dosing methods. *Crit Care Med.* 1988;16(9):840–843.
290. Chelluri L, Jastremski MS. Inadequacy of standard aminoglycoside loading doses in acutely ill patients. *Crit Care Med.* 1987;15(12):1143–1145.
291. Tegeder I, Schmidtko A, Brautigam L, et al. Tissue distribution of imipenem in critically ill patients. *Clin Pharmacol Ther.* 2002;71(5):325–333.
292. Moore RD, Smith CR, Lietman PS. The association of aminoglycoside plasma levels with mortality in patients with gram-negative bacteremia. *J Infect Dis.* 1984;149(3):443–448.
293. Moore RD, Smith CR, Lietman PS. Association of aminoglycoside plasma levels with therapeutic outcome in gram-negative pneumonia. *Am J Med.* 1984;77(4):657–662.
294. Forrest A, Nix DE, Ballow CH, et al. Pharmacodynamics of intravenous ciprofloxacin in seriously ill patients. *Antimicrob Agents Chemother.* 1993;37(5):1073–1081.
295. Preston SL, Drusano GL, Berman AL, et al. Pharmacodynamics of levofloxacin: a new paradigm for early clinical trials. *JAMA.* 1998;279(2): 125–129.

296. Drusano GL, Preston SL, Fowler C, et al. Relationship between fluoroquinolone area under the curve: minimum inhibitory concentration ratio and the probability of eradication of the infecting pathogen, in patients with nosocomial pneumonia. *J Infect Dis.* 2004;189(9):1590–1597.
297. Moore RD, Lietman PS, Smith CR. Clinical response to aminoglycoside therapy: importance of the ratio of peak concentration to minimal inhibitory concentration. *J Infect Dis.* 1987;155(1):93–99.
298. Kashuba AD, Nafziger AN, Drusano GL, et al. Optimizing aminoglycoside therapy for nosocomial pneumonia caused by gram-negative bacteria. *Antimicrob Agents Chemother.* 1999;43(3):623–629.
299. Schentag JJ, Smith IL, Swanson DJ, et al. Role for dual individualization with cefmenoxime. *Am J Med.* 1984;77(6A):43–50.
300. Craig WA. Pharmacokinetic/pharmacodynamic parameters: rationale for antibacterial dosing of mice and men. *Clin Infect Dis.* 1998;26(1):1–10.
301. Lodise TP, Lomaestro BM, Drusano GL. Piperacillin-tazobactam for *Pseudomonas aeruginosa* infection: Clinical implications of an extended-infusion dosing strategy. *Clin Infect Dis.* 2007;44:357–363.
302. Craig WA, Ebert SC. Continuous infusion of beta-lactam antibiotics. *Antimicrob Agents Chemother.* 1992;36(12):2577–2583.
303. Craig WA. Once-daily versus multiple-daily dosing of aminoglycosides. *J Chemother.* 1995;7(Suppl 2):47–52.
304. Kashuba AD, Bertino JS Jr, Nafziger AN. Dosing of aminoglycosides to rapidly attain pharmacodynamic goals and hasten therapeutic response by using individualized pharmacokinetic monitoring of patients with pneumonia caused by gram-negative organisms. *Antimicrob Agents Chemother.* 1998;42(7):1842–1844.
305. Bodey GP, Ketchel SJ, Rodriguez V. A randomized study of carbenicillin plus cefamandole or tobramycin in the treatment of febrile episodes in cancer patients. *Am J Med.* 1979;67(4):608–616.
306. Daenen S, Vries-Hospers H. Cure of *Pseudomonas aeruginosa* infection in neutropenic patients by continuous infusion of ceftazidime. *Lancet.* 1988;1(8591):937.
307. Egerer G, Goldschmidt H, Hensel M, et al. Continuous infusion of ceftazidime for patients with breast cancer and multiple myeloma receiving high-dose chemotherapy and peripheral blood stem cell transplantation. *Bone Marrow Transplant.* 2002;30(7):427–431.
308. Benko AS, Cappelletty DM, Kruse JA, et al. Continuous infusion versus intermittent administration of ceftazidime in critically ill patients with suspected gram-negative infections. *Antimicrob Agents Chemother.* 1996; 40(3):691–695.
309. Thalhammer F, Traunmuller F, El Manyawi I, et al. Continuous infusion versus intermittent administration of meropenem in critically ill patients. *J Antimicrob Chemother.* 1999;43(4):523–527.
310. Sfeir T, Saha DC, Astiz M, et al. Role of interleukin-10 in monocyte hyporesponsiveness associated with septic shock. *Crit Care Med.* 2001;29(1):129–133.
311. Haupt W, Riese J, Mehler C, et al. Monocyte function before and after surgical trauma. *Dig Surg.* 1998;15(2):102–104.
312. Brandtzaeg P, Osnes L, Ovstebo R, et al. Net inflammatory capacity of human septic shock plasma evaluated by a monocyte-based target cell assay: identification of interleukin-10 as a major functional deactivator of human monocytes. [Erratum in *J Exp Med.* 1996;184(5):2075.]. *J Exp Med.* 1996;184(1):51–60.
313. Williams MA, Withington S, Newland AC, et al. Monocyte anergy in septic shock is associated with a predilection to apoptosis and is reversed by granulocyte-macrophage colony-stimulating factor ex vivo. *J Infect Dis.* 1998;178(5):1421–1433.
314. Tavares-Murta BM, Zaparoli M, Ferreira RB, et al. Failure of neutrophil chemotactic function in septic patients. *Crit Care Med.* 2002;30(5):1056–1061.
315. Holzer K, Konietzny P, Wilhelm K, et al. Phagocytosis by emigrated, intra-abdominal neutrophils is depressed during human secondary peritonitis. *Eur Surg Res.* 2002;34(4):275–284.
316. Benjamim CF, Ferreira SH, Cunha FQ. Role of nitric oxide in the failure of neutrophil migration in sepsis. *J Infect Dis.* 2000;182(1):214–223.
317. Barriere SL. Monotherapy versus combination antimicrobial therapy: a review. *Pharmacotherapy.* 1991;11(2 Pt 2):64S–71S.
318. Hughes WT, Armstrong D, Bodey GP, et al. 2002 guidelines for the use of antimicrobial agents in neutropenic patients with cancer. *Clin Infect Dis.* 2002;34(6):730–751.
319. Bochud PY, Glauser MP, Calandra T, et al. Antibiotics in sepsis. *Intensive Care Med.* 2001;27(Suppl 1):S33–S48.
320. Safdar N, Handelsman J, Maki DG, et al. Does combination antimicrobial therapy reduce mortality in Gram-negative bacteraemia? A meta-analysis [see comment]. *Lancet Infect Dis.* 2004;4(8):519–527.
321. Hilf M, Yu VL, Sharp J, et al. Antibiotic therapy for *Pseudomonas aeruginosa* bacteremia: outcome correlations in a prospective study of. 200 patients. *Am J Med.* 1989;87(5):540–546.
322. Chow JW, Fine MJ, Shlaes DM, et al. *Enterobacter* bacteremia: clinical features and emergence of antibiotic resistance during therapy. *Ann Intern Med.* 1991;115(8):585–590.
323. Korvick JA, Bryan CS, Farber B, et al. Prospective observational study of *Klebsiella* bacteremia in 230 patients: outcome for antibiotic combinations versus monotherapy. *Antimicrob Agents Chemother.* 1992;36(12):2639–2644.
324. Anderson ET, Young LS, Hewitt WL. Antimicrobial synergism in the therapy of gram-negative rod bacteremia. *Chemotherapy.* 1978;24(1):45–54.
325. Baddour LM, Yu VL, Klugman KP, et al. Combination antibiotic therapy lowers mortality among severely ill patients with pneumococcal bacteremia. *Am J Resp Crit Care Med.* 2004;170(4):440–4.
326. Waterer GW, Somes GW, Wunderink RG. Monotherapy may be suboptimal for severe bacteremic pneumococcal pneumonia. *Arch Intern Med.* 2001;161(15):1837–1842.
327. Martinez JA, Horcajada JP, Almela M, et al. Addition of a macrolide to a beta-lactam-based empirical antibiotic regimen is associated with lower in-hospital mortality for patients with bacteremic pneumococcal pneumonia [see comment]. *Clin Infect Dis.* 2003;36(4):389–395.
328. Rodriguez A, Mendia A, Sirvent JM, et al. Combination antibiotic therapy improves survival in patients with community-acquired pneumonia and shock. *Crit Care Med.* 2007;35(6):1493–1498.
329. Sprung CL, Finch RG, Thijs LG, et al. International sepsis trial (INTERSEPT): role and impact of a clinical evaluation committee. *Crit Care Med.* 1996;24(9):1441–1447.
330. Sudarsky LA, Laschinger JC, Coppa GF, et al. Improved results from a standardized approach in treating patients with necrotizing fasciitis. *Ann Surg.* 1987;206(5):661–665.
331. Moss RL, Musemeche CA, Kosloske AM. Necrotizing fasciitis in children: prompt recognition and aggressive therapy improve survival. *J Pediatr Surg.* 1996;31(8):1142–1146.
332. Kumar A, Wood K, Gurka D, et al. Outcome of septic shock correlates with duration of hypotension prior to source control implementation. *ICAAC Proceedings.* 2004;350:K–1222.
333. Kumar A, Parrillo JE. Shock: pathophysiology, classification and approach to management. In: Parrillo JE, Dellinger RP, eds. *Critical Care Medicine: Principles of Diagnosis and Management in the Adult.* 3rd ed. St. Louis, MO: Mosby; 2007:379–422.
334. Bond RF. Peripheral macro- and microcirculation. In: Schlag G, Redl H, eds. *Pathophysiology of Shock, Sepsis and Organ Failure.* Berlin, Germany: Springer-Verlag; 1993:893–907.
335. Desjars P, Pinaud M, Potel G, et al. A reappraisal of norepinephrine therapy in human septic shock. *Crit Care Med.* 1987;15(2):134–137.
336. Desjars P, Pinaud M, Bugnon D, et al. Norepinephrine therapy has no deleterious renal effects in human septic shock. *Crit Care Med.* 1989;17(5):426–429.
337. Fukuoka T, Nishimura M, Imanaka H, et al. Effects of norepinephrine on renal function in septic patients with normal and elevated serum lactate levels. *Crit Care Med.* 1989;17(11):1104–1107.
338. Hesselvik JF, Brodin B. Low dose norepinephrine in patients with septic shock and oliguria: effects on afterload, urine flow, and oxygen transport. *Crit Care Med.* 1989;17(2):179–180.
339. Meadows D, Edwards JD, Wilkins RG, et al. Reversal of intractable septic shock with norepinephrine therapy. *Crit Care Med.* 1988;16(7):663–666.
340. Redl-Wenzl EM, Armbruster C, Edelmann G, et al. The effects of norepinephrine on hemodynamics and renal function in severe septic shock states. *Intensive Care Med.* 1993;19(3):151–154.
341. Neviere R, Mathieu D, Chagnon JL, et al. The contrasting effects of dobutamine and dopamine on gastric mucosal perfusion in septic patients. *Am J Resp Crit Care Med.* 1996;154(6 Pt 1):1684–1688.
342. Marin C, Eon B, Saux P, et al. Renal effects of norepinephrine used to treat septic shock patients. *Crit Care Med.* 1990;18(3):282–285.
343. Marik PE, Mohedin M. The contrasting effects of dopamine and norepinephrine on systemic and splanchnic oxygen utilization in hyperdynamic sepsis. *JAMA.* 1994;272(17):1354–1357.
344. Ruokonen E, Takala J, Kari A, et al. Regional blood flow and oxygen transport in septic shock. *Crit Care Med.* 1993;21(9):1296–1303.
345. Meier-Hellmann A, Specht M, Hannemann L, et al. Splanchnic blood flow is greater in septic shock treated with norepinephrine than in severe sepsis. *Intensive Care Med.* 1996;22(12):1354–1359.
346. Levy B, Bollaert PE, Charpentier C, et al. Comparison of norepinephrine and dobutamine to epinephrine for hemodynamics, lactate metabolism, and gastric tonometric variables in septic shock: a prospective, randomized study [see comment]. *Intensive Care Med.* 1997;23(3):282–287.
347. De Backer D, Creteur J, Silva E, et al. Effects of dopamine, norepinephrine, and epinephrine on the splanchnic circulation in septic shock: which is best? *Crit Care Med.* 2003;31(6):1659–1667.
348. Martin C, Papazian L, Perrin G, et al. Norepinephrine or dopamine for the treatment of hyperdynamic septic shock? *Chest.* 1993;103(6):1826–1831.
349. Devins SS, Miller A, Herndon BL, et al. The effects of dopamine on T-cell proliferative response and serum prolactin in critically ill patients. *Crit Care Med.* 1992;20:1644–1649.
350. Kumar A, Schupp E, Bunnell E, et al. The cardiovascular response to dobutamine in septic shock. *Clin Invest Med.* 1994;17, B18 Abstract #107.
351. Rhodes A, Lamb FJ, Malagon R, et al. A prospective study of the use of a dobutamine stress test to identify outcome in patients with sepsis, severe sepsis or septic shock. *Crit Care Med.* 1999;27(11):2361–2366.
352. Barton P, Garcia J, Kouatli A, et al. Hemodynamic effects of i.v. milrinone lactate in pediatric patients with septic shock. A

prospective, double-blinded, randomized, placebo-controlled, interventional study. *Chest.* 1996;109:1302–1312.
353. Gattinoni L, Brazzi L, Pelosi P, et al. A trial of goal-oriented hemodynamic therapy in critically ill patients. SvO_2 Collaborative Group. *N Engl J Med.* 1995;333:1025–1032.
354. Hayes MA, Timmins AC, Yau EHS, et al. Elevation of systemic oxygen delivery in the treatment of critically ill patients. *N Engl J Med.* 1994; 330:1717–1722.
355. Shoemaker WC, Appel PL, Kram HB, et al. Temporal hemodynamic and oxygen transport patterns in medical patients. Septic shock. *Chest.* 1993; 104(5):1529–1536.
356. Shoemaker WC, Appel PL, Kram HB, et al. Sequence of physiologic patterns in surgical septic shock. *Crit Care Med.* 1993;21(12):1876–1889.
357. Ivanov R, Allen J, Calvin JE. The incidence of major morbidity in critically ill patients managed with pulmonary artery catheters: a meta-analysis. *Crit Care Med.* 2000;28(3):615–619.
358. Tuchschmidt J, Fried J, Astiz M, et al. Elevation of cardiac output and oxygen delivery improves outcome in septic shock. *Chest.* 1992;102:216–220.
359. Yu M, Levy MM, Smith P, et al. Effect of maximizing oxygen delivery on morbidity and mortality rates in critically ill patients: a prospective, randomized, controlled study. *Crit Care Med.* 1993;21(6):830–838.
360. Yu M, Burchell S, Hasaniya NW, et al. Relationship of mortality to increasing oxygen delivery in patients > or = 50 years of age: a prospective, randomized trial. *Crit Care Med.* 1998;26(6):1011–1019.
361. Alia I, Esteban A, Gordo F, et al. A randomized and controlled trial of the effect of treatment aimed at maximizing oxygen delivery in patients with severe sepsis or septic shock. *Chest.* 1999;115(2):453–461.
362. Heyland DK, Cook DJ, King D, et al. Maximizing oxygen delivery in critically ill patients: a methodologic appraisal of the evidence. *Crit Care Med.* 1996;24(3):517–524.
363. Bussolino F, Camussi G, Baglioni C. Synthesis and release of platelet activating factor by human vascular endothelial cells treated with tumor necrosis factor or interleukin-1. *J Biol Chem.* 1988;263:11856–11861.
364. Landry DW, Levin HR, Gallant EM, et al. Vasopressin pressor sensitivity in vasodilatory septic shock. *Crit Care Med.* 1997;25:1279–1282.
365. Patel BM, Chittock DR, Russell JA, et al. Beneficial effects of short-term vasopressin infusion during severe septic shock. *Anesthesiology.* 2002; 96(3):576–582.
366. Russell JA, Walley KR, Singer J, et al. Vasopressin versus norepinephrine infusion in patients with septic shock. *N Engl J Med.* 2008;358: 877–887.
367. Schaer GL, Fink MP, Parrillo JE. Norepinephrine alone versus norepinephrine plus low-dose dopamine: enhanced renal blood flow with combination pressor therapy. *Crit Care Med.* 1985;13:492–496.
368. Hoogenberg K, Smit AJ, Girbes AR. Effects of low-dose dopamine on renal and systemic hemodynamics during incremental norepinephrine infusion in healthy volunteers. *Crit Care Med.* 1998;26(2):260–265.
369. Olson D, Pohlman A, Hall JB. Administration of low-dose dopamine to nonoliguric patients with sepsis syndrome does not raise intramucosal gastric pH nor improve creatinine clearance. *Am J Resp Crit Care Med.* 1996;154(6 Pt 1):1664–1670.
370. Ichai C, Passeron C, Carles M, et al. Prolonged low-dose dopamine infusion induces a transient improvement in renal function in hemodynamically stable, critically ill patients: a single-blind, prospective, controlled study. *Crit Care Med.* 2000;28(5):1329–1335.
371. Bellomo R, Chapman M, Finfer S, et al. Low-dose dopamine in patients with early renal dysfunction: a placebo-controlled randomised trial. Australia New Zealand Intensive Care Society (ANZICS) Clinical Trials Group. *Lancet.* 2000;356(9248):2139–2143.
372. Marik PE, Iglesias J. Low-dose dopamine does not prevent acute renal failure in patients with septic shock and oliguria. NORASEPT II Study Investigators. *Am J Med.* 1999;107(4):387–390.
373. Mimoz O, Rauss A, Rekik N, et al. Pulmonary artery catheterization in critically ill patients: a prospective analysis of outcome changes associated with catheter-prompted changes in therapy. *Crit Care Med.* 1994;22(4):573–579.
374. Connors AF Jr, McCaffree DR, Gray BA. Evaluation of right-heart catheterization in the critically ill patient without acute myocardial infarction. *N Engl J Med.* 1983;308:263–267.
375. Weisel RD, Vito L, Dennis RC, et al. Myocardial depression during sepsis. *Am J Surg.* 1977;133:512–521.
376. Cohn JN. Central venous pressure as a guide to volume expansion. *Ann Intern Med.* 1967;66(6):1283–1287.
377. Connors AF Jr, Dawson NV, Shaw PK, et al. Hemodynamic status in critically ill patients with and without acute heart disease. *Chest.* 1990; 98(5):1200–1206.
378. Kumar A, Anel R, Bunnell E, et al. Pulmonary artery occlusion pressure and central venous pressure fail to predict ventricular filling volume, cardiac performance, or the response to volume infusion in normal subjects. *Crit Care Med.* 2004;32(3):691–699.
379. Robin ED. The cult of the Swan-Ganz catheter. Overuse and abuse of pulmonary flow catheters. *Ann Intern Med.* 1985;103(3):445–449.
380. Dalen JE, Bone RC. Is it time to pull the pulmonary artery catheter [see comment]? *JAMA.* 1996;276(11):916–918.
381. Pronovost PJ, Jenckes MW, Dorman T, et al. Organizational characteristics of intensive care units related to outcomes of abdominal aortic surgery. *JAMA.* 1999;281:1310–1317.
382. Carson SS, Stocking C, Podsadecki T, et al. Effects of organizational change in the medical intensive care unit of a teaching hospital: a comparison of 'open' and 'closed' formats. *JAMA.* 1996;276:322–328.
383. Pronovost PJ, Angus DC, Dorman T, et al. Physician staffing patterns and clinical outcomes in critically ill patients: a systematic review. *JAMA.* 2002;288(17):2151–2162.
384. Li TC, Phillips MC, Shaw L, et al. On-site physician staffing in a community hospital intensive care unit. Impact on test and procedure use and on patient outcome. *JAMA.* 1984;252(15):2023–2027.
385. Pollack MM, Katz RW, Ruttimann UE, et al. Improving the outcome and efficiency of intensive care: the impact of an intensivist. *Crit Care Med.* 1988;16(1):11–17.
386. Reynolds HN, Haupt MT, Thill-Baharozian MC, et al. Impact of critical care physician staffing on patients with septic shock in a university hospital medical intensive care unit. *JAMA.* 1988;260:3446–3450.
387. Hutton P, Dye J, Prys-Roberts C. An assessment of the Dinamap. *Anaesthesia.* 1984;39:261–267.
388. Cohn JN. Blood pressure measurement in shock. Mechanism of inaccuracy in ausculatory and palpatory methods. *JAMA.* 1967;199(13):118–122.
389. Connors AF Jr, Dawson NV, McCaffree DR, et al. Assessing hemodynamic status in critically ill patients: do physicians use clinical information optimally? *J Crit Care.* 1987;2:174–180.
390. Michard F, Teboul JL. Predicting fluid responsiveness in ICU patients: a critical analysis of the evidence. *Chest.* 2002;121(6):2000–2008.
391. Marik PE. Pulmonary artery catheterization and esophageal Doppler monitoring in the ICU. *Chest.* 1999;116(4):1085–1091.
392. Humphrey H, Hall J, Sznajder I, et al. Improved survival in ARDS patients associated with a reduction in pulmonary capillary wedge pressure. *Chest.* 1990;97(5):1176–1180.
393. Mitchell JP, Schuller D, Calandrino FS, et al. Improved outcome based on fluid management in critically ill patients requiring pulmonary artery catheterization. *Am Rev Resp Dis.* 1992;145(5):990–998.
394. Connors AF Jr, Speroff T, Dawson NV, et al. The effectiveness of right heart catheterization in the initial care of critically ill patients. *JAMA.* 1996;276:889–897.
395. Richard C, Warszawski J, Anguel N, et al. Early use of the pulmonary artery catheter and outcomes in patients with shock and acute respiratory distress syndrome: a randomized controlled trial. *JAMA.* 2003;290(20):2713–2720.
396. Rhodes A, Cusack RJ, Newman PJ, et al. A randomised, controlled trial of the pulmonary artery catheter in critically ill patients. *Intensive Care Med.* 2002;28(3):256–264.
397. Polanczyk CA, Rohde LE, Goldman L, et al. Right heart catheterization and cardiac complications in patients undergoing noncardiac surgery: an observational study. *JAMA.* 2001;286(3):309–314.
398. Sandham JD, Hull RD, Brant RF, et al. A randomized, controlled trial of the use of pulmonary-artery catheters in high-risk surgical patients. *N Engl J Med.* 2003;348(1):5–14.
399. Ivanov RI, Allen J, Sandham JD, et al. Pulmonary artery catheterization: a narrative and systematic critique of randomized controlled trials and recommendations for the future. *New Horiz.* 1997;5(3):268–276.
400. Zanotti S, Kumar A, Kumar A. Cytokine modulation in sepsis and septic shock. *Expert Opin Investig Drugs.* 2002;11(8):1061–1075.
401. Anel RL, Kumar A. Experimental and emerging therapies for sepsis and septic shock. *Expert Opin Investig Drugs.* 2001;10(8):1471–1485.
402. Ely EW, Bernard GR, Vincent JL. Activated protein C for severe sepsis. *N Engl J Med.* 2002;347(13):1035–1036.
403. Beale R, Wright TJ, Wong K, et al. Safety of drotrecogin alfa (activated) in adult patients with severe sepsis: comparison of global ENHANCE to PROWESS. *Chest.* 2003;124:102S.
404. Vincent JL, Bernard GR, Beale R, et al. Drotrecogin alfa (activated) treatment in severe sepsis from the global open-label trial ENHANCE: further evidence for survival and safety and implications for early treatment. *Crit Care Med.* 2005;33(10):2266–2277.
405. Siegel JP. Assessing the use of activated protein C in the treatment of severe sepsis. *N Engl J Med.* 2002;347(13):1030–1034.
406. Nadel S, Goldstein B, Williams MD, et al. Drotrecogin alfa (activated) in children with severe sepsis: a multicentre phase III randomised controlled trial [see comment]. *Lancet.* 2007;369(9564):836–843.
407. Alejandria MM, Lansang MA, Dans LF, et al. Intravenous immunoglobulin for treating sepsis and septic shock. *Cochrane Database Syst Rev.* 2002; (1):CD001090.
408. Douzinas EE, Pitaridis MT, Louris G, et al. Prevention of infection in multiple trauma patients by high-dose intravenous immunoglobulins. *Crit Care Med.* 2000;28(1):8–15.
409. Darenberg J, Ihendyane N, Sjolin J, et al. Intravenous immunoglobulin G therapy in streptococcal toxic shock syndrome: a European randomized, double-blind, placebo-controlled trial. *Clin Infect Dis.* 2003;37(3):333–340.
410. Pitcairn M, Schuler J, Erve PR, et al. Glucocorticoid and antibiotic effect on experimental gram-negative bacteremic shock. *Arch Surg.* 1975;110(8): 1012–1015.

411. Sprung CL, Caralis PV, Marcial EH, et al. The effects of high-dose corticosteroids in patients with septic shock. A prospective, controlled study. *N Engl J Med.* 1984;311(18):1137–1143.
412. Bone RC, Fisher CJ Jr, Clemmer TP, et al. A controlled clinical trial of high-dose methylprednisolone in the treatment of severe sepsis and septic shock. *N Engl J Med.* 1987;317(11):653–658.
413. Luce JM, Montgomery AB, Marks JD, et al. Ineffectiveness of high-dose methylprednisolone in preventing parenchymal lung injury and improving mortality in patients with septic shock. *Am Rev Resp Dis.* 1988;138(1):62–68.
414. The Veterans Administration Systemic Sepsis Cooperative Study Group. Effect of high-dose glucocorticoid therapy on mortality in patients with clinical signs of systemic sepsis. *N Engl J Med.* 1987;317(11):659–665.
415. Schiffl H, Lang SM, Fischer R. Daily hemodialysis and the outcome of acute renal failure. *N Engl J Med.* 2002;346(5):305–310.
416. Ronco C, Bellomo R, Homel P, et al. Effects of different doses in continuous veno-venous haemofiltration on outcomes of acute renal failure: a prospective randomised trial. *Lancet.* 2000;356(9223):26–30.
417. Phu NH, Hien TT, Mai NT, et al. Hemofiltration and peritoneal dialysis in infection-associated acute renal failure in Vietnam. *N Engl J Med.* 2002; 347(12):895–902.
418. Krinsley JS. Association between hyperglycemia and increased hospital mortality in a heterogeneous population of critically ill patients. *Mayo Clin Proc.* 2003;78(12):1471–1478.
419. Vanden Berghe G, Wouters P, Weekers F, et al. Intensive insulin therapy in the critically ill patients. *N Engl J Med.* 2001;345(19):1359–1367.
420. Latham R, Lancaster AD, Covington JF, et al. The association of diabetes and glucose control with surgical-site infections among cardiothoracic surgery patients. *Infect Control Hosp Epidemiol.* 2001;22(10):607–612.
421. Vanden Berghe G, Wilmer A, Hermans G, et al. Intensive insulin therapy in the medical ICU. *N Engl J Med.* 2006;354(5):449–461.
422. Hermans G, Wilmer A, Meersseman W, et al. Impact of intensive insulin therapy on neuromuscular complications and ventilator dependency in the medical intensive care unit. *Am J Resp Crit Care Med.* 2007;175(5):480–489.
423. Cooper MS, Stewart PM. Corticosteroid insufficiency in acutely ill patients. *N Engl J Med.* 2003;348(8):727–734.
424. Annane D, Bellissant E, Sebille V, et al. Impaired pressor sensitivity to noradrenaline in septic shock patients with and without impaired adrenal function reserve. *Br J Clin Pharmacol.* 1998;46:589–597.
425. Briegel J, Forst H, Haller M, et al. Stress doses of hydrocortisone reverse hyperdynamic septic shock: a prospective randomized, double-blind, single-center study. *Crit Care Med.* 1999;27(4):723–732.
426. Bollaert PE, Charpentier C, Levy B, et al. Reversal of late septic shock with supraphysiologic doses of hydrocortisone. *Crit Care Med.* 1998;26(4):645–650.
427. Keh D, Boehnke T, Weber-Cartens S, et al. Immunologic and hemodynamic effects of "low-dose" hydrocortisone in septic shock: a double-blind, randomized, placebo-controlled, crossover study. *Am J Resp Crit Care Med.* 2003;167(4):512–520.
428. Annane D, Sebille V, Charpentier C, et al. Effect of treatment with low doses of hydrocortisone and fludrocortisone on mortality in patients with septic shock. *JAMA.* 2002;288(7):862–871.
429. Hamrahian AH, Oseni TS, Arafah BM. Measurements of serum free cortisol in critically ill patients. *N Engl J Med.* 2004;350(16):1629–1638.
430. Sprung C, Annane D, Keh D, et al. Hydrocortisone therapy for patients with septic shock. *N Engl J Med.* 2008;358:111–124.
431. Ranieri VM, Suter PM, Tortorella C, et al. Effect of mechanical ventilation on inflammatory mediators in patients with acute respiratory distress syndrome: a randomized controlled trial. *JAMA.* 1999;282(1):54–61.
432. Tremblay L, Valenza F, Ribeiro SP, et al. Injurious ventilatory strategies increase cytokines and c-fos m-RNA expression in an isolated rat lung model. *J Clin Invest.* 1997;99(5):944–952.
433. International consensus conferences in intensive care medicine: Ventilator-associated Lung Injury in ARDS. This official conference report was cosponsored by the American Thoracic Society, The European Society of Intensive Care Medicine, and The Societe de Reanimation de Langue Francaise, and was approved by the ATS Board of Directors, July, 1999. *Am J Resp Crit Care Med.* 1999;160(6):2118–2124.
434. Bernard GR, Artigas A, Brigham KL, et al. The American-European Consensus Conference on ARDS. Definitions, mechanisms, relevant outcomes, and clinical trial coordination. *Am J Resp Crit Care Med.* 1994;149(3 Pt 1): 818–824.
435. Amato MB, Barbas CS, Medeiros DM, et al. Effect of a protective-ventilation strategy on mortality in the acute respiratory distress syndrome. *N Engl J Med.* 1998;338(6):347–354.
436. The Acute Distress Syndrome Network. Ventilation with lower tidal volumes as compared with traditional tidal volumes for acute lung injury and the acute respiratory distress syndrome. *N Engl J Med.* 2000;342(18):1301–1308.
437. Stewart TE, Meade MO, Cook DJ, et al. Evaluation of a ventilation strategy to prevent barotrauma in patients at high risk for acute respiratory distress syndrome. Pressure- and Volume-Limited Ventilation Strategy Group. *N Engl J Med.* 1998;338(6):355–361.
438. Hussain SN, Graham R, Rutledge F, et al. Respiratory muscle energetics during endotoxic shock in dogs. *J Appl Physiol.* 1986;60(2):486–493.
439. Leon A, Boczkowski J, Dureuil B, et al. Effects of endotoxic shock on diaphragmatic function in mechanically ventilated rats. *J Appl Physiol.* 1992;72(4):1466–1472.
440. Marik PE, Zaloga GP. Early enteral nutrition in acutely ill patients: a systematic review. *Crit Care Med.* 2001;29(12):2264–2270.
441. Heyland DK. Nutritional support in the critically ill patients. A critical review of the evidence. *Crit Care Clin.* 1998;14(3):423–440.
442. Heyland DK, MacDonald S, Keefe L, et al. Total parenteral nutrition in the critically ill patient: a meta-analysis. *JAMA.* 1998;280(23):2013–2019.
443. Moore FA, Feliciano DV, Andrassy RJ, et al. Early enteral feeding, compared with parenteral, reduces postoperative septic complications. The results of a meta-analysis. *Ann Surg.* 1992;216(2):172–183.
444. Cooper DJ, Walley KR, Wiggs BR, et al. Bicarbonate does not improve hemodynamics in critically ill patients who have lactic acidosis. A prospective, controlled clinical study *Ann Intern Med.* 1990;112:492–498.
445. Mathieu D, Neviere R, Billard V, et al. Effects of bicarbonate therapy on hemodynamics and tissue oxygenation in patients with lactic acidosis: a prospective, controlled clinical study. *Crit Care Med.* 1991;19(11):1352–1356.
446. van der Poll T, van Deventer SJ. Cytokines and anticytokines in the pathogenesis of sepsis. *Infect Dis Clin North Am.* 1999;13(2):413–426.
447. Leaver SK, Finney SJ, Burke-Gaffney A, et al. Sepsis since the discovery of Toll-like receptors: disease concepts and therapeutic opportunities. *Crit Care Med.* 2007;35(5):1404–1410.
448. Van Amersfoort ES, Van Berkel TJ, Kuiper J, et al. Receptors, mediators, and mechanisms involved in bacterial sepsis and septic shock. *Clin Micro Rev.* 2003;16(3):379–414.
449. Arcaroli J, Fessler MB, Abraham E, et al. Genetic polymorphisms and sepsis. *Shock.* 2005;24(4):300–312.
450. Lin MT, Albertson TE, Lin MT, et al. Genomic polymorphisms in sepsis. *Crit Care Med.* 2004;32(2):569–579.
451. Texereau J, Pene F, Chiche JD, et al. Importance of hemostatic gene polymorphisms for susceptibility to and outcome of severe sepsis. *Crit Care Med.* 2004;32(5 Suppl):S313–S319.
452. Papathanassoglou ED, Giannakopoulou MD, Bozas E, et al. Genomic variations and susceptibility to sepsis. *AACN Advanced Critical Care.* 2006;17(4):394–422.
453. Sharma S, Mink S. Septic shock. http://www.emedicine.com/MED/topic2101.htm. 2007. Accessed Dec. 1, 2007.

CHAPTER 58 ■ HEMORRHAGIC SHOCK

MARIANNE E. CINAT • DAVID B. HOYT

The definition of *shock* describes the final common pathway of many disease states: ineffective tissue perfusion, resulting in severe dysfunction of organs vital to survival. The most commonly used classification system for shock includes four categories based on hemodynamic characteristics (1):

1. *Hypovolemic shock* resulting from a decreased circulating blood volume in relation to the total vascular capacity and characterized by a reduction of diastolic filling pressures and volumes
2. *Cardiogenic shock* related to cardiac pump failure caused by loss of myocardial contractility/functional myocardium or structural/mechanical failure of the cardiac anatomy characterized by elevations of diastolic filling pressures and volumes
3. *Extracardiac obstructive shock* involving obstruction to flow in the cardiovascular circuit and characterized by either impairment of diastolic filling or excessive afterload
4. *Distributive shock* caused by loss of vasomotor control, resulting in arteriolar and venular dilation and characterized by increased cardiac output and decreased systemic vascular resistance after fluid resuscitation.

Although the hemodynamic characteristics of the various forms of shock may vary, the final common pathway—inadequate cellular perfusion—must be addressed early to prevent long-term sequelae and death (Fig. 58.1).

Hemorrhagic shock is a form of hypovolemic shock. It is a common, yet complicated, clinical condition that physicians are frequently called upon to evaluate and treat. Etiologies include trauma, postoperative bleeding, medical conditions, and iatrogenic causes. Diagnosis must be accurate and expedient. Therapy must be direct, efficient, and multifactorial in order to avoid the potential multisystem sequelae.

The purpose of this chapter is to address the immediate concerns for patients with hemorrhagic shock, as well as the etiology and epidemiology of this clinical condition, and to describe the pathophysiology, clinical features, and diagnostic and therapeutic approach to hemorrhagic shock. New and experimental therapies will also be introduced.

IMMEDIATE CONCERNS

The key steps in the approach to patients with hemorrhagic shock are listed in Table 58.1.

1. **Early recognition.** Early recognition requires astute clinical acumen to identify early systemic signs of hemorrhage and hypovolemic shock. Signs and symptoms include restlessness, anxiety, altered level of consciousness, shortness of breath, tachypnea, pallor, tachycardia, and oliguria. A decreased pulse pressure may also be observed along with decreased capillary refill due to peripheral vasoconstriction. Hypotension indicates significant volume depletion and may be a late clinical manifestation.
2. **Important aspects in the patient history.** An accurate history should be obtained expediently. For patients with traumatic injury, a thorough understanding of the mechanism of injury should be obtained, including the magnitude of blunt force trauma and/or the trajectory of the missile or object in penetrating trauma. In postoperative or postprocedural patients, the exact nature of the surgical procedure should be defined and potential sites of hemorrhage identified. In patients without recent surgery, risk factors for nonpostoperative, nontraumatic etiologies should also be sought (gastritis, peptic ulcer disease, atherosclerosis with aneurysmal disease). Significant comorbidities should also be delineated including coagulation disorders (von Willebrand, hemophilia), medical conditions associated with altered coagulation (cirrhosis, renal failure, iatrogenic vitamin K deficiency from parenteral nutrition or antimicrobials), or use of medications such as antiplatelet therapy and anticoagulants (Coumadin, heparin, low-molecular-weight heparin, or antimicrobials).
3. **Initial action and intervention.** The initial action taken in each case of hemorrhagic shock, regardless of etiology, should be directed at restoring circulating volume to ensure adequate tissue perfusion. Once the airway is secured and adequate ventilation is ensured, two peripheral large-bore intravenous catheters should be placed and fluid resuscitation begun. A blood sample should also be sent immediately for type and cross-match per institutional protocol. Initial resuscitation can include crystalloid, but should quickly be changed to blood products if signs of hypovolemia and ongoing hemorrhage persist. If a patient is in extremis and cross-matched blood products are not immediately available, type O blood (universal donor) should be immediately requested and transfused. For massive hemorrhage, clotting factors such as fresh frozen plasma, platelets, and cryoprecipitate should be prepared. The value of massive transfusion protocols to include predetermined ratios of clotting factors will be discussed later in this chapter.
4. **Directed physical examination.** Physical examination should be directed at obvious sources of external bleeding such as lacerations, extremity fractures, or surgical incisions. If identified, these should be immediately controlled. Physical signs of underlying liver disease should also be identified such as petechia, jaundice, ascites, angiomas, or testicular atrophy. Previous cardiac or carotid surgical incisions may hint toward concurrent antiplatelet or anticoagulant therapy. Evidence of retroperitoneal bleeding in patients with pancreatitis is marked by flank or periumbilical contusions.

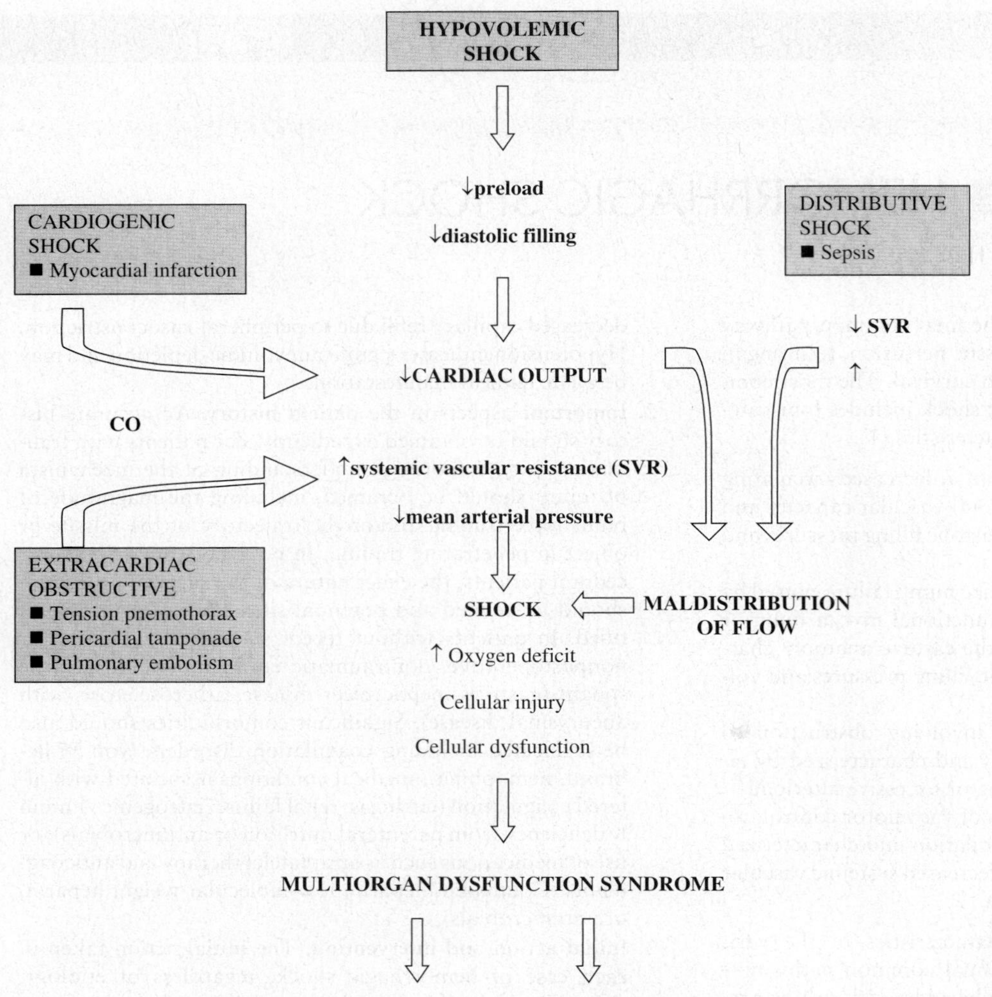

FIGURE 58.1. Final common pathway of shock. Hemorrhagic shock results in acute changes in circulating blood volume that culminates in a final common pathway shared by all classifications of shock.

5. **Identify occult source of hemorrhage.** If no obvious source of external bleeding is identified, a rapid evaluation should be performed to identify likely occult sources of bleeding. In the trauma patient, significant internal hemorrhage can occur in four defined regions: the thoracic cavity, the peritoneal cavity, the retroperitoneum, and extremity fractures. These areas can be rapidly assessed by chest radiograph, pelvic radiograph, a focused abdominal sonographic examination for trauma (FAST), and physical examination of extremities along with appropriate radiographs. In nontrauma patients without clear evidence of bleeding, the gastrointestinal tract should be rapidly evaluated via nasogastric tube, rectal examination, and endoscopy where appropriate. Additional diagnostic tests can be obtained based on clinical history, patient background, and condition. Abdominal aortic aneurysms can be identified on physical examination, by ultrasound, or by calcifications on abdominal radiograph. In rare selected instances, angiography may be used to identify and treat sources of hemorrhage not otherwise apparent (pelvic fractures, pancreatitis, lower gastrointestinal bleeding). This should only be instituted when a specific source of hemorrhage is highly likely and therapeutic intervention is sought. Computed tomography should never be sought in hemodynamically unstable patients with hemorrhage.
6. **Expedite treatment.** Once a source of bleeding is identified, a swift and directed treatment plan should be formulated and implemented without delay. Prolonged untreated hemorrhagic shock can lead to rapid decompensation and death if not appropriately identified and treated. Rapid intervention with surgical, angiographic, or endoscopic control of the hemorrhage is indicated, along with rapid correction of the underlying coagulopathy.

EPIDEMIOLOGY AND ETIOLOGY

Hypovolemic shock can be due to hemorrhagic and nonhemorrhagic sources. Hemorrhage is the most frequent cause of hypovolemic shock and is most commonly due to blood loss after trauma or major surgery (Table 58.2). Following trauma, obvious external signs of injury and hemorrhage should be rapidly identified and controlled. As described above, the thoracic cavity, peritoneal cavity, and retroperitoneum should all be evaluated for occult hemorrhage.

TABLE 58.1

KEY STEPS IN THE APPROACH TO A PATIENT WITH HEMORRHAGIC SHOCK

1. Early recognition
   a. Signs and symptoms may be subtle.
   b. Astute clinical acumen is necessary to identify hemorrhage prior to hemodynamic collapse.
2. Obtain an accurate patient history
   a. Trauma
   b. Recent surgical procedures
   c. Medical history
      (i) Gastrointestinal disease (peptic ulcer disease, varices, etc.)
      (ii) Atherosclerosis (aneurysmal disease)
      (iii) Coagulation disorders
   d. Medication use
      (i) Antiplatelet therapy
      (ii) Anticoagulants
3. Initiate intervention
   a. "ABCs"—airway, breathing, circulation
   b. Initiate resuscitation
      (i) Crystalloid
      (ii) Blood products
         1. Type O uncross-matched blood if *in extremis*
         2. Cross-matched blood when available
         3. Clotting factors
4. Directed physical examination
   a. External sources of bleeding
   b. Internal sources of bleeding
5. Expedite definitive treatment
   a. Surgical control
   b. Endoscopic control
   c. Angiographic control
6. Correct coagulopathy

TABLE 58.2

MAJOR ETIOLOGIES OF HEMORRHAGIC SHOCK

I. **Trauma (blunt or penetrating)**
- Intrathoracic
- Intraperitoneal
- Retroperitoneal
- Soft tissue or fractures

II. **Gastrointestinal**
- Upper gastrointestinal tract
  - Peptic ulcer disease, reflux esophagitis, variceal bleeding, erosive gastritis, aortoduodenal fistula
- Lower gastrointestinal tract
  - Hemorrhoids, tumor, arteriovenous malformation, diverticulitis, ulcerative colitis, Crohn disease, ischemia
- Hemobilia
  - Biliary tumor, iatrogenic injury or manipulation, penetrating trauma
- Pancreatic
  - Pancreatitis, iatrogenic injury or manipulation

III. **Retroperitoneal (nontrauma)**
- Abdominal aortic aneurysm

Causes of hemorrhagic shock not due to trauma include a ruptured abdominal aortic aneurysm and gastrointestinal bleeding. Gastrointestinal bleeding can be caused by peptic ulcer disease, reflux esophagitis, variceal bleeding, erosive gastritis (stress ulcers), or an aortoduodenal fistula after vascular surgery. Prior manipulation by endoscopy or sphincterotomy can also lead to upper gastrointestinal bleeding. Lower gastrointestinal bleeding can result from diverticular disease, carcinoma, polyps, arteriovenous malformations, ischemia, or colitis. Pulmonary sources of hemorrhage can occur from tumor, tuberculosis, fungal infection, bronchiectasis, or tracheoinnominate fistula following tracheostomy. Hematuria from a tumor, trauma, or polycystic kidney disease is rare but can lead to hemorrhagic shock.

Nonhemorrhagic sources of hypovolemic shock can also occur. Although not the focus of this chapter, these are due to external fluid losses such as dehydration, vomiting, diarrhea, polyuria, uncontrolled diabetes mellitus leading to osmotic diuresis, and acute adrenocortical insufficiency. Disorders that lead to interstitial fluid redistribution such as thermal injury, trauma, and anaphylaxis can also lead to hypovolemic shock. Finally, disorders that cause increased vascular capacitance (venodilation) can lead to a relative hypovolemia and include sepsis, anaphylaxis, and the release of toxins/drugs leading to vasodilation.

CLASSIFICATION OF HEMORRHAGIC SHOCK

Early diagnosis of hemorrhagic shock is imperative to avoid delay in treatment. However, clinical signs are relatively insensitive for small amounts of blood loss (2). There is a progressive hemodynamic deterioration with ongoing blood loss. This classic progression is delineated in Table 58.3. Total blood volume is estimated at approximately 70 mL/kg in the average adult, or nearly 5 L for a 70-kg person.

Class I

Class I hemorrhage is marked by a less than 750 mL estimated blood loss, or less than 15% of total circulating blood volume. There are minimal physical signs associated with this volume of blood loss. The patient may not have tachycardia, with a heart rate remaining less than 100 beats per minute; the systolic blood pressure and pulse pressure remain normal; the respiratory rate remains at 14 to 20 breaths per minute; and urine output remains adequate (>30 mL/hour). Only subtle physical signs such as delayed capillary refill and slight anxiety may exist.

Class II

Class II hemorrhage is marked by an estimated blood loss of 750 to 1,500 mL (or 15% to 30% of the total circulating blood volume). Physical signs begin to manifest during this stage of hemorrhage. Although the systolic blood pressure may be maintained, the patient usually becomes tachycardic (heart rate greater than 100 beats per minute), the pulse pressure begins to decrease, and capillary refill is delayed. The respiratory rate begins to increase (20–30 breaths per minute), urine output

TABLE 58.3

CLINICAL CLASSES OF HEMORRHAGIC SHOCK

	Class I	Class II	Class III	Class IV
Blood loss	<750 mL <15%	750–1,500 mL 15%–30%	>1,500–2,000 mL >30%–40%	>2,000 mL >40%
Heart rate (beats per minute)	<100	>100	>120	>140
Systolic blood pressure	Normal	Normal	Decreased	Decreased
Pulse pressure	Normal	Decreased	Decreased	Decreased
Capillary refill	Delayed	Delayed	Delayed	Delayed
Respiratory rate (breaths per minute)	14–20	20–30	30–40	>35
Urine output (mL/h)	>30	20–30	5–15	Minimal
Mental status	Slightly anxious	Anxious	Confused	Confused and lethargic

becomes diminished (20–30 mL/hour), and the patient becomes very anxious.

Class III

Class III hemorrhage is marked by an estimated blood loss of >1,500 to 2,000 mL (or >30%–40% of total circulating blood volume). During this phase, significant hemodynamic compromise becomes apparent. Heart rate increases to >120 beats per minute, systolic blood pressure decreases, pulse pressure decreases, capillary refill decreases, tachypnea worsens with a respiratory rate of 30 to 40 breaths per minute, urine output drops to 5 to 15 mL/hour, and the patient becomes confused, showing further evidence of decreased perfusion of the central nervous system.

Class IV

Class IV hemorrhage is marked by an estimated blood loss of >2,000 mL (or >40% of total circulating blood volume). During this phase, most compensatory cardiovascular mechanisms have been maximized and total hemodynamic collapse is imminent. Signs of class IV hemorrhage include severe tachycardia with a heart rate >140 beats per minute, a decreased systolic blood pressure, a decreased pulse pressure, delayed capillary refill, significant tachypnea with a respiratory rate of >35 breaths per minute, minimal to no urine output, and severely altered mental status as marked by confusion and/or lethargy.

Potential Pitfalls

Despite these guidelines, several potential pitfalls exist that can make the diagnosis more difficult. Concurrent medication, such as β-blockers, may attenuate the physiologic response to hemorrhage. In the presence of β-blockade, tachycardia may be blunted or may not occur at all. Prior hydration status and use of diuretics can also alter the rate at which these signs present. Pregnant patients have a significantly increased total blood volume, and thus can lose up to 1,000 mL of blood before presenting with any clinical signs of hemorrhage. Blood is diverted from the placenta via vasoconstriction; the mother's total blood circulation is maintained at the expense of the fetus. Elderly patients may have atrial arrhythmias leading to a high ventricular response, making tachycardia less sensitive in this patient population. Concurrent use of antiplatelet or anticoagulant medication can cause relatively small injuries to bleed excessively, and identification and intervention may be delayed. Although unloading of the baroreceptors and activation of the sympathetic nervous system usually lead to tachycardia, some patients may respond to traumatic hemorrhage with bradycardia as a result of a vagal nerve–mediated transient sympathoinhibition due to acute and sudden blood loss (3–9). Finally, a significant reduction in skin blood flow (i.e., cool, clammy skin) is an early ominous sign of shock in view of selective cutaneous vasoconstriction (10). Intervention and resuscitation must be imminent upon presentation of these signs and symptoms.

PATHOPHYSIOLOGY

Circulatory Changes

Hemorrhage results in a predictable pattern of events that begins with acute changes in circulating blood volume and culminates in a final common pathway shared by all classifications of shock (Fig. 58.1). Hemodynamically, hypovolemic shock is characterized by a fall in ventricular preload, resulting in decreased ventricular diastolic filling pressures and volumes. This in turn leads to a decrease in cardiac output and stroke volume (3–5,11–15). Following unloading of the cardiac baroreceptors and activation of the sympathetic nervous system, tachycardia ensues in an attempt to compensate for the decrease in cardiac output and stroke volume (12). The sympathetic output also results in vasoconstriction, leading to a decrease in pulse pressure. Greater variations in blood pressure will occur with the respiratory cycle due to an increased sensitivity of the underfilled heart to changes in venous return with varying intrathoracic pressure (16–18). The increased sympathetic tone may prevent a severe drop in arterial blood pressure initially. However, continued blood loss will ultimately result in hypotension and shock (3). Due to compensatory vasoconstriction, systemic vascular resistance rises early after the development of hypovolemic shock, but may fall in later stages, potentially heralding irreversibility and death (3,19,20).

The response to blood loss is a dynamic process that involves competing adaptive (compensatory) and maladaptive responses at each stage of development. Although intravascular volume replacement is always a necessary component of resuscitation in hypovolemic shock, the complex biologic response to the insult may progress to a point at which such resuscitation is insufficient to reverse the progression of the shock syndrome. For instance, patients who have sustained greater than a 40% loss of blood volume for 2 hours or more may not be able to be effectively resuscitated. Severe hemorrhage leads to a series of inflammatory mediator, cardiovascular, and organ responses that supersede the injury itself and ultimately drive recovery or death (3,19–25).

Oxygen Balance

Shock is characterized by an oxygen deficit in tissues and cells. The significance of the deficit and the extent of cellular injury can be quantified as a function of both the severity and the duration of the deficit—the greater the severity, the longer the duration, the worse the outcome of shock.

Oxygen delivery to tissues is determined by cardiac output and the oxygen content in arterial blood. *Oxygen content* refers to the number of milliliters of oxygen contained in 100 mL of blood (mL/dL) and is a function of the hemoglobin concentration, the oxygen saturation of hemoglobin, and the amount of oxygen dissolved in plasma (the calculation is [Hgb $\times$ 1.34 $\times$ O_2 saturation] + [PaO_2 $\times$ 0.0003]). During hemorrhage, as the cardiac output falls, oxygen delivery to the tissues also falls. Initially, the body will maintain sufficient uptake of oxygen by extracting more from the arterial blood. This will result in a fall in the mixed venous oxygen saturation (SvO_2) with an increase in the arteriovenous oxygen content gradient (CaO_2 – CvO_2). Eventually, this compensatory mechanism also fails, and tissue hypoxia with lactic acidosis ensues. Cerebral and cardiac functions are maintained by diversion of blood flow from other organs (skin, muscle, and kidneys) (26). However, when these compensatory mechanisms are maximized, cardiac function and tissue oxygen delivery deteriorates further, and irreversible shock may develop (27).

Critical oxygen delivery is a function of cellular needs for oxygen and the ability of cells to extract oxygen from the arterial blood. Many factors contribute to this equation. During hemorrhage, tissue oxygen needs may increase due to increased respiratory muscle activity and increased catecholamine circulation (28). However, some evidence suggests that catecholamines down-regulate the metabolic needs of cells during hypovolemic shock (4,5,28–30). Regional blood flow is modified during hypovolemic shock in an attempt to maintain oxygen delivery to critical tissues (26,31). In addition, the individual needs of various tissues may vary during hemorrhagic shock. For instance, the oxygen needs of the kidney may decline during hemorrhage because a fall in renal perfusion leads to a fall in glomerular filtration and a decrease in energy-consuming tubular absorption (26). In contrast, the gut may experience an increased oxygen debt early due to the high oxygen need of the mucosa, along with redistribution of blood away from the gut to more critical tissues. This is the physiologic basis for gastric tonometry as a means of measuring the adequacy of resuscitation early following hemorrhage (32,33).

Oxygen extraction in tissues is influenced by the position of the oxyhemoglobin dissociation curve (34–37). Factors that improve the ability of tissues to extract oxygen from hemoglobin (i.e., shift the curve to the right) include acidosis, hypercarbia, hyperthermia, and decreased blood viscosity. However, in any extreme, each of these factors can be overcome by inadequate oxygen delivery and cardiovascular collapse. Interestingly, the oxyhemoglobin curve has been shown to shift to the left in critically ill patients (38). The presence of 2,3-diphosphoglycerate (DPG) in transfused blood has also been associated with a left shift of the oxyhemoglobin dissociation curve (39). Thus, although transfusions may increase the hemoglobin level, theoretically improving oxygen delivery, they may negatively affect the ability of tissues to extract oxygen from the hemoglobin.

The severity of oxygen debt during hypovolemic shock has been shown to be a major determinant of survival in animals and in patients following trauma, hemorrhage, and major surgery (20,27,40,41). A large oxygen debt has been associated with the development of acute respiratory distress syndrome (ARDS) and multiple organ dysfunction syndrome (MODS) (33,40–44). Conversely, a high oxygen delivery and uptake during resuscitation has been associated with improved survival (27,41–46). Whether increasing oxygen delivery to supranormal levels ultimately improves survival during resuscitation in critical illness remains controversial, and the medical literature has produced mixed results (27,33,43,44,47–50).

Cellular Response

During hypovolemic shock, the oxygen deficit in the tissues causes a fall in the mitochondrial production and concentration of high-energy phosphates because of greater breakdown than production (51–57). This led many researchers to evaluate the utility of adenosine triphosphate (ATP) in the resuscitation of hemorrhagic shock (58,59). In the presence of sufficient oxygen, aerobic combustion of 1 mol of glucose yields 38 mol of energy-rich ATP. However, in the absence of sufficient oxygen, glucose taken up by the cells cannot be combusted because of insufficient uptake of pyruvate into the mitochondrial tricarboxylic acid cycle. Pyruvate is then converted to lactate within the cytoplasm. Anaerobic glycolysis yields only 2 mol of ATP, which is then hydrolyzed into hydrogen ion, ultimately leading to intracellular and extracellular metabolic acidosis (51,52,60–62) (Fig. 58.2). This process is ultimately a function of the severity and duration of regional hypoperfusion relative to oxygen demand and is more pronounced in some tissues (diaphragm, liver, kidney, gut) than in others (heart, skeletal muscle). Ultimately, a significant fall in the high-energy phosphates for a prolonged duration will lead to irreversible cellular injury and death.

The sequelae of low ATP production are profound. About 60% of the energy produced by respiring cellular mitochondria is needed to fuel the sodium-potassium (Na^+-K^+) pump of the cell. This pump controls the gradient in electrolyte concentrations and electric potential over the cell membrane. In the absence of sufficient ATP, the Na^+-K^+ pump is inhibited, resulting in an influx of sodium into the cell and efflux of potassium out of the cell. This in turn leads to cellular fluid uptake (51,53,63–66). Hyperkalemia may result due to potassium exchange between cells, the interstitial fluid, and vascular space.

Independent of the Na^+-K^+ pump, there may be a selective increase in cell membrane permeability for ions during hemorrhagic shock. Hypovolemic shock has been shown to lead to a

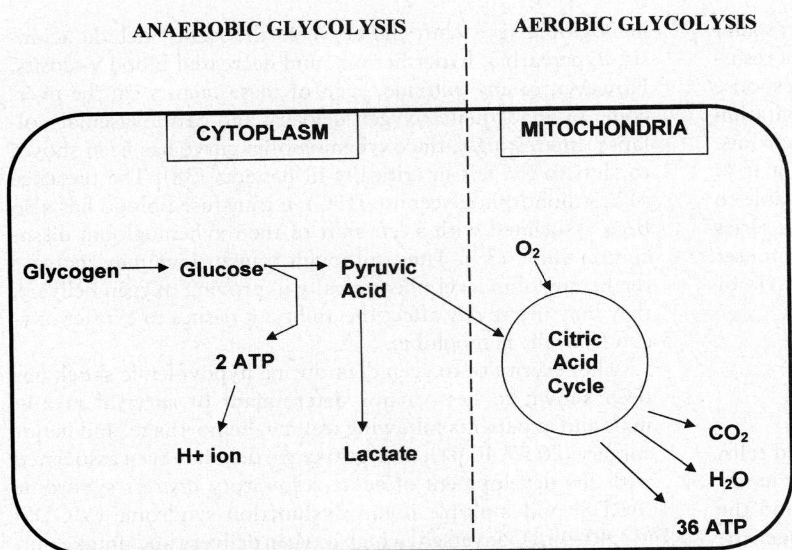

FIGURE 58.2. Cellular mechanisms during anaerobic and aerobic glycolysis. In anaerobic conditions, pyruvic acid cannot enter the citric acid cycle within the mitochondria and is instead shunted to the production of lactate. This process produces only two molecules of adenosine triphosphate (ATP), as opposed to the 36 molecules of ATP produced from glucose in the mitochondria during aerobic glycolysis. Hydrolysis of ATP molecules in anaerobic conditions results in the production of hydrogen ions that cannot be cleared, leading to intracellular acidosis. (Adapted from Mizock BA, Falk JL. Lactic acidosis in critical illness. *Crit Care Med.* 1992;20[1]:80.)

rapid decrease in the transmembrane potential (with a less negative inner membrane potential), resulting in rapid electrolyte and fluid shifts across the membrane. Circulating heat shock proteins may also contribute to these changes independent of energy deficit (66–71).

Finally, calcium (Ca^{2+}) influx into cells and their mitochondria inhibits cellular respiration and ultimately contributes to cellular damage and swelling. Plasma levels of free Ca^{2+} may also fall. This may have profound consequences on the function of several organs during shock including the liver, kidney, heart, and vascular smooth muscle (64,65,72–82). Intracellular lysosomes lose their integrity, and proteolytic enzymes are released and contribute to cellular dysfunction and cell death.

The sum of the intracellular changes and alterations in signaling transduction pathways described above ultimately leads to the development of cellular dysfunction and multiple organ dysfunction syndrome, which may be irreversible (82). Laboratory investigations are aimed at novel resuscitation techniques involving substances that attenuate abnormalities of cellular signaling following hemorrhagic shock (58,59, 77–82).

Neurohumoral Response

In response to hemorrhage and hypovolemia, a complex neurohumoral response is initiated in an attempt to maintain blood pressure and retain fluid. Decreased intravascular volume stimulates baroreceptors in the carotid body and aortic arch, along with mechanoreceptors in the right atrium. This stimulation leads to several neurohumoral responses (Fig. 58.3). Circulating catecholamines are liberated by activation of the sympathetic nervous system and the adrenal medulla. Direct sympathetic stimulation of the vessel wall leads to vasoconstriction. Angiotensin II is liberated via the renin–angiotensin–aldosterone system. Vasopressin (antidiuretic hormone [ADH]) is released by the pituitary in hypovolemic shock and leads to vasoconstriction. Finally, decreased cardiac filling pressures reduce cardiac secretion of α-atrial natriuretic peptide (ANP), thereby reducing the vasodilatory and diuretic effects of ANP.

Macrocirculation

During loss of circulating blood volume, mechanisms are initiated to counteract the fall in cardiac output and oxygen delivery by facilitating a redistribution of peripheral blood flow (26). Regional autoregulation takes place via a delicate balance of endogenous vasodilators and vasoconstrictors. Endothelial cells produce potent vasodilators such as endothelium-derived relaxing factor (nitric oxide [NO]), heme oxygenation–derived carbon monoxide (CO), and metabolic byproducts in tissues, including carbon dioxide (CO_2), potassium, and adenosine (25, 83–89). Some authors describe that inhibition of NO early following hemorrhage ameliorates early hypotension and improves mortality (90–94). Conversely, other authors describe endothelial dysfunction in organs with diminished NO production (95–96). Endothelin is a potent endothelial cell–derived vasoconstrictor that is released upon catecholamine stimulation or hypoxia (97). The overall increase in systemic peripheral vascular resistance is distributed differently among various organs in the body (31). Vasoconstriction also occurs in the venous vasculature, increasing return of available blood to the heart (14,98). The complex interplay of these mechanisms for vasodilation and vasoconstriction ultimately determines the regional redistribution of blood flow to organs following hemorrhagic shock. The redistribution of blood flow results in a greater share of oxygen delivery to organs with high obligatory metabolic demands (heart and brain), and a lesser share to those with fewer demands including the skin, skeletal muscle, kidney, intestine, and pancreas (5,31,86,99–101).

Microcirculation

One of the most important determinants of tissue perfusion during shock is the response and function of the microvasculature, which is defined as vessels less than 100 to 150 μm in diameter. Although arteries and medium-sized arterioles constrict in response to the extrinsic control mechanisms described above, terminal arterioles, venules, and capillaries remain unaffected and are more controlled by local metabolic factors.

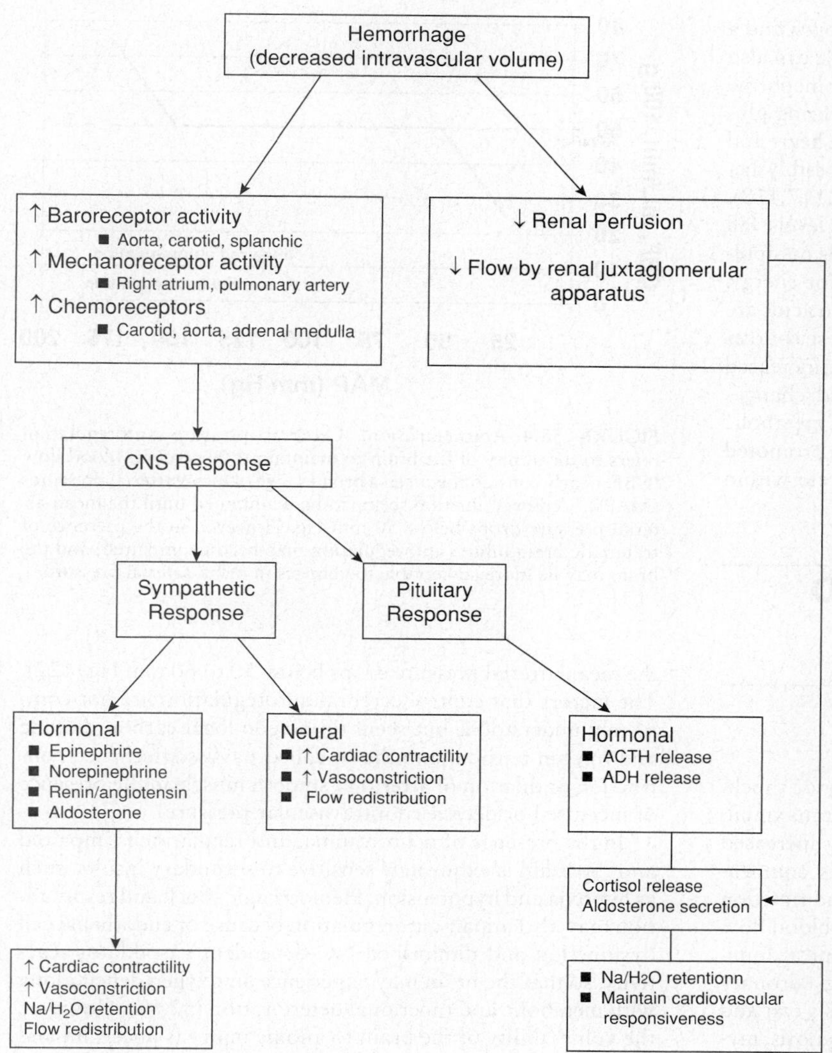

FIGURE 58.3. Neurohormonal response to hemorrhage. Hemorrhage results in a decrease in the circulating intravascular volume, which initiates a complex cascade of compensatory events. CNS, central nervous system; ACTH, adrenocorticotropic hormone; ADH, antidiuretic hormone.

Alterations in microvascular function and flow are effected through precapillary and postcapillary sphincters, which are sensitive to both extrinsic and intrinsic control mechanisms. Exchange of metabolites and compartmental regulation of fluids occurs at the capillary level. Therefore, alteration of tone of the pre- and postcapillary sphincters can have significant effects on microcirculatory function (102–104). Failure to dilate sphincters supplying metabolically active tissues may result in ischemia and anaerobic metabolism with lactate production. Increased precapillary tone, as seen with sympathetic stimulation, results in increased blood pressure systemically and decreased hydrostatic pressure locally. In fact, the microvascular arterioles may even dilate in response to the above vasoconstriction due to release of metabolic byproducts of underperfusion (carbon dioxide, hydrogen ion, etc.). The decrease in hydrostatic pressure locally then leads to redistribution of fluid from the interstitium to the circulation. Conversely, increased postcapillary tone (relative to precapillary tone) results in vascular pooling of blood and loss of fluid to the interstitium (as a result of increased hydrostatic pressure). This increased hydrostatic pressure may become accentuated in response to crystalloid resuscitation, leading to interstitial edema (104). Finally, hemorrhage and shock have also been shown to induce increased permeability of capillaries, leading to interstitial fluid leak during resuscitation (105,106).

Hypovolemic shock and hemorrhage also induce the expression of endothelial adhesion molecules on neutrophils and endothelium (63,107). This results in neutrophil adherence and "rolling" of cells within the capillary bed (108–113). Capillary flow then diminishes and may also impair red blood cell flow. While this decrease in transit time may augment the ability of tissue to extract oxygen, it may also lead to microvascular thrombosis and further tissue ischemia (114,115).

Metabolic and Hormonal Response

The early hyperglycemic response to trauma/hemorrhage is the combined result of enhanced glycogenolysis, caused by the hormonal response to stress including elevated epinephrine, cortisol, and glucagon levels; increased gluconeogenesis in the liver, partly mediated by glucagon; and peripheral resistance to the action of insulin (51,116). Increased gluconeogenesis in the liver, and to a lesser extent in the kidneys, follows increased efflux of amino acids, such as alanine and glutamine from the muscle to the liver, due to a breakdown of muscle protein. The latter is evidenced by increased urinary losses of nitrogen and a negative nitrogen balance. Lactate produced in muscle can also be converted to glucose in the liver (117). Increased epinephrine also results in skeletal muscle insulin resistance, sparing glucose for use by glucose-dependent organs such as the heart and brain. Later in shock, hypoglycemia may ensue, possibly because of glycogen depletion or hepatic ischemia (51,117,118). Fatty acids are increased early in shock, but later levels fall (116). Without energy for glycolysis, the cell depends on lipolysis and the autodigestion of intracellular protein for energy. Initially, ketone bodies and the branched-chain amino acids are used as alternative fuel sources. Without oxygen, these sources become inefficient, leading to hypertriglyceridemia, increased β-hydroxybutyric acid and acetoacetate levels, and changes in the amino acid concentration pattern. As these metabolic changes occur, set in motion by cellular hypoxia and promoted by systemic hormonal changes, structural changes occur within individual cells (119).

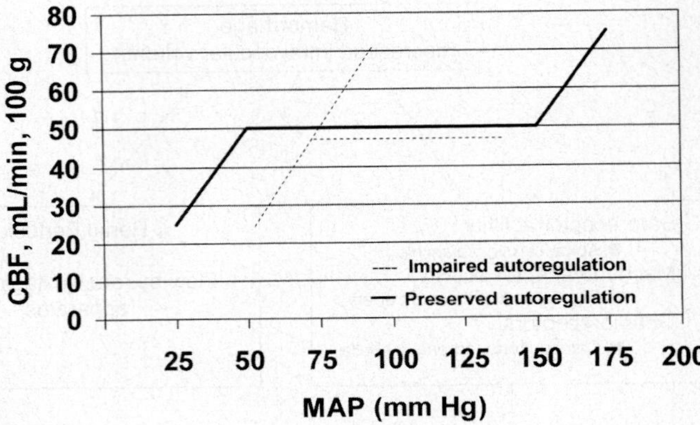

FIGURE 58.4. Autoregulation. Cerebral pressure autoregulation refers to the ability of the brain to maintain total cerebral blood flow (CBF) nearly constant between a broad range of mean arterial pressures (MAPs). Cerebral function seems to be maintained until the mean arterial pressure drops below 50 mm Hg. However, in the presence of traumatic brain injury, autoregulation may become impaired, and the brain may be more susceptible to changes in mean arterial pressure.

ORGAN PERFUSION AND FUNCTION DURING HEMORRHAGE

Heart

The heart is a critical organ in the pathophysiology of shock. At baseline, myocardial oxygen extraction is almost maximal; therefore, increased cardiac work must be met by increased coronary blood flow. When coronary perfusion is compromised, as it is during systemic hypotension, cardiac function suffers. In the presence of sympathetic stimulation, blood flow from the endocardium is redistributed toward the epicardium, impairing cardiac performance (120). Underlying coronary artery disease, arrhythmias, hypoxemia, and acidosis can add to cardiac dysfunction. In the absence of coronary stenosis, myocardial necrosis/infarction is unusual in hypovolemic shock. Rather, the heart plays a participatory role in which it is unable to compensate fully for arterial hypotension caused by hypovolemia, vasodilation, and other factors.

Under basal aerobic conditions, 60% of energy comes from fat (free fatty acids and triacylglycerides), 35% from carbohydrates, and 5% from amino acids and ketone bodies. However, during anaerobic conditions imposed by hypoxemia or ischemia, the myocardium shifts to glycolysis. Anaerobic glycolysis, however, is insufficient to meet cardiac work demands for any length of time because the myocardial glycogen stores, as an alternative fuel source, are minimal and rapidly depleted.

Brain

Like the heart, the brain almost exclusively depends on perfusion, rather than changes in extraction, to meet its oxidative metabolic needs. Protective mechanisms, collectively referred to as *autoregulation*, have evolved to guard perfusion. *Pressure autoregulation* refers to the ability of the brain to maintain total and regional cerebral blood flow (CBF) nearly constant despite large changes in systemic arterial blood pressure (Fig. 58.4) (121). Cerebral function seems to be maintained until the mean arterial pressure drops below 50 to 60 mm Hg (122). The factors that control cerebral autoregulation are not completely understood, but seem to include local carbon dioxide and oxygen tension, and the so-called Bayliss effect (i.e., contraction or dilation of arteriolar smooth muscle in the presence of increased or decreased intravascular pressure).

In the presence of neurotrauma, autoregulation is impaired and the brain is exquisitely sensitive to secondary insults, such as hypoxia and hypotension. Hemorrhagic shock and resuscitation may also impair autoregulation because of endothelial cell dysfunction and diminished NO-dependent vasodilator reactivity, so that the brain may experience an oxygen deficit along with metabolic and functional deterioration (52,87). However, the vulnerability of the brain to anoxic injury is uncertain and appears variable. The adequacy and the method of resuscitation can critically influence postischemic recovery. These observations have motivated investigation of specific brain resuscitation regimens (123–126). However, there are no conclusive data that one modality provides improved outcomes.

Lungs

Hypovolemic shock is associated with a rise in minute ventilation marked by tachypnea, hyperventilation, and a fall in arterial PCO_2 (28,30,127–130). These changes are usually due to a decrease in pulmonary perfusion, leading to an increase in dead space ventilation. Thus, a higher minute ventilation is necessary for a given CO_2 production (28,30,127). In addition, minute ventilation may need to increase further in order to compensate for a metabolic acidosis following accumulation of lactic acid in the blood. The imbalance between the increased demands of the diaphragm and reduced blood flow in shock may finally lead to respiratory muscle fatigue and respiratory failure, requiring intubation (28). Therefore, early airway control is imperative in patients with severe hemorrhagic shock.

Hemorrhagic shock requiring massive transfusion also increases the risk of acute respiratory distress syndrome (129,130–132). Contributing factors include release of proinflammatory mediators; activation of neutrophils in the lungs and other organs after reperfusion; contusion and/or ischemia-reperfusion of the lung; pulmonary microemboli of neutrophils, platelets, and fat particles from long bone fractures; and induction of transfusion-related acute lung injury (TRALI), which is discussed later in this chapter.

Kidney

Oliguria, as defined by a urinary output of less than 0.5 mL/kg/hour, is a cardinal manifestation of shock. However, the pathogenesis of shock-related oliguria is more complex than mere renal hypoperfusion (133–135). Blood flow to the kidney is rarely reduced below 40% to 50% of normal levels, even in the face of more severe reductions in overall cardiac output. Thus, the decreased glomerular filtration rate results from additional mechanisms. Sympathetic stimulation, circulating catecholamines, angiotensin, and locally produced prostaglandins contribute to afferent arteriolar vasoconstriction. These compounds promote the redistribution of blood flow away from cortical glomeruli toward the renal medulla (65). Vasodilation of the efferent arteriole may amplify these changes. The net effect is a decreased glomerular filtration rate and a decrease in the energy needs of the kidney. Additional fluid (and salt) conservation is promoted by the effects of aldosterone and antidiuretic hormone.

If renal hypoperfusion persists, the cortical kidney will become ischemic. Three pathologic changes are observed: (a) tubular necrosis with back-diffusion of glomerular infiltrate, (b) tubular obstruction by casts or other cellular debris, and (c) tubular epithelial damage with consequent interstitial edema and tubular collapse. Following hypovolemia and renal ischemia, these pathologic changes may be secondary events (i.e., reperfusion injury) that can amplify but rarely initiate acute renal failure. The presence of these pathologic changes partially explains why restoration of normal hemodynamic function does not often lead to an immediate improvement in renal function. Although irreversible renal failure from shock alone is rare, fluid and electrolyte balance are often supported by dialysis although normal perfusion has been restored.

Intestine

During hypovolemic shock, blood flow from intestine is redistributed to other organs. The decrease in blood flow to the gut is relatively greater than the decrease in cardiac output due to the local vasoconstriction caused by catecholamines, vasopressin, and angiotensin II (4,5,26,136–139). Ischemic injury to the gut is manifested primarily by interstitial fluid sequestration and hemorrhage or necrosis of the mucosal lining, and is most prominent in the stomach (139). Ulcer formation (140) with exsanguinating hemorrhage can occur several days after normal hemodynamic function has been restored (141). Breakdown of the gut epithelium creates a port of entry for translocation of bacteria or deleterious bacterial products (endotoxin) (142,143). These factors may be important in the pathogenesis of irreversible shock (144) by releasing mediators to the systemic circulation. The determination of mucosal pH via tonometry has been described as a potential indicator of the therapeutic response and a marker of MODS (145,146).

Liver

Hepatic perfusion declines during hypovolemic shock because of diminished portal and hepatic arterial blood flow, roughly in proportion to the fall in cardiac output (57,61,109,147–150). Clinical manifestations of ischemic liver injury are not usually apparent in the early stages of hemorrhagic shock, as the organ participates in the release of acute-phase reactants. As hepatic cells die, they release characteristic enzymes (i.e., aspartate aminotransferase, alanine aminotransferase) (151). Occasionally, an obstructive picture with elevated bilirubin and alkaline phosphatase predominates. Later, the synthesis of coagulation factors, albumin, and prealbumin may deteriorate (152,153). Less clinically obvious is the impairment in the reticuloendothelial system function. Impaired hepatic clearance functions and reticuloendothelial system failure contribute to continued circulation of vasoactive substances that can perpetuate shock. Hepatic ischemia may result in a diminished capacity for metabolism of drugs and for gluconeogenesis from lactate and amino acids, contributing to hypoglycemia in the late stages of hypovolemic shock. The capacity to clear gut-derived endotoxin and lactate may also decrease, and the ischemic liver produces lactate (154). The appearance of "shock liver" with massive hepatocellular necrosis is unusual and presents mainly in patients with pre-existing liver conditions (155).

Spleen

The spleen contracts during hypovolemic shock, probably due to an increased sympathetic tone, which results in the release of red blood cells into the circulation (5,26). Changes in hematocrit during the early phase of bleeding probably underestimate the severity of plasma losses. The spleen also releases stored platelets.

Pancreas

The importance of the pancreas in the clinical picture in hemorrhagic shock has not been fully established. Older studies have demonstrated that the pancreas becomes severely ischemic during hypovolemic shock (156). Recently, much work has been done to better elucidate the role of the pancreas following hemorrhage and reperfusion. Preliminary data suggest that following hemorrhage, the mucosal barrier of the intestine becomes ischemic and therefore has increased permeability to pancreatic enzymes. These digestive enzymes then gain access to the wall of the intestine, initiating self-digestion of submucosal extracellular matrix proteins and interstitial cells. This initiates the generation and release of a host of strong inflammatory mediators, which may contribute to the multiorgan dysfunction syndrome. Recent investigations are focusing on protease inhibition in the intestinal lumen as a means of attenuating the inflammatory response following hemorrhage (157–163).

INFLAMMATORY RESPONSE AND TISSUE INJURY

A detailed discussion of the inflammatory and immune response to trauma and hemorrhage is beyond the scope of this chapter. However, several general concepts can be introduced. Following hemorrhage and resuscitation, macrophages, including lung macrophages and Kupffer cells in the liver, may release proinflammatory cytokines including tumor necrosis factor (TNF)-α and interleukin (IL)-1, -6, and -8. During reperfusion, cytokines may induce and amplify the inflammatory response to ischemia and may further induce local and remote organ damage (148,164–174). The reperfused gut, for example, may, together with the liver, be a source of systemically circulating cytokines, and possibly endotoxin. Release of mediators into the mesenteric lymph, portal, or systemic circulations during reperfusion may have deleterious effects on remote organs, such as the lungs, due to neutrophil activation and adherence, leading to pulmonary vascular injury with increased permeability (165,168,169). Circulating levels of proinflammatory cytokines may thus be of predictive value for remote organ damage, including ARDS, after trauma and hemorrhage in patients (167,170).

Arachidonic acid makes up 20% of cell membranes and is released from these membranes in response to a multitude of stimuli that activate phospholipase A_2 and C, and is then metabolized via one of two major enzyme systems. The *cyclo-oxygenase pathway* results in the production of thromboxanes and prostaglandins, while the *lipoxygenase pathway* produces leukotrienes. Thromboxane has potent vasoconstricting properties on both the pulmonary and splanchnic circulation, promotes aggregation of thrombocytes and neutrophils, causes bronchoconstriction, and can lead to increased vascular permeability. The prostaglandins have varied effects. Prostacyclin (prostaglandin I_2 [PGI_2]) has potent vasodilating properties and inhibits thrombocyte and neutrophil aggregation (175). PGE_2 and PGD_2 also have vasodilating properties, while other prostaglandins ($PGF_{2\alpha}$) are potent vasoconstrictors. Leukotrienes, which are produced by the lipoxygenase pathway, cause vasoconstriction and increased capillary permeability and attract neutrophils (175). Thromboxane, prostaglandins, and leukotrienes interact with other mediators in a complex fashion (175–179). Vasoconstricting prostaglandins may be involved in the tissue damage during ischemia/reperfusion. Vasodilating prostaglandins may be involved in the vasodilated state of terminal hypovolemic shock (3,175–179).

Platelet-activating factor (PAF) is a nonprotein phospholipid, which is secreted by many cells including platelets, endothelial cells, and inflammatory cells. It is a major mediator of the pulmonary and hemodynamic effects of endotoxin. The major systemic effects of PAF are vasodilatation, cardiac depression, and enhancement of capillary leak. Its complex interactions with other mediators are still poorly understood (180).

Antigen–antibody complexes activate the complement cascade, and complement fragments thus generated can interact with other cytokines to promulgate the inflammatory response. Complement activation can yield potent vasodilating and leukoattractant substances (175,177,181,182).

Oxygen radicals, such as hydrogen peroxide and superoxide anion, are released by activated neutrophils in response to a variety of stimuli. They are also released when xanthine oxidase is activated after reperfusion in ischemia-reperfusion models. These highly reactive products lead to cell membrane dysfunction, increased vascular permeability, and release of eicosanoids (183–186).

This inflammatory process results in the local accumulation of activated inflammatory cells, which release various local toxins such as oxygen radicals, proteases, eicosanoids, platelet-activating factor, and other substances. When unregulated, such accumulations can cause tissue injury. The initial attachment of neutrophils to the vascular endothelium at an inflammatory site is facilitated by the interaction of adherence molecules on the neutrophil and endothelial cell surfaces (108,187–192).

IMMUNE FUNCTION FOLLOWING HEMORRHAGE AND RESUSCITATION

Despite the initiation of the inflammatory cascade, hypovolemic shock and resuscitation depress the immune system by suppressing the function of lymphocytes, macrophages, and neutrophils, depressing both humoral and cellular immune responses, decreasing antigen presentation and delayed hypersensitivity to skin-test antigens, and increasing susceptibility to sepsis (63,166,193–198). The immune consequences of hemorrhage and resuscitation differ among cell populations, however, with some cells expressing enhanced (199–201) and others diminished inflammatory responses (202,203). Hormone may also influence immune response (204,205). The immunosuppression after hypovolemic shock may also be potentiated by the release of anti-inflammatory cytokines (IL-10) (206–208) and soluble cytokine receptors (receptor antagonists) for the proinflammatory cytokines (203,209,210).

MANAGEMENT OF HEMORRHAGIC SHOCK

Trauma is by far the most common etiology for hemorrhagic shock. While other causes do exist, management priorities are similar regardless of the source of bleeding. Diagnosis, evaluation, and management must often occur simultaneously. A methodical approach is necessary to optimize outcome. Unique to hemorrhagic shock, as opposed to other forms of shock, is that definitive management frequently requires surgical or procedural intervention to cease bleeding. The diagnostic pathway and interventions pursued become part of the resuscitation pathway. What follows is a summary of the interventions, diagnostic studies, monitoring strategies, and resuscitation techniques for hemorrhagic shock.

Immediate Management

Airway and Breathing

When approaching any patient in shock, the sequence of events should be to address the issues of airway, breathing, and circulation—also known as the "ABCs" (211). Most patients with fully developed shock require tracheal intubation and mechanical ventilation, even if acute respiratory failure has not yet developed. Studies have shown that during shock, the respiratory muscles require a disproportionate percent of the cardiac output (28). Failure to mount a hyperventilatory response to a metabolic acidosis is a significant predictor of the need for subsequent intubation in trauma patients (212). Mechanical ventilation allows flow to be redistributed, lessens the work of breathing, may help reverse lactic acidosis, and supports the patient's airway until other therapeutic measures can be effective. Tracheal intubation is also required if there is evidence of mental status changes, such that airway protection is questionable. Evidence of hypoxemia and/or hypoventilation is also an absolute requirement for early intubation.

Perhaps most complex is the patient with evidence of compensated hemorrhagic shock whose mental status is still intact. In this type of patient, clinical acumen is imperative. If the initial response to resuscitation is sustained (i.e., "a responder"—see below), then close observation of the airway may be appropriate while additional workup and treatment are pursued. However, in a patient who is not responsive or has a transient response (see below) to fluid resuscitation, control of the airway early is necessary prior to respiratory collapse (212). In addition, if diagnostic and therapeutic interventions, such as angiography and embolization, are required during resuscitation to control hemorrhage, early airway control should be obtained.

Once the airway is secured, it is important to closely monitor techniques of ventilation. Studies have shown that there is a tendency of rescue and medical personnel to hyperventilate patients during resuscitation (213,214). Hyperventilated patients have been shown to have an increased mortality when compared to nonhyperventilated patients in the setting of severe traumatic brain injury (214). Animal studies have supported this information, showing that cardiac output increases with hypoventilation and decreases with hyperventilation and positive end-expiratory pressure (PEEP) (215,216). Thus, adequate appropriate ventilator strategies are imperative early in hemorrhagic shock to optimize tissue perfusion and outcome.

Circulation

The management steps to restore adequate circulation are threefold:

1. Secure access to the bloodstream in order to initiate infusion of fluids and blood products
2. Control obvious sources of hemorrhage and prevent ongoing hemorrhage
3. Assess extent of shock and hemorrhage

Intravenous Access. Access to the bloodstream should be obtained expediently. Two peripheral large-bore intravenous catheters (18 gauge or larger) are necessary. If cannulation of a peripheral vein is difficult due to collapse, then central venous access should be secured. In the presence of trauma to the torso, venous access above and below the diaphragm is preferable. When obtaining intravenous access, it is important to note that the maximal rate of infusion via a catheter is directly proportional to the diameter of the catheter and indirectly proportional to the length. Therefore, a 9 French percutaneous introducer sheath will infuse fluids more rapidly than a 7 French triple-lumen catheter. A large-bore peripheral intravenous catheter will also infuse fluids more rapidly than a 7 French triple lumen catheter due to a shorter length and less resistance. In pediatric patients, an intraosseous access may be necessary. This is only recommended for children under the age of 6 and should only be used until an alternative source of venous access is obtained.

Control Obvious Hemorrhage Immediately. Resuscitation of the bleeding patient requires early identification of potential bleeding sources followed by prompt action to minimize blood loss, restore tissue perfusion, and achieve hemodynamic stability. This is particularly important in the trauma patient where multiple sources may be involved. Wound compression is the initial maneuver to control an exsanguinating wound. For massive soft tissue injuries, placing a tourniquet proximally may decrease hemorrhage and allow resuscitation prior to definitive control. Fractures should be splinted or placed in traction. Evidence of pelvic instability or hemorrhage may be temporized by a sheet, a pelvic binder, an external fixator, or a pelvic C-clamp (217–220). In the presence of massive trauma, patients may present with coagulopathy in the emergency department and this should be preemptively addressed. The same principles should be applied to nontraumatic hemorrhagic shock, such as gastrointestinal bleeding and ruptured aortic aneurysms: rapidly identify and attenuate the obvious sources of hemorrhage.

Initiate Resuscitation and Assess Extent of Bleeding: Responders and Nonresponders. The traditional classification of hemorrhagic shock was discussed earlier (Table 58.3). While this is a useful guideline for determining the extent of blood loss for a given patient, perhaps more important in determining an appropriate treatment algorithm is the patient's response to resuscitation. Following hemorrhage, resuscitation should be initiated with 2 L of lactated Ringer solution or isotonic crystalloid solution. The response to this initial fluid bolus will provide critical insight as to the presence of ongoing hemorrhage and need for surgical intervention (Table 58.4) (221).

Rapid responders become hemodynamically normal and remain this way following the initial fluid bolus. This group of patients has likely lost <20% of their total circulating blood volume, and ongoing aggressive resuscitation is not necessary. Intravenous fluids can be lowered to maintenance rates while additional workup proceeds. Blood should still be sent for type and cross-match and should be made available. Retrospective studies have shown that patients with field hypotension who become normotensive on arrival to the emergency department have increased morbidity, mortality, need for operation, and admission rate to the intensive care unit (ICU) (222–224). Approximately 15% of these patients will need transfusion, with 37% requiring therapeutic surgery (224). Hence, even a brief episode of hypotension can be a marker for significant underlying injury.

Transient responders represent a group of patients who initially respond to a 2-L bolus of crystalloid, but then begin to show signs of deterioration when intravenous fluid infusion is lowered to maintenance levels. These patients have likely lost 20% to 40% of their circulating blood volume, and either have ongoing blood loss or inadequate resuscitation. Continued fluid resuscitation and initiation of blood transfusion are indicated. A transient response to blood infusion indicates ongoing hemorrhage. Rapid surgical intervention or angioembolization (225–228) to control hemorrhage is immediately indicated.

Nonresponders represent patients who fail to respond to crystalloid and blood administration in the emergency department. These patients have likely lost >40% of their circulation blood volume and have ongoing hemorrhage. Immediate control of hemorrhage is necessary via surgical intervention

TABLE 58.4

RESPONSE TO INITIAL FLUID RESUSCITATION AND PATIENT MANAGEMENT

	Rapid response	Transient response	No response
Vital signs	Return to normal	Transient response, recurrent hypotension, and/or tachycardia	Remains abnormal
Estimated blood loss	Minimal (10%–20%)	Moderate (20%–40%)	Severe (>40%)
Additional crystalloid	Unlikely	Yes	Yes
Need for blood transfusion	Unlikely	Moderate to high	Immediate
Blood preparation	Type and cross-match (30–60 min)	Type-specific (10–20 min)	Emergency blood release (immediate type O Rh-negative blood)
Operative intervention	Possible	Likely	Highly likely
Early presence of surgeon	Yes	Yes	Yes

Adapted from American College of Surgeons Committee on Trauma. Shock. In: *Advanced Trauma Life Support*. 7th ed. American College of Surgeons Chicago, IL; 2004:79.

or angioembolization in the face of significant pelvic fractures (225–228). On rare occasions, failure to respond to fluid administration may be due to pump failure as a result of blunt cardiac injury, cardiac tamponade, tension pneumothorax, or myocardial infarction. Central venous pressure monitoring and cardiac ultrasonography may help differentiate between various etiologies in this setting.

Emergency Department Resuscitative Thoracotomy. Resuscitative thoracotomy is occasionally indicated for exsanguinating hemorrhage. In trauma, indications for resuscitative thoracotomy include (a) patients with penetrating thoracic injuries who arrive pulseless, but with myocardial electrical activity, and (b) blunt trauma patients who have vital signs on arrival but then sustain a witnessed arrest or onset of pulseless electrical activity. Specific recommendations are listed in Table 58.5. Therapeutic maneuvers that can be attained with a resuscitative thoracotomy include (a) evacuation of pericardial blood causing tamponade, (b) direct control of exsanguinating thoracic or cardiac hemorrhage, (c) open cardiac massage, and (d) cross-clamping of the descending aorta to slow blood loss below the diaphragm and improve perfusion to the heart and brain.

Depending on the cause of injury, the overall mortality rate in these situations is extremely high (229–231). The highest survival rates are found in patients with isolated cardiac injury without loss of vital signs (approximately 35%). Some reports of thoracic aortic cross-clamping for exsanguinating intra-abdominal hemorrhage have reported survival rates of nearly one third (231,232), but this is mainly in the setting of penetrating abdominal trauma. Survival rates following resuscitative thoracotomy in blunt trauma are dismal, ranging from 0% to 5%. Aortic cross-clamping should be viewed as an adjunct to other initial hemorrhage control measures. It has not been established whether thoracic aortic clamping should be performed before or after the abdominal incision, or whether thoracic or intra-abdominal aortic cross-clamping is more effective (233). However, when aortic cross-clamping is deemed necessary for continuous bleeding or low blood pressure, the prognosis is generally poor (234). No clinical data exist for the use of emergency room thoracotomy in nontrauma infradiaphragmatic bleeding.

Adjunctive Measures. Historical teachings have been that tilting a patient into head-down position (i.e., Trendelenburg) diverts blood volume into the central circulation and improves venous return, thereby improving stroke volume and cardiac output in hypovolemic shock. However, recent studies do not show any significant redistribution of blood volume centrally (235). In fact, the head-down position can worsen gas exchange and cardiac function. Therefore, the Trendelenburg position is no longer recommended as a resuscitative technique. If this type of measure is deemed desirable, raising the legs above the level of the heart should be adequate (13).

TABLE 58.5

INDICATIONS AND CONTRAINDICATIONS FOR EMERGENCY DEPARTMENT RESUSCITATIVE THORACOTOMY

INDICATIONS

Salvageable postinjury cardiac arrest

- Patients sustaining witnessed penetrating trauma with <15 min of prehospital cardiopulmonary resuscitation (CPR)
- Patients sustaining witnessed blunt trauma with <5 min of prehospital CPR

Persistent severe postinjury hypotension (systolic blood pressure ≤60 mm Hg) due to:

- Cardiac tamponade
- Hemorrhage—intrathoracic, intra-abdominal, extremity, cervical
- Air embolism

CONTRAINDICATIONS

■ Penetrating trauma:	CPR >15 min, and No signs of life[a]
■ Blunt trauma:	CPR >5 min, and No signs of life[a] or asystole

[a]No signs of life = no pupillary response, respiratory effort, or motor activity.

Adapted from Cothren CC, Moore EE. Emergency department thoracotomy for the critically injured patient: objectives, indications, and outcomes. *World J Emerg Surg*. 2006;1:4.

The use of pneumatic antishock garments (PASGs, previously military antishock trousers [MAST]) currently has a limited role in the management of hypotensive trauma patients. Although their use was almost universal for hemorrhage control in the late 1970s and 1980s, recent studies have demonstrated that they have no effect on patients with thoracic injury. In fact, some evidence suggests that mortality is higher when PASGs are applied (236,237). No survival advantage has been demonstrated in the pediatric population, although there may be a small survival benefit in children with a systolic blood pressure of less than 50 mm Hg (238). The main utility of PASGs currently is as a temporizing agent to stabilize pelvic fractures.

Fluid Resuscitation

Careful attention to fluid resuscitation is necessary during management of hemorrhagic shock to optimize outcome. It is still unclear which type of fluid should be employed in the initial treatment of the bleeding patient.

Colloids versus Crystalloids

Several meta-analyses have shown an increased risk of death in patients resuscitated with colloids as compared with crystalloids (239–243) during hemorrhagic shock. While three of these studies suggested that the effect was particularly significant in the trauma population (239,242,243), the results of a recent meta-analysis showed no significant difference (244). A recent trial evaluating 4% albumin versus 0.9% normal saline in nearly 7,000 ICU patients showed that albumin administration was not associated with worse outcome. There was a trend, however, toward higher mortality in the trauma subgroup that received albumin ($p = 0.06$) (245). The difficulty with interpreting these meta-analyses and the individual studies is that they are very heterogenous. Each evaluates different patient populations and resuscitation strategies, and mortality may not always be a primary end point. However, given these results, crystalloid resuscitation is currently the accepted standard as initial therapy for hemorrhagic shock.

Many synthetic colloid solutions such as hetastarch and dextran have also been associated with coagulopathy. Recent research suggests that hetastarch solutions with a high mean molecular weight and a high C2/C6 ratio suppress coagulation more than solutions with rapidly degradable low-molecular-weight colloids (246–248). This coagulopathy may be produced by one of several potential mechanisms including a reduction in von Willebrand factor, platelet dysfunction, reduced factor VII levels, and an interaction with fibrinogen (249,250).

Crystalloid solutions are not without side effects. Resuscitation with fluids that contain supraphysiologic concentrations of chloride can lead to hyperchloremic acidosis. This can be significant in patients where lactic acidosis may already be present. Lactated Ringer solution contains a more physiologic concentration of chloride (109 mEq/L) than normal saline (NS 154 mEq/L), and therefore may be the preferred choice. Animal studies have also shown that resuscitation with normal saline can lead to more coagulopathy and increased blood loss than resuscitation with lactated Ringer solution (251).

Massive resuscitation with crystalloid fluids alone can lead to several significant complications including cardiac and pulmonary complications, gastrointestinal dysmotility, coagulation abnormalities, and immunologic dysfunction (252). Reports of lactated Ringer solution and normal saline increasing reperfusion injury and leukocyte adhesion suggest that crystalloid resuscitation may worsen acidosis and coagulopathy in severely injured patients and possibly increases the risk of ARDS, systemic inflammatory response syndrome (SIRS), and multiorgan failure (MOF) (252–256). Abdominal compartment syndrome has been clearly associated with excessive use of crystalloid resuscitation (50,257–261). Recently, there has been increased focus on early use of blood products in order to minimize crystalloid use in the resuscitation of hemorrhagic shock (262). Finally, resuscitation strategies that focus on early aggressive fluid resuscitation to normalize blood pressure before bleeding is controlled may result in increased hemorrhage and increased mortality. This has led some authors to suggest that "hypotensive resuscitation" should be the goal until the source of hemorrhage is controlled (263–265). However, the exact goals for mean arterial pressure and trigger points for bleeding have not been established. The potential adverse sequelae when used in patients with associated injuries or comorbidities (i.e., severe closed head injury) have not been clearly established (266).

In light of these potential sequelae of resuscitation, future research should focus on improvement in fluid composition and adjuncts to the administration of large volumes of fluid (266). Current strategies should focus on the type of fluid delivered, the rate of delivery, the timing of delivery, and the prevention of sequelae from large-volume resuscitation.

Preventing Hypothermia

All fluids during resuscitation from hemorrhagic shock should be warmed to prevent hypothermia. Equipment is now available that allows the rapid infusion of blood and/or crystalloids at warmed temperatures (i.e., up to 750 mL fluid per minute warmed to over 37°C). This newer equipment is more effective and efficient and results in fewer complications associated with earlier models (such as air embolism and bacterial contamination) (267). Other techniques during resuscitation that can be used to prevent hypothermia in the acutely hemorrhaging patient include warming the circuit on the ventilator in ventilated patients, ensuring the patient is covered with warm blankets at all times following exposure and thorough examination, warming the resuscitation and operating rooms, using external warming blankets such as the Baer hugger during resuscitation and in the operating room, and using warm water blankets on the operating room table during exploratory operations. Hypothermia is clearly associated with increased mortality following resuscitation from hemorrhagic shock (268), and every attempt to prevent or minimize its occurrence and severity should be employed.

DIAGNOSTIC APPROACH

If no obvious source of external bleeding is identified, a rapid evaluation should be performed to identify likely occult sources of bleeding. In the trauma patient, significant internal hemorrhage can occur in four defined regions: the thoracic cavity, the peritoneal cavity, the retroperitoneum, and extremity fractures. These areas can be rapidly assessed via chest radiograph, a pelvic radiograph, FAST, and physical examination of extremities along with appropriate radiographs. In-depth coverage of the diagnosis of abdominal trauma is provided in a later chapter of this book. In nontrauma patients without clear evidence of bleeding, the gastrointestinal tract should be rapidly evaluated via nasogastric tube, rectal examination, and endoscopy where appropriate. Additional diagnostic tests can be obtained based on clinical history, patient background, and condition. Abdominal aortic aneurysms can be identified on physical examination, by ultrasound, or by calcifications on abdominal radiograph. In selected instances, angiography may be used to identify and treat sources of hemorrhage not otherwise apparent (pelvic fractures, pancreatitis, lower gastrointestinal bleeding) (225–228,269–277). This should only be instituted when a specific source of hemorrhage is highly likely and therapeutic intervention is sought. Computed tomography should never be sought in hemodynamically unstable patients with hemorrhage.

Laboratory Testing and Monitoring of Resuscitation

Measurement of Bleeding

Hematocrit/Hemoglobin. Hemoglobin and hematocrit measurements have long been part of the basic diagnostic workup of patients with hemorrhage and/or trauma. However, in patients with rapid bleeding, a single hematocrit measurement on presentation to the emergency department may not reflect the degree of hemorrhage. In a short transport or presentation time, prior to initiation of resuscitation, the body's compensatory mechanisms for fluid retention and resorption into the vascular space have not taken place, and initial hematocrit levels may remain stable despite significant blood loss. A retrospective study of 524 trauma patients (278) determined that the initial hematocrit had a sensitivity of only 0.50 for detecting patients with an extent of traumatic hemorrhage requiring surgery. The diagnostic value is further confounded by the administration of intravenous fluids and red cell concentrates during resuscitation (278–281).

Two prospective observational studies determined the sensitivity of serial hematocrit measurements for detecting patients with severe injury (282,283). In the first study (282), the authors compared values of hematocrit at admission and 15 minutes and 30 minutes following arrival to the emergency department. A normal hematocrit on admission did not preclude significant injury. The mean change in hematocrit levels between arrival and 15 minutes, and 15 minutes and 30 minutes was not significantly different in patients with or without serious injuries. However, a decrease of hematocrit by >6.5% at 15 and 30 minutes had a high specificity for injury (0.93–1.0), but a low sensitivity (0.13–0.16).

Another prospective observational study examined the utility of serial hematocrit measurements during the initial 4 hours following admission (283). A significant limitation to this study is that they removed patients who required a blood transfusion in order to eliminate confounding variables. In the remaining 494 patients, a decrease in hematocrit of more than 10% between admission and 4 hours was highly specific for severe injury (0.92–0.96), but again, it was not sensitive (0.09–0.27).

Overall, decreasing hematocrit levels over time may reflect continued bleeding. However, patients with significant bleeding may maintain their hematocrit level, especially in the absence of resuscitation. Conversely, hematocrit levels may also be confounded by aggressive fluid resuscitation early during resuscitation (278–281). An initial hematocrit level will help to identify patients who present with pre-existing anemia who may have a lower threshold for hemorrhage. The hematocrit level should be used in conjunction with other measures of perfusion in order to determine the presence of occult hemorrhage.

Measurements of Perfusion

Lactate. Lactate was initially suggested as a diagnostic parameter and prognostic indicator of hemorrhagic shock in the 1960s (284). Substantial data exist that lactate levels as a marker of tissue oxygen debt can predict outcome in various forms of shock (60,285–288). In 1983, Vincent et al. performed a prospective study on 27 patients with circulatory shock and concluded that changes in lactate concentrations provided an early and objective evaluation of a patient's response to therapy (289). However, its overall utility has been questioned by some because it is felt to be a late marker of tissue hypoperfusion, can be affected by hepatic function, and can be influenced by glycolysis and alkalosis (290–293).

Despite these concerns, data do exist showing that the amount of lactate produced by anaerobic glycolysis is an accurate indirect marker of oxygen debt, tissue hypoperfusion, and the severity of hemorrhagic shock (294–305). In many forms of shock, arterial lactate levels above 2 mEq/L have been associated with increased mortality (286,287,300,305). However, during hemorrhage, not only is the initial lactate level important, but also the rate of clearance (298,299). Two prospective studies confirm this. In one prospective observational study (298), 76 patients with multiple trauma were analyzed with respect to clearance of lactate between survivors and nonsurvivors over 48 hours. If lactate normalized within 24 hours, survival was 100%. Survival decreased to 77.8% if normalization occurred within 48 hours, and to 13.6% in those in whom lactate levels remained elevated above 2 mEq/L for more than 48 hours. This was confirmed in another prospective study of 129 trauma patients (299) in which initial lactate levels were higher in nonsurvivors. A prolonged time to normalization (>24 hours) was associated with the development of posttraumatic organ failure. Finally, venous lactate has been shown to be an excellent approximation for arterial lactate in acute trauma patients and is a useful marker for significant injury (306).

Taken together, these studies suggest that both the initial lactate level and the rate of clearance are reliable indicators of morbidity and mortality following trauma. However, whether lactate should be used as an end point of resuscitation or is merely a marker of tissue ischemia has not been clearly established.

Base Deficit. Base deficit values derived from arterial blood gas analysis have also been shown to provide an indirect estimation of tissue acidosis due to impaired perfusion (294,296,297, 300–303). However, base deficit can be affected by resuscitation fluids (hyperchloremic metabolic acidosis) and exogenous administration of sodium bicarbonate. Despite these potential drawbacks, initial base deficit has been shown in several retrospective studies to correlate with transfusion requirements, organ dysfunction, morbidity, and mortality following trauma (307–313). The magnitude and severity of the base deficit also correlates to outcome, and is useful in both pediatric and elderly patients (307,310–312). Base deficit has been shown to be a better predictor of outcome than pH alone following traumatic injury (309). Recently, serum bicarbonate levels have been shown to be an appropriate surrogate for arterial base deficit in the ICU (314–315).

Lactate versus Base Deficit. Although many studies have shown that both base deficit and serum lactate levels correlate with outcome following trauma and hemorrhage, these two parameters do not always correlate with each other (304,316). In fact, lactate has been found to be a superior predictor of mortality as compared to base deficit in a recent study of patients in the intensive care unit following trauma (304). Both base deficit and lactate have been shown to correlate to outcome in nontraumatic etiologies of hemorrhagic shock (268,317). Given that there are confounding variables following trauma that can affect measured levels of both lactate and base deficit, independent assessment of both parameters along with the patient's clinical condition is recommended for the evaluation of shock in trauma patients.

Measurement of Coagulopathy

Standard Coagulation Studies. Coagulopathy associated with hemorrhagic shock may be due to one of several etiologies: (a) *iatrogenic,* in which a dilutional coagulopathy develops due to inadequate resuscitation with clotting factors and blood products; (b) *premorbid,* in which some patients may have a pre-existing coagulopathy due to underlying disease (such as cirrhosis, hemophilia, von Willebrand, renal failure, etc.); and (c) *acute traumatic coagulopathy,* in which coagulopathy after trauma is common. Traditional teachings have been that this coagulopathy is not inherent, but rather iatrogenic, due to dilution from intravenous fluid therapy, massive blood transfusions, progressive hypothermia, and acidosis. Recent literature has now determined that an inherent acute traumatic coagulopathy is present in up to 30% of patients who present to the emergency department immediately following trauma and is an independent predictor of morbidity and mortality (318–321). Therefore, acute measurement of coagulation parameters during resuscitation from hemorrhagic shock is indicated.

Traditional studies of coagulation include prothrombin time (PT), activated partial thromboplastin time (aPTT), fibrinogen level, and platelet count. Although no tightly controlled trials have been performed, current recommendations for therapeutic end points in hemorrhagic shock include maintaining PT and aPTT at less than 1.5 times the normal value, maintaining a platelet count of >100 in patients with active bleeding or traumatic brain injury, and maintaining a fibrinogen level of >1 g/L (229,322,323) (Table 58.6).

While these laboratory studies are standard, they do present several drawbacks. To begin, *in vivo* coagulation depends on the interaction between platelets and coagulation factor enzymes. Laboratory values of PT and aPTT are performed on platelet-poor plasma and fail to evaluate the cellular interactions of clotting. PT and aPTT measurements also do not take into account hypothermia-induced coagulopathy because samples are warmed prior to measurement. Platelet and fibrinogen assays give numerical values, but fail to assess function. Finally, each of these tests takes time, up to 30 to 45 minutes. This lag time makes these studies clinically inefficient because when the results become available, they may not truly reflect the patient's clinical condition. During resuscitation, actively bleeding patients are in a constant state of flux. Alternative point-of-care testing such as the iSTAT handheld analyzer can provide rapid bedside results, but is currently limited to activated clotting time (ACT) and PT/international normalized ratio (INR) (250). The clinical implications of acute trauma coagulopathy and clinical testing are discussed further later in this chapter.

Thromboelastograph Analyzer. The thromboelastograph (TEG) analyzer is a bedside machine that provides a functional evaluation of overall coagulation on whole blood at the same temperature as the patient. The TEG has been shown to be a more sensitive measure of coagulation disorders than standard coagulation measures (324). The thromboelastograph assay provides a tracing that measures clotting (R value), clot formation (α angle), clot strength (maximum amplitude [MA]), and clot lysis (LY 30) (Fig. 58.5). Elongation of the R value represents a deficiency in coagulation factors. The α angle

TABLE 58.6

TRANSFUSION GUIDELINES FOR PATIENTS WITH COAGULOPATHY AND HEMORRHAGE OR TRAUMATIC INJURY

GOALS **Hematologic/coagulation parameters**	RECOMMENDED THERAPY **Blood products**
Hemoglobin/hematocrit ■ Hgb >7.0 g/dL ■ Hemodynamic stability	Packed red blood cells
Prothrombin time <1.5 times normal	Fresh frozen plasma Prothrombin complex concentrate
Activated partial prothrombin time <1.5 times normal	Fresh frozen plasma
Fibrinogen >100 g/dL	Cryoprecipitate
Platelets $>50 \times 10^9$ per liter (stable, nonbleeding patient)	Platelet transfusion
Platelets $>100 \times 10^9$ per liter (acute, bleeding patient)	

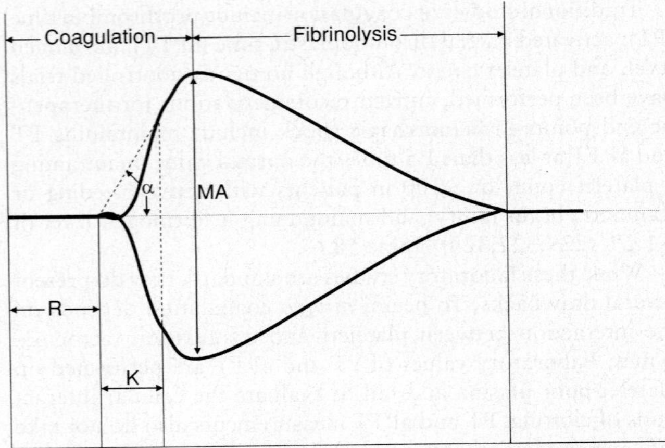

FIGURE 58.5. Thromboelastogram. The thromboelastograph (TEG) analyzer is a bedside machine that provides a functional evaluation of overall coagulation on whole blood at the same temperature as the patient. The thromboelastograph assay provides a tracing that measures time to clot formation (R value), speed to a certain clot strength (K value), rate of clot formation (α angle), overall clot strength (maximum amplitude [MA]) and clot lysis (LY 30).

represents the rate of fibrin accumulation and cross-linking, which can be affected by fibrinogen function and, to a lesser degree, platelet function. The MA is a measure of clot strength and is affected primarily by platelets and, to a lesser degree, fibrinogen. A study investigating the utility of the TEG in trauma patients found that 65% of patients were hypercoagulable and 10% were hypocoagulable. Of the seven hypocoagulable patients, only one had an elevated PT and PTT, but six of seven required blood transfusion (325). Only the Injury Severity Score (ISS) and TEG were predictive of early transfusion.

A large volume of literature exists describing the use of the TEG in various settings including trauma, transplant, and cardiac surgery (250,325–330). However, despite its many advantages, the TEG has not become the standard of care for measurement of coagulopathy. Using the TEG, whole blood samples must be run within 3 to 4 minutes of collection, necessitating the presence of multiple machines in critical areas of the hospital. Quality control of each of these machines is work intensive. Differences due to age, gender, blood collection sites, and sample stability have been raised (331–336). Finally, accurate readings require appropriate processing, and intensive ongoing education of hospital staff would be necessary to ensure accurate results. Although the real-time functional results of routine TEG analysis would be clinically useful, the current processing and maintenance requirements make it impractical for routine use.

RAPID DEFINITIVE CONTROL OF BLEEDING

Multiple studies have confirmed that patients in need of emergency surgery for ongoing hemorrhage have a better survival if the elapsed time to definitive care is minimized (337–347). Those patients with unnecessary delays in diagnosis and definitive treatment will have increased morbidity and mortality (344). Although there are no prospective randomized trials confirming this, multiple retrospective studies provide ample data to confirm the validity of this strategy. In trauma, early surgical control of hemorrhage has been associated with improved survival in penetrating vascular injuries (337), duodenal injuries (338), and polytrauma patients in extremis (339). A multicenter retrospective review of over 500 deaths in the operating room concluded that delayed transfer to the operating room was a cause of death that could be avoided by shortening the time to diagnosis and resuscitation (348). Similar results have been documented in the treatment of patients with ruptured abdominal aortic aneurysms who are hemodynamically unstable (345–347). The benefit for rapid transport time to the operating room is not as dramatic for patients who are hemodynamically stable following ruptured abdominal aortic aneurysm (AAA), implying that ongoing hemorrhage has been arrested in this group of patients.

The development of trauma systems has significantly contributed to improved trauma outcomes by triaging more severely injured patients to hospitals that have systems in place to rapidly diagnose, resuscitate, and definitively treat patients with hemorrhagic shock (340–343). The implementation of trauma systems has resulted in improved outcomes in severely injured patients, decreased time to operating room in hypotensive patients, decreased complications, decreased hospital length of stay, and decreased mortality, especially in patients with severe injury as measured by an ISS of >15 (343). Definitive prompt care is critical to optimize outcomes in patients with trauma and hemorrhage.

LETHAL TRIAD OF RESUSCITATION: HYPOTHERMIA, ACIDOSIS, AND COAGULOPATHY

Patients with severe hemorrhagic shock requiring massive resuscitation are at risk for exhaustion of their physiologic reserves, leading to irreversible shock and the inability to recover despite ongoing resuscitation. The common denominator in these patients is the development of the "lethal triad," "bloody vicious cycle," or "spiral of death"—terms used to describe the combination of profound acidosis, hypothermia, and coagulopathy (Fig. 58.6). Each of these factors has been independently associated with increased risk of death

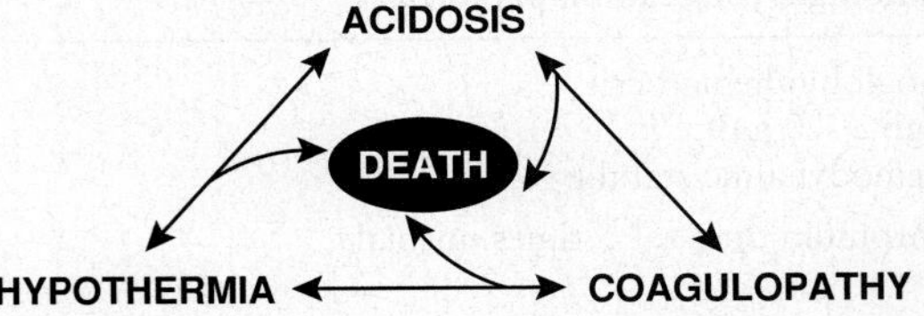

FIGURE 58.6. Lethal triad of hemorrhagic shock. The development of acidosis, hypothermia, and coagulopathy during resuscitation from hemorrhagic shock is described as the "lethal triad," "bloody vicious cycle," or "spiral of death." Each of these factors has been independently associated with mortality. There is a cumulative synergistic effect for each of these variables, such that irreversible shock may develop if all factors are present.

(268,303,319,349–354). There also seems to be a cumulative synergistic effect for each of these risk factors in patients with hemorrhagic shock. In one retrospective study of 39 patients with abdominal packing for surgically uncontrollable bleeding (351), five risk factors for death were identified: pH <7.18, temperature ≤33°C, PT ≥16, PTT ≥50, and transfusion greater than 10 units of blood. Patients with zero to one risk factor had an 18% mortality, two to three risk factors 83% mortality, and four to five risk factors 100% mortality. Similar findings were reported by Cosgriff et al., who identified risk factors for the development of life-threatening coagulopathy (352). Patients with an ISS of >25, pH <7.1, temperature less than 34°C, and systolic blood pressure ≤70 mm Hg had a 98% chance of developing life-threatening coagulopathy, whereas patients with none of these risk factors had a 1% chance of developing coagulopathy.

The development of profound acidosis, hypothermia, and coagulopathy is a lethal combination in patients during the resuscitation from hemorrhagic shock. Resuscitation strategies should be designed at limiting the development of these complications.

Damage Control Laparotomy

Damage control laparotomy (355) is a concept that was initially introduced by Pringle in 1908 when he described the use of hepatic sutures over packs to control bleeding. In 1913, Halsted detailed the procedure and modified its techniques. During World War II, damage control laparotomy fell out of favor and was not reintroduced until 1955 when Madding et al. reported the use of packs to temporize intraoperative bleeding, but felt that they needed to be removed prior to abdominal closure. In the 1970s, Ledgerwood had successful case reports using abdominal packing to control bleeding following trauma. However, the modern era of damage control laparotomy is attributed to Stone et al. who, in 1983, described the techniques of abbreviated laparotomy, packing to control hemorrhage, and deferred definitive surgical repair of injuries until coagulation had been established (356). Since then, a number of authors have described the beneficial effects of damage control laparotomy (357–366). Although retrospective, studies have documented a nearly 50% decrease in operative times for the most severely injured patients treated by this approach and salvage rates of 20% to 60% in patients who would have formerly died in the operating room (351,353,358,367).

The principle of damage control surgery is to obtain rapid control of hemorrhage and contamination, with early completion of the operation, with a goal to restore normal physiology as opposed to normal anatomy (Table 58.7). The ultimate goal is to prevent patients from exhausting their physiologic reserves by developing the "lethal triad of death," or profound hypothermia, acidosis, and coagulopathy. Damage control surgery has three basic components. First, an abbreviated laparotomy for control of bleeding, control of contamination, and restitution of blood flow are necessary. The goal is to achieve these end points as quickly as possible without spending unnecessary time on traditional organ repairs that can be performed at a later time. The abdomen is packed and a temporary abdominal closure is performed (Fig. 58.7). The second component involves treatment in the intensive care unit that is focused on core rewarming, correction of acidosis, and reversal of coagulopathy, as well as optimizing ventilation and

TABLE 58.7

DAMAGE CONTROL LAPAROTOMY AND DAMAGE CONTROL RESUSCITATION

DAMAGE CONTROL LAPAROTOMY

1. **Abbreviated laparotomy (initial procedure)**
   - Control of bleeding
   - Control of contamination
   - Restitution of blood flow
2. **Resuscitation in the intensive care unit (24–48 h)**
   - Core rewarming
   - Correction of acidosis
   - Reversal of coagulopathy
   - Optimization of ventilation and hemodynamics
3. **Definitive surgical repair (days to weeks)**
   - Restoration of continuity
   - Completion of resection
   - Removal of packs
   - Closure of abdomen

DAMAGE CONTROL RESUSCITATION

- ■ Hypotensive resuscitation[a]
- ■ Hemostatic resuscitation

[a]Hypotensive resuscitation is still considered experimental and requires experienced physician oversight and careful patient selection.

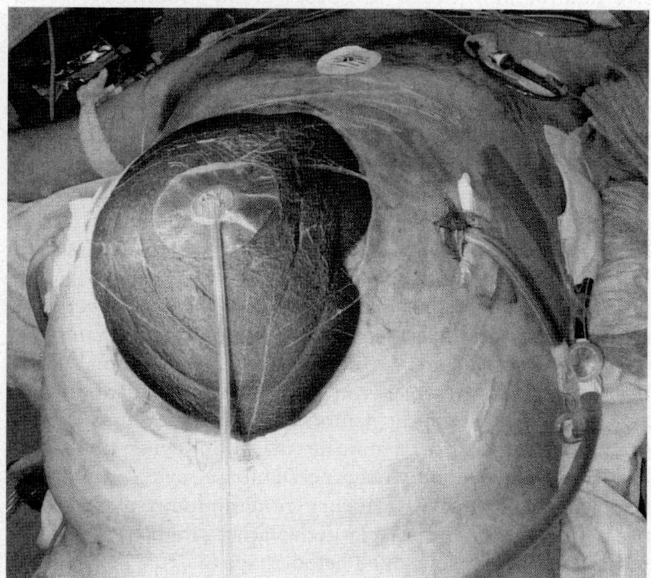

FIGURE 58.7. Open abdomen with temporary abdominal closure. A key component to damage control laparotomy is to perform an abbreviated laparotomy for control of bleeding, control of contamination, and restitution of blood flow. The goal is to achieve these end points as quickly as possible to avoid the development of irreversible shock and the lethal triad of acidosis, hypothermia, and coagulopathy. Frequently, the abdomen is temporarily closed and the fascia left open to prevent the development of abdominal compartment syndrome during resuscitation. Re-exploration usually takes place 24 to 48 hours later, and every few days thereafter until the fascia is closed. Occasionally, the fascia cannot be reapproximated due to loss of domain. In this circumstance, a ventral hernia remains, which can be repaired at a later date (usually 6–12 months postinjury).

hemodynamic status. This phase will typically last for 24 to 48 hours. The third component is definitive surgical repair that is performed only when target parameters have been achieved. This sequence may require several operative interventions to attain definitive repair, each with a goal of preserving the physiologic reserve of the patient.

Damage Control Resuscitation

Damage control resuscitation (DCR) is a term that has recently been coined to describe a specific strategy during the resuscitation phase of trauma care (250,368,369). It should be initiated within minutes of presentation and is meant to preemptively address issues associated with resuscitating critically injured patients: prevention of hypothermia, acidosis, and coagulopathy. Damage control resuscitation involves two components: hypotensive resuscitation and hemostatic resuscitation (Table 58.7).

Hypotensive Resuscitation

Hypotensive resuscitation refers to the concept that fluid should be administered at a rate that returns the systolic blood pressure to a safe but lower than normal pressure until operative control of bleeding can be established. The traditional treatment of hemorrhaging patients has used early and aggressive fluid administration to restore blood volume. However, this approach may increase hydrostatic pressure on the wound or injured vessel, leading to dislodgement of blood clots, a dilution of coagulation factors, and undesirable cooling of the patient. Low-volume fluid resuscitation, or "permissive hypotension," may avoid the adverse effects of early aggressive resuscitation while maintaining a level of tissue perfusion adequate for short periods. This strategy has been suggested historically for the management of ruptured abdominal aortic aneurysm patients (370), and has recently regained attention in the trauma population (263–266,371–375). It has shown promise in animal and human trials (263,265), but has yet to be confirmed in large-scale prospective randomized human clinical trials. Overall, data have been mixed (264). A recent animal trial suggests that increases in blood pressure are well tolerated without exacerbating hemorrhage when they are achieved gradually and with a significant delay following the injury (376). Finally, a recent Cochrane Database review found that there was not conclusive evidence from randomized controlled trials for or against early or larger volumes of intravenous fluid resuscitation in uncontrolled hemorrhage (377).

Although the concept of permissive hypotension seems promising in some circumstances, further work needs to be done. In addition, it requires extraordinarily tight control by an experienced physician who is guiding fluid resuscitation moment to moment. Hypotensive resuscitation should not be considered in patients with traumatic brain injury and spinal cord injury where adequate cerebral perfusion pressure is crucial to ensure tissue oxygenation (229,375). It should also be carefully considered in elderly patients and may be contraindicated in patients with a history of chronic hypertension (229). At the present time, it is considered experimental, and should be employed only in specific circumstances with experienced physicians.

Hemostatic Resuscitation

Conventional resuscitation practice for damage control has focused on rapid reversal of acidosis and prevention of hypothermia. Surgical techniques are aimed at controlling hemorrhage and contamination rapidly, with definitive repair occurring following hemodynamic stabilization. However, direct treatment of coagulopathy early has been relatively neglected, and has been viewed as a byproduct of resuscitation, hemodilution, and hypothermia. Delay in availability of blood products due to current blood banking techniques has also hindered the ability to employ immediate resuscitation with clotting factors.

It has now been demonstrated that *acute traumatic coagulopathy* is present in 25% to 30% of critically injured patients on arrival to the emergency department (318–321). The presence of coagulopathy may be even higher in patients with severe closed head injury, with an incidence of 21% to 79% when stratified by ISS (378). It has also been shown that the presence of early coagulopathy is an independent predictor of mortality following trauma (319). Early acute traumatic coagulopathy appears to be due to alterations in the thrombomodulin–protein C pathway rather than consumption of coagulation factors (321); however, additional work needs to be done to clarify these mechanisms.

Hemostatic resuscitation employs blood components *early* in the resuscitation process to restore both perfusion and normal coagulation function while minimizing crystalloid use. Lactated Ringer solution and normal saline resuscitation have been shown to increase reperfusion injury and leukocyte adhesion (252–256,379). As such, standard crystalloid resuscitation may worsen, presenting acidosis and coagulopathy in severely injured patients. Several retrospective studies in trauma have shown that survival is associated with an increased use of clotting factors (352,367). Many other studies have recommended more aggressive use of clotting factors to treat and correct underlying coagulopathy (380–388).

Although additional prospective studies need to be completed, there seems to be increased literature supporting early aggressive resuscitation with clotting factors while minimizing crystalloid use during massive resuscitation. Current military experience has moved to using thawed plasma as the primary resuscitation fluid in at least a 1:1 or 1:2 ratio with packed red blood cells (368,387–389). Continued resuscitation occurs with a massive transfusion protocol at a ratio of 6 units of plasma, 6 units of packed red blood cells, 6 units of platelets, and 10 units of cryoprecipitate. Recombinant factor VIIa is occasionally used along with early red cell transfusion to promote early hemostasis (368,389).

Massive Transfusion

Definition

In the 1970s, *massive transfusion* was defined as greater than 10 units of blood transfused in a 24-hour period of time, and survival rates were dismal (6.6%) (390). Over the last two decades, however, survival rates have improved, and the criteria to define massive transfusion have evolved (367,383,384,391–396). Recent reports use variable end points, increasing the number of transfusions to greater than 20 units in 24 hours (383) or defining transfusions during the entire hospital stay

TABLE 58.8

SURVIVAL FOLLOWING MASSIVE TRANSFUSION

Study/year	No. of patients	Transfusion volume (avg. units)	Overall survival (%)
Wilson et al., 1971 (390)	45	>25	7
Phillips et al., 1987 (383)	56	35	39
Kivioja et al., 1991 (391)	29	56	38
Wudel et al., 1991 (392)	92	33	52
Harvey et al., 1995 (384)	43	19	60
Velmahos et al., 1998 (393)	141	31	31
Cinat et al., 1999 (367)	46	63	45
Hakala et al., 1999 (394)	23	79	69
Vaslef et al., 2002 (395)	44	75	43
Huber-Wagner et al., 2007 (396)	148	41	40

(392). Most recently, investigators have reported outcomes on patients receiving over 50 units of blood in 48 hours (367).

Survival

As technology and blood banking procedures have improved, patient outcomes following massive transfusion have also improved (397). Although early survival rates were dismal, recent reviews report survival rates as high as 60% in patients requiring over 50 units of blood in the early resuscitation period (Table 58.8). Moreover, many of these patients can ultimately return to work (75% of survivors), and survival in elderly patients has also been reported in several studies (367,392,394,395). This dramatic improvement in survival over the past several decades can be attributed to many factors including an improved understanding of the consequences of massive resuscitation (268,349,352), improved technology for massive resuscitation (i.e., rapid transfusion with warmed fluids) (267), increased use of damage control techniques (353,367), improved trauma systems (343), improved transfusion practices during resuscitation (367), and improved blood banking techniques (367). Based on these results, massive transfusion in trauma patients receiving over 50 units of blood in the acute period following injury is justified, with acceptable survival and functional capacity following discharge (367,383,384,391–397).

Transfusion Protocols

Historically, massive transfusion protocols have been developed to assist clinicians in the resuscitation of hemorrhaging patients. However, a recent review of massive transfusion protocols globally revealed wide variation in practice (389). Most protocols recommend empiric strategies of 1 unit of fresh frozen plasma (FFP) for every 4 to 10 units of packed red blood cells (PRBCs) and 1 plateletpheresis for every 10 to 20 units of PRBCs (380). Organizational guidelines recommended transfusing to laboratory end points (322). However, recent literature suggests that a more aggressive approach is warranted (368,380,387,388). During ongoing hemorrhage, the clinical situation of the patient changes too rapidly to depend on laboratory values sent 20 to 45 minutes prior. Thus, empiric strategies to correct or avoid coagulopathy need to be employed. These strategies need to be modified for two clinical conditions: (a) ongoing hemorrhage and (b) coagulopathy following hemorrhage control.

Resuscitation during Ongoing Hemorrhage. Recent data have established that a significant number of patients have an acute traumatic coagulopathy on presentation to the emergency department immediately following injury. Moreover, it appears that traditional strategies for resuscitation have been inadequate and unable to reverse this coagulopathy early following trauma (387). Several retrospective clinical studies suggest that aggressive early transfusion of clotting factors (fresh frozen plasma, platelets, and cryoprecipitate) is associated with increased survival (352,367,380,385,388).

Randomized prospective controlled trials evaluating therapy for massive hemorrhage are challenging. However, recently two studies utilizing computer modeling have suggested that more aggressive resuscitation is necessary to correct coagulopathy. In the first study, the optimal replacement ratios were 2:3 of FFP to PRBCs and 8:10 of platelets to PRBCs (398). Interestingly, a second computer model found similar results, suggesting a transfusion rate of 1:1 for FFP per unit of blood transfused if there is no pre-existing coagulopathy, and a ratio of 1.5 units of FFP per unit of PRBCs if coagulopathy exists on presentation (399). Moreover, both of these mathematical models underestimate the potential need for clotting factor replacement because only dilutional coagulopathy is taken into account; there is no assessment for the relative contributions of consumption, acidosis, and hypothermia, which are frequently seen in the acute trauma patient.

Based on these data, old transfusion strategies appear to be fundamentally flawed in the acutely hemorrhaging patient. Current recommendations suggest that, in patients with ongoing hemorrhage, empiric transfusion should occur in the ratio of 1:1:1 (1 unit of fresh frozen plasma to 1 unit of packed red blood cells to 1 unit of platelets) (Table 58.9) (368,380,387,388). Since platelets are usually supplied pooled as 6 to 10 units or as a plateletpheresis, which is equivalent to 6 to 10 units, patients should receive a platelet transfusion for every 6 to 10 units of PRBCs. When blood products are available, crystalloids should be avoided in the acutely hemorrhaging patients as they can worsen coagulopathy.

It is important to note that while this is the recommended transfusion protocol for patients with traumatic injury and hemorrhage, it is unclear if the same blood products and clotting factors are necessary in nontrauma patients with acute hemorrhage (i.e., intra-operative, gastrointestinal, ruptured aneurysm) (322,400–403). In blood loss during elective

TABLE 58.9

RECOMMENDED EMPIRIC MASSIVE TRANSFUSION PROTOCOL FOR ACUTE ONGOING HEMORRHAGE

CURRENT SUGGESTED PROTOCOL FOR TRAUMATIC HEMORRHAGE
- 6 units packed red blood cells
- 6 units of fresh frozen plasma
- 1 plateletpheresis (or 6–10 units of platelets)
- Cryoprecipitate as indicated

TRADITIONAL PROTOCOL–INADEQUATE FOR TRAUMA
- 10–20 units packed red blood cells
- 1–4 units fresh frozen plasma
- 1 plateletpheresis
- Cryoprecipitate as indicated

surgery, the situation is more controlled and resuscitation can be initiated immediately. A premorbid coagulopathy may or may not exist. Goals in resuscitation in this circumstance are similar: maintain adequate tissue perfusion to avoid acidosis, correct coagulopathy, and prevent hypothermia.

Resuscitation Once Hemorrhage Is Controlled. Once hemorrhage is controlled, goal-directed transfusion can be pursued based on laboratory data and clinical variables. Many clinicians will work to achieve normal coagulation parameters for 24 hours post injury and control of hemorrhage (PT INR <1.5, platelet count >100 × 10^9 per liter) (387). In a patient who no longer shows evidence of medical or surgical bleeding, traditional guidelines for transfusion therapy can be employed (322). These include using red blood cell transfusion for symptomatic anemia or a hemoglobin concentration of less than 7 g/dL; FFP or prothrombin complex concentrate for a prothrombin time >1.5 times normal; fresh frozen plasma for an activated partial thromboplastin time >1.5 times normal; cryoprecipitate for a fibrinogen level <80 to 100 mg/dL; and platelet transfusion for a platelet count <50 × 10^9 per liter (Table 58.6).

Complications of Massive Transfusion. Despite acceptable survival rates, there are several known complications to massive transfusion (Tables 58.10 and 58.11) (397,404–409). Physicians caring for patients who require massive transfusion must anticipate, identify, and rapidly treat these potential complications in order to optimize outcome.

Disordered hemostasis following massive transfusion is a known complication of massive blood transfusion (397,400,401). Stored blood is lacking in factors V and VIII. These factors degrade over time in stored blood, and thus become deficient in the massively transfused patient. This can contribute to the coagulopathy seen following massive transfusion. Dilutional thrombocytopenia also occurs during massive transfusion, and is more common after 1.5 times the normal blood volume is transfused. However, thrombocytopenia can occur earlier, especially if there is disseminated intravascular coagulation, pre-existing thrombocytopenia, or a consumptive coagulopathy. As discussed previously, resuscitation of hemorrhagic shock must include clotting factors and platelets to avoid ongoing coagulopathy.

TABLE 58.10

NONINFECTIOUS TRANSFUSION-ASSOCIATED COMPLICATIONS

ACUTE (WITHIN 24 H OF TRANSFUSION)
Hemolytic reactions
Febrile nonhemolytic reactions
Allergic reactions
Transfusion-related acute lung injury (TRALI)
Hypothermia
Hypocalcemia
Hypo- or hyperkalemia
Acid-base derangements

DELAYED (MORE THAN 24 H AFTER TRANSFUSION)
Alloimmunization
Immunosuppression
Posttransfusion purpura
Graft vs. host disease
Multiple organ dysfunction syndrome

Oxygen delivery to tissues is also affected by blood transfusion. Transfused blood tends to have a higher affinity for oxygen, thus leading to decreased oxygen delivery to tissues. Longer storage periods for blood lead to a reduction in red cell deformability, altered red cell adhesiveness, and other red cell storage lesions. These changes reduce red blood cell viability after transfusion, reduce tissue oxygen availability, and promote the inflammatory response, specifically neutrophil priming and pulmonary endothelial cell activation.

Systemic inflammation and potential tissue injury may also be induced by the transfusion of aged blood. Transfusion of aged blood (>14 days of storage) in the first 6 hours of resuscitation has been shown to be an independent risk factor for postinjury multiorgan failure (410) and is associated with

TABLE 58.11

INFECTIOUS TRANSFUSION-ASSOCIATED COMPLICATIONS

Type of infectious complication	Incidence per all transfused components
Bacterial contamination (PRBCs + platelets)	1 per 2,000
Hepatitis B transmission	1 per 205,000
PRBC-related bacterial sepsis	1 per 500,000–786,000
Hepatitis A transmission	1 per 1,000,000
Hepatitis C transmission	1 per 1,600,000
HIV transmission	1 per 2,135,000

PRBC, packed red blood cell; HIV, human immunodeficiency virus. Adapted with data from Silliman CC, Moore EE, Johnson JL, et al. Transfusion of the injured patient: proceed with caution. *Shock.* 2004;21(4):291; McIntyre LA, Hebert PC. Can we safely restrict transfusion in trauma patients? *Curr Opin Crit Care.* 2006;12:575; Dodd RY, Notari EP, Stramer SL. Current prevalence and incidence of infectious disease markers and estimated window-period risk in the American Red Cross donor population. *Transfusion.* 2002;42:975; and Kleinman S, Chan P, Robillard P. Risks associated with transfusion of cellular blood components in Canada. *Transfus Med Rev.* 2003;17:120.

delayed apoptosis of neutrophils (411), increased infection rates (412), and a longer ICU stay (413). This may be particularly significant in large trauma centers and transplantation centers where older blood is preferentially distributed because of their high-volume use.

Alloimmunization can occur when an immunocompetent host develops an immune response to donor antigens. The antigens most often involved include the human leukocyte antigen (HLA) class I and II on platelets and leukocytes, granulocyte-specific antigens, platelet-specific antigens, and red blood cell–specific antigens. Consequences of alloimmunization include a refractory response to platelet transfusion, posttransfusion purpura, neonatal alloimmune thrombocytopenia, acute intravascular hemolytic transfusion reaction, hemolytic disease in newborns, and febrile nonhemolytic reactions against granulocytes. Clinical manifestations can be minor, such as fever, leading to active bleeding and hemolysis, which can be fatal. Workup and treatment vary, depending on the severity of the reaction (414,415).

Metabolic and electrolyte disturbances can also occur following massive transfusion (397). Citrate toxicity can occur in patients with abnormal liver function or in whom the administration of blood is very rapid. The healthy adult liver will metabolize 3 g of citrate every 5 minutes. Each unit of blood contains approximately 3 g of citrate. Therefore, transfusion rates higher than 1 unit every 5 minutes can exceed the liver's capacity to handle this overload. Citrate then binds to calcium and can lead to clinical hypocalcemia. Patients may exhibit temporary tetany and hypotension. Calcium replacement should occur concurrently during massive transfusion.

Electrolyte disturbances such as hyperkalemia or hypokalemia can occur with massive transfusion. The longer the shelf life, the higher the potassium concentration; sometimes concentrations may even exceed 30 mmol/L. Unless very large amounts of blood are transfused, hyperkalemia is generally not a problem. On the other hand, as red cells begin active metabolism, intracellular uptake of potassium begins, and hypokalemia may result.

Acid-base disturbances can also occur with massive blood transfusions. Stored blood contains lactate at levels up to 30 to 40 mmol/L. In addition, citric acid is present and may be metabolized to bicarbonate, resulting in severe metabolic alkalosis. Conversely, the patient's overall condition and tissue hypoperfusion may actually lead to metabolic acidosis.

Although rare, blood transfusion can also result in the induction of acquired inhibitors of coagulation. The most common antibodies are directed against coagulation factor VIII. This can result in massive bleeding, which is difficult and costly to treat. The main goals of treatment are to stop hemorrhage and remove the inhibitor. Factor VIII concentrate is used only for life-threatening circumstances. Successful elimination of the anti-VIII antibody has been accomplished with the use of oral immunosuppressants such as cyclophosphamide and prednisone (416).

Transfusion-related acute lung injury. TRALI is a devastating complication of transfusion that consists of a syndrome that includes dyspnea, hypotension, bilateral pulmonary edema, and fever. Its incidence is reported to be between 0.04% and 0.06% (or approximately 1 in 2,000). Clinically, it resembles acute respiratory distress syndrome. Criteria for the diagnosis of TRALI include:

- Acute lung injury (ALI) as defined by acute onset, hypoxemia (PaO_2:FiO_2 ratio ≤300), bilateral infiltrates on frontal chest radiograph, and no evidence of left atrial hypertension or circulatory overload
- No pre-existing ALI before transfusion
- Occurs during or within 6 hours of transfusion
- No temporal relationship to an alternative risk factor for ALI (i.e., burns, aspiration, multiple trauma, cardiopulmonary bypass, sepsis, etc.)

If an additional risk factor exists, then possible TRALI is diagnosed (Table 58.12) (417–420).

The pathogenesis can be either immune (antibody) mediated or nonimmune mediated (Table 58.13) (418–422). *Immune-mediated TRALI* is most common and is due to the presence of leukocyte antibodies in the donor transfusion (421,422). These antibodies form immune complexes that are deposited in the pulmonary vascular bed, leading to release of vasoactive substances, leakage of fluid into alveolar spaces, activation of complement, leukostasis, and activation of polymorphonuclear neutrophils. Immune-mediated TRALI occurs more commonly with fresh frozen plasma than with platelet concentrates, is associated with multiparous female donors (423), can occur in healthy recipients, and is usually severe, requiring mechanical ventilation in 70% of individuals. *Non–immune-mediated TRALI* is thought to be due to the presence of biologically active lipids in the donor transfusion (418–420). It occurs with stored platelet concentrates more commonly than stored red cells, occurs predominantly in critically ill patients with a primed immune system, and is usually mild and transient, requiring only supplemental oxygen support. Treatment of TRALI is generally supportive and includes ventilatory and hemodynamic assistance. There are no data to support the use of corticosteroids, and additional blood component therapy should be given only if transfusion needs exist. The diagnosis of TRALI in the patients requiring massive transfusion is

TABLE 58.12

CRITERIA FOR TRANSFUSION-RELATED ACUTE LUNG INJURY (TRALI)

CRITERIA FOR TRALI

- Acute lung injury (ALI)
  - Acute onset
  - Hypoxemia
    - PaO_2:FiO_2 ratio ≤300
    - SpO_2 <90% on room air
- No pre-existing ALI before transfusion
- Occurs during or within 6 h of transfusion
- No temporal relationship to an alternative risk factor for ALI

CRITERIA FOR POSSIBLE TRALI

- ALI
- No pre-existing ALI before transfusion
- Occurs during or within 6 h of transfusion
- A clear temporal relationship to an alternative risk factor for ALI

Adapted from Kleinman S, Caulfield T, Chan P, et al. Toward an understanding of transfusion-related acute lung injury: statement of a consensus panel. *Transfusion.* 2004;44:1774.

TABLE 58.13

CHARACTERISTICS OF IMMUNE AND NONIMMUNE TRANSFUSION-RELATED ACUTE LUNG INJURY (TRALI)

	Immune TRALI	Nonimmune TRALI
Trigger	Leukocyte antibodies	Biologically active lipids
Blood components implicated	Fresh frozen plasma > platelet concentrates	Stored platelet concentrates > stored red blood cells
Host	Healthy or critically ill	Predominantly in critically ill
Clinical course	Severe, often life threatening Mechanical ventilation	Mild, self-limiting Supplemental oxygen

Adapted from Bux J. Transfusion-related acute lung injury (TRALI): a serious adverse event of blood transfusion. *Vox Sang.* 2005;89:1.

difficult because of the many other etiologies also present that can lead to acute lung injury (424,425).

RECOMBINANT FACTOR VIIA IN MASSIVE TRANSFUSION AND HEMORRHAGE

New developments in transfusion therapy include the discovery and use of recombinant coagulation factor VIIa (rFVIIa). Recombinant factor VIIa is a synthesized analog of human factor VII that has been used effectively in the treatment of patients with hemophilia as well as other congenital and acquired coagulopathies. Recently, there have been reports of the successful use of rFVIIa in treating coagulopathic trauma patients (426). In this study, patients with active hemorrhage and clinical coagulopathy from diverse causes such as traumatic hemorrhage, traumatic brain injury, warfarin use, congenital factor VII deficiency, and other acquired hematologic defects were administered rFVIIa as a last resort. Coagulopathy was reversed in 75% of patients, with an associated decrease in prothrombin time. Forty-two percent of patients survived to discharge.

Recently, two randomized, prospective, placebo-controlled, double-blind clinical trials were conducted simultaneously to evaluate the efficacy and safety of recombinant factor VIIa as adjunctive therapy for the control of bleeding in patients with severe blunt ($N = 143$) or penetrating ($N = 134$) trauma (427). In blunt trauma, the red blood cell transfusion requirement was significantly reduced by 2.6 units ($p = 0.02$) and the need for massive transfusion (>20 units of packed red blood cells) was reduced (14% vs. 33%, $p = 0.03$). In patients with penetrating trauma, the trends were similar, but not significant (reduction in red cell transfusion 1.0 unit, $p = 0.10$; massive transfusion 7% vs. 19%, $p = 0.08$). Trends toward reduction in mortality and critical complications were also observed. A subgroup analysis from this trial found particular benefit in those patients who were coagulopathic on presentation to the emergency department, with a significant decrease in transfusion of packed red blood cells, fresh frozen plasma, platelets, and need for massive transfusion. In addition, treatment with rFVIIa was also associated with a significant reduction in multiorgan failure and/or acute respiratory distress syndrome (3% vs. 20%, $p = 0.004$), without an increase in thromboembolic events (428).

Recombinant factor VIIa, however, must be used responsibly. Recent studies have shown that early administration following trauma is more effective than late administration (429,430). Furthermore, the presence of profound acidosis, coagulopathy, and signs of irreversible hemorrhagic shock predict failure of rFVIIa therapy (431). Current recommendations suggest that optimal preconditions should be present prior to administration of rFVIIa, which include a fibrinogen concentration of >50 mg/dL, a platelet count of $>50 \times 10^9$ per liter, and a pH ≥ 7.2 (432,433). Although early results in traumatic hemorrhage appear promising, rFVIIa should still be considered experimental and further investigation is warranted. Recombinant factor VIIa has shown promise for perioperative bleeding during liver transplantation (434) and in patients undergoing cardiac surgery (435,436). Investigations for its utility in perioperative bleeding for other surgical procedures have been mixed (437–442).

A prospective randomized trial investigating the use of rFVIIa in patients with cirrhosis and upper gastrointestinal bleeding who were treated with standard endoscopic therapy and pharmacologic interventions showed that the administration of rFVIIa was not more effective than placebo with respect to the primary end point of failure to control bleeding within 24 hours and failure to prevent rebleeding or death within 5 days (443). However, subgroup analysis of patients with more severe cirrhosis showed that rFVIIa showed a reduction in the composite primary end point (8% vs. 23%, $p = 0.03$). None of the rFVIIa patients had rebleeding within the first 24 hours, whereas rebleeding occurred in 11% of the placebo group ($p = 0.01$) (443).

As with any hemostatic agent, there are concerns over the potential thrombogenicity of rFVIIa (444). Although preliminary evidence shows a favorable safety profile (445,446), thrombogenic effects are being followed closely in ongoing clinical trials.

PREVENTION OF HEMORRHAGIC SHOCK

Antifibrinolytic Therapy

Antifibrinolytic therapy has been shown to significantly reduce the risk of bleeding following cardiac surgery in several randomized controlled trials. Aprotinin has been studied most extensively (447–451), followed by tranexamic acid, then aminocaproic acid. However, recent information raises concern for the risk of renal failure following use of aprotinin with cardiac surgery (448,449) and a potential for increased mortality at 5 years following use of aprotinin (450). Although clearly the risk of postoperative bleeding following cardiac surgery is reduced, further investigation into these potential side effects is warranted.

A recent systematic review of randomized controlled trials of antifibrinolytic agents (mainly aprotinin or tranexamic acid) in elective surgical procedures identified 89 trials including 8,580 randomized patients (74 cardiac, eight orthopedic, four liver, three vascular). Results demonstrated that these treatments reduced the number of patients needing transfusion by one third, reduced the volume needed per patient by 1 unit, and halved the need for further surgery to control bleeding. These differences were all statistically significant. There was also a trend toward a reduction in the risk of death (risk ratio = 0.85; 95% confidence interval, 0.63–1.14), although this was not statistically significant (452).

To date, there are limited data on the use of antifibrinolytic agents in other clinical scenarios (453). However, at this time, the CRASH-2 trial (Clinical Randomization of an Anti-fibrinolytic in Significant Hemorrhage) is ongoing in Europe and is designed to evaluate the utility of antifibrinolytic agents in the management of acute traumatic injury (454).

Experimental Therapy

Red Cell Substitutes

Although the blood supply in the United States is safe and currently has sufficient capacity to meet most patient needs, there is room for considerable improvement. The current system is dependent on blood donors on a regular basis, and the blood supply is subject to seasonal shortages due to holidays and convenience. The gap between the donor pool and the increasing transfusion requirements of an aging population is narrowing, and shortages are becoming more frequent. The risk of transmission of known infectious diseases still exists (Table 58.11), while the threat of new and emerging infections such as West Nile virus and Creutzfeldt-Jakob disease underscore the risk of a tainted blood supply (455).

The ideal red cell substitute should have several characteristics including an ability to deliver (and potentially enhance) oxygen delivery, no risk of disease transmission, no immunosuppressive effects, available in abundant supply, universally compatible, prolonged shelf life, similar *in vivo* half-life to the red blood cell, available at a reasonable cost, easy to administer, able to access all areas of the human body (including ischemic tissues), and effective at room air or ambient conditions (455–457). There have been many attempts to develop red cell substitutes since 1934 when Amberson first reported the successful use of a bovine hemolysate for exchange transfusions in cats and dogs (455). However, this work could not be replicated.

The two main types of oxygen carriers that are used as red blood cell substitutes are hemoglobin-based oxygen carriers (HBOCs) and perfluorocarbons (PFCs). Based on previous clinical trials, many obstacles still need to be overcome. Adverse effects associated with HBOCs include (a) severe vasoconstriction due to binding of nitric oxide and dysregulation of endothelin; (b) nephrotoxicity; (c) interference of macrophage function; (d) antigenicity; (e) oxidation on storage; (f) activation of complement, kinin, and coagulation; (g) iron deposition with concerns of hemochromatosis and iron overload; (h) gastrointestinal distress; (i) neurotoxicity; (j) free radical generation; and (k) interference with diagnosis of transfusion reaction. Adverse effects of PFCs include (a) limited shelf life, (b) flulike symptoms during infusion, (d) complement and phagocytic activation, and (d) short circulation time (456).

Despite much research, no product to date has been able to fulfill all of the previously mentioned criteria or meet the U.S. Food and Drug Administration's requirements of purity, potency, and safety. At the time of this publication, three HBOC products continue in advanced clinical trials (455).

Hypertonic Saline

Hypertonic saline (7.5% saline ± 6% dextan-70) has been investigated as an alternative resuscitation strategy in critically injured patients (458–464). Hypertonic resuscitation evokes an increase in serum osmolarity, which results in the redistribution of fluid from the interstitial and intracellular space to the intravascular space. This leads to a rapid restoration of circulating intravascular volume with a small amount resuscitation fluid. Hypertonic saline has also been shown to decrease intracranial pressure via its osmotic effects (125,126). This is particularly beneficial in patients with hypovolemic shock and closed head injury due to the ability of hypertonic saline resuscitation to concurrently restore circulating blood volume, improve tissue (including cerebral) perfusion, and lower intracranial pressure (126,465–466).

Hypertonic saline resuscitation has also been shown to have significant immunomodulatory effects that could mitigate the dysfunctional inflammatory response seen after traumatic injury (108,109,111,150,253,467–472). The hypertonicity associated with hypertonic saline resuscitation is associated with significant effects on the innate and adaptive immune systems. There is suppression of the neutrophil oxidative burst, potentially leading to an attenuation of inflammatory organ injury (150,473).

Several clinical trials and meta-analyses have suggested improved outcome in patients resuscitated with hypertonic saline (474–477). Despite these results, hypertonic saline resuscitation has not gained widespread acceptance in North America. However, in 1999, the U.S. Navy, through the Office of Naval Research, requested that the Institute of Medicine (IOM) recommend that hypertonic saline be used as the initial resuscitation fluid for combat casualty (256,478). The rapid restoration of intravascular volume and possible immunomodulatory effects associated with hypertonic saline resuscitation make it an attractive alternative for the resuscitation of severe hemorrhagic shock. However, it is still considered experimental and prospective randomized trials are needed to confirm its utility.

SUMMARY

Hemorrhagic shock is a common, yet complicated, clinical condition that physicians are frequently called upon to evaluate and treat. Diagnosis must be accurate and expedient. Therapy must be direct, efficient, and multifactorial in order to avoid the potential multisystem sequelae. Metabolism and function of all organs are altered during hemorrhagic shock. A better understanding of the pathophysiology of hemorrhagic shock has led to improved resuscitation techniques and improved survival over recent years. Damage control laparotomy and damage control resuscitation have changed the approach to management in patients with multisystem trauma and hemorrhagic shock. Staged resuscitation and operative intervention to avoid irreversible shock are now the mainstays of care. Recognition of acute traumatic coagulopathy has improved the composition of massive transfusion protocols to include increased use of clotting factors early during resuscitation. New experimental therapies for resuscitation are being evaluated and appear promising. Overall, survival following hemorrhagic shock has improved. Early diagnosis, definitive cessation of bleeding, and comprehensive hemostatic resuscitation are the key elements to successful outcome.

References

1. Weil MH, Shubin H. Proposed reclassification of shock states with special reference to distributive effects. In: Hinshaw LB, Cox BG, eds. *The Fundamental Mechanisms of Shock*. New York: Plenum Press; 1972:13.
2. Hamilton-Davies C, Mythen MG, Salmon JB, et al. Comparison of commonly used clinical indicators of hypovolaemia with gastrointestinal tonometry. *Intens Care Med*. 1997;23(3):276.
3. Bond RF, Johnson G III. Vascular adrenergic interactions during hemorrhagic shock. *Fed Proc*. 1985;44:281.
4. Schadt JC, Ludbrook J. Hemodynamic and neurohumoral responses to acute hypovolemia in conscious mammals. *Am J Physiol*. 1991;260:H305.
5. Koyama S, Sawano F, Matsuda Y, et al. Spatial and temporal differing control of sympathetic activities during hemorrhage. *Am J Physiol*. 1992;262:R579.
6. Wisbach G, Tobias S, Woodman R, et al. Preserving cardiac output with beta-adrenergic receptor blockade and inhibiting the Bezold-Jarisch reflex during resuscitation from hemorrhage. *J Trauma*. 2007;63(1):26.
7. Victorino GP, Battistella FD, Wisner DH. Does tachycardia correlate with hypotension after trauma? *J Am Coll Surg*. 2003;196(5):679.
8. Demetriades D, Chan LS, Bhasin P, et al. Relative bradycardia in patients with traumatic hypotension. *J Trauma*. 1998;45:534.
9. Sander-Jensen K, Secher NH, Bie P, et al. Vagal slowing of the heart during hemorrhage: observations from 20 consecutive hypotensive patients. *Br J Med*. 1986;292:364.
10. Vincent JL, Moraine JJ, Van der Linden P. Toe temperature versus transcutaneous oxygen tension monitoring during acute circulatory failure. *Intensive Care Med*. 1988;14:64.
11. Van Leeuwen AF, Evans RG, Ludbrook J. Haemodynamic responses to acute blood loss: new roles for the heart, brain, and endogenous opioids. *Anaesth Intensive Care*. 1989;17(3):312.
12. Ludbrook J, Ventura S. Roles of carotid baroreceptor and cardiac afferents in hemodynamic responses to acute central hypovolemia. *Am J Physiol*. 1996;270(5 Part 2):H1538.
13. Wong DH, O'Connor D, Tremper KK, et al. Changes in cardiac output after acute blood loss and position change in man. *Crit Care Med*. 1989;17(10):979.
14. Bressack MA, Raffin TA. Importance of venous return, venous resistance, and mean circulatory pressure in the physiology and management of shock. *Chest*. 1987;92:906.
15. Shen YT, Knight DR, Thomas JX Jr, et al. Relative roles of cardiac receptors and arterial baroreceptors during hemorrhage in conscious dogs. *Circ Res*. 1990;66(2):397.
16. Westphal G, Garrido Adel P, de Almeida DP, et al. Pulse pressure respiratory variation as an early marker of cardiac output fall in experimental hemorrhagic shock. *Artif Organs*. 2007;31(4):284.
17. Magder S, Lagonidis D, Erice F. The use of respiratory variations in right atrial pressure to predict the cardiac output response to PEEP. *J Crit Care*. 2001;16(3):108–114.
18. Rooke GA, Schwid HA, Shapira Y. The effect of graded hemorrhage and intravascular volume replacement on systolic pressure variation in humans during mechanical and spontaneous ventilation. *Anesth Analg*. 1995;80(5):925.
19. Zweifach BW, Fronek A. The interplay of central and peripheral factors in irreversible hemorrhagic shock. *Prog Cardiovasc Dis*. 1975;18(2):147.
20. Schwartz S, Frantz RA, Shoemaker WC. Sequential hemodynamic and oxygen transport responses in hypovolemia, anemia, and hypoxia. *Am J Physiol*. 1981;241(6):H864.
21. Alyono D, Ring WS, Chao RY, et al. Characteristics of ventricular function in severe hemorrhagic shock. *Surgery*. 1983;94(2):250.
22. Sarnoff SJ, Case RB, Waithe PE, et al. Insufficient coronary flow and myocardial failure as a complication factor in late hemorrhagic shock. *Am J Physiol*. 1954;176(3):439.
23. Rush BF Jr. Irreversibility in the post-transfusion phase of hemorrhagic shock. *Adv Exp Med Biol*. 1971;23:215.
24. Secher NH, Sander-Jensen K, Werner C, et al. Bradycardia during severe but reversible hypovolemic shock in man. *Circ Shock*. 1984;14:267.
25. Thiemermann C, Szabo C, Mitchell JA, et al. Vascular hyporeactivity to vasoconstrictor agents and hemodynamic decompensation in hemorrhagic shock is medicated by nitric oxide. *Proc Natl Acad Sci*. 1993;90:267.
26. Vatner SF. Effects of hemorrhage on regional blood flow distribution in dogs and primates. *J Clin Invest*. 1974;54:225.
27. Shoemaker WC. Relation of oxygen transport patterns to the pathophysiology and therapy of shock states. *Intensive Care Med*. 1987;13(4):230.
28. Aubier M, Viires N, Syllie G, et al. Respiratory muscle contribution to lactic acidosis in low cardiac output. *Am Rev Respir Dis*. 1982;126(4):648.
29. Revelly JP, Gardaz JP, Nussberger J, et al. Effect of epinephrine on oxygen consumption and delivery during progressive hemorrhage. *Crit Care Med*. 1995;23(7):1272.
30. Hannon JP, Wade CE, Bossone CA, et al. Oxygen delivery and demand in conscious pigs subjected to fixed-volume hemorrhage and resuscitated with 7.5% NaCl in 6% Dextran. *Circ Shock*. 1989;29(3):205.
31. Edouard AR, Degremont AC, Duranteau J, et al. Heterogeneous regional vascular responses to simulated transient hypovolemia in man. *Intensive Care Med*. 1994;20(6):414.
32. Groeneveld AB, Kolkman JJ. Splanchnic tonometry: a review of physiology, methodology, and clinical implications. *J Crit Care*. 1994;9(3):198.
33. Kirton OC, Windsor J, Wedderburn R, et al. Failure of splanchnic resuscitation in the acutely injury trauma patient correlates with multiple organ failure and length of stay in the ICU. *Chest*. 1998;113:1064.
34. Riggs TE, Shafer AW, Guenter CA. Acute changes in oxyhemoglobin affinity: effects on oxygen transport and utilization. *J Clin Invest*. 1973;52:2660.
35. Malmberg PO, Hlastala MP, Woodson RD. Effect of increased blood-oxygen affinity on oxygen transport in hemorrhagic shock. *J Appl Physiol*. 1979;47(4):889.
36. Woodson RD. Physiologic significance of oxygen dissociation curve shifts. *Crit Care Med*. 1979;7(9):368.
37. Woodson RD. Functional consequences of altered blood oxygen affinity. *Acta Biol Med Ger*. 1981;40:733.
38. Myburgh JA, Webb RK, Worthley LI. The P50 is reduced in critically ill patients. *Intensive Care Med*. 1991;17(6):355.
39. Herman CM, Rodkey FL, Valeri CR, et al. Changes in the oxyhemoglobin dissociation curve and peripheral blood after acute red cell mass depletion and subsequent red cell mass restoration in baboons. *Ann Surg*. 1971;174:734.
40. Sauaia A, Moore FA, Moore EE, et al. Early predictors of postinjury multiple organ failure. *Arch Surg*. 1994;129(1):39.
41. Shoemaker WC, Appel PL, Kram HB. Role of oxygen debt in the development of organ failure sepsis, and death in high-risk surgical patients. *Chest*. 1992;102(1):208.
42. Abou-Khalil B, Scalea TM, Trooskin SZ, et al. Hemodynamic responses to shock in young trauma patients: need for invasive monitoring. *Crit Care Med*. 1994;22(4):633.
43. Shoemaker WC, Appel PL, Kram HB, et al. Prospective trial of supranormal values of survivors as the therapeutic goals in high-risk surgical patients. *Chest*. 1988;94:1176–1186.
44. Bishop MH, Shoemaker WC, Appel PL, et al. Prospective randomized trial of survivor values of cardiac index, oxygen delivery, and oxygen consumption as resuscitation endpoints in severe trauma. *J Trauma*. 1995;38(5):780.
45. Shoemaker WC, Appel PL, Kram HB. Measurement of tissue perfusion by oxygen transport patterns in experimental shock and in high-risk surgical patients. *Intensive Care Med*. 1990;16(Suppl 2):S135.
46. Chang MC, Mondy JS, Meredith JW, et al. Redefining cardiovascular performance during resuscitation: ventricular stroke work, power, and the pressure-volume diagram. *J Trauma*. 1998;45(3):470.
47. Velmahos GC, Demetriades D, Shoemaker WC, et al. Endpoints of resuscitation of critically injured patients: normal or supranormal? A prospective randomized trial. *Ann Surg*. 2000;232(3):409.
48. Kern JW, Shoemaker WC. Meta-analysis of hemodynamic optimization in high-risk patients. *Crit Care Med*. 2002;30(8):1686.
49. Yu M, Levy MM, Smith P, et al. Effect of maximizing oxygen delivery on morbidity and mortality rates in critically ill patients: a prospective, randomized, controlled study. *Crit Care Med*. 1993;21(6):830.
50. Balogh Z, McKinley BA, Cocanour CS, et al. Supranormal trauma resuscitation causes more cases of abdominal compartment syndrome. *Arch Surg*. 2003;138:637.
51. Chaudry IH. Cellular mechanisms in shock and ischemia and their correction. *Am J Physiol*. 1983;245(2):R117.
52. Mongan PD, Fontana JL, Chen R, et al. Intravenous pyruvate prolongs survival during hemorrhagic shock in swine. *Am J Physiol*. 1999;277(6 Part 2):H2253.
53. Amundson B, Jennische E, Haljamae H. Correlative analysis of

microcirculatory and cellular metabolic events in skeletal muscle during hemorrhagic shock. *Acta Physiol Scand.* 1980;108(2):147.

54. Ratcliffe PJ, Moonen CT. Holloway PA, et al. Acute renal failure in hemorrhagic hypotension: cellular energetics and renal function. *Kidney Int.* 1986;30(3):355.
55. Zager RA. Adenine nucleotide changes in kidney, liver, and small intestine during different forms of ischemic injury. *Circ Res.* 1991;68(1):185.
56. Pellicane JV, DeMaria EJ, Abd-Elfattah A, et al. Interleukin-1 receptor antagonist improves survival and preserves organ adenosine-5-triphosphate after hemorrhagic shock. *Surgery.* 1993;114(2):278.
57. Salzman AL, Vromen A, Denenberg A, et al. K(ATP)-channel inhibition improves hemodynamics and cellular energetics in hemorrhagic shock. *Am J Physiol.* 1997;272(2 Part 2):H688.
58. Robinson DA, Wang P, Chaudry IH. Administration of ATP-MgCl2 after trauma-hemorrhage and resuscitation restores the depressed cardiac performance. *J Surg Res.* 1997;69(1):159.
59. Kline JA, Maiorano PC, Schroeder JD, et al. Activation of pyruvate dehydrogenase improves heart function and metabolism after hemorrhagic shock. *J Mol Cell Cardiol.* 1997;29(9):2465.
60. Mizock BA, Falk JL. Lactic acidosis in critical illness. *Crit Care Med.* 1992;20(1):80.
61. Nakatani T, Sakamoto Y, Ando H, et al. Bile and bilirubin excretion in relation to hepatic energy status during hemorrhagic shock and hypoxemia in rabbits. *J Trauma.* 1995;39(4):665.
62. Sjoberg F, Gustafsson U, Lewis DH. Extracellular muscle surface pO2 and pH heterogeneity during hypovolemia and after reperfusion. *Circ Shock.* 1991;34(3):319.
63. Davis JM, Stevens JM, Peitzman A, et al. Neutrophil migratory activity in severe hemorrhagic shock. *Circ Shock.* 1983;10(3):199.
64. Sayeed MM. Ion transport in circulatory and/or septic shock. *Am J Physiol.* 1987;252(5 Part 2):R809.
65. Horton JW. Calcium-channel blockade in canine hemorrhagic shock. *Am J Physiol.* 1989;257(5 Part 2):R1012.
66. Eastridge BJ, Darlington DN, Evans JA, et al. A circulating shock protein depolarizes cells in hemorrhage and sepsis. *Ann Surg.* 1994;219(3):298.
67. Kiang JG. Inducible heat shock protein 70kD and inducible nitric oxide synthase in hemorrhage/resuscitation-induced injury. *Cell Res.* 2004;14(6):450.
68. Menezes JM, Hierholzer C, Watkins SC, et al. The modulation of hepatic injury and heat shock expression by inhibition of inducible nitric oxide synthase after hemorrhagic shock. *Shock.* 2002;17(1):13.
69. DeMaio A. Heat shock proteins: facts, thoughts, and dreams. *Shock.* 1999;11(1):1.
70. Kregel KC. Heat shock proteins: modifying factors in physiological stress responses and acquired thermotolerance. *J Appl Physiol.* 2002;92:2177.
71. DeMaio A. The heat-shock response. *New Horizons.* 1995;3(2):198.
72. Zhao Q, Zhao KS. Inhibition of L-type calcium channels in arteriolar smooth muscle cells is involved in the pathogenesis of vascular hyporeactivity in severe shock. *Shock.* 2007; accepted for print.
73. Carlson DE, Nguyen PX, Soane L, et al. Hypotensive hemorrhage increases calcium uptake capacity and Bcl-XL content of liver mitochondria. *Shock.* 2007;27(2):192.
74. Zhao K, Liu J, Jin C. The role of membrane potential and calcium kinetic changes in the pathogenesis of vascular hyporeactivity during severe shock. *Chin Med J.* 2000;113:59.
75. Maitra SR, Geller ER, Pan W, et al. Altered cellular calcium regulation and hepatic glucose production during hemorrhagic shock. *Circ Shock.* 1992;38(1):14.
76. Xu J, Liu L. The role of calcium desensitization in vascular hyporeactivity and its regulation after hemorrhagic shock in the rat. *Shock.* 2005;23(6):576.
77. Yang G, Liu L, Xu J, et al. Effect of arginine vasopressin on vascular reactivity and calcium sensitivity after hemorrhagic shock in rats and its relationship to Rho-kinase. *J Trauma.* 2006;61(6):1336.
78. Silomon M, Rose S. Effect of sodium bicarbonate infusion on hepatocyte Ca2+ overload during resuscitation from hemorrhagic shock. *Resuscitation.* 1998;37(1):27.
79. Silomon M, Pizanis A, Larsen R, et al. Pentoxyfilline prevention of altered hepatocyte calcium regulation during hemorrhagic shock/resuscitation. *Crit Care Med.* 1998;26(3):494.
80. Zhong Z, Enomoto N, Connor HD, et al. Glycine improves survival after hemorrhagic shock. *Shock.* 1999;12(1):54.
81. Wang G, Zhao M, Wang EH. Effects of glycine and methylprednisolone on hemorrhagic shock in rats. *Chin Med J.* 2004;117(9):1334.
82. Jarrar D, Chaudry IH, Wang P. Organ dysfunction following hemorrhage and sepsis: mechanisms and therapeutic approaches (review). *Int J Mol Med.* 1999;4(6):575.
83. Lieberthal W, McGarry AE, Sheils J, et al. Nitric oxide inhibition in rats improves blood pressure and renal function in hypovolemic shock. *Am J Physiol.* 1991;261(5 Part 2):F868.
84. Szabo C, Farago M, Horvath I, et al. Hemorrhagic hypotension impairs endothelium-dependent relaxations in the renal artery of the cat. *Circ Shock.* 1992;36(3):238.
85. Dignan RJ, Wechsler AS, DeMaria EJ. Coronary vasomotor dysfunction following hemorrhagic shock. *J Surg Res.* 1992;52(4):382.
86. Bitterman H, Brod V, Weisz G, et al. Effects of oxygen on regional hemodynamics in hemorrhagic shock. *Am J Physiol.* 1996;271(1 Part 2): H203.
87. Szabo C, Csaki C, Benyo Z, et al. Role of L-arginine-nitric oxide pathway in the changes in cerebrovascular reactivity following hemorrhagic hypotension and retransfusion. *Circ Shock.* 1992;37(4):307.
88. Guarini S, Bini A, Bazzani C, et al. Adrenocorticotropin normalizes the blood levels of nitric oxide in hemorrhage-shocked rats. *Eur J Pharmacol.* 1997;336(1):15.
89. Pannen BH, Kohler N, Hole B, et al. Protective role of endogenous carbon monoxide in hepatic microcirculatory dysfunction after hemorrhagic shock in rats. *J Clin Invest.* 1998;102(6):1220.
90. Szabo C, Billiar TR. Novel roles of nitric oxide in hemorrhagic shock. *Shock.* 1999;12(1):1.
91. Kiang JG, Bowman PD, Lu X, et al. Geldanamycin inhibits hemorrhage-induced increases in caspase-3 activity: role of inducible nitric oxide synthase. *J Appl Physiol.* 2007;103:1045.
92. Ng KC, Moochhala SM, Md S, et al. Preservation of neurological functions by nitric oxide synthase inhibitors following hemorrhagic shock. *Neuropharmacology.* 2003;44(2):244.
93. Hierbolzer C, Billiar TR, Tweardy DJ, et al. Reduced hepatic transcription factor activation and expression of IL-6 and ICAM-1 after hemorrhage by NO scavenging. *Arch Orthop Trauma Surg.* 2003;123(2–3):55.
94. Hierbolzer C, Menezes JM, Ungeheuer A, et al. A nitric oxide scavenger against pulmonary inflammation following hemorrhagic shock. *Shock.* 2002;17(2):98.
95. Kobara M, Tatsumi T, Takeda M, et al. The dual effects of nitric oxide synthase inhibitors on ischemia-reperfusion injury in rat hearts. *Basic Res Cardiol.* 2003;98(5):319.
96. Adachi T, Hori S, Miyazaki K, et al. Inhibition of nitric oxide synthesis aggravates myocardial ischemia in hemorrhagic shock in constant pressure model. *Shock.* 1998;9(3):204.
97. Thompson A, Valeri CR, Lieberthal W. Endothelin receptor A blockade alters hemodynamic response to nitric oxide inhibition in rats. *Am J Physiol.* 1995;269(2 Part 2):H743.
98. Rothe CF, Drees JA. Vascular capacitance and fluid shifts in dogs during prolonged hemorrhagic hypotension. *Circ Res.* 1976;38(5):347.
99. Schlichtig R, Kramer DJ, Pinsky MR. Flow redistribution during progressive hemorrhage is a determinant of critical O_2 delivery. *J Appl Physiol.* 1991;70(1):169.
100. Chien S. Role of the sympathetic nervous system in hemorrhage. *Physiol Rev.* 1967;47(2):214.
101. Forsyth RP, Hoffbrand BI, Melmon KL. Redistribution of cardiac output during hemorrhage in the unanesthetized monkey. *Circ Res.* 1970;27(3):311.
102. Rothe CF, Drees JA. Vascular capacitance and fluid shifts in dogs during prolonged hemorrhagic hypotension. *Circ Res.* 1976;38(5):347.
103. Zweifach BW. Mechanisms of blood flow and fluid exchange in microvessels: hemorrhagic hypotension model. *Anesthesiology.* 1974;41(2):157.
104. Prist R, Rocha-e-Silva M, Scalabrini A, et al. A quantitative analysis of transcapillary refill in severe hemorrhagic hypotension in dogs. *Shock.* 1994;1(3):188.
105. Childs EW, Udobi KF, Hunter FA, et al. Evidence of transcellular albumin transport after hemorrhagic shock. *Shock.* 2005;23(6):565.
106. Schumacher J, Binkowski K, Dendorfer A, et al. Organ-specific extravasation of albumin-bound Evans blue during non-resuscitated hemorrhagic shock in rats. *Shock.* 2003;20(6):565.
107. Boyd AJ, Rubin BB, Walker PM, et al. A CD18 monoclonal antibody reduces multiple organ injury in a model of ruptured abdominal aortic aneurysm. *Am J Physiol.* 1999;277(1 Part 2):H172.
108. Pascual JL, Ferri LE, Seely AJ, et al. Hypertonic saline resuscitation of hemorrhagic shock diminishes neutrophil rolling and adherence to endothelium and reduces in vivo vascular leakage. *Ann Surg.* 2002;236(5):634.
109. Corso CO, Okamoto S, Ruttinger D, et al. Hypertonic saline dextran attenuates leukocyte accumulation in the liver after hemorrhagic shock and resuscitation. *J Trauma.* 1999;46(3):417.
110. Childs EW, Udobi KF, Wood JG, et al. In vivo visualization of reactive oxidants and leukocyte-endothelial adherence following hemorrhagic shock. *Shock.* 2002;18(5):423.
111. Yada-Langui MM, Anjos-Valotta EA, Sannomiya P, et al. Resuscitation affects microcirculatory polymorphonuclear leukocyte behavior after hemorrhagic shock: role of hypertonic saline and pentoxyfilline. *Exp Biol Med (Maywood).* 2004;229(7):684.
112. Childs EW, Udobi KF, Wood JG, et al. In vivo visualization of reactive oxidants and leukocyte-endothelial adherence following hemorrhagic shock. *Shock.* 2002;18(5):423.
113. Botha AJ, Moore FA, Moore EE, et al. Early neutrophil sequestration after injury: a pathogenic mechanism for multiple organ failure. *J Trauma.* 1995;39(3):411.
114. Barroso-Aranda J, Schmid-Schonbein GW, Zweifach BW, et al. Granulocytes and no-reflow phenomenon in irreversible hemorrhagic shock. *Circ Res.* 1988;63(2):437.
115. Connolly HV, Maginniss LA, Schumacker PT. Transit time heterogeneity in canine small intestine: significance for oxygen transport. *J Clin Invest.* 1997;99(2):228.

116. Douglas RG, Shaw JHF. Metabolic response to sepsis and trauma. *Br J Surg.* 1989;76:115.
117. Pearce FJ, Connett RJ, Drucker WR. Extracellular-intracellular lactate gradients in skeletal muscle during hemorrhagic shock in the rat. *Surgery.* 1985;98:625.
118. Alibegovic A, Ljungqvist O. Pretreatment with glucose infusion prevents fatal outcome after hemorrhage in food-deprived rats. *Circ Shock.* 1993;39:1.
119. Barton R, Cerra FB. The hypermetabolism of multiple organ failure syndrome. *Chest.* 1989;96:1153.
120. Miyazaki K, Hori S, Inoue S, et al. Characterization of energy metabolism and blood flow distribution in myocardial ischemia in hemorrhagic shock. *Am J Physiol.* 1997;273(2 Pt 2):H600.
121. Paulson OB, Strandgaard S, Edvinsson L. Cerebral autoregulation. *Cerebrovasc Brain Metab Rev.* 1990;2:161.
122. Harper AM. Autoregulation of cerebral blood flow: influence of the arterial blood pressure on the blood flow through the cerebral cortex. *J Neurol Neurosurg Psychiatry.* 1966;29:398.
123. Meybohm P, Cavus E, Bein B, et al. Cerebral metabolism assessed with microdialysis in uncontrolled hemorrhagic shock after penetrating liver trauma. *Anesth Analg.* 2006;103(4):948.
124. Meybohm P, Renner J, Boening A, et al. Impact of norepinephrine and fluid on cerebral oxygenation in experimental hemorrhagic shock. *Pediatr Res.* 2007;62(4):1.
125. Filho JA, Machado MA, Nani RS, et al. Hypertonic saline solution increases cerebral perfusion pressure during clinical orthotopic liver transplantation for fulminant hepatic failure: preliminary results. *Clinics.* 2006;61(3): 231.
126. Pinto FC, Capone-Neto A, Prist R, et al. Volume replacement with lactated Ringer's or 3% hypertonic saline solution during combined experimental hemorrhagic shock and traumatic brain injury. *J Trauma.* 2006;60(4):758.
127. Steenblock U, Mannhart H, Wolff G. Effect of hemorrhagic shock on intrapulmonary right-to-left shunt (QS/QT) and dead space (VD/VT). *Respiration.* 1976;33(2):133.
128. Adrogue HJ, Rashad MN, Gorin AB, et al. Arteriovenous acid-base disparity in circulatory failure: studies on mechanism. *Am J Physiol.* 1989;257(6 Pt 2):F1087.
129. Pretorius JP, Schlag G, Redl H, et al. The "lung in shock" as a result of hypovolemic-traumatic shock in baboons. *J Trauma.* 1987;27(12):1344.
130. Garber BG, Hebert PC, Yelle JD, et al. Adult respiratory distress syndrome: a systemic overview of incidence and risk factors. *Crit Care Med.* 1996;24(4):687.
131. Pallister I, Dent C, Topley N. Increased neutrophil migratory activity after major trauma: a factor in the etiology of acute respiratory distress syndrome? *Crit Care Med.* 2002;30(8):1717.
132. Pallister I, Gosling P, Alpar K, et al. Prediction of post-traumatic adult respiratory distress syndrome by albumin excretion rate eight hours after admission. *J Trauma.* 1997;42(6):1056.
133. Wardle EN. Acute renal failure and multiorgan failure. *Nephron.* 1994; 66(4):380.
134. Myers BD, Moran SM. Hemodynamically mediated acute renal failure. *N Engl J Med.* 1986;314(2):97.
135. Brenner BM. Hemodynamically mediated glomerular injury and the progressive nature of kidney disease. *Kidney Int.* 1983;23(4):647.
136. Toung T, Reilly PM, Fuh KC, et al. Mesenteric vasoconstriction in response to hemorrhagic shock. *Shock.* 2000;13(4):267.
137. Reilly PM, Bulkly GB. Vasoactive mediators and splanchnic perfusion. *Crit Care Med.* 1993;21(2 Suppl):S55.
138. Yilmaz EN, Vahl AC, van Rij GL, et al. The renin-angiotensin system in swine during hypovolaemic shock combined with low-flow ischaemia of the sigmoid colon. *Cardiovasc Surg.* 1999;7(5):539.
139. Reilly PM, Wilkins KB, Fuh KC, et al. The mesenteric hemodynamic response to circulatory shock: an overview. *Shock.* 2001;15(5):329.
140. Fusamoto H, Hagiwara H, Meren H, et al. A clinical study of acute gastrointestinal hemorrhage associated with various shock states. *Am J Gastroenterol.* 1991;86(4):429.
141. Schuster DP, Rowley H, Feinstein S, et al. Prospective evaluation of the risk of upper gastrointestinal bleeding after admission to a medical intensive care unit. *Am J Med.* 1984;76(4):623.
142. Van Leeuwen PAM, Boermeester MA, Houdijk APJ, et al. Clinical significance of translocation. *Gut.* 1994;35 (Suppl 1):S28.
143. Berg RD. Bacterial translocation from the gastrointestinal tract. *Adv Exp Med Biol.* 1999;473:11.
144. Haglund U. Systemic mediators released from the gut in critical illness. *Crit Care Med.* 1993;21(Suppl 2):S15.
145. Fiddian-Green RG. Associations between intramucosal acidosis in the gut and organ failure. *Crit Care Med.* 1993;21(Suppl 2):S103.
146. Hameed SM, Cohn SM. Gastric tonometry: the role of mucosal pH measurement in the management of trauma. *Chest.* 2003;123:475S.
147. Wang P, Ba ZF, Burkhardt J, et al. Measurement of hepatic blood flow after severe hemorrhage: lack of restoration despite adequate resuscitation. *Am J Physiol.* 1992;262(1 Part 1):G92.
148. Nordin A, Mildh L, Makisalo H, et al. Hepatosplanchnic and peripheral tissue oxygenation during treatment of hemorrhagic shock: the effects of pentoxifylline administration. *Ann Surg.* 1998;228(6):741.
149. Tadros T, Traber DL, Herndon DN. Trauma- and sepsis-induced hepatic ischemia and reperfusion injury: role of angiotensin II. *Arch Surg.* 2000;135:766.
150. Hoppen RA, Corso CO, Grezzana TJ, et al. Hypertonic saline and hemorrhagic shock: hepatocellular function and integrity after six hours of treatment. *Acta Cir Bras.* 2005;20(6):414.
151. Kitai T, Tanaka A, Tokuka A, et al. Changes in the hepatic oxygenation state during hemorrhage and following epinephrine or dextran infusion as assessed by near-infrared spectroscopy. *Circ Shock.* 1993;41(3):197.
152. Bor NM, Alvur M, Ercan MT, et al. Liver blood flow rate and glucose metabolism in hemorrhagic hypotension and shock. *J Trauma.* 1982;22(9): 753.
153. Hawker F. Liver dysfunction in critical illness. *Anaesth Intensive Care.* 1991;19(2):165.
154. Tashkin DP, Goldstein PJ, Simmons DH. Hepatic lactate uptake during decreased liver perfusion and hypoxemia. *Am J Physiol.* 1972;223(4):968.
155. Champion HR, Jones RT, Trump BF, et al. A clinicopathologic study of hepatic dysfunction following shock. *Surg Gynecol Obstet.* 1976;142(5):657.
156. Lefer AM, Spath JA. Pancreatic hypoperfusion and the production of a myocardial depressant factor in hemorrhagic shock. *Ann Surg.* 1974;179(6):868.
157. Schmid-Schonbein GW, Hugli TE, Kistler EB, et al. Pancreatic enzymes and microvascular cell activation in multiorgan failure. *Microcirculation.* 2001;8(1):5.
158. Mitsuoka H, Kistler EB, Schmid-Schonbein GW. Protease inhibition in the intestinal lumen: attenuation of systemic inflammation and early indicators of multiple organ failure in shock. *Shock.* 2002;17(3):205.
159. Waldo SW, Rosario HS, Penn AH, et al. Pancreatic digestive enzymes are potent generators of mediators for leukocyte activation and mortality. *Shock.* 2003;20(2):138.
160. Fitzal F, DeLano FA, Young C, et al. Improvement in early symptoms of shock by delayed intestinal protease inhibition. *Arch Surg.* 2004;139:1008.
161. Ishimaru K, Mitsuoka H, Unno N, et al. Pancreatic proteases and inflammatory mediators in peritoneal fluid during splanchnic arterial occlusion and reperfusion. *Shock.* 2004;22(5):467.
162. Schmid-Schonbein GW, Hugli TE. A new hypothesis for microvascular inflammation in shock and multiorgan failure: self-digestion by pancreatic enzymes. *Microcirculation.* 2005;12:71.
163. Penn AH, Hugli TE, Schmid-Schonbein GW. Pancreatic enzymes generate cytotoxic mediators in the intestine. *Shock.* 2007;27(3):296.
164. Ramos-Kelly JR, Toledo-Pereyra LH, Jordan JA, et al. Upregulation of lung chemokines associated with hemorrhage is reversed with a small molecule multiple selectin inhibitor. *J Am Coll Surg.* 1999;189(6):546.
165. Upperman JS, Deitch EA, Guo W, et al. Post-hemorrhagic shock mesenteric lymph is cytotoxic to endothelial cells and activates neutrophils. *Shock.* 1998;10(6):407.
166. Chaudry IH, Ayala A, Ertel W, et al. Hemorrhage and resuscitation: immunological aspects. *Am J Physiol.* 1990;259(4 Part 2):R663.
167. Nast-Kolb D, Waydhas C, Gippner-Steppert C, et al. Indicators of the posttraumatic inflammatory response correlate with organ failure in patients with multiple injuries. *J Trauma.* 1997;42(3):446.
168. Hierholzer C, Kalff JC, Omert L, et al. Interleukin-6 production in hemorrhagic shock is accompanied by neutrophil recruitment and lung injury. *Am J Physiol.* 1998;275(3 Part 1):L611.
169. Hierholzer C, Kalff JC, Chakraborty A, et al. Impaired gut contractility following hemorrhagic shock is accompanied by IL-6 and G-CSF production and neutrophil infiltration. *Dig Dis Sci.* 2001;46(2):230.
170. Roumen RMH, Hendriks T, van der Ven-Jongekrijg J, et al. Cytokine patterns in patients after major vascular surgery, hemorrhagic shock and severe blunt trauma: relation with subsequent adult respiratory distress syndrome and multiple organ failure. *Ann Surg.* 1993:218(6):769.
171. Meng X, Ao L, Song Y, et al. Signaling for myocardial depression in hemorrhagic shock: roles of toll-like receptor 4 and p55 TNF-alpha receptor. *Am J Physiol Regul Integr Comp Physiol.* 2005;288(3):R600.
172. Prince JM, Levy RM, Yang R, et al. Toll-like receptor-4 signaling mediates hepatic injury and systemic inflammation in hemorrhagic shock. *J Am Coll Surg.* 2006;202(3):407.
173. Watters JM, Tieu BH, Todd SR, et al. Fluid resuscitation increases inflammatory gene transcription after traumatic injury. *J Trauma.* 2006;61(2):300.
174. Lee CC, Chang IJ, Yen ZS, et al. Delayed fluid resuscitation in hemorrhagic shock induces proinflammatory cytokine response. *Ann Emerg Med.* 2007;49(1):37.
175. Turnage RH, Kadesky KM, Rogers T, et al. Neutrophil regulation of splanchnic blood flow after hemorrhagic shock. *Ann Surg.* 1995;222(1):66.
176. Gonzalez RJ, Moore EE, Ciesla DJ, et al. Phospholipase A(2)-derived neutral lipids from post-hemorrhagic shock mesenteric lymph prime the neutrophil oxidative burst. *Surgery.* 2001;130(2):198.
177. Patel JP, Beck LD, Briglia FA, et al. Beneficial effects of combined thromboxane and leukotriene receptor antagonism in hemorrhagic shock. *Crit Care Med.* 1995;23(2):231.
178. Yokoyama Y, Nimura Y, Nagino M, et al. Role of thromboxane in producing hepatic injury during hepatic stress. *Arch Surg.* 2005;140:801.
179. Vanlersberghe C, Lauwers MH, Camu F. Prostaglandin synthetase inhibitor treatment and the regulatory role of prostaglandins on organ perfusion. *Acta Anaesthesiol Belg.* 1992;43(4):211.
180. Yamakawa Y, Takano M, Patel M, et al. Interaction of platelet-activating

factor, reactive oxygen species generated by xanthine oxidase, and leukocytes in the generation of hepatic injury after shock/resuscitation. *Ann Surg.* 2000;231(3):387.
181. Fruchterman TM, Spain DA, Wilson MA, et al. Complement inhibition prevents gut ischemia and endothelial cell dysfunction after hemorrhage/resuscitation. *Surgery.* 1998;124(4):782.
182. Spain DA, Fruchterman TM, Matheson PJ, et al. Complement activation mediates intestinal injury after resuscitation from hemorrhagic shock. *J Trauma.* 1999;46(2):224.
183. Childs EW, Udobi KF, Hunter FA. Hypothermia reduces microvascular permeability and reactive oxygen species expression after hemorrhagic shock. *J Trauma.* 2005;58(2):271.
184. Szabo C. The pathophysiological role of peroxynitrite in shock, inflammation, and ischemia-reperfusion injury. *Shock.* 1996;6(2):79.
185. Kapoor R, Prasad K. Role of oxyradicals in cardiovascular depression and cellular injury in hemorrhagic shock and reinfusion: effect of SOD and catalase. *Circ Shock.* 1994;43(2):79.
186. Prasad K, Kalra J, Buchko G. Acute hemorrhage and oxygen free radicals. *Angiology.* 1988;39(12):1005.
187. Ahmed N, Christou N. Systemic inflammatory response syndrome: interactions between immune cells and the endothelium. *Shock.* 1996;6(Suppl 1):S39.
188. van Meurs M, Wulfert FM, Knol AJ, et al. Early organ-specific endothelial activation during hemorrhagic shock and resuscitation. *Shock.* 2008;29:291.
189. Martinez-Mier G, Toledo-Pereyra LH, Ward PA. Adhesion molecules and hemorrhagic shock. *J Trauma.* 2001;51(2):408.
190. Horgan MJ, Ge M, Gu J, et al. Role of ICAM-1 in neutrophil-mediated lung vascular injury after occlusion and reperfusion. *Am J Physiol.* 1991;261(5 Part 2):H1578.
191. Adams CA, Sambol JT, Xu DZ, et al. Hemorrhagic shock induced upregulation of P-selectin expression is mediated by factors in mesenteric lymph and blunted by mesenteric lymph duct interruption. *J Trauma.* 2001;51(4):625.
192. Xu DZ, Lu Q, Adams CA, et al. Trauma-hemorrhagic shock-induced upregulation of endothelial cell adhesion molecules is blunted by mesenteric lymph duct ligation. *Crit Care Med.* 2004;32(3):760.
193. Jarrar D, Chaudry IH, Wang P. Organ dysfunction following hemorrhage and sepsis: mechanisms and therapeutic approaches. *Int J Mol Med.* 1999;4(6):575.
194. Guillou PJ. Biological variation in the development of sepsis after surgery or trauma. *Lancet.* 1993;342(8865):217.
195. O'Mahony JB, Palder SB, Wood JJ, et al. Depression of cellular immunity after multiple trauma in the absence of sepsis. *J Trauma.* 1984;24(10):869.
196. Stephan RN, Kupper TS, Geha AS, et al. Hemorrhage without tissue produces immunosuppression and enhances susceptibility to sepsis. *Arch Surg.* 1987;122(1):62.
197. Walz CR, Zedler S, Schneider CP, et al. Depressed T cell-derived IFN-gamma following trauma-hemorrhage: a potential mechanism for diminished APC responses. *Langenbecks Arch Surg.* 2007;392(3):339.
198. Ertel W, Morrison MH, Ayala A, et al. Insights into the mechanisms of defective antigen presentation after hemorrhage. *Surgery.* 1991;110(2):440.
199. Fan J, Li Y, Levy RM, et al. Hemorrhagic shock induces NAD(P)H oxidase activation in neutrophils: role of HMGB1-TLR4 signaling. *J Immunol.* 2007;178(10):6573.
200. Lomas-Neira J, Chung CS, Perl M, et al. Role of alveolar macrophage and migrating neutrophils in hemorrhage-induced priming for ALI subsequent to septic challenge. *Am J Physiol Lung Cell Mol Physiol.* 2006;290(1):L51.
201. Fan J, Li Y, Vodovotz Y, et al. Hemorrhagic shock-activated neutrophils augment TLR4 signaling-induced TLR2 upregulation in alveolar macrophages: role in hemorrhage-primed lung inflammation. *Am J Physiol Lung Cell Mol Physiol.* 2006;290(4):L738.
202. Schneider CP, Schwacha MG, Chaudry IH. Influence of gender and age on T-cell responses in a murine model of trauma-hemorrhage: differences between circulating and tissue-fixed cells. *J Appl Physiol.* 2006;100(3):826.
203. Faist E, Schinkel C, Zimmer S. Update on the mechanisms of immune suppression of injury and immune modulation. *World J Surg.* 1996;20(4):454.
204. Angele MK, Chaudry IH. Surgical trauma and immunosuppression: pathophysiology and potential immunomodulatory approaches. *Langenbeck Arch Surg.* 2005;390(4):333.
205. Knoferl MW, Angele MK, Diodato MD, et al. Female sex hormones regulate function after trauma-hemorrhage and prevent increased cell death rate from subsequent sepsis. *Ann Surg.* 2002;235(1):105.
206. Schneider CP, Schwacha MG, Chaudry IH. The role of interleukin-10 in the regulation of the systemic inflammatory response following trauma-hemorrhage. *Biochim Biophys Acta.* 2004;1689(1):22.
207. Yokoyama Y, Kitchens WC, Toth B, et al. Role of IL-10 in regulating proinflammatory cytokine release by Kupffer cells following trauma-hemorrhage. *Am J Physiol Gastrointest Liver Physiol.* 2004;286(6):G942.
208. Lyons A, Kelly JL, Rodrick ML, et al. Major injury induces increased production of interleukin-10 by cells of the immune system with a negative impact on resistance to infection. *Ann Surg.* 1997;226(4):450.
209. Cinat ME, Waxman K, Granger GA, et al. Trauma causes sustained elevation of soluble tumor necrosis factor receptors. *J Am Coll Surg.* 1994;179(5):529.
210. Cinat M, Waxman K, Vaziri ND, et al. Soluble cytokine receptors and receptor antagonists are sequentially released after trauma. *J Trauma.* 1995;39(1):112.
211. American College of Surgeons Committee on Trauma. Initial assessment and management. In: *Advanced Trauma Life Support.* 7th ed. American College of Surgeons, Chicago, IL; 2004:11.
212. Daniel SR, Morita SY, Yu M, et al. Uncompensated metabolic acidosis: an underrecognized risk factor for subsequent intubation requirement. *J Trauma.* 2004;57:993.
213. Aufderheide TP, Sigurdsson G, Pirrallo RG, et al. Hyperventilation-induced hypotension during cardiopulmonary resuscitation. *Circulation.* 2004;109:1960.
214. Davis DP, Hoyt DB, Ochs M, et al. The effect of paramedic rapid sequence intubation on outcome in patients with severe traumatic brain injury. *J Trauma.* 2003;54:444.
215. Pepe PE, Lurie KG, Wigginton JG, et al. Detrimental hemodynamic effects of assisted ventilation in hemorrhagic states. *Crit Care Med.* 2004;32:S414.
216. Krismer AC, Wenzel V, Lindner KH, et al. Influence of negative expiratory pressure ventilation on hemodynamic variables during severe hemorrhagic shock. *Crit Care Med.* 2006;34:2175.
217. Miller PR, Moore PS, Mansell E, et al. External fixation or arteriogram in bleeding pelvic fracture: initial therapy guided by markers of arterial hemorrhage. *J Trauma.* 2003;54:437.
218. Heetveld MJ, Harris I, Schlaphoff G, et al. Guidelines for the management of haemodynamically unstable pelvic fracture patients. *ANZ J Surg.* 2004;74:520.
219. Ertel W, Keel M, Eid K, et al. Control of severe hemorrhage using C-clamp and pelvic packing in multiply injured patients with pelvic ring disruption. *J Orthop Trauma.* 2001;15:468.
220. Giannoudis PV, Pape HC. Damage control orthopaedics in unstable pelvic ring fractures. *Injury.* 2004;35:671.
221. American College of Surgeons Committee on Trauma. Shock. In: *Advanced Trauma Life Support.* 7th ed. American College of Surgeons, Chicago, IL; 2004:69.
222. Codner P, Obaid A, Porral D, et al. Is field hypotension a reliable indicator of significant injury in trauma patients who are normotensive on arrival to the emergency department? *Am Surg.* 2005;71(9):768.
223. Chan L, Bartfield JM, Reilly KM. The significance of out-of-hospital hypotension in blunt trauma patients. *Acad Emerg Med.* 1997;4:785.
224. Lipsky AM, Gausche-Hill M, Henneman PL, et al. Prehospital hypotension is a predictor of the need for an emergent, therapeutic operation in trauma patients with normal systolic blood pressure in the emergency department. *J Trauma.* 2006;61:1228.
225. Hagiwara A, Minakawa K, Fukushima H, et al. Predictors of death in patients with life-threatening pelvic hemorrhage after successful transcatheter arterial embolization. *J Trauma.* 2003;55:696.
226. Hoffer EK, Borsa JJ, Bloch RD, et al. Endovascular techniques in the damage control setting. *Radiographics.* 1999;19:1340.
227. Shapiro M, McDonald AA, Knight D, et al. The role of repeat angiography in the management of pelvic fractures. *J Trauma.* 2005;58:227.
228. Panetta T, Sclafani SJ, Goldstein AS, et al. Percutaneous transcatheter embolization for massive bleeding from pelvic fractures. *J Trauma.* 1985;25:1021.
229. Spahn DR, Cerny V, Coats TJ, et al. Management of bleeding following major trauma: a European guideline. *Crit Care.* 2007;11:R17.
230. Hunt PA, Greaves I, Owens WA. Emergency thoracotomy in thoracic trauma—a review. *Injury.* 2006;37:1.
231. Cothren CC, Moore EE. Emergency department thoracotomy for the critically injured: objectives, indications, and outcomes. *World J Emerg Surg.* 2006;1:4.
232. Millikan JS, Moore EE. Outcome of resuscitative thoracotomy and descending aortic occlusion performed in the operating room. *J Trauma.* 1984;24:387.
233. Richardson JD, Bergamini TM, Spain DA, et al. Operative strategies for management of abdominal aortic gunshot wounds. *Surgery.* 1996;120:667.
234. Nicholas JM, Rix EP, Easley KA, et al. Changing patterns in the management of penetrating abdominal trauma: the more things change, the more they stay the same. *J Trauma.* 2003;55:1095.
235. Reich DL, Konstadt SN, Raissi S, et al. Trendelenburg position and passive leg raising do not significantly improve cardiopulmonary performance in the anesthetized patient with coronary artery disease. *Crit Care Med.* 1989;17:313.
236. Mattox KL, Bickell W, Pepe PE, et al. Prospective MAST study in 911 patients. *J Trauma.* 1989;29(8):1104.
237. Mattox KL, Bickell WH, Pepe PE, et al. Prospective randomized evaluation of antishock MAST in post-traumatic hypotension. *J Trauma.* 1986;26(9):779.
238. Cayten CG, Berendt BM, Byrne DW, et al. A study of pneumatic antishock garments in severely hypotensive trauma patients. *J Trauma.* 1993;34(5):728.
239. Velanovich V. Crystalloid versus colloid fluid resuscitation: a meta-analysis of mortality. *Surgery.* 1989;105:65.
240. Bisonni RS, Holtgrave DR, Lawler F, et al. Colloids versus crystalloids in fluid resuscitation: an analysis of randomized controlled trials. *J Fam Pract.* 1991;32:387.

241. Schierhout G, Roberts I. Fluid resuscitation with colloid or crystalloid solutions in critically ill patients: a systematic review of randomized trials. *BMJ.* 1998;316:961.
242. Human albumin administration in critically ill patients: systematic review of randomized controlled trials. Cochrane Injuries Group Albumin Reviewers. *BMJ.* 1998;317:235.
243. Choi PT, Yip G, Quinonez LG, et al. Crystalloids vs. colloids in fluid resuscitation: a systematic review. *Crit Care Med.* 1999;27:200.
244. Roberts I, Alderson P, Bunn F, et al. Colloids vs crystalloids for fluid resuscitation in critically ill patients. *Cochrane Database Syst Rev.* 2004;CD000567.
245. Finfer S, Bellomo R, Boyce N, et al. A comparison of albumin and saline for fluid resuscitation in the intensive care unit. *N Engl J Med.* 2004;350:2247.
246. Entholzner EK, Mielke LL, Calatzis AN, et al. Coagulation effects of a recently developed hydroxyethyl starch (HES 130/0.4) compared to hydroxyethyl starches with higher molecular weight. *Acta Anesth Scand.* 2000;44:1116.
247. Jamnicki M, Zollinger A, Seifert B, et al. Compromised blood coagulation: an in vitro comparison of hydroxyethyl starch 130/0.4 and hydroxyethyl starch 200/0.5 using thromboelastography. *Anesth Analg.* 1998;87:989.
248. Langeron O, Doelberg M, Ang ET, et al. Voluven, a lower substituted novel hydroxyethyl starch (HES 130/0.4) causes fewer effects on coagulation in major orthopedic surgery than HES 200/0.5. *Anesth Analg.* 2001;92:855.
249. Fenger-Eriksen C, Anker-Moller E, Heslop J, et al. Thromboelastographic whole blood clot formation after ex vivo addition of plasma substitutes: improvements of the induced coagulopathy with fibrinogen concentrate. *Br J Anaesth.* 2005;94:324.
250. Tieu BH, Holcomb JB, Schreiber MA, et al. Coagulopathy: its pathophysiology and treatment in the injured patient. *World J Surg.* 2007;31:1055.
251. Kiraly LN, Differding JA, Enomoto TM, et al. Resuscitation with normal saline versus lactated ringers modulates hypercoagulability and leads to increased blood loss in an uncontrolled hemorrhagic shock swine model. *J Trauma.* 2006;61:57.
252. Cotton BA, Guy JS, Morris JA, et al. The cellular, metabolic, and systemic consequences of aggressive fluid resuscitation strategies. *Shock.* 2006;26:115.
253. Coimbra R, Hoyt DB, Junger WG, et al. Hypertonic saline resuscitation decreases susceptibility to sepsis after hemorrhagic shock. *J Trauma.* 1997;42:602.
254. Rhee P, Wand D, Ruff P, et al. Human neutrophil activation and increased adhesion by various resuscitation fluids. *Crit Care Med.* 2000;28:74.
255. Ayuste EC, Chen H, Koustova E, et al. Hepatic and pulmonary apoptosis after hemorrhagic shock in swine can be reduced through modifications of conventional Ringers solution. *J Trauma.* 2006;60:52.
256. Rhee P, Koustova E, Alam HB. Searching for the optimal resuscitation method: recommendations for the initial fluid resuscitation of combat casualties. *J Trauma.* 2003;54(Suppl.):S52.
257. Raeburn CD, Moore EE, Biffl WL, et al. The abdominal compartment syndrome is a morbid complication of post injury damage control surgery. *Am J Surg.* 2001;182:542.
258. Biffl WL, Moore EE, Burch JM, et al. Secondary abdominal compartment syndrome is a highly lethal event. *Am J Surg.* 2001;182:645.
259. Maxwell RA, Fabian TC, Croce MA, et al. Secondary abdominal compartment syndrome: an underappreciated manifestation of severe hemorrhagic shock. *J Trauma.* 1999;47:995.
260. Miller RS, Morris JA, Diaz JJ, et al. Complications after 344 damage control open celiotomies. *J Trauma.* 2004;57:436.
261. Gracias VH, Braslow B, Johnson J, et al. Abdominal compartment syndrome in the open abdomen. *Arch Surg.* 2002;137:1298.
262. Kauvar DS, Holcomb JB, Norris GC, et al. Fresh whole blood transfusion: a controversial military practice. *J Trauma.* 2006;61:181.
263. Owens TM, Watson WC, Prough DS, et al. Limiting initial resuscitation of uncontrolled hemorrhage reduces internal bleeding and subsequent volume requirements. *J Trauma.* 1995;39:200.
264. Dutton RP, Mackenzie CF, Scalea TM. Hypotensive resuscitation during active hemorrhage: impact on in-hospital mortality. *J Trauma.* 2002;52:1141.
265. Bickell WH, Wall MJ, Pepe PE, et al. Immediate versus delayed fluid resuscitation for hypotensive patients with penetrating torso trauma. *N Engl J Med.* 1994;331:1105.
266. Hirschberg A, Hoyt DB, Mattox KL. From "leaky buckets" to vascular injuries: understanding models of uncontrolled hemorrhage. *J Am Coll Surg.* 2007;204:665.
267. Iserson KV, Huestis DW. Blood warming: current applications and techniques. *Transfusion.* 1991;31:558.
268. Janczyk RJ, Howells GA, Bair HA, et al. Hypothermia is an independent predictor of mortality in ruptured abdominal aortic aneurysms. *Vasc Endovascular Surg.* 2004;38:37.
269. Strate LL, Syngal S. Predictors of utilization of early colonoscopy versus radiography for severe lower intestinal bleeding. *Gastrointest Endosc.* 2005;61:46.
270. Gady JS, Reynolds H, Blum A. Selective arterial embolization for control of lower gastrointestinal bleeding: recommendations for a clinical management pathway. *Curr Surg.* 2003;60(3):344.
271. Kuo WT, Lee DE, Saad WE, et al. Superselective microcoil embolization for the treatment of lower gastrointestinal hemorrhage. *J Vasc Intern Radial.* 2003;14(12):1503.
272. DeBarros J, Rosas L, Cohen J, et al. The changing paradigm for the treatment of colonic hemorrhage: superselective angiographic embolization. *Dis Colon Rectum.* 2002;45(6):802.
273. Johnston C, Tuite D, Pritchard R, et al. Use of provocative angiography to localize site in recurrent gastrointestinal bleeding. *Cardiovasc Intervent Radiol.* 2007;30:1042.
274. Lin S, Rockey DC. Obscure gastrointestinal bleeding. *Gastroenterol Clin North Am.* 2005;34(4):679.
275. Hyare H, Desigan S, Brookes JA, et al. Endovascular management of major arterial hemorrhage as a complication of inflammatory pancreatic disease. *J Vasc Interv Radiol.* 2007;18(5):591.
276. Zyromski NJ, Vieira C, Stecker M, et al. Improved outcomes in postoperative and pancreatitis-related visceral pseudoaneurysms. *J Gastrointest Surg.* 2007;11(1):50.
277. Nicholson AA, Patel J, McPherson S, et al. Endovascular treatment of visceral aneurysms associated with pancreatitis and a suggested classification with therapeutic implications. *J Vasc Interv Radiol.* 2006;17(8):1279.
278. Snyder HS. Significance of the initial spun hematocrit in trauma patients. *Am J Emerg Med.* 1998;16:150.
279. Greenfield RH, Bessen HA, Henneman PL. Effect of crystalloid infusion on hematocrit and intravascular volume in healthy nonbleeding subjects. *Ann Emerg Med.* 1989;18:51.
280. Kass LE, Tien IY, Ushkow BS, et al. Prospective crossover study of the effect of phlebotomy and intravenous crystalloid on hematocrit. *Acad Emerg Med.* 1997;4:198.
281. Stamler KD. Effect of crystalloid infusion on hematocrit in non-bleeding patients with application to clinical traumatology. *Ann Emerg Med.* 1989;18:747.
282. Paradis NA, Balter S, Davison CM, et al. Hematocrit as a predictor of significant injury after penetrating trauma. *Am J Emerg Med.* 1997;15:224.
283. Zehtabchi S, Sinert R, Goldman M, et al. Diagnostic performance of serial hematocrit measurements in identifying major injury in adult trauma patients. *Injury.* 2006;37:46.
284. Broder G, Weil MH. Excess lactate: an index of reversibility of shock in human patients. *Science.* 1964;143:1457.
285. Bakker J, Coffemils M, Leon M, et al. Blood lactate levels are superior to oxygen-derived variables in predicting outcome in human septic shock. *Chest.* 1992;99:956.
286. Weil MH, Atiti AA. Experimental and clinical studies on lactate and pyruvate as indicators of the severity of acute circulatory failure (shock). *Circulation.* 1970;41:989.
287. Hemming RJ, Weil MH, Weiner F. Blood lactate as a prognostic indicator of survival in patients with acute myocardial infarction. *Circ Shock.* 1982;9:307.
288. Vincent JL, Roman A, Kahn RJ. Dobutamine administration in septic shock: addition to a standard protocol. *Crit Care Med.* 1990;18: 689.
289. Vincent JL, Dufaye P, Berre J, et al. Serial lactate determinations during circulatory shock. *Crit Care Med.* 1983;11:449.
290. Levy B. Lactate and shock state: the metabolic review. *Curr Opin Crit Care.* 2006;12:315.
291. Fall PJ, Szerlip HM. Lactic acidosis: from sour milk to septic shock. *J Intens Care Med.* 2005;20(5):255.
292. Madias NE. Lactic acidosis. *Kidney Int.* 1986;29:752.
293. Eldridge F, Sulzer J. Effect of respiratory alkalosis on blood lactate and pyruvate in humans. *J Appl Physiol.* 1967;22:461.
294. Wilson M, Davis DP, Coimbra R. Diagnosis and monitoring of hemorrhagic shock during the initial resuscitation of multiple trauma patients: a review. *J Emerg Med.* 2003;24:413.
295. Baron BJ, Scalea TM. Acute blood loss. *Emerg Med Clin North Am.* 1996;14:35.
296. Porter JM, Ivatury RR. In search of the optimal endpoints of resuscitation in trauma patients: a review. *J Trauma.* 1998;44:908.
297. Bilkovski RN, Rivers EP, Horst HM. Targeted resuscitation strategies after injury. *Curr Opin Crit Care.* 2004;10:529.
298. Abramson D, Scalea TM, Hitchcock R, et al. Lactate clearance and survival following injury. *J Trauma.* 1993;35:584.
299. Manikis P, Jankowski S, Zhang H, et al. Correlation of serial blood lactate levels to organ failure and mortality after trauma. *Am J Emerg Med.* 1995;13:619.
300. Rixen D, Siegel JH. Bench-to-bedside review: oxygen debt and its metabolic correlates as quantifiers of the severity of hemorrhagic and post-traumatic shock. *Crit Care.* 2005;9:441.
301. Aslar AK, Kuzu MA, Elhan AH, et al. Admission lactate level and the APACHE II score are the most useful predictors of prognosis following torso trauma. *Injury.* 2004;35:746.
302. Dunne JR, Tracy K, Scalea TM, et al. Lactate and base deficit in trauma: does alcohol or drug use impair their predictive accuracy? *J Trauma.* 2005;58:959.
303. Kaplan LJ, Kellum JA. Initial pH, base deficit, lactate, anion gap, strong ion difference, and strong ion gap predict outcome from major vascular injury. *Crit Care Med.* 2004;32:1120.
304. Martin MJ, FitzSullivan E, Salim A, et al. Discordance between lactate and

base deficit in the surgical intensive care unit: which one do you trust? *Am J Surg.* 2006;191:625.

305. Waxman K, Nolan LS, Shoemaker WC. Sequential perioperative lactate determination. Physiological and clinical implications. *Crit Care Med.* 1982;10:96.
306. Lavery RF, Livingston DH, Tortella BJ, et al. The utility of venous lactate to triage injured patients in the trauma center. *J Am Coll Surg.* 2000;190(6):656.
307. Rutherford EJ, Morris JA, Reed GW, et al. Base deficit is stratifies mortality and determines therapy. *J Trauma.* 1992;33:417.
308. Davis JW, Parks SN, Kaups KL, et al. Admission base deficit predicts transfusion requirements and risk of complications. *J Trauma.* 1996;41:769.
309. Davis JW, Kaups KL, Parks SN. Base deficit is superior to pH in evaluating clearance of acidosis after traumatic shock. *J Trauma.* 1998;44:114.
310. Davis JW, Kaups KL. Base deficit in the elderly: a marker of severe injury and death. *J Trauma.* 1998;45:873.
311. Randolph LC, Takacs M, Davis KA. Resuscitation in the pediatric trauma population: admission base deficit remains an important prognostic indicator. *J Trauma.* 2002;53:838.
312. Peterson DL, Schinco MA, Kerwin AJ, et al. Evaluation of initial base deficit as a prognosticator of outcome in the pediatric trauma population. *Am Surg.* 2004;70(4):326.
313. Sauaia A, Moore FA, Moore EE, et al. Early risk factors for post-injury multiple organ failure. *World J Surg.* 1996;20:392.
314. Martin MJ, FitzSullivan E, Salim A, et al. Use of serum bicarbonate measurement in place of arterial base deficit in the surgical intensive care unit. *Arch Surg.* 2005;140:745.
315. FitzSullivan E, Salim A, Demetriades D, et al. Serum bicarbonate may replace the arterial base deficit in the trauma intensive care unit. *Am J Surg.* 2005;190:961.
316. Mikulaschek A, Henry SM, Donovan R, et al. Serum lactate is not predicted by anion gap or base excess after trauma resuscitation. *J Trauma.* 1996;40:218.
317. Singhal R, Coghill JE, Guy A, et al. Serum lactate and base deficit as predictors of mortality after ruptured abdominal aortic aneurysm repair. *Eur J Vasc Endovasc Surg.* 2005;30(3):263.
318. Brohi K, Singh J, Heron M, et al. Acute traumatic coagulopathy. *J Trauma.* 2003;54:1127.
319. MacLeod JBA, Lynn M, McKenney MG, et al. Early coagulopathy predicts mortality in trauma. *J Trauma.* 2003;55:39.
320. Hess JR, Lawson JH. The coagulopathy of trauma versus disseminated intravascular coagulation. *J Trauma.* 2006;60:S12.
321. Brohi K, Cohen MJ, Ganter MT, et al. Acute traumatic coagulopathy: initiated by hypoperfusion. Modulated through the protein C pathway? *Ann Surg.* 2007;245:812.
322. Practice guidelines for perioperative blood transfusion and adjuvant therapies: an updated report by the American Society of Anesthesiologists Task Force on Perioperative Blood Transfusion and Adjuvant Therapies. *Anesthesiology.* 2006;105:198.
323. Roissant R, Cerny V, Coats TJ, et al. Key issues in advanced bleeding care in trauma. *Shock.* 2006;26(4):322.
324. Zuckerman L, Cohen E, Vagher JP, et al. Comparison of thromboelastography with common coagulation tests. *Thromb Haemost.* 1981;46:752.
325. Kaufmann CR, Dwyer KM, Crews JD, et al. Usefulness of thromboelastography in assessment of trauma patient coagulation. *J Trauma.* 1997;42:716.
326. Rugeri L, Levrat A, David JS, et al. Diagnosis of early coagulation abnormalities in trauma patients by rotation thrombelastography. *J Thromb Haemost.* 2007;5(2):289.
327. Coakley M, Reddy K, Mackie I, et al. Transfusion triggers in orthotopic liver transplantation: a comparison of the thromboelastometry analyzer, the thromboelastogram, and conventional coagulation tests. *J Cardiothorac Vasc Anesth.* 2006;20(4):548.
328. Ronald A, Dunning J. Can the use of thromboelastography predict and decrease bleeding and blood and blood product requirements in adult patients undergoing cardiac surgery? *Interact Cardiovasc Thorac Surg.* 2005;4(5):456.
329. Spalding GJ, Hartrumpg M, Sierig T, et al. Cost reduction of perioperative coagulation management in cardiac surgery: value of "bedside" thromboelastography (ROTEM). *Eur J Cardiothorac Surg.* 2007;31(6):1052.
330. Hobson AR, Agarwala RA, Swallow RA, et al. Thromboelastography: current clinical applications and its potential role in interventional cardiology. *Platelets.* 2006;17(8):509.
331. Zambruni A, Thalheimer U, Leandro G, et al. Thromboelastography with citrated blood: comparability with native blood, stability of citrate storage, and effect of repeated sampling. *Blood Coagul Fibrinolysis* 2004;15:103.
332. Pivalizza EG, Pivalizza PJ, Gottschalk LI, et al. Celite-activated thromboelastography in children. *J Clin Anesth.* 2001;13:20.
333. Gorton HJ, Warren ER, Simpson NS, et al. Thromboelastography identifies sex-related differences in coagulation. *Anesth Analg.* 2000;91:1279.
334. Camenzind V, Bombeli T, Seifert B, et al. Citrate storage affects thromboelastograph analysis. *Anesthesiology.* 2000;92:1242.
335. Vig S, Chitolie A, Bevan DH, et al. Thromboelastography: a reliable test? *Blood Coagul Fibrinolysis.* 2001;12:555.
336. Rajwal S, Richards M, O'Meara M. The use of recalcified citrated whole blood—a pragmatic approach for thromboelastography in children. *Paediatr Anaesth.* 2004;14:656.
337. Jackson MR, Olson DW, Beckett WC Jr, et al. Abdominal vascular trauma: a review of 106 injuries. *Am Surg.* 1992;58:622.
338. Blocksom JM, Tyburski JG, Sohn RL, et al. Prognostic determinants in duodenal injuries. *Am Surg.* 2004;70:248.
339. Ertel W, Eid K, Keel M, et al. Therapeutic strategies and outcome of polytraumatized patients with pelvic injuries: a six year experience. *Eur J Trauma.* 2000;26:278.
340. Hill DA, West RH, Roncal S. Outcome of patients with haemorrhagic shock: an indicator of performance in a trauma centre. *J R Coll Surg Edinb.* 1995;40:221.
341. Thoburn E, Norris P, Flores R, et al. System care improves trauma outcome: patient care errors dominate reduced preventable death rate. *J Emerg Med.* 1993;11:135.
342. Alberts KA, Brismar B, Nygren A. Major differences in trauma care between hospitals in Sweden: a preliminary report. *Qual Assur Health Care.* 1993;5:13.
343. Peitzman AB, Courcoulas AP, Stinson C, et al. Trauma center maturation: quantification of process and outcome. *Ann Surg.* 1999;230(1):87.
344. Harrington DT, Connolly M, Biffl WL, et al. Transfer times to definitive care facilities are too long: a consequence of an immature trauma system. *Ann Surg.* 2005;241(6):961.
345. Moore R, Nutley M, Cina CS, et al. Improved survival after introduction of an emergency endovascular therapy protocol for ruptured abdominal aortic aneurysms. *J Vasc Surg.* 2007;45:443.
346. Bounoua F, Schuster R, Grewal P, et al. Ruptured abdominal aortic aneurysm: does trauma center designation affect outcome? *Ann Vasc Surg.* 2007;21(2):133.
347. Salhab M, Farmer J, Osman I. Impact of delay on survival in patients with ruptured abdominal aortic aneurysm. *Vascular.* 2006;14(1):38.
348. Hoyt DB, Bulger EM, Knudson MM, et al. Death in the operating room: an analysis of a multicenter experience. *J Trauma.* 1994;37:426.
349. Jurkovich GJ, Greiser WB, Luterman A, et al. Hypothermia in trauma victims: an ominous predictor of survival. *J Trauma.* 1987;27(9):1019.
350. Garrison JR, Richardson JD, Hilakos AS, et al. Predicting the need to pack early for severe intra-abdominal hemorrhage. *J Trauma.* 1996;40(6):923.
351. Sharp KW, Locicero RJ. Abdominal packing for surgically uncontrollable hemorrhage. *Ann Surg.* 1992;215(5):467.
352. Cosgriff N, Moore EE, Sauaia A, et al. Predicting life-threatening coagulopathy in the massively transfused trauma patient: hypothermia and acidosis revisited. *J Trauma.* 1997;42(5):857.
353. Gentilello LM, Pierson DJ. Trauma critical care. *Am J Respir Crit Care Med.* 2001;604.
354. Lee JC, Peitzman AB. Damage control laparotomy. *Curr Opin Crit Care.* 2006;12:346.
355. Morris JA, Eddy VA, Rutherford EJ. The trauma celiotomy: the evolving concepts of damage control. *Curr Probl Surg.* 1996;33:611.
356. Stone HH, Strom PR, Mullins RJ, et al. Management of the major coagulopathy with onset during laparotomy. *Ann Surg.* 1983;197:532.
357. Burch JM, Ortiz VB, Richardson RJ, et al. Abbreviated laparotomy and planned reoperation for critically injured patients. *Ann Surg.* 1992;215:476.
358. Morris JA, Eddy VA, Blinman TA, et al. The staged celiotomy for trauma: issues in packing and reconstruction. *Ann Surg.* 1993;217:576.
359. Moore EE, Burch JM, Franciose RJ, et al. Staged physiologic restoration and damage control surgery. *World J Surg.* 1998;22:1184.
360. Johnson JW, Gracias VH, Schwab CW, et al. Evolution in damage control for exsanguinating penetrating abdominal injury. *J Trauma.* 2001;51:261.
361. Grotz MR, Gummerson NW, Gansslen A, et al. Staged management and outcome of combined pelvic and liver trauma: an international experience of the deadly duo. *Injury.* 2006;37:642.
362. Rotondo MF, Schwab CW, McGonigal MD, et al. "Damage control": an approach for improved survival in exsanguinating penetrating abdominal injury. *J Trauma.* 1993;35:375.
363. Carrillo EH, Spain DA, Wilson MA, et al. Alternatives in the management of penetrating injuries to the iliac vessels. *J Trauma.* 1998;44:1024.
364. Moore EE. Thomas G. Orr Memorial Lecture. Staged laparotomy for the hypothermia, acidosis, and coagulopathy syndrome. *Am J Surg.* 1996;172:405.
365. Rotondo MF, Zonies DH. The damage control sequence and underlying logic. *Surg Clin North Am.* 1997;77:761.
366. Shapiro MB, Jenkins DH, Schwab CW, et al. Damage control: collective review. *J Trauma.* 2000;49:969.
367. Cinat ME, Wallace WC, Nastanski F, et al. Improved survival following massive transfusion in patients who have undergone trauma. *Arch Surg.* 1999;134:964.
368. Holcomb JB, Jenkins D, Rhee P, et al. Damage control resuscitation: directly addressing the early coagulopathy of trauma. *J Trauma.* 2007;62:307.
369. Holcomb JB, Hoyt DB. Damage control resuscitation: the need for specific blood products to treat the coagulopathy of trauma. *Transfusion.* 2006;46:685.
370. Roberts K, Revell M, Youssef H, et al. Hypotensive resuscitation in patients with ruptured abdominal aortic aneurysm. *Eur J Vasc Endovasc Surg.* 2006;31(4):339.

371. Stern SA. Low-volume fluid resuscitation for presumed hemorrhagic shock: helpful or harmful? *Curr Opin Crit Care.* 2001;7(6):422.
372. Kauvar DS, Wade CE. The epidemiology and modern management of traumatic hemorrhage: US and international perspectives. *Crit Care.* 2005;9(Suppl 5):S1.
373. Sondeen JL, Coppes VG, Holcomb JB. Blood pressure at which rebleeding occurs after resuscitation in swine with aortic injury. *J Trauma.* 2003;54(Suppl):S110.
374. Wade CE, Holcomb JB. Endpoints in clinical trials of fluid resuscitation of patients with traumatic injuries. *Transfusion.* 2005;45:4S.
375. Deitch EA, Dayal SD. Intensive care unit management of the trauma patient. *Crit Care Med.* 2006;34:2294.
376. Burris D, Rhee P, Kaufmann C, et al. Controlled resuscitation for uncontrolled hemorrhagic shock. *J Trauma.* 1999;46(2):216.
377. Kwan I, Bunn F, Roberts I. Timing and volume of fluid administration for patients with bleeding. *Cochrane Database Syst Rev.* 2003;CD002245.
378. May AK, Young JS, Butler K, et al. Coagulopathy in severe closed head injury: is empiric therapy warranted? *Am Surg.* 1997;63:233.
379. Alam HB, Stanton K, Koustova E, et al. Effect of different strategies on neutrophil activation in a swine model of hemorrhagic shock. *Resuscitation.* 2004;60(1):91.
380. Ho AM, Karmakar MK, Dion PW. Are we giving enough coagulation factors during trauma resuscitation? *Am J Surg.* 2005;190:479.
381. Faringer PD, Mullins RJ, Johnson RL, et al. Blood component supplementation during massive transfusion of AS-1 red cells in trauma patients. *J Trauma.* 1993;34:481.
382. Hewson JR, Neame PB, Kumar N, et al. Coagulopathy related to dilution and hypotension during massive transfusion. *Crit Care Med.* 1985;13:387.
383. Phillips TF, Soulier G, Wilson RF. Outcome of massive transfusion exceeding two blood volumes in trauma and emergency surgery. *J Trauma.* 1987;27:903.
384. Harvey MP, Greenfield TP, Sugrue ME, et al. Massive blood transfusion in a tertiary referral hospital: clinical outcomes and haemostatic complications. *Med J Aust.* 1995;163:356.
385. Mitchell KJ, Moncure KE, Onyeije C, et al. Evaluation of massive volume replacement in the penetrating trauma patient. *J Natl Med Assoc.* 1994;86:926.
386. Spahn DR, Rossaint R. Coagulopathy and blood component transfusion in trauma. *Br J Anaesth.* 2005;95:130.
387. Gonzalez EA, Moore FA, Holcomb JB, et al. Fresh frozen plasma should be given earlier to patients requiring massive transfusion. *J Trauma.* 2007;62:112.
388. Ketchum L, Hess JR, Hiippala S. Indications for early fresh frozen plasma, cryoprecipitate, and platelet transfusion in trauma. *J Trauma.* 2006;60(6):S51.
389. Malone L, Hess JR, Fingerhut A. Massive transfusion practices around the globe and a suggestion for a common massive transfusion protocol. *J Trauma.* 2006;60(6):S91.
390. Wilson RF, Mammen E, Walt AJ. Eight years experience with massive blood transfusion. *J Trauma.* 1971;11(4):275.
391. Kivioja A, Myllynen P, Rokkanen P. Survival after massive transfusion exceeding four blood volumes in patients with blunt injuries. *Am Surg.* 1991;57(6):398.
392. Wudel JH, Morris JA, Yates K, et al. Massive transfusion: outcome in blunt trauma patients. *J Trauma.* 1991;31(1):1.
393. Velmahos GC, Chan L, Chan M, et al. Is there a limit to massive blood transfusion after severe trauma? *Arch Surg.* 1998;133:947.
394. Hakala P, Hiippala S, Syrjala M, et al. Massive blood transfusion exceeding 50 units of plasma poor red cells or whole blood: the survival rate and the occurrence of leucopenia and acidosis. *Injury.* 1999;30:619.
395. Vaslef SN, Knudsen NW, Neligan PJ, et al. Massive transfusion exceeding 50 units of blood products in trauma patients. *J Trauma.* 2002;53(2):291.
396. Huber-Wagner S, Qvick M, Mussack T, et al. Massive blood transfusion and outcome in 1062 polytrauma patients: a prospective study based on the trauma registry of the German Trauma Society. *Vox Sang.* 2007;92:69.
397. Codner P, Cinat ME. Massive transfusion for trauma is appropriate. *Trauma Care, The Official Publication of ITACCS.* 2005;15(3):148.
398. Hirschberg A, Dugas M, Banez EI, et al. Minimizing dilutional coagulopathy in exsanguinating hemorrhage: a computer simulation. *J Trauma.* 2003;54:454.
399. Ho AM, Dion PW, Cheng CAY, et al. A mathematical model for fresh frozen plasma transfusion strategies during major trauma resuscitation with ongoing hemorrhage. *Can J Surg.* 2005;48(6):470.
400. Hardy JF, de Moerloose P, Samama CM. The coagulopathy of massive transfusion. *Vox Sang.* 2005;89:123.
401. Hardy JF, Moerloose P, Samama CM, et al. Massive transfusion and coagulopathy: pathophysiology and implications for clinical management. *Can J Anesth.* 2006;53(6):S40.
402. Erber WN. Massive blood transfusion in the elective surgical setting. *Transfus Apheresis Sci.* 2002;27:83.
403. Kozek-Langenecker S. Management of massive operative blood loss. *Minerva Anesthesiol.* 2007;73:1–15.
404. Silliman CC, Moore EE, Johnson JL, et al. Transfusion of the injured patient: proceed with caution. *Shock.* 2004;21(4):291.
405. McIntyre LA, Hebert PC. Can we safely restrict transfusion in trauma patients? *Curr Opin Crit Care.* 2006;12:575.
406. Dodd RY, Notari EP, Stramer SL. Current prevalence and incidence of infectious disease markers and estimated window-period risk in the American Red Cross donor population. *Transfusion.* 2002;42:975.
407. Kleinman S, Chan P, Robillard P. Risks associated with transfusion of cellular blood components in Canada. *Transfus Med Rev.* 2003;17:120.
408. Blajchmann MA. Incidence and significance of the bacterial contamination of blood components. *Dev Biol (Basel).* 2002;108:59.
409. Schreiber GB, Busch MP, Kleinman SH, et al. The risk of transfusion-transmitted viral infections: the retrovirus epidemiology donor study. *N Engl J Med.* 1996;334:1685.
410. Zallen G, Offner PJ, Moore EE, et al. Age of transfused blood is an independent risk factor for postinjury multiple organ failure. *Am J Surg.* 1999;178:570.
411. Biffl WL, Moore EE, Offner PJ, et al. Plasma from aged stored red blood cells delays neutrophil apoptosis and primes for cytotoxicity: abrogation by poststorage washing by not prestorage leukoreduction. *J Trauma.* 2001;50:426.
412. Offner PJ, Moore EE, Biffl WL, et al. Increased rate of infection associated with transfusion of old blood after severe injury. *Arch Surg.* 2002;137:711.
413. Murrell Z, Haukoos JS, Putnam B, et al. The effect of older blood on mortality, need for ICU care, and the length of stay after major trauma. *Am Surg.* 2005;71:781.
414. Heddle NM, Soutar RI, Ohoski PL, et al. A prospective study to determine the frequency and clinical significance of alloimmunization post-transfusion. *Br J Haematol.* 1995;91:1000.
415. Dutton RP, Shih D, Edelman BB, et al. Safety of uncrossmatched Type-O red cells for resuscitation from hemorrhagic shock. *J Trauma.* 2005;59:1445.
416. Shaffer LG, Phillips MD. Successful treatment of acquired hemophilia with oral immunosuppressive therapy. *Ann Intern Med.* 1997;127:206.
417. Kleinman S, Caulfield T, Chan P, et al. Toward an understanding of transfusion-related acute lung injury: statement of a consensus panel. *Transfusion.* 2004;44:1774.
418. Bux J, Sachs UJH. The pathogenesis of transfusion-related acute lung injury. *Br J Haematol.* 2007;136:788.
419. Bux J. Transfusion-related acute lung injury (TRALI): a serious adverse event of blood transfusion. *Vox Sang.* 2005;89:1.
420. Triulzi DJ. Transfusion-related acute lung injury: an update. *Hematol Am Soc Hematol Educ Program.* 2006;497.
421. Curtis BR, McFarland JG. Mechanisms of transfusion-related acute lung injury (TRALI): anti-leukocyte antibodies. *Crit Care Med.* 2006; 34(Suppl):S118.
422. Zupanska B, Uhrynowska M, Michur H, et al. Transfusion-related acute lung injury and leucocyte-reacting antibodies. *Vox Sang.* 2007;93:70.
423. Eder AF, Herron R, Strupp A, et al. Transfusion-related acute lung injury surveillance (2003-2005) and the potential impact of the selective use of plasma from male donors in the American Red Cross. *Transfusion.* 2007;47:599.
424. Gajic O, Gropper MA, Hubmayr RD. Pulmonary edema after transfusion: how to differentiate transfusion-associated circulatory overload from transfusion-related acute lung injury. *Crit Care Med.* 2006;34(Suppl):S109.
425. Swanson K, Dwyre DM, Krochmal J, et al. Transfusion-related acute lung injury (TRALI): current clinical and pathophysiologic considerations. *Lung.* 2006;184:177.
426. Dutton RP, McCunn M, Hyder M, et al. Factor VIIa for correction of traumatic coagulopathy. *J Trauma.* 2004;57(4):709.
427. Boffard KD, Riou B, Warren B, et al. Recombinant factor VIIa as adjunctive therapy for bleeding control in severely injured trauma patients: two parallel randomized, placebo-controlled, double-blind clinical trials. *J Trauma.* 2005;59:8.
428. Rizoli SB, Boffard KD, Riou B, et al. Recombinant activated factor VII as an adjunctive therapy for bleeding control in severe trauma patients with coagulopathy: subgroup analysis from two randomized trials. *Crit Care.* 2006;10:R178.
429. Perkins JG, Schreiber MA, Wade CE, et al. Early versus late recombinant factor VIIa in combat trauma patients requiring massive transfusion. *J Trauma.* 2007;62:1095.
430. Harrison TD, Laskosky J, Jazaeri O, et al. "Low dose" recombinant activated factor VII results in less blood and blood product use in traumatic hemorrhage. *J Trauma.* 2005;59:150.
431. Stein DM, Dutton RP, O'Connor J, et al. Determinants of futility of administration of recombinant factor VIIa in trauma. *J Trauma.* 2005;59:609.
432. Martinowitz U, Michaelson M. Guidelines for the use of recombinant activated factor VII (rFVIIa) in uncontrolled bleeding: a report by the Israeli Multidisciplinary rFVIIa Task Force. *J Thromb Haemost.* 2005;3:640.
433. Rizoli SB, Nascimento B, Osman F, et al. Recombinant activated coagulation factor VII and bleeding trauma patients. *J Trauma.* 2006;61:1419.
434. Lodge JPA, Jonas S, Jones RM, et al. Efficacy and safety of repeated perioperative doses of recombinant factor VIIa in liver transplantation. *Liver Transpl.* 2005;11:973.
435. Filsoufi F, Castillo JG, Rahmanian PB, et al. Effective management of refractory postcardiotomy bleeding with the use of recombinant activated factor VII. *Ann Thorac Surg.* 2006;82:1779.
436. Diprose P, Herbertson MJ, O'Shaughnessy D, et al. Activated recombinant

factor VII after cardiopulmonary bypass reduces allogeneic transfusion in complex non-coronary cardiac surgery: randomized double-blind placebo controlled pilot study. *Br J Anaesth.* 2005;95(5):596.
437. Grounds RM, Seebach C, Knothe C, et al. Use of recombinant factor VII (Novoseven) in trauma and surgery: analysis of outcomes reported to an international society. *J Intensive Care Med.* 2006;21:27.
438. Vincent JL, Rossaint R, Riou B, et al. Recommendations on the use of recombinant activated factor VII as an adjunctive treatment for massive bleeding—a European perspective. *Crit Care.* 2006;10:R120.
439. Scarpelini S, Rizoli S. Recombinant factor VIIa and the surgical patient. *Curr Opin Crit Care.* 2006;12:351.
440. Kaw LL, Coimbra R, Potenza BM, et al. The use of recombinant factor VIIa for severe intractable bleeding during spine surgery. *Spine.* 2004;29:1384.
441. Shao YF, Yang JM, Chau GY, et al. Safety and hemostatic effect of recombinant activated factor VII in cirrhotic patients undergoing partial hepatectomy: a multicenter, randomized, double-blind, placebo-controlled trial. *Am J Surg.* 2006;191:245.
442. Friederich PW, Henry CP, Messelink EJ, et al. Effect of recombinant activated factor VII on perioperative blood loss in patients undergoing retropubic prostatectomy: a double-blind placebo-controlled randomized trial. *Lancet.* 2003;361:201.
443. Bosch J, Thabut D, Bendtsen F, et al. Recombinant factor VIIa for upper gastrointestinal bleeding in patients with cirrhosis: a randomized, double-blind, trial. *Gastroenterology.* 2004;127:1123.
444. Aledort LM. Comparative thrombotic event incidence after infusion of recombinant factor VIIa versus factor VIII inhibitor bypass activity. *J Thromb Haemost.* 2004;2:1700.
445. Roberts HR, Monroe DM III, Hoffman M. Safety profile of recombinant factor VIIa. *Semin Hematol.* 2004;41(1 Suppl 1):101.
446. Levi M, Peters M, Buller HR. Efficacy and safety of recombinant factor VIIa for treatment of severe bleeding: a systematic review. *Crit Care Med.* 2005;33:883.
447. Mannucci PM, Levi M. Prevention and treatment of major blood loss. *N Engl J Med.* 2007;356:2301.
448. Brown JR, Birkmeyer NJO, O'Connor GT. Meta-analysis comparing the effectiveness and adverse outcomes of antifibrinolytic agents in cardiac surgery. *Circulation.* 2007;115:2801.
449. Mangano DT, Tudor JC, Dietzel C, et al. The risk associated with aprotinin in cardiac surgery. *N Engl J Med.* 2006;354:353.
450. Mangano DT, Miao Y, Vuylsteke A, et al. Mortality associated with aprotinin during 5 years following coronary artery bypass graft surgery. *JAMA.* 2007;297(5):471.
451. Bridges CR. Valid comparisons of antifibrinolytic agents used in cardiac surgery. *Circulation.* 2007;115:2790.
452. Henry DA, Moxey AJ, Carless PA, et al. Anti-fibrinolytic use for minimizing perioperative allogeneic blood transfusion. *Cochrane Database Syst Rev.* 2001;1:CD001886.
453. Coats T, Roberts I, Shakur H. Antifibrinolytic drugs for acute traumatic injury (review). *Cochrane Database Syst Rev.* 2004;4:CD004896.
454. Coats T, Hunt B, Roberts I, et al. Antifibrinolytic agents in traumatic hemorrhage: a large-scale randomized controlled trial is needed. *PLoS Med.* 2005;2(3):e64.
455. Ness PM, Cushing MM. Oxygen therapeutics: pursuit of an alternative to the donor red blood cell. *Arch Pathol Lab Med.* 2007;131:734.
456. Jahr JS, Walker V, Manoochehri K. Blood substitutes as pharmacotherapies in clinical practice. *Curr Opin Anaesthesiol.* 2007;20:235.
457. Moore EE, Johnson JL, Cheng AM, et al. Insights from studies of blood substitutes in trauma. *Shock.* 2005;24(3):197.
458. Bulger EM, Cuschieri J, Warner K, et al. Hypertonic resuscitation modulates the inflammatory response in patients with traumatic hemorrhagic shock. *Ann Surg.* 2007;245(4):635.
459. Holcroft JW, Vassar MJ, Perry CA. Use of 7.5% NaCl/6% Dextran 70 solution in the resuscitation of injured patients in the emergency room. *Prog Clin Biol Res.* 1989;299:331.
460. Mattox KL, Maningas PA, Moore EE, et al. Prehospital hypertonic saline/dextran infusion for post-traumatic hypotension: the USA multicenter trial. *Ann Surg.* 1991;213:482.
461. Vassar MJ, Perry CA, Gannaway WL, et al. 7.5% sodium chloride/dextran for resuscitation of trauma patients undergoing helicopter transport. *Arch Surg.* 1991;126:1065.
462. Younes RN, Aun F, Accioly CQ, et al. Hypertonic solutions in the treatment of hypovolemic shock: a prospective randomized study in patients admitted to the emergency room. *Surgery.* 1992;111:380.
463. Vassar MJ, Fischer RP, O'Brien PE, et al. A multicenter trial for resuscitation of injured patients with 7.5% sodium chloride: the effect of added dextran 70. The Multicenter Group for the Study of Hypertonic Saline in Trauma Patients. *Arch Surg.* 1993;128:1003.
464. Cooper DJ, Myles PS, McDermott FT, et al. Prehospital hypertonic saline resuscitation of patients with hypotension and severe traumatic brain injury: a randomized controlled trial. *JAMA.* 2004;291:1350.
465. Tyagi R, Donaldson K, Loftus CM. Hypertonic saline: a clinical review. *Neurosurg Rev.* 2007;30:277.
466. Tseng MY, Al-Rawi PG, Czosnyka M, et al. Enhancement of cerebral blood flow using systemic hypertonic saline therapy improves outcome in patient with poor-grade spontaneous subarachnoid hemorrhage. *J Neurosurg.* 2007;107(2):274.
467. Kolsen-Petersen JA. Immune effect of hypertonic saline: fact or fiction? *Acta Anaesthesiol Scand.* 2004;48:667.
468. Junger WG, Coimbra R, Liu FC, et al. Hypertonic saline resuscitation: a tool to modulate immune function in trauma patients? *Shock.* 1997;8:235.
469. Homma H, Deitch EA, Feketeova E, et al. Small volume resuscitation with hypertonic saline is more effective in ameliorating trauma-hemorrhagic shock-induced lung injury, neutrophil-activation, and red blood cell dysfunction than pancreatic protease inhibition. *J Trauma.* 2005;59:266.
470. Coimbra R, Loomis W, Melbostad H, et al. Role of hypertonic saline and pentoxifylline on neutrophil activation and tumor necrosis factor-alpha synthesis: a novel resuscitation strategy. *J Trauma.* 2005;59(2):257.
471. Rotstein O. Novel strategies for immunomodulation after trauma: revisiting hypertonic saline as a resuscitation strategy for hemorrhagic shock. *J Trauma.* 2000;49:580.
472. Deree J, Martins JO, Leedom A, et al. Hypertonic saline and pentoxifylline reduces hemorrhagic shock resuscitation-induced pulmonary inflammation through attenuation of neutrophil degranulation and proinflammatory mediator synthesis. *J Trauma.* 2007;62(1):104.
473. Cryer HM, Gosche J, Harbrecht J, et al. The effect of hypertonic saline resuscitation on responses to severe hemorrhagic shock by the skeletal muscle, intestinal, and renal microcirculation systems: seeing is believing. *Am J Surg.* 2005;190:305.
474. Wade C, Grady J, Kramer G. Efficacy of hypertonic saline dextran (HSD) in patients with traumatic hypotension: meta-analysis of individual patient data. *Acta Anaesthesiol Scand Suppl.* 1997;110:77.
475. Wade CE, Grady JJ, Kramer GC. Efficacy of hypertonic saline dextran fluid resuscitation for patient with hypotension and penetrating trauma. *J Trauma.* 2004;54(Suppl 5):144.
476. Wade CE, Grady JJ, Kramer GC. Individual patient cohort analysis of the efficacy of hypertonic saline/dextran in patients with traumatic brain injury. *J Trauma.* 1997;42(Suppl 5):61.
477. Wade CE, Kramer GC, Grady JJ, et al. Efficacy of hypertonic 7.5% saline and 6% dextran-70 in treating trauma: a meta-analysis of controlled clinical studies. *Surgery.* 1997;122:609.
478. Alam HB, Koustova E, Rhee P. Combat casualty care research: from bench to the battlefield. *World J Surg.* 2005;29:S7.

CHAPTER 59 ■ NEUROGENIC SHOCK

SUSANNE MUEHLSCHLEGEL • DAVID M. GREER

Neurologically injured patients, regardless of the nature of the injury, frequently experience hypotension and shock. *Neurogenic shock* refers to a neurologically mediated form of circulatory system failure that can occur with acute brain, spinal cord, or even peripheral nerve injuries. In this chapter, we will explain the epidemiology, pathophysiology, clinical presentation, and management strategies for this special form of shock.

Contrary to common belief, neurogenic shock is not a single entity due to one single pathologic mechanism. The term is sometimes used in nonneuroscience intensive care units to explain hypotension occurring in any brain-injured patient, but neurogenic shock should be considered only after systemic causes of shock have been carefully ruled out. Just like other critically ill patients, neurologically ill patients are prone to developing systemic conditions, such as dehydration, congestive heart failure, acute blood loss, sepsis, pericardial tamponade, or massive pulmonary embolism.

SUBTYPES OF NEUROGENIC SHOCK

Once other systemic reasons for shock have been ruled out, neurogenic shock should be considered. Three mechanisms can lead to neurogenic shock (Fig. 59.1):

- *Vasodilatory (distributive) shock* from autonomic disturbance with interruption of sympathetic pathways, with associated parasympathetic excitation, which causes profound vasodilatation and bradycardia, as seen in spinal cord injury or diseases of the peripheral nervous system (Guillain-Barré syndrome)
- *Cardiogenic shock*, as frequently seen in subarachnoid hemorrhage (SAH) with stunned myocardium after a catecholamine surge or ischemic stroke, especially those involving the right insula
- Hypopituitarism/adrenal insufficiency.

Although some subtypes of neurogenic shock occur more frequently with certain disease entities—for example, cardiogenic neurogenic shock after SAH, vasodilatory neurogenic shock with spinal cord injury—significant overlap exists between different disease entities (intracerebral hemorrhage [ICH], SAH, traumatic brain injury [TBI], ischemic stroke), and one cannot establish a firm rule by which neurogenic shock occurs. Interestingly, only some patients with neurologic injuries experience true neurogenic shock, and it remains difficult to predict in whom this will be seen.

INCIDENCE OF NEUROGENIC SHOCK

Due to the small number of prospective epidemiologic studies, it is difficult to establish the natural incidence of neurogenic shock. In a retrospective review of cervical spinal cord injuries, Bilello et al. (1) reported a 31% incidence of neurogenic shock with hypotension and bradycardia after high cervical spinal cord injury (C1–C5) and 24% after low cervical spinal cord injury (C6–C7).

Cardiogenic neurogenic shock has been studied foremost in SAH and ischemic stroke. Banki et al. (2) prospectively studied the incidence of left ventricular (LV) dysfunction with transthoracic echocardiography (TTE) in the first 7-day period after SAH in 173 patients. Thirteen percent had a normal ejection fraction (EF) but had regional wall motion abnormalities that did not correlate with coronary artery territories, and 15% had an LVEF of less than 50%. Others report a 9% incidence of LV wall motion abnormalities, resulting in hypotension requiring vasopressor therapy, as well as pulmonary edema in most (80%) of these patients (3). The spectrum of injury can range from mild to severe systolic dysfunction—the latter defined as an EF less than 30%. Polick et al. (4) observed LV abnormalities on TTE in 4 of 13 patients (31%) studied within 48 hours of SAH. Resolution of these neurologically mediated wall motion abnormalities is usually seen (2,3,5).

The third subtype of neurogenic shock, adrenal insufficiency, has been studied primarily in traumatic brain injury. In the largest study to date, adrenal insufficiency occurred in about 50% of patients and led to hypotension in 26% (6). Although it has been documented in other cases of acute brain injury, the exact incidence and relationship to outcome is not clear (7).

PATHOPHYSIOLOGY OF NEUROGENIC SHOCK

Vasodilatory Neurogenic Shock

This variation of neurogenic shock is commonly seen with spinal cord injuries and Guillain-Barré syndrome (acute demyelinating peripheral neuropathy) but also with traumatic brain injuries, large hemispheric ischemic strokes, and intracerebral hemorrhages. The hallmark of vasodilatory neurogenic shock is the combination of bradycardia with fluctuating blood pressures and heart rate variability due to interruption of sympathetic output and excitation of parasympathetic fibers.

The sympathetic fibers originate in the hypothalamus, giving rise to neurons projecting to autonomic centers in the

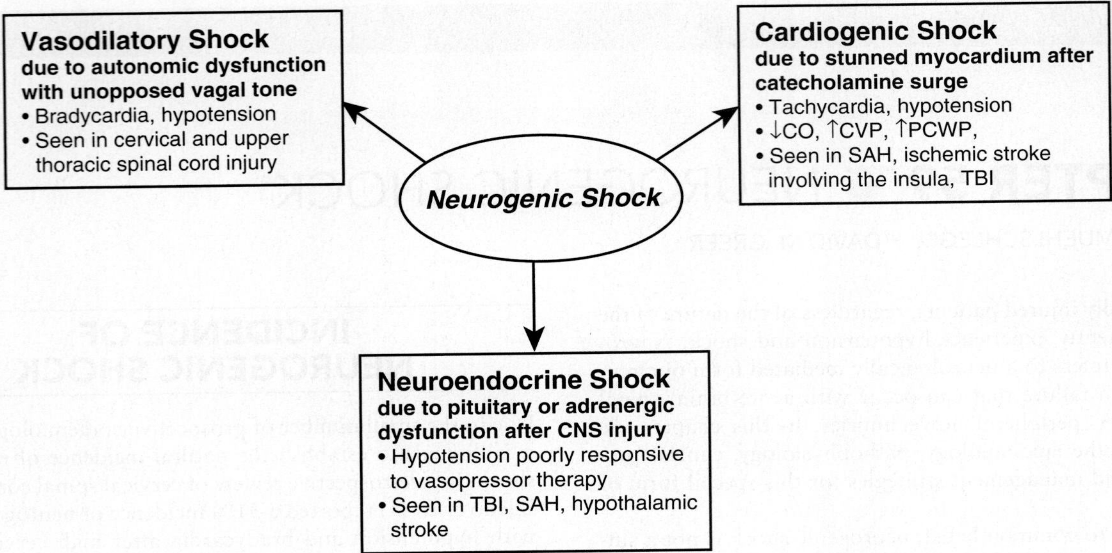

FIGURE 59.1. Neurogenic shock consists of three pathomechanisms. CNS, central nervous system; CO, cardiac output; CVP, central venous pressure; PCWP, pulmonary capillary wedge pressure; SAH, subarachnoid hemorrhage; TBI, traumatic brain injury.

brainstem—the periaqueductal gray matter in the midbrain, the parabrachial regions in the pons, and the intermediate reticular formation located in the ventrolateral medulla. From here, neurons project to nuclei in the spinal cord. The sympathetic preganglionic neurons originate in the intermediolateral cell column within the spinal cord gray matter between T1 and L2 and are therefore called the thoracolumbar branches. From here, they exit the spinal cord and project to 22 pairs of paravertebral sympathetic trunk ganglia next to the vertebral column. The main ganglia within the sympathetic trunk are the cervical and stellate ganglia. The adrenal medulla receives preganglionic fibers and thus is equivalent to a sympathetic ganglion. Blood pressure control depends on tonic activation of the sympathetic preganglionic neurons by descending input from the supraspinal structures (8).

The parasympathetic nervous system consists of cranial and sacral aspects. The cranial subdivision originates from the parasympathetic brainstem nuclei of cranial nerves III, VII, IX, X, and XI. The cranial parasympathetic neurons travel along the cranial nerves until they synapse in the parasympathetic ganglia in close proximity to the target organ. The sacral subdivision originates in the sacral spinal cord (S2–S4), forming the lateral intermediate gray zone where preganglionic neurons travel with the pelvic nerves to the inferior hypogastric plexus and synapse on parasympathetic ganglia within the target organs.

Following a spinal cord injury, the sympathetic pathways are interrupted with dissociation of the sympathetic supply from higher control below the level of transection (9,10). Parasympathetic fibers are usually spared. This results in autonomic hyperreflexia with associated hypertension or hypotension with bradycardia, all observed in human studies as well as in animal models (10–13). Loss of supraspinal control of the sympathetic nervous system leads to unopposed vagal tone with relaxation of vascular smooth muscles below the level of the cord injury, resulting in decreased venous return, decreased cardiac output, hypotension, loss of diurnal fluctuations of blood pressure, reflex bradycardia, and peripheral adrenoreceptor hyperresponsiveness (14). The latter accounts for the excessive vasopressor response repeatedly seen in this clinical scenario. The acute phase, also known as *spinal shock*, more frequently consists of periods of hypotension. After the acute phase, starting about 2 months after the injury, autonomic dysreflexia occurs in patients with lesions above T5 (15). This state is characterized by sympathetically mediated vasoconstriction in muscular, skin, renal, and presumably gastrointestinal vascular beds, induced by afferent peripheral stimulation below the level of the lesion. For example, stimuli such as urinary catheterization, dressing changes, or surgical stimulation can lead to severe blood pressure spikes out of proportion to the stimulus. In Guillain-Barré syndrome, the autonomic dysregulation is likely caused by acute demyelination not only of sensory and motor fibers, but also of autonomic fibers.

Injury to the brain can also lead to vasodilatory neurogenic shock. Certain cerebral structures, such as the insular cortex, amygdala, lateral hypothalamus, and medulla, have great influence on the autonomic nervous system. Cortical asymmetry is present and is reflected in a higher incidence of tachycardia, ventricular arrhythmias, and hypertension with lesions of the right insula—resulting in loss of parasympathetic input and thus sympathetic predominance—and a higher incidence of bradycardia and hypotension with injuries to the left insula—resulting in a loss of sympathetic input and subsequent parasympathetic predominance (16–18) (Fig. 59.2).

Cardiogenic Neurogenic Shock

This form of neurogenic shock is primarily encountered in SAH and TBI but is also seen in ischemic stroke and intracerebral hemorrhage. Cardiac dysfunction is a well-known complication of ischemic and hemorrhagic stroke, first described over 50 years ago (19). It is most often recognized on the electrocardiogram (ECG) as arrhythmias, QRS, ST-segment, and

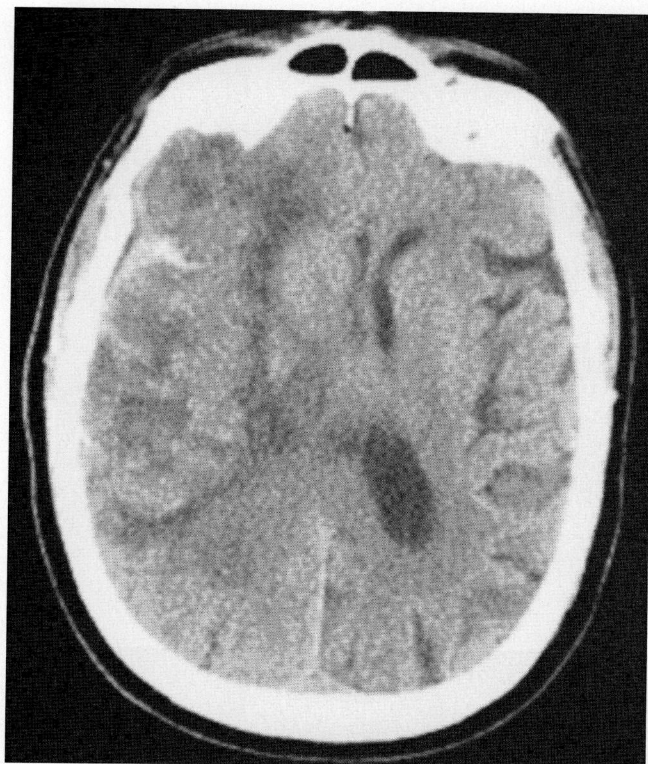

FIGURE 59.2. Example of a right ischemic stroke resulting in ventricular arrhythmias and cardiogenic shock. A 61-year-old man presents with sudden onset of left hemiparesis affecting his face and arm, left-sided neglect, and a left hemianopia. He presented outside of any acute treatment window and did not undergo thrombolysis. He was admitted to the neurointensive care unit (NICU) for close monitoring of his cardiac and respiratory function. The noncontrast head CT shows a right middle cerebral artery stroke and incidental hemorrhagic conversion. Electrocardiogram on admission showed diffuse T-wave inversion in all leads. Telemetry monitoring revealed frequent premature ventricular complexes and intermittent nonsustained ventricular tachycardia of 4 to 8 beats for the first 72 hours after stroke onset. His systolic blood pressure on admission was elevated at 190 mm Hg but then dropped to 85 mm Hg several hours after admission to the NICU, requiring vasopressor support for 2 days. Troponin T levels were elevated in the emergency room and peaked at 12 hours after stroke onset. Echocardiogram showed global hypokinesis and no regional wall motion abnormalities. No other causes for shock were found, so that the stroke involving the right insula was the most likely cause. The shock slowly resolved over 72 hours, and vasopressor infusion was weaned off successfully. A repeat echocardiogram 2 weeks later showed resolution of the abnormalities.

T-wave abnormalities (20,21). Studies of SAH and cardiac injury have shown that the severity of SAH is an independent predictor of cardiac injury, supporting the hypothesis that cardiac neurogenic shock is a neurally mediated process (22). Based on the similarities observed between pheochromocytoma crisis and SAH, the cardiovascular changes have been linked to a catecholamine surge.

This hypothesis has been confirmed by many studies. Patients with SAH can have a threefold increase in norepinephrine levels that are sustained for 10 days or longer after SAH but that normalize after the acute phase of injury (23). In an animal model, an increase in plasma catecholamines after experimental SAH causes specific lesions on electron microscopy within 4 hours of SAH (24). Selective myocardial cell necrosis, also known as contraction band necrosis, is the hallmark of catecholamine exposure (25–27). The same lesions can be found in patients with pheochromocytoma (28) and SAH (29), underlining the pathologic mechanism of cardiac injury in SAH or other neurologic injuries (Fig. 59.3). The cardiac dysfunction is not related to coronary atherosclerosis, as normal coronary arteries have been documented in these patients studied at autopsy or by coronary angiography (5,29–31). In fact, it appears that pre-existing heart disease, such as hypertensive heart disease, might even be *protective* of this form of neurogenic shock (32). In a case series of 54 consecutive SAH deaths, 42 had myocardial lesions consisting of foci of necrotic muscle fibers, hemorrhages, and inflammatory cells, none of which were found in the control group. Patients with a wider range of heart rate and blood pressure fluctuations were more likely to have myocardial lesions. Pre-existing hypertensive heart disease led to significantly fewer myocardial lesions, possibly reflecting a decreased sensitivity of these patients to the catecholamine surge (32).

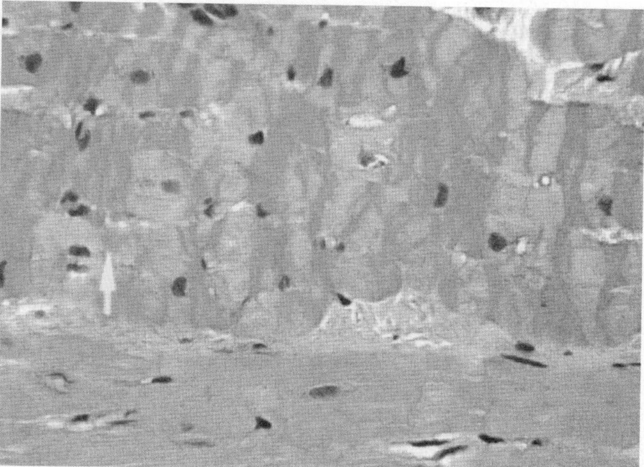

FIGURE 59.3. Contraction band necrosis. Histologic examination of the myocardium, showing contraction band necrosis, see *arrow*. (Courtesy of Dr. James R. Stone, M.D., Ph.D., Department of Pathology, Massachusetts General Hospital, Boston, MA.)

Pathologic studies link the central catecholamine release to the posterior hypothalamus. Postmortem studies have found microscopic hypothalamic lesions consisting of small hemorrhages and infarctions in those patients with typical myocardial lesions as noted above (29,32–34). However, it appears that raised intracranial pressure (ICP) is not responsible for these hypothalamic changes, as the control group with elevated ICP did not have any hypothalamic injury (32).

Overall, by the described pathomechanism, the catecholamine surge results in direct myocardial injury resulting in decreased inotropy, and in addition an increase in cardiac preload due to venous constriction and increased cardiac afterload by peripheral arterial constriction. As a consequence, stroke volume diminishes, which cannot be compensated for by reflex tachycardia, thus resulting in decreased cardiac output and shock. This transient LV dysfunction with loss of myocardial compliance (stunning of the myocardium) is reflected by a characteristic shape of the cardiac silhouette on a ventriculogram and on chest radiograph, which has given this disease

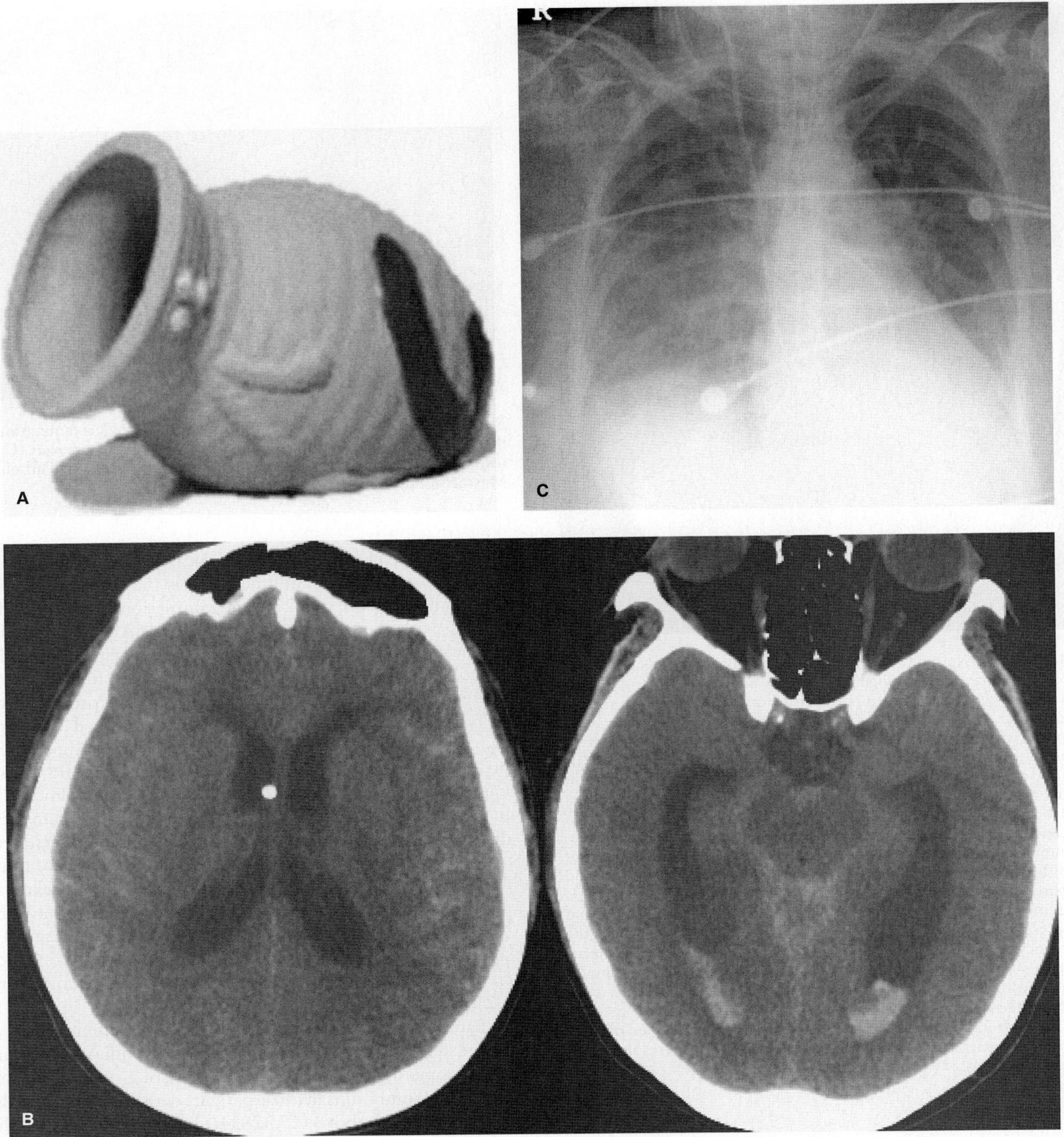

FIGURE 59.4. Takotsubo cardiomyopathy. **A:** Japanese octopus fishing pot. **B:** CT brain of a 47-year-old woman with subarachnoid hemorrhage (SAH). **C:** Chest x-ray view of the same patient with typical cardiac silhouette of Takotsubo cardiomyopathy. An echocardiogram revealed an ejection fraction of 29 degrees with apical ballooning, global hypokinesis, and sparing of the apex. The chest radiograph and echocardiogram became normal within 1 week after her SAH.

entity its other name, Takotsubo cardiomyopathy, derived from the Japanese word for the Japanese octopus fishing pot, *takotsubo* (35–37) (Fig. 59.4).

Pulmonary edema with concomitant hypoxia is frequently encountered in this context and may result from cardiac congestion but can occur independently from the cardiac dysfunction as its own entity: neurogenic pulmonary edema. Massive increases in pulmonary capillary pressures lead to pulmonary edema and hypoxia, which in turn decreases the uptake of oxygen in a high demand state, contributing to hemodynamic instability. The Vietnam war era head injury series (38) reported the rapid onset of acute pulmonary edema after severe head injury. In addition, experimental models as well as multiple human case reports of TBI and SAH have shown massive

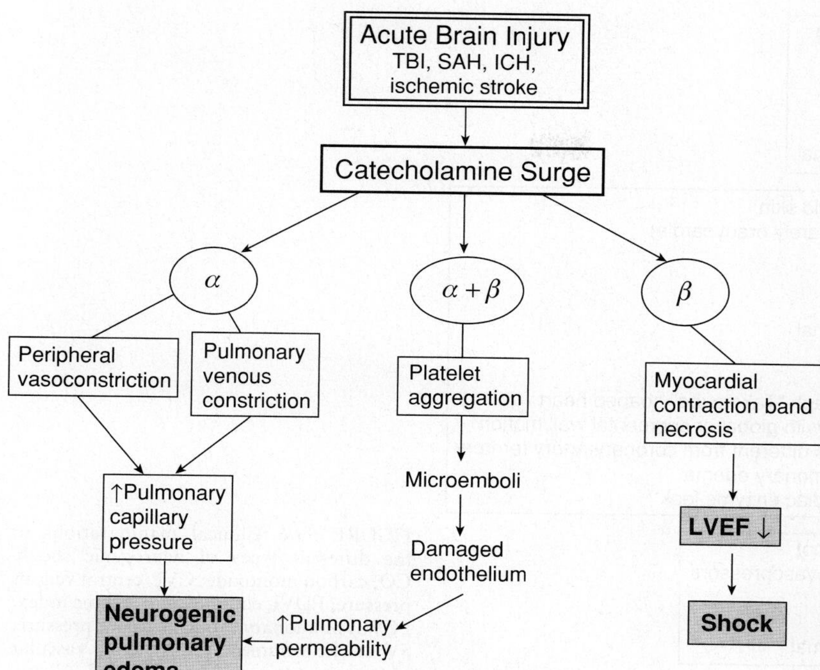

FIGURE 59.5. Summary of the pathophysiology of the cardiogenic type of neurogenic shock. ICH, intracerebral hemorrhage; LVEF, left ventricular ejection fraction; SAH, subarachnoid hemorrhage; TBI, traumatic brain injury.

sympathetic discharges as the primary cause of neurogenic pulmonary edema (39–41). Figure 59.5 summarizes the pathophysiology of cardiogenic neurogenic shock.

Overall, cardiac neurogenic shock, with or without neurogenic pulmonary edema, is usually transient, with resolution within several days to 2 weeks (2–4). Prevention of secondary brain injury from hypoxia and decreased cerebral perfusion pressures should be the focus of care in the management of this neurally mediated complication.

Neuroendocrine Neurogenic Shock

Insufficiency of the hypothalamic-pituitary-adrenal axis has been recognized as an important cause for shock. Inappropriately reduced release of cortisol in stress situations can lead to decreased systemic vascular resistance, reduced cardiac contractility, hypovolemic shock, or hyperdynamic shock that can mimic septic shock. Secondary adrenal insufficiency due to injury to the hypothalamic-hypopituitary feedback loop can cause neuroendocrine neurogenic shock. Acute brain injury, particularly TBI and SAH, can commonly lead to injury of the hypothalamus, pituitary gland, or the connecting structures (42). Cohan et al. (6) revealed that adrenal insufficiency after traumatic brain injury occurred in about half of all patients and led to a significantly higher rate of hypotension in these patients. Most cases of adrenal insufficiency developed within 4 days of injury. Importantly, the authors defined adrenal insufficiency using a low random serum cortisol value and highlight the fact that an increase in the cortisol level after a stimulation test does not rule out the presence of adrenal insufficiency. This issue is particularly relevant in TBI patients, in whom the hypothalamus and the pituitary gland are the likely affected organs, and the adrenal glands might well be expected to mount an appropriate response when stimulated. When recognized, primary and secondary adrenal insufficiency can easily be treated.

In septic shock, a low-dose vasopressin infusion has been shown to successfully restore blood pressure in hypotension refractory to standard catecholamine therapy (43,44). Recent studies in SAH have shown that endogenous vasopressin serum levels are elevated during the first 2 days after SAH but decrease to subnormal levels after 4 days (45–47). Arginine vasopressin supplementation in SAH at low dose (0.01–0.04 units/min) has been studied in only one single retrospective study (48). The role of vasopressin in the setting of neurogenic shock remains to be studied in a prospective manner, but the changes in endogenous vasopressin levels might indicate neuroendocrine changes in neurogenic shock and potential new treatment options in SAH.

CLINICAL MANIFESTATIONS

Figure 59.6 illustrates the clinical manifestations and symptoms seen in neurogenic shock. Acutely, *vasodilatory neurogenic shock* presents with a “warm and dry” hemodynamic profile. The patient is hypotensive and frequently bradycardic; however, the peripheral vessels are dilated, leading to warm limbs and a normal capillary refill time. Central venous pressure (CVP) is normal or low, and systemic venous resistance (SVR) is always low. Stroke volume and cardiac output are low due to the unopposed vagal tone. When a spinal cord injury is present, a difference in smooth muscle and vasculature tone can be observed between the body parts above and below the level of the injury. For example, in an injury at thoracic level 7 (T7), normal upper limb perfusion might be observed, while vasodilatation below T7 leads to warm and dry lower extremities. Orthostatic hypotension without reflex tachycardia on changing from a supine to an upright position—by standing

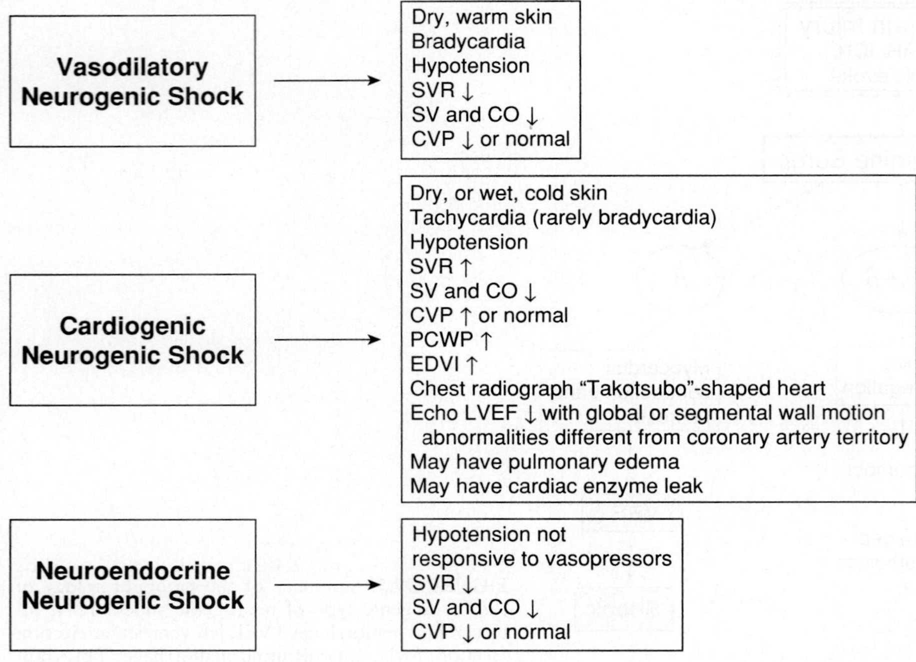

FIGURE 59.6. Clinical manifestations of the different types of neurogenic shock. CO, carbon monoxide; CVP, central venous pressure; EDVI, end-diastolic volume index; PCWP, pulmonary capillary wedge pressure; SV, stroke volume; SVR, systemic vascular resistance.

or with reverse Trendelenburg position—is common. When treating this form of neurogenic shock with a vasopressor infusion (such as phenylephrine or other pressors), extreme caution should be applied, as vasopressor hypersensitivity can lead to severe rebound hypertension, which can be difficult to control.

Cardiogenic neurogenic shock manifests as hypotension and tachycardia, with bradycardia seen rarely. Peripheral vessels are often vasoconstricted, leading to a high SVR and cold and wet skin. Vascular filling, as measured by CVP, pulmonary capillary wedge pressure (PCWP), and end-diastolic volume index (EDVI), is normal or high, with low stroke volumes and cardiac output due to global myocardial dysfunction. Leaking of cardiac enzymes—troponin, creatine kinase (CK), CK-MB—may be seen, but frequently the peak levels are not as high as one would find in myocardial infarction. It is difficult to establish a cutoff value that differentiates stunned myocardium from myocardial infarction with atherosclerotic coronary artery disease. A retrospective study in SAH measuring troponin-I levels has reported an appropriate cutoff value to be 2.8 ng/mL (49), whereas CK-MB did not help differentiate between the two kinds of myocardial injury. Higher levels of troponin should raise the suspicion of true myocardial infarction, and ECG and echocardiography correlation is important.

Neuroendocrine neurogenic shock presents with hypotension that does not respond well to vasopressor infusion. Hemodynamic signs of this category of neurogenic shock are low CVP, SVR, stroke volume, and cardiac output. Low baseline cortisol levels are the hallmark. A cosyntropin stimulation test frequently leads to an appropriate increase in the cortisol level, which *does not* rule out the presence of neuroendocrine neurogenic shock, as the adrenal gland is usually not the primarily affected organ (6). For this reason, we do not find any clinical utility in this test when neuroendocrine neurogenic shock is suspected. Resolution of the hypotension with the use of hydrocortisone clinically confirms the presence of this shock form.

DIAGNOSTIC CONSIDERATIONS

In any case of hypotension and shock in the neurointensive care unit, systemic causes for shock must be ruled out first. Especially in the paralyzed patient (for example, one with a high spinal cord injury), recognition of other life-threatening injuries can be quite difficult. Signs of hypovolemic shock may be absent, even in a patient with profound internal bleeding, because of the absence of sympathetic tone below the level of injury. The usual pallor from vasoconstriction and reflex tachycardia might also be absent. The patient may even be bradycardic while continuing to bleed. For the same reason, signs of peritoneal irritation may be absent in patients with abdominal injuries. The reported incidence of pulmonary embolism (PE) varies tremendously in the neurocritical care patient population—ranging from 0.5% to 20% in ischemic stroke (50,51), to 1% in intracranial hemorrhage (52), to 8.4% in brain tumors (53)—and there are only limited data during the acute phase of subarachnoid hemorrhage, traumatic brain injury, and spinal cord injury (51). Interestingly, according to the study by Skaf et al. (50) using the National Hospital Discharge Survey, the incidence of PE did not change in patients with ischemic and hemorrhagic stroke between 1979 and 2003. However, the death rate from PE in the subgroup with ischemic stroke decreased, likely due to an increased use of antithrombotic prophylaxis over the last 20 years (54). Additionally, over the last two decades, the methods of PE detection have improved immensely—for example, pulmonary CT-angiogram versus nucleotide scan—and autopsy studies report additional asymptomatic cases. In our opinion, the true incidence of PE is underestimated. Pulmonary embolism should always be considered in cases of refractory shock. If profound hypotension is present, or hypotension becomes progressive, reasons other than neurogenic shock should be suspected and thoroughly ruled out.

Every patient should undergo serial ECGs, serial cardiac enzyme measurements, and a chest radiograph. As previously mentioned, pulmonary edema and neurocardiogenic injury may occur together or separately, making chest x-ray films important diagnostic tools. In particular, one should look for pulmonary vascular congestion and evaluate the size and shape of the cardiac silhouette. Hemodynamic monitoring with continuous blood pressure and central venous pressure (CVP) monitoring with an arterial line and central venous line (CVL) should be undertaken. Blood pressure measurements should be done continuously with an arterial line. Arteriosclerosis of the upper extremities is common and should be kept in mind either when there is a large discrepancy between right- and left-sided pressures or when the clinical appearance of the patient does not match the readings from the arterial line. Central venous access is key for determining CVP and for the administration of fluids and medications, especially vasopressors. The site of the placement of the central venous line (CVL) may play an important role in the management of shock in a neurologically injured patient. Subclavian vein catheters are the preferred site in patients with elevated intracranial pressure (ICP), as there is a theoretical risk of venous stasis within the internal jugular vein with venous congestion and higher risk for venous sinus thrombosis, which could result in increased ICP (55). In addition, trauma patients frequently have cervical spine injuries and require cervical collars, making the internal jugular vein accessible only with difficulty.

In patients with cardiogenic neurogenic shock, more extensive hemodynamic monitoring may be necessary with either noninvasive cardiac monitoring devices or a pulmonary artery catheter (PAC). Echocardiography is very important to understanding the etiology of shock. In most cases, a transthoracic echocardiogram is sufficient. The typical echocardiographic appearance is that of apical ballooning, which results from global hypokinesis sparing the apex (56). This part of the heart is devoid of sympathetic nerve terminals, supporting the hypothesis that cardiac injury in SAH is neurally mediated by a sympathetic storm. Segmental wall motion abnormalities not conforming to distinct coronary artery territories is another characteristic echocardiographic finding. However, myocardial infarction from ischemic coronary disease is frequently seen in brain-injured patients, just as in any critically ill patient, and should always be ruled out first as a cause of shock. In the setting of fever and shock, blood cultures must be obtained and the patient appropriately covered with antibiotics until the cultures yield results. However, older and immunosuppressed patients may not mount an appropriate febrile response, and thus sepsis should still be considered in these patients even when they are afebrile, especially in the setting of a rising white blood cell (WBC) count. Cerebral spinal fluid cultures are very important in the neurointensive care unit, with antibiotic coverage of potential central nervous system CNS infections, especially in patients after head trauma with skull fracture or sinus disease, after instrumentation of the head or spinal canal, or in immunocompromised patients. Placement of intracranial pressure measurement devices do not contribute to the diagnostic workup of shock, but they are important tools in the management of neurogenic shock, such as when the goal mean arterial pressure (MAP) is being titrated to the cerebral perfusion pressure. Finally, adrenal insufficiency should always be considered. Random serum cortisol levels should be obtained in the early stages of shock, keeping in mind that in some forms of brain injury, low random serum cortisol levels, and thus adrenal insufficiency, may be encountered for several days after injury (6).

Many neurologically injured patients, especially those with spinal cord injuries, receive steroids while in the neurointensive care unit. The doses administered may be high enough to alter the result of a random serum cortisol level, but often the dose is not enough to treat true adrenal insufficiency appropriately. In these cases, one could either empirically treat with higher doses of steroids that also treat adrenal insufficiency—hydrocortisone, with or without fludrocortisone—or, keeping the potential adverse effects of steroids in acute injury in mind, one could withhold the administration of steroids for 12 hours, then obtain a random cortisol level and resume steroid treatment right after the blood draw. However, hypotension is frequently severe enough that immediate treatment is warranted, and withholding steroids often is not an option. Dexamethasone, which is frequently used in the neurointensive care unit, is the steroid that interferes the least with the cortisol assay after a corticotropin stimulation test and therefore allows for such a test. In cases of high suspicion, a random cortisol level is often preferred because of its simplicity. The cortisol level should be drawn immediately before the steroid dose. However, given the lack of mineralocorticoid activity of dexamethasone, changing to hydrocortisone with or without fludrocortisone is recommended when adrenal insufficiency is suspected.

MANAGEMENT

Two important reasons for early and proactive treatment of patients in neurogenic shock are as follows:

1. Prevention of secondary brain injury from hypoxia and hypotension
2. The fact that neurogenic shock, especially cardiogenic and neuroendocrine forms, is easily treatable and transient, with potentially good outcomes despite the moribund appearance of the patient in the acute phase.

Identifying patients at risk has been very difficult, but at least in SAH it appears that poor neurologic grade, age older than 30 years, and ventricular repolarization abnormalities are risk factors for neurogenic shock (57).

Once the diagnosis of neurogenic shock has been established and the pathophysiology (subtype) has been understood, treatment tailored to the specific subtype is initiated. In all cases, euvolemia is of utmost importance and must be achieved before any other treatment can be successful. In general, vasopressor treatment as a continuous infusion is initiated and titrated to a goal MAP and cerebral perfusion pressure (CPP). As an important management tool, an intracranial pressure measurement device is very helpful, allowing the indirect measurement of CPP. We recommend a goal CPP of greater than or equal to 65 mm Hg. The optimal CPP is not known. Data regarding the minimum tolerable CPP comes from TBI patients, in whom the ICP is often elevated. Several studies have suggested an improved outcome when CPP is maintained at greater than 70 mm Hg (58,59). Other studies using physiologic measurements, such as cerebral blood flow and brain tissue PO_2 ($P_{bt}O_2$), indicate that adverse changes do not occur unless the CPP is below 50 to 60 mm Hg (60,61).

Vasodilatory neurogenic shock can be difficult to treat. In general, vagal tone predominates; however, in this state, patients frequently have peripheral α-adrenoceptor hyperresponsiveness, limiting the use of norepinephrine, epinephrine, ephedrine, and phenylephrine. In fact, sympathomimetics should be avoided as they can lead to severe blood pressure fluctuations. Since arginine vasopressin (AVP) does not affect α- or β-adrenergic receptors, but acts on V1 receptors, AVP may have an advantage over catecholamines or phenylephrine in this form of neurogenic shock. It has not been studied in neurogenic shock, however, and it remains unclear whether AVP may have adverse effects on neurologically ill patients. This concern is based on animal studies indicating that vasopressin may promote the development of vasospasm in SAH, and indirect experimental studies showing a reduction in brain edema with vasopressin antagonists. No prospective human study has been undertaken to confirm or dismiss this concern, and the only retrospective study on the use of vasopressin in SAH did not show any of these potentially adverse effects (48). In addition to vasopressors, a temporary demand pacemaker and/or atropine may be required in cases of refractory bradycardia and hypotension.

In cardiogenic neurogenic shock, some form of inotropic support may be necessary, either in the form of a dobutamine, milrinone, or norepinephrine infusion. Dopamine is generally avoided because of its proarrhythmic properties. Dobutamine and milrinone also have vasodilatory effects, frequently leading to more hypotension, requiring additional therapy with an α-receptor agonist, such as phenylephrine or norepinephrine. Afterload increases in the former, and tachycardia in the latter, might be limiting factors and need careful monitoring. Cardiac output monitoring may be undertaken with the guidance of a PAC. Beta-blockade is usually not recommended. In neurogenic cardiogenic shock, coronary artery disease is typically not present, and compensatory tachycardia is necessary to maintain cardiac output. Afterload reduction with cautious use of angiotensin-converting enzyme (ACE) inhibitors should be attempted, but further hypotension must be avoided to maintain tenuous cerebral perfusion pressures. Short-acting agents should be used whenever possible. Repeating an echocardiogram several days after the initial one is recommended to monitor the progression/resolution of cardiac dysfunction. The need for an intra-aortic balloon pump to mechanically reduce afterload and improve coronary perfusion pressure may be considered, albeit rarely used.

Once diagnosed, neuroendocrine neurogenic shock from primary, or more often secondary, adrenal insufficiency is treated with steroid replacement therapy. We use the same dosing as in adrenal insufficiency in septic shock: hydrocortisone, 50 mg intravenously every 6 hours. As previously discussed, a cortisol stimulation test is usually not helpful, and empiric treatment after a random cortisol level should be initiated.

SUMMARY

Neurogenic shock is not a single entity, but rather is composed of three subtypes and pathophysiologies: vasodilatory, cardiac, and neuroendocrine. Other causes of hypotension should be ruled out first, prior to making the diagnosis of neurogenic shock. In most cases, neurogenic shock is transient and reversible, making this entity very treatable. Diagnosis and treatment should be tailored to the subtype of neurogenic shock. Maintenance of cerebral perfusion pressures is the key principle of management to prevent secondary brain injury and improve outcome.

References

1. Bilello JF, Davis JW, Cunningham MA, et al. Cervical spinal cord injury and the need for cardiovascular intervention. *Arch Surg.* 2003;138(10):1127–1129.
2. Banki N, Kopelnik A, Tung P, et al. Prospective analysis of prevalence, distribution, and rate of recovery of left ventricular systolic dysfunction in patients with subarachnoid hemorrhage. *J Neurosurg.* 2006;105(1):15–20.
3. Mayer SA, Lin J, Homma S, et al. Myocardial injury and left ventricular performance after subarachnoid hemorrhage. *Stroke.* 1999;30(4):780–786.
4. Pollick C, Cujec B, Parker S, et al. Left ventricular wall motion abnormalities in subarachnoid hemorrhage: an echocardiographic study. *J Am Coll Cardiol.* 1988;12(3):600–605.
5. Kono T, Morita H, Kuroiwa T, et al. Left ventricular wall motion abnormalities in patients with subarachnoid hemorrhage: neurogenic stunned myocardium. *J Am Coll Cardiol.* 1994;24(3):636–640.
6. Cohan P, Wang C, McArthur DL, et al. Acute secondary adrenal insufficiency after traumatic brain injury: a prospective study. *Crit Care Med.* 2005;33(10):2358–2366.
7. Dimopoulou I, Tsagarakis S, Douka E, et al. The low-dose corticotropin stimulation test in acute traumatic and non-traumatic brain injury: incidence of hypo-responsiveness and relationship to outcome. *Intensive Care Med.* 2004;30(6):1216–1219.
8. Calaresu FR, Yardley CP. Medullary basal sympathetic tone. *Ann Rev Physiol.* 1988;50:511–524.
9. Osborn JW, Taylor RF, Schramm LP. Determinants of arterial pressure after chronic spinal transection in rats. *Am J Physiol.* 1989;256(3 Pt 2):R666–673.
10. Maiorov DN, Weaver LC, Krassioukov AV. Relationship between sympathetic activity and arterial pressure in conscious spinal rats. *Am J Physiol.* 1997;272(2 Pt 2):H625–631.
11. Osborn JW, Taylor RF, Schramm LP. Chronic cervical spinal cord injury and autonomic hyperreflexia in rats. *Am J Physiol.* 1990;258(1 Pt 2):R169–174.
12. Krassioukov AV, Weaver LC. Episodic hypertension due to autonomic dysreflexia in acute and chronic spinal cord-injured rats. *Am J Physiol.* 1995;268(5 Pt 2):H2077–2083.
13. Sutters M, Wakefield C, O'Neil K, et al. The cardiovascular, endocrine and renal response of tetraplegic and paraplegic subjects to dietary sodium restriction. *J Physiology.* 1992;457:515–523.
14. Teasell RW, Arnold JM, Krassioukov A, et al. Cardiovascular consequences of loss of supraspinal control of the sympathetic nervous system after spinal cord injury. *Arch Phys Med Rehab.* 2000;81(4):506–516.
15. Karlsson AK. Autonomic dysfunction in spinal cord injury: clinical presentation of symptoms and signs. *Prog Brain Res.* 2006;152:1–8.
16. Lane RD, Wallace JD, Petrosky PP, et al. Supraventricular tachycardia in patients with right hemisphere strokes. *Stroke.* 1992;23(3):362–366.
17. Oppenheimer SM, Gelb A, Girvin JP, et al. Cardiovascular effects of human insular cortex stimulation. *Neurology.* 1992;42(9):1727–1732.
18. Zamrini EY, Meador KJ, Loring DW, et al. Unilateral cerebral inactivation produces differential left/right heart rate responses. *Neurology.* 1990;40(9):1408–1411.
19. Burch GE, Meyers R, Abildskov JA. A new electrocardiographic pattern observed in cerebrovascular accidents. *Circulation.* 1954;9(5):719–723.
20. Davies KR, Gelb AW, Manninen PH, et al. Cardiac function in aneurysmal subarachnoid haemorrhage: a study of electrocardiographic and echocardiographic abnormalities. *Br J Anaesth.* 1991;67(1):58–63.
21. Macrea LM, Tramer MR, Walder B. Spontaneous subarachnoid hemorrhage and serious cardiopulmonary dysfunction–a systematic review. *Resuscitation.* 2005;65(2):139–148.
22. Tung P, Kopelnik A, Banki N, et al. Predictors of neurocardiogenic injury after subarachnoid hemorrhage. *Stroke.* 2004;35(2):548–551.
23. Naredi S, Lambert G, Eden E, et al. Increased sympathetic nervous activity in patients with nontraumatic subarachnoid hemorrhage. *Stroke.* 2000;31(4):901–906.
24. Elrifai AM, Bailes JE, Shih SR, et al. Characterization of the cardiac effects of acute subarachnoid hemorrhage in dogs. *Stroke.* 1996;27(4):737–741; discussion 741–732.
25. Cowan MJ, Giddens WE Jr, Reichenbach DD. Selective myocardial cell necrosis in nonhuman primates. *Arch Pathol Lab Med.* 1983;107(1):34–39.
26. Baroldi G, Mittleman RE, Parolini M, et al. Myocardial contraction bands. Definition, quantification and significance in forensic pathology. *Intern J Legal Med.* 2001;115(3):142–151.
27. Todd GL, Baroldi G, Pieper GM, et al. Experimental catecholamine-induced myocardial necrosis, I: morphology, quantification and regional distribution of acute contraction band lesions. *J Molecular Cell Cardiol.* 1985;17(4):317–338.
28. Kline IK. Myocardial alterations associated with pheochromocytomas. *Am J Pathol.* 1961;38:539–551.

29. Hammermeister KE, Reichenbach DD. QRS changes, pulmonary edema, and myocardial necrosis associated with subarachnoid hemorrhage. *Am Heart J* 1969;78(1):94–100.
30. Koskelo P, Punsar S, Sipilae W. Subendocardial haemorrhage and E.C.G. Changes in Intracranial Bleeding. *Br Med J.* 1964;1(5396):1479–1480.
31. Smith RP, Tomlinson BE. Subendocardial haemorrhages associated with intracranial lesions. *J Pathol Bacteriol.* 1954;68(2):327–334.
32. Doshi R, Neil-Dwyer G. A clinicopathological study of patients following a subarachnoid hemorrhage. *J Neurosurg.* 1980;52(3):295–301.
33. Crompton MR. Hypothalamic lesions following the rupture of cerebral berry aneurysms. *Brain.* 1963;86:301–314.
34. Greenhoot JH, Reichenbach DD. Cardiac injury and subarachnoid hemorrhage. A clinical, pathological, and physiological correlation. *J Neurosurg.* 1969;30(5):521–531.
35. Kawai S, Suzuki H, Yamaguchi H, et al. Ampulla cardiomyopathy ('Takotsubo' cardiomyopathy)–reversible left ventricular dysfunction: with ST segment elevation. *Jpn Circ J.* 2000;64(2):156–159.
36. Akashi YJ, Nakazawa K, Sakakibara M, et al. Reversible left ventricular dysfunction "takotsubo" cardiomyopathy related to catecholamine cardiotoxicity. *J Electrocardiol.* 2002;35(4):351–356.
37. Akashi YJ, Nakazawa K, Sakakibara M, et al. The clinical features of takotsubo cardiomyopathy. *QJM* 2003;96(8):563–573.
38. Simmons RL, Martin AM Jr, Heisterkamp CA 3rd, et al. Respiratory insufficiency in combat casualties, II: pulmonary edema following head injury. *Ann Surg.* 1969;170(1):39–44.
39. Pender ES, Pollack CV Jr. Neurogenic pulmonary edema: case reports and review. *J Emerg Med.* 1992;10(1):45–51.
40. Hoff JT, Nishimura M, Garcia-Uria J, et al. Experimental neurogenic pulmonary edema, 1: the role of systemic hypertension. *J Neurosurg.* 1981; 54(5):627–631.
41. Lang SA, Maron MB, Signs SA. Oxygen consumption after massive sympathetic nervous system discharge. *Am J Physiol.* 1989;256(3 Pt 1):E345–351.
42. Aimaretti G, Ambrosio MR, Di Somma C, et al. Traumatic brain injury and subarachnoid haemorrhage are conditions at high risk for hypopituitarism: screening study at 3 months after the brain injury. *Clin Endocrinol.* 2004;61(3):320–326.
43. Dunser MW, Wenzel V, Mayr AJ, et al. Management of vasodilatory shock: defining the role of arginine vasopressin. *Drugs.* 2003;63(3):237–256.
44. Landry DW, Levin HR, Gallant EM, et al. Vasopressin pressor hypersensitivity in vasodilatory septic shock. *Crit Care Med.* 1997;25(8):1279–1282.
45. Isotani E, Suzuki R, Tomita K, et al. Alterations in plasma concentrations of natriuretic peptides and antidiuretic hormone after subarachnoid hemorrhage. *Stroke.* 1994;25(11):2198–2203.
46. Huang WD, Yang YM, Wu SD. Changes of arginine vasopressin in elderly patients with acute traumatic cerebral injury. *Chinese J Traumatol.* 2003;6(3):139–141.
47. Barreca T, Gandolfo C, Corsini G, et al. Evaluation of the secretory pattern of plasma arginine vasopressin in stroke patients. *Cerebrovasc Dis.* 2001; 11(2):113–118.
48. Muehlschlegel S, Dunser MW, Gabrielli A, et al. Arginine vasopressin as a supplementary vasopressor in refractory hypertensive, hypervolemic, hemodilutional therapy in subarachnoid hemorrhage *Neurocrit Care.* 2007; 6(1):3–10.
49. Bulsara KR, McGirt MJ, Liao L, et al. Use of the peak troponin value to differentiate myocardial infarction from reversible neurogenic left ventricular dysfunction associated with aneurysmal subarachnoid hemorrhage. *J Neurosurg.* 2003;98(3):524–528.
50. Skaf E, Stein PD, Beemath A, et al. Venous thromboembolism in patients with ischemic and hemorrhagic stroke. *Am J Cardiol.* 2005;96(12):1731–1733.
51. Hamilton MG, Hull RD, Pineo GF. Venous thromboembolism in neurosurgery and neurology patients: a review. *Neurosurgery.* 1994;34(2):280–296; discussion 296.
52. Maramattom BV, Weigand S, Reinalda M, et al. Pulmonary complications after intracerebral hemorrhage. *Neurocrit Care.* 2006;5(2):115–119.
53. Brisman R, Mendell J. Thromboembolism and brain tumors. *J Neurosurg.* 1973;38(3):337–338.
54. Skaf E, Stein PD, Beemath A, et al. Fatal pulmonary embolism and stroke. *Am J Cardiol.* 2006;97(12):1776–1777.
55. Stephens PH, Lennox G, Hirsch N, et al. Superior sagittal sinus thrombosis after internal jugular vein cannulation. *Br J Anaesth.* 1991;67(4):476–479.
56. Zaroff JG, Rordorf GA, Ogilvy CS, et al. Regional patterns of left ventricular systolic dysfunction after subarachnoid hemorrhage: evidence for neurally mediated cardiac injury. *J Am Soc Echocardiogr.* 2000;13(8):774–779.
57. Mayer SA, LiMandri G, Sherman D, et al. Electrocardiographic markers of abnormal left ventricular wall motion in acute subarachnoid hemorrhage. *J Neurosurg.* 1995;83(5):889–896.
58. Eisenberg HM, Frankowski RF, Contant CF, et al. High-dose barbiturate control of elevated intracranial pressure in patients with severe head injury. *J Neurosurg.* 1988;69(1):15–23.
59. Narayan RK, Kishore PR, Becker DP, et al. Intracranial pressure: to monitor or not to monitor? A review of our experience with severe head injury. *J Neurosurg.* 1982;56(5):650–659.
60. Bullock R, Chesnut RM, Clifton G, et al. Guidelines for the management of severe head injury. Brain Trauma Foundation. *Eur J Emerg Med.* 1996;3(2):109–127.
61. Czosnyka M, Guazzo E, Iyer V, et al. Testing of cerebral autoregulation in head injury by waveform analysis of blood flow velocity and cerebral perfusion pressure. *Acta Neurochirurgica.* 1994;60:468–471.

CHAPTER 60 ■ ANAPHYLACTIC SHOCK

MEGHAVI S. KOSBOTH • ERIC S. SOBEL

Anaphylaxis is severe, has a rapid onset, and is potentially fatal—a systemic allergic reaction that occurs after contact with an allergy-causing substance (1,2). Activation of mast cell and basophil populations by either IgE-dependent (i.e., anaphylactic reactions) or IgE-independent (i.e., anaphylactoid reactions) mechanisms results in the release of multiple mediators capable of altering vascular permeability and vascular and bronchial smooth muscle tone, as well as recruiting and activating inflammatory cell cascades. Because the clinical presentations of anaphylactic and anaphylactoid reactions are indistinguishable, they will be referred to as anaphylaxis for the purposes of this chapter. Initial sequelae, which occur within minutes to an hour after exposure to an inciting stimulus, include generalized hives, tachycardia, flushing, pruritus, faintness, and a sensation of impending doom. Dermatologic (i.e., urticaria and angioedema), respiratory (i.e., dyspnea, wheeze, stridor, bronchospasm, and hypoxemia), and gastrointestinal (i.e., abdominal distension, nausea, emesis, and diarrhea) manifestations are common. Involvement of the cardiovascular and respiratory systems may result in potentially life-threatening manifestations, such as cardiovascular collapse caused by vasodilation and capillary leak, myocardial depression, myocardial ischemia and infarction, and atrial fibrillation (3). Prompt recognition and effective intervention are essential to prevent the fatal manifestations of anaphylactic and anaphylactoid reactions.

INCIDENCE

The incidence of anaphylaxis is difficult to determine accurately due to underdiagnosis and underreporting. In the United States, fatal anaphylaxis causes 500 to 1,000 fatalities per year and accounts for 1% of emergency department visits (1,4,5). The anaphylaxis rate was found to be 21 per 100,000 person-years in a study of nonhospitalized individuals in Olmsted County, Minnesota, between 1983 and 1987 (6). A subsequent analysis of the General Practice database in the United Kingdom noted the incidence to be 8.4 per 100,000 person-years (7). An epidemiologic study involving 481,752 individuals suggested that hospitalized patients are at increased risk of anaphylaxis, but these reactions are rarely fatal (8).

ETIOLOGY

The most common causes of anaphylaxis include insect stings, foods, drugs, and physical factors/exercise. Idiopathic anaphylaxis (where no causative agent is identified) accounts for up to two thirds of patients referred to allergy/immunology specialty clinics (9,10). Foods such as shellfish, eggs, nuts, and milk account for one third of food-induced anaphylactic episodes (10–13) (Tables 60.1 and 60.2). There is a syndrome of food-dependent, exercise-induced anaphylaxis (FDEIA) that develops only if food is ingested prior to exercise or exertion (14). Seafood, nuts, celery, wheat, and grains have been implicated as allergens in this syndrome. It is important to note that these foods are tolerated by the patient in the absence of exertion (14,15).

Anaphylactic reactions to stings or bites of various insects, such as members of the order Hymenoptera (yellow jackets, bees, wasps, hornets, and saw flies) are commonly reported. A positive venom skin test along with a systemic reaction to the insect sting predicts a 50% to 60% risk of reaction to future stings (16). Medications can cause anaphylactic (IgE-mediated) and anaphylactoid (non–IgE-mediated) reactions. Previous exposure to drugs is required for IgE production and anaphylactic reactions, but anaphylactoid reactions can occur upon first administration. Penicillin is one of the most common causes of anaphylaxis, with 1 to 5 per 10,000 courses with penicillin resulting in allergic reactions and 1 in 50,000 to 1 in 100,000 courses with a fatal outcome (17–19). Nonsteroidal anti-inflammatory drugs (NSAIDs) and aspirin are the second most common class of drugs implicated in anaphylaxis (20). Some hypersensitivity reactions will occur with different NSAID agents, while others are specific to a single drug (21).

With widespread adoption of universal precautions against infections, latex allergy has become a significant problem. The development of low-protein, powder-free gloves has been associated with reduction in occupational-contact urticaria caused by latex rubber gloves (22). Despite this, latex allergy is still a concern since latex is found in gloves, catheters, and tubing (23–25). Iodinated radiocontrast media can cause anaphylaxis; however, life-threatening reactions are rare (26). A history of a previous reaction to radiocontrast media, asthma or atopic disease, treatment with β-blockers, and cardiovascular disease are risk factors for developing anaphylaxis to radiocontrast media (27–29).

CLINICAL MANIFESTATIONS

The clinical syndromes associated with systemic anaphylactic and anaphylactoid reactions represent medical emergencies, as they are associated with a rapid, critical destabilization of vital organ systems. These syndromes, which are, again, clinically indistinguishable, may become rapidly fatal if appropriate therapy is not instituted *immediately*. Initial symptoms can appear within seconds to minutes but may be delayed by as much as 1 (or rarely more) hour after exposure to an inciting agent (30), and are often nonspecific (31). These symptoms include tachycardia, faintness, cutaneous flushing, urticaria, diffuse or palmar pruritus, and a sensation of impending doom (32). Of these, generalized urticaria is the most common, occurring in approximately 90% of patients (Table 60.3) (33,34). Subsequent manifestations indicate involvement of the cutaneous, gastrointestinal, respiratory, and cardiovascular systems. Involvement of the cardiovascular and respiratory systems is responsible for the fatal

TABLE 60.1

ETIOLOGIC AGENTS FOR ANAPHYLAXIS (IGE-MEDIATED)

HAPTENS **β-Lactam antibiotics** Sulfonamides Nitrofurantoin Demethylchlortetracycline Streptomycin Vancomycin Local anesthetics Others	VENOM Stinging insects, particularly **Hymenoptera**, fire ants, deer flies, jelly fish, kissing bugs (triatoma), and rattlesnakes
SERUM PRODUCTS γ-Globulin Immunotherapy for allergic diseases Heterologous serum	HORMONES Insulin Adrenocorticotropic hormone Thyroid-stimulating hormone
FOODS **Nuts** (peanuts, brazil nuts, hazelnuts, cashews, pistachios, almonds, soy nuts) **Shellfish** Buckwheat **Egg white** Cottonseed **Cow's milk** Corn Potato Rice Legumes Citrus fruits Chocolate Others	ENZYMES Chymopapain L-Asparaginase MISCELLANEOUS Seminal fluid Others

Boldface: Relatively common causes
Modified from Austen KF. Systemic anaphylaxis in man. *JAMA*. 1965; 192:108; and Kaliner M. Anaphylaxis. *NER Allergy Proc*. 1984;5: 324.

TABLE 60.2

ETIOLOGIC AGENTS FOR ANAPHYLACTOID REACTIONS

COMPLEMENT-MEDIATED REACTIONS	ARACHIDONIC ACID MODULATORS
Blood	Nonsteroidal anti-inflammatory drugs
Serum	Tartrazine (possible)
Plasma	
Plasmate (but not albumin)	IDIOPATHIC
Immunoglobins	Most common conclusion after thorough evaluation
NONIMMUNOLOGIC MAST CELL ACTIVATORS	UNKNOWN
Opiates and narcotics	Sulfites
Radiocontrast media	Others
Dextrans	
Neuromuscular blocking agents	THERMOREGULATORY MECHANISM
	Cold temperature, exercise

Boldface: Relatively common causes.
Adapted from Kaliner M. Anaphylaxis. *NER Allergy Proc.* 1984;5:324.

complications of anaphylactic/anaphylactoid reactions. An unsettling sensation—including hoarseness, dysphonia, or dyspnea—may precede acute upper airway obstruction secondary to laryngeal edema. Other pulmonary manifestations include acute bronchospasm, intra-alveolar pulmonary hemorrhage, bronchorrhea, and a noncardiogenic, high permeability–type pulmonary edema (17,35). Tachycardia and syncope may precede the development of hypotension and frank cardiovascular collapse (36,37). Anaphylactic shock occurs as a consequence of diminished venous return secondary to systemic vasodilation and intravascular volume contraction caused by capillary leak. Although transient increases in cardiac output may occur at the onset of anaphylaxis, hemodynamic parameters later reveal decreases in cardiac output, systemic vascular resistance, stroke volume, pulmonary artery occlusion, and central venous pressures (38–44). In addition, the acute onset of a lactic acidosis and diminished oxygen consumption have been noticed after an anaphylactoid reaction (45). Other potentially serious cardiovascular manifestations are myocardial ischemia and acute myocardial infarction, atrioventricular and intraventricular conduction abnormalities such as prolonged PR interval, transient left bundle branch block, and supraventricular arrhythmias such as atrial fibrillation. Severe, but reversible, myocardial depression also has been reported (37). Hematologic manifestations, such as disseminated intravascular coagulation and hemoconcentration secondary to volume contraction, also may complicate anaphylactic and anaphylactoid reactions (32). Gastrointestinal manifestations include nausea, bloating, abdominal cramps, and diarrhea.

In 1% to 20% of patients, there is a recurrence of symptoms after a period of recovery, termed *biphasic anaphylaxis* (46). In most cases, the symptoms recurred 1 to 8 hours after the initial

TABLE 60.3

CLINICAL MANIFESTATIONS OF ANAPHYLACTIC AND ANAPHYLACTOID REACTIONS

System	Symptom	Frequency	Sign/clinical manifestation
RESPIRATORY		60%–80%	
Upper	Dyspnea, dysphonia, cough, "lump in throat"		Upper airway obstruction caused by laryngeal edema and spasm; bronchorrhea
Lower	Dyspnea, cyanosis		Noncardiogenic pulmonary edema, bronchospasm, acute hyperinflation, alveolar hemorrhage
CARDIOVASCULAR	Palpitations, faintness, weakness	20%	Shock, tachycardia, capillary leak, syncope, supraventricular arrhythmias, conduction disturbances, myocardial ischemia and infarction
CUTANEOUS	Flushing, pruritus, rash	90%	Urticaria, angioedema, diaphoresis
GASTROINTESTINAL	Abdominal pain, bloating, cramps, nausea	30%	Emesis, diarrhea, hepatosplenic congestion; rarely hematemesis and bloody diarrhea
NEUROLOGIC	Dizziness, disorientation, hallucinations, headache, feeling of impending doom	5%–10%	Syncope, lethargy, seizures
NASAL	Pruritus, sneezing	16%–20%	Rhinorrhea, nasal congestion
OCULAR	Conjunctival pruritus, periorbital edema	10%–15%	Conjunctival suffusion, lacrimation
HEMATOLOGIC			Hemoconcentration, DIC

DIC, disseminated intravascular coagulation.

presentation, although there have been reports of recurrence up to 72 hours later. There were no features of the primary response that predicted the occurrence of a secondary response (47).

DIAGNOSIS

The diagnosis of anaphylaxis is established on the basis of clinical grounds alone because expedient institution of appropriate therapy is mandatory. These diagnoses should be considered when typical multisystem manifestations occur in a direct temporal relationship with exposure to an inciting agent. Recently, the National Institute of Allergy and Infectious Diseases (NIAID) and the Food Allergy and Anaphylaxis Network (FAAN) proposed clinical criteria for the diagnosis of anaphylaxis (Fig. 60.1) (1). Because of the multisystem nature of anaphylactic and anaphylactoid reactions, the list of differential diagnoses that must be considered is extensive. Diagnostic possibilities include cardiac dysrhythmias, myocardial infarction, distributive or hypovolemic shock, vasovagal syncope, asthma, pulmonary embolism, upper airway obstruction secondary to ingestion of a foreign body, hypoglycemia, and the carcinoid syndrome (Table 60.4).

Demonstration of acute elevations of markers specific to mast cell activation such as histamine and tryptase have been proposed to help confirm the diagnosis of anaphylaxis (48,49). However, in a series of 97 patients presenting to an emergency department and given the diagnosis of anaphylaxis, only 42% were found to have elevated plasma histamine levels, and 24% had increased plasma tryptase levels (50). Skin testing or serum antibody tests can help demonstrate the presence of IgE against a specific allergen. Skin testing should be delayed for up to 4 weeks to allow the dermal mast cells to replenish intracellular mediators (51).

PATHOPHYSIOLOGY

The systemic manifestations of anaphylactic and anaphylactoid reactions represent sequelae that result from the release of inflammatory mediators by mast cells and basophils. The classic anaphylactic response occurs through allergen-induced crosslinking of IgE tightly bound to the high-affinity FcϵR1 receptor constitutively expressed by mast cells (52). Release of histamine from preformed mast cell granules seems to be the primary pathophysiologic mediator, resulting in systemic vasodilation, increased vascular permeability, bronchoconstriction, pruritus, and increased mucus production. However, a number of other preformed mediators are released, including heparin, serotonin, and mast cell proteases such as chymase and tryptase (53). In addition, other important mediators of anaphylaxis are generated by the metabolism of membrane phospholipids. Activation of the 5-lipoxygenase pathway results in synthesis of leukotrienes, including leukotrienes C_4, D_4, E_4 (termed the slow-reacting substance of anaphylaxis), and B_4. Leukotrienes C_4, D_4, and E_4, along with the intermediary products 5-hydroxyeicosatetraenoic acid and 5-hydroperoxyeicosatetraenoic acid, elicit increases in vascular permeability and bronchoconstriction, whereas leukotriene B_4 possesses eosinophil and neutrophil chemotactic properties. Activation of the cyclooxygenase pathway leads to the production of prostaglandin D_2, which produces bronchoconstriction. Platelet-activating factor is also newly synthesized by activated mast cells and can result in bronchoconstriction, increased vascular permeability, platelet aggregation, and neutrophil chemotaxis. It also leads to further production of platelet-activating factor through stimulation of nuclear factor (NF)-κB, a positive feedback mechanism involving the cytokines interleukin-1 (IL-1) and tumor necrosis factor (TNF)-α, and contributes to a biphasic pattern seen in some patients (54). Combined, these primary mediators then facilitate the production of a diverse number of secondary mediators by platelets, neutrophils, eosinophils, and other cells, resulting in activation of the complement, coagulation, and fibrinolytic pathways (55).

Many of these mediators have complicated effects, and their relative roles in mediating anaphylaxis *in vivo* have been difficult to evaluate. Mouse models of anaphylaxis using strains with targeted deletions of specific mediators have been useful in elucidating the importance of different effector molecules, such as the leukotrienes (56–58), and in identifying regulatory

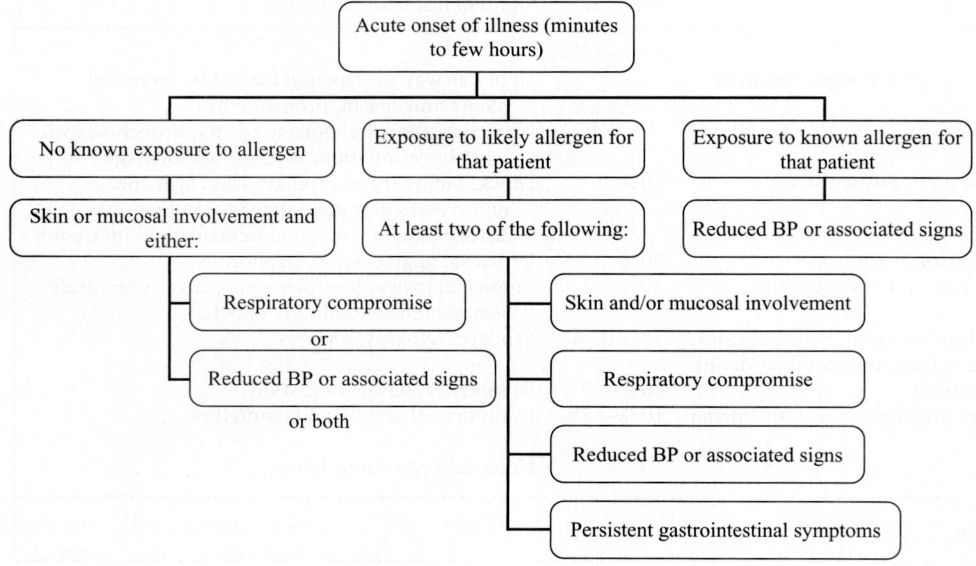

FIGURE 60.1. Clinical criteria for diagnosing anaphylaxis. Fewer signs are required for diagnosis as the history of allergen exposure becomes more certain. ***Signs or symptoms of skin involvement:*** Generalized hives, pruritus, or flushing. ***Signs of mucosal involvement:*** Swollen lips, tongue, and/or uvula. ***Signs of respiratory compromise:*** Dyspnea, wheeze, bronchospasm, stridor, reduced peak expiratory flow, and/or hypoxemia. ***Definition of reduced blood pressure (BP):*** Adults—systolic BP less than 90 mm Hg or greater than 30% decrease from that person's baseline; children—systolic BP less than 70 mm Hg from 1 month to 1 year, less than (70 mm Hg + [2 × age]) from 1 to 10 years, and less than 90 mm Hg from 11 to 17 years or ***associated signs:*** Hypotonia, syncope, incontinence. ***Persistent gastrointestinal symptoms:*** Crampy abdominal pain and vomiting.

TABLE 60.4

DIFFERENTIAL DIAGNOSIS OF ANAPHYLAXIS

FLUSH SYNDROME Carcinoid Pheochromocytoma Peri-postmenopausal hot flushes Medullary carcinoma of thyroid Red man syndrome (vancomycin)	**POSTPRANDIAL COLLAPSE** Airway foreign body Monosodium glutamate ingestion Sulfite Scombroid fish poisoning
HYPOTENSION Septic shock Hemorrhagic shock Cardiogenic shock Hypovolemic shock Vasovagal reaction	**MISCELLANEOUS** Panic attacks Systemic mastocytosis Basophilic leukemia Hereditary angioedema Hyper-IgE syndrome
RESPIRATORY DISTRESS Status asthmaticus Airway foreign body Epiglottitis Pulmonary embolism Asthma and COPD exacerbation Vocal cord dysfunction	

IgE, immunoglobulin E; COPD, chronic obstructive pulmonary disorder.

pathways, such as IL-10 (59), but have also provided some surprises that may lead to clinically useful information. For example, mice with targeted deletions of either the high-affinity FcϵR1 receptor or IgE, not surprisingly, had a markedly decreased susceptibility to IgE-mediated anaphylaxis (53,60). This pathway can also be blocked with targeted deletion of histamine receptor 1 and, to a lesser extent, platelet-activating factor (52,53). However, such mice also revealed the presence of an alternate IgE-independent pathway of anaphylaxis (61). This pathway was mediated largely through platelet-activating factor, which was triggered by the binding of IgG to FcγRIII receptors present on macrophages (52,62). Like the classic IgE-mediated pathway, this alternative pathway required prior exposure to antigen, but differed in that much higher concentrations of antigen were required. The importance of this pathway in humans is as yet unclear (52). However, the administration of biologic agents, such as the anti-TNF antibody infliximab, has been reported to cause an IgE-independent anaphylactic response (63), and may be an example of this alternative pathway. The use of these biologic agents is expected to continue to increase.

MANAGEMENT

The clinician must have a high index of suspicion for anaphylactic and anaphylactoid reactions because they require a prompt clinical diagnosis and a rapid therapeutic response. Because anaphylactic and anaphylactoid reactions both represent sequelae of mast cell and basophil degranulation, the therapeutic approaches to these disorders are identical. Initial attention should be given to assessment and stabilization of the pulmonary and cardiovascular manifestations of anaphylaxis, because these are the major causes of death.

Epinephrine is the mainstay of initial management and should be administered immediately. It decreases mediator synthesis and release by increasing intracellular concentrations of cyclic adenosine monophosphate (cAMP) and antagonizes many of the adverse actions of the mediators of anaphylaxis (41). Aqueous epinephrine, 0.01 mg/kg (maximum dose 0.5 mg) administered intramuscularly every 5 to 15 minutes as necessary to control symptoms and maintain blood pressure, is recommended (41,64). The participants of the NIAID/FAAN symposium concluded that the intramuscular administration of epinephrine in the anterior lateral thigh is preferred over subcutaneous injection (1,2). In cases of severe laryngospasm or frank cardiovascular collapse, or when there is an inadequate response to subcutaneous epinephrine administration and fluid resuscitation, intravenous epinephrine is an option. There is no established dosage regimen for intravenous epinephrine in anaphylaxis, but suggested dosages are 5 to 10 μg bolus (0.2 μg/kg) for hypotension and 0.1 to 0.5 mg in the setting of cardiovascular collapse (1,2,65). When epinephrine is administered IV, the clinician should be aware of the potential adverse consequences of severe tachycardia, myocardial ischemia, hypertension, severe vasospasm, and gangrene—the latter when infused by peripheral venous access (66).

Blood pressure measurements should be obtained frequently, and an indwelling arterial catheter should be inserted in cases of moderate to severe anaphylaxis. High-flow oxygen given via endotracheal tube or a nonrebreather mask should be administered to patients experiencing hypoxemia, respiratory distress, or hemodynamic instability (1,2). Orotracheal intubation may be attempted if the airway obstruction compromises effective ventilation despite pharmacologic intervention; however, attempts may be unsuccessful if laryngeal edema is severe. If endotracheal intubation is unsuccessful, then either needle-catheter cricothyroid ventilation, cricothyrotomy, or surgical tracheostomy is required to maintain an adequate airway. Clinicians must be familiar with at least one of these techniques in the event that endotracheal intubation cannot be accomplished. It has been suggested that inhaled β_2-agonists such as albuterol may be useful for bronchospasm refractory to epinephrine (1,2,67). Patients should be placed in the recumbent position, with lower extremities elevated to increase fluid return centrally, thereby increasing cardiac output (68). Airway protection should be ensured in the event of vomiting.

Antihistamines (H_1 and H_2 antagonists) are considered second-line treatment for anaphylaxis (1,2). They are useful in the treatment of symptomatic urticaria-angioedema and pruritus. Recent studies suggest that treatment with a combination of H_1 and H_2 antagonists is more effective in attenuating the cutaneous manifestations of anaphylaxis than H_1 antagonists alone (50,69). Diphenhydramine hydrochloride (25 to 50 mg IV or IM for adults and 1 mg/kg, up to 50 mg, for children) and ranitidine (50 mg IV over 5 minutes) are commonly used in this setting. If hypotension persists despite administration of epinephrine and H_1 and H_2 blockers, aggressive volume resuscitation should be instituted. Up to 35% of the blood volume may extravasated in the first 10 minutes of a severe reaction, with subsequent reduction in blood volume due to vasodilatation, causing distributive shock (70). Persistent hypotension may require multiple fluid boluses (10 to 20 mL/kg under pressure) as well as colloid and crystalloid infusions (1,2). Vasopressors such as norepinephrine, vasopressin, Neo-Synephrine, or even metaraminol may be useful in persistent hypotension (31).

There have been no placebo-controlled trials evaluating the efficacy of corticosteroids in anaphylaxis, but their contribution in other allergic diseases has led to their inclusion in anaphylactic management. Due to their slow onset of action, they are not useful in acute management. However, it has been suggested that they may prevent protracted or biphasic reactions (67,71). The usual dose is 100 to 250 mg of hydrocortisone IV every 6 hours (39).

The management of anaphylaxis in a patient receiving β-antagonist medications, such as β blockers, represents a special circumstance in which the manifestations of anaphylaxis may be exceptionally severe (72). β Blockade increases mediator synthesis and release, as well as end-organ sensitivity. In addition, β-blockade antagonizes the beneficial β-mediated effects of epinephrine therapy, thereby resulting in unopposed α-adrenergic and reflex vagotonic effects: vasoconstriction, bronchoconstriction, and bradycardia. Therapy of anaphylaxis occurring in patients receiving β-antagonist drugs, however, is similar to that of other patients. In addition, atropine may be useful for heart block and refractory bronchospasm, whereas glucagons—which increase cAMP levels through a β-receptor–independent mechanism—have been reported to reverse the cardiovascular manifestations of anaphylaxis in patients receiving β-antagonists (72). Glucagon can be administered as a 1- to 5-mg (20–30 μg/kg with maximum dose of 1 mg in children) intravenous infusion over 5 minutes, followed by an infusion of 5 to 15 μg/minute titrated to a clinical response (1,2). Furthermore, these patients may require extended periods of observation because of the long duration of action of many β-antagonist medications.

An emergent evaluation for the inciting etiologic agent must accompany initial therapeutic interventions. After the etiologic agent is identified, the clinician should attempt to prevent further access to the circulation or limit further absorption. Infusions of possible etiologic agents should be stopped and the contents saved for analysis. If a Hymenoptera sting is responsible, the stinger should be removed. Small amounts of local epinephrine—0.1 to 0.2 mL of a 1:1,000 solution—should be injected next to a subcutaneous or intramuscular injection site that is dispersing the inciting agent. A tourniquet also should be placed proximal to the injection site and pressure applied to occlude venous return. After successful pharmacologic therapy, the tourniquet may be cautiously removed and the patient carefully observed for recurrent adverse sequelae. In cases where the offending agent was ingested, consideration may be given to insertion of a nasogastric tube to perform gastric lavage and gastric instillation of activated charcoal.

THERAPEUTIC PEARLS

1. *Rapidly assess and maintain the airway, breathing, and circulation.* If airway obstruction is imminent, perform endotracheal intubation; if unsuccessful, consider needle-catheter cricothyroid ventilation, cricothyrotomy, or tracheostomy. Patients in anaphylactic shock should be placed in a recumbent position with the lower extremities elevated, unless precluded by shortness of breath or vomiting.
2. *Remove the inciting agent* (i.e., remove Hymenoptera stinger) and follow with an intramuscular epinephrine injection in the anterior lateral thigh. Consider gastric lavage and administration of activated charcoal if the inciting agent was ingested.
3. *Administer aqueous epinephrine*, 0.01 mg/kg (maximum dose, 0.5 mg) intramuscularly every 5 to 15 minutes as necessary for controlling symptoms and maintaining blood pressure.
4. *Establish intravenous access* for hydration and provide supplemental oxygen.
5. *Administer histamine antagonists* to block vasodilation, capillary leak, and shock (H_1 blockade, 25–50 mg of diphenhydramine IV or IM for adults, and 1 mg/kg—up to 50 mg—for children; H_2 blockade, 50 mg of ranitidine IV).
6. *Administer vasopressors* for persistent hypotension and titrate to a mean arterial pressure of 60 mm Hg.
7. *Consider aggressive fluid resuscitation* with multiple fluid boluses (10–20 mL/kg under pressure), including colloid as well as crystalloid, in patients who remain hypotensive despite epinephrine.
8. *Administer inhaled β_2-agonists* such as albuterol for bronchospasm refractory to epinephrine (73).
9. *Consider corticosteroid therapy* for protracted anaphylaxis or to prevent biphasic anaphylaxis (1.0–2.0 mg/kg methylprednisolone IV every 6 hours). Oral prednisone at 1.0 mg/kg, up to 50 mg, may be used for milder attacks. Corticosteroids are not effective therapy for the acute manifestations of anaphylaxis.
10. *Consider glucagon* administration (1–5 mg IV over 1 minute, then 1–5 mg/hour in a continuous infusion) in the setting of prior β-blockade because of its positive inotropic and chronotropic effects mediated by a β-receptor–independent mechanism.

11. *Prevent recurrent episodes* by avoidance of the inciting agent, desensitization, or premedication with corticosteroids and H_1 and H_2 blockade.
12. *Admission to the intensive care unit* is warranted for invasive monitoring with arterial and pulmonary artery catheters, electrocardiography, pulse oximetry, and frequent arterial blood gas measurements.

OBSERVATION

An observation period should be considered for all patients following treatment of an anaphylactic reaction. On the basis of clinical data available to date, the NIAID/FAAN symposium recommends that observation periods be individualized on the basis of severity of initial reaction, reliability of the patient, and access to care. A reasonable time would be 4 to 6 hours for most patients, with prolonged observation or hospital admission for severe or refractory symptoms and patients with reactive airway disease (1,2).

FOLLOW-UP, MANAGEMENT, AND PREVENTION

The ideal method for managing severe systemic anaphylactic and anaphylactoid reactions is by preventing their occurrence. Persons with a known sensitivity should avoid re-exposure to the inciting etiologic agents. Patients who have experienced respiratory or cardiovascular symptoms of anaphylaxis should receive self-injectable epinephrine for use if anaphylaxis develops. These patients should also have an emergency action plan detailing its use and follow-up management (1,2). If a precipitating allergen is known or identified, patients should receive information about avoiding it in the future, prior to their discharge from the emergency facility. They should be encouraged to obtain prompt follow-up with their primary care physician as well as an allergist (1,2).

IMPLICATIONS AND OUTCOME

Anaphylactic/anaphylactoid reactions represent important, potentially reversible, acute respiratory and cardiovascular emergencies. Although the optimal management method is that of prevention, prompt diagnosis and institution of therapy are crucial after these reactions have been initiated in order to prevent the fatal cardiovascular and pulmonary manifestations. Factors associated with improved survival include the sensitivity of the person to the inciting agent, the duration between the exposure and the onset of symptoms (short latency periods are associated with more severe manifestations), the route and dose of the offending agent (larger doses and parenteral administration are associated with more severe manifestations), and the interval between onset of symptoms and subsequent diagnosis and institution of appropriate therapy (74). Optimal management of acute systemic reactions includes appropriate pharmacologic intervention, support of pulmonary and cardiovascular function, and removal of the offending agent. Expeditious institution of these measures helps to reduce the morbidity and mortality associated with these potentially life-threatening syndromes.

SUMMARY

1. Anaphylactic reactions represent type I immune responses mediated by IgE bound to mast cells or basophils. Common inciting agents include β-lactam antibiotics and Hymenoptera stings. Other common causes include foods, local anesthetics, and serum products.
2. Anaphylactoid reactions represent IgE-independent activation of mast cells or basophils, with resultant degranulation and mediator release. Common inciting agents include iodinated radiocontrast media, neuromuscular depolarizing agents, and opiates, all of which induce direct mast cell activation; nonsteroidal anti-inflammatory agents acting through cyclooxygenase inhibition; and blood products acting through complement activation.
3. A history of a previous reaction to radiocontrast media, asthma or atopic disease, treatment with β-blockers, and cardiovascular disease are risk factors for developing anaphylaxis to radiocontrast media (27–29).
4. The differential diagnosis of anaphylactic and anaphylactoid reactions includes cardiac arrhythmias, myocardial infarction and cardiogenic shock, distributive or hypovolemic shock, vasovagal syncope, asthma, pulmonary embolism, upper airway obstruction secondary to a foreign body, vocal chord dysfunction, hypoglycemia, carcinoid syndrome, systemic mastocytosis, hereditary angioedema, and leukemia with excess histamine production.
5. Epinephrine is the initial drug of choice for the management of anaphylactic or anaphylactoid reactions. H_1- and H_2-blocking agents also should be administered. Corticosteroids are not effective for the acute management of anaphylactic or anaphylactoid reactions, but may prevent biphasic anaphylaxis or attenuate prolonged reactions. Glucagon may be used for persistent hypotension in patients taking β-blockers.

References

1. Sampson HA, Munoz-Furlong A, Campbell RL, et al. Second symposium on the definition and management of anaphylaxis: summary report–second National Institute of Allergy and Infectious Disease/Food Allergy and Anaphylaxis Network symposium. *J Allergy Clin Immunol.* 2006;117:391–397.
2. Sampson HA, Munoz-Furlong A, Campbell RL, et al. Second symposium on the definition and management of anaphylaxis: summary report–second National Institute of Allergy and Infectious Disease/Food Allergy and Anaphylaxis Network symposium. *Ann Emerg Med.* 2006;47:373–380.
3. Brown SG. Anaphylaxis: clinical concepts and research priorities. *Emerg Med Australas.* 2006;18:155–169.
4. Clark S, Long AA, Gaeta TJ, et al. Multicenter study of emergency department visits for insect sting allergies. *J Allergy Clin Immunol.* 2005;116:643–649.
5. Neugut AI, Ghatak AT, Miller RL. Anaphylaxis in the United States: an investigation into its epidemiology. *Arch Intern Med.* 2001;161:15–21.
6. Yocum MW, Butterfield JH, Klein JS, et al. Epidemiology of anaphylaxis in Olmsted County: a population-based study. *J Allergy Clin Immunol.* 1999; 104:452–456.
7. Peng MM, Jick H. A population-based study of the incidence, cause, and severity of anaphylaxis in the United Kingdom. *Arch Intern Med.* 2004;164: 317–319.
8. An epidemiologic study of severe anaphylactic and anaphylactoid reactions among hospital patients: methods and overall risks. The International Collaborative Study of Severe Anaphylaxis. *Epidemiology.* 1998;9:141–146.
9. Webb LM, Lieberman P. Anaphylaxis: a review of 601 cases. *Ann Allergy Asthma Immunol.* 2006;97:39–43.
10. Tang AW. A practical guide to anaphylaxis. *Am Fam Physician.* 2003;68: 1325–1332.
11. Thong BY, Cheng YK, Leong KP, et al. Anaphylaxis in adults referred to a

clinical immunology/allergy centre in Singapore. *Singapore Med J.* 2005;46: 529–534.
12. Novembre E, Cianferoni A, Bernardini R, et al. Anaphylaxis in children: clinical and allergologic features. *Pediatrics.* 1998;101:E8.
13. Kaliner MA. Anaphylaxis. *NER Allergy Proc.* 1984;5:324.
14. Chong SU, Worm M, Zuberbier T. Role of adverse reactions to food in urticaria and exercise-induced anaphylaxis. *Int Arch Allergy Immunol.* 2002; 129:19–26.
15. Dohi M, Suko M, Sugiyama H, et al. Food-dependent, exercise-induced anaphylaxis: a study on 11 Japanese cases. *J Allergy Clin Immunol.* 1991;87:34–40.
16. Graham DM, McPherson H, Lieberman P. Skin testing in the evaluation of Hymenoptera allergy and drug allergy. *Immunol Allergy Clin North Am.* 2001;21:301–320.
17. Delage C, Irey NS. Anaphylactic deaths: a clinicopathologic study of 43 cases. *J Forensic Sci.* 1972;17:525–540.
18. Joint Task Force on Practice Parameters, American Academy of Allergy, Asthma and Immunology, American College of Allergy, Asthma and Immunology, and the Joint Council of Allergy, Asthma and Immunology. The diagnosis and management of anaphylaxis. *J Allergy Clin Immunol.* 1998;101: S465–S528.
19. Idsoe O, Guthe T, Willcox RR, et al. Nature and extent of penicillin side-reactions, with particular reference to fatalities from anaphylactic shock. *Bull World Health Organ.* 1968;38:159–188.
20. Brown AF, McKinnon D, Chu K. Emergency department anaphylaxis: a review of 142 patients in a single year. *J Allergy Clin Immunol.* 2001;108:861–866.
21. Stevenson DD. Approach to the patient with a history of adverse reactions to aspirin or NSAIDs: diagnosis and treatment. *Allergy Asthma Proc.* 2000;21:25–31.
22. Allmers H, Schmengler J, John SM. Decreasing incidence of occupational contact urticaria caused by natural rubber latex allergy in German health care workers. *J Allergy Clin Immunol.* 2004;114:347–351.
23. Schwartz HA, Zurowski D. Anaphylaxis to latex in intravenous fluids. *J Allergy Clin Immunol.* 1993;92:358–359.
24. Mitsuhata H, Horiguchi Y, Saitoh J, et al. An anaphylactic reaction to topical fibrin glue. *Anesthesiology.* 1994;81:1074–1077.
25. Laxenaire MC, Mata-Bermejo E, Moneret-Vautrin DA, et al. Life-threatening anaphylactoid reactions to propofol (Diprivan). *Anesthesiology.* 1992;77:275–280.
26. Katayama H, Yamaguchi K, Kozuka T, et al. Adverse reactions to ionic and nonionic contrast media. A report from the Japanese Committee on the Safety of Contrast Media. *Radiology.* 1990;175:621–628.
27. Greenberger PA, Halwig JM, Patterson R, et al. Emergency administration of radiocontrast media in high-risk patients. *J Allergy Clin Immunol.* 1986; 77:630–634.
28. Enright T, Chua-Lim A, Duda E, et al. The role of a documented allergic profile as a risk factor for radiographic contrast media reaction. *Ann Allergy.* 1989;62:302–305.
29. Bush WH, Swanson DP. Acute reactions to intravascular contrast media: types, risk factors, recognition, and specific treatment. *AJR Am J Roentgenol.* 1991;157:1153–1161.
30. Inomata N, Osuna H, Yamagimachi M, et al. Late-onset anaphylaxis to fermented soybeans: the first confirmation of food-induced, late-onset anaphylaxis by provocation test. *Ann Allergy Asthma Immunol.* 2005;94:402–406.
31. Brown SG. Cardiovascular aspects of anaphylaxis: implications for treatment and diagnosis. *Curr Opin Allergy Clin Immunol.* 2005;5:359–364.
32. Smith PL, Kagey-Sobotka A, Bleecker ER, et al. Physiologic manifestations of human anaphylaxis. *J.Clin Invest.* 1980;66:1072–1080.
33. Kemp SF, Lockey RF, Wolf BL, et al. Anaphylaxis. A review of 266 cases. *Arch Intern Med.* 1995;155:1749–1754.
34. Kemp SF, Lockey RF. Anaphylaxis: a review of causes and mechanisms. *J Allergy Clin Immunol.* 2002;110:341–348.
35. Carlson RW, Schaeffer RC Jr, Puri VK, et al. Hypovolemia and permeability pulmonary edema associated with anaphylaxis. *Crit Care Med.* 1981;9:883–885.
36. Simon MR. Anaphylaxis associated with relative bradycardia. *Ann Allergy.* 1989;62:495–497.
37. Raper RF, Fisher MM. Profound reversible myocardial depression after anaphylaxis. *Lancet.* 1988;1:386–388.
38. Wasserman SI. The heart in anaphylaxis. *J Allergy Clin Immunol.* 1986; 77:663–666.
39. Nicolas F, Villers D, Blanloeil Y. Hemodynamic pattern in anaphylactic shock with cardiac arrest. *Crit Care Med.* 1984;12:144–145.
40. Serafin WE, Austen KF. Mediators of immediate hypersensitivity reactions. *N Engl J Med.* 1987;317:30–34.
41. Perkin RM, Anas NG. Mechanisms and management of anaphylactic shock not responding to traditional therapy. *Ann Allergy.* 1985;54:202–208.
42. Silverman HJ, Van Hook C, Haponik EF. Hemodynamic changes in human anaphylaxis. *Am J Med.* 1984;77:341–344.
43. Moss J, Fahmy NR, Sunder N, et al. Hormonal and hemodynamic profile of an anaphylactic reaction in man. *Circulation.* 1981;63:210–213.
44. Hanashiro PK, Weil MH. Anaphylactic shock in man. Report of two cases with detailed hemodynamic and metabolic studies. *Arch Intern Med.* 1967; 119:129–140.
45. Fawcett WJ, Shephard JN, Soni NC, et al. Oxygen transport and haemodynamic changes during an anaphylactoid reaction. *Anaesth Intensive Care.* 1994;22:300–303.
46. Brazil E, MacNamara AF. "Not so immediate" hypersensitivity–the danger of biphasic anaphylactic reactions. *J Accid Emerg Med.* 1998;15:252–253.
47. Lieberman P. Biphasic anaphylactic reactions. *Ann Allergy Asthma Immunol.* 2005;95:217–226.
48. Bochner BS, Lichtenstein LM. Anaphylaxis. *N Engl J Med.* 1991;324:1785–1790.
49. Yocum MW, Khan DA. Assessment of patients who have experienced anaphylaxis: a 3-year survey. *Mayo Clin Proc.* 1994;69:16–23.
50. Lin RY, Schwartz LB, Curry A, et al. Histamine and tryptase levels in patients with acute allergic reactions: an emergency department-based study. *J Allergy Clin Immunol.* 2000;106:65–71.
51. Weiss ME, Adkinson NF. Immediate hypersensitivity reactions to penicillin and related antibiotics. *Clin Allergy.* 1988;18:515–540.
52. Finkelman FD, Rothenberg ME, Brandt EB, et al. Molecular mechanisms of anaphylaxis: lessons from studies with murine models. *J Allergy Clin Immunol.* 2005;115:449–457.
53. Strait RT, Morris SC, Yang M, et al. Pathways of anaphylaxis in the mouse. *J Allergy Clin Immunol.* 2002;109:658–668.
54. Choi IW, Kim YS, Kim DK, et al. Platelet-activating factor-mediated NF-kappaB dependency of a late anaphylactic reaction. *J Exp Med.* 2003;198: 145–151.
55. Kaplan AP, Joseph K, Silverberg M. Pathways for bradykinin formation and inflammatory disease. *J Allergy Clin Immunol.* 2002;109:195–209.
56. Goulet JL, Snouwaert JN, Latour AM, et al. Altered inflammatory responses in leukotriene-deficient mice. *Proc Natl Acad Sci USA.* 1994; 91:12852–12856.
57. Haribabu B, Verghese MW, Steeber DA, et al. Targeted disruption of the leukotriene B(4) receptor in mice reveals its role in inflammation and platelet-activating factor-induced anaphylaxis. *J Exp Med.* 2000;192:433–438.
58. Kanaoka Y, Maekawa A, Penrose JF, et al. Attenuated zymosan-induced peritoneal vascular permeability and IgE-dependent passive cutaneous anaphylaxis in mice lacking leukotriene C4 synthase. *J Biol Chem.* 2001;276: 22608–22613.
59. Mangan NE, Fallon RE, Smith P, et al. Helminth infection protects mice from anaphylaxis via IL-10-producing B cells. *J Immunol.* 2004;173:6346–6356.
60. Dombrowicz D, Brini AT, Flamand V, et al. Anaphylaxis mediated through a humanized high affinity IgE receptor. *J Immunol.* 1996;157:1645–1651.
61. Oettgen HC, Martin TR, Wynshaw-Boris A, et al. Active anaphylaxis in IgE-deficient mice. *Nature.* 1994;370:367–370.
62. Miyajima I, Dombrowicz D, Martin TR, et al. Systemic anaphylaxis in the mouse can be mediated largely through IgG1 and Fc gammaRIII. Assessment of the cardiopulmonary changes, mast cell degranulation, and death associated with active or IgE- or IgG1-dependent passive anaphylaxis. *J Clin Invest.* 1997;99:901–914.
63. Cheifetz A, Mayer L. Monoclonal antibodies, immunogenicity, and associated infusion reactions. *Mt Sinai J Med.* 2005;72:250–256.
64. Project Team of the Resuscitation Council (UK). Emergency medical treatment of anaphylactic reactions. *Resuscitation.* 1999;41:93–99.
65. Hepner DL, Castells MC. Anaphylaxis during the perioperative period. *Anesth Analg.* 2003;97:1381–1395.
66. Taneli Vayrynen MJ, Luurila HO, Maatta TK, et al. Accidental intravenous administration of racemic adrenaline: two cases associated with adverse cardiac effects. *Eur J Emerg Med.* 2005;12:225–229.
67. Lieberman P, Kemp SF, Oppenheimer J, et al. The diagnosis and management of anaphylaxis: an updated practice parameter. *J Allergy Clin Immunol.* 2005;115(Suppl 2):S483–S523.
68. Boulain T, Achard JM, Teboul JL, et al. Changes in BP induced by passive leg raising predict response to fluid loading in critically ill patients. *Chest.* 2002;121:1245–1252.
69. Simons FE. Advances in H1-antihistamines. *N Engl J Med.* 2004;351:2203–2217.
70. Fisher MM. Clinical observations on the pathophysiology and treatment of anaphylactic cardiovascular collapse. *Anaesth Intensive Care.* 1986;14:17–21.
71. Sampson HA, Mendelson L, Rosen JP. Fatal and near-fatal anaphylactic reactions to food in children and adolescents. *N Engl J Med* 1992;327:380–384.
72. Thomas M, Crawford I. Best evidence topic report. Glucagon infusion in refractory anaphylactic shock in patients on beta-blockers. *Emerg Med J.* 2005;22:272–273.
73. Sampson HA. Anaphylaxis and emergency treatment. *Pediatrics.* 2003; 111:1601–1608.
74. Sheffer AL. Anaphylaxis. *J Allergy Clin Immunol.* 1985;75:227–233.

CHAPTER 61 ■ SPLANCHNIC FLOW AND RESUSCITATION

JOHN W. MAH • ORLANDO C. KIRTON

Ischemia signifies failure to satisfy the metabolic needs of the cell secondary to either impaired oxygen delivery or the impairment of cellular oxygen extraction and utilization. Incomplete splanchnic cellular resuscitation has been associated with the development of multiple organ system failure and increased mortality in the critically ill patient (1,2). For many years, the merits of augmenting systemic oxygen delivery and consumption and attainment of supranormal levels have been examined and debated as primary treatment goals (3–6). There is convincing evidence that systemic hemodynamic and oxygen transport variables fail to accurately portray the complex interaction between energy requirements and the energy supply at the tissue level (7–9), and that achieving supranormal cardiovascular oxygen transport and utilization indices does not reliably confer improved outcome (i.e., decreased mortality rates and diminished multiple organ system failure) in several clinical conditions (e.g., sepsis, acute respiratory distress syndrome [ARDS]) (10–13). These findings have led to the search for monitoring techniques that directly measure changes in regional tissue bioenergetics.

Intestinal tonometry has been proposed as a relatively noninvasive index of the adequacy of aerobic metabolism in organs whose superficial mucosal lining is extremely vulnerable to low flow and hypoxemia, and in which blood flow is sacrificed first in both shock and the cytokine milieu of the systemic inflammatory response (1,14,15). The gastrointestinal tract, therefore, acts like the "canary," displaying early metabolic changes before other indices of adequate oxygen utilization (16). This chapter reviews the fundamental and clinical underpinnings of splanchnic ischemia and resuscitation, intestinal and subsequently sublingual tonometry, the potential applications and limitations of this technology, its use as a prognostic and treatment end point, and, finally, a consideration of potential future directions.

THE INTESTINAL MICROCIRCULATION

The gastrointestinal tract has three major functions: motility, secretion, and absorption. Blood flow is important for each of these functions, being highest in the small intestines and lowest in the colon. The splanchnic circulation contains approximately 30% of the circulating blood volume at any given moment with the bulk of this volume held in the postcapillary venous capacitance vessels (17). Resting blood flow in the intestine is ten times higher than in skeletal muscle. Most of the blood flow is delivered to the mucosa and submucosa, reflecting the varying demands for oxygen within the intestinal wall, being highest in the mucosal layer. The arterial supply emanates from an extensive arterial plexus in the submucosa. A *countercurrent* blood flow exchange system exists within the superficial mucosal layer between the arterial and venous circulation, rendering this tissue particularly sensitive to neuronal and systemic vasoconstrictors (18). The arterioles, which run in parallel with the venules in the stalk of the intestinal villus, allow diffusion of oxygen from the arterioles down a concentration gradient to the venules, bypassing the capillary bed at the villus tip; thus, the mucosa at the villus tip is rendered vulnerable to changes in oxygen content. Water also diffuses from arterioles to venules because of an osmotic gradient caused by the absorption of sodium in the capillary bed at the villus tip. Therefore, the sodium concentration is higher in the venules. Plasma water content is then lowered at the villus tip compared with the base of the stalk, predisposing this area to low or absent flow in states of compensated or uncompensated shock when splanchnic circulation is compromised.

Mesenteric vasoconstriction is mediated by α-adrenergic postganglionic sympathetic fibers, but, even more dramatically, by the effects of circulating hormones and peptides (Table 61.1). Endogenous vasoconstrictors known to be released in major injury, sepsis, and other physiologically stressful circumstances include catecholamines, angiotensin, vasopressin, myocardial depressant factor, leukotriene D_4, thromboxane A_2, and serotonin. The high concentration of receptors for these systemically released vasoconstrictors, which affect the splanchnic circulation more than any other tissue beds, has a substantial effect on peripheral (systemic) vascular resistance and, hence, on systemic blood pressure by redistributing blood from the splanchnic organs (as well as the peripheral circulation) to the central circulation (i.e., heart and brain). This effect may be compounded by tissue edema and atheroma in the splanchnic arteries. The peptides, angiotensin II and vasopressin, are the most potent splanchnic vasoconstrictors (14). The splanchnic vasoconstriction induced by these two peptides alone accounts for most of the increase in total vascular resistance recorded in animal models of cardiogenic and hemorrhagic shock. The adequacy of gut mucosal oxygenation cannot be reliably inferred from measurements of tissue oxygenation in the skin or of subcutaneous tissue because of their different response to endogenous vasoconstrictors.

TABLE 61.1

ENDOGENOUS VASOCONSTRICTORS KNOWN TO BE RELEASED IN STRESSFUL CIRCUMSTANCES AND THEIR ACTIONS ON DIFFERENT TISSUE BEDS

Vasoconstrictor	Gut	Renal	Brain	Coronary	Pulmonary	Muscle	Skin
Catecholamines	+	+	0	+	±	±	+
Angiotensin II	+	+	0	0	0	0	0
Vasopressin	+	+	?0	+	?	?	+
Myocardial depressant factor	+	0	0	0	0	0	0
Leukotriene D_4	+	+	0	+	?	0	0
Thromboxane A_2	+	+	+	+	+	+	+
Serotonin	+	+	?	?	+	–	±

+, vasoconstriction; –, vasodilatation; 0, no effect; ±, effect varies; ?, undefined.
From Fiddian-Green RG. Studies in splanchnic ischemia and multiple organ failure. In: Marston A, Bulkley GR, Fiddian-Green RG, et al., eds. *Splanchnic Ischemia and Multiple Organ Failure*. London: Edward Arnold/St. Louis: CV Mosby; 1989:349.

PATHOPHYSIOLOGY OF MESENTERIC ISCHEMIA AND REPERFUSION

Tissues with a high perfusion-to-extraction (demand) ratio, such as skeletal muscle, have high capillary densities that act as a microvascular reserve to produce an increase in local blood flow. These organs, in situations of low flow, use a disproportionate share of the cardiac output as increased capillary recruitment lowers local vascular resistance. These tissues are characterized by low oxygen extraction ratios and high mixed venous oxygen saturations. Less "fortunate" tissues, which include the intestinal tract, possess a lower capillary density and are unable to recruit capillaries to augment local blood flow to match increases in metabolic needs. This results in low perfusion-to-oxygen demand ratios and subsequent tissue hypoxia (the "trickle down economy" of systemic oxygenation) (15). The gastrointestinal tract is characterized by a high oxygen extraction ratio, lactate release, and low mixed venous oxygen saturation; it can tolerate severe hypoxemia without a decrease in oxygen consumption but is limited in its ability to respond to decreased blood flow.

Intestinal tissue injury can be induced by the initial ischemia (either from inadequate oxygen content or inadequate flow) or by the generation of oxygen-derived free radicals during reperfusion (1,7). Ischemic injury may be progressive, spanning a spectrum from mild injury characterized by increased capillary permeability with no microscopic changes to transmural infarction, depending on the severity and duration of the ischemia (1,2,19,20). Inadequate oxygen supply results in anaerobic glycolysis and systemic lactic acidosis. In the anoxic cell, uncompensated adenosine triphosphate (ATP) hydrolysis is associated with the intracellular accumulation of adenosine diphosphate (ADP), inorganic phosphate, and hydrogen ions with resultant intracellular acidosis (7,21). These hydrogen ions lead to tissue acidosis as well, with unbound hydrogen ions combining with interstitial bicarbonate to form the weak acid, carbonic acid, that disassociates to produce carbon dioxide (CO_2) plus water.

Hypoxia renders the superficial gastrointestinal mucosa susceptible to the cytolytic effects of gastric acid, proteolytic enzymes, and bacteria already present in the intestine by impairing cellular mucus and bicarbonate secretion. Disruption of the mucosal barrier is associated with the generation of myocardial depressant factors that cause a low cardiac output syndrome in animals (14,22,23). Commonly, in low flow and hypoxic states, tissue oxygen consumption ($\dot{V}O_2$) is maintained by adaptive mechanisms that are activated when oxygen delivery ($\dot{D}O_2$) falls below a critical level and oxygen consumption becomes delivery dependent.

Intracellular acidosis impairs cellular function by one of several mechanisms: (a) the loss of adenosine nucleotides from mitochondria by the inhibition of the ATP–magnesium/inorganic phosphate carrier; (b) inhibition of sodium–calcium exchange, resulting in the intracellular sequestration of calcium ions; (c) increases in the activity of cyclic adenosine monophosphate (AMP) deaminase and loss of adenine nucleotide precursors from the cell; (d) decreases in the nicotinamide adenine nucleotide pool by the acid-catalyzed destruction of nicotinamide adenine dinucleotide (NAD); and (e) the conversion of intracellular inorganic phosphate to its inhibitory deproteinated form (7).

Hypoxia also results in intracellular calcium overload by inhibiting ATP-driven membrane transport pumps and sodium–calcium exchange. Increases in intracellular calcium are a pivotal event in cellular dysfunction during hypoxia, because calcium-activated proteases can destroy the sarcolemma and the cellular cytoskeleton (7). Cellular membrane degradation seems to be related to calcium influx. Calcium stimulates phospholipase A_2 (PLA_2) and phospholipase C, which are known to degrade membrane phospholipids (24,25). The resultant imbalance between the rate of membrane synthesis and the rate of membrane breakdown results in the accumulation of arachidonic acid, the precursor of thromboxane, prostaglandins, and leukotrienes, substances that produce further cellular damage and profound alterations in microvascular control.

THE SPLANCHNIC MODEL OF MULTIPLE ORGAN FAILURE

Multiple system organ failure (MSOF) (defined as failure of two or more vital organs or systems, in sequence or simultaneously, irrespective of the primary disease) and sepsis are distressingly familiar to surgeons who perform major elective cases, as well as to those involved in transplantation and trauma (26). Uncompensated or compensated shock leading to progressive oxygen debt, ischemia/reperfusion injury, and cellular dysfunction is the underlying unifying pathophysiologic mechanism (1). Throughout the world, MSOF has become the most common cause of death in the intensive care unit: The reported mortality rates vary from 30% to 100% with a mean of 50%, depending on the number of organ systems involved; the patients' intensive care unit (ICU) stay lasts for 6 weeks to many months and, in prior studies, these patients have used nearly 40% of the available ICU days (26–30). Many hypotheses link the noxious event, whether surgery or trauma, to the development of MSOF and sepsis. There have also been many attempts to use single agents (e.g., antibiotics, monoclonal antibodies against cytokines and endotoxin) or combinations of these agents to affect the process; unfortunately, no significant progress has been made with these approaches. This may result from the many redundancies in the initiation and promulgation of MSOF, so that attacking a single pathway is ineffective or, perhaps, efforts have been started too late in the sequence of events. Bacterial endotoxin in the gut may translocate across the semipermeable mucosa as a result of ischemia/reperfusion. Besides endotoxins, the products of the damaged mucosa also may contribute to the systemic inflammatory response and subsequent MSOF and death of the ICU patient. The translocation of enteric bacteria across the ischemic gut seems to be an important cause of nosocomial infection in the critically ill (14,26). However, reducing the number of nosocomial infections from enteric organisms by selective decontamination does not seem to have a dramatic effect on outcome; that is, "again, the horse is already out of the barn" (31).

While representing an oversimplification, we believe the current hypotheses can be combined. Most current thinking can be categorized as the *gut starter* hypothesis popularized by Moore et al. (32) and the *gut motor* hypothesis as described by Deitch (27) and Marshall et al. (28,29).

In the gut starter hypothesis, the noxious stimulus leads to a neurohumoral response. High levels of catecholamines cause splanchnic vasoconstriction and a decrease in splanchnic flow. This leads to gut ischemia and, depending on the length of ischemic time, allows various reactions that prime tissue to develop a reperfusion injury once flow is restored. During reperfusion, PLA_2 is activated, which in turn activates platelet-activating factor (PAF). PAF attracts and primes polymorphonuclear leukocytes (PMNs) in the gut; thereafter, they are released into the systemic circulation, where they undergo activation (the *two-hit* model) and cause end-organ injury (32). Therefore, the PMN is implicated as the major effector of cellular damage attributed to ischemia/reperfusion through its respiratory burst and activation of cytokines and arachidonic acid metabolites.

In the gut motor hypothesis, the steps leading to ischemia are the same. During reperfusion, gut mucosal injury results from the accumulation of intracellular calcium, activation of PLA_2, and generation of free oxygen radicals. This leads to bacterial translocation and initial production and amplification of numerous systemic cytokines (33,34). The end result again is MSOF. It is likely that these hypotheses are correct, although they are still incomplete explanations.

SYSTEMIC OXYGEN DELIVERY, UTILIZATION, AND MONITORING

The determinants of arterial oxygenation include hemoglobin content, inspired oxygen tension, alveolar oxygen tension, pH, temperature, mixed venous oxygen tension, ventilation/perfusion ($\dot{V}/\dot{Q}$) mismatch, physiologic shunting, and cellular–interstitial diffusion abnormalities. Indices of adequacy of systemic perfusion include the following: (a) global systemic parameters, such as blood pressure, heart rate, central venous pressure measurements, and urine output; (b) tissue markers, including arterial pH (pHa), base excess, and serum lactate level; and (c) pulmonary artery catheter measurements and derivations, such as cardiac output, oxygen delivery, oxygen consumption, and oxygen extraction. In fact, Rivers et al. demonstrated that goal-directed resuscitation using certain systemic measures (mean arterial pressure [MAP], urine output [UOP], central venous pressure [CVP]) including improving oxygen delivery to an $ScVO_2 > 70\%$ can improve mortality in patients in severe sepsis and septic shock (35). Nonetheless, the interpretation of oxygen delivery and oxygen consumption measurements is challenging because (a) these parameters are global markers and do not provide any direct information regarding the oxygen requirements of specific tissues, (b) the distribution of oxygen delivery is impacted by local microvascular and neurogenic responses, (c) the effect of cytokines and endogenous peptides is unpredictable, and (d) the disease process may affect cellular metabolism directly (i.e., sepsis and ARDS) (36–38). Several prospective studies suggest that failure to achieve supranormal oxygen delivery and utilization parameters in the acute phase of major injury or physiologic stress is associated with increased mortality and shock-related complications, including multiple organ system dysfunction syndrome. The failure to reverse pathologic flow dependency, tissue hypoxia, and oxygen debt has been inferred as the cause of these adverse outcomes (3–6,39,40). In these prospective studies, both responders and nonresponders achieved normal or hyperdynamic cardiovascular function; however, more cardiovascular interventions were often used in patients who died, so, ultimately, failure of patient response to achieve therapeutic objectives could be considered as the cause of the observed increased mortality and morbidity. Several reports failed to identify either an optimal or a critical value of oxygen delivery or consumption to distinguish survivors from nonsurvivors in critically ill patients (10–13,23). Adequate or supranormal oxygen delivery may not be tantamount to effective tissue oxygen utilization.

"Critical oxygen delivery" purportedly marks the transition from aerobic to anaerobic metabolism; however, the relationship between oxygen delivery and consumption obtained in critically ill patients with ARDS, sepsis, and heart failure has been linear (23). The lack of a clearly defined inflection point in a linear $\dot{D}O_2$–$\dot{V}O_2$ function makes it impossible to determine a critical level of oxygen delivery that aerobically satisfies cellular energy requirements.

REGIONAL OXYGEN DELIVERY, UTILIZATION, AND MONITORING

A Historical Review of Gastric Tonometry

A tonometer is composed of a semipermeable silicone balloon, which is filled with either air or fluid and allowed to equilibrate with the surrounding tissue. The fluid/air is then accessed and the pressure of CO_2 can be directly measured. Tonometry was first used by Bergofsky (41) and Dawson et al. (42) in 1964 to demonstrate that the gas tension within a hollow viscus approximates that within the mucosa of the viscus. Grum et al. (21) extended this concept to the intestinal tract of adults. Antonsson et al. (43) and Hartmann et al. (44) performed validation studies demonstrating that both the stomach and small intestine could be used as suitable sites to measure intraluminal PCO_2. They confirmed that intraluminal PCO_2 equaled that measured within the intestinal mucosa as well as approximated hepatic vein PCO_2. Moreover, it has been validated that the intramucosal PCO_2 rises and falls in parallel with changes in PCO_2 in arterial blood (45). This indirect method of measuring the pH within the intestinal mucosa (pHi) is based on the fact that CO_2 is a highly permeable gas and on the assumption that this generated CO_2 is the end result of ATP hydrolysis, with neutralization of generated hydrogen ions by intestinal interstitial bicarbonate (46).

The measurement of pHi depends also on the assumption that the bicarbonate concentration in the wall of the organ is the same as that which is delivered to it by arterial blood, and that the dissociation constant (pK) is the same as that in the plasma. Using the Henderson-Hasselbalch equation, pHi is calculated as follows:

$$\text{pHi} = 6.1 + \log(\text{HCO}_3{}^-/0.03 \times \text{PCO}_2)$$

pKa is 6.1, and 0.03 is the solubility coefficient for CO_2. The pK in plasma is not the same as that in the cytosol, but the value 6.1 is the best approximation of the pK within the intestinal fluid of the superficial layers of the mucosa (14,47,48).

Doglio et al. (49) demonstrated that gastric pHi was a predictor of ICU mortality at the time of admission to the ICU and at 12 hours later. Patients admitted with a pHi <7.36 had a greater ICU mortality rate, 65% versus 44% ($p < 0.04$). Furthermore, patients with persistently low pHi at 12 hours after ICU admission had the highest mortality rate (87%). Maynard et al. (50) repeated the study in patients with acute circulatory failure and found remarkably similar outcomes. In addition, there were significant differences in mean gastric pHi values between survivors and nonsurvivors on admission (7.40 vs. 7.28) and at 24 hours (7.40 vs. 7.24), respectively ($p < 0.001$). There was no difference in cardiac index, oxygen delivery, and oxygen uptake, suggesting that pHi is a more specific marker of resuscitation than our common global parameters.

We also confirmed that failure of splanchnic resuscitation correlated with MSOF and increased length of ICU stay in the hemodynamically unstable trauma patient (51). The relative risk of death in patients whose pHi was less than 7.32 was 4.5-fold higher and the relative risk of developing multiple organ system failure was 5.4 times higher compared with those having a pHi of 7.32 or more. Global parameters of oxygen transport utilization did not distinguish survivors from nonsurvivors nor those patients who developed MSOF from those who did not.

Chang et al. (52) then conducted a prospective study of 20 critically ill patients and were able to demonstrate that correction of an abnormal admission pHi correlated with better outcomes. Patients with pHi less than 7.32 on admission, who did not correct within the initial 24 hours, had a higher mortality (50% vs. 0%; $p = 0.03$) and more frequent MSOF (2.6 vs. 0.62 organs/patient; $p = 0.02$) than those whose pHi corrected.

Ivatury et al. (53) compared correction of pHi versus supranormal oxygen delivery (as defined by Shoemaker et al. [3] in 27 critically ill trauma patients). Seventy-five percent of the patients who developed MSOF had pHi less than 7.3. Interestingly, four of the five patients who died in the supranormal oxygen group achieved supranormal oxygen delivery and consumption goals, but had a pHi less than 7.3 at 24 hours. Moreover, they observed that a late fall in pHi was often associated with a physiologic catastrophe (e.g., intestinal leak, gangrene, bacteremia).

There have been only two prospective controlled interventional studies in which therapy was instituted because the pHi was low. Neither of these studies, however, attempted to normalize the pHi, but rather focused on increasing oxygen delivery and utilization. Gutierrez et al. (54) observed that the hospital mortality rate was significantly greater in control patients whose pHi was normal on admission (pHi ≥7.35) and then became abnormal during their ICU stay compared with those whose abnormal pHi prompted interventions to increase oxygen delivery. Unfortunately, if admission pHi was low, the mortality rates were the same in both treatment and control groups. The authors chose to increase oxygen delivery rather than restore pHi to normal values.

We also specifically studied ICU patients with persistent uncorrected gastric pHi who had pulmonary artery catheters to guide resuscitation (55). We observed a significant reduction in the incidence of MSOF per patient (1.9 ± 0.4 to 0.9 ± 0.2; $p = 0.02$), length of ICU stay (35 ± 9 to 18 ± 4 days; $p = 0.03$), and total hospital stay (51 ± 12 to 29 ± 5 days; $p = 0.03$) in patients with persistent gastric intramucosal acidosis who were administered agents that increased splanchnic perfusion and that were intended to prevent free radical damage during reperfusion. We conclude that efforts to correct gastrointestinal intramucosal acidosis related to splanchnic hypoperfusion are warranted because MSOF and mortality were increased in those patients whose pHi never corrected (i.e., pHi <7.25).

Despite the potential benefits of regional monitoring, gastric tonometry has fallen out of favor for multiple reasons. The monitoring itself is labor intensive and time consuming, often requiring multiple attempts to ensure proper positioning and frequent catheter adjustments, lengthy equilibration times, and need for frequent troubleshooting of abnormal results. Gastric acid must be neutralized (pH >4.5), requiring pH litmus paper analysis and adjustments to the peptic ulcer prophylaxis regimen in the ICU patient. Tube feedings also must be held. In addition, one must use a dedicated blood gas analyzer for all pHi determinations. Periodic calibration of the analyzer with 10 to 20 ampules at three different PCO_2 levels must be done. The saline sample must be transported immediately on ice because of rapid loss of CO_2 from the sample and overestimation of the pHi.

SECTION VII ■ PHARMACOLOGY, NUTRITION, TOXICOLOGY, AND THE ENVIRONMENT

CHAPTER 62 ■ PHARMACOLOGIC PRINCIPLES

AIMÉE C. LeCLAIRE • DALE H. WHITBY

Pharmacotherapy is an essential component in the successful treatment of the critically ill patient. Thus, critical care practitioners must possess a good working knowledge and understanding of pharmacokinetic and pharmacodynamic principles as well as altering or confounding factors. Clinical application of these principles in the clinical setting is equally important.

Critical care therapeutics often involves the use of multiple pharmacologic agents, each having a therapeutic purpose, toxicity, and side effects. Many agents are affected by acute or chronic impairment of metabolic organs such as the liver, kidney, and lungs; changes in fluid balance; drug–drug and drug–nutrient interactions; and other factors.

The goal of pharmacotherapy is the attainment of a desired therapeutic response without untoward toxicity. The goal of this chapter is to present principles that will be clinically useful in developing a practical approach to pharmacotherapy in the critically ill patient. Pharmacokinetic principles, special population considerations, drug–drug interactions, adverse drug reactions, and the role of the clinical pharmacist are reviewed.

PHARMACOKINETICS AND PHARMACODYNAMICS

Pharmacokinetics can be defined as the quantitative study of the processes of absorption, distribution, metabolism, and elimination of a drug in the body (1). The use of mathematical models describing these processes allows predictions to be made about drug concentrations in various parts of the body as a function of dosage, route of administration, clearance, and time.

Pharmacodynamics is the study of the relationship between the concentration of a drug and the biochemical or physiologic response obtained by that drug in a given patient (2). Some drugs exhibit a linear dose–response relationship through the entire range of clinically used doses; that is, doubling the dose doubles the response. Others may exhibit a linear dose–response relationship to a response ceiling, where increases in drug dose do not elicit any additional response. Some agents do not behave in a linear fashion at all. A decrease in heart rate during beta-antagonist or calcium channel antagonist therapy and decrease in ectopy during antiarrhythmic therapy are examples of quantifiable pharmacodynamic measurements. Some pharmacodynamic responses are more difficult to measure, such as the response to corticosteroid or anticonvulsant therapies.

A pharmacokinetic-pharmacodynamic relationship exists in most cases, as demonstrated in Figure 62.1. In general, because it crosses tissues and elicits a pharmacodynamic response, free or unbound drug in the plasma is considered to be the pharmacologically active component in achieving efficacy or producing toxicity. The free drug fraction is also the only portion available to be metabolized and eliminated.

Pharmacokinetics

As stated, pharmacokinetics is the study of the absorption, distribution, metabolism, and elimination of drugs. Much of our knowledge of this subject has resulted from the development of sensitive and specific assays for determining drug concentrations in biologic fluids. Conceptual models and mathematical equations have been devised to describe these behaviors (3); however, the pharmacokinetic parameters described in the literature often are based on data from small numbers of patients or normal volunteers, which may not accurately reflect the behavior of a drug in a critically ill patient. In individualizing a patient's drug therapy, appropriate interpretation of accurately obtained plasma level measurements of a given drug in a specific patient provides significantly more information than any empiric calculation could provide.

The simplest pharmacokinetic model describes the body as a singular "compartment" or one-compartment model. Drugs enter the compartment at rates determined by routes of administration (e.g., intravenous bolus, intravenous infusion, intramuscular, oral, or transdermal) and leave the compartment at rates determined by routes of elimination (e.g., renal, hepatic, or pulmonary).

A two-compartment model reasonably describes the behavior of most drugs in humans (4). In this model, a small central compartment consists of the rapidly perfused organs (heart, lungs, kidney, and endocrine glands), and a larger peripheral compartment consists of the less rapidly perfused organs (skin, muscle, bone, and fat). After administration, drugs initially distribute into the central compartment and then redistribute into the peripheral compartment, reaching equilibrium between compartments at a rate dependent on the perfusion of peripheral compartment tissues and the tissue affinity for the drug.

The two-compartment model assumes that the drug obeys first-order or linear kinetics, where a constant proportion of the drug is removed per unit of time. Rate of elimination of the drug is proportional to the serum concentration and diminishes logarithmically over time. However, the fraction of drug removed per unit of time remains constant and independent of dose. In first-order elimination, both clearance and volume of distribution also remain constant. Thus, serum concentration can be affected by changing the dose in relation to the desired

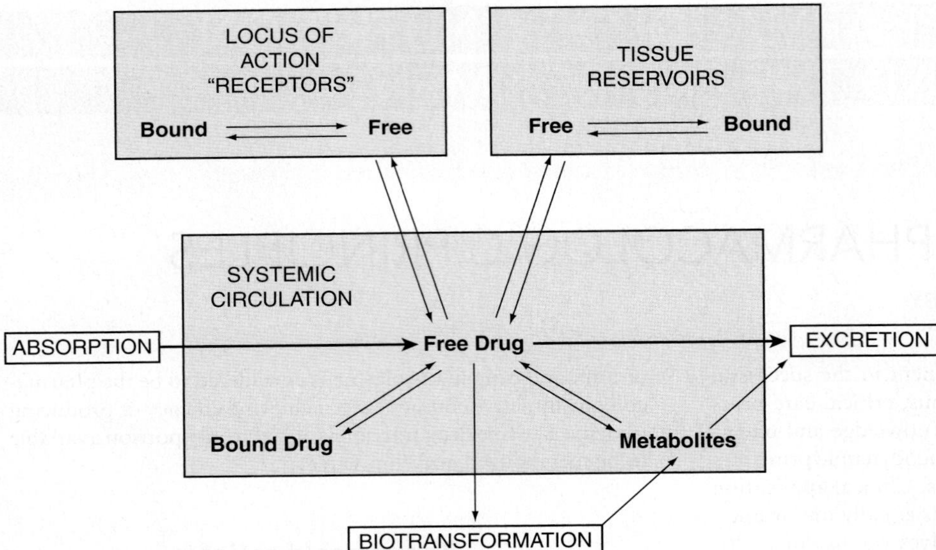

FIGURE 62.1. Schematic representation of the interrelationship of the absorption, distribution, binding, metabolism, and excretion of a drug and its concentration at its locus of action. Possible distribution and binding of metabolites are not depicted. (From Benet LZ, Kroetz DL, Sheiner LB. Pharmacokinetics: the dynamics of drug absorption, distribution and elimination. In: Hardin JG, Limbird LE, Gilman AG, et al., eds. *Goodman and Gilman's The Pharmacologic Basis of Therapeutics*. 9th ed. New York, NY: McGraw-Hill; 1996:3, with permission.)

change in concentration; in simplest terms, doubling the dose doubles the concentration.

However, some drugs follow zero-order kinetics, where a constant amount of drug is eliminated per unit of time, irrespective of serum concentration. Other medications obey nonlinear or saturable kinetics. Drugs having saturable kinetics exhibit capacity-limited metabolism, and elimination may not be proportional to serum concentration. For example, phenytoin exhibits Michaelis-Menten kinetics and demonstrates linear elimination to a point where the patient's hepatic enzyme system is functioning at the maximum rate. Subsequently, phenytoin serum levels increase out of proportion to dose, meaning an increase in dose from 300 to 400 mg/day may result in an exponentially greater increase in serum level.

In first-order kinetics, a plot of the logarithm of serum concentration after initial distribution versus time is a straight line. As seen in Figure 62.2, the intravenous injection of a drug

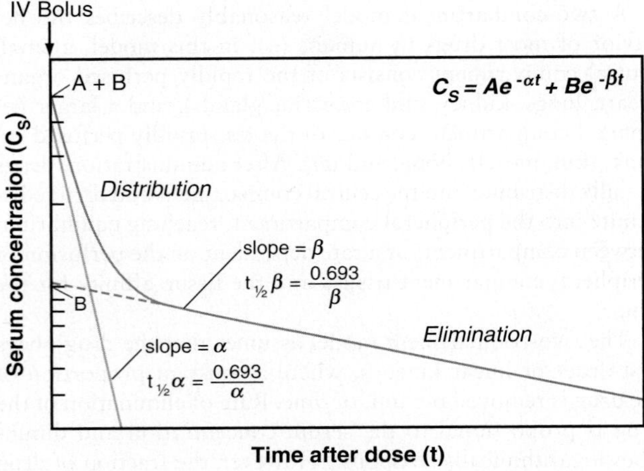

FIGURE 62.2. Schematic graph of serum drug concentrations (C_s) plotted on a logarithmic scale versus time after a single intravenous bolus injection. (From Greenblatt DJ, Koch-Weser J. Clinical pharmacokinetics. *N Engl J Med*. 1975;293:703, with permission.)

results in an initially high serum drug concentration, followed by a rapid decrease because of drug distribution. After the distribution (or alpha) phase, the serum concentration further decreases because of the drug elimination (or beta) phase. At any point in time, the serum drug concentration (C_s) can be calculated from the biexponential disappearance function:

$$C_s = Ae^{-\alpha t} + Be^{-\beta t}$$

where α and β are the first-order rate constants for the alpha and beta phases, respectively (5).

Pharmacokinetic parameters of particular value in the application of pharmacokinetic principles to clinical practice include the volume of distribution, clearance, half-life, and bioavailability.

Volume of distribution (Vd) is the apparent volume of fluid in which a given dose would have to be distributed to achieve the observed serum concentration as mathematically described by the following equations:

$$C_s = \text{dose}/\text{Vd} \quad \text{or} \quad \text{Vd} = \text{dose}/C_s$$

Clinically, the volume of distribution is useful for estimating the initial loading dose required to achieve a desired serum concentration or for calculating an incremental bolus dose required to raise a serum level by a desired amount. For instance, theophylline has a volume of distribution of approximately 0.5 L/kg in most patients; thus a 60-kg person would have an apparent volume of distribution of 30 L. If the desired serum concentration is 15 mg/L, the loading dose required to achieve this goal may be calculated as follows:

$$\text{Dose} = (\text{Vd})(C_s) = (30\text{L})(15\text{ mg/L}) = 450\text{ mg}$$

Clearance (Cl) is defined as the volume of blood or serum from which all drug is removed per unit of time. Clearance can be affected by alterations in distribution, metabolism, or excretion. Specific issues relating to changes in clearance from impairment of renal or hepatic function are discussed later in this chapter. At steady-state, the drug administration rate equals the drug elimination rate (6). Based on this principle, drug clearance can be useful in determining the amount of drug required to

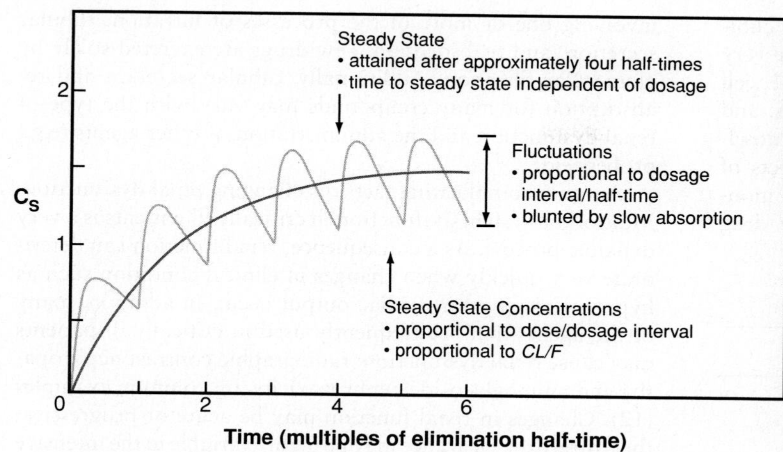

FIGURE 62.3. Fundamental pharmacokinetic relationships for repeated administration of drugs. (From Benet LZ, Kroetz DL, Sheiner LB. Pharmacokinetics: the dynamics of drug absorption, distribution and elimination. In: Hardin JG, Limbird LE, Gilman AG, et al., eds. *Goodman and Gilman's The Pharmacologic Basis of Therapeutics*. 9th ed. New York, NY: McGraw-Hill; 1996:23, with permission.)

maintain a therapeutic drug level. With an intravenously administered or completely absorbed oral agent, the steady-state serum concentration (C_{ss}) can be determined by the following equations:

$$C_{ss} = \frac{\text{dose}}{(\text{dosage interval})\ (\text{Cl})}$$

Half-life ($t_{1/2}$) is a function of both drug volume of distribution and clearance:

$$t_{1/2} = \frac{(0.693)\ (\text{Vd})}{\text{Cl}}$$

In most cases, this variable refers to elimination half-life, meaning the time required to reduce the initial serum concentration by 50% after the initial distribution phase. The drug half-life can be useful in determining the amount of time required to reach steady-state serum concentration. Four elimination half-lives are required to achieve approximately 94% of steady state. The time required to reach steady-state serum concentration is independent of dose and dosage interval. As seen in Figure 62.3, drug accumulation occurs with repeated dosing until equilibrium or steady state is reached at approximately four to five half-lives. If, in this example, the desired pharmacologic response is observed at a serum concentration of 1 to 2 units, a period of time after the initiation of therapy exists during which the serum concentration is subtherapeutic. To ascertain therapeutic levels at the initiation of therapy, a loading dose may be given, followed by maintenance doses.

For example, digoxin has an elimination half-life of 36 hours in a patient with normal renal function. Therefore, a period of 6 days is required to achieve a steady-state drug level with daily dosing. If a loading dose of 1 mg is incrementally given over 24 hours, therapeutic digoxin concentrations may be achieved more rapidly.

The bioavailability of a drug is defined as the fraction of a drug dose that reaches the systemic circulation. Bioavailability is a consideration primarily with orally administered agents. Absorption can be affected by many factors relating to the pharmaceutical dosage form (e.g., tablet, capsule, oral liquid, suspension, or sustained-release product), gastric pH and emptying time, intestinal motility, and drug complex formation with other drugs or nutrients (7). Many orally absorbed drugs demonstrate a first-pass effect with significant metabolism in the liver before the drug enters the systemic circulation. Examples are propranolol, hydralazine, verapamil, and lidocaine. Lidocaine's first-pass effect is so great that it must be administered by the parenteral route. For other drugs like propranolol and verapamil, oral doses need to be substantially higher than parenteral doses to account for this effect. For these drugs, the fraction of drug available to the systemic circulation or bioavailability (F) must be included in the calculation of steady-state serum concentration as follows:

$$C_{ss} = \frac{(\text{F})(\text{dose})}{(\text{dosage interval})(\text{Cl})}$$

Pharmacodynamics

Whereas pharmacokinetics is a detailed, often mathematical, approach to the way that the body handles a drug, pharmacodynamics deals with the mechanism of action of drugs and their biochemical and physiologic effects on the patient (8). Although frequently discussed separately, in reality, pharmacokinetics and pharmacodynamics are closely interconnected. For example, along with the dosing regimen, the pharmacokinetic properties of a drug determine the concentration of that drug in the body, and in many situations, the drug concentration is directly related to the effects experienced by the patient. In addition, the degree of protein binding that a particular drug exhibits is typically considered a pharmacokinetic property. However, in many cases, it is only the unbound drug that is pharmacologically active and therefore responsible for the pharmacodynamic effects.

Drugs produce desired effects through various types of mechanisms of action. Some drugs demonstrate a relatively direct mechanism of action, such as mannitol administered for osmotic diuresis. When mannitol is administered intravenously, the osmolarity of the blood and other body fluids is increased, causing shifts in the distribution of water. Other medications, such as epinephrine and beta-blockers, act by agonizing or antagonizing physiologic receptors. The effect of the drug is, therefore, directly related to the physiologic action of the associated receptor. Continued stimulation of some receptors with agonists frequently results in a state of down-regulation. In the intensive care unit (ICU), where exogenous catecholamines are commonly used, receptor down-regulation is important given that the continued or subsequent exposure to the same concentration of a particular agonist may have a lesser clinical effect over time. Other drugs, such as steroids, have very complex mechanisms of action involving crossing the cell membrane, regulating the transcription of specific genes, and ultimately altering protein synthesis. A practitioner's knowledge of the mechanisms of action and physiologic effects of drugs will help in determining the appropriate therapy, monitoring treatment, and anticipating pharmacodynamic drug interactions.

SPECIAL POPULATIONS

Renal Impairment

Whether a pre-existing disease state or a new condition developed in the ICU, renal dysfunction is often present in critically ill patients. Reduced renal function may be related to a disease state, either iatrogenic or age related. Acute and chronic renal impairment can have profound effects on the pharmacokinetics and pharmacodynamics of many commonly used agents. In addition, the degree of renal dysfunction and resulting degree of fluid retention and uremia determine the degree of pharmacokinetic and pharmacodynamic changes. For example, a drug may exhibit no clinically significant changes in a patient with mild renal dysfunction, or the medication may be contraindicated in a patient with renal failure. The practitioner must evaluate each drug individually in relation to the degree of renal dysfunction present.

Renal dysfunction has been shown to alter bioavailability, protein binding, volume of distribution, and excretion of certain compounds (9). There are relatively few data providing details regarding the alteration of bioavailability of most drugs in patients with renal dysfunction. However, certain conditions that are more common among uremic patients, including a higher gastric pH, altered gastric emptying time, vomiting, and intestinal edema, are known to alter the absorption and bioavailability of enterally administered drugs.

The distribution of some drugs may also be significantly altered in renal dysfunction. Because patients with significant renal dysfunction have a higher percentage of their body mass as water, the apparent volume of distribution for water-soluble drugs is often increased. In addition, the protein binding of drugs is often altered in the presence of uremia, which changes the apparent volume of distribution. In general, the plasma protein binding of acidic drugs, like phenytoin, is decreased (10). Because there is a larger percentage of unbound (free) drug available for pharmacologic activity, uremic patients may experience toxicity with total drug concentrations in the therapeutic range. For this reason, some practitioners prefer to measure free phenytoin concentrations instead of total phenytoin concentrations in patients with renal failure. Altered tissue binding also may affect the apparent volume of distribution of a drug. For example, digoxin's volume of distribution has been reported to be significantly reduced in patients with renal disease (11). As a result, in patients with renal dysfunction, digoxin loading doses should be used cautiously and serum concentrations should be monitored carefully.

The major pharmacokinetic effect seen in renal dysfunction is the impaired elimination of drugs and their metabolites by the kidney. Renal clearance of pharmacologic agents is complex, involving one or more of the processes of filtration, tubular secretion, and reabsorption. Few drugs are excreted solely by glomerular filtration. Additionally, tubular secretion and reabsorption for many compounds may vary with the type of renal dysfunction and the administration of other agents (e.g., probenecid).

Another complicating factor is changing renal dysfunction. Multiorgan system dysfunction in critically ill patients is a very dynamic process. As a consequence, renal function can deteriorate very quickly when changes in clinical condition such as hypotension or poor cardiac output occur. In addition, many of the agents that are frequently used in critically ill patients may cause renal dysfunction; radiographic contrast nephropathy and aminoglycoside nephrotoxicity are common examples (12). Changes in renal function may be acute or progressive; therefore, drug clearance may be highly variable in the intensive care setting and requires constant reassessment of the patient's clinical condition.

In evaluating medication use in renal impairment, the first step is to estimate the degree of dysfunction. Most medications that require dosage adjustment in patients with renal dysfunction are adjusted based on creatinine clearance. Although many hospital laboratories now report estimated GFR (eGFR) along with serum creatinine values, The National Kidney Disease Education Program recommends the use of equations, such as the Cockcroft-Gault equation, which is designed to estimate creatinine clearance for drug dosage adjustments (13).

When evaluating a medication profile, the intensivist must evaluate each drug individually and determine if a dosage adjustment or additional monitoring is necessary. Although for most medications, initial or loading dose does not need to be altered in renal dysfunction, maintenance dosing regimens may need to be adjusted by prolonging dosing intervals, reducing the standard maintenance dose, or both, depending on the particular agent and degree of renal dysfunction. In cases of drugs with a narrow therapeutic index, serum concentrations should be monitored carefully to avoid potential toxicity. In general, drug administration steady state should be achieved before a serum concentration is obtained, unless the patient rapidly progresses to renal failure, in which case an earlier sample may be warranted prior to reaching steady state to assess the appropriateness of redosing at current interval. For example, in patients with normal renal function, a vancomycin trough is typically obtained before the third or fourth dose; however, in the setting of renal dysfunction, a trough level prior to the second dose may be beneficial to help determine the patient's ability to clear the drug before further dosing.

In addition to the parent drug, practitioners also have to consider the route of elimination of any metabolites. For example, the active metabolite of morphine, morphine-6-glucuronide, is renally excreted and may exert important clinical effects when it accumulates in patients with renal failure (14). Although this does not prohibit the use of morphine in patients with renal dysfunction, practitioners may want to consider another agent, such as fentanyl, that does not have an active metabolite (15). If morphine is the preferred drug, a longer duration of action should be expected in a patient with renal impairment when compared to the same dose in a patient with normal renal function. Frequent assessment of morphine use by pain score and sedation level should be planned.

Critical care practitioners may also have to consider the effect of renal replacement therapy on drug clearance. The degree of drug clearance is determined by both drug-specific factors and the type of renal replacement therapy used. Drug-specific factors include molecular weight, solubility, degree of ionization, protein binding, and volume of distribution (9). For example, standard modes of dialysis are relatively ineffective in significantly clearing phenytoin, a highly protein-bound drug, from the body. However, more complicated techniques such as high-flux dialysis with charcoal hemoperfusion have been reported to remove considerable amounts of drug in a patient with phenytoin toxicity (16). Dialysis-specific factors that can affect the degree of drug clearance include the mode of dialysis, type of filter used, filter pore size, ultrafiltration rate, and blood and dialysate flow rates (17). As a general rule, peritoneal dialysis is less efficient in drug removal compared to intermittent hemodialysis and continuous renal replacement therapies (such as continuous venovenous hemodiafiltration) (9). Due to the potential complexity of drug dosing in the presence of renal replacement therapy, consulting a clinician who is readily familiar with the pharmacokinetic implications of intermittent or continuous renal replacement is advisable.

Hepatic Disease

Like renal insufficiency, hepatic disease can also significantly alter the pharmacokinetic profile of a drug and the ultimate effect on the patient. Unfortunately, data relating the degree of hepatic dysfunction in relation to drug metabolism and elimination is limited, and dosage adjustment guidelines for hepatic dysfunction are available for only some medications.

Because patients with severe liver failure often suffer from secondary gastrointestinal problems, the bioavailability of some orally administered drugs may be altered (18). Severe liver failure and cirrhosis have been associated with delayed gastric emptying and delayed absorption (18). For example, enteral furosemide has been shown to have delayed absorption in patients with mild and severe cirrhosis irrespective of the presence of ascites (19). In addition, patients with cirrhosis are at increased risk for severe upper gastrointestinal tract bleeding, which can limit enteral medication tolerance (20).

Liver failure also affects the volume of distribution of some drugs. Patients with significant ascites comprise a larger portion of their body weight as water. Therefore, the volume of distribution of hydrophilic drugs is increased (18). Most patients with significant liver dysfunction are also hypoalbuminemic, leading to a higher free fraction of highly protein-bound drugs.

Finally, while useful in evaluating long-term prognosis, liver cirrhosis severity scores, such as the Child-Pugh score, are less helpful in assessing the need for dosage adjustments of drugs (18). Many factors influence hepatic drug clearance; however, the most significant characteristics are hepatic blood flow and enzyme activity.

High extraction drugs are significantly removed (>60%) during the first passage across the liver, and the clearance of these drugs is significantly dependent on hepatic blood flow (18). In significant liver disease, such as cirrhosis, hepatic blood flow is decreased or totally shunted if portosystemic shunt is present (21). When a drug is administered enterally in these patients, drug enters the systemic circulation with minimal or no first-pass effect (22). Thus, the bioavailability of some orally administered drugs with extensive first-pass effect is greatly increased, and dosages should be appropriately reduced to prevent adverse side effects (23). Table 62.1 lists some of the high extraction drugs that may be used in the ICU.

TABLE 62.1

HIGH EXTRACTION DRUGS COMMONLY USED IN THE INTENSIVE CARE UNIT

Buspirone	Nicardipine
Chlorpromazine	Promethazine
Cyclosporine	Propranolol
Fluvastatin	Quetiapine
Isosorbide dinitrate	Sertraline
Labetalol	Sildenafil
Lovastatin	Sirolimus
Metoprolol	Tacrolimus
Midazolam	Venlafaxine
Morphine	Verapamil

Low extraction drugs are those that experience a relatively minimal first-pass effect (<30%), and initial bioavailability is not largely affected by liver disease (18). The clearance of hepatically metabolized, low extraction drugs may be influenced by the effects of liver disease on the enzyme system responsible for the metabolic process. Research has shown that a reduction in the activity of drug-metabolizing enzymes in livers from cirrhotic patients is associated with increasing disease severity (24,25). However, a large variation in the degree of enzyme activity impairment exists, probably due to the heterogeneity of the enzymes involved in drug metabolism processes. Numerous enzymes are affected differently by liver disease. For example, oxidation reactions tend to be more sensitive than glucuronidation (26).

Low extraction ratio drugs are less dependent on hepatic blood flow but are highly dependent on protein binding and the level of enzymatic capacity of the liver. These drugs are susceptible to changing clearance because of the induction or inhibition of liver enzymes and are sometimes referred to as enzyme limited or capacity limited (27). The hepatic clearance of some enzyme-limited drugs is termed binding sensitive or binding restrictive when only the circulating free drug is removed. Therefore, a decrease in drug binding causes an increase in the hepatic clearance of the drug. Drugs that are highly protein bound, such as phenytoin and warfarin, are most sensitive to this change in clearance.

Unfortunately, multiple factors determine the degree of impairment for the hepatic clearance of drugs, and no standard guidelines aid practitioners in the dosage adjustments of these medications. In addition, most available data that addresses the effect of liver disease on drug clearance are from studies evaluating patients with a single organ dysfunction (e.g., alcoholic cirrhosis); this is frequently not the case in critically ill patients. Therefore, any degree of other organ dysfunction, such as renal impairment or low cardiac output state, could further alter the pharmacokinetics and pharmacodynamics of the drug. The critical care team must initially evaluate the extent of organ dysfunction and determine whether a dosage reduction for a given drug is likely to be needed, and then monitor the patient carefully for early signs of toxicity. When possible, blood concentrations of the affected medications should be monitored.

Pregnancy

Because pregnant females represent a subset of critically ill patients with special needs and characteristics, considerations beyond the predicted physiologic changes to risk/benefit therapy assessment for both mother and fetus apply. Each subspecialty discipline must share their expertise with the intensivist team, and when possible, decisions should be made collaboratively with both the mother and fetus in mind. A fine balance must be obtained between avoiding undertreating the mother and presenting unnecessary risks to the fetus. Even in the otherwise healthy pregnant female, determining the optimal dosing regimen presents a considerable challenge due to the significant pharmacokinetic changes that occur during pregnancy.

Few gastrointestinal tract changes may affect drug absorption during pregnancy (28). With the exception of the active labor period, gastric emptying time appears to be unchanged (29). However, due to a decrease in gastrin secretion, pregnant women have a higher gastric pH and slower intestinal motility (30). The clinical significance of these changes in relation to drug absorption is not known. Some women experience significant nausea and vomiting, especially during the first trimester, which may affect their ability to tolerate some enteral medications. Noxious stimuli of any kind should be minimized.

Unlike absorption, the volume of distribution of certain drugs can be significantly changed by pregnancy. Most impressively, blood volume increases by approximately 40% to 50% during pregnancy (31). The exception is patients with severe pre-eclampsia or eclampsia; blood volume may expand very little in this population (28). Changes in plasma protein concentrations, such as a decrease in albumin concentration, can affect the free fraction of some drugs. Some examples of drugs that have a higher free fraction during pregnancy include diazepam, valproic acid, and phenytoin (32).

Pregnancy can also affect the metabolism and elimination of drugs as well. Interestingly, hepatic metabolism via the cytochrome P450 (CYP) system may be increased or decreased, depending on the specific enzyme. Specifically, pregnancy decreases the activity of CYP1A2 and CYP2C19. However, the activities of CYP3A4, CYP2D6, CYP2C9, and CYP2A6 are increased (30). The renal clearance of some drugs is also significantly increased during pregnancy due to an increase in glomerular filtration rate (GFR) of approximately 50% (30). For example, several β-lactam antibiotics, such as ampicillin, cefazolin, and piperacillin, have been shown to have increased clearance in pregnant women (33–35). Alterations in tubular secretion/reabsorption may also occur; however, few data are available in this area. Based on the available pharmacokinetic studies of renally excreted drugs, the effect of pregnancy on drug clearance varied widely from 20% to 65% above the clearance in nonpregnant females (30). For this reason, drugs that are primarily renally excreted unchanged may require a dosage increase of 20% to 65% to maintain prepregnancy blood concentrations (30).

In addition to pharmacokinetic changes that occur during pregnancy, the critical care practitioner also has to consider other physiologic changes that may affect the patient's need for drug therapy. For example, pregnant females are normally hypercoagulable and are at risk for venous thrombosis. The addition of other factors commonly seen in the ICU, such as immobility and endothelial injury, may put them at even higher risk. Unfractionated heparin and low-molecular-weight-heparins (LMWHs) are the drugs of choice for the prevention or treatment of thrombosis during pregnancy. Practitioners should be aware that many pregnant females require higher doses of heparin compared to nonpregnant females due to increased concentrations of heparin-binding proteins, increased volume of distribution, and increased clearance (36). In fact, the dose required for therapeutic anticoagulation may be as much as twice the typical weight-based dose (37). LMWHs are considered to be a safe alternative to unfractionated heparin during pregnancy, but their use in the acute setting for the treatment of venous thrombosis is controversial. Similar to unfractionated heparin, the clearance of LMWHs is increased during pregnancy, making dosing less straightforward than in the nonpregnant patient. Pregnant females have been shown to require higher than standard doses of LMWH to maintain goal anti–factor Xa concentrations (37,38). Therefore, frequent monitoring of anti–factor Xa concentrations is recommended, and multiple dosage adjustments may be required. With this increase in monitoring and related potential dosage adjustments, some argue that many of the advantages, both clinical and financial, of LMWHs are lost in this setting.

In conclusion, when the critical care practitioner is faced with determining the drug regimen for a pregnant patient, several steps should be taken. Most important, a multidisciplinary approach, including experts in the area of obstetrics and drug therapy, is invaluable. Next, the need to prescribe any drug must be carefully considered prior to the ordering process, and standard protocols should be modified as appropriate. Once the need for a drug is determined, the practitioner must consider the implications on fetal development and choose the safest drug available that will appropriately treat the mother. In considering the safety of a drug during pregnancy, the practitioner must go beyond simply identifying the "Pregnancy Risk Factor" that is included in the drug package labeling. A thorough search for information should be conducted, and the current trimester of the pregnancy should be considered. Some medications are safer for use during certain periods of the pregnancy. For example, nonsteroidal anti-inflammatory drugs (NSAIDs) are thought to carry the most risk during the first and third trimesters (39). In addition to primary literature, a medical reference that specifically addresses medication use in pregnancy should be consulted (39). In summary, once the treatment has been chosen, the practitioner must also consider the physiologic changes during pregnancy that may lead to a need for a dosage adjustment and monitor both the drug level, when possible, and the clinical picture.

ADVERSE DRUG REACTIONS

The term adverse drug reactions (ADRs) encompasses a broad range of drug effects, ranging from exaggerated but predictable pharmacologic actions of the drug to toxic effects unrelated to intended pharmacologic effects (40). As such, the true incidence rate of ADRs is difficult to determine, with estimates ranging from 5% to 47% (41–43). Only by maintaining a high index of clinical suspicion, keeping the drug therapy to the minimum necessary, and stopping the suspect drug, if possible, could one minimize the incidence of ADRs, thereby decreasing patient morbidity, perhaps even mortality, and also keeping the cost of therapy low.

A small group of widely used drugs account for a disproportionate number of ADRs; aspirin, anticoagulants, diuretics, digoxin, antimicrobials, steroids, and hypoglycemic agents account for 90% of reactions (40).

The most frequent ADRs result from the exaggerated but predicted pharmacologic actions of the drug, and, as such, are readily identifiable and often are preventable. Examples include hemorrhagic complications caused by anticoagulants or hypoglycemia caused by oral hypoglycemic agents or insulin. The most important determinant for such adverse effect is the abnormally high drug concentration at the receptor site. This can occur for various reasons, ranging from errors in calculating drug dosage or administration to an alteration in the pharmacokinetics (such as reduction in the volume of distribution, rate of metabolism, or rate of excretion), or because of a drug interaction resulting in increased concentration of free drug at the receptor site, leading to untoward effects.

Other ADRs result from toxic effects unrelated to the intended pharmacologic actions. Such events, therefore, often are unpredictable and frequently are severe. Various mechanisms are involved: genetic, immunologic and nonimmunologic, or idiosyncratic. A list of genetic susceptibilities leading to ADRs with certain drugs is presented in Table 62.2. The most relevant examples are succinylcholine-induced prolonged apnea (suxamethonium sensitivity) and drug-induced malignant hyperthermia (MH).

Succinylcholine is a depolarizing muscle relaxant that is rapidly metabolized by plasma pseudocholinesterase, with a duration of paralysis for 2 to 4 minutes. Approximately 1 in 3,200 patients is homozygous for a defective pseudocholinesterase, which has an autosomal recessive transmission and demonstrates markedly prolonged block with succinylcholine in the range of 3 to 8 hours (44).

MH is a clinical syndrome of muscle rigidity, tachycardia, tachypnea, rapidly increasing temperature, hypoxia, hypercapnia, hyperglycemia, hyperkalemia, hypercalcemia, lactic acidosis, and eventual cardiovascular collapse that occurs during or after general anesthesia (45). Several drugs have been implicated in triggering MH, particularly the halogenated inhalational agents (halothane, enflurane, and isoflurane), succinylcholine, and possibly an amino amide local anesthetic (lidocaine or bupivacaine) (46,47).

The cause of MH seems to be an inability of the sarcoplasmic reticulum of skeletal muscle to take up released myoplasmic calcium. When a MH episode is triggered, the myoplasmic levels of calcium rise tremendously, accelerating muscle metabolism and contraction, and leading to the clinical manifestations of the syndrome (45). The manifestation of MH may appear in the operating room or in the ICU shortly after the end of the surgical procedure.

Dantrolene is the cornerstone of therapy for MH (48). It reduces rigidity and restores muscle function by preventing calcium release from the sarcoplasmic reticulum and antagonizes its effects on muscle contraction (49). Treatment of MH is initiated by discontinuing the anesthetic and other possible triggering agents, ventilating the patient with 100% oxygen, providing hemodynamic support as needed, and administering dantrolene. The mortality rate from the fulminant syndrome was approximately 70% before the use of dantrolene (50). With early recognition and optimal therapy, reported mortality rates decreased from 10% to 7% (50).

An immunologically mediated ADR is epitomized by the classic anaphylactic reaction, which is IgE mediated, and a serum sickness–like condition. A similar reaction, but not immunologically mediated, known as anaphylactoid reaction, is sometimes seen as an indirect histamine release from the mast cells by morphine, or a complement activation leading to mediator release from the mast cell and basophil by aspirin and radiographic contrast media. There are a host of drug reactions for which the exact underlying mechanism of toxicity is not well understood, which are termed idiosyncratic reactions. Every organ system can potentially be adversely affected by drug exposures, or ADRs can present with effects on multiple organ systems. Of the multisystem manifestations of ADRs, drug fever, drug withdrawal reactions, and anaphylaxis are worth elaborating.

Drug-induced fever should always be considered in the workup of pyrexia in the intensive care unit, and more so when

TABLE 62.2

EXAMPLES OF INHERITED DISORDERS INVOLVING AN ABNORMAL RESPONSE TO DRUGS

	Disorder		
Characteristic	**Suxamethonium sensitivity**	**Malignant hyperthermia**	**Warfarin insensitivity**
Molecular abnormality	Pseudocholinesterase in plasma	Unknown	Altered receptors
Mode of inheritance	Autosomal recessive	Autosomal dominant	Autosomal dominant
Clinical effects	Apnea	Hyperpyrexia, muscle rigidity	Inability to achieve anticoagulation
Drugs producing abnormal response	Succinylcholine	Halothane, succinylcholine, cyclopropane	Warfarin

From Goldstein JL, Brown MS. Genetics and disease. *Harrison's Principles of Internal Medicine*. 13th ed. New York, NY: McGraw-Hill; 1994:349, with permission.

no other obvious source is apparent. Fever is thought to be relatively rare as a primary or sole manifestation of a drug reaction and is usually associated with other hypersensitivity type reactions like anaphylaxis, serum sickness, rash, or eosinophilia. Yet, sometimes fever may be the only manifestation of an ADR. Antibiotics, cardiovascular drugs, and central-acting agents are the largest categories of drugs causing fever (51). Patients with hypersensitivity-induced drug fever have been observed to have fevers as high as 40°C and yet generally appear well, which can be an important clue to the presence of a drug-related fever (52).

Medication withdrawal can trigger fever. Opiate and benzodiazepine tolerance and dependence can develop over a short period, and subsequent attempts at withdrawing these medications might be associated with hypermetabolism and "sympathetic overdrive" characterized by fever, hypertension, mental confusion, seizures, and cardiac arrhythmias, a clinical picture that may be confused with an underlying disease process (53). Management consists of the gradual withdrawal of the drug and substitution of longer-acting agents; clonidine, a centrally acting drug, has been used with some success in these conditions (54). The pathophysiology of anaphylactic shock from drug reactions has been described elsewhere in this text.

Mental confusion is a common problem in the ICU, and the cause is often multifactorial (55). Drugs that have been reported to alter mood and increase mental confusion, especially in the elderly, include corticosteroids, histamine-2 receptor antagonists, fluoroquinolones, theophylline, barbiturates, benzodiazepines, digoxin, antidepressants, penicillin, lidocaine, antihistamines, quinidine, opiates, and phenothiazines. Occasionally, confusion is associated with discontinuation of one of the aforementioned medications if used for a long period of time. Drugs like imipenem-cilastatin have been implicated as an inducer or promoter of seizure-like activity (56).

Some of the antiarrhythmic drugs, particularly procainamide, have a strong proarrhythmic effect, and drug levels should be closely monitored during use. Torsade de pointes, a form of polymorphic ventricular tachyarrhythmia caused by drugs that can prolong the QTc interval (like phenothiazines and tricyclic antidepressants), can be fatal. Treatment with intravenous magnesium and overdrive pacing has been used with some success to reverse cardiac arrest associated with this dysrhythmia.

Drug-induced renal injury remains a major cause of increased morbidity, and contributes to the overall mortality of the critically ill. The aminoglycoside antibiotics and radiographic contrast agents are the leading causes of acute nephrotoxicity in the ICU. Other risk factors that make patients prone to develop nephrotoxicity include advanced age, prior renal disease, intravascular volume depletion, simultaneous use of other nephrotoxic agents, and certain disease states such as congestive heart failure, liver cirrhosis, and diabetes mellitus (57).

Drugs can cause abnormalities in any of the formed elements of blood, which can lead to diagnostic confusion in separating these from primary disease processes. Drug-induced pancytopenia, hemolytic anemia, thrombocytopenia, and granulocytopenia all have been well described (57). Some of these conditions are more pertinent to ICU patients than others; heparin-induced thrombocytopenia (HIT) is an example. The mechanism is believed to be the induction of platelet-specific IgG antibody by heparin, with subsequent aggregation of platelets causing vascular thrombosis and fall in circulating platelets (58). Once the syndrome occurs, even trivial amounts of heparin can perpetuate the pathology. Heparin-containing flush solutions, indwelling catheters, and even heparin-coated pulmonary artery catheters have been reported to sustain the syndrome.

Generalized skin reactions of various forms occur as a part of a hypersensitivity reaction to various drugs. The drugs frequently involved are sulfonamides, the penicillins, and phenytoin. Of concern to the intensivists are the three major types of drug-induced skin diseases with the potential for life-threatening complications, including erythema multiforme (Stevens-Johnson syndrome), toxic epidermal necrolysis, and exfoliative erythroderma (40). The lesions range from typical target-shaped eruptions to extensive bullous eruptions and large areas of skin sloughing. These conditions are usually associated with hypovolemic shock, a hypercatabolic state, and multisystem organ dysfunction; the management is mainly supportive.

DRUG INTERACTIONS

Conventionally, a drug interaction is regarded as the modification of the effect of one drug by prior or concomitant administration of another (59). Several textbooks (60–64) and reviews (65) have compiled extensive listings of potential interactions. Most drug interaction studies report on small numbers of noncritically ill patients or volunteers, and thus, extrapolation of these studies to the ICU setting is undesirable, possibly leading to an unnecessary restriction of useful medications. This section reviews clinically significant drug interactions encountered in the ICU.

Drug interactions can result from pharmacokinetic or pharmacodynamic causes. Pharmacokinetic interactions affect the process of drug absorption, distribution, metabolism, and excretion. Pharmacodynamic interactions alter the biochemical or physiologic effect of a drug.

Pharmacokinetic Interactions

Absorption

Many drug interactions affect the bioavailability of drugs through their effects on absorption. These include adsorption and formation of drug complexes, changes in gastric emptying time and pH, alteration in intestinal motility and mucosal function, and reduction in splanchnic perfusion. Phenytoin absorption has been found to vary with type of enteral feeding (66). Anion exchange resin (cholestyramine) aluminum-containing drugs such as sucralfate and antacids, kaolin pectin, activated charcoal, and iron-containing preparations impair the absorption of various drugs such as digoxin, warfarin, and levothyroxine by forming insoluble complexes. In response, the safest action is to not give any oral medication within 2 hours of administering these chelating agents.

Drug incompatibilities in intravenous preparations also can present as drug interaction or absorption problems. Precipitation or chemical alteration may occur before parenteral dosing. Knowledge of *in vitro* drug incompatibilities is, therefore, essential, and in-depth resources are available (66,67). The

TABLE 62.3

DRUGS WITH HIGH PLASMA PROTEIN BINDING AFFINITY

Digoxin	Quinidine	Valproic acid
Hydralazine	Salicylates	Warfarin
NSAIDs	Sulfonamides	
Phenytoin	Tolbutamide	

NSAIDs, nonsteroidal anti-inflammatory drugs.

precipitation of phenytoin in glucose-containing solution is a relevant example (68).

Distribution

Many drugs circulate in the plasma partly bound to plasma proteins. Because the free or unbound serum concentration of a drug determines its biologic activity, changes in protein binding induced by another agent can have an important effect on the drug's pharmacologic response (69–72). Displacement from a protein of one drug by another depends on the concentration and relative binding affinities of the drugs. A drug with a higher serum concentration and higher protein-binding affinity displaces a second drug more readily. For example, warfarin's displacement by another drug can result in clinical bleeding complications. The acute elevation of free drug concentration in serum often is accompanied by an increased distribution to other tissues or increased elimination by metabolism and excretion until a new steady state is reached. Thus, when a new steady state is reached, the total drug level in the blood will be lower because of less protein-bound drug, whereas the free drug level will be in the therapeutic range. Individualization of drug therapy should be based on the clinical response or the plasma concentration of unbound drug, if available. Highly protein-bound drugs are particularly susceptible to these interactions (Table 62.3).

Metabolism

The metabolism of most drugs occurs largely in the liver. Quantitatively, the cytochrome P450 microsomal enzyme system containing mixed-function oxidases present in smooth endoplasmic reticulum is most important for initial metabolic conversion. The activity of these enzymes can be profoundly influenced by genetic factors and the coadministration of many drugs. These enzymes can be induced or inhibited by various agents (73,74).

Some common enzyme-inducing agents include the anticonvulsants, phenytoin, phenobarbital, and carbamazepine; ethanol; phenylbutazone; and rifampin (Table 62.4). Cigarette smoking has been shown to be an excellent inducer of isoenzymes responsible for theophylline metabolism. Enzyme induction increases the rate of elimination of various drugs, leading to lower plasma levels (Table 62.5).

Several compounds (Table 62.4) inhibit microsomal enzyme function, inhibiting the metabolism of many of the same drugs affected by enzyme induction (Table 62.5). For example, cimetidine is a potent inhibitor of oxidative metabolism of warfarin, quinidine, nifedipine, lidocaine, theophylline, and phenytoin. Erythromycin inhibits the metabolism of cyclosporine, warfarin, carbamazepine, and theophylline.

Excretion

The most important route of drug excretion is renal and involves the processes of filtration, secretion, and reabsorption (75,76). All of these aspects of renal handling of compounds can potentially lead to drug interactions.

Several drugs, such as the aminoglycoside antibiotics, are eliminated almost completely by glomerular filtration. Furosemide, a potent loop diuretic, by causing intravascular

TABLE 62.5

DRUGS COMMONLY AFFECTED BY ENZYME-INDUCING OR ENZYME-INHIBITING AGENTS

Carbamazepine	Lidocaine	Quinidine
Chlorpropamide	Metoprolol	Rifampin
Cyclosporine	Phenobarbital	Tolbutamide
Digoxin	Phenytoin	Theophylline
Glucocorticoids	Propranolol	Warfarin

TABLE 62.4

DRUGS COMMONLY AFFECTING METABOLIZING ENZYMES IN LIVER

INDUCING AGENTS	Acetaminophen	Cyclosporine	Metoprolol
	Barbiturates	Digoxin	Phenytoin
	Carbamazepine	Glucocorticoids	Quinidine
	Cimetidine	Methadone	Rifampin
	Clonazepam		Theophylline
INHIBITING AGENTS	Allopurinol	Erythromycin	Propranolol
	Amiodarone	Ethyl alcohol (acute)	Quinidine
	Chlorpromazine		Sulfonamide
	Cimetidine	INH	Tolbutamide
	Ciprofloxacin	Ketoconazole	Trimethoprim
	Diltiazem	Oral contraceptives	Verapamil

INH, isoniazid.
From Chernow B, ed. *The Pharmacologic Approach to the Critically Ill Patient.* Baltimore, MD: Williams & Wilkins, 1983, with permission.

volume depletion, can decrease renal perfusion pressure and filtration rate, thereby reducing elimination of gentamicin.

Many drugs are actively secreted in the proximal tubule. The most important of these agents include the organic acids, captopril, cephalosporins, sulfonamides, sulfonylureas, penicillins, diuretics, probenecid, and nonsteroidal anti-inflammatory agents. These compounds can block each others' secretions, thus decreasing their urinary excretion. Also, quinidine decreases the tubular secretion of digoxin. Thus, the coadministration of quinidine and digoxin approximately doubles the serum digoxin concentration. Inhibition of the tubular cation transport system by cimetidine impedes the renal clearance of procainamide and its active metabolite, *N*-acetyl procainamide.

The reabsorption of filtered or secreted compounds occurs in the distal tubule or collecting duct as a function of drug concentration, urinary flow, and pH of the urine. Alteration in distal urine pH can cause ion trapping of certain weak acids or bases and reduce passive reabsorption. Thus, alkalinization of urine by sodium bicarbonate facilitates the excretion of acidic drugs such as phenobarbital, salicylates, and amphetamines (40).

Lithium is reabsorbed with sodium in the kidney by the same renal mechanism. In case of volume depletion from chronic diuretic use, renal increases in sodium and lithium reabsorption occur, leading to a potentially toxic lithium level (40).

Pharmacodynamic Interactions

Unlike pharmacokinetic interactions, pharmacodynamic interactions occur when a pharmacodynamic effect of one medication affects the actions or effects of a second medication. Because critically ill patients are frequently on many medications for multiple indications, they are at high risk for these types of interactions. In some cases, pharmacodynamic interactions may be purposely used to achieve a desired therapeutic end point. For example, opioids and benzodiazepines are frequently used in combination to take advantage of their synergistic effects, possibly allowing for lower doses of each to be used (77,78). More frequently in the ICU, however, the pharmacodynamic interactions experienced are not desired and may lead to suboptimal therapy and adverse events.

Because of the numerous drug combinations and disease states that are seen in critical care units, the number of potential pharmacodynamic drug interactions is infinite and continues to grow as more medications are developed. For example, the chronic use of some antiepileptic medications may cause resistance to nondepolarizing neuromuscular blocking agents due to both enzyme induction, a pharmacokinetic interaction, and an up-regulation of acetylcholine receptors—namely, a pharmacodynamic interaction (79). In addition, the fluoroquinolone gatifloxacin has been reported to cause severe hypoglycemia when used in combination with oral hypoglycemic medications (80). Perhaps one of the most well-recognized pharmacodynamic interactions is the increased risk of torsade de pointes and death when two drugs that are known to cause QT prolongation are used in combination (81).

The principles of pharmacokinetics and pharmacodynamics are key to optimizing drug therapy of all types. If practitioners are unfamiliar with a medication, they should investigate the pharmacokinetic and pharmacodynamic characteristics of that drug to avoid subtherapeutic or supratherapeutic dosing, maximize efficacy, and minimize adverse events. Practitioners must be particularly careful in the ICU because critically ill patients frequently have some degree of organ dysfunction and may be receiving numerous medications.

A PRACTICAL APPROACH TO PHARMACOLOGICAL MANAGEMENT IN ICU

Pharmacotherapy is a complex science in the management of the critically ill patient. However, knowledge of pharmacokinetic principles, drug–drug interactions, changes related to systemic diseases, and possible drug toxicities permits the critical care clinician to design an appropriate medication regimen. The considerations listed below are recommended:

1. Review the medication administration record daily.
2. Monitor therapeutic end points and toxic effects for each drug.
3. Be knowledgeable of the pharmacokinetics of each drug (e.g., first-order versus zero-order kinetics, serum elimination half-life).
4. Remember that systemic disease (e.g., renal, hepatic) may create the need to alter the dosage regimen: an increase in volume of distribution may increase the required loading dose; and a decrease in clearance may decrease the required maintenance dose.
5. Look for possible drug–drug interactions.
6. Minimize the number of drugs.
7. Substitute equally effective, less expensive medications when possible.
8. Plan an approach to monitoring therapeutic and toxic effects. Check serum levels as appropriate, allowing four to five half-lives for steady-state achievement.

THE CLINICAL PHARMACIST'S ROLE IN CRITICAL CARE

In the multidisciplinary approach to care of the critically ill patient, the pharmacist is an essential member of the health-care team (77–79). The impact of a pharmacist on the delivery of cost-effective care has been established in multiple settings, including the spectrum of intensive care units (80–91). In addition to affecting economics, the critical care pharmacist directly influences clinical outcomes. Pharmacist involvement in critically ill patient care has been associated with optimal fluid and neuromuscular blockade management as well as significant reductions in adverse drug events, medication errors, unnecessary serum drug measurements, and ventilator-associated pneumonia rates (92–104).

As outlined by the Society of Critical Care Medicine and American College of Clinical Pharmacy Task Force on Critical Care Pharmacy Services position paper, fundamental critical care pharmacist activities include: prospective medication therapy evaluation; prevention, management, and reporting of adverse drug events; pharmacokinetic monitoring; drug information and education services; medication policy and procedure implementation and maintenance; cost-effectiveness analyses; and quality assurance measures and reviews (79). With departmental and service support, many critical care pharmacists participate in didactic and clinical teaching programs as well as clinical critical care pharmacotherapy research endeavors.

SUMMARY

Pharmacotherapy in the critically ill patient is extremely complex. A good understanding of pharmacologic principles, special population considerations, impact of single or multiple organ dysfunction, drug–drug interactions, and adverse drug reactions is paramount to maximize good outcome and minimize iatrogenic complications. Although the exact role and activities may vary in any given institution and patient population, the inclusion of a critical care pharmacist in daily patient care is recommended given the demonstrated cost savings and morbidity and mortality reductions.

References

1. Benet LZ, Kroetz DL, Sheiner LB. Pharmacokinetics: the dynamics of drug absorption, distribution, and elimination. In: Hardin JG, Limbird LE, Gilman AG, eds. *Goodman and Gilman's The Pharmacologic Basis of Therapeutics*. New York, NY: McGraw-Hill; 1996:3.
2. Bauer LA. Individualization of drug therapy: clinical pharmacokinetics and pharmacodynamics. In: DiPiro JT, ed. *Pharmacotherapy: A Pathophysiologic Approach*. New York, NY: Elsevier; 1992:15.
3. Winter ME. Clinical pharmacokinetics. In: *Applied Therapeutics: The Clinical Use of Drugs*. Vancouver, WA: Applied Therapeutics; 1992.
4. Riegelman S, Loo JC, Rowland M. Shortcomings in pharmacokinetic analysis by conceiving the body to exhibit properties of a single compartment. *J Pharm Sci*. 1968;57(1):117–123.
5. Greenblatt DJ, Kock-Weser J. Drug therapy. Clinical Pharmacokinetics (first of two parts). *N Engl J Med*. 1975;293(14):702–705.
6. Winter ME. *Basic Clinical Pharmacokinetics*. 6th ed. Vancouver, WA: *Applied Therapeutics*; 1999.
7. Koch-Weser J. Bioavailability of drugs (first of two parts). *N Engl J Med*. 1974;291(5):233–237.
8. Ross EM, Kennakin TP. Pharmacodynamics mechanisms of drug action and the relationship between drug concentration and effect. In: Hardman JG, Limbird LE, Gilman AG, eds. *Goodman and Gilman's The Pharmacological Basis of Therapeutics*. New York, NY: McGraw-Hill; 2001:31–43.
9. Frye RF, Matzke GK. Drug therapy individualization for patients with renal insufficiency. In: DiPiro JT, et al., eds. *Pharmacotherapy: A Pathophysiologic Approach*. New York, NY: McGraw-Hill; 1999:939–952.
10. Vanholder R, Van Landschoot N, De Smet R, et al. Drug protein binding in chronic renal failure: evaluation of nine drugs. *Kidney Int*. 1988;33(5):996–1004.
11. Cheng JW, Charland SL, Shaw LM, et al. Is the volume of distribution of digoxin reduced in patients with renal dysfunction? Determining digoxin pharmacokinetics by fluorescence polarization immunoassay. *Pharmacotherapy*. 1997;17(3):584–590.
12. Taber SS, Mueller BA. Drug-associated renal dysfunction. *Crit Care Clin*. 2006;22(2):357–374.
13. National Kidney Disease Education Program. Creatinine standardization program: recommendations for pharmacists and authorized drug prescribers. July 2006. http://www.nkdep.nih.gov/labprofessionals/Pharm_Recommendations_508.pdf. Accessed August 2, 2007.
14. Lötsch J. Opioid metabolites. *J Pain Symptom Manage*. 2005;29(5 Suppl):S10–24.
15. Jacobi J, Fraser GL, Coursin DB, et al. Clinical practice guidelines for the sustained use of sedatives and analgesics in the critically ill adult. *Crit Care Med*. 2002;30(1):119–141.
16. De Schoenmakere G, De Waele J, Terryn W, et al. Phenytoin intoxication in critically ill patients. *Am J Kidney Dis*. 2005;45(1):189–192.
17. Veltri MA, Neu AM, Fivush BA, et al. Drug dosing during intermittent hemodialysis and continuous renal replacement therapy: special considerations in pediatric patients. *Paediatr Drugs*. 2004;6(1):45–65.
18. Delcò F, Tchambaz L, Schlienger R, et al. Dose adjustment in patients with liver disease. *Drug Saf*. 2005;28(6):529–545.
19. Fredrick MJ, Pound DC, Hall SD, et al. Furosemide absorption in patients with cirrhosis. *Clin Pharmacol Ther*. 1991;49(3):241–247.
20. Schemmer P, Decker F, Dei-Anane G, et al. The vital threat of an upper gastrointestinal bleeding: risk factor analysis of 121 consecutive patients. *World J Gastroenterol* 2006;12(22):3597–3601.
21. Vyas K, Gala B, Sawant P, et al. Assessment of portal hemodynamics by ultrasound color Doppler and laser Doppler velocimetry in liver cirrhosis. *Indian J Gastroenterol*. 2002;21(5):176–178.
22. Rodighiero V. Effects of liver disease on pharmacokinetics. An update. *Clin Pharmacokinet*. 1999;37(5):399–431.
23. Hoyumpa AM, Schenker S. Influence of liver disease on the disposition and elimination of drugs. In: Schiff L, Schiff ER, eds. *Diseases of the Liver*. Philadelphia, PA: JB Lippincott Co; 1993.
24. George J, Murray M, Byth K, et al. Differential alterations of cytochrome P450 proteins in livers from patients with severe chronic liver disease. *Hepatology*. 1995;21(1):120–128.
25. Iqbal S, Vickers C, Elias E. Drug metabolism in end-stage liver disease. In vitro activities of some phase I and phase II enzymes. *J Hepatol*. 1990;11(1):37–42.
26. McLean AJ, Morgan DJ. Clinical pharmacokinetics in patients with liver disease. *Clin Pharmacokinet*. 1991;21(1):42–69.
27. Blaschke TF. Protein binding and kinetics of drugs in liver diseases. *Clin Pharmacokinet*. 1977;2(1):32–44.
28. Yeomans ER, Gilstrap LC III. Physiologic changes in pregnancy and their impact on critical care. *Crit Care Med*. 2005;33(10 Suppl):S256–258.
29. Cunningham FG, MacDonald PC, Gant NF, eds. *Williams Obstetrics*. 18th ed. Norwalk, CO: Appleton & Lange; 1989.
30. Anderson GD. Pregnancy-induced changes in pharmacokinetics: a mechanistic-based approach. *Clin Pharmacokinet*. 2005;44(10):989–1008.
31. Pritchard JA. Changes in the blood volume during pregnancy and delivery. *Anesthesiology*. 1965;26:393–399.
32. Loebstein R, Lalkin A, Koren G. Pharmacokinetic changes during pregnancy and their clinical relevance. *Clin Pharmacokinet*. 1997;33(5):328–343.
33. Philipson A. Pharmacokinetics of ampicillin during pregnancy. *J Infect Dis*. 1977;136(3):370–376.
34. Philipson A, Stiernstedt G, Ehrnebo M. Comparison of the pharmacokinetics of cephradine and cefazolin in pregnant and non-pregnant women. *Clin Pharmacokinet*. 1987;12(2):136–144.
35. Heikkilä A, Erkkola R. Pharmacokinetics of piperacillin during pregnancy. *J Antimicrob Chemother*. 1991;28(3):419–423.
36. Stone SE, Morris TA. Pulmonary embolism during and after pregnancy. *Crit Care Med*. 2005;33(10 Suppl):S294–300.
37. Barbour LA, Smith JM, Marlar RA, et al. Heparin levels to guide thromboembolism prophylaxis during pregnancy. *Am J Obstet Gynecol*. 1995;173(6):1869–1873.
38. Jacobsen AF, Qvigstad E, Sandset PM. Low molecular weight heparin (dalteparin) for the treatment of venous thromboembolism in pregnancy. *BJOG*. 2003;110(2):139–144.
39. Briggs GG, Freeman RK, Yaffe SJ, eds. *Drugs in Pregnancy and Lactation*. 7th ed. Philadelphia, PA: Lippincott Williams & Wilkins; 2005.
40. Oates JA, Wood AJ. Adverse reaction to drugs. In: *Harrison's Principles of Internal Medicine*. New York, NY: McGraw-Hill; 1991:373.
41. Gray TK, Adams LL, Fallon HJ. Short-term intense surveillance of adverse drug reactions. *J Clin Pharmacol New Drugs*, 1973;13(2):61–67.
42. Jick H. Adverse drug effects in relation to renal function. *Am J Med*. 1977;62(4):514–517.
43. Leape LL, Cullen DJ, Dempsey Clapp M, et al. Pharmacist participation on physician rounds and adverse drug events in the intensive care unit. *JAMA*. 1999;281(3):267–270.
44. Whittaker M. Plasma cholinesterase variants and the anaesthetist. *Anaesthesia* 1980;35(2):174–197.
45. Nelson TE, Flewellen EH. Current concepts. The malignant hyperthermia syndrome. *N Engl J Med*. 1983;309(7):416–418.
46. Gronert GA. Malignant hyperthermia. *Anesthesiology*. 1980;53(5):395–423.
47. Gronert GA. Malignant hyperthermia. In: Miller RD, ed. *Anesthesia*. New York, NY: Churchill Livingstone; 1986:1971.
48. Kolb ME, Horne ML, Martz R. Dantrolene in human malignant hyperthermia. *Anesthesiology*. 1982;56(4):254–262.
49. Morgan KG, Bryant SH. The mechanism of action of dantrolene sodium. *J Pharmacol Exp Ther*. 1977;201(1):138–147.
50. Gronert GA. Malignant hyperthermia. *Semin Anesth*. 1983;2:197.
51. Norwood S. An approach to the febrile patient. In: Civetta JM, Taylor RW, Kirby RR, eds. *Critical Care*. Philadelphia, PA: JB Lippincott Co; 1992:992.
52. Mackowiak PA, LeMaistre CF. Drug fever: a critical appraisal of conventional concepts. An analysis of 51 episodes in two Dallas hospitals and 97 episodes reported in the English literature. *Ann Intern Med*. 1987;106(5):728–733.
53. George CF, Robertson D. Clinical consequences of abrupt drug withdrawal. *Med Toxicol Adverse Drug Exp*, 1987;2(5):367–382.
54. Bohrer H, et al. Clonidine as a sedative adjunct in intensive care. *Intensive Care Med*. 1990;16(4):265–266.
55. Easton C, MacKenzie F. Sensory-perceptual alterations: delirium in the intensive care unit. *Heart Lung*. 1988;17(3):229–237.
56. Messing RO, Closson RG, Simon RP. Drug-induced seizures: a 10-year experience. *Neurology*. 1984;34(12):1582–1586.
57. Albertson TE, Foulke GE, Tharratt S. Pharmacokinetics and iatrogenic drug toxicity in the intensive care unit. In: Hall JB, Schmidt GA, Wood LH, eds. *Principles of Critical Care*. New York, NY: McGraw-Hill; 1992:2061.

58. Warkentin TE, Kelton JG. Heparin and platelets. *Hematol Oncol Clin North Am.* 1990;4(1):243–264.
59. McInnes GT, Brodie MJ. Drug interactions that matter. A critical reappraisal. *Drugs.* 1988;36(1):83–110.
60. Chernow B, ed. *The Pharmacologic Approach to the Critically Ill Patient.* Baltimore, MD: Williams & Wilkins; 1988.
61. Hardman JG, Limbird LE, Gilman AG, eds. *The Pharmacologic Basis of Therapeutics.* 10th ed. New York, NY: Mc-Graw-Hill; 2001.
62. Hansen PD, Horn JR. *Drug Interaction.* St. Louis, MO: Wolters Kluwer Health; 2006.
63. Morselli PL, Garattinni S, Cohen SN. *Drug Interactions.* New York, NY: Raven Press; 1974.
64. Stockley I. *Drug Interactions.* 3rd ed. Oxford, UK: Blackwell Science; 1995.
65. Prescott LF. Pharmacokinetic drug interactions. *Lancet.* 1969;2(7632): 1239–1243.
66. Guidry JR, Eastwood TF, Curry SC. Phenytoin absorption in volunteers receiving selected enteral feedings. *West J Med.* 1989;150(6):659–661.
67. Trissel LA. *Handbook of Injectable Drugs.* 13th ed. Bethesda, MD: American Society of Health-System Pharmacists; 2005.
68. Cloyd JC, Bosch DE, Sawchuk RJ. Concentration-time profile of phenytoin after admixture with small volumes of intravenous fluids. *Am J Hosp Pharm.* 1978;35(1):45–48.
69. Koch-Weser J, Sellers EM. Binding of drugs to serum albumin (first of two parts). *N Engl J Med.* 1976;294(6):311–316.
70. MacKichan JJ. Pharmacokinetic consequences of drug displacement from blood and tissue proteins. *Clin Pharmacokinet.* 1984;9(Suppl 1):32–41.
71. McElnay JC, D'Arcy PF. Protein binding displacement interactions and their clinical importance. *Drugs.* 1983;25(5):495–513.
72. Wood M. Plasma drug binding: implications for anesthesiologists. *Anesth Analg.* 1986;65(7):786–804.
73. Burns JJ, Conney AH. Enzyme stimulation and inhibition in the metabolism of drugs. *Proc R Soc Med.* 1965;58(11 Pt 2):955–960.
74. Gelehrter TD. Enzyme induction (first of three parts). *N Engl J Med.* 1976;294(10):522–526.
75. Prescott LF. Mechanisms of renal excretion of drugs (with special reference to drugs used by anaesthetists). *Br J Anaesth,* 1972;44(3):246–251.
76. Weiner IM, Mudge GH. Renal tubular mechanisms for excretion of organic acids and bases. *Am J Med.* 1964;36:743–762.
77. Gilliland HE, Prasad BK, Mirakhur RK, et al. An investigation of the potential morphine sparing effect of midazolam. *Anaesthesia.* 1996;51(9):808–811.
78. Richman PS, Baram D, Varela M, et al. Sedation during mechanical ventilation: a trial of benzodiazepine and opiate in combination. *Crit Care Med.* 2006;34(5):1395–1401.
79. Perucca E. Clinically relevant drug interactions with antiepileptic drugs. *Br J Clin Pharmacol.* 2006;61(3):246–255.
80. LeBlanc M, Bélanger C, Cossette P. Severe and resistant hypoglycemia associated with concomitant gatifloxacin and glyburide therapy. *Pharmacotherapy.* 2004;24(7):926–931.
81. Allen LaPointe NM, Curtis LH, Chan KA, et al. Frequency of high-risk use of QT-prolonging medications. *Pharmacoepidemiol Drug Saf.* 2006;15(6):361–368.
82. Brilli RJ, Spevetz A, Branson RD, et al. Critical care delivery in the intensive care unit: defining clinical roles and the best practice model. *Crit Care Med.* 2001;29(10):2007–2019.
83. Haupt MT, Bekes CE, Brilli RJ, et al. Guidelines on critical care services and personnel: recommendations based on a system of categorization of three levels of care. *Crit Care Med.* 2003;31(11):2677–2683.
84. Rudis MI, Brandl KM. Position paper on critical care pharmacy services. Society of Critical Care Medicine and American College of Clinical Pharmacy Task Force on Critical Care Pharmacy Services. *Crit Care Med.* 2000;28(11):3746–3750.
85. Baldinger SL, Chow MS, Gannon RH, et al. Cost savings from having a clinical pharmacist work part-time in a medical intensive care unit. *Am J Health Syst Pharm.* 1997;54(24):2811–2814.
86. Gandhi PJ, Smith BS, Tataronis GR, et al. Impact of a pharmacist on drug costs in a coronary care unit. *Am J Health Syst Pharm.* 2001;58(6):497–503.
87. Krupicka MI, Bratton SL, Sonnenthal K, et al. Impact of a pediatric clinical pharmacist in the pediatric intensive care unit. *Crit Care Med.* 2002;30(4):919–921.
88. Patel NP, Brandt CP, Yowler CJ. A prospective study of the impact of a critical care pharmacist assigned as a member of the multidisciplinary burn care team. *J Burn Care Res.* 2006;27(3):310–313.
89. Hatoum HT, Hutchinson RA, White KW, et al. Evaluation of the contribution of clinical pharmacists: inpatient care and cost reduction. *Drug Intell Clin Pharm.* 1988;22(3):252–259.
90. Herfindal ET, Bernstein LR, Kishi DT. Impact of clinical pharmacy services on prescribing on a cardiothoracic/vascular surgical unit. *Drug Intell Clin Pharm.* 1985;19(6):440–444.
91. Katona BG, Ayd PR, Walters JK, et al. Effect of a pharmacist's and a nurse's interventions on cost of drug therapy in a medical intensive-care unit. *Am J Hosp Pharm.* 1989;46(6):1179–1182.
92. McMullin ST, Hennenfent JA, Ritchie DJ, et al. A prospective, randomized trial to assess the cost impact of pharmacist-initiated interventions. *Arch Intern Med.* 1999;159(19):2306–2309.
93. Miyagawa CI, Rivera JO. Effect of pharmacist interventions on drug therapy costs in a surgical intensive-care unit. *Am J Hosp Pharm.* 1986;43(12):3008–3013.
94. Montazeri M, Cook DJ. Impact of a clinical pharmacist in a multidisciplinary intensive care unit. *Crit Care Med.* 1994;22(6):1044–1048.
95. Schumock GT, Meek PD, Ploetz PA, et al. Economic evaluations of clinical pharmacy services—1988–1995. The Publications Committee of the American College of Clinical Pharmacy. *Pharmacotherapy.* 1996;16(6): 1188–1208.
96. Smythe MA, Shah PP, Spiteri TL, et al. Pharmaceutical care in medical progressive care patients. *Ann Pharmacother.* 1998;32(3):294–299.
97. Broyles JE, Brown RO, Vehe KL, et al. Pharmacist interventions improve fluid balance in fluid-restricted patients requiring parenteral nutrition. *DICP.* 1991;25(2):119–122.
98. Calabrese AD, Erstad BL, Brandl K, et al. Medication administration errors in adult patients in the ICU. *Intensive Care Med.* 2001;27(10):1592–1598.
99. Devlin JW, Holbrook AM, Fuller HD. The effect of ICU sedation guidelines and pharmacist interventions on clinical outcomes and drug cost. *Ann Pharmacother.* 1997;31(6):689–695.
100. Kaye J, Ashline V, Erickson D, et al. Critical care bug team: a multidisciplinary team approach to reducing ventilator-associated pneumonia. *Am J Infect Control.* 2000;28(2):197–201.
101. Lazarou J, Pomeranz BH, Corey PN. Incidence of adverse drug reactions in hospitalized patients: a meta-analysis of prospective studies. *JAMA.* 1998;279(15):1200–1205.
102. Leape LL, Cullen DJ, Clapp MD, et al. Pharmacist participation on physician rounds and adverse drug events in the intensive care unit. *JAMA.* 1999;282(3):267–270.
103. Rudis MI, Sikora CA, Angus E, et al. A prospective, randomized, controlled evaluation of peripheral nerve stimulation versus standard clinical dosing of neuromuscular blocking agents in critically ill patients. *Crit Care Med.* 1997;25(4):575–583.
104. Dager WE, Albertson TE. Impact of therapeutic drug monitoring of intravenous theophylline regimens on serum theophylline concentrations in the medical intensive care unit. *Ann Pharmacother.* 1992;26(10):1287–1291.

CHAPTER 63 ■ SEDATION AND NEUROMUSCULAR BLOCKADE

MICHAEL J. MURRAY • ERIC L. BLOOMFIELD

PERSPECTIVE

Anxiety is one of the human emotions that help us anticipate and prepare for real or perceived threats. Anxiety results in the release of endogenous catecholamines with an accompanying increase in heart rate, blood pressure, tremulousness, and so on. In some critically ill patients, anxiety can lead to agitation, i.e., anxiety coupled with confusion and movement and, if the confusion is severe enough, delirium. Increasingly, there is recognition that the spectrum of anxiety, agitation, and delirium may be a manifestation of the effects of the systemic inflammatory response syndrome (SIRS) and multiple organ dysfunction syndrome (MODS), with the brain being the end organ affected. With this recognition of the significance of anxiety has come an increasing attention to monitoring its severity, as well as treatment and assessment of the effects of therapy.

The lung is the most frequently injured organ in patients with MODS, resulting in acute respiratory distress syndrome (ARDS) or acute lung injury (ALI). Patients with ALI and ARDS require intubation and mechanical ventilation, and, with modes of mechanical ventilation adjusted to deliver low tidal volumes with resultant hypercarbia, patients are more likely to become agitated. In such patients in whom sedation is inadequate, neuromuscular blocking agents (NMBAs) may be required. These medications should always be administered cautiously, with daily drug "holidays," which permit the clinician caring for the patient to determine if the NMBA is still required.

FEATURES

Anxiety

Anxiety is often described as a heightened sense of awareness, apprehension, dread, or anticipation. The latter is an important characteristic, for anxiety is an emotional state; the individual "anticipates" a threat, and anxiety prepares the individual for "fight or flight." Anxiety has its anatomic construct in the limbic system and is associated with the release of catecholamines, which lead to the tremulousness, sweating, tachycardia, and tachypnea—all the hallmarks of anxiety. In its extreme, an individual may have a "panic attack."

Oftentimes when clinicians round on patients in the ICU, they find a patient who looks distressed, and blood pressure and heart rate are elevated. We commonly assume that the patient is in pain, and yet frequently, anxiety is the problem. Interestingly, the easiest way to separate these two perceptions is to ask the patient. As part of the daily evaluation of patients in the ICU, they should be asked if they are anxious, if they are in pain, and if they are "getting enough air to breathe?" The latter two complaints are likely to exacerbate anxiety, along with several other experiences that ICU patients may have (Table 63.1). The treatment for pain and anxiety are often the same, but for patients without pain, the treatment algorithm is different (see below). However, anxiety and pain are often a continuum, with the perception of one increasing the perception of the other.

Anxiety may lead to insomnia, a common problem in the ICU, and insomnia (and sleep deprivation) can increase the perception of anxiety (1). Sleep interruption occurs for several reasons, starting with excessive noise levels in many ICUs at night, patient care activities, measurement of vital signs, laboratory tests, radiographs, and so on. Patients who are intubated and mechanically ventilated are even more likely to have interrupted sleep, along with experiencing discomfort from the mode of mechanical ventilation and/or tracheal suctioning, as well as hypercarbia and hypoxia. In surveys of patients discharged from the ICU, patients recall feelings of terror, nervousness, and insomnia (2). Older patients, because they have less organ reserve, are more at risk of developing problems; depending on the extent of chronic health problems, the acute illness, and medications the patients receive, they are more at risk of cognitive dysfunction (3), which increases the risk of developing agitation and delirium (4).

Agitation

In the 2001 Agitation Consensus Conference, agitation was described as "continual movement characterized by constant fidgeting, moving from side to side, pulling at dressings and bed sheets, and attempting to remove catheters or other tubes" (5). Agitation is associated with some degree of cognitive impairment—disorientation, confusion, confabulation, and so on. Agitation is different from anxiety because the agitated patient displays purposeless movement and has some degree of cognitive dysfunction. For the reasons mentioned about removal of invasive devices, agitated patients are at risk of injuring themselves and, in some circumstances, injuring health care providers. Factors associated with agitation (6) include advanced age, neuropsychiatric comorbidities, seriousness of illness, pain, and some drugs that, when given to ICU patients, have unrecognized interactions and side effects. Agitation is associated with an increased length of stay, iatrogenic infections,

TABLE 63.1

EXPERIENCES THAT INCREASE PATIENT ANXIETY IN THE INTENSIVE CARE UNIT

Pain	Physical restraints
Insomnia	Tracheal suctioning
Dyspnea	Hypoxia/hypercarbia
Temperature extremes	Distended bladder
Loneliness	Invasive lines/devices
Clinical outlook	Loss of control/autonomy

TABLE 63.2

SEDATION SCALES

ATICE	Adaptation to the Intensive Care Environment (7)
MSAT	Minnesota Sedation Assessment Tool (8)
RSS	Ramsay Sedation Scale (9)
RASS	Richmond Agitation-Sedation Scale (10)
SAS	Sedation Agitation Scale (11)
VICS	Vancouver Interaction and Calmness Scale (12)

and self-extubation (6). Many believe that prolonged anxiety, depending on the cause, if left untreated, can lead to agitation (5). Most of the tools to monitor agitation and the effects of therapeutic interventions are listed in Table 63.2 (7–12). However, because patient movement is one of the hallmarks of agitation, some clinicians use a variant of the Ramsay Sedation Scale and the Motor Activity Assessment Scale (Table 63.3) to monitor for agitation (13).

Delirium

The hallmark of delirium is cognitive dysfunction, most commonly manifested as disorientation in a patient who is critically ill. In the past, such patients were diagnosed as having "ICU syndrome," a diagnosis of exclusion. Heightened awareness has resulted in several studies that have examined the prevalence (14), types (15), consequences (16), and the diagnosis and management (17) of delirium.

In a coronary care unit, the prevalence of delirium can run as low as 7% (14), whereas in a medical ICU, it may run as high as 70% to 80% (15). Delirious patients may manifest a variety of psychomotor behavior, from hypoactive (listlessness) to hyperactive (combative behavior), with a mixed picture also seen (15). Independent of the motor type, the delirious patient is at risk for developing long-term cognitive impairment (18), a greater length of ICU and hospital stay, and an increased mortality (16). Patients frequently cycle between overly sedated states to hyperactive, agitated states. Management can be difficult, as some medications commonly given to sedate patients have also been associated with an increased incidence of delirium (19).

Anxiety, agitation, and delirium require recognition (20) and education of health care professionals (17) so we can identify at-risk patients and improve treatment.

EVALUATION

Although anxiety is a valid emotional response to hospitalization in an ICU, an overexuberant response to the stressors in the ICU environment can be detrimental. Anxious patients have an increase in the incidence of several disease states/processes (Table 63.4) (21–25).

Patients should be examined on a daily basis, particularly to look for certain signs that increase the likelihood of anxiety (Table 63.5). The laboratory evaluation (Table 63.6) is also helpful in determining if the patient is, indeed, hypercapnic, septic, or has increased or decreased concentrations of electrolytes in the blood that often correlate with an increased risk of neurologic dysfunction.

TABLE 63.3

MOTOR ACTIVITY ASSESSMENT SCALE

Score	Description	Definition
0	Unresponsive	Does not move with noxious stimulus
1	Responsive only to noxious stimuli	Opens eyes *or* raises eyebrows *or* turns head toward stimulus *or* moves limbs with noxious stimulus
2	Responsive to touch or name	Opens eyes *or* raises eyebrows *or* turns head toward stimulus *or* moves limbs when touched or name is loudly spoken
3	Calm and cooperative	No external stimulus is required to elicit movement, *and* the patient is adjusting sheets or clothes purposefully and follows commands
4	Restless and cooperative	No external stimulus is required to elicit movement, *and* patient is picking at sheets or clothes or uncovering self and follows commands
5	Agitated	No external stimulus is required to elicit movement, *and* patient is attempting to sit up *or* moves limbs out of bed *and* does not consistently follow commands
6	Dangerously agitated, uncooperative	No external stimulus is required to elicit movement, *and* patient is pulling at tubes or catheters *or* thrashing side to side *or* striking at staff *or* trying to climb out of bed *and* does not calm down when asked

Reprinted from Devlin JW, Boleski G, Mlynarek M, et al. Motor Activity Assessment Scale: a valid and reliable sedation scale for use with mechanically ventilated patients in an adult surgical intensive care unit. *Crit Care Med.* 1999;27:1271–1275, with permission.

TABLE 63.4

ANXIETY ASSOCIATED WITH AN INCREASED INCIDENCE OF SEVERAL DISEASE STATES/PROCESSES

Myocardial ischemia (21)
Asthma (22)
Pain (23)
Agitation (24)
Delirium (25)

TABLE 63.5

PHYSICAL EXAMINATION

Tachypnea
Tachycardia
Confusion
Abdominal distention (ileus, full bladder)
Movement

TABLE 63.6

LABORATORY EVALUATION

Complete blood count (anemia, leukocytosis/leukopenia)
Arterial blood gases (hypoxia, hypocarbia/hypercapnia)
Electrolytes[a]
Glucose
Creatinine/blood urea nitrogen

[a]To include calcium and magnesium.

TABLE 63.7

NONPHARMACOLOGIC THERAPY FOR ANXIETY-PRODUCING EVENTS

Thorough explanation of situation/findings
Reassurance
Increased presence of family members (26)
Decreased noise (27)
Decreased nocturnal interruptions
Assisted ventilation for hypercarbia
Cardioversion for hemodynamically significant tachyarrhythmias
Decrease/stop tube feedings if (partial) ileus
Foley catheter for bladder distention
Re-establishment of sleep cycle (28)

TABLE 63.8

THERAPY FOR ANXIETY-PRODUCING EVENTS

Supplemental oxygen for hypoxia
Minimize dose of supplemental catecholamines
Continue any of patients' psychotropic medications, if appropriate
Opioids
Benzodiazepines
Haloperidol
Propofol
Dexmedetomidine
Ketamine

When a patient admits to excessive anxiety, one should first attempt to decrease the anxiety through nonpharmacologic means (Table 63.7) (26–28). First and foremost is the recognition that the environment in the ICU must be calm and nurturing, with attention to such details as room temperature, noise levels, and sleep disturbance—the bane of most modern ICUs.

Approximately 60% to 70% of patients who reside in the ICU for greater than 48 hours will require pharmacologic therapy (Table 63.8). Of the possible agents, opioids, benzodiazepines, haloperidol, propofol, and dexmedetomidine are the mainstays of treatment.

TREATMENT

Nonsteroidal Anti-inflammatory Drugs

Nonsteroidal anti-inflammatory drugs (NSAIDs) do not have sedative properties, but to the extent that they decrease pain, they do decrease pain-associated anxiety. NSAIDs would most likely be contraindicated in ICU patients because of their side effects. However, when cyclo-oxygenase (COX)-2 inhibitors, which have fewer side effects, are coupled with gabapentin or its precursor, pregabalin, they have analgesic and sedative properties if given preoperatively *per os* to patients who are anticipated to be admitted postoperatively to the ICU. In one study, a combination of 400 mg of celecoxib and 150 mg of pregabalin improved patients' sedation levels by approximately 33% for up to 24 hours postoperatively (29).

Opioids

Because pain or discomfort (from tracheal tube suctioning, nasogastric tubes, or Foley catheters) is a frequent, confounding factor for anxious patients, analgesics are often administered, usually via continuous intravenous infusions. Importantly, opioids have not only analgesic but also anxiolytic properties (30). Morphine has anxiolytic properties, but is not nearly as effective as newer opioids, and, because of the buildup of active metabolites in patients with renal insufficiency, it is not recommended for patients in the ICU. Fentanyl and remifentanil are over 90% effective in providing adequate sedation for intubated and mechanically ventilated patients in the ICU (31). Because of equal efficacy and differences in cost, fentanyl is recommended in most patients, except those with significant renal/hepatic impairment (Table 63.9).

TABLE 63.9

OPIOIDS AS SEDATIVE DRUGS IN THE INTENSIVE CARE UNIT

	Bolus dose	Infusion
Fentanyl	1 μg/kg	1–2 μg/kg/h
Remifentanil	—	9 μg/kg/h

Side effects: Hypotension, nausea and vomiting, respiratory depression.

Benzodiazepines

Benzodiazepines, which potentiate the effects of gamma-aminobutyric acid via the benzodiazepine receptor and suppress central nervous system (CNS) activity (32), are administered to provide sedation in the ICU. They were observed to have sedative properties in animals (33), which led to their use because of their hypnotic, muscle-relaxant, anticonvulsive, and antegrade and variable retrograde amnestic properties. The benzodiazepines do not have analgesic properties, but similar to the opioids, they can and do produce respiratory depression in a dose-dependent fashion.

In critically ill patients, many of whom have MODS, because benzodiazepines are metabolized in the liver with the metabolites excreted by the kidneys, the half-lives ($t^1/_2$) are prolonged, and active metabolites may accumulate. Most commonly, benzodiazepines are administered by continuous infusion, so the context-sensitive $t^1/_2$ is more germane but independent of the method of administration because of the potential prolonged effect; a daily "off" period should be established to avoid overdosage (see below). The most commonly used benzodiazepines in the ICU are diazepam, midazolam, and lorazepam (Table 63.10).

Diazepam

Diazepam is an effective sedative-hypnotic with amnestic properties. Because diazepam is irritating when injected intramuscularly or intravenously and due to its long half-life, it is not often administered in the ICU.

Lorazepam

Lorazepam is an intermediate-acting benzodiazepine with a $t^1/_2$ of 10 to 12 hours. Respiratory and cardiovascular effects of lorazepam are no different than those for diazepam and midazolam. Lorazepam is recommended for long-term (greater than 24 hours) administration for patients who are critically ill (34). This may seem surprising because of its $t^1/_2$, but because its metabolites have no clinical activity and there is less intraindividual variability (35), recovery from lorazepam, compared to midazolam, following long-term administration is no different (36) and is associated with pharmacoeconomic benefits (37).

Midazolam

Midazolam is the shortest acting of those benzodiazepines used in the ICU, with a $t^1/_2$ of 1 to 5 hours. Midazolam causes no pain or phlebitis following intravenous administration and is two to four times more potent than diazepam. These characteristics make midazolam an ideal drug for continuous intravenous infusion, as it has rapid onset and relatively rapid offset. It is recommended for short-term use (34); long-term (>24–48 hours) use is problematic because gamma-hydroxy midazolam, the main metabolite, with sedative properties almost identical to the parent compound, accumulates in critically ill patients with decreased albumin levels and decreased renal function, leading to prolonged sedation once the infusion is discontinued. Typically, when administering midazolam for anxiolysis or sedative-hypnotic reasons, 1-mg increments are given intravenously as a bolus, with repeated boluses administered every 5 minutes to effect. A continuous infusion of 0.5 to 5 mg/hour can then be started and continued for as long as necessary.

Additional Cautions and Recommendations Regarding Benzodiazepine Use

The United States Food and Drug Administration (FDA) has administered black box warnings for benzodiazepines to the effect that anyone administering these respiratory depressants must be skilled in airway management and resuscitation. Similarly, one must have the benzodiazepine antagonist flumazenil—a drug that reverses all known CNS effects of benzodiazepines—available in the ICU. Flumazenil has maximum effect within 5 to 10 minutes after intravenous administration and has a mean $t^1/_2$ of approximately 1 hour. Typically, it is given in 0.1- to 0.2-mg increments, repeated every 5 to 10 minutes, to a total dose of 1 mg. Because of the active metabolites of diazepam and midazolam, these benzodiazepines should be used with extra caution in patients with renal insufficiency, as the active metabolites will accumulate. Furthermore, although these medications are often given as intravenous infusions, because of the increasing emphasis on cost efficacy in our ICUs, patients who are able to take medications *per os* should, when feasible, have their intravenous medication discontinued and an oral benzodiazepine started (38).

Furthermore, despite the guidelines that have previously been established (34), not all studies have shown a benefit of lorazepam compared to midazolam for long-term administration; Barr et al. (39) found in 24 patients that those who received midazolam for greater than 72 hours had emergence times from their drug-induced hypnotic state that were shorter than those patients who received lorazepam. Additional research in this area of finding the best short-term and long-term sedative agents is recommended (40).

It is further recommended and supported by clinical studies that patients who are on long-term (greater than 24 hours)

TABLE 63.10

BENZODIAZEPINES USED FOR ANXIOLYSIS IN THE INTENSIVE CARE UNIT

Drug (classification)	$t_{1/2}$ (h)	Active metabolite(s) ($t^1/_2$)	Intermittent IV bolus	Continuous IV infusion
Diazepam (long-acting)	20–50	Desmethyldiazepam (30–200)	1–2 mg (max 0.1–0.2 mg/kg)	—
Lorazepam (intermittent-acting)	10–20	None[a]	0.5–2 mg (max 4 mg)	Up to 0.025 mg/kg/h
Midazolam (short-acting)	1–2.5	1-hydroxy midazolam	0.5–2 mg (max 0.1 mg/kg)	Up to 0.05 mg/kg/h

[a] 3-0-phenolic glucuronide is the inactive metabolite.

TABLE 63.11

RAMSEY SEDATION SCALE

Patient:	
Awake	1. Anxious or agitated
	2. Cooperative/tranquil
	3. Responds to commands only, response to glabellar tap
Asleep	4. Brisk
	5. Sluggish
	6. None

From Ramsay MAE, Savege TM, Simpson BRJ, et al. Controlled sedation with alphaxalone-alphadolone. *Br Med J*. 1974;2:656–659, with permission.

infusions of benzodiazepines benefit from a daily drug "holiday" (41), i.e., infusion stopped typically every morning around 7:00 or 8:00 a.m., and the infusion remains off until the patient exhibits symptoms or signs that warrant restarting the infusion. The possibility of overdosing is decreased if patients are assessed on a regular basis for their degree of sedation. There are several tools that can be used to monitor the adequacy of sedation, beginning with the Ramsey Sedation Scale (Table 63.11) (9), although there are several others that may be more comprehensive (Table 63.2) (7–12).

The team that manages patients in the ICU who require intravenous administration of benzodiazepines should follow a protocol for the administration of these drugs and use a tool with which they are familiar to monitor the degree of sedation. As a final caveat, once these medications are completely discontinued, up to one third of the patients will exhibit signs of withdrawal (42). In these patients, it is common practice to discontinue the benzodiazepines slowly over several days, treating the side effects of withdrawal—tachycardia and hypertension—with a beta-blocker or an alternative drug, including chronic low doses of benzodiazepines in those patients in whom beta-blockers are contraindicated.

Propofol

Propofol (di-isopropylphenol) is a highly lipophilic compound formulated in an isotonic oil in water emulsion (Intralipid) that is unrelated to other sedative/anesthetic agents (43). Because it is formulated in lipid emulsion, side effects include hypertriglyceridemia and bacterial contamination of infusions. The addition of ethylenediaminetetraacetic acid (EDTA) or bisulfite as preservatives decreases the incidence of bacterial overgrowth. A rare side effect is the propofol infusion syndrome (44), metabolic acidosis, and ventricular fibrillation in children and in young adults with neurologic injury receiving greater than 100 μg/kg per minute of propofol for greater than 12 to 24 hours. Propofol is now probably the most commonly used intravenous anesthesia induction agent, and is being advocated by some for use in moderate sedation (endoscopy suite) protocols (45). Because of its rapid onset and offset, few residual aftereffects, and low side-effect profile, it is often used for short-term sedation in the ICU. As the cost of the product has decreased, it is more commonly administered for long-term sedation in the ICU. Propofol has no analgesic properties, so for patients with pain, an analgesic drug should be coadministered. Propofol has also been used to treat status epilepticus (46) and to induce sleep in the ICU (47).

Dexmedetomidine

Alpha-2 (α_2) agonists, such as methyldopa and clonidine, have long been known to have sedative properties; in fact, clonidine is administered epidurally for its antinociceptive effects in the spinal cord. Dexmedetomidine is an α_2 agonist that acts by binding to α_2 receptors in the locus ceruleus with a high α_2/α_1 ratio of approximately 1,620:1, approximately seven times more avidly than clonidine. Binding to the α_2 receptor releases norepinephrine and decreases sympathetic activity; the net effect is sedation, analgesia, and amnesia. Dexmedetomidine is unique compared to the other anxiolytic drugs because patients are not only calm but appear to be sleeping (48). It is commonly used to sedate patients following cardiac surgery (49) and after neurosurgical procedures (50). Whether it is superior to propofol for these patients has not been determined (51). Patients who abuse alcohol, cocaine, and marijuana may benefit the most because dexmedetomidine treats many of the symptoms and signs of withdrawal (52). Many clinicians prefer dexmedetomidine to opioids or benzodiazepines because it is not associated with respiratory depression. However, because of its central alpha agonist, hypotension can and does occur. Fortunately, low-dose dexmedetomidine (6 μg/kg per hour for 10 minutes followed by an infusion of 0.2 μg/kg per hour) is as effective as higher doses (0.6 μg/kg per hour), with fewer side effects (48,53). There is concern that if dexmedetomidine is used for greater than 24 hours and discontinued abruptly, that a hyperdynamic state will ensue similar to the one that develops when clonidine is stopped abruptly following long-term use; but cases of cardiac arrest, though reported, are uncommon. Dexmedetomidine has been approved by the FDA for 24-hour use (54), although many clinicians are using it for longer than 24 hours. Of the currently used anxiolytic medications, dexmedetomidine is the most expensive.

Butyrophenones

Butyrophenones are neuroleptic drugs that are also known as antipsychotic drugs or major tranquilizers. They induce apathy, a state of mental detachment in patients with psychoses or delirium. By inhibiting dopamine-mediated neurotransmissions in the CNS, they decrease the frequency of hallucinations, delusions, and other abnormal thoughts. Patients become so detached from their environment that they develop a characteristic flat affect. Butyrophenones are active in the chemoreceptor trigger zone in the brainstem and thus are effective antiemetics; they are also used to treat hiccups and are used as synergistic anxiolytic drugs when used with benzodiazepines.

Of the butyrophenones, haloperidol is the drug used most often to treat delirium in the ICU. Haloperidol has a wide therapeutic margin but has important side effects including hypotension, extrapyramidal symptoms, anticholinergic effects (tachycardia, urinary retention, ileus), neuroleptic malignant syndrome, and seizures. These side effects are rare. Hypotension following a dose of haloperidol is almost always seen in patients who are hypovolemic. Extrapyramidal symptoms are more often seen in younger patients and in patients with depleted dopamine stores, e.g., patients with Parkinson disease.

The initial dose of haloperidol is usually 0.5 to 2 mg administered parenterally, although depending on the patient's size, age, and degree of agitation/delirium, 5 mg can be given. Haloperidol has a slow onset, so peak effects may not be seen for 15 to 30 minutes. Repeat doses then should be administered at 30- to 60-minute intervals. Recurrence of agitation or an increase in delirium is an indication for repeat doses, which may be increased if the initial dose was inadequate. Tardive dyskinesia or neuroleptic malignant syndrome can occur even during the short duration of therapy used in the ICU.

Haloperidol, because of its anticholinergic effects, may prolong the QT in a dose-dependent fashion, resulting in arrhythmias and torsades de pointes. Patients receiving haloperidol should have their electrocardiogram monitored.

A recent retrospective study of 989 patients who were mechanically ventilated in the ICU found that those patients who received haloperidol had significantly lower mortality than those who did not (55). Although not an indication for increased use of haloperidol, the results should be reassuring to those who have concerns about its use.

Other Agents

Several anesthetic agents have been tried to sedate patients in the ICU, with unanticipated results. When nitrous oxide was used, anemia developed and led to the realization that nitrous oxide interfered with vitamin B_{12} metabolism. Similarly, when etomidate was used for sedation, patients developed adrenocortical insufficiency because we now know that etomidate interferes with cortisol metabolism. However, a few anesthetic agents have withstood the test of time with respect to their use in the ICU.

Barbiturates

Barbiturates have pronounced effects on the CNS, lowering intracranial pressure and raising the seizure threshold. They have been used in the past to induce a "barbiturate coma" in patients with increased intracranial pressure and terminate seizures. Barbiturates administered by intravenous bolus produce hypotension and because of their lipid solubility, if given by continuous infusion, accumulate in fat stores and, therefore, have a duration of action that can be significantly long, i.e., days to weeks. In current practice, they are infrequently administered by continuous infusion for long-term use.

Ketamine

Ketamine is a phencyclidine derivative that is a nonbarbiturate, rapid-acting, general anesthetic that is administered parenterally to induce anesthesia. Ketamine induces "dissociative anesthesia" because it interrupts association pathways of the brain before blocking sensory pathways—patients may perceive pain, but it does not bother them. However, because it is a phencyclidine derivative, 10% to 20% of adult patients may have psychologic sequelae including hallucinations.

Ketamine is used as a general anesthetic because it raises cardiac output, pulse rate, and arterial and venous pressures. Ketamine maintains pharyngeal and laryngeal reflexes without suppressing respiration. Ketamine is also a bronchodilator and has been advocated as the anesthetic agent of choice in patients with reactive airways disease. Twenty to 30 years ago, it was commonly used. Because of the increasing incidence of reactive airways disease, there is renewed interest in ketamine for sedation of patients with lung disease. A 1-mg/kg bolus of ketamine can be administered, followed by an infusion of 1.0 mg/kg per hour, titrated up to 4.5 mg/kg per hour; many administer a benzodiazepine to reduce the frequency of psychologic sequelae. Ketamine is contraindicated in patients with cardiac ischemia or raised intracranial pressure.

NEUROMUSCULAR BLOCKADE

Despite what should be effective doses of anxiolytic drugs, some patients remain delirious and agitated, and a further increase in the dose of anxiolytic drugs is proscribed because of side effects. Such patients, along with those with closed-head injuries, tetanus, and ALI, may require other therapeutic modalities. If the patient is tracheally intubated, mechanically ventilated, and receiving adequate sedation, chemical paralysis with a NMBA is an option (Table 63.12).

Patients with ARDS are often difficult to ventilate and are commonly agitated, hemodynamically unstable, and have a decreased mixed venous oxygen saturation that is life threatening. Additional sedative drugs will only worsen hemodynamics, so NMBAs may be the only (life-saving) alternative that have been shown to improve gas exchange (56).

TABLE 63.12

INDICATIONS FOR THE MANAGEMENT OF PATIENTS WITH NEUROMUSCULAR BLOCKING AGENTS

Closed-head injury with raised intracranial pressure
Tetanus
Decreased $S\bar{v}O_2$ in hypermetabolic, agitated states
Modes of mechanical ventilation that produce agitation, which in turn interferes with ventilation/oxygenation, e.g., pressure-controlled inverse ratio ventilation, jet/high-frequency ventilation.

Purpose:

To describe the process of utilizing a nerve stimulator to stimulate the ulnar nerve, usually with tactile assessment of a neuromuscular twitch, usually tactile assessment of an abducted thumb, to assess the degree of neuromuscular block.

Definitions:

Neuromuscular block: the process by which the postsynaptic acetylcholine receptor is depressed and variably response to release of acetylcholine in the neuromuscular junction cleft
Peripheral nerve stimulation: electrical stimulation, usually from 40 to 120 mA at a peripheral nerve, usually the ulnar, either at the elbow or at the wrist
Train-of-four: a specific type of nerve stimulation in which the nerve stimulator delivers an electrical stimulus to the nerve lasting 10 ms and repeated every 500 ms for a total of 4 stimuli

Equipment:

1. Peripheral nerve stimulator
2. Two electrode pads (electrocardiogram pads may be used)

Procedure:

1. Clean the area where the electrode pads will be placed with alcohol to remove any skin oils. This will reduce the resistance at the skin and decrease the amount of current needed to stimulate the nerve. If the resistance of the skin is still high, then an abrasive compound can be used to remove dead skin.
2. Place two electrodes over the ulnar nerve, usually 3 to 5 cm apart.
3. Attach electrodes to the leads, usually the positive electrode proximally.
4. Cover the fingers and abduct the thumb. Increase the amperage of the stimulator until 4 twitches of the thumb are palpated by tactile assessment. Stimuli should not be delivered more frequently than every 20 seconds. Once 4 twitches are palpated, a supramaximal stimulus can be delivered by increasing the amperage 10% to 30% over the amperage required to palpate 4 twitches.

Goals:

1. To achieve a level of train-of-four of 2 to 4. If with 3 or 4 twitches the patient either spontaneously triggers the ventilator or exhibits muscular activity that adversely affects oxygenation or airway or intracranial pressure, then increased neuromuscular block is required.
2. A train-of-four of 1 to 0 indicates that the degree of neuromuscular block is too great, and the dosage of neuromuscular blocking agent should be decreased.

FIGURE 63.1. Protocol for monitoring degree of neuromuscular block using a nerve stimulator and assessment of the train-of-four twitch. (Reproduced from Murray MJ, Oyen L, Bazzell CM. Use of sedatives, analgesics, and neuromuscular blockers. In: Parillo JE, Dellinger RP, eds. *Critical Care Medicine: Principles of Diagnosis and Management.* 2nd ed. St. Louis, MO: Mosby; 2001:296–311, with permission.)

Monitoring

Before administering NMBAs to patients, certain requirements must be met. Patients must be mechanically ventilated, sedated, and monitored.

Obviously, if patients are going to be paralyzed, they must be mechanically ventilated. Similarly, they must be sufficiently sedated that they will have no recall of the experience; most patients who are not adequately sedated will have terrifying dreams/recall (57). Most practitioners will first implement sedation therapy to the point that the patient is unconscious before initiating NMBA therapy. Finally, the use of NMBAs is associated with many adverse side effects. Monitoring the depth of blockade and the necessity of blockade is essential in minimizing these side effects.

Assessing the degree of blockade by measuring the amount of block of the neuromuscular receptor with a twitch monitor is the preferred technique. An electrical stimulus is applied to a peripheral motor nerve, and the effects of the stimulus on the motor group supplied by that nerve are observed (Fig. 63.1). This is most often performed using a twitch stimulator that generates a stimulus of up to 160 mA intensity that lasts 10 ms and is repeated every 500 ms so that four stimuli (train-of-four [TOF]) are delivered (Fig. 63.2). The effects can be visualized, but the preferred technique is for the observer to palpate the response. In the ICU, it is probably easiest to measure the TOF response by stimulating the ulnar nerve at the wrist. The goal of therapy is to provide a sufficient amount of drug so that the patient has only one to two twitches, as opposed to none (overblocked) or three to four (possibly underblocked) twitches.

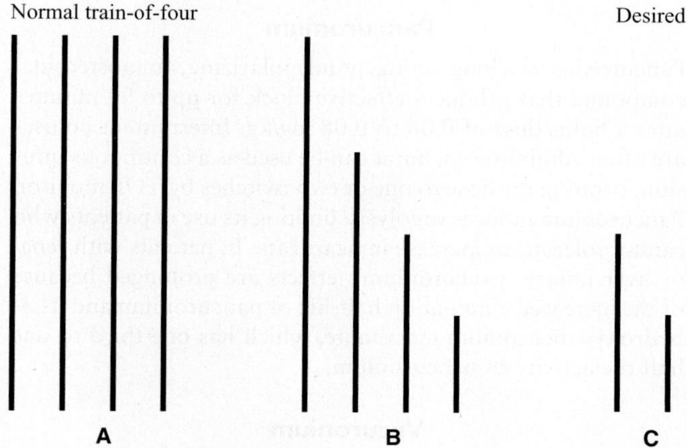

FIGURE 63.2. Train-of-four monitoring. **A:** With the twitch stimulator at 40 to 10 mA, four twitches are measured. **B:** As the neuromuscular blocking agent (NMBA) takes effect, the second, third, and fourth twitches are weaker/fade. **C:** The goal with additional time or drug is to have one to two twitches.

Complications of NMBA

One of the most feared complications of neuromuscular block is accidental extubation. Should a paralyzed patient become accidentally extubated, time is of the essence, especially in patients with ARDS. Ventilation must begin immediately with a mask and anesthesia bag using 100% oxygen while steps are taken to reintubate the patient.

Another feared complication is profound weakness once the drug is discontinued. This may seem counterintuitive—the NMBA is administered to produce profound weakness. This is true, but when the NMBA is discontinued, we anticipate that the patient will recover normal neuromuscular function within hours. One study of two of the longest-lasting NMBAs (pancuronium and doxacurium) in which 40 critically ill patients were paralyzed an average of two to three days found that once doxacurium was discontinued, patients recovered their strength within 4 hours; the patients receiving pancuronium recovered their strength within 24 hours (58).

Though not seen in this study, approximately 10% of patients who receive NMBAs will develop a myopathy from which it takes days or weeks to recover (59). Weakness is a common problem in the ICU and, when secondary to muscle weakness per se, is known as CIM (critical illness myopathy). The cause of CIM in the ICU is multifactorial (60), but most studies indicate that prolonged use of NMBAs in the ICU is one of the causative factors (59). Because corticosteroids are also known to produce myopathy, many intensivists are very cautious when infusing NMBAs in patients who are also receiving corticosteroids (61), a common scenario. Caution is appropriate and should be the norm when infusing NMBAs in patients who are critically ill. Daily assessments must be made to determine if NMBA use is justified, and the TOF should be maintained at one to two twitches.

TREATMENT

Aminosteroidal Compounds (Fig. 63.3)

Pancuronium

Pancuronium is a long-acting, nondepolarizing, aminosteroidal compound that produces effective block for up to 90 minutes after a bolus dose of 0.06 to 0.08 mg/kg. Intermittent boluses are often administered, but it can be used as a continuous infusion, titrating the dose to one or two twitches by TOF monitor. Pancuronium induces vagolysis, limiting its use in patients who cannot tolerate an increase in heart rate. In patients with renal or liver failure, pancuronium's effects are prolonged because of the increased elimination half-life of pancuronium and its 3-hydroxypancuronium metabolite, which has one third to one half the activity of pancuronium.

Vecuronium

With the deletion of the methyl group at one of pancuronium's two N-methyl-piperidine moieties (leaving vecuronium with a single [monoquaternary] piperidine group at the R-2 position), scientists were able to produce an intermediate-acting NMBA without the vagolytic properties of pancuronium. An intravenous bolus dose of 0.08 to 0.10 mg/kg produces block within $2\frac{1}{2}$ to 3 minutes that typically lasts 35 to 45 minutes. After a bolus dose, it can be given as a continuous infusion of 0.8 to 1.4 μg/kg per minute, titrating the rate to the degree of block desired. The 3-desacetylvecuronium metabolite has 50% of the pharmacologic activity of the parent compound (62) so that patients with hepatic dysfunction may have increased plasma concentrations of both the parent compound and the active metabolite, causing prolonged block. Renal dysfunction also prolongs the duration of block. Vecuronium is associated with CIM, especially in patients receiving corticosteroids. Vecuronium is being used with decreased frequency in ICU patients.

Rocuronium

Rocuronium is a newer aminosteroidal NMBA, with an intermediate duration of action and a rapid onset that has been tested in the ICU (63). When given as a bolus of 0.6 to 0.1 mg/kg, block is almost always achieved within 2 minutes, with maximum block occurring within 3 minutes; continuous infusions are administered at 8 to 10 μg/kg per minute (64) and usually produce a fairly dense block. Rocuronium's metabolite, 17-desacetylrocuronium, has approximately only 5% to 10% activity compared to the parent compound. Renal failure should not have an effect on duration of action, but hepatic failure may prolong rocuronium's duration of action.

Benzylisoquinolinium Compounds

Atracurium

Atracurium is an intermediate-acting NMBA with minimal cardiovascular side effects but is associated with histamine release at higher doses. Atracurium has a unique metabolism (ester hydrolysis and Hofmann elimination) so that renal or hepatic dysfunction does not affect its duration of block. Atracurium has been associated with persistent neuromuscular weakness as has been reported with other NMBAs.

Cisatracurium

Cisatracurium, one of atracurium's 16 isomers, is an intermediate-acting benzylisoquinolinium NMBA that is increasingly used in lieu of atracurium. It produces few, if any, cardiovascular effects and has fewer tendencies to produce mast cell degranulation than does atracurium. Bolus doses with a 0.10 to 0.2 mg/kg result in paralysis in an average of 2.5 minutes, and recovery begins at approximately 25 minutes; maintenance infusion rates should be started at 2.5 to 3.0 μg/kg per minute. Cisatracurium is also metabolized by ester hydrolysis and Hofmann elimination, so duration of block should not be affected by MODS. There have not yet been reports of significantly prolonged recovery associated with cisatracurium. The mean peak plasma laudanosine concentrations are lower in patients receiving cisatracurium compared to patients receiving clinically equivalent doses of atracurium. Laudanosine at high doses produces seizures in animals; a case of seizures in a human receiving atracurium or cisatracurium has not been reported.

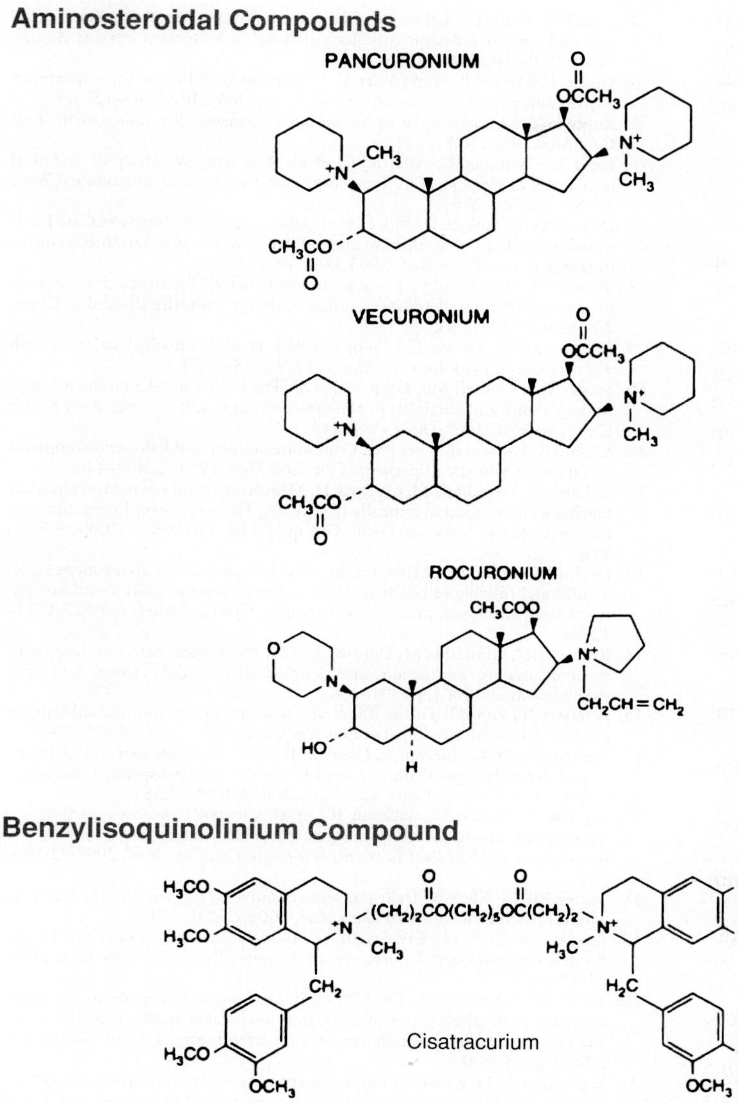

Aminosteroidal Compounds

PANCURONIUM

VECURONIUM

ROCURONIUM

Benzylisoquinolinium Compound

Cisatracurium

FIGURE 63.3. Chemical structures of neuromuscular blocking agents. Cisatracurium is the 1R-cis 1′R-cis isomer, one of the 10 isomers found in atracurium.

RECOVERY

Patients receiving an NMBA should have daily drug holidays. If the NMBA is no longer required, it is discontinued. It is anticipated that with all the NMBAs, the TOF should normalize (four twitches) within 3 to 4 hours. If not, the patient may have a CIM associated with the NMBA (with an increased incidence in patients receiving corticosteroids and patients with sepsis, etc.). If, after 24 hours, the patient has inadequate strength, additional studies should be done to include an assessment of the antibiotics the patient is receiving, electrolytes (calcium, magnesium, phosphorus), and temperature (hypothermia prolongs neuromuscular block). If no comorbid condition accounts for the degree of neuromuscular block, a neurology consult should be considered. In this context, an electromyography is typically performed (to rule out critical illness polyneuropathy) and, in some circumstances, a muscle biopsy is obtained. Patients with CIM secondary to the neuromuscular blockade will have loss of myosin. Treatment is supportive with maintenance of sedation, mechanical ventilation, physical therapy, skin care, eye care, and so on.

SUMMARY

Over the past 30 years, there is increased recognition that patients in the ICU are anxious, and as patients become older, have more comorbid conditions, and are more critically ill, they will increasingly exhibit agitation and delirium. These factors increase morbidity and mortality, prolonging the length of stay and worsening the outcome. Even patients who survive have memories that are disturbing and, in some circumstances, lead to the equivalent of a posttraumatic stress syndrome. Practitioners in an ICU must recognize when their patients become anxious, agitated, and delirious; identify contributing factors; and treat the disorders with anxiolytic medications. The effects of therapy must be monitored with the use of a standard scale, one that is used throughout the institution's ICUs. In some patients in whom the sedation is inadequate, NMBAs may be indicated. Appropriate sedation, monitoring, securing of the airway, and monitoring the adequacy of mechanical ventilation must be ensured. Patients receiving any of these medications are at risk for side effects, which must be monitored as well. An effective sedation and paralysis protocol will improve patient outcome and patient satisfaction.

Stress Points

1. Anxiety and pain are different emotional states, and most patients who are oriented can differentiate between anxiety and pain.
2. Before relying on pharmacologic interventions to treat pain or anxiety, first assess possible confounding factors such as a distended bladder in a patient who does not have a Foley catheter; hypercapnia in someone with impending respiratory failure; or someone who is becoming septic, which is manifested by encephalopathy.
3. Anxiety can lead to agitation, which in turn can result in self-injury and injury to care providers.
4. Delirium is an increasingly recognized problem in the intensive care unit (ICU), which can result in long-term cognitive impairment.
5. Physiologic derangements must first be ruled out before treating anxiety, agitation, or delirium.
6. Opioids and benzodiazepines are the pharmacologic mainstays of treating anxiety.
7. Midazolam, propofol, or dexmedetomidine are the preferred short-term (24–48 hours) treatments of anxiety.
8. Lorazepam and fentanyl are the preferred long-term anxiolytic agents.
9. Haloperidol is an effective therapy for older patients with delirium.
10. Mechanically ventilated patients who remain agitated despite adequate anxiolytic therapy are candidates for an NMBA.
11. Patients must be adequately sedated before an NMBA is administered.
12. Patients receiving NMBAs must be mechanically ventilated, with precautions taken to ensure that the tracheal tube or tracheostomy tube is protected.
13. The primary NMBAs used for mechanically ventilated patients are the aminosteroidal compounds (pancuronium or rocuronium) and the benzylisoquinolinium compounds (atracurium or cisatracurium).
14. Daily drug "holidays" should be implemented when using anxiolytic drugs or NMBAs.
15. Patients who have received anxiolytic drugs for greater than 3 to 7 days are at risk of becoming dependent and may exhibit signs of withdrawal when the drug(s) is/are discontinued.
16. Patients who have received NMBAs for greater than 12 to 24 hours are at increased risk of developing critical illness myopathy (CIM) when the NMBA is discontinued.

References

1. Treggiari-Venzi M, Borgeat A, Fuchs-Buder T, et al. Overnight sedation with midazolam or propofol in the ICU: effects on sleep quality, anxiety and depression. *Intensive Care Med.* 1996;22:1186–1190.
2. Rotondi A, Lakshmipathi C, Sirio C, et al. Patients' recollections of stressful experiences while receiving prolonged mechanical ventilation in an intensive care unit. *Crit Care Med.* 2002;30:746–752.
3. Fong HK, Sands LP, Leung JM. The role of postoperative analgesia in delirium and cognitive decline in elderly patients: a systematic review. *Anesth Analg.* 2006;102:1255–1266.
4. Vaurio L, Sands LP, Wang Y, et al. Postoperative delirium: the importance of pain and pain management. *Anesth Analg.* 2006;102:1267–1273.
5. Anonymous. Management of the agitated intensive care unit patient. *Crit Care Med.* 2002;30:S97–S123.
6. Jaber S, Chanques G, Altairac C, et al. A prospective study of agitation in a medical-surgical ICU. Incidence, risk factors, and outcomes. *Chest.* 2005;128:2749–2757.
7. De Jonghe B, Cook D, Griffith L, et al. Adaptation to the Intensive Care Environment (ATICE): development and validation of a new sedation assessment instrument. *Crit Care Med.* 2003;31:2344–2354.
8. Weinert C, McFarland L. The state of intubated ICU patients: development of a two-dimensional sedation rating scale for critically ill adults. *Chest.* 2004;126:1727–1730.
9. Ramsay MAE, Savege TM, Simpson BRJ, et al. Controlled sedation with alphaxalone-alphadolone. *Br Med J.* 1974;2:656–659.
10. Sessler CN, Gosnell MS, Grap MJ, et al. The Richmond Agitation-sedation Scale. Validity and reliability in adult intensive care unit patients. *Am J Respir Crit Care Med.* 2002;166:1338–1344.
11. Riker RR, Graser GL, Cox PM; Continuous infusion of haloperidol controls agitation in critically ill patients. *Crit Care Med.* 1994;22:433–440.
12. de Lemos J, Tweeddale M, Chittock D. Measuring quality of sedation in adult mechanically ventilated critically ill patients. The Vancouver Interaction and Calmness Scale. Sedation Focus Group. *J Clin Epidemiol.* 2000;53:908–919.
13. Devlin JW, Boleski G, Mlynarek M, et al. Motor Activity Assessment Scale: a valid and reliable sedation scale for use with mechanically ventilated patients in an adult surgical intensive care unit. *Crit Care Med.* 1999;27:1271–1275.
14. Rincon HG, Granados M, Unutzer J, et al. Prevalence, detection and treatment of anxiety, depression, and delirium in the adult critical care unit. *Psychosomatics.* 2001;42:391–396.
15. Peterson JF, Pun BT, Dittus RS, et al. Delirium and its motoric subtypes: a study of 614 critically ill patients. *J Am Geriatr Soc.* 2006;54:479–484.
16. Thomason JWW, Shintani A, Peterson JF, et al. Intensive care unit delirium is an independent predictor of longer hospital stay: a prospective analysis of 261 non-ventilated patients. *Crit Care.* 2005;9:R375–R381.
17. Ely EW, Stephens RK, Jackson JC, et al. Current opinions regarding the importance, diagnosis, and management of delirium in the intensive care unit: a survey of 912 healthcare professionals. *Crit Care Med.* 2004;32:106–112.
18. Miller RR III, Ely EW. Delirium and cognitive dysfunction in the intensive care unit. *Semin Respir Crit Care Med.* 2006;27:210–220.
19. Pandharipande P, Ely EW. Sedative and analgesic medications: risk factors for delirium and sleep disturbances in the critically ill. *Crit Care Clin.* 2006; 22:313–327.
20. McNicoll L, Pisani MA, Ely EW, et al. Detection of delirium in the intensive care unit: comparison of confusion assessment method for the intensive care unit with confusion assessment method ratings. *J Am Geriatr Soc.* 2005;53:495–500.
21. Rosengren A, Hawken S, Ôunpuu S, et al. Association of psychosocial risk factors with risk of acute myocardial infarction in 11119 cases and 13648 controls from 52 countries (the INTERHEART study): case-control study. *Lancet.* 2004;364:953–962.
22. Rosenkranz MA, Busse WW, Johnstone T, et al. Neural circuitry underlying the interaction between emotion and asthma symptom exacerbation. *Proc Natl Acad Sci U S A.* 2005;102:13319–13324.
23. Ploghaus A, Narain C, Beckmann C, et al. Exacerbation of pain by anxiety is associated with activity in a hippocampal network. *J Neurosci.* 2001; 21:9896–9903.
24. Crippen D. Agitation in the ICU: part one. Anatomical and physiologic basis for the agitated state. *Crit Care.* 1999;3R35–R46.
25. Kain ZN, Caldwell-Andrews AA, Maranets I, et al. Preoperative anxiety and emergence delirium and postoperative maladaptive behaviors. *Anesth Analg.* 2004;99:1648–1654.
26. Fumagalli S, Boncinelli L, Lo Nostro A, et al. Reduced cardiocirculatory complications with unrestrictive visiting policy in an intensive care unit. *Circulation.* 2006;113:946–952.
27. Baker CF. Sensory overload and noise in the ICU: sources of environmental stress. *Crit Care Q.* 1984;6:66–80.
28. Parthasarathy S. Sleep in the intensive care unit: sleepy doctors and restless patients. *Clin Intensive Care.* 2005;16:129–136.
29. Reuben SS, Buvanendran A, Kroin JS, et al. The analgesic efficacy of celecoxib, pregabalin, and their combination for spinal fusion surgery. *Anesth Analg.* 2006;103:1271–1777.
30. Park G, Lane M, Rogers S, et al. A comparison of hypnotic and analgesic based sedation in a general intensive care unit. *Br J Anaesth.* 2007;98:76–82.
31. Muellejans B, López A, Cross MH, et al. Remifentanil versus fentanyl for analgesia based sedation to provide patient comfort in the intensive care unit: a randomized, double-blind controlled trial [ISRCTN43755713]. *Crit Care* 2004;8:R1–R11.
32. Haefely W. The biological basis of benzodiazepine actions. *J Psychoactive Drugs.* 1983;15:19–39.

33. Zbinden G, Randall LO. Pharmacology of benzodiazepines: laboratory and clinical correlations. *Adv Pharmacol.* 1967;5:213–291.
34. Jacobi J, Fraser GL, Coursin DB, et al. Clinical practice guidelines for the sustained use of sedatives and analgesics in the critically ill adult. *Crit Care Med.* 2002;30:119–141.
35. Swart EL, van Schijndel RJ, van Loenen AC, et al. Continuous infusion of lorazepam versus midazolam in patients in the intensive care unit: sedation with lorazepam is easier to manage and is more cost-effective. *Crit Care Med.* 1999;27:1461–1465.
36. Swart EL, Zuideveld KP, de Jongh J, et al. Comparative population pharmacokinetics of lorazepam and midazolam during long-term continuous infusion in critically ill patients. *Br J Clin Pharmacol.* 2004;57:135–145.
37. MacLaren R, Sullivan PW. Pharmacoeconomic modeling of lorazepam, midazolam, and propofol for continuous sedation in critically ill patients. *Pharmacotherap.y* 2005;25:1319–1328.
38. Cigada M, Pezzi A, Di Mauro P, et al. Sedation in the critically ill ventilated patient: possible role of enteral drugs. *Intensive Care Med.* 2005;31:482–486.
39. Barr J, Zomorodi K, Bertaccini EJ, et al. A double-blind, randomized comparison of i.v. lorazepam versus midazolam for sedation of ICU patients via a pharmacologic model. *Anesthesiology.* 2001;95:286–298.
40. Izurieta R, Rabatin JT. Sedation during mechanical ventilation: a systematic review. *Crit Care Med.* 2002;30:2644–2648.
41. Schweickert WD, Gehlbach BK, Pohlman AS, et al. Daily interruption of sedative infusions and complications of critical illness in mechanically ventilated patients. *Crit Care Med.* 2004;32:1272–1276.
42. Cammarano WB, Pittet J-F, Weitz S, et al. Acute withdrawal syndrome related to the administration of analgesic and sedative medications in adult intensive care unit patients. *Crit Care Med.* 1998;26:676–684.
43. Barr J. Propofol: a new drug for sedation in the intensive care unit. *Int Anesthesiol Clin.* 1995;33:131–154.
44. Fudickar A, Bein B, Tonner PH. Propofol infusion syndrome in anaesthesia and intensive care medicine. *Curr Opin Anaesthesiol.* 2006;19:404–410.
45. Riphaus A, Gstettenbauer T, Frenz MB, et al. Quality of psychomotor recovery after propofol sedation for routine endoscopy: a randomized and controlled study. *Endoscopy.* 2006;38:677–683.
46. Brown LA, Levin GM. Role of propofol in refractory status epilepticus. *Ann Pharmacothe.r* 1998;32:1053–1059.
47. Kelly DF, Goodale DB, Williams J, et al. Propofol in the treatment of moderate and severe head injury: a randomized, prospective double-blinded pilot trial. *J Neurosurg.* 1999;1042–1052.
48. Hall JE, Uhrich TD, Barney JA, et al. Sedative, amnestic, and analgesic properties of small-dose dexmedetomidine infusions. *Anesth Analg.* 2000; 90:699–705.
49. Herr DL, Sum-Ping STJ, England M. ICU sedation after coronary artery bypass graft surgery: dexmedetomidine-based versus propofol-based sedation regimens. *J Cardiothorac Vasc Anesth.* 2003;17:576–584.
50. Bekker A, Sturaitis MK. Dexmedetomidine for neurological surgery. *Neurosurgery.* 2005;57(1 Suppl):1–10; discussion 1–10.
51. Corbett SM, Rebuck JA, Greene CM, et al. Dexmedetomidine does not improve patient satisfaction when compared with propofol during mechanical ventilation. *Crit Care Med.* 2005;33:940–945.
52. Steadman JL, Birnbach DJ. Patients on party drugs undergoing anesthesia. *Curr Opin Anaesthesiol.* 2003;16:147–152.
53. Ingersoll-Weng E, Manecke GR Jr, Thistlethwaite PA. Dexmedetomidine and cardiac arrest. *Anesthesiology.* 2004;100:738–739.
54. Chang NS, Simone AF, Schultheis LW. From the FDA: what's in a label? A guide for the anesthesia practitioner. *Anesthesiology.* 2005;103:179–185.
55. Milbrandt EB, Kersten A, Kong K, et al. Haloperidol use is associated with lower hospital mortality in mechanically ventilated patients. *Crit Care Med.* 2005;33:226–229.
56. Gainnier M, Roch A, Forel J-M, et al. Effect of neuromuscular blocking agents on gas exchange in patients presenting with acute respiratory distress syndrome. *Crit Care Med.* 2004;32:113–119.
57. Ballard N, Robley L, Barrett D, et al. Patients' recollections of therapeutic paralysis in the intensive care unit. *Am J Crit Care.* 2006;16:86–95.
58. Murray MJ, Coursin DB, Scuderi PE, et al. Double-blind, randomized, multicenter study of doxacurium vs. pancuronium in intensive care unit patients who require neuromuscular-blocking agents. *Crit Care Med.* 1995;23:450–458.
59. Murray MJ, Brull SJ, Bolton CF. Brief review: nondepolarizing neuromuscular blocking drugs and critical illness myopathy. *Can J Anaesth.* 2006; 53:1148–1156.
60. Bolton CF. Neuromuscular manifestations of critical illness. *Muscle Nerve.* 2005;32:140–163.
61. Larsson L, Xiapeng L, Edström L, et al. Acute quadriplegia and loss of muscle myosin in patients treated with nondepolarizing neuromuscular blocking agents and corticosteroids: mechanisms at the cellular and molecular levels. *Crit Care Med.* 2000;28:34–45.
62. Segredo V, Caldwell JE, Matthay MA, et al. Persistent paralysis in critically ill patients after long-term administration of vecuronium. *N Engl J Med.* 1992;327:524–528.
63. Stene J, Murray M, DeRuyter M, et al. Selective rocuronium pharmacodynamics and kinetics during ICU infusion. *Anesthesiology.* 1998;89:477A.
64. Khuenl-Brady KS, Sparr H, Pühringer F, et al. Rocuronium bromide in the ICU: dose finding and pharmacokinetics. *Eur J Anesthesiol Suppl.* 1995;11: 79–80.

CHAPTER 64 ■ NUTRITIONAL ISSUES

JOHN K. STENE • THOMAS C. VARY

IMMEDIATE CONCERNS

The care of critically ill patients usually focuses on the immediate concerns of cardiorespiratory resuscitation, ventilatory support, maintenance of adequate hemodynamic parameters, and antibiotics to control infectious processes. Despite the increase in metabolic substrate utilization, as critically ill patients become catabolic, nutritional support is frequently overlooked. The extreme catabolism and negative nitrogen balance from critical illness has been well recognized for decades, as described in a 1976 review by Cuthbertson (1), but there still exists a conventional wisdom that starvation is not harmful to critically ill patients and no attempts to reverse it with nutrition support should be undertaken (1). However, there is no medical evidence that starvation is therapeutic. In fact, Kinney (2) pointed out more than 25 years ago that the catabolic response to multiple injuries resulted in loss of up to 20% of normal body weight within 3 weeks despite some oral intake started during the first week. Kinney also noted the catabolic melting (rapid wasting) of large weight-bearing muscle groups of critically injured patients in a hospital setting (2).

Critical illness leads to a change in the hormonal milieu in response to cytokines released from injured tissues; this change increases the demands for energy substrates. In addition, cytokines promote break down of muscle proteins to provide amino acids that are deaminated and carbon chains utilized for energy (3). The tidal metaphor of Cuthbertson has long been used to describe the metabolic response to acute injury. In this metaphor, the initial response to shock is a

TABLE 64.1

EBB FLOW PHASE OF RESPONSE TO INJURY

	Ebb	Catabolic flow	Anabolic flow
O_2 consumption	↓	↑↑	↑
Nitrogen balance	↓	↓↓	↑
Cortisol	↑	↑	↔
Epinephrine	↑↑↑	↔	↔
Insulin	↑	↑	↑↑
Glucagon	↑↑	↑↑	↑
Glucose	↑	↑	↔

marked reduction in metabolic rate, termed the *ebb phase*, conjuring up an image of the patient's life ebbing away like the receding tide. The flow phase suggests the image of the returning tide, which involves the patient mounting a compensatory response to shock and tissue injury.

Further refinement of this concept has described an early catabolic period of the flow phase when muscle protein is mobilized to provide energy and substrate for tissue repair (4). This is followed in the late flow phase, a period of anabolic activity and a tissue healing component of the flow phase. Both subintervals of the flow phase increase the patient's need for nutritional supplementation to optimize healing and reduce the length of the critical illness. The flow phase is associated with an increased metabolic rate as measured by oxygen consumption/heat production, which gradually returns to normal (Table 64.1). Nutritional support prescriptions need to change throughout the patient's period of critical illness to provide adequate protein-energy substrates during the flow phase and to prevent overfeeding when the patient's convalescence is complete. Although critical illness most frequently compromises a patient's ability to normally intake adequate nutrition, critical care technology offers several alternative routes of providing nutritional support. These routes of nutrition support include intravenous routes—total parenteral nutrition (TPN) and peripheral parenteral nutrition—and enteral routes with various formulae tailored to the patient's unique requirements (Table 64.2).

NUTRITIONAL SUPPORT SERVICE

A nutritional support service aids those caring for critically ill patients in providing appropriate nutritional prescriptions. The nutritional support service is also responsible for evaluating the patients' responses to nutrition prescriptions. These monitored evaluations range from the patients' actual calorie expenditure to protein requirements so as to prevent catabolism with profoundly negative nitrogen balance. Finally, the nutritional support service should be a focus for research concerning the improvement of nutritional care of critically ill patients.

Classically, the nutritional support service consisted of a registered dietitian (RD) with advanced training in the biochemical aspects of critical illness, a physician consultant, and assistants who provide nutritional consults to metabolically unstable patients (Table 64.3). One of the team's duties is screening patients for risks of malnutrition and diagnosing various nutritional deficiency states. The team consults on patients either by specific request or on a systematic protocol-driven basis—such as for patients in the critical care unit—according to local hospital policy.

The nutritional consult includes estimates of the patient's metabolic rate and calorie expenditure, estimated either with the Harris-Benedict equation or actually measured via indirect calorimetry. The nutritional support team may collaborate with respiratory care professionals to perform indirect calorimetry measurements.

Protein requirements are estimated from the patient's critical illness diagnosis and monitored via visceral protein analysis or 24-hour nitrogen-balance measurements. The nutritional support service incorporates such measurements into their daily nutritional prescriptions to provide the patients with optimum nutritional support.

TABLE 64.2

COMMONLY USED ROUTES OF NUTRITION

	Parenteral	
Enteral	Central	Peripheral
ADVANTAGES		
Uses gut barrier to control water and electrolyte absorption; natural relationship for hepatic "first pass" metabolism; cost-effective	Uninterrupted nutrient administration; can be continued in OR; rapid change in formula possible; doesn't interfere with oral drug administration; doesn't depend on gut motility	Avoids central venous catheter
DISADVANTAGES		
Frequent interruptions for NPO status; interference with drug absorption (e.g., phenytoin); frequent feeding tube complications	Hyperosmolar, hyperglycemic coma; expensive; central venous line complications/infections	Partial nutritional support to supplement low levels of enteral intake

NPO, nothing by mouth.

TABLE 64.3

ORGANIZATION OF A NUTRITION SUPPORT SERVICE

OPTIMAL ORGANIZATION
Physician: Provides consults for nutrition support; needs critical care experience
Nurse: Expertise in managing tubes, i.v. catheters, and delivery of nutrition support to patients
Pharmacist: Expertise in compounding and mixtures for nutrition support
Nutritionist: Expert in nutritional needs
Respiratory therapist: Performs indirect calorimetry

PRAGMATIC ORGANIZATION
Nutritionist: Expert in critical care nutrition support dedicated to nutrition support service
Physician consultant: Intensivist overseeing care of the patients, writes orders to follow up nutrition recommendations
Respiratory therapist consultant: Performs indirect calorimetry

Alternatives to Nutrition Support Services

The author (JKS) has participated as a physician member of a nutrition support service that rounded on all patients receiving artificial nutrition support, both parenteral and enteral, and participated in the redesigning of the service when physician shortages precluded using a dedicated physician. Currently, the author's institution uses a RD with an advanced degree and extensive critical care experience to oversee a team of RDs who see patients by request and estimate nutritional needs. The team works with the physicians in the various critical care units to provide recommended nutritional prescriptions.

The nutritional support service also provides an educational service to critical care physicians in training, advises attending critical care physicians on nutritional issues, and spearheads nutritional research projects in the various intensive care units (ICUs). This service appears to work as well as the service organized with an obligatory physician consultant and is more cost effective in terms of physician time.

NUTRITIONAL ASSESSMENT

Critically ill patients are at risk for nutritional deficiencies. The diagnostic criteria for various protein and calorie-deficient states are noted in Table 64.4. It is wise for critical care practitioners to remember that kwashiorkor can be seen in the critically ill patient following prolonged fasting, not just in famine-stricken developing countries.

In general, protein-energy malnutrition, commonly known as *protein-caloric malnutrition* (PCM), has been classified as marasmus, kwashiorkor, and marasmic kwashiorkor (5). The differentiation has been the presence of edema and severe serum protein depletion in kwashiorkor as compared with body wasting without edema and preservation of plasma proteins in marasmus. Marasmic kwashiorkor exhibits features of both severe wasting (marasmus) and protein depletion with edema (kwashiorkor). Typically, marasmic kwashiorkor occurs when a chronically malnourished patient is subjected to added catabolic stress such as trauma or sepsis.

Because of the risk that a critically ill patient with underlying nutritional deficiency will develop marasmic kwashiorkor, they are screened for chronic undernutrition on admission to the hospital/intensive care unit. One such screening tool, the Malnutrition Universal Screening Tool (MUST), provides a numerical index: 0, minimal risk; 1, medium risk; or 2, high risk of malnutrition (6). The urgency of instituting nutritional support increases for patients with a score of 1 and especially 2. The MUST evaluates patients' body mass index (weight in kilograms [kg] divided by height in meters squared [m^2]), prehospital involuntary weight loss as a percent of body weight, and the potential for critical illness-induced starvation for the next 5 days.

TABLE 64.4

INDICES OF MALNUTRITION: PROTEIN-ENERGY MALNUTRITION

% IBW	Undernutrition 80%	Marasmus less than 60%	Kwashiorkor 60%–80% with edema	Obesity
BMI	18.5–20	Less than 18.5	Less than 18.5	Greater than 30
Unplanned weight loss past 3–6 mo	5%–10%			Less than 5%
Acute disease effect	Iatrogenic starvation	Prolonged underfeeding with catabolic illness	Severe protein-energy deprivation, usually prolonged fasting with catabolic diseases	Eating
Arm circ. (cm)	23.5	Less than 23.5	Less than 23.5	32.0
MUST score	1	2	2	0
Edema	–	–	+	–
Cause	Low nutrition intake, chronic illness	Low protein calorie intake	Low protein intake	Excess energy intake
T-lymphocyte count (cells/μL)	Less than 1,800	Less than 800	Less than 800	More than 2,000

IBW, ideal body weight; BMI, body mass index; circ., circumference; MUST, Malnutrition Universal Screening Tool.

Anthropometric indices such as MUST are useful for identifying patients who need aggressive nutritional support. However, a more precise diagnosis of a critically ill patient's current nutritional state as well as a tool to monitor the patient's response to nutritional support requires a combination of anthropometric, serum chemical analysis, and physiologic measurements (7). Charting the patient's daily weight is one of the simplest anthropometric measurements that can identify both long-term loss of lean body mass and the development of edema. The body mass index, mid–upper arm circumference, and estimate of body fat from triceps skin fold are other measurements to track the critically ill patient's nutritional state (7).

Many biochemical markers are available to track a patient's nutritional state. These include albumin concentration, estimates of whole body potassium, water balance, and visceral proteins such as prealbumin, transferrin, and retinol-binding protein. Albumin concentration is a good prognostic marker of a patient's *chronic* nutritional state. Perioperative mortality has been shown to increase when albumin concentration is less than 30 gm/L (8). However, serum albumin has a long serum half-life and, hence, does not reflect acute responses to nutritional therapy.

Total body potassium represents lean cellular mass and can be a useful measurement of changes in lean tissue mass that occur rather slowly. In a similar fashion, 24-hour creatinine production is a marker of total skeletal muscle mass. However, both of these markers change relatively slowly and may not be useful to monitor the patient's response to nutritional therapy for critical illness.

Visceral proteins—prealbumin, transferrin, and retinol-binding protein—with their short half-lives, can be useful to monitor protein synthetic response to nutritional support therapy (7). Measuring nitrogen (N) balance via a 24-hour urine urea nitrogen excretion is a very useful technique to monitor response to nutritional support. *Nitrogen balance*, defined as protein N intake minus protein N excretion, is approximately zero (balanced) in the healthy, free-living state. The catabolism triggered by critical illness will lead to increased loss of protein N and a negative nitrogen balance. The goal of the intensivist is to provide nutritional support to lead to a positive N balance until the patient's depleted protein state is replenished.

The most direct method to monitor N balance is to measure 24-hour protein intake, divide the number by 6.25, which is the average ratio of molecular weight of amino acid to nitrogen content, then subtract protein loss, represented by the excretion of urine urea N (UUN) over the same 24-hour period. Usually, an empiric constant of 4 gm N per day is added to the UUN measurement to account for nonurinary losses of proteins (Table 64.5). If the patient's blood urea nitrogen (BUN) is not stable, corrections for retained N must be performed (Table 64.5).

Energy expenditure may be calculated by the Harris-Benedict equation or measured directly with an indirect calorimeter. The Harris-Benedict equation is fairly accurate if the patient's weight is near his or her ideal body weight. Because lipid has a metabolic rate different from lean body, the Harris-Benedict equation may not accurately estimate the patient's actual caloric expenditure, especially in the obese.

Indirect calorimetry takes advantage of the fact that oxygen consumption (VO_2) and carbon dioxide production (VCO_2) are stoichiometric products of aerobic metabolism. Thus, the patient's pulmonary gas exchange is measured over a several-hour period and converted to the patient's actual energy expenditure by empiric equation (9) (Table 64.6). The longer the time period over which the measurements occur, the closer to the patient's actual average daily metabolic rate. Because patients have a diurnal variation, as well as an activity variation, in metabolic rate, short time periods of indirect calorimetry may overestimate or underestimate the average 24-hour energy expenditure. Indirect calorimetry also provides information that is useful for managing a patient's respiratory status, because a high oxygen consumption and carbon dioxide production is associated with obligatory mechanical ventilatory support. Furthermore, mean expired carbon dioxide, a value required for accurate measurement of pulmonary dead space, is directly measured by indirect calorimetry.

TABLE 64.5

ASSESSMENT OF DAILY NITROGEN BALANCE

Nitrogen intake = protein administered in g/day divided by 6.25 = g N/day
[0.1 g protein = 0.16 g N (6.25 g protein contains 1 g N)]
Urine urea nitrogen = 80% of total urine nitrogen
1 g (16.6 mMol) urea = 28/60 g nitrogen[a]

1) 24-h urine urea N in g/day = (A) in g
2) Measure of proteinuria, if any = Y
   Y × 0.16 = (B) in g
3) Correction for any rise of BUN assuming no change in body weight in kg
   Rise in blood urea (in 24 h) = Z in g · L^{-1}
   Z in g × 60% body weight × 28/60 = Z × body weight × 0.28 = (C) in g

(A) + (B) + (C) = nitrogen loss
N balance = (nitrogen intake – nitrogen loss)

[a]28 is mol weight of N in urea and 60 is total mol weight of urea, i.e., 1 g urea = 0.47 g N.

TABLE 64.6

INDIRECT CALORIMETRY—DAILY ENERGY EXPENDITURE

$$\text{Kcal/day} = 3.94 \times VO_2\ (\text{L/24 h}) + 1.11 \times VCO_2\ (\text{L/24 h}) \times 2.17\ \text{UN (g/24 h)}$$

$$VO_2 = [(F_IO_2 \times V_I) - (F_EO_2 \times V_E)] \times 1{,}440\ \text{min/24 hrs}$$

$$VCO_2 = (F_ECO_2 \cdot V_E - F_ICO_2 \cdot V_I) \times 1{,}440\ \text{min/24 h}$$

$$V_I = \frac{V_E[(1 - F_EO_2) - F_ECO_2]}{(1 - F_IO_2)} \quad \text{Haldane correction}$$

VO_2 = oxygen consumption (L/24 h)
VCO_2 = carbon dioxide production (L/24 h)
V_I = inspired ventilation (L/min)
V_E = expired ventilation (L/min)
F_IO_2 = mole fraction inspired oxygen
F_EO_2 = mole fraction expired oxygen
F_ICO_2 = mole fraction inspired carbon dioxide (assumed to be 0)
F_ECO_2 = mole fraction expired carbon dioxide
UN = 24-hour urinary nitrogen loss (g/24 h)

Overall, monitoring of a patient's response to nutrition support is performed by a battery of the tests described above. Daily weights are tracked to monitor a patient's response to nutritional support. Initially, weight gain will represent an increase in total body water, which will start decreasing (diuresing) as the patient becomes anabolic. During the anabolic phase, the patient will initially lose weight via diuresis of water, then gain weight as lean body mass. Obese patients may continue to lose weight from fat stores if they are fed a high-protein, restricted calorie diet. Repeated indirect calorimetry can follow the respiratory quotient (VCO_2/VO_2) that provides a measure of whether a patient is being underfed or overfed. Utilization of protein intake can be tracked by repeated 24-hour N balances via urine urea nitrogen measurements and nutrition intake.

Beyond direct physiologic measurements of adequacy of nutritional intake, functional measurements that indirectly depend on the nutrition response, such as immunologic function, can be followed. The severely malnourished patient exhibits immunocompromise by skin test anergy, low absolute lymphocyte count, low T-cell lymphocyte count, difficulty mounting a fever, and increased susceptibility to infections; these functions should improve with aggressive nutritional support.

TIMING OF NUTRITIONAL SUPPORT

Nutritional evaluation of the critically ill frequently reveals patients admitted to the ICU who exhibit signs of marasmic kwashiorkor and who have an urgent need for nutritional support. Once the decision is made to provide nutritional support for the critically ill, one has to decide on the best route of administration—parenteral or enteral. Data from one to two decades ago suggested that parenteral nutrition (total parenteral nutrition or TPN) was associated with a higher mortality rate than enteral nutrition (total enteral nutrition or TEN) in patients who had abdominal trauma (10,11). However, more recent studies in other patient populations have failed to confirm these results (12,13). In several studies comparing the administration routes of nutritional support, the major difference between TEN and TPN was the fact that enteral-fed patients had more frequent interruptions of nutrition (14,15). Therefore, TEN patients received somewhat less nutritional substrate than TPN patients.

Historically, there has been grave concern that TPN puts a patient at risk for serious infection complications. However, recent studies reveal that bloodstream infections are relatively rare during TPN, and TEN patients have a significantly higher incidence of feeding tube complications than TPN patients have from central venous catheter complications.

In one review of infectious complications in the ICU, it was noted that inadequate nutritional intake—less than 7 kcal/kg per day—was associated with sepsis. In this group of underfed patients, those who received TEN were equally likely to have infectious complications as those who received TPN (16). This study supports the practice of starting early and adequate nutrition support to prevent infectious morbidity.

One of the alleged benefits of early enteral feeding is to maintain the integrity of the gut mucosal lining and thus limit translocation of microorganisms from intestinal lumen to bloodstream. This hypothesis was tested using a macromolecular marker of gut permeability in two groups of patients: those with early enteral feedings and those kept NPO (nothing by mouth) (17). There was no demonstrated difference in permeability between the two groups, which suggests that bacterial translocation from the gut to the bloodstream is not the source of bloodstream infections in patients who are fed parenterally.

TEN does have some demonstrated advantages over TPN, including lower cost, using gut absorption to regulate total body water balance, and the ability to utilize larger molecules as a food source. TPN has advantages over TEN that include fewer interruptions for NPO status prior to procedures and no interference with drug absorption.

We recommend that patients receive early nutritional support to help reduce infectious complications. Because patients need adequate protein and calorie intake to prevent complications from infections, those patients who cannot tolerate TEN should be immediately switched to TPN. It is clearly an error to withhold TPN for the notion that the risks of TPN outweigh the risks of starvation for several days.

The marked improvement in managing central venous access that developed in recent years has markedly reduced the risk of infectious complications of TPN. Furthermore, accurate and widespread assessment of actual metabolic needs with indirect calorimetry and N balance has led to a significant reduction in TPN calorie load that has decreased metabolic complications of TPN (18,19).

NUTRITION SUPPORT FOR SPECIFIC ORGAN DYSFUNCTION

Nutritional support is often modified for specific organ dysfunction because certain pathophysiologic conditions lead to changes in the metabolic handling of nutrient substrates. These disease states include liver failure, kidney failure, diabetes/glycemic control, and brain injury.

Hepatic Failure

Liver failure is one of the most vexing morbidities requiring prescriptions for nutritional support. In severe hepatic failure, nitrogen from amino acid metabolism remains as ammonia because it is not metabolized to urea. Hyperammonemia leads to secondary neurologic dysfunction including hepatic coma. Thus, protein needs to be administered in amounts to replace catabolic losses, but not high enough to lead to high levels of ammonia. Sorbitol may be administered enterally to try to lower ammonia by increasing gut motility and decreasing intestinal transit time to decrease the absorption of proteins and ammonia from bacterial metabolism of intraluminal amino acids. However, sorbitol has no effect on hepatic amino acid metabolism.

Hepatic glycogen stores are also depleted in end-stage hepatic failure, making the maintenance of normoglycemia extremely difficult. High glucose feedings may be required to compensate for lack of hepatic glucose production. The bottom line in end-stage hepatic failure is that nutritional support needs to be modified to minimize plasma ammonia levels and maintain normal glucose levels; nutritional support will not, of course, reverse significant hepatic injury.

Renal Failure

Rising blood levels of the nitrogenous waste product urea and creatinine are the hallmarks of renal failure. Acute renal failure is, unfortunately, rather common in critically ill patients in response to intrarenal insults from circulating inflammatory mediators as well as changes in renal perfusion. Although past nutritional efforts for acute renal failure have focused on limiting protein intake to reduce urea production or using only essential amino acids to recycle amines to reduce urea production, modern critical care uses renal replacement therapy (20,21). Either hemodialysis or continuous venovenous hemoperfusion is used to maintain acceptable levels of urea, creatinine, and electrolytes until the kidney regains its function. One of the few evidence-based therapies that enhances the repair of acute renal failure is nutritional support with adequate protein for renal healing. Thus, efforts to restrict protein intake in patients with acute renal failure are misguided and should be discouraged. Renal replacement therapy should be instituted to maintain acceptable levels of urea while the healing kidney is supported by adequate protein replacement. Prior to the commencement of renal replacement therapy, serum electrolytes need to be carefully monitored because renal failure often leads to excess water (H_2O), low sodium (Na), and high potassium (K). Nutrition support may have to be modified to correct serum electrolyte disorders.

Glycemic Control

Hyperglycemia is a common occurrence in critically ill patients. Not all hyperglycemic critically ill patients have diabetes, but the hormonal milieu of the stress response tends to cause hyperglycemia. Among the hormones that increase plasma glucose are growth hormone, cortisol, glucagon, and epinephrine (22). Furthermore, one of the diagnostic hallmarks of sepsis is glucose intolerance/insulin resistance. Some authors have postulated that hyperglycemia has survival advantages in providing energy substrate for collagen synthesis for wound healing. A large randomized trial compared glucose levels of 180 to 200 mg/dL in the control group, consistent with the survival advantage hypothesis, to normoglycemia of 80 to 110 mg/dL in the experimental group (23). The normoglycemic group had a significant improvement in outcome effects that persisted for several months post recovery. These effects included decreased ICU length of stay, reduced infectious complications, and survival.

Despite fears that tight glucose control might expose patients to risks of dangerous hypoglycemic episodes, it is recommended that critically ill patients be managed with normal glucose levels (23,24). Furthermore, in the controlled environment of the critical care unit, where it is feasible to monitor glucose levels every hour, an insulin infusion is the best method to manage glucose concentrations. Infusions of regular insulin can be rapidly changed to respond to hourly, or more frequent, bedside glucometer measurements that may vary widely in unstable critically ill patients. To protect patients from hypoglycemia from the insulin infusion, patients receive either nutritional support (TPN or TEN at goals) or, if needed, a 10% dextrose infusion (23–25).

Brain Injury

The injured brain is characterized by an impairment of the blood–brain barrier, which causes increased susceptibility to changes in plasma concentrations of glucose and electrolytes. The prevention of edema in the injured brain, an essential requirement to allow the brain to heal and reorganize neural pathways, places demands on the composition of nutritional support. Nutritional goals for the head-injured patient include avoidance of hyperglycemia, hyperosmolar state, and maintenance of normal sodium and potassium. Hyperosmolar coma, a known complication of TPN, is usually caused by extreme hyperglycemia and can be treated with insulin. This is certainly another good reason to accurately assess a patient's metabolic rate and calorie requirement from nutrition support. Hyperglycemia, even with normal osmolality, is detrimental to the injured brain by causing cerebral edema in ischemic areas of the brain. This occurs when one glucose molecule diffuses into the brain and is anaerobically metabolized to two lactic acid molecules that are highly polar and do not diffuse out into the bloodstream. Thus, the interior of the cell increases in osmolality (more nondiffusable particles) relative to plasma and attracts increased cell water. The above effect is magnified by hyperglycemia in patients who have brain lesions associated with low perfusion/O_2 delivery (26,27).

Besides adjusting nutritional support to maintain euglycemia, with appropriate calorie administration and insulin use, sodium replacement is important in brain-injured patients. Many patients with brain injuries develop hyponatremia, which tends to increase the risk of cerebral edema from excess plasma water and decreased serum osmolality. Cerebral salt-wasting syndrome or inability to conserve sodium in the kidney needs to be differentiated from syndrome of inappropriate antidiuretic hormone (ADH) secretion (SIADH). Cerebral salt-wasting patients tend to be hypovolemic and need extra sodium replacement in their nutrition support, whereas patients with SIADH tend to be hypervolemic and generally need fluid restriction to correct their serum sodium levels.

Brain-injured patients will require adequate protein intake to compensate for their increased demands to provide brain healing. The metabolic rate should be measured directly and caloric needs met by appropriate amounts of nutritional support. There is some concern about excitatory amino acids having deleterious effects on the injured brain, but it is unclear that nutritional support affects the CNS concentration of these amino acids.

SUMMARY

Nutritional support for critically ill patients is often overlooked by clinicians concerned with the immediate concerns of hemodynamic instability and respiratory failure. However, starvation is not therapeutic, and prolonged inadequate energy intake will lead to malnutrition states in critically ill patients. Increased metabolic activity stimulated by stress hormonal response and a generalized inflammatory state may accelerate the appearance of malnutrition. Adequate protein-energy intake reduces critical care unit–acquired bloodstream infections, and aggressive insulin management to maintain euglycemia will reduce mortality as well as infectious complications of critical illness. Supported in part by NIH GM 39277 (TCV).

References

1. Cuthbertson DP. Surgical metabolism: historical and evolutionary aspects. In: Wilkinson AW, Cuthbertson D, eds. *Metabolism and the Response to Injury*. Chicago, IL: Year Book Medical; 1976:1–34.
2. Kinney JM. The application of indirect calorimetry to clinical studies. In: Kinney JM, Buskirk ER, Munrot N, eds. *Assessment of Energy Metabolism in Health and Disease*. Columbus, OH: Ross Laboratories; 1980:42–48.
3. Vary TC, Siegel JH. Sepsis, abnormal metabolic control and multiple organ failure syndrome. In: Siegel JS, ed. *Trauma: Emergency Surgery and Critical Care*. New York, NY: Churchill Livingstone; 1987:411.
4. Kinney JM, Gump FE. The metabolic response to injury in American College of Surgeons Committee on Pre and Post Operative Care: *Manual of Preoperative and Postoperative Care*, ed 3. Philadelphia, PA: WB Saunders; 1983;15–37.
5. Odigwe C, Ejibe DK. Malnutrition. *Student BMJ*. 2005;13:404–405.
6. Malnutrition Advisory Group: Malnutrition Universal Screening Tool ('MUST'). www.bapen.org.uk. Accessed August 30, 2007.
7. Halder M, Halder SQ. Assessment of protein-calorie malnutrition. *Clin Che*. 1984;30:1286–1299.
8. Mullen JL, Buzby GP, Waldman MT, et al. Prediction of operative morbidity and mortality by pre-operative nutritional assessment. *Surg Forum*. 1979;30:80–82.
9. Bursztein S, Elwyn DH, Askanazi J, et al. Energy metabolism, indirect calorimetry, and nutrition. Baltimor, MD: Williams & Wilkins; 1989.
10. Kudsk KA, Croce MA, Fabian TG, et al. Enteral versus parenteral feeding. Effects on septic morbidity after blunt and penetrating abdominal trauma. *Ann Surg*. 1992;215:503–513.
11. Heyland DK, MacDonald S, Keefe L, et al. Total parenteral nutrition in the critically ill patient: a meta-analysis. *JAMA*. 1998;280:2013–2019.
12. Lipman TO. Grains or veins: is enteral nutrition really better than parenteral nutrition? A look at the evidence. *JPEN J Parenter Enteral Nutr*. 1998;22:167–182.
13. Woodcock W, Zeigler D, Palmer M, et al. Enteral versus parenteral nutrition: a pragmatic study. *Nutrition*. 2001;17:1–12.
14. Jeejebhory KN. Total parenteral nutrition: potion or poison? *Am J Clin Nutr*. 2001;74:160–163.
15. Pacelli F, Bossola M, Papa V, et al. Enteral vs. parenteral nutrition after major abdominal surgery: an even match. *Arch Surg*. 2001;136:933–936.
16. Rubinson L, Diette GB, Song X, et al. Low caloric intake is associated with nosocomial blood stream infections in patients in the medical intensive care unit. *Crit Care Med*. 2004;32:350–357.
17. Reynolds JV, Kanwar S, Welsh FKS, et al. Does the route of feeding modify gut barrier function and clinical outcome in patients after major upper gastrointestinal surgery? *JPEN J Parenter Enteral Nutr*. 1997;21:196–201.
18. McCowen KC, Friel C, Sternberg J, et al. Hypocaloric total parenteral nutrition: effectiveness in prevention of hyperglycemia and infections complications—a randomized clinical trial. *Crit Care Med*. 2000;28:3606–3611.
19. Lowry SF, Brennan MF. Abnormal liver function during parenteral nutrition: relation to infusion excess. *J Surg Res*. 1979;26:300.
20. Giordano C. Use of exogenous and endogenous urea for protein synthesis in normal and uremic subjects. *J Lab Clin Med*. 1963;62:231.
21. Grovanetti S, Neaggiore Q. A low nitrogen diet with protein of high biologic value for severe chronic uremia. *Lancet*. 1964;1:1000.
22. Bone RC. Toward an epidemiology and natural history of SIRS (systemic inflammatory response syndrome). *JAMA*. 1992;268:3452–3455.
23. Vanden Berghe G, Wouters P, Weekers F, et al. Intensive insulin therapy in critically ill patients. *N Engl J Med*. 2001;345:1359–1367.
24. Vanden Berghe G, Wilmer A, Hermans G, et al. Intensive insulin therapy in medical ICU. *N Engl J Med*. 2006;359:449–461.
25. Inzucchi SE. Management of hyperglycemia in the hospital setting. *N Engl J Med*. 2006;355:1903–1911.
26. Young B, Ott L, Haack D, et al. Effect of total parenteral nutrition upon intracranial pressure in severe head injury. *J Neurosurg*. 1987;67:76–80.
27. Sieber FE, Smith DS, Traystman RJ, et al. Glucose: a re-evaluation of its intraoperative use. *Anesthesiology*. 1987;67:72.

CHAPTER 65 ■ PRACTICAL ASPECTS OF NUTRITIONAL SUPPORT

CHRISTOPHER D. TAN

"If the gut works, use it. If it isn't working, make it work." This adage summarizes how a clinician should approach nutritional support in the intensive care unit. Although it may seem intuitive that parenteral nutrition should improve morbidity and mortality because the patient is "being fed," conclusive data are sparse. On the contrary, much has been published on the benefits of enteral feeds, especially if the patient is fed early (1,2).

Being familiar with nutrition support is not just about calories and proteins the patient needs, but requires familiarity with the ordering, initiating, monitoring, and discontinuing processes of nutrition support as well. This chapter is meant to complement the previous chapter by taking the clinician through the practical aspects of nutritional support.

WRITING A TOTAL PARENTERAL NUTRITION ORDER

In 2003, the American Society for Parenteral and Enteral Nutrition (A.S.P.E.N.) assembled a task force to look into the safe practice of parenteral nutrition practice. Out of this task force emerged the 2004 A.S.P.E.N. guidelines on Safe Practice for Parenteral Nutrition (3), as well as the 2005 A.S.P.E.N. *Nutrition Support Practice Manual* (2nd ed.) (4). The latter is considered to be one of the primary resources for nutritional support.

Life-threatening errors continue to occur in the preparation and delivery of parenteral nutrition (PN) admixtures to patients. Many of these errors are related to the ordering process. One solution to this problem is to use a standardized PN form that is institution specific. Research has demonstrated the benefit of a standardized order-writing process in reducing prescription errors (5). These forms, however, are not perfect themselves, as shown by one study, which reported an increase in prescriber errors after a standardized PN order form was introduced (5).

Providing nutrition support to critically ill patients is a complex but important task. The ultimate goal should be to minimize loss of lean body mass, especially in patients with burns, sepsis, acute respiratory distress syndrome, and trauma. Energy expenditure of the critically ill patient depends on the underlying disease state, as well as the nutritional status of the patient before the injury or illness. Although the Harris-Benedict equation is widely used to estimate the basal energy expenditure, the stress and activity factors used to adjust for the severity of illness may be excessive, and can lead to overfeeding (4). One recommendation from the A.S.P.E.N. guidelines, as well as from the American College of Chest Physicians (ACCP), is using a total energy requirement of 25 kcal/kg/day (4,6). If the patient is obese, then an adjusted body weight should be used in the calculation (4).

Protein requirements for critically ill patients with normal renal function can range from 1.3 to 2 g/kg/day (moderate to severe stress), using the premorbid body weight or the adjusted body weight if obese (4). In patients with acute renal failure, the following amounts of protein are recommended: 0.8 to 1.2 g/kg/day if patients are not dialyzed, 1 to 1.4 g/kg/day in patients receiving dialysis, and 1.5 and 2.5 g/kg/day in patients undergoing continuous renal replacement therapy (CRRT) (4). For chronic kidney disease, the A.S.P.E.N. recommends 0.5 to 0.6 g of protein/kg/day (4). The ACCP, on the other hand, recommends no change in the amount of protein given to patients with acute renal failure versus patients with normal kidney function (i.e., 1.2–2 g/kg/day) (6). In chronic renal failure, the ACCP recommends 0.5 to 0.8 g of protein/kg/day (6).

There are at least three different ways PN can be ordered. If the patient has only peripheral venous access, peripheral parenteral nutrition (PPN) is used. Compared to total parenteral nutrition (TPN), PPN is lower in osmolarity (<900 mOsm/L) to minimize thrombophlebitis (7). For formulas to be given via central line, TPN can be administered in two ways. One is a two-in-one TPN formula, which is protein and dextrose in one bag, with the intravenous fat emulsions (IVFEs) hung separately. The other method is a three-in-one TPN formula, in which all three fuel substrates (amino acids [AAs], dextrose, and fats) are mixed in one bag. Each has advantages and disadvantages. The two-in-one formula allows visualization of particulate matter but takes up more nursing time and requires two different intravenous lines. The three-in-one is more user friendly since only one bag needs to be hung, but the cloudiness of the solution will not allow visualization of particulate matter. The A.S.P.E.N. guidelines do not favor one formula over another.

Most institutions have premixed PN formulas with known amounts of protein (g/L) and calories (kcal/L) to make it easier for order writing. For three-in-one formulas, once the caloric and protein needs have been assessed, the volume of PN needed is calculated to match the assessed needs. For instance, if 2 L of formula X from your institution is needed to meet needs, then the PN rate should be 83 mL/hour (i.e., 2,000 mL/day ÷ 24 hours/day). If your institution does not have premixed PN formulas or none of the formulas is appropriate for your patient, then a customized mixture will be necessary. This will be discussed later in the chapter.

For two-in-one formulas, fat is administered separately, usually three times a week. To calculate the total caloric contributions, the amount of calories per week from fat is totaled and then divided by 7 days per week to obtain the calories per day. For example, Intralipid 20% 500 mL containing 1,000 kcal is given three times a week. The caloric contribution per day would be 3,000 kcal/week ÷ 7 days/week, which equals 429 kcal/day from fat. This amount is then added to the known calories provided by the dextrose and amino acids in the two-in-one formula.

Most institutions have default amounts of additives (electrolytes) to facilitate the ordering process. The amounts are based on guidelines and may not suit every patient. For example, using default additives with potassium and phosphorus in a renal failure patient can lead to hyperkalemia and hyperphosphatemia, respectively.

Ordering electrolytes and other additives is as much an art as it is a science. With practice, one can develop a "feel" for how patients will respond to the additives depending on their condition. The most difficult part of the ordering process is how much electrolyte to add initially. The subsequent adjustments are easier with adjustments to increase, decrease, or keep the additives the same, depending on the laboratory values. Table 65.1 summarizes how to determine the quantity of electrolytes to add to PN solutions.

INITIATING PARENTERAL NUTRITION

The A.S.P.E.N. guidelines suggest no more than 150 to 200 g/day of glucose initially to ensure tolerance of PN (4). Thus, it may be prudent to infuse only 1 L of the TPN on the first day (i.e., 42 mL/hour) and reaching goal rate on day 2 or 3, depending on the patient's tolerance of volume and macronutrients. It is imperative that central line placement be verified by radiography before initiating TPN, and that TPN be administered through a dedicated infusion port via an infusion pump that is equipped with protection from "free flow" and has reliable alarms. To reduce the chance for infusing particulates, microorganisms, and pyrogens, a 1.2-micron filter may be used (anything smaller than 1.2 micron may filter out the fat emulsions in a three-in-one formula). Alternatively, a 0.22-micron filter may be used for a two-in-one formula. PPN formula is not as calorie dense and contains less protein; therefore, it may be initiated at goal rate (assuming the patient is able to tolerate the fluid load). The PN administration set must be changed every 24 hours using aseptic techniques and universal precautions. An exception is if the PN does not contain fat emulsions (i.e., the two-in-one formulation); then the administration set may be changed every 72 hours (4). However, the administration set used in infusing the IVFE separately must be discarded after use or at least every 12 hours (4).

TABLE 65.1

PARENTERAL NUTRITION (PN) ADDITIVES AND SUGGESTED AMOUNTS

Electrolytes/additives	Suggested amounts	Comments
Sodium	1–2 mEq/kg/d	Assess the current IV fluid the patient is receiving and how the sodium level is responding (i.e., if the patient is receiving lactated Ringer solution [130 mEq/L], and Na^+ is within desired range, then add 130 mEq/L in the PN). Patients no longer requiring fluid resuscitation will need 1/2 normal saline or 80 mEq/L of Na^+ in PN.
Potassium	1–2 mEq/kg/d	Major intracellular cation. There is obligatory daily loss. Assess current repletion and patient's response as this will guide the clinician on how much to add to the PN.
Chloride	Default salt	This is the "acidifying" salt; acidemia is preferable in most situations to alkalemia (improved unloading of O_2 to the tissues). It can be given as either NaCl or KCl.
Acetate (Ac)	Add if patient has metabolic acidosis	May be useful in patients with metabolic acidosis secondary to renal failure; acetate is metabolized into bicarbonate in the body. Bicarbonate is not compatible in the PN solution. It can be given as NaAc or KAc.
Calcium gluconate	10–15 mEq/d	Use ionized calcium as a guide rather than total calcium.
Magnesium sulfate	8–20 mEq/d	Intracellular cation. It can accumulate in renal failure; 1 g = 8 mEq.
Phosphorus	20–40 mmol/d	Major intracellular anion. May be given as KPO_4 (4.4 mEq K^+/3 mmol PO_4^-) or $NaPO_4$ (4 mEq Na^+/3 mmol PO_4^-) depending on cation deficiency. Amount of calcium or phosphorus in total PN is limited by the calcium-phosphate solubility curve.
Trace elements	Standard amount daily	Adjust to twice a week in patients with severe renal failure and severe hepatic failure.
Insulin	Add 50%–70% of insulin sliding scale needs	Use amounts of insulin used by the sliding scale used in the last 24 h to guide how much to add to the PN bag. Start conservatively with 50%–70% of total insulin used during last 24 h.
H_2 blocker	Add total daily dose	Continuous infusion of H_2 blocker is superior in keeping pH elevated compared to intermittent dosing.[a] Protein pump inhibitors are not compatible in total PN.

[a]Ballesteros MA, Hogan DL, Koss MA, et al. Bolus or intravenous infusion of ranitidine: effects on gastric pH and acid secretions. A comparison of efficacy and cost. *Ann Intern Med.* 1990;112:334–339.
From Merritt R, ed. *The A.S.P.E.N. Nutrition Support Practice Manual.* 2nd ed. Silver Spring, MD: A.S.P.E.N; 2005.

TRANSITIONAL FEEDING AND WEANING PARENTERAL NUTRITION

The transitional period is the time during which enteral feeding is started and PN is discontinued. Patients who are young, have no history of malignancy, and were well nourished before PN was started can have their PN discontinued as soon as they are able to tolerate solid food. In general, PN can be discontinued once 60% of energy needs is met enterally (4). In older debilitated patients who have a history of malnutrition and malignancy, transitioning to enteral feeds may be more challenging. Calorie counts help to guide the reduction or discontinuation of PN. Factors such as aspiration risk, appetite, strength, and ileus play a role in whether patients successfully transition to enteral feeds.

Terminating TPN is just the opposite of initiating. The major concern is rebound hypoglycemia from rapid cessation of PN. It is recommended that the TPN be decreased by half for 1 to 2 hours before discontinuation if the current infusion rate is >42 mL/hour (4). This will allow time for the body to adjust its insulin secretion to decreasing amounts of circulating dextrose and avoid hypoglycemia. Weaning of PN is not necessary in patients receiving oral nutrition.

If problems occur with the TPN bag that render it not usable (e.g., a leak in the bag) and the patient is on a rate >42 mL/hour, dextrose 10% (D10W) or dextrose 10% with 0.9% sodium chloride (D10NS) should be infused at the same rate as the TPN to avoid rebound hypoglycemia. In the same scenario, dextrose 5% (D5W) may be substituted in place of PPN, not because of rebound hypoglycemia, but more for maintaining caloric intake.

CYCLIC PARENTERAL NUTRITION

PN that is infusing 24 hours a day means that the patient is tethered to the intravenous pole, limiting mobility. Getting the patient who is receiving PN to eat more may be problematic because the satiety center is constantly being stimulated. A reduced oral intake can be expected if more than 25% of caloric needs is provided by PN (9). In these two scenarios, transitioning over to cyclic PN may be a good option. Cyclic or nocturnal PN is almost like regular PN except that instead of infusing the PN over 24 hours, the same volume is infused over a shorter period (12 or 14 hours), starting in the evening and finishing in the morning. Cyclic PN allows patients to be more mobile during the day, as well as have more of an appetite. Other benefits of cyclic PN include less deterioration of liver function (10).

Before transitioning to cyclic PN, the nutritional goal needs to be defined: Full support versus supplemental to a diet. Full support means that the total amount of protein and calories will be provided. In this case, it is important to make sure that the TPN is already concentrated, since the patient will be receiving the same volume that was previously given over 24 hours over a shorter period of time. If the goal is to have the patient eat more but not get behind in nutrition, then one can provide 50% of assessed needs as cyclic PN while the patient is fed orally or enterally. An important aspect of cyclic TPN is calculating the tapered flow rate to minimize harmful fluctuations of blood sugar (i.e., hyperglycemia during initiation of PN and rebound hypoglycemia during cessation of PN). One simplified method of calculating the tedious cyclic PN rate comes from Stanford University (11):

$$v = r + 2r + 4r(t - 4) + 2r + r, \text{ where } t = \text{cyclic PN time},$$
$$v = \text{volume infused, and } r = \text{rate of PN}$$
$$v = 6r + 4rt - 16r$$
$$v = 4rt - 10r$$
$$v = r(4t - 10)$$
$$r = v/(4t - 10)$$
$$r = 1{,}500\ \text{mL}/(4[12\ \text{hours}] - 10)$$
$$r = 39.47 \text{ or } \sim 40\ \text{mL/hour}$$

For example, the patient will be receiving a total of 1,500 mL ("v") of PN formula X over 12 hours ("t"). To calculate the cyclic TPN rate ("r"), the formula uses the model (r mL/hour × 1 hour) + (2r mL/hour × 1 hour) + [4r mL/hour × (cyclic PN time – 4)] + (2r mL/hour × 1 hour) + (r mL/hour × 1 hour). Therefore, the cyclic TPN will be ordered as follows: 40 mL/hr × 1 hour, then 80 mL/hour × 1 hour, then 160 mL/hour × 8 hour, then 80 mL/hour × 1 hour, then 40 mL/hour × 1 hour, then stop. It is important that there be a "ramp up" and "ramp down" during cyclic TPN infusion to avoid significant glucose fluctuations. Glucose may be drawn 60 minutes after the maximal infusion rate, or 60 minutes after discontinuation of cyclic PN to make sure the patient is tolerating (4).

HIDDEN SOURCES OF KCALS

Inadvertent hypercaloric feeding can result in increased carbon dioxide production, hyperglycemia, and hepatomegaly, all of which may be detrimental to the critically ill patient. It is important to pay attention to medications that can inadvertently lead to excessive calories. Propofol, which is suspended in 10% Intralipid, contributes 1.1 kcal/mL. A patient on a relatively high dose of 50 μg/kg/minute (assuming a 70-kg patient) can easily receive an extra 554 kcal/day.

Another hidden source of calories is the dextrose concentration in the dialysate fluid of patients receiving CRRT. Diffusion greatly influences dextrose absorption across the hemofilter. It has been reported that the daily caloric contribution ranges from 123 to 2,388 kcal depending on the dextrose concentration of 0.5% to 4.25% in the dialysate solution. Approximately 43% to 45% of dextrose can be absorbed by the body across the hemofilter (12). Other factors that affect the degree of dextrose absorption are the dialysis flow rate, blood flow rate, ultrafiltration rate, arterial blood glucose concentration, and integrity of the hemofilter (12–14). Using the lowest possible concentration of dextrose in the dialysate is the best way to avoid hyperglycemia.

FLUID RESTRICTION

In institutions that use electronic admixing equipment (e.g., Baxter's Automix/Micromix), formulating the TPN is virtually just a touch of a button. Reformulating PN formulas to maximize caloric density and minimize fluids is not labor intensive. Although mixing standard or nonstandard formulas makes little difference from an admixture standpoint when using the automatic mixing machines, the calculation of a nonstandard PN formula can be tedious and requires knowledge of base solution stabilities used by the pharmacy to admix the PN (see calculations below).

ESTIMATING PROTEIN, FAT, AND CARBOHYDRATE REQUIREMENTS

As discussed earlier, most institutions will likely have premixed standard PN formulas for ease of ordering. However, there are times when the clinician has to formulate a PN formula for special cases. One instance could be if the assessed calories and proteins do not match up to any of the premixed formulas. Another instance could be if the patient has hypertriglyceridemia, and the PN formula has to be adjusted so that the fat is taken out and the dextrose is increased to compensate for the absence of fat. To better understand how to formulate a three-in-one TPN formula, a sample case will be presented.

Base Solutions (may vary with different institutions)

Amino acids base solution:	Travasol 10%
Dextrose base solution	70%
Intralipid base solution	20%

Assessed caloric needs: 2,000 kcal/day
Assessed protein needs: 130 g/day

STEP 1: Assess calories and volume provided by protein (4 kcal/g).

$$4\ \text{kcal}/1\ \text{g} = x/130\ \text{g (see Table 65.2)}$$
$$x = 520\ \text{kcal (from protein)}$$
$$\text{Travasol } 10\% = 10\ \text{g}/100\ \text{mL} = 130\ \text{g}/xx$$
$$xx = 1300\ \text{mL(volume of 130 g protein)}$$

STEP 2: Assess amount of nonprotein calories required. Nonprotein calories should be 15% to 30% fat based, and

TABLE 65.2

RESPIRATORY QUOTIENT (RQ) AND CALORIES PER GRAM OF DIFFERENT FUEL SUBSTRATES

Fuel substrates	RQ	Kcal per gram
Fats	0.7	9 kcal/g; Intralipid 10% contains 1.1 kcal/mL and 20% contains 2 kcal/mL due to the presence of phospholipids
Proteins	0.8	4 kcal/g
Carbohydrates	1	3.4 kcal/g

the rest (70%–85% of nonprotein calories) should be dextrose based (4).

2,000 kcal (total caloric needs) − 520 kcal (calories from proteins) = y
y = 1,480 kcal (nonprotein calories needed)
1,480 kcal × 0.2 (i.e., 20% calories from fat) ~ 300 kcal (fat calories)
1,480 kcal − 300 kcal = 1,180 kcal (dextrose calories)

STEP 3: Assess volume contributed by dextrose (3.4 kcal/g) and fat calories, rounding up the numbers.

Fat calories = 300 kcal
Intralipid = 20% or 2 kcal/mL (see Table 65.2)
Therefore, 300 kcal = 150 mL fat volume
Since 20% is 20 g/100 mL, 150 mL = 30 g fat
Dextrose calories = 1,180 kcal ÷ 3.4 kcal/g = 347 g (see Table 65.2)
Dextrose 70% = 70 g/100 mL = 347 g/z
z = 495.7 or ~ 496 mL (volume from dextrose)

STEP 4: Add up the protein, fat, and dextrose volume to calculate minimum amount of fluid needed to make the TPN formula.

1,300 mL (from AA) + 150 mL (from fat) + 496 mL (from dextrose) = 1,946 mL
1,946 mL/day ÷ 24 hour/day = ~81 mL/hour.
The 1,946-mL volume represents the minimum amount of volume needed to make the TPN (i.e., the TPN is "concentrated").

STEP 5: Put it all together. The PN order would look something like this:

Amino acids = 130 g
Dextrose = 347 g
Fat emulsion = 30 g
Rate = 81 mL/hour (i.e., 1,946 mL over 24 hours)
This formula will provide 1,997 kcal + 130 g protein over 24 hours

If the clinician wanted 100 mL/hour of fluids, the rate can simply be changed to 100 mL/hour (i.e., 2,400 mL over 24 hours; sterile water is added to make up the balance) without affecting the amount of calories and proteins given to the patient. Since 81 mL/hour (1,946 mL) represents the minimum volume needed to make the above TPN, it is not possible to go below 81 mL/hour without decreasing the calories and proteins given to the patient.

ELECTROLYTE ABNORMALITIES

Refeeding syndrome is an imbalance of electrolytes as well as vitamins, micronutrients, and fluids that occurs within the first few days of refeeding malnourished patients as nutrients replete the intracellular space (15). The hallmark biochemical findings include hypophosphatemia (intracellular shift plus depletion of phosphorus substrate to synthesize adenosine triphosphate [ATP]), hypomagnesemia (intracellular shift plus magnesium is a cofactor in many enzymatic functions), and hypokalemia (intracellular shift of potassium with insulin secretion as a response to dextrose infusion). Patients may exhibit respiratory distress, cardiac arrhythmias, congestive heart failure, hemolytic anemia, or paresthesias, or they may die (16). The three most important steps in preventing refeeding are (a) high-risk patients (chronic alcoholism, kwashiorkor, marasmus, rapid refeeding) and those receiving high TPN rates must be identified (17); (b) baseline electrolytes must be checked before the initiation of PN (4,17), and low magnesium, phosphorus, or potassium levels must be corrected immediately; (c) the TPN rate should be advanced slowly (<150 g/day of carbohydrates) as tolerated over several days before going to the goal rate (4,17). In patients receiving enteral nutrition (EN), the rate could be advanced more aggressively if needed, provided that electrolytes are monitored closely and repleted in a timely manner (18).

Replacing electrolytes is both a science and an art, because patients respond differently. Table 65.3 will help guide the clinician in managing electrolyte imbalances that occur. There are two things to remember when adjusting the electrolytes in PN: First, the degree of metabolic derangements must be determined before any adjustments are made. Second, PN should not be used to replace electrolytes rapidly, but should be used for maintenance.

MONITORING

The potential for serious complications is high in patients receiving PN unless careful monitoring is conducted by clinicians. Furthermore, appropriate monitoring can be cost effective by avoiding complications. Suggested protocols for monitoring PN in adults are shown in Table 65.4.

WRITING ENTERAL ORDERS

Ordering enteral feedings is less complex than ordering PN, but it could be just as confusing with many different formulas. Enteral feeding should be started as early as possible since it is a "pharmacotherapy" for the gut (improves mesenteric blood flow and maintains gut integrity). Feeding early, which is defined as 48 hours within mechanical ventilation onset, is associated with a 20% decrease in intensive care unit (ICU) mortality and a 25% decrease in hospital mortality, according to a recent retrospective, multi-institutional study looking at 4,409 patients (1). When choosing enteral formulas, consideration depends on the patient's digestive capability, fluid restriction status, electrolyte balance, nutrient requirements, disease state, and possible routes available for administration.

Enteral formulas may be categorized into the monomeric (which contain free amino acids with or without peptides, with modified fat) and the polymeric formulas. Most enteral formulas fall in the semi-synthetic polymeric formulas, which are more cost effective but require patients to have digestive capability. Monomeric formulas are for patients with malabsorption, such as short-gut syndrome. Because of the cost associated with monomeric formulas, polymeric formulas should be tried first. For instance, in patients with pancreatitis, instead of using monomeric formulas, adding pancreatic enzyme tablets may help with polymeric tube feed tolerance. If the patient

TABLE 65.3

AN EXAMPLE OF MANAGEMENT GUIDELINES FOR METABOLIC COMPLICATIONS IN ADULTS INDUCED BY PARENTERAL NUTRITION

Hyperglycemia	>200 mg/dL	Once daily requirements of insulin are known from the insulin sliding scale, add 50%–75% into TPN. Consider insulin drip if blood sugar is uncontrolled, or if patient is edematous with unreliable absorption of subcutaneous insulin. Goal blood sugar is 80–110 mg/dL in critically ill surgical patients.
Hypoglycemia	<80 mg/dL	If related to sudden discontinuance of TPN, administer D10W or D10NS at the same rate as the TPN. If related to insulin in TPN, initiate continuous glucose supplement (e.g., D10W). If glucose is still below desirable level, discontinue TPN and hang D10W or D10NS at the same rate as the TPN.
Hypernatremia	>150 mEq/L	If hypovolemic, give isotonic or hypotonic fluid depending on degree of hypovolemia. If euvolemic or hypervolemic, reduce sodium from TPN and/or other source. If patient is symptomatic, consider discontinuing TPN and starting D10W at the same rate as the TPN.
Hyponatremia	<130 mEq/L	If hypervolemic, restrict fluid intake ± diuretics; if euvolemic/hypovolemic, increase sodium content in TPN; if hypovolemic, give additional isotonic fluid.
Hyperkalemia	>5 mEq/L	If TPN related and patient symptomatic, discontinue TPN and initiate D10W or D10NS at the same rate as the TPN. If patient is asymptomatic, decrease K^+ in TPN and other sources.
Hypokalemia	<3.5 mEq/L	Give KCl bolus either IV or enterally (4 mEq for each 0.1 <4.5 of K^+; maximum IV KCl concentration is 20 mEq/50 mL via central venous access and 10 mEq/50 mL via peripheral vein). Add K^+ in TPN.
Hypermagnesemia	>2.6 mEq/L	If TPN related and patient is symptomatic, discontinue TPN and start D10W or D10NS at the same rate as the TPN. If patient is asymptomatic, decrease Mg^{2+} in TPN.
Hypomagnesemia	<1.8 mEq/L	Give magnesium bolus either IV or enterally (1 g $MgSO_4$ = 8 mEq; 1 tablet magnesium oxide = 6 mEq). Maximum rate of IV infusion is 1 g in 7 min. (If level is <1, give 4–6 g IV or enteral equivalent; if level is >1 but <1.8, give 2–4 g IV or enteral equivalent). Increase Mg^{2+} in TPN.
Hypercalcemia	>10.2 mg/dL	If TPN related and patient is symptomatic, discontinue TPN and initiate D10W or D10NS at the same rate as the TPN. If patient is asymptomatic, decrease Ca^{2+} in TPN. Check ionized calcium in critically ill patients.
Hypocalcemia	<8.5 mg/dL	Correct for hypoalbuminemia [True Ca^{2+} = Ca^{2+} observed + 0.8 (4 – albumin observed)]. Increase Ca^{2+} in TPN if corrected Ca^{2+} is trending low. If hemodynamically unstable and/or critically ill, obtain an ionized calcium level (normal range 1.05–1.35 mg/dL). Give calcium chloride bolus via slow IV push if ionized calcium is low (<1.05) and patient is symptomatic (e.g., hypotensive). 1 g $CaCl_2$ = 13.6 mEq; 1 g calcium gluconate = 4.7 mEq.
Hyperphosphatemia	>4.8 mg/dL	If TPN related and patient is symptomatic, discontinue TPN and run D10W or D10NS at the same rate as the TPN. If patient is asymptomatic, decrease phosphate (PO_4^-) in TPN.
Hypophosphatemia	<2.4 mg/dL	Phosphorus replacement should be given over 6 h to avoid hypotension. If level is <1, give 30 mmol PO_4^- × 2 doses IV plus check phosphorus level 1 h after end of infusion; if level is ≥1 but <1.8, give 30 mmol PO_4^- × 1 dose or enteral equivalent and check phosphorus level 1 h after end of infusion; if level is ≥1.8 but <2.4, give 15 mmol PO_4^- or enteral equivalent. One packet of Neutra-Phos enterally = 8 mmol of PO_4^-. Increase phosphorus in TPN.
Metabolic acidosis	pH <7.4 HCO_3^- <23	Consider increasing acetate-to-chloride ratio.
Metabolic alkalosis	pH >7.4 HCO_3^- >29	Consider increasing chloride-to-acetate ratio.

TPN, total parenteral nutrition; D10W, dextrose 10%; D10NS, dextrose 10% with 0.9% sodium chloride.

continues to have absorption issues, then monomeric formulas could be substituted.

Enteral formulas also vary by caloric density. In patients with chronic renal failure who require fluid restrictions, choosing polymeric formulas with high caloric density (high caloric-to-fluid ratio) may be helpful. Enteral formulas also differ in the amount of protein, the carbohydrate-to-fat ratio, and the fiber content.

Each enteral feed formula has known amounts of kcal/mL, as well as g/L of protein. Once caloric and protein needs are assessed, the volume needed can be calculated. Unlike PN, in which the amounts of protein, dextrose, and fat can be easily modified, enteral feeding formulas are fixed. However, there are protein powders available if supplemental protein is necessary.

Before starting any enteral feeds, feeding tube placement must be confirmed by abdominal radiography and documented

TABLE 65.4

MONITORING PARAMETERS FOR CRITICALLY ILL ADULT PATIENTS ON PARENTERAL NUTRITION

Parameter	Frequency
Na^+, K^+, Cl^-, HCO_3^-, BUN, serum creatinine	Daily
Ca^{2+}, Mg^{2+}, phosphorus, liver function tests	Two to three times per week
Serum triglycerides	Weekly
CBC with differential	Weekly
Input/output	Daily
Prealbumin	Weekly
Indirect calorimetry	As needed. Highly recommended in the following patients: Difficult to estimate accurately caloric requirements, inadequate response to nutrition support, and clinical signs of over- or underfeeding
24-h urine urea nitrogen	As needed. Highly recommended in the following patients: Difficult to estimate accurately protein requirements, inadequate response to nutrition support, and clinical signs of over- or underfeeding
Weight	Daily
Serum glucose	As needed to keep blood sugar control of 80–110 mg/dL

BUN, blood urea nitrogen; CBC, complete blood count.
From Merritt R, ed. *The A.S.P.E.N. Nutrition Support Practice Manual.* 2nd ed. Silver Spring, MD: A.S.P.E.N; 2005.

in the orders. Once the enteral feeding formula has been selected, indicate initial strength (e.g., full or half-strength), initial rate in mL/hour, and desired progression regimen, followed by the goal rate. The rate can be started at 10 to 20 mL/hour and be advanced by 10- to 20-mL/hour every 8 hours as tolerated until goal (as long as residual is <200 mL via nasogastric tube or <100 mL via gastrostomy tube in 4 hours) (19). Many institutions have converted to a "closed system" to reduce the risk of microbial contaminations by minimizing the number of times the formula is manipulated. Enteral feedings start at full strength since a "closed system" will make it difficult to order partial-strength formulas.

When the patient is ready to transition over to a regular diet, similar strategies employed with the cyclic PN can be used. The patient may be converted to bolus feeding of the full-strength enteral formula with increases of 60 to 120 mL every 8 to 12 hours as tolerated up to goal volume. This simulates meals plus snacks (4). Bolus feedings are more physiologic, allowing the brain to stimulate sensations of hunger and satiety. When the patient is able to consume 60% of nutritional needs by mouth, the tube feeding can be discontinued (4).

"DESIGNER" ENTERAL FEEDINGS: FACTS AND MYTHS

Designer enteral feedings or specialized formulas contain modified protein and other ingredients to assist patients in stressed states. Sometimes the ratio of carbohydrate to fat, and the sources of fat, may also be altered to achieve desired effects.

Hepatic Formula

Specialized hepatic formulas (e.g., NutriHep) differ from the standard formulas in two ways: the actual protein content is usually lower (around 40–46 g/L) and the ratio of branched-chain amino acids (BCAAs) to aromatic and ammonia-forming amino acids (AAAs) is higher in the hepatic formula. The theory is that in patients with liver dysfunction, depletion of BCAAs might enhance the passage of AAAs across the blood–brain barrier, resulting in the synthesis of false neurotransmitters (20). By giving a higher BCAA formula, the altered ratio is returned to a more normal state.

Although there are conflicting data, there is evidence of the beneficial effects of "special hepatic formulas" to support their use in the treatment of malnourished patients with advanced cirrhosis. A relatively recent multicenter, randomized, nutrient-controlled trial from 2003 demonstrated improved survival, serum albumin concentration, and quality of life in patients with cirrhosis when given BCAAs (21). A meta-analysis from 2003 reviewed 11 randomized trials and concluded that BCAAs improved hepatic encephalopathy in patients with chronic encephalopathy (22). There is evidence that in patients with acute overt encephalopathy, restriction or withdrawal of proteins may be necessary. Once encephalopathy has been reversed, adequate protein may be administered to target a positive nitrogen balance. Based on the available studies, and cost consideration of up to 20 times more, the "hepatic formula" should be restricted to patients who present with grade II or higher encephalopathy, or whose grade of encephalopathy worsens with the advancement standard enteral formulation.

Renal Formula

Enteral formulas in this class (e.g., Nepro) tend to be more calorie dense and low in electrolytes and mineral contents (especially potassium and phosphorus). The purpose of these modifications is to provide adequate nutrients but at the same time minimize complications such as uremia, fluid overload, and electrolyte accumulation. The older renal formulas differ from standard amino acids in that they were designed for patients who could not tolerate dialysis or for whom dialysis was being avoided; thus, the formulas tend to be enriched with essential amino acids (EAAs). The rationale with this admixture is that the urea from EAAs would be recycled to produce nonessential amino acids.

Evidence supporting the use of the older renal formulas is scant and of poor quality. In addition, the cost of the older renal formulas is 10 to 15 times that of standard polymeric formulas. These formulas have now been replaced with standard polymeric proteins since most patients with acute renal failure are now being dialyzed or are receiving CRRT. The new renal formulas continue to be more calorie dense (usually 2 kcal/mL) with minimal electrolytes or additives (K^+, Mg^{2+}, PO_4^-) that could accumulate in renal failure. They are appropriate for patients whose serum electrolyte and mineral levels are difficult to control.

Pulmonary Formula

Respiratory quotient (RQ) is defined as the molecule of carbon dioxide produced per molecule of oxygen consumed (VCO_2/VO_2). Pulmonary formulas (e.g., PulmoCare) are designed to decrease carbon dioxide by providing the fuel substrate with the lower respiratory quotient (see Table 65.2). To achieve this, the manufacturer decreases the carbohydrate-to-fat ratio to achieve fat calories of about 38% to 55%. By decreasing the carbohydrates (RQ = 1)–to–fat (RQ = 0.7) ratio, the assumption is that the carbon dioxide production is reduced as well.

Studies looking at the benefit of high-fat enteral feeds have been criticized as having a small sample size. One trial looking at high-fat enteral formula in 12 patients with chronic airflow obstruction suggests that the higher-fat formulas may be less likely to impair work performance in patients with chronic airflow obstruction (23). Another trial looking at 20 artificially ventilated patients demonstrated that the high-fat group spent 62 hours less time on the ventilator and the result was clinically significant (24). More recent evidence suggests that reducing total calories is more important than the source of calories, in terms of reducing carbon dioxide production (since the RQ of lipogenesis or overfeeding is 1–1.2) (25).

The source of fat has also changed over the years. Many formulas marketed today list canola oil and medium-chain triglyceride (MCT) oil as the primary sources of fat, compared to fat formulas containing higher omega-6 fatty acids (precursor of arachidonic acid) that were used in the clinical trials. Whether the data from the earlier studies can be extrapolated to reflect the effect of the modern formulas on CO_2 remains to be answered.

Metabolic Stress (Critical Care) Formula

The critical care formulas (e.g., Perative) are somewhat similar to the hepatic formulas in that both have a high percentage of BCAAs, which are the preferred substrate of muscles during critical illness. Differences include higher protein content and fewer aromatic amino acids in the critical care formulas compared to the hepatic formulas. The clinical trials looking at these formulas are small, and have been equivocal from the standpoint of nutritional markers. Overall, BCAA-enriched enteral formulas are not the current standard of practice. Because this class of enteral formula, like the immunomodulating formulas, may contain immune-enhancing agents (i.e., arginine), they must be used cautiously in critically ill septic patients (see next section on immunonutrition timing).

Immunomodulating Formula

This class of enteral feedings is a subset of the metabolic stress formulas. Compared to the hepatic, renal, or pulmonary formulas, the formula designed to reduce inflammatory response (e.g., acute respiratory distress syndrome [ARDS]) is a more recent development. These so-called immunomodulating formulas are standard enteral formulas fortified with omega-3 fatty acids, nucleotides, arginine, and/or glutamine. The enteral feeding Oxepa contains no glutamine and arginine, but does contain 55% of calories as fat, of which the omega-6–to–omega-3 ratio is optimized to 2:1. Formula Impact has 25% of calories as fat, has arginine and glutamine, and contains 17.1% BCAAs in protein, and the omega-3–to–omega-6 ratio is 1.4:1. Formula Immun-Aid has 36% protein as BCAAs, contains arginine and glutamine, has 20% fat calories, and has an omega-6–to–omega-3 ratio of 2.1:1 (ratio similar to Oxepa). The theory behind this class of enteral feeds is that by minimizing omega-6 fatty acids and optimizing the ratio of omega-6 to omega-3 fatty acids, the inflammatory response is reduced, resulting in less lung injury.

Based on the early clinical trials and meta-analyses, which have mainly looked at Immun-Aid and Impact, it appears that surgical patients benefited most from this class of enteral formula. There was no effect on mortality in the meta-analyses, but there were significant reductions in infection rate, ventilator days, and hospital length of stay (26). More recent trials in this class of enteral feeds have focused on formula (i.e., Oxepa) enriched with eicosapentaenoic acid (EPA) from sardine oil and γ-linolenic acid (GLA) from borage oil plus antioxidants (vitamin E, vitamin C, β-carotene, taurine). One prospective, double-blind, placebo-controlled, randomized trial in 165 critically ill patients with severe sepsis found that this formula decreased mortality (19.4% absolute risk reduction), as well as decreased the number of days on the ventilator (27). Another prospective, randomized, controlled trial looking at enteral diet enriched with EPA + GLA in 100 patients with acute lung injury concluded that the formula reduced the length of time on the ventilator (28). Despite the many pieces of evidence pointing toward the benefit of immunomodulating formulas, it does have to be used with caution and at the right time. This will be discussed later in the chapter.

Glycemic Control Formula

The glycemic control enteral formulas are very similar to the pulmonary formulas in their design. The carbohydrate (35%–40%)–to–fat (40%–50%) ratio is reduced compared to standard formulas, with varying ratios of omega-6 to omega-3 fatty acids (e.g., Glucerna). This modification results in a greater proportion of fat calories than recommended (American Heart Association recommends $\leq$30% of calories from fat [29]). Various soluble fibers and/or soy polysaccharides are also added to the glycemic enteral formulas.

Clinical trials looking into the use of these specialty formulas in critically ill patients are limited. As with the pulmonary formulas, the high fat content in the glycemic formulas can decrease stomach emptying, which could decrease tolerance to these formulas even more in patients with diabetic gastroparesis. If glycemic control is needed, consider insulin drip. More studies are needed before these formulas can be recommended.

TIMING OF SPECIALIZED ENTERAL FEEDING (IMMUNONUTRITION) AND MANIPULATION OF IMMUNE AND INFLAMMATORY SYSTEM

Immunonutrition enteral feedings (e.g., Impact and Immun-Aid) are formulas containing nutrients that have been shown to influence immunologic and inflammatory responses in humans. These so-called immune-enhancing agents usually include the following: glutamine, arginine, omega-3 fatty acids, nucleotides, and antioxidants. Heyland et al. did an extensive meta-analysis to determine whether immunonutrition is safe and effective in critically ill patients (30). Although they were not able to find any mortality benefit, immunonutrition was associated with a statistically significant decrease in infectious complications and shorter length of hospital stay. When subgroup analyses of critically ill patients versus elective surgical patients were done, the results were surprising. There was a trend toward higher mortality in the critically ill patients, leading to the recommendation that immunonutrition not be used in critically ill patients until more clinical trials are conducted.

Bertolini et al. conducted a randomized multicenter trial comparing parenteral and early enteral nutrition containing immune-enhancing formula (Perative) in patients with and without severe sepsis (31,32). Results of an interim analysis indicated that mortality in severely septic patients receiving immune-enhancing enteral formulas was significantly higher than in those receiving parenteral nutrition (44.4% vs. 14.3%), and the study was aborted. Interestingly, in patients without sepsis, there was no 28-day mortality difference between the patients receiving parenteral nutrition versus immune-enhancing enteral formulas. However, those receiving immunonutrition had fewer episodes of septic shock, and the ICU length of stay was 4 days shorter.

Based on these studies, immunonutrition formulas should be used with caution in critically ill septic patients. Based on expert opinions, the immune-modulating nutrient likely to be responsible for the excess harm is arginine (see later), which has not been well studied in a randomized, clinical fashion in critically ill patients (33). In the critically ill nonseptic patients, immune-enhancing formulas appear to be beneficial if started within 48 hours.

IMMUNOMODULATORS

Glutamine

Normally nonessential, glutamine becomes conditionally essential during times of high stress as evidenced by a decrease in glutamine concentration in the body during this period (34). Glutamine comes in the free form (unstable in solution, so only found in dried form) and protein-bound form as seen in all protein sources used in enteral formulas. Glutamine is an important amino acid because of its involvement in many vital functions, such as (a) gluconeogenesis; (b) synthesis of glycogen, nucleotides, nucleic acid, and urea; (c) ammoniagenesis; and (d) ammonia reduction (34). Glutamine is also the preferred fuel substrate for rapidly dividing cells in both the small intestine mucosa and the immune system (34). Furthermore, glutamine plays a big part in the antioxidation process, since it is the precursor of glutathione, a strong antioxidant (35). In critically ill patients, about 30 g/day or 0.5 g/kg/day of glutamine is needed to meet both basal and increased enterocyte requirements (35).

A meta-analysis looking at 14 randomized trials concluded that glutamine supplementation in critically ill patients may be associated with a reduction in complication and mortality rates (35). In the same meta-analysis, glutamine supplementation in surgical patients may be associated with a reduction in infectious complication rates and shorter hospital stay without any adverse effect on mortality. Evidence from this meta-analysis also suggests that parenteral glutamine is more effective than enteral glutamine.

The effectiveness and benefits of glutamine supplementation are still not conclusive. A recent prospective but unblended study examining the benefit of enteral glutamine supplementation in 185 surgical ICU patients failed to detect a mortality difference between the control and treatment group (36).

Arginine

Like glutamine, many would consider arginine also to be a conditionally essential amino acid. About 5% to 6% of arginine comes from intake of proteins, and the rest is synthesized by the body via the urea cycle. Arginine is important in ammonia detoxification, as well as producing nitric oxide, which, among other things, mediates vasodilatory effects of endotoxin (37). Arginine supplementation has been purported to enhance wound healing in humans, mainly via improvements in *in vitro* markers of immune function (e.g., CD4 count), rather than outcome measures like infection rates (38).

Most human studies have largely been conducted using immune-enhancing diets containing relatively high amounts of L-arginine. The optimal dose of arginine in the critically ill patient is unknown, but a dose of up to 30 g/day is generally well tolerated by relatively healthy people (39).

Although evidence is not robust, arginine supplementation is capable of promoting an increase in nitric oxide production, which can lead to vascular smooth muscle dilation (36). Given this theoretical potential for harm, the clinician should use arginine-containing formulas with caution in critically ill septic patients (31,33,40).

Nucleotides

Nucleotides are structural units for nucleic acids and various enzymes involved in energy transfer. They are essential for the formation of new cells (e.g., intestinal epithelium) and in the synthesis of protein, lipids, and carbohydrates. Nucleotides are of interest because supplementation of infant formulas with nucleotides was noted to enhance bifidobacteria growth in the gastrointestinal tract. Bifidobacteria decrease the colonic lumen pH and inhibit growth of enteric bacteria (41).

Studies involving nucleotide use in humans are very limited, and like arginine, the studies available often involve immune-enhancing diets fortified with nucleotides, making it difficult to determine the effects of the nucleotides per se. One prospective, controlled trial studied the effects of nucleotide-supplemented formula in 26 severely malnourished children (younger than 4 years old). Insulin-like growth factor (IGF-1), growth factor binding protein-3 (IGFBP-3), leptin, soluble leptin receptor (sOB-R), and other hormonal biomarkers were measured. Enteral formulas enriched with nucleotides were shown to have a notable effect on IGF-1 and IGFBP-3, which could stimulate the catch-up growth of severely malnourished infants and toddlers (42).

Structured Lipids

Triglycerides are three fatty acid chains attached to a glycerol backbone. Structured lipids are triglycerides with combinations of long-, medium-, and short-chain fatty acids on a single glycerol backbone not found in nature. The intent of this chemical manipulation is to make a product that has improved absorption (compared to long-chain triglycerides), minimizes immune dysfunction, and can provide essential fatty acids (43). Structured lipids are not yet commercially available in intravenous forms, although it has been a component of immunomodulating enteral formulas.

Antioxidant Therapy

Antioxidants such as vitamin C, vitamin E, selenium, and β-carotene are often found in immunomodulating formulas. The role of antioxidant supplementation during critical illness is unclear. Studies have shown that critically ill patients often have low serum concentrations of some antioxidants, the significance of which is still not clear (44,45). However, there is good evidence now to suggest that reactive oxygen species (ROS) induce direct oxidative tissue injury by means of peroxidation of cellular membranes, oxidation of critical enzymatic and structural proteins, and induction of apoptosis (44,45). Thus, the importance of antioxidants seems obvious. Nathens et al. conducted a prospective, observational clinical trial looking at 595 critically ill surgical patients (91% trauma patients) who were administered with vitamin E 1,000 international units every 8 hours via nasogastric tube and vitamin C 1 g intravenously every 8 hours (46). This study found that early administration of vitamin E and vitamin C reduced the incidence of organ failure by 57% and shortened the ICU stay by 1 day. Another randomized study looking at 37 burned patients (>30% of body surface area) concluded that high-dose vitamin C (66 mg/kg/hour) for 24 hours reduced resuscitation fluid volume requirements, body weight gain, wound edema, and the severity of respiratory dysfunction (47).

References

1. Artinian V, Krayem H, DiGiovine B. Effects of early enteral feeding on the outcome of critically ill mechanically ventilated medical patients. *Chest.* 2006;129:960–967.
2. Heyland DK, Dhaliwal R, Drower JW, et al. Canadian clinical practice guidelines for nutrition support in mechanically ventilated, critically ill adult patients. *J Parenter Enteral Nutr.* 2003;27:355–373.
3. Mirtallo J, Canada T, Johnson D, et al. Safe practices for parenteral nutrition. *J Parenter Enteral Nutr.* 2004;28:S39–S70.
4. Merritt R, ed. *The A.S.P.E.N. Nutrition Support Practice Manual.* 2nd ed. Silver Spring, MD: A.S.P.E.N; 2005.
5. Michell KA, Jones EA, Meguid MM, et al. Standardized TPN order form reduces staff time and potential for error. *Nutrition.* 1990;6:457–460.
6. Cerra FB, Benitez, MR, Blackburn GL. Applied Nutrition in ICU Patients: a consensus statement of the American College of Chest Physicians. *Chest.* 1997;111:769–778.
7. Isaacs JW, Millikan WJ, Stackjouse J, et al. Parenteral nutrition of adults with 900-milliosmolar solution via peripheral vein. *Am J Clin Nutr.* 1977;30:552–559.
8. Ballesteros MA, Hogan DL, Koss MA, et al. Bolus or intravenous infusion of ranitidine: effects on gastric pH and acid secretion. A comparison of efficacy and cost. *Ann Intern Med.* 1990;112:334–339.
9. Gil KM, Skeie B, Kvetan V, et al. Parenteral nutrition and oral intake: effect of glucose and fat infusions. *J Parenter Enteral Nutr.* 1991;15:426–432.
10. Hwang TL, Lue MC, Chen LL. Early use of cyclic TPN prevents further deterioration of liver functions for the TPN patients with impaired liver function. *Hepatograstroenterology.* 2000;47(35):1347–1350.
11. Longhurt C, Naumovski L, Garcia-Careaga M, et al. A practical guideline for calculating parenteral nutrition cycles. *Nutr Clin Pract.* 2003;18:517–520.
12. Monson P, Mehta RL. Nutritional considerations in continuous renal replacement therapies. *Semin Dial.* 1996;9:152–160.
13. Palevsky PM. Continuous renal replacement therapy component selection: replacement fluid and dialysis. *Semin Dial.* 1996;9:107–111.
14. Bellomo R, Martin H, Parkin G, et al. Continuous arteriovenous hemodiafiltration in the critically ill: influence on major nutrient balances. *J Intensive Care Med.* 1991;17:399–402.
15. Brooks MJ, Melnik G. The refeeding syndrome: an approach to understanding its complications and preventing its occurrence. *Pharmacotherapy.* 1995;15:713–726.
16. Weinsier RL, Krumdieck CL. Death resulting from overzealous total parenteral nutrition: the refeeding syndrome revisited. *Am J Clin Nutr.* 1981; 393–399.
17. Kraft MD, Btaiche IF, Sacks GS. Review of the refeeding syndrome. *Nutr Clin Pract.* 2005;20:625–633.
18. Flesher ME, Archer KA, Leslie BD, et al. Assessing the metabolic and clinical consequences of early enteral feeding in the malnourished patient. *J Parenter Enteral Nutr.* 2005;29:108–117.
19. McClave SA, Snider HI, Lowen CC, et al. Use of residual volume as a marker for enteral feeding tolerance: prospective blinded comparison with physical examination and radiographic findings. *J Parenter Enteral Nutr.* 1992;16:99–105.
20. Munoz SJ. Nutritional therapies in liver disease. *Semin Liver Dis.* 1991; 11:279–291.
21. Marchesini G, Bianchi G, Merli M, et al. Nutritional supplementation with branched-chain amino acids in advanced cirrhosis: a double-blind, randomized trial. *Gastroenterology.* 2003;124:1792–1801.
22. Als-Nielsen B, Koretz RL, Kjaegard LL, et al. Branched-chain amino acids for hepatic encephalopathy. *Cochrane Database Syst Rev.* 2003;2:CD001939.
23. Franfort JD, Fischer CE, Stansbury DW, et al. Effects of high- and low-carbohydrate meals on maximum exercise performance in chronic airflow obstruction. *Chest.* 1991;792:795.
24. Al-Saady NM, Blackmore CM, Bennett ED. High fat, low carbohydrate, enteral feeding lowers $PaCO_2$ and reduces the period of ventilation in artificially ventilated patients. *Intensive Care Med.* 1989;15:290–295.
25. Talpers SS, Romberger DJ, Bunce SR, et al. Nutritionally associated increased carbon dioxide production. Excess of total calories vs. high proportion of carbohydrate calories. *Chest.* 1992;15:551–555.
26. Beale RJ, Bryg DJ, Bihari DJ. Immunonutrition in the critically ill: a systematic review of clinical outcome. *Crit Care Med.* 1999;27:2799–2805.
27. Pontes-Arruda A, Albuquerque-Aragao AM, Albuquerque JD. Effects of enteral feeding with eicosapentaenoic acid, gamma-linolenic acid, and antioxidants in mechanically ventilated patients with severe sepsis and septic shock. *Crit Care Med.* 2006;34:2325–2333.
28. Singer P, Theilla M, Fisher H. Benefit of an enteral diet enriched with eicosapentaenoic acid and gamma-linolenic acid in ventilated patients with acute lung injury. *Crit Care Med.* 2006;34:1033–1038.
29. Krauss RM, Eckel RH, Howard B, et al. AHA dietary guidelines. Revision 2000: a statement for healthcare professionals from the nutrition committee of the American Heart Association. *Circulation.* 2000;102:2284–2299.
30. Heyland DK, Novak F, Drover JW, et al. Should immunonutrition become

routine in critically ill patients?: a systematic review of the evidence. *JAMA.* 2001;286:944–953.
31. Bertolini G, Iapichino G, Radrizzani D, et al. Early enteral immunonutrition in patients with severe sepsis. *Intensive Care Med.* 2003;29:834–840.
32. Radrizzani D, Bertolini G, Facchini R, et al. Early enteral immunonutrition vs. parenteral nutrition in critically ill patients without severe sepsis: a randomized clinical trial. *Intensive Care Med.* 2006;32:1191–1198.
33. Heyland DK, Samis A. Does immunonutrition in patients with sepsis do more harm than good? [Editorial]. *Intensive Care Med.* 2006;32:669–671.
34. Wilmore DW, Shabert JK. Role of glutamine in immunologic responses. *Nutrition.* 1998;618–626.
35. Novak F, Heyland DK, Avenell A. Glutamine supplementation in serious illness: a systematic review of the evidence. *Crit Care Med.* 2002;30:2022–2029.
36. Schulman AS, Willcutts KF, Claridge JA. Does the addition of glutamine to enteral feeds affect patient mortality? *Crit Care Med.* 2005;33:2501–2506.
37. Bruins MJ, Soeters PB, Lamers WH. L-Arginine supplementation in hyperdynamic endotoxemic pigs: Effect on nitric oxide synthesis by the different organs. *Crit Care Med.* 2002;30:508–517.
38. Tong BC, Barbul A. Cellular and physiologic effects of arginine. *Mini Rev Med Chem.* 2004;4:823–832.
39. Braverman MD. *The Healing Nutrients Within.* New Canaan, CT: Keats Publishing, Inc.; 1997.
40. Stechmiller JK, Childress B, Porter T. Arginine immunonutrition in critically ill patients: a clinical dilemma. *Am J Crit Care.* 2004;12:17–23.
41. Uauy R. Nonimmune system responses to dietary nucleotides. *J Nutr.* 1994;124:1575–1595.
42. Vasquez-Garibay E, Kratzch J, Romero-Velarde E, et al. Effect of nucleotide intake and nutritional recovery on insulin-like growth factor 1 and other hormonal biomarkers in severely malnourished children. *Br J Nutr.* 2006;96:683–690.
43. Osborn HT, Akoh CC. Structured lipids- novel fats with medical, nutraceutical, and food applications. *Compr Rev Food Sci Food Saf.* 2002;1:93–103.
44. Goode HF, Cowley HC, Walker BE, et al. Decreased antioxidant status and increased lipid peroxidation in patients with septic shock and secondary organ dysfunction. *Crit Care Med.* 1995;23:646–651.
45. Metnitz PG, Bartens C, Fischer M, et al. Antioxidant status in patients with acute respiratory distress syndrome. *Intensive Care Med.* 1999;25:180–185.
46. Nathens AB, Neff MJ, Jurkovich GJ, et al. Randomized, prospective trial of antioxidant supplementation in critically ill surgical patients. *Ann Surg.* 2002;236:814–822.
47. Tanaka H, Matsuda T, Miyagantani Y. Reduction of resuscitation fluid volumes in severely burned patients using ascorbic acid administration: a randomized, prospective study. *Arch Surg.* 2000;135:326–331.

CHAPTER 66 ■ TOXICOLOGY

ANDREW STOLBACH • LEWIS R. GOLDFRANK

HISTORY

Poisonings are recognized in the earliest recorded history. The word *toxicology* is derived from the Greek terms *toxikos* ("bow") and *toxikon* ("poison into which arrowheads are dipped") (1, 2). In the 16th century, scientist Paracelsus made the astute observation that still holds strong: "What is there that is not poison? All things are poison and nothing [is] without poison. Solely, the dose determines that a thing is not a poison" (3). Today, we share Paracelsus' appreciation of the dose-response relationship. One need not look farther than basic elements such as oxygen or water to see that all substances can act as a poison at a specified dose. In modern medicine, the unique challenges posed by poisoned patients were recognized with the opening of the first poison control center in Chicago in 1953 (4); today, all 50 states are served by poison control centers. Medical toxicology, the care of poisoned patients, was recognized as a subspecialty by the American Board of Medical Subspecialties in 1992.

The American Association of Poison Control Centers (AAPCC) maintains the National Poisoning and Exposure Database (NPED), consisting of data from every case reported to poison centers in the United States. This database suffers from many obvious limitations. Many exposures go unreported. One investigator found that only 12% of poisoning deaths identified by the medical examiner were reported to poison centers (5). Those that are reported are usually unconfirmed. Nevertheless, the database is a useful source of epidemiologic information, giving us an estimation of the incidence of various exposures. The NPED categorizes exposures based on outcome, designating effects as minor, moderate, or major. *Major effects* are those where the patient exhibits signs or symptoms as a result of exposure that is life threatening or results in significant disability or disfigurement; this category constitutes a large portion of intensive care unit (ICU) toxicology cases. In 2005, the AAPCC received nearly 2.5 million reports of exposures, including 16,545 major effects and 1,261 deaths (6). Thus, while fatalities are 0.005% of total exposures, a rough estimate of the incidence of poisoning in the United States represents 7% of the sum of major exposures and fatalities.

Throughout this chapter, any substance introduced to the body will be referred to as a *xenobiotic*. The terms *drug* and *pharmaceutical* identify the subgroup of xenobiotics that are commercially produced, while a *toxin* is a xenobiotic produced by a biologic system, such as plant, animal, or fungi. An *exposure* occurs whenever a human comes into contact with a xenobiotic. Exposures may be dermal, oral, ophthalmic, or inhalational. *Poisoning*, *intoxication*, and *toxicity* characterize the harmful consequences of a xenobiotic exposure. Consistent use of these definitions should enhance the clarity of our discussion.

DIAGNOSIS AND GENERAL APPROACH TO THE POISONED PATIENT

By the time the patient has reached a critical care unit, initial stabilization should already have occurred. Nevertheless, the initial approach to the poisoned patient deserves mention because the clinician should respond to any deterioration in the patient's condition by going back to the basic principles of diagnostic and therapeutic approaches. A key principle in managing poisoned patients is summarized by the phrase "treat the patient, not the poison." The management of the poisoned patients begins with addressing airway compromise, breathing difficulty, and circulatory problems. Vital signs should be obtained, and cardiac and respiratory monitoring should be applied and given supplemental oxygen. Significant vital sign abnormalities or oxygen desaturation should be addressed immediately.

Bedside serum glucose concentration should be rapidly obtained in any patient with altered sensorium or an abnormal neurologic examination. In fact, hypoglycemia may present with almost any altered mental status including agitation, delirium, coma, seizure, or focal neurologic deficit. This condition, while common and easy to correct, can be life threatening if diagnosis is delayed or missed (see section on antidiabetics).

A thorough physical examination will identify the presence of a toxic syndrome, or "toxidrome." The classic toxic syndromes (Table 66.1) can be differentiated based on vital signs, mental status, pupil size, and presence (or absence) of peristalsis, diaphoresis, and urinary retention. The physician should keep in mind that these toxic syndromes are archetypes. Because of coexisting assumption of other poisons or coexisting disease processes, patients do not always demonstrate the typical symptoms of a particular syndrome. For example, the practice of "speedballing" (concurrent heroin and cocaine abuse) might result in small, normal, or large pupils. Though identification of a toxic syndrome will not specifically identify the exact poison responsible, it will somewhat guide therapy. For instance, the presence of a sedative-hypnotic toxic syndrome (overdose) warrants support of the airway, whether the condition is a result of ethanol or diazepam abuse.

Electrocardiogram (ECG) should be obtained in most cases of suspected poisoning. In fact, several well-defined exposures (such as tricyclic antidepressants) will be identified based on a characteristic ECG. Xenobiotics such as cocaine or lidocaine can produce life-threatening dysrhythmias via direct myocardial effect. Xenobiotics can also produce dysrhythmias by causing an electrolyte abnormality. Exposure to hydrofluoric acid, even dermally, can result in hypocalcemia, resulting in QTc prolongation and torsades de pointes.

While most poisoned patients can be managed appropriately by physical examination and judicious use of laboratory studies alone, history should attempt to identify the specific xenobiotic exposure, the amount, the time and reason for exposure, and general medical history. At times, a specific antidote may be warranted based on the history (see Appendix).

A thoughtful use of laboratory studies is important in the management of poisoned patients. Electrolyte abnormalities complicate many severe poisonings. Therefore, serum chemistries are warranted for all critically ill patients. Blood gases and aminotransferases should be judiciously used as well.

In contrast with the fundamental information provided in blood samples, a routine urine toxicologic screen rarely aids in management and is therefore not recommended. A urine toxicologic screen generally focuses on select drugs of abuse and omits the vast majority of potential toxins. Moreover, the assays included in the commonly used qualitative urine screen have either too many false positives or false negatives. For example, fentanyl, a synthetic opioid, will not produce a positive result on an opiate screen, while dextromethorphan may yield a positive result for phencyclidine. Even a true positive result on a toxicologic screen is not necessarily helpful. The cocaine assay, while remarkably specific, will remain positive for days after the clinical effects have subsided.

TABLE 66.1

TOXIDROMES

Group	BP	P	R	T	Mental status	Pupil size	Peristalsis	Diaphoresis	Primary treatment
Anticholinergic	–/↑	↑	+/–	↑	Delirium	↑	↓	↓	Benzodiazepines
Cholinergic	+/–	+/–	–/↑	–	Normal/depressed	+/–	↑	↑	Atropine, oximes
Ethanol, sedative-hypnotic	↓	↓	↓	–/↓	Depressed	+/–	↓	–	Airway support
Opioid	↓	↓	↓	↓	Depressed	↓	↓	–	Naloxone
Sympathomimetic	↑	↑	↑	↑	Agitated	↑	–/↑	↑	Benzodiazepines
Withdrawal from ethanol or sedative-hypnotic	↑	↑	↑	↑	Agitated, disoriented	↑	↑	↑	Benzodiazepines
Withdrawal from opioids	↑	↑	–	–	Normal, anxious	↑	↑	↑	Opioids

BP, blood pressure; P, pulse; R, respirations; T, temperature.
Adapted with permission from Flomenbaum NE, Goldfrank LR, Hoffman RS, et al. Initial evaluations of the patient: vital signs and toxic syndromes. In: Flomenbaum NE, Goldfrank LR, Hoffman RS, et al., eds. *Goldfrank's Toxicologic Emergencies.* 8th ed. New York: McGraw-Hill; 2006:37–41.

In contrast to "shotgun" urine toxicologic screening, the acetaminophen concentration should be obtained following all overdoses where self-harm was intended. In one series, 1 in 365 individuals with suicidal ingestion and a history negative for acetaminophen ingestion had a potentially hepatotoxic acetaminophen concentration (7).

DETERMINING THE NEED FOR INTENSIVE CARE UNIT ADMISSION

Criteria that are traditionally used to determine whether patients need critical care do not necessarily apply to poisoned patients. For most patients, disposition is determined by how "sick" the patient is. In contrast, patients poisoned by dangerous xenobiotics but who appear well may require precautionary ICU admission and monitoring.

The factors that influence the need for critical care can be divided into three general categories: (a) patient characteristics, (b) xenobiotic characteristics, and (c) hospital unit capabilities (8).

All unstable poisoned patients require ICU care. Patients with significant laboratory abnormalities, unresponsiveness, inability to protect the airway, hypotension, dysrhythmias, or conduction abnormalities should be admitted to the ICU. Preexisting medical conditions such as severe liver or renal insufficiency, congestive heart failure, or pregnancy may also influence disposition.

The disposition for minimally symptomatic patients is often determined by the xenobiotic involved rather than the clinical status of the patient. The most important considerations are the potential for deterioration or the requirement for a therapeutic agent with potentially adverse effects. Sustained-release products, potentially lethal doses, or xenobiotics that may cause dysrhythmias have the potential to cause rapid clinical deterioration. For this reason, asymptomatic patients with exposure to calcium channel blockers or sulfonylureas are often admitted to an ICU for observation. Similarly, when xenobiotics require a therapy that has the potential for adverse effects, such as high-dose atropine for organic phosphorus insecticides, ICU admission is appropriate.

Finally, the capabilities of the hospital as a whole influence the disposition of the patient. Time-consuming nursing activities, such as hourly bedside glucose checks or the administration of drug infusions, that may not be possible on general inpatient units are indications for ICU admission. When the admitting team or nursing staff is not familiar with the complications associated with a particular xenobiotic exposure, ICU admission may also be indicated.

NONOPIOID ANALGESICS: ACETAMINOPHEN, NONSTEROIDAL ANTI-INFLAMMATORY DRUGS, AND SALICYLATES

In 2005, the American Association of Poison Centers NPED received 227,496 reports of exposures to analgesics (6).

The extensive availability of these drugs contributes to their prevalence in both suicidal ingestions and unintentional pediatric ingestions. Although they are generally safe when used correctly, the widely held misconception that these pharmaceuticals are harmless undoubtedly contribute to their potential for causing harm.

Acetaminophen

Over 100,000 reports of acetaminophen exposure were received by the NPED in 2005 (6). The vast majority of exposures do not result in significant morbidity, and only 333 were fatal and another 3,310 considered major. Although the data set is controversial, acetaminophen is estimated to be responsible for 51% of all cases of acute liver failure in the United States (9). Acetaminophen ingestions require ICU admission when hepatotoxicity is established.

Acetaminophen is an analgesic and antipyretic with less anti-inflammatory activity than the nonsteroidal anti-inflammatory drugs. The analgesic effects of acetaminophen are mediated by central cyclo-oxygenase (COX)-2 and prostaglandin synthase (10) inhibition. Less than 5% of acetaminophen is eliminated unchanged in the urine. The metabolism of acetaminophen occurs principally in the liver. Ninety percent of absorbed acetaminophen undergoes hepatic conjugation with either glucuronide or sulfate to produce inactive metabolites. The remainder (5%–15%) is oxidized by the cytochrome P450, forming *N*-acetyl-p-benzoquinoneimine (NAPQI), a toxic oxidant (11). Thiol-containing compounds, such as reduced glutathione, are used as electron donors to detoxify NAPQI.

The single dose of acetaminophen generally thought to be required to produce toxicity is ≥150 mg/kg (11). In overdose, absorption of acetaminophen may be delayed, although peak absorption generally occurs at 2 hours, and rarely after 4 hours (12,13). Absorption may be expected to be further delayed in the presence of peristalsis-decreasing opioid or anticholinergic coingestants, or if the acetaminophen is formulated for extended release. In overdose, metabolism by sulfation becomes saturated, and the formation of NAPQI exceeds that which can be detoxified by available glutathione (14). Because the toxic metabolite is formed in the liver, hepatic toxicity is the key clinical feature. *N*-acetylcysteine (NAC), the key to management of acetaminophen poisoning, acts as a precursor to glutathione synthesis, a substrate for sulfation; it directly binds to NAPQI itself; and enhances the reduction of NAPQI to acetaminophen (15).

Clinical Manifestations

Acute acetaminophen toxicity has been divided into four clinical stages (16). Not every untreated patient will advance through each of these stages. Spontaneous improvement is possible at any point, but the stages of toxicity serve as a useful guide to the progression of symptoms. During *stage I,* the patient is either asymptomatic or has nonspecific clinical findings (nausea, vomiting, malaise), and no laboratory abnormalities are recognized. *Stage II* begins with the onset of liver injury, generally within 24 hours but always within 36 hours of ingestion (17). Symptoms are similar to other causes of hepatitis.

Initial laboratory findings include elevated aminotransferases (aspartate aminotransferase [AST]/alanine aminotransferase [ALT]), but progress to signs of hepatic dysfunction, including prolonged prothrombin time (PT), metabolic acidosis, and hypoglycemia. *Stage III* represents the time of peak hepatotoxicity, usually 72 to 96 hours from ingestion. While AST and ALT may ultimately exceed 10,000 IU/L, creatinine, lactate, phosphate, and PT are better indicators of prognosis. Fatalities usually occur within 3 to 5 days of ingestion. When death does not occur, hepatic recovery is referred to as *stage IV*. Hepatic regeneration will be histologically and functionally complete in survivors.

Management

N-acetylcysteine is the key to managing acetaminophen poisoning. Because of its proven efficacy, decontamination with activated charcoal should only be considered if significant coingestants are expected. NAC is available for both oral and intravenous administration. The oral protocol for acute ingestions is a 140 mg/kg loading dose, followed by 17 doses of 70 mg/kg every 4 hours for a total of 72 hours. The intravenous regimen is 150 mg/kg over 45 minutes, followed by 50 mg/kg over 4 hours, and then 100 mg/kg over 16 hours. Both regimens have equal efficacy for simple acute ingestion, but the intravenous regimen has the advantage of a shorter course, and is the only route that has been studied adequately in patients with hepatic failure. Unlike oral NAC, parenteral NAC carries the risk of anaphylactoid reactions. The duration and route of treatment are determined by the type of presentation.

The simple, acute ingestion occurs when a single dose of acetaminophen is ingested over a short period of time, within 24 hours of presentation. There is little controversy in managing this type of ingestion. The serum acetaminophen concentration should be plotted against the number of hours following ingestion on the Rumack-Matthew nomogram to determine whether treatment with NAC is necessary (18). The treatment line is a sensitive, but not specific, predictor of hepatotoxicity. The currently recommended line intersects 150 μg/mL at 4 hours, incorporating a 25% safety margin over the original nomogram line, which was itself nearly 100% sensitive for predicting hepatotoxicity. When the concentration at a specific time is plotted above the line, treatment is required. When treatment is initiated within 8 hours of ingestion, NAC has complete efficacy in preventing hepatotoxicity (19). NAC should be started immediately in any patient with suspected acetaminophen poisoning when the laboratory result for the acetaminophen concentration is not expected to be available within 8 hours of the initial ingestion. Once the serum acetaminophen concentration is available, the decision whether to continue the NAC can be made based on the nomogram (Fig. 66.1). When there is uncertainty with regard to the exact time of ingestion, the physician should use the most conservative estimate (i.e., the earliest possible time) when using the nomogram. The risk of inadvertently failing to treat because of an incorrect history is mitigated by the safety margin associated with the nomogram.

The literature is less clear on the indications for the use of NAC for hepatotoxicity following suspected chronic acetaminophen use. The vast majority of people who take acetaminophen have no adverse clinical manifestations. Clinical trials involving daily dosing of 4 g of acetaminophen in both alcoholics and nonalcoholics showed that patients either have normal aminotransferase concentrations or very minor increases (20,21). Despite its safety, hepatoxicity from chronic use occurs. Because chronic acetaminophen use often occurs in the setting of comorbid conditions, the diagnosis can be difficult to establish with certainty. NAC should be administered to all patients with suspected acetaminophen hepatotoxicity until the diagnosis has been excluded.

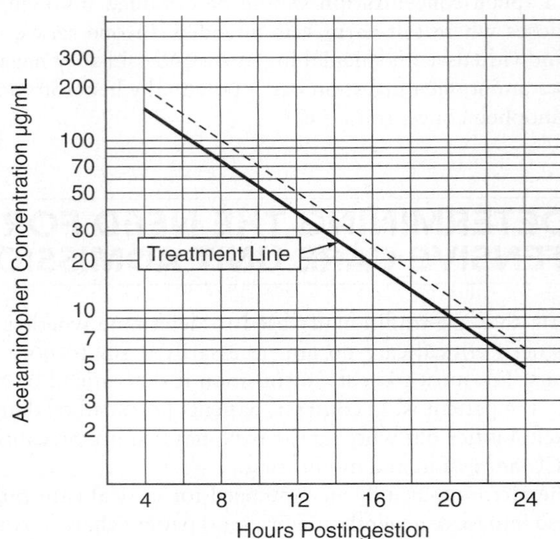

FIGURE 66.1. Acetaminophen nomogram. (Adapted with permission from Hendrickson RG, Bizovi KE. Acetaminophen. In: Flomenbaum NE, Goldfrank LR, Hoffman RS, et al., eds. *Goldfrank's Toxicologic Emergencies*. 8th ed. New York: McGraw-Hill; 2006:523–543.)

The nomogram cannot be used for patients who present more than 24 hours after ingestion. In such cases, NAC should be started immediately upon presentation. If the patient has both an undetectable acetaminophen concentration and normal aminotransferases, acetaminophen overdose is highly unlikely, and NAC need not be continued. If either acetaminophen or aminotransferase concentrations are elevated (even minimally so), the patient should be administered 20 hours of IV NAC. Following the treatment period, aminotransferase and acetaminophen concentrations should be obtained again. At this point, if the aminotransferase concentrations are only minimally elevated, the patient was either minimally poisoned or acetaminophen was not the cause of the liver damage.

When acetaminophen-induced hepatoxicity is encountered, intravenous NAC should be administered as described above, but the maintenance dose should be continued until clinical improvement, liver transplantation, or death occur. Even in the presence of fulminant hepatic failure, IV NAC has been shown to decrease mortality, cerebral edema, and the need for vasopressors (22).

Hepatic Transplantation

Generally, patients with significant acetaminophen poisoning will have AST and ALT concentrations >1,000 IU/L by 24 to 48 hours after ingestion. The decision to perform hepatic transplantation is particularly difficult in these patients, because those who survive without a transplant will make a complete recovery, while the long-term complications of a transplant are significant. Under ideal conditions, the clinician could immediately determine which patients would survive without transplant and which would not, so that the appropriate patients could be listed for a liver transplant and the procedure could be performed before irreversible clinical deterioration. In practice, it is not always clear. Several prognostic criteria are available. The King's College Hospital Criteria suggest that pH <7.3 after resuscitation or the combination of PT >100, creatinine >3.3 mg/dL, and grade III or IV encephalopathy are predictive of death in the absence of a transplant (23). Serum phosphate has also been shown to be a good predictor. A 48-hour serum phosphate concentration >1.2 mmol/L has been shown to be sensitive and specific for predicting the need for transplant and the probability of death from acetaminophen hepatotoxicity (24). Presumably, a low or normal phosphate concentration is evidence that the phosphate is being utilized by hepatocytes for adenosine triphosphate (ATP) generation.

SALICYLATES AND OTHER NONSTEROIDAL ANTI-INFLAMMATORY DRUGS

The nonsteroidal anti-inflammatory drugs (NSAIDs) are widely available both with and without prescription for relief of inflammation, pain, and fever. Salicylates are a subgroup of NSAIDs that have unique features of toxicity and require distinct management. In this chapter, we will use the term *NSAID* in reference to the *nonsalicylate* NSAIDs. ICU admission is required when patients present with metabolic acidosis and hemodynamic instability, or if they require bicarbonate infusion or frequent measurements of salicylate concentration.

The therapeutic effects of salicylates and NSAIDs result from the inhibition of cyclo-oxygenase (COX), a mediator of prostaglandin synthesis. The myriad medications in this class preclude discussion of the individual pharmacokinetic characteristics. In general, they are renally eliminated. Because they are designed to promote fast relief, therapeutic doses of the immediate-release drugs produce significant concentrations within an hour. However, when taken in overdose or as enteric-coated or sustained-release formulations, absorption may be greatly delayed, and maximal serum concentrations may not be observed for hours after the ingestion.

In addition to these effects, salicylates also uncouple oxidative phosphorylation, meaning that some of the proton gradient across the mitochondrial matrix is dissipated in the formation of heat, rather than ATP, forcing the production of lactate.

Clinical Manifestations of Salicylate Poisoning

Acute salicylate poisoning may cause epigastric pain, nausea, and vomiting. Salicylates induce hyperventilation (both tachypnea and hyperpnea) by direct stimulation of the brainstem respiratory center (25). Neurologic signs and symptoms of salicylate poisoning range from mild to severe, and include tinnitus, delirium, coma, and seizure. The initial feature of toxicity is primary respiratory alkalosis. A primary metabolic acidosis is characterized by the presence of lactic acid, ketoacids, and salicylic acids (26). The net result is an increased anion gap metabolic acidosis. The simultaneous presence of a respiratory alkalosis and metabolic acidosis can be difficult to interpret. Because the respiratory alkalosis initially predominates in adults, the presence of an acidemia or even normal pH indicates advanced poisoning.

Chronic salicylate poisoning presents with the same signs and symptoms as acute poisoning, but typically occurs in elderly patients taking supratherapeutic amounts of salicylate to treat a chronic condition. Chronic poisoning can be a challenging diagnosis to establish because it is often not suspected. Elderly salicylate-poisoned patients presenting with metabolic acidosis and an altered sensorium may be initially misdiagnosed with sepsis, dehydration, or cerebrovascular accident (CVA) if a salicylate concentration is not obtained.

Serum salicylate concentrations only correlate loosely with toxicity because the principal site of poisoning is the central nervous system. The threshold for toxicity is usually considered to be 30 mg/dL when tinnitus develops. Chronically poisoned patients have a lower salicylate concentration for the same degree of illness because much of their total body burden has redistributed into the central nervous system. The degree of poisoning is determined by evaluating the serum concentration in the context of the patient's clinical appearance, laboratory results, and acuity of the ingestion.

Management of Salicylate Poisoning

The key principles for management of salicylate poisoning are to minimize absorption, speed elimination, and minimize redistribution to tissues. Gastric emptying should only be attempted if a significant amount of drug is expected to be present in the stomach. Activated charcoal, 1 g/kg, should be administered every 4 hours if it can be given safely. Salicylates cause pylorospasm and may form concretions in overdose, leading to delayed absorption. Multiple-dose activated charcoal (MDAC) not only prevents delayed absorption, but also may speed elimination of salicylates by disrupting the enteroenteric circulation of the drug (27). Serum chemistry, venous or arterial blood gas, and salicylate concentration should be obtained every 2 hours until the salicylate concentration demonstrates an interval decrease.

Moderately poisoned patients (increased anion gap or a salicylate concentration greater than 40 mg/dL) should also have blood and urine alkalinized with sodium bicarbonate. As a weak acid (pKa 3.5), salicylates will be ionized in an alkaline environment and "trapped" (i.e., unable to passively move through lipid membranes). Ionization prevents salicylate in the proximal tubule from diffusing into the plasma and salicylate in the plasma from diffusing into tissues, such as the brain (28). Alkalinization can be achieved with an infusion of sodium bicarbonate of 150 mEq in 1 L of D5W at twice the maintenance rate. The urine pH should be maintained from 7.5 to 8.0 and systemic arterial pH between 7.45 and 7.55. Close attention should be paid to potassium repletion, as low serum potassium will cause preferential reabsorption of potassium over hydrogen ions in the proximal tubule and compromise attempts to alkalinize the urine (29). Endotracheal intubation and sedation should be avoided whenever possible. The tachypnea and

TABLE 66.2

INDICATIONS FOR HEMODIALYSIS IN SALICYLATE POISONING

Renal failure
Congestive heart failure (relative)
Acute lung injury
Persistent CNS disturbances
Progressive deterioration in vital signs
Severe acid-base or electrolyte imbalance, despite appropriate treatment
Hepatic compromise with coagulopathy
Salicylate concentration (acute) >100 mg/dL or (chronic) >60 mg/dL

CNS, central nervous system.
Adapted with permission from Flomenbaum NE. Salicylates. In: Flomenbaum NE, Goldfrank LR, Hoffman RS, et al., eds. *Goldfrank's Toxicologic Emergencies*. 8th ed. New York: McGraw-Hill; 2006:550–564.

hyperpnea of salicylate poisoning does not necessarily represent "tiring," and produces a helpful alkalosis. When intubation is unavoidable, patients should be administered 1 to 2 mEq/kg of bicarbonate prior to the procedure, intubated quickly, and hyperventilated afterward to avoid respiratory acidosis.

Early consultation with a nephrologist is recommended for seriously ill patients. Extracorporeal elimination is reserved for patients who are very ill, those who cannot tolerate alkalinization, or those with serum concentrations so elevated that their clinical status is expected to deteriorate. We recommend hemodialysis for severe acid-base disturbances, mental status changes, inability to tolerate alkalinization (renal failure or congestive heart failure), and serum concentrations of 100 mg/dL after acute poisoning and 60 mg/dL in chronic poisoning (Table 66.2).

Clinical Manifestations of Nonsteroidal Anti-inflammatory Drug Poisoning

NSAIDs are considered safer than salicylates in therapeutic dosing. An acute overdose of NSAIDs can cause gastric injury. While chronic NSAID use is associated with interstitial nephritis, nephritic syndrome, or analgesic nephropathy, acute overdose is sometimes accompanied by a reversible azotemia caused by vasoconstriction from decreased prostaglandin production (30). In severe overdose, the most consequential effects are elevated anion gap metabolic acidosis, coma, and hypotension (31).

Management of Nonsteroidal Anti-inflammatory Drug Poisoning

Activated charcoal should be administered if the patient presents within several hours of overdose. Good supportive care is the mainstay of therapy after NSAID overdose. NSAID elimination is not increased with alkalinization, and NSAIDs' high degree of protein binding precludes removal with hemodialysis. Hemodialysis has been used to correct acidemia and electrolyte abnormalities in patients with multiorgan system failure.

PSYCHIATRIC MEDICATIONS

Psychiatric medications represent a disproportionate number of poisonings in the United States. Antidepressants, antipsychotics, and sedative-hypnotics accounted for more than half of all deaths reported to poison control centers in 2005 (6). This high mortality figure is a function of the prevalence of these ingestions, as these drugs do not have a high case-fatality rate. With sound supportive care, most patients can be managed successfully.

Antipsychotic Medications

The antipsychotics are categorized as either typical or atypical. The typical antipsychotics, which include haloperidol, chlorpromazine, and thioridazine, antagonize dopamine primarily at the D_2 receptor. The newer medications, the atypical drugs, are exemplified by clozapine, olanzapine, quetiapine, risperidone, and ziprasidone, which have less dopaminergic antagonism and more serotonergic effects than the typical antipsychotics. When antipsychotic medications produce coma, conduction abnormalities, or hyperthermia, these patients require ICU admission.

Clinical Manifestations of Overdose

The antipsychotics are a diverse group of medications, although useful generalizations can be made about their clinical manifestations. All produce sedation in overdose, though respiratory depression is usually not consequential. The drugs have varying degrees of muscarinic and α-adrenergic antagonism, often resulting in tachycardia and moderate hypotension (32). Many of the typical antipsychotics have type IA antidysrhythmic properties. Most of the typical and a few of the atypical drugs (notably ziprasidone) can cause QTc prolongation and torsades de pointes (33,34). Management of overdose of the antipsychotics generally only requires supportive care.

Clinical Manifestations of the Neuroleptic Malignant Syndrome

The dopamine antagonism required for control of psychosis can cause a group of distinct movement disorders that range in severity from mild to life threatening. These conditions—dystonia, akathisia, parkinsonism, tardive dyskinesia, and neuroleptic malignant syndrome (NMS)—are more likely to occur in the presence of the typical antipsychotics, although the atypical antipsychotics can cause them as well. The first four conditions mentioned above are of less concern to the intensivist than NMS, and will not be discussed.

NMS is the most consequential of the movement disorders associated with the antipsychotics. The syndrome is characterized by the presence of altered mental status, muscular rigidity, hyperthermia, and autonomic dysfunction (35). While symptoms usually begin within weeks of starting treatment, they do occur in individuals that are taking the drug on a chronic basis. Risk factors include young age, male gender, extracellular fluid volume contraction, use of high-potency antipsychotics, depot drug preparations, concomitant lithium use, rapid increase in dose, or simultaneous use of multiple drugs (34). Diagnosis is not always clear because there is no reference standard. The differential diagnosis of hyperthermia and altered mental status is very broad. Other diagnoses to consider include infection, environmental hyperthermia, hyperthyroidism, serotonin syndrome, ethanol and sedative-hypnotic withdrawal, sympathomimetic intoxication, and anticholinergic intoxication.

Management of NMS begins with immediate treatment of life-threatening hyperthermia. Ice-water immersion and paralysis by neuromuscular blockade should not be delayed if temperature is >106°F (41.1°C). In instances of environmental hyperthermia, a delay of cooling longer than 30 minutes has been associated with significant morbidity and mortality (36). Benzodiazepines should be titrated to sedation and muscle relaxation. When present, rhabdomyolysis, electrolyte disorders, and hypotension should be aggressively treated.

Bromocriptine, a centrally acting dopamine agonist given at 2.5 to 10 mg three to four times a day, may be of theoretical benefit even though it is not well studied. NMS may not be controlled for days after the introduction of bromocriptine. After signs and symptoms begin to improve, bromocriptine should be decreased by no more than 10% a day since decreasing the dose too rapidly may precipitate a relapse of NMS.

There is no evidence for the antidotal use of dantrolene in the management of NMS. Dantrolene is the drug of choice in malignant hyperthermia, a disorder affecting the sarcoplasmic reticulum that occurs in susceptible individuals receiving inhalational anesthetics or succinylcholine that some confuse with neuroleptic malignant syndrome because of their similar names and clinical manifestations.

Benzodiazepines

In 2005, the AAPCC received reports of 3,018 major effects and 243 fatalities from benzodiazepines (6). Benzodiazepines are widely used for their sedative, anxiolytic, and anticonvulsant properties. All these effects result from increasing the frequency of opening of γ-aminobutyric acid (GABA)-mediated chloride channels in the central nervous system (CNS) (37). In overdose, these drugs produce somnolence, coma, and minimal decreases in blood pressure, heart rate, and respiratory rate.

Management of benzodiazepine overdose is supportive. Care of the comatose patient should focus on supporting the airway and blood pressure while waiting for the drug to be eliminated. There is a limited role for flumazenil, a competitive benzodiazepine antagonist; flumazenil can precipitate withdrawal in individuals who are tolerant to benzodiazepines and induce seizures in those with seizure disorders (38,39). Flumazenil may be indicated in patients without tolerance to benzodiazepines who suffer from a pure benzodiazepine overdose. Benzodiazepine overdoses in children may meet these criteria. When indicated, flumazenil should be given intravenously, 0.1 mg/minute, up to 1 mg. The dose can be repeated if the clinical response is inadequate. Because the duration of the effect of flumazenil is shorter than the effect of the benzodiazepine, recurrence of symptoms should be expected. Alternatively, redosing or a continuous IV infusion at 0.1 to 1.0 mg/hour may be administered. The clinician should determine that the risk–benefit analysis of flumazenil favors administration of the drug.

If there is any doubt as to whether the patient has tolerance to benzodiazepines, flumazenil should not be administered. Benzodiazepine poisoning can be managed effectively and safely with supportive care only, but benzodiazepine withdrawal precipitated by flumazenil can be life threatening.

Cyclic Antidepressants

Until the introduction of the selective serotonin reuptake inhibitors (SSRIs), the cyclic antidepressants were the principal pharmacologic treatment available for depression. Roughly, 12% of the 11,198 cyclic antidepressant exposures reported to the AAPCC in 2005 had either a major outcome or fatality. While the cyclic antidepressants (CAs) differ slightly from each other in their receptor affinities, they can be treated as a group.

The CAs are usually absorbed within hours of ingestion, although the antimuscarinic effects may delay absorption in overdose. The drugs also exhibit α-adrenergic antagonism, inhibition of reuptake of norepinephrine, and anticholinergic properties. Acting as type IA antidysrhythmics, CAs block sodium entry into myocytes during phase 0 of depolarization.

Clinical Manifestations

Important CNS effects include lethargy, delirium, coma, and seizures. Tachycardia and hypotension develop early in toxicity. The IA antidysrhythmic properties cause prolongation of the QRS interval. CAs also produce a characteristic rightward shift of the axis in the terminal portion of the QRS, best seen as an R wave in the terminal 40 msec of lead aVR (40) (Fig. 66.2).

Management

Gastrointestinal decontamination should be considered in every patient. If the history suggests a recent large ingestion, gastric lavage may be attempted. Acute ingestions of 10 to 20 mg/kg of most CAs can cause significant poisoning (41). Activated charcoal should be administered. Serum drug concentrations may be obtained but do not correlate well with toxicity (42).

The ECG is the most important diagnostic test when managing CA overdose. A terminal 40-msec QRS axis of 130 to

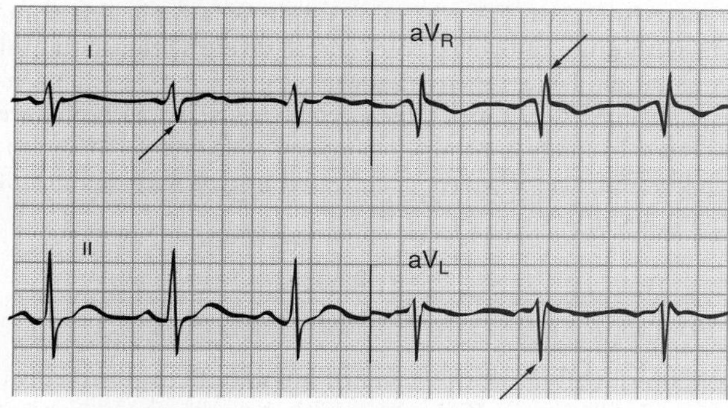

FIGURE 66.2. Terminal elevation of aVR and QRS prolongation. (Adapted with permission from Clancy C. Electrocardiographic principles. In: Flomenbaum NE, Goldfrank LR, Hoffman RS, et al., eds. *Goldfrank's Toxicologic Emergencies.* 8th ed. New York: McGraw-Hill; 2006:51–62.)

270 degrees discriminated patients with CA toxicity from those without toxicity in one study (43). While the terminal 40-msec QRS toxicity is a good indicator of exposure, QRS duration is a better indicator of severity of poisoning. In another series, no patients with QRS <160 msec had ventricular dysrhythmias and no patients with a QRS duration <100 msec had seizures (42).

The decision to administer sodium bicarbonate should be based on the ECG. Sodium bicarbonate should be administered if the QRS duration is ≥100 msec. Both the high sodium concentration and alkaline pH of sodium bicarbonate solution are responsible for its salutary effects. The sodium load increases the sodium gradient across the poisoned myocardial sodium channel, resulting in a narrowing of the QRS complex. The bicarbonate raises the pH, reducing CA binding to the sodium channel. Sodium bicarbonate should be administered as a 1 to 2 mEq/kg bolus during continuous ECG monitoring. If the complex narrows, sodium bicarbonate can be administered as an infusion. If the complex remains unchanged, the diagnosis of CA poisoning should be reconsidered. The sodium bicarbonate infusion may be performed by adding 150 mEq of bicarbonate to 1 L of D5W and infusing at twice the maintenance rate. The arterial pH should be targeted to 7.50 to 7.55. Occasional repeat boluses of 1 to 2 mEq/kg may be necessary. Hypertonic sodium chloride (3% NaCl) may be indicated when the QRS complex widens and the serum pH precludes further alkalinization. Hyperventilation may be used to induce alkalemia in intubated CA-poisoned patients. Hyperventilation may be utilized in those patients who cannot tolerate the fluid or sodium load from sodium bicarbonate. Although hyperventilation did not have an effect in one experimental model, it has been used clinically with success (44,45).

If hypotension persists despite fluid resuscitation and vasopressors become necessary, the direct-acting drug, norepinephrine, may be superior to the indirect-acting dopamine, because intracellular catecholamines may be depleted.

Seizures should be rapidly controlled. Convulsions will result in a metabolic acidosis, causing even more avid binding of the CA to the cardiac sodium channels, potentially resulting in more cardiotoxicity. Benzodiazepines can be safely administered, and propofol or barbiturates are also appropriate. Phenytoin, a type IA antidysrhythmic, may worsen cardiac toxicity and is therefore not indicated (46).

Therapy should continue until vital signs and ECG improve. In most instances, CA poisoning results in a rapid deterioration within hours of overdose—most severe within hours of presentation. Unless there has been a significant secondary injury (such as from shock), those who survive to 24 hours are expected to make a complete recovery. Because of their protein binding, hemodialysis is ineffective at removing significant quantities of CAs.

Lithium

Lithium is used in the treatment of bipolar affective disorders. Patients will require ICU admission when they have signs of CNS toxicity, do not tolerate fluid therapy, or have serum concentrations >2 mmol/L, which may result in rapid deterioration. Of 5,559 exposures reported to the AAPCC, 5.7% were classified as major or fatal.

Pharmacology

Lithium is thought to increase serotonin release and increase receptor sensitivity to serotonin, as well as modulate the effects of norepinephrine on its second-messenger system (47). Like sodium, lithium is a monovalent cation. The kidney handles lithium and sodium similarly. Lithium is freely filtered by the glomerulus, and 80% is reabsorbed, with 60% occurring in the proximal tubule (48). Immediate-release lithium preparations produce peak serum concentrations within hours, but sustained-release lithium may not peak for 6 to 12 hours. The generally accepted therapeutic range of lithium is 0.6 to 1.2 mmol/L, although in both overdose and therapeutic dosing, clinical signs and symptoms may serve as a better guide than the serum concentration.

Clinical Manifestations of Overdose

Acute and chronic lithium toxicity have similar neurologic features, although acute toxicity is usually associated with significant gastrointestinal manifestations. Acute toxicity occurs when an individual without a body burden of lithium takes a supratherapeutic dose of the drug. Chronic toxicity is usually the result of decreased elimination of the drug in a patient who is receiving a fixed dose (e.g., after developing renal insufficiency). Acute-on-chronic toxicity occurs when a patient with a pre-existent total body drug takes a supratherapeutic dose. In acute toxicity, a large ingestion of lithium—a gastrointestinal irritant—will initially cause gastrointestinal symptoms, such as vomiting and diarrhea. Neurotoxicity (which is clinically more significant) will be delayed until the drug has been absorbed and is redistributed into the CNS. In chronic lithium toxicity, gastrointestinal symptoms may be completely absent. Neurotoxicity manifests itself as disorders of movement and alterations in mental status. In very mild toxicity, only a fine tremor will be present, but in more advanced poisoning, fasciculations, hyperreflexia, dysarthria, and nystagmus may be seen as well (48). Mental status changes range from confusion to coma and seizures (49).

Nephrogenic diabetes insipidus and hypothyroidism occur following chronic therapeutic lithium use but are not features of overdose. The syndrome of irreversible lithium-effectuated neurotoxicity (SILENT) is a chronic neurologic disorder with many of the same features of lithium neurotoxicity. The distinction is that SILENT persists even when the body burden of lithium is eliminated. The mechanism is not completely elucidated but may involve demyelination. SILENT has been reported both as a result of chronic therapeutic use and as a sequela of lithium intoxication (50).

Management

Gastrointestinal decontamination should be considered after acute lithium toxicity. Since lithium does not bind to activated charcoal, activated charcoal should only be considered when a mixed overdose is suspected (51). When sustained-release preparations are ingested, whole bowel irrigation has been shown to decrease serum lithium concentration (52). Whole bowel irrigation can be performed by administering 2 liters of polyethylene glycol orally every hour (25 mL/kg/hour in children) until the rectal effluent is clear. After both acute and chronic toxicity, intravenous fluids should be given to optimize intravascular volume. The volume-depleted patient will have a decreased glomerular filtration rate and increased reabsorption of lithium. When fluid deficits are restored, 0.9% saline can be administered at twice the maintenance rate or approximately 200 mL/hour in adults to aid in elimination of lithium.

Extracorporeal elimination may be necessary to treat lithium toxicity. Lithium can be removed by hemodialysis due to its low volume of distribution and limited protein binding. Although hemodialysis can only remove the lithium residing in the vascular compartment, the elimination of serum lithium will allow the remaining intracellular lithium to redistribute into the plasma. Thus, although lithium concentrations may rebound following dialysis, the tissue burden has actually decreased. The indications for dialysis are not universally agreed upon. Hemodialysis should be performed when there are signs of significant end-organ damage, when lithium cannot be eliminated without dialysis, or when the serum concentration is elevated such that severe toxicity is highly likely. We recommend dialysis when there is significant CNS toxicity such as clonus, obtundation, coma, or seizures; when a patient with milder toxicity cannot eliminate lithium efficiently (renal insufficiency) or tolerate saline resuscitation (congestive heart failure); or in the presence of a serum lithium concentration >4.0 mmol/L following acute poisoning or >2.5 mmol/L following chronic poisoning. Since repeat dialysis may be necessary, the clinician should reapply the above criteria 4 hours after dialysis is completed to determine if dialysis should be repeated.

A common clinical pitfall is to deny dialysis to patients with an elevated lithium concentration and signs of toxicity because consecutive lithium concentrations have shown a small decrease. The clinician concludes that the lithium will eventually be eliminated without dialysis, so dialysis should not be helpful. Unfortunately, duration of exposure to the toxic lithium levels may predispose the patient to SILENT. In other words, it is better to be exposed to a neurotoxin for a few hours than a few days. While this area is not adequately studied, it seems prudent to hemodialyze these patients.

TOXICOLOGIC BRADYCARDIA: DIGOXIN, β-ADRENERGIC ANTAGONISTS, AND CALCIUM CHANNEL BLOCKERS

In 2005, the AAPCC NPED reported more than 30,000 exposures to cardioactive steroids (including digoxin), β-adrenergic antagonists, and calcium channel blockers. This figure includes 1,085 major outcomes and 167 fatalities (6). These xenobiotics have a narrow therapeutic index, drawing a fine line between therapeutic dosing and poisoning. The individuals who take these medications usually have underlying cardiovascular disease, making management of overdose even more challenging.

Digoxin

Digoxin is a cardioactive steroid derived from the foxglove plant. Though digoxin and digitoxin are the only pharmaceuticals in the class, plants such as oleander, yellow oleander, dogbane, and red squill contain cardioactive steroids with similar toxicity. While some of these plants cause a great deal of morbidity worldwide, this chapter will deal primarily with digoxin, which causes more morbidity than any other cardioactive steroid in North America. Of 2,828 reported exposures to cardiac steroid medications in 2005, 7.4% were classified as major or fatal (6).

Digoxin has multiple therapeutic and toxic cardiovascular effects, all of which result from inhibition of the Na^+-K^+-ATPase. The Na^+-K^+-ATPase extrudes sodium from the myocardial cell, creating a sodium gradient that drives an Na^+-Ca^{2+}-antiporter that moves calcium extracellularly. The inhibition of the Na^+-K^+-ATPase by digoxin increases intracellular Ca^{2+}, which therapeutically triggers Ca^{2+}-mediated Ca^{2+} release from the sarcoplasmic reticulum (Fig. 66.3). Ca influx through the cell membrane triggers Ca release through sarcoplasmic reticulum (SR); this is commonly called Ca-mediated Ca release.

Digoxin also slows conduction through the sinoatrial (SA) and atrioventricular (AV) nodes, probably through direct and vagally mediated mechanisms (53). In therapeutic use, digoxin decreases heart rate and increases inotropy. In overdose, the increased intracellular Ca^{2+} brings the cell closer to threshold, resulting in increased automaticity.

Digoxin does not exert its therapeutic and toxic effects until it redistributes from the serum into the myocardium. Digoxin has a large volume of distribution, precluding elimination by hemodialysis. Digoxin is mostly eliminated renally, although there is some hepatic metabolism. The maximal effect from a therapeutic dose of digoxin is seen at 4 to 6 hours when administered orally and 1.5 to 3 hours when given intravenously.

Clinical Manifestations

Digoxin poisoning can be either acute or chronic. Acute toxicity occurs when an individual without a tissue burden of digoxin ingests a supratherapeutic dosage of the drug. Chronic toxicity usually occurs when an individual on a fixed dose of the drug loses the ability to excrete it effectively. Both syndromes have similar cardiovascular manifestations, but acute toxicity may feature more prominent gastrointestinal symptoms. Acute poisoning may result in nausea, vomiting, and abdominal pain, whereas chronic poisoning develops more insidiously. In addition to gastrointestinal symptoms, chronic poisoning may present with weakness, confusion, or delirium (54,55).

Bradycardia with a preserved blood pressure typically occurs in digoxin toxicity. The ECG is the most important test in establishing the diagnosis. Because digoxin has multiple cardiac effects, there is no single ECG manifestation that is consistently seen in patients with digoxin toxicity. Almost any rhythm is possible, with the exception of a rapidly conducted supraventricular rhythm. The most common rhythm disturbance on initial ECG is the presence of ventricular ectopy (56). The ECG could potentially exhibit increased automaticity from elevated resting potential, conduction disturbance from AV and SA nodal block, both, or neither. The ectopy may degrade into ventricular tachycardia or ventricular fibrillation. If conduction disturbance predominates, the ECG may demonstrate sinus bradycardia or varying degrees of AV block.

The laboratory provides clues to toxicity. The therapeutic range for digoxin is usually reported as 0.5 to 2.0 ng/mL. Serum digoxin concentration should be interpreted in the context of the history and ECG. Digoxin is a cardiotoxin, and serum concentrations do not necessarily reflect the degree of poisoning. Digoxin requires several hours to redistribute from the serum to the tissues. Shortly after an acute ingestion, the serum concentration may overestimate toxicity, while a mild increase in

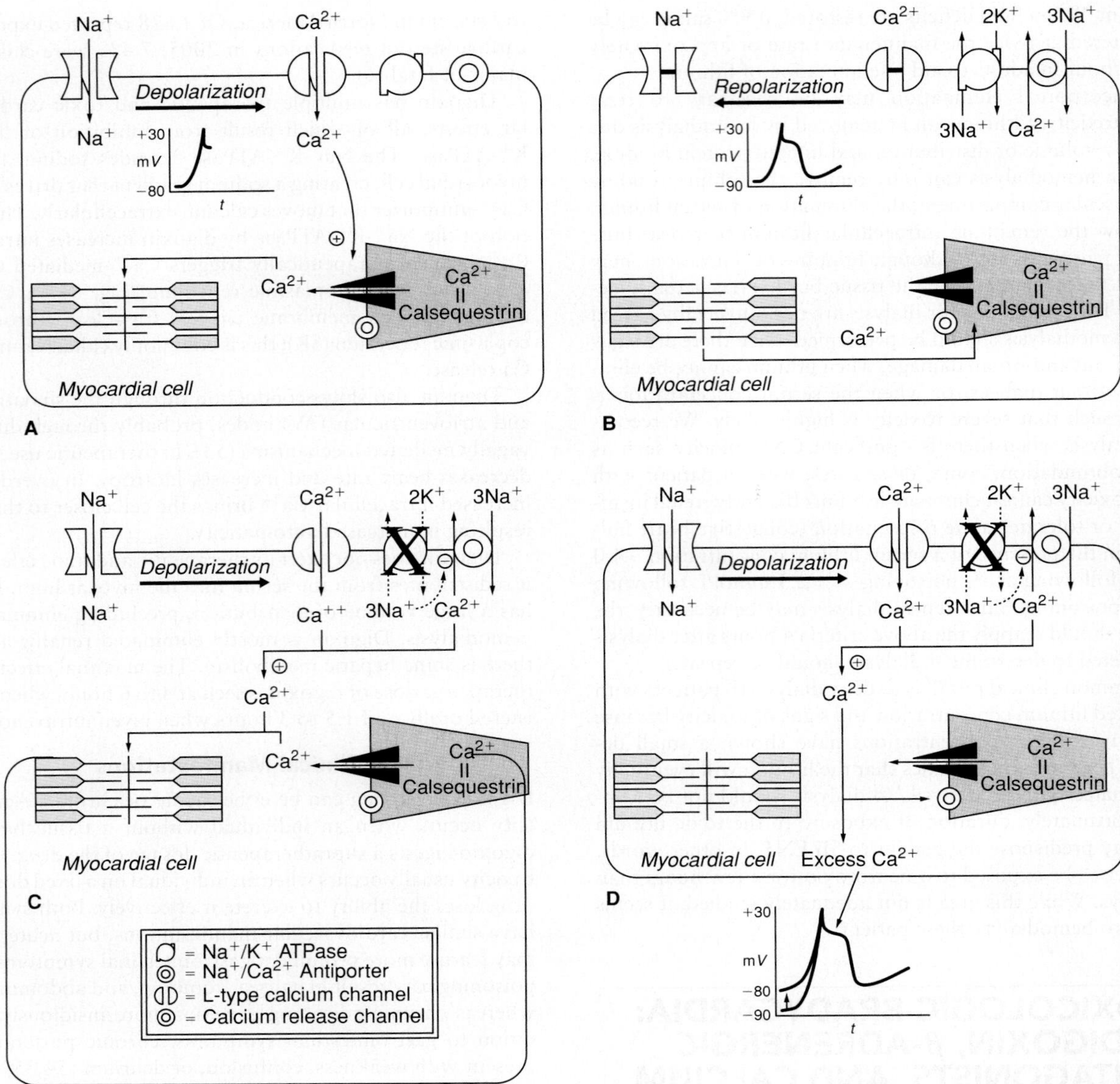

FIGURE 66.3. Normal depolarization. (Adapted with permission from Hack JB, Lewin NA. Cardioactive steroids. In: Flomenbaum NE, Goldfrank LR, Hoffman RS, et al., eds. *Goldfrank's Toxicologic Emergencies.* 8th ed. New York: McGraw-Hill; 2006:971–982.)

serum concentration of a patient chronically on digoxin may underestimate the high extent of the increased tissue burden.

Serum potassium concentration is a better predictor of illness following acute ingestions. A study of 91 digitoxin-poisoned patients performed in the pre–digoxin-specific antibody fragment era found no mortality when the potassium concentration was less than 5.0 mEq/L and 50% mortality when the potassium concentration was 5.0 to 5.5 mEq/L (57).

Management of Toxicity

Because acute toxicity can cause vomiting, activated charcoal and gastric lavage may be of limited value.

Atropine can be given intravenously in 0.5-mg doses for bradycardia, although it is probably not important to "correct" the heart rate if the blood pressure is preserved. If necessary, potassium should be supplemented. Hypokalemia inhibits the function of the Na^+-K^+-ATPase, and thereby exacerbates digoxin poisoning. A pitfall in managing digoxin-poisoned patients is the administration of calcium in response to the recognition of hyperkalemia. When hyperkalemia is the result of an increase in total body burden of potassium, such as in renal failure, calcium is the treatment of choice. However, calcium administration is not recommended in the setting of digoxin poisoning where extracellular distribution of potassium is the result of a poisoned Na^+-K^+-ATPase, not an increase in total body potassium. Under these circumstances, increasing extracellular calcium may accentuate toxicity.

Digoxin-specific Immune Fragments

Administration of digoxin-specific antibody fragments (Fab) is the most important intervention in digoxin-poisoned patients. Fab are prepared by cleaving the Fc fragment from IgG. The resulting Fab fragments are much less immunoreactive than the whole IgG antibodies. In a large series, digoxin-specific

TABLE 66.3

DIGOXIN-SPECIFIC FAB DOSE CALCULATION

When serum digoxin concentration (SDC) known:
No. of vials = [SDC (ng/mL) × patient weight (kg)]/100
When SDC unknown, dose known:
No. of vials = Amount ingested (mg)/0.5 mg/vial
When both SDC and dose unknown (acute poisoning)
Empiric therapy
10–20 vials (adult or pediatric)
When both SDC and dose unknown (chronic poisoning)
Empiric therapy
Adult: 3–6 vials
Pediatric: 1–2 vials

antibody fragments caused allergic reaction in 0.8% of patients (58).

Digoxin-specific Fab should be administered to anyone with digoxin-induced cardiotoxicity, a serum potassium concentration ≥5.0 mEq/L after an acute overdose, or a serum digoxin concentration ≥15 ng/mL at any time or ≥10 ng/mL at 6 hours postingestion (59).

Digoxin-specific Fab are given by intravenous infusion and dosed according to serum concentration (Table 66.3). In the presence of suspected severe toxicity, treatment should not be dependent on nor await serum digoxin concentration results. The first clinical effect of Fab should be seen within 20 minutes and a maximal response within several hours (60). Following immune-specific antibody fragment administration, the serum digoxin concentration determined by most laboratories will be a total digoxin concentration, which will include the antibody-bound digoxin. The result will be a very elevated value without clinical utility. The determination of free digoxin concentration, which is available at some institutions, would not be affected.

β-Adrenergic Antagonists and Calcium Channel Blockers

In 2005, the National Poisoning and Exposure Database received 18,207 reports of exposures to β-adrenergic antagonists (including 60 fatalities and 525 major outcomes) and 10,500 reports of exposures to calcium channel blockers (75 fatalities and 384 major outcomes) (6).

The β-adrenergic antagonists and calcium channel blockers represent a diverse group of medications with a wide range of clinical indications. There is, however, an overlap in the clinical effects and the management of overdose of these medications. The description of each class is described individually, whereas the discussion of appropriate management is integrated.

β-Adrenergic Antagonists

β-Adrenergic receptors are coupled to G proteins, which activate adenyl cyclase, resulting in increased production of ATP from cyclic adenosine monophosphate (cAMP). The cAMP activates protein kinase A (PKA), which initiates a series of phosphorylations. Phosphorylation of L-type calcium channels on cell membranes increases intracellular calcium, which allows more activation of the SR and further calcium release from the SR, causing muscle contraction. The calcium influx also brings pacemaker cells closer to threshold. The net result is increased inotropy and chronotropy (61).

Most of the β-adrenergic antagonists are exclusively metabolized or biotransformed in the liver and then renally eliminated. The exception to the rule is atenolol, which is exclusively renally eliminated.

Clinical Manifestations of Overdose

All β-adrenergic antagonists have the potential to produce bradycardia and hypotension in a dose-dependent fashion. However, there are subtle differences among the agents in terms of receptor selectivity, lipid solubility, membrane-stabilizing activity, and potassium channel blockade that result in varied clinical manifestations.

β-Adrenergic antagonists differ from each other in their selectivity for α-, β_1-, and β_2-adrenergic receptors. Drugs with α- and β-adrenergic antagonist effects, such as labetalol and carvedilol, produce more hypotension and afterload reduction. The more β_1-selective drugs, including metoprolol and atenolol, have less potential for β_2-related adverse effects such as bronchospasm. The more lipid-soluble β-adrenergic antagonists, such as propranolol, penetrate the CNS more readily, causing obtundation or seizures prior to hemodynamic collapse (62). Membrane-stabilizing activity, similar to type I antidysrhythmic activity, produces lengthening of the QRS interval, tachydysrhythmias, and hypotension. The membrane-stabilizing effect is usually associated with propranolol and other lipid-soluble drugs, although it has been observed after overdose with others (63,64). Sotalol and acebutolol can produce QTc prolongation due to potassium channel blockade, which may result in torsades de pointes (65).

Calcium Channel Blockers

The calcium channel blockers (CCBs) are formulated as both immediate and sustained release, but in overdose, the effects of either type may be prolonged. The CCBs undergo hepatic metabolism.

There are three major classes of CCBs: Dihydropyridines (including amlodipine, nifedipine, and others ending with the suffix "-pine"), phenylalkylamines (verapamil), and benzothiazepine (diltiazem). In practice, it is more clinically useful to divide them into two classes: the dihydropyridines and the nondihydropyridines. All of the drugs inhibit the function of L-type calcium channels. The dihydropyridines have greater affinity for calcium channels in vascular smooth muscle than the myocardium (66).

Clinical Manifestations of Overdose

The most consequential clinical features of CCB overdose are cardiovascular. All of the CCBs produce hypotension, but effects on heart rate and contractility vary based on the class of the particular drug. As a result, they cause hypotension with a reflex tachycardia. Diltiazem, in contrast, produces little peripheral blockade, but does suppress contractility and conduction through the SA and AV nodes, resulting in bradycardia and decreased inotropy. These cardiac effects can be much more difficult to treat than the peripheral vasodilation of the dihydropyridines. In severe poisoning, heart block or complete cardiovascular collapse results. Verapamil, which is active in the peripheral vasculature and in the myocardium, produces a combination of the effects of the dihydropyridines and diltiazem. For this reason, verapamil is considered to be the most dangerous of the CCBs, although any of them can cause death in overdose.

CCBs have effects outside the cardiovascular system. The blockade of L-type calcium channels in pancreatic β-islet cells, where they trigger the blockade of insulin release, may result in hyperglycemia (67).

Management of Overdose of β-adrenergic Antagonists and Calcium Channel Blockers

Patients who initially present without symptoms may rapidly become very ill. Patients with these overdoses should be taken very seriously and treated aggressively. Many antidotes have been investigated, with varying degrees of clinical success. Patients with β-adrenergic antagonist and CCB overdose do not benefit from removal with hemodialysis. There is no single antidote for either β-adrenergic antagonists or CCBs. The optimal treatment consists of a combination of the treatments described below.

Gastrointestinal decontamination should be considered in all patients. Gastric lavage may be indicated if there are pills still expected to be in the stomach (usually in the first hour or two after ingestion). Activated charcoal should be administered. Whole bowel irrigation with polyethylene glycol is indicated for patients with a history of ingesting sustained-release drugs.

The initial management for hypotension will be intravenous crystalloid fluid. Although intravenous atropine, 0.5 mg to 1 mg, may be given for bradycardia, studies of atropine efficacy in CCB toxicity are not definitive (68).

Calcium has a role not only in calcium channel blocker toxicity, but also for β-adrenergic antagonist poisoning (69,70). Increasing extracellular calcium helps to overcome calcium channel blockade and increase intracellular calcium, typically with greater improvement in blood pressure than heart rate. The ideal dosing of calcium is not yet established. An intravenous bolus of 13 to 25 mEq of Ca^{2+} (10–20 mL of 10% calcium chloride or 30–60 mL of 10% calcium gluconate) can be followed by repeat boluses or an infusion of 0.5 mEq/kg/hour of Ca^{2+} (71). Calcium concentration should be closely monitored.

Glucagon, an endogenous polypeptide hormone released by pancreatic α cells, has significant inotropic effects mediated by its ability to activate myocyte adenylate cyclase by itself, effectively bypassing the β-adrenergic receptor (72). Because calcium channel opening occurs "downstream" from adenylate cyclase, glucagon may not be as effective for overcoming calcium channel blockade. Glucagon should be given intravenously, at an initial dose of 3 to 5 mg (50 μg/kg in children), up to 10 mg. The total initial dose that produces a response should be given hourly as an infusion (73). Glucagon may cause hyperglycemia or vomiting, but neither complication should limit the therapy if it is effective.

Hyperinsulemia/euglycemia therapy should be instituted early in patients with moderate to severe poisoning. Insulin is a positive inotrope and may independently increase Ca^{2+} entry into cells (74). Insulin may allow the myocardium, which usually relies on fatty acids, to use more carbohydrate for metabolism (75). As with other therapies for poisoning with these agents, the ideal dose is not known. We recommend an intravenous bolus of 1 unit/kg, followed by an infusion of 0.5 to 1 unit/kg/hour. The initial bolus should be preceded by a 1 g/kg bolus of dextrose, followed by an infusion to maintain euglycemia. An initial infusion of 0.5 g/kg/hour of dextrose can be instituted and then adjusted based on the subsequent glucose concentration. Although some clinicians are understandably apprehensive about using a dose of insulin that is 10-fold greater than the typical diabetic ketoacidosis regimen, the regimen has been successfully used clinically and in animal models of both β-adrenergic antagonists and calcium channel blocker poisoning (76,77).

In severe poisoning, all of the above measures should be performed, as well as institution of inotropes and vasoactive drugs. Intra-aortic balloon counterpulsation should also be considered if cardiac output is severely compromised. These patients may be ideal for this procedure because, unlike with most other causes of cardiogenic shock, their cardiac output can recover in a relatively short period of time.

TOXIC ALCOHOLS

The term *toxic alcohols* refers in particular to methanol and ethylene glycol, which are the most important chemicals in the class because they are both of high potential toxicity and wide availability. In 2005, the NPED received 6,220 reports of exposure to ethylene glycol, including 5.4% classified as major or fatal, and 2,276 exposures to methanol, with 3.2% major or fatal (6).

The toxic alcohols have numerous industrial and consumer uses. Methanol is commonly found in windshield wiper fluid and ethylene glycol in automobile antifreeze, and isopropanol is a ubiquitous topical disinfectant. Since specific laboratory testing is usually not available for these chemicals, establishment of the diagnosis of toxic alcohol poisoning will necessitate skilled use of the serum osmolarity and anion gap.

The toxic alcohols are readily absorbed and have a volume of distribution similar to total body water. Both the parent compounds and the toxic metabolites are dialyzable. It is not the toxic alcohols themselves that produce significant toxicity, but their metabolites. Methanol and ethylene glycol are metabolized in a stepwise fashion by alcohol dehydrogenase (ADH) and aldehyde dehydrogenase (ALDH) to the clinically important metabolites formic acid (methanol) and glycolic, glycoxylic, and oxalic acid (ethylene glycol) (Figs. 66.4 and 66.5). Isopropanol is less clinically consequential, as it is converted by ADH to acetone, which is an end product rather than a substrate of ALDH.

Because ADH preferentially metabolizes ethanol over all other alcohols, no significant metabolism of toxic alcohols will occur while high concentrations of ethanol are present. When ADH is inhibited, the parent compounds are eliminated very slowly without metabolism. In the absence of ADH, ethylene glycol is renally eliminated with a half-life of 8.5 hours while methanol, which is eliminated as a vapor, has a half-life of 30 to 54 hours (78–80).

When suspected, toxic alcohol poisoning requires ICU admission. Patients may be obtunded and require therapeutic medication infusions and hemodialysis that cannot be accomplished in general inpatient units.

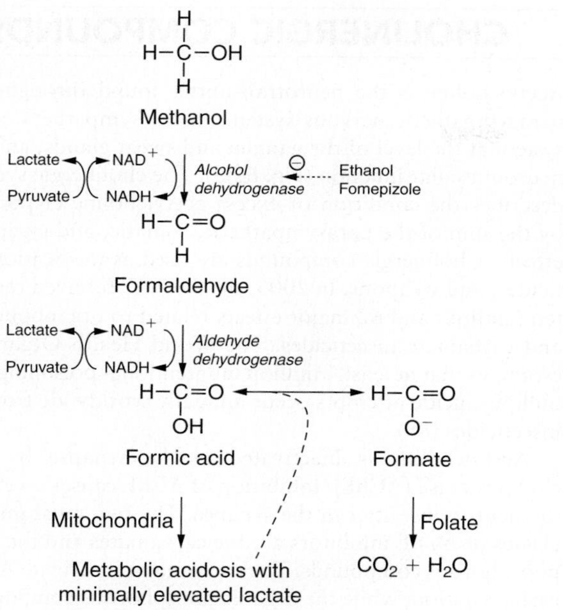

FIGURE 66.4. Metabolism of methanol. (Adapted with permission from Wiener SW. Toxic alcohols. In: Flomenbaum NE, Goldfrank LR, Hoffman RS, et al., eds. *Goldfrank's Toxicologic Emergencies.* 8th ed. New York: McGraw-Hill; 2006:1447–1459.)

Clinical Manifestations

The physical examination may be unremarkable. All of the toxic alcohols can produce significant CNS depression, and a compensatory tachypnea may be present if there is a metabolic acidosis. Acetone, generated from ADH metabolism of isopropanol, produces nausea, hypotension, hemorrhagic gastritis, and tachycardia, but these are not usually life threatening (81). Formate, a methanol metabolite, can produce blindness from toxicity to the retina and optic nerve (82).

Laboratory studies can suggest—but not establish or exclude—the diagnosis of toxic alcohol poisoning. Metabolites of methanol or ethylene glycol may cause an elevated anion gap metabolic acidosis. The hallmark laboratory finding of isopropanol poisoning is ketonemia without acidosis. Ethylene glycol may cause nephrotoxicity when the primary metabolite oxalic acid precipitates as calcium oxalate crystals in the renal tubules (83).

The osmolar gap, the difference between the measured and unmeasured osmoles, may be increased when the serum contains toxic alcohol osmoles. A very high osmolar gap does suggest the presence of toxic alcohol, whereas a low or normal gap does not exclude the presence of ethylene glycol or methanol. There is a great population variation in the "normal" osmolar gap, from −10 to 10, such that very high concentrations of toxic alcohols might not be apparent when the gap is calculated (84).

Other tests, such as fluorescence of the urine or presence of calcium oxalate crystals in the presence of ethylene glycol poisoning, are neither sensitive nor specific (85). Since fluorescein is added to some brands of ethylene glycol–based antifreeze in order to facilitate detection of radiator leaks, some authors suggest the use of a Woods lamp to detect urine for fluorescence as a screen for ethylene glycol. However, in one study of a large group of children not exposed to ethylene glycol, almost all of them had urinary fluorescence (86). Because of the limitations in these laboratory studies, treatment should be started empirically as soon as the diagnosis is considered.

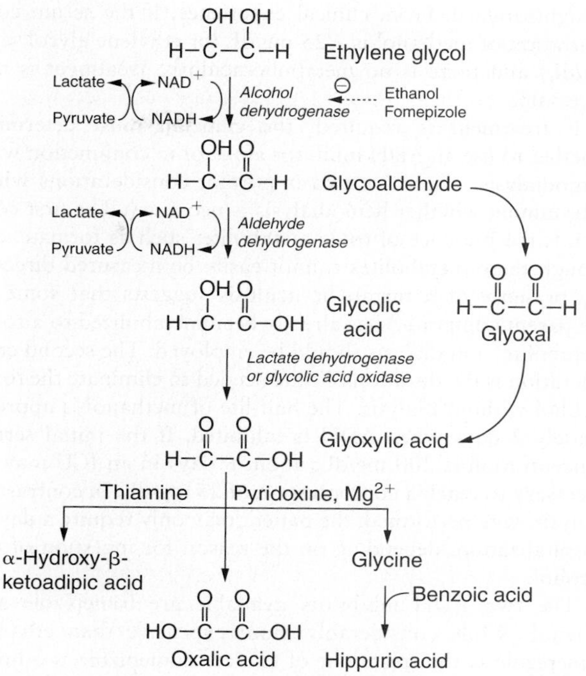

FIGURE 66.5. Metabolism of ethylene glycol. (Adapted with permission from Wiener SW. Toxic alcohols. In: Flomenbaum NE, Goldfrank LR, Hoffman RS, et al., eds. *Goldfrank's Toxicologic Emergencies.* 8th ed. New York: McGraw-Hill; 2006:1447–1459.)

Management

There are several clinical presentations that suggest poisoning with a toxic alcohol, and each requires different management considerations. The first type of patient presents without acidosis and either a history of ingesting ethylene glycol or methanol or a very elevated osmolar gap. The physician should immediately begin an ADH inhibitor and obtain toxic alcohol concentrations (when available). Later, the decision to continue treatment or begin hemodialysis can be made based on the presence of a toxic alcohol in a high concentration. If the result is not expected in a timely manner, dialysis should be presumptively performed.

The second scenario is the patient who presents with an unexplained elevated anion gap metabolic acidosis that is not explained by the presence of lactate, ketoacids, or uremia. In such cases, the diagnosis should be considered, and ADH inhibition and hemodialysis should be instituted. One test that is very helpful in this scenario is a serum ethanol concentration. As long as there is elevated ethanol concentration present in the serum, toxic alcohols cannot be converted into their metabolites. Therefore, if a patient has a very elevated ethanol concentration, his or her elevated anion gap metabolic acidosis cannot be explained by toxic alcohol poisoning, unless the ethanol was consumed only hours after the ingestion of the toxic alcohol.

If a serum toxic alcohol concentration is available, the diagnosis can be established rapidly, and management is straightforward. From clinical experience, if the serum concentration of methanol is <25 mg/dL (or ethylene glycol <50 mg/dL) and there is no metabolic acidosis, treatment is not necessary.

If treatment is required, the clinician must determine whether to use an ADH inhibitor alone or in conjunction with hemodialysis. There are two important considerations when determining whether hemodialysis is necessary. The first concern is the presence of toxic metabolites such as formate. Although these metabolites cannot easily be measured directly, the presence of a metabolic acidosis suggests that some of the parent compound has already been metabolized to a toxic metabolite, and dialysis should be employed. The second consideration is the duration of time needed to eliminate the toxic alcohol without dialysis. The half-life of methanol is approximately 2 days when ADH is inhibited. If the initial serum concentration is 200 mg/dL, about 6 days in an ICU may be necessary to reach a concentration of 25 mg/dL. In contrast, if dialysis were performed, the patient may only require a day of hospitalization, depending on the reason for ingestion of the alcohol.

The two ADH inhibitors available are fomepizole and ethanol. While considerably more expensive than ethanol, fomepizole is the treatment of choice. Fomepizole is administered by empiric weight-based dosing, while ethanol infusion requires serum concentrations to be obtained frequently. Unlike ethanol, fomepizole does not cause CNS or respiratory depression. Fomepizole should be given as a 15 mg/kg intravenous loading dose, followed in 12 hours by 10 mg/kg every 12 hours for 48 hours. If continued dosing is required, the infusion rate should be increased to 15 mg/kg. When fomepizole is unavailable, ethanol should be given intravenously, or orally if necessary. We recommend a loading dose of ethanol at 0.8 g/kg over 20 to 60 minutes, followed by an initial infusion of 100 mg/kg/hour (87). The goal of ethanol therapy is to maintain an ADH inhibitory concentration of 100 mg/dL. The serum ethanol concentration should be obtained frequently and the rate adjusted accordingly.

As stated above, hemodialysis should be performed for patients with concentrations of methanol >25 mg/dL or ethylene glycol >50 mg/dL when toxic metabolites are shown to be present (indicated by metabolic acidosis), or when ADH inhibition alone would require an unreasonable amount of time. ADH blockade should continue during hemodialysis; fomepizole should be dosed every 4 hours and ethanol should be administered at a rate of 250 to 350 mg/kg/hour (87).

Several hemodialysis sessions may be needed to remove the toxic alcohol, depending on the initial concentration. Symptoms of isopropanol can usually be managed with fluids and supportive care alone, although rarely, hemodialysis may be indicated.

Folate is a cofactor in the conversion of formic acid to a nontoxic metabolite, and thiamine and pyridoxine assist in transforming toxic metabolites following ethylene glycol poisoning. Therefore, 1 to 2 mg/kg of folic acid should be given every 4 to 6 hours in the first 24 hours of methanol poisoning, and thiamine hydrochloride (100 mg IM or IV) and pyridoxine (100 mg/day IV) should be administered for ethylene glycol poisoning.

It is reasonable to administer sodium bicarbonate to a target pH of 7.2 to shift the equilibrium from formic acid to the less toxic formate.

CHOLINERGIC COMPOUNDS

Acetylcholine is the neurotransmitter found throughout the parasympathetic nervous system, in the sympathetic nervous system at the level of the ganglia and sweat glands, and at the neuromuscular junction (Fig. 66.6). The cholinergic syndrome describes the condition of excess acetylcholine characterized by the sum of the parasympathetic, somatic, and sympathetic effects. Cholinergic compounds are used as medications, pesticides, and weapons. In 2005, the AAPCC received reports of ten fatalities and 62 major effects related to organophosphate and carbamate insecticides. The World Health Organization estimates that at least 1 million unintentional poisonings and 2 million suicide attempts occur annually worldwide from these insecticides (88).

Acetylcholine is inactivated in the synapse by acetylcholinesterase (AChE). Inhibition of AChE causes an excess of the neurotransmitter in the synapse. The two most important classes of AChE inhibitors are the carbamates and the organic phosphorous compounds. The carbamates inactivate AChE by carbamylation, while the organic phosphorous compounds do so by phosphorylation. The carbamates and organic phosphorous compounds are both absorbed by ingestion, by inhalation, and through skin.

There are some generalizations that can be made about the two classes. Organic phosphorous compounds have a greater delay to onset of action. After ingestion, peak concentrations have been reported at 6 hours (89). Many of the organic phosphorous agents are activated in the liver, resulting in a further delay to peak action. In contrast, many of the carbamates have peak concentrations within 40 minutes following ingestion (90). The organic phosphorous compounds are generally very lipophilic. Redistribution from fat allows measurable serum concentrations for up to 48 days, while carbamates may be almost completely eliminated within days (91,92). Organic phosphorous compounds exhibit peripheral and CNS effects, while the carbamates do not readily cross into the CNS, resulting in a predominance of peripheral symptoms (93). Most importantly, organic phosphorous compounds exhibit "aging," whereby the reversible inhibition of AChE becomes permanent. Aging can take minutes to days, depending on the particular compound. Carbamates, in contrast, spontaneously hydrolyze from the active site of AChE and do not age.

ICU admission is required for those with respiratory compromise, hemodynamic instability, or the need for administration of large amounts of atropine.

Clinical Manifestations

Diagnosis is often established by recognition of the muscarinic signs: salivation, lacrimation, urination, defecation, bradycardia, bronchorrhea, and bronchospasm. Acetylcholine initially acts as an agonist, but in excess becomes an antagonist at the neuromuscular junction, producing weakness, fasciculations, and paralysis. Simulation of nicotinic receptors at the sympathetic ganglia produces tachycardia and mydriasis.

Management

The first management priorities involve securing the airway when necessary and decontaminating the patient's skin to

concentration is less than 5%, but smokers may have a concentration of up to 10% (124). Carboxyhemoglobin concentrations are an indicator of exposure, but do not correlate with the degree of toxicity (125). When there is a delay from exposure to measurement of carboxyhemoglobin, the concentration loses further value as a clinical tool. This is more likely if the patient has been receiving supplemental oxygen, which decreases the half-life of carboxyhemoglobin.

Chronic Sequelae

For those who survive an acute CO exposure, there may be significant chronic neurologic and cardiovascular effects. Delayed neurologic sequelae (DNS) follow the resolution of initial symptoms, sometimes days to weeks later, and include dementia, movement disorders, and memory impairment (126).

Diagnostic Studies

In patients with chest pain, shortness of breath, palpitations, or neurologic deficits indicating severe exposure, an electrocardiogram should be performed, and serum cardiac markers should be obtained. Pregnancy status should be determined in women of childbearing age.

Elevated serum cardiac markers during moderate and severe acute toxicity predict long-term mortality (127). The pathophysiology of chronic cardiovascular effects of carbon monoxide poisoning probably involves CO poisoning of cardiac myoglobin, but needs further study.

Within 12 hours of exposure, loss of consciousness occurs, and changes on a computed tomography (CT) scan of the brain may be seen. Characteristic findings include symmetric, low-density changes in the globus pallidus, putamen, and caudate nuclei (128). A normal CT scan is a good prognostic indicator. In a series of 18 patients, a negative CT within 1 week of admission was associated with good outcome (129).

Management

As soon as the diagnosis is considered, the patient should be administered 100% oxygen, and the carboxyhemoglobin concentration should be obtained. Without supplemental oxygen, studies have found that the half-life of carboxyhemoglobin in blood is 4 to 6 hours. With oxygen, it has been found to range from 1 to 2 hours (130).

The most important decision is whether to administer hyperbaric oxygen (HBO). While HBO decreases the half-life of carbon monoxide even more rapidly than 100% normobaric oxygen, this is not a clinically important objective. Most patients who are brought to a hospital will survive whether or not they receive HBO. The value of HBO is its potential to decrease morbidity, not mortality. Specifically, HBO may reduce delayed neurologic sequelae. In animal models, HBO prevents brain lipid peroxidation and regenerates CNS cytochrome oxidase after CO exposure (131,132).

The use of HBO for CO poisoning is controversial. Many clinicians do not advocate its use. Whereas the animal data and case series suggest a benefit, large randomized clinical trials report mixed results. Some trials show a benefit for HBO in preventing neurologic sequelae, and some do not indicate any difference. (For a detailed review of the literature, see Tomaszewski C. Carbon monoxide. In: Flomenbaum NE, Goldfrank LR, Hoffman RS, et al., eds. *Goldfrank's Toxicologic Emergencies*. 8th ed. New York: McGraw-Hill; 2006:1689–1704.)

All of the trials conducted to date have limitations, and the ideal trial may never be performed because of the ethical concerns of randomizing patients to nonhyperbaric therapy. In light of the demonstrable benefit of HBO and the relative safety of the therapy, we recommend HBO in patients with moderate to severe poisoning. The patient should receive the therapy as early as safely possible; in one series, a delay greater than 6 hours was associated with a worse outcome (133). The following are indications for HBO: (a) syncope, coma, seizure, or any other hard neurologic findings; (b) signs of cardiac ischemia or dysrhythmias; and (c) carboxyhemoglobin >20%.

Pregnancy and Carbon Monoxide

Because fetal circulation relies on maternal oxyhemoglobin for oxygenation, any disturbance in maternal oxygen delivery will be magnified in the fetus. Even though fetal hemoglobin has less affinity for CO than adult hemoglobin, there is a high incidence of fetal CNS damage and spontaneous abortion after severe maternal poisoning (134,135). In contrast, pregnant women who have lesser exposures have normal pregnancies and deliver healthy children (136). Because all prospective trials of HBO have excluded pregnant patients, the literature is not clear as to whether this population would benefit from the therapy. We recommend treating these patients similarly to those who are not pregnant.

CAUSTICS

Caustics are chemicals that produce damage during contact with tissues. They are generally acid or alkali, and are commercially available as toilet bowl cleaners, drain cleaners, and other products. There are myriad caustics available in both the home and work environment. Commonly encountered alkalis include ammonium hydroxide (ammonia) and sodium hydroxide (lye, found in drain cleaners). Hydrochloric acid and sulfuric acid are both used as drain cleaners, with the latter used in automobile batteries as well. Alkali drain cleaners accounted for more than 3,677 reported exposures in 2005, more than any other caustic chemical. Of these, 46 were major and 5 fatal (6).

The amount of damage caused by caustics is determined by pH, quantity, duration of contact, and the titratable alkaline (or acid) reserve (TAR). Ingested caustics can potentially produce damage to the oropharynx, esophagus, stomach, and respiratory tract. Acid and alkali produce different types of injury. Alkaline exposure produces dissociated OH^- ion, resulting in fat saponification, membrane dissolution, and cell death—a process known as liquefactive necrosis (137). Acid exposure releases H^+ ions, producing an eschar and desiccation, a process referred to as *coagulation necrosis*. Both acid and alkali produce stomach and esophageal injury (138).

Esophageal burns can be described by a commonly used classification system (139,140). Grade I burns demonstrate hyperemia without ulceration; grade II burns demonstrate ulcers, but do not damage periesophageal tissues; grade II lesions are subdivided into IIa (noncircumferential) and IIb (circumferential) lesions; and grade III describes burns with deep ulceration and damage to surrounding tissues. The classification of the burn predicts chronic sequelae. Grade IIb and III injuries may heal with strictures and dysphagia, and may perforate. When esophageal perforation is suspected, or when there is airway injury, patients should be admitted to the ICU.

Clinical Manifestations

The lack of oral burns does not exclude significant esophageal injury, nor does the presence of oral lesions guarantee visceral burns. The physical examination following caustic ingestion can be deceiving. A series of pediatric patients found visceral burns in 37.5% of patients without oral burns and 50% of patients with oral burns (141). Drooling, odynophagia, and abdominal pain are common findings following significant caustic exposure. However, a series of acid ingestions noted abdominal pain or tenderness in less than half of patients with gastric injury (138).

Pulmonary aspiration may lead to coughing and respiratory distress. Absorption of acid from the stomach may cause acidemia following ingestion. Alkalis are not systemically absorbed in consequential amounts, but a metabolic acidosis may be present if significant injury has occurred.

Management

Endoscopy should be performed in all adult patients presumed to have significant exposures in order to establish the severity of the burn. If endoscopy is normal, the patient can be safely discharged, while patients with severe injury are rapidly stabilized and referred for surgical care before their condition worsens. Endoscopy should be performed as early as possible, ideally within 12 hours. Wound strength is weakest between 5 days and 2 weeks postingestion, when the perforation risk is greatest. The exception to universal endoscopy may be a subset of pediatric exposures based upon a series of 79 patients younger than 20 years of age when no serious esophageal injuries were found in patients who lacked stridor or the combination of vomiting and drooling (142). Another group of investigators found no lesions in asymptomatic pediatric patients (143).

The presence of endoscopic evidence of perforation mandates immediate surgery. Other indications for operative repair include pleural effusions, ascites, and a serum pH <7.2 (144). If endoscopy demonstrates grade I injury, the patient can be started on a soft diet and the diet advanced as tolerated. The presence of grade II esophageal burns with gastric sparing warrants placement of a nasogastric tube under direct visualization. More severe injury may require parenteral nutrition or a jejunostomy. Silicone rubber esophageal stents have been used to prevent stricture (145).

Administer antibiotics that cover anaerobic bacteria and Gram-positive and Gram-negative aerobic organisms as soon as perforation is considered. Piperacillin/tazobactam are appropriate choices, or levofloxacin and clindamycin. Corticosteroids have been recommended to help prevent scarring and stricture formation in grade II lesions. Randomized controlled trials have provided conflicting results. The most recent meta-analysis could not find a benefit for the administration of corticosteroids following exposure to caustics (146).

HYDROFLUORIC ACID

Hydrofluoric acid (HF) is a weak acid, and does not have important tissue-corrosive properties. HF and ammonium bifluoride have numerous industrial uses. HF dissolves metal oxides and glass, making it useful in rust removal and glass etching. Because of these properties, HF is stored in plastic, not glass.

HF is an important dermal, ophthalmic, pulmonary, and systemic toxin. HF penetrates deeply into tissues before dissociating into protons and fluoride ions. Although the protons cause some damage, the most important toxic effects result from fluoride ions binding the divalent cations calcium and magnesium (147). The consumption of these cations leads to neuropathic pain and cell death. HF ingestions and exposures resulting in electrolyte abnormalities require ICU admission.

Clinical Manifestations

HF produces a clinical syndrome distinct from the caustic agents and requires specific therapy. In small dermal exposures, HF produces severe pain with limited dermal findings. Large exposures by any route, including dermal, can produce severe hypocalcemia and death.

Most unintentional HF exposures are dermal. The severity of HF exposure is determined by the duration of exposure, concentration, and extent of surface area exposed. Solutions with low fluoride concentration may cause severe pain beginning hours after the exposure, with a very unremarkable physical examination. An area that appears normal or merely mildly erythematous may be extremely painful. High-concentration industrial preparations may cause immediate pain, with hyperemia and ulceration (148). Similarly, ophthalmic exposures result in pain, chemosis, and damage to conjunctiva and corneal epithelium (149).

The most consequential effects of HF poisoning are systemic. Systemic toxicity can result from ingestions or dermal exposures. Dermal exposures to concentrated HF covering as little as 2.5% body surface area have resulted in systemic toxicity, although typical fatal dermal exposures are larger (150,151). Fluoride ions scavenge divalent cations, causing life-threatening hypocalcemia and hypomagnesemia. Hyperkalemia may be seen as well (152). The electrocardiogram may reflect these electrolyte abnormalities. Lengthening of the QRS and QT intervals or presence of peaked T waves may be early indicators of toxicity. The proximal cause of death is usually dysrhythmias; ventricular fibrillation and sudden cardiac arrest have been described (153,154).

Management

The most important concern in small dermal injuries is pain control. The mainstay of therapy is calcium gluconate. The calcium derives its efficacy from binding fluoride ions. Calcium chloride should only be used topically. Should calcium extravasate, the solution itself can cause tissue damage. Other analgesics and regional anesthesia are not contraindicated, but calcium has the advantage of halting tissue damage in addition to providing pain relief. Following decontamination with water, calcium gluconate gel should be applied to the injured area. If the hands are involved, the gel can be held in contact by placing it in a sterile glove and putting the glove on the hand. Prepare the gel by mixing 25 mL of 10% calcium gluconate in 75 mL of water-based lubricant (155). If the wound is located in an area where compartment syndrome is not a concern, 0.5% calcium gluconate can be injected intradermally, 0.5 mL/cm^2 (151).

If these techniques fail to give relief, there is a role for careful use of intra-arterial calcium gluconate. The obvious advantage of this route is that calcium can be administered directly and by continuous infusion to the affected area. Add 10 mL of 10% calcium chloride to 40 mL of 0.9% sodium chloride and infuse over 4 hours (156). A nasogastric tube should be carefully placed, and any material in the stomach should be aspirated and followed by instillation of a calcium solution. The benefits of this practice are not established, but it seems reasonable in view of the severity of the ingestion and the relative safety of the intervention.

Intravenous calcium and magnesium should be given liberally, and electrolytes should be obtained hourly. Calcium can be administered as calcium gluconate or calcium chloride. One gram of calcium gluconate contains 4.5 mEq of elemental calcium, and 1 g of calcium chloride contains 13.6 mEq. Both calcium salts can produce vasodilation and dysrhythmias when administered too quickly. Intravenous calcium should be administered no faster than 0.7 to 1.8 mEq/minute (157). One patient required 267 mEq of calcium over 24 hours (158,159). Dysrhythmias should be expected in severely poisoned patients. Place defibrillator pads on the patient and perform continuous cardiac monitoring. In animal models, quinidine was protective after lethal doses of intravenous fluoride (160). When systemic toxicity occurs, electrolyte abnormalities are most severe in the first several hours of toxicity. Those who have no signs or symptoms of systemic toxicity for 24 hours can be transferred to a lower level of care.

ANTIDIABETIC AGENTS

Diabetes is characterized by an inability to maintain normal blood glucose concentration due to deficiency of insulin, resistance to insulin, or a combination of both. The medications used to treat diabetes are collectively known as *antidiabetic agents*, while a subset of these drugs are properly called *hypoglycemic agents*. The hypoglycemics include insulin and those drugs that promote the release of endogenous insulin. The terms hypoglycemic agents and antidiabetic agents are not synonymous, because many diabetic medications (metformin, thiazolidinediones) cannot produce hypoglycemia. In 2005, the AAPCC received reports of 8,695 exposures to sulfonylureas and biguanides, including 244 major exposures and 28 deaths (6).

The antidiabetics are a diverse group of drugs, but some important generalizations can be made. The sulfonylureas, meglitinides, and thiazolidinediones are very highly protein bound, and thus not amenable to extracorporeal removal. Insulin and metformin are completely renally eliminated, while most of the sulfonylureas have active hepatic metabolites with urinary excretion of both active metabolites and the parent drug. By far, the most important pharmacokinetic parameter of the hypoglycemics is duration of action. Of great clinical importance, the duration of action of insulin and the sulfonylureas is greatly increased in overdose. Insulin is available in multiple forms. Short-acting insulin preparations are designed to reduce postprandial hyperglycemia, while long-acting forms are intended to create a constant basal level of insulin. In therapeutic subcutaneous doses, lispro has onset of action within an hour and duration of action of less than 5 hours. Ultralente insulin, the longest-acting insulin commonly used, does not take effect for 4 to 6 hours but lasts as long as 36 hours (161). Regular insulin, lente, and NPH fall in between lispro and ultralente insulin. In overdose, the formation of depots of the drug in tissues can slow release and greatly prolong the duration of action. The vascularity of the site of injection will also influence the duration of hypoglycemia. The sulfonylureas generally have a duration of action of 12 to 24 hours in therapeutic doses. Chlorpropamide, a first-generation sulfonylurea, may promote insulin release for up to 72 hours (162). As in the case of insulin, the duration of action is prolonged in overdose, resulting in delayed hypoglycemia (163). Meglitinides, intended to prevent postprandial hyperglycemia, induce insulin release for only 1 to 4 hours. There is not yet enough data on their pharmacokinetics in overdose, but it appears likely that duration of action would be increased in overdose.

Clinical Manifestations

The most important signs and symptoms of the aptly classified hypoglycemics are manifestations of decreased serum glucose. The diagnosis of hypoglycemia is established by interpreting a serum glucose concentration in the context of a patient's clinical status. In one study, the serum glucose threshold for symptoms of hypoglycemia was 78 mg/dL in poorly controlled diabetics and 53 mg/dL in nondiabetics (164). Manifestations of hypoglycemia can be classified as either autonomic or neuroglycopenic. The former result from an increase in counterregulatory hormones (e.g., epinephrine), while the latter are due to a lack of glucose substrate available for the brain. The autonomic symptoms include tremor, diaphoresis, hunger, and nausea. Neuroglycopenic features of hypoglycemia can manifest as almost any conceivable neurologic deficit, including coma, agitation, seizure, hemiplegia, or mild confusion. Typically, the autonomic symptoms precede neuroglycopenic symptoms, thereby serving as a warning of hypoglycemia before the brain is deprived of a critical level of glucose. However, the autonomic symptoms may be blunted or absent in diabetics or patients taking β-adrenergic antagonists (165). The onset and duration of hypoglycemia is unpredictable after overdose.

Of less clinical importance, the hypoglycemics can also produce electrolyte abnormalities such as hypokalemia, hypomagnesemia, and hypophosphatemia (166). These are reported more frequently in very large insulin overdoses (167).

Metformin does not produce hypoglycemia itself, but is often formulated with drugs that do, such as glipizide or glyburide. Metformin and its biguanide predecessor, phenformin, are associated with lactic acidosis. The biguanides promote anaerobic metabolism and inhibit lactate metabolism (168). Lactic acidosis is rare, but is more likely in the setting of liver disease, renal insufficiency, heart failure, other acute illness, or acute overdose (169,170). Hepatotoxicity is reported from therapeutic use of thiazolidinediones and acarbose, but there are limited data on acute overdose of these drugs (171,172).

Management

A rapid bedside serum glucose concentration should be obtained as soon as hypoglycemia is considered. If the diagnosis of hypoglycemia is established, 1 g/kg intravenous dextrose should be given. Because high concentrations of dextrose can be irritating, children should receive 25% dextrose solution and infants 10% dextrose solution. As soon as a normal mental status is restored, the patient should be fed. Each 50-mL vial of 50% dextrose supplies 100 kcal of short-lived simple carbohydrate. In contrast, a meal will supply hundreds of "sustained-release" kilocalories. Glucagon should not be administered unless intravenous access is delayed and the patient cannot be fed. Glucagon will not be effective in patients with depleted glycogen stores.

If hypoglycemia recurs after it is initially corrected, the treatment is determined by the causative agent. Recurrent insulin-induced hypoglycemia should be treated with a dextrose infusion. Administer a 10% to 20% solution and titrate to maintain glucose in a normal range. A 5% dextrose solution is inappropriate for glucose maintenance.

Octreotide, a somatostatin analogue, is indicated for hypoglycemia following sulfonylurea use. Octreotide should be given subcutaneously, 50 μg every 6 hours (4–5 μg/kg/day in divided doses in children). Dextrose alone might not be sufficient to manage sulfonylurea-induced hypoglycemia. Because sulfonylureas potentiate endogenous β-islet cell insulin release, supplemental dextrose will induce more insulin release, with transient corrections and subsequent recurrence of hypoglycemia. Octreotide inhibits the β-islet cell calcium channel, inhibiting sulfonylurea-induced insulin release (173,174). There are no significant adverse effects of short-term octreotide use. Octreotide should be continued for 24 hours. After octreotide is discontinued, the patient should be observed for 24 hours. There are limited data in the literature regarding meglitinide toxicity. With a mechanism of action similar to the sulfonylureas, the meglitinides are shorter acting. Based on their shorter duration of action, we would expect they would be less likely to produce recurrent hypoglycemia, but we have no data to support this assumption. Until we have more experience with overdose of these drugs, it is prudent to manage meglitinide overdose similarly to sulfonylureas.

Metformin-associated lactic acidosis should be considered in patients taking an overdose of metformin, children exposed to more than one or two tablets, and those patients who take metformin therapeutically who also have renal insufficiency, hepatic insufficiency, heart failure, or another acute illness. The diagnosis is established by obtaining a serum chemistry, lactate concentration, and serum pH. The primary therapy is supportive. Although the role of bicarbonate in metformin-associated lactic acidosis is unclear, supplemental bicarbonate should be used to maintain the pH above 7.1. Although metformin is highly protein bound, hemodialysis can be used to correct refractory acidosis (175).

Adults who present with a history of sulfonylurea overdose and children who may have been exposed to sulfonylureas should be observed for 24 hours, even in the absence of hypoglycemia. Similarly, patients who present with hypoglycemia from long-acting forms of insulin should be observed for 24 hours as well.

NATURAL TOXINS

Plants

This brief discussion focuses on a few important plants that might necessitate intensive care management. In 2005, there were 76 major outcomes resulting from plant exposure that were reported to the AAPCC.

Belladonna Alkaloids

Plants such as jimsonweed (*Datura stramonium*) contain numerous anticholinergic compounds. They are used recreationally, often in the form of teas, for their hallucinatory effects. Toxicity is identified by the presence of anticholinergic symptoms: tachycardia; hyperthermia; dry, flushed skin; urinary retention; and agitation. One hundred jimsonweed seeds contain nearly 6 mg of atropine and similar alkaloids (176). In addition to supportive care, physostigmine can be given when the diagnosis is relatively certain. Physostigmine is administered 1 to 2 mg IV slowly over 5 minutes. Physostigmine should be discontinued and the diagnosis reconsidered if cholinergic symptoms develop. If there is improvement or no change in the patient's condition, physostigmine can be readministered after a 10- or 15-minute delay.

Nicotine and Nicotinelike Alkaloids

Nicotine poisoning occurs from inhaled, transdermal, and ingested nicotine. A dose of 1 mg/kg can be lethal in an adult (177). A cigarette contains 13 to 30 mg of nicotine, but most of it is not delivered to the smoker when the cigarette is used as intended. The largest portion of the nicotine is pyrolyzed but not inhaled. As much as 5 to 7 mg of nicotine remains in the cigarette butt, a potentially lethal dose for a child (178). Workers handling tobacco can be poisoned from nicotine as well (179). Signs and symptoms of nicotine toxicity result from activation and then inhibition (from overstimulation) of nicotinic receptors. Gastrointestinal signs include nausea, vomiting, and diarrhea. Early cardiovascular toxicity involves hypertension from nicotinic stimulation of the sympathetic ganglia, but hypotension eventually occurs. The most important signs and symptoms result from nicotinic agonist effects at the neuromuscular junction. Early toxicity causes fasciculation, which gives way to paralysis. Management is supportive. Vasoactive agents may be necessary to maintain blood pressure, and intubation may be indicated to support respiration during paralysis.

Cicutoxin

Cicutoxin is found in *Cicuta* spp. such as water hemlock. The toxin is found throughout the plant, which is often eaten by adults who misidentify it as wild parsley, turnip, or parsnip (180). The mechanism of cicutoxin poisoning is unclear. Early symptoms are primarily gastrointestinal and begin soon after ingestion. Later, cicutoxin can cause status epilepticus, renal failure, and rhabdomyolysis (181).

Sodium Channel–altering Plants

Aconitine, from *Aconitum* spp., opens sodium channels, increasing cellular excitability (180,182). Increased sodium influx delays repolarization, which in turn delays conduction. Slow conduction of peripheral nerves can lead to decreased sensation, weakness, paralysis, and CNS seizures. Vagal and cardiac myocyte sodium channel effects lead to bradycardia, atrioventricular blockade, increased automaticity, or asystole. Aconitine is found in *Aconitum napellus* (monkshood) and Chinese herbal remedies. Management is supportive. Gastrointestinal decontamination should be performed. Cardiac complications have been successfully managed with a ventricular assist device (183).

Mushrooms

Forty-six major outcomes and six deaths from mushroom ingestions were reported to poison control centers in 2005 (6). The vast majority of mushroom exposures do not result in significant morbidity, and most of the fatalities that occur are caused by only a few of the many mushroom species in North America. Identification of mushrooms is challenging and best left to the mycologist. However, because each of the clinically important toxic mushrooms causes a distinct clinical syndrome, the physician should be able to identify the toxicologic manifestations of several mushrooms. Mushroom toxins have been divided into ten groups (184). We will discuss the most common exposures and those most likely to require ICU care.

Gastrointestinal Toxin–containing Mushrooms

Most reported exposures are to mushrooms containing gastrointestinal toxins. Hundreds of types of mushrooms fall into this category. The most notable clinical feature of ingestion of these mushrooms is the development of vomiting and diarrhea within several hours of ingestion. With few exceptions, mushrooms that cause gastrointestinal symptoms within 6 hours belong to this category and will not cause life-threatening symptoms. The early onset of vomiting following exposure to gastrointestinal toxin–containing mushrooms clinically differentiates them from the cyclopeptide-containing mushrooms. Treatment of exposure to these mushrooms is supportive, and symptoms are generally self-limited. These mushrooms rarely lead to toxicity requiring ICU admission.

Cyclopeptide-containing Mushrooms

Three of five fatalities from mushrooms in 2004 were related to cyclopeptide-containing mushrooms. Historically, mortality from these mushrooms is high, although improvements in critical care have improved the prognosis. The most prominent member of this group is *Amanita phalloides* and other *Amanita* species. *Amanita phalloides* contains numerous cyclopeptides, but the most important are a group called the amatoxins. Amatoxins are heat stable and present in lethal concentrations in mushrooms as small as 20 g (184).

Clinical Manifestations and Management. Amatoxins cause endocrine, renal, and CNS injury, but the hepatic effects are the most consequential. Patients will be asymptomatic for the first few hours after ingestion. In 5 to 24 hours, patients will have watery diarrhea. Hepatic toxicity is evident on day 2 with elevations in bilirubin, AST, and ALT. Signs of fulminant hepatic failure such as encephalopathy and coagulopathy follow. Hypoglycemia results not just from hepatic failure, but from direct pancreatic toxicity (185). Cyclopeptides may also cause decreased levels of thyroid hormone and increased calcitonin.

Because patients do not seek help until symptoms develop, it is not uncommon for patients to present to a healthcare facility with volume depletion and early hepatic injury. Good supportive care and prevention of secondary complications are the keys to management. Activated charcoal should be administered 1 g/kg every 2 to 4 hours in order to adsorb any toxin remaining in the gut and interrupt the potential enterohepatic circulation (186). Many therapies to mitigate hepatotoxicity have been investigated, with no substantial or reproducible evidence of efficacy.

Although there are no data to support its use in *Amanita* poisoning, NAC effectively treats hepatic failure from other hepatotoxins, such as acetaminophen. Administer NAC intravenously, according to the acetaminophen protocol: 150 mg/kg over 45 minutes, 50 mg/kg over 4 hours, and 100 mg/kg over 16 hours. Continue the final infusion until the patient expires, definitively recovers, or receives liver transplant.

Silibinin, extracted from milk thistle, improved hepatic markers and mortality in a dog model of *Amanita* poisoning, but was not found beneficial in a meta-analysis of human studies (187). Because a clinical trial will likely never be conducted, and in light of its experimental benefits, we recommend orally administered silibinin, 20 to 50 mg/kg/day. Silibinin is not a Food and Drug Administration–approved drug, but is available at health food stores.

High-dose penicillin had some effectiveness in a dog model of *Amanita* poisoning, possibly by blocking hepatocyte uptake of amatoxin (188). Therapy includes intravenous penicillin G, 1 million units/kg/day in divided doses (189).

The criteria for liver transplantation have not been clearly established. Transplantation is not without risk, and those who survive fulminant hepatic failure from *Amanita* without transplantation are expected to make a full recovery. Ideally, the decision to transplant should be delayed until it is clear the patient will not recover. Some consider transplantation for those with encephalopathy and prolonged PT, persistent hypoglycemia, metabolic acidosis, increased serum ammonia, aminotransferases, and hypofibrinogenemia (184). Patients should be referred to transplantation centers early in their clinical course so that they may be listed early, and transport should be avoided when they are gravely ill.

Gyromitrin-containing Mushrooms

Gyromitra mushrooms are found throughout the United States. These mushrooms contain gyromitrin (*N*-methyl-*N*-formyl hydrazone), which is hydrolyzed to monomethylhydrazine (MMH). MMH inhibits the formation of pyridoxal-5′-phosphate (PLP), an enzyme cofactor synthesized from pyridoxine (vitamin B_6). Of great importance, PLP is a cofactor for glutamic acid decarboxylase, the enzyme in the CNS that converts glutamate to GABA. Inhibition of PLP by monomethylhydrazine results in excessive excitation relative to inhibition.

Clinical Manifestations and Management. The initial phase of toxicity, occurring 5 to 10 hours after ingestion, is manifest by nonspecific clinical features including nausea, vomiting, diarrhea, and headache, and ultimately leads to intractable seizures (184). Patients ingesting *Gyromitra* spp. should receive activated charcoal, 1 g/kg. Seizures may not respond to benzodiazepines alone. If *Gyromitra* spp. ingestion is considered, or if a patient presents with seizures after mushroom ingestion, pyridoxine 70 mg/kg IV should be given. Pyridoxine serves as substrate for pyridoxine phosphokinase, allowing some PLP to be generated despite inhibition by MMH.

Allenic Norleucine–containing Mushrooms

The nephrotoxic *Amanita smithiana* contains the amino acid toxins allenic norleucine (amino-hexadienoic acid) and possibly 1-2-amino-4-pentynoic acid (184). All known exposures to these mushrooms have occurred in the Pacific Northwestern United States. These serve as important exceptions to the "rule" that mushrooms that cause early gastrointestinal toxicity do not cause significant end-organ damage later.

Clinical Manifestations and Management. Initial symptoms, which include nausea, vomiting, diarrhea, and abdominal cramping, may begin within an hour of ingestion. The most important clinical features of toxicity develop later. Acute renal failure, indicated by elevations in blood urea nitrogen (BUN) and creatinine, manifest 4 to 6 days following ingestion (190).

Activated charcoal should be administered when patients present after ingesting mushrooms from the Pacific Northwest. Management of nephrotoxicity is supportive. Patients who required hemodialysis underwent the procedure two to three times per week for approximately 1 month (184).

Orellanine- and Orellinine-containing Mushrooms

Cortinarius orellanus, found in North America, contains the toxin orellanine, which is converted by photochemical degradation to another toxin, orellinine (184). Orellanine and orellinine are important causes of mushroom-induced nephrotoxicity. Orellanine is activated by the P450 system. These molecules generate oxidative damage by sustained redox cycling.

Clinical Manifestations and Management. Symptoms begin 24 to 36 hours after ingestion. Patients report headache, chills, polydipsia, nausea, and vomiting. Early laboratory findings of hematuria, leukocyturia, and proteinuria indicate interstitial nephritis. Later, renal failure develops, characterized histologically by tubular damage and fibrosis of tubules with relative glomerular sparing (191,192). Hepatotoxicity is an uncommon feature.

Management is supportive. Administer activated charcoal if patients present early. Some patients will rapidly improve, whereas others require chronic hemodialysis (193).

TREATMENT REFUSAL

Patents with toxicologic emergencies are often suicidal and self-destructive, and may have an altered level of consciousness. We have an ethical obligation to our patients to allow them to guide their own treatment. At times, this means that the patient will decide against the physician's recommendation. In order to refuse care, the patient must demonstrate the capacity to understand his or her condition and the implications of treatment refusal. The refusal must be voluntary in the absence of a medical or psychiatric condition precluding the ability to make such a decision. The hospital has the right to physically restrain a person who has an altered level of consciousness for the purpose of evaluation and intervention (194).

There is a potential for legal liability whenever the medical staff physically restrain a patient, retain a patient against his or her will, or allow a patient to refuse a life-saving therapy. The physician and hospital staff can reduce liability by thoroughly documenting the patient's decision-making process and by involving psychiatric consultation in determining the patient's capacity. When in doubt, the physician should consult the hospital's legal department.

OTHER RESOURCES

This chapter is intended to be a review of common and consequential xenobiotic exposures. *Goldfrank's Toxicologic Emergencies* (McGraw-Hill, 2006) contains a more comprehensive review of all the substances discussed here. The regional poison center (1-800-222-1222) is an excellent resource for further information and recommendations specific to your patient.

Owing a great deal to the success of prevention measures, significant poisonings are relatively rare events. In 2005, there were fewer than 20,000 patients with major effects and deaths reported to the AAPCC. Although this figure underestimates total poisoning, it represents a very small number of patients per hospital per year. Because each ICU sees a paucity of these patients, many critical care physicians do not see enough of them to develop familiarity with their care. We encourage close collaboration between ICU physicians, regional poison centers, and toxicologists to provide the best possible care to poisoned patients.

References

1. Timbrell JA. *Introduction to Toxicology.* London: Taylor & Francis; 1989.
2. Anonymous. *American Heritage Dictionary.* 2nd college ed. Boston: Houghton Mifflin; 1991.
3. Deichmann WB, Henschler D, Holmsted B, et al. What is there that is not poison? A study of the Third Defense by Paracelsus. *Arch Toxicol.* 1986; 58:207–213.
4. Press E, Mellins RB. A poisoning control program. *J Psychedelic Drugs.* 1954;44:1515–1525.
5. Linakis JG, Frederick KA. Poisoning deaths not reported to the regional poison control center. *Ann Emerg Med.* 1993;22:1859–1860.
6. Lai MW, et al. 2005 Annual Report of the American Association of Poison Control Centers' National Poisoning and Exposure Database. *Clin Toxicol.* 2006;44:803–932.
7. Ashbourne JF, Olson KR, Khayam-Bashi H. Value of rapid screening for acetaminophen in all patients with intentional drug overdose. *Ann Emerg Med.* 1989;18(10):1035–1038.
8. Kirk MA, Pope JS. Use of the intensive care unit. In: Flomenbaum NE, Goldfrank LR, Hoffman RS, et al., eds. *Goldfrank's Toxicologic Emergencies.* 8th ed. New York: McGraw-Hill; 2006:173–181.
9. Larson AM, Polson J, Fontana RJ, et al. Acetaminophen-induced acute liver failure: results of a United States multicenter, prospective study. *Hepatology.* 2005;42:1364–1372.
10. Graham GG, Kieran FS. Mechanism of action of paracetamol. *Am J Ther.* 2005;12:46–55.
11. Hendrickson RG, Bizovi KE. Acetaminophen. In: Flomenbaum NE, Goldfrank LR, Hoffman RS, et al., eds. *Goldfrank's Toxicologic Emergencies.* 8th ed. New York: McGraw-Hill; 2006:523–543.
12. Prescott LF. Absorption of paracetamol. In: Prescott LF, et al. *Paracetamol (Acetaminophen). A Critical Bibliographic Review.* London: Taylor & Francis; 1996:33–59.

13. Tighe TV, Walter FG. Delayed toxic acetaminophen level after initial four hour nontoxic level. *J Toxicol Clin Toxicol.* 1994;32:431–434.
14. Prescott LF. Kinetics and metabolism of paracetamol and phenacetin. *Br J Clin Pharmacol.* 1980;10(Suppl 2):291S–298S.
15. Howland MA. Antidotes in depth: N-acetylcysteine. In: Flomenbaum NE, Goldfrank LR, Hoffman RS, et al., eds. *Goldfrank's Toxicologic Emergencies.* 8th ed. New York: McGraw-Hill; 2006:544–549.
16. Rumack BH, Peterson RG, Koch GG, et al. Acetaminophen overdose. 662 cases with evaluation of oral acetylcysteine treatment. *Arch Intern Med.* 1981;141:380–385.
17. Singer AJ, Carracio TR, Mofenson HC. The temporal profile of increased transaminase levels in patients with acetaminophen-induced liver dysfunction. *Ann Emerg Med.* 1995;26:49–53.
18. Rumack BH, Matthew H. Acetaminophen poisoning and toxicity. *Pediatrics.* 1975;55:871–876.
19. Smilkstein MJ, Rumack BH. Efficacy of oral N-acetylcysteine in the treatment of acetaminophen overdose: analysis of the national multicenter study (1976–1985). *N Engl J Med.* 1988;3190:1557–1562.
20. Kuffner EK, Dart RC, Bogdan GM, et al. Effect of maximal daily doses of acetaminophen on the liver of alcoholic patients: a randomized, double-blind, placebo-controlled trial. *Arch Intern Med.* 2001;161:2247–2252.
21. Watkins PB, Kaplowitz N, Slattery JT, et al. Aminotransferase elevations in healthy adults receiving 4 grams of acetaminophen daily. *JAMA.* 2006;296:87–93.
22. Keays R, Harrison PM, Wendon JA, et al. Intravenous acetylcysteinein paracetamol induced fulminant hepatic failure: a prospective controlled trial. *BMJ.* 1991;202:1026–1029.
23. O'Grady JG, Alexander GJM, Hayllar KM, et al. Early indicators of prognosis in fulminant hepatic failure. *Gastroenterology.* 1989;97:439–445.
24. Schmidt LE, Dalhoff K. Serum phosphate is an early predictor of outcome in severe acetaminophen-induced hepatotoxicity. *Hepatology.* 2002;36:659–665.
25. Tenney SM, Miller RM. The respiratory and circulatory action of salicylate. *Am J Med.* 1955;19:498–508.
26. Krebs HG, Woods HG, Alberti KG. Hyperlactemia and lactic acidosis. *Essays Med Biochem.* 1975;1:81–103.
27. Johnson D, Eppler J, Giesbrecht E, et al. Effect of multiple-dose activated charcoal on the clearance of high-dose intravenous aspirin in a porcine model. *Ann Emerg Med.* 1995;26:569–574.
28. Morgan AG, Polak A. The excretion of salicylate in salicylate poisoning. *Clin Sci.* 1971;41:475–484.
29. Wax PM. Antidotes in depth: sodium bicarbonate. In: Flomenbaum NE, Goldfrank LR, Hoffman RS, et al., eds. *Goldfrank's Toxicologic Emergencies.* 8th ed. New York: McGraw-Hill; 2006:565–572.
30. Perazella MA, Eras J. Are selective COX-2 inhibitors nephrotoxic? *Am J Kidney Dis.* 2000;35:937–940.
31. Seifert SA, Bronstein AC, McGuire T. Massive ibuprofen ingestion with survival. *Clin Toxicol.* 2000;38:55–57.
32. Lutz EG. Cardiotoxic effects of psychotropic drugs. *J Med Soc NJ.* 1976; 73:105–112.
33. Wech R, Chue P. Antipsychotic agents and QT changes [review]. *J Psychiatry Neurosci.* 2000;25:154–160.
34. Juurilink D. Antipsychotics. In: Flomenbaum NE, Goldfrank LR, Hoffman RS, et al., eds. *Goldfrank's Toxicologic Emergencies.* 8th ed. New York: McGraw-Hill; 2006:1039–1051.
35. Velamoor VR, Norman RM, Caroff SN, et al. Progression of symptoms in neuroleptic malignant syndrome. *J Nerv Ment Dis.* 1994;3:168–173.
36. Dematte JE, O'Mara K, Buescher J, et al. Near-fatal heat stroke during the 1995 heat wave in Chicago. *Ann Intern Med.* 1998;129:173–181.
37. Allan AM, Zhang X, Baier LD. Barbiturate tolerance: effects on GABA-operated chloride channel function. *Brain Res.* 1992;588:255–260.
38. Höjer J, Baehrendtz S. The effect of flumazenil (Ro15-1788) in the management of self-induced benzodiazepine poisoning: a double-blind controlled study. *Acta Med Scand.* 1988;224:357–365.
39. Amrein R, Leishman B, Bentzinger C, et al. Flumazenil in benzodiazepine antagonism: actions and clincal use in intoxications and anaesthesiology. *Med Toxicol.* 1987;2:411–429.
40. Wolfe TR, Caravati EM, Rollins DE, et al. Terminal 40-ms frontal plane QRS axis as a marker for tricyclic antidepressant overdose. *Ann Emerg Med.* 1989;18:348–351.
41. Liebelt EL. Cyclic antidepressants. In: Flomenbaum NE, Goldfrank LR, Hoffman RS, et al., eds. *Goldfrank's Toxicologic Emergencies.* 8th ed. New York: McGraw-Hill; 2006:1083–1097.
42. Boehnert M, Lovejoy FH. Value of the QRS duration versus the serum drug level in predicting seizures and ventricular arrhythmias after an acute overdose of tricyclic antidepressants. *N Engl J Med.* 1985;313:474–479.
43. Niemann JT, Bessen HA, Rothstein RJ, et al. Electrocardiographic criteria for tricyclic antidepressant cardiotoxicity. *Am J Cardiol.* 1986;57:1154–1159.
44. Kingston ME. Hyperventilation in tricyclic antidepressant poisoning. *Crit Care Med.* 1979;7:550–551.
45. McCabe JL, Cobaugh DJ, Menegazzi JJ, et al. Experimental tricyclic antidepressant toxicity: a randomized controlled comparison of hypertonic saline solution, sodium bicarbonate, and hyperventilation. *Ann Emerg Med.* 1998;32:329–333.
46. Callaham M, Schumaker H, Pentel P. Phenytoin prophylaxis of cardiotoxicity in experimental amitryptiline poisoning. *J Pharmacol Exp Ther.* 1988; 245:216–220.
47. Brunello N, Tascedda F. Cellular mechanisms and second messengers: relevance to the psychopharmacology of bipolar disorders. *Int J Neuropsychopharmacol.* 2003;6:181–189.
48. Timmer RT, Sands JM. Lithium intoxication. *J Am Soc Nephrol.* 1999; 10:666–674.
49. Brust JC, Hammer JS, Challenor Y, et al. Acute generalized polyneuropathy accompanying lithium poisoning. *Ann Neurol.* 1989;6:360–362.
50. Adityanjee, Munshi KR, Thampy A. The syndrome of irreversible lithium-effectuated neurotoxicity. *Clin Neuropharmacol.* 2005;28:38–49.
51. Linakis JG, Lacouture PG, Eisenberg MS, et al. Administration of activated charcoal or sodium polystyrene sulfonate (kayexelate) as gastric decontamination for lithium intoxication: an animal model. *Pharmacol Toxicol.* 1989;65:387–389.
52. Smith SW, Ling LJ, Haltenson CE. Whole-bowel irrigation as a treatment for acute lithium overdose. *Ann Emerg Med.* 1991;20:536–539.
53. Goodman DJ, Rossen RM, Ingham R, et al. Sinus node function in the denervated human heart. Effect of digitalis. *Br J Heart.* 1975;37:612–618.
54. Cooke D. The use of central nervous system manifestations in the early detection of digitalis toxicity. *Heart Lung.* 1993;22:477–481.
55. Gorelick DA, Kussin SZ, Kahn I. Paranoid delusions and auditory hallucinations associated with digoxin intoxication. *J Nerv Ment Dis.* 1978;166: 817–819.
56. Rosen MR, Wit AL, Hoffman BF. Cardiac antiarrhythmic and toxic effects of digitalis. *Am Heart J.* 1975;89:391–399.
57. Bismuth C, Gaultier M, Conso F, et al. Hyperkalemia in acute digitalis poisoning: prognostic significance and therapeutic implications. *Clin Toxicol.* 1973;6:153–162.
58. Hickey AR, Wenger TL, Carpenter VP, et al. Digoxin Immune Fab therapy in the management of digitalis intoxication: safety and efficacy results of an observational surveillance study. *J Am Coll Cardiol.* 1991;17:590–598.
59. Hack JB, Lewin NA. Cardioactive steroids. In: Flomenbaum NE, Goldfrank LR, Hoffman RS, et al., eds. *Goldfrank's Toxicologic Emergencies.* 8th ed. New York: McGraw-Hill; 2006:971–982.
60. Curd J, Smith TW, Jaton J, et al. The isolation of digoxin specific antibody and its use in reversing the specific effects of digoxin. *Proc Natl Acad Sci U S A.* 1971;68:2401–2406.
61. Brubacher J. β-Adrenergic antagonists. In: Flomenbaum NE, Goldfrank LR, Hoffman RS, et al., eds. *Goldfrank's Toxicologic Emergencies.* 8th ed. New York: McGraw-Hill; 2006:924–941.
62. Reith DM, Dawson AH, Epid D, et al. Relative toxicity of beta blockers in overdose. *J Toxicol Clin Toxicol.* 1996;34:273–278.
63. Henry JA, Cassidy SL. Membrane stabilizing activity: a major cause of fatal poisoning. *Lancet.* 1986;1:1414–1417.
64. Love JN, Elshami J. Cardiovascular depression resulting from atenolol intoxication. *European J Emerg Med.* 2002;9:111–114.
65. Neuvonen PJ, Elonen E, Vuorenmaa T, et al. Prolonged QT interval and severe tachyarrhythmias, common features of sotalol intoxication. *Eur J Clin Pharmacol.* 1981;20:85–89.
66. Pitt B. Diversity of calcium antagonists. *Clin Ther.* 1997;19(Suppl A):3–17.
67. Enyeart JJ, Price WA, Hoffman DA, et al. Profound hyperglycemia and metabolic acidosis after verapamil overdose. *J Am Coll Cardiol.* 1983;2: 1228–1231.
68. Ramoska EA, Spiller HA, Myers A. Calcium channel blocker toxicity. *Ann Emerg Med.* 1990;19:649–653.
69. Hariman RJ, Mangiardi LM, McAllister RG. Reversal of cardiovascular effects of verapamil by calcium and sodium: differences between electrophysiologic and hemodynamic responses. *Circulation.* 1979;59:797–804.
70. Love JN, Hanfling D, Howell JM. Hemodynamic effects of calcium chloride in a canine model of acute propranolol intoxication. *Ann Emerg Med.* 1996;28:1–6.
71. DeRoos F. Calcium channel blockers. In: Flomenbaum NE, Goldfrank LR, Hoffman RS, et al., eds. *Goldfrank's Toxicologic Emergencies.* 8th ed. New York: McGraw-Hill; 2006:911–923.
72. Yagami T. Differential coupling of glucagon and beta-adrenergic receptors with the small and large forms of the stimulatory G protein. *Mol Pharmacol.* 1995;48:849–854.
73. Brubacher J. β-adrenergic antagonists. In: Flomenbaum NE, Goldfrank LR, Hoffman RS, et al., eds. *Goldfrank's Toxicologic Emergencies.* 8th ed. New York: McGraw-Hill; 2006:924–940.
74. Farah AE, Alousi AA. The actions of insulin on cardiac contractility. *Life Sci.* 1981;29:975–1000.
75. Kline JA, Raymond RM, Leonova E, et al. Insulin improves heart function and metabolism during non-ischemic cardiogenic shock in awake canines. *Cardiovasc Res.* 1997;34:289–298.
76. Yuan TH, Kerns WP, Tomaszewski CA, et al. Insulin-glucose as adjunctive therapy for severe calcium channel antagonist poisoning. *J Toxicol Clin Toxicol.* 1999;37:463–474.
77. Kerns W 2nd, Schroeder D, Williams C, et al. Insulin improves survival in a canine model of acute beta-blocker toxicity. *Ann Emerg Med.* 1997; 29:748–757.

78. Sivilotti MLA, Burns MJ, McMartin KE, et al. Toxicokinetics of ethylene glycol during fomepizole therapy: implications for management. *Ann Emerg Med.* 2000;36:114–124.
79. Brent J, McMartin K, Phillips S, et al. Fomepizole for the treatment of methanol poisoning. *N Engl J Med.* 2001;344:424–429.
80. Palatnick W, Redman LW, Sitar DS, et al. Methanol half life during ethanol administration: implications for management of methanol poisoning. *Ann Emerg Med.* 1995;26:202–207.
81. Dyer S, Mycyk MB, Ahrens WR, et al. Hemorrhagic gastritis from topical isopropanol exposure. *Ann Pharmacother.* 2002;36:1733–1735.
82. Treichel JL, Murray TG, Lewandowski MF, et al. Formate, the toxic metabolite of methanol, in cultured ocular cells. *Neurotoxicology.* 2003;2: 825–834.
83. McMartin KE, Cenac TA. Toxicity of ethylene glycol metabolites in normal human kidney cells. *Ann N Y Acad Sci.* 2000;919:315–317.
84. Hoffman RS, Smilkstein MJ, Howland MA, et al. Osmol gaps revisited: normal values and limitations. *J Toxicol Clin Toxicol.* 1993;31:81–93.
85. Jacobsen D, Hewlett TP, Webb R, et al. Ethylene glycol intoxication: evaluation of kinetics and crystalluria. *Am J Med.* 1988;84:145–152.
86. Casavant MJ, Shah MN, Battels R. Does fluorescent urine indicate antifreeze ingestion by children? *Pediatrics.* 2001;107:113–114.
87. Howland MA. Antidotes in depth: ethanol. In: Flomenbaum NE, Goldfrank LR, Hoffman RS, et al., eds. *Goldfrank's Toxicologic Emergencies.* 8th ed. New York: McGraw-Hill; 2006:1465–1468.
88. Chaudry R, Lall SB, Baijayantimal M, et al. A foodborne outbreak of organophosphate poisoning. *BMJ.* 1998;17:268–269.
89. Nolan RJ, Rick DL, Freshour NL, et al. Chlorpyrifos: pharmacokinetics in human volunteers. *Toxicol Appl Pharmacol.* 1984;73:8–15.
90. Casper HH, Pekas JC. Absorption and excretion of radiolabeled 1-naphthyl-N-methylcarbamate (carbaryl) by the rat. *NY Acad Sci.* 1971; 24:160–161.
91. Nye DE, Dorough HW. Fate of insecticides administered endotracheally to rats. *Bull Environ Contam Toxicol.* 1976;15:291–296.
92. Clark RF. Insecticides: organic phosphorous compounds and carbamates. In: Flomenbaum NE, Goldfrank LR, Hoffman RS, et al., eds. *Goldfrank's Toxicologic Emergencies.* 8th ed. New York: McGraw-Hill; 2006:1497–1512.
93. Gallo MA, Lawryk NJ. Organic phosphorous pesticides. In: Hayes WJ, Laws ER, eds. *Handbook of Pesticide Toxicology.* San Diego, CA: Academic Press; 1991:917–100.
94. Harris LW, Talbot BG, Lennox WJ, et al. The relationship between oxime-induced reactivation of carbamylated anticholinesterase and antidotal efficacy against carbamate intoxication. *Toxicol Appl Phamacol.* 1989;98:128–133.
95. Howland MA. Antidotes in depth: pralidoxime. In: Flomenbaum NE, Goldfrank LR, Hoffman RS, et al., eds. *Goldfrank's Toxicologic Emergencies.* 8th ed. New York: McGraw-Hill; 2006:1513–1522.
96. Murphy MR, Blick DW, Dunn MA, et al. Diazepam as a treatment for nerve agent poisoning in primates. *Aviat Space Environ Med.* 1993;64:110–115.
97. De Luca CJ, Buccafusco JJ, Roy SH, et al. The electromyographic signal as a presynaptic indicator of organophosphates in the body. *Muscle Nerve.* 2006;33:369–376.
98. Senanayake N, Karalliedde L. Neurotoxic effects of organophosphate insecticides: an intermediate syndrome. *N Engl J Med.* 1987;316:761–763.
99. He F, Xu H, Qin F, et al. Intermediate myasthenia syndrome following acute organophosphate poisoning—an analysis of 21 cases. *Human Exp Toxicol.* 1998;17:40–45.
100. Merrill DG, Mihm FG. Prolonged toxicity of organophosphate poisoning. *Crit Care Med.* 1982;10:550–551.
101. Way JL. Cyanide intoxication and its mechanism of antagonism. *Annu Rev Pharmacol Toxicol.* 1984;24:451–481.
102. Baud FJ, Borron SW, Megarbane B, et al. Value of lactic acidosis in the assessment of the severity of acute cyanide poisoning. *Crit Care Med.* 2002;30:2044–2050.
103. Chen KK, Rose C. Nitrite and thiosulfate therapy in cyanide poisoning. *JAMA.* 1952;149:113–119.
104. Howland MA. Sodium and amyl nitrites. In: Flomenbaum NE, Goldfrank LR, Hoffman RS, et al., eds. *Goldfrank's Toxicologic Emergencies.* 8th ed. New York: McGraw-Hill; 2006:1725–1727.
105. Marrs TC. Antidotal treatment of acute cyanide poisoning. *Adverse Drug React Acute Poisoning Rev.* 1988;7:179–206.
106. Hall AH, Rumack BH. Hydroxycobalamin/sodium thiosulfate as a cyanide antidote. *J Emerg Med.* 1987:115–121.
107. Agarwal PK, Kumari R. Nitroprusside in critically ill patients with aortic stenosis. 2003;349:811–813.
108. Pahl MV, Vaziri ND. In-vivo and in-vitro hemodialysis studies of thiocyanate. *J Toxicol Clin Toxicol.* 1982;19:965–974.
109. Prchal JT, Borgese N, Moore MR, et al. Congenital methemoglobinemia due to methemoglobin reductase deficiency in two unrelated American black families. *Am J Med.* 1990;89:516–522.
110. Greer FR, Shannon M. Infant methemoglobin: the role dietary nitrate in food and water. *Pediatrics.* 2005;116:784–786.
111. Price D. Methemoglobin inducers. In: Flomenbaum NE, Goldfrank LR, Hoffman RS, et al., eds. *Goldfrank's Toxicologic Emergencies.* 8th ed. New York: McGraw-Hill; 2006:1734–1745.
112. Barker SJ, Tremper KK, Hyatt J. Effects of methemoglobinemia on pulse oximetry and mixed venous oximetry. *Anesthesiology.* 1989;70:112–117.
113. Yano SS, Danish EH, Hsia YE. Transient methemoglobinemia with acidosis in infants. *J Pediatr.* 1982;100:415–418.
114. Hanukoglo A, Danon PN. Endogenous methemoglobinemia associated with diarrheal disease in infancy. *J Pediatr Gastroenterol Nutr.* 1996;23:1–7.
115. Ash-Bernal R, Wise R, Scott M. Acquired methemoglobinemia: a retrospective series of 138 cases at two teaching hospitals. *Medicine.* 2004;83:265–273.
116. Rhodes LE, Tingle MD, Park BK, et al. Cimetidine improves the therapeutic/toxic ratio of dapsone in patients on chronic dapsone therapy. *Br J Dermatol.* 1995;132:257–262.
117. Miro O, Casademont J, Barrientos A, et al. Mitochondrial cytochrome c oxidase inhibition during acute carbon monoxide poisoning. *Pharmacol Toxicol.* 1998;82:199–202.
118. Thom SR, Ohnishi ST, Ischiropoulos H. Nitric oxide release by platelets inhibits neutrophil B2 integrin function following acute carbon monoxide poisoning. *Toxicol Appl Pharmacol.* 1994;128:105–110.
119. Thom SR. Carbon monoxide-mediated brain lipid peroxidation in the rat. *J Appl Physiol.* 1990;68:997–1003.
120. Coburn RF, Ploegmakers P, Gondrie P, et al. Myocardial myoglobin oxygen tension. *Am J Physiol.* 1973;224:870.
121. Stewart RD. Paint remover hazard. *JAMA.* 1976;235:398–401.
122. Marius-Nunez AL. Myocardial infarction with normal coronary arteries after acute exposure to carbon monoxide. *Chest.* 1990;97:491–494.
123. Bozeman WP, Myers RA, Barish RA. Confirmation of the pulse oximetry gap in carbon monoxide poisoning. *Ann Emerg Med.* 1997;30: 608–611.
124. Stewart R, Baretta ED, Platte LR, et al. Carboxyhemoglobin levels in American blood donors. *JAMA.* 1974;229:1187–1195.
125. Raphael JC, Elkharrat D, Jars-Guincestre MC, et al. Trial of normobaric and hyperbaric oxygen for acute carbon monoxide intoxication. *Lancet.* 1989;8660:414–419.
126. Choi IS. Delayed neurologic sequelae in carbon monoxide intoxication. *Arch Neurol.* 1983;40:433–435.
127. Henry CR, Satran D, Lindgren B, et al. Myocardial injury and long-term mortality following moderate to severe carbon monoxide poisoning. *JAMA.* 2006;295:398–402.
128. Nardizzi LR. Computerized tomographic correlate of carbon monoxide poisoning. *Arch Neurol.* 1979;36:38–39.
129. Tom T, Abedon S, Clark RI, et al. Neuroimaging characteristics in carbon monoxide toxicity. *J Neuroimag.* 1996;6:161–166.
130. Tomaszewski C. Carbon monoxide. In: Flomenbaum NE, Goldfrank LR, Hoffman RS, et al., eds. *Goldfrank's Toxicologic Emergencies.* 8th ed. New York: McGraw-Hill; 2006:1689–1704.
131. Thom SR. Antagonism of carbon monoxide-mediated brain lipid peroxidation in the rat. *J Appl Physiol.* 1990;68:997–1003.
132. Brown SD, Piantodosi CA. Recovery of energy metabolism in rat brain after carbon monoxide hypoxia. *J Clin Invest.* 1991;89:666–672.
133. Goulon M, Barios A, Raphin M, et al. Carbon monoxide poisoning and acute anoxia due to breathing coal gas and hydrocarbons. *Ann Med Intern.* 1969;120:335–349.
134. Engel RR, Rodkey FL, O'Neal JD, et al. Relative affinity of human fetal hemoglobin for carbon monoxide. *Blood.* 1969;33:37–45.
135. Van Hoesen KB, Camporesi EM, Moon RE, et al. Should hyperbaric oxygen be used to treat the pregnant patient for acute carbon monoxide poisoning? A case report and literature review. *JAMA.* 1989;261:1039–1043.
136. Koren G, Sharav T, Patuszak A, et al. A multicenter, prospective study of fetal outcome following accidental maternal carbon monoxide poisoning in pregnancy. *Reprod Toxicol.* 1991;5:397–403.
137. Ashcraft KW, Padula RT. The effect of dilute corrosives on the esophagus. *Pediatrics.* 1974;53:226–232.
138. Zargar SA, Kochlar R, Nagi B, et al. Ingestion of corrosive acids: spectrum of injury to upper gastrointestinal tract and natural history. *Gastroenterology.* 1989;97:702–707.
139. Kirsch MM, Peterson A, Brown JW, et al. Treatment of caustic injuries of the esophagus: a ten-year experience. *Ann Surg.* 1978;188:675–678.
140. Christensen BT. Prediction of complications following unintentional caustic ingestion in children. Is endoscopy always necessary? *Acta Paediatr.* 1995; 84:1178–1182.
141. Previtera C, Guisti F, Guglielmi M. Predictive value of visible lesions (cheeks, lips, oropharynx) in suspected caustic ingestion: may endoscopy be reasonably omitted in completely negative pediatric patients? *Pediatr Emerg Care.* 1990;6:176–178.
142. Crain EF, Gershel JC, Mezey AP. Caustic ingestions—symptoms as predictors of esophageal injury. *Am J Dis Child.* 1984;138:863–865.
143. Lamireau T, Rebouissoux L, Denis D, et al. Accidental caustic ingestion in children: is endoscopy always mandatory? *J Pediatr Gastroenterol Nutr.* 2001;33:81–84.
144. Wu MH, Lai WW. Surgical management of extensive corrosive injuries of the alimentary tract. *Surg Gynecol Obstet.* 1993;177:12–16.
145. Berkovits RN, Bos CE, Wijburg FA, et al. Caustic injury of the oesophagus. Sixteen years' experience and introduction of a new model oesophageal stent. *J Laryngol Otol.* 1996;110:1041–1045.

146. Pelclova D, Navratil T. The evidence base. Are steroids still indicated in second- and third-degree corrosive burns of the oesophagus? *J Toxicol Clin Toxicol.* 2004;42:414–416.
147. Boink AB, Wemer J, Meulenbelt J, et al. The mechanism of fluoride-induced hypocalcemia. *Hum Exp Toxicol.* 1994;13:149–155.
148. Sheridan RL, Ryan CM, Quinby WC Jr, et al. Emergency management of major hydrofluoric acid exposures. *Burns.* 1990;83:698–700.
149. Kirkpatrick JJ, Enion DS, Burd DAR. Hydrofluoric acid burns: a review. *Burns.* 1995;21:483–493.
150. Tepperman PB. Fatality due to acute systemic fluoride poisoning following a hydrofluoric acid skin burn. *J Occup Med.* 1980;22:691–692.
151. Su M. Hydrofluoric acid and fluorides. In: Flomenbaum NE, Goldfrank LR, Hoffman RS, et al., eds. *Goldfrank's Toxicologic Emergencies.* 8th ed. New York: McGraw-Hill; 2006:1417–1423.
152. Baltazar RF, Mower MM, Reider R, et al. Acute fluoride poisoning leading to fatal hyperkalemia. *Chest.* 1980;78:660–663.
153. Mullett T, Zoeller T, Bingham H, et al. Fatal hydrofluoric acid cutaneous exposure with refractory ventricular fibrillation. *J Burn Care Rehabil.* 1987; 8:216–219.
154. McIvor ME, Cummings CE, Mower MM, et al. Sudden cardiac death from acute fluoride intoxication: the role of potassium. *Ann Emerg.* 1987; 16:777–781.
155. Burkhart KK, Brent J, Kirk MA, et al. Comparison of topical management and calcium treatment for dermal hydrofluoric acid burns. *Ann Emerg Med.* 1994;24:9–13.
156. Pegg SP, Siu S, Gillett G. Intra-arterial infusions in the treatment of hydrofluoric acid burns. *Burns.* 1985;11:440–443.
157. Howland MA. Antidotes in depth: calcium. In: Flomenbaum NE, Goldfrank LR, Hoffman RS, et al., eds. *Goldfrank's Toxicologic Emergencies.* 8th ed. New York: McGraw-Hill; 2006:1424–1428.
158. Stremski ES, Grande GA, Ling LJ. Survival following hydrofluoric acid ingestion. *Ann Emerg Med.* 1992;21:1396–1399.
159. Greco RJ, Hartford CE, Haith LR, et al. Hydrofluoric acid-induced hypocaclcemia. *J Trauma.* 1988;28:1593–1596.
160. Cummings CC, McIvor ME. Fluoride-induced hyperkalemia—the role of calcium-dependent potassium channels. *Am J Emerg Med.* 1986;6: 1–3.
161. Bosse GM. Antidiabetics and hypoglycemics. In: Flomenbaum NE, Goldfrank LR, Hoffman RS, et al., eds. *Goldfrank's Toxicologic Emergencies.* 8th ed. New York: McGraw-Hill; 2006:749–763.
162. Davis SN. Insulin, oral hypoglycemic agents, and the pharmacology of the endocrine pancreas. In: Brunton LL, Lazo JS, Parker KL, eds. *Goodman & Gilman's The Pharmacological Basis of Therapeutics.* 11th ed. New York: McGraw Hill; 2006:1613–1645.
163. Quadrani DA, Spiller HA, Widder P. Five-year retrospective evaluation of sulfonylurea ingestion in children. *J Toxicol Clin Toxicol.* 1996;34:267–270.
164. Boyle PJ, Schwartz NS, Shah SD, et al. Plasma glucose concentrations at the onset of hypoglycemic symptoms in patients with poorly controlled diabetes and in nondiabetics. *N Engl J Med.* 1988;318:1487–1492.
165. Cryer PE. Diverse causes of hypoglycemia-associated autonomic failure in diabetes. *N Engl J Med.* 2004;350:2272–2279.
166. Tofade TS, Liles EA. Intentional overdose with insulin glargine and insulin aspart. *Pharmacotherapy.* 2004;24:1412–1418.
167. Matsumura M, Nakashima A, Tofuku Y. Electrolyte disorders following massive insulin overdose in a patient with type 2 diabetes. *Intern Med.* 2000;39:55–57.
168. Radziuk J, Zhang Z, Wiernsperger N, et al. Effects of metformin on lactate uptake and gluconeogenesis in the perfused rat liver. *Diabetes.* 1997;46: 1406–1413.
169. Lalau JD, Mourlhon C, Bergeret A, et al. Consequences of metformin intoxication. *Diabetes Care.* 1998;21:2036–2037.
170. Chan NN, Brain HP, Feher MD. Metformin-associated lactic acidosis: a rare or very rare clinical entity. *Diabet Med.* 1999;16:273–281.
171. Carrascosa M, Pascual F, Aresti S. Acarbose-induced severe hepatotoxicity. *Lancet.* 1997;349:698–699.
172. Gitlin N, Julie NL, Spurr CL, et al. Two cases of severe clinical and histologic toxicity associated with troglitazone. *Ann Emerg Med.* 1998;129:36–38.
173. Hsu W, Xiang H, Rajan A, et al. Somatostatin inhibits insulin secretion by a G-protein-mediated decrease in Ca^{2+} channels in the beta cell. *J Biol Chem.* 1991;206:837–843.
174. Boyle PJ, Justice K, Krentz AJ, et al. Octreotide reverses hyperinsulinemia and prevents hypoglycemia induced by sulfonylurea overdoses. *J Clin Endocrinol Metab.* 1993;76:752–756.
175. Lalau JD, Andrejak M, Moriniere P, et al. Hemodialysis in the treatment of lactic acidosis in diabetics treated by metformin: a study of metformin elimination. *Int J Clin Pharmacol Ther Toxicol.* 1989;27:285–288.
176. Boumba VA, Mitselou A, Vougiouklakis T. Fatal poisoning from ingestion of Datura stramonium seeds. *Vet Hum Toxicol.* 2004;46:81–82.
177. McGee D, Brabson T, McCarthy J, et al. Four-year review of cigarette ingestion in children. *Pediatr Emerg Care.* 1995;11:13–16.
178. Salomon ME. Nicotine and tobacco preparations. In: Flomenbaum NE, Goldfrank LR, Hoffman RS, et al., eds. *Goldfrank's Toxicologic Emergencies.* 8th ed. New York: McGraw-Hill; 2006:1564–1576.1221–1230.
179. Quandt SA, Arcury TA, Preisser JS, et al. Migrant farmworkers and green tobacco sickness: new issues for an understudied disease. *Am J Ind Med.* 2000;37:307–315.
180. Palmer M, Betz JM. Plants. In: Flomenbaum NE, Goldfrank LR, Hoffman RS, et al., eds. *Goldfrank's Toxicologic Emergencies.* 8th ed. New York: McGraw-Hill; 2006:1577–1602.
181. Heath KB. A fatal case of apparent water hemlock poisoning. *Vet Hum Toxicol.* 2001;43:35–36.
182. Ameri A. The effects of Aconitum alkaloids on the central nervous system. *Prog Neurobiol.* 1998;56:211–235.
183. Fitzpatrick AJ, Crawford M, Allan RM, et al. Aconite poisoning managed with a ventricular assist device. *Anaesth Intensive Care.* 1994;22:714–717.
184. Goldfrank LR. Mushrooms. In: Flomenbaum NE, Goldfrank LR, Hoffman RS, et al., eds. *Goldfrank's Toxicologic Emergencies.* 8th ed. New York: McGraw-Hill; 2006:1564–1576.
185. Kelner MJ, Alexander NM. Endocrine hormone abnormalities in *Amanita* poisoning. *J Toxicol Clin Toxicol.* 1987;25:21–37.
186. Faulstich H. New aspects of *Amanita* poisoning. *Klin Wochenschr.* 1979; 57:1143–1152.
187. Jacobs BP, Dennehy C, Ramirez G, et al. Milk thistle for the treatment of liver disease: a systematic review and meta-analysis. *Am J Med.* 2002;113: 506–515.
188. Floersheim GL, Eberhard M, Tschumi P, et al. Effects of Penicilli
189. Klein AS, Hart J, Brems JJ, et al. *Amanita* poisoning: treatment and the role of liver transplantation. *Am J Med.* 1989;86:187–193.
190. Warden CR, Benjamin DR. Acute renal failure associated with suspected *Amanita smithiana* mushroom ingestions: a case series. *Acad Emerg Med.* 1998;5:808–812.
191. Schumacher T, Hoiland K. Mushroom poisoning caused by species of the genus Cortinarius Fries. *Arch Toxicol.* 1983;53:87–106.
192. Carder CA, Wojciechlowski NJ, Skoutakis VA. Management of mushroom poisoning. *Clin Toxicol Consult.* 1983;5:103–118.
193. Bouget J, Bousser J, Pats B, et al. Acute renal failure following collective intoxication by *Cortinarius orellanus*. *Intensive Care Med.* 1990;16:506–510.
194. *Gonzalez vs. State* 110, AD 2d 810, 488, NY 2d 231, 67, NY 2d 647(1985).

APPENDIX

SELECTED ANTIDOTES WITH COMMON DOSES

Xenobiotic	Antidote and dose
Acetaminophen	***N*-acetylcysteine- IV:** 150 mg/kg infused over 60 min, followed by 50 mg/kg over 4 h, then 100 mg/kg over 16 h **Oral:** 140 mg/kg, followed by 70 mg/kg every 4 h for 17 doses
β-Adrenergic antagonists	**Atropine (for bradycardia):** 0.5–1 mg IV **Glucagon:** 3–5 mg IV (50 μg/kg in children) up to 10 mg/h **Calcium:** 13–25 mEq of Ca^{2+} IV bolus (10–20 mL of 10% calcium chloride or 30–60 mL of 10% calcium gluconate) **Hyperinsulinemia/euglycemia:** Insulin 0.5–1 U/kg/h accompanied by 0.5 g/kg/h dextrose, titrated to maintain euglycemia
Calcium channel blockers	**Atropine (for bradycardia):** 0.5–1 mg IV **Calcium:** 13–25 mEq of Ca^{2+} IV bolus (10–20 mL of 10% calcium chloride or 30–60 mL of 10% calcium gluconate) **Glucagon:** 3–5 mg IV (50 μg/kg in children) up to 10 mg/h **Hyperinsulinemia/euglycemia:** Insulin 0.5–1 U/kg/h accompanied by 0.5 g/kg/h dextrose, titrated to maintain euglycemia
Cholinergic compounds	**Atropine:** 1 mg IV (0.05 mg/kg in children) doubled every 2 min until muscarinic symptoms are controlled **Pralidoxime:** Adults: 1–2 g IV over 30 min followed by 500 mg/g infusion for sickest patients. Children: 20–50 mg/kg (max 1–2 g) infused IV over 30–60 min and then 10–20 mg/kg/h (max 500 mg/h)
Cyanide	**Adults:** 1. Sodium nitrite: 300 mg (10 mL of a 3% conc.) infused IV over 2–5 min 2. Sodium thiosulfate: 12.5 g (50 mL of a 25% conc.) infused IV over 10–20 min or as a bolus 3. Hydroxocobalamin IV 70 mg/kg (up to 5 g) **Children:** 1. Sodium nitrite: 6–8 mL/m^2 (0.2 mL/kg of a 3% conc., up to adult dose) infused IV over 2–5 min 2. Sodium thiosulfate: 7 g/m^2 (0.5 g/kg, up to adult dose) infused over 10–30 min or as a bolus
Cyclic antidepressants	**Sodium bicarbonate:** 1 mEq/kg IV bolus, followed by infusion of 150 mEq in 1 L of D5W, infused at twice maintenance rate
Digoxin	**Digoxin-specific Fab:** Known level: # of vials = [wt (kg) × level (ng/mL)/100] rounded up to nearest vial. Empiric dosing: Acute: 10–20 vials. Chronic: Adults 3–6 vials; children: 1–2 vials. Usually given as IV infusion over 30 min (administer as IV bolus for asystole)
Ethylene glycol, methanol	**Fomepizole:** 15 mg/kg infused IV over 30 min; next 4 doses at 10 mg/kg every 12 h; additional doses at 15 mg/kg every 12 h if needed **Ethanol (when fomepizole not available):** 0.8 g/kg infused IV over 20 to 60 min, followed by initial infusion of 100 mg/kg/h
Methemoglobin	**Methylene blue:** 1–2 mg/kg IV over 5 min followed by a 30-mL fluid flush
Salicylates	**Sodium bicarbonate:** 150 mEq in 1 L of D5W, infused at twice maintenance rate. Activated charcoal, 1g/kg every 4 h
Sulfonylurea-related hypoglycemia	**Octreotide:** 50 μg SQ every 6 h. Children: 1.25 μg/kg (up to adult dose) SQ every 6 h

Adapted with permission from Flomenbaum NE, Goldfrank LR, Hoffman RS, et al., eds. *Goldfrank's Toxicologic Emergencies.* 8th ed. New York: McGraw-Hill; 2006.

CHAPTER 67 ■ SUBSTANCE ABUSE AND WITHDRAWAL: ALCOHOL, COCAINE, OPIOIDS AND OTHER DRUGS

S. SUJANTHY RAJARAM • JANICE L. ZIMMERMAN

Ethanol, illicit drugs, and prescription drugs used for nonmedical purposes are a significant medical as well as social problem. The 2005 National Survey on Drug Use and Health found that 22.7% of Americans, or 55 million individuals, were binge drinkers, which includes 16 million heavy drinkers (five or more drinks on the same occasion at least 5 different days in the prior 30 days) (1). Pain relievers were used nonmedically by 4.7 million Americans, and 3.5 million used stimulants or cocaine. Casual or habitual use of these drugs contributes to acute and chronic illness. Substance abuse also underlies many forms of injury, including vehicular accidents, falls, near-drowning, thermal injuries, homicide, and suicide. Other critical illnesses may be impacted by either substance use or substance withdrawal. This chapter will cover acute toxicity and withdrawal syndromes related to ethanol, cocaine, opioids, and other selected drugs likely to be of importance to the critical care practitioner.

ETHANOL

Alcohol abuse and alcoholism (a dependence on alcohol) are major social, economic, and public health problems throughout the world. Alcoholism is the third leading cause of death in the United States and it reduces life expectancy by 10 to 12 years. Men who imbibe more than 14 drinks per week or four drinks at one time or women who have more than seven drinks per week or three drinks at one time are at risk for alcohol abuse and dependence (a standard drink is one 12-ounce beer or wine cooler, one 5-ounce glass of wine, or 1.5 ounces of 80-proof distilled spirits).

Ethanol is rapidly absorbed in unaltered form from the stomach and small intestine. The presence of food (especially milk and fatty foods) in the stomach delays absorption, whereas the presence of water enhances absorption. Ethanol diffuses freely into body tissues. It is primarily metabolized in the liver. Less than 10% is excreted by the lungs or kidneys or through the skin. Several hepatic enzyme systems independently metabolize ethanol to acetaldehyde. The primary degradation pathway is in the hepatic cytosol by alcohol dehydrogenase, with nicotinamide adenine dinucleotide (NAD) as a cofactor. Acetaldehyde generated by this process is in turn metabolized through the Krebs cycle to carbon dioxide and water with 7 kcal/g liberated in this process. Most people can metabolize about 150 mg of ethanol per kilogram body weight per hour. This is equivalent to about 12 ounces of beer or 1 ounce of 90-proof whiskey.

Acute Toxicity

Common features of acute ethanol intoxication are shown in Table 67.1. Intoxication with ethanol depends on the rate of rise of the blood alcohol level and the length of time the level is maintained. Blood alcohol levels of 20 to 30 mg/dL are often associated with a mild euphoria, delayed reaction time, decreased inhibition, and alteration in judgment. Most people exhibit gross intoxication at levels above 150 mg/dL. Obtundation often develops at levels above 300 mg/dL, and death may result from respiratory depression, aspiration, or cardiovascular collapse when levels exceed 400 to 500 mg/dL (2).

Ethanol is a sedative-hypnotic drug and exerts its primary effects on the central nervous system (CNS). Patients can present with altered consciousness, agitation, euphoria, slurred speech, ataxia, stupor, and coma. Awareness of the environment (e.g., heat or cold exposure) and perception of pain are diminished. Ethanol may depress the respiratory center and lead to hypoventilation and respiratory arrest. Although seizures are more common in alcohol withdrawal, they may also occur with acute intoxication.

Acute ethanol intoxication is often associated with an increased heart rate and cardiac output, whereas prolonged intoxication may be associated with depressed myocardial contractility (3). Acute intoxication can also be associated with a variety of cardiac arrhythmias, especially atrial fibrillation ("holiday heart" syndrome). Cutaneous vessels dilate, whereas splanchnic vessels constrict. Increased sweating associated with cutaneous vasodilation may account for the decrease in core temperature often associated with acute ethanol intoxication.

Metabolic problems related to alcohol ingestion can be life threatening. Alcohol enhances the urinary excretion of phosphate and magnesium that can result in clinically significant hypophosphatemia and hypomagnesemia. The chronic alcoholic patient often has decreased glycogen stores, and because alcohol also inhibits hepatic gluconeogenesis, profound hypoglycemia may occur. A variety of acid-base disturbances are seen in acute alcoholic intoxication. Depression of the respiratory center in the severely intoxicated person may result in respiratory acidosis. Nausea and vomiting may cause hypokalemia and metabolic alkalosis. The presence of a

TABLE 67.1

CLINICAL MANIFESTATIONS OF ALCOHOL INTOXICATION

CENTRAL NERVOUS SYSTEM
Decreased inhibition
Slowed reaction time
Visual disturbance
Incoordination
Slurred speech
Diplopia
Nystagmus
Lethargy, stupor, coma
CARDIOVASCULAR
Vasodilation
Cardiac dysrhythmias
Myocardial depression
RESPIRATORY
Hypoventilation
Aspiration
METABOLIC
Hypoglycemia
Electrolyte abnormalities
Hypophosphatemia
Hypomagnesemia
Acid-base disturbance
Respiratory acidosis
Metabolic alkalosis (vomiting)
Metabolic acidosis (alcoholic ketoacidosis)
GASTROINTESTINAL
Gastritis
Increased incidence of peptic ulcer
Pancreatitis
Alcoholic hepatitis
HEMATOLOGIC
Suppression of all bone marrow cell lines
OTHER
Suppression of antidiuretic hormone (diuresis)
Increased sweating
Altered temperature regulation

significant metabolic acidosis or elevated lactate should prompt a search for conditions other than alcohol intoxication.

Ethanol ingestion may cause acute gastritis and gastrointestinal (GI) bleeding. Alcoholics have an increased incidence of peptic ulcer disease and pancreatitis. Acute alcohol intoxication may precipitate alcoholic hepatitis in the chronic user. All bone marrow cell lines are suppressed by alcohol ingestion. Suppression of antidiuretic hormone by ethanol causes diuresis and may lead to profound hypovolemia, especially if there is associated nausea, vomiting, or diarrhea.

Assessment and Treatment of Acute Intoxication

Treatment of acute ethanol intoxication is primarily supportive, but a careful examination is needed to detect complications. The first priority is assessment and stabilization of the airway and ventilation. The respiratory rate, depth of respirations, SpO_2, mental status, gag reflex, and presence of vomitus should be rapidly evaluated. An arterial blood gas should be obtained if hypoventilation is a concern but is not obvious on clinical examination. Intubation is indicated in the obtunded or comatose patient who is unable to protect his or her airway and when aspiration has occurred or is likely. Positive pressure ventilation should be instituted to correct alveolar hypoventilation and hypoxemia. If the patient presents with altered mental status, 50 to 100 mg of thiamine and 25 g of glucose should be administered intravenously. If the patient responds to the administration of glucose or if blood glucose levels are low, a continuous infusion of glucose should be given. Intravenous naloxone may be administered if concomitant opioid use is suspected. Hypotension should be treated initially with volume resuscitation. GI bleeding should be considered in the hypotensive patient and further assessment may include a rectal examination and insertion of a nasogastric tube. GI decontamination is of limited utility because the majority of alcohol is already absorbed. Ethanol is not adsorbed by activated charcoal, but charcoal may be administered if ingestion of other toxic drugs is suspected. Hypothermia should be corrected. Fluid, electrolyte, and acid-base disturbances are corrected, depending on the clinical presentation. A creatine phosphokinase (CPK) level may be warranted in the patient with trauma or prolonged muscle compression to evaluate for rhabdomyolysis. An ethanol blood level may be helpful in documenting the severity of intoxication and estimating the duration of impairment. A low ethanol level in the setting of a patient with a depressed level of consciousness should prompt an evaluation for other etiologies. A chest radiograph is often necessary to assess for evidence of aspiration or other complications such as pneumonia. Consider obtaining computed tomography of the head if there is any suspicion of subdural hematoma or other intracranial injury. Hemodialysis has been used in cases of massive ethanol ingestion (4).

The chronic alcoholic may also develop alcoholic ketoacidosis (5). This condition is typically preceded by binge drinking followed by a period of abstinence for 1 to 3 days with nausea, vomiting, and insufficient nutrient intake. The liver produces excessive ketones in response to starvation, which results in an anion gap acidosis. Pancreatitis is frequently present in these patients. The blood glucose may be low or high in this setting but is rarely above 300 mg/dL unless chronic glucose intolerance is present. The condition responds to volume replacement and administration of glucose. Insulin is not needed. Thiamine should be administered before glucose to avoid precipitation of acute beriberi and Wernicke-Korsakoff syndrome.

Alcohol Withdrawal

Chronic excessive alcohol ingestion depresses central α and β receptors and potentiates the inhibitory neurotransmitter γ-aminobutyric acid (GABA). The brain adapts with a functional increase in *N*-methyl D-aspartate (NMDA) receptors, which are part of an excitatory system. When alcohol consumption stops, the excess excitatory receptors and removal of the inhibitory effects mediated by GABA contribute to the hyperadrenergic state that causes the symptoms seen in alcohol withdrawal.

Alcohol withdrawal syndromes occur in dependent patients during the initial period of abstinence. In hospitalized patients,

TABLE 67.2

STAGES OF ALCOHOL WITHDRAWAL AND TREATMENT

Symptoms	Time frame[a]	Treatment
Tremulousness Hyperactivity, tremor Diaphoresis, nausea Mild tachycardia, hypertension Clear sensorium	Onset within hours Peak 10–30 h Subside in ∼40 h	Benzodiazepines (oral or IV) Supportive measures Fluid and electrolytes PRN Quiet environment Thiamin, folate, vitamins
Seizures	Onset 6–48 h Peak 13–24 h	Lorazepam 2–4 mg IV; repeat as needed Diazepam 10–20 mg IV Supportive measures as above
Hallucinations Auditory Visual Tactile	Onset 8–48 h May last 1–6 d	Benzodiazepines (oral or IV) Supportive measures as above
Delirium Tremens Coarse tremors, agitation Altered sensorium (delusions, hallucinations, confusion) Fever, tachycardia Hypertension Circulatory collapse	Onset 60–96 h 48–72	Benzodiazepines IV as needed Diazepam Lorazepam Midazolam Alternative treatments Propofol Barbiturates β Blockers

[a]Time after last drink.

symptoms of alcohol withdrawal may occur in up to 40% of those who drink excessive amounts of alcohol (6). Prevention of alcohol withdrawal syndromes has been shown to improve morbidity and mortality and shorten hospital and intensive care unit (ICU) length of stay (7). Four stages of alcohol withdrawal have been described (8), but symptoms are a continuum of neuropsychiatric and hemodynamic manifestations. Patients may manifest one or more of these syndromes on presentation or develop additional manifestations and progress from less severe to more severe stages while hospitalized (Table 67.2). A key distinction is to determine if the patient has an intact or altered sensorium.

Assessment of the severity of withdrawal is needed to determine appropriate treatment. Although the revised Clinical Institute Withdrawal Assessment-Alcohol Scale (CIWA-Ar) is often used for assessment, it has less applicability in critically ill patients (9). Patients with minor withdrawal symptoms can usually be treated with intravenous or oral benzodiazepines. Benzodiazepines act as an alcohol substitute to dampen the excitatory neuronal activity, and additional benefits include prevention of seizures and delirium tremens. The choice of benzodiazepine in hospitalized patients may depend on severity of hepatic dysfunction, desired duration of action, and available routes of administration. All benzodiazepines are effective when appropriate doses are used. Fixed dosing and symptom-triggered regimens have been used effectively. Fixed dosing may be more appropriate in critically ill patients until other conditions have stabilized. Treatment duration beyond 7 days is seldom required.

Although benzodiazepines are clearly superior to placebo in treating alcohol withdrawal, it is difficult to draw conclusions regarding the efficacy of benzodiazepines compared to β blockers, clonidine, carbamazepine, and valproic acid due to heterogeneity of clinical trials. Many trials are conducted in outpatients and have limited applicability to hospitalized and critically ill patients (10,11). Hallucinosis also responds well to benzodiazepines. Intravenous ethanol may be an option for alcohol withdrawal treatment or prophylaxis (12). However, it is not recommended for routine use due to dosing variability and lack of established efficacy (13). Other agents such as clonidine and β blockers have been reported to be effective for minor withdrawal symptoms but their use is less common. Clonidine and β blockers do not prevent the development of delirium. All patients with alcohol withdrawal should receive supportive measures in addition to pharmacologic intervention. Thiamine (vitamin B_1) should be given intravenously or orally to prevent Wernicke encephalopathy. Magnesium sulfate may be needed to correct hypomagnesemia.

Seizures

Approximately 5% to 10% of patients with untreated mild alcohol withdrawal symptoms progress to seizures. Patients who have been drinking heavily for only a few years but have several detoxification admissions are at higher risk of seizures than patients with long drinking histories but fewer detoxification admissions. Previous nonalcohol-related admissions also increase the risk of alcohol withdrawal seizures. This association has been termed the "kindling effect." According to the kindling hypothesis, each withdrawal episode is an irritative phenomenon to the brain. The accumulation of multiple episodes lowers the seizure threshold (14). Most alcohol withdrawal seizures are brief and self-limited in duration. Alcohol withdrawal seizures are usually generalized tonic-clonic but focal seizures may also occur. Multiple seizures (two to six episodes) occur in approximately 60% of patients and within a 12-hour period. It may be difficult to distinguish withdrawal seizures from a pre-existing seizure disorder or new onset of a nonalcohol-related seizure. Other causes of seizures such as hypoglycemia, metabolic abnormalities, trauma, infection, and other drug intoxication must be considered. A computed tomography (CT) scan of the head should be obtained for new-onset seizure, persistent neurologic deficits, or evidence or suspicion of trauma. Alcohol withdrawal seizures can be terminated with benzodiazepines (15). Intravenous lorazepam or midazolam is commonly used. If the seizure terminates without intervention, a benzodiazepine should be administered as soon as possible to prevent subsequent seizures. The risk of a recurrent seizure is 13% to 24% (16). Lorazepam (2 mg) significantly reduces the risk of recurrent seizure, whereas phenytoin has no effect (16,17). Less than 3% of patients develop status epilepticus and they should be treated with benzodiazepines or propofol. Phenytoin is not as effective.

Delirium Tremens

Delirium tremens (DT) is the most severe manifestation of alcohol withdrawal and these patients should be cared for in an ICU setting. Untreated DT carries a mortality of 15%, but mortality declines to 1% if treated. The accumulation of multiple prior withdrawal episodes leads to more severe DT with each episode (14). Patients with DT have more severe autonomic hyperactivity than milder stages of withdrawal and manifest delirium that may fluctuate. Some patients with severe withdrawal symptoms may need intubation during treatment. Fluid requirements may be increased due to increased insensible losses (fever, diaphoresis) and lack of oral intake. High-dose intravenous benzodiazepines (diazepam, lorazepam, midazolam) administered at frequent intervals or as a continuous infusion are needed to control the hyperadrenergic symptoms. Dosing should be individualized to achieve light somnolence (18). Benzodiazepines bind at the GABA–benzodiazepine receptor, and once these receptors are saturated, additional drug cannot bind. Patients may tolerate high doses of benzodiazepines but do not necessarily benefit from them (19). Caution is advised when administering high doses of intravenous lorazepam or diazepam over long periods of time as the propylene glycol diluent may result in a lactic acidosis (20). Daily dose reductions of 25% can be initiated after the second or third day of treatment. Propofol infusions may be useful for patients who are refractory to benzodiazepines. Propofol has dual activity similar to alcohol (GABA agonist and NMDA antagonist properties) that may explain its efficacy. Propofol has a rapid onset of action, sedation, and anticonvulsive properties (6,21). Other sedative-hypnotic drugs such as paraldehyde and barbiturates are effective in treating DT but are not commonly used. Neuroleptic agents are inferior to benzodiazepines and should not be used as single agents for treatment of DT (18). Neuromuscular blockers may be considered to control agitation when high-dose sedatives are not effective. Cardiac monitoring is necessary to detect arrhythmias early and institute therapy. Torsade de pointes may develop due to hypomagnesemia or prolongation of the QTc interval and should be treated aggressively with intravenous magnesium sulfate. Beta blockers may be needed to treat hypertension or tachycardia but they should not be administered to treat delirium. Propranolol may worsen delirium. Thiamine supplementation (100 mg/day) is recommended for 3 days.

DT usually lasts 2 to 5 days, but in 5% to 10% of cases, DT lasts greater than a week. Elderly alcoholics have a longer withdrawal period with more symptoms than younger alcoholics (23). A small percentage of patients remain delirious for several weeks and require continuing treatment. Be aware, however, that after head trauma, a subdural hematoma can evolve subacutely in the alcoholic patient. Repeat imaging of the brain may be warranted 7 to 10 days into a course of protracted delirium to rule out a slowly accumulating subdural hematoma (19).

COCAINE

Cocaine (benzoylmethylecgonine) is an alkaloid derived from leaves of *Erythroxylon coca*. It is the second most commonly used illicit drug and the most frequent cause of drug-related deaths. Eighteen- to twenty-five-year-olds are the most common users, although it is abused by younger and older individuals (1).

Cocaine is available in two forms. Cocaine hydrochloride is prepared by dissolving alkaloidal cocaine in hydrochloric acid resulting in a white water-soluble powder, crystals, or granules. This form of cocaine is used intranasally (snorting), orally, or intravenously. The other available form of cocaine is free base or crack cocaine. Heating cocaine hydrochloride in sodium bicarbonate or ammonia makes the hard crystallized cocaine base called crack because of the popping sound it makes when heated (24). Smoking crack cocaine has become a widespread practice due to the rapid absorption across the alveolar surface. Both forms of cocaine are readily absorbed from all body mucosal surfaces. The peak effects of cocaine range from 1 to 90 minutes depending on the route of administration. Inhalational and intravenous use result in the most rapid peak effects and shortest duration of action. Cocaine is rapidly metabolized by hepatic and plasma cholinesterases and nonenzymatic hydrolysis to ecgonine methyl ester and benzoylecgonine, which are excreted in urine. The urinary excretion of unchanged cocaine ranges from 1% to 15%. The route of administration does not affect metabolic excretion patterns appreciably and half-lives of most metabolites range from 45 to 90 minutes (25). Subjective rating of euphoria declines within minutes after constant concentrations are achieved, demonstrating rapid desensitization and acute tolerance (26). Duration of positive urinary metabolites is somewhat dependent on the assay technique, the activity of plasma cholinesterases, and the duration and dosing of cocaine use.

Cocaine's lipophilic nature, compounded with rapid distribution into and out of the CNS, suggests a highly abusive profile (rush and crash) and increased incidence of kindling. The major neurochemical actions of cocaine are CNS stimulation with release of dopamine; inhibition of neuronal norepinephrine and dopamine uptake, resulting in generalized sympathetic nervous system stimulation; release of serotonin or blockade of serotonin reuptake; and inhibition of sodium current in neuronal tissue, resulting in a local anesthetic effect (27).

Toxicity

Numerous morbidities have been associated with acute and chronic cocaine use (Table 67.3). Complications of particular interest to intensivists are discussed below.

Cardiovascular

Cocaine increases the heart rate, blood pressure, and left ventricular contractility, leading to an increase in myocardial oxygen demand (28). The increased demand may combine with underlying coronary artery disease, vasoconstriction, platelet aggregation, or *in situ* thrombus formation to produce ischemia and infarction. Chronic cocaine use also accelerates atherosclerosis (29). Apart from structural changes in epicardial vessels, wall thickening is described in the intramyocardial small coronary arteries in people with cocaine-induced chest pain (30).

Chest pain is the most common cocaine-associated complication in patients who present for medical care. All patients presenting with chest pain should be questioned regarding cocaine use. Myocardial ischemia can occur with all routes of abuse with no relation to the dose or chronicity of use. The onset of chest pain often occurs temporally related to the use of cocaine. However, chest pain may occur hours to days after the last use of cocaine. Electrocardiograms are often abnormal in patients presenting with cocaine-associated chest pain (31, 32). Myocardial infarction may be present with a normal or abnormal electrocardiogram. Conversely, electrocardiograms may suggest acute ischemia in the absence of infarction due to J-point elevation or repolarization changes (32). Cardiac troponins are more specific for assessing myocardial injury than creatine kinase-MB, which may be elevated due to skeletal muscle injury (33). Myocardial infarction is reported to occur in approximately 6% to 7% of patients and occurs with normal coronary arteries and in the presence of significant atherosclerotic disease (32,34,35). Periods of silent ischemia are common in chronic users of cocaine, as shown by Holter tests and during periods of withdrawal (36). Dilated cardiomyopathy, myocarditis, and congestive heart failure can occur secondary to chronic cocaine use (37).

Cocaine is arrhythmogenic when taken in large quantities because of catecholamine effects. The arrhythmias are usually transient and resolve when cocaine is metabolized. Sinus tachycardia, supraventricular tachycardia, atrial fibrillation, premature ventricular beats, ventricular tachycardia, ventricular

TABLE 67.3

CLINICAL MANIFESTATIONS OF COCAINE USE

ANESTHETIC EFFECTS	**RESPIRATORY**
Localized numbness	Pulmonary edema
Central neuronal depression	Pulmonary hypertension
Coma	Respiratory arrest
	Pulmonary vascular occlusion, pulmonary infarction
CENTRAL NERVOUS SYSTEM	Pneumothorax
Euphoria	Pneumomediastinum
Alertness	Hemoptysis
Tremor	
Sleeplessness	**GASTROINTESTINAL**
Paranoia	Mesenteric ischemia, infarction
Psychosis	Gastrointestinal perforations
Headache	
Seizures	**METABOLIC**
Stroke	Weight loss
Transient ischemic events	Hyperthermia
Intracerebral hemorrhage	Rhabdomyolysis
Cerebral vasculitis	
Cognitive dysfunction	**OTHER COMPLICATIONS**
	Nasal mucosal injury
CARDIOVASCULAR	Nasal septal perforation
Tachycardia	Chronic rhinitis
Arrhythmias	Deep venous thrombosis
Hypertension	Dystonic reaction
Myocardial ischemia and infarction	Skin ischemia
Myocarditis	
Aortic dissection or rupture	**OBSTETRIC**
Sudden death	Spontaneous abortions
Cardiomyopathy	Abruptio placentae
Atherosclerosis	Intrauterine growth retardation
Vasculitis	Prematurity
RENAL	
Induction of renal atherogenesis	
Renal failure	
Renal infarction	
Scleroderma renal crisis	

fibrillation, bundle branch block, asystole, and torsade de pointes may occur.

Elevation of blood pressure occurs due to the acute effects of cocaine, but it is usually self-limited. Sustained elevations of blood pressure suggest the presence of chronic hypertension or another complication (e.g., intracranial process). The elevations of blood pressure may contribute to other catastrophic complications such as stroke and intracranial hemorrhage. Rupture of the ascending aorta in previously healthy men has been reported as well as aortic dissection (38).

Central Nervous System

In large doses, cocaine may cause a generalized impairment of neuronal impulse transmission leading to CNS depression, coma, respiratory depression, and respiratory arrest. At low doses, stimulation is the common feature of cocaine use. The euphoria produced by cocaine is the principal reason for its abuse. Excessive CNS stimulation can occur and is manifested by tremulousness, agitation, sleeplessness, paranoia, and frank psychosis. Aggressive and assaultive behavior can occur in cocaine overdose.

Seizures can be induced, even on the first exposure, because cocaine lowers the threshold for seizures. Cocaine-related seizures are usually brief and self-limited, occurring soon after taking cocaine, although the interval between last use of cocaine and onset of seizures can be several hours (39). Sustained or repeated seizure activity suggests an additional complication such as hyperthermia, intracranial hemorrhage, metabolic abnormality, or massive intake of cocaine.

Cocaine use is associated with ischemic cerebrovascular accidents as well as transient ischemic attacks (39–41). Radiologic studies have demonstrated cerebral vasoconstriction as well as vessel thrombosis with cocaine (41,42). Although most symptoms occur during or immediately after cocaine use, neurologic symptoms may occur within hours to several days after the last use. Subarachnoid, parenchymal, and intraventricular hemorrhage may occur within moments of drug use, possibly related to blood pressure elevation. Some patients have anatomic abnormalities such as vascular malformation or aneurysm that may be amenable to specific therapy (39,43,44). Cerebral atrophy, predominantly in the temporofrontal regions, has been noted in patients with chronic cocaine abuse (45).

Pulmonary

Pulmonary complications associated with cocaine are much less common than cardiovascular and cerebrovascular events but include a variety of conditions (46,47). Inhalation of cocaine, in contrast to IV use, has been demonstrated to cause bronchoconstriction (48). This response may be due to an irritant effect and may contribute to wheezing and exacerbations of asthma in cocaine users (49,50). Barotrauma (pneumothorax and pneumomediastinum) is reported secondary to snorting cocaine and crack inhalation (51). Noncardiogenic pulmonary edema may occur and is described more commonly with intravenous use of cocaine. Massive hemoptysis with diffuse alveolar hemorrhage is a rare complication of unknown etiology and has been reported with smoking free-base cocaine and other routes of abuse. Other rare pulmonary toxicities, more commonly reported after inhalation of cocaine, include interstitial pneumonitis, pulmonary infiltrates with peripheral and/or lung eosinophil prominence, and bronchiolitis obliterans (52). Septic pulmonary emboli and pulmonary vascular obstruction resulting from foreign body granulomas or angiothrombosis may develop as a consequence of IV cocaine use similar to IV heroin use (53).

Hyperthermia/Rhabdomyolysis

Hyperthermia may result from muscle hyperactivity or as a direct effect of cocaine on the hypothalamic temperature regulatory center. High ambient temperatures are associated with increased mortality from cocaine and hyperthermia is probably one of several factors that play a role (54). Cocaine impairs sweating and cutaneous vasodilation as well as heat perception under conditions of heat stress (55).

Cocaine-induced rhabdomyolysis is common and can lead to acute renal failure. Multiple factors such as hyperthermia, seizures, vasoconstriction with ischemia, excessive motor activity, concomitant use of other drugs, and even a direct toxic effect of cocaine may contribute to muscle injury. Myalgias and muscle tenderness are infrequently present. Seizures, hypotension or hypertension, arrhythmia, coma, and cardiac arrest identify a subgroup of patients who are prone to severe rhabdomyolysis (56,57).

Other Toxicities

Intestinal ischemia, infarction, and perforation have been reported following ingested, intravenous, and inhaled cocaine (58,59). Patients may present with complaints of acute or chronic abdominal pain. Acute renal failure may be precipitated by rhabdomyolysis, but other etiologies may include accelerated hypertension and glomerulonephritis (60). Rare cases of renal infarction have also been reported.

Diagnosis of Acute Intoxication

Patients with cocaine intoxication may present with a variety of primary complaints such as altered mental status, chest pain, syncope, palpitations, seizures, or attempted suicide (61). Characteristic findings of CNS stimulation such as agitation, mydriasis, sweating, hypertension, and tachycardia are often present. However, the effects of other drugs, the presence of complications, and delays in presentation may obscure the typical sympathomimetic manifestations. Other medical conditions such as meningitis, encephalopathy, epilepsy with status, and thyrotoxicosis may mimic cocaine intoxication (27). Confirmation of acute or recent cocaine exposure is made by urine toxicology testing.

Treatment for Acute Intoxication

Benzodiazepines are the pharmacologic agents of choice for control of cocaine-induced agitation. The agitation and psychosis of cocaine overdose usually can be managed with titrated doses of IV diazepam, 5 to 20 mg; lorazepam, 2 to 4 mg; or midazolam, 5 to 10 mg slowly. Haloperidol is not recommended as a first-line agent because of the lack of experimental support (62) and potential to lower the seizure threshold. Adequate hydration and correction of electrolyte abnormalities are important.

Cardiovascular

No large clinical trials have evaluated treatment strategies for cocaine-associated ischemia. Treatment of cardiac toxicity due to cocaine is directed at reversing physiologic effects that cause ischemia or arrhythmias. Aspirin should be administered as an antiplatelet agent for suspected myocardial ischemia unless there is evidence of cerebral hemorrhage. Oxygen may also help to limit myocardial ischemia. Benzodiazepines and nitroglycerin are considered first-line agents for relief of chest pain, but small clinical studies have yielded conflicting results on the benefit of combining the agents (63,64). Benzodiazepines decrease the blood pressure and heart rate, thus decreasing myocardial oxygen demand, and nitroglycerin may dilate coronary arteries or relieve vasoconstriction. Alpha blockers such as phentolamine have been recommended as a second-line treatment for unrelieved pain, but are rarely needed (65). The use of β blockers in the management of myocardial ischemia is debated. There is a potential concern of worsening vasospasm or hypertension due to unopposed stimulation of α receptors. Intracoronary propranolol results in a small decrease in coronary artery diameter following intranasal cocaine, but β blockers are not administered by this route or as soon after cocaine use in most patients (66). However, β blockers have been used, particularly in the setting of myocardial infarction, without complications. Administration of β blockers might be avoided in patients manifesting acute sympathomimetic findings, but the benefits of these agents should be considered in other patients with ongoing myocardial ischemia.

Most patients with cocaine-associated chest pain will not have infarction. Patients can be managed in chest pain or observation units similar to other chest pain patients (67). Low-risk patients with normal cardiac markers can be risk stratified safely with stress testing.

Early therapy for cocaine-induced myocardial infarction should consist of oxygen, aspirin, and nitroglycerin as required for pain relief. If pain persists, patients with cocaine-induced myocardial infarction are candidates for reperfusion therapy. Primary percutaneous angiography is preferred in patients with evidence of ST-elevation myocardial infarction, especially when the diagnosis may be in doubt (65,68). Thrombolytic therapy has been safely used in cocaine-associated myocardial infarction and may be considered if invasive reperfusion is not available (69).

Arrhythmias associated with cocaine use are usually transient. Standard therapy should be considered for sustained arrhythmias unresponsive to control of pain and agitation. Although lidocaine is seldom used for ventricular arrhythmias, theoretical concerns of enhancing cocaine toxicity do not appear to be clinically significant (70).

Sustained hypertension in acute cocaine intoxication is not common due to the short physiologic effects of the drug. Control of agitation with benzodiazepines often results in resolution of hypertension. Intravenous labetalol is a reasonable option if the blood pressure needs to be lowered due to its α- and β-blocking effects. Cocaine-intoxicated patients should be considered to have acute elevations in blood pressure, and unless there is documentation or clinical evidence of long-standing hypertension, there should be little concern about cerebral hypoperfusion with immediate lowering of blood pressure to normal levels (71).

Central Nervous System

Seizures induced by cocaine are best controlled with IV benzodiazepines. Other standard antiepileptics can be added for refractory cases. If neuromuscular blockers are used, brain seizure activity may persist unrecognized and, hence, warrants continuous electroencephalographic monitoring.

Interventions for ischemic strokes associated with cocaine use should be carefully considered. Since the etiology may involve vasoconstriction as well as thrombosis, the decision to use thrombolytic agents in patients presenting within 3 hours of symptom onset may be more difficult. Vascular imaging, if readily available, may be helpful. Blood pressure is not usually severely elevated, but if sustained hypertension is present, current guidelines should be followed for lowering blood pressure. Neurosurgical consultation should be sought for intracranial hemorrhages to evaluate for possible interventions. Patients with subarachnoid hemorrhage should be evaluated for vascular malformations that may be amenable to treatment.

Pulmonary

Most pulmonary toxicities associated with cocaine are managed with usual care or supportive care (46,47). Bronchospasm and asthma should be treated with inhaled β agonists and corticosteroids if indicated. Pneumomediastinum can be followed without hospital admission for most patients. Small pneumothoraces may also resolve without intervention, whereas large pneumothoraces will require thoracostomy. Noncardiogenic pulmonary edema may require supplemental oxygen and mechanical ventilation but resolves within a few days unless other complications occur.

Hyperthermia/Rhabdomyolysis

Hyperthermia associated with cocaine use should be treated aggressively by rapid cooling (please see chapter discussing heat stroke). Control of coexisting agitation, psychosis, or seizures is essential to achieve and maintain cooling while avoiding brain, hepatic, and muscle cell destruction. There is no evidence that pharmacologic agents such as dantrolene are of benefit in cooling patients with life-threatening hyperthermia.

Patients with hyperthermia, severe agitation or motor activity, seizures, and obtundation should be evaluated for rhabdomyolysis. Aggressive fluid resuscitation to replete the intravascular volume and enhance urine output should often be initiated prior to definitive diagnosis. Serial tests of electrolytes, renal function, and creatine kinases are needed to monitor the severity and response of rhabdomyolysis.

Body Packers/Stuffers

Individuals may ingest packets of cocaine or any illicit drug for the purpose of transport or concealment. Body stuffers swallow small amounts of drug (wrapped or unwrapped) in order to avoid arrest. In this circumstance, drugs are not prepared for passage through the GI tract and drug is frequently absorbed. Due to the smaller quantities of drug, toxicity is usually mild (71). In contrast, body packers swallow larger quantities of drug in multiple packets that are specially prepared for smuggling to withstand transit through the GI tract. Abdominal radiographs often show the location of the packets and allow tracking as they move through the GI tract. However, a negative result on plain abdominal radiograph does not rule out body packing, and an abdominal CT scan may be needed to visualize the packets (72).

Most body packers are asymptomatic and can be managed conservatively until the packets have been completely evacuated (72,73). Activated charcoal given every 4 to 6 hours can reduce the lethality of oral cocaine. Whole bowel irrigation may assist with passage of the packets. Body packers with signs and symptoms of drug toxicity, *in vivo* degradation, or gastrointestinal obstruction require emergent surgical intervention (72).

Cocaine Withdrawal

Psychological and biochemical dependency on cocaine may be intense. Cocaine causes activation of the dopamine system and blocks dopamine uptake, especially in the pleasure centers of the brain (74). The brain becomes dopamine deficient, and even a short period of cocaine abstinence can result in a withdrawal state.

The clinical effects of cocaine withdrawal include depression, fatigue, irritability, sleep and appetite dysfunction, psychomotor agitation or retardation, and craving for more cocaine (25). A period of prolonged somnolence and decreased arousal can occur after binge use of cocaine and often necessitates evaluations to rule out complications associated with cocaine use (75). A supportive environment and professional drug counseling are warranted.

OPIOIDS

Opioids include all drugs (synthetic as well as natural) that have morphine-like properties and/or bind to opioid receptors. There are at least five opioid receptors with various physiologic roles including analgesia, ventilatory depression, drug dependence, bradycardia, dysphoria, hallucinations, sedation, and miosis. Opioids are classified as receptor agonists or antagonists. Some have combined properties because they stimulate one type of receptor and antagonize another. A classification of opioids is found in Table 67.4. Opioid dependence is characterized by repeated self-administration of drug and encompasses physiologic dependence and addictive behavior. Exposure to opioids causes neural changes that produce tolerance, dependence, and withdrawal (76).

Toxicity

Although all opioids are associated with toxicity, heroin use has been increasing and the purity has increased, resulting in overdoses and fatalities (77). Heroin is rapidly absorbed by all routes of administration, including intravenous, intranasal, intramuscular, subcutaneous (skin popping), and inhalation. Most fatal overdoses occur with IV administration. Intravenous fentanyl extracted from analgesic patches is also associated with fatalities (78). Oral opioids are available illicitly or by prescription and toxicity depends on the potency of the agent, dose ingested, and tolerance of the individual. Codeine elixir ("syrup") is abused by adolescents and young adults. The diagnosis of opioid toxicity is made by characteristic clinical findings, exposure history, qualitative toxicology assay, and response to naloxone. Qualitative urine assays may not detect all opioid derivatives (e.g., fentanyl).

Opioid intoxication is characterized by a clinical syndrome of depressed level of consciousness, respiratory depression, and miosis. However, manifestations may be variable depending on the drug used and presence of other drugs or alcohol. Miosis is not seen with meperidine and propoxyphene toxicity. The primary toxic manifestations of opioids are mediated by the

TABLE 67.4

CLASSIFICATION OF OPIOID AGENTS

OPIOID AGONISTS
Natural opium derivatives
Codeine
Morphine
Semisynthetic opioids
Heroin
Hydrocodone
Hydromorphone
Oxymorphone
Oxycodone
Synthetic opioids
Diphenoxylate
Fentanyl
Levorphanol
Loperamide
Meperidine
Methadone
Propoxyphene
Tramadol
PURE OPIOID ANTAGONISTS
Nalmefene
Naloxone
Naltrexone
AGONISTS–ANTAGONISTS
Butorphanol
Nalbuphine
Pentazocine

μ and κ receptors in the brain, which cause CNS depression. Common clinical effects of these drugs are shown in Table 67.5.

The most worrisome feature of CNS depression is hypoventilation. Tidal volume decreases first, and then respiratory rate falls. Although less common, seizures may be associated with meperidine, propoxyphene, and tramadol toxicity or result from hypoventilation and hypoxemia due to other opioids. Arteriolar and venous dilatation with opioid use can precipitate preload reduction, a fall in cardiac output, and hypotension.

An opioid-induced release of histamine from mast cells can precipitate bronchospasm, urticaria, and pruritus. Other respiratory complications include aspiration of gastric contents, noncardiogenic pulmonary edema, asthma exacerbation (heroin), pulmonary hypertension, acute respiratory distress syndrome, and septic pulmonary emboli (53,79). Intravenously injected illicit opioids may be mixed with microcrystalline cellulose, talc, or cellulose. These fillers are capable of producing angiothrombosis and a foreign body granulomatous reaction in the lung.

A pronounced decrease in gastrointestinal peristalsis and increased ileocecal and anal sphincter tone are responsible for the constipation frequently seen with opioid use. Urinary retention may be caused by increased detrusor muscle tone. Local infections, endocarditis, and other systemic infections are especially common in the IV user.

Treatment for Acute Intoxication

The most common cause of death in opioid overdose is ventilatory failure, and the immediate priority in acute opioid

TABLE 67.5

CLINICAL MANIFESTATIONS OF OPIOID INTOXICATION

CENTRAL NERVOUS SYSTEM
Analgesia
Apathy
Lethargy
Seizures
Coma
Ventilatory depression
Nausea
Emesis
Miosis
RESPIRATORY
Histamine release—bronchospasm
Pulmonary edema
CARDIOVASCULAR
Arteriolar and venous dilation
Preload reduction
Hypotension
GASTROINTESTINAL
Decreased peristalsis
Decreased hydrochloric acid secretion
Constipation
OTHER
Histamine release—urticaria, pruritus
Muscle rigidity (fentanyl)
Urinary retention

intoxication is airway management and ventilation. If reversal of respiratory depression cannot be accomplished quickly with naloxone, intubation may be necessary. Naloxone, a pure opioid antagonist, reverses all of the opioid-induced CNS and ventilatory depressant effects. The dose required to reverse opioid effects depends on the amount and type of opioid administered. The initial dose of naloxone is 0.4 to 2 mg; the lower dose should be administered initially in patients suspected of chronic addiction to avoid precipitating acute withdrawal symptoms. Additional doses of naloxone can be given based on the patient's response. Although intravenous administration is preferred, naloxone can be administered intramuscularly, by sublingual injection, or through an endotracheal tube. The goal of therapy is to restore adequate spontaneous respirations rather than complete arousal. Doses of naloxone up to 10 to 20 mg may be required in patients who have administered large quantities of opioids or opioids such as propoxyphene, pentazocine, methadone, and fentanyl. If CNS depression is not reversed by 20 mg of naloxone, alternate causes should be aggressively addressed (e.g., hypoglycemia, hypothermia, head trauma). Close observation of the patient after naloxone administration is warranted because its effects last approximately 60 to 90 minutes. The patient may require repeated bolus injections of naloxone or a continuous infusion to maintain adequate respirations, particularly with long-acting opioids. The dose for infusion is one half to two thirds of the initial naloxone dose that reversed respiratory depression given on an hourly basis. Adjustments of the dose should be made to achieve clinical end points and avoid withdrawal symptoms. Additional boluses may be required as the infusion is started. Nalmefene, a long-acting opioid antagonist, has also been used to treat opioid overdoses, but prolonged withdrawal symptoms are a concern (80).

Isotonic fluids should be administered for hypotension due to opioids. Patients with significant opioid toxicity should be observed for other potential complications including aspiration pneumonitis and noncardiogenic pulmonary edema. Noncardiogenic pulmonary edema is usually self-limited (24–36 hours) and managed with supportive care that may include intubation and mechanical ventilation (81). Seizures unresponsive to naloxone should be treated with intravenous benzodiazepines. Refractory seizures may suggest either body packing or another complication. The potential for acetaminophen toxicity should be considered in patients ingesting opioids formulated with acetaminophen.

Acute Opioid Withdrawal

The chronic administration of exogenous opiates is thought to lead to diminished endogenous opioid peptides. When these exogenous opiates are discontinued, the patient can develop opioid withdrawal. The clinical manifestations of opioid withdrawal are outlined in Table 67.6. The onset of symptoms varies with the drug abused. Symptoms can begin within 6 to 12 hours of the last dose with short-acting opioids such as heroin and within 36 to 48 hours with long-acting opioids such as methadone. Opioid withdrawal is rarely life threatening and usually does not require intensive care.

TABLE 67.6

CLINICAL MANIFESTATIONS OF OPIOID WITHDRAWAL

EARLY
Yawning
Lacrimation
Rhinorrhea
Sneezing
Sweating
INTERMEDIATE
Restless sleep
Piloerection
Restlessness
Irritability
Anorexia
Flushing
Tachycardia
Tremor
Hyperthermia
LATE
Fever
Nausea
Vomiting
Abdominal pain
Diarrhea
Difficulty sleeping
Muscle spasm
Joint pain
Involuntary ejaculation
Suicidal ideation

If it is necessary to control withdrawal symptoms, most opioids in sufficient dosage will alleviate symptoms. Methadone, buprenorphine, and clonidine have been used to treat acute opioid withdrawal. In addition, methadone and buprenorphine have been used to treat opioid addiction chronically. Methadone can cause constipation, respiratory depression, dizziness, sedation, nausea, and diaphoresis. Oral buprenorphine use is restricted in the United States to qualified physicians who treat opioid dependence. It has low toxicity in high doses, partly because its μ-antagonistic effects limit the opioid effects of sedation, respiratory depression, and hypotension. Buprenorphine is more effective than clonidine and similar to methadone for management of opioid withdrawal (82).

Clonidine has also been used to suppress the autonomic effects of opioid withdrawal. Doses of 0.1 to 0.3 mg orally can suppress the signs and symptoms of opiate withdrawal within 24 hours and shorten acute withdrawal reactions by 3 to 4 days (83). Side effects are hypotension, drowsiness, dry mouth, and bradycardia.

Heroin Body Packers

Heroin body packers should be managed similar to cocaine body packers (see above). If there is evidence of systemic absorption from leaking packets, opioid toxicity should be treated with a continuous infusion of naloxone.

AMPHETAMINES AND DERIVATIVES

Amphetamines, methamphetamines, and similar derivatives are the most commonly abused CNS stimulants along with cocaine. Although there are limited medical uses for these drugs (narcolepsy, attention deficit disorder, obesity), they are usually abused for the euphoric effects or to enhance performance. Amphetamines act by increasing release and inhibiting reuptake of dopamine and serotonin in the brain. Minor chemical substitutions can enhance the hallucinogenic properties of the drug. The ease of production of these drugs from readily available ingredients in clandestine laboratories has resulted in increased supply throughout the United States. Methamphetamine can be made from common ingredients such as rock salt, paint thinner, lantern fuel, battery acid, lye, ammonia, lithium, ether, rubbing alcohol, iodine, and cold medicines containing pseudoephedrine (84).

Methamphetamine in a crystalline form (commonly called ice, crank, glass, or crystal) is one of the most popular drugs in this class. It can be orally ingested, smoked, snorted, or injected intravenously. An amphetamine-like drug, 3–4-methylenedioxymethamphetamine, is a designer drug (commonly known as Ecstasy, XTC, or MDMA) that acts simultaneously as a stimulant and hallucinogen (85). It results in greater serotonin release in the brain with inhibition of serotonin reuptake. It is abused in pill or capsule forms that are orally ingested. MDMA use has been associated with rave parties and is more commonly abused by adolescents and young adults. Most amphetamines are detected on qualitative urine toxicology assays but a negative result does not rule out amphetamine intoxication or abuse.

Toxicity

In general, these drugs cause release of catecholamines, which result in a sympathomimetic/adrenergic syndrome. Compared to cocaine, the "high" and physiologic effects last longer (hours to several days depending on the agent used). The clinical presentation is characterized by tachycardia, hyperthermia, agitation, hypertension, and mydriasis. Hallucinations (visual and tactile), hypervigilance, and acute psychoses (often paranoia) are frequently observed. MDMA leads to increased verbosity and sociability. MDMA use is associated with bruxism that is often countered by sucking on a pacifier or lollipop. Amphetamine use is often associated with behaviors resulting in trauma and risky sexual encounters. The acute adverse medical consequences are similar to those seen with cocaine abuse (see above) and include myocardial ischemia and arrhythmias, seizures, intracranial hemorrhage, stroke, hyperthermia, rhabdomyolysis, necrotizing vasculitis, and death (86). Long-term use of these drugs may result in dilated cardiomyopathy and "meth mouth." Meth mouth refers to a pattern of oral signs and symptoms of methamphetamine abuse, thought to include rampant caries and tooth fracture, leading to multiple tooth loss and edentulism (84). Burn injuries from methamphetamine laboratory explosions are associated with a higher incidence of inhalational injury and greater use of critical care resources (87).

Complications of MDMA use are usually a result of the drug effects and nonstop physical activity. The effects of MDMA last 4 to 6 hours. Medical complications include hyperthermia, hyponatremia, rhabdomyolysis, seizures, renal failure, arrhythmias, syncope, cerebral infarction/hemorrhage, hepatotoxicity, serotonin syndrome, and death (88). Hyponatremia and hepatoxicity are relatively unique with this agent and the mechanisms leading to these complications are unknown.

Management

Management of amphetamine intoxication is primarily supportive. Gastric lavage is not recommended because absorption after oral ingestion is usually complete when patients present. Activated charcoal may be considered if a recent oral ingestion is known to have occurred. Further interventions are dependent on patient complaints and clinical findings. A careful assessment for complications should be made, including measurement of core temperature, obtaining an electrocardiogram (ECG), searching for evidence of trauma, and evaluating laboratory data for evidence of renal or hepatic dysfunction and rhabdomyolysis. IV hydration for possible rhabdomyolysis is warranted in individuals with known exertional activities pending CPK results. Patients should be placed in a quiet, calm environment and benzodiazepines, often in high doses, are used for controlling agitation. Haloperidol should be reserved for patients who do not have an adequate response to benzodiazepines.

Withdrawal

Acute withdrawal from amphetamines is similar to cocaine and symptoms include fatigue, depression, anxiety, motor retardation, hypersomnia (followed by insomnia), increased eating, and drug craving (89). Although withdrawal is uncomfortable, the manifestations are not dangerous. Patients may become suicidal during withdrawal and should be evaluated for this possibility. Symptoms may persist for months.

γ-HYDROXYBUTYRATE

γ-Hydroxybutyrate (GHB), a naturally occurring metabolite of GABA found in the brain, has limited clinical use in narcolepsy but is more commonly a drug of recreational abuse. It is one of several agents characterized as a "date rape" drug and it has been promoted to build muscle, improve performance, produce euphoria, and enhance sleep. The drug is usually available as a colorless, odorless liquid with a mild salty taste that is easy to mask in drinks. GHB is rapidly absorbed from the stomach (usually within 10–15 minutes) and readily crosses the blood–brain barrier where it interacts with GHB and γ-aminobutyric acid type B ($GABA_B$) receptors. Stimulatory effects occur from resulting increased dopamine levels in the brain and sedative effects by potentiation of endogenous opioids. γ-Butyrolactone (GBL), also known as 2(3H)-furanone-di-hydro, and 1,4 butanediol (BD), also called tetramethylene glycol, have been abused with the same adverse effects as GHB (90). Both agents are metabolized systemically to GHB.

Acute Toxicity

The manifestations of GHB toxicity are dose related and include agitation, coma, seizures, respiratory depression, and vomiting. Other effects include amnesia, tremors, myoclonus, hypotonia, hypothermia, decreased cardiac output, and bradycardia. A dose of 20 to 30 mg/kg can produce euphoria and sleepiness and coma may result from doses of ≥40 to 60 mg/kg (91). Concomitant use of ethanol results in synergistic CNS and respiratory depressant effects. Deaths attributed to GHB and related agents usually result from respiratory depression, hypoxemia, or aspiration. GHB is not routinely detected by urine toxicology assays but can be detected in plasma or urine by gas chromatographic-mass spectrophotometric techniques. Rapid clearance precludes detection beyond 12 hours after a dose (91). Diagnosis is usually determined by the clinical course and history of exposure elicited after the patient recovers. A hallmark of GHB intoxication is rapid onset of toxicity and sudden, rapid recovery rather than a gradual recovery usually seen with ethanol or benzodiazepine intoxication.

Assessment and Treatment of Acute Intoxication

There is no antidote for GHB, GBL, or BD toxicity. The primary management for ingestion of these drugs is supportive care with particular attention to airway protection. In some cases, intubation and mechanical ventilation are required. Gastric lavage and activated charcoal are not warranted because of the small amounts involved and the rapid absorption. Naloxone and flumazenil are of no benefit. Atropine may be needed for symptomatic bradycardia. Patients with mild intoxication may be observed in the emergency department and released after symptoms resolve. A rapid recovery of consciousness from an obtunded condition in a few hours is frequently observed. In patients requiring intubation and mechanical ventilation, symptoms can be expected to resolve within 2 to 96 hours unless complications such as aspiration or anoxic injury have occurred. The concomitant use of alcohol may prolong the CNS depression. Although physostigmine has been reported to awaken patients with GHB intoxication, its use is not recommended (92).

γ-Hydroxybutyrate Withdrawal

A sedative withdrawal syndrome following high-dose frequent use (every 1–3 hours) of GHB, GBL, and BD has been described (91, 93). Mild symptoms such as anxiety, insomnia, nausea, vomiting, and tremors begin within 6 hours of the last dose and may progress to severe delirium with autonomic instability (usually mild) requiring hospitalization and sedation. Patients may experience auditory, visual, and tactile hallucinations. The duration of symptoms requiring treatment may be as long as 2 weeks. Benzodiazepines are the initial choice for management and high doses may be required. Propofol and barbiturates have also been used successfully (91,93).

PHENCYCLIDINE

Phencyclidine (PCP) is a psychoactive drug used as a hallucinogen that can be administered by oral ingestion, nasal insufflation, smoking, or intravenous injection. PCP is a dissociative agent that blocks the NMDA receptors leading to an inhibition of sensory perception. Sympathomimetic effects result from inhibition of norepinephrine and dopamine reuptake.

Clinical Manifestations

Signs and symptoms reported with PCP use are variable depending on the route of abuse, susceptibility of the user, and concomitant drug use (94). Behavioral effects of PCP include coma, catatonia, psychosis, and confusion. Agitation may be intermittent and unexpected. Misperception of reality can lead to violent behavior, risk-taking behavior, and accidents resulting in trauma. Nystagmus (horizontal, vertical, and/or rotatory) and miosis are characteristic findings with PCP intoxication along with ataxia. Medical complications can include hyperthermia, rhabdomyolysis, and seizures. Dystonic reactions occur rarely. PCP is usually detected on urine qualitative toxicology tests.

Management

Management of a patient with PCP intoxication includes control of agitation using a quiet, nonstimulatory environment and benzodiazepines as needed. Haloperidol may be beneficial for frank psychosis. Physical restraints are often needed until adequate sedation is achieved. Tachycardia and hypertension, if present, usually respond to control of agitation. Activated charcoal does adsorb PCP but most patients present after GI absorption is complete following oral ingestion. Although urinary acidification enhances PCP excretion, that intervention is not recommended. The possibility of rhabdomyolysis should be evaluated and early fluid therapy should be considered while awaiting test results.

References

1. Department of Health and Human Services. Results from the 2005 National Survey on Drug Use and Health: national findings. http://www.drugabusestatistics.samhsa.gov/NSDUH/2k5NSDUH/2k5results.htm. Accessed March 22, 2008.
2. Johnston RE, Reier CE. Acute respiratory effects of ethanol in man. *Clin Pharmacol Ther.* 1973;14:503.
3. Friedman HS, Lieber CS. Cardiotoxicity of alcohol. *Cardiovasc Med.* 1977; 2:111.
4. Marc Aurcle J, Schreier GE. The dialysance of ethanol and methanol: a proposed method of treatment for massive intoxication by ethyl or methyl alcohol. *J Clin Invest.* 1960;39:802.
5. Wrenn KD, Slovis CM, Minion GE, et al. The syndrome of alcoholic ketoacidosis. *Am J Med.* 1991;91:119.
6. Sharma AN, Hoffman RS. Withdrawal syndromes. In: Brent J. (ed) *Critical Care Toxicology: Diagnosis and Management of the Critically Poisoned Patient*. Philadelphia: Elsevier Mosby; 2005:363–371.
7. Spies C, Tonnesen HS, Andreasson S. Perioperative morbidity and mortality in chronic alcoholic patients. *Alcohol Clin Exp Res.* 2001;25:164s–170s.
8. Victor M, Adams RD. The effect of alcohol on the nervous system. *Res Publ Assoc Res Nerv Ment Dis.* 1953;32.
9. Sullivan JT, Sykora K, Schneiderman J, et al. Assessment of alcohol withdrawal: the revised Clinical Institute Assessment for Alcohol scale (CIWA-Ar). *Br J Addict.* 1989;84:1353.
10. Ntais C, Pakos E, Kyzas P, et al. Benzodiazepines for alcohol withdrawal. *Cochrane Database Syst Rev.* 2005;3:CD005063.
11. Polycarpou A, Papanikolaou P, Ioannidis JPA, et al. Anticonvulsants for alcohol withdrawal. *Cochrane Database Syst Rev.* 2005;3:CD005064.
12. Dissanaike S, Halldorsson A, Frezza EE, et al. An ethanol protocol to prevent alcohol withdrawal syndrome. *J Am Coll Surg.* 2006;203:186–191.
13. Hodges B, Mazur JE. Intravenous ethanol for the treatment of alcohol withdrawal syndrome in critically ill patients. *Pharmacotherapy.* 2004;24:1578.
14. Lechtenberg R, Worner TM. Relative kindling effect of detoxification and non-detoxification admissions in alcoholics. *Alcohol.* 1991;26:221.
15. Brathen G, Ben-Menachem F, Brodtkorb E, et al. EFNS guideline on the diagnosis and management of alcohol-related seizures: report of an EFNS task force. *Eur J Neurol.* 2005;12:575.
16. Hillbom M, Pieninkeroinen I, Leone M. Seizures in alcohol dependent patients. Epidemiology, pathophysiology and management. *CNS Drugs.* 2003; 17:1013.
17. D'Onofrio G, Rathlev NK, Ulrich AS, et al. Lorazepam for the prevention of recurrent seizures related to alcohol. *N Engl J Med.* 1999;340:915.
18. Mayo-Smith MF, Beecher LH, Fischer TL, et al. Management of alcohol withdrawal delirium, an evidence-based practice guideline. *Arch Intern Med.* 2004;164:1405.
19. Miller FT. Protracted alcohol withdrawal delirium. *J Subst Abuse Treat.* 1994;11:127.
20. Wilson KC, Reardon C, Theodore AC, et al. Propylene glycol toxicity: a severe iatrogenic illness in ICU patients receiving IV benzodiazepines. *Chest.* 2005;128:1674.
21. McCowan C, Marik P. Refractory delirium tremens treated with propofol. *Crit Care Med.* 2000;28:1781–1784.
22. Cuculi F, Kobza R, Ehmann T, et al. ECG changes amongst patients with alcohol withdrawal seizures and delirium tremens. *Swiss Med Wkly.* 2006;136:223.
23. Brower KJ, Mudd S. Severity and treatment of alcohol withdrawal in elderly vs younger patients. *Alcohol Clin Exp Res.* 1994;18:196.
24. Olmedo R, Hoffman RS. Cocaine. In: Brent J. (ed) *Critical Care Toxicology: Diagnosis and Management of the Critically Poisoned Patient*. Philadelphia: Elsevier Mosby; 2005:3785–3797.
25. Hall WC, Talbert RL. Cocaine abuse and its treatment. *Pharmacotherapy.* 1990;10:47.
26. Ambre JJ, Belknap SM, Nelson J. Acute tolerance to cocaine in humans. *Clin Pharmacol Ther.* 1988;44:1.
27. Mueller PD, Olson KR. Cocaine. *Emerg Med Clin North Am.* 1990;8:481.
28. Lange RA, Hills LD. Cardiovascular complications of cocaine use. *N Engl J Med.* 2001;345:351–358.
29. Eichhorn EJ, Peacock E, Grayburn PA, et al. Chronic cocaine abuse in association with accelerated atherosclerosis in human coronary arteries. *J Am Coll Cardiol.* 1992;19:105A.
30. Majid PA, Patel B. An angiographic and histologic study of cocaine induced chest pain. *Am J Cardiol.* 1990;65:812.
31. Zimmerman JL, Dellinger RP, Majid PA. Cocaine associated chest pain. *Ann Emerg Med.* 1991;20:611–615.
32. Gitter MJ, Goldsmith SR, Dunbar DN, et al. Cocaine and chest pain: clinical features and outcome of patients hospitalized to rule out myocardial infarction. *Ann Intern Med.* 1991;115:277–282.
33. Hollander JE, Levitt A, Young GP, et al. Effect of recent cocaine use on the specificity of cardiac markers for diagnosis of acute myocardial infarction. *Am Heart J.* 1998;135:245–252.
34. Hollander JE, Hoffman RS, Gennis P, et al. Prospective multicenter evaluation of cocaine associated chest pain. *Acad Emerg Med.* 1994;1:330–339.
35. Kontos MC, Jesse RL, Tatum JL, et al. Coronary angiographic findings in patients with cocaine-associated chest pain. *J Emerg Med.* 2003;24:9–13.
36. Nademanee K, Gorelick DA, Josephson MA, et al. Myocardial ischemia during withdrawal. *Ann Intern Med.* 1989;111:876.
37. Kloner RA, Hale S, Alker K, et al. The effects of acute and chronic cocaine use on the heart. *Circulation.* 1992;85:407–419.
38. Barth CW III, Bray M, Roberts WC. Rupture of the ascending aorta during cocaine intoxication. *Am J Cardiol.* 1986;57:496.
39. Lowenstein DH, Massa SM, Rowbothem MC. Acute neurological and psychological complications associated with cocaine. *Am J Med.* 1987;87:841.
40. Kaku DA. Emergence of recreational drug use as a risk factor for stroke in young adults. *Ann Intern Med.* 1990;113:821.
41. Levine SR, Brust JCM, Futrell N. Cerebrovascular complications of the use of the "crack" form of alkaloidal cocaine. *N Engl J Med.* 1990;323:699.
42. Kaufman MJ, Levin JM, Ross MH, et al. Cocaine-induced cerebral vasoconstriction detected in humans with magnetic resonance angiography. *JAMA.* 1998;279:376–380.
43. Oyesiku NM, Colohan ART, Barrow DL, et al. Cocaine-induced aneurysmal rupture: an emergent negative factor in the natural history of intracranial aneurysms? *Neurosurgery.* 1993;32:518–526.
44. Fessler RD, Esshaki CM, Stankewitz RC, et al. The neurovascular complications of cocaine. *Surg Neurol.* 1997;47:339–345.
45. Leone AP, Dhuna A. Cerebral atrophy in habitual cocaine abusers: a planimetric CT study. *Neurology.* 1991;41:34.
46. Haim DY, Lippmann ML, Goldberg SK, et al. The pulmonary complications of crack cocaine. A comprehensive review. *Chest.* 1995;107:233–240.
47. Albertson TE, Walby WF, Derlet RW. Stimulant-induced pulmonary toxicity. *Chest.* 1995;108:1140–1149.
48. Tashkin DP, Kleerup KC, Koyal SN, et al. Acute effects of inhaled and i.v. cocaine on airway dynamics. *Chest.* 1996;110:904–910.
49. Osborn HH, Tang M, Bradley K, et al. New-onset bronchospasm or recrudescence of asthma associated with cocaine abuse. *Acad Emerg Med.* 1997;4:689–692.
50. Levine M, Iliescu ME, Margellos-Anast H, et al. The effects of cocaine and heroin use on intubation rates and hospital utilization in patients with acute asthma exacerbations. *Chest.* 2005;128:1951–1957.
51. Matthew E, Seaman M. Barotrauma related to inhalational drug abuse. *J Emerg Med.* 1990;8:141.
52. Forrester JM, Steele AW, Waldron JA, et al. Crack lung: an acute pulmonary syndrome with a spectrum of clinical and histological findings. *Am Rev Respir Dis.* 1990;142:462.
53. Zimmerman JL, Dellinger RP. Septic pulmonary emboli in the intravenous substance abuser. In: Dellinger RP, ed. *The Substance Abuser: Problems in Critical Care*. Philadelphia: J.B. Lippincott; 1987.
54. Marzuk PM, Tardiff K, Leon AC, et al. Ambient temperature and mortality from unintentional cocaine overdose. *JAMA.* 1998;279:1795–1800.
55. Crandall CG, Vongpatanasin W, Victor RG. Mechanism of cocaine-induced hyperthermia in humans. *Ann Intern Med.* 1992;136:785–791.
56. Dwelch R, Todd K. Incidence of cocaine associated rhabdomyolysis. *Ann Emerg Med.* 1991;20:154.
57. Brody S, Wrenn KD. Predicting the severity of cocaine associated rhabdomyolysis. *Ann Emerg Med.* 1990;19:1137.
58. Muniz AE, Evans T. Acute gastrointestinal manifestations associated with use of crack. *Am J Emerg Med.* 2001;19:61–63.
59. Feliciano DV, Ojukwu JC, Rozycki GS, et al. The epidemic of cocaine-related juxtapyloric perforations. *Ann Surg.* 1999;6:801–806.
60. Nzerue CM, Hewan-Lowe K, Riley LJ. Cocaine and the kidney: a synthesis of pathophysiologic and clinical perspectives. *Am J Kid Dis.* 2000;35:783–795.
61. Derlet RN, Albertson TE. ED presentation of cocaine intoxication. *Ann Emerg Med.* 1989;18:182.
62. Derlet RN, Albertson TE, Rice P. Effect of haloperidol in cocaine and amphetamine intoxication. *J Emerg Med.* 1989;7:633.
63. Baumann BM, Perrone J, Hornig SE, et al. Randomized, double-blind, placebo-controlled trial of diazepam, nitroglycerin, or both for treatment of patients with potential cocaine-associated acute coronary syndromes. *Acad Emerg Med.* 2000;7:878–885.
64. Honderick T, Williams D, Seaberg D, et al. A prospective, randomized, controlled trial of benzodiazepines and nitroglycerine or nitroglycerine alone in the treatment of cocaine-associated acute coronary syndromes. *Am J Emerg Med.* 2003;21:39–42.
65. Braunwald E, Antman EM, Beasley JW, et al. ACC/AHA 2002 guideline update for the management of patients with unstable angina and non-ST-segment elevation myocardial infarction. *J Am Coll Cardiol.* 2002;40:1366–1374.
66. Lange RA, Cigarroa RG. Potentiation of cocaine-induced coronary vasoconstriction by beta-adrenergic blockade. *Ann Intern Med.* 1990;112:897.
67. Weber JE, Shofer FS, Larkin GL, et al. Validation of a brief observation period for patients with cocaine-associated chest pain. *N Engl J Med.* 2003;348:510–517.

68. Hollander JE. The management of cocaine induced myocardial ischemia. *N Engl J Med.* 1995;333:1267–1272.
69. Hollander JE, Burstein JL, Hoffman RS, et al. Cocaine-associated myocardial infarction. Clinical safety of thrombolytic therapy. *Chest.* 1995;107:1237–1241.
70. Shih RD, Hollander JE, Burstein JL, et al. Clinical safety of lidocaine in patients with cocaine-associated myocardial infarction. *Ann Emerg Med.* 1995;26:702–706.
71. Goldfrank LR, Hoffman RS. The cardiovascular effects of cocaine. *Ann Emerg Med.* 1991;20:165.
72. Traub SJ, Hoffman RS, Nelson LS. Body packing—the internal concealment of illicit drugs. *N Engl J Med.* 2004;349:2519–2526.
73. Das D, Ali B, Mackway-Jones K. Conservative management of asymptomatic cocaine body packers. *Emerg Med J.* 2003;20:172–174.
74. Dackis CA, Gold MS. New concepts in cocaine addiction: the dopamine depletion hypothesis. *Neurosci Biobehav Rev.* 1985;9:469.
75. Roberts JR, Greenberg MI. Cocaine washout syndrome. *Ann Intern Med.* 2000;132:679–680.
76. Fiellin DA, O'Connar PG. Office based treatment of opioid dependent patients. *N Engl J Med.* 2002;347:817–823.
77. Sporer KA. Acute heroin overdose. *Ann Intern Med.* 1999;130:584.
78. Tharp AM, Winecker RE, Winston DC. Fatal intravenous fentanyl abuse. *Am J Forensic Med Pathol.* 2004;25:178.
79. Wolff AJ, O'Donnell AE. Pulmonary effects of illicit drug use. *Clin Chest Med.* 2004;25:203.
80. Kaplan JL, Marx JA, Calabro JJ, et al. Double blind, randomized study of nalmefene and naloxone in emergency department patients with suspected narcotic overdose. *Ann Emerg Med.* 1999;34:42.
81. Sporer KA, Dorn E. Heroin-related noncardiogenic pulmonary edema. *Chest.* 2001;120:1628.
82. Growing L, Ali R, White J. Buprenorphine for the management of opioid withdrawal. *Cochrane Database Syst Rev.* 2006;2:CD002025.
83. Cuthill JD, Beroniade V. Evaluation of clonidine suppression of opiate withdrawal reactions: a multidisciplinary approach. *Can J Psychiatry.* 1990;35:377.
84. Curtis EK. Meth mouth: a review of methamphetamine abuse and its oral manifestations. *General Dentistry.* 2006;54:125–129.
85. de la Torre R, Farré M, Roset PN, et al. Human pharmacology of MDMA, pharmacokinetics, metabolism, and disposition. *Ther Drug Monit.* 2004;26:137.
86. Lineberry TW, Bostwick JM. Methamphetamine abuse: a perfect storm of complications, *Mayo Clin Proc.* 2006;81:77.
87. Santos AP, Wilson AK, Hornung CA, et al. Methamphetamine laboratory explosions: a new and emerging burn injury. *J Burn Care Rehabil.* 2005;26:228.
88. Kalant H. The pharmacology and toxicology of "ecstasy" (MDMA) and related drugs. *CMAJ.* 2001;165:917.
89. McGregor C, Srisurapanont M, Jittiwutikarn J, et al. The nature, time course, and severity of methamphetamine withdrawal. *Addiction.* 2005;100:1320.
90. Zvosec DL, Smith SW, McCutcheon JR, et al. Adverse events, including death, associated with the use of 1,4-butanediol. *N Engl J Med.* 2001;344:87–94.
91. Snead OC, Gibson KM. γ-Hydroxybutyric acid. *N Engl J Med.* 2005;352:2721–2732.
92. Traub SJ, Nelson LS, Hoffman RS. Physostigmine as a treatment for gamma-hydroxybutyrate toxicity: a review. *J Toxicol Clin Toxicol.* 2002;40:781.
93. Dyer JE, Roth B, Hyma BA. Gamma-hydroxybutyrate withdrawal syndrome. *Ann Emerg Med.* 2001;37:147–153.
94. McCarron MM, Schulze BW, Thompson GA, et al. Acute phencyclidine intoxication: incidence of clinical findings in 1,000 cases. *Ann Emerg Med.* 1981;10:237–242.

CHAPTER 68 ■ ENVENOMATION

CRAIG S. KITCHENS – Snakes Native to the United States • STEVEN A. SEIFERT – Snakes Non-Native to the United States • CLAUDIA L. BARTHOLD – Spiders and Scorpions • JENNIFER A. OAKES – Marine Envenomation

This review will discuss envenomation by snakes (both native and non-native to the United States), spiders, scorpions, and marine animals. Clinical and laboratory manifestations of envenomations are due to a spectacular array of substances that gain entry into the victim and cause symptoms. A great deal of attention has been paid to the biochemistry and mechanisms regarding venoms. As complex and varied as these are, one should expect that the symptoms and severity can range from mild to serious, or even be fatal, and the treatment can range from supportive to the administration of various substances (antivenoms) meant to neutralize the activity of the venoms. Over the past 50 years, the scientific approach to understanding venoms and their manifestations has converted the approach to envenomation syndromes from folklore and anecdotal first-aid nostrums to an ever-growing and sophisticated scientific discipline.

SNAKES NATIVE TO THE UNITED STATES

Man has had a long and storied relationship with snakes, with references several millennia ago found in the third chapter of Genesis. Despite most references' depiction of dread, the medical profession's positive regard for snakes is attested by the universally accepted sign of the medical profession: a snake intertwined on the staff of Aesculapius.

This portion of the chapter will deal with our management style regarding snake envenomation by snakes native to the United States; other physicians' styles may be less conservative; few will be more so. First, these facts not only underscore differences in therapeutic philosophy, but also acknowledge that there exists a considerable range in morbidity and mortality in envenomation based partly on the bitten host, but especially on the species of the offending reptile—we treat what we see. Second, one can deduce that there is no clear "standard of care."

The second part of the chapter will address envenomation by snakes not native to the United States. Unfortunately, this separation sometimes is blurred by the increasing number of exotic snakes kept either professionally by herpetologists who work in zoos, research, or the pharmaceutical industry, or by amateurs who collect a variety of exotic poisonous snakes. Accordingly, the health care professional must be prepared to deal with a broad range of snake envenomations.

A mere century ago, the treatment of North American snakebites was shrouded in mystery, folklore, and old wives' tales, and indeed, was not even considered a medical problem. As clinical observation followed by clinical investigation became more commonplace in the study of snake envenomation syndromes, snake bite management has become an important area of clinical medicine (1).

In the United States, there are two broad categories of venomous snakes. The first, and the less common, is the coral snake, members of the family Elapidae, with two genera and several species. This snake represents the only venomous snake in North America that is not a pit viper, does not have "cat eye"–shaped pupils, and has a rather small head. Only 1% to 2% of all U.S. snakebite envenomations involve coral snakes, yet this small number accounts for a somewhat disproportionate amount of human morbidity and mortality. As the epidemiology, symptomatology, and treatment of coral snake envenomation is entirely different and apart from pit viper envenomation, it will be discussed separately.

The pit vipers account for about 95% of U.S. snakebites. These are members of the family Crotalidae and comprise rattlesnakes, water moccasins, and copperheads. Pit vipers are composed of three genera and numerous species, which will be briefly discussed separately. As pit vipers, they have two heat-sensing pits approximately halfway between their nostrils and eyes. Because of their considerable venom apparatus, they appear to have heads significantly larger than one might expect, given the size of their bodies. Rattlesnakes have a series of distal specialized skin attachments that cause the rattlesnake to generate the distinctive rattle when its tail is shaken. The remaining 2% to 3% of all U.S. snakebites are inflicted by exotic venomous snakes, which will be covered in the second section of this chapter, "Snakes Non-native to the United States."

Identification of offending animals should be done if possible, but without undue risk of further bites to the victim or others. Because the U.S. pit viper and coral snake antivenoms are polyvalent, it is only necessary to identify a snake to the family level. Identification charts are available and experts such as local herpetologists may be consulted in certain cases.

Coral Snake Envenomation

Coral snakes are rather small and brilliantly colored secretive reptiles. As opposed to most snakes, which prefer isolation, they are often found around newer housing projects and may be encountered in one's garden or yard. By habit, they are not aggressive, supporting stories that children may play with them for hours to days without being bitten. Additionally, their anatomy is such that they cannot open their mouths as widely as the pit vipers, so they typically bite only at the tips of fingers or the webbed space between the thumb and first finger. Lacking long fangs, envenomation requires hanging on to this small anatomic part for 10 to 30 seconds in order to work venom into the skin, an activity most victims will not tolerate, again accounting for the rather small number of victims.

This colorful snake has several nonpoisonous distant look-alikes with which it is sometimes confused. In the United States, the coral snake has a black nose, with alternating rings of red, yellow (sometimes white), and black encircling the entire body of the snake. Hospitals should have a snake identification chart, but identification of snakes from pictures by patients, let alone by younger patients and/or patients in an inebriated state, is notoriously poor.

Coral snake envenomation is complicated by the fact that, in direct contradistinction to pit viper envenomation, there is little or no local tissue damage; therefore, the characteristic triad of immediate local pain, swelling, and discoloration characteristic of pit viper envenomation does not develop. It is accordingly possible to misconstrue a serious bite from a coral snake as one from either a "dry bite" by a venomous snake or a bite by a nonvenomous snake. This can lead to an unfortunate outcome.

Symptoms and Manifestations

Symptoms may be delayed up to 12 hours, yet are dangerous and can progress rapidly should they occur; therefore, patients should be observed for 24 hours to determine whether an envenomation has occurred.

As the venom is chiefly neurotoxic, neurologic signs and symptoms are declared in approximately the following ascending order and frequency: a mild numbness in the bitten extremity; and euphoria, often precipitously followed by cranial nerve symptoms, with diplopia being the one that the patient most often first notices, whereas a distinct flat dysarthria (similar to patients with myasthenia gravis) is the one that health care professionals usually first notice. Stridor, inability to swallow, and, finally, respiratory arrest may rapidly ensue. During progression from dysarthria to respiratory arrest, aspiration pneumonia is extremely common and comprises one of the major morbidities and mortalities of coral snake envenomation. Should cranial nerve involvement be noted to develop, it is important to prophylactically and preemptively intubate the patient in order to protect the airway.

Lacking the large fangs characteristic of pit vipers, puncture wounds are notoriously not prominent. Rather, if one squeezes the bite site, one may see minute, pinpoint accumulations of blood welling up from the tissue, indicating that the teeth of the coral snake have successfully worked their way into the subcutaneous tissue, thereby allowing the deposition of venom. We have reported (2) a triad of risk factors that, in our opinion, if any two are present, warrant strong consideration for the infusion of three to five vials of antivenom: (a) the snake is positively identified as a coral snake; (b) there is a history of the snake "hanging on" the bitten site for at least 15 to 30 seconds, thus allowing sufficient time to work the venom under the skin; and/or (c) one can observe pinpoints of blood following applied pressure to the bitten area. We typically do not administer antivenom for the presence of only one feature of this triad but typically observe the patient for about a day.

The primary manifestation of envenomation is paralysis of the entire nervous system, with the primary threat to life being respiratory arrest, with or without aspiration pneumonia. Our local experience suggests that the natural history of those patients who develop respiratory arrest do so for approximately 7 to 10 days before the effects of the venom naturally abate. Mentation is not affected. One must be able to support a totally flaccid patient for this period of time, with particular attention to maintenance of respiratory care and respiratory hygiene. Long-term sequelae following either successful treatment or the natural history of the envenomation syndrome may include several months of dysesthesias and paresthesias in the bitten extremity, but generally fade after several months to a year.

Antivenom Administration

The antivenom for coral snake envenomation supplied by Wyeth (Antivenin [Micrurus fulvius] [equine origin]) unfortunately is no longer being manufactured. As there are limited and dwindling supplies available, present statements and future predictions on how to treat envenomation by coral snake are most difficult. If antivenom can be procured, and if symptoms are deemed either imminent or present, usually three to five vials of the antivenom are given intravenously about every 8 to 12 hours until symptoms stop progressing. Typically, a single treatment is sufficient. If symptoms develop an hour or more before antivenin administration, it is notoriously difficult to reverse the neurologic blockade, and repeated administration of antivenom is not only futile, but in this time of extremely limited supplies, is probably unwise for society in general. Skin testing has been suggested prior to intravenous administration of the antivenom, but is imperfect in predicting safety or reaction to this antivenom, and should not delay administration in life-threatening situations in any case.

With the impending collapse of the supply of coral snake antivenom presently in the United States, it is unclear what course of action to recommend. It appears that antivenom prepared for South American members of the Micrurus family is not very effective for the Micrurus species in the northern hemisphere (3). A coral snake antivenom, prepared in Mexico (Coralmyn, Bioclon), is available in emergencies. Presently, it is recommended to call your regional poison center (1-800-222-1222) to assist in acquisition, as most of the Mexican product in the United States is held by zoos. See the section on Snakes Non-native to the United States for further information.

Pit Viper Envenomation

Genera

1. *Crotalus:* This family, Crotalidae, consists of three genera found within the United States. The largest genus, composed of some 15 to 20 species and subspecies, is *Crotalus*, the rattlesnakes. Rattlesnakes are distinctly New World animals. The rattle is composed of specialized scales that produce a rattling sound when the reptile shakes its tail. The most serious bites are those of the two largest snakes, namely the eastern diamondback rattlesnake (*Crotalus adamanteus*) and the western diamondback rattlesnake (*Crotalus atrox*). Some special comments will also be made about specific effects of the venoms of the canebrake rattlesnake (*Crotalus horridus atricaudatus*) and the Mojave rattlesnake (*Crotalus scutulatus*). The remaining rattlesnakes tend to be smaller and located mostly in the desert southwest and California.
2. *Sistrurus:* Two other species of rattlesnakes are in the second genus, *Sistrurus*. *Sistrurus catenatus* (also known as the massasauga) is mostly encountered in the upper Midwest from western Pennsylvania and New York across to Michigan and Iowa. *Sistrurus miliarius* (also known as the pygmy rattlesnake) is seen chiefly in Florida and up into the Atlantic coast states. Both species of *Sistrurus* are smaller rattlesnakes with poorly developed rattles. Their bites are characterized by a very low morbidity and virtually zero mortality (4–6). We use antivenom only occasionally (approximately 10% of the time) in pygmy rattlesnake bites.
3. *Agkistrodon:* The third genus of the family Crotalidae is *Agkistrodon*, which is composed of two species. The copperhead (*Agkistrodon contortrix*) is the most common pit viper from Georgia up through the Atlantic Coast states. In three reviews (7–9), antivenom was administered to only 0% to 11% of victims. Some practitioners may infuse antivenom more liberally in bites adjudged to be more serious than most. *Agkistrodon piscivorus* (commonly known as the water moccasin) is also in the Atlantic Coast states, in Florida, and westward through Alabama and Mississippi and into eastern Texas. Neither species of *Agkistrodon* is extremely venomous. Bites characteristically cause significant edema but virtually no mortality (7–9). Significant *in vitro* coagulation abnormalities are rare (9,10). We employ antivenom in only about 25% of victims of water moccasin envenomations and those chiefly for patients either at the extremes of age or with significant comorbidities.

Range of Venom Effects

Bites from these species of pit vipers vary enormously, from the least lethal with no documented deaths (*Sistrurus miliarius*—pygmy rattlesnake) to the most lethal (*Crotalus adamanteus*—eastern diamondback rattlesnake). The variability of the virulence is due to the variability of the venom. All pit viper venoms are very complex, containing upwards to 20 to 40 proteinaceous substances, about half of which are enzymes that are designed to help spread the venom throughout the prey's tissues and to predigest the intended prey, and another equal number of nonenzymatic proteins that have many other effects, including those on the autonomic nervous system. Indeed, pit viper venom is one of the most complex mixtures of poisons known to exist. Snake venom is best regarded as an offensive weapon to assist the animal rather than regarded as a defensive weapon against an accidental prey.

The complexity of the venom is demonstrated by its multiple effects. At one time, it was fashionable to describe venom as "neurotoxic" or "hematotoxic," but those notions tend to break down. It is fair to regard the venom of the coral snake to be chiefly, if not exclusively, neurotoxic. Several excellent reviews exist regarding the complex nature of pit viper venoms (11–19).

This mixture of venom components vary enormously not only within the family, but also within the genus and species. In fact, even within the same subspecies, there is considerable variation in the relative concentrations of various components in the venom. Even individual members of a species, kept over time, display variability in their venom pattern (20).

This is important when one considers the antivenom that is currently available. CroFab (Crotalidae polyvalent immune Fab [ovine] [FabAV], Therapeutic Antibodies, Inc., Nashville TN) is a mixture of Fab fragments prepared from purified immunoglobulins, produced by healthy sheep that have been repeatedly injected with venom from one of the following four snakes: *Crotalus atrox*, *Crotalus adamanteus*, *Crotalus scutulatus*, or *Agkistrodon piscivorus*. The Fab fragments from all four preparations are then mixed together to produce a polyvalent mixture. As there are variable degrees of immunogenicity and responses from the sheep to the injection of multiple and variable components (antigens) within the venom of these four pit vipers, it should be realized that not all venom components will be neutralized to exactly the same degree. Because many of the venom principles within other species of this genus may be shared with other genera, there is a variable degree of crossover of the Fab antivenom against the venom of species to which the sheep was never exposed, such as *Crotalus horridus atricaudatus*, *Sistrurus miliarius*, and others. This no doubt explains, in part, the variability of the response of some envenomation syndromes from other snake bites to the same Fab antivenom. As an example, the author has had experience (unpublished data) with a patient envenomated by a pet mottled rock rattlesnake (*Crotalus lepidus lepidus*), a small and rather rarely offending reptile. The victim of this bite had essentially no salubrious response to repeated administrations of FabAV. One may deduce that there exist few Fab fragments directed against that snake's individual venom pattern. On the other hand, the venom of the Southern Pacific rattlesnake (*Crotalus helleri*) is not injected into those sheep, yet envenomation by this reptile seems to respond well to FabAV (21).

Symptoms and Manifestations

The near-immediate onset of the triad of symptoms occurring in human victims of pit viper envenomation—namely, pain, swelling, and discoloration—supports the concept of disruption and digestion due to the venom. Digestive enzymes such as phosphatases, hyaluronidases, proteinases, phospholipases, and other substances dissolve connective tissue and proteins, and attack nerve endings (17,19). Edema is largely brought about by disruption of the endothelium of capillaries and lymphatics due to a variety of proteins that directly attack the endothelial integrity of the microcirculation. Discoloration results from extravasation of red cells through the disrupted microcirculation (19). A far smaller role in local hemorrhage is played by disruptions of the coagulation system, which is discussed in more detail below. Evidence for this concept is that while hemorrhage within soft tissues may be spreading and progressive, it is typically confined to the bitten extremity and hemorrhage only rarely occurs systemically in victims of bites from snakes native to the United States; this is not always the case with bites from many snakes not native to this country.

Pain, swelling, and discoloration (immediate to approximately 2 hours at the latest) serve as excellent signs of envenomation. On the other hand, lack of pain, swelling, and discoloration usually indicate that the victim has been fortunate to be one of the 15% to 30% of pit viper victims in which the reptile did not inject venom. These victims of so-called "dry bites" clearly not only have been fortunate, but also do not require antivenom. One pitfall and caveat is that some patients may be envenomated by a pit viper but fail to have any local signs of pain, swelling, or discoloration, yet may be clearly ill as attested by their profuse weakness, fasciculations, diaphoresis, hypotension, nausea, vomiting, diarrhea, mental status alterations (which include confusion and stupor), and the oft-mentioned "metallic taste" experienced by several victims. This situation occurs in approximately 5% to 10% of envenomations, and is best attributed to injection of the venom more or less directly into a vessel or a muscular bed rich in capillaries such that local pain, swelling, and discoloration are bypassed as the venom goes more directly into the circulatory system. In this situation, local signs and symptoms are nonexistent, or at least are far outweighed by a very obvious systemic envenomation syndrome. Sites in which such situations occur are the muscular areas within the hands (thenar or hypothenar eminences) as well as the calf, or even more proximally in the great muscles of the legs or arms. It is often striking how few local signs there are other than puncture marks over these muscular areas in a patient who is clearly extremely ill.

Many of the venom components that cause pain, swelling, and discoloration are neutralized by the currently available FabAV. A great many of these principles are shared within the Crotalid family; however, not all are. The venom of some native snakes contains a principle that is quite myotoxic and this appears to be less promptly neutralized by FabAV. Reptiles that characteristically cause massive rhabdomyolysis with large elevations of the serum creatine phosphokinase (CPK)—including the CPK-MB band, but with negative troponin assays—include the canebrake rattlesnake (*Crotalus horridus atricaudatus*) (22) of the eastern United States and the Mojave rattlesnake (*Crotalus scutulatus*) (23) of the desert southwest. Additionally, neurologic symptoms are more pronounced in the Mojave rattlesnake victim than in victims of most other Crotalid species (24).

Clinical and Laboratory Findings

Coagulopathic findings, both clinical and laboratory, have always been of great interest to those who treat pit viper envenomations. Whereas some laboratory coagulation defects may be seen to some extent in most of the pit viper envenomations, they are by far most pronounced within the *Crotalus* genus and rarely encountered in the *Agkistrodon* (9,10) and rarely, if ever, in the *Sistrurus* genera (10).

Laboratory coagulation abnormalities that have been described in bite victims of *Crotalus* subspecies have been most thoroughly studied in the bites from the eastern diamondback (*Crotalus adamanteus*) (10) and the western diamondback (*Crotalus atrox*) (16). The venom of these snakes contains a thrombin-like enzyme that has been referred to as crotalase. This enzyme rapidly and efficiently, yet only partially, cleaves fibrinogen by cleaving the B-peptide off the β-subunit as does thrombin but, unlike thrombin, does not complete fibrinogen cleavage as it neither cleaves the A-peptide from the α-subunit nor activates factors V, VIII, or XIII. This partially clotted fibrinogen forms a loose gel that is exquisitely sensitive to any proteolytic activity, so visible thromboses or organ manifestations of systemic thromboses are not encountered. Also different from thrombin's actions, crotalase neither activates platelets nor consumes antithrombin III. These are distinct and durable differentiating points from disseminated intravascular coagulation (DIC). In DIC, consumption of fibrinogen is typical but it is accompanied by severe depletion of platelets, factor V, factor VIII, occurs from the bite of some exotic snakes (15).

Crotalase does not activate plasminogen directly (i.e., *in vitro* or *in vivo*) but does so indirectly, most likely by release of endothelial-secreted tissue plasminogen activator (tPA). Plasma levels of tPA spike in a reflex response to the deposition of the partially formed fibrin on the endothelial surface, and a brisk fibrinolysis occurs, attacking the extremely labile non-crosslinked, partially formed clot that produces massive quantities of circulating fibrin degradation products (FDPs), as essentially the total body fibrinogen complement (some 15 g) is nearly totally converted into FDPs within an hour (10).

Crotalase is necessary in only extremely small amounts to totally defibrinogenate an adult human. This hypothesis is supported by three lines of evidence. The first is that even the most trivial bite from the smallest of eastern diamondbacks may be associated with total defibrinogenation, resulting in plasma fibrinogen levels less than 50 mg/dL. Therefore, the coagulation end point (visible fibrin clot) of routine coagulation tests, such as prothrombin time (PT) and partial thromboplastin time (PTT), is so impaired that many interpret this as the blood being "incoagulable," which only seems true. Thrombin generation via the intact coagulation cascade is totally retained save for the lack of the visible clot. Intact thrombin generation serves to afford intact hemostasis, despite incoagulable *in vitro* PTs and PTTs. Thrombin generation is sufficient to affect platelet adhesion at sites of wounds and, with even limited amounts of remaining fibrinogen, to secure a reasonable clot. This is also supported by the lack of systemic bleeding in the vast majority of defibrinogenated patients, as well as the impunity of insertion of central lines or even surgical procedures at the wound site.

A second line of evidence that crotalase need be present in only very small amounts is evidenced by an event termed "recurrence" (25,26). In this clinical situation, despite total arrest of the envenomation syndrome—as defined by a lack of progression of present swelling at the bite site, a lack of new swelling, cessation of nausea and vomiting, normalization of vital signs, and, at least temporarily, total correction of the PT and PTT (27)—after several days, the PT and PTT may revert to incoagulability as defibrinogenation recurs, most likely as a result of a pharmacodynamic and pharmacokinetic mismatch between venom principles and Fab antivenom. That is, antivenom fails to neutralize all of the injected venom, and also is cleared from circulation much more rapidly than venom components.

The third line of evidence is the astounding efficacy of readministration of FabAV to re-reverse the recurrence of coagulopathy. It would appear that the circulatory release of crotalase with sudden defibrinogenation may be among the most sensitive markers of envenomation by either the eastern or western diamondback rattlesnake.

There is great and healthy debate of whether or not the recurrence syndrome should be treated (26). Patients who have been clinically stable for several days following prompt administration of FabAV may and usually do remain totally free of any symptoms, including any clinical signs of abnormal hemostasis, only to be found to have incoagulable PTs and PTTs as they are being prepared for hospital discharge.

A stumbling block for the majority of clinicians is drawing interpretations and conclusions based on their prior clinical experiences from clinical situations resulting in equally impaired PTs and PTTs, and then comparing those situations to this fairly benign defibrinogenation syndrome. Such examples may include the true, real, and quite obvious hemostatic disarray that may accompany greatly prolonged PTs and PTTs in patients with liver disease, warfarin overdosage, DIC, hemophilia, or administration of heparin or other anticoagulants (28). These situations in which hemorrhage is quite obvious do not translate into the patient who is merely defibrinogenated. Defibrinogenation in this situation is rather most analogous to defibrinogenation following the therapeutic administration of plasminogen activators such as streptokinase or tPA. Whereas hemorrhage is experienced in approximately 1% of all patients who receive these therapeutic thrombolytic agents, it is highly concentrated among older patients, hypersensitive patients, or those with prior central nervous system lesions such as strokes, trauma, metastatic disease, or primary tumors.

Treatment of true DIC is rather difficult and hinges on successful elimination of the underlying cause. Rather, the defibrinogenation syndrome is very easily and promptly reversed by the administration of fibrinogen in the form of approximately 8 to 10 units of cryoprecipitate and/or the readministration of FabAV. However, recurrence may happen yet again if unneutralized venom principles continue to enter the general circulation after the clearance of the additional antivenom. The clinical significance of recurrence, particularly as manifest by return of coagulation abnormalities from victims of North American pit vipers, is not at all evident. These recurrences have been best studied and defined as the result of study and follow-up of patients bitten by, particularly, rattlesnakes and administered FabAV. This was enabled because of the research, development, and observation from clinical protocol-driven prospective studies of patients treated with FabAV, which garnered the largest and most extensively followed group of patients (29). In fact, in retrospective studies, Bogdan et al. (30) found data showing that, among 354 consecutive patients treated for North American Crotalid bites, 112 exhibited coagulopathy. Of these, 31 had undergone coagulation testing sufficient to detect whether a recurrence occurred; of these 31, 14 (45%) had a recurrence of the coagulopathy to include severe hypofibrinogenemia or thrombocytopenia. Apparently, none of these patients experienced spontaneous hemorrhage despite these laboratory recurrences.

Boyer et al. (29), in studying FabAV-treated Crotalid envenomations in 38 patients, found that 20 (53%) had recurrent, persistent, or late coagulopathy, some occurring 13 days following envenomation and treatment. No patient experienced significant spontaneous bleeding. The most common severe, if not even dramatic, abnormality was incoagulable and/or extremely prolonged PTs or PTTs, all of which were due to severe selective defibrinogenation. Of their 20 patients, 16 were observed with no further FabAV treatment, and all fared well. Two patients who received supplemental doses of FabAV had prompt normalization of laboratory findings. Of interest, all their patients with defibrinogenation on presentation showed significant increases in their plasma fibrinogen levels following FabAV treatment, which is a major laboratory criterion for a therapeutic response to FabAV. One patient who was hypofibrinogenemic underwent a minor surgical procedure at a time that his fibrinogen was undetectable, and experienced hemorrhage limited to this surgical site. No blood products were administered. They suggested that for patients whose envenomation syndrome had included significant coagulopathy, repeat testing of the coagulation system for up to 2 weeks seemed appropriate, although which tests to order, what to do with these data, and whether the patient should remain hospitalized were not addressed.

Ruha et al. (31) studied 28 cases of rattlesnake envenomation in Arizona, noting that in some cases, despite initial control of coagulopathy, there was return of either coagulation defects and/or thrombocytopenia. As this was fairly benign, it was their opinion that one need not wait for total normalization of all the coagulation and platelet studies as a therapeutic end point for FabAV therapy. Odeleye et al. (32) noted, in two cases of rattlesnake envenomation, that thrombocytopenia was difficult to reverse either with FabAV and/or platelet transfusions, and suggested that unless bleeding occurs, transfusion of platelets and blood products might best be withheld. Camilleri et al. (33) reported a crotaline envenomation with profound coagulopathy that was resistant to therapy, which they curtailed after 4 days of FabAV therapy, suggesting only close observation without further therapeutic intervention. Their patient was discharged home on day 12 with severe defibrinogenation, and apparently underwent spontaneous resolution sometime between day 17 and 37. They concluded that despite "critical value" coagulopathies, if a patient is not bleeding and systemic and local manifestations of the bite have already been controlled, close observation without further therapeutic intervention is appropriate. Similar conservative conclusions were made from South American pit viper experiences by de Oliveira et al. (34) regarding their experience with Bothrops, and by Sano-Martins et al. (35) regarding the South American cascabel (*Crotalus durissus*), with both reports noting that, despite severe coagulation abnormalities, the clinical outcome did not seem to be linked to blood incoagulability; what few deaths occurred apparently were not thought due to venom-induced coagulation disturbances.

Postmortem Findings

Death from American pit viper envenomation is rare, and full autopsies are even rarer. Dart et al. (36) reviewed the few reports regarding 16 deaths out of about 1,000 cases of North American envenomations reported up to 1989. Central nervous system edema and hemorrhage were reported in a few cases, but cerebral hemorrhage was deemed the cause of death in only one. They speculated that the mortality rate from severe, complicated rattlesnake envenomation was approximately 1.4%, but were unable to more precisely construct an overall figure because so many cases, particularly mild cases, are not reported. They also opined that the exact cause of death may be difficult to determine, deducing that the most common cause was progressive shock leading to multiorgan failure and death hours to a few days later. Generalized edema from extravasation of fluid into the heart, lung, and brain was implicated. It appeared that edema is a result not of frank hemorrhage, but of direct effect of the toxin on the circulatory endothelial integrity and the microcirculation in particular. It was frequently noted in their review that delayed therapy and/or inadequate therapy, or even no antivenom therapy, seemed to be disproportionately encountered among fatal cases. They also opined that in patients to whom antivenom had been administered and died hours to days later, the primary cause included severe alteration in capillary permeability.

Prehospital Treatment

The key to good and effective therapy with minimal chance of loss of life, limb, or function is prompt transportation to a medical care facility. In areas where snakes are endemic, almost all hospitals have at least a modicum of antivenom available or close at hand. Calling the emergency room prior to arrival is reasonable if such does not delay transport.

Initial scene management is to prevent further bites and to calm the patient. If successful transport is anticipated within an hour, it is probably best to forgo any local therapy other than to gently splint the bitten extremity, keeping it at or slightly below heart level, and transport the patient to an appropriate health care facility. The use of topical cold packs may provide some relief of severe pain, if properly applied. Incising or excising the wound, the application of electrical currents, or other traumatic manipulations are contraindicated. Suction devices remove at best 2% of the venom load, are likely to be clinically insignificant, and, if used, should not delay transport. The use of a tourniquet with pressure sufficient to impede either arterial or venous flow is contraindicated. A lymphatic constriction band (ideally a blood pressure cuff inflated to 15 to 25 mm Hg, a band that allows a finger to pass easily beneath) or a properly applied pressure immobilization bandage may be considered if there are immediate life-threatening effects or a prolonged (greater than 1 hour) transport time. Any procedure that concentrates venom and slows its clearance from the bitten extremity, while used theoretically to decrease systemic manifestations, is likely to worsen local morbidity.

Hospital Treatment

Treatment of victims who have been envenomated by North American snakes will not be encountered by most physicians. If encountered, particularly if physicians are approaching their initial treatment of such victims, there is often an undue amount of anxiety, which is not well founded.

Approximately 5,000 to 10,000 bites occur in the United States each year. Death from envenomation by North American pit vipers occurs only about five to ten times (0.1%) per year, representing approximately a 99.9% survival rate. Reasons for this fairly enviable situation, especially when compared to higher mortalities in other countries, include three facts. The first of these is that medical care is far more accessible than it is in many countries in which envenomations occur and for which survival is much less favorable, including the continents of Australia, South America, and the Indian subcontinent. Nearly anyone in the United States is within an hour of emergent care as opposed to many hours or several days in some parts of the world, and most facilities, at least in endemic areas, have antivenom on hand. A second reason is that the venoms of North American pit vipers do not cause true DIC with thrombosis and/or DIC-type bleeding, which may cause multiorgan failure, as is seen with many snakes, including those on the Indian subcontinent and especially Australia. Third is the employment of prompt and sound medical care, including fluid resuscitation and monitoring of vital signs, to maximize morbidity. Table 68.1 outlines the essentials of appropriate management of such patients.

Immediate Management

1. *Confirm the bite*: First, confirm that the patient was bitten by a snake and, particularly, a venomous snake. With the exception of coral snake envenomation, this usually includes the presence of puncture wounds. Whereas snakes normally have two fangs, it is not uncommon to see snakes with one fang or even three or four, as their fangs maturate and move

TABLE 68.1

INITIAL EVALUATION AND DIAGNOSTIC POINTS

- Confirm patient was bitten by a venomous snake; determine snake species if possible.
- Evaluate for local signs of envenomation:
  - ☐ Pain
  - ☐ Swelling
  - ☐ Discoloration
- Evaluate for systemic signs of envenomation:
  - ☐ Alterations in vital signs, nausea, vomiting, diarrhea
  - ☐ Fasciculations
  - ☐ Coagulation abnormalities
  - ☐ Altered mental status

TABLE 68.2

CLINICAL CHARACTERISTICS OF ENVENOMATION THAT POTENTIALLY AID IN IDENTIFICATION OF OFFENDING CROTALUS SPECIES

Common name	Scientific name	Distribution	Neurologic symptoms	Coagulopathic findings	Rhabdomyolysis
Eastern Diamondback	*Crotalus adamanteus*	Southeastern United States	+	Prolonged PT/PTT; minimal thrombocytopenia	+
Canebrake	*Crotalus horridus atricaudatus*	Eastern United States	nil	nil	++++
Mojave	*Crotalus scutulatus*	Desert southwest United States	+++	nil	++++
Timber	*Crotalus horridus horridus*	Eastern United States	nil	Prolonged PT/PTT; moderate to severe thrombocytopenia	nil

PT, prothrombin time; PTT, partial prothrombin time.
+ = usually minimally present; ++ = usually moderately present; + + + = usually extensively present; + + ++ = always present.

forward, replacing one another with time. Similarly, a single puncture wound may be present on a smaller part of the body (such as a finger) with the other fang missing the target altogether. Some victims may have three or even four puncture wounds per bite. The vast majority of patients will have the prompt triad of pain, swelling, and discoloration confined to the bite site almost within minutes of the event, but up to 2 hours later in unusual cases. If a patient does have puncture wounds consistent with pit viper envenomation, and does *not* have pain, swelling, and discoloration, or any systemic symptoms such as hypotension, nausea, vomiting, diarrhea, constipation, mental status changes, fasciculations, or diaphoresis, one may strongly consider that the patient has been bitten yet not envenomated. A caveat for this pronouncement is that many children, when anxious, frequently vomit, which may be a misleading sign. An alarming number of victims of snakebites are not at their normal mental status, given the frequency of concomitant inebriation from alcohol or other substances. This impedes obtaining a detailed history and the patient's full cooperation. In many locales, a minority of bites are accidents in the true sense of the word.

2. *Determine the genus and species*: Next, one should try to determine the family and/or genus and species of snake if at all possible. The majority of victims know not only precisely that they were in the same area as a venomous snake, but also the snake's common name, yet still are compelled to taunt, toy with, kiss, or otherwise handle the venomous animal for reasons that are not clear. In such patients, snake identification is not difficult. Another 25% to 30% will bring the snake to the health care facility in conditions ranging from badly mutilated to quite alive. Identification by charts or consulting herpetologists or other experts is quite useful in determining the species of the snake, whereas it is not of much benefit for the victim if he or she cannot identify the type of snake that inflicted the bite. Whether by confusion or the desire to please, children will agree that the picture of nearly any snake presented to them is indeed the offending reptile. Several online links, such as http://www.pitt.edu/~mcs2/herp/SoNA.html, are available to assist identification.

   One can occasionally augment identification of an offending snake by the symptom complex its bite produces, as is demonstrated in Table 68.2. The prognosis is generally species dependent, but also related to the time to presentation, time to antivenom administration, the health of the host, and other factors. Management will be based on a mixture of observed and anticipated symptoms and physical findings, as well as one's prior experience in handling this emergency.

3. *Determine systemic signs and manifestations*: Assuming the patient does have signs of local envenomation, next in order is to determine whether there are any systemic signs of envenomation, remembering the fact that no one dies of local envenomation, but only from systemic manifestations. As a general rule, in mild and moderate envenomations, the symptoms are due primarily to the local pain, swelling, and discoloration, which, while quite alarming, are not usually of a life-threatening nature. Systemic symptoms such as nausea, vomiting, diarrhea, and diaphoresis, as well as fasciculations—particularly in *Crotalus* envenomations—do portend the possibility of a more serious outcome. Many coagulation abnormalities seen in *Crotalus* envenomations are often spectacular in their laboratory manifestations. Altered mental status to include a noticeable stupor and a metallic taste is often reported in serious envenomations.
4. *Assign degree of severity*: In attempting to assign a degree of severity from mild to moderate to severe, one must recognize several principles. The first is that the envenomation syndrome is progressive and, secondly, evaluation is ongoing and time dependent. Two patients may be bitten in the same manner. If the first patient is seen in 15 or 20 minutes after the bite, very few local signs of pain, swelling, or discoloration will be seen, whereas a similar patient requiring 2 hours to arrive for emergent care will have much more advanced and obvious pain, swelling, and discoloration, although with exactly the same prognosis. The corollary to that adage is that it is the *rate of change* in signs, symptoms, and other manifestations that is important. It is important not only in grading the severity of the bite, but also in grading the effect—or lack of effect—of the administration of antivenom.

Antivenom Administration

Because of the present lack of prospective, outcome-based studies, practices regarding perceived indications for the use of antivenom vary. Most practitioners will not administer antivenom to anyone without envenomation ("dry bites") or to those who have minimal envenomation, particularly if it is by the *Sistrurus* species. Bites by the copperhead (*Agkistrodon contortrix*) are usually not treated (7–9) with antivenom unless the patient is at the extremes of age or with many comorbid conditions. Envenomation by the water moccasin (*Agkistrodon piscivorus*) is notorious for a large amount of local edema but not much in the way of systemic symptoms and laboratory manifestations (10), and even less in the way of mortality. Their swelling can be so massive that, if untreated for any reason, bites of the hand may progress up the arm, chest wall, neck, face, and even abdomen; this is all reversible.

Severe envenomations are often apparent by the time they arrive at emergency care, primarily because of the rapidity with which the venom initially gains entry into the circulatory system. The corollary with that adage is that while it is common to see someone progress from minimum envenomation to moderate envenomation, it is quite rare to see one, in our experience, progress from moderate envenomation to severe envenomation. Rather, when they arrive—even within minutes of the event—severely envenomated patients may be considerably hypotensive with lethargy, nausea, and vomiting, and require immediate and aggressive therapy (Table 68.3). Suggested therapy is outlined in Table 68.4. At least one large-bore intravenous access site must be obtained and blood drawn for a variety of tests.

While one is evaluating the rate and degree of swelling, it is useful to outline the leading edge of proximal progression of the swelling with some type of ink pen. This may be more apparent by tactile rather than visual means. In this manner, one can observe whether the swelling is progressive. Whereas some relatively slow progression is tolerated—particularly if one elects not to treat the patient or if antivenom is not immediately available—more rapid swelling, particularly with concomitant systemic symptoms, usually justifies prompt and aggressive therapy.

In a situation involving our native reptiles, we do not administer antivenom in patients who have no envenomation; about 10% to 15% of people with minimal envenomation, half of those patients with moderate envenomation, and all patients with severe envenomation are administered antivenom.

TABLE 68.4

SUMMARY OF THERAPEUTIC MEASURES FOR PIT VIPER ENVENOMATION

- Obtain IV access and administer crystalloid as indicated.
- Obtain CBC, PT, PTT, and platelet count every 6–12 h
- Estimate severity of envenomation:
  - ☐ Species of snake
  - ☐ Age, health status of victim
  - ☐ Rate of progression of signs/symptoms
- Administer FabAV per Table 68.3.
- Follow rate of progression of signs/symptoms after FabAV administration.
- Determine tetanus vaccination status.
- Seek consultation from experts or a poison center (1-800-222-1222), especially if one is less experienced in treating snake envenomation.

CBC, complete blood count; PT, prothrombin time; PTT, partial thromboplastin time.

The offending reptiles in one's locale and the experience of those evaluating the patient will often override this simplification. Reasons for not administering antivenom to all, or nearly all, victims are several: (a) the extremely low mortality rate of envenomation by snakes native to the United States, (b) the—admittedly very low—rate (less than 0.01%) of serious and mild (14%) allergic reactions, (c) the modest rate (15%) of serum sickness–like late reactions (occurring typically 8–12 days after administration) to FabAV (1), and (d) the cost of antivenom treatment can easily exceed $50,000.

As antivenom is more efficacious the earlier it is administered, if the decision has been made to employ the drug, it should be done promptly. Control of the envenomation syndrome is adjudged by the slowing, or preferably the cessation, of progressive local swelling (27). One should not expect extant swelling to regress or any areas of local damage to the bite site such as a swollen or discolored area to regress, as such damage has already been done prior to the patient's treatment. Hemorrhagic bleb formation at the site of the bite is *not* an important sign in and of itself, although it generates much attention. These should be left alone or, if one thinks that bursting is imminent, the blebs should be topically sterilized and lanced, although this usually does not occur until the second or third day of the envenomation.

TABLE 68.3

SEVERITY OF ENVENOMATION BY PIT VIPERS

Grade	Frequency	Initial findings	FabAV vials in first 24 h
No envenomation	15%–30%	No local, systemic, or laboratory abnormalities 2 h after bite	0
Minimal envenomation	20%–40%	Local and slowly progressive swelling without systemic or severe laboratory abnormalities	0–6
Moderate envenomation	20%–40%	Rapidly progressive local swelling; systemic symptoms of nausea, vomiting, diarrhea, diaphoresis, fasciculations, moderate hypotension, and moderate hemostatic abnormalities, but without bleeding	6–18
Severe envenomation	5%–10%	Severe systemic symptoms as above plus severe hypotension and lethargy; severe hemostatic abnormalities and possible bleeding	12–24 or more

Compartment syndromes are seen very rarely, and indications for surgical intervention are justified by pressure measurements in only about 1% to 2% of all envenomated U.S. patients. The degree of swelling in and of itself is not a reliable sign of compartment syndrome given the elasticity of skin. More reliable signs are total lack of function and exquisite pain of the muscles contained within a compromised compartment, and often an intense hardness of the site owing to the nonelasticity of fascial tissue, which, while limiting swelling, allows pressure to increase as it is locked beneath the fascial plane. The palmar aspect of the hand and lateral compartment of the tibia may be so involved. Direct measurement of pressure within an anatomic compartment may be of use, and adequate antivenom therapy and elevation will usually result in normalization of pressures. Orthopedic consultation may be indicated, but in animal models, fasciotomy has not been shown to result in improved outcomes.

The mainstay for treatment for North American pit viper envenomation is ovine FabAV for bites in both adults and children (26,27). The Fab portions of sheep immunoglobulins are made by enzyme cleavage and elimination of the Fc fragment, which is regarded as the more immunogenic part of the intact immunoglobulin molecule, and by further enzymatic cleavage of the resulting $F(ab')_2$. Pretreatment skin or conjunctival testing is neither required nor recommended prior to the administration of FabAV.

The small FabAV molecule has the theoretical advantage of a larger volume of distribution and the potential to neutralize more venom at the bite site. This has not been demonstrated clinically, however. On the other hand, as it has a more rapid distribution and shorter half-life than IgG, periodic readministration during the initial treatment period is important. Research and development of a $Fab(ab')_2$ antivenom is currently under way. $Fab(ab')_2$ has a smaller volume of distribution and a longer circulating half-life, and thus may decrease the recurrence syndrome.

Another general rule of thumb for pit viper envenomation is that approximately half of the total swelling expected to occur does so within the first 2 hours of envenomation, and nearly all of it occurs by 12 hours after envenomation. This seems congruent with one study that involved timed rate of change in swelling (9). Accordingly, if a patient presents over 12 hours after the bite, it would be unusual to experience significantly more swelling, and most systemic symptoms should have occurred and abated. We rarely *initiate* administration of antivenom treatment more than 12 hours after a bite, and essentially never after 24 hours of the bite. One may initiate or continue antivenom administration after 24 hours in selected situations, such as in the management of continued coagulopathic effects or in the management of recurrence.

We hold that the defibrinogenation syndrome itself is not such a clear and present risk for spontaneous hemorrhage that its presence alone requires administration of antivenom, nor that its recurrence represents an established reason to readminister antivenom (10,26). As the literature and experience garnered thus far supports that defibrinogenation alone seems benign, the administration of blood products such as fresh frozen plasma (FFP) or cryoprecipitate is usually not warranted, even prior to a surgical procedure, as the risks of these blood products probably outweigh their (unproven) benefit. If one does encounter a patient with systemic hemorrhage, or should unacceptable bleeding follow a surgical procedure, administration of additional antivenom plus cryoprecipitate (eight to ten bags in an adult) is the treatment of choice. Likewise, other isolated, noncritical coagulation abnormalities without bleeding do not in and of themselves, in our opinion, demand antivenom treatment (10).

Some species of snakes, particularly the timber rattlesnake (*Crotalus horridus horridus*), have a principle in their venom that causes significant thrombocytopenia, which appears rather resistant to reversal by antivenom therapy (37). If platelet counts are significantly falling and/or are less than 10,000 to 20,000 cells/μL, administration of (additional) antivenom and infusion of platelets may be indicated, particularly if there is evidence for systemic bleeding. In general, with most Crotalid envenomation, there is a mild thrombocytopenia in the range of 50,000 to 150,000 cells/μL that is thought to be due to passive entrapment of platelets within the previously described soft fibrin network and, as mentioned, does not support a diagnosis of DIC. The platelet count often will rebound within the day as the soft fibrin network is quickly cleaved by endogenously generated plasmin.

Surgical Procedures

A surgical procedure for the wound is rarely indicated, and there are several case series and experimental studies suggesting that surgical procedures correlate with a delayed outcome, some with a paradoxic increase in permanent loss of tissue, loss of anatomic function, and nonspecific stiffness (38–40). Antibiotics are generally not employed as they are of questionable assistance, and their routine use is not recommended (41,42). If there has been significant surgical manipulation of the wound in the field, such as with repeated knife wounds, that stance may need to be reconsidered. Tetanus vaccination status should be ascertained as being up to date.

Observation

When observing the wound for any changes, it is best to have the extremity clearly visible so as not to compromise the evaluation; we do not advocate any covering dressings or wraps. Once the patient is at the hospital and receiving antivenom, the extremity should be elevated above the level of the heart. Monitoring is usually best performed in the emergency department, with subsequent admission to the intensive care unit (ICU), although ICU therapy should not be considered, in our opinion, as necessarily a standard of care. The usual length of hospitalization required is 4 to 6 days.

For up to 24 hours, we often observe patients—either in the emergency department or in the hospital—who are deemed to have no envenomation or mild envenomations, and who do not receive antivenom because of the very high incidence of concurrent inebriation, which would allow for the possibility of inadequate history or incomplete evaluation and follow-up.

Prognosis

Nearly all North American pit viper bites result in some near-instantaneous local tissue destruction, which should not be expected to be totally absent or to resolve, even with the very best and most rapid care. Most edema and swelling that does occur after antivenom treatment lasts only for a month or two, with longer recovery times seen in older or debilitated patients. In general, there is a total return of function to the bitten extremity, although some patients can experience mild stiffness, atrophy, and weakness for up to a year or more (43,44). The loss of tissue, including fingers or limbs, is very rare, and often occurs with the injudicious prehospital use of ice or tourniquets or, perhaps, very delayed care. Unfortunately, patients who are bitten by snakes tend to continue their risky behavior, resulting in the finding that re-envenomation is not rare.

SNAKES NON-NATIVE TO THE UNITED STATES

This section summarizes the epidemiology, pathophysiology, diagnosis, and treatment of non-native snake envenomations in the United States.

Envenomations by reptile, amphibian, arthropod, or marine species not native to the United States pose special challenges to the provider. Clinicians are likely to be unfamiliar with the clinical spectrum of exotic envenomation and its current management. Antivenoms, if they exist, may not be available or may take many hours to locate and acquire. Zoos, aquaria, and academic institutions may possess non-native species for research and display. The problem is compounded by private collectors, whose existence is not usually known to their regional health care system until an exposure occurs. Policies and procedures governing acquisition, storage, handling, antivenom, and preparations for managing envenomations range from comprehensive to nonexistent.

Immediate Concerns

Major Problems

The severity and spectrum of effects in envenomation varies widely. A significant number of bites and stings do not result in envenomation. However, life-threatening effects may be seen and fatalities do occur. Identification to the species level of the envenomating organism is important in anticipation of effects and the selection of nonspecific and specific therapies. Antivenom may or may not be available for non-native species, and identification of the appropriate antivenom and its acquisition may require many hours. Other specific therapies may be available, and nonspecific therapies are directed at general classes of venom effects.

Epidemiology

There are about 3,000 snake species in the world, of which fewer than 300 are dangerous to humans (45). Venomous reptiles include the families Atractaspididae Colubridae, Crotalidae, Elapidae, Helodermatidae, and Hydrophiidae (46).

Between 40 and 50 non-native snake envenomations occur per year in the United States. Although non-native envenomations in the United States involved at least 77 separate species over the past decade, certain families, genera, and species are more commonly encountered. Cobras (family Elapidae) account for one third of all non-native venomous snake exposures, and 86% of Elapids. *Naja naja, Naja nigricollis*, and *Ophiophagus hannah* are the most commonly involved Elapid species. Viperids account for 46% of all non-native venomous snake exposures, with *Bothrops*, *Bitis*, and *Lachesis* genera accounting for 33%, 19%, and 11% of these, respectively. *Bothrops goodmanni, Bothrops schlegeli, Bitis gabonica,* and *Lachesis mutus* are the most commonly encountered viperid species (47).

Compared with other etiologies of critical illness, venomous snake bites account for few ICU admissions per year. Nevertheless, almost one third of non-native envenomations develop major to moderate symptoms and signs of disease, and are admitted to an ICU. The case fatality rate of approximately 1% is significantly greater than in native snakebites. Males are involved in 84% of bites, a similar percentage to that in native bites. Almost 15% are aged 17 years or less, and approximately 7% are aged 5 years or younger, most likely as a result of private collections in home settings (47). Identification of the snake in non-native bites is usually not difficult, as zoos, aquaria, and academic institutions will know their collections to the species or subspecies level and have procedures in place to identify the biting snake. The private collector is also usually well informed. However, the bitten individual with a private collection may not be capable of communication, and potential penalties for possession of venomous animals in some jurisdictions may result in the withholding of critical information (48). A qualified herpetologist should be consulted for the identification of non-native snakes that are otherwise unidentified. The presence of a puncture and typical appearance of the site, progression of findings, and consistent laboratory abnormalities of a snakebite, indicate the possibility even when the history is not available.

Pathophysiology

The venom glands of poisonous snakes are modifications of salivary glands (49). The venom of a single snake is a complex mixture of enzymes, nonenzymatic proteins and peptides, and other substances (50,51). These substances exert simultaneous toxic or lethal effects on the integumentary, hematologic, nervous, respiratory, muscular, and cardiovascular systems. The clinical picture also can be complicated by the effects of endogenous mediator release, such as histamine, cytokines, and nitric oxide (52). Some of these components may be found in all venomous snakes, with mixed clinical effects. The most important deleterious components of snake venom are shown in Table 68.5. Hyaluronidase is found in all venoms and produces hydrolysis of connective tissue stroma, allowing the dispersion of other toxic components (53). Zinc-dependent metalloprotease enzymes damage vascular membranes and produce local and systemic hemorrhage (54,55). Phospholipases are found in most snake venoms, with a variety of effects (50), including destabilizing biologic membranes and abolishing the selective membrane ion channel permeability to ions such as calcium (56,57). Crotalid venom is rich in proteinases, amino acidases, and phospholipases, and typically produces findings of cellular destruction, increased membrane permeability, and coagulation impairment. Coagulation abnormalities may result from multiple mechanisms, including consumption, aggregation or inhibition of platelets, or effects on the coagulation cascade, such as activation or inhibition of coagulation factors, procoagulant activity, defibrinogenation, prothrombin action, collagenase-like activity, and other effects (58–60). Elapid venoms vary widely among species but contain more neurotoxins and cardiotoxins (51), resulting in various expressions of nerve and cardiac toxicity. Sea snakes have venom similar to elapids.

TABLE 68.5

SOME COMPONENTS OF SNAKE VENOM

Component	Viperid	Elapid	Effect
Proteinases	+++	+	Tissue destruction; hematologic effects
Hyaluronidase	++	++	Hydrolyzes connective tissue stroma; promotes spread
Cholinesterase	+	++	Catalyzes hydrolysis of acetylcholine
Phospholipase A_2	+++	+	Hemolysis; may potentiate neurotoxins; myonecrosis
Phosphodiesterase	+	+++	Unknown
Neurotoxins	+	+++	Flaccid paralysis; muscle fasciculation
Cardiotoxins	+	+++	Depolarizing/depression/rhythm disturbances

+ = usually minimally present; ++ = usually moderately present; + + + = usually extensively present.

Diagnosis and Monitoring

The spectrum of symptoms and signs produced in a victim by a given venomous snakebite varies with the species of snake, the natural variability in venom composition between snakes, and, in any given snake over time, the quantity of venom injected, bite location, and the age and health of the victim.

Size and Species

In general, larger snakes contain and deliver more venom, but fatal envenomations may result from juvenile snakes. Toxicities of the venom will depend on the species and other factors that affect venom production.

Quantity Injected

As many as 30% of Crotalid bites and 50% of Elapid bites may result in no envenomation (46,61). When venom is injected, the amount may be reduced by poor penetration of the fang or high tissue pressures, as in fingertips. The volume of available venom may also be reduced by recent previous feedings.

Bite Location

Tissues and anatomic areas with a low capacity for swelling, or which are functionally important, such the fingers or hand, are particularly at risk of both short- and long-term impairment. The destructive effects of proteolytic enzymes may directly damage tissues. Also, even where no true compartments exist, tissue pressures may be significantly elevated and vascular compromise may occur. True muscle compartments may be subject to elevated pressures, either because of direct injection of venom with intracompartmental edema, from passage of venom into a compartment via direct spread or lymphatics, or as a result of extrinsic pressure on a compartment secondary to subcutaneous edema. Lower extremity bites may damage venous valves and produce long-term dependent edema. Decreased mobility and mobilization after a bite may predispose to deep venous thrombosis or other morbidities.

Age and Health of the Victim

Those at greatest risk of morbidity and mortality include patients with long delays to treatment, those with significant comorbid conditions, and those at the extremes of age. Because of smaller body mass, children receive a relatively greater dose of venom. As with native envenomations, some private collectors may be under the influence of alcohol at the time of envenomation, which may affect their ability to avoid envenomation, predispose to multiple bites, and delay seeking care.

Symptoms and Manifestations

Since snakes can, to some extent, control whether and how much venom to deliver, and as other factors may affect the quantity and specific components available and delivered, it is difficult to make an *a priori* determination of the clinical potential of the envenomation. The manifestations of snake envenomations can be divided into local and systemic effects.

Local Effects. Snake venom that produces local effects causes pain and edema at the bite site, erythema, ecchymosis, and occasional bleb formation. Later, the increased membrane permeability and cellular destruction produced by proteases result in spreading edema both distally and proximally, and may cause tissue necrosis. If the bite is on an extremity, elevated tissue pressures may compromise vascular supply or result in elevated compartmental pressures. Periodically marking the extent over time of proximal spread of edema directly on the skin is useful in documenting the progression of local venom effects and response to treatment. The leading edge is usually palpable as a sharply demarcated ridge and differs from later redistribution of tissue edema, which more gradually transitions to normal tissue. Edema may spread from an extremity onto the trunk or involve the head and neck, compromising the airway (62,63). Pain, possibly requiring opioid-level management, is common and cannot be used to diagnose compartment syndrome. Because of the similarity of findings with compartment syndrome, if there is concern for elevated tissue or compartmental pressures, they should be measured directly (Stryker Intra-Compartmental Pressure Monitor System, Stryker United Kingdom; COACH Transducer, MIPM GmbH, Mammendorf, Germany). Local venom effects will respond to adequate amounts of antivenom with cessation of progression of proximal edema and reduced tissue pressures. Recurrence of progression of local effects may occur, particularly with Fab antivenoms, which have a larger volume of distribution and, thus, its circulating concentrations fall more quickly than $F(ab')_2$ or IgG antivenoms. Locally acting venom components are usually exhausted by 24 to 36 hours, although the resulting tissue injury may continue to develop over days to weeks. Starting on the second day post envenomation, the clinical appearance of the bitten extremity, with increased heat and inflammation of the lymphatics, may be difficult to distinguish from an infective process. Overall, the incidence of infection is low, but will vary depending on the snake, the host, and factors such as the development of necrosis and wound manipulation. Potentially life-threatening infections such as necrotizing fasciitis and disseminated osteomyelitis, have been reported following snakebites (64–66).

Hematologic Effects. Coagulation alterations result from proteases acting on various parts of the coagulation cascade and may occur singly or in any combination. Fibrinogenolysis may occur, resulting in decreased levels of fibrinogen and increased levels of fibrin degradation products (60,66–69). Platelet inhibition, aggregation, or consumption may occur with abnormal function and/or decreased platelet counts (60,70). Intravascular hemolysis has also been reported with some snake venoms (71). The coagulation defects may result in local or systemic bleeding, including life-threatening hemorrhage (71–76). Laboratory tests, including a complete blood count (CBC) with platelet count, PT/international normalized ratio (INR), PTT, fibrinogen, and fibrin degradation products (or d-dimers), should be obtained on arrival and periodically reassessed. Most patients who will develop hematologic abnormalities will demonstrate them within 1 to 2 hours, although early use of antivenom may mask this finding; normal hematologic values at 6 hours suggests an absence of such effects. If abnormalities are present, the use of antivenom may halt (e.g., fibrinogenolysis) or reverse (e.g., platelet aggregation) venom effects. The timing of repeat labs is based on the use of antivenom, clinical findings, and laboratory trends. Unneutralized venom components responsible for hematologic effects may remain active in the body for up to 3 weeks, resulting in delayed, persistent, or recurrent hematologic abnormalities (29,77,78).

Neurologic Effects. These may result from Atractaspid, Elapid, Helodermid, Hydrophiid, or Viperid envenomations. Clinical effects can include sweating, numbness, paresthesias, convulsions, coma, muscle fasciculation, muscle weakness, and respiratory arrest. Respiratory muscle paralysis is the primary cause of death with most Elapid and Hydrophiid venoms. Viperid snakes rarely cause clinically significant respiratory compromise. Coma may be secondary to hypovolemia or to a direct effect of the toxin (68). Neurologic effects may develop rapidly, with respiratory arrest occurring within 15 to 30 minutes, but also may be delayed by many hours (79,80). Measures such as the application of a pressure immobilization bandage (PIB) may also delay the onset of neurotoxicity (81). Even with delayed onset, once neurologic effects occur, they may progress very rapidly. Patients should be observed for a sufficient period of time, and preparations to manage the airway should be readily available. It should be kept in mind that some Elapids produce little to no local effects, and therefore, their absence cannot be relied upon to confirm nonenvenomation. Once muscle weakness or paralysis has occurred, it may be difficult to reverse, although both antivenom and cholinergic agonists will generally stop the progression of effects and have been reported to result in either dramatic or more rapid improvement than would otherwise be expected (82–84). Extubation criteria are based on standard tests of respiratory sufficiency.

Nonhematologic Systemic Effects. These include effects on the cardiovascular, respiratory, and neurologic systems. In general, snakes from any family may produce any of these effects, although certain effects predominate within families. Type I hypersensitivity reactions to venom (IgE or non–IgE mediated) with or without hypotension may occur. The incidence is believed to be approximately 1% (85). Type I hypersensitivity reactions are characterized by wheezing, urticaria, laryngeal edema, and/or hypotension. Airway compromise from laryngeal edema may also occur, and direct myocardial depression, injury, or dysrhythmic effects of venom have been reported (85–90). The clinical picture may be complicated by possible adverse reactions to antivenom. The incidence of type I hypersensitivity to antivenoms varies from less than 5% to 25%. Other systemic findings common in snakebites are nausea, vomiting, diaphoresis, and pulmonary edema, especially in more severe cases. These usually resolve in response to antivenom and rarely persist beyond the immediate postbite period. Adverse reactions to antivenoms can complicate care. Type III hypersensitivity reactions—"serum sickness"—may occur in any patient who has received antivenom and are the result of circulating immune complexes. The frequency of occurrence is dependent on the amount of antivenom received as well as the type (e.g., source animal, immunoglobulin fragment). Type III reactions usually occur between 5 and 21 days after receiving antivenom and vary widely in incidence by antivenom utilized, from less than 5% to 100% (91–95). Symptoms and signs usually consist of muscle and joint aches, low-grade fever, and/or a urticarial rash; severe cases may have severe symptoms, including renal insufficiency.

Diagnosis

The diagnosis of snakebite may be a clinical one and should be suspected in any unknown presentation with any of the above clinical manifestations. Although immunoassays and bioassays have been used to identify various snake venoms in tissue within endemic areas, such tests are not available in the United States (96,97). In the United States, envenomations are likely to occur in zoo, academic, and private collector settings (47). Snake identification may be inaccurate in noninstitutional settings, yet obtaining an accurate identification of the snake is of utmost importance in order to select the appropriate antivenom. When dealing with private collectors, consideration should be given to independently verifying the snake species. A local zoo or aquarium may be of assistance in identifying the snake.

Management

The management of clinically significant snake envenomation can be divided into first aid, specific antivenin therapy, and supportive therapy (Table 68.6).

Online Antivenom Index. Initiation of efforts to obtain the appropriate antivenom should not wait until symptoms or signs develop; rather, this should be done immediately following the bite. The Online Antivenom Index is a resource for determining the appropriate antivenom(s) for any given snake and maintains a continuously updated listing of zoo antivenom stocks and contact information. It is accessible by regional poison centers (1-800-222-1222), which can assist in the identification and acquisition of an appropriate antivenom and in the clinical management of a snake envenomation.

First Aid. In general, the patient should get away from the snake and the snake should be secured by a qualified individual. Pre-existing medical information, information regarding the biting species, and any available antivenom should be transported with the patient. The bitten body part should be splinted

TABLE 68.6

DIAGNOSTIC PEARLS

- Up to 30% of Viperid and 50% of Elapid bites do not result in envenomation.
- Signs and symptoms of envenomation may be delayed by many hours.
- Identification of the snake to the species level is required for antivenom selection.
- Viperid venoms usually produce (a) local tissue injury and (b) hematologic abnormalities, and may also include (c) cardiovascular effects and (d) neurologic effects.
- Elapid venoms usually produce (a) neurologic toxicity, progressing to respiratory muscle paralysis, and may also include (b) local tissue injury and (c) hematologic abnormalities.
- Type I hypersensitivity reactions (anaphylaxis) may occur to venom or antivenom.
- Anaphylaxis, cardiotoxins, or fluid loss may produce hypotension.
- Local tissue injury may result in severe swelling, pain, and elevated tissue and/or compartmental pressures. Functional impairment, necrosis, and tissue loss may occur.
- Hematologic effects include impairment or consumption of platelets, fibrinogenolysis, hypofibrinogenemia, prolongation of PT/PTT, procoagulant effects, and other abnormalities, either singly or in combination; also, significant bleeding may occur.
- Neurologic effects include diplopia, ptosis, fasciculations, respiratory muscle paralysis, and arrest. Viperids may cause weakness, but usually not respiratory compromise.
- Other venom effects include tachycardia, nausea, vomiting, diaphoresis, and anxiety.
- Wound infection is uncommon, documented in less than 5% of cases.
- Local effects may continue or recur for the first 24–36 h, and hematologic effects may continue or recur for up to 3 wk.

PT, prothrombin time; PTT, partial thromboplastin time.

TABLE 68.7

PREHOSPITAL MANAGEMENT

- A pressure immobilization bandage (PIB, a crepe bandage wrapped at lymphatic pressure tension from the distal to proximal aspects of an extremity) or lymphatic constriction band (a blood pressure cuff inflated to 15 to 25 mm Hg) will retard progression of venom into the general circulation.
  - □ Indicated prehospital with Elapids; in Viperids with early, severe, systemic effects; and possibly when there are long transport times
- The bitten body part should otherwise be kept gently splinted, slightly below heart level. It may be lowered further if systemic effects are seen, and elevated for excessive swelling.
- At least one large-bore IV should be initiated.
- The offending snake should be identified to the species level, if possible.
- If available, antivenom should accompany the patient.
- The victim should be rapidly transported by emergency medical services to a health care facility.
- CONTRAINDICATED MANAGEMENTS
  - □ Arterial or venous tourniquets
  - □ Incision, excision, heat, cold, electricity, or other local wound manipulations
  - □ Suction devices are not effective and should not delay transport to definitive care.

to slow the passage of venom into circulation (98). With envenomations from known neurotoxic snakes, generally the Elapids and sea snakes, the application of a PIB (a wide crepe bandage wrapping the entire extremity from distal to proximal at lymphatic compression pressures) or a lymphatic constriction band (LCB; i.e., a blood pressure cuff inflated to 15–25 mm Hg) has been shown to slow central compartment spread of venom and reduce the risk of out-of-hospital respiratory arrest, and thus should be routinely employed (99,100). With Viperid envenomations, the risk of rapidly developing life-threatening systemic effects is generally less. Although the use of a PIB prolonged survival in an animal model, it also resulted in increased tissue pressures; thus, the potential benefits must be weighed against the risk of increased local injury in Viperid envenomations (101). Hypotension, airway compromise, or other signs of a severe type I hypersensitivity reaction would be examples of appropriate indications for the use of a PIB or LCB in a Viperid bite. In general, prior to arrival at a hospital and administration of antivenom, the bitten area should be kept at or slightly below the level of the heart. A dependent position may be used if rapid, severe systemic effects are occurring. These measures can be instituted on arrival at the hospital if they have not been done previously. Transport to a health care facility should be by paramedic ambulance. The initiation of two, large-bore intravenous lines is a sensible precaution. The PIB or LCB should not be removed until antivenom has been obtained and is infusing, if nonenvenomation appears to be the case, or a decision has been made to observe the patient without specific treatment (Table 68.7).

Hospital Care. At the hospital, basic wound care should be provided, including updating the tetanus status, if needed. If, after a sufficient period of observation, which varies from 8 to 24 hours depending on the species of the snake, the victim demonstrates no signs or symptoms of envenomation, the person can be released from the hospital (Tables 68.8 through 68.10).

Pain Control. Opioid analgesics are best deferred until after hospital evaluation because of the risk of potentiating respiratory depression. An ice pack applied to the bite site, with customary precautions, may provide some pain relief without risking additional tissue injury (98,102). Opioid-level analgesia, however, may be required and its judicious use can be considered.

Antibiotics. Most authors recommend against routine prophylactic antibiotics. Antibiotics are suggested only for those with necrosis or clinical or laboratory evidence of infection (103).

Antivenom. Antivenom is composed of antibodies raised in an animal such as a sheep or horse to the venom of one or more species of snakes. A single snake's venom may be used to produce a monovalent antivenom, effective only against that snake or other snakes with the same or a subset of venom components. Since, in their endemic areas, it may not always be possible to identify the biting species, many antivenoms

TABLE 68.8

HOSPITAL BITE SITE AND WOUND MANAGEMENT

- If previously applied, a pressure immobilization bandage (PIB) or lymphatic constriction band (LCB) should not be removed until antivenom is being administered or a decision has been made to observe without antivenom.
- Wash the bite site, apply antibiotic ointment, leave it otherwise uncovered, and provide tetanus immunization updating as needed.
- Once antivenom has been initiated, or a decision has been made not to administer it, keep a bitten extremity elevated with periodic assessment of edema (and tissue pressures if indicated), and monitor for development or progression of systemic symptoms.
- Management of progressive tissue edema and elevated tissue or compartmental pressures is by adequate amounts of antivenom and elevation, if tolerated.
- Frankly necrotic tissue should be debrided.
- There is little to no role for dermotomy or fasciotomy.

are polyvalent; that is, they are designed to provide neutralizing efficacy for a number of different snake species. Venoms range from those that are relatively unpurified—whole IgG immunoglobulins, containing other proteins and immunoglobulin fractions—to highly purified specific IgG, $F(ab')_2$, or Fab immunoglobulin fragments. In general, horse serum–based products are more immunogenic than sheep-based antivenoms. IgG has a smaller volume of distribution, longer half-life, and higher rates of type I and type III hypersensitivity reactions, while Fab antivenoms have the largest volume of distribution, shortest half-lives, and lowest rates of allergic reactions. There is both considerable overlap and considerable variation of venom components within genera and species. When possible, species-specific antivenom that claims efficacy for the particular snake should be used. Antivenoms effective against other snakes in the same genus may be tried if species-specific antivenom is not available.

TABLE 68.9

HOSPITAL ANTIVENOM MANAGEMENT

- Antivenom is the definitive management of snake envenomation, when it is available.
- Antivenom for an exotic species can be located via the Online Antivenom Index. Poison centers (1-800-222-1222) can assist.
- When available, species-specific antivenom should be used.
- Skin testing is indicated if recommended by the manufacturer.
    - Skin tests are neither sensitive nor specific to predict hypersensitivity reactions.
    - A positive reaction does not preclude antivenom administration.
    - Skin testing should not delay administration of antivenom in a life- or limb-threatening envenomation.
- Exotic antivenoms are imported under Investigational New Drugs licenses and if used, appropriate reports need to be made to the hospital's institutional review board (IRB) and the Food and Drug Administration (FDA).

TABLE 68.10

HOSPITAL SYMPTOMATIC MANAGEMENT

- Hypotension
    - May be due to a type I hypersensitivity reaction to venom or to antivenom, cardiotoxins, or fluid loss.
    - Management is with Trendelenburg positioning, crystalloid fluid expansion, pressors, anaphylaxis treatments (epinephrine, H_1 and H_2 blockers), and antivenom (if believed to be secondary to venom).
- Neurologic effects
    - Should be managed with antivenom and mechanical airway support as needed.
    - Cholinergic agonists, such as neostigmine, may be used as adjunctive or substitute managements of muscle weakness in some Elapid envenomations.
- Hematologic effects
    - Severe or multicomponent abnormalities are managed primarily with antivenom.
    - Blood products are reserved for clinically significant hemorrhage, and given with additional antivenom if needed.
    - Some effects (e.g., platelet aggregation) may be readily reversed, while other processes (e.g., fibrinogenolysis) may be stopped, with components returning to normal levels by their natural replenishment.
- Other systemic effects are managed with symptomatic and supportive care.
    - Parenteral opioids may be required for pain.
- Recurrence of local and/or hematologic venom effects may occur.
    - Patients at high risk should be closely monitored, especially postdischarge.
    - Additional antivenom should be considered for recurrent local effects in the first 24 h or recurrent severe or multicomponent hematologic abnormalities.

Antivenoms for non-native snakes are imported into the United States under Investigational New Drug (IND) application. As such, their use carries additional Food and Drug Administration (FDA) and institutional review board (IRB) reporting requirements. As no U.S. hospital routinely stocks antivenoms for non-native species, such antivenoms are generally acquired by zoos and other institutions against the species they have in their collection for use in the event of one of their workers being envenomated. Zoos have traditionally made their antivenoms available to physicians on a compassionate basis. Since an IND antivenom will usually be brought into a hospital from an outside, nonhospital source, questions may be raised by the pharmacy regarding storage conditions, expiration dates, and other issues relating to its administration. If the potential for a non-native envenomation can be anticipated, such as a known zoo or university collection, it is prudent to have a pre-existing protocol as well as having obtained prior IRB approval (104).

Antivenom is considered the definitive treatment for all clinical effects of snake venom, although for a variety of reasons, such as incorrect snake identification, geographic variation of venom components, irreversible or time-dependent toxicity, and so forth, it may have limited to no observable efficacy against any particular venom effect (105–108). In addition, there are rarely prospective, controlled clinical trials to document appropriate indications, efficacy, and safety or to establish optimal dose and dosing regimens. Since antivenoms carry a risk of allergic reactions, potential benefits must be weighed against the risks of administration. Skin tests are neither sensitive nor specific enough to predict type I hypersensitivity reactions, but if recommended by the manufacturer, they should be administered. Their result, however, should not serve as a contraindication to administration when indicated, and preparations to manage an allergic reaction should always be immediately available. Regardless, skin testing should not delay administration of antivenom in a life-threatening envenomation.

Treatment with antivenom alters venom component distribution pharmacokinetics. Venom components bound to antibody become inaccessible to target tissues and are thus neutralized. Therefore, the dose of antivenom should be great enough to theoretically bind/neutralize the entire venom dose injected by the snake. These doses have been determined by knowledge of typical snake venom loads, neutralization properties of antivenoms in animal studies, and clinical studies. In most cases, it would be best to give doses of antivenom to ensure adequate venom neutralization on the assumption of a severe envenomation, since the degree of envenomation is difficult to appreciate early in the course. Such neutralization, however, occurs predominantly in the vascular compartment, and there may be unneutralized venom components remaining in the tissues. Venom may thus redistribute from target tissues and continue to produce toxicity if the antivenom dose is inadequate or if unbound antivenom has been eliminated. These pharmacokinetic relationships illustrate why antivenom administration as soon as possible following envenomation is beneficial and why the use of shorter-acting antivenoms may result in recurrent hematologic effects. Also, because of difficulty reaching damaged tissue and despite the use of antivenom early in the course of a snake envenomation, there may still be limitations as to the effectiveness of antivenom in preventing worsening of local tissue damage, and it will not benefit already devitalized tissue.

Indications, timing, and doses of antivenom will vary and expert guidance should be sought. Since the required dose of antivenom is that needed to neutralize a given amount of venom in the body, it is not dosed by patient weight, and children may require larger doses than adults. Over a 10-year period in the United States, antivenom was only used in 26% of non-native snake envenomations, possibly because of difficulties in determining, locating, and obtaining appropriate antivenom in a timely manner (47,104). Antivenom is most effective in preventing or ameliorating local venom effects when given early in the course. Since most local reactions have stopped progressing within 24 to 36 hours, giving an initial dose of antivenom after this time frame is not likely to be of any benefit. Antivenom is also most effective at preventing or reversing hematologic effects when given early, but may still be beneficial for weeks after an envenomation if there are still circulating venom components (67,77,109). Clinically significant hemorrhage is managed with additional antivenom as well as blood component therapy. Large doses may be required to stop or reverse some effects.

Finally, zoos may only have or choose to send expired antivenom. Expired antivenoms may have decreased efficacy and thus may require higher doses, but barring discoloration or frank contamination, there is otherwise no contraindication to their use (Warrell, personal communication). The regional poison center should be contacted for further assistance (1-800-222-1222).

Surgical Management. Frankly devitalized tissue, usually becoming evident several days following an envenomation, should be debrided. Because high concentrations of venom have been found in blisters overlying the bite area, unroofing these should be considered. Fasciotomy or dermotomy have been advocated for compartment syndrome or tense tissue edema potentially affecting blood flow. Unfortunately, a true compartment syndrome is difficult to diagnose by clinical means, since the typical signs and symptoms of snake envenomation mimic classic compartment syndrome findings, and early surgical intervention often leads to prolonged convalescence, increased tissue damage, decreased function, and greater scarring. Finally, there is no evidence of improved outcome, and there is animal-model evidence of increased myotoxicity with fasciotomy (110). Reported fasciotomy rates vary by geographic region and historical practice, ranging from 0% to greater than 10%. Fasciotomy should only be considered in patients with objective evidence of a compartment syndrome (i.e., a documented significant increase in intracompartmental pressures), vascular impairment, unusual entrapment syndromes, or other tissue threats unresponsive to an adequate trial of antivenom and elevation (111–115). Mannitol and hyperbaric oxygen have also been used in conjunction with antivenom (116). Noninvasive vascular studies may identify patients at risk for ischemia (117).

Other Supportive Therapies. These include basic wound care and updating tetanus status. Blood products should be reserved for significant hemorrhage or hemolysis and administered with additional antivenom. Ventilatory support and hemodialysis may be necessary for pulmonary and renal complications of severe envenomation. Corticosteroids may be used for hypersensitivity reactions to venom or antivenom. Antibiotics are indicated for documented infection or in the presence of frank necrosis.

Hypersensitivity Reactions. If a type I hypersensitivity reaction develops, the antivenom infusion should be stopped. Anaphylactoid reactions are primarily related to rate of infusion, and stopping the infusion often results in rapid improvement. Anaphylactic reactions (i.e., those IgE mediated) are often dramatic and continue to progress after the infusion has been stopped. There is, as one might expect, considerable clinical overlap between the reactions (118). Standard managements should be used. If symptoms persist, the patient should be treated with H_1 (e.g., diphenhydramine, 50 mg IV) and H_2 (e.g., ranitidine, 50 mg IV) blockers. Wheezing may respond to β-adrenergics by nebulizer (e.g., albuterol). If there is hypotension or laryngeal edema, epinephrine, either subcutaneously or intravenously, should be considered (119). Antivenom should be withheld until the reaction has subsided and then a determination made whether to restart it. If restarted, the patient should receive pretreatment with H_1 and H_2 blockers and the infusion begun more slowly.

Type III reactions are usually managed with nonsteroidal anti-inflammatory drugs (NSAIDs) and H_1 and H_2 blockers. More severe cases may require opioid-level pain relief, as well as corticosteroids. All patients receiving antivenom should be

TABLE 68.11

POSTDISCHARGE MANAGEMENT

- Physical therapy may be helpful in minimizing the extent and duration of functional impairment.
- Type III hypersensitivity reactions ("serum sickness"):
  - They usually develop between 5 and 14 d following antivenom administration.
  - The incidence varies from less than 5% to greater than 80% of cases depending on the antivenom, host, and other factors.
  - Nonsteroidal anti-inflammatory drug analgesics and antihistamines are usually sufficient for symptomatic care.
  - Severe reactions may have renal involvement and require steroids and, in rare cases, rehospitalization.
- Patients with significant hematologic abnormalities, especially those treated with Fab antivenoms, may be at risk of recurrent effects postdischarge.
  - Close follow-up is necessary for at least 2 to 4 d to detect recurrence.
  - Consider readministration of antivenom for clinical bleeding or multicomponent or severe hematologic abnormalities, especially with comorbid conditions.

cautioned regarding the possibility of a type III reaction occurring after discharge.

Post discharge Considerations. It is desirable to see patients at least once post discharge in order to monitor for persistent or recurrent hematologic effects if indicated or tissue injury and its sequelae, and to refer for physical or occupational therapy in order to maximize functional recovery. Patients should also be cautioned about the possible risk of sensitization to snake venoms or antivenoms regarding possible future envenomations (Table 68.11).

Treatments *Not* Recommended

1. There is no evidence for efficacy, and there is potential for additional injury with arterial or venous tourniquets, incision or excision of the wound, or the application of heat, cold, or electricity.
2. Suction apparatuses remove only a small amount of venom, have not been shown to improve outcome, and may only serve to delay transport and definitive care (120,121).
3. Although some snake venoms also contain procoagulant factors, and the overall clinical picture is DIC-like, the conditions are not identical, so heparinization and other treatments for DIC are not applicable in snakebites.
4. In the absence of necrosis, prophylactic antibiotics also are of no proven value.
5. Corticosteroids are of no proven value for acute venom effects.

SPIDERS AND SCORPIONS

Spiders

Spiders of medical significance can be found worldwide (122), while in the United States, only two groups of spiders are typically considered medically significant. These are the widow or *Latrodectus* spiders and the brown spiders belonging to the *Loxosceles* genus.

Widow Spiders (*Latrodectus* Genus)

Widow spiders, including the well-known black widow, belong to the *Latrodectus* genus. These spiders are among the most medically important spiders, and representatives are found almost worldwide. In the United States, the widow spiders are found throughout most of the country but are most common in the southeast, with the black widow (*Lactrodectus mactans*) believed to cause most envenomations. The female black widow, more harmful to humans than the male, as her fangs are longer and better able to penetrate human skin, has a shiny black round abdomen and a characteristic bright red hourglass marking on her underside (123). Other species of widow spiders can also be found in the United States. Widow spiders are considered shy spiders and can be found in dark, secluded areas such as under leaf litter (124). All widow spiders worldwide are believed to have similar venom characteristics and similar clinical symptoms.

Pathophysiology. The primary component of widow spider venom that causes human clinical effects is α-latrotoxin. It binds to neuronal tissue and causes neurotransmitter release in at least two ways: (a) it binds to and helps form ion channels, which allow calcium and other ions to leak, causing a calcium-dependent release of neurotransmitter; and (b) it binds to the latrophilin receptor on neuronal tissue, and causes a calcium-independent release of synaptic vesicles (125). This neurotransmitter release, either through calcium-dependent or -independent means, is believed to cause the clinical symptoms seen after widow spider envenomation.

Diagnosis. Diagnosis is primarily clinical and historical, as there are no laboratory tests to confirm envenomation. Typically, bite victims will recall a painful pin prick-like bite, but the bite can be painless. Bites can occur in dark, outdoor places such as leaf litter or woodpiles and, historically, are associated with outhouse use. Bites can also occur when dressing or putting on shoes, especially if they are left outside, or even while in bed (126).

Clinical Effects: Local. Bites from the widow spiders can produce mild local irritation. The bite is classically described as two small punctures with a small area of erythema surrounding a minimally blanched area centrally, producing a "halo" or "target" effect (126). Local injection of venom is not believed to cause necrotic wounds and, while superinfection is possible, it is uncommon.

Clinical Effects: Systemic. The more medically significant effects following widow envenomation are the constellation of systemic symptoms known as *latrodectism*. Typically, symptoms begin within an hour after the bite. What may begin as local muscle cramps can progress to involve larger muscle groups, spreading continuously from the site of the bite. Abdominal muscles can be involved, leading to abdominal rigidity that can imitate the peritoneal signs of a perforated viscus and which may result in an incorrect diagnosis in the young child or uncommunicative adult. Priapism (127), compartment syndrome (128), elevations in creatine kinase (126), and myocarditis (129) have been reported as associated with a *Latrodectus* bite. Though no reported cases of spontaneous abortion have been reported in pregnant patients (130), concern exists for premature delivery given the intense muscle cramping and hypertension that can occur following a widow spider envenomation. Hypertension has been reported (126) and could be life threatening in susceptible populations.

Management. While the *Latrodectus* venom is very potent, the volume of venom is minuscule. There is no role for tourniquets, incision, or excision at the venom injection site. Initial control of pain and muscle contraction should be accomplished through administration of opiates and benzodiazepines. Benzodiazepines are preferred as muscle relaxants, given their wide therapeutic window and minimal hemodynamic and cardiac side effects when compared to agents such as cyclobenzaprine or methocarbamol. Intravenous calcium has not been shown to provide significant benefit (123,126) and is no longer considered a first-line agent.

An antivenom specific to *L. mactans* is available ([*L. mactans*] Black Widow Spider Antivenin, Equine Origin, Merck & Co., Inc). As with administration of other IgG antivenoms, there is a risk of hypersensitivity reactions, including anaphylaxis (126) and serum sickness (131). While skin testing is recommended by the manufacturer, it is insufficiently sensitive or specific to either predict or exclude the likelihood of a type I hypersensitivity reaction (123). Type III hypersensitivity reactions ("serum sickness") have been reported, (131) though they are believed to be a rare complication given the small volume of antivenom necessary to neutralize the injected venom.

The use of antivenom is controversial. Most would agree that when dealing with patients in the extremes of age, pregnant patients, or those with intractable muscle cramping and pain, the use of antivenom should be strongly considered. For those with mild to moderate envenomations, clinicians can attempt a trial of benzodiazepine and opioid therapy. Moss and Binder (131) found that most bite effects were self-limited and needed only minimal pharmacologic intervention, while others found that antivenom was associated with minimal adverse events and rapid resolution of symptoms, and should therefore be considered early in the course after moderate to severe envenomations (123,126,132). The clinician at the bedside must weigh the small risk of hypersensitivity reactions to the possible benefit from reversal of the venom's effects. If administered, the antivenom should be administered in a controlled, monitored environment, with treatments for acute reactions available such as steroids, histamine blockers, and epinephrine immediately available. There is no evidence that pretreatment with any of these agents is efficacious in preventing a reaction, and caution should be used before administering antivenom in anyone with risk factors for immediate hypersensitivity reactions (126). The dose for adults or children is the contents of one restored vial (2.5 mL) of antivenom. It can be given as an intramuscular injection (133) but is typically administered as a slow intravenous infusion (134). It can be redosed if needed, but one vial of antivenom is usually sufficient (133).

There is evidence for cross-reactivity of antivenoms produced to various *Latrodectus* species, including a purified $F(ab')_2$ antivenom produced in Australia to the red-backed spider (*Latrodectus hasselti*) by CSL Limited and which possesses an improved safety profile compared with the U.S. product (135). As this antivenom is not currently approved for use in the United States, consultation with a regional poison center (1-800-222-1222) can be beneficial.

Follow-up. Unless antivenom is administered, in which case monitoring for serum sickness should be arranged, there are no long-term sequelae expected from a widow spider envenomation (131). Local wound care should be satisfactory for the bite site, and prophylactic antibiotics are not warranted. Standard recommendations for any secondary sequelae such as rhabdomyolysis are appropriate.

Brown Spiders (*Loxosceles* Genus)

Loxosceles spiders are found primarily in the southern half of the United States. While at least 50 species of *Loxosceles* can be found on several continents, the *Loxosceles reclusa* species ("brown recluse") is the most common and medically important in the United States (123,136). As their name implies, these are considered shy spiders, hiding in woodpiles and dark corners, only biting when threatened. Bites are more common in warmer months and are often presumed to occur when a spider is caught next to skin by clothing or linens (136). True epidemiology is difficult, as necrotic wounds, which can occur because of *Loxosceles* envenomations, are often inaccurately attributed to spider bites when other insect bites, skin infections, or other dermatologic conditions are truly responsible.

Pathophysiology. Venom from *Loxosceles* spiders is a complex mixture of cytotoxic components that indirectly cause impressive, delayed local symptoms and have the potential for causing human systemic toxicity. Hyaluronidase in the venom causes significant tissue destruction, allowing spread of other venom components in the soft tissues following an envenomation (137). Sphingomyelinase D in *Loxosceles* venom is believed responsible for the dermal inflammation seen after bites (138). Venom injected in the skin starts a cascade of cellular reactions including neutrophil migration and degranulation, which leads to potentially severe local tissue injury (139).

Diagnosis. Because the bite is usually painless and thus unnoticed at the time, unless a *Loxosceles* bite is witnessed and positive identification of the spider occurs, the diagnosis is typically a historical and clinical one. The necrotic wounds found with *Loxosceles* spider bites can mimic numerous other common cutaneous conditions, such as bites by other spiders or other insects, soft tissue bacterial infections, or a vasculitis. A broad differential, including these, as well as conditions such as erythema nodosum, pyoderma gangrenosum, pyogenic granuloma, and herpes infections, should be reviewed before a necrotic wound is attributed to a *Loxosceles* spider in the absence of a known bite (140). Cases of necrotic wounds have been linked to other U.S. spiders such as the hobo spider (141), though clear and well-accepted causation between these spiders and dermonecrotic wounds is still not established (135, 142). Positive laboratory identification by enzyme-linked immunosorbent assay (ELISA) or hemagglutination is possible to confirm *Loxosceles* envenomation in research settings (143), but is not at this time clinically useful. Results are not available in a clinically relevant time frame, and specific therapeutic interventions are not available.

Clinical Effects: Local. Unlike the widow spiders, the majority of clinical effects seen from *Loxosceles* spiders are a result of local tissue injury. The characteristic necrotic wounds are described as having a "red, white, and blue" appearance, though clearly demarcated color rings are rare and not needed to make a diagnosis. Local tissue inflammation occurs over the first day after envenomation, causing skin erythema. In the center of this reddened skin, a small necrotic or "blue" area develops that is surrounded by a halo of blanched tissue appearing gray or "white." Often the wound is not noted until it begins to cause significant pain or the necrotic area becomes prominent.

Clinical Effects: Systemic. Rarely, a *Loxosceles* spider bite can lead to a clinical syndrome known as *systemic loxoscelism*. Cases, many of them in children, begin as low-grade febrile illness with arthralgias and other nonspecific symptoms (144). Within 24 to 48 hours after the bite, these symptoms can progress to a potentially life-threatening illness characterized by hemolysis and shock (136,144,145). Systemic loxoscelism should be in the differential of unexplained hemolysis associated with shock (145).

Management. Many pharmacologic and surgical treatments have been proposed in the management of the necrotic dermal wounds associated with *Loxosceles* spiders, but none has been proven to have significant effects in preventing or reversing damage. These include hyperbaric oxygen (146,147), steroids (148), dapsone (146–150), nitroglycerin (151), and early surgical debridement, and are not recommended. The venom spreads rapidly after a bite, and early attempts to "core" out affected areas to prevent venom spread result in poor wound healing and worsened scarring (149). If significant cosmetic defects occur as a result of the necrotic wound, surgical intervention, including skin grafting, should be delayed at least 4 to 12 weeks (152).

Systemic loxoscelism should be treated with symptomatic and supportive care. Successful treatment of proven loxoscelism cases has included aggressive fluid resuscitation, blood product transfusion, and vasopressor use. While there is no antivenom available in the United States for *Loxosceles* bites, antivenoms to *Loxosceles* spiders exist in South America. Although *Loxosceles* venoms of a variety of species share many antigenic components (153), cross-reactivity data are lacking, and it is unknown whether such antivenoms would confer any benefit in a U.S. *Loxosceles* envenomation.

Non-native Spiders

The funnel web spiders (*Hadronyche* and *Atrax* spp.), native to Australia, and the banana spider (*Phoneutria* spp.), native to South America, are considered far more dangerous than the native *Latrodectus* and *Loxosceles* spiders. In the United States, these can be found through collectors or as accidental stowaways in goods transported internationally. The funnel web spider venom contains a potent neurotoxin that can cause fasciculations, weakness, and autonomic instability, with coma and pulmonary edema complicating the clinical course. An antivenom available in Australia has been successfully used in severe envenomations (154).

The South American spiders belonging to the genus *Phoneutria* have a neurotoxic venom that can cause pain and neurologic and gastrointestinal symptoms, as well as shock and pulmonary edema in severe cases (155). An equine antivenom is available in South America.

These antivenoms may be located in the United States through the Online Antivenom Index, with the assistance of a regional poison center (1-800-222-1222).

Scorpions

In the United States, there is only one medically significant species of scorpion, *Centruroides exilicauda* (formerly *Centruroides sculpturatus*). Found in the southwestern United States, primarily in southern Arizona, it is commonly known as the bark scorpion. Stings occur by the tail, with the venom containing neurotoxins and other components.

Pediatric patients are at greatest risk of having clinically significant symptoms associated with such a scorpion sting. Symptoms can be minor with only some local paresthesias, but, for some, symptoms can be severe, including cardiac manifestations such as tachycardia and hypertension, neurologic manifestations such as roving eye movements and agitation, and respiratory manifestations, including tachypnea and stridor (156,157). Cholinergic symptoms such as hypersalivation have also been reported (158).

Treatment options in the past have included a goat-derived antivenom, limited to use within the state of Arizona. This antivenom is no longer produced, however, and existing supplies are rapidly dwindling. A $F(ab')_2$ antivenom is currently in clinical trials. A continuous midazolam infusion, ventilatory support, and otherwise supportive and symptomatic care are current mainstays of treatment (159,160). Atropine for excessive cholinergic signs has been recommended (158).

MARINE ANIMALS

This review will cover marine envenomations. Organisms that are poisonous when ingested will not be covered. Marine envenomations can occur from interaction with both vertebrate and invertebrate organisms. In the vertebrate category are stingrays, sea snakes, catfish, scorpionfish and leatherjacks, among others. Invertebrates encompass a much larger grouping, including coelenterates, echinoderms, annelid worms, and mollusks.

Stingray

Eleven different species of stingray are found in U.S. waters, seven of which are found in the Atlantic Ocean (161). These animals have long, sharp, serrated barbs along the dorsal surface of their tails, which can cause significant tissue damage and death, even without envenomation (162). They often will bury themselves in the sandy bottom of temperate shallow waters where they may be inadvertently stepped on or otherwise startled to lash out with their tail. The tail barbs are covered in an integumentary sheath that covers two ventrolateral venom glands. Their venom is a complex mixture that includes phosphodiesterase, nucleosidases, and serotonin (161,163).

Clinical Effects

Burning pain at the wound site typically intensifies with time, and local symptoms may last up to 48 hours (162). Venom can cause initial vasodilation and edema at the bite site, then vasoconstriction with hemorrhagic necrosis of tissue and inflammatory infiltrate (163,164). Cardiac conduction abnormalities ranging from bradycardia to atrioventricular nodal blocks with dysrhythmias and cardiac arrest from asystole have been reported. Venom effects also include nausea/vomiting/diarrhea and abdominal pain, as well as ataxia, seizure, coma, hypotension, and respiratory distress (161,163).

Treatment

Treatment is symptomatic and supportive. Radiographic imaging as well as local wound exploration is necessary to evaluate for retained foreign body in the wound. Tetanus prophylaxis should be administered if needed. Prophylactic antibiotics to cover marine microorganisms should be considered, as secondary bacterial infections are common (161,165). Pain control with narcotic analgesia is often required, and immersion of the limb in hot water (110°F, 43°C) may aid in pain relief (162,166,167). Care should be taken to not produce thermal injury. Consider an observation period of at least 4 hours to ensure that symptoms do not progress to systemic effects.

Scorpaenoidea

This group is composed of a number of venomous fish, and is the most common marine source of human envenomation, both in the wild and in home aquaria. They are found in the warm waters of the Gulf of Mexico and Florida Keys, as well as the Pacific, including around Hawaii, and the Indian Ocean. Fish in this group include lionfish (*Pterois*), zebrafish (*Danio*), scorpionfish (*Scorpaena*), and stonefish (*Synanceja*) among many others. Venom apparatus is a collection of spines along the body of the fish, each composed of paired venom glands covered by an integumentary sheath. The dorsal spines are typically the most numerous and can inject the most venom (163). The venom of the fish in this phylum is a complex mixture, and most contain significant amounts of inflammatory mediators such as thromboxane and prostaglandins (161,163). The chemical makeup and potency of venom varies by species within this group, and clinical effects range from very severe (stonefish) to mild (lionfish). The stonefish is by far the deadliest of this group; however, outside of zoos, educational institutions, and private aquaria, it is not likely to be encountered in the United States. It lives in the temperate and warm waters of the Australian and Indo-Pacific and east African coast. There is the potential for envenomation by stonefish in private collections. Of more relevance in this group are the lionfish, zebrafish, and scorpionfish since, although not found wild in U.S. coastal waters, they are a favorite of exotic fish collectors, and stings can result from pets kept in home aquaria (168–171).

Clinical Effects

The majority of reported stings occur on hands and fingers, followed by local, excruciating pain. Local swelling was common, with few reported vesicular lesions at the bite site (163,172). Systemic symptoms are much less commonly reported but include nausea, sweats, chest and abdominal pain, and rarely hypotension (162,167,173–175). Local effects, especially numbness, may persist long after the sting, and often wounds are very slow to heal, usually resulting in granulomatous and fibrous scarring (166,167).

Treatment

Treatment is primarily by symptomatic and supportive care, with the exception of the stonefish, for which there is an antivenom (176). Antivenom can be located by contacting a regional poison center (1-800-222-1222). Good wound care is also essential. Spines may break off during envenomation, and the wound should be closely inspected for any retained foreign body. Immersion of the limb in nonscalding hot water (110°F, 43°C) may aid in pain relief (162,166,167,169). Unroofing of any blisters that form at the envenomation site is indicated as the vesicle may contain venom and contribute to persistent effects. Tetanus immunization or booster should be administered as needed. Antibiotics should be given if secondary infection develops.

Sea Snakes

There are approximately 50 species of sea snakes in several subfamilies. They are found primarily in the warm tropical waters of the Indo-West Pacific. None are found in the Atlantic Ocean or Caribbean Sea. Envenomations are likely the result of such snakes being kept in zoos or academic institutions or kept by private collectors. Their venom is similar to Elapid venom, with neurotoxicity—and potentially respiratory arrest—as the primary clinical effect. See the section on non-native snake envenomations for management considerations.

Invertebrates

Five phyla—Cnidaria, Porifera (sponges), Echinodermata (sea urchins, starfish), Mollusca (octopi and cone snails), and Annelida (bristle worms)—constitute the venomous invertebrates. There are over 10,000 species in the phylum Cnidaria (formerly Coelenterata), and several hundred are dangerous to humans. This grouping includes jellyfish (class Scyphozoa), the Portuguese man-of-war and other sea hydroids (class Hydrozoa), and the sea anemones and fire corals (class Anthozoa). All possess envenoming apparatus in the form of nematocysts (161,163,177).

In jellyfish and hydroids, nematocysts are primarily on the tentacles, and each tentacle can contain thousands. Each nematocyst is a spiral-coiled dart-like structure within venom sacs. Venom is injected when the barb penetrates the flesh of its prey. Nematocysts that have become detached from the tentacle, tentacles of dead jellyfish, or detached tentacles can all still cause envenomation upon contact. The popularity of scuba diving and snorkeling has increased the chances of contact with the nematocysts of sessile Cnidaria, such as sea anemones and soft and true corals (178). The Portuguese man-of-war (*Physalia physalis*) is found in the Atlantic waters off the southern coast of the United States, especially from July through September, and is actually a complex colony of multiple hydroids (179). The body is pale blue and bell or bottle shaped and the tentacles may grow to more than 100 feet in length. The venom is especially complex and also contains neurotoxins.

The severity of the sting depends on the organism, the number of successful discharges, and the composition of the venom. Like the majority of venoms, Cnidaria venoms are complex mixtures of many substances. Commonly found chemicals include histamine, serotonin, alkaline and acid phosphatases, proteases, hyaluronidase, nucleosidases, hemolysins, and inflammatory mediators, among others (167,180).

Clinical Effects

Most organisms in this grouping, with the exception of the Portuguese man-of-war, cause only mild local effects in humans. These local effects consist of burning pain at the site of the sting, which may be severe, with swelling, erythema, and possible vesicle formation and ulceration of the area (181,182). Regional lymphadenopathy may be seen, and secondary infection and scarring are common.

Anaphylactoid reactions can occur as well. Systemic effects, if any, are mild, but immune reactions such as erythema nodosum and reactive arthritis have been reported (183–185). Irukandji syndrome is a constellation of both local and systemic symptoms that occur in a delayed fashion after envenomation by an Australian jellyfish (*Carukia barnsi*). There have been reports of a similar syndrome occurring in swimmers and divers off the coast of southern Florida, likely after exposure to another organism in the same genus, although the responsible organism has not yet been identified (185).

With envenomation by the Portuguese man-of-war, there is immediate intense local pain at the sting site, with development of large, linear, erythematous welts where tentacles have contacted the skin. These welts often leave significant scarring. Systemic effects include nausea and vomiting, headache, and myalgias, and may progress to muscle weakness, respiratory distress, and cardiovascular collapse in severe envenomations (161,167,186). The intense pain and occasional paralysis caused by many stings from this jellyfish can result in drowning. Multiple stings can be fatal.

Fire coral (*Millepora*) is not a true coral, rather a relative of fresh water hydra, but has nematocysts to envenomate its prey. The stings cause local burning pain, urticaria, and intense pruritus (179). These wheals may take weeks to heal completely and may leave hyperpigmented scars.

The Scyphozoa contain the "true" jellyfish, including the deadly box jellyfish (*Chironex fleckeri* or sea wasp), which is not found in U.S. waters, and is present here in zoo, institutional, and possibly private collections only. It is usually found in tropical climates of the Indian and Pacific Oceans, including the coastal waters of Australia. The box jellyfish is so named because of its four translucent panels that roughly form a box. The sting of the box jellyfish is painful and can cause death within minutes, and the mortality rate in native settings is 15% to 20% (161,187,188). An antivenom is available and should be stocked by the institutions that house these creatures; antivenom can be located by contacting the regional poison center (1-800-222-1222).

The Scyphozoa also include sea nettles (*Dactylometra quinquecirrha*), which pose a greater chance of exposure to swimmers of this country, but the sting in most cases is a minor annoyance, although systemic symptoms similar to those seen with Physalia envenomations have been reported (179).

Treatment

Swimmers and divers in waters endemic for venomous animals and health care providers caring for victims of envenomations should wear gloves and clothing for personal protection. If stung, any nematocysts still on the skin should be inactivated with 5% acetic acid (vinegar) and then removed by "shaving" the area with a dull-edged knife or the edge of a credit card (179,189,190). Shaving cream may aid in the shaving process. Adhesive tape may also be effective at removing unseen nematocysts. Papain meat tenderizer has been reported to improve symptoms and may be used with caution (167). Alcohol or fresh water may cause the remaining nematocysts to fire and should not be used. A few species' nematocysts will fire in the setting of acetic acid, including the American sea nettle, the little mauve stinger jellyfish, and the hairy or lion's mane jellyfish. For these few, a slurry of baking soda should be applied for at least 10 minutes over the affected area. If tentacles remain attached to the skin, a vinegar or baking soda slurry should be applied, then shaving cream and scraping as for nematocysts to remove the tentacles. Many components of the venoms of these organisms are heat-labile, and immersion of the affected area in nonscalding hot water (110°F, 43°C) may aid in pain relief (162,166,167,169,189,190).

Tetanus prophylaxis should be given as needed and a third-generation cephalosporin used for secondary infection. Pain should be treated with both NSAIDs and opioids as needed. Persistent pruritus and swelling should be treated with antihistamines. Systemic steroids have not been shown to be of any benefit.

Sea Lice (Seabather's Eruption)

The prolific time period for the appearance of sea lice is March through June on the southeast coast of Florida. A contact dermatitis can develop with exposure to the larvae of sea lice (*Linuche unguiculata*). The larvae attach to the fibers in bathing suits and cause a rash in the distribution of the swimwear, thus "seabather's eruption." The rash is pruritic, erythematous, and maculopapular, and typically resolves spontaneously in hours to days without sequelae (178,191–193). Topical treatment with antihistamines and calamine lotion may give relief.

Sponges

Some sponges contain spicules composed of calcium carbonate and silica, which can cause local irritation and itching of skin upon contact. This is also known as "skin diver's" or "sponge fisherman's" disease. The fire, red, and bun sponges also have toxins in their coatings that can cause local irritation, which may be painful and pruritic and produce erythema (178,194). Pain and paresthesias after contact may persist for weeks (161,194).

Treatment

Remove spicules with adhesive tape or the edge of a dull knife or credit card. Washing the area with 5% acetic acid may aid in symptom control (161,178,194). Antihistamines and NSAIDs may be used for symptom control.

Mollusca

Conus Snails

Cone shell snails have an ejectable tooth at the end of a long flexible proboscis, and envenomate their prey by sinking this tooth deep into the flesh (194). The venom contains primarily neurotoxins that act by ion channel effects (167,195).

Clinical Effects. Clinical effects include local burning pain, numbness, and paresthesias, as well as systemic effects of perioral paresthesias, cranial nerve palsies, coma, respiratory muscle paralysis, and cardiovascular collapse (161). Although the majority of human envenomations are mild and limited to local effects, at least 15 deaths have been reported (194).

Treatment. Treatment is primarily symptomatic and supportive.

Toxic Octopi

Other marine animals may cause serious, and at times fatal, envenomations. The bite of the blue-ringed octopus introduces tetrodotoxin, a potent neurotoxin also found in the puffer fish, as well as several other neurotoxins, including maculotoxin (167,179). This organism is of importance, as it may be found in zoo aquaria and the home aquaria of private collectors in the United States. The giant monster octopus should not be of concern in the United States.

Clinical Effects

Clinical effects include local pain, numbness, and paresthesias, which may also involve distant sites such as the lips and tongue. Cranial nerve palsies can be seen and, in severe envenomations, muscle weakness progressing to respiratory paralysis and cardiovascular collapse occurs (163,167,196).

Treatment

Treatment is primarily symptomatic and supportive care. Respiratory and cardiovascular support may be required. No antivenom is available.

Echinodermata

Crown of thorns (*Acanthaster planci*) is found primarily in the Indo-Pacific Oceans and should be of little concern in the United States except when encountered in zoo, academic institution, and private collector aquaria. Sharp, rigid spines over the dorsum of the organism can cause deep puncture wounds, even through gloves, and the venom delivered is a complex mixture of inflammatory mediators, histamine, and others including toxic saponins, with hemolytic and anticoagulant effects (163,194,197).

Clinical Effects

Local effects predominate, such as burning pain and local hemorrhagic injury. Secondary infection and retained foreign body from broken spines are not uncommon. Systemic symptoms are rarely reported but may include nausea and vomiting. Immersion of the limb in nonscalding hot water (110°F, 43°C) may aid in pain relief, as the venom components are heat-labile (162,166,167,169,197).

Sea Urchins

Many sea urchins have long, sharp spines composed of calcium carbonate that cause local injury, but most are not venomous. Deep tissue injury and extension of spines into organs and joint spaces may cause tissue destruction and morbidity from secondary infection. If it is a venom-containing species, the gland is located at the end of the spines and in their pedicellaria (the mouthlike apparatus at the end of a stalk used to gather food). Venom is composed of a mixture of steroid glycosides, serotonin, proteases, and others (198).

Clinical Effects

Local pain, erythema, and edema are typically self-limited. Partial paralysis of the envenomated limb has been reported with exposure to some species (194,197). Rare systemic symptoms are noted in the literature.

Treatment

The affected area should be immersed in nonscalding hot water (110°F, 43°C), with oral analgesics and local wound care, and removal of any embedded spines as needed. Care is otherwise symptomatic and supportive.

Annelid Worms

The common bristle worm, found in Floridian and Caribbean waters, causes intense local inflammation with edema, erythema, and urticaria (163). No systemic reactions have been reported, and the toxin is unknown. Removal of any bristles adherent to the skin and otherwise simple symptomatic and supportive care are the mainstays of treatment.

References

1. Kitchens CS. From ETOH to FAB: the medicalization of therapy for pit viper envenomation. *Trans Am Clin Climatol Assn.* 2001;112:117–137.
2. Kitchens CS, van Mierop LHS. Envenomation by the Eastern coral snake (Micrurus fulvius vulvius). A study of 39 victims. *JAMA.* 1987;258:1615–1618.
3. de Roodt AR, Paniagua-Solis JF, Dolab JA, et al. Effectiveness of two common antivenoms for North, Central, and South American Micrurus envenomations. *J Toxicol Clin Toxicol.* 2004;42:171–178.
4. van Mierop LHS. Poisonous snakebite: a review. 2. Symptomatology and treatment. *J Fla Med Assn.* 1976;63:191–120.
5. Hankin FM, Smith MD, Penner JA, et al. Eastern massasauga rattlesnake bites. *J Pediatr Orthop.* 1987;7:201–205.
6. Christiansen J, Fieselmann J. Massasauga rattlesnake bites in Iowa. *Iowa Med.* 1993;83:187–191.
7. Whitley RE. Conservative treatment of copperhead snakebites without antivenin. *J Trauma.* 1996;41:219–221.
8. Lavonas EJ, Gerardo CJ, O'Malley G, et al. Initial experience with Crotalidae polyvalent immune Fab (ovine) antivenom in the treatment of copperhead snakebite. *Ann Emerg Med.* 2004;43:200–206.
9. Scharman EJ, Noffsinger VD. Copperhead snakebites: clinical severity of local effects. *Ann Emerg Med.* 2001;38:55–61.
10. Kitchens CS, van Mierop LHS. Mechanism of defibrination in humans after envenomation by the eastern diamondback rattlesnake. *Am J Hematol.* 1983;14:345–353.
11. Lewis RL, Gutmann L. Snake venoms and the neuromuscular junction. *Semin Neurol.* 2004;24:175–179.
12. Mounier CM, Bon C, Kini RM. Anticoagulant venom and mammalian secreted phospholipases A(2): protein-versus phospholipid-dependent mechanism of action. *Haemostasis.* 2001;31:279–287.
13. Lu Q, Clemetson JM, Clemetson KJ. Snake venoms and hemostasis. *J Thromb Haemost.* 2005;3:1791–1799.
14. Kini RM, Rao VS, Joseph JS. Procoagulant proteins from snake venoms. *Haemostasis.* 2001;31:218–224.
15. Parkin JD, Ibrahim K, Dauer RJ, et al. Prothrombin activation in eastern tiger snake bite. *Pathology.* 2002;34:162–166.
16. Budzynski AZ, Pandya BV, Rubin RN, et al. Fibrinogenolytic afibrinogenemia after envenomation by western diamondback rattlesnake (Crotalus atrox). *Blood.* 1984;63:1–14.

17. Markland FS. Snake venoms and the hemostatic system. *Toxicon.* 1998;36:1749–1800.
18. White J. Snake venoms and coagulopathy. *Toxicon.* 2005;45:951–967.
19. Gutierrez JM, Rucavado A, Escalante T, et al. Hemorrhage induced by snake venom metalloproteinases: biochemical and biophysical mechanisms involved in microvessel damage. *Toxicon.* 2005;45:997–1011.
20. Reid HA, Theakston RD. Changes in coagulation effects by venoms of Crotalus atrox as snakes age. *Am J Trop Med Hyg.* 1978;27:1053–1057.
21. Bush SP, Green SM, Moynihan JA, et al. Crotalidae polyvalent immune Fab (ovine) antivenom is efficacious for envenomations by Southern Pacific rattlesnakes (Crotalus helleri). *Ann Emerg Med.* 2002;40:619–624.
22. Carroll RR, Hall EL, Kitchens CS. Canebrake rattlesnake envenomation. *Ann Emerg Med.* 1997;30:45–48.
23. Farstad D, Thomas T, Chow T, et al. Mojave rattlesnake envenomation in southern California: a review of suspected cases. *Wilderness Environ Med.* 1997;8:89–93.
24. Clark RF, Williams SR, Nordt SP, et al. Successful treatment of Crotalid-induced neurotoxicity with a new polyspecific Crotalid Fab antivenom. *Ann Emerg Med.* 1997;30:54–57.
25. Boyer LV, Seifert SA, Cain JS. Recurrence phenomena after immunoglobulin therapy for snake envenomations: part 2. Guidelines for clinical management with Crotaline Fab antivenom. *Ann Emerg Med.* 2001;32:196–201.
26. Yip L. Rational use of Crotalidae polyvalent immune Fab (ovine) in the management of Crotaline bite. *Ann Emerg Med.* 2002;39:648–650.
27. Dart RC, McNally JT, Spaite DW, et al. Validation of a severity score for the assessment of Crotalid snakebite. *Ann Emerg Med.* 1996;27:321–326.
28. Kitchens CS. To bleed or not to bleed? Is that the question for the PTT? *J Thromb Haemost.* 2005;3:2607–2611.
29. Boyer LV, Seifert SA, Clark RF, et al. Recurrent and persistent coagulopathy following pit viper envenomation. *Arch Intern Med.* 1999;159:706–710.
30. Bogdan GM, Dart RC, Falbo SC, et al. Recurrent coagulopathy after antivenom treatment of crotalid snakebite. *South Med J.* 2000;93:562–566.
31. Ruha AM, Curry SC, Beuhler M, et al. Initial postmarketing experience with crotalidae polyvalent immune Fab for treatment of rattlesnake envenomation. *Ann Emerg Med.* 2002;39:648–650.
32. Odeleye AA, Presley AE, Passwater ME, et al. Report of two cases: rattlesnake venom-induced thrombocytopenia. *Ann Clin Lab Sci.* 2004;34:467–470.
33. Camilleri C, Offerman S, Gosselin R, et al. Conservative management of delayed, multicomponent coagulopathy following rattlesnake envenomation. *Clin Toxicol.* 2005;43:201–206.
34. de Oliveira RB, Ribeiro LA, Jorge MT. Risk factors associated with coagulation abnormalities in Bothrops envenoming. *Rev Soc Bras Med Trop.* 2003;36:657–663.
35. Sano-Martins IS, Tomy SC, Campolina D, et al. Coagulopathy following lethal and non-lethal envenoming of humans by the South American rattlesnake (Crotalus durissus) in Brazil. *QJM.* 2001;94:551–559.
36. Dart RC, McNally JR, Spaite DW, et al. The sequelae of pitviper poisoning in the United States. In: Campbell JA, Brodie ED Jr, eds. *Biology of Pit Vipers.* Tyler, TX: Selva Publications; 1992:395–404.
37. Bond RG, Burkhart KK. Thrombocytopenia following timber rattlesnake envenomation. *Ann Emerg Med.* 1997;30:40–41.
38. Offerman SR, Bush SP, Moynihan JA, et al. Crotaline Fab antivenom for the treatment of children with rattlesnake envenomation. *Pediatrics.* 2002;110:968–971.
39. Shaw BA, Hosalkar HS. Rattlesnake bites in children: antivenin treatment and surgical indications. *J Bone Joint Surg Am.* 2002;84:1624–1629.
40. Stewart RM, Carey PP, Schwesinger WH, et al. Antivenin and fasciotomy/debridement in the treatment of the severe rattlesnake bite. *Am J Surg.* 1989;158:543–547.
41. Clark RF, Selden BS, Furbee B. The incidence of wound infection following Crotalid envenomation. *J Emerg Med.* 1993;11:583–586.
42. LoVecchio F, Klemens J, Welch S, et al. Antibiotics after rattlesnake envenomation. *J Emerg Med.* 2002;23:327–328.
43. Cowin DJ, Wright T, Cowin JA. Long-term complications of snake bites to the upper extremity. *J South Ortho Assn.* 1998;7:205–211.
44. Spiller HA, Bosse GM. Prospective study of morbidity associated with snakebite envenomation. *J Toxicol Clin Toxicol.* 2003;41:125–130.
45. Russell FE, Carlson RW, Wainschel J, et al. Snake venom poisoning in the United States: experiences with 550 cases. *JAMA.* 1975;233:341.
46. Kunkel DB, Curry SC, Vance MV, et al. Reptile envenomations. *J Toxicol Clin Toxicol.* 1983–84;21:503.
47. Seifert SA, Audi J, Boyer LV. Toxic Exposure Surveillance System (TESS)-based characterization of US non-native venomous snake exposures, 1995–2004. *Clin Toxicol. (Phila).* 2007; 45(5):571–578. (Abstract: Seifert SA. TESS-based characterization of non-native snake envenomation in the United States. *J Med Toxicol.* 2006;2(1):35–36.)
48. Bey TA, Boyer LV, Walter FG, et al. Exotic snakebite: envenomation by an African puff adder (Bitis arietans). *J Emerg Med.* 1997;15(6):827–831.
49. Kochva E, Gans C. Salivary glands of snakes. *Clin Toxicol.* 1970;3:363.
50. Chacur M, Gutierrez JM, Milligan ED, et al. Snake venom components enhance pain upon subcutaneous injection: an initial examination of spinal cord mediators. *Pain.* 2004;111(1–2):65–76.
51. Saha A, Gomes A, Giri B, et al. Occurrence of non-protein low molecular weight cardiotoxin in Indian King Cobra (*Ophiophagus hannah*) Cantor 1836, venom. *Indian J Exp Biol.* 2006;44(4):279–285.
52. Petricevich VL. Cytokine and nitric oxide production following severe envenomation. *Curr Drug Targets Inflamm Allergy.* 2004;3(3):325–332.
53. Girish KS, Kemparaju K. Inhibition of Naja naja venom hyaluronidase: role in the management of poisonous bite. *Life Sci.* 2006;78(13):1433–1440. Epub 2005 Oct 25.
54. Escalante T, Shannon J, Moura-da-Silva AM, et al. Novel insights into capillary vessel basement membrane damage by snake venom hemorrhagic metalloproteinases: a biochemical and immunohistochemical study. *Arch Biochem Biophys.* 2006;455(2):144–153. Epub 2006 Oct 6.
55. Mazzi MV, Magro AJ, Amui SF, et al. Molecular characterization and phylogenetic analysis of BjussuMP-I: A RGD-P-III class hemorrhagic metalloprotease from *Bothrops jararacussu* snake venom. *J Mol Graph Model.* 2007;26(1)69–85.
56. Daniele JJ, Bianco ID, Fidelio GD. Kinetic and pharmacologic characterization of phospholipase A_2 from *Bothrops neuwiedi* venom. *Arch Biochem Biophys.* 1995;65:65–70.
57. Gutierrez JM, Lomonte B. Phopholipase A_2 myotoxins from *Bothrops* snake venoms. *Toxicon.* 1995;33:1405–1424.
58. Kamiguti AS, Cardoso JLC, Theakston RDG, et al. Coagulopathy and haemorrhage in human victims of *Bothrops jararaca* envenoming in Brazil. *Toxicon.* 1991;29:961–972.
59. Milani R Jr, Jorge MT, Ferraz De Campos FP, et al. Snake bites by the jararacussu (*Bothrops jrararacussu*): clinicopathological studies of 29 proven cases in Sao Paulo, Brazil. *Q J Med.* 1997;90:323–334.
60. White J. Snake venoms and coagulopathy. *Toxicon.* 2005;45(8):951–967. Epub 2005 Apr 12.
61. Jelinek GA, Hamilton T, Hirsch RL. Admissions for suspected snake bite to the Perth adult teaching hospitals, 1979 to 1988. *Med J Aust.* 1991;155(11–12):761–764.
62. Bentur Y, Cahana A. Unusual local complications of Vipera palaestinae bite. *Toxicon.* 2003;41(5):633–635.
63. Richardson WH 3rd, Barry JD, Tong TC, et al. Rattlesnake envenomation to the face of an infant. *Pediatr Emerg Care.* 2005;21(3):173–176.
64. Hofer M, Hirschel B, Kirschner P, et al. Brief report: disseminated osteomyelitis from Mycobacterium ulcerans after a snakebite. *N Engl J Med.* 1993;328(14):1007–1009.
65. Wu CH, Hu WH, Hung DZ, et al. Snakebite complicated with Vibrio vulnificus infection. *Vet Hum Toxicol.* 2001;43(5):283–285.
66. Angel MF, Zhang F, Jones M, et al. Necrotizing fasciitis of the upper extremity resulting from a water moccasin bite. *South Med J.* 2002;95(9):1090–1094.
67. Russel FE, Picchioni AL. Snake venom poisoning. *Clin Toxicol Consultant.* 1983;5:73.
68. Ekenback K, Hulting J, Persson H, et al. Unusual neurological symptoms in a case of severe crotalid envenomation. *Clin Toxicol.* 1985;23:357.
69. Li QB, Huang GW, Kinjoh K, et al. Hematological studies on DIC-like findings observed in patients with snakebite in south China. *Toxicon.* 2001;39(7):943–948.
70. Kamiguti AS, Laing GD, Lowe GM, et al. Biological properties of the venom of the Papuan black snake (Pseudechis papuanus): presence of a phospholipase A2 platelet inhibitor. *Toxicon.* 1994;32(8):915–925.
71. Joseph JK, Simpson ID, Menon NC, et al. First authenticated cases of life-threatening envenoming by the hump-nosed pit viper (Hypnale hypnale) in India. *Trans R Soc Trop Med Hyg.* 2007;101(1):85–90. Epub 2006 Jul 12.
72. Hantson P, Verhelst D, Wittebole X, et al. Defibrination and systemic bleeding caused by an imported African snakebite. *Eur J Emerg Med.* 2003;10(4):349–352.
73. Benvenuti LA, Franca FO, Barbaro KC, et al. Pulmonary haemorrhage causing rapid death after Bothrops jararacussu snakebite: a case report. *Toxicon.* 2003;42(3):331–334.
74. Mosquera A, Idrovo LA, Tafur A, et al. Stroke following *Bothrops* spp. Snakebite. *Neurology.* 2003;60(10):1577–1580.
75. Bartholdi D, Selic C, Meier J, et al. Viper snakebite causing symptomatic intracerebral haemorrhage. *J Neurol.* 2004;251(7):889–891.
76. Top LJ, Tulleken JE, Ligtenberg JJ, et al. Serious envenomation after a snakebite by a Western bush viper (*Atheris chlorechis*) in the Netherlands: a case report. *Neth J Med.* 2006;64(5):153–156.
77. Seifert SA, Boyer LV, Dart RC, et al. Relationship of venom effects to venom antigen and antivenom serum concentrations in a patient with *Crotalus atrox* envenomation treated with a Fab antivenom. *Ann Emerg Med.* 1997;30(1):49–53.
78. Khadwal A, Bharti B, Poddar B, et al. Persistent coagulopathy in snake bite. *Indian J Pediatr.* 2003;70(5):439–441.
79. Blaylock RS, Lichtman AR, Potgieter PD. Clinical manifestations of Cape cobra (*Naja nivea*) bites. A report of 2 cases. *S Afr Med J.* 1985;68(5):342–344.
80. Watt G, Padre L, Tuazon L, et al. Bites by the Philippine cobra (*Naja naja philippinensis*): prominent neurotoxicity with minimal local signs. *Am J Trop Med Hyg.* 1988;39(3):306–311.
81. Watt G, Padre L, Tuazon ML, et al. Tourniquet application after cobra bite: delay in the onset of neurotoxicity and the dangers of sudden release. *Am J Trop Med Hyg.* 1988;38(3):618–622.
82. Lalloo DG, Trevett AJ, Black J, et al. Neurotoxicity, anticoagulant activity

and evidence of rhabdomyolysis in patients bitten by death adders (*Acanthophis sp.*) in southern Papua New Guinea. *QJM.* 1996;89(1):25–35.
83. Gold BS. Neostigmine for the treatment of neurotoxicity following envenomation by the Asiatic cobra. *Ann Emerg Med.* 1996;28(1):87–89.
84. Jones RG, Lee L, Landon J. The effects of specific antibody fragments on the 'irreversible' neurotoxicity induced by Brown snake (*Pseudonaja*) venom. *Br J Pharmacol.* 1999;126(3):581–584.
85. Brooks DE, Graeme KA. Airway compromise after first rattlesnake envenomation. *Wilderness Environ Med.* 2004;15(3):188–193.
86. Weiser E, Wollberg Z, Kochva E, et al. Cardiotoxic effects of the venom of the burrowing asp, *Atractaspis engaddensis* (*Atractaspididae, Ophidia*). *Toxicon.* 1984;22(5):767–774.
87. de Siqueira JE, Higuchi Mde L, Nabut N, et al. Myocardial lesions after snake bites by the *Crotalus durissus terrificus* species (rattlesnake). A case report. *Arq Bras Cardiol.* 1990;54(5):323–325.
88. Hinze JD, Barker JA, Jones TR, et al. Life-threatening upper airway edema caused by a distal rattlesnake bite. *Ann Emerg Med.* 2001;38(1):79–82.
89. Hafeez S, Majeed I. Cardiac arrhythmia as presentation of snakebite. *J Coll Physicians Surg Pak.* 2004;14(1):48–49.
90. Thewjitcharoen Y, Poopitaya S. Ventricular tachycardia, a rare manifestation of Russell's viper bite: case report. *Med Assoc Thai.* 2005;88(12):1931–1933.
91. Chippaux JP, Lang J, Eddine SA, et al. Clinical safety of a polyvalent F(ab')2 equine antivenom in 223 African snake envenomations: a field trial in Cameroon. VAO (Venin Afrique de l'Ouest) Investigators. *Trans R Soc Trop Med Hyg.* 1998;92(6):657–662.
92. Shemesh IY, Kristal C, Langerman L, et al. Preliminary evaluation of Vipera palaestinae snake bite treatment in accordance to the severity of the clinical syndrome. *Toxicon.* 1998;36(6):867–873.
93. Tokish JT, Benjamin J, Walter F. Crotalid envenomation: the southern Arizona experience. *J Orthop Trauma.* 2001;15(1):5–9.
94. LoVecchio F, Klemens J, Roundy EB, et al. Serum sickness following administration of Antivenin (*Crotalidae*) Polyvalent in 181 cases of presumed rattlesnake envenomation. *Wilderness Environ Med.* 2003;14(4):220–221.
95. Bentur Y, Raikhlin-Eisenkraft B, Galperin M. Evaluation of antivenom therapy in Vipera palaestinae bites. *Toxicon.* 2004;44(1):53–57.
96. Frethewie ER. Detection of snake venom in tissue. *Clin Toxicol.* 1970; 3:445.
97. Minton SA, Weinstein SA, Wilde CE. An enzyme-linked immunoassay for detection of North American pit viper venoms. *Clin Toxicol.* 1984;22:303.
98. McKinney PE. Out-of-hospital and interhospital management of crotaline snakebite. *Ann Emerg Med.* 2001;37(2):168–174.
99. Hodgson PS, Davidson TM. Biology and treatment of the mamba snakebite. *Wilderness Environ Med.* 1996;7(2):133–145.
100. German BT, Hack JB, Brewer K, et al. Pressure-immobilization bandages delay toxicity in a porcine model of eastern coral snake (*Micrurus fulvius fulvius*) envenomation. *Ann Emerg Med.* 2005;45(6):603–608.
101. Bush SP, Green SM, Laack TA, et al. Pressure immobilization delays mortality and increases intracompartmental pressure after artificial intramuscular rattlesnake envenomation in a porcine model. *Ann Emerg Med.* 2004;44(6):599–604.
102. Glass TG. *Management of Poisonous Snakebite.* San Antonio, TX: Thomas G. Glass; 1976.
103. Blaylock RS. Antibiotic use and infection in snakebite victims. *S Afr Med J.* 1999;89(8):874–876.
104. Seifert SA, Keyler D, Isbister G, et al. ACMT Position statement: institutions housing venomous animals. *J Med Toxicol.* 2006;2(3):118–119.
105. Warrell DA, Greenwood BM, Davidson NM, et al. Necrosis, haemorrhage and complement depletion following bites by the spitting cobra (*Naja nigricollis*). *Q J Med.* 1976;45(177):1–22.
106. Tilbury CR. Observations on the bite of the Mozambique spitting cobra (*Naja mossambica mossambica*). *S Afr Med J.* 1982;61(9):308–313.
107. Gillissen A, Theakston RD, Barth J, et al. Neurotoxicity, haemostatic disturbances and haemolytic anaemia after a bite by a Tunisian saw-scaled or carpet viper (*Echis 'pyramidum'-complex*): failure of antivenom treatment. *Toxicon.* 1994;32(8):937–944.
108. Trevett AJ, Lalloo DG, Nwokolo NC, et al. The efficacy of antivenom in the treatment of bites by the Papuan taipan (*Oxyuranus scutellatus canni*). *Trans R Soc Trop Med Hyg.* 1995;89(3):322–325.
109. Tiwari I, Johnston WJ. Blood coagulability and viper envenomation. *Lancet.* 1986;i:613.
110. Tanen DA, Danish DC, Grice GA, et al. Fasciotomy worsens the amount of myonecrosis in a porcine model of crotaline envenomation. *Ann Emerg Med.* 2004;44(2):99–104.
111. Whitesides TE, Haney TC, Morimoto K, et al. Tissue pressure measurements as a determinant for the need of fasciotomy. *Clin Orthop.* 1975;113:43.
112. Mars M, Hadley GP, Aitchison JM. Direct intracompartmental pressure measurement in the management of snakebites in children. *S Afr Med J.* 1991;80(5):227–228.
113. Blaylock RS. Femoral vessel entrapment and compartment syndromes following snakebite. *S Afr J Surg.* 2003;41(3):72–73.
114. Chattopadhyay A, Patra RD, Shenoy V, et al. Surgical implications of snakebites. *Indian J Pediatr.* 2004;71(5):397–399.
115. Hardy DL Sr, Zamudio KR. Compartment syndrome, fasciotomy, and neuropathy after a rattlesnake envenomation: aspects of monitoring and diagnosis. *Wilderness Environ Med.* 2006;17(1):36–40.
116. Gold BS, Barish RA, Dart RC, et al. Resolution of compartment syndrome after rattlesnake envenomation utilizing non-invasive measures. *J Emerg Med.* 2003;24(3):285–288.
117. Curry SC, Kraner JC, Kunkel DB, et al. Noninvasive vascular studies in management of rattlesnake envenomations to extremities. *Ann Emerg Med.* 1985;14:1081.
118. Schwartz LB. Effector cells of anaphylaxis: mast cells and basophils. *Novartis Found Symp.* 2004;257:65–74; discussion 74–79, 98–100, 276–285.
119. Alberts MB, Shalit M, LoGalbo F. Suction for venomous snakebite: a study of "mock venom" extraction in a human model. *Ann Emerg Med.* 2004;43(2):181–186.
120. Bush SP, Hegewald KG, Green SM, et al. Effects of a negative pressure venom extraction device (Extractor) on local tissue injury after artificial rattlesnake envenomation in a porcine model. *Wilderness Environ Med.* 2000;11(3):180–188.
121. Kularatne SA, Kumarasiri PV, Pushpakumara SK, et al. Routine antibiotic therapy in the management of the local inflammatory swelling in venomous snakebites: results of a placebo-controlled study. *Ceylon Med J.* 2005;50(4):151–155.
122. White J. Overview of spider envenoming. In: Brent J, Wallace KL, Burkhart KK, et al., eds. *Critical Care Toxicology.* Philadelphia: Mosby Inc.; 2005:1179–1185.
123. White J, Cardoso JL, Fan HW. Clinical toxicology of spider bites. In: Meier J, White J, eds. *Handbook of Clinical Toxicology of Animal Venoms and Poisons.* New York: CRC Press; 1995:259–330.
124. Foster S, Caras R. *Venomous Animals & Poisonous Plants.* New York: Houghton Mifflin Company; 1994.
125. Grishin EV. Black widow spider toxins: the present and the future. *Toxicon.* 1998;36:1693–1701.
126. Clark RF, Wethern-Kestner S, Vance MV, et al. Clinical presentation of black widow spider envenomation: a review of 163 cases. *Ann Emerg Med.* 1992;210:782–787.
127. Hoover NG, Fortenberry JD. Use of antivenom to treat priapism after a black widow spider bite. *Pediatrics.* 2004;114:e128–e129.
128. Cohen J, Bush S. Case report: compartment syndrome after a suspected black widow spider bite. *Ann Emerg Med.* 2005;45:414–416.
129. Pneumatikos IA, Galiatsou E, Goe D, et al. Acute fatal myocarditis after black widow spider envenomation. *Ann Emerg Med.* 2003;41: 158.
130. Langley RL. A review of venomous animal bites and stings in pregnant patients. *Wilderness Environ Med.* 2004;15:207–215.
131. Moss HS, Binder LS. A retrospective review of black widow spider envenomations. *Ann Emerg Med.* 1987;16:188–191.
132. Jelinek GA. Widow spider evenomation (latrodectism): a worldwide problem. *Wilderness Environ Med.* 1997;8:226–231.
133. Package Insert Black Widow Spider Antivenom. Available at: http://www.merck.com/product/usa/pi_circulars/a/antivenin/antivenin_pi.pdf. Accessed January 29, 2007.
134. Bond GR. Black widow spider envenomation. In: Ford MD, Delaney KA, Long EJ, et al., eds. *Clinical Toxicology.* Philadelphia: WB Saunders Co.; 2001:885–889.
135. Isbister GK, White J, Currie BJ, et al. Spider bites: addressing mythology and poor evidence. *Am J Trop Med Hyg.* 2005;72:361–364.
136. Hogan CJ, Barbaro KC, Winkel K. Loxoscelism: old obstacles, new directions. *Ann Emerg Med.* 2004;44:608–624.
137. DeSilveira RB, Chaim OM, Mangili OC, et al. Hyaluronidases in Loxosceles intermedia (Brown spider) venom are endo-β-N-acetyl-D-hexosaminidases hydrolases. *Toxicon.* 2007;49(6):758–768.
138. Tambourgi DV, Magnoli FC, van den Berg CW, et al. Sphingomyelinases in the venom of the spider Loxosceles intermedia are responsible for both dermonecrosis and complement-dependent hemolysis. *Biochem Biophys Res Comm.* 1998;251:366–373.
139. Gomez HF, Greenfield DM, Miller MJ, et al. Direct correlation between diffusion of Loxosceles recluse venom and extent of dermal inflammation. *Acad Emerg Med.* 2001;8:309–314.
140. Osterhoudt KC, Zaoutis T, Zorc JJ. Lyme disease masquerading as a brown recluse spider bite. *Ann Emerg Med.* 2002;39:558–561.
141. Vest DK. Envenomation by Tegenaria agrestis (walckenaer) spiders in rabbits. *Toxicon.* 1987;25:221–224.
142. Vetter RS, Isbister GK. Do hobo spider bites cause dermonecrotic injuries? *Ann Emerg Med.* 2004;44:605–607.
143. Gomez HF, Krywko DM, Stoecker WV. A new assay for the detection of Loxosceles species (brown recluse) spider venom. *Ann Emerg Med.* 2002;39:469–474.
144. Bey TA, Walter FG, Lobre W, et al. Loxosceles arizonica bite associated with shock. *Ann Emerg Med.* 1997;30:701–703.
145. Blackall DP. Intravascular hemolysis with brown recluse spider envenomation. *Transfusion.* 2004;44:1543.
146. Hobbs GD, Anderson AR, Grene TJ, et al. Comparison of hyperbaric oxygen and dapsone therapy for loxosceles envenomation. *Acad Emerg Med.* 1996;3:758–761.

147. Phillips S, Kohn M, Baker D, et al. Therapy of brown spider envenomation: a controlled trial of hyperbaric oxygen, dapsone and cyprohepatadine. *Ann Emerg Med.* 1995;25:363–368.
148. Elston DM, Miller SD, Young RJ, et al. Comparison of colchicine, dapsone, triamcinolone, and diphenhydramine therapy for the treatment of brown recluse spider envenomation. *Arch Dermatol.* 2005;141:595–597.
149. Rees RS, Altenbern DP, Lynch JB, et al. Brown recluse spider bites: a comparison of early surgical excision versus dapsone and delayed surgical excision. *Ann Surg.* 1985;202:659–663.
150. Rees RS, Campbell D, Rieger E, et al. The diagnosis and treatment of brown recluse spider bites. *Ann Emerg Med.* 1987;16:945–949.
151. Lowry BP, Bradfield JF, Carroll RG, et al. A controlled trial of topical nitroglycerin in a New Zealand white rabbit model of brown recluse spider envenomation. *Ann Emerg Med.* 2001;37:161–165.
152. Wasserman GS. Wound care of spider and snake envenomation. *Ann Emerg Med.* 1988;17:1331–1335.
153. Barbaro KC, Eickstedt VR, Mota I. Antigenic cross-reactivity of venoms from medically important Loxosceles (Araneae) species in Brazil. *Toxicon.* 1994;32:113–120.
154. Isbister GK, Gray MR, Balit CR, et al. Funnel web spider bite: a systematic review of recorded clinical cases. *Med J Aust.* 2005;182:407–411.
155. Bucaretchi F, Deus Reinaldo CR, Hyslop S, et al. A clinico-epidemiological study of bites by spiders of the genus Phoneutria. *Rev Inst Med Trop Sao Paulo.* 2000;42:17–21.
156. Berg RA, Tarantino MD. Envenomation by the scorpion Centruroides exilicauda (C sculpturatus): severe and unusual manifestations. *Pediatrics.* 1991;87:930–933.
157. LoVecchio F, McBride C. Scorpion envenomations in young children in Central Arizona. *J Toxicol Clin Toxicol.* 2003;41:937–940.
158. Suchard JR, Hilder R. Atropine use in Centruroides scorpion envenomation. *J Toxicol Clin Toxicol.* 2001;39:595–598.
159. Gibley R, Williams M, Walter FG, et al. Continuous intravenous midazolam infusion for Centruroides exilicauda scorpion envenomation. *Ann Emerg Med.* 1999;34:620–625.
160. Riley BD, LoVecchio F, Pizon AF. Lack of scorpion antivenom leads to increased pediatric ICU admissions. *Ann Emerg Med.* 2006;47:398–399.
161. Auerbach PS. Hazardous marine animals. *Emerg Med Clin North Am.* 1984;2(3):531–544.
162. McGoldrick J, Marx JA. Marine envenomations; part 1: vertebrates. *Emerg Med Rev.* 1991;9:497–502.
163. Auerbach PS. Marine envenomations. *N Engl J Med.* 1991;325:486–493.
164. Barass P. Wound necrosis caused by the venom of stingrays: pathological findings and surgical management. *Med J Aust.* 1984;141:854–855.
165. Klontz KC, Lieb S, Schreiber M, et al. Syndromes of vibrio vulnificus infections. Clinical and epidemiologic features in Florida cases 1981–1987. *Ann Intern Med.* 1988;109:318–323.
166. Kizer KW, McKinney HE, Auerbach PS. Scorpaenidae envenomation. A five year poison center experience. *JAMA.* 1985;253:807–810.
167. Brown CK, Shepard SM. Marine trauma, envenomations and intoxications. *Emerg Med Clin North Am.* 1992;10(2):385–408.
168. Trestrial JH III, Al Mahasneh QM. Lionfish sting experiences of an inland poison center: a retrospective study of 23 cases. *Vet Hum Toxicol.* 1989;31:173–175.
169. Aldred B, Erickson T, Lipscomb J. Lionfish envenomations in an urban wilderness. *Wilderness Environ Med.* 1996;7:291–296.
170. Garyfallou GT, Madden JF. Lionfish envenomation. *Ann Emerg Med.* 1996;28(4):456–457.
171. deHaro L, Pommier P. Envenomation: a real risk of keeping exotic house pets. *Vet Hum Toxicol.* 2003;45(4):214–216.
172. Hanley M, Tomaszewski C, Kerns W. The epidemiology of aquatic envenomations in the US: most common symptoms and animals [Abstract]. *J Toxicol Clin Toxicol.* 2000;38(5):512.
173. Lehmann DF, Hardy JC. Stonefish envenomation. *N Engl J Med.* 1993; 329(7):510–511.
174. Church JE, Hodgson WC. The pharmacological activity of fish venoms. *Toxicon.* 2002;40:1083–1093.
175. Church JE, Hodgson WC. Dose-dependent cardiovascular and neuromuscular effects of stonefish (Synanceja trachynis) venom. *Toxicon.* 2000;38:391–407.
176. Currie BJ. Marine antivenoms. *J Toxicol Clin Toxicol.* 2003;41(3):301–308.
177. Auerbach PS. Trauma and envenomaitons from marine fauna. *Emerg Med.* 1992;119:666–669.
178. Preuss JM. Marine envenomations and toxidromes. *Topics Emerg Med.* 2000;22(2):44–73.
179. McGoldrick J, Marx JA. Marine envenomations part 2: Invertebrates. *Emerg Med Rev.* 1992;10:71–77.
180. Burnett JW, Calton GJ. The chemistry and toxicology of some venomous pelagic coelenterates. *Toxicon.* 1977;15(3):177–196.
181. Burnett JW, Calton GJ. Jellyfish envenomation syndromes updated. *Ann Emerg Med.* 1987;16(9):1000–1005.
182. Fisher AA. Water-related dermatoses. II. Nematocyst dermatitis. *Cutis.* 1980;25:242.
183. Fisher AA. Toxic and allergic cutaneous reactions to jellyfish with special reference to delayed reactions. *Cutis.* 1987;40:303.
184. Russo AJ, Calton GJ, Burnett JW. The relationship of the possible allergic response to jellyfish envenomation and serum antibody titers. *Toxicon.* 1983;21:475–480.
185. Grady JD, Burnett JW. Irukandji-like syndrome in South Florida divers. *Ann Emerg Med.* 2003;42:763–766.
186. Stein MR, Marraccini JV, Rothschild NE, et al. Fatal Portuguese man-of-war (*Phsyalia phsyalia*) envenomation. *Ann Emerg Med.* 1989;18:312–315.
187. Fenner PJ, Williamson JA. Worldwide deaths and severe envenomation from jellyfish stings. *Med J Aust.* 1996;2(16):658–661.
188. Williamson JA, Le Ray LE, Wohlfahrt M, et al. Acute management of serious envenomation by box-jellyfish (Chironex fleckeri). *Med J Aust.* 1984;141:851.
189. Lopez EA, Weisman RS, Bernstein J. A prospective study of the acute therapy of jellyfish envenomations [Abstract]. *J Toxicol Clin Toxicol.* 2000;38(5):513.
190. Burnett JW, Rubinstein H, Calton GJ. First aid for jellyfish envenomation. *South Med J.* 1983;76:870.
191. Freudenthal AR, Joseph PR. Seabather's eruption. *N Engl J Med.* 1993;329:542–544.
192. Tomchik RS, Russell MT, Szmant AM, et al. Clinical perspectives on seabather's eruption, also known as "sea lice." *JAMA.* 1993;269:1669–1672.
193. Wong DE, Meinking TL, Rosen LB, et al. Seabather's eruption. *J Am Acad Dermatol.* 1994;30:399–406.
194. Auerbach PS. Marine envenomations. *Wilderness Med.* 1998;52:1327–1374.
195. Terlau H, Olivera BM. Conus venoms: a rich source of novel ion channel-targeted peptides. *Physiol Rev.* 2004;84:41–68.
196. Kizer KW. Marine envenomations. *J Toxicol Clin Toxicol.* 1983;21:527–555.
197. Otten EJ. Venomous animal injuries. *Emerg Med.* 1992;43:875–893.
198. Halstead BW. *Coelenterata: Poisonous and Venomous Marine Animals of the World.* Princeton, NJ: Darwin Press; 1978.

CHAPTER 69 ■ PERIOPERATIVE PULMONARY FUNCTION TESTING AND CONSULTATION

PHILIP BOYSEN

Measurement of pulmonary function is an important adjunct to the symptoms exhibited by a patient, as well as the findings on physical examination. The quantification of pulmonary function has specific applications to clinical medicine in the intensive care unit setting, such as the following:

- Confirming a clinical diagnosis of obstructive versus restrictive ventilatory defects in a patient with respiratory insufficiency or failure
- Following the course of the patient's disease and the response to treatment
- Enhancing decision making for patients about to undergo thoracoabdominal surgery
- Developing an anesthetic and postoperative plan for a patient with pulmonary disease

This chapter will outline the pulmonary function tests that are now considered routine and will address the interpretation of the tests. The timing and nature of the effects of thoracic and abdominal surgery and the clinical implications of the anesthetic and surgical procedures will also be considered.

The evaluation of a patient who is being considered for resectional lung surgery is an important issue for the anesthesiologist, surgeon, and intensivist. Finally, there are some aspects of pulmonary function measurement that are particularly applicable to practitioners of intensive care medicine.

ROUTINE PULMONARY FUNCTION TESTING

Although it might be argued that no form of testing can be considered routine, when clinicians refer to "routine pulmonary function testing" there are three types of measurement and assessment of lung function that define the pulmonary status of a patient: (i) spirometry, (ii) measurement of lung volumes, and (iii) measurement of lung diffusing capacity.

Spirometry

Spirometry remains the most basic technique to assess lung function, and the most valuable. The concept is simple, but the assessment of the results can be complex. In essence, the patient is asked to inhale to total lung capacity (TLC) and then to forcefully exhale into a device that measures volume versus time. The ability to perform a forceful exhalation is key to obtaining an adequate study. Maximal forced exhalation from TLC to residual volume (RV) results in a spirogram with a smooth and reproducible curve that defines a maximal forced expiratory volume envelope. To ensure that patient effort and cooperation is maximal and approaches the envelope that the patient cannot penetrate, the procedure is repeated three times, and the spirometric curves are superimposed and compared.

Performance of a forced vital capacity maneuver is not problematic for a normal person, but a patient with pulmonary impairment is greatly distressed by this procedure. It may take some time for the technician to achieve the performance needed. Once this occurs, the patient is asked to use a metered dose inhaler ($beta_2$ agonist) and then repeat the forced vital capacity maneuver three more times, as the technician again assesses the results for maximal performance and its response to bronchodilators (Fig. 69.1).

The evaluation of a spirogram is straightforward, compares the results to data provided by examining a normal population of men and women, and seeks to answer two additional questions. From a physiologic standpoint, the spirogram defines patients with an obstructive or a restrictive physiologic defect or impairment. Restrictive defects are associated with a decrease in the forced vital capacity (FVC) of at least 20% of the predicted value. Obstructive ventilatory defects are revealed when the ratio of the forced expiratory volume in 1 second (FEV_1) divided by the FVC (the FEV_1/FVC ratio) is less than 85%. Other indications of obstructive lung disease available from the spirogram include the peak expiratory flow rate (PEFR), a useful method of following airflow obstruction due to asthma, and the maximal midexpiratory flow rate. With the latter measurement taken at the midpoint of the FVC, the slope of the line between 25% and 75% of the FVC (FEF 25%–75%) is a better indication of obstructive lung disease due to chronic bronchitis (Fig. 69.2).

Another method of representing a maximal forced expiratory maneuver depicts the FVC versus flow rather than versus time (Fig. 69.3).

The forced exhaled volume between TLC and RV is the maximal expiratory flow curve. If the patient is asked to fully inhale back to TLC once the expiratory maneuver is completed, the flow–volume relationship is referred to as a flow–volume loop. This study is especially useful for diagnosing intrathoracic and extrathoracic upper airway obstruction.

Whereas the FVC measures exhaled volume versus time, and therefore gives an index of airflow, the maximum voluntary ventilation (MVV) is a test that involves repeated breaths and vigorous breathing for 10 to 12 seconds. The MVV is reported in L/minute, which means that the 10- or 12-second effort is multiplied by 6 or 5 respectively. Although it is only a rough

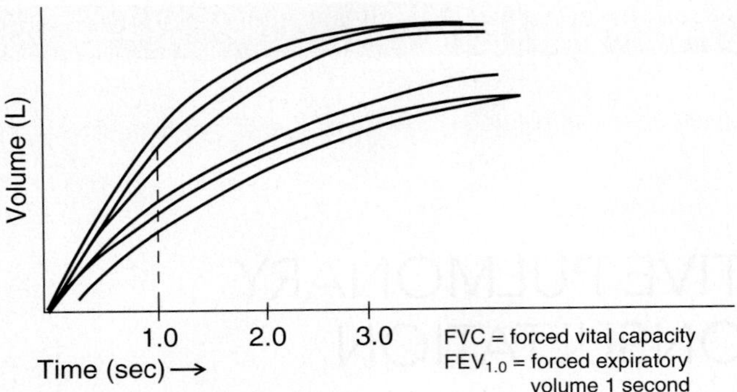

FIGURE 69.1. Three forced exhalations are performed before and after bronchodilator inhalation to assess immediate response. The maximum measured exhaled volume is FVC. The exhaled volume at 1 second is $FEV_{1.0}$. The $FEV_{1.0}$/FVC ratio is reduced with an obstructive ventilatory deficit.

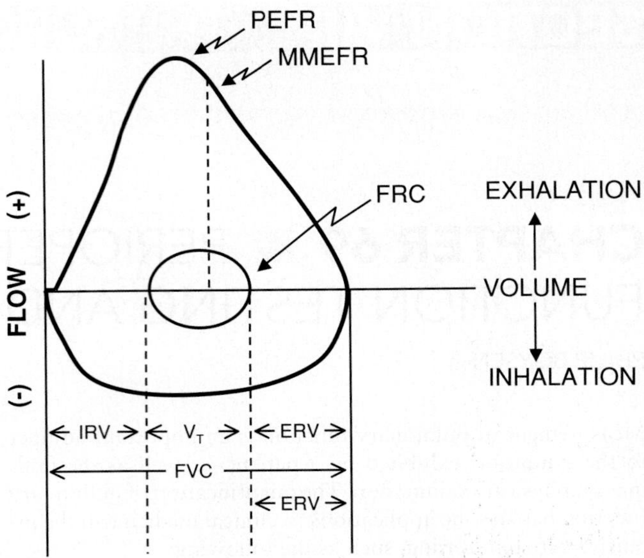

FIGURE 69.3. The relationship between a recording of flow and volume during a forced vital capacity (FVC) maneuver. ERV, expiratory reserve; FRC, functional residual capacity; IRV, inspiratory reserve; MMEFR, maximal midexpiratory flow rate; PEFR, peak expiratory flow rate; V_T, tidal volume.

index, the MMV assesses both airway status and respiratory muscle endurance.

Lung Volumes

Whereas spirometry is a simple test and widely available, measurement of lung volumes requires more complex instrumentation. Lung volume determinations add another dimension to spirometry as a means of defining pathophysiologic changes in lung function.

Several methods are available to measure lung volumes, two of which depend on analysis of a specific gas—one physiologic and one inert. The first method, requiring a nitrogen analyzer, is easily performed over a 7- to 10-minute period of spontaneous breathing of 100% oxygen. With each breath, a certain percentage of nitrogen in the lungs is replaced by oxygen until a certain point where very little nitrogen remains in the lungs, although the nitrogen level never reaches absolute zero. The log of the exhaled nitrogen concentration over time is displayed until no further decrement is noted. Since 79% of the resident lung volume is elemental nitrogen (N_2), measuring the total amount of nitrogen exhaled allows calculation of the volume from which it came. In the lung with significant ventilation perfusion mismatch, the log N_2 versus time is not a straight slope, and it takes longer to reach the equilibration end point.

In the operating room, this phenomenon can be demonstrated in the patient with asthma or chronic bronchitis if the gas analyzer is able to measure nitrogen in addition to the other physiologic or anesthetic gasses.

Rather than "wash out" a physiologic gas, the "wash in" of an inert gas can also be used to determine lung volumes, and helium is used for this purpose. Fitted with a nose clip and a one-way valve in the breathing circuit, the patient is asked to breathe quietly with normal tidal volumes and is then connected to the circuit with a reservoir containing a known volume and concentration (10%) of helium. Measuring helium

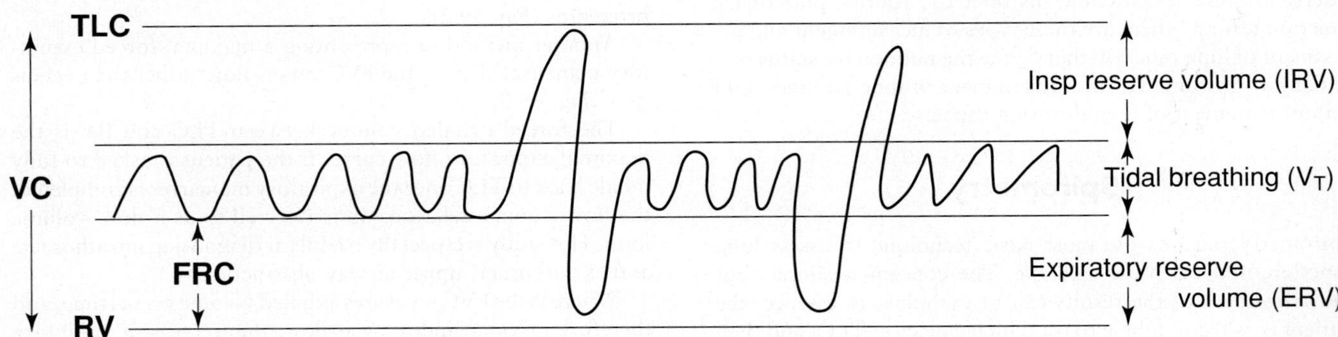

FIGURE 69.2. Compartmentalization of lung volume is achieved by noting the volume excursion during tidal breathing and repeated inhalation and exhalation. The functional residual capacity is measured using gas wash-in or wash-out techniques. TLC, total lung capacity; VC, vital capacity; FRC, functional residual capacity; RV, residual volume.

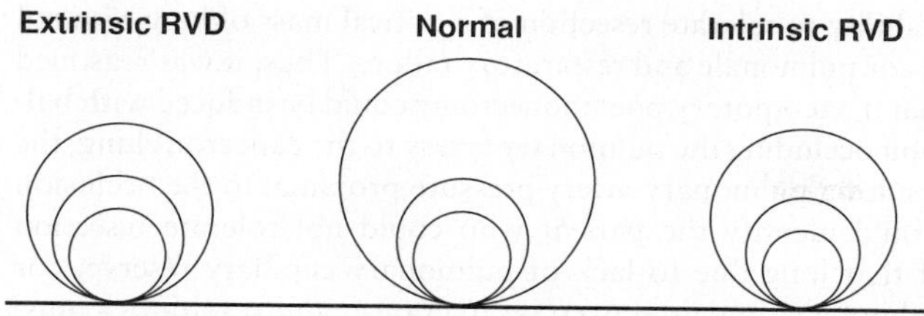

FIGURE 69.4. Changes in lung volumes with extrinsic and intrinsic restriction ventilatory defects (RVD) are compared to normal. An extrinsic RVD mainly alters the total lung capacity (TLC) with minimal alteration of the functional residual capacity (FRC) and the residual volume (RV). An intrinsic RVD results in concentric reduction of the TLC, FRC, and RV.

breath by breath, the technician records the point at which the decline in helium concentration reaches a steady state. Using the formula $V_1C_1 = V_2C_2$, the total volume of the helium black box and the patient's lungs is calculated, and the black box volume is subtracted, yielding the lung volume of the patient. The volume that is measured with either of these techniques depends on the point at which the patient is linked continuously into the breathing circuit. The intent is to begin the measurement at the end of a tidal breath, at functional residual capacity (FRC). Using either a solenoid that detects flow reversal at the end of the tidal breath, or simply using direct observation of tidal breathing, this is usually easily accomplished.

The lung volume study is completed by once again using the spirometer and coaching the patient to a full respiratory maneuver. Then, after quiet tidal breathing, the patient is asked to exhale to residual volume (RV), then inspire fully to total lung capacity (TLC), and after a second interval of quiet tidal breathing, fully inspire to TLC and expire to RV. Knowing the FRC from the dilution studies, all of the lung volume compartments can be calculated (Fig. 69.2).

Residual volume, functional residual capacity, and total lung capacity can be viewed as a system of concentric circles (Fig. 69.4).

An obstructive ventilatory defect is characterized by hyperinflation, with a greater effect on RV and FRC than on TLC. A restrictive ventilatory defect can be either intrinsic or extrinsic. An intrinsic restrictive ventilatory defect is characterized by a concentric reduction (each volume decreases by the same percentage). An extrinsic restrictive ventilatory defect shows a disproportionate loss of volume "off the top"; the major change is in TLC. The postoperative patient who has had a surgical procedure in the thorax or upper abdomen shows the latter change in physiology. Though transient, the extrinsic restrictive ventilatory change, especially when superimposed on a patient with obstructive physiology, can be significant.

Diffusing Capacity

The third pulmonary function study of importance is aimed at assessing gas transfer at the alveolocapillary membrane. Oxygen is the gas transfer of interest, but making this measurement is difficult because there is always a back pressure or gas tension in the blood that must be compared to alveolar gas. This problem can be overcome by introducing a gas that is not normally in the bloodstream, specifically small amounts of carbon monoxide (CO). Since CO is not a physiologic gas, this measurement is referred to as the *diffusing* capacity, not *diffusion* capacity.

The measurement can be made in two ways, and there is controversy over which test gives superior information. The two methods include introducing CO into a breathing circuit and measuring the change in tidal breathing to a steady state, and similarly inhaling CO with a single breath. With the second technique, a further piece of information is obtained by relating the gas transfer to the size of the breath, reported as the KCO. This is an indication of diffusing capacity "where the gas goes," and is considered another method of evaluating both restrictive and obstructive changes in physiology.

If the tissue of an adult lung were microdissected and spread out, it would cover the space of a football field. Thus, one of the reasons for a decrease in diffusing capacity (as opposed to a thickened alveolar-capillary membrane) is loss of effective surface area for gas transfer. This is a pathognomonic change seen in patients with emphysema.

When spirometry, lung volumes, and diffusing capacity are all evaluated, there is a characteristic pattern of physiologic changes that identifies patient status and diagnosis, which is important in the care of the perioperative patient (Table 69.1).

TABLE 69.1

PATTERNS OF PULMONARY PATHOLOGY MEASURED BY PULMONARY FUNCTION TESTS

		OVD_E	OVD_{CBR}	OVD_A	RVD_I	RVD_E
Spirometer	FVC	NL or ↓	NL or ↓	NL or ↓	↓	↓
	$FEV_{1.0}/FVC$	↓	↓	↓	NL or ↑	NL
	BD responder	0	10%	25%	0	0
	TLC	↑	NL or ↑	NL or ↑	↓	↓
	RV/TLC	↑	↑	NL or ↑	N	↑
	DLCO	↓	NL	NL or ↑	↓	NL
	PaO_2	NL or ↓	↓	NL or ↓	↓	NL or ↓
	$PaCO_2$	NL	↑	NL or ↑	NL	NL

OVD_E, emphysema; OVD_{CBR}, chronic bronchitis; OVD_A, asthma; RVD_I, intrinsic restrictive vent defect; RVD_E, extrinsic restrictive vent defect.

Arterial Blood Gas Analysis

Arterial blood gas analysis (ABG) is usually included in the panoply of routine pulmonary function testing. In preparing a patient for surgery, ABG analysis is often ordered, but the usefulness is limited to an analysis of trends and diagnosis of underlying chronic disease. Prognostic value is limited, and for resectional lung surgery, postoperative ABGs are often improved. However, there is value in identifying the patients with obstructive lung disease who have emphysema, as opposed to chronic bronchitis, in assessing and designing postoperative therapy. Table 69.1 summarizes the findings for the various physiologic states.

PREOPERATIVE PULMONARY FUNCTION TESTING

Resectional Lung Surgery

The main indication for lung resection remains the removal of a lung cancer (1). Since both the presence of obstructive lung disease and the incidence of cancer are related to smoking, it is not surprising that patients being evaluated for surgical resection of a lung tumor also suffer from chronic bronchitis or emphysema. Imaging studies have advanced such that the extent of the disease is well documented before surgery; imaging to guide biopsies also identifies the cell type during early evaluation. However, until the surgeon explores the open chest, the extent of the necessary resection for cure is not known. Thus the evaluation should always determine whether the patient can tolerate a pneumonectomy and subsequently live with one lung. Thus, the first step is to measure overall pulmonary function as shown in Table 69.2 (2).

If the patient meets *all* of these criteria, one can assume that the loss of the cancerous lung will result in pulmonary function that is at least half of the $FEV_{1.0}$, i.e., the postoperative $FEV_{1.0}$ will exceed 1.0 (3,4).

If the criteria are not met, and surgical resection, including pneumonectomy, is still being considered, the next step is to perform split lung function testing, and ascertain the contribution of the right versus the left lung to overall pulmonary function. The first method used to perform such an analysis was invasive but based on sound physiologic concepts. It had been observed, in both humans and animal models, that the inability to tolerate resection of a critical mass of lung resulted in cor pulmonale and respiratory failure. Thus, it was reasoned that if a temporary pneumonectomy could be induced with balloon occluding the pulmonary artery to the cancerous lung, the resulting pulmonary artery pressure proximal to the occlusion would identify the patient who could not tolerate resection of that lung due to lack of pulmonary capillary reserve, cor pulmonale, impaired exercise tolerance, and respiratory muscle fatigue (5–7). Other studies not only predicted survival but also morbidity and mortality and identified obstructive lesions of the trachea and larynx (8,9).

A second technique, bronchospirometry, is also invasive but yielded the desired information. An awake patient underwent tracheal intubation with a double-lumen tube, and each port was connected to a separate spirometer. When the patient performed a forced vital capacity maneuver, the right contribution to the FVC could be distinguished from the left.

In the 1970s, investigators noted that most of these patients had abnormal ventilation perfusion lung scans, but for each lung as a whole, the radionuclide scans were fairly well matched. Reasoning that a perfusion scan, or even a ventilation scan, could be used to determine split lung function, they studied a series of patients preoperatively who then went on to surgical resection and had pulmonary function measured after recovery from surgery months later (10). Since that time, clinicians have found this to be a useful method of preparing the patient for surgery and predicting remaining lung function following pneumonectomy. For example, if the preoperative $FEV_{1.0} = 1.6$ L, and the scan reveals 60%/40% left lung versus right lung, and the right lung is being considered for resection, then:

$$1.6\,\text{L} \times .60 = .96\,\text{L}, \text{ the calculated postoperative } FEV_{1.0}$$

The same investigators made two other early observations. First, the diseased lung often made little or no contribution to overall lung function, and if the calculation was incorrect, it was usually because postoperative lung function was *better* than predicted. Second, they suggested that the requirement for the predicted postoperative $FEV_{1.0}$ be lowered from 1.0 L to 800 mL, the level below which they noted that respiratory failure and cor pulmonale usually occurred in the chronic obstructive pulmonary disease (COPD) patient.

TABLE 69.2

PULMONARY FUNCTION INDICATING PHYSIOLOGICAL TOLERANCE FOR SURGERY UP TO AND INCLUDING PNEUMONECTOMY

Pulmonary function	Physiologic tolerance
FVC	>50% Predicted, or >3.0 L
$FEV_{1.0}$	>2.0 L
$FEV_{1.0}$/FVC	>50%
RV/TLC	<59%
DLCO	>50% Predicted
MVV	>50% Predicted

Noncardiothoracic Surgery

Whereas quantitative assessment of pulmonary function is useful for thoracic surgery patients, there is little evidence to suggest that measurement of pulmonary function should be obtained solely for the purpose of perioperative management of an individual patient. Although certain types of surgery, such as upper abdominal surgery, nonresectional thoracic surgery, and cardiac surgery, often cause severe alterations in pulmonary function (the FVC may be reduced as much as 50% the first postoperative day), little is added to the history and physical examination in terms of considering risk.

PREDICTING POSTOPERATIVE PULMONARY COMPLICATIONS

Postoperative pulmonary complications (PPCs) are usually defined as newly developed atelectasis, pneumonia, pulmonary thromboembolism, and acute respiratory failure requiring mechanical ventilation following surgery. Because of the difficulty of making predictions based solely on the measurement of pulmonary function, other strategies for assessment are continually being developed and analyzed. Early studies sought to first identify normal pulmonary function criteria for large populations and then demonstrate changes due to other changes in lung function, such as aging and cigarette smoking (11,12). The next step included identifying risk factors and determining if a preoperative therapeutic regimen would alter outcome, or if alterations in anesthetic technique improved or lessened postoperative pulmonary complications (13,14).

Most studies have been limited by the number of patients entered into the study protocol, but the accumulated evidence would indicate that preoperative testing would identify patients at risk for postoperative pulmonary complications (15–18). The efficacy of strategies to reduce postoperative pulmonary complications is not so well defined (19–24). Recently, the National Veterans Surgical Quality Improvement Program, in developing a multifactorial risk index for predicting postoperative pneumonia and respiratory failure after major noncardiac surgery, has reported large numbers of patients. The consistent risk factors in this population include the following (25):

- *Smoking status:* The duration of smoking cessation to achieve benefit appears to be at least 4 weeks, possibly as long as 8 weeks.
- *Chronic obstructive lung disease,* as defined by history and physical examination (spirometry has not been shown to be useful in prognosis)
- *Measures of general health status:* includes the presence/measures of comorbid conditions, functional status, recent weight loss.
- *Cognitive impairment,* for whatever reason
- *Previous stroke*
- *Type and location of the anticipated surgical procedure*
- *Age:* a risk factor when controlled for comorbid conditions
- *Long-term steroid therapy*
- *Recent moderate-to-heavy alcohol intake*
- *Impaired renal function*
- *Large transfusion:* generally >6 units of packed red blood cells, plus other blood products

In this study, the authors were not able to analyze the importance of serum albumin, spirometry, use of prophylactic antibiotics, and body mass index or obesity. Other studies have suggested that a low serum albumin carries a higher risk for PPC, and the outcome is not changed by administering intravenous hyperalimentation, but risk is possibly lessened by feeding through the gut. As mentioned, spirometry is diagnostically accurate, but is not useful for prognosis; and obesity in the absence of comorbid conditions is not a significant risk factor for PPCs.

The use of general anesthesia for surgical procedures, and the duration of the anesthetic and surgical procedures (greater than 4 hours) were reported to increase the risk of PPCs. A common consultant comment has been, "OK for spinal, avoid general anesthesia," implying that the volatile anesthetic agent had some negative impact on postoperative pulmonary function. Advances in anesthesia technology and skills have allowed investigators to reframe the question. Does the presence of adequate neuroaxial blockade during a surgical procedure reduce risk? The anesthetic plan can include spinal anesthesia, epidural anesthesia, combined spinal/epidural anesthesia, and these can also be combined with light levels of general anesthesia (the "epigeneral"). Further, neuroaxial blockade can be continued into the postoperative period for pain management. Postoperative pain management is an important goal that also enables a patient to complete deep breathing maneuvers. It does appear that the presence of neuroaxial blockade, either alone or in combination with general anesthesia, is associated with fewer deaths and complications.

STRATEGIES TO REDUCE PPCS AFTER NONCARDIOTHORACIC SURGERY

The general approach to the patient with impaired pulmonary function has included cessation of smoking and an attempt to maximize pulmonary function with the use of bronchodilators, both beta-2-agonists and parasympatholytic agents, treatment of underlying infections or purulent sputum, and coaching to learn deep-breathing exercises. Bronchodilators are continued throughout the anesthetic and surgical procedure.

A recent publication reviewed the available literature on interventions to prevent PPCs after noncardiothoracic surgery. A synthesis of the evidence indicates the following:

- *Studies with good evidence:* The evidence indicates that lung expansion interventions are useful in preventing PPCs. This includes incentive spirometry, deep breathing exercises, and continuous positive airway pressure.
- *Studies with fair evidence:* The evidence indicates that selective rather than routine use of nasogastric tubes after abdominal surgery is beneficial, given that it decompresses the stomach, allowing for better diaphragmatic excursion. The use of short-acting, intraoperative neuromuscular blocking agents (e.g., rocuronium vs. pancuronium) is associated with improved outcomes.
- *Studies with conflicting evidence:* The evidence is conflicting or insufficient for cessation of smoking, epidural anesthesia, epidural analgesia, and laparoscopic versus open abdominal surgery. As noted above, the presence or absence of neuroaxial blockade—not the anesthetic choice—may be the determining factor. Also, laparoscopic procedures result in less pain and a lesser reduction in the FVC. Finally, although malnutrition is associated with increased risk, routine total enteral or parenteral nutrition does not reduce risk.

In summary, for noncardiothoracic surgery, there has been substantial investigation for decades aimed at performing a preoperative assessment to identify risk (26) early with invasive techniques (27). The value of preoperative pulmonary function testing has been repeatedly called into question (28,29) owning to the added time and expense. Preoperative pulmonary function testing is safe and noninvasive, but should not be routinely performed; rather, it should be limited to a specific indication supported by changes in the anesthetic or surgical procedure (30). Furthermore, the incidence of postoperative pulmonary dysfunction is influenced by the surgical site and the propensity to cause diaphragmatic dysfunction (31,32).

ADDITIONAL PULMONARY FUNCTION TESTS PERTINENT TO THE INTENSIVE CARE UNIT

Lung–Thorax Compliance and Airway Resistance

Physiologists described lung–thorax pressure relationships in normal subjects by defining elastic recoil pressure. With a nose clip and mouthpiece in place, the subject inhaled deeply to TLC and, with an open glottis and no airflow, relaxed against a pressure monitor. The process was repeated in decrements of 200 mL to record the pressure–volume curve of the lung and thorax.

The same process can be adapted to the mechanically ventilated patient. In the ventilated patient who is not breathing spontaneously, changes in transpulmonary pressure—and thus lung volume—are achieved by positive pressure applied at the airway by the ventilator. Although some clinicians have suggested the construction of the pressure–volume relationship throughout the tidal breath, the common approach is to deliver a tidal breath—under positive pressure in the range of 8 mL/kg body weight—and measure the resulting airway pressure at two points: the peak inspiratory pressure (flow) and the relaxation pressure with the tidal breath held in the lungs with no airflow. Measurement of these two pressures, the second measurement accomplished with a short inspiratory hold, allows the calculation of lung–thorax compliance and airway resistance (33).

Clt = V/P in mL/cm H_2O, where V = tidal volume and P = relaxation pressure

Raw = PIP/inspiratory flow, where inspiratory flow is constant during lung inflation

Since Raw is measured in cm H_2O/mL/second, the product of lung–thorax compliance and airway resistance is the time constant for the lungs to achieve improved distribution of inspired gas.

$$\text{Clt (mL/cm H}_2\text{O)} = \text{Raw (cm H}_2\text{O/mL/second)}$$
$$= \text{seconds (or time constant for the lung)}$$

Testing Respiratory Muscle Strength

The ability to separate a patient from mechanical ventilation depends on respiratory muscle function—both strength and endurance. Respiratory muscle strength is assessed in clinical settings by measuring a pressure resulting from the generation of a forcing pressure due to activation of the respiratory muscle. Pressure measurements can be obtained at many different sites (e.g., the distal or proximal end of the endotracheal tube) or esophageal pressure measurements, as a reflection of changes in pleural pressure, can be obtained using various devices. Pressure measurements can also be made across structures. Thus, transdiaphragmatic pressures can be obtained by simultaneously measuring esophageal and gastric pressures. As yet, baseline measurements indicating the ability to separate a patient from mechanical ventilation have yet to be defined (34).

Tests of Respiratory Muscle Endurance

From the standpoint of a working muscle, endurance is defined as the ability of a muscle to develop tension and sustain it over time; the time–tension index is, therefore, the physiologic manifestation of muscle endurance. For the respiratory muscles, pressure is a manifestation of the ability to generate tension, and the pressure–time product, therefore, correlates with respiratory muscle endurance in the normal subject breathing against a resistive load. Measurement of tidal volume, mean inspiratory mouth pressure, and the duty cycle determine the pressure–time product. Similarly, in the intubated patient, pressures can be measured at the proximal end of the endotracheal tube as an index of the energy necessary to move the lung to a higher volume during positive pressure ventilation (35).

Breathing Patterns

Normal tidal breathing begins at FRC, a point where the tendency for the chest wall to spring outward is balanced by the tendency of the lung to collapse. The balance of these two forces occurs when there is complete apposition of the pleural surfaces. A tidal breath is an energy-transferring mechanism, the reason why exhalation is usually a passive phenomenon returning the lung volume to the normal FRC. Tidal excursions occur within the TL-to-RV envelope, and both an inspiratory reserve volume and an expiratory reserve volume are maintained. Patients in respiratory distress alter their tidal breathing patterns according to the added load placed on the respiratory system. Patients with a resistive load will slow inspiratory or expiratory flows and diminish the respiratory rate, in an effort to attain searching for the best combination of rate and tidal volume/flow to work against the imposed load. Patients with alterations in compliance, in a similar manner, reach the best combination of rate and tidal volume, which results in a rapid respiratory rate and smaller tidal volumes.

In the latter patients, tracheal intubation, mechanical ventilation, and the addition of positive end expiratory pressure (PEEP) are used to support the patient. This is often instituted with the observation of rapid, shallow breathing patterns, owing to the propensity to respiratory failure and collapse, a high oxygen cost of breathing, and, finally, hypoxemia and carbon dioxide retention.

The reoccurrence of rapid, shallow breathing is used to assess the ability to wean a patient from positive pressure ventilation. The so-called *spontaneous breathing trial* involves watching the patient breathe with very low levels of positive pressure support, presumably enough to overcome the endotracheal tube resistance prior to extubation. Thus, rapid shallow breathing patterns, which can be measured by the rapid shallow breathing index (RSBI), are used to assess the feasibility of weaning from ventilatory support (36,37).

SUMMARY

Pulmonary evaluation is a critical step in managing patients with lung disease who are undergoing elective surgeries or are admitted to the ICU for respiratory insufficiency or failure. A few examples of this evaluation are indicated below:

- Confirming a clinical diagnosis of obstructive versus restrictive ventilatory defects in a patient with respiratory insufficiency or failure
- Following the course of patient disease and the response to treatment
- Enhancing decision making for patients about to undergo thoracoabdominal surgery
- Developing an anesthetic and postoperative plan for a patient with pulmonary disease

Although there are few effective strategies for preventing complications in the postoperative period, it is still not clear if risk stratification can be assessed with the use of sophisticated or simple exercise tests and measurements. Efforts should be directed to an accurate prediction caused by respiratory impairment in high-risk patients to anticipate and correct their physiologic response to surgery and improve outcome.

References

1. Boysen PG, Block AJ, Olsen GN, et al. Prospective evaluation for pneumonectomy using the Tc99 quantitative perfusion lung scan. *Chest.* 1977; 72:422.
2. Boysen PG, Clark CA, Block AJ. Graded exercise testing and post-thoracotomy complications. *J Cardiovasc Anesth.* 1980;4:68.
3. Olsen GN, Block AJ, Tobias JA. Prediction of postpneumonectomy pulmonary function using quantitative macro aggregate lung scanning. *Chest.* 1974;66:13.
4. Olsen GN, Block AJ, Swenson EQ, et al. Pulmonary function evaluation of the lung resection candidate: a prospective study. *Am Rev Resp Dis.* 1975; 111:379.
5. Roussas C. Function and fatigue of respiratory muscles. *Chest.* 1985;88:124.
6. Smith TP, Kinasewitz GT, Tucker WY, et al. Exercise capacity as a predictor of post-thoracotomy morbidity. *Am Rev Resp Dis.* 1984;129:730.
7. Uggla LG. Indication for and results of thoracic surgery with regard to respiratory and circulatory function tests. *Acta Chir Scand.* 1956;111:197.
8. Miller RD, Hyatt RE. Evaluation of obstructive lesions of the trachea and larynx by flo-volume loops. *Am Rev Resp Dis.* 1973;108:476.
9. Markos J, Mullin BP, Mittman DR, et al. Preoperative assessment as a predictor of morbidity and mortality after lung resection. *Am Rev Resp Dis.* 1989;139:902.
10. Kristerrson S, Lindell S, Stranberg L. Prediction of pulmonary function loss due to pneumonectomy using Xe133 radiospirometry. *Chest.* 1972;62:694.
11. Knudson RJ, Kalterborn WT, Knudson DE, et al. The single breath carbon monoxide diffusing capacity reference equations derived from a healthy non-smoking population and the effects of hematocrit. *Am Rev Resp Dis.* 1987;135:805.
12. Knudson RJ, Lebowitz MD, Hobberg CJ, et al. Changes in the maximal expiratory flow volume curve with growth and aging. *Am Rev Resp Dis.* 1983;127:725.
13. Gracey DR, Divertie MB, Didier EP. Preoperative pulmonary preparation of patients with chronic obstructive pulmonary disease. *Chest.* 1979;76:123.
14. Rodgers A, Walker N, Shug S, et al. Reduction of postoperative morbidity and mortality with spinal or epidural anaesthesia: results from overview of randomized trials. *BMJ.* 2000;321:1493.
15. Warner MA, Offord KT, Warner ME, et al. Role of preoperative cessation of smoking and other factors in postoperative pulmonary complications: a blinded prospective study of coronary artery bypass patients. *Mayo Clin Thor.* 1989;64:609.
16. Nagasawa M, Tanaki H, Tsukurna H, et al. Relationship between the duration of preoperative smoke-free period and the incidence of postoperative pulmonary complications after pulmonary surgery. *Chest.* 2006;120:705.
17. Ramsay SJ. Postoperative pulmonary complications. *Ann Intern Med.* 2002; 137:550.
18. Lawrence VA, Connell JE, Smetana GW. Strategies to reduce postoperative pulmonary complications after noncardiothoracic surgery: systematic review for the American College of Physicians. *Ann Intern Med.* 2006;144:596.
19. Bapoje SR, Whitaker JF, Schulz T, et al. Preoperative evaluation of the patient with pulmonary disease. *Chest.* 2007;132:1637.
20. Cohn SL, Smetana GW. Update in perioperative medicine. *Ann Intern Med.* 2007;147:263.
21. Arozullah AM, Daley J, Henderson WG, et al. Multifactorial risk index for predicting postoperative respiratory failure in men after major noncardiac surgery. *Ann Surg.* 2000;232:243.
22. Arozullah AM, Khuri SF, Henderson WG, et al. Development and validation of a multifactorial risk index for predicting postoperative pneumonia after major noncardiac surgery. *Ann Intern Med.* 2001;135:847.
23. Qaseem A, Snow V, Fitterman N, et al. Risk assessment for strategies to reduce perioperative pulmonary complications for patients undergoing noncardiothoracic surgery: a guideline from the American College of Physicians. *Ann Intern Med.* 2006;144:575.
24. Lawrence VA. Predicting post-operative pulmonary complications: the sleeping giant stirs. *Ann Intern Med.* 2007;135:919.
25. Khuri SF, Daley J, Henderson W, et al. The National Veterans Administration Surgical Risk Study: risk adjustment for the comparative assessment of the quality of surgical care. *J Am Coll Surg.* 1995;180:519.
26. Smetana GW. Preoperative pulmonary evaluation. *N Engl J Med.* 1999;340: 937.
27. Carlena E, Hanson HE, Nordenstrom B. Temporary unilateral balloon occlusion of the pulmonary artery. *J Thorac Surg.* 1961;22:527.
28. Celli BR. What is the value of preoperative pulmonary function testing? *Med Clin North Am.* 1993;77:309.
29. Crapo RO. Pulmonary function testing. *N Engl J Med.* 1994;331:25.
30. Gardner RM. ATS Statement. Snowbird workshop standardization of spirometry. *Am Rev Resp Dis.* 1979;119:831.
31. Ford GT, Whitelaw WA, Rosenal TW, et al. Diaphragm function after upper abdominal surgery in humans. *Am Rev Resp Dis.* 1983;127:431
32. Simmoneau G, Viven A, Sartene R, et al. Diaphragm dysfunction induced by upper abdominal surgery: role of postoperative pain. *Am Rev Resp Dis.* 1983;128:899.
33. Jubran W, Toban M. Passive mechanics of lung and chest wall in patients who failed or succeeded in trials of weaning. *Am J Respir Crit Care Med.* 1997;155:916–921.
34. Hubmayr RD, Rehder K. Respiratory muscle failure in critically ill patients. *Semin Respir Med.* 1992;13:14–21.
35. Tobin MJ, Laghi F, Jubran W. A respiratory muscle dysfunction in mechanically ventilated patients. *Mol Cell Biochem.* 1998;179:87–98.
36. Stroetz RW, Hubmayr RD. Tidal volume maintenance during weaning with pressure support. *Am J Respir Crit Care Med.* 1995;152:1034–1040.
37. Capdevila X, Perrigault PF, Ramonatxo M, et al. Changes in breathing pattern and respiratory muscle performance parameters during difficult weaning. *Crit Care Med.* 1998;26:79–87.

CHAPTER 70 ■ PREOPERATIVE EVALUATION OF THE HIGH-RISK SURGICAL PATIENT

BHIKEN I. NAIK • DEANE MURFIN • LISA THANNIKARY

OVERVIEW

The perioperative mortality rate for elective surgical procedures is low, ranging from 0.001% to 1.9% (1). This incidence increases, however, depending on the type of surgery, whether it is emergent in nature, the severity of concurrent disease, and the patient's age. Browner et al. (2), in a prospective cohort study of 474 men between 38 and 89 years of age at a Veterans Medical Center, reported a mortality rate of 5% during major noncardiac surgery. Multivariate analysis demonstrates that hypertension, limited functional capacity, and renal dysfunction are independently associated with increased perioperative mortality. Other studies have shown that both age and the American Society of Anesthesiologist (ASA) physical status classification systems are good predictors of perioperative complications (Table 70.1). Specifically, age greater than 70 years and ASA physical status greater than or equal to II are strong predictors of postoperative pulmonary complications (3).

The ASA physical status classification remains the most widely used perioperative patient classification. Its simplicity is both its strength and weakness. Its strength is based on its ability to be applied to all age groups, medical conditions, and degrees of health. The weakness of the ASA classification system is its inability to distinguish among disorders of different systems and to cumulate risk based on multiple disorders.

In an attempt to provide a multidimensional model of perioperative risk, Holt and Silverman (4) have devised an integrative model using various risk factors. In its simplest form, it provides a successive listing of the ASA physical status, surgical risk/invasiveness, physical factors affecting mask ventilation, intubation predictors, and a list of optional risk indicators. The acronym ASPIRIN is applied to this model. Although not validated in large studies, the ASPIRIN model provides an integrated framework for the assessment of the perioperative patient.

The approach to the high-risk patient begins with preoperative identification, stratification, and modification of risk factors. This is achieved initially by the preoperative history and physical examination, which may be cursory in the event of a life-threatening emergency or more thorough if an elective procedure is planned. The data obtained from the history and physical examination allow for the application of *Bayesian decision making*—that is, using preoperative testing based on clinical risk categorization. As a result, rational use of preoperative testing, particularly in this era of cost containment, can be achieved. Almanaseer et al. (5) demonstrated a 6.7% and 9.4% absolute reduction in stress thallium/echocardiogram and dobutamine echocardiogram testing, respectively, following the implementation of the American College of Cardiology/American Heart Association (ACC/AHA) guidelines for preoperative cardiac risk assessment. They also demonstrated a 19% increase in the use of beta-blockers following implementation of the ACC/AHA guidelines. Froehlich et al. (6) analyzed the impact of implementing the ACC/AHA guideline on resources utilization for aortic surgery. Initiation of the preoperative guideline reduced mean preoperative evaluation cost from $1,087 to $171, with no change in the incidence of myocardial infarction or death.

Evidence-based preoperative evaluation allows for appropriate and cost-effective resource use, without increasing the risk of perioperative complications (6).

CARDIOVASCULAR SYSTEM

Noncardiac Surgery

Of the approximately 44 million patients undergoing noncardiac surgery in the United States yearly, 30% either have, or are at risk for, coronary artery disease (CAD). The presence of CAD increases the incidence of perioperative myocardial ischemia, with a 2.8-fold increase in adverse postoperative cardiac events (7). Therefore, in an attempt to identify high-risk cardiac patients presenting for noncardiac surgery, both Goldman et al. (8) and Lee et al. (9) devised cardiac risk indices. Based on the points accrued during risk stratification, patients have either no testing performed or are referred for noninvasive testing or angiography. However, the predictive value of the cardiac risk index is poor in patients undergoing major vascular surgery.

Vascular surgery patients represent a unique cohort, as the incidence of CAD in this population group is disproportionately higher than in the general population. Hertzer et al. (10), in a landmark study, evaluated 1,000 patients with coronary angiography prior to vascular surgery. The primary vascular diagnoses were abdominal aortic aneurysm, cerebrovascular disease, and lower extremity ischemia. Severe correctable CAD was demonstrated in 25% of the cohort whereas 6% of the study group demonstrated severe inoperable CAD; only 8% of the patients had no evidence of CAD. Furthermore, over the last decade, the management of the patient presenting with an ST-segment elevation myocardial infarction (STEMI) has evolved. Early aggressive reperfusion therapy and post-MI risk stratification are the current cornerstones of therapy.

In an attempt to provide current evidence-based recommendations to manage the cardiac patient presenting for noncardiac surgery, the ACC/AHA Task Force on Practice Guidelines convened a panel of experts and published guidelines

TABLE 70.1

AMERICAN SOCIETY OF ANESTHESIOLOGIST PHYSICAL STATUS CLASSIFICATION

Physical status	Definition
I	Healthy patient
II	Mild systemic disease; no functional limitation
III	Severe systemic disease; definite functional limitation
IV	Severe systemic disease that is constant threat to life
V	Moribund patient; unlikely to survive 24 hours with or without surgery
VI	Brain-dead patient; organ donor
E	Emergency procedure

on the perioperative cardiovascular evaluation for noncardiac surgery (11). The guideline was subsequently revised in March 2002; the update is available at the following Web site: www.acc.org/qualityandscience/clinical/statements.htm

The important aspects of the guideline are to identify high-risk patients, appropriately stratify them according to their risk category, and perform preoperative testing in a rational and cost-effective manner. The guideline emphasizes that no test should be performed unless it is likely to influence patient treatment.

The ACC/AHA guideline is an eight-step algorithm that incorporates clinical predictors based on the patient's history and physical examination, surgery-specific risk, and the functional capacity or exercise tolerance (Fig. 70.1). In the event of an emergency procedure, patients should be taken to surgery with risk stratification performed after the surgical procedure is completed. No preoperative testing is warranted under these circumstances. If an elective or urgent procedure is planned, the decision making proceeds down steps 2 and 3 of the algorithm. If the patient has had a coronary revascularization procedure, either coronary artery bypass grafting (CABG) or percutaneous coronary intervention (PCI) performed within the last 5 years with no recurrent symptoms or signs, then no further workup is necessary. A cardiac evaluation performed within the last 2 years with no deterioration in cardiac status also negates the need for further workup.

Steps 5 to 8 of the algorithm integrate the clinical predictor, surgery-specific risk, and the functional capacity to determine whether the patient warrants further cardiac workup.

The presence of major clinical predictors demands intense further workup and may result in delay or cancellation of elective surgery. Intermediate clinical predictors increase the risk of perioperative cardiovascular complications, whereas minor clinical predictors have not been proven to independently increase cardiac risk (Table 70.2).

The nature and duration of the surgical procedure is a strong predictor of cardiovascular morbidity and mortality. Aortic, major vascular, and prolonged procedures associated with significant fluid shifts have a greater than 5% cardiac risk. Intermediate-risk procedures, which include intrathoracic, major orthopedic, intraperitoneal, head and neck, and prostate surgery, have a cardiac risk that is less than 5%. Endoscopic procedures, and cataract, breast, and superficial procedures are associated with minimal risk (less than 1%), and further workup is necessary only if the patient has major clinical predictors (Table 70.3).

It is important to factor institutional and surgical expertise when evaluating the surgery-specific risk. Pronovost et al. (12) analyzed outcomes from abdominal aortic surgery in nonfederal acute care hospitals in Maryland. Mortality varied among hospitals from 0% to 66%, based on several factors including hospital and surgeon volume. Postoperatively, the absence of daily rounds by an ICU physician increased the risk of cardiac arrest, acute renal failure, sepsis, and reintubation (12).

Finally, the functional capacity of the patient must be evaluated, as it is a strong predictor of perioperative outcome (13). Functional capacity is expressed in metabolic equivalents (METs), where one MET is 3.5 mL/kg/min of oxygen consumption in a 70 kg, 40-year-old man at rest. Increasing levels of activity correlate with increasing METs, with strenuous sports requiring greater than 10 METs, whereas activities of daily living require between 1 and 3 METs (Table 70.4). According to the ACC/AHA guidelines, the inability to perform at least 4 METs is associated with increased perioperative cardiac risk.

Based on the aforementioned triad of clinical predictors, functional capacity, and surgery-specific risk, a decision is made whether the patient can proceed to surgery or whether additional investigations to delineate the ischemic burden are required (Table 70.5) (14).

Delineation of the ischemic burden can be broadly achieved by two methods. The first method involves coronary vasodilatation and induction of a "steal" phenomenon by pharmacologic agents, followed by a nuclear imaging technique to determine the degree of myocardial ischemia. The second method involves increasing myocardial oxygen demand and evaluating electrocardiographic or echocardiographic data for evidence of ischemia. Myocardial oxygen demand can be increased either by exercise stress testing or pharmacologically with dobutamine or atropine.

In light of their limited functional capacity, vascular patients can rarely complete exercise stress testing. Therefore, dipyridamole-thallium nuclear imaging or dobutamine stress echocardiography remains the mainstay of noninvasive testing for this cohort of patients. The negative-predictive value of both tests is high. However, the positive-predictive value of dobutamine stress echocardiography is higher (14). To increase the predictive value of nuclear imaging, several criteria have been proposed that help to differentiate the low-risk scan from the high-risk scan. These include the size of the defect, increased lung uptake, and the presence of left ventricular cavity dilation (15).

Once the degree of myocardial ischemia is quantified, patients can either undergo perioperative medical optimization or revascularization by either percutaneous coronary intervention or surgery. It is important to note that to obtain benefit from a preoperative coronary intervention, the risk of noncardiac surgery must supersede the combined risk of both coronary catheterization and subsequent revascularization procedure. Eagle et al. (16) evaluated the Coronary Artery Surgery Study (CASS) database for patients requiring noncardiac surgery. CASS registry enrollees had coronary artery disease and were randomized to either optimal medical therapy or CABG. In patients undergoing high-risk surgery, prior CABG was associated with fewer postoperative deaths (1.7% versus 3.3%, $p = 0.03$) and MIs (0.8% versus 2.7%, $p = 0.002$) compared to medical management. In patients undergoing vascular surgery, the

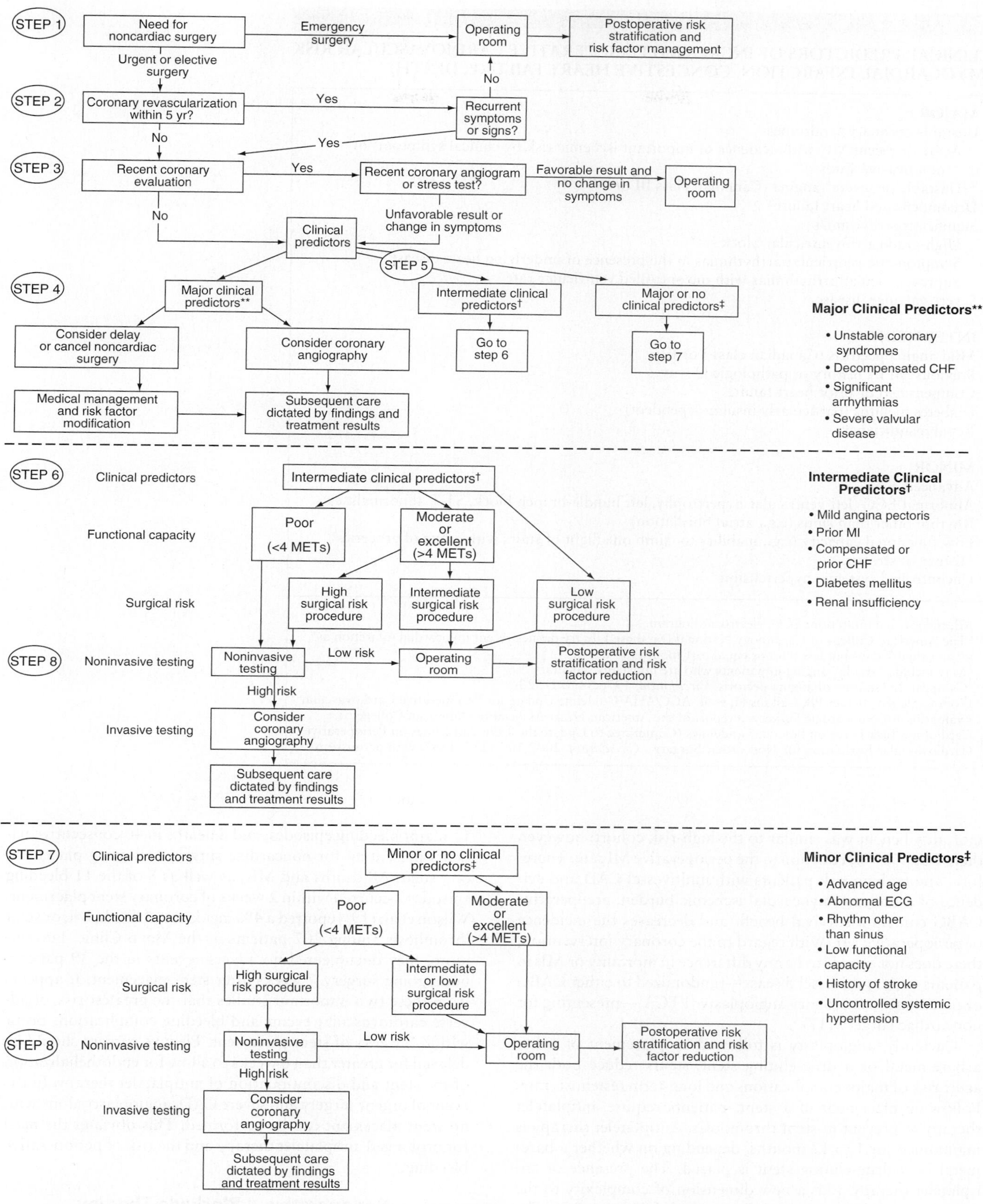

FIGURE 70.1. Stepwise approach to preoperative cardiac assessment. (Reproduced with permission from Eagle KA, Berger PB, Calkins H, et al. ACC/AHA Guideline Update for Perioperative Cardiovascular Evaluation for Noncardiac Surgery: a report of the American Heart Association/American College of Cardiology Task Force on Practice Guidelines (Committee to Update the 1996 Guidelines on Perioperative Cardiovascular Evaluation for Noncardiac Surgery). *Circulation.* 2002;105:1257–1267.

TABLE 70.2

CLINICAL PREDICTORS OF INCREASED PERIOPERATIVE CARDIOVASCULAR RISK (MYOCARDIAL INFARCTION, CONGESTIVE HEART FAILURE, DEATH)

MAJOR
Unstable coronary syndromes
Acute or recent MI[a] with evidence of important ischemic risk by clinical symptoms or noninvasive study
Unstable or severe[b] angina (Canadian class III or IV)[c]
Decompensated heart failure
Significant arrhythmias
High-grade atrioventricular block
Symptomatic ventricular arrhythmias in the presence of underlying heart disease
Supraventricular arrhythmias with uncontrolled ventricular rate
Severe valvular disease
INTERMEDIATE
Mild angina pectoris (Canadian class I or II)
Previous MI by history or pathologic Q waves
Compensated or prior heart failure
Diabetes mellitus (particularly insulin-dependent)
Renal insufficiency
MINOR
Advanced age
Abnormal ECG (left ventricular hypertrophy, left bundle-branch block, ST-T abnormalities)
Rhythm other than sinus (e.g., atrial fibrillation)
Low functional capacity (e.g., inability to climb one flight of stairs with a bag of groceries)
History of stroke
Uncontrolled systemic hypertension

MI, myocardial infarction; ECG, electrocardiogram.
[a]The American College of Cardiology National Database Library defines recent myocardial infarction as greater than 7 days but less than or equal to 1 month (30 days).
[b]May include "stable" angina in patients who are unusually sedentary.
[c]Campeau L. Grading of angina pectoris. *Circulation*. 1976;54:522–523.
From Eagle KA, Berger PB, Calkins H, et al. ACC/AHA Guideline Update for Perioperative Cardiovascular Evaluation for Noncardiac Surgery: a report of the American Heart Association/American College of Cardiology Task Force on Practice Guidelines (Committee to Update the 1996 Guidelines on Perioperative Cardiovascular Evaluation for Noncardiac Surgery). *Circulation*. 2002;105:1257–1267, with permission

mortality benefit was similar to the high-risk cohort; however, there was a 7.9% reduction in the perioperative MI rate. Therefore, among high-risk patients with multivessel CAD and evidence of significant myocardial ischemic burden, preoperative CABG confers a survival benefit and decreases the incidence of perioperative MI. With regard to the coronary intervention, there does not appear to be any difference in mortality or MIs in patients with multivessel disease—randomized to either CABG or percutaneous coronary angioplasty (PTCA)—presenting for noncardiac surgery (17).

Currently, angioplasty is followed by placement of either a bare-metal or a drug-eluting stent; stents reduce both the acute risk of major complications and long-term restenosis rate. Following placement of a stent, patients require antiplatelet therapy to prevent in-stent thrombosis. Antiplatelet therapy is maintained for 1 to 12 months, depending on whether a bare-metal or a drug-eluting stent is placed. The presence of antiplatelet therapy adds a new dimension of complexity to the patient presenting for noncardiac surgery following PCI. The risk–benefit ratio of preventing thrombosis of the stent versus the risk of catastrophic perioperative bleeding must be carefully weighed. Kaluza et al. (18) reported 7 myocardial infarctions, 11 major bleeding episodes, and 8 deaths in 40 consecutive patients presenting for noncardiac surgery following placement of a stent. All deaths and MIs, as well as 8 of the 11 bleeding episodes, occurred within 2 weeks of coronary stent placement. Wilson et al. (19) reported a 4% incidence of death, MI, or stent thrombosis among 207 patients at the Mayo Clinic. Furthermore, they documented no adverse events in the 39 patients undergoing surgery 7 weeks after stent placement. It appears from these two important studies that the greatest risk of adverse cardiovascular events and bleeding complications occur within 2 weeks of stent placement. Elective surgery should be delayed for greater than 6 weeks to allow for endothelialization of the stent and discontinuation of antiplatelet therapy. In the event of urgent surgery and severe CAD, angioplasty alone with no stent placement can be performed. This obviates the need for prolonged antiplatelet therapy and the risk of perioperative bleeding.

Perioperative β-Blockade Therapy

Of the pharmacologic agents that have been used during the perioperative period, β-blockade therapy remains the most studied. β-Blockers have several salutary effects that decrease the

TABLE 70.3

CARDIAC RISK[a] STRATIFICATION FOR NONCARDIAC SURGICAL PROCEDURES

High (Reported cardiac risk often greater than 5%)
- Emergent major operations, particularly in the elderly
- Aortic and other major vascular surgery
- Peripheral vascular surgery
- Anticipated prolonged surgical procedure associated with large fluid shifts and/or blood loss

Intermediate (Reported cardiac risk generally less than 5%)
- Carotid endarterectomy
- Head and neck surgery
- Intraperitoneal and intrathoracic surgery
- Orthopedic surgery
- Prostate surgery

Low[b] (Reported cardiac risk generally less than 1%)
- Endoscopic procedures
- Superficial procedures
- Cataract surgery
- Breast surgery

[a]Combined incidence of cardiac death and nonfatal myocardial infarction.
[b]Do not generally require further preoperative cardiac testing.
From Eagle KA, Berger PB, Calkins H, et al. ACC/AHA Guideline Update for Perioperative Cardiovascular Evaluation for Noncardiac Surgery: a report of the American Heart Association/American College of Cardiology Task Force on Practice Guidelines (Committee to Update the 1996 Guidelines on Perioperative Cardiovascular Evaluation for Noncardiac Surgery). *Circulation.* 2002;105:1257–1267, with permission

TABLE 70.4

ESTIMATED ENERGY REQUIREMENTS FOR VARIOUS ACTIVITIES

1 MET	Can you take care of yourself? Eat, dress, or use the toilet? Walk indoors around the house? Walk a block or two on level ground at 2 to 3 mph (3.2 to 4.8 km/h)?
4 METs	Do light work around the house like dusting and washing dishes? Climb a flight of stairs or walk up a hill? Walk on level ground at 4 mph (6.4 km/h)? Run a short distance? Do heavy work around the house like scrubbing floors or lifting or moving heavy furniture? Participate in moderate recreational activities like golf, bowling, dancing, doubles tennis, or throwing a baseball or football?
>10 METs	Participate in strenuous sports like swimming, singles tennis, football, basketball, or skiing?

MET, metabolic equivalent.
Adapted from the Duke Activity Status Index and AHA Exercise Standards.
From Eagle KA, Berger PB, Calkins H, et al. ACC/AHA Guideline Update for Perioperative Cardiovascular Evaluation for Noncardiac Surgery: a report of the American Heart Association/American College of Cardiology Task Force on Practice Guidelines (Committee to Update the 1996 Guidelines on Perioperative Cardiovascular Evaluation for Noncardiac Surgery). *Circulation.* 2002;105:1257–1267, with permission.

risk for cardiovascular morbidity and mortality in a select cohort of patients.

β-Blockers help to correct the imbalance between myocardial oxygen demand and supply. They have additional plaque-stabilizing, antiarrhythmic, anti-inflammatory, and altered gene expression effects (20). Their beneficial effects on perioperative mortality has been assessed in two much-discussed studies (21,22). Although both studies have design flaws, they demonstrate both short-term and potentially long-term beneficial effects of perioperative β-blockade. However, two recent trials have failed to demonstrate a beneficial effect with β-blockade therapy. The **Di**abetic **Po**stoperative **M**ortality and Morbidity (DIPOM) trial, involving 921 diabetic patients undergoing noncardiac surgery, did not demonstrate a significantly decreased risk of death and cardiac complications with metoprolol use (23). In the **M**etoprolol **a**fter **V**ascular **S**urgery (MaVS) trial, vascular patients scheduled for abdominal aortic aneurysm reconstruction or infrainguinal or extra-anatomic revascularization were randomized to either metoprolol or placebo 2 hours prior to surgery (24). The study drug was continued until hospital discharge or a maximum of 5 days. This trial demonstrated no difference in cardiac mortality, nonfatal MI, or new congestive heart failure between the two groups.

Although the aforementioned trials demonstrated no benefit in certain cohorts of patients, is there potential harm in initiating perioperative β-blockade? Lindenauer et al. (25) conducted a retrospective cohort study of patients 18 years of age or older undergoing noncardiac surgery at 329 hospitals. Propensity score matching was used to adjust for differences between patients who received perioperative. β-blockade and those who did not receive such therapy. In-hospital mortality was compared using multivariable logistic modelling. The Revised Cardiac Risk Index (RCRI) score was used to assess the association between β-blocker therapy and the risk of in-hospital death. In patients with a RCRI of 0 or 1, perioperative β-blockade was associated with no benefit and possible harm (RCRI 0: odds ratio [OR] 1.43; 95% confidence interval [CI] 1.29–1.58). The beneficial effects of β-blockade were seen only in patients with a RCRI of 2 or more (OR 0.9; 95% CI 0.75–1.08). In this study, β-blockade therapy appears to have a beneficial effect only in a select high-risk patient group.

Currently, the best evaluation of the level of evidence for perioperative β-blockade is the ACC/AHA 2006 Guideline Update on Perioperative Cardiovascular Evaluation for Noncardiac Surgery: Focused Update on Perioperative Beta-Blocker Therapy (26). Based on the patient's cardiac risk and the nature of the surgery, three classes of recommendations are made from the current evidence. Insufficient data is available regarding the use of β-blockade therapy in low cardiac risk patients undergoing intermediate or high-risk surgery. In addition, the role of β-blockade therapy in low-risk surgery has not been defined.

TABLE 70.5

SUMMARY OF AMERICAN COLLEGE OF CARDIOLOGY AND AMERICAN HEART ASSOCIATION GUIDELINES FOR CARDIAC EVALUATION BEFORE NONEMERGENT, NONCARDIAC SURGERY

	Clinical predictors				
		Intermediate clinical predictors		Minor clinical predictors	
Risk of surgery	Major clinical predictors	Poor functional capacity	Good functional capacity	Poor functional capacity	Good functional capacity
High Emergent major operations, particularly in the elderly Aortic and other major vascular surgery Peripheral vascular surgery Anticipated prolonged surgical procedures associated with large fluid shift and/or anticipated blood loss	Postpone or delay surgery	Testing indicated	Testing indicated	Testing indicated	Testing not indicated
Intermediate Carotid endarterectomy Head and neck surgery Intraperitoneal and intrathoracic surgery Orthopedic surgery Prostate surgery	Postpone or delay surgery	Testing indicated	Testing not indicated	Testing not indicated	Testing not indicated
Low Doscopic procedure Superficial procedures Cataract surgery Breast surgery	Postpone or delay surgery	Possible testing	Testing not indicated	Testing not indicated	Testing not indicated

From Akhtar S, Silverman DG. Assessment and management of patients with ischemic heart disease. *Crit Care Med.* 2004;32(Suppl):S126, with permission.

In an attempt to clarify the role of β-blockade therapy in these groups of patients, two randomized controlled trials are in their recruitment phase. The **P**eri**O**perative **IS**chemic Evaluation trial (POISE) is designed to evaluate the efficacy of 30 days of controlled-release metoprolol to prevent major perioperative cardiovascular events in patients undergoing all types of noncardiac surgery (27); a total recruitment of 10,000 patients is planned. The DECREASE IV trial is designed to evaluate the efficacy of combination therapy with fluvastatin and bisoprolol in 6,000 patients scheduled to undergo noncardiac, nonvascular surgery (28). It is hoped that these trials with large study samples will clarify the role of β-blockade therapy in the low- and intermediate-risk patient.

Cardiac Surgery

Perioperative and long-term risk evaluation in cardiac surgery is complicated by several factors. These include procedural factors, patient factors, and data collection.

Cardiac surgery, with its many confounding variables, requires large patient numbers for studies to be statistically relevant. Appropriate and meaningful data collection is a relatively recent phenomenon (29,30). However, this collection effort has been hampered by the reluctance to publish data on high-risk subgroups and the inclusion of data from low-output centers that are not part of a larger data collection network. Risk factors for cardiac surgery are identified by examining multiple databases and large case series. In one large database, 19 independent variables have been identified (31). However, there are no standardized definitions for risk thresholds; many of the assessments of statistical risk are based on odds ratios. In addition, multiple risk factors frequently coexist, making risk profiling for the individual patient difficult.

Patients are presenting cumulatively with more risk factors; however, the impact of the individual risk factor appears to be decreasing. Data accrued over the last two decades suggest a steady improvement in cardiac surgical outcomes (32). This improvement is attributed to improving surgical technique, perioperative care, and patient selection. There is still, however, large variation in surgical technique across the spectrum of cardiac surgical procedures, which may explain the significant interunit variation in outcomes (32–34).

Preoperative Evaluation

Cardiac risk profiling begins with a thorough clinical examination and a review of the completed special investigations. Additional investigations will be guided by the presence and severity of other organ dysfunction.

Cardiac risk evaluation can be performed by risk assessment tools. These tools are based on large databases, such as the EuroSCORE and the Society for Thoracic Surgeons (STS) database (29,31). The value of these databases is that standardized definitions are used to classify patients. The risk assessment tools have two important objectives:

1. Identifying independent risk factors for morbidity and mortality in valvular, coronary, and thoracic aortic surgery.
2. Risk prediction modelling through multivariate logistic regression analysis with a view to assessing individual patient risk, comparing and auditing individual units, and appropriate resource allocation.

The STS database working group has recently published their analysis of independent risk factors in valvular surgery (31). Table 70.6 represents the information submitted by North American centers for 409,904 cardiac valvular procedures for the decade starting in 1994 and ending 2003. The risk factors are stratified according to procedural risk and patient-related factors.

Statistical analysis techniques have been used to generate scoring systems. The Parsonnet score, developed in the late 1980s, predicts risk for CABG and valvular surgery based on an additive score of weighted risk factors (35). This score tends to overestimate mortality in modern clinical practice (32). In 1999, Nashef et al. (29) published an additive-weighted scoring system called EuroSCORE based on and validated using the EuroSCORE database. This system has an improved correlation with modern practice but still overestimates the mortality in higher-risk patients. The Parsonnet and EuroSCORE have modified versions applicable at the bedside.

Recently, a score based on Bayesian modeling has been advocated by the United Kingdom's Society of Cardiothoracic Surgeons (32). This system uses only nine weighted variables and has the best correlation and receiver operator curve of all three systems tested.

Scoring systems have a role in predicting both perioperative and long-term mortality and intensive care unit (ICU) resource use (30,32,36–38). Furthermore, they provide a framework to direct clinical examination and special investigations, thereby facilitating the process of identifying and modifying preoperative risk. Patients with a prohibitive perioperative risk can be better identified by these scoring systems. EuroSCORE is a compilation of risk factors as weighted by the Parsonnet, EuroSCORE, and Society of Cardiothoracic Surgeons databases. The percentages quoted in Table 70.7 are for *individual* risk factors in each section. Risk factors may be additive and/or synergistic.

Preoperative Risk Modification

Preoperative risk modification involves optimization of comorbidity and limiting cardiopulmonary bypass-related myocardial injury.

Comorbidity. Cardiac patients have multiple comorbidities; the most common are renal dysfunction, diabetes mellitus, and congestive cardiac failure. Renal dysfunction and failure are significant risk factors in both valvular and CABG surgery (39). The severity of renal dysfunction preoperatively correlates well with mortality postoperatively. Kuitunen et al. (40)

TABLE 70.6

PERIOPERATIVE RISK FACTORS FOR VALVULAR CARDIAC SURGERY

Surgical factors		Patient factors	
High risk	**Odds ratio**		**Odds ratio**
Aortic root replacement	2.78		
Isolated tricuspid replacement	2.26	4 Comorbidities	2
Emergent operation	2.11		
Multiple valve replacement	2.06		
Moderate risk			
Concurrent operation	1.58		
Reoperation	1.61	Age ≥70 years	1.88
Valve replacement vs. repair	1.52	3 Comorbidities	1.68
		Endocarditis	1.59
Low risk		Coronary artery disease	1.58
Isolated mitral replacement	1.47		
Year <1999	1.34	2 Comorbidities	1.41
Isolated pulmonic replacement	1.29	CHF	1.39
Isolated aortic replacement	1	Female gender	1.37
		Ejection fraction <0.35	1.34
		Average per comorbidity	1.19
Procedural risk is compared to the lowest-risk procedure—Isolated Aortic valve replacement The odds ratio for perioperative mortality during valvular surgery is compared to the lowest risk valvular procedure (aortic valve replacement; odds ratio 1, mortality 5.6 %).			

CHF, congestive heart failure.
From Rankin JS. Determinants of operative mortality in valvular heart surgery. *J Thorac Cardiovasc Surg.* 2006;131:547, with permission.

TABLE 70.7

PERIOPERATIVE RISK FACTORS FOR CABG ACCORDING TO SCORING SYSTEM

Parsonnet Score	EuroSCORE	UKSCTS complex Bayes
HIGH RISK (17%–40% MORTALITY)		
Cardiogenic shock Acute renal failure Acute structural defect, e.g., VSD >80 y old	Postinfarct septal rupture Thoracic aortic surgery LV EF <30% ARF Preop IABP or inotropes Preop ventilation Active endocarditis Reoperation Age ≥75 y	Emergency surgery LV EF <30% Dialysis Creatinine >200 μmol/L (2.3 mg/dL)
SIGNIFICANTLY ELEVATED RISK (9%–17% MORTALITY)		
75–79 y old Third reoperation Dialysis dependency Rare circumstances Recently failed intervention <24 h PA pressure ≥60 mm Hg AV pressure gradient ≥120 mm Hg	CABG plus major symptoms Emergency Systolic PAP >60 mm Hg Recent MI <90 days IVI nitrates on arrival in theatre Serum creatinine >200 μmol/L (2.3mg/dL) Neurology affecting ADL Peripheral vascular disease Age 70–74 y	Age >75 y One or more previous operations BSA <1.70 m^2
ELEVATED RISK (3%–9% MORTALITY)		
MV surgery PAP <60 mm Hg AV surgery gradient <120 mm Hg Recently failed intervention >24 h Aneurysmectomy Second reoperation Age 70–74 y LV EF <30% Hypertension BMI >35 IABP preoperative Female	LV EF 30%–50% Chronic pulmonary disease Female Age 65–69 y	Age 71–75 y Left main stem disease Diabetes Urgent surgery LV EF 30%–49% Hypertension

UKSCTS, United Kingdom Society of Cardiothoracic Surgeons; VSD, ventricular septal defect; LV EF, left ventricular ejection fraction; IABP, intra-aortic balloon counter pulsation; CABG, coronary artery bypass grafting; PAP, pulmonary artery pressure; BSA, body surface area; MI, myocardial infarction; PA, pulmonary artery; IVI, intravenous infusion; AV, atrioventricular; ADL, activities of daily living; MV, mitral valve; BMI, body mass index.

reported that patients with an increase in plasma creatinine of one and half times from baseline with short periods of oliguria had a 90-day mortality of 8%. However, in the anuric patient with a threefold increase in creatinine, mortality increased to 32%.

Patients with cardiogenic shock or an emergent indication for surgery often have acute renal failure; these patients have a high risk of death perioperatively. All scoring systems categorize their mortality above 40%, irrespective of the reason for the cardiogenic shock or the surgery required (30–32). These poor outcomes make it difficult to ascertain the beneficial effects that preoperative dialysis will confer.

Patients presenting for coronary revascularization with dialysis-dependent end-stage kidney disease have been extensively studied (41,42). These patients appear to have a major survival benefit when coronary revascularization is performed under cardiopulmonary bypass. This survival advantage is lost when either off-pump CABG or percutaneous coronary intervention is performed (42). Survival rates at 8 years in dialysis-dependent patients were 45.9% for CABG, 32.7% for PCI, and 29.7% for no surgical intervention. Patients with non–dialysis-dependent renal insufficiency have a significant incidence of postbypass renal failure (43). The STS CABG database suggests that they have higher perioperative mortality than patients with dialysis-dependent kidney failure (44). Prophylactic dialysis in nondialysis-dependent renal insufficiency may decrease the incidence of postbypass acute renal failure (45). In addition, these patients are fluid restricted and are often on diuretic therapy. Marathias et al. (46) reported that preoperative rehydration, with 1 mL/kg/hour of 0.45% saline, nearly halved the incidence of acute renal failure and decreased the need for postoperative dialysis.

Diabetics undergoing cardiac surgery are at increased risk of prolonged ventilation, postoperative sepsis, renal failure, and cognitive dysfunction (47). The perioperative management of diabetes and hyperglycemia in cardiac surgery is controversial. Insulin has been used in two strategies: tight glycemic control and as part of glucose-insulin-potassium regimens (GIK). The studies evaluating these strategies have concentrated on the intraoperative and postoperative periods.

The implementation of tight glycemic control in the postoperative setting improves mortality significantly: 8.0% versus 4.6% for tight glycemic control (48). This study, by Van den Berghe et al., was performed on predominantly postoperative cardiac patients and revealed significant reductions in length of stay, renal failure, and nosocomial sepsis. Intraoperative insulin infusion has also been shown to reduce postoperative complications in diabetic CABG patients (49,50). The use of a GIK infusion in the setting of ongoing myocardial ischemia and infarction results in significant improvements in myocardial preservation and contractile function (51). The technique has been applied to both coronary and valvular surgery with mixed results. The trials showing modest benefit initiated GIK preoperatively, used high doses of insulin, and continued the infusion through cardiopulmonary bypass and reperfusion (51). Meta-analysis of GIK therapy indicates that trials using tight glycemic control gave the best results. This observation needs validation by other randomized trials.

Clinical experience indicates that ongoing myocardial ischemia and poor diabetic control frequently occur preoperatively. Evidence from the intraoperative and postoperative periods suggests that preoperative initiation of GIK, combined with tight glycemic control, may significantly decrease postoperative complications.

Congestive cardiac failure represents a complex neurohumoral syndrome that develops in response to altered cardiac function. The stages of this condition have been classified by the ACC/AHA (Table 70.8) (52). In the perioperative period, decompensated stage C or D heart failure represents an independent risk factor for cardiac complications (31). The syndrome covers a spectrum of patients: from those with cardiogenic shock and an ejection fraction less than 30% to those with stable but inotrope-dependent cardiac function. These patients are at high risk for postoperative complications (29–32,35).

Decompensated cardiac failure in valvular or coronary heart disease may represent a progression of the primary disease process. Under these circumstances, surgery offers the only chance to improve the biomechanical cardiac dysfunction and attenuate the maladaptive myocardial response. Mortality in medically managed decompensated cardiac failure can be improved by using new classes of drugs such as β-type natriuretic peptide and the calcium channel sensitizers (53–56). These agents have an inotrope-sparing effect, shorten hospital stay, and improve medium-term survival. The role of these agents in the perioperative setting has not been assessed, although small studies show promising results. The role of nonsurgical therapy is in the long-term prevention of progression of structural heart disease, prevention of remodeling, and modification of underlying risk factors (57).

TABLE 70.9

INDICATIONS FOR INTRA-AORTIC BALLOON COUNTERPULSATION

- Ongoing unstable angina refractory to medical therapy
- Acute myocardial ischemia/infarction associated with percutaneous transluminal angioplasty (PTCA)
- Perioperative low cardiac output syndrome
- Cardiogenic shock after myocardial infarction
- Congestive heart failure
- Bridge to transplant
- Ischemic ventricular septal defect
- Acute mitral valve insufficiency
- Poorly controlled perioperative ventricular arrhythmias

Myocardial Preservation Interventions. Several nonpharmacologic and pharmacologic interventions can be initiated preoperatively to improve intraoperative and postoperative outcomes. Intra-aortic balloon counter pulsation (IABP) is a nonpharmacologic intervention that can be commenced preoperatively in the appropriate group of patients (Table 70.9). Pharmacologic therapies include preoperative statins, β-type natriuretic peptide, calcium channel sensitizers, and antioxidant therapy.

Intra-aortic balloon counterpulsation (IABP). The optimal use of the IABP in cardiac surgery is controversial. Preoperative IABP may offer improved myocardial perfusion and stability during induction and maintenance of anesthesia, prior to cardiopulmonary bypass. Good evidence exists for IABP in CABG patients with ischemia or with an ejection fraction less than 25% undergoing nonelective operation or reoperation, or who have New York Heart Association (NYHA) class III to IV symptoms. The evidence is less clear for patients without ongoing ischemia but who are undergoing reoperation, have isolated left main disease or a low ejection fraction, or who are undergoing procedures other than an isolated CABG (58). The efficacy of IABP for valvular surgery is poor and is associated with a twofold increase in mortality regardless of timing of use.

TABLE 70.8

ACC/AHA CLASSIFICATION OF HEART FAILURE

Stage A	Patients at high risk of developing heart failure (HF) because of the presence of conditions that are strongly associated with the development of HF. Such patients have no identified structural or functional abnormalities of the pericardium, myocardium, or cardiac valves and have never shown signs or symptoms of HF
Stage B	Patients who have developed structural heart disease that is strongly associated with the development of HF but who have never shown signs or symptoms of HF
Stage C	Patients who have current or prior symptoms of HF associated with underlying structural heart disease
Stage D	Patients with advanced structural heart disease and marked symptoms of HF at rest despite maximal medical therapy and who require specialized interventions

This probably reflects the fact that the ventricular dysfunction is either nonreversible or only partially reversible (59).

IABP improves cardiac output by approximately 20% *if* set to maximal efficiency. However, the insertion and use of an IABP is not a benign procedure. Limb ischemia occurs in 8% to 42% of patients, and 30% of those will require a surgical intervention. Limb ischemia is more common when a Seldinger technique is used for insertion as opposed to surgical exposure of the femoral vessels and placement under direct vision (59).

In conclusion, the best 5-year results for IABP are in patients undergoing isolated CABG (51%), whereas those undergoing CABG with aortic valve replacement have the lowest actuarial survival (34%). Further research is required to better define the role of this intervention in cardiac surgery (59).

HMG CoA reductase inhibitors. HMG CoA reductase inhibitors, commonly known as statins, have several beneficial effects on arteriosclerosis and vascular graft disease. Their mechanism of action is via a lipid-dependent and a lipid-independent pathway. Inhibition of atherogenesis, thrombosis, and inflammation and maintenance of endothelial integrity are all attributed to this class of drug (60,61). The efficacy of statins in the reduction of graft stenosis and progression of atheroma in native vessels post-CABG is well documented (62). However, in many of these trials, statin therapy was initiated after surgery. The early beneficial effects of statins are on endothelium recovery and in inflammation in coronary vessels (63). In a large prospective longitudinal study, Collard et al. (64) evaluated the effect of preoperative statin therapy on cardiac mortality following CABG. Preoperative statin therapy was associated with a 1.1% absolute reduction in mortality (OR 0.25; CI 0.07–0.87). Interestingly, cessation of statin therapy after surgery was associated with an increased in-hospital and late cardiac mortality. This suggests that preoperative statin therapy must be considered prior to CABG and may become a standard of care in the future.

Brain natriuretic peptide. Nesiritide is a recombinant form of brain natriuretic peptide that decreases pulmonary artery pressures and myocardial oxygen consumption, and increases coronary blood flow and urine output. Nesiritide is used in two clinical settings: inotrope-resistant cardiac failure and post-cardiac surgery patients with high pulmonary pressures and low cardiac output syndrome. Salzberg et al. (53) published a case series of 14 patients with severe mitral regurgitation and pulmonary pressures above 60 mm Hg undergoing cardiac surgery. Their predicted mortality based on EuroSCORE was 26%. These patients received a nesiritide infusion preoperatively, with the goal of reducing pulmonary pressures by 25%. The infusion was discontinued intraoperatively and restarted on return to the ICU. There was no reported mortality among the patients receiving nesiritide (53). These results need to be confirmed in a properly powered study, but the evidence for preoperative use in heart failure patients with pulmonary hypertension is promising.

Calcium sensitizers. Levosimendan is a calcium-sensitizing inodilator that improves myocardial contractility without increasing oxygen demand. It also decreases pulmonary vascular resistance in patients with heart failure. The LIDO trial showed it to be more effective than dobutamine in the management of severe congestive heart failure insofar as hemodynamic and mortality benefit (54). These findings have been verified by other large double-blind randomized trials (55).

Experience with levosimendan in cardiac surgery is currently limited to small studies. These studies looked at the physiologic effects of levosimendan in patients with good left ventricular function, poor ventricular function, or acute myocardial ischemia with hemodynamic compromise. In all three groups, low-dose levosimendan infusions improved cardiac output and decreased systemic vascular resistance, myocardial oxygen demand, and inotropic requirements coming off bypass (54). This drug offers enormous promise in the preoperative period in patients with severe congestive cardiac failure and poor cardiac output.

Antioxidants. Reactive oxygen species (ROS), both within myocardial cells and those derived from the systemic circulation, are thought to overwhelm local endogenous antioxidant systems during bypass. They initiate cellular damage, necrosis, and apoptosis during cardiopulmonary bypass and reperfusion. There have been many attempts to provide external sources of antioxidants or to improve endogenous antioxidant systems, and these approaches are supported by a large body of animal studies (65).

Allopurinol, which inhibits xanthine oxidase, a significant source of ROS outside the myocardium, has been studied in ten human CABG trials. Eight of these trials showed improved hemodynamic markers and less cardiac enzyme release (65). However, despite these encouraging data, allopurinol has not received widespread support. Superoxide dismutase, desferrioxamine, mannitol, vitamins C and E, and N-acetylcysteine are additional antioxidants with encouraging results in small human trials. They demonstrate decreased surrogate markers of tissue damage, although no outcome improvements have been shown. More research is required to define the role of antioxidant therapy in cardiac surgery.

There has been an improvement in the ability to identify and categorize the high-risk cardiac patient presenting for cardiac surgery. As more data are accrued, risk profiling is becoming more accurate. This will allow for cost-effective implementation of promising preoperative interventions in the appropriate patient.

PULMONARY SYSTEM

The risk of postoperative pulmonary complications varies widely and according to the definitions applied. The risk evaluation process also differs between cardiothoracic and noncardiothoracic surgery. In elective noncardiothoracic surgery, postoperative pulmonary complications vary between 1.7% and 2.6%, whereas in valvular heart surgery, the Society of Thoracic Surgeons database reports a pulmonary complication rate of 8.9% (66–68). The definition of pulmonary complications in these studies included respiratory failure, atelectasis, pneumonia, and pulmonary edema. Pulmonary thromboembolic disease has been specifically excluded in these studies.

The contribution of postoperative pulmonary complications to morbidity, mortality, and length of stay is not dissimilar to the cardiac complication profile (66,67,69–71). However, in the subgroup of patients older than 70 years of age, pulmonary complication is a better predictor of long-term mortality than cardiac risk factors (72). Predicting the likelihood of postoperative pulmonary complications requires preoperative pulmonary risk stratification. Smetana et al. (3) in a systematic review identified and categorized preoperative risk factors that predicted postoperative pulmonary complications following noncardiothoracic surgery.

Preoperative Evaluation

The initial evaluation for risk factors requires a thorough history and clinical examination. Following the history and clinical examination, patients can be classified into two groups: those with known pulmonary disease and those with suspected pulmonary disease. Both groups require an assessment of their functional classification and the degree of pulmonary reversibility.

Following the history and physical examination, laboratory and special investigations are guided by the database established from the clinical evaluation. Laboratory investigations with a good predictive value for postoperative pulmonary complications include blood urea nitrogen greater than 7.5 mMol/L (21 mg/dL) and creatinine level greater than 133 μmol/L (1.5mg/dL) (73–75). However, the most powerful predictor of pulmonary outcome is a serum albumin level. Albumin less than 3.0 g/dL correlates with an increased 30-day perioperative morbidity and mortality (76).

The utility and cost effectiveness of routine preoperative chest radiography has been extensively debated. An abnormal chest radiograph does predict postoperative complications; however, only 4.9% of radiographs in patients younger than 50 years of age will be abnormal. Among routine preoperative chest radiographs ordered, only 0.1% to 3% will alter management (77,78). A focused history and physical examination should identify the patient who is likely to have an abnormal preoperative chest radiograph; this is supported by a recent practice guideline issued by the American College of Physicians suggesting that (3):

1. Only patients with known cardiopulmonary disease should have a *routine* preoperative chest radiograph.
2. Patients older than 50 years undergoing procedures with high pulmonary risk should have a preoperative chest radiograph. These procedures include aortic surgery (thoracic or abdominal), neurosurgery, abdominal surgery, and prolonged surgery.

Spirometry has been evaluated as a predictive tool for pulmonary disorders in noncardiothoracic surgery. There are, unfortunately, no studies to guide spirometry evaluation in the perioperative period for restrictive pulmonary disorders. In obstructive pulmonary disorders, there are conflicting data on the utility of spirometry; however, it may identify patients at higher risk for postoperative pulmonary complications (3). No threshold or prohibitive value has been defined for spirometry indices in obstructive pulmonary disease, probably related to the evidence that long-term prognosis for chronic obstructive pulmonary disease (COPD) is better predicted by the BODE severity scoring system (79). This system uses a holistic approach assessing the body mass index, degree of airway obstruction, symptom scoring, and exercise testing to assess severity and predict outcome.

In lung resection surgery, however, spirometry forms the cornerstone of the evaluation process in both Europe and North America (80,81). Here, the perioperative risk of morbidity and mortality is directly related to a three-legged physiologic testing algorithm. Spirometry data are an integral part of the respiratory mechanics evaluation process. Other parameters evaluated are the cardiopulmonary reserve and the lung parenchymal function (Fig. 70.2). A simplified algorithm integrating these parameters assists in the preoperative workup for lung resection surgery (Fig. 70.3).

A forced expiratory volume (FEV_1) greater than 80% of predicted or greater than 2 L allows pneumonectomy without further investigation. An FEV_1 greater than 1.5 liters allows lobectomy without further investigation. If any of these criteria are not met, then a predicted postoperative FEV_1 ($ppoFEV_1$) and carbon monoxide diffusion capacity (ppoDLCO) need to be calculated. This allows for further risk stratification:

1. Patients with $ppoFEV_1$ and ppoDLCO greater than 40% can be resected.
2. If the $ppoFEV_1$ or ppoDLCO is less than 40% *and* >30%, then a VO_{2max} needs to be assessed. If the VO_{2max} is greater than 15 mL/kg/min, then resection can continue.
3. If the VO_{2max} is less than 15 mL/kg/min, then the risk is prohibitive unless V:Q scanning indicates that the lung pathology is predominantly involving the area to be resected.
4. A VO_{2max} less than 10 mL/kg/min or $ppoFEV_1$ less than 30%, and ppoDLCO less than 30% are all prohibitive risks (79,80).

When the information gathered from history, physical examination, and special investigations is examined, a risk profile can be constructed from the guidelines published by the American College of Physicians (Table 70.10) (3,82).

Important points that need to be highlighted from Table 70.10 are as follows:

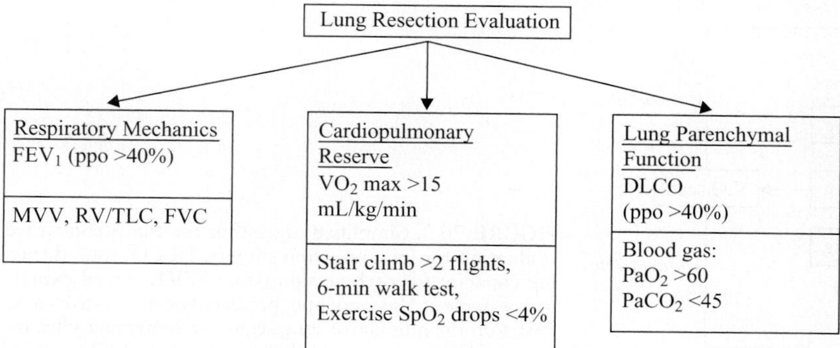

FIGURE 70.2. The best validated test is shown in the first box. Alternative tests are shown below. DLCO, total diffusing capacity for carbon monoxide; FEV1, forced expiratory volume at 1 second; FVC, forced vital capacity; MVV, maximal voluntary ventilation; PaO_2, arterial partial pressure of oxygen; $PaCO_2$, arterial partial pressure of carbon dioxide; ppo, predicted postoperative value based on the number of lung segments remaining after resection; RV/TLC, residual volume divided by total lung capacity; SpO_2, pulse oximetric oxygen saturation; VO_2, oxygen uptake/consumption.

TABLE 70.10

RISK FACTORS FOR RESPIRATORY COMPLICATIONS

High risk	OR	Strength of evidence	Indeterminate risk	OR	Strength of evidence
PATIENT-RELATED RISK FACTORS					
Age 60–69 years	2.09				
Age 70–79 years	3.04	A	Diabetes		C
ASA class ≥2	2.55–4.87	A	Obesity		D
CHF	2.93	A	Asthma		D
Functionally dependent	1.65–2.51	A	Obstructive sleep apnea		I
			Corticosteroid use		I
Moderate risk			HIV infection		I
COPD	1.79	A	Arrhythmia		I
Weight loss	1.62	B	Poor exercise capacity		I
Low Risk					
Impaired sensorium	1.39	B			
Cigarette use	1.26	B			
Alcohol use	1.21	B			
Abnormal findings on chest exam	NA	B			
PROCEDURE-RELATED RISK FACTORS					
High risk			**Indeterminate risk**		
Aortic aneurysm repair	6.9	A			
Thoracic surgery	4.24	A	Hip surgery		D
Abdominal surgery	3.01	A	Gynecologic or urologic surgery		D
Upper abdominal surgery	2.91	A	Esophageal surgery		I
Neurosurgery	2.53	A			
Prolonged surgery	2.26	A			
Moderate risk					
Head and Neck surgery	2.21	A			
Emergency surgery	2.21	A			
Vascular surgery	2.1	A			
General anesthesia	1.83	A			
Low risk					
Perioperative transfusion >4 units	1.47	B			
SPECIAL INVESTIGATIONS					
High risk			**Indeterminate risk**		
Albumin level <3.5 g/dL	2.53	A	BUN level >7.5 mmol/L (21 mg/dL)	NA	B
Chest radiography	4.81	B	Spirometry		I

A = Good evidence that the factor is an independent predictor, B = At least fair evidence that the factor is an independent predictor, C = At least fair evidence that the factor is *not* a predictor, D = Good evidence that the factor is *not* a predictor, I = Evidence is lacking, conflicting, or indeterminate
OR, odds ratio; ASA, American Society of Anesthesiologists; CHF, congestive heart failure; HIV, human immunodeficiency virus; COPD, chronic obstructive pulmonary disease; BUN, blood urea nitrogen; NA, not available.
Adapted from Smetana G. Preoperative pulmonary risk stratification for noncardiothoracic surgery: systematic review for the American College of Physicians. *Ann Int Med.* 2006;144:581, with permission.

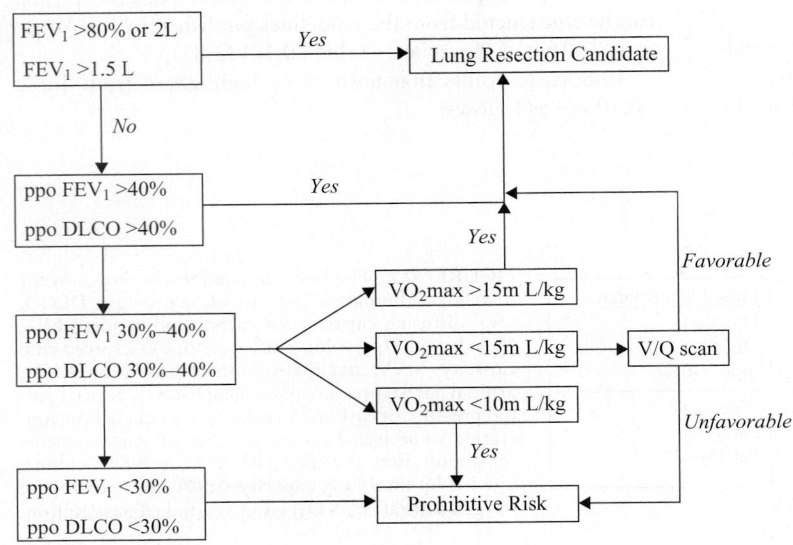

FIGURE 70.3. Simplified algorithm for the preoperative evaluation for lung resection surgery. DLCO, total diffusing capacity for carbon monoxide; FEV1, forced expiratory volume at 1 second; ppo, predicted postoperative value based on the number of lung segments remaining after resection; VO$_2$, oxygen uptake/consumption; V/Q, ventilation/perfusion ratio.

- Advanced age is reported with differing definitions. The multivariate analyses shown on the table represent odds ratios for ages 60 to 69 and 70 to 79 years.
- *Functional dependence* refers to both total dependence for activities of daily living, and partial dependence when equipment is required to perform activities of daily living. This is distinct from exercise capacity, which has not been evaluated as an independent risk factor in the setting of noncardiothoracic surgery.
- COPD has been poorly investigated as a risk factor, but evidence consistently suggests an independent risk.
- Impaired sensorium refers to patients with mental status changes, delirium, or both who are able to respond to verbal cues or light tactile stimulation.
- Cigarette use refers to ongoing smoking. *Recent cessation, within an 8-week period, carries an increased risk of perioperative pulmonary complications over and above that associated with continued smoking* (83).
- When eight multivariate trials were examined, only one trial suggested that obesity was an independent pulmonary predictor. This is indirectly verified by evidence that increasing levels of morbid obesity is not associated with increased pulmonary complications following surgery (84).
- Obstructive sleep apnea is associated with airway management difficulty and an increased all-cause admission to the intensive care. An increased pulmonary complication rate has not been elucidated.
- Asthmatic patients have a pulmonary complication rate of only 3%, which is similar to the general surgical population. This is probably related to pulmonary optimization before elective and emergency surgery (3).
- Studies of diabetes mellitus are of poor quality and are unadjusted univariate analyses, which makes them difficult to interpret.

The relationships between individual risk factors in each risk category have not been fully elucidated; they may be either additive or synergistic. Once a risk profile is formulated, risk modification strategies should be implemented.

Preoperative Management

The management of pulmonary disorders in the preoperative period fall into two categories, which include restrictive and obstructive disorders. Characteristics of restrictive disorders include the presence of mechanical volume limitations, the occasional presence of bronchial hyperreactivity, and the static nature of the disease. Obstructive pulmonary disorders are recognized by fixed airway obstruction, the presence of bronchial hyperreactivity, and a predisposition to infection.

Restrictive Pulmonary Disorders

Restrictive pulmonary disorders are substantially less common than obstructive disorders. Furthermore, they are an uncommon cause of complication or death postoperatively (3). These disorders are static in nature unless bronchial hyperreactivity coexists (e.g., hypersensitivity pneumonitis). The restriction can be either pulmonary or extrapulmonary (Table 70.11). In the extrapulmonary group, management of the mechanical volume effects can improve the perioperative pulmonary status of the patient. Drainage of a pleural effusion and re-expansion of a collapsed lung are interventions that optimize ventilation-perfusion matching. An improvement in oxygenation and ventilation can be expected. Another strategy associated with an improvement in outcome is lung protective ventilation using positive end-expiratory pressures (PEEP) and low tidal volumes of 6 to 8 mL/kg (85). This ventilator strategy has become the standard of care for acute respiratory distress syndrome (ARDS) and other disorders of static compliance found in this group of conditions. It must be emphasized that the ideal low tidal volume and appropriate PEEP strategy have still not been resolved.

TABLE 70.11

CAUSES OF RESTRICTIVE PULMONARY DISEASE

Pulmonary/Parenchymal	Extrapulmonary
Pulmonary edema	Pleural effusion
ARDS	Pneumothorax
Atelectasis	Kyphoscoliosis
Sarcoidosis	Increased abdominal pressure (ascites, pregnancy, obesity)
Hypersensitivity pneumonitis	
Silicosis	
Tuberculosis	
Lung resection	

ARDS, acute respiratory distress syndrome.

Obstructive Airways Disease

Chronic obstructive pulmonary disease (COPD) is differentiated from asthma on the basis of having a chronic fixed component of airway obstruction. In nonoptimized patients with COPD, a component of reversible airway obstruction or bronchial hyperreactivity, similar to asthma, is present. Furthermore, both asthmatics and COPD patients are prone to acute exacerbations of airway obstruction triggered by upper and lower airway infections (86).

Obstructive pulmonary disorders are associated with increased risk of postoperative pulmonary complications (3). When reversible airway obstruction is present, this risk is amplified (87,88). However, Milledge and Nunn (89) demonstrated that even patients with severe airway obstruction—defined as an FEV_1 less than 1 L—can safely be operated on without an increase in postoperative complications. The key element in the management of patients with COPD is the identification and appropriate treatment of the reversible component of the airway disease.

β_2-Agonists have a salutary effect on airway hyperreactivity in obstructive airway disease. When symptom-free mild asthmatic volunteers were intubated under local anesthesia, FEV_1 decreased by 50%. In the group pretreated with a β_2-agonist, the FEV_1 decreased by only 20% (90). However, it is important to note that the incidence of postintubation bronchospasm is still significant, even when β_2-agonists are used as monotherapy (91,92).

Preoperative steroid therapy, even of short duration, has been shown to decrease the incidence of wheezing post intubation (91,93,94). The concern for negative effects on wound healing and increased infection rates have not been borne out in the literature (95). With regard to the use of methylxanthines, a Cochrane review in 2001 showed that neither theophylline

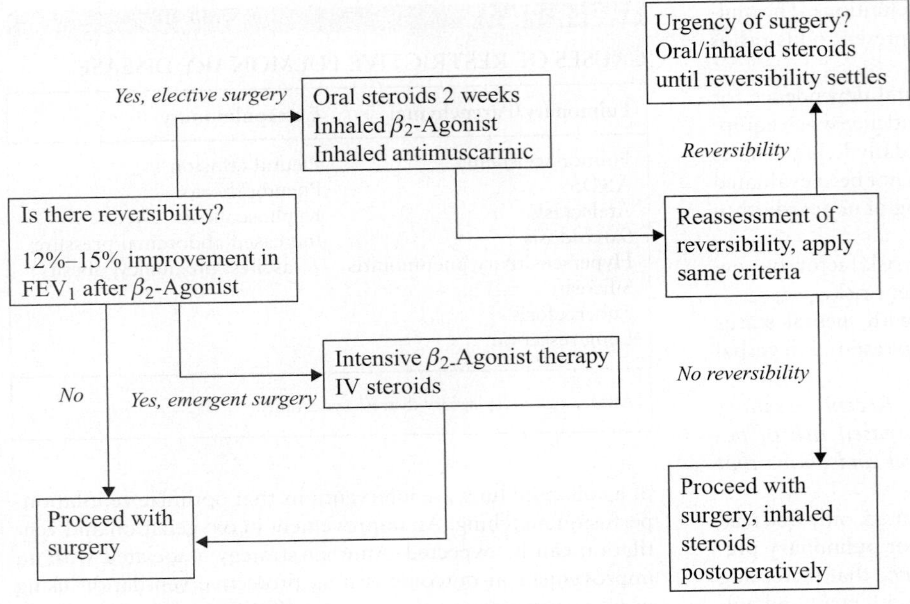

FIGURE 70.4. Preoperative optimization of obstructive airways disease. FEV_1, forced expiratory volume at 1 second; IV, intravenous.

nor aminophylline offered any advantage over β_2-agonists in the setting of acute bronchospasm (96).

Finally, there is good evidence in adults that upper and lower airway infections increase airway reactivity and result in demonstrable spirometry abnormalities for 6 to 8 weeks post infection (97). Elective surgery should ideally be delayed in patients with underlying bronchial hyperreactivity. The American Thoracic Society and the Global Initiative for Chronic Obstructive Lung Disease (GOLD) have issued guidelines for the assessment and management of obstructive lung disorders and their acute exacerbations (86,98). This approach can be modified for the patient presenting for surgery (Fig. 70.4). The most important intervention on a global scale is smoking cessation and prevention of exposure to second-hand smoke. Epidemiology studies have shown that a patient who successfully stops smoking will have a life table mortality rate that comes to parallel that of someone who has never smoked (86).

Another intervention that can be started in the preoperative period is nutritional support, which can be administered either enterally or parenterally. Preoperative enteral nutrition with an immune-repleting diet improves outcomes in malnourished elective gastroenterology oncology patients; they experience a significant decrease in nosocomial sepsis and hospital length of stay (99,100). Enthusiasm for total parenteral nutrition has waned due to the increased rates of infection associated with long-term central venous access and hyperglycemia (99).

In conclusion, the Practice Guideline published by the American College of Physicians helps generate a risk profile for noncardiothoracic surgery. Risk modification strategies can then be applied to optimize the patient.

RENAL SYSTEM

Acute and chronic renal failure are important medical problems worldwide. The incidence of ICU-associated acute renal failure (ARF) varies between 15% and 35%, whereas the incidence of ARF requiring renal replacement therapy approximates 1%. In the United States, the incidence of end-stage kidney disease (ESKD) varies between 331 and 343 cases per million population, whereas more than 104,000 new patients began therapy for ESKD in 2004. The economic burden of ESKD continues to rise and currently exceeds 20 billion dollars, approximately 6.7% of the Medicare budget (101).

The preoperative evaluation and management of the patient with renal disease is complicated by the coexistence of multiple medical and surgical problems. Therefore a stepwise logical approach to these patients is required to ensure that important data are not omitted.

Chronic Renal Failure

Risk Evaluation and Stratification

Preoperative renal risk evaluation and stratification are based on the comorbid medical condition of the patient, pre-existing renal function, and the procedure-specific renal risk (Fig. 70.5).

Comorbid Status. Comorbid conditions that increase the risk of chronic renal insufficiency include a spectrum of

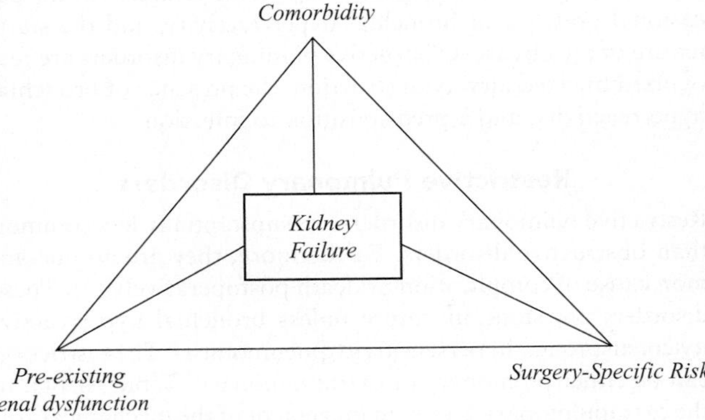

FIGURE 70.5. Triad of factors that collectively increases the risk of perioperative kidney failure

TABLE 70.12

CAUSES OF CHRONIC KIDNEY DISEASE

- Advanced age
- Hypertension
- Renovascular atherosclerotic disease
- Poorly controlled diabetes
- Hepatorenal syndrome
- Autoimmune disorders (systemic lupus erythematosus)
- Pregnancy-induced hypertension
- Congenital (polycystic kidney disease)

cardiovascular, endocrine, hepatic, autoimmune, and congenital disorders (Table 70.12). The severity, duration, and appropriate management of the conditions determine the degree of renal dysfunction a patient will develop.

Diabetes mellitus (DM) is the leading cause of ESKD, with hypertension, glomerulonephritis, and polycystic kidney disease being the other major diagnoses (101). The incidence of diabetes mellitus–related ESKD has risen over the past three decades from 28% in 1980 to approximately 50% currently (101). Diabetes affects the kidney by several mechanisms, resulting in proteinuria, the nephrotic syndrome, and progressive renal failure. Patients with diabetes mellitus who have microalbuminuria (30–300 mg/24 hours) have not yet begun to lose glomerular filtration but they are at high risk of renal complications. The introduction of ACE inhibitors in this group of patients has a powerful renoprotective effect and slows the progression to overt renal failure (102).

Coronary artery disease is common in patients with diabetes mellitus and may be asymptomatic due to an associated autonomic neuropathy. A high index of suspicion for untreated CAD should be maintained for patients with diabetic nephropathy. Danaei et al. (103) reported that 21% of deaths from ischemic heart disease and 13% from stroke worldwide are attributable to higher-than-optimum blood glucose concentrations. The ACC/AHA guidelines for the preoperative evaluation of the cardiac patient presenting for noncardiac surgery list DM as an intermediate clinical predictor for perioperative cardiovascular events (11). Therefore, the preoperative workup of the diabetic patient with renal dysfunction should be done within the framework of the ACC/AHA algorithm discussed previously (11).

Hypertension is the second leading cause of ESKD in the United States. Rates of ESKD caused by hypertension show dramatic variation when comparing African American patients with those of other races and ethnicities (101). The 2004 rate of hypertensive ESKD in African American patients aged 30 to 39 years is 149 cases per million population, approximately 15 times higher than in Caucasian counterparts. Hypertension is both a cause and a consequence of ESKD. Aggressive control of the blood pressure to approximately 125/75 mm Hg in patients with diabetic renal disease is recommended by the National Kidney Foundation. The Modification of Diet in Renal Disease study provided convincing evidence that lower blood pressure reduces the rate of loss of renal function in patients with proteinuric renal disease (104). Polycystic kidney disease is an inherited disorder that is characterized by multiple cysts in the kidney as well as the liver. It is responsible for 4% to 5% of ESKD in the United States (101). Important extrarenal manifestations of polycystic kidney disease include intracranial aneurysm in approximately 10% of patients, whereas 26% of patients have evidence of mitral valve prolapse.

TABLE 70.13

STAGES OF CHRONIC KIDNEY DISEASE

Stage	Definition
1	GFR $\geq$90 mL min/1.73 m^2 with evidence of kidney damage
2	GFR 60–89 mL/min/1.73 m^2 with evidence of kidney damage
3	GFR 30–59 mL/min/1.73 m^2
4	GFR 15–29 mL/min/1.73 m^2
5	GFR $\leq$15 mL/min/1.73 m^2 or dialysis dependent

GFR, glomerular filtration rate.

Once comorbid conditions and their related complications are identified, an attempt must be made to quantify the degree of renal dysfunction.

Pre-existing Renal Dysfunction. The National Kidney Foundation-Kidney Disease Outcomes Quality Initiative recently proposed a standardized classification system to assess the severity of pre-existing chronic renal disease. It is based on an estimation of the glomerular filtration rate (GFR) and the documentation of renal injury (Table 70.13) (105). The GFR can be estimated using either mathematical models or by determining the clearance of inulin or other filtration markers. To estimate the GFR, either the Cockroft-Gault equation or the formula derived from the Modification of Diet in Renal Disease Study can be used. The latter formula, although mathematically more complex, uses readily available data to provide a more accurate estimate of the GFR than the Cockroft-Gault equation (106):

$$\begin{aligned} \text{GFR}\,(\text{mL/min/1.73 m}^2) &= 170 \times [P_{Cr}]^{-0.999} \times [\text{age}]^{-0.176} \\ &\times [0.762 \text{ if patient is female}] \\ &\times [1.18 \text{ if patient is black}] \times [\text{SUN}]^{-0.17} \\ &\times [\text{Alb}]^{+0.318} \end{aligned}$$

where SUN is serum urea nitrogen and Alb is albumen. The presence of pre-existing renal dysfunction increases the incidence of perioperative morbidity and mortality in high-risk surgery. Safi et al. (107) analyzed factors responsible for developing acute renal failure following thoracoabdominal repair. On multivariate analysis, preoperative creatinine (P_{Cr}) greater than or equal to 2.8 mg/dL was strongly associated with postoperative ARF (OR 10.3; 95% CI 12–411, p <0.0001). Of the patients who developed ARF, the mortality rate was 49%. This elevated operative mortality risk associated with renal failure is reflected by Kashyap et al. (108) in their study of thoracoabdominal aortic surgery (OR 9.2; 95% CI 2.6–33; p < 0.005).

Procedure-related Risk. Procedure-related renal risk is an important determinant of perioperative renal failure. Cardiac and major vascular procedures are associated with a high incidence of ARF. For example, cardiopulmonary bypass (CPB) has several negative effects on renal function. The use of nonpulsatile flow, inadequate renal perfusion pressure, and the induction of an inflammatory response all contribute to renal dysfunction. The incidence of ARF following cardiac surgery varies between 1% and 30% (109). The development of renal failure is associated with increased mortality, hospital length of stay, and cost. Conlon et al. (109) studied 2,672 consecutive patients undergoing CABG and reported a 7.9% incidence of ARF and 0.7% incidence of ARF requiring renal replacement therapy. The mortality for patients who developed ARF was 14% compared with 1% among those who did not develop ARF.

Off-pump CABG, by avoiding cardiopulmonary bypass, has been shown to have a protective effect on renal function post surgery. Ascione et al. (110) randomized patients with normal renal function prior to cardiac surgery to either an on-pump or off-pump group. Postoperatively, the off-pump group had better preservation of renal function as evidenced by the creatinine clearance, albumin-creatinine ratio, and the N-acetyl-β-glucosamine levels. The same group evaluated 253 patients with preoperative renal insufficiency undergoing CABG. ARF occurred in 15.8% of patients who underwent on-pump CABG compared to 5.9% of those who had off-pump CABG (111). It appears that off-pump CABG has a renoprotective effect in patients with both normal and impaired renal function. Furthermore, it highlights the positive influence that modification of a surgical technique can have on organ protection.

Renal insufficiency or failure exists in many patients presenting for major vascular surgery. Swaminathan and Stafford-Smith (112) analyzed data from eight studies and reported an incidence between 4% and 24% of pre-existing renal insufficiency in patients with aortic disease. The broad range of reported incidence is attributed to the lack of consensus for the definition of renal insufficiency.

In vascular surgery, the location of the arterial reconstruction, the duration of the aortic cross-clamp, and the emergent nature of the procedure are all strong predictors of postoperative renal complications. Reported incidence of acute postoperative renal dysfunction for thoracoabdominal reconstruction varies between 13% and 25%, whereas renal failure rates for abdominal aortic reconstruction are much lower at approximately 1.5% to 2% (113). The hypothesized mechanisms of postoperative renal injury are ischemia-reperfusion of the kidneys, atheroembolic injury, nephrotoxin, and inflammatory damage.

Measures aimed at modifying surgical technique to reduce the incidence of postoperative renal dysfunction in aortic surgery have been met with mixed success. The most significant advance recently has been the widespread adoption of endovascular techniques for aortic aneurysm repair. Several small studies have suggested that the reduced aortic manipulation and renal ischemia that accompany the endovascular technique is associated with reduced inflammation and postoperative renal injury (114,115). However, a recent large study comparing endovascular to open repair for abdominal aortic aneurysm (AAA) demonstrated no difference in renal outcome between the two groups. Renal complications were 1.1% and 1.2% in the open and endovascular group, respectively (116). In patients with baseline chronic renal insufficiency, endovascular aortic repair does not confer a renal benefit compared to open AAA surgery. Parmer et al. (117) reviewed 98 patients undergoing endovascular and open aortic repair at a single institution with baseline renal insufficiency. Postoperative renal failure rates were 28% and 29% for the open and endovascular group, respectively. Further research will be required to establish whether endovascular surgery is truly renoprotective.

Acute Renal Failure

Definition

Acute renal failure (ARF) is a common complication of critical illness and is associated with significant morbidity and mortality. There is no consensus definition of ARF in critically ill patients. More than 30 definitions have been used in the literature, making it difficult to compare data from different studies. In order to standardize the definition of ARF, the Acute Dialysis Quality Initiative (ADQI) group proposed the RIFLE classification of ARF (Table 70.14) (118). The classification system includes criteria for serum creatinine, GFR, and urine output. The RIFLE classification is a valuable tool in determining the extent of acute renal dysfunction and helps to prognosticate outcome

TABLE 70.14

THE RIFLE CLASSIFICATION SCHEME FOR ACUTE RENAL FAILURE

	GFR criteria	Urine output criteria	Mortality
Risk	Increased plasma creatinine × 1.5 or GFR decrease >25%	<0.5 mL/kg/h × 6 h	8%
Injury	Increased plasma creatinine × 2 or GFR decrease >50%	<0.5 mL/kg/h × 12 h	21.40%
Failure	Increased plasma creatinine × 3 or acute plasma creatinine ≥350 μmol/L (4 mg/dL) or acute rise ≥44 μmol/L (0.5 mg/dL)	<0.3 mL/kg/h × 24 h or anuria × 12 h	32.50%
Loss	Persistent acute renal failure with complete loss of kidney function × 4 weeks		
ESKD	End-stage kidney disease (× 3 mo)		

GFR, glomerular filtration rate; ESKD, end-stage kidney disease.

in the face of ARF. Kuitunen et al. (40) used the RIFLE classification to categorize postoperative renal impairment following cardiac surgery. Patients with RIFLE-F (failure) had a 90-day mortality of 32.5% compared with 8% for those in the RIFLE-R (risk) and 21.4% for RIFLE-I (injury) patients (Table 70.14). Multivariate logistic regression analysis demonstrates that the RIFLE classification is an independent risk factor assessment for 90-day mortality.

Classification of ARF

ARF is divided into three categories based on its pathophysiology. They are prerenal, postrenal, and intrarenal ARF.

1. **Prerenal ARF:** Prerenal ARF is reversible renal insufficiency due to renal hypoperfusion. If the renal hypoperfusion is left untreated, acute tubular necrosis (ATN) secondary to ischemia will develop. Prerenal ARF is characterized by clinical evidence of hypovolemia such as systemic hypotension, low central venous pressures, low cardiac output, or systolic pulse variation on positive pressure ventilation. Laboratory data that indicate prerenal ARF include low urine Na^+, fractional excretion of Na^+ less than 1%, and bland urine sediment.
2. **Postrenal ARF:** Postrenal ARF is due to obstruction of urine flow at any level of the urine collecting system. Postrenal ARF can be diagnosed promptly by either ultrasound or CT scan, and relief of the obstruction usually results in prompt reversal of the renal insufficiency. Postrenal ARF must be excluded in every patient presenting with ARF.
3. **Intrarenal ARF:** Intrarenal ARF is divided into five groups based on the underlying pathology. *Acute tubular necrosis (ATN)* is injury and subsequent death of the tubular epithelium. ATN is caused by either ischemia or nephrotoxic agents. *Acute interstitial nephritis* is an inflammation of the renal interstitium and the tubules. It may occur secondary to infections or drugs, such as the penicillins or cephalosporins. Other causes of intrarenal ARF include *acute glomerulonephritis, acute vascular syndromes,* and *intratubular obstruction.* The differential diagnosis of intrarenal ARF should be guided by the clinical history and physical examination. Examination of the urine sediment helps to narrow the differential diagnosis. The presence of tubular epithelial cells and granular cast is suggestive of ATN, whereas the presence of red cell cast indicates glomerulonephritis. Eosinophiluria suggests the presence of interstitial nephritis; however, it is not diagnostic.

ARF is characterized by retention of nitrogenous waste products, fluid and electrolyte abnormalities, acid-base disorders, and impairment of the hematologic and coagulation systems. The preoperative evaluation of these patients must therefore take into account these specific changes and the increased risk they pose during the perioperative period.

Preoperative Evaluation of Renal Failure

As highlighted previously, both acute and chronic renal failure affect multiple organ systems. The history and physical examination should be directed toward evaluating the severity of the comorbid conditions and the complications related to the acute renal dysfunction. Signs and symptoms of uncompensated cardiac failure and pericarditis should be elicited. Uremic patients are at risk for the development of large pericardial effusions, which can be hemodynamically compromising. The presence of an elevated jugular venous pressure and pulsus paradoxus of greater than 10 mm Hg should alert the clinician to the presence of a pericardial effusion.

Uremia is associated with nausea, vomiting, and recurrent episodes of hiccoughing. Severe nausea and vomiting may result in dehydration, and a thorough evaluation of the patient's volume status must be performed. These patients may either be on intermittent hemodialysis or peritoneal dialysis. Records of the last dialysis, fluid balance, and body weight must be obtained to help with the assessment of the fluid status.

Anemia in renal failure is multifactorial in nature. Bleeding from platelet dysfunction, malnutrition, and decreased erythropoietin production all contribute toward the low red cell mass. Electrolyte abnormalities are common in renal failure. Hyperkalemia, hyperphosphatemia, and hypocalcemia is the typical electrolyte profile seen in renal failure. Hypocalcemia may manifest as cramps, paraesthesia, and, in severe cases, with mental status changes.

Diagnostic Testing. The diagnostic studies in patients with renal dysfunction are determined by the findings on the history and physical examination. Complete blood count helps to assess the severity of the anemia, morphology of the red blood cells, and the platelet count. Although uremic patients may have normal platelet numbers, they develop an acquired platelet dysfunction that results in an increased risk of bleeding. The pathogenesis of this hemostatic dysfunction is multifactorial and includes the effects of circulating toxins, alteration of the vessel wall, and anemia. To assess the degree of platelet function, either a bleeding time, or more accurately, a platelet function assay can be performed.

The basic metabolic panel helps to determine the electrolyte profile and allows the anion gap to be calculated. ARF is characterized by an increased anion gap metabolic acidosis. The BUN and creatinine can be tracked to assess the efficacy of renal replacement therapy.

An electrocardiogram must be performed to determine whether ischemia, ventricular hypertrophy, or strain pattern is present. Hyperkalemia is characterized by tall peaked T waves, widened QRS complex, and shortened QT interval. The ECG of patients with pericardial effusion may demonstrate small QRS complexes and the presence of electrical alternans (change in QRS amplitude with each heartbeat). A chest radiograph may reveal signs of pulmonary edema, cardiomegaly, or a large pericardial effusion.

Examination of the urine and determination of the urine indices provides invaluable data in helping to differentiate prerenal from intrarenal ARF (Table 70.15). The fractional

TABLE 70.15

CRITERIA TO DIFFERENTIATE PRERENAL FROM INTRARENAL FAILURE

	Prerenal	Intrarenal
Urine Na^+	<20 mEq/L	>40 mEq/L
FE_{Na+}	<1%	>2%
FE_{UN}	<35%	>50%
Urine/plasma creatinine	>40	<20
Urine/plasma osmolarity	>1.3	<1.1
Urine/plasma urea	>8	<3

excretion of urea is a useful index to differentiate prerenal from intrarenal failure if diuretic therapy has been initiated:

$$FE_{UN} = [(\text{urine nitrogen}/\text{blood urea nitrogen})/(\text{urine creatinine}/\text{plasma creatinine})] \times 100$$

Fractional excretion of urea nitrogen is primarily dependent on passive forces and is therefore less influenced by diuretic therapy. In contrast, diuretic therapy will falsely raise the FE_{Na+} under prerenal conditions.

Primary and Secondary Prevention of ARF

Primary prevention of ARF refers to clinical strategies that reduce the occurrence of ARF in patients with or without chronic renal disease. Secondary injury is additional renal injury developing in the face of a primary insult to the renal system. Various nonpharmacologic and pharmacologic strategies have been developed to reduce both primary and secondary renal injury. However, these have been met with mixed success, and no pharmacologic agent has been approved in the United States as a sole renoprotective agent.

The principles of management of patients with ARF are to maintain an adequate mean arterial pressure, maintain an appropriate cardiac output, ensure euvolemia, and avoid nephrotoxic agents. The mean arterial pressure required to maintain adequate renal perfusion pressure, however, may vary according to the patient's underlying medical condition. Patients with hypertension have an autoregulatory curve that is shifted to the right; therefore, they may require a higher mean arterial pressure. Low cardiac output states induce renal ischemia and reduce the glomerular filtration rate. It is important to restore cardiac output to normal levels to prevent secondary injury to the kidney. This may require placement of monitors such as a pulmonary artery catheter or a transesophageal echocardiography probe to determine cardiac output.

Volume expansion has been shown to prevent contrast-induced nephropathy and attenuate the tubular injury associated with rhabdomyolysis (119,120). Furthermore, Mertens et al. (121) compared the incidence of contrast-induced nephropathy with either isotonic saline or bicarbonate hydration. Patients received an intravenous bolus of 3 mL/kg of the study solution over an hour, before radiocontrast injection. This was followed by a continuous infusion of 1 mL/kg/hour during the procedure and for 6 hours after the procedure. The incidence of contrast-induced nephropathy was 13.6% in the saline group but only 1.7% in the bicarbonate arm. These are low-cost, high-yield interventions that can significantly affect the outcome of patients with marginal renal function.

In conclusion, the best evidence to date suggests that nonpharmacologic therapy strategies are more effective than drugs in reducing the risk of ARF. High-risk patients should be identified early and secondary renal injury aggressively prevented.

NEUROLOGIC SYSTEM

Ischemic Cerebrovascular Disease

The incidence of perioperative stroke in patients undergoing nonvascular surgery under general anesthesia is less than 0.5%. However, the mortality associated with a perioperative stroke may be as high as 26% (122).

Carotid Stenosis

The risk of a perioperative stroke increases in the presence of carotid stenosis or a history of transient ischemic attack (TIA). In a retrospective study, Evans et al. (123) studied 284 patients with ultrasound-documented evidence of carotid stenosis undergoing general surgical procedures. The presence of carotid stenosis of at least 50% was associated with a perioperative stroke rate of approximately 3.6%. Although higher than the general population stroke rate, this risk does not appear sufficient to mandate prophylactic carotid endarterectomy (CEA). The cumulative risk for stroke in asymptomatic patients is the sum of the perioperative stroke risk for CEA and the residual perioperative stroke risk for the general surgical procedure. This cumulative risk must be significantly lower than 3.6% to justify preemptive CEA. Therefore, asymptomatic carotid stenosis discovered during general surgical procedure workup does not require carotid endarterectomy. Patients with carotid disease who present with TIAs have a 10% risk of stroke during the subsequent year. Of the patients who develop a stroke, 20% will have their stroke within the first month and about 50% within 1 year of the TIA. After the first year, the stroke rate decreases to about 5% per year (124). Carotid stenosis can be managed both surgically and pharmacologically.

Two large randomized studies have defined the role of CEA in symptomatic patients with carotid stenosis. The North American Symptomatic Carotid Endarterectomy Trial (NASCET) and the European Carotid Surgery Trial (ESCT) validated the role of CEA among symptomatic patients with severe (70%–99%) and moderate (50%–69%) carotid stenosis (125). Two criteria must be met for CEA to have a beneficial effect. First, surgical skills with a low complication rate are essential; second, the surgical benefit must persist for several years to justify the perioperative risk.

The benefit of antiplatelet therapy in reducing perioperative stroke during CEA is unresolved. However, based on the current level of evidence, patients should receive aspirin prior to surgery unless there are obvious contraindications. The optimal dose of aspirin is uncertain; however, a dose range of 50 to 1,300 mg/day has been used in various studies (126).

Surgery-specific Risk

Perioperative stroke rates vary depending on the surgery-specific risk. Currently, the noncarotid procedure associated with the highest risk of perioperative neurologic injury is cardiac surgery. Contemporary prospective studies report a 3% incidence of stroke in CABG procedures, 8% in isolated valve surgery, and 11% in combined CABG-valve surgery. Advanced age and female gender are additional risk factors for perioperative neurologic injury (127). The single most important factor for cerebral injury during cardiac surgery is macroembolization of atheromatous debris during aortic manipulation. Every attempt should be made to identify the high-risk patient with a large atheromatous burden by using epiaortic echocardiography and minimizing manipulation of the aorta (128).

Preoperative Evaluation

The history and physical examination of the patient with cerebrovascular disease requires a thorough assessment of the cardiovascular and neurologic system. Patients with carotid artery stenosis are at an increased risk of coronary artery disease. Severe correctable CAD is evident in approximately 26% of patients with cerebrovascular disease, whereas only 9% of patients have normal coronary anatomy (10). Despite the increased incidence of CAD in patients with carotid stenosis, the rate of medical complications in patients undergoing CEA is low. Paciaroni et al. (129) recorded medical complications that occurred within 30 days after CEA in 1,415 patients enrolled in the NASCET trial. Perioperative medical complications occurred in less than 10% of patients who underwent CEA, and only 0.4% had severe complications. Of note, perioperative nonfatal and fatal MI occurred in only 1% of the patients and was associated with a mortality rate of approximately 0.2%. Therefore, recommending a CABG procedure to a patient with symptomatic carotid disease and asymptomatic CAD is not justified, as the combined mortality and stroke rate after CABG is higher than an expertly performed CEA.

The ACC/AHA guidelines for noncardiac surgery list CEA as an intermediate-risk procedure where the perioperative cardiac risk is less than 5% (11). The cardiac workup of patients presenting for CEA can be performed within the framework of the ACC/AHA algorithm.

Hypertension is another chronic condition that needs to be evaluated during the history and physical examination. Hypertension is a prevalent and treatable risk factor for stroke. Treatment of systolic and diastolic hypertension results in a 36% and 42% stroke reduction, respectively (126). The preoperative blood pressure is important in determining the hemodynamic management strategies intraoperatively. Patients with long-standing hypertension have their cerebral autoregulatory curve shifted to the right; therefore, a higher mean arterial pressure may be required during periods of cerebral ischemia to ensure adequate cerebral perfusion. Poor control of blood pressure following CEA increases the risk of cerebral hyperperfusion syndrome. This complication occurs due to impairment of cerebral autoregulation and can result in intracerebral hemorrhage and white matter edema. Patients with severe preoperative carotid stenosis and chronic hypertension are at greatest risk for this complication. Blood pressure should be carefully monitored and aggressively treated if symptoms of hyperperfusion syndrome develop (126).

Hemorrhagic Cerebrovascular Disease

Aneurysmal Subarachnoid Hemorrhage

The prevalence of cerebral aneurysm in the general population ranges between 0.2% and 7.9% (130). Subarachnoid hemorrhage (SAH) accounts for 2% to 5% of all new strokes in the United States (131). The incidence increases with age, with a higher preponderance in females and the African American population. The vast majority of deaths occur within 2 weeks of the rupture, with 10% occurring in the prehospital area. The risk of re-rupture is greatest within 24 hours, and thereafter decreases to approximately 1% to 1.5% per day for the initial 14 days. The cumulative re-rupture risk during the first 14 days is about 25% (132).

Preoperative Evaluation. The preoperative evaluation of the patient with an intracranial bleed must begin with a thorough history and physical examination. Patients with an aneurysmal SAH will complain of a severe sudden headache following the ictus. Features of meningeal irritation including neck stiffness and photophobia can be elicited. An altered level of consciousness, seizures, and coma are found in the higher grades of SAH. Aneurysmal subarachnoid hemorrhage is graded according to the Hunt-Hess classification or the World Federation of Neurologic Surgeons Scale. The amount of subarachnoid blood is evaluated using the Fischer grading system. The quantity of blood in the subarachnoid space determines the risk of developing delayed cerebral ischemia or vasospasm (Table 70.16).

The initial diagnostic modality of choice is a CT scan of the brain, which can detect SAH in approximately 95% of cases. Once the diagnosis of a SAH is made, either a CT angiogram or a four-vessel cerebral angiogram is performed to delineate the cause of the SAH. A four-vessel cerebral angiogram remains the gold standard for diagnosing an intracranial aneurysm; however, it has the disadvantage of being highly invasive and time consuming. Furthermore, the incidence of microembolism during this procedure is high and the risk of rebleeding is increased (133).

The sensitivity and specificity of CT angiogram for aneurysm detection are 87% and 100%, respectively (134).

TABLE 70.16

WFNS, HUNT-HESS, AND FISCHER GRADING SYSTEM FOR SUBARACHNOID HEMORRHAGE

Grade	World Federation of Neurologic Surgeons Scale	Hunt-Hess	Fischer
0	Unruptured aneurysm		
I	Glasgow Coma Score of 15	Asymptomatic or mild headache	No subarachnoid blood detected
II	Glasgow Coma Score of 13–14 without focal deficit	Moderate to severe headache, nuchal rigidity, cranial nerve palsy	Diffuse or vertical layers ≤1 mm thick
III	Glasgow Coma Score of 13–14 with focal deficit	Lethargy, confusion, mild focal deficit	Localized clot and/or vertical layer ≥1 mm
IV	Glasgow Coma Score of 7–12	Stupor, moderate to severe hemiparesis, early decerebrate rigidity	Intracerebral or intraventricular clot with diffuse or no SAH
V	Glasgow Coma Score of 3–6	Deep coma, decerebrate rigidity, moribund	

SAH, subarachnoid hemorrhage.

The advantages of a CT angiogram compared with four-vessel angiogram include its rapidity, decreased invasiveness, and substantially lower cost. The disadvantages include its difficulty in detecting small and unusually located aneurysms and the use of an iodinated contrast medium. However, in the era of cost-consciousness, CT angiogram remains a viable option for the diagnostic workup for aneurysmal SAH.

Magnetic resonance (MR) angiography conversely does not require radiation exposure, and its contrast material has a substantially lower allergic and renal complication rate. MR angiography has a 74% to 98% detection rate for aneurysms greater than 3 mm. However, in aneurysms smaller than 3 mm, the detection rate is generally low (133). An advantage that MR angiography has over CT angiography is its ability to locate aneurysms close to the cranial base. With continual improvement in technology, the role of noninvasive cerebral angiography is rapidly being defined and may eventually supersede four-vessel cerebral angiography.

Complications of Aneurysmal SAH

Central nervous system. Vasospasm or delayed cerebral ischemia occurs in 60% to 70% of patients following SAH, half of whom will develop symptomatic ischemia (130). The exact cause of vasospasm is not fully understood, but the breakdown products of subarachnoid blood are probably responsible for initiating the ischemia. Vasospasm begins within 4 days following the ictus and may last for as long as 14 to 16 days. Vasospasm is diagnosed clinically and confirmed by transcranial Doppler or angiography. The treatment of delayed cerebral ischemia is broadly classified into preventative measures, triple-H therapy (hypertension, hemodilution, hydration), and endovascular intervention. The only useful pharmacologic agent available for vasospasm is the calcium channel blocker nimodipine. It is given orally or by nasogastric tube. A Cochrane database review of eight trials demonstrated a reduction in poor neurologic outcome, secondary ischemia, and mortality with oral nimodipine (135).

With aggressive multimodal therapy, morbidity from vasospasm can be reduced to 5% (130). Triple-H therapy involves inducing hypertension to systolic blood pressures between 180 and 200 mm Hg. This is achieved initially with fluids and with pressors such as phenylephrine when needed. Rheologic benefits are achieved by keeping the hematocrit at approximately 30%. Care must be taken not to induce severe anemia, which can decrease cerebral oxygen delivery and worsen ischemia. Hydration is optimized with either a colloid or an isotonic crystalloid. Given that the central venous pressure is a poor indicator of intravascular volume status (136), these patients may require placement of a pulmonary artery catheter to better manage their fluid status (137).

Endovascular therapy for vasospasm consists of balloon angioplasty and intra-arterial infusions of nimodipine or verapamil; papaverine has fallen out of favor. Balloon angioplasty is best used for large vessel spasm whereas vasodilator therapy is useful for distal branch vasospasm.

Cardiovascular. Rupture of an intracranial aneurysm is associated with substantial cardiovascular and hemodynamic changes. The myocardial injury following SAH is related to the massive sympathetic discharge and is characterized by subendocardial contraction band necrosis. ECG abnormalities are detected in 50% to 80% of patients following aneurysmal SAH. The spectrum of ECG changes includes repolarization abnormalities, ST-T wave changes, and conduction alterations. Myocardial injury and enzyme leaks are found in 20% to 50% of patients with abnormal postictal ECGs, whereas echocardiographic evidence of myocardial dysfunction is found in two thirds of patients with elevated levels of troponin I (138).

The cardiac workup of patients with aneurysmal SAH is determined by their premorbid cardiovascular status and the degree of hemodynamic compromise following rupture of the aneurysm. An ECG, cardiac enzymes, and echocardiography should be considered for patients presenting with hemodynamic instability. In our experience, patients with mild-to-moderate cardiac dysfunction often require no specific cardiac intervention, and tolerate surgery and neurointerventional procedures well. The patient with severe cardiac dysfunction may require placement of invasive monitors such as a pulmonary artery catheter to optimize cardiac output and cerebral perfusion pressure. In a retrospective study of 453 patients, Kim et al. (137) showed that pulmonary artery catheter-guided hemodynamic management reduced the incidence of pulmonary complications and sepsis by 8%.

Pharmacologic and mechanical intervention, such as intra-aortic balloon counterpulsation, may also be required to support the severely dysfunctional myocardium (139). Intra-aortic balloon counterpulsation has the added advantage of possibly improving cerebral blood flow in patients with severe vasospasm that is refractory to traditional triple-H and neurointerventional therapy (140).

Pulmonary. Pulmonary complications occur in approximately 22% of aneurysmal SAHs and are associated with a substantial risk of mortality (141,142). The most frequent pulmonary complications are nosocomial pneumonia and pulmonary edema. Patients at risk for nosocomial pneumonia are those with an altered level of consciousness and with aspiration of gastric contents. Neurogenic pulmonary edema occurs from the massive sympathetic discharge following the ictus and is characterized by disruption of the pulmonary epithelial-endothelial barrier. Protein-rich fluid leaks into the alveoli and results in alveoli instability and atelectasis. Pulmonary edema can also be triggered secondary to aggressive triple-H therapy. Friedman et al. (141), using logistic regression analysis, showed a strong and independent association between pulmonary complications and the development of symptomatic vasospasm. The likely explanation for this phenomenon is that patients with pulmonary compromise are treated less aggressively with triple-H therapy than their counterparts with normal pulmonary function.

Evaluation of the pulmonary system begins with an assessment of the neurologic status of the patient and the determination of whether he or she is able to protect the airway. Patients with a GCS score of less than or equal to 8 require intubation to protect the lower respiratory tract from aspiration. A chest radiograph and arterial blood gas assessment help to assess the degree of pulmonary dysfunction and the need for intubation and ventilation. Ventilation strategies that should be used include a lung-protective ventilation strategy and the appropriate use of positive end expiratory pressure.

Electrolytes. The most common electrolyte abnormality following SAH is hyponatremia, occurring in 30% to 40% of

TABLE 70.17

CLINICAL AND BIOCHEMICAL FEATURES OF SIADH AND CSW

	SIADH	CSW
Extracellular fluid volume	↑	↓
Sodium balance	↑ to normal	↓
Serum sodium	↓	↓
Serum osmolality	↓	Normal to ↑
Hematocrit	Normal	↑
Plasma BUN/creatinine	↓	↑

SIADH, syndrome of inappropriate antidiuretic hormone secretion; CSW, cerebral salt-wasting syndrome; BUN, blood urea nitrogen.

patients (142). The two major mechanisms of hyponatremia are either the syndrome of inappropriate antidiuretic hormone (SIADH) or cerebral salt-wasting syndrome (CSW). It is important to differentiate these two conditions, as the management strategies are markedly different. Table 70.17 shows the clinical and biochemical features of SIADH and CSW. The most important feature between the two syndromes is the extracellular volume, which is elevated in SIADH and decreased in CSW. Either clinical or hemodynamic data such as pulmonary artery occlusion pressure and ventricular end-diastolic volume must be assessed to determine the volume status of the hyponatremic patient. SIADH is treated with fluid restriction whereas cerebral salt-wasting syndrome is treated with hypertonic fluid and salt replacement.

Other electrolyte abnormalities commonly encountered in patients with SAH include hypomagnesemia and hypokalemia in 37% and 27% of patients, respectively (142). Magnesium has been shown to have a neuroprotective effect in numerous stroke models and reverses vasospasm and infarct volume in rat models of SAH (143,144). Van den Bergh et al. (145) conducted a prospective human trial on the use of magnesium prior to the onset of vasospasm following SAH. The study demonstrated that magnesium infusion during the vasospasm period decreased the incidence of "poor outcome" by 23%. Magnesium levels were kept between 1 and 2 mMol/L by means of a continuous magnesium infusion. Although based on a small cohort, this low-cost, high-yield intervention holds great promise for the future.

Hyperglycemia. The incidence of hyperglycemia following SAH is 30% (142). This is due to the activation of the sympathoadrenal system and the increase in stress hormones following the ictus. Hyperglycemia is associated with a poor prognosis in the face of cerebral ischemia (146). Blood glucose levels must be monitored regularly, and an insulin infusion should be initiated if blood glucose exceeds 110 mg/dL. The salutary effects of "tight" glucose control are not limited to only the central nervous system. Van den Berghe et al. (48) randomized 1,548 postcardiac surgery patients to either an intensive insulin (80–110 mg/dL) or conventional therapy (180–200 mg/dL). Intensive insulin therapy was associated with a lower mortality and a decreased incidence of acute renal failure requiring renal replacement therapy. Critical illness polyneuropathy and documented bacteremia rates were also lower in the intensive insulin therapy arm. Tight glucose control should therefore be an integral part of the management algorithm for the patient with a SAH.

The proportion of deaths directly attributed to medical complications following SAH is 23% (142). This is comparable to the death rate following vasospasm and rebleeding. Therefore, medical complications following SAH should be aggressively sought and treated. A stepwise systematic approach to the various organ systems will help identify and treat complications related to SAH.

SUMMARY

High-risk surgical patients present a unique challenge to the perioperative physician. Due to their multiple comorbidities and the increasing complexity of surgery being performed, their perioperative risk is disproportionately higher than the general surgical population. To appropriately manage these patients, risk factors must be identified and stratified following completion of the clinical, laboratory, and special investigations. Risk-modification strategies may be implemented preoperatively if they are likely to have a beneficial effect during the operative course. Otherwise, they can be initiated postoperatively as part of the long-term care plan for the patient.

PEARLS

- Assessment of the high-risk patient begins with preoperative identification, stratification, and modification of risk factors.
- No preoperative test should be performed unless it is likely to influence patient treatment.
- In noncardiac surgery, the ACC/AHA algorithm provides a structured and cost-effective evaluation strategy.
- Dobutamine stress echocardiography is a useful preoperative test to detect ischemia in patients with a limited ability to perform exercise testing.
- Scoring systems in cardiac surgery assist with risk profiling, predicting mortality, and resource use.
- Promising interventions exist for the optimization of the severely dysfunctional ventricle.
- Systematic reviews have now defined patient and surgery-specific risk for postoperative pulmonary complications.
- It is very important to assess and treat reversible airway obstruction in chronic obstructive airway disease.
- The risk of acute renal failure in patients with chronic renal insufficiency is determined by comorbidities, baseline renal function, and procedure-specific risk.
- The RIFLE classification categorizes the severity and prognosticates the outcome of acute renal failure.
- Nondialysis-dependent chronic renal insufficiency patients are at a high risk for perioperative renal complications; aggressive management of secondary renal injury is advised.
- The prevention of secondary neuronal injury must be the focus of perioperative intervention.
- Medical complications are a significant contributor to perioperative morbidity and mortality in aneurysmal SAH. Aggressive investigation and treatment of these complications improves outcome.

References

1. Brown DL, Heard SO, Stevens DS, et al. Preoperative Evaluation of High-Risk Surgical Patients. In: Civetta JM, ed. *Critical Care.* 3rd ed. Philadelphia, PA: Lippincott-Raven; 1997:999.
2. Browner WS, Li J, Mangano DT. In-hospital and long term mortality in male veterans following noncardiac surgery. The Study of Perioperative Ischemia Research Group. *JAMA.* 1992;268:252.
3. Smetana GW, Lawrence VA, Comell JE. Preoperative pulmonary risk stratification for noncardiothoracic surgery: systematic review for the American College of Chest Physicians. *Ann Intern Med.* 2006;144:581.
4. Holt NF, Silverman DG. Modeling perioperative risk: can numbers speak louder than words? *Anesthesiology Clin.* 2006;24:427.
5. Almanaseer Y, Mukherjee D, Kline-Rogers EM, et al. Implementation of the ACC/AHA Guidelines for Preoperative Cardiac Risk Assessment in a general medicine preoperative clinic: improving efficiency and preserving outcomes. *Cardiology.* 2005;103:24.
6. Froehlich JB, Karavite D, Russman PL, et al. American College of Cardiology/American Heart Association preoperative assessment guidelines reduce resource utilization before aortic surgery. *J Vasc Surg.* 2002;36:758.
7. Mangano DT, Browner WS, Hollenberg M, et al. Association of perioperative myocardial ischemia with cardiac morbidity and mortality in men undergoing noncardiac surgery. The Study of Perioperative Ischemia Research Group. *N Engl J Med.* 1990;323:1781.
8. Goldman L, Caldera DL, Southwick FS, et al. Cardiac risk factors and complications in non-cardiac surgery. *Medicine (Baltimore).* 1978;57:357.
9. Lee TH, Marcantonio ER, Mangione CM, et al. Derivation and prospective validation of a simple index for prediction of cardiac risk of major noncardiac surgery. *Circulation.* 1999;100:1043.
10. Hertzer NR, Beven EG, Young JR, et al. Coronary artery disease in peripheral vascular patients. A classification of 1000 coronary angiograms and results of surgical management. *Ann Surg.* 1984;2:223.
11. Eagle KA, Berger PB, Calkins H, et al. ACC/AHA Guideline Update for Perioperative Cardiovascular Evaluation of Noncardiac Surgery: Executive Summary. A report of the American College of Cardiology/American Heart Association Task Force on Practice Guidelines (Committee to Update the 1996 Guidelines on Perioperative Cardiovascular Evaluation for Noncardiac Surgery). *Anesth Analg.* 2002;94:1052.
12. Pronovost PJ, Jenckes MW, Dorman T, et al. Organizational characteristics of intensive care units related to outcomes of abdominal aortic surgery. *JAMA.* 1999;281:1310.
13. Morris CK, Ueshima K, Kawaguchi T, et al. The prognostic value of exercise capacity: a review of the literature. *Am Heart J.* 1991;122:1423.
14. Akhtar S, Silverman DG. Assessment and management of patients with ischemic heart disease. *Crit Care Med.* 2004;32(Suppl):S126.
15. Fleisher LA. Preoperative cardiac evaluation. *Anesthesiology Clin N Am.* 2004;22:59.
16. Eagle KA, Rihal CS, Mickel MC, et al. Cardiac risk of noncardiac surgery: influence of coronary disease and type of surgery in 3368 operations. *Circulation.* 1997;96:1882.
17. Hassan SA, Hlatky MA, Boothroyd DB, et al. Outcomes of noncardiac surgery after coronary bypass surgery or coronary angioplasty in the Bypass Angioplasty Revascularization Investigation (BARI). *Am J Med.* 2001;110:260.
18. Kaluza GL, Joseph J, Lee JR, et al. Catastrophic outcomes of noncardiac surgery soon after coronary stenting. *J Am Coll Cardiol.* 2000;35:1288.
19. Wilson SH, Fasseas P, Orford JL, et al. Clinical outcome of patients undergoing non-cardiac surgery in the two months following coronary stenting. *J Am Coll Cardiol.* 2003;42:234.
20. Preibe HJ. Perioperative myocardial infarction-aetiology and prevention. *Br J Anaesth.* 2005;95:3.
21. Poldermans D, Boersma E, Bax JJ, et al. The effect of bisoprolol on perioperative mortality and myocardial infarction in high-risk patients undergoing vascular surgery. Dutch Echocardiographic Cardiac Risk Evaluation Applying Stress Echocardiography Study Group. *N Engl J Med.* 1999;341:1789.
22. Mangano DT, Layug EL, Wallace A, et al. Effect of atenolol on mortality and cardiovascular morbidity after noncardiac surgery. Multicenter Study of Perioperative Ischemia Research Group. *N Engl J Med.* 1996;335:1713.
23. Juul AB, Wetterslev J, Gluud C, et al. Effect of perioperative beta blockade in patients with diabetes undergoing major non-cardiac surgery: randomised placebo controlled, blinded multicentre trial. *BMJ.* 2006;332:1482.
24. Yang H, Raymer K, Butler R, et al. Metoprolol after vascular surgery (MaVS) (Abstract). *Can J Anaesth.* 2004;51.
25. Lindenauer PK, Pekow P, Wang K, et al. Perioperative beta-blocker therapy and mortality after major noncardiac surgery. *N Engl J Med.* 2005;353:349.
26. Fleisher LA, Beckman JA, Brown KA, et al. ACC/AHA 2006 Guideline Update on Perioperative Cardiovascular Evaluation for Noncardiac Surgery: Focused Update on Perioperative Beta-blocker Therapy. A Report of the American College of Cardiology/American Heart Association Task Force on Practice Guidelines (Writing Committee to Update the 2002 Guidelines on Perioperative Cardiovascular Evaluation for Noncardiac Surgery). *J Am Coll Cardiol.* 2006;47:2343.
27. Devereaux PJ, Yusuf S, Yang H, et al. Are the recommendations to use perioperative beta-blocker therapy in patients undergoing noncardiac surgery based on reliable evidence? *CMAJ.* 2004;171:245–247.
28. Schouten O, Poldermans D, Visser L, et al. Fluvastatin and bisoprolol for the reduction of perioperative cardiac mortality and morbidity in high-risk patients undergoing non-cardiac surgery: rationale and design of the DECREASE-IV study. *Am Heart J.* 2004;148:1047.
29. Nashef SA, Roques F, Michel P, et al. European system for cardiac operative risk valuation (EuroSCORE). *Eur J Cardiothorac Surg.* 1999;16:9.
30. Roques F, Nashef SA, Michel P, et al. Risk factors and outcome in European cardiac surgery: analysis of the EuroSCORE multinational database of 19030 patients. *Eur J Cardiothorac Surg.* 1999;15:816.
31. Rankin J, Hammill B, Ferguson T, et al. Determinants of operative mortality in valvular heart surgery. *J Thorac Cardiovasc Surg.* 2006;131:547.
32. National Adult Cardiac Surgical Database Report 2000–2001. Available at: www.ctsnet.org. Accessed November 30, 2006.
33. Edwards FH, Grover FL, Shroyer AL, et al. The Society of Thoracic Surgeons national cardiac surgery database: current risk assessment. *Ann Thorac Surg.* 1997;63:903.
34. Shroyer AL, Grover FL, Edwards FH. 1995 Coronary artery bypass risk model: The Society of Thoracic Surgeons adult cardiac national database. *Ann Thorac Surg.* 1998;65:879.
35. Parsonnet V, Dean D, Bernstein AD. A method of uniform stratification of risk for evaluating the results of surgery in acquired heart disease. *Circulation.* 1989;79;I3.
36. Parsonnet V, Bernstein A. Bedside estimation of risk as an aid for decision-making in cardiac surgery. *Ann Thorac Surg.* 2000;69:823.
37. Biancari F, Kangasniemi OP, Luukkonen J, et al. EuroSCORE predicts immediate and late outcome after coronary artery bypass surgery. *Ann Thorac Surg.* 2006;82:57.
38. Nilsson J, Algotsson L, Hoglund P, et al. EuroSCORE predicts intensive care unit stay and costs of open heart surgery. *Ann Thorac Surg.* 2004;78:1528.
39. Chertow GM, Levy EM, Hammermeister KE, et al. Independent association between acute renal failure and mortality following cardiac surgery. *Am J Med.* 1998;104:343.
40. Kuitunen A, Vento A, Suojaranta-Ylinen R, et al. Acute renal failure after cardiac surgery: evaluation of the RIFLE classification. *Ann Thorac Surg.* 2006;81:542.
41. Dewey TM, Herbert MA, Prince SL, et al. Does coronary artery bypass graft surgery improve survival among patients with end-stage renal disease? *Ann Thorac Surg.* 2006;81:591.
42. Hemmelgarn BR, Southern D, Culleton BF, et al. Survival after coronary revascularization among patients with kidney disease. *Circulation.* 2004;110:1890.
43. Rao V, Weisel RD, Buth KJ, et al. Coronary artery bypass grafting in patients with non-dialysis-dependent renal insufficiency. *Circulation.* 1997;96(Suppl 2):38.
44. Cooper WA, O'Brien SM, Thourani VH, et al. Impact of renal dysfunction on outcomes of coronary artery bypass surgery. *Circulation.* 2006;113:1063.
45. Durmaz I, Yagdi T, Calkavur T, et al. Prophylactic dialysis in patients with renal dysfunction undergoing on-pump coronary artery bypass surgery. *Ann Thorac Surg.* 2003;75:859.
46. Marathias K, Vassli M, Robola A, et al. Preoperative intravenous hydration confers renoprotection in patients with chronic kidney disease undergoing cardiac surgery. *Artif Organs.* 2006;30:615.
47. Ouattara A, Lecomte P, Le Manach Y, et al. Poor intraoperative blood glucose control is associated with a worsened hospital outcome after cardiac surgery in diabetic patients. *Anesthesiology.* 2005;103:687.
48. Van den Berghe G, Wouters P, Weekers F, et al. Intensive insulin therapy in critically ill patients. *N Eng J Med.* 2001;345:1359.
49. Furnary AP, Gao G, Grunkemeier GL, et al. A continuous insulin infusion reduces mortality in patients with diabetes undergoing coronary artery bypass grafting. *J Thorac Cardiovasc Surg.* 2003;125:985.
50. Lazar HL, Chipkin SR, Fitzgerald CA, et al. Tight glycemic control in diabetic coronary artery bypass graft patients improves perioperative outcomes and decreases recurrent ischemic events. *Circulation.* 2004;109:1497.
51. Doenst T, Bothe W, Beyersdorf F. Therapy with insulin in cardiac surgery: controversies and possible solutions. *Ann Thorac Surg.* 2003;75:S721.
52. Hunt SA, Baker DW, Chin MH, et al. ACC/AHA guidelines for the evaluation and management of chronic heart failure in the adult: executive summary: a report of the American College of Cardiology/American Heart Association Task Force on Practice Guidelines (Committee to revise the 1995 Guidelines for the Evaluation and Management of Heart Failure). *J Am Coll Cardiol.* 2001;38:2101.
53. Salzberg SP, Filsoufi F, Anyanwu A, et al. High-risk mitral valve surgery: perioperative hemodynamic optimization with Nesiritide (BNP). *Ann Thorac Surg.* 2005;80:502.
54. Follath F, Cleland JG, Just H, et al. Efficacy and safety of intravenous levosimendan compared with dobutamine in severe low-output heart failure (the LIDO study): a randomised double-blind trial. *Lancet.* 2002;360:196.
55. Raja SG, Rayen BS. Levosimendan in cardiac surgery: current best available evidence. *Ann Thorac Surg.* 2006;81:1536.
56. Mills RM, Hobbs RE, Young JB. "BNP" for heart failure: role of nesiritide in cardiovascular therapeutics. *Congest Heart Fail.* 2002;8:270.
57. Jessup M, Brozena S. Heart failure. *N Engl J Med.* 2003;348:2007.

58. McCarthy P, Golding L. Temporary mechanical circulatory support. In: Edmunds L, ed. *Cardiac Surgery in the Adult.* New York, NY: McGraw-Hill; 1997:319.
59. Baskett RJF, Ghali WA, Maitland A, et al. The intraaortic balloon pump in cardiac surgery. *Ann Thorac Surg.* 2002;74:1276.
60. Corsini A, Raiteri M, Soma MR, et al. Pathogenesis of atherosclerosis and the role of drug intervention: focus on HMG-CoA reductase inhibitors. *Am J Cardiol.* 1995;76:21A.
61. Bellosta S, Ferri N, Arnaboldi L, et al. Pleiotropic effects of statins in atherosclerosis and diabetes. *Diabetes Care.* 2000;23(Suppl 2):B72.
62. Hindler K, Shaw AD, Samuels J, et al. Improved postoperative outcomes associated with preoperative statin therapy. *Anesthesiology.* 2006;105:1260.
63. Werba JP, Tremoli E, Massironi P, et al. Statins in coronary bypass surgery: rationale and clinical use. *Ann Thorac Surg.* 2003;76:2132.
64. Collard CD, Body SC, Shernan SK, et al. Preoperative statin therapy is associated with reduced cardiac mortality after coronary artery bypass graft surgery. *J Thorac Cardiovasc Surg.* 2006;132:392.
65. Kevin LG, Novalija E, Stowe DF. Reactive oxygen species as mediators of cardiac injury and protection: the relevance to anesthesia practice. *Anesth Analg.* 2005;101:1275.
66. Thomas EJ, Goldman L, Mangione CM, et al. Body mass index as a correlate of postoperative complications and resource utilization. *Am J Med.* 1997;102:277.
67. Rosen AK, Geraci JM, Ash AS, et al. Postoperative adverse events of common surgical procedures in the Medicare population. *Med Care.* 1992;30:753.
68. Rankin J, Hammill B, Ferguson T, et al. Determinants of operative mortality in valvular heart surgery. *J Thorac Cardiovasc Surg.* 2006;131:3:547.
69. Lawrence VA, Hilsenbeck SG, Noveck H, et al. Medical complications and outcomes after hip fracture repair. *Arch Intern Med.* 2002;162:2053.
70. Escarce JJ, Shea JA, Chen W, et al. Outcomes of open cholecystectomy in the elderly: a longitudinal analysis of 21,000 cases in the prelaparoscopic era. *Surgery.* 1995;117:156.
71. Pedersen T. Complications and death following anaesthesia. A prospective study with special reference to the influence of patient-, anaesthesia-, and surgery-related risk factors. *Dan Med Bull.* 1994;41:319.
72. Manku K, Bacchetti P, Leung JM. Prognostic significance of postoperative in-hospital complications in elderly patients, I: long-term survival. *Anesth Analg.* 2003;96:583.
73. Arozullah AM, Daley J, Henderson WG, et al. Multifactorial risk index for predicting postoperative respiratory failure in men after major noncardiac surgery. The National Veterans Administration Surgical Quality Improvement Program. *Ann Surg.* 2000;232:242.
74. Arozullah AM, Khuri SF, Henderson WG, et al. Development and validation of a multifactorial risk index for predicting postoperative pneumonia after major noncardiac surgery. *Ann Intern Med.* 2001;135:847.
75. O'Brien MM, Gonzales R, Shroyer AL, et al. Modest serum creatinine elevation affects adverse outcome after general surgery. *Kidney Int,* 2002;62:585.
76. Gibbs J, Cull W, Henderson W, et al. Preoperative serum albumin level as a predictor of operative mortality and morbidity: results from the National VA Surgical Risk Study. *Arch Surg.* 1999;134:36.
77. Smetana GW, Macpherson DS. The case against routine preoperative laboratory testing. *Med Clin North Am.* 2003;87:7.
78. Archer C, Levy AR, McGregor M. Value of routine preoperative chest x-rays: a meta-analysis. *Can J Anaesth.* 1993;40:1022.
79. Celli B, Cote C, Marin J, et al. The body-mass index, airflow obstruction, dyspnoea and exercise capacity index in chronic obstructive pulmonary disease. *N Eng J Med.* 2004;350:1005.
80. Mazzone P, Aroliga A. Preoperative pulmonary evaluation of the lung resection candidate. *Am J Med.* 2005;118:578.
81. Slinger P, Johnston M. Preoperative assessment for pulmonary resection. *J Cardiothorac Vasc Anesth.* 2000;14:202.
82. Qaseem A, Snow V, Fitterman N, et al. Risk assessment for and strategies to reduce perioperative pulmonary complications for patients undergoing noncardiothoracic surgery: a Guideline from the American College of Physicians. *Ann Int Med.* 2006;144:575.
83. Bluman LG, Mosca L, Newman N, et al. Preoperative smoking habits and postoperative pulmonary complications. *Chest.* 1998;113:883.
84. Blouw E, Rudolph A, Narr B, et al. The frequency of respiratory failure in patients with morbid obesity undergoing gastric bypass. *AANA J.* 2003;71:45.
85. Acute Respiratory Distress Syndrome Network. Ventilation with lower tidal volumes as compared with traditional tidal volumes for acute lung injury and the acute respiratory distress syndrome. *N Eng J Med.* 2000;342:1301.
86. Pauwels RA, Buist AS, Calverley PM, et al. Global strategy for the diagnosis, management, and prevention of chronic obstructive pulmonary disease. NHLBI/WHO Global Initiative for Chronic Obstructive Lung Disease (GOLD) Workshop summary. *Am J Resp Crit Care Med.* 2001;163:1256.
87. Warner DO, Warner MA, Offord KP, et al. Airway obstruction and perioperative complications in smokers undergoing abdominal surgery. *Anesthesiology.* 1999;90:372.
88. Warner DO, Warner MA, Barnes RD, et al. Perioperative respiratory complications in patients with asthma. *Anesthesiology.* 1996;85:460.
89. Milledge JS, Nunn JF. Criteria of fitness for anaesthesia in patients with chronic obstructive lung disease. *BMJ.* 1975;3:670.
90. Groeben H, Schlicht M, Stieglitz S, et al. Both local anesthetics and salbutamol pretreatment affect reflex bronchoconstriction in volunteers with asthma undergoing awake fiberoptic intubation. *Anesthesiology.* 2002; 97:1445.
91. Silvanus MT, Groeben H, Peters J. Corticosteroids and inhaled salbutamol in patients with reversible airway obstruction markedly decrease the incidence of bronchospasm after tracheal intubation. *Anesthesiology.* 2004;100:1052.
92. Maslow AD, Regan MM, Israel E, et al. Inhaled albuterol, but not intravenous lidocaine, protect against intubation-induced bronchoconstriction in asthma. *Anesthesiology.* 2000;93:1198.
93. Sauder RA, Lenox WC, Tobias JD, et al. Methylprednisolone increases sensitivity to β-adrenergic agonists within 48 hours in Basenji greyhounds. *Anesthesiology.* 1993;79:1278.
94. Barnes PJ. Mechanisms of action of glucocorticoids in asthma. *Am J Resp Crit Care Med.* 1996;154:S21.
95. Pien LC, Grammer LC, Patterson R. Minimal complications in a surgical population with severe asthma receiving prophylactic corticosteroids. *J Allergy Clin Immunol.* 1988;82:696.
96. Belda J, Parameswaran K, Rowe BH. Addition of intravenous aminophylline to beta 2-agonists in adults with acute asthma. The Cochrane Library 2001;2:1.
97. Tait A, Malviya S. Anesthesia for the child with an upper respiratory tract infection: still a Dilemma? *Anesth Analg.* 2005;100:59.
98. Ferguson GT. Recommendations for the management of COPD. *Chest.* 2000;117:23S.
99. Braunschweig CL, Levy P, Sheean PM, et al. Enteral compared with parenteral nutrition: a meta-analysis. *Am J Clin Nutr.* 2001;74:534.
100. Sacks GS, Genton L, Kudsk KA. Controversy of immunonutrition for surgical critical-illness patients. *Curr Opin Crit Care.* 2003;9:300.
101. U.S. Renal Data System, USRDS 2006 Annual Data Report: Atlas of End-Stage Renal Disease in the United States. Bethesda, MD: National Institutes of Health, National Institute of Diabetes and Digestive and Kidney Diseases; 2006.
102. Ritz E, Orth SR. Nephropathy in patients with type 2 diabetes mellitus. *N Engl J Med.* 1999;341:1127.
103. Danaei G, Lawes CMM, Vander Hoorn S, et al. Global and regional mortality from ischaemic heart disease and stroke attributable to higher-than-optimum blood glucose concentration: comparative risk assessment. *Lancet.* 2006;368:1651.
104. Peterson JC, Adler S, Burkart JM, et al. Blood pressure control, proteinuria, and the progression of renal disease. The Modification of Diet in Renal Disease Study. *Ann Intern Med.* 1995;123:754.
105. National Kidney Foundation. K/DOQI clinical practice guidelines for chronic renal disease: evaluation, classification and stratification. *Am J Kidney Dis.* 2002;39:S1.
106. Levey AS, Bosch JP, Lewis JB, et al. A more accurate method to estimate glomerular filtration rate from serum creatinine: a new prediction equation. *Ann Intern Med.* 1999;130:461.
107. Safi HJ, Harlin SA, Miller CC, et al. Predictive factors for acute renal failure in thoracic and thoracoabdominal aortic aneurysm surgery. *J Vasc Surg.* 1996;24:338.
108. Kashyap VS, Cambria RP, Davison K, et al. Renal failure after thoracoabdominal aortic surgery. *J Vasc Surg.* 1997;26:949.
109. Conlon PJ, Stafford-Smith M, White WD, et al. Acute renal failure following cardiac surgery. *Nephrol Dial Transplant.* 1999;14:1158.
110. Ascione R, Lloyd CT, Underwood MJ, et al. On-pump versus off-pump coronary revascularization: evaluation of renal function. *Ann Thorac Surg.* 1999;68:493.
111. Ascione R, Nason G, Al-Ruzzeh S, et al. Coronary revascularization with or without cardiopulmonary bypass in patients with preoperative non-dialysis-dependent renal insufficiency. *Ann Thorac Surg.* 2001;72: 2020.
112. Swaminathan M, Stafford-Smith M. Renal dysfunction after vascular surgery. *Curr Opin Anaesthesiol.* 2003;16:45.
113. Hertzer N, Mascha EJ, Karafa MT, et al. Open infrarenal abdominal aortic aneurysm repair: the Cleveland Clinic experience from 1989 to 1998. *J Vasc Surg.* 2002;35:1145.
114. Sweeney KJ, Evoy D, Sultan S, et al. Endovascular approach to abdominal aortic aneurysms limits the postoperative systemic immune response. *Eur J Vasc Endovasc Surg.* 2002;23:303.
115. Wijnen MHWA, Cuypers P, Buth J, et al. Differences in renal response between endovascular and open repair of abdominal aortic aneurysms. *Eur J Vasc Endovasc Surg.* 2001;21:171.
116. Prinssen M, Verhoeven ELG, Buth J, et al. A randomized trial comparing conventional and endovascular repair of abdominal aortic aneurysms. *N Engl J Med.* 2004;351:1607.
117. Parmer SS, Fairman RM, Karmacharya J, et al. A comparison of renal function between open and endovascular aneurysm repair in patients with baseline chronic renal insufficiency. *J Vasc Surg.* 2006;44:706.
118. Bellomo R, Ronco C, Kellum JA, et al. Acute renal failure-definition, outcome measures, animal models, fluid therapy and information technology needs: the second international consensus conference of the Acute Dialysis Quality Initiative (ADQI) group. *Crit Care.* 2004;8:R204.
119. Trivedi HS, Moore H, Nasr S, et al. A randomized prospective trial to assess

the role of saline hydration on the development of contrast nephrotoxicity. *Nephron Clin.* 2003;93:C29.
120. Gunal AL, Celiker H, Dogukan A, et al. Early and vigorous resuscitation prevents acute renal failure in the crush victims of catastrophic earthquakes. *J Am Soc Nephrol.* 2004;15:1862.
121. Mertens GJ, Burgess WP, Gray LV, et al. Prevention of contrast-induced nephropathy with sodium bicarbonate. *JAMA.* 2004;291:2328.
122. Parikh S, Cohen JR. Perioperative stroke after general surgical procedures. *N Y State J Med.* 1993;93:162.
123. Evans BA, Wijdicks EFM. High-grade carotid stenosis detected before general surgery: is endarterectomy indicated? *Neurology.* 2001;57:1328.
124. Ellis JE, Roizen MF, Mantha S, et al. Anesthesia for vascular surgery. In: Barash PG, ed. *Clinical Anesthesia.* 3rd ed. Philadelphia, PA: Lippincott Williams & Wilkins; 1997:880.
125. Naylor AR, Rothwell PM, Bell PRF. Overview of the principal results and secondary analyses from the European and North American randomized trials of endarterectomy for symptomatic carotid stenosis. *Eur J Vasc Endovasc Surg.* 2003;26:115.
126. Biller J, Feinberg WM, Castaldo JE, et al. Guidelines for carotid endarterectomy. A statement for healthcare professionals from a special writing group of the Stroke Council, American Heart Association. *Stroke.* 1998;29:554.
127. Taggart DP, Westaby S. Neurological and cognitive disorders after coronary artery bypass grafting. *Curr Opin Cardiol.* 2001;16:271.
128. Djaiani GN. Aortic arch atheroma: stroke reduction in cardiac surgical patients. *Semin Cardiothorac Vasc Anesth.* 2006;10:143.
129. Paciaroni M, Eliasziw M, Kappelle J, et al. Medical complications associated with carotid endarterectomy. *Stroke.* 1999;30:1759.
130. Jabbour PM, Awad IA, Huddle D. Hemorrhagic cerebrovascular disease. In: Layon AJ, ed. *Textbook of Neurointensive Care.* 1st ed. Philadelphia, PA: WB Saunders; 2004:155.
131. Suarez JI, Tarr RW, Selman WR. Aneurysmal subarachnoid hemorrhage. *N Engl J Med.* 2006;354:387.
132. Berkow LC, Mirski M, Kirsch JR. Subarachnoid hemorrhage and cerebrovascular accident. In: Murray MJ, ed. *Critical Care Medicine. Perioperative Management.* 2nd ed. Philadelphia, PA: Lippincott Williams & Wilkins; 2002:264.
133. Sato M, Nakano M, Sasanuma J, et al. Preoperative cerebral aneurysm assessment by three-dimensional magnetic resonance angiography: feasibility of surgery without conventional catheter angiography. *Neurosurgery.* 2005;56:903.
134. Karamessini MT, Kagadis GC, Petsas T, et al. CT angiography with three-dimensional techniques for the early diagnosis of intracranial aneurysm. Comparison with intra-arterial DSA and the surgical findings. *Eur J Radiol.* 2004;49:212.
135. Rinkel GJ, Feigin VL, Algra A, et al. Calcium antagonist for aneurysmal subarachnoid hemorrhage. *Cochrane Database Syst Rev.* 2005;1:CD000277.
136. Kuntscher MV, Germann G, Hartmann B. Correlation between cardiac output, stroke volume, central venous pressure, intra-abdominal pressure and total circulating blood volume in resuscitation of major burns. *Resuscitation.* 2006;70:37.
137. Kim DH, Haney CL, Van Ginhoven G. Reduction of pulmonary edema after SAH with pulmonary artery catheter-guided hemodynamic management protocol. *Neurocrit Care.* 2005;3:11.
138. Lobato EB, Sulek CA. Cardiac care in neurosurgery. In: Layon AJ, ed. *Textbook of Neurointensive Care.* 1st ed. Philadelphia, PA: WB Saunders; 2004:533.
139. Apostolides PJ, Greene KA, Zambramski JM, et al. Intraaortic balloon pump counterpulsation in the management of concomitant cerebral vasospasm and cardiac failure after subarachnoid hemorrhage. Technical case report. *Neurosurgery.* 1996;38:1056.
140. Nussbaum ES, Sebring LA, Ganz WF, et al. Intra-aortic balloon counterpulsation augments cerebral blood flow in the patient with cerebral vasospasm: a xenon-enhanced computed tomography study. *Neurosurgery.* 1998;42:206.
141. Friedman JA, Pichelmann MA, Piepgras DG, et al. Pulmonary complications of aneurysmal subarachnoid hemorrhage. *Neurosurgery.* 2003;52:1025.
142. Wartenberg KE, Mayer SA. Medical complications after subarachnoid hemorrhage: new strategies for prevention and management. *Curr Opin Crit Care.* 2006;12:78.
143. van Den Bergh WM, Zuur JK, Kamerling NA, et al. Role of magnesium in the reduction of ischemic depolarization and lesion volume after experimental subarachnoid hemorrhage. *J Neurosurg.* 2002;97:416.
144. Ram Z, Sadeh M, Shacked I, et al. Magnesium sulfate reverses experimental delayed cerebral vasospasm after subarachnoid hemorrhage in rats. *Stroke.* 1991;22:922.
145. van den Bergh WM, Algra A, van Kooten F, et al. Magnesium sulfate in aneurysmal subarachnoid hemorrhage. *Stroke.* 2005;36:1011.
146. Bruno A, Biller J, Adams HP, et al. Acute blood glucose level and outcome from ischemic stroke. *Neurology.* 1999;52:280.

CHAPTER 71 ■ ANESTHESIA: PHYSIOLOGY AND POSTANESTHESIA PROBLEMS

ERAN SEGAL • A. JOSEPH LAYON

IMMEDIATE CONCERNS

Major Problems

Modern anesthesia is a complex art and science that involves exposing patients to various drugs and procedures in a controlled and safe environment. Even under the best of circumstances, some complications occur. The overall risk of death from anesthesia is between 1 in 112,000 and 1 in 450,000 (1). Anesthetic-related morbidity is even more common, with respiratory depression noted between 1 in 500 and 1 in 1,100 patients receiving epidural narcotics, and 1 in 100 patients given parenteral opioids (1). Studies reviewing adverse incidents and claims due to anesthetic mishaps have shown that the most common reasons for adverse events are due to respiratory problems, followed by neural injury and damage due to regional anesthesia (2). The characteristics of anesthetic injuries have changed over the past years, with an increase in problems related to cardiovascular issues and a decrease in those related to the respiratory system (3). Patients who sustain an anesthetic complication may require treatment in the intensive care unit (ICU).

Airway problems are still extremely common causes for critical perioperative anesthetic mishaps, as maintaining an adequate airway is the first priority in all anesthetic management. An algorithm for airway management during anesthesia has been formulated by the American Society of Anesthesiologists (4) (Fig. 71.1).

In the immediate postoperative period, effects from residual anesthetic and muscle relaxants may result in airway obstruction, which should be quickly diagnosed and treated.

AMERICAN SOCIETY OF ANESTHESIOLOGISTS

DIFFICULT AIRWAY ALGORITHM

1. Assess the likelihood and clinical impact of basic management problems:
   - A. Difficult Ventilation
   - B. Difficult Intubation
   - C. Difficulty with Patient Cooperation or Consent
   - D. Difficult Tracheostomy
2. Actively pursue opportunities to deliver supplemental oxygen throughout the process of difficult airway managemen
3. Consider the relative merits and feasibility of basic management choices:

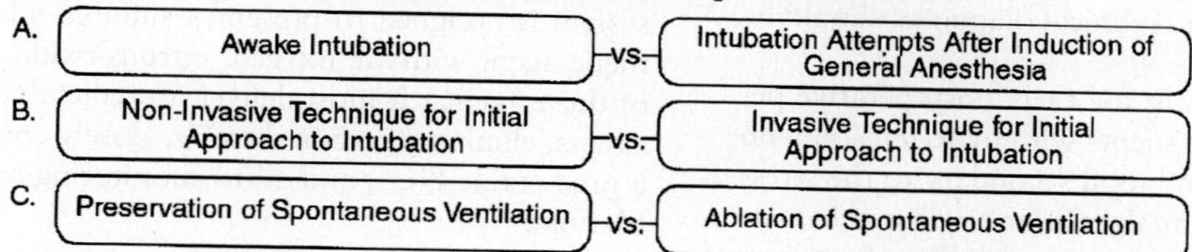

4. Develop primary and alternative strategies:

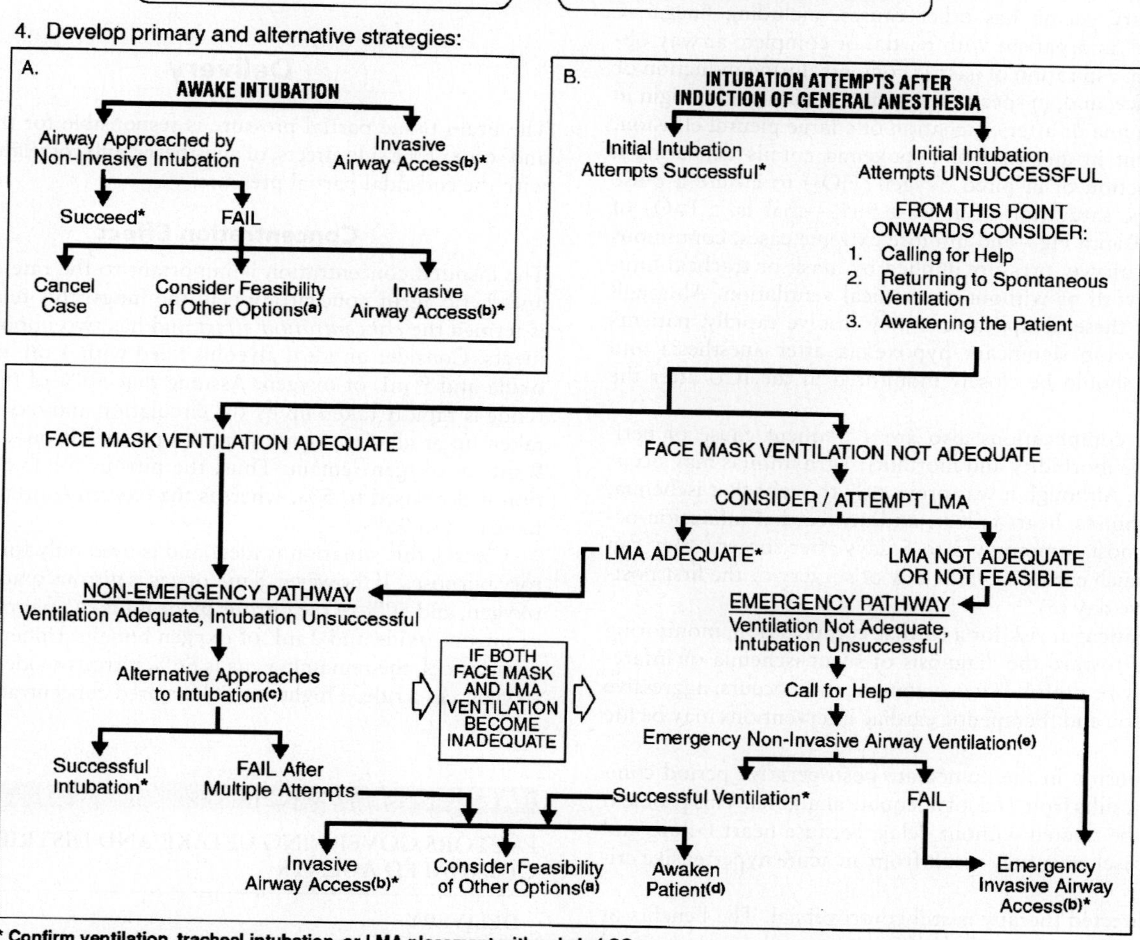

* **Confirm ventilation, tracheal intubation, or LMA placement with exhaled CO_2**

a. Other options include (but are not limited to): surgery utilizing face mask or LMA anesthesia, local anesthesia infiltration or regional nerve blockade. Pursuit of these options usually implies that mask ventilation will not be problematic. Therefore, these options may be of limited value if this step in the algorithm has been reached via the Emergency Pathway.

b. Invasive airway access includes surgical or percutaneous tracheostomy or cricothyrotomy.

c. Alternative non-invasive approaches to difficult intubation include (but are not limited to): use of different laryngoscope blades, LMA as an intubation conduit (with or without fiberoptic guidance), fiberoptic intubation, intubating stylet or tube changer, light wand, retrograde intubation, and blind oral or nasal intubation.

d. Consider re-preparation of the patient for awake intubation or canceling surgery.

e. Options for emergency non-invasive airway ventilation include (but are not limited to): rigid bronchoscope, esophageal-tracheal combitube ventilation, or transtracheal jet ventilation.

FIGURE 71.1. American Society of Anesthesiologists difficult airway algorithm.

Hypoventilation is also a common problem. Patients should be aggressively monitored with pulse oximetry and capnography, and oxygen should be given to postoperative patients until they are shown to have adequate ventilatory drive and pulmonary function.

STRESS POINTS

1. Postoperative acute respiratory failure is an uncommon but dramatic complication. Several clinical diagnoses should be explored in these situations.
2. Pulmonary edema can occur in the early postoperative period. It is more common in patients with hypertension who develop an acute elevation in blood secondary to the stress response, lack of significant analgesia, or cardiac ischemia.
3. Pulmonary edema has other causes, including "negative pressure" in a patient with partial or complete airway obstruction, aspiration of gastric contents during induction or emergence, and, in special situations, a neurogenic origin in head trauma or after evacuation of a large pleural effusion.
4. Treatment in any case of hypoxemia entails delivering a high fraction of inspired oxygen (FiO_2) to ensure a pulse oximetric saturation of at least 90%—that is, a PaO_2 of about 60 mm Hg—and in more extreme cases, continuous positive airway pressure applied by mask or tracheal intubation, with or without mechanical ventilation. Although some of these complications may resolve rapidly, patients who develop significant hypoxemia after anesthesia and surgery should be closely monitored in the ICU after the event.
5. Cardiac complications also are a frequent cause of perioperative morbidity and mortality. Arrhythmias may occur anytime. Although it was previously thought that ischemia, dysrhythmias, heart failure, and myocardial infarction occurred most commonly 3 to 5 days after surgery, they can occur much earlier—on the day of surgery or the first postoperative day (5).
6. In the patient at risk for a cardiac complication, monitoring directed toward the diagnosis of silent ischemia or infarction may be useful. When a complication occurs, aggressive diagnostic and therapeutic cardiac interventions may be life saving.
7. Hypertension in the immediate postoperative period commonly results from lack of adequate analgesia. This problem should be treated without delay, because heart failure and cardiac ischemia may result from an acute hypertensive crisis.
8. Goal-directed therapy is still controversial. The benefits of aggressive monitoring and achieving normal or supranormal hemodynamic values in patients undergoing major surgery, who have suffered trauma, or who are septic are unclear. At the same time, it makes sense to monitor patients at least to a degree that allows the rapid identification and prompt therapy of disturbed respiratory and hemodynamic function.
9. Patients with malignant hyperthermia (MH) may develop the syndrome at any time after exposure to a triggering agent (e.g., potent inhalational agents or succinylcholine). When MH is suspected, all triggering agents must be stopped. If possible, surgery should be canceled, and dantrolene administered (6). An MH hotline is available in many countries and can be contacted for assistance in caring for these patients.

UPTAKE AND DISTRIBUTION OF INHALATIONAL AGENTS

The goal of inhalational anesthesia is to develop a critical partial pressure of the agent within the brain. Brain levels are determined by several discrete steps (7) (Table 71.1). The anesthesia system is designed to present a suitable mixture of the anesthetic agent with air, oxygen, nitrous oxide, or a combination of these agents. It must deliver a predictable concentration of agents, eliminate carbon dioxide, closely control and maintain a predictable FiO_2, and allow monitoring and control of ventilation.

Delivery

The brain tissue partial pressure is responsible for the depth, and some of the side effects, of anesthesia, and correlates closely with the end-tidal partial pressure.

Concentration Effect

The inspired concentration is important to the rate of rise of anesthetic agent concentration in the lungs; this relationship is termed the *concentration effect* and has two important elements. Consider an ideal alveolus filled with 1 mL of nitrous oxide and 9 mL of oxygen. Assume that 50% of the nitrous oxide is rapidly taken up by the circulation and oxygen is not taken up at all. On completion, 0.5 mL of nitrous oxide and 9 mL of oxygen remain. Thus, the nitrous oxide concentration is decreased to 5%, whereas the oxygen concentration is increased to 95%.

Clearly, this situation is ideal and is used only for explanatory purposes. If, however, 8 mL of gas is nitrous oxide, 2 mL is oxygen, and 50% of the nitrous oxide is taken up rapidly, 4 mL of nitrous oxide and 2 mL of oxygen remain. Under these circumstances, the remaining gas is 66% nitrous oxide and 33% oxygen. As a rule, a higher initial inspired concentration of the

TABLE 71.1

FACTORS GOVERNING UPTAKE AND DISTRIBUTION OF INHALED AGENTS

DELIVERY
Inspired concentration
Concentration effect
Second gas effect
Ventilation
UPTAKE FROM LUNGS
Solubility
Cardiac output
Alveolar–mixed venous partial pressure gradient
DISTRIBUTION TO TISSUES
Solubility of agent in tissue
Blood flow to tissue

agent results in a higher alveolar level in spite of uptake from the lung.

Second Gas Effect

When large amounts of an anesthetic agent such as nitrous oxide are rapidly taken up, the lungs do not collapse. Instead, a subatmospheric alveolar pressure is generated as a result of the rapid removal of this gas by the pulmonary blood flow, and a passive inflow of additional gas from the anesthesia circuit replaces that which is taken up. This second gas effect may have important consequences and can be used to clinical advantage. When another anesthetic agent is administered, its partial pressure increase is also more rapid than when it is administered alone because it is drawn into the lungs with the first agent.

Alveolar Ventilation

Another primary factor influencing the delivery of the anesthetic agent is alveolar ventilation ($\dot{V}_A$). In other words, a greater $\dot{V}_A$ increases the rate at which the alveolar partial pressure approaches the inspired partial pressure. This factor is limited only by lung volume; that is, a larger functional residual capacity decreases the "wash-in" rate of the agent.

Uptake from the Lungs

Solubility

Solubility describes the extent to which the anesthetic agent dissolves in blood and tissues (Tables 71.1 and 71.2); the more soluble the agent is in blood, the more is dissolved in the pulmonary blood and the longer it takes to reach a necessary partial pressure of agent in the lungs and brain. This fact represents the key difference between inhaled agents and other commonly used drugs. For example, 2 g of ampicillin given intravenously is dissolved in blood, carried to the site of infection, and produces the desired pharmacologic effect. The partial pressure of the anesthetic agent reaching the brain is the determinant of its desired effect, but is controlled by the partial pressure achieved in the alveoli. Thus, the greater the amount of anesthetic dissolved in the blood—taken away from the alveoli—the longer it takes to develop the necessary alveolar and brain partial pressures to produce anesthesia.

TABLE 71.2

PARTITION COEFFICIENTS OF SELECTED INHALATIONAL AGENTS (AT 37°C ± 0.5°C)

Agent	Blood/gas	Tissue/blood
Nitrous oxide	0.47	Brain: 1.06
Isoflurane	1.41	Brain: 2.6 Fat: 45.0
Enflurane	1.78	Brain: 1.45 Fat: 36.2
Halothane	2.36	Brain: 2.6 Fat: 60
Sevoflurane	0.69	Brain: 1.7 Fat: 48
Desflurane	0.42	Brain: 1.3 Fat: 27

An agent such as nitrous oxide, with a blood/gas partition coefficient of 0.47, is relatively insoluble, and its alveolar partial pressure increases rapidly compared with that of halothane, which has a blood/gas partition coefficient of 2.36. The speed of induction of a more soluble agent can be increased by increasing the inspired fraction to a level well in excess of that required for maintenance of anesthesia (7).

Cardiac Output

A high cardiac output increases uptake, thereby decreasing the alveolar partial pressure of the agent. This effect is greater with more soluble inhalational anesthetics. Thus, a longer induction time is required for a patient with a high cardiac output, as in thyrotoxicosis. Conversely, a patient with a low cardiac output, as with compensated congestive cardiomyopathy, has a rapid increase of alveolar partial pressure, resulting in a rapid induction and possible overdose if care is not taken.

Alveolar–Mixed Venous Anesthetic Partial Pressure Gradient

The last major factor of importance is the influence of the alveolar–to–central mixed venous anesthetic partial pressure gradient. This factor relates the size of the anesthetic "sink" to the increase or decrease in uptake from the lungs. At the beginning of induction when the tissue anesthetic level is zero, most of the anesthetic in the arterial blood is removed. Thus, the venous anesthetic partial pressure is much lower than that in the arterial blood, and a large uptake of anesthetic occurs as the venous blood passes through the lungs. The alveolar partial pressure of the anesthetic agent, accordingly, is reduced. However, as the tissue sinks become filled, the alveolar to venous anesthetic partial pressure difference decreases, and this effect is minimized.

Distribution

Tissue Solubility and Blood Flow

The tissue distribution (delivery) of the anesthetic is dependent on two major factors (Table 71.1). The greater the solubility of an anesthetic in a tissue, the larger the capacity of that tissue for the agent. If the tissue has a large capacity but low blood flow, equilibration takes a long time; if the tissue has a small capacity and large blood flow, equilibration is rapid. Tissues can be categorized according to the blood flow they receive. The vessel-rich group is composed of the brain, liver, heart, and kidneys. An intermediate group includes muscle and skin. The vessel-poor group incorporates skeletal elements, ligaments, and cartilage, all of which have minimal blood supply. Finally, fat has a poor blood supply but a great capacity.

Based on this division, one can easily determine when the different groups equilibrate with the inspired fraction of anesthetic agent, that is, when they cease removing appreciable amounts of the anesthetic. Nitrous oxide equilibration with the vessel-rich group occurs within 5 to 15 minutes from the beginning of induction. The muscle group equilibrates within approximately 1 hour, and the vessel-poor group and fat group equilibrate within 2 to 3 hours. When a highly fat-soluble agent such as halothane is used for a long case in an obese patient, significant amounts of agent are stored in fat and are released slowly after the agent is discontinued; emergence from anesthesia is thereby prolonged. At the end of surgery, the factors that affect elimination of the agent from the body are the same as those that govern the uptake and distribution at the beginning. Hypoventilation lengthens the period of emergence, as do increased cardiac output, use of a highly soluble anesthetic agent, and an increased alveolar-to-venous anesthetic concentration gradient.

Diffusion Hypoxia

Diffusion hypoxia may be apparent at the conclusion of an anesthetic if the patient is allowed to breathe room air while large quantities of nitrous oxide diffuse into the alveoli and dilute the oxygen that is present. This problem is significant only for approximately 10 minutes and can be alleviated by having the patient breathe 100% oxygen after discontinuation of the nitrous oxide.

Effects of Illness

Changes in Ventilation

Organ system dysfunction can affect the uptake and distribution of inhaled anesthetic agents. For example, to control intracranial pressure (ICP) in brain-injured patients, tracheal intubation and mechanical hyperventilation may be used. For each 1 mm Hg decrease in the $PaCO_2$ caused by an increase in $\dot{V}_A$, an approximate 3% to 4% decrease in cerebral blood flow (CBF) occurs. If the patient is taken to the operating room, and if hyperventilation is continued, a change in the length of time of anesthetic induction results from three factors: increased $\dot{V}_A$, decreased CBF, and solubility of the inhaled agents used for induction. The induction time for a moderately soluble agent like halothane is decreased because the increased $\dot{V}_A$ produces a more rapid rise in end-tidal halothane partial pressure that offsets the decrease in CBF. For a relatively nonsoluble agent such as nitrous oxide, induction time is increased because the modest increase in end-tidal nitrous oxide partial pressure obtained by hyperventilation is more than offset by the decrease in CBF.

Changes in Cardiac Output

This particular example can become complicated by a decrease in cardiac output, secondary to hyperventilation-induced alkalemia, and a decrease in venous return, resulting from fluid restriction and the effects of mechanical ventilation. The decrease in cardiac output yields an increase in the agent's end-tidal partial pressure, whereas a decrease in CBF decreases transfer of the agent from the lungs to the brain. With halothane, the increase in the end-tidal partial pressure is sufficient to balance the decrease in CBF; thus, the initial rise in brain partial pressure may be normal. Eventually, no matter what agent is used, the increased end-tidal partial pressure resulting from the decrease in cardiac output and increase in $\dot{V}_A$ is enough to overcome the decrease in CBF.

INHALATION AGENTS AND ORGAN SYSTEM FUNCTION

The differential effects of various inhalation agents on organ system function must be compared at equipotent doses. The minimum alveolar concentration (MAC) is the amount of an inhalational agent that prevents movement in 50% of patients in response to surgical incision (Table 71.3). In neonates, the MAC is less than in children, adolescents, and young adults. After approximately 31 years of age, the MAC value begins to decrease; theoretically, the value for a patient 100 years of age is only 25% to 50% that of a young adult.

TABLE 71.3

MINIMUM ALVEOLAR CONCENTRATION IN PATIENTS AGED 31–55 YRS

Halothane	0.75%
Isoflurane	1.15%
Enflurane	1.68%
Nitrous oxide	110%[a]
Desflurane	6%
Sevoflurane	2.05%

[a] Obtainable only under hyperbaric conditions.

Circulatory Effects

Blood pressure is decreased with the use of all inhalational agents. This may be due to decreased contractility as with halothane, or due to decreased systemic vascular resistance as with isoflurane or desflurane (7). There is some concern regarding the effect of inhalational anesthetics on the coronary circulation. Isoflurane and desflurane lead to coronary vasodilatation and may cause ischemia, although desflurane probably has a significantly lesser effect on coronary blood flow than the other inhalational agents (8). The effect of both isoflurane and desflurane on contractility is less than halothane and enflurane (8).

Cardiac Rhythm

Of the several methods for evaluation of the effects of inhalational agents on cardiac rhythm, a common procedure is to determine the dose of epinephrine required to produce three or more premature ventricular contractions in 50% of normal patients breathing oxygen and anesthetized at 1.25 MAC (Table 71.4). With halothane, 2.1 μg of epinephrine/kg body weight is required to produce rhythm abnormalities; if the epinephrine is given with 0.5% lidocaine, the required dose increases to 3.7 μg/kg. With isoflurane, 6.7 μg/kg of epinephrine is needed, and with enflurane, approximately 10.9 μg/kg is required. Desflurane and sevoflurane have properties similar to those of enflurane. Thus, halothane is the most and enflurane, desflurane, and sevoflurane are the least arrhythmogenic of the potent inhalation anesthetic agents. Inhalational agents may lead to prolongation of the QT segment; desflurane at a concentration of 6% led to a significant increase in QTc in children, whereas 2% sevoflurane did not (9).

Hypoxic Pulmonary Vasoconstriction

Hypoxic pulmonary vasoconstriction (HPV) may be impaired when potent agents are used. If inhaled concentrations of halothane or enflurane are increased *in vitro* from 1 to 2 MAC and $PaCO_2$ is held constant, the local response to hypoxia is

TABLE 71.4

RESPIRATORY AND CIRCULATORY EFFECTS OF THE INHALATION AGENTS

	N_2O	Halothane	Enflurane	Isoflurane
Respiratory				
$\dot{V}_E$	↓	↓	↓↓↓	↓↓
% awake response to CO_2	↓↓	↓↓	↓↓	↓↓
% awake response to hypoxia	—	↓	↓↓	↓↓
Circulatory				
% awake ballistocardiogram	—	↓	↓↓	θ
% awake cardiac output	θ	↓	↓	θ
% awake stroke volume	θ	↓	↓↓	↓
μg/kg epinephrine for three or more PVCs	—	2.1–3.7	10.9	6.7

—, no data; θ, no change; ↓, decrease of ≤33%; ↓↓, decrease of ≤66%; ↓↓↓, decrease of ≥66%; PVCs, premature ventricular contractions; N_2O, nitrous oxide; $\dot{V}_E$, expired volume per min; CO_2, carbon dioxide.

unchanged. Under these same conditions using isoflurane, HPV seems to be significantly impaired; with desflurane, HPV is inhibited in a concentration-dependent fashion (10). However, the clinical significance of the difference between the anesthetic agents in this regard is not clear. When looking at a porcine model of one-lung anesthesia, neither isoflurane nor desflurane were found to have a deleterious effect on oxygenation (11).

Respiratory Effects

All inhalational agents are respiratory depressants. Decreases in minute ventilation at 1 MAC are 20% with nitrous oxide, 28% with halothane, 34% with isoflurane, and 71% with enflurane. The ventilatory response to an elevation in $PaCO_2$ at 1 MAC is decreased by 50% with nitrous oxide, 60% with halothane, 35% with isoflurane, and 45% with enflurane (Table 71.4). The response to hypoxia is depressed by 30% with halothane, 40% with isoflurane, and 45% with enflurane. There is probably some genetic predisposition in the sensitivity to the different anesthetic agents. It has been shown in animal models that subjects may respond differently to the different anesthetics, but at a dose of 0.5 MAC, all anesthetics blunt the response to hypercapnia (12).

Hepatic Effects

Up to 20% of patients may demonstrate mild disturbances in liver function following anesthesia with halothane; these effects present as mild abnormalities of liver function tests (7). They may also be due to other physiologic disturbances such as hemodynamic abnormalities during surgery or blood transfusion. The incidence is lower when other inhalational agents are used, and to some degree this has been one of the reasons for the marked reduction in the use of halothane as a common anesthetic agent, which is the concern regarding halothane hepatitis.

Patients who underwent surgery and anesthesia with isoflurane and halothane manifested a slight increase in alanine aminotransferase (ALT), aspartate aminotransferase (AST), and lactate dehydrogenase. The changes seen with halothane may be greater than those observed with isoflurane. A comparison of low-dose sevoflurane, high-dose sevoflurane, and isoflurane showed comparable mild increases in liver enzymes following a prolonged (greater than 10 hours) exposure in patients undergoing orthopedic surgery (13). A statistically significant increase in bromsulphthalein retention on the second postoperative day also was seen with halothane and isoflurane. The increase was greater with halothane. Neither desflurane nor sevoflurane seems to have hepatotoxic properties (14).

Renal Effects

All potent inhalation agents result in a dose-dependent decrease in renal blood flow from 25% to 50%, glomerular filtration rate from 23% to 40%, and urine flow from 35% to 67%. No change in creatinine clearance or ability to concentrate urine in response to subcutaneous injection of vasopressin occurs after the use of isoflurane, halothane, or enflurane. However, when comparing high- and low-dose sevoflurane to isoflurane, no significant changes in renal functions were observed in any of the groups (13). In patients with preoperative renal impairment, anesthesia with either desflurane or isoflurane did not lead to worsened renal function (15).

Immune Function

Anesthesia and surgery may impair immune system function, at least *in vitro* (Table 71.5) (16). Serious questions as to cause and effect and the relevance to clinical outcome have been raised. There are many effects on nonspecific immune system components (17).

An element of immune dysfunction may be caused by stress, with elevations in norepinephrine, epinephrine, steroids, inflammatory mediators, and other mediators of the stress response. If this supposition is true, perhaps different anesthetic techniques (18,19), or even the use of sympathetic blockade, might ameliorate these responses perioperatively and thus decrease some of the reported abnormalities.

TABLE 71.5

EFFECTS OF INHALATION AGENTS ON IMMUNE FUNCTION

	N_2O	Halothane	Enflurane	Isoflurane
Monocyte function	?	↓	?	?
Natural killer cell activity	↑[a]	↓, ?	?	?
ADCC K-cell activity	?	?	?	?
Neutrophil function	?	↓	↓	↓
Lymphocyte function	θ[a]	↓, ?	↓, ?	?

θ, no change; ↑, activity/function increased; ↓, activity/function decreased; ?, needs study; ADCC, antibody-dependent cellular cytotoxicity; N_2O, nitrous oxide.
[a]Used with intravenous anesthesia.

Phagocytosis

Phagocytosis reportedly is depressed perioperatively, perhaps because of surgical stress and the direct effects of inhalation anesthetic agents (17). Everson et al. (20) showed increased monocytic function in the first 24 hours postoperatively in patients who had undergone an operative procedure for nonmalignant disease. Patients who underwent surgery for carcinoma had no change in monocytic function. Shennib et al. (21) believe that some members of the mononuclear phagocytic system are affected by the stress of nutritional depletion and may take up to 3 weeks to recover. How standard measures of immunocompetence correlate with the functioning of the alveolar macrophage, abnormalities of which may put the patient at risk for pulmonary infection, is unclear.

Killer Cells

Natural Killer Cells. Natural killer (NK) cells are cytotoxic to target cells and do not require the presence of complement or specific antibody to perform their killing function. The effect of surgery—laparotomy versus laparoscopy in patients undergoing surgery for benign disease—was shown to have an effect on cell-mediated immunity, but not on NK cell function (22) (Table 71.5). Tonnesen et al. (23) showed that NK cell activity increased in the perioperative period, returning toward normal by the second postoperative day after intravenous anesthesia. The reasons for and significance of these changes are unclear. The same group showed that the use of epidural anesthesia abolished the suppressive effect of surgery and anesthesia on NK cells (24). On the other hand, Katzav et al. (25) showed that mice exposed to ketamine or halothane, but not to nitrous oxide or sodium thiopental, had significantly decreased NK cell function 5 days after exposure. This decrement in NK cell function was significantly improved by treatment of exposed mice with polyinosinic-polycytidylic acid (100 μg intraperitoneally). This agent is an NK cell modulator that augments activity through interferon induction. Page et al. (26) also found that surgical stimulation depleted NK cell number and decreased NK activity; the use of morphine for pain control mitigated the measured immunologic effects of surgical stress.

Neutrophils

Data on neutrophil function during and after surgery and anesthesia are more abundant but also conflicting (Table 71.5). Nakagawara et al. (27) reported that halothane, enflurane, and isoflurane depress *superoxide production*—the reactive oxygen species produced by neutrophils during phagocytosis—in part because of a decrease in the mobilization of intracellular calcium. In an accompanying editorial, Welch (28) suggested that calcium-blocking properties of potent inhalational agents may cause neutrophil dysfunction. He noted that the volatile anesthetics, whose potency is correlated with lipid solubility, may prevent the release of membrane-bound intracellular calcium, as well as calcium influx, by occupying hydrophobic sites in the cellular membranes.

In patients undergoing various types of surgery, Ciepichal and Kubler found a decrease in chemotactic, phagocytic, and bactericidal activity after both regional and general anesthesia (29). In contrast, using intravenous anesthetic agents, van Dijk et al. (30) found no changes in neutrophil phagocytosis, chemotaxis, or chemoluminescence. Perttila et al. (31), using "balanced" anesthesia, consisting of both intravenous and relatively small doses of inhalation anesthetic agents, found minimally depressed neutrophil function that returned to preinduction values by the third postoperative day.

Lymphocytes

Lymphocyte function is believed to be impaired in the critically ill. Surgical procedures, including corneal transplantation, dilation and curettage, transurethral resection of the prostate, arthroplasty, open heart procedures, cholecystectomy, nephrectomy, herniorrhaphy, and others, show a decrease in lymphocyte response to mitogens, such as phytohemagglutinin and concanavalin A, which stimulate most T cells, and pokeweed mitogen, which stimulates proliferation of T cells and B cells. The suppressive effect of surgery on lymphocyte function is dependent to a degree on the anesthetic technique chosen. Volk et al. showed that postoperative epidural analgesia can reduce the effect of surgery on lymphocytes but not on monocytes (32).

Hemorrhagic Stress-induced Serum Factor

Abraham and Chang (33) reported a hemorrhagic stress-induced serum factor that depresses lymphocyte proliferation, is heat stable and dialyzable, and has a molecular weight between 13,000 and 23,000 daltons. This factor, or group of factors, seems to suppress lymphocyte proliferation in a rapid and irreversible manner, and may have some significance in the suppression of cell-mediated immunity in response to the stress of anesthesia and surgery. Recently, extension of this work showed that after an approximate 30% loss of calculated blood volume, mice exposed to bacterial antigen produce significantly less antigen-specific antibody than did exposed but nonhemorrhaged animals (34). Potent inhalation agents also may cause lymphocyte dysfunction. However, this area is poorly studied and controversial.

INTRAVENOUS AGENTS

Narcotics

General Properties

Although opiates have been used for thousands of years, morphine sulfate was first isolated from opium in 1803. Near the end of the 19th century, morphine and scopolamine, in doses of 1 to 3 mg/kg, were used intramuscularly or intravenously to provide "complete" anesthesia. Because of the increasing operative morbidity and mortality seen with this technique, it rapidly fell into disfavor. However, the use of high-dose narcotics for anesthesia again was popularized in the 1970s.

In 1973 Pert and Snyder demonstrated the specific binding sites for opiates in the central nervous system (35). Since then, the opiate receptor complex has been delineated and three major receptor groups have been described: μ, δ, and κ. The main drugs available for pain relief are relatively selective for the μ-receptor. These drugs also affect the respiratory, cardiovascular, gastrointestinal, and neuroendocrine systems (36).

Modern anesthesia practice has a diverse group of narcotic drugs at its disposal, including morphine, meperidine, methadone, fentanyl, alfentanil, sufentanil, and more recently remifentanil. Problems with morphine include recall, histamine release, prolonged postoperative respiratory depression, hypertension, and increased blood and fluid requirements because of vasodilation. Synthetic drugs related to the phenylpiperidines, such as fentanyl, sufentanil, alfentanil, and remifentanil, do not induce histamine release, nor do they increase blood and fluid requirements. Their use in anesthetic practice is common—less so for alfentanil and increasingly so for remifentanil—because of a rapid time to onset; a short duration of effect, which allows titration to effect; and relative hemodynamic stability (36). Remifentanil, in particular, has a time to effect that is very rapid, and since it is metabolized by plasma esterases, it has a half-life of 8 to 20 minutes independent of liver or renal function. This makes the drug ideal for situations in which rapid discontinuation of a drug is required to enable assessment of consciousness, such as in patients following neurosurgical procedures or head injury.

Generally speaking, healthier patients require larger doses of drugs than sicker, older patients. If 30 μg/kg of fentanyl is given to patients ages 18 to 31 years, 57% lose consciousness; if, however, the same dose is given to patients over 60 years, 100% lose consciousness. Narcotic drugs, though, cannot be depended upon to provide complete anesthesia, which requires amnesia, hypnosis, and muscle relaxation to enable safe surgery without awareness or patient discomfort. To this end, the addition of intravenous hypnotics and muscle relaxants, or inhaled agents, is required.

Pharmacokinetics/Pharmacodynamics

Selected pharmacokinetic data for four commonly used opioids are summarized in Table 71.6. Similarities between the redistribution and elimination half-lives and the clearance and steady-state volume of distribution are noteworthy. The major difference is in lipid solubility, which correlates with potency. Interestingly, the peak respiratory depressant effect of morphine is 15 to 30 minutes after injection, but with fentanyl, it occurs at 5 to 10 minutes. The depressant effect from morphine usually lasts longer, although that of fentanyl can be seen even after the analgesic effect of that drug has dissipated. Remifentanil is unique in that it has a rapid onset and offset of effect, even when delivered for a prolonged infusion. Because of these traits, it is very useful as an adjunct in different types of anesthesia (37,38).

Hemodynamic Effects

Hypotension can be a significant problem with morphine in a dose of 1 to 4 mg/kg. During induction of anesthesia with morphine, systolic blood pressure may decrease to less than 70 mm Hg in 10% of patients. Possible mechanisms include vagal-induced bradycardia, vasodilation, and splanchnic blood sequestration. The rate of infusion seems to be important, because hypotension seldom occurs at rates of 5 mg/minute or

TABLE 71.6

SELECTED PHARMACOKINETIC DATA FOR FOUR OPIOIDS

	Morphine	Fentanyl	Sufentanil	Remifentanil
Lipid solubility[a]	1	580	1778	50
$t^1/_2\ \pi$ (min)[b]	0.9–2.4	1–3	0.5–2	1
$t^1/_2\ \alpha$ (min)[c]	10–20	5–20	5–15	6
$t^1/_2\ \beta$ (h)[d]	2–4	2–4	2–3	0.06
Clearance (mL/kg/min)	10–20	10–20	10–12	40–70
Vd_{ss} (L/kg)[e]	3–5	3–5	2.5	0.2–0.3

[a]Proportional to ease with which agent crosses blood–brain barrier and, hence, potency.
[b]$t^1/_2\ \pi$, rapid redistribution half-life.
[c]$t^1/_2\ \alpha$, slow redistribution half-life.
[d]$t^1/_2\ \beta$, elimination half-life.
[e]Vd_{ss}, steady-state volume of distribution.

less, but is frequently seen at rates of 10 mg/minute. Morphine as an induction agent in anesthesia is not common today because of the availability of other narcotic drugs with more stable hemodynamic profiles.

Some of the effects of morphine seem to result from histamine release. After a 1 mg/kg intravenous dose of morphine, histamine increases four to nine times above the control values. Treatment with H_1 (diphenhydramine) and H_2 (cimetidine) blockers attenuates the cardiovascular response to histamine. Fentanyl, 30 to 100 μg/kg, rarely causes hypotension, even in patients with poor left ventricular function, perhaps because it does not cause histamine release. No significant changes in contractility, heart rate, cardiac output, or systemic or pulmonary artery occlusion pressure occur. When blood pressure decreases with fentanyl, it is often secondary to a decrease in heart rate and is attenuated with a vagolytic agent. Remifentanil has a beneficial hemodynamic profile, similar to fentanyl. When induction of anesthesia using fentanyl was compared with remifentanil, the incidence of bradycardia, hypotension, and ischemia was the same between the two drugs (39).

Respiratory Effects

Significant dose-dependent respiratory depression can occur with opioids. Both the end-tidal partial pressure of carbon dioxide and the apneic threshold—defined as the $PaCO_2$ below which spontaneous ventilation is not initiated unless hypoxia is present—are increased. Hypoxic ventilatory drive is decreased and the increase in ventilatory drive seen with increased airways resistance is blunted. The pontine and medullary centers for respiratory rhythmicity also are impaired, resulting in increased respiratory pauses and delayed exhalation, producing irregular and periodic breathing.

A possible concern with the use of morphine is the possible triggering or worsening of bronchospasm due to histamine release. This does not occur with fentanyl, sufentanil, or remifentanil. Another issue to consider is the possible effect of fentanyl and its derivatives to cause chest wall rigidity. This is probably a condition of hypertonicity of striated muscle, which can occur during induction of anesthesia using fentanyl or similar drugs. While the mechanism is not well understood, it apparently does not result from a direct effect of the opioid on muscle fibers or on the neural components of muscle. Rather, it may result from stimulation of γ-aminobutyric acid (GABA) receptors located on interneurons. When it occurs, it can lead to difficulties in ventilating the patient; treatment is commonly with a muscle relaxant.

Neurologic Effects

Alterations in neurophysiology are common with opioids. Morphine, at a dose of 1 to 3 mg/kg with 70% nitrous oxide, has no effect on CBF, cerebral metabolic rate for oxygen ($CMRO_2$), or cerebral metabolic rate for glucose (CMR_G). In a rat model of subarachnoid hemorrhage, morphine 1 mg/kg led to a decrease in cerebral blood flow, but autoregulation was better maintained than in the control group (40). Fentanyl, in a model of traumatic brain injury, did not lead to a reduction in CBF despite a decrease in arterial blood pressure (41).

Gastrointestinal Effects

The effects of analgesic doses of opioids on the gastrointestinal system are well known and include emesis secondary to stimulation of the chemoreceptor trigger zone in the area postrema of the medulla; increased gastrointestinal secretions; decreased motility that also may affect emetic action; and increased smooth muscle tone of the gastrointestinal tract and the sphincter of Oddi. Reports suggesting that the agonist–antagonist narcotics, nalbuphine or butorphanol, cause a lesser increase in gastrointestinal tract tone are controversial.

TABLE 71.7

OPIOID EFFECT ON STRESS RESPONSE

	Morphine (1–4 mg/kg)	Fentanyl (50–100 μg/kg)
Catecholamines	↑ ↓	θ to ↑
Cortisol	θ to ↑	↓
HGH	θ	↓
ADH	↑	θ

θ, no change; ↑, activity/function increased; ↓, activity/function decreased; HGH, human growth hormone; ADH, antidiuretic hormone.

Stress

The effect to which a given drug ameliorates the surgical stress response may be important to immune system function and nutritional balance; however, the associated clinical relevance, as with the potent inhalational agents, remains controversial. High-dose, as compared to low-dose, fentanyl for abdominal surgery can suppress the stress response with regard to catecholamines and corticosteroids (42). When comparing high-dose alfentanil to balanced anesthesia with fentanyl and droperidol, Moller et al. found that the increase in cortisol and hyperglycemia associated with surgery were decreased for the duration of surgery and the 1 to 3 hours following surgery (43). The effects of morphine and fentanyl on metabolic responses are shown in Table 71.7; these data are drawn from several series, including those with patients undergoing cardiac surgery.

Immune Function

As is the case with inhalational agents, controversy exists concerning the narcotic effects on cellular immune system function. In a rat model inoculated with lung tumor cells, high-dose fentanyl suppressed NK function and led to an increase in the number of metastases (44). This type of immune suppression is not due to the impairment of ventilation. Fentanyl led to suppressed NK cells in rats that were ventilated to the same degree as rats breathing spontaneously (45).

McDonough et al. (46) and Brown et al. (47) suggest that a transient impairment of *in vitro* cellular immunity is demonstrable in opiate addicts. After treatment of lymphocytes with naloxone, or after cessation of intravenous opiate administration, the response to mitogen stimulation returns toward normal. Whether this apparent impairment of cellular immune function is caused by contaminants in the intravenous opioid obtained by drug abusers or whether it is a more specific effect of opioids in general is unclear. Balanced anesthesia, including fentanyl, has no depressive effects on the mitogen responses of lymphocytes. But large-dose fentanyl impairs NK cell activity following abdominal surgery (48). When atropine and

TABLE 71.8

SELECTED PHARMACOKINETIC DATA FOR NONOPIOID INTRAVENOUS ANESTHETICS

	Thiopental	Propofol	Diazepam	Lorazepam	Midazolam	Ketamine
t½ α (min)[a]	2–4	2–4	10–15	3–10	7–15	7–17
t½ β (h)[b]	10	1–3	20–40	10–20	2–4	2–3
Clearance (mL/kg/min)[c]	2.6–2.8	20–40	0.2–0.5	0.7–1	4–8	18–20
Vd_{ss}(L/kg)[c,d]	1.4–2.8	2.8–7.1	0.85–1.4	0.7–1.3	1–1.8	2.8–3.6

[a]t½ α, slow redistribution half-life.
[b]t½ β, elimination half-life.
[c]Vd_{ss}, steady-state volume of distribution.
[d]Assume a 70-kg person.
Modified from White PF. Propofol: pharmacokinetics and pharmacodynamics. *Semin Anesth.* 1988;7(Suppl):4.

meperidine are used as premedication, a small number of patients show a decrease in lymphocyte response to mitogens.

Barbiturates

Thiobarbiturates (e.g., sodium thiopental and methohexital) are frequently used. In contradistinction to other barbiturates, the thiopental ring structure has a sulfur atom in place of the oxygen atom at carbon-2. Methohexital, while retaining its carbon-2 oxygen atom, has a methyl group that replaces the hydrogen at the nitrogen-1 position of the ring. These chemical changes confer ultrashort onset and offset action compared with other barbiturates. Sodium thiopental usually comes in a 2.5% solution with a pH greater than 10, causing the drug to be irritating if accidentally extravasated. Methohexital is two to three times more potent than thiopental.

Pharmacokinetics/Pharmacodynamics

The pharmacokinetics of thiopental, as well as other commonly used nonnarcotic, intravenous anesthetic agents, are summarized in Table 71.8. Thiopental is a highly lipophilic agent with a pKa of 7.6 and is 60% nonionized at pH 7.4. With a standard clinical dose of 3 to 5 mg/kg, loss of consciousness occurs within one arm–brain circulation time, that is, 10 to 15 seconds. The short duration of action of this drug—5 to 10 minutes—is secondary to its redistribution from the brain to muscle, skin, and, to a lesser extent, fat. The elimination half-life of the drug is long, making thiopental into a long-acting drug when a large enough dose has been given to saturate the redistribution compartment. Less than 1% of the administered drug appears unchanged in the urine; hepatic metabolism is important for its inactivation. Seventy to eighty-five percent of thiopental is albumin bound in the blood. Thus, factors that decrease albumin binding also decrease the amount of drug needed for the appropriate anesthetic effect. Renal and hepatic impairment also decrease the amount of drug necessary as a result of decreased albumin.

Methohexital is only slightly less lipid soluble than sodium thiopental and is somewhat less ionized at pH 7.4. The onset and duration of loss of consciousness are approximately the same as with thiopental because of its rapid redistribution, with an elimination half-life of 3 to 5 minutes. Because it is more dependent on hepatic blood flow for clearance, any changes in flow are more significant for its final elimination.

Neurologic Effects

The mechanisms of action of the barbiturates are multiple and dose related. At clinically relevant doses, two effects are seen: facilitation of action of inhibitory—GABA—neural transmitters and inhibition of excitatory neural transmitter action. A barbiturate-induced increase in GABA neuronal hyperpolarization is believed to be related to an increase in the time that chloride (Cl^-) ion channels remain open. Specifically, barbiturates seem to decrease the frequency of channel opening while increasing the duration of opening. Within the central nervous system (CNS), sodium thiopental results in a decrease in $CMRO_2$, CBF, and ICP. It is thus used sometimes as a drug to reduce intracranial pressure and improve cerebral hemodynamics while providing a degree of brain protection.

Cardiorespiratory Effects

Cardiovascular effects of thiopental are of some significance. Increases in coronary blood flow, heart rate, and myocardial oxygen consumption occur, together with a decrease in the inotropic state of the myocardium. The result is a 10% to 25% decrease in cardiac output, blood pressure, and stroke volume at clinically relevant doses. Venous tone may also decrease, resulting in decreased preload. At doses of 3 to 5 mg/kg, the responses to carbon dioxide elevation and hypoxia are impaired. After injection of thiopental, patients usually take two to three deep breaths—and often yawn—and then become apneic.

In an *in vitro* model of peripheral blood monocytes, barbiturates were found to decrease the ability to proliferate and produce cytokines (49). In patients who are given continuous barbiturate infusion, there may be an effect on immune function and they may be more prone to develop infections (50).

Propofol

Propofol is an intriguing intravenous anesthetic agent. It is a sedative–hypnotic agent, similar to the thiobarbiturates and benzodiazepines that may be used for induction and maintenance of anesthesia. The agent is not antianalgesic—as are the thiobarbiturates—but is reported to have minimal amnestic effects (51). An alkylphenol, propofol is virtually insoluble in aqueous media and thus is provided in a 1% weight/volume (Intralipid) emulsion. The emulsion is composed of 1% diisopropylphenol (propofol), 10% soybean oil, 2.25% glycerol, and 1.2% purified egg phosphatide. Histamine release is not a problem with this formulation. Propofol is 95% to 99% plasma protein bound; whereas the pH of the emulsion is 7 to 8.5, the drug itself is slightly acidic. A newer formulation of 2% propofol is used for prolonged sedation in critically ill patients (52).

Pharmacokinetics/Pharmacodynamics

The basic pharmacokinetic data of propofol are shown in Table 71.8. Like the thiobarbiturates, propofol is extensively distributed into vessel-rich tissues, and ultimately redistributed to lean muscle and fat. The pharmacokinetic data suggest that accumulation occurs with repeated bolus injections or continuous infusion. Propofol is metabolized to water-soluble, highly polar glucuronide and sulfate conjugates; the metabolites are not thought to be active and are excreted in the urine. Almost none of the parent drug is found in urine (less than 0.3%) or stool (less than 2%); extrahepatic metabolism or extrarenal elimination might occur.

In comparing propofol with the other agents in Table 71.8, one observes the high clearance and the short elimination half-life. This profile, one of the reasons that the agent is so appealing, may be increased by age (decreased clearance and dose requirement), obesity (increased clearance and volume of distribution), and type of procedure; with major intra-abdominal surgery, volume of distribution increases and the elimination half-life is prolonged, as well as with the use of narcotics and potent inhaled anesthetic agents (decreased hepatic blood flow with a prolonged elimination half-life).

With intravenous injection in a non–premedicated patient, a propofol dose of 2 to 2.5 mg/kg results in loss of consciousness in less than 60 seconds; rapid intravenous injection of 1 to 1.5 mg/kg in the elderly or a patient who has been given narcotic or benzodiazepine premedication is often sufficient for induction.

Anesthetic depth is assessed by changes in the respiratory rate in spontaneously breathing patients or by increases in heart rate, blood pressure, and autonomic activity in those receiving a balanced anesthetic technique. A need to increase the anesthetic depth may be met by increasing the infusion rate or augmenting with 20- to 40-mg boluses intravenously. A relatively linear relationship exists between maintenance infusion rate of propofol and the resultant blood levels of the agent. Nonetheless, as with other intravenous agents, interpatient variability is such that a given dosage rate can result in levels that vary by three- to sixfold.

A fairly predictable relationship also exists between the adequacy of anesthetic depth and the blood levels of propofol. For example, to achieve an adequate level of anesthesia, blood levels of the drug must be higher (3–6 μg/mL) for major as opposed to superficial (2–4 μg/mL) surgical procedures. The former blood level is frequently obtained, notwithstanding interpatient variability, with infusion rates between 100 and 150 μg/kg/minute.

Finally, the probability of awakening is reasonably predicted by observing blood levels. More than 50% of persons are awake with a level of 1 μg/mL, over 95% are awake and oriented with a level of 0.5 μg/mL, and most will have recovered baseline psychomotor function when the propofol level is 0.2 μg/mL. For propofol, the effective dose in 50% of patients studied (ED_{50}), which is analogous to MAC for potent inhalation agents, is 53.5 μg/kg/minute (95% confidence limits; 39.9–63 μg/kg/minute) (53).

Neurologic Effects

The mechanisms of action of propofol are unclear. Propofol can cause desynchronization of the awake electroencephalographic (EEG) pattern when a loading dose of 2.5 mg/kg followed by an infusion of 100 to 200 μg/kg/minute are used; this effect is seen within 60 seconds of intravenous administration. Propofol in a dosage of more than 150 μg/kg/minute results in EEG burst suppression lasting 15 seconds or longer; the EEG returns to the awake state within about 11 minutes after the drug infusion is discontinued.

Some evoked potentials are altered by the drug. The latency of the primary complex may be increased and its amplitude decreased in median nerve and posterior tibial nerve somatosensory-evoked potentials. Propofol leads to a dose-related decrease in CBF and $CMRO_2$, and leads to progressive EEG suppression with increasing dose of propofol (54). For this reason, propofol is used in patients with intracranial disease and is frequently employed in the ICU for long-term sedation.

Cardiovascular Effects

Like thiopental, propofol produces a dose-dependent decrease in systolic, diastolic, and mean arterial blood pressure; this effect is enhanced by narcotic premedication. Profound cardiovascular depression may be seen when propofol is used in elderly or hypovolemic patients and those with impaired ventricular function. Despite the decrease in blood pressure, heart rate remains relatively stable; this response is thought to be caused by a central sympatholytic or vagotonic effect rather than by impaired baroreceptor sensitivity.

The agent is a negative inotrope and, when used in patients with ischemic heart disease, has been associated with an increase in myocardial lactate production. Yet, a recent study described the hemodynamic effects of propofol infusion on critically ill adults and reported no significant reductions in cardiac output, oxygen delivery, oxygen consumption, or arterial blood lactate concentrations (55).

Respiratory Effects

Apnea is seen on induction with propofol in 30% to 60% of unpremedicated patients, and in virtually 100% of those premedicated with narcotics. Whereas the incidence of apnea is about the same as that seen with the thiobarbiturates, the duration tends to be somewhat longer. When breathing resumes, the tidal volume is decreased and the slope of the carbon dioxide response curve is decreased by 40% to 60%. The response to hypoxia is also significantly blunted by propofol (56). Adjuvant use of narcotics further depresses respiratory drive.

Other Effects

Propofol does not seem to have any clinically relevant adverse effect on the production of cortisol, although intravenous anesthesia with propofol and remifentanil does lead to a decreased stress response including cortisol production compared to balanced anesthesia with inhalational agents (57). It does not affect the coagulation profile as measured by the thrombin time, prothrombin time, partial thromboplastin time, fibrinogen level, titer of fibrin degradation products, and platelet number and function.

Up to 58% of patients with an intravenous catheter in the dorsum of the hand reported pain on injection of propofol;

this number decreased to about 10% if the drug was injected through a vein in the antecubital fossa. Administration of lidocaine through the cannula just before injection of propofol may decrease the pain. Younger patients require a higher dose of lidocaine to suppress the injection pain of propofol (58).

Although for the most part propofol is a very safe drug, in recent years a syndrome of severe hemodynamic compromise with bradycardia up to asystole combined with severe metabolic acidosis. This entity has been termed *propofol infusion syndrome* and has been described initially in children and then in adults undergoing anesthesia but also during propofol administration for sedation in the ICU (59). An association with acute lung injury has also been reported (60). The pathophysiology of the propofol infusion system is unclear and various theories have been suggested, such as an effect on mitochondrial function leading to extreme metabolic acidosis and rhabdomyolysis. Other theories include a genetic predisposition of mitochondria to dysfunction induced by the propofol or problems with lipid metabolism, particularly in patients who have a low carbohydrate input (61). Risk factors include a high dose of drug and its prolonged administration. Most patients described had a neurologic etiology for their critical illness such as trauma or status epilepticus (62), but other clinical settings such as sepsis or nonneurologic trauma have also been described (63,64).

Benzodiazepines

The benzodiazepines of most significance in anesthesia and critical care are diazepam, lorazepam, and midazolam (Table 71.8). Diazepam and lorazepam are insoluble in water. Midazolam, because of its imidazole ring, is water soluble at a pH of less than 4. Lorazepam is less lipid soluble than diazepam, and its slow entry into the CNS may be significant to its slower onset of action.

Pharmacokinetics/Pharmacodynamics

Diazepam. The sedative properties of diazepam make it useful as a premedicant; peak plasma levels are seen 30 to 60 minutes after an oral dose. Intramuscular injection is painful, and absorption is erratic. Clearance involves oxidation to active metabolites. The free fraction of diazepam is only 1% to 2%; the rest is bound to albumin. Therefore, changes in albumin binding affect the clearance and half-life of this drug.

With hepatic disease, the volume of distribution increases and metabolism decreases, resulting in an increase in the half-life from 40 to 80 hours. With significant renal disease, an increase in the unbound fraction of diazepam results in a twofold to threefold increase in hepatic clearance and a resultant decrease in the half-life. The significance of these changes is hard to document, however, because no simple relationship can be demonstrated between the plasma levels of diazepam, its metabolites, and the clinical effect.

Lorazepam. Lorazepam is useful in oral, intramuscular, and intravenous forms. This agent is directly metabolized in the liver to inactive, glucuronide-conjugated metabolites. The kinetics of this drug are unaltered by age or renal disease, but hepatic disease increases the half-life.

Midazolam. Midazolam also can be administered by intramuscular, intravenous, or oral routes. The drug undergoes extensive metabolism to active and inactive metabolites. We have extensive experience using this drug as an induction agent in thermally injured patients. Loss of consciousness is rapid after an intravenous loading dose of 300 μg/kg followed by either ketamine or, more often, a narcotic such as fentanyl in a dose of 2 to 5 μg/kg/hour after a loading dose of 5 to 10 μg/kg.

Neurologic Effects

Like barbiturates, the benzodiazepines have multiple, dose-dependent effects on the CNS and potentiate inhibitory GABA neurotransmission. They increase the frequency but not the duration of chloride channel opening. In addition, at least two specific benzodiazepine receptors have been identified: type 1, which is a postsynaptic receptor found in the cerebellum, and type 2, which is a presynaptic receptor found in the hippocampus and descending GABA pathways from the caudate nucleus to the substantia nigra. The clinical significance of these receptors is under investigation.

Loss of consciousness occurs 2 to 3 minutes after an intravenous induction dose of diazepam, lorazepam, or midazolam. Antegrade amnesia is seen with all of the benzodiazepines, but more so with lorazepam.

Cardiorespiratory Effects

When the benzodiazepines are used alone, cardiovascular effects are reported to be insignificant; however, cardiovascular depression has been observed when they are used in conjunction with other anesthetic agents. Respiratory effects are also minimal. Some decrease in the ventilatory response to carbon dioxide may occur after the use of these agents, but data are conflicting in this regard. No difference in recovery time or duration of action of either depolarizing or nondepolarizing muscle relaxants occurs when the benzodiazepines are used.

Ketamine

Pharmacokinetics/Pharmacodynamics

Ketamine is the only arylcyclohexylamine used in anesthesia. It is structurally related to phencyclidine, known in street vernacular as "angel dust." The pKa of ketamine is 7.5, and it is about ten times more water soluble than thiopental. Its pharmacokinetics are summarized in Table 71.8. Ketamine is approximately ten times more lipid soluble than thiopental; however, its onset of action is somewhat slower. After an intravenous dose of 2 mg/kg, consciousness is lost in little more than one arm–brain circulation time and returns 10 to 15 minutes later. Ketamine is 45% to 50% protein bound.

Recovery of consciousness probably results from rapid drug redistribution into muscle and other tissues. However, 95% of the injected drug ultimately is metabolized by the liver, and less than 5% is recovered unchanged in the urine. At least eight different metabolites of the parent compound have been identified, the most important of which is norketamine, which has approximately one-third the potency of ketamine.

Neurologic Effects

The exact mechanism of action of ketamine is not well understood. Apparently it does not facilitate GABA inhibitory neurotransmitters, as do the benzodiazepines and barbiturates. Like barbiturates, however, ketamine blocks ion channels in the open position. Specific arylcyclohexylamine receptors in the brain may be related to the μ subclass of opioid receptors. Ketamine increases CBF and so must be used with caution in individuals with elevated ICP.

Cardiovascular Effects

Ketamine causes an increase in systemic blood pressure and cerebrovasodilation, resulting in increased ICP. It also causes central stimulation of the sympathetic arm of the autonomic nervous system. The cardiovascular effects are primarily related to CNS stimulation. Ketamine inhibits the uptake of catecholamines by the postganglionic adrenergic neurons and the uptake of extraneuronal norepinephrine.

Because of the dose-related increase in arterial blood pressure, heart rate, and coronary vasodilation, and overall unchanged peripheral vascular resistance associated with ketamine administration, the drug often is thought not to be a myocardial depressant. Nonetheless, with sympathetic blockade or in patients in prolonged shock with a significantly stressed autonomic nervous system, cardiac depression can be seen with ketamine. Pulmonary vascular resistance and right ventricular stroke work also are frequently increased.

Respiratory Effects

Although ketamine is not commonly thought of as a respiratory depressant when used in anesthetic doses of 1 to 2 mg/kg, a moderate decrease in the PaO_2 may occur. The ventilatory response to carbon dioxide is maintained, and ketamine potentiates the bronchodilatory effects of catecholamines. It also increases oral secretions so that an anticholinergic agent may be necessary.

Other Effects

Ketamine enhances the effect of depolarizing and nondepolarizing neuromuscular blocking drugs. The drug has been used safely in patients with MH. Postanesthetic emergence reactions—nightmares and hallucinations—may occur in 5% to 30% of patients. A benzodiazepine and 2 mg/kg (or less) maximal doses of ketamine seem to decrease the incidence of this problem.

Immune System Function

As with the potent inhalation and opioid anesthetics, controversy exists regarding the effects of barbiturates, benzodiazepines, and ketamine on immune function. Sodium thiopental, at clinically relevant doses *in vitro*, decreases the mitogenic response of lymphocytes to phytohemagglutinin and inhibits cytotoxicity. Ketamine attenuates the proinflammatory response following abdominal surgery (65). In experimental animals, both thiopental in tumor-bearing mice and pentobarbital in dogs decrease lymphocyte function. The *in vivo* response of lymphocytes in patients exposed to thiopental, nitrous oxide, oxygen, droperidol, fentanyl, and muscle relaxants shows no adverse effect. However, balanced anesthesia, including inhaled and intravenous agents, leads to greater reduction of lymphocyte function than a purely intravenous technique (18).

Etomidate

An induction agent that maintains hemodynamic stability, etomidate is commonly used in the induction of anesthesia or for intubation of critically ill patients suspected of cardiac dysfunction or hemodynamic instability from other causes. Etomidate causes a dose-dependent reduction in contractility in both normal and failing heats, but this decrease is minimal and most likely does not have any clinical significance (66).

The major problem with etomidate is the adrenal suppression it induces when used in a prolonged infusion. It has also been demonstrated following a single dose for induction of anesthesia (67). Concern about the effect of adrenal suppression in patients in the ICU leads some clinicians to avoid the use of etomidate in patients at risk for adrenal insufficiency (68,69). On the other hand, it has been suggested that the benefits of hemodynamic stability may overcome any concerns about adrenal dysfunction and its consequences (70).

Dexmedetomidine

Dexmedetomidine is a novel, new, highly selective, short-acting central α_2-agonist. It is used in the ICU for providing sedation and some degree of analgesia. It is used primarily for sedation in the ICU. It provides a dose-dependent degree of sedation, analgesia, anxiolysis, and sympatholysis. When used in postoperative patients in the ICU, dexmedetomidine can provide better sedation with fewer narcotics than propofol (71). Siobal et al. used dexmedetomidine to facilitate a weaning trial and extubation in patients who were ventilated and did not tolerate a weaning trial prior to the drug (72). The place of this agent in intensive care medicine practice is still being evaluated.

PREFERRED ANESTHETIC TECHNIQUES FOR SPECIFIC CLINICAL SCENARIOS

Should any agent or technique be used or, conversely, avoided in critically ill patients? Almost no data conclusively support one technique over another. Yet, although we prefer not to muddy the waters, we believe it makes sense in a hemodynamically unstable patient to shy away from the potent inhalation agents and to use in their place an intravenous technique of either ketamine or one of the phenylpiperidine narcotics. Furthermore, in patients with traumatic brain injury, we use intravenous benzodiazepines, barbiturates, and narcotics with isoflurane; ketamine and the other potent inhaled anesthetic agents are avoided.

The options for total intravenous anesthesia available today with the short-acting narcotics and propofol allow for an easily titratable anesthesia without the disadvantages of inhalational anesthesia. It is now possible to administer anesthesia without any significant hemodynamic embarrassment, which is easily controlled and rapidly reversed. An issue to be considered is that of respiratory function of the critically ill or injured patient undergoing surgery. If the patient has a component of respiratory failure, the need of delivering high oxygen concentration may require avoiding inhaled agents. Closed gas space such as pneumothorax, pneumocephalus, or bowel obstruction demands that nitrous oxide be withheld.

The less than adequate data suggest avoidance of potent inhalation anesthetic agents in patients with questionable perioperative immune function. In such cases, intravenous narcotics or ketamine may be useful. However, no outcome studies show that potent inhalation agents increase morbidity or mortality more than agents with no demonstrated adverse effects on *in vitro* immune function. Emerging data indicate the significance of regional anesthesia on immune function and behavior of tumors. For example, when patients undergoing breast surgery for cancer were anesthetized with general anesthesia or a regional technique, the disease-free survival was significantly greater in the patients with regional technique (73).

The Patient with Acute Respiratory Distress Syndrome

Patients with acute respiratory distress syndrome (ARDS) present with difficulties in mechanical ventilation, particularly with regard to hypoxemia. Current approach to mechanical ventilation dictates the use of low tidal volumes of 6 to 8 mL/kg ideal body weight (74,75). This can be coupled with a higher respiratory rate to maintain adequate ventilation and tolerance of a higher than normal $PaCO_2$, so called "permissive hypercapnia." The approach of lung protective strategy has been shown to improve outcome in patients with ARDS and should probably be maintained in patients undergoing surgery. The effect of sepsis on the development of acute lung injury can be affected by anesthesia, and in an animal model it has been shown that use of barbiturates (76) and ketamine (77) can attenuate the development of acute lung injury due to sepsis. Some intraoperative parameters such as hemodynamic instability, the need for vasopressors, fluid and blood requirements, and hypoxemia are related to the development of acute lung injury (78).

Providing adequate mechanical ventilation can now be done with most modern anesthesia ventilators. Older ventilators, on the other hand, could not provide the flows and pressures required by patients with severe lung injury. These patients may need to be ventilated with an ICU ventilator, and anesthesia maintained with intravenous anesthetic agents (79). Fluid management of patients with ARDS should be directed at the maintenance of adequate hemodynamics without fluid overload (80,81).

The Patient with a Head Injury

Patients with head injury present with multiple neurologic, respiratory, and hemodynamic problems. The anesthesiologist should be vigilant about maintaining optimal cerebral perfusion pressure—generally considered to be "optimized" at 60 to 65 mm Hg—by providing anesthesia directed at reducing intracerebral pressure, barbiturates, maintenance of normo- or mild hypothermia, increasing serum osmolarity, and judicious use of diuretics, while vasopressors and inotropes can improve cardiac output and blood pressure; at times, hyperventilation will be necessary. On occasion, the therapeutic dilemma of giving priority to the ICP *versus* a lung protective strategy may arise. Another clinical dilemma is the fluid status of the patient: Is optimizing preload going to increase cerebral edema? Our approach is to direct therapy to optimize cerebral blood flow by improving central perfusion pressure. To prevent hypovolemia, these patients should be monitored aggressively. There are many options for measuring cardiac output: invasively, as with a pulmonary artery catheter, or semi-invasively with pulse contour cardiac output, such as is done with the PiCCO, FloTrak, or LiDCO systems. Indeed, these systems can provide additional information that can be beneficial in the hemodynamic management of the patient as indicators of fluid responsiveness such as pulse pressure variation, systolic pressure variation, or stroke volume variation and, in the case of the PiCCO system, measurement of extravascular lung water.

The Patient with Shock

Patients in shock require therapy directed at the cause of the shock state, as well as avoidance of therapies that may be specifically problematic in this patient population. All anesthesiologists are aware of the deleterious effects of mechanical ventilation on patients with hypovolemia and shock. In these patients, it is important to keep intrathoracic pressures as low as possible while fluid resuscitation is being administered. Drugs that depress heart function and lead to vasodilation should be avoided and, in extreme cases, even drugs that are considered to maintain hemodynamic stability, such as ketamine, can lead to hemodynamic collapse.

In patients with a cardiac source of shock, intrathoracic pressure will usually not have a detrimental, and may even have a beneficial, effect on cardiac output. Still, most anesthetics are cardiac depressants and, thus, should be used with extreme caution in patients in shock. All patients in shock should be monitored invasively to assess the degree of both hypovolemia and responsiveness to therapy (82,83).

The Patient Requiring Tight Glucose Control

The significance of tight glucose control in critically ill patients has become clear in recent years. The adherence to glucose levels between 80 and 110 mg/dL has been shown to improve outcome in surgical critically ill patients. This effect of controlling glucose has also been shown to be significant during surgery. In patients undergoing cardiac surgery, poor intraoperative glucose control was associated with worse outcome (84). While less clear in medical ICU patients, it appears that those in the unit for longer than 3 to 5 days are benefited by tight control of glucose.

POSTANESTHESIA PROBLEMS

Difficulties in the early postoperative period are common. Postanesthetic complications have been found to occur in 5% to 30% of patients; the wide range results from lack of uniform criteria defining complications, different practices in individual institutions, differences in the strictness of observational practice, and possible significant differences in populations studied.

Hypoxemia

Postoperative hypoxemia may result from diverse etiologies. Hypoventilation caused by residual anesthetic or muscle relaxant and atelectasis, which may have resulted from a one-lung intubation during surgery, are diagnoses to be considered and treated aggressively in the immediate postoperative period. Upper airway obstruction due to a decreased level of consciousness is a common reason for hypoxemia and hypercarbia. Consideration should be given to pulmonary edema resulting from heart failure in susceptible patients, noncardiogenic pulmonary edema from aspiration, acute respiratory distress syndrome, infection, trauma, a transfusion reaction, or a head injury resulting in neurogenic pulmonary edema.

Postoperative hypoxemia can lead to acute complications such as cardiac ischemia, and may also have an effect on the patient's immunity. Supplemental oxygen decreased the rate of wound infections in patients following colonic resection (85) as well as the incidence of nausea and vomiting following surgery (86).

Negative-pressure Pulmonary Edema

Pulmonary edema may develop after a strenuous inspiratory effort against an obstructed airway. This type of pulmonary edema may appear immediately or up to 10 hours after the episode of airway obstruction. It most commonly is associated with laryngospasm during anesthetic induction of or emergence from anesthesia; therefore, it frequently is diagnosed in the postanesthesia care unit or ICU.

The pathophysiologic mechanism of negative-pressure pulmonary edema is not completely understood, although a common explanation is that the massive negative intrapleural pressure generated during airway obstruction shifts the balance in the Starling forces toward a large fluid transudation from the intravascular to the interstitial space. The increase in extravascular lung water causes a reduction in lung compliance and an increase in shunt.

The diagnosis of negative-pressure pulmonary edema is based on the history and clinical picture of pulmonary edema in patients without heart failure or predisposition for acute respiratory distress syndrome from other causes. Typically, the patient is a young, vigorous adult who sustains an episode of laryngospasm either before intubation or after tracheal decannulation (87). The radiologic picture in negative-pressure pulmonary edema has been described as alveolar and interstitial edema, which rarely occur unilaterally. The heart size is normal, but the vascular pedicle is enlarged.

Treatment of negative-pressure pulmonary edema is mainly supportive. Patients should be given oxygen to maintain an arterial saturation of at least 90%. Some patients require reintubation and mechanical ventilation with positive pressure to ensure oxygenation and to reduce work of breathing; diuretics may be used judiciously in these cases. In most cases, the edema resolves within 24 hours.

Pain and Perioperative Stress

Early postoperative pain remains a serious concern. Up to 75% of patients receiving parenteral narcotics for moderate to severe pain have significant residual pain after the drug is administered. Uncontrolled pain can lead to serious physiologic consequences. For example, sympathetic nervous system stimulation that accompanies uncontrolled pain leads to elevated plasma catecholamine levels, tachycardia, hypertension, increased systemic vascular resistance, and an increase in myocardial oxygen requirements. In the patient with underlying coronary artery disease, this increased oxygen demand may not be met, resulting in ischemia or infarction.

Surgical procedures on the upper abdomen and thorax may have profound effects on the respiratory system. Because of the pain and surgery-induced muscular alterations, vital capacity and functional residual capacity may be decreased by as much as 60% and 20%, respectively. Although these changes may not be evident with resting tidal respiration, the ability to deep breathe (sigh) and cough is impaired, resulting in atelectasis and retained secretions. Decreased oxygenation and the potential for pulmonary parenchymal infection may follow.

Stress Response

An area less clearly understood and described, but likely no less important with regard to postoperative pain, is the stress response to surgery. Weissman (88) reviews the intriguing and manifold physiologic changes observed with an operative intervention. Surgery, as any trauma, was classically described as being composed of two stages: an initial *ebb phase* is characterized by a shock state with low metabolic activity and cardiac output, and a second period termed the *flow phase* is characterized by a hyperdynamic state from the endocrine, metabolic, and cardiovascular standpoints.

The endocrine parameters of the latter stage are evidenced by an increase in catecholamine levels, an increased secretion of corticotropin and steroids, and resultant hyperglycemia. An increase in antidiuretic hormone (ADH) secretion enables conservation of water by the kidneys. Other aspects of the response to surgery and anesthesia are an increase in growth hormone and a slight increase in thyroxine, with a decrease in triiodothyronine levels. β-Endorphin levels are increased, as is the plasma level of prolactin.

The systemic response to trauma also includes an important component of immune depression, which can appear early after the stressful event (89,90) and is mediated through several different pathways (91,92). Traditionally, the stress response was thought to be beneficial for homeostatic stability and, indeed, there was perhaps an evolutionary advantage accrued to the organism that could mount this response to major trauma, blood loss, and organ dysfunction. Currently, however, data show that the metabolic response to trauma may often be exaggerated and thus disadvantageous.

In the otherwise well-controlled diabetic patient, for example, one may see hyperglycemia that is extremely difficult to regulate. An increase in catecholamine secretion that increases myocardial work and oxygen consumption may result in ischemia in patients with coronary artery disease. Increased ADH secretion may result in a picture similar to the syndrome of inappropriate ADH (SIADH) secretion with significant hyponatremia, particularly in patients treated with hypotonic solutions after surgery (93). The significant hyponatremia seen in this syndrome can present with convulsions, respiratory arrest, and permanent brain damage. The hyponatremic syndrome has been described in children after spinal surgery (94,95) as well as in adults (96) and in thermally injured patients (97).

These data suggest—although we note that significant controversy exists—that the stress response to surgery should at least be attenuated if the detrimental effects are to be avoided. Different anesthetic techniques may affect this response in various ways; thus, the choice of an anesthetic may affect the patient's course in the postoperative period and in the surgical ICU.

General Anesthesia. Patients studied under a variety of general anesthetics show an increase in corticotropin, corticosteroids, β-endorphins, and catecholamines in response to intubation, skin incision, and intra-abdominal manipulation, and on emergence (98). Nevertheless, some researchers believe that a well-maintained general anesthetic can blunt the stress response or, at least, some of its components. Roizen et al. (99) have used the acronym MAC-BAR, indicating the minimal alveolar concentration at which the adrenergic response is blocked; it is usually observed at approximately 2 MAC for most inhalational agents. Furthermore, others have shown that graded surgical stress causes minimal endocrine response (100). Thus, patients who undergo relatively less stressful surgery under adequate anesthesia do not mount a deleterious stress response.

High-dose narcotic techniques, commonly used in cardiac anesthesia or for patients with ischemic heart disease, have been shown to blunt the endocrine response to stress inasmuch as plasma levels of various stress hormones are not increased (101). The difference between the different types of narcotics is probably insignificant. With any general anesthetic technique, the metabolic response is triggered on emergence, even if attenuated during the surgical procedure itself. In the surgical ICU, patients may begin to mount the metabolic–endocrine response in the postoperative period (102).

Regional Anesthesia. The stress response to surgery is triggered by several mechanisms. Among these, an important one is that of direct neural activation by transmission of noxious stimuli from the traumatized area. This event occurs even when patients receive a general anesthetic and, therefore, are not consciously aware of the noxious stimulus. Blunting the response can be achieved by blocking this neural pathway.

Analgesia and anesthesia achieved with a regional technique do attenuate the stress response when compared with general techniques. Kehlet et al. (103,104) have studied this relationship extensively and found major differences in levels of corticosteroids, catecholamines, aldosterone, renin, growth hormone, prolactin, and ADH in patients undergoing surgery with epidural anesthesia compared with those given general anesthesia. Some aspects of the immune depression after surgery also have been shown not to occur with regional as opposed to general anesthesia (32).

Combined Anesthesia. The advantages of regional anesthesia may be put to use in surgery on the extremities and lower abdomen. A purely regional technique is seldom used for upper abdominal surgery; some anesthesiologists do not use regional techniques in a prolonged surgical procedure if it involves uncomfortable positioning or if immobility is important. In the latter procedures, a common approach is to use regional anesthesia, with control of the airway by intubation, inhalational agents, and positive-pressure ventilation; this approach is called *combined anesthesia*. The term was coined by Crile in 1921 and involves the block of surgical stimulus by a regional technique, combined with loss of consciousness achieved by light general anesthesia (105).

Applications. Whereas combined anesthesia usually refers to a general anesthetic combined with a spinal or epidural technique, the regional anesthetic might also be a brachial plexus or any other nerve block. Proving that combined anesthesia is successful in obtunding the stress response to trauma is more difficult than in studies comparing regional anesthesia with general anesthetic techniques. This observation probably results from several factors: (a) obtaining control of the airway (the intubation) may itself elicit a strong stress response, (b) the surgical field may include areas that are not well anesthetized, and (c) part of the stress response may be mediated by the release of humoral factors from the locally injured area.

Potential advantages. The possible advantages of combined anesthesia over a purely general technique are controversial. Yeager et al. (106) compared major abdominal and vascular procedures done under a general anesthetic technique with those done under combined general and epidural techniques. They found significant differences in the ICU course and in outcome between the two patient groups. The combined group required less time to tracheal decannulation and a shorter ICU stay; they had fewer infectious complications and a lower mortality. Expense per patient was considerably lower. Thus, the anesthetic choice becomes an important ICU issue. Some studies did not find an advantage to this approach (107), whereas one found specific benefits of epidural anesthesia, such as a reduced propensity for thrombosis of vascular grafts (108).

An extreme case of stress-induced hypermetabolism is burn injury. In these patients, it has been shown that decreasing the sympathetic response with β-blockers can improve the metabolic response and reverse catabolism (109). Decreasing the sympathetic response with β-blockers following high-risk surgery has been shown in a number of studies to reduce cardiac ischemia and the incidence of perioperative myocardial infarction; this has been particularly noted in patients undergoing vascular surgery (110). Despite this fact, a meta-analysis of studies looking at β-blockade in the perioperative period did not find a significant consistent effect on outcome, although ischemia and arrhythmias decreased in frequency (111).

Cardiac output and oxygen delivery. An important body of data regarding the significance of the stress response in terms of outcome has been generated by Shoemaker (112). He demonstrated that patients surviving high-risk surgery, sepsis, and shock states are those in whom measured parameters of cardiac function and oxygen delivery are highest. Moreover, patients with low oxygen delivery developed an oxygen deficit during surgery that was more pronounced in those who developed complications and died. Thus, hemodynamic values may be of use in predicting outcome.

Other investigators have shown that the early use of invasive monitoring may be helpful in the management of elderly (113) and young (114) trauma patients using goal-directed therapy. In a prospective study (115), three groups of general surgical patients were followed. The first group was managed with central venous pressure monitoring; the second group had a pulmonary artery catheter inserted, but therapy was directed by the surgical service according to conventional clinical criteria; and the third group was managed with a pulmonary artery catheter using a rigid protocol to maintain oxygen delivery at supranormal values; the results reported are of interest. The mortality rate decreased from about 30% in both control

TABLE 71.9

ETIOLOGY OF POSTOPERATIVE MENTAL STATUS ALTERATION

Drugs	In the patient emergently anesthetized from the ED, street drugs such as alcohol, narcotics, and cocaine may have been present on induction; residual neuromuscular blockade must also be considered.
Postseizure	A seizure under anesthesia may be easily missed. One must consider the delayed emergence as a possible postictal event.
Glucose	Hyperglycemia or hypoglycemia can result in altered mental status.
Metabolic causes	Hypoxia, hypercarbia, hypernatremia or hyponatremia, hypercalcemia, and hypothermia (usually at or below 31°C) are several examples.
Trauma	Again, in the patient emergently anesthetized from the ER, head trauma must be considered.
Infection	Agitation in an infected patient is sometimes seen; this is no less so in the postoperative period.
Psychogenic causes	Rarely, a patient will feign unconsciousness for some secondary gain. This may only be diagnosed after other life-threatening and treatable causes have been ruled out.
Hemodynamic instability	Hypotension, and sometimes severe hypertension, may cause mental status changes. The former may result from hypovolemia, anaphylaxis, sepsis, or ischemia.
Pain	Pain at the operative site, a full bladder, or gastric distention can result in agitation.

ED, emergency department.

groups to 4% in the protocol group. Other indicators such as length of hospital stay, utilization of resources, and hospital charges per patient were also significantly lower in the protocol group compared with either the central venous pressure–monitored or conventional criteria groups. Other researchers, however, did not find the same results. Gattinoni et al. did not find an advantage to goal-directed therapy designed to increase either cardiac index or mixed venous saturation (116). Sandham et al. looked at the significance of a protocolized treatment with a pulmonary artery catheter and found no advantage compared to standard care without invasive monitoring (117). In contrast, Rivers et al. found that, in the early hours of sepsis, goal-directed therapy that is delivered in the emergency room can improve outcome and decrease hospital mortality (118). Perhaps the effectiveness of goal-directed therapy is dependent on the time frame and will only be effective in the early hours of the insult, particularly when treating a patient population with a high incidence of hypovolemia and unrecognized shock. The surviving sepsis guidelines that endorsed the conclusions from the Rivers' study advocate early goal-directed therapy in septic patients. The goals of this therapy are increasing central venous pressure (CVP) to 8 to 12 cm H_2O, MAP to 65 mm Hg, urine output to 0.5 mL/kg/hour, and central venous saturation to 70%. These goals are probably of great importance in the hypovolemic patient in the early stages of ***un***resuscitated septic shock. There are questions regarding the incidence of these clinical scenarios in other settings (119).

In conclusion, although the data in this section, at first glance, seem to contradict the concept of the beneficial effects of stress reduction, a unified view is that, in the postoperative period, monitoring and therapy should be aggressive and appropriate to ensure adequate systemic oxygen delivery on the one hand, with strict control of the patient's stress on the other. Modifying risk by blunting the stress response should not lead to a compromise in terms of hemodynamic function and oxygen delivery. Thus, although some reduction of the stress response should reduce postoperative adverse events, prospective randomized studies are necessary to confirm this view.

Delirium

Delirium and acute confusional states (Table 71.9) can be very disturbing for patients and family members as well as impose a significant risk to patients with regard to line disconnections, dressing management, and risk of falling from the gurney or bed. The patients require additional nursing care and may require an unplanned ICU admission. The reasons for postoperative delirium are many. Dyer et al. reviewed 80 articles that studied the issue of postoperative delirium. They found that some studies described a diverse incidence from 0% to 73%, and found that age, preoperative cognitive impairment, and use of anticholinergic agents were associated with an increase in the occurrence of delirium (120). Lepouse et al. studied a group of patients following general anesthesia and found that 4.7% of them developed postoperative delirium in the postanesthesia care unit (121). The risk factors for developing delirium were benzodiazepines as premedication, breast surgery, abdominal surgery, and particularly long surgical procedures. Marcantonio et al. found that postoperative delirium was not related to the type of anesthetic used. They did find that intra- and postoperative bleeding and increasing transfusion requirements led to an increase in postoperative delirium (122). In children, some increase in the incidence has been related to the introduction of newer inhalational agents (123). The treatment of delirium is multifactorial. It is probably accepted that the best approach is prevention and should start with exclusion of treatable physical disorders such as pain, electrolyte abnormalities, and urinary retention—a kink in the urinary drainage catheter can be an easily resolved reason for agitation.

Treatment

When treatment is considered, several previously discussed therapeutic modalities are available. Propofol is an attractive drug for continuous sedation, and its cost has decreased markedly in the last years. A comparison of propofol with midazolam for continuous sedation of postoperative, mechanically ventilated patients found similar results for both drugs, although some advantages were claimed for propofol in terms of tolerance of the ICU environment and duration to complete wakefulness after discontinuation of sedation (124).

For continuous propofol sedation, a loading dose of 1 to 2 mg/kg is administered over 1 to 2 minutes, followed by an infusion of 50 to 100 μg/kg/minute; the dose is titrated up or down so that, with gentle stimulation, the patient awakens. Midazolam is dosed at 0.25 to 3 mg/hour in a 70-kg adult. The use of neuromuscular blocking agents without sedation to abort nonpurposeful movement is wrong, and will lead to pain with awareness.

Residual Neuromuscular Blockade

Residual neuromuscular blockade usually presents in one of three ways: (a) delayed return to consciousness, which should have been noted in the operating room by both the surgeon and anesthesiologist; (b) respiratory difficulty with hypercapnia (Table 71.10); and (c) muscle weakness (Table 71.11). The major point in the diagnosis of this entity is to consider it; the major point in treatment is to protect the airway—if necessary, by replacing the endotracheal tube—while the differential diagnosis is worked through.

Diagnosis

Most anesthesiologists monitor the depth of neuromuscular blockade with a twitch-stimulating device or a group of clinical signs. Nevertheless, some persons arrive in the surgical ICU with residual neuromuscular blockade. This condition may take the form of an apparent alteration in mental status (Table 71.9), hypoventilation with hypercapnia, or a seemingly awake and alert status with adequate breathing but a weak or "floppy" appearance. The effect of muscle relaxants can be monitored by applying a supramaximal electrical stimulus to a motor nerve; in the operating room, the ulnar nerve is stimulated to contract the adductor pollicis brevis. If the equipment is properly set up, a single supramaximal stimulus at 50 Hz for 5 seconds that produces contraction without fade correlates with signs of clinical recovery from neuromuscular blockade.

Other more quantitative estimations of neuromuscular blockade use the train-of-four stimulus (four supramaximal stimuli in 2 seconds with each stimulus lasting 0.2 seconds), or double-burst stimulation. With the train-of-four stimulus, when the ratio of the fourth contraction to the first is more than 60%, patients are able to sustain a head lift for over 3 seconds; when the ratio is more than 75%, adequate clinical recovery is present (Table 71.12).

TABLE 71.10

ETIOLOGY OF POSTOPERATIVE HYPERCAPNIA

I. **Central respiratory depression**
   - Intravenous (narcotic) anesthetics
   - Inhaled anesthetic agents

II. **Respiratory muscle dysfunction**
   - Site of incision (upper abdominal, thoracic)
   - Residual neuromuscular blockade
     - Use of drugs that enhance neuromuscular blockade (gentamicin, clindamycin, neomycin, furosemide)
     - Physiologic factors that prevent reversal of neuromuscular blockade (hypokalemia, respiratory acidosis) or enhance the blockade (hypothermia, hypermagnesemia)

III. **Physical factors**
   - Obesity
   - Gastric dilation
   - Tight dressings
   - Body cast

IV. **Increased production of carbon dioxide**
   - Sepsis
   - Shivering
   - Malignant hyperthermia

V. **Underlying hyperthermia**
   - Chronic obstructive pulmonary disease with CO_2 retention
   - Neuromuscular—chest cage dysfunction (kyphoscoliosis)
   - Acute or chronic respiratory failure of any etiology

Modified from Feeley TW. The recovery room. In: Miller RD, ed. *Anesthesia.* 2nd ed. New York: Churchill Livingstone; 1986:1921; and Wyngaarden JB, Smith LH Jr, eds. *Cecil Textbook of Medicine.* 18th ed. Philadelphia: WB Saunders; 1988:417, 472, 474.

Treatment

If residual neuromuscular blockade is present, an attempt to reverse it may be in order. If blockade results from succinylcholine, which can occur in patients with pseudocholinesterase deficiency, reversal agents will not be of any benefit. The diagnosis is made by measuring pseudocholinesterase activity in plasma, and the options are either to keep the patient mechanically ventilated and sedated until neuromuscular function returns or to administer fresh frozen plasma that has the missing enzyme. If a nondepolarizing blocking agent was used, reversal may be attempted with anticholinesterases and anticholinergics (Table 71.13).

An important issue with regard to neuromuscular blocking agents is that of prolonged paralysis in patients who have received neuromuscular blockers for a long period in the ICU. Although controlled studies addressing this problem have not been published, several risk factors for the development of prolonged paralysis have been delineated. Among these are renal failure, concomitant drug use, length of administration, monitoring technique used, and the use of steroids in patients receiving steroid-based drugs such as pancuronium or vecuronium. The best way to prevent this distressing complication is to avoid neuromuscular blockers as much as possible, and to monitor all patients receiving these drugs with a peripheral nerve stimulator. It should also be noted that patients may develop critical illness neuropathy, which can be difficult to differentiate from the residual effects of prolonged administration and in fact

TABLE 71.11

ETIOLOGY OF PROLONGED NEUROMUSCULAR BLOCKADE

I. Nondepolarizing neuromuscular blocking agents
Intensity of neuromuscular blockade
Renal failure (decreased metocurine and pancuronium excretion)
Hepatic failure (decreased pancuronium and vecuronium excretion)
Residual potent inhaled anesthetic agent
Inadequate dose of reversal agents
Hypothermia
Acid-base state
Hypokalemia, hypermagnesemia
Drugs
Antibiotics (gentamicin, clindamycin, and multiple other drugs with several mechanisms)
Local anesthetics
Antiarrhythmics (quinidine)
Furosemide
Dantrolene
Trimethaphan (possibly)
Underlying diseases (myasthenia gravis, myasthenic syndrome, familial periodic paralysis)
II. Depolarizing neuromuscular blocking agents (succinylcholine)
Decreased effective pseudocholinesterase
Phase II block
Hypermagnesemia
Local anesthetics

Modified from Miller RD, Savarese JJ. Pharmacology of muscle relaxants and their antagonists. In: Miller RD, ed. *Anesthesia.* 2nd ed. New York: Churchill Livingstone; 1986:889.

could be pathophysiologically related (125). The use of neuromuscular blocking agents and the effect they may have on development of critical illness neuropathy has also been linked to an increased cost of illness (126).

Malignant Hyperthermia

Manifestations of malignant hyperthermia may be divided into early, late, and postcrisis (Table 71.14). The differential diagnosis of MH includes sepsis, light anesthesia, thyrotoxicosis, myotonias, neuroleptic malignant syndrome, and pheochromocytoma.

Background

Malignant hyperthermia is a pharmacogenetic clinical syndrome that usually occurs during general anesthesia. Its onset may be delayed for several hours; thus, the initial presentation may be in the surgical ICU. The hallmark of the syndrome is rapidly increasing temperature caused by uncontrolled skeletal muscle metabolism that can result in rhabdomyolysis and death. After exposure to a triggering agent, a dramatic increase in aerobic metabolism occurs in the skeletal muscle of susceptible persons. Oxygen consumption can increase threefold, whereas blood lactate may increase 15- to 20-fold. The mechanism for this entity involves myoplasmic calcium accumulation and a failure of calcium uptake by the sarcoplasmic reticulum.

TABLE 71.12

CLINICAL SIGNS OF RECOVERY FROM NEUROMUSCULAR BLOCKADE

I. Awake patient
Opens eyes widely
Coughs effectively
Sustains tongue protrusion
Sustains hand grip
Sustains head lift for more than 5 sec
Vital capacity of greater than or equal to 15 mL/kg
PNP of greater than or equal to 20 cm H_2O
Sustained 50-Hz tetanic stimulation for 5 sec
II. Patient who is asleep or unable to follow commands
Tidal volume of 5–10 mL/kg
PNP of greater than or equal to 25 cm H_2O
Sustained 50-Hz tetanic stimulation for 5 sec

PNP, peak negative pressure.
Modified from Ali HH, Miller RD. Monitoring of neuromuscular function. In: Miller RD, ed. *Anesthesia.* 2nd ed. New York: Churchill Livingstone; 1986:871.

The incidence of MH varies; fulminant cases are seen from 1 in 250,000 to 1 in 62,000 anesthetics, the latter incidence when triggering agents are used; suspected MH occurs in 1 in 6,000 anesthetics overall and 1 in 4,200 anesthetics with triggering agents. A 24-hour per day emergency phone number for consultations has been set up by the Malignant Hyperthermia Association of the United States (1-209-634-4917).

Evaluation of susceptibility includes the family history and measurement of baseline creatine kinase level; it is elevated in 70% of those affected. The definitive test is a muscle biopsy for contracture studies after exposure to halothane, caffeine, halothane plus caffeine, or potassium. Although laboratory standardization of contracture testing is not complete, patients who have negative *in vitro* contracture tests for MH appear to have no adverse anesthetic outcome when subsequently exposed to triggering anesthetic agents. However, this test is invasive and not available in all medical facilities. A new approach is that of genetic testing—the mutation conferring the susceptibility for MH is recognized and can be mapped. The future of diagnosis of MH susceptibility probably lies in genetic diagnosis (127).

TABLE 71.13

REVERSAL AGENTS USED WITH NEUROMUSCULAR BLOCKING AGENTS

Anticholinesterase	Anticholinergic
Neostigmine 35–70 μg/kg (maximum, 5 mg)	Atropine 20 μg/kg
	or
Edrophonium 500–1,000 μg/kg	Glycopyrrolate 10 μg/kg
Pyridostigmine 175–350 μg/kg (maximum, 20 mg)	

Modified from Miller RD, Savarese JJ. Pharmacology of muscle relaxants and their antagonists. In: Miller RD, ed. *Anesthesia.* 2nd ed. New York: Churchill Livingstone; 1986:889.

TABLE 71.14

SIGNS OF MALIGNANT HYPERTHERMIA

Early signs	Late signs	Postcrisis signs
Skeletal muscle rigidity	Hyperpyrexia—may exceed 43°C (109.4°F)	Muscle pain, edema
Tachycardia and hypertension	Cyanosis	Central nervous system damage
Elevated $PetCO_2$	Serum electrolyte abnormalities	Renal failure
Acidosis	Elevated serum creatinine phosphokinase	Continued electrolyte imbalance
Dysrhythmias	Myoglobinuria Coagulopathy Cardiac failure and pulmonary edema	

$PetCO_2$, end tidal partial pressure of carbon dioxide.

Diagnosis

Treating MH is easier than making the clinical diagnosis because the presenting signs may be mistaken for benign conditions, and MH is relatively uncommon. When triggering anesthetic drugs—potent inhaled anesthetic agents, succinylcholine—are used, MH must be considered in the presence of unexplained tachycardia, tachypnea, arrhythmias, mottling, cyanosis, hyperthermia, muscle rigidity, diaphoresis, or hemodynamic instability. The presence of more than one sign must initiate arterial and central venous blood gas analysis for metabolic and respiratory acidosis and hyperkalemia. Central venous oxygen and carbon dioxide partial pressures change more dramatically than do those of arterial blood.

TABLE 71.15

ACUTE THERAPY FOR MALIGNANT HYPERTHERMIA

I. **Discontinue all anesthetic agents.**
   Hyperventilate with an FiO_2 of 1.0.
   CO_2 is increased so hyperventilate to achieve a normal $PaCO_2$.
II. **Dantrolene**
   Intravenously 2 mg/kg every 5 min to a total of 10 mg/kg
   Effective dosage should be repeated every 10–15 h for at least 48 h
III. **Sodium bicarbonate**
   Initial dose (mEq) = (base excess × [body weight in kg])/4
   Give half the calculated dose; repeat as determined by arterial blood gas studies.
IV. **Control fever**
   Iced fluids
   Surface cooling
   Cooling of body cavities with sterile iced saline
   Heat exchanger with a pump oxygenator
   Dantrolene
V. **Monitor urinary output**
   At least 0.5 mL/kg/h
   If myoglobinuria is present, at least 1 mL/kg/h
VI. **Further therapy**
   Guided by blood studies, temperature, and urine output
   (Blood studies include blood gases, electrolytes, liver profile, coagulation studies [including DIC studies], serum hemoglobin and myoglobin, and urine hemoglobin and myoglobin.)

DIC, disseminated intravascular coagulation; FiO_2, fraction of inspired oxygen.
Modified from Askanazi J. Principles of nutritional support. In: Barash PG, Deutsch S, Tinker J, eds. *Refresher Courses in Anesthesiology.* Vol. 14. Philadelphia: JB Lippincott; 1986:1.

Treatment

The mortality rate of MH has decreased from 70% to less than 5% when recognized and treated appropriately because of improved therapy (Table 71.15) (6). After brief administration of a triggering agent, discontinuation may abort the attack. With fulminant MH—$PaCO_2$ above 60 mm Hg and increasing; base excess more than –5 mEq/L; and a body temperature that is increasing by approximately 1°C every 15 minutes—specific therapy with dantrolene is required. The mechanism of action of dantrolene is not completely clear, but it is known to affect the ryanodine receptor, which is a major calcium release channel of the skeletal muscle sarcoplasmic reticulum, thus decreasing the intracellular calcium. Dantrolene is the key to successful MH treatment. Because of its poor water solubility, the preparation of dantrolene for intravenous use requires the full attention of at least one person. Thus, help must be requested as soon as the diagnosis is tentatively made (128).

References

1. Brown D. Risk and outcome analysis: myths and truths. In: Kirby RR, Gravenstein N, ed. *Clinical Anesthesia Practice.* Philadelphia: JB Lippincott; 1994:62.
2. Aders A, Aders H. Anaesthetic adverse incident reports: an Australian study of 1,231 outcomes. *Anaesth Intensive Care.* 2005;33(3):336–344.
3. Cheney FW, Posner KL, Lee LA, et al. Trends in anesthesia-related death and brain damage: a closed claims analysis. *Anesthesiology.* 2006;105(6): 1081–1086.
4. Benumof JL. Management of the difficult adult airway. With special emphasis on awake tracheal intubation. *Anesthesiology.* 1991;75(6):1087–1110.
5. Badner NH, Gelb AW. Postoperative myocardial infarction (PMI) after noncardiac surgery. *Anesthesiology.* 1999;90(2):644.
6. Ali SZ, Taguchi A, Rosenberg H. Malignant hyperthermia. *Best Pract Res Clin Anaesthesiol.* 2003;17(4):519–533.
7. Evers A, Koblin D. Inhalational anesthetics. In: Evers A, Maze M, eds. *Anesthetic Pharmacology: Physiologic Principles and Clinical Practice.* Philadelphia: Churchill Livingstone; 2004:369–393.

8. Pagel PS, Kampine JP, Schmeling WT, et al. Comparison of the systemic and coronary hemodynamic actions of desflurane, isoflurane, halothane, and enflurane in the chronically instrumented dog. *Anesthesiology.* 1991;74(3): 539–551.
9. Aypar E, Karagoz AH, Ozer S, et al. The effects of sevoflurane and desflurane anesthesia on QTc interval and cardiac rhythm in children. *Paediatr Anaesth.* 2007;17(6):563–567.
10. Loer SA, Scheeren TW, Tarnow J. Desflurane inhibits hypoxic pulmonary vasoconstriction in isolated rabbit lungs. *Anesthesiology.* 1995;83(3):552–556.
11. Schwarzkopf K, Schreiber T, Bauer R, et al. The effects of increasing concentrations of isoflurane and desflurane on pulmonary perfusion and systemic oxygenation during one-lung ventilation in pigs. *Anesth Analg.* 2001;93(6): 1434–1438, table of contents.
12. Groeben H, Meier S, Tankersley CG, et al. Influence of volatile anaesthetics on hypercapnoeic ventilatory responses in mice with blunted respiratory drive. *Br J Anaesth.* 2004;92(5):697–703.
13. Fukuda H, Kawamoto M, Yuge O, et al. A comparison of the effects of prolonged (>10 hour) low-flow sevoflurane, high-flow sevoflurane, and low-flow isoflurane anaesthesia on hepatorenal function in orthopaedic patients. *Anaesth Intensive Care.* 2004;32(2):210–218.
14. Reichle FM, Conzen PF. Halogenated inhalational anaesthetics. *Best Pract Res Clin Anaesthesiol.* 2003;17(1):29–46.
15. Litz RJ, Hubler M, Lorenz W, et al. Renal responses to desflurane and isoflurane in patients with renal insufficiency. *Anesthesiology.* 2002;97(5):1133–1136.
16. Kelbel I, Weiss M. Anaesthetics and immune function. *Curr Opin Anaesthesiol.* 2001;14(6):685–691.
17. Walton B. Effects of anaesthesia and surgery on immune status. *Br J Anaesth.* 1979;51(1):37–43.
18. Schneemilch CE, Ittenson A, Ansorge S, et al. Effect of 2 anesthetic techniques on the postoperative proinflammatory and anti-inflammatory cytokine response and cellular immune function to minor surgery. *J Clin Anesth.* 2005;17(7):517–527.
19. Beilin B, Shavit Y, Trabekin E, et al. The effects of postoperative pain management on immune response to surgery. *Anesth Analg.* 2003;97(3):822–827.
20. Everson NW, Neoptolemos JP, Scott DJ, et al. The effect of surgical operation upon monocytes. *Br J Surg.* 1981;68(4):257–260.
21. Shennib H, Mulder DS, Chiu RC. Replenishing the starved patient. When do lung immune cells recover? *Chest.* 1985;87(2):138–139.
22. Bolla G, Tuzzato G. Immunologic postoperative competence after laparoscopy versus laparotomy. *Surg Endosc.* 2003;17(8):1247–1250.
23. Tonnesen E, Mickley H, Grunnet N. Natural killer cell activity during premedication, anaesthesia and surgery. *Acta Anaesthesiol Scand.* 1983;27(3): 238–241.
24. Tonnesen E, Wahlgreen C. Influence of extradural and general anaesthesia on natural killer cell activity and lymphocyte subpopulations in patients undergoing hysterectomy. *Br J Anaesth.* 1988;60(5):500–507.
25. Katzav S, Shapiro J, Segal S, et al. General anesthesia during excision of a mouse tumor accelerates postsurgical growth of metastases by suppression of natural killer cell activity. *Isr J Med Sci.* 1986;22(5):339–345.
26. Page GG, Ben-Eliyahu S, Liebeskind JC. The role of LGL/NK cells in surgery-induced promotion of metastasis and its attenuation by morphine. *Brain Behav Immun.* 1994;8(3):241–250.
27. Nakagawara M, Takeshige K, Takamatsu J, et al. Inhibition of superoxide production and Ca2+ mobilization in human neutrophils by halothane, enflurane, and isoflurane. *Anesthesiology.* 1986;64(1):4–12.
28. Welch WD. Inhibition of neutrophil cidal activity by volatile anesthetics. *Anesthesiology.* 1986;64(1):1–3.
29. Ciepichal J, Kubler A. Effect of general and regional anesthesia on some neutrophil functions. *Arch Immunol Ther Exp (Warsz).* 1998;46(3):183–192.
30. van Dijk WC, Verbrugh HA, van Rijswijk RE, et al. Neutrophil function, serum opsonic activity, and delayed hypersensitivity in surgical patients. *Surgery.* 1982;92(1):21–29.
31. Perttila J, Lilius EM, Salo M. Effects of anaesthesia and surgery on serum opsonic capacity. *Acta Anaesthesiol Scand.* 1986;30(2):173–176.
32. Volk T, Schenk M, Voigt K, et al. Postoperative epidural anesthesia preserves lymphocyte, but not monocyte, immune function after major spine surgery. *Anesth Analg.* 2004;98(4):1086–1092, table of contents.
33. Abraham E, Chang YH. Cellular and humoral bases of hemorrhage-induced depression of lymphocyte function. *Crit Care Med.* 1986;14(2):81–86.
34. Abraham E, Chang YH. Effects of intravenous immunoglobulin on hemorrhage-induced alterations in plasma cell repertoires. *Crit Care Med.* 1990; 18(11):1252–1256.
35. Pert CB, Snyder SH. Opiate receptor: demonstration in nervous tissue. *Science.* 1973;179(77):1011–1014.
36. Gutstein H, Huda A. Opioid analgesics. In: Brunton L, Lazo J, Parker K, eds. *Goodman and Gilman's the Pharmacological Basis of Therapeutics.* 11th ed. San Diego: McGraw-Hill Companies; 2006:547–590.
37. Scott LJ, Perry CM. Remifentanil: a review of its use during the induction and maintenance of general anaesthesia. *Drugs.* 2005;65(13):1793–1823.
38. Richardson SP, Egan TD. The safety of remifentanil by bolus injection. *Expert Opin Drug Saf.* 2005;4(4):643–651.
39. Joo HS, Salasidis GC, Kataoka MT, et al. Comparison of bolus remifentanil versus bolus fentanyl for induction of anesthesia and tracheal intubation in patients with cardiac disease. *J Cardiothorac Vasc Anesth.* 2004;18(3):263–268.
40. Ma XD, Hauerberg J, Pedersen DB, et al. Effects of morphine on cerebral blood flow autoregulation CO2-reactivity in experimental subarachnoid hemorrhage. *J Neurosurg Anesthesiol.* 1999;11(4):264–272.
41. Bedell EA, DeWitt DS, Prough DS. Fentanyl infusion preserves cerebral blood flow during decreased arterial blood pressure after traumatic brain injury in cats. *J Neurotrauma.* 1998;15(11):985–992.
42. Giesecke K, Hamberger B, Jarnberg PO, et al. High- and low-dose fentanyl anaesthesia: hormonal and metabolic responses during cholecystectomy. *Br J Anaesth.* 1988;61(5):575–582.
43. Moller IW, Krantz T, Wandall E, et al. Effect of alfentanil anaesthesia on the adrenocortical and hyperglycaemic response to abdominal surgery. *Br J Anaesth.* 1985;57(6):591–594.
44. Shavit Y, Ben-Eliyahu S, Zeidel A, et al. Effects of fentanyl on natural killer cell activity and on resistance to tumor metastasis in rats. Dose and timing study. *Neuroimmunomodulation.* 2004;11(4):255–260.
45. Beilin B, Shavit Y, Cohn S, et al. Narcotic-induced suppression of natural killer cell activity in ventilated and nonventilated rats. *Clin Immunol Immunopathol.* 1992;64(2):173–176.
46. McDonough RJ, Madden JJ, Falek A. Alteration of T and null lymphocyte frequencies in the peripheral blood of human opiate addicts. *J Immunol.* 1980;125:2539.
47. Brown SM, Stimmel B, RN T. Immunologic dysfunction in heroin addicts. *Arch Int Med.* 1974;134:1001.
48. Beilin B, Shavit Y, Hart J, et al. Effects of anesthesia based on large versus small doses of fentanyl on natural killer cell cytotoxicity in the perioperative period. *Anesth Analg.* 1996;82(3):492–497.
49. Schneemilch CE, Hachenberg T, Ansorge S, et al. Effects of different anaesthetic agents on immune cell function *in vitro*. *Eur J Anaesthesiol.* 2005;22(8):616–623.
50. Frenette A, Perreault M, Lam S, et al. Thiopental-induced neutropenia in two patients with severe head trauma. *Pharmacotherapy.* 2007;27(3):464–471.
51. White P. Propofol: pharmacokinetics and pharmacodynamics. *Semin Anesth.* 1988;7(Suppl 1):4.
52. Barrientos-Vega RM, Sanchez-Soria MMR, Morales-Garcia CR, et al. Pharmacoeconomic assessment of propofol 2% used for prolonged sedation. *Crit Care Med.* 2001;29(2):317–322.
53. Coates D. Diprivan (propofol) infusion anesthesia. *Semin Anesth.* 1988; 7(Suppl 1):73.
54. Ramani R, Todd MM, Warner DS. A dose-response study of the influence of propofol on cerebral blood flow, metabolism and the electroencephalogram in the rabbit. *J Neurosurg Anesthesiol.* 1992;4(2):110–119.
55. Nimmo GR, Mackenzie SJ, IS G. Haemodynamic and oxygen transport effects of propofol infusion in critically ill adults. *Anaesthesia.* 1994;49(6): 485–489.
56. Blouin RT, Seifert HA, Babenco HD, et al. Propofol depresses the hypoxic ventilatory response during conscious sedation and isohypercapnia. *Anesthesiology.* 1993;79(6):1177–1182.
57. Ledowski T, Bein B, Hanss R, et al. Neuroendocrine stress response and heart rate variability: a comparison of total intravenous versus balanced anesthesia. *Anesth Analg.* 2005;101(6):1700–1705.
58. Fujii Y, Shiga Y. Influence of aging on lidocaine requirements for pain on injection of propofol. *J Clin Anesth.* 2006;18(7):526–529.
59. Kam PC, Cardone D. Propofol infusion syndrome. *Anaesthesia.* 2007; 62(7):690–701.
60. Chondrogiannis KD, Siontis GC, Koulouras VP, et al. Acute lung injury probably associated with infusion of propofol emulsion. *Anaesthesia.* 2007;62(8):835–837.
61. Fudickar A, Bein B, Tonner PH. Propofol infusion syndrome in anaesthesia and intensive care medicine. *Curr Opin Anaesthesiol.* 2006;19(4):404–410.
62. Kumar MA, Urrutia VC, Thomas CE, et al. The syndrome of irreversible acidosis after prolonged propofol infusion. *Neurocrit Care.* 2005;3(3):257–259.
63. De Waele JJ, Hoste E. Propofol infusion syndrome in a patient with sepsis. *Anaesth Intensive Care.* 2006;34(5):676–677.
64. Eriksen J, Povey HM. A case of suspected non-neurosurgical adult fatal propofol infusion syndrome. *Acta Anaesthesiol Scand.* 2006;50(1):117–119.
65. Beilin B, Rusabrov Y, Shapira Y, et al. Low-dose ketamine affects immune responses in humans during the early postoperative period. *Br J Anaesth.* 2007.
66. Sprung J, Ogletree-Hughes ML, Moravec CS. *The Effects of Etomidate on the Contractility of Failing and Nonfailing Human Heart Muscle.* Vol 91. 2000:68–75.
67. Lundy JB, Slane ML, Frizzi JD. Acute adrenal insufficiency after a single dose of etomidate. *J Intensive Care Med.* 2007;22(2):111–117.
68. Bloomfield R, Noble DW. Etomidate, pharmacological adrenalectomy and the critically ill: a matter of vital importance. *Crit Care.* 2006;10(4):161.
69. Jackson WL Jr. Should we use etomidate as an induction agent for endotracheal intubation in patients with septic shock?: a critical appraisal. *Chest.* 2005;127(3):1031–1038.

70. Ray DC, McKeown DW. Effect of induction agent on vasopressor and steroid use, and outcome in patients with septic shock. *Crit Care.* 2007;11(3):R56.
71. Gerlach AT, Dasta JF. Dexmedetomidine: an updated review. *Ann Pharmacother.* 2007;41(2):245–252.
72. Siobal MS, Kallet RH, Kivett VA, et al Use of dexmedetomidine to facilitate extubation in surgical intensive-care-unit patients who failed previous weaning attempts following prolonged mechanical ventilation: a pilot study. *Respir Care.* 2006;51(5):492–496.
73. Exadaktylos AK, Buggy DJ, Moriarty DC, et al. Can anesthetic technique for primary breast cancer surgery affect recurrence or metastasis? *Anesthesiology.* 2006;105(4):660–664.
74. Ventilation with lower tidal volumes as compared with traditional tidal volumes for acute lung injury and the acute respiratory distress syndrome. The Acute Respiratory Distress Syndrome Network. *N Engl J Med.* 2000;342(18):1301–1308.
75. Amato MB, Barbas CS, Medeiros DM, et al. Effect of a protective-ventilation strategy on mortality in the acute respiratory distress syndrome. *N Engl J Med.* 1998;338(6):347–354.
76. Kao SJ, Su CF, Liu DD, et al. Endotoxin-induced acute lung injury and organ dysfunction are attenuated by pentobarbital anaesthesia. *Clin Exp Pharmacol Physiol.* 2007;34(5-6):480–487.
77. Yang J, Li W, Duan M, et al. Large dose ketamine inhibits lipopolysaccharide-induced acute lung injury in rats. *Inflamm Res.* 2005;54(3): 133–137.
78. Tandon S, Batchelor A, Bullock R, et al. Peri-operative risk factors for acute lung injury after elective oesophagectomy. *Br J Anaesth.* 2001;86(5):633–638.
79. Katz JA, Kallet RH, Alonso JA, et al. Improved flow and pressure capabilities of the Datex-Ohmeda SmartVent anesthesia ventilator. *J Clin Anesth.* 2000;12(1):40–47.
80. Wiedemann HP, Wheeler AP, Bernard GR, et al. Comparison of two fluid-management strategies in acute lung injury. *N Engl J Med.* 2006; 354(24):2564–2575.
81. Nisanevich V, Felsenstein I, Almogy G, et al. Effect of intraoperative fluid management on outcome after intraabdominal surgery. *Anesthesiology.* 2005;103(1):25–32.
82. Michard F. Changes in arterial pressure during mechanical ventilation. *Anesthesiology.* 2005;103(2):419–428; quiz 449–445.
83. Michard F, Teboul JL. Predicting fluid responsiveness in ICU patients: a critical analysis of the evidence. *Chest.* 2002;121(6):2000–2008.
84. Ouattara A, Lecomte P, Le Manach Y, et al. Poor intraoperative blood glucose control is associated with a worsened hospital outcome after cardiac surgery in diabetic patients. *Anesthesiology.* 2005;103(4):687–694.
85. Belda FJ, Aguilera L, Garcia de la Asuncion J, et al. Supplemental perioperative oxygen and the risk of surgical wound infection: a randomized controlled trial. *JAMA.* 2005;294(16):2035–2042.
86. Greif R, Laciny S, Rapf B, et al. Supplemental oxygen reduces the incidence of postoperative nausea and vomiting. *Anesthesiology.* 1999;91(5):1246–1252.
87. Patton WC, Baker CL Jr. Prevalence of negative-pressure pulmonary edema at an orthopaedic hospital. *J South Orthop Assoc.* 2000;9(4):248–253.
88. Weissman C. The metabolic response to stress: an overview and update. *Anesthesiology.* 1990;73(2):308–327.
89. Abraham E. Physiologic stress and cellular ischemia: relationship to immunosuppression and susceptibility to sepsis. *Crit Care Med.* 1991;19(5): 613–618.
90. Abraham E, Freitas AA. Hemorrhage in mice induces alterations in immunoglobulin-secreting B cells. *Crit Care Med.* 1989;17(10):1015–1019.
91. Schmand JF, Ayala A, Chaudry IH. Effects of trauma, duration of hypotension, and resuscitation regimen on cellular immunity after hemorrhagic shock. *Crit Care Med.* 1994;22(7):1076–1083.
92. Knoferl MW, Angele MK, Diodato MD, et al. Female sex hormones regulate macrophage function after trauma-hemorrhage and prevent increased death rate from subsequent sepsis. *Ann Surg.* 2002;235(1):105–112.
93. Arieff AI. Hyponatremia, convulsions, respiratory arrest, and permanent brain damage after elective surgery in healthy women. *N Engl J Med.* 1986; 314(24):1529–1535.
94. Burrows FA, Shutack JG, Crone RK. Inappropriate secretion of antidiuretic hormone in a postsurgical pediatric population. *Crit Care Med.* 1983;11(7): 527–531.
95. Lieh-Lai MW, Stanitski DF, Sarnaik AP, et al. Syndrome of inappropriate antidiuretic hormone secretion in children following spinal fusion. *Crit Care Med.* 1999;27(3):622–627.
96. Amini A, Schmidt MH. Syndrome of inappropriate secretion of antidiuretic hormone and hyponatremia after spinal surgery. *Neurosurg Focus.* 2004;16(4):E10.
97. Shirani KZ, Vaughan GM, Robertson GL, et al. Inappropriate vasopressin secretion (SIADH) in burned patients. *J Trauma.* 1983;23(3):217–224.
98. Kouraklis G, Glinavou A, Raftopoulos L, et al. Epidural analgesia attenuates the systemic stress response to upper abdominal surgery: a randomized trial. *Int Surg.* 2000;85(4):353–357.
99. Roizen MF, Horrigan RW, Frazer BM. Anesthetic doses blocking adrenergic (stress) and cardiovascular responses to incision–MAC BAR. *Anesthesiology.* 1981;54(5):390–398.
100. Chernow B, Alexander HR, Smallridge RC, et al. Hormonal responses to graded surgical stress. *Arch Intern Med.* 1987;147(7):1273–1278.
101. Stanley TH, Berman L, Green O, et al. Plasma catecholamine and cortisol responses to fentanyl–oxygen anesthesia for coronary-artery operations. *Anesthesiology.* 1980;53(3):250–253.
102. Roth-Isigkeit A, Brechmann J, Dibbelt L, et al. Persistent endocrine stress response in patients undergoing cardiac surgery. *J Endocrinol Invest.* 1998; 21(1):12–19.
103. Holte K, Kehlet H. Effect of postoperative epidural analgesia on surgical outcome. *Minerva Anestesiol.* 2002;68(4):157–161.
104. Kehlet H, Brandt MR, Hansen AP, et al. Effect of epidural analgesia on metabolic profiles during and after surgery. *Br J Surg.* 1979;66(8):543–546.
105. Boltz MG, Krane EJ. Combined regional and light general anesthesia: are the risks increased or minimized? *Curr Opin Anaesthesiol.* 1999;12(3):321–323.
106. Yeager MP, Glass DD, Neff RK, et al. Epidural anesthesia and analgesia in high-risk surgical patients. *Anesthesiology.* 1987;66(6):729–736.
107. Baron JF, Bertrand M, Barre E, et al. Combined epidural and general anesthesia versus general anesthesia for abdominal aortic surgery. *Anesthesiology.* 1991;75(4):611–618.
108. Tuman KJ, McCarthy RJ, March RJ, et al. Effects of epidural anesthesia and analgesia on coagulation and outcome after major vascular surgery. *Anesth Analg.* 1991;73(6):696–704.
109. Herndon DN, Hart DW, Wolf SE, et al. Reversal of catabolism by beta-blockade after severe burns. *N Engl J Med.* 2001;345(17):1223–1229.
110. Venkataraman R. Vascular surgery critical care: perioperative cardiac optimization to improve survival. *Crit Care Med.* 2006;34(9 Suppl):S200–207.
111. Wiesbauer F, Schlager O, Domanovits H, et al. Perioperative beta-blockers for preventing surgery-related mortality and morbidity: a systematic review and meta-analysis. *Anesth Analg.* 2007;104(1):27–41.
112. Shoemaker WC. Pathophysiology, monitoring, outcome prediction, and therapy of shock states. *Crit Care Clin.* 1987;3(2):307–357.
113. Scalea TM, Simon HM, Duncan AO, et al. Geriatric blunt multiple trauma: improved survival with early invasive monitoring. *J Trauma.* 1990;30(2): 129–134; discussion 134–136.
114. Abou-Khalil B, Scalea TM, Trooskin SZ, et al. Hemodynamic responses to shock in young trauma patients: need for invasive monitoring. *Crit Care Med.* 1994;22(4):633–639.
115. Shoemaker WC, Appel PL, Kram HB, et al. Prospective trial of supranormal values of survivors as therapeutic goals in high-risk surgical patients. *Chest.* 1988;94(6):1176–1186.
116. Gattinoni L, Brazzi L, Pelosi P, et al. A trial of goal-oriented hemodynamic therapy in critically ill patients. SvO2 Collaborative Group. *N Engl J Med.* 1995;333(16):1025–1032.
117. Sandham JD, Hull RD, Brant RF, et al. A randomized, controlled trial of the use of pulmonary-artery catheters in high-risk surgical patients. *N Engl J Med.* 2003;348(1):5–14.
118. Rivers E, Nguyen B, Havstad S, et al. Early goal-directed therapy in the treatment of severe sepsis and septic shock. *N Engl J Med.* 2001;345(19):1368–1377.
119. Ho BC, Bellomo R, McGain F, et al. The incidence and outcome of septic shock patients in the absence of early-goal directed therapy. *Crit Care.* 2006;10(3):R80.
120. Dyer CB, Ashton CM, Teasdale TA. Postoperative delirium. A review of 80 primary data-collection studies. *Arch Intern Med.* 1995;155(5):461–465.
121. Lepouse C, Lautner CA, Liu L, et al. Emergence delirium in adults in the post-anaesthesia care unit. *Br J Anaesth.* 2006;96(6):747–753.
122. Marcantonio ER, Goldman L, Orav EJ, et al. The association of intraoperative factors with the development of postoperative delirium. *Am J Med.* 1998;105(5):380–384.
123. Vlajkovic GP, Sindjelic RP. Emergence delirium in children: many questions, few answers. *Anesth Analg.* 2007;104(1):84–91.
124. Ronan KP, Gallagher TJ, George B, et al. Comparison of propofol and midazolam for sedation in intensive care unit patients. *Crit Care Med.* 1995; 23(2):286–293.
125. Gorson KC. Approach to neuromuscular disorders in the intensive care unit. *Neurocrit Care.* 2005;3(3):195–212.
126. Kress JP, Hall JB. Cost considerations in sedation, analgesia, and neuromuscular blockade in the intensive care unit. *Semin Respir Crit Care Med.* 2001;22(2):199–210.
127. Litman RS, Rosenberg H. Malignant hyperthermia: update on susceptibility testing. *JAMA.* 2005;293(23):2918–2924.
128. Krause T, Gerbershagen MU, Fiege M, et al. Dantrolene—a review of its pharmacology, therapeutic use and new developments. *Anaesthesia.* 2004;59(4):364–373.

CHAPTER 72 ■ INITIAL MANAGEMENT OF THE TRAUMA PATIENT

SCOTT R. KARLAN • DANIEL R. MARGULIES

The many chapters of this book testify to the many facets of critical care. Most are applicable to trauma patients in the intensive care unit (ICU). In contrast, the initial management of the trauma patient requires a different focus and prioritization. This chapter presents common life-threatening problems that face all critical care physicians who care for trauma victims.

Trauma patients look different. Most start out younger and healthier than other ICU patients but the severity of many of their injuries mandates expert critical care management. How does initial trauma care differ from other critical care treatment? Time is the key. Many of the more common traumatic injuries are rapidly lethal. One's desire to thoroughly evaluate a trauma patient must therefore be tempered by a need to prioritize within available time. This prioritization, aided by careful planning and a team approach, contributes to patient survival.

THE TEAM

Your treatment plan needs to start before the next trauma patient arrives. A multiply injured patient may require several simultaneous interventions. Having a team of physicians, nurses, technicians, therapists, and aides allows for parallel rather than sequential treatment. Adding personnel (e.g., x-ray technicians, respiratory therapists, surgical specialists) to your team encourages these individuals (and their departments) to commit to trauma care, potentially reducing treatment delays. Noise rises exponentially with the size of the team, making it difficult to communicate or to auscultate breath sounds and heart tones. Having a common paging system for all members of the team is essential to reduce redundancy and activate the necessary team prior to the arrival of the patient at your hospital. This activation system can be a tiered response depending on the facility you work in. Regardless, critically reviewing prior trauma resuscitations in your facility will reveal any needed additions or deletions of members to your team.

Take a lesson from the National Association for Stock Car Auto Racing (NASCAR). To function as a team, you need to practice as a team. Mock trauma drills allow you to do it over until you do it right. Do you have more than one chest tube set? How long does it take to get the drugs for a rapid sequence induction and intubation? Do you even have a pediatric endotracheal tube? A NASCAR team can change four tires and fill the gas tank in about a minute. Your team will need to establish IV access and administer fluid, gather baseline vital signs, and complete the primary survey in this time frame. Do team members understand the big picture (what needs to be done for the patient) beyond their specific assignments? Are they prepared to shift roles when necessary (e.g., when a patient needs intubation, or when IV access is problematic)? If you have team members trained in the medical intensive care unit, can they "think surgically," as intervention may be needed without a clear diagnosis?

As you build a team, think outside the hospital. Organized trauma networks reduce preventable deaths (1,2). By joining such a network, your hospital integrates paramedics and other field triage personnel into your team. Although the number of trauma centers has risen from 471 in 1991 to 1,154 in 2002 (including 190 level I and 263 level II centers) (3), 46 million Americans still live more than an hour from a level 1 or 2 center (4). Committing the resources to become a level I or level II trauma center will optimize care at your hospital and in the community. These resources include on-site trauma surgeons, immediately available operating rooms, rapidly available surgical specialists, a trauma manager, quality improvement processes, and other benefits.

TRIAGE

Called to the scene of an accident, paramedics initially triage the victims. They determine who to transport and when and where to take them (following established community protocols). In all cases, the number of patients and severity of their injuries are weighed against available resources. Ideally the most severely injured are taken to the center most capable of treating that patient, so when many injuries occur at the same time they may be divided between available hospitals. Blunt and penetrating urban trauma typically involves relatively few patients at a time. Several simultaneous incidents may occur and may overwhelm a community. September 11 has taught us that we need to prepare for multiple victims.

In a mass casualty event, you may need to evacuate the emergency department (ED) to make room for incoming patients. The seriously injured will be brought in slowly as patients with minor injuries flood into your waiting room. ED physicians normally stay with the ED patients as they are moved elsewhere in the hospital. Although surgeons will be needed in the operating room, it is important that the vital role of making these initial triage decisions be filled by someone who is experienced in trauma management and understands the physiology of traumatic injury.

Triage is most effective at "ground zero," a site in the field where patients are gathered prior to transport. If roads and communications are disrupted, much of the initial trauma care may need to be provided at that site. Ideally, a physician with trauma experience and knowledge of community resources goes to the field to oversee triage rather than waiting in the emergency department.

Paramedics play a critical role even when triage is not an issue. Their observations may be the only medical history that is ever available. Did they speak to witnesses of a shooting? How far did a patient fall? Was extrication necessary after a car crash? How much blood was at the scene? Paramedics will communicate most of this information to the trauma team upon arrival, along with any other observations (patient stability, apparent injuries). Radio communication provides much of this prehospital information, but direct communication with the paramedics before they leave is important. Knowing about likely injuries allows you to focus on treating the patient, rather than listening to paramedics, when the patient arrives. If paramedics have already started two large-bore IVs, intubated the patient, and given 2 liters of fluid, your priorities will change. Every minute of advance warning can save critical seconds later on.

PRIORITIZATION

The American College of Surgeons, through its Advanced Trauma Life Support (ATLS) course (5), has taught generations of physicians and nurses to focus on the ABCDE's of trauma. "Airway, breathing, and circulation" is worth repeating over and over as you struggle to revive a trauma victim. When circumstances go from bad to worse (e.g., multiple simultaneous life-threatening injuries, in a deteriorating patient not responding to resuscitation), remember the ABC's. An obstructed airway is lethal within minutes. Securing an airway can buy enough time to address many other injuries. For this reason, it is more important to look for airway obstruction (even in intubated patients) than for intracerebral bleeding, aortic dissection, pancreatic transection, or virtually any other injury.

After ensuring the ABCs, "D" is a reminder to consider disability or, more specifically, to perform a rapid neurologic assessment. At the bare minimum, this should include an assessment of the patient's pupils (size and reaction to light), extremity motion (looking for lateralizing signs), and Glasgow coma scale. Assessing strength and sensation requires an awake, cooperative patient. In an unstable patient or patient with an altered mental status (from alcohol, drugs, or head trauma), you may need to complete the neurologic examination later that day or the following day. The Glasgow coma scale is primarily used as a tool for sequential assessment. Patients with head trauma or an altered mental status should be rescored every few hours. Their score should improve as they recover (or sober up), and deterioration warrants prompt re-evaluation and/or repeat computed tomography (CT) scanning.

"E" reminds you to expose the patient. Cutting off clothes may seem wasteful until you miss an unsuspected wound, or find a knife, by radiography, in pants that should have been removed. Slight tracheal deviation may be the only sign of a tension pneumothorax. The odds of identifying this are vastly improved if the patient is exposed.

Placing a blanket warmer in the emergency room allows you to quickly cover and uncover a patient. This mitigates the hypothermia caused by cold IV fluid, field exposure, and ED exposure. Blunt trauma, in particular, causes bleeding from both small and large vessels. Platelets and clotting factors normally control the small-vessel bleeding, allowing the surgeon to focus on the large vessels. Coagulopathy vastly complicates the surgeon's task, adversely affecting survival. In the ICU setting, coagulopathy is most often caused by a drug overdose (e.g., heparin) or an adverse drug reaction. In trauma, coagulopathy is multifactorial. Ongoing bleeding, attempted clotting, and crystalloid resuscitation lead to the direct loss, consumption, and dilution of platelets and clotting factors. With mild hypothermia, platelets adhere poorly. Below 33°C, coagulation enzymes fail. Once the core body temperature drops below 32°C, trauma patients have a 100% mortality (6). Hypothermia is a preventable cause of death mitigated by simple measures like warming the ED trauma bay and operating room.

THE PRIMARY SURVEY

ATLS divides the patient's initial evaluation into a primary and secondary survey. The primary survey focuses on high-priority injuries: those that are *rapidly lethal and rapidly correctable.* Many common injuries are rapidly lethal. Rapidly correctable implies that you can fix (or temporize) the problem using simple tools (a laryngoscope, a chest tube, direct pressure, etc.) kept in an ambulance or in the ED. The primary survey is designed to identify such injuries (Table 72.1).

Airway Obstruction and Airway Management

Airway management is a common cause for anxiety. Failure in airway maintenance rapidly leads to death. Apart from the rare patient with severe facial trauma who requires an immediate cricothyroidotomy, trauma patients should be approached in a standardized fashion. Assume that all patients are at risk for a respiratory arrest, and for a cervical spine injury, and are likely to have a full stomach.

Patients are categorized into three groups: (a) those who are awake, alert, and breathing with no difficulty at all; (b) those in respiratory distress who need immediate intubation; and (c) everyone else. The first group should be treated with periodic reassessment. With the second group, check for airway obstruction while setting up for a rapid sequence induction and intubation. Simple measures, like a jaw thrust or

TABLE 72.1

THE FOCUS OF THE PRIMARY SURVEY

Rapidly lethal and rapidly correctable injuries	Initial treatment
Airway obstruction	Obtain a secure airway
Tension pneumothorax	Needle thoracostomy
Open pneumothorax	Support ventilation
Cardiac tamponade	Decompression
Peripheral arterial injuries	Direct pressure

chin lift, or an oral or nasal airway, rarely allow you to avoid intubation. However, these maneuvers may convert an emergent intubation into a semi-elective intubation. The third group includes all of the patients who don't need intubation at that moment, but who may be close to needing it or who may need it in the future. This is the group that requires judgment. Trauma patients with an altered mental status but with no respiratory distress will be sent for a head CT scan. Some will stop breathing in radiology, a suboptimal place for an emergent intubation. If you try to intubate every patient prior to CT, you will fail 2% to 3% of the time (7). Failure to obtain an airway can be managed if you have a backup plan (8), including cricothyroidotomy. Generally, intubate patients with a Glasgow coma scale score of 8 or less. If a patient has no mental status changes but needs to go to the operating room, consider early intubation prior to transport, particularly if the patient has been hypotensive. If you have any doubt, err on the side of intubating the patient.

The best way to intubate a patient is the way that works best for you. Be consistent. Pick one set of drugs and your favorite Macintosh or Miller blade. If you develop a routine, you will be reminded to use suction and to apply cricoid pressure. Your success depends less on your speed and more on your skill with mask ventilation. Preoxygenation is critical. Several minutes of effective mask ventilation with 100% oxygen will create a luxurious amount of time to inspect the airway and place an endotracheal tube without disturbing the spine. Not every patient needs sedation. In an unresponsive patient, you can bypass the rapid sequence induction unless you have selected the drugs to reduce intracranial pressure during intubation.

Airway Management and the Cervical Spine

Any patient who rapidly decelerates (e.g., motor vehicle accident, fall) requires spinal stabilization. Such a patient should arrive on a backboard with a collar. Also consider spinal injuries after direct trauma to the head, neck, or back. Clearing the cervical spine requires more than a radiograph as ligamentous injuries can occur in the absence of radiologic findings. In an alert, cooperative patient who has no neck tenderness, no distracting injury, and a normal neurologic examination, the collar may be safely removed (9). Unfortunately, neck tenderness and mental status changes are common. In such patients, clearing the C-spine is not an immediate priority and should be delayed until they are stable. Clearance criteria are controversial and may require a C-spine series or CT of the neck, to rule out fractures, followed by flex/ex (flexion/extension) views or magnetic resonance imaging (MRI) of the neck, to rule out ligamentous injuries.

Protecting the spine is occasionally at odds with needed intervention. This occurs most often during intubation, although there are other circumstances where it may be necessary to transiently remove the front of the collar. This conflict is best overcome by assigning one team member to maintain in-line stabilization (not traction) while other team members perform necessary interventions. Although direct laryngoscopy will angulate the spine despite in-line stabilization (10), orotracheal intubation can be performed safely in patients with cervical spine fractures when reasonable precautions are taken (11). Fiberoptic intubation can be done without any movement of the neck and should be considered in high-risk patients when time permits. While nasotracheal intubation also avoids spinal manipulation, it is rarely used in trauma because it requires an awake, breathing patient; takes time to perform; can cause nasal bleeding; and can lead to vomiting and aspiration.

Pneumothorax and Tension Pneumothorax

Pneumothorax is one of the most common thoracic injuries. As a consequence, any physician caring for trauma patients should be comfortable placing a chest tube. Air usually enters the pleural space from a lung injury, although it may also enter through a chest wound. During normal inspiration, the diaphragm contracts, intrapleural pressure falls, and the lung expands via the bellows effect. If the pleural space contains trapped air, the lung cannot fully expand. Blood then circulates through nonaerated alveoli, leading to hypoxia. Despite this, healthy patients can generally tolerate the complete collapse of one lung.

Tension pneumothorax starts in a similar manner; however, the pathophysiology soon diverges. Some lung injuries act as a one-way valve. Inspiration pulls air into the pleural space. Expiration compresses the lung and obstructs air egress. As pleural pressure builds, the mediastinum is pushed to the contralateral side (shifting the trachea), eventually kinking the superior vena cava and inferior vena cava. Venous pressure then rises (distending the neck veins) and venous return falls. As preload drops, cardiac output drops, and then blood pressure drops. Patients die from cardiogenic shock, not hypoxia, although hypoxia may also be present. If a patient with a chest injury becomes hypotensive after intubation, consider tension pneumothorax. Positive pressure ventilation can rapidly raise the intrapleural pressure in these patients.

Tension pneumothorax is both rapidly lethal and rapidly correctable. There are several mandatory treatments. The first should be decompression. If you suspect tension pneumothorax, perform needle thoracostomy (or expeditiously place a chest tube). Do not wait for chest radiograph confirmation. Use the largest IV catheter immediately available (ideally 14 or 16 gauge). Place the catheter in the second or third intercostal space, in the midclavicular line, aiming toward the back. This will decompress the pleural space. Whether or not the patient had a tension pneumothorax, the outcome will be a simple pneumothorax. A chest tube should be placed at the earliest opportunity. A small chest tube (e.g., 20 French) placed anteriorly will work, but most chest injuries involve some degree of bleeding and a large chest tube (e.g., 36 French) is preferable. Place it in the fifth intercostal space in the midaxillary line high enough to avoid hitting the liver or spleen. Although tube thoracostomy is optimal treatment, it takes a few minutes to complete. As death can occur rapidly, needle thoracostomy should be considered first unless you have all the equipment actually in your hands.

Volume loading should be done simultaneously for treating a tension pneumothorax. If you have a patient who is hypotensive and hypoxic with distended neck veins and tracheal shift, turn up the IV as you look for a catheter for needle thoracostomy. Increasing the venous volume (and pressure) will overcome the venous obstruction (until the mediastinum shifts further). This will not treat the hypoxia, but it will raise the blood pressure for a few minutes. As with other interventions, the goal of initial trauma care is to buy time for definitive treatment.

Open Pneumothorax and Flail Chest

In an open pneumothorax, there is a large hole into the chest. As the patient tries to breathe, air moves in and out through the hole. For this reason, an open pneumothorax is also known as a sucking chest wound. Intrapleural pressure never falls, so the ipsilateral lung never expands. There are two treatment options. If you cover the hole, you create a simple pneumothorax, which can then be treated with tube thoracostomy. If you intubate the patient, positive pressure ventilation will expand both lungs regardless of the presence of an open pneumothorax.

Flail chest has similar pathophysiology. If three or more ribs are broken in two places, the "flail" segment moves in and out as the patient tries to breathe. As with open pneumothorax, there are three choices: you can place a chest tube, intubate the patient, or both. Unfortunately, the force needed to cause these injuries usually damages the adjacent lung. Although treating the flail segment is easy, patients may still die from the associated pulmonary contusion and hypoxia.

Cardiac Tamponade

Beck's triad (hypotension, jugular venous distention, and muffled heart sounds) and pulsus paradoxus (an exaggerated drop in systolic blood pressure of >10 mm Hg with inspiration) are the hallmarks of cardiac tamponade. These clinical signs are less reliable in trauma. Hypotension is nearly universal, hypovolemia may prevent jugular venous distention, and ED noise obscures heart sounds. Clinical suspicion (any wound near the heart) is essential to making this diagnosis, although cardiac tamponade has been rarely reported after minor chest trauma (12). The widespread adoption of focused abdominal sonography for trauma (FAST) has made it easier to identify cardiac tamponade.

Cardiac tamponade is both rapidly lethal and rapidly correctable. For this reason, patients who present in shock after chest trauma have a better chance of survival if they present with cardiac tamponade (13). As blood enters the rigid pericardial sack, it prevents the heart from filling during diastole. Venous return is obstructed, venous pressure rises, and cardiac output falls. The rapid infusion of IV fluid will transiently raise the blood pressure (14), but decompression is key, followed by definitive correction of the underlying injury. The pathophysiology is similar to tension pneumothorax. Although rare, tension pneumomediastinum presents (15) in an identical fashion and can also be treated with mediastinal decompression.

In the nontrauma setting, pericardiocentesis, done with a pigtail catheter under ultrasound guidance, is the treatment of choice. Pericardiocentesis has been used effectively for trauma (16). However, the preferred treatment is subxiphoid pericardial window (17) or emergency room thoracotomy (with pericardial fenestration) whenever a surgeon is available. Decompression buys time but rarely addresses the underlying injury. Most trauma patients with cardiac tamponade should therefore be expeditiously taken to the operating room for median sternotomy or anterolateral thoracotomy.

Peripheral Arterial Injuries

Significant arterial bleeding from extremity laceration is sometimes "audible." Direct pressure is the treatment of choice, particularly with peripheral arterial injuries. Tourniquets cut off collateral circulation and are best reserved for those situations where you need to stop bleeding while carrying the victim to safety. Direct clamping is instantaneously effective, but may be difficult in the emergency room with limited light, suction, and retraction. Even when applied properly, a clamp may crush the artery, reducing the length available for a primary anastomosis. As arteries travel with nerves and veins, direct clamping may damage adjacent structures. For these reasons, direct pressure is preferred, even though it may fully occupy one person.

Resuscitation

Resuscitation starts in the field and continues after arrival. Administer fluid rapidly if justified by the mechanism of injury. It is rare for a patient to develop congestive heart failure from resuscitation in the emergency room even if they have underlying cardiac disease. In contrast, underresuscitation is common (18). Young, athletic patients may be able to compensate for significant blood loss without tachycardia or hypotension. Essential hypertension and heart block also make it difficult to interpret vital signs in the elderly. As a sign of shock, tachycardia is more sensitive than hypotension; however, tachycardia may reflect pain rather than blood loss. With the foregoing caveats, continuously monitoring the vital signs is the best way to gauge the efficacy of ongoing resuscitation (Table 72.2).

If you can palpate a pulse, you can estimate the blood pressure. As a general guide, a palpable carotid pulse implies that the blood pressure is at least 60 mm Hg; a femoral pulse implies that the blood pressure is over 70 mm Hg; and a radial pulse implies 80 mm Hg.

Intravenous Access

"Two large-bore IVs, placed at different sites" is a tenet of trauma resuscitation. With too many IVs, the tubing tangles and hampers patient transfers. "Large bore" implies that the line can be used to rapidly transfuse blood. The infusion rate depends on pressure and resistance. Commercial warming equipment (e.g., Level 1 or Rapid Infusion System) as well as simple pressure bags can greatly increase the transfusion pressure. Resistance varies with blood viscosity (which increases with refrigeration) and line (tubing plus IV catheter) impedance. Large IV catheters (6 or 8 French) are readily available and can be placed easily using the Seldinger technique. With large IV catheters, the transfusion rate is limited by the tubing itself. A shorter length and larger diameter are advantageous. Catheter impedance increases exponentially (to the fourth power of the radius) as the catheter gets smaller. For this reason, 18-gauge catheters can be problematic and smaller catheters should not be used.

If you place femoral lines in patients with pelvic trauma, you may find one of your lines infusing into the peritoneal cavity through a lacerated iliac vein. Whenever possible, place IV lines

TABLE 72.2

ESTIMATED FLUID AND BLOOD LOSSES BASED ON PATIENT'S INITIAL PRESENTATION

	Class I	Class II	Class III	Class IV
Blood loss (mL)	Up to 750	750–1,500	1,500–2,000	>2,000
Blood loss (% blood volume)	Up to 15%	15%–30%	30%–40%	>40%
Pulse rate	<100	>100	>120	>140
Blood pressure	Normal	Normal	Decreased	Decreased

From American College of Surgeons Committee on Trauma. *ATLS Advance Trauma Life Support for Doctors*. Chicago: American College of Surgeons; 2004:74 (Table 1).

away from the site of trauma. Choose a different extremity for the second line. If the first is in the arm, place the second in the groin or leg (and vice versa). Separating IV lines maximizes the likelihood that infused fluid will reach the heart.

Colloid, Crystalloid, and Blood Substitutes

How best to replace lost blood has been a perennial topic of controversy. Restoring volume can be achieved with colloid or crystalloid. Restoring oxygen-carrying capacity requires red cells.

Crystalloid should be used first in trauma resuscitation. It is readily available, inexpensive, and free of viruses and allergic reactions. As rapid infusion may be necessary, it must be isotonic. Normal saline (0.9% NaCl) is the preferred solution if you need to administer blood through the same line. Since normal saline contains 154 mEq of sodium and no potassium, large amounts lead to hyperchloremia and hypokalemia. Ringer lactate and Ringer acetate avoid this problem by reducing the sodium and adding potassium (and calcium).

Unlike blood, which is confined to the vasculature, crystalloid equilibrates throughout the interstitial and intracellular spaces. As a consequence, 3 liters of crystalloid is needed to replace 1 liter of blood. ATLS recommends starting O-negative or type-specific blood (if available) after 2 liters of crystalloid have been given and the patient remains hypotensive. Nonetheless, a huge volume of crystalloid may be needed in a badly injured patient. This inevitably leads to peripheral edema and if the heart cannot pump the fluid forward, pulmonary edema may develop (19). In order to reduce the time and volume of fluid needed for resuscitation and to reduce the associated edema, several alternatives have been studied. Small-volume resuscitation has been attempted with hypertonic saline (7.5% saline), colloid (albumin, dextran, gelatins, hydroxyethyl starch), and hypertonic saline plus colloid (20,21). Despite the potential advantages of these small-volume resuscitations, which have been of particular interest to the military, crystalloid appears to be associated with a lower mortality in trauma (22,23).

Blood substitutes have advanced from theory to phase 3 clinical trials. Perfluorocarbons and hemoglobin-based oxygen carriers (HBOCs) share many of the benefits of crystalloid: they can be produced in large quantities with a long shelf life, they are universally compatible, and they are free of viruses and allergic reactions (24). Early formulations were plagued by toxicity (vasoconstriction, neurotoxicity, renal dysfunction, and impaired immunity). However, new polymerized HBOC formulations should reduce the volume needed for resuscitation with fewer adverse reactions (25).

As you contemplate your choices among crystalloid, colloid, and blood substitutes, it is worth emphasizing that pressors should never be used as the therapy for traumatic shock and should only be used in spinal shock after volume resuscitation. Spinal cord injuries occur in patients with occult intra-abdominal or intrathoracic bleeding. If your patient has any degree of hemorrhagic shock, volume expansion is essential. Patients with neurogenic shock may respond to a lesser extent, as volume expansion improves cardiac output, which helps to compensate for the loss of vascular tone.

Permissive Hypotension

The goal of resuscitation is to restore normal perfusion and oxygen delivery. In experimental models of uncontrolled hemorrhagic shock, aggressive resuscitation actually increased mortality by increasing the bleeding from injured vessels (26). Human studies (27,28), including one prospective study in patients with penetrating torso trauma (29), have also suggested that fluid resuscitation should be delayed until bleeding can be controlled. These studies done in younger patients with penetrating torso trauma should not be extrapolated to other types of patients until further studies are done. Permissive hypotension, where patients are resuscitated to a less than normal blood pressure, is also supported by animal and human studies (30). Underresuscitating a patient may be lethal. Overresuscitation may also be detrimental. Ultimately, the degree of resuscitation may be less important than the time it takes to get definitive control of bleeding.

THE SECONDARY SURVEY

This chapter has explored the initial management of the trauma patient. After ruling out injuries that are *rapidly lethal and rapidly correctable*, many other injuries remain. Some are severe, contributing to death and disability. To avoid missing these injuries, the secondary survey should be thorough, detailed, and compulsive, similar to the critical care detailed elsewhere in this book. Building on lessons from the primary survey and resuscitation, the next chapter reviews the secondary and tertiary surveys, diagnostic evaluation, and definitive treatment.

References

1. West JG, Trunkey DD, Lim RC. Systems of trauma care. A study of two counties. *Arch Surg.* 1979;114(4):455–460.
2. Shackford SR, Hollingworth-Fridlund P, Cooper GF, et al. The effect of regionalization upon the quality of trauma care as assessed by concurrent audit before and after institution of a trauma system: a preliminary report. *J Trauma.* 1986;26(9):812–820.
3. MacKenzie EJ, Hoyt DB, Sacra JC, et al. National inventory of hospital trauma centers. *JAMA.* 2003;289(12):1515–1522.
4. Branas CC, MacKenzie EJ, Williams JC, et al. Access to trauma centers in the United States. *JAMA.* 2005;293(21):2626–2633.
5. American College of Surgeons Committee on Trauma. *ATLS Advance Trauma Life Support for Doctors.* Chicago: The American College of Surgeons; 2004:13.
6. Wolberg AS, Meng ZH, Monroe DM 3rd, et al. A systematic evaluation of the effect of temperature on coagulation enzyme activity and platelet function. *J Trauma.* 2004;56(6):1221–1228.
7. Bushra JS, McNeil B, Wald DA, et al. A comparison of trauma intubations managed by anesthesiologists and emergency physicians. *Acad Emerg Med.* 2004;11(1):66–70.
8. Carley SD, Gwinnutt C, Butler J, et al. Rapid sequence induction in the emergency department: a strategy for failure. *Emerg Med J.* 2002;19(2):109–113.
9. Hoffman JR, Mower WR, Wolfson AB, et al. Validity of a set of clinical criteria to rule out injury to the cervical spine in patients with blunt trauma. *N Engl J Med.* 2000;343(2):94–99.
10. Lennarson PJ, Smith D, Todd MM, et al. Segmental cervical spine motion during orotracheal intubation of the intact and injured spine with and without external stabilization. *J Neurosurg.* 2000;92(2 Suppl):201–206.
11. Patterson H. Emergency department intubation of trauma patients with undiagnosed cervical spine injury. *Emerg Med J.* 2004;21(3):302–305.
12. Ombrellaro M, Hagedorn F. Cardiac tamponade: a covert source of hypotension after minor blunt chest trauma. *Am J Emerg Med.* 1994;12(4):507–509.
13. Tyburski JG, Astra L, Wilson RF, et al. Factors affecting prognosis with penetrating wounds of the heart. *J Trauma.* 2000;48(4):587–590; discussion 590–591.
14. Gascho JA, Martins JB, Marcus ML, et al. Effects of volume expansion and vasodilators in acute pericardial tamponade. *Am J Physiol.* 1981;240(1):H49–53.
15. Cummings RG, Wesly RL, Adams DH, et al. Pneumopericardium resulting in cardiac tamponade. *Ann Thorac Surg.* 1984;37(6):511–518.
16. Breaux EP, Dupont JB Jr, Albert HM, et al. Cardiac tamponade following penetrating mediastinal injuries: improved survival with early pericardiocentesis. *J Trauma.* 1979;19(6):461–466.
17. Kurimoto Y, Hase M, Nara S, et al. Blind subxiphoid pericardiotomy for cardiac tamponade because of acute hemopericardium. *J Trauma.* 2006;61(3):582–585.
18. Deane SA, Gaudry PL, Woods P, et al. The management of injuries—a review of deaths in hospital. *Austr NZ J Surg.* 1988;58(6):463–469.
19. Rackow EC, Falk JL, Fein IA, et al. Fluid resuscitation in circulatory shock: a comparison of the cardiorespiratory effects of albumin, hetastarch, and saline solutions in patients with hypovolemic and septic shock. *Crit Care Med.* 1983;11(11):839–850.
20. Wade CE, Kramer GC, Grady JJ, et al. Efficacy of hypertonic 7.5% saline and 6% dextran-70 in treating trauma: a meta-analysis of controlled clinical studies. *Surgery.* 1997;122(3):609–616.
21. Boldt J. Fluid choice for resuscitation of the trauma patient: a review of the physiological, pharmacological, and clinical evidence. *Can J Anaesth.* 2004;51(5):500–513.
22. Velanovich V. Crystalloid versus colloid fluid resuscitation: a meta-analysis of mortality. *Surgery.* 1989;105(1):65–71.
23. Choi PT, Yip G, Quinonez LG, et al. Crystalloids vs. colloids in fluid resuscitation: a systematic review. *Crit Care Med.* 1999;27(1):200–210.
24. Proctor KG. Blood substitutes and experimental models of trauma. *J Trauma.* 2003;54(5 Suppl):S106–109.
25. Moore EE, Johnson JL, Cheng AM, et al. Insights from studies of blood substitutes in trauma. *Shock.* 2005;24(3):197–205.
26. Bickell WH, Bruttig SP, Millnamow GA, et al. The detrimental effects of intravenous crystalloid after aortotomy in swine. *Surgery.* 1991;110(3):529–536.
27. Hambly PR, Dutton RP. Excess mortality associated with the use of a rapid infusion system at a level 1 trauma center. *Resuscitation.* 1996;31(2):127–133.
28. Sampalis JS, Tamim H, Denis R, et al. Ineffectiveness of on-site intravenous lines: is prehospital time the culprit? *J Trauma.* 1997;43(4):608–615; discussion 615–617.
29. Bickell WH, Wall MJ Jr, Pepe PE, et al. Immediate versus delayed fluid resuscitation for hypotensive patients with penetrating torso injuries. *N Engl J Med.* 1994;331(17):1105–1109.
30. Dutton RP, Mackenzie CF, Scalea TM. Hypotensive resuscitation during active hemorrhage: impact on in-hospital mortality. *J Trauma.* 2002;52(6):1141–1146.

CHAPTER 73 ■ SECONDARY AND TERTIARY TRIAGE OF THE TRAUMA PATIENT

ROBERT D. WINFIELD • LAWRENCE LOTTENBERG

The previous chapter covered the initial assessment and care of the injured trauma patient. Following the period of stabilization and the management of immediately life-threatening injuries described therein, the patient will make the transition to the more comprehensive capabilities of the inpatient setting. This chapter is focused on that critical period of time that begins with transfer to the intensive care unit, in which transport, transfer of care to the intensive care unit team, the gathering of additional information, continued resuscitation, and a more complete and thorough assessment of the patient's injuries are undertaken. Additionally, this chapter will address some of the more common injuries that are associated with delayed presentations, and cover current diagnosis and management strategies in these situations.

RDW was supported by a T32 training grant (T32 CA-XXXXX-02) in surgical oncology from the National Cancer Institute, NIH.

IMMEDIATE CONCERNS

Patient Transport to the Intensive Care Unit

Of immediate concern following stabilization is safe transport of the critically injured patient from the emergency department

TABLE 73.1

AMERICAN COLLEGE OF CRITICAL CARE MEDICINE/SOCIETY OF CRITICAL CARE MEDICINE GUIDELINES FOR INTRAHOSPITAL TRANSFER OF THE CRITICALLY ILL PATIENT

Pretransport coordination	Continuity of care ensured by physician-to-physician and/or nurse-to-nurse communication to review patient condition and the treatment plan Confirmation by the receiving location that it is ready to receive the patient Coordination of appropriate hospital personnel (e.g., respiratory therapy) to be available on patient arrival
Accompanying personnel	Minimum of two people In unstable patients, a physician with training in airway management, advanced cardiac life support (ACLS), and critical care training or equivalent
Accompanying equipment	A blood pressure monitor (or standard blood pressure cuff), pulse oximeter, and cardiac monitor/defibrillator accompany every patient without exception When available, a memory-capable monitor with capacity for storing and reproducing patient bedside data Airway management equipment and oxygen source to supply for projected needs and 30-minute reserve Basic resuscitation medications (epinephrine, antiarrhythmic agents) If a transport ventilator is to be employed, it must have alarms to indicate disconnection and excessively high airway pressures and must have a backup battery power supply
Monitoring during transport	At a minimum, continuous electrocardiographic monitoring, continuous pulse oximetry, and periodic measurement of blood pressure, pulse rate, and respiratory rate

Adapted from Warren J, Fromm RE Jr, Orr RA, et al. 2004. Guidelines for the inter- and intrahospital transport of critically ill patients. *Crit Care Med.* 2004;32:256.

or trauma bay to the intensive care unit setting. While the practice of moving the patient between these two settings would seem to be quite simple, numerous authors have described the pitfalls associated with the transfer of patients within a given facility (1–4). In 2004, the American College of Critical Care Medicine and the Society of Critical Care Medicine released specific guidelines for appropriate intrahospital transfer of critically ill patients (5). These guidelines are summarized in Table 73.1. Briefly, they highlight the need for appropriate pretransport communication between the transporting and receiving teams, the presence of appropriate numbers of adequately trained personnel in the transport, the equipment and medications that should accompany the patient on the transfer, and the minimal level of monitoring that the patient should receive during transport.

Communication between Trauma Team and Intensive Care Unit Providers

Upon the arrival of a critically injured trauma patient, communication should begin between the trauma team and intensive care unit (ICU) providers. Initial impressions of the extent and severity of injuries, known medical and surgical history, and immediate surgical plans can all be helpful to the ICU team in making arrangements for appropriate equipment, medications, and personnel to be available upon patient transfer to the ICU.

Physician-to-physician communication will vary depending on whether or not the ICU is an open or closed unit. In an open ICU, the trauma surgeon responsible for admitting the patient will remain primarily responsible for the patient's care throughout his or her hospitalization, including all moment-to-moment ICU decisions. This clearly precludes the need for a handoff of care responsibilities. In a closed ICU, a designated physician intensivist or intensivist team will assume primary responsibility over the patient's care. In the latter situation, concise yet complete discussions should ensue between the trauma surgeon and intensivist regarding the patient's status in order to minimize disruption upon transfer of care.

Additionally, the need to communicate with nursing staff and hospital administration regarding needs for bed space cannot be underestimated. In busy tertiary care centers, particularly level I trauma centers, intensive care unit bed space is at a premium. Unidirectional flow of trauma patients (from the emergency department to radiology to the ICU, without a return to the emergency department) is dependent on keeping the bed control coordinator informed of needs. In single or dual traumas, this unidirectional flow is highly desirable, but in mass casualty situations, it is essential to the successful triage and management of the injured patients.

OBTAINING THE PATIENT'S HISTORY AND HISTORY OF INJURY

Communication with Patients/ Family Members

Oftentimes, communication with patients is not possible in critically ill trauma patients, and much of the information that will subsequently be known about the trauma victim is obtained through discussion with family. Interaction with the family of a recently injured patient can pose incredible challenges for the trauma or intensive care unit provider. In a brief period of time, the physician must explain the circumstances that led to the patient's injuries, what has been done for the patient up to this point, injuries that have been identified, the prognosis (if this can be estimated), and immediate plans for the patient's care. Additionally, this will be a time to obtain family contact information and valuable background information about the patient and his or her relevant health history, as well as discuss informed consent for any pending invasive procedures. While this can be a daunting task, a sensitive and systematic approach will ensure effective and thorough communication that engenders trust among the loved ones of the patient and allows the care providers to obtain needed information.

The time following notification of a severe injury to a loved one is a time of intense emotion. Many authors have reported that signs and symptoms of anxiety, depression, and even posttraumatic stress disorder (PTSD) are present in family members of trauma victims and intensive care unit patients (6–8). It has been suggested that some of these symptoms may be lessened by early communication with the family as this allows the family members to transition to an emotional state where they are capable of dealing with the issues at hand (9,10). Cross et al. performed a study in which they observed the time that elapsed between the arrival of family members and the time when a physician member of the trauma team held a discussion with the family (9). They found that families waited an average of 37 minutes in the hospital before being approached by a trauma physician. They concluded that this was an unacceptable wait time, as it was added to an average 38-minute transport time to the hospital. The study indicated that this wait time was often prolonged because of failure to notify the physician that the family had arrived, and physician delays in approaching the family secondary to patient care issues, awaiting radiologic studies, and simply forgetting that the family was waiting. They recommended the designation of a member of the caregiving team to be the liaison to the family as soon as possible to prevent undue emotional duress.

On approaching the family, Epperson recommends three steps in alleviating anxiety: the provision of brief and accurate information about patient status, an explanation of procedures currently being performed, and allowing time for the family members to communicate their initial impressions regarding the trauma and its impact (9,10). This should promote open discussion and a sense of trust for the health care providers in the trauma team. Interestingly, the satisfaction and comprehension of the family under these circumstances appears not to be dependent on communication with an attending or fellow, indicating that a resident may be designated to perform this important task (11).

Following adequate time for the family to voice concerns, as thorough a history as may be obtained should be undertaken in order to plan for special care needs of the individual patient. Particular attention should be paid to chronic diseases with known end-organ dysfunction, anticoagulation agents (aspirin, warfarin, clopidogrel, etc.), and patient allergies. Finally, with the arrival of appropriate family members, informed consent should be obtained for any planned invasive procedures. This allows for the possibility of early involvement of the family in the patient's care plans, and maximizes the chances that the patient will receive care that is in keeping with his or her personal beliefs. One method that we have found helpful in our institution's intensive care unit is the use of a standardized ICU "universal" consent form, which covers many of the commonly performed procedures in the ICU (Fig. 73.1). This allows us to obtain consent for many procedures simultaneously, allowing us to rapidly perform life-saving procedures with the knowledge that the family has agreed to their performance. Additionally, it promotes consideration of, and discussion about, the opinion of the family regarding the patient's desires for life-sustaining measures.

The Role of the Social Worker

The social worker has unique training that focuses on the concept of the patient as a member of a family system, and this makes him or her an invaluable part of an optimally functioning trauma team. Oftentimes, the social worker is the first member of the team to meet with the family following a traumatic injury and he or she continues to play an integral role in the patient's care plan throughout the patient's hospital course. The social worker has the ability to obtain insight into family dynamics and resources, and is likely the first individual that truly begins discharge planning on admission of a patient to the hospital. Additionally, the social worker will have the opportunity many times to interact with law enforcement officials and get a thorough description of the circumstances surrounding the issue, even as the acute resuscitation and management phase is taking place.

Interaction with Law Enforcement

Traumatic injury often involves interaction with officers of the law. In circumstances of motor vehicle collisions and assaults in particular, law enforcement officials may be present in the trauma bay and the intensive care unit to provide and gather additional information as well as obtain blood samples for alcohol and drug testing. Cooperation is obviously encouraged; however, the patient's care must remain the priority under these circumstances. Additionally, there will be situations in which patients are found after proven or suspected assault. Under these conditions, reporting of a suspected assault and relevant details should be communicated with law enforcement officials in keeping with state and local reporting standards.

SHANDS
at the University of Florida

This form provided by Shands at UF as a courtsey to patients and their physicians

Patient Name: MR#:

Consent for Commonly Performed Procedures in the Adult Critical Care Units

Date______ Time______

I, the undersigned, understand that the adult intensive and intermediate care units ("critical care units") are places where seriously ill patients are cared for by specially trained staff. The critical care staff works closely together as a team to provide the best possible care. The critical care team uses a number of specialized machines and devices, called monitors, to frequently check the heartbeat, blood pressure, and breathing. Machines that help the patient breathe, called mechanical ventilators, may also be used.

I have been informed that patients in the adult critical care units often undergo certain medical procedures and/or treatments, either to help determine what is wrong, or to relieve symptoms or resolve problems.

I understand that some of these procedures may be performed more than once during a patient's admission. These commonly performed procedures, their use in diagnosis and treatment, as well as the substantial risks and possible complications involved, have been explained to me by Dr.__________.

I have also read, or had read to me, the information sheet entitled "Commonly Performed Procedures and Related Complications," a copy of which is attached to this form and which briefly describes each of these commonly performed procedures, and their substantial risks, potential benefits and medically reasonable alternative treatments.

I have had an opportunity to ask questions of Dr.__________ regarding the commonly performed procedures and I have had all my questions answered to my satisfaction.

I understand the potential benefits and drawbacks, potential problems related to recuperation, the likelihood of success, the possible results of non-treatment, and any medically resonable alternatives associated with these commonly performed procedures.

I understand that the information I have recieved about risks is not exhaustive, and there may be other, more remote risks. I have received no guarantees from anyone regarding the results that may be obtained from any of these treatments or procedures.

I,__________, consent to the treatments and/or procedures indicated by my initials below, which in
Name or Person Consenting
the judgment of my critical care units physicians may be considered necessary or advisable for __________'s diagnosis or treatment, and which may be performed by any of the adult critical
Patient's Name
care units' physicians and their associates and assistants (including resident physicians). I understand that this consent will be considered good for my/the patient's critical care unit admission, up to 60 days, and that I may at any time withdraw my consent to any treatment or procedure.

I also understand that a refusal to consent to any of these procedures may have a serious adverse impact on my health and/or ability to recuperate.

Procedures	Initials of patient or representative	Procedures	Initials of patient or representative
Arterial Line Insertion	______	Sedation Maintenance or Procedural	______
Pulmonary Artery Catheter Placement	______	Intubation & Mechanical Ventilation	______
Central Venous Line Insertion	______	Bronchoscopy	______
Peripherally Inserted Central Catheter	______	Chest Tube Insertion	______

Consent for Commonly Performed Procedures in the Adult Critical Care Units

Rev. 7/20/05 PS50371-0705

FIGURE 73.1. The "universal" intensive care unit consent of Shands Hospital at the University of Florida.

REASSESSING THE ABCs WHILE MAINTAINING VITAL FUNCTION

Assessment Methods

As previously mentioned, the transport of the patient from the trauma bay to the ICU can be a time of potential peril. As such, arrival in the ICU represents a time for reassessment of patient status, particularly the ABCs. None of the methods subsequently listed should, in any way, disrupt the continued resuscitation or care of the patient.

The airway may be assessed in standard fashion in the awake, nonintubated patient by confirming that the patient is able to speak. In circumstances where the patient was intubated during resuscitation, confirmation of endotracheal or nasotracheal tube placement should be undertaken using confirmation of end-tidal carbon dioxide and capnography. The patient's care record should indicate the depth of tube placement. Should this be in question, or if a variation is present, an anteroposterior (AP) chest radiograph can quickly confirm tube position.

Assessment of breathing should consist of both auscultation of the lungs bilaterally and confirmation of adequate saturation via pulse oximetry. If the patient is being mechanically ventilated, confirmation of appropriate ventilator settings should be established, and if an arterial blood gas has not been performed recently, this may be used to guide changes in ventilator settings.

Finally, evaluation of circulatory status should include auscultation of the heart, confirmation of pulses, measurement of blood pressure, and verification of adequate intravenous access. If blood pressure measurements are felt to be inaccurate, and an arterial line was not placed previously during initial resuscitation, this may serve as a useful adjunct in circulatory management. It may also provide a stable line for the obtaining of arterial blood gas measurements in the ventilated patient. The authors prefer the use of percutaneous lower extremity access for arterial lines in an attempt to avoid the monitoring devices commonly placed on the upper extremities, and due to the frequent occurrence of upper extremity injuries. If the patient has a previously placed arterial line, the line should be zeroed, and appropriate pressure tracing confirmed. With regard to venous access, two large-bore intravenous lines should be adequate, although a large-bore central venous line (e.g., a 9 French introducer) may be preferred in the critically injured patient as it is less likely to become dislodged and has the potential to offer the benefits of central venous pressure measurements as well as superior vena cava mixed venous oxygen saturation measurements; both of these may have the added benefits of assisting in guidance of fluid resuscitation. Furthermore, large-bore central access may be used for rapid infusion of crystalloid and blood products, and can provide a port of entry for a right heart catheter should this be desired. The authors recommend a subclavian approach due to the greater incidence of catheter-related bloodstream infections in alternate sites, as well as the difficulty in accessing the internal jugular vein in the patient with suspected cervical spine injury (12). The femoral vein may also be utilized for rapid access; however, femoral venous catheters should be removed within 24 hours due to the risk of deep vein thrombosis (12).

Pitfalls

The intubated patient can have his or her airway disrupted by any number of usual and customary motions during transfer, and in certain cases, loss of airway represents a potentially catastrophic complication. As such, it is generally good practice to have an appropriately trained individual responsible for maintenance of airway at all times. This person should monitor the position and security of the tube, as well as the connection of the tube to the Ambu-bag or ventilator. Ideally, this person should be comfortable with intubation and surgical airway management. Pharmacologic agents can be of great assistance in preventing loss of airway, as analgesics, anxiolytics, and paralytics can alleviate patient agitation. In our experience, intermittent administration of paralytic agents has decreased the incidence of tube dislodgement during transport.

Dislodgement of the tube should be dealt with emergently. The simplest solution is to perform bag-mask ventilation until such time as a controlled reintubation may take place. Should this fail, a laryngeal mask airway or Combitube may provide a temporary alternative. Finally, should these methods be unsuccessful, a cricothyrotomy or tracheostomy should be undertaken immediately.

While dislodgement of the endotracheal tube represents the issue that requires attention most urgently, it is important to remember that advancement of the tube may pose a problem as well. In this circumstance, the patient may be experiencing a right mainstem intubation, and is undergoing single lung ventilation only. This can be detected quickly by physical examination, noting absent left-sided breath sounds and absence of left-sided chest movement on inspiration. Additionally, a chest radiograph may aid in identification of this problem.

When assessing the adequacy of ventilation in the patient, it was mentioned previously that pulse oximetry may be used to evaluate oxygen saturation. This has limitations, though, as adequate oxygen saturation may not reflect adequate oxygen tension (13), and in hypotensive patients, tremendous error may be seen in pulse oximetry measurements (14). As such, should there be any question regarding the sufficiency of ventilation, an appropriately obtained arterial blood gas should provide the needed information.

PERSISTENT SHOCK

Persistent Shock in the Multisystem Trauma Patient

The patient arriving in the ICU in persistent shock poses a challenge for caregivers, who are attempting to quickly gain hemodynamic and ventilatory stability. In the trauma patient, it is essential to remember that persistent shock is hemorrhage until proven otherwise, and a meticulous search for hidden sources of bleeding is indicated. There are a number of sources that may not have been considered during initial evaluation and resuscitation (but always should be). Open wounds can ooze a large amount of blood, and should be managed with pressure dressings. Should the wound involve an open fracture, it should be placed in anatomic continuity and fixed with a temporary splint. Scalp lacerations can bleed profusely, but a quickly performed locked running suture with a large monofilament nylon followed by a securely applied pressure dressing will quell the hemorrhage. A mangled extremity presents a potentially difficult challenge, but a simple one-stage tourniquet can provide a temporizing measure until definitive management can be pursued. Finally, hemorrhage may also result from other hidden sources; these will be covered in the subsequent section of this chapter on missed injuries.

Management of the Patient in Persistent Hemorrhagic Shock

Patients may experience persistent hemorrhagic shock not only through a discrete bleeding injury, but also as a result of the vascular permeability that results from the inflammatory response to injury and the coagulopathy that occurs when large volumes

Schedule for Massive Transfusion Protocol
Shands at the University of Florida

Shipment	Red Blood Cells	Plasma	Platelet Dose	**Cryo	***rFVIIa
*1	10 (O-Neg)	4(AB)			
2	10	4	1	10	rFVIIa
3	10	4	1		
4	10	4	1	10	rFVIIa
5	10	4	1		
6	10	4	1	10	

The shipment number refers to the allotment of blood components (Red Blood Cells, Plasma, Platelets, Cryoprecipitate, and rFVIIa) provided at each step of massive transfusion. At the conclusion of each step, the decision must be made by the team providing care whether or not to order the next shipment of blood products.

Definition of massive transfusion

Massive transfusion at Shands at the University of Florida is defined as a presumed need for the transfusion of at least 10 units of packed red blood cells (PRBC) in an adult patient or at least five (5) units of PRBC in a child within a short time frame (i.e. two (2)-hour time period).

Adult	Greater than 10 units
6-12 year old child	Greater than or equal to 5 units
4-5 year old child	Greater than or equal to 3 units
2-3 year old child	Greater than or equal to 2 units
0-1 year old child	Greater than or equal to 1 unit

*Shipment 1 is located in the Satellite Blood Bank Refrigerator, located in the Emergency Department and Operating Room.
**Cryo=Cryoprecipitate
***Recombinant Factor VIIa (rFVIIa) is not routinely shipped and must be ordered from Pharmacy. These are recommended intervals if rFVIIa is clinically warranted.

FIGURE 73.2. The massive transfusion protocol of the Acute Care Surgery Service of Shands Hospital at the University of Florida, Appendix A.

of resuscitation are administered. Recently, it has been advocated that resuscitation of the critically injured trauma patient in shock is best performed with blood and fresh frozen plasma in a 1:1 ratio (15). In patients who have experienced significant blood loss, are in persistent shock, and require greater than 10 units of blood replacement, it is helpful for a trauma center to have a massive transfusion protocol in place to guide management. This will ensure the most efficient and effective use of blood products. An example of the massive transfusion protocol used at the authors' institution is seen in Figure 73.2.

As mentioned, an additional concern in the patient with severe injury and large resuscitations, particularly in the setting of a massive transfusion, is coagulopathy. Some authors have advocated the use of recombinant factor VIIA (rFVIIA) as an adjunct measure in the control of ongoing hemorrhage in this setting. Martinowitz et al. performed an early look at the use of rFVIIA in seven trauma patients, noting a significant decrease in transfusion requirements, concluding that rFVIIA could be a useful adjunct treatment in trauma patients (16). Dutton et al. at Maryland reviewed their experience using rFVIIA in 81 trauma patients with coagulopathy and hemorrhage, noting that there was a reversal in coagulopathy, but not an improvement in mortality; however, they pointed to the fact that rFVIIA was often used as a "therapy of last resort" and indicated that more information was needed regarding the timing of administration (17). Perkins et al. recently looked at combat-injured patients who received "early" (before 8 units of blood) or "late" (after 8 units of blood) rFVIIA during massive transfusion, again demonstrating a decrease in red blood cell use (a 20% decrease in their series) without a decrease in mortality (18). Finally, there has been a set of parallel, randomized, double-blinded clinical trials reported on the subject (19). Once again, a decrease in transfusion requirements was noted, but without a significantly improved mortality. So, while there have been some promising results in that patients who have received rFVIIA require less transfusions, there has yet to be a study demonstrating a survival benefit or improved outcome with its use. There is currently an ongoing trial evaluating this issue.

Goal-directed Therapy

Goal-directed therapy refers to the use of resuscitation end points to guide management of the patient in shock, and has been the source of controversy in the medical and surgical literature for greater than a decade. While there is a general consensus that maintenance of tissue oxygenation is beneficial in preventing the sequelae of shock, debate has centered on the specific end points that should be utilized, whether a pulmonary artery catheter should be used, and whether normal or supranormal values should be pursued in these patients. This section reviews the concept of goal-directed therapy in the traumatically injured patient, along with an overview of some of the broad concepts within goal-directed therapy.

Goal-directed Therapy in the Trauma Patient

Gattinoni et al., as part of the SvO_2 Collaborative Group, were among the first to assess outcome in patients utilizing goal-directed therapy, performing a multicenter study of critically ill patients, including those with multiple injuries secondary to trauma (20). In their study, they randomized hospitalized critically ill patients into groups designed to achieve one of three ends: a normal cardiac index, a supranormal cardiac index, or a normal SvO_2. In 762 patients divided between the three groups, the authors found no differences in organ dysfunction, intensive care unit length of stay, or mortality. They concluded that there is no benefit in achieving supranormal hemodynamic parameters in critically ill patients. The problems with this study were (a) late entry into the study protocol (by 48 hours), (b) infrequent hemodynamic measurements (every 12 hours), and (c) only 45% of subjects reaching the cardiac index goal and 67% of patients reaching the SvO_2 goal.

In a similar study with a slightly different design, Baue's group in St. Louis performed a prospective, randomized trial evaluating a group of critically ill patients that included those who were involved in acute trauma (21). Their desired end points in the experimental group included goals of resuscitation including oxygen consumption index (VO_2I) of greater than 150 mL/minute/m^2 or oxygen delivery index (DO_2I) of greater than 600 mL/minute/m^2. The control group underwent standard resuscitation using urine output, heart rate, pulmonary capillary wedge pressure, mean arterial pressure, and cardiac index as end points. They showed no difference in mortality or organ failure in patients engaged in goal-directed therapy. They did a subgroup analysis of their trauma patients and demonstrated identical findings. Interestingly, in their experience, they noted a longer length of stay in the experimental group despite similar measures of critical illness, and this approached significance. As with Gattinoni's paper, this study was undertaken in patients already admitted to the intensive care unit.

Around the same time, Bishop et al. further evaluated this issue, focusing solely on severely injured trauma patients in a single-center, prospective, randomized trial at the King/Drew Medical Center in Los Angeles (22). They enrolled study patients into a standardized care pathway in which patients were resuscitated to achieve a supranormal cardiac index, DO_2I, and VO_2I. Control subjects were resuscitated using standard physiologic end points for normal blood pressure, hemoglobin, urine output, and central venous pressure. They showed a decreased incidence of organ failure, as well as a decreased mortality in protocol patients when compared to control, and thus concluded that attaining supranormal hemodynamic characteristics provided a benefit in both morbidity and mortality in severely injured trauma patients. Of significance in this study is that patient resuscitation began on admission, as opposed to the studies by Gattinoni and Durham, where goal-directed therapy began following identification of patients in organ failure already in the intensive care unit.

In a multicenter study that included 139 trauma patients, Shoemaker et al. took a different approach, performing a prospective study of noninvasive methods for monitoring hemodynamic parameters, including bioelectric impedance, pulse oximetry, and transcutaneous oxygen (tcO_2) and carbon dioxide ($tcCO_2$) measurements (23). They found that in the trauma population, over half had reduced cardiac index (CI) measurements and reduced transcutaneous oxygen measurements, half had decreased oxygen consumption, and nearly half had high transcutaneous carbon dioxide values. Not surprisingly, most had more than one abnormality. Comparing the noninvasive methods to standard pulmonary artery catheter measurements, they found similar disturbances, and showed that regardless of the method used to monitor hemodynamic status, patterns were seen relative to the nadir of the CI that were associated with survival versus nonsurvival, with higher blood pressures and heart rates, as well as lower oxygen saturation preceding and following the nadir in nonsurvivors. Conversely, survivors demonstrated higher initial CI and tcO_2 values, which they speculated might represent lower blood volume deficits or better compensation. They concluded that either noninvasive or invasive methods could be utilized to measure resuscitation status, and could potentially provide data on early identification of low flow and poor tissue perfusion states that precede the nadir of CI that is seen in nonsurvivors. Additionally, they suggested that use of this noninvasive equipment could be helpful in guiding early goal-directed resuscitation for the critically ill patient, beginning in the emergency department or upon admission.

A group that consisted of many of the same investigators as the studies by Bishop and Shoemaker attempted to clarify the issue of supranormal versus normal values in resuscitation of trauma patients (24). In this effort, the authors randomized 75 consecutive patients on admission to either "optimal" resuscitation (CI $>$4.5, tcO_2 to fraction of inspired oxygen ratio $>$200, DO_2I $>$600, and VO_2I $>$170) or a standard resuscitation with normalization of blood pressure, urine output, base deficit, hemoglobin, and cardiac index. They utilized bioimpedance to begin estimating these values prior to ICU admission. They reached "optimal" levels in 70% of the optimal group and 40% of the standard group. While they found no difference in mortality, organ failure, sepsis, or ICU length of stay between the two groups, they performed an additional comparison in which they analyzed patients based on whether or not they reached "optimal" levels and found that both outcome and mortality rates were significantly improved in patients achieving "optimal" resuscitation. Interestingly, they noted that the only factor associated with achieving "optimal" levels was age younger than 40. They suggested that differences in being able to achieve optimal resuscitation indicated a superior physiologic reserve, rather than an effect of the resuscitation efforts themselves, and thus concluded that early goal-directed therapy in trauma patients does not improve outcome.

Finally, Balogh et al. in Houston noted that achieving supranormal resuscitation end points requires additional fluid, and indicated that this led to a greater incidence of intra-abdominal hypertension and abdominal compartment syndrome (25). They performed a retrospective analysis of patients in their trauma intensive care unit, looking at patients who underwent supranormal resuscitation versus those undergoing standard resuscitation. They found that patients in the supranormal group received more fluid, had higher gastric partial carbon dioxide minus end-tidal carbon dioxide (GAPCO_2) measurements, and had greater incidences of intra-abdominal hypertension and abdominal compartment syndrome. Additionally, they found a significantly increased incidence of organ failure and death in the supranormal resuscitation group. They concluded that supranormal resuscitation was deleterious when compared with standard resuscitation.

Goal-directed Therapy: Other Considerations

Obviously, shock may result from any of a number of insults; thus, this issue has been examined in a number of settings, primarily in that of septic shock. In 2001, Rivers et al. released a landmark paper describing early goal-directed therapy in septic shock (26). In this randomized, controlled trial, in which patients were treated with 6 hours of goal-directed or standard resuscitation therapy in the emergency department, they demonstrated improvements in organ dysfunction and in-hospital mortality. Despite their striking findings, and the findings of previous and subsequent authors, questions exist about the validity and applicability of the data, particularly when extrapolated to other settings (27). Judging by the ongoing debate in the literature at present, it is safe to say that no consensus has yet been reached on whether or not early goal-directed therapy is necessary in the resuscitation of the critically ill patient.

Another area of contention in the trauma literature for decades has been the use of crystalloid versus colloid resuscitation fluids. The Cochrane Library performed a recent meta-analysis on the randomized controlled studies covering this topic, and determined that there is no survival advantage to using colloid resuscitation fluids (albumin, hydroxyethyl starch, modified gelatin, or dextran) and thus concluded that at this time, there is no justification for their use outside of clinical trials (28). Despite this, debate continues on the subject, and there are ongoing trials evaluating this topic.

With regard to end points and the equipment utilized to measure them, there is again no true consensus. The use of pulmonary artery catheters to guide management is a particularly controversial one, particularly in light of studies such as that by Connors et al., which demonstrated an increased mortality in critically ill patients undergoing right heart catheterization (29). While authors such as Shoemaker have attempted to address this issue, even they recognize the limitations of noninvasive monitoring (23). There are a number of methods and end points that may be used to monitor ongoing resuscitation, and these will be touched on briefly here.

Laboratory Testing

Lactate and base deficit are two levels commonly used to evaluate the adequacy of resuscitation. Elevated lactate levels have been correlated with both morbidity and mortality in critically ill patients, and both absolute levels and clearance of lactate are considered appropriate end points for use in resuscitation (30–33). Base deficit has been shown to be associated with volume of resuscitation fluid and blood following injury, and elevated levels have additionally been shown to correlate with increased mortality (30,34,35).

Right Heart Catheterization Levels

Values obtained through right heart catheterization are considered the "gold standard" physiologic measurements to that which noninvasive cardiovascular measurements are compared. The primary end point obtained through right heart catheterization that is referred to in the literature is DO_2I, which is a function of cardiac index, hemoglobin, and oxygen saturation. The previously mentioned articles provide a sampling of the mixed data regarding the use of DO_2I as an indicator of resuscitation in the critically ill (20,21,23–25). Utilizing a new-generation pulmonary artery catheter, the right ventricular ejection fraction (or right ventricular end-diastolic volume index [RVEDVI]) may be used as a surrogate marker for assessment of preload. Maintenance of RVEDVI greater than 120 mL/m^2 has been associated with improved outcome in trauma patients (30,36,37).

Alternative Methods

Thoracic electrical bioimpedance (TEB) was used in the previously mentioned study by Shoemaker et al., and in an additional study of noninvasive monitoring of blunt trauma patients by Velmahos at the same institution (23,38). In each of these, good correlation between TEB and simultaneously obtained right heart catheter cardiac output measurements existed, and its use was recommended as a noninvasive alternative to right heart catheterization.

Lithium dilution cardiac output (LiDCO) utilizes a venous lithium chloride injection, which is then measured at an arterial catheter site and used to calculate cardiac output. It has been shown to correlate well with standard right heart catheter values, even when the lithium is injected peripherally (30,39), although it has not been studied in the traumatically injured. It does carry the benefit of not requiring calibration with an existing right heart catheter (30).

Esophageal Doppler monitoring (EDM) is a less invasive method (the Doppler probe is placed within the esophagus) for measuring both preload and continuous cardiac output that has shown benefit in the reduction of postoperative recovery time following surgery and in septic patients, although its use has not been evaluated in trauma patients (30,40–42).

Near-infrared spectroscopy (NIRS) uses near-infrared light absorption by hemoglobin, myoglobin, and cytochrome aa3 oxidase to calculate tissue oxygen saturation (StO_2) (30). NIRS has been shown to correlate with systemic oxygen delivery (43), in severely injured trauma patients showed a parallel with DO_2I values (44), and using cytochrome aa3 measurements in 24 severely injured trauma patients, illustrated that early evidence of mitochondrial dysfunction suggested a predisposition for progression to multisystem organ failure (45).

BLUNT CARDIAC INJURY

Definition/Discussion

In 1992, Mattox et al. proposed that the broad term *myocardial contusion* and *myocardial concussion* be replaced with the phrase *blunt cardiac injury* (46). They further suggested that blunt cardiac injury (BCI) be classified according to descriptors of the specific abnormalities associated with the injury, thus the terms that follow:

Blunt cardiac injury with minor electrocardiogram (ECG) or enzyme abnormality
Blunt cardiac injury with complex arrhythmia
Blunt cardiac injury with coronary artery thrombosis
Blunt cardiac injury with free wall rupture
Blunt cardiac injury with septal rupture
Blunt cardiac injury with cardiac failure

This new terminology allowed for improved description of the injuries, more consistent monitoring and management of each specific type of injury, and descriptions of the short- and long-term effects of having sustained such an injury. It is estimated that 20% of patients who die in the prehospital setting have sustained cardiac injuries, and an additional 30,000 patients per year with BCI survive to hospital discharge (47).

Clinical Suspicion

BCI must be suspected in any case involving blunt thoracic trauma. In most cases, this will involve a motor vehicle collision, but any of a number of mechanisms may lead to these injuries, including bicycle crashes, falls, blast injuries, sports-related trauma, and assaults (48). Because of the nature of these injuries, other concomitant injuries will be seen, with head injury, rib fracture, extremity injuries, hemothorax, sternal fracture, pulmonary contusion, aortic or great vessel injury, pneumothorax, solid abdominal organ injuries, and flail chest most commonly noted (47,48). In the conscious patient, complaints of chest pain may heighten suspicion, but due to the severe multisystem nature of these injuries and concurrent head injuries, BCI patients are often in a state of altered consciousness. In this latter group of patients, the presence of refractory hypotension should suggest the possibility of BCI.

Diagnosis/Monitoring

There are currently no specific diagnostic criteria for BCI (46–48). In cases of suspected or possible BCI, it is essential to perform a systematic evaluation. Again, mechanism of injury is important to obtain from the patient, those present at the scene, or first responders. A complete thoracic and cardiovascular exam will yield hints of the diagnosis, with hypotension, visual sequelae of chest trauma (abrasions, bruising, seatbelt sign, or steering wheel imprint), flail chest, rib fractures, sternal fractures, abnormal heart sounds (muffling, distance, S_3, S_4, murmurs, bruits, or rubs), and jugular venous distention all suggestive (47). Following the history and physical exam, and during the trauma evaluation, the Focused Assessment with Sonography in Trauma (FAST) exam should be performed to look for fluid in the pericardium. It has been suggested by more than one series that the pericardium can be evaluated with tremendous accuracy during a trauma evaluation using this technology (49,50).

Simultaneously, or in the ICU, ECG and chest radiograph may be obtained, both of which may provide findings that are nonspecific for, but suggestive of, this injury. The utility of ECG in BCI has been evaluated by a number of authors, all of whom found that abnormal ECG findings on admission or early in the hospital course were associated with complications, or that absence of findings was associated with a lack of complications and warranted no further studies (51–56). There are no ECG findings that are pathognomonic for BCI; however, the finding of any abnormality on ECG should prompt further workup. With regard to the chest radiograph, there are no findings that will definitively demonstrate cardiac injury, but they often prove useful by demonstrating some of the associated injuries that may accompany a BCI.

Should the ECG and mechanism of injury heighten suspicion for a BCI, obtaining a troponin I level should be considered. Troponin I has been shown in BCI patients to have a sensitivity ranging from 23% to 100% and a specificity of 85% to 97% (47,57–59). In perhaps the most important look at this topic, Velmahos et al. reviewed a series of 333 BCI patients over a 2½-year period, and found that in all cases, a normal admission ECG and troponin I followed by a normal ECG and troponin I at 8 hours completely ruled out BCI, and they suggested that in the absence of other injuries, patients with these findings could be discharged safely (60).

Formal echocardiography has been looked at by several authors in BCI (55,61–63). In each circumstance, the authors have noted that echocardiography has no role in the screening of the stable patient with suspected BCI. In the patient with hemodynamic instability, it is felt that transthoracic echocardiography may provide diagnostic information; however, transesophageal echocardiography offers improved images and evaluation of the aorta, making it of greater value (47,64,65).

Monitoring of the patient with diagnosed BCI is largely dependent on the type of injury sustained. In the patient with ECG and/or enzyme abnormalities with normal blood pressure, continuous monitoring is recommended, but a stay in the intensive care unit is not required (47). The patient with BCI accompanied by hypotension should be continuously monitored in the intensive care unit, with use of right heart catheterization an option in critically ill patients.

Management

Like monitoring, management is dependent on the type of injury sustained. Blunt chest injury sequelae may range from benign ECG abnormalities to mortal hemorrhage. Management must be tailored to the pattern of injury.

The majority of patients will be categorized as having BCI with minor ECG or enzyme abnormality. While these findings may be initially benign, both Maenza et al. and Velmahos et al. found in their respective series that ECG and/or enzyme irregularities on admission and at subsequent points were more likely to predict cardiac complications (hypotension, arrhythmias, pump failure) and interventions during hospitalization (53,60). Thus, patients with these abnormalities should be observed for complications with management dependent upon the presenting symptoms.

Complex arrhythmia with BCI is the next most common injury pattern, and may consist of atrial dysrhythmia, ventricular dysrhythmia, or commotio cordis (myocardial concussion). These are seen to occur in anywhere from 2% to 30% of patients (47,48,53) and are managed in accordance with the rhythm disturbance seen. Commotio cordis is a seldom seen injury in which it is postulated that a blow to the chest results in an immediate rhythm disruption, and is unusual due to its lack of association with myocardial structural damage (66). Despite its rare occurrence, commotio cordis is the second most common cause of sudden death in young athletes due to its association with the generation of ventricular fibrillation (67).

Cardiac failure with BCI is less commonly seen, but should be on the list of differential diagnoses in any patient with persistent hypotension in the absence of a defined injury. Although the diagnosis is suggested by hypotension, tachycardia, jugular venous distention, and an abnormal ECG, definitive diagnosis is often made using echocardiography or right heart catheterization. Supportive care is the mainstay of management in these patients, although there have been reports of successful use of intra-aortic balloon counterpulsation pump (IABP) (68,69). The use of this modality would require weighing the benefits and risks of heparinization, a requirement of IABP use.

Myocardial wall rupture is even more seldom seen than cardiac failure, primarily because the majority of these patients expire at the scene or en route to the trauma center. It is possible to see a patient with one of these injuries when there is rupture of an atrium, a delayed rupture of a ventricle, or a small, contained pericardial tear (70,71). Should this injury be suspected, or the diagnosis confirmed with echocardiography, immediate operation via open thoracotomy is the sole management option.

Coronary artery thrombosis with BCI is also infrequently seen. The diagnosis is made via findings of ST-segment changes consistent with myocardial ischemia following blunt chest trauma. Management is similar to that employed when a patient presents with a myocardial infarction of another etiology, with percutaneous angioplasty, stenting, and bypass among available options (47).

EXTREMITY COMPARTMENT SYNDROME

Definition/Discussion

The upper and lower extremities are divided into several fascial compartments that contain the musculature, blood vessels, and nerves that supply the respective limbs. During traumatic injury, fluid (as a result of the combination of leaking capillaries and large volumes of resuscitation) or blood (as a result of direct injury and/or coagulopathy) may accumulate in these closed fascial spaces, leading to an increase in pressure within the compartment. This increased pressure causes impaired lymphatic, venous, and arterial flow, and may lead to nerve compression. This may lead to palsies, permanent nerve damage, and, if allowed to continue unchecked, ischemic injury and tissue necrosis in the affected extremity.

Clinical Suspicion

Extremity compartment syndrome should be considered in any patient who has presented with extremity trauma. McQueen et al. reported that compartment syndrome most commonly occurs in patients with an extremity fracture (usually of the tibial shaft or distal radius), followed by patients with soft tissue injuries without fracture (72). While compartment syndrome is most commonly associated with fracture within a closed space, an open fracture does not preclude the presence of a compartment syndrome. Suspicion should also be heightened in patients taking any anticoagulant medications (73). It must be remembered that while injury to the extremity often causes these injuries, at times therapeutic measures may exacerbate this condition with wraps and dressings, traction splinting, use of the lithotomy position or abduction of the leg during surgery, or even intramedullary nailing in a tibial fracture repair all having been associated with the development of extremity compartment syndrome (73).

Diagnosis/Monitoring

Diagnosis of extremity compartment syndrome is primarily clinical, and requires a high index of suspicion. It is frequently suggested that the presence of the "six P's" (pain, pulselessness, pallor, pressure, paresthesias, and paralysis) are the keys to diagnosis (73), although in the authors' experience, this correlates better with acute arterial occlusion than compartment syndrome. Pain during passive range-of-motion exercises is often the first sign of a developing problem; unfortunately, this has clear limitations in the patient with mental status changes, and can be a limited finding. Pulselessness is found occasionally, although usually as a late finding once compartmental pressures have become great enough to overcome arterial pressure. An increase in compartment pressure is a potentially objective finding, as the extremity may feel tense and swollen, although it can often be difficult, particularly for the inexperienced examiner, to distinguish this from the edema that follows a significant traumatic injury to the affected extremity. Paresthesias are potentially ominous signs, as they may represent muscle or nerve ischemia; conversely, they may be only a manifestation of pain and are thus not reliable indicators of compartment syndrome (73). Additionally, as with pain, paresthesias cannot be assessed in the unconscious or sedated patient. Finally, paralysis is a late finding that is resultant from prolonged nerve ischemia or irreversible muscle damage.

Since the clinical diagnosis can sometimes be difficult and/or unclear, monitoring devices have been developed to evaluate intracompartmental pressures. Both slit catheter and side port needle techniques have been described for this purpose with equal efficacy and accuracy reported in the literature (74). Regardless of method utilized for measurement, it has been recommended that patients demonstrating a ΔP value of 20 mm Hg between measured compartment pressure and diastolic blood pressure should undergo fasciotomy (73).

Management

Once diagnosed, management of extremity compartment syndrome is straightforward, depending on the etiology. In cases where therapeutic measures have led to the compartment syndrome, loosening bandages, repositioning the patient, or reducing the degree of traction may provide relief. If these are inadequate, the patient should undergo immediate fasciotomy of the affected compartment. Performance of fasciotomy in the lower extremity is accomplished through either a single incision on the anterolateral calf or incisions on the medial and lateral calf, with subsequent division of the fascial compartments. On the upper extremity, fasciotomy may be likewise performed through single or double incisions. Following fasciotomy, the patient should be adequately decompressed. A currently popular method of dressing the patient is with vacuum-assisted closure (V.A.C., KCI, San Antonio, TX), although wet-to-dry dressings with saline will provide adequate coverage. In cases where the patient has developed muscle necrosis, debridement will be necessary at an interval operation between fasciotomy and closure. Closure may be accomplished primarily, if tension allows, or by secondary intention. Skin grafting is the final option, and should be considered any time that tension precludes closure by the first two techniques.

ABDOMINAL COMPARTMENT SYNDROME

Definition/Discussion

Abdominal compartment syndrome (ACS) occurs from increased intra-abdominal pressure. Richardson and Trinkle described elevated end-inspiratory pressures and hypoperfusion secondary to a low cardiac output (CO) associated with ACS (75). Impaired venous return and high peak inspiratory pressure with hypercarbia were present, causing hypoperfusion and severe pulmonary dysfunction. Early surgical decompression is mandatory, and a better outcome is associated with early detection. Release of the restrictive abdominal pressure will result in the correction of organ dysfunction. Oliguria is an early sign of ACS, but the most reliable clinical indicator is progressive failure of ventilation. A typical case of ACS has a peak inspiratory pressure in the range of 85 cm H_2O, with a rise in $PaCO_2$. A decompressive celiotomy is indicated in the presence of abdominal distention, hypercarbia, and high peak inspiratory pressures. This procedure may be performed either at bedside or in the operating room.

The surgical technique performed for damage control is a continuum that includes primary resuscitation, damage control celiotomy, secondary resuscitation, and delayed reconstruction (76). Patients in extremis usually do not tolerate reconstruction. In summary, ACS is a surgical emergency that requires the damage control technique to prevent organ dysfunction. If ACS is recognized late or goes unrecognized, it can lead to multiple organ failure and death.

Clinical Suspicion/Diagnosis/Monitoring

Intra-abdominal pressure is that pressure concealed within the abdominal cavity which varies with respiration. A normal intra-abdominal pressure is approximately 5 mm Hg, but may be higher with obesity. Intra-abdominal pressure should be expressed in mm Hg and measured at end-expiration with the patient in the supine position, without abdominal contractions. The pressure transducer should be zero-referenced to the level of the midaxillary line. Direct intra-abdominal measurement is obtained with direct needle puncture and transduction of the pressure within the abdominal cavity. Indirect intra-abdominal pressure measurement is accomplished via transduction of the pressure within the bladder. Bladder pressure may be measured by injecting 50 to 100 mL of sterile saline into the aspiration port of the Foley drainage tube. The catheter is then clamped distal to the aspiration port, and a 16-gauge needle is used to connect a pressure transducer to the aspiration port of the catheter. The top of the symphysis pubis (or the midaxillary line) is used as the zero point on the supine patient.

For continuous, indirect intra-abdominal pressure measurement, a balloon-tipped catheter in the stomach or a continuous bladder irrigation method is recommended (Fig. 73.3). ACS is not seen as long as the intra-abdominal pressure is normal. The group at Denver Health Medical Center has proposed a grading system based on urinary bladder pressure measurements (77). A pressure of 25 mm Hg or higher is associated with organ dysfunction and considered clinical intra-abdominal hypertension. At or above this pressure, surgical decompression is justifiable.

The old saw "If it's not in your differential, you can't make the diagnosis" applies to ACS. A high index of suspicion is of utmost importance if ACS is to be prevented. Early identification of high-risk groups mandates early and aggressive monitoring of intra-abdominal compartment pressures in order to initiate appropriate treatment if needed. In the nonmonitored patient, clinical findings of elevated intra-abdominal pressure include an abnormal increase in abdominal girth associated with an increase in peak airway pressures and/or hypercarbia, increased central venous pressure (in euvolemic patients), and oliguria. In patients who are monitored with a urinary bladder catheter, early detection of intra-abdominal hypertension can direct aggressive treatment to prevent ACS. Indirect measurement of intra-abdominal pressure, through the monitoring of bladder pressure, is a very important tool that, after proper calibration, can provide vital information used to direct therapy. Urinary bladder pressures greater than 25 mm Hg in the high-risk patient are strongly associated with the presence of ACS and suggest the need for initiation of aggressive treatment to prevent clinical deterioration.

The inaugural World Conference on Abdominal Compartment Syndrome held in Australia in December 2004 produced consensus definitions as follows (78,79):

> Intra-abdominal hypertension is defined by either one or both of the following: (a) an intra-abdominal pressure of 12 mm Hg or greater, recorded by a minimum of three standardized measurements conducted 4 to 6 hours apart; (b) an abdominal perfusion pressure (abdominal perfusion pressure = mean arterial pressure − intra-abdominal pressure) of 60 mm Hg or less, recorded by a minimum of two standardized measurements conducted 1 to 6 hours apart.

Intra-abdominal hypertension is graded as described in Table 73.2.

Abdominal perfusion pressure—defined as mean arterial pressure minus intra-abdominal pressure—was compared with intra-abdominal pressure, arterial pH, base deficit, arterial lactate, and urinary output as an end point of resuscitation and predictor of survival (80). An abdominal perfusion pressure of 50 mm Hg was a potential end point for resuscitation in the patient with an elevated intra-abdominal pressure, and was superior to other end points listed in predicting survival for patients with intra-abdominal hypertension and ACS. The ACS was defined as the presence of an intra-abdominal pressure of 20 mm Hg or greater, with or without an abdominal perfusion pressure below 50 mm Hg, recorded by a minimum of three standardized measurements conducted 1 to 6 hours apart, and

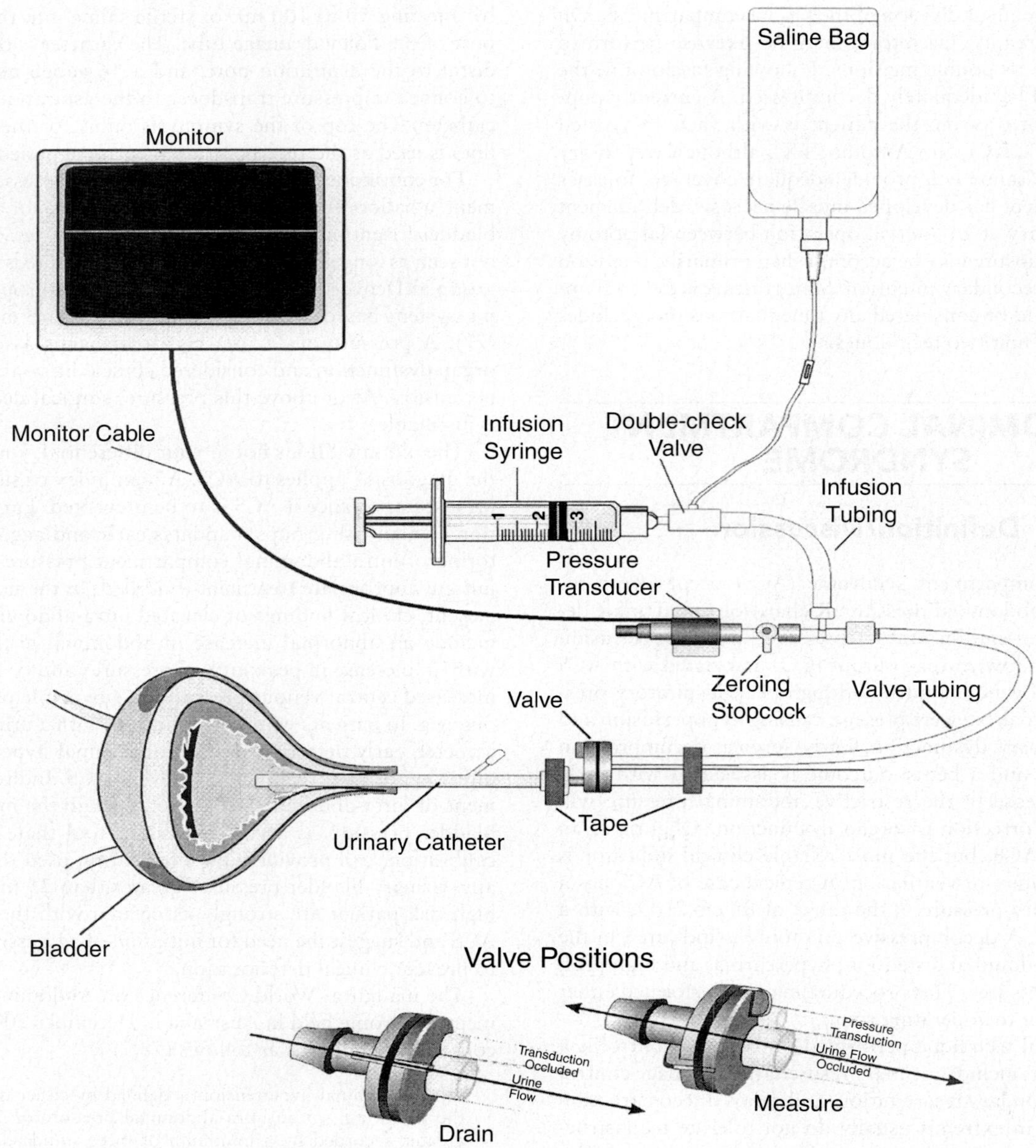

FIGURE 73.3. Intra-abdominal pressure monitoring device. The device is placed into the urinary drainage circuit. By changing the valve from "drain" to "measure," intermittent measurements may be taken. This device allows measurement of intra-abdominal pressure without breaking or interrupting the urinary drainage circuit.

single or multiple organ system failure that was not previously present (78,79).

Management

Aggressive, nonsurgical, critical care support is of utmost importance to prevent the complications of ACS, and should include continuous cardiorespiratory monitoring and aggressive intravascular fluid replacement, especially when associated with blood loss (81). *Excessive* fluid resuscitation, however, is detrimental. Oda et al. studied 36 thermally injured patients, with 40% or greater total body surface area burned and without inhalation injuries, who were treated with a fluid resuscitation protocol using hypertonic lactated saline or lactated Ringer solution (82). Their results showed that the total fluid volume infusion requirement and intra-abdominal and peak inspiratory pressure at 24 hours postinjury were significantly lower than those in the lactated Ringer group. The hypertonic lactated saline group developed intra-abdominal hypertension in 14% of patients compared with 50% in the lactated Ringer group, suggesting that hypertonic lactated saline resuscitation may reduce the risk of secondary ACS due to lower fluid volume requirements during the acute resuscitation phase. Nonsurgical management of ACS is listed in Table 73.3.

A pilot study performed by Latenser et al. compared percutaneous decompression versus decompressive laparotomy with a diagnostic peritoneal lavage catheter for acute ACS

TABLE 73.2

GRADING OF INTRA-ABDOMINAL HYPERTENSION

Grade	Intra-abdominal pressure (mm Hg)
I	12–15
II	16–20
III	21–25
IV	>25

Adapted from World Society of Abdominal Compartment Syndrome. http://www.wsacs.org/. Accessed.

in thermally injured patients (83). Of nine patients who developed intra-abdominal hypertension, five were successfully treated with catheter decompression using a diagnostic peritoneal lavage catheter. The other four—with more than 80% total body surface burn area and severe inhalation injuries—did not respond to percutaneous decompression and required laparotomy. These findings suggest an important role for percutaneous decompression as an alternative treatment prior to decompressive laparotomy.

Decompressive laparotomy is the gold standard for treatment of ACS. Restoration of volume status, restoration and correction of poor perfusion, and correction of hypothermia, acidosis, and coagulopathy are priorities during the acute phase of resuscitation. Decompression of the abdominal cavity may be performed at bedside if necessary; the surgical suite may be used when more complex procedures are needed. Decompressive laparotomy is followed by temporary abdominal closure, the selected method depending upon whether the abdominal wall fascial layer is left open or closed. When the abdominal wall fascia is closed, primary closure with a synthetic material or polytetrafluoroethylene is recommended. If the fascia is to be left open, the skin may be closed or left open. Mesh can be used for temporary abdominal closure, and is sutured to the skin or fascia and covered with moist sterile dressings, thus preserving the fascia for later definitive closure. Skin closure itself may be associated with increased intra-abdominal pressure, so care must be taken when selecting this option. Permanent abdominal closure is usually planned for a time after the acute phase of resuscitation, with primary closure of the fascia and then skin.

TABLE 73.3

COMPONENTS OF NONSURGICAL MANAGEMENT OF THE ABDOMINAL COMPARTMENT SYNDROME

Gastric decompression
Rectal enemas
Colonic prokinetic agents (neostigmine)
Continuous venovenous hemofiltration with aggressive ultrafiltration
Paralysis
Botulinum toxin into the internal anal sphincter
Paracentesis
Gastrointestinal prokinetic agents (cisapride, metoclopramide, domperidone, erythromycin)
Furosemide with or without use of human albumin 20%
Sedation
Body positioning

Adapted from Sugrue M. Abdominal compartment syndrome. *Curr Opin Crit Care.* 2005;11:333.

Scott et al. described the results of a retrospective review of 37 patients with open abdomens who underwent definitive abdominal closure, using a combination of vacuum pack, vacuum-assisted wound management, human acellular dermal matrix (HADM, Alloderm, Lifecell Corporation, Branchburg, NJ), and skin advancement (84). The mean duration of the open abdomen was 21.7 days (range 6–45). No major complications (intra-abdominal infections, fistulae, or failed graft) other than two superficial wound infections were reported, and all 37 patients survived (84).

What Are the Complications if the Abdominal Compartment Syndrome Is Not Diagnosed in a Timely Manner?

Multiple organ dysfunction results from prolonged intra-abdominal hypertension. Forced abdominal wall fascial closure should be avoided. Physiologic exhaustion can lead to multiple organ failure and death if ACS is allowed to progress. Prolonged bowel ischemia is associated with intestinal necrosis. Kinking of the bowel mesentery is associated with necrosis of the bowel, followed by intra-abdominal abscess. Respiratory failure and cardiovascular collapse will follow. Bowel torsion causes ischemia and can lead to necrosis. In this situation, delayed diagnosis may allow progression to diffuse peritonitis with the attendant large fluid resuscitation requirement unassociated to blood loss. Abdominal wall compliance will determine the degree of distention prior to development of ACS signs. Once the intra-abdominal pressure reaches 25 mm Hg, the major concerns are extensive ischemia and necrosis of the small bowel. Short bowel syndrome may result from radical resections of dead bowel; this will require evaluation of nutritional status to prevent malnutrition. Missed colonic injuries may be associated with diffuse peritonitis. In this situation, intestinal diversion is mandatory. Temporary abdominal closure requires the open technique; an occlusive dressing may be used to contain the intra-abdominal contents, along with a suction system composed of two drain catheters to remove the excessive fluid accumulation associated with ACS. Indirect measurement of pressures from the urinary bladder is important in order to prevent recurrent ACS.

PELVIC FRACTURES

Definition/Discussion

Patients who sustain injury secondary to blunt mechanisms, particularly in vehicular or pedestrian trauma, are at risk for pelvic fractures. These fractures often are indicative of a high-energy blunt impact, as the pelvic ring is an extremely stable bony structure; thus, pelvic fractures rarely occur in isolation (85). They are estimated to occur in about 9% of all patients who are injured via blunt trauma (86). While about 91% of these fractures are neither deforming nor displaced, 9% can be considered "severe" pelvic fractures, defined by a pelvic injury with substantial deformation and displacement (86). The so-called "nonsevere" pelvic fractures do not typically pose much risk to patients in and of themselves, are not generally associated with other injuries, and tend to be managed conservatively with rest, non–weight-bearing status, and bracing, depending on the specific injury. This section of the chapter will focus on the diagnosis and management of "severe" pelvic injuries, which are associated with injuries to abdominal or pelvic organs as well as life-threatening hemorrhage and hemodynamic instability, and carry a mortality of about 10% in all patients, and up to 80% when hemodynamic instability is seen (87–89).

Clinical Suspicion

As mentioned previously, patients involved in blunt traumas are at risk for pelvic fractures. As such, the diagnosis should be considered in any patient sustaining blunt trauma. Regarding specific mechanisms of injury, Demetriades et al. performed a retrospective review of 16,630 blunt trauma patients, and found that patients involved in motorcycle crashes, sustaining pedestrian injuries, falling from heights greater than 15 feet, and involved in automobile crashes represented the most likely groups of patients to suffer pelvic injuries, with patients in motorcycle crashes the most likely to have severe pelvic injuries (86). In the conscious patient, complaints of pelvic pain, pain on hip rotation, pain on pelvic compression, the presence of blood at the urethral meatus, and finding a perineal and/or scrotal hematoma have all been associated with pelvic fracture and warrant further investigation (90). Most importantly, though, pelvic fractures represent another potential "hidden" source of hemorrhage, as patients may bleed into the retroperitoneum; thus, a patient with an appropriate mechanism of injury and unexplained hypotension should have the diagnosis of pelvic fracture considered.

Diagnosis

In situations where clinical suspicion is raised due to mechanism or physical examination findings, radiologic imaging confirms the diagnosis. Advanced Trauma Life Support (ATLS) guidelines suggest that plain film radiographs should be performed in all trauma patients sustaining blunt torso trauma, regardless of mechanism (91). The absolute requirement for these films has been called into question by many authors, most recently Gonzalez et al. in Birmingham (90). In their prospective analysis of blunt trauma patients, they determined that physical examination in the trauma resuscitation room carried a greater sensitivity for pelvic injuries (93%) than did anteroposterior radiographs of the pelvis (87%).

With the advent of increasingly rapid computerized tomography (CT), these scans are being routinely performed for patients with blunt trauma. Obaid et al. compared CT and plain films in a retrospective review, determining that CT scans are superior to plain films for the detection of pelvic fracture, although they determined that plain films maintain a role as a screening tool in the hemodynamically unstable patient, and may allow for early notification of interventional radiology of the need for embolization (92). In addition to being more sensitive than plain films for the detection of fracture alone, CT scans offer the advantage of identifying active hemorrhage at the site of pelvic fracture, in the form of a contrast "blush" on arterial phase imaging. This is discussed further in the subsequent section, as the finding of a blush has significant implications for management.

Based on the history of injury, physical exam, and radiologic findings, pelvic fractures may be classified by type, each with predictive value for subsequent management, morbidity, and mortality. Pennal et al. developed one of the initial classification systems for pelvic fractures, correlating them with particular vascular injury patterns: type 1, anteroposterior compression with transverse opening of the pelvic ring (open book fracture, risk of internal iliac artery lesions); type 2, lateral compression (risk of iliac vessel and retropubic plexus injuries); and type 3, vertical instability (risk of posterior structural lesions) (93). Burgess et al. at Maryland Shock Trauma reviewed their experience with 210 pelvic fracture patients, classifying them into groups based on the original classification system of Pennal; additionally, they added a group for patients with combined mechanical injury (94). In their series, they demonstrated that type I injuries predicted greater transfusion requirements (mean 14.8 units) and a mortality risk of 20%, while lateral compression injuries were associated with much lower use of blood products (mean 3.6 units) and a mortality of 7%. Furthermore, they indicated that no patient with an isolated pelvic fracture or a vertical shear injury in their series died. They developed a system of management based on these classifications, elements of which are found in the discussion on management below.

Management

Beyond the usual components of the trauma resuscitation, management of the patient with severe pelvic fracture is aimed at control of hemorrhage and fixation of fractures (Table 73.4). A description of the orthopedic maneuvers and procedures for permanent fixation of pelvic fractures is beyond the scope of this chapter; thus, this section will focus on rapid measures for control of bleeding.

One of the first and fastest ways to gain control following pelvic fracture is through external compression of the pelvis. A simple, rapid method to achieve this end was proposed in 2002 by both Routt et al. and Simpson et al., in separate articles (95,96). They proposed circumferential wrapping of the pelvis with a bed sheet and clamping the sheet anteriorly. This is a widely available, inexpensive method for temporary control under these circumstances, and is the recommended method of the ATLS guidelines (91). To achieve a similar end, the authors utilize a commercially available pelvic circumferential compression device ("pelvic binder") placed during trauma resuscitation. The pelvic binder has been shown in a prospective trial to be a safe and effective method for the management of pelvic fractures, particularly those of the "open book" type (97). Pneumatic antishock garments (PASGs) are a final measure that have been utilized in the management of these injuries, although they carry the disadvantages of being large, being not readily available, preventing lower extremity access, and being associated with worsened outcomes in patients with thoracic trauma (98).

While stopping blood loss is the earliest goal in the patient with pelvic fractures and hemodynamic instability, it should be

TABLE 73.4

MANAGEMENT PEARLS IN ABDOMINAL COMPARTMENT SYNDROME

Early identification of intra-abdominal hypertension may prevent abdominal compartment syndrome.
Intra-abdominal perfusion pressure (IAPP) goal is ≥60 mm Hg [IAPP = Mean arterial pressure – Intra-abdominal pressure].
Forced abdominal wall fascial closure should be avoided.
Perioperative correction of hypothermia, acidosis, and coagulopathy is of utmost importance during the acute resuscitation phase.
Damage control surgery consists of control of hemorrhage and contamination and identification of injuries, utilizing an abbreviated laparotomy. Reoperation is indicated with refractory hypoperfusion associated with ongoing resuscitation.
Increased intra-abdominal girth combined with high ventilatory peak airway pressures and oliguria are common manifestations of abdominal compartment syndrome.
Oliguria is an early sign of abdominal compartment syndrome. Urinary bladder pressure monitoring is strongly recommended.
Temporary abdominal closure is an essential component of the management of abdominal compartment syndrome. Permanent closure is considered during the postresuscitation phase, and deferred until after secondary resuscitation is completed.

remembered that fixation is often one of the best ways to accomplish this, as restoration of anatomic alignment may stop bleeding from small veins and cancellous bone. An external fixator may be applied reasonably rapidly, particularly in the case of a posterior ring disruption, where a C-clamp may be used; fixations involving anterior disruptions may require the additional transport time as well as the conditions and resources of the operating room to be accomplished (85).

In cases of major vascular injury, surgical techniques including exploration and internal iliac artery ligation have not been shown to be effective; thus, they cannot be recommended (99,100). In cases of combined abdominal and pelvic injury, a damage control laparotomy with pelvic packing may provide a quick method for dealing with multiple injuries that include bleeding pelvic fractures. Additionally, preperitoneal and retroperitoneal packing have recently been receiving attention in the trauma literature (101,102). Of particular interest is the paper by Cothren et al., in which the authors retrospectively analyzed their series of 28 patients undergoing preperitoneal packing (102). They demonstrated that the procedure could be performed rapidly and decreased the need for emergent angioembolization. Additionally, they showed decreased transfusion requirements and a reduction in mortality secondary to these injuries. This method, while needing additional validation, should be strongly considered in situations where angioembolization is not immediately available for hemodynamically unstable patients with pelvic fractures.

Following the initial resuscitation of the patient with pelvic fracture, CT scanning will often be pursued as a diagnostic means. As previously mentioned, CT has shown excellent sensitivity for identification of arterial pelvic hemorrhage through the identification of a contrast "blush." In cases where CT demonstrates a potential arterial source for bleeding, or in cases where this injury is suspected, arteriography with possible angioembolization typically represents the next step in management. These techniques involve the obtaining of arterial access, selective cannulation of the iliac vessels, and instillation of contrast dye with the intent to locate the bleeding source within the pelvis under fluoroscopic visualization. Upon identification of an actively bleeding site (noted by extravasation of contrast), embolization is performed through the injection of Gelfoam or coils, which occlude the bleeding artery. Angioembolization is extremely successful in the control of hemorrhage, and is currently considered the treatment of choice in pelvic fractures with hemodynamic instability where appropriately trained staff and the necessary equipment are available (85). It should be noted that there are complications particular to angioembolization that should be watched for in the postprocedural period. As with any percutaneous arterial access, access site injuries may occur; however, a number of authors have also pointed out the complications associated with the embolization itself, including gluteal, skin, bladder, and femoral head necrosis (85).

DELAYED DIAGNOSIS

Discussion

Under ideal circumstances, the primary and secondary surveys allow for the identification of all injuries sustained by the trauma patient. Unfortunately, the evaluation of the critically injured patient does not always allow for the immediate identification of all injuries. Limitations in the examination of the patient due to mental status changes secondary to head trauma or intoxication as well as the presence of distracting injuries often make detection of these injuries difficult. Although rapid, high-quality imaging techniques are now widely used in trauma evaluations, some findings are sufficiently subtle to evade early recognition. Finally, some injuries simply do not manifest themselves in a meaningful way until time has passed and signs or symptoms are present. Some of these injuries were described in previous sections. This section highlights some commonly missed injuries, situations in which suspicion might be heightened for these injuries, and the role of the tertiary survey instrument in avoiding missed injuries.

Commonly Missed Injuries

Musculoskeletal injuries are among the most commonly missed injuries in multisystem trauma patients. In a retrospective review of 111 multisystem trauma patients, Ward and Nunley noted that 6% of orthopedic injuries were not detected (103). They found that most injuries were eventually discovered on the basis of physical exam and plain film radiographs alone, and identified several risk factors for missed orthopedic injuries: significant multisystem trauma with another more readily apparent injury in the same extremity; physiologic instability; altered sensorium; quickly applied splints for a less serious injury; poor-quality initial radiographs; and inadequate significance being applied to minor signs and symptoms. Laasonen and Kivioja reported a similar phenomenon, with 4% of orthopedic injuries missed and similar risk factors noted, with the significant addition of missed injuries on existing radiographs also implicated (104). Findings such as these prompted Mackersie et al. to recommend routine plain film screening to include the lower extremities in obtunded blunt trauma patients (105). At our own institution, we have noted missed musculoskeletal injuries in obese trauma patients. Physical examination of these patients can be difficult, even when the patient's sensorium is completely intact; we have thus begun to perform routine plain film extremity surveys in these patients in order to decrease the incidence of missed injuries.

Injuries involving retroperitoneal structures have a strong potential for presenting in delayed fashion. While CT scan has allowed for early and ready detection of retroperitoneal hematomas, pancreatic and duodenal injuries can sometimes be difficult, if not impossible, to identify in the early moments following injury. Pancreatic injuries occur in less than 5% of blunt abdominal traumas; however, they carry with them substantial morbidity and mortality risks (106). Suspicion should be raised in cases where the victim sustained a blow to the central abdomen. Since pancreatic injuries rarely occur in isolation, injuries to surrounding solid organs and other structures should prompt consideration of pancreatic trauma. In the alert patient, exam findings are typically nonspecific, with vague abdominal pain, epigastric discomfort, nausea, vomiting, and fever commonly seen. Laboratory testing provides equally imprecise findings as an elevated amylase may hint at the diagnosis, but is not specific for pancreatic injury (107). Imaging may provide clues to the diagnosis; however, CT findings are often subtle, and may be delayed following injury (108). In the days that follow injury, the patient may progress to develop any number of manifestations, including pancreatitis, pancreatic leak secondary to a fracture, or a pancreatic pseudocyst. Early identification of the injury may help to guide the most appropriate management. As there are no physical exam, laboratory, or imaging findings that reliably make the diagnosis, the onus falls to the trauma and intensive care unit provider to take into account the mechanism and the soft findings that suggest the injury, and to maintain awareness of the possibility of pancreatic trauma as the patient's hospital course progresses.

Duodenal injuries resulting from blunt trauma are equally challenging to diagnose, and possess many of the same features of pancreatic injury. These uncommon injuries (they occur in less than 5% of blunt abdominal traumas [109]) often result from forces similar to those leading to pancreatic trauma, the most common mechanism being a blow to the central abdomen leading to compression of intra-abdominal contents against the spine. Duodenal tears have also been reported to result from deceleration injuries (110). As with pancreatic injuries, associated trauma is common, with concurrent liver injuries occurring most often. Physical exam is also similar to that seen in pancreatic injuries, with ambiguous abdominal pain being the most common symptom, and nausea, vomiting, and the development of progressively increasing tachycardia and fever also seen (109). Laboratory findings are once again nonspecific, with elevated amylase levels suggestive of, but not diagnostic for, duodenal injury. CT scan is a sensitive modality for detection of retroperitoneal air and extravasated oral contrast, both of which may be seen in duodenal injury, although neither is specific for this condition. Additionally, CT scan is able to detect duodenal wall thickening and hematoma formation, signs of injury that would require different management than a frank perforation. Progression of an undetected duodenal injury with leakage into the retroperitoneum may either be walled off and contained or communicate with the peritoneal cavity, resulting in a life-threatening peritonitis (109). Once again, early diagnosis is often difficult with only soft findings pointing to the identification of a duodenal injury, and only maintenance of a high index of suspicion will allow the physician to make the diagnosis early and allow for the most appropriate management.

Jejunal or ileal injuries may go undetected because, as in the case of pancreatic or duodenal trauma, the findings may be subtle. In the recent EAST multi-institutional hollow viscus injury trial, small bowel injuries affected only 0.9% of blunt trauma victims; however, the authors noted significant increases in both morbidity (29% vs. 14%) and mortality (19% vs. 12%) when patients with small bowel injuries were compared to similar patients without them (111). As with pancreatic and duodenal injuries, physical examination is only of suggestive benefit, with abdominal pain, nausea, vomiting, and potentially signs and symptoms of peritonitis (in the case of a perforation) pointing to the diagnosis. CT scan may show unexplained free abdominal fluid, bowel wall thickening, or in the case of a perforation, free air or extravasated gastrointestinal contrast material. These findings are not always seen and CT scan is estimated to have a reasonable sensitivity of about 88% with a specificity of 99% (112). Malhotra et al. in Memphis were concerned about the grave prognosis that was previously reported by Fakhry in association with as little as an 8-hour delay in diagnosis of small bowel injury (113). In their review of patients with proven or suspected blunt bowel or mesenteric injury, the group in Memphis proposed an algorithm for management of patients with findings suggestive of these injuries (112). They found that hemodynamically stable patients with multiple CT findings suggestive of bowel or mesenteric injury showed a high likelihood of having such injuries, and should undergo exploratory laparotomy. They felt that the rarity of the injury and the lack of sensitivity of CT scan precluded laparotomy in patients with only one finding, but given the potentially devastating complications of a missed injury, suggested that diagnostic peritoneal lavage (DPL) be performed in this group of patients. They recommended that patients with positive microscopic, cell count, or biochemical criteria on DPL undergo exploratory laparotomy. We have adopted this approach at our institution and recommend it, with the additional caveat that we believe diagnostic laparoscopy is warranted in patients with equivocal findings on DPL.

The Role of the Tertiary Survey Instrument

As mentioned in the introductory segment of this section, the primary and secondary surveys do not always allow for the identification of all injuries. In 1990, Enderson et al. reported their experience with the prospective performance of a formal trauma tertiary survey, finding that this simple step allows for the detection of missed injuries (114). It is notable that in their series, they performed the survey in the first 24 hours following injury. Janjua et al. followed this up with a prospective study demonstrating that tertiary survey done within 24 hours detected 56% of all missed injuries and 90% of all clinically significant missed injuries (115). Biffl et al. described their experience following implementation of a formal tertiary survey form and policy at the Rhode Island Hospital, showing a decrease of 36% in missed injuries (116). In their discussion, they called attention to the fact that a limitation of their policy and practice was that many times, within 24 hours, patients were still in an altered mental state and at times were not yet ambulatory, and that this could potentially lead to missed injuries. They proposed that the tertiary survey be performed once within 24 hours and then once again in patients who were nonambulatory or comatose when these situations had subsided. It is the practice at our institution to follow this recommendation. An example of our Acute Care Surgery Service's tertiary survey form is seen in Figures 73.4 and 73.5. At our institution, we take advantage of the tertiary survey instrument to review and record the patient's mechanism of injury, medical history, physical examination findings, laboratory trends, final radiologist reads on imaging findings, the interventions that have been performed up to that point in time, and the patient's immediate plan of care. We feel that this approach leads to a thorough evaluation that allows for an appropriate tailoring of care in the patient with medical comorbidities and minimizes missed injuries. Additionally, we find that it provides a succinct summary of the patient's admission, with the benefit of a time lapse for review of key findings and interventions, to which all care providers may refer for patient information.

SHANDS
at the University of Florida

Trauma and Emergency Surgery
Tertiary Survey Form *(page 1 of 2)*

Patient Name: MR#:

Date:

Admission Date: Admission Time:

HPI Recap (MOI, Interventions, Hospital Course):

Past Med / Surg Hist:

Social Hist:

Physcial Examination	Lacerations / Abrasions / Burns *(Document Location / Size)*
VS:	R L L R
T: P: BP: R:	
GCS:	
Eyes: Verbal: Motor:	
HEENT:	
Neck:	
CV:	
Resp / Chest:	
Abd / Rectal:	
GU:	
Extremities:	
Neuro (CN, Extremities):	

Rev. 4/1/05 *(continued on next page)* PS57995-0405

FIGURE 73.4. The tertiary survey instrument of the Acute Care Surgery Service of Shands Hospital at the University of Florida, Page 1.

SHANDS
at the University of Florida

Trauma and Emergency Surgery
Tertiary Survey Form *(page 2 of 2)*

Patient Name: MR#:

Consults / Interventions (include dates):

Neurosurgery:

Orthopaedics:

Plastics / ENT / OMFS:

Urology:

Others:

Radiologic Findings (Please provide *FINAL READS*):

Plain Films

CXR:

Pelvis:

T/L/S Spine:

Extremities:

CT / MR

Chest:

Abdomen / Pelvis:

Other:

Laboratory Trends:

Plan:

MD Signature ____________ MD# ____________ Date / Time ____________

TRE Attending:
I have seen this patient with ____________ *and agree with plan and assessment.*

FIGURE 73.5. The tertiary survey instrument of the Acute Care Surgery Service of Shands Hospital at the University of Florida, Page 2.

References

1. Andrews PJ, Piper IR, Dearden NM, et al. Secondary insults during intrahospital transport of head-injured patients. *Lancet.* 1990;335:327.
2. Braman SS, Dunn SM, Amico CA, et al. Complications of intrahospital transport in critically ill patients. *Ann Intern Med.* 1987;107:469.
3. Ehrenwerth J, Sorbo S, Hackel A. Transport of critically ill adults. *Crit Care Med.* 1986;14:543.
4. Waydhas C. Intrahospital transport of critically ill patients. *Crit Care.* 1999;3:R83.
5. Warren J, Fromm RE Jr, Orr RA, et al. Guidelines for the inter- and intrahospital transport of critically ill patients. *Crit Care Med.* 2004;32:256.
6. Auerbach SM, Kiesler DJ, Wartella J, et al. Optimism, satisfaction with needs met, interpersonal perceptions of the healthcare team, and emotional distress in patients' family members during critical care hospitalization. *Am J Crit Care.* 2005;14:202.
7. Perez-San Gregorio MA, Blanco-Picabia A, Murillo-Cabezas F, et al. Psychological problems in the family members of gravely traumatised patients admitted into an intensive care unit. *Intensive Care Med.* 1992;18:278.
8. Pochard F, Azoulay E, Chevret S, et al. Symptoms of anxiety and depression in family members of intensive care unit patients: ethical hypothesis regarding decision-making capacity. *Crit Care Med.* 2001;29:1893.
9. Cross ML, Wright SW, Wrenn KD, et al. Interaction between the trauma team and families: lack of timely communication. *Am J Emerg Med.* 1996;14:548.
10. Epperson MM. Families in sudden crisis: process and intervention in a critical care center. *Soc Work Health Care.* 1977;2:265.

11. Moreau D, Goldgran-Toledano D, Alberti C, et al. Junior versus senior physicians for informing families of intensive care unit patients. *Am J Respir Crit Care Med.* 2004;169:512.
12. Merrer J, De Jonghe B, Golliot F, et al. Complications of femoral and subclavian venous catheterization in critically ill patients: a randomized controlled trial. *JAMA.* 2001;286:700.
13. Van de Louw A, Cracco C, Cerf C, et al. Accuracy of pulse oximetry in the intensive care unit. *Intensive Care Med.* 2001;27:1606.
14. Hinkelbein J, Genzwuerker HV, Fiedler F. Detection of a systolic pressure threshold for reliable readings in pulse oximetry. *Resuscitation.* 2005;64:315.
15. Gonzalez EA, Moore FA, Holcomb JB, et al. Fresh frozen plasma should be given earlier to patients requiring massive transfusion. *J Trauma.* 2007;62:112.
16. Martinowitz U, Kenet G, Segal E, et al. Recombinant activated factor VII for adjunctive hemorrhage control in trauma. *J Trauma.* 2001;51:431.
17. Dutton RP, McCunn M, Hyder M, et al. Factor VIIa for correction of traumatic coagulopathy. *J Trauma.* 2004;57:709.
18. Perkins JG, Schreiber MA, Wade CE, et al. Early versus late recombinant factor VIIa in combat trauma patients requiring massive transfusion. *J Trauma.* 2007;62:1095.
19. Boffard KD, Riou B, Warren B, et al. Recombinant factor VIIa as adjunctive therapy for bleeding control in severely injured trauma patients: two parallel randomized, placebo-controlled, double-blind clinical trials. *J Trauma.* 2005;59:8.
20. Gattinoni L, Brazzi L, Pelosi P, et al. A trial of goal-oriented hemodynamic therapy in critically ill patients. SvO2 Collaborative Group. *N Engl J Med.* 1995;333:1025.
21. Durham RM, Neunaber K, Mazuski JE, et al. The use of oxygen consumption and delivery as endpoints for resuscitation in critically ill patients. *J Trauma.* 1996;41:32.
22. Bishop MH, Shoemaker WC, Appel PL, et al. Prospective, randomized trial of survivor values of cardiac index, oxygen delivery, and oxygen consumption as resuscitation endpoints in severe trauma. *J Trauma.* 1995;38:780.
23. Shoemaker WC, Belzberg H, Wo CC, et al. Multicenter study of noninvasive monitoring systems as alternatives to invasive monitoring of acutely ill emergency patients. *Chest.* 1998;114:1643.
24. Velmahos GC, Demetriades D, Shoemaker WC, et al. Endpoints of resuscitation of critically injured patients: normal or supranormal? A prospective randomized trial. *Ann Surg.* 2000;232:409.
25. Balogh Z, McKinley BA, Cocanour CS, et al. Supranormal trauma resuscitation causes more cases of abdominal compartment syndrome. *Arch Surg.* 2003;138:637.
26. Rivers E, Nguyen B, Havstad S, et al. Early goal-directed therapy in the treatment of severe sepsis and septic shock. *N Engl J Med.* 2001;345:1368.
27. Peake S, Webb S, Delaney A. Early goal-directed therapy of septic shock: we honestly remain skeptical. *Crit Care Med.* 2007;35:994.
28. Roberts I, Alderson P, Bunn F, et al. Colloids versus crystalloids for fluid resuscitation in critically ill patients. *Cochrane Database Syst Rev.* 2004;CD000567.
29. Connors AF Jr, Speroff T, Dawson NV, et al. The effectiveness of right heart catheterization in the initial care of critically ill patients. SUPPORT Investigators. *JAMA.* 1996;276:889.
30. Bilkovski RN, Rivers EP, Horst HM. Targeted resuscitation strategies after injury. *Curr Opin Crit Care.* 2004;10:529.
31. Broder G, Weil MH. Excess lactate: an index of reversibility of shock in human patients. *Science.* 1964;143:1457.
32. Nguyen HB, Rivers EP, Knoblich BP, et al. Early lactate clearance is associated with improved outcome in severe sepsis and septic shock. *Crit Care Med.* 2004;32:1637.
33. Husain FA, Martin MJ, Mullenix PS, et al. Serum lactate and base deficit as predictors of mortality and morbidity. *Am J Surg.* 2003;185:485.
34. Davis JW, Shackford SR, Mackersie RC, et al. Base deficit as a guide to volume resuscitation. *J Trauma.* 1998;28:1464.
35. Rutherford EJ, Morris JA Jr, Reed GW, et al. Base deficit stratifies mortality and determines therapy. *J Trauma.* 1992;33:417.
36. Chang MC, Meredith JW. Cardiac preload, splanchnic perfusion, and their relationship during resuscitation in trauma patients. *J Trauma.* 1997;42:577.
37. Miller PR, Meredith JW, Chang MC. Randomized, prospective comparison of increased preload versus inotropes in the resuscitation of trauma patients: effects on cardiopulmonary function and visceral perfusion. *J Trauma.* 1998;44:107.
38. Velmahos GC, Wo CC, Demetriades D, et al. Invasive and non-invasive physiological monitoring of blunt trauma patients in the early period after emergency admission. *Int Surg.* 1999;84:354.
39. Garcia-Rodriguez C, Pittman J, Cassell CH, et al. Lithium dilution cardiac output measurement: a clinical assessment of central venous and peripheral venous indicator injection. *Crit Care Med.* 2002;30:2199.
40. Gan TJ, Soppitt A, Maroof M, et al. Goal-directed intraoperative fluid administration reduces length of hospital stay after major surgery. *Anesthesiology.* 2002;97:820.
41. Sinclair S, James S, Singer M. Intraoperative intravascular volume optimisation and length of hospital stay after repair of proximal femoral fracture: randomised controlled trial. *BMJ.* 1997;315:909.
42. Eachempati SR, Young C, Alexander J, et al. The clinical use of an esophageal Doppler monitor for hemodynamic monitoring in sepsis. *J Clin Monit Comput.* 1999;15:223.
43. Beilman GJ, Groehler KE, Lazaron V, et al. Near-infrared spectroscopy measurement of regional tissue oxyhemoglobin saturation during hemorrhagic shock. *Shock.* 1999;12:196.
44. McKinley BA, Marvin RG, Cocanour CS, et al. Tissue hemoglobin O2 saturation during resuscitation of traumatic shock monitored using near infrared spectrometry. *J Trauma.* 2000;48:637.
45. Cairns CB, Moore FA, Haenel JB, et al. Evidence for early supply independent mitochondrial dysfunction in patients developing multiple organ failure after trauma. *J Trauma.* 1997;42:532.
46. Mattox KL, Flint LM, Carrico CJ, et al. Blunt cardiac injury. *J Trauma.* 1992;33:649.
47. Elie MC. Blunt cardiac injury. *Mt Sinai J Med.* 2006;73:542.
48. Schultz JM, Trunkey DD. Blunt cardiac injury. *Crit Care Clin.* 2004;20:57.
49. Rozycki GS, Feliciano DV, Schmidt JA, et al. The role of surgeon-performed ultrasound in patients with possible cardiac wounds. *Ann Surg.* 1996;223:737.
50. Mandavia DP, Hoffner RJ, Mahaney K, et al. Bedside echocardiography by emergency physicians. *Ann Emerg Med.* 2001;38:377.
51. Foil MB, Mackersie RC, Furst SR, et al. The asymptomatic patient with suspected myocardial contusion. *Am J Surg.* 1990;160:638.
52. Biffl WL, Moore FA, Moore EE, et al. Cardiac enzymes are irrelevant in the patient with suspected myocardial contusion. *Am J Surg.* 1994;168:523.
53. Maenza RL, Seaberg D, D'Amico F. A meta-analysis of blunt cardiac trauma: ending myocardial confusion. *Am J Emerg Med.* 1996;14:237.
54. Dubrow TJ, Mihalka J, Eisenhauer DM, et al. Myocardial contusion in the stable patient: what level of care is appropriate? *Surgery.* 1989;106:267.
55. Nagy KK, Krosner SM, Roberts RR, et al. Determining which patients require evaluation for blunt cardiac injury following blunt chest trauma. *World J Surg.* 2001;25:108.
56. Feghali NT, Prisant LM. Blunt myocardial injury. *Chest.* 1995;108:1673.
57. Adams JE 3rd, Davila-Roman VG, Bessey PQ, et al. Improved detection of cardiac contusion with cardiac troponin I. *Am Heart J.* 1996;131:308.
58. Bertinchant JP, Polge A, Mohty D, et al. Evaluation of incidence, clinical significance, and prognostic value of circulating cardiac troponin I and T elevation in hemodynamically stable patients with suspected myocardial contusion after blunt chest trauma. *J Trauma.* 2000;48:924.
59. Salim A, Velmahos GC, Jindal A, et al. Clinically significant blunt cardiac trauma: role of serum troponin levels combined with electrocardiographic findings. *J Trauma.* 2001;50:237.
60. Velmahos GC, Karaiskakis M, Salim A, et al. Normal electrocardiography and serum troponin I levels preclude the presence of clinically significant blunt cardiac injury. *J Trauma.* 2003;54:45.
61. Karalis DG, Victor MF, Davis GA, et al. The role of echocardiography in blunt chest trauma: a transthoracic and transesophageal echocardiographic study. *J Trauma.* 1994;36:53.
62. Christensen MA, Sutton KR. Myocardial contusion: new concepts in diagnosis and management. *Am J Crit Care.* 1993;2:28.
63. Lindstaedt M, Germing A, Lawo T, et al. Acute and long-term clinical significance of myocardial contusion following blunt thoracic trauma: results of a prospective study. *J Trauma.* 2002;52:479.
64. Chirillo F, Totis O, Cavarzerani A, et al. Usefulness of transthoracic and transoesophageal echocardiography in recognition and management of cardiovascular injuries after blunt chest trauma. *Heart.* 1996;75:301.
65. Weiss RL, Brier JA, O'Connor W, et al. The usefulness of transesophageal echocardiography in diagnosing cardiac contusions. *Chest.* 1996;109:73.
66. Link MS, Estes NA 3rd. Mechanically induced ventricular fibrillation (commotio cordis). *Heart Rhythm.* 2007;4:529.
67. Maron BJ. Sudden death in young athletes. *N Engl J Med.* 2003;349:1064.
68. Penney DJ, Bannon PG, Parr MJ. Intra-aortic balloon counterpulsation for cardiogenic shock due to cardiac contusion in an elderly trauma patient. *Resuscitation.* 2002;55:337.
69. Snow N, Lucas AE, Richardson JD. Intra-aortic balloon counterpulsation for cardiogenic shock from cardiac contusion. *J Trauma.* 1982;22:426.
70. Pevec WC, el-Hillel M, McArdle DQ, et al. Rupture of the left ventricle and interventricular septum by blunt trauma. *Crit Care Med.* 1989;17:837.
71. Pevec WC, Udekwu AO, Peitzman AB. Blunt rupture of the myocardium. *Ann Thorac Surg.* 1989;48:139.
72. McQueen MM, Gaston P, Court-Brown CM. Acute compartment syndrome. Who is at risk? *J Bone Joint Surg Br.* 2000;82:200.
73. Olson SA, Glasgow RR. Acute compartment syndrome in lower extremity musculoskeletal trauma. *J Am Acad Orthop Surg.* 2005;13:436.
74. Moed BR, Thorderson PK. Measurement of intracompartmental pressure: a comparison of the slit catheter, side-ported needle, and simple needle. *J Bone Joint Surg Am.* 1993;75:231.
75. Richardson JD, Trinkle JK. Hemodynamic and respiratory alterations with increased intra-abdominal pressure. *J Surg Res.* 1976;20:401.
76. Rotondo MF, Schwab CW, McGonigal MD, et al. 'Damage control': an approach for improved survival in exsanguinating penetrating abdominal injury. *J Trauma.* 1993;35:375.
77. Meldrum DR, Moore FA, Moore EE, et al. Prospective characterization and selective management of the abdominal compartment syndrome. *Am J Surg.* 1997;174:667.

78. The World Society on Abdominal Compartment Syndrome. Abdominal compartment syndrome. http://www.wsacs.org/. Accessed 2006.
79. Sugrue M. Abdominal compartment syndrome. *Curr Opin Crit Care.* 2005;11:333.
80. Cheatham ML, White MW, Sagraves SG, et al. Abdominal perfusion pressure: a superior parameter in the assessment of intra-abdominal hypertension. *J Trauma.* 2000;49:621.
81. Simon RJ, Friedlander MH, Ivatury RR, et al. Hemorrhage lowers the threshold for intra-abdominal hypertension-induced pulmonary dysfunction. *J Trauma.* 1997;42:398.
82. Oda J, Ueyama M, Yamashita K, et al. Hypertonic lactated saline resuscitation reduces the risk of abdominal compartment syndrome in severely burned patients. *J Trauma.* 2006;60:64.
83. Latenser BA, Kowal-Vern A, Kimball D, et al. A pilot study comparing percutaneous decompression with decompressive laparotomy for acute abdominal compartment syndrome in thermal injury. *J Burn Care Rehabil.* 2002;23:190.
84. Scott BG, Welsh FJ, Pham HQ, et al. Early aggressive closure of the open abdomen. *J Trauma.* 2006;60:17.
85. Geeraerts T, Chhor V, Cheisson G, et al. Clinical review: initial management of blunt pelvic trauma patients with haemodynamic instability. *Crit Care.* 2007;11:204.
86. Demetriades D, Karaiskakis M, Toutouzas K, et al. Pelvic fractures: epidemiology and predictors of associated abdominal injuries and outcomes. *J Am Coll Surg.* 2002;195:1.
87. Gilliland MD, Ward RE, Barton RM, et al. Factors affecting mortality in pelvic fractures. *J Trauma.* 1982;22:691.
88. Smejkal R, Izant T, Born C, et al. Pelvic crush injuries with occlusion of the iliac artery. *J Trauma.* 1988;28:1479.
89. Mucha P Jr, Welch TJ. Hemorrhage in major pelvic fractures. *Surg Clin North Am.* 1988;68:757.
90. Gonzalez RP, Fried PQ, Bukhalo M. The utility of clinical examination in screening for pelvic fractures in blunt trauma. *J Am Coll Surg.* 2002;194:121.
91. *ATLS: Advanced Trauma Life Support for Doctors: Student Course Manual.* Chicago: American College of Surgeons; 2004.
92. Obaid AK, Barleben A, Porral D, et al. Utility of plain film pelvic radiographs in blunt trauma patients in the emergency department. *Am Surg.* 2006;72:951.
93. Pennal GF, Tile M, Waddell JP, et al. Pelvic disruption: assessment and classification. *Clin Orthop Relat Res.* 1980;12.
94. Burgess AR, Eastridge BJ, Young JW, et al. Pelvic ring disruptions: effective classification system and treatment protocols. *J Trauma.* 1990;30:848.
95. Routt ML Jr, Falicov A, Woodhouse E, et al. Circumferential pelvic antishock sheeting: a temporary resuscitation aid. *J Orthop Trauma.* 2002;16:45.
96. Simpson T, Krieg JC, Heuer F, et al. Stabilization of pelvic ring disruptions with a circumferential sheet. *J Trauma.* 2002;52:158.
97. Krieg JC, Mohr M, Ellis TJ, et al. Emergent stabilization of pelvic ring injuries by controlled circumferential compression: a clinical trial. *J Trauma.* 2005;59:659.
98. Mattox KL, Bickell W, Pepe PE, et al. Prospective MAST study in 911 patients. *J Trauma.* 1989;29:1104.
99. Seavers R, Lynch J, Ballard R, et al. Hypogastric artery ligation for uncontrollable hemorrhage in acute pelvic trauma. *Surgery.* 1964;55:516.
100. Goins WA, Rodriguez A, Lewis J, et al. Retroperitoneal hematoma after blunt trauma. *Surg Gynecol Obstet.* 1992;174:281.
101. Smith WR, Moore EE, Osborn P, et al. Retroperitoneal packing as a resuscitation technique for hemodynamically unstable patients with pelvic fractures: report of two representative cases and a description of technique. *J Trauma.* 2005;59:1510.
102. Cothren CC, Osborn PM, Moore EE, et al. Preperitonal pelvic packing for hemodynamically unstable pelvic fractures: a paradigm shift. *J Trauma.* 2007;62:834.
103. Ward WG, Nunley JA. Occult orthopaedic trauma in the multiply injured patient. *J Orthop Trauma.* 1991;5:308.
104. Laasonen EM, Kivioja A. Delayed diagnosis of extremity injuries in patients with multiple injuries. *J Trauma.* 1991;31:257.
105. Mackersie RC, Shackford SR, Garfin SR, et al. Major skeletal injuries in the obtunded blunt trauma patient: a case for routine radiologic survey. *J Trauma.* 1998;28:1450.
106. Cirillo RL Jr, Koniaris LG. Detecting blunt pancreatic injuries. *J Gastrointest Surg.* 2002;6:587.
107. Jurkovich GJ, Carrico CJ. Pancreatic trauma. *Surg Clin North Am.* 1990; 70:575.
108. Akhrass R, Kim K, Brandt C. Computed tomography: an unreliable indicator of pancreatic trauma. *Am Surg.* 1996;62:647.
109. Carrillo EH, Richardson JD, Miller FB. Evolution in the management of duodenal injuries. *J Trauma.* 1996;40:1037.
110. Degiannis E, Boffard K. Duodenal injuries. *Br J Surg.* 2000;87:1473.
111. Watts DD, Fakhry SM. Incidence of hollow viscus injury in blunt trauma: an analysis from 275,557 trauma admissions from the East multi-institutional trial. *J Trauma.* 2003;54:289.
112. Malhotra AK, Fabian TC, Katsis SB, et al. Blunt bowel and mesenteric injuries: the role of screening computed tomography. *J Trauma.* 2000;48: 991.
113. Fakhry SM, Brownstein M, Watts DD, et al. Relatively short diagnostic delays (<8 hours) produce morbidity and mortality in blunt small bowel injury: an analysis of time to operative intervention in 198 patients from a multicenter experience. *J Trauma.* 2000;48:408.
114. Enderson BL, Reath DB, Meadors J, et al. The tertiary trauma survey: a prospective study of missed injury. *J Trauma.* 1990;30:666.
115. Janjua KJ, Sugrue M, Deane SA. Prospective evaluation of early missed injuries and the role of tertiary trauma survey. *J Trauma.* 1998;44:1000.
116. Biffl WL, Harrington DT, Cioffi WG. Implementation of a tertiary trauma survey decreases missed injuries. *J Trauma.* 2003;54:38.

CHAPTER 74 ■ SURGICAL AND POST-SURGICAL BLEEDING

DANNY M. TAKANISHI, JR.

It is of critical importance that clinicians who provide care to surgical patients understand the dynamic interplay of the coagulation and fibrinolytic systems. An appreciation for the relevant underlying biologic mechanisms is central to the diagnosis and appropriate management of patients who present with bleeding diatheses in both the operative and the postoperative setting. Surgery provides the most significant challenge to the integrity of the hemostatic system, and the fidelity of the coagulation system serves as the homeostatic defense mechanism that abrogates the proclivity for bleeding in this context.

INITIAL APPRAISAL OF HEMOSTATIC IMPAIRMENT: GENERAL OVERVIEW AND IMMEDIATE CONCERNS

To expeditiously manage a critically ill patient experiencing life-threatening hemorrhage, it is crucial that a defined approach for prompt recognition of the underlying cause is used. First, attention is directed toward stabilizing the patient. This includes securing an adequate airway, ventilation, vascular access, and restoring intravascular volume. Second, there should be immediate dialogue with individuals involved in the intraoperative management of the patient. This may provide pertinent information regarding the intraoperative course of the patient, specifically regarding any observed characteristics of bleeding that may suggest an underlying coagulation disorder. A generalized slow oozing of blood from raw surfaces (often termed "nonsurgical bleeding") is often a manifestation of a systemic disorder of hemostasis (1–3). On the other hand, bleeding related to technical factors that can be associated with the conduct of any surgical procedure (often termed "surgical bleeding") is localized and is the most common cause of postoperative bleeding. Dialogue with the surgical team should include consideration for re-exploration. The evolving coagulopathy may proceed swiftly in critically ill patients. Qualitative abnormalities of platelet function, depletion of both platelets and plasmatic coagulation factors, and hypothermia are major contributors to the underlying pathophysiology responsible for the coagulopathy that manifests in the critical care setting (2–9). Moreover, previously undiagnosed, rare, at times clinically latent, congenital coagulation disorders may be unmasked by the physiologic stress resulting from a surgical procedure. Familial coagulation defects that may be encountered in a bleeding postoperative patient include von Willebrand disease, factor VIII deficiency (hemophilia A, or classic hemophilia), and factor IX deficiency (hemophilia B or Christmas disease) (10–14).

The initial phase of assessment must include an immediate reconciliation of intravascular volume status to appropriately guide resuscitation and to assist in decision making for early operative intervention. Although signs of an expanding hematoma or saturated dressings are indicative of localized bleeding, there is considerable overlap, and coagulation system defects may present in a similar fashion postoperatively. In terms of management, however, early recognition of the clinical symptoms and signs attributable to hypovolemia (restlessness, anxiety, shortness of breath, pallor, tachycardia, and oliguria) is compulsory. Adjunctive estimates of intravascular volume status may be obtained using both noninvasive and invasive monitoring, as is common in the critical care setting. Systemic hypotension is a late sign of significant hypovolemia, and expeditious resuscitation is paramount to avert the disastrous consequences of an unrecognized and inappropriately triaged patient with ongoing, potentially life-threatening hemorrhage.

It is important to differentiate the inherited (primary) coagulation disorders, which are associated with a history of bleeding diatheses, from the more commonly acquired (secondary) coagulation disorders, which are the consequence of pathologic conditions and numerous medications (1,3,15). This nomenclature (primary vs. secondary) is distinct from and should not be confused with the traditional nomenclature used to describe the hemostatic *process* itself. In the formation of a stable clot, the hemostatic process was classically described as comprising two phases, a primary phase (also called *primary hemostasis*) and a secondary phase (also called *secondary hemostasis*). The primary phase of hemostasis involves vascular or tissue injury, initiating platelet adhesion and aggregation to form the platelet plug. The secondary phase involves the activation of the plasmatic coagulation protein cascade (both the extrinsic and the intrinsic systems), which results in formation of the stable fibrin clot. Disorders involving platelet number or function, or vascular interactions, are classified as disorders of primary hemostasis, and disorders involving the plasmatic coagulation factors are classified as disorders of secondary hemostasis. This serves the purpose of an operational definition, since *in vivo* these events are not separate processes but highly integrated.

Hemostatic disorders, whether primary (inherited) or secondary (acquired), can both be manifest by diffuse bleeding from the operative site, puncture wounds, vascular access sites, or traumatized tissue outside of the operative field. Surgical and postsurgical bleeding may therefore result from either quantitative (thrombocytopenia) or qualitative (abnormal function) platelet disorders.

Thrombocytopenia may be further attributed to a decrease in production of platelets (aplastic anemia, hypoplastic bone marrow, chemotherapy, space-occupying lesions of the bone marrow as seen with malignancy), ineffective production (vitamin B_{12} or folic acid deficiency states), platelet sequestration (primary or secondary hypersplenism), increased destruction or consumption of platelets (hemorrhagic conditions; microangiopathic processes such as thrombotic thrombocytopenic purpura [TTP]; disseminated intravascular coagulation [DIC]; hemolytic-uremic syndrome [HUS]; immune destruction due to antiplatelet antibodies, such as in posttransfusion purpura or idiopathic thrombocytopenic purpura), or dilution of circulating platelet volume (massive blood transfusion) (1–4,6–9,16–18).

Qualitative platelet disorders may be inherited (Bernard-Soulier syndrome, abnormal release mechanism, Glanzmann thrombasthenia, storage pool disease, or von Willebrand disease) or acquired (uremia, drug interactions, myeloproliferative disorders). Disorders involving plasmatic coagulation factors are generally caused by either a decrease in production of clotting factors (commonly associated with hepatic insufficiency, cirrhosis, vitamin K deficiency, obstructive jaundice) or by an increase in consumption of circulating coagulation factors (such as in DIC) (3,6–9,18,19). Coagulopathy manifested in the critically ill patient is often a result of a combination of both platelet and plasmatic coagulation factor defects. Well-known examples include obstructive biliary tract disease or chronic liver disease, which results in diminished production of coagulation factors given that the liver is the major site of synthesis of all coagulation factors with the exception of factor VIII. In addition, platelet sequestration may occur from secondary hypersplenism (18). Massive trauma often results in decreases of both platelets and coagulation factors as a result of consumption secondary to ongoing bleeding or hemorrhage (4). If shock and acidosis develop, there is further decrease in coagulation factor synthesis due to impairment in liver function that results from low perfusion, in addition to impairment of both coagulation factor and platelet function from the acidemic state (20,21). Additionally, well-described sequelae of massive blood transfusion, often associated with multiple trauma and hemorrhagic shock, is the development of a coagulopathy (22). This results from a combination of dilution of plasmatic coagulation factors and platelets, chelating of ionized calcium (a necessary component of the coagulation cascade) by the anticoagulant (citrate) present in banked blood, acidosis that often attends the underlying disease, hypothermia, or the condition that made massive blood transfusion necessary in the first place. Hypothermia significantly impairs both platelet and plasmatic coagulation function (5,21). Last, transient platelet dysfunction, responsive to desmopressin (DDAVP, 1-desamino-8-d-arginine vasopressin), is a well-recognized phenomenon in patients after cardiopulmonary bypass (23–26).

In parallel with the ongoing resuscitation of the bleeding patient, attention must be directed toward expeditiously determining the need for surgical re-exploration. All bleeding patients must be considered candidates for reoperation. A comprehensive assessment must take into account the degree and the duration of active bleeding, the anatomic site of involvement, and the potential for additional morbidity or mortality (for example, evolving acidosis, myocardial ischemia, diminished mental status, oliguria, or a progressive neck wound hematoma with impending acute airway obstruction). Physiologic reserve is also a compelling variable to consider, for patients with significant comorbidities, such as the elderly, pediatric, obese and diabetic patients are attended by less reserve. Hence, vigilant observation to recognize early postoperative bleeding is crucial, before hemodynamic instability and shock become manifest. In these patients, consideration for early operative intervention may be necessary because this cohort may not be able to readily tolerate even mild degrees of anemia, hypovolemia, and hypoperfusion. Consideration of other modalities of hemorrhage control (interventional radiology and embolization) may be entertained in appropriate situations.

An important caveat is that not every instance of bleeding requires surgical intervention, and conversely, patients who may initially appear to have clinically self-limited bleeding postoperatively may still require reoperation for control of bleeding. Major pelvic fractures are contemporaneously managed by either fracture stabilization or arteriography with embolization of the culprit bleeding pelvic vessels. In contrast, the natural history of a contained perioperative vascular anastomotic dehiscence is characterized by the evolution of a false aneurysm. In this setting, immediate re-exploration with operative repair is indicated to avert the potentially catastrophic consequence of free rupture and death from exsanguinating hemorrhage.

EVALUATION OF BLEEDING: CLINICAL HISTORY AND THE UTILITY OF DIAGNOSTIC TESTING

A detailed history and physical examination is the most important preliminary step in elucidating the cause of surgical bleeding and should be done simultaneously with resuscitative efforts (1). Collateral history from family members and previous medical records is a helpful adjunct to determine if a primary, congenital defect in the coagulation system is present. A history of easy bruisability, excessive gingival bleeding after brushing of teeth, bleeding diathesis with dental extractions, hypermenorrhagia, frequent spontaneous epistaxis, melenic stools or spontaneous hematuria, petechiae or purpura, hemarthroses, and a family history of bleeding disorders may indicate a congenital or familial coagulation disorder, such as hemophilia A or B or von Willebrand disease. The family pedigree may provide important clues as to the presumptive disease process based on the pattern of inheritance, whether autosomal or sex linked, dominant or recessive. Suspicion for a congenital disorder of coagulation is further raised by a history of blood transfusions required for common ambulatory procedures such as dental extractions, circumcisions, tonsillectomies, or biopsies. Due to differences in gene penetrance, not all individuals afflicted with inherited coagulation disorders are diagnosed at an early age, and clinically latent, attenuated bleeding disorders may be unmasked when confronted by a major surgical procedure or trauma. A past history of liver disease or heavy ethanol consumption should alert the clinician to the possibility of acquired plasmatic factor deficiencies, in addition to thrombocytopenia resulting from secondary hypersplenism with platelet sequestration.

A thorough medication history is essential (including soliciting information on the use of dietary supplements or herbal tonics, and over-the-counter medications), to determine if the patient has been on any medication that interferes with hemostasis (common examples include aspirin, other nonsteroidal anti-inflammatory agents, ticlopidine, clopidogrel, or semisynthetic penicillins) (16,23–26). Popular supplements that may aggravate bleeding are ginkgo, garlic, ginger, ginseng, feverfew, and vitamin E. A history of anticoagulation therapy is equally important in this regard (19,27). Nutritional assessment is paramount, and careful evaluation for the presence of a vitamin K deficiency is obligatory, as this may occur in patients on parenteral nutrition or with cancer cachexia in those with malignancies. Other variables that may affect the integrity of the coagulation system include previous irradiation, renal failure, and sepsis, which affect the coagulation cascade at multiple points.

Physical examination often provides an index of the severity and the extent of the disease and may provide additional clues that assist in distinguishing localized surgical bleeding from systemic bleeding resulting from a coagulopathy. For example, the presence of petechiae, purpura, and mucosal bleeding is often indicative of thrombocytopenia, a qualitative functional disorder of platelets, or increased vascular fragility. Ecchymoses or spontaneous, nontraumatic hemarthrosis is consistent with plasmatic coagulation factor abnormalities or deficiencies such as hemophilia. Both platelet and plasmatic coagulation disorders are associated with hematomas. Hepatic insufficiency or failure can be presumptively identified by recognizing jaundice, ascites, angiomas, palmar erythema, asterixis, congestive splenomegaly, and testicular atrophy. Splenomegaly itself may also be associated with hematologic dyscrasias and malignancies associated with hemostatic abnormalities (lymphomas and leukemias). Connective tissue or collagen vascular disorders that result in increased vascular fragility may manifest with petechiae, joint abnormalities, and a history of delayed wound healing. These conditions focus attention on the increased risk for a perioperative bleeding complication, which underscores the need for vigilance both intraoperatively and postoperatively. Last, the possibility of sepsis as an underlying cause for the development of a coagulopathy must always be entertained in the postoperative, critically ill patient (9).

The establishment of a definitive diagnosis of a coagulation disorder rests on selective use of a limited battery of laboratory tests guided by information derived from the history and physical examination. These assays are selected to broadly screen the hemostatic system. These tests are, for the most part, automated (except for the bleeding time), readily available, and amenable to point-of-care testing methodology. The tests most commonly used include the template bleeding time, quantitative platelet count, prothrombin time (PT), activated partial thromboplastin time (PTT), fibrinogen level, and thrombin time (TT). The template bleeding time is the only test that screens for qualitative platelet function abnormalities, a frequent cause of abnormal bleeding. This test also evaluates platelet number and vascular fragility, demonstrating abnormal prolongation in thrombocytopenic states and in conditions associated with increased vascular fragility (examples include connective tissue disorders such as senile purpura, Ehlers-Danlos syndrome, steroid-induced purpura, or Marfan syndrome; scurvy; amyloidosis; or hereditary hemorrhagic telangiectasia/Osler-Weber-Rendu disease). Therefore, if both the platelet count and the template bleeding time are normal, the presumptive differential diagnosis is directed toward a plasmatic coagulation factor abnormality. Measurement of both the PT and PTT will serve to further define the abnormality, given that each test is more sensitive to changes in procoagulants in the initial phases of the extrinsic and intrinsic pathways, respectively. The PTT provides a global measure of the activity of factors XII, XI, IX, and VIII in addition to the common pathway factors shared by the extrinsic system (factors X, V, II, and I) and, therefore, identifies many of the inherited disorders of bleeding, typically a deficiency of factor VIII (hemophilia A), IX (hemophilia B), or von Willebrand factor, vWF (von Willebrand disease). It is worth noting that factor XII deficiency is not associated with any significant bleeding tendency despite abnormal prolongation of the PTT. Enzymatically active vWF is a necessary cofactor for optimum functioning of the factor VIII procoagulant protein. The PT exclusively evaluates factor VII, which is one of the vitamin K–dependent factors (in addition to factors II, IX, and X). Therefore, the PT is prolonged in individuals on Coumadin (warfarin) therapy, and this test is used to measure therapeutic efficacy of this form of oral anticoagulation therapy. Liver disease is another common cause for a prolonged PT, perhaps most notably because factor VII has the shortest half-life of the plasmatic coagulation factors. Liver disease, by virtue of the diminished synthesis of all plasmatic coagulation factors (with the exception of vWF) also results in prolongation of the PTT in addition to the PT. Due to the sensitivity of factors XII, XI, IX, VIII, and X to the effects of heparin (in the presence of antithrombin III), heparin therapy primarily is reflected by abnormal prolongation of the PTT. In conditions associated with prolongation of both the PT and the PTT, quantitative measurement of the fibrinogen (factor I) level may be useful to determine if the coagulation disorder is a result of a defect or deficiency of multiple coagulation factors, which may be associated with liver disease, sepsis, and DIC, or if an inhibitor is present (3,6–9,18). Examples of circulating inhibitors include heparin, paraproteinemias associated with monoclonal gammopathies (multiple myeloma or Waldenstrom macroglobulinemia), fibrin/fibrinogen degradation products, or other circulating anticoagulants (such as antibodies to factor VIII or IX, and the lupus anticoagulant). Factor levels reflect a dynamic equilibrium, and fibrinogen is an acute-phase protein that increases in response to stress. Fibrinogen consumption may not be apparent based solely on measurement of levels because of the propensity for the liver to increase synthesis of this protein in response to the same stressors responsible for fibrinogen consumption. This fact is important to bear in mind for proper interpretation of laboratory results. The thrombin time is a qualitative measure of fibrinogen levels and will be prolonged if the fibrinogen level is less than 100 mg/dL, by the presence of dysfibrinogenemia associated with liver disease, and also by circulating inhibitors similar to the PT and PTT (28). Its most useful role clinically is in the detection of circulating heparin not detectable by changes in the PTT.

The therapeutic approach to hemostatic abnormalities must be reasonably guided by the patient's clinical condition and the outcome of appropriately selected laboratory tests, as outlined above (14). An important concept is not to fall behind in factor replacement. Due to the lag time in receiving laboratory values, in clinical conditions where the patient is actively bleeding, initiation of fresh frozen plasma (FFP) and platelets should be started early with red cell transfusion. In patients with known warfarin use and a small bleed in an uncompromising area (skull), FFP should be used *before* patients develop increasing intracranial hemorrhage. In general, FFP is the most commonly used blood component for plasmatic coagulation abnormalities since it provides all necessary coagulation factors in concentrations that approach those found in normal plasma (3,10,11,14). Cryoprecipitate, a component made from thawing FFP in the cold under specialized conditions, is rich in factors XIII, VIII, I, vWF, and fibronectin. It has been used in factor VIII–deficient states (hemophilia A) if virally inactivated plasma-derived or recombinant factor VIII concentrates are not readily available; in von Willebrand disease recalcitrant to desmopressin and if virally inactivated plasma derived factor VIII concentrate rich in vWF is not readily available; in hypofibrinogenemic or dysfibrinogenemic conditions; in hemorrhage associated with massive blood transfusions; in DIC; in factor XIII deficiency (FFP is also used); in bleeding uremic patients with qualitative platelet function defects unresponsive to desmopressin therapy; or as a topically applied surgical sealant ("fibrin glue") (10,14,29). For specific coagulation disorders, such as hemophilia A, hemophilia B (deficiencies of factor VIII and IX, respectively), and von Willebrand disease, virally inactivated plasma-derived factor concentrates are commercially available, as are recombinant products, and these are the blood components of choice if available for use. These concentrates (and the recombinant product) also have a lower risk for virally transmitted disease because of a processing procedure that results in viral inactivation. For deficiencies of the vitamin K–dependent factors (II, VII, IX, X), prothrombin complex concentrates are also commercially available, as is recombinant factor VII for isolated factor VII deficiency states. Platelet concentrates are used for both quantitative (thrombocytopenias) and qualitative platelet disorders associated with significant bleeding (3,10,12,14). Patients transfused with any blood component, whether FFP, cryoprecipitate, plasma-derived factor concentrates, or platelet concentrates, incur similar risks of complications attributed to all types of blood component therapy such as febrile and allergic reactions, transmission of blood-borne pathogens (human immunodeficiency virus, hepatitis B and C), immunosuppression, transfusion-related pulmonary injury, and hemolytic transfusion reactions if a substantial volume of ABO-incompatible units are transfused. Therefore, judicious use of blood component therapy must always be adhered to.

CAUSES OF POST-OPERATIVE BLEEDING

Post-operative bleeding, often termed local hemostatic failure or surgical bleeding, is a known potential complication of any surgical procedure. When associated with evolving hypovolemia, mental status changes, restlessness, anxiety, tachycardia, dyspnea, and oliguria are commonly associated manifestations. Hypotension is a late finding, and aggressive attempts must be made to avert this serious consequence with expeditious concurrent resuscitation as identification of the source of bleeding is confirmed. The vast majority of patients affected typically present within the immediate perioperative period. Subtle signs may be evident in the postanesthesia care unit, and generally become apparent within the first 8 hours after surgery. A high index of suspicion is necessary to render an early diagnosis of post-operative bleeding, and meticulous attention to look for any evidence of bleeding must be applied, given that many signs of evolving hypovolemia are nonspecific and may also be observed in nonbleeding patients after major thoracic or abdominal procedures (tachycardia associated with post-operative pain, anxiety and restlessness, mental status changes secondary to narcotic analgesic administration, or oliguria resulting from anticipated third-space fluid sequestration after major abdominal surgery). Blood in the peritoneal cavity ordinarily does not result in a significant inflammatory response unless associated with secondary bacterial contamination and therefore is not associated with obvious peritoneal signs. On occasion, localized symptoms may be elicited that are attributable to irritation caused by a collection of blood, exemplified by the Kehr sign. This is referred pain to the right shoulder ascribed to an accumulation of blood under the right hemidiaphragm. Serial hemoglobin and hematocrit levels may assist in determining the degree of bleeding, but isolated, single values can be difficult to interpret. It is difficult to quantitatively account for the effects of isotonic fluid sequestration (third-spacing) after major abdominal procedures that may result in hemoconcentration and elevated hemoglobin and hematocrit levels, or the effects of isotonic fluid administration in the perioperative period that may contribute to hemodilution and lower hemoglobin and hematocrit levels.

Certain surgical procedures are not associated with exsanguinating hemorrhage or hypotension but can be life threatening. Prototypic examples include neck operations for endocrine diseases (thyroid, parathyroid surgery), lymphadenectomies (radical neck dissections), major composite resections for tumors of the neck, and carotid surgery. From a pathophysiologic perspective, an expanding neck hematoma results in airway obstruction from both mechanical compression and from mural edema caused by lymphatic obstruction. The cause is frequently venous bleeding, compounded by hypertension and liberal preoperative use of antiplatelet medications in those undergoing carotid surgery. Acutely reopening the incision and evacuating the hematoma is often life-saving, although endotracheal intubation or cricothyroidotomy may be required as a temporizing measure until the airway edema resolves. Nearly all patients who develop neck hematomas require operative re-exploration. It is common practice to place drains in the operative field at the time of surgery prior to closure, and surgical procedural anthologies are replete with instructions substantiating this approach. Caution must be exercised in interpreting drain output as an accurate index of early perioperative bleeding, and it is correspondingly crucial to recognize that placement of a drain is not an appropriate substitute for ensuring meticulous surgical hemostasis (30).

There is no single criterion available to direct re-exploration for control of post-operative bleeding, and this decision is based on considering a number of variables. The timing of the active bleed relative to the operative procedure, its duration, its rate, the potential for additional morbidity, the patient's age as a surrogate for physiologic reserve, and other comorbid diseases (such as underlying cardiac or pulmonary disease, renal disease, diabetes, or obesity) must all be taken into consideration when deciding on the need for reoperation. Timing of re-exploration is of significant concern in conditions associated with limited or poor physiologic reserve as these patients are often quite ill and require judicious resuscitation and expeditious definitive surgical intervention prior to the inception of irreversible shock. The most conservative treatment is to return to the operating room with early control of surgical bleeding. Often times the need to return emergently to the operating room is quite obvious, as in the case of exsanguinating hemorrhage resulting from a coronary artery bypass graft dehiscence attended by brisk bleeding from the mediastinal drain. There are two caveats for consideration. First, it is desirable to correct any coagulopathy prior to returning to the operating room, and in some instances with minimal or mild bleeding this may be all that is necessary. It is important to recognize, however, that situations characterized by exsanguinating hemorrhage from failure of local surgical hemostasis may not allow for correction of the coagulopathy because of rapid ongoing consumption of coagulation factors and platelets. In these instances, operative intervention is paramount, and the decision to reoperate must not be unduly delayed while awaiting normalization of coagulation parameters. Second, as stated earlier, some subscribe to the notion that drains placed at the time of surgery are a useful adjunct to alert the surgical team to early signs of postoperative bleeding and to gauge the amount and rate of bleeding when it does occur. Caution with this practice must be promulgated, as it is a well-accepted observation that the absence of blood in a drain is not conclusive evidence that bleeding is not occurring, because the drain tip may be dislodged or may have migrated from its original position and this may not be readily apparent externally, or the drain may be obstructed with clot.

There are certain circumstances where operative re-exploration is obligatory, despite the fact that the bleeding may be self-limiting. A vascular anastomosis with a contained leak, even if seemingly small and hemodynamically inconsequential, must be repaired to avert the consequences of false aneurysm formation and later rupture. Small contained leaks may be difficult to recognize and pose a diagnostic dilemma. A duplex study may be helpful in further elucidating anastomotic integrity, but an arteriogram should be performed if any doubt exists.

Last, the surgeon must also be cognizant of the fact that there are some instances where bleeding is optimally addressed without surgical intervention. The prototypic illustration is the severe pelvic fracture with signs of ongoing hemorrhage, as alluded to earlier. In accordance with the Advanced Trauma Life Support protocol, associated injuries and additional sources of obvious bleeding must first be excluded. Once hemoperitoneum and hemothorax have been excluded, the pelvis is stabilized by external fixation, followed by arteriography with embolization of any bleeding pelvic or retroperitoneal blood vessels.

Disorders of Plasmatic Coagulation Factors: Overview

Hemostasis involves a complex interplay between elements of the vascular endothelium, plasmatic coagulation factors, platelets, and the fibrinolytic system. Primary isolated disorders of the fibrinolytic system as a cause of major bleeding are rare in the critically ill patient and are covered elsewhere (31,32). Disorders of the clotting system can be broadly classified as congenital or acquired, and a comprehensive history and physical examination often assists in determining the nature of a coagulation disorder in this regard. Acquired coagulopathies are relatively common in the post-operative ICU patient, and these disorders can be operationally separated in those involving platelets, the plasmatic coagulation factors, or both (3).

Thus, post-operative bleeding can be a result of quantitative abnormalities (thrombocytopenia), due to decreased production, ineffective thrombopoiesis (production), sequestration, increased destruction or consumption, and dilution; or qualitative platelet function abnormalities. Post-operative bleeding can also occur with acquired disorders of the coagulation system, which encompasses decreased production, impairment of function, or increased consumption of coagulation factors.

Quantitative Platelet Disorders: Thrombocytopenia

Thrombocytopenia, defined as a platelet count less than 140×10^9/L, results from decreased production, ineffective thrombopoiesis, sequestration particularly in the spleen, increased destruction or consumption, and dilution of circulating platelets associated with massive blood transfusion (1,10,12,14). Petechiae, purpura, and mucosal oozing is characteristic of thrombocytopenic states, although these findings may also be observed in qualitative platelet disorders and in conditions associated with increased vascular fragility. Platelet counts of 50×10^9/L or higher are generally considered adequate for surgical hemostasis in the absence of an associated qualitative functional defect, but below 20×10^9/L there is increased risk for spontaneous hemorrhages (10,12,14). Particularly lethal in this regard are those involving the central nervous system.

Cytotoxic chemotherapy and radiation therapy (total body) produce thrombocytopenia by suppression of bone marrow megakaryocytes, the progenitor cell for platelets. Together these are the most common causes of bleeding in patients undergoing therapy for malignancies. Marrow aplasia, hypoplasia, and space-occupying diseases of the bone marrow (such as metastatic carcinoma, leukemias, lymphomas) also result in decreased production of platelets. Certain drugs, including alcohol, have been associated with decreased production of platelets via a direct toxic effect on megakaryocytes. Ineffective thrombopoiesis is a characteristic trait of megaloblastic anemia resulting from either vitamin B_{12} or folate deficiency. Although there is an increase in the megakaryocytic mass, platelet production is impaired. Notwithstanding, hemorrhagic diatheses manifest in a few of these individuals (33).

The most frequent cause of thrombocytopenia resulting from increased destruction of circulating platelets is post-operative infection (9,34). Significantly, thrombocytopenia may be the first presenting sign of an occult infection and may herald impending sepsis. Consequently, in the post-operative setting, thrombocytopenia of unclear cause must promptly direct attention toward uncovering a potential source of occult sepsis.

Thrombocytopenia caused by increased destruction of platelets is also observed in microangiopathic hemolytic states, such as in thrombotic thrombocytopenic purpura (TTP) and hemolytic-uremic syndrome (HUS) (35,36). Mechanical injury occurs when platelets traverse the small capillary beds in the peripheral circulation. TTP is characterized by fever, fluctuating neurologic symptoms (headaches, confusion, seizures, or coma), and acute renal failure, in addition to a microangiopathic hemolytic anemia and thrombocytopenia. HUS manifests similarly to TTP, with the notable exceptions that the pediatric population is more commonly affected, neurologic manifestations are minimal, but the renal impairment is more pronounced. Central to the treatment of both these entities is supportive care, with particular attention given to management of the renal dysfunction (35–37). Plasma exchange is often efficacious in treating these diseases, and hemodialysis may also be required in some instances for support of renal failure.

Immune-mediated destruction of platelets is observed in several clinical conditions. Alloimmune antibodies are believed to account for posttransfusion purpura observed primarily in women, who may have been previously immunized by fetal-derived platelets since there is a significant association with a prior history of pregnancy (38). Immunizations to a number of candidate alloantigens have been reported in the literature, the most common being the PL^{A1} antigen. The antibodies induced are generally of the IgG class and therefore are also able to cross the placenta, as a described cause of neonatal thrombocytopenia. The purpura becomes apparent approximately 7 to 10 days after blood transfusion, presumably attributed to an anamnestic response, and can last several months. The population at risk has been estimated to be approximately 1% to 3%, and the condition tends to be self-limiting and responds to intravenous immune globulin. Idiopathic thrombocytopenic purpura is one of the more common examples of immune-mediated platelet destruction (17). It tends to occur in otherwise healthy individuals, and both an acute and a chronic form have been described. Mechanistically, platelets coated with autoantibodies are removed by the reticuloendothelial cells in the spleen (and to an extent in the liver). The diagnosis is one of exclusion after other causes of thrombocytopenia have been ruled out. A similar mechanism may account for the thrombocytopenia associated with collagen vascular diseases, such as systemic lupus erythematosus, lymphoreticular diseases, and in some infectious diseases, such as infectious mononucleosis or human immunodeficiency virus infections. It is noteworthy in this regard that the acute form, often observed in the pediatric population, is often preceded by a viral syndrome. Splenectomy is required in a third of patients if immune globulin, corticosteroids, or plasmapheresis is unable to control the condition (17,39,40). In this condition, significant bleeding may not occur until platelet counts decrease as low as 10×10^9/L because most of the circulating platelet pool consists of younger, more functionally active platelets. The significance of this impacts on the operative approach traditionally adopted during splenectomy. During splenectomy, platelets are hung by the anesthesiologist but not administered until the splenic artery is clamped or splenectomy completed. There is by and large minimal bleeding encountered despite the pronounced degree of thrombocytopenia, and if platelets are infused prior to control of the splenic arterial inflow, the infused platelets will merely be consumed by the spleen and not available for the hemostatic process. Immune-mediated destruction of platelets can also be caused by several drugs that can induce antibodies to platelets via hapten-mediated, or by immune complex–mediated, "innocent bystander" mechanisms. Quinine, amiodarone, sulfa drugs, cimetidine, ranitidine, phenytoin, and semisynthetic penicillins are some examples that may be encountered in the critical care environment (3). Heparin-induced thrombocytopenia is an unusual example of drug-induced thrombocytopenia in this context because a hypercoagulable condition is actually created characterized by thrombotic complications with the manifestation of the "white clot syndrome" (41). This syndrome typically becomes apparent after 1 week of therapy but may present within a few hours after implementing heparin therapy in already sensitized patients. Discontinuation of the offending agent is the appropriate treatment approach central to all causes of drug-induced, immune mediated thrombocytopenia.

Qualitative Platelet Function Disorders

Acquired disorders are the leading cause of qualitative platelet function abnormalities in the critically ill patient. It is vital to be aware that qualitative bleeding disorders are not measured by the standard battery of coagulation tests described above, with the exception of the template bleeding time. This test is not commonly used, given that this does not lend itself to automation and still requires the laboratory technologist to remain at the patient's bedside. Furthermore, this test has been attended by poor reproducibility, particularly in conditions associated with significant peripheral edema. Nevertheless, when a qualitative platelet function abnormality is suspected, the bleeding time is an appropriate first screening test to guide discriminate use of additional testing to further elucidate the underlying cause.

Ingestion of numerous drugs has been associated with inhibition of platelet function (3,16,42). Among these, aspirin is the most well described and best characterized. Aspirin interferes with cyclo-oxygenase–mediated prostaglandin and thromboxane synthesis and has profound effects at multiple steps in the formation of the hemostatic platelet plug. It decreases the platelet response to aggregation in response to collagen, inhibits the second phase of aggregation in response to adenosine diphosphate (ADP) and epinephrine, and irreversibly injures platelets for the duration of their lifespan. It is generally recommended that antiplatelet medications, such as aspirin, ticlopidine, and clopidogrel, are discontinued approximately 7 to 10 days prior to surgery. For nonsteroidal anti-inflammatory agents other than aspirin, ticlopidine, or clopidogrel, some investigators advocate 2 days of abstinence. It is important to recognize that many over-the-counter medications contain aspirin (e.g., Alka-Seltzer, Ecotrin, Anacin) and many patients are not aware of this, so it is imperative to obtain a comprehensive drug history, specifically querying for use of aspirin-containing products. Discontinuing the antiplatelet drug combined with use of desmopressin and platelet transfusions have been beneficial in treating bleeding encountered in these situations (10,12,14,16).

Another common cause of acquired qualitative defects in platelet function is hypothermia (5,21,43). Massive blood transfusions or crystalloid infusions without attention to use of blood warmers, lack of attention to maintaining a warm ambient environment in the operating room, especially during long procedures and for individuals at the extremes of age, and prolonged extrications and exposure time in the field in the patient with multiple traumatic injuries are all too familiar causes of hypothermia. Vigilant awareness must be directed toward maintaining normothermia to avert the potentially disastrous consequences of hypothermia in the already bleeding critically ill patient. Rewarming patients reverses the effects of hypothermia on the hemostatic system.

Renal failure is not uncommon in the critical care setting. In its acute form, bleeding is a common manifestation, most often from the gastrointestinal tract. The underlying mechanism is probably multifactorial, as there clearly is a qualitative platelet function defect related to the degree of uremia, in combination with abnormalities in the plasmatic coagulation system (44–46). The presence of acidosis also contributes to both the platelet and coagulation factor dysfunction. The fundamental approach to therapy centers on dialysis, which results in abatement of the bleeding diathesis. Use of desmopressin and cryoprecipitate, as temporizing measures to transiently stop the bleeding while awaiting institution of dialysis, have been reported to be successful. Conjugated estrogens have also been used with some success, albeit the effects are not as rapid but more durable, but any positive outcomes are balanced by undesirable consequences of hormonal side effects. In its chronic form, renal failure is still attended by a mild qualitative platelet function defect, but significant impact on hemostatic homeostasis is usually not seen.

Acquired Disorders of the Coagulation System Decreased Production

Decreased production of circulating plasmatic coagulation factors occurs secondary to liver failure (with the exception of factor VIII), vitamin K deficiency (seen with oral antibiotic usage, which depresses gut flora in the setting of nutritional deficiency; malabsorption syndromes, such as celiac sprue or chronic diarrheal conditions; or obstructive jaundice), and use of warfarin (Coumadin) (18,19). In these situations, therapy is acutely centered on replacement of coagulation factors, most commonly with use of FFP. Vitamin K is administered parenterally in patients with deficient states or to reverse the effects of Coumadin. Appreciable effects on coagulation factor synthesis (in the presence of normal hepatic synthetic function) is not generally seen for 24 to 36 hours after administration of parenteral vitamin K (19,27).

Impaired Function

The effect of hypothermia on antagonizing normal functioning of the hemostatic mechanism globally has been described under qualitative platelet abnormalities (2,5,21,43). It is important to bear in mind that all enzymatic processes in biologic systems are governed to an extent by the necessity to function in an optimal, typically narrow, temperature range. The coagulation factors are enzymes, and therefore function best under normothermic conditions. Platelets, too, function optimally under normothermic conditions. The implication of this is that the clinician must always remain alert to the effects of hypothermia as the origin of a coagulopathy, particularly in the critical care environment. Reliance solely on the values of the PT, PTT, or TT is misleading, understanding that these assays are performed by both manual and automated laboratory methods at 37°C and results may thus fall within the reference range *in vitro*, despite ongoing coagulopathy clinically. External warming measures include blankets generating heated air, warming of all fluid infusions, heated humidifier in ventilated patients, and warming the environment. In extreme conditions, Gentilello et al. (47) reported that continuous arteriovenous rewarming, which does not require heparinization of the patient and hence does not exacerbate the coagulopathy, improves hemostasis more rapidly than any other method with the exception of cardiopulmonary bypass.

Normal physiologic processes (fibrinolytic system) exist to control for unremitting clot formation and are described in several reviews (1,31,32). Impaired function of the coagulation cascade may be the result of various disorders that are characterized by the genesis of circulating anticoagulants, abnormal protein products, or accumulation of proteinaceous breakdown products that affect the normal function of coagulation proteins. Collagen vascular diseases, such as systemic lupus erythematosus, is one example (48,49). In these patients an antibody is produced (lupus anticoagulant) that affects the coagulation cascade at the juncture of the intrinsic and extrinsic systems, resulting in prolongation of both the PT and PTT *in vitro*. Paradoxically, these patients tend to be hypercoagulable, and if clinically significant bleeding is noted, it is attributable to associated thrombocytopenia and increased vascular fragility. When there are elevated titers of either the lupus anticoagulant or anticardiolipin antibodies, or both, these patients may present with manifestation of the antiphospholipid antibody syndrome with generalized microvascular thrombosis, thrombocytopenia, gangrene of the extremities, multiorgan failure, and death. Plasmapheresis, anticoagulation, and immunosuppressive therapy serve as the foundation of treatment (48,49). Other commonly acquired inhibitors or circulating anticoagulants include factor VIII inhibitors and factor IX inhibitors, related primarily to prior frequency of transfusion with plasma-derived blood concentrates and alloimmunization (50–52). Exogenously administered heparin, the prototype for anticoagulation therapy, binds to circulating antithrombin III and catalyzes its ability to neutralize the action of a number of coagulation factors. The end result is interference with the normal coagulation cascade. Disorders characterized by the production of abnormal globulins, often referred to collectively as the paraproteinemias (associated with multiple myeloma and Waldenstrom macroglobulinemia), also result in interference with coagulation proteins and inhibition of fibrin polymerization. In these conditions the PT, PTT, and TT are prolonged. Fibrinogen/fibrin degradation products also inhibit fibrin polymerization, as does uremia, with prolongation of the PT, PTT, and TT. Treatment of the coagulopathy associated with all of these conditions consists of replacement of deficient coagulation factors when bleeding is dominant and definitive treatment directed at the underlying disease process.

Increased Destruction or Consumption

The most common cause of increased destruction of plasmatic coagulation factors has been variously termed DIC, defibrination syndrome, or consumptive coagulopathy (6–9). This syndrome is characterized by a hemorrhagic diathesis with unrestrained clotting and fibrinolysis in the vascular microcirculation, initiated by activation of the intrinsic or the extrinsic system, or both (6–9,37). Release of tissue thromboplastin, from injured tissue or from leukocytes, activates the extrinsic system, whereas damage to vascular endothelium (in addition to releasing tissue thromboplastin) results in activation of the intrinsic system via collagen exposure (8). Exposed collagen initiates platelet aggregation with release of platelet factor III and also activates factor XII directly. The net result is deposition of fibrin in the microvasculature. This results in a microangiopathic hemolytic anemia with fragmentation of red blood cells as they traverse these vascular beds. These fragmented red blood cells, or schistocytes, seen on the peripheral blood smear are a classic finding in this syndrome. Additionally, microthrombi cause stasis and ischemia in a number of capillary beds, manifesting as renal insufficiency or failure with kidney involvement, pulmonary insufficiency with lung involvement, mental status changes with brain involvement, or dermal necrosis with skin involvement. Stasis itself can result in further activation of clotting factors. Fibrin deposition and endothelial wall damage both bring about the release of plasminogen activator, which catalyzes the conversion of circulating plasminogen to plasmin. Plasmin proteolytically hydrolyzes both fibrinogen and fibrin (secondary fibrinolysis), resulting in fibrinogen and fibrin degradation (or "split") products. These degradation products then interfere with fibrin polymerization through the formation of complexes, further contributing to the hemorrhagic state. Additionally, these degradation products also interfere with platelet function, impairing both adhesion and aggregation. The number of disorders associated with DIC is substantial, but the unifying approach to management is supportive therapy with replacement of coagulation factors and platelets with attention focused on treating the underlying disease process. The end point is normalization of the PT, PTT, TT, and platelet count. Both acute and chronic forms have been identified. In the acute form patients are critically ill, whereas in the chronic form the natural history is more indolent and protracted, and thrombotic complications may be the predominant feature.

In the post-operative patient in the ICU, infection is the principle cause for DIC (9). Several causative organisms have been implicated, including Gram-negative bacteria, such as the Enterobacteriaceae as well as the nonlactose fermenters; Gram-positive bacteria; rickettsial organisms (Rocky Mountain spotted fever); mycotic infections, such as disseminated aspergillosis; parasitic agents, such as malaria; and viruses. The underlying pathophysiology has been best elucidated with Gram-negative infections, with endotoxin (cell wall lipopolysaccharide) triggering the intrinsic system by activation of factor XII directly and by factor XII exposure to subendothelial collagen, as a result of endotoxin-mediated damage to vascular endothelium. Endotoxin may also trigger the coagulation cascade by inducing expression of procoagulant activity in circulating leukocytes, hepatic macrophages, and endothelial cells, and by activating the extrinsic system mediated by the release of tissue thromboplastin from damaged leukocytes and vascular endothelium (53–55).

Traumatic injuries (particularly involving brain, bone, or liver), thermal injuries, and severe crush injuries, as well as surgical procedures may produce a consumptive coagulopathy (6–9,56–58). Secondary infection and hemorrhagic shock further serve to aggravate the coagulopathy, especially if acidosis, hypothermia, or tissue ischemia and necrosis develops.

Acute pancreatitis, arising from various causes, may be associated with DIC due to release of enzymes that may directly activate a number of coagulation factors (59). In many instances, there is associated multiorgan dysfunction involving cardiopulmonary, renal, and hepatic function. In addition, pyogenic sequelae, such as the development of infected pancreatic necrosis or abscess formation, may result in DIC attributable to sepsis. Treatment is primarily supportive, with aggressive resuscitation, replacement of deficient coagulation factors if there is associated bleeding, appropriate use of broad-spectrum antibiotics, and surgical debridement and drainage for control of infectious complications.

Obstetric complications can result in some of the most profound and challenging instances of DIC. Well-recognized examples include amniotic fluid embolism, abruptio placentae, retained dead fetus, and eclampsia (6–8). In these circumstances, the culprit is massive systemic release of tissue thromboplastin that generates a fulminant course characterized by bilateral renal cortical necrosis to frank cardiopulmonary collapse, shock, multiorgan failure, and, at times, death even if aggressive attempts are made to treat these individuals.

The laboratory diagnosis of DIC is readily established with routinely available tests. The PT, PTT, and TT are all prolonged, and the platelet count is decreased. Depending on the severity of the disease process, fibrinogen may not be detectable. Fibrinogen/fibrin degradation products are elevated, and the peripheral blood smear often reveals the presence of schistocytes. Factors I (fibrinogen), V, VIII, and XIII tend to be markedly depressed. In milder forms, fibrinogen levels may not be significantly decreased, particularly in the presence of adequate hepatic function. Radioimmunoassays of fibrinopeptide A, a by-product of the action of thrombin on fibrinogen, may be useful in these situations to establish the correct diagnosis and management approach (60). Although rare, primary fibrinolysis differs from DIC (where secondary fibrinolysis occurs) in the following ways. In primary fibrinolysis, (a) platelet count is normal, (b) soluble fibrin monomers are not present (measured by the plasma paracoagulation test), (c) schistocytes (red cell fragments) are not seen, and (d) tests for increased levels of plasmin activity are strongly positive (euglobulin clot lysis time, whole blood clot lysis time).

Optimum management of DIC requires aggressive treatment of the underlying disease process and supportive therapy with coagulation factor and platelet replacement. FFP and platelet concentrates are the two most common blood products used as a temporizing measure (10–12,14). Stored or banked whole blood is a reasonable source of most clotting factors if the units are less than 24 hours old (10,14,61). The biologic half-life of factors V, VII, VIII, and IX are on the order of 24 hours or less; hence whole blood stored for longer than 24 hours may not provide adequate amounts of these coagulation factors. Heparin had been used in the past in a theoretical attempt to abrogate the clotting cascade, but its contemporaneous use for this purpose is at best controversial, may be contraindicated in the perioperative period, and is not supported by evidence-based data (6–8,62). In septic patients with or without DIC, treatment with recombinant activated protein C reduces mortality, and this may be attributable in part to its profibrinolytic, anti-inflammatory, and anticoagulant effects (6,63).

COMPLEX POST-OPERATIVE BLEEDING PROBLEMS

Hepatobiliary Disease

Hepatic parenchymal and biliary obstructive disease results in diverse manifestations of hemostatic abnormalities (18). Extrahepatic biliary obstruction results in diminished absorption of vitamin K due to lack of bile salts necessary for gastrointestinal absorption of lipid soluble vitamins. Decreased synthesis of the vitamin K–dependent factors II, VII, IX, and X occurs with abnormal prolongation of the PT and eventually the PTT.

Parenchymal diseases such as cirrhosis, chronic active hepatitis, fulminant hepatic failure, or metastatic carcinoma impact on the hemostatic system in a heterogeneous manner. Most coagulation factors, naturally occurring anticoagulants (such as antithrombin III), fibrinolysin precursors (plasminogen), and inhibitors of the fibrinolytic system (antiplasmins) are synthesized by the liver. In severe liver disease, acquired dysfibrinogenemia has also been reported (18,28). This impairs polymerization of soluble fibrin monomers and is suggested by a prolonged TT on purified fibrinogen, which is generally done in a research laboratory. The liver also removes activated coagulation factors from the circulation, but it is speculative to conclude that this results in a coagulopathy by itself, despite the fact that this increased consumption of activated factors by the liver lowers coagulation factors already depressed by decreased production in a diseased liver. Clearance of fibrinogen/fibrin degradation products is reduced in chronic liver disease. These breakdown products inhibit both fibrin polymerization and platelet function and thus contribute to a defective hemostatic system, as discussed earlier. Thrombocytopenia occurs secondary to hypersplenism, potentially exacerbated by vitamin deficiencies associated with decreased thrombopoiesis. Additionally, alcohol has a direct toxic effect on megakaryocytes, which contributes to prevailing vitamin deficiencies and decreased bone marrow production of platelets. Treatment of bleeding in liver failure with vitamin K usually is not successful given the lack of hepatic synthetic function. Whole blood both corrects the red blood cell deficit and is as effective as fresh frozen plasma in correcting coagulation factor deficits if the units of blood have not been banked for an extended period of time (14,61). Platelet transfusions should be judiciously used to raise the platelet count to above 100×10^9/L if bleeding is encountered in this setting, and FFP should be provided to correct deficits in plasmatic coagulation factors (10,11,12,14).

Transfusion-Induced Bleeding

Major trauma, major orthopedic (spine, hip, or pelvis) or hepatic procedures (major hepatic resections, liver transplantation), or other causes of potentially life-threatening, exsanguinating hemorrhage is often associated with the need for what has been termed massive blood transfusion (21,22,61). This term has been variously defined but generally refers to administering the equivalent of one total blood volume or more to a patient in less than a 24-hour period. Due to consumption of coagulation factors and platelets, release of inflammatory mediators, dilution of elements necessary for the optimal function of the coagulation cascade, hypocalcemia, hypothermia, fibrinolysis, and alterations in acid-base homeostasis, a coagulopathy often develops in this scenario (21,22,61,64). Banked blood is a negligible source of viable platelets, which rapidly deteriorate under conditions of cold storage (10,12,14). Additionally, depending on the age of the unit, plasmatic coagulation factors may also be diminished in activity. The derangement in clotting represents nonlocalized, nonsurgical bleeding that is characterized by sanguinous oozing from all raw surfaces, including any wounds, mucosal or peritoneal surfaces, and percutaneous entry sites. Numerous risk factors for the development of this condition (particularly in the setting of trauma) include high injury severity score, acidosis, hypothermia, and hypotension (2,4,20,21). Prophylactic administration of platelets during massive blood transfusion in an attempt to prevent the development of a coagulopathy has been advocated by many centers, but the efficacy of this policy is unproven. Studies have failed to demonstrate conclusively a benefit to this approach (10,12,14,22,61,65–67). It is reasonable, however, to administer platelets to a bleeding patient or one with DIC if the platelet count is less than 50×10^9/L. For those patients with rapid bleeding or with multiple traumatic injuries undergoing surgery or other high-risk procedures, a goal of at least 100×10^9/L has been recommended, albeit in the absence of high-level evidence-based data. One unit of platelet concentrate typically raises the platelet count by 5×10^9/L, whereas one apheresis concentrate raises the platelet count by 20 to 25×10^9/L in an average 70-kg adult. Despite plasmatic coagulation factor activity deteriorating with storage, dilution of these factors below levels required for adequate hemostasis is rare. Therefore, routine administration of FFP after an arbitrary number of units of banked blood has been transfused is not supported by stringent investigations (2,4,10,11,14,67–71). If there is bleeding due to a coagulopathy with concomitant prolongation of the PT and PTT of more than 1.5 times normal, FFP should be infused (to normalize the PTT and achieve a PT international normalized ratio [INR] <1.5). There is emphasis on early correction since timid replacement of coagulation products will lead to more bleeding and being more coagulopathic, leading to a vicious cycle. Cryoprecipitate should be considered if the fibrinogen level is less than 0.8 g/dL. Recombinant activated factor VIIa has demonstrated promise in significantly reducing bleeding and blood transfusion requirements in patients with traumatic injuries, or surgical procedures attended by significant hemorrhage, in addition to liver transplantation (72–78).

Complications directly attributable to blood transfusions have been described earlier. However, in the setting of massive blood transfusion, numerous points are warranted. Hemolytic transfusion reactions may occur as a result of ABO incompatibility between the actual units of blood transfused, or potentially because of clerical error, magnified by the volume of units required in a relatively short period of time. Red blood cells are a rich source of tissue thromboplastin, and hemolysis results in a massive release of this extrinsic system activator. This manifests as a generalized oozing from all raw surfaces, similar to the coagulopathy seen with massive blood transfusions, rendering this a difficult diagnosis to make. Hemoglobinuria may be observed due to filtration of plasmafree hemoglobin into the urine. Consistent with other types of transfusion reactions, the coagulation abnormality corrects rapidly once the offending transfusion is terminated. Treatment must be directed toward prevention of hemoglobin casts precipitating in the acidic environment of the collecting tubules, resulting in acute tubular necrosis and acute renal failure. Appropriate fluid resuscitation to maintain intravascular volume and to initiate a diuresis is paramount. Mannitol, an osmotic diuretic and free radical scavenger, is administered intravenously as an adjunct to maintain urine flow, and intravenous sodium bicarbonate may be considered to alkalinize the urine to avoid further precipitation of hemoglobin in the renal tubules.

Cardiopulmonary Bypass

Post-operative bleeding is a frequent impediment of cardiopulmonary bypass. Numerous mechanisms are apparently involved, which include contact factor (factors XII and XI) activation, elevations of tissue plasminogen activator level and tissue thromboplastin, dilution of plasmatic coagulation factors, residual effects of systemic heparinization, hypothermia, platelet function defects, and failure of surgical hemostasis (23–26). Some investigations have demonstrated a 30% to 50% decrement in platelet count attributable to the shearing forces that are encountered in the bypass apparatus. The routine use of antiplatelet agents in patients with cardiac disease, such as aspirin and thienopyridine derivatives (clopidogrel or ticlopidine), also contributes to the increased risk for bleeding. The combined effects of aspirin and a thienopyridine derivative, such as clopidogrel, on bleeding complications is synergistic and not additive. In approximately 4% to 5% of patients, surgical re-exploration of the mediastinum is necessary, which varies based on the original procedure performed (23,25,79). Several criteria for re-exploration have been proposed that have in common the rate of blood loss from mediastinal or chest tubes. Criteria variably used include blood loss from chest or mediastinal tubes of 300 mL/hour within the first 3 hours; total blood loss of 1,000 mL after 4 hours; a sudden increase in bleeding (>300 mL/hour) in a patient who previously had minimal drainage; or evidence of cardiac tamponade. A coagulopathy must never be presumed to be the cause of bleeding postoperatively unless surgical causes of bleeding have first been excluded. A site of localized bleeding (surgical failure) is identified in more than 50% of patients re-explored based on these types of criteria (23,25,80).

Despite multiple contributing factors to the bleeding that occurs in these patients, the prime offender is collectively believed to be secondary to qualitative platelet function defects (1,23–26,79,80). The bypass circuitry results in platelet activation with degranulation and aggregation. Although this functional deficit is transient, increased time on bypass, hypothermia, and antiplatelet medications significantly exacerbates this condition. Laboratory analysis reveals a prolongation of the bleeding time with impaired adhesion and aggregation, particularly in the presence of adenosine diphosphate (ADP) and ristocetin. This latter finding is believed to be linked to low levels of vWF found in plasma after cardiopulmonary bypass. Hence, some investigators have proposed use of desmopressin in this circumstance (and in patients with a history of preoperative use of aspirin), to increase levels of vWF by stimulating release from endothelial cells, increasing the glycoprotein receptors on platelets, and increasing the level of factor VIII and tissue plasminogen activator. However, others believe that this practice increases the risk of graft thrombosis and coronary occlusion (2,79,80). Additionally, peer-reviewed, reported outcome data in this circumstance are indeterminate (2). Usually the acquired qualitative platelet function defect resolves within 4 hours of completion of cardiopulmonary bypass without any intervention. In instances where there is prolonged nonsurgical postoperative bleeding, platelet transfusions are often beneficial (10,14,80).

Many pharmacologic agents have proven efficacy in the management of nonsurgical bleeding, particularly in the post–cardiopulmonary bypass setting. Desmopressin has already been described. Antifibrinolytic agents constitute a heterogenous group of drugs with proven efficacy in cardiac surgery patients. Aprotinin, a bovine serine protease inhibitor, inhibits plasmin and has been shown to reduce the need for red blood cell transfusions in several randomized trials and reduces the need for reoperation for nonsurgical bleeding (1,2,4,26,80–82). There are several adverse side effects that limit its usefulness. Thromboembolic phenomena, renal insufficiency, and allergic reactions (probably due to its bovine origin) have all been reported. The occurrence of serious anaphylactic reactions has been the impetus for use of a test dose prior to full implementation of the agent (2,80). Aprotinin has been removed from FDA approval until further studies are done confirming safety. Epsilon aminocaproic acid (EACA) and tranexamic acid are lysine analogues that inhibit binding of plasmin to fibrin. EACA appears to have the weakest antifibrinolytic effect compared to tranexamic acid and aprotinin, but nevertheless has been used in the cardiopulmonary bypass patient with some success. Tranexamic acid has met with considerable success in the reduction of postoperative blood loss and the reduced need for red blood cell transfusion in cardiac surgery, total knee arthroplasty, transurethral prostate surgery, and in oral surgery procedures. Neither EACA nor tranexamic acid are associated with thrombotic complications or anaphylactic reactions. The most commonly reported adverse reactions include nausea, diarrhea, and orthostatic reactions (83). Considering efficacy, side effect profile, and lower cost, tranexamic acid has several advantages over aprotinin (26,80–83).

Monitoring for increased risks of hemorrhage commences during surgery (84–86). The activated clotting time, which measures the effect of heparin on fibrin clot formation, has been traditionally used for intraoperative management of anticoagulation therapy. Thromboelastography, an assay popularized in Europe, can be used to determine if there is a platelet function abnormality, a deficit in plasmatic coagulation factors, the presence of circulating anticoagulants, or fibrinolysins in patients undergoing cardiopulmonary bypass (4,16,85,86). This technique evaluates clot formation and continually evaluates clot firmness in an integrated manner and is amenable to point-of-care testing, hence its usefulness both intraoperatively and postoperatively. No specific specimen processing is required, and whole blood is used for testing. This technology is rapidly gaining attention as a valuable adjunct to managing complex coagulation disorders. It has been efficacious in decreasing blood transfusion requirements during cardiac surgery and in liver transplantation (87,88). The effect of hypothermia on a patient's coagulation profile can also be determined simply by adjusting the temperature of the apparatus to correspond with the patient's core body temperature. Several automated analyzers are available commercially.

SUMMARY

Postoperative bleeding requires immediate recognition of early shock, resuscitation, and differentiation between surgical and nonsurgical bleed. Knowledge of coagulation and appropriate replacement of blood and blood products is essential. Careful evaluation of the patient to identify primary or secondary coagulation disorders is necessary.

References

1. Adams GL, Manson RJ, Turner I, et al. The balance of thrombosis and hemorrhage in surgery. *Hematol Oncol Clin N Am.* 2007;21:13.

2. Rossaint R, Cerny V, Coats TJ, et al. Key issues in advanced bleeding care in trauma. *Shock*. 2006;26:322.
3. Staudinger T, Locker GJ, Frass M. Management of acquired coagulation disorders in emergency and intensive care medicine. *Semin Thromb Hemost*. 1996;22:93.
4. Fries D, Innerhofer P, Schobersberger W. Coagulation management in trauma patients. *Curr Opin Anaesthesiol*. 2002;15:217.
5. Rohrer M, Natale A. Effect of hypothermia on the coagulation cascade. *Crit Care Med*. 1992;20:1402.
6. Dempfle C. Disseminated intravascular coagulation and coagulation disorders. *Curr Opin Anaesthesiol*. 2004;17:125.
7. Levi M, Ten Cate H. Disseminated intravascular coagulation. *N Eng J Med*. 1999;341:586.
8. Bick RL. Disseminated intravascular coagulation: current concepts of etiology, pathophysiology, diagnosis, and treatment. *Hematol Oncol Clin North Am*. 2003;17:149.
9. Zeerleder S, Hack CE, Wuillemin WA. Disseminated intravascular coagulation in sepsis. *Chest*. 2005;128:2864.
10. Practice Guidelines Development Task Force of the College of American Pathologists. Practice parameters for the use of fresh frozen plasma, cryoprecipitate, and platelets. *JAMA*. 1994;271:777.
11. British Committee for Standards in Haematology. Guidelines for the use of fresh frozen plasma. *Transfusion Med*. 1992;2:57.
12. British Committee for Standards in Haematology Blood Transfusion Task Force. Guidelines for the use of platelet transfusions. *Br J Haematol*. 2003;122:10.
13. Shortt J, Dunkley S, Rickard K, et al. Efficacy and safety of a high purity, double virus inactivated factor VIII/von Willebrand factor concentrate (Biostate) in patients with von Willebrand disorder requiring invasive or surgical procedures. *Hemophilia*. 2007;13:144.
14. American Society of Anesthesiologists Task Force on Blood Component Therapy: practice guidelines for blood component therapy. *Anesthesiology*. 1996;84:732.
15. Kearon C, Hirsh J. Management of anticoagulation before and after elective surgery. *N Engl J Med*. 1997;336:1506.
16. Shore-Lesserson L. Platelet inhibitors and monitoring platelet function: implications for bleeding. *Hematol Oncol Clin North Am*. 2007;21:51.
17. George JN, Woolf SH, Raskob GE, et al. Diagnosis and treatment of idiopathic thrombocytopenic purpura: recommendations of the American Society of Hematology. *Ann Intern Med*. 1997;126:319.
18. Senzolo M, Burra P, Cholongitas E, et al. New insights into the coagulopathy of liver disease and liver transplantation. *World J Gastroenterol*. 2006;12:7725.
19. Ansell J, Hirsh J, Poller L, et al. The pharmacology and management of the vitamin K antagonists: the seventh ACCP conference on antithrombotic and thrombolitic therapy. *Chest*. 2004;126:204.
20. MacLeod JB, Lynn M, McKenney MG, et al. Early coagulopathy predicts mortality in trauma. *J Trauma*. 2003;55:39.
21. Cosgrif N, Moore EE, Sauaia A, et al. Predicting life-threatening coagulopathy in the massively transfused trauma patient: hypothermia and acidosis revisited. *J Trauma*. 1997;42:857.
22. Levy JH. Massive transfusion coagulopathy. *Semin Hematol*. 2006;43:S59.
23. Despotis GJ, Filos KS, Zoys TN, et al. Factors associated with excessive postoperative blood loss and hemostatic transfusion requirements: a multivariate analysis in cardiac surgical patients. *Anesth Analg*. 1996;82:13.
24. Khuri SF, Wolfe JA, Josa M, et al. Hematologic changes during and after cardiopulmonary bypass and their relationship to the bleeding time and nonsurgical blood loss. *J Thorac Cardiovasc Surg*. 1992;104:94.
25. Dacey LJ, Munoz JJ, Baribeau YR, et al. Reexploration for hemorrhage following coronary artery bypass grafting: incidence and risk factors. *Arch Surg*. 1998;133:442.
26. Levi M, Cromheecke ME, de Jonge E, et al. Pharmacological strategies to decrease excessive blood loss in cardiac surgery: a meta-analysis of clinically relevant endpoints. *Lancet*. 1999;354:1940.
27. Dentali F, Ageno W, Crowther M. Treatment of coumarin-associated coagulopathy: a systematic review and proposed treatment algorithms. *J Thromb Haemost*. 2006;4:1853.
28. Martinez J, MacDonald KA, Palascak JE: The role of sialic acid in the dysfibrinogenemia associated with liver disease: distribution of sialic acid on the constituent chains. *Blood*. 1983;61:1196.
29. MacGillivray TE. Fibrin sealants and glues. *J Card Surg*. 2003;18:480.
30. Kunkel JM, Gomez ER, Spebar MJ, et al. Wound hematomas after carotid endarterectomy. *Am J Surg*. 1984;148:844.
31. Kwaan HC, Nabhan C. Hereditary and acquired defects in the fibrinolytic system associated with thrombosis. *Hematol Oncol Clin N Am*. 2003;17:103.
32. Wolberg AS. Thrombin generation and fibrin clot structure. *Blood Rev*. 2007;21:131.
33. Murphy S. Disorders of platelet production. In: Colman RW, Hirsch J, Marder VJ, et al., eds. *Hemostasis and Thrombosis*. Philadelphia, PA: JB Lippincott Co, 1982:259.
34. Jacobson MA, Young LS. New developments in the treatment of gram-negative bacteremia. *West J Med*. 1986;144:185.
35. George JN. Evaluation and management of patients with thrombotic thrombocytopenic purpura. *J Intensive Care Med*. 2007;22:82.
36. Franchini M. Thrombotic microangiopathies: an update. *Hematology*. 2006;11:139.
37. Harlan JM. Thrombocytopenia due to non-immune platelet destruction. *Clin Haematol*. 1983;12:39.
38. McCrae KR, Herman JH. Posttransfusion purpura: two unusual cases and a literature review. *Am J Hematol*. 1996;52:205.
39. Koene HR. Critical issues of current and future developments in the treatment of immune thrombocytopenic purpura. *Pediatr Blood Cancer*. 2006;47(5 Suppl):705.
40. Bussel J. Treatment of immune thrombocytopenic purpura in adults *Semin Hematol* 2006;43(3 Suppl 5):S3.
41. Warkentin T, Greinacher A. Heparin-induced thrombocytopenia: recognition, treatment, and prevention. The seventh ACCP conference on antithrombotic and thrombolytic therapy. *Chest*. 2004;126:311.
42. Mielke CH Jr. Influence of aspirin on platelets and the bleeding time. *Am J Med*. 1985;74:72.
43. Valeri CR, Feingold H, Cassidy G, et al; Hypothermia-induced reversible platelet dysfunction. *Ann Surg*. 1987;205:175.
44. Escolar G, Diaz-Ricart M, Cases A. Uremic platelet dysfunction: past and present. *Curr Hematol Rep*. 2005;4:359.
45. Boccardo P, Remuzzi G, Galbusera M. Platelet dysfunction in renal failure. *Semin Thromb Hemost*. 2004;30:579.
46. Kaw D, Malhotra D. Platelet dysfunction and end-stage renal disease. *Semin Dial*. 2006;19:317.
47. Gentilello LM, Cortes V, Moujaes S, et al. Continuous arteriovenous rewarming: experimental results and thermodynamic model simulation of treatment for hypothermia. *J Trauma*. 1990;30:1436.
48. Galli M, Barbui T. Antiphospholipid syndrome: clinical and diagnostic utility of laboratory tests. *Semin Thromb Hemost*. 2005;31:17.
49. Galli M, Luciani D, Bertolini G, et al. Lupus anticoagulants are stronger risk factors for thrombosis than anticardiolipin antibodies in the antiphospholipid syndrome: a systematic review of the literature. *Blood*. 2003;101: 1827.
50. Sultan Y. Acquired hemophilia and its treatment. *Blood Coagul Fibrinolysis*. 1997;8(Suppl 1):S15.
51. Franchini M. Acquired hemophilia A. *Hematology*. 2006;11:119.
52. Lusher JM. Inhibitor antibodies to factor VIII and factor IX: management. *Semin Thromb Hemost*. 2000;26:179.
53. Thiagarajan P, Niemetz J. Procoagulant-tissue factor activity of circulating peripheral blood leukocytes: results of *in vivo* studies. *Thromb Res*. 1980;17:891.
54. Maier RV, Ulevitch RJ. The induction of a unique procoagulant activity in rabbit hepatic macrophages by bacterial lipopolysaccharides. *J Immunol*. 1981;127:1596.
55. Schorer AE, Rick PD, Swaim WR, et al. Structural features of endotoxin required for stimulation of endothelial cell tissue factor production: exposure of preformed tissue factor after oxidant-mediated endothelial cell injury. *J Lab Clin Med*. 1985;106:38.
56. Bennett B, Towler HM. Haemostatic response to trauma. *Br Med Bull*. 1985;41:274.
57. Kaufman HH, Hui KS, Mattson JC, et al. Clinicopathological correlations of disseminated intravascular coagulation in patients with head injury. *Neurosurgery*. 1984;15:34.
58. Risberg B, Medegard A, Heideman M, et al. Early activation of humoral proteolytic systems in patients with multiple trauma. *Crit Care Med*. 1986;14:917.
59. Lasson A, Ohlsson K. Consumptive coagulopathy, fibrinolysis and protease-antiprotease interactions during acute human pancreatitis. *Thromb Res*. 1986;41:167.
60. Leeksma OC, Meijer-Huizinga F, Stoepman-van Dalen EA, et al. Fibrinopeptide A and the phosphate content of fibrinogen in venous thromboembolism and disseminated intravascular coagulation. *Blood*. 1986;67: 1460.
61. Counts RB, Haisch C, Simon TL, et al. Hemostasis in massively transfused trauma patients. *Ann Surg*. 1979;190:91.
62. Feinstein DI: Diagnosis and management of disseminated intravascular coagulation: the role of heparin therapy. *Blood*. 1982;60:284.
63. Bernard GR, Vincent JL, Laterre PF, et al. Efficacy and safety of recombinant human activated protein c for severe sepsis. *N Engl J Med*. 2001;344: 699.
64. Spahn DR. Hypocalcemia in trauma: frequent but frequently undetected and underestimated. *Crit Care Med*. 2005;33:2124.
65. Reed RLD, Ciavarella D, Heimbach DM, et al. Prophylactic platelet administration during massive transfusion: a prospective, randomized, double-blind clinical study. *Ann Surg*. 1986;203:40.
66. Segal JB, Dzik WH. Paucity of studies to support that abnormal coagulation test results predict bleeding in the setting of invasive procedures: an evidence-based review. *Transfusion*. 2005;45:1413.
67. Gajic O, Dzik WH, Toy P. Fresh frozen plasma and platelet transfusion for nonbleeding patients in the intensive care unit: benefit or harm? *Crit Care Med*. 2006;34(5 Suppl):S170.
68. Holland L, Sarode R. Should plasma be transfused prophylactically before invasive procedures? *Curr Opin Hematol*. 2006;13:447.
69. Dara SI, Rana R, Afessa B, et al. Fresh frozen plasma transfusion in critically ill medical patients with coagulopathy. *Crit Care Med*. 2005;33:2667.

70. Gonzalez EA, Moore FA, Holcomb JB, et al. Fresh frozen plasma should be given earlier to patients requiring massive transfusion. *J Trauma.* 2007; 62:112.
71. Abdel-Wahab OI, Healy B, Dzik WH. Effect of fresh-frozen plasma transfusion on prothrombin time and bleeding in patients with mild coagulation abnormalities. *Transfusion.* 2006;46:1279.
72. Dutton RP, McCunn M, Hyder M, et al. Factor VIIa for correction of traumatic coagulopathy. *J Trauma.* 2004;57:709.
73. Gala B, Quintela J, Aguirrezabalaga J, et al. Benefits of recombinant activated factor VII in complicated liver transplantation. *Transplantation Proc.* 2005;37:3919.
74. Rossaint R, Boffard K, Warren B, et al. Decreased transfusion utilization using recombinant factor VIIa as an adjunct in trauma. *Intensive Care Med.* 2004;30(Suppl):S199.
75. Boffard KD, Riou B, Warren B, et al. Recombinant factor VIIa as adjunctive therapy for bleeding control in severely injured trauma patients: two parallel randomized, placebo-controlled, double-blind clinical trials. *J Trauma.* 2005;59:8.
76. Rizoli SB, Boffard KD, Riou B, et al. Recombinant activated factor VII as an adjunctive therapy for bleeding control in severe trauma patients with coagulopathy: subgroup analysis from two randomized trials. *Crit Care.* 2006;10:R178.
77. Filsoufi F, Castillo JG, Rahmanian PB, et al. Effective management of refractory postcardiotomy bleeding with the use of recombinant activated factor VII. *Ann Thor Surg.* 2006;82:1779.
78. Levi M, Peters M, Buller HR. Efficacy and safety of recombinant factor VIIa for treatment of severe bleeding: a systematic review. *Crit Care Med.* 2005;33:883.
79. Woodman RC, LA Harker: Bleeding complications associated with cardiopulmonary bypass. *Blood.* 1990;76:1680.
80. Royston D. Blood-sparing drugs: aprotinin, tranexamic acid, and epsilon-aminocaproic acid. *Int Anesthesiol Clin.* 1995;33:155.
81. Levy JH. Anti-inflammatory strategies and hemostatic agents: old drugs, new ideas. *Hematol Oncol Clin N Am.* 2007;21:89.
82. Harker LA. Bleeding after cardiopulmonary bypass [editorial]. *N Engl J Med.* 1986;314:1446.
83. Dunn CJ, Goa KL. Tranexamic acid: a review of its use in surgery and other indications. *Drugs.* 1999;57:1005.
84. Spiess BD, Davalle M. Coagulation monitoring in the surgical intensive care unit. *Crit Care Clin.* 1988;4:605.
85. Despotis GJ, Santoro SA, Spitznagel E, et al. Prospective evaluation and clinical utility of on-site monitoring of coagulation in patients undergoing cardiac operations. *J Thorac Cardiovasc Surg.* 1994;107:271.
86. Bracey AW, Grigore AM, Nussmeier NA. Impact of platelet testing on presurgical screening and implications for cardiac and noncardiac surgical procedures. *Am J Card.* 2006;98(Suppl 1):S25.
87. Shore-Lesserson L, Manspeitzer HE, Deprio M, et al. Thrombelastography-guided transfusion algorithm reduces transfusion in complex cardiac surgery. *Anesth Analg.* 1999;88:312.
88. Kang YG, Martin DJ, Marquez J. Intraoperative changes in blood coagulation and thromboelastographic monitoring in liver transplantation. *Anesth Analg.* 1995;64:888.

CHAPTER 75 ■ ABDOMINAL TRAUMA: NONOPERATIVE MANAGEMENT AND POSTOPERATIVE CONSIDERATIONS

C. CLAY COTHREN • ERNEST E. MOORE

Multiply injured patients admitted to the intensive care unit (ICU) have an array of physiologic derangements that may include metabolic failure and cardiopulmonary embarrassment. In addition to the seeming routine care of the critically ill patient, the intensivist should be able to recognize the inherent differences in care of the postinjury patient. The intensivist should be familiar with the implications of specific injuries including guidelines for nonoperative management, postoperative care, and expected postinjury complications and their sequelae. This chapter will focus on specific issues encountered in the acute resuscitation and overall ICU management of the trauma patient, rather than the initial evaluation of the patient in the emergency department (ED). Initial therapy in the trauma bay, precise indications for operation, and intraoperative decision making for particular injury patterns is beyond the scope of this chapter.

INITIAL EVALUATION IN THE INTENSIVE CARE UNIT

Although some patients may arrive in the ICU *in extremis* necessitating continued resuscitation without a thorough history and physical examination, the majority should undergo a complete assessment promptly, and it should not be assumed that the ED evaluation was comprehensive and accurate. Such an evaluation, often termed the tertiary survey, is a repeated history and physical examination performed in light of imaging studies and pertinent intraoperative findings (1,2). Additionally, the evaluation is more detailed than that performed in the ED, because all the diagnostic results should be available, further information is obtained from family members, and the physician has time for a more meticulous physical examination. Key elements include the patient's past medical history, specifically issues such as cardiopulmonary disease; hypertension including past myocardial infarction; use of β-blockers, steroids, angiotensin-converting enzyme (ACE) inhibitors, and bronchodilators; and other elements that may acutely impact the patient's ongoing care. Discovering minor injuries on the tertiary survey such as subtle extremity injuries overlooked on the initial ED evaluation is common (3–5). Documentation of this evaluation, particularly of final imaging results, can be done through a standardized form and facilitates communication among care providers (Fig. 75.1).

The reliability of clinical examination in these patients after ICU admission is often questioned. The clinical exam is

Name, MR#, Pat#, DOB

DENVER HEALTH MEDICAL CENTER

TERTIARY SURVEY OF THE CRITICALLY ILL PATIENT

Attending: ____________ **SICU Resident:** ____________

Date: ____ / ____ / ____ Time: ____
MM DD YY

Injuries Identified:

1. ____
2. ____
3. ____
4. ____
5. ____

Operations:

1. ____
2. ____
3. ____
4. ____
5. ____

New Information re: PMHx/Comorbidities: ____

Physical Exam

Mental Status: GCS ____ Best exam: ____

HEENT

Scalp: ☐ WNL, or describe: ____

Eyes: ☐ WNL, or describe: ____

Ears: ☐ WNL, or describe: ____

Nose: ☐ WNL, or describe: ____

Mouth/Throat: ☐ WNL, or describe: ____

Facial (step offs, swelling, etc.): ☐ WNL, or describe: ____

Neck: ☐ WNL, or describe: ____

Chest: ☐ WNL, or describe: ____

Abdomen: ☐ WNL, or describe: ____

Back: ☐ WNL, or describe: ____

Pelvis: ☐ WNL, or describe: ____

Extremities:

RUE: ☐ WNL, or describe: ____

LUE: ☐ WNL, or describe: ____

RLE: ☐ WNL, or describe: ____

LLE: ☐ WNL, or describe: ____

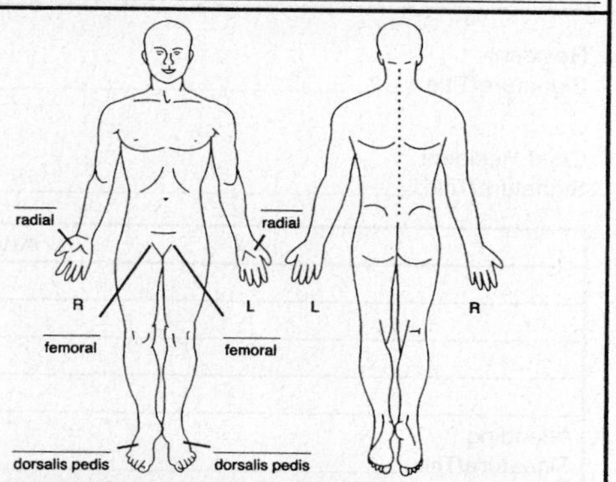

radial radial
R L L R
femoral femoral
dorsalis pedis dorsalis pedis

TRAUMA SITES

1. LACERATION / SW
2. PUNCTURE / GSW
3. FRACTURE
4. ABRASION
5. BURN
6. DEFORMITY
7. AVULSION
8. CONTUSION
9. CREPITUS
10. ECCHYMOSIS
11. HEMATOMA
12. OPEN FX
13. PAIN

A F50-091 (2/05) Pg 1 of 2

FIGURE 75.1. A thorough history and physical examination in the intensive care unit including imaging, termed the tertiary survey, can be documented on a standardized form to facilitate communication among care providers. (*Continued*)

Trauma Studies (Big 3 - Plus)		
	Date Completed	Findings
FAST		
Head CT		
Chest CT		
Abdominal CT		
Aortogram		

Diagnostic Studies				
	Ordered	Date Done	WNL	Abnormal - Findings
Repeat Head CT				
4-vessel Angio				
Extremity 1				
Extremity 2				

Status of Spine		
	Radiographically Cleared	Clinically Cleared
Cervical	Name: Date/Time:	Name: Date/Time:
TLS	Name: Date/Time:	Name: Date/Time:

Consultants Involved:
☐ Neurosurgery ☐ Orthopedics ☐ Plastics ☐ GU ☐ Other: ____

Change/New symptoms since ED evaluation: None or describe: ____

Drains (include site): ____

Lines (include site): ____
(Change ED Lines within 24 hours)

Diagnosis	Plan
1.	
2.	
3.	
4.	
5.	
6.	

Resident Signature/Title: ____ ID #: ____ Date: ____ / ____ / ____ Time: ____
MM DD YY

Chief Resident Signature/Title: ____ ID #: ____ Date: ____ / ____ / ____ Time: ____
MM DD YY

Attendings Only Below This Line
Attending Signature/Title: ____ ID #: ____ Date: ____ / ____ / ____ Time: ____ (MM DD YY)

B F50-091 (2/05) Pg 2 of 2

FIGURE 75.1. (*Continued*)

TABLE 75.1

INDICATIONS FOR SURGEON EVALUATION IN THE INTENSIVE CARE UNIT FOR POSSIBLE EXPLORATORY LAPAROTOMY

- Persistent drop in hemoglobin
- Hypotension and associated abdominal distension or free fluid on bedside ultrasound
- Overt peritonitis on physical examination
- Computed tomography (CT) scan with evidence of free air or gastrointestinal contrast extravasation
- CT scan with free fluid without associated solid organ injury
- Intra-abdominal hypertension

important, even in injured patients who are intoxicated or who have sustained a head injury; in addition to external evidence of trauma, the patient's reported pain or discomfort, particularly whether this is increasing or decreasing in nature with time, is paramount. Only in the intubated patient is the clinical examination more limited from a patient response standpoint; specific signs of injury such as ecchymosis, distention, and crepitus are still critical to recognize. Similar to the physician evaluation in the ED, there are clear indications in the ICU for surgeon evaluation for possible laparotomy (Table 75.1).

Some patients will require imaging upon arrival to ICU; patients with intracranial or thoracic injury may go emergently to the operating room prior to computed tomography (CT) scanning of the abdomen. These patients, once hemodynamically stable in the ICU, should undergo CT scanning to delineate any associated intra-abdominal injuries. Even in patients who undergo exploratory laparotomy, CT of the abdomen may be necessary to diagnose spine fractures and to evaluate the retroperitoneum. Routine postadmission studies include repeat chest film and laboratory studies. A chest film is important to determine central line catheter, tube thoracostomy, and endotracheal tube positions, as any of these could become dislodged with transport. The chest radiograph may also show interval change in a patient's hemothorax, pneumothorax, or pulmonary contusion. Based upon physical exam findings in the tertiary survey, further imaging of extremities may also be required.

Once the patient has been fully evaluated by the treating ICU physicians and associated imaging and laboratory results obtained, the therapeutic plan is initiated to optimize the patient's cardiopulmonary and metabolic status. In addition to the patient's ongoing cardiopulmonary resuscitation, there is concurrent treatment of known injuries, ongoing evaluation for missed injuries, and monitoring for the sequelae of recognized injuries.

POSTINJURY RESUSCITATION

ICU management of the trauma patient, either with direct admission from the ED or following emergent operative intervention, is considered in distinct phases because there are differing goals and priorities. The period of acute resuscitation, typically lasting for the first 12 to 24 hours following injury, combines several principles: optimizing tissue perfusion, ensuring normothermia, and restoring coagulation. There are a multitude of management algorithms aimed at accomplishing these goals—the majority involves goal-directed resuscitation with initial volume loading to attain adequate preload, followed by judicious use of inotropic agents or vasopressors (6). Although the optimal hemoglobin (Hb) level remains debated, during shock resuscitation an Hb >10 g/dL optimizes oxygen delivery (6). A more judicious transfusion trigger of Hb <7 g/dL in the euvolemic patient after the first 24 hours of resuscitation limits adverse inflammatory effects and improves mortality (7,8). The optimum hemoglobin level may vary depending on the patient's underlying cardiac function. The resuscitation of the severely injured trauma patient may require what appears to be an inordinate amount of crystalloid resuscitation. Infusion volumes upwards of 10 liters during the initial 6 to 12 hours may be required to attain an adequate central venous pressure (CVP) above 8 mm Hg. In fact, this is a challenging aspect of early care (i.e., balancing cardiac preload vs. promoting an abdominal compartment syndrome or tissue edema). During this initial treatment period, a low urine output is usually suggestive of a low preload and not an indication for diuretics. Moreover, the use of diuretics during a patient's initial resuscitation should be carefully considered, even if the patient is on such medications as an outpatient.

Invasive monitoring with pulmonary artery catheters may be a critical adjunct in the multiply injured patient (6,9). Not only do such devices allow minute-to-minute monitoring of the patient, but also the added information on the patient's volume status, cardiac function, peripheral vascular tone, and metabolic response to injury permits appropriate therapeutic intervention. With added information on the patient's cardiac function, cardiac indices (CIs) and oxygen delivery (DO_2) become important variables in the ongoing ICU management. Resuscitation to values of $DO_2I > 500$ mL/minute/m^2 and CI >3.8 L/minute/m^2 are the goals (6,10,11). Pulmonary artery catheters also enable the physician to monitor response to vasoactive agents. Although norepinephrine is the agent of choice for patients with low systemic vascular resistance (SVR) unable to maintain a mean arterial pressure (MAP) >60 mm Hg (6), patients may have an element of myocardial dysfunction requiring inotropic support. In patients with ongoing need for pressors, one should evaluate for adrenal insufficiency (12,13).

Adequate resuscitation is mandatory, and often determines when the surgeon can safely return the patient to the operating room (OR) after initial operative intervention. Specific goals of resuscitation prior to repeated "semi-elective" transport include a core temperature $>35°$C, base deficit less negative than 6, and normal coagulation indices. Even those patients who do not require repeat operations should be monitored for resolution of physiologic perturbations; specific indices monitored over time include lactate and base deficit levels as well as temperature. Although correction of base deficit and lactate values is desirable, how quickly this should be accomplished requires careful consideration. Adverse sequelae of aggressive crystalloid resuscitation include increased intracranial pressure, worsening pulmonary edema, and intra-abdominal visceral and retroperitoneal edema resulting in secondary abdominal compartment syndrome (14,15). Therefore, it should be the overall trend of the resuscitation rather than a rapid reduction of the base deficit to less than 5 during the first 4 hours of treatment that is the goal. Exogenous bicarbonate, occasionally given to improve cardiovascular function and response to vasoactive agents if the serum pH is below 7.2, obfuscates the acid-base balance and lactate may be a more reliable indicator of adequate perfusion.

NONOPERATIVE MANAGEMENT OF TRAUMA

Blunt Liver and Spleen Injuries

The liver and spleen are the most commonly injured solid organs following trauma, occurring in approximately 10% to 15% of all trauma admissions. The liver's large size makes it the most susceptible organ injured in blunt trauma, and it is frequently involved in upper torso penetrating trauma. Similarly, blunt trauma to the left upper quadrant, often with associated rib fractures, should raise the concern for a splenic injury. Although the liver is more often injured, splenic injuries tend to be more precarious clinically. Nonoperative management of solid organ injuries is pursued in hemodynamically stable patients who do not have overt peritonitis or other indications for laparotomy (16–25). Since its initial use in the early 1980s, CT scanning has largely supplanted diagnostic peritoneal lavage in the initial evaluation of trauma patients (Fig. 75.2). Key questions when looking at the CT scan include how extensive the injury is by the American Association for the Surgery of Trauma (AAST) solid organ injury grading scale (Table 75.2), how much associated free fluid is within the abdomen, whether there is free contrast extravasation indicating ongoing arterial bleeding, and whether there are pseudoaneurysms of the arteries (Fig. 75.3). High-grade injuries, a large amount of hemoperitoneum, contrast extravasation, and pseudoaneurysms are not absolute contraindications for nonoperative management; however, these patients are at high risk for failure and are more likely to need angioembolization (26–29). Likewise, there is not an age cutoff for patients for the nonoperative management of solid organ injuries (30–32).

The AAST developed a grading scale to provide a uniform definition of solid organ injuries based upon the magnitude of anatomic disruption (33–35). The grading of solid organ injuries permits accurate relay of information between care providers, a predictive value on the incidence of nonoperative failure, and information for appropriate monitoring (Table 75.3). The vast majority of patients with liver or spleen injuries, regardless of grade, can be managed nonoperatively (18,19). Predictors of failure include increasing grade of injury, evidence of blush on CT scan (particularly if this involves free extravasation into the peritoneal cavity rather than pooling within the organ), and a large amount of hemoperitoneum (18,19,27,29,36).

A multidisciplinary approach including angiography with selective angioembolization and endoscopic retrograde

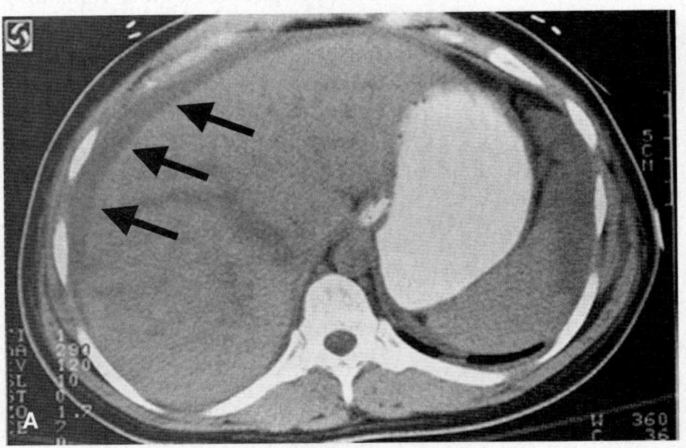

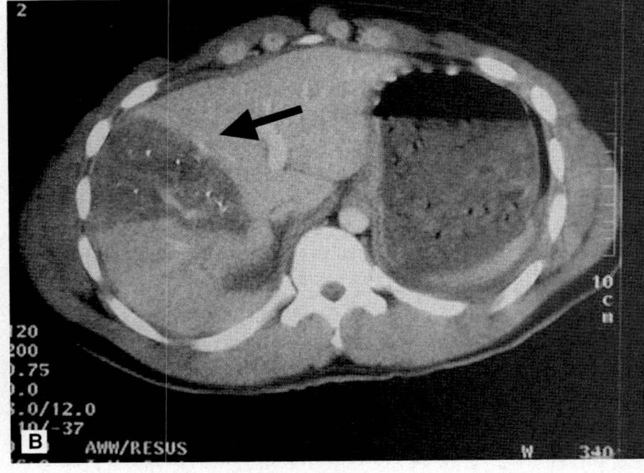

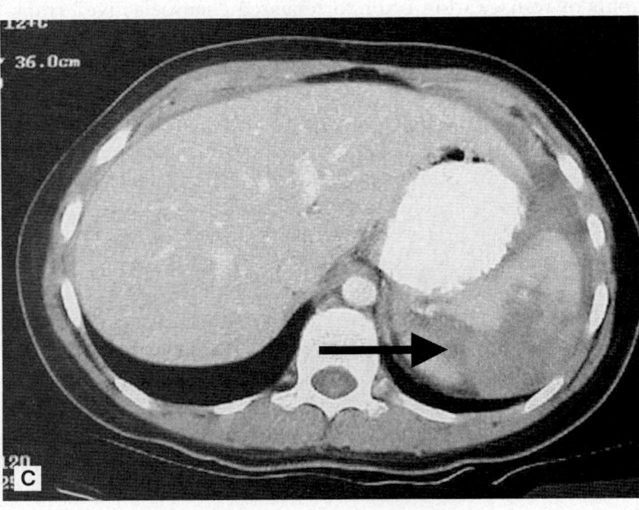

FIGURE 75.2. Representative solid organ injuries; American Association for the Surgery of Trauma grading includes evidence of subcapsular hematomas (A) and parenchymal lacerations (B, C).

TABLE 75.2

AMERICAN ASSOCIATION FOR THE SURGERY OF TRAUMA SOLID ORGAN INJURY GRADING SCALES

	Subcapsular hematoma	Laceration
LIVER INJURY GRADE		
I	<10% surface area	<1 cm in depth
II	10%–50% surface area	1–3 cm
III	>50% or >10 cm	>3 cm
IV	25%–75% of a hepatic lobe	
V	>75% of a hepatic lobe	
VI	Hepatic avulsion	
SPLEEN INJURY GRADE		
I	<10% surface area	<1 cm in depth
II	10%–50% surface area	1–3 cm
III	>50% surface area	>3 cm
IV	>25% devascularization	Hilar injury
V	Shattered spleen	

cholangiopancreatography (ERCP) with stenting has resulted in decreased nonoperative failure rates and improved survival in liver (37,38) and splenic injuries (39). Splenic angioembolization has been employed since 1995 as an adjunct to nonoperative therapy, with reported salvage rates of 98% (40). Patients with significant hemoperitoneum or overt contrast extravasation who are hemodynamically stable should be considered for possible splenic embolization. Additionally, patients with splenic artery pseudoaneurysms or arteriovenous (AV) fistulae within the spleen are also candidates (41). If a patient is going to fail nonoperative management (Fig. 75.4), the time to failure is different for liver versus spleen injuries. Typically liver injuries rebleed within the first hours of admission, while splenic laceration may have delayed rupture or bleeding weeks following the original injury. General guidelines for operative or angioembolization are noted in Table 75.4. Repeat imaging in patients with complex hepatic injuries can be performed with bedside ultrasound. Patients with evidence of right upper quadrant fluid collections or clinical deterioration (increasing abdominal pain, worsening liver function tests, unexplained fever) should undergo CT scanning (42,43).

Pancreatic Injuries

Historically, injuries to the pancreas were managed with operative intervention (44). With the recent evolution of nonoperative management for solid organ injuries, a nonresectional management schema has been developed for select pancreatic injuries (45,46). Observation of pancreatic contusions, particularly those in the head of the pancreas that may involve ductal disruption, includes serial exams and monitoring of serum amylase. Patients with pancreatic injuries involving the major ducts, originally a strict indication for operative intervention,

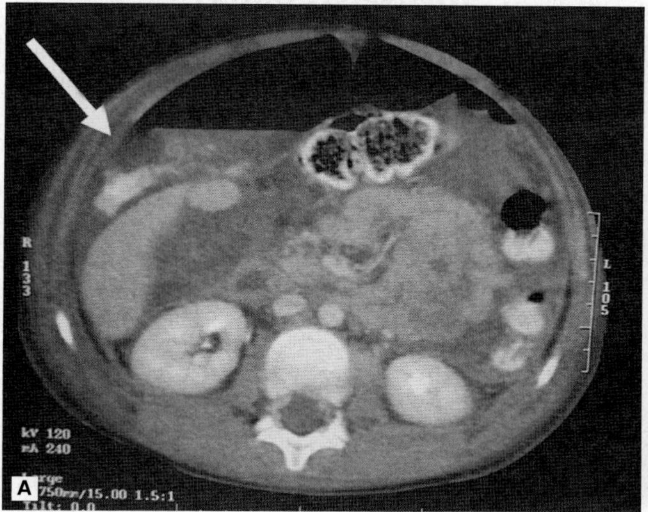

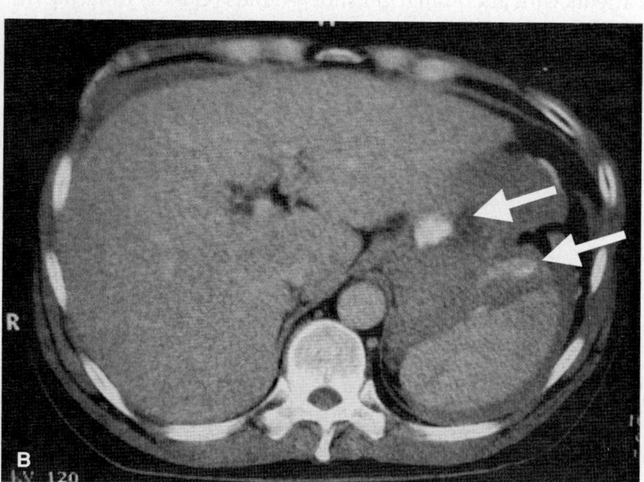

FIGURE 75.3. Free contrast extravasation noted on computed tomography scan imaging of the liver (A) and spleen (B).

TABLE 75.3

APPROPRIATE MONITORING AND NONOPERATIVE MANAGEMENT FAILURE RATES FOR SOLID ORGAN INJURIES BY GRADE

Grade of injury	Admission	Monitoring	Failure rate
I	Floor	Exam/Hct every 12°	2%–5%
II	Floor	Exam/Hct every 6° × 4	8%–10%
III	ICU	Exam/Hct every 4° × 6	6%–20%
IV	ICU	Exam/Hct every 2–4° × 6	15%–34%
V	ICU	Exam/Hct every 2–4° × 8	22%–75%

Hct, hematocrit; ICU, intensive care unit; °, hour.

may be managed with ERCP and stenting in select patients; durability of this approach is currently under investigation (47).

Duodenal Hematomas

Following blunt trauma, patients may develop hematomas in the duodenal wall that obstruct the lumen. Clinical exam findings include epigastric pain associated with either emesis or high nasogastric tube (NGT) output; CT scan imaging with oral contrast failing to pass into the proximal jejunum is diagnostic (Fig. 75.5). Patients with suspected associated perforation, suggested by clinical deterioration or imaging with retroperitoneal free air or contrast extravasation, should be explored operatively. Nonoperative management includes continuous NGT decompression and nutritional support with total parenteral nutrition (TPN) (48,49). A marked drop in NGT output heralds resolution of the hematoma, which typically occurs within 2 weeks; repeat imaging to document these clinical findings is optional. If the patient does not improve clinically or radiographically within 4 weeks, operative evaluation is warranted.

Penetrating Wounds

Patients with abdominal gunshot wounds (GSWs) violating the peritoneum undergo emergent laparotomy due to an approximate 90% visceral injury rate. Select patients with isolated low-energy GSWs to the right upper quadrant are observed (50,51); CT scan imaging must delineate the tract of the bullet, which should be confined to the parenchyma of the liver, and the patient must be hemodynamically stable with a benign clinical examination. Patients with abdominal stab wounds (SWs) to the back or flank with negative CT imaging or an isolated kidney injury are also managed nonoperatively (52). Similar to patients with right upper quadrant GSWs, individuals with SWs and a CT scan showing the tract of injury confined to the liver are usually observed (53). In some cases, laparoscopy will be done to assess the penetrating liver injury and ensure the viscera are not violated. Regardless of the trauma surgeon's decision for operative versus nonoperative management, it is essential that these patients undergo repeated abdominal examination. Observation for a missed small or large bowel injury is critical; clinical findings in such patients include a rising white blood cell count, fever, tachycardia, and increasing abdominal pain or frank peritonitis. In patients with isolated liver injuries, complications are similar to those for patients with blunt injuries, namely bleeding and bile leaks or biliary sepsis.

COMPLICATIONS OF NONOPERATIVE INJURY MANAGEMENT

Following hepatic injuries, the most common complication is a bile leak or biloma, occurring in up to 20% of patients

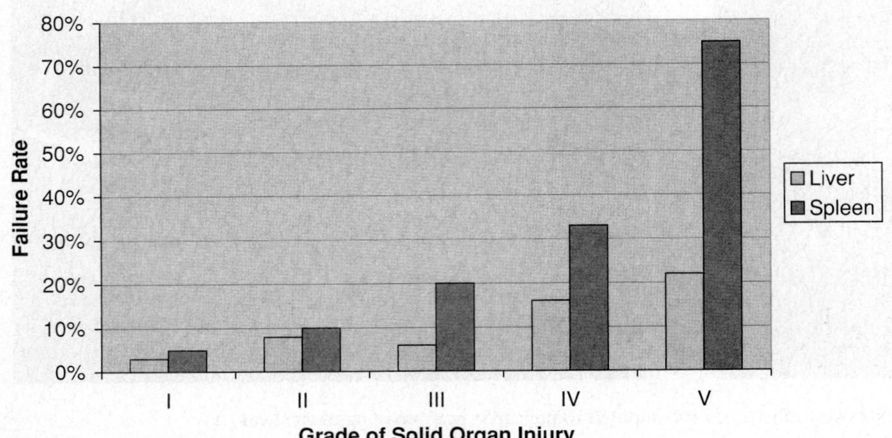

FIGURE 75.4. Rates of nonoperative failure for solid organ injuries.

TABLE 75.4

GENERAL GUIDELINES FOR OPERATIVE OR INTERVENTIONAL RADIOLOGY INTERVENTION DURING NONOPERATIVE MANAGEMENT OF SOLID ORGAN INJURIES

LIVER: Hemodynamically unstable with 4 units of packed red blood cells (PRBCs) in 6 h or 6 units PRBCs in 24 h
SPLEEN: Hemodynamically unstable with need for initial transfusion related to splenic injury rather than associated trauma

(Fig. 75.6) (54,55). Clinical presentation includes abdominal distention, intolerance of enteral feeds, and elevated liver functions tests. CT scanning effectively diagnoses the underlying problem, and the vast majority is treated with percutaneous drainage and ERCP with sphincterotomy. Occasionally, laparoscopy or laparotomy with drainage of biliary ascites is indicated, particularly if the patient fails to resolve his or her ileus and fever (56). Hemobilia, manifested by the triad of right upper quadrant pain, jaundice, and upper gastrointestinal bleeding, is a rare complication. Delayed rupture of a subcapsular hematoma with hemorrhage is another infrequent complication but the diagnosis is usually obvious. Patients undergoing

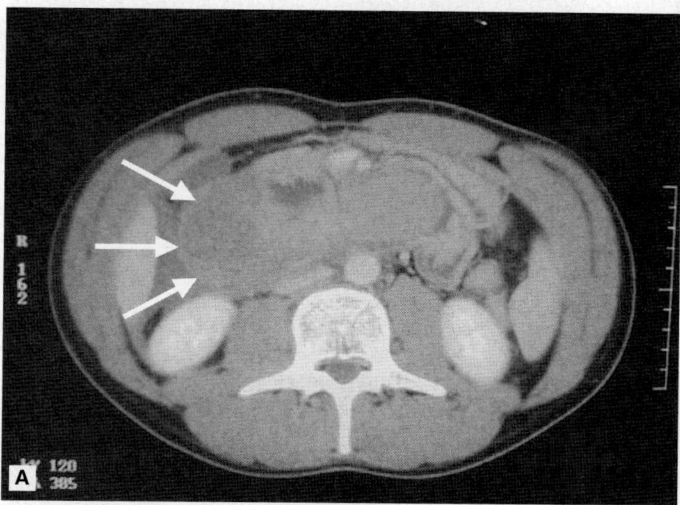

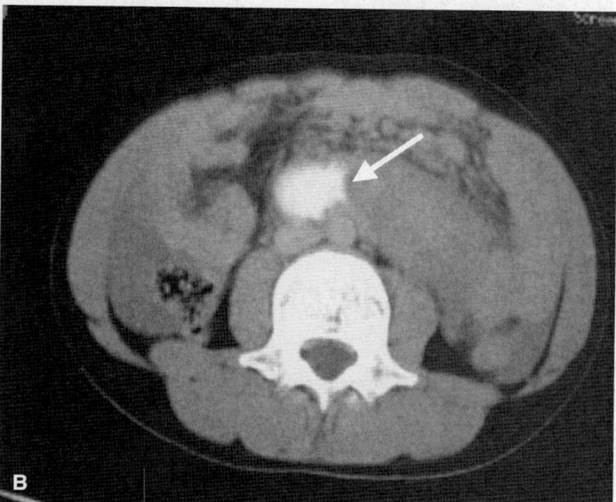

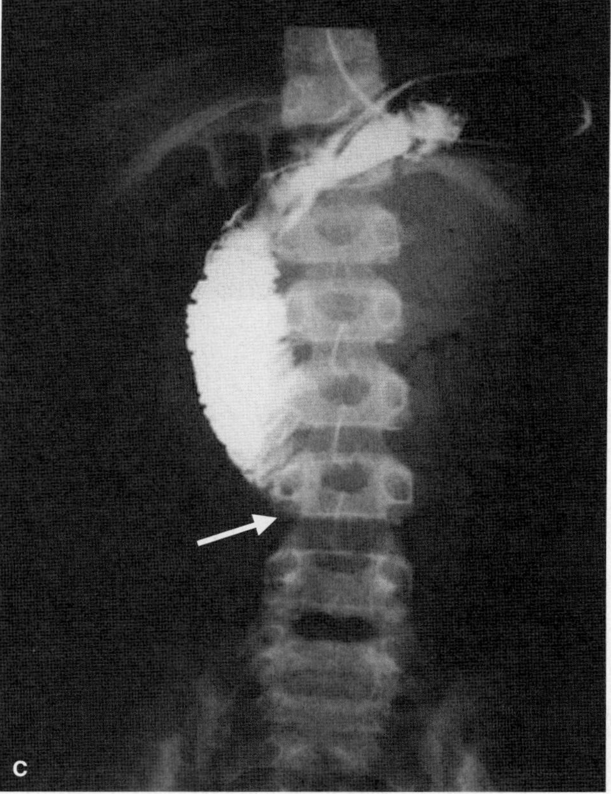

FIGURE 75.5. Duodenal hematomas are diagnosed radiographically by direct identification of a hematoma (**A**) or failure to pass oral contrast past the third portion of the duodenum on computed tomography scan (**B**) or upper gastrointestinal series (**C**).

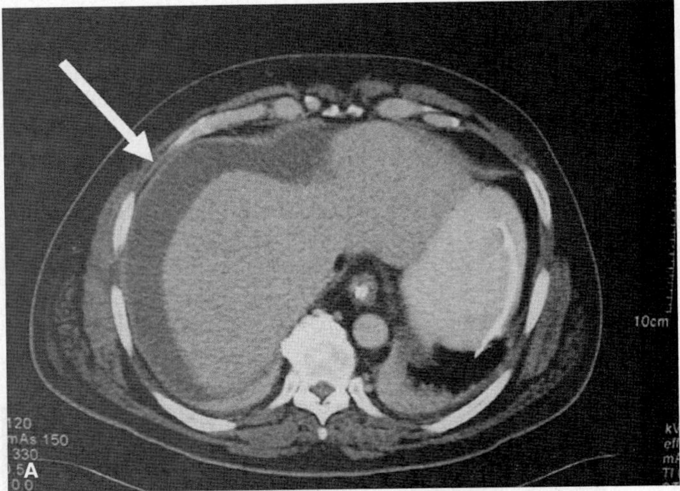

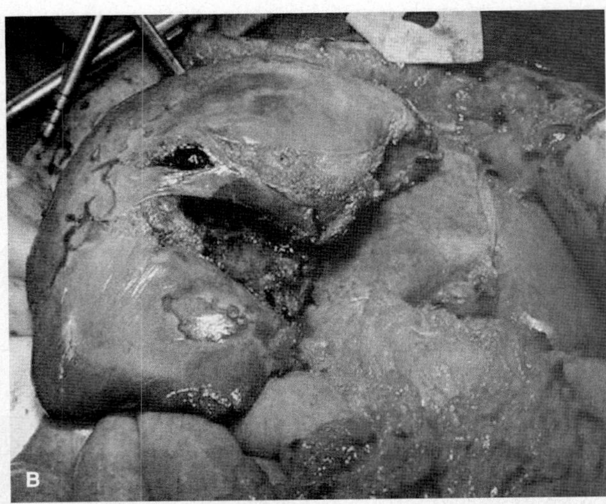

FIGURE 75.6. Bilomas are the most common complication following hepatic trauma (**A**), while angioembolization for unremitting postinjury liver hemorrhage may result in partial hepatic necrosis (**B**).

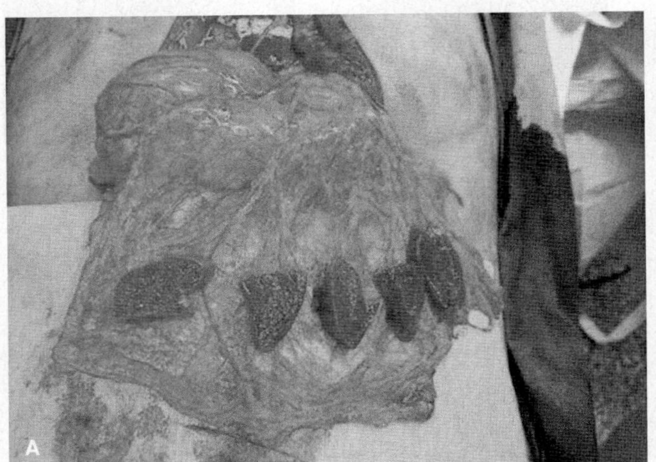

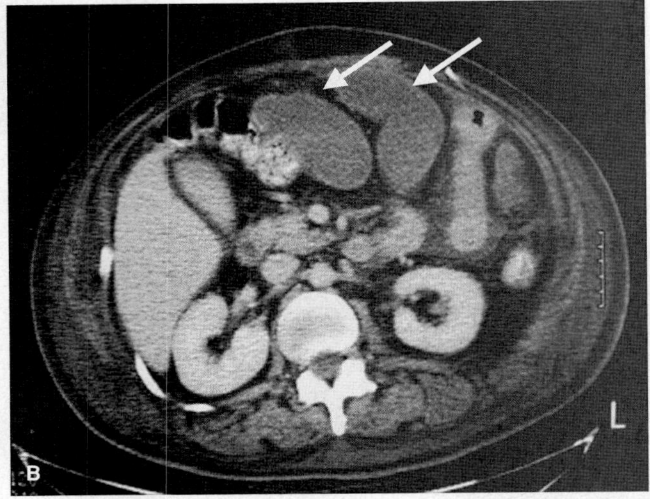

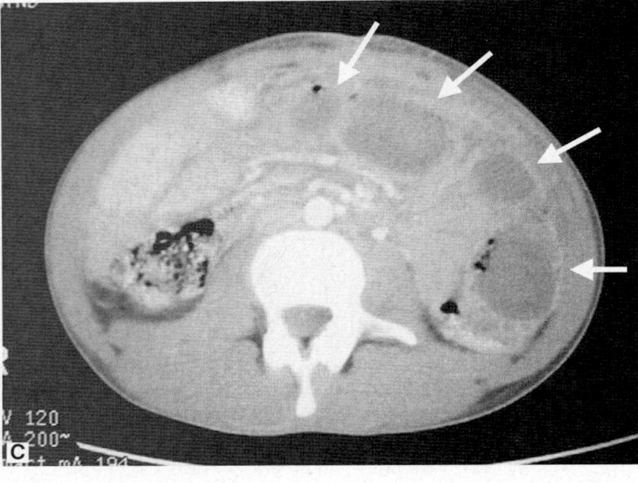

FIGURE 75.7. Splenic implants are autotransplanted into the greater omentum to prevent overwhelming postsplenectomy sepsis (**A**); follow-up computed tomography scan imaging can differentiate between "normal" implants (**B**) versus infected implants (**C**).

angioembolization for liver trauma must be carefully monitored for hepatic necrosis, and may occasionally require delayed formal hepatic resection (Fig. 75.6). Although some clinicians repeat CT scans on all patients with grade IV and V injuries, typically, only patients with symptoms or persistent altered liver function tests should be reimaged (43).

The most common problem in patients with splenic injuries is delayed bleeding, although as noted previously, the majority fails over an established timeframe. Patients undergoing splenic embolization can fail with rebleeding with 13% of patients requiring splenectomy (57). Moreover, those undergoing successful angioembolization typically have significant pain associated with their "splenic infarct," and up to 20% develop splenic abscesses. In centers that advocate splenic autotransplantation to prevent overwhelming postsplenectomy sepsis (OPSS), recognition of CT scan findings of normal splenic implants versus infected splenic implants is critical in patients with clinical deterioration (Fig. 75.7) (58).

ONGOING EVALUATION FOR INJURIES (HOW TO AVOID A MISSED INJURY)

With the paradigm shift from operative to nonoperative management of trauma, the clinician must have a heightened sense of awareness to avoid missing an occult injury. This is particularly true in multiply injured blunt trauma patients, especially those who are intubated without a reliable abdominal examination. CT scan imaging is not 100% accurate; repeat CT scan imaging, diagnostic peritoneal lavage (DPL), ultrasound, and even laparotomy may be necessary for definitive evaluation.

Missed bowel injuries are the most commonly pursued injury, not due to their frequency (less than 5% of blunt trauma) but rather their associated morbidity. Diagnosing a hollow viscus injury is notoriously difficult (59), and even short delays in diagnoses result in increased morbidity (60,61). If a patient's initial CT scan of the abdomen shows free fluid without evidence of a solid organ injury to explain such fluid, evaluation for a bowel injury should be performed (62–64). DPL should also be considered in a patient if there is increasing intra-abdominal fluid on bedside ultrasound in patients with a solid organ injury but a stable hematocrit, and/or in patients with unexplained clinical deterioration. Typically, the DPL at the bedside is done, with specific laboratory values indicating need for laparotomy (Table 75.5) (65,66); particular attention should be paid to elevations in bilirubin, alkaline phosphatase, and amylase when pursuing a diagnosis of bowel injury. The specific type of injury may be either bowel perforation due to ischemia from an avulsed mesentery, a direct antimesenteric blowout injury, or a blunt serosal injury (Fig. 75.8). One should not assume that drugs, alcohol, or their associated withdrawal syndromes are the primary source of a patient's clinical deterioration.

TABLE 75.5

A POSITIVE DIAGNOSTIC PERITONEAL LAVAGE FOLLOWING BLUNT TRAUMA DEFINED BY SPECIFIC LABORATORY VALUES

Laboratory study	Positive value
White blood cell	>500 cells/μL
Red blood cell	>100,000 cells/μL
Amylase	>19 IU/L
Alkaline phosphatase	>2 IU/L
Bilirubin	>0.1 mg/dL

Missing a rectal injury may be life threatening in patients with pelvic fractures. While some patients have clear findings on physical examination, ranging from hematochezia to overt degloving of the perineum, others may have occult injuries that are missed on initial evaluation in the trauma bay. In fact, the rectal exam may have been omitted in the trauma bay, so the intensivist should ensure that this has been adequately done. Flexible sigmoidoscopy is the easiest diagnostic procedure for the clinician to perform at the bedside in the ICU; endoscopic evaluation should rule out blood within the canal, clear intestinal perforation, or ischemic mucosa (67).

Pancreatic contusions, with or without associated ductal disruption, are difficult to diagnose in patients with blunt abdominal trauma (68). Patients clearly at risk include those with significant mechanisms including high force, a seatbelt sign on physical examination, or a blow to the epigastrium (69). The initial CT scan may show nonspecific stranding of the pancreas. Associated fluid around the pancreas should prompt further invasive studies such as ERCP or magnetic resonance cholangiopancreatography (MRCP) to rule out a biliary or pancreatic duct injury. With a tentative diagnosis of a pancreatic contusion, one may consider following serial determinations of amylase/lipase; although these lab studies do not have a reliable sensitivity (70), increasing values over time combined with an alteration in clinical exam should prompt a repeat CT scan, a duodenal C-loop study, a DPL, or an ERCP depending upon the suspected lesion.

POSTOPERATIVE MANAGEMENT OF SPECIFIC INJURIES

In addition to the global resuscitation of the trauma patient, ICU oversight must include management of injuries found at operative exploration. Communication between the operating surgeon and the intensivist is critical, and should include intraoperative findings and procedures, any tenuous operative repairs, anticipated problems or complications, the need for repeat operative exploration, and location of drains. The intraoperative estimated blood loss (EBL) and associated blood product transfusion requirements are essential data to anticipate events in the postoperative period. The transfusion information should include whether a massive transfusion protocol was initiated, entailing a 1:1 ratio of packed red blood cells to FFP, or any objective evidence of clinical coagulopathy during operative treatment. Finally, all clinicians caring for the patient should remember that injuries can be missed even with prior operative intervention.

Liver and Spleen Injuries

Although the majority of patients are successfully managed with nonoperative treatment, hemodynamically unstable patients or those with associated injuries may require urgent operative temporization of their solid organ injuries.

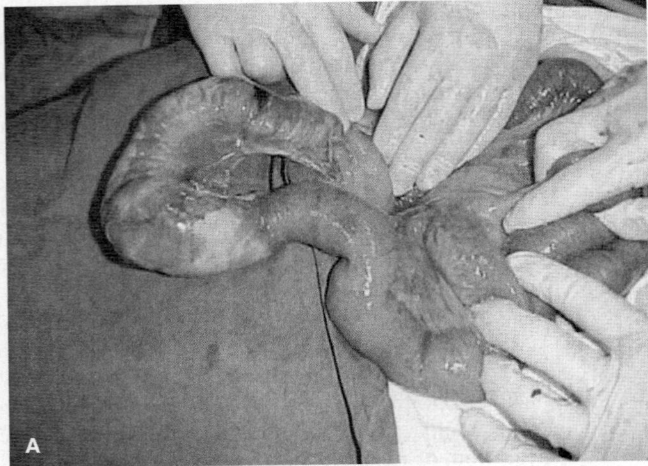

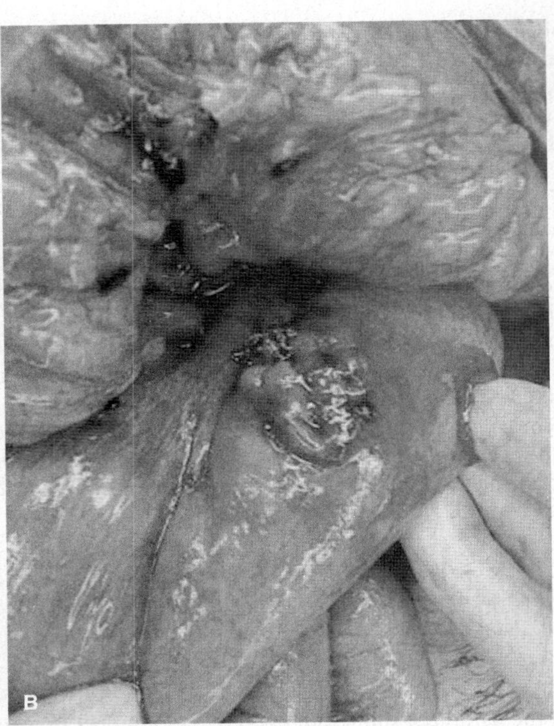

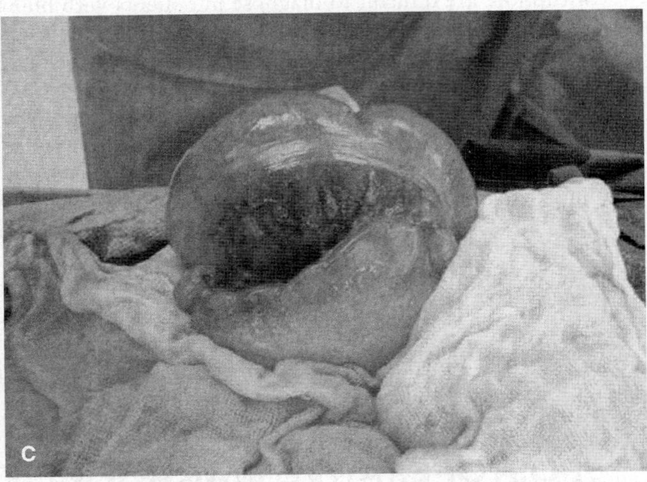

FIGURE 75.8. Bowel injuries following blunt trauma include perforation due to ischemia from an avulsed mesentery (**A**), a direct antimesenteric blowout injury (**B**), and a blunt serosal injury (**C**).

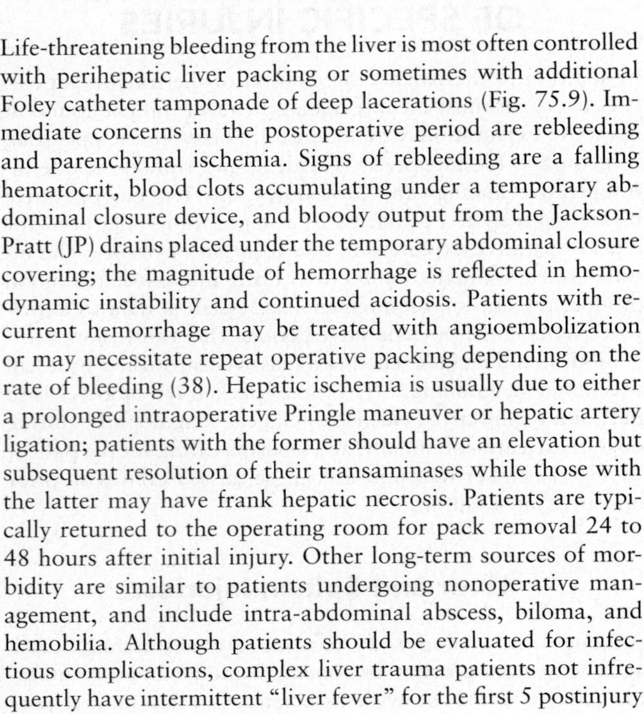

Life-threatening bleeding from the liver is most often controlled with perihepatic liver packing or sometimes with additional Foley catheter tamponade of deep lacerations (Fig. 75.9). Immediate concerns in the postoperative period are rebleeding and parenchymal ischemia. Signs of rebleeding are a falling hematocrit, blood clots accumulating under a temporary abdominal closure device, and bloody output from the Jackson-Pratt (JP) drains placed under the temporary abdominal closure covering; the magnitude of hemorrhage is reflected in hemodynamic instability and continued acidosis. Patients with recurrent hemorrhage may be treated with angioembolization or may necessitate repeat operative packing depending on the rate of bleeding (38). Hepatic ischemia is usually due to either a prolonged intraoperative Pringle maneuver or hepatic artery ligation; patients with the former should have an elevation but subsequent resolution of their transaminases while those with the latter may have frank hepatic necrosis. Patients are typically returned to the operating room for pack removal 24 to 48 hours after initial injury. Other long-term sources of morbidity are similar to patients undergoing nonoperative management, and include intra-abdominal abscess, biloma, and hemobilia. Although patients should be evaluated for infectious complications, complex liver trauma patients not infrequently have intermittent "liver fever" for the first 5 postinjury days (71).

Operative intervention for splenic injuries includes splenectomy and splenorrhaphy. Postoperative hemorrhage may be due to the splenic hilar vessel tie loosening, a missed short gastric artery, or recurrent bleeding from the spleen if splenic repair was used. An immediate postsplenectomy increase in platelets and white blood cells (WBCs) is normal; however, beyond postoperative day 5 a WBC count above 15,000 should prompt a thorough search for underlying infection (72). Additional sources of morbidity include a concurrent but unrecognized iatrogenic injury to the pancreatic tail during rapid splenectomy resulting in pancreatic ascites or fistula. Patients have an increased incidence of intra-abdominal abscesses in the left upper quadrant following splenectomy with concomitant gastrointestinal injury, but presumptive drainage does not prevent this complication. Routine care also includes immunizations for encapsulated organisms (*Streptococcus pneumoniae, Haemophilus influenzae,* and *Meningococcus*) usually just prior to discharge, optimally at 2 to 3 weeks postsplenectomy (73).

Gastrointestinal Injuries

Operative intervention for either penetrating or blunt gastrointestinal injuries entails primary repair, resection with primary

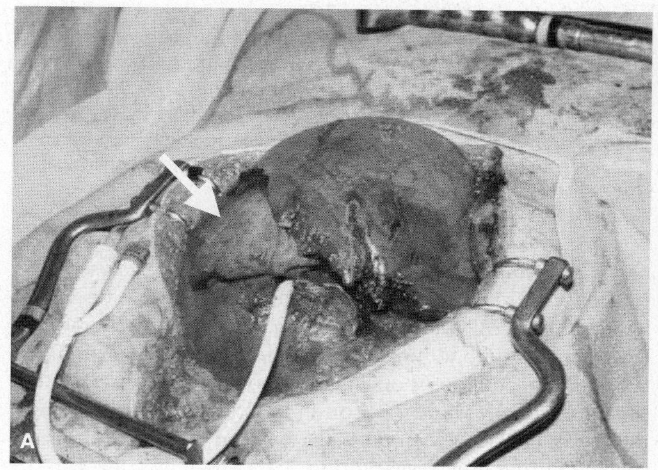

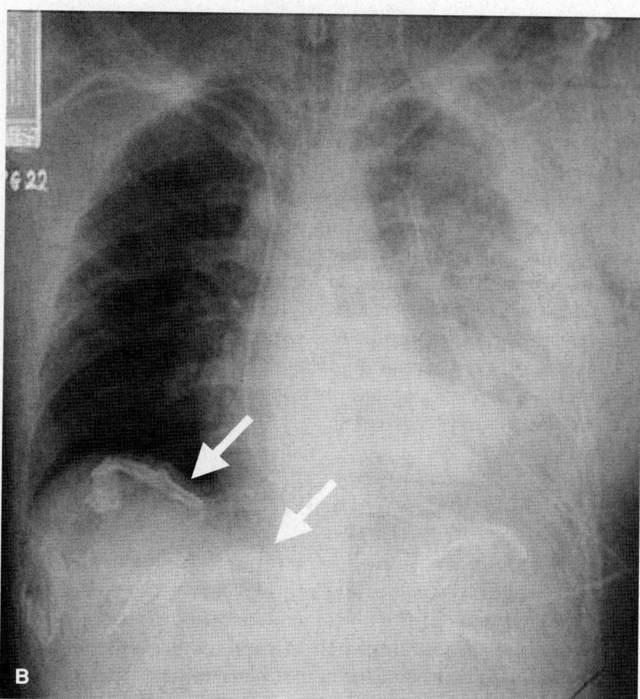

FIGURE 75.9. Perihepatic liver packing or Foley catheter tamponade of deep lacerations is employed to halt hepatic hemorrhage (**A**); subsequent abdominal imaging shows the radiopaque markers of operatively placed laparotomy pads around the liver (**B**).

anastomosis, or resection with a stoma diversion. Regardless of the type of operation or the type of anastomosis (stapled vs. sewn) (74), one should await resolution of the patient's expected postoperative ileus. Return of bowel function is noted by a decrease in gastrostomy or NGT output and the passing of flatus or stool. If an ileostomy or colostomy was required, one should inspect it daily to ensure it is pink without evidence of necrosis. Postoperative complications include anastomotic leak, prolonged ileus, and bowel obstruction. A leak with intra-abdominal contamination or sepsis presents with increasing abdominal pain, fevers, and respiratory compromise in the extubated patient, or persistent fevers and intolerance of enteral feeding in the intubated patient. CT scan is diagnostic and repeat operation is often required.

Important questions for the intensivist following operative intervention for pancreatic injuries include how much of the pancreas was resected, is there a pancreaticoenteric anastomosis, was the pancreatic stump closed with either staples and/or fibrin glue, was the spleen preserved, and where were drains placed (77)? Closed suction drains should remain in place until the patient is tolerating an oral diet or enteral nutrition with the associated drain output being less than 30 mL/day. Postoperative complications include pancreatic fistula, pseudocyst, abscess, pancreaticoenteric leak, and pancreatitis. The most common of these is a pancreatic fistula, occurring in 7% to 20% of patients with isolated pancreatic trauma including the major duct, and in up to 35% of patients with combined pancreatic and duodenal injuries (76). Diagnosis in patients with drains in place is defined as output greater than 30 mL/day with an amylase level three times greater than serum value after postoperative day 5 (77). In patients without drains in place who have persistent abdominal pain, fevers, or intolerance of oral intake, CT scan imaging should be performed to evaluate for an intra-abdominal fluid collection. Drainage by interventional radiology (IR) is performed for fistula diagnosis and control. Pancreatic fistulae following trauma are managed in an identical fashion to those occurring following elective pancreatic resection (77).

Abdominal Vascular Injuries

Vascular injuries can produce rapid exsanguination and threaten extremities, or may be a clinically silent time bomb due to temporary retroperitoneal tamponade. Few result in a delayed diagnosis, particularly with CT scanning, and hence the focus of the intensivist is postoperative management. In general, outcome following vascular injuries is related to the technical success of the operation; the main causes of patient morbidity and mortality are associated soft tissue and nerve injuries once the vascular repair has been accomplished. Therefore, optimizing the patient's hemodynamic status, maintaining euthermia, and correcting coagulopathy are critical points of resuscitation. Prosthetic graft infections are rare complications (78) but preventing bacteremia is imperative; administration of perioperative antibiotics and treatment of secondary infections are indicated. Long-term arterial graft complications such as stenosis or pseudoaneurysms are uncommon, and routine graft surveillance is rarely performed. Consequently, long-term antiplatelet agents or antithrombotics are not routine.

There are specific injuries that require additional care. Abdominal aortic injuries are repaired using either a polytetrafluoroethylene (PTFE) patch or interposition grafting; the patient's systolic blood pressure should not exceed 120 mm Hg for at least the first 72 hours postoperatively. Patients requiring ligation of an inferior vena cava injury often develop marked bilateral lower extremity edema; to limit the associated morbidity the patient's legs should be wrapped with ACE bandages from the toes to the hips and elevated at a 45- to 60-degree angle. For superior mesenteric vein injuries, either ligation or thrombosis following venorrhaphy results in marked bowel edema; fluid resuscitation should be aggressive and abdominal pressure monitoring routine in these patients. In complex hepatic trauma, the right or left hepatic artery, or in urgent situations, the portal vein may be selectively ligated; persistent elevation in liver transaminases indicates secondary liver parenchymal necrosis and may necessitate delayed resection. Of note, if the right hepatic artery is ligated intraoperatively, cholecystectomy is performed concurrently.

Abdominal Wounds

In general, wounds sustained from trauma should be examined daily for progression of healing and signs of infection. Complex soft tissue wounds of the abdomen, such as degloving injuries following blunt trauma (termed Morel-Lavallee lesions), shotgun wounds, and other destructive blast injuries, are particularly difficult to manage. Following initial debridement of devitalized tissue, wound care includes wet-to-dry dressing changes twice daily, or application of the wound vacuum-assisted closure (VAC). One should carefully watch for infection, development of necrotizing fasciitis, subcutaneous abscess, or associated undrained hematoma. Repeated operative débridements may be necessary, and early involvement of the reconstructive surgery service for possible flap coverage is advised.

Midline laparotomy wounds are inspected 48 hours postoperatively by removing the sterile surgical dressing. If the patient develops high-grade fevers, inspection of the wound should be done sooner to exclude an early necrotizing infection. If a wound infection is identified—evidenced by erythema, pain along the wound, or purulent drainage—the wound should be widely opened by removing skin staples. After ensuring that the midline fascia is intact with digital palpation, the wound is managed with wet-to-dry dressing changes.

DAMAGE CONTROL SURGERY

Damage control surgery (DCS) is an abbreviated operation whose goals are to control hemorrhage, limit contamination from enteric sources, and enable rapid transport to the ICU for correction of adverse physiology (79,80). There are standard indications for performing the DCS abbreviated laparotomy in patients with unresolved metabolic failure (Table 75.6). Intraoperative techniques of DCS include perihepatic packing, balloon tamponade of deep liver lacerations, segmental stapled bowel resection left in discontinuity, ligation of abdominal venous injuries, shunting of abdominal arterial injuries, and pancreatic drainage.

Following DCS, the surgeon will "close" the abdomen with a temporary closure device. Options for temporary closure include Bogotá bag closure (a 3-L Urology irrigation bag), 1010 Steri-Drape (3M Health Care, St. Paul, MN) and Ioban closure, and wound VAC dressing (Fig. 75.10). In the majority of major trauma centers, the patient's abdomen is closed with the 1010 Steri-Drape and Ioban closure after the first operation and with the VAC following additional operative explorations. The temporary abdominal closure allows egress of abdominal contents and contains the edematous bowel while providing excellent decompression. Jackson-Pratt drains are placed under the Ioban covering to control the marked effluent from third spacing during fluid resuscitation.

TABLE 75.6

INTRAOPERATIVE INDICATIONS TO PERFORM DAMAGE CONTROL SURGERY

Factor	Level
Body temperature	Temperature <35°C
Acid-base status	
Arterial pH	pH <7.2
Base deficit (BD)	BD < −15 mmol/L in patient <55 y BD < −8 mmol/L in patient >55 y
Serum lactate	Lactate >5 mmol/L
Coagulopathy	PT or PTT >50% of normal

T, temperature; PT, prothrombin time; PTT, partial thromboplastin time; BD, base deficit.

Upon transfer to the ICU, aggressive resuscitation of the patient is performed to reverse metabolic failure (81). This includes vigorous rewarming through heating the room, infusion of fluids and blood products through a warming device, and use of a warming device such as the Bair Hugger (Augustine Medical, Inc., Eden Prairie, MN); more aggressive measures may include warm saline irrigation of the stomach, chest, and abdominal cavities via an NGT, thoracostomy tubes, and DPL catheters. Continuous arteriovenous rewarming may be warranted for refractive temperatures <34°C. Restoration of a normal cardiovascular state is attained by infusion of fluids and blood products, as well as judicious use of vasopressor agents. Finally, the patient's coagulopathy must be reversed with appropriate blood products including fresh frozen plasma, cryoprecipitate, and platelets. Occasionally recombinant activated factor VII (rFVIIa; NovoSeven, NovoNordisk, Denmark) is needed. Ideally, physiologic correction should occur within 12 to 24 hours of admission to the ICU, with planned return to the operating room for definitive repair.

There are several specific management points of the patient with an open abdomen that deserve mention. Despite a widely open abdomen, patients can develop abdominal compartment syndrome (ACS) (82); therefore, bladder pressures should be monitored every 4 hours, with significant increases in pressures alerting the clinician to the possible need for repeat operative intervention and abdominal decompression. Patients with an open abdomen lose between 500 and 2,500 mL/day of abdominal effluent. Appropriate volume compensation for this albumin-rich fluid remains controversial, both in the amount administered (replacement based on clinical indices vs. routine 1/2-mL replacement for every milliliter lost) as well as the type of replacement (crystalloid vs. colloid/blood products). Patients with abdominal packing in place, particularly for liver lacerations, may rebleed from such injuries. In these situations, the patient may begin to exsanguinate from the abdomen through the JP drains placed under the Ioban covering. Rapid clamping

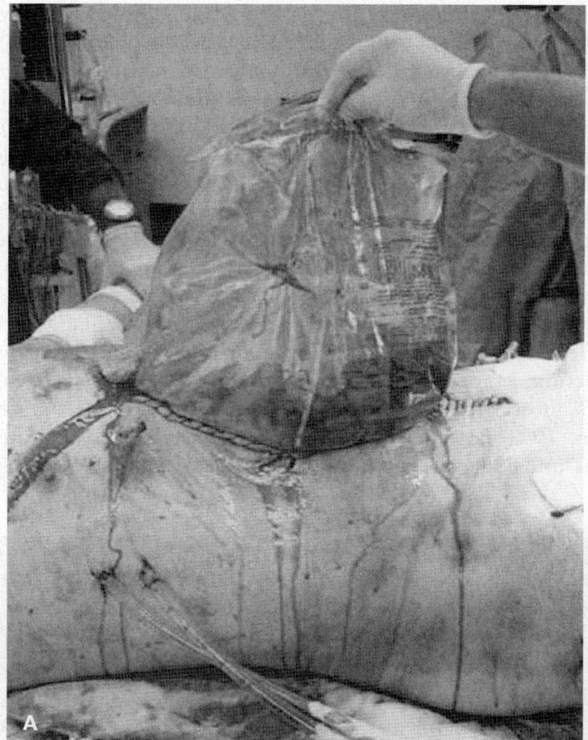

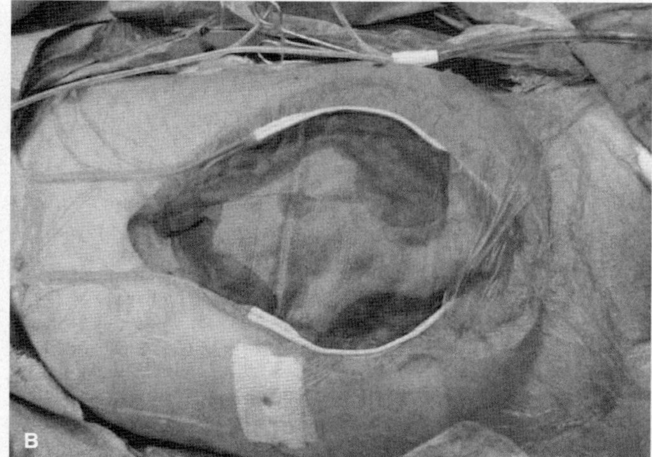

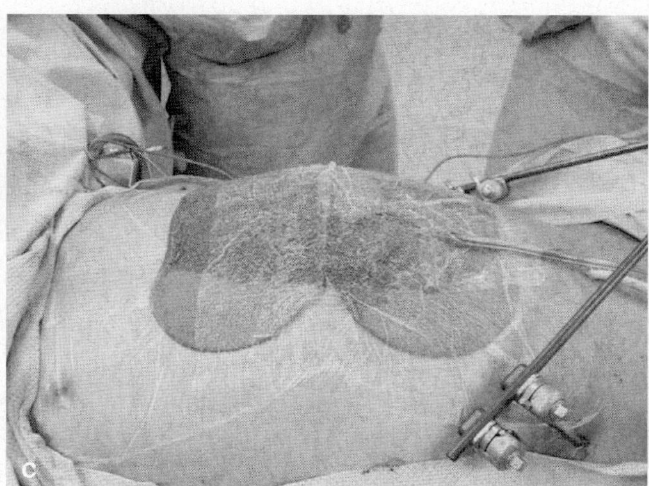

FIGURE 75.10. Methods of temporary abdominal closure following damage control surgery or operative decompression for abdominal compartment syndrome: Bogotá bag closure (**A**), 1010 Steri-Drape and Ioban closure (**B**), and vacuum-assisted closure dressing (**C**).

of the abdominal JP drains with blood product resuscitation may provide enough intra-abdominal pressure and subsequent tamponade to stabilize the patient for reoperation. Alternatively, bedside laparotomy with repacking of the liver is an option. In patients suffering cardiac arrest from hemorrhage, removing the temporary abdominal closure dressing at the bedside with aortic and portal triad clamping is warranted.

ABDOMINAL COMPARTMENT SYNDROME

The abdominal compartment syndrome is typified by intra-abdominal hypertension due to either intra-abdominal injury (primary) or following massive resuscitation (secondary) (83–87). Secondary ACS may be due to any etiology requiring such a resuscitation, including extremity trauma, isolated head injury, chest trauma, or even following postinjury related sepsis (88). The large volumes of crystalloid required to manage multiply injured patients results in resuscitation-associated bowel edema, retroperitoneal edema, or large quantities of ascitic fluid. A diagnosis of intra-abdominal hypertension cannot be definitively made by physical examination, but is obtained by measuring bladder pressures. To measure a patient's bladder pressure, 50 mL of saline is instilled into the bladder via the aspiration port of the Foley catheter with the drainage tube clamped; a three-way stopcock and water manometer is placed at the level of the pubic symphysis (89). Bladder pressures are then measured on the manometer in centimeters of water (Table 75.7) and correlate with the physiologic impact of ACS. Conditions in which the bladder pressure is unreliable include bladder rupture, external compression from pelvic packing, neurogenic bladder, and adhesive disease.

TABLE 75.7

ABDOMINAL COMPARTMENT SYNDROME GRADING SYSTEM BASED UPON BLADDER PRESSURE MEASUREMENTS

ACS grade	Bladder pressure (cm H_2O)
I	10–15
II	16–25
III	26–35
IV	>35

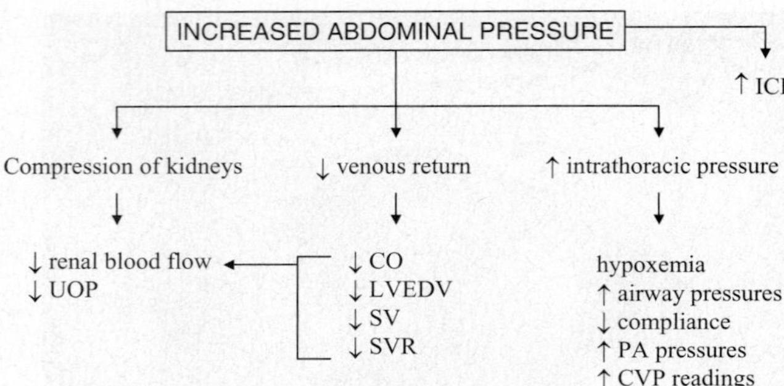

FIGURE 75.11. Physiologic derangements associated with intra-abdominal hypertension leading to abdominal compartment syndrome. ICP, intracranial pressure; UOP, urine output; CO, cardiac output; VEDV, ventricular end-diastolic volume; SV, stroke volume; SVR, systemic vascular resistance; PA, pulmonary artery; CVP, central venous pressure.

Increased abdominal pressure affects multiple organ systems (Fig. 75.11). The ACS, however, is defined by intra-abdominal hypertension causing such end organ sequelae as decreased urine output, increased pulmonary pressures, decreased preload and subsequent cardiac dysfunction, and even elevated intracranial pressure (ICP) (83). As any of these clinical manifestations of ACS may be attributed to the primary injury, a heightened awareness of this entity must be maintained. Organ failure can occur over a wide range of recorded bladder pressures; there is not a single measurement of bladder pressure that prompts therapeutic intervention, except >35 cm H_2O. Rather, emergent decompression is warranted in the patient with intra-abdominal hypertension with end organ dysfunction. Mortality is directly affected by decompression, with 64% mortality in patients undergoing presumptive decompression, 70% mortality in patients with a delay in decompression, and 89% mortality in those without decompression (90).

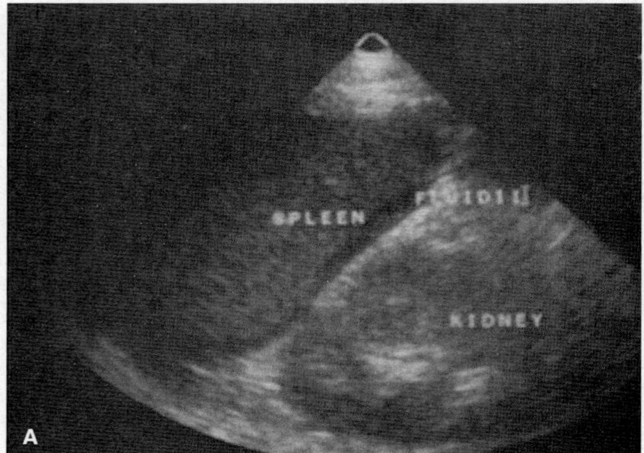

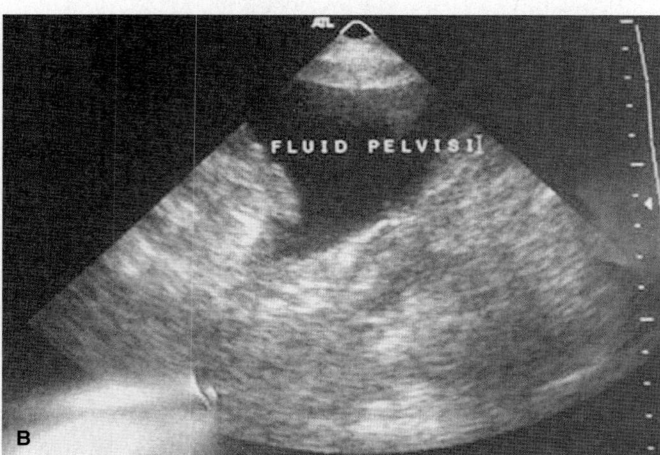

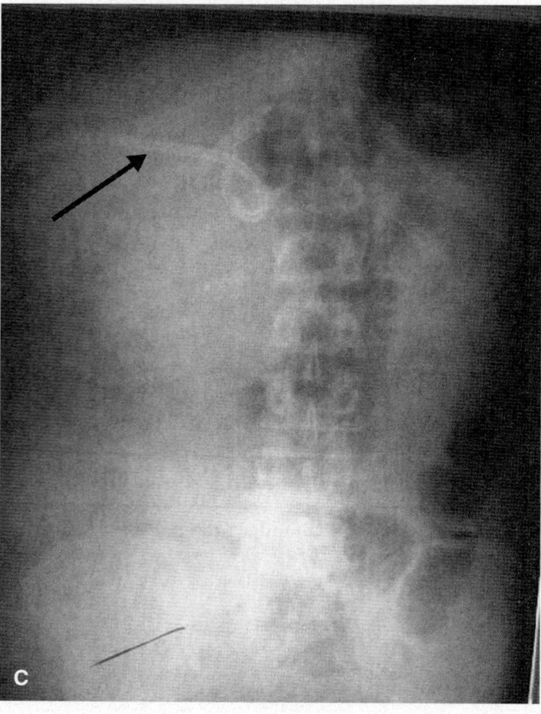

FIGURE 75.12. Bedside ultrasound of the abdomen demonstrates resuscitation-induced ascites (A, B); placement of a pigtail drain (C) over the liver may evacuate enough fluid to reduce the intra-abdominal pressure and associated abdominal compartment syndrome organ failure.

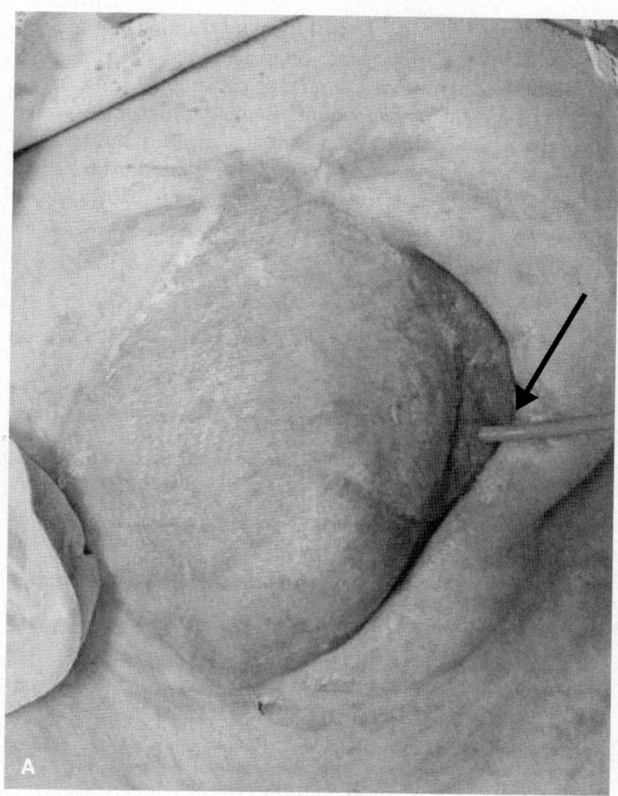

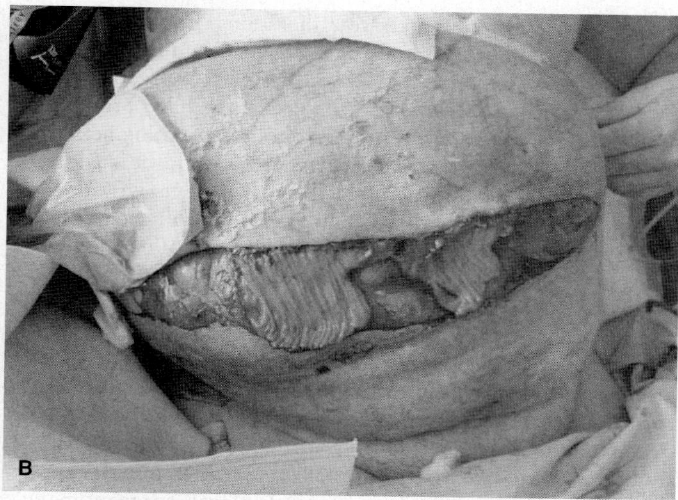

FIGURE 75.13. Complications of the open abdomen include intra-abdominal abscess, bile leaks, enteric fistula (A), and bowel perforations (B).

Decompression is typically performed operatively either at the bedside in the ICU if the patient is hemodynamically unstable, or in the operating room. Bedside laparotomy is easily accomplished, precludes transport in hemodynamically compromised patients, and requires minimal equipment (scalpel, suction, cautery, and abdominal temporary closure dressings). Patients with significant intra-abdominal fluid as the primary component of their ACS, rather than bowel or retroperitoneal edema, may be candidates for decompression via a percutaneous drain (91,92). Differentiation of those amenable to such drainage is determined by bedside ultrasound, hence obviating a trip to the operating room for a critically ill patient (Fig. 75.12).

With morbidity and mortality rates exceeding 50% (82,86, 93), patients at risk for development of ACS, particularly those receiving large amounts of crystalloid and blood products during shock resuscitation, should be evaluated closely. Development of secondary ACS is a particularly indolent process; decreasing urine output and increasing peak airway pressures may herald the onset of intra-abdominal hypertension. Moreover, despite prior decompression with temporary abdominal closure, patients may develop recurrent ACS, which impacts overall morbidity and mortality (82). Some clinicians have queried aggressive intervention to prevent the development of ACS, such as the role of limiting unnecessary volume resuscitation and the use of alternative fluids such as colloids (15); however, the choice of albumin for fluid resuscitation in the intensive care unit has always been questioned (94). Supranormal trauma resuscitation has been shown to require more crystalloid administration and to cause more cases of ACS (86); therefore, goal-directed therapy should aim for an oxygen delivery index of $\geq$500 mL/minute/m^2 (10). Although perhaps counterintuitive in the acute resuscitation of patients, early administration of vasoactive agents to reduce the volume of crystalloid administered might be a therapeutic alternative in these patients at risk for ACS. In patients with acute renal failure, with minimal to no urine output, judicious fluid administration, early use of pressors, and institution of renal replacement therapy prior to fluid overload may also be warranted.

Damage control surgery and the recognition of the abdominal compartment syndrome have improved patient outcomes but at the cost of an open abdomen. Over 20% of patients with an open abdomen suffer a significant number of gastrointestinal complications that prolong their hospital course. Reported complications include intra-abdominal abscess, bile leaks, enteric fistula, and bowel perforations (Fig. 75.13) (95). Management includes operative or percutaneous drainage of abscesses, ERCP and drainage of bilomas, and control of fistulae and nutritional support for bowel complications. Current research is under way to develop techniques to minimize complications and reduce morbidity in patients with these devastating injuries.

ANCILLARY CARE ISSUES

Tubes and Drains

Following operative or nonoperative management of abdominal injuries, patients may have a variety of tubes and drains. Intra-abdominal drains are typically closed suction drains such as JP or Blake drains; the amount from the drain should be quantified every 8-hour shift, and the character of the output (bilious, succus, bloody, etc.) from the drains should be monitored daily. Although general guidelines for drain removal are <30 to 50 mL/day, one should consult with the surgeon prior to removal. Patients with rectal injuries may have presacral drains placed, which consist of Penrose drains exiting next to the rectum; these are passive drains, and should be covered with ABD pads for appropriate coverage. Patients with open abdomens and temporary abdominal closure will often have drains of some type; again, quantity and quality of the effluent may guide treatment options such as intravenous fluid replacement and need for return to the operating room.

Enteral access for nutrition is acquired through multiple techniques. NGTs, placed for gastric decompression, can be used for enteral nutrition once NGT output drops off. Gastrostomy tubes, either percutaneously or operatively placed, exit the abdominal cavity in the left upper quadrant. These should be placed to gravity for 24 hours after initial insertion. Jejunal feeding tubes are operatively placed; surgeons may choose to use needle catheter jejunostomy (NCJ) tubes or red rubber catheters. The primary issues with jejunal feeding tubes are those encountered with NCJs. Due to the small caliber of the feeding tube, there is the propensity for clogging. The NCJ should be flushed every 6 hours with saline, and only NCJ compatible enteral formulas should be used. Additionally, no medications should be placed down the NCJ. Nasojejunal tubes, often called nasobiliary feeding tubes, may be placed in the ICU using upper endoscopy.

Nutrition

Although the topic of nutrition could encompass an entire textbook, a few issues warrant mention (96). Multiple studies have illustrated the importance of early total enteral nutrition (TEN) in the trauma population, particularly its impact in reducing septic complications (97–100). The route of enteral feedings, stomach versus small bowel, tends to be less important as gut tolerance appears equivalent unless there is upper gastrointestinal pathology (101,102). Although early enteral nutrition is the goal, one should be cognizant of any bowel anastomoses; typically, evidence of bowel function should be present prior to advancing to goal tube feeds. Overzealous jejunal feeding can lead to small necrosis, a devastating complication (103). Patients undergoing monitoring for nonoperative management of solid organ injuries should remain NPO in the first 24 to 48 hours in case they require an operation. There is some residual concern about TEN in patients with an open abdomen; tube feeding, by any route, may be started within 24 hours of abdominal closure, as over 90% of patients will tolerate TEN (104, 105). Moreover, in patients relegated to an open abdomen, TEN should be started. The role of trophic tube feeds (10–20 mL/hour) while actively attempting to close fascia remains controversial.

Prophylaxis

A critical component of the overall care of the multiply injured patient in the ICU includes prevention of secondary complications, such as deep venous thrombosis (DVT) and stress gastritis. Administration of heparinoids for the prevention of DVT following trauma or surgical intervention is the current standard of care (106). Issues following abdominal trauma include timing of such administration in patients with either active bleeding from traumatic injury or those with solid organ injuries. Typically, heparin products are held until patients have resolved their hemorrhagic diathesis or until 24 hours after their hemoglobin has stabilized. Carafate is the current drug of choice for the prevention of stress gastritis (107,108). In patients who have had specific gastric surgery, H_2 blockers may be used as an alternative.

References

1. Janjua KJ, Sugrue M, Deane SA. Prospective evaluation of early missed injuries and the role of tertiary trauma survey. *J Trauma.* 1998;44:1000–1006; discussion 1006–1007.
2. Biffl WL, Harrington DT, Cioffi WG. Implementation of a tertiary trauma survey decreases missed injuries. *J Trauma.* 2003;54:38–43; discussion 43–44.
3. Enderson BL, Reath DB, Meadors J, et al. The tertiary trauma survey: a prospective study of missed injury. *J Trauma.* 1990;30:666–669; discussion 669–670.
4. Brooks A, Holroyd B, Riley B. Missed injury in major trauma patients. *Injury.* 2004;35:407–410.
5. Buduhan G, McRitchie DI. Missed injuries in patients with multiple trauma. *J Trauma.* 2000;49:600–605.
6. Moore FA, McKinley BA, Moore EE, et al. Inflammation and the Host Response to Injury, a large-scale collaborative project: patient-oriented research core—standard operating procedures for clinical care. III. Guidelines for shock resuscitation. *J Trauma.* 2006;61:82–89.
7. Herbert PC, Wells G, Blajchman MA, et al. A multicenter, randomized, controlled trial of transfusion requirements in critical care. *N Engl J Med.* 1999;340:409–417.
8. Moore FA, Moore EE, Sauaia A. Blood transfusion. An independent risk factor for postinjury multiple organ failure. *Arch Surg.* 1997;132:620–624; discussion 624–625.
9. Abou-Khalil B, Scalea TM, Trooskin SZ, et al. Hemodynamic responses to shock in young trauma patients: need for invasive monitoring. *Crit Care Med.* 1994;22:633–639.
10. McKinley BA, Kozar RA, Cocanour CS, et al. Normal versus supranormal oxygen delivery goals in shock resuscitation: the response is the same. *J Trauma.* 2002;53:825–832.
11. Velmahos GC, Demetriades D, Shoemaker WC, et al. Endpoints of resuscitation of critically injured patients: normal or supranormal? A prospective randomized trial. *Ann Surg.* 2000;232:409–418.
12. Cooper MS, Stewart PM. Corticosteroid insufficiency in acutely ill patients. *N Engl J Med.* 2003;348:727–734.
13. Offner PJ, Moore EE, Ciesla D. The adrenal response after severe trauma. *Am J Surg.* 2002;184:649–653.
14. Balogh Z, McKinley BA, Holcomb JB, et al. Both primary and secondary abdominal compartment syndrome can be predicted early and are harbingers of multiple organ failure. *J Trauma.* 2003;54:848–859.
15. Balogh Z, McKinley BA, Cocanour CS, et al. Secondary abdominal compartment syndrome is an elusive early complication of traumatic shock resuscitation. *Am J Surg.* 2002;184:538–543.
16. Carrillo EH, Wohltmann C, Richardson JD, et al. Evolution in the treatment of complex blunt liver injuries. *Curr Probl Surg.* 2001;38:1–60.
17. Hurtuk M, Reed RL, Espositio TJ, et al. Trauma surgeons practice what they preach: the NTDB story on solid organ injury management. *J Trauma.* 2006;61:243–255.
18. Peitzman AB, Heil B, Rivera L, et al. Blunt splenic injury in adults: multi-institutional study of the Eastern Association for the Surgery of Trauma. *J Trauma.* 2000;49:177–187.
19. Richardson DJ, Franklin GA, Lukan JK, et al. Evolution in the management of hepatic trauma: a 25-year perspective. *Ann Surg.* 2000;232:324–330.
20. Velmahos GC, Toutouzas KG, Radin R, et al. Nonoperative treatment of blunt injury to solid abdominal organs: a prospective study. *Arch Surg.* 2003;138:844–851.
21. Malhotra AK, Fabian TC, Croce MA, et al. Blunt hepatic injury: a paradigm shift from operative to nonoperative management in the 1990s. *Ann Surg.* 2000;231:804–813.
22. Pachter HL, Guth AA, Hofstett SR, et al. Changing patterns in the management of splenic trauma: the impact of nonoperative trauma. *Ann Surg.* 1998;227:708–717; discussion 717–719.
23. Christmas AB, Wilson AK, Manning B, et al. Selective management of blunt hepatic injuries including nonoperative management is a safe and effective strategy. *Surgery.* 2005;138:606–610.
24. Velmahos GC, Toutousas K, Radin R, et al. High success with nonoperative management of blunt hepatic trauma: the liver is a sturdy organ. *Arch Surg.* 2003;138:475–480; discussion 480–481.

25. Rojani RR, Claridge JA, Yowler CJ, et al. Improved outcome of adult blunt splenic injury: a cohort analysis. *Surgery.* 2006;140:625–631; discussion 631–632.
26. Goan YG, Huang MS, Lin JM. Nonoperative management for extensive hepatic and splenic injuries with significant hemoperitoneum in adults. *J Trauma.* 1998;45:360–364; discussion 365.
27. Nwomeh BC, Nadler EP, Meza MP, et al. Contrast extravasation predicts the need for operative intervention in children with blunt splenic trauma. *J Trauma.* 2004;56:537–541.
28. Malhotra AK, Latifi R, Fabian TC, et al. Multiplicity of solid organ injury: influence on management and outcomes after blunt abdominal trauma. *J Trauma.* 2003;54:925–929.
29. Schurr MJ, Fabian TC, Gavant M, et al. Management of blunt splenic trauma: computed tomographic contrast blush predicts failure of nonoperative management. *J Trauma.* 1995;39:507–512; discussion 512–513.
30. Falimirski ME, Provost D. Nonsurgical management of solid abdominal organ injury in patients over 55 years of age. *Am Surg.* 2000;66:631–635.
31. Myers JG, Dent DL, Stewart RM, et al. Blunt splenic injuries: dedicated trauma surgeons can achieve a high rate of nonoperative success in patients of all ages. *J Trauma.* 2000;48:801–805; discussion 805–806.
32. Harbrecht BG, Peitzman AB, Rivera L, et al. Contribution of age and gender to outcome of blunt splenic injury in adults: multicenter study of the Eastern Association for the Surgery of Trauma. *J Trauma.* 2001;51:887–895.
33. Moore EE, Cogbill TH, Jurkovich GJ, et al. Organ injury scaling: spleen and liver (1994 revision). *J Trauma.* 1995;38:323–324.
34. Moore EE, Cogbill TH, Malangoni MA, et al. Organ injury scaling. *Surg Clin North Am.* 1995;75:293–303.
35. Moore EE, Cogbill TH, Malangoni MA, et al. Organ injury scaling, II: pancreas, duodenum, small bowel, colon, and rectum. *J Trauma.* 1990;30:1427–1429.
36. Watson GA, Rosengart MR, Zenati MS, et al. Nonoperative management of severe blunt splenic injury: are we getting better? *J Trauma.* 2006;61:1113–1118.
37. Johnson JW, Gracias VH, Gupta R, et al. Hepatic angiography in patients undergoing damage control laparotomy. *J Trauma.* 2002;52:1102–1106.
38. Denton JR, Moore EE, Coldwell DM. Multimodality treatment for grade V hepatic injuries: perihepatic packing, arterial embolization, and venous stenting. *J Trauma.* 1997;42:964–967.
39. Haan JM, Biffl WL, Knudson MM, et al. Splenic embolization revisited: a multicenter review. *J Trauma.* 2004;56:542–547.
40. Dent D, Alsabrook G, Erickson BA, et al. Blunt splenic injuries: high nonoperative management rate can be achieved with selective embolization. *J Trauma.* 2004;56:1063–1067.
41. Davis KA, Fabian ATC, Croce MA, et al. Improved success in nonoperative management of blunt splenic injuries: embolization of splenic artery pseudoaneurysms. *J Trauma.* 1998;44:1008–1013; discussion 1013–1015.
42. Lyass S, Sela T, Lebensart PD, et al. Follow-up imaging studies of blunt splenic injury: do they influence management? *Isr Med Assoc.* 2001;10:731–733.
43. Cox JC, Fabian TC, Maish GO 3rd, et al. Routine follow-up imaging is unnecessary in the management of blunt hepatic injury. *J Trauma.* 2005;59:1175–1178; discussion 1178–1180.
44. Patton JH Jr, Lyden SP, Croce MA, et al. Pancreatic trauma: a simplified management guideline. *J Trauma.* 1997;43:234–239; discussion 239–241.
45. Wales PW, Shuckett B, Kim PC. Long-term outcome after nonoperative management of complete traumatic pancreatic transection in children. *J Pediatr Surg.* 2001;36:823–827.
46. Jobst MA, Canty TG, Lynch FP. Management of pancreatic injury in pediatric blunt abdominal trauma. *J Pediatr Surg.* 1999;34:818–823.
47. Lin BC, Liu NJ, Fang JF, et al. Long-term results of endoscopic stent in the management of blunt major pancreatic duct injury. *Surg Endosc.* 2006;20:1551–1555.
48. Cogbill TH, Moore EE, Feliciano DV. Conservative management of duodenal trauma: a multicenter perspective. *J Trauma.* 1990;30:1469–1475.
49. Huerta S, Bui T, Porral D, et al. Predictors of morbidity and mortality in patients with traumatic duodenal injuries. *Am Surg.* 2005;71:763–767.
50. Demetriades D, Gomez H, Chahwan S, et al. Gunshot injuries to the liver: the role of selective nonoperative management. *J Am Coll Surg.* 1999;188:343–348.
51. Moore EE. When is nonoperative management of a gunshot wound to the liver appropriate? *J Am Coll Surg.* 1999;188:427–428.
52. Chiu WC, Shanmuganathan K, Mirvis SE, et al. Determining the need for laparotomy in penetrating torso trauma: a prospective study using triple-contrast enhanced abdominopelvic computed tomography. *J Trauma.* 2001;51:860–868; discussion 868–869.
53. Demetriades D, Hadjizacharia P, Constantinou C, et al. Selective nonoperative management of penetrating abdominal solid organ injuries. *Ann Surg.* 2006;244:620–628.
54. Kozar RA, Moore FA, Cothren CC, et al. Risk factors for hepatic morbidity following nonoperative management: multicenter study. *Arch Surg.* 2006;141:451–459.
55. Giss SR, Dobrilovic N, Brown RL, et al. Complications of nonoperative management of pediatric blunt hepatic injury: diagnosis, management, and outcomes. *J Trauma.* 2006;61:334–339.
56. Goldman R, Zilkowski M, Mullins R, et al. Delayed celiotomy for the treatment of bile leak, compartment syndrome, and other hazards of nonoperative management of blunt liver injury. *Am J Surg.* 2003;185:492–497.
57. Cocanour CS, Moore FA, Ware DN, et al. Delayed complications of nonoperative management of blunt adult splenic trauma. *Arch Surg.* 1998;133:619–624; discussion 624–625.
58. Cothren CC, Biffl WL, Moore EE, et al. Characteristic radiographic findings of post-injury splenic autotransplantation: avoiding a diagnostic dilemma. *J Trauma.* 2004;57(3):537–541.
59. Fakhry SM, Watts DD, Luchette FA; EAST Multi-Institutional Hollow Viscus Injury Research Group. Current diagnostic approaches lack sensitivity in the diagnosis of perforated blunt small bowel injury: analysis from 275,557 trauma admissions from the EAST multi-institutional HVI trial. *J Trauma.* 2003;54:295–306.
60. Fakhry SM, Brownstein M, Watts DD, et al. Relatively short diagnostic delays (<8 hours) produce morbidity and mortality in blunt small bowel injury: an analysis of time to operative intervention in 198 patients from a multicenter experience. *J Trauma.* 2000;48:408–414.
61. Niederee MJ, Byrnes MC, Helmer SD, et al. Delay in diagnosis of hollow viscus injuries: effect on outcome. *Am Surg.* 2003;69:293–298.
62. Ng AK, Simons RK, Torreggiani WC, et al. Intra-abdominal free fluid without solid organ injury in blunt abdominal trauma: an indication for laparotomy. *J Trauma.* 2002;52:1134–1140.
63. Miller PR, Croce MA, Bee TK, et al. Associated injuries in blunt solid organ trauma: implications for missed injury in nonoperative management. *J Trauma.* 2002;53:238–242.
64. Rodriguez C, Barone JE, Wilbanks TO, et al. Isolated free fluid on computed tomographic scan in blunt abdominal trauma: a systematic review of incidence and management. *J Trauma.* 2002;53:79–85.
65. McAnena OJ, Marx JA, Moore EE. Peritoneal lavage enzyme determinations following blunt and penetrating abdominal trauma. *J Trauma.* 1991;31:1161–1164.
66. Heneman PL, Marx JA, Moore EE, et al. Diagnostic peritoneal lavage: accuracy in predicting necessary laparotomy following blunt and penetrating trauma. *J Trauma.* 1990;30:1345–1355.
67. Velmahos GC, Gomez H, Falabella A, et al. Operative management of civilian rectal gunshot wounds: simpler is better. *World J Surg.* 2000;24:114–118.
68. Leppaniemi AK, Haapiainen RK. Risk factors of delayed diagnosis of pancreatic trauma. *Eur J Surg.* 1999;165:1134–1137.
69. Arkovitz MS, Johnson N, Garcia VF. Pancreatic trauma in children: mechanisms of injury. *J Trauma.* 1997;42:49–53.
70. Takishima T, Sugimoto K, Hirata M, et al. Serum amylase level on admission in the diagnosis of blunt injury to the pancreas: its significance and limitations. *Ann Surg.* 1997;226:70–76.
71. Cogbill TH, Moore EE, Feliciano DV, et al. Hepatic enzyme response and hyperpyrexia after severe liver injury. *Am Surg.* 1992;58:395–399.
72. Weng J, Brown CVR, Rhee P, et al. White blood cell and platelet counts can be used to differentiate between infection and the normal response after splenectomy for trauma: prospective validation. *J Trauma.* 2005;59:1076–1080.
73. Howdieshell TR, Heffernan D, Dipiro JT. Therapeutic Agents Committee of the Surgical Infection Society. Surgical infection society guidelines for vaccination after traumatic injury. *Surg Infect.* 2006;7:275–303.
74. Demetriades D, Murray JA, Chan L, et al. Penetrating colon injuries requiring resection: diversion or primary anastomosis? An AAST prospective multicenter study. *J Trauma.* 2001;50:765–775.
75. Conlon KC, Labow D, Leung D, et al. Prospective randomized clinical trial of the value of intraperitoneal drainage after pancreatic resection. *Ann Surg.* 2001;234:487–493; discussion 493–494.
76. Ridgeway MG, Stabile BE. Surgical management and treatment of pancreatic fistulas. *Surg Clin North Am.* 1996;76:1159–1173.
77. Howard TJ, Stonerock CE, Sarkar J, et al. Contemporary treatment strategies for external pancreatic fistulas. *Surgery.* 1998;124:627–632.
78. Wolford HY, Cothren CC, Moore EE. Postinjury abdominal aortic graft infection: documentation and successful management. *J Trauma.* 2006;61:1274–1276.
79. Moore EE, Burch JM, Franciose RJ, et al. Staged physiologic restoration and damage control surgery. *World J Surg.* 1998;22:1184–1190; discussion 1190–1191.
80. Hirshberg A, Walden R. Damage control for abdominal trauma. *Surg Clin North Am.* 1997;77:813–820.
81. Sagraves SG, Toschlog EA, Rotondo MF. Damage control surgery—the intensivist's role. *J Intensive Care Med.* 2006;21:5–16.
82. Raeburn CD, Moore EE, Biffl WL, et al. The abdominal compartment syndrome is a morbid complication of postinjury damage control surgery. *Am J Surg.* 2001;182:542–546.
83. Burch JM, Moore EE, Moore FA, et al. The abdominal compartment syndrome. *Surg Clin North Am.* 1996;76:833–842.
84. Meldrum DR, Moore FA, Moore EE, et al. Prospective characterization and selective management of the abdominal compartment syndrome. *Am J Surg.* 1997;174:667–672.
85. Ivatury RR, Porter JM, Simon RJ, et al. Intra-abdominal hypertension after life-threatening penetrating abdominal trauma: prophylaxis, incidence,

and clinical relevance to gastric mucosal pH and abdominal compartment syndrome. *J Trauma.* 1998;44:1016–1021.
86. Balogh Z, McKinley BA, Cox Jr CS, et al. Abdominal compartment syndrome: the cause or effect of postinjury multiple organ failure. *Shock.* 2003;20:483–492.
87. Maxwell RA, Fabian TC, Croce MA, et al. Secondary ACS: an underappreciated manifestation of severe hemorrhagic shock. *J Trauma.* 1999;47:995–999.
88. McNelis J, Marini CP, Jurkiewicz A, et al. Predictive factors associated with the development of abdominal compartment syndrome in the surgical intensive care unit. *Arch Surg.* 2002;137:133–136.
89. Kron IL. A simple technique to accurately determine intra-abdominal pressure. *Crit Care Med.* 1989;17:714–715.
90. Cheatham ML, White MW, Sagraves SG, et al. Abdominal perfusion pressure: a superior parameter in the assessment of intra-abdominal hypertension. *J Trauma.* 2000;49:621–626.
91. Corcos AC, Sherman HF. Percutaneous treatment of secondary abdominal compartment syndrome. *J Trauma.* 2001;51:1062–1064.
92. Latenser BA, Kowal-Vern A, Kimball D, et al. A pilot study comparing percutaneous decompression with decompressive laparotomy for acute abdominal compartment syndrome in thermal injury. *J Burn Care Rehabil.* 2002;23:190–195.
93. Biffl WL, Moore EE, Burch JM, et al. Secondary abdominal compartment syndrome is a highly lethal event. *Am J Surg.* 2001;182:645–648.
94. Finfer S, Norton R, Bellomo R, et al. The SAFE study: saline vs. albumin for fluid resuscitation in the critically ill. *Vox Sang.* 2004;87(Suppl 2):123–131.
95. Miller RS, Morris JA Jr, Diaz JJ Jr, et al. Complications after 344 damage-control open celiotomies. *J Trauma.* 2005;59:1365–1371.
96. Jacobs DG, Jacobs DO, Kudsk KA, et al. Practice management guidelines for nutritional support of the trauma patient. *J Trauma.* 2004;57:660–678.
97. Moore FA, Moore EE, Jones TN, et al. TEN versus TPN following major abdominal trauma—reduced septic morbidity. *J Trauma.* 1989;29:916–922.
98. Moore FA, Feliciano DV, Andrassy RJ, et al. Early enteral feeding, compared with parenteral, reduces postoperative septic complications. The results of a meta-analysis. *Ann Surg.* 1992;216:172–183.
99. Moore FA, Moore EE, Haenel JB. Clinical benefits of early post-injury enteral feeding. *Clin Intensive Care.* 1995;6:21–27.
100. Hasenboehler E, Williams A, Leinhase I, et al. Metabolic changes after polytrauma: an imperative for early nutritional support. *World J Emerg Surg.* 2006;1:29.
101. Neumann DA, DeLegge MH. Gastric versus small-bowel tube feeding in the intensive care unit: a prospective comparison of efficacy. *Crit Care Med.* 2002;30:1436–1438.
102. Reignier J, Bensaid S, Perrin-Gachadoat D, et al. Erythromycin and early enteral nutrition in mechanically ventilated patients. *Crit Care Med.* 2002;30:1237–1241.
103. Melis M, Fichera A, Ferguson MK. Bowel necrosis associated with early jejunal tube feeding: a complication of postoperative enteral nutrition. *Arch Surg.* 2006;141:701–704.
104. Cothren CC, Moore EE, Ciesla DJ, et al. Post-injury abdominal compartment syndrome does not preclude early enteral feeding following definitive closure. *Am J Surg.* 2004;188:653–658.
105. Kozar RA, McQuiggan MM, Moore EE, et al. Postinjury enteral tolerance is reliably achieved by a standardized protocol. *J Surg Res.* 2002;104:70–75.
106. Rogers FB, Cipolle MD, Velmahos G, et al. Practice management guidelines for the prevention of venous thromboembolism in trauma patients: the EAST practice management guidelines work group. *J Trauma.* 2002;53:142–164.
107. Maier RV, Mitchell D, Gentilello L. Optimal therapy for stress gastritis. *Ann Surg.* 1994;220:353–360.
108. Eddleston JM, Vohra A, Scott P, et al. A comparison of the frequency of stress ulceration and secondary pneumonia in sucralfate- or ranitidine-treated intensive care unit patients. *Crit Care Med.* 1991;19:1491–1496.

CHAPTER 76 ■ EVALUATING THE ACUTE ABDOMEN

H. DAVID REINES • HANI SEOUDI

An *acute abdomen* is any problem in which the patient's pain or other physical findings originates from an abdominal lesion resulting in serious morbidity or mortality without appropriate therapy.

As sicker patients are admitted to our intensive care units (ICUs), the challenge of diagnosis and treatment of the acute abdomen becomes more important. Patients who are immunocompromised from diseases such as HIV, posttransplant, or chemotherapy frequently present with a nonclassic sign of pain and inflammation. Patients who are post–cardiac surgery have a well-recognized constellation of intra-abdominal catastrophes. Bariatric surgery presents ICU physicians with a whole new set of intra-abdominal problems, which if not recognized early, can lead to death or significant morbidity.

Patients admitted to respiratory care units are subject to various acute abdominal problems. Aranha and Goldberg reported that 32 of 175 (18%) patients on ventilators had acute abdominal problems in the following order of frequency (1): gastrointestinal bleeding, ileus, bowel obstruction, and peritonitis that required operation. Acute abdominal problems are frequent sources of admission and complications in ICUs (2). Early recognition of the acute abdomen and initiation of definitive surgical or medical therapy often determines the outcome. Therefore, knowledge of common abdominal problems and appropriate diagnostic modalities are essential parts of the armamentarium of all ICU physicians. A high index of suspicion that an abdominal problem is causing a patient's critical illness is important to stimulate the necessary diagnostic and therapeutic responses.

Searching for a cause of abdominal signs and symptoms is difficult in the critically ill patient. The patient may not be able to give a lucid history, especially if intubated or sedated. Physical findings may be masked by narcotics, steroids, and other therapy administered.

ANATOMY

The peritoneal cavity is a potential space with less than 100 mL of free fluid to lubricate the bowel, liver, and other abdominal organs. Knowledge of the sensory nerve supply of the abdomen is particularly important in evaluating the abdomen in critically ill patients. Deep visceral pain is transmitted via autonomic nerves, both sympathetic and parasympathetic. Visceral pain is poorly localized as pain receptors are much sparser than somatic receptors. The pain is typically unpleasant and is associated with autonomic symptoms such as tachycardia, bradycardia, and diaphoresis. The primary stimulus to visceral pain is stretching of hollow viscera or solid organ capsules. Visceral pain signals share common pathways with somatic pain in the spinothalamic tracts. Visceral pain signals are received in areas of the sensory cortex where somatic structures that originated from the same embryonic segment are represented. This is the reason why visceral pain tends to be referred to remote dermatomes, e.g., shoulder pain caused by diaphragmatic irritation. Abdominal pain becomes more localized when the parietal peritoneum is affected by the underlying inflammatory process. The parietal peritoneum has a rich somatic sensory supply.

Knowledge of the blood supply of the abdomen is also important given the extensive diagnostic and therapeutic applications of angiography in acute abdominal pathology. The foregut (esophagus to duodenum) is supplied by branches of the celiac trunk, the midgut (duodenum to distal transverse colon) is supplied by branches of the superior mesenteric artery (SMA), and the hindgut (descending colon and rectum) is supplied by branches of the inferior mesenteric artery (IMA). The right hepatic artery is replaced (arises from the SMA) in about 10% of the population. An embolus tends to lodge distal to the origins of the most proximal branches of the SMA, namely, the inferior pancreaticoduodenal, the middle colic, and the proximal jejunal branches. The proximal jejunum and the transverse colon are typically spared in acute ischemia due to SMA embolism compared to thrombosis. Collateral circulation exists between branches of the three mesenteric vessels. The marginal artery of Drummond is formed by the anastomosing branches of the SMA and IMA along the mesenteric border of the colon. The arc of Riolan connects the middle colic artery with the ascending branch of the left colic artery. The internal iliac artery contributes to colonic circulation through the anastomosis between the middle and superior rectal arteries.

HISTORY

A detailed review of abdominal symptoms should be obtained from either the patient or a family member. The history should include previous surgery, family history, and a list of medications. It should also include allergies, immunosuppressive drugs, and a history of human immunodeficiency virus (HIV), hepatitis, or chemotherapy. As we become more globalized, awareness of infectious disease from emerging countries is necessary for evaluation of disparate symptoms. A complete surgical history is likewise necessary to help focus on the diagnostic and therapeutic interventions. Previous abdominal surgery and hernias are the two most common causes of bowel obstruction. The presence of a percutaneous endoscopic gastrostomy (PEG) or other tubes should alert the physician to the possibility of a problem related to tube misplacement or obstruction.The history should detail any nausea and vomiting, hematemesis, hematochezia, and constipation. Symptoms of biliary disease, especially pain, and jaundice, and a history of ethanol use should be noted. Alcohol abuse and cholelithiasis are the two most common causes of acute pancreatitis.

A careful evaluation of the characteristics of abdominal pain is essential. Its nature, onset, associated symptoms, radiation, and other characteristics are useful in localizing and delineating the cause. Abdominal symptoms can be masked by other disease processes. A diabetic patient who presents with diabetic ketoacidosis may have an underlying abdominal catastrophe as a precipitating factor. Syncope is a symptom that can be caused by ruptured aneurysm, a ruptured spleen, an ectopic pregnancy, or any severe abdominal catastrophe, as well as by neurologic and metabolic problems.

Inferior myocardial infarction, pericarditis, and lower lobe pneumonia may present with upper abdominal pain. Diabetic and immune-suppressed patients, particularly those on steroids, can present with advanced intra-abdominal sepsis before peritoneal signs become obvious. Arthritic patients who are taking steroids or nonsteroidal anti-inflammatory agents and whose conditions suddenly deteriorate must be suspected of harboring an intra-abdominal problem, such as gastrointestinal bleeding or perforation, as a consequence of their medications. Severe bleeding can occur when a posterior ulcer in the first portion of the duodenum erodes into the gastroduodenal artery. Syncope at the onset of abdominal pain may signify a perforated ulcer or intra-abdominal hemorrhage such as from a ruptured aneurysm, spleen, or ectopic pregnancy. Although porphyria and sickle cell crises can mimic abdominal catastrophes, they rarely cause admission to the intensive care unit.

PHYSICAL EXAMINATION

Abdominal examination in the critically ill patient can be challenging as many patients will be unconscious or intubated. Examination of the abdomen in the critically ill patient who may be combative, comatose, narcotized, or paralyzed is difficult. The standard routine of inspection, palpation, percussion, and auscultation should be followed. Vital signs, including blood pressure (with the patient sitting if possible), pulse, respiratory rate, and rectal or core temperature, should be taken. Too often, oral or axillary temperatures are normal because of peripheral cooling, nasal oxygen administration, or nasogastric (NG) tubes.

Inspection of the abdomen can give many clues. The Gray-Turner sign, flank ecchymosis, was initially described with hemorrhagic pancreatitis but can occur with other causes of retroperitoneal bleeding. The Sister Mary Joseph nodule indicates abdominal or breast malignancy that spread along the round ligament to the umbilicus. Dilated abdominal wall veins indicated advanced portal hypertension. A large abdominal aortic aneurysm may be discerned as a pulsating upper abdominal mass in a thin patient. Absent or hypoactive bowel sounds is a nonspecific sign as many patients will have ileus associated with their critical illness. Bowel sounds are frequently absent in paralyzed patients, despite the fact that muscular paralysis should not eliminate autonomic bowel function. Hyperactive sounds or "rushes" are most common with small bowel obstruction. The presence of bowel sounds, however, does not always correlate with normal bowel function.

The presence of guarding or rigidity indicates peritoneal irritation. Rebound may not be present in a postoperative patient with significant abdominal pathology. It is important to note, however, that patients' response to the presence of blood in the peritoneal cavity is variable. Some patients will have guarding or rigidity whereas others will have a soft abdomen. Assessment of obese patients for abdominal wall rigidity is also unreliable. Obese patients may also have groin or incisional hernias that are not easily discerned. Patients with mesenteric ischemia have pain that is out of proportion to the findings of the physical exam. Rectal and pelvic examinations are frequently avoided in the ICU; however, they are mandatory to discover low pelvic abscesses and masses, prostatic infection, and bloody stools.

The physical examination of the acute abdomen should be performed by an experienced physician on a regular basis. Serial examinations are essential to carefully document any progression of tenderness, muscular rigidity, and the overall trend toward improvement or deterioration. An isolated examination is not nearly as useful as sequential examinations by the same observer. The physician who will ultimately make the decision whether surgical intervention is required should be involved as early as possible.

The presence of abdominal distention in the setting of decreased urine output and increased ventilator pressures should lead to a possible diagnosis of abdominal compartment syndrome and immediately to a measurement of intra-abdominal pressures using bladder pressure manometry.

LABORATORY EVALUATION

Laboratory tests should be viewed as adjuncts in the evaluation of patients. They often provide useful information but are rarely diagnostic. Depending excessively on laboratory findings is costly and occasionally misleading. A complete hemogram, including hematocrit, hemoglobin, and complete white blood cell (WBC) count, is routine. A decreasing WBC count may give a false sense of improvement, because severe sepsis can cause a leukopenia with a shift to the left that will be missed without a differential count. Urinalysis, including specific gravity and analysis for bacteria, bile, and reducing substances, should be performed. Patients with indwelling Foley catheters often have asymptomatic bacteriuria and mild hematuria. A full workup of "benign bacteriuria" may delay the diagnosis of the true cause of sepsis. The serum amylase concentration, especially fractionated into isoenzymes, is helpful in diagnosing intra-abdominal catastrophe when it is elevated but is not specific. Amylase may be increased in ischemic bowel disease, facial trauma, perforated ulcer, and pancreatitis, or without apparent cause (3). The serum lipase is a more specific marker of acute pancreatitis than amylase and is less influenced by other intra-abdominal problems. Calcium and phosphorus values are also helpful in determining the severity of pancreatitis.

An elevated serum bilirubin level is associated with sepsis, resolving hematoma, hemolysis, and hepatobiliary disease. Likewise, the lactate dehydrogenase concentration may be elevated in numerous disease processes. Liver enzymes, such as serum glutamate oxaloacetic transaminase, serum glutamic pyruvic transaminase, and alkaline phosphatase may be helpful but are rarely diagnostic by themselves.

Laboratory data are most useful in the management and correction of fluids, electrolytes, and acid-base derangements. Persistent acidosis and arterial hypoxemia suggest severe metabolic problems that may be a reflection of unresolved third-space losses from untreated abdominal sepsis or ischemia. These causes are frequently overlooked in the early workup of these problems.

RADIOGRAPHIC STUDIES

Although plain portable radiographs of the abdomen are obtained on most patients with suspicious abdominal findings, their yield is relatively low and their quality is frequently suboptimal. They are most useful to determine the position of intra-abdominal tubes such as NG and drains. Plain abdominal films are useful to examine abnormal gas patterns intraluminally and extraluminally. The absence of gas may be found with ischemic bowel, whereas small bowel obstruction and colonic volvulus present with massive gaseous distention. An upright abdominal film is desirable; however, many patients in an ICU cannot tolerate this procedure, and therefore, a left lateral decubitus film to discover air-fluid levels and free air above the liver should be obtained. Free air from perforated viscus is best seen in an upright chest radiograph, which is usually possible to obtain in the critically ill patient by sitting the patient up in bed and elevating the head of the bed 75 to 90 degrees.

A retrospective study of 1,000 patients presenting to the emergency room (ER) with acute abdominal pain compared the use of plain films to computed tomography (CT) scans. The majority, 588 of 871 (68%), of abdominal radiographs were interpreted as nonspecific, whereas 83 demonstrated specific diagnostic abnormalities, including bowel obstruction (4%), urolithiasis (2%), ileus (2%), and abnormal foreign bodies (1%) (4). No free air was found. Films were most sensitive for foreign bodies (90%) and bowel obstruction (49%). Only 38 of 188 CT scans were normal. Of these, 120 of 188 had undergone plain films. CT was predictive of bowel obstruction in 75% and pancreatitis in 60%. Of the 120 patients who had both exams, abdominal films were negative in 20%, nonspecific in 76%, and abnormal in 4%. These data could be extrapolated to ICU patients although there are no studies to confirm similar findings.

Ultrasonography has emerged as a dependable adjunctive diagnostic tool. It can be brought to the bedside and give data on acalculous cholecystitis, fluid collection, and blood flow. Ultrasound is useful in demonstrating intra-abdominal blood or fluid and to perform percutaneous abscess drainage. It is less invasive and less expensive than CAT scan and does not require transporting patients. However, in patients who have been in an ICU for extended periods, the gallbladder can be expected to be distended with poor contractility, and the ultrasound is not specific for acalculous cholecystitis unless a radionuclide study using a HIDA (hepatobiliary iminodiacetic acid) scan confirms abnormal gallbladder filling. Ultrasound is also difficult to interpret in patients with distended bowel gas. Ultrasound can also be used as a therapeutic tool to help perform procedures such as percutaneous cholecystostomy (Fig. 76.1).

The CT scan has become the most widely used tool to examine the abdomen for abnormalities, and CT scanning is more accurate for diagnosing intra-abdominal fluid collections than any other modality. It is especially useful in liver, splenic, renal, and retroperitoneal abscesses but may not be as useful as ultrasound in the diagnosis of right upper quadrant and pelvic masses.

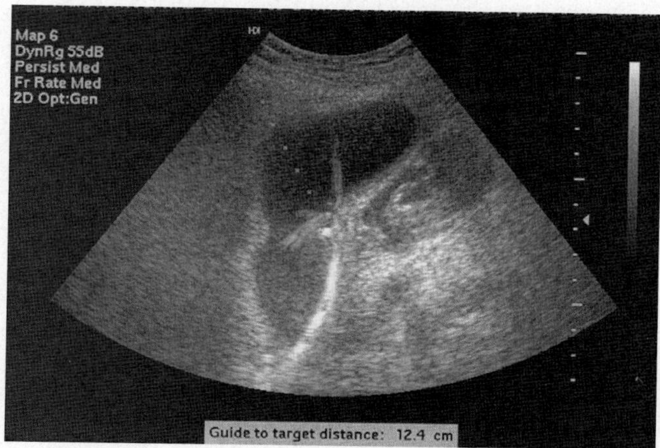

FIGURE 76.1. Ultrasound-guided percutaneous cholecystectomy.

Optimal use of CT scan requires oral contrast, which may be difficult for the critically ill patient to ingest and retain and may be an aspiration risk. It also requires transporting the patient to the scanner accompanied by the nurse, therapist, and physician, and the possibility exists of an untoward event during transport.

Despite the significant increase in accuracy and decrease in time of the actual scan, recent studies by Hendershot et al. (5) demonstrated that the time for a scan was significantly longer than imagined, because of the efforts to get patients ready, transport patients, transfer them to the table, and then repackage them and return them to the ICU.

The enthusiasm for CT scanning must also be tempered by an evaluation of the efficacy of scans in critically ill patients. In a study by Norwood and Civetta (6), scans were found to be helpful in only 23% of patients, most of whom had been examined because of postoperative sepsis. This study has not been repeated, and therefore it is difficult to determine the efficacy of the CT scan in ICU patients. The CT scan not only has become part of the diagnostic armamentarium, it can be increasingly useful as a therapeutic modality. CT drainage of abscesses, aspiration of pancreatic collections, CT-guided nephrostomy tube insertions, and aspiration of ascites are now easily performed.

A Gastrografin swallow is still an excellent tool to differentiate a gastric leak following gastric bypass surgery or persistent leak from a perforated ulcer.

Diagnostic peritoneal lavage (DPL) has long been a tool to help differentiate abdominal collections from intra-abdominal blood (7). Ultrasonography has largely obviated the need to perform bedside DPL, but the technique is still useful to drain tense ascites and determine the source and infectious nature of the fluid.

THERAPY

The treatment of intra-abdominal problems in the acutely ill frequently requires surgical intervention. Surgical consultation should be obtained early in the evaluation. In the preoperative patient, adequate volume resuscitation and electrolyte correction are vital to prepare the patient for surgical repair of the underlying problem. Most fluid losses in preoperative surgical patients are isotonic. Patients who are volume contracted may be hyponatremic, hypochloremic, hypokalemic, and alkalotic because of vomiting, nasogastric suctioning, and third-space losses. These patients require normal saline resuscitation to prevent anesthetic disaster. Only after volume and salt repletion will their chloride-dependent alkalosis resolve. Although hypokalemia may exist, potassium should be administered cautiously until oliguria is resolved.

Acute abdominal catastrophe may be the first event in the precipitous cascade of multiple organ system failure (MOSF). Unrecognized abdominal sepsis is associated with MOSF in 44% of cases (8,9). Early aggressive surgical therapy, vigorous fluid replacement, and appropriate antibiotic regimens are necessary.

The specific management of disease entities should be based on well-established surgical principles. However, the explosion of minimally invasive surgery has lead to a new era in surgical intervention. Many acute abdominal procedures can now be performed either via an open or laparoscopic technique. Most acute cholecystitis can be treated conservatively for 24 to 48 hours. If the signs and symptoms do not improve within 48 hours or if cholangitis appears, an endoscopic retrograde cholangiopancreatography (ERCP) can be performed to drain the common duct. A percutaneous cholecystostomy or a laparoscopic cholecystectomy can then be performed in most cases. Perforated ulcers can now be treated laparoscopically in some surgeons' hands. A true "sea change" in the treatment of ruptured abdominal aneurysm has taken place with the improvements in endovascular aortic repair (EVAR) (10). A significant number of patients can now be treated under local anesthesia with bilateral groin cutdown, avoiding the significant morbidity of open procedures. Although it is too early to determine how much the minimally invasive procedure can affect early and late mortality, initial studies imply that the overall mortality for EVAR, as well as ICU stay and morbidity, may be lower than that of open procedures (11).

Stress ulceration without perforation may be prophylactically treated with antacids, H2 blockers, and sucralfate, although aggressive pH control may lead to an increase in nosocomial pneumonia (12–14). Stress ulcer bleeding is rare, but the best treatment is prevention. If bleeding cannot be contained with conservative measures, an operative intervention should be undertaken, which carries with it a high mortality rate of 50% (15,16). Do not wait until multiple transfusions have created dilutional or hypothermic coagulopathies, because mortality rates will approach 100%.

The use of CT scan and ultrasonic-guided drainage and catheter decompression of intra-abdominal abscesses had revolutionized care in some postoperative patients. This procedure results in excellent control of the septic source with a low morbidity (17). It is often preferable to secondary exploratory laparotomy. However, if a patient persists in a downward clinical course, exploration with wide drainage of abscesses may be necessary. In patients with diffuse persistent peritonitis or necrotizing pancreatitis, conversion to an open abdomen with zipper technique may be needed to control the infection (18).

Antibiotics are not panacea for intra-abdominal sepsis, and abscesses will form despite adequate coverage. The use of antibiotics in acute abdominal problems is usually adjunctive to prevent systemic sepsis. The prolonged use of antibiotics for localized abscesses instead of surgical or radiologic drainage can lead to morbidity and increased mortality.

In patients with diffuse peritonitis or necrotizing infected pancreatitis, conversion from a closed abdomen into an open abdomen may be necessary to control the process (19).

Specific Disease States

Any stable patient in an ICU developing sudden shock or sepsis must be examined closely for an intra-abdominal cause. Several conditions that are common causes of abdominal symptoms in critically ill patients are presented in the following sections.

Although appendicitis is the most common abdominal condition requiring surgery, it is rarely seen in the ICU. Pancreatitis and acalculous cholecystitis are more common, especially after open heart surgery. Abdominal distention in elderly patients after orthopedic procedures is frequently caused by ileus and colonic pseudo-obstruction. Patients receiving mechanical ventilation are at high risk for gastrointestinal bleeding, ileus, and unrecognized perforation (2). Stress ulcer perforation and ileus are insidious causes of respiratory failure and sepsis in any patient with a spinal injury (20).

Acquired Immunodeficiency Syndrome (AIDS)

Immunocompromised hosts require special attention when presenting either with abdominal pain or sepsis of unknown origin. Since the advent of antiretroviral medication therapy, the incidence of severe abdominal problems in HIV-positive patients has decreased. Patients presenting with overt AIDS have a constellation of problems that are unique to this population. The frequency of pulmonary, cardiac, gastrointestinal, and renal disease that is not directly related to the underlying HIV has increased (21).

Acute abdominal pain is a complaint in 12% to 45% of patients with HIV infection presenting to the emergency room (22). Earlier studies have noted that cytomegalovirus (CMV), gastroenteritis, followed by lymphoma, Kaposi sarcoma, and mycobacterial disease were frequent causes of abdominal pain in HIV patients. There has been a significant reduction in these opportunistic infections, especially peritonitis secondary to atypical mycobacterium and fungi (23,24).

The clinician must be aware that the HIV patient continues to present with non–HIV-related problems, such as appendicitis, diverticulitis, and pancreatitis. Only 11% of acute abdominal pain in HIV patients is caused by HIV/AIDS, whereas opportunistic infection results in surgery in only 0.9% of patients (25). Surgery should be considered early because of the difficulty in interpreting findings in these patients and the importance of differentiating true surgical from nonsurgical abdominal problems. Earlier studies reported increased morbidity and mortality in patients with AIDS (26), whereas recent data yield 10% to 19% operative mortality for emergency surgery (24).

Fever and nonspecific abdominal pain are frequently noted although peritoneal signs may be lacking in severely immunocompromised patients (27). Prognosis of patients is somewhat dependent on the CD4 count and viral loads. CD4 counts less than 200 cells/mm^3, total lymphocyte count less than 1,000 cells/mm^3, and viral loads greater than 75,000 RNA copies/mL are associated with higher morbidity and mortality (24).

Plain films have a low yield compared to CT scan in the diagnoses of processes such as pneumatosis intestinalis. This finding on CT is very suggestive of bowel necrosis. Intraperitoneal collections associated with opportunistic infections can be aspirated under CT guidance (4,28).

Acute appendicitis in AIDS patients may be routine or secondary to opportunistic organisms. Although fever and pain are frequent, white blood cell count may be low or normal (29).

There has been a decrease in bowel perforation secondary to CMV or Kaposi sarcoma since the advent of retroviral therapy. However, diligence is required to ensure perforation has not occurred. Recent data point to lymphoma and disseminated mycobacterial disease as causes for perforation (25). CMV perforations are more common in the ileum and colon secondary to ischemic lesions, which require aggressive surgical therapy and diversion of the fecal stream (23). Acute bowel obstruction suggests disseminated disease and has a poor prognosis if the cause is age related.

Colonic disease, especially toxic megacolon, has been seen with *Clostridium difficile* colitis, especially in patients with CMV infection. Megacolon can be a significant prognostic indicator in advanced age and may best be treated with colonoscopy for short-term management of the severely ill (30).

Acute hepatobiliary disease secondary to opportunistic disease can present difficult diagnostic problems in patients with CD4 counts less than 100 cells/mm^3. Acalculous cholecystitis is more common in HIV/AIDS patients than in the normal population (31–33).

Neutropenic patients with cancer also present a diagnosis and therapeutic challenge. In patients who underwent emergency celiotomy for suspected intra-abdominal disease, the most common disease has been reported to be neutropenic enteropathy (61%) with postoperative mortality up to 32% (34).

BILIARY DISEASE

Primary biliary tract disease in critically ill patients appears as calculous or acalculous cholecystitis. Calculous disease may present as acute cholecystitis, cholangitis, or pancreatitis. Acute acalculous biliary disease is a concomitant of critical illness and has been reported in 1% of surgical patients and 0.2% of postoperative cardiac patients (35).

The differentiation of calculous from acalculous disease can be difficult. Several risk factors are associated with the development of acalculous cholecystitis, including use of narcotics for more than 6 days, gastric suction, prolonged ileus with nothing by mouth, ventilatory support longer than 24 hours, multiple recent operations, more than ten blood transfusions, open wound or abscesses, and intravenous hyperalimentation for more than 3 days. The presence of five of these risk factors in a patient with acute abdominal findings should lead to a search for acalculous biliary disease (35,36).

The typical presentation of right upper quadrant pain, a positive Murphy sign, and fever may be absent in critically ill patients. Symptoms of right upper quadrant pain were present in only 30% of patients with acalculous disease, although all exhibited fever. Peritonitis was an inconsistent finding and present in only 24%. Persistent fever was the most consistent finding (37).

The laboratory findings of biliary disease are variable. Leukocytosis is common, although nonspecific. Up to 65% of patients with acalculous cholecystitis have elevated bilirubin; however, a control group of patients receiving multiple transfusions had similar hyperbilirubinemia. Liver enzymes are elevated in less than 50% (35).

Acute cholecystitis can mimic numerous other disease processes in the abdomen. Conversely, the presence of stones in the gallbladder in patients with nonspecific symptoms is not pathognomonic of acute biliary disease. Improved ultrasonography can be supplemented by radionucleotide imaging techniques that can distinguish cystic duct obstruction in acute cholecystitis from other causes of abdominal pain have markedly increased our diagnostic acumen. Derivatives of iminodiacetic acid are rapidly taken up by the hepatocytes and excreted into the bile even in patients with elevations of bilirubin up to 6 g/dL. The test has proved to be 95% accurate in the diagnosis of acute cholecystitis. The presence of fever, mild elevation of bilirubin, sludge on ultrasound, and nonvisualization on HIIDA are accurate indications of acute acalculous cholecystitis in critically ill patients. Caution is urged in patients receiving hyperalimentation, which severely limits the usefulness of the test (38,39). Furthermore, HIDA scan requires moving the critically ill patient to the radiology suite for up to 4 hours, and the risk–benefit ratio requires a high degree of clinical suspicion. The treatment of choice has been surgical drainage, either cholecystostomy or cholecystectomy, if the patient is able to tolerate a major procedure. The use of percutaneous cholecystostomy has been reported in severely ill patients. The mortality rate associated with acalculous cholecystitis is as high as 40% secondary to the multiplicity of the patient's problems (37,40).

ABSCESS

Intra-abdominal abscesses develop as a complication of secondary peritonitis that is the result of a perforation of a hollow viscus. They usually occur postoperatively, particularly after colonic resection complicated by anastomotic leak (41). This is followed in frequency by diverticular disease, appendicitis, inflammatory bowel disease, and malignancy. Patients undergoing gastric bypass procedures for obesity are also a potential population to develop abscess accompanied by an anastomotic leak. Abscesses can also develop retroperitoneally. This can be the result of retroperitoneal visceral perforation, e.g., cecal perforation or lymphatic and hematogenous spread of bacteria, e.g., infected pancreatic necrosis. Peritonitis and abscess should be suspected in any patient deteriorating following abdominal surgery.

Making the diagnosis of intra-abdominal abscess requires a high index of suspicion as the clinical picture can be vague. Peritonitis is rare, and bowel function may be normal. Physical examination is rarely helpful. Abscesses that have the anterior abdominal wall as part of their walls are associated with a palpable tender mass. Nonspecific manifestations such as fever, chills, malaise, and leukocytosis should raise the suspicion. Hiccup, unexplained pleural effusion, and a raised hemidiaphragm on chest radiograph may indicate subphrenic abscess. Diarrhea and urinary retention may indicate a pelvic abscess. CT scanning, preferably with oral and intravenous contrast, is the standard diagnostic modality. Bedside ultrasonography may be used in patients who are too unstable to move out of the ICU.

The bacterial flora are related to the organ involved, the host defenses, and the duration of the critical illness. The flora of the normal stomach and duodenum is very sparse and is composed mainly of swallowed oral organisms such as microaerophilic streptococci and *Streptococcus viridans*, lactobacillus, fusiform bacteria, and *Candida* species. The flora grows and changes remarkably if there is gastric outlet obstruction, achlorhydria, or acid-suppressive therapy. Small bowel flora consists mainly of Enterobacteriaceae, *Enterococcus* species, and anaerobic species. The flora becomes gradually more dense distally. Colonic flora is extremely dense; it accounts for one sixth of the dry weight of stools and contains both aerobic and anaerobic bacteria with the former much more abundant than the latter. Aerobic bacteria are primarily Gram-negative, e.g., *Escherichia* coli, *Klebsiella* species, *Enterococcus* species, and *Proteus* species. Anaerobic bacteria include *Bacteroides fragilis*, *Eubacterium* species, and *Bifidobacterium* species. Intra-abdominal abscesses are typically polymicrobial, but anaerobes are difficult to grow on cultures.

Whenever possible the source of infection should be dealt with surgically, e.g., appendectomy or resection of necrotic or perforated intestine. Open surgical management is not always possible or necessary. Surgical consultation should be obtained, and the decision to operate is based on individual patient conditions. Open surgical drainage does not always entail a celiotomy. Drainage of subphrenic abscess can be performed through the bed of the 12th rib, and extra peritoneal drainage of lower quadrant abscesses may be done. The efficacy of CT-guided percutaneous drainage of intra-abdominal abscesses (Fig. 76.2) has long been established (17,42,43). This minimally invasive technique is quite helpful, particularly when operative intervention carries a high risk of morbidity as in the case of Crohn disease (44). In a retrospective study of 38 patients with intra-abdominal abscesses due to colorectal disease both postoperative and primary, the overall success rate of percutaneous drainage was 89% (45). Antibiotic therapy is based on empiric coverage of bacteria that is normally present within the gut rather than culture results. Antibiotics are adjunctive in treating intra-abdominal sepsis. The antibiotic regimen should cover Gram-positive, Gram-negative, and anaerobic bacteria. Antifungal agents are not given even if fungi are seen on cultures unless the patient is immunosuppressed or has recurrent intra-abdominal infection. Guidelines for the use of antimicrobial agents are published by several medical societies (46).

Mortality from intra-abdominal sepsis ranges from 7.5% for single abscess to 43% for patients with multiple abscesses and peritonitis (47). Overall mortality from intra-abdominal infection is 24%. Mortality correlates directly with acute physiology score, malnutrition, age, and shock. Only early recognition, appropriate use of antibiotics, and prompt drainage can improve on these data.

PNEUMOPERITONEUM

The most common cause of pneumoperitoneum is laparotomy or laparoscopy. After abdominal surgery, free air may persist for weeks, although air from laparoscopy is frequently absent at 48 hours.

Pneumoperitoneum in a patient who does not have a recent history of laparotomy or laparoscopy should be presumed to be due to a perforated viscus until proven otherwise. Perforation of the stomach or duodenum due to peptic ulcer disease is more

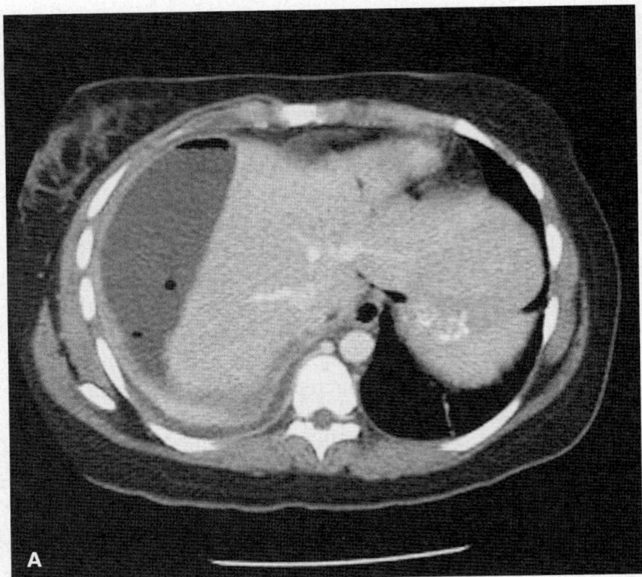

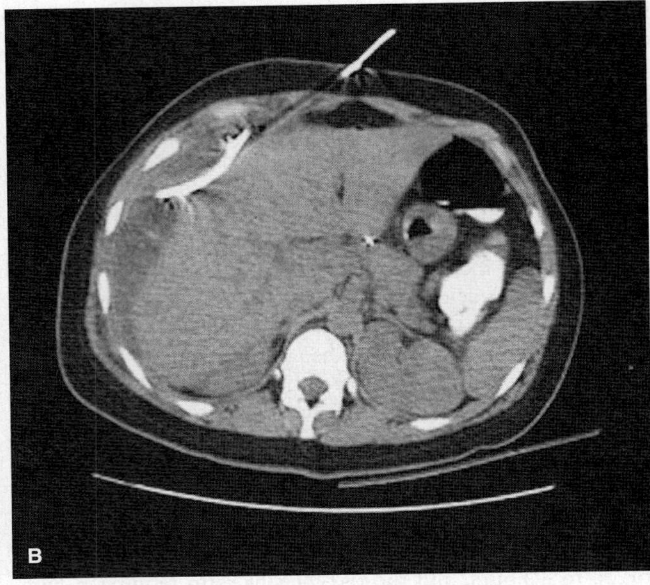

FIGURE 76.2. Right subphrenic abscess is drained percutaneously under computed tomography guidance.

likely to cause an obvious pneumoperitoneum than perforation of the colon due to diverticular disease. Other conditions that may cause pneumoperitoneum are a recent percutaneous endoscopic gastrostomy and barotrauma to the lung (48,49). The latter, however, occurs much less frequently with today's lung-protective strategies whereby peak airway pressures are not allowed to exceed 40 cm H_2O. Patients who suffer severe chest trauma with pneumothorax and pneumomediastinum can also have pneumoperitoneum.

Pneumoperitoneum has been observed in up to 10% of patients who have demonstrated other evidence of extra alveolar air. Macklin and Macklin (49) postulated that air first ruptures though distended alveoli and dissects toward the mediastinum. From there, it dissects down the mediastinum and ruptures into the peritoneal cavity. The diagnosis of perforated viscus may be difficult in paralyzed, mechanically ventilated patients who cannot complain of tenderness and who will have a soft abdomen and absent bowel sounds.

Pneumoperitoneum should be evaluated in the context of the patient's overall condition. In unconscious or paralyzed septic patients with no obvious source of sepsis, pneumoperitoneum should prompt an exploratory laparotomy. Diagnostic peritoneal lavage may be considered if the risk of operative exploration is too high or the index of suspicion is low. The presence of bacteria, bile, more than 500 WBCs/mm^3 can be inferred to indicate an acute abdominal process requiring immediate laparotomy.

PSEUDO-OBSTRUCTION OF THE COLON

Isolated colonic ileus without mechanical obstruction was first described by Ogilvie (50). Patients at risk are the elderly and those requiring bed rest, prolonged narcotic use, and mechanical ventilation. Massive colonic distention presents a perplexing dilemma in the ICU. The cause is unknown, but the condition typically occurs in patients with associated illness who are bedridden for a long time. The most common risk factors are old age, multiple trauma, abdominal and pelvic operations, orthopedic operations, and spinal cord injuries (50,51). Hyponatremia and hypokalemia may play a role in the development of this condition. The abdomen is distended and tympanitic without signs of peritonitis, fever, or leukocytosis.

On radiograph the colon appears diffusely distended, including the rectum, and the small bowel is usually not seen. The cecum, being the widest segment of the colon, is at risk for necrosis and perforation if the diameter reaches 12 cm. Mechanical obstruction should be ruled out with a Hypaque enema. This is a hyperosmolar water-soluble enema that helps to cleanse the colon and, unlike barium, does not interfere with a subsequent colonoscopy.

Initial management consists of decompressing the stomach and colon with nasogastric and rectal tubes. Electrolyte abnormalities, especially hypokalemia, should be promptly corrected. If there is no response to these measures, neostigmine, a parasympathomimetic, should be given to stimulate colonic motility (52). Neostigmine is given in a dose of 1 to 2 mg intravenously and can be repeated in 3 hours. This should be done under cardiac monitoring as it may result in severe bradycardia. Neostigmine should not be given if the patient's baseline heart rate is less than 60 beats per minute, the systolic blood pressure is less than 90 mm Hg, or if there is a significant heart block or bronchospasm. The next step in management, if the previous measures fail, is colonoscopic decompression. This is associated with a higher-than-normal risk of perforation and therefore should be used gently and with the goal of decompression only. It is not necessary to advance the colonoscope all the way to the cecum. Recurrence is seen in up to 40% of patients, and colonoscopy can be repeated. Surgery is reserved for patients who fail all other measures and those with complications or impending cecal rupture, i.e., diameter more than 12 cm. The operation of choice is right hemicolectomy with primary ileocolic anastomosis if there is no evidence of necrosis or perforation, in which case an ileostomy with mucus fistula should be performed.

MANAGEMENT OF THE OPEN ABDOMEN IN THE ICU

The abdominal compartment syndrome (ACS) is a condition in which the intra-abdominal pressure rises to a point that impairs respiratory, renal, and cardiovascular function (53). The condition is described mainly in the trauma population but can occur in any patient who receives a massive resuscitation for a profound shock state. The abdomen is not necessarily the site where the original pathology occurs, e.g., severe burns (54). This is sometimes described as secondary ACS. It is believed that severe edema of the abdominal wall, bowel wall, and the retroperitoneum occurs as a result of massive fluid shifts associated with the severe systemic inflammation that accompanies reperfusion of tissues after shock states. The diagnosis of ACS is made when there is abdominal distention associated with high ventilator pressures, oliguria, and elevated urinary bladder pressures (>25–30 cm H_2O). Treatment consists of abdominal decompression using a midline celiotomy and keeping the abdomen open using various dressing mechanisms over the bowel. For a detailed discussion of the ACS, see the section on abdominal trauma.

The treatment principles in trauma patients have been extrapolated to general surgery patients. More abdomens are now kept open if fascial closure is expected to increase abdominal pressure. By keeping the abdomen open, renal and pulmonary functions are not compromised and the integrity of fascial edges is preserved. The open abdomen also gives the opportunity for frequent bedside washouts and debridements such as with infected pancreatic necrosis. Once the swelling has resolved, the abdomen should be closed as soon as possible either by primary fascial closure or using one of the commercially available biologic or synthetic grafts. Prolongation of the open abdomen management is associated with increased risk of fistula formation.

BARIATRIC SURGERY

It is estimated that over 130,000 bariatric procedures will be performed in the United States each year (55). Many of these patients have sleep apnea, hypoventilation, or other physiologic abnormalities that require ICU care in the immediate postoperative period. Since anastomotic leaks following gastric bypass and duodenal switch are potentially fatal, rapid recognition, diagnosis, and treatment are necessary to minimize patient risk. Likewise, acute gastric dilatation requires immediate treatment. The hallmarks of dilatation and leak are persistent tachycardia, tachypnea, fever, anxiety, and hiccups, usually accompanied by a mild leukocytosis with or without fever (56). Because this is also found in patients with pulmonary emboli, it is vital that the diagnosis of leak be made early.

Abdominal pain is frequently not a major symptom, although shoulder (referred) pain may be present. In the absence of hypoxemia in the first 48 hours, the above symptoms should suggest leak and immediate Gastrografin swallow with adequate volume of contrast should be performed. The presence of a large gastric bubble without leak requires immediate decompression via either a percutaneous or surgical therapy (56). This will prevent gastric perforation or an anastomotic disruption from pressure. A leak must be addressed immediately with drainage either percutaneously for small and contained leaks, or operative intervention to attempt to repair and drain the area of concern.

ACUTE MESENTERIC ISCHEMIA

Numerous causes exist for acute intestinal ischemia. Embolus (50%–60%) or thrombus (25%–35%) of the superior mesenteric artery (SMA) must be differentiated from nonmesenteric thrombosis (10%–20%) and acute mesenteric venous occlusions (5%) (57–60). Colonic and rectal ischemias have been reported after abdominal aortic aneurysmectomy in which the inferior mesenteric artery was ligated (61).

A characteristic of gut ischemia is the disparity between the patient's pain and abdominal findings. Pain is found in 75% to 90% of patients. Nausea and vomiting are present in 50% to 60% of patients, whereas upper gastrointestinal bleeding is less common (62,63). Abdominal distention is present in 56% to 80%, peritoneal signs in 60%, ileus in 50%, and shock and fever in 30% of patients. Leukocytosis (WBC count of 20,000/mm^3) is seen in less than 50% of patients. A mild elevation in amylase is common (59,64).

The presence of physical signs indicating peritoneal irritation is extremely important because they portend impending or progressive gangrene and are associated with significant mortality. Leukocytosis out of proportion to the physical findings, elevated hematocrit, unexplained acidosis, and blood-tinged fluid on peritoneal lavage are all signs of advancing intestinal necrosis (62).

Plain radiographs are useful to exclude the other processes that can stimulate the symptoms. Signs of intestinal ischemia on plain radiographs is a grave prognosticator with 90% mortality (62).

Patients at highest risk are those older than 50 years of age with either valvular or atherosclerotic heart disease, congestive

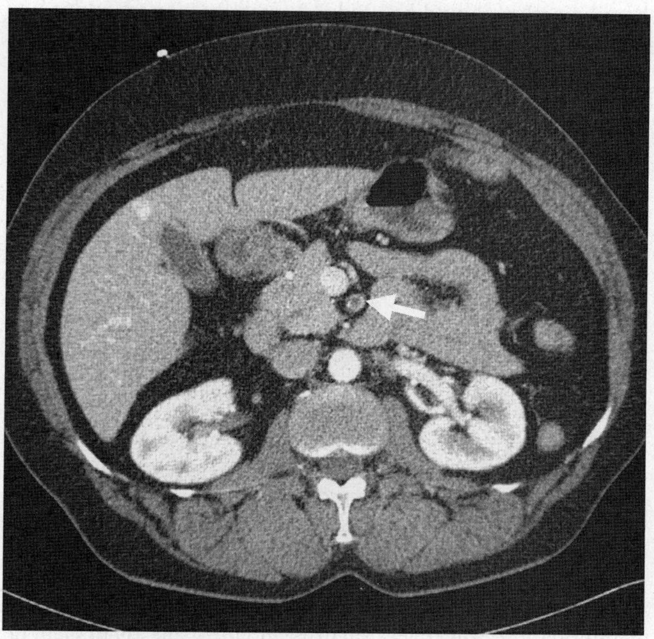

FIGURE 76.3. Superior mesenteric artery embolus (*white arrow*).

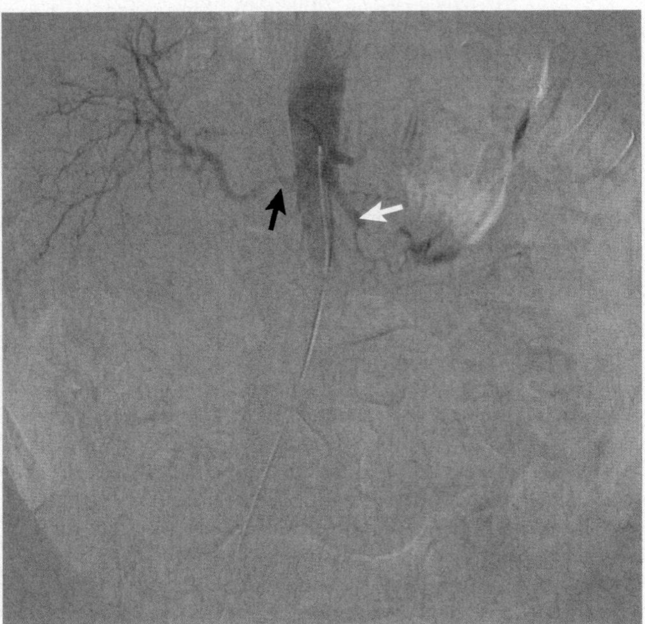

FIGURE 76.4. Superior mesenteric artery angiogram showing an embolus distal to the proximal jejunal branches (*white arrow*) and a replaced right hepatic artery (*black arrow*).

heart failure (especially if there is poor control with digitalis and diuretics), hypovolemia, hypotension of any cause, recent myocardial infarction or cardiogenic shock, or cardiac arrhythmias (58,59,62). Dialysis patients seem to be at added risk for right colon ischemia. The use of sigmoid tonometry also has been suggested to detect colonic ischemia (65).

Once the diagnosis is suspected, vigorous fluid resuscitation is necessary to maintain adequate blood flow and pressure head in the mesenteric vessels. Gastrointestinal decompression with a NG tube and proper hemodynamic monitoring are necessary to adequately resuscitate these precarious patients. Early heparinization should be used if immediate surgery is not undertaken.

CAT scans have improved in both availability and reliability and may demonstrate clot or ischemia (Fig. 76.3). Emergency selective arteriography is still the keystone of the diagnostic and therapeutic approach to acute mesenteric ischemia (Fig. 76.4). Arteriography can differentiate occlusive from nonocclusive disease. Although there are reports of successful thrombolysis of clot in the SMA (66), acute occlusion is best treated by immediate surgical restoration of circulation by embolectomy or aortosuperior mesenteric artery bypass. Examination of the bowel for ischemia, which will require resection, is essential to avoid unnecessary morbidity and mortality.

Nonocclusive mesenteric ischemia is diagnosed when mesenteric vasoconstriction on angiogram is seen in the patient with a clinical picture suggestive of intestinal ischemia. Shock and vasopressors make interpretation of the arteriogram difficult. Treatment of this disease is begun in the radiology suite by the administration of papaverine (30–60 mg/hour) through a catheter placed selectively in the SMA. If peritoneal signs are present and abdominal exploration is necessary to examine the viability of the bowel, vasodilators and local anesthetics can be injected directly into the base of the mesentery.

When papaverine is the primary treatment for nonocclusive ischemia, it is continued for 24 hours and an arteriogram is repeated. Heparin may be used concomitantly.

Maintaining adequate plasma volume and blood pressure is essential to maintain perfusion of the splanchnic vessels. Occasionally, dextran has been used to expand plasma and to decrease sludging. Digitalis should be used cautiously.

Systemic antibiotics are indicated because of the high incidence of positive blood cultures resulting from compromised bowel. Antibiotics may mask peritoneal signs. Decompression by NG suction can decrease bowel distention.

The mortality rate for acute mesenteric ischemia has remained at 70% to 80% (59,63). Embolus in the SMA is still associated with a 44% to 90% mortality rate whereas nonocclusive ischemia without peritoneal signs has a more favorable outcome. Peritonitis is associated with mortality rates of 60% to 90% (59,62). Logistic regression yields an odds ratio of 22 for peritonitis and 14.9 for hypotension as independent predictors of mortality (59).

The early workup of a suspicion of ischemia followed by aggressive and rapid diagnostic workup seems to be the only method for improving this abysmal mortality rate (63). Death occurs from MSOF secondary to ischemia (65%), sepsis (25%), pulmonary failure (8%), and stroke (2%) (59). Although second-look operations are frequently used at 24 to 48 hours to determine viability of remaining bowel, survival is not necessarily improved by this technique (67).

SUMMARY

Acute abdominal problems are frequent among ICU patients. The physician must maintain a high level of suspicion that an abdominal problem is present when faced with a deteriorating critically ill patient. History and physical examination must be used to guide the use of more invasive and expensive tests. Laboratory tests are usually adjunctive and rarely diagnostic. Radiographic procedures, especially ultrasound and CT scans, when appropriately used, can be helpful. Surgical consultation should be obtained early in a patient's course, because treatment frequently requires surgical intervention. Only by maintaining constant vigilance can critical care practitioners guide their patients through the multiple perturbations created by acute abdominal problems.

PEARLS

- Patients admitted to an ICU with abdominal pain, fever, evidence of multiorgan failure, unexplained acidosis, or jaundice should have an acute abdominal source ruled out early in their course.
- The absence of obvious signs and symptoms in an acutely ill patient does not rule out an acute abdominal problem.
- Resuscitation of acute abdominal problems frequently requires large volumes of isotonic crystalloid fluids and broad-spectrum antibiotics.
- Common postoperative abdominal problems include abscess, leak from anastomoses or perforated bowel, acalculous cholecystitis, and ileus.

- Acute abdominal pain in an immunocompromised patient requires a high index of suspicion and rapid diagnosis of uncommon infectious causes.
- The diagnostic approach to acute abdominal symptoms includes radiologic examinations—ultrasound or CT scan (with oral contrast when indicated) early in the workup.
- Abdominal distension associated with low urine output and high ventilatory pressures should prompt measurement of abdominal compartment pressures and surgical consult.
- Acute mesenteric embolus is the most common cause for intestinal ischemia (50%–60%). It may present as severe pain out of proportion to the physical signs and requires immediate diagnosis and surgical treatment to prevent significant morbidity/mortality.

References

1. Aranha GV, Goldberg NB. Surgical problems in patients on ventilators. *Crit Care Med.* 1981;9:478.
2. Brewer RJ, Golden GT, Hitch DD, et al. Abdominal pain: an analysis of 1,000 consecutive cases in a university hospital emergency room. *Am J Surg.* 1976;131:219.
3. Weaver DW, Busuito MJ, Bouwman DL, et al. Interpretation of serum amylase levels in the critically ill patient. *Crit Care Med.* 1985;13:532.
4. Ahn SH, Mayo-Smith WW, Murphy BL, et al. Acute nontraumatic abdominal pain in adult patients: abdominal radiography compared with CT evaluation. *Radiology.* 2002;225:159.
5. Hendershot KM, Fakhry SM, Haikman H, et al. Duration and safety of computed tomography in severely injured blunt trauma patients. Paper presented at: 56th Annual Meeting of the Association for the Surgery of Trauma; September 28–30, 2006; New Orleans, LA.
6. Norwood SH, Civetta JM. Abdominal CT scanning in critically ill surgical patients. *Ann Surg.* 1985;202:166.
7. Larson FA, Haller C, Delcore R, et al. Diagnostic peritoneal lavage in acute peritonitis. *Am Surg.* 1992;164:449.
8. Fry DE, Pearlstein L, Fulton RL, et al. Multiple system organ failure: the role of uncontrolled infection. *Arch Surg.* 1980;115:136.
9. Knaus WA, Draper EA, Wagner DP, et al. Prognosis in acute organ-system failure. *Ann Surg.* 1985;202:685.
10. Lifeline Registry of EVAR Committee. Lifeline registry of endovascular aneurysm repair: long-term primary outcome measures. *J Vasc Surg.* 2005;42:1.
11. EVAR Trial Participants. Endovascular aneurysm repair versus repair in patients with abdominal aortic aneurysm (EVAR trial 1): randomized controlled trial. *Lancet.* 2005;365:2179.
12. Hastings PR, Skillman JJ, Bushnell LS, et al. Antacid titration in the prevention of acute gastrointestinal bleeding: a controlled, randomized trail in 100 critically ill patients. *N Engl J Med.* 1978;298:1041.
13. Shuman RN, Schoster DP, Zuckerman GR. Prophylactic therapy for stress ulcer feeding: a reappraisal. *Ann Intern Med.* 1987;106:562.
14. Tryba M. Risk of acute stress bleeding and nosocomial pneumonia in ventilated intensive care unit patients: sucralfate vs. antacids. *Am J Med.* 1987;83:117.
15. Cook DJ, Fullder HD, Guyatt, et al. Risk factors for gastrointestinal bleeding in critically ill patients. *N Engl J Med.* 1994;330:377.
16. Hubert JP, Kiernan PD, Weld JS, et al. The surgical management of bleeding stress ulcers. *Ann Surg.* 1980;191:672.
17. Levison MA. Percutaneous versus open operative drainage of intra-abdominal abscesses. *Infect Dis Clin North Am.* 1992;6:25.
18. Mismatsu K, Oida T, Kanou H, et al. Open abdomen management after massive bowel resection for superior mesenteric arterial occlusion. *Surg Today.* 2006;36:241.
19. Ashley SW, Perez A, Pierce EA, et al. Necrotizing pancreatitis: contemporary analysis of 99 consecutive cases. *Ann Surg.* 2001;234:572.
20. Reines HD, Harris RC. Pulmonary complications of acute spinal cord injuries. *Neurosurgery.* 1987;21:193.
21. Huang l, Quartin A, Jones D, et al. Intensive care of patient with HIV Infection. *N Engl J Med.* 2006;355:173.
22. Barone JE, Gingold BS, Arvanitis ML, et al. Abdominal pain in patients with acquired immune deficiency syndrome. *Ann Surg.* 1986;204:619.
23. Saltzman DJ, Williams RA, Gelfand DV, et al. The surgeon and AIDS. *Arch Surg.* 2005;140: 961.
24. Tran HS, Moncure M, Tarnoff M, et al. Predictors of operative outcome in patients with human immunodeficiency virus infection and acquired immunodeficiency syndrome. *Am J Surg.* 2000;180:228.
25. Yoshida D, Caruso JM. Abdominal pain in the HIV infected patient. *J Emerg Med.* 2002;23:111.
26. Davidson T, Allen-Mersh TG, Miles AJ, et al. Emergency laparotomy in patients with AIDS. *Br J Surg.* 1991;78:924.
27. Lowy AM, Barie PS. Laparotomy in patients infected with human immunodeficiency virus: indications and outcome. *Br J Surg.* 1994;81:942.
28. Wiesner W, Mortele KJ, Glickman JN, et al. Pneumatosis intestinalis and portomesenteric venous gas in intestinal ischemia: correlation of CT findings with severity of ischemia and clinical outcome. *AJR Am J Roentgenol.* 2001;177:1319.
29. Binderow SR, Shaked AA. Acute appendicitis in patients with AIDS/HIV infection. *Am J Surg.* 1991;162:9.
30. Beaugerie L, Ngo Y, Goujard F, et al. Etiology and management of toxic megacolon in patients with human immunodeficiency virus infection. *Gastroenterology.* 1994;107:858.
31. French AL, Beaudet LM, Benator DA, et al. Cholecystectomy in patients with AIDS: clinicopathologic correlations in 107 cases. *Clin Infect Dis.* 1995;21:852.
32. Flum DR, Wallack MK. Cholecystectomy and AIDS. *J Am Coll Surg.* 1997:184:669.
33. LaRaja RD, Rothenberg RE, Odom JW, et al. The incidence of intra-abdominal surgery in acquired immunodeficiency syndrome: a statistical review of 904 patients. *Surgery.* 1989;105:175.
34. Glenn J, Funkhouser WK, Schneider PS. Acute illnesses necessitating urgent abdominal surgery of neutropenic cancer patients: description of 14 cases and review of the literature. *Surgery.* 1989;105:778.
35. Savino JA, Scalea TM, Del Guercio LRM: Factors encouraging laparotomy in acalculous cholecystitis. *Crit Care Med.* 1985;13:377.
36. Petersen SR, Sheldon GF. Acute acalculous cholecystitis: a complications of hyperalimentation. *Am J Surg.* 1979;138:814.
37. Long TN, Heimbach DM, Carrico CJ. Acalculous cholecystitis in critically ill patients. *Am J Surg.* 1978;136:31.
38. Shuman WP, Gibbs P, Rudd TG, et al. PIPIDA scintigraphy for cholecystitis: false positives in alcoholism and total parenteral nutrition. *Am J Radiol.* 1982;138:1.
39. Kalff V, Froelich JW, Lloyd R, et al. Predictive value of an abdominal hepatobiliary scan in patients with severe intercurrent illness. *Radiology.* 1983;146:191.
40. Longmaid HE, Bassett JG, Gottlieb H. Management of gallbladder perforation by percutaneous cholecystostomy. *Crit Care Med.* 1985;13:686.
41. Deveney CW, Lurie K, Deveny KE. Improved treatment of intra-abdominal abscess. *Arch Surg.* 1988;123:1126.
42. Wright HK, Dunn E, MacArthur JD, et al. Specific but limited role of new imaging techniques in decision-making intra-abdominal abscesses. *Am J Surg.* 1982;143:456.
43. Montgomery RS, Wilson SE. Intra-abdominal abscesses: image-guided diagnosis and therapy. *Clin Infect Dis.* 1996;23:8.
44. Sahai A, Belair M, Fianfelice D, et al. Percutaneous drainage of intra-abdominal abscesses in Crohn's disease: short and long term outcome. *Am J Gastroenterol.* 1997;92:75.
45. Eng M, Hyman N, Osler T. The role of computed tomography-guided percutaneous drainage of intraabdominal abscesses in colon and rectal disease. *J Pelvic Surg.* 2002;8(3):163.
46. Solomkin JS, Mazuski JE, Baron EJ, et al. Guidelines for the selection of anti-infective agents for complicated intra-abdominal infections. *Clin Infect Dis.* 2003;37:99.
47. Dellinger EP, Wertz MJ, Meakins JL, et al. Surgical infection stratification system for intra-abdominal infection: multicenter trial. *Arch Surg.* 1985:120:21.
48. Hillman KM. Pneumoperitoneum: a review. *Crit Care Med.* 1982;10:476.
49. Macklin MT, Macklin CC. Malignant interstitial emphysema of the lungs and mediastinum as an important occult complication in many respiratory diseases and other conditions: an interpretation of the clinical literature in the light of laboratory experiment. *Medicine.* 1944;23:281.
50. Ogilvie H. Large intestine colic due to sympathetic deprivation: a new clinical syndrome. *Br J Med.* 1948;2:671.
51. Jetmore AB, Timmcke AE, Gathright JB, et al. Ogilvie's syndrome: colonoscopic decompression and analysis of predisposing factors. *Dis Colon Rectum.* 1992;35:1135.
52. Ponec RJ, Saunders MD, Kimmey MB. Neostigmine for the treatment of acute colonic pseudo-obstruction. *N Engl J Med.* 1999;341:137.
53. Burch JM, Moore EE, Moore FA, et al. The abdominal compartment syndrome. *Surg Clin North Am.* 1996;76:88.
54. Ivy ME, Atweh NA, Palmer J, et al. Intra-abdominal hypertension and abdominal compartment syndrome in burn patients. *J Trauma.* 2000;49: 387.
55. Santry HP, Gillen DL, Lauderdale DS. Trends in bariatric surgical procedures. *JAMA.* 2005;294:1909–1917.
56. DeMaria E. Morbid obesity. In: Mulholland MW, ed. *Greenfield's Surgery.* 4th ed. Philadelphia, PA: Lippincott Williams & Wilkins; 2006:741.
57. Stoney RJ, Cunningham CG. Acute mesenteric ischemia. *Surgery.* 1993;114:489.
58. Safioleas MC, Moulakakis KG, Papavassiliou VG, et al. Acute mesenteric ischaemia, a highly lethal disease with a devastating outcome. *Vasa.* 2003;35:106.

59. Edwards MS, Cherr GS, Craven TE, et al. Acute occlusive mesenteric ischemia: surgical management and outcomes. *Ann Vasc Surg.* 2003;17:72.
60. Endean ED, Barnes SL, Kwolek CJ, et al. Surgical management of thrombotic acute intestinal ischemia. *Ann Surg.* 2001;233:801.
61. Birnabaum W, Rudy L, Wylie EJ. Colonic and rectal ischemia following abdominal aneurysmectomy. *Dis Colon Rectum.* 1964;7:293.
62. Boley SJ, Brandt LJ, Veith FJ. Ischemic disorders of the intestine. *Curr Probl Surg.* 1978;15:1.
63. Birnabaum W, Rudy L, Wylie EJ. Colonic and rectal ischemia following abdominal aneurysmectomy. *Dis Colon Rectum.* 1964;7:293.
64. Ottinger LW. The surgical management of acute occlusion of the superior mesenteric artery. *Ann Surg.* 1978;188:721.
65. Montgomery A, Hartmann M, Jonsson K, et al. Intramucosal pH measurements with tonometers for detecting gastrointestinal ischemia in porcine hemorrhage shock. *Circ Shock.* 1989;29:319.
66. Nishida A, Fukui K. Transcatheter treatment of thromboembolism in the superior mesenteric artery. *N Engl J Med.* 2005;353:4.
67. Kaminsky O, Yampolski I, Aranovich D, et al. Does a second-look operation improve survival in patients with peritonitis due to acute mesenteric ischemia? A five-year retrospective experience. *World J Sur.* 2005;29:645.

CHAPTER 77 ■ THE DIFFICULT POST-OPERATIVE ABDOMEN

STEPHANIE A. SAVAGE • TIMOTHY C. FABIAN

The practice of surgery inevitably carries the risk of postoperative complications and difficult therapeutic choices. Some of the most vexing operative dilemmas result from managing a difficult postoperative abdomen. Routine intra-abdominal therapies will result in adhesion formation, which may plague the patient with recurrent episodes of abdominal pain and partial or complete bowel obstruction. Enterocutaneous, intra-abdominal, or pancreatic fistulas may result from the natural progression of intra-abdominal pathology or may be the sequelae of invasive procedures. Abdominal catastrophes may result in a compartment syndrome mandating aggressive management decisions including temporary abdominal closures and planned ventral hernias. Less common issues, including radiation enteritis and short bowel syndrome, may significantly impact lifestyle and health, requiring surgical attention.

In this chapter, we will address many of these difficult postoperative issues. Our discussion will include etiology, diagnosis, and therapeutic approaches. The core principles of careful surgical technique and meticulous patient management, including wound care, nutritional management, and timing of recurrent interventions, are key in treating these obstacles.

ADHESIONS

Intra-abdominal adhesions are an unavoidable consequence of operative therapy. Intra-abdominal adhesions are the primary cause for postoperative bowel obstruction, accounting for approximately 75% of cases (1). Adhesions intrinsically play a crucial role in postoperative healing. Formation of adhesive tissue protects an anastomosis and prevents leaks, in addition to assisting in the body's attempt to isolate intra-abdominal catastrophes like abscesses. When adhesive bands become too dense, kink, or encompass loops of bowel, they may result in negative consequences such as bowel obstruction and persistent abdominal pain. In this chapter, we will discuss the development of adhesions, their natural history, and methods of prevention.

Adhesion formation occurs in the course of repairing an injury site, anastomosis, or incision. Within the first 48 to 72 hours of injury, macrophages converge to form a protective layer over the injured tissue. These macrophages further differentiate into mesothelial cells, while additional fibroblasts and mesothelial cells are recruited from nearby locales. These cell populations complete the initial stages of healing over a period of 7 to 10 days (2,3). Ultimately, these healing cell populations will not only continue the process of restoring tissue integrity but may form unnatural connections. Adhesive connections may occur between loops of bowel, intra-abdominal structures and the abdominal wall, and between the pelvis and nearby structures (bowel, gynecologic organs, etc.) resulting in intra-abdominal pathology and patient morbidity.

Most (94%–98%) of abdominal adhesions are acquired, either from operative therapy or via inflammatory processes (i.e., Crohn's disease, cancer, etc.). The remaining 2% to 6% of adhesions are congenital and largely consist of Ladd bands. In the reoperative abdomen, adhesions are present in 30% to 40% of patients. The most frequent morbidity in those with postoperative adhesions is small bowel obstruction, which accounts for 12% to 17% of hospital admissions following previous abdominal surgery. One quarter of these admissions occur within the first year following surgery, and 2% to 5% of small bowel obstructions due to adhesions will require operative adhesiolysis (2). The degree of morbidity related to adhesion formation is profoundly affected by the type of surgery performed. Laparoscopic surgeries have been shown to have a 15% adhesion rate as opposed to open laparotomies, in which 50% result in adhesion formation. Adhesion formation tends to follow predictable patterns. Adhesions form more commonly following surgery to the small and large bowel than with other intra-abdominal organs, especially in surgeries involving bowel distal to the transverse colon or involving gynecologic organs (1). The areas most frequently affected are the under surface of the midline incision and the operative site, for example at an anastomosis. Due to its tendency to migrate to regions of inflammation, the omentum is the most frequently involved organ (57%). Small and large bowel adhesions continue to result in the highest morbidity (4).

The cost of adhesion-related disease, both regarding morbidity and monetarily, has resulted in extensive research focused on developing methods to avoid adhesion formation. Adhesions result from trauma to tissues, relative ischemia, infection within the abdominal cavity, inflammatory processes, or by the presence of foreign bodies such as suture, talc from gloves, and lint from sponges. To minimize adhesions, principles of good surgical technique are the best defense. Gentle tissue handling with strict hemostasis and minimization of intraperitoneal trauma are core principles. In addition, frequent irrigation to dilute or to remove contaminants and the use of small, nonreactive suture material will diminish the contribution to adhesiogenesis. Raw surfaces or anastomoses should be protected by autologous tissue, either with a tongue of omentum or via mobilized local tissue flaps. Perhaps the most effective method of preventing serious adhesions is via the use of the omentum. As is well known, the omentum is key to protecting areas of inflammation and infection within the abdomen. In a similar manner, the omentum may be used to wrap anastomoses or to protect abdominal contents from a healing midline incision. Unfortunately, the omentum is often too limited by prior inflammatory processes or surgery to be of use.

Barriers to Adhesiogenesis

Despite meticulous technique and conscientious efforts to prevent adhesions, they will continue to form with attendant postoperative morbidity and mortality. Research efforts have focused on developing materials to minimize the occurrence and severity of adhesions. The most common method of decreasing the number and strength of adhesions is with one of a variety of barrier materials. Seprafilm (Seprafilm Adhesion Barrier, Genzyme Corporation, Cambridge, MA) is an FDA-approved material composed of hyaluronic acid and carboxymethylcellulose. Applied to regions at risk for adhesions, it forms a deposit that acts as a mechanical barrier to adhesion formation. It is eventually reabsorbed by the body after 7 to 10 days. One large study demonstrated no difference in rates of small bowel obstruction with Seprafilm; however, the need for operative therapy to treat adhesions was significantly reduced (1). Of note, Seprafilm should not be used to wrap anastomoses to decrease adhesions at these sites, as this has resulted in higher rates of fistula formation (1). Interceed (Gynecare Interceed, Johnson & Johnson, New Jersey) is an older option that is a mechanical barrier designed to be placed over injured surfaces and operative sites. It is composed of oxidized regenerated meshlike cellulose; data have been mixed on its effectiveness. Although some studies have demonstrated that Interceed is safe and effective in reducing adhesions, other studies have shown no clinical benefit from its use (4). Additionally, it requires a completely hemostatic field, and the region in question must be completely covered for effective results, not always practical especially in laparoscopic surgery. Other methods to decrease adhesion formation have been shown to be less effective in adhesion prevention and are not used commonly in clinical practice. Gore-Tex Surgical Membrane (W.L. Gore and Associates, Flagstaff, AZ), a thin PTFE (polytetrafluoroethylene) membrane that prevents cellular penetration, must be secured in place and removed at a later date. This method is cumbersome, has not shown significant clinical benefit in preventing adhesions, and is not commonly used. Streptokinase infusion has shown no benefit in reducing adhesions. The use of tissue plasminogen activator to break down adhesions has shown some promise in animal studies but has not been proven in humans to date (4,5). These latter methods are of interest, either historically or in a research perspective, but are not commonly used in clinical practice.

Regardless of which product is ultimately chosen, the ideal barrier would be nonreactive *in vivo*, would be active during the key healing stages, and then be reabsorbed by the body when no longer needed. Locales that remain prime candidates for adhesion barriers include around temporary stomas, around the Hartman pouch after colectomy, beneath the midline incision, and in the pelvis following surgery in that region, especially in patients prone to inflammation. Research interest in this area remains high as adhesion-related morbidity continues to plague surgical patients.

FISTULAS

A fistula is an abnormal communication between two spaces. In the abdomen, varieties of fistulas differ tremendously and include such types as pancreatic fistulas, biliary fistulas, fistulas between two intra-abdominal organs (i.e., colovesical fistulas), and enterocutaneous fistulas. The natural history of a fistula begins as a leak from bowel or other intra-abdominal organ. The ultimate type of fistula depends on whether the leak is uncontrolled, partially controlled, or well controlled. An uncontrolled leak will result in peritonitis, which immediately results in surgical exploration and correction. A partially controlled leak may result in an intra-abdominal abscess, which will require definitive therapy. Controlled leaks result in fistulas, and the most dreaded of these is the enterocutaneous fistula. Management of fistulas can be a long-term challenge for surgeon and patient.

An enterocutaneous fistula is an abnormal communication between lumen of bowel and the skin. Fistulas are postoperative complications in 71% to 90% of cases, though they may occur spontaneously (2,6). Spontaneous causes of fistulas are uncommon but may include malignancy, inflammatory processes such as Crohn's disease, or vascular insufficiency, as seen in radiation enteritis. The iatrogenic fistula is the most common and presents a difficult management problem. Iatrogenic fistulas may result from inadvertent enterotomies, intra-abdominal infections, direct injury or bowel desiccation in the open abdomen, misplaced stitches, or anastomotic breakdown. Impaired tissue perfusion from hypotension or vascular disease may predispose to this complication, as will infections, steroids, and malnutrition.

An enterocutaneous fistula typically presents as discolored, watery drainage from the midline incision. A seeming wound infection opened at bedside will result in copious drainage of discolored, watery material or frank succus. Passage of gas from the midline wound is diagnostic of an enterocutaneous fistula. Patients will usually demonstrate signs of advancing infection including increasing temperature, white blood cell count, and persistent ileus. In less common cases, patients may develop profound shock due to electrolyte imbalances and sepsis. In these cases, emergent re-exploration is necessary. However, if the patient presents with drainage or an obvious fistula but is hemodynamically stable, conservative management is warranted, at least in the short term.

Conservative Management of the Enterocutaneous Fistula

Management is predicated on controlling output, managing electrolyte fluxes and nutritional deficiencies, and maximizing the potential for spontaneous closure (Fig. 77.1). In the immediate care of the patient, aggressive fluid resuscitation and close monitoring of electrolyte balance are mandatory to maintain stability. If the patient remains stable without the need for emergent operative intervention, nutritional replacement should begin immediately. This patient population is exceptionally prone to malnutrition from protein losses, increased metabolic demands, and limited or no oral intake. Parenteral nutrition is nearly mandatory to provide early and aggressive nutritional repletion, to allow close management of electrolyte and protein balances, and to decrease volume transit past the fistula in the gastrointestinal tract. Perhaps a greater challenge in this patient population is control of fistula output. Enteric contents are extremely caustic to the skin and surrounding tissues. An immediate goal in caring for patients with fistulas is to create some method to isolate enteric contents from the skin. For a simple enterocutaneous fistula, a stoma appliance may be all that is needed. However, many fistulas present in open wound beds, including on granulating abdomens. These tissue fields are not amenable to the placement of a simple stoma appliance. In these situations, a close association between the surgeon, patient, and wound care nurse/enterostomal therapist is mandatory to control fistula output. Once initial control is achieved, it may be possible to close fistulas surgically or to skin graft the region. These surgical options will be discussed in more detail later in this section

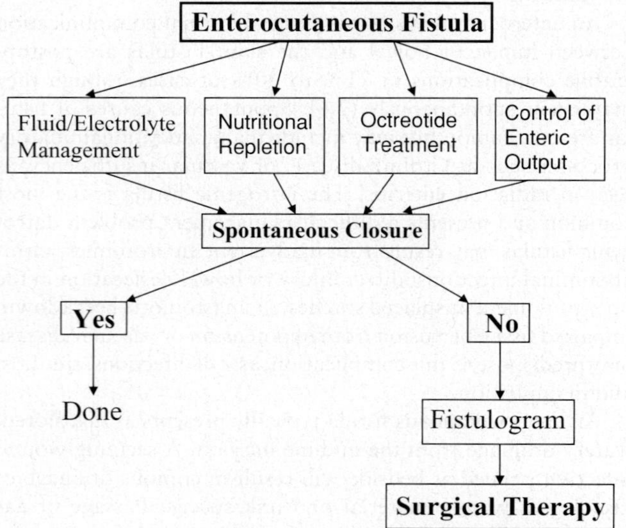

FIGURE 77.1. Management strategy for managing enterocutaneous fistulas.

Spontaneous Closure

The goal of conservative therapy is to achieve spontaneous closure of the fistula. Spontaneous closure is dependent largely on inherent characteristics of the fistula. Most fistulas that close without intervention will do so in the first 3 to 6 weeks after appearance. Fistulas with long tracts and narrow mouths are most likely to resolve independently. Additionally, low-output fistulas, defined as having an output less than 500 mL per day, have a higher likelihood of closure than high-output fistulas. A fistula that is not closed by 3 months is unlikely to close without surgical therapy. Additionally, many patient factors have been associated with failure of the fistula to close spontaneously. Factors that will virtually ensure patency of the fistula include the presence of a foreign body in the fistula tract, close association between the fistula and an abscess, association with a malignancy, distal bowel obstruction leading to increased pressure and transit through the fistulous tract, epithelialization of the tract, and a short neck with wide fistula mouth. As noted, long-standing fistulas with high outputs are unlikely to close spontaneously.

The patient and surgeon are not completely at the mercy of physiology and chance while awaiting spontaneous closure. At least in the short term, parenteral nutrition is pursued to decrease the volume transiting the gastrointestinal tract and through the fistula. A positive nitrogen balance and a transferrin level greater than 200 mg/dL are also associated with successful closure (7). The use of octreotide or other somatostatin analogue (100 μg intravenously every 8 hours) may decrease secretion in the gastrointestinal tract as well. Somatostatin inhibits the secretion of most gastrointestinal hormones and enhances fluid and electrolyte absorption, thereby decreasing intraluminal volume and potentially decreasing fistula output. Despite the theoretical benefits of somatostatin use, clinical studies have revealed mixed results on effectiveness. Although some studies have demonstrated a decreased fistula output and higher rate of spontaneous closure, an equivalent literature reveals no statistical difference in output or closure rates (8). As side effects are relatively mild, including gastrointestinal discomfort and increased biliary sludge, we recommend trying a somatostatin analogue in conjunction with other conservative therapies while waiting for a fistula to close spontaneously. However, somatostatin analogues should not be relied on as a primary therapy to close fistulas.

Surgical Therapy for Enterocutaneous Fistulas

If after approximately 3 months a fistula has failed to resolve, the likelihood of closure without operative intervention is poor. The first step in surgical closure is defining the fistula. The best method of defining a fistula tract is via fistulogram. In the standard method, Gastrografin is injected into the tract and fluoroscopy is used to follow the progress of the contrast. A fistulogram is useful to define the length of the tract, tortuosity, tract diameter, and which segment of the gastrointestinal tract is involved. An alternative method described in the litrature supports the use of hydrogen peroxide–enhanced ultrasound. The fistula is injected with hydrogen peroxide and ultrasound is used to define the tract. This method has no associated radiation, and ultrasound allows inspection of other intra-abdominal organs. A computed tomography (CT) scan may also be helpful in defining intra-abdominal abscesses, malignancy, and hernias (9).

In addition to defining the nature of the fistula, it is imperative that the patient's nutrition be maximized at the time of repair. Attention should be paid to control of fistula output, as healthy skin at the time of operation will improve the success of abdominal wall reconstruction (8). Essentially, by delaying operative repair until all criteria are met (nutrition, fistula definition, wound care), the morbidity and mortality may be decreased from 50% mortality and 50% recurrence in early surgeries to 94% successful closure and a 4% mortality rate with careful planning and delayed surgery (2,10).

Laparotomy with formal surgical repair is typically not the first surgery performed for these patients. A particular challenge for surgeons attempting to address enterocutaneous fistulas operatively is the condition of intra-abdominal adhesions. Extensive, dense adhesions may make access to the fistula very difficult, and there is a real risk of multiple enterotomies in approaching the segment involved in fistulization. A common initial attempt is to oversew the fistula primarily. Indeed, this technique may even be attempted at formal laparotomy. Although it may be appealing due to simplicity and avoidance of an anastomosis, it has a dismal failure rate and often results in a larger fistula. Simply oversewing fistulas should be avoided whenever possible. The preferred method for definitive surgical therapy remains complete lysis of intra-abdominal adhesions and resection of the involved segment. With this method, the diseased portion of bowel is removed and the anastomosis is performed between two healthy segments of intestine. The complete lysis of adhesions allows careful inspection of small bowel to rule out downstream obstruction or other pathology. Although potentially time consuming and technically demanding, this approach provides the highest likelihood of recovery without recurrent fistulization.

Enterocutaneous fistulas are unfortunately common in the open, granulating abdomen. These fistulas are an especially challenging management problem as it is difficult to control output on the granulating abdominal bed. A superior option for the patient with a fistula in the face of the granulating, open abdomen is the split-thickness skin graft. Although the skin graft rarely results in fistula closure, the adherence of the graft to the remainder of the granulation bed is excellent. The skin graft will decrease the metabolic demands of a granulating abdomen in an already stressed body and provide a good base for appliances placed for control of fistula output. For patients who may not tolerate an extensive repeat laparotomy, local mobilization of the fistula tract may allow for definitive closure. The fistula and the bowel are mobilized circumferentially proximally and distally by local dissection. The fistula portion is resected and closed, and the entire abdomen is covered with a split-thickness skin graft. Advocates claim a 56% success rate for this technique, and it may indeed be a better choice for some patients (2). In general, the split-thickness skin graft, with or without fistula closure, is more successful in low-output fistulas. High-output fistulas will stress a fistula repair leading to recurrent fistulization. Additionally, high fistula outputs will interfere with adherence of the grafted skin and ultimately digest the skin graft. Therefore, as with most procedures, careful patient selection will improve the success rate.

The Pancreatic Fistula

The pancreatic fistula is of an entirely different nature. In surgical patients, these fistulas most often result from trauma or iatrogenic injury, though a small percentage will be the result of pancreatitis. The cardinal principles of management are diagnosis of the fistula and wide drainage. A pancreatic fistula may drain from 100 to 1,000 mL of fluid per day. The resulting pancreatic ascites may cause abdominal pain, fevers, and a plethora of vague symptoms including abdominal bloating, hiccups, intolerance to oral intake, and abscess. Pancreatic fluid contains a large amount of bicarbonate compared to plasma (70–90 mEq/L), and inadequate replacement of bicarbonate may lead to nonanion gap metabolic acidosis. All patients respond differently to a pancreatic leak, and whereas some may present in profound shock, other patients may tolerate large-output pancreatic fistulas with few signs or symptoms. The source of this variability in clinical presentation is poorly understood but is likely due to the degree of enzymatic activation of the leaking fluid. The most common method of diagnosis is by CT scan. If the patient is of reasonable body habitus and transport is hazardous, an ultrasound may provide equivalent information.

For most patients, the initial treatment for a pancreatic fistula is simply drainage. In the modern era, interventional radiology is invaluable in placing these drains. However, if at initial operation there is concern for postoperative leak, wide drainage with a closed-system drain should be established before closing the patient's abdomen. Wide drainage of pancreatic secretions should allow time for the patient to stabilize and prevent damage to other abdominal organs. Frequently, patience to allow long-term drainage to resolve will permit spontaneous closure of the pancreatic fistula. In addition to drains, adjuncts such as total parenteral nutrition and octreotide may be helpful in decreasing secretory stimulation to the pancreas. A multiseries review demonstrated that the octreotide group (administered 100 μg subcutaneously every 8 hours begun immediately after procedures deemed at high risk for pancreatic fistulas) had reduced fistula outputs, lower serum amylase and lipase levels, and an earlier return of positive nitrogen balance than in control groups (8). As in many areas of research, there is an opposing literature demonstrating no statistically significant improvement in patient outcomes with octreotide therapy. However, it is reasonable to pursue this therapy for a time-limited course (approximately 1 week) to improve chances of nonoperative resolution.

Conservative management with drains is generally pursued for up to 6 months and has a success rate of upto 97% in some studies (11). Depending on the cause of the fistula, intervention may be indicated on an earlier basis. If drainage fails to resolve the fistula, an imaging study should be pursued to define the duct and to determine if an obstructive process is mandating fistula patency. Although both magnetic resonance cholangiopancreatography (MRCP) and endoscopic retrograde cholangiopancreatography (ERCP) may provide equivalent information, ERCP is preferred. ERCP allows the opportunity to identify pathology of the pancreatic duct and also allows the opportunity to intervene. Stenting of a proximal obstruction may be adequate to allow prograde drainage of pancreatic secretions and closure of the fistula, thereby avoiding surgical therapy (12). When all less invasive therapies fail, however, exploratory laparotomy remains the gold standard for definitive therapy. Options at laparotomy depend on the level of the injury. Primary duct repair is unlikely in most circumstances. Rather, a fistula resulting from the distal duct (perhaps secondary to a splenectomy) is well treated by distal pancreatectomy. If the leaking duct is sufficiently large, as is seen in relation to a ductal obstruction, a pancreaticojejunostomy may be performed to allow for a low-resistance drainage pathway. Pancreatic fistulas involving the proximal duct are most often iatrogenic or related to trauma and are troublesome to deal with, in light of other major structures in the region. For these patients, a pancreaticoduodenectomy (Whipple procedure) will resect the leaking portion of pancreas and allow reconstruction. The Whipple procedure should be entertained only in patients with good physiologic reserve. As noted, an attempt at conservative therapy and complete preoperative imaging and optimization are mandatory as these procedures are a major commitment for surgeon and patient. Despite the wealth of surgical options, most pancreatic fistulas will resolve with appropriate drainage, and thus, surgical correction is an end-stage option for correction of the fistula (11).

ABDOMINAL COMPARTMENT SYNDROME

Abdominal compartment syndrome has historically been a source of significant patient morbidity and mortality. First described in 1984, abdominal compartment syndrome was the result of an intra-abdominal catastrophe (ruptured abdominal aortic aneurysm) resulting in elevated pressure and multiple highly morbid sequelae (13). More recently, secondary abdominal compartment syndrome has resulted from massive resuscitations required by major trauma, burns, and pancreatitis. Regardless of the source of the compartment syndrome, those requiring decompressive laparotomy have a mortality rate of 19% to 33% (14). Occurrence of abdominal compartment syndrome has been lessened somewhat within the last decade due to increased recognition of the phenomenon and prophylactic use of the open abdomen technique. In operative cases requiring large-volume resuscitations, the abdomen is frequently left open postoperatively until edema decreases enough to allow tension-free primary closure. In this way, compartment syndrome and its sequelae are avoided. In the following section, diagnosis and management of abdominal compartment syndrome will be addressed, including methods to care for the open abdomen.

Since its first description in the 1980s, abdominal compartment syndrome has become an increasingly recognized clinical entity. Although classically described as a primary entity, in current surgical therapy it is usually seen following a massive fluid resuscitation from trauma, burns, intraoperative resuscitation, pancreatitis, or sepsis. Capillary leak occurs secondary to sepsis or reperfusion injury in the splanchnic circulation and results in massive interstitial edema. As the abdomen is a limited potential space, increasing interstitial edema and free fluid in the abdomen result in increased intra-abdominal pressure, which is transmitted to organs in both the thorax and abdomen. The physiologic effects range from cardiovascular to pulmonary to renal. Compression of the inferior vena cava by abdominal contents and fluid results in decreased preload and a subsequent decrease in cardiac output. This ultimately leads to increased systemic vascular resistance and decreased stroke volume. Clinically, patients will become increasingly tachycardic and hypotensive. Increased abdominal volume also places pressure on the diaphragm, limiting intrathoracic space. This results in increasing peak ventilatory pressures (greater than 30–35 mm Hg) and decreased ventilation with hypercapnia and hypoxemia. Compression of the ureters and bladder, as well as renal vein compression, leads to diminished urine output and renal injury, as well as elevated bladder pressures (greater than 25–30 mm Hg) (15,16).

Clinically, the key to diagnosis is a high index of suspicion. Multiple clinical factors, as noted above, will establish the diagnosis. The first clue to abdominal compartment syndrome is a distended and tense abdomen. These patients will frequently demonstrate hemodynamic instability with difficulty ventilating and poor urine output. Examination of the patient's ventilatory status will reveal elevated peak inspiratory pressures, often well above 30 mm Hg. If the patient is ventilated with a pressure-control ventilatory method, he or she will alternatively demonstrate low tidal volumes. As clinical suspicion increases, a bladder pressure may be transduced for definitive diagnosis. An arterial pressure line is attached to the patient's Foley catheter, and approximately 60 mL of sterile saline is introduced. Abdominal pressures greater than 15 mm Hg are indicative of abdominal compartment syndrome. When the transduced pressure reaches 25 to 30 mm Hg, a decompressive laparotomy is indicated as therapy for abdominal compartment syndrome (16,17). Of importance, decompressive laparotomy may be indicated at lower intra-abdominal pressures depending on the patient's clinical condition (18). After decompressing the abdominal contents, the abdomen is left open with a temporary abdominal closure until swelling diminishes enough to allow closure. Although decompressive laparotomy for abdominal compartment syndrome is life-saving, it continues to be associated with a 42% to 68% mortality rate (15) although a lower mortality rate has been reported and is dependent on the severity score (19).

The Open Abdomen

Over the last two decades, management strategies for abdominal domain have changed drastically. Even as few as 15 to 20 years ago, the surgical bias was that the abdomen must be closed at all costs. Two increasingly recognized trends in surgery have led to a change in perspective, where the open abdomen is no longer a catastrophe but rather a tool in the surgeon's armamentarium. First, the increasing recognition of primary and secondary abdominal compartment syndrome has led many surgeons to choose the open abdomen as a management strategy for the short term. Second, "damage control laparotomies" have become increasingly common in treating major abdominal trauma. Although the idea of abbreviated laparotomy was first described by Stone et al. in 1983 (20), the formal nomenclature and increasing popularity are credited to Rotondo et al. in 1993 (21). Damage control laparotomy is aimed at limiting intraoperative times for deteriorating patients, allowing transfer to the intensive care unit for vigorous resuscitation. Intraoperatively, major vascular hemorrhage is controlled, either by ligation or packing, and gross bowel contamination is controlled through ligation, often leaving the gastrointestinal tract in discontinuity. The patient's abdomen is then closed in a rapid and temporary manner, with a plan to return when the patient is more stable to effect definitive repair. Damage control laparotomy remains an aggressive strategy for treatment of patients who develop the deadly triad of coagulopathy, hypothermia, and metabolic acidosis (Fig. 77.2). By definition, it requires use of the open abdomen technique, at least until definitive surgical repair is possible.

The open abdomen, while an appropriate management technique, may ultimately become a Gordian knot. The questions of how to manage an open abdomen, and how and when to close it, may be difficult. Continuing management of the open abdomen involves three primary decision-making stages—initial operative management, decision to close primarily versus a planned ventral hernia, and definitive closure of the planned ventral hernia. At the time of the initial damage control laparotomy, the surgeon must choose to temporarily close the abdomen. The original temporary abdominal dressing is known as the *Bogota bag*. Initially described from its use in Colombia during the 1980s, it consists of covering the abdominal contents with a sterile saline bag to protect the bowel until reexploration. A derivation of the Bogota bag is a widely used method of temporary abdominal closure in current practice. A plastic drape, such as a sterile cassette cover, is placed over the bowels to prevent them from injury and to allow drainage of fluid. A sponge or blue towel, with two large Jackson-Pratt drains (Cardinal Health, McGaw Park, IL), is then placed over the plastic drape. The entire system is folded under the

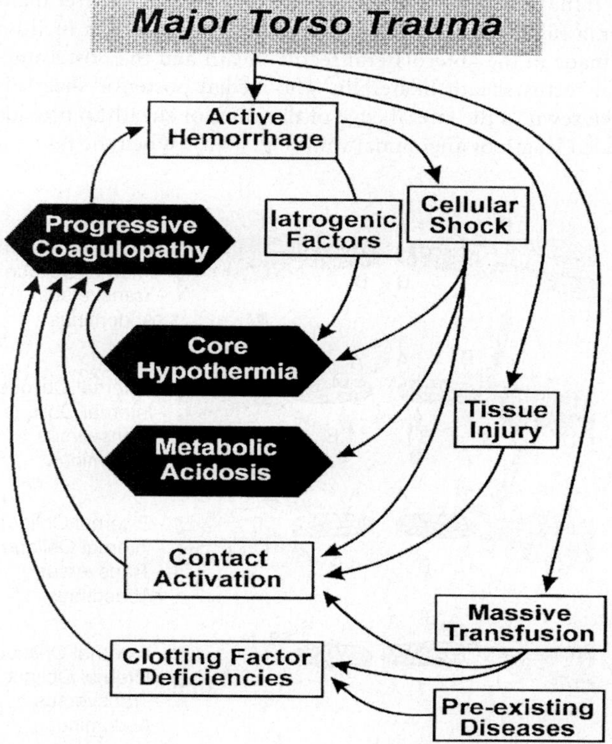

FIGURE 77.2. The "bloody vicious cycle" of coagulopathy, hypothermia, and metabolic acidosis.

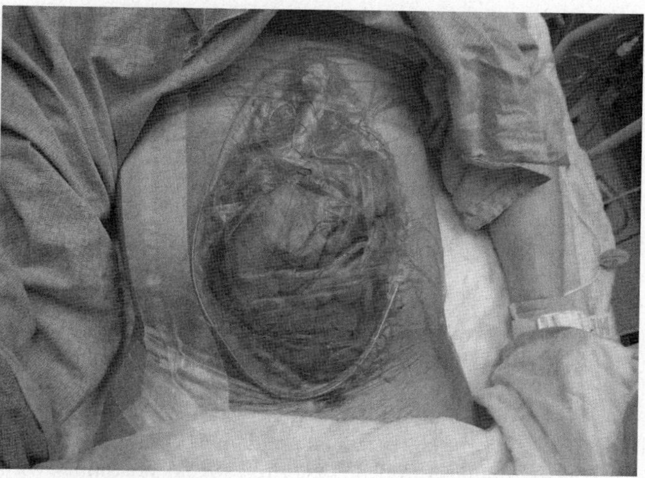

FIGURE 77.3. A temporary abdominal closure, using a sterile cassette cover and drains, as used in our practice.

fascia to contain the abdominal contents. An adhesive drape is placed over the abdomen to maintain sterility, contain contents, and prevent free drainage of fluid (Fig. 77.3). The drains are placed to suction to allow egress of blood and edema fluid. This dressing is then left intact until return to the operating room (22). This method is preferred to a traditional Bogotà bag, as it allows control of abdominal edema with no significant additional investment in time or supplies in the operating room. Regardless of method, the primary goal at this stage is rapid closure with protection of intra-abdominal contents. The exact technique is the surgeon's choice (19,23).

After an appropriate resuscitation period, typically 24 to 48 hours, the patient is returned to the operating room. If definitive therapy is complete, the decision to close primarily depends on the quantity of intra-abdominal edema and the quality of the fascia. Whenever possible, primary closure of fascia is ideal. The goal of every closure is to minimize tension on the fascia. High-tension closures not only result in elevated intra-abdominal pressures, but also lead to ischemia of the involved fascia with subsequent breakdown and the risk of dehiscence. If it is not possible to close the fascia, or if further trips to the operating room are indicated, the surgeon should choose a temporary closure that prevents lateral retraction of the fascia and facilitates later primary closure. Vicryl mesh sewn directly to the fascia is a form of temporary abdominal closure that may be pleated later in the intensive care unit. Mesh pleating and wound care may continue until intra-abdominal swelling diminishes and the fascia is near enough to close (15). Alternatively, vacuum-assisted fascial closure may be pursued. The most commonly used system is made by KCI (KCI Wound VAC System, Kinetic Concepts, Inc., San Antonio, TX) and involves a pie-crusted plastic drape with incorporated sponge, a separate wound sponge, and adhesive dressing with suction tubing. In this method, the bowels are protected with the plastic drape containing the incorporated sponge. A specially designed drainage sponge with constant suction is then placed, and the abdomen is covered with an adhesive dressing. The sponge suction provides constant medial tension, without disrupting the fascia, to prevent lateral retraction (22,23). Regardless of which method is chosen, most studies have indicated a high rate of primary closure if the patient has a net negative fluid balance at the time of operation. Therefore, management of the patient's volume status may be as important as the method of temporary closure in allowing later reapproximation of the fascia. However, net negative volume balance is extremely difficult to achieve in critically ill trauma patients requiring large-volume resuscitations. Therefore, a large percentage of these patients will go on to planned giant ventral hernias. In a study by Jernigan et al. (24) in 2003, 42% of patients with temporary closures for hemorrhagic shock ultimately were managed with planned, giant ventral hernias.

Closure of the Giant Ventral Hernia

For those who are not closed primarily, the ultimate management may be with the creation of a giant ventral hernia. These patients are managed for the first 1 to 2 weeks postinjury with Vicryl mesh and dressing changes or vacuum-assisted abdominal closures. Once the abdominal contents display a healthy bed of granulation tissue, the abdomen is given a split-thickness or full-thickness skin graft. The patient is then observed for 6 to 12 months as she or he undergoes rehabilitation and nutritional repletion.

As the ventral hernias are somewhat debilitating and cosmetically displeasing, most patients will be eager for definitive closure of the hernia (Fig. 77.4). The surgeon must consider the patient's nutritional status, as well as the laxity of the skin graft, prior to offering closure. Over time, the skin graft and intra-abdominal adhesions will soften, allowing easier graft removal and adhesiolysis. Rushing to repair a giant ventral hernia will result in operating in a hostile abdomen, with the risk of enterotomies and injury to the patient. As noted above, the ideal window for most patients appears to be at 6 to 12 months (Table 77.1) (25). The repair of the giant ventral hernia is also a good time for repair of any fistulas and reversal of stomas.

Most giant ventral hernias will not be amenable to primary closure. Therefore, the surgeon must decide the best method of restoring abdominal domain. The use of mesh is one option but may not be possible if enterotomies are made during the lysis stage or if stoma reversal is necessary. An increasingly popular option for these patients is a full or modified components

TABLE 77.1

MANAGEMENT OPTIONS FOR THE OPEN ABDOMEN

Initial Surgery	Cassette cover for damage control laparotomy
24–48 degrees	Primary closure→if hemorrhage controlled, resuscitated, no elevation of abdominal pressures
Unable to close primarily	Vicryl mesh: for 2–3 weeks until adequate granulation bed
	Wound vac: until adequate granulation bed
2–3 weeks, granulation	Split-thickness skin graft
	Planned ventral hernia
6–12 months	Closures of planned ventral hernia: with mesh
	Separation of components

separation. After sharply removing the skin graft, adhesed small bowel is freed from the overlying fascia for a distance of 4 to 6 cm. Skin flaps are raised laterally on both sides to the level of the midaxillary line to allow placement of relaxing incisions and full mobility of the fascia. When the skin flaps are fully raised, a relaxing incision is made in the external oblique fascia just lateral to the semilunar line. The incision is taken from above the ribs, often requiring division of some muscle, to the level of the pubis. Some additional medial mobility may be gained by dividing the filmy tissue between the external oblique muscle and the overlying fascia. This limited release may be adequate to allow reapproximation of the fascia at the midline. Aggressive closure under tension may lead to respiratory compromise and all the complications associated with abdominal compartment syndrome.

If the fascia will still not come together in a tensionfree manner, a full separation of components is indicated. An incision is made in the anterolateral rectus sheath and the posteromedial rectus sheath bilaterally. The medial posterior sheath is then sewn to the lateral edge of the anterior sheath to provide added length of abdominal wall (Fig. 77.5). When the fascia is

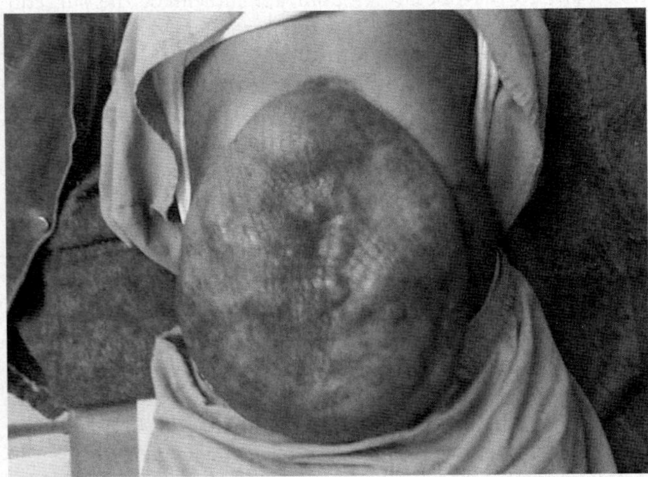

FIGURE 77.4. A planned ventral hernia, quite large, ready for definitive repair.

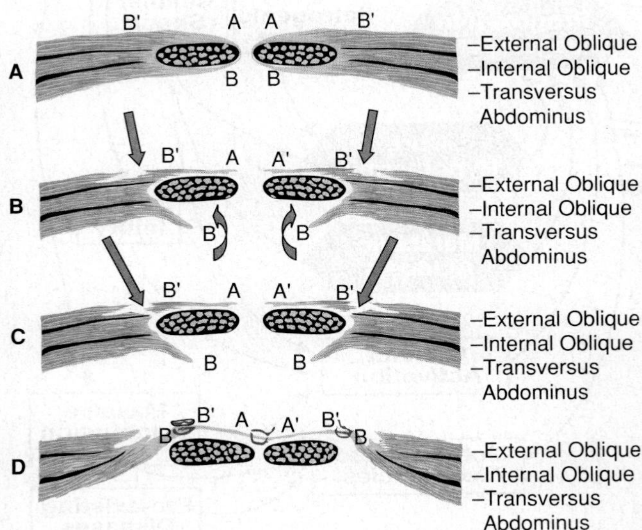

FIGURE 77.5. Depiction of a separation of components repair of a giant ventral hernia.

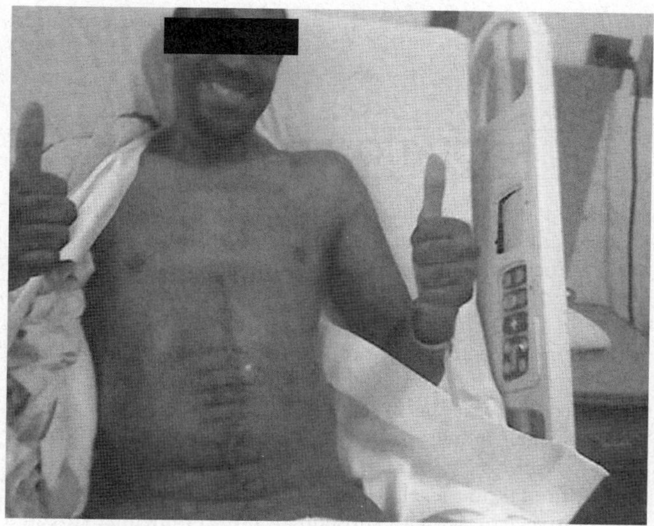

FIGURE 77.6. Definitive closure of a giant ventral hernia.

closely approximated, it is closed with interrupted PDS (polydioxanone sutures). Four Jackson-Pratt drains are then placed, one superior and one inferior bilaterally, and the skin is closed. Postoperatively, nasogastric suction is maintained until output decreases and drains are left in until output drops to less than 20 mL per day.

Occasionally, despite full separation, the fascia is still not close enough for a tensionfree repair. In these patients, a mesh or AlloDerm interposition may be necessary to achieve closure. This is most commonly seen in the upper portion of the closure where the rib cage may provide some increased lateral tension. Overall, patients tolerate closure well and long-term success is excellent with only a 5% recurrent hernia rate in experienced hands (Fig. 77.6) (24,25).

SHORT BOWEL SYNDROME

Short bowel is defined as a gastrointestinal length of 2 m, or less, and the cause may vary greatly between children and adults. Short bowel is an outcome of intra-abdominal catastrophe resulting in extensive surgical resection. Children most commonly end with short gut syndrome following a congenital or neonatal process such as necrotizing enterocolitis, intestinal atresia, volvulus, or gastroschisis. Adults acquire short gut syndrome following extensive surgical resection necessitated by malignancy, trauma, obstruction, or vascular insufficiency. Regardless of the cause, a patient's ultimate outcome is largely determined by the length of remaining small bowel and the presence or absence of the colon. Presence of the colon can extend the functional capacity of the remaining bowel. To have the potential for enteral autonomy, a patient requires at least 150 cm of small bowel, or 60 to 90 cm if the colon is present (26). Presence of the ileocecal valve is also important in maintaining hydration and modulating gastrointestinal transit time.

Short gut syndrome is most obviously defined by difficulty meeting nutritional requirements and dependence on parenteral nutrition. Patients will complain of weight loss, diarrhea, and steatorrhea. On a physiologic level, patients develop gastric emptying abnormalities and rapid transit times due to short intestinal length. Dehydration is a constant threat if the colon is absent due to an inability to reabsorb the approximately 4 L of gastrointestinal secretions per day. Loss of absorption results in deficiencies in B_{12}, fat-soluble vitamins, and bile salts. Short gut patients are also prone to cholelithiasis and nephrolithiasis due to altered absorption of bile salts and oxalate, peptic ulcers due to increased gastric secretions, line sepsis from deep catheters for delivery of parenteral nutrition, and liver dysfunction from that same parenteral nutrition (27).

A surgeon's role in managing short gut starts in the operating room with the very first incision. At the initial operation, the surgeon should make every effort to preserve bowel length, as well as the ileocecal valve. In some cases, it may be safest to limit resection and return at a later date to inspect marginally viable bowel. Initial postoperative therapy is often supportive, as this patient population is critically ill after emerging from the operating room. Early central venous access with immediate institution of parenteral nutrition aids in healing and prevents malnutrition. The long-term management of short gut patients then requires a multidisciplinary team involving physicians and nurses, nutritionists, patients, and their families.

Patients with short gut generally fall into two groups—those with insufficient length (usually less than 45–60 cm) who require lifelong parenteral nutrition and those with adequate length to potentially adapt and become partially or totally enterally independent. Adaptation is a process whereby the absorptive surface of the gut alters to increase digestive capacity and improve nutritional potential. In most cases, the ability is dependent on time and the nature of the remaining bowel. The ileum is capable of adapting to many jejunal functions, but the reverse is less successful (27). Some studies advocate the use of recombinant growth hormone to improve adaptation. In patients who are nutritionally maximized, growth hormone promotes mucosal hyperplasia and increases villous surface area. The process is further enhanced by high-carbohydrate, low-fat diets. Although minimal evidence exists in humans, animal studies have shown enhanced adaptation and nutritional repletion with selective use of growth hormone. Glutamine has also been proven beneficial and works synergistically with growth hormone. Glutamine, and trophic feeds, stimulate enterocytes and enhance cell proliferation. Even in patients who are completely parenterally dependent, low-rate trophic feeds maintain mucosal health (28). Additionally, preservation of colonic length improves fluid reabsorption. This improves patient hydration, leading to a more normal bowel regimen and improving the success of adaptation and weaning from parenteral nutrition. With these facts in mind, surgeons have a number of adjuncts to improve intestinal performance once bowel length is defined.

Occasionally, surgical therapy is required to deal with the sequelae of short gut or to promote adaptation. In patients with enteral continuity who are increasing oral intake, rapid transit due to inadequate length for absorption may result in persistent and disabling diarrhea and worsening of malnutrition. In these cases, conservative therapies such as medication and diet modification are the first line of therapy. If these are inadequate, segmental interposition may be attempted. Ideally, approximately 10 cm of small bowel is reversed and interposed in the gastrointestinal tract. When intraluminal contents reach the reversed segment, the antiperistaltic flow slows transit time. In cases where small bowel length is inadequate, a colonic limb may be interposed. This option is much less favored and rarely performed. Creation of an artificial valve is also a possibility for those lacking a native ileocecal valve. The key to creation of a successful valve is an appropriate length, as one that is too short will have minimal impact on transit time and one that is too long may cause obstruction. An ideal length is felt to be 2 cm although evidence regarding effectiveness is limited, as this is not a commonly performed procedure (29). Of note, surgical therapy for short bowel syndrome is pursued infrequently and is generally referred to tertiary centers with extensive experience managing these challenging patients.

In some cases, patients may have adequate remaining length for enteral independence but suffer from poor function secondary to obstruction, pseudo-obstruction, or dilation. Initial focus should be on relief of the obstruction. Obviously, adhesive bands obstructing the bowel lumen should be dealt with by simple lysis. In some cases, however, the small bowel may demonstrate one or multiple strictures. As bowel length in short gut patients is obviously at a premium, resection with anastomosis is not a good option. To preserve length and relieve obstruction, a stricturoplasty remains a reasonable alternative. In standard Heineke-Mikulicz stricturoplasty, a longitudinal incision is made along the length of the stricture. The enterotomy is then closed in one or two layers in a transverse direction. More involved stricturoplasties may be indicated depending on the specific details of the situation. However, a standard stricturoplasty should be adequate for most circumstances. Alternatively, a dilated, poorly functioning segment of bowel may exist in short gut patients due to distal obstructions, like strictures. When the distal obstruction has been dealt with, the dilated segment(s) may be treated by tapering enteroplasty. In this situation, interrupted Lembert stitches are placed on intact bowel to imbricate the wall and to decrease the caliber of the lumen. All of these procedures have specific indications and are pursued to maximize function of minimal bowel length.

When bowel length is too short, additional centimeters may be gained via a lengthening procedure. This may mean the difference between total parental nutrition dependence and partial enteral autonomy. In lengthening procedures, the antimesenteric border is incised, as well as the mesenteric border. Care must be taken to preserve the blood supply to both sides. Each side is then closed to form parallel tubes. These tubes are anastomosed end to end to create a segment that is twice as long but with a narrower lumen (2). A final option in pursuit of enteral independence is small bowel transplantation. Depending on the patient's hepatic function, a complete small bowel and liver transplant may be required. Small bowel transplantation remains an area of growth and continued challenge in the transplant community. Indications for small bowel transplantation include permanent intestinal failure as demonstrated by occlusion of two or more major veins, frequent episodes of line sepsis, unacceptable quality of life, or liver failure. With current induction and maintenance therapies, the 1-year survival for small bowel transplantation is approximately 65% and is only slightly lower at 59% when liver transplantation is included (30). With early evaluation and referral, specialized centers are achieving much better 2-year survival after small bowel transplantation with less morbidity related to immunosuppressive dosing. Transplant centers have been able to maintain good graft function while weaning patients off steroids and minimizing dosing of the most toxic immunosuppressive agents. Transplant remains an imperfect choice for short gut patients but has increasing promise for patients who have exhausted alternatives.

RADIATION ENTERITIS

Radiation damage to the gastrointestinal organs can be a particularly vexing problem for the surgeon and the patient. Ionizing radiation is delivered neoadjuvantly or adjuvantly for neoplastic processes occurring in organs of the pelvis. Radiation damages mitotically active cells of the mucosal surface epithelium, especially crypt cells. The incidence of injury is dependent on such factors as volume of irradiated small bowel, total dose delivered as well as dose per fraction, and type of radiation being delivered (31). In addition, radiation causes production of oxygen free radicals which further damages tissues at the cellular level. These cellular disruptions manifest as obliterative arteritis with subsequent bowel ischemia. Affected bowels may develop strictures, perforate, or develop fistulas (Fig. 77.7). Additionally, inflammation resulting from injury causes formation of dense local adhesions. Of patients undergoing abdominal and pelvic radiation, 50% to 75% will have some symptoms related to the therapy in the months to years following treatment. The most common symptoms are vague abdominal pain, diarrhea, rectal bleeding, and tenesmus. In 1% to 15%, bothersome symptoms will progress into actual radiation enteritis. Although symptoms most commonly occur during therapy, and may be abrogated by decreasing the radiation dose by 10%, patients may develop chronic radiation enteritis years after treatment. In the case of late radiation enteritis, workup should include dismissing recurrence of the initial neoplasm (2,32).

Initial management of radiation enteritis should embrace conservative measures. Sitz baths and stool softeners are effective initial treatments for rectal and anal symptoms. Opiates, antispasmodics, and anticholinergics will decrease transit time if diarrhea is the primary problem. Steroid enemas and sucralfate (by mouth or by rectum) can diminish irritation of the mucosa, which results in rectal pain and bleeding. If the patient is malnourished from chronic enteritis, total parenteral nutrition

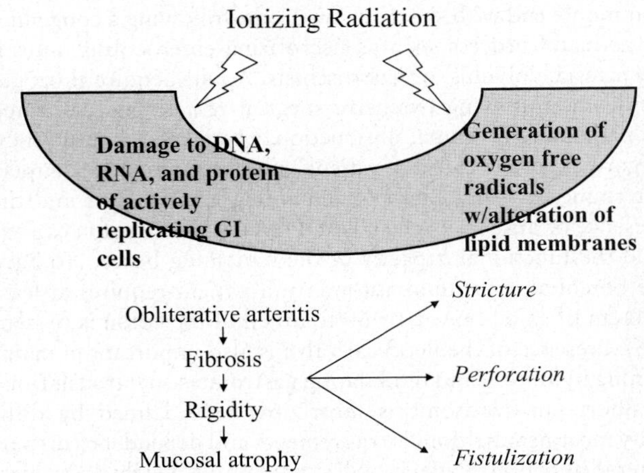

FIGURE 77.7. The effects of ionizing radiation on gastrointestinal cells and overall small bowel.

(TPN) may be necessary, especially if operative intervention is entertained.

Surgical Therapy for Radiation Enteritis

Surgical therapy for radiation enteritis encompasses two phases—prevention and therapy. If radiation is planned as an adjuvant therapy following surgery, some techniques may be used to diminish radiation injury. Simple nonsurgical methods to diminish radiation injury include patient positioning, multiple field techniques, and bladder distention (31). Following pelvic surgery, reperitonealizing the operative field will diminish local adhesions, which may serve to draw small bowel into the radiation field. Intra-operative efforts are designed to decrease the volume of small bowel included in the radiation field postoperatively. Use of mesh to construct a sling for exclusion of small bowel from the pelvis has had some success. However, this increases the risk of mesh-related hernias with the attendant risk of obstruction or strangulation, the rate of deep venous thrombosis, and the incidence of pelvic fluid collections. Using omentum to exclude the pelvis is rarely an option. This alternative is not available for most patients but has a lower incidence of the aforementioned mesh-related complications. Small bowel displacement systems, though not commonly used, have had some success in physically excluding up to 50% of small bowel volume from the radiation field (31).

The second role of surgery is in the treatment of complications of radiation enteritis. The most common indication for surgery remains obstruction, but other indications include excessive bleeding, intractable diarrhea, pain, fistulas, and persistent abscess. Any surgical intervention should use the least invasive procedure required to address the issue. Excessive handling of radiated tissues commonly results in unplanned enterotomies and may interrupt an already tenuous blood supply. Any suspicious-appearing areas should be biopsied to evaluate for recurrent neoplasm. The diseased segment, if involved in obstruction or fistula, should be excised, and the anastomosis should attempt to include nonradiated bowel. Minimal lysis of adhesions should be pursued to prevent disruption of tenuous blood supplies. If dense adhesions prevent access to the involved segment, a gastrointestinal bypass may be necessary. This option will predispose a patient to blind loop syndrome and bleeding but may be a better option than attempting to mobilize frozen bowel (32).

Approximately 2% to 5% of patients with a history of pelvic radiation therapy will develop chronic proctopathy, which may include rectal pain and bleeding (33). First-line therapies of sucralfate and steroid enemas are of limited benefit. Endoscopic coagulation of bleeding with electrocautery or laser has been successful for limited bleeding sites. Laser photocoagulation has a low morbidity rate of 5% to 15% but requires multiple treatment sessions. The most effective nonoperative therapy remains the topical application of 4% formalin, with 85% of patients responding after two instillations or less (33). When these measures fail, invasive therapy is pursued. If there is a component of stricture, initial therapy should include serial dilation. However, if this is unsuccessful or the indication is intractable pain, severe incontinence, or profound bleeding, a diverting colostomy may be necessary. In worst case situations, abdominoperineal resection may be pursued. In the event of fistulas, the fistula tract and involved tissue at either end must be resected and the sites closed. An interposition flap of omentum or muscle should then be placed to protect the repair sites. Again, prevention is truly the best option for the problem of radiation enteritis. New radiation regimens with lower doses and more specific direction potentially provide the most benefit for this patient population.

SUMMARY

Even the most routine abdominal surgery has the potential for a difficult postoperative course. When postoperative patients do not progress as anticipated, or when complications develop, a high index of suspicion is important for rapid diagnosis and treatment. The cornerstone of every difficult postoperative problem is meticulous and careful technique at the time of the original surgery. Once the problem is manifest, attention to the patient's condition and conservative management are widely favored initial approaches. Ultimate therapeutic choices may have a profound effect on the patient's eventual recovery and quality of life. Whether the final cure is by careful manipulation of patient physiology or by surgical intervention, the critical care surgeon must be well versed in a multitude of complex postoperative issues to provide exceptional and appropriate therapy.

PEARLS

- Routes to provide enteral feedings should be considered at the time of surgery for patients in whom oral intake is not anticipated for some time. Either surgical jejunostomy or manual placement of small nasoenteric feeding tubes past the pylorus will help the patients with early nutrition and possible avoidance of parenteral nutrition.
- All tubes and drains must be secured to minimize inadvertent dislodgement. Loss of carefully placed tubes and drains can lead to significant morbidity.
- Avoid re-entering the abdomen in the first 2 to 3 weeks after previous surgery (if possible). This is the peak time for dense adhesions and iatrogenic injury may occur.
- Carefully assess the patient's general condition before entering a hostile abdomen. Cardiovascular and pulmonary status, nutritional support, blood sugar control, and coagulation profile should be optimized if possible.

References

1. Fazio VW, Cohen Z, Fleshman JW, et al. Reduction in adhesive small-bowel obstruction by Seprafilm Adhesion Barrier after resection. *Dis Colon Rectum*. 2006;49(1):1–11.
2. Cameron JL, ed. *Current Surgical Therapy*. 7th ed. St. Louis, MO: Mosby; 2001.
3. ten Raa S, van den Tol MP, Sluiter M, et al. The role of neutrophils and oxygen free radicals in post-operative adhesions. *J Surg Res*. 2006;136(1):45–52.
4. Johns A. Evidence based prevention of post-operative adhesions. *Hum Reprod Update*. 2001;7(6):577–579.
5. Van't Rient M, de Vos van Steenwijk PJ, Bonthuis F, et al. Prevention of adhesions to prosthetic mesh: comparison of different barriers using incisional hernia model. *Ann Surg*. 2003;237(1):123–128.
6. Memon AS, Siddiqui FG. Causes and management of postoperative enterocutaneous fistulas. *J Coll Physicians Surg Pak*. 2004;14(1):25–28.

7. Li J, Ren J, Zhu W, et al. Management of enterocutaneous fistulas: 30-year clinical experience. *Chinese Med J*. 2003;116(2):171–175.
8. Gray M, Jacobson T. Are somatostatin analogues (octreotide and lanreotide) effective in promoting healing of enterocutaneous fistulas? *J Wound Ostomy Continence Nurs*. 2002;29(5):228–233.
9. Maconi G, Parente F, Porro GB. Hydrogen peroxide enhanced ultrasound-fistulography in the assessment of enterocutaneous fistulas complicating Crohn's disease. *Gut*. 1999;45(6):874–878.
10. Draus JM Jr, Huss SA, Harty NJ, et al. Enterocutaneous fistula: are treatments improving? *Surgery*. 2006;140(4):570–578.
11. Pannegeon V, Pessaux P, Sauvanet A, et al. Pancreatic fistula after distal pancreatectomy: predictive risk factors and value of conservative treatment. *Arch Surg*. 2006;141(11):1071–1076.
12. Kaman L, Behera A, Singh R, et al. Internal pancreatic fistulas with pancreatic ascites and pancreatic pleural effusions: recognition and management. *ANZ J Surg*. 2001;71(4):221–225.
13. Kron IL, Harman PK, Nolan S. The measurement of intra-abdominal pressure as a criterion for abdominal reexploration. *Ann Surg*. 1984;199(1):28–30.
14. Reed SF, Britt RC, Collins J, et al. Aggressive surveillance and early catheter-directed therapy in the management of intra-abdominal hypertension. *J Trauma*. 2006;61(6):1359–1365.
15. Maxwell RA, Fabian TC, Croce MA, et al. Secondary abdominal compartment syndrome: an underappreciated manifestation of severe hemorrhagic shock. *J Trauma*. 1999;47(6):995.
16. Crandall M, West MA. Evaluation of the abdomen in the critically ill patient: opening the black box. *Curr Opin Crit Care*. 2006;12(4):333–339.
17. Ivatury RR. Abdominal compartment syndrome: a century later, isn't it time to accept and promulgate? *Crit Care Med*. 2006;34(9):2494–2495.
18. DeWaele JJH, Malbrain EA, Lng M. Decompressive laparotomy for abdominal compartment syndrome—a critical analysis. *Crit Care*. 2006;10(2):R51.
19. Malbrain MLNG, Chiumello D, Pelosi P, et al. Incidence and prognosis of intraabdominal hypertension in a mixed population of critically ill patients: a multiple-center epidemiological study. *Crit Care Med*. 2005;33:315.
20. Stone HH, Strom PR, Mullins RJ. Management of the major coagulopathy with onset during laparotomy. *Ann Surg*. 1983;197:532–535.
21. Rotondo M, Schwab CW, McGonigal MD, et al. Damage control: an approach for improved survival in exsanguinating penetrating abdominal injury. *J Trauma*. 1993;35:375–383.
22. Stone PA, Hass SM, Flaherty SK, et al. Vacuum-assisted fascial closure for patients with abdominal trauma. *J Trauma*. 2004;57(5):1082–1086.
23. James C, Stawicki SP, Hoff WS, et al. A proposed algorithm for managing the open abdomen. *Am Surg*. 2005;71(3):202–207.
24. Jernigan TW, Fabian TC, Croce MA, et al. Staged management of giant abdominal wall defects: acute and long-term results. *Ann Surg*. 2003;238(3):349–357.
25. Fabian TC. Damage control in trauma: laparotomy wound management acute to chronic. *Surg Clin North Am*. 2007;87:73–93.
26. DiBaise JK, Matarese LE, Messing B, et al. Strategies for parenteral nutrition weaning in adult patients with short bowel syndrome. *J Clin Gastroenterol*. 2006;40(Suppl 2):S94–98.
27. Nightingale J, Woodward JM. Guidelines for management of patients with a short bowel. *Gut*. 2006;55(Suppl 4):1–12.
28. Steiger E, DiBaise JK, Messing B, et al. Indications and recommendations for the use of recombinant human growth hormone in adult short bowel syndrome patients dependent on parenteral nutrition. *J Clin Gastroenterol*. 2006;40(Suppl 2):S99–106.
29. Thompson JS. Surgical aspects of the short-bowel syndrome. *Am J Surg*. 1995;170(6):532–536.
30. Dijkstra GR, Rings EHHM, van Dullemen HM, et al. Small bowel transplantation as a treatment option for intestinal failure in children and adults. *Ned Tijdschr Geneeskd*. 2005;149(8):391–398.
31. Park W, Huh SJ, Lee JE, et al. Variation of small bowel sparing with small bowel displacement system according to the physiological status of the bladder during radiotherapy for cervical cancer. *Gynecol Oncol*. 2005;99(3):645–651.
32. Onodera H, Nagayama S, Mori A, et al. Reappraisal of surgical treatment for radiation enteritis. *World J Surg*. 2005;29(4):459–463.
33. Cullen SN, Frenz M, Mee A. Treatment of hemorrhagic radiation-induced proctopathy using small volume topical formalin instillation. *Aliment Pharmacol Ther*. 2006;23(11):1575–1579.

CHAPTER 78 ■ CRITICAL CARE OF HEPATOPANCREATOBILIARY SURGERY PATIENTS

ROBIN D. KIM • KRISTIN L. MEKEEL • ALAN W. HEMMING

Patients are admitted to the intensive care unit (ICU) for a variety of reasons following hepatopancreatobiliary (HPB) surgery, including maintenance or restoration of normal physiology immediately after extensive surgery and the subsequent management of complications that develop. Many of the issues that require ICU management are common to all ICU patients and will not be discussed in this chapter; however, there are recurring issues that are relatively specific to HPB surgery patients that will be discussed. The role of normal liver physiology and its alteration during HPB surgery and disease states will be discussed, as well as the management of common problems that arise after HPB surgery.

HPB surgery is composed of surgery of the liver, bile duct, and pancreas, and may include portal decompressive procedures for complications of portal hypertension. Surgical procedures on the pancreas and bile duct alone generally do not require care in a critical care setting immediately after leaving the operating room unless complications occur. Liver resections, particularly when extensive, can require admission to a critical care unit immediately following surgery due to the alterations in normal physiology that occur during the procedure itself. An understanding of normal liver physiology and the alterations it undergoes during surgery is important when managing these patients.

LIVER ANATOMY AND PHYSIOLOGY

The liver is approximately 4% to 5% of total body weight and has multiple complex functions. The anatomy of the liver

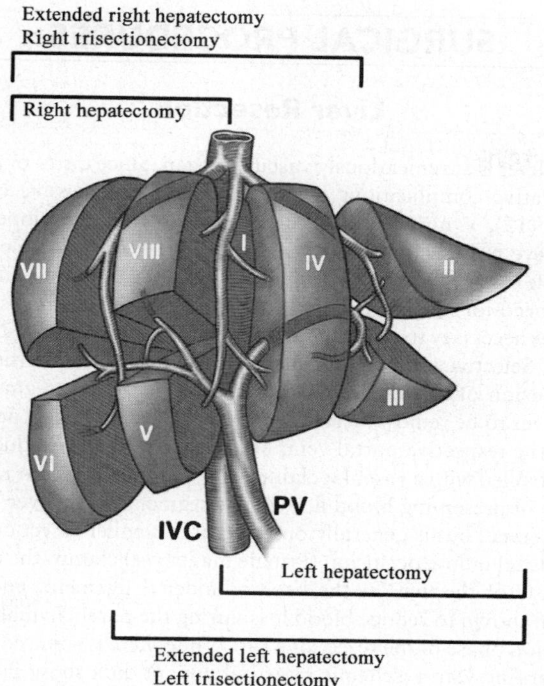

FIGURE 78.1. Diagrammatic representation of liver segments with standard liver resections demonstrated. IVC, inferior vena cava; PV, pulmonary vein.

has been described using various and different methods (1–5); however, surgical anatomy is based on the segmental nature of vascular and bile duct distribution. The liver receives a dual blood supply from both the portal vein and hepatic artery that run, along with the bile duct, within the glissonian sheath or main portal pedicle. The portal pedicle divides into right and left branches and then supplies the liver in a segmental fashion. Venous drainage is via the hepatic veins, which drain directly into the inferior vena cava. Hepatic segmentation is based on the distribution of the portal pedicles and their relation to the hepatic veins (Fig. 78.1). The three hepatic veins run in the portal scissurae and divide the liver into four sectors, which are, in turn, divided by the portal pedicles running in the hepatic scissurae. The liver is divided into right and left hemilivers by the middle hepatic vein. The right hemiliver is divided by the right hepatic vein into anterior and posterior sectors. The anterior sector is divided by the plane of the portal pedicle into an inferior segment V and a superior segment VIII. The posterior sector is divided by the plane of the portal pedicle into an inferior segment VI and a superior segment VII. The left hemiliver lies to the left of the middle hepatic vein and is divided into anterior and posterior sectors by the left hepatic vein. The anterior sector is divided by the umbilical fissure into segment IV medially and segment III laterally. The segment posterior to the left hepatic vein is segment II. Segment IV can be divided by the plane of the portal pedicle into a superior segment IVa and an inferior segment IVb. Segment I is the caudate lobe, which lies between the inferior vena cava and the hepatic veins. The caudate lobe has variable portal venous, hepatic arterial and biliary anatomy, and is essentially independent of the portal pedicle divisions and hepatic venous drainage.

Segmental anatomy becomes important in considering surgical resection when essentially any segment or combination of segments can be resected if attention is paid to maintaining vascular and biliary continuity to the remaining segments.

Common liver resections performed that may require ICU admission after surgery are left or right hepatectomies, in which approximately 50% of liver volume is removed, or more extensive procedures such as right or left trisectionectomy, in which up to 80% of the liver is removed (Fig. 78.1). If less than 40% of the liver is resected in patients with normal underlying liver function, then relatively little derangement of liver physiology is noted.

The liver performs many functions, including uptake, storage, and eventual distribution of nutrients from the blood or gastrointestinal tract, as well as synthesis, metabolism, and elimination of a variety of endogenous and exogenous substrates and toxins (including narcotics and other drugs). Although the liver is only 4% to 5% of total body weight, it is responsible for 20% to 25% of body oxygen consumption and 20% of total energy expenditure (6). The liver receives a dual blood supply, with 75% of flow from the portal vein and 25% from the hepatic artery. Total blood flow (7) to the liver is approximately 1.5 L/minute/1.73 m^2. While decreasing portal venous flow causes a subsequent increase in hepatic arterial flow, with complete portal occlusion or diversion, hepatic arterial flow does not completely compensate, and total liver blood flow is diminished (8). The opposite is not true, however (i.e., decreasing flow in the hepatic artery does not increase flow in the portal vein). There is autoregulation of hepatic arterial flow but not of the portal venous system. Portal flow is increased by food intake, bile salts, secretin, pentagastrin, vasoactive intestinal peptide (VIP), glucagon, isoproterenol, prostaglandin E_1 and E_2, and papaverine. Portal flow is decreased by serotonin, angiotensin, vasopressin, nitrates, and somatostatin.

Bile, composed of inorganic ions and organic solutes, is formed at the canalicular membrane of the hepatocyte, as well as in the bile ductules, and is secreted by an active process that is relatively independent of blood flow (9). The major organic components of bile are the conjugated bile acids, cholesterol, phospholipid, bile pigments, and protein. Under normal conditions, 600 to 1,000 mL of bile is produced per day (10). Bile secretory pressure is approximately 10 to 20 cm saline, with maximal secretory pressures of 30 to 35 cm in the presence of complete biliary obstruction.

Bilirubin, a degradation product of heme, is eliminated almost entirely in the bile. Bilirubin circulates bound to albumin and is removed from plasma by the liver via a carrier-mediated transport system. In the hepatocyte, bilirubin is bound to glucuronic acid before being secreted in bile. The liver maintains the ability to clear bilirubin with partial duct obstruction. Complete obstruction of one of the right or left hepatic ducts alone will cause marked liver enzyme abnormalities, but rarely causes jaundice.

The liver synthesizes many of the major human plasma proteins including albumin, γ-globulin, and many of the coagulation proteins. Liver dysfunction can have a profound effect on coagulation through the decreased production of coagulation proteins or, in the case of obstructive jaundice, there is decreased activity of factors II, V, VII, IX, and X, secondary to a lack of vitamin K–dependent posttranslational modification. Reversal of coagulation abnormalities by exogenous administration of vitamin K allows differentiation between synthetic dysfunction and lack of vitamin K absorption secondary to obstructive jaundice.

After liver resection, liver function is altered through both a reduction in functional liver mass and potential ischemia/reperfusion injury to the liver remnant. With extensive liver resection in patients with normal presurgical underlying liver function, reduction of functional liver volume below 25% has been associated with an increased risk of both liver failure and mortality (11). To reduce the risk of liver failure in this setting, preoperative portal vein embolization (PVE) has been developed. During PVE, the portal vein of the side of the liver to be resected is embolized percutaneously. Diversion of portal flow and its hepatotrophic factors to the future liver remnant (FLR) causes growth and hypertrophy of the FLR of about 30% (Fig. 78.2) over a 6-week period and has been shown to reduce the complications associated with subsequent extended liver resections (12).

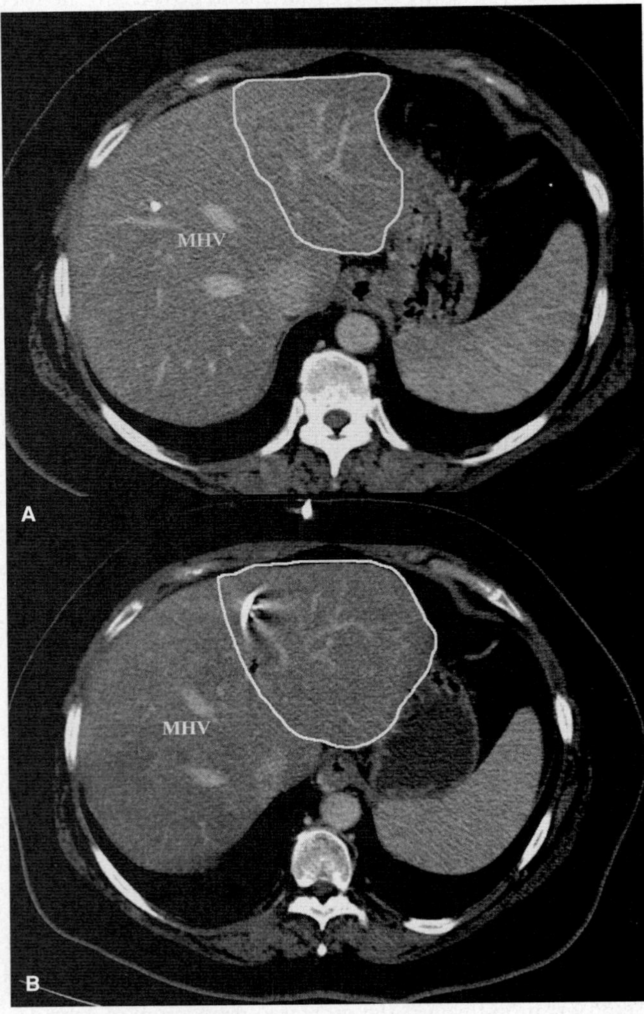

FIGURE 78.2. Right portal vein embolization preoperatively allows an increase of functional liver remnant of approximately 30% from prior to embolization (A) to postembolization (B). MHV, middle hepatic vein. (Reused with permission from Hemming AW, Reed AI, Howard RJ, et al. Preoperative portal vein embolization for extended hepatectomy. *Ann Surg.* 2003;237[5]:686–691.)

SURGICAL PROCEDURES

Liver Resection

The liver is a tremendously vascular organ. Since intra- or postoperative complications are often related to excessive blood loss (13), a number of techniques have been developed to achieve preresection vascular control and decreased bleeding. While liver resection may be performed, in many cases without the need for interruption of blood flow to the liver, it is sometimes necessary to reduce blood flow to prevent excessive blood loss. Selective inflow control can be established by division or occlusion of the vascular structures supplying the segment(s) of liver to be removed. The right or left portal pedicle containing the respective portal vein, hepatic artery, and bile duct are controlled with a vascular clamp. This technique has the advantage of preserving blood flow to the segment of the liver being preserved, but is generally only useful in smaller resections.

Total inflow occlusion (Pringle maneuver) clamps the entire inflow of the liver at the hepatoduodenal ligament, and has been shown to reduce blood loss during the parenchymal transection phase of the resection (14). While there is some concern regarding warm ischemic injury, abundant data show that the normal liver can tolerate inflow occlusion for up to 1 hour, and there are reports suggesting that some cirrhotic livers can safely tolerate 60 minutes of inflow occlusion as well (15). We use total inflow occlusion when selective occlusion provides insufficient control. Clamp times are expected to be less than 30 minutes for formal hepatectomies, but may be higher for more complex parenchymal transections. In such cases, total occlusion is carried out in 15-minute increments with 5-minute reperfusion intervals. An alternative to the intermittent clamping technique is to use ischemic preconditioning, during which the liver inflow is occluded for 10 minutes, after which it is allowed to reperfuse for 15 minutes prior to clamping again for a sustained time period up to 1 hour. Intermittent clamping is associated with more blood loss than ischemic preconditioning; however, the protective results of ischemic preconditioning in ischemia reperfusion injury have not been uniform across age groups, and may not be as effective in livers that have been exposed to preoperative chemotherapy (16).

Total vascular isolation of the liver with both inflow occlusion and occlusion of the supra- and infrahepatic vena cava can be useful for technically demanding cases where the vena cava or proximal hepatic veins are involved with tumor (Fig. 78.3). Total isolation has been shown to be safe for up to 60 minutes in normal liver, but can be accompanied by varying degrees of hemodynamic instability (17). In cases where this is required, we carry out as much of the operation as possible prior to isolation of the liver to reduce the ischemic time and the period of hemodynamic instability.

The most troublesome bleeding sources during liver resection are usually from hepatic vein branches, which may be minimized by maintaining the central venous pressure (CVP) below 5 mm Hg during the period of hepatic transection. Cooperation of the anesthetist in minimizing volume loading, and occasionally using pharmacologic agents to reduce CVP, is essential. However, if total vascular isolation is to be used, volume loading prior to caval clamping is required to avoid an acute decrease in cardiac output at the time the clamps are applied.

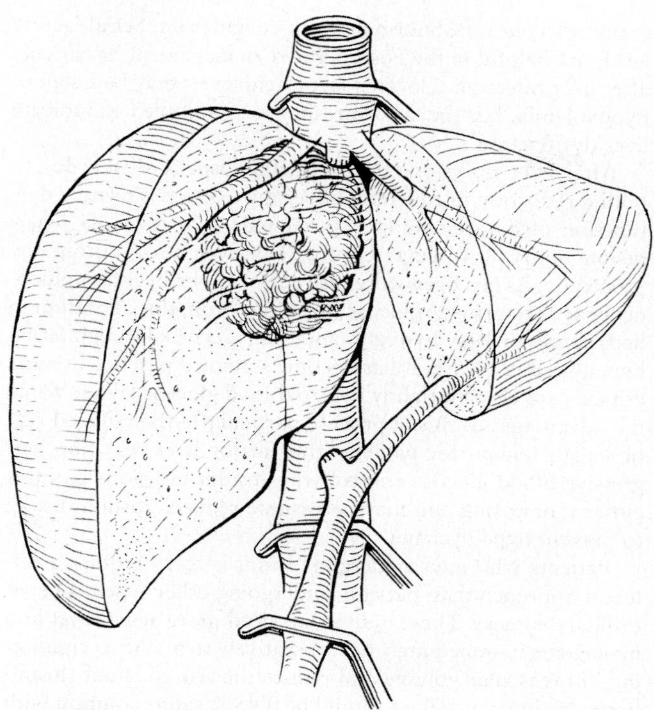

FIGURE 78.3. Tumors that involve the inferior vena cava or hepatic veins may require total vascular isolation of the liver. Both the infrahepatic and suprahepatic inferior vena cava are clamped along with the portal vein and hepatic artery. (Reused with permission from Hemming AW, Reed AI, Langham MR, et al. Combined resection of the liver and inferior vena cava for hepatic malignancy. *Ann Surg.* 2004;239[5]:712–721.)

Knowledge of the details of intraoperative conduct of the operation is therefore important to the physicians who are to manage the postoperative care of the liver resection patient in the ICU setting. Was inflow occlusion or vascular isolation required, and for how long? Prolonged clamp times are associated with greater liver dysfunction. Was the patient maintained with a low CVP throughout the course of the surgery? If so, then the patient may need volume expansion on arrival to the ICU. How much liver remains, and is it normal? If the percentage of remaining liver is less than 25% in normal livers or less than 40% in cirrhotic livers or livers with bile duct obstruction, then the chance of liver failure and the need for its management are higher. Was there significant blood or fluid requirements? Patients may need a period of ventilation while fluid shifts and equilibrates.

Pancreatic and Bile Duct Surgery

The majority of patients who undergo pancreatic or bile duct surgeries do not require admission to an ICU setting in the immediate postoperative period because of issues specific to the pancreaticobiliary surgery itself. In general, procedures on the pancreas or biliary tree should not be associated with major intraoperative hemodynamic changes or alterations in physiology. Tumors of the head of the pancreas or bile duct may involve the portal vein or cause extensive fibrotic reaction in the area. Technical difficulties can arise in which damage occurs to, or resection is required of, the portal vein (Fig. 78.4). If portal vein resection or repair is required, it is more likely that the patient will require ICU care. Portal vein resection, when planned, requires variable durations of portal venous outflow obstruction from the gut, which are usually short and well tolerated, but can increase the amount of fluid third-spaced into the bowel wall. Portal vein injury, however, can lead to massive transfusion requirements and hypotension that can require postoperative ICU care. The more common indications for admission to the ICU after pancreatic or biliary surgery are either an underlying medical condition or the development of a postoperative complication. Pancreatic or bile leaks, which can lead to sepsis, will be discussed later in the chapter.

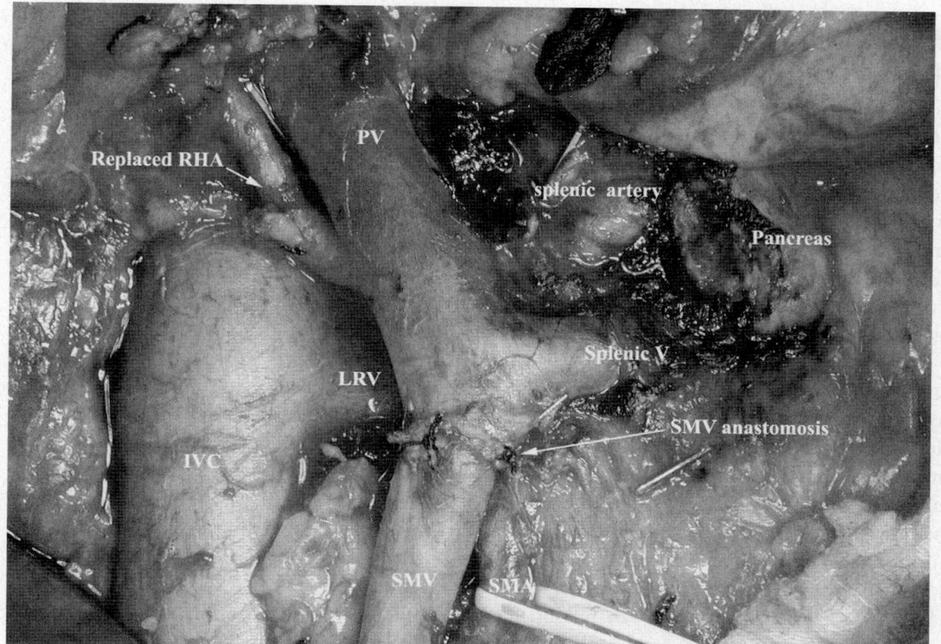

FIGURE 78.4. Pancreaticoduodenectomy demonstrating resection of the portal vein. IVC, inferior vena cava; LRV, left renal vein; PV, portal vein; RHA, right hepatic artery; SMA, superior mesenteric artery; SMV, superior mesenteric vein; splenic V, splenic vein. (Reused with permission from Hemming AW, Reed AI, Langham MR, et al. Combined resection of the liver and inferior vena cava for hepatic malignancy. *Ann Surg.* 2004;239[5]:712–721.)

Portal Decompressive Procedures

Surgical portal decompressive procedures, although a rarity since the introduction of the transjugular intrahepatic portosystemic shunt (TIPS), remain indicated in select patients with variceal bleeding and preserved liver function who have failed medical management and are not transplant candidates. The myriad technical variations of surgical portosystemic shunts are beyond the scope of this chapter, but certain commonalities exist. Whether total or partial shunts, selective or nonselective, patients will have had the high-pressure portal system surgically connected to the low-pressure caval circulation to lower the pressure in the portal venous system and stop variceal bleeding. Reduction of portal flow in patients who have borderline liver function can precipitate liver dysfunction or failure. Additionally, the fraction of portal flow that is diverted into the systemic circulation through the shunt is not cleared by the liver until it returns to the liver via the arterial circulation. This may induce encephalopathy; shunts that divert most or all of the portal flow into the systemic circulation are more likely to induce encephalopathy than those shunts that are selective or partial. One special case scenario is Budd-Chiari syndrome, in which the hepatic venous outflow is obstructed, usually due to thrombosis secondary to a hypercoagulable state. In this disorder, blood flow perfuses the hepatic sinusoids from both the hepatic artery and portal vein but cannot exit through the blocked hepatic veins. A functional side-to-side shunt is performed (portacaval, mesocaval) that allows hepatic arterial blood to flow into the sinusoids and then exit via the portal vein, and through the shunt into the systemic circulation. It is not uncommon for liver function to deteriorate initially after the shunt is performed, with subsequent gradual improvement and liver regeneration. Support of liver function may be required immediately after the shunt while liver function stabilizes. In some cases, the shunt may precipitate acute liver failure, making urgent liver transplantation the only option.

IMMEDIATE POSTOPERATIVE MANAGEMENT

Postoperative fluid management is important in the care of patients after major hepatobiliary surgery. In particular, postoperative fluid shifts in patients who have had major liver resection can be difficult to manage. Intraoperatively, most liver resections are performed with low central venous pressure and low intravascular volume. While this practice minimizes bleeding during the hepatic parenchymal transection phase of the procedure, it may pose some difficulty postoperatively, as these patients may have signs of hypovolemia with low urine output and low blood pressure. Volume reexpansion should be gentle, as partial liver resection leads to hypoalbuminemia, and pulmonary edema and ascites can develop with aggressive resuscitation. Although the use of albumin infusions is generally frowned upon in critical care medicine, albumin and fresh frozen plasma may be useful in the resuscitation of patients after liver resection, as the physiology is similar to patients with cirrhosis. We use albumin-containing fluids for volume expansion if the serum albumin is less than 2.9 mg/dL. Fresh frozen plasma can be used for volume expansion; however, it is generally reserved for abnormalities in coagulation. Serial lactate levels are helpful in the postoperative management of patients after liver resection. Elevated lactic acid levels may be a sign of hypovolemia, but the lack of response to volume can indicate liver dysfunction.

After liver resection, glucose metabolism is altered due to both a reduction in functional liver mass and the relative dysfunction of the remaining liver secondary to ischemia reperfusion injury if vascular control has been used during the procedure. As glycogen stores are depleted, the liver uses gluconeogenesis to provide glucose. Resulting from this alteration in hepatic physiology, hypoglycemia may occur, although lethal hypoglycemia is rare. It has become standard practice in most critical care units to tightly control blood glucose levels. While the advantages of this approach, particularly the reduced risk of sepsis, remain for patients after major liver resection, aggressive blood glucose control with insulin infusions requires closer monitoring and may necessitate reduced insulin dosing to prevent hypoglycemia.

Patients who have undergone shunt surgery require a different approach than patients undergoing other types of hepatobiliary surgery. These individuals need more aggressive fluid management immediately postoperatively to maintain circulating intravascular volume and reduce the risk of shunt thrombosis. Maintenance fluid should be 0.45% saline solution with 5% dextrose to provide the liver with carbohydrate. After the immediate postoperative period, patients are also at risk for ascites formation, so excessive sodium should be minimized and additional volume expansion—if needed—should be albumin or fresh frozen plasma. Diuretics can be reinstituted after the immediate postoperative period. A general rule is to use a combination of Lasix and spironolactone, with 100 mg of spironolactone for every 40 mg of Lasix. Antibiotics are administered for 48 hours postoperatively to minimize infection from bacterial translocation.

Encephalopathy is rare in patients after liver resection, unless they are in liver failure or have pre-existing liver disease. The presence of asterixis can be an early sign of encephalopathy. Encephalopathy is treated with lactulose and dietary protein restriction, as in other patients with end-stage liver disease. Infection, dehydration, and bleeding, as well as narcotic use, must be evaluated, as they can trigger decompensation that leads to encephalopathy.

Hypophosphatemia

While the exact mechanism of the hypophosphatemia seen after hepatic resection remains unclear, care must be taken to aggressively replace the low serum phosphate, since increased utilization during liver regeneration and a renal wasting mechanism have been proposed (18).

Regardless of the etiology, the clinical consequences of hypophosphatemia are well established and include respiratory depression, diaphragmatic insufficiency, seizures, and cardiac irritability. In addition, hepatocellular regeneration is dependent on adenosine triphosphate (ATP), and after liver resection, regeneration may be impaired if phosphate is not repleted (19). In a series of 35 liver resections, 21% had significant postoperative hypophosphatemia (less than 2.5 mg/dL) after surgery. This group had a significant increase in complications (80%) compared to the normophosphatemic group (28%) (20).

Phosphate should be replaced with potassium or sodium phosphate preparations, or added to parenteral nutrition solutions. Recent data in living donor right hepatic lobectomies suggest that replacement up to two times the recommended daily allowance (60 mmol) is necessary to replete severe hypophosphatemia and prevent complications associated with hypophosphatemia (21).

Liver Function: Assessment and Support

Liver function should be carefully monitored after major liver resections and shunt surgery, as liver failure is a risk in any major hepatobiliary surgery. The risk of liver failure increases with the extent of hepatectomy and in patients with preoperative liver disease or cirrhosis (22,23). Although standard liver function tests are helpful after major liver resection or shunt surgery, they may not show elevation until the patient has significant liver failure. Transaminases are frequently elevated into the 200 to 300 units/dL range post resection due to the direct effect of mechanical injury to the liver during transection, as well as to partial devascularization of areas of the liver. Measurements of liver function, including the prothrombin time and lactate, are more helpful in evaluating early postoperative liver dysfunction.

Elevated total and indirect bilirubin are also useful indicators of postoperative liver dysfunction. However, isolated elevation of total bilirubin in the presence of normal liver function can have other etiologies. Perioperative blood transfusions can lead to hemolysis and hyperbilirubinemia, with a predominance of direct hyperbilirubinemia, and can be diagnosed with a standard hemolytic workup. Bile leaks or obstruction can also lead to an elevated serum bilirubin. The diagnosis and treatment of bile leaks is covered later in this chapter. Many popular anesthetics, antibiotics, and other drugs can cause hepatotoxicity and elevation of the serum bilirubin and need to be reduced or stopped if liver failure occurs.

When postoperative liver dysfunction does develop, it is important to exclude sepsis and anatomic causes of liver failure. A postoperative ultrasound can evaluate for portal vein, hepatic arterial, or hepatic vein thrombosis or obstruction, which may be amenable to surgical intervention. If the patient does not have sepsis, drug toxicity, biliary obstruction or leak, or vascular occlusion, liver failure is likely related to a pre-existing liver disease and/or the extent of resection. Treatment is then supportive, with correction of coagulopathy, encephalopathy, and ascites as described above. Systemic antibiotics or gut decontamination may be beneficial, since the liver Kupffer cells play a role in decreasing bacterial translocation from the portal blood flow, and patients with liver failure or biliary leak or obstruction may have an increased risk of bacteremia and sepsis.

N-acetylcysteine has been shown to decrease liver injury after acetaminophen overdose (24) and lessen ischemia reperfusion injury of the liver (25). Intravenous infusions of prostaglandin have also been linked to improvement of ischemia reperfusion injury and liver damage (26). Although definitive clinical data are lacking, both *N*-acetylcysteine and prostaglandin (PG) E_1 have been used to ameliorate postoperative liver damage in both liver resection and transplant patients. *N*-acetylcysteine is given as a continuous infusion of 40 mL of 10% solution mixed in 250 mL of D5W and given over 16 hours. Prostaglandin is also given as a continuous intravenous infusion, starting at 0.15 μg/kg/hour. It is titrated up to 1 μg/kg/hour based on systemic hypotension.

Coagulopathy

Coagulopathy is common after liver resection, and several studies have demonstrated an increase in prothrombin time directly proportional to the extent of liver resection (27,28). This coagulopathy has been attributed to impaired synthesis and clearance of clotting factors, inhibitors, and regulatory proteins (29,30). Patients with underlying liver disease and cirrhosis also often have thrombocytopenia and qualitative platelet defects. In addition, intraoperative hypothermia and perioperative transfusions, while not routine, are not uncommon during major hepatobiliary surgery, and can contribute to postoperative coagulopathy.

Serial hemoglobin and prothrombin levels should be measured. Because of the vascular nature of hepatobiliary surgery combined with postoperative coagulopathy from decreased liver function, as well as the frequent need for intravascular volume expansion, serial hemoglobin levels should be followed for postoperative bleeding. In general, we would obtain a hematocrit and international normalized ratio (INR) on ICU arrival and then repeat them, every 6 hours, for the next 24 hours. The surgeon should be notified of excessive bloody output from the drains, increasing abdominal distention, or hemodynamic instability. If coagulopathy does develop, it should be corrected if the INR goes above 2.0 (31), both with vitamin K and fresh frozen plasma. Any patient who is bleeding should have his or her coagulopathy completely corrected. For severe bleeding, both aprotinin and activated factor VII are safe in patients during and after liver resection (30,32). Patients who fail to stop bleeding after correction of their coagulopathy require return to the operating room for exploration. The surgical team should be made aware of any patient immediately postsurgery who requires transfusion. Once the postoperative coagulopathy has resolved or stabilized, all patients should be given subcutaneous heparin or low-molecular-weight heparin with sequential compression devices to prevent the formation of deep venous thrombosis.

Pain Management and Sedation

The large subcostal incision needed for major hepatobiliary surgery can result in significant pain after surgery. However, altered pharmacokinetics and coagulopathy, in particular after partial liver resection or shunt surgery, can make postoperative pain management a challenging proposition. Patients with liver failure or compromised liver function secondary to hepatectomy have altered metabolism of many common medications, in particular narcotics and sedatives that require hepatic clearance.

One of the more common problems that arises in the ICU after liver resection is oversedation of patients. A standard dose of narcotics given to a patient who has had 80% of the liver resected may well cause prolonged respiratory depression and signs and symptoms of encephalopathy. Narcotics and benzodiazepines should be used at the minimum dose required to achieve pain control. After liver resection, it is recommended that basal rates on patient-controlled anesthesia pumps be avoided, as metabolism of narcotics is difficult to forecast. Benzodiazepines also have altered clearance after liver resection, and should be administered at a lower dose or, if possible, avoided altogether. In patients requiring ongoing endotracheal intubation and mechanical ventilation, we have found it useful to use sedative agents such as propofol rather than narcotics since the level of sedation can be more easily titrated and reversed. Our institution has, at present, no experience with dexmedetomidine.

Epidural pain management may be the optimal analgesic technique after liver resection. Unfortunately, it is contraindicated in many patients because of postoperative coagulopathy. Recent literature has examined the use of epidural catheters in patients undergoing living donor partial hepatic resection. In a review of eight patients with epidural catheters, good pain control was achieved, with only one case of oversedation requiring naloxone. Although postoperative coagulopathy did occur, it was not to the extent that factor transfusion was needed prior to catheter removal, and there were no cases of hemorrhage (33). Epidural analgesia may be useful in select patients who do not have underlying liver disease and who are not undergoing extensive resections.

Nutrition

Although nutrition plays an important role in the care of any critically ill patient, the role of the liver in protein and carbohydrate metabolism makes proper postoperative nutrition imperative in the management of patients after major hepatobiliary surgery, in particular after partial liver resection when liver function is temporarily reduced. Patients with preoperative biliary obstruction, malignancy, and cirrhosis are at a higher risk for nutrition-related complications after major liver or bile duct surgery. Preoperative nutritional risk factors associated with postoperative complications in hepatobiliary surgery include weight loss greater than 14% lean body mass over 6 months, serum albumin less than 3 g/dL, hematocrit of less than 30%, total body potassium less than 85% of normal, less than the 25th percentile for midarm circumference, and skin test anergy (34). Preoperative bilirubin, albumin, prealbumin, prothrombin time, transferrin, as well as replacement of vitamin and trace mineral deficits may also be important preoperatively.

As with most critically ill patients, early enteral nutrition has been associated with improved outcomes. In hepatobiliary surgery, both enteral and parenteral nutrition have been associated with improved outcomes, especially in high-risk patients (34,35). However, parenteral nutrition has been clearly associated with an increased risk of infection (36). Enteral nutrition has been shown to improve gut flora, preventing gastrointestinal atrophy and loss of immunocompetence. A review of five prospective randomized trials on enteral and parenteral nutrition in patients after liver resection found a decrease in wound infection and catheter sepsis in patients receiving enteral nutrition (37). As one might expect, there were no mortality differences.

In patients who have undergone routine liver resection or shunt surgery, low-volume enteral feeds can be started almost immediately post surgery. Those patients having undergone hepaticojejunostomies or pancreatic surgery must await return of bowel function prior to starting feeds, unless the feeding tube is placed distal to the anastomosis. It is best to consult with the operating surgeon before starting enteral feeds in any patient, particularly those with enteric reconstruction. Patients with major pancreatic surgery (pancreaticoduodenectomy, subtotal or total pancreatectomy) may require pancreatic enzyme supplementation with enteral feeds or when resuming oral intake.

Patients with chronic liver disease or cirrhosis often have severe metabolic derangements that make nutritional management difficult. The depletion of the fat-soluble vitamins, in particular a loss of vitamin K, leads to coagulopathy and diminished antioxidant response. Chronic liver disease also stimulates a catabolic state with proteolysis and cachexia. Protein loss can be exacerbated by dietary restriction to help decrease encephalopathy. Branched-chain amino acids were initially thought to reduce the development of encephalopathy in catabolic patients with advanced liver failure, but this has not borne out in clinical data. Patients with cirrhosis also have abnormal glucose tolerance and insulin levels, along with elevated ammonia levels, hypophosphatemia, and hypoalbuminemia, all which influence perioperative nutrition. All Child's B or C cirrhotic patients should be fed enterally when hospitalized. The caloric needs of these patients are increased, and goal kcal is 25 to 25 kcal/kg/day, with administration of protein at 1 to 1.5 g/kg dry weight in nonencephalopathic patients and 0.5 g/kg dry weight in encephalopathic patients (37). Patients with ascites need sodium restriction of 2 g/day and a fluid restriction of 1 to 1.5 L/day, in combination with diuretics if tolerated.

Patients with preoperative obstructive jaundice often have chronic, low-grade endotoxemia and sepsis. This can lead to weight loss and anorexia, often due to malabsorption of fat and fat-soluble vitamins from obstruction of bile flow, which leads to coagulopathy and a diminished antioxidant response. Endotoxemia also results in decreased hepatic protein synthesis and catabolism (38). Most patients with biliary obstruction and resultant sepsis should undergo biliary decompression prior to major hepatobiliary surgery to allow malnutrition secondary to biliary obstruction and sepsis to resolve. Although it is controversial as to whether preoperative biliary decompression is required prior to surgery, one prospective, randomized trial looked at patients with obstructive jaundice who underwent biliary decompression and then were randomized to immediate operation or 2 weeks of alimentation (both parenteral and enteral) followed by operation. The second group had a lower risk of infection, morbidity, and mortality (39). Since these patients usually do not have hepatic dysfunction, standard enteral or parenteral nutrition is acceptable. Patients in whom bile flow has not been restored should have a low-fat diet—as fat absorption is impaired—and replacement of the fat-soluble vitamins. Medium-chain triglycerides may be helpful, because their absorption is not bile salt-dependent and may avoid diarrhea until bile flow is reestablished.

Partial liver resections also cause metabolic abnormalities secondary to the regenerating liver. Hepatic mitochondria switch to fat from glucose as their preferred energy source in hepatic regeneration (40). As a result, hypertonic glucose and insulin infusions should be avoided immediately after resection, as hyperglycemia and insulinemia suppress fatty acid release and decrease ketone body production by the liver. Some investigators have advocated administering fat and/or ketone bodies after liver resection to accelerate regeneration, although conclusive evidence that this is beneficial is lacking. Similarly, infusions of glucose and insulin directly into the portal vein have also been investigated in their role to improve regeneration, although, again, conclusive evidence is lacking. Adequate liver regeneration is also dependent on protein and calories. Postoperative parenteral nutrition should be supplemented with protein and fat, but low on glucose to improve hepatic regeneration. General goals are 30 kcal/kg/day, with 1.0 to 1.5 g/kg protein; glucose approximating 5 mg/kg/minute, and fat should not exceed 30% of the calories. Patients with cancer may need an increase of up to 35 kcal/kg/day and 2 g/kg protein.

Renal Failure

Acute renal failure occurs after major hepatobiliary surgery in 10% of patients (41) and, similar to other critically ill patients, significantly increases postoperative mortality (42). Risk factors for perioperative renal failure include postoperative sepsis, preoperative uremia, preoperative anemia, malignant disease, and preoperative jaundice (41,43,44). In particular, preoperative obstructive jaundice appears to be a significant risk factor, with an estimated 10% of patients developing postoperative renal failure (45). Both dehydration and endotoxin production from bile duct obstruction have been postulated to cause renal failure in these patients (46). Many studies have been done to try to decrease this risk, including using mannitol, bile salts, hydration, and lactulose (45–48).

In all patients with acute renal failure, adequate hydration, treatment of sepsis, and avoidance of nephrotoxic drugs are mandatory. However, in patients with obstructive jaundice, lactulose and bile salts may decrease endotoxin absorption, and have been shown in some studies to be beneficial in the prevention of renal failure (44,45). Preoperative biliary drainage to help lessen the perioperative inflammatory response is also an important adjunct to prevent postoperative renal failure. Once acute renal failure does occur, supportive care and dialysis are needed until renal function returns.

Patients with advanced cirrhosis or postoperative liver failure can develop hepatorenal syndrome (HRS). This is more significant in the acute care of patients with liver failure or after liver transplantation. Hepatorenal syndrome is a diagnosis of exclusion, with decreased renal function associated with a urine sodium less than 10 mg/dL combined with a urine osmolality greater than plasma osmolality that does not respond to volume administration. The cause of hepatorenal syndrome is likely multifactorial, but is primarily related to circulatory disturbances in patients with advanced liver disease, reduced liver function, and portal hypertension. Systemic vasodilatation and low mean arterial pressure results in renal vasoconstriction and a reduction in the glomerular filtration rate (49). Although liver transplantation remains the only cure for HRS, vasoconstrictors, albumin infusions, and transhepatic portosystemic shunts are able to reduce HRS and may prevent its development in patients with spontaneous bacterial peritonitis (50).

POSTOPERATIVE COMPLICATIONS FOLLOWING LIVER RESECTION

The morbidity associated with liver resection is reported to range between 30.7% and 47.7% (51–54). In addition to the standard complications associated with all major operations, liver resection is associated with specific problems including bleeding, bile leaks, liver insufficiency, ascites, pleural effusions, and infections.

Risk factors of complications following liver resection include increased blood loss, increased number of segments resected, increased preoperative bilirubin, increased prothrombin time, prolonged operative time, resection of segment VIII, diabetes, and concomitant surgical procedures (53,55–59).

Mortality

The in-hospital mortality due to liver resection has decreased over the last two decades, and high-volume centers have reported rates of 0% to 5% (51–53,60–62). The decrease in mortality is attributed to improved surgical technique, intraoperative anesthesia management, and perioperative care. These changes have helped decrease in-hospital mortality in liver resection patients despite their increased mean age and comorbidities (51).

Risk factors associated with increased mortality include hypoalbuminemia, thrombocytopenia, preoperative total bilirubin greater than 6 mg/dL, serum creatinine greater than 1.5 mg/dL, cholangitis, major hepatic resection, increased number of segments resected, synchronous abdominal procedure, major comorbid illness, diabetes mellitus, and blood transfusion requirements (51,52,59,62–65).

Specific surgical strategies to decrease mortality include minimizing blood loss and transfusions, and avoiding ischemic injury to the remnant liver. Specific posthepatectomy strategies include minimizing ongoing liver injury by maintaining tissue oxygenation, early nutritional support to facilitate liver regeneration, and replenishing phosphate levels (60).

Bleeding

Bleeding was once the "Achilles heel" of liver resection surgery, but has decreased dramatically over the last two decades due to a better appreciation of liver anatomy, surgical technique, and improved anesthesia management (60). As a result, centers routinely performing liver resections have noted decreased estimated blood loss of 300 mL to 750 mL and perioperative transfusion rates of 17.3% to 28.3% (51,52,62). Risk factors for increased bleeding from liver resection include cirrhosis, portal hypertension, increased segments resected, coagulopathy, thrombocytopenia, and elevated central venous pressure during resection (59,66).

Strategies to minimize blood loss during liver resection include appropriate patient selection—especially avoiding resection in patients with portal hypertension—and maintenance of central venous pressure under 6 mm Hg, Pringle maneuver, preoperative correction of coagulopathy and thrombocytopenia, use of fibrin sealant on raw liver surfaces, use of intraoperative ultrasound to locate the hepatic venous branches, and utilization of selective hepatic vascular exclusion (66–70).

Bile Leak

Biliary leaks occur in 3.6% to 17% of liver resection cases (71–74), and are associated with increased mortality and concomitant complications (71,72,75). Risk factors associated with biliary leaks following liver resection include older age, preoperative leukocytosis, left-sided hepatectomy, prolonged operative time, resection for peripheral cholangiocarcinoma, and resection of segment IV (71,74). When liver resections were performed for hepatocellular carcinoma (HCC), risk factors for bile leaks included central tumor location and preoperative transarterial chemoembolization (TACE) (72).

Various strategies have been described to prevent bile leaks following resection. A few groups have shown that the use of fibrin glue on the cut surface of the liver results in such a reduction (74); others have combined fibrin glue with bioabsorbable polyglycolic acid to significantly reduce bile leaks (76). While these small studies may indicate some effect of fibrin glue in reducing biliary leaks, there are at least as many studies that show no difference in bile leak rate when fibrin glue is employed.

Most bile leaks following liver resections without biliary reconstructions are small and can be managed nonoperatively. If a drain was not placed during the surgical procedure, a percutaneous drain is placed to prevent abdominal sepsis from an undrained biloma and to control the leak (71), and broad-spectrum antibiotics are started for fevers, leukocytosis, or positive bile cultures. Persistent drainage for 2 to 3 days of more than 100 mL of bilious fluid confirms an active leak, and is managed with endoscopic retrograde cholangiopancreatography (ERCP), sphincterotomy, and stent placement. This procedure may define the location of the leak and facilitate enteric biliary drainage and leak closure. When leaks are at the resected hepatic duct stump, a stent traversing the leak may further facilitate leak closure, although the main principle of treatment is to reduce the pressure in the biliary tree and allow spontaneous closure (71). Early endoscopic management of biliary leaks can minimize hospital length of stay and are not associated with late biliary complications (73). Others have used endoscopically placed nasobiliary tubes to decompress the biliary system, as it allows easy repeat cholangiograms and later removal (73,77). Although most leaks will close with time with these measures, they may persist for months (78).

From 0% to 32% of patients ultimately require reoperation because the leak cannot be controlled, and these procedures are associated with a high mortality rate (71,73,77). Biliary enteric drainage is performed on patients in whom ERCP cannot be performed for technical reasons, or with persistent on leaking despite ERCP. Important factors contributing to a good outcome are early reoperation, control of the biliary fistula before surgery, and utilization of healthy bile duct edges for enteric anastomosis.

Hemobilia may complicate bile leaks or liver resections or may occur secondary to trauma. Open communication from a branch of the hepatic artery to the biliary tree occurs and leads to intermittent, and sometimes exsanguinating, gastrointestinal (GI) bleeding. Identification is made when blood is seen exiting the ampulla when endoscopy is performed for upper GI bleeding. Computed tomography (CT) scanning with arterial phase contrast can localize the bleeding within the liver; however, management is by angiographic embolization.

Liver Failure and Dysfunction

Liver failure complicates liver resection in up to 12% of cases (57), and occurs when inadequate functional liver volume is left after resection. This complication occurs primarily in patients undergoing resection for hepatocellular carcinoma with underlying liver disease, and is often a consequence of patient selection and choice of operation.

Risk factors for hepatic insufficiency in cirrhotics include major resections, especially right lobectomy, portal hypertension, long-standing jaundice, Childs-Pugh Turcotte (CPT) score greater than A, and hepatic steatosis (79). More recently, preoperative chemotherapy has become routine in patients with colorectal cancer metastatic to the liver. While there is no doubt that the addition of newer agents such as irinotecan, oxaliplatin, and Avastin have improved long-term results, they also cause an increase in both hepatic steatosis as well as steatohepatitis, which can contribute to postoperative liver dysfunction.

By assessing the patient's functional liver status, the surgeon can estimate the maximum amount of liver mass that can be resected while preserving adequate functional liver volume. In patients with a normal liver, up to 75% of total liver volume can be resected safely. It is patients with abnormal livers, such as those with cirrhosis, who need careful assessment. In general, Child-Pugh class C is a contraindication to any sort of resection. Early Child's class B patients without portal hypertension may undergo minor resections—from wedge resection to a single segmentectomy. However, these patients may be better served by nonsurgical local ablation techniques. Child-Pugh class A patients who are considered for major hepatectomy—resection of four or more segments—should undergo assessment of both liver and physiologic status (80,81). Others have found that a Model for End-Stage Liver Disease (MELD) score equal to or greater than 11 predicts liver failure following HCC resection (82). Portal hypertension, defined as a hepatic vein pressure gradient (HVPG) greater than 10 mm Hg, and as suggested by signs such as esophageal varices, anatomic portosystemic shunts, and ascites (83), has been associated with increased morbidity and mortality following major resection (84). Thrombocytopenia with platelet counts less than 100,000 cells/μL is one laboratory indicator of portal hypertension and has been associated with in-hospital mortality following liver resection (80).

Although various tests exist to assess liver function in Child-Pugh class A and B patients before a possible major liver resection—defined as greater than or equal to four segments—none has been uniformly adopted. The indocyanine green (ICG) clearance test, commonly used in Asia, is one method of quantifying liver function (85–87). Early studies have shown that an ICG retention at 15 minutes (ICGR15) of less than 20% allows safe, limited liver resection, and a value of less than 14% is associated with near-zero operative mortality (88–90).

In Child-Pugh class A patients with right-sided lesions curable by major resection but whose liver reserve may be inadequate, preoperative ipsilateral portal vein embolization increases the remnant contralateral liver volume (91). Portal vein embolization is generally performed in patients with a predicted function liver remnant of less than 25% in noncirrhotics or less than 40% in patients with significant fibrosis and/or cirrhosis.

Liver failure following liver resection presents clinically with encephalopathy and asterixis. In severe cases, these patients appear similar to those with fulminant liver failure, presenting with marked acidosis, jaundice, and hemodynamic instability. The patient ultimately succumbs to multiorgan failure and sepsis. In mild cases, treatment is supportive, with judicious fluid management, optimization of tissue oxygenation, infection prophylaxis, and nutritional support if recovery is prolonged. The goal in the mild and salvageable cases is to promote immediate liver functional recovery from the insults inherent to liver resection; to promote liver regeneration with nutritional and electrolyte repletion, particularly phosphate; and to minimize the chance of infectious complications. Although early studies demonstrated a significantly improved hepatic oxygen delivery and extraction in patients receiving N-acetylcysteine for nonacetaminophen-induced liver failure (92,93), subsequent conflicting studies have failed to support a definite role in patients following liver resection (94). Nonetheless, many centers, including our own, selectively administer *N*-acetylcysteine in patients with marginal liver function following resection, based mainly on a favorable small series and anecdotal benefits (95). This practice may be reasonable because of the sheer number of favorable outcome reports and the good drug safety profile, but controlled trials are needed.

Ascites and Pleural Effusion

Ascites occurs in up to 9% of liver resections (57) and is associated with decreased survival, as it is a surrogate marker of liver insufficiency and because of its potential contribution to prerenal insufficiency (75). Pleural effusion, usually occurring on the right side and frequently accompanying ascites, is found following liver resection in 3.8% to 21% of cases (57, 96) and is usually asymptomatic, requiring no treatment. Effusion may develop from underlying ascites that crosses the diaphragm. In addition, the same pathophysiologic processes of fluid overload and hypoproteinemia that cause ascites may also contribute to the development of pleural effusion.

Risk factors for both ascites and pleural effusion include right lobectomy, diabetes mellitus, poor nutritional status and hypoalbuminemia, left-sided cardiac insufficiency, and liver and renal insufficiency (79,97). In addition, risk factors specifically associated with pleural effusion have been found to include resection for hepatocellular carcinoma with underlying liver disease, subphrenic collections, postoperative liver insufficiency with ascites, and duration of inflow occlusion (96).

Strategies to prevent postresection ascites and pleural effusion include avoiding overhydration, including gentle diuresis; preventing renal insufficiency by avoiding nephrotoxic drugs and hypotension; early detection and treatment of infection; maintaining adequate nutrition; and the use of perioperative drains (97). The appropriate selection of patients and resection to maintain adequate liver function, especially in patients with hepatomas and underlying liver disease, will minimize the risk of liver failure and subsequent ascites.

COMPLICATIONS FOLLOWING BILE DUCT RESECTION/ RECONSTRUCTION

Perhaps the most extensive hepatobiliary operations are performed for proximal extrahepatic cholangiocarcinomas. With mounting evidence demonstrating significantly improved survival following extended liver and bile duct resections and reconstructions versus local bile duct resections, centers with experienced hepatobiliary surgeons are presenting series with improved outcomes (98–101). Nonetheless, significant complications remain associated with these procedures.

Perioperative mortality following extended liver and biliary resections ranges from 1.3% to 16% (101–104). Complications following these procedures occur in 51% to 81%, and many patients have multiple complications (100–103). Complications include bile duct leaks, bleeding, liver failure, pleural effusions, wound infection, and sepsis (102,104–106). Each of these complications can also be found in liver resections alone and share the same risk factors. In addition, each complication can be approached with the same preventative strategy and treatment.

Liver failure following extended resections for obstructive cholangiocarcinoma may have a unique pathophysiology and, hence, preventative strategy. Interestingly, prolonged biliary obstruction causes significant hepatocellular dysfunction, with liver failure occurring in up to 27.6% of patients who undergo extended liver and biliary resections and reconstructions for cholangiocarcinoma. Further, this is frequently fatal (102,106). Resection of up to 75% of the liver, along with possible vascular reconstruction that requires an increased duration of ischemic injury to the liver, is often necessary to resect hilar cholangiocarcinoma, and, in the setting of pre-existing liver dysfunction, liver failure can be problematic. Strategies to optimize functional liver volume prior to extended liver resections for hilar cholangiocarcinomas are essential to preventing postoperative liver failure. One strategy is to promote hepatocellular functional recovery by preoperatively decompressing the biliary tree using percutaneous transhepatic cholangiocatheterization. This practice is somewhat controversial, as it may introduce infectious agents into an otherwise sterile biliary tree, and so may be avoided in patients who can undergo surgery within 2 to 3 weeks after the onset of jaundice. Another strategy is to perform contralateral portal vein embolization to increase the remnant liver volume prior to resection. A number of centers have demonstrated decreased liver failure rates when these strategies were employed (98,104,107).

COMPLICATIONS FOLLOWING PANCREATIC SURGERY

The mortality rate following pancreaticoduodenectomy (PD) ranges between 2.7% and 6.9% (108–112). Risk factors for perioperative mortality include elevated serum bilirubin, the diameter of the pancreatic duct, increased intraoperative blood loss, pancreatic fistulae, and older age (109). Complications are seen to occur in 22.1% to 30.2% of PDs, and include pancreatic fistulae, delayed gastric emptying, bleeding, abdominal abscesses, and wound infections (108,109).

Pancreatic fistulae are a dreaded complication of PD, occurring in 12% to 18% of patients (108,110,111,113–116). Pancreatic fistulae are associated with a mortality rate ranging to 19% (104,106,108,111). These patients often die secondary to massive erosive *bleeding* from sepsis and pancreatic enzyme accumulation. These bleeding episodes occur in 1% to 8.8% of PD patients and carry a mortality rate of 47% to 50% (112,117,118).

Risk factors for pancreatic fistulae include small duct size, soft pancreas texture, duration of surgery greater than 8 hours, diabetes mellitus, lower creatinine clearance, preoperative jaundice, and increased intraoperative blood loss (108,114,116,119). Despite numerous studies evaluating potential strategies to prevent pancreatic fistulae following

PD, including the use of octreotide, fibrin sealants, pancreatic stents, and different methods and sites of pancreatic anastomosis, none has proven effective (113,120–124).

Pancreatic fistulae are initially detected on postoperative day 6 as abdominal pain, fever, nausea/vomiting, and leukocytosis. Fistulae are then confirmed by CT scan demonstrating fluid collection behind the pancreatic anastomosis, elevated serum amylase, drain output greater than 50 mL/day, and drain amylase 10-fold greater than serum amylase (113,122). Management is initially conservative, with bowel rest, total parenteral nutrition, antibiotics, and monitoring of clinical signs and symptoms and drain output. If repeat imaging demonstrates increased accumulation of fluid and the patient does not respond to conservative measures, another drain may be placed percutaneously to prevent progression to abdominal sepsis. Eighty to ninety percent of patients seal pancreatic fistulae with these measures (110,115). However, those patients who develop uncontrolled leaks and abdominal sepsis may require surgery, usually for completion pancreatectomy. In addition, a smaller group of patients with fistulae will suffer life-threatening erosive intra-abdominal bleeding, usually from the stump of the gastroduodenal artery, small arterial branches to the pancreas, or, rarely, the portal vein. These patients will present with signs and symptoms of sepsis and hypovolemia, such as fever, abdominal pain, hypotension, anemia, and bloody drain output. These patients are treated by rapid resuscitation and angiography for potential embolization of the bleeding arterial branch. If arterial bleeding cannot be controlled in this manner, or if the bleeding is venous, the patient is explored for hemostasis and completion pancreatectomy. However, surgery in this setting is associated with a high mortality, with up to 36% of such patients dying if they require surgery for bleeding after PD (112,118).

References

1. Bismuth H. Surgical anatomy and anatomical surgery of the liver. *World J Surg.* 1982;6:3–9.
2. Botero AC, Strasberg SM. Division of the left hemiliver in man- segments, sectors or sections. *Liver Transpl Surg.* 1998;4:226–231.
3. McCluskey DA 3rd, Skandalakis LJ, Colburn GL, et al. Hepatic surgery and hepatic surgical anatomy: historical partners in progress. *World J Surg.* 1997;21:330–342.
4. Strasberg SM. Terminology of liver anatomy and liver resections: coming to grips with hepatic Babel. *J Am Coll Surg.* 1997;184:413–434.
5. Couinaud C. Surgical anatomy of the liver. Several new aspects. *Chirurgie.* 1986;112:337–342.
6. Baldwin RL, Smith NE. Molecular control of energy metabolism. In: Sink, ed. *The Control of Metabolism.* University Park, PA: Pennsylvania State University Press; 1974:17.
7. Bradley EL III. Measurement of hepatic bloodflow in man. *Surgery.* 1974;75:783.
8. Kock NG, Hahnloser P, Roding B, et al. Interaction between portal venous and hepatic arterial bloodflow: an experimental study in the dog. *Surgery.* 1972;72:414.
9. Brauer RW. Hepatic blood supply and the secretion of bile. In: Taylor RW, ed. *The Biliary System.* Oxford, England: Blackwell Scientific Publishers; 1965:41.
10. Prandi D, Erlinger S, Glasinovic JC, et al. Cannilicular bile production in man. *Eur J Clin Invest.* 1975;5:1.
11. Abdalla EK, Barnett CC, Doherty D, et al. Extended hepatectomy in patients with hepatobiliary malignancies with and without preoperative portal vein embolization. *Arch Surg.* 2002;137(6):675–680; discussion 680–681.
12. Hemming AW, Reed AI, Howard RJ, et al. Preoperative portal vein embolization for extended hepatectomy. *Ann Surg.* 2003;237(5):686–691; discussion 691–693.
13. Takenaka K, Kanematsu T, Fuzawa K, et al. Can hepatic failure after surgery for hepatocellular carcinoma in cirrhotic patients be prevented? *World J Surg.* 1990;14:123–127.
14. Man MB, Fan ST, Ng I, et al. Prospective evaluation of Pringle maneuver in hepatectomy for liver tumors by a randomized study. *Ann Surg.* 1997;6:704–713.
15. Nagasue N, Yukaya H, Suehiro S, et al. Tolerance of the cirrhotic liver to normothermic ischemia. A clinical study of 15 patients. *Am J Surg.* 1984; 147:772–775.
16. Clavien PA, Selzner M, Rudiger HA, et al. A prospective randomized study in 100 consecutive patients undergoing major liver resection with versus without ischemic preconditioning. *Ann Surg.* 2003;238(6):843–850; discussion 851–852
17. Huguet C, Addario-Chieco P, Gavelli A, et al. Technique of hepatic vascular exclusion for extensive liver resection. *Am J Surg.* 1992;163:602–605.
18. Salem RR, Tray K. Hepatic resection-related hypophosphatemia is of renal origin as manifested by isolated hyperphosphaturia. *Ann Surg.* 2005; 241(2):343–348.
19. Campbell KA, Wu YP, Chacko VP, et al. In vivo 31P NMR spectroscopic changes during liver regeneration. *J Surg Res.* 1990;49:244–247.
20. Buell JF, Berger AC, Plotkin JS, et al. The clinical implications of hypophosphatemia following major hepatic resection or cryosurgery. *Arch Surg.* 1998;133:757–761.
21. Pomposelli JJ, Pomfret EA, Burns DL, et al. Life-threatening hypophosphatemia after right hepatic lobectomy for live donor adult liver transplantation. *Liver Transpl.* 2001;7:637–642.
22. Nanashima A, Yamaguchi H, Shibasaki S, et al. Comparative analysis of postoperative morbidity according to type and extent of hepatectomy. *Hepatogastroenterology.* 2005;52:844–848.
23. Midorikawa Y, Kubota K, Takayama T, et al. A comparative study of postoperative complications after hepatectomy in patients with and without chronic liver disease. *Surgery.* 1999;126:484–491.
24. Riordan SM, Williams R. Fulminant hepatic failure. *Clin Liver Dis.* 2000; 4:25–45.
25. Glantzounis GK, Yang W, Koti RS, et al. The role of thiols in liver ischemia-reperfusion injury. *Curr Pharm Des.* 2006;12:2891–2901.
26. Hossain MA, Wakabayashi H, Izuishi K, et al. The role of prostaglandins in liver ischemia-reperfusion injury. *Curr Pharm Des.* 2006;12:2935–2951.
27. Suc B, Panis Y, Belghiti J, et al. 'Natural history' of hepatectomy. *Br J Surg.* 1992;79:39–42.
28. Vishnevskii VA, Titova MI, Sivkov VV, et al. [Hemostasis disorders after resection of liver and approaches to their prevention and correction]. *Klin Med (Mosk).* 1996;74:32–34.
29. Borromeo CJ, Stix MS, Lally A, et al. Epidural catheter and increased prothrombin time after right lobe hepatectomy for living donor transplantation. *Anesth Analg.* 2000;91:1139–1141.
30. Silva MA, Muralidharan V, Mirza DF. The management of coagulopathy and blood loss in liver surgery. *Semin Hematol.* 2004;41:132–139.
31. Martin RC, Jarnagin WR, Fong Y, et al. The use of fresh frozen plasma after major hepatic resection for colorectal metastasis: is there a standard for transfusion? *J Am Coll Surg.* 2003;196(3):402–409.
32. Shao YF, Yang JM, Chau GY, et al. Safety and hemostatic effect of recombinant activated factor VII in cirrhotic patients undergoing partial hepatectomy: a multicenter, randomized, double-blind, placebo-controlled trial. *Am J Surg.* 2006;191:245–249.
33. Schumann R, Zabala L, Angelis M, et al. Altered hematologic profiles following donor right hepatectomy and implications for perioperative analgesic management. *Liver Transpl.* 2004;10:363–368.
34. Fan ST, Lo CM, Lai EC, et al. Perioperative nutritional support in patients undergoing hepatectomy for hepatocellular carcinoma. *N Engl J Med.* 1994;331:1547–1552.
35. Richter B, Schmandra TC, Golling M, et al. Nutritional support after open liver resection: a systematic review. *Dig Surg.* 2006;23:139–145.
36. Gramlich L, Kichian K, Pinilla J, et al. Does enteral nutrition compared to parenteral nutrition result in better outcomes in critically ill adult patients? A systematic review of the literature. *Nutrition.* 2004;20:843–848.
37. McCullough AJ, Tavill AS. Disordered energy and protein metabolism in liver disease. *Semin Liver Dis.* 1991;11:265–277.
38. Curran RD, Billiar TR, Stuehr DJ, et al. Multiple cytokines are required to induce hepatocyte nitric oxide production and inhibit total protein synthesis. *Ann Surg.* 1990;212:462–469; discussion 70–71.
39. Foschi D, Cavagna G, Callioni F, et al. Hyperalimentation of jaundiced patients on percutaneous transhepatic biliary drainage. *Br J Surg.* 1986;73:716–719.
40. Nakatani T, Ozawa K, Asano M, et al. Changes in predominant energy substrate after hepatectomy. *Life Sci.* 1981;28:257–264.
41. Thompson JN, Edwards WH, Winearls CG, et al. Renal impairment following biliary tract surgery. *Br J Surg.* 1987;74:843–847.
42. Schroeder RA, Marroquin CE, Bute BP, et al. Predictive indices of morbidity and mortality after liver resection. *Ann Surg.* 2006;243:373–379.
43. Dixon JM, Armstrong CP, Duffy SW, et al. Factors affecting morbidity and mortality after surgery for obstructive jaundice: a review of 373 patients. *Gut.* 1983;24:845–852.
44. Uslu A, Cayci M, Nart A, et al. Renal failure in obstructive jaundice. *Hepatogastroenterology.* 2005;52:52–54.
45. Pain JA, Cahill CJ, Gilbert JM, et al. Prevention of postoperative renal dysfunction in patients with obstructive jaundice: a multicentre study of bile salts and lactulose. *Br J Surg.* 1991;78:467–469.

46. Evans HJ, Torrealba V, Hudd C, et al. The effect of preoperative bile salt administration on postoperative renal function in patients with obstructive jaundice. *Br J Surg.* 1982;69:706–708.
47. Cahill CJ, Pain JA, Bailey ME. Bile salts, endotoxin and renal function in obstructive jaundice. *Surg Gynecol Obstet.* 1987;165:519–522.
48. Gubern JM, Sancho JJ, Simo J, et al. A randomized trial on the effect of mannitol on postoperative renal function in patients with obstructive jaundice. *Surgery.* 1988;103:39–44.
49. Gines P, Guevara M, Arroyo V, et al. Hepatorenal syndrome. *Lancet.* 2003;362:1819–1827.
50. Arroyo V, Terra C, Gines P. New treatments of hepatorenal syndrome. *Semin Liver Dis.* 2006;26:254–264.
51. Poon RT, Fan ST, Lo CM, et al. Improving perioperative outcome expands the role of hepatectomy in management of benign and malignant hepatobiliary diseases: analysis of 1222 consecutive patients from a prospective database. *Ann Surg.* 2004;240:698–708.
52. Vauthey JN, Pawlik TM, Abdalla EK, et al. Is extended hepatectomy for hepatobiliary malignancy justified? *Ann Surg.* 2004;239:722–730.
53. Sitzmann JV, Greene PS. Perioperative predictors of morbidity following hepatic resection for neoplasm. A multivariate analysis of a single surgeon experience with 105 patients. *Ann Surg.* 1994;219:13–17.
54. Benzoni E, Cojutti A, Lorenzin D, et al. Liver resective surgery: a multivariate analysis of postoperative outcome and complication. *Langenbecks Arch Surg.* 2006.
55. Imamura H, Seyama Y, Kokudo N, et al. One thousand fifty-six hepatectomies without mortality in 8 years. *Arch Surg.* 2003;138:1198–1206.
56. Wu CC, Yeh DC, Lin MC, et al. Improving operative safety for cirrhotic liver resection. *Br J Surg.* 2001;88:210–215.
57. Pol B, Campan P, Hardwigsen J, et al. Morbidity of major hepatic resections: a 100-case prospective study. *Eur J Surg.* 1999;165:446–453.
58. Shimada M, Matsumata T, Akazawa K, et al. Estimation of risk of major complications after hepatic resection. *Am J Surg.* 1994;167:399–403.
59. Jarnagin WR, Gonen M, Fong Y, et al. Improvement in perioperative outcome after hepatic resection: analysis of 1,803 consecutive cases over the past decade. *Ann Surg.* 2002;236:397–406.
60. Fan ST, Lo CM, Liu CL, et al. Hepatectomy for hepatocellular carcinoma: toward zero hospital deaths. *Ann Surg.* 1999;229:322–330.
61. Miyagawa S, Makuuchi M, Kawasaki S, et al. Criteria for safe hepatic resection. *Am J Surg.* 1995;169:589–594.
62. Belghiti J, Hiramatsu K, Benoist S, et al. Seven hundred forty-seven hepatectomies in the 1990s: an update to evaluate the actual risk of liver resection. *J Am Coll Surg.* 2000;191:38–46.
63. Melendez J, Ferri E, Zwillman M, et al. Extended hepatic resection: a 6-year retrospective study of risk factors for perioperative mortality. *J Am Coll Surg.* 2001;192:47–53.
64. Wei AC, Tung-Ping PR, Fan ST, et al. Risk factors for perioperative morbidity and mortality after extended hepatectomy for hepatocellular carcinoma. *Br J Surg.* 2003;90:33–41.
65. Little SA, Jarnagin WR, DeMatteo RP, et al. Diabetes is associated with increased perioperative mortality but equivalent long-term outcome after hepatic resection for colorectal cancer. *J Gastrointest Surg.* 2002;6:88–94.
66. Smyrniotis V, Kostopanagiotou G, Theodoraki K, et al. The role of central venous pressure and type of vascular control in blood loss during major liver resections. *Am J Surg.* 2004;187:398–402.
67. Nakajima Y, Shimamura T, Kamiyama T, et al. Control of intraoperative bleeding during liver resection: analysis of a questionnaire sent to 231 Japanese hospitals. *Surg Today.* 2002;32:48–52.
68. Wang WD, Liang LJ, Huang XQ, et al. Low central venous pressure reduces blood loss in hepatectomy. *World J Gastroenterol.* 2006;12:935–939.
69. Schwartz M, Madariaga J, Hirose R, et al. Comparison of a new fibrin sealant with standard topical hemostatic agents. *Arch Surg.* 2004;139:1148–1154.
70. Frilling A, Stavrou GA, Mischinger HJ, et al. Effectiveness of a new carrier-bound fibrin sealant versus argon beamer as haemostatic agent during liver resection: a randomised prospective trial. *Langenbecks Arch Surg.* 2005;390:114–120.
71. Lo CM, Fan ST, Liu CL, et al. Biliary complications after hepatic resection: risk factors, management, and outcome. *Arch Surg.* 1998;133:156–161.
72. Lee CC, Chau GY, Lui WY, et al. Risk factors associated with bile leakage after hepatic resection for hepatocellular carcinoma. *Hepatogastroenterology.* 2005;52:1168–1171.
73. Bhattacharjya S, Puleston J, Davidson BR, et al. Outcome of early endoscopic biliary drainage in the management of bile leaks after hepatic resection. *Gastrointest Endosc.* 2003;57:526–530.
74. Capussotti L, Ferrero A, Vigano L, et al. Bile leakage and liver resection: where is the risk? *Arch Surg.* 2006;141:690–694.
75. Yamashita Y, Hamatsu T, Rikimaru T, et al. Bile leakage after hepatic resection. *Ann Surg.* 2001;233:45–50.
76. Hayashibe A, Sakamoto K, Shinbo M, et al. New method for prevention of bile leakage after hepatic resection. *J Surg Oncol.* 2006;94:57–60.
77. Tanaka S, Hirohashi K, Tanaka H, et al. Incidence and management of bile leakage after hepatic resection for malignant hepatic tumors. *J Am Coll Surg.* 2002;195:484–489.
78. Reed DN Jr, Vitale GC, Wrightson WR, et al. Decreasing mortality of bile leaks after elective hepatic surgery. *Am J Surg.* 2003;185:316–318.
79. Nanashima A, Yamaguchi H, Shibasaki S, et al. Comparative analysis of postoperative morbidity according to type and extent of hepatectomy. *Hepatogastroenterology.* 2005;52:844–848.
80. Poon RT, Fan ST, Lo CM, et al. Improving perioperative outcome expands the role of hepatectomy in management of benign and malignant hepatobiliary diseases: analysis of 1222 consecutive patients from a prospective database. *Ann Surg.* 2004;240:698–708.
81. Llovet JM, Schwartz M, Mazzaferro V. Resection and liver transplantation for hepatocellular carcinoma. *Semin Liver Dis.* 2005;25:181–200.
82. Cucchetti A, Ercolani G, Vivarelli M, et al. Impact of model for end-stage liver disease (MELD) score on prognosis after hepatectomy for hepatocellular carcinoma on cirrhosis. *Liver Transpl.* 2006;12:966–971.
83. Llovet JM. Updated treatment approach to hepatocellular carcinoma. *J Gastroenterol.* 2005;40:225–235.
84. Bruix J, Castells A, Bosch J, et al. Surgical resection of hepatocellular carcinoma in cirrhotic patients: prognostic value of preoperative portal pressure. *Gastroenterology.* 1996;111:1018–1022.
85. Poon RT, Fan ST. Assessment of hepatic reserve for indication of hepatic resection: how I do it. *J Hepatobiliary Pancreat Surg.* 2005;12:31–37.
86. Takayama T, Sekine T, Makuuchi M, et al. Adoptive immunotherapy to lower postsurgical recurrence rates of hepatocellular carcinoma: a randomised trial. *Lancet.* 2000;356:802–807.
87. Hemming AW, Scudamore CH, Shackleton CR, et al. Indocyanine green clearance as a predictor of successful hepatic resection in cirrhotic patients. *Am J Surg.* 1992;163:515–518.
88. Miyagawa S, Makuuchi M, Kawasaki S, et al. Criteria for safe hepatic resection. *Am J Surg.* 1995;169:589–594.
89. Poon RT, Fan ST. Hepatectomy for hepatocellular carcinoma: patient selection and postoperative outcome. *Liver Transpl.* 2004;10:S39–S45.
90. Fan ST, Lai EC, Lo CM, et al. Hospital mortality of major hepatectomy for hepatocellular carcinoma associated with cirrhosis. *Arch Surg.* 1995;130:198–203.
91. Sugawara Y, Yamamoto J, Higashi H, et al. Preoperative portal embolization in patients with hepatocellular carcinoma. *World J Surg.* 2002;26:105–110.
92. Harrison PM, Wendon JA, Gimson AE, et al. Improvement by acetylcysteine of hemodynamics and oxygen transport in fulminant hepatic failure. *N Engl J Med.* 1991;324:1852–1857.
93. Devlin J, Ellis AE, McPeake J, et al. N-acetylcysteine improves indocyanine green extraction and oxygen transport during hepatic dysfunction. *Crit Care Med.* 1997;25:236–242.
94. Sklar GE, Subramaniam M. Acetylcysteine treatment for non-acetaminophen-induced acute liver failure. *Ann Pharmacother.* 2004;38:498–500.
95. Ben Ari Z, Vaknin H, Tur-Kaspa R. N-acetylcysteine in acute hepatic failure (non-paracetamol-induced). *Hepatogastroenterology.* 2000;47:786–789.
96. Bilimoria MM, Chaoui AS, Vauthey JN. Postoperative liver failure. *J Am Coll Surg.* 1999;189:336–338.
97. Matsumata T, Taketomi A, Kawahara N, et al. Morbidity and mortality after hepatic resection in the modern era. *Hepatogastroenterology.* 1995;42:456–460.
98. Hemming AW, Reed AI, Fujita S, et al. Surgical management of hilar cholangiocarcinoma. *Ann Surg.* 2005;241:693–699.
99. Shimada K, Sano T, Sakamoto Y, et al. Safety and effectiveness of left hepatic trisegmentectomy for hilar cholangiocarcinoma. *World J Surg.* 2005;29:723–727.
100. Kawarada Y, Das BC, Naganuma T, et al. Surgical treatment of hilar bile duct carcinoma: experience with 25 consecutive hepatectomies. *J Gastrointest Surg.* 2002;6:617–624.
101. Jarnagin WR, Fong Y, DeMatteo RP, et al. Staging, resectability, and outcome in 225 patients with hilar cholangiocarcinoma. *Ann Surg.* 2001;234:507–517.
102. Zervos EE, Pearson H, Durkin AJ, et al. In-continuity hepatic resection for advanced hilar cholangiocarcinoma. *Am J Surg.* 2004;188:584–588.
103. IJitsma AJ, Appeltans BM, de Jong KP, et al. Extrahepatic bile duct resection in combination with liver resection for hilar cholangiocarcinoma: a report of 42 cases. *J Gastrointest Surg.* 2004;8:686–694.
104. Kawasaki S, Imamura H, Kobayashi A, et al. Results of surgical resection for patients with hilar bile duct cancer: application of extended hepatectomy after biliary drainage and hemihepatic portal vein embolization. *Ann Surg.* 2003;238:84–92.
105. Meunier B, Lakehal M, Tay KH, et al. Surgical complications and treatment during resection for malignancy of the high bile duct. *World J Surg.* 2001;25:1284–1288.
106. Nagino M, Kamiya J, Uesaka K, et al. Complications of hepatectomy for hilar cholangiocarcinoma. *World J Surg.* 2001;25:1277–1283.
107. Sano T, Shimada K, Sakamoto Y, et al. One hundred two consecutive hepatobiliary resections for perihilar cholangiocarcinoma with zero mortality. *Ann Surg.* 2006;244:240–247.
108. Yang YM, Tian XD, Zhuang Y, et al. Risk factors of pancreatic leakage after pancreaticoduodenectomy. *World J Gastroenterol.* 2005;11:2456–2461.
109. Bottger TC, Engelmann R, Junginger T. Is age a risk factor for major pancreatic surgery? An analysis of 300 resections. *Hepatogastroenterology.* 1999;46:2589–2598.

110. Grobmyer SR, Rivadeneira DE, Goodman CA, et al. Pancreatic anastomotic failure after pancreaticoduodenectomy. *Am J Surg*. 2000;180:117–120.
111. Cullen JJ, Sarr MG, Ilstrup DM. Pancreatic anastomotic leak after pancreaticoduodenectomy: incidence, significance, and management. *Am J Surg*. 1994;168:295–298.
112. Rumstadt B, Schwab M, Korth P, et al. Hemorrhage after pancreatoduodenectomy. *Ann Surg*. 1998;227:236–241.
113. Hashimoto N, Yasuda C, Ohyanagi H. Pancreatic fistula after pancreatic head resection; incidence, significance and management. *Hepatogastroenterology*. 2003;50:1658–1660.
114. Aranha GV, Aaron JM, Shoup M, et al. Current management of pancreatic fistula after pancreaticoduodenectomy. *Surgery*. 2006;140:561–568.
115. Srivastava S, Sikora SS, Pandey CM, et al. Determinants of pancreaticoenteric anastomotic leak following pancreaticoduodenectomy. *ANZ J Surg*. 2001;71:511–515.
116. Yeh TS, Jan YY, Jeng LB, et al. Pancreaticojejunal anastomotic leak after pancreaticoduodenectomy–multivariate analysis of perioperative risk factors. *J Surg Res*. 1997;67:119–125.
117. Koukoutsis I, Bellagamba R, Morris-Stiff G, et al. Haemorrhage following pancreaticoduodenectomy: risk factors and the importance of sentinel bleed. *Dig Surg*. 2006;23:224–228.
118. Santoro R, Carlini M, Carboni F, et al. Delayed massive arterial hemorrhage after pancreaticoduodenectomy for cancer. Management of a life-threatening complication. *Hepatogastroenterology*. 2003;50:2199–2204.
119. Tien YW, Lee PH, Yang CY, et al. Risk factors of massive bleeding related to pancreatic leak after pancreaticoduodenectomy. *J Am Coll Surg*. 2005;201:554–559.
120. Lillemoe KD, Cameron JL, Kim MP, et al. Does fibrin glue sealant decrease the rate of pancreatic fistula after pancreaticoduodenectomy? Results of a prospective randomized trial. *J Gastrointest Surg*. 2004;8:766–772.
121. Levy MJ, Chari S, Adler DG, et al. Complications of temporary pancreatic stent insertion for pancreaticojejunal anastomosis during pancreaticoduodenectomy. *Gastrointest Endosc*. 2004;59:719–724.
122. Barnett SP, Hodul PJ, Creech S, et al. Octreotide does not prevent postoperative pancreatic fistula or mortality following pancreaticoduodenectomy. *Am Surg*. 2004;70:222–226.
123. Lowy AM, Lee JE, Pisters PW, et al. Prospective, randomized trial of octreotide to prevent pancreatic fistula after pancreaticoduodenectomy for malignant disease. *Ann Surg*. 1997;226:632–641.
124. Mansueto G, D'Onofrio M, Iacono C, et al. Gastroduodenal artery stump haemorrhage following pylorus-sparing Whipple procedure: treatment with covered stents. *Dig Surg*. 2002;19:237–240.

CHAPTER 79 ■ CRITICAL CARE OF THE THORACIC SURGICAL PATIENT

THOMAS L. HIGGINS • PATRICK MAILLOUX

IMMEDIATE CONCERNS

Thoracic surgical patients are among the most complicated admissions to intensive care due to their challenging preoperative status, the variety of possible operative procedures, airway and pleural appliances, and requirements for postoperative interventions, including airway management, mechanical ventilation, and pain control. Information transfer is key: the ICU physicians and nurses must have a clear understanding of the operative procedure accomplished, the patient's expected medical course, and the predictable potential complications. More time than usual must be allotted for briefing of the ICU team by the operative team.

Immediate concerns include assessment of oxygenation, cardiovascular support to ensure adequate oxygen delivery, provision of ventilation support if needed, and transferral of monitors and drains that accompany the patient from the operating room. Special concerns apply to fluid management (discussed in detail below) and pain control, which is especially important, as pain will limit respiratory effort and can precipitate delirium and agitation. Table 79.1 provides a checklist for immediate interventions.

In operations where the pleural space has been opened, the patient will arrive with at least one—but usually two or more—chest tubes. Complete lung expansion helps to force out any remaining extrapleural air, which exits through an apical chest tube. Removal of air from the thorax is demonstrated when bubbling is seen in the water seal bottle. The posterior/inferior tube(s) should be draining blood, and some clots are expected; however, a large quantity of clots suggests continued bleeding. An immediate chest radiograph will confirm both the absence of significant pneumothorax or effusions as well as properly placed invasive lines and chest tube.

PREOPERATIVE CONSIDERATIONS: IDENTIFYING THE HIGH-RISK PATIENT

The patient undergoing thoracic surgery is frequently older, with concurrent medical problems and often debilitated due to cancer and associated malnutrition. Pulmonary abnormalities commonly arise from prior occupational exposure, tobacco use, or a primary disease process. Prior history of asthma, wheezing, or allergic airway responses are risk factors and serve to identify patients in whom bronchodilator management may be needed in the postoperative period.

Many thoracic surgical patients have preoperative pulmonary function tests (PFTs), particularly if lung resection is contemplated. However, these tests by themselves are not reliable predictors of postoperative pulmonary function. The FEV_1 (forced expiratory volume in 1 second) provides a reasonable indicator of a patient's postoperative ability to cough effectively and clear secretions. A postoperative FEV_1 is affected by inspiratory muscle strength, elastic recoil, and degree of obstructive air trapping, as well as any surgical removal of lung tissue. However, the decrease in FEV_1 after lung resection for cancer is not necessarily a simple proportional relationship if an obstructed lobar or mainstem bronchus was present. A cutoff value for a postpneumonectomy FEV_1 of 800 mL is commonly used as a criterion of resectability, since this amount is required to generate a sufficient cough to clear secretions.

TABLE 79.1

IMMEDIATE ICU CONSIDERATIONS IN THE THORACIC SURGICAL PATIENT

Preparation:
- Supplemental oxygen or mechanical ventilator ready
- Bedside monitoring: ECG, pulse oximetry; possible arterial, central, or PA line
- Infusion pumps if inotropes, vasopressors, or vasodilators in use
- Wall suction to connect to pleural drainage system

On Arrival in ICU:
- Connect patient to bedside monitors and ventilator (if needed)
- Check and secure all connections to chest tubes and assess function
- Auscultate breath sounds and observe chest excursion; suction if necessary
- Assess adequacy of circulation (BP, HR, pulse oximetry)
- Assess adequacy of oxygenation and ventilation (via ABG or noninvasive devices)
- Consider need for lung-protective ventilation if trauma/sepsis/operative issues
- Fluid management: confirm need for continued maintenance fluid; generally keep "dry"
- Monitor inputs and outputs; label all chest tubes and chart outputs
- Control pain with intravenous analgesics and/or regional anesthetics/analgesics
- Order any necessary laboratory studies and chest radiograph

Information to Be Obtained from Operating Room Team:
- Patient name, age, gender, and brief history
- Operation performed and any major problems encountered
- Circulatory and ventilatory requirements as determined in OR
- Current drug infusions and titration plans; timing and dose antibiotics
- Anesthetic agents given and plans for awakening/extubation (if relevant)
- Fluids and blood products given; urine output during case
- Estimated blood loss, assessment of hemostasis at closing, and blood products available including surgical salvage if any
- Laboratory results (e.g., ABGs, Hct) obtained during operating room

ABG, arterial blood gas; BP, blood pressure; ECG, electrocardiogram; Hct, hematocrit; HR, heart rate; OR, operating room; PA, pulmonary artery.

Surgical entry to the chest cavity, even if tissue is not resected, produces substantial changes in lung function, with lateral thoracotomy producing greater postoperative impairment than median sternotomy. Following thoracotomy, forced vital capacity (FVC) and functional residual capacity (FRC) can fall to less than 60% of their preoperative values on the first postoperative day. Subsequent return to baseline can take up to 14 days. Any decline in FRC is especially important, because the resulting atelectasis contributes to physiologic shunting and hypoxemia.

In patients with severe chronic obstruction, the best predictors of postoperative ventilation requirements are arterial pO_2 less than 70% of that predicted for age and the presence of dyspnea at rest (1). Factors associated with postoperative pneumonia after elective surgery include low preoperative serum albumin values, high American Society of Anesthesiologists (ASA) physical status classification, smoking history, prolonged preoperative stay, longer operative procedure, and thoracic or upper abdominal site for surgery (2).

Advanced age is frequently cited as a surgical risk factor. Elderly patients have a number of age-related changes in pulmonary function, including decreased elastic recoil and progressive stiffening of the chest wall, increase in the ratio of FRC to total lung capacity, and diminished vital capacity and FEV1 (3). The activity of upper airway reflexes is blunted, which may result in impaired clearance of secretions and the ability to protect the airway.

Obesity results in decreases in FRC and expiratory reserve volume (ERV), causing the ERV to drop below closing volume, resulting in perfused, unventilated segments of lung and a widened alveolar-arterial (A-a) pO_2 gradient. Obese patients are more likely to cough poorly, retain secretions, and develop basilar atelectasis.

Cigarette smoking is well recognized for its contribution to perioperative morbidity via its effects on the cardiovascular system, mucus secretion and clearance, and small airway narrowing. Although patients are invariably counseled to stop smoking prior to elective surgery, data from coronary artery bypass patients suggests this should occur at least 8 weeks prior to surgery, because smoking cessation *just prior* to surgery may actually increase the risk of postoperative pulmonary complications (4), probably due to transient increases in sputum volume. Expectations as to the duration of postoperative respiratory failure allow the caregiver to heighten his or her awareness if the patient develops unanticipated cardiovascular or respiratory deterioration. A very large patient population from the Veterans Affairs Medical Centers provided a database for researchers to learn what factors play a role in predicting

TABLE 79.2

RESPIRATORY FAILURE RISK INDEX

Preoperative predictor	Point value
Type of surgery	
Abdominal aortic aneurysm	27
Thoracic procedure	21
Neurosurgery, upper abdominal, or peripheral vascular	14
Neck procedure	11
Emergency surgery	11
Albumin (<30 g/L)	9
Blood urea nitrogen (>30 mg/dL)	8
Partially or fully dependent functional status	7
History of chronic obstructive pulmonary disease	6
Age (years)	
≥70	6
60–69	4

Adapted from Arozullah AM, Daley J, Henderson WG, et al. Multifactorial risk index for predicting postoperative respiratory failure in men after major noncardiac surgery. *Ann Surg.* 2000;332:242–253.

TABLE 79.3

RESPIRATORY FAILURE RISK INDEX SCORES AND OUTCOMES

Class	Point total	N (%)	Predicted probability of PRF (%)	Observed phase I (% RF)	PRF phase II (% RF)
1	≤10	39,567 (48%)	0.5	0.5	0.5
2	11–19	18,809 (23%)	2.2	2.1	1.8
3	20–27	13,865 (17%)	5.0	5.3	4.2
4	28–40	7,976 (10%)	11.6	11.9	10.1
5	>40	1,502 (2%)	30.5	30.9	26.6

Phase I indicates patients enrolled between October 1, 1991, and December 31, 1993, and phase II indicates patients enrolled between January 1, 1994, and August 31, 1995.
Adapted from Arozullah AM, Daley J, Henderson WG, et al. Multifactorial risk index for predicting postoperative respiratory failure in men after major noncardiac surgery. *Ann Surg*. 2000;332:242–253.

postoperative respiratory failure (5). Factors negatively influencing outcome included the type of surgery, emergency surgery, low preoperative albumin, high preoperative blood urea nitrogen, partial or full dependent status, chronic obstructive pulmonary disease (COPD), and age older than 60 years (5). These factors are all assigned a point status (Table 79.2); more points increase the probability of postoperative respiratory failure (Table 79.3). It is important to realize that women were excluded from data collection in this study, but the factors noted do not have gender specificity.

OPERATING ROOM EVENTS THAT IMPACT ICU CARE

The pace of postoperative recovery depends on the amount and types of anesthetic agents given as premedication and during the operative procedure. Anesthetic delivery is constrained by patient factors. The need for high inspired oxygen concentrations, particularly during one-lung anesthesia, limits the ability to use nitrous oxide. A goal of early extubation limits the use of opioids. Regional techniques (spinal, epidural) can supplement general anesthesia but are generally not applicable to operative anesthesia for thoracic procedures because of the difficulty in providing a high enough spinal level. Controlled ventilation is necessary to sustain respiration during open thorax procedures. For most procedures, the plan is to have the patient awake, comfortable, and extubated at the end of the procedure, thus avoiding the potential stress on fresh suture lines from positive pressure ventilation and coughing or bucking on the endotracheal tube.

Selective endobronchial intubation with isolation of the right and left lung permits the surgeon to operate on a quiet, collapsed lung while the other side is ventilated. Disposable polyvinyl double-lumen tubes are available in odd sizes between 35 and 41 French in both right-sided and left-sided configurations. The nonoperative bronchus is usually chosen for selective intubation in lobectomies and pneumonectomies, so that surgical manipulation does not displace the tube, and to allow resection of the mainstem bronchus if necessary. When selective endobronchial intubation is impossible (as in pediatric patients, very small adults, and laryngectomy patients), a bronchial blocker can be placed under fiberoptic guidance to selectively occlude a bronchus.

One-lung ventilation alters the ventilation/perfusion relationship, as blood passing through the unventilated lung effectively causes a right-to-left shunt, thus reducing arterial saturation. Perfusion of the unventilated lung will be reduced somewhat by the physical collapse of the lung and hypoxic pulmonary vasoconstriction. The double-lumen endotracheal tube (DLETT) is large and has the potential to cause airway trauma and edema. It may shift its position, and suctioning through it is difficult. The DLETT is generally removed at the end of the operation and replaced by a single-lumen tube when continued mechanical ventilation is required. Specific indications for continued postoperative selective endobronchial intubation include the need to protect against soilage (pus or blood) and provision of different levels of positive end-expiratory pressure to a lung of different compliance in emphysematous patients undergoing single-lung transplantation. A flexible tube changer and a pediatric (small-diameter) fiberoptic bronchoscope are essential tools that should be available in the ICU for placement and adjustment of double-lumen tubes.

The choice of postoperative recovery location depends on the degree of patient illness and the ability of a particular nursing unit to deal with postoperative ventilation and/or hemodynamic monitoring. At many hospitals, patients undergoing bronchoscopy, mediastinoscopy, esophageal dilatation, esophagoscopy, gastrostomy, jejunostomy, laryngoscopy, pleuroscopy, or scalene node biopsy can spend a short time in the postanesthesia care/recovery unit (PACU) and then be transferred to a step-down or general nursing floor, or even sent home. Patients undergoing lobectomy, segmental or wedge pulmonary resections, hiatal hernia repairs, or Heller myotomy can generally be recovered in the PACU and then sent to a step-down unit if there are no complications. Patients undergoing esophagectomy, esophagogastrectomy, and pneumonectomy are likely to have ongoing monitoring or postoperative ventilation needs and generally are managed in an intensive care setting.

IMMEDIATE POSTOPERATIVE ISSUES

Usual postoperative monitoring includes intermittent blood pressure determinations, continuous electrocardiography, and pulse oximetry. In selected patients, assessing intravascular volume status and cardiopulmonary function may be facilitated with central venous pressure or pulmonary artery catheters.

Chest tubes are usually inserted to drain the surgical site at the end of the procedure, except in pneumonectomy patients where the standard practice is to avoid a chest tube unless there is the need to monitor the pneumonectomy space postoperatively. Chest tubes should never be clamped during patient transport because of the dangers of unrecognized bleeding and tension pneumothorax. Chest tubes, except for those in pneumonectomy spaces, are usually connected to a vacuum regulator to provide –20 cm H_2O of suction. A chest radiograph will confirm endotracheal, nasogastric, and chest tube placement, as well as identify any pneumothorax, mediastinal shift, or significant atelectasis. Routine chest radiographs are not necessary after an uncomplicated removal of chest tubes, and the decision to reinsert a chest tube is usually based on clinical appearance rather than radiologic findings (6).

Commercially available chest tube systems vary in their appearance, but all provide calibrated drainage chambers, a method to release excess positive pressure, and regulated amounts of negative pressure. Air bubbles are normally expected in the chamber that limits the amount of applied suction; air bubbles in the water seal chamber represent an active leak.

Hourly output from chest tubes should be recorded and the operative team notified if drainage is greater than 100 mL/hour for more than 4 hours, or if greater than 200 mL of drainage is recorded in any 1-hour observation period. Expected chest tube drainage from major procedures in the first 24 hours is roughly 300 to 600 mL, tapering to less than 200 mL by the second day. Daily chest radiographs are usually obtained while chest tubes are in place. The level of fluid in the water seal chamber should fluctuate with each respiration (assuming no air leak) and serves as confirmation of chest tube patency. Most pulmonary resection patients will return with mild to moderate air leaks, which become problematic only if the underlying lung parenchyma does not completely expand to fill the pleural space, or if a significant percentage of tidal volume is lost through the chest tubes with mechanical ventilation. Additional pleural drainage may then be required or changes in ventilation made to minimize the air leak and optimize ventilation. Leaks may occur only above a given inflation pressure, and ventilation techniques such as smaller volumes at higher rates, pressure-controlled inverse ratio ventilation, or high-frequency oscillation (HFO) may sometimes minimize leaks and allow a seal to develop. Once all air leaks resolve and drainage is minimal (less than 100 mL/24 hours), chest tubes may be removed during the expiratory phase of ventilation or while the patient performs a Valsalva maneuver.

Prophylactic positive end-expiratory pressure (PEEP) is sometimes used in an effort to decrease postoperative drain output, especially from mediastinal drains in cardiac surgery patients. The evidence, however, suggests that higher PEEP levels do not affect chest tube output or transfusion requirements (7).

Intensive insulin therapy, defined as maintaining blood glucose between 80 and 110 mg/dL, leads to improved survival in patients admitted to a surgical ICU when compared to the conventional therapy of initiating insulin once the glucose level exceeds 215 mg/dL (8).

EXTUBATION AND AIRWAY CONCERNS

Extubation can often be accomplished in the operating room, but continued ventilation may be necessary in the presence of concurrent cardiac illness, inability to protect the airway, malnutrition, or coexisting lung disease. Silent aspiration of gastric contents is an important complication following pulmonary resections, and maintenance of endotracheal intubation for 24 hours postoperatively has been shown to decrease the occurrence of pneumonia and the operative mortality rate (9) in high-risk patients.

Measurement of maximal inspiratory pressure (MIP, often called negative inspiratory force, NIF) is helpful in determining respiratory muscle strength, particularly in patients recovering from thymectomy for myasthenia gravis, and in those who received long-acting neuromuscular blocking agents in the operating room. Residual neuromuscular blockade can be assessed using a train-of-four monitor and reversed, if necessary, with small doses of neostigmine plus vagolytic agents such as atropine or glycopyrrolate. Ideally, the patient should be awake and following instructions, and have an adequate gag reflex (signifying airway protection) and cough (for secretion clearance). Measured parameters suggesting readiness for extubation include a respiratory rate to tidal volume (f/Vt) ratio of <100, a MIP of greater than 25 cm H_2O, and adequate oxygen saturation (>92%) on FiO_2 <50% at PEEP <5 cm H_2O. Although many patients will not strictly meet these criteria for extubation, it is usually best to attempt weaning and extubation rather than risk the complications of continued ventilation. Specific indications to delay extubation are in Table 79.4.

Laryngeal and glottic edema frequently occurs after airway manipulation or intubation with a large double-lumen endotracheal tube. The presence of serious laryngeal edema can be detected (after first suctioning the posterior pharynx) by deflating the endotracheal tube cuff and occluding the endotracheal tube, and watching for evidence of airway obstruction. Endotracheal intubation may need to be maintained while edema resolves. Racemic epinephrine and corticosteroids are traditionally used, although the literature support for this is sparse. If there is any doubt about airway patency, the endotracheal tube should be removed only under direct laryngoscopic or fiberoptic observation, with a percutaneous tracheostomy set immediately at hand to provide airway access should reintubation be impossible because of airway swelling.

Only a few thoracic surgery patients require postoperative ventilation. In thoracic surgery patients, reduction of barotrauma becomes an additional consideration. Low tidal volumes (6 mL/kg) are recommended in the population at risk for acute respiratory distress syndrome (ARDS) (10), but this approach has not been well studied in routine thoracotomy

TABLE 79.4

INDICATIONS FOR CONTINUED POSTOPERATIVE VENTILATION

Airway compromise due to edema or bleeding
Inadequate pulmonary reserve post surgery
Compromised myocardial function, especially with perioperative infarction
Expected large fluid shifts with thoracoabdominal procedures
Severe neurologic impairment
Continued bleeding with likelihood of return to operating room
Esophageal surgery patients (risk for reflux and aspiration—delay extubation until airway reflexes have fully recovered as for full stomach intubation)

patients. The normal inspiratory-to-expiratory ratio is about 1:2, and inspiratory times longer than 1 second are poorly tolerated in awake patients. Longer inspiratory times reduce peak airway pressure but require addition of sedative agents and, in patients with significant airway obstruction, may not allow sufficient time for exhalation, resulting in auto-PEEP with consequent hemodynamic compromise.

Intermittent mandatory ventilation or continuous positive airway pressure (CPAP) with pressure support can be used. The FiO_2 in the early postoperative period is generally set at 50% to 60% and reduced as clinically appropriate. The combination of pulse oximetry and end-tidal carbon dioxide monitoring will reduce the need for frequent arterial blood gas sampling. Controversy still exists as to the optimal level of PEEP in the thoracic surgery patient. Low levels of PEEP (3–5 cm) may be helpful in restoring functional residual capacity and substituting for the "physiologic PEEP" of the glottis.

High-frequency jet ventilation (HFJV) has a role in the operating room during "shared airway" procedures (i.e., laryngoscopy, bronchoscopy, microlaryngeal procedures, and airway surgery). The role of high-frequency jet ventilation in the intensive care unit, particularly for management of hypoxemic respiratory failure, is poorly defined, the one exception being ventilation of a patient with a bronchopleural fistula. In theory, HFJV allows ventilation at lower airway pressures than conventional ventilation. The reduction in ventilation pressure will minimize the amount of air passing through the fistula and may promote healing by allowing adjacent tissues to approximate and possibly seal the fistula. In the face of decreased pulmonary compliance, the beneficial effect of HFJV in lowering airway pressure may be lost (11).

POSTOPERATIVE FLUID MANAGEMENT

Thoracic surgery patients present unique issues in terms of fluid management in the postoperative period due to the heightened potential for pulmonary edema. Postpneumonectomy pulmonary edema occurs in approximately 4% to 27% of patients (12,13) and pulmonary edema from all causes in 27% of pneumonectomy patients (13). Understanding the contribution of insensible (600–1,200 mL/day in a 70-kg adult) and measured fluid loss during the surgical procedure provides valuable information when anticipating the patient's needs in the postoperative period. Thoracic surgery patients may also lose an additional 6 to 8 mL/kg per hour of third-space fluid from the interstitial space and intracavitary areas (14). The choice of fluid for resuscitation is left to the discretion of the caregiver, as there is no known difference in outcome with use of either isotonic crystalloid or colloid.

During their procedures, patients are exposed to intraoperative handling of the lung, fresh frozen plasma (FFP), prolonged one-lung ventilation, collapse and re-expansion of the lung, as well as increases in postresection pulmonary artery pressures (15). These factors all contribute to the lung parenchyma being primed for a more profound inflammatory response and potential fluid accumulation. Patients undergoing procedures involving the mediastinum, such as esophagectomies or tumor excision, experience even more profound fluid shifts and likely pose a greater management challenge in the postoperative period.

There is no one formula applicable across the broad spectrum of patient types seen in this population to adequately predict fluid needs. Traditional markers of perfusion help determine if a patient is adequately volume-resuscitated. These include urine output (usually >0.5 mL/kg per hour), mental status, blood pressure, heart rate, blood lactate level, capillary refill time, venous oxygen saturation, filling pressures, and cardiac performance.

Resection patients, especially those with a right-sided pneumonectomy who experienced high ventilatory pressures during surgery (13), require greater scrutiny when determining fluid needs due to the increased risk for postpneumonectomy pulmonary edema. Ideally, the clinician will limit crystalloid infusion to 20 mL/kg for the first 24 hours in this cohort (12). If a state of poor perfusion persists, invasive devices allowing for precise hemodynamic monitoring and oxygen consumption need consideration in an effort to accurately establish goals of therapy.

PAIN MANAGEMENT

The pain associated with thoracotomy is considered one of the most intense of any surgical procedure (16). Adequate pain control is important not only to ensure patient comfort, but also to avoid potential cardiac and pulmonary complications. Early pain management is also important in an effort to reduce the chances of developing long-term postthoracotomy pain (17). The reasons for pain in this setting are many and include the skin incision, dissection of the intercostal muscles and pleura, pleural irritation, chest tube insertion, and prolonged rib retraction leading to ligamentous and muscle injury (14). Without satisfactory pain relief, the patient is exposed to adverse effects, including the inability to breathe deeply, which decreases vital capacity and functional residual capacity. Splinting also occurs, making it more difficult to clear secretions. These factors increase the likelihood of developing respiratory failure in the postoperative period. The cardiovascular system is at risk, as pain is associated with elevated circulating levels of catecholamines, which act on the myocardium to increase oxygen consumption.

Various options exist for pain management. They include systemic analgesics, neuraxial opioids, and local anesthetics via the epidural or intrathecal route; regional anesthesia such as intercostal and paravertebral nerve blocks; and adjuvant therapies such as transcutaneous electrical nerve stimulation (TENS) or applied heat.

The mainstay of postoperative pain control is systemic analgesics in the form of opioids. Agents such as morphine, fentanyl, and hydromorphone are frequently used and can be administered intravenously, subcutaneously, or intramuscularly, with the intravenous route providing the most predictable responses. Opioid side effects remain the greatest issue, with respiratory depression, nausea, vomiting, and ileus being a few examples. Nonopiate medications such as nonsteroidal anti-inflammatory drugs (NSAIDs)—including the parenteral prostaglandin inhibitor, ketorolac (18)—are reasonable adjuncts to the opioids. Because NSAIDs may exacerbate renal dysfunction, it is necessary to exercise caution when using them in the presence of underlying renal insufficiency. Also, NSAIDs may pose a risk with postoperative healing; one animal model demonstrated less effective pleural adhesions following pleurodesis (19).

Neuraxial opioids and local anesthetics via the epidural or intrathecal route provide excellent regional pain control. Epidural catheters are the preferred route, and when local anesthetics, either with or without opioids, are infused in this manner, the incidence of pulmonary complications decreases relative to that with systemic opioids (20). The initiation of epidural catheters prior to the operation appears to be the ideal approach, as it allows for better management of pain in the postoperative setting (21). Hypotension due to sympathetic blockade is a potential side effect when local anesthetics such as bupivacaine are administered. Therefore, it may be necessary to either decrease the dose or eliminate the local anesthetic completely from the infusion and use opioids exclusively.

Intercostal and paravertebral nerve blocks provide regional pain control. These blocks may be performed either intraoperatively or postoperatively and can provide relief lasting up to 12 hours; repetitive dosing may be needed and can even be accomplished with cryoablation of the intercostal nerves during the surgery (22). Chest tube insertion sites are potential sites of discomfort and may be blocked either directly or proximally. Intercostal nerve blocks are relatively contraindicated in postpneumonectomy patients due to the risks of entering and contaminating the empty chest cavity; the presence of splinting on the pneumonectomy side may actually be beneficial in reducing atelectasis in the remaining lung.

Intrapleural catheters can be used to deliver local anesthetic. These catheters are inserted in the posterior pleural cavity and threaded toward the lung apex; local anesthetics, such as bupivacaine or lidocaine, can be administered via intermittent bolus or continuous infusion. They are not a viable option in the setting of pleural effusion (the anesthetic is diluted) or pleural fibrosis; complications include technical difficulties during placement, pneumothorax, toxicity to the anesthetic, and tachyphylaxis to the local anesthetic with time.

The described methods are some of the traditional modalities used when controlling pain in the thoracic surgery patient. TENS, heat and cold application, music therapy, and relaxation techniques are additional means of providing a comfortable setting (22). In addition, patients requiring prolonged postoperative mechanical ventilation may benefit from the centrally acting α-adrenergic agonist, dexmedetomidine. In the coronary artery bypass grafting population, this agent decreased the amount of narcotics needed to achieve adequate pain control and may thereby decrease the untoward side effects of excessive narcotic use (23).

SPECIFIC PATIENT POPULATIONS

Thoracic Trauma

Trauma patients are typically evaluated and treated for acute, life-threatening injuries prior to their arrival in the ICU. The role of the critical care physician is to understand the nature of the injuries—whether blunt or penetrating—and the anticipated clinical course. In addition, maintaining a high degree of vigilance is paramount for diagnosing potential missed injuries.

Typical blunt injuries to the chest include rib fractures, flail chest, hemothorax, pneumothorax, tension pneumothorax, pulmonary contusion, cardiac contusion, and aortic disruption. Penetrating trauma such as gunshots and stabbings are less predictable in terms of the injuries generated and therefore require a case-by-case assessment in terms of management issues. Uncontrolled hemoptysis or cavitary lesions following penetrating injury require emergent surgical intervention.

Mortality increases in thoracic trauma with increasing age, lower Glasgow coma scale scores, liver injury, splenic injury, more than five rib fractures, and long bone fractures. Mortality rates typically are between 9% and 20% in the United States (24). If the patient suffers an out-of-hospital cardiac arrest in relation to his or her trauma, the chances of survival diminish even further, with less than 10% of patients in this group surviving to hospital discharge (25). A proposed therapeutic algorithm is illustrated in Figure 79.1 and will be discussed below in detail.

Rib Fractures

Rib fractures are the most common type of chest trauma, with ribs five through nine being the most susceptible. Rib fractures by themselves are rarely life threatening but may serve as indicators for more severe intrathoracic or intra-abdominal injuries. Pain may be significant and impairs usual respiratory mechanics, leading to splinting, hypoventilation, atelectasis, and potentially pneumonia as pulmonary toilet is compromised. First and/or second rib fractures indicate a large transfer of energy to the thoracic cage and should raise further suspicion for other intrathoracic problems such as aortic rupture or tear (26). The elderly, defined in this instance as 65 years of age and older, pose a particular problem when faced with these types of injuries; mortality increases by 19% with each rib fracture and the risk of pneumonia by 27% (27). The implications of age begin at 45 years, given that those with four or more rib fractures in this group show more in-hospital complications, such as increased ventilator and ICU days (28).

One intervention, however, may prove valuable in improving the outcome of patients with multiple rib fractures. Provided patients are suitable candidates for epidural analgesia, this method of pain control is associated with a decreased incidence of nosocomial pneumonia and shorter duration of mechanical ventilation in those with three or more rib fractures (29).

Flail Chest

Flail chest occurs when two or more adjacent ribs are fractured at two or more sites. This leads to a paradoxical movement of that segment during inspiration, manifested as an inward collapse. As with rib fractures, pain control is important to avoid splinting and to facilitate pulmonary toilet. Positive pressure ventilation, whether invasive or noninvasive, may be required to stent open the affected lung region and thereby avoid atelectasis.

Hemothorax

Hemothorax is a collection of blood in the pleural cavity. Patients potentially experience chest pain, dyspnea, and tachycardia along with dullness to percussion and decreased or absent breath sounds to auscultation on the affected side. Chest radiographs help to confirm the diagnosis if the collection of blood is large enough (i.e., >200 mL) to be seen radiographically. The mainstays of therapy are ensuring adequate circulating blood volume and tube thoracostomy to drain blood from the pleural space. Thoracotomy is required if bleeding continues at a

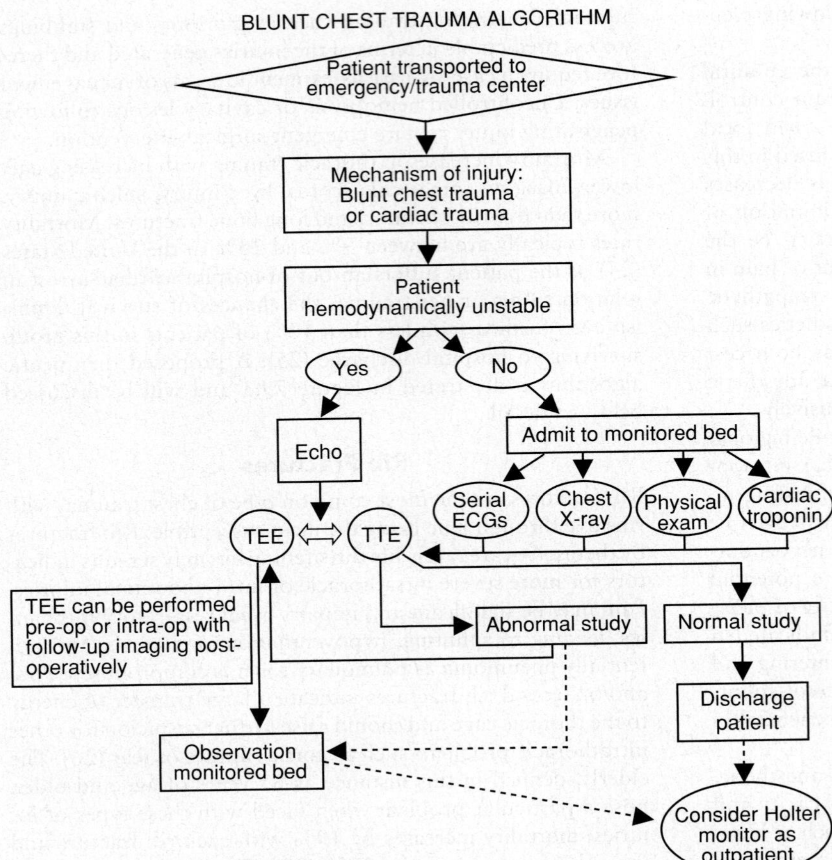

FIGURE 79.1. Therapeutic algorithm. ECGs, electrocardiograms; TEE, transesophageal echocardiography; TTE, transthoracic echocardiography.

significant rate, defined as 1,500 mL of blood output with initial tube placement or continuous bleeding of at least 250 mL/hour for 4 hours or if the patient's vital signs suddenly decompensate (26). Failure to adequately drain the hemothorax potentially leads to a condition of retained clot. This is problematic, as it may progress to empyema or fibrothorax. Options for therapy include further large-diameter tube thoracostomy, open thoracotomy, video-assisted thoracoscopy (VATS), or intrapleural fibrinolytic therapy. Further tube thoracostomy likely has a limited role, as it does not consistently liberate clotted blood products, and early surgical drainage with VATS decreases the duration of tube drainage, length of hospital stay, and hospital cost (30). VATS is the surgical intervention of choice because it is less invasive than open thoracotomy and just as effective, unless there are extensive adhesions (31). Fibrinolytic therapy offers a possible alternative to thoracoscopy or decortication, especially if the time from injury to therapy is delayed, with a response rate of up to 92% in terms of resolution (32).

Pneumothorax

Pneumothorax is the accumulation of air, originating from the lung, between the visceral and parietal pleura, and is the most common intrathoracic finding following blunt or penetrating trauma. The size of the pneumothorax is expressed as a percentage, determined by its size relative to the entire lung on an anterior-posterior chest radiographic film. Treatment with tube thoracostomy is indicated when the size is >20%, the patient is on positive pressure ventilation, and there are signs and symptoms of hypoxia and dyspnea. If following tube placement the lung does not completely re-expand and there is a persistent air leak, it is important to search for a more severe tracheal or bronchial injury, as this situation would require surgical intervention.

Tension Pneumothorax

Tension pneumothorax is a life-threatening condition requiring immediate therapy. It occurs when air accumulates in a hemithorax under pressure, causing impaired venous return and cardiac output. The absence of breath sounds on the affected side, along with deviation of the trachea and mediastinum away from that side, are the hallmarks of this condition, especially in the presence of severe hypotension. Initial therapy includes relief of the pressure by placing a large-bore (14-gauge) intravenous catheter into the second intercostal space in the midclavicular line on the affected side, followed by tube thoracostomy to treat the pneumothorax.

Pulmonary Contusion

Pulmonary contusion is a result of blunt force transmitted across the thorax. The mechanism for its development is not completely understood but is felt to be related to compression and re-expansion of the lung tissue, leading to capillary disruption with interstitial and intra-alveolar edema, decreased compliance, and hypoxemia due to a shunt physiology (26). Care is largely supportive in this population, with close

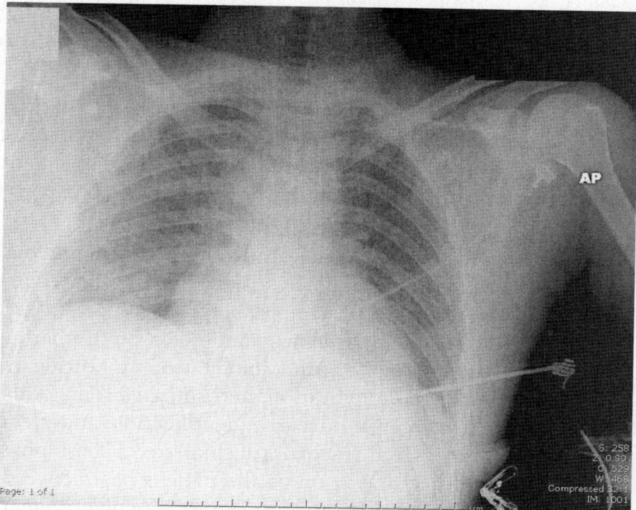

FIGURE 79.2. There are multiple fractured ribs on the right with several fractured in more than one place. This leads to a flail segment with inspiration.

attention to pain management and pulmonary toilet. Typical chest radiographic findings are shown in Figure 79.2.

Cardiac Contusion

Cardiac contusion is a potential complication of blunt chest trauma (Fig. 79.3.) Its exact incidence is unclear, as different studies used varying criteria to make the diagnosis (33). It is typically well tolerated in mildly injured patients but may lead to fatal arrhythmias or cardiogenic shock if severe. Rapid deceleration, as occurs in motor vehicle accidents, is the most common cause since, in this situation, the heart moves freely and can strike the internal sternum with a substantial amount of force (33). Electrocardiography findings in cardiac contusion are summarized in Table 79.5. Biomarkers, such as creatine kinase (CK) or troponin I and T, are potentially helpful in the diagnosis, as the histologic changes associated with contusion are similar to those seen with infarction. Troponin I and T are specific to the myocardium and may avoid false positives by relying solely on CK, as trauma patients often have diffuse muscular damage leading to massive CK release from many tissues. Electrocardiography may show nonspecific findings, such as sinus tachycardia and premature atrial or ventricular systoles, and not provide further clarification of the diagnosis (33). Echocardiography, whether transthoracic (TTE) or transesophageal (TEE), offers the best insight into cardiac damage from contusion due to its ability to directly visualize wall motion abnormalities (Table 79.6). Treatment involves cardiac monitoring and stabilization of the traumatically induced injuries, supporting blood pressure and cardiac output as indicated. (See algorithm, Fig. 79.1.)

TABLE 79.5

ELECTROCARDIOGRAPHIC FINDINGS IN CARDIAC CONTUSION

Nonspecific abnormalities
Pericarditis-like ST-segment elevation or PTa depression
Prolonged QT interval
Myocardial injury
New Q wave
ST-T segment elevation or depression
Conduction disorders
Right bundle branch block
Fascicular block
Atrioventricular (AV) nodal conduction disorders (1st-, 2nd-, and 3rd-degree AV block)
Arrhythmias
Sinus tachycardia
Atrial and ventricular extrasystoles
Atrial fibrillation
Ventricular tachycardia
Ventricular fibrillation
Sinus bradycardia
Atrial tachycardia

Adapted from Sybrandy KC, Cramer MJM, Burgersdijk C. Diagnosing cardiac contusion: old wisdom and new insights. *Heart.* 2003;89:485–489.

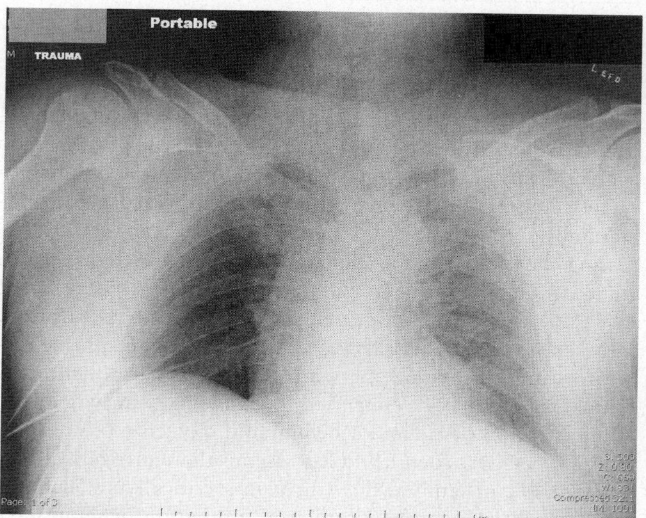

FIGURE 79.3. Diffuse infiltrative pattern on the left side is consistent with findings seen following pulmonary contusion.

Aortic Disruption

Aortic disruption leads to a high mortality, as only 13% to 15% of these patients reach the hospital alive. Those surviving that

TABLE 79.6

ECHOCARDIOGRAPHIC FINDINGS IN ACUTE CARDIAC CONTUSION

Transthoracic Echocardiography
- Regional wall motion abnormalities
- Pericardial effusion
- Valvular lesions
- Right and left ventricular enlargement
- Ventricular septal rupture
- Intracardiac thrombus

Transesophageal Echocardiography
- Aortic endothelial laceration or aortic dissection
- Aortic rupture

long have a 30% chance of subsequent rupture and death (34). Diagnostic modalities include findings on chest radiograph of a widened mediastinum, aortography (the gold standard), CT scanning, and TEE. Treatment is immediate surgery by a cardiothoracic surgeon to repair the injury.

Posttraumatic empyema occurs in up to 2% of the thoracic trauma population and is most often caused by *Staphylococcus aureus* (35). Factors increasing the likelihood of developing empyema include retained hemothorax, pulmonary contusion, and multiple chest tube placement (36). Of note, since most empyemas are of a parapneumonic etiology (37), pneumonia has little impact on the development of pleural space infection in this population. Treatment includes removal of the infected fluid or collection and may be accomplished by guided drainage, VATS, or open thoracotomy.

Lung Volume Reduction Surgery

Lung volume reduction surgery (LVRS) is used in an effort to improve the pulmonary dynamics of patients with severe emphysema by palliating dyspnea and improving functional status. This population is prone to more postsurgical complications than most other thoracic surgery patients due to their underlying fragile nature. Anticipated complications include arrhythmias, prolonged respiratory failure, air leaks, pneumonia, and ICU readmission. Air leaks occur in 90% of patients and rarely require surgical intervention (38). The prevalence of air leaks correlates with a more prolonged, complicated hospital course, and severity is predicted by patient characteristics such as worsened pulmonary function, use of inhaled steroids, distribution of disease (lower lobe disease is less frequent and has shorter duration), and presence of adhesions (38). Management involves chest tube drainage with efforts to minimize or eliminate suction so the tissue has the greatest chance to heal.

Esophageal Surgery

Esophageal surgery patients undergo procedures that traumatize the lung, the interposed stomach, and the diaphragm. Patients who undergo esophageal resection for carcinoma tend to be malnourished. Pulmonary complications, including atelectasis, pneumonia, aspiration, and retained secretions, are all possible. Up to 29% of patients experience respiratory complications (39) with increasing patient age and decreasing performance on spirometry, which is predictive of increased risk (40). Aspiration risk is minimized by having patients undergo a thorough swallowing evaluation, including radiographic testing, prior to initiating oral intake.

The most dangerous complication of esophageal surgery is leakage from the surgical site. Anastomotic leak occurs in as many as 11% of patients, and factors impacting the incidence include high estimated intraoperative blood loss, cervical location of the anastomosis, and the development of postoperative ARDS (41). Interestingly, the use of thoracic epidural analgesia is associated with a decreased occurrence of anastomotic leakage (41). Mortality associated with anastomotic leaks is historically high, but with improved surgical techniques, the patients now face a more promising outcome. One center showed a reduction in mortality with intrathoracic leaks from 43% to 3.3% over a 34-year period (42). Early identification is important, and endoscopy provides a safe method for determining the integrity of the graft and whether surgery is necessary to avoid loss of the graft (43).

RESPIRATORY THERAPY

Thoracic surgical patients often have significant underlying COPD, impaired mucociliary clearance, excessive secretions, and/or increased closing volumes, all of which predispose to atelectasis. The respiratory therapist plays an important role in providing secretion management and chest physiotherapy (percussion and vibration). Other modalities supporting recovery include adequate hydration, aerosolized bronchodilators, humidified oxygen, and early identification and treatment of infection of the tracheobronchial tree. Chest physiotherapy should begin as soon as the patient has recovered sufficiently from anesthesia to cooperate. Mucolytic agents (such as N-acetylcysteine) are helpful in solubilizing thick secretions, but may cause bronchospasm. Oral or nasotracheal suctioning is used in selected extubated patients, but discomfort and the possibility of complications (hypoxemia, vagal-mediated bradycardia, or cardiac arrest) limit routine use. A mini-tracheostomy (bedside percutaneous cricothyroidotomy for suctioning) can provide access to the lower airway in patients with thick secretions. Inadequate clearance of secretions often requires flexible bronchoscopy, which is of greatest benefit in the extubated patient who cannot adequately be suctioned. If pulmonary parenchymal involvement is confined to one lung, altering body position can improve gas exchange by changing the relationships between ventilation and perfusion. The lateral decubitus position, with the *un*involved lung down, allows maximal blood flow to ventilated areas during spontaneous ventilation. This relationship may be altered with mechanical breaths and application of PEEP. Specialized beds can be set to supine, lateral, or rotating modes to optimize oxygenation (44).

COMPLICATIONS

Complications common to all thoracic surgical patients are listed in Table 79.7. Those more likely to occur following specific procedures are listed in Table 79.8.

Airway complications can be precipitated by prolonged intubation with large or double-lumen endotracheal tubes, passage of bronchial blockers, use of rigid bronchoscopes, or frequent reintubation. Edema of the larynx or trachea can substantially narrow the cross-sectional area of the airway. Assessing the patient for an air leak around an occluded endotracheal tube just prior to extubation may identify significant laryngeal and supraglottic edema. Upright or sitting position, intravenous corticosteroids (45), and racemic epinephrine respiratory treatments are the mainstay of edema reduction. A critical airway may be converted to an adequate airway by the administration of Heliox, a helium and oxygen mixture (46). Helium, being less dense and less viscous than nitrogen, allows maintenance of laminar flow through a critically swollen upper airway. Prolonged endotracheal intubation or temporary tracheostomy may be required to allow resolution of airway edema.

TABLE 79.7

POSTOPERATIVE COMPLICATIONS FOLLOWING ANY THORACIC PROCEDURE

Airway edema/stridor
Arrhythmias (especially atrial fibrillation, multifocal atrial tachycardia)
Arytenoid dislocation
Aspiration of gastric contents
Atelectasis
Bronchospasm
Bronchopleural fistula
Chylothorax
Congestive heart failure
Deep venous thrombosis
Empyema
Hemorrhage
Hemothorax
Infection (superficial, deep)
Lobar collapse
Lobar torsion
Myocardial infarction
Pain and splinting
Pleural effusion
Pneumothorax
Pulmonary embolus
Re-expansion pulmonary edema
Respiratory failure
Retaining secretions
Subcutaneous emphysema
Tension pneumothorax

From Higgins TL. Selected issues in postoperative management. In: American College of Chest Physicians: *The ACCP Critical Care Board Review*. Northbrook IL; 1998:323–334, with permission.

The recurrent laryngeal nerves branch from the vagus nerves as they enter the chest. The right recurrent laryngeal nerve arises high in the apex of the right chest and loops around the right subclavian artery to travel back to the larynx in the tracheoesophageal groove. The left recurrent laryngeal nerve, which is more susceptible to injury, wraps around the aortic arch in the left chest before it enters the tracheoesophageal groove. Injury can result from excessive traction, aggressive dissection about these nerves, or the operative sacrifice of these nerves. Mediastinoscopy, anterior mediastinotomy, left pulmonary resection with subaortic exenteration, and resections of mediastinal tumors are common operations in which the recurrent laryngeal nerve may be damaged. Associated airway and laryngeal edema may allow for adequate coaptation of the vocal cords for the first days postextubation, often preventing identification of cord injury until after discharge from the ICU, when ineffective cough or aspiration of secretions will become apparent. If there is permanent damage or division of the recurrent laryngeal nerve, injection of the vocal cord with a long-lasting substance such as Teflon may be considered. In many instances, aggressive chest physiotherapy, careful airway management, and temporary avoidance of oral feeding may eliminate the need for any intervention until recovery of the nerve function has occurred. Intermittent noisy inspiration and painful swallowing suggest arytenoid dislocation, an uncommon cause of postextubation respiratory failure (47). Treatment consists of surgical reduction, which must be accomplished before the cricoarytenoid joint becomes fibrosed in poor position.

Retained secretions and blood in the airway are especially common if the airway was opened, such as during a bronchoplastic procedure or closure of a bronchial stump. Mechanical airway obstruction secondary to secretions may be aggravated by bronchospasm, and preoperative bronchodilators should be continued in patients with reactive airways, as secretions can precipitate coughing and bronchospasms.

Postoperative air leaks most often result from very distal fistulae between tiny bronchioles or respiratory units and the pleural cavity. One of the main functions of the chest tube is to evacuate air from these small air leaks to ensure complete expansion of the lung and coaptation of the cut surface of the lung to the parietal pleura, which will seal these leaks. Repositioning of the chest tubes or insertion of further chest tubes into undrained spaces, adequate suction applied to the pleural cavity, and full expansion of the lung with vigorous chest physiotherapy help to close these small distal fistula. A substantial persistent air leak from the chest tube, or incomplete expansion of the lung, suggests a significant bronchopleural fistula. Major proximal airway problems such as failure of the anastomosis, disruption of a bronchial closure, or retained secretions or foreign bodies can be identified by bronchoscopy. Within the first 7 postoperative days, any fistula is likely to be due to a technical problem. More than 1 week after the operation, but usually within the first 6 weeks, fistulae are more often due to an empyema or local peribronchial abscess. Late occurrence of a bronchopleural fistula, (more than 6 months after the operation) is frequently due to recurrent lung carcinoma.

Early postoperative bronchopleural fistula in a pneumonectomy patient is a surgical emergency. The typical presentation is sudden expectoration of copious amounts of pink, frothy sputum, which may be misdiagnosed as pulmonary edema. The patient should be positioned with the operated or pneumonectomy side down to trap remaining fluid in the pneumonectomy space and prevent drowning. A chest radiograph will show loss of fluid from the pneumonectomy space. Further management will likely include both bronchoscopy to assess the stump closure and immediate reoperation.

Empyema is initially treated with closed tube drainage and antibiotic therapy. After the patient has been stabilized and any bronchopleural fistula identified and treated, drainage of the empyema cavity is converted from closed tube drainage to open tube drainage. A chest radiograph helps to determine if the mediastinum is fixed or whether it has shifted and compressed the contralateral remaining lung. If the mediastinum is stable, drainage of the cavity may be permanently converted to open drainage. This may take the form of rib resection and marsupialization of the pneumonectomy cavity (Clagett window or Eloesser flap). With time, the pneumonectomy cavity shrinks in size, and the window or flap may be closed.

Postoperative hypoxemia is common and may be due to sepsis, ARDS, pneumonia, or pulmonary embolization. If pulmonary emboli are suspected, ventilation/perfusion scanning, spiral computed tomography, and pulmonary angiography should be done, and treatment initiated with anticoagulation or lytic therapy, depending on timing and indications. If these measures are contraindicated, an inferior vena caval filter should be placed. Systemic tumor emboli, though uncommon, may be seen after pulmonary resections for primary bronchogenic carcinomas or metastatic sarcomas.

TABLE 79.8

COMPLICATIONS OF SPECIFIC THORACIC PROCEDURES

Procedure	Complications
Anterior mediastinotomy (Chamberlain)	Damage to recurrent laryngeal nerve (particularly left)
Bronchoscopy/mediastinoscopy	Bleeding from major vessels if torn, air leak with biopsy of bronchus
Bronchopleural fistula repair	Persistent leak, dehiscence
Bronchopulmonary lavage	Respiratory distress/contralateral spillage
Bullectomy	Tension pneumothorax, air leak
Chest wall reconstruction	Blood loss, altered chest wall compliance, unstable chest, infection prosthetic material
Clagett window	Air leak
Collis-Belsey	Gastric leak, splenic injury
Decortication	Blood loss, air leak(s)
Esophageal dilatation	Esophageal perforation, pleural effusion, airway obstruction
Esophagoscopy	Esophageal perforation
Esophagogastrectomy	Third-spacing of fluids, anastomotic leak, gastric devasculatization, splenic injury, gastric torsion
Heller myotomy	Esophageal tear
Lobectomy	Bronchial leak, lobar collapse, lobar torsion
Mediastinal tumor excision	Airway obstruction with sedation/anesthesia, damage to recurrent laryngeal nerve
Nissen fundoplication	Esophageal obstruction (with tight wrap), splenic injury
Pectus repair	Costochondritis, unstable sternum
Pleuroscopy	Pharyngeal laceration, air leak
Pneumonectomy	Atrial arrhythmias (atrial fibrillation, MAT), mediastinal shift, cardiac torsion, air embolism, disrupted bronchus
Thoracic aortic aneurysm	Paraplegia, bleeding, aortobronchial fistula, esophageal injury
Thymectomy	In myasthenics, possible weakness and respiratory failure
Lung transplant	Rejection (day 5), reperfusion injury, infection, overdistention of native lung, dehiscence
Tracheal resection	Fixed neck flexion postoperatively, dehiscence, air leak

From Higgins TL. Selected issues in postoperative management. In: American College of Chest Physicians: *The ACCP Critical Care Board Review*. Northbrook, IL; 1998:323–334, with permission.

Massive postoperative hemorrhage can present as significant shock and occasionally occurs during transfer of the patient to the recovery room or ICU. This potentially lethal condition can be the result of a slipped tie from the pulmonary vein—or, less commonly, the pulmonary artery—and requires emergent reoperation. Slower postoperative hemorrhage usually results from small bleeding arteries or veins in the mediastinum or chest wall. Reoperation is required for control of bleeding and to evaluate the hemothorax to prevent future fibrothorax or restrictive lung disease.

PULMONARY PARENCHYMAL COMPLICATIONS

Tracheoesophageal Fistula

A communication may occur between the anterior esophageal wall and membranous (posterior) wall of the trachea following prolonged intubation due to pressure exerted from the cuff of the endotracheal or tracheostomy tube, which can lead to potential tissue necrosis. Tracheoesophageal fistula should be suspected when feedings are aspirated from the airway. Surgical revision of the damaged area is the definitive therapy but may not be practical in patients still requiring positive pressure ventilation, and may need to be delayed until the patient has been weaned off mechanical ventilation (48). Stenting of the esophagus, performed at the bedside in the ICU, allows for temporary sealing of the fistula until the patient is a suitable candidate for final surgical repair (49).

Tracheoinnominate Fistula

Bleeding seen 48 hours or greater following tracheostomy raises concern about the presence of a tracheoinnominate fistula. Even though this occurs rarely, it is a life-threatening complication and requires urgent action. Most cases arise when pressure necrosis on the posterior aspect of the blood vessel occurs due to overinflation of the endotracheal cuff. Initial steps include hyperinflation of the tracheostomy cuff or direct arterial compression with a finger to tamponade the bleeding. Bronchoscopy is the diagnostic procedure of choice, followed by surgery to divide the innominate artery, with subsequent separation of the trachea from the divided artery by viable tissue (50).

Atelectasis

The most common complication following thoracic surgery is atelectasis. Potential contributors include hypoventilation, splinting, bronchospasm, poor cough, retained secretions, pneumothorax, and trauma to the lung during the surgical procedure. Most patients in the ICU will tolerate some degree of atelectasis with symptoms including fever, tachypnea, arrhythmias, hypoxia, or respiratory failure. More severe atelectasis or a compromised host can present with respiratory failure requiring mechanical ventilation. Auscultation of the lungs may identify the impaired areas due to the diminished air movement, and a chest radiograph may further highlight the portions of collapsed lung. Atelectasis is not limited to the lung on the operative side, although it is more likely to occur in that parenchyma.

Efforts to avoid atelectasis include frequent suctioning of the tracheobronchial tree, chest percussion and postural drainage, humidification of inspired gases, frequent patient rotation, bronchodilators, pain control, coughing, deep breathing, bronchoscopy for removal of mucus plugs or secretions, invasive or noninvasive positive pressure ventilation, and early ambulation (14). Chest physiotherapy uses physical therapy such as clapping and vibration to stimulate coughing and thereby move secretions out of the lungs. Incentive spirometry, often used following surgical procedures, does not provide the same benefit of chest physiotherapy in the recovery phase, as physiotherapy potentially decreases hospital costs due to shorter lengths of stay (51).

Lobar Collapse and Torsion

Lobar collapse most commonly occurs in either the right upper lobe following surgery that uses a double-lumen endotracheal tube or in the right middle lobe after right upper lobectomy, which alters the anatomy, allowing the horizontal fissure to rise. This results in compression on the right middle lobe bronchus and subsequent occlusion.

Lobar torsion occurs as the result of a lung segment twisting about its hilar structures. This twisting occludes the bronchial, arterial, and venous supply to the affected segment, with infarction occurring if the process is not recognized and treated. The right middle lobe and lingula are at greatest risk following thoracotomy (14). The patient may initially present as simply having atelectasis, but over time, the chest radiograph shows opacification of the affected lobe. As ischemia progresses to infarction, there will be signs of tissue necrosis, such as bloody or malodorous secretions and foul chest tube drainage. Bronchoscopy is the initial tool for evaluation, followed by thoracotomy for an urgent detorsion and lobectomy if necrotic tissue is found.

PLEURAL COMPLICATIONS

Pneumothorax is the second most frequent postoperative complication after atelectasis (14). Signs and symptoms of a pneumothorax range from subtle to severe and include increased work of breathing, decreased breath sounds and chest movement, wheezing, hypoxia, increased airway pressures if still on the ventilator, and hemodynamic instability if tension pneumothorax occurs. A chest radiograph is the first modality used in the diagnosis of pneumothorax, save for the instance when tension is present and chest tube placement must occur immediately to prevent further clinical deterioration of the patient. If a pneumothorax develops on the surgical side and chest tubes are already present, it is necessary to ensure that the tubes are functioning properly. This involves inspecting the entire system for any evidence of leaks, inadequate suction, or loss of tubing patency due to blood clots. It is possible to declot chest tubes with vigorous stripping or by placing a balloon occlusion catheter to physically remove the obstruction.

Pleural effusions persisting in the postoperative period should be evaluated via thoracentesis to determine if there is an intrathoracic or extrathoracic cause. If the fluid is transudative, the underlying cause needs to be addressed. If the fluid is exudative, a high suspicion for empyema must be maintained. If pleural effusions and pneumothoraces do not resolve over time, the decision for more definitive therapy, such as pleurodesis, needs to be entertained.

Thoracic duct injury is a known complication following any surgery involving dissection in the posterior mediastinum and may result in chylothorax. Confirmation of the diagnosis includes testing the pleural fluid which is high in triglycerides and chylomicrons. The leakage site is localized with lymphangiography or CT scanning, and the clinical situation will dictate the type of management. It occurs in approximately 4% of patients undergoing esophageal surgery with the transthoracic approach as compared to transhiatal; an increased number of positive nodes are predictive of its incidence (52). Management initially includes chest tube drainage and parenteral nutrition to decrease the thoracic duct output. If the drainage resolves with conservative management, surgical intervention can likely be reserved for those not decreasing their chylous output (53).

OTHER COMPLICATIONS

Postoperative Infections

The incidence of developing nosocomial infection following lung surgery increases with a history of COPD, duration of surgery (with an increased risk for each additional minute), and ICU admission (54). Surgical site infection occurs rarely due to the use of prophylactic perioperative antibiotics. Factors increasing the risk of infection at the incision site include emergent thoracotomy in the trauma patient and procedures for treatment of empyema, lung abscess, mediastinitis, or perforated esophagus. Any unexplained fever requires careful inspection of the surgical site.

When air tracks into the subcutaneous space via the path of least resistance, it generates subcutaneous emphysema. The air is forced along these pathways with positive pressure ventilation and instances of increased intrathoracic pressure during spontaneous breathing. Coughing and forced exhalation are two examples. Subcutaneous air may be striking in appearance but rarely affects patient outcome in a detrimental way. If the collection of air is massive enough to compromise the airway, endotracheal intubation may be indicated, realizing the pitfalls of instituting positive pressure ventilation in such a situation. Following sterile preparation, puncturing the skin with small-gauge (no. 25) needles provides a conduit for the subcutaneous air to escape and decrease the cosmetic deformation.

SUMMARY

The thoracic patient presents unique management issues due to the complexities of fluid management, preoperative morbidities, the need for specialized pain control to preserve respiratory function, and nature of drainage devices left in place postoperatively. As a critical care physician, it is important to understand the interplay of these circumstances when anticipating the patient's postoperative needs in the ICU. The pulmonary system is more susceptible to adverse events if fluid management is not judiciously managed. Patients undergoing thoracotomies for lung or esophageal surgery tend to have an impaired functional status and nutrition at baseline, negatively impacting their postoperative course. If pain control is inadequate, the patient will have impaired pulmonary function, which potentially delays recovery. Chest tubes require extra vigilance due to the potential complications should they malfunction.

With a well thought out care plan, the outcome for thoracic surgery patients will be positive and the road to recovery smooth.

References

1. Nunn JF, Miledge S, Chen D, et al. Respiratory criteria for fitness for surgery and anesthesia. *Anaesthesia.* 1988;43:543–611.
2. Garibaldi RA, Britt MR, Coleman ML, et al. Risk factors for postoperative pneumonia. *JAMA.* 1981;70:677–680.
3. Wahba WM. Influence of aging on lung function—clinical significance of changes from age twenty. *Anesth Analg.* 1983;62:764–776.
4. Warner MA, Offord KP, Warner ME, et al. Role of preoperative cessation of smoking and other factors in postoperative pulmonary complications: a blinded, prospective study of coronary artery bypass patients. *Mayo Clin Proc.* 1989;64:609–616.
5. Arozullah AM, Daley J, Henderson WG, et al. Multifactorial risk index for predicting postoperative respiratory failure in men after major noncardiac surgery. *Ann Surg.* 2000;332:242–253.
6. Palesty JA, McKelvey AA, Dudrick SJ. The efficacy of x-rays after chest tube removal. *Am J Surg.* 2000;179:13–16.
7. Collier B, Kolff J, Devineni R, et al. Prophylactic positive end-expiratory pressure and reduction of postoperative blood loss in open-heart surgery. *Ann Thorac Surg.* 2002;74(4):1191–1194.
8. Van den Berghe G, Wouters P, Weekers F, et al. Intensive insulin therapy in critically ill patients. *N Engl J Med.* 2001;345:1359–1367.
9. DeHaven CB, Hurst JM, Branson RD. Evaluation of two different extubation criteria: attributes contributing to success. *Crit Care Med.* 1986;14:92.
10. The Acute Respiratory Distress Syndrome Network. Ventilation with lower tidal volumes as compared with traditional tidal volumes for acute lung injury and the acute respiratory distress syndrome. *N Engl J Med.* 2000;342:1301–1308.
11. Baumann MH, Sahn SA. Medical management and therapy of bronchopleural fistulas in the mechanically ventilated patient. *Chest.* 1990;97:721.
12. Slinger PD. Perioperative fluid management for thoracic surgery: the puzzle of postpneumonectomy pulmonary edema. *J Cardiothorac Vasc Anesth.* 1995;9(4):442–451.
13. van der Werff YD, van der Houwen HK, Heijmans P, et al. Postpneumonectomy pulmonary edema, a retrospective analysis of incidence and possible risk factors. *Chest.* 1997;111:1278–1284.
14. Amini S, Gabrielli A, Caruso LJ, et al. The thoracic surgical patients: initial postoperative care. *Semin Cardiothorac Vasc Anesth.* 2002;6(3):169–188.
15. Jordan S, Mitchell JA, Quinlan GJ, et al. The pathogenesis of lung injury following pulmonary resection. *Eur Respir J.* 2000;15:790–799.
16. Loan WB, Morrison JD. The incidence and severity of postoperative pain. *Br J Anaesth.* 1967;39:695–698.
17. Katz J, Jackson M, Kavanagh BP. Acute pain relief after thoracic surgery predicts long term post-thoracotomy pain. *Clin J Pain.* 1996;12(1):50–55.
18. Yee JP, Koshiver JE, Allbon C, et al. Comparison of intramuscular ketorolac tromethamine and morphine sulfate for analgesia of pain after major surgery. *Pharmacotherapy.* 1986;6(5):253–261.
19. Lardinois D, Vogt P, Yang L, et al. Non-steroidal anti-inflammatory drugs decrease the quality of pleurodesis after mechanical pleural abrasion. *Eur J Cardiothorac Surg.* 2004;25(5):865–871.
20. Ballantyne JC, Carr DB, deFerranti S, et al. The comparative effects of postoperative analgesic therapies on pulmonary outcome: cumulative meta-analyses of randomized, controlled trials. *Anesth Analg.* 1998;86:598–612.
21. Yegin A, Erdogan A, Kayacan N, et al. Early postoperative pain management after thoracic surgery; pre and postoperative versus postoperative epidural anesthesia: a randomized study. *Eur J Cardiothorac Surg.* 2003;24(3):420–424.
22. Peeters-Asdourian C, Gupta S. Choices in pain management following thoracotomy. *Chest.* 1999;115:122S–124S.
23. Herr DL, Sum-Ping ST, England M. ICU sedation after coronary artery bypass graft surgery: dexmedetomidine-based versus propofol-based regimens. *J Cardiothoracic Vasc Anesth.* 2003;17(5):576–584.
24. Kulshrestha P, Munshi I, Wait R. Profile of chest trauma in a level I trauma center. *J Trauma.* 2004;57:576–581.
25. Lockey D, Crewsdon K, Davies G. Traumatic cardiac arrest: who are the survivors? *Ann Emerg Med.* 2006;48(3):240–244.
26. Munshi IA. Thoracic trauma. In: Higgins TL, ed. *Cardiopulmonary Critical Care.* Oxford, UK: BIOS Scientific Publishers Ltd.; 2002.
27. Bulger EM, Arneson MA, Mock CN, et al. Rib fractures in the elderly. *J Trauma.* 2000;48(6):1040–1046.
28. Holcomb JB, McMullin NR, Kozar RA, et al. Morbidity from rib fractures increases after age 45. *J Am Coll Surg.* 2003;196(4):549–555.
29. Bulger EM, Edwards T, Klotz P, et al. Epidural analgesia improves outcome after multiple rib fractures. *Surgery.* 2004;136(2):426–430.
30. Meyer DM, Jessen ME, Wait MA, et al. Early evacuation of traumatic retained hemothoraces using thoracoscopy: a prospective, randomized trial. *Ann Thorac Surg.* 1997;64:1396–1400.
31. Navsaria PH, Vogel RJ, Nicol AJ. Thoracoscopic evacuation of retained posttraumatic hemothorax. *Ann Thorac Surg.* 2004;78:282–285.
32. Inci I, Ozcelik C, Ulku R, et al. Intrapleural fibrinolytic treatment of traumatic clotted hemothorax. *Chest.* 1998;114:160–165.
33. Sybrandy KC, Cramer MJM, Burgersdijk C. Diagnosing cardiac contusion: old wisdom and new insights. *Heart.* 2003;89:485–489.
34. Fabian TC, Richardson JD, Croce MA, et al. Prospective study of blunt aortic injury: multicenter trial of the American Association for the Surgery of Trauma. *J Trauma.* 1997;42(3):1128–1143.
35. Mandal AK, Thadepalli H, Chettipalli U. Posttraumatic empyema thoracis: A 24-year experience at a major trauma center. *J Trauma.* 1997;43(5):764–771.
36. Aguilar MM, Battistella FD, Owings JT, et al. Posttraumatic empyema. Risk factor analysis. *Arch Surg.* 1997;132(6):647–650.
37. Hoth JJ, Burch PT, Bullock Tk, et al. Pathogenesis of posttraumatic empyema: the impact of pneumonia on pleural space infections. *Surg Infect.* 2003;4(1):29–35.
38. DeCamp MM, Blackstone EH, Naunheim KS, et al. Patient and surgical factors influencing air leak after lung volume reduction surgery: lessons learned from the national Emphysema Treatment Trial. *Ann Thorac Surg.* 2006;82:197–207.
39. Atkins BZ, Shah AS, Hutcheson KA, et al. Reducing hospital morbidity and mortality following esophagectomy. *Ann Thor Surg.* 2004;78(4):1170–1176.
40. Ferguson MK, Durkin AE. Preoperative prediction of the risk of pulmonary complications after esophagectomy for cancer. *J Thorac Cardiovasc Surg.* 2002;123(4):661–669.
41. Michelet P, D'Journo KB, Roch A, et al. Perioperative risk factors for anastomotic leakage after esophagectomy: influence of thoracic epidural analgesia. *Chest.* 2005;128(5):3461–3466.
42. Martin LW, Swisher SG, Hofstetter W, et al. Intrathoracic leaks following esophagectomy are no longer associated with increased mortality. *Ann Surg.* 2005;242:392–402.
43. Maish MS, DeMeester SR, Choustoulakis E, et al. The safety and usefulness of endoscopy for evaluation of the graft and anastomosis early after esophagectomy and reconstruction. *Surg Endosc.* 2005;19(8):1093–1102.
44. Nelson LD, Anderson HB. Physiologic effects of steep positioning in the surgical intensive care unit. *Arch Surg.* 1989;124:352–355.
45. Cheng K-C, Hou C-C, Huang H-C, et al. Intravenous injection of methylprednisolone reduces the incidence of postextubation stridor in intensive care unit patients. *Crit Care Med.* 2006;34:1345–1350.
46. Skrinskas GJ, Hyland RH, Hutcheon MA. Using helium-oxygen mixtures in the management of acute upper airway obstruction. *Can Med Assoc J.* 1983;128:555–558.
47. Castella X, Gilabert J, Perez C. Arytenoid dislocation after tracheal intubation: an unusual cause of acute respiratory failure? *Anesthesiology.* 1991;74:613–615.
48. Athanassiadi K, Gerazounis M. Repair of postintubation tracheoesophageal fistula in polytrauma patients. *Injury.* 2005;36(8):897–899.
49. Eleftheriadis E, Kotzampassi K. Temporary stenting of acquired benign tracheoesophageal fistulas in critically ill ventilated patients. *Surg Endosc.* 2005;19(6):811–815.
50. Allan JS, Wright CD. Tracheoinnominate fistula: diagnosis and management. *Chest Surg Clin N Am.* 2003;13(2):331–341.
51. Varela G, Ballesteros E, Jimenez MF, et al. Cost-effectiveness of prophylactic respiratory physiotherapy in pulmonary lobectomy. *Eur J Cardiothorac Surg.* 2006;29:216–220.
52. Lagarde SM, Omloo JM, de Jong K, et al. Incidence and management of chyle leakage after esophagectomy. *Ann Thor Surg.* 2005;80(2):449–454.
53. Shimizu K, Yoshida J, Nishimura M, et al. Treatment strategy for chylothorax after pulmonary resection and lymph node dissection for lung cancer. *J Thorac Cardiovasc Surg.* 2002;124(3):499–502.
54. Nan DN, Fernandez-Ayala M, Farinas-Alvarez C, et al. Nosocomial infection after lung surgery. *Chest.* 2005;128:2647–2652.

CHAPTER 80 ■ POSTOPERATIVE MANAGEMENT OF ADULT CARDIOVASCULAR SURGERY PATIENTS

HOWARD K. SONG • MATTHEW S. SLATER

Adult patients undergoing cardiovascular surgery procedures all pass through a period of critical illness during their recovery. These patients present intensivists with unique critical care management challenges because of the hemodynamic changes that occur as a result of the surgery itself and the broad inflammatory after-effects of cardiopulmonary bypass. The specialized nature of the critical care of adult cardiovascular surgery patients is apparent in the proliferation of heart centers, specialized units, treatment protocols, and pathways designed to optimize patient outcomes by standardizing care and focusing provider expertise. Optimal outcomes for adult cardiovascular surgery patients are most likely to occur where critical care systems are designed to support this specific patient population and practitioners have strong familiarity with normal recovery milestones and complications that can interrupt this process.

CARDIOPULMONARY BYPASS

A significant portion of adult cardiovascular surgery procedures are performed with the use of cardiopulmonary bypass. The development of the heart–lung machine over the past 50 years represents one of the major achievements of modern medicine and has made complex repairs of intracardiac structures and the great vessels feasible. Cardiopulmonary bypass techniques allow the surgeon to interrupt blood flow through the heart and lungs, providing a relatively bloodless and motionless field for the conduct of the operation. The most basic components of a cardiopulmonary bypass system are a venous cannula, a venous reservoir, a pump, an oxygenator, a heat exchanger, a filter, and an arterial cannula (Fig. 80.1). Other components that are commonly used are a cardioplegia delivery system, an ultrafiltration unit, a cardiotomy suction system, a left ventricular vent, and a cell saver system.

Although cardiopulmonary bypass is an indispensable tool for the intraoperative care of the cardiovascular surgery patient, it incites a broad inflammatory cascade that can have far-reaching consequences on the subsequent intensive care unit (ICU) course of the patient. The primary trigger for this inflammatory cascade is the interaction between the patient's blood components and the large plastic surface area represented by the cardiopulmonary bypass circuit (1). This interaction activates plasma enzyme systems and blood cells, dilutes plasma proteins, causes coagulopathy, produces emboli, and leads to release of an array of vasoactive mediators that affect vascular motor tone and endothelial permeability (Table 80.1). Because of the systemic nature of this response, nearly every end organ is susceptible to at least temporary inflammatory-mediated dysfunction in the postoperative period.

Fortunately, the post-cardiopulmonary bypass inflammatory cascade is typically self-limited (Fig. 80.2). Circulating levels of vasomotor mediators peak within 24 hours of surgery and subside over ensuing days (2). Although cardiovascular surgery patients frequently have temporary mild end organ dysfunction postoperatively, rates of major complications for elective routine cases are low. Much of the critical care of cardiovascular surgery patients is oriented toward supporting patients through the early period during which they are subject to the temporary effects of cardiopulmonary bypass.

IMMEDIATE CONCERNS

The patient's admission to the ICU is a hectic transition period during which the patient is physically transported, monitoring and mechanical ventilation is re-established, intravenous medications are titrated, diagnostic tests are performed, and patient information is transferred from providers on the perioperative team to providers on the postoperative ICU team. In the midst of all this activity, almost all patients arriving in the ICU after cardiovascular surgery are in a state of controlled shock because of fluid shifts and changes in vascular tone. Cardiovascular surgery patients are therefore especially vulnerable to lapses in monitoring or distractions that divert the attention of providers at the bedside. A checklist is useful to ensure that essential tasks are accomplished within the first 30 minutes of a patient's arrival in the ICU (Table 80.2).

The first step on the patient's arrival to the ICU should be a quick assessment of the ABCs (airway, breathing, circulation). The arterial pressure monitoring unit is transferred from the portable setup accompanying the patient to the ICU monitor. The systemic arterial pressure waveform allows you to assess adequate systemic perfusion pressure and provides a means to detect arrhythmias while the electrocardiogram (ECG) and other pressure measurement catheters are connected and calibrated. Next, connect the hemodynamic monitoring catheters that provide some measure of central circulatory volume status, including the central venous pressure (CVP) catheter, pulmonary artery catheter, or both. The ECG leads are then switched from the transport unit to the ICU system. After these monitors are established, others can be connected and calibrated including the mixed venous oxygen saturation ($S\bar{v}O_2$), and pulse oximetry waveform.

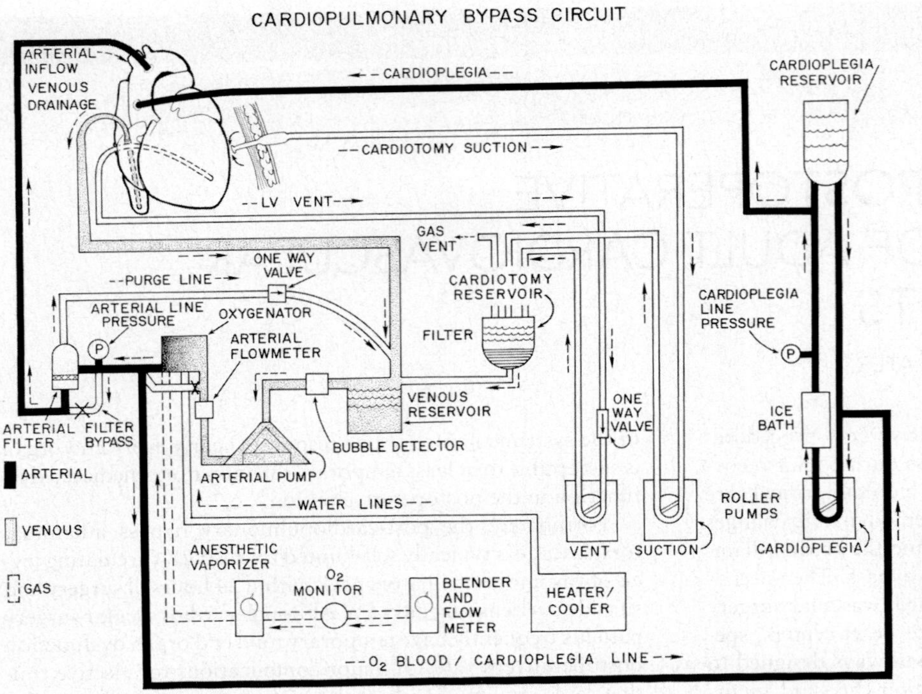

FIGURE 80.1. Schematic of a typical cardiopulmonary bypass circuit. (Reproduced from Wellons HA Jr, Zacour RK. Cardiopulmonary bypass. In: Kaiser LR, Kron IL, Spray TL, eds. *Mastery of Cardiothoracic Surgery*. 2nd ed. Philadelphia, PA: Lippincott Williams & Wilkins; 2007:312, with permission.)

Mechanical ventilation is continued using the ICU ventilator. Significant arterial-alveolar (A-a) gradients are common following cardiopulmonary bypass so patients should routinely be given high concentrations of oxygen (70%–80%) until adequate oxygenation is confirmed. Tidal volume in the absence of acute lung injury is set at 8 mL/kg of predicted body weight and respiratory rate is set at 14 breaths per minute. If the patient is not synchronized with the ventilator, analgesia and sedation are assessed for adequacy.

Once stable hemodynamic function is confirmed, pressure monitoring can be interrupted to obtain blood samples for various tests, including arterial blood gas, complete blood count, serum potassium, ionized calcium, hematocrit, platelet count, and coagulation studies. Rezeroing of all pressure monitors and calibration of the venous saturation monitor should be performed. For patients with a pulmonary artery catheter, baseline measurements of cardiac output and calculations of systemic vascular resistance (SVR) and pulmonary vascular resistance (PVR) are obtained.

A physical exam is performed. Particular attention is given to adequacy of airway control and ventilation and assessment

TABLE 80.1

VASOACTIVE SUBSTANCES RELEASED FOLLOWING CARDIOPULMONARY BYPASS

Aldosterone
Angiotensin II
Atrial natriuretic peptide
Complement: C3a, C4a, C5a, C5b-9
Electrolytes: Ca^{2+}, Mg^{2+}, K^+
Endothelin-1
Epinephrine
Glucagon
Histamine
Interleukins: IL-1, IL-6, IL-8, IL-10
Leukotrienes: LTB_4, LTC_4, LTD_4
Lysosomal enzymes
Nitric oxide
Norepinephrine
Oxygen free radicals
Platelet-activating factor
Prostacyclins
Prostaglandin E_2
Proteases
Renin
Serotonin
Thromboxane A_2
Thyroid hormones: T_3, T_4
Vasopressin

ECG, electrocardiogram; FiO_2, fraction of inspired oxygen.

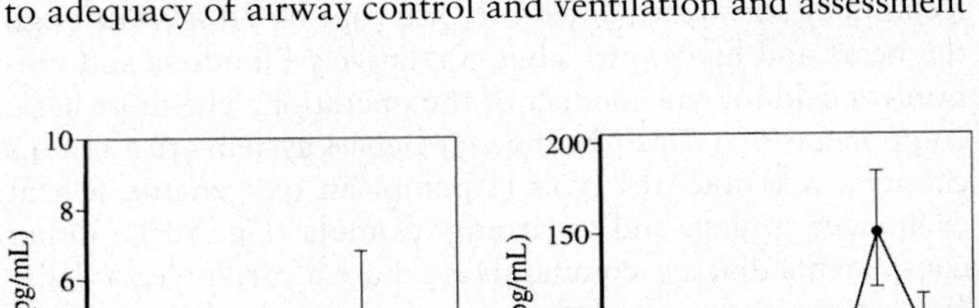

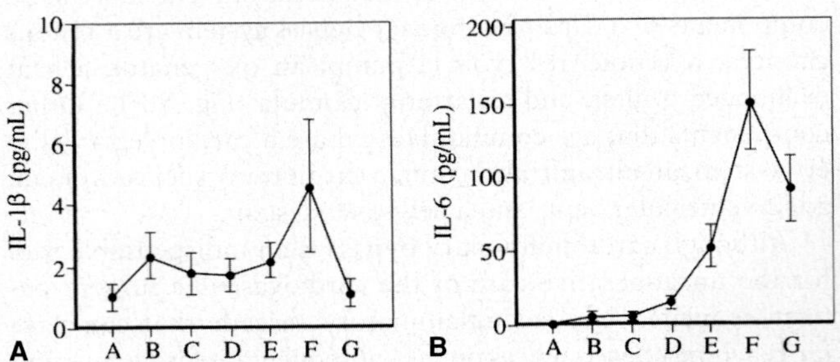

FIGURE 80.2. Changes in IL-1β (A) and IL-6 (B) in 30 patients who had elective first-time myocardial revascularization. Letters on x-axis represent the following events: A, induction of anesthesia; B, 5 minutes after heparin; C, 10 minutes after starting cardiopulmonary bypass (CPB); D, end of CPB; E, 20 minutes after protamine; F, 3 hours after CPB; G, 24 hours after CPB. (Redrawn from Steinberg JB, Kapelanski DP, Olson JD, et al. Cytokine and complement levels in patients undergoing cardiopulmonary bypass. *J Thorac Cardiovasc Surg.* 1993;106:1008.)

TABLE 80.2

TASKS TO BE COMPLETED WITHIN THE FIRST 30 MINUTES OF A PATIENT'S ARRIVAL TO THE ICU FOLLOWING CARDIOVASCULAR SURGERY

Establish monitoring
- Arterial waveform
- Central venous and pulmonary artery waveforms
- ECG
- Mixed venous oxygen saturation
- Pulse oximetry
- Mark and record urometer and mediastinal drains

Re-establish mechanical ventilation
- Assess airway control and bilateral air entry
- 70%–100% FiO_2
- Tidal volume 8 mL/kg of predicted body weight
- Respiratory rate 14 breaths/min

Directed physical exam
- Airway
- Ventilation
- Adequacy of blood pressure and cardiac output
- Abdomen
- Peripheral pulse exam

Studies
- Arterial blood gas, electrolytes, ionized calcium, hematocrit, platelet count, coagulation studies
- Chest radiograph

Transfer responsibility of patient care from perioperative team to ICU team
- Verbal sign-out of patient's clinical history and perioperative course

of peripheral pulses in all extremities. Although affected sometimes by the presence of severe atherosclerosis, skin temperature, pulse amplitude, and capillary refill time provide essential clinical information about the adequacy of cardiac output. Palpable peripheral pulses are an excellent indicator of systemic perfusion. Mental status and central nervous system assessment is also part of the initial exam.

A portable chest radiograph is obtained to determine the proper placement of the endotracheal tube, monitoring catheters, and nasogastric tube. Examine this radiograph closely for evidence of a pneumothorax, hemopneumothorax, and areas of lung collapse or atelectasis.

A word of caution is necessary about obtaining chest radiographs immediately after the patient arrives in the ICU, particularly if the body temperature is below 35.5°C and hemodynamic instability is present. In this situation, the chest radiograph should be deferred until the temperature rises to above 35.5°C to avoid the occurrence of life-threatening arrhythmias during placement of the film cassette. Sudden movement may induce ventricular tachycardia or fibrillation resulting from the reduced fibrillation threshold caused by hypothermia and electrolyte imbalance, especially hypokalemia.

As the physical process of patient admission to the ICU is taking place, a transfer of responsibility for the patient's care is also occurring. This usually involves a verbal sign-out of patient information from providers on the perioperative team to providers on the ICU team. The patient's clinical history is reviewed, and the perioperative course is described. This information is particularly important to ensure the safe transition from perioperative to postoperative care. Important details may include information on ease of intubation, perioperative ventricular function, inotropic and vasopressor requirement, optimal volume status, completeness of revascularization, and suspected coagulopathy.

Initial Therapy

The first hour after admission to the ICU following cardiovascular surgery is a critical and unstable time. The goals in this first hour are to maintain adequate systemic perfusion, adequate oxygenation and respiration, and control cardiac rate and rhythm. Patients who experience intravascular volume shifts during transport to the ICU require intravascular volume expansion, bolus dosages of intravenous calcium chloride if ionized calcium is low, or both to maintain adequate systemic blood pressure and flow during the crucial 15 to 30 minutes required to settle the patient in the ICU.

In this early period of stabilization, especially when the patient is mildly to moderately hypothermic, serum potassium levels should be assessed rapidly and supplemented to maintain levels in the 4.5- to 5.0-mmol/L range. This intervention helps protect the heart against ventricular irritability. At times, patients arrive to the ICU in an acidemic state. Avoid attempting to correct acidosis with rapid intravenous infusions of sodium bicarbonate. Serum potassium can be acutely lowered, which may increase ventricular irritability. Once the potassium level is adequate, moderate to severe metabolic acidosis (base deficit >5 mmol/L) can be corrected with resuscitation and if necessary with sodium bicarbonate.

Urine output is monitored closely to detect inappropriate diuresis, which occurs commonly in patients after cardiopulmonary bypass. Patients exhibiting this may require especially rapid replacement of crystalloid and electrolyte losses. Mediastinal drain output is also closely observed to detect excessive blood loss. If rapid hemorrhage is suspected, transfusion therapy is initiated early to replace red blood cell mass and correct coagulopathy as directed by postoperative studies and clinical findings. The operating team should be made aware of any patient who has massive hemorrhage so that mediastinal exploration can be undertaken expeditiously when indicated.

The First 8 Hours after Cardiopulmonary Bypass

After initial stabilization, a period frequently follows when the patient's hemodynamics are adequate and the patient is relatively stable. This period of time is designated the *golden period* and lasts for approximately 8 hours after cessation of cardiopulmonary bypass (CPB). Pay careful attention to optimizing cardiac function, because the initial 8 to 14 hours are characterized by decreasing cardiac function. The nadir of this decline occurs approximately 12 hours after CPB. Particularly notable is a decrease in ventricular compliance leading to reduced cardiac output at any given filling pressure. This condition generally persists over the next 12 to 24 hours, followed by a gradual improvement in cardiopulmonary performance over the next 48 hours. In the golden period, the goal is to optimize cardiorespiratory performance so that the ensuing decrease in cardiac function from 8 to 24 hours after CPB does not jeopardize end organ perfusion. Caution should be used in weaning inotropes rapidly during this period despite adequate hemodynamics in anticipation of the deterioration that typically follows.

Despite this caution, stable patients undergoing non-emergent cardiovascular surgery can usually be extubated safely during this period. The major criteria for proceeding with extubation during this early period are adequate central nervous system function, stable hemodynamics without malignant arrhythmias, normothermia, low A-a gradient, adequate pulmonary mechanics, and no ongoing mediastinal hemorrhage. If these screening criteria are met, patients can be observed for a brief period on minimal ventilatory support followed by extubation. Intravenous narcotics are useful to treat incisional pain during the period that sedative drugs are weaned just prior to extubation. Anesthetic technique should also be tailored to allow patients who can reasonably be expected to be extubated early to emerge from the effects of anesthesia during this period. In our institution the majority of patients undergoing non-emergent cardiovascular surgery are extubated within the first 6 hours of admission to the ICU using this strategy. Patients who have undergone a period of deep hypothermic circulatory arrest or long cardiopulmonary bypass periods, patients with poor ventricular function or unstable hemodynamics, and patients with hemorrhage or coagulopathy and large anticipated transfusion requirement are not suitable for early extubation.

The Next 16 Hours after Cardiopulmonary Bypass

The next 16 hours is probably the most challenging time, especially for the patients whose cardiac performance was not optimized during the golden period. The cause of the decline in cardiac performance during this time period is unclear. It is notable that many of the vasoactive factors that are released after cardiopulmonary bypass reach their peak concentrations during this period (2). The effects of cardiac reperfusion injury peak during this period in patients who have had aortic cross-clamping and obligatory global myocardial ischemia during their operation (3).

Changes in Heart Compliance

Clinically, the heart seems to become noncompliant or "stiff." In this situation, one usually observes a rise in pulmonary artery pressure and pulmonary artery occlusion pressure (PAOP), and a reduction in the systemic arterial pressure, cardiac output, and mixed venous oxygen saturation (4). If the patient is doing extremely well before the onset of compliance changes, alterations in these parameters may go unnoticed. However, patients with a low cardiac output syndrome before the onset of changes in compliance often develop hemodynamic instability.

Time Course

The usual time course is a steady deterioration in cardiac performance between the 8th to 12th hours following cardiopulmonary bypass. This condition seems to stabilize near the 12th hour and remains stable for the next 6 to 8 hours. Once a patient becomes unstable, far more interventions are required to return to a steady state than if problems are anticipated and appropriate changes made to help maintain stability. Even if patients remain in a relatively low cardiac output state during these 16 hours, they tolerate this condition better than those who are subjected to marked swings in hemodynamics.

Optimizing the Determinants of Cardiac Output

As patients enter this period, all parameters of cardiac performance should be evaluated individually. A strategy of optimizing cardiac rate and rhythm, preload, afterload, and contractility is useful. Heart rate and rhythm play a particularly important role in determining cardiac output in post-cardiopulmonary bypass patients. This is because the ventricles are stiff and noncompliant with limited capacity to increase stroke volume. In this situation, slower heart rates do not necessarily lead to increased filling and improved stroke volume. Rates of 90 to 110 beats per minute are typically necessary to optimize this component of cardiac output. In addition, atrial fibrillation may also be poorly tolerated during this period as the noncompliant ventricles may be dependent on atrial contraction to be adequately filled. Measures such as those described below should be taken to maintain sinus rhythm and restore it if atrial arrhythmias occur.

During this period, volume loading to achieve a PAOP beyond 12 to 14 mm Hg is unlikely to lead to significant increases in stroke volume due to noncompliance (unless the patient has an underlying stiff myocardium). Therefore, once a PAOP in this range is achieved, attention should be turned to other determinants of cardiac output to improve cardiac performance.

Afterload reduction is an efficient way to improve cardiac performance without increasing myocardial oxygen consumption ($\dot{M}VO_2$) (5). Afterload reduction should be instituted cautiously during this period to avoid hypotension. Renal function in older patients may be particularly sensitive to decreases in perfusion pressure. Patients with recent right ventricular infarcts and right ventricular stunning are also sensitive to hypotension.

Patients with a relatively normal cardiac output before surgery often poorly tolerate a cardiac index below 2.0 L/minute per m^2, a venous PO_2 below 30 mm Hg, or an $S\bar{v}O_2$ below 50% after surgery. Although costly to the heart in terms of $M\dot{V}O_2$, enhancement of cardiac contractility is an effective method to augment cardiac output by increasing the ejection fraction. In this period, inotropic support is a useful and frequently necessary means to achieve an adequate cardiac output until reversible cardiac dysfunction related to cardiopulmonary bypass and reperfusion effects have resolved. Moderate doses of inotropes are generally well tolerated by patients with ischemic heart disease who have been completely revascularized and by patients with valvular heart disease. Inotropes can cause myocardial ischemia in patients with ischemic heart disease who have been incompletely revascularized and should be used with caution in this setting.

Myocardial Ischemia

Increases in heart rate, filling pressures, and contractility to support patients during this period may cause myocardial ischemia from increased $M\dot{V}O_2$. An electrocardiogram should be obtained immediately after surgery and as clinically indicated thereafter. Continuous telemetry should be monitored closely for ischemic changes in the ST segment. Cardiac enzymes are usually not helpful in diagnosing myocardial ischemia during this early period because they typically rise in all cardiovascular surgery patients. Although an unusually high enzyme level or a sudden change in the usual pattern of enzyme leak may be useful. If acute graft closure is suspected following a coronary artery bypass procedure, echocardiography should show a new segmental wall motion abnormality. Comparison with intraoperative transesophageal studies, if performed, is particularly useful. If bypass graft failure of a large myocardial territory is suspected, coronary angiography with either percutaneous or open surgical reintervention may be indicated. In the absence of ischemia, cardiac performance will stabilize, usually by the 12th post-cardiopulmonary bypass hour.

The Second 24 Hours after Cardiopulmonary Bypass

During the second 24 postoperative hours, cardiovascular function typically improves. Small increases in the $S\bar{v}O_2$ and cardiac output, together with a noticeable decrease in fluid requirements, herald this recovery phase. Patients who preoperatively have normal systolic ventricular function usually tolerate weaning of inotropes. In these patients, the amount of active intervention is largely determined by the function of other organ systems such as the lungs and kidneys. If supraphysiologic cardiac output is desired to facilitate diuresis and optimize lung and kidney function, moderate inotropic support may be continued. For patients who preoperatively have decompensated left ventricular function, weaning of inotropic support should be slower. During this process, active diuresis and substitution of oral afterload-reducing drugs, particularly angiotensin-converting enzyme (ACE) inhibitors, may be useful.

Invasive monitoring with arterial and pulmonary artery catheters should be maintained until patients demonstrate recovery. If not extubated in the early postoperative period, the patient should be continuously re-evaluated for extubation to limit their risk for ventilator-associated complications. For patients who have undergone routine elective procedures, transfer to a step-down telemetry ward may be considered. Important criteria for transfer include adequate central nervous system (CNS) function, no or trivial requirement for inotropes, no dependence on temporary pacemaker leads, and good pulmonary toilet. Patients who have required maximum support during the first 24 hours after surgery may require an additional 24 hours to see progress, which warrants longer ICU stay.

The Third 24 Hours after Cardiopulmonary Bypass

During this period, patient care is focused on the transition from ICU care to ward care. Compliance in the left ventricle should improve rapidly accompanied by a decrease in interstitial pulmonary water. Lower pulmonary artery pressures and improved cardiac performance at lower filling pressure can be anticipated. Mobilization of third-spaced fluid occurs, and active diuresis should be instituted. Oral medications oriented more toward long-term cardiovascular risk reduction, such as beta-blockers, aspirin, and statins, are started. ACE inhibitors are favored in patients with valvular heart disease, particularly those who have had adverse left ventricular remodeling preoperatively. Physical rehabilitation with emphasis on pulmonary toilet and early ambulation is instituted. Intravenous insulin protocols are transitioned to long-acting subcutaneous regimens. Most patients who have undergone elective surgical procedures are able to be transferred to the step-down telemetry unit by the third postoperative day.

Catheters and Tubes

Mediastinal drains, pacing wires, arterial lines, Foley catheters, and pulmonary artery catheters often can be removed. If continuous invasive cardiac monitoring is still considered necessary, a CVP catheter positioned in the superior vena cava will provide a measurement of right ventricular filling pressure. Venous saturation readings from the superior caval–atrial junction correlate closely with the $S\bar{v}O_2$ in the absence of a left-to-right shunt (6,7). The association of the CVP and PAOP will be known by this point (although this relationship may change), and left heart filling pressures can thus be estimated.

Arrhythmias

Despite rapid improvements in the third 24-hour period, this is a time when atrial arrhythmias are prominent, including atrial flutter and atrial fibrillation. These may be significant problems because the atrial contribution to cardiac output remains high and a rapid heart rate may not be well tolerated.

Prophylaxis and treatment strategies for atrial fibrillation vary from institution to institution (8–12). Patients undergoing elective cardiovascular procedures frequently are already on beta-blockers preoperatively. At our institution, beta-blockers are instituted the week prior to surgery if patients are not already on them. Amiodarone and atorvastatin have also shown promise for prophylaxis against atrial fibrillation (9,11,12). Postoperatively, all patients are begun on low-dose metoprolol as soon as inotropes are discontinued. The dose of metoprolol is up-titrated as the patient's blood pressure and heart rate permit. For patients with depressed left ventricular function who require prolonged inotropic support, amiodarone may be used for arrhythmia prophylaxis.

The mainstays of atrial fibrillation treatment in the hemodynamically stable patient include diuresis, aggressive repletion of serum potassium and magnesium, intravenous amiodarone loading, and intravenous beta-blockers. Beta-blockers should be used with caution in patients still requiring inotropic support. Intravenous calcium channel blockers and procainamide are used occasionally in certain circumstances. For instance, procainamide is useful in heart transplant recipients who are still on inotropic support because of the desire to avoid long-acting agents such as amiodarone, which may have a prolonged slowing effect on sinus and atrioventricular node function. Of course, patients who deteriorate hemodynamically with the onset of atrial fibrillation should be treated with synchronized direct-current cardioversion. Whenever feasible, rapid atrial pacing should be attempted to suppress by overdrive pacing atrial flutter with a 2:1 block.

Monitoring and Managing Cardiovascular Performance

No single physiologic parameter reliably predicts adequacy of a patient's hemodynamic performance early in the postoperative course after cardiovascular surgery. We therefore rely on several physiologic measurements and clinical signs to assess hemodynamic performance and end organ perfusion.

Arterial Blood Pressure

For all critically ill patients, a minimum arterial blood pressure is required for overall systemic perfusion and especially for cerebral and renal perfusion. Most adults require a mean arterial pressure of at least 50 to 55 mm Hg (13). Older patients, particularly those with severe atherosclerotic disease, may require a mean arterial pressure of 65 mm Hg or greater depending on their baseline.

Pulse pressure is a useful indicator of systemic perfusion. We recommend display of the arterial waveform at full scale on the patient monitor. Determination of the systolic, diastolic, and mean pressures as well as the height of the dicrotic notch provides an indication of left ventricular ejection volume. Poorer ventricular ejection is observed when the dicrotic notch is at the base of the arterial pressure trace. Better ventricular output is found when the dicrotic notch is located midway up the down slope of the tracing, resulting in a greater area under the arterial pressure curve (14). The arterial pressure waveform also provides an indication of peripheral vascular tone. Harmonic augmentation in peripheral arteries suggests an increase in peripheral vascular tone and is characterized by a sharp, spiked arterial pressure tracing with virtually no dicrotic notch.

Normally, the arterial blood pressure is continuously monitored in a peripheral vessel such as the radial artery. However, any doubt concerning the pressure waveform from a peripheral artery should lead to measurement in a more central vessel, such as the femoral artery. A central arterial pressure reading provides better and more reliable assessment of overall hemodynamic function and cardiac output and is closer to the pressure that the heart sees.

Heart Rate and Rhythm

Sinus rhythm is extremely important in the first 24 hours, and efforts should be focused on maintaining sequential atrioventricular (AV) activity for better loading of the ventricles and optimal cardiac output. Normally, the atrial contraction or atrial "kick" contributes approximately 5% of the cardiac output. However, in the postoperative patient, the atrial contribution to cardiac output may be as high as 30%. Minimizing the incidence of atrial fibrillation using prophylaxis regimens as described above is an important component of rhythm management after cardiovascular surgery.

Pacemakers. Temporary epicardial atrial and ventricular pacing wires are commonly placed at the completion of cardiovascular procedures and can be invaluable both diagnostically and therapeutically. Heart rates of 90 to 110 beats per minute are generally well tolerated, even in patients who have undergone revascularization procedures. This is an important strategy to optimize cardiac output because of the poor compliance of the ventricles immediately following cardiovascular surgery. In addition, premature ventricular beats can frequently be suppressed by pacing to this heart rate range. Patients with temporary heart block following surgery can have A-V synchrony restored with dual-mode pacing/sensing (DDD) pacemakers.

In certain situations, an atrial pacing wire may be needed to determine the cardiac rhythm and differentiate supraventricular tachycardia. To perform an atrial ECG, simply connect the atrial pacing wire to the right arm ECG limb lead and observe the rhythm of leads I, II, or III on the patient monitor. Observation of the contour of the left and right atrial waveforms is another useful way of determining sinus rhythm.

Ventricular Preload

Ventricular preload, the load on the muscle that determines resting muscle length, is primarily manipulated in the postoperative period by fluid administration. Generally, we try to maintain cardiac preload at an adequate but not excessive level. For the left ventricle, this means maintaining the left ventricular end-diastolic pressure between 12 and 14 mm Hg as assessed by PAOP.

Fluid Administration. A common tendency is the desire to increase right and left ventricular filling pressures to their upper limits (16 to 20 mm Hg) to ensure adequate volume resuscitation. This approach exacerbates several problems that are difficult to manage later in the postoperative period, especially pulmonary dysfunction. Immediately after cardiopulmonary bypass, colloid oncotic pressure is reduced by as much as 50% and returns to normal over a 2-week period of time (Fig. 80.3) (15). In addition, neutrophil and endothelial activation following cardiopulmonary bypass increase pulmonary vascular permeability, resulting in a higher loss of intravascular fluids at lower hydrostatic pressures, promoting increased pulmonary interstitial water accumulation and pulmonary edema (16). We therefore caution against trying to maximize cardiac output by moving toward the upper pressure–volume limits along the Starling curve. Attempts to reach venous pressures greater than 16 mm Hg result in administration of excess fluids accompanied by increased pulmonary interstitial water.

Crystalloids and Colloids. Controversy persists concerning which type of fluids are most effective for volume resuscitation in post–cardiopulmonary bypass patients. The focus of this debate concerns the administration of crystalloid versus colloid (blood products, albumin, or hydroxyethyl starch) solutions (17). We have used multiple fluid combinations for maintaining adequate preload, all of which have advantages and disadvantages. Sole reliance on crystalloid solutions such as Ringer lactate for volume expansion may result in an inordinate amount of fluid administration to maintain adequate preload. Our current practice for volume resuscitation in patients without ongoing hemorrhage is to use up to 2 L of crystalloid solution after which 5% albumin may be used.

When the hematocrit is low (<22%) and the patient is bleeding or hemodynamically unstable, blood products are indicated. If red cell mass is adequate but coagulation factors are abnormal and bleeding continues, fresh frozen plasma and platelets should be considered. The threshold to give blood is lowered in patients with incomplete revascularization, low cardiac output, and signs of inadequate oxygen delivery such as low mixed venous oxygen saturation ($S\bar{v}O_2$).

Ventricular Afterload

Afterload reduction offers the most efficient means to improve cardiac output at little or no expense to myocardial oxygen demand. Following afterload reduction, ventricular volume, wall tension, and $M\dot{V}O_2$ usually are not increased. In some patients, the ejection fraction can be dramatically improved by a reduction in systemic vascular resistance (SVR) and peripheral vascular resistance (PVR). Afterload reduction should be

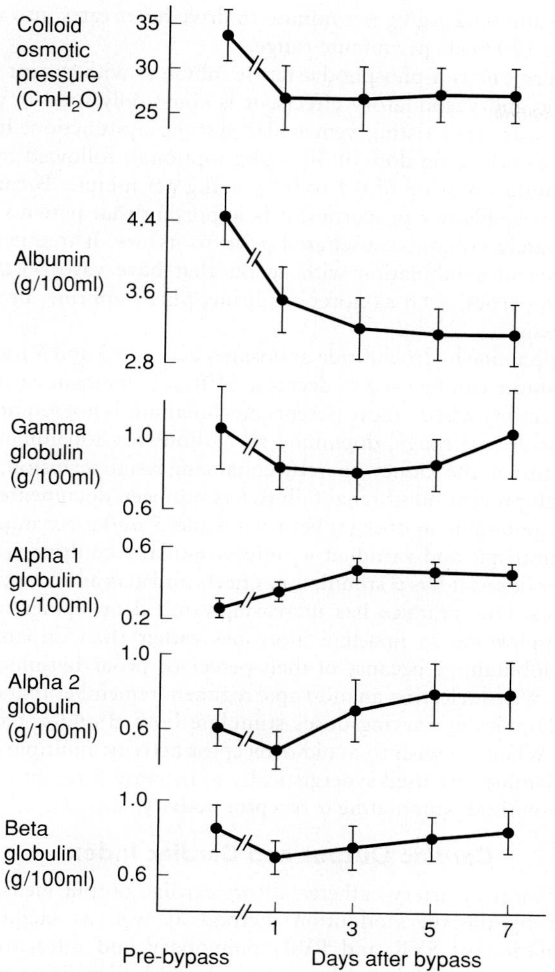

FIGURE 80.3. The relationship between colloid osmotic (oncotic) pressure and plasma proteins during and after cardiopulmonary bypass. (Reproduced from Webber CE, Garnett ES. The relationship between colloid osmotic pressure and plasma proteins during and after cardiopulmonary bypass. *J Thorac Cardiovasc Surg.* 1973;65:234, with permission.)

performed after judicious volume loading to avoid hypotension and hemodynamic collapse. Afterload reduction typically begins in the operating room after the cessation of cardiopulmonary bypass (CPB) with the release of vasoactive mediators and with systemic rewarming. The extent of afterload reduction that is necessary greatly depends on ventricular performance. Patients with severely depressed systolic ventricular function benefit the most from afterload reduction.

Vasodilators. Nicardipine hydrochloride, a peripheral acting calcium channel blocker, acts as a direct systemic arterial vasodilator. Its dose range is 1 to 15 mg per hour. It is our primary afterload-reducing agent because it is reasonably evanescent and avoids problems with cyanide toxicity associated with sodium nitroprusside. In our experience, it is less associated with pulmonary artery shunting and ventilation–perfusion (V-Q) mismatch (resulting in low PaO_2) than sodium nitroprusside.

Sodium nitroprusside remains as an alternative agent for afterload reduction. It increases venous capacitance and directly vasodilates the systemic and pulmonary arterioles. Its advantage is its fast onset of action (15–20 seconds), allowing rapid titration (0.3–10 μg/kg per minute). It can be associated with cyanide toxicity as well as pulmonary artery shunting and V-Q mismatch.

Nitroglycerin (NTG) is a venous and arterial vasodilator but is primarily a preload-reducing agent with mild afterload-reducing effects including on the coronary arterial tree. An additional advantage in patients with right ventricular failure is its vasodilatory effects on the pulmonary vasculature. The intravenous dosage of NTG ranges between 0.5 and 2 μg/kg per minute. It decreases myocardial oxygen consumption and may be especially useful in patients with incomplete revascularization.

Pulmonary Artery Vasodilators. Certain patients benefit from vasodilators that act specifically on the pulmonary artery tree. Right ventricular failure is common in patients who have suffered right ventricular myocardial infarction and in patients who have undergone orthotopic heart transplantation as the implanted organ adjusts to its new setting of increased pulmonary artery vascular resistance. Patients who have had pulmonary endarterectomy may have reactive pulmonary artery constriction. Patients with a long-standing history of congestive heart failure also may have a component of reactive pulmonary artery hypertension following cardiopulmonary bypass in addition to fixed changes. In these scenarios, isolated right ventricular failure may be the primary cause of low cardiac output because of inadequate left ventricular filling.

The inhaled prostacyclin analogue iloprost is our preferred specific pulmonary artery vasodilator. An important advantage is its ease of administration. It can be delivered intermittently via a nebulizer to either intubated or extubated patients. Inhaled nitric oxide also has vasodilatory activity restricted to the pulmonary artery tree because of its short half-life. It requires continuous delivery via a specialized system and can be used only in intubated patients.

It is important to keep in mind the pulmonary vasoconstrictive effects of hypercapnia and hypoxia when managing patients with severe right ventricular dysfunction. Hypercapnia and hypoxia should be strictly avoided in patients with marginal right ventricular function, even if this requires prolonging the period of intubation. High FiO_2 can be considered a form of pulmonary vasodilator in this subset of patients.

Vasoconstrictors. Cardiopulmonary bypass causes release of numerous vasoactive substances, many of which have vasodilatory effects (1). Vasodilation following cardiovascular surgery is especially common in patients who have had prolonged cardiopulmonary bypass, a period of circulatory arrest, or who have been treated with ACE inhibitors preoperatively (18,19). Various agents, including steroids and methylene blue, have been studied for the treatment of vasoplegic shock following cardiopulmonary bypass (20). Vasoconstrictors remain the first-line treatment for patients with low SVR and adequate volume status and contractile state, however (21). It is crucial that prior to instituting vasoconstrictor treatment, patients must be adequately volume resuscitated and their hypotension determined to be related to vasodilation rather than pump failure. Treatment of hypotension related to pump failure with a pure vasoconstrictor can lead to permanent end organ damage.

Patients ideally treated with vasoconstrictors are in a high cardiac output state with low SVR.

Phenylephrine hydrochloride, an α-specific catecholamine, acts as a pure peripheral vasoconstrictor. Its dose range is 20 to 180 μg/minute. It has a relatively short half-life, and its primary advantage is that it can be easily titrated for goal parameters, such as mean arterial blood pressure.

Vasopressin also acts as a pure peripheral vasoconstrictor. Because of its longer half-life, it is less suited for minute-to-minute changes in response to blood pressure changes. It may be particularly useful in patients treated preoperatively with ACE inhibitors. Its usual dose range is 1 to 10 units/hour. Its mechanism of action is synergistic with norepinephrine. Vasopressin in combination with norepinephrine is therefore useful in patients who have profound vasodilatory shock.

Contractility

The contractile state of the heart is a determinant of cardiac output, and patients with reversible myocardial stunning after aortic cross-clamping and cardiopulmonary bypass or pre-existing decompensated left ventricular function frequently benefit from a period of inotropic support. When required, inotropes are usually begun in the operating room at the time of weaning from CPB under guidance of intraoperative transesophageal echocardiography and are continued into the postoperative period. In the ICU, if cardiac performance is marginal and does not respond to other measures, we quickly institute inotropes and continue them throughout the first 24 to 48 hours. Remember that the specific conditions under which the operation was conducted, including repairs performed, completeness of revascularization, length of cardiopulmonary bypass, and quality of myocardial preservation can profoundly influence postoperative myocardial contractility.

Inotropes. Few pharmacologic agents affect only one determinant of cardiac performance, and this is especially true of inotropes. When selecting drugs, individually or in combination, bear in mind that a major goal after CPB is to gain cardiac output with as little increase in myocardial oxygen consumption as possible. The choice of drugs varies with the patient's condition.

Epinephrine, in the 0.01 to 0.10 μg/kg per minute range, is our principle choice. These dosage levels are not exceeded unless absolutely necessary to maintain an acceptable mean arterial perfusion pressure. Epinephrine also has vasoconstrictor and chronotropic effects; however, its inotropic effects predominate in this dose range. Epinephrine can be particularly useful when used to support right ventricular function.

Norepinephrine, also in the 0.01 to 0.10 μg/kg per minute range, is also frequently used. Because of increased α agonist, norepinephrine has stronger vasoconstrictor effects in this range and has been associated with improved coronary and splanchnic blood flow (22,23). Because of its vasoconstrictor properties, it can be especially useful in patients with vasodilatation after cardiopulmonary bypass who also require inotropic support.

Isoproterenol is a relatively weak inotrope with primarily chronotropic properties. In our ICU, its primary use is in heart transplant recipients in whom we are trying to cause relative tachycardia because of the normal coronary arteries, diastolic dysfunction, and right ventricular distention commonly encountered in this population. It can be used in dosages between 0.005 and 0.02 μg/kg per minute to drive heart rates into the 100 to 120 beats per minute range.

Milrinone is a phosphodiesterase inhibitor with potent inotropic and vasodilatory effects. It is commonly used in patients with pre-existing ventricular systolic dysfunction. It is given as a loading dose of 50 μg/kg (optional) followed by a continuous infusion of 0.1 to 0.75 μg/kg per minute. Because of its vasodilatory properties, it is important that patients be adequately volume resuscitated prior to its use. It frequently is given in combination with agents that have vasoconstrictor properties, such as norepinephrine, phenylephrine, or vasopressin.

Dopamine hydrochloride at dosages between 3 and 5 μg/kg per minute can be used to decrease SVR and augment cardiac contractility when a more potent catecholamine is not required. In this dosage range, dopamine also stimulates dopaminergic receptors in the kidney, thereby enhancing renal perfusion, although prevention of renal failure has not been documented.

Dobutamine in dosages between 3 and 5 μg/kg per minute has inotropic and vasodilatory effects similar to milrinone. At higher doses, it has α stimulatory effects and acts as a vasoconstrictor. Our practice has increasingly relied on epinephrine and milrinone as first-line inotropes rather than dopamine and dobutamine because of their perceived proarrhythmic effects. When selecting an inotropic regimen, remember that catecholamines at varying doses stimulate both β and α receptors. When we wish to avoid α receptor activity, multiple catecholamines are used synergistically to increase β receptor activity without stimulating α receptor activity.

Cardiac Output and Cardiac Index

A pulmonary artery catheter allows cardiac output measurement by the thermodilution method as well as facilitates calculation of SVR and PVR, pulmonary and intracardiac shunts, and estimation of left ventricular end-diastolic pressure (LVEDP) by PAOP. Cardiac output readings should always be normalized by conversion to cardiac index (cardiac output divided by the body surface area). This adjusts cardiac output for the size of the individual patient and therefore is a better estimate of adequacy of tissue perfusion. A cardiac index of 2.0 L/minute per m^2 or greater is usually sufficient to maintain end organ performance. Exceptions exist in certain pathologic conditions, however. For example, patients with long-standing mitral valve disease and in a low cardiac output state preoperatively may well tolerate a cardiac index of less than 2.0 L/minute per m^2 in the immediate postoperative period. In contrast, higher body temperature and agitation, or other concomitant conditions such as sepsis, may lead to cardiac index requirements of greater than 2.0 L/minute per m^2. Bear in mind that these indices are at the lower limits for providing adequate organ function and that postoperative stress normally produces cardiac indices approaching 3.5 to 4.0 L/minute per m^2. Cardiac output should not be the sole criterion used to determine adequacy of end organ oxygen delivery.

Mixed Venous Saturation

Continuous display of the $S\bar{v}O_2$ affords one the opportunity to observe acute as well as gradual changes in cardiac performance, increasing oxygen consumption ($\dot{V}O_2$), or both. Based on the Fick method of determining cardiac output, changes in the $S\bar{v}O_2$ reflect changes in systemic blood flow as long as $\dot{V}O_2$ remains stable. Acute changes in $\dot{V}O_2$ and cardiac performance are especially demonstrable during episodes of agitation, tracheal suctioning, and rapid extracellular volume shifts. $S\bar{v}O_2$ monitoring is particularly helpful in tracking the gradual deterioration of cardiac performance during the second 8-hour period after cardiopulmonary bypass. $S\bar{v}O_2$ varies with cardiac output, hemoglobin, SaO_2, and oxygen consumption and is a balance between oxygen delivery and oxygen consumption.

Equipment used to measure physiologic parameters such as the arterial pressure and $S\bar{v}O_2$ must be calibrated regularly. $S\bar{v}O_2$ monitors are calibrated using venous saturation readings from a mixed venous blood sample from the pulmonary artery. The accuracy of any single measure of cardiac performance should always be evaluated in the context of other measures. For example, if the arterial pressure waveform is dampened, it may be compared against readings from an oscillometric, Doppler, or return-to-flow technique. Incongruent readings should always be evaluated with a suspicion for the accuracy of measurement.

Serum Lactate

As an indicator of anaerobic metabolism, serum lactate can provide information about the adequacy of cardiac performance in meeting the body's oxygen requirement. Several problems, however, limit the usefulness of serum lactate as a means to assess cardiac performance. On arrival to the ICU, lactate values may range between normal (<2.0 mmol/L) to as high as 8 to 9 mmol/L. As body temperature rises to normal, serum lactate may actually rise despite improving hemodynamics because underperfused vascular beds open and release lactate into the systemic circulation. The difficulty in this situation is whether to attribute a rise in serum lactate to a washout phenomenon or to a diminution of cardiac performance. Evaluation of the cardiac index, $S\bar{v}O_2$, and SVR in conjunction with serial serum lactate determinations helps to resolve this dilemma. Lactate levels should decrease after 8 hours if perfusion is adequate.

Serum Ionized Calcium and Potassium

Rapid access (5–10 minutes) to laboratory determinations or bedside point-of-care testing is essential for guiding therapy, especially in the first 24 hours. Important serum values include ionized calcium (Ca^{2+}), potassium, hematocrit, glucose, and sodium. Serial measurement of Ca^{2+} is especially helpful when solutions containing protein such as blood, fresh frozen plasma, albumin, or plasma protein solutions are administered. Protein binds calcium and may diminish that which is available for myocardial function. Clinically, this phenomenon can be recognized during the rapid infusion of protein-containing solutions by noting a rise in cardiac filling pressures, a drop in blood pressure, and a drop in the $S\bar{v}O_2$, all indicative of worsening performance despite volume resuscitation. In certain situations, particularly in hemodynamically unstable patients, simultaneous infusion of calcium chloride markedly improves cardiac performance.

Postoperative maintenance of adequate serum potassium is crucial, especially after the usually brisk diuresis following CPB and in conjunction with diuretic therapy. Potassium chloride should be considered a first-line agent for prevention and treatment of arrhythmias after cardiovascular surgery. Potassium chloride should be given as a standing medication to actively diuresing patients with normal renal function, and serum potassium values should be measured frequently to guide replacement therapy toward a normal to high-normal range (4.5–5 mmol/L).

Urine Output

In the initial postoperative period, urine output is typically brisk but then diminishes dramatically between the 8th and 12th post-CPB hours. Initially, urine output alone should not be relied on to judge cardiac performance, because it is influenced by numerous variables including high serum glucose, denatured plasma protein fractions, and diuretics such as furosemide and mannitol used during cardiopulmonary bypass. In later stages of the postoperative period, urine output may be influenced by various stress hormones such as antidiuretic hormone, aldosterone, and cortisol, which generally cause conservation of intravascular volume. Similarly, conservation of intravascular volume occurs in patients who enter surgery with high ventricular end-diastolic filling pressures but return to the ICU after surgery with lower filling pressures. In patients who are conditioned to higher filling pressures, the sudden reduction in atrial pressure usually sets off a strong antidiuretic hormone–mediated response designed to correct perceived hypovolemia and leads to fluid retention and low urine output.

Almost all patients return from the operating room with excess total body water because of the hemodilution and obligate volume load caused by the bypass circuit. These effects have been partially ameliorated by cell saver systems and ultrafiltration units that reconcentrate red cell mass. Despite the usual excess in total body water, intravascular volume status is variable because of third-spacing related to increased capillary permeability and post-cardiopulmonary bypass inflammation. Diuretic therapy should therefore be guided by cardiac filling pressures. Our practice is to diurese patients to low normal filling pressures as long as hemodynamics are not compromised to minimize interstitial lung water and improve pulmonary function. Diuresis should be performed cautiously during the early postoperative period when ventricular compliance is poor and cardiac function may be especially preload dependent. This is particularly true in patients with concentric ventricular hypertrophy, such as those with long-standing hypertension or aortic stenosis.

Special Concerns

Bleeding

Bleeding after cardiovascular operations with cardiopulmonary bypass is a major destabilizing complication. Severe postoperative bleeding occurs in 3% to 5% of patients who undergo cardiopulmonary bypass (24). Significant progress has been made in understanding its causes and optimal treatment.

Causes. Although inadequate surgical hemostasis should always be suspected, at least half of patients with severe postoperative bleeding have acquired hemostatic defects (25,26). These include activation of fibrinolysis, decreased levels of clotting factors due to dilution and consumption, and transient platelet dysfunction. Therapeutic protocols may influence postoperative bleeding. For example, chronic preoperative use of antiplatelet agents such as clopidogrel and aspirin are associated with increased postoperative transfusion requirements.

Treatment. Antifibrinolytic agents, such as epsilon aminocaproic acid and aprotinin, have been shown to decrease the need for transfusion in high-risk subpopulations (27,28). Aprotinin is currently not available until further studies are done to determine its side effects. These agents are begun intraoperatively and discontinued shortly on arrival to the ICU. There is no evidence supporting initiation of their use in the postoperative period. When bleeding does occur, blood component replacement is guided by laboratory studies. Red blood cell transfusions should be initiated promptly when massive hemorrhage is suspected. Clotting factor deficiencies demonstrated by prolonged prothrombin and activated partial thromboplastin times are treated with fresh frozen plasma. Cryoprecipitate is usually reserved for patients with low fibrinogen levels. Factor replacement therapy with recombinant clotting factors such as activated factor VII and factor XIII is an emerging strategy under current study (29,30).

Isolated elevation of the activated partial thromboplastin time may indicate heparin rebound and should be reversed with protamine sulfate administration (25). Circulating heparin levels are also useful in guiding protamine administration (31).

Platelet counts of greater than 100,000 may seem reassuring; however, the function of these platelets is frequently inadequate in patients with clinical coagulopathy. Point-of-care platelet function assays may be useful for directing platelet transfusion in patients without thrombocytopenia.

Our threshold for returning the patient to the operating room is a blood loss rate through the chest tubes of greater than 3 mL/kg per hour for several consecutive hours. Patients who experience bleeding at this rate cannot be stabilized hemodynamically, irrespective of the amount of volume replacement. Patients with brisk hemorrhage should be returned to the operating room even before coagulopathy is corrected to stop presumed surgical bleeding prior to development of cardiac tamponade and hemodynamic collapse. Even when no source of surgical bleeding is identified on mediastinal re-exploration, clinical coagulopathy frequently improves after evacuation of the mediastinal hematoma.

Cardiac Tamponade. Mediastinal drains may fail to adequately evacuate blood after cardiovascular surgery, leading to cardiac tamponade. Abrupt cessation of bleeding from the mediastinal drains warrants close attention to the cardiac filling pressures and to overall cardiac performance. When flexible drains have been used, they should be periodically milked to prevent clotting off.

Two fairly reliable signs of cardiac tamponade are increased or exaggerated cycling of the systolic blood pressure during positive pressure ventilation, and equalization of right and left atrial and pulmonary artery diastolic pressures. A reduction in $S\bar{v}O_2$ and a decrease in urine output will also be observed. The diagnosis may be confirmed by echocardiography.

In cardiac tamponade, equalization of the atrial pressures does not always occur. Blood clots on the acute margin of the right ventricle may substantially affect cardiac performance without atrial pressure equalization. In severe low-output states, cardiac tamponade must be ruled out by either mediastinal exploration in the operating room or a limited opening of the lower portion of the chest incision at the bedside. Percutaneous drainage is not useful in the immediate postoperative period because the hematoma is generally clotted.

Thrombocytopenia

Thrombocytopenia is common following cardiovascular surgery (25). Causes include platelet activation and consumption during cardiopulmonary bypass, mechanical destruction by intravascular devices including prosthetic heart valves and intra-aortic balloon pumps (IABPs), inadequate production caused by malnutrition and drugs such as milrinone, and heparin-induced thrombocytopenia. Platelet counts of less than 100,000/μl are quite typical and are generally managed conservatively by removal of offending agents as soon as is feasible. If the platelet count falls by greater than 50% or a thrombotic event occurs between 4 and 14 days of heparin exposure, a diagnosis of heparin-induced thrombocytopenia (HIT) should be excluded by testing for HIT antibody seroconversion. If HIT is diagnosed or is strongly suspected, anticoagulation with a nonheparin anticoagulant such as lepirudin or bivalirudin should be considered because of the risk of thrombotic complications (32). Patients should be screened for deep vein thrombosis (DVT) with ultrasonography. For patients who require long-term anticoagulation for DVT, warfarin can be started once platelet levels return to a normal range. Warfarin is not recommended for initial therapy of HIT due to the risk of thrombotic complications.

Ventilator Management

Ventilator management after cardiac surgery is directed toward optimizing pulmonary function without compromising hemodynamics. On patient admission to the ICU in our institution, the synchronous intermittent mandatory ventilation (SIMV) rate is set at 14 breaths per minute with a tidal volume of 8 mL/kg of predicted body weight. We do not pressure-limit the ventilator, and we carefully monitor hemodynamic function throughout the period of assisted ventilation. Acute hemodynamic changes may be indicative of patient distress, a blocked endotracheal tube, the need for suctioning, or a bronchodilator such as albuterol. Patient dyssynchrony with the ventilator should prompt assessment of the patient's level of sedation and analgesia.

Caution is advised when using positive end-expiratory pressure (PEEP) above 8 to 10 cm H_2O, because cardiac chamber filling may be affected causing cardiac performance to decrease. When high PEEP is used, intravascular volume augmentation may be necessary to raise the effective LVEDP. Although some use the estimate that one half the PEEP subtracted from the PAOP is the effective LVEDP, this assumption may not be correct since the amount of pressure transmitted through diseased lungs may vary.

Administration of nitroprusside and to a lesser extent nicardipine to patients who are heavy smokers or have severe chronic lung disease may increase the amount of pulmonary shunting and cause hypoxia due to V-Q mismatch. Bronchodilators and PEEP as high as 15 to 20 cm H_2O rarely correct this problem. In such cases, these vasodilators should be discontinued and substituted with another drug such as nitroglycerin (3 to 5 μg/kg per minute) or hydralazine.

The appearance of the acute respiratory distress syndrome (ARDS) after cardiac surgery is much less frequent due, in part, to shorter CPB times and the use of membrane oxygenators. Unfortunately, when ARDS does occur in the postoperative period, it may be accompanied by multiple organ dysfunction syndrome or sepsis (33).

Diuretics

Diuresis is desirable during the recovery period to reverse hemodilution and improve pulmonary function, but should always be closely monitored. Excessive diuretic therapy rapidly depletes intravascular volume if the renal response to these drugs is brisk. Forced diuresis that results in a urine output of 500 to 1,500 mL over several hours may significantly reduce cardiac performance and promote increased SVR.

Smaller and more frequent doses of diuretics produce a more constant diuresis and the ability to maintain a gradual negative fluid balance throughout the second 24-hour postoperative period. A sustained diuresis that prevents large hourly urine loss spares the patient rapid volume shifts. To accomplish a stable diuresis in patients with normal ventricular and renal function, our practice is to use frequent doses of relatively small doses of furosemide (10–20 mg) every 4 to 8 hours as needed. In patients with marginal ventricular or renal function, particularly those who have been treated with furosemide chronically, more aggressive treatment is necessary. In this situation we use a continuous furosemide infusion at doses of 0 to 20 mg/hour. We state a 24-hour diuresis goal and titrate the infusion to meet this goal over the course of the day with reassessments to avoid hypovolemia. Intermittent doses of thiazide diuretics are a useful adjunct in patients who have an inadequate response to the infusion.

Renal Failure

Patients who experience an extremely low cardiac output or hypotension during the first 24 hours after cardiopulmonary bypass may develop acute tubular necrosis. Most respond to adequate volume maintenance and diuretic therapy and can be maintained in a nonoliguric renal failure. However, some, especially those with a preoperative creatinine clearance of less than 50 mL/minute, may develop oliguric or anuric renal failure.

Diuretics. Patients with oliguria should be given a test bolus of furosemide (60–120 mg) and then be evaluated for a urine response of greater than 50 mL/hour. A continuous furosemide infusion at doses of 0 to 20 mg/hour can then be maintained with intermittent doses of thiazide diuretics as necessary. This regimen usually maintains urine output and avoids gross volume overload after surgery, even if acute tubular necrosis is present. Avoiding hypovolemia is also essential.

Ultrafiltration. Patients with renal failure and volume overload may be candidates for ultrafiltration to remove excess salt and water (34). There are several advantages to this approach for patients who fail initial diuretic therapy. Commercially available systems are highly automated and allow device-based removal of salt and water from the circulation without clinically significant effects on hemodynamics or electrolyte balance. Standard central or peripheral venous catheters can be used for access, frequently avoiding the need for invasive procedures to place specialized hemodialysis catheters. We reserve this approach for patients with adequate electrolyte and urea clearance who require removal of excess water.

Dialysis. Intravascular volume overload and inadequate clearance of potassium levels are the principal indications for dialyzing a patient with acute renal failure in the immediate postoperative period. The overall goal of dialysis is to remove excess water and solutes while maintaining cardiovascular stability. For the postoperative cardiovascular surgery patient, this is best achieved with the use of continuous venovenous hemodialysis (CVVHD). This technique is easily initiated, offers good clearance, and allows accurate control of ultrafiltration that is adaptable to the patient's hemodynamic requirements. Fluid removal can therefore usually be accomplished while maintaining stable hemodynamics. CVVHD does require placement of a dedicated double-lumen central venous catheter. If postoperative bleeding is not a concern, heparin should be administered to prolong filter life. Without heparin, the average filter life ranges from 16 to 24 hours.

Patients should be transitioned to conventional hemodialysis only after a significant period of myocardial recovery. Conventional hemodialysis requires blood flow rates of at least 200 mL/hour and results in large volumes of fluid removal over a several-hour period. The fluid shifts associated with this technique are inappropriate for patients early in their recovery from cardiopulmonary bypass.

Central Nervous System Complications

After operations with cardiopulmonary bypass, the historical incidence of cerebrovascular accidents (CVAs) with focal neurologic sequelae is 2% to 5% (35). The contemporary rate may be lower because of advancements in intraoperative technique including routine use of epiaortic ultrasound (36). Advanced age, history of CVA, peripheral vascular disease, valvular heart surgery, and procedures requiring a period of circulatory arrest are associated with a higher incidence of central nervous system events. Patients with a history of CVA whose focal deficits have resolved prior to operation may have unmasking of their old symptoms in the immediate postoperative period. Untoward psychological and cognitive sequelae are more prevalent than focal CVAs (37,38). The precise cause of neuropsychological complications remains unclear, however recent data suggest that microemboli, especially air, are related to both severe and subtle postoperative neuropsychological deficits (39,40).

Patients should be continuously monitored for the appearance of neuropsychological complications in the postoperative period. From the time of their emergence from anesthesia, patients should be assessed for focal motor deficits and the ability to comprehend and follow simple commands. Focal deficits should be evaluated promptly with noncontrast computed tomography (CT) of the brain to rule out hemorrhagic mass lesions that may require intervention. Magnetic resonance imaging (MRI) may be useful to identify smaller embolic foci that are not apparent on head CT. Fresh post-cardiopulmonary bypass patients are usually poor candidates for thrombolysis because of their risk for bleeding. The treatment for major embolic CNS events is usually supportive. Higher blood pressures may lead to greater perfusion via collaterals in patients with severe occlusive cerebrovascular disease.

Delirium. Postcardiotomy delirium is typically preceded by a lucid interval, usually 36 to 48 hours from the time patients awaken from anesthesia. This syndrome is characterized by confusion, disorientation, and disordered thinking and perception (37). Severe manifestations may include visual and auditory illusions, hallucinations, and paranoid ideation (41). Treatment consists of undisturbed rest, frequent reorientation, ensuring patient safety, reassurance to both the patient and family, and treatment with haloperidol. It is our practice to avoid the use of benzodiazepines in this situation because of their paradoxical excitatory response seen occasionally in the elderly population. Subtle changes in mentation and thinking processes occur frequently during the first few weeks after surgery. They may be frightening to the patient and may interfere with the immediate recovery process. However, most of these problems are temporary and usually resolve by the sixth postoperative month (37,38,42).

Sedation and Paralysis

In addition to the pain and discomfort characteristic of any major surgical procedure, several conditions occurring after cardiac operation warrant sedation and, in rare instances, complete paralysis. As the patient emerges from anesthesia, a perceived reduction in cardiac performance may result, in part, from shivering, agitation, or both. Shivering can produce a marked increase in $\dot{V}O_2$, a reduction in $S\bar{v}O_2$, and an overall imbalance of oxygen supply and demand in the body, especially in low cardiac output states. Once gross neurologic function is assessed (e.g., movement and sensation in the extremities and the ability to follow simple commands), shivering or agitation in the immediate postoperative period is best treated with narcotic agents. Our preference is to use fentanyl to control shivering or agitation, although these conditions can be managed with morphine or other narcotics. Meperidine is particularly efficacious, although the mechanism by which it acts is unknown.

For patients who have undergone elective procedures and are expected to be extubated early in the postoperative course, a propofol infusion is started soon on arrival to the ICU. This agent is useful in this setting because once hemodynamics and bleeding are assessed and the patient is warm, the patient's sedation can be stopped quickly because of the agent's short half-life. The patient's neurologic function can be assessed, and the patient can be extubated after a brief spontaneous breathing trial.

When a patient is expected to require a prolonged period of mechanical ventilation, we typically use a combination of narcotic and benzodiazepine infusions. Fentanyl is our preferred narcotic because of its limited effects on myocardial contractility and the peripheral vasculature. In rare instances, such as severe pulmonary artery hypertension and right heart failure, a paralytic agent may be indicated to prevent any respiratory effort by the patient, which can trigger increased pulmonary artery pressures and precipitate hemodynamic collapse. Because of their association with critical illness neuropathy, we prefer to avoid paralytic agents and treat these patients with deep sedation. When paralytics are required, our practice is to use vecuronium, which has a lesser chronotropic effect than pancuronium.

Mechanical Cardiac Assistance

Mechanical cardiac assist devices include IABPs, centrifugal blood pumps, ventricular assist devices, and total artificial hearts. In some cases, extracorporeal membrane oxygenation (ECMO) is indicated for profound cardiorespiratory failure.

Intra-aortic Balloon Pumps. An IABP should be considered when patients fail to respond to moderately high-dose inotropic drug combinations such as epinephrine and milrinone. The IABP improves cardiac performance primarily by afterload reduction and augmentation of systemic diastolic pressure, thereby increasing coronary artery perfusion pressure. IABP therapy should be considered earlier rather than later and can be instituted quickly at the bedside via a percutaneous technique. Its main contraindications are aortic insufficiency and aortoiliac occlusive disease. Complications and adverse effects include platelet consumption, catheter sepsis, and lower extremity ischemic complications.

Ventricular Assist Devices and Total Artificial Hearts. Ventricular assist devices (VADs) replace the pumping function of the right or left ventricle, or both. VADs may be used to support patients until myocardial recovery occurs or until cardiac transplantation can be performed. For patients with end-stage congestive heart failure who are not candidates for transplantation, a VAD may be placed as destination therapy. Several different VAD systems are FDA-approved and marketed for these various applications. Currently, total artificial heart therapy remains experimental and is limited to patients who are treated on research protocols.

Blood Glucose Control

There has been increasing emphasis on maintaining tight blood glucose control in critically ill patients because of demonstrated reductions in morbidity and mortality. The benefits of tight glucose control have been demonstrated in cardiac surgery patients specifically (43–45). Maintenance of tight glucose control reduces the incidence of mediastinitis, atrial fibrillation, ischemia, length of stay, hospital costs, and mortality and has been shown to benefit both diabetic and nondiabetic patients following cardiovascular surgery. In our practice, we have instituted an intensive intravenous insulin therapy protocol with a goal of maintaining normoglycemia (blood glucose 80–110 mg/dL). A continuous insulin infusion is typically started intraoperatively, and we have found all adult patients to require intravenous insulin at least through the immediate postoperative period if normoglycemia is to be maintained.

The requirement for intravenous insulin is reduced as inotropes, particularly epinephrine, are weaned. Once patients begin taking an oral diet, we supplement the intravenous insulin infusion with a fast-acting insulin formulation given subcutaneously. The dose of insulin aspart is based on the patient's oral intake and intravenous insulin requirement over the preceding 12 hours. Patients are subsequently transitioned to a long-acting insulin formulation, such as NPH, given subcutaneously three times a day to cover basal needs in addition to fast-acting insulin, which is still based on percentage of meals consumed. Nondiabetic patients typically have a progressively decreasing insulin requirement during their hospital recovery and are not discharged on any insulin. We have found this regimen to provide improved blood glucose control while also decreasing the frequency and severity of episodes of hypoglycemia and hyperglycemia.

Catheter Sepsis

Bloodstream infections have particularly significant implications in cardiovascular surgery patients as prosthetic intravascular devices, such as heart valves and arterial conduits, are frequently implanted during surgery. Patients typically return from the operating room following cardiovascular surgery with multiple invasive monitoring catheters including central lines, pulmonary artery catheters, arterial lines, and urinary catheters. The incidence of sepsis increases when invasive monitoring catheters are left in place for longer than 72 hours (46). For straightforward cases, our goal is to have all monitoring catheters removed by this time. All peripheral intravenous lines are also removed at the time of the patient's transfer to the intermediate care floor and a new peripheral intravenous line is placed. If a patient remains critically ill and still requires invasive monitoring, we observe the patient closely for signs of sepsis such as fever and leukocytosis, and have a low threshold to remove old lines. We avoid rewiring catheters and prefer to insert new catheters at a different site. Cultures are drawn at this time, and vancomycin is started if clinical suspicion for catheter sepsis is high. Antibiotic coverage is narrowed or discontinued based on subsequent culture results.

Clinical Pathways

Clinical pathways have been increasingly used by health care systems to improve the continuity and coordination of care for patients being treated for many diseases. They frequently are developed around procedures, and patients undergoing coronary artery bypass grafting (CABG) procedures were among the first to benefit from their implementation. CABG procedures are common, usually elective, have typical recovery milestones, and require coordination of multidisciplinary provider teams. These characteristics make CABG pathways extremely useful to support both clinical and administrative management.

Many institutions have implemented clinical pathways for other cardiovascular procedures including heart valve repair or replacement and heart transplantation. Clinical pathways typically are based around a timeline, categories of care such as nursing and physical therapy, and a variance record that allows deviations to be incorporated. When successfully implemented, they encourage the use of clinical guidelines, improve multidisciplinary teamwork, reduce variations in patient care, and improve clinical outcomes. It is important that clinical pathways not discourage personalized care and that they function well even in the face of unexpected changes in a patient's condition.

Cardiac Surgery Databases

Institutional and multi-institutional databases are useful tools with which to track outcomes following cardiovascular operations, conduct clinical research, and guide continuous quality improvement. These data are also used by various regulatory bodies and third-party payers to monitor health care quality and costs. It will also be used for pay-for-performance initiatives in the future. The data collected in these databases is clinical, administrative, or a combination of both. The Society of Thoracic Surgeons Cardiac Database is the largest clinical cardiothoracic surgery database in the world and currently has more than 500 participating sites. The large volume of clinical information collected allows risk modeling for common procedures and provides individual institutions with comparative outcomes data and national benchmarks. All cardiac databases are limited by the variable quality of collected data, which in many instances is self-reported. Comparison of outcomes is also subject to selection bias not corrected by imprecise risk models.

Special Clinical Scenarios

Off-pump Coronary Artery Bypass Surgery

Over the last 10 years, there has been increasing interest in performing CABG surgery without the use of cardiopulmonary bypass. This growth has been largely driven by increasing recognition of the deleterious effects of cardiopulmonary bypass and the desire to avoid the diffuse inflammatory response, multiorgan dysfunction, and neurocognitive complications that may follow (Table 80.3) (47–55). Approximately 25% of CABGs performed in the United States are performed off-pump, and some centers report a significantly higher percentage of off-pump coronary artery bypass procedures (OPCABs). Even among surgeons not routinely performing coronary revascularization off-pump, there are newly recognized clinical scenarios, such as a patient with severe atherosclerosis of the ascending aorta, for whom use of OPCAB techniques is strongly favored. OPCAB itself is a facilitating technology for surgeons developing minimally invasive approaches to coronary revascularization. OPCAB has therefore evolved into a requisite component of modern cardiovascular surgery practice.

TABLE 80.3

BENEFITS OF OFF-PUMP CORONARY ARTERY BYPASS GRAFTING DEMONSTRATED IN PROSPECTIVE, RANDOMIZED STUDIES

Myocardial protection
Reduced release of cardiac enzymes
Decreased need for inotropic support
Fewer postoperative arrhythmias
Pulmonary function
Decreased requirement for mechanical ventilation
Renal protection
Improved preservation of glomerular filtration and renal tubular function
Coagulation
Decreased coagulopathy
Decreased transfusion requirement
Inflammation
Reduced release of cytokines
Reduced complement activation
Decreased incidence of postoperative infections
Neurocognitive function
Improved early postoperative neurocognitive function
Resource utilization
Decreased total resource utilization

Reproduced from Song HK, Puskas JD. Off-pump coronary artery bypass surgery. In: Kaiser LR, Kron IL, Spray TL, eds. *Mastery of Cardiothoracic Surgery*. 2nd ed. Philadelphia, PA: Lippincott Williams & Wilkins; 2007:455, with permission.).

The postoperative care of patients who have undergone OPCAB surgery does not differ in many respects from that of patients undergoing conventional CABG surgery. There are several important differences, however, that providers must be aware of to take advantage of the opportunity for expedited care that OPCAB surgery can offer. Patients who have undergone OPCAB surgery have a decreased need for inotropic support in the postoperative period, most likely because of avoidance of global ischemia and reduced myocardial stunning. The intravenous fluid requirement for patients who have undergone OPCAB surgery is also reduced because the systemic inflammatory response and capillary leak related to CPB is avoided. Massive volume resuscitation in the early postoperative period should be avoided in favor of low-dose vasopressors that may be necessary secondary to intravenous sedation. OPCAB patients typically are volume loaded intraoperatively and are more likely to be euvolemic in the immediate postoperative period than conventional CABG patients.

Postoperative hemorrhage and transfusion requirements are reduced in OPCAB patients because of reduced fibrinolytic pathway activation and coagulation factor and platelet consumption. We do not routinely check platelet counts or clotting times in these patients in the immediate postoperative period for this reason. Persistent or massive hemorrhage in the postoperative period should prompt early evaluation for surgical bleeding because this is unlikely to be related to factor or platelet deficiency in an OPCAB patient.

Patients who have undergone OPCAB surgery are in a relatively hypercoagulable state as opposed to manifesting the coagulopathy that is typical after CPB. This state has the potential to adversely affect graft patency in the postoperative period. After surgery we continue aspirin administration daily as with patients undergoing conventional CABG surgery. In addition, we start clopidogrel, 75 mg/day, in the immediate postoperative period once chest tube drainage has been low for 3 consecutive hours.

One of the major benefits of OPCAB surgery to the healthcare system is the potential for OPCAB patients to have reduced resource use. An area where this advantage can be exploited is in reducing length of mechanical ventilation and ICU stay. To realize this benefit for the patient and the health system, providers should be cognizant of this and be immediately prepared to wean and extubate patients as their need for mechanical assistance is diminished. With appropriate anesthesia planning and staffing, patients can generally be extubated in the operating room after an OPCAB procedure or within 30 minutes of arrival in the ICU. When this is not feasible, clinical pathways that set objective criteria and goals facilitate the timely progression of ventilator weaning and extubation that minimize patient exposure to ventilator-related complications and maximize efficiency and cost-effectiveness.

Thoracic Aortic Surgery

Patients undergoing surgery for disorders of the thoracic aorta present critical care providers with several unique challenges, including neurologic complications, hemodynamic disturbances, and malperfusion syndromes. Several of these conditions are caused by the period of circulatory arrest that the patient undergoes during the conduct of the surgical repair whereas others are caused by the specific anatomy of the underlying thoracic aortic pathology.

Circulatory Arrest Sequelae. Patients undergoing aortic arch procedures usually have a period of circulatory arrest during their operation. This increases their risk for neurologic complications, particularly psychological and cognitive disorders. It is typical for elderly patients who require prolonged hypothermic circulatory arrest (greater than 30 minutes) to have neurologic dysfunction resulting in agitation and delirium. Although this finding is usually transient, it may necessitate a several-day period of supportive care during which the patient requires mechanical ventilation.

Circulatory arrest is also associated with increased bleeding and transfusion requirement related to profound coagulopathy (56,57). Profound coagulopathy is especially problematic in this patient group because of the long suture lines used in large-vessel surgery. Patients presenting with acute aortic dissections have attenuated and friable aortic tissue, making vascular anastomoses potentially tenuous. Coagulopathy following emergency thoracic aortic surgery for dissection should be treated aggressively as described earlier in this chapter. Surgical bleeding should always be suspected in patients with brisk hemorrhage. Avoidance of hypertension is desirable in patients with long suture lines and friable aortic tissue.

Patients who have undergone complex vascular repairs with long bypass times and circulatory arrest also may develop profound vasodilatory shock that is recalcitrant to combination therapy with multiple vasopressors. The cause for this is unclear but may be related to bacterial translocation of intestinal flora (58–60). Patients who exhibit this should be adequately volume resuscitated and supported with vasopressors and inotropes if poor myocardial contractility is contributing to the hypotension. We have also used intravenous steroids and methylene blue in patients with profound vasodilation (20,61–63). Addition of these agents has allowed reduction of high doses of vasopressors that can lead to ischemic complications.

Spinal Cord Ischemia. Spinal cord ischemia and paralysis is a particularly devastating complication following thoracoabdominal aneurysm repair. Spinal cord ischemia occurs at the time of thoracoabdominal aneurysm repair and is exacerbated by postoperative hypoperfusion, particularly when the variable origin of the artery of Adamkiewicz is not adequately reconstituted. This results in an anterior spinal artery syndrome with impaired lower extremity motor function and, to a lesser degree, impaired sensory function. Patients should be monitored closely for these findings in the immediate postoperative period. When spinal cord ischemia is suspected, a lumbar drain should be placed if one was not already placed intraoperatively. Cerebrospinal fluid (CSF) should be drained for a CSF pressure of 10 mm Hg or greater, and the mean arterial blood pressure should be raised to 85 to 100 mm Hg using vasopressors to increase the perfusion pressure to the spinal cord. These maneuvers have led to reversal of acute lower extremity neurologic findings in patients following thoracoabdominal aneurysm repair. MRI is useful for confirming the diagnosis of spinal cord ischemia. Treatment as outlined above should not be delayed until after MRI scanning if spinal cord ischemia is suspected.

Malperfusion Syndromes. Malperfusion syndromes occur in patients with aortic dissection as a result of obstruction of arterial branch orifices by the dissected intimal flap or inadequate perfusion via the false lumen of the aorta. Patients presenting with aortic dissection can develop malperfusion of virtually any limb or end organ, depending on the anatomic extent of the dissection. Patients with ascending aorta involvement (Stanford type A) typically undergo emergency surgery whereas patients with only descending aorta involvement (Stanford type B) are treated initially with medical therapy. Even patients who have undergone repair of ascending aortic dissection are frequently left with residual dissection involving the descending aorta. Therefore, providers must remain vigilant for the development of malperfusion syndromes in both patient groups. Patients admitted to the ICU with dissection should undergo serial peripheral pulse, neurologic, and abdominal exams for evidence of malperfusion. Serial arterial blood gases, liver enzymes, and lactate levels are useful when visceral malperfusion is suspected.

We have a low threshold for performing angiography when malperfusion is suspected. If confirmed by this study, interventional techniques such as fenestration or stenting can frequently be used to treat malperfusion during the same procedure. Laparotomy may be occasionally required for patients with visceral malperfusion who progress to bowel infarction.

References

1. Hall RI, Smith MS, Rocker G. The systemic inflammatory response to cardiopulmonary bypass: pathophysiological, therapeutic, and pharmacological considerations. *Anesth Analg.* 1997;85:766.
2. Steinberg JB, Kapelanski DP, Olson JD, et al. Cytokine and complement levels in patients undergoing cardiopulmonary bypass. *J Thorac Cardiovasc Surg.* 1993;106:1008.
3. Miller BE, Levy JH. The inflammatory response to cardiopulmonary bypass. *J Cardiothor Vasc Anesth.* 1997;11:355.
4. Lobato EB, Gravenstein N, Martin TD. Milrinone, not epinephrine, improves left ventricular compliance after cardiopulmonary bypass [see comment]. *J Cardiothor Vasc Anesth.* 2000;14:374.
5. Kouchoukos NT, Karp RB. Management of the postoperative cardiovascular surgical patient. *Am Heart J.* 1976;92:513.
6. Reinhart K, Kersting T, Fohring U, et al. Can central-venous replace mixed-venous oxygen saturation measurements during anesthesia? *Adv Exp Med Biol.* 1986;200:67.
7. Reinhart K, Rudolph T, Bredle DL, et al. Comparison of central-venous to mixed-venous oxygen saturation during changes in oxygen supply/demand. *Chest.* 1989;95:1216.
8. Halonen J, Hakala T, Auvinen T, et al. Intravenous administration of metoprolol is more effective than oral administration in the prevention of atrial fibrillation after cardiac surgery. *Circulation.* 2006;114:I1.
9. Katariya K, DeMarchena E, Bolooki H. Oral amiodarone reduces incidence of postoperative atrial fibrillation. *Ann Thor Surg.* 1999;68:1599.
10. Kurz DJ, Naegeli B, Kunz M, et al. Epicardial, biatrial synchronous pacing for prevention of atrial fibrillation after cardiac surgery. *Pacing Clin Electrophysiol.* 1999;22:721.
11. Patti G, Chello M, Candura D, et al. Randomized trial of atorvastatin for reduction of postoperative atrial fibrillation in patients undergoing cardiac surgery: results of the ARMYDA-3 (Atorvastatin for Reduction of Myocardial Dysrhythmia After cardiac surgery) study. *Circulation.* 2006;114:1455.
12. Stamou SC, Hill PC, Sample GA, et al. Prevention of atrial fibrillation after cardiac surgery: the significance of postoperative oral amiodarone. *Chest.* 2001;120:1936.
13. Spaan JA, Piek JJ, Hoffman JI, Siebes M. Physiological basis of clinically used coronary hemodynamic indices. *Circulation.* 2006;113:446.
14. Kouchoukos NT, Sheppard LC, McDonald DA, et al. Estimation of stroke volume from the central arterial pressure contour in postoperative patients. *Surg Forum.* 1969;20:180.
15. Webber CE, Garnett ES. The relationship between colloid osmotic pressure and plasma proteins during and after cardiopulmonary bypass. *J Thor Cardiovasc Surg.* 1973;65:234.
16. Ng CS, Wan S, Yim AP, et al. Pulmonary dysfunction after cardiac surgery. *Chest.* 2002;121:1269.
17. Gallagher JD, Moore RA, Kerns D, et al. Effects of colloid or crystalloid administration on pulmonary extravascular water in the postoperative period after coronary artery bypass grafting. *Anesth Analg.* 1985;64:753.
18. Morales DL, Garrido MJ, Madigan JD, et al. A double-blind randomized trial: prophylactic vasopressin reduces hypotension after cardiopulmonary bypass. *Ann Thorac Surg.* 2003;75:926.
19. Weis F, Kilger E, Beiras-Fernandez A, et al. Association between vasopressor dependence and early outcome in patients after cardiac surgery. *Anaesthesia.* 2006;61:938.
20. Shanmugam G. Vasoplegic syndrome—the role of methylene blue. *Eur J Cardiothorac Surg.* 2005;28:705.
21. Masetti P, Murphy SF, Kouchoukos NT. Vasopressin therapy for vasoplegic syndrome following cardiopulmonary bypass. *J Cardiac Surg.* 2002;17:485.
22. Di Giantomasso D, Morimatsu H, May CN, et al. Increasing renal blood flow: low-dose dopamine or medium-dose norepinephrine. *Chest.* 2004;125:2260.
23. Nikolaidis LA, Trumble D, Hentosz T, et al. Catecholamines restore myocardial contractility in dilated cardiomyopathy at the expense of increased coronary blood flow and myocardial oxygen consumption (MvO_2 cost of catecholamines in heart failure). *Eur J Heart Fail.* 2004;6:409.
24. Eagle KA, Guyton RA, Davidoff R, et al; American Heart Association Task Force on Practice, and American Society for Thoracic Surgery and the Society of Thoracic Surgeons. ACC/AHA 2004 guideline update for coronary artery bypass graft surgery: summary article: a report of the American College of Cardiology/American Heart Association Task Force on Practice Guidelines (Committee to Update the 1999 Guidelines for Coronary Artery Bypass Graft Surgery) [erratum in *Circulation.* 2005 Apr 19;111(15):2014]. *Circulation.* 2004;110:1168.
25. Linden MD. The hemostatic defect of cardiopulmonary bypass. *J Thromb Thrombolys.* 2003;16:129.
26. Woodman RC, Harker LA. Bleeding complications associated with cardiopulmonary bypass. *Blood.* 1990;76:1680.
27. Slaughter TF, Faghih F, Greenberg CS, et al. The effects of epsilon-aminocaproic acid on fibrinolysis and thrombin generation during cardiac surgery. *Anesth Analg.* 1997;85:1221.
28. Smith PK, Datta SK, Muhlbaier LH, et al. Cost analysis of aprotinin for coronary artery bypass patients: analysis of the randomized trials. *Ann Thorac Surg.* 2004;77:635.
29. Bishop CV, Renwick WE, Hogan C, et al. Recombinant activated factor VII: treating postoperative hemorrhage in cardiac surgery. *Ann Thorac Surg.* 2006;81:875.
30. Halkos ME, Levy JH, Chen E, et al. Early experience with activated recombinant factor VII for intractable hemorrhage after cardiovascular surgery. *Ann Thorac Surg.* 2005;79:1303.
31. Hayward CP, Harrison P, Cattaneo M, et al. The Platelet Physiology Subcommittee of the Scientific and Standardization Committee of the International Society on Thrombosis and Haemostasis. Platelet function analyzer (PFA)-100 closure time in the evaluation of platelet disorders and platelet function. *J Thromb Haemost.* 2006;4:312.
32. Holmes-Ghosh E. Heparin-induced thrombocytopenia and thrombosis syndrome after cardiopulmonary bypass. *Am J Crit Care.* 2000;9:276.
33. Asimakopoulos G, Smith PL, Ratnatunga CP, et al. Lung injury and acute respiratory distress syndrome after cardiopulmonary bypass. *Ann Thorac Surg.* 1999;68:1107.
34. Jaski BE, Miller D. Ultrafiltration in decompensated heart failure. *Curr Heart Fail Rep.* 2005;2:148.
35. Gardner TJ, Horneffer PJ, Manolio TA, et al. Stroke following coronary artery bypass grafting: a ten-year study. *Ann Thorac Surg.* 1985;40:574.
36. Hogue CW Jr, Palin CA, Arrowsmith JE. Cardiopulmonary bypass management and neurologic outcomes: an evidence-based appraisal of current practices. *Anesth Analg.* 2006;103:21.
37. Gao L, Taha R, Gauvin D, et al. Postoperative cognitive dysfunction after cardiac surgery. *Chest.* 2005;128:3664.
38. O'Brien DJ, Bauer RM, Yarandi H, et al. Patient memory before and after cardiac operations. *J Thorac Cardiovasc Surg.* 1992;104:1116.
39. Clark RE, Brillman J, Davis DA, et al. Microemboli during coronary artery bypass grafting. Genesis and effect on outcome [see comment]. *J Thorac Cardiovasc Surg.* 1995;109:249.
40. Stump DA. Embolic factors associated with cardiac surgery. *Semin Cardiothor Vasc Anesth.* 2005;9:151.
41. Vasquez E, Chitwood WR Jr. Postcardiotomy delirium: an overview. *Int J Psych Med.* 1975;6:373.
42. Townes BD, Bashein G, Hornbein TF, et al. Neurobehavioral outcomes in cardiac operations. A prospective controlled study. *J Thorac Cardiovasc Surg.* 1989;98:774.
43. Ouattara A, Lecomte P, Le Manach Y, et al. Poor intraoperative blood glucose control is associated with a worsened hospital outcome after cardiac surgery in diabetic patients [see comment]. *Anesthesiology.* 2005;103:687.
44. Rassias AJ, Givan AL, Marrin CA, et al. Insulin increases neutrophil count and phagocytic capacity after cardiac surgery [see comment]. *Anesth Analg.* 2002;94:1113.
45. Shann KG, Likosky DS, Murkin JM, et al. An evidence-based review of the practice of cardiopulmonary bypass in adults: a focus on neurologic injury, glycemic control, hemodilution, and the inflammatory response. *J Thor Cardiovasc Surg.* 2006;132:283.
46. Eggimann P, Sax H, Pittet D. Catheter-related infections. *Microbes Infect.* 2004;6:1033.
47. Angelini GD, Taylor FC, Reeves BC, et al. Early and midterm outcome after off-pump and on-pump surgery in Beating Heart Against Cardioplegic Arrest Studies (BHACAS 1 and 2): a pooled analysis of two randomised controlled trials [see comment]. *Lancet.* 2002;359:1194.
48. Ascione R, Lloyd CT, Gomes WJ, et al. Beating versus arrested heart revascularization: evaluation of myocardial function in a prospective randomized study. *Eur J Cardiothorac Surg.* 1999;15:685.
49. Ascione R, Lloyd CT, Underwood MJ, et al. Economic outcome of off-pump coronary artery bypass surgery: a prospective randomized study. *Ann Thor Surg.* 1999;68:2237.
50. Ascione R, Williams S, Lloyd CT, et al. Reduced postoperative blood loss and transfusion requirement after beating-heart coronary operations: a prospective randomized study. *J Thorac Cardiovasc Surg.* 2001;121:689.
51. Puskas JD, Williams WH, Duke PG, et al. Off-pump coronary artery bypass grafting provides complete revascularization with reduced myocardial injury, transfusion requirements, and length of stay: a prospective randomized comparison of two hundred unselected patients undergoing off-pump versus conventional coronary artery bypass grafting. *J Thorac Cardiovasc Surg.* 2003;125:797.
52. Puskas JD, Williams WH, Mahoney EM, et al. Off-pump vs conventional coronary artery bypass grafting: early and 1-year graft patency, cost, and quality-of-life outcomes: a randomized trial [see comment]. *JAMA.* 2004;291:1841.

53. Van Dijk D, Jansen EW, Hijman R, et al. Cognitive outcome after off-pump and on-pump coronary artery bypass graft surgery: a randomized trial [see comment]. *JAMA.* 2002;287:1405.
54. van Dijk D, Nierich AP, Jansen EW, et al. Early outcome after off-pump versus on-pump coronary bypass surgery: results from a randomized study [see comment]. *Circulation.* 2001;104:1761.
55. Zamvar V, Williams D, Hall J, et al. Assessment of neurocognitive impairment after off-pump and on-pump techniques for coronary artery bypass graft surgery: prospective randomised controlled trial. *BMJ.* 2002;325:1268.
56. Westaby S. Coagulation disturbance in profound hypothermia: the influence of anti-fibrinolytic therapy. *Semin Thorac Cardiovasc Surg.* 1997;9:246.
57. Wilde JT. Hematological consequences of profound hypothermic circulatory arrest and aortic dissection. *J Cardiac Surg.* 1997;12:201.
58. Rossi M, Sganga G, Mazzone M, et al. Cardiopulmonary bypass in man: role of the intestine in a self-limiting inflammatory response with demonstrable bacterial translocation. *Ann Thorac Surg.* 2004;77:612.
59. Ryan T, Mc Carthy JF, Rady MY, et al. Early bloodstream infection after cardiopulmonary bypass: frequency rate, risk factors, and implications. *Crit Care Med.* 1997;25:2009.
60. Tsunooka N, Maeyama K, Hamada Y, et al. Bacterial translocation secondary to small intestinal mucosal ischemia during cardiopulmonary bypass. Measurement by diamine oxidase and peptidoglycan. *Eur J Cardiothorac Surg.* 2004;25:275.
61. Callister ME, Evans TW. Haemodynamic and ventilatory support in severe sepsis. *J R Coll Physicians Lond.* 2000;34:522.
62. Maslow AD, Stearns G, Batula P, et al. The hemodynamic effects of methylene blue when administered at the onset of cardiopulmonary bypass. *Anesth Analg.* 2006;103:2.
63. Sparicio D, Landoni G, Zangrillo A. Angiotensin-converting enzyme inhibitors predispose to hypotension refractory to norepinephrine but responsive to methylene blue [comment]. *J Thorac Cardiovasc Surg.* 2004;127:608.

CHAPTER 81 ■ MANAGEMENT OF THE PEDIATRIC CARDIAC SURGICAL PATIENT

KAREN L. BOOTH • STEPHEN J. ROTH

Pediatric cardiac surgery and postoperative care has undergone significant advancements over the past several decades. The successful collaboration of numerous disciplines including pediatric cardiac surgery, anesthesia, cardiology, and intensive care have led to an increase in the complexity of cardiac lesions repaired with a simultaneous reduction in surgical mortality. There has been a shift away from palliative procedures to primary repair as early as possible, even in the very premature neonate (1–3). The heterogeneity of congenital heart disease and the individualized care these patients require has led to the emergence of dedicated pediatric cardiac intensive care units. This chapter focuses on the key principles for successful management of the pediatric cardiac surgical patient including assessment of the preoperative status and operative course, postoperative stabilization, subsequent evaluation of the repair, and support of myocardial function.

CARDIAC INTENSIVE CARE: A SPECIALIZED ENVIRONMENT

The pediatric cardiac intensive care unit (CICU) shares many of the common features of a generalized intensive care unit. Bedside monitors with the ability to display heart rate, arterial blood pressure, central venous pressure, pulse oximetry, and respiratory rate are essential. Additionally, the monitor should be capable of transducing several pressures simultaneously, including right atrial pressure, left atrial pressure, and pulmonary artery or right ventricular pressure, as many pediatric cardiac patients have several intracardiac catheters placed for postoperative hemodynamic monitoring. There should be central monitoring capable of storing at least 24 hours of individual patient hemodynamic data and alarms. This is often important for reconstructing critical events and trending a patient's recovery or deterioration over time.

Ventilators capable of supporting patients of all sizes (from premature neonates through adults) should be readily available. Specialized ventilators such as the oscillator should be also available for patients with coexisting lung disease. Inhaled nitric oxide has become an essential therapy in the treatment of the postoperative cardiac patient with pulmonary hypertension (4,5). There should be several ventilators capable of delivering inhaled nitric oxide, as it is common for more than one patient to be receiving this therapy simultaneously. Bedside blood gas analysis with hand-held point-of-care testing devices is the norm at many institutions. If this is not available, rapid blood gas analysis with a laboratory turnaround time of less than 15 to 30 minutes is necessary.

Many postoperative cardiac patients have dysrhythmias, including tachycardias, bradycardias, and heart block. Thus, the cardiac intensive care unit must be equipped with the equipment to provide temporary cardiac pacing. Most contemporary battery-operated temporary pacemakers also have the ability to deliver rapid atrial pacing, which can terminate tachyarrhythmia including re-entrant supraventricular tachycardia and atrial flutter. A portable electrocardiogram (ECG) machine and defibrillator are essential devices for bedside diagnosis, cardioversion, and emergency defibrillations.

Echocardiography should be accessible for rapid assessment of the postoperative patient for important residual lesions or tamponade. Equipment for emergent bedside sternotomies for tamponade is required. This is accomplished with a mediastinal cart or tray stored in the CICU and stocked with all the necessary instruments. This cart will also facilitate emergency cannulation for extracorporeal membrane oxygenation (ECMO) if mechanical support of the myocardium is necessary.

POSTOPERATIVE ASSESSMENT AND STABILIZATION

The admission of a pediatric patient to the CICU after congenital heart surgery is a complex undertaking. Considerable advanced preparation is required for successful transition of a patient from the operative environment to the intensive care unit. The first several hours after separation from cardiopulmonary bypass (CPB) is the time when patients are the most vulnerable to decompensation as they are physically moved and care is transferred to a new team. Preparations should begin before the patient is admitted to the hospital. Most cardiovascular surgical programs have multidisciplinary conferences to review each patient's history and data. Important components of the preoperative review include the precise anatomic diagnosis, prior operative procedures, coexisting medical conditions, medication regimen, and current preoperative echocardiographic and catheterization findings. In this venue, the surgical approach as well as the initial postoperative care should be planned. For example, if a patient is known to have pulmonary hypertension by preoperative catheterization data, the team can plan to have nitric oxide available in the operating room and/or CICU. If additional studies or subspecialty consultations are required, ample time should be allotted to accomplish a complete preoperative evaluation.

Transition from the Operating Room

As the surgery concludes, a patient report should be formulated by the operating room team and called to the receiving nurse and physician in the CICU. This report includes information on the procedure performed, the hemodynamic status, current vasoactive infusions, and ventilator settings. This allows the CICU sufficient time to prepare the appropriate personnel, equipment, and medications. The patient is transferred to the CICU by the anesthesia and surgical team. Upon arrival the initial goal is to transition from portable monitoring and transport equipment to the bedside CICU monitor and ventilator as efficiently as possible while maintaining gas exchange and patient stability. It is prudent to use the same infusion pumps from the operating room so as to not interrupt any vasoactive infusions. During this critical time, the medical decision making and management of the patient should continue to be provided by the anesthesia and surgical team until a complete exchange of information occurs.

The key operative events are details of the repair, length of CPB including any special techniques used such as deep hypothermic circulatory arrest or low-flow regional perfusion, abnormal rhythms, or significant bleeding after CPB. The initial assessment of the repair typically includes transesophageal or epicardial echocardiography, intraoperative intracardiac saturation measurements to assess for residual shunts, and initial hemodynamic pressure measurements. If a second CPB run is required to correct residual lesions, this can have important effects on myocardial function in the initial postoperative period. If the sternum is left open, it is important to know the exact surgical reason for this decision. For example, was there excessive chest bleeding, poor myocardial function, or difficulty with ventilation (6)? Each would have different implications for management strategies in the first postoperative hours.

The anesthesia team can provide a wealth of information regarding patient course and stability. The key anesthesia events are airway issues such as difficulty with bag-mask ventilation or tracheal intubation, type of anesthesia given including cumulative dose of narcotics and benzodiazepines, current vasoactive and inotropic support, and blood and colloid products administered. The anesthesia team should be able to predict the initial course and readiness for extubation.

After patient transfer and the exchange of information have occurred, the CICU team performs their initial assessment. The physical exam should focus on clinical cardiac output and evidence for residual lesions. Patients often emerge from the operating room hypothermic, and perfusion may be affected by the need to rewarm slowly. Some murmurs are expected (e.g., after a procedure that includes an aortopulmonary shunt). Other patients should have a silent precordial exam, such as repair of a ventricular septal defect (VSD). Patients with cavopulmonary connections such as the bidirectional Glenn or Fontan procedure should also have a quiet precordial exam. Murmurs in these patients may indicate outflow tract obstruction or atrioventricular valve regurgitation, each of which can adversely affect the function of the single ventricle.

Initial laboratory evaluation should include immediate arterial blood gas (ABG) analysis. Ideally, the anesthesia and surgical team should remain in the CICU until the first ABG has been measured to ensure that the patient has adequate gas exchange. Interpretation of the initial ABG requires understanding of the patient's physiology. Patients with two-ventricle physiology are often receiving 100% oxygen (O_2) and, in the absence of significant pulmonary pathology, should have a high arterial partial pressure of O_2 (PaO_2) to reflect this. Patients with large left-to-right shunts preoperatively may have significant alveolar–arterial gradients from pulmonary edema. Patients undergoing right ventriculotomies, as in tetralogy of Fallot repairs, may have right ventricular dysfunction and elevated central venous pressures. This may cause a right-to-left shunt at the atrial level if a patent foramen ovale (PFO) is preserved, and a PaO_2 <100 mm Hg regardless of the fraction of inspired oxygen (FIO_2) delivered. Single-ventricle patients receive a lower FIO_2 to prevent pulmonary overcirculation and systemic undercirculation (see Single Ventricle Physiology). The PaO_2 in these patients should be 35 to 45 mm Hg. In general, patients should be ventilated to a normal arterial partial pressure of carbon dioxide ($PaCO_2$), which is 35 to 45 mm Hg. An indication for mildly hyperventilating a patient ($PaCO_2$ 30–35 mm Hg) would include pulmonary hypertension to reduce pulmonary vascular resistance (PVR) (7).

Pulmonary overcirculation may be treated with hypoventilation to increase PVR ($PaCO_2$ 45–50 mm Hg). Evaluation of a metabolic acidosis with low pH and bicarbonate levels should raise concern for low cardiac output syndrome. This should be treated immediately by providing judicious intravascular volume supplementation, providing increased inotropic support, and maximizing oxygen-carrying capacity with a blood transfusion for anemia. If the cause of the low cardiac syndrome is unclear or is unresponsive to initial measures to improve cardiac output, urgent bedside echocardiography to evaluate the repair and myocardial function and to look for possible tamponade should be performed.

Additional laboratory evaluations to be performed are blood chemistries, complete blood count with platelet count, coagulation studies, and lactate level. Serial postoperative lactate levels after congenital heart surgery have been predictive of outcomes. Higher initial ICU lactate levels (9.4 vs. 5.6 mmol/L) and lactates that continue to rise greater than 0.75 mmol/L/hour are associated with poorer outcome (death or use of ECMO) (8,9). Coagulation parameters including prothrombin time (PT), partial thromboplastin time (PTT), fibrinogen, and platelet count should be normal. Any abnormalities in the setting of excessive chest bleeding should be aggressively corrected. Additional doses of protamine can be given in the CICU if the PTT is prolonged and there is excessive chest bleeding. If all coagulation parameters are corrected and there is still excessive bleeding, an antifibrinolytic such as aprotinin, tranexamic acid, or ε-aminocaproic acid may be considered (10). Aprotinin is currently not available until further studies are done regarding its side effects. Activated factor VIIa has been successfully used for refractory surgical bleeding in the setting of post-CPB ECMO (11). If bleeding remains pronounced despite aggressive pharmacologic and blood product transfusion, it may be a surgical bleed requiring chest exploration. Similarly, brisk chest bleeding that abruptly stops with a concurrent rise in intracardiac pressures is likely due to cardiac tamponade; chest exploration is also typically required in this situation.

An admission chest radiograph should be performed minutes after arrival. This study will verify tracheal tube, nasogastric tube, pacing wire, and intracardiac catheter placement. An assessment of cardiac size and the lungs is essential to rule out a significant pneumothorax or hemothorax, both of which should be evacuated immediately. In some procedures such as unifocalization of aortopulmonary collaterals, there can be alveolar infiltrates from increased blood flow or hemorrhage, and the early use of positive end-expiratory pressure on the ventilator can improve oxygenation. Assessing the placement of intracardiac catheters is important in interpreting pressure and saturation data (see Hemodynamic Monitoring). The right atrial catheter or common atrial catheter typically enters the heart through the right atrial appendage and is directed inferiorly toward the inferior vena cava. The left atrial catheter usually enters the heart through a right pulmonary vein and is directed to the left atrium with a horizontal course. Alternatively, the left atrial catheter may enter the heart through the left atrial appendage and course inferiorly toward the mitral valve. A pulmonary artery catheter enters the heart through the right ventricular outflow tract and is directed superiorly across the pulmonary valve into the main pulmonary artery. A right ventricular catheter enters the heart through the right atrium and crosses the tricuspid valve with the tip in the body of the right ventricle.

A 12- or 15-lead ECG should be performed to assess rhythm and atrioventricular (AV) conduction. Lack of AV synchrony can contribute to a low cardiac output state, so every effort should be made to preserve AV synchrony with temporary pacing if there is AV nodal block or an ectopic junctional rhythm (see Postoperative Rhythm and Pacing). The QRS complex should be compared to baseline to assess for new abnormalities including bundle branch block. Complete right bundle branch block is common after VSD closure for tetralogy of Fallot or truncus arteriosus repairs, but usually it is not of hemodynamic significance. The ST segment should be assessed for signs of ischemia, especially after procedures that include coronary artery reimplantation.

After the initial assessment and stabilization, a plan may be made for weaning both inotropic support and ventilatory support over the subsequent hours to days. Analgesia and sedation will be tailored to this assessment and plan. Older children with short CPB support times, stable hemodynamics, and minimal chest bleeding (e.g., conduit revisions, subaortic membrane resections, septal defect closures) can be extubated almost immediately when they awaken from anesthesia (12). Neonates and younger infants often undergo more complex repairs (e.g., the arterial switch operation, truncus arteriosus repair, AV canal repair, tetralogy of Fallot repair) and will need more gradual weaning of support over 24 to 48 hours. Those undergoing complex neonatal single-ventricle palliation (e.g., stage I palliation for hypoplastic left heart syndrome [HLHS]) often have open sternums; these patients will require several days of stabilization and diuresis before their sternums can be closed.

Hemodynamic Monitoring

Patients undergoing congenital heart surgery will have intravascular or transthoracic intracardiac catheters placed for postoperative hemodynamic monitoring. These catheters are invaluable for the continual assessment of the patient and have a low risk of complications (13,14). Virtually every patient will have an arterial catheter placed for ABG sampling and blood pressure monitoring. Monitoring the central venous pressure is routine as well except for the simplest procedures performed via a thoracotomy (e.g., patent ductus arteriosus ligation or coarctation repair). The most common transthoracic intracardiac catheter placed is a right atrial catheter. This catheter may have more than one lumen, thus allowing for simultaneous central venous pressure measurement and vasoactive medication delivery. Patients may have a second central venous catheter placed by the anesthesiologist to manage the patient in the operating room before CPB is initiated. Often this catheter is inserted into the internal jugular vein with the tip at the superior vena cava–right atrial junction. This catheter may be placed in lieu of a right atrial catheter in older children. Young infants with complex two-ventricle repairs or a mitral valve repair will typically have a transthoracic left atrial intracardiac catheter placed. This catheter is valuable in assessing left ventricular function, mitral valve function, and intravascular volume status.

In single-ventricle patients, a common atrium is either congenitally present or created at the first stage of the procedure. Therefore, transthoracic intra-atrial catheters in these patients are referred to as common atrial catheters. Transthoracic pulmonary artery catheters are placed for selected repairs including truncus arteriosus and tetralogy of Fallot repairs. However, with the increased use of intraoperative transesophageal echocardiography, these catheters are less common and are reserved for procedures where the incidence of postoperative pulmonary hypertension is high, such as repair of obstructed total anomalous pulmonary venous return. More commonly used are transthoracic right ventricular catheters that enter the heart through the right atrial appendage and are positioned with the tip crossing the tricuspid valve. These catheters are useful in assessing right ventricular and pulmonary artery pressures after complex pulmonary artery reconstructions such as in tetralogy of Fallot with pulmonary atresia and aortopulmonary collaterals. In contrast to adults, children rarely have flow-directed pulmonary artery (Swan Ganz) catheters placed for postoperative monitoring. This is due to both small patient size and the need for unobstructed access for intracardiac repairs.

TABLE 81.1

CAUSES OF ELEVATED OR REDUCED RIGHT ATRIAL PRESSURE

ELEVATED
Volume overload
Right ventricular dysfunction
Systolic dysfunction
Diastolic dysfunction or noncompliance
Tricuspid stenosis
Tricuspid regurgitation
Tamponade
Loss of AV synchrony from heart block, junctional rhythm
Tachyarrhythmia
Catheter or transducer malposition or malfunction
REDUCED
Volume depletion
Inadequate preload
Bleeding
Catheter or transducer malposition or malfunction

AV, atrioventricular.

There are multiple causes of abnormal right and left atrial pressures (Tables 81.1 and 81.2). Typically, the mean right atrial pressure ranges from 0 to 8 mm Hg, and the mean left atrial pressure is 1 to 2 mm Hg higher than the right atrial pressure (15). In postoperative patients, these mean pressures are higher due to the effects of CPB on the myocardium and the volume of fluid received in the operating room. In general, mean right and left atrial pressures should not exceed 15 mm Hg; when they are elevated, the etiology should be addressed. In determining the cause of high atrial pressures, the onset is important. Gradually increasing pressures often indicate that a clinical problem such as low cardiac output or tamponade physiology is evolving. A sudden change in the pressure without a change in heart rhythm or other vital signs may indicate a technical problem with the catheter or transducer (e.g., the transducer fell off the bed). Rezeroing a transducer is always indicated if the numbers are not compatible with the clinical status. The morphology of the atrial tracing is also helpful in determining the etiology of a pressure elevation. Large a waves, referred to as cannon a waves, occur when the atrium is contracting against a closed AV valve. This occurs with loss of AV synchrony as in AV block or junctional rhythm. Large v waves occur during ventricular contraction with an incompetent AV valve. Severe AV regurgitation in a low cardiac output state may require surgical consultation and possible reoperation. Low atrial filling pressures in the setting of low arterial blood pressure or cardiac output should be treated with volume expansion. Typically 5 to 10 mL/kg of colloid or crystalloid fluid is the initial dose to restore preload. Chest bleeding with low atrial pressure should prompt correction of any coagulopathy and/or anemia with blood products.

TABLE 81.2

CAUSES OF ELEVATED OR REDUCED LEFT ATRIAL PRESSURE

ELEVATED
Volume overload
Left ventricular dysfunction
Systolic dysfunction
Diastolic dysfunction or noncompliance
Mitral stenosis
Mitral regurgitation
Left-to-right shunt
Tamponade
Loss of AV synchrony from heart block, junctional rhythm
Tachyarrhythmia
Catheter or transducer malposition or malfunction
REDUCED
Volume depletion
Catheter or transducer malposition or malfunction

AV, atrioventricular.

TABLE 81.3

CAUSES OF ELEVATED OR REDUCED PULMONARY ARTERY PRESSURE

ELEVATED
Primary pulmonary hypertension
Anatomical obstruction
Pulmonary artery stenosis
Pulmonary vein stenosis
Mitral stenosis
Left atrial hypertension
Ventricular dysfunction
Mitral valve disease
Hypoxia
Lung disease (edema, atelectasis)
Pleural effusion
Pneumothorax
Acidosis
Hypoventilation
Metabolic
Left-to-right shunt
Hyperviscosity (polycythemia)
Catheter or transducer malposition or malfunction
REDUCED
Intravascular volume depletion
Obstruction to pulmonary blood flow
Catheter or transducer malposition or malfunction

Causes of abnormal pulmonary artery or right ventricular pressures are listed in Table 81.3. Normal mean pulmonary artery pressures are 10 to 20 mm Hg (15). There can be considerable variation in the postoperative patient, but the mean should not exceed 25 to 30 mm Hg in repaired patients. The right ventricular systolic pressure is often expressed as a percentage of the systemic systolic pressure, as both may be transiently elevated in response to high catecholamine states such as agitation. The right ventricular pressure should be less than 30% to 50% systemic. Elevated pulmonary pressures are generally not well tolerated for long periods of time. Correcting associated hypocarbia and acidosis, both of which elevate PVR, should be accomplished quickly. Inhaled nitric oxide as a selective pulmonary vasodilator is useful for pulmonary hypertension and low cardiac output (5,16).

Saturation data from intracardiac catheters are also valuable in assessing the postoperative cardiac patient. The causes of abnormal right atrial, left atrial, and pulmonary arterial saturations are listed in Table 81.4. Accurate interpretation of this saturation data relies on precise knowledge of the location

TABLE 81.4

CAUSES OF ABNORMAL RIGHT ATRIAL, LEFT ATRIAL, AND PULMONARY ARTERY SATURATION

Location	Elevated	Reduced
RA	Left-to-right atrial shunt Anomalous pulmonary venous return Increased venous oxygen content Decreased oxygen extraction Catheter tip position (near IVC)	Low cardiac output (increased O_2 extraction) Increased oxygen consumption (fever, high catecholamines) Decreased arterial saturation with normal O_2 extraction Catheter tip position (near coronary sinus) Anemia
LA	Normal is fully saturated	Right-to-left atrial shunt Decreased pulmonary vein saturation (lung disease, arteriovenous malformation)
PA	Left-to-right cardiac shunt Catheter tip wedged (LA sample)	Low cardiac output (increased O_2 extraction) Increased oxygen consumption (fever, high catecholamines) Decreased arterial saturation with normal O_2 extraction Anemia

RA, right atrium; LA, left atrium; PA, pulmonary artery; IVC, inferior vena cava.

of the catheter tip for sampling and the patient's physiology. Right atrial and pulmonary artery saturation data are a useful assessment of the patient's cardiac output and oxygen extraction. Normal superior vena cava, right atrial, and pulmonary arterial saturations in a patient with two-ventricle physiology and no intracardiac shunts are approximately 70% to 80%. If the patient has a normal cardiac output and fully saturated systemic arterial blood, the arteriovenous O_2 saturation difference will be normal at approximately 25% to 30% (17). It is common for the right atrial saturation to be in the 60% range after CPB with adequate oxygen delivery and perfusion. Lower right atrial saturations are expected in patients with single-ventricle physiology because of intracardiac right-to-left shunting and systemic O_2 desaturation. As long as the arteriovenous saturation difference is $\leq$30%, the cardiac output should be normal. In patients with two-ventricle physiology, the true mixed venous saturation is in the pulmonary arteries where complete mixing of systemic venous blood occurs. An elevation in the pulmonary artery saturation after atrial or ventricular septal defect repair is indicative of a residual left-to-right shunt. An absolute pulmonary artery saturation of >80% while receiving an FIO_2 <0.4 is predictive of a residual intracardiac shunt of greater than 1.5:1 (18). The most common causes of decreased left atrial saturation and concurrent systemic desaturation are right-to-left atrial shunting (common after tetralogy of Fallot repair when the PFO is left open) and pulmonary disease.

Transthoracic intracardiac catheters should be maintained in the postoperative period only until the necessary data are obtained. Typically, left atrial and pulmonary artery catheters are removed within the first 48 hours while the patient is still intubated and the chest tubes are in place in case there is bleeding (the coagulation profile should be normal) upon catheter removal. Although significant bleeding is rare, catheters are removed with blood available at the bedside. Right atrial catheters may remain in place up to 2 weeks but should be removed as soon as clinically indicated.

Postoperative Rhythm and Pacing

Arrhythmias are common after congenital heart surgery (19). Postoperative electrolyte imbalances, myocardial stress and dysfunction, and intracardiac incisions and suture lines all play a role in the etiology of new rhythm disturbances. Both bradycardias and tachycardias occur, but fortunately most are self-limited.

The most common bradycardia is sinus bradycardia. Sinus bradycardia is normal in children during sleep and with high vagal tone and is generally benign. Patients returning from the operating room may be hypothermic with core temperatures of 32°C to 34°C; they will remain bradycardic until their temperature rises closer to normal. Patients at risk for sinus bradycardia are those undergoing atrial baffles such as a lateral tunnel-type Fontan for a single-ventricle defect or atrial switch procedures for transposition of the great arteries. Patients with sinus venosus and primum atrial septal defect repairs also commonly have slower sinus rates. Extremely bradycardic patients can be treated with pacing with temporary epicardial wires placed in the operating room, but in the absence of long sinus pauses, sinus bradycardia tends to be well tolerated.

Surgeries near the AV node such as ventricular septal defect repairs, AV canal repairs, resection of subaortic muscle, and tetralogy of Fallot repairs create risk for injury to the conduction system. Usually this is manifest as bundle branch block, most commonly right bundle branch block after tetralogy of Fallot repair. Left bundle branch block can occur with subaortic surgeries. Rarely there is more significant block such as complete heart block. Fortunately, it resolves in the majority of patients (<2% incidence overall, with recovery in two thirds of affected patients) without need for permanent pacemaker placement (20).

Common tachyarrhythmias include supraventricular tachycardia and junctional tachycardia. Patients with accessory

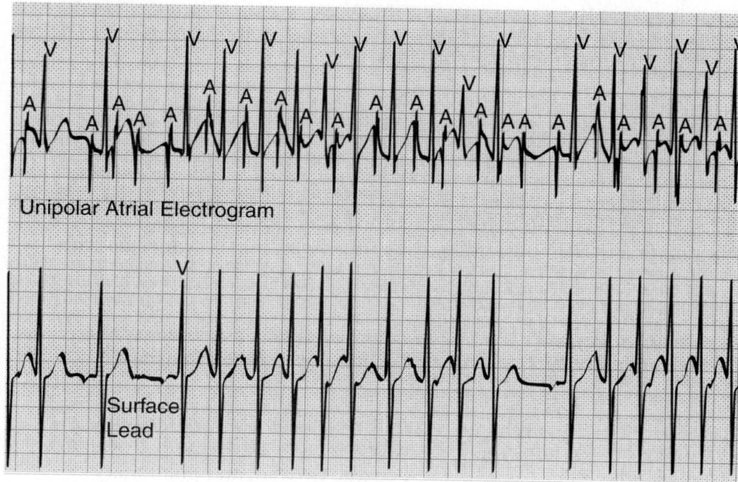

FIGURE 81.1. The use of an atrial electrocardiogram to diagnose ectopic atrial tachycardia. The surface electrocardiogram (*lower tracing*) reveals an irregular, narrow complex rhythm. Atrial depolarizations (P waves) are not easily discernible. The unipolar atrial electrocardiogram (*upper tracing*) reveals a rapid ectopic atrial tachycardia with many blocked atrial premature beats. Atrial depolarization is denoted by "A" and ventricular depolarization is denoted by "V."

pathways will often first develop a tachyarrhythmia in the postoperative period. Ectopic tachycardias are also common after congenital heart surgery (21). High catecholamine states, intracardiac catheters and suture lines, and electrolyte abnormalities all contribute to the appearance of postoperative tachyarrhythmias in previously asymptomatic patients. The onset of tachycardia may provide useful information regarding its etiology. Tachycardias with a sudden onset that generate a sustained heart rate with minimal variability are likely to be re-entrant in nature. Tachycardias with a gradual increase in heart rate with some beat-to-beat variability are likely to be automatic in nature. Temporary epicardial atrial wires can be used to obtain intracardiac atrial electrograms to examine the relationship of the P waves to the QRS complex to further aid in diagnosis (see Fig. 81.1). Atrial wires can also be used to terminate re-entrant rhythms by overdrive pacing. The indication for treatment is a hemodynamic change causing low cardiac output or blood pressure, as most tachyarrhythmias will improve with time. A summary of common antiarrhythmics used after congenital heart surgery is provided in Table 81.5.

For re-entrant and ectopic supraventricular tachycardias, β-blockers, such as esmolol, are usually the first-line therapy and are well tolerated. Digoxin can be considered in patients with apparent accessory pathways that are not pre-excited or for rate control in rapid atrial rhythms. Second-line agents include procainamide and amiodarone. Amiodarone should be used with caution, as the incidence of serious side effects including circulatory collapse and proarrhythmia is high (22). Once the tachycardia is controlled and the patient has progressed to extubation, intravenous agents can be transitioned to oral agents (e.g., the β-blocker propranolol can be substituted for esmolol). More refractory supraventricular tachycardias may be treated with the class III agent sotalol, or class IC agents flecainide or propafenone. The length of oral treatment will vary with the nature of the tachycardia, but should be considered for at least 1 to 3 months postoperatively.

Junctional ectopic tachycardia (JET) is a narrow complex rhythm that arises just below the AV node. It is most common after ventricular septal defect closure in tetralogy of Fallot and AV canal repairs. JET usually occurs in the first 24 to 48 hours postoperatively and is almost always self-limited. The typical electrocardiographic finding is AV dissociation (Fig. 81.2) with a more rapid ventricular rate (typically >180 bpm), but there can be retrograde P waves with a 1:1 relationship. Because of the lack of AV synchrony, this rhythm can lead to elevated atrial pressures and low cardiac output with hypotension. Treatment is directed toward reducing catecholamine states by weaning vasoactive infusions such as dopamine; providing sedation, analgesia, and possibly paralysis; and avoiding hyperthermia with active cooling. Atrial pacing above the junctional rate (if <180 bpm) can restore AV synchrony and improve hemodynamics. The most efficacious pharmacologic therapy includes procainamide in combination with cooling (23). Amiodarone has been reported to be successful in the treatment of JET (24), but it should be used with caution due to acute cardiac side effects such as hypotension and proarrhythmia (22). Because JET is a self-limited tachycardia, once the patient has regained normal sinus rhythm, a gradual reduction in therapy starting with rewarming and removal of deep sedation and/or paralysis can occur. Pharmacologic support should then be weaned over 24 to 48 hours.

Ventricular ectopy after congenital heart surgery can occur, especially in the setting of electrolyte abnormalities. Monomorphic premature ventricular beats or ventricular bigeminy or trigeminy is usually benign and self-limited. Sustained ventricular tachycardia that is rapid and polymorphic is dangerous and concerning for myocardial ischemia. Treatment with lidocaine and cardioversion should be attempted, but an urgent evaluation of myocardial function and perfusion must be pursued or a cardiac arrest may be imminent.

Respiratory and Ventilatory Management

Postoperative ventilation should take into consideration the important cardiopulmonary interactions that occur after congenital heart surgery. Each patient's ventilatory support and weaning plan should be individualized to his or her physiology and hemodynamic status using a set of guiding principles. Frequent reassessment and ventilatory adjustments should be expected.

Positive pressure ventilation has effects on preload. Increasing tidal volumes and positive end-expiratory pressure (PEEP) increase intrathoracic pressure and limit systemic venous return. Increased lung volume and intrathoracic pressure also increase afterload to the right (pulmonary) ventricle (25).

TABLE 81.5

COMMON ANTIARRHYTHMIC AGENTS USED AFTER CONGENITAL HEART SURGERY

Drug name	Class/mechanism/indications	Dosing	Considerations/side effects
Adenosine	Blocks AV node; termination of re-entrant SVT	0.1–0.2 mg/kg rapid IV push (max 6 mg)	Sinus arrest (have pacing available), hypotension, bronchospasm
Procainamide	IA, prolongs atrial refractory period; atrial tachycardia (re-entrant SVT, atrial fib/flutter)	5–15 mg/kg IV load (30 min) 20–80 μg/kg/min IV infusion	Myocardial depressant, vasodilator, monitor levels, lupus syndrome with long term use
Esmolol	II, β-blocker; re-entrant SVT, ectopic atrial tachycardia, ventricular tachycardia	0.1–0.5 mg/kg IV load 50–250 μg/kg/min IV infusion	Myocardial depressant, bradycardia, hypotension, bronchospasm
Amiodarone	III, prolongs atrial and ventricular refractory periods; atrial, junctional, ventricular tachycardia	5 mg/kg IV load (60 min) 5–15 μg/kg/min IV infusion 5–10 mg/kg/day PO	Potent vasodilator and myocardial depressant, proarrhythmic (torsades), hepatic, thyroid, and pulmonary toxicity
Lidocaine	IB, prolongs ventricular refractory period; prevents ventricular ectopy, tachycardia, and fibrillation	1 mg/kg slow IV push 20–50 μg/kg/min IV infusion	Monitor levels, seizures at toxic levels
Verapamil	IV, Ca channel blocker, prolongs AV node refractory period; re-entrant SVT	0.1 mg/kg/dose slow IV push 3–4 mg/kg/day PO divided Q8h	Myocardial depressant, avoid in infants, do not use concurrently with β-blockers
Digoxin	Prolongs AV node refractory period; atrial tachycardia except WPW syndrome	20–60 μg/kg IV/PO digitalizing 4–10 μg/kg IV/PO divided Q12h	Multiple medication interactions, AV block and proarrhythmic at toxic levels
Propanolol	II, β-blocker; oral treatment atrial tachycardia	2–4 mg/kg/day PO divided Q6–8h	Hypotension, hypoglycemia, bronchospasm
Sotalol	III, β-blocker, prolongs atrial and ventricular refractory period; oral treatment atrial and ventricular tachycardia	80–200 mg/m^2/day PO divided Q8–12h	Myocardial depressant
Flecainide, Propafenone	IC, prolongs atrial and ventricular refractory period; oral treatment of atrial tachycardia	Flec: 2–6 mg/kg/day divided q8h Prop: 150–300 mg/m^2 day	Myocardial depressant, proarrhythmic, monitor QRS prolongation

AV, atrioventricular; SVT, supraventricular tachycardia; PO, per os; Ca, calcium; WPW, Wolf-Parkinson-White; Flec, flecainide; Prop, propafenone.

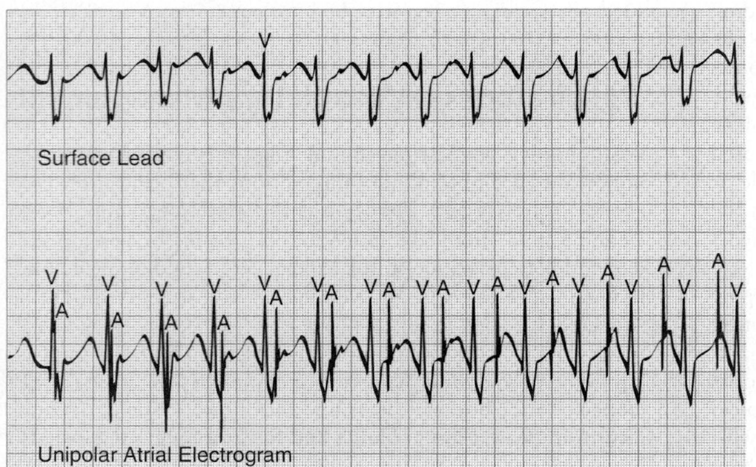

FIGURE 81.2. The use of an atrial electrocardiogram to diagnose junctional ectopic tachycardia. The surface electrocardiogram (*upper tracing*) reveals a regular, narrow complex rhythm with possible atrioventricular (AV) disassociation. The unipolar atrial electrocardiogram (*lower tracing*) demonstrates AV dissociation with a ventricular rate that is more rapid than the atrial rate. This is junctional ectopic tachycardia. Atrial depolarization is denoted by "A" and ventricular (or junctional) depolarization is denoted by "V."

Therefore, in patients with limited right ventricular function, such as patients undergoing tetralogy of Fallot repair with a ventriculotomy, right ventricular output may be compromised by elevated mean airway pressures. This can result in high right-sided filling pressure, poor right ventricular function, hepatomegaly, ascites, and pleural effusions. As the patient becomes fluid overloaded and gas exchange is impaired, the temptation is to increase ventilatory support. However, this may worsen the patient's clinical status. Patients with cavopulmonary connections and passive pulmonary blood flow also have compromised pulmonary blood flow and cardiac output with positive pressure ventilation (26,27). A strategy of a larger tidal volume (15 mL/kg) with a lower ventilatory rate may minimize afterload and give the right ventricle an opportunity to eject or the pulmonary arteries additional filling time during a longer expiratory phase. The patient should be allowed to breathe spontaneously with less mandatory ventilator breaths. Ideally, if the patient will tolerate it, he or she should be extubated as soon as possible after surgery.

Positive pressure has the opposite effect on the left (systemic) ventricle. The higher-pressure aorta is not as affected by the lung volumes. The increased intrathoracic pressure decreases left ventricular afterload due to the decreased transmural pressure across the myocardium (28). Therefore, patients with left ventricular dysfunction can improve with the initiation of positive pressure ventilation (29). Patients with ventricular dysfunction also have increased work of breathing due to increased pulmonary edema and decreased lung compliance. Positive pressure ventilation helps these patients by decreasing the work of breathing and oxygen consumption. A judicious amount of PEEP at 3 to 5 cm H_2O maintains lung volumes at functional residual capacity. This keeps alveoli recruited and minimizes increases in pulmonary vascular resistance caused by atelectasis.

The mode of ventilation used to support cardiac patients often depends on the experience of the team members in the cardiac intensive care unit. Many units will ventilate in a pressure mode, acknowledging that the lung compliance in most postoperative cardiac patients is normal and not rapidly changing as it is in patients with primary lung disease. Volume ventilation is equally acceptable, and newer ventilators are capable of volume ventilation with deceleration flow patterns, which is more comfortable for spontaneously breathing patients. More novel techniques employing higher airway pressures such as high-frequency oscillatory ventilation and airway pressure release ventilation have been used successfully in pediatric patients with primary lung disease (30,31). These modes of ventilation have limited use after congenital heart surgery due to reductions in cardiac output that occur at higher mean airway pressures in infants (32,33). Fortunately, significant lung disease after cardiac surgery is uncommon. There are selected cases where the degree of lung disease outweighs the cardiac disease and high-frequency oscillatory ventilation has been anecdotally beneficial. Scenarios such as pulmonary hemorrhage after collateral unifocalization procedures, severe pulmonary edema after repair of obstructed total anomalous pulmonary return, and respiratory distress syndrome in premature infants undergoing cardiac surgery are examples.

Timing of extubation is contingent upon several factors. The patient should be evaluated for significant residual cardiac lesions and the adequacy of myocardial function. Hemostasis should be achieved. The patient should be weaned to a low mandatory ventilatory rate (4–6 breaths per minute) or to a pressure support mode with no mandatory breaths and a FIO_2 of ≤ 0.4. The patient should be awake, not tachypneic for age, and able to generate spontaneous tidal volumes of 6 to 8 mL/kg per breath. Problems encountered postextubation include atelectasis, stridor, and diaphragm paresis or paralysis. Atelectasis is most common in neonates, larger but immobile children, or chronically malnourished patients. Chest physiotherapy and occasionally bronchoscopy may be employed to re-expand atelectatic segments of lung. Stridor is usually self-limited and can be treated with nebulized racemic epinephrine and steroids, which reduce mucosal swelling. Persistent stridor or a weak cry can also be a manifestation of a recurrent laryngeal nerve injury with vocal cord paresis or paralysis (34).

Formal assessment of swallowing function to prevent recurrent aspiration of oral feeds may be required if vocal cord injury is identified. Phrenic nerve injury with associated hemidiaphragm dysfunction is challenging to treat. The postextubation chest radiograph typically reveals an elevated hemidiaphragm with collapse of the ipsilateral lung. Fluoroscopy demonstrating decreased (paretic) or paradoxical (paralyzed) movement of the diaphragm will confirm the diagnosis. Ultrasound can also be used to assess diaphragm function, but it is less reliable in distinguishing a paretic from a paralyzed diaphragm, which may impact treatment (35). Usually the injured phrenic nerve will recover with time. Older children can often tolerate the phrenic nerve injury and compensate with the use of accessory muscles of breathing. Neonates and infants may require a hemidiaphragm plication, especially if the diaphragm is paralyzed, to wean successfully from mechanical ventilation (36).

Noninvasive forms of respiratory support are being used more commonly after congenital heart surgery. Continuous positive airway pressure (CPAP) delivered with nasal prongs or a mask and bilevel positive airway pressure (BiPAP) also delivered with nasal or full face masks provides respiratory support using positive pressure without a tracheal tube. In patients who have been extubated but have increased work of breathing or have developed atelectasis, these methods will often avert the need for reintubation. In patients with ventricular dysfunction and marginal hemodynamics, a planned extubation to noninvasive support such as CPAP will provide continued afterload reduction of the systemic ventricle (37). Also, for those patients with prolonged ventilator courses and respiratory muscle deconditioning, a planned extubation directly to CPAP or BiPAP with subsequent weaning can successfully transition a patient to unassisted breathing. Children often require additional sedation to tolerate CPAP and BiPAP masks for longer periods of time.

Sedation, Analgesia, and Neurologic Monitoring

Sedation and analgesia are important components of postoperative care of pediatric cardiac surgical patients. The strategy of sedation and analgesia should be tailored to the age and anatomy of the patient; type of repair and operative course, including rhythm and bleeding concerns; and anticipated postoperative course, including timing of sternal closure (if delayed) and initial hemodynamics. A patient following atrial septal defect closure requires different sedation and analgesia management than a patient following stage 1 palliation who has an open sternum and labile blood pressure. Analgesia is initiated in the operating room, and most agents used are narcotic based. High-dose narcotics have been shown to alleviate the stress response associated with cardiac surgery and CPB (38,39). High-dose fentanyl (up to 25 μg/kg) can be administered to neonates with minimal hemodynamic effect (40). As a continuation of operative anesthesia, patients with marginal hemodynamics and complex repairs or palliations are deeply sedated with continuous fentanyl infusions and usually paralyzed as well for the initial postoperative course to minimize the stress response and oxygen consumption. Interventions in the intensive care unit that may provoke stress such as tracheal tube suctioning should be managed with anticipatory doses of fentanyl (41).

Common muscle relaxants used in the pediatric cardiac intensive care unit are rocuronium, vecuronium, pancuronium, and cisatracurium. Rocuronium has the shortest onset of action and is often used for intubation, but not continuous paralysis. Vecuronium is commonly employed as an infusion for continuous paralysis. Pancuronium is the longest-acting agent and is cleared by the kidneys, so it should be used with caution in patients with renal insufficiency. Cisatracurium is cleared by Hofmann degradation (i.e., independent of renal and hepatic function), so it may be the best choice in patients with multisystem organ failure. The significant side effects of succinylcholine, including severe bradycardia, have limited its routine use in the pediatric cardiac population.

Patients who have achieved hemodynamic stability but may require a longer ventilatory course for diuresis or pulmonary recovery, such as after a unifocalization procedure, benefit from sedation with continuous infusions of a narcotic and benzodiazepine. This provides a more continuous level of sedation and analgesia than intermittent bolus dosing of these agents. As the patient develops tolerance to these agents over several days, doses must be increased to achieve the same effect. The most common narcotic used is morphine, but fentanyl (shorter acting) and hydromorphone can be considered. Caution should be used with bolus dosing of fentanyl because of an idiosyncratic chest wall rigidity reaction that can occur with rapid infusion (42,43). Chest wall rigidity can prevent effective ventilation, and rapid muscle relaxation may be required to treat it.

Midazolam is the most common benzodiazepine used and is desirable due to its amnestic properties. Lorazepam and diazepam are other sedating benzodiazepines employed in the cardiac intensive care unit, but they are administered in bolus doses rather than as infusions. Patients typically develop tolerance to narcotics and benzodiazepine infusions after 5 to 7 days and will need to be transitioned to methadone and lorazepam for a weaning taper after extubation. The advantage to these agents is that they are longer acting and can be administered orally. Therefore, recovered patients can continue narcotic and benzodiazepine tapering as outpatients. Patients who have been successfully extubated can be transitioned to oral agents including acetaminophen, ibuprofen, and oxycodone. Older patients can benefit from the use of narcotic-based patient-controlled analgesia pumps. Short courses of the nonsteroidal anti-inflammatory drug ketorolac (eight doses or less) can be used in patients with normal coagulation and renal function.

Propofol has become a popular sedating agent in adult ICUs (44). It has a rapid onset of action and clearance, and it is an ideal agent in patients for whom rapid awakening is desired. Of note, propofol has no analgesic properties. Because it is a potent vasodilator and negative inotrope, it has limited use in cardiac patients with decreased myocardial function. There also have been reports of myocardial failure and acidosis in children (45). Therefore, propofol has generally been restricted to short-term use in older patients with two-ventricle physiology and normal myocardial function who are anticipated to extubate within 6 to 12 hours.

A promising new agent for sedation in the pediatric population is dexmedetomidine (46). It is an α_2 agonist used as a continuous infusion in addition to a narcotic and benzodiazepine. Patients treated with a dexmedetomidine infusion require fewer rescue doses of other agents for sedation. The infusion does not depress respiration, and patients do not develop tolerance. Thus far, this agent appears safe and effective in pediatric cardiac patients, although data are limited to older infants and children (47). Some patients develop bradycardia, which resolves when the infusion is discontinued. A relative contraindication to dexmedetomidine may be high-grade AV nodal block or concurrent administration of medications that slow conduction at the AV node such as digoxin (48).

Procedural anesthesia in the cardiac intensive care unit for intubations, chest thoracentesis, and catheter placement is commonly required. For many patients, ketamine is an excellent agent for this indication. It is a dissociative anesthetic agent with rapid onset and excellent analgesic properties. Heart rate and blood pressure are preserved through central stimulation and diminished postganglionic reuptake. It has minimal effects on respiratory drive at lower doses, although airway secretions can be increased. A benzodiazepine should be given concurrently for hallucinations in older children. Another effective agent for procedural anesthesia is etomidate. It causes minimal cardiovascular depression and is an ideal agent for tracheal intubation in a hemodynamically compromised patient. Chloral hydrate is a hypnotic agent that can be safely given by mouth or per rectum for nonpainful procedures such as echocardiography.

The practice of neurologic monitoring in postoperative patients is evolving as more information about the neurologic sequelae of cardiac surgery becomes available. The incidence of neurologic abnormalities following CPB surgery is likely to be higher than reported. Postoperative electroencephalographic (EEG) seizures occur in up to 11% to 20% of neonates undergoing contemporary CPB techniques (49,50). The duration of deep hypothermic circulatory arrest appears to have a role in the incidence of seizures (50). Periventricular leukomalacia (as a marker of brain injury) is found on brain magnetic resonance imaging (MRI) in greater than 50% of neonates after congenital heart surgery (51). Most of these lesions appear to resolve over time, but the long-term implications on cognition and development are still being determined (52).

Neurologic surveillance in the cardiac intensive care unit is increasing. Routine EEG monitoring and a brain MRI for every patient are not practical. These tests tend to be reserved for patients with a high clinical suspicion of neurologic injury. The increasing use of near-infrared spectroscopy (NIRS) to monitor transcutaneous cerebral oxygen saturation in the intensive care unit may help identify periods of vulnerability to central nervous system injury. The cerebral oxygen saturation is measured by an oximeter probe placed on the forehead below the hairline. The measured saturation is a combination of mixed venous saturation (approximately 85%) and arterial saturation (approximately 15%). Normal cerebral oxygen saturation varies with cardiac defect but is approximately 70% in acyanotic lesions. A decrease of cerebral oxygen saturation of 20% from baseline was associated with an increased incidence of seizures and coma (53), and prolonged cerebral oxygen desaturation <45% has been associated with an increased incidence of periventricular leukomalacia on brain MRI (54). This technology may be used to monitor cerebral oxygen saturation as a surrogate for cerebral oxygen delivery. Studies demonstrating that interventions that raise the cerebral oxygen saturation lead to a reduction in neurologic injury have not been published to date.

Fluids and Nutrition

The body's inflammatory response to CPB results in significant increases in total body water and edema with diffuse capillary leak. Operative strategies to minimize this process include ultrafiltration on CPB and steroid administration (55). High-risk patients such as neonates and young infants may have peritoneal dialysis catheters placed electively in the operating room. Fluid management and diuretic therapy in the first 24 to 48 hours after cardiac surgery have a significant impact on the patient's hemodynamic status and recovery. During the first 24 hours, many patients are oliguric despite adequate atrial filling pressures. Longer CPB times, increased complexity of the repair, and preoperative renal dysfunction contribute to the duration of oliguria. Intravenous fluids should be restricted to one half of calculated maintenance fluids for at least 24 hours (or longer) if the patient does not have improved urine output. Preload should be maintained with crystalloid or colloid solutions using intermittent boluses of 5 to 10 mL/kg. Albumin (5% solution) priming of CPB circuits results in less requirement for volume expansion and less weight gain during and after CPB when compared to crystalloid solutions (56). This is likely due to increased intravascular oncotic pressure with albumin administration. Anecdotally, neonates benefit from volume expansion with 5% albumin over crystalloid, although there are no controlled trials comparing colloid and crystalloid in the postoperative setting. Older children with less complex repairs can receive normal saline or lactated Ringer solution to avoid blood product exposure.

Electrolytes should be normalized; potassium replacement should be performed cautiously in patients who are oliguric to avoid hyperkalemia. Calcium is a potent inotrope and ionized calcium levels should be maintained at the higher end of the normal range for age (1.2–1.3 mmol/L) (57). This strategy is particularly useful in neonates, patients with 22q11.2 deletions (DiGeorge syndrome) with hypoparathyroidism, and patients with myocardial dysfunction. Calcium can be repleted with bolus dosing (10 mg/kg calcium chloride or 100 mg/kg calcium gluconate) or with a continuous infusion. Magnesium should be repleted to avoid the development of ventricular dysrhythmias, which is more common with hypomagnesemia.

After 12 to 24 hours, diuretics can be introduced as bolus doses or as a continuous infusion. Diuretics can be considered earlier in patients with large left-to-right shunts and pulmonary edema to encourage clearance of excess lung water and weaning from the ventilator. Diuretics should be held longer than 24 hours in hemodynamically unstable patients who need frequent preload repletion with volume boluses. The diuretic initiated first at most institutions is the loop diuretic furosemide; it is administered at a 1 to 2 mg/kg dose intravenously every 6 to 12 hours. A continuous furosemide infusion of 0.1 to 0.3 mg/kg/hour (after an initial loading dose of 1 mg/kg) may be more desirable in hemodynamically fragile patients, or in patients with significant fluid overload (58). If urine output is not adequate, a second agent can be added. Common agents include the thiazide diuretic chlorothiazide, which can be given at a 5 to 10 mg/kg dose intravenously every 6 to 12 hours, and metolazone, which can be given at a 0.1 to 0.4 mg/kg dose enterally once daily. Newer agents including fenoldopam (Table 81.6), a selective dopamine receptor agonist, and nesiritide (Table 81.7), a natriuretic peptide, are additional choices (59,60).

It is common for patients to develop a significant hypochloremic metabolic alkalosis, as well as hypokalemia and hyponatremia, when receiving furosemide and/or chlorothiazide. Chloride can be repleted with arginine chloride, potassium chloride, or sodium chloride (only if hyponatremic from sodium loss and not congestive heart failure). Neonatal patients with shunted single-ventricle physiology can develop high serum bicarbonate levels and a compensatory respiratory acidosis with hypochloremia; their electrolytes should be normalized prior to extubation. Their reduced ventilatory drive and potential for apnea may impact the balance of pulmonary and systemic blood flow if not corrected prior to extubation.

Significant renal dysfunction beyond 72 hours after cardiac surgery is uncommon. Renal replacement therapy should be considered when renal function continues to worsen despite maximizing cardiac output. Often a peritoneal dialysis catheter inserted into the peritoneum and placed to gravity drainage can improve fluid balance without dialysis. Indications for dialysis include life-threatening electrolyte abnormalities including hyperkalemia, persistent metabolic acidosis, severe fluid overload impairing ventilation or sternal closure (if open), and rising blood urea nitrogen levels >100 mg/dL. If required, dialysis can be accomplished with peritoneal exchanges or with continuous venovenous hemofiltration (61). Conventional hemodialysis is usually not well tolerated in postoperative cardiac patients with myocardial dysfunction. Significant ongoing renal dysfunction carries a poor prognosis with >50% mortality in some reports (62,63).

Adequate nutrition after cardiac surgery is required for adequate wound healing and recovery. Unfortunately, nutrition is often compromised for several days due to hemodynamic instability and fluid intake restrictions. Enteral feedings should be restarted as soon as feasible. The use of promotility agents such as metoclopramide and postpyloric feeding tubes can enable enteral feeding in nearly all postoperative cardiac patients. An absolute contraindication for enteral feeding is the presence of necrotizing enterocolitis. Relative contraindications are the presence of an umbilical artery catheter, high-dose vasoconstrictive agents, and paralysis. Patients at increased risk for necrotizing enterocolitis are neonates with left-sided obstructive lesions, aortopulmonary shunts, and cyanotic lesions (64). Enteral feedings can be introduced in these patients but should advance slowly with close observation for signs of feeding intolerance such as emesis and abdominal distention. In

TABLE 81.6

SUMMARY OF CATECHOLAMINES AND DOPAMINERGIC AGENTS

Name	IV dose range	Peripheral vascular effect			Cardiac effect		Comment
		Alpha	Beta2	Dopa	Beta1	Beta2	
Dopamine	2–4 μg/kg/min 4–10 μg/kg/min 10–20 μg/kg/min	0 0 2–4+	0 2+ 0	2+ 2+ 0	0 1–2+ 1–2+	0 1+ 2+	Increasing doses produce increasing alpha effect, splanchnic vasodilator
Epinephrine	0.01–0.05 μg/kg/min 0.1–0.5 μg/kg/min	1+ 4+	1–2+ 0	0 0	2–3+ 4+	2+ 3+	Increasing doses produce increasing alpha effect
Dobutamine	2–10 μg/kg/min	1+	2+	0	3–4+	1–2+	Dose-dependant effect similar to dopamine, increasing doses associated with tachycardia and dysrhythmias
Isoproterenol	0.1–0.5 μg/kg/min	0	4+	0	4+	4+	Potent inotrope and chronotrope, vasodilator, increasing doses produce tachycardia and increased oxygen consumption
Norepinephrine	0.01–0.1 μg/kg/min	4+	1+	0	2+	1+	Moderate inotrope, increases systemic vascular resistance
Phenylephrine	0.01–0.5 μg/kg/min	4+	0	0	0	0	Increases systemic vascular resistance, no inotropy
Fenoldopam	0.05–1 μg/kg/min	0	0	yes	0	0	Dopaminergic receptor agonist. Little chronotopic or inotropic effect. May increase renal blood flow

IV, intravenous; kg, kilogram; min, minute
From Castanada AR. *Cardiac Surgery of the Neonate and Infant*. Philadelphia: W. B. Saunders, 1994.

patients for whom enteral feedings are not feasible, total parenteral nutrition should be used to avoid a catabolic state. Ranitidine or another histamine-2 antagonist should be routinely prescribed for protection against gastric mucosal bleeding from stress and nasogastric tubes until full-volume enteral feeds are re-established. Extubated patients with nausea should be treated with antiemetics such as ondansetron to encourage oral intake and weaning of intravenous fluids.

Infectious Issues

In the first 24 hours following surgery, it is common for patients to have fever. This is presumably related to the inflammatory response after CPB and does not represent infection. Early postoperative fevers should be treated to help minimize oxygen consumption, but the patient may be observed for additional signs of infection prior to starting antibiotic treatment. All patients receive at least three doses of a second-generation cephalosporin (e.g., cefazolin) intravenously in the first 24 hours after surgery as prophylaxis. Treatment is extended in high-risk patients such as those with an open sternum, with immune deficiency, or receiving mechanical circulatory support. Fevers that persist or arise after the first 24 hours should be evaluated with a physical exam focused on the sternal incision, blood cultures obtained from indwelling intravascular catheters, and a urine culture. If tracheal secretions are copious and/or discolored, suggesting a respiratory source for fever, a tracheal aspirate may be obtained for Gram stain and culture. Chronically ventilated patients are often colonized with bacteria in their trachea, so a qualitative change in their secretions or increase in white blood cells on Gram stain may indicate a new respiratory infection. If the clinical suspicion for infection is high, intravenous antibacterial coverage should be broadened while awaiting culture results. Nosocomial infections are a significant cause of morbidity in the ICU (65,66). Every effort should be made to insert intravascular catheters using sterile technique, to enter and manipulate catheters using meticulous care, and to remove intravascular catheters as soon as feasible. Mediastinitis is a serious postoperative infection that occurs in approximately 2% of patients, with *Staphylococcus aureus* as the most common bacterial agent. Risk factors include prolonged open sternum and need for multiple chest re-explorations (67). Prompt antibiotic treatment with open debridement and use of muscle flaps has decreased the morbidity and mortality from mediastinitis (68).

LOW CARDIAC OUTPUT SYNDROME

Low cardiac output syndrome (LCOS) is a common problem after congenital heart surgery with CPB, especially in neonates

TABLE 81.7

SUMMARY OF NONCATECHOLAMINE VASOACTIVE AGENTS

Name	IV dose range	Peripheral vascular effect	Cardiac effect	Comment
Calcium		Vasoconstrictor	Inotropic effect; depends on iCa level	Slows sinus node and AV node conduction
Chloride	10–20 mg/kg			
Gluconate	50–100 mg/kg			
Milrinone	50 μg/kg load 0.25–1 μg/kg/min	Systemic and pulmonary vasodilator	Diastolic relaxation, decreases afterload	Minimal tachycardia
Amrinone	1–3 mg/kg load 5–20 μg/kg/min	Systemic and pulmonary vasodilator	Diastolic relaxation, decreases afterload	Minimal tachycardia, lowers platelet count, longer half life than milrinone
Nitroprusside	0.5–5 μg/kg/min	NO donor, relaxes smooth muscle, dilates pulmonary and systemic vessels	Decreases afterload	Reflex tachycardia
Nitroglycerin	0.5–10 μg/kg/min	NO donor, venodilator, more preload effect than nitroprusside	Decreases preload and afterload, may decrease myocardial wall stress	Minimal tachycardia, sometimes used as a coronary vasodilator
Vasopressin	0.0003–0.003 U/kg/min	Potent vasoconstrictor	Weak inotrope	Used to increase systemic blood pressure
Tri-iodothyronine	0.05–0.1 μg/kg/hour	Vasodilation	Inotrope	Tachycardia
Nesiritide	0.01–0.03 μg/kg/min	Natriuresis	Diastolic relaxation	Hyponatremia
Digoxin	6–10 μg/kg/day	Increases systemic vascular resistance	Inotrope	Slows sinus node and AV node conduction

IV, intravenous; mg, milligram; kg, kilogram; min, minute; iCa, ionized calcium; U, units; NO, nitric oxide; AV, atrioventricular; μg, microgram.

and young infants (69). Many factors are thought to contribute to decreased cardiac output including myocardial ischemia from aortic cross-clamping and associated reperfusion injury, inflammation from CPB, ventriculotomies (when performed), and the existence of hemodynamically significant residual lesions. There is an expected decrease in cardiac output that occurs over the first 6 to 12 hours after CPB with a nadir of <2 L/minute/m^2 in the youngest patients (70). With appropriate recognition, the significant morbidities and occasional mortality related to LCOS can be prevented.

Recognition of Low Cardiac Output

There are several clinical symptoms and signs of LCOS that should be immediately recognized (Table 81.8). On physical exam, early findings of low cardiac output include tachycardia, cool extremities, delayed capillary refill time, and diminished pulses. Decreased urine output, elevated filling pressures, and low mixed venous oxygen saturation are important signs. Hypotension and metabolic acidosis are later findings; they require immediate attention or a cardiac arrest may be imminent. Evaluation of LCOS should begin with physical exam. For example, auscultation for pathologic murmurs caused by residual obstructions, shunts, or valvar regurgitation is important. Hepatomegaly and ascites may indicate right heart failure, especially in surgeries involving right ventriculotomies. An echocardiogram should be obtained promptly to assess ventricular systolic function and to rule out tamponade. The quality of the repair should be assessed to look for residual lesions that can be corrected by reoperation or catheter-based intervention. Large residual shunts, severe valvular regurgitation, outflow

TABLE 81.8

SIGNS OF LOW CARDIAC OUTPUT SYNDROME

PHYSICAL EXAM/SIGNS
Tachycardia
Hypotension
Narrowed pulse pressure/diminished pulses
Cool extremities
Central hyperthermia
Diminished heart sounds
Hepatomegaly
Pleural effusion and ascites
Oliguria
Elevated central venous pressure/left atrial pressure

LABORATORY
Anion gap acidosis
Elevated lactate
Low mixed venous saturation
Indices of abnormal end organ function
Cardiomegaly on chest radiograph

tract obstructions, and venous baffle obstructions are generally poorly tolerated in the postoperative patient. If the patient has an open sternum, or if chest dressings obstruct transthoracic echocardiographic windows, a transesophageal echocardiogram should be performed. Occasionally, the etiology of the low cardiac output is not obvious by echocardiography or needs additional clarification before considering reoperation. There should be a low threshold to progress to cardiac catheterization in these patients. Catheterization in this population can be accomplished safely, even in patients supported with ECMO, and facilitates the diagnosis of important lesions in a majority of the patients (55%–76%) that can be addressed with interventional catheter procedures or reoperation (71,72).

Treatment of Low Cardiac Output Syndrome

Once LCOS is recognized, and concurrent with ruling out correctible residual lesions, immediate therapy should be initiated. The goals of therapy are to maximize oxygen delivery and minimize oxygen consumption of the recovering myocardium. Anemic patients should be transfused with packed red blood cells to increase oxygen-carrying capacity. Cardiac output is a function of preload, contractility, and afterload. Intravascular volume should be repleted either with a colloid solution such as 5% albumin or alternatively with a crystalloid solution. Pharmacologic agents can be used to increase inotropy and decrease afterload (see Tables 81.6 and 81.7). Fevers should be actively prevented (e.g., by cooling the patient) to minimize oxygen consumption. The most unstable patients should receive neuromuscular blockade, deep sedation or anesthesia, and active cooling to minimize oxygen consumption. Continual reassessment of the response to therapy by physical exam focused on perfusion, and monitored parameters such as urine output and acidosis, is required.

Pharmacologic Therapy

Catecholamines (Table 81.6) have been the first-choice pharmacologic agents for increasing cardiac output. Almost all patients who undergo congenital heart surgery receive dopamine immediately after CPB. Dopamine stimulates β receptors in the heart and increases contractility; typical initial dosing is 3 to 7 μg/kg/minute via continuous infusion. Higher doses (>10 μg/kg/minute) will also stimulate α receptors in the peripheral vasculature and cause vasoconstriction. Epinephrine is another commonly used catecholamine. Low to moderate doses of epinephrine (0.02–0.1 μg/kg/minute) increase contractility and cause mild peripheral vasoconstriction, both of which tend to increase blood pressure. Dobutamine primarily stimulates β receptors in the heart. Higher doses have been associated with arrhythmias and tachycardia. This synthetic catecholamine is most often used in pediatric patients with chronic congestive heart failure (e.g., dilated cardiomyopathy) rather than in the postoperative setting. Isoproterenol stimulates β receptors in the heart and is both an inotrope and chronotrope. Because it causes tachycardia, which increases oxygen consumption, and peripheral vasodilation, which can lower blood pressure, it is not commonly used to treat LCOS. Norepinephrine and phenylephrine (pure α agonist) are predominantly α-receptor agonists; norepinephrine possesses reduced inotropic activity compared to dopamine and epinephrine, and their use is limited to patients with profound hypotension. Arginine vasopressin is a noncatecholamine vasoconstrictor that increases blood pressure by promoting vascular smooth muscle constriction without causing tachycardia. Its use has been described in patients with vasodilatory shock, but its role in cardiogenic shock is unclear and it has not improved outcomes in pediatric patients with poor myocardial function (73–75). Patients requiring continued high doses of these potent vasoconstricting agents to support systemic blood pressure should be considered for mechanical circulatory support. Catecholamines should also be used judiciously in postoperative neonates. While these agents do increase cardiac output, the relatively noncompliant neonatal myocardium may be more susceptible to catecholamine-driven increases in tachycardia, afterload, and oxygen consumption. Animal data show actual necrosis of neonatal piglet myocardium exposed to high-dose epinephrine (76). Fortunately, alternative pharmacologic options are available.

Afterload reduction is increasingly recognized as the principal form of pharmacologic support for the myocardium after CPB. The type III phosphodiesterase inhibitors milrinone and amrinone inhibit the breakdown of cyclic adenosine monophosphate (AMP), thus increasing the intracellular Ca^{2+} concentration, which enhances myocyte contractility, peripheral vasodilation, and diastolic relaxation (77). Milrinone has a shorter half-life than amrinone and less antiplatelet side effects, thus making it the more desirable alternative. Milrinone is tolerated well by postoperative neonates, and it promotes increased cardiac output, lower atrial pressures, and decreased pulmonary and systemic vascular resistance (78). A large, multicenter trial of milrinone after congenital heart surgery investigated the prophylactic use of milrinone in preventing LCOS. Patients treated with 0.75 μg/kg/minute of milrinone had a relative risk reduction of 55% for LCOS compared to patients treated with placebo (79). Based on these data and anecdotal experience, milrinone combined with dopamine is currently the combination therapy most commonly used to prevent and treat LCOS after congenital heart surgery. The vasodilators nitroprusside and nitroglycerine, both of which are nitric oxide donors, can decrease afterload and improve cardiac output, but they have no direct inotropic effects on the heart.

Other agents used to treat LCOS include thyroid hormone, B-type natriuretic peptide (BNP), and glucocorticoids. All patients exposed to CPB develop low thyroid hormone levels in the blood approximately 24 hours after bypass; this typically recovers by 5 to 7 days. Data are mixed, but there is some evidence that replacing tri-iodothyronine, the biologically active form of thyroid hormone, after congenital heart surgery increases cardiac output, blood pressure, and time to negative fluid balance and extubation (80–82). The natriuretic hormone system is important in regulating fluid balance and is normally activated in response to atrial stretch receptors. Data from adult patients with heart failure suggest that infusions of nesiritide, a synthetic form of BNP, decreases atrial pressures and systemic vascular resistance, and improves cardiac output (83). Preliminary pediatric data are less convincing for improved cardiac output, although diuresis was enhanced (60). Lastly, glucocorticoids in the form of hydrocortisone have been shown to decrease the inotrope requirements in neonates and infants receiving high-dose catecholamines (>0.15 μg/kg/minute epinephrine) after congenital heart surgery (84). The mechanism of the effect is not clear, but may be due to increased expression of β receptors on myocytes. Inflammation after CPB may produce relative adrenal insufficiency and vasodilation that is partially reversed with additional steroids in the postoperative course. However, many of the patients studied did not have cortisol levels measured prior to glucocorticoid administration.

Extracorporeal Membrane Oxygenation

When all interventions to maximize oxygen delivery are performed but the patient remains in a low cardiac output state with metabolic acidosis and end organ dysfunction, mechanical circulatory support should be considered. The principal mode of mechanical circulatory support in the postoperative pediatric cardiac patient is venoarterial (cardiac) ECMO. The overall goal of ECMO is to provide myocardial rest that allows for recovery. The indications for cardiac ECMO are listed in Table 81.9. Ideally, the patient should be placed on ECMO before the development of severe end organ dysfunction or cardiac arrest. In the event of an unexpected cardiac arrest, a patient can be supported using a crystalloid-primed circuit following rapid arterial and venous cannulation. Survival to hospital discharge as high as 64% has been reported for such patients (85). Cannulation can be initiated via an open sternum with direct atrial and aortic cannulation when the patient fails to wean from CPB or suffers a postoperative cardiac arrest. Alternatively, the neck or groin vessels can be accessed if there is more time for cannulation.

The expected course of myocardial recovery after CPB is 3 to 5 days (86,87). If the patient is unable to wean from ECMO after this time, and there are no residual cardiac lesions to be corrected, the possibility of cardiac transplantation should be explored, since most patients cannot be supported with ECMO for longer than 2 to 4 weeks due to complications. Smaller ventricular assist devices are becoming available to bridge infants and young children to transplant when indicated (88). Patient populations with poor outcomes are those who fail to wean from CPB, those with cavopulmonary connections, and adult congenital patients (89,90). The results of cardiac ECMO for all indications through July 2006 as reported to the international registry of the Extracorporeal Life Support Organization (ELSO) were 60% survival through decannulation and 42% survival to discharge (89).

TABLE 81.9

INDICATIONS FOR VENOARTERIAL EXTRACORPOREAL MEMBRANE OXYGENATION

LOW CARDIAC OUTPUT
Cardiomyopathy with progressive dysfunction
Myocarditis
Failure to wean from cardiopulmonary bypass
Sudden cardiac arrest
CYANOSIS
Marked intracardiac shunting with inadequate oxygenation
Acute obstruction to pulmonary flow (shunt thrombosis)
Pulmonary hemorrhage from pulmonary venous hypertension
Respiratory failure
ARRHYTHMIA
Refractory primary arrhythmias
Postoperative arrhythmia
SUPPORT DURING INTERVENTIONAL PROCEDURES
Intervention that creates life-threatening physiology

Support of the Myocardium after Cardiac Transplantation

Pediatric cardiac transplant recipients are a unique population in the postoperative period because both donor and recipient considerations are relevant to outcomes. Myocardial function of the donated heart will depend on donor factors including the circumstances leading to donor status, the level of vasoactive support preharvest, and the ischemic time. Recipient factors include preoperative pulmonary vascular resistance and its impact on donor right heart function, end organ function, and the overall condition of the patient. Patients with congenital heart disease often have pre-existing adhesions and variant anatomy that may complicate and lengthen transplant surgery. Because the transplanted heart is denervated and tends to be bradycardic in the immediate postoperative period, pacing wires should be placed to allow control of the heart rate. If pacing wires do not exist or do not capture, isoproterenol can be used as a chronotrope. This is less desirable because isoproterenol increases oxygen consumption and can cause arrhythmias and systemic hypotension at higher doses. All cardiac transplant patients should have both right and left heart atrial pressures monitored. In infants and young children, this will necessitate the placement of an intracardiac left atrial catheter. Monitoring both right and left heart filling pressures is critical in differentiating right heart failure caused by elevated PVR (only right atrial pressures elevated) from biventricular failure due to graft ischemia or acute rejection (both right and left atrial pressures elevated). Right heart failure is an important cause of morbidity and mortality after cardiac transplantation and should be treated aggressively (see next section) (91).

Pulmonary Hypertension and Right Heart Failure

Primary right heart failure and pulmonary hypertension leading to secondary right heart failure are significant causes of morbidity in postoperative pediatric cardiac patients. Primary right heart failure should be anticipated in patients undergoing right ventriculotomies for right ventricular outflow tract reconstruction (e.g., tetralogy of Fallot repair) or conduit placement (e.g., truncus arteriosus repair). Those at risk for pulmonary hypertension and secondary right heart failure include patients with pulmonary venous or pulmonary arterial obstruction, heart transplant recipients with elevated PVR from preoperative left atrial hypertension, and patients with preoperative pulmonary hypertension from large left-to-right shunts (16). Anticipatory postoperative care and early recognition of right ventricular dysfunction will optimize recovery.

Patients who are expected to have a reactive pulmonary vascular bed should have a transthoracic pulmonary artery or right ventricular catheter placed intraoperatively for monitoring in the ICU. In the absence of direct measurement of pulmonary artery pressures, signs of pulmonary hypertension include elevated right-sided filling pressures with normal or low left-sided filling pressures and tachycardia. Patients with right-to-left shunts can become more cyanotic. As the right heart fails, physical exam will reveal poor perfusion, hepatomegaly, and possibly a loud tricuspid regurgitation murmur. In a pulmonary hypertensive crisis, signs of poor left heart filling occur and include systemic hypotension and bradycardia. In the immediate postoperative period, a patient with pulmonary hypertension should be evaluated for residual anatomic problems. Residual pulmonary venous obstruction, pulmonary artery stenosis, or significant left-to-right shunts can all cause pulmonary hypertension and may not be responsive to medical therapies.

Patients who undergo an extensive right ventriculotomy or who are anticipated to have pulmonary hypertension can benefit from an intraoperative strategy that allows right-to-left shunting at the atrial level. Typically, these are patients with tetralogy of Fallot or truncus arteriosus who have hypertrophied and noncompliant right ventricles. With an incision as part of the repair, the right ventricle may develop both systolic and diastolic dysfunction (92). If a transannular patch across the right ventricular outflow tract is required to relieve obstruction, pulmonary regurgitation creates a volume load on the struggling right ventricle as well. It is helpful to leave the foramen ovale patent, or even to create a new atrial level communication, to allow the right ventricle to decompress with a right-to-left shunt. In this physiology, systemic cardiac output will be preserved at the expense of mild cyanosis, which is usually well tolerated and transient (93).

Postoperative care should focus on minimizing the reactivity of the pulmonary vascular bed. The post-CPB inflammatory response, pulmonary arterial endothelial dysfunction, and alveolar hypoxia from edema and atelectasis all contribute to pulmonary hypertension (16). These should be time-limited processes as the patient recovers. The strategies for medical treatments are outlined in Table 81.10. The initial approach is to minimize the factors that increase PVR. Acidosis, agitation, and hypoxia all increase PVR and can provoke a pulmonary hypertensive crisis. Therefore, patients with pulmonary hypertension should be pain free, deeply sedated, and possibly paralyzed. They should be maintained with a mild alkalosis using either mild hyperventilation or sodium bicarbonate administration. Oxygen is a pulmonary vasodilator, so patients should receive supplemental oxygen and not be weaned to room air even if the arterial oxygen saturation is normal. Patients not responding to these initial maneuvers should be treated with vasodilators.

TABLE 81.10

TREATMENT OF POSTOPERATIVE PULMONARY HYPERTENSION

ENCOURAGE/ADMINISTER

Investigate for residual shunts, obstructions to pulmonary blood flow
Supplemental oxygen
Mild alkalosis (pH 7.45–7.5)
Mild hyperventilation (pH 7.45–7.5)
Sedation and analgesia, consider paralysis
Inotropic support of right ventricle
Intravenous vasodilators
Inhaled nitric oxide

AVOID

Metabolic acidosis (pH <7.30)
Hypoventilation or respiratory acidosis
Agitation and pain
Alveolar hypoxia
Atelectasis or alveolar overdistention
Polycythemia

Nitric oxide (NO) is a selective pulmonary vasodilator when inhaled. It crosses the alveolar wall where it acts on vascular smooth muscle by increasing levels of cyclic guanosine monophosphate (cGMP) to cause relaxation. It is usually delivered via a tracheal tube but can also be delivered via a face mask or nasal cannula. A reduction in pulmonary artery pressure is usually seen at doses of up to 40 parts per million; higher doses may increase toxicity (from methemoglobinemia) without any additional reduction in the pulmonary pressure (94). The uses of inhaled nitric oxide (iNO) in the treatment of pulmonary hypertension after congenital heart surgery are extensive (95,96). Its selective pulmonary vasodilation occurs without significant systemic hemodynamic effects, which is desirable in tenuous postoperative patients. The most responsive patients appear to be those who have relief of pulmonary venous obstruction such as with repair of obstructed total anomalous pulmonary venous return or congenital mitral stenosis (97). iNO is also an ideal agent to prevent right ventricular failure in a transplanted heart not accustomed to elevated PVR (91,98).

After the patient's pulmonary artery pressures have normalized and diuresis has been achieved, iNO can be slowly weaned off. If the dose of iNO is decreased too rapidly (e.g., dose lowered at intervals <4 to 6 hours), and especially below doses of 5 parts per million, pulmonary hypertension can recur. This is called "rebound" pulmonary hypertension (99). If the patient fails to wean off due to rebound, he or she can be transitioned to sildenafil (a phosphodiesterase type V inhibitor, which reduces the degradation of cGMP) to mitigate this phenomenon and as a transition to oral therapy (100,101). Caution should be used in administering iNO to patients with pulmonary hypertension caused by severe left ventricular dysfunction. Pulmonary vasodilation can increase pulmonary blood flow and left atrial pressures, which may volume overload the left ventricle, causing further dysfunction (102).

Intravenous vasodilators are not selective for the pulmonary vasculature, but some agents still have a role in treating pulmonary hypertension and right ventricular dysfunction. Milrinone (a phosphodiesterase type III inhibitor) is used to afterload reduce the right ventricle and provide inotropic support and diastolic relaxation. Prostaglandin derivatives such as prostacyclin, delivered either nebulized or as an intravenous infusion, can be beneficial but are dose limited by their systemic vasodilatory side effects. Prostacyclin is now commonly prescribed as a long-term outpatient therapy for pulmonary hypertension associated with congenital heart disease in children (103). Given the extensive literature supporting the benefits of iNO, the nonspecific vasodilators such as nitroprusside, tolazoline (an α-receptor agonist), and isoproterenol should be used infrequently for the treatment of postoperative pulmonary hypertension (104). Oral therapies for adults with chronic primary pulmonary hypertension, including calcium channel blockers and endothelin receptor blockers, have not been adequately studied in children in the postoperative setting, but may have a future role.

SINGLE-VENTRICLE PHYSIOLOGY

Patients with single-ventricle physiology are among the most challenging to care for in the pediatric cardiac intensive care unit. There are many variations of single-ventricle anatomy, but the defects can be broadly divided into those with a single left ventricle and obstruction to pulmonary blood flow, such as tricuspid or pulmonary atresia, and those with a single right ventricle and obstruction to systemic blood flow, such as HLHS. Most neonates with single-ventricle anatomy require prostaglandin E_1 to maintain adequate pulmonary or systemic blood flow via the ductus arteriosus. The single ventricle's output occurs in parallel to the lungs and body, rather than in series as in normal (two-ventricle) physiology. The output to the systemic and pulmonary circulations is dependent on the vascular resistance in each circulation. The single ventricle's workload is the sum of the outputs to these two circulations, so that the single ventricle does the work of two ventricles. During the postnatal transition, PVR falls rapidly, so these patients often develop excessive pulmonary blood flow and compromised systemic flow within a few days of birth. This is commonly referred to as pulmonary overcirculation.

Most neonates with single-ventricle anatomy will need a palliative operation. This will be either an aortopulmonary shunt when pulmonary flow is obstructed or a stage I (Norwood) operation with aortic arch reconstruction and an aortopulmonary shunt or right ventricle–pulmonary artery conduit when systemic flow is obstructed. Occasionally, a single-ventricle patient will have unobstructed pulmonary and systemic blood flow through two well-developed outflow tracts. These patients usually require a pulmonary artery band shortly after birth to limit pulmonary blood flow as their first-stage palliation.

Shunted Single-ventricle Physiology

Irrespective of whether a stage I palliation, aortopulmonary shunt alone, or pulmonary artery band is the first palliative operation, the principles of balancing the systemic and pulmonary circulations are the same in the postoperative period. The operation does not alter the basic physiology of parallel circulations. An acceptable balance of pulmonary-to-systemic blood flow can be defined as sufficient pulmonary blood flow to provide adequate systemic oxygenation without pulmonary overcirculation. The newer modification of the stage I palliation that includes a right ventricle–to–pulmonary artery conduit is less likely to create overcirculation compared to an aortopulmonary shunt, since pulmonary blood flow occurs only in systole (105). However, depending on the size of the patient and the conduit, overcirculation from a right ventricle–to–pulmonary artery conduit can still occur. Assuming normal pulmonary venous saturations of 100% and normal oxygen extraction with a mixed venous saturation of 60%, a systemic and pulmonary artery saturation of 80% would result in a pulmonary blood flow (Qp)–to–systemic blood flow (Qs) ratio of 1:1, which represents balanced circulations (106). This would correlate with an arterial PaO_2 of approximately 40 mm Hg. Typically, the Qp:Qs ratio is higher than this, and as it progresses toward 2:1, the single ventricle becomes volume overloaded. A Qp:Qs ratio of greater than 2:1 may be associated with low systemic output, hypotension, and acidosis.

The ability to monitor Qp:Qs accurately at the bedside is limited. Arterial saturations and mixed venous saturations (using superior vena caval saturation as a representative value) can be measured, but pulmonary venous saturations are assumed (107). Since the degree of postoperative lung disease is highly variable, assuming that pulmonary venous saturations are normal can erroneously underestimate pulmonary blood flow and the degree of overcirculation in patients with low systemic oxygen saturations (108). In patients with complete cardiac mixing, high systemic saturations are likely to represent pulmonary overcirculation. A patient with high systemic saturations (>90%) and high arterial PaO_2 (>50 mm Hg) with low blood pressure and metabolic acidosis should be treated for pulmonary overcirculation.

Strategies to treat pulmonary overcirculation focus on increasing PVR and decreasing pulmonary blood flow. Transfusing the patient to a hematocrit of 45% to 50% will increase blood viscosity and PVR. Minimizing inspired oxygen to a room air level and/or even lower (e.g., FIO_2 of 17%–19%) with the addition of nitrogen also increases PVR. Allowing the $PaCO_2$ to rise (e.g., to 45–50 mm Hg with a pH <7.34) with hypoventilation or by the addition of carbon dioxide to the ventilator circuit has a similar effect (7). A cross-over trial comparing hypoxic gas mixtures to inhaled carbon dioxide in preoperative neonates with HLHS for increasing PVR was performed (109). Both methods increased the resistance and decreased the pulmonary blood flow, but carbon dioxide administration increased oxygen delivery to the brain as measured by increased mixed venous saturations in the superior vena cava and decreased arteriovenous saturation difference. In addition, high systemic vascular resistance should be avoided, as it increases pulmonary blood flow and the afterload on the single ventricle (110). High upper extremity blood pressures and oxygen saturations should raise the suspicion of residual coarctation of the aorta in single-ventricle patients and aortic arch obstruction. Large-dose catecholamines should be avoided, and afterload reduction with milrinone should be optimized. If a patient remains in a low cardiac output state despite ventilatory and pharmacologic strategies to limit pulmonary blood flow, surgical options such as narrowing the pulmonary conduit or aortopulmonary shunt with clips should be considered.

Excessive cyanosis is less common after patients are palliated with an aortopulmonary shunt, but it does occur. Possible etiologies include lung disease, elevated PVR, obstruction to pulmonary blood flow, and low mixed venous saturation from increased oxygen consumption or low cardiac output. Lung disease should be detectible by chest radiograph, and interventions can be performed in an effort to improve gas exchange. Elevated PVR is less common but may be seen in a patient with HLHS who has an intact or highly restrictive atrial septum and pulmonary venous hypertension before surgery (111). Despite decompression of atrial hypertension by opening the atrial septum, PVR can remain elevated postoperatively; it may respond to a brief course of iNO, similar to other patients who undergo relief of left atrial hypertension (16). The mortality rate of patients with HLHS and intact atrial septum is high despite strategies for emergent decompression and operation (112). When a shunt-dependent postoperative patient suddenly develops oxygen desaturation and bradycardia, it should raise the suspicion of acute shunt thrombosis. These patients need emergent cannulation for ECMO and shunt revision. Many patients with shunted single-ventricle physiology have labile hemodynamics for the first several postoperative hours to days. Delayed sternal closure is an accepted strategy that provides rapid access for additional procedures such as clipping of the shunt and emergent ECMO cannulation, if needed (6).

Cavopulmonary Connections

The transition to a superior vena cava–to–pulmonary artery connection, which is called a bidirectional Glenn shunt (BDG), is typically performed when a single-ventricle patient is 3 to 6 months old. The BDG is the first of a two-stage conversion to a total cavopulmonary circulation with separation of pulmonary and systemic blood flow (Fontan circulation). The advantage of a BDG is a reduced volume load and work for the single ventricle. The patient usually undergoes a cardiac catheterization to assess the pulmonary artery anatomy and measure PVR prior to the BDG. A PVR of less than approximately 3 to 4 Woods units is considered optimal. This operation is usually well tolerated by patients. It is common to observe systemic hypertension after the BDG; this may be secondary to intracranial hypertension from elevated superior vena cava pressures. Patients are often irritable in the first postoperative days, perhaps due to headache. Mild hypertension should be tolerated, as this preserves cerebral blood flow during the transition to passive pulmonary blood flow through the BDG. Systemic hypertension associated with bleeding or marked hypertension (>120 mm Hg systolic blood pressure) should be treated.

Cyanosis associated with elevated superior vena cava pressure occasionally occurs after BDG. If there is a low transpulmonary gradient with elevated atrial pressures, ventricular function should be optimized with inotropes. If the atrial pressures are low and the transpulmonary gradient is greater than 10 mm Hg, this suggests either anatomic obstruction to pulmonary blood flow or elevated PVR. The role of carbon dioxide and its effects on PVR and pulmonary blood flow is complex in BDG patients. Modest hypoventilation with elevated carbon dioxide increases arterial PaO_2, presumably by increasing pulmonary blood flow via greater cerebral blood flow from cerebral autoregulation (113). The vasodilatory role of carbon dioxide in the brain predominates over any increase in PVR from hypoventilation and lower blood pH (114). The data for use of nitric oxide in these patients are mixed. In one study it appeared to lower superior vena cava pressures and improve oxygenation (115). However, in another study, it had no impact on oxygenation (116). Positive pressure ventilation and increased intrathoracic pressures may play a role in limiting passive pulmonary blood flow, so early extubation is advocated (117). A superior vena cava pressure of >20 mm Hg that is unresponsive to medical therapies is concerning for the successful transition to BDG physiology. Postoperative cardiac catheterization to assess for reversible causes and consideration of possible takedown of the BDG should be pursued.

The final stage in the single-ventricle palliation is the completion of the cavopulmonary connection with a Fontan operation. This can be performed with either a lateral tunnel baffle through the common atrium or an extracardiac conduit, usually when the patient is 2 to 3 years old and weighs 10 to 15 kg. Patients again undergo a preoperative cardiac catheterization to assess pulmonary artery anatomy and PVR. It is common at this catheterization to discover both aortopulmonary collaterals and decompressing venovenous collaterals from systemic to pulmonary veins. Large aortopulmonary collaterals are typically eliminated (by coil embolization) to lower pulmonary artery pressure, and venovenous collaterals are occluded to increase pulmonary blood flow from systemic veins into the pulmonary arteries (118, 119). Postoperative concerns after a Fontan are usually focused on PVR and cardiac output. An ideal Fontan baffle pressure is 10 to 15 mm Hg with a transpulmonary gradient of <10 mm Hg. A Fontan baffle pressure >20 mm Hg is worrisome. Elevated Fontan baffle and atrial pressures indicate low cardiac output or tamponade physiology. An elevated Fontan baffle pressure with a low atrial pressure indicates either high PVR or obstruction in the Fontan pathway; these patients should be promptly investigated and treated. Low Fontan baffle and atrial pressures indicate inadequate intravascular volume status (106). The passive pulmonary blood flow of the Fontan circulation is preload dependent, so hypovolemia will quickly lead to low cardiac output and hypotension. Patients undergoing Fontan operations often have sinus node dysfunction with junctional rhythm. AV synchrony should be preserved with mechanical pacing to maximize cardiac output. Surgical fenestration of the Fontan baffle has a positive impact on the early recovery Fontan patients. In the immediate postoperative hours, the fenestration allows for a right-to-left shunt. This shunt decompresses the Fontan baffle and causes mild oxygen desaturation; however, it preserves cardiac output by increasing preload to the ventricle. The PVR is transiently elevated due to the inflammatory response after CPB. The Fontan circulation is highly sensitive to elevations in PVR, so acidosis, alveolar hypoxia, and atelectasis should be avoided. As the patient diureses and is extubated from positive pressure ventilation, PVR decreases and the arterial oxygen saturation improves as less blood is shunted right to left. The duration of pleural effusions, which are common after the Fontan operation, is also reduced by the fenestration (120). The fenestration may be electively closed with an occluder device during cardiac catheterization at a later time with good intermediate functional outcomes (121).

Pediatric cardiac surgery patients can be challenging. With specialized care, vigilant monitoring, and good communication between teams, outcomes may be rewarding.

References

1. Jonas RA. *Comprehensive Surgical Management of Congenital Heart Disease.* New York: Oxford University Press; 2004:3–10.
2. Tweddell JS, Spray TL. Newborn heart surgery: reasonable expectations and outcomes. *Pediatr Clin North Am.* 2004;51(6):1611–1623, ix.
3. Wernovsky G, Rubenstein SD, Spray TL. Cardiac surgery in the low-birth weight neonate. New approaches. *Clin Perinatol.* 2001;28(1):249–264.
4. Curran RD, et al. Inhaled nitric oxide for children with congenital heart disease and pulmonary hypertension. *Ann Thorac Surg.* 1995;60(6):1765–1771.
5. Wessel DL. Inhaled nitric oxide for the treatment of pulmonary hypertension before and after cardiopulmonary bypass. *Crit Care Med.* 1993;21(9 Suppl):S344–345.
6. Tabbutt S, et al. Delayed sternal closure after cardiac operations in a pediatric population. *J Thorac Cardiovasc Surg.* 1997;113(5):886–893.
7. Chang AC, et al. Pulmonary vascular resistance in infants after cardiac surgery: role of carbon dioxide and hydrogen ion. *Crit Care Med.* 1995;23(3):568–574.

8. Charpie JR, et al. Serial blood lactate measurements predict early outcome after neonatal repair or palliation for complex congenital heart disease. *J Thorac Cardiovasc Surg.* 2000;120(1):73–80.
9. Munoz R, et al. Changes in whole blood lactate levels during cardiopulmonary bypass for surgery for congenital cardiac disease: an early indicator of morbidity and mortality. *J Thorac Cardiovasc Surg.* 2000;119(1):155–162.
10. Jonas RA. *Comprehensive Surgical Management of Congenital Heart Disease.* New York: Oxford University Press; 2004:61–62.
11. Dominguez TE, et al. Use of recombinant factor VIIa for refractory hemorrhage during extracorporeal membrane oxygenation. *Pediatr Crit Care Med.* 2005;6(3):348–351.
12. Marianeschi SM, et al. Fast-track congenital heart operations: a less invasive technique and early extubation. *Ann Thorac Surg.* 2000;69(3):872–876.
13. Flori HR, et al. Transthoracic intracardiac catheters in pediatric patients recovering from congenital heart defect surgery: associated complications and outcomes. *Crit Care Med.* 2000;28(8):2997–3001.
14. Gold JP, et al. Transthoracic intracardiac monitoring lines in pediatric surgical patients: a ten-year experience. *Ann Thorac Surg.* 1986;42(2):185–191.
15. Lock JE. Hemodynamic evaluation of congenital heart disease. In: Lock JE, Keane JF, Perry SB, eds. *Diagnostic and Interventional Catheterization in Congenital Heart Disease.* 2nd ed. Boston: Kluwer Academic Publishers; 2000:37–72.
16. Wessel DL. Current and future strategies in the treatment of childhood pulmonary hypertension. *Prog Pediatr Cardiol.* 2001;12(3):289–318.
17. Barratt-Boyes BG, Wood EH. The oxygen saturation of blood in the venae cavae, right-heart chambers, and pulmonary vessels of healthy subjects. *J Lab Clin Med.* 1957;50(1):93–106.
18. Lang P, et al. Early assessment of hemodynamic status after repair of tetralogy of Fallot: a comparison of 24 hour (intensive care unit) and 1 year postoperative data in 98 patients. *Am J Cardiol.* 1982;50(4):795–799.
19. Lan YT, Lee JC, Wetzel G. Postoperative arrhythmia. *Curr Opin Cardiol.* 2003;18(2):73–78.
20. Weindling SN, et al. Duration of complete atrioventricular block after congenital heart disease surgery. *Am J Cardiol.* 1998;82(4):525–527.
21. Rosales AM, et al. Postoperative ectopic atrial tachycardia in children with congenital heart disease. *Am J Cardiol.* 2001;88(10):1169–1172.
22. Saul JP, et al. Intravenous amiodarone for incessant tachyarrhythmias in children: a randomized, double-blind, antiarrhythmic drug trial. *Circulation.* 2005;112(22):3470–3477.
23. Walsh EP, et al. Evaluation of a staged treatment protocol for rapid automatic junctional tachycardia after operation for congenital heart disease. *J Am Coll Cardiol.* 1997;29(5):1046–1053.
24. Perry JC, et al. Pediatric use of intravenous amiodarone: efficacy and safety in critically ill patients from a multicenter protocol. *J Am Coll Cardiol.* 1996;27(5):1246–1250.
25. Shekerdemian L, Bohn D. Cardiovascular effects of mechanical ventilation. *Arch Dis Child.* 1999;80(5):475–480.
26. Penny DJ, Hayek Z, Redington AN. The effects of positive and negative extrathoracic pressure ventilation on pulmonary blood flow after the total cavopulmonary shunt procedure. *Int J Cardiol.* 1991;30(1):128–130.
27. Shekerdemian LS, et al. Cardiopulmonary interactions after Fontan operations: augmentation of cardiac output using negative pressure ventilation. *Circulation.* 1997;96(11):3934–3942.
28. Pinsky MR, et al. Augmentation of cardiac function by elevation of intrathoracic pressure. *J Appl Physiol.* 1983;54(4):950–955.
29. Grace MP, Greenbaum DM. Cardiac performance in response to PEEP in patients with cardiac dysfunction. *Crit Care Med.* 1982;10(6):358–360.
30. Arnold JH, et al. High-frequency oscillatory ventilation in pediatric respiratory failure: a multicenter experience. *Crit Care Med.* 2000;28(12):3913–3919.
31. Courtney SE, et al. High-frequency oscillatory ventilation versus conventional mechanical ventilation for very-low-birth-weight infants. *N Engl J Med.* 2002;347(9):643–652.
32. Gullberg N, Winberg P, Sellden H. Changes in mean airway pressure during HFOV influences cardiac output in neonates and infants. *Acta Anaesthesiol Scand.* 2004;48(2):218–223.
33. Simma B, et al. Conventional ventilation versus high-frequency oscillation: hemodynamic effects in newborn babies. *Crit Care Med.* 2000;28(1):227–231.
34. Khariwala SS, Lee WT, Koltai PJ. Laryngotracheal consequences of pediatric cardiac surgery. *Arch Otolaryngol Head Neck Surg.* 2005;131(4):336–339.
35. Miller SG, Brook MM, Tacy TA. Reliability of two-dimensional echocardiography in the assessment of clinically significant abnormal hemidiaphragm motion in pediatric cardiothoracic patients: comparison with fluoroscopy. *Pediatr Crit Care Med.* 2006;7(5):441–444.
36. Joho-Arreola AL, et al. Incidence and treatment of diaphragmatic paralysis after cardiac surgery in children. *Eur J Cardiothorac Surg.* 2005;27(1):53–57.
37. Midelton GT, Frishman WH, Passo SS. Congestive heart failure and continuous positive airway pressure therapy: support of a new modality for improving the prognosis and survival of patients with advanced congestive heart failure. *Heart Dis.* 2002;4(2):102–109.
38. Anand KJ, Hansen DD, Hickey PR, Hormonal-metabolic stress responses in neonates undergoing cardiac surgery. *Anesthesiology.* 1990;73(4):661–670.
39. Anand KJ, Hickey PR. Halothane-morphine compared with high-dose sufentanil for anesthesia and postoperative analgesia in neonatal cardiac surgery. *N Engl J Med.* 1992;326(1):1–9.
40. Hickey PR, et al. Pulmonary and systemic hemodynamic responses to fentanyl in infants. *Anesth Analg.* 1985;64(5):483–486.
41. Hickey PR, et al. Blunting of stress responses in the pulmonary circulation of infants by fentanyl. *Anesth Analg.* 1985;64(12):1137–1142.
42. Muller P, Vogtmann C. Three cases with different presentation of fentanyl-induced muscle rigidity—a rare problem in intensive care of neonates. *Am J Perinatol.* 2000;17(1):23–26.
43. Fahnenstich H, et al. Fentanyl-induced chest wall rigidity and laryngospasm in preterm and term infants. *Crit Care Med.* 2000;28(3):836–839.
44. McKeage K, Perry CM. Propofol: a review of its use in intensive care sedation of adults. *CNS Drugs.* 2003;17(4):235–272.
45. Bray RJ. Propofol infusion syndrome in children. *Paediatr Anaesth.* 1998;8(6):491–499.
46. Tobias JD, Berkenbosch JW. Initial experience with dexmedetomidine in paediatric-aged patients. *Paediatr Anaesth.* 2002;12(2):171–175.
47. Chrysostomou C, et al. Use of dexmedetomidine in children after cardiac and thoracic surgery. *Pediatr Crit Care Med.* 2006;7(2):126–131.
48. Berkenbosch JW, Tobias JD. Development of bradycardia during sedation with dexmedetomidine in an infant concurrently receiving digoxin. *Pediatr Crit Care Med.* 2003;4(2):203–205.
49. Helmers SL, et al. Perioperative electroencephalographic seizures in infants undergoing repair of complex congenital cardiac defects. *Electroencephalogr Clin Neurophysiol.* 1997;102(1):27–36.
50. Gaynor JW, et al. Increasing duration of deep hypothermic circulatory arrest is associated with an increased incidence of postoperative electroencephalographic seizures. *J Thorac Cardiovasc Surg.* 2005;130(5):1278–1286.
51. Mahle WT, et al. An MRI study of neurological injury before and after congenital heart surgery. *Circulation.* 2002;106(12 Suppl 1):I109–114.
52. Gaynor JW, et al. The relationship of postoperative electrographic seizures to neurodevelopmental outcome at 1 year of age after neonatal and infant cardiac surgery. *J Thorac Cardiovasc Surg.* 2006;131(1):181–189.
53. Austin EH 3rd, et al. Benefit of neurophysiologic monitoring for pediatric cardiac surgery. *J Thorac Cardiovasc Surg.* 1997;114(5):707–715, 717; discussion 715–716.
54. Dent CL, et al. Brain magnetic resonance imaging abnormalities after the Norwood procedure using regional cerebral perfusion. *J Thorac Cardiovasc Surg.* 2005;130(6):1523–1530.
55. Gaynor JW. The effect of modified ultrafiltration on the postoperative course in patients with congenital heart disease. *Semin Thorac Cardiovasc Surg Pediatr Card Surg Annu.* 2003;6:128–139.
56. Russell JA, Navickis RJ, Wilkes MM. Albumin versus crystalloid for pump priming in cardiac surgery: meta-analysis of controlled trials. *J Cardiothorac Vasc Anesth.* 2004;18(4):429–437.
57. Langer GA. Role of sarcolemmal-bound calcium in regulation of myocardial contractile force. *J Am Coll Cardiol.* 1986;8(1 Suppl A):65A–68A.
58. Singh NC, et al. Comparison of continuous versus intermittent furosemide administration in postoperative pediatric cardiac patients. *Crit Care Med.* 1992;20(1):17–21.
59. Costello JM, et al. Fenoldapam after pediatric cardiac surgery: what is conventional diuretic therapy? *Pediatr Crit Care Med.* 2006;7(4):399–400.
60. Mahle WT, et al. Nesiritide in infants and children with congestive heart failure. *Pediatr Crit Care Med.* 2005;6(5):543–546.
61. Fleming F, et al. Renal replacement therapy after repair of congenital heart disease in children. A comparison of hemofiltration and peritoneal dialysis. *J Thorac Cardiovasc Surg.* 1995;109(2):322–331.
62. Giuffre RM, et al. Acute renal failure complicating pediatric cardiac surgery: a comparison of survivors and nonsurvivors following acute peritoneal dialysis. *Pediatr Cardiol.* 1992;13(4):208–213.
63. Shaw NJ, et al. Long-term outcome for children with acute renal failure following cardiac surgery. *Int J Cardiol.* 1991;31(2):161–165.
64. McElhinney DB, et al. Necrotizing enterocolitis in neonates with congenital heart disease: risk factors and outcomes. *Pediatrics.* 2000;106(5):1080–1087.
65. Stover BH, et al. Nosocomial infection rates in US children's hospitals' neonatal and pediatric intensive care units. *Am J Infect Control.* 2001;29(3):152–157.
66. Slonim AD, et al. The costs associated with nosocomial bloodstream infections in the pediatric intensive care unit. *Pediatr Crit Care Med.* 2001;2(2):170–174.
67. Huddleston CB. Mediastinal wound infections following pediatric cardiac surgery. *Semin Thorac Cardiovasc Surg.* 2004;16(1):108–112.
68. Tortoriello TA, et al. Mediastinitis after pediatric cardiac surgery: a 15-year experience at a single institution. *Ann Thorac Surg.* 2003;76(5):1655–1660.
69. Wessel DL. Managing low cardiac output syndrome after congenital heart surgery. *Crit Care Med.* 2001;29(10 Suppl):S220–230.
70. Wernovsky G, et al. Postoperative course and hemodynamic profile after the arterial switch operation in neonates and infants. A comparison

of low-flow cardiopulmonary bypass and circulatory arrest. *Circulation.* 1995;92(8):2226–2235.
71. Booth KL, et al. Cardiac catheterization of patients supported by extracorporeal membrane oxygenation. *J Am Coll Cardiol.* 2002;40(9):1681–1686.
72. Zahn EM, et al. Interventional catheterization performed in the early postoperative period after congenital heart surgery in children. *J Am Coll Cardiol.* 2004;43(7):1264–1269.
73. Dunser MW, et al. Cardiac performance during vasopressin infusion in postcardiotomy shock. *Intensive Care Med.* 2002;28(6):746–751.
74. Rosenzweig EB, et al. Intravenous arginine-vasopressin in children with vasodilatory shock after cardiac surgery. *Circulation.* 1999;100(19 Suppl):II182–186.
75. Rozenfeld V, Cheng JW. The role of vasopressin in the treatment of vasodilation in shock states. *Ann Pharmacother.* 2000;34(2):250–254.
76. Caspi J, et al. Age-related response to epinephrine-induced myocardial stress. A functional and ultrastructural study. *Circulation.* 1991;84(5 Suppl):III394–399.
77. Young RA, Ward A. Milrinone. A preliminary review of its pharmacological properties and therapeutic use. *Drugs.* 1988;36(2):158–192.
78. Chang AC, et al. Milrinone: systemic and pulmonary hemodynamic effects in neonates after cardiac surgery. *Crit Care Med.* 1995;23(11):1907–1914.
79. Hoffman TM, et al. Efficacy and safety of milrinone in preventing low cardiac output syndrome in infants and children after corrective surgery for congenital heart disease. *Circulation.* 2003;107(7):996–1002.
80. Bettendorf M, et al. Tri-iodothyronine treatment in children after cardiac surgery: a double-blind, randomised, placebo-controlled study. *Lancet.* 2000;356(9229):529–534.
81. Chowdhury D, et al. Usefulness of triiodothyronine (T3) treatment after surgery for complex congenital heart disease in infants and children. *Am J Cardiol.* 1999;84(9):1107–1109, A10.
82. Mackie AS, et al. A randomized, double-blind, placebo-controlled pilot trial of triiodothyronine in neonatal heart surgery. *J Thorac Cardiovasc Surg.* 2005;130(3):810–816.
83. Mills RM, et al. Sustained hemodynamic effects of an infusion of nesiritide (human b-type natriuretic peptide) in heart failure: a randomized, double-blind, placebo-controlled clinical trial. Natrecor Study Group. *J Am Coll Cardiol.* 1999;34(1):155–162.
84. Shore S, et al. Usefulness of corticosteroid therapy in decreasing epinephrine requirements in critically ill infants with congenital heart disease. *Am J Cardiol.* 2001;88(5):591–594.
85. Duncan BW, et al. Use of rapid-deployment extracorporeal membrane oxygenation for the resuscitation of pediatric patients with heart disease after cardiac arrest. *J Thorac Cardiovasc Surg.* 1998;116(2):305–311.
86. Black MD, et al. Determinants of success in pediatric cardiac patients undergoing extracorporeal membrane oxygenation. *Ann Thorac Surg.* 1995;60(1):133–138.
87. Duncan BW, et al. Mechanical circulatory support in children with cardiac disease. *J Thorac Cardiovasc Surg.* 1999;117(3):529–542.
88. Hetzer R, et al. Mechanical cardiac support in the young with the Berlin Heart EXCOR pulsatile ventricular assist device: 15 years' experience. *Semin Thorac Cardiovasc Surg Pediatr Card Surg Annu.* 2006:99–108.
89. *ECLS Registry Report.* Ann Arbor, MI: Extracorporeal Life Support Organization.
90. Booth KL, et al. Extracorporeal membrane oxygenation support of the Fontan and bidirectional Glenn circulations. *Ann Thorac Surg.* 2004;77(4):1341–1348.
91. Stobierska-Dzierzek B, Awad H, Michler RE. The evolving management of acute right-sided heart failure in cardiac transplant recipients. *J Am Coll Cardiol.* 2001;38(4):923–931.
92. Cullen S, Shore D, Redington A. Characterization of right ventricular diastolic performance after complete repair of tetralogy of Fallot. Restrictive physiology predicts slow postoperative recovery. *Circulation.* 1995;91(6):1782–1789.
93. Laudito A, et al. Complete repair of conotruncal defects with an interatrial communication: oxygenation, hemodynamic status, and early outcome. *Ann Thorac Surg.* 2006;82(4):1286–1291; discussion 1291.
94. Journois D, et al. Inhaled nitric oxide as a therapy for pulmonary hypertension after operations for congenital heart defects. *J Thorac Cardiovasc Surg.* 1994;107(4):1129–1135.
95. Adatia I, et al. Diagnostic use of inhaled nitric oxide after neonatal cardiac operations. *J Thorac Cardiovasc Surg.* 1996;112(5):1403–1405.
96. Russell IA, et al. The effects of inhaled nitric oxide on postoperative pulmonary hypertension in infants and children undergoing surgical repair of congenital heart disease. *Anesth Analg.* 1998;87(1):46–51.
97. Atz AM, et al. Inhaled nitric oxide in children with pulmonary hypertension and congenital mitral stenosis. *Am J Cardiol.* 1996;77(4):316–319.
98. Auler Junior JO, et al. Low doses of inhaled nitric oxide in heart transplant recipients. *J Heart Lung Transplant.* 1996;15(5):443–450.
99. Atz AM, Adatia I, Wessel DL. Rebound pulmonary hypertension after inhalation of nitric oxide. *Ann Thorac Surg.* 1996;62(6):1759–1764.
100. Atz AM, Wessel DL. Sildenafil ameliorates effects of inhaled nitric oxide withdrawal. *Anesthesiology.* 1999;91(1):307–310.
101. Knoderer CA, Ebenroth ES, Brown JW. Chronic outpatient sildenafil therapy for pulmonary hypertension in a child after cardiac surgery. *Pediatr Cardiol.* 2005;26(6):859–861.
102. Loh E, et al. Cardiovascular effects of inhaled nitric oxide in patients with left ventricular dysfunction. *Circulation.* 1994;90(6):2780–275.
103. Rosenzweig EB, Kerstein D, Barst RJ. Long-term prostacyclin for pulmonary hypertension with associated congenital heart defects. *Circulation.* 1999;99(14):1858–1865.
104. Drummond WH, Lock JE. Neonatal 'pulmonary vasodilator' drugs. Current status. *Dev Pharmacol Ther.* 1984;7(1):1–20.
105. Cua CL, et al. Early postoperative outcomes in a series of infants with hypoplastic left heart syndrome undergoing stage I palliation operation with either modified Blalock-Taussig shunt or right ventricle to pulmonary artery conduit. *Pediatr Crit Care Med.* 2006;7(3):238–244.
106. Wernovsky G, Bove E. Single ventricle lesions. In: Chang AC, Hanley FL, Wernovsky G, et al., eds. *Pediatric Cardiac Intensive Care.* Baltimore: Williams & Wilkins; 1998:271–287.
107. Rossi AF, et al. Usefulness of intermittent monitoring of mixed venous oxygen saturation after stage I palliation for hypoplastic left heart syndrome. *Am J Cardiol.* 1994;73(15):1118–1123.
108. Taeed R, et al. Unrecognized pulmonary venous desaturation early after Norwood palliation confounds Gp:Gs assessment and compromises oxygen delivery. *Circulation.* 2001;103(22):2699–2704.
109. Tabbutt S, et al. Impact of inspired gas mixtures on preoperative infants with hypoplastic left heart syndrome during controlled ventilation. *Circulation.* 2001;104(12 Suppl 1):I159–164.
110. Wright GE, et al. High systemic vascular resistance and sudden cardiovascular collapse in recovering Norwood patients. *Ann Thorac Surg.* 2004;77(1):48–52.
111. Atz AM, et al. Preoperative management of pulmonary venous hypertension in hypoplastic left heart syndrome with restrictive atrial septal defect. *Am J Cardiol.* 1999;83(8):1224–1228.
112. Vlahos AP, et al. Hypoplastic left heart syndrome with intact or highly restrictive atrial septum: outcome after neonatal transcatheter atrial septostomy. *Circulation.* 2004;109(19):2326–2330.
113. Bradley SM, Simsic JM, Mulvihill DM. Hypoventilation improves oxygenation after bidirectional superior cavopulmonary connection. *J Thorac Cardiovasc Surg.* 2003;126(4):1033–1039.
114. Fogel MA, et al. Brain versus lung: hierarchy of feedback loops in single-ventricle patients with superior cavopulmonary connection. *Circulation.* 2004;110(11 Suppl 1):II147–152.
115. Agarwal HS, et al. Inhaled nitric oxide use in bidirectional Glenn anastomosis for elevated Glenn pressures. *Ann Thorac Surg.* 2006;81(4):1429–1434.
116. Adatia I, Atz AM, Wessel DL. Inhaled nitric oxide does not improve systemic oxygenation after bidirectional superior cavopulmonary anastomosis. *J Thorac Cardiovasc Surg.* 2005;129(1):217–219.
117. Tabbutt S. Systemic oxygenation in patients with a bilateral cavopulmonary anastomosis. *Pediatr Crit Care Med.* 2006;7(4):396–397.
118. Spicer RL, et al. Aortopulmonary collateral vessels and prolonged pleural effusions after modified Fontan procedures. *Am Heart J.* 1996;131(6):1164–1168.
119. Sugiyama H, et al. Characterization and treatment of systemic venous to pulmonary venous collaterals seen after the Fontan operation. *Cardiol Young.* 2003;13(5):424–430.
120. Bridges ND, et al. Effect of baffle fenestration on outcome of the modified Fontan operation. *Circulation.* 1992;86(6):1762–1769.
121. Goff DA, et al. Clinical outcome of fenestrated Fontan patients after closure: the first 10 years. *Circulation.* 2000;102(17):2094–2099.

CHAPTER 82 ■ VASCULAR SURGERY IN THE INTENSIVE CARE UNIT

ROBERT J. FEEZOR • TIMOTHY C. FLYNN

Patients requiring vascular intervention—whether open surgery or endovascular procedures—are elderly and have comorbidities that make their overall care complicated. To achieve a successful outcome, the perioperative care of the vascular surgery patient requires meticulous attention to detail and knowledge about the possible pitfalls these patients can encounter. Even the most seemingly innocuous clinical symptom must be thoroughly investigated and potentially treated in order to achieve acceptable perioperative outcomes. Despite meticulous attention to detail, vascular patients often fall victim to their comorbidities.

A key element in the care of the vascular patient is the recognition of vascular pathology as a systemic disease and not just a focal anatomic problem regardless of the procedure that brings the patient to the intensive care unit (ICU). The main exception to this is the young patient who sustains vascular injury. The nature of atherosclerosis is that it affects the blood vessels of all circulatory beds: cardiac, peripheral, and cerebral. Thus, patients who present with leg ischemia are at significantly higher risk than the general population for having both myocardial infarctions as well as cerebrovascular accidents. In fact, the average patient with claudication has an estimated mortality rate of 50% at 5 years, with the predominant cause of death being cardiovascular (1). Furthermore, there is progressing evidence that the vascular occlusive process is proinflammatory in nature. These patients have elevated levels of C-reactive protein (CRP), interleukin (IL)-6, and soluble intercellular adhesion molecule-1. Elevated CRP has recently been shown to be a predictor of cardiovascular events among patients with peripheral artery disease (PAD) (2). Up-regulation of inflammatory mediators may contribute to complications in the ICU.

In most series, patients with vascular occlusive disease have a high incidence of chronic obstructive pulmonary disease, occult cardiac disease, diabetes, and renal insufficiency. The adverse pulmonary sequelae of arterial revascularization are frequently related to the ravages of smoking. In most reports of operative repair of peripheral arterial disease, the incidence of tobacco use among patients exceeds 50%, and often approaches 90%. In a study looking at femoral atherosclerosis using duplex ultrasound, smoking was the largest risk factor, more influential than exercise tolerance, hypertension, or hypercholesterolemia (3). We may choose a potentially less durable endovascular therapy for patients based on their condition and ability to tolerate general anesthesia. Although general endotracheal anesthesia (GETA) is still the most common type of anesthesia used in vascular patients, increasing evidence suggests that spinal or epidural anesthesia may be more appropriate. In a review of 14,788 patients in the National Surgical Quality Improvement Program (NSQIP) of the Department of Veterans Affairs, GETA was associated with a higher incidence of cardiac, pulmonary, and graft complications when compared to spinal or epidural anesthesia (4).

Patients with known vascular disease are assumed to have associated coronary artery disease, even though they may be asymptomatic. In a landmark study by Hertzer et al., greater than 90% of patients undergoing peripheral vascular reconstruction had coronary artery disease evident by cardiac catheterization, and nearly one third had multivessel disease (5). The goals of the American Heart Association/American College of Cardiology should be targeted, including a blood pressure less than 140/90 mm Hg, serum low-density lipoprotein (LDL) <100 mg/dL, and hemoglobin A_{1C} less than 7% (6). To achieve these goals, patients should be on an aspirin, a β-blocker dosed to a target heart rate of 70 to 75, an angiotensin-converting enzyme (ACE) inhibitor or other antihypertensive therapy, and probably a statin (independent of baseline cholesterol levels). Despite recent reports questioning the use of β-blockers, judicious use that avoids excessive hypotension or bradycardia may still be reasonable (7).

There is increasing evidence that patients with vascular disease should all be treated with a statin regardless of cholesterol levels (8). Statins have numerous effects other than reduction of cholesterol including anti-inflammatory, immunomodulatory, and anticoagulant effects. Moreover, abrupt discontinuation may lead to a rebound effect and possibly increase cardiovascular complications (9). It is our practice to routinely start patients on a statin preoperatively and continue it throughout the postoperative period. The antiplatelet drug clopidogrel is frequently used in vascular patients. Preoperatively we review the indications for this drug, and if the indications are compelling, such as the patient with a recent coronary stent placement, we will continue the drug through the perioperative period, recognizing that there may be a slightly increased incidence of wound complications. We do not hesitate to start the drug in patients who exhibit cardiac ischemia in the postoperative period.

The electrocardiogram (ECG) should be monitored continuously for any changes suggestive of ischemia. For the diabetic population, angina may present as nausea and must be interpreted as signs of myocardial ischemia until proven otherwise. Lastly, cardiac dysrhythmias are often caused by ischemia, electrolyte disturbances, or fluid shifts in the postoperative period, and patients should be monitored closely for such events.

In order to decrease the risk of perioperative cardiac events in the vascular surgery patient population, much attention has been given to preoperative risk stratification. In the surgical and anesthesia literature, most vascular surgery procedures for occlusive or aneurysmal disease are placed in the "high-risk" category. The question is how to minimize the risk of perioperative cardiac complications. Data from several randomized, multicenter trials have shown that coronary revascularization (percutaneous or open) before elective major vascular surgery does not decrease the overall mortality (10). Nevertheless, many clinicians request preoperative cardiology consultation to help determine existing cardiac function, usually with an ECG, an echocardiogram, or a chemical cardiac stress test.

Even without prior known elevated serum creatinine, many vascular patients have renal insufficiency as determined by creatinine clearance. Nephrotoxic effects of the IV contrast commonly used in revascularization procedures make postoperative renal dysfunction a constant threat. Moreover, perioperative mortality after most vascular procedures is significantly increased in patients with renal failure (11). Strict monitoring of fluid balance, maintenance of serum electrolytes, appropriate dosing of nephrotoxic medications, adequate hydration, and resumption of chronic diuretics will all help to minimize the chance of postoperative renal dysfunction.

A majority of vascular patients have diabetes mellitus and this group is at higher risk for postoperative complications, both vascular and nonvascular. From a vascular perspective, patients with diabetes have a higher rate of postoperative amputations after peripheral bypass surgery for tissue loss (11). Diabetics are also at risk for other postoperative morbidities including postoperative wound infections. They should be maintained euglycemic, even if that requires a constant intravenous infusion of insulin, with a target blood glucose of 80 to 110 mg/dL.

There is a subset of patients with vascular disease with underlying hypercoagulable states. The concern for a hypercoagulable state should be raised with patients with seemingly advanced atherosclerotic disease at a younger age. A careful history can assist with determining these patients, but when identified, they should be started on appropriate anticoagulation. Hematology consultation should be obtained, but may be of somewhat limited value in the setting of the acute thrombotic event.

VASCULAR CARE IN THE INTENSIVE CARE UNIT

All patients in an ICU have a propensity for developing venous thromboembolic events. Virchow's triad dictates that patients at risk include those with stasis, endothelial injury, and a hypercoagulable state. In the postsurgical population, venous stasis is inevitable due to the patients' relative immobility. Endothelial injury occurs during the course of the surgical procedure. It is our practice that all patients receive chemical and/or mechanical prophylaxis; we routinely use low-molecular-weight or unfractionated heparin and/or sequential compression devices when there is no existing contraindication. We avoid lower extremity sequential compression devices in patients with severe peripheral arterial occlusive disease, although the data for this practice are anecdotal. The incidence of heparin-induced thrombocytopenia is relatively rare, and when suggested by a decline in platelet count, we promptly cease all systemic or local heparin and transition to purely mechanical prophylaxis.

Stress gastritis is a constant threat in the vascular ICU patient. Patients are routinely placed on either histamine-receptor blockers or proton pump inhibitors, irrespective of any clinically detected gastrointestinal hemorrhage. Opponents of this practice suggest that in doing so, one of the body's natural defense mechanisms (gastric acidity) is altered, but we find that the risk of stress gastritis exceeds the diminution in host defenses.

Ventilator-associated pneumonia has been well documented to increase in-hospital mortality, length of stay, and overall cost of hospitalization. We employ routine suctioning, aggressive bronchoscopy to control secretions, and head elevation for all our intubated patients. Once extubated, activity is encouraged and adequate pain control is important for patients with an abdominal or a thoracic incision.

The routine assessment of the vascular ICU patient includes not only all the usual cardiovascular, pulmonary, and metabolic parameters, but also frequent and detailed physical exams. All incisions should be inspected for signs of early wound complications such as infection, separation, or hematoma. Objective assessment of distal perfusion should be performed regularly, even hourly, in the immediate postoperative period. This assessment includes looking at the extremity for cutaneous signs of malperfusion, assessing motor function, and palpating the major muscle groups for tenseness, which may signify compartment syndrome in patients who are too sedated to relate the classic "pain with passive motion." The best exam, in our opinion, is to elevate the lower extremity by placing the hand behind the Achilles tendon and palpating the anterior calf compartment with the posterior leg off the bed. A patient should be alert enough to follow commands of simple dorsiflexion, again ensuring that the posterior knee is off the bed. (Dorsiflexing the foot with the heel resting on the bed can be achieved with flexion of the quadriceps muscles, thereby not testing the anterior calf compartment, which is the muscle group of interest.)

Some centers have advocated use of pressure monitoring devices to measure compartment pressures, but it has been our practice that if compartment syndrome is even suspected, it is imperative to perform fasciotomies emergently. This is best accomplished by the two-incision technique with a medial infrageniculate incision releasing the pressure within the deep and posterior compartments, and a lateral incision releasing the anterior and lateral compartments. Fasciotomies can be performed in the ICU setting using Bovie electrocautery and sterile scissors. The underlying muscle should bulge when released, thereby confirming the diagnosis. The wound should be left open and treated with routine dressing changes with subsequent closure in several days to weeks when the swelling abates. The metabolic sequelae of compartment syndrome may consist of cellular lysis with release of potassium and myoglobin that may cause systemic hyperkalemia and possibly acute renal failure. We routinely check urine myoglobin and administer aggressive intravenous fluids to ensure brisk urine output of at least 100 mL/hour. Electrolytes are checked frequently and continuous telemetric cardiac monitoring is employed.

Each extremity should be assessed by checking for palpable pulses; if none is found, Doppler signals must be auscultated to assess the perfusion. Ample quantity of Doppler gel should be used and the Doppler probe should be positioned at 60 degrees from the long axis of blood flow to maximize the signal. Normal Doppler signals are described as triphasic: the initial forward flow of blood is due to left ventricular systolic ejection; the second (reversal) flow is due to the intrinsic resistance of the arterioles in the circulation; the third phase again is forward-directed flow, and is largely attributed to the elasticity of the aorta. Doppler signals distal to an obstruction may be characterized as biphasic or monophasic signals with the latter suggesting significantly diminished blood flow. Sometimes it is difficult to tell if the sound is venous or arterial. If the sound disappears with gentle pressure on the Doppler probe, it is likely a venous sound. Also, if the sound in one of the pedal pulses disappears with gentle compression around the forefoot, it may be a venous and not arterial sound. At the conclusion of any vascular procedure, extremity perfusion is assessed prior to leaving the operating room. The operating surgeon should relay to the ICU team of physicians and nurses the quality and location of each Doppler signal or palpable pulse, as well as the frequency that he or she wants the perfusion assessed. Any change in the exam or inability of the examiner to detect the signal may potentially constitute an emergent trip back to the operating room to restore perfusion. Loss of a palpable pulse even if the pulse remains by Doppler should always be cause for alarm and the operating team should be alerted.

As an objective marker of extremity perfusion, we advocate bedside ankle-brachial index (ABI) measurements. This is done by inflating blood pressure cuffs on each arm and listening to the Doppler signal of the brachial arteries and comparing the values to the Doppler signals auscultated at the dorsalis pedis (DP) and posterior tibial (PT) arteries after inflating the cuff on the calves. The pressure at which arterial perfusion is restored as the cuff deflates is noted in each location. The ABI is the quotient of the pressure in the higher of the DP or PT pressures and the higher of the arm pressures. Each leg has a single ABI. Any change of greater than 0.15 is significant and should be reported, independent of any other clinical event.

All vascular surgery wounds should be examined daily for signs of infection. Of particular difficulty are the incisions made in the groins. The incidence of groin wound complications in the vascular surgery patient has been estimated to be up to 44% in some series (12,13). Although most surgeons try to close groin wounds with several layers of suture, any breakdown of the wound can be a significant complication. Groin wound breakdown is especially common in obese patients and efforts should be directed toward keeping this area dry and covered with sterile gauze. We tend to keep Foley catheters in place in the questionably mobile patient to avoid contamination of the wound, or at the least, maceration of the skin surrounding the surgical site. Most breakdowns can be treated with local therapy, usually routine dressing changes at the bedside.

Although there has been a great deal of interest in new techniques and agents to expedite wound healing, few advances have impacted the overall rate of wound complications, possibly owing to the patient's underlying systemic illnesses that translate into slow healing. The most disastrous complication of groin, or any other wound, breakdown is the exposure of the underlying vascular graft or anastomosis with the devastating potential for anastomotic disruption. When the bypass graft is noted to be exposed, patients should be scheduled for the operating room for exploration and attempted reclosure of the wound, preferably with autogenous tissue such as a sartorius or rectus flap. Until the patient can go back to the operating room (OR), it is imperative that all health care personnel treating the patient be aware of exposed vasculature. We have instituted a "blowout precaution" protocol wherein patients are kept at bedrest and blood typed and crossed. Any bleeding from the wound is a potential emergency. Immediate pressure should be held on the wound, the patient stabilized, and the operating team notified. We have on occasion had to rush back to the operating room with a member of the team holding direct pressure on the wound until the patient is intubated and anesthetized, the surgeon scrubbed in, and the operative field prepped (even if this includes the team member's gloved hand being prepped into the field).

For the vascular patient, meticulous care of the skin is mandatory, and even modest duration of pressure on the heel by the bed mattress can lead to skin breakdown and turn a successful revascularization into an amputation. Since the vast majority of vascular patients have compromised distal perfusion, we try to keep the heels off of the bed by placing the extremity on pillows, which allows the weight of the leg to be borne over a larger surface area. There is no substitute for frequent inspection of all pressure-sensitive areas and this should be part of the physician's and nurse's practice.

Pharmacologic prophylaxis against thromboembolic events is the routine. However, many patients require systemic anticoagulation after vascular surgical procedures (14) such as with distal bypasses when there is compromised outflow or less than ideal conduit. The need for systemic anticoagulation must be balanced with the risk of bleeding complications, and usually we hold off full anticoagulation until postoperative day 2 or 3. In most patients we will give subtherapeutic heparin (400–500 U/hour) in the early postoperative period. Patients are monitored for any decline in platelet counts, and if seen, a heparin antibody panel is sent. If the clinical suspicion is high, we stop all heparin and switch to anticoagulation with other agents. Regardless of the agent chosen, it is imperative that the anticoagulation be monitored closely and is best accomplished with protocol-driven therapy (15).

Acute limb ischemia in the ICU setting can have disastrous consequences. The pathologic differential includes embolic events (usually from cardiac or aortic sources) or *in situ* thrombosis of pre-existing atherosclerotic lesions that likely is a consequence of plaque instability and the aggregation of platelets, which then occludes the vessel. If identified acutely, there may be a role for intra-arterial thrombolysis, although in the setting of the postsurgical patient, this role is limited due to excessive bleeding risk. When an ischemic extremity is identified, patients should immediately be fully anticoagulated while resources are being mobilized to further evaluate the problem. More aggressive intervention, either catheter-based therapy or open surgical thrombectomy, should be entertained. In general, if the acute arterial occlusion is associated with motor or sensory deficits, then an emergent exploration is indicated. On rare occasions, patients present with acute lower extremity paralysis secondary to acute infrarenal aortic occlusion. There is often a delay in diagnosis owing to an investigation of neurologic causes of the paraplegia. Absence of femoral pulses is a clue to the vascular nature of the paralysis. These patients typically require emergent procedures, and despite operative success, the perioperative mortality rate exceeds 50% (16).

Common ICU causes of arterial occlusion include sequelae of invasive monitoring, usually intra-arterial lines. In a recent review of brachial artery cannulations for cardiac catheterizations, the overall complication rate was an astonishing 36% (17). Not infrequently we are called to assess lack of distal perfusion in an extremity with an indwelling arterial line. The first step is to remove the catheter and to observe for restoration of perfusion. The collateral blood supply should also be assessed (usually the ulnar pulse in the event of radial artery occlusion) as well as the distal perfusion, including motor and sensory assessment. Choices of therapy include observation, systemic anticoagulation, local thrombolysis, and operative thrombectomy with the potential for bypass.

The choice of invasive arterial and venous monitoring can represent a continuous challenge in any ICU patient, but in particular the vascular ICU patient. Lower extremity intravenous and arterial lines are contraindicated in patients with peripheral arterial occlusive disease. Furthermore, patients with dialysis access fistulae should have that extremity kept free of IVs, central venous catheters, invasive arterial lines, and noninvasive blood pressure cuffs. If a patient is identified as likely to require permanent vascular access in the future, duplex ultrasonography should be used to identify a potential arm for future access, and the identified extremity should be preserved.

Various bleeding complications can occur in the postoperative vascular wound. These can range from simple "skin edge" bleeding to frank exsanguination. Skin edge bleeding may be a nuisance, and may be treated with manual compression, application of silver nitrate, or a simple suture. Hematomas are monitored closely. Recurrent blood transfusion requirements, overlying skin or wound compromise, deleterious mass effects, and hemodynamic instability are all indications for operative evacuation of the hematoma. Patients who have had percutaneous interventions (usually through the groin at the common femoral artery) should also be monitored for hematomas, and in these instances, simple manual compression may be adequate. Attempted femoral artery punctures that are aimed more cephalad may in fact be external iliac artery punctures. Compression for hemostasis may be ineffective due to the retroperitoneal location of the arteriotomy. A progressive hematoma in such a location more often requires surgical repair (open or endovascular).

SPECIFIC CONDITIONS

Aneurysmal Disease

Infrarenal Abdominal Aortic Aneurysm

Approximately 90% of the extracranial aneurysms found in the human body involve the infrarenal aorta. The natural history of aneurysms of the aorta is to expand and rupture. The tension felt by the thinning aortic wall can be estimated by the Law of Laplace, which describes the relationship between aortic diameter and wall tension. The results of randomized trials and observational studies have led vascular surgeons to recommend operative repair when the diameter of the aorta reaches 5.5 cm in asymptomatic patients (18), but the numeric value varies, especially with female patients. Most aneurysms are asymptomatic and are discovered during radiographic workup of other problems. Patients who have symptomatic aneurysms generally complain of back or abdominal pain. These symptoms should be interpreted as a sign of impending rupture necessitating urgent repair. We no longer place pulmonary artery catheters routinely, but all patients have arterial lines and Foley catheters and most have central lines. All patients get a single dose of preoperative antibiotics, which are not continued postoperatively.

Endovascular Repair. Depending on patient anatomy and institutional expertise, abdominal aortic aneurysm repair can be performed either via an open or endovascular approach. The endovascular approach holds great appeal in terms of reduced physiologic insult to the patient. Typically, both common femoral arteries are accessed either percutaneously or via an open groin exposure, and the device is placed from within the arterial lumen using fluoroscopic guidance. The weakened arterial wall is bolstered from within with stents made of a malleable metal alloy and a woven fabric. These patients rarely require admission to the ICU but are monitored for hematomas and lower extremity pulses. The devices used to deploy endovascular stents can be as large as 26 French, and these are introduced through femoral or external iliac arteries. There is a possibility of local arterial damage or dislodging of plaque that may embolize distally.

Open Repair. Open aneurysms, on the other hand, require surgical ICU monitoring postoperatively. The overall perioperative mortality is approximately 5% (19). Because a prosthetic graft has been sewn to the abdominal aorta, the main concern is bleeding. Furthermore, because the blood supply to the lower extremities is occluded intraoperatively during the aortic repair, it is vital to objectively assess and document lower extremity perfusion. Lower extremity ischemic events after open abdominal aortic aneurysm repairs occur in 2% to 5% of patients (20). Any inability to detect a Doppler signal or palpate a pulse when there previously was one is a potential surgical emergency.

A major complication of open abdominal aortic aneurysm surgery is gastrointestinal problems. A large retrospective study estimated the incidence of postoperative prolonged ileus to be 11% and nonischemic diarrhea to be 7.1% (20). All patients will have a brief period of postoperative ileus that may be shortened by use of a retroperitoneal approach to aneurysmorrhaphy (21). However, the dreaded complication is colonic ischemia with an estimated prevalence of 0.6% (20). Most instances present as bloody stools 3 to 5 days postoperatively but may occur as early as the first 24 hours after surgery and are cause for considerable concern. Warning signs include fever, abdominal pain, thrombocytopenia, unexplained leukocytosis, or lactic acidosis. Any suspicion of colonic ischemia should prompt endoscopic evaluation, with the obvious caveat that endoscopy will only view the mucosal changes, and cannot evaluate for transmural ischemia. However, in the appropriate clinical setting, mucosal ischemia may justify operative exploration with possibly colon resection and end colostomy. These patients require intensive invasive ICU monitoring, as they often progress to multisystem organ failure as a result of their colonic ischemia. Routine broad-spectrum antibiotics to include Gram-negative and anaerobic coverage are used.

Other potential gastrointestinal complications known to occur include cholecystitis and pancreatitis. The latter is probably related to direct surgical trauma during aortic exposure and is usually self-limited. Cholecystitis may be ischemia related or may be a variant of acalculous cholecystitis seen in ICU patients. Treatment options range from percutaneous cholecystostomy to surgical cholecystectomy. Much like the problem of colon ischemia in the setting of an aortic graft, an infected gallbladder should not be overlooked or minimized.

The incidence of postoperative renal dysfunction can be as high as 5.4% after open infrarenal aortic surgery, but dialysis requirement is much less at 0.6% (20). Renal dysfunction is significantly lower in patients who have undergone infrarenal aortic cross-clamp, thereby avoiding the obligate renal ischemia-reperfusion. The exact etiology of the renal dysfunction after infrarenal clamping is largely speculative, but may involve migration of atheroemboli leading to acute tubular necrosis. In the early postoperative period, oliguria is most frequently due to intravascular depletion and not intrinsic renal dysfunction. However, patients with baseline renal insufficiency, those more than 2 days postoperative, or those who do not respond appropriately to intravenous fluid challenges should be investigated for acute tubular necrosis or other intrinsic (nonprerenal) cause of oliguria.

In the absence of other causes (e.g., colon ischemia), patients may experience postoperative thrombocytopenia. Although an inciting event or agent is not always identifiable, there are several likely etiologies. Before occluding the aorta in the operating room, all patients are systemically heparinized, and although our practice is to reverse the anticoagulant effects of heparin toward the end of the case, the drug's side effects may persist. Unless there is evidence of ongoing bleeding, mild thrombocytopenia is usually well tolerated.

The cohort of patients who get abdominal aneurysms may have coronary artery disease and are at risk for postoperative myocardial infarctions, dysrhythmias, and episodes of congestive heart failure. Johnston reported an incidence of myocardial infarctions (5.2%), heart failure (8.9%), and dysrhythmia requiring treatment (10.5%). The overall incidence of any perioperative cardiac event was 15.1% (20). Unless contraindicated, patients undergoing open aneurysm repair should be on a medical regimen consisting of a β-blocker with a target heart rate of 70 to 75, a statin (independent of serum cholesterol levels), and some form of antiplatelet therapy, usually aspirin.

Ruptured Aortic Aneurysms

A meta-analysis found the operative mortality rate of ruptured abdominal aortic aneurysm (AAA) to be 48%, with a small decline in mortality for each decade from the 1950s to the 1990s (22) (much higher than an elective AAA repair of <5% mortality). With ruptured AAA, there are impressive fluid shifts that transpire during such an emergent operation, independent of overt blood loss. These fluid shifts, associated with the hypotension and the physiologic strain of an emergent procedure, contribute to a tenuous postoperative course. The incidence of colonic ischemia is significantly higher after ruptured aneurysm repair compared to elective open aneurysmorrhaphy, and some authors recommend empiric and routine endoscopic evaluation of the colonic mucosa.

Juxtarenal or Suprarenal Aortic Aneurysms

Most aortic aneurysms are infrarenal, meaning that the proximal extent of the dilated segment of aorta is caudal to the lowest renal artery. Therefore, operative repair usually can be performed with infrarenal aortic occlusion in the operating room. If the aneurysm extends to the level of the renal arteries, or involves the para-visceral aorta, the repair becomes technically more challenging. The postoperative complications escalate dramatically due to renal and possibly mesenteric ischemia-reperfusion. Depending on the length of intraoperative ischemia, there is a resultant release of pro- and anti-inflammatory cytokines that drives a systemic inflammatory reaction resulting in multisystem organ failure (23). There is considerable third spacing of fluid in the first 24 hours as edema collects in the interstitial spaces. Attempts to improve mortality and morbidity by a hybrid approach involving multiple visceral bypasses and endovascular repair of the aneurysm have met with mixed results (24).

If the thoracic cavity is violated as a part of the aneurysm repair, the patient will have an even greater risk of pulmonary complications. Routinely a chest tube is placed intraoperatively to drain any pleural fluid that may accumulate. Adequate pain control is key in these patients.

Infected Aortic Graft

One of the more dreaded complications of aortic surgery is infection of the prosthesis. This rarely happens in the early postoperative period, and the majority occurs months to years later with unexplained fevers and a computed tomography (CT) scan that shows fluid around an aortic graft. Other patients present with gastrointestinal bleeding (a manifestation of an aortoenteric fistula) or a draining sinus in the groin. These are serious surgical problems, and patients should be treated aggressively. Broad-spectrum antibiotics (although the causative organism is usually *Staphylococcus*), IV resuscitation, and close hemodynamic monitoring should be undertaken. Patients should be medically optimized and prepared for a staged procedure. The initial step is usually an extra-anatomic bypass in the form of an axillobifemoral bypass, with subsequent laparotomy and excision of the aortic graft. In patients who are good operative candidates, a single-stage aortic replacement using autogenous tissue (syndactylized bilateral femoral veins) of cadaveric vessels can be entertained. These patients are routinely sent to the ICU since some may become floridly septic after manipulation of the infected retroperitoneum.

Despite the misnomer of a "dissecting aneurysm," aneurysms do not dissect. Rather, dissections may become aneurysmal. Dissections start as an intimal flap and blood escapes the true lumen and channels down the aorta, shearing apart the layers of the wall. Dissections that involve the ascending aorta (Stanford type A) are cardiac surgical emergencies for fear of retrograde dissection, causing coronary malperfusion or cardiac tamponade. Aortic dissections that do not involve the ascending aorta (Stanford type B) are usually treated medically with aggressive blood pressure control. The four indications for operative intervention are branch vessel malperfusion (usually celiac, superior mesenteric, renal, or iliac), inability to control hypertension, persistent pain related to the dissection, or aneurysmal degeneration. Dissections can be repaired via open techniques or endovascularly. The postoperative implications and precautions are the same as with any thoracic aortic intervention, with the additional caveat that blood pressure control is paramount.

Arterial Occlusive Disease

Many patients experience narrowing or occlusion of their aortoiliac arterial tree. This can be detected by the absence of a palpable femoral pulse and symptoms of lower extremity vascular compromise: claudication, tissue loss, or ischemic rest pain. The specific diagnosis and management of these problems are beyond the scope of this chapter. The most durable surgical solution for aortoiliac occlusive disease is an aortobifemoral (ABF) bypass. This is accomplished using a celiotomy incision as well as two groin incisions. The prosthetic graft (usually Dacron) is sewn to the aorta just below the renal arteries with similar complications as with open aneurysmorrhaphy (i.e., bleeding, postoperative ileus, colonic ischemia, renal dysfunction, lower extremity ischemia, cholecystitis, pancreatitis). The limbs of the bifurcated graft are then tunneled beneath the ureters and sewn into the femoral bifurcation, usually hooded onto the profunda femoris. The groin incisions, similar to those used for infrainguinal bypasses, should be monitored for wound breakdown, infection, and drainage. Peripheral pulses are regularly monitored and any deviation from the immediate postoperative result is a potential emergency as it may represent a graft thrombosis. Another complication is distal embolization with ischemia of the toes (trash foot). Management is expectant and most often this resolves with minimal or no permanent tissue loss.

As endovascular technology evolves, many iliac lesions are treated with angioplasty and possible stent placement. Although better tolerated by patients, the stents may not be as durable as the surgical bypass procedures. The wound is much smaller in stent placement (puncture sites) compared to the larger abdominal and groin incisions seen in ABF. A small subset of patients, namely patients under the age of 55, are believed to have better long-term vascular durability for infrarenal aortic reconstruction with autogenous tissue rather than Dacron (25). Femoral veins can be harvested and syndactylized to be used as aortic replacement. This requires more extensive operations with longer OR times and larger leg incisions, which can be a cause of significant morbidity.

As with any surgical procedure, redo aortic surgery is fraught with intraoperative and postoperative complications. Patients generally require longer recovery periods. If the decision is made to avoid operating in the same surgical field (abdomen and retroperitoneum), extra-anatomic bypasses may be performed, usually axillobifemoral. These procedures are considered to be less invasive but less durable and still require the same vascular monitoring as any other bypass procedures. Although abdominal complications are not seen, patients still require groin and axillary incisions and there is significant subcutaneous tunneling for the graft placement. With rehabilitation, trapeze devices are contraindicated to avoid undue stress on a fresh arterial axillary anastomosis.

Infrainguinal Bypasses

Infrainguinal bypasses are commonly performed to alleviate symptoms of vascular compromise. The principles for vascular surgery are simple: the patient must have adequate inflow (from the femoral artery), adequate outflow (of the popliteal, tibial, peroneal, or pedal arteries), and conduit ("pipe" to perform the bypass). The incisions that are made are significant, and may not only be located on the extremity being reperfused, but also may be on either leg or either arm as a site of vein harvest. We are particularly aggressive about harvesting autogenous tissue for vein conduit as the patency of infrainguinal bypass grafts using autogenous tissue, especially the greater saphenous vein, is clearly superior to that using prosthetic tissue (e.g., polytetrafluoroethylene [PTFE]) (26). The main sources of morbidity from these procedures are arterial occlusion (which can be detected with routine close pulse/Doppler monitoring), bleeding, and wound complications. The mortality from peripheral bypasses is estimated to be between 2% and 8%, and the cause of mortality is primarily cardiac, so aggressive cardiac medical management, judicious use of antiplatelet therapy, and careful fluid status monitoring are essential (27,28).

Any revascularization procedure is associated with a reperfusion syndrome that is usually mild and well tolerated. However, the reperfused extremity should always be monitored for compartment syndrome and acted upon early. Details about the technique of detecting compartment syndrome and fasciotomies have been described above. Electrolytes and cardiac rhythm should be monitored, and the urine assessed for myoglobinuria, even if that means a simple visual inspection of the urine color.

A major complication of any revascularization procedure is graft thrombosis with the highest risk in the immediate postoperative period most likely due to platelet aggregation on a surgically damaged endothelium. Patients with "high-risk" grafts (i.e., multiple segments of vein sewn together as a conduit, small distal target arteries, or poor-quality arteries) are routinely systemically anticoagulated postoperatively with heparin (14). At our institution, there has been a slight increase in the incidence of postoperative wound hematomas, but the fraction that need operative evacuation is small. In addition to full anticoagulation, patients with endovascular stents are routinely placed on clopidogrel to decrease the incidence of in-stent restenosis. All patients should be on aspirin unless otherwise contraindicated.

Carotid Endarterectomy

Carotid endarterectomy has been shown to decrease the chance of a future cerebrovascular accident in certain patients with carotid stenosis. The procedure involves a neck incision along the anterior border of the sternocleidomastoid muscle, and occlusion of the carotid artery to attain vascular control. Once occluded, the operating surgeon then may place a plastic shunt to reroute blood flow and allow distal perfusion while the endarterectomy is being performed. Although there are many intraoperative variables in technique (mode of anesthesia, whether or not to shunt, and type of shunt), the key outcome variable is perioperative stroke related to disruption of cerebral blood flow or embolic event from clamping an atherosclerotic vessel. Aspirin should be continued in the recovery phase, but full anticoagulation is seldom indicated unless carotid occlusion has occurred. Neurologic deficit may manifest itself upon awakening or occur in the early postoperative period. Any change in neurologic function that occurs after awakening with a normal neurologic examination should be reported to the operating team. Opinions vary whether to investigate with imaging or return directly to the operating room depending on whether the deficit is transient or seems to be dense and progressive.

Due to the baroreceptors in the carotid bulb, patients often experience large fluctuation in blood pressures, which should be targeted to the "normal range" of 120 to 140 mm Hg. Additionally, any wound hematoma, because the neck is a relative closed space, can cause carotid compression and resultant bradycardia or potentially airway compression. The operating team should be alerted if hematoma is suspected. Because the field of dissection is intimately associated with the cranial nerves, a detailed head and neck exam is mandatory at regular intervals. Particular attention should be paid to assessing the function of the marginal mandibular nerve and the hypoglossal nerve. Headache and even seizure activity may be a manifestation of cerebral reperfusion syndrome. This is rarely seen in the immediate postoperative period, but may cause readmission for blood pressure control in the weeks after carotid endarterectomy. These patients should also have a

CT scan because of the incidence of intracranial bleeding that accompanies these symptoms.

Mesenteric Revascularization

Mesenteric ischemia, whether acute or chronic, can have lethal consequences. The restoration of intestinal perfusion sets in motion a cascade of inflammatory cytokines that frequently progresses to the systemic inflammatory response syndrome, multisystem organ failure, and even death. After restoration of blood flow, patients typically have a period of hemodynamic stability for 24 to 48 hours after the procedure, but then progress to retaining more fluid and show signs of systemic inflammation. Subtle early changes such as a diminution in platelet count should elicit concern. To date, despite numerous anticytokine therapies, the treatment of the systemic inflammation is largely supportive (29). As this response is not uniform, efforts to predict which patient will progress to clinical deterioration have been unsuccessful. As with any other revascularization bypass, the patency of the mesenteric graft should be assessed objectively. Duplex ultrasound is noninvasive and is highly sensitive. Despite all the usual supportive measures, the average postoperative length of stay is over 3 weeks (30).

VASCULAR TRAUMA

The care of the trauma patient with vascular injuries shares many of the same principles as care of other vascular surgery patients with the exception that this cohort frequently, but not always, lacks the systemic comorbidities of the typical atherosclerotic vascular patient. Most extremity vascular injuries are associated with orthopedic fractures and dislocations; some injuries are nearly synonymous with vascular injuries, such as a posterior knee dislocation and popliteal artery injury. In the secondary survey as part of the Advanced Trauma Life Support (ATLS) evaluation of the trauma patient, extremity pulses should be assessed and clearly documented. For any patient recovering from an orthopedic procedure, the same attention to distal perfusion is merited. Any change in pulse exam or hard sign of vascular injury mandates radiographic evaluation, usually with an arteriogram, although a CT angiogram is sufficient.

Although most surgeons no longer explore extremities when a penetrating injury is in proximity to a vessel, penetrating trauma associated with hard signs of vascular injury (decreased distal perfusion, active arterial hemorrhage, or a rapidly expanding hematoma) should be evaluated immediately after lifesaving measures are undertaken. Often, the area of interest is operatively explored and the vessel visually inspected. If injured, it is either repaired or blood is rerouted around the "blast field" (e.g., an external iliac artery injury in a contaminated field may be repaired with vessel ligation and a femoral-femoral bypass to perfuse the ipsilateral leg). Venous injuries are ligated unless easily repaired. Revascularization of an extremity that has been malperfused for greater than 6 hours increases the likelihood of a reperfusion syndrome and at the least, compartment syndromes should be considered. Most surgeons will perform fasciotomies if there is any question of reperfusion injury.

Naturally, vascular injury to an extremity that has too extensive musculoskeletal damage to be salvageable can be treated with simple ligation and amputation. Lastly, trauma to an artery and adjacent vein can result in a traumatic arteriovenous fistula. This can occur even months after the inciting trauma, and unexplained extremity swelling, distal ischemic symptoms, heart failure, or an audible bruit over an extremity should alert the clinician to the presence of a fistula.

The perceived incidence of aortic trauma is increasing, possibly due to the increased use of CT scans in trauma management. In the abdomen, any central periaortic hematoma should be operatively evaluated. With the resolution of the current scanners we are seeing a number of intimal injuries and short segments of dissection in the infrarenal aorta and iliac vessels that previously were not detected. In the absence of hemodynamic compromise most of these can be observed. Thoracic aortic injuries are increasingly treated with endovascular devices. Initial care is directed toward treating the urgent life-threatening injuries and controlling blood pressure with β-blockers. Open surgical repair is still a viable option, though in most series the morbidity is clearly greater.

Penetrating neck trauma can involve the carotid artery, which can be exposed readily in certain locations (zone 2) or require more extensive operations to expose adequately (zones 3 and 1). Our current management of neck trauma in the stable patient with a zone 2 injury is to cover the wound in the trauma bay, perform the global assessment of the patient including abdominal sonography and intravenous resuscitation, and then take the patient to the OR for exploration. Only then is the injury exposed since unroofing a clot and losing hemostasis is best done with good exposure in the OR. For more proximal or distal injuries, angiography (standard contrast angiography or CT angiography) plays a vital role in both diagnosing and planning either open or endovascular treatment.

Blunt trauma to the head can result in injury to the carotid or vertebral arteries. Because these injuries are relatively rare (<1% of blunt trauma patients), controversy remains about the best way to diagnose and treat these patients. The Eastern Association for the Surgery of Trauma (EAST) has recently published practice management guidelines on blunt cerebrovascular injury (31). They recommended screening, preferably with angiography, for blunt trauma patients who present with or develop an unexplained neurologic deficit or who have cervical spine fractures, LeFort II or III fractures, petrous bone fracture, or fracture through the foramen transversum, and for those with a Glasgow coma scale score <8 or diffuse axonal injury. While CT angiography has been reportedly used as screening, some have questioned its sensitivity, although it is likely that the newest generation of devices may eventually be accurate enough for diagnosis in this situation (32). The most common lesion discovered is a dissection or intramural hematoma. The general consensus is that these lesions should be treated with either full anticoagulation or an antiplatelet agent that should continue for 3 to 6 months. Occasionally pseudoaneurysms are seen and endovascular repair seems to be the evolving treatment modality for this lesion. Morbidity from this lesion remains high since many patients present with a deficit. In one large series there was a 26% mortality and only 31% of patients were discharged to home. However, in the asymptomatic group that was treated with either anticoagulation or antiplatelet therapy, the failure rate was only 9% (33).

Traumatic amputations, although grossly impressive, typically are not life threatening. Traumatic amputations of a major extremity (digits not included) should be wrapped with warm gauze, and manual pressure applied while the protocol-driven trauma evaluation proceeds. Once other life-threatening injuries have been evaluated, the amputated stump may be examined. The treatment priority should be hemostasis and local debridement to remove large debris. Patients should be given tetanus toxoid if there are no other contraindications. Dressing changes should be initiated, and when stabilized, a formal, closed amputation can be undertaken, with an emphasis on leaving a functional stump for the patient to use.

HEMODIALYSIS

Although the annual mortality of patients on hemodialysis approaches 25%, many patients in the ICU are on chronic hemodialysis with functional fistulae. The extremity with the fistula should be preserved from invasive and noninvasive monitoring devices, and all IVs and central lines should be placed away from that extremity unless there are no other options. Because of the presence of the fistula, the extremity distal to it is at risk of ischemic events, and should be monitored closely. Additionally, tunneled catheters already in place should not be routinely used as a convenient intravenous line except in dire circumstances. These lines can often be a source of infection, and limiting their use to their intended purpose will decrease the chance of infection. When they are accessed for dialysis purposes, it is routine practice to "lock" the catheter with concentrated heparin to minimize the chance of a mechanical catheter complication. Flushing this heparin "lock" will systemically anticoagulate the patient, even if transiently.

SUMMARY

The care of the vascular patient in the ICU setting can be complex and challenging; it requires not only meticulous attention to detail, but also comprehensive knowledge of cardiovascular anatomy and physiology. As vascular disease is a systemic process, the patients typically have comorbidities that are symptomatic before surgery or unmasked with the stress of a surgical intervention. Regular and careful assessment of the patient can minimize, but not eliminate, the risks of perioperative complications.

PEARLS

- Peripheral vascular disease is one manifestation of a systemic process that is proinflammatory in nature and affects the coronary, cerebral, and peripheral vasculature.
- Ninety-three percent of patients undergoing the most common vascular procedures (AAA repair, carotid endarterectomy, peripheral bypass) have documented coronary artery disease; all patients should be managed accordingly.
- Patients with diabetes can manifest angina as nausea, diaphoresis, or "indigestion."
- Any objective change in the assessment of distal perfusion—either by palpation of pulses or auscultation of Doppler signals—is a potential surgical emergency.
- All patients with obstructive or aneurysmal vascular disease should be placed on a β-blocker, an aspirin, and a statin, unless otherwise contraindicated.
- Compartment syndrome may be subtle, especially in the sedated ICU patient. The disappearance of pulses is a late finding. Clinicians should have a low threshold to perform fasciotomies.
- Colon ischemia after aortic surgery may present as hematochezia or melena, or may be more insidious: leukocytosis, thrombocytopenia, or fevers.

References

1. Muluk SC, Muluk VS, Kelley ME, et al. Outcome events in patients with claudication: a 15-year study in 2,777 patients. *J Vasc Surg.* 2001;33:251–257; discussion 7–8.
2. Rossi E, Biasucci LM, Citterio F, et al. Risk of myocardial infarction and angina in patients with severe peripheral vascular disease: predictive role of C-reactive protein. *Circulation.* 2002;105:800–803.
3. Leng GC, Papacosta O, Whincup P, et al. Femoral atherosclerosis in an older British population: prevalence and risk factors. *Atherosclerosis.* 2000;152:167–174.
4. Singh N, Sidawy AN, Dezee K, et al. The effects of the type of anesthesia on outcomes of lower extremity infrainguinal bypass. *J Vasc Surg.* 2006;44:964–968; discussion 8–70.
5. Hertzer NR, Beven EG, Young JR, et al. Coronary artery disease in peripheral vascular patients. A classification of 1,000 coronary angiograms and results of surgical management. *Ann Surg.* 1984;199:223–233.
6. Smith SC Jr, Allen J, Blair SN, et al. AHA/ACC guidelines for secondary prevention for patients with coronary and other atherosclerotic vascular disease: 2006 update: endorsed by the National Heart, Lung, and Blood Institute. *Circulation.* 2006;113:2363–2372.
7. Perioperative Ischemia Evaluation (POISE). http://www.cardiosource.com/clinicaltrials/trial.asp?trialID=1629. Accessed December 4, 2007.
8. Durazzo AE, Machado FS, Ikeoka DT, et al. Reduction in cardiovascular events after vascular surgery with atorvastatin: a randomized trial. *J Vasc Surg.* 2004;39:967–975; discussion 75–76.
9. Weant KA, Cook AM. Potential roles for statins in critically ill patients. *Pharmacotherapy.* 2007;27:1279–1296.
10. McFalls EO, Ward HB, Moritz TE, et al. Coronary-artery revascularization before elective major vascular surgery. *N Engl J Med.* 2004;351:2795–2804.
11. Seeger JM, Pretus HA, Carlton LC, et al. Potential predictors of outcome in patients with tissue loss who undergo infrainguinal vein bypass grafting. *J Vasc Surg.* 1999;30:427–435.
12. Kent KC, Bartek S, Kuntz KM, et al. Prospective study of wound complications in continuous infrainguinal incisions after lower limb arterial reconstruction: incidence, risk factors, and cost. *Surgery.* 1996;119:378–383.
13. Wengrovitz M, Atnip RG, Gifford RR, et al. Wound complications of autogenous subcutaneous infrainguinal arterial bypass surgery: predisposing factors and management. *J Vasc Surg.* 1990;11:156–161; discussion 61–63.
14. Sarac TP, Huber TS, Back MR, et al. Warfarin improves the outcome of infrainguinal vein bypass grafting at high risk for failure. *J Vasc Surg.* 1998;28:446–457.
15. Baird RW. Quality improvement efforts in the intensive care unit: development of a new heparin protocol. *Proc (Bayl Univ Med Cent).* 2001;14:294–296; discussion 6–8.
16. Babu SC, Shah PM, Nitahara J. Acute aortic occlusion–factors that influence outcome. *J Vasc Surg.* 1995;21:567–572; discussion 73–75.
17. Hildick-Smith DJ, Khan ZI, Shapiro LM, et al. Occasional-operator percutaneous brachial coronary angiography: first, do no arm. *Catheter Cardiovasc Interv.* 2002;57:161–165; discussion 6.
18. Lederle FA, Wilson SE, Johnson GR, et al. Immediate repair compared with surveillance of small abdominal aortic aneurysms. *N Engl J Med.* 2002;346:1437–1444.
19. Johnston KW, Scobie TK. Multicenter prospective study of nonruptured abdominal aortic aneurysms. I. Population and operative management. *J Vasc Surg.* 1988;7:69–81.
20. Johnston KW. Multicenter prospective study of nonruptured abdominal aortic aneurysm. Part II. Variables predicting morbidity and mortality. *J Vasc Surg.* 1989;9:437–447.
21. Cinar B, Goksel O, Kut S, et al. Abdominal aortic aneurysm surgery: retroperitoneal or transperitoneal approach? *J Cardiovasc Surg (Torino).* 2006;47:637–641.
22. Bown MJ, Sutton AJ, Bell PR, et al. A meta-analysis of 50 years of ruptured abdominal aortic aneurysm repair. *Br J Surg.* 2002;89:714–730.
23. Welborn MB, Oldenburg HS, Hess PJ, et al. The relationship between visceral ischemia, proinflammatory cytokines, and organ injury in patients undergoing thoracoabdominal aortic aneurysm repair. *Crit Care Med.* 2000;28:3191–3197.
24. Lee WA, Brown MP, Martin TD, et al. Early results after staged hybrid repair of thoracoabdominal aortic aneurysms. *J Am Coll Surg.* 2007;205:420–431.

25. Jackson MR, Ali AT, Bell C, et al. Aortofemoral bypass in young patients with premature atherosclerosis: is superficial femoral vein superior to Dacron? *J Vasc Surg.* 2004;40:17–23.
26. Gentile AT, Lee RW, Moneta GL, et al. Results of bypass to the popliteal and tibial arteries with alternative sources of autogenous vein. *J Vasc Surg.* 1996;23:272–279; discussion 9–80.
27. Abou-Zamzam AM Jr, Lee RW, Moneta GL, et al. Functional outcome after infrainguinal bypass for limb salvage. *J Vasc Surg.* 1997;25:287–295; discussion 95–97.
28. Nicoloff AD, Taylor LM Jr, McLafferty RB, et al. Patient recovery after infrainguinal bypass grafting for limb salvage. *J Vasc Surg.* 1998;27:256–263; discussion 64–66.
29. Huber TS, Gaines GC, Welborn MB 3rd, et al. Anticytokine therapies for acute inflammation and the systemic inflammatory response syndrome: IL-10 and ischemia/reperfusion injury as a new paradigm. *Shock.* 2000;13:425–434.
30. Rectenwald JE, Huber TS, Martin TD, et al. Functional outcome after thoracoabdominal aortic aneurysm repair. *J Vasc Surg.* 2002;35:640–647.
31. Blunt Cerebrovascular Injury Practice Management Guidelines. http://www.east.org/tpg/archive/html/BluntCVInjury.html. Accessed December 4, 2007.
32. Malhotra AK, Camacho M, Ivatury RR, et al. Computed tomographic angiography for the diagnosis of blunt carotid/vertebral artery injury: a note of caution. *Ann Surg.* 2007;246:632–642; discussion 42–43.
33. Edwards NM, Fabian TC, Claridge JA, et al. Antithrombotic therapy and endovascular stents are effective treatment for blunt carotid injuries: results from longterm followup. *J Am Coll Surg.* 2007;204:1007–1013; discussion 14–15.

CHAPTER 83 ■ NEUROLOGIC INJURY: PREVENTION AND INITIAL CARE

CHERYLEE W. J. CHANG

HEAD INJURY

The Problem

Each year in the United States, nearly 1.4 million people sustain a traumatic brain injury (TBI) (1). Of those, an estimated 235,000 are hospitalized, and approximately 50,000 die. In children younger than 14 years, TBI results in 2,685 deaths per year with 37,000 hospitalizations and 435,000 emergency department visits. Worldwide, an estimated 57 million people are hospitalized with TBI with 10 million deaths annually (2).

Compared to females, males have at least double the risk of TBI (1). In 1994, the National Center for Health Statistics (NCHS) reported that the TBI death rate for males was 3.3 times higher than for females (30.7 per 100,000 males vs. 9.3 per 100,000 females). Death rates were highest in persons aged 75 years or older (46.3 per 100,000) (3).

The leading causes of TBI are falls (28%), motor vehicle collisions (MVC) (20%), "struck by/against" events, which include colliding with a moving or stationary object (19%) and assaults (11%) (4). The rate of falls is highest with children younger than 4 years and adults age 75 years and older. MVC-related TBI is highest in adolescents age 15 to 19 years and results in the greatest number of TBI-related hospitalizations (1). Firearm-inflicted TBI has the highest mortality of 90.4% compared with 10.2% associated with falls (3,5). In the military population, TBI is often due to blast injuries with concussion, contusion, subdural hematoma, and axonal shear injury as the primary injuries (6). The Defense and Veterans Brain Injury Coalition estimates that during the recent wars, 40% of injured soldiers suffer from mild TBI (7).

Over 5.3 million Americans require assistance with activities of daily living as a consequence of the long-term effects on cognition and behavior with emotional and physical impairment following TBI (3,8). In the United States, lifetime costs of TBI, which include medical costs and lost productivity, are estimated at $60 billion annually (9).

Although outcome is chiefly determined by the severity of the initial injury, with appropriate neurologic support, secondary brain injury from hypotension, hypoxia, hyperthermia, and hyperglycemia may be prevented and decrease morbidity and mortality.

Prevention

Primary prevention of TBI includes strategies to increase public awareness to wear seat belts, use child safety seats, wear helmets, avoid driving while intoxicated, and install window guards and safety gates. For the elderly, available exercise programs, appropriate lighting, and handrails may prevent injury (10).

PRIMARY BRAIN INJURY

Primary focal neurologic injury following TBI includes hemorrhage into the subdural or epidural spaces, intraparenchymal hematomas (IPH) and cerebral contusions and lacerations. Primary diffuse injury includes subarachnoid (SAH) and intraventricular hemorrhage (IVH) and diffuse axonal injury (DAI).

Subdural Hematoma

Subdural hematomas (SDH) are more common than epidural hematomas (EDH) and were seen in 25% of patients with severe head injury entered into the Traumatic Coma Data Bank (TCDB) supported by the National Institute of Neurological Disorders and Stroke (NINDS) between 1980 and 1988 (11,12). SDH typically results from tearing of the bridging veins between the brain and the draining venous sinuses. The mechanism usually involves high-velocity acceleration and deceleration forces.

Imaging shows a crescent-shaped hyperdensity that follows the contours of the brain. Hyperacute hemorrhages or SDH in anemic patients are isointense on initial CT and may be overlooked. Acute SDH carries a poor prognosis and is one of the most lethal of all head injuries. Fifty to 60% of patients with SDH die, and only 19% to 38% will achieve functional recovery despite surgical treatment (13,14). Early evacuation within the first 4 hours of injury decreased mortality from 90% to 30% in a single study of 82 consecutive comatose patients. This suggested that preventable secondary injury was the cause of the high mortality, despite multiple studies, these findings have not been replicated. More likely the high mortality is a result of the severity of initial forces from the primary mechanism of injury (15,16).

Epidural Hematomas

Epidural hematoma was found in 9% of 1,030 patients in the TCDB (17). An EDH requires a great impact force and is often associated with a skull fracture that disrupts the middle meningeal artery in the supratentorial space or causes injury to the venous sinuses in the posterior fossa (18). Classically, patients present awake and alert, known as the lucid interval, and quickly lapse into unconsciousness. Imaging shows a lenticular-shaped hyperdensity. With rapid evacuation, EDH has a relatively good prognosis, and the mortality rate is 5% to 10% (19). Factors determining mortality and functional outcome include age, best motor response on the Glasgow coma score (GCS), hematoma volume, and degree of midline shift (19–21). In patients with EDH who are comatose with either a very short or no period of wakefulness following injury, mortality can be as high as 40%. The motor score immediately before surgical evaluation is predictive; two thirds of patients with scores of 3 or less become vegetative or die (22).

Cerebral Contusions

Cerebral contusions result from direct impact of the brain on the skull. These are known as coup injuries. Alternatively, acceleration/deceleration injury of the brain against the contralateral side of the direct impact causes contrecoup injuries. The most common areas of contusion are the frontal, temporal lobes and occipital regions. These lesions are hyperintense areas within the parenchyma on CT scan and are more diffuse than IPH. As discussed below, secondary injury can result when contusions enlarge, which causes cerebral edema and intracranial hypertension (23). Clinical deterioration or elevation in ICP requires urgent repeat cerebral imaging.

Intraparenchymal Hemorrhage

Intraparenchymal hemorrhage (IPH), similar to a contusion, is hyperintense on CT scan. It is a focal process and less diffuse than a contusion as it is caused by direct vascular injury or by stretching of the vessels with brain shift and distortion. Hemorrhage in the upper brainstem (midbrain and pons), known as Duret hemorrhages, can also occur with rapidly evolving transtentorial herniation and may be due to stretching of the perforating arterioles or from venous thrombosis and infarction. Spontaneous causes of IPH are hypertensive hemorrhagic stroke, or hemorrhaging due to arteriovenous malformation, aneurysm, amyloid angiopathy, or tumor. In the setting of hemorrhage in the basal ganglia, cerebellum, or thalamus, the clinician should consider the differential of spontaneous IPH as a possible cause of the traumatic event, rather than the result.

Subarachnoid Hemorrhage

Trauma is the most common cause of subarachnoid hemorrhage. It occurs in 21% to 53% of patients with severe TBI and worsens outcome (24,25). In contrast to aneurysmal SAH, traumatic SAH (tSAH) is less likely concentrated in the basal cisterns and is usually found over the hemispheric convexities. The presence of tSAH in the basal cisterns carries a positive predictive value of unfavorable outcome of up to 70% (26).

Intraventricular Hemorrhage

Intraventricular hemorrhage (IVH) in isolation is not commonly seen in closed head injury (CHI). However, like traumatic SAH, it has been associated with worsened outcome (25). Obstructive hydrocephalus may result and may require cerebrospinal fluid (CSF) diversion by external ventricular drainage.

Diffuse Axonal Injury

Diffuse axonal injury (DAI) occurs in approximately half of patients with severe CHI (12). Sudden acceleration-deceleration impact causes rotational forces and shear injury to axons. The axon may not be entirely transected, but axoplasmic transport is disrupted causing swelling and disconnection (27). A retraction ball forms, and the axon undergoes Wallerian degeneration. Since axonal degeneration may be a secondary injury process, eventually pharmacologic strategies to intervene may be developed. Outcome is worsened with severe DAI (28,29). Although microscopic neuronal injury cannot be seen on imaging studies, the diagnosis is best made with MR imaging with gradient echo and susceptibility-weighted sequences that detect blood products from the capillary injury and leak that accompanies DAI (30).

PHYSIOLOGIC PRINCIPLES

The Monro-Kellie hypothesis describes the skull as a semi-closed compartment containing brain and interstitial fluid (80%), CSF (10%), and blood (10%). Compensatory mechanisms to decrease cerebral blood or CSF volume become active in pathologic conditions where intracranial volume and pressure increase. For example, with hemorrhage or edema after TBI, reductions in CSF production and cerebral blood flow (CBF) are seen. Once these compensatory mechanisms are overwhelmed, depending on the compliance (volume/pressure relationship) of the intracranial contents, pressure will increase. Patients with atrophy are able to tolerate larger volumes before the intracranial pressure (ICP) increases. A young patient without much atrophy has low cerebral compliance, which increases the risk for early intracranial hypertension and potential cerebral herniation.

Cerebral perfusion pressure (CPP) is determined by the difference of the mean arterial pressure (MAP) and ICP. When ICP monitoring is used, the CPP supplants MAP goals in the intensive care unit (ICU). Normal ICP is less than 10 mm Hg. In a study in which ICP and CPP were closely evaluated with respect to outcome, the most powerful predictor of neurologic worsening was the presence of intracranial hypertension defined as an ICP of 20 mm Hg or greater. As long as CPP was maintained greater than 60 mm Hg, CPP did not correlate with neurologic worsening (31). Current Brain Trauma Foundation (BTF) guidelines recommend CPP greater than 60 mm Hg and ICP between 20 and 26 mm Hg. Prior to placement of an intracranial monitor, recommendations are to maintain a MAP of 90 mm Hg or greater (32,33).

EVALUATION

On arrival at the ICU, the initial focus is on respiratory and hemodynamic stability. This will be discussed below. In addition to the usual general examination, in the neurologically injured patient, the evaluation includes an examination of the head for scalp lacerations, which can be a major source of bleeding and orbital, facial, and depressed skull fractures. Evidence for basilar skull fractures include periorbital ecchymoses known as raccoon eyes indicative of frontal skull base injury or postauricular ecchymosis known as the Battle sign seen with middle fossa or temporal bone fractures. Cervical spine precautions are maintained in these patients and will be discussed later.

During the evaluation and observation of the TBI patient, repeated neurologic monitoring includes the vital signs with special attention to extremes in blood pressure. Hypotension may result in secondary injury, whereas hypertension, not always associated with bradycardia, can be a sign of impending cerebral herniation. If ICP rises, cerebral autoregulation elevates MAP to maintain an adequate CPP.

A rapid neurologic assessment includes level of consciousness and ability to speak or understand language by assessing the ability to follow simple commands or to at least mimic clear hand signals. Vision is assessed by asking the patient to count fingers placed in the right or left visual field with one eye covered, or to mimic finger movements. In patients with a lower level of consciousness, vision is assessed by blinking to a visual threat. Pupillary response to light (cranial nerves [CN] II, III), corneal reflex (CN V, VII), and gag and cough (CN IX, X) responses assess cranial nerve and brainstem function. Oculocephalic maneuvers (CN III, VI, VIII) should not be performed in patients who have a risk of cervical spine fracture. Ice water caloric response (CN III, VI, VIII) can be performed if the tympanic membranes are intact. The head of the bed should be up at 30 degrees, and 60 to 90 mL of ice water instilled into the otic canal. A normal response is a slow lateral deviation to the side stimulated with ice water and nystagmus with the fast phase to the opposite ear. Absence may be caused by medications or brainstem injury. Motor response is assessed by verbal commands to move the limbs. In patients with lower levels of consciousness, motor responses are elicited by painful stimuli delivered to the sternum or fingernail bed. During painful stimulation, the examiner should also reassess facial movement for asymmetry. If flexion is noted, pain is applied to the supraorbital ridge or by trapezius squeeze to test for localization. In the lower extremities, it is important to recognize a triple flexion response, which is described by the flexion of the ankle, knee, and hip. Triple flexion is a spinal reflex to painful stimulation of the legs or feet. It is stereotyped in appearance independent of the location of pain delivery on the lower extremity. It does not reflect brainstem or upper spinal cord function. Patients who are brain dead or with higher cord complete lesions can triple-flex lower extremities.

The clinical evaluation in TBI includes a GCS, which was first developed and introduced in 1974 to assess the depth and duration of impaired consciousness (34). The GCS has been divided into three categories: (i) A GCS of 8 or less is defined as severe head injury, (ii) a GCS of 9 to 12 represents moderate head injury, and (iii) a GCS of 13 to 15 is mild or minor (Table 83.1). The best GCS following adequate fluid resuscitation and stabilization has previously been shown to be predictive of outcome (35). Interrater variability is often minimal, but can exist (36). In unintubated patients, field and arrival GCS correlate highly. A change between the field and arrival GCS can be predictive of outcome (37).

Laboratory evaluation of patients with head injury include complete blood count with platelet counts, partial thromboplastin time (PTT), prothrombin time (PT), electrolytes with

TABLE 83.1

GLASGOW COMA SCALE

Score	Eye opening	Best verbal	Best motor
1	No response	No response	No response
2	To pain	Incomprehensible	Extensor
3	To speech	Inappropriate	Flexor
4	Spontaneous	Disoriented	Withdraws to pain
5	—	Oriented	Localizes pain
6	—	—	Obeys command

From Teasdale G, Jennett B. Assessment of coma and impaired consciousness: a practical scale. *Lancet.* 1974;2:81–84.

blood urea nitrogen, creatinine, glucose, and liver function tests to assess for renal insufficiency or liver dysfunction, which may impair clotting ability. A toxicology screen including a blood alcohol level is essential to assist in evaluating for other causes of altered mental status and to determine whether delirium tremens may be a factor in the following days of ICU care. Arterial blood gas (ABG) and lactic acid levels help assess volume status and whether ventilation is adequate.

Imaging

The initial imaging, often coupled with the neurologic exam, determines the need for acute neurosurgical intervention. Neurosurgical guidelines have been established for focal intracranial lesions (38–40). Noncontrast head CT is the fastest, most widely available noninvasive imaging technique to determine this. All patients with altered mental status and/or focal neurologic findings should have an initial CT scan performed. In minor head injury, a CT scan may not be necessary if the exam is normal and the GCS is 15 unless the patient is older than 60 years, has a headache, emesis, drug or alcohol intoxication, deficits in short-term memory, physical evidence of trauma above the clavicles, or seizures (41).

Evolving Injury and Repeat Head CT

Progressive intracranial hemorrhage consistent with an evolving contusion is seen in 14% to 38% (42–44). Although worsening CT findings does not necessarily require treatment, 54% of patients may require neurosurgical intervention including ICP monitoring or craniotomy subsequent to the findings on a repeat scan (23,45–50). A significant risk factor is early initial imaging within 2 hours of injury (24,42,50), and often community standards are to repeat a CT scan within 12 to 24 hours of the initial imaging. In stable patients without clinical neurologic deterioration, the utility of repeat imaging is debated since it is unlikely that neurosurgical intervention will be necessary (24,47,50). Other independent risk factors for progression include associated tSAH, SDH, older age, and prolonged partial thromboplastin (23,42,44,50,51). A large initial contusional or intraparenchymal hemorrhage size and effacement of cisterns is strongly predictive of failure of nonoperative management (44).

SECONDARY BRAIN INJURY PREVENTION: TREATMENT AND MANAGEMENT

Following immediate impact and anatomic damage, secondary damage at the cellular level from inflammation, edema, free radicals, and excitatory neurotransmitters can worsen outcome. Contributing factors include hypoxemia, hypotension, seizures, fever, and intracranial hypertension. Immediate postinjury care focuses on the prevention of these problems.

Hypoxemia and Respiratory Management

Hypoxia, defined as a PaO_2 less than 60 mm Hg or O_2 saturation less than 90% can independently increase mortality from 27% to 50% and increase poor outcome from 28% to 71% (52,53). Early intubation can prevent aspiration and minimize hypoxic and hypercapnic events (54) and is recommended by the Advanced Trauma Life Support (ATLS) guidelines from the American College of Surgeons (55) and the Brain Trauma Foundation Traumatic Brain Injury prehospital guidelines (56). A GCS of 8 or less is the usual threshold for endotracheal intubation.

In the prehospital setting, rapid sequence intubation has been associated with increased mortality (57,58). This may result from decreased cerebral perfusion due to hyperventilation-induced hypocapnia. Positive pressure ventilation may cause hypotension in a hypovolemic patient if central venous return is impeded by high intrathoracic pressures (59). Intubation presents a high-risk procedure for secondary neurologic injury. Sedative/hypnotic medications and bag/mask ventilation with positive pressure ventilation contribute to hypotension and hypercapnia and hypocapnia during induction. In addition, direct laryngoscopy causes a marked, transient increase in ICP. Intravenous lidocaine may blunt this ICP response (60).

Hyperventilation with resultant hypocapnia causes cerebral vasoconstriction and a reduction in CBF (61–63). Prolonged hypocapnia appears to slow neurologic recovery (64). Prophylactic hyperventilation of $PaCO_2$ less than 35 mm Hg should be avoided, although $PaCO_2$ as low as 30 mm Hg may be necessary for brief periods for immediate treatment of intracranial hypertension. Options to identify cerebral ischemia in the setting of hyperventilation include the use of jugular venous oxygen saturation, arterial jugular venous oxygen content differences, brain tissue oxygen monitoring (see below), or cerebral blood flow monitoring (32).

To achieve adequate ventilation, positive end-expiratory pressure (PEEP) may be necessary. Positive end-expiratory pressure affects CPP and ICP when the lung is compliant and the chest wall is not. The high lung compliance allows for an increased intrathoracic volume, which in the setting of a low compliant chest wall increases intrathoracic pressures. The high intrathoracic pressure decreases cerebral venous outflow, which will increase ICP (65,66). When intrathoracic pressure is elevated, cardiac venous return is diminished and results in lowered mean arterial pressure and CPP.

Pulmonary infections were seen in 41% of patients registered in the Traumatic Coma Data Bank and were an independent predictor of unfavorable outcome (67). Bedside management includes adequate pulmonary toilet and strategies such as elevation of the head of the bed (HOB) to decrease the risk for ventilator-associated pneumonia (VAP). In patients with intracranial hypertension, during endotracheal suctioning, adequate sedation is necessary to prevent an increase in ICP (68).

Neurogenic Pulmonary Edema

In addition to hypoventilation and aspiration from poor airway protection, a less frequently recognized cause of hypoxemia following TBI is neurogenic pulmonary edema (NPE). Neurogenic pulmonary edema results from central sympathetic stimulation. Pretreatment with adrenergic-blocking agents prevents experimental NPE (69). Experimental lesions in the hypothalamus (70), bilateral nucleus tractus solitarius (71), and the ventrolateral medulla (72) can produce NPE. Traumatic brain injury causes a sympathetic discharge, which increases systemic and pulmonary vascular pressures. The resultant increase in pulmonary capillary pressure increases the hydrostatic pressure and causes pulmonary capillary injury; this in turn causes leakage of fluid and protein, and pulmonary hemorrhages (73–75).

Clinical signs include dyspnea, tachypnea, tachycardia, and chest pain if the patient is awake. Rales are present on chest auscultation. Laboratory results show hypoxemia and a mild leukocytosis. Chest radiography shows a bilateral alveolar filling process (76). Pulmonary capillary wedge pressures and pulmonary artery pressures can be elevated or normal. There are two distinct forms of NPE. The classic form appears early, within minutes to a few hours after acute brain injury. A delayed form of NPE slowly progresses over 12 to 72 hours following injury. Treatment is supportive and often requires supplemental oxygen and positive pressure ventilation. Dobutamine may be effective by decreasing cardiac afterload and increasing cardiac contractility (77).

Hypotension

Hypotension, defined as systolic blood pressure (SBP) less than 90 mm Hg, independently worsens mortality (78,79). Traumatic Coma Data Bank reports hypotension was present in 29% of patients and doubled mortality from 27% to 55% (67,78). If the patient presented in shock, mortality was 65% independent of age, admission GCS motor score, hypoxia, or associated severe extracranial trauma. Adequate fluid resuscitation with euvolemia is essential. Independent of ICP, mean arterial pressure or CPP or negative fluid balance of nearly 600 mL was associated with poorer outcome (80). Guidelines recommend adequate fluid resuscitation and blood pressure support to maintain MAPs greater than 90 mm Hg (33). Once an ICP monitor is placed, the optimal blood pressure is determined by a CPP of 60 mm Hg or greater.

Contraction Band Necrosis

Following head trauma, subarachnoid hemorrhage, seizures, or stroke, patients may have cardiogenic shock with global hypokinesis associated with transient cardiac arrhythmias and repolarization changes (81–84). Arrhythmias may include supraventricular tachycardias, sinus bradycardia, atrioventricular (AV) block, AV dissociation, nodal rhythms, and paroxysmal ventricular tachycardia. These changes are cerebrally mediated and are recognized as myofibrillar degeneration (also known as contraction band necrosis [CBN] or coagulative myocytolysis). The histologic appearance of CBN contrasts to the coagulation necrosis seen with ischemic injury where there are cytoplasmic degenerative changes with cloudy swelling, hyaline droplets, and fatty change. With CBN, the myocardium instead shows loss of definition of the linear arrangement of myofibrils and the appearance of prominent dense eosinophilic transverse bands (contraction bands), and intervening granularity throughout the cytoplasm (85). This injury pattern was first described with pheochromocytoma and has been associated with the administration of catecholamines including cocaine abuse (86,87). It is postulated that centrally mediated sympathetic or exogenous catecholamine stimulation of the myocardium results in cellular calcium overload and results in the formation of the contraction bands (88). Contraction band necrosis is predominantly located in the subendocardium with the cardiac conducting system, which results in the associated arrhythmias (89).

In CBN, cardiac enzymes are often elevated and may be difficult to differentiate from an acute coronary syndrome. However, the treatment for CBN is vastly different and typically includes observation for arrhythmias and blood pressure support in contrast to reperfusion therapy with an acute ischemic myocardial infarction. Clinical differentiation typically relies on the recognition of patients with higher risk for coronary artery disease such as older age, hypertension, diabetes, and hyperlipidemia rather than a young patient with massive head injury.

Posttraumatic Vasospasm

Following TBI, focal cerebral ischemia as a result of posttraumatic vasospasm can occur in 24% to 36% of patients (90,91) and may manifest as lateralizing neurologic deficits such as hemiparesis and aphasia between 2 to 37 days following injury (92,93). In patients with severe TBI, small studies have reported incidence as high as 82% (94). Transcranial Doppler, while reasonably specific, is not a sensitive test for vasospasm. If vasospasm is suspected, cerebral angiography can confirm the diagnosis. The effectiveness of treatment of posttraumatic vasospasm with modalities used following aneurysmal SAH (e.g., hypervolemic, hypertensive therapy or nimodipine) has not been assessed.

Fever

Hyperthermia accelerates neuronal injury by increasing basal energy requirements (neuronal discharges), excitatory neurotransmitters, free radial production, calcium-dependent protein phosphorylation, ICAM-1 and inflammatory responses, DNA fragmentation, and apoptosis, causing blood–brain barrier changes as seen by extravasation of protein tracers (95,96). Despite this, previous TBI studies of prophylactic moderate hypothermia (32°C to 33°C) and their meta-analyses were not able to show improved outcome (97–99). This may be due to significant intercenter variability in the management of MAP, CPP, fluids, and vasopressors (97,100).

In the individual patient, therapeutic hypothermia lowers ICP by reducing the cerebral metabolic rate 7% for each degree Celsius decrease. This treatment can be life-saving and result in reasonable neurologic recovery (101). Pentobarbital coma and/or neuromuscular blockade may be necessary to achieve cooling without shivering. New techniques for intravascular and topical cooling are available. Although complications of hypothermia can include increased risk of cardiac arrhythmias, hypotension, bradycardia, thrombocytopenia, and pneumonia, in studies evaluating hypothermia in cardiac arrest patients, there was no statistical increase in these adverse events (102,103).

Hyperglycemia

Hyperglycemia causes brain tissue acidosis (104), and early hyperglycemia has been associated with worsened neurologic outcome following TBI (105,106). It is not fully understood whether the hyperglycemia is causative or is a marker for severity of injury and subsequent poor outcome. Although tighter glucose control with TBI is theoretically reasonable, based on current evidence, it is not clear that aggressive treatment of hyperglycemia in the neurologic and neurosurgical population improves outcome.

In the ICU setting, where glycemic control often uses insulin infusion or injection, patients with acutely altered mental status should be urgently evaluated for hypoglycemia.

Coagulopathy

Brain is rich in tissue thromboplastin and following head injury, increased tissue thromboplastin activity in the frontal, parietal, and temporal lobes activates the coagulation cascade and causes a disseminated intravascular coagulopathy (107). The Traumatic Coma Data Bank reported that 19% of patients were coagulopathic (67). Although initial evaluation may show thrombocytopenia in 14% and coagulopathy in 21% of TBI patients, in ensuing days, disseminated intravascular coagulation can be seen in 41% to 60% of patients with blunt brain injury (108,109). It is more common in patients with penetrating head trauma (110).

Abnormalities in PT, PTT, or platelet count have been associated with 55% of patients with progressing hemorrhage after TBI (111,112). Associated coagulopathy and thrombocytopenia increases mortality in TBI (108,109,112). Although there are no guidelines for correction of coagulopathy or thrombocytopenia, usual practice is to transfuse platelets for values <100,000 per mL and fresh frozen plasma for an elevated PTT or a PT international ratio (INR) of 1.5 or more. Other alternatives such as activated factor VII or prothrombin complex concentrate may be effective emergently (110).

Intracranial Pressure Monitoring and Management

Normal ICP is less than 10 mm Hg. The Traumatic Coma Data Bank reports that 72% of patients with severe TBI had ICPs above 20 mm Hg (113). Since multiple studies show worsened outcome with ICP above 20 to 25 mm Hg, published guidelines use this as the threshold to treat (32,33).

Maneuvers for management of ICP begin with those with fewer potential side effects and progress to more invasive treatments with higher complication risk (Fig. 83.1). Elevation of the head of bed to greater than 30 to 45 degrees not only decreases the risk of ventilator-associated pneumonia but can facilitate cerebral venous drainage and lower ICP. In orthostatic, hypovolemic patients, however, head of bed elevation can lower MAP. Adequate fluid resuscitation is necessary.

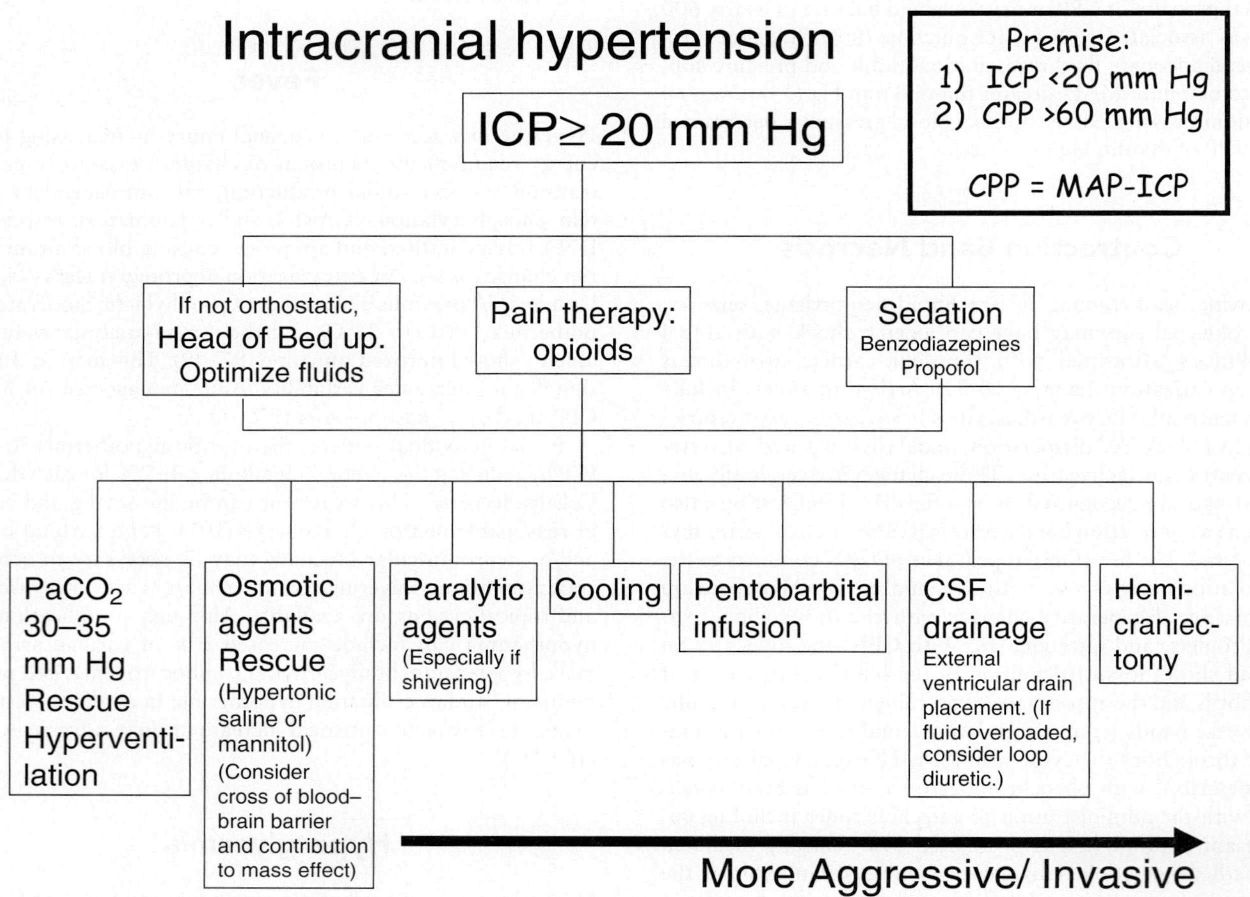

FIGURE 83.1. Algorithm for management of intracranial hypertension. CCP, cerebral perfusion pressure; CSF, cerebrospinal fluid; ICP, intracranial pressure.

Adequate pain therapy with opioids and adequate sedation with sedative-hypnotics decrease ICP. Constant infusion may be hemodynamically better tolerated than bolus administration.

Prophylactic or sustained hyperventilation of $PaCO_2$ less than 35 mm Hg may be harmful and should be avoided. In the situation of impending herniation or refractory intracranial hypertension, decreasing $PaCO_2$ to 30 mm Hg for transient "rescue" therapy will give the practitioner time to initiate other maneuvers to lower ICP.

Osmotic therapy is a mainstay in ICP management. Mannitol or hypertonic saline are both effective. However, repetitive dosing by the above agents may worsen the volume of injured brain (114–116). To avoid this, osmotic therapy similarly to hyperventilation, may also be best used as rescue therapy until more definitive therapy is implemented. Doses of 0.25 g/kg to 1 g/kg of mannitol are effective. The lower dose drops ICP and may decrease the risk of vasogenic edema seen with multiple dosing (114). Due to potential renal damage, maximal mannitol dosing traditionally has been when serum osmolarity reaches 320 mosm/kg, but this convention is under debate. An osmolar gap of greater than 10 from baseline may be a better indicator for maximizing mannitol administration (117,118). Hypertonic saline may be more effective and have a longer duration of action on lowering ICP than mannitol (116,119). Doses include 250 mL of 3% or 7.5% saline or 30 mL of 23.42% saline (120).

Osmotic therapy is best administered through a central venous access as it may sclerose veins. When deciding which osmotic agent to use, elevated ICP with low fluid status would be best treated with hypertonic saline. Studies evaluating the use of hypertonic saline compared to conventional fluids for prehospital or emergency department resuscitation have not shown outcome improvement (121,122).

Neuromuscular blockade (NMB) lowers ICP by decreasing muscle tone, especially during shivering. Shivering increases the metabolic rate and generates carbon dioxide. After administering neuromuscular blockade, an ABG should be obtained to ensure that the $PaCO_2$ has not dropped below 35 mm Hg. The minute ventilation should be adjusted accordingly. Rapid increases in $PaCO_2$ may result in rebound vasodilation and ICP elevation. Ventilator manipulation should be performed in small increments when adjusting to increase the $PaCO_2$.

Neuromuscular blockade also assists in cooling the patient. As noted above, hypothermia is useful in refractory intracranial hypertension. Temperatures of 32°C to 33°C can be well tolerated. The combination of neuromuscular blockade and cooling appears to have a high risk for pneumonia. The patient is unable to effectively clear secretions, and empiric pulmonary toilet with frequent suctioning is often necessary.

Barbiturate-induced coma lowers the cerebral metabolic rate. This results in lowered cerebral blood volume and ICP. Thiopental or pentobarbital infusions can be used. Thiopental in long-term infusion, because of its lipophilicity, may take over a week to clear after the infusion is stopped. For pentobarbital, 20 mg/kg is given as a slow loading dose followed by a maintenance infusion of 1 mg/kg/hour. The loading dose may significantly lower mean arterial pressure. Often fluids and vasopressor administration may be necessary. Electroencephalography (EEG) is critical to titrating the dose during barbiturate coma. Although the infusion can be titrated to ICP effect, if the EEG is isoelectric, there is little to be gained in the way of ICP control by increasing the infusion. At this point, worsening side effects result from increasing the infusion. These include hypotension from peripheral vasodilation, decreased cardiac inotropy, and ileus. Also cough reflex is diminished and decreased bronchociliary activity and slowed leukocyte chemotaxis increase the risk for pneumonia. A benefit of barbiturate coma is a quiescent hypothalamus that no longer modulates body temperature. Hypothermia can often be achieved without the need for neuromuscular blockade since shivering is diminished.

Loop diuretics have been used to help manage ICP by decreasing CSF production in the choroids plexus. Loop diuretics will decrease volume status. Unless the patient is hypervolemic, CSF diversion is a more effective method of lowering ICP.

Other therapy for refractory intracranial hypertension requires neurosurgical intervention. Placement of an external ventricular drainage allows for CSF drainage. Hemicraniectomy may be life-saving and a viable option depending on the patient. Case series of 19, 23, and 51 children at three different centers had mortalities of 30% to 31.4%. Favorable outcome with return to school and functional independence was reported in 68% to 81%. Eighteen percent to 21% were severely disabled and dependent on caregivers (123–125). To date, there are no randomized controlled trials to evaluate its effectiveness and outcome in the setting of TBI.

Brain Tissue Oxygenation

Hypoxic brain injury causes secondary damage. To monitor and help prevent this injury, new modalities to evaluate cerebral oxygenation have been developed. Jugular bulb oximetry ($SjvO_2$) is a global measure of the balance between oxygen delivery to the brain and oxygen consumption. Local brain tissue partial pressure oxygen ($PBtO_2$) is measured by a polarographic Clark-type microcatheter. An increase in cerebral oxygen delivery is reflected by increases in $SjvO_2$ and $PBtO_2$. Oxygen delivery to the brain is manipulated by increases in blood pressure, cardiac output, and red blood cell transfusion (126). Normobaric hyperoxia has not shown to improve cerebral oxygen metabolism on PET imaging, and the use of 100% oxygen is not supported by the available literature (127). Optimal $SjvO_2$ is generally accepted as 50% oxygen saturation (128). The optimal $PBtO_2$ has not been established. Various studies show worsened outcome in patients with mean $PBtO_2$ less than 15 mm Hg. Other thresholds include 25 mm Hg (129–132). Mortality was significantly decreased and functional outcomes improved in one study comparing 25 patients treated by traditional ICP/CPP-guided therapy to 28 patients with therapy targeted to a $PBtO_2$ greater than 25 mm Hg (133). No randomized controlled trials of $SjvO_2$ or $PBtO_2$-targeted therapy have been performed to establish effectiveness. Current guidelines for management of TBI do not recommend the use of these modalities. Cerebral microdialysis evaluating the biochemical byproducts of ischemia such as increased lactate and glutamate and lactate-pyruvate ratio is another potential technology to assist bedside care, but has not yet reached practical clinical use (134).

Antibiotic Prophylaxis

Fractures of the skull base and severe facial trauma can result in a CSF leak. Various studies report incidences of 2.6% to 4.6%

of all patients with basilar or facial fractures (135,136). In one study, otorrhea was three times more common than rhinorrhea (135). Approximately 50 percent of CSF leaks stop within 5 days (137). The risk of bacterial meningitis is approximately 12% to 21%. Studies conflict as to whether prophylactic antibiotics decrease the risk of infection, and there are no guidelines or recommendations (137,138). Constant surveillance for meningitis is essential.

In the setting of CSF leak, if the spine is stable and blood pressure is adequate, the head of the bed should be elevated to facilitate leak closure. Stool softeners help avoid vigorous Valsalva maneuvers that may worsen the leak. Neurosurgical intervention with CSF diversion (i.e., lumbar drain or external ventricular drain) or surgical closure may be necessary if the leak persists.

Following penetrating head trauma, a CSF leak is the primary predictor of intracranial infection. Infection is seen in 38% to 63% of CSF leaks after military-related penetrating cerebral injury (139–141). Current recommendations are to treat with empiric broad-spectrum antibiotics following penetrating brain injury (141,142). Optimum duration and regimen are unknown.

For clean neurosurgical procedures, such as external ventricular drain placement or craniotomy, guidelines have been established by the Surgical Infection Prevention and Surgical Care Improvement Projects that recommend cefazolin within 1 hour prior to surgical incision (143).

Posttraumatic Seizures

Early posttraumatic seizures occur within 7 days of injury. Three percent to 6 percent of patients with closed head injury suffer early posttraumatic seizures compared to 8% to 10% with penetrating brain injury (144–146). Late posttraumatic seizure by definition manifests at least 7 days postinjury and is seen in 30% of patients with penetrating brain injury. Late posttraumatic seizures can occur up to 5 years after injury. There is adequate evidence to recommend antiseizure medications, e.g., phenytoin and carbamazepine, for the first week after closed and penetrating brain injury to prevent early posttraumatic seizures (33,147–149). Of note, valproate showed no benefit for seizures following brain injury and had a trend to higher mortality (150). There is no evidence that continuing prophylactic antiseizure medications beyond a week prevents late seizures, and it is not recommended for closed or penetrating head injury (33,149).

Thromboprophylaxis

In the general postoperative neurosurgical population, the risk for deep venous thrombosis (DVT) is 3% to 14% (151–154). Following major head injury, the risk for DVT is as high as 54% (155). The Brain Trauma Foundation has no recommendations for thromboprophylaxis (33). However, current recommendations from the seventh conference of the American College of Chest Physicians (ACCP) are that patients undergoing major neurosurgical procedures receive thromboprophylaxis in the form of intermittent pneumatic compression (IPC) devices with or without graduated compression stockings (GPC) (grade 1A) (154). Acceptable alternatives include subcutaneous unfractionated heparin (grade 2B) or postoperative low-molecular-weight heparin (LMWH) (grade 2A). In high-risk neurosurgery patients, the combination of mechanical and pharmacologic prophylaxis is recommended (grade 2B). In patients who are not neurosurgical candidates, a grade 1A recommendation is that trauma patients receive LMWH as soon as it is considered safe to do so. In the meantime, mechanical prophylaxis with intermittent pneumatic compression and/or graded compression stockings should be used (grade 1B). Inferior vena cava filters are not considered acceptable primary prophylaxis in trauma patients (grade 1C).

Nutrition

Following severe traumatic brain injury, patients have a hypermetabolic, catabolic state with rapid weight loss associated with a negative nitrogen balance and protein wasting. In experimental models of TBI, 3 hours after injury morphologic changes are seen in the gut mucosa that include shedding of epithelial cells, fracture of villi, focal ulcers, fusion of adjacent villi, mucosal atrophy, and edema in the villous interstitium and lamina propria. On electron microscopy, there is a loss of tight junctions between enterocytes, damage of mitochondria and endoplasm, and apoptosis of epithelial cells (156). These changes in gut permeability increase bacteria translocation and endotoxin, which increases the risk of the systemic inflammatory response. Arginine and glutamine modulate gut permeability. There is some debate whether glutamine should be used in brain injury patients due to the potential increase in cerebral glutamate with neuroexcitatory properties and cell damage.

Early parenteral or enteral nutrition can speed neurologic recovery and decrease disability and mortality (157–160). Early enteral feeding may have benefit over parenteral feeding by protecting against intestinal apoptosis and atrophy (161) and decreasing infection clinically (162). Early enteral nutrition with glutamine and probiotics may decrease the infection rate and length of ICU stay (163).

Current guidelines in severe TBI are to replace 140% of resting metabolism in nonparalyzed patients and 100% of resting metabolism expenditure in paralyzed patients within 7 days. Either enteral or parenteral nutrition should contain at least 15% of calories from protein (32).

Stress Gastritis

Stress gastritis was seen in 91% of 44 comatose mechanically ventilated patients within 24 hours of head injury. Lesions were most commonly seen in the fundus and body of the stomach (164). Mucosal ulceration is typically prevented by maintaining intraluminal pH above 5 or by H_2 receptor blockade (165). In TBI patients, stress ulcer bleeding prophylaxis is typically given. Sucralfate, H_2-antagonists, proton pump inhibitors, or antacids in patients with mechanical ventilation may be effective; none are recommended over another with regard to risk of ventilator-associated pneumonia.

Prognosis

Survivors of traumatic brain injury variably suffer from long-term cognitive, motor, sensory, and emotional deficits. These manifest as weakness, incoordination, emotional lability, impulsivity, and difficulty with vision, concentration, memory, judgment, and mood. Nearly 5.3 million in the United States live with disabilities as a result of TBI (3). When the postresuscitation GCS is not complicated by medications or intubation, approximately 20% of patients with GCS 3 will survive and 8% to 10% will have moderate to good recovery such that they are able to live independently (166). Despite this, 34% to 47% of "minor" head injury patients cannot return to work or their previous lifestyle (167,168). Independent predictors of outcome include older age at time of injury, the postresuscitation Glasgow coma score, injury severity score (ISS), pupillary response on admission, and CT scan findings of diffuse edema, subarachnoid hemorrhage, subdural hematoma, partial obliteration of the basal cisterns, or midline shift (169–174). The Traumatic Coma Data Bank reports a mortality rate of severe TBI patients with postresuscitation GCS of 3 to be 76% and 18% for patients with GCS of 6 to 8, respectively. Overall mortality was 36% in 746 patients (12). In another study of 1,311 head-injured patients, the highest mortality was associated with spinal cord injury, obstructed airway, difficulty breathing, and shock, although none of these was independently predictive of survival when adjusted for GCS (175).

SPINAL CORD INJURY

The annual incidence of acute spinal cord injury (ASCI) in North America is between 27 and 47 cases per million (176). The United States has approximately 11,000 cases per year (177). Those at highest risk are young males. ACSI is most commonly caused by MVC (46.9%) followed by falls, acts of violence, particularly gunshot wounds, and recreational sporting activities (177).

Management

Primary spinal cord injury (SCI) results from cord compression from discs, bone, ligament, or hematoma or from distractional forces such as flexion, extension, dislocation, or rotation, which cause shearing of the neuronal axons or vasculature. Similar to head injury, the spinal cord undergoes both primary and secondary injury. Secondary injury results from systemic and local vascular insults, which may be a result of hypotension, electrolytes changes, edema, and excitotoxicity (178).

Immobilization

Three percent to 25% of spinal cord injuries may occur after the initial traumatic event, and nearly 20% of ACSI includes multiple noncontiguous vertebral levels (179,180). For this reason, early management of patients with SCI includes immediate immobilization of the entire spine. Spine immobilization can be uncomfortable and carries potential morbidity of pressure sores and risk of aspiration, and may limit respiratory function; however, it is the usual treatment for all patients with a mechanism of injury that may cause spinal injury (179). Various methods for complete spine immobilization can be used, but a rigid cervical collar with supportive blocks on a rigid backboard is effective.

Radiologic Evaluation

No cervical radiologic evaluation is recommended in awake, alert, nonintoxicated trauma patients who have no neck pain or tenderness unless there are significant associated injuries that would interfere with their history and physical examination (181). In patients with neck pain or tenderness, a combination of radiologic techniques may be necessary to clear the cervical spine of significant injury. The CT scan is better than MRI for evaluating bones; however, flexion/extension radiographs in an awake patient or MR within 48 hours of injury can best detect ligamentous injury. Newer-generation CT scanners are sensitive, and some centers no longer perform plain radiographs. However, current American Association of Neurological Surgeons (AANS) standards are for an anteroposterior, lateral, and odontoid cervical spine series supplemented with CT scan in the initial evaluation. In an awake patient with neck pain, options to clear the cervical spine include normal flexion/extension films or a normal MRI within 48 hours of injury. In obtunded patients with normal cervical spine films, options to clear the spine include (a) dynamic flexion/extension studies under fluoroscopy, (b) normal MRI obtained within 48 hours of injury, or (c) the discretion of the treating physician (182).

Hemodynamic Support

Systemic hypotension, which contributes to secondary spinal cord injury, can result from trauma-related hypovolemia and from neurogenic shock (183–186). Neurogenic shock is defined as the loss of sympathetic innervation that causes loss of peripheral vasoconstriction and cardiac compensatory mechanisms of tachycardia and increased stroke volume and cardiac output. In experimental models, microvascular spasm, thrombosis, and rupture disrupt spinal cord vascular autoregulation and make the spinal cord more susceptible to systemic hypotension. This worsens spinal cord ischemia several hours after injury (186).

Augmentation of mean arterial pressures to 85 to 90 mm Hg for 5 to 7 days postinjury has been shown to reduce morbidity and mortality and shorten length of stay (187–190).

Treatment typically includes volume resuscitation with crystalloid or red blood cell transfusion if the patient is anemic. Vasoactive medications such as norepinephrine, dopamine, and phenylephrine are used as needed. Volume-resistant hypotension is fivefold more common among patients with complete spinal cord injury above the thoracic sympathetic innervation (188). In the subset of patients requiring vasopressors and inotropes, central venous catheters and invasive monitoring with arterial catheters should be used. Some investigators use pulmonary artery catheters to establish volume status. No studies have been performed to compare these modalities.

Surgical Intervention

The timing of surgical decompression, reduction of bony structions, and fusion in the treatment of acute spinal cord injury remains in debate. A multicenter retrospective study of 585 patients at 36 North American centers applied decompression traction in 47% of patients with cervical injury and successfully decompressed the cord in 42% of patients. Neurologic deterioration occurred in 8.1% of cases with traction. Surgical intervention was undertaken in 65.4% of patients. Surgery was performed within 24 hours of trauma in 23.5%, between 25 to 48 hours in 15.8%, between 48 and 96 hours in 19%, and more than 5 days in 41.7% (191). This wide variation confirmed that there is little agreement on optimal timing. Early surgery may be associated with shorter hospitalizations and reduced pulmonary complications (192–194).

A meta-analysis of studies performed between 1966 to 2000 of 1,687 eligible patients comparing early decompression to conservative management or later decompression concluded that there was weak evidence that surgery within 24 hours improved neurologic outcome (195). Multicenter studies attempting to evaluate outcome of early decompression within 8 or 12 hours are much needed but have been difficult to perform due to the barriers to operative treatment within this time frame (196). At this time, surgical intervention of patients with incomplete injury with persisting compression from dislocation with bilateral locked facets, burst fracture, or disc rupture, especially in patients with neurologic deterioration, is considered a practice option (193).

Pharmacologic Intervention

Following acute spinal cord injury, a cascade of biochemical processes is activated that produces excitatory amino acids, calcium fluxes, free radicals, acidosis, protein phosphorylation, phospholipases, and apoptosis, which can further injure surrounding tissue (186). Pharmacologic agents targeted to interrupt this cascade may provide neuroprotection by preventing secondary injury.

Naloxone, GM-1 ganglioside, and methylprednisolone have undergone randomized clinical trials to examine their effects following spinal cord injury. Despite multiple trials evaluating the use of methylprednisolone, meta-analyses do not agree with respect to recommendations for its use (197,198). A multicenter National Acute Spinal Cord Injury Study (NASCIS) II trial in 1985 of 30 mg/kg bolus followed by 5.4 mg/kg per hour infusion for 23 hours given within 8 hours of injury reported significant improvement in motor function and pin and light touch at 6 months compared to those treated after 8 hours and those treated with naloxone or placebo (199). Criticism of this study include the use of only the right side for motor scores, the lack of anatomic level injury limit or required motor deficit (i.e., injury below T12 and normal motor examination were included), and lack of functional outcome measures. NASCIS III, which compared methylprednisolone to a free radical scavenger, tirilazad mesylate, for 2–4 or 48-hour infusions, showed that a 48-hour infusion initiated within 3 to 8 hours improved motor scores at 6 weeks and 6 months (200).

Multiple trials have failed to show the benefit seen in the NASCIS trials (201), and increased complications such as a higher rate of respiratory complications including pneumonia, gastrointestinal hemorrhage, sepsis, and longer hospital stays have been reported (202–204). The NASCIS III trial showed a higher rate of sepsis and pneumonia in the patients treated for 48 hours. For this reason, the American Association of Neurosurgical Surgeons CNS guidelines offer it as an option, but suggest that harmful side effects may be more consistent with the data than actual clinical benefit. Medical evidence also does not support the use of GM-1 ganglioside in acute spinal cord injury (205).

Pulmonary Support

The most common cause of death in patients with spinal cord injury is due to pneumonia, pulmonary emboli, and septicemia. In patients with tetraplegia, pneumonia and other respiratory complications occur in 40% to 70% of patients (206,207). Aggressive pulmonary toilet is essential. Although diaphragmatic innervation arises from the cervical levels of 3 through 5, an effective cough and deep inspiration requires intercostal musculature and thoracic innervation to splint the chest wall while the diaphragm descends. Patients with high-level cervical injuries (C3–5) may fatigue over the first few hours to days. Also, patients such as smokers with lower cervical injuries with increased pulmonary secretions or those who have aspirated fluid such as blood, water, or stomach contents may have difficulty clearing their airway and should be monitored closely for failing pulmonary reserve. Early measurements indicating the need for elective endotracheal intubation include the use of vital capacity ($<$20 mL/kg) and negative inspiratory forces (less negative than −20 cm H_2O). Hypoxia and hypercapnia are late signs of respiratory failure, and intubation should not await these findings.

Associated Vascular Injury

Blunt cervical spinal trauma can result in vertebral artery injury and cause posterior circulation ischemia (208). Incidence varies from 0.05% to 1% and may depend on screening methods (209,210). Mortality ranges from 23% to 28%, whereas 48% to 58% of survivors have significant neurologic deficits (211). The most common mechanism of injury is MVC, followed by falls and pedestrian and motorcycle crashes. Patients at risk include those with cervical fractures with subluxation or with a fracture through the transverse foramen, especially those with displaced or complex midface or mandibular fracture, a basilar skull fracture involving the carotid canal or sphenoid sinus, near-hanging resulting in cerebral hypoxia, and cervical vertebral body fraction or distraction injury (209). Suspicion should be high if the patient develops a lateralizing neurologic deficit with normal initial CAT scan, or evidence of a recent ischemic stroke on cerebral imaging. Although CT angio with a 16-channel detector shows high sensitivity for screening, the gold standard is four-vessel cerebral angiography (212,213).

A grading system of injury has been described by Biffl (214) (Table 83.2). Fifty-seven percent of grade I injuries heal spontaneously in 10 days independent of therapy (215); therefore, they can be treated with aspirin. Retrospective studies of grade II through IV injuries show no difference between antiplatelet agent or heparin therapy although heparinization increases hemorrhage risk (216,217).

TABLE 83.2

GRADING SCALE FOR BLUNT CERVICAL VASCULAR INJURY

Grade I: Luminal irregularity or dissection $<$25% luminal narrowing
Grade II: Dissection or intramural hematoma with $\geq$25% luminal narrowing, intraluminal thrombus, or raised intimal flap
Grade III: Pseudoaneurysm
Grade IV: Occlusion
Grade V: Transection with free extravasation

Adapted from: Biffl WL, Moore EE, Offner PJ, et al. Blunt carotid arterial injuries: implications of a new grading scale. *J Trauma.* 1999;47:845, with permission.

Thromboprophylaxis

Deep venous thrombosis detection with ^{131}I-fibrinogen scans of patients with acute spinal cord injury and paralysis is as high as 100% (218). The Consortium for Spinal Cord Medicine recommends ultrasound for the initial screening for DVT and venography if suspicion remains high and the ultrasound is negative (219).

Prophylactic anticoagulation for all patients with acute SCI is a grade 1A recommendation from the American College of Chest Physicians (154). The recommended anticoagulation is LMWH once primary hemostasis is achieved or a combination of intermittent pneumatic compression and either low-dose unfractionated heparin or LMWH. If anticoagulation is contraindicated, it is recommended that intermittent pneumatic compression with or without graduated compression stockings be used (grade 1C). The period of highest risk for DVT is in the first few months following injury. For this reason, duration of treatment is recommended for at least 6 to 12 weeks. Warfarin is recommended for the rehabilitative phase of SCI (220).

Vena caval filters are not recommended as primary prophylaxis against pulmonary embolus. However, in conjunction with intermittent pneumatic compression and/or graduated compression stockings, the vena caval filter is a useful option for patients who are at high risk for anticoagulation such as patients with concurrent severe head injury (221). Removable filters are important for patients with SCI. "Quad" coughing is a Heimlich maneuver used for pulmonary toilet to clear secretions in SCI patients with a poor cough (222). Caval filters have been reported to embolize or perforate with quad coughing, and quad coughing probably should be avoided until the filter is removed.

Following trauma, full anticoagulation may be indicated for patients who have undergone spinal surgery. This may occur in the setting of acute pulmonary embolism or myocardial ischemia or infarction. There are no prospective randomized studies of the safety of anticoagulation following spinal surgery (223). In this setting, an open discussion of the risks and benefits with the patient and his or her decision makers is necessary. If anticoagulation is used, close neurologic checks are essential as early evacuation of an acute epidural hematoma can impact neurologic outcome if the injury to the spinal cord is incomplete (224,225).

Nutritional Support and Metabolic Changes

As described above, traumatic injury is associated with a hypermetabolic, catabolic state with nitrogen loss. In spinal cord injury victims, indirect calorimetry will be more accurate than the Harris-Benedict equation to determine metabolic needs (157,226). Although metabolic needs may be increased, the resting energy expenditure may be lower than expected.

Autonomic Dysreflexia

Autonomic dysreflexia (AD) is a life-threatening hypertensive emergency that typically occurs in patients with motor-complete SCI above the T6 neurologic level (227,228). Autonomic dysreflexia is typically seen in the rehabilitative phase of SCI; it has been recognized as early as 4 days after injury (229). Noxious stimuli including fecal impaction, bladder distention, or pain to the lower extremities increases sympathetic outflow below the injury level. Resultant vasoconstriction of the splanchnic bed forces blood into the system circulation and increases blood pressure. Reflex parasympathetic outflow rostral to the injury allows flushing of the skin above the level of the lesion and bradycardia. Recognition of this entity and detection and removal of the inciting noxious stimulus is primary. Blood pressure treatment traditionally included ganglionic blockers, although intravenous antihypertensives such as nicardipine or nitroprusside can be effective.

Prognosis

To better standardize the language used to describe SCI, the American Spinal Injury Association developed the ASIA Spinal Cord Injury Classification (Table 83.3) (230), which has shown good interrater reliability, making the classification useful for studies and comparison of outcome (231). Incomplete injury has a better prognosis than those that are complete. The ASIA Impairment Scale severity on presentation of injury is one of the strongest predictors for outcome (232,233). Those in group A are unlikely to have significant recovery (233) whereas those in groups C and D recover better than those in B. Magnetic resonance imaging shows that complete spinal cord injury was associated with more substantial maximum canal compromise, spinal cord compression, length of lesion, hemorrhage, and cord edema. Substantial canal compromise, intramedullary hemorrhage, and cord edema at time of presentation were predictive of a poorer prognosis (234).

Two clinical entities described in SCI are pertinent to prognosis. The first, spinal shock, is a transient loss of spinal cord sensorimotor function. Patients present with flaccid paralysis and loss of all spinal cord reflexes including the bulbocavernosus, cremasteric, and deep tendon reflexes. Priapism can be seen due to local unopposed parasympathetic outflow. If there is no anatomic injury, function returns within hours to days.

TABLE 83.3

AMERICAN SPINAL INJURY ASSOCIATION IMPAIRMENT SCALE

A: Complete: No motor or sensory function is preserved in the sacral segments S4–S5.

B: Incomplete: Sensory but not motor function is preserved below the neurologic level and includes the sacral segments S4–S5.

C: Incomplete: Motor function is preserved below the neurologic level, and more than half of key muscles below the neurologic level have a muscle grade less than 3.

D: Incomplete: Motor function is preserved below the neurologic level, and at least half of key muscles below the neurologic level have a muscle grade of 3 or more.

E: Normal: Motor and sensory function are normal.

From Krassioukov AV, Furlan JC, Fehlings MG. Autonomic dysreflexia in acute spinal cord injury: an under-recognized clinical entity. *J Neurotrauma*. 2003;20:707–716.

The second is the central cord syndrome (CCS) in which the motor deficit in the upper extremities is disproportionately worse than that in the lower extremities, with bowel and bladder dysfunction and variable sensory loss below the level of injury (235,236). Typically, central cord syndrome results from hyperextension injury without a fracture in older patients as a result of a stenotic spondylotic cervical canal (238). Motor recovery is improved when there is a higher motor score at the time of injury (236). The natural history of central cord syndrome is good neurologic recovery, although some patients have persistent neurologic deficits. Conservative nonsurgical treatment is the usual course. Another group predisposed to central cord syndrome includes a younger population with acute central cervical disc herniation or with spinal instability that may require surgical decompression or stabilization.

SUMMARY

Primary prevention and avoidance of neurologic injury would be ideal. Once neurologic injury ensues, a key principle is that the primary injury helps determine prognosis; however, secondary injury will also play a significant role in the overall functional outcome. Preventable significant secondary neurologic injury can occur in the ICU. The role of the intensivist is to identify these mechanisms of injury and to optimize management. Priority concerns are adequate cerebral perfusion pressure, maintenance of adequate blood pressure and euvolemia, good oxygenation, fever control, adequate nutrition, and avoiding complications of critical care.

References

1. Langlois JA, Rutland-Brown W, Thomas KE. *Traumatic Brain Injury in the United States: Emergency Department Visits, Hospitalizations, and Deaths*. Atlanta, GA: Centers for Disease Control and Prevention, National Center for Injury Prevention and Control; 2004.
2. Murray CJ, Lopez AD. *Global Health Statistics*. Geneva, Switzerland: World Health Organization; 1996.
3. Thurman D, Alverson C, Dunn K, et al. Traumatic brain injury in the United States: a public health perspective. *J Head Trauma Rehabil*. 1999;14:602–615.
4. Langlois JA, Rutland-Brown W, Wald MM. The epidemiology and impact of traumatic brain injury: a brief overview. *J Head Trauma Rehabil*. 2006;21:375–378.
5. Centers for Disease Control and Prevention (CDC), National Center for Injury Prevention and Control. *Traumatic Brain Injury in the United States—A Report to Congress*. Atlanta, GA: Centers for Disease Control and Prevention; 1999.
6. Warden D. Military TBI during the Iraq and Afghanistan Wars. *J Head Trauma Rehabil*. 2006;21:398–402.
7. The neurological burden of the war in Iraq and Afghanistan. *Ann Neurol*. 2006;60:A13–15.
8. US Dept of Health and Human Services. National Institutes of Health. Office of the Director. Rehabilitation of Persons with Traumatic Brain Injury: *NIH Consens Statement*. 1998;16:1–41.
9. Finkelstein E, Corso P, Miller T. *The Incidence and Economic Burden of Injuries in the United States*. New York, NY: Oxford University Press; 2006.
10. Gardner MM, Robertson MC, Campbell AJ. Exercise in preventing falls and fall related injuries in older people: a review of randomised controlled trials. *Br J Sports Med*. 2000;34:7–17.
11. Hlatky R, Valadka AB, Goodman JC, et al. Evolution of brain tissue injury after evacuation of acute traumatic subdural hematomas. *Neurosurgery*. 2004;55:1318–1324.
12. Marshall LF, Gautille T, Klauber MR, et al. The outcome of severe closed head injury. *J Neurosurg*. 1991;75:S28–S39.
13. Koc RK, Akdemir H, Oktem IS, et al. Acute subdural hematoma: outcome and outcome prediction. *Neurosurg Rev*. 1997;20:239–244.
14. Seelig JM, Becker DP, Miller JD, et al. Traumatic acute subdural hematoma: major mortality reduction in comatose patients treated within four hours. *N Engl J Med*. 1981;304:1511–1518.
15. Jamieson KG, Yelland JD. Surgically treated subdural hematomas. *J Neurosurg*. 1972;37:137–149.
16. Wilberger JE, Harris M, Diamond DL. Acute subdural hematoma: morbidity, mortality, and operative timing. *J Neurosurg*. 1991;74:212–218.
17. Foulkes MA, Eisenberg HM, Jane JA, et al. The Traumatic Coma Data Bank: design, methods and baseline characteristics. *J Neurosurg*. 1991;75:S8–S13.
18. Ford LE, McLaurin RL. Mechanisms of extradural hematomas. *J Neurosurg*. 1963;20:760–769.
19. Servadei F, Piazza G, Seracchioli A, et al. Extradural haematomas: an analysis of the changing characteristics of patients admitted from 1980 to 1986. Diagnostic and therapeutic implications in 158 cases. *Brain Inj*. 1988;2:87–100.
20. Servadei F. Prognostic factors in severely head injured adult patients with epidural haematomas. *Acta Neurochir (Wien)*. 1997;139:273–278.
21. Lee EJ, Hung YC, Wang LC, et al. Factors influencing the functional outcome of patients with acute epidural hematomas: analysis of 200 patients undergoing surgery. *J Trauma*. 1998;45:946–952.
22. Seelig JM, Marshall LF, Toutant SM, et al. Traumatic acute epidural hematoma: unrecognized high lethality in comatose patients. *Neurosurgery*. 1984;15:617–620.
23. Oertel M, Kelly DF, McArthur D, et al. Progressive hemorrhage after head trauma: predictors and consequences of the evolving injury. *J Neurosurg*. 2002;96:109–116.
24. Kaups KL, Davis JW, Parks SN. Routinely repeated computed tomography after blunt head trauma: does it benefit patients? *J Trauma*. 2004;56:475–481.
25. Maas A, Hukkelhoven C, Marshall LF, et al. Prediction of outcome in traumatic brain injury with computed tomographic characteristics: a comparison between the computed tomographic classification and combinations of computed tomographic predictors. *Neurosurgery*. 2005;57:1173–1182.
26. Chestnut R, Ghajar J, Maas A, et al. Early indicators of prognosis in severe traumatic brain injury. *J Neurotrauma*. 2000;17:535–627.
27. Povlishock JT, Pathobiology of traumatically induced axonal injury in animals and man. *Ann Emerg Med*. 1993;22:980–986.
28. Jennett B, Hume Adams J, Murray LS, et al. Neuropathology in vegetative and severely disabled patients after head injury. *Neurology*. 2001;56:486–490.
29. de la Plata CM, Ardelean A, Koovakkattu D, et al. Magnetic resonance imaging of diffuse axonal injury: quantitative assessment of white matter lesion volume. *J Neurotrauma*. 2007;24:591–598.
30. Ezaki Y, Tsutsumi K, Morikawa M, et al. Role of diffusion-weighted magnetic resonance imaging in diffuse axonal injury. *Acta Radiol*. 2006;47:733–740.
31. Juul N, Morris GF, Marshall SB, et al. Intracranial hypertension and cerebral perfusion pressure: influence on neurological deterioration and outcome in severe head injury. The Executive Committee of the International Selfotel Trial. *J Neurosurg*. 2000;92:1–6.
32. Brain Trauma Foundation, American Association of Neurological Surgeons, Joint Section on Neurotrauma and Critical Care. Guidelines for the management of severe head injury. *J Neurotrauma*. 1996;13:641–734.
33. Brain Trauma Foundation, American Association of Neurological Surgeons, Joint Section on Neurotrauma and Critical Care. Guidelines for the management of severe traumatic brain injury. *J Neurotrauma*. 2000;17:457–554.
34. Teasdale G, Jennett B. Assessment of coma and impaired consciousness: a practical scale. *Lancet*. 1974;2:81–84.
35. Gennarelli TA, Champion HR, Copes WS, et al. Comparison of mortality, morbidity, and severity of 59,713 head injured patients with 114,447 patients with extracranial injuries. *J Trauma*. 1994;37:962–968.
36. Marion DM, Carlier PM. Problems with initial Glasgow Coma Scale assessment caused by prehospital treatment of patients with head injuries: results of a national survey. *J Trauma*. 1994;36:89–95.
37. Davis DP, Serrano JA, Vilke GM, et al. The predictive value of field versus arrival Glasgow Coma Scale Score and TRISS calculations in moderate-to-severe traumatic brain injury. *J Trauma*. 2006;60:985–990.
38. Bullock MR, Chestnut R, Ghajar J, et al. Surgical management of acute epidural hematomas. *Neurosurgery*. 2006;58(3 Suppl):S7–S15.
39. Bullock MR, Chestnut R, Ghajar J, et al. Surgical management of acute subdural hematomas. *Neurosurgery*. 2006;58(3 Suppl):S16–S24.
40. Bullock MR, Chestnut R, Ghajar J, et al. Surgical management of traumatic parenchymal lesions. *Neurosurgery*. 2006;58(3 Suppl):S25–S46.
41. Haydel MJ, Preston CA, Mills TJ, et al. Indication for computed tomography in patients with minor head injury. *N Engl J Med*. 2000;343:100–105.
42. Servadei F, Murray GD, Penny K, et al. The value of the "worst" computed tomographic scan in clinical studies of moderate and severe head injury. *Neurosurgery*. 2000;46:70–77.
43. Lee TT, Aldana PR, Kirton OC, et al. Follow-up computerized tomography (CT) scans in moderate and severe head injuries: correlation with Glasgow Coma scores (GCS) and complication rate. *Acta Neurochir (Wien)*. 1997;139:1042–1048.
44. Chang EF, Meeker M, Holland MC, et al. Acute traumatic intraparenchymal hemorrhage: risk factors for progression in the early post-injury period. *Neurosurgery*. 2006;58:647–656.

45. Hurst JM, Davis K, Johnson DJ, et al. Cost and complications during in-hospital transport of critically ill patients: a prospective cohort study. *J Trauma.* 1992;33:582–585.
46. Givner A, Guerney J, O'Connor D, et al. Reimaging in pediatric neurotrauma: factors associated with progression of intracranial injury. *J Pediatr Surg.* 2002;37:381–385.
47. Sifri ZC, Homnick AT, Vaynman A, et al. A prospective evaluation of the value of repeat cranial computed tomography in patients with minimal head injury and an intracranial bleed. *J Trauma.* 2006;61:862–867.
48. Schuster R, Waxman K. Is repeated head computed tomography necessary for traumatic intracranial hemorrhage? *Am Surg.* 2005;71:701–704.
49. Wang MC, Linnau KF, Tirschwell DL, et al. Utility of repeat head computed tomography after blunt head trauma: a systematic review. *J Trauma.* 2006;61:226–233.
50. Velmahos GC, Gervasini A, Petrovick L, et al. Routine repeat head CT for minimal head injury is unnecessary. *J Trauma.* 2006;60:494–501.
51. Chieregato A, Fainardi E, Morselli-Labate AM, et al. Factors associated with neurological outcome and lesion progression in traumatic subarachnoid hemorrhage patients. *Neurosurgery.* 2005;56:671–680.
52. Chestnut RM, Marshall LF, Klauber MR, et al. The role of secondary brain injury in determining outcome from severe head injury. *J Trauma.* 1993;34:216–222.
53. Chi JH, Knudson MM, Vassar, et al. Prehospital hypoxia affects outcome in patients with traumatic brain injury: a prospective multicenter study. *J Trauma.* 2006;61:1134–1141.
54. Singbartl G. Significance of preclinical emergency treatment for the prognosis of patients with severe craniocerebral trauma [in German]. *Anasth Intensivther Notfallmed.* 1985;20:251–260.
55. *Advanced Trauma Life Support for Doctors.* Chicago, IL: American College of Surgeons; 1997.
56. Gabriel EJ, Ghajar J, Jacoda A, et al. Guidelines for Prehospital Management of Traumatic Brain Injury. New York, NY: Brain Trauma Foundation, U. S. Department of Transportation National Highway Traffic Safety Administration; 2000.
57. Bernard SA. Paramedic intubation of patients with severe head injury: a review of current Australian practice and recommendations for change. *Emerg Med Australas.* 2006;18:221–228.
58. Davis DP, Fakhry SM, Wang HE, et al. Paramedic rapid sequence intubation for severe traumatic brain injury: perspectives from an expert panel. *Prehosp Emerg Care.* 2007;11:1–8.
59. Shafi S, Gentilello L. Pre-hospital endotracheal intubation and positive pressure ventilation is associated with hypotension and decreased survival in hypovolemic trauma patients: an analysis of the National Trauma Data Bank. *J Trauma.* 2005;59:1140–1147.
60. Yano M, Nishiyama H, Yokota H, et al. Effect of lidocaine on ICP response to endotracheal suctioning. *Anesthesiology.* 1986;64:651–653.
61. Coles JP, Minhas PS, Fryer TD, et al. Effect of hyperventilation on cerebral blood flow in traumatic head injury: clinical relevance and monitoring correlates. *Crit Care Med.* 2002;30:1950–1959.
62. Diringer MN, Videen TO, Yundt K, et al. Regional cerebrovascular and metabolic effects of hyperventilation after severe traumatic brain injury. *J Neurosurg.* 2002;96:103–108.
63. Imberti R, Bellinzona G, Langer M. Cerebral tissue PO2 and SjvO2 changes during moderate hyperventilation in patients with severe traumatic brain injury. *J Neurosurg.* 2002;96:97–102.
64. Muizelaar JP, Marmarou A, Ward JD, et al. Adverse effects of prolonged hyperventilation in patients with severe head injury: a randomized clinical trial. *J Neurosurg.* 1991;75:731–739.
65. Luce JM, Huseby JS, Kirk W, et al. Mechanism by which positive end-expiratory pressure increases cerebrospinal fluid pressure in dogs. *J Appl Physiol.* 1982;52:231–235.
66. Huseby JS, Pavlin EG, Butler J. Effect of positive end-expiratory pressure on intracranial pressure in dogs. *J Appl Physiol.* 1978;44:25–27.
67. Piek J, Chestnut RM, Marshall LF, et al. Extracranial complications of severe head injury. *J Neurosurg.* 1992;77:901–907.
68. Gemma M, Tommasino C, Cerri M, et al. Intracranial effects of endotracheal suctioning in the acute phase of head injury. *J Neurosurg Anesthesiol.* 2002;14:50–54.
69. Bean JW, Beckman DL. Centrogenic pulmonary pathology in mechanical head injury. *J Appl Physiol.* 1969;27:807–812.
70. Marie FW, Patton HD. Neural structures involved in the genesis of preoptic pulmonary edema, gastric erosions, and behavior changes. *Am J Physiol.* 1956;184:345–350.
71. Talman WT, Perrone MH, Reis DJ. Acute hypertension after the local injection of kainic acid in to the nucleus tractus solitarii of rats. *Circulation Res.* 1981;48:292–298.
72. Blessing WW, West MJ, Chalmers J. Hypertension, bradycardia and pulmonary edema in the conscious rabbit after brainstem lesions coinciding with the A1 group of catecholamine neurons. *Circulation Res.* 1981;49:949–958.
73. Schraufnagel DE, Patel KR. Sphincters in pulmonary veins. *Am Rev Respir Dis.* 1990;141:721–726.
74. Simon RP. Neurogenic pulmonary edema. *Neurol Clin.* 1993;11:309–323.
75. Theodore J, Robin ED. Speculation on neurogenic pulmonary edema (NPE). *Am Rev Resp Dis.* 1976;113:405–411.
76. Colice GL. Neurogenic pulmonary edema. *Clin Chest Med.* 1985;6:473–489.
77. Knudsen F, Jensen HP, Petersen PL. Neurogenic pulmonary edema: treatment with dobutamine. *Neurosurgery.* 1991;29:269–270.
78. Chestnut RM, Marshall SB, Piek J, et al. Early and late systemic hypotension as a frequent and fundamental source of cerebral ischemia following severe brain injury in the Traumatic Coma Data Bank. *Acta Neurochir Suppl (Wien).* 1993;59:121–125.
79. Manley G, Knudson MM, Morabito D, et al. Hypotension, hypoxia, and head injury. Frequency, duration, and consequences. *Arch Surg.* 2001;136:1118–1123.
80. Clifton GL, Miller ER, Choi SC, et al. Fluid thresholds and outcome from severe brain injury. *Crit Care Med.* 2002;30:739–745.
81. Britton M, de Faire U, Helmers C, et al. Arrhythmias in patients with acute cerebrovascular disease. *Acta Med Scand.* 1979;205:425–428.
82. Andreoli A, di Pasquale G, Pinelli G, et al. Subarachnoid hemorrhage: frequency and severity of cardiac arrhythmia: a survey of 70 cases studied in the acute phase. *Stroke.* 1987;18:558–564.
83. Blumhardt LD, Smith PEM, Owen L. Electrocardiographic accompaniments of temporal lobe epileptic seizures. *Lancet.* 1986;8489:1051–1055.
84. Jachuck SJ, Ramani PS, Clark F, et al. Electrocardiographic abnormalities associated with raised intracranial pressure. *BMJ.* 1975;1:242–244.
85. Reichenbach DD, Benditt EP. Catecholamines and cardiomyopathy: the pathogenesis and potential importance of myofibrillar degeneration. *Hum Pathol.* 1970;1:125–150.
86. Fineschi V, Wetli CV, Di Paolo M, Baroldi G. Myocardial necrosis and cocaine. A quantitative morphologic study in 26 cocaine-associated deaths. *Int J Legal Med.* 1997;110:193–198.
87. Kline IK. Myocardial alterations associated with pheochromocytomas. *Am J Pathol.* 1961;38:539.
88. Arnold G, Fischer R. Myocardial "contraction bands." *Hum Pathol.* 1987;18:99–100.
89. Samuels MA. Neurogenic heart disease: a unifying hypothesis. *Am J Cardiol.* 1987;60:15J–19J.
90. Taneda M, Kataoka K, Akai F, et al. Traumatic subarachnoid hemorrhage as a predictable indicator of delayed ischemic symptoms. *J Neurosurg.* 1996;84:762–768.
91. Zubkov AY, Pilkington AS, Parent AD, et al. Morphological presentation of posttraumatic vasospasm. *Acta Neurochir Suppl.* 2000;76:223–226.
92. Martin NA, Doberstein C, Alexander M, et al. Posttraumatic cerebral arterial spasm. *J Neurotrauma.* 1995;12:897–901.
93. Kohta M, Minami H, Tanaka K, et al. Delayed onset massive oedema and deterioration in traumatic brain injury. *J Clin Neurosci.* 2007;14:167–170.
94. Gomez CR, Backer RJ, Bucholz RD. Transcranial Doppler ultrasound following closed head injury: vasospasm or vasoparalysis. *Surg Neurol.* 1991;35:30–35.
95. Noor R, Wang CX, Shuaib A. Effects of hyperthermia on infarct volume in focal embolic model of cerebral ischemia in rats. *Neurosci Lett.* 2003;349:130–132.
96. Olsen TS, Weber UJ, Kammersgaard LP. Therapeutic hypothermia for acute stroke. *Lancet Neurol.* 2003;2:410–416.
97. Clifton GL, Miller E, Choi SC, et al. Lack of effect of induction of hypothermia after acute brain injury. *N Engl J Med.* 2001;344:556–563.
98. Henderson WR, Dhingra VK, Chittock DR, et al. Hypothermia in the management of traumatic brain injury: a systematic review and meta-analysis. *Intensive Care Med.* 2003;29:1637–1644.
99. McIntyre LA, Fergusson DA, Hebert PC, et al. Prolonged therapeutic hypothermia after traumatic brain injury in adults: a systematic review. *JAMA.* 2003;289:2992–2999.
100. Clifton GL, Choi SC, Miller ER, et al. Intercenter variance in clinical trials of head trauma—experience of the National Acute Brain Injury Study: Hypothermia. *J Neurosurg.* 2001;95:751–755.
101. Shiozaki T, Sugimoto H, Eaneda M, et al. Effect of mild hypothermia on uncontrollable intracranial hypertension after severe head injury. *J Neurosurg.* 1993;79:363–368.
102. Bernard SA, Gray TW, Buist MD, et al. Treatment of comatose survivors of out-of-hospital cardiac arrest with induced hypothermia. *N Engl J Med.* 2002;346:557–563.
103. The Hypothermia after Cardiac Arrest Study Group. Mild therapeutic hypothermia to improve the neurologic outcome after cardiac arrest. *N Engl J Med.* 2002;346:549–556.
104. Zygun DA, Steiner LA, Johnston AJ, et al. Hyperglycemia and brain tissue pH after traumatic brain injury. *Neurosurgery.* 2004;55:877–882.
105. Cochran A, Scaife ER, Hansen KW, et al. Hyperglycemia and outcomes from pediatric traumatic brain injury. *J Trauma.* 2003;55:1035–1038.
106. Jeremitsky E, Omert LA, Dunham CM, et al. The impact of hyperglycemia on patients with severe brain injury. *J Trauma.* 2005;58:47–50.
107. Ashis P, Marwaha DS, Singh D, et al. Change in tissue thromboplastin content of brain following trauma. *Neurology India.* 2005;53:178–182.
108. Carrick MM, Tyrock AH, Youens CA, et al. Subsequent development of thrombocytopenia and coagulopathy in moderate and severe head injury: support for serial laboratory examination. *J Trauma.* 2005;58:725–730.
109. Hulka F, Mullins RJ, Frank EH. Blunt brain injury activates the coagulation process. *Arch Surg.* 1996;131:923–928.

110. Aiyagari V, Menendez JA, Diringer MN. Treatment of severe coagulopathy after gunshot injury to the head using recombinant activated factor VII. *J Crit Care.* 2005;20:176–180.
111. Stein S, Young G, Talucci R, et al. Delayed brain injury after head trauma: significance of coagulopathy. *Neurosurgery.* 1992;30:160–165.
112. Engstrom M, Romner B, Schalen W, et al. Thrombocytopenia predicts progressive hemorrhage after head trauma. *J Neurotrauma.* 2005;22:291–296.
113. Marmarou A, Anderson RL, Ward JD, et al. NINDS Traumatic Coma Data Bank: intracranial pressure monitoring methodology. *J Neurosurg.* 1991;75:S21–S27.
114. Kaufmann AM, Cardoso ER. Aggravation of vasogenic cerebral edema by multiple-dose mannitol. *J Neurosurg.* 1992;77:584–589.
115. Bhardwaj A, Harukuni I, Murphy SJ, et al. Hypertonic saline worsens infarct volume after transient focal ischemia in rats. *Stroke.* 2000;31:1694–1701.
116. Wakai A, Roberts I, Schierhout G. Mannitol for acute traumatic brain injury. *Cochrane Database Syst Rev.* 2007;1:CD001049.
117. Kruse JA, Cadnapaphornchai P. The serum osmole gap. *J Crit Care.* 1994;9:185–197.
118. Garcia-Morales EJ, Cariappa R, Parvin CA, et al. Osmole gap in neurologic-neurosurgical intensive care unit: its normal value, calculation, and relationship with mannitol serum concentrations. *Crit Care Med.* 2004;32:986–991.
119. Mirski AM, Denchev ID, Schnitzer SM, et al. Comparison between hypertonic saline and mannitol in the reduction of elevated intracranial pressure in a rodent model of acute cerebral injury. *J Neurosurg Anesthesiol.* 2000;12:334–344.
120. Harutjunyan L, Holz C, Rieger A, et al. Efficiency of 7.2% hypertonic saline hydroxyethyl starch 200/0.5 versus mannitol 15% in the treatment of increased intracranial pressure in neurosurgical patients—a randomized clinical trial. *Crit Care.* 2006;9:R530–R540.
121. Shackford SR, Bourguignon PR, Wald SL, et al. Hypertonic saline resuscitation of patients with head injury: a prospective, randomized clinical trial. *J Trauma.* 1998;44:50–58.
122. Cooper DJ, Myles PS, McDermott FT, et al. Prehospital hypertonic saline resuscitation of patients with hypotension and severe traumatic brain injury: a randomized controlled trial. *JAMA.* 2004;291:1350–1357.
123. Kan P, Amini A, Hansen K, et al. Outcomes after decompressive craniectomy for severe traumatic brain injury in children. *J Neurosurg.* 2006;105:337–342.
124. Jagannathan J, Okonkwo DO, Dumont AS, et al. Outcome following decompressive craniectomy in children with severe traumatic brain injury: a 10-year single-center experience with long-term follow up. *J Neurosurg.* 2007;106(Suppl 4):268–275.
125. Skoglund TS, Eriksson-Ritzen C, Jensen C, et al. Aspects on decompressive craniectomy in patients with traumatic head injuries. *J Neurotrauma.* 2006;23:1502–1509.
126. Nortje J, Gupta AK. The role of tissue oxygen monitoring in patients with acute brain injury. *Br J Anaesth.* 2006;97:95–106.
127. Diringer MN, Aiyagari V, Zazulia AR, et al. Effect of hyperoxia on cerebral metabolic rate for oxygen measured using positron emission tomography in patients with acute severe head injury. *J Neurosurg.* 2007;106:526–529.
128. Kiening KL, Unterberg AW, Bardt TF, et al. Monitoring of cerebral oxygenation in patients with severe head injuries: brain tissue PO2 versus jugular vein oxygen saturation. *J Neurosurg.* 1996;85:751–757.
129. Doppenberg EMR, Zauner A, Bullock PD, et al. Correlations between brain tissue oxygen tension, carbon dioxide tension, pH, and cerebral blood flow—a better way of monitoring the severely injured brain? *Surg Neurol.* 1998;49:650–654.
130. Zauner A, Doppenberg EM, Woodward JJ, et al. Continuous monitoring of cerebral substrate delivery and clearance: initial experience in 24 patients with severe acute brain injuries. *Neurosurgery.* 1997;41:1082–1091.
131. Vladka AB, Gopinath SP, Contant CF, et al. Relationship of brain tissue PO2 to outcome after severe head injury. *Crit Care Med.* 1998;26:1576–1581.
132. van den Brink WA, van Santbrink H, Steyerberg Ew, et al. Brain oxygen tension in severe head injury. *Neurosurgery.* 2000;46:868–876.
133. Stiefel MF, Spiotta A, Gracias VH, et al. Reduced mortality rate in patients with severe traumatic brain injury treated with brain tissue oxygen monitoring. *J Neurosurg.* 2005;103:805–811.
134. Sarrafzadeh AS, Sakowitz OW, Callsen TA, et al. Bedside microdialysis for early detection of cerebral hypoxia in traumatic brain injury. *Neurosurg Focus.* 2000;9:e2.
135. Bell RB, Dierks EJ, Homer L, et al. Management of cerebrospinal fluid leak associated with craniomaxillofacial trauma. *J Oral Maxillofac Surg.* 2004;62:676–684.
136. Bernal-Sprekelsen M, Bleda-Vazquez C, Carrau RL. Ascending meningitis secondary to traumatic cerebrospinal fluid leaks. *Am J Rhinol.* 2000;14:257–259.
137. Friedman JA, Ebersold MJ, Quast LM. Post-traumatic cerebrospinal fluid leakage. *World J Surg.* 2001;25:1062–1068.
138. Choi D, Spann R. Traumatic cerebrospinal fluid leakage: risk factors and the use of prophylactic antibiotics. *Br J Neurosurg.* 1996;10:571–575.
139. Arendall RE, Meirowsky AM. Air sinus wounds: an analysis of 163 consecutive cases incurred in the Korean War: 1950-1952. *Neurosurgery.* 1983;13:377–380.
140. Gonul E, Baysefer A, Kahraman S, et al. Causes of infections and management results in penetrating craniocerebral injuries. *Neurosurg Rev.* 1997;20:177–181.
141. Meirowsky AM, Caveness WF, Dillon JD, et al. Cerebrospinal fluid fistulas complicating missile wounds of the brain. *J Neurosurg.* 1981;54:44–48.
142. Antibiotic prophylaxis for penetrating brain injury. *J Trauma.* 2001; 51:S34–S40.
143. Bratzler DW, Hunt DR. The Surgical Infection Prevention and Surgical Care Improvement Projects: national initiatives to improve outcomes for patients having surgery. *Clin Infect Dis.* 2006;43:322–330.
144. Lee S, Lui T. Early seizures after mild closed head injury. *J Neurosurg.* 1992;76:435–439.
145. Jennett B. Early traumatic epilepsy: incidence and significance after nonmissile injuries. *Arch Neurol.* 1974;30:394–398.
146. Annegers JF, Hauser WA, Coan SP, et al. A population-based study of seizures after traumatic brain injuries. *N Engl J Med.* 1998;338:20–24.
147. Temkin NR, Dikmen SS, Wilensky AJ, et al. A randomized, double-blind study of phenytoin for the prevention of post-traumatic seizures. *N Engl J Med.* 1990;323:497–502.
148. Temkin NR. Antiepileptogenesis and seizure prevention trials with antiepileptic drugs: meta-analysis of controlled trials. *Epilepsia.* 2001; 42:515–524.
149. Antiseizure prophylaxis for penetrating brain injury. *J Trauma.* 2001; 51:S41–S43.
150. Temkin NR, Dikmen SS, Anderson GD. Valproate therapy for prevention of posttraumatic seizures: a randomized trial. *J Neurosurg.* 1999;91: 593–600.
151. Dickinson LD, Miller LD, Patel CP, et al. Enoxaparin increases the incidence of postoperative intracranial hemorrhage when initiated preoperatively for deep venous thrombosis prophylaxis in patients with brain tumors. *Neurosurgery.* 1998;43:1074–1079.
152. Constantini S, Kornowski R Pomeranz S, et al. Thromboembolic phenomena in neurosurgical patients operated upon for primary and metastatic brain tumors. *Acta Neurochir (Wien).* 1991;109:93–97.
153. Auguste KI, Quinones-Hinojosa A, Gadkary C, et al. Incidence of venous thromboembolism in patients undergoing craniotomy and motor mapping for glioma without intraoperative mechanical prophylaxis to the contralateral leg. *J Neurosurg.* 1003;99:680–684.
154. Geerts WH, Pineo GF, Heit JA, et al. Prevention of venous thromboembolism: the Seventh ACCP Conference on Antithrombotic and Thrombolytic Therapy. *Chest.* 2004;126(3 Suppl):338S–400S.
155. Geerts WH, Code KI, Jay RM, et al. A prospective study of venous thromboembolism after major trauma. *N Engl J Med.* 1994;331:1601–1606.
156. Hang C, Shi J, Li J, et al. Alterations of intestinal mucosa structure and barrier function following traumatic brain injury in rats. *World J Gastroenterol.* 2003;9:2776–2781.
157. Young B, Ott L, Twyman D, et al. The effect of nutritional support on outcome from severe head injury. *J Neurosurg.* 1987;67:668–676.
158. Rapp RP, Young B, Twyman D, et al. The favorable effect of early parenteral feeding on survival in head-injured patients. *J Neurosurg.* 1983;58:906–912.
159. Perel P, Yanagawa T, Bunn F, et al. Nutritional support for head-injured patients. *Cochrane Database Syst Rev.* 2006;4:1–17.
160. Grahm TW, Zadrozny DB, Harrington T. The benefits of early jejunal hyperalimentation in the head-injured patient. *Neurosurgery.* 1989;25:729–735.
161. Aydin S, Ulusoy H, Usul H, et al. Effects of early versus delayed nutrition on intestinal mucosal apoptosis and atrophy after traumatic brain injury. *Surg Today.* 2005;35:751–759.
162. Taylor SJ, Fettes SB, Jewkes C, et al. Prospective, randomized, controlled trial to determine the effect of early enhanced enteral nutrition on clinical outcome in mechanically ventilated patients suffering head injury. *Crit Care Med.* 1999;27:2525–2531.
163. Falcao de Arruda IS, de Aguilar-Nascimento JE. Benefits of early enteral nutrition with glutamine and probiotics in brain injury patients. *Clin Sci.* 2004;106:287–292.
164. Brown TH, Davidson PF, Larson GM. Acute gastritis occurring within 24 hours of severe head injury. *Gastrointest Endosc.* 1989;35:37–40.
165. Thompson JC, Walker JP. Indications for the use of parenteral H2-receptor antagonists. *Am J Med.* 1984;77:111–115.
166. The Brain Trauma Foundation. The American Association of Neurological Surgeons. The Joint Section on Neurotrauma and Critical Care. Glasgow Coma scale score. *J Neurotrauma.* 2000;17:563–571.
167. Rimel RW, Giordani B, Barth JT, et al. Disability caused by minor head injury. *Neurosurgery.* 1981;9:221–228.
168. Thornhill S, Teasdale GM, Murray GD, et al. Disability in young people and adults one year after head injury: prospective cohort study. *BMJ.* 2000;320:1631–1635.
169. Marshall LF, Marshall SB, Kauber MR, et al. A new classification of head injury based on computerized tomography. *J Neurosurg.* 1991;75(Suppl):S14–20.

170. Mosenthal AC, Lavery RF, Addis M, et al. Isolated traumatic brain injury: age is an independent predictor of mortality and early outcome. *J Trauma.* 2002;52:907–911.
171. Livingston DH, Lavery RF, Mosenthal AC, et al. Recovery at one year following isolated traumatic brain injury: a Western Trauma Association prospective multicenter trial. *J Trauma.* 2005;59:1298–1304.
172. Fearnside MR, Cook RJ, McDougall P, et al. The Westmead head injury project outcome in severe head injury: a comparative analysis of prehospital, clinical and CT variables. *Br J Neurosurg.* 1993;7:267–279.
173. Wardlaw JM, Easton VJ, Statham P. Which CT features help predict outcome after head injury? *J Neurol Neurosurg Psychiatry.* 2002;72:188–192.
174. Maas AI, Steyerberg EW, Butcher I, et al. Prognostic value of computerized tomography scan characteristics in traumatic brain injury: results from the IMPACT study. *J Neurotrauma.* 2007;24:303–314.
175. Klauber MR, Marshall LR, Barrett-Connor E, et al. Prospective study of patients hospitalized with head injury in San Diego County 1978. *Neurosurgery.* 1981;9:236–241.
176. Fisher CG, Noonan VK, Dvorak MF. Changing face of spine trauma care in North America. *Spine.* 2006;31:S2–S8.
177. National Spinal Cord Injury Statistical Center. Spinal cord injury: facts and figures at a glance-June 2006. http://www.spinalcord.uab.edu. Accessed May 7, 2007.
178. AANS/CNS Joint Committee on Acute Spinal Cord Injury. Guidelines for management of acute spinal cord injuries. *Neurosurgery.* 2002;50:S1–S179.
179. [No author listed.] Cervical spine immobilization before admission to the hospital. *Neurosurgery.* 2002;50:S7–S17.
180. Hachen HJ. Emergency transportation I the event of acute spinal cord lesion. *Paraplegia.* 1974:12:33–37.
181. [No author listed.] Radiographic assessment of the cervical spine in asymptomatic trauma patients. *Neurosurgery.* 2002;50:S30–S35.
182. [No author listed.] Radiographic assessment of the cervical spine in symptomatic trauma patients. *Neurosurgery.* 2002;50:S36–S43.
183. Tator CH. Update on the pathophysiology and pathology of acute spinal cord injury. *Brain Pathol.* 1995;5:407–413.
184. Tator CH. Experimental and clinical studies on the pathophysiology and management of acute spinal cord injury. *J Spinal Cord Med.* 1996;19:206–214.
185. Tator CH, Fehlings, MG. Review of the secondary injury theory of acute spinal cord trauma with emphasis on vascular mechanisms. *J Neurosurg.* 1991;75:15–26.
186. Amar AP, Levy ML. Pathogenesis and pharmacological strategies for mitigating secondary damage in acute spinal cord injury. *Neurosurgery.* 1999;44:1027–1040.
187. Levi L, Wolf A, Rigamonti D, et al. Anterior decompression in cervical spine trauma: does the timing of surgery affect the outcome? *Neurosurgery.* 1991;29:216–222.
188. Levi L, Wolf A, Belzberg H. Hemodynamic parameters in patients with acute cervical cord trauma: description, intervention and prediction of outcome. *Neurosurgery.* 1993;33:1007–1017.
189. Vale FL, Burns J, Jackson AB, et al. Combined medical and surgical treatment after acute spinal cord injury: results of a prospective pilot study to assess the merits of aggressive medical resuscitation and blood pressure management. *J Neurosurg.* 1997;87:239–246.
190. Wolf A, Levi L, Mirvis S, et al. Operative management of bilateral facet dislocation. *J Neurosurg.* 1991;75:883–890.
191. Tator CH, Fehlings MG, Thorpe K, et al. Current use and timing of spinal surgery for management of acute spinal surgery in North America: results of a retrospective multicenter study. *J Neurosurg.* 1999;91(Suppl 1):12–18.
192. Duh MS, Shepard MJ, Wilberger JE, et al. The effectiveness of surgery on the treatment of acute spinal cord injury and its relation to pharmacological treatment. *Neurosurgery.* 1994;35:240–248.
193. Tator CH. Review of treatment trials in human spinal cord injury: issues, difficulties, and recommendations. *Neurosurgery.* 2006;59:957–987.
194. McKinley W, Meade MA, Kirshblum S, et al. Outcomes of early surgical management versus late or no surgical intervention after acute spinal cord injury. *Arch Phys Med Rehabil.* 2004;85:1818–1825.
195. La Rosa G, Conti A, Cardali S, et al. Does early decompression improve neurological outcome of spinal cord injured patients? Appraisal of the literature using a meta-analytical approach. *Spinal Cord.* 2004;42:503–512.
196. Ng WP, Fehlings MG, Cuddy B, et al. Surgical treatment for acute spinal cord injury study pilot study #2: evaluation of protocol for decompressive surgery within 8 hours of injury. *Neurosurg Focus.* 1999;15:e3.
197. Short DJ, El Masry WS, Jones PW: High dose methylprednisolone in the management of acute spinal cord injury: a systematic review from a clinical perspective. *Spinal Cord.* 2000;38:273–286.
198. Bracken MB. Steroids for acute spinal cord injury. *Cochrane Database Syst Rev.* 2002;3:CD001046.
199. Bracken MB, Shepard MJ, Collin, et al. A randomized, controlled trial of methylprednisolone or naloxone in the treatment of acute spinal-cord injury. Results of the Second National Acute Spinal Cord Injury Study. *N Engl J Med.* 1990;322:1405–1411.
200. Bracken MB, Shepard MJ, Holford TR, et al. Administration of methylprednisolone for 24 or 48 hours or tirilazad mesylate for 48 hours in the treatment of acute spinal cord injury. Results of the Third National Acute Spinal Cord Injury Randomized Controlled Trial. National Acute Spinal Cord Injury Study. *JAMA.* 1997;277:1597–1604.
201. Poynton AR, O'Farrell DA, Shannon F, et al. An evaluation of the factors affecting neurological recovery following spinal cord injury. *Injury.* 1997;28:545–548.
202. Galandiuk S, Raque G, Appel S, et al. The two-edged sword of large-dose steroids for spinal cord trauma. *Ann Surg.* 1993;218:419–427.
203. Gerndt SJ, Rodriguez JL, Pawlik JW, et al. Consequences of high-dose steroid therapy for acute spinal cord injury. *J Trauma.* 1997;42:279–284.
204. Pointillart V, Petitjean ME, Wiart L, et al. Pharmacological therapy of spinal cord injury during the acute phase. *Spinal Cord.* 2000;38:71–76.
205. Pharmacological therapy after acute cervical spinal cord injury. *Neurosurgery.* 2002;50:S63–S72.
206. Bellamy R, Pitt RW, Stauffer ES. Respiratory complications in traumatic quadriplegia. *J Neurosurg.* 1973;39:596–600.
207. Kiwerski J. Respiratory problems in patients with high lesion quadriplegia. *Int J Rehabil Res.* 1992;15:49–52.
208. Management of vertebral artery injuries after nonpenetrating cervical trauma. *Neurosurgery.* 2002;50:S173–S178.
209. Biffl WL. Diagnosis of blunt cerebrovascular injuries. *Curr Opin Crit Care.* 2003;9:530–534.
210. Mayberry JC, Brown CV, Mullins RJ, et al. Blunt carotid artery injury: the futility of aggressive screening and diagnosis. *Arch Surg.* 2004;139:609–613.
211. Biffl WL, Moore EE, Ryu RK, et al. The unrecognized epidemic of blunt carotid arterial injuries: early diagnosis improves neurologic outcome. *Ann Surg.* 1998;228:462–470.
212. Eastman A, Chason D, Perez CL, et al. Computed tomographic angiography for the diagnosis of blunt cervical vascular injury: is it ready for prime time? *J Trauma.* 2006;60(5):925–929.
213. Biffl WL, Egglin T, Gibbs F. Sixteen-slice CT-angiography is a reliable noninvasive test that allows liberal screening for blunt cerebrovascular injuries. *J Trauma.* 2006;60(4):745–751.
214. Biffl WL, Moore EE, Offner PJ, et al. Blunt carotid arterial injuries: implications of a new grading scale. *J Trauma.* 1999;47:845–853.
215. Biffl WL, Ray CE, Moore EE, et al. Treatment-related outcomes from blunt cerebrovascular injuries: importance of routine follow-up arteriography. *Ann Surg.* 2002;235:699–707.
216. Wahl WL, Brandt MM, Thompson BG, et al. Antiplatelet therapy: an alternative to heparin for blunt carotid injury. *J Trauma.* 2002;52:896–901.
217. Eachempati SR, Vaslef SN, Sebastian MW, et al. Blunt vascular injuries of the head and neck: is heparinization necessary?. *J Trauma.* 1998;45:997–1004.
218. Myllynen P, Kammonen M, Rokkanen P, et al. Deep venous thrombosis and pulmonary embolism in patients with acute spinal cord injury: a comparison with nonparalyzed patients immobilized due to spinal fractures. *J Trauma.* 1985;25:541–542.
219. Consortium for Spinal Cord Medicine. Prevention of thromboembolism in spinal cord injury. *J Spinal Cord Med.* 1997;20:259–83.
220. [Guidelines for management of acute cervical spine injuries.] Deep venous thrombosis and thromboembolism in patients with cervical spinal cord injuries. *Neurosurgery.* 2002;50(3 Suppl):S73–S80.
221. Johns JS, Nguyen C, Sing RF. Vena cava filters in spinal cord injuries: evolving technology. *J Spinal Cord Med.* 2006;29:183–190.
222. Kinney TB, Rose SC, Valji K, et al. Does cervical spinal cord injury induce a higher incidence of complications after prophylactic Greenfield interior vena cava filter usage? *J Vasc Interv Radiol.* 1996;7:907–915.
223. Barnes B, Alexander JT, Branch CL. Postoperative level I anticoagulation therapy and spinal surgery: practical guidelines for management. *Neurosurg Focus.* 2004;17:E5–10.
224. Lawton MT, Porter RW, Heiserman JE, et al. Surgical management of spinal epidural hematoma: relationship between surgical timing and neurological outcome. *J Neurosurg.* 1995;83:1–7.
225. Spanier DE, Stambough JL. Delayed postoperative epidural hematoma formation after heparinization in lumbar spinal surgery. *J Spinal Disord.* 200;13:46–49.
226. [Guidelines for management of acute cervical spinal injuries.] Nutritional support after spinal cord injury. *Neurosurgery.* 2002;50:S81–S84.
227. Khastgir J, Drake MJ, Abrams P. Recognition and effective management of autonomic dysreflexia in spinal cord injuries. *Expert Opin Pharmacother.* 2007;8:945–956.
228. Helkowski WM, Ditunno JF, Boninger M. Autonomic dysreflexia: incidence in persons with neurologically complete and incomplete tetraplegia. *J Spinal Cord Med.* 2003;26:244–247.
229. Krassioukov AV, Furlan JC, Fehlings MG. Autonomic dysreflexia in acute spinal cord injury: an under-recognized clinical entity. *J Neurotrauma.* 2003;20:707–716.
230. Young W. Spinal cord injury levels and classification. http://www.sci-info-pages.com/levels.html. Published June 25, 2006. Accessed May 22, 2007.
231. Savic G, Bergstrom EM, Frankel HL, et al. Inter-rater reliability of motor and sensory examinations performed according to American Spinal Injury

Association standards. *Spinal Cord.* 2007;45(6):444–451; Epub 2007 Mar 27.
232. Cifu DX, Huang ME, Kolakowsky-Hayner SA, et al. Age, outcome, and rehabilitation costs after paraplegia caused by traumatic injury of the thoracic spinal cord, conus medullaris, and cauda equina. *J Neurotrauma.* 1999;16:805–815.
233. Coleman WP, Geisler FH. Injury severity as primary predictor of outcome in acute spinal cord injury: retrospective results from a large multicenter clinical trial. *Spine J.* 2004;4:373–378.
234. Miyanji F, Furlan JC, Aarabi B, et al. Acute cervical traumatic spinal cord injury: MR imaging findings correlated with neurologic outcome—prospective study with 100 consecutive patients. *Radiology.* 2007;243(3):820–827. Epub 2007 Apr 12.
235. Schneider RC, Cherry G, Pantek H. The syndrome of acute central cervical spinal cored injury, with special reference to the mechanisms involved in hyperextension injuries of cervical spine. *J Neurosurg.* 1954;11:546–577.
236. Dvorak MF, Fisher CG, Hoekema J, et al. Factors predicting motor recovery and functional outcome after traumatic central cord syndrome: a long-term follow-up. *Spine.* 2005;30:2303–2311.
237. Harrop JS, Sharan A, Ratliff J. Central cord injury: pathophysiology, management and outcomes. *Spine J.* 2006;6:198S–206S.

CHAPTER 84 ■ CNS VASCULAR DISEASE

DAVID A. DECKER • BRIAN L. HOH • MICHAEL F. WATERS

IMMEDIATE CONCERNS

Major Problems

The first concern is to establish the diagnosis of stroke and determine if the patient is a candidate for thrombolytic therapy.

Stress Points

1. Strokes may be ischemic, resulting from the occlusion of small or large arteries, or hemorrhagic, resulting from the rupture of a conducting artery or an intraparenchymal arteriole.
2. An abrupt focal lateralizing neurologic deficit attributable to a cerebrovascular distribution is the hallmark of ischemic stroke.
3. A depressed level of consciousness is rarely the presenting symptom of ischemic stroke and much more commonly occurs in the setting of a hemorrhagic event.
4. Patients with acute ischemic stroke may be candidates for thrombolytic therapy, but the therapeutic window is extremely narrow, so timely diagnosis and evaluation is of the utmost importance.

Essential Diagnostic Tests and Procedures

1. A computed tomography (CT) scan of the brain is critical for the initial evaluation and management of the stroke patient. Additionally, when available, CT angiography and perfusion studies may aid in diagnosis and management.
2. Magnetic resonance imaging (MRI) is more sensitive than CT, but it is usually less available urgently, and patients must remain still for a much longer period of time.
3. Vascular ultrasound allows rapid bedside assessment of abnormal flow within the major intracranial and extracranial arteries and can provide valuable immediate information about the vascular physiology to supplement the anatomic information provided by the CT scan.
4. A transthoracic or transesophageal echocardiogram may identify potential cardiac sources of cerebral emboli.
5. An electrocardiogram (ECG) followed by continuous cardiac telemetry monitoring is often necessary to identify arrhythmias associated with stroke.
6. A lumbar puncture may be necessary to rule out subarachnoid hemorrhage (SAH) in patients in whom the diagnosis is strongly suspected but CT is unrevealing.

Initial Therapy

1. Thrombolytics are the mainstay of treatment of acute ischemic stroke in eligible patients.
2. Careful attention to blood pressure may reduce complications such as hemorrhage.
3. Supportive care, with special attention paid to prevention of aspiration pneumonia and deep vein thromboses, is essential to reduce mortality associated with stroke.
4. Rapid initiations of secondary preventive therapies are effective in reducing risk for recurrent stroke.
5. Certain patients, such as those with large ischemic or hemorrhagic strokes, will require monitoring of intracranial pressure and, potentially, decompressive surgery.

DIFFERENTIAL DIAGNOSIS

Most patients who suddenly develop a lateralized focal neurologic problem have, in fact, had a stroke. It is by far the most common acute, focal, nontraumatic brain disease. When the presentation differs from this definition, further investigation and supportive evidence should be sought before establishing the diagnosis. As shown in Table 84.1, there are many stroke symptoms that may occur alone, unaccompanied by other

TABLE 84.1

SYMPTOMS SELDOM RESULTING FROM CEREBROVASCULAR DISEASE

Vertigo alone	Confusion
Dysarthria alone	Memory loss
Dysphagia alone	Delirium
Diplopia alone	Coma
Headache	Syncope
Tremor	Incontinence
Tonic-clonic motor activity	Tinnitus

evidence of neurologic damage, that are not an expression of vascular disease. Most of the errors in the diagnosis of stroke occur in patients with altered mental status. Beware of attributing such nonfocal symptoms to strokes without corroborating historic or diagnostic evidence.

Table 84.2 lists the diseases most commonly mistaken for stroke. Epilepsy mimics stroke more often than any other condition. In one study of 821 consecutive patients admitted to a stroke unit, only 13% had a disease other than stroke, but almost 40% of these misdiagnosed patients had seizures (1). Focal onset seizures may leave a portion of the ictal brain dysfunctional for a prolonged period (hours or more), and the deficits may be indistinguishable from those of ischemic stroke. Often, the only clues will be a history of seizures or absence of diagnostic evidence of ischemia.

Intracranial hemorrhage, encephalitis, or other structural brain lesions, such as tumors, may produce focal deficits identical to ischemic stroke. However, headache and altered or depressed level of consciousness are more likely to be the primary complaint in these cases. Findings consistent with infection or demonstration of a hemorrhage on CT are usually all that is required to differentiate these disorders from ischemic stroke. The next largest group of mistaken diagnoses occurs in patients suffering confusion and neurologic deficits from drug intoxication, alcohol, or metabolic abnormalities. Extreme electrolyte or serum glucose derangements can produce temporary focal deficits.

Migraine may produce several transient neurologic symptoms that may be misinterpreted as stroke. Visual phenomena, such as bright lines, and blurriness or loss of vision are commonly described. Sensory disturbances, and particularly well-demarcated regions on the upper extremity and periorally often occur. These symptoms may occur with or without the associated head pain but do not respect laterality or vascular

TABLE 84.2

CONDITIONS MOST FREQUENTLY MISTAKEN FOR STROKE

Seizures	Peripheral neuropathy and Bell palsy
Metabolic encephalopathy	Multiple sclerosis
Cerebral tumor	Hypoglycemia
Subdural hematoma	Encephalitis
Cerebral abscess	Migraine
Vertigo, Meniere disease	Psychogenic illness

territories as ischemic strokes do. People who suffer migraines, however, are at increased risk for ischemic stroke, so a thorough evaluation is warranted before dismissing the symptoms, particularly if it is the first occurrence. Motor deficits only very rarely result from migraine, so they should be attributed to stroke until proven otherwise.

Occasionally, peripheral nerve lesions, such as Bell palsy, may appear suddenly and mimic an ischemic stroke. Careful differentiation between upper and lower motor signs will most often clarify the diagnosis, but incomplete presentations can be confusing. In general, dense paralysis in the absence of other neurologic signs or complaints is more likely the result of a peripheral lesion. Although uncommon, stroke may present with bizarre or otherwise unbelievable symptoms, so the diagnosis of a psychogenic disorder should remain one of exclusion.

Establishing a correct diagnosis of these stroke mimics usually depends heavily on the patient's history, and the physician must specifically probe for characteristics of these diseases. A thorough history and physical examination, combined with appropriate laboratory testing and brain imaging such as MRI or CT scan, can usually exclude most conditions that mimic a stroke.

ISCHEMIC STROKE

Pathogenesis

Ischemic stroke occurs when the supply of blood to brain tissue is acutely interrupted. Normal cerebral blood flow in gray matter is about 80 mL/100 g tissue per minute, whereas white matter is about 20 mL/100 g tissue per minute. A global average in cortical mantle (assuming a 50:50 mix of gray and white matter) is about 50 mL/100 g tissue per minute. Modest perturbations of the amount of cerebral blood flow can be accommodated by the autoregulatory capacity of the cerebral vasculature. When systemic blood pressure drops, resistance vessels in the brain dilate to increase flow. Once these vessels are maximally dilated, further drops in systemic pressure will reduce cerebral blood flow. If the average cerebral blood flow drops below 35 mL/100 g tissue per minute, protein synthesis stops; below 20 mL/100 g tissue per minute, synaptic failure occurs and neurons cease to function. As this threshold is crossed, patients become suddenly symptomatic. When cerebral blood flow drops below 10 mL/100 g tissue per minute, metabolic failure and irreversible cell death occur.

Disruption of blood flow to the brain does not affect all tissues within the vascular distribution equally. Most often, there is a region with markedly reduced flow that quickly undergoes infarction; surrounding that area are regions with diminished flow that will survive longer, but not indefinitely. This potentially salvageable area is referred to as the *penumbra*. The purpose of acute stroke therapies is to salvage the penumbra.

In the general adult population, the causes of disruptions of arterial flow can be separated into three major categories based on cause: (i) large vessel atherothrombotic disease, (ii) small vessel (lacunar) infarction, and (iii) cardiogenic embolism. This categorization will focus the diagnostic evaluation and therapy and has prognostic implications. Determining the cause will also guide the clinician in administering the appropriate level of care based on the possibility of progression and anticipated complications. For example, subtle speech changes and right hand weakness could be the presenting symptoms of any of the three stroke subtypes outlined above. If a lacunar infarction is the cause, symptoms will most likely be maximal at onset and rarely will the patient experience complications compromising respiration or circulation. The volume of brain tissue involved is by definition small, and the risk for progression or recurrence in the acute period is quite small. A cardiogenic embolus would also be expected to cause symptoms maximal at onset, but the infarct volume could be large enough to cause mass effect and, depending on the underlying cardiac pathology, the risk for complications could be substantial.

Large Vessel Atherothrombosis

Large vessel atherothrombosis encompasses approximately 15% of all strokes; of these, two thirds are of extracranial internal carotid artery (ICA) origin, and one third are due to intracranial atheromatous disease (2). Atheromatous disease of large vessels is a slowly degenerative process, but as the disease progresses, the chance for lesion instability increases. Vascular plaques may fragment, exposing an ulcerated surface that is highly thrombogenic and leading to local occlusion or creation of emboli material. Thus, in large vessel disease, thrombosis or artery-to-artery embolism are often parts of the same underlying pathologic process. Atherosclerotic lesions tend to occur at bifurcations or sharp turns in the vessel, both of which are associated with increased blood flow turbulence. The prototypic example of this is carotid stenosis at the origin of the ICA. Other common extracranial sites include the origin of the vertebral artery and the other great vessels. Intracranially, common sites include the distal vertebral artery, the midbasilar artery, the siphon of the ICA, and the proximal middle cerebral artery (MCA).

Lacunar Strokes

Lacunar strokes represent approximately one quarter of all such events. They are caused by occlusion of a single perforating arteriole, such as those that supply deep brain structures like the thalamus, pons, or basal ganglia (Fig. 84.1). The result is a small infarction—by most definitions, less than 1 cm^3—that undergoes liquefaction necrosis with time, leaving a tiny fluid-filled space for which they are named. The primary risk factor for lacunar infarction is hypertension, which results in lipohyalinosis of the vessel wall with progressive concentric stenosis and eventual thrombosis (3).

Cardiogenic Embolism

Approximately 60% of all ischemic strokes are caused by cerebral embolism, of which only one third have a definitively known clinical source (4). Cerebral emboli may be composed of atherosclerotic plaque material, clotted blood, or, in rare cases, air or fat. Once free in the arterial circulation, the emboli will tend to follow the straightest path formed by the most blood. Therefore, most emboli will affect distal branches of the MCA, although other locations are possible; the larger the embolus, the more proximal it will lodge.

Cerebral emboli may originate from atheromatous disease of more proximal large vessels, such as the aortic arch, as outlined above, or the heart (5). Atrial fibrillation is the most common cardiac cause, but others include valvular heart disease, intracardiac thrombus, atrial myxoma, dilated cardiomyopathy, patent foramen ovale (PFO), especially when accompanied by an atrial septal defect, and endocarditis. Air emboli are usually iatrogenic and result when a large amount of air enters the venous circulation (e.g., through a central venous catheter) and bypasses the lungs through a PFO, thereby entering the arterial circulation. Fat emboli are generally the result of long-bone fractures in severe trauma. It is important to seek out the definitive source whenever possible, as it may have a profound impact on the management of secondary stroke prevention. For example, although most sources of cardiogenic emboli are treated with oral anticoagulation, several conditions may contraindicate it, such as bacterial endocarditis (6) or atrial myxoma (7).

Arterial Dissections

Although arterial dissections may occur at any age, they are probably the most common cause of stroke in young patients (younger than 50 years old) who are unlikely to have typical risk factors. Arterial dissections may arise spontaneously or following a traumatic head or neck injury (8). These lesions typically arise at the petrous portion of the ICA or at the cervical 1–2 level in the vertebral artery. Thrombus may form at the site of intimal tear, extending into the media, with subsequent artery-to-artery embolism. If a large intimal flap or intramural hematoma forms, occlusion of the affected vessel may occur. Dissection may also lead to subarachnoid hemorrhage when a pseudoaneurysm forms after the artery passes intradurally (9).

Clinical Evaluation

History

The history, when available, is the key instrument in diagnosing neurologic disease. If the patient is unable to provide a reliable history, which is often the case in acute brain dysfunction, then historic details should be sought from witnesses, family, EMS records, or whatever sources are available; no other diagnostic tool will so quickly narrow the differential diagnosis.

The key historic element in ischemic cerebrovascular disease is *sudden* onset of symptoms, which are typically maximal at onset. Under certain circumstances, the symptoms may follow a stuttering or stepwise progression, but in each instance there is a sudden change. Contrast this with the waxing and waning character of delirium or the symptoms that may develop over days to weeks from a brain tumor. There is an unfortunate tendency to dismiss symptoms of short duration, but this is a serious mistake, as the duration of the symptoms speaks little to the underlying pathogenesis. For example, a patient with occult atrial fibrillation may suffer transient neurologic deficits from an embolus that happens to spontaneously lyse before infarction has completed. Without addressing the underlying cause, the patient is unlikely to continue to be so fortunate, and an opportunity to prevent a devastating neurologic injury will have been lost.

If the ictal event is consistent with a stroke, the remainder of the initial history should be focused on determining if the patient is a candidate for thrombolytic therapy and identifying possible risk factors. Whereas other details not elucidated in the initial history can be revisited at a later time, it is of

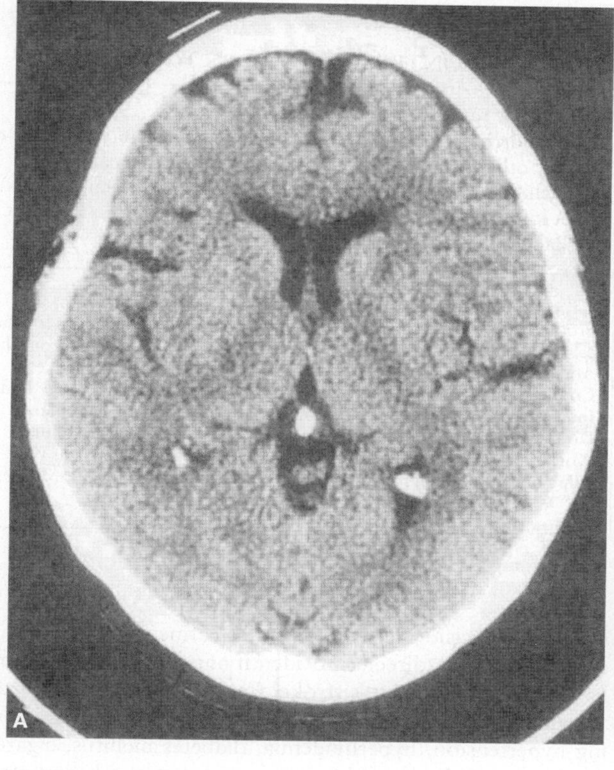

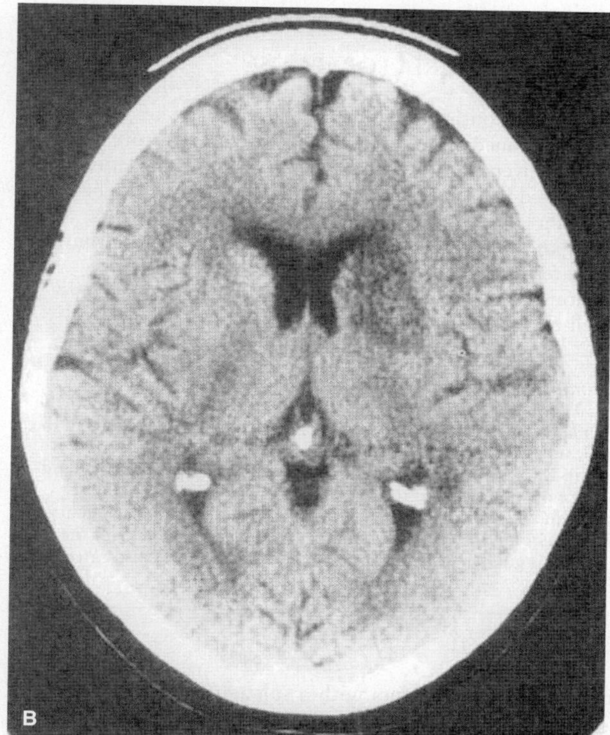

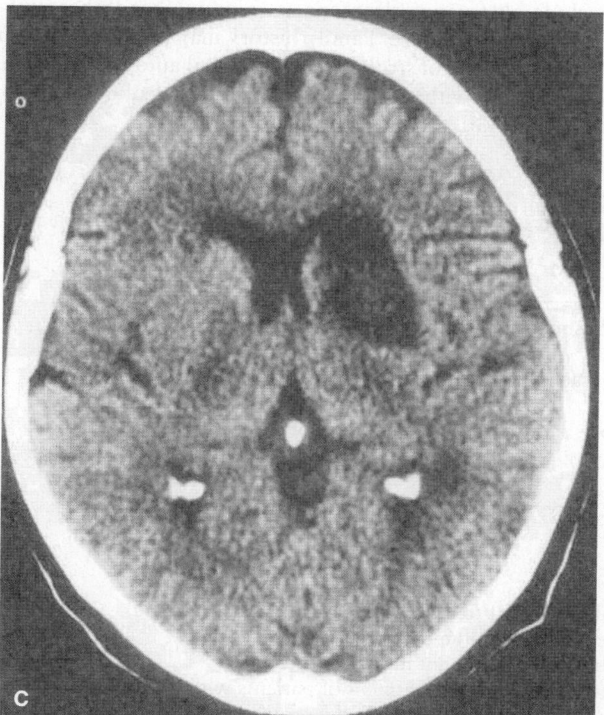

FIGURE 84.1. Intracerebral hemorrhage of the left basal ganglia. Hyperdense appearance of blood on the CT scan easily defines the extent of hemorrhage.

the utmost importance to obtain the exact time of symptom onset, as current acute stroke treatment protocols depend on this for inclusion. If the onset was not witnessed, then the time when last known to be normal is used. For example, if the patient awakes with symptoms, then the time when the patient retired is used (assuming he or she was asymptomatic then). The reason time of onset is so important is that it is used as a surrogate marker for the likelihood that salvageable tissue remains. Additionally, the risk of intracerebral hemorrhage associated with thrombolytics increases with time after onset of symptoms. Current research is focused on using multimodal imaging to generate physiologic data that may be used in lieu

TABLE 84.3

INCLUSION CRITERIA FOR tPA USE

1. Symptoms consistent with acute ischemic stroke, with a clearly defined onset of less than three hours before rt-PA will be given (if the onset was not witnessed, the ictus is measured from the time the patient was last seen to be at baseline);
2. A significant neurological deficit is expected to result in long-term disability
3. A non-contrast CT with no evidence of hemorrhage or well-established infarction.

CT, computed tomography.
From Adams HP Jr, Del Zoppo G, Albert MJ, et al. Guidelines for the early management of adults with ischemic stroke: a guideline from the American Heart Association/American Stroke Association Stroke Council, Clinical Cardiology Council, Cardiovascular Radiology and Intervention Council, and the Atherosclerotic Peripheral Vascular Disease and Quality of Care Outcomes in Research Interdisciplinary Working Groups: the American Academy of Neurology affirms the value of this guideline as an educational tool for neurologists. *Stroke.* 2007;38(5):1655–1711, with permission.

TABLE 84.4

ABSOLUTE CONTRAINDICATIONS TO tPA USE

1. Mild or rapidly improving deficits
2. Hemorrhage on CT, well-established acute infarct on CT, or any other CT diagnosis that contraindicates treatment, including abscess or tumor (excluding small meningiomas)
3. A known CNS vascular malformation or tumor
4. Bacterial endocarditis

CT, computed tomography; CNS, central nervous system.
From Adams HP Jr, Del Zoppo G, Albert MJ, et al. Guidelines for the early management of adults with ischemic stroke: a guideline from the American Heart Association/American Stroke Association Stroke Council, Clinical Cardiology Council, Cardiovascular Radiology and Intervention Council, and the Atherosclerotic Peripheral Vascular Disease and Quality of Care Outcomes in Research Interdisciplinary Working Groups: the American Academy of Neurology affirms the value of this guideline as an educational tool for neurologists. *Stroke.* 2007;38(5):1655–1711, with permission.

of time to identify patients with a salvageable penumbra, but these techniques have yet to mature.

Aside from time of onset, factors that may place the patient at increased risk for bleeding must be sought. Tables 84.3 through 84.5 list common inclusion and exclusion criteria for intravenous (IV)-tPA (tissue plasminogen activator), which are based on those used in the pivotal trials. Most institutions have their own protocols, which may vary somewhat from those used in the trials.

Once a decision regarding acute treatment has been made, attention can be directed to identifying conditions that may have caused the patient's stroke. Cerebrovascular and cardiovascular diseases share many of the same risk factors, including hypertension, hyperlipidemia, diabetes mellitus, cigarette smoking, and obesity. Other risk factors that may be important include obstructive sleep apnea, migraine headaches with an aura, and drug abuse. Family history may provide insight into heritable causes of stroke such as cerebral autosomal dominant arteriopathy with subcortical infarcts and leukoencephalopathy (CADASIL) or Fabry disease.

TABLE 84.5

RELATIVE CONTRAINDICATIONS TO tPA USE

1. Significant trauma within the past 3 months (including CPR with chest compressions within the past 10 days)
2. Ischemic stroke within 3 months
3. History of intracranial hemorrhage, or symptoms suggestive of subarachnoid hemorrhage
4. Major surgery within the past 14 days
5. Minor surgery within past 19 days, including liver and kidney biopsy, thoracentesis, and lumbar puncture
6. Arterial puncture at a noncompressible site within past 14 days
7. Pregnancy (and ≤10 days postpartum)
8. Gastrointestinal, urologic, or respiratory hemorrhage within past 21 days
9. Known bleeding diathesis (includes renal and hepatic insufficiency)
10. Peritoneal dialysis or hemodialysis
11. PTT >40 sec, PT >15 (INR >1.7), platelet count <100,000
12. Seizure at onset of stroke (This relative contraindication is intended to prevent treatment of patients with a deficit due to postictal Todd paralysis or with seizure due to some other CNS lesion that precludes thrombolytic therapy. If rapid diagnosis of vascular occlusion can be made, treatment may be given.)
13. Glucose <50 or >400 mg/dL (This relative contraindication is intended to prevent treatment of patients with focal deficits due to hypoglycemia or hyperglycemia. If the deficit persists after correction of the serum glucose, or if rapid diagnosis of vascular occlusion can be made, treatment may be given.)
14. Systolic BP >180 mm Hg *or* diastolic BP >110 mm Hg, despite basic measures to lower it acutely
15. Consideration should be given to the increased risk of hemorrhage in patients with severe deficits (NIHSS >20), age >75, or early edema with mass effect on CT.

CPR, cardiopulmonary resuscitation; PTT, partial thromboplastin time; PT, prothrombin time; INR, international normalized ratio; CNS, central nervous system; BP, blood pressure; NIHSS, National Institutes of Health Stroke Scale; CT, computed tomography.

Neurologic Examination

The neurologic examination will allow the clinician to quickly determine which brain areas are dysfunctional and further narrow the differential diagnosis. The neurologic deficits caused by ischemic cerebrovascular disease are expected to be lateralizing and confined to a vascular distribution. For example, the triad of language disturbance and right face and arm motor deficits is typical for occlusion of the left MCA. However, sudden-onset motor and sensory deficit of both arms is not lateralizing, nor readily explained by a cerebrovascular occlusion, and thus is more likely due to spinal cord pathology.

The first step in localization of vascular lesions is determining, based on the signs and symptoms, whether they arise from the anterior circulation (carotid artery and its main branches, the anterior and middle cerebral arteries) or the posterior circulation (vertebral, basilar, and posterior cerebral arteries). This finding will guide the remainder of the diagnostic evaluation, therapy, and prognosis. Ideally, these two separate circulations would be robustly connected such that a failure in one could be compensated by the other, but this is rarely the case.

The two symptoms that most accurately reflect carotid circulation disease are aphasia and monocular blindness. Aphasia is a deficit in either the expression or comprehension of language and may involve both in the acute period. Aphasia must be distinguished from dysarthria, which is the inability to correctly produce words due to motor impairment of facial, lingual, or pharyngeal muscles; dysarthria may result from either anterior or posterior circulation infarcts. The areas responsible for language reside in the dominant (nearly always left) hemispheric cortex, within the territory of the MCA; a stroke causing aphasia must, therefore, involve this circulation. Similarly, the blood supply of the eye arises largely from the ophthalmic artery, a direct branch from the carotid artery, and monocular ischemia therefore implicates the carotid circulation. The prototypic example of this process is amaurosis fugax, or transient monocular blindness in which vision is lost in *one eye* for minutes. This must be contrasted with a visual field deficit, which affects one field of *both eyes*, as this is more likely the result of posterior circulation ischemia. Pain is rarely a significant complaint, but when present, especially if following the course of a major blood vessel, arterial dissection should be considered. Involvement of the carotid artery may cause a Horner syndrome.

Because of the density of discrete populations of neurons supplied by the posterior circulation, the clinical syndromes that result from strokes in this area are usually more complex than those in the cerebral hemispheres. The medulla, pons, midbrain, cerebellum, parts of the thalami, and the visual cortices are the major structures involved. Strokes involving the brainstem often manifest with cranial nerve dysfunction (dysarthria, dysphagia, diplopia). Crossed signs, with motor or sensory deficits affecting one side of the face and the opposite side of the body, may occur as major decussations in these pathways and occur in the pons and medulla. The unique vascular anatomy of the basilar artery, with a single midline vessel supplying both sides of the pons and the posterior cerebral arteries, may lead to bilateral neurologic deficits.

Lacunar infarctions also have a set of clinical features that may be used to differentiate them from other stroke subtypes. Classic lacunar syndromes include pure motor hemiparesis (caused by infarction in the internal capsule or *basis pontis*), pure hemisensory symptoms (caused by infarction in the ventral posterolateral [VPL] thalamic nucleus), dysarthria–clumsy hand syndrome (with pontine or internal capsule infarcts), and ataxia-hemiparesis (pontine infarct).

Vascular System Examination

Physical examination of the vascular system itself is usually surprisingly unrewarding. Atherosclerosis may present few outward signs. Although carotid bruits were classically emphasized, modern ultrasound techniques have proven them to be of low sensitivity and specificity for predicting vascular disease. No characteristic feature, including the volume, pitch, or duration of the bruit, reliably indicates the degree or the nature of constriction of the vascular lumen. Many bruits reflect benign conditions. The clinical significance of carotid bruits is minimized because they are audible in many asymptomatic persons without atherosclerosis who never suffer from cerebrovascular disease, but may be absent in severely diseased vessels. Therefore, even if a carotid bruit is detected, it may be difficult to decide whether it is relevant to the patient's symptoms, and it should not be given undue emphasis in the overall evaluation. Clinical decisions should be based on definitive assessment of blood vessels using ultrasound or angiography.

Examination of the heart should focus on detecting thrombogenic diseases, including myocardial infarction, congestive heart failure, arrhythmias, prosthetic valves, and bacterial endocarditis. Heart disease is a key risk factor for stroke and may complicate the acute period. Patients with stroke may also present concurrently with a myocardial infarction (MI) and, without careful examination, the less dramatic of the two may go undetected. Elevation of serum troponin levels is a very sensitive and specific indicator of an MI. Isolated creatine kinase (CK)-MB elevations should be interpreted with caution, however, as the MB fraction is expressed in brain tissue, and small elevations are not uncommon in stroke (10).

Laboratory Studies

Laboratory studies will also help narrow the differential diagnosis and may reveal relevant comorbid conditions. Some studies need to be obtained immediately to determine a patient's candidacy for thrombolytic therapy, including an electrolyte battery, glucose, platelet count, cardiac enzymes, beta-HCG (human chorionic gonadotropin), and coagulation parameters. Severe electrolyte (specifically hyponatremia or hypernatremia) or glucose disturbances can cause neurologic dysfunction that may mimic stroke. Cardiac enzymes will determine if cardiac ischemia is part of the current presentation, and a beta-HCG will reveal occult pregnancy, both of which may be contraindications to systemic thrombolytics. Coagulation parameters and a platelet count will identify patients who may be at greater risk for bleeding.

Other laboratory studies will help determine the cause and identify risk factors but do not need to be obtained immediately. A fasting lipid profile should be obtained for potential vascular risk factor modification. In patients older than 50 years of age, an erythrocyte sedimentation rate and C-reactive protein are essential if giant cell arteritis is suspected. In patients for whom an unusual cause of stroke is suspected (young patients or minimal vascular risk factors), laboratory investigation of prothrombotic states could be considered. The interpretation of these tests is very complex and should be performed in consultation with a hematologist (11). Toxicology screening should be performed on hospital admission, with attention

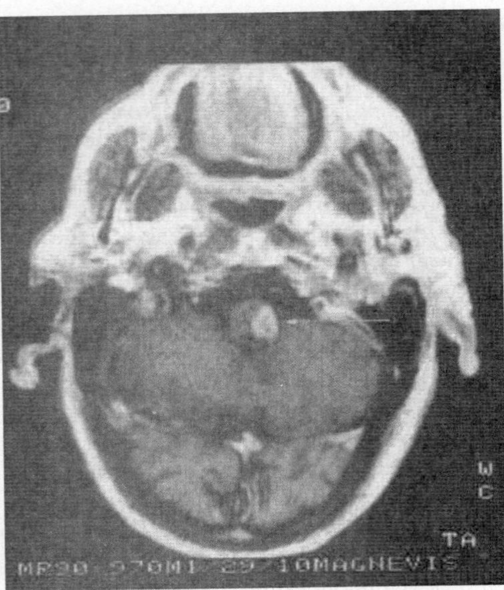

FIGURE 84.2. Evolving radiographic evidence of cerebral infarction. CT scan at 3 hours (A) shows little evidence of acute ischemia. At 3 days, damaged brain is indicated by hypodensity in the left subcortical region (B). At 8 days, frank infarction is now clearly demonstrated by CT (C).

directed to amphetamines, phencyclidine, ephedrine, and cocaine.

Imaging Studies

CT Scan. Several imaging studies are used in the evaluation of acute stroke. A noncontrasted CT scan of the brain is the standard initial evaluation for stroke. CT is very sensitive to the presence of hemorrhage, which is the primary reason for its use in the acute setting, and is the only radiologic test necessary to determine eligibility for IV-tPA. CT is not sensitive for detection of an acute cerebral infarction (Fig. 84.2), and the lack of abnormality within the first 24 hours should be expected. The view of the posterior fossa is also quite limited, and any changes (with the exception of hemorrhage) seen within the brainstem or cerebellum should be confirmed with MRI. When available, CT angiography and perfusion studies can be obtained with very little additional time and provide valuable additional information regarding the patency of blood vessels and blood flow to individual large vessel territories. Pathologic changes on these studies are visible immediately, but they require iodinated contrast, which may be a limiting factor for some patients. The angiographic results from CTA are closest to the traditional gold standard exam: digital subtraction catheter angiography (CTA). When examining the carotid arteries, the results from CTA are often sufficient to differentiate a high-grade stenosis (60%–99%) that is treatable from complete occlusion that is not.

MRI. MRI is far more sensitive for acute infarction than CT. Diffusion MR sequences can detect ischemia within, perhaps, minutes of onset. MRI is of special value in brainstem and posterior circulation strokes, since the images it produces are not obscured by bony artifacts as with CT (Fig. 84.3). The combination of multiple MRI sequences allows for much more specific differentiation between ischemic brain and other structural abnormalities. In addition, MRI can display flow-related enhancement of the vasculature, resulting in a magnetic resonance angiogram (MRA). The resulting image can be manipulated in three dimensions, allowing for more accurate interpretation of small abnormalities. However, MRA tends to slightly overestimate the degree of stenosis, and thus is not usually sufficient to differentiate high-grade stenosis from occlusion (12). MRA uses gadolinium as a contrast agent instead of an iodinated material, making the study available to more patients. Perfusion studies, very similar to those performed with CT, may also be obtained if the right equipment is available. Disadvantages of MRI and MRA include reduced availability and substantially longer scanning times, which place some limitations on their use.

Digital Subtraction Catheter Angiography. Digital subtraction catheter angiography is an invasive imaging technique in which the artery of interest is selectively catheterized under fluoroscopy and dye injection enables a high resolution view of the vessel that can be obtained in multiple planes. As the quality of noninvasive imaging techniques has improved and the associated morbidity has decreased to approximately 1% (11), catheter angiography is no longer used as a routine screening test. Indications now include precisely delimiting critical vascular stenoses and examination of arterial dissections, arteriovenous malformations, and aneurysms.

Carotid Ultrasound. Carotid ultrasound provides a rapid noninvasive assessment of carotid artery disease, based on abnormalities of either flow (Doppler) or morphology (B-mode). As with any ultrasound technique, sensitivity is to some degree operator dependent, but with experienced technicians and interpreters, duplex scanning provides a reproducible, accurate screening examination for carotid disease. However, this technique suffers from the same limitation as MRA in differentiating high-grade stenosis and occlusion. Lesions of the more distal internal carotid artery may also be difficult to visualize in some patients.

Transcranial Doppler. Transcranial Doppler (TCD) allows rapid bedside assessment of abnormal flow within the distal ICA and major intracranial arteries. It is primarily a functional study that provides information about blood flow velocity and vascular resistance rather than structural features. The 2-MHz ultrasonic signal can penetrate various bony "windows" in most patients, and its gated character allows identification of arteries by "depth" of the reflected signal. TCD can examine proximal portions of all major branches of the circle of Willis, but is insensitive for pathology beyond the A1, M1, or P1 segments. Newer applications include detection of microemboli and online monitoring of arterial flow during invasive procedures, such as carotid endarterectomy (Fig. 84.4). TCD may also be useful as an adjunctive therapy to tPA, as continuous insonation may enhance thrombolysis (13). Disadvantages include major dependency on operator skill and the prevalence of acoustically inadequate bony windows.

Transthoracic Echocardiography. Transthoracic echocardiography (TTE) is essential to evaluate cardiac function. Physicians must attend not only to a visualized thrombus, but also to other pathologic states associated with systemic embolization,

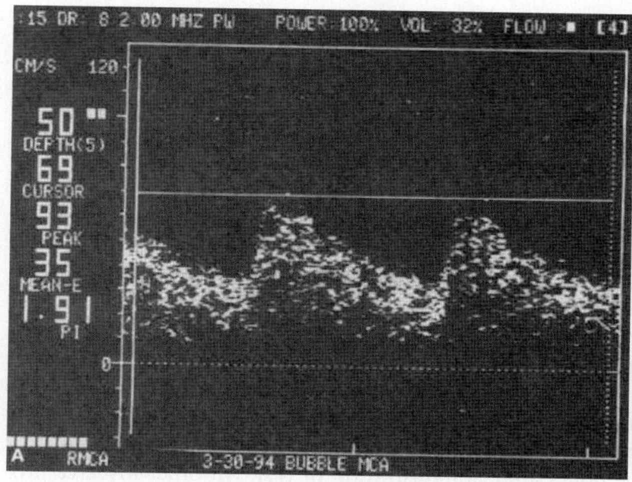

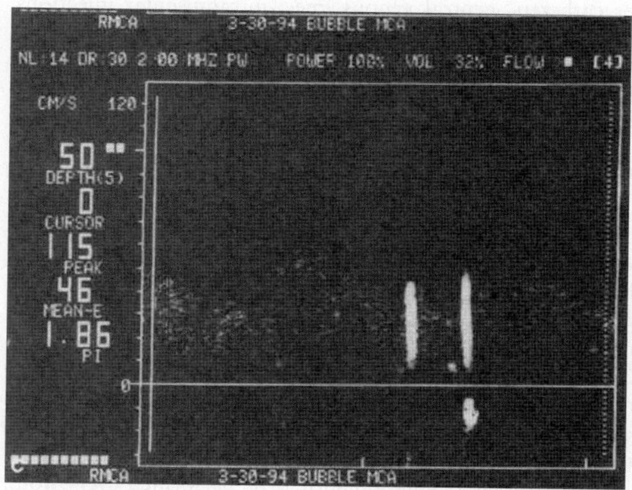

including left ventricular wall motion abnormalities, chamber dilatation, valvular disease, ejection fraction, and septal defects. TTE can be routinely performed and is a superior study for the detection of ventricular apex pathology, left ventricle thrombus, and views of prosthetic valves. Transesophageal echocardiography (TEE) provides much greater resolution and is more sensitive for pathology of the left atrial appendage, intra-atrial septum, atrial aspect of mitral-tricuspid valves, and the ascending aorta. TEE is an invasive procedure that requires sedation but can be performed safely on most patients (14).

Management

Acute Therapy

As with any acutely ill patient, attention should initially be focused on the evaluation of airway, breathing, and circulation. A secure airway should be established for patients with a depressed consciousness. Supplemental oxygen or mechanical ventilation should be used as needed to treat any degree of hypoxia. Circulation assessment includes evaluation of blood pressure and cardiac electrical activity with an ECG, as coexistent MI is not uncommon. Patients with acute stroke are often markedly hypertensive, and one should be cautious in

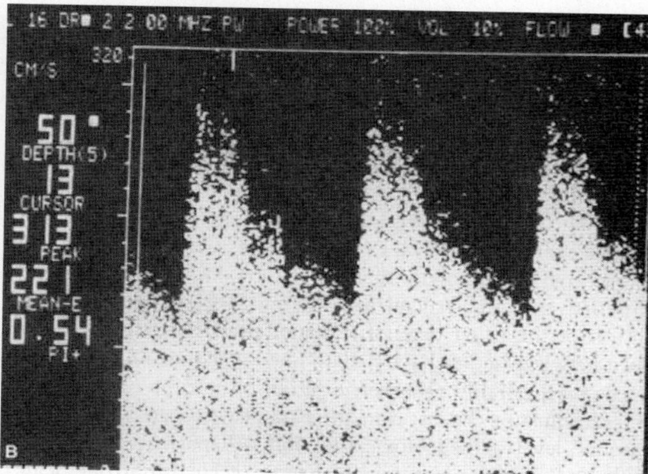

FIGURE 84.3. MRI demonstrates enhancing left lateral medullary infarction in a patient with Wallenberg syndrome.

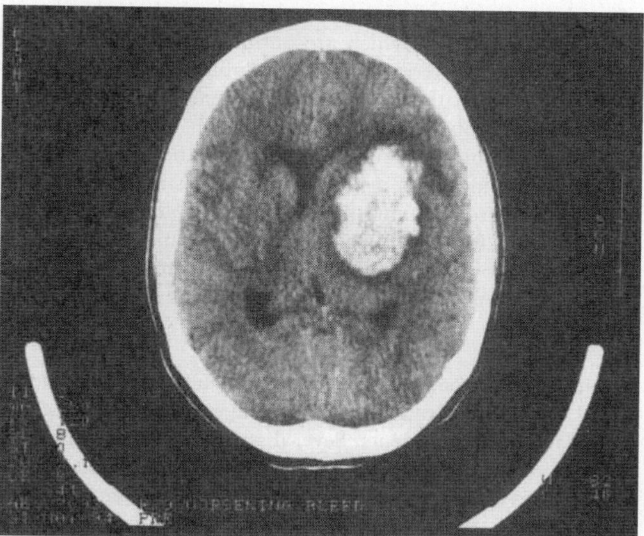

FIGURE 84.4. Transcranial Doppler. **A:** The normal flow-velocity profile through the middle cerebral artery (velocity plotted over time during three cardiac cycles) is demonstrated. **B:** Elevated flow velocities as a result of the arterial spasm associated with subarachnoid hemorrhage is demonstrated. **C:** Two microemboli are detected through the middle cerebral artery as transient high-intensity signals.

aggressively treating elevated blood pressure before a more complete assessment of the patient has been completed (15). Blood pressure goals are determined by type of stroke, cause, and the presence of comorbid conditions, such as coronary artery disease; this will be discussed in the following sections.

The immediate goal will be to determine if the patient is a candidate for thrombolytic therapy; thus attention should be focused on obtaining the relevant history and performing a neurologic examination. The care of patients who will ultimately not receive thrombolytic therapy will be discussed below (see Supportive Care*)*. Crucial for therapy is the proper determination of the exact time of onset of the stroke. The patient must be witnessed to have had an abrupt change in neurologic status by a reliable observer; otherwise the time of onset, by default, must be the last time the patient was seen at his or her baseline level of neurologic function. All patients should be evaluated with the National Institutes of Health Stroke Scale (NIHSS), which can help to exclude a patient from potentially harmful therapy on the basis of the stroke being too small or too severe.

Thrombolytic Therapy. Currently, thrombolytic treatment with recombinant tissue plasminogen activator (tPA) in eligible stroke patients is the standard of care based on the results of four large trials: the National Institute of Neurological Disorders and Stroke (NINDS) recombinant t-PA study (16–18), the European Cooperative Acute Stroke Study (ECASS)-I (19), ECASS-II (20), and the ATLANTIS tPA (Alteplase) Acute Stroke Trial (parts A and B) (21,22). The collective results indicate that patients treated with tPA within 3 hours of onset were ≥30% more likely to have minimal or no disability at 3 months compared with placebo-treated patients (23). The average disability across all groups was, additionally, decreased in the treatment group. The benefit seen by the tPA-treated group existed regardless of patient age or stroke subtype.

To maximize the possible benefit and minimize the risk for hemorrhage, the NINDS study helped to establish strict inclusion criteria for the administration of thrombolytic therapy in acute stroke patients, which are outlined in Table 84.3. Absolute exclusion criteria have been established as well (Table 84.4). In addition, there is a long list of *relative* contraindications to thrombolytic therapy (Table 84.5), which often vary slightly in institutional protocols. These can be summarized as risks for bleeding from a noncompressible site, the presence of potential stroke mimics, or uncontrollable hypertension. The rationale for excluding patients with improving symptoms is to avoid giving a potentially harmful treatment to patients with epileptic postictal presentations or spontaneous recovery.

Tissue Plasminogen Activator (tPA). When the protocol is followed, the administration of tPA is safe relative to other commonly accepted treatments. Several studies have attempted to examine the risk, but perhaps the most clinically relevant is the number needed to harm. For every 100 patients treated with tPA who match the NINDS trials populations across all levels of final global disability, approximately 32 will receive benefit, and approximately 3 will be harmed (24). The risk–benefit ratio, thus, strongly favors treatment. Many of the hemorrhages that occur are asymptomatic, and of those that are symptomatic, not all symptoms persist to discharge. Most patients who experience intercerebral hemorrhage (ICH) after tPA therapy have severe baseline insults and were already destined for a poor outcome; thus the hemorrhage does little to alter the final outcome (25). One should keep in mind that, although excluding a patient from treatment will mitigate the risk for hemorrhage, it also denies the patient a significantly better chance of recovery.

The dose of tPA is 0.9 mg/kg, with a maximum dose of 90 mg; 10% is given as a bolus over 1 minute, and the remaining 90% is infused over 60 minutes. Following treatment, patients should be monitored in an ICU for more than 24 hours. While many post-tPA patients will not need ventilatory or pressor support, as do many other patients in the ICU, blood pressure monitoring and frequent neurologic exams are critical for a favorable outcome, as hypertension dramatically increases the risk for hemorrhage. Blood pressure must initially be monitored noninvasively as arterial puncture is contraindicated for 24 hours after administration of tPA. All other invasive procedures, such as placement of nasogastric tubes, urinary bladder catheters, central venous lines, intramuscular injections, and rectal temperature must be avoided for 24 hours as well. Also, any drug that impairs hemostasis such as heparin, or antiplatelet or nonsteroidal anti-inflammatory agents, are contraindicated during this 24-hour period.

Vital Signs. Vital signs should be checked every 15 minutes for the first 2 hours, then every 30 minutes for 6 hours, and then every hour for 16 hours. Blood pressure should be strictly controlled for 24 hours, keeping the systolic blood pressure less than 180 mm Hg and the diastolic blood pressure less than 105 mm Hg (Table 84.6). Labetalol is recommended for control of hypertension; 10 mg should be given intravenously over 1 to 2 minutes, and the dose repeated or doubled every 10 to 20 minutes, up to a total of 150 mg. If the blood pressure remains refractory despite these measures, consideration can be given to a continuous infusion of nicardipine or sodium nitroprusside. Neurologic evaluation should be performed every hour. Oxygenation should be checked by continuous pulse oximetry and oxygen provided to keep saturation >95%. The benefit of therapeutic hypothermia is yet to be confirmed, but euthermia is clearly associated with better outcome (26). Acetaminophen, 650 mg every 4 hours orally or rectally, should be given for any temperature higher than 37.4°C, and a cooling blanket used for temperatures over 38.9°C.

STAT Head CT. A STAT head CT should be performed for any worsening neurologic status. Should an intracerebral hemorrhage develop following thrombolysis, several steps must be taken emergently. Neurosurgery should be contacted for possible hematoma evacuation, and anticoagulation should be reversed according to the protocol outlined in Table 84.7.

Intra-arterial Approach for Thrombolytic Therapy. The use of thrombolytic interventions outside of the 3-hour time window is controversial. Trials that have extended the therapeutic window beyond 3 hours for intravenous therapy have failed to show convincing benefit (19,20,22), as the risk of hemorrhage rapidly increases with time. However, there have been several attempts to prove the benefit of catheter-directed therapy via an intra-arterial approach for focal clot lysis. The most studied agent was prourokinase (27), but it was unfortunately removed from the market in 1999 due to concerns with its preparation. The agent most commonly used today is tPA.

TABLE 84.6

BLOOD PRESSURE CONTROL AFTER tPA

1. Management of blood pressure during and after treatment with tPA or other acute reperfusion intervention:
   a. Monitor blood pressure every 15 minutes during treatment and then for another 2 hours, then every 30 minutes for 6 hours, and then every hour for 16 hours;
   b. For systolic 180 to 230 mm Hg or diastolic 105 to 120 mm Hg:
      i. Labetalol 10 mg IV over 1 to 2 minutes, may repeat every 10 to 20 minutes, maximum dose of 300 mg; or
      ii. Labetalol 10 mg IV followed by an infusion at 2 to 8 mg/min
   c. For systolic greater than 230 mm Hg or diastolic 121 to 140 mm Hg:
      i. Labetalol 10 mg IV over 1 to 2 minutes, may repeat every 10 to 20 minutes, maximum dose of 300 mg; or
      ii. Labetalol 10 mg IV followed by an infusion at 2 to 8 mg/min; or
      iii. Nicardipine infusion, 5 mg/h, titrate up to desired effect by increasing by 2.5 mg/h every 5 minutes to maximum of 15 mg/h
      iv. If blood pressure not controlled, consider sodium nitroprusside.

From Adams HP Jr, Del Zoppo G, Albert MJ, et al. Guidelines for the early management of adults with ischemic stroke: a guideline from the American Heart Association/American Stroke Association Stroke Council, Clinical Cardiology Council, Cardiovascular Radiology and Intervention Council, and the Atherosclerotic Peripheral Vascular Disease and Quality of Care Outcomes in Research Interdisciplinary Working Groups: the American Academy of Neurology affirms the value of this guideline as an educational tool for neurologists. *Stroke*. 2007;38(5):1655–1711, with permission.

Theoretically, there are several potential benefits to treatment of stroke via an intra-arterial approach. First, angiographic confirmation of vessel occlusion can be obtained at the time of treatment. Second, high concentrations of thrombolytic agents can be given directly at the site of thrombosis, thereby minimizing systemic exposure. Third, the response to lysis can be monitored by direct visualization. Fourth, mechanical disruption of the clot (e.g., via balloon angioplasty, MERCI device) may accelerate thrombolysis (28).

According to the American Stroke Association guidelines (29), intra-arterial thrombolysis is an option for treatment of selected patients who have major stroke of <6 hours' duration due to occlusion of the MCA and who are not otherwise candidates for intravenous tPA. The availability of intra-arterial thrombolysis should not preclude the administration of IV-tPA in otherwise eligible patients. Treatment requires immediate access to cerebral angiography and qualified interventionalists.

Supportive Care

Supportive care lacks the excitement and drama of acute therapy, but nonetheless is critical to patient outcomes. Since the 1970s, mortality from stroke has markedly diminished from a rate of 156 to 56/100,000 cases (30), with only 3% to 10% of stroke patients receiving thrombolytic therapy; this trend

TABLE 84.7

MANAGEMENT OF POST-tPA HEMORRHAGE

1. Blood should be sent STAT for CBC, PT, PTT, platelets, fibrinogen and D-dimer (this should be repeated every two hours until bleeding is controlled).
2. Give two units of fresh frozen plasma every six hours for 24 hours after the thrombolytic agent was given.
3. Give cryoprecipitate (20 units); if the fibrinogen level is <200 mg/dL at one hour, repeat the cryoprecipitate dose.
4. Give 4 units of platelets.
5. Give protamine sulfate (1 mg per 100 units of heparin given in the past 3 hours);
   a. A test dose of 10 mg slow IV push over 10 minutes should be given while observing for anaphylaxis;
   b. Then the remaining dose by slow IV push, up to a maximum dose of 50 mg.
6. Institute frequent neuro checks, as well as management of increased ICP, as needed.
7. Aminocaproic acid (Amicar) can be given as a last resort, in a dose of 5 g in 250 mL normal saline IV over 1 hour.

CBC, complete blood count; PT, prothrombin time; PTT, partial thromboplastin time; IV, intravenous; ICP, intracranial pressure.
From Adams HP Jr, Del Zoppo G, Albert MJ, et al. Guidelines for the early management of adults with ischemic stroke: a guideline from the American Heart Association/American Stroke Association Stroke Council, Clinical Cardiology Council, Cardiovascular Radiology and Intervention Council, and the Atherosclerotic Peripheral Vascular Disease and Quality of Care Outcomes in Research Interdisciplinary Working Groups: the American Academy of Neurology affirms the value of this guideline as an educational tool for neurologists. *Stroke*. 2007;38(5):1655–1711, with permission.

TABLE 84.8

SUGGESTED RECOMMENDED GUIDELINES FOR TREATING ELEVATED BLOOD PRESSURE IN SPONTANEOUS ICH

1. If SBP is >200 mm Hg or MAP is >150 mm Hg, then consider aggressive reduction of blood pressure with continuous intravenous infusion, with frequent blood pressure monitoring every 5 minutes.
2. If SBP is >180 mm Hg or MAP is >130 mm Hg and there is evidence of or suspicion of elevated ICP, then consider monitoring ICP and reducing blood pressure using intermittent or continuous intravenous medications to keep cerebral perfusion pressure >60 to 80 mm Hg.
3. If SBP is >180 mm Hg or MAP is >130 mm Hg and there is not evidence of or suspicion of elevated ICP, then consider a modest reduction of blood pressure (e.g., MAP of 110 mm Hg or target blood pressure of 160/90 mm Hg) using intermittent or continuous intravenous medications to control blood pressure, and clinically re-examine the patient every 15 minutes.

SBP, systolic blood pressure; MAP, mean arterial pressure; ICP, intracranial pressure.
From Broderick J, Connolly S, Feldmann E, et al. Guidelines for the management of spontaneous intracerebral hemorrhage in adults: 2007 update: a guideline from the American Heart Association/American Stroke Association Stroke Council, High Blood Pressure Research Council, and the Quality of Care and Outcomes in Research Interdisciplinary Working Group. *Circulation*. 2007;116(16):e391–413, with permission.

cannot be explained by tPA (31,32). Rather, it is the advancements made in the prevention of medical complications that has reduced mortality.

Motor Deficits

Dysphagia is common after stroke, whether it be from upper or lower motor neuron deficits. All patients with stroke should be screened for dysphagia before being allowed to take anything by mouth, as aspiration pneumonia is a substantial contributor to mortality after stroke (33). Any impairment in level of consciousness or motor function of mouth, tongue, palate, or muscles of facial expression should alert the physician to a high risk for dysphagia. Coarse breath sounds may indicate that aspiration has already occurred. A preserved gag reflex may not indicate safety with swallowing (34). If any of these signs are present, a formal swallowing evaluation is indicated. Enteral access can be achieved by placement of a nasogastric or Dobhoff tube. Feeding and hydration should be initiated immediately (35). Dysphagia often improves rapidly, but placement of a percutaneous endoscopic gastrostomy (PEG) tube may be necessary for prolonged feeding.

Before the advent of routine prophylaxis, deep vein thromboses and resulting pulmonary emboli were common in stroke patients who frequently have profound lower extremity immobility; pulmonary embolism presently accounts for approximately 10% of deaths in stroke patients (36). Recent trials, including PREVAIL (37), have shown low-molecular-weight heparin to be safe and more effective than unfractionated heparin. Early mobilization not only prevents deep vein thromboses (DVTs), but also speeds rehabilitation.

Blood Pressure Maintenance

Blood pressure goals in the acute period after ischemic stroke are often a source of confusion for many practitioners. Ischemic stroke patients are often quite hypertensive, and, while the reflex may be to aggressively lower the blood pressure, this may cause more harm than benefit. When blood flow is impaired, the resulting change in pressure gradients will allow circulation through alternative or collateral paths. Through autoregulation, these collateral vessels maximally dilate, and thus flow becomes entirely dependent on cerebral perfusion pressure. Some even advocate the induction of therapeutic hypertension with pressors, but insufficient evidence exists to recommend this practice. Therefore, lowering blood pressure potentially reduces blood flow to the potentially salvageable penumbra. Determining the exact pressure required for adequate blood flow is not readily accomplished, so one must err on the side of hypertension. For most stroke patients with acute hypertension, the general practice is to refrain from intervening until the pressure exceeds an arbitrary limit of 220 mm Hg systolic or 120 mm Hg diastolic (29). Patients with coronary artery disease or those with another comorbidity that may preclude tolerance of such pressures may require a careful decrement in blood pressure. In these cases, it is recommended that blood pressure be lowered slowly, using frequent smaller doses of drug rather than larger ones that may cause rapid changes; patients should be carefully observed for acute worsening as pressure is lowered. In patients having received thrombolytics, the tolerable limit is lower, as the risk for intracerebral hemorrhage increases with increasing blood pressure. In this case, pressures greater than 180 mm Hg systolic or greater than 105 mm Hg diastolic require treatment according to the protocol (Table 84.8).

Hyperglycemia

Hyperglycemia will be detected on admission in approximately one third of patients with stroke (38). Predictions for patients with persistent hyperglycemia (blood glucose level >200 mg/dL) during the first 24 hours after stroke are expansion of the volume of ischemic stroke and poor neurologic outcomes (39). Our practice is to aggressively control glucose—keeping it between 80 and 140 mg/dL—but care must be taken to avoid hypoglycemia, as the morbidity from that may abolish the benefit obtained from treating hyperglycemia.

Although most patients eventually improve substantially after a stroke, early clinical deterioration is not uncommon. Neurologic causes of clinical deterioration include progressive or recurrent stroke, hemorrhagic transformation of the infarct, and local cerebral edema. The latter is the most common cause of deterioration, and may well cause fatal herniation in large MCA infarctions, especially in the young, women, and in patients with involvement of additional vascular territories (40). Brain swelling typically appears about 4 days after the stroke onset (41). Dramatic early swelling has been described; the term *malignant MCA infarction* is used to delineate a group of patients with large territorial infarcts that swell within 24 hours (42).

Ischemia-related edema is cytotoxic and unresponsive to treatments useful for vasogenic edema. Corticosteroids, in particular, do not appear helpful, and hyperglycemia associated with their use may worsen clinical outcome (29,43,44). Although no evidence exists that ultimate outcome is improved, certain treatments are often used to reduce intracranial pressure: mannitol (1 g/kg bolus, then 0.3 g/kg every 6 hours) dehydrates viable brain tissue (45) to create more space for swelling tissue, and is primarily useful as a temporizing measure for patients destined for decompressive surgery, as the effects of this medication are transient and associated with eventual rebound. Other measures such as mechanical hyperventilation (to a $PaCO_2$ of 25–30 mm Hg), or use of albumin and furosemide to raise colloid oncotic pressure (to 25–30 mm Hg) are used, but, again, their efficacy in improving outcome remains to be demonstrated.

Decompressive Surgery

Decompressive surgery, including hemicraniectomy and durotomy with temporal lobe resection, for treatment of brain edema after stroke has been a controversial topic. Many studies in the past have shown conflicting results, but these trials enrolled mixed age groups, and surgery was often not performed until symptomatic herniation occurred (46). Three large European trials (HAMLET, DESTINY, and DECIMAL) (47–49) that enrolled patients younger than 60 years of age and treated within 48 hours of onset were prematurely terminated after it became clear that decompressive craniotomy was associated with a dramatic survival and outcome benefit. In elderly patients, the results have generally shown that, while mortality may be decreased, outcomes remained poor (50).

The likelihood of hemorrhagic transformation of a stroke increases as stroke volume increases. Often, this transformation may be limited to petechial transudation of blood products into the ischemic tissue bed. Generally, this phenomenon occurs in a delayed fashion with no associated clinical deterioration. Specific therapy is not usually required, although any ongoing anticoagulation is generally held for 1 to 2 weeks. If the hemorrhage is associated with clinical deterioration, management should follow those principles outlined in the intracerebral hemorrhage section below.

Early initiation of physical, occupational, and speech therapy services hastens functional recovery from stroke. Each patient requires individualized assessment for potential benefit from these services. Speech therapists are also commonly involved in formal assessment of aspiration risk. A video fluoroscopy swallowing study is the most sensitive measure and should be a consideration for most patients with a stroke. At the least, bedside swallowing function should be observed by a trained technician, nurse, or physician before oral intake is resumed.

INTRACEREBRAL HEMORRHAGE

Pathogenesis

In contrast to ischemic stroke, primary intracerebral hemorrhage (ICH) involves bleeding, usually of arterial origin, into normally perfused brain, and thus must be distinguished from hemorrhagic transformation of an initially ischemic stroke. The expanding hematoma causes direct injury to local brain tissue and dysfunction in surrounding regions. The onset is typically very sudden, although continued bleeding often progresses over minutes or hours. Very often, there is either depression or loss of consciousness due to an abrupt increase in intracranial pressure (ICP) from the sudden outpouring of blood into the brain. In addition to the initial cerebral insult caused by the hemorrhage, secondary injury can occur by various means, including seizures, hydrocephalus, and edema, all of which can lead to a further increase in ICP.

In younger patients, hypertension is by far the more common cause, and, as such, ICH tends to occur in the same brain areas where other hypertensive pathologies occur, specifically brainstem, cerebellum, and deep supratentorial structures (51). In contrast, lobar ICHs occur more commonly in the elderly population and are often associated with cerebral amyloid angiopathy in the absence of hypertension (52). ICH may also occur in the setting of trauma, use of illicit drugs (e.g., cocaine) or over-the-counter medications (e.g., phenylpropanolamine) (53), excessive alcohol consumption (54), an underlying vascular abnormality (e.g., arteriovenous malformation, cerebral aneurysm), brain tumor (primary or secondary), or a bleeding diathesis.

ICH causes approximately 10% of first-time strokes. The 30-day mortality rate is high at 35% to 50%, with half of the deaths occurring within the first 2 days (12). Outcome in ICH is dependent on several factors, including the location and size of the hemorrhage (55), the age of the patient, the Glasgow Coma Scale (GCS) on presentation (56), and the cause of the hemorrhage. When intraventricular blood is present, the mortality substantially increases (57) and worsens further with increasing volume (58). The presence of hydrocephalus also confers a poor prognosis (59).

Clinical Evaluation

Rapid diagnosis of ICH is essential, as progression during the first several hours is the norm. The hallmark is sudden onset focal neurologic deficit, which progresses over minutes to hours. Steady symptomatic progression of a focal deficit is rare in either ischemic stroke or subarachnoid hemorrhage. Headache, increased blood pressure, and impaired level of consciousness are common features that complete the presentation. History gathering should be directed at elucidating the presence of risk factors as outlined above. Other considerations include the use of antithrombotic medications (e.g., aspirin or warfarin) or hematologic disorders that predispose to bleeding, such as severe liver disease. The initial physical examination is similar to that of patients with ischemic stroke, focusing on airway, breathing, and circulation before assessing the level of consciousness and neurologic deficits. The patient's coagulation parameters should be checked immediately and corrected if abnormal.

Once stabilized, the patient should undergo a noncontrast head CT immediately to verify brain hemorrhage. CT angiography may also be helpful in detecting aneurysms, arteriovenous malformations (AVMs), underlying tumors, or abscesses. Contrast extravasation into the hematoma is thought to represent ongoing bleeding (60). MRI will also provide information

TABLE 84.9

INTRAVENOUS MEDICATIONS THAT MAY BE CONSIDERED FOR CONTROL OF ELEVATED BLOOD PRESSURE IN PATIENTS WITH ICH

Drug	Intravenous bolus dose	Continuous infusion rate
Labetalol	5 to 20 mg every 15 min	2 mg/min (maximum 300 mg/day)
Nicardipine	NA	5 to 15 mg/h
Esmolol	250 μg/kg IVP loading dose	25 to 300 $\mu g \cdot kg^{-1} \cdot min^{-1}$
Enalapril	1.25 to 5 mg IVP every 6 h*	NA
Hydralazine	5 to 20 mg IVP every 30 min	1.5 to 5 $\mu g \cdot kg^{-1} \cdot min^{-1}$
Nipride	NA	0.1 to 10 $\mu g \cdot kg^{-1} \cdot min^{-1}$
Nitroglycerin	NA	20 to 400 μg/min

NA, not applicable; IVP, intravenous push.
*Because of the risk of precipitous blood pressure decrease, the first test dose of enalapril should be 0.625 mg.
From Broderick J, Connolly S, Feldmann E, et al. Guidelines for the management of spontaneous intracerebral hemorrhage in adults: 2007 update: a guideline from the American Heart Association/American Stroke Association Stroke Council, High Blood Pressure Research Council, and the Quality of Care and Outcomes in Research Interdisciplinary Working Group. *Circulation.* 2007;116(16):e391–413, with permission.

about the hemorrhage but is time consuming and potentially dangerous for an unstable patient. When it can be obtained safely, MRI is most useful for dating the time course of the hemorrhage if the history is in doubt, detecting areas of prior hemorrhage (with the use of gradient-echo imaging) (61), and diagnosing cavernous malformations. Catheter angiography should be considered in a young patient with an ICH with no history of hypertension, as an occult AVM or aneurysm may be responsible.

Cardiac arrhythmias represent another potentially catastrophic secondary complication of ICH, especially those that occur in the right hemisphere insular region. Dysfunction of this area has a propensity for causing abnormal cardiac electrical activity and "cerebrogenic sudden death" (62). Patients with such lesions must have close cardiac monitoring in the intensive care unit during their first several days after hemorrhage.

Management

The mainstays of medical treatment of acute ICH are correction of any coagulopathy and avoidance of hypertension. Most studies suggest that hematoma expansion occurs within the first several hours of onset, and therefore treatment must begin as soon as possible (63). If the patient recently received heparin, protamine sulfate (1 mg/100 units of heparin) should be administered; this drug is given carefully to avoid hypotension. Patients anticoagulated with warfarin with an elevated international normalized ratio (INR) should be reversed with vitamin K (10 mg intravenously administered over 15–20 minutes to prevent anaphylactoid reaction), as well as fresh frozen plasma to normalize the prothrombin time (PT).

Beyond the first few hours after onset, aggressive lowering of blood pressure may be potentially harmful. Large hemorrhages will lead to increased ICP, and attention must be focused on maintaining the cerebral perfusion pressure (mean arterial pressure–intracranial pressure [MAP-ICP]) >70 mm Hg to avoid secondary ischemia (64). Despite several clinical trials, a definitive guideline has yet to emerge. The American Stroke Association guidelines regarding blood pressure, presented in Table 84.8, are based on the best available, albeit incomplete, evidence. Table 84.9 lists recommended antihypertensives.

Seizures—occasionally nonconvulsive—occur commonly after ICH. The published incidence rates vary from 4% in unmonitored populations (65) to 28% in patients with continuous electrophysiologic monitoring in a neurocritical care unit (66). Prophylactic anticonvulsant medications may be considered for patients, especially for those with cortical involvement. If seizures are confirmed, they should be treated aggressively. Phenytoin remains the preferred first-line agent, as it is nonsedating, and loading doses can be given intravenously. Loading doses are 15 to 20 mg/kg and should be given as fosphenytoin if needed quickly to avoid hypotension and potential toxic infusion reactions. Maintenance doses are often 4 to 5 mg/kg and may be given slowly. Total serum levels of phenytoin should be followed daily, at least initially. Free levels may be necessary, as phenytoin is protein bound, and critically ill patients are very frequently protein depleted. Additional antiepileptics should be added as necessary. The duration of therapy with anticonvulsants is unclear, but in seizurefree nonepileptic patients, antiepileptic medications are often arbitrarily withdrawn after 4 to 6 weeks of therapy.

Other general supportive care measures are similar to those described above for ischemic stroke, including attention to DVT prophylaxis, and treatment of hyperthermia and hyperglycemia. Patients with increased intracranial pressure often develop disturbances of free water homeostasis in the form of either hyponatremia or hypernatremia. As with ischemic stroke, corticosteroids for treatment of edema are of no benefit and actually increase morbidity (67).

Treatment of increased ICP should initially focus on more conservative noninvasive measures, such as keeping the head of the bed at 30 degrees, hyperventilation if intubated, and osmolar therapy with hypertonic saline or mannitol. An implanted ICP monitor should be considered for those patients with large hematomas. This will inform the decision to place an intraventricular drain or perform a surgical evacuation.

In general, patients with a GCS of 4 or more have a uniformly poor outcome, whether or not surgery is performed,

TABLE 84.10

SEVERITY GRADE OF SUBARACHNOID HEMORRHAGE

Grade 1: Fully conscious, no neurologic deficit, headache only Grade 2: Mild drowsiness, no neurologic deficits other than cranial nerve dysfunction Grade 3: Drowsy, mild neurologic deficit Grade 4: Stuporous, moderate to severe neurologic deficits Grade 5: Coma
From Hunt WE, Hess RM. Surgical risk as related to the time of intervention in the repair of intracranial aneurysms. *J Neurosurg.* 1968;28:14.

and thus these patients should be treated medically. Patients with cerebellar hemorrhages >3 cm in diameter should be considered for emergency decompression, especially if there are signs of brainstem compression, hydrocephalus, or neurologic deterioration (64); whether surgery is indicated in most other patients is not clear. Clinicians treating patients who deteriorate despite maximal medical therapy may turn to surgical decompression, but results from clinical trials have been mixed (68,69). Patients with lobar hemorrhages secondary to amyloid angiopathy have exceptionally friable cortical blood vessels and are poor surgical candidates.

SUBARACHNOID HEMORRHAGE

Subarachnoid hemorrhage (SAH) is a relatively uncommon but often devastating type of stroke. Incidence is estimated at 30,000 patients per year in the United States, with a mortality that exceeds 50%. Whereas head trauma is the most frequent cause of subarachnoid hemorrhage, aneurysmal rupture results in the greatest morbidity and mortality. Clinically, this is an apoplectic disorder. Most commonly, patients perceive a sudden severe headache with rapid impairment of consciousness, both symptoms related to the sudden release of irritating blood products into the meningeal spaces surrounding the brain. Focal neurologic symptoms such as hemiparesis, sensory loss, or diplopia may occur if loculation of subarachnoid blood or intraparenchymal extension of the hemorrhage develops. The most important features of the neurologic examination are the assessment of level of consciousness, cranial nerve function, and motor function. Clinical severity of SAH is graded on these findings (70) (grades I to V, Table 84.10) and can be rough prognostic indicators.

Diagnosis

Diagnosis of SAH is based on neuroimaging or cerebrospinal fluid (CSF) analysis. Brain CT scan is a very sensitive indicator of the presence of subarachnoid blood, although close examination must be paid to the subarachnoid spaces surrounding the brainstem and over the cerebral convexities (Fig. 84.5). Brain parenchyma itself most commonly displays no acute abnormalities. Erythrocyte concentration in CSF below approximately 30,000 cells/μL may not result in the diagnostic increased density within CSF on CT scans. In approximately 10% of patients, diagnosis therefore requires CSF analysis through lumbar puncture. In addition to elevated erythrocyte count, CSF xanthochromia and elevation of CSF D-dimer can often be detected in true subarachnoid hemorrhage. The latter two findings may help distinguish bloody CSF from a "traumatic tap," as these serve as markers of the breakdown of thrombosis or blood products. Serial cell counts should always be obtained, however, whenever SAH is suspected. Cell counts in SAH should be roughly equivalent in all tubes, whereas a declining count is usual in traumatic punctures. It should be stressed that lumbar puncture should be avoided in any patient with a depressed level of consciousness until CT scan excludes a focal mass (such as intraparenchymal or subdural hemorrhage). If bacterial meningitis is a concern, blood

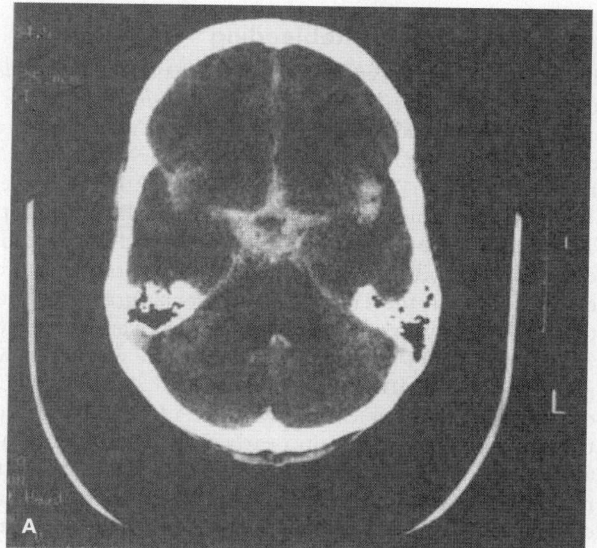

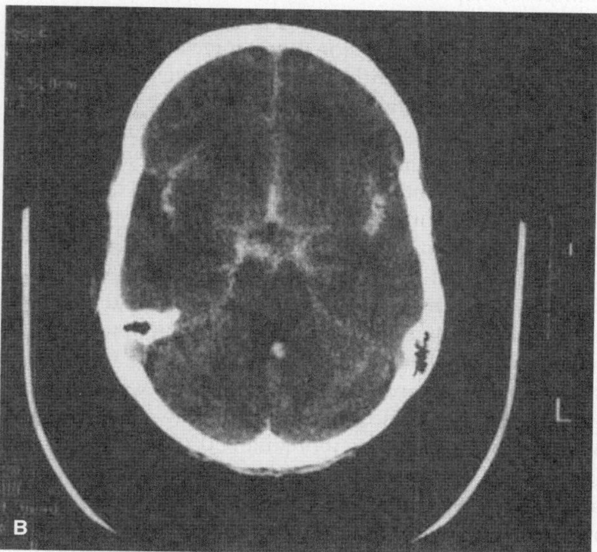

FIGURE 84.5. Subarachnoid hemorrhage. Blood is imaged as hyperdense fluid within the cisterns surrounding the brainstem and within bilateral sylvian fissures.

TABLE 84.11

COMPLICATIONS OF SUBARACHNOID HEMORRHAGE

Complication	Clinical features	Diagnostic tests	Therapy
Increased ICP	Decreased alertness, worsened headache, herniation syndrome	ICP monitor	Mannitol, steroids, hyperventilation
Hydrocephalus	Decreased alertness, worsened headache, herniation syndrome	CT scan	Ventriculostomy drainage or shunt
Vasospasm	Delayed focal neurologic deficit	TCD, angiography	Nimodipine, hypervolemia, hypertension, angioplasty
Rebleed	Worsened neurologic condition, especially level of consciousness	CT scan, lumbar puncture	Ablation of aneurysm
Seizure	Sudden behavioral change or uncontrolled motor activity	EEG	Anticonvulsants
Hyponatremia	Confusion, seizure	Serum electrolytes	Isotonic fluids to achieve euvolemia or hypervolemia
Infection	Confusion, lethargy	Panculture, chest radiograph, urinalysis	Appropriate antibiotic

ICP, intracranial pressure; CT, computed tomography; TCD, transcranial Doppler; EEG, electroencephalogram.

cultures should be obtained and antibiotics started while awaiting results of the CT scan.

Management

Patients with acute SAH are at high risk for a multitude of complications (71) (Table 84.11) that usually mandate admission to an intensive care facility. All patients should be placed on strict bed rest, with appropriate precautions for deep venous thrombosis and aspiration. Patients with progressive lethargy may require intubation for airway protection and mechanical ventilation. Until the aneurysm has been ablated, blood pressure should be kept in the normotensive range, and isotonic intravenous fluids should be used to maintain normovolemia. All patients should be started on nimodipine at 60 mg every 4 hours (duration 21 days), either orally or through a nasogastric tube, for prevention of vasospasm (see below).

Historically, patients were placed on prophylactic anticonvulsants; this practice has recently come into question, as patients enrolled in the international tirilazad trials who were on prophylactic anticonvulsants had significantly more in-hospital complications and worse clinical outcomes (72).

ECG changes and elevations in cardiac enzymes, troponin, and CK-MB are commonly seen in SAH patients and may represent the phenomenon of stunned myocardium, in which case management should be aimed at optimizing left ventricular function to support cardiovascular and cerebrovascular perfusion (73–76). Serum electrolytes are closely monitored, as hyponatremia may be seen in more than 30% of patients after SAH; however, hypernatremia can occur as well and is significantly associated with clinical outcome (77). The cause of hyponatremia after SAH is most commonly reported to be due to syndrome of inappropriate antidiuretic hormone (SIADH) but can also be due to cerebral salt-wasting (CSW) syndrome and other causes (78). One theory links SAH-induced hyponatremia to levels of serum brain natriuretic peptide, which is thought to be associated with delayed ischemic neurologic deficits (79). It is intuitive that SIADH and CSW are *not* treated in the same manner.

Serum glucose levels should also be closely monitored, as hyperglycemia has been significantly associated with mortality and poor functional outcome in SAH patients (80). Because fever in SAH patients has been associated with mortality and poor clinical outcome (80), and has even been linked to vasospasm (81), patients should be kept normothermic. Platelet levels should be monitored, as a relatively significant incidence of heparin-induced thrombocytopenia has been reported in SAH patients (82).

Rebleeding

In those patients surviving the initial hemorrhage, *the leading factor associated with mortality is rebleeding from the aneurysm*. A second bleed from an aneurysm is associated with a 74% mortality rate (83). Untreated aneurysms rebleed at a rate of 4% on day 1, then 1% to 2% a day for the next 4 weeks. Thus, early treatment to secure a ruptured aneurysm is critical. This can be done either via a craniotomy and clipping, or by endovascular coiling. The findings of the International Cooperative Study on the Timing of Aneurysm Surgery concluded that aneurysmal clipping was best performed either early (0 to 3 days) or late (11 to 14 days), but outcome was worse when performed at 7 to 10 days after the onset of SAH (84). Because of the concern for rebleeding, we have adopted a protocol of treating aneurysms in the ultra-early period (less than 24 hours after presentation). The advent of endovascular therapy to treat ruptured aneurysms may bypass the risks associated with open clipping during the 7- to 10-day period; thus we recommend treatment for the ruptured aneurysm as soon as it is found, and not waiting until the late 11- to 14-day period. Early treatment of the ruptured aneurysm also allows aggressive management

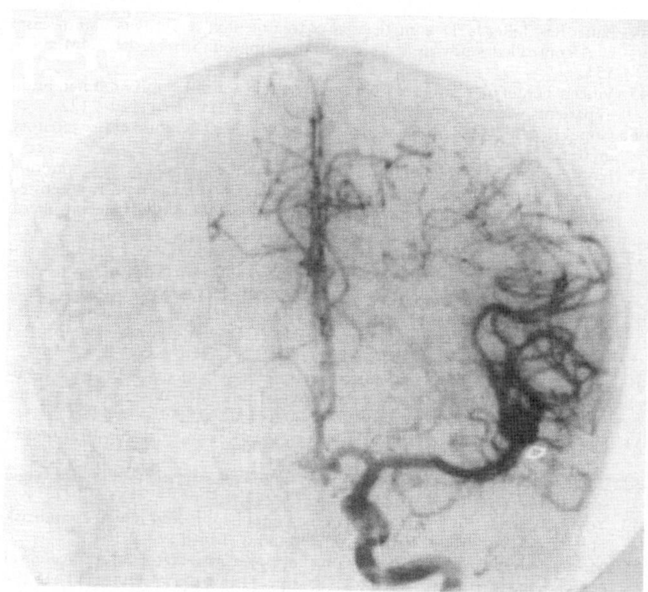

FIGURE 84.6. Aneurysm at the bifurcation of the left middle cerebral artery demonstrated by angiography. (Courtesy of R. Nick Bryan, MD, Baylor College of Medicine, Houston, TX.)

of vasospasm, manipulations that would increase the risk of rebleeding from an unsecured aneurysm.

Vasospasm

After rebleeding, vasospasm is the next leading cause of mortality and morbidity from a SAH (85,86). The exact cause of arterial vasospasm following SAH is unknown, but its incidence does appear to be correlated with the density of blood products seen on CT scan, the basis for the Fisher score to predict vasospasm (87,88). Severe vasospasm may result in cerebral infarction within the vascular distribution of the involved artery. The risk for vasospasm begins about 3 days after the bleed and may persist for 3 weeks. Transcranial Doppler is a sensitive, noninvasive indicator of the presence and degree of vasospasm within proximal arteries, although it may not detect vasospasm restricted to smaller peripheral vessels. This technique may be used daily to guide and monitor management strategies. Modern techniques, such as CT angiography and CT perfusion studies, have been reported to be successful in diagnosing vasospasm (89) (Fig. 84.6).

The calcium channel blockers nimodipine and nicardipine can reduce the incidence of vasospasm as well as associated cerebral infarction. Trials with magnesium sulfate have yielded promising results in reducing vasospasm (90–92) or achieving better clinical outcomes in patients (93). Studies with statin therapy (HMG Co-A inhibitors), such as pravastatin and simvastatin, have demonstrated promising results with reduced rates of vasospasm and better clinical outcomes (94–97).

Once the aneurysm is secured, vasospasm can be managed aggressively. Triple-H therapy—hypertension, hypervolemia, hemodilution—is the first-line therapy against vasospasm. Once vasospasm occurs, IV fluids should be pushed to the tolerance of the patient (below 400 mL/hour). Since congestive heart failure is a potential complication, central pressure monitoring—at a minimum—should be used in patients at risk; optimal central venous pressure is 8 to 12 mm Hg. Other modalities of monitoring, from pulse-waveform variability (FlowTrak, PICCO, LiDCO) to placement of a pulmonary artery catheter, may be necessary to properly care for these patients. If hypervolemic therapy is not adequate to control vasospasm, hypertension can be initiated by cessation of antihypertensives or use of vasopressors (e.g., phenylephrine, 0.1–5 μg/kg per minute, or vasopressin, 0.01–0.04 units per minute), targeting mean arterial pressures of 120 to 140 mm Hg (systolic blood pressure [BP] 180–200 mm Hg). Triple-H therapy does not increase the risk of rupture of other, incidentally found, aneurysms in patients with multiple aneurysms (98).

For symptomatic vasospasm refractory to these therapies, endovascular interventions can be performed, such as percutaneous transluminal balloon angioplasty, and/or intra-arterial administration of calcium channel blockers or other vasodilating agents (99) may be considered in experienced hands. Even using the most aggressive management strategies, vasospasm remains a leading cause of morbidity and mortality after subarachnoid hemorrhage.

Acute Hydrocephalus

Acute hydrocephalus occurs in approximately 20% of survivors of SAH, either as a result of direct obstruction of CSF channels or by impeding CSF absorption at arachnoid granulations. The likelihood of hydrocephalus increases with worsening grade of hemorrhage. Ventriculostomy drainage is recommended for patients with acute hydrocephalus and decreased level of consciousness; improvement can be expected in >50% of patients.

References

1. Norris JW, Hachinski VC. Misdiagnosis of stroke. *Lancet.* 1982;1(8267): 328–331.
2. Inzitari D, et al. The causes and risk of stroke in patients with asymptomatic internal-carotid-artery stenosis. North American Symptomatic Carotid Endarterectomy Trial Collaborators. *N Engl J Med.* 2000;342(23):1693–1700.
3. Fisher CM. The arterial lesions underlying lacunes. *Acta Neuropathol.* 1968; 12(1):1–15.
4. Bogousslavsky J, Van Melle G, Regli F. The Lausanne Stroke Registry: analysis of 1,000 consecutive patients with first stroke. *Stroke.* 1988;19(9):1083–1092.
5. Mohr JP, et al. The Harvard Cooperative Stroke Registry: a prospective registry. *Neurology.* 1978;28(8):754–762.
6. Pruitt AA, et al. Neurologic complications of bacterial endocarditis. *Medicine (Baltimore).* 1978;57(4):329–343.
7. Roeltgen DP, Weimer GR, Patterson LF. Delayed neurologic complications of left atrial myxoma. *Neurology.* 1981;31(1):8–13.
8. Bogousslavsky J, Pierre P. Ischemic stroke in patients under age 45. *Neurol Clin.* 1992;10(1):113–124.
9. Kalb R. Spontaneous dissection of the carotid and vertebral arteries. *N Engl J Med.* 2001;345(6):467.
10. Ay H, Arsava EM, Saribas O. Creatine kinase-MB elevation after stroke is not cardiac in origin: comparison with troponin T levels. *Stroke.* 2002; 33(1):286–289.
11. Hankey GJ, et al. Inherited thrombophilia in ischemic stroke and its pathogenic subtypes. *Stroke.* 2001;32(8):1793–1799.
12. Anderson CS, et al. Spectrum of primary intracerebral haemorrhage in Perth, Western Australia, 1989–90: incidence and outcome. *J Neurol Neurosurg Psychiatry.* 1994;57(8):936–940.
13. Alexandrov AV, et al. Ultrasound-enhanced systemic thrombolysis for acute ischemic stroke. *N Engl J Med.* 2004;351(21):2170–2178.
14. DeRook FA, et al. Transesophageal echocardiography in the evaluation of stroke. *Ann Intern Med.* 1992;117(11):922–932.
15. Johannessen KA, et al. Risk factors for embolisation in patients with left ventricular thrombi and acute myocardial infarction. *Br Heart J.* 1988;60(2): 104–110.
16. Tissue plasminogen activator for acute ischemic stroke. The National Institute of Neurological Disorders and Stroke rt-PA Stroke Study Group. *N Engl J Med.* 1995;333(24):1581–1587.

17. Generalized efficacy of t-PA for acute stroke. Subgroup analysis of the NINDS t-PA Stroke Trial. *Stroke.* 1997;28(11):2119–2125.
18. Intracerebral hemorrhage after intravenous t-PA therapy for ischemic stroke. The NINDS t-PA Stroke Study Group. *Stroke.* 1997;28(11):2109–2118.
19. Hacke W, et al. Intravenous thrombolysis with recombinant tissue plasminogen activator for acute hemispheric stroke. The European Cooperative Acute Stroke Study (ECASS). *JAMA.* 1995;274(13):1017–1025.
20. Hacke W, et al. Randomised double-blind placebo-controlled trial of thrombolytic therapy with intravenous alteplase in acute ischaemic stroke (ECASS II). Second European-Australasian Acute Stroke Study Investigators. *Lancet.* 1998;352(9136):1245–1251.
21. Clark WM, et al. The rtPA (alteplase) 0- to 6-hour acute stroke trial, part A (A0276g): results of a double-blind, placebo-controlled, multicenter study. Thrombolytic therapy in acute ischemic stroke study investigators. *Stroke.* 2000;31(4):811–816.
22. Clark WM, et al. Recombinant tissue-type plasminogen activator (Alteplase) for ischemic stroke 3 to 5 hours after symptom onset. The ATLANTIS Study: a randomized controlled trial. Alteplase Thrombolysis for Acute Noninterventional Therapy in Ischemic Stroke. *JAMA.* 1999;282(21):2019–2026.
23. Kwiatkowski TG, et al. Effects of tissue plasminogen activator for acute ischemic stroke at one year. National Institute of Neurological Disorders and Stroke Recombinant Tissue Plasminogen Activator Stroke Study Group. *N Engl J Med.* 1999;340(23):1781–1787.
24. Saver JL. Number needed to treat estimates incorporating effects over the entire range of clinical outcomes: novel derivation method and application to thrombolytic therapy for acute stroke. *Arch Neurol.* 2004;61(7):1066–1070.
25. Saver JL. Hemorrhage after thrombolytic therapy for stroke: the clinically relevant number needed to harm. *Stroke.* 2007;38(8):2279–2283.
26. Olsen TS, Weber UJ, Kammersgaard LP. Therapeutic hypothermia for acute stroke. *Lancet Neurol.* 2003;2(7):410–416.
27. del Zoppo GJ, et al. PROACT: a phase II randomized trial of recombinant pro-urokinase by direct arterial delivery in acute middle cerebral artery stroke. PROACT Investigators. Prolyse in Acute Cerebral Thromboembolism. *Stroke.* 1998;29(1):4–11.
28. Smith WS, et al. Safety and efficacy of mechanical embolectomy in acute ischemic stroke: results of the MERCI trial. *Stroke.* 2005;36(7):1432–1438.
29. Adams HP Jr., et al. Guidelines for the early management of adults with ischemic stroke: a guideline from the American Heart Association/American Stroke Association Stroke Council, Clinical Cardiology Council, Cardiovascular Radiology and Intervention Council, and the Atherosclerotic Peripheral Vascular Disease and Quality of Care Outcomes in Research Interdisciplinary Working Groups: the American Academy of Neurology affirms the value of this guideline as an educational tool for neurologists. *Stroke.* 2007; 38(5):1655–1711.
30. Jemal A, et al. Trends in the Leading Causes of Death in the United States, 1970–2002. *JAMA.* 2005;294(10):1255–1259.
31. Heuschmann PU, et al. Frequency of Thrombolytic Therapy in Patients With Acute Ischemic Stroke and the Risk of In-Hospital Mortality: The German Stroke Registers Study Group. *Stroke.* 2003;34(5):1106–1112.
32. Koennecke H-C, et al. Intravenous tPA for Ischemic Stroke Team Performance Over Time, Safety, and Efficacy in a Single-Center, 2-Year Experience. *Stroke.* 2001;32(5):1074–1078.
33. Aslanyan S, et al. Pneumonia and urinary tract infection after acute ischaemic stroke: a tertiary analysis of the GAIN International trial. *Eur J Neurol.* 2004;11(1):49–53.
34. Addington WR, Stephens RE, Gilliland KA. Assessing the laryngeal cough reflex and the risk of developing pneumonia after stroke: an interhospital comparison. *Stroke.* 1999;30(6):1203–1207.
35. Choi-Kwon S, et al. Nutritional status in acute stroke: undernutrition versus overnutrition in different stroke subtypes. *Acta Neurol Scand.* 1998;98(3): 187–192.
36. Wijdicks EF, Scott JP. Pulmonary embolism associated with acute stroke. *Mayo Clin Proc.* 1997;72(4):297–300.
37. Sherman DG, et al. The efficacy and safety of enoxaparin versus unfractionated heparin for the prevention of venous thromboembolism after acute ischaemic stroke (PREVAIL Study): an open-label randomised comparison. *Lancet.* 2007;369(9570):1347–1355.
38. Williams LS, et al. Effects of admission hyperglycemia on mortality and costs in acute ischemic stroke. *Neurology.* 2002;59(1):67–71.
39. Baird TA, et al. Persistent poststroke hyperglycemia is independently associated with infarct expansion and worse clinical outcome. *Stroke.* 2003;34(9): 2208–2214.
40. Maramattom BV, Bahn MM, Wijdicks EF. Which patient fares worse after early deterioration due to swelling from hemispheric stroke? *Neurology.* 2004;63(11):2142–2145.
41. Ropper AH, Shafran B. Brain edema after stroke. Clinical syndrome and intracranial pressure. *Arch Neurol.* 1984;41(1):26–29.
42. Qureshi AI, et al. Timing of neurologic deterioration in massive middle cerebral artery infarction: a multicenter review. *Crit Care Med.* 2003;31(1):272–277.
43. Tellez H, Bauer RB. Dexamethasone as treatment in cerebrovascular disease. 1. A controlled study in intracerebral hemorrhage. *Stroke.* 1973;4(4):541–546.
44. Bauer RB, Tellez H. Dexamethasone as treatment in cerebrovascular disease. 2. A controlled study in acute cerebral infarction. *Stroke.* 1973;4(4):547–555.
45. Videen TO, et al. Mannitol bolus preferentially shrinks non-infarcted brain in patients with ischemic stroke. *Neurology.* 2001;57(11):2120–2122.
46. Gupta R, et al. Hemicraniectomy for massive middle cerebral artery territory infarction: a systematic review. *Stroke.* 2004;35(2):539–543.
47. Hofmeijer J, et al. Hemicraniectomy after middle cerebral artery infarction with life-threatening edema trial (HAMLET). Protocol for a randomised controlled trial of decompressive surgery in space-occupying hemispheric infarction. *Trials.* 2006;7:29.
48. Vahedi K, et al. Sequential-design, multicenter, randomized, controlled trial of early decompressive craniectomy in malignant middle cerebral artery infarction (DECIMAL Trial). *Stroke.* 2007;38(9):2506–2517.
49. Juttler E, et al. Decompressive surgery for the treatment of malignant infarction of the middle cerebral artery (DESTINY): a randomized, controlled trial. *Stroke.* 2007;38(9):2518–2525.
50. Holtkamp M, et al. Hemicraniectomy in elderly patients with space occupying media infarction: improved survival but poor functional outcome. *J Neurol Neurosurg Psychiatry.* 2001;70(2):226–228.
51. Flaherty ML, et al. Racial variations in location and risk of intracerebral hemorrhage. *Stroke.* 2005;36(5):934–937.
52. Tonk M, Haan J. A review of genetic causes of ischemic and hemorrhagic stroke. *J Neurol Sci.* 2007;257(1–2):273–279.
53. Yoon BW, et al. Phenylpropanolamine contained in cold remedies and risk of hemorrhagic stroke. *Neurology.* 2007;68(2):146–149.
54. Monforte R, et al. High ethanol consumption as risk factor for intracerebral hemorrhage in young and middle-aged people. *Stroke.* 1990;21(11):1529–1532.
55. Broderick JP, et al. Volume of intracerebral hemorrhage. A powerful and easy-to-use predictor of 30-day mortality. *Stroke.* 1993;24(7):987–993.
56. Tuhrim S, et al. Prediction of intracerebral hemorrhage survival. *Ann Neurol.* 1988;24(2):258–263.
57. Tuhrim S, et al. Validation and comparison of models predicting survival following intracerebral hemorrhage. *Crit Care Med.* 1995;23(5):950–954.
58. Tuhrim S, et al. Volume of ventricular blood is an important determinant of outcome in supratentorial intracerebral hemorrhage. *Crit Care Med.* 1999; 27(3):617–621.
59. Diringer MN, Edwards DF, Zazulia AR. Hydrocephalus: a previously unrecognized predictor of poor outcome from supratentorial intracerebral hemorrhage. *Stroke.* 1998;29(7):1352–1357.
60. Becker KJ, et al. Withdrawal of support in intracerebral hemorrhage may lead to self-fulfilling prophecies. *Neurology.* 2001;56(6):766–772.
61. Greenberg SM, Finklestein SP, Schaefer PW. Petechial hemorrhages accompanying lobar hemorrhage: detection by gradient-echo MRI. *Neurology.* 1996;46(6):1751–1754.
62. Cheung RT, Hachinski V. The insula and cerebrogenic sudden death. *Arch Neurol.* 2000;57(12):1685–1688.
63. Kazui S, et al. Enlargement of spontaneous intracerebral hemorrhage. Incidence and time course. *Stroke.* 1996;27(10):1783–1787.
64. Broderick J, et al. Guidelines for the management of spontaneous intracerebral hemorrhage in adults: 2007 update: a guideline from the American Heart Association/American Stroke Association Stroke Council, High Blood Pressure Research Council, and the Quality of Care and Outcomes in Research Interdisciplinary Working Group. *Circulation.* 2007;116(16):e391–e413.
65. Passero S, et al. Seizures after spontaneous supratentorial intracerebral hemorrhage. *Epilepsia.* 2002;43(10):1175–1180.
66. Vespa PM, et al. Acute seizures after intracerebral hemorrhage: a factor in progressive midline shift and outcome. *Neurology.* 2003;60(9):1441–1446.
67. Poungvarin N, et al. Effects of dexamethasone in primary supratentorial intracerebral hemorrhage. *N Engl J Med.* 1987;316(20):1229–1233.
68. Morgenstern LB, et al. Surgical treatment for intracerebral hemorrhage (STICH): a single-center, randomized clinical trial. *Neurology.* 1998;51(5): 1359–1363.
69. Auer LM, et al. Endoscopic surgery versus medical treatment for spontaneous intracerebral hematoma: a randomized study. *J Neurosurg.* 1989;70(4):530–535.
70. Hunt WE, Hess RM. Surgical risk as related to the time of intervention in the repair of intracranial aneurysms. *J Neurosurg.* 1968;28:14.
71. Mayberg MR, Batjer HH, Dacey R, et al. Guidelines for the management of aneurysmal subarachnoid hemorrhage. *Circulation.* 1994;90:2592.
72. Rosengart AJ, Huo JD, Tolentino J, et al. Outcome in patients with subarachnoid hemorrhage treated with antiepileptic drugs. *J Neurosurg.* 2007; 107:253–260.
73. Urbaniak K, Merchant AI, Amin-Hanjani S, Roitberg B. Cardiac complications after aneurysmal subarachnoid hemorrhage. *Surg Neurology.* 2007; 67:21–28.
74. Banki NM, Kopelnik A, Dae MW, et al. Acute neurocardiogenic injury after subarachnoid hemorrhage. *Circulation.* 2005;112:3314–3319.
75. Naidech AM, Kreiter KT, Janjua N, et al. Cardiac troponin elevation, cardiovascular morbidity, and outcome after subarachnoid hemorrhage. *Circulation.* 2005;112:2851–2856.
76. Deibert E, Barzilai B, Braverman AC, et al. Clinical significance of elevated troponin I levels in patients with nontraumatic subarachnoid hemorrhage. *J Neurosurg.* 2003;98:741–746.

77. Qureshi AI, Suri MF, Sung GY, et al. Prognostic significance of hypernatremia and hyponatremia among patients with aneurysmal subarachnoid hemorrhage. *Neurosurgery.* 2002;50:749–755.
78. Sherlock M, O'Sullivan E, Agha A, et al. The incidence and pathophysiology of hyponatremia after subarachnoid haemorrhage. *Clin Endocrinol* (Oxf). 2006;64:250–254.
79. McGirt MJ, Blessing R, Nimjee SM, et al. Correlation of serum brain natriuretic peptide with hyponatremia and delayed ischemic neurologic deficits after subarachnoid hemorrhage. *Neurosurgery.* 2004;54:1369–1373.
80. Wartenberg KE, Schmidt JM, Claassen J, et al. Impact of medical complication on outcome after subarachnoid hemorrhage. *Crit Care Med.* 2006; 34:617–623.
81. Oliveira-Filho J, Ezzeddine MA, Segal AZ, et al. Fever in subarachnoid hemorrhage—relationship to vasospasm and outcome. *Neurology.* 2001; 56:1299–1304.
82. Hoh BL, Aghi M, Pryor JC, et al. Heparin-induced thrombocytopenia Type II in subarachnoid hemorrhage patients—incidence and complications. *Neurosurgery.* 2005;57:243–248.
83. Juvela S. Rebleeding from ruptured intracranial aneurysms. *Surgical Neurol.* 1989;32:323–326.
84. Kassell NF, Torner JC, Jane JA, et al. The international cooperative study on the timing of aneurysm surgery Part 2—Surgical results. *J Neurosurg.* 1990;73:37–47.
85. Hoh BL, Topcuoglu MA, Singhal AB, et al. Effect of clipping, craniotomy, or intravascular coiling on cerebral vasospasm and patient outcome after aneurysmal subarachnoid hemorrhage. *Neurosurgery.* 2004;55:779–786.
86. Hoh BL, Rabinov JD, Pryor JC, et al. A modified technique for using elastase to create saccular aneurysms in animals that histologically and hemodynamically resemble aneurysms in human. *Acta Neurochir (Wien).* 2004;146:1177–1183.
87. Fisher CM, Kistler JP, Davis JM. Relation of cerebral vasospasm to subarachnoid hemorrhage visualized by computer tomographic scanning. *Neurosurgery.* 1980;6:1–9.
88. Kistler JP, Crowell RM, Davis KR, et al. The relation of cerebral vasospasm to the extent and location of subarachnoid blood visualized by CT scan—a prospective study. *Neurology.* 1983;33:424–436.
89. Binaghi S, Colleoni ML, Maeder P, et al. CT angiography and perfusion CT in cerebral vasospasm after subarachnoid hemorrhage. *AJNR Am J Neuroradiol.* 2007;28:750–758.
90. van den Bergh WM, Algra A, van Kooten F, et al. Magnesium sulfate in aneurysmal subarachnoid hemorrhage—a randomized controlled trial. *Stroke.* 2005;36:1011–1015.
91. Stippler M, Crago E, Levi EI, et al. Magnesium infusion for vasospasm prophylaxis after subarachnoid hemorrhage. *J Neurosurg.* 2006;105:723–729.
92. Schmid-Elsaesser R, Kunz M, Zausinger S, et al. Intravenous magnesium versus nimodipine in the treatment of patients with aneurysmal subarachnoid hemorrhage—a randomized study. *Neurosurgery.* 2006;58:1054–1065.
93. Muroi C, Terzic A, Fortunati M, et al. Magnesium sulfate in the management of patients with aneurysmal subarachnoid hemorrhage—a randomized, placebo-controlled, dose-adapted trial. *Surg Neurol.* 2008;69:33–39.
94. McGirt MJ, Blessing R, Alexander MJ, et al. Risk of cerebral vasospasm after subarachnoid hemorrhage reduced by statin therapy. A multivariate analysis of an institutional experience. *J Neurosurg.* 2006;105:671–674.
95. Lynch JR, Wang H, McGirt MJ, et al. Simvastatin reduces vasospasm after aneurysmal subarachnoid hemorrhage—results of a pilot randomized clinical trial. *Stroke.* 2005;36:2024–2026.
96. Tseng MY, Czosnyka M, Richards H, et al. Effects of acute treatment with pravastatin on cerebral vasospasm, autoregulation and delayed ischemic deficits after aneurysmal subarachnoid hemorrhage—a phase II randomized, placebo controlled trial. *Stroke.* 2005;36:1627–1632.
97. Tseng MY, Hutchinson PJ, Czosnyka M, et al. Effects of acute pravastatin treatment on intensity of rescue therapy, length of inpatient stay, and 6 month outcome in patients after aneurysmal subarachnoid hemorrhage. *Stroke.* 2007;38:1545–1550.
98. Hoh BL, Carter BS, Ogilvy CS. Risk of hemorrhage from unsecured, unruptured aneurysms during and after hypertensive, hypervolemic therapy. *Neurosurgery.* 2002;50:1207–1211.
99. Hoh BL, Ogilvy CS. Endovascular treatment of cerebral vasospasm—transluminal balloon angioplasty, intra-arterial papaverine, and intra-arterial nicardipine. *Neurosurg Clin North Am.* 2005;16:501–516.

CHAPTER 85 ■ ORTHOPEDIC CRITICAL CARE

DEBORAH STERN • ANDREW POLLAK • THOMAS M. SCALEA

Bony and soft tissue injuries often complicate trauma. Optimal treatment of these injuries is essential for good overall patient care. Patients treated suboptimally are at risk for myriad complications such as fat embolism syndrome, pulmonary embolus, soft tissue infection, and multiple organ failure. There is little prospective randomized data to guide treatment decisions in patients with bony injuries. However, certain treatment principles have emerged. These must, of course, be interpreted in the context of the total patient.

Fracture stabilization is an operative procedure of significance. Some patients may be too critically ill or injured at the time of initial presentation to tolerate definitive fracture fixation. The critical care staff must be well versed in the management principles that govern musculoskeletal injuries as they will often have important roles to play in decision making. Orthopedic surgeons and/or anesthesiologists may not have sufficient information on total patient physiology in order to make these decisions without input from the critical care staff.

DIAGNOSING MUSCULOSKELETAL INJURY

Patients presenting after injury should typically have either signs or symptoms to guide diagnosis of their injuries. Pain, swelling, and soft tissue discoloration often accompany musculoskeletal injury, particularly in badly displaced or comminuted fractures. However, the initial presentation of many fractures may be far more subtle. Patients who have fractures that are not badly displaced may actually have only modest soft tissue swelling and discoloration or none at all at the time of presentation. Patients who are multiply injured often undergo endotracheal intubation at the time of emergency department presentation and are unable to complain of pain. Multiply injured patients may have other injuries that distract them from the pain of a minor fracture. Patients with brain injury and/or intoxication may not complain of pain. The authors are constantly impressed how the signs and symptoms of fractures can be subtle or completely absent initially. Fractures missed at the time of initial presentation can cause significant morbidity or mortality. While these data on missed injuries are sparse, estimates are that fractures are missed up to 10% of the time in multiply injured patients (1). Several options exist to try to reduce that number.

Certainly any patient with any signs, symptoms, or suspicion of fractures should undergo evaluation both by physical exam and plain radiographs. While the yield is low, obtaining radiographs on every area of soft tissue contusions will yield unsuspecting fractures in a small number of cases. Thus, screening algorithms should be broad to avoid missing fractures. Technologic advances have helped. The Lodox Corporation has produced the Statscan, a total body screening x-ray machine (Fig. 85.1). Using low-dose radiation developed in the diamond mine industry, it is possible to obtain both anteroposterior (AP) and lateral total body images of the skeleton (Fig. 85.2). These can be obtained in 13 seconds and the images available for viewing 15 seconds later. This allows the clinician to obtain an entire skeletal survey rapidly (2).

Another option is to perform a "tertiary survey" somewhere between 12 and 24 hours postadmission (1). Patients with fractures that have been missed generally develop some signs or symptoms in the ensuing hours after admission. The tertiary survey is a careful head-to-toe physical examination attempting to identify areas of missed injuries. Diagnostic imaging can be obtained to diagnose injuries that had been initially missed.

As with any injury, fractures are dynamic. It is not simply that a bone is broken. X-ray images are static and will not allow the clinician to appreciate the degree of energy transfer at the time of impact. Bones may be substantially displaced at the time of impact and then be spontaneously reduced or be reduced by actions of the local muscle and appear relatively undisplaced in the emergency department. Fractures are a source of significant bleeding, either from the fracture fragments themselves, muscle bleeding, or accompanied major vascular injury.

Physical examination should be able to identify blood loss in the extremity. The generally accepted rule is that closed long bone fractures each bleed up to 2 units of blood. Thus, bilateral femur fractures and a tibia fracture in a 70-kg person will result in a 3-liter blood loss, which produces class III hemorrhage.

Neurovascular injury can be diagnosed relatively simply in patients who are awake and alert. Careful neurovascular exam directed by patient complaints should pick up virtually every injury. The same is not true for patients who are multiply injured, intubated, and in the intensive care unit (ICU). In addition, neurovascular injury may evolve over time. For instance, nerve contusion can progress to neurapraxia or paralysis. Swelling around the fracture site can progress and compress the nerve, producing neurologic dysfunction. Compartment syndrome often occurs 6 to 24 hours postinjury as a result of muscular swelling within the noncompliant fascial envelope following crush injuries and/or fractures. Partial thickness vascular injuries can go on to vascular thrombosis hours or even days after injury, producing limb-threatening ischemia.

Critical care practitioners must be cognizant of all of these. Careful ongoing assessment is critical in order to make these diagnoses as early as possible. A delayed diagnosis can produce substantial disability that is lifelong. Even worse, unrecognized

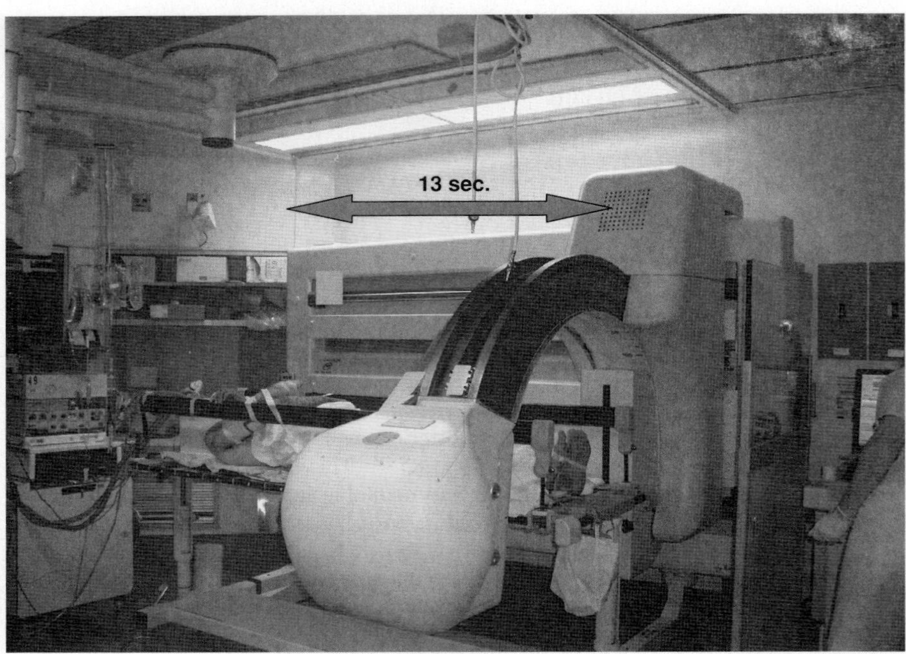

FIGURE 85.1. Statscan in trauma bay.

ischemia and/or compartment syndrome can place a limb at jeopardy, requiring amputation later. Unrecognized ischemia can also produce life-threatening electrolyte abnormalities such as hyperkalemia and/or be the source of multiple organ failure, either one of which can prove to be fatal.

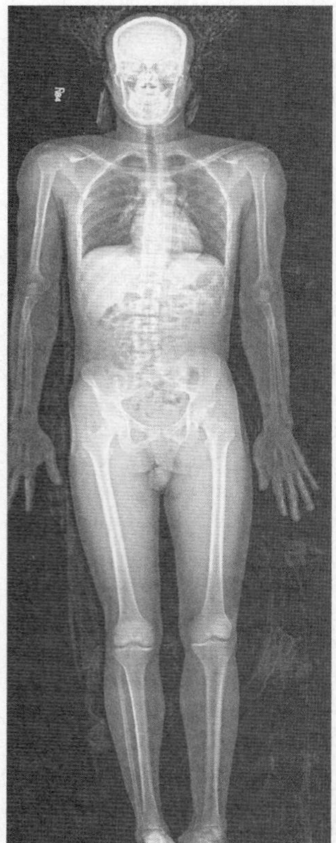

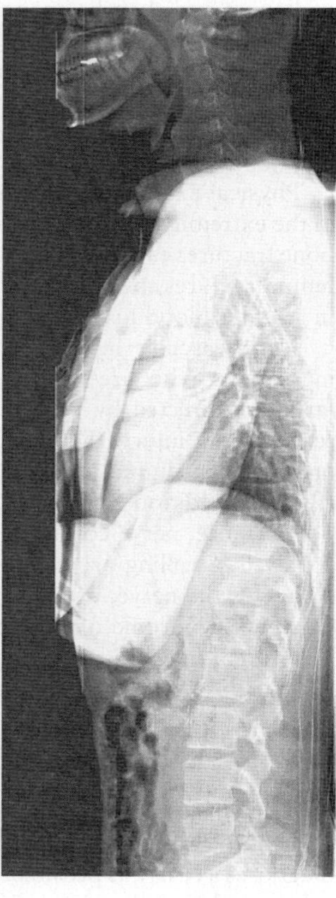

FIGURE 85.2. Normal anterior total body and lateral spine.

TREATMENT OPTIONS FOR FRACTURES

Clearly, fractures that are not associated with life-threatening bleeding are not the highest priority following initial patient presentation. However, all long bone fractures should be splinted as part of the initial management. Every time the patient is transferred or moved in any way, unsplinted fractures are displaced, producing additional blood loss and pain and risking secondary nerve or vascular injury. Splinting can be accomplished simply by utilizing several IV boards and some rolled gauze to fashion a makeshift splint. There are commercially available molded metal splints that can also be used short term. These two methods can lead to skin breakdown if applied for long periods of time. Once time permits, more definitive, lightweight plaster splints can be made to restore stability and decrease the risk of skin breakdown.

It is also important for the critical care practitioner to understand the various options for more definitive fracture fixation. Rigid fracture fixation is generally obtained via open reduction/internal fixation (ORIF) or closed intramedullary (IM) nail fixation. ORIF involves directly exposing the fracture fragments. They are then manually reduced and rigid fixation is achieved utilizing a number of techniques such as plates and screws or rods. Overlying muscles must often be divided in order to obtain adequate exposure. This also allows for debridement of nonviable and/or contused muscle and irrigation of the fracture hematoma. Depending on the particular fracture, ORIF can be a substantial operative procedure with significant soft tissue injury and blood loss from the procedure itself. Fractures often treated with ORIF include proximal and distal tibial fractures, acetabular fractures, periarticular humerus, elbow fractures, and distal radius fractures (Fig. 85.3).

Approximately 70 years ago, the technique of closed IM nailing was developed. This technique involves making a small incision proximally or distally in the extremity. The fracture

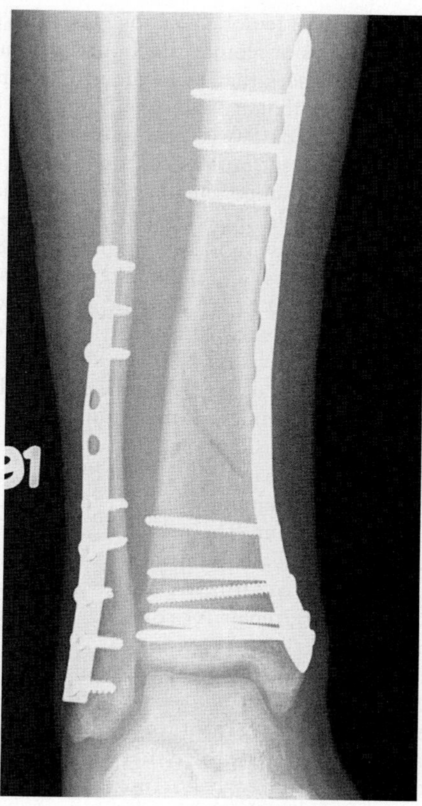

FIGURE 85.3. This 17-year-old female sustained a high-energy distal tibial fracture as a result of a motorcycle crash. Open reduction with plate fixation offers the best chance of achieving anatomic restoration of articular congruity and reduction of the risk of posttraumatic arthritis.

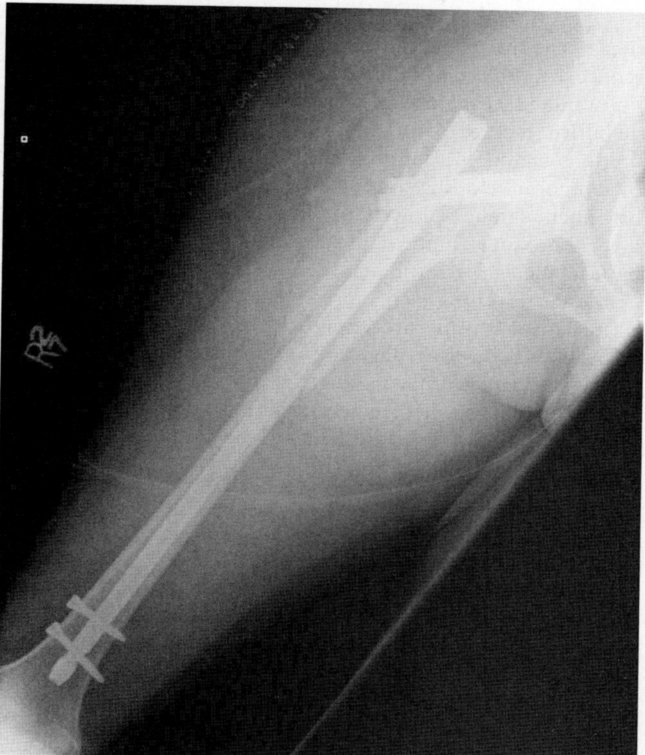

FIGURE 85.4. The fracture was treated with early intramedullary nail fixation. With early fixation of femoral fractures in multiply injured patients, many pulmonary problems can be avoided. Stable fixation of even complex, comminuted injuries can allow early weight bearing and facilitate functional rehabilitation despite polytrauma.

fragments are then reduced manually under fluoroscopic visualization. The medullary canal is accessed and a guidewire is placed across the fracture. A nail is then driven up the medullary canal over the guidewire to sterilize the bone. If desired, the canal can be reamed before the nail is placed. The nail can be locked in place by placing several screws in the very proximal or distal portion of the nail through a secondary small incision. These screws are placed under fluoroscopic control (Fig. 85.4).

IM nailing does not typically require direct exposure of the fracture fragment. Theoretically, there is less soft tissue injury and less blood loss associated with IM nailing as compared to ORIF of fractures. Passage of a nail through the medullary canal is, however, associated with liberation of a number of mediators and/or fat globules into the systemic circulation. Either of these can produce systemic inflammatory response syndrome (SIRS) and/or acute lung injury (ALI). In addition, passage of the nail can produce significant bleeding around the fracture itself, which may not be appreciated as it is not directly visualized in the operative field. IM nailing is generally used for most midshaft femur and tibia fractures. It is necessary to have adequate bone on either side of the fracture in order to achieve sufficient fixation to restore stability.

External fixation involves placing an external frame that spans the fracture, limiting fracture movement (Fig. 85.5). External fixation achieves relatively good fracture stabilization, though it may not produce optimal fracture reduction, particularly with periarticular injuries. It can be rapid and noninvasive and result in substantially less blood loss than ORIF or IM nailing. Pins are placed into the bone on either side of the fracture connected to a frame. This can be used as definitive fixation for some fractures if acceptable restoration of length, alignment, and stability have been achieved.

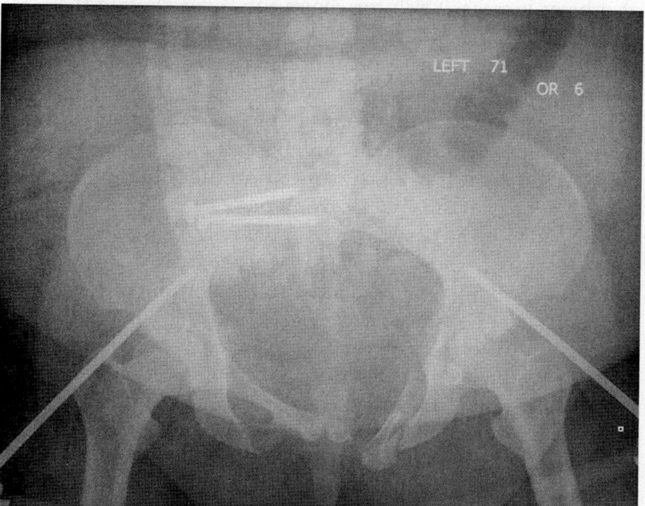

FIGURE 85.5. This patient's pelvic ring injury was treated with posterior screw fixation and an anterior external fixator.

Open fractures require an initial debridement and irrigation of the fracture fragments as a minimum. This is done to reduce the rate of early soft tissue infection and late osteomyelitis. While ideal therapy involves irrigation, debridement, and definitive fracture fixation, this is not always the wisest course. Options include irrigation, and debridement can be followed by temporary external fixation. In addition, irrigation and debridement can be followed by simple splinting of the fractures if there are more immediate patient care priorities. This technique is ideally performed in the operating room and involves debridement followed by pulse lavage. Patients can be temporized with a bedside procedure if that is all they are able to tolerate initially or if there are other more urgent priorities. While the data supporting any treatment algorithm are not definitive, most studies suggest that rates of infection are similar provided operative debridement is accomplished within 24 hours of injury (3).

OPTIMAL TIMING OF FRACTURE FIXATION

There are a significant number of advantages to early definitive fracture fixation. Ideally, this should take place as soon as possible following patient presentation. While the definition of early fracture fixation has varied over the years, most would agree that fracture fixation within 24 hours is early. These advantages may be most pronounced in patients with multiple system injury. Obviously, these are the patients most at risk for systemic complications from a significant operative procedure. Thus, judgment must be key in weighing the various risks and benefits to early fracture fixation.

Patients who are treated nonoperatively initially are often treated in some type of balanced traction, particularly for femoral and acetabular fractures. This requires that the patient remain supine in bed. Patients are at risk for developing dependent atelectasis resulting in worsening respiratory failure. Patients with brain injury and intracranial hypertension may have worsening of their intracranial pressures as they cannot have the head of the bed elevated as easily. These patients may also be at increased risk for aspiration. Even though the fracture is somewhat reduced by the traction apparatus or by a splint, as with any fracture, motion at the fracture site worsens bleeding and produces pain and such motion is only reduced by traction and splinting, not eliminated. Either bleeding or pain can increase the systemic inflammatory response. Any immobilized patient is at risk for thromboembolic complications such as deep vein thrombosis or pulmonary embolus. Those in traction may be at particular risk. Patients kept at bed rest in traction cannot be rolled from side to side, producing pressure ulcerations on areas in contact with the bed. Finally, the incidence of fat embolism syndrome may be higher in patients who undergo delayed fracture repair.

In 1985, Seibel et al. published a prospective nonrandomized cohort study of patients with femoral shaft fractures or acetabulum fractures who also had additional injury (4). All aspects of care of the patients were reportedly controlled except fracture management. Their patient population was divided into four groups. The first group underwent immediate operative fixation of their femoral or acetabular fracture (defined as less than 24 hours after injury). The second group underwent an average of 10 days of femoral traction. The third group underwent up to 30 days of femoral traction. The fourth group had special circumstances that were predicted to potentially contribute to their pulmonary failure septic state. Ventilator days and intensive care days were both substantially greater in the groups that underwent prolonged traction than in the immediate fixation group, supporting the conclusion that femoral traction was detrimental in the setting of blunt multiple trauma.

This led the authors to propose a number of principles governing the care of patients with multisystem trauma and fractures. They proposed that the fracture hematoma was itself a metabolically active organ, capable of producing multiple organ failure. Early fracture fixation allowed for irrigation of the fracture hematoma. They also included the orthopedic surgeon as one of the frontline members of the trauma team, emphasizing the need for early consultation. In addition, they strongly advocated for fracture repair on the night of admission including using two teams to simultaneously repair fractures if that was available and prudent. They argued that all efforts must be made to support the patient through early fracture fixation as they had demonstrated far better results with this technique as opposed to delaying repair for some days to allow patient stabilization.

Following this report, others also demonstrated better results with early fracture fixation (5–7). Fracture fixation within 24 hours became the standard of care. However, in the early 1990s, data began being published that suggested that not every patient benefited from early fracture fixation. In fact, these studies strongly suggested that patient outcome was much more a function of underlying injury and not so much the timing of fracture fixation. Poole et al. published a series of patients with long bone fracture and brain injury (8). They were unable to demonstrate any advantage to early fracture fixation, and instead argued that the severity of the brain injury was the ultimate determinate of final outcome. Rogers et al. addressed the cost of performing early fracture fixation, particularly on off hours in hospitals that did not have in-house operating room resources (9). Outcomes were the same when femur fractures were repaired in the middle of the night as compared to a group of patients who were placed on the operating room schedule for the next day. The cost, however, was significantly higher in patients who underwent emergency fracture fixation.

It is unclear as to why these authors were unable to substantiate the findings that seemed to show clear benefit to early operative fixation. One possibility is that the care during the critical care phase of these multiply injured patients improved over the late 1980s and early 1990s. End points of resuscitation were defined (10). The role of invasive monitoring was made more clear (11). Specific needs for patient populations such as geriatric trauma patients were defined (12). Thus, it is possible that the time taken to stabilize the patient in the ICU preoperatively was now, in fact, time well spent.

In the mid- to late 1990s, several papers were published that strongly suggested that early fracture fixation was, in fact, dangerous, particularly in patients who sustained traumatic brain injury. The group from Yale reported on 32 patients treated over a 5-year period with brain injury and long bone fractures (13). Those who underwent early fracture fixation, defined as within the first 24 hours of admission, had statistically significant worse neurologic outcome at the time of discharge. This was thought to be secondary to the increased rate of intraoperative hypotension and hypoxia seen in patients with early fracture fixation. Townsend et al. observed similar findings (14). In their study, episodes of intracranial hypertension were more common in patients who underwent early fracture fixation. They also noted an increased rate of intraoperative hypotension and hypoxia. This risk seemed to persist for approximately 24 hours.

Scalea et al., however, reported different findings (15). They studied over 180 patients with long bone fracture and traumatic brain injury over the same 5-year period as studied by the group at Yale. They found no difference in neurologic outcome in the group of patients treated with early fracture fixation.

How, then, should a critical care physician decide when a patient ought to have fracture fixation? It would seem reasonable to address a number of issues. The first would be to assess the risk of anesthesia and the magnitude of the operative procedure. There certainly are scoring systems that can be applied to assess perioperative risk. Careful clinical assessment may be equally good. The second issue would be to examine operative options. For instance, does the patient have a reasonable nonoperative option? Would a lesser procedure, while perhaps not ideal, at least be adequate? This obviously would require a discussion between the critical care service and the orthopedic surgeons, trauma team, and anesthesiologist. Finally, one must ask whether the patient is in optimal condition. Can we reduce perioperative risk with a reasonable period of preoperative optimization? Can cardiac performance be improved with volume and/or inotropes? Will 1 to 2 days allow ventilatory requirements to be reduced? Would a delay improve renal function? Only when all of these questions are answered can an intelligent decision about the optimal time and fracture fixation be made.

DAMAGE CONTROL ORTHOPEDICS

Damage control was a technique developed in the late 1980s and early 1990s in early urban American trauma centers. This shift in approach coincided with a period of time when penetrating trauma became much more common. Not only was penetrating trauma more common, but also multiple high-velocity missiles became the norm, rather than the exception. Traditional teaching was to repair all injuries at the time of initial surgical procedure. Unfortunately, this often required prolonged operative care. Patients developed what was termed the lethal triad of acidosis, coagulopathy, and hypothermia, only to arrive in the ICU and die of acute organ failure, usually 6 to 24 hours postoperatively.

Many trauma centers began using a staged approach with encouraging results. In 1993, Rotundo et al. published the series that named the technique damage control, and demonstrated statistically significant better outcomes in a group of patients treated with the new techniques (16).

The principles that govern damage control are listed in Table 85.1 when damage control is used for abdominal injuries. In essence, only life-saving procedures are performed at the time of the initial procedure. Important but non–life-threatening injuries such as gastrointestinal injuries are simply temporized. The patient is then packed and the fascia left open to avoid the potential of developing abdominal compartment syndrome. The patient is then admitted to the ICU and resuscitated. Between 1 and 3 days later, the patient can be brought back to the operating room for re-exploration, gastrointestinal reconstruction, and an attempt at fascial closure.

TABLE 85.1

PRINCIPLES OF DAMAGE CONTROL

- It is easy to miss an injury if you rush
- Hypothermia, acidosis, and coagulopathy only lead to more of the same
- The best place for a sick person is in the ICU
- Only blood loss kills early
- GI injuries cause problems much later
- Everything takes longer than you think

The same principles can be applied to bony injuries. Fractures are common and occur in over 75% of multiply injured patients. There are clear advantages to early fracture fixation. Yet, some patients may not be best served by such technique. A technique that would achieve many of the advantages of fracture fixation without the disadvantages of definitive surgery would be advantageous for some patients.

It is important to recognize that remote organ injury occurs not only in association with, but also as a direct consequence of long bone fractures. In addition to the fracture itself, soft tissue injury, compartment syndrome, infection, and extremity ischemia-reperfusion injury can all be associated with release of toxic mediators that can cause remote endothelial cell damage. The primary target of this remote organ injury appears to be the lungs, but secondary targets include the gut, kidney, and brain. The resultant injury is a progressive one and can lead to multiple organ dysfunction syndrome. This understanding led to the development of the concept of damage control orthopedics (DCO). DCO is the process by which temporary stabilization of long bone fractures is accomplished using techniques not associated with secondary systemic injury. Secondary definitive stabilization is delayed until after physiologic stabilization has been achieved (Figs. 85.6 through 85.8). The goal of damage control therefore is to provide the patient with the benefits of early stabilization of long bones without exposing him or her to the risks associated with definitive stabilization procedures.

For that subset of patients whose physiologic condition precludes primary definitive operative stabilization of fractures (early total care), external fixation can be a useful technique for temporary stabilization of long bone fractures. Such external fixation is advantageous because it can be applied rapidly, with minimal blood loss, and with sufficient restoration of stability to prevent ongoing soft tissue injury and to prevent ongoing release of inflammatory mediators. Effective limitation of secondary effects of shock has been demonstrated with this type of initial DCO approach.

The disadvantages to employing this type of technique in all patients with even questionable polytrauma are at least twofold. First, employing temporizing external fixation techniques necessitates a return to the operating room for delayed definitive fixation, thus exposing the patient to two separate operative interventions. This is obviously warranted if the benefit is prevention of a serious secondary consequence such as acute respiratory distress syndrome (ARDS). In the absence of a clear decrease in the risk of ARDS, it is harder to justify exposing polytrauma patients to a need for secondary surgical procedures.

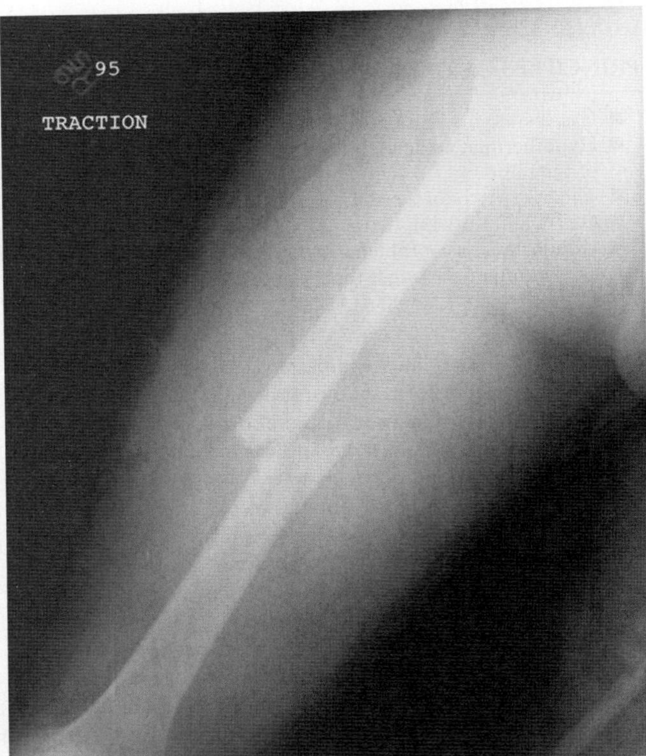

FIGURE 85.6. Damage control orthopedics case example. This 27-year-old motorcyclist sustained multiple injuries including an open right femoral shaft fracture. He presented in physiologic extremis. Laparotomy demonstrated a grade 5 hepatic injury and a retrohepatic caval injury. Right hepatic lobectomy and repair of a vena caval laceration were performed as part of a damage control laparotomy procedure.

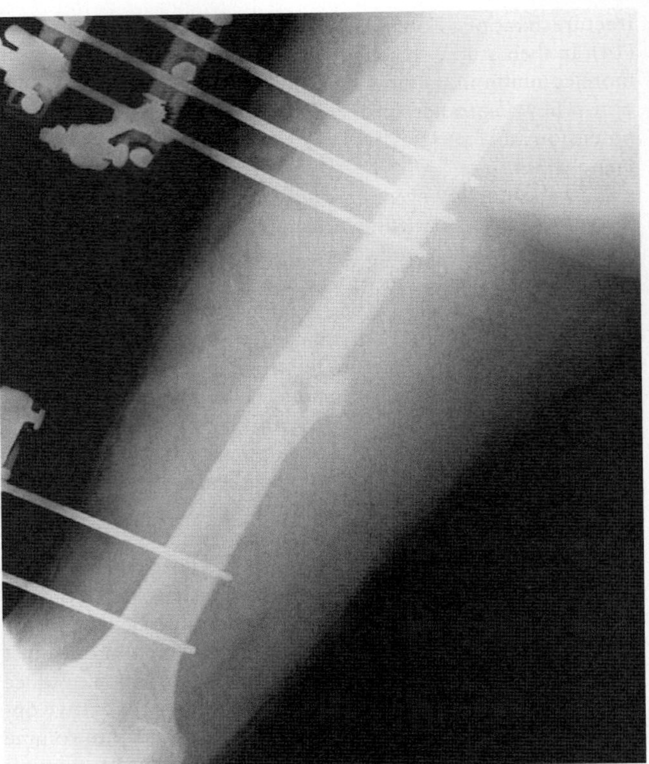

FIGURE 85.7. Damage control orthopaedics consisted of rapid debridement of the open femoral fracture plus temporizing external fixation to achieve restoration of femoral length and alignment and decrease ongoing injury secondary to release of inflammatory mediators.

A second major disadvantage to external fixation (a temporary device) is the risk of complications with conversion from external fixation to intramedullary nailing or other definitive treatment. Experience in the tibia has suggested that if external fixation is in place for less than 2 weeks, the risk of infection with definitive fixation is lower, particularly if there is no history of pin tract infection at any point (17). In the femur, conversion from external fixation to definitive nailing appears safe within the first 4 weeks following application of the initial frame (18).

Advantages of external fixation include rapid application with minimal blood loss and simultaneous stabilization of multiple limbs expeditiously.

The issues that led to the use of DCO have been debated for some time. In 1989, Bone et al. published a prospective randomized trial of early (less than 24 hours after injury) versus late (greater than 72 hours after injury) nail fixation of femoral shaft fractures (19). They found that in patients with an overall Injury Severity Score (ISS) of greater than 18 (indicative of polytrauma), intensive care days and pulmonary complications were reduced with early fixation as compared to late fixation. They concluded that stabilization of femoral fractures within 24 hours of injury in multiply injured patients decreases pulmonary morbidity as compared to stabilization after 72 hours. The study was flawed in that it was not blinded, that parameters of resuscitation were not defined, and that very few patients with severe pulmonary injury were included in the early fixation group.

In 1993, Pape et al. published a worrisome report implicating primary nail fixation of femoral shaft fractures (reamed) as a potential cause of posttraumatic ARDS (20). They reviewed patients admitted over a period of 10 years with an ISS greater than 18 and midshaft femoral fractures. Those with and without chest injury and those who underwent femoral nailing less than 24 hours and greater than 24 hours after injury were compared. They found a higher incidence of ARDS and death in patients with severe chest trauma who were treated with early reamed nailing as compared to those with severe chest trauma treated with delayed reamed nailing. They concluded that early reamed nail stabilization of femoral shaft fractures in "borderline" patients may increase the risk of secondary pulmonary injury and development of ARDS. They recommended that definitive fracture fixation be delayed in these patients and that temporizing techniques such as external fixation be employed.

The problem with Pape's study was that the early nailing group included eight patients with pulmonary contusions as compared to only two in the late nailing group. Both Pape et al. (20) and Bone et al. (19) failed to report on any parameters of resuscitation within their patient populations.

What was becoming obvious as trauma surgeons became more aggressive with early nailing of femoral (and to a certain extent tibial) shaft fractures in polytrauma patients was that the operative procedure for intramedullary stabilization of long bone fractures was associated with some component of pulmonary injury (21,22). While fracture fixation–associated pulmonary injury appeared to be well tolerated in the majority of patients including polytrauma patients, certain susceptible

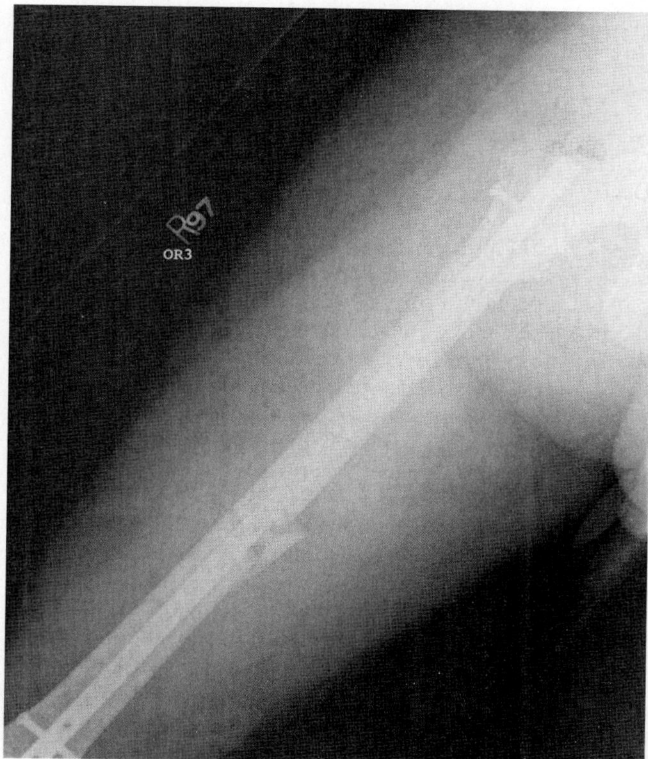

FIGURE 85.8. On postinjury day 5, after adequate restoration of physiologic stability, the patient underwent removal of the temporary external fixator and definitive fixation of the femoral fracture using a reamed intramedullary nail. He was discharged to a rehabilitation facility 19 days after injury.

polytrauma patients seemed to be at risk for worsening lung injury. Paradoxically, these are likely the same patients who are at greatest risk for developing secondary pulmonary injury from a nonoperative management of their long bone fractures and the most in need of early fracture stabilization.

Several groups of surgeons have engaged in the process of temporary stabilization of long bone fractures in polytrauma patients using techniques associated with minimal systemic consequences. Scalea et al. published their experience with external fixation as a temporary tool for stabilization of long bone fractures in polytrauma patients in 2000 (23). They reported that as part of DCO, external fixation was an alternative mechanism of achieving temporary stabilization in multiply injured patients and that it was rapid, associated with minimal blood loss, and safely convertible to better definitive fixation after appropriate delayed physiologic stabilization of the patient. Other authors have expanded on the DCO concept and reported more specifically on its efficacy (24).

The physiologic rationale for DCO is based upon the timing and extent of the initial inflammatory response that follows a major injury. In most individuals, that initial inflammatory response is followed by a counterregulatory anti-inflammatory response that leads to spontaneous recovery. In situations where the initial inflammatory response is excessive, secondary remote organ injury such as acute lung injury related to increased pulmonary capillary membrane permeability can occur. The likelihood of this secondary remote organ injury developing may be increased in situations associated with substantial ischemia-reperfusion injury (such as prolonged shock), continued loss of body temperature, tourniquet-mediated ischemia-reperfusion injury, a surgical blood loss with failure of resuscitation, and embolization of fat and marrow contents secondary to instrumentation of the femoral or tibial canal. This secondary remote organ injury is characterized by increased capillary membrane permeability, acute lung injury, gut bacterial translocation, and acute tubular necrosis. It can be mediated by cytokines, complement, activated neutrophils, eicosanoids, and reactive oxygen products.

Thus, both early total care and ongoing long bone instability can serve as second hits that lead to the development of severe secondary remote organ injury. In the "at-risk" patient population, early DCO can limit ongoing release of inflammatory mediators and allow for further physiologic stabilization prior to proceeding with definitive stabilization (25).

Hildebrand et al. evaluated the association between the timing of secondary definitive surgical intervention, inflammatory changes, and systemic outcome (26). They reviewed a prospective cohort of patients treated with DCO. They compared those treated with early secondary surgery (2–4 days after initial injury) to those treated with late secondary surgery (5–8 days after initial injury). They found that early secondary surgery was associated with a higher incidence of organ dysfunction and concluded that there was no particular advantage to early secondary surgery. They recommended that if DCO is selected, secondary surgery should be delayed more than 5 days after the initial DCO procedure.

In a prospective randomized trial, Pape et al. compared nailing to DCO with regard to immunoinflammatory parameters in patients with tibial or femoral shaft fractures, and ISS greater than 16 (27). Patients with a thoracic abbreviated injury scale score (AIS) greater than 3, ongoing shock, or elevated intracranial pressure were excluded. They found that primary femoral nailing was associated with significantly higher systemic interleukin (IL)-6 and IL-8 levels for 48 hours postoperatively compared to either initial DCO procedures or secondary femoral nailing after initial damage control. This suggested that the secondary release of inflammatory mediators associated with femoral nailing can be effectively mitigated by initial DCO with delayed femoral nailing.

O'Toole et al. looked at the effect of resuscitation prior to femoral nailing on the development of ARDS in multiply injured patients (28). They found that a practice of resuscitation protocol that included normalization of lactate prior to IM nailing resulted in rare need of damage control and development of ARDS.

DCO, the practice of utilizing temporary external fixation to limit ongoing injury secondary to long bone fractures in situations where definitive operative stabilization is contraindicated, may be effective in patients with polytrauma and lung or brain injury. For the majority of patients with femoral shaft fractures, including most polytrauma patients, primary reamed femoral nailing within 24 hours of injury remains the gold standard of treatment (21). Defining the "at-risk" patients who are unable to tolerate early reamed nailing is difficult, but if adequate resuscitation and normalization of serum lactate is achieved, damage control should rarely be necessary (28). In borderline patients who are physiologically unstable because of severe chest or head injury or inadequate resuscitation, temporizing external fixation and damage control orthopedics may be advantageous.

COMPARTMENT SYNDROME

Compartment syndrome occurs when there is increased tissue pressure within a confined osseofascial space. This increased pressure compromises blood flow and subsequently results in tissue damage if left untreated. The fascia of muscle compartments is stiff and does not expand to accommodate significant swelling. Increases in compartment volume and subsequent pressure can be caused by fractures, soft tissue crush injury, hemorrhage, reperfusion following arterial revascularization, and increased capillary permeability as may occur in the setting of burns or shock states. Compartment syndrome was first recognized as a causative factor in ischemia of the hand by Richard von Volkmann in 1881 (29). Other investigators subsequently described and confirmed that ischemia of muscle in a fascial compartment was caused by an increase in pressure from compromised venous outflow and edema secondary to reperfusion (30,31). Although most typically found in the leg, compartment syndrome of the arm and hand is well recognized as is compartment syndrome of the buttock, thigh, and foot (32–35). The reported incidence of compartment syndrome varies widely. Rates of 6% in patients with open tibial fractures and 1% in patients with closed fractures have been reported, but much higher percentages have been published in association with concomitant vascular injury (36,37). In children, rates of up to 20% have been reported with open forearm fractures (32).

Any increase in compartment volume elevates compartment pressures, which, in turn, compromises lymphatic and venous outflow. This leads to additional edema and ultimately arterial insufficiency. Compromised arterial inflow causes tissue ischemia and cellular edema, which only serves to increase compartment pressures further (38,39). Experimental studies have shown that the longer pressure remains elevated, the more severe the muscle and nerve damage (39). Additionally, episodes of hypotension increase the extent of muscle ischemia.

External restriction of an extremity may also lead to compartment syndrome. Compartment syndrome has been described as a result of constrictive casting or dressings and with the use of pneumatic antishock garments (military antishock trousers) (40). Regardless of the underlying cause, if left untreated, the end result of compartment syndrome is muscle and nerve injury from infarction and necrosis.

The clinical diagnosis of compartment syndrome can be elusive. Symptoms may often be ascribed to other causes (41,42). In the alert patient, pain is typically the first symptom. Pain is typically worsened with palpation of the affected compartment and ameliorated with passive stretch of the muscle group. Pain or physical findings are frequently attributed to the associated fracture, however. Sensory deficits may occur late and are typically in the distribution of the sensory nerve traversing the affected compartment. The classic description of sensory loss is in the first web space of the foot secondary to elevated anterior leg compartment pressures and the effect on the deep peroneal nerve. Motor weakness is a late and ominous sign. Loss of palpable pulses is typically associated with vascular injury and is a very late and rare finding in the extremity with compartment syndrome.

In the patient who is not awake and alert, the diagnosis of compartment syndrome requires extreme vigilance and a high degree of clinical suspicion. The diagnosis in these patients requires frequent physical examination and tissue pressure measurements. Tissue pressure measurements are typically accomplished via accessing the affected compartment with a needle or catheter and recording pressure measurements via manometry or pressure transduction. Many techniques have been described, but the simplest and most widely used is the STIC Device (Stryker Corporation, Kalamazoo, MI). The handheld STIC catheter utilizes a disposable syringe and needle and after zeroing the monitor, insertion of the needle through the fascia of the compartments. It allows for rapid and reliable assessment of compartment pressures (43). Alternatively, a 16-gauge needle attached to a transduction system also can produce reliable measurements (44). Some have advocated continuous pressure monitoring using systems designed specifically for that purpose, although recent data do not support the use of continuous monitoring in the alert patient (45,46). Several researchers have attempted to develop noninvasive methods of compartment pressure measurements with limited success in the setting of acute compartment syndrome (47,48).

There is some debate in the literature concerning the measured pressure at which the diagnosis of compartment syndrome should be made and fasciotomy performed. Many advocate the use of absolute values of greater than 30 to 35 mm Hg as an indication for fasciotomy (45,49). Others have stressed the importance of the difference between systemic diastolic pressure and measured compartment pressure (50,51). This difference in pressures has been shown to be a more reliable indicator of impending compartment syndrome. A Δp of less than 30 mm Hg is used by many as an indication for fasciotomy. This highlights the concern that patients who are hypotensive are at significantly greater risk of compartment syndrome than normotensive patients with comparable absolute compartment pressure measurements. Therefore, intraoperative Δp should be calculated based on the preoperative diastolic blood pressure and compartment pressures should be measured early in the postoperative period (51).

In the patient who is at risk of compartment syndrome, there are some steps that can be taken that may minimize the development of compartment syndrome. First, tight casts, splints, and dressings should be avoided and promptly removed if the patient complains of pain out of proportion to the underlying injury or fracture. There is some controversy about the optimal extremity position in patients at risk for compartment syndrome. Elevation of the extremity may lead to a reduction of arterial perfusion pressure and subsequent blood flow (52). Alternatively, placing the limb in a dependent position may exacerbate edema and reduce venous outflow. The optimal position for the patient at risk of compartment syndrome is to place the affected extremity at the level of the heart to optimize both arterial and venous flow.

Surgical decompression is the treatment of compartment syndrome. Care must be taken to ensure that all affected osseofascial compartments are widely opened. The fasciotomy wounds should be left open, as any attempt to provide tissue coverage over the at-risk muscle may lead to additional muscle injury. A variety of techniques have been described for fasciotomy of the various compartments of the extremities.

In the patient at high risk for the development of compartment syndrome, prophylactic fasciotomy may be appropriate. If the patient will be unexaminable, unable to complain of symptoms, or unavailable for serial or continuous measurements of compartment pressures, prophylactic fasciotomy may be indicated to prevent the morbid sequelae of untreated compartment syndrome. In patients with prolonged hypotension or arterial vascular repairs, prophylactic fasciotomy should be performed if the affected extremity was poorly vascularized or unvascularized for more than a few hours. In the setting of concomitant venous injury, fasciotomy should not be delayed because venous insufficiency may exaggerate edema and increase the risk of the development of compartment syndrome.

Once fasciotomies are performed, sterile dressings or a closed vacuum suction device should be applied and the wounds re-examined in about 48 hours. If fasciotomy was done late in the course of compartment syndrome, frankly necrotic muscle should be debrided at the time of decompression. Muscle with borderline or questionable viability should be left and re-examined in 24 to 48 hours. There are a number of techniques available for delayed muscle coverage following fasciotomy that have been described. Closure by secondary intention is an option, as is split-thickness skin grafting. Other techniques of delayed coverage include the "Op-Site roller," the "shoelace technique," the STAR (suture tension adjustment reel) method, and vacuum-assisted closure (53–56).

Complications of untreated compartment syndrome include muscle necrosis, irreparable nerve damage, and limb loss (57,58). Delay in therapy may also result in these morbid sequelae (50,57,58). When irreversible ischemia in an affected extremity occurs, there is a depreciable decrease in functional recovery (59,60). Additionally, delay in fasciotomy causes an increase in infection rates, which may lead to sepsis and multiple organ system failure (57,60). When treatment is delayed more than 12 hours, amputation rates may be over 20%.

Massive necrosis of muscle also has significant systemic effects. Myonecrosis can result in the release of large amounts of myoglobin. Myoglobin is released from damaged muscle, particularly during the reperfusion phase following fasciotomy, causing rhabdomyolysis. Myoglobin can precipitate renal failure via three mechanisms: decreased renal perfusion, renal tubular obstruction due to cast formation, and direct toxic effects of myoglobin on the kidney (61,62). The incidence of renal failure in the setting of rhabdomyolysis is estimated at 4% to 33% and carries a mortality of 3% to 50% (62,63). Early diagnosis is critical to prevention of renal failure, and all patients who have compartment syndrome should be monitored with serial creatine kinase (CK) levels. Generally, CK levels of greater than 5,000 U/L are diagnostic of rhabdomyolysis, although renal failure is usually seen at higher levels (63). The mainstay of treatment of rhabdomyolysis is aggressive hydration and maintenance of high-volume urine output. Some have advocated the use of mannitol and urine alkalinization with bicarbonate-containing solutions, although others have demonstrated no benefit of these therapies over high-volume normal saline hydration alone. Continuous renal replacement therapies can also be used to clear myoglobin from the blood and are advantageous if renal failure occurs due to greater hemodynamic stability and tolerance in critically ill patients.

In addition to poor long-term functional recovery following late or untreated compartment syndrome, a Volkmann contracture may occur. A Volkmann contracture is the chronic limb deformity arising from untreated compartment syndrome causing muscular ischemia and subsequent fibroblastic proliferation, contraction, and adhesion formation. Additionally, nerve ischemia leads to loss of denervation of the muscle, muscle paresis, and paralysis. A Volkmann contracture causes significant long-term morbidity and may lead to a need for amputation or extensive reconstruction to regain function of the affected extremity.

FAT EMBOLISM SYNDROME

Fat embolism syndrome (FES) has been reported to occur in bone marrow transplant, pancreatitis, fatty liver, and liposuction (64,65). However, FES is most commonly associated with long bone fractures. Although fat embolism may occur in up to 90% of trauma patients, FES occurs in only 2% to 5% of patients with long bone fractures (66,67). FES is characterized by both pulmonary and systemic fat embolism and includes a spectrum from subclinical to mild and fulminate presentations (65,68,69). Clinical FES typically involves multiple organ systems; however, involvement of the pulmonary, neurologic, hematologic, and dermatologic systems is the most common.

Fat embolization can occur at the time of fracture. Long bone fixation may result in additional embolization and FES. Elevated pressures during reaming of the intramedullary canal appear to be temporally associated with embolization to the pulmonary circulation when studied with echocardiography (70). Once fat is liberated into the circulation and embolizes, the pulmonary microvasculature becomes occluded.

Depending on the size of fat globules, smaller globules may traverse the pulmonary microvasculature and reach the systemic circulation, leading to the common neurologic manifestation of FES. Although the pulmonary, cerebral, retinal, and skin microcirculations are typical clinical manifestations of FES, fat embolization can affect any microcirculatory bed.

Acute lung injury (ALI) and ARDS may result from fat emboli occluding pulmonary capillaries, and biochemical alterations directly damage the pulmonary capillary endothelium (65,71–73).

Although many patients with long bone fractures develop fat embolism, far fewer develop FES, suggesting that additional factors may be necessary in the development of lung injury. Biochemical fat embolization is associated with the release of free fatty acids (FFAs) (74). FFAs in the lung are locally hydrolyzed in pulmonary circulation by lipoprotein lipase, which releases toxic substances that injure the capillary endothelium. The release of FFAs increases vascular permeability, producing alveolar hemorrhage, edema, and inactivation of the surfactant molecules (75,76). Ultimately, these pulmonary alterations lead to ALI and ARDS. As fat accumulates in the pulmonary microcirculation and lipoprotein lipase liberates FFAs, disseminated intravascular coagulation (DIC) and platelet aggregation further compound capillary disruption and systemic inflammation.

Fat emboli that pass through the pulmonary vasculature result in systemic embolization, most commonly in the brain and kidneys (77). Cerebral FES is a rare, yet potentially lethal, complication of long bone fractures. Neurologic symptoms vary from confusion to encephalopathy with coma and seizures. A clinical diagnosis may be difficult as cerebral FES may be masked by other clinical scenarios (78). Diffuse encephalopathy, petechial hemorrhages, localized cerebral edema, and white matter changes have also been seen in patients diagnosed with FES. Magnetic resonance imaging (MRI) may be necessary to show the characteristic cerebral lesions of the acute state of

FES as opposed to a computed tomography (CT) scan, which often may appear normal (79).

A specific treatment for FES does not currently exist. Treatments with heparin, dextran, and corticosteroids have not been shown to reduce the morbidity or mortality (64,80). However, when given prophylactically, corticosteroids (methylprednisolone) may have beneficial effects (81,82). The mainstay of treatment for FES is supportive; therefore, prevention, early diagnosis, and adequate symptom management are paramount. Although long bone fracture fixation is the main cause of fat embolism and FES, early fracture fixation may be critical in reducing recurrent liberation of fat into the circulation as a result of fracture movement and decreases the incidence of FES (83).

Patients with polytrauma are at risk of other forms of respiratory failure (atelectasis, pneumonia) and multiple system organ failure (MSOF). Early fixation and patient mobilization may reduce those complications (84). Methods to reduce intramedullary pressure and embolization during reaming have been developed, which include venting or applying a vacuum during reaming to limit the elevation of intramedullary pressure and thus reduce the incidence of fat embolization (85,86).

Respiratory failure from FES is characterized as permeability edema with decreased compliance similar to oleic acid lung injury. Gas exchange abnormalities include shunt and increased dead space from atelectasis and alveolar flooding comparable to ALI and ARDS from other causes (87,88). The general goals of ALI and ARDS management focus on maintaining acceptable gas exchange while limiting ventilator-associated lung injury (VALI).

Patients with FES may develop cerebral edema, leading to rapid deterioration (89). In such cases, intracranial pressure (ICP) monitoring may be beneficial (90). In general, trauma patients should not have their neurologic examination obscured by excessive sedation or neuromuscular blocking agents in order to allow them to tolerate mechanical ventilation (91).

The outcome in patients with FES who receive supportive care is generally favorable, with mortality rates of less than 10% (92). Pulmonary, neurologic, and retinal abnormalities generally resolve completely. General management is supportive in nature and focuses on early fixation and mobilization. Organ support includes shock resuscitation and gas exchange support, which balances lung recruitment and limits the potential for VALI. Ideally, neurologic support would include the ability to conduct a clinical neurologic examination.

PELVIC FRACTURES

Pelvic fractures occur from high-impact trauma and are associated with mortality rates ranging from 10% to 50% (93). The principles of pelvic fracture management after the initial assessment of "airway, breathing, and circulation" include detection of associated injuries (especially intraperitoneal bleeding source), stabilization of pelvic fracture in patients who demonstrate signs of hemorrhage (external compression devices), early embolization of pelvic arterial bleed, and avoiding coagulopathy and hypothermia by vigilant monitoring and treatment. Older patients (≥60 years) have a higher likelihood of arterial bleeding with more transfusion requirement (94). After control of life-threatening issues such as bleeding, careful assessment of other injuries that may cause significant morbidity such as rectal and vaginal tears and bladder and urethral injuries need to be assessed. Missed open pelvic fractures will lead to sepsis. Adequate hydration, monitoring for abdominal compartment syndrome, and vigilant secondary and tertiary survey are necessary. Some patients require more than one embolization to control hemorrhage (95). A newer concept adopted from the European trauma groups is the method of preperitoneal packing, which can be done expeditiously and save time in transporting patients to the radiology suite and waiting for angiographers (96). Due to the high-energy impact required to cause pelvic fractures, these patients have multiple sites of injury and remain a challenge.

References

1. Enderson BL, Reath DB, Meadors J. The tertiary trauma survey: a prospective study of missed injury. *J Trauma.* 1990;30:666–670.
2. Miller LA, Mirvis SE, Harris L, et al. Total-body digital radiography for trauma screening: Initial experience. *Appl Radiol.* 2004;33:8–14.
3. Pollak A. Timing of debridement of open fractures. *J Am Acad Orthopaed Surg.* 2006;14:548–551.
4. Seibel R, LaDuca J, Hassett JM, et al. Blunt multiple trauma (ISS 36), femur traction, and the pulmonary failure-septic state. *Ann Surg.* 1985;202:283–295.
5. Charash WE, Fabian TC, Croce MA. Delayed surgical fixation of femur fractures is a risk factor for pulmonary failure independent of thoracic trauma. *J Trauma.* 1994;37:663–672.
6. Behrman SW, Fabian TC, Kudsk KA, et al. Improved outcome with femur fractures: early versus delayed fixation. *J Trauma.* 1994;37:667–672.
7. Johnson KD, Cadambi A, Seibert B. Incidence of adult respiratory distress syndrome in patients with multiple musculoskeletal injuries: effect of early operative stabilization of fractures. *J Trauma.* 1985;25:375–384.
8. Poole GV, Miller JD, Agnew SG, et al. Lower extremity fracture fixation in head-injured patients. *J Trauma.* 1992;32:654–659.
9. Rogers FB, Shackford SR, Vane DW, et al. Prompt fixation of isolated femur fractures in a rural trauma center: a study examining the timing of fixation and resource allocation. *J Trauma.* 1994;36:774–777.
10. Abrahamson D, Scalea T, Hitchcock R, et al. Lactate clearance and its effects on survival. *J Trauma.* 1992;32:951.
11. Abou-Khalil B, Scalea T, Trooskin S. Hemodynamic responses to shock in young trauma patients. The need for invasive monitoring. *J Trauma.* 1991;31:1713.
12. Scalea TM, Simon HM, Duncan AO, et al. Geriatric blunt trauma: improved survival with early invasive monitoring. *J Trauma.* 1990;30:129–136.
13. Jaicks RR, Cohn SM, Moller BA. Early fracture fixation may be deleterious after head injury. *J Trauma.* 1997;42P:1–6.
14. Townsend RN, Lheureau T, Protetch J, et al. Timing fracture repair in patients with severe brain injuries. *J Trauma.* 1998;44:977–981.
15. Scalea TM, Scott JD, Brumback RJ, et al. Early fracture fixation may be "just fine" after head injury: no difference in central nervous system outcomes. *J Trauma.* 1999;46:839–846.
16. Rotondo M, Schwab CW, McGonigal M, et al. Damage control: an approach for improved survival in exsanguinating penetrating abdominal injury. *J Trauma.* 1993;35:375–382.
17. Bhandari M, Zlowodzki M, Tornetta P, et al. Intramedullary nailing following external fixation in femoral and tibial shaft fractures. *J Orthopaed Trauma.* 2005;19:140–144.
18. Nowotarski PJ, Turen CH, Brumback RJ, et al. Conversion of external fixation to intramedullary nailing for fractures of the shaft of the femur in multiply injured patients. *J Bone Joint Surg.* 2000;6:781–787.
19. Bone LB, Johnson KD, Weigelt J, et al. Early versus delayed stabilization of femoral fractures—a prospective randomized study. *J Bone Joint Surg.* 1989;3:336–340.
20. Pape HC, Auf m'Koolk M, Paffrath T, et al. Primary intramedullary femur fixation in multiple trauma patients with associated lung contusion—a cause of posttraumatic ARDS? *J Trauma.* 1993;34:540–548.
21. Bosse MJ, MacKenzie EJ, Riemer BL, et al. Adult respiratory distress syndrome, pneumonia and mortality following thoracic injury and a femoral fracture treated either with intramedullary nailing with reaming or with a plate. *J Bone Joint Surg.* 1997;6:799–809.
22. Pape HC, Regel G, Dwenger A, et al. The risk of early intramedullary nailing of long bone fractures in multiply traumatized patients. *Complications Orthop.* 1995;15–23.
23. Scalea TM, Boswell SA, Scott JD, et al. External fixation as a bridge to intramedullary nailing for patients with multiple injuries and with femur fractures: damage control orthopaedics. *J Trauma.* 2000;48:613–623.
24. Pape HC, Hildebrand F, Pertschy S, et al. Changes in the management of femoral shaft fractures in polytrauma patients. From early total care to damage control orthopedic surgery. *J Trauma.* 2002;53:452–462.
25. Roberts CS, Pape HC, Jones AL, et al. Damage control orthopaedics—evolving concepts in the treatment of patients who have sustained orthopaedic trauma. *J Bone Joint Surg.* 2005;2:434–449.

26. Hildebrand F, Giannoudis PV, Griensven M, et al. Management of polytraumatized patients with associated blunt chest trauma: a comparison of two European countries. *Injury.* 2005;36:293–302.
27. Pape HC, Grimme K, Van Griensven M, et al.; EPOFF study group. Impact of intramedullary instrumentation versus damage control for femoral fractures on immunoinflammatory parameters: prospective randomized analysis by the EPOFF study group. *J Trauma.* 2003;55:7–13.
28. O'Toole R, O'Brien M, Habashi N, et al. Resuscitation prior to stabilization of femoral shaft fractures limits ARDS in polytrauma patients despite low utilization of damage control orthopaedics. Presented at the Annual Meeting of the Orthopaedic Trauma Association, Phoenix, AZ, October 5, 2006.
29. Volkmann R. Die ischaemischen muskellahmungen und kontrakturen. *Zentrabl Chir.* 1881;8:801.
30. Murphy JB. Myositis. *JAMA.* 1914;63:1249.
31. Brooks B, Johnson JS, Kirtley JA. Simultaneous vein ligation. *Surg Gynecol Obstet.* 1934;59:496.
32. Haasbeek JF, Cole WG. Open fractures of the arm in children. *J Bone Joint Surg.* 1995;77:576–581.
33. Hayden G, Leung M, Leong J. Gluteal compartment syndrome. *ANZ J Surg.* 2006;76:668–670.
34. Schwartz JT, Brumback RJ, Lakatos R, et al. Acute compartment syndrome of the thigh. *J Bone Joint Surg.* 1989;71:392.
35. Meyerson M. Acute compartment syndromes of the foot. *Bull Hosp J Dis Orthop.* 1987;47:251.
36. DeLee JC, Stiehl JB. Open tibia fracture with compartment syndrome. *Clin Orthop.* 1981;160:175–184.
37. Rorabeck CH, Clarke KM. The pathophysiology of the anterior tibial compartment syndrome: an experimental investigation. *J Trauma.* 1978;18:299.
38. Heppenstall RB, Scott R, Sapiga A, et al. A comparative study of the tolerance of skeletal muscle to ischemia. *J Bone Joint Surg.* 1986;68:820.
39. Geary N. Late surgical decompression for compartment syndrome of the forearm. *J Bone Joint Surg.* 1984;66:745.
40. Kunkel JM. Thigh and leg compartment syndrome in the absence of lower extremity trauma following MAST application. *Am J Emerg Med.* 1987;5:118.
41. Rorabeck CH. The treatment of compartment syndromes of the leg. *J Bone Joint Surg.* 1984;66:93.
42. Boody AR, Wongworawat MD. Accuracy in the measurement of compartment pressures: a comparison of three commonly used devices. *J Bone Joint Surg.* 2005;87:2415–2422.
43. Wilson SC, Vrahas MS, Berson L, et al. A simple method to measure compartment pressures using an intravenous catheter. *Orthopedics.* 1997;20:403.
44. Rorabeck CH, Castle GSP, Hardie R, et al. Compartment pressure measurements: an experimental investigation using the slit catheter. *J Trauma.* 1981;21:446.
45. Harris IA, Kadir A, Donald G. Continuous compartment pressure monitoring for tibia fractures: does it influence outcome? *J Trauma.* 2006;60:1330–1335.
46. Abraham P, Leftheriotis G, Saumet JL. Laser Doppler flowmetry in the diagnosis of chronic compartment syndrome. *J Bone Joint Surg.* 1998;80:365.
47. Weimann JM, Ueno T, Leek BT, et al. Noninvasive measurements of intramuscular pressure using pulsed phase-locked loop ultrasound for detecting compartment syndrome. *J Orthop Trauma.* 2006;20:458–463.
48. Amendola A, Twaddle BC. Compartment syndrome. In: Browner: *Skeletal Trauma: Basic Science, Management and Reconstruction.* 3rd ed. WB Saunders St. Louis, MO; 2003.
49. McQueen JMM, Court-Brown CM. Compartment monitoring in tibial fractures. *J Bone Joint Surg.* 1995;78:99.
50. Whitesides TE, Haney TC, Morimoto K, et al. Tissue perfusion measurements as a determinant for the need for fasciotomy. *Clin Orthop.* 1975;113: 43.
51. Kakar S, Firoozabadi R, McKean J, et al. Diastolic blood pressure in patients with tibia fractures under anaesthesia: implications for the diagnosis of compartment syndrome. *J Orthop Trauma.* 2007;21:99–103.
52. Matsen FA, Wyss CR, Krugmire RB, et al. The effects of limb elevation and dependency on local arteriovenous gradients in normal human limbs with particular reference to limbs with increased tissue pressure. *Clin Orthop.* 1980;150:187.
53. Bulstrode CK, King JB, Worpole R, et al. A simple method for closing fasciotomies. *Ann R Coll Surg.* 1985;67:119.
54. Bermann SS, Schnilling JD, McIntyre KE, et al. Shoelace technique for delayed primary closure of fasciotomies. *Am J Surg.* 1994;167:435–436.
55. McKenney MG, Nir I, Fee T, et al. A simple device for closure of fasciotomy wounds. *Am J Surg.* 1995;172:275.
56. Yang CC, Chang DS, Webb LX. Vacuum-assisted closure of fasciotomy following compartment syndrome of the leg. *J Surg Orthop Adv.* 2006;15:19–23.
57. Frink M, Klaus AK, Kuther G, et al. Long term results of compartment syndrome of lower limb in polytraumatized patients. *Injury Int J Care Injured.* 2007;38:607–613.
58. Mithoefer K, Lhowe DW, Vrahas MS, et al. Functional outcome after acute compartment syndrome of the thigh. *J Bone Joint Surg.* 2006;88:729–737.
59. Bradley EL. The anterior tibial compartment syndrome. *Surg Gynecol Obstet.* 1973;136:289–297.
60. Sheridan GW, Matsen FA. Fasciotomy in the treatment of the acute compartment syndrome. *J Bone Joint Surg.* 1976;58:112–115.
61. Slater M, Mullins R. Rhabdomyolysis and myoglobinuric renal failure in trauma and surgical patients. A review. *J Am Coll Surg.* 1998;186:693–716.
62. Ward MM. Factors predictive of acute renal failure in rhabdomyolysis. *Arch Intern Med.* 1998;148:1553–1557.
63. Homsi E, Barreiro MF, Orlando JM, et al. Prophylaxis of acute renal failure in patients with rhabdomyolysis. *Ren Fail.* 1997;19:283–288.
64. Dudney TM, Elliott CG. Pulmonary embolism from amniotic fluid, fat and air. *Prog Cardiovasc Dis.* 1994;36:447–474.
65. Levy D. The fat embolism syndrome. A review. *Clin Orthop Relat Res.* 1990;261:281–286.
66. Riska EB, Myllynen P. Fat embolism in patients with multiple injuries. *J Trauma.* 1982;22:891–894.
67. Glover P, Worthley L. Fat embolism. *Crit Care Resus.* 1999;1:276–284.
68. Peltier LF. Fat embolism. A perspective. *Clin Orthop Relat Res.* 1988;232: 263–207.
69. Fabian TC, Hoots AV, Stanford DS, et al. Fat embolism syndrome: prospective evaluation in 92 fracture patients. *Crit Care Med.* 1990;18:42–26.
70. Mellor A, Soni N. Fat embolism. *Anesthesia.* 2001;56:145–154.
71. Riseborough EJ, Herndon JH. Alterations in pulmonary function, coagulation and fat metabolism in patients with fractures of the lower limbs. *Clin Orthop Relat Res.* 1976;115:248–267.
72. Fonte DA, Hausberger FX. Pulmonary free fatty acids in experimental fat embolism. *J Trauma.* 1971;11:668–672.
73. Hofmann S, Huemer G, Slazer M. Pathophysiology and management of the fat embolism syndrome. *Anaesthesia.* 1998;2:35–37.
74. Nakata Y, Tanaka H, Kuwagata Y, et al. Triolein-induced pulmonary embolization and increased microvascular permeability in isolated perfused rat lungs. *J Trauma.* 1999;47:111–119.
75. Brow PJ, Toung T, Margolis S, et al. Pulmonary injury caused by free fatty acid: evaluation of steroid and albumin therapy. *Surgery.* 1981;89:582–587.
76. Gemer M, Dunegan LJ, Lehr JL, et al. Pulmonary insufficiency induced by oleic acid in the sheep: a model for investigation of extracorporeal oxygenation. *J Thorac Cardiovasc Surg.* 1975;69:793–799.
77. Richards RR. Fat embolism syndrome. *Can J Surg.* 1997;40:334–339.
78. Parizel PM, Demey HE, Veeckmans G, et al. Early diagnosis of cerebral fat embolism syndrome by diffusion-weighted MRI (starfield pattern). *Stroke.* 2001;32:2942–2944.
79. Satoh H, Kurisu K, Ohtani M, et al. Cerebral fat embolism studied by magnetic resonance imaging, transcranial Doppler sonography, and single photon emission computed tomography: case report. *J Trauma.* 1997;43:345–348.
80. Worthley LI, Fisher MM. The fat embolism syndrome treated with oxygen, diuretics, sodium restriction and spontaneous ventilation. *Anaesth Intensive Care.* 1979;7:136–142.
81. Alho A, Saikku K, Eerola P, et al. Corticosteroids in patients with a high risk of fat embolism syndrome. *Surg Gynecol Obstet.* 1978;147:358–362.
82. Shier MR, Wilson RF, James RE, et al. Fat embolism prophylaxis: a study of four treatment modalities. *J Trauma.* 1977;17:621–629.
83. Gossling HR, Donohue TA. The fat embolism syndrome. *JAMA.* 1979;241: 2740–2742.
84. Brundage SI, McGhan R, Jurkovich GJ, et al. Timing of femur fracture fixation: effect on outcome in patients with thoracic and head injuries. *J Trauma.* 2002;52:299–307.
85. Pitto RP, Schramm M, Hohmann D, et al. Relevance of the drainage along the linea aspera for the reduction of fat embolism during cemented total hip arthroplasty. A prospective, randomized clinical trial. *Arch Orthop Trauma Surg.* 1999;119:146–150.
86. Pitto RP, Koessler M, Kuehle JW. Comparison of fixation of the femoral component without cement and fixation with use of a bone-vacuum cementing technique for the prevention of fat embolism during total hip arthroplasty. A prospective, randomized clinical trial. *J Bone Joint Surg Am.* 1999;81:831–843.
87. Peltier LF. Fat embolism. III. The toxic properties of neutral fat and free fatty acids. *Surgery.* 1956;40:665–670.
88. Gossling Hr, Pellegrini VD Jr. Fat embolism syndrome: a review of the pathophysiology and physiological basis of treatment. *Clin Orthop Relat Res.* 1982;165:68–82.
89. Meeke RI, Fitzpatrick GJ, Phelan DM. Cerebral edema and the fat embolism syndrome. *Intensive Care Med.* 1987;15:147–148.
90. Sie MY, Toh KW, Rajeev K. Cerebral fat embolism: an indication for ICP monitor? *J Trauma.* 2003;55:1185–1186.
91. Habashi N. Other approaches to open-lung ventilation: airway pressure release ventilation. *Crit Care Med.* 2005;33:228–240.
92. Fulde GW, Harrison P. Fat embolism—a review. *Arch Emerg Med.* 1991;8: 233–239.
93. Durkin A, Sagi HC, Durham R, et al. Contemporary management of pelvic fractures. *Am J Surg.* 2006;192:211.
94. Kimbrell BJ, Velhamos GC, Chan LS et al. Angiographic embolization for pelvic fractures in older patients. *Arch Surg.* 2004;139:728.
95. Gourlay D, Hoffer E, Routt M et al. Pelvic angiography for recurrent traumatic pelvic arterial hemorrhage. *J Trauma.* 2005;59:1168.
96. Cothren CC, Osborn PM, Moore EE et al. Preperitoneal pelvic packing for hemodynamically unstable pelvic fractures: a paradigm shift. *J Trauma.* 2007;62:834.

CHAPTER 86 ■ UROLOGIC SURGERY AND TRAUMA

MICHAEL COBURN

IMMEDIATE CONCERNS

Primary emergency considerations in urology from the critical care perspective include hemorrhagic, obstructive, infectious, and ischemic processes, in addition to a wide variety of general postoperative difficulties that may warrant emergent intervention. Oncologic emergencies also arise in urology and may require urgent critical care management. Urologic trauma (addressed in a separate section, below) encompasses a wide variety of injuries that may vary from life threatening issues to those impacting functional outcomes.

Gross hematuria is an alarming symptom to the patient and the medical practitioner, and may mandate immediate critical care intervention depending on the magnitude of the hematuria and details of the individual case (1). Patients presenting with gross hematuria to the emergency center may have a defined cause (e.g., known radiation cystitis, recurrent benign prostatic hypertrophy [BPH]-related bleeding) or may be reporting a new sign not previously evaluated. Immediate urologic intervention is necessary if the patient has clot retention (unable to void or empty adequately due to the presence of clots in the bladder), is bleeding severely (which may be difficult to judge), has significant pain, is infected, has coagulopathy, or has other underlying medical factors with increased risk of further complications. Vital sign measurement, physical examination, and basic laboratory studies including complete blood count (CBC), coagulation functions, electrolyte and renal function testing, urinalysis, and culture will often answer the above questions and determine the need for immediate intervention. Palpation and percussion of the bladder may reveal bladder distention with or without tenderness. Bladder ultrasound units (BladderScan) or other readily available ultrasound instruments may rapidly answer the question of whether the bladder is distended. In the setting of gross hematuria and a distended bladder, a catheter must be inserted. Often too small a catheter is placed, which does not allow adequate irrigation of clots; clots must be fully evacuated to allow proper catheter drainage as well as to determine the degree of bleeding and continuation of bleeding. Small clots may be evacuated via an 18 to 20 French catheter; large clots require a bigger catheter (22–24 French) for satisfactory evaluation. The catheter should be irrigated to and fro with a piston syringe using 60 to 120 mL of normal saline. When no more clots can be retrieved, the irrigation efflux should become clear if bleeding is not ongoing. If the efflux remains bloody despite complete clot evacuation or if new clots continue to form, there is ongoing bleeding and input from the urologist is needed. One can change the patient to a three-way catheter in the setting of continuing bleeding in order to keep the catheter patent, but this decision is best made along with urologic consultation. There are risks involved in the implementation of continuous bladder irrigation, including bladder rupture if the outflow lumen becomes occluded without recognition and the inflow of irrigant continues. It is preferable to diagnose early with definitive intervention as cystoscopic examination and fulguration may solve the problem with less morbidity and less blood replacement than more conservative approaches. Gross hematuria in the urologic postoperative setting will be addressed in more detail below.

Other hemorrhagic urologic problems requiring immediate critical care intervention include renal or perirenal bleeding (e.g., spontaneous hematoma in the anticoagulated patient or the renal tumor patient) or scrotal hematoma. Bleeding in these sites is often trauma related (see below).

Urosepsis is another concern. Sepsis of the urinary tract or urogenital origin may present in a most precipitous and potentially life-threatening manner, or may be indolent (2). It is essential to understand the importance of the combination of infection and obstruction in producing a dangerous septic state. A common scenario is the patient presenting with an obstructing ureteral calculus. Typical symptoms of ureteral colic include flank pain (often radiating to the lower quadrant, and ipsilaterally to the genitalia with distal stones), irritative voiding symptoms (when the stone is distal in the intramural ureter), nausea, vomiting, or distention (due to ileus). These symptoms can be extremely distressing and require urgent medical attention, but the most critical emergency seen in such a setting occurs when these symptoms are accompanied by infection and sepsis. The combination of infection and obstruction of the urinary tract (upper or lower) is a veritable surgical emergency requiring immediate action. Septic shock may unfold rapidly in such situations with a significant mortality rate, even in the otherwise healthy host. We teach our residents that the sun should never set on an undrained, infected obstructed urinary tract.

Other infectious states requiring urgent critical care intervention include renal or perirenal abscess, scrotal abscess, acute epididymo-orchitis, and Fournier gangrene (see below).

Obstruction of the urinary tract and urinary retention may require critical care intervention independent of the presence or absence of hematuria or infection. Upper or lower tract obstruction can result in acute or chronic renal failure, mandating prompt drainage to control metabolic instability. Acute urinary retention with bladder distention is a miserable experience for the patient, and must be promptly relieved by introduction of a catheter into the bladder, preferably by a transurethral route, or alternatively by a suprapubic route if the urethra is impassable.

Ischemic states represent another form of pathology for which immediate intervention is essential (3,4). The quintessential example in our discipline is that of testicular torsion. Delayed diagnosis of torsion is a common cause of unnecessary testicular loss (as well as avoidable litigation). After 8 hours, the likelihood of testicular salvage decreases significantly. A high index of suspicion is necessary when addressing "the acute scrotum," with accurate history and physical examination forming the core of this assessment, with diagnostic imaging (mainly scrotal ultrasound, occasionally computed tomography [CT] scanning when extension from an intra-abdominal process is suspected). When clinical suspicion of acute testicular torsion is high, surgical exploration should not be delayed to obtain confirmatory imaging that is not readily and rapidly available. The outcome with regard to testicular salvage is critically time sensitive. The occasional negative exploration or the finding of some other cause of the acute scrotum is appropriate, similar to the principles of exploration for the acute abdomen and for acute appendicitis. Naturally, proper patient education is important preoperatively in addressing the differential diagnosis and both the possibility of finding a lesion, which might have been manageable without surgery, as well as the possibility of orchiectomy. The differential diagnosis of the acute scrotum includes incarcerated or strangulated inguinal hernia for which urgent surgical management is also critical. Physical and sonographic findings are usually diagnostic preoperatively.

Other ischemic states of critical care relevance in urology include the ischemic kidney (due to atherosclerotic or embolic disease or pedicle injury from trauma). The kidney begins to undergo irreversible loss of function following approximately 30 minutes of warm ischemia time; thus, rapid action is necessary.

Oncologic emergencies in urology often involve hemorrhagic, obstructive, and infectious problems. Other emergencies include neurologic compromise and pain management issues. Prostate cancer may metastasize preferentially to the skeletal system. In prior eras, presentation with extensive spinal involvement was much more common than in current practice; however, sudden neurologic compromise from spinal cord compression due to prostate cancer is still seen. Sensory loss, paralysis, and loss of urinary, bowel, and sexual function may be manifestations of neurologic compromise from malignant involvement of the central nervous system. When observed, immediate neurosurgical consultation should be obtained to determine if corticosteroids, emergency radiation therapy, or decompressive laminectomy is indicated. In addition, medical oncology input is valuable. Commencing antiandrogen therapy emergently may be of great value when prostate cancer patients present with complications such as neurologic or urinary obstructive compromise. Intramuscular leuteinizing hormone–releasing hormone (LH-RH) agonists such as leuprolide acetate may be started immediately; to prevent transient worsening from the androgen flare that accompanies the initiation of such regimens, an antiandrogen drug such as bicalutamide should be commenced simultaneously or prior to the LH-RH analog.

POSTOPERATIVE MANAGEMENT

Both major and minor urologic surgery may present critical care issues that require rapid and accurate assessment and intervention. While the postoperative considerations following major retroperitoneal or pelvic surgery will be familiar to the surgical critical care specialist as they mirror the issues relevant to general and vascular surgery, there are special considerations in urologic patients. Patients undergoing endoscopic surgery and genital surgery may present with postoperative issues less familiar to the critical care teams, and it is important to understand the anatomy and the issues that may require expeditious intervention. Currently, many urologic procedures that have traditionally been performed through open surgical approaches are now commonly being approached via laparoscopic, robotic, and other minimally invasive techniques, which bring with them their own set of postoperative challenges. We will address the more common and important types of urologic procedures with relevance to the critical care provider.

Upper abdominal surgery in urology usually involves extirpative procedures on the adrenal gland, kidney, or ureter and/or reconstructive procedures on these structures.

Patient position and selection of incision are relevant to the postoperative management. While the anterior midline incision is often favored by general surgeons for intraperitoneal procedures, urologists often prefer to operate through the flank or through other incisional approaches to the upper abdomen. Flank surgery is an art that is mastered through extensive experience: exactly how and where to make an incision reflect one's training and the task to be accomplished. Large renal tumors are often approached through a thoracoabdominal incision, which may enter the chest through the bed of the 8th to 11th rib through a rib resection or intercostal technique. Smaller or lower pole tumors are commonly approached through a subcostal flank or anterior incision, which generally does not enter the thoracic cavity. Such incisions may be developed as extraperitoneal exposure or through a transperitoneal route. The critical care provider in these postoperative patients should know how the patient was positioned, what kind of incision was made, and whether it was transthoracic and intra- or extraperitoneal. These details allow one to anticipate the types of problems that may arise postoperatively. In flank surgery, it is not uncommon to encounter a "down-lung" syndrome, with postoperative atelectasis involving the lung positioned downward against the operating table, particularly when the operation is prolonged and the patient is large. Occasionally lobar or complete lung atelectasis may be noted and may require bronchoscopic intervention. If a tube thoracostomy is placed following urologic surgery, the standard problems typical of the use of such tubes can occur; rarely, lung resection is performed as part of a urologic procedure (e.g., wedge resection of a solitary metastasis from renal cell carcinoma) and problems related to air leak or postoperative intrathoracic bleeding may be encountered. Excellent pulmonary toilet is critical following upper abdominal and flank urologic surgery and ideally should be initiated preoperatively, with patients being medically optimized and being taught to use an incentive spirometer, and then being closely monitored for pulmonary difficulties with early intervention as indicated. Postoperative pain from flank surgery can be a major problem and can require expert pain management intervention, continuous epidural analgesic strategies, subcutaneous pain pumps, and patient-controlled intravenous analgesic. Appropriate pain control is also key to minimizing pulmonary complications by aiding respiratory and coughing efforts.

Following surgery that involves removal or manipulation of the adrenal gland, the possibility of an early postoperative hypoadrenal state should be considered, including the potential for addisonian crisis. These entities may be unsuspected and may be missed or noted with a delay in diagnosis when assessing postoperative electrolyte and hemodynamic abnormalities and other nonspecific signs that may be consistent with acute adrenal dysfunction or deficiency. The critical care specialist should know if the adrenal was removed along with a nephrectomy procedure and whether there is any reason to suspect hypofunction or absence of the contralateral gland.

Acute renal insufficiency may occur following any major surgery, and is of particular concern following renal surgery. Partial nephrectomies may be performed using warm or cold ischemia techniques. When the latter approach is used, the patient's kidney is packed in saline slush following noncrushing occlusion of the renal artery and the excisional procedure is completed in a setting of local hypothermia. While the objective in such surgery is to minimize the negative impact on the function of the operated kidney, some degree of postoperative acute tubular necrosis (ATN) may still occur. Whether this is clinically noted or relevant depends largely on the state of the contralateral kidney, and standard management principles for acute renal insufficiency are applicable.

Bleeding following renal or other upper abdominal urologic surgery is of vital importance. Postoperative bleeding may be manifested by hemodynamic changes, acute anemia, physical findings such as palpable flank hematoma or ecchymosis, or radiologic findings of blood in the renal fossa, chest (after a transthoracic procedure) or peritoneal cavity (after a transperitoneal procedure). If a drain is left in place following surgery, elevated output of bloody fluid is important to monitor. Following a partial nephrectomy, significant postoperative bleeding most commonly arises from arterial branch vessels within the renal parenchyma at the resection site. An effort is made intraoperatively to suture significant parenchymal bleeding points, often supplemented by the use of additional bolstering sutures, hemostatic agents, and coagulation instruments (e.g., Argon beam coagulator). If significant bleeding occurs following renal surgery, expectant management with transfusion and correction of any coagulopathy, return to the operating room for re-exploration, angiographic embolization, or CT scanning to assess the specific anatomic site of bleeding and judge the size of the hematoma are options to consider. The choice between these measures is individualized based on the severity of the bleeding, patient condition and physiologic reserve, and access to imaging, interventional radiologic, and surgical resources. If there is evidence that major early postoperative bleeding occurs that may be due to an uncontrolled renal pedicle, rapid surgical re-exploration is the best approach. If bleeding occurs subacutely and renal parenchymal bleeding is suspected, interventional radiology (IR) is usually favored. The patient should be maintained in a fluid-resuscitated state when a renal bleeding issue is evolving, with the hemoglobin at a level that would allow the patient to tolerate continued blood loss without catastrophic decompensation.

Urinary extravasation following upper urinary tract surgery may be manifested by increased drainage from suction drains for which creatinine determination confirms the fluid's identity as urine. Urologic input should be sought as to whether the region is well drained, whether the leak is expected, and whether intervention versus observation is indicated.

Pelvic surgery procedures requiring postoperative critical care include exenterative procedures for malignancies (radical prostatectomy or cystectomy), simple open prostatectomy for benign prostatic hyperplasia, and reconstructive pelvic surgeries for incontinence. Critical care issues typically relate to standard postoperative abdominal surgical concerns such as pain, bleeding, and ileus. Specifically with pelvic urologic procedures, management of tubes and drains and recognizing when urinary extravasation arising in the postoperative period requires urgent attention or can be managed expectantly is important. Patients that have undergone major surgery involving an open bladder (open prostatectomy, bladder stone removal, etc.) may have significant bladder spasms postoperatively requiring anticholinergic medication. Bleeding following major urologic pelvic surgery may result in Foley catheter occlusion with clot, and it should be established with the urologist how much hematuria is acceptable and what measures should be taken if failure of catheter drainage develops. Catheter manipulation should be pursued only with the input of the urologist. Significant bleeding from the catheter is relatively uncommon following radical prostatectomy, while dramatic hematuria is much more common following an open simple prostatectomy performed for BPH, in which the adenoma is enucleated from the prostatic capsule by finger dissection, leaving a raw, vascular tissue bed. Urologic input is needed for problematic bleeding in such patients.

The possibility of anastomotic leakage or a missed injury to the ureter exists in the radical prostatectomy patient. If inordinately high pelvic suction drainage is noted, the fluid should be sent for creatinine level to determine if a urine leak is present. If well drained, no immediate intervention may be necessary, but radiographic studies may be indicated to localize the site of extravasation and plan definitive management.

Following radical cystectomy for bladder cancer, complications may include urinary extravasation from the urinary diversion reconstruction, pelvic bleeding, ileus, bowel obstruction or anastomotic leak, and pelvic lymphocele accumulation. These patients invariably require stays in the intensive care unit (ICU) postoperatively, due to the length and complexity of the surgery, potential for postoperative bleeding, and general medical management. Patients undergoing major urologic surgery, and especially patients undergoing cystectomy and urinary diversion, may require nutritional support. These patients, who have had both a major exenterative procedure as well as complex bowel surgery, may have a prolonged ileus, develop partial small bowel obstruction, and be depressed, and will often require aggressive nutritional supplementation, which should be begun early when a prolonged recovery is anticipated, to avoid the healing problems seen with development of a progressive catabolic state.

Deep venous thrombosis (DVT) and pulmonary embolism are risks of many urologic surgical procedures, and urologists are acutely aware of the issues related to DVT prophylaxis. Because major retroperitoneal or pelvic surgery also presents significant risks for postoperative bleeding, a judicious approach to postoperative anticoagulation is applied, with careful assessment of DVT risk factors and risk–benefit analysis. Radical cystectomy is the procedure with the greatest DVT risk of the urologic operations, as an extensive pelvic lymphadenectomy is also typically included, and many urologic oncologists will start low-molecular-weight heparin regimens 24 hours following surgery if there are no bleeding issues.

Other pelvic surgical procedures the critical care provider may encounter include the wide range of pelvic floor reconstructive operations performed for management of prolapse or stress incontinence. The traditional pubovaginal sling or retropubic bladder neck suspension procedures, and particularly some of the newer procedures that involve passage of artificial tape and mesh materials either via the retropubic space, through a transobturator foramen approach, or through other transvaginal techniques, may introduce the risks of enteric pelvic injury or major pelvic vascular injury. If major bleeding occurs following these types of procedures, either via the surgical incisions or resulting in large pelvic hematoma and hemodynamic instability, pelvic exploration or angiographic study may be indicated and vascular surgical expertise may be necessary.

Endoscopic upper and lower urinary tract surgery encompasses a wide variety of commonly performed procedures, including diagnostic cystoscopy (rigid, flexible), cystoscopic surgery (bladder biopsy, transurethral resection of prostate or bladder tumor [TURP, TURBT]), ureteroscopy (rigid, flexible, diagnostic alone, or with stone manipulation or biopsy/fulguration), and percutaneous renal access surgery (percutaneous nephrostolithotripsy). Each of these varieties of urologic instrumentation can be simple or complicated, and can raise problems for the critical care provider.

Lower tract endoscopy for diagnostic purposes is usually performed in an office setting, using a flexible cystoscope (some urologists use the rigid cystoscope in the female, as it is well tolerated due to short length and straight orientation of the female urethra; most male cystoscopy utilizes the flexible cystoscope). Lidocaine jelly is usually used as a local anesthetic, typically instilled with a prepackaged applicator (Uro-jet). The procedure causes minimal discomfort. Postprocedure infection can occur, but the risk is small if the urine is sterile preprocedure. Prophylactic oral antibiotics are often administered for all endourologic procedures to minimize the infection risk. Gross hematuria can occur following simple diagnostic cystoscopy, but is usually self-limiting and minimal, especially when the flexible cystoscope is used. Cystoscopic surgery, on the other hand, is generally performed under regional or general anesthesia, and specific issues exist.

When cutting or resection is required, a resectoscope is used, which is a rigid instrument that employs a cutting loop or cutting blade. When performing a traditional TURP, normal saline is not used as an irrigant, as the electrolyte solution will cause dissipation of electric current and prevent effective cutting or coagulation. The most common irrigant used for TURP in the United States is 1.5% glycine, which is nonelectrolyte and isotonic to plasma. This irrigant allows the electroresection system to function properly while avoiding hemolysis if intravascular extravasation occurs, a problem seen historically when sterile water was used. Cystoscopic surgery using glycine can result in significant hyponatremia if major absorption occurs, either directly into the vasculature (as with cutting into a periprostatic venous sinus during a TURP) or into interstitial tissues (as with fluid entering the retropubic space or infiltrating under the bladder trigone). As hyponatremia develops, the patient may develop altered mental status, bradycardia, hypertension, and respiratory compromise. If under general endotracheal anesthesia, foamy material may be noted in the breathing circuit. Severe hyponatremia may cause cerebral edema and grand mal seizures, and may be life threatening. Some interstitial extravasation has been shown to occur during TURP even without capsular or venous perforation but it does not cause morbidity if minimal. If this problem is recognized intraoperatively, the procedure may need to be prematurely terminated. Diuretics with normal saline or hypertonic saline administered intravenously may be indicated, depending on the clinical manifestations. The more abrupt the development of the hyponatremia and the lower the serum sodium, the more dramatic the clinical manifestations are. TURBT procedures are sometimes performed using sterile water as the irrigant of choice in order to minimize cell implantation risk, but there is a lack of data to support this concept, and extravasation of sterile water can introduce both a hyponatremia and a hemolysis risk. We strongly recommend avoiding sterile water as an irrigant for operative cystoscopy, confining its use to simple diagnostic cystoscopy. If bladder perforation occurs during TURBT or bladder biopsy procedures, there is the potential for significant irrigant extravasation to occur rapidly. If the perforation is extraperitoneal, management with catheter drainage will suffice and the fluid is usually reabsorbed without sequelae unless the volume is very large, in which case placing a drain in the retropubic space to evacuate the fluid may be indicated. Minimal intraperitoneal resectoscopic injuries may be manageable with catheter drainage alone. If problems arise (abdominal distention, persistent extravasation) with this nonoperative approach to intraperitoneal bladder perforation, laparoscopic or open surgical repair should be performed. (This situation is very different from the intraperitoneal bladder rupture due to blunt trauma, which typically results in a large defect in the bladder dome, consistently requiring suture repair to prevent urinary ascites and sepsis.)

Bleeding may be a problem following either TURP or TURBT. Urologists are well trained to deal with this problem and distinguish arterial bleeding, which will likely warrant return to the operating room for a second look and fulguration attempt, from acceptable venous bleeding, which is self-limiting. Often three-way catheter continuous bladder irrigation is employed following these procedures to maintain catheter patency and prevent clot formation postoperatively. While these devices are valuable adjuncts in our management of such patients, they introduce the potential for postoperative difficulties with occlusion of the outflow channel from clot, while irrigant inflow continues. Bladder distention and bladder rupture can result in this situation. When managing any continuous bladder irrigation system, the critical care provider must closely monitor the inflow and output, and palpate the lower abdomen on a regular basis to be certain that occlusion does not occur. If uncertain as to whether the three-way catheter is draining properly, the inflow should be turned off while the catheter is irrigated or urologic assistance is obtained. Only normal saline should be used as irrigant for continuous bladder irrigation systems. For TURP procedures, catheter traction may help control bleeding from within the prostatic fossa. Only the urologist should implement or adjust the traction system. For TURBT procedures, catheter traction is of no value, as the bladder body cannot be compressed, so a lower threshold to take the patient back to surgery for a second look is safer for post-TURBT bleeding. If a catheter needs to be changed in the early postoperative period following a TURP or TURBT, this should be done by the operating urologist's team or on their specific order. Newer technologies for TURP and TURBT employ laser energy to ablate, vaporize, or coagulate tissue endoscopically. These approaches usually result in less bleeding than the traditional electroresection approaches. Complications usually relate to obstruction following catheter removal or to iatrogenic injury from the laser energy being misdirected.

Upper tract endoscopy (ureteroscopy, percutaneous nephroscopy) has progressed greatly in the last two decades, with the current instrumentation allowing complex upper tract procedures to be performed with low morbidity. Ureteroscopy is often performed for hematuria evaluation, treatment of ureteral or renal stones, endoscopic assessment, and treatment of upper tract urothelial neoplasms, and for addressing obstructive lesions with laser or other incision procedures. Normal saline is used for most such procedures, although glycine may be needed when electrofulguration in the upper tract is planned. Problems that the critical care provider may encounter usually relate to ureteral perforation, gross hematuria with stent occlusion or "clot colic," or obstructive problems related to retained stone fragments. Percutaneous renal surgery may be accompanied by problems related to having surgery in the prone position, a high access traversing or affecting the chest, and postoperative bleeding. Percutaneous nephrostolithotomy or nephrolithotomy (PCNL) involves gaining access to the collecting system through the flank with the patient in the prone position. A needle, guidewire, and balloon or other dilating system is utilized to place a hollow plastic working sheath through the renal parenchyma into the collecting system, through which a flexible or rigid working nephroscope can be advanced. Laser, electrohydraulic, ultrasonic, or pneumatic devices are used to fragment and remove stone, or resection, incision, or fulguration instruments can be introduced to deal with neoplastic or obstructive lesions. Depending on the task to be accomplished, the access for percutaneous renal surgery may be obtained by the interventional radiologist or by the urologist. If entry into the upper pole calyx is needed for stone access, a supracostal puncture may be required (above the 12th rib). The risk exists to traverse the chest cavity resulting in pneumothorax or hydrothorax, which may require tube thoracostomy postoperatively. If elevated airway pressures and difficulty with ventilation occur intraoperatively, these possibilities should be entertained and managed acutely. As the kidney is a very vascular organ and the access traverses the renal parenchyma, significant bleeding can occur intraoperatively, perioperatively, or days or weeks postoperatively at the time of nephrostomy removal. Occasionally angiographic embolization may be necessary for major renal bleeding associated with PCNL. If brisk bleeding with hemodynamic instability occurs via an indwelling nephrostomy tube, the tube can be clamped while urologic input is urgently obtained. When removing a nephrostomy tube following PCNL, a tamponade catheter should be immediately available to place into the tract and inflate if dangerous bleeding ensues following tube removal.

While not strictly endoscopic surgery, extracorporeal shock wave lithotripsy (ESWL) is another common procedure for stone management that the critical care provider may encounter. This approach involves the noninvasive fragmentation of renal or ureteral calculi with a shock wave generator system under fluoroscopic or ultrasound guidance. The procedure commonly produces transient gross hematuria, which is rarely troublesome, as ESWL does result in some mild blunt trauma to the kidney. The typical procedure involves administering approximately 3,000 shocks to the stone(s). Following ESWL, colic can occur due to passage of fragments. Whether manageable expectantly or requiring stent insertion depends on the stone burden, the amount of debris created, the size of residual fragments, the degree of symptoms, and whether there are signs of infection and septic shock.

Laparoscopy in urologic surgery has come into its own in recent years and has become a major element of our approach to a wide range of surgical tasks that previously were performed solely through major open approaches. In many centers, the open radical retropubic prostatectomy (RRP) has been nearly replaced by the robotic-assisted laparoscopic prostatectomy (RALP), and kidney surgery done through a flank incision has been largely replaced by laparoscopic approaches. The same special considerations that are relevant to all laparoscopic surgeries are important to urologic laparoscopy. Such common issues include postoperative ileus, CO_2 retention, venous CO_2 embolism, postoperative bleeding, unrecognized intraoperative iatrogenic injury, and trochar and port-site complications (5).

In laparoscopy for renal surgery, there are two potential major sites of postoperative bleeding: the renal pedicle and the renal parenchyma (relevant for partial nephrectomy). The traditional means of controlling vessels in open surgery, using suturing and ligation, is often replaced in laparoscopic surgery with vascular stapling devices and instruments like the harmonic scalpel. The technology has advanced rapidly with these tools, and they are generally reliable and secure. There are, however, user-dependent factors and there is a learning curve involved in mastering the use of these devices. Bleeding can occur immediately postoperatively or in a more delayed fashion, and be manifested by hemodynamic and laboratory changes or visible bleeding from instrument ports or incisions. When precipitous and life threatening, a quick return to the operating room with either laparoscopic or open re-exploration may be the most appropriate course. When more gradual and when the luxury of the opportunity for further evaluation is appropriate, postoperative CT scanning to determine if there is a renal or perirenal hematoma may be relevant prior to a surgical effort. If bleeding occurs from the cut surface of the kidney following either open or laparoscopic partial nephrectomy, angiography with subselective embolization is often the preferred approach.

Drains left within the abdomen following laparoscopic procedures are often placed intraperitoneally, as opposed to the case in extraperitoneal flank surgery, where the drain is often not within the peritoneal cavity. As such, intraperitoneal drains may drain retained irrigant or peritoneal fluid in copious amounts following surgery. If there is uncertainty as to the significance of increased drain output, fluid may be sent for chemical analysis (creatinine to determine if fluid is urine, amylase to rule out pancreatic fluid leak). Leakage of urine following laparoscopic urologic surgery may not require immediate intervention if the leak is well drained. If action is needed, postoperative ureteral stent insertion (along with a urethral Foley catheter or in some cases nephrostomy insertion) will often allow the collecting system to heal without sequelae. In general, drains should be removed as early as possible, as they have the downside of potentially allowing the entry of bacteria into the abdominal cavity.

In the course of dissection during laparoscopic urologic surgery, especially if electrocautery is extensively utilized, the risk of unrecognized bowel injury must be appreciated. The presentation of such complications may be subtle, with low-grade fever; minimal diffuse tenderness, which may be consistent with the expected postsurgical state; or delayed return of bowel function or persistent anorexia. A high degree of suspicion is important when patients fail to thrive following laparoscopic surgery, and postoperative CT scanning may demonstrate a fluid collection in an unexpected location or inflammatory changes in or near the intestine that would not be otherwise anticipated.

As robotic surgery for radical prostatectomy is rapidly becoming commonplace, the critical care provider may encounter such patients in the postoperative period. The same considerations noted above apply to the RALP patient with regard to suspecting and identifying inadvertent injuries. Gross hematuria causing catheter occlusion is important to recognize, as the vesicourethral anastomosis in these patients is quite delicate and usually performed with a running suture. Clot retention from catheter occlusion can result in bladder distention, which may strain or cause dehiscence of the anastomosis. Clear instructions from the urologist should be noted regarding catheter management, what to expect regarding volume and appearance of efflux, and appropriate interventions. If a catheter fails to drain following RALP, judicious irrigation with normal saline is generally safe, using no more that 60 mL. If a small clot is present and this maneuver results in normal clear efflux, no further action is necessary. Otherwise, the urologist should be informed and should provide specific intervention instructions or deal with the situation personally. Under no circumstances should anyone but the operating urologist ever remove and attempt replacement of an indwelling urethral catheter during the early perioperative period following major lower tract urologic surgery, especially when a fresh anastomosis or reconstructive site is present; such manipulation without direct visualization may disrupt the reconstruction site and cause major additional complications.

Genital surgery issues that may arise in the critical care setting may relate to penile, sphincter, and testicular prosthetic implants; neurologic stimulater implants; or complications of the wide range of other genital procedures urologists perform. Dressings on the genitalia should be inspected for bleeding or excessive tightness, which can cause vascular compromise, especially if applied circumferentially around the penis. Any major local complaint by a patient following genital surgery should be referred to the urologic surgeon for input. It is important for the critical care provider to know when a patient has a genitourinary prosthesis implanted. Obviously, there should never be any needle placement or incisional procedure performed by a nonurologist in the region of the genitalia in the setting of a prosthetic implant, as the fluid-filled components are prone to damage. If a patient with an artificial urinary sphincter (AUS) device needs a Foley catheter inserted, it is important that the device be deactivated (i.e., locked in an open position) by cycling the device and pressing the deactivation button on the pump once the pump has cycled full of fluid. Forcibly passing a Foley catheter into the urethra of an AUS patient risks damage to the urethra and the device. Infection and erosion can occur with any of the urologic prostheses, rarely resulting in abscess formation and major soft tissue infections and sepsis. Explantation and drainage procedures may be necessary, which require urologic surgical expertise. If uncertain as to how to approach any genitourinary prosthesis, obtain urologic expertise. Other genital surgery procedures such as vasectomy, testicular biopsy, reconstructive microsurgery for fertility treatment, and orchiectomy for tumor or benign disease can be complicated by bleeding or infection. If marked swelling occurs following genital surgery, the urologist should be immediately made aware. Orchiectomy for tumor is performed through a groin incision and involves removing the testis, its investing tunics (intact), and the spermatic cord to the level of the internal inguinal ring. If bleeding occurs from the stump of the spermatic cord, the hematoma can develop in the retroperitoneum and require high exploration for control.

UROLOGIC TRAUMA

Trauma centers vary markedly with regard to the role played by the urologist in trauma management. Some highly respected trauma centers utilize the urologist's expertise on a regular basis for assistance with the management of genitourinary injuries, while others rarely include the urologist. At our trauma center, the urology service plays a central role in the assessment and management of urologic injuries, participating in the selection and interpretation of imaging studies, the decision of when to operate, and the operative intervention itself (6). As such, we have achieved a high level of cooperation between our service and the trauma surgery and critical care services. This discussion will address the basic approach to the diagnosis and management of urologic trauma, with a recommendation that the urologist be included whenever possible in management decisions (7). The urologist's experience in elective urologic surgery; endoscopic, radiologic, and open surgical intervention; reconstructive approaches; and management of complications may be very helpful to the trauma and critical care teams when faced with the multiply injured patient or with solitary urologic organ trauma. When no urologist is available, however, or critical care decisions need to be made in the absence of urologic input, the critical care provider must have a working knowledge of the approach to the most common and important types of urologic trauma. We will address management of iatrogenic urinary tract trauma, followed by trauma from external violence for renal, ureteral, bladder, urethral, and genital injuries with regard to assessment and management, and discuss the relevance of damage control strategies in urologic trauma.

Iatrogenic Injury Management

The occurrence of an iatrogenic urologic injury provokes significant anxiety in the surgical team. Having a basic concept of the standard approach to management is essential in maintaining a focus on prompt resolution of the problem.

For bladder injuries, simple closure is feasible as long as the injury involves the upper bladder segment, the trigone is uninvolved, and there is not significant tissue loss. We try to perform a running, two-layer closure using heavy absorbable suture. A generously sized Foley catheter should be used (20 French or larger) to allow drainage of bloody efflux and allow efficient irrigation when needed. If the bladder wall surrounding the injury is markedly abnormal (fibrotic, friable, irradiated), a two-layer closure may not be feasible. In these cases, we prefer a one-layer, interrupted closure with heavy suture, with a plan to leave the bladder catheterized for a longer period of time.

If there is involvement of the trigone, ureteral orifices, or intramural ureters, the situation is more complex, and ureteral stent insertion or ureteral reimplantation may be needed. This is best accomplished with urologic support, and may involve placing an externalized single-J or internalized double-J ureteral stent, then suturing the bladder injury, taking care not to include the ureter in the sutures. If a stricture ultimately forms, endoscopic management or delayed elective ureteral reimplantation is always an option. Feeding tubes may also be temporarily passed up the ureters during the bladder repair to identify and potentially protect the ureters and support performing a safe cystorrhaphy. Prophylactic insertion of externalized ureteral catheters prior to complex pelvic or retroperitoneal surgery may be helpful in avoiding surgical injury to the ureter (8).

For iatrogenic ureteral injuries, the repair approach depends on the level of injury, whether there is loss of ureteral length, the condition of the ureter and surrounding tissue, and the comfort of the surgeon. Traditional urologic teaching states that if the ureter is transected caudal to the crossing of the internal iliac artery, a reimplant rather than a primary anastomosis should be performed. This policy reflects the concern for the viability of the distal ureteral stump in the setting of abnormal pelvic anatomy and surgical insult. The reimplant can be performed with or without a psoas hitch depending on ureteral length and bladder status. For injuries in the mid- or upper ureter, primary, spatulated anastomosis performed over an indwelling stent is the preferred solution. As long as one is dissecting outside the ureteral adventitial sheath, substantial length can be gained by mobilizing the ureter toward the kidney and deep into the pelvis with devascularization unlikely to be a concern. If primary repair is not possible, the options include ligation followed by nephrostomy insertion and planned delayed reconstruction, transureteroureterostomy, renal autotransplantation (seldom appropriate in the acute care surgery setting), or ileal ureteral replacement (also seldom appropriate in the acute care surgery setting).

When dissecting in the groin, especially in the setting of a redo hernia, the spermatic cord is at risk for injury. If there is injury to cord vasculature, precise suture ligation of bleeding points should occur, as a hematoma around the cord is very problematic. If there is concern for devascularization of the testis, use of a fine-tipped Doppler probe to detect an arterial pulse distal to the area of dissection or over the testis itself is helpful. Even if one is quite concerned that most of the cord vasculature has been lost, we would generally recommend leaving the testis alone and observing it. The testis has redundant blood supplies (internal spermatic, external spermatic, and vasal arteries, which come from aortic, external iliac, and internal iliac sources, respectively) and may survive on collateral blood supply. The status of the testis can be addressed postoperatively.

Penetrating and Blunt Trauma to the Genitourinary System

General Evaluation

Diagnosis of urinary tract injury is typically based on history and mechanism of injury, physical examination, laboratory assessment, and the findings on imaging studies. Any patient with a history of gross hematuria following trauma should be imaged, unless of course he or she is unstable and/or must be taken directly to surgery (9). In addition, current literature supports also obtaining imaging studies for patients with microscopic hematuria and hypotension at any time following trauma, as well as those patients with significant deceleration mechanisms of injury and other injury factors that portend a high risk of urinary tract injury such as lower posterior rib fracture, transverse spinal process fracture, or pelvic or femur fracture. The contrast-enhanced CT scan of the abdomen and pelvis has become the standard study of choice for assessment of hematuria, for staging of injuries in the trauma setting, and for the evaluation of renal or ureteral injuries. The "shock room intravenous pyelogram (IVP)" has fallen out of favor and provides much less information than the CT scan. Bladder injuries may be suspected based on the presence of gross hematuria following pelvic trauma with confirmation by either standard radiographic or CT cystography. Adequate bladder filling must be accomplished to demonstrate extravasation and minimize false-negative studies. When urethral injury is suspected (following pelvic fracture or perineal or genital trauma), especially when blood is exiting from the urethra or present at the urethral meatus, retrograde urethrography should be performed prior to any attempt at urethral catheterization. For genital trauma, scrotal ultrasonography may be of great value in diagnosing testicular rupture from blunt forces; in penetrating genital trauma, surgical exploration is usually necessary and one can usually forego imaging studies.

Urethral injuries should be suspected in cases of pelvic fracture, particularly with severe pubic diastasis and vertical shear injuries. A urethrogram that demonstrates contrast extravasation is diagnostic (10). Some urologists may be comfortable with a careful attempt at catheter insertion under cystoscopic guidance or a fluoroscopically and endoscopically guided catheter realignment procedure, though whether this approach provides advantages over traditional suprapubic diversion remains controversial. The standard approach remains suprapubic (SP) tube insertion; certainly any nonurologist should handle such injuries with placement of a suprapubic catheter, obtaining urologic consultation when available. Suprapubic cystostomy insertion may be accomplished using trochar-based percutaneous systems if the bladder is adequately distended. If not, an open surgical approach in the operating room is preferable. Blunt trauma to the perineum with complete urethral rupture is also best handled with suprapubic diversion. Penetrating injuries to the urethra can also be managed in a delayed fashion with suprapubic diversion, or, if the injury is readily apparent, direct suture repair with fine absorbable suture may be attempted in the stable patient. All such injuries can be managed in a delayed fashion as long as proximal urinary diversion is achieved acutely.

Bladder injuries from blunt trauma are diagnosed on cystography (11), and can usually be managed with catheter drainage alone, if the injury is **extraperitoneal**. Adequate-bore catheters (20 French or larger) are preferable to evacuate grossly bloody efflux. If there is failure of catheter management (continued profuse hematuria with repeated occlusion of the catheter, continued urinary extravasation), surgical repair may be necessary. If it is necessary to surgically repair such an injury, a high midline cystotomy should be made to avoid entering into a fresh retropubic hematoma, which may produce problematic bleeding. The laceration may be sutured in a single layer transvesically by placing retractors into the bladder and exposing the injury. Other cases of extraperitoneal bladder injury that benefit from surgical repair include those which involve communication with a vaginal or rectal injury. A suprapubic tube, in addition to the urethral Foley catheter, may be left indwelling in cases in which the repair is tenuous or prolonged tube drainage is anticipated (e.g., closed head or spinal cord injury). In the uncomplicated case, performing a contrast cystogram at approximately 10 to 14 days postinjury and prior to catheter removal ensures complete healing before stressing the bladder.

For **intraperitoneal** bladder injuries, direct suture repair is required. These injuries invariably occur in the bladder dome, and result from sudden compression of the full bladder. Transabdominal suture repair is straightforward. We generally do not use suprapubic tubes in such cases.

Ureteral injury is usually noted upon abdominal exploration in the penetrating trauma setting, or may be noted on preoperative CT scanning (12). It is necessary to obtain a delayed excretory phase on the CT such that the excreted contrast column has transited the entire ureter, or the risk of missing a ureteral injury is significant. Injuries from penetrating trauma are managed similarly to the approach described above for iatrogenic injuries, or by applying damage control techniques when necessary (see below). For gunshot wounds to the mid- and upper ureter, limited debridement to viable ureter, careful extra-adventitial mobilization, and spatulated suture anastomosis is appropriate. For distal ureteral injuries, reimplantation into the bladder ("ureteroneocystostomy") is a more dependable approach, as the problem of the distal stump having impaired vascularity is avoided. Ureteral injuries from blunt trauma are rare. Exceptions would include the pediatric population, where ureteropelvic avulsion injuries or renal pelvic lacerations may occur following blunt injuries. When major injury occurs to the urinary tract following seemingly trivial trauma, one should be suspicious of the presence of previously existent underlying pathology of the urinary tract such as neoplasm or ureteropelvic junction obstruction.

Renal injuries are typically staged by contrast-enhanced CT using the American Association for the Surgery of Trauma (AAST) Organ Injury Scaling system (13,14). Renal injuries are managed according to a multifactorial decision process that considers grade and whether they are due to blunt or penetrating forces, and is based on patient clinical status and hemodynamic stability. In general, for **blunt renal injury**, grade I, II, and III injuries are routinely managed nonoperatively. Grade IV injuries, which involve deeper, significant parenchymal injury and laceration to the collecting system, require a selective approach, largely influenced by hemodynamic parameters and degree of progressive blood loss, and often warrant monitoring to address whether continued bleeding or urinoma formation occurs, which may warrant delayed intervention (15). The majority of such injuries in most series do not require early exploration, and the observation of extravasation from the collecting system is not, in itself, a strong indication for surgical exploration. If there is extensive medial extravasation on CT, retrograde pyelography may be indicated to exclude a major injury to the renal pelvis or proximal ureter. Grade V injuries from blunt trauma routinely require surgical exploration and often nephrectomy, and most reported results of attempts to manage true grade V injuries nonoperatively have not resulted in good outcomes. Renal pedicle injuries, which are considered in both the grade IV and V groups, require careful consideration to select appropriate management. When the kidney suffers a pedicle stretch injury from deceleration trauma, resulting in arterial intimal disruption, the artery can thrombose, resulting in renal devascularization (16). This can be diagnosed on CT scan with the finding of renal nonperfusion. If the vessels are thrombosed but not avulsed or lacerated, the decision of whether to operate to revascularize the kidney depends on how much time has elapsed, which predicts renal salvage, as well as the patient's other injuries and ability to tolerate a laparotomy. After 30 minutes of warm ischemia, irreversible renal damage begins; by 3 hours, the kidney is not retrievable. If there is a pedicle avulsion injury, surgery is mandatory to prevent delayed catastrophic bleeding.

For **penetrating renal trauma**, the standard approach traditionally has been surgical exploration and repair or nephrectomy. This view has evolved over the past two decades, however, with reports demonstrating favorable outcomes from nonoperative management of carefully selected penetrating injuries. It has been reported that up to 50% of renal stab wounds and over 20% of renal gunshot wounds may be successfully managed nonoperatively. When comparing the approach to blunt versus penetrating trauma, one must consider the high likelihood of there being associated injuries in penetrating trauma. Still, a fully staged penetrating kidney injury (based on CT) may be appropriately managed nonoperatively if certain conditions are met. These include, in our view, a lateral or polar parenchymal injury, which spares the renal sinus or deep central region of the kidney; in a hemodynamic stable patient; and with low suspicion of injury to the extrarenal collecting system or ureter. The larger the renal hematoma, the less comfortable we are with nonoperative management of a penetrating renal injury. Proactive angiography may be considered when weighing the safety of a nonoperative approach to the penetrating renal injury in selected cases, and admission to the ICU is essential to monitor for renewed bleeding. It should be stated for the critical care provider that the default mode for penetrating trauma to genitourinary organs is operative exploration and repair; departure from this approach is appropriate when complete staging information is available that predicts a favorable outcome for a specific injury with a nonoperative approach, the patient is hemodynamically stable, and careful monitoring for failure of nonoperative management can be carried out. Criteria and a plan for changing to an operative strategy should exist.

Genital injuries require specialized care and should be handled by practitioners experienced in genital surgery. As a general principle, a very conservative approach to genital debridement should be maintained, with tissues of questionable viability reassessed in a delayed fashion. Nearly all penetrating genital injuries should be surgically explored acutely assuming the patient is sufficiently stable to undergo a reconstructive effort. Penetrating penile injuries are repaired surgically by closing lacerations in the corpus cavernosum, urethral repair, and skin and soft tissue reconstruction. Penetrating testicular injuries can usually be repaired by closing the tunica albuginea of the testis after debriding nonviable testicular parenchyma. Blunt fracture of the penis, which results from forcible flexing of the penile shaft during erection (often due to trauma during intercourse), should be explored and repaired acutely, upon presentation, to achieve the most favorable cosmetic and functional outcome. For blunt scrotal injury, it is often useful to assess the patient with scrotal ultrasonography to determine if testicular rupture is present, as it may be difficult to determine this on physical exam if there is scrotal wall swelling, which makes identification of internal structures difficult. Ultrasound is quite accurate for detecting testicular rupture: loss of capsular continuity or marked heterogeneity of testicular parenchyma is predictive of rupture. Testicular salvage is enhanced by early exploration and repair.

Damage Control Strategies for the Management of Urologic Injury in the Unstable Patient

Damage control approaches to the management of the unstable trauma patient have become well accepted in the trauma center setting. This concept refers to abbreviating the initial operative effort in order to minimize the effects of prolonged surgery, which results in progressive metabolic deterioration. Critical injuries (surgical bleeding, fecal contamination sources) are addressed, while noncritical injuries are handled in a delayed fashion, on a subsequent visit to the operating room after stabilization in the ICU. This approach avoids development of the "lethal triad" of progressive acidosis, hypothermia, and coagulopathy, which occurs in critically injured patients when initial surgical efforts are prolonged. Many urologic injuries are quite amenable to initial management by applying damage control strategies (17). With the exception of severe renal or bladder bleeding cases, urinary tract injuries do not directly result in early mortality. When, in the surgeon's judgment, the patient would not tolerate the magnitude of reconstructive effort needed to deal definitively with a urologic injury at initial laparotomy (due to pattern of injury, hypothermia, acidosis, coagulopathy, or other parameters that mandate a damage control approach), certain temporary solutions may be very desirable (18). We have gained substantial experience with such approaches in our center and have achieved an effective working relationship with the trauma surgeons in patient selection and technical approach for such cases.

Renal injuries that are incompletely staged or unstaged may be approached with delayed assessment and exploration, as long as a determination is made that early exsanguinating bleeding from the injury is unlikely. In the absence of significant bleeding from the renal fossa into the peritoneal cavity, a large midline hematoma, or an expanding or pulsatile renal hematoma, one can elect to leave the perinephric hematoma undisturbed and either obtain postoperative imaging during the resuscitation phase following initial laparotomy or explore at the time of a second-look procedure. If the kidney is already surgically exposed, hemostasis for major bleeding from parenchyma or branch renal vessels can be rapidly obtained. If a major reconstructive effort is still needed in the unstable patient, packing the kidney and returning for reconstructive interventions later is also an option.

Ureteral injuries may be initially managed with externalized stenting, ligation, or simple local drainage. Of these options, we favor externalized stenting, as it allows control of the urinary output, minimizes ongoing urinary extravasation, and can be maintained for several days until the patient is stable enough to return to surgery for definitive reconstruction. A 7 French or 8.5 French single-J urinary diversion stent can be placed into the ureter through the injury site and advanced proximally into the kidney, then externalized through the abdominal wall. The stent should be tied to the very end of the injured ureter at the injury site, so as not to lose ureteral length by ligating it more proximally and making later reconstruction more challenging. The distal ureteral limb is best left undisturbed; ligating it requires subsequent debridement and causes further tissue loss.

A similar approach can be utilized for extensive bladder injuries: the ureteral orifices can be catheterized, the catheters externalized, and the pelvis packed, leaving bladder reconstruction to be performed at a more suitable time, following appropriate resuscitation. Urethral and genital injuries are also amenable to damage control approaches, generally involving tube urinary diversion, placement of moistened dressings, and tissue preservation until definitive reconstruction following appropriate resuscitation.

UROLOGIC TUBES AND DRAINS FOR THE CRITICAL CARE PROVIDER

Tube drainage and diversion of the urinary tract and adjacent areas constitute important and commonly employed strategies in urologic care and urologic surgery. The safe insertion, maintenance, and management of such tubes are essential to avoid preventable morbidity and support appropriate medical and surgical management. The frequently utilized tubes that may be encountered by the critical care provider include nephrostomy, suprapubic cystostomy, urethral Foley catheter, and internal ureteral stents. In addition, externalized drains are often placed near the site of urologic surgery or injuries and employed for various purposes including drainage of blood, infectious fluid, lymph, or extravasated urine. The general principles behind urologic tube drainage along with specific management considerations for the different types of tube mentioned above will be addressed in this section (19).

Tubes placed within the urinary tract may be intended as temporary or permanent solutions to various urologic problems, including bladder muscle failure and obstructive upper or lower tract lesions. Patients with detrusor muscle failure require regular bladder emptying, which may be managed by intermittent catheterization (typically utilizing a clean/nonsterile technique) or by an indwelling catheter. In the case of indwelling catheters, the options include a transurethral Foley catheter or a suprapubic cystostomy tube. In the male, due to the potential morbidity of a long-term indwelling urethral catheter (including urethral erosion, periurethral abscess, epididymitis, and traumatic hypospadias), the SP tube is often favored. All patients with indwelling bladder catheters of either variety will become bacteriuric, but patients with SP tubes are less likely to develop the list of catheter-related complications noted above. In women, long-term urethral catheters are better tolerated, though the urethra may gradually become dilated and capacious, resulting in troublesome leakage around the tube.

Urethral catheter placement techniques are well known. If a standard Foley catheter is needed but resistance is met during placement, it is important not to force the catheter into the urethra, which risks urethral mucosal perforation, creation of a false passage, and bleeding, which greatly complicates further catheterization attempts. This principle is relevant both to the trauma and nontrauma setting. A catheter balloon should not be inflated until urine return is ensured; if no urinary drainage occurs upon catheter insertion, aspiration of the catheter using a piston syringe should occur before balloon inflation. In general, most catheter balloons should be inflated with a full 10 mL of saline or water, to avoid inadvertent migration into the urethra. Some balloons are rated to 30-mL inflation volume or greater; this information is clearly printed on the catheter inflation hub. If a standard catheter will not advance into the bladder, options include trying a smaller catheter, using a coude catheter, or requesting urologic consultation. If obstruction is met deep in the urethra in the male, the coude catheter is particularly helpful, as the curved tip will often navigate over the prostate and bladder neck and solve the problem. If resistance is met more distally in the penile or distal bulbar urethra, a stricture may be present for which a smaller catheter may be of benefit. Beyond these measures, the safest approach is to seek urologic expertise to assist with bladder access.

In the female, urethral catheter insertion is seldom difficult; true urethral strictures are uncommon (seen occasionally following radiation therapy or local surgery) and the urethra is generally straight and short. At times, due to atrophic changes, the female urethral meatus may be difficult to identify visually. In such cases, the meatus is often retracted onto the distal anterior vaginal wall. We can typically palpate it with a gloved fingertip and guide a catheter into the appropriate location. Problems in placing a female urethral catheter not solved by the above technique or by using a smaller tube may indicate significantly abnormal anatomy and should prompt urologic consultation.

In the hospital setting, patients often arrive in the critical care venue already with an indwelling catheter in place. It is important to verify that, on arrival, the catheter is properly positioned and is draining properly. It is remarkable how often we are consulted for a mysteriously malfunctioning catheter only to find that the balloon is easily palpable in the perineum or penis, plainly indicative of malposition. If a catheter fails to drain, it should be irrigated with 60 to 120 mL of normal saline or water. It should be possible to infuse and withdraw the instilled irrigant. If the catheter is not draining spontaneously and one can infuse but not withdraw fluid, the catheter is probably malpositioned and will likely require repositioning or replacement. When changing an indwelling catheter for routine purposes (generally monthly is advised), choose a convenient time when help is readily available if difficulty is encountered, not in the middle of the night shift. If a patient forcibly removes a catheter with the balloon inflated, dramatic urethral bleeding often occurs. Catheter replacement is typically necessary, and may be difficult due to deep laceration of the urethral mucosa. We would recommend trying to pass a coude catheter with the tip pointed cephalad; if not successful, obtain urologic assistance.

Suprapubic (SP) cystostomy tubes are straightforward devices that may be used as a temporary bladder drain or as a permanent strategy as noted above. SP tubes can be placed in the awake patient under local anesthesia using trochar-based kits, or can be placed through an open surgical approach under anesthesia in the operating room. If placed percutaneously, it is essential that the bladder be well distended prior to insertion. If the bladder is not well distended, the trochar, over which the catheter is advanced, can penetrate fully through the bladder lumen and pierce the posterior bladder wall, causing bladder injury and potentially injuring the vagina or rectum, or can injure intraperitoneal structures. Signs of such adjacent organ injury should prompt immediate surgical and urologic consultation. Once in place, a SP tube should generally be left indwelling for at least a week so that an established track forms between the skin and the bladder lumen. If prematurely removed, extravasation of urine into the retropubic and perivesical space may occur, which can result in urine absorption, azotemia, or urosepsis. A long-term indwelling SP tube through an established track is usually easy to change by simple removal and replacement with the same caliber and type of tube. Occasionally the track may be oblique or tortuous and direct visualization with a flexible cystoscope by a urologist and placement of the new tube over a guidewire may be necessary. If a SP tube is inadvertently removed or displaced, the track may close within a matter of hours or certainly over the course of a day, even when the tube has been in place long term. It is important that tube replacement be accomplished promptly to avoid track closure and the need to re-establish access in a more invasive manner.

It is important to realize, as noted above, that nearly all indwelling urinary tract tubes that communicate with the external environment will result in bacteriuria, often within about 10 days of tube placement (20). In most cases this is a harmless process and does not result in clinical infection. If, however, urinary tract manipulation or an invasive urinary tract procedure is planned, instrumentation in the face of such bacteriuria may precipitate urosepsis, and the tissues are vulnerable to intravasation of bacteria when a chronic catheter has been present. It is beneficial to obtain urine culture data and institute therapy with culture-specific agents prior to significant instrumentation of the chronically catheterized urinary tract, to minimize the risk of iatrogenically induced clinical infection or urosepsis.

The same principle applies when considering removal of an indwelling bladder tube, especially when there is the potential for the patient failing a voiding trial and developing urinary retention following catheter removal (as in BPH patients with episodic retention who may or may not pass a voiding trial). If a patient with catheter-related bacteriuria develops urinary retention upon catheter removal, the risk of clinical infection or urosepsis is significant. These patients as well should have coverage with culture-specific antibiotics whenever possible, or at least have the provision of empiric broad-spectrum urinary antibiotics (fluoroquinolone or extended-spectrum penicillin derivative) prior to a voiding trial. Such patients are likely to have resistant organisms, as they have often been in the hospital environment.

Nephrostomy tubes are placed directly through the renal parenchyma into the collecting system to provide proximal ipsilateral urinary tract drainage and diversion. They may be placed percutaneously under fluoroscopic, CT, or ultrasound guidance in an interventional radiology suite, or in the operating room as part of a urologic surgical procedure through radiologic, endoscopic, or open techniques. Several types of tube are available and critical care practitioners should know what type of tube they are dealing with. Most commonly used are the loop nephrostomy tubes, which have some type of retention system, usually consisting of a pull-string that is deployed upon tube placement to allow it to be retained effectively within the collecting system. Percutaneously placed tubes are usually in the range of 8 to 12 French in size and are attached to drainage bags with connector tubing. Tubes placed as part of percutaneous stone or other upper tract surgical procedures may be larger; often Foley catheters ranging from 16 to 24 French in size are often employed. In such cases the tube is usually sutured to the skin for retention, as inflating the balloon is problematic in the renal collecting system and may impair drainage or stress or tear the delicate collecting system wall. Critical care practitioners should be entirely clear as to what is expected with regard to such tubes under their care; a conversation with the urologist or whomever is responsible for the tube insertion and familiar with its specific purpose is desirable. Is it expected to drain continuously? What action should be taken if it fails to drain? How should bloody efflux be interpreted or acted upon? The purposes of these tubes may vary from providing a large-bore drain after a bloody percutaneous lithotripsy to a small tube placed only to drain urine for an obstructed ureter. It may be safe to irrigate nephrostomy tubes if they fail to drain, but again, this should be arranged by specific order, and assumptions regarding the purpose and management approach to such tubes introduce unnecessary risk. When irrigating a nephrostomy when it is determined that doing so is safe and appropriate, a small volume of saline (5 to 10 mL) should be utilized. If, in the postoperative urologic surgery setting, a nephrostomy tube begins to drain blood at an alarming rate, the best course of action may be to clamp the tube, address hemodynamics urgently, and urgently call the urologist for instructions. As for other tubes mentioned above, the collecting system will become colonized with bacteria after being indwelling for a week, and clamping trials, manipulation, or tube removal is best done following institution of culture-specific antibiotics.

Internal ureteral stents are commonly used in urology, often for the purpose of relieving ureteral obstruction, but also following urologic surgery or trauma to allow low-pressure drainage or provide urinary diversion while the trauma of surgery or local edema or inflammatory changes are allowed to resolve. The most common variety of stent is the double-J or pigtail stent. These stents have a loop in the bladder and a loop in the kidney. They are placed either retrograde via cystoscopy or antegrade during open or percutaneous surgery, over a guidewire. The proximal and distal coils form upon removal of the guidewire. Typical sizes in adults are 6 to 7 French caliber and 22 to 28 cm length, depending on the patient's height and ureteral length and tortuosity. Some stents include a pull-string on the distal coil, which, at the urologist's discretion, may be either cut short or allowed to exit the external urethral meatus to aid in subsequent removal without requiring repeat cystoscopy. Patient care personnel should be instructed as to the presence of a pull-string and should be aware of the importance of not pulling on it or allowing the patient to do so. Stents are of great value in urologic surgery but they do have their pitfalls, mainly related to their small caliber and proneness to obstruction, the potential for them to migrate and become malpositioned, their tendency to cause unpleasant flank or bladder symptoms, and the risk that they may be forgotten and lost to follow-up. In the critical care setting, the major issues relate to obstruction, migration, or infection. Significant flank pain, chills or fever, or a change in stent position on serial abdominal radiographs should prompt urologic consultation to address these stent-related complications. As discussed in the Immediate Concerns section above, stent occlusion in the setting of obstruction is a surgical emergency that may result in septic picture and require immediate urologic intervention in the form of endoscopic stent replacement or urgent nephrostomy insertion. Stents are typically certified for a 3- to 6-month maximum indwelling time, after which they need to be changed to avoid calcification and obstruction.

Some stents are specifically designed for long indwelling times (e.g., persistent obstructive states such as benign or malignant retroperitoneal fibrosis or postradiation strictures) of up to 12 months. There are stents that combine the function of an externalized nephrostomy and an internal stent; these are usually termed nephrostents or "universal stents." They can be capped at the flank entry point and made to drain internally, or may be uncapped to drain as an externalized nephrostomy tube.

Nephrostomy change or removal and stent change or removal should only be performed by a urologist or interventional radiologist or upon his or her specific direction.

For a patient presenting with upper tract obstruction, the option often exists to observe, or provide relief with stent insertion or nephrostomy placement (21). The decision of how to manage such patients acutely depends on the ability to get the patient to either the cystoscopy suite or the IR suite more expeditiously, the expertise available, and the clinical picture. For patients seriously ill with an obstructed, infected upper tract, many urologists prefer to have IR place a nephrostomy tube percutaneously, control the infection, and then reserve any retrograde instrumentation for an elective setting. If the patient is coagulopathic or anticoagulated, a retrograde cystoscopic approach may be safer, as the radiologist will be quite reticent to enter the kidney percutaneously when the coagulation functions are abnormal for fear of creating a major hemorrhagic complication.

Closed suction drains or Penrose drains may be left in place following urologic surgery to allow external drainage of blood, urine, lymph, or infectious fluid. From the critical care viewpoint, the urologist should be asked specifically what should be expected regarding appropriate function of the drain and exactly what parameters should be a cause for concern. Is significant blood output expected? Is continuous drainage important? Under what circumstances should the surgeon be informed urgently? Urine leaks following certain types of urologic surgery, such as some partial nephrectomies for trauma, may be expected, and if adequately drained externally, seldom constitute an emergency. Elevated blood output may be an indication of internal bleeding and should prompt a call to the surgeon if there is any doubt as to whether the situation is acceptable.

As a general statement to the critical care team, urologic drainage tubes have widely varying purposes and specifications and should be managed in concert with the surgeon who placed them or is responsible for them to avoid confusion and preventable complications.

Any of these tubes may become malpositioned or occluded (often with blood clots or mucus from the bowel segment), requiring intervention.

URINARY DIVERSION MANAGEMENT FROM THE CRITICAL CARE PERSPECTIVE

Beyond the considerations regarding tube diversion or drainage, some patients under the critical care team's care may have undergone, either acutely or remotely, a surgical urinary diversion procedure. The variety of such diversions is considerable, and the critical care team deserves a full explanation of the patient's anatomy and how to deal with any problems that may arise. Problems include urinary outflow obstruction, intra-abdominal urinary extravasation, infectious complications, and problems with the intestinal anastomosis.

One can divide urinary diversion procedures into conduits and reservoirs (and reservoirs into cutaneous and orthotopic). Conduits are simple surgical reconstructions that allow urine to exit to the outside and do not involve an internal urinary reservoir (22).

An **ileal conduit** is one of the most commonly encountered urinary diversions, often performed following cystectomy for lower urinary tract cancer, but also at times for neurogenic or inflammatory disease. In this procedure, a segment of distal ileum is isolated from the fecal stream, followed by a small bowel anastomosis to re-establish intestinal continuity. One end of the isolated segment is closed, and the other end is brought to the skin of the abdominal wall as a stoma. The ureters are sutured into the conduit intra-abdominally to route the urinary stream externally. Most ileal conduits seen acutely by the critical care team in the immediate postsurgical period have indwelling tube drainage present—often externalized stents that enter the stoma, travel up each ureter to allow the ureteroileal anastomosis to heal, and avoid obstruction or urinary extravasation in the early postoperative period. A second tube, often a simple straight catheter segment, may also be placed from outside the stoma to inside the conduit beneath the abdominal wall fascia to allow conduit drainage.

Other conduits employed in urologic surgery may utilize other bowel segments, including jejunum and descending or transverse colon, especially when there has been extensive pelvic irradiation that has damaged the ileum and lower small intestine.

Reservoirs (neobladders) involve the use of larger segments of intestine to fashion a neobladder internally, along with some form of urinary efflux mechanism, often designed to create a continent diversion that the patient can catheterize (and not wear a urinary collection appliance) or that is sutured to the native urethra (in the male or female) to allow restoration of voiding (an "orthotopic neobladder").

While conduits may be complicated by obstruction or urinary leakage as noted above, and the same issues can arise in neobladder reservoirs, the reservoir urinary diversions can develop certain other potentially serious problems including "pouchitis," pouch rupture, and formation of pouch calculi. These issues require specialty input and prompt urologic consultation. The issue of pouch rupture, however, deserves specific mention as this must be promptly recognized. Any patient with signs of abdominal infection or sepsis who has a neobladder should raise the suspicion of pouch rupture. This entity can also be seen in patients who have had an augmentation cystoplasty, in which a segment of bowel is added to the native bladder to increase capacity or deal with severe and intransigent overactive bladder symptoms. Such patients should have urgent urologic assessment, which may involve contrast imaging studies (CT or "pouchography") to rule out urinary leakage intra-abdominally. Broad-spectrum antibiotics should be instituted early in such cases, as the urine is often colonized and intra-abdominal infection may be developing. Many such cases can be managed with tube drainage of the neobladder alone, though in some cases surgical exploration and repair, and/or evacuation of infectious fluid from the abdominal cavity are necessary.

Depending on the type of urinary diversion and the specific segment of the gastrointestinal tract used for the reconstruction, these patients may be at risk for dehydration, and specific electrolyte and metabolic disturbances may be seen (23,24). The significance of these problems is related to the portion of the gastrointestinal tract utilized for the diversion and the length of time the urine is exposed to the bowel surface. Jejunal conduits may result in hyponatremic, hypochloremic metabolic acidosis; this process may be clinically manifested by nausea, vomiting, anorexia, and muscular weakness. When ileum and colon are utilized for the urinary diversion, hyperchloremic metabolic acidosis may be seen. Clinically this may produce weakness, anorexia, vomiting, or Kussmaul breathing, and may progress to coma. This type of process was seen more commonly in the past when ureterosigmoidostomy was a commonly used form of diversion. With appropriate metabolic management, it is much less commonly noted with contemporary conduit or continent diversions. When gastric segments are utilized for urinary diversion, dehydration and hyponatremic metabolic alkalosis may occur, requiring replacement of sodium and chloride through intravenous salt administration.

Other metabolic abnormalities seen with urinary diversion procedures include bile salt metabolism following ileal resection, which can affect fat digestion and uptake of vitamins A and D. Malabsorption and steatorrhea and a propensity to develop cholelithiasis may also be associated with ileal resection. Gastric or ileal resection may cause vitamin B_{12} deficiency, which can lead to megaloblastic anemia and peripheral nerve dysfunction; B_{12} nutritional supplementation may be indicated.

Other complications include stomal complications, recurrent upper tract urinary infection and deteriorating renal function, and calculus formation in the upper tract or the diversion conduit or reservoir. Stomal stenosis may cause obstructive uropathy requiring catheterization and stomal revision. Catheter insertion into a conduit or reservoir construct may be challenging; if difficulty is encountered, a small-bore coude catheter may be useful, as may use of fluoroscopy to guide catheter positioning. Stomal bleeding is usually superficial and manageable with local compression or minimal cautery when necessary. Parastomal hernias may occasionally become incarcerated requiring urgent surgical intervention. Azotemia and upper tract dilation may be problematic, especially when more than 10 years have elapsed since the diversion. Upper tract deterioration is seen in at least 50% of patients who have undergone urinary diversion during childhood or young adult years, and the risk of developing chronic renal insufficiency is increased in such patients. Calculi occur in roughly 8% to 10% of urinary diversion or bladder substitution patients, where urease-producing organisms (*Proteus, Pseudomonas, Klebsiella,* etc.) are common affecting organisms.

UROSEPSIS AND COMPLEX UROGENITAL INFECTION IN THE CRITICAL CARE SETTING

Urosepsis has been addressed in several sections within this chapter, related to immediate concerns, urologic tubes and drains, and below in renal failure management. It is also addressed elsewhere in this text with regard to general management principles for sepsis and septic shock (2,25,26). In addition, there are several specific urologic infectious disease phenomena that warrant specific mention.

Specific Infectious Processes of the Upper and Lower Urinary Tract

The combination of obstruction and infection of the upper and lower urinary tract requires urgent drainage, antibiotic therapy, and supportive care. Initial empiric antibiotic therapy for presumed urosepsis must address the likely offending organisms and must consider the "worst-case scenario" from the bacteriologic standpoint. While awaiting culture data, Gram stain findings can also be very helpful in selecting initial therapy. Broad-spectrum antibiotics that cover aerobic Gram-negative rods and the typical Gram-positive cocci that appear as uropathogens are critical. If the patient has been recently instrumented, has been recently hospitalized, or has other risk factors for having sepsis due to atypical or resistant pathogens, coverage should be expanded accordingly. The newer-generation cephalosporins, imipenem and related drugs, aminoglycosides, and vancomycin are commonly used in such circumstances. It may be necessary in certain situations to consider the presence of anaerobic infections of the genitourinary system. Sepsis following transrectal prostate biopsy procedures (typically ultrasound guided and office based) may introduce the risk of anaerobic infection. We are aware of mortality cases where a patient presented with urosepsis and retroperitoneal cellulitis following a needle biopsy of the prostate, in which anaerobic coverage was not provided and ultimately death from *Bacteroides fragilis* infection occurred. Anaerobic infection of the urinary tract has also been described outside the setting of iatrogenic rectal violation, so this uncommon scenario is worth bearing in mind (27). Staphylococcal infections of the urinary system do also occur, particularly in the elderly or immunocompromised population, or in patients who have iatrogenic manipulation, which may result in the entry of skin flora into the urinary system (percutaneous lithotripsy, suprapubic cystostomy tube presence). When a Gram-positive coccus is noted on stained urine or infectious fluid, vancomycin is an appropriate empiric choice for sepsis of urinary tract origin, as both *Enterococcus* and *Staphylococcus* species are usually covered. Fungal organisms should be considered especially in the diabetic patient and in the patient who has had extensive antibiotic therapy. Fluconazole is an appropriate empiric coverage agent pending culture results.

In addition to supportive care and antibiotic management, prompt drainage of the urinary tract is critical in certain conditions of urinary infection and urosepsis (28). When either upper or lower tract obstruction is present with urosepsis, prompt imaging of the urinary tract should be obtained (noncontrast CT of the abdomen and pelvis or renal ultrasound, bladder ultrasound to exclude retention) (29). Rapid decline in clinical status may ensue if there is a delay in instituting prompt drainage of an infected, obstructed system (30). We encourage our medical colleagues to practice the principle that the "sun never sets" on an obstructed, infected urinary tract. Uncertainty occasionally arises when there is incomplete obstruction (evidenced by contrast passing beyond a stone on an imaging study) and the patient is clinically stable. The goal is to provide low-pressure drainage of the infected system since the patient can still deteriorate even when some urine is progressing beyond the point of obstruction. Whether to drain the upper tract through cystoscopy and stent placement versus percutaneous nephrostomy, or the lower tract through transurethral catheter placement or suprapubic tube insertion, reflects a set of clinical judgments that varies from case to case. The available facilities and expertise, promptness of access to resources, coagulation status, and clinical instability and mobility all come into play in selecting the best approach to draining the urinary tract emergently. One major potential diagnostic pitfall occurs when a patient has complete unilateral upper tract obstruction with a negative urinalysis, as no urine from the obstructed system enters the bladder, and the urinary tract origin of sepsis is therefore not suspected. While one can argue the cost effectiveness of routine abdominal imaging of septic patients with an unknown source, such a policy does avoid the potential for missing upper tract obstruction, potentially with a preventable poor outcome.

Certain specific infectious processes of the urinary tract deserve mention with regard to their relevance to the critical care provider (31,32). Emphysematous pyelonephritis and cystitis are infections of the kidney and bladder, respectively, which result in gas formation within the tissues. The presence of gas in the urinary tract may be due to gas-forming infection, previous instrumentation, or fistula. The clinical situation will usually lead to the correct etiology. Gas-forming infections in the upper tract may represent a range of infectious processes: emphysematous pyelitis describes infection that results in gas within the collecting system, whereas emphysematous pyelonephritis describes gas within the renal parenchyma (which may progress into the perinephric space or other sites in the retroperitoneum). The most commonly seen organism in such infections is not the classic anaerobes, but *Escherichia coli*, which may enter into a state of facultative anaerobic metabolism, especially in a diabetic when severe hyperglycemia is present. These patients may become severely ill and require aggressive resuscitation and sometimes drainage procedures or occasionally urgent nephrectomy; urologic consultation is essential. Emphysematous cystitis reflects the same bacteriologic basis and propensity for the diabetic patient as for the renal counterpart. Bladder catheter drainage and aggressive antibiotic management will usually correct the process.

Acute papillary necrosis may also be seen in a diabetic due to microvascular renal disease that affects the vasculature of the renal papillae and pyramids, though other underlying conditions include excessive use of certain analgesics. When accompanied by infection, these patients behave like those with ureteral colic from calculous disease, and will often require drainage and decompression of the urinary tract along with aggressive medical management. Sloughed papillae may dwell within the renal collecting system and undergo surface calcification, often resembling typical calculous disease, though the changes in the appearance of the calyces due to the sloughed papilla are indicative.

Renal and perinephric abscesses are important causes of urosepsis, and one must have a high index of suspicion in the setting of incomplete resolution of upper tract urinary infection with standard antibiotic regimens, prompting imaging to detect an undrained source of relapsing or persistent infection. CT scanning is significantly superior to ultrasound for imaging the perinephric space, and is preferable when an abscess is suspected. Small renal parenchymal abscesses not causing a septic picture may resolve with antibiotic treatment alone. Large parenchymal abscesses or perinephric collections usually require drainage, which in most cases can be appropriately attempted by CT- or ultrasound-guided percutaneous drainage. When multiloculated or when inadequately drained by the percutaneous route, an open surgical drainage procedure may be necessary.

Acute prostatitis may be categorized by etiology (bacterial, abacterial) or clinical course and manifestations (acute, chronic) (33,34). Acute bacterial prostatitis can present with a septic picture. Common symptoms include dysuria, frequency, urgency, chills and fever, elevated white blood count on CBC, and infected urine. Some urologists believe that urethral catheterization and instrumentation should be avoided in such patients due to concern of worsening sepsis. If the patient is emptying adequately, antibiotic administration is usually adequate without catheter drainage. If the patient is in acute urinary retention, bladder drainage is needed; one can proceed either with a gentle attempt at Foley catheter passage per urethra or with percutaneous suprapubic cystostomy placement. Our view is that urethral catheterization is usually preferable and is less invasive. For patients presenting with acute prostatitis or other complex lower tract infection who do not respond appropriately to antibiotic therapy, or for those with suspicious findings on a digital rectal examination (DRE), prostatic abscess should be suspected. The findings of concern on DRE would include unusual tenderness and/or an area of fluctuance on prostatic palpation. One should avoid an aggressive prostate exam on such patients, and it is generally ill-advised to put significant digital pressure on the tender, acutely infected prostate to obtain a sample of expressed prostatic secretion as is often done in the chronic prostatitis patient. Acute prostatitis patients usually have infected urine and culture information from prostatic secretions is usually not necessary. Transrectal ultrasound or CT scanning of the pelvis will usually confirm the presence of a prostatic abscess when present, and can also guide therapy by revealing whether the abscess cavity may be best drained through a transurethral, transperineal, or transrectal route. We usually prefer the transurethral approach if the cavity is abutting the prostatic urethral lumen. A transperineal drainage procedure can be performed under ultrasound guidance if the abscess is deep and a transurethral approach is deemed too risky. Unless the abscess has already started to drain spontaneously into the rectal lumen, we do not favor this approach to prostatic abscess drainage.

Acute infectious conditions involving the genitalia and perineum are important both with regard to the challenges sometimes faced in differential diagnosis (e.g., epididymitis vs. torsion, trauma, or incarcerated hernia) and systemic management as in some conditions (e.g., Fournier gangrene). Acute epididymitis or epididymo-orchitis may be due to standard enteric bacteria (more common in patients over age 35 and those with obstructive urethral or prostatic disease) or to venereal transmission of chlamydial or gonococcal infection. Mild epididymitis can be treated on an ambulatory basis with antibiotics (often fluoroquinolone if enteric infection is suspected, tetracycline derivative if venereal transmission is more likely, or a combination of two drugs if coverage for both entities is desired while awaiting culture data). Severe epididymo-orchitis is manifested by global enlargement of the hemiscrotal contents and loss of palpable anatomic landmarks, often with skin fixation and marked redness and tenderness. Such patients find it very painful to walk or stand, and may be best managed by hospitalization, bedrest, scrotal elevation, anti-inflammatory drugs, and broad-spectrum antibiotics until improvement is observed. Scrotal ultrasound examination may be useful for clarifying the diagnosis and excluding the presence of abscess formation, which may require surgical drainage and sometimes orchiectomy.

Urologic Involvement in Complex Soft Tissue Infectious Processes

Urologic involvement with such entities as perirectal abscess or Fournier gangrene is common. Fournier gangrene may be idiopathic with no identifiable point of origin, or may be due to extension from primary rectal, urinary, intra-abdominal, or retroperitoneal processes. Diabetics are at increased risk for this disease. When there is genital, perineal, or groin involvement in such processes, several applicable management principles may be of value to the critical care provider or acute care surgeon. Such patients should be treated with broad-spectrum ("triple antibiotic") regimens that cover aerobes, anaerobes, and Gram-positive and -negative organisms, as polymicrobial infection is the norm. These patients require a combination of aggressive antibiotic therapy, metabolic and fluid resuscitation, and prompt and aggressive surgical debridement and drainage. These infectious processes can progress very rapidly, and delays in bringing the patient to surgery may result in loss of otherwise salvageable tissues and increased mortality. The surgical approach for this entity in our institution is based on the areas of involvement and typically includes the urology and general surgery teams in a close collaboration to address our areas of anatomic specialty expertise (surgery performing proctoscopy and addressing debridement of involved abdominal wall, rectal, ischiorectal fossa, thigh, or buttock tissues; urology performing cystoscopy as indicated and addressing genital and perineal debridement). We believe the advantages of this specialty focus assists in functional and organ preservation, and subsequent reconstructive efforts. When an abscess or necrotizing process extends into the region of the perineum or genital soft tissues, incision or debridement of scrotal or penile skin and underlying dartos may be necessary. In the scrotum, we try to establish a dissection plan just superficial to the parietal tunica vaginalis and keep this membrane, which surrounds the testes, intact. The testes are rarely involved in these soft tissue infections, and not directly exposing the testes to the wound will aid in subsequent wound management and avoid the pain and dessication that occurs when the testis is exposed externally. On the penis, necrotic skin and dartos may be debrided up to the coronal sulcus when necessary, taking care to stay superficial to the Buck fascia (deep fascial layer) of the penis, to avoid injury to the corpora and the dorsal neurovascular bundle, which lies in a wide band across the center on the top of the penis. Fournier gangrene may occasionally arise from a urethral source (such as a periurethral abscess or perforated stricture or diverticulum). Debridement of urethral tissue should be avoided unless it is grossly necrotic, as a superficial exudate may create the appearance of marginally perfused tissue; such changes can be reassessed on take-back to the operating room and allowed to declare themselves further into the course of the disease. If the surgeon must enter the scrotal wall for drainage of a local abscess, it is best to avoid deep incision into the tunica vaginalis compartment to avoid preventable injury to the scrotal contents.

As general considerations for the patient with urosepsis, there is the potential that the patient's hemodynamics and degree of severity of sepsis may transiently worsen following needed urinary tract drainage or manipulation. A low threshold to have such patients in an ICU setting is appropriate even if they are not so critically ill that they initially clearly need ICU management. For example, if we perform percutaneous nephrostomy insertion or ureteral stent placement in a patient with infection, an obstructing stone, tachycardia, and fever, especially when addressed "after hours," we will arrange ICU observation overnight to ensure that any deterioration is promptly recognized and managed. When culture data become available, broad-spectrum empiric antibiotic regimens should be simplified based on bacteriologic identification and sensitivities. Tubes that are placed into the urinary tract to drain infected spaces must be appropriately secured to the patient to avoid inadvertent malposition or removal and observed to avoid kinking or occlusion of outflow systems, which may prevent low-pressure drainage and exacerbate sepsis.

UROLOGIC CAUSE OF RENAL FAILURE

The urologist's view of renal failure is usually focused on "postrenal" factors, as this is the setting in which we are typically consulted. At times, however, it is unclear whether a patient with acute renal failure is suffering from an obstructive process, whether the process is remediable, and how best to approach therapy.

Assessment and management of acute renal failure are covered in detail elsewhere in this text. The urologist is typically consulted when there is suspicion or evidence that the state of renal failure is due to a mechanical or vascular etiology usually manifested by significant oliguria and distention of some level of the urinary tract.

If a Foley catheter is in place in a patient with impaired urine output, palpation of the lower abdomen to detect bladder distention, ultrasound assessment of bladder volume, and/or irrigation of the catheter to ensure patency are appropriate initial steps. Management of catheter-related dysfunction is discussed in detail above. If uncertainty remains as to the appropriate positioning or function of an indwelling catheter, urologic consultation should be obtained.

If lower tract or bladder catheter malfunction has been excluded, one must exclude upper urinary tract obstruction. Renal ultrasound or noncontrast CT scanning is commonly employed for this purpose. The findings of hydronephrosis or ureteral dilatation raise concerns about the possibility of postrenal failure. It is important to appreciate that ureteral obstruction can exist without significant collecting system dilation in some cases, particularly if the obstructive process is of very recent onset. Patients with two normally functioning kidneys should not develop renal failure in the face of unilateral upper tract obstruction; in fact, complete obstruction of one ureter often causes little or no change in serum creatinine if the contralateral kidney is functionally normal. Unilateral upper tract obstruction involving a solitary kidney (or marked hypofunction of the contralateral kidney) may result in anuria and renal failure. In most such cases, radiographic evidence of underlying inadequacy of the contralateral kidney is evident (atrophy, long-standing obstruction with hydronephrosis and marked parenchymal thinning). In entities that can cause asymmetric and asynchronous development of obstructive uropathy (advancing prostate cancer with trigonal invasion, progressive pelvic lymphadenopathy, asymmetric retroperitoneal fibrosis with extrinsic ureteral compression), unrecognized loss of function of one kidney may result from obstruction without symptoms or much change in serum creatinine. Only when the remaining kidney becomes obstructed and renal failure ensues is the entire process recognized.

When evidence of upper tract obstruction is noted, one must expeditiously implement a strategy to determine definitively if postrenal obstruction is present, and choose the least morbid means of relieving it. The gold standard for such determination is to perform cystoscopy and retrograde pyelography. This procedure can be performed in the operating room setting using static or fluoroscopic imaging capability, or at the bedside in the ICU. We have successfully performed flexible cystoscopy, retrograde pyelography, guidewire insertion and manipulation past a point of obstruction, and internal or externalized stent placement in the ICU. This approach is especially applicable in the hemodynamically unstable patient for whom movement to the operating room may be hazardous. The newer digital X-ray units are ideally suited for such procedures, as the digital plate is placed beneath the patient once, allowing multiple images to be obtained and viewed on the monitor almost immediately. If an obstructed or tortuous ureter is encountered, the area of difficulty may often be navigated using a 5 French open-ended catheter through which an angle-tipped guidewire is advanced. Rotating the guidewire may allow passage across an area of ureter that is not possible using straight wires or catheters. Once a guidewire has been advanced past the complex ureter into the kidney, either an open-ended catheter or a double-J type internal stent may be inserted over the wire. Open-ended catheters may be tied to a Foley catheter for stability and attached to an external drainage appliance.

An alternative to achieving upper tract drainage cystoscopically is to have a percutaneous nephrostomy tube placed through interventional radiology techniques. It is important that the patient's coagulation functions be normal when pursuing such an approach, and it is also important to verify that there is, in fact, upper tract obstruction present, before introducing the risk of a percutaneous puncture. In the appropriate clinical setting, where there is certainty that upper tract drainage is needed, PCNL is an important option, and may be preferable to achieving drainage through lower tract instrumentation when dealing with urosepsis or challenging lower tract anatomy where manipulation may be difficult (gross hematuria, some cases of prior lower tract surgery, permanent urinary diversion states). It is usually necessary for the patient to be prone on the radiology table to accomplish PCNL placement, and one must determine if such a position is safe or advisable. Respiratory compromise, recent abdominal surgery, or body habitus may create major challenges in placing the patient prone for such a procedure.

When lower or upper tract drainage is achieved in the setting of postrenal failure, one must observe the patient closely for transient worsening of urosepsis and for the possibility of pathologic postobstructive diuresis. Worsening of sepsis can result from instrumenting the infected urinary tract, and supportive measures may be necessary, including the institution of pressor support. Adequate hydration prior to urinary tract manipulation and provision of prophylactic antibiotics will minimize the risk of worsening sepsis with instrumentation. Pathologic postobstructive diuresis may occur when there is a major solute load and severe obligatory water loss occurs following relief of obstruction. This can be seen with lower tract or bilateral upper tract obstruction. Fluid and electrolyte monitoring and judicious fluid replacement may be necessary during the diuresis period.

Acute papillary necrosis may result in acute renal failure. Papillary necrosis may develop as a gradually progressive, indolent process, recognized by the classic cavitary appearance of the renal calyces on contrast studies, or may present as a fulminant, infectious course with urosepsis and obstruction from sloughed papillae. Relief of obstruction, treatment of infection, and supportive care are indicated.

Other entities for which urologic input may be valuable when acute renal failure occurs include vasculogenic renal failure (due to renal artery or renal vein thrombosis) and abdominal compartment syndrome–related renal failure. Both are covered elsewhere in this text. An important pitfall in diagnosis occurs when a patient presents with abrupt onset of flank pain, nonfunction of the ipsilateral kidney is noted in intravenous pyelography, and the presumptive diagnosis of renal colic from stone is declared. In fact, complete nonfunction is as uncommon as an IVP finding from ureteral obstruction; more commonly, a persistent nephrogram with delayed excretion is observed. Complete nonfunction may be due to vascular compromise of the kidney either from primary arterial occlusion or renal vein thrombosis, which leads to microvascular occlusion and nonfunction. One should be suspicious of renovascular compromise whenever acute onset of flank pain occurs. Contrast-enhanced CT scanning is diagnostic, as the affected kidney will fail to opacify. When vascular compromise of the kidney occurs, urgent vascular surgical and interventional radiologic consultation should be obtained to determine if immediate revascularization is feasible and warranted.

SUMMARY

Critical care issues in urology are many and varied. The critical care provider must be familiar with the anatomic and physiologic factors that are relevant to urologic disease, and must have a low threshold to request urologic consultation when specialty expertise may be of value to the patient. Recognition of obstructive, infectious, and ischemic entities for which time-sensitive intervention is important is most essential for the critical care provider. In the postoperative setting, issues common to other surgical specialties are relevant to urology patients, and various specialty-specific problems may also arise, often related to renal dysfunction, the complexities of endoscopic and reconstructive surgery, and perioperative infection. Urologic residency training in the United States provides a strong background in critical care knowledge and skills, as all urology residents spend 1 to 2 years in general surgery and related specialties, including exposure to surgical intensive care experience. The field of critical care requires an enormous breadth of knowledge and capability, however, and the practicing urologist and his or her patients may benefit greatly from the input and expertise of those specializing in the care of critical care patients. A close collaboration between these specialties greatly enhances the quality of urologic patient care.

References

1. Hicks D, Li CY. Management of macroscopic haematuria in the emergency department. *Emerg Med J*. 2007;24:385–390.
2. Coburn M, Zimmerman JL. Sepsis and septic shock in the urology patient. *Am Urol Assoc Update Series*. 2002;XXI(14).
3. Cummings JM, et al. Adult testicular torsion. *J Urol*. 2002;167:2109.
4. Marcozzi D, Suner S. The nontraumatic acute scrotum. *Emerg Med Clin North Am*. 2001;19:547.
5. Philips P, Amaral J. Abdominal access complications in laparoscopic surgery. *J Am Coll Surgeons*. 2001;192:525.
6. Coburn M. Genitourinary Trauma. In: Moore EE, Feliciano DV, Mattox KL, eds. *Trauma*. 5th ed. New York: McGraw Hill; 2004.
7. Coburn M, Guerriero WG. Complications in genitourinary trauma. In: Mattox KL, ed. *Complications of Trauma*. New York: Churchill Livingstone; 1994.
8. Kuno K, Menzin A, Kauder HH, et al. Prophylactic ureteral catheterization in gynecologic surgery. *Urology*. 1998;52:1004–1008.
9. Ahn JH, Morey AF, McAninch JW. Workup and management of traumatic hematuria. *Emerg Med Clin North Am*. 1998;15:145.
10. Chapple CR, Png D. Contemporary management of urethral trauma and post-traumatic stricture. *Curr Opin Urol*. 1999;9:253.
11. Gomez RG, Ceballos L, Coburn M, et al. Consensus statement of bladder injuries. *Br J Urol Int*. 2004;94:27.
12. Brandes S, Coburn M, Armenakas N, et al. Diagnosis and management of ureteric injury: an evidenced-based analysis. *Br J Urol Int*. 2004;94:277.
13. Kawashima A, et al. Imaging of renal trauma: a comprehensive review. *Radiographics*. 2001;21:557.
14. Moore EE, et al. Organ injury scaling: spleen, liver, kidney. *J Trauma*. 1989; 29:1664.
15. Santucci RA, McAninch JW. Grade IV renal injuries: evaluation, treatment and outcome. *World J Surg*. 2001;25:1562.
16. Knudson MM, et al. Outcome after major renovascular injuries: a Western Trauma Association multicenter report. *J Trauma*. 2000;49:1116.
17. Coburn M. Damage control for urologic injuries. *Surg Clin North Am*. 1997;77:821–834.
18. Coburn M. Genitourinary trauma—minimally invasive alternatives. In: Moore RG, Bischoff JT, Loening S, et al., eds. *Minimally Invasive Urologic Surgery*. New York: Taylor & Francis Group; 2005.
19. Bloom DA, McGuire EJ, Lapides J. A brief history of urethral catheterization. *J Urol*. 1994;151:317.
20. Bjerklund TE, Cek M, Naber K, et al. Prevalence of hospital-acquired urinary tract infections in urology departments. *Eur Urol*. 2007;51:1100–1111.
21. Lopez Cubillana P. What is the best method for urgent urinary diversion in patients with obstruction and infection due to ureteral colic? *Urol Int*. 2001; 66:178.
22. Bloom DA, Grossman HB, Konnak JW. Stomal construction and reconstruction. *Urol Clin North Am*. 1986;13:275.
23. Hall MC, Koch MO, McDougal WS. Metabolic consequences of urinary diversion through intestinal segments. *Urol Clin N Am*. 1991;18:25.
24. Stein R, et al. Long-term metabolic effects in patients with urinary diversion. *World J Urol*. 1998;16:292.
25. Nicolle L. AMMI Canada Guideline Committee: complicated urinary tract infection in adults. *Can J Infect Dis Med Microbiol*. 2005;16:349–360.
26. Wagenlehner FM, Weidner W, Naber KG. Optimal management of urosepsis from the urological perspective. *Int J Antimicrob Agents*. 2007;30:390–397.
27. Brook I. Urinary tract and genito-urinary suppurative infections due to anaerobic bacteria. *Int J Urol*. 2004;11:133–141.
28. Watson RA, Esposito M, Richter F, et al. Percutaneous nephrostomy as adjunct management in advanced upper urinary tract infection. *Urology*. 1999; 54:234–239.
29. Rubenstein JN, Schaeffer AJ. Managing complicated urinary tract infections: the urologic view. *Infect Dis Clin North Am*. 2003;17:333–351.
30. Abramson S, et al. Impact in the emergency department of unenhanced CT on diagnostic confidence and therapeutic efficacy in patients with suspected renal colic. A prospective study. *Am J Roentgenol*. 2000;175:1689.
31. Stapleton A. Urinary tract infections in patients with diabetes. *Am J Med*. 2002;113(Suppl 1A):80S–84S.
32. Wan YL, et al. Predictors of outcome in emphysematous pyelonephritis. *J Urol*. 1998;159:369.
33. Ludwig M. Diagnosis and therapy of acute prostatitis, epididymitis and orchitis. *Andrologia*. 2008;40:76–80.
34. Barozzi L, et al. Prostatic abscess: diagnosis and treatment. *Am J Roentgenol*. 1998;170:753.

CHAPTER 87 ■ FACIAL TRAUMA

M. BARBARA HONNEBIER

Facial trauma is any injury of the midface, including the maxillary complex. Panfacial injuries involve trauma to the upper, middle, and lower facial bones. Although injuries to the mandible often accompany other facial injuries, mandibular trauma is usually discussed as a separate entity. Injuries to the frontal bone and frontal sinus are also discussed separately since they are often complicated by injuries to the cranial vault and violate the intracranial space. Often, such distinctions based on anatomic boundaries (1) are used for the sake of organization, as injuries to the nasal cavity or sinuses, orbits, and ethmoids may also involve violations of the cranium and cranial space.

Facial trauma may present in clinically different ways: with lacerations of skin and soft tissues, obstruction of the nasal cavity or sinuses, problems with vision, and problems with occlusion, which often are more outward manifestations of underlying facial fractures. Maxillofacial injury may result from both penetrating and blunt trauma. Comprehensive management and treatment of facial trauma involves airway control, control of bleeding, reduction of swelling, prevention of infection, repair of soft tissue lacerations, and repair of bone fractures to restore function and esthetic form to the face. The aim of this chapter is to discuss the potential pitfalls and problems that facial injuries may create. The operative management of facial fractures has undergone many changes in the last decade. With the advent of rigid fixation and continued new technologies, detailed discussions of methods of operative reconstruction of different types of facial fractures are best discussed in specialty textbooks.

PATHOPHYSIOLOGY

In the treatment of a patient with multiple maxillofacial injuries, it is critical to differentiate injuries that require immediate operative intervention from those for which operation can be deferred. However, immediate intervention may be indicated for stabilization. Procedures that require an extensive workup are delayed until the patient is clinically stable.

The most essential component of initial care begins with the ABC's (airway, breathing, circulation), as well as cervical spine assessment. As with any other trauma patient, the facial trauma patient should be evaluated in a systematic and comprehensive fashion in cooperation with the trauma team. Although rare, isolated facial trauma may be severe and life threatening. Critical facial injuries are usually obvious upon presentation (e.g., gunshot wound to the face, profuse bleeding from orifices). Abdominal, thoracic, cervical spine, and neurosurgical emergencies take priority over maxillofacial injury. If possible, a detailed history of the event and past medical history should be obtained from the patient, paramedics, and/or family members. Dental records are typically difficult to obtain but very helpful in diagnosis and treatment planning.

Particularly in the facial trauma patient, early airway control and neurologic assessment of a potential head injury are critical because the eyes and oropharynx are the "shock organs" of the face and development of facial edema will obscure the pupils and obstruct the upper airway. Immediate treatment of maxillofacial trauma patients is indicated in the following situations: (a) airway compromise, (b) severe hemorrhage, (c) large open wounds, (d) superior orbital fissure and orbital apex syndrome, (e) mandibular condylar impaction into the cranial fossa, and (f) if urgent surgical procedures need to be performed by other services.

CONTRAINDICATIONS

Definitive treatment of maxillofacial injuries is delayed if the patient has severe, concomitant, and/or undetermined systemic trauma. Definitive treatment of facial fractures can be delayed as much as 2 weeks after injury as long as the fractures do not violate the cranial space (2). Patients with neurologic or cranial injury are operated on when stable. Blood volume, electrolytes, and acid-base problems should all be addressed prior to the surgical procedure. In addition, the resolution of facial edema and perineural contusion during this period of time allows for a much more accurate evaluation and simplifies surgical planning and operative treatment.

EPIDEMIOLOGY: CAUSES, INCIDENCE, AND RISK FACTORS

Facial trauma is multifactorial with a variety of etiologies ranging from sports, falls, penetrating injuries, assaults, and violence, to motor vehicle accidents. The incidence and frequency of any specific etiology varies with culture and within geographic regions. Prominent factors include lifestyle, population density, and socioeconomic status. Urban trauma centers evaluate and treat many facial trauma patients on a daily basis. Many university hospitals are well known for their high volume of facial fracture management (3). Oral and maxillofacial surgery, plastic surgery, and otolaryngology services are heavily consulted by the emergency department and trauma team to assist with management of facial injuries. A large body of research has focused on data collection regarding types of facial trauma and studies on the outcome and morbidity associated with the treatment of facial fractures. Data regarding age, race, gender, social habits, mechanism of injury, and incidence of previous facial trauma are available from many centers in many countries (4). In most urban areas, mandible fractures account for the majority of injuries, followed by lacerations and miscellaneous facial injuries. Interpersonal violence is the primary cause of injury and motor vehicle accidents are the next most frequent culprit. Half of the patients who experience facial injuries as victims of assault are likely to have interpersonal violence and have a high likelihood for a future injury (5).

AIRWAY MANAGEMENT

The possibility of cervical spine injury makes airway management more complex in the facial trauma patient. Spinal injuries are increased fourfold if there is a clinically significant head injury (Glasgow coma scale [GCS] score <9). A cervical spine injury should be suspected in all patients involving forced blunt trauma. Cervical spine injury may be occult, in which case secondary injury to the spinal cord must be avoided. Immobilization of the cervical spine must be instituted immediately until a complete clinical and radiologic evaluation has excluded injury (6).

A fully conscious, coherent patient is maintaining his or her own airway. Because overall status may deteriorate at any time, the ABC's must constantly be reassessed. The following subsets of patients require immediate securement of airway to prevent respiratory failure: (a) patients with GCS score <9, (b) patients with sustained seizure activity, (c) patients with unstable midface trauma, (d) patients with direct injuries to the airway, (e) patients with aspiration risk or unable to maintain an airway, and (f) patients with oxygenation problems. In the facial trauma patient, the clinical urgency of airway maintenance may interfere with the proper planning of the safest and most appropriate technique to use for securing the airway, but airway must take precedence.

The airway should be cleared of debris, foreign bodies (teeth), blood, and secretions. The classic "chin lift" or "jaw thrust" maneuvers are commonly employed for assessment of airway patency and to remove obstruction of the tongue base. However, jaw thrust and chin lift may cause distraction of at least 5 mm in a cadaver with C5–6 instability that is unaffected by the use of a rigid collar (6). Manual in-line axial stabilization must therefore be maintained throughout. Bag and mask ventilation also produce significant degrees of cervical spine movement at zones of instability. The "sniffing the morning air" position for standard endotracheal intubation should similarly be avoided as it flexes the lower cervical spine and extends the occiput on the atlas. Atlanto-occipital extension is necessary to visualize the vocal cords. Patients with unstable C1 or C2 injuries might therefore be at more risk from this technique. The hard C-collar may interfere with intubation efforts. If necessary, the front part of the collar can be removed to facilitate intubation as long as manual stabilization remains in effect.

The safest method of securing an endotracheal tube remains debatable. The Advanced Trauma Life Support (ATLS) recommends a nasotracheal tube in the spontaneously breathing patient, and orotracheal intubation in the apneic patient. Orotracheal intubation is the fastest and surest method of intubating the trachea and therefore the more commonly used method. At Shock Trauma in Baltimore, Maryland, more than 3,000 patients were intubated orally with a modified rapid sequence induction technique with preoxygenation and cricoid pressure. Ten percent of these patients were found to have cervical spine injury and none deteriorated neurologically following intubation (7). Blind nasal intubation is ultimately successful in 90% of patients but requires multiple attempts in up to 90% of these. Nasotracheal intubation is (relatively) contraindicated in patients with potential skull base fractures or unstable midface injuries that typically involve the naso-orbito-ethmoid (NOE) complex. The same holds true for the use of nasogastric tube placement. Any paranasal manipulation may notoriously produce or recreate local hemorrhage, making airway manipulations difficult or impossible. Inadvertent placement and contamination/violation of the cranial space is a theoretical possibility.

Nasotracheal intubation in nontrauma patients is often accomplished by rotating or flexing the neck to align the tube correctly. In the trauma patient, this requires prior cervical spine clearance. Local anesthetic preparation of the airway is also time consuming and might increase the risk of aspiration. Laryngeal mask airway (LMA) does not protect the airway from aspiration, and by acting as a bolus in the pharynx, may increase esophageal reflux. The need for a surgical airway should be recognized and obtained without delay. A percutaneous needle cricothyroidotomy with high-flow oxygen is indicated in emergency situations when standard tracheotomy is not feasible or advisable. The potential for carbon dioxide retention with this technique must be remembered and the levels in arterial samples monitored. Studies on movement of the neck during cricothyroidotomy, ease of cricothyroidotomy with neck immobilization, or neurologic deterioration following cricothyroidotomy are lacking. If identification of anatomic landmarks is ambiguous, one should proceed with standard tracheotomy or needles, if time is of the essence. Cricothyroidotomy is contraindicated in laryngeal or tracheal trauma, cervical infection, and young children, but unfortunately is necessary if unable to intubate. A standard tracheotomy is essential in unstable patients who require prolonged maxillomandibular fixation for fracture stabilization and management.

LIFE-THREATENING HEMORRHAGE AND BLEEDING FROM FACIAL FRACTURES

In the multisystem-injured patient, hemorrhage is the most common cause of hypovolemia. Hemorrhage can be external or internal into body cavities. Because the face and neck have a rich vascular supply, injuries in these areas can lead to substantial blood loss. Major hemorrhage can result from large scalp wounds, nasal or midface fractures, and penetrating wounds. As opposed to bleeding into body cavities, hemorrhage in the head and neck area is almost always immediately detectable in the trauma bay on clinical examination and often external in nature. Hence, external hemorrhage can usually be controlled by direct pressure to the wound and/or bleeding areas. Pressure can also be applied proximal to major arteries if direct pressure to the wound is not effective.

Scalp wounds are notorious for large amounts of blood loss in a short time if the galea is involved. Scalp wounds can be rapidly approximated with 2.0 nonabsorbable sutures (nylon, Prolene) or staples if available. Sutures should be placed away from the wound edge to ensure hemostasis as the galea tends to retract. Direct pressure over the wound can be applied as well. The patient can be stabilized first before continuing with further diagnostic studies.

Nasal fractures and midface fractures can result in tearing of the ethmoidal arteries. Most of these can be controlled with direct pressure or packing. Nasal packing can be made of gauze, foam, or cotton. The term "packing" refers to commercially available gauze strips or cotton pledgets that are packed as they are inserted into the nasal cavity via the nares to form a compression plug. Packings may be made by cutting the fingers of a sterile examination glove and stuffing with gauze. Nasal packing may be coated with petrolatum, antibiotic ointment, or agents such as lidocaine and thrombin that aid in hemostasis and clot formation. Preformed foam nasal packs may have small tubes in the center of the pack to allow nasal breathing while the packing is in place as nasal packing prevents air exchange through the nose. Nonintubated patients with nasal packing in place should have the head of the bed elevated 30 degrees and be observed and monitored for respiratory distress. Continued bleeding may not be apparent on the nasal side of the packing. Nasal packing easily slips posteriorly with swallowing or out with movement or sneezing. The posterior oropharynx should be checked regularly.

Fractures of the posterior maxillary wall, as in LeFort I and II fractures, may be associated with profuse bleeding from the internal maxillary artery. Bleeding from this artery can be very difficult to control by gauze packing. Epinephrine and liquid thrombin can be added to the packing and the head elevated to help achieve hemostasis. However, a postnasal pack has to be used to treat the bleeding in the postnasal area. This is a difficult area to pack. A balloon catheter can be passed through the nose and pulled out through the mouth. The safety and length of nasal packing is not evidence based. In rhinoplasty surgery, nasal stents and packs are routinely left in place for 7 to 10 days. Complications can be packing related. The most common complication of nasal packing is that removal of the packing dislodges healing tissue and causes recurrent hemorrhage. Hypoxemia and hypercarbia can cause respiratory and cardiac complications. Airway obstruction and asphyxiation can occur if the nasal packing slips back into the airway, particularly during sleep. Complications may occur if a pack compresses the eustachian tube. Rarely, infections can develop in the nose, sinus, or middle ear after nasal packing and lead to toxic shock syndrome (TSS). Risk factors for TSS include any wound and respiratory infections, such as sinusitis, sore throat (pharyngitis), laryngitis, tonsillitis, or pneumonia. Foul odor is alarming as the nasal pack ages over the next 48 hours. Bruising or swelling of the eyelids secondary to nasal packing may develop. Therefore, packing is best removed within 24 to 48 hours following placement provided the patient's clinical condition has stabilized.

When tight nasal/oral packing fails in unstable patients, supraselective arteriography and embolization is the treatment of choice in institutions where this modality is available (8). Ligation of the external carotid artery is a last resort in the unstable multitrauma patient who cannot be transported. However, due to collateral circulation of the face, ligation is seldom truly effective. Best control of hemorrhage is obtained by exploratory surgery and fixation of fractures. In patients with isolated LeFort fractures, open reduction/internal fixation (ORIF) is the first line of treatment (9).

WOUND MANAGEMENT

The management of facial soft tissue injuries depends on the area of injury. However, there are some basic rules that apply in treating soft tissue injuries. Soft tissue injuries are only properly evaluated after the wound is cleaned of dirt, foreign bodies, debris, and dry blood. A local anesthetic is usually necessary to properly clean the wound and perform a thorough examination. In the awake patient, most local infiltrative anesthetics cause great discomfort, which may compromise spinal precautions. Very slow injection using a fine needle (30 gauge) as well as adding bicarbonate in a 1:10 ratio may help. Facial nerve function should be assessed in all patients with facial lacerations and nerve function should be documented *prior* to anesthetic use. Anatomic landmarks are of great importance: if facial nerve paralysis results from a laceration anterior to a line perpendicular to the lateral canthus of the eye, the terminal nerve branches are involved. If facial nerve paralysis results from a laceration posterior to this imaginary line, the facial nerve should be explored. Ideally, repair of the facial nerve should occur as soon as possible, but no later than 72 hours unless the wound is heavily contaminated. In this case, the nerve endings are tagged with a permanent suture and repair is performed when the wound is clean. In patients with deep lacerations of the cheek, the wound should also be explored for injury to the parotid duct (Stensen duct). One may see saliva in the wound if the duct is lacerated. The parotid duct is repaired over a stent to prevent stenosis. Lacerations and contusions of specialized three-dimensional structures such as the eyelid, nasal alae, and ear are often best referred to a specialist, especially if flaps show signs of devascularization.

Optimum timing of facial laceration repair is a topic of debate. After tetanus prophylaxis, soft tissue repair can be performed within 12 to 24 hours provided the wounds are irrigated, cleaned, and kept moist. Because of the abundant blood supply, definite wound closure can be delayed and, in general, requires minimal debridement. "Traumatic tattooing" is a greater problem in the face than skin loss. A perfect repair is difficult to obtain in the acute setting as areas of contusion have to declare themselves and often leave irregularities later on. As long as important anatomic landmarks are aligned (e.g., vermillion border of the lip, gray line of the eyelid) and like tissues are approximated (mucosa to mucosa, muscle to muscle, cartilage to cartilage, and skin to skin), revisions can be done later. Deep sutures are used to close dead space to avoid hematomas and to remove tension from the skin closure, preventing an unsightly scar. Good esthetic results depend less on suture technique than on proper redraping of tissues. Scars are noticeable as a result of reflection of light and creation of shadow. For cosmesis, it is of importance to create an "even" closure and, if possible, to place scars in areas of shadow and along lines perpendicular to facial muscle pull. Photographic documentation is important so that the patient may later realize the extent of the original injury, to follow healing, to document subsequent revisions, and for medical-legal reasons.

CRANIAL NERVE EXAM

Olfaction (cranial nerve [CN] I): Olfaction is typically not examined in the acute trauma bay setting but reserved for later trauma surveys (e.g., tertiary survey). Damage to CN I should be considered with NOE fractures and frontal sinus fractures if disruption of the cribriform plate is present.

Pupillary responses (CN II, III): Examine the pupil size and shape at rest. This can be difficult in patients with extensive orbital trauma as the eyelid swells rapidly and is difficult to open. Next, examine with a flashlight. Note the direct constriction of the illuminated pupil, as well as the consensual constriction of the opposite pupil. In an afferent pupillary defect there is decreased direct response in the affected eye. This can be demonstrated by moving the flashlight back and forth between the two eyes, with a lag of 2 to 3 seconds. The afferent defect becomes evident when the flashlight is moved from the normal to the affected eye because the affected eye will dilate in response to light. Brief pupillary oscillations of the stimulated pupil (hippus) are normal and should be distinguished from pathologic response. Finally, test the pupillary response to accommodation, by moving an object (e.g., finger) from far to near. The pupils should constrict. The direct response of the ipsilateral pupil is absent in lesions to the ipsilateral optic nerve, the pretectal area, the ipsilateral sympathetic nerves traveling with CN III, or the pupillary constrictor muscle of the iris. The consensual response is impaired (contralateral pupil illuminated) in lesions of the contralateral optic nerve, the pretectal area, the sympathetic nerves, or the pupillary constrictor of the iris. Accommodation is affected for the same reasons and in pathways from optic nerve to the visual cortex. Accommodation is spared in injury to the pretectal area (10).

Extraocular movements (CN III, IV, VI): Extraocular movement is readily checked by asking patients to look in all directions without moving their head and asking them if they experience any diplopia in any direction. Test "smooth pursuit" by slowly moving an object or finger up and down and sideways. Test convergence by asking the patient to fixate on an object that is moved toward a point between the eyes. During these tests, look closely for nystagmus and dysconjugate gaze.

Facial sensation and muscles of mastication (CN V): Test facial sensation using a soft object or finger in the forehead, cheek, and lower jaw line to capture all three branches of the nerve. Test the masseter muscles during jaw clench. In facial fractures, the most commonly affected nerve is the Vb branch, which may indicate maxillary, orbital, or zygomaticomaxillary complex (ZMC) fractures.

Muscles of facial expression and taste (CV II): Look for asymmetries in spontaneous facial expressions and blinking, smiling, and squinting. Taste testing is usually not performed. Facial weakness can be caused by lesions of upper motor neuron in the contralateral cortex or in descending nerve pathways (ipsilateral). Upper motor neurons to the upper face cross over to both facial nuclei so in intracranial injury or stroke, motor functions of the upper face remain intact. Lower motor neuron lesions typically cause weakness to the entire ipsilateral face.

Hearing and vestibular sense (CN VIII): Hearing and vestibular sense are seldom checked in the acute setting. Vestibular sense is typically not tested except in patients with vertigo.

Palate elevation and gag reflex (CN IX, X): Perform an intraoral exam and observe palatal motion when the patient says "aaah." Observe the gagging motion when the posterior pharynx is touched. The gag reflex is usually checked in patients with suspected brainstem pathology.

Sternocleidomastoid and trapezius muscles (CN XI): These muscles are examined by asking the patient to shrug the shoulders and turn the head from side to side. Of note is that bilateral upper motor neuron projections control the sternocleidomastoid, analog to the bilateral CN VII projections controlling the upper face.

Tongue (CN XII): The tongue will deviate toward the weak side. Lesions of the motor cortex cause contralateral tongue weakness as opposed to lower motor lesions or lesions of the tongue muscles.

SPECIFIC SIGNS AND SYMPTOMS OF FACIAL FRACTURES

Nasal Bones

The clinical features of an isolated nasal fracture are as follows:

- Tenderness over nasal bones
- Mobility
- Swelling
- Flattened or deviated nose
- Epistaxis
- Septal deviation
- Septal hematoma
- Mouth breathing

Due to the prominence of the nose, nasal injuries are fairly common and the nose is the most commonly fractured bone in the facial skeleton. Nasal fracture diagnosis is often a clinical, and not a radiologic, diagnosis. External nasal deformities are usually obvious during examination. Crepitus will distinguish recent trauma from a nasal deformity due to a previous injury. Septal hematoma must be ruled out in every patient. A septal hematoma forms between the septal cartilage and perichondrium from which it gets its blood supply. It appears as edema and ecchymosis of the septum with narrowing of the nasal airway on speculum exam. Septal hematoma is treated with incision and drainage. Failure to treat can lead to a septal abscess, intracranial complications, or delayed saddle nose deformity due to cartilage loss.

Leakage of cerebrospinal fluid (CSF) indicates a fracture through the cribriform plate of the ethmoid bone. This potentially carries a risk of meningitis. There is controversy on the use of prophylactic antibiotics. Epistaxis is treated by packing the nose as discussed above. If this is not successful, an epistaxis catheter can be inserted to control bleeding from branches of the anterior ethmoidal artery. Treatment of most noncomminuted nasal fractures is closed reduction. Manipulation is required to restore an obstructed nasal airway and for restoration of facial cosmesis. The ideal timing for manipulative treatment varies. If reduction is not performed within the first few hours following injury, treatment is delayed 3 to 5 days for swelling to resolve. After a prolonged period (7–14 days), manipulation becomes increasingly difficult as the nasal bones will be difficult to move into place without osteotomies and a formal rhinoplasty may be required.

Naso-orbito-ethmoid Fractures

The clinical features of a nasoethmoidal fracture are as follows:

- Flat nasal bridge with splaying of nasal complex and crepitus
- Saddle-shaped deformity of nose ("punched-in" look)
- Telecanthus (increased distance between the medial canthi)
- Circumorbital edema and ecchymosis ("raccoon eyes")
- Subconjunctival hemorrhage
- Epistaxis
- CSF rhinorrhea
- Supraorbital/supratrochlear nerve paresthesia

With true nasoethmoidal fractures, a CSF leak should be assumed even if not clinically evident. Classically, an increased intercanthal distance (greater than 35 mm) and depression of the nasal root are unequivocal clinical signs of traumatic telecanthus. Closed manipulation of naso-orbito-ethmoid injuries notoriously gives a poor result, with a high incidence of persistent or recurrent deformity postoperatively. The results of secondary surgery of this deformity are seldom satisfactory. ORIF, often with bone grafting to the nose, is usually necessary as the NOE complex is a very difficult area of the facial skeleton to reconstruct. Access to the nasoethmoidal region can be obtained through an existing laceration, if present, or through a coronal incision for adequate access to the frontal bone, nasal root, and orbits (11).

The evaluation of the stability of the medial canthal ligament forms an integral part of the clinical assessment. The clinical classification of status of the medial canthal ligament and its attachment to underlying bone can be classified according to Gruss et al. (12) or Markowitz et al. (13). The medial canthus must be stabilized usually by wiring to the opposite anterior lacrimal crest (transnasal canthopexy). If both canthal ligaments are detached, then the telecanthus can be addressed by means of wiring the two medial canthal ligaments to each other (transnasally).

Orbital Blowout Fracture

The term *orbital blowout fracture* is reserved for a fracture of the bones of the orbit. This may involve the orbital floor, walls, or roof. The majority of cases involve the orbital floor and medial wall, as these areas comprise the thinnest bone of the orbit. An isolated orbital blowout fracture is usually secondary to a blunt blow. Smith and Regan demonstrated that when an object of slightly greater diameter than the orbital rim strikes the orbit and incompressible eyeball, a fracture results in the middle orbit likely due to increased intraorbital pressure (14). Often, the thin bone of the floor displaces downward into the maxillary antrum, remaining attached to the orbital periosteum as one fragment ("trap door"). The periorbital fat herniates through the defect, thereby interfering with the inferior rectus and inferior oblique muscles, which are contained within the same fascia sheath. This prevents upward movement and outward rotation of the eye and the patient experiences diplopia on upward gaze. This clinical finding should be distinguished from true "entrapment," which indicates impingement of the ocular muscles. Those patients will present with pain, tenderness around the eye, swelling, and subjective diplopia in all outer fields of gaze. Painful eye movement is common with significant swelling and hemorrhage in the orbit, and restriction of eye motility and double vision are not necessarily an indication for surgical repair of the fracture. Ophthalmologic evaluation is advised if significant eye trauma is detected. If the patient is unresponsive, an afferent pupillary defect may uncover occult visual loss. If indicated clinically, tonometry may be used to assess intraocular pressure. This may serve as a baseline for serial examinations. Also, forced duction testing can be done to check extraocular movements. This is done by grasping the sclera in the fornix and mechanically moving the globe. To test inferior rectus entrapment, the globe is moved superiorly. Inhibition of this motion would indicate need for exploration. A computed tomography (CT) scan will determine the presence or absence and size of the fracture. Surgical repair of orbital fractures depends on symptoms and largely on the size of the fracture itself. Small fractures (less than 50% of the floor or <2 cm^2), even if associated with double vision, can be observed for 1 to 2 weeks to assess if repair is indicated if symptoms do not resolve. Patients are instructed to avoid blowing their nose and to use nasal decongestants. Should symptoms persist and/or if the fracture is large, surgical intervention is required to return the orbital contents to their correct position and to restore orbital volume. This is done by placement of a graft in the orbital floor. Many different graft materials can be used but autologous bone remains the gold standard and may be required if the defect is large enough, especially in a young patient (15).

Complications of unrecognized orbital floor fracture are as follows:

- Posttraumatic persistent enophthalmos
- Hypoglobus (inferior displacement of the orbit)
- Persistent diplopia
- Lower eyelid retraction (ectropion) and scleral show
- Persistent edema of the lower eyelid

Zygoma Fractures

Clinical features of ZMC fractures are as follows:

- Swelling and bruising over the cheek/flattening
- Step-off deformity at the orbital rim
- Periorbital ecchymosis
- Subconjunctival hemorrhage
- Para-/anesthesia of the infraorbital nerve
- Trismus and restricted lateral excursion
- Para-/anesthesia of Z-facial/temporal nerves

The zygomaticomaxillary complex is both a functional and esthetic unit of the facial skeleton and the prominent zygoma is the second most commonly fractured facial bone. Zygomatic fractures usually result from high-impact trauma. Leading causes of fractures include assault, motor vehicle or motorcycle accidents, sports injuries, and falls. The majority of zygomatic fractures occur in men in the third decade of life. The zygoma separates the orbit from the maxillary sinus and temporal fossa. Because the zygoma articulates superficially with the maxilla, frontal, and temporal bones, zygomatic fractures in the past have been referred to as tripod or trimalar fractures. However, the fourth articulation with the sphenoid really makes it a quadripod fracture. The ZMC can be defined by two arcs: a vertical arc from the zygomaticofrontal suture down to the lateral antrum, and a horizontal arc from the zygomatic arch to the inferior orbital rim. The intersection of these two arcs defines the malar prominence (1). The zygoma itself is a relatively strong bone, and isolated fractures of the body of the zygoma are rare unless there is a direct blow to the zygomatic arch. Due to traction on the infraorbital nerve, patients often complain of upper lip/tooth numbness. Trismus may be present as the masseter muscle pulls the malar fragment down, which impinges on the mandible. Radiologic imaging remains an important step in the evaluation of orbitozygomaticomaxillary fractures. CT scanning offers advantages over plain films that justify the increased cost. Important areas to evaluate on CT scanning include the buttresses, the orbital walls, the zygomatic arch, the palate, and the mandibular condyles (16).

For the zygoma, timing of repair is 5 to 7 days postinjury to allow tissue edema and swelling to subside. After 10 days, masseter contracture may complicate closed reduction of the zygoma. If the zygomatic arch is minimally displaced and there is no comminution, the patient is a candidate for "simple" reduction. If there is moderate displacement or comminution of the maxillary wall, the maxilla will have to be plated for stability. For true ZMC fractures, ORIF is typically necessary at the lateral maxilla, the inferior orbital rim, the zygomaticofrontal (ZF) suture, the zygomatic arch, and commonly the orbital floor as well. Full access to the arch unfortunately requires a coronal approach (17).

The Midfacial Skeleton: LeFort Fractures

LeFort fractures tend to result from anterior forces. The fracture possibilities and combinations thereof are numerous; hence, classification schemes fail to describe them all. The original fracture patterns described by LeFort in 1901 are based on experimentally induced midface trauma. LeFort established that midface fractures tend to occur in reproducible patterns along weaker areas of the craniofacial skeleton. The LeFort I fracture essentially separates the lower maxilla, including the alveolar ridge and teeth, from the rest of the midface. The fracture classically travels through the inferior portion of the piriform aperture across the maxilla to the pterygoid fissure. This fracture pattern may occur as a single entity or in association with LeFort II and II fractures. The LeFort II fracture is a pyramidal fracture that includes the entire piriform aperture in the distracted midface. The fracture line includes the frontonasal suture, passes through the inferomedial orbit, and runs between the zygoma and maxilla for a larger area of dissociation. The LeFort III fracture is a suprazygomatic fracture through the lateral orbit. The fracture line extends from the dorsum of the nose and the cribriform plate along the medial and lateral wall of the orbit to the ZF suture line. This is also known as craniofacial dissociation as the bones of the midface are essentially completely disarticulated from the cranium (18).

Signs and Symptoms of LeFort Fractures

All complete LeFort fractures will create mobility of the maxilla, especially the upper alveolus (tooth-bearing portion of the maxilla). Hence, all will lead to subjective (and objective) malocclusion in varying degrees of severity. Infraorbital nerve paresthesia may be present. There can be palpable crepitus in the upper buccal sulcus from the fracture line. An intraoral hematoma or ecchymosis is likely. In LeFort II and III fractures, the nose is often involved and epistaxis common. In LeFort III fractures, this should be distinguished from CSF rhinorrhea. Periorbital ecchymosis and edema, subconjunctival hemorrhage, and visual disturbance occur only in LeFort III fractures.

MANAGEMENT OF MAXILLARY FRACTURES

Minimally displaced fractures can be clinically observed provided no malocclusion is present. The patient is allowed oral intake but only full liquid/soft foods as load bearing (chewing) may displace fracture fragments. Comminuted fractures and fractures with malocclusion are treated with maxillomandibular fixation (MMF) and/or by ORIF. Truly rigid fixation of the midface, unlike the mandible, is unattainable due to the thin bones and correspondingly thin plates.

For comminuted or displaced fractures, the status of the mandible is critical for management. If the mandible is intact, it serves as a guide for placing the upper dentition into occlusion. MMF is placed, and then the midface is treated with appropriate ORIF. Intraoperatively used MMF can be released after fracture fixation and the patient allowed range of motion (soft diet only). If the mandible is also fractured, the patient is placed in MMF for 2 to 3 weeks (19).

SUMMARY OF PATIENT EVALUATION

Evaluating the facial trauma patient can be challenging. The basics of ATLS courses apply to the facial trauma patient as well. Airway stabilization and securement may be difficult in extensive facial trauma with the possibility of basilar skull base injury where endotracheal intubation is relatively contraindicated and one must consider a surgical airway. Any patient who has sustained forces adequate to cause facial fractures must be assumed to have a cervical spine injury until proven otherwise. Epistaxis can be troublesome and hemodynamically significant. In the clinical evaluation of facial fractures, subjective data that the patient is able to provide offer clues to facial fracture diagnosis and include pain, malocclusion, numbness in portions of the face, trismus, and diplopia. Malocclusion is a very sensitive indicator of injury due to the high sensitivity of the periodontal ligaments. Numbness often indicates disruption or compression of a peripheral nerve. Trismus may result from mandibular trauma or from an impacted zygoma impinging on the temporalis muscle. Diplopia may result from entrapment of the extraocular muscles or gross globe malposition. Of special note, monocular diplopia indicates an intrinsic globe problem and mandates prompt ophthalmologic evaluation.

Unfortunately, many trauma patients are obtunded or intoxicated and unable to provide any subjective information. Physical examination alone is inconclusive in the majority of cases. On physical examination the examiner should note presence and location of lacerations, ecchymoses, and gross asymmetry. Palpation is done to assess instability, crepitus, tenderness, bony stepoffs, and canthal tendon disruption. The trigeminal nerve should be tested. Ophthalmologic examination deserves special mention. Many authors believe that it is impractical to expect ophthalmologic consultation on every patient with facial injury (15). Most physicians are able to test visual acuity (subjective and objective), pupillary function, ocular motility, anterior chamber exam (to look for hyphema), and funduscopic exam. Ophthalmologic consultation should then be obtained as indicated. Last but not least: although cosmesis is not an immediate concern, it is of great concern to patients, especially once the acute trauma experience has worn off. Long-term goals and appearance outcomes should therefore be discussed with every patient on an individual basis to avoid misunderstandings and misconceptions. Facial fracture management aims to restore facial height, width, and projection. Newer techniques of rigid fixation are constantly being developed to optimize treatment outcomes for facial fracture management. Bioresorbable plates have come onto the market with particular utility in the pediatric population, where there is concern that rigid fixation with hardware may get incorporated in growing bone and inhibit facial growth. However, the behavior of the soft tissue envelope is much more difficult to predict depending on age, gender, race, and soft tissue trauma sustained at the injury. In general, the abatement of swelling and soft tissue adjustment takes at least 3 months, and neurapraxia substantially longer. In general, patients should be told that it takes about a year before final settling and a stable end result. This helps dissuade requests for interventions as the tissues continue to improve (20).

References

1. Frost DE, Kendell BD. Applied surgical anatomy of the head and neck. In: Fonseca RJ, Walker RV, eds. *Oral and Maxillofacial Trauma.* 3rd ed. Philadelphia: WB Saunders; 2005.
2. Hohlrieder M, Hinterhoelzl J, Ulmer H, et al. Traumatic intracranial hemorrhages in facial fracture patients: review of 2, 195 patients. *Intensive Care Med.* 2003;29(7):1095–1100.
3. Clark N, Birely B, Manson PN, et al. High-energy ballistic and avulsive facial injuries: classification, patterns, and an algorithm for primary reconstruction. *Plastic Reconstr Surg.* 1996;98(4; Suppl 1):583–601.
4. Sahlin GF, Guimaraes-Ferreira J, Lauritzen C. Orbital fractures in craniofacial trauma in Goteborg: trauma scoring, operative techniques, and outcome. *Scand J Plast Reconstr Surg Hand Surg.* 2003;37:69–74.
5. Ford K (commentator). A hospital-based violence prevention intervention reduced hospital recidivism for violent injury and arrests for violent crimes. *Evid Based Med.* 2007;12(4):110.
6. Manoach S, Paladino L. Manual in-line stabilization for acute airway management of suspected cervical spine injury: historical review and current questions. *Ann Emerg Med.* 2007;50(3):236–245.
7. Kwok H, McCormack J, Cece R, et al. Controlled trial of oronasal versus nasal mask ventilation in the treatment of acute respiratory failure. *Crit Care Med.* 2003;31(2):468–473.
8. Chen C-C, Jeng S-F, Tsai HH, et al. Life threatening bleeding of bilateral maxillary arteries in maxillofacial trauma: report of two cases. *J Trauma Inj.* 2006;61:1–5.
9. Janus SC, MacLeod SP, Odland R. Analysis of results in early versus late midface fracture repair. *Otolaryngology—Head and Neck Surgery.* 2008;138(4):464–467.
10. Wang BH, Robertson BC, Girotto JA, et al. Traumatic optic neuropathy: a review of 61 patients. *Plastic Reconstr Surg.* 2001;107(7):1655–1664.
11. Sargent LA. Nasoethmoid orbital fractures: diagnosis and treatment. *Plastic Reconstr Surg Craniofac Trauma.* 2007;120(7; Suppl 2):16S–31S.
12. Gruss JS, Hurwitz JJ, Nik NA, et al. The pattern and incidence of nasolacrimal injury in naso-orbital-ethmoid fractures: the role of delayed assessment and dacryocystorhinostomy. *Br J Plast Surg.* 1985;38:116–121.
13. Markowitz BL, Manson PN, Sargent L, et al. Management of the canthal tendon in nasoethmoid orbital fractures: the importance of the central fragment in classification and treatment. *Plast Reconstr Surg.* 1991;87:843–853.
14. Smith B, Regan WF Jr. Blow-out fracture of the orbit; mechanism and correction of internal orbital fracture. *Am J Ophthalmol.* 1957;44(6):733–739.
15. Cole P, Boyd V, Banerji S, et al. Comprehensive management of orbital fractures. *Plastic Reconstr Surg Craniofac Trauma.* 2007;120(7; Suppl 2):57S–63S.
16. Ellis E. Fractures of the zygomatic complex and arch. In: Fonseca RJ, Walker RV, eds. *Oral and Maxillofacial Trauma.* 3rd ed. Philadelphia: WB Saunders; 2005:569.
17. Stanley RB. The zygomatic arch as a guide to reconstruction of comminuted malar fractures. *Arch Otolaryngol.* 1989;115:1459–1462.
18. Manson PN, Clark N, Robertson B, et al. Subunit principles on midface fractures: the importance of sagittal buttresses, soft-tissue reductions, and sequencing treatment of segmental fractures. *Plastic Reconstr Surg.* 1999;103(4):1287–1306.
19. Lew D, Sinn DP. Diagnosis and treatment of midface fractures. In: Fonseca RJ, Walker RV, eds. *Oral and Maxillofacial Trauma.* Philadelphia: WB Saunders; 1991.
20. Girotto JA, MacKenzie E, Fowler C, et al. Long-term physical impairment and functional outcomes after complex facial fractures. *Plastic Reconstr Surg.* 2001;108(2):312–327.

CHAPTER 88 ■ BURN INJURY: THERMAL AND ELECTRICAL

WINSTON T. RICHARDS • DAVID W. MOZINGO

Burn injury accounts for 40,000 hospital admissions per year, including 25,000 admissions to hospitals with specialized burn centers. More than 60% of the 40,000 hospitalizations for burn injuries in the United States each year are now admitted to 125 hospitals with specialized burn centers. Over one third of the admissions—38%—exceeded 10% total body surface area (TBSA), and 10% exceeded 30% TBSA involvement. Most included severe burns of such vital body areas as the face, hands, and feet; interestingly, 70% of burn patients were male. Data from the National Hospital Discharge survey of 2003, as well as the Agency for Healthcare Research and Quality health care cost and utilization project national inpatient sample 2003, selected state hospital data systems from 2002 through 2004, and the American Burn Association National Burn Repository

2005 report suggest that the causes of the burns include fire (46%), scald burns (32%), contact with a hot object (8%), electrical (4%), and chemical burns 3%.

Burn injury has a systemic effect on the patient, and each organ system responds to this injury in a predictable manner proportional to the extent of burn. The current literature supports the following physiologic responses in each organ system.

BURN PHYSIOLOGY AND THE EFFECTS ON ORGAN SYSTEMS

Cardiovascular System

The cardiovascular system is affected in several ways after burn injury. Cardiac output becomes depressed, peripheral vascular resistance increases, and the patient's capillary permeability is altered. Each of these occurs in a burn size- and time-dependent fashion.

During the late 1960s and early 1970s, studies by Moncrief, Asch, and Wilmore clearly defined the physiologic response of the heart and systemic and pulmonary vasculature to burn injury (1–3). These animal experiments showed a burn size- and severity-dependent depression in cardiac output, which resolved over time and could be altered with fluid resuscitation and the addition of vasoactive medications. They also showed a time-dependent increase in systemic and pulmonary vascular resistance, which was resolved with fluid resuscitation as well as with the administration of vasoactive medication.

Burn injury causes loss of the skin's fluid barrier function. These resultant fluid losses, as well as increased capillary permeability, lead to hypovolemia and burn shock. The loss of fluid leads to decreased cardiac preload and, ultimately, decreased cardiac output. Integumentary fluid losses and tissue edema drive the cardiovascular response to burn injury, but improvement in cardiac function parameters achieved by fluid resuscitation do not fully resolve this deficit. There is also evidence for a myocardial depressant factor being linked to multiple inflammatory mediators (4–7).

Cardiac depression after a thermal injury is mediated by the interaction of multiple inflammatory and anti-inflammatory molecular signals. Early and late inflammatory mediators influence myocardial contraction and relaxation in the first 24 to 48 hours after burn injury (8,9). Factors including tumor necrosis factor–α (TNF-α), Fas ligand, interleukin-1, interleukin-18, interleukin-6, macrophage migration inhibitory factor, high mobility group box 1 chemokines, and caspase-1 have been implicated in the loss of cardiac contractility as well as myocardial relaxation, leading to decreased cardiac output after injury. By contrast, the anti-inflammatory pathways involving interleukin-10, transforming growth factor–β, and soluble TNF receptor lead to the resolution of the initial myocardial depression.

Resuscitation of the burn patient addresses the cardiac depression, with administered fluid bolstering the intravascular volume by replacing losses and anticipating future deficits. Multiple formulas exist for fluid management in the burn patient, which are discussed separately below. Myocardial depression can be marginally supported pharmacologically with the use of inotropic agents. Further research toward more direct management of the decreased contractility could target the inflammatory mediators released after burn injury (7).

Pulmonary System

Burn injury has multiple effects on the pulmonary system. Depending on the mode of injury, including inhalation and direct burns to the chest wall, these effects may be manifest as alterations in respiratory rate, tidal volume, gas exchange, and even long-term effects on pulmonary function. Burn injury not only affects the lungs in a direct manner, but the complications of these injuries may add to the dysfunction manifested. Pneumonia and tracheal irritation from prolonged intubation are some of the complicating factors that affect the burn patient (1).

The pulmonary response to burn injury is characterized by transient pulmonary hypertension, decreased lung compliance, and hypoxia. These functional changes are mediated by multiple factors including inflammation, acid-base imbalance, airway injury, and chest wall restriction. The body's pH balance highlights the close interaction of the pulmonary system and the renal system in addressing disturbances caused by burn injury. Anti-inflammatory treatment preburn has been noted to alter the pattern of decreased compliance, pulmonary hypertension, and hypoxia, suggesting a cause-and-effect relationship.

With relatively small TBSA burns, increases in the patients' respiratory rate, peaking by postburn day 8 and returning to control levels by about 3 weeks postburn, have been noted. Along with these respiratory rate changes, an increase in tidal volume and minute ventilation were also recorded; these returned to control levels in approximately 3 weeks.

Chest burns with their concurrent edema formation showed notable restrictive effects on pulmonary function during the first 3 days postinjury; these effects resolved over time. During the patient's initial resuscitation, decreased chest wall compliance may lead to restricted ventilation and increased airway pressures; burn wound escharotomy of the chest wall is indicated in these situations to improve chest wall compliance.

Further effects of burn injury on pulmonary function have been attributed to burn wound infection, which may lead to lung dysfunction secondary to inflammatory mediator release from the periburn, possibly mediated by thromboxane A2. Management of the inflammatory process initiated by burn injury may prove to be helpful in modulating this effect.

Complications associated with intubation after burn injuries include ventilator-associated pneumonia (VAP) and tracheal stenosis. Protocols for the reduction/prevention of VAP have been extensively reviewed and are currently being used in many hospitals. The judicious management of ventilator support and endotracheal intubation addresses postinjury tracheal stenosis. Extubation at the earliest opportunity afforded by the patient's physiology—and his or her operative schedule—is important in reducing this complication. At this time, a generalized benefit from the VAP bundle has not been clearly defined in the burn patient population, and requires further study.

Smoke inhalation injury affects between 10% and 30% of burn patients. This injury is caused by the inhalation of hot gases and products of incomplete combustion. When present, an inhalation injury is associated with increased mortality over that predicted by age and extent of burn alone. Although in the past, increased fluid resuscitation was advocated for patients with inhalation injury, this did not correlate well with fluid requirements during resuscitation; interestingly, a low initial

PaO_2/FiO_2 ratio does so correlate. An increased TBSA injury is associated with increased pneumonia rates, and the presence of pneumonia in patients with an inhalation injury results in a higher mortality rate. Pneumonia and inhalation injury increases length of stay over inhalation injury alone; this is discussed further below.

In the late 1980s, high-frequency percussive ventilation (HFPV) was used to treat patients with severe inhalation injury; the results were promising, and further studies followed. By 2007, it had been noted that HFPV for inhalation injury did not change mean ventilator days, intensive care unit (ICU) length of stay, hospital length of stay, or incidence of pneumonia. Despite the similarities in the HFPV and conventional ventilator groups, a decrease in both overall morbidity and mortality in a subset of patients with less than or equal to 40% TBSA burned was noted. This finding led to the recommendation for further study in a randomized and controlled fashion (10–22).

Renal System

Renal failure has been reported in up to 20% of burn injury patients, with a clinical picture related to the size and severity of burn injury. Multifactorial in nature, the time course of renal failure falls into early or late categories. The mortality of patients developing severe renal failure with burn injury approaches 80%.

Early acute renal failure appears to be directly associated with clinical events such as delayed resuscitation, underresuscitation, hypotension, and rhabdomyolysis.

More extensive and deeper burns are associated with a higher incidence of acute renal failure. Rhabdomyolysis, a rare consequence of flame burns, but often associated with electrical injury, has a direct association with renal failure. Late episodes of acute renal failure are more commonly associated with sepsis, toxic drugs, and pre-existing medical conditions.

Treatment of acute renal failure in the burn patient and other patient populations involves multiple steps. Adequate fluid resuscitation initiated as early as possible during the time course of the burn injury will reduce the presentation of early acute renal failure. Monitoring urine output as a measure of renal perfusion will allow the clinician to maintain adequate fluid input. Late episodes of acute renal failure can be addressed by treating the underlying cause. Sepsis from lines, wound, pneumonia, or urinary tract should be controlled by replacing the lines, excising the burn wound, and providing adequate antibiotic therapy for pneumonia and urinary tract infection. When needed, renal replacement therapy should be instituted.

Gastrointestinal Tract and Liver

Ileus presents in patients with burns exceeding 20% TBSA. Despite this problem, using the gut with some—even minimal—level of feeding is advocated early after injury, and is usually well tolerated. Tube feeding should be instituted for patients with large burns where the patient is unable to tolerate sufficient intake by mouth to sustain the markedly increased nutritional requirements.

Gastroduodenal stress ulceration has been a hallmark of early burn care, with significant bleeding or perforation complicating the care of extensively burned individuals. This complication markedly decreased with the use of antacids, H_2-antagonists, and proton pump inhibiting medications. Their use has become routine in the management of the thermally injured patient.

Perforation

Poor perfusion of the gut during resuscitation may lead to segmental ischemia in the watershed areas of the intestine. With this condition, there is a risk for developing necrosis and subsequent perforation. The use of vasoactive medications during burn resuscitation or during prolonged septic events may increase this risk (23).

Normal gut flora has been identified as an infection source in the burn patient as well as in other critically injured patients (24–26). Maintaining gut integrity with nutritional support in the form of glutamine supplementation has been proposed and studied in the burn patient. A second approach to this problem, selective gut decontamination, has been proposed and tested in animal models (27–29). Selective gut decontamination has been shown to reduce bacterial translocation from the gut in burned rats (30). With this reduction in translocation, immunosuppression was reduced and the cardiac response to subsequent septic challenge was improved. Clinical success with this approach is not well documented (31–35).

Intra-abdominal hypertension, as defined by a bladder pressure of 30 mm Hg or greater is the precursor to the abdominal compartment syndrome. Respiratory compromise with increasing peak airway pressures, renal compromise with decreased renal perfusion and urine output, and increased mortality among burn patients are the features of this syndrome (36). Burn patients with 30% or greater TBSA injury requiring fluid resuscitation over and above the standard calculated rates are at risk for this complication (37). We recommend monitoring bladder pressures in each patient with burns greater than 30% and initiating therapeutic maneuvers for those patients with pressures of greater than 30 mm Hg (38).

Therapy for intra-abdominal hypertension follows a graded response. Reduced fluid administration, sedation, and chemical paralysis of the patient are the initial treatments. Escharotomies and peritoneal drainage make up the next most invasive line of management, and ultimately, abdominal decompression through a laparotomy incision may be needed to relieve the symptoms. In the severely burned population, abdominal compartment syndrome has a high mortality rate and should be addressed urgently when recognized (39,40).

Central Nervous System

Burn injury and resuscitation in an ovine model showed that cerebral autoregulation adjusted to the hemodynamic changes caused by burn injury. Autoregulation of cerebral blood flow was effective to a point and then began to fail as resuscitation proceeded, suggesting that the cerebrovascular system has a limited reserve to tolerate the effects of burn injury (41,42).

Endocrine System

There is a graded response of the endocrine system after burn injury. Hormone levels are directly related to the TBSA involved; these levels rise and fall in a time-dependent fashion from the onset of injury. Burn injury is characterized by a painful incident followed by a significant inflammatory response, with fluid losses and shifts occurring both near the burn wound itself and systemically. Each part of the endocrine system reacts to regain or maintain its preburn state.

The hypothalamus responds by secreting antidiuretic hormone (ADH) which acts on the collecting ducts of the kidney to facilitate the reabsorption of water into the blood. This reduces the volume of urine formed while retaining water in response to losses of fluid from the intravascular space. The anterior pituitary releases adrenal corticotropic hormone (ACTH), which stimulates the release of the mineralocorticoid aldosterone and glucocorticoid cortisol. Aldosterone acts on the kidney to promote retention of sodium ions in the blood. Water follows the salt and helps maintain normal blood volume and pressure. Glucocorticoids increase blood sugar levels through the stimulation of gluconeogenesis. This elevation in the blood glucose levels is thought necessary to supply the increased metabolic demand of the injured body. Cortisol and other glucocorticoids also have a potent anti-inflammatory effect on the body (43–51). They depress the immune response, especially cell-mediated immune responses.

The adrenal medulla releases the tyrosine-derived neurotransmitters adrenaline and noradrenaline into the blood. This response is associated with the autonomic nervous system—sometimes called the fight or flight response—and leads to multiple effects, some of which are an increase in the rate and strength of the heartbeat, resulting in increasing blood pressure; and the shunting of blood from the skin to the skeletal muscles, coronary arteries, liver, and brain. With the release of adrenaline and noradrenaline, blood sugar rises and the metabolic rate is increased; bronchial dilation occurs; pupils dilate; and blood clotting time is decreased. This autonomic response also leads to increased ACTH secretion from the anterior lobe of the pituitary.

The elevations in stress-related hormones are noted in a time- and burn size–dependent manner after injury. This hormone response follows a pattern associated with the ebb and flow of the burn injury process. An initial increase in the hormone levels in response to fluid shifts and inflammation resolves over time as the patient's fluid balance returns to normal, and the burn wounds close.

Several medications are available that can modify the endocrine response to burn injury. A recent prospective, double-blind, randomized single-center study on the effect of oxandrolone on the endocrine, inflammatory, and hypermetabolic responses during the acute phase of burn injury suggested that this treatment shortened the length of acute hospital stay, maintained lean body mass, and improved body composition and hepatic protein synthesis while having no adverse effects on the endocrine axis postburn. This study and another using beta-blockade to modify the metabolic response after burn injury are at the heart of attempts to improve the outcome of patients after a severe burn injury (52,53).

Hematopoietic System

Typically, the red blood cell (RBC) mass in the burn patient declines in a burn size- and severity-dependent fashion. This is initially related to the burn injury itself and thereafter can be attributed to the therapeutic interventions of the treating service. Although surgery and phlebotomy account for the iatrogenic loss of red blood cells, several possible causes have been explored for the injury-related loss of blood in the burn patient. Initial heat injuries to the RBCs, as well as sequestration of blood in the burn eschar, are early factors in the loss of RBCs and the decline in hemoglobin and hematocrit. Damage to RBCs secondary to the inflammatory response to the burn wound is a later developing cause for blood loss in these patients (54–60).

In 1973, a paper by Loebl (58) described studies of RBC half-life in burn victims and healthy volunteers. Red blood cells from the burn patient had a normal half-life when transfused into healthy volunteers. The same red blood cells had a decreased half-life in the burn victim and, when normal red blood cells were transfused into a burn victim, they acquired a similar decrease in their half-life. This study suggested a humoral or inflammatory process driving the loss of red cells.

Later studies have linked this loss in red cells to a process mediated by inflammation and the release of toxic oxygen free radicals, representing a nonspecific mechanism for the destruction of red cells. Immune system–mediated processes for the destruction of red cells in burn patients have also been postulated, but Coombs testing in these patients has failed to reveal a definite link to immune-mediated blood loss.

Immune System

Infection remains a major complicating factor of burn injury (61–63). Burned skin loses its barrier function against the environment, and normal skin flora and environmental pathogens are able to gain access to the system. The risk of infection and its complications are directly related to the size of the burn injury and additional factors such as inhalation injury and preexisting medical conditions. Burn injury leads to compromised immune function, resulting in increased susceptibility to subsequent sepsis and multiple organ system failure.

Immune system dysfunction occurs on the cellular and humoral levels. Multiple avenues for this effect have been investigated. Currently, macrophages, T cells, other lymphocyte subpopulations, and humoral factors such as opsonins, immunoglobulins, protease inhibitors, and chemotactic factors have been implicated in the process. Some combination of all of the above factors, related to their natural interaction, produces a weakened immune system susceptible to infection entering through multiple avenues.

In general, burn patients are assailed by bacteria from multiple directions. Damaged skin, its barrier function destroyed, is the most obvious portal. Burn-related hypotension and peripheral vasoconstriction may permit intestinal hypoperfusion and translocation of normal gastrointestinal flora into the systemic circulation. Other clinically relevant pathways are associated with current treatment modalities used in thermally injured patients: intubations of the respiratory, vascular, and genitourinary systems provides ready access for bacteria into the compromised host.

Musculoskeletal System

Loss of muscle mass and bone are notable in severely burned patients. Bone loss is, in part, due to an increase in glucocorticoids that inhibit bone formation and osteoblast differentiation; hypercalciuria secondary to hypoparathyroidism; and vitamin-D deficiency. Muscle loss is secondary to an intense catabolic state initiated by the inflammatory response to burn injury and is fueled by the need to repair the surface injury suffered. Current research has identified possible treatment avenues in each of these systems (64–67).

A randomized, double-blind, placebo-controlled study by Klein and Herndon (64) suggested that intravenous pamidronate administration may help preserve bone mass in children with >40% TBSA burns. Follow-up to that study 2 years later showed a sustained improvement in bone mineral content as measured by dual-energy radiograph absorptiometry (66). This effect was attributed to a decrease in the glucocorticoid-mediated effect on bone mass.

FLUID RESUSCITATION

Fluid resuscitation addresses the clinical picture of burn shock. Whereas multiple resuscitation regimens have been developed to overcome the cardiac depression, vasoconstriction, and hypovolemia associated with acute burn injury, most, if not all, of the current formulae have been developed through retrospective review of the fluid requirements of burn patients. Aided by the use of the rule of nines and Lund-Browder charts, a patient's TBSA burn and weight measurements are used to determine his or her initial fluid requirement. One half of the fluid requirements calculated are given in the first 8 hours after the burn injury, with the remaining amount administered over the subsequent 16 hours. A slight variation in the composition of the resuscitation fluid is present in the different formulae; there are also differences in the addition of colloid to the initial resuscitation scheme (68–79). The most commonly used formulae are noted in Table 88.1.

Colloid infusion during the resuscitation of acutely injured patients has been debated for some time. Acute burn injury leads to capillary permeability, which allows loss of intravascular albumin into the interstitial spaces of the acutely injured patient. This particular problem has been studied at length, and, although the infusion of colloid after completion of the acute resuscitation phase increases plasma oncotic pressure, it has not shown any improvement in clinical outcome. Currently, the application of albumin or fresh frozen plasma is considered after the initial 8-hour period postburn in an attempt to avoid loss of the colloid secondary to capillary permeability.

Adequate resuscitation is measured by end organ perfusion. Currently, exact measures of end organ perfusion are being developed and tested. A surrogate measure of the success of fluid administration is the measurement of urine output. Renal function is highly dependent on renal blood flow, which can be adequately assessed by the rate of urine output. Most practitioners view a urine production rate of 0.5 to 1.0 mL/kg ideal (or adjusted) body weight per hour as adequate. Secondary measures of perfusion are also important in the resuscitation plan. The combination of blood pressure, heart rate, oxygenation, and central venous pressure are used in tandem to determine the adequacy of treatment.

Other measures of adequate resuscitation, such as blood pressure, heart rate, and central venous pressure, must be monitored cautiously. Postburn tissue edema will decrease the accuracy of cuff blood pressure measurements, and the vasoconstriction caused by catecholamine release will adversely affect the accuracy of indwelling arterial lines. Central venous pressure measurements require the interaction of multiple physiologic and environmental parameters to provide the practitioner with meaningful measurements.

Patients who begin to lag in their urine output during resuscitation should have their fluid rates adjusted. Urinary rates of one third the predicted value, or less, of the patient's body weight over 2 consecutive hours should prompt an increase in intravenous fluid administration. On the other hand, patients running one third or more over their expected urine output may benefit from decreased fluid administration. A graded increase or decrease of the intravenous fluid rate of 20% per hour is a measured and conservative response to these situations. Those patients who do not respond as expected to calculated fluid administration or who require more than 6 mL/kg per percent TBSA fluid administration should be considered for more invasive monitoring, such as pulse-waveform analysis (FlowTrack, PICCO, LiDCO, among others) or pulmonary artery catheter monitoring. With measurements obtained through this more advanced monitoring, a decision can be made to either support the cardiac output or reduce the peripheral vascular resistance, or both. Small doses of hydralazine may be used to reduce peripheral resistance in situations where the cardiac output remains low. Hydralazine doses on the order of 0.5 mg/kg have been shown to be effective when used in this situation. In animal models of burn injury, sodium nitroprusside and verapamil decreased peripheral resistance and supported cardiac output with good effect. This approach should be used with caution in the severely burn-injured patient to avoid further tissue hypoperfusion, which may exacerbate the condition of the partially burned tissues.

Insensible water losses become more significant with larger total body surface area burns. Evaporative water losses from the open wounds/burns usually peak on the third day postburn and then trail off until the wounds are completely closed. An estimation of insensible water losses may be calculated as follows:

$$\text{Insensible water loss (in mL/h)} = (125 + \%\text{TBSA burned}) \times \text{TBSA (in m}^2\text{)}.$$

The total body surface area involved may be estimated using the formula of DuBois and DuBois as follows:

$$\text{BSA} = (\text{W}^{0.425} \times \text{H}^{0.725}) \times 0.007184$$

where W is the weight in kilograms and H is the height in centimeters. Initially, the replacement fluid should free water and then be altered based on electrolyte measurements.

TABLE 88.1

THE COMMON RESUSCITATION FORMULAE

	Common burn formulae		
	Evans formula	Brooke formula	Parkland formula
Colloid	1.0 mL/kg/%	0.5 mL/kg/%	None
Crystalloid	1.0 mL/kg/%	1.5 mL/kg/%	4.0 mL/kg/%
Free Water	2,000 mL	2,000 mL	None

ELECTRICAL INJURY

Electrical injuries can be divided into those due to low voltage—less than 1,000 volts—and those due to high voltage—greater than or equal to 1,000 volts (80). These injuries have varying patterns. Low-voltage injuries range from the circumoral injuries noted in children who have bitten home electrical cables to deaths caused by dropping electrical appliances in a bathtub full of water. High-voltage injuries have a range that includes the more severe episodes of instant death, massive tissue loss, and secondary clothing ignition. Some of the less dramatic injuries include thermal injury, central nervous system related trauma, and fractures. With high-voltage injuries, there is a high ratio of limb amputations, highlighting the danger of this modern-day source of power. Herein, we will concentrate on high-voltage injuries.

Electrical energy interacts with human anatomy following the basic principles of physics. Current flowing through tissue is related to the voltage drop across the resistance of that tissue. Heat produced by this current can be represented mathematically as follows:

$$J \text{ (heat in Joules)} = I^2 \times R \times T$$

where I is current, R resistance, and T time in seconds. Body tissues have differing electrical resistances. Given the above equation, it appears that differing tissues would create varying degrees of heat and subsequent damage; interestingly, clinical findings do not wholly support this concept. The highest resistance is found in the bone, fat, and tendons, whereas the lowest resistance has been identified in the muscles, blood, and nerves; skin has an intermediate resistance. Clinical findings in electrically injured patients support the idea that the body represents a volume conductor with a resistance on the order of 500 to 1,000 ohms. In this model, the relative differences in tissue resistance are small enough that the body is considered a single resistor. Heat generated by the current flowing through the resistor is related to the cross-sectional area of the entry or exit wound and the local anatomy.

Contact wounds on the hands and feet are common. Each of the contact areas might have a low cross section, releasing more heat in that area; as the current crosses the "bottleneck" areas of the ankles and wrists, there may be more tissue damage generated at those sites. At its most extreme, heat released by high-voltage injuries produces coagulation necrosis of the tissues and varying other effects on the organs as the electricity passes through.

Arc injuries are less common but just as destructive. Electricity can travel 2 to 3 cm/10,000 volts, and may travel 10 feet or more to its target. Temperatures at the contact points range from 2,000 to 4,000°C, with spikes of up to 20,000°C; this intense temperature leads to severe and deep tissue damage.

Electrical injuries have specific organ effects in addition to the thermal injury described above. With high-voltage injuries, cardiac standstill and ventricular fibrillation are the most lethal cardiac injuries. Other electrocardiograph (ECG) findings and rhythm changes that have been reported include atrial fibrillation, focal ectopic arrhythmias, supraventricular tachycardia, right bundle branch block, and nonspecific ST-T segment changes. These clinical findings are thought to be associated with direct myocardial muscle damage, coronary vasospasm, and coronary endarteritis.

Renal injury may be direct, although this is rare, or may take on the more familiar form of acute renal failure secondary to rhabdomyolysis. Large quantities of muscle protein, hemoglobin, and other tissue proteins released from the tissues coagulated by high voltage and current are filtered into the renal tubules, causing acute renal failure with oliguria or polyuria. Up to 15% of patients injured in high-voltage accidents will suffer from this type of renal injury.

Central nervous system injury ranges from the devastating effect of high voltage and current on the brain and brainstem, leading to instant death, to more subtle findings. Altered levels of consciousness with varying degrees of recovery have been reported, while progressive neurologic deterioration has been noted in both the central and the peripheral nervous systems. With high-voltage injuries, progressive deterioration of the microvascular nutrient vessels to the nerves has been identified, and is thought to lead to ischemia, necrosis, and fibrosis of the injured nerve; progressive loss of function can be seen as a late developing problem.

Other organ systems may be directly affected by the passage of current through them. Each is susceptible to both the current and the resistance-induced production of high temperatures and tissue damage. Cataracts may form in the eyes of a patient who has had an electrical injury in which the current pathway is through the orbits; this complication has been reported in ≤30% of patients suffering from this injury.

INHALATION INJURY

The pathophysiology associated with smoke inhalation injury falls into three broad categories: (i) upper airway injury, (ii) asphyxiant gases and hypoxic environments, and (iii) carbonaceous particle deposition. These areas are all involved in an inhalational injury (81–84).

The diagnosis of inhalation injury is based on several site-specific and clinical findings surrounding each burn patient. For example, closed space injuries or explosions are some of the circumstances surrounding inhalation injury. Noxious fumes noted at the scene by the scene responders, as well as facial burns noted on the patient, are other findings consistent with inhalation injury. Clinical findings on examination, such as large burns, carbonaceous sputum, hoarseness, or an abnormal lung exam, are associated with this injury, and elderly patients are more susceptible to inhalation injury.

Once inhalation injury is suspected, upper airway pathology should be expected. Heated smoke or ambient air may injure the supraglottic airway from the lips to the vocal cords. This injury may occur abruptly, leading to significant edema and swelling of the face and oropharynx, as well as affecting the region around the vocal cords.

True heat injury below the cords is rare, with the exception of steam injuries or ignition of flammable gases in the airway. Signs and symptoms of a true airway burn injury include hoarseness; stridor and/or wheezing; carbonaceous sputum; singed nasal hair, eyebrows, or facial hair; and edema or inflammatory changes in the upper airway. The resultant upper airway edema formation can threaten the airway and the patient's breathing.

Asphyxiant gases and hypoxic environments lead to the second area of pathology associated with inhalation injury. In fires involving structures, the ambient oxygen level markedly decreases; this lack of oxygen may lead to carbon monoxide generation, as this molecule is a byproduct of incomplete combustion in the burning structure. Carbon monoxide binds tightly to hemoglobin, reducing the amount of oxygen delivered to end organs, which may cause a hypoxic injury. Aside from carbon monoxide, other toxic gases can be released by the flames. Cyanide generation is associated with burning plastics; this molecule is highly lethal. Treatment of carbon monoxide intoxication includes a high concentration of oxygen and, sometimes, hyperbaric oxygen. Cyanide poisoning treatment includes delivery of oxygen, as well as a three-part regimen to bind the cyanide compound in the blood.

The third broad area of pathology associated with smoke inhalation injury is related to the deposition of carbonaceous particles in the airway. The flame-generated toxins that are bound to the carbon particles will slowly be released after the latter are deposited in the lungs, inducing a chemical tracheal bronchitis. This effect is manifested by impaired ciliary function and edema, significant inflammation, and ulceration or necrosis of the respiratory epithelium. The clinical sequelae of tracheal bronchial injury include bronchorrhea, bronchospasm, distal airway obstruction, and atelectasis, as well as pneumonia. Epithelial injury leads to sloughing of the mucosa and blockage of the airways with this cellular debris. Air trapping in this situation leads to atelectasis and the development of barotrauma and pneumonia.

Treatment for each area of pathology is based on standard clinical practice. When presented with a patient who is suspected of having an inhalation injury and upper airway edema, endotracheal intubation to protect the airway should be performed early to avoid the consequences of airway compromise. Patients suffering from carbon monoxide exposure, and showing clinical signs of intoxication, should be treated with 100% oxygen to displace the molecule from hemoglobin. If immediately available, and if the patient is stable, high levels of carboxy hemoglobin and severe neurologic symptoms should be treated with hyperbaric oxygen therapy. The tracheal-bronchial injury associated with inhalational injury and carbonaceous particle deposition should be treated with humidified oxygen by face mask, and frequent examination of the airway should be performed to evaluate for signs of compromise that may require endotracheal intubation.

Cyanide toxicity presents clinically with lethargy, nausea, headache, weakness, and coma. Cyanide combines with cytochrome oxidase, thereby blocking oxygen use and inhibiting high-energy phosphate compound production. Cyanide toxicity begins at 0.1 μg/mL of serum and quickly leads to death at concentrations of 1 μg/mL. Laboratory studies show a decreased arterial-venous oxygen difference with severe metabolic acidosis; this acidosis is unresponsive to fluids and oxygen administration.

S-T segment elevations may be seen on the patient's electrocardiogram, mimicking a myocardial infarction. Treatment of this condition includes the administration of 100% oxygen and a three-part medication regimen. Initially, the administration of amyl nitrate pearls, by inhalation for 15 to 30 seconds every minute, is followed by 10 mL 3% sodium nitrate solution (300 mg) intravenously over 3 minutes, repeated at one-half the dosage in 2 hours if symptoms persist or recurrent signs of toxicity are present. Sodium thiosulfate is the final medication, given in a dose of 50 mL of a 25% solution (12.5 gm) intravenously over 10 minutes, repeated at one-half the dosage in 2-hour intervals if persistent or recurrent signs of toxicity are present.

INFECTION CONTROL

Historically, mortality from burn injury was associated with burn shock (85–87); the loss of fluid through the burned and damaged skin, as well as fluid shifts related to the release of inflammatory mediators, led to hypovolemia and unrecoverable end organ failure. As our understanding of the injury suffered during burns improved, so did the survivability of these injuries. Currently, burn shock is well controlled by our fluid resuscitation regimens. The new challenge in burn injury is the concurrent development of infection in a compromised host. Burn injury is associated with a burn size–dependent depression in the immune system in which bacterial, fungal, and viral elements are better able to breach the defense mechanisms of the body, thereby worsening the injury.

As fluid resuscitation techniques advanced, wound colonization and sepsis became a leading factor in morbidity and mortality. The advent of topical antibiotic/anti-infective agents addressed this new area of pathology. Subsequent movement toward early wound excision and skin grafting led to improvements in the rates of wound sepsis and its complications. Although the burn wound has become less of a risk for infection, other portals of entry have persisted in plaguing the burn patient. With our current methods of intubating the respiratory, vascular, and genitourinary systems, we expose the burn patient to other portals of entry for pathogens.

NUTRITION

Burn patients present to the ICU in a severe inflammatory state. This state, along with a wide variety of prehospital factors and premorbid conditions, provides the practitioner with a challenging nutritional problem. Nutritional support for the burn patient can be addressed in several steps: first, an assessment of the patient's initial nutritional status, and second, monitoring of his or her nutritional status throughout the hospital course, and adjustments based on the monitoring measures. By using a combination of variables, including burn size and severity, time from injury, physical parameters such as age, weight, and the presence of other medical factors, nutrition support can be tailored to each burn patient.

Nutritional assessment should begin with measurement of the patient's weight, estimation of the patient's calorie and protein needs, measurement of the patient's serum albumin, prealbumin, and C-reactive protein levels (88–101). Pre-existing illnesses should prompt the practitioner to make adjustments in the rate of feeding, use of additional medications, and the need for additional nutrient support.

Glutamine supplementation has been shown to improve morbidity and mortality when administered to critically ill patients. This response appears to improve with increasing doses of the amino acid, and parenteral administration appears to have an improved response over enteral administration. Not all of the trials reported to date have shown a definitive benefit, and the general consensus is that a large randomized controlled trial would be needed to confirm or refute the benefits of glutamine administration.

Physiologically, glutamine affects the immune system, the anti-oxidant status, glucose metabolism, and heat shock protein response. These physiologic effects appear to provide benefit with regard to gastrointestinal mucosal integrity, wound healing, Gram-negative bacteremia and infection—including with *Pseudomonas*—as well as a reduction in mortality, and possibly cost savings to burn patients. At the time of this writing, a consensus has not been reached on the length of time for glutamine therapy, the optimum dose, and definite safety aspects of the supplementation of glutamine in critically ill and burn patients. Most studies suggest that clinically important differences appear to commence at doses greater than 0.2 gm/kg body weight per day, and most trials have used 15 to 30 gm per day glutamine supplementation.

WOUND MANAGEMENT

With the exception of chemical burns, for which prompt water irrigation to remove the offending agent is required, no specific treatment of the thermal burn wound is needed in the prehospital setting (81,102,103). The patient should be covered with a clean sheet and blanket to conserve body heat and minimize burn wound contamination during transport to the hospital. The application of ice or cold water soaks, when initiated within 10 minutes after burning, may reduce tissue heat content and lessen the depth of thermal injury. If cold therapy is used, care must be taken to avoid causing hypothermia; this is accomplished by limiting this form of therapy to 10% or less of the body surface and only for the time required to produce analgesia.

Following admission to the burn center, definitive care of the burn wound can begin. Daily wound care involves cleansing, debridement, and dressing of the burn wound. On the day of injury, the burn wound is best cleansed by means of hydrotherapy, a practice that has been used in the treatment of burn patients for many years and remains an integral part of current treatment plans. Hydrotherapy is accomplished by means of showering, immersion, or use of a spray table. Showering is often used for ambulatory patients who remain capable of independent, or near-independent, wound care. Patients who are near to discharge are encouraged to use the shower, especially if showering is to be used at home.

Use of a spray table is generally reserved for newly admitted patients, those with limited mobility, or those with large open wounds. The patient is placed on the table, and the wounds are washed and rinsed with running water. As an alternative, a stretcher or plinth can be placed over a Hubbard tank. The patient is placed on the stretcher, and the wounds are washed and rinsed as described previously.

Immersion hydrotherapy often is used for patients in a less acute stage who have a moderate or smaller injury and who will benefit from soaking in a tub. Soaking promotes removal of therapeutic creams and exudate, debridement of loose eschar, and active participation by the patient in range-of-motion exercises. Immersion hydrotherapy should be avoided in patients with an extensive thermal injury, since this process may spread contamination from one site to the entire burn surface. Also, if the water becomes contaminated with fecal material, the entire wound would be exposed.

The consensus is that a hydrotherapy session of 30 minutes or less is optimal for patients with acute burns. Longer sessions may cause excessive sodium loss through the burn wound—remember that water is hypotonic—as well as heat loss, pain, and stress. Adequate cleansing is achieved by using a mild soap or surgical detergent such as chlorhexidine gluconate, although very dilute solutions of sodium hypochlorite and povidone iodine have also been used. Care must be taken in selecting a wound cleanser; skin cleansers that contain cytotoxic chemicals should not be used. Studies have shown that most wound cleansers need to be diluted to maintain cell viability. Body hair within the burned area and within about 2.5 cm of the wound periphery should be shaved, with the exception of the eyebrows. Gentle cleansing and debridement of the burn wound are important because bacteremia has been demonstrated in up to 21% of wound debridements or manipulations. The incidence of bacteremia increases with increase in the size of the burn and with the extent of wound manipulation. To prevent infection and cross-contamination between patients, single-use, plastic tub liners are used and discarded after each hydrotherapy session.

Hydrotherapy may be contraindicated for some patients because of a recent grafting procedure or because of cardiopulmonary instability and the need for continuous monitoring and support. For these patients, the burn wounds are washed with a mild soap or surgical detergent and thoroughly rinsed while the patient remains in bed.

Wound debridement involves the removal of all loose tissue, wound debris, and eschar (nonviable tissue); debridement of a burn wound is accomplished through mechanical, chemical (enzymatic), or surgical means.

Mechanical debridement is accomplished through application and removal of gauze dressings, hydrotherapy, irrigation, and use of scissors and tweezers. Wet-to-dry or wet-to-moist dressings are sometimes used to debride exudative wounds. Wet dressings of coarse, meshed gauze are applied to the wound surface. A wet dressing is made by saturating an all-gauze dressing with the prescribed solution, wringing the dressing out until it is just moist, and applying it to the wound surface. The dressing material is allowed to dry (wet-to-dry dressing) or to become less moist (wet-to-moist dressing). As the dressing dries, drainage, exudate, and necrotic debris adhere to the gauze, and on careful removal, the wound is mechanically debrided. However, this process is nonselective, and new granulating and epithelial tissue can be removed along with the necrotic tissue; therefore care must be taken in removing the dressing. Bleeding should not occur when the dressing is removed. If the dressing is too dry and adherent to remove, it can be moistened with sterile normal saline or the patient can soak the area before attempts are made to remove it. This method of debridement can be extremely painful, necessitating adequate analgesia.

Hydrotherapy aids in mechanical wound debridement. As discussed earlier, hydrotherapy promotes the removal of loose wound exudate and debris through gradual softening of the eschar.

Wound irrigation using the hydraulic force created by water pressure is another method of debridement useful for wounds without hard eschar. High-pressure irrigation, defined as water pressure above 8 pounds per square inch (psi), removes wound debris, bacteria, and necrotic tissue. Low-pressure irrigation (less than 8 psi) is useful in removing foreign bodies and exudate. Regardless of the irrigation system and force used, irrigation must be done gently so as not to damage healing tissue. It should be discontinued once the wound has begun to granulate unless there are still significant areas of necrosis.

Surgical, or sharp, debridement requires the use of scalpels and scissors to debride wounds of loose, necrotic tissue. Care must be taken to avoid excessive debridement that results in bleeding and pain. Bleeding may indicate injury to the healthy underlying tissue. In most instances, sharp debridement should be carried out in the operating room to ensure adequate debridement and hemostasis.

Mafenide acetate (Sulfamylon), silver sulfadiazine (Silvadene), and silver nitrate are the three most commonly used topical antimicrobial agents for burn wound care. Each agent has specific limitations and advantages with which the physician must be familiar to ensure patient safety and optimal benefit. Mafenide acetate and silver sulfadiazine are available as topical creams to be applied directly to the burn wound, whereas silver nitrate is applied as a 0.5% solution in occlusive dressings. Either cream is applied in a half-inch (about one-third of a centimeter) layer to the entire burn wound in an aseptic manner after initial debridement, and reapplied at 12-hour intervals or as required to maintain continuous topical coverage. Once daily, all of the topical agents should be cleansed from the patient using a surgical detergent disinfectant solution and the burn wounds examined by the attending physician. Silver nitrate is applied as a 0.5% solution in multilayered occlusive dressings that are changed twice daily.

Mafenide acetate burn cream is an 11.1% suspension in a water-soluble base. This compound diffuses freely into the eschar, owing to its high degree of water solubility. Mafenide is the preferred agent if the patient has heavily contaminated burn wounds or has had burn wound care delayed by several days. This agent has the added advantage of being highly effective against Gram-negative organisms, including most *Pseudomonas* species. Physicians using this agent must be aware of several potential clinical limitations associated with its use. Hypersensitivity reactions occur in 7% of patients, and pain or discomfort of 20 to 30 minutes duration is common when it is applied to partial-thickness burn wounds. This agent is also an inhibitor of carbonic anhydrase, and a diuresis of bicarbonate is often observed after its use. The resultant metabolic acidosis may accentuate postburn hyperventilation, and significant acidemia may develop if compensatory hyperventilation is impaired. Inhibition of this enzyme rarely persists for >7 to 10 days, and the severity of the acidosis may be minimized by alternating applications of mafenide with silver sulfadiazine cream every 12 hours.

Silver sulfadiazine burn cream is a 1% suspension in a water-miscible base. Unlike mafenide, silver sulfadiazine has limited solubility in water and, therefore, limited ability to penetrate into the eschar. The agent is most effective when applied to burns soon after injury to minimize bacterial proliferation on the wound's surface. This agent is painless on application, and serum electrolytes and acid-base balance are not affected by its use. Hypersensitivity reactions are uncommon; an erythematous maculopapular rash sometimes seen subsides on discontinuation of the agent. Silver sulfadiazine occasionally induces neutropenia by a mechanism thought to involve direct bone marrow suppression; white blood cell counts usually return to normal following discontinuation. With continual use, resistance to the sulfonamide component of silver sulfadiazine is common, particularly in certain strains of *Pseudomonas* and many *Enterobacter* species. However, the continued sensitivity of microorganisms to the silver ion of this compound has maintained its effectiveness as a topical antimicrobial agent.

A 0.5% silver nitrate solution has a broad spectrum of antibacterial activity imparted by the silver ion. This agent does not penetrate the eschar, since the silver ions rapidly precipitate on contact with any protein or cationic material. Use of this agent is not associated with more intense wound pain, except from the mechanical action required for dressing changes. The dressings are changed twice daily and moistened every 2 hours with the silver nitrate solution to prevent evaporation from increasing the silver nitrate concentration to cytotoxic levels within the dressings. Transeschar leaching of sodium, potassium, chloride, and calcium should be anticipated, and these chemical constituents should be appropriately replaced. Hypersensitivity to silver nitrate has not been described. Mafenide acetate, silver sulfadiazine, and 0.5% silver nitrate are effective in the prevention of invasive burn wound infection; however, because of their lack of eschar penetration, silver nitrate soaks and silver sulfadiazine burn cream are most effective when applied soon after burn injury.

Acticoat is a new burn wound dressing. It consists of a urethane film onto which nanocrystalline elemental silver is deposited. When moistened, application of this dressing to the wound results in a sustained release of elemental silver, which is bactericidal and fungicidal. The mechanism of action is probably much like that of silver nitrate dressings; however, Acticoat does not cause transeschar leaching of electrolytes. The silver does not penetrate the eschar, limiting its use on infected or heavily contaminated wounds. Transient mild pain may be noted occasionally after application. The use of Acticoat is currently limited to partial-thickness burns.

Aquacel Ag hydrofiber is another dressing containing elemental silver, though at a much lower concentration. When compared to silver sulfadiazine on partial-thickness burns, this dressing was associated with an increased rate of reepithelization and was slightly more cost-effective. This study was limited due to sample size; however, the replacement of burn cream pharmaceuticals with silver-containing barrier dressings is occurring in certain settings, namely those of superficial burns.

PAIN MANAGEMENT

Because burn pain is variable in its degree and time course, reliance on a single analgesic regimen is unreliable at best and unsuccessful at worst. Conversely, the diverse spectrum of burn patients—adult versus children, large burns versus small, intensive care unit nursing versus ward setting—makes the routine individualization of analgesic plans overwhelming and impractical. Our recommendation is to determine an analgesic regimen for each individual patient based on two broad categories: the assessed clinical need for analgesia and the limitations imposed by the patient.

The first step is to address background, procedural, postoperative, and breakthrough pain treatment separately, and then consider individual drug choices based on patient limitations. To reinforce this type of approach to analgesic management, detailed institutional guidelines to help physicians and nurses choose and administer specific analgesics are recommended.

Background Pain

In general, because it is a pain of continuous nature, background pain is best treated with mild-to-moderately potent, longer-acting analgesics administered so that plasma drug concentrations remain relatively constant throughout the day. Examples include the continuous IV infusion of fentanyl or morphine (with or without patient-controlled analgesia [PCA]), oral administration of long-acting opioids with prolonged elimination (methadone) or prolonged enteral absorption (sustained-release morphine, sustained-release oxycodone), or oral administration on a regular schedule of short-acting oral analgesics (oxycodone, hydromorphone, codeine, acetaminophen). Such analgesics should almost never be administered on an as-needed (PRN) basis during the early and middle phases of hospitalization.

Procedural Pain

In contrast, procedural pain is significantly more intense but shorter in duration; therefore, analgesic regimens for procedural pain are best composed of more potent opioids that have a short duration of action. Intravenous access is helpful in this setting, with short-acting opioids (fentanyl) offering a potential advantage over more longer-acting agents (morphine, hydromorphone). When intravenous access is not present, orally administered opioids (morphine, hydromorphone, oxycodone, codeine) are commonly used, although their relatively long duration of action (2–6 hours) may potentially limit postprocedure recovery for other rehabilitative or nutritional activities. Oral transmucosal fentanyl and nitrous oxide are useful agents when IV access is not present due to their rapid onset and short duration of action.

Postoperative Pain

Postoperative pain deserves special mention because increased analgesic needs should be anticipated following burn wound excision and grafting. This is particularly true when donor sites have been harvested, as these are often the source of increased postoperative pain complaints. In contrast, pain from excised/grafted burns may increase, decrease, or not change postoperatively compared to preoperatively. Typically, this increased analgesic need in the postoperative period is limited to 1 to 4 days following surgery before returning to, or falling below, preoperative levels.

Breakthrough Pain

Breakthrough pain occurs at rest when background analgesic therapy is inadequate. Breakthrough pain occurs commonly in burn patients, particularly in early stages of hospitalization until a stable, appropriate, and individualized pharmacologic regimen can be determined for each patient. Analgia for breakthrough pain can be provided with IV or oral opioids. When breakthrough pain occurs repeatedly, it is an indication to reevaluate and likely increase the patient's background pain analgesic regimen, as it may be inadequate in terms of analgesic dose and/or frequency. Tolerance develops rapidly in these patients and may initially manifest as breakthrough pain.

Patient Limitations

As stated above, the presence of intravenous access directly influences analgesic drug choice, particularly in children. Similarly, patients who are endotracheally intubated and ventilated are somewhat protected from the risk of opioid-induced respiratory depression; thus, opioids may be more generously administered in these individuals, as is often required for painful burn debridements. Also, individual differences in opioid efficacy should be considered in all patients, including opioid tolerance in patients requiring prolonged opioid analgesic therapy or in those with pre-existing substance abuse histories.

An appropriate rationale is to titrate the drug dose to the desired effect, rather than to rely on a particular textbook dose for all patients. Due to the development of drug tolerance with prolonged medical use or recreational abuse of opioids (i.e., increasing drug doses are required to attain adequate levels of analgesia), opioid analgesic doses needed for burn analgesia may exceed those recommended in standard dosing guidelines. Furthermore, because of cross-tolerance, tolerance to one opioid analgesic usually implies tolerance to all opioid analgesics. One clinically relevant consequence of drug tolerance is the potential for opioid withdrawal to occur during inpatient burn treatment. Thus, the period of inpatient burn care is not an appropriate time to institute deliberate opioid withdrawal or detoxification measures in tolerant patients, because such treatment ignores the very real analgesic needs—background pain and procedural pain—of these patients. Similarly, when reductions in analgesic therapy are considered as burn wounds close, reductions should occur by careful tapering, rather than abrupt discontinuation of opioids, to prevent the acute opioid withdrawal syndrome.

Anxiolysis in the Treatment of Burn Pain

Current aggressive therapies for cutaneous burns, together with the qualities of background and wound care pain, make burn care an experience that normally induces anxiety in a large proportion of adult and pediatric patients. Anxiety, in itself, can exacerbate acute pain. This has led to the common practice in many burn centers of using anxiolytic drugs in combination with opioid analgesics. Intuitively, this practice seems particularly useful in premedicating patients for wound care, to diminish the anticipatory anxiety experienced by these patients prior to and during debridement. Low-dose benzodiazepine administration significantly reduces burn wound care pain scores and narcotic requirements. It appears that the patients most likely to benefit from this therapy are not those with *high trait* or premorbid anxiety, but rather those with *high state* or the time of the procedure anxiety, or those with high baseline pain scores. Other nonpharmacologic anxiolysis techniques, such as hypnosis and behavioral therapy, could also be considered.

TEAM APPROACH TO BURN PATIENTS

The management of the burned patient is a multidisciplinary effort of burn care professionals to provide optimal care to the burn patient. This multidisciplinary care spans the early resuscitative phases of care through the long-term rehabilitation and reconstructive phases. The Burn Center Director coordinates all activities of the multidisciplinary care of the critically ill burn patients. Team members include burn surgeons, plastic and reconstructive surgeons, critical care specialists, anesthesiologists, critical care burn nurses, physical therapists, occupational therapists, clinical nutritional specialists, psychologists, social workers, and pastoral care support personnel. This multidisciplinary approach affords the patients and their families state-of-the-art resources for optimal outcome, education, and rehabilitation. This concept of team care, originating in the 1950s when the first burn centers opened, has persisted to this day and is a model of coordinated, interdisciplinary, outcome-driven patient care.

References

1. Moncrief JA. Effect of various fluid regimens and pharmacologic agents on the circulatory hemodynamics of the immediate postburn period. *Ann Surg.* 1966;164(4):723–750.
2. Asch MJ, Feldman RJ, Walker HL, et al. Systemic and pulmonary hemodynamic changes accompanying thermal injury. *Ann Surg.* 1973;178(2):218–221.
3. Wilmore DW, Aulick LH, Mason AD, Pruitt BA. Influence of the burn wound on local and systemic responses to injury. *Ann Surg.* 1977;186(4):444–456.
4. Kuntscher MV, Germann G, Hartmann B. Correlations between cardiac output, stroke volume, central venous pressure, intra-abdominal pressure and total circulating blood volume in resuscitation of major burns. *Resuscitation.* 2006;70(1):37–43.
5. Cioffi WG, DeMeules JE, Gamelli RL. Vascular reactivity following thermal injury. *Circ Shock.* 1988;25(4):309–317.
6. Lund T, Reed RK. Acute hemodynamic effects of thermal skin injury in the rat. *Circ Shock.* 1986;20(2):105–114.
7. Hilton JG. Effects of verapamil on the thermal trauma depressed cardiac output in the anaesthetized dog. *Burns Incl Therm Inj.* 1984;10(5):313–317.
8. Carlson DL, Horton JW. Cardiac molecular signaling after burn trauma. *J Burn Care Res.* 2006;27:669–675.
9. Horton JW, Sanders B, White DJ, Maass DL. The effects of early excision and grafting on myocardial inflammation and function after burn injury. *J Trauma.* 2006;61(5):1069–1077.
10. Nieminen S, Fraki J, Niinikoski J, et al. Acute effects of burn injury on tissue gas tensions in the rabbit. *Scand J Plast Reconstr Surg.* 1977;11(1):69–74.
11. Tripathi FM, Pandey K, Paul PS, et al. Blood gas studies in thermal burns. *Burns Incl Therm Inj.* u 1983;Sep;10(1):13–16.
12. Mlcak R, Desai MH, Robinson E, et al. Lung function following thermal injury in children—an 8-year follow up. *Burns.* 1998;24(3):213–216.
13. Whitener DR, Whitener LM, Robertson KJ, et al. Pulmonary function measurements in patients with thermal injury and smoke inhalation. *Am Rev Respir Dis.* 1980;122(5):731–739.
14. Tripathi FM, Pandey K, Paul PS, et al. Respiratory functions in thermal burns. *Burns Incl Therm Inj.* 1983;9(6):401–408.
15. Demling RH, Wenger H, Lalonde CC, et al. Endotoxin-induced prostanoid production by the burn wound can cause distant lung dysfunction. *Surgery.* 1986;99(4):421–431.
16. Demling RH, Wong C, Jin LJ, et al. Early lung dysfunction after major burns: role of edema and vasoactive mediators. *J Trauma.* 1985;25(10):959–966.
17. Demling RH. Effect of early burn excision and grafting on pulmonary function. *J Trauma.* 1984;24(9):830–834.
18. Tasaki O, Goodwin CW, Saitoh D, et al. Effects of burn on inhalation injury. *J Trauma.* 1997;43(4):603–607.
19. Teixidor HS, Novick G, Rubin E. Pulmonary complications in burn patients. *J Can Assoc Radiol.* 1983;34(4):264–270.
20. Pruitt BA Jr, Erickson DR, Morris A. Progressive pulmonary insufficiency and other pulmonary complications of thermal injury. *J Trauma.* 1975;15(5):369–379.
21. Endorf FW, Gamelli RL. Inhalation injury, pulmonary perturbations, and fluid resuscitation. *J Burn Care Res.* 2007;28(1):80–83.
22. Petroff PA, Hander EW, Mason AD Jr. Ventilatory patterns following burn injury and effect of sulfamylon. *J Trauma.* 1975;15(8):650–656.
23. Moore LJ, Kowal-Vern A, Latenser BA. Cecal perforation in thermal injury: case report and review of the literature. *J Burn Care Rehabil.* 2002;23(6):371–374.
24. Manson WL, Klasen HJ, Sauer EW, Olieman A. Selective intestinal decontamination for prevention of wound colonization in severely burned patients: a retrospective analysis. *Burns.* 1992;19(2):98–102.
25. Mackie DP, van Hertum WA, Schumburg TH, et al. Reduction in staphylococcus aureus wound colonization using nasal mupirocin and selective decontamination of the digestive tract in extensive burns. *Burns.* 1994;20(Suppl 1):S14–17.
26. Mackie DP, van Hertum WA, Schumburg T, et al. Prevention of infection in burns: preliminary experience with selective decontamination of the digestive tract in patients with extensive injuries. *J Trauma.* 1992;32(5):570–575.
27. Horton JW, Maass DL, White J, Minei JP. Reducing susceptibility to bacteremia after experimental burn injury: a role for selective decontamination of the digestive tract. *J Appl Physiol.* 2007;102(6):2207–2216.
28. Yao YM, Lu LR, Yu Y, et al. Influence of selective decontamination of the digestive tract on cell-mediated immune function and bacteria/endotoxin translocation in thermally injured rats. *J Trauma.* 1997;42(6):1073–1079.
29. Yao YM, Yu Y, Sheng ZY, et al. Role of gut-derived dedotoxaemia and bacterial translocation in rats after thermal injury: effects of selective decontamination of the digestive tract. *Burns.* 1995;21(8):580–585.
30. Baron P, Traber LD, Traber DL, et al. Gut failure and translocation following burn and sepsis. *J Surg Res.* 1994;57(1):197–204.
31. Taylor N, van Saene HK, Abella A, et al. Selective digestive decontamination. why don't we apply the evidence in the clinical practice? *Med Intensiva.* 2007;3193:136–145.
32. de La Cal MA, Cerda E, Garcia-Hierro P, et al. Survival benefit in critically ill burned patients receiving selective decontamination of the digestive tract: a randomized, placebo-controlled, double-blind trial. *Ann Surg.* 2005;241(3):424–430.
33. Szanto Z, Pulay I, Kotsis L, Dinka T. Selective bowel decontamination. *Orv Hetil.* 2006;147(14):643–647.
34. Barrett JP, Jeschke MG, Herndon DN. Selective decontamination of the digestive tract in severely burned pediatric patients. *Burns.* 2001;27(5):439–445.
35. Verwaest C, Verhaegen J, Ferdinande P, et al. Randomized, controlled trial of selective digestive decontamination i 600 mechanically ventilated patients in a multidisciplinary intensive care unit. *Crit Care Med.* 1997;25(1):63–71.
36. Tuggle D, Skinner S, Garza J, et al. The abdominal compartment syndrome in patients with burn injury. *Acta Clin Belg Suppl.* 2007;(1):136–140.
37. Oda J, Yamashita K, Inoue T, et al. Resuscitation fluid volume and abdominal compartment syndrome in patients with major burns. *Burns.* 2006;32(2):151–154.
38. Meldrum DR, Moore FA, Moore EE, et al. Prospective characterization and selective management of the abdominal compartment syndrome. *Am J Surg.* 1997;174(6):667–672.
39. Hobson KG, Young KM, Ciraulo A, et al. Release of abdominal compartment syndrome improves survival in patients wit burn injury. *J Trauma.* 2002;53(6):1129–1133.
40. Hershberger RD, Hunt JL, Arnoldo BD, Purdue GF. Abdominal compartment syndrome in the severely burned patient. *J Burn Care Res.* 2007;28(5):708–714.
41. Khedr EM, Khedr T, El-Oteify MA, Hassan HA. Peripheral neuropathy in burn patients. *Burns.* 1997;23(7–8):579–583.
42. Shin C, Kinsky MP, Thomas JA, et al. Effect of cutaneous burn injury and resuscitation on the cerebral circulation in an ovine model. *Burns.* 1998;24(1):39–45.
43. Finfer S. Corticosteroids in septic shock. *N Engl J Med.* 2008;358(2):188–190.
44. Jeschke MG, Boehning EF, Finnerty CC, Herndon DN. Effect of insulin on the inflammatory and acute phase response after burn injury. *Crit Care Med.* 2007;35(9 Suppl):S519–523.
45. Matsui M, Kudo T, Kudo M, et al. The endocrine response after burns. *Agressologie.* 1991;32(4):233–235.
46. Murton SA, Tan ST, Prickett TCR, et al. Hormone responses to stress in patients with major burns. *Br J Plast Surg.* 1998;51:388–392.
47. Smith A, Barclay C, Quaba A, et al. The bigger the burn, the greater the stress. *Burns.* 1997;23(4):291–294.
48. Sprung CL, Annane D, Keh D, et al., for the CORTICUS Study Group. Hydrocortisone therapy for patients with septic shock. *N Engl J Med.* 2008;358(2):111–124.
49. Sedowofia K, Barclay C, Quaba A, et al. The systemic stress response to thermal injury in children. *Clin Endocrinol.* 1998;49:335–341.
50. Jeschke MG, Finnerty CC, Suman OE, et al. The effect of xyandrolone on the endocrinologic, inflammatory, and hypermetabolic responses during the acute phase postburn. *Ann Surg.* 2007;246(3):351–362.
51. Wick S. Endocrinology: Hormone Effects. August 1997. Human Physiology and Anatomy Laboratories, Allwine Hall 211E, University of Nebraska at Omaha.
52. Jeschke MG, Norbury WB, Finnerty CC, et al. Propranolol does not increase inflammation, sepsis, or infectious episodes in severely burned children. *J Trauma.* 2007;62(3):676–681.
53. Norbury WB, Jesche MG, Herndon DN. Metabolism modulators in sepsis: propranolol. *Crit Care Med.* 2007;35(9 Suppl):S616–620.
54. Wong CH, Song C, Heng KS, et al. Plasma free hemoglobin: a novel diagnostic test for assessment of the depth of burn injury. *Plast Reconstru Surg.* 2006;117(4):1206–1213.

55. Lawrence C, Atac B. Hematologic changes in massive burn injury. *Crit Care Med.* 1992;20(9):1284–1288.
Endoh Y, Kawakami M, Orringer EP, et al. Causes and time course of acute hemolysis after burn injury of the rat. *J Burn Care Rehabil.* 1992;13(2 Pt 1): 203–209.
56. Wong CH, Song C, Heng KS, et al. Plasma free hemoglobin: a novel diagnostic test for assessment of the depth of burn injury. *Plast Reconstr Surg.* 2006;117(4):1206–1213.
57. Hatherill JR, Till GO, Bruner LH, Ward P. Thermal injury, intravascular hemolysis, and toxic oxygen products. *J Clin Invest.* 1986;78:629–636.
58. Loebl EC, Baxter CR, Curreri PW. The mechanism of erythrocyte destruction in the early post-burn period. *Ann Surg.* 1973;178(6):681–686.
59. Kawakami EY, Orringer EP, Peterson HD, Meyer AA. Causes and time course of acute hemolysis after burn injury in the rat. *J Burn Care Rehabil.* 1992;12(2 Pt 1):203–209.
60. Griswold JA. White blood cell response to burn injury. *Semin Nephrol.* 1993;13(4):409–415.
61. Oberbeck R, Schmitz D, Wilsenack K, et al. Adrenergic modulation of survival and cellular immune functions during polymicrobial sepsis. *Neuroimmunomodulation.* 2004;11(4):214–223.
62. Schmitz D, Wilsenack K, Lendemanns S, et al. Beta-adrenergic blockade during systemic inflammation: impact on cellular immune functions and survival in a murine model of sepsis. *Resuscitation.* 2007;72(2):286–294.
63. Klein GL. Burn-induced bone loss: importance, mechanisms, and management. *J Burns Wounds* 2006;5:32–38.
64. Klein GL, Herndon DN, Goodman WG, et al. Histomorphometric and biochemical characterization of bone following acute severe burns in children. *Bone.* 1995;17(5):455–460.
65. Przkora R, Herndon DN, Sherrard DJ, et al. Pamidronate preserves bone mass for at least 2 years following acute administration for pediatric burn injury. *Bone.* 2007;41:279–302.
66. Klein GL, Wimalawansa SJ, Kulkarni G, et al. The efficacy of acute administration of pamidronate on the conservation of bone mass following severe burn injury in children: a double-blind, randomized, controlled study. *Osteoporos Int.* 2005;16(6):631–635.
67. Tanaka H, Matsuda T, Miyagantani Y, et al. Reduction of resuscitation fluid volumes in severely burned patients using ascorbic acid administration. *Arch Surg.* 2000;135:326–331.
68. Klein MB, Hayden D, Elson C, et al. The association between fluid administration and outcome following major burn. *Ann Surg.* 2007;245(4):622–628.
69. Hoskins SL, Elgjo GI, Lu J, et al. Closed-loop resuscitation of burn shock. *J Burn Care Res.* 2006;27(3):377–385.
70. Berger MM, Bernath MA, Chiolero RL. Resuscitation, anesthesia and analgesia of the burned patient. *Curr Opin Anaesthesiol.* 2001;14:431–435.
71. Mansfield MD. Resuscitation and monitoring. *Balliere's Clinical Anesthesiology* 1997;11(3):369–384.
72. Demling RH. The burn edema process: current concepts. *J Burn Care Rehab.* 2005;26:207–277.
73. Bert J, Gyenge C, Bowen B, et al. Fluid resuscitation following a burn injury: implications of a mathematical model of microvascular exchange. *Burns.* 1997;23(2):93–105.
74. Ampratwum RT, Bowen BD, Lund T, et al. A model of fluid resuscitation following burn injury: formulation and parameter estimation. *Comput Methods Programs Biomed.* 1995;47:1–19.
75. Lund T, Bert JL, Onarheim H, et al. Microvascular exchange during burn injury. I: A review. *Circ Shock.* 1989;28(3):179–197.
76. Bert JL, Bowen BD, Gu X, et al. Microvascular exchange during burn injury: ii. formulation and validation of a mathematical model. *Circ Shock.* 1989;28(3):199–219.
77. Bowen BD, Bert JL, Gu X, et al. Microvascular exchange during burn injury: iii. implications of the model. *Circ Shock.* 1989;28(3):221–233.
78. Bert JL, Bowen BD, Reed RK, Onarheim H. Microvascular exchange during burn injury: iv, fluid resuscitation model. *Circ Shock.* 1991;34(3):285–297.
79. Remensnyder JP. Acute electrical injuries. In: Martyn JAJ, ed. *Acute Management of the Burned Patient.* Philadelphia: W.B. Saunders Company, 1990:66–86.
80. Mozingo DW, Cioffi WG Jr, Pruitt BA Jr. Burns. In: Bongard FS, Sue DY, eds. *Current Critical Care Diagnosis &Treatment.* 2nd ed.: New York: Lange Medical Books/McGraw-Hill, 2002, pp. 799–828.
81. Elderman DA, Khan N, Kempf K, White MT. Pneumonia after inhalation injury. *J Burn Care Res.* 2007;28(2):241–246.
82. Cioffi WB, Graves TA, McManus WF, Pruitt BA Jr. High-frequency percussive ventilation in patients with inhalation injury. *J Trauma.* 1989;29(3): 350–354.
83. Hall JJ, Hunt JL, Arnoldo BD, Purdue GF. Use of high-frequency percussive ventilation in inhalation injuries. *J Burn Care Res.* 2007;28(3):396–400.
84. O'grady NP, Alexander M, Dellinger EP, et al. Healthcare infection control practices advisory committee: guidelines for the prevention of intravascular catheter-related infections. *Am J Infect Control.* 2002;30(8):476–489.
85. Tompkins RG, Burke JF, Schoenfeld DA, et al. Prompt eschar excision: a treatment system contributing to reduced burn mortality. *Ann Surg.* 1986;204(3):272–280.
86. Gastmeier P, Geffers C. Prevention of ventilator-associated pneumonia: analysis of studies published since 2004. *J Hosp Infect.* 2007;67(1):1–8.
87. Purdue GF. American Burn Association Presidential Address 2006 on Nutrition: Yesterday, Today, and Tomorrow. *J Burn Care Res.* 2006;28(1):1–5.
88. Juang P, Fish DN, Jung R, MacLaren R. Enteral glutamine supplementation in critically ill patients with burn injuries: a retrospective case-control evaluation. *Pharmacotherapy.* 2007;27(1):11–19.
89. Peng YZ, Yuan ZQ, Ciao GX. Effects of early enteral feeding on the prevention of enterogenic infection in severely burned patients. *Burns.* 2001;27(2):145–149.
90. Chen Z, Wang S, Yu B, Li A. A comparison study between early enteral nutrition and parenteral nutrition in severe burn patients. *Burns.* 2007;33(6):708–712.
91. Prelack K, Dylewski M, Sheridan RL. Practical guidelines for nutritional management of burn injury and recovery. *Burns.* 2007;33:14–24.
92. Berger MM, Shenkin A. Trace element requirements in critically ill burned patients. *J Trace Elements.* 2007;SI:44–48.
93. Wolf SE. Nutrition and metabolism in burns: state of the science, 2007. *J Burn Care Res.* 2007;28(4):572–576.
94. Windle EM. Glutamine supplementation in critical illness: evidence, recommendations, and implications for clinical practice in burn care. *J Burn Care Res.* 2006;27(6):764–772.
95. Bongers T, Griffiths RD, McArdle A. Exogenous glutamine: the clinical evidence. *Crit Care Med.* 2007;35(9):S545–S552.
96. Druml W. Protein metabolism in acute renal failure. *Miner Electrolyte Metab.* 1998.
97. Druml W. Nutritional management of acute renal failure. *Am J Kidney Dis.* 2001;37(1 Suppl 2):S89–94.
98. Chan L. Nutritional support in acute renal failure. *Curr Opin Clin Nutr Metab Care.* 2004;7:207–212.
99. Cynober L. Amino acid metabolism in thermal burns. *J Parenter Enteral Nutr.* 1989;12(2):196–205.
100. Windle EM. Glutamine supplementation in critical illness: evidence, recommendations, and implications for clinical practice in burn care. *J Burn Care Res.* 2006;27(6):764–672.
101. Nguyen TT, Gilpin DA, Meyer NA, Herndon DN. Current treatment of severely burned patients. *Ann Surg.* 1996;223(1):14–25.
102. Murphy KD, Lee JO, Herndon DN. Current pharmacotherapy for the treatment of severe burns. *Exp Opin Pharmacother.* 2003;4(3):369.
103. Rue LW, Cioffi WG, Rush R, et al. Thromboembolic complications in thermally injured patients. *World J Surg.* 1992;16:1151–1155.

CHAPTER 89 ■ TEMPERATURE-RELATED INJURIES

TAKERU SHIMIZU • TARO MIZUTANI

Human body temperature is maintained within tight limits by a balance between heat production and dissipation. Heat is normally generated by muscular activity and metabolic reactions, the latter mainly by the liver. It is dissipated by a combination of radiation, convection, conduction, and evaporation. This balance between heat generation and dissipation is the key to maintaining optimal body temperature. Under normal circumstances, body temperature is 37°C under the tongue, 38°C in the rectum, 32°C at the skin, and 38.5°C in the central liver. Significant deviation from normal body temperature is a critical condition that requires prompt diagnosis, treatment, and normalization of the temperature alteration. Herein, we discuss hypothermia, hyperthermia, and malignant hyperthermia and the neuroleptic malignant hyperthermia.

HYPOTHERMIA

Hypothermia is generally defined as a core temperature below 35°C (95° F) (1–3). In a more detailed manner, the literature classifies hypothermia as mild, moderate, or severe: mild hypothermia is that between 35°C and 32°C, moderate hypothermia between 32°C and 28°C, and severe hypothermia below 28°C (4). Table 89.1 outlines the classification of severity and clinical manifestations.

Hypothermia may be precipitated by various acute and chronic medical conditions, environmental exposure, or drugs. Hypothermia caused without exposure to the extreme temperatures is generally limited to mild to moderate in degree. Interestingly, however, with equivalent body temperature, patients found indoors were more severely affected and died more frequently than those found outdoors (5).

Hypothermia is considered to be an underrecognized condition, especially in the aged (2,3). Elderly patients who develop hypothermia are more likely to live alone, have other intercurrent diseases, to have their home heating turned off or inadequate home heating, and to wear inappropriate clothing for actual ambient temperatures (6).

Several confounding factors can further impair temperature control. Intoxicants, medications, extremes of age, and the general state of health—including intercurrent diseases—can modify the heat loss. Hypothermia occurs in various clinical settings; Table 89.2 outlines the clinical causes and disorders associated with this finding.

Accidental hypothermia is defined as a spontaneous decrease in core temperature. It is often caused by a cold environment and associated with an acute problem, but without any primary disorder of the temperature regulatory center. This is most commonly observed in neonates; the elderly; unconscious, immobile, or drugged persons; and workers in an extremely cold environment. Mortality rates for accidental hypothermia have been reported to range between 10% and 80%. A multicenter review of 428 cases of accidental hypothermia reported an overall mortality of 17% (7–9). Intercurrent diseases or infection seem to contribute to most deaths, as it was shown that patients with sepsis had a markedly worse mortality rate when they presented with hypothermia, as opposed to fever (10).

Temperature Regulation and Mechanism of Heat Loss

Hypothermia presents when heat generation cannot keep up with heat dissipation. Heat generation depends on the metabolic process at rest and on skeletal muscle metabolism during exercise. Humans have a high capacity to dissipate heat, with four primary means of heat dissipation or transmission. It is important to know these mechanisms to prevent hypothermia and to develop effective rewarming strategies.

1. *Conduction:* Conduction is the transfer of heat between two masses in contact with one another. The rate of heat transfer depends on the temperature gradient at the interface and the size of the contact area. It is also determined by the thermal conductivity of the materials. Metals and liquids are most conductive, and gases are most insulating. For example, water has a 25- to 30-fold larger conductivity than air. This means that contacting a wet surface is one of the fastest ways to dissipate body temperature.
2. *Convection:* Convection is the transfer of heat due to the flow of liquids or gases over a surface. Convective heat loss occurs when air around a patient is continuously swept away, and it is directly proportional to the body surface area, the temperature gradient, and the air velocity.
3. *Radiation:* Transfer of radiant energy is due to electromagnetic transmission.
4. *Evaporation:* Evaporation is the process whereby atoms or molecules in a liquid state gain sufficient energy to enter the gaseous state. Evaporation proceeds more quickly at higher temperature and/or at higher flow rates between the gaseous and liquid phase. Therefore, the heat loss by this mechanism is proportional to the change of the vapor pressure from the surface to ambient air and the velocity of air movement. Approximately 30% of evaporative heat loss occurs in the lung, and the rest is from the skin surface at usual room temperature. Evaporation accounts for 10% to 15% of total body

TABLE 89.1

CLASSIFICATION OF HYPOTHERMIA

Core temperature	Consciousness	Shivering	Heart rate	ECG	Respiration
Mild (35°C–33°C)	Normal	+	Normal	Normal	Normal
Moderate (33°C–30°C)	Depressed (stupor)	–	Slight decrease	Prolongation	Depressed
Severe (30°C–25°C)	Confusion	–	Decreased	Osborne J-wave	Apneic/agonal
25°C–20°C	Coma	Muscle rigidity	Decreased	Atrial fibrillation	Apneic
Below 20°C	Coma	Muscle rigidity	Asystole	Ventricular fibrillation	Apneic

heat loss. The heat of evaporation of water is 0.58 kcal/g H_2O. Given that 30 g of water is lost during the breathing of dry room air per hour, about 18 kcal, which is nearly half of an anesthetized patient's hourly heat production, is lost.

Clinical Syndromes

Cardiovascular

A sympathetic response increases myocardial oxygen consumption and causes tachycardia and peripheral vasoconstriction—that is, diminished pulses, pallor, acrocyanosis, and cold extremities—in patients with mild hypothermia (core temperature of 32°C–35°C). Blood pressure and heart rate are initially increased, followed by bradycardia, which further deteriorates at 32°C, and consequently, cardiac output, myocardial contractility, and arterial pressure fall.

Electrocardiographic (ECG) findings include the Osborne J-wave after the QRS complex as hypothermia becomes more severe (Fig. 89.1) The Osborne J-wave is an important diagnostic feature, which can be observed in other pathologic conditions such as central nervous system lesions and sepsis, but it is frequently absent (3,11). Atrial and ventricular fibrillation are common, and electrical defibrillation during hypothermia is often ineffective. It is important to remember that the hypothermic myocardium is irritable, making placement of pulmonary artery or other central catheters dangerous.

Respiratory System

Respiratory rate falls. The patient becomes apneic or has an agonal respiratory pattern when the body temperature is less than 28°C.

Central Nervous System

The electroencephalogram (EEG) becomes flat at 19°C to 29°C (12). Cerebrovascular autoregulation remains intact until the core temperature falls to below 25°C, but mentation starts to drop at 30°C. Dysarthria and hyperreflexia occur below 35°C, and hyporeflexia occurs below 32°C.

Coagulation

Hypothermia produces coagulopathy via three major mechanisms (13,14). First, the enzymatic coagulation cascade is impaired; second, platelet dysfunction occurs; and third, plasma fibrinolytic activity is enhanced. Because coagulation tests, such as prothrombin time (PT) or partial thrombin time (PTT), are performed at 37°C in the laboratory, a major disparity between clinical coagulopathy and the reported values is frequently observed (15). A disseminated intravascular coagulation (DIC) type of syndrome is also reported (16). Clinically significant coagulopathies occur and are often associated with trauma (17,18).

Renal System

Exposure to cold induces a diuresis irrespective of the state of hydration. Centralization of the blood volume—due to the

TABLE 89.2

CAUSES OF HYPOTHERMIA

Clinical cause	Associated disorders
Central Nervous System	Head trauma, tumor, stroke, Wernicke encephalopathy, Shapiro syndrome, Parkinson disease, multiple sclerosis, sarcoidosis, acute spinal cord transection, paraplegia
Metabolic	Hypoglycemia, hypothyroidism, hypoadrenalism, panhypopituitarism, diabetic ketoacidosis, anorexia nervosa
Integument	Burns, erythroderma, ichthyosis, psoriasis, exfoliative dermatitis
Infection	Sepsis
Chronic Diseases	Chronic heart failure, chronic renal failure, chronic hepatic insufficiency, advanced age
Environmental Exposure	Outdoor activities and physical or metabolic exhaustion, cold water immersion, inadequate indoor heating (particularly in the elderly and infirm), operating room
Pharmaceuticals/Drugs	Ethanol, muscle relaxants, phenothiazines, barbiturates, tricyclic antidepressants, lithium (toxic dose), α-adrenergic agonist (clonidine), anticholinergic drugs, β-adrenergic blocker

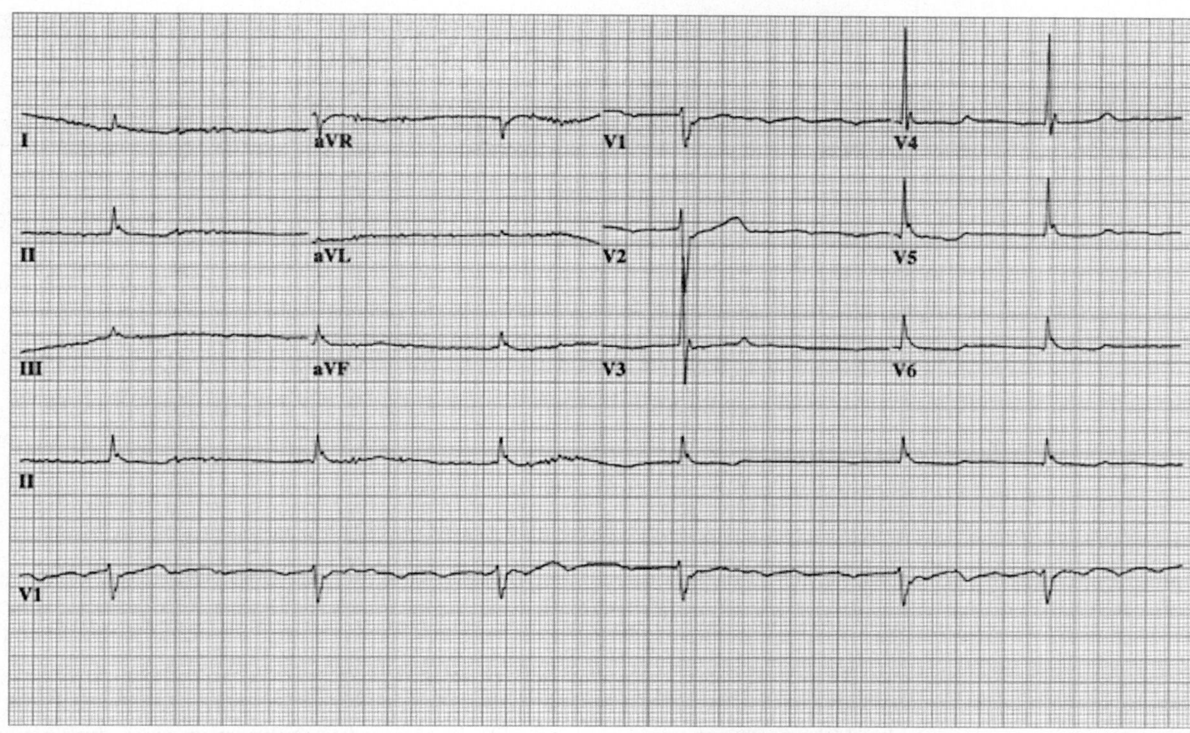

FIGURE 89.1. The electrocardiogram (ECG) shows atrial fibrillation with a very slow ventricular response, prominent J (Osborne) waves (late, terminal upright deflection of QRS complex; best seen in leads V3–V6), and nonspecific QRS widening. (Adapted from O'Keefe J, Hammill S, Freed M, et al. *The Complete Guide to ECGs.* 2nd ed. Royal Oak, MI: Physicians' Press; 2002.)

initial peripheral vasoconstriction—stimulates the diuresis. Hypothermia depresses renal blood flow by 50% at 27°C to 30°C, and the renal cellular basal metabolic rate decreases (2). As a result, renal tubular cell reabsorptive function decreases and the kidney excretes a large amount of dilute urine. This is termed *cold diuresis*, resulting in a decreased blood volume and progressive hemoconcentration (19).

Glucose Metabolism

Blood glucose concentration commonly increases because pancreatic function, insulin activity, and/or response to insulin decrease, along with activated function of the autonomic nervous system in hypothermia. At the same time, hemoconcentration results in elevated serum glucose concentration.

Therapeutic Approach

While rewarming is the common goal in the clinical treatment of the hypothermic patient, it is both difficult and controversial to treat. At the same time as treatment is initiated, a search for and discovery of the mechanism of heat loss will play a key role in achieving a better outcome. Treatment includes that delivered by prehospital providers as well as inpatient care.

Prehospital Treatment

Hypothermia is often combined with mental and physical exhaustion. Even if a patient is found down, cold, stiff, and cyanotic, the patient is not necessarily dead and may make a recovery even when signs of life are initially absent. Thus, rescue efforts should not be given up while the patient is cold. Since ventricular fibrillation or asystole may be induced by any stimuli, such as tracheal intubation, comatose patients should be treated with extreme care.

The initial primary focus of prehospital treatment is to avoid further loss of heat. Removal of wet clothing and applying dry insulating covers such as blankets, pads, coats, and sleeping bags are effective in treating all the mechanisms of heat loss described above. During transportation, an aluminized space blanket may be used. To make the most of its effect, the patient should be carefully wrapped with additional blankets. The patient should be kept horizontal to minimize the circulatory and sympathetic change. Vigorous rubbing should be avoided because it induces vasodilation, which may be followed by hypotension or "rewarming shock." Hot water bottles or hot packs may be used if available but should be used cautiously to avoid burn injury.

Resuscitation using the ABCs—airway, breathing, circulation—of basic life support are implemented if needed. Warmed (42°C–46°C), humidified oxygen during bag/mask ventilation (20) and warmed intravenous fluids should be given if possible. Death should not be declared below 32°C.

In-hospital Treatment

Indicated monitoring includes an ECG, Doppler evaluation of pulses, and temperature. General laboratory studies include electrolytes, complete blood count, coagulation studies (prothrombin time and partial thromboplastin time), blood urea nitrogen, creatinine, amylase, calcium, magnesium, and glucose concentrations. Radiologic examinations are indicated. Patients with hypothermia are usually dehydrated, which should be corrected with IV fluids warmed to 43°C (20). The

TABLE 89.3

REWARMING METHODS

Classification		Methods	Effects
Passive	External	Adding an insulating layer (e.g., blanket, sleeping bag)	0.1°C–0.7°C increase/h
		Increasing ambient temperature	Effective when body temperature is above 32°C
Active	External	Hot water bottles Heating blanket Infrared lamp	1°C–4°C increase/h Internal rewarming should be applied to avoid rewarming shock
		Submersion in a warm water tank	5°C–7°C increase/h
	Internal (core)	Warmed crystalloid fluids or blood transfusion	1.5°C–2°C increase/h
		Gastric lavage Rectal lavage Cystic lavage Airway rewarming	Warmed fluids administration required due to loss of circulatory blood volume caused by cold diuresis
	(invasive)	Peritoneal dialysis Thoracic cavity lavage Hemodialysis Cardiopulmonary bypass Percutaneous cardiopulmonary support	3°C–15°C increase/h

use of glucose-containing solutions should be used with caution as hypothermic patients are usually hyperglycemic due to hypoactivity of insulin.

The various options for therapeutic approaches can be considered, and rewarming should be performed along with other supportive therapy. Techniques of rewarming include active and passive methods, and external and internal (core) methods (Table 89.3). Although no difference in survival and clinical or histopathologic morbidity has been demonstrated by some prospective studies comparing active and external rewarming versus core rewarming methods (21,22), percutaneous or open chest cardiopulmonary bypass is recommended for pulseless hypothermic patients if it is available (23–31).

Bronchopneumonia secondary to aspiration is a common complication. Oral intake of warm or hot drink should be avoided because obtunded, hypothermic patients may have suppressed airway protective mechanisms, including cough or gag reflexes. Prophylactic tracheal intubation may be considered if suppression of these reflexes is present. When the trachea is intubated, warmed (42°C–46°C), humidified oxygen should be administered (20).

HYPERTHERMIA

There are many conditions that elevate the body temperature. Table 89.4 outlines the major causes, which may be classified as hyperthermia or fever. In this section, we discuss environmental hyperthermia as well as malignant hyperthermia and the neuroleptic malignant syndrome.

Environmental Hyperthermia—Heat Stroke

Heat stroke is a medical emergency, characterized by a high body temperature, altered mental status, and hot dry flushed skin (32). It may lead to multisystem organ dysfunction with hemorrhage and necrosis in the lungs, heart, liver, kidneys, brain, and intestines (33). Heat stroke is thought to be relatively uncommon in temperate climates. The documented body temperature with this disorder is 41.1°C or more. There has been no obvious decrease in mortality in the last 50 years, which is variably quoted as ranging between 10% and 50% (33).

There are several heat-related illnesses, which may take the form of heat syncope, heat cramps, heat exhaustion, and heat stroke. Heat stroke may be further classified as exertional and nonexertional (classic heatstroke). Table 89.5 outlines the syndromes.

- *Heat syncope:* Heat syncope is fainting due to peripheral vasodilation secondary to high ambient temperature.
- *Heat cramp:* Heat cramp refers to muscular cramping occurring during exercise in heat, which is related to electrolyte deficiency; it is usually benign.
- *Heat exhaustion:* This is often referred to as heat prostration. Heat exhaustion occurs when the individual becomes dehydrated and weak. The patient collapses from dehydration, salt depletion, and hypovolemia. Anorexia, nausea, and vomiting frequently occur. Excessive sweating leads to a loss of water and/or electrolytes. There are two mechanisms for this disorder: salt-depletion and water-depletion heat exhaustion. Salt-depletion heat exhaustion usually occurs when an unacclimatized person exercises and replaces only water. Water-depletion heat exhaustion is usually observed in an acclimatized person who has inadequate water intake during exposure to extreme heat. Serum sodium concentration may be normal or mildly elevated. The core temperature may or may not be raised (usually mild to moderate, less than 38°C) and tissue damage does not occur.
- *Heat stroke:* Heat stroke occurs when the core body temperature rises against a failing thermoregulatory system (32). The core temperature most often quoted is a rectal temperature exceeding 40.6°C (34). Heat stroke may be divided into

TABLE 89.4

HYPERTHERMIA AND FEVER

HYPERTHERMIA		
Environmental exposure		
Malignant hyperthermia		
Neuroleptic malignant syndrome		
Thyroid storm		
Pheochromocytoma		
Serotonin syndrome		
Iatrogenic hyperthermia		
Brainstem/hypothalamic injury		
Drugs:		
Diuretics	Anticholinergics	Phenothiazines
Antidepressants	Lithium	Antihistamines
Ethanol	Salicylates	β-adrenergic blockers
FEVER		
Inflammatory disorders		
Infection		
Allergic reactions		
Collagen diseases		
Neoplasm		
Inherited and metabolic diseases		
Factitious fever		

exertional and nonexertional (classic) heat stroke (34). Exertional heat stroke occurs in previously healthy young people exercising in hot and humid climates without being acclimatized. Nonexertional heat stroke occurs during extreme heat waves, the elderly being particularly vulnerable (Table 89.6).

Temperature Regulation

Normal heat production is primarily due to metabolic activity in the liver and skeletal muscle, with the liver generating most body heat at rest and muscle being the major source with exercise or shivering. Skeletal muscle heat production ranges from 65 to 85 kcal/hour at basal level, but it may increase up to 900 kcal/hour (35). Heat elimination occurs by four major mechanisms as we have discussed in hypothermia. Convection and radiation are normally the most important mechanisms for heat elimination. Evaporation becomes a major mechanism for heat dissipation with incremental skeletal muscle metabolic activity. If the ambient temperature exceeds body temperature, heat loss may depend only on evaporation. However, sweating produces only 400 to 650 kcal/hour of heat dissipation. Therefore, blood flow regulation to skin and sweat gland activity are critical in maintaining thermal balance. There is a distinction made between exertional and nonexertional heat stroke at this point; failure of thermoregulation (lack of sweating) may be more important in nonexertional (classic) heat stroke and less so in exertional heat stroke (36).

The process of thermoregulation consists of three parts: (i) afferent thermal sensing, (ii) hypothalamic processing, and (iii) efferent responses through the sympathetic system. Heat stimuli are carried by C fibers from the skin to the spinal cord. Central temperature sensors in the abdominal and thoracic viscera, spinal cord, and brain may play a significant role in preventing hyperthermia, although peripheral sensors in the skin seem to be most important. The hypothalamus integrates all afferent temperature input to alter body temperature by regulating vasomotor tone to the skin and inducing sweat formation. Neural output to the cerebral cortex is also important in modifying behavior to compensate for changes in temperature. The efferent hypothalamic response to heat consists of cutaneous

TABLE 89.5

HEAT SYNDROMES

Syndrome	Temperature	Manifestation
Heat syncope	Normal	Faintness
Heat cramps	Normal	Muscle cramps
Heat exhaustion	Normal to 39°C	Faintness, weakness
Heat stroke	>40.6°C	Gross neurologic impairment

TABLE 89.6

EXERTIONAL AND NONEXERTIONAL HEAT STROKE SYNDROMES

	Exertional	Nonexertional
Age	Young	Elderly
Precipitating event	Heat, strenuous activity	Heat
Underlying process	None	Medical illness, drug therapy
Onset	Rapid	Slow
Sweating	Present	Absent

vasodilation, sweat formation, and inhibition of muscle tone. Vasomotor tonic changes result in cutaneous dilation and shunting of blood away from the liver and splanchnic circulation, facilitating heat transfer from the core to skin. Sweat formation is under cholinergic sympathetic control. Removing clothes, limiting physical activity, and moving to a cooler place are important behaviors.

Acclimatization is a physiologic process whereby an individual adapts to work in a hot environment (35). Acclimatization to sustained increases in body temperature is slow and requires 1 to 2 weeks for peak effect. Sweat volume increases from 1.5 L/hour up to 4 L/hour. The sweating threshold decreases over an extended period of time. Sweat sodium concentration decreases from 30 to 60 mEq/L to about 5 mEq/L. Plasma antidiuretic hormone, growth hormone, and aldosterone levels increase. Cardiovascular mechanisms include a 10% to 25% increase in plasma volume and an increased stroke volume and cardiac output with a slowing of heart rate.

Clinical Syndrome

Heat stroke is mostly defined as a core temperature above 40.6°C, but neurologic impairment may occur at lower temperatures in some cases; indeed, neurologic dysfunction is a cardinal feature of heat stroke (37). Neurologic manifestations include slurred speech, delirium, stupor, lethargy, coma, and seizures (38). Seizures occur more commonly at temperatures above 41°C. Ataxia, dysmetria, and dysarthria may also be observed.

The cardiovascular system is commonly compromised in the presence of heat stroke. Tachydysrhythmia and hypotension frequently occur (38). Hypotension may result from translocation of blood from the central circulation to the periphery to dissipate heat, or the increased production of nitric oxide may result in vasodilation (37,39). A study of Doppler and echocardiographic findings in patients with classic heat stroke and heat exhaustion reported a circulation that was hyperdynamic, with tachycardia, resulting in high cardiac output (34). It also reported that hypovolemia was more pronounced in heat stroke patients with signs of peripheral vasoconstriction. Heat exhaustion patients were more likely to demonstrate peripheral vasodilation.

Lactic acidosis may occur. Since patients in heat stroke are in shock, the mechanism by which lactate is cleared by the liver and converted to glucose is less effective, and restoration of the circulating volume may lead to worsening lactic acidosis as skeletal muscle is reperfused and the elevated lactate cleared. Patients typically hyperventilate to compensate for the acute acidosis with an acute respiratory alkalosis. This may lead to heat-induced tetany. After several hours, a mixed acid-base disorder may occur because of sustained tissue damage.

Significant dehydration is noted in most patients with exertional heat stroke and may be reflected as elevated blood urea nitrogen and creatinine levels or hemoconcentration. Sodium, potassium, phosphate, calcium, and magnesium serum concentrations are frequently low in the early period (35,40–44). Sodium, potassium, and magnesium are lost through increased sweating. Hypokalemia may be as a result of catecholamine release or may occur secondary to hyperventilation. Hypokalemia decreases sweat secretion and skeletal muscle blood flow, which may impair heat dissipation. Cellular death begins to occur throughout the body at temperatures above 42°C. Hyperkalemia may occur if significant skeletal muscle damage or cellular lysis develops. If significant rhabdomyolysis develops, injured cells release phosphate, which reacts with serum calcium and may lead to hypocalcemia.

Renal dysfunction is well documented in exertional heat stroke, with the incidence of acute renal failure approximately 25% (45). The cause is usually multifactorial, including direct thermal injury, the prerenal insults of volume depletion, and renal hypotension, rhabdomyolysis, and disseminated intravascular coagulation (DIC) (38).

Liver damage is very frequently seen and is probably related to splanchnic redistribution (46,47). Elevated liver enzymes are common.

Hemorrhagic complications may be observed. These may be petechial hemorrhages and ecchymoses, which may represent direct thermal injury or may be related to the development of DIC. Damatte et al. (38) reported that 45% of patients had laboratory evidence of DIC. This consumption coagulopathy may be further compounded by hepatocellular damage.

Complications

Cardiac complications include myocardial pump failure, tachydysrhythmia, high cardiac output, and myocardial infarction. ECG abnormalities are also observed (48). Sinus tachycardia and QT prolongation are followed by nonspecific ST-T wave changes, suggesting cardiac ischemia.

Neurologic complications include seizures, cerebral edema, and localized brain hemorrhages. Irreversible brain damage occurs above 42°C. Cerebellar impairment may persist after recovery.

Pulmonary edema may be caused by a limited cardiac function or may develop secondary to the acute respiratory distress syndrome (ARDS) (49). Pulmonary aspiration may be observed in obtunded patients.

Acute renal failure may be caused by direct heat damage, renal hypoperfusion, or rhabdomyolysis. The incidence of renal failure is about 35% with exertional heat stroke and about 5% in classic nonexertional heat stroke, with which rhabdomyolysis is less likely to coexist.

Liver damage and dysfunction occur in most patients with heat stroke. Cholestasis and centrilobular necrosis elevate bilirubin and liver enzymes, which may not be apparent until 48 to 72 hours after injury (44).

Hematologic complications include hemolysis, thrombocytopenia, and DIC (49). DIC is triggered by diffuse endothelial and organ damage, has an onset delay of 2 to 3 days after the initiating event, and is associated with high mortality.

Therapeutic Approach

Heat stroke requires prompt and effective treatments. Oxygen therapy, rapid cooling, and cautious hydration should be immediately instituted to avoid complications and achieve recovery. Tracheal intubation should be considered if the patient is obtunded or in respiratory distress. Oxygen delivery is often less than normal, and pulmonary shunt fraction is increased (50).

Rapid cooling is accomplished by external techniques. These include immersion in ice water or application of cooling blankets above and below the patient (conductive cooling technique), and wetting the skin with water or alcohol, followed by the use of fans to facilitate evaporation and heat dissipation (evaporative-convective cooling technique). Both techniques usually reduce core temperature below 40°C in 1 hour. A significant disadvantage of immersion is impairment of access to the patient and limited monitoring. Another disadvantage of immersion is that intense vasoconstriction can slow the rate of heat loss (51). Vasoconstriction may also have adverse cardiovascular effects in patients with limited cardiac function because it increases cardiac afterload. Vasoconstriction may be reduced by skin massage, which prevents dermal stasis of cooled blood. More aggressive cooling techniques include gastric lavage with iced saline, cold hemodialysis, and cardiopulmonary bypass. They are only rarely required, being used in cases of refractory temperature elevation or malignant hyperthermia, in which thermogenesis is ongoing. In addition, the efficacy of rapid infusion of large-volume ice-cold intravenous fluid (LVICF)—using either lactated Ringer solution or normal saline—has been implicated in clinical trials of induced hypothermia. Bernard et al. (52) showed that 30 mL/kg of LVICF (lactated Ringer solution at 4°C) over 30 minutes decreased core temperature by 1.7°C immediately after infusion, with improvements in acid-base and renal function.

Core body temperature should be monitored closely at the rectum, bladder, or tympanic membrane. Vital signs, neurologic functions, urine output, and laboratory measurements should also be monitored closely. Laboratory measurements include arterial blood gas and serum electrolyte concentrations, especially potassium, which may increase significantly and result in life-threatening hyperkalemia. Glucose–insulin therapy should be instituted emergently in patients with ECG changes.

Intravenous volume repletion should be individualized. Volume deficit is not a prominent feature in classic nonexertional heat stroke. Central venous catheter and pulmonary artery catheter placement may be invaluable to assess volume depletion, peripheral vascular vasodilation, or primary myocardial dysfunction, especially in patients with limited cardiac reserve. Hypotension usually responds to intravenous fluids, but if an inotropic drug is needed, dobutamine is the drug of choice for heat stroke.

Seizures occur commonly in heat stroke patients and should be treated with intravenous diazepam or other benzodiazepines. The efficacy or clinical rationale for the administration of dehydrating drugs is uncertain, but these drugs may be potentially beneficial for some patients at risk of acute renal failure secondary to rhabdomyolysis, as acute renal failure can be a major cause of patient morbidity. This may be prevented by prompt repletion of intravascular volume and restabilizing adequate renal perfusion pressure. Hemodialysis may be required if hyperkalemia or other metabolic disturbances exist.

DIC may be treated with continuous infusion heparin therapy. Although this therapy brings some benefit, its utility seems uncertain (40,42,44).

Malignant Hyperthermia and the Neuroleptic Malignant Syndrome

Malignant hyperthermia (MH) and the neuroleptic malignant syndrome (NMS) are disorders of rising body temperature related to an imbalance between heat production and heat dissipation. MH was not clearly described as a syndrome until 1960 (53,54). NMS was first described by Delay et al. (55) after the introduction of neuroleptics in 1960. These disorders are uncommon but life-threatening complications related to the administration of anesthetic or neuroleptic drugs. Their main features include hyperthermia, muscle rigidity, metabolic acidosis, and autonomic disturbances. Endogenous heat production resulting from impaired physiologic heat-dissipating mechanisms and hypothalamic temperature regulation is responsible for elevation of core body temperature in NMS. On the other hand, it usually appears intact in MH (56). Both of them are uniquely characterized by their association with various drugs, although they are distinctive from each other; associated drugs are listed in Table 89.7 (56–65). An additive in commercial succinylcholine, chlorocresol, has been reported as an additional trigger in MH (66). The *in vitro* halothane–caffeine contracture test on skeletal muscle helps to identify susceptible individuals and to establish with certainty the genetic nature of the disorder in most individuals (67).

TABLE 89.7

DRUGS ASSOCIATED WITH MALIGNANT HYPERTHERMIA AND THE NEUROLEPTIC MALIGNANT SYNDROME

Classification	Associated drugs
MALIGNANT HYPERTHERMIA	
Volatile anesthetics	Halothane, cyclopropane, enflurane, methoxyflurane, isoflurane, sevoflurane, desflurane, diethyl ether
Depolarizing muscle relaxants	Succinylcholine, decamethonium
Antidysrhythmics	Lidocaine
NEUROLEPTIC MALIGNANT SYNDROME	
Phenothiazines	Fluphenazine, chlorpromazine, levomepromazine, thioridazine, trimeprazine, methotrimeprazine, trifluoperazine, prochlorperazine, promethazine, alimemazine
Butyrophenones	Haloperidol, bromperidol, droperidol
Thioxanthenes	Thiothixene, zuclopenthixol
Dibenzazepines	Loxapine
Dopamine-depleting drugs	Alpha-methyltyrosine, tetrabenazine, amoxapine
Dopamine agonist withdrawal	Levodopa, levodopa/carbidopa, amantadine
Serotonin dopamine antagonists	Risperidone
Serotonin-depleting drugs	Paroxetine

Incidence

A Danish survey indicates an incidence of fulminant MH of 1 in 250,000 patients. The overall incidence of MH is between 1 in 50,000 and 1 in 100,000 patients receiving general anesthesia (68–70). Suspected MH occurred in 1 in 16,000 anesthetics overall and 1 in 4,200 anesthetics involving potent volatile agents and succinylcholine. Incidence rates of MH reported vary by country. The mortality rate was initially 70%; earlier diagnosis and use of dantrolene have reduced it to less than 5% (71).

The incidence of NMS ranges from 0.07% to 2.2% among patients receiving neuroleptic agents (72–74). A decrease in mortality has been reported; NMS has had a 76% mortality before 1970, a 22% mortality from 1970 to 1980, and a 15% mortality since 1980 (75).

Temperature Regulation

Most patients with an episode of MH have a history of relatives with a similar episode or an abnormal response to the halothane–caffeine contracture test. Genetic inheritance patterns reflect the complexity of the responsible genes of MH. Genes on chromosomes 1, 3, 5, 7, 17, and 19 (1q32, 3q13, 5p, 7q21–24, 17q21–24) have been indicated (76–78). The exact mechanisms of MH are poorly understood. The initial focus was on an abnormal calcium channel receptor, ryanodine RYR1 receptor, in patients with MH, which is responsible for calcium release from the sarcoplasmic reticulum and plays a critical role in muscle depolarization. Further studies have shown that many patients with MH have a normal ryanodine receptor. However, mutations in RYR1 occur in at least 50% of susceptible subjects and almost all families. More than 30 missense mutations and one deletion have been associated with a positive contracture test result or clinical MH (79). Other than RYR1, only two other genes—α1s-subunit of DHPR, and CACNL1A3 in MHS3—are implicated, and they are responsible for less than 1% of the cases (80). For practical purposes, the RYR1 gene remains the target for genetic analysis.

Resultant from this mutation, free inbound ionized calcium can be released from the storage sites, which normally maintain skeletal muscle relaxation by sequestering calcium from the muscle contractile apparatus (56). The administration of anesthetics may unpredictably trigger rapid calcium release into the myoplasm, followed by the development of muscle contracture, rigidity, and increased muscle metabolic activity. This process can cause core body temperature to rise vigorously at a rate of 1°C every 5 minutes.

The administration of certain neuroleptic drugs may induce a similar elevation of body core temperature. A common pathophysiology of NMS and MH has been suggested (81,82). This suggestion is based mainly on three points: (i) NMS and MH have clinical features in common, such as hyperthermia, rigidity, an elevated creatine kinase concentration, and a mortality rate of 10% to 30%; (ii) sodium dantrolene has been used successfully in both syndromes; and (iii) abnormal findings have been observed in *in vitro* contractility tests in patients with either of the syndromes. Caroff et al. (83) suggested that patients with a genetic predisposition for MH might also be at risk for developing NMS. However, Adnet et al. (84) reported that abnormal sarcolemmal calcium permeability was not shared in the pathogenesis of these disorders. The mechanism of hyperthermia and muscle rigidity is not yet defined, but two major theories have been postulated, which are central dopamine receptor blockade and the direct toxic effect of skeletal muscle induced by neuroleptics. Hypothalamic thermoregulation involves noradrenergic, serotoninergic, cholinergic, and central dopaminergic pathways (85). Dopamine plays a role in central thermoregulation in mammals. A dopamine injection into the hypothalamus causes a reduction in core temperature (86). Since neuroleptics block dopamine receptors, the hyperthermia associated with NMS may result from a blockade of

TABLE 89.8A

SCORING RULES FOR THE MALIGNANT HYPERTHERMIA (MH) CLINICAL GRADING SCALE

MH INDICATORS

Review the list of clinical indicators. If any indicator is present, add the points applicable for each indicator while observing the double-counting rule below, which applies to multiple indicators representing a single process.

If no indicator is present, the patient's MH score is zero.

DOUBLE-COUNTING

If more than one indicator represents a single process, *count only the indicator with the highest score*. Application of this rule prevents double-counting when one clinical process has more than one clinical manifestation.

Exception: The score for any relevant indicators in the final category of Table 89.8B ("other indicators") *should* be added to the total score without regard to double-counting.

MH SUSCEPTIBILITY INDICATORS

The italicized indicators listed below apply only to MH susceptibility. Do not use these indicators to score an MH event. To calculate the score for MH susceptibility, add the score of the italicized indicators below to the score for the highest-ranking MH event.

Positive family history of MH in relative of first degree

Positive family history of MH in relative not of first degree

Resting elevated serum creatinine kinase

Positive family history of MH together with another indicator from the patient's own anesthetic experience other than elevated serum creatine kinase

Interpreting the raw score: MH rank and qualitative likelihood

Raw score range	MH rank	Description of likelihood
0	1	Almost never
3–9	2	Unlikely
10–19	3	Somewhat less than likely
20–34	4	Somewhat greater than likely
35–49	5	Very likely
50+	6	Almost certain

hypothalamic dopamine sites. In addition, the blockade of dopamine receptors in the corpus striatum is thought to cause muscular rigidity and heat generation. Muscle contracture has been induced *in vitro* by chlorpromazine (87), which is reported to influence calcium ion transport across the sarcoplasmic reticulum and the contractile system (88). However, other studies that do not support the mechanism have also been reported (83,84).

Clinical Syndrome

MH may occur shortly after induction of anesthesia, at any time during the administration of anesthetics, or postoperatively. Trismus is the initial event in 50% of patients, and other early signs are tachycardia and hypercapnia due to increased metabolism (89). These are followed by whole-body rigidity and a marked increase in core body temperature. Trismus may occur in up to 1% of normal patients, and it has been also reported that fewer than 50% of patients prove to be susceptible to MH by muscle testing (90). Tachypnea is obvious when muscle relaxants are not administered. Sympathetic system overactivity produces tachycardia, hypertension, and mottled cyanosis. These symptoms precede hyperthermia, hyperkalemia, hypercalcemia, and lactic acidosis. Capnography may provide an early warning, since carbon dioxide production is remarkably increased while MH is in progress (91). Core body temperature can rise at a rate of 1°C every 5 minutes when hyperthermia occurs. Hypertension may be rapidly followed by hypotension as cardiac depression occurs. Anesthesia should be aborted if these signs appear or if MH is suspected. Laboratory evaluation reveals increased serum myoglobin, creatine kinase (CK, greater than 20,000 U/L), lactate dehydrogenase, and aldolase levels. Dark urine reflects myoglobinemia and myoglobinuria. However, elevation of both myoglobin and CK levels can be observed in some normal patients after succinylcholine administration without MH. The recent most significant study on a clinical grading scale for the prediction of MH was reported and is summarized in Table 89.8A and B (89).

NMS should be suspected in patients given any neuroleptic drugs who subsequently develop signs of muscular rigidity,

TABLE 89.8B

CLINICAL INDICATORS FOR USE IN DETERMINING THE MALIGNANT HYPERTHERMIA (MH) RAW SCORE

Process	Indicator	Points
Process I: Rigidity	Generalized muscular rigidity (in absence of shivering due to hypothermia, or during or immediately following emergence from inhalational general anesthesia)	15
	Masseter spasm shortly following succinylcholine administration	15
Process II: Muscle breakdown	Elevated creatine kinase >20,000 IU after anesthetic that included succinylcholine	15
	Elevated creatine kinase >10,000 IU after anesthetic without succinylcholine	15
	Cola-colored urine in perioperative period	10
	Myoglobin in urine >60 μg/L	5
	Myoglobin in serum >170 μg/L	5
	Blood/plasma/serum K >6 mEq/L (in absence of renal failure)	3
Process III: Respiratory acidosis	$PETCO_2$ >55 mm Hg with appropriately controlled ventilation	15
	Arterial $PaCO_2$ >60 mm Hg with appropriately controlled ventilation	15
	$PETCO_2$ >60 mm Hg 15 with spontaneous ventilation	
	Arterial $PaCO_2$ >65 mm Hg with spontaneous ventilation	15
	Inappropriate hypercarbia (in anesthesiologist's judgment)	15
	Inappropriate tachypnea	10
Process IV: Temperature increase	Inappropriately rapid increase in temperature (in anesthesiologist's judgment)	15
	Inappropriately increased temperature >38.8°C (101.8°F) in the preoperative period (in anesthesiologist's judgment)	10
Process V: Cardiac involvement	Inappropriate sinus tachycardia	3
	Ventricular tachycardia or ventricular fibrillation	3
Process VI: Family history (used to determine MH susceptibility only)	*Positive MH family history in relative of first degree*[a]	15
	Positive MH family history in relative not of first degree[a]	5
Other indicators that are not part of a single process[b]	Arterial base excess more negative than −8 mEq/L	10
	Arterial pH <7.25	10
	Rapid reversal of MH signs of metabolic and/or respiratory acidosis with IV dantrolene	5
	Positive MH family history together with another indicator from the patient's own anesthetic experience other than elevated resting serum creatine kinase[a]	10
	Resting elevated serum creatine kinase[a] *(in patient with a family history of MH)*	10

[a]These indicators should be used only for determining MH susceptibilty.
[b]These should be added without regard to double-counting.

TABLE 89.9

CRITERIA FOR GUIDANCE IN THE DIAGNOSIS OF NEUROLEPTIC MALIGNANT SYNDROME

Category	Manifestations
Major	Fever, rigidity, elevated creatine kinase concentration
Minor	Tachycardia, abnormal arterial pressure, tachypnea, altered consciousness, diaphoresis, leukocytosis

dystonia, or unexplained catatonic behavior, followed by hyperpyrexia. Other symptoms include unstable blood pressure, confusion, coma, and delirium. Although laboratory data may vary, a raised CK may be observed in patients who develop rhabdomyolysis. Some authors incline to make a diagnosis of NMS if certain signs are present. Levenson (92), for example, suggested that the presence of all three major signs, or two major and four minor signs (Table 89.9), indicates a high probability of NMS. These criteria are commonly used in clinical research studies (83,84).

Complications

Complications arising from MH and NMS are in general parallel to those of heat stroke syndrome, but complications associated with MH may be more severe because of extreme elevation of temperature. Rhabdomyolysis and hepatic necrosis may be fulminant, and DIC is more common (56). Renal failure is seen almost exclusively in patients with severe rhabdomyolysis. Ventricular fibrillation can occur, and cerebral edema with seizures is uncommon but may be seen. Patients with NMS are at risk for aspiration pneumonia because of dystonia and the inability to handle secretions (93).

Therapeutic Approach

Successful treatment of MH and NMS depend on early clinical recognition and prompt withdrawal of the suspected drugs. In MH, discontinuation alone is effective if the syndrome is not well established (56). NMS may be similarly aborted with discontinuation of the drugs. It may take 5 to 7 days to return to the patient's baseline (89) because neuroleptics cannot be removed by dialysis and blood concentrations decline slowly. General symptomatic treatment, such as hydration, nutrition, and reduction of fever, is essential.

Dantrolene should be administered emergently to prevent further release of calcium from the sarcoplasmic reticulum. The dose is 2 mg/kg intravenously every 5 minutes to a total dose of 10 mg/kg until the episode terminates (94). Dantrolene also decreases temperature in NMS and thyroid storm.

Acidosis should be treated aggressively with intravenous administration of bicarbonate, 2 to 4 mEq/kg. Hyperkalemia should be treated with insulin and glucose infusion, and diuresis.

Fever should be controlled by iced fluids, surface cooling, and cooling of body cavities with sterile iced fluids. Cold dialysis and cardiopulmonary bypass may also be applicable if other measures fail.

Mannitol infusion—0.5 g/kg—with or without furosemide should be used to establish a diuresis and prevent the onset of acute renal failure from myoglobinuria.

Further therapy is guided by blood gases, electrolytes, temperature, arrhythmia, muscle tone, and urinary output. Blood chemical analyses include electrolytes, CK concentrations, liver enzymes, blood urea nitrogen, lactate, glucose, serum hemoglobin and myoglobin, and urine hemoglobin and myoglobin. Coagulation studies also should be done.

SUMMARY

In general, when significant deviation from normal body temperature exists, prompt diagnosis, treatment, and normalization of the temperature alteration are required immediately, followed by careful review of each patient's condition. Therapeutic approaches vary from conservative to invasive methods, and thus risk–benefit balance always should be taken into consideration for a better outcome.

References

1. Moss J. Accidental severe hypothermia. *Surg Gynecol Obstet.* 1986;162:501.
2. Larach MG. Accidental hypothermia. *Lancet.* 1995;345:493.
3. Danzl DF, Pozos RS. Accidental hypothermia. *N Engl J Med.* 1994;331:1756.
4. Maclean D, Emslie-Smith D. *Accidental hypothermia.* Edinburgh, Scotland: Blackwell Scientific Publications; 1977.
5. Megarbane B, Axler O, Chary I, et al. Hypothermia with indoor occurrence is associated with a worse outcome. *Intensive Care Med.* 2000;26:1843–1849.
6. Woodhouse P, Keatinge WR, Coleshaw SR. Factors associated with hypothermia in patients admitted to a group of inner city hospitals. *Lancet.* 1989;2:1201–1205.
7. Fox RH, Brooke OG, Collins JC, et al. Measurement of deep body temperature from the urine. *Clin Sci Mol Med.* 1975;48:1–7.
8. Miller JW, Danzl DF, Thomas DM. Urban accidental hypothermia: 135 cases. *Ann Emerg Med.* 1980;9:456–461.
9. Koutsavlis AT, Kosatsky T. Environmental-temperature injury in a Canadian metropolis. *J Environ Health.* 2003;66:40–45.
10. Clemmer TP, Fisher CJ Jr, Bone RC, et al. Hypothermia in the sepsis syndrome and clinical outcome. The Methylprednisolone Severe Sepsis Study Group. *Crit Care Med.* 1992;20:1395–1401.
11. Solomon A, Barish RA, Browne B, et al. The electrocardiographic features of hypothermia. *J Emerg Med.* 1989;7:169–173.
12. Ehrmantraut WR, Fazekas JF, Ticktin HE. Cerebral hemodynamics and metabolism in accidental hypothermia. *AMA Arch Intern Med.* 1957;99:57–59.
13. Ferrara A, MacArthur JD, Wright HK, et al. Hypothermia and acidosis worsen coagulopathy in the patient requiring massive transfusion. *Am J Surg.* 1990;160:515–518.
14. Ferraro FJ Jr, Spillert CR, Swan KG, et al. Cold-induced hypercoagulability in vitro: a trauma connection? *Am Surg.* 1992;58:355–357.
15. Rohrer MJ, Natale AM. Effect of hypothermia on the coagulation cascade. *Crit Care Med.* 1992;20:1402–1405.
16. Patt A, McCroskey BL, Moore EE. Hypothermia-induced coagulopathies in trauma. *Surg Clin North Am.* 1988;68:775–785.
17. Kashuk JL, Moore EE, Millikan JS, et al. Major abdominal vascular trauma–a unified approach. *J Trauma.* 1982;22:672–679.
18. Cosgriff N, Moore EE, Sauaia A, et al. Predicting life-threatening coagulopathy in the massively transfused trauma patient: hypothermia and acidoses revisited. *J Trauma.* 1997;42:857–861.
19. Cupples WA, Fox GR, Hayward JS. Effect of cold water immersion and its combination with alcohol intoxication on urine flow rate of man. *Can J Physiol Pharmacol.* 1980;58:319–321.
20. American Heart Association. Hypothermia. 2005 American Heart Association (AHA) guidelines for cardiopulmonary resuscitation (CPR) and emergency cardiovascular care (ECC). *Circulation.* 2005;112:IV136–IV138.
21. Ledingham IM, Mone JG. Treatment of accidental hypothermia: a prospective clinical study. *Br Med J.* 1980;280:1102–1105.
22. Moss JF, Haklin M, Southwick HW, et al. A model for the treatment of accidental severe hypothermia. *J Trauma.* 1986;26:68–74.
23. Gregory JS, Bergstein JM, Aprahamian C. Comparison of three methods of rewarming from hypothermia: advantages of extracorporeal blood warming. *J Trauma.* 1991;31:1247–1251.
24. Wong PS, Pugsley WB. Partial cardiopulmonary bypass for the treatment of profound accidental hypothermic circulatory collapse. *J R Soc Med.* 1992;85:640.

25. Gentilello LM, Cobean RA, Offner PJ, et al. Continuous arteriovenous rewarming: rapid reversal of hypothermia in critically ill patients. *J Trauma.* 1992;32:316–325.
26. Vretenar DF, Urschel JD, Parrott JC, et al. Cardiopulmonary bypass resuscitation for accidental hypothermia. *Ann Thorac Surg.* 1994;58:895–898.
27. Antretter H, Dapunt OE, Mueller LC. Portable cardiopulmonary bypass: resuscitation from prolonged ice-water submersion and asystole. *Ann Thorac Surg.* 1994;58:1786–1787.
28. Mair P, Schwarz B, Komberger E, et al. Case 5-1997. Successful resuscitation of a patient with severe accidental hypothermia and prolonged cardiocirculatory arrest using cardiopulmonary bypass. *J Cardiothorac Vasc Anesth.* 1997;11:901–904.
29. Dobson JA, Burgess JJ. Resuscitation of severe hypothermia by extracorporeal rewarming in a child. *J Trauma.* 1996;40:483–485.
30. Roeggla G, Wagner A, Roeggla M, et al. Immediate use of cardiopulmonary bypass in patients with severe accidental hypothermia in the emergency department. *Eur J Emerg Med.* 1994;1:155.
31. Mayor Pleines AF, Guyot E, Yersin B. Accidental hypothermia: an extreme case of successful resuscitation [in German]. *Schweiz Rundsch Med Prax.* 2006;95:1075–1079.
32. Duthie DJ. Heat-related illness. *Lancet.* 1998;352:1329–1330.
33. Bouchama A. Heatstroke: a new look at an ancient disease. *Intensive Care Med.* 1995;21:623–625.
34. Shahid MS, Hatle L, Mansour H, et al. Echocardiographic and Doppler study of patients with heatstroke and heat exhaustion. *Int J Card Imaging.* 1999;15:279–285.
35. Porter AM. Heat illness and soldiers. *Mil Med.* 1993;158:606–609.
36. Knochel JP. Exertional heat stroke—pathophysiology of heat stroke. In: Hopkins PM, Ellis FR, eds. *Hyperthermic and Hypermetabolic Disorders.* Cambridge, UK: Cambridge University Press; 1996:42–46.
37. Alzeer AH, Al-Arifi A, Warsy AS, et al. Nitric oxide production is enhanced in patients with heat stroke. *Intensive Care Med.* 1999;25:58–62.
38. Dematte JE, O'Mara K, Buescher J, et al. Near-fatal heat stroke during the 1995 heat wave in Chicago. *Ann Intern Med.* 1998;129:173–181.
39. Howorth PJN. The biochemistry of heat illness. *J R Army Med Corps.* 1995;141:40–41.
40. Knochel JP. Environmental heat illness. An eclectic review. *Arch Intern Med.* 1974;133:841–864.
41. Hart GR, Anderson RJ, Crumpler CP, et al. Epidemic classical heat stroke: clinical characteristics and course of 28 patients. *Medicine (Baltimore).* 1982;61:189–197.
42. O'Donnell TF. Acute heat stroke. Epidemiologic, biochemical, renal, and coagulation studies. *JAMA.* 1975;234:824–828.
43. Tucker LE, Stanford J, Graves B, et al. Classical heatstroke: clinical and laboratory assessment. *South Med J.* 1985;78:20–25.
44. Hassanein T, Razack A, Gavaler JS, et al. Heatstroke: its clinical and pathological presentation, with particular attention to the liver. *Am J Gastroenterol.* 1992;87:1382–1389.
45. Yu F, Lu K, Lin S, et al. Energy metabolism in exertional heat stroke with acute renal failure. *Nephrol Dial Transplant.* 1997;2087–2092.
46. Giercksky T, Boberg KM, Farstad IN, et al. Severe liver failure in exertional heat stroke. *Scand J Gastroenterol.* 1999;34:824–827.
47. Saissy JM. Liver transplantation in a case of fulminant liver failure after exertion. *Intensive Care Med.* 1996;22:831.
48. Akhtar MJ, Al-Nozha M, Al-Harthi S, et al. Electrocardiographic abnormalities in patients with heat stroke. *Chest.* 1993;104:411–414.
49. El Kassimi FA, Al-Mashhadani SA, Akhtar J. Adult respiratory distress syndrome and disseminated intravascular coagulation complicating heat stroke. *Chest.* 1986;90:571–574.
50. Dahmash NS, Al-Harthi SS, Akhtar J. Invasive evaluation of patients with heat stroke. *Chest.* 1993;103:1210–1214.
51. Gonzalez-Alonso J, Mora-Rodriguez R, Below PR, et al. Dehydration markedly impairs cardiovascular function in hyperthermic endurance athletes during exercise. *J Appl Physiol.* 1997;82:1229–1236.
52. Bernard S, Buist M, Monteiro O, et al. Induced hypothermia using large volume, ice-cold intravenous fluid in comatose survivors of out-of-hospital cardiac arrest: a preliminary report. *Resuscitation.* 2003;56:9–13.
53. Denborough MA, Lovell RR. Anaesthetic deaths in a family. *Lancet.* 1960;2:45.
54. Denborough MA, Forster JF, Lovell RR, et al. Anaesthetic deaths in a family. *Br J Anaesth.* 1962;34:395–396.
55. Delay J, Pichot P, Lemperiere T, et al. A non-phenothiazine and non-reserpine major neuroleptic, haloperidol, in the treatment of psychoses. *Ann Med Psychol.* 1960;118:145–152.
56. Urwyler A, Censier K, Kaufmann MA, et al. Genetic effects on the variability of the halothane and caffeine muscle contracture tests. *Anesthesiology.* 1994;80:1287–1295.
57. Gronert GA. Malignant hyperthermia. *Anesthesiology.* 1980;53:395–423.
58. Neuroleptic malignant syndrome. *Lancet.* 1984;1:545–546.
59. Smego RA, Durack DT. The neuroleptic malignant syndrome. *Arch Intern Med.* 1982;142:1183–1185.
60. Morris HH 3rd, McCormick WF, Reinarz JA. Neuroleptic malignant syndrome. *Arch Neurol.* 1980;37:462–463.
61. Guze BH, Baxter LR. Current concepts. Neuroleptic malignant syndrome. *N Engl J Med.* 1985;313:163–166.
62. Kemperman CJ. Zuclopenthixol-induced neuroleptic malignant syndrome at rechallenge and its extrapyramidal effects. *Br J Psychiatry.* 1989;154:562–563.
63. van Maldegem BT, Smit LM, Touw DJ, et al. Neuroleptic malignant syndrome in a 4-year-old girl associated with alimemazine. *Euro J Pediatr.* 2002;161:259–261.
64. Webster P, Wijeratne C. Risperidone-induced neuroleptic malignant syndrome. *Lancet.* 1994;344:1228–1229.
65. Heinemann F, Assion HJ, Hermes G, et al. Paroxetine-induced neuroleptic malignant syndrome [in German]. *Nervenarzt.* 1997;68:664–666.
66. Tegazzin V, Scutari E, Treves S, et al. Chlorocresol, an additive to commercial succinylcholine, induces contracture of human malignant hyperthermia-susceptible muscles via activation of the ryanodine receptor Ca2+ channel. *Anesthesiology.* 1996;84:1380–1385.
67. Rosenberg H, Reed S. In vitro contracture tests for susceptibility to malignant hyperthermia. *Anesth Analg.* 1983;62:415–420.
68. Ording H. Incidence of malignant hyperthermia in Denmark. *Anesth Analg.* 1985;64:700–704.
69. Ording H. Investigation of malignant hyperthermia susceptibility in Denmark. *Dan Med Bull.* 1996;43:111–125.
70. Halliday NJ. Malignant hyperthermia. *J Craniofac Surg.* 2003;14:800–802.
71. Gronert GA, Pessah IN, Muldoon SM, et al. Malignant hyperthermia. In: Miller RD, ed. *Miller's Anesthesia.* 6th ed. Philadelphia, PA: 2005:1169.
72. Gelenberg AJ, Bellinghausen B, Wojcik JD, et al. A prospective survey of neuroleptic malignant syndrome in a short-term psychiatric hospital. *Am J Psychiatry.* 1988;145:517–518.
73. Hermesh H, Aizenberg D, Lapidot M, et al. Risk of malignant hyperthermia among patients with neuroleptic malignant syndrome and their families. *Am J Psychiatry.* 1988;145:1431–1434.
74. Hermesh H, Aizenberg D, Weizman A, et al. Risk for definite neuroleptic malignant syndrome. A prospective study in 223 consecutive in-patients. *Br J Psychiatry.* 1992;161:254–257.
75. Adnet P, Lestavel P, Krivosic-Horber R. Neuroleptic malignant syndrome. *Br J Anaesth.* 2000;85:129–135.
76. Fletcher JE, Tripolitis L, Hubert M, et al. Genotype and phenotype relationships for mutations in the ryanodine receptor in patients referred for diagnosis of malignant hyperthermia. *Br J Anaesth.* 1995;75:307–310.
77. Wallace AJ, Wooldridge W, Kingston HM, et al. Malignant hyperthermia–a large kindred linked to the RYR1 gene. *Anaesthesia.* 1996;51:16–23.
78. Serfas KD, Bose D, Patel L, et al. Comparison of the segregation of the RYR1 C1840T mutation with segregation of the caffeine/halothane contracture test results for malignant hyperthermia susceptibility in a large Manitoba Mennonite family. *Anesthesiology.* 1996;84:322–329.
79. McWilliams S, Nelson T, Sudo RT, et al. Novel skeletal muscle ryanodine receptor mutation in a large Brazilian family with malignant hyperthermia. *Clin Genet.* 2002;62:80–83.
80. Robinson RL, Brooks C, Brown SL, et al. RYR1 mutations causing central core disease are associated with more severe malignant hyperthermia in vitro contracture test phenotypes. *Hum Mutat.* 2002;20:88–97.
81. Denborough MA, Collins SP, Hopkinson KC. Rhabdomyolysis and malignant hyperpyrexia. *Br Med J.* 1984;288:1878.
82. Tollefson G. A case of neuroleptic malignant syndrome: in vitro muscle comparison with malignant hyperthermia. *J Clin Psychopharmacol.* 1982;2:266–270.
83. Caroff SN, Rosenberg H, Fletcher JE, et al. Malignant hyperthermia susceptibility in neuroleptic malignant syndrome. *Anesthesiology.* 1987;67:20–25.
84. Adnet PJ, Krivosic-Horber RM, Adamantidis MM, et al. The association between the neuroleptic malignant syndrome and malignant hyperthermia. *Acta Anaesthesiol Scand.* 1989;33:676–680.
85. Bligh J, Cottle WH, Maskrey M. Influence of ambient temperature on the thermoregulatory responses to 5-hydroxytryptamine, noradrenaline and acetylcholine injected into the lateral cerebral ventricles of sheep, goats and rabbits. *J Physiol.* 1971;212:377–392.
86. Cox B, Kerwin R, Lee TF. Dopamine receptors in the central thermoregulatory pathways of the rat. *J Physiol.* 1978;282:471–483.
87. Kelkar VV, Doctor RB, Jindal MN. Chlorpromazine-induced contracture of frog rectus abdominis muscle. *Pharmacology.* 1974;12:32–38.
88. Takagi A. Chlorpromazine and skeletal muscle: a study of skinned single fibers of the guinea pig. *Exp Neurol.* 1981;73:477–486.
89. Larach MG, Localio AR, Allen GC, et al. A clinical grading scale to predict malignant hyperthermia susceptibility. *Anesthesiology.* 1994;80:771–779.
90. O'Flynn RP, Shutack JG, Rosenberg H, et al. Masseter muscle rigidity and malignant hyperthermia susceptibility in pediatric patients. An update on management and diagnosis. *Anesthesiology.* 1994;80:1228–1233.
91. Meier-Hellman A, Romer M, Hannemann L, et al. Early recognition of malignant hyperthermia using capnometry. *Anaesthesist.* 1990;39:41–43.
92. Levenson JL. Neuroleptic malignant syndrome. *Am J Psychiatry.* 1985;142:1137–1145.
93. Wedel DJ, Quinlan JG, Iaizzo PA. Clinical effects of intravenously administered dantrolene. *Mayo Clin Proc.* 1995;70:241–246.
94. Brandom BW, Larach MG, North American MH registry. Reassessment of the safety and efficacy of dantrolene. *Anesthesiology.* 2002;97:A1199.

CHAPTER 90 ■ TRANSPLANTATION: AN OVERVIEW OF PROBLEMS AND CONCERNS

DAVID M. LEVI • JOSEPH FERREIRA • ANDREAS G. TZAKIS

IMMEDIATE CONCERNS

Critical care and clinical organ transplantation have developed in parallel over the past several decades. While organ transplantation has emerged as the treatment of choice for an ever-growing number of patients with end-stage organ failure, the intensive care unit (ICU) has become the venue where much of this care is rendered. The modern intensivist plays an important role in the care of the critically ill patient awaiting transplant, the postoperative management of the transplant recipient, and the identification and management of the potential deceased organ donor.

The success of organ transplantation can be attributed to a number of factors. These include better patient selection and preoperative preparation, standardization of surgical techniques, advances in immunosuppression and graft surveillance, and improved postoperative care. This success, in part reflective of advances in critical care medicine, poses a great challenge to the skills of the intensivist and the resources of the ICU. The continuing shortage of organs available for transplantation translates into longer waiting times for recipients, during which their condition may further deteriorate. Additionally, organ allocation algorithms—especially heart, lung, liver, and intestine—in the United States emphasize the "sickest first" philosophy, which states that the highest priority for organs should go to those most in danger of imminent death. Finally, the shortage of organs has forced the transplant community to consider the use of organs from less than ideal donors. The organs from these marginal or "expanded criteria" donors (ECDs), while used with caution, must be considered in order to minimize deaths on the waiting list. The impact on the ICU is clear: more transplants are being performed on critically ill patients with an organ pool that now includes compromised organs.

A prerequisite to the success of organ transplantation is the availability of suitable organs. Deceased organ donors are, and will continue to be in the foreseeable future, our most important organ source. A crucial consideration of the ICU staff should be the timely recognition of the potential organ donor, both those who are brain dead and those for whom death is imminent, and the early involvement of organ procurement organization (OPO) personnel to facilitate the process. The assessment of the potential organ donor, a clear understanding of donation after brain death and cardiac death protocols, and donor management are skills of the intensivist that are fundamental to the organ procurement process and the subsequent transplants performed.

TRANSPLANT ACTIVITY, RESULTS, AND TRENDS

Organ procurement and transplantation are highly regulated endeavors governed in the United States by the federal Organ Procurement and Transplant Network (OPTN). The OPTN contract is managed by the United Network for Organ Sharing. Each OPO and transplant center (TC) collects and reports data regarding their activity and results. The Scientific Registry of Transplant Recipients (SRTR), administered by the Arbor Research Collaborative for Health with the University of Michigan, analyzes these data and continually evaluates the status of clinical organ transplantation in the United States. This comprehensive analysis is periodically updated and is available to the public through the SRTR Web site (www.ustransplant.org). Data and figures in this chapter regarding transplant activity, results, and trends are from the SRTR (1).

In 2002, in an effort to promote organ donation and procurement, and ultimately increase the number and quality of transplants performed, the U.S. Secretary of Health launched the Health Resources and Services Administration (HRSA) Organ Donation Breakthrough Collaborative. The goal of this nationwide endeavor was to identify the best operational and clinical practices of the most successful OPOs and share these "best practices" with the rest of the health care community. The result of these efforts has been the steady increase, in recent years, in the number of organ donors, the number of organs procured, and the number of transplants performed. As discussed below, the increasing quality of these transplants has manifested as better graft and patient survival.

Kidney

Over 46,000 patients were on the active waiting list for a kidney transplant in 2005. In that year, approximately 16,000 kidney transplants were performed. The total number of kidney transplants has gradually increased, as has the fraction of those kidneys transplanted with other organs. Living donor kidneys accounted for approximately 41% of those transplants, while the remainder of transplanted kidneys originated from deceased donors. Policy changes continue to refine deceased donor kidney allocation to better utilize this scarce resource. Additionally, novel living donor–recipient matching strategies have been developed that offer the prospect of some relief to this shortage (2). As shown in Figure 90.1, the disparity between the number

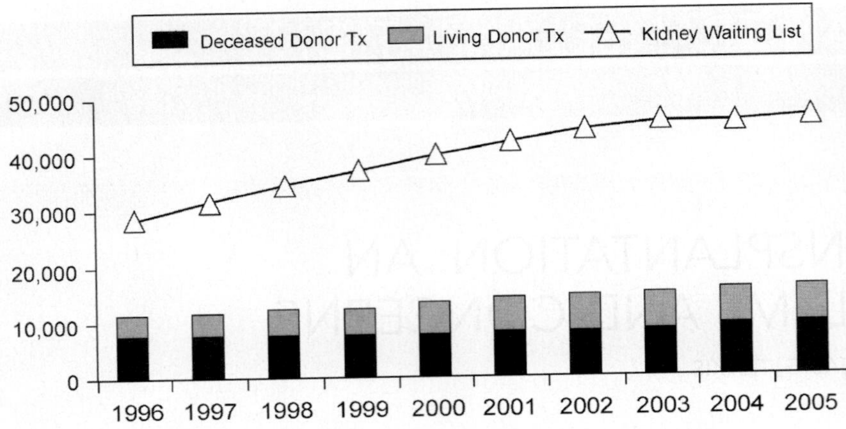

FIGURE 90.1. Number of kidney transplants and size of active waiting list per year. TX, transplant. (Source: 2006 Annual Report of the U.S. Organ Procurement and Transplantation Network and the Scientific Registry of Transplant Recipients: Transplant Data 1996–2005. Rockville, MD: Health Resources and Services Administration, Healthcare Systems Bureau, Division of Transplantation, Tables 1.7 and 5.1a. The data and analyses reported in the 2006 Annual Report of the U.S. Organ Procurement and Transplantation Network and the Scientific Registry of Transplant Recipients have been supplied by UNOS and Arbor Research under contract with HHS. The authors alone are responsible for reporting and interpreting these data; the views expressed herein are those of the authors and not necessarily those of the U.S. Government.)

of those waiting for a kidney and those transplanted continues to increase despite increases in both living and deceased organ donation over the past decade.

Kidney transplantation confers a clear survival advantage for patients with end-stage renal failure compared to long-term hemodialysis (3). For living donor kidney recipients, 5-year patient and graft survival are 90% and 80%, respectively (Fig. 90.2).

Pancreas

Pancreas transplantation offers selected diabetic patients the prospect of glucose control, avoiding—and, in some cases, reversing—the devastating complications of the disease. Most pancreata are transplanted simultaneously with a kidney (SPK), although a significant fraction is transplanted alone (PTA) or at some time after a kidney (PAK) transplant. Deceased donor pancreata remain a relatively underutilized organ resource; only 19% of available deceased donor pancreata are recovered and transplanted. A few percent are procured, processed, and transplanted as islet cell transplants. The reasons for this underutilization are multifactorial, and include regional variation in the number of potential recipients, donor and organ quality, and competition for kidneys with other patients.

In 2005, 903 SPK transplants, 344 PAK transplants, and 195 PTA transplants were performed. These totals have changed little over the last several years. Figure 90.3 depicts the trend for SPK transplants over the past decade. Similarly, patient and graft survival has improved, with 5-year patient survival approaching 90% (Fig. 90.4).

Liver

Liver transplantation remains the only therapy for end-stage, chronic liver disease and irreversible, fulminant liver failure. It is increasingly being performed for patients with localized, unresectable hepatocellular carcinoma with promising results

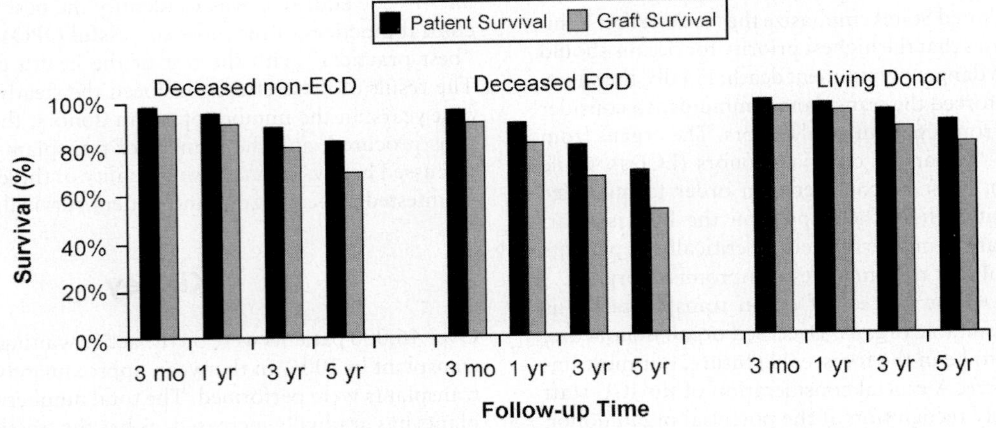

FIGURE 90.2. Kidney transplant patient and graft survival by donor type. ECD, expanded criteria donor. (Source: 2006 Annual Report of the U.S. Organ Procurement and Transplantation Network and the Scientific Registry of Transplant Recipients: Transplant Data 1996–2005. Rockville, MD: Health Resources and Services Administration, Healthcare Systems Bureau, Division of Transplantation, Tables 5.10a, 5.10b, 5.10c, 5.14a, and 5.14b. The data and analyses reported in the 2006 Annual Report of the U.S. Organ Procurement and Transplantation Network and the Scientific Registry of Transplant Recipients have been supplied by UNOS and Arbor Research under contract with HHS. The authors alone are responsible for reporting and interpreting these data; the views expressed herein are those of the authors and not necessarily those of the U.S. Government.)

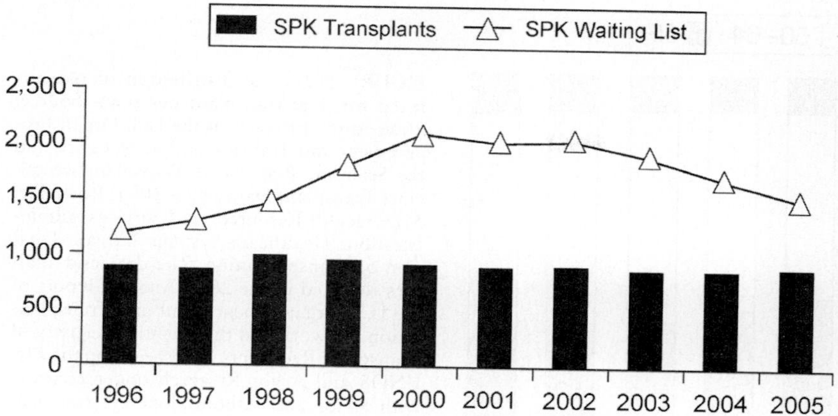

FIGURE 90.3. Number of simultaneous pancreas kidney transplants (SPK) and size of active waiting list per year. (Source: 2006 Annual Report of the U.S. Organ Procurement and Transplantation Network and the Scientific Registry of Transplant Recipients: Transplant Data 1996–2005. Rockville, MD: Health Resources and Services Administration, Healthcare Systems Bureau, Division of Transplantation, Tables 1.7 and 8.1a. The data and analyses reported in the 2006 Annual Report of the U.S. Organ Procurement and Transplantation Network and the Scientific Registry of Transplant Recipients have been supplied by UNOS and Arbor Research under contract with HHS. The authors alone are responsible for reporting and interpreting these data; the views expressed herein are those of the authors and not necessarily those of the U.S. Government.)

(4). Since 2002, the number of patients waiting for liver transplantation has slowly increased to near 13,000. The age distribution of those waiting has changed more dramatically, with ages between 50 and 64 making up the majority (Fig. 90.5).

The total number of liver transplants performed has steadily increased over the past decade, with 6,441 transplants in 2005. This increase is due primarily to the increase in deceased donor livers available for transplant. Living donor liver transplantation (LDLT) accounted for 5% of liver transplants performed in 2005, down from a peak of 10% in 2001 (Fig. 90.6). This decrease may be due in part to the increased utilization of ECD livers and concerns about the morbidity and mortality risks associated with living donor liver transplantation.

Liver allocation for adults depends primarily on disease severity as determined by the Model for End-Stage Liver Disease (MELD). The MELD formula uses easily obtained laboratory data—total bilirubin, serum creatinine, and international normalized ratio—and is highly predictive of death on the waiting list (5). Important exceptions are made for selected patients with hepatocellular carcinoma and other groups of patients for whom the MELD score does not reflect disease severity. Despite performing transplants in more older patients, utilizing more ECD livers, and employing an allocation system that gives priority to the sickest patients, the results of liver transplantation continue to be encouraging (Fig. 90.7).

Heart

The number of patients on the waiting list for a heart and the number of transplants performed has decreased significantly over the past decade (Table 90.1). Over the same time, deaths on the waiting list have declined and survival results after heart transplantation remain high (Fig. 90.8). These data reflect the improvements in transplantation, better medical management of interventional techniques for patients with heart disease, and the development of more effective mechanical support devices.

Limitations to heart preservation require that geographic location be a significant factor in the heart allocation system. Also, determining the urgency remains difficult because it is

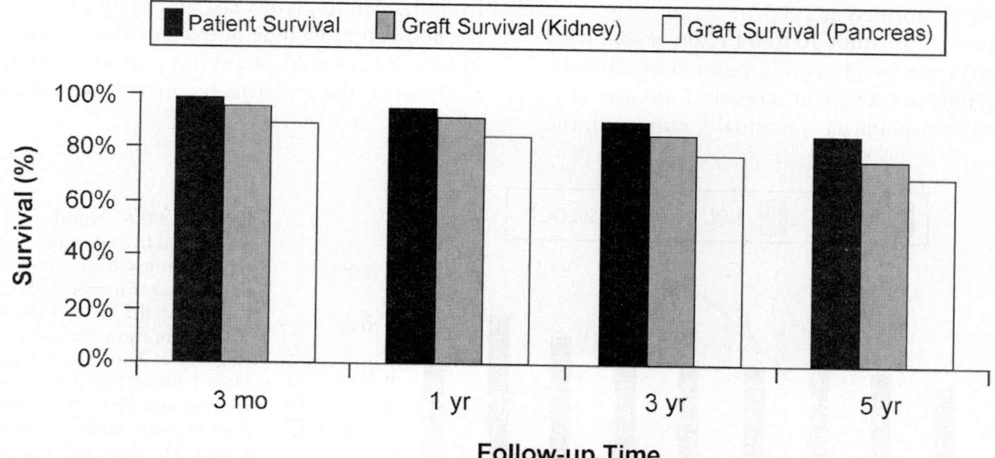

FIGURE 90.4. Patient and graft survival for simultaneous pancreas kidney transplantation. (Source: 2006 Annual Report of the U.S. Organ Procurement and Transplantation Network and the Scientific Registry of Transplant Recipients: Transplant Data 1996–2005. Rockville, MD: Health Resources and Services Administration, Healthcare Systems Bureau, Division of Transplantation, Tables 8.10 and 8.14. The data and analyses reported in the 2006 Annual Report of the U.S. Organ Procurement and Transplantation Network and the Scientific Registry of Transplant Recipients have been supplied by UNOS and Arbor Research under contract with HHS. The authors alone are responsible for reporting and interpreting these data; the views expressed herein are those of the authors and not necessarily those of the U.S. Government.)

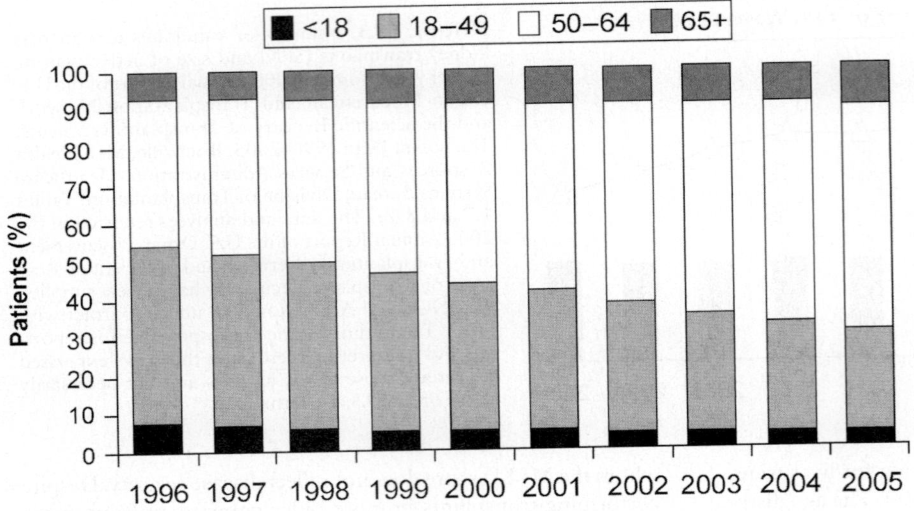

FIGURE 90.5. Age distribution of patients listed for liver transplant per year. (Source: 2006 Annual Report of the U.S. Organ Procurement and Transplantation Network and the Scientific Registry of Transplant Recipients: Transplant Data 1996–2005. Rockville, MD: Health Resources and Services Administration, Healthcare Systems Bureau, Division of Transplantation. The data and analyses reported in the 2006 Annual Report of the U.S. Organ Procurement and Transplantation Network and the Scientific Registry of Transplant Recipients have been supplied by UNOS and Arbor Research under contract with HHS. The authors alone are responsible for reporting and interpreting these data; the views expressed herein are those of the authors and not necessarily those of the U.S. Government.)

based on qualitative factors, including the "need" for hospitalization, inotropes, and mechanical support by the potential recipient.

Lung

There were more than 3,000 patients awaiting lung transplants at the end of 2005. The past decade has seen a steady increase in the percentage of older patients on the waiting list (Fig. 90.9). Over the past several years, the average waiting time to transplant has decreased, the number of deaths on the list has decreased, and the number of transplants has increased, with a peak of 1,407 lung transplants in 2005 (Fig. 90.10). These data are the product of changes in lung allocation policy, better patient management while on the list, and the efforts of OPOs and hospitals to recognize and optimize potential lung donors. Of note, the number of combined heart–lung transplants has declined, with just 45 performed in 2005.

The typical recipient is an adult 50 to 64 years of age, with a diagnosis of emphysema or idiopathic pulmonary fibrosis. The median waiting time to transplant is nearly 7 months. Survival rates after lung transplant have gradually improved, the main determinants of outcome including recipient age, diagnosis, history of prior transplant, and severity of illness at the time of transplant. Adjusted survival rates at 1, 3, and 5 years are currently 85%, 66%, and 51%, respectively.

Intestine

Intestinal transplantation has emerged as an accepted therapy for complicated intestinal failure. Standardization of surgical techniques, better management of the intestinal failure patient, improvements in immunosuppression, and advances in graft surveillance have led to better patient and graft survival (6). Survivors are almost always able to be completely tapered from parenteral nutrition.

The intestine can be transplanted as an isolated organ or as part of a composite graft depending on the needs of the patient. The multivisceral graft includes, en bloc, the stomach, liver, duodenum, pancreas, and small intestine. This graft can be modified to include or exclude the liver, spleen, colon, or a kidney. Each modification has critical care implications, especially when the recipient requires a liver as part of the transplant.

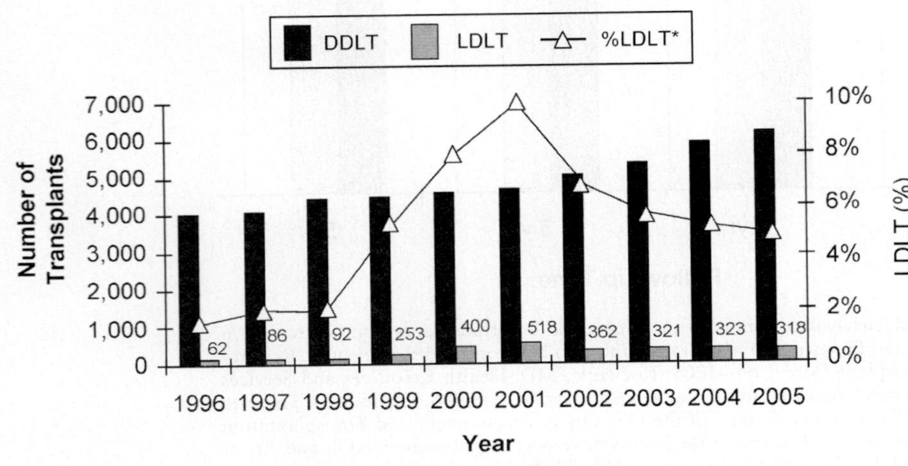

FIGURE 90.6. Number of liver transplants performed by donor type per year. DDLT, deceased donor liver transplant; LDLT, living donor liver transplant. (Source: 2006 Annual Report of the U.S. Organ Procurement and Transplantation Network and the Scientific Registry of Transplant Recipients: Transplant Data 1996–2005. Rockville, MD: Health Resources and Services Administration, Healthcare Systems Bureau, Division of Transplantation. The data and analyses reported in the 2006 Annual Report of the U.S. Organ Procurement and Transplantation Network and the Scientific Registry of Transplant Recipients have been supplied by UNOS and Arbor Research under contract with HHS. The authors alone are responsible for reporting and interpreting these data; the views expressed herein are those of the authors and not necessarily those of the U.S. Government.)

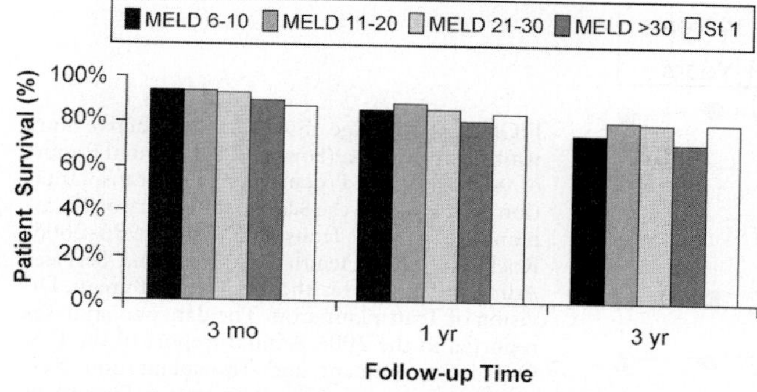

FIGURE 90.7. Patient survival after deceased donor liver transplant over time by decrease severity. St 1 represents status 1 patients—these patients have the highest priority. The Model for End-Stage Liver Disease (MELD) ranges from 6 to 40. A higher MELD reflects a greater disease severity and a higher place on the waiting list. (Source: 2006 Annual Report of the U.S. Organ Procurement and Transplantation Network and the Scientific Registry of Transplant Recipients: Transplant Data 1996–2005. Rockville, MD: Health Resources and Services Administration, Healthcare Systems Bureau, Division of Transplantation. The data and analyses reported in the 2006 Annual Report of the U.S. Organ Procurement and Transplantation Network and the Scientific Registry of Transplant Recipients have been supplied by UNOS and Arbor Research under contract with HHS. The authors alone are responsible for reporting and interpreting these data; the views expressed herein are those of the authors and not necessarily those of the U.S. Government.)

TABLE 90.1

NUMBER OF PATIENTS ON HEART WAITING LIST BY YEAR

Year	Patients active[a]
1996	2,436
1997	2,414
1998	2,525
1999	2,478
2000	2,421
2001	2,257
2002	2,055
2003	1,809
2004	1,590
2005	1,334

[a] *Patients listed as active at end of each year.
From the 2006 Annual Report of the U.S. Organ Procurement and Transplantation Network and the Scientific Registry of Transplant Recipients: Transplant Data 1996–2005. Rockville, MD: Health Resources and Services Administration, Healthcare Systems Bureau, Division of Transplantation, Chapter V. The data and analyses reported in the 2006 Annual Report of the U.S. Organ Procurement and Transplantation Network and the Scientific Registry of Transplant Recipients have been supplied by UNOS and Arbor Research under contract with HHS. The authors alone are responsible for reporting and interpreting these data; the views expressed herein are those of the authors and not necessarily those of the U.S. Government.

The number of intestinal transplants has been increasing, as illustrated in Figure 90.11. Many variables affect outcome, and, in recent years, patient and graft survival have been improving. Patient survival from data over the past 15 years is shown in Figure 90.12.

DONOR RECOGNITION AND ASSESSMENT

Transplantation depends on organ donation. OPOs are charged with the responsibility of deceased organ donor recognition and assessment. Medical professionals are required to cooperate with OPO personnel to ensure that all potential organ and tissue donors are identified and afforded the opportunity to donate (7,8). It is recommended that OPO and hospital staff collaborate by establishing criteria as to when it is the earliest appropriate time to consult the OPO.

The critical care physician's first priority is to provide excellent patient care. Additionally, he or she should recognize, when brain death is imminent or when withdrawal of support measures are considered, that there is an opportunity through organ donation to help other patients. Timing is critical: approaching

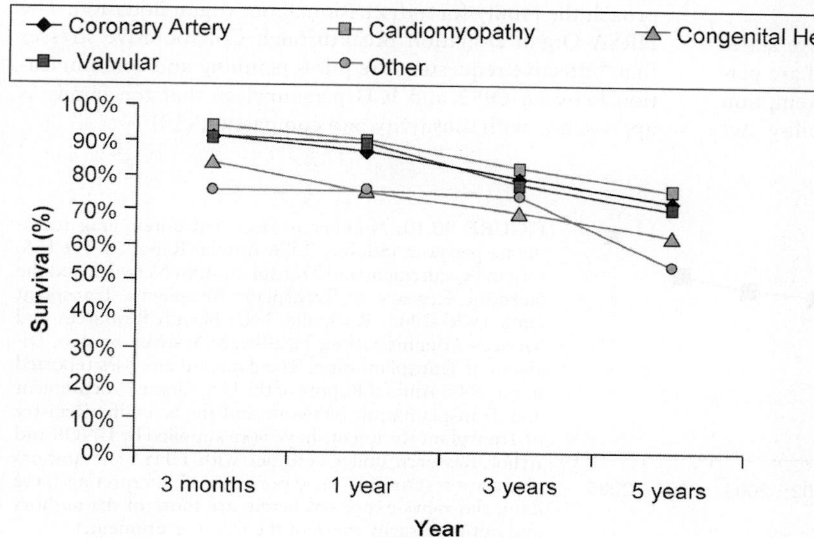

FIGURE 90.8. Patient survival after heart transplant by diagnosis. (Source: 2006 Annual Report of the U.S. Organ Procurement and Transplantation Network and the Scientific Registry of Transplant Recipients: Transplant Data 1996–2005. Rockville, MD: Health Resources and Services Administration, Healthcare Systems Bureau, Division of Transplantation. The data and analyses reported in the 2006 Annual Report of the U.S. Organ Procurement and Transplantation Network and the Scientific Registry of Transplant Recipients have been supplied by UNOS and Arbor Research under contract with HHS. The authors alone are responsible for reporting and interpreting these data; the views expressed herein are those of the authors and not necessarily those of the U.S. Government.)

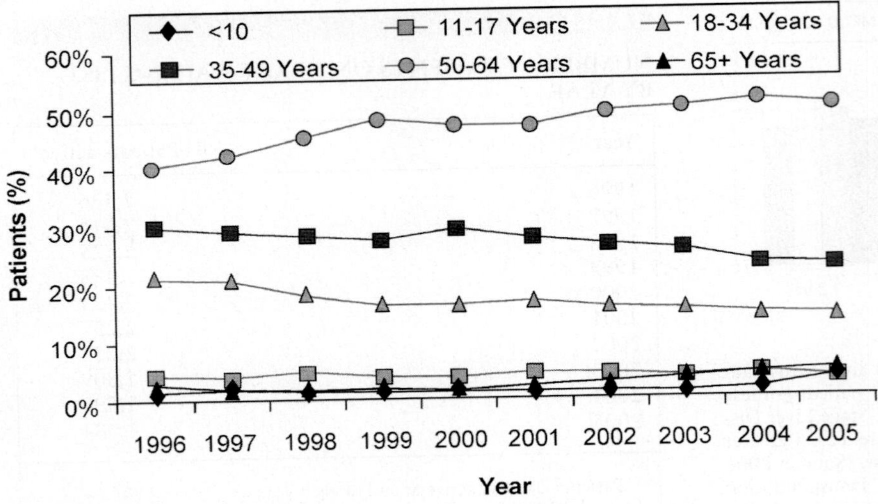

FIGURE 90.9. Age distribution of active lung waiting list by year. (Source: 2006 Annual Report of the U.S. Organ Procurement and Transplantation Network and the Scientific Registry of Transplant Recipients: Transplant Data 1996–2005. Rockville, MD: Health Resources and Services Administration, Healthcare Systems Bureau, Division of Transplantation. The data and analyses reported in the 2006 Annual Report of the U.S. Organ Procurement and Transplantation Network and the Scientific Registry of Transplant Recipients have been supplied by UNOS and Arbor Research under contract with HHS. The authors alone are responsible for reporting and interpreting these data; the views expressed herein are those of the authors and not necessarily those of the U.S. Government.)

a family too early is inappropriate and too late threatens the potential for organ donation.

To assist in defining the appropriate time to consider OPO involvement, UNOS has devised the term *imminent neurologic death*. This term describes the patient with an irreversible brain injury who may fit the general criteria of a potential organ donor but has not been legally declared brain dead. It is appropriate to notify the OPO when a patient meets this definition and displays an absence of at least three of the following neurologic functions as a result of the brain injury (not pharmacologic sedation or other confounding variables):

- Pupillary reaction
- Response to cold calorics
- Gag reflex
- Cough reflex
- Corneal reflex
- Doll's eyes reflex
- Response to painful stimuli
- Spontaneous breathing

In short, when the diagnosis of brain death is being considered, and the clinical assessment has begun to confirm that diagnosis, the OPO should be notified.

There are two important implications of the above statement that warrant clarification. First, OPO personnel are permitted access to patients' medical records per an exemption in the Health Insurance Portability and Accountability Act (HIPAA) (9). Second, the critical care provider is not required to notify the patient's family that the OPO has been consulted. If they wish, critical care providers can inform the family and/or introduce the idea of organ donation. It is not recommended that they discuss the process and options in detail. That task should be left to OPO personnel who are specially trained to approach grieving families and are qualified to obtain informed consent for organ and tissue donation.

DONATION CONSENT REQUEST

Informed consent is required for organ donation. Signed organ donor cards, living wills, and driver's license organ donor designation are recognized as legal "first-person consent" documents. More often, informed consent is obtained by trained OPO personnel from the potential donor's legal next-of-kin or designated health care surrogate. Before the family is approached for consent, it is appropriate that the ICU team inform the family as to the patient's condition and prognosis. Once brain death has been declared and confirmed or, alternatively, once care efforts have been deemed futile and a decision has been made to withdraw support, OPO personnel can approach the family for a discussion about organ donation. The HRSA Organ Donation Breakthrough Collaborative stresses that "effective requesting" requires planning and communication between OPO and ICU personnel so that the family is approached with sensitivity and compassion (10).

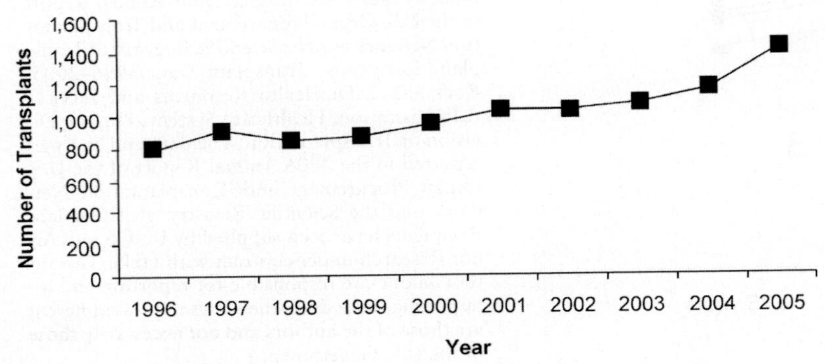

FIGURE 90.10. Number of deceased donor lung transplants per year. (Source: 2006 Annual Report of the U.S. Organ Procurement and Transplantation Network and the Scientific Registry of Transplant Recipients: Transplant Data 1996–2005. Rockville, MD: Health Resources and Services Administration, Healthcare Systems Bureau, Division of Transplantation. The data and analyses reported in the 2006 Annual Report of the U.S. Organ Procurement and Transplantation Network and the Scientific Registry of Transplant Recipients have been supplied by UNOS and Arbor Research under contract with HHS. The authors alone are responsible for reporting and interpreting these data; the views expressed herein are those of the authors and not necessarily those of the U.S. Government.)

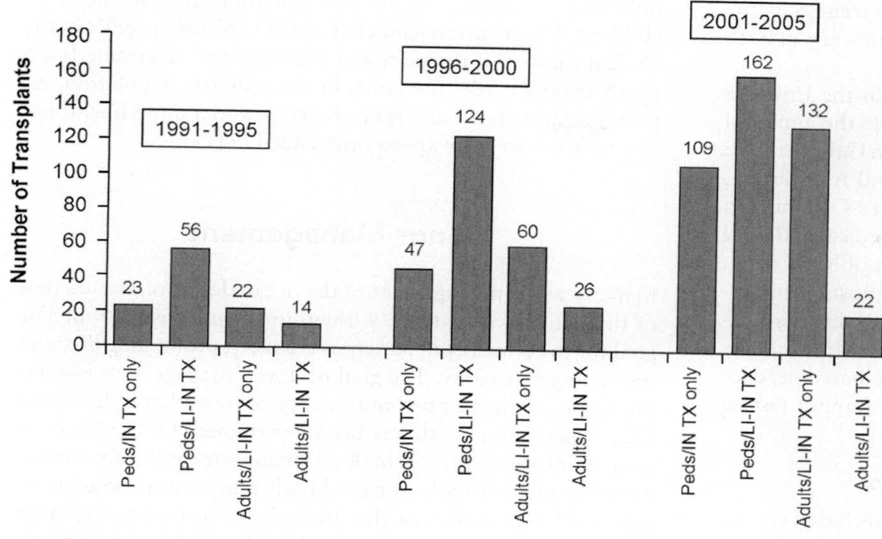

FIGURE 90.11. Number of intestinal transplants by age group and era. TX, transplant; LI, liver; IN, intestine; Peds, pediatric patients. (Source: 2006 Annual Report of the U.S. Organ Procurement and Transplantation Network and the Scientific Registry of Transplant Recipients: Transplant Data 1996–2005. Rockville, MD: Health Resources and Services Administration, Healthcare Systems Bureau, Division of Transplantation. The data and analyses reported in the 2006 Annual Report of the U.S. Organ Procurement and Transplantation Network and the Scientific Registry of Transplant Recipients have been supplied by UNOS and Arbor Research under contract with HHS. The authors alone are responsible for reporting and interpreting these data; the views expressed herein are those of the authors and not necessarily those of the U.S. Government.)

ORGAN DONATION PROCESS

There are fundamentally two types of potential donors that can be considered from the critical care population: ventilator-dependent patients who will be withdrawn from life-sustaining measures and patients who are declared clinically brain dead. In the former circumstance, it is possible to offer the option of organ donation after cardiac death (DCD), provided certain criteria are met. In the latter, donation may occur in the presence of circulation after the patient has been declared clinically brain dead. This is termed *organ donation after brain death* (DBD). As guidelines, UNOS has published the Critical Pathway for the Organ Donor and the Critical Pathway for Donation After Cardiac Death (11).

Brain Death

History and Legislation

For centuries, the timing of death coincided with the cessation of circulation. Advances in cardiopulmonary resuscitation and techniques such as hypothermic total circulatory arrest demand a re-examination of this definition. Death, by definition, is permanent. Also, the advent of prolonged mechanical ventilation showed that respiration and circulation could be supported even in cases of complete, irreversible cessation of brain function. Medical advancements over the past century have required that the definition and timing of death be reconsidered. It is out of this milieu that the concept of brain death has emerged and evolved.

In 1956, Löfstedt and Von Reis described six mechanically ventilated patients with lethal brain injuries. On examination, all were unarousable and unresponsive, flaccid, areflexic, and apneic. Spontaneous respiratory effort had ceased abruptly. Cerebral angiography demonstrated no blood flow to the brain. Autopsy revealed cerebral necrosis (12). In 1959, Wertheimer et al. described "the death of the nervous system," which they concluded should be regarded in the same accord as death by cardiopulmonary arrest (13). In the same year, Mollaret and Goulon introduced the term *coma dépassé* (beyond coma), an irreversible condition of coma and apnea (14). These observations, as well as those by others over the next decade, culminated in the well-known review of the Harvard Committee, which, in 1968, described brain death as being characterized by "unresponsiveness and lack of receptivity, the absence of movement and breathing, the absence of brainstem reflexes, and coma whose cause has been identified" (15).

In the years that followed, the criteria were revised to exclude the need for a 24-hour period between brain death evaluations and that an electroencephalogram (EEG) is useful in the diagnosis but not required (16). In 1971, Mohandas and

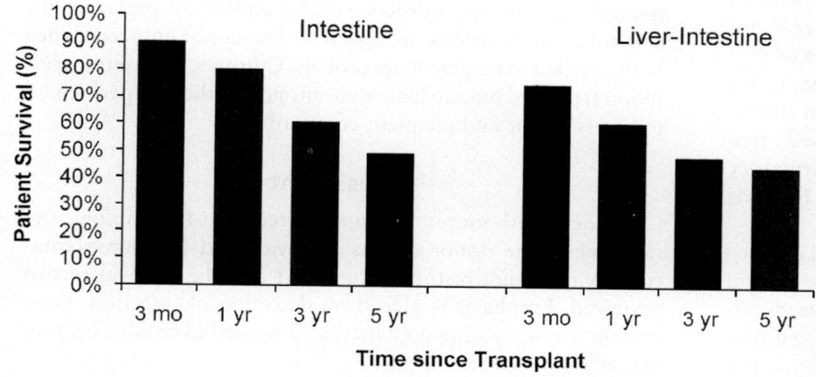

FIGURE 90.12. Patient survival after intestinal transplant, 1991–2005. (Source: 2006 Annual Report of the U.S. Organ Procurement and Transplantation Network and the Scientific Registry of Transplant Recipients: Transplant Data 1996–2005. Rockville, MD: Health Resources and Services Administration, Healthcare Systems Bureau, Division of Transplantation. The data and analyses reported in the 2006 Annual Report of the U.S. Organ Procurement and Transplantation Network and the Scientific Registry of Transplant Recipients have been supplied by UNOS and Arbor Research under contract with HHS. The authors alone are responsible for reporting and interpreting these data; the views expressed herein are those of the authors and not necessarily those of the U.S. Government.)

Chou specifically identified damage to the brain stem as a critical component of brain death. This point remains key in both clinical and legal brain death definitions (17).

Key legislation was introduced in 1980 with the Uniform Determination of Death Act (UDDA), which met the approval of the National Conference of Commissioners on Uniform State Laws in cooperation with the American Medical Association, the American Bar Association, and the President's Commission on Medical Ethics. This law has served as the medical and legal communities' foundation for the determination of brain death in all situations (18). In the United States, the most recent appraisal and comprehensive guide to assist clinicians in the evaluation of brain death was published by the American Academy of Neurology in 1995, which provided evidence-based practice measures along with a very practical version of apnea testing (19).

Brain Death Determination

Brain death is fundamentally a clinical diagnosis based on key physical examination features in the context of a specific history and in the absence of confounding factors. Important considerations in a precise brain death evaluation include a history of an acute, irreversible catastrophic event involving the cerebral hemispheres and brain stem, ruling out any conditions that may confound the determination. Confounding factors that prohibit a diagnosis of brain death include acid-base, electrolyte, or endocrine disturbances; severe hypothermia; hypotension; drug intoxication; poisoning; or the presence of neuromuscular blocking agents.

The clinical physical examination remains the gold standard for brain death evaluation. The key examination features include no motor response to pain, no pupillary response to light, absent oculocephalic reflex, absent corneal reflex, absent cough and gag reflex, and apnea (20). If the patient does not exhibit any of these neural reflexes, the clinician may document the diagnosis of clinical brain death in accordance with state law. Each state specifies who is qualified to make the determination of brain death. A given hospital may have a policy stating who can determine brain death and whether a time interval or second exam is needed to verify the diagnosis.

Confirmatory tests can serve a complementary role in the determination of brain death, but are not routinely required; though at times helpful, their availability and utility vary from institution to institution. Commonly used diagnostic tests to confirm brain death include cerebral angiography, cerebral nuclear imaging with contrast, and EEG. These tools can be especially useful in pediatric patients or those patients in whom the neurologic examination findings may be difficult to assess. Examples of the latter include the patient with severe facial trauma or spinal cord injury. Cerebral angiography and nuclear imaging serve to assess intracranial perfusion. The absence of perfusion supports the diagnosis of brain death but, alone, is not sufficient to make the diagnosis. The use of the EEG can also be complementary, but must be used with caution. It is used often because of its wide availability relative to other confirmatory studies, but is subject to artifact and interference in the ICU environment.

Although the same principles for the evaluation and diagnosis of brain death are used in the pediatric patient, the clinical examination may be difficult because of the patient's size, developmental differences, and course of treatment. In 1987, a group composed of several prominent medical societies convened and published guidelines for the determination of brain death in children. The group concluded that although the specifics of the clinical exam and the pertinent findings that determine brain death are essentially the same, in the pediatric population, repeat assessments by different observers and a more liberal use of confirmatory tests are recommended (21).

Donor Management

In many ways, management of the organ donor resembles that of the critically ill patient, with an important distinction. The goal for the critically ill patient is recovery, prolonging life, and improving its quality. The goal of donor management is maximization of the number and quality of transplantable organs (22). Once brain death has been determined, OPO personnel play an instrumental role in donor management. Brain death is associated with grossly impaired body temperature regulation, profound hypernatremia due to diabetes insipidus, impaired blood pressure regulation, coagulopathy, endocrine dysfunction, and electrolyte and acid-base disturbances. Physiologic derangement may have been the manifestation of the inciting injury or insult; this is often worse at the time of cerebral edema, herniation, and brain death (23–28).

Monitoring and Maintenance

Donor maintenance has become more sophisticated in recent years. Each OPO has detailed protocols and care pathways for organ donor optimization. Each has a medical director and/or critical care physician as a consultant or as an active participant in the process. The OPO community under the direction of the HRSA has developed its "best practices" for donor monitoring and maintenance. Fluids administered, urine output, and any other fluid losses are measured. Monitoring routinely includes the use of arterial catheters for blood pressure monitoring, central venous pressure monitoring, and sometimes pulmonary artery (PA) catheter placement. Arterial oxygenation is monitored via continuous pulse oximetry.

Fluid warmers and other warming devices are utilized as needed to maintain normothermia. Mechanical ventilation modalities geared toward maintaining oxygenation and ventilation while minimizing pulmonary injury are utilized. Hemodynamic derangement is addressed with fluids (crystalloid, colloid, and blood products) and the administration of vasopressors, inotropes, or antihypertensives as indicated. A standardized battery of laboratory tests is obtained, and detected abnormalities are corrected, if possible. Acid-base abnormalities are corrected, and hypernatremia and hyperglycemia are treated. Antibiotics, corticosteroids, endocrine replacement, and other medications are given to the donor in accordance with detailed management protocols. Cultures, viral serologies, blood type, and human leukocyte antigen studies are performed to assess donor and recipient compatibility.

Assessment

Coincident with monitoring and correction of physiologic derangement, the donor organs are evaluated for transplantation. A thorough history is obtained and the medical record reviewed. Emphasis is placed on detection of infection, presence or a history of malignancy, and comorbid conditions that can affect organ viability.

Each organ is considered individually, and specific tests are available to measure function or detect impairment (29). The heart is evaluated by an assessment of the donor's hemodynamic status, sometimes with the aid of a PA catheter, need for vasopressors or inotropic drugs, transthoracic echocardiography, and, in selected cases, coronary angiography. Lung assessment includes serial arterial blood gas measurement, chest radiography, and flexible bronchoscopy. The kidneys are evaluated by urine output, serum creatinine measurement, and, for some OPOs, a calculation of the glomerular filtration rate. After procurement, a renal cortical biopsy can yield important information regarding organ quality. Some OPOs and TCs preserve kidneys with a pulsatile perfusion machine. Some transplant surgeons use the performance parameters of the kidney(s) on the pump as an adjunct measure of quality. There are few specific indicators of pancreas viability and quality. Euglycemia without the need for significant amounts of exogenous insulin is preferable. Elevated serum amylase may raise concern that the gland is not suitable because of pancreatitis. The liver is assessed by transaminase and bilirubin measurements. Serum albumin and coagulation studies are measures of liver function. A liver biopsy obtained percutaneously before procurement, or in the operating room at the time of organ recovery, can be useful for detecting inflammation, necrosis, fibrosis, or steatosis. There are no specific standardized methods for the evaluation of the donor intestine.

While organ evaluation has improved, nothing has approached the judgment of the experienced transplant surgeon visually inspecting the organs at the time of organ recovery. It is this important evaluation, in conjunction with the donor's history and physiologic condition and the results of organ-specific studies, that is ultimately used to decide whether an organ is suitable for transplant.

ORGAN RECOVERY AND PRESERVATION

Like donor maintenance and assessment, the surgical recovery and preservation of organs for transplant has become a highly orchestrated process directed by the OPO. The procurement procedure often occurs at a hospital with otherwise little contact with transplant procedures or patients. The procedure is usually added to an already busy operating room schedule and is often given little priority. Yet, procurement is a time in which multiple surgeons—sometimes from multiple institutions—convene to assess, remove, and preserve those organs suitable for transplantation. While the procurement takes place, specialized OPO personnel support a grieving family, and critically ill patients are being mobilized and prepared for transplant surgery. The procurement is a time-sensitive, highly orchestrated procedure.

The organ recovery operation has become standardized. The procedure is performed in the operating room using a standard sterile technique. The donor's identity, informed consent, blood type, brain death certification, and medical record are again reviewed. The chest and abdomen are opened. The donor is inspected for malignancy or occult disease. The organs to be procured are visually inspected. Some dissection is done to mobilize the organs. The donor is heparinized, followed by the insertion of cannulas for the administration of cold preservation fluid. The time is recorded, and the aorta is clamped, initiating the start of cold ischemia. The donor organs are flushed with specialized preservation solutions to exsanguinate the organs and instill preservation fluid. Three commonly used solutions are the University of Wisconsin (UW) solution, histidine-tryptophan-ketoglutarate (HTK) solution, and Celsior solution. The organs are removed sequentially, with the thoracic organs being removed first, followed by the abdominal organs, then the kidneys. Finally, various vessels are taken for vascular conduits if needed, and lymph nodes and the spleen are taken for immunologic studies.

Our ability to preserve organs for transplant is rather limited. Optimally, the cold ischemia time for transplanted organs should be less than 4 hours for hearts and lungs, less than 10 hours for the abdominal viscera, and less than 24 hours for kidneys. Certainly, organs have been successfully transplanted with many more hours of ischemia, but the risk of delayed graft function and graft nonfunction rises rapidly as time elapses.

The brain-dead organ donor remains the preferred donor type, since circulation and supportive interventions continue until the moment hypothermic preservation is initiated. This type of donor is relatively controlled, and allows time for confirmation of death, informed consent, optimization, assessment, organ allocation, and coordinating the recovery. Finally, the quantity and quality of the organs recovered from this donor type are typically greater than that obtained from DCD donors.

In the DCD donor, there is a time interval between the withdrawal of support from the patient, cardiopulmonary arrest, determination and pronouncement of death, the start of the recovery procedure, and initiation of cold preservation. The amount of time this takes is difficult to predict, but certainly adds to the ischemic injury to the organs, and limits the surgeon's ability to assess the organs for transplant (30). Logistically, the process is more difficult than that for the brain-dead organ donor. The process is emotionally sensitive and must be handled with the utmost sensitivity and care (31).

The DCD donor concept is simple: some patients with lethal insults or injuries for whom supportive measures are to be withdrawn are candidates for organ donation if the organ recovery can take place within minutes of the cessation of circulation. The logistics of the process are complex. OPO personnel must be consulted prior to the withdrawal of support, but they do not participate in the withdrawal process or pronouncement of death (32). The task of the OPO personnel is to explain the options regarding organ donation to the patient's family or designee, obtain informed consent, and coordinate the assembling of a surgical recovery team to be present and immediately available at the time of death.

The withdrawal of support usually takes place in, or near, the operating suite. The family may be present, but must be willing to leave immediately upon declaration of death. It is preferred that the patient be heparinized prior to cessation of circulation. The physician authorized and designated to assess and pronounce death is present. This physician must not be affiliated with the OPO, the transplant team, or potential recipient(s). The surgical recovery team prepares to begin, but waits in an adjacent room beyond view for two reasons: (a) in deference to any family members present and (b) to ensure that they in no way influence the protocol for the withdrawal of life support, nor the physician's assessment and determination of death. Once death has been declared, the recovery must begin after 2 minutes but before 5 minutes have elapsed. If the patient does not expire in 30 to 60 minutes, he or she is brought back to the ICU, and the procurement is cancelled. This possibility should be explained when consent is obtained. Recently, the issue of DCD organ donation has been addressed separately by a consensus conference of experts in transplantation, the Institute of Medicine, and UNOS (33–35).

FUTURE EXPECTATIONS

The past several years have generated dramatic advances in transplantation, and the future promises much more. The transplant community will continue to investigate methods for expanding the pool of organs available for transplantation. Multiple modalities, ranging from public education to increasing organ donation awareness to the use of living donors and ECDs, will continue. The problems related to the long-term use of immunosuppressive drugs, disease recurrence, and organ donor disease transmission will pose important challenges in the years to come. The development of comprehensive centers designed to treat the spectrum of patients with end-stage organ failure, and not just those patients who are potentially transplant recipients, will likely continue. Strategies are evolving that may take us closer to the lofty goal of immunologic tolerance. Finally, advances in tissue engineering and cell transplantation give us a glimpse of a future where organs can be repaired or produced in the laboratory to the recipient's exact specifications.

References

1. 2006 Annual Report of the U.S. Organ Procurement and Transplantation Network and the Scientific Registry of Transplant Recipients: Transplant Data 1996. Rockville, MD: Health Resources and Services Administration, Healthcare Systems Bureau, Division of Transplantation. (The data and analyses reported in the 2006 Annual Report of the U.S. Organ Procurement and Transplantation Network and the Scientific Registry of Transplant Recipients have been supplied by UNOS and Arbor Research under contract with HHS. The authors alone are responsible for reporting and interpreting these data; the views expressed herein are those of the authors and not necessarily those of the U.S. Government.)
2. Segev DL, Gentry SE, Warren DS, et al. Kidney paired donation and optimizing the use of live donor organs. *JAMA*. 2005;293:1883.
3. Wolfe RA, Ashby VA, Milford EL, et al. Comparison of mortality in all patients on dialysis, patients on dialysis awaiting transplantation, and recipients of a first cadaveric transplant. *N Engl J Med*. 1999;341:1725.
4. Kim RD, Reed AI, Fujita S, et al. Consensus and controversy in the management of hepatocellular carcinoma. *J Am Coll Surg*. 2007;205:108.
5. Kamath PS, Kim WR. The model for end-stage liver disease (MELD). *Hepatology*. 2007;45:797.
6. Ruiz P, Kato T, Tzakis AG. Current status of transplantation of the small intestine. *Transplantation*. 2007;83:1.
7. Department of Health and Human Services, Centers for Medicare and Medicaid Services Conditions of Participation CFR 42, Parts 405, 482, 488, 498, Volume 72:61, March 30, 2007, Rules and Regulations.
8. United Network for Organ Sharing (UNOS). Policies and Procedures 7.0. http://www.unos.org/PoliciesandBylaws2/policies/docs/policy_23.doc. Accessed February 10, 2007.
9. Joint Commission on Accreditation of Health Care Organizations. Healthcare at the Crossroads: Strategies for Narrowing the Organ Donation Gap and Protecting Patients. Federal Register § 164.512(h), December 28, 2000.
10. U.S. Department of Health and Human Services, Health Resources and Services Administration, Office of Special Programs, Division of Transplantation. *The Organ Donation Breakthrough Collaborative: Best Practices Final Report*. Washington, DC: U.S. Department of Health and Human Services; 2003. Contract: 240–94-0037, Task Order No. 12.
11. United Network for Organ Sharing (UNOS). Critical Pathway for the Organ Donor and the Critical Pathway for Donation After Cardiac Death. http://www.unos.org/resources/donorManagement.asp?index=2. Accessed February 10, 2007.
12. Löfstedt S, Von Reis G. Intracranial lesions with abolished passage of x-ray contrast through the internal carotid arteries. *Opuscula Med*. 1956;8:199.
13. Wertheimer P, Jouvet M, Descotes J. A propos du diagnostic de la mort du système nerveux dans les comas avec arrêt respiratoire traites par respiration artficielle. *Presse Med*. 1959;67:87.
14. Mollaret P, Goulon M. Le coma dépassé. *Rev Neurol*. 1959;101:3.
15. A definition of irreversible coma. Report of the Ad Hoc Committee of the Harvard Medical School to examine the definition of brain death. *JAMA*. 1968;205:337.
16. Beecher HK. After the definition of irreversible coma. *N Engl J Med*. 1969; 281:1070.
17. Mohandas A, Chou SN. Brain death: a clinical and pathological study. *J Neurosurg*. 1971;35:211.
18. Uniform Determination of Death Act, 12 Uniform Laws Annotated (U.L.A.) 589 (West 1993 and West Supp. 1997).
19. The Quality Standards Subcommittee of the American Academy of Neurology. Practice parameters for determining brain death in adults (summary statement). *Neurology*. 1995;45:1012.
20. Wijdicks EFM. The diagnosis of brain death. *N Engl J Med*. 2001;344: 1215.
21. Guidelines for the determination of brain death in children. American Academy of Pediatrics Task Force on Brain Death in Children. *Pediatrics*. 1987;80:298.
22. Rudow DL, Ohler L, Shafer T. *A Clinician's Guide to Donation and Transplantation*. Lenexa, KS: Applied Measurement Professionals Inc; 2006.
23. Grossman MD, Reilly PM, McMahon DJ, et al. Loss of potential solid organ donors due to medical failure. *Crit Care Med*. 1996;24: A76.
24. Powner D, Darby J. Management of variations in blood pressure during care of organ donors. *Prog Transplant*. 2000;10:25.
25. Powner D, Kellum J, Darby J. Abnormalities in fluids, electrolytes, and metabolism of organ donors. *Prog Transplant*. 2000;10:88.
26. Powner D, Kellum J. Maintaining acid-base balance in organ donors. *Prog Transplant*. 2000;10:98.
27. Powner D, Reich H. Regulation of coagulation abnormalities and temperature in organ donors. *Prog Transplant*. 2000;10:146.
28. Powner D, Darby J, Stuart S. Recommendations for mechanical ventilation during donor care. *Prog Transplant*. 2000;10:33.
29. United Network for Organ Sharing (UNOS). Policies and Procedures 2.0. http://www.unos.org/PoliciesandBylaws2/policies/docs/policy-2.doc. Accessed February 10, 2007.
30. Lewis J, Peltier J, Nelson H, et al. Development of the University of Wisconsin donation after cardiac death evaluation tool. *Prog Transplant*. 2003;13:265.
31. McVearry-Kelso C, Lyckholm LJ, Coyne PJ, et al. Palliative care consultation in the process of organ donation after cardiac death. *J Palliative Med*. 2007;10:118.
32. United Network for Organ Sharing (UNOS). OPTN Bylaws, Appendix B, Attachment III-1 of the OPTN bylaws. Model elements for controlled DCD recovery protocols. http://www.unos.org/policiesandBylaws2/bylaws/UNOSByLaws/DOCs/ bylaw_145.doc. Accessed July 1, 2007.
33. Bernat JL, D'Alessandro AM, Port FK, et al. Report of a national conference on donation after cardiac death. *Am J Transplant*. 2006;6: 281.
34. Institute of Medicine, National Academy of Sciences. *Non-Heart Beating Organ Transplantation: Medical and Ethical Issues in Procurement*. Washington, DC: National Academy Press; 1997.
35. Institute of Medicine, National Academy of Sciences. *Non-Heart Beating Organ Transplantation: Practice and Protocols*. Washington, DC: National Academy Press; 1997.

CHAPTER 91 ■ HEART TRANSPLANTATION

CHARLES W. HOOPES

Cardiac allotransplantation is now an established therapeutic modality for end-stage heart disease (1). Although the operative procedure remains essentially unchanged, recent advances in mechanical assist technology and significant advances in the medical therapy of congestive heart failure have changed heart transplantation from an "operation" to a definitive therapy among competing therapies in integrated heart failure management programs. Ventricular assist devices (VAD), cardiac resynchronization therapy, nontransplant surgical procedures, and novel molecular strategies have further complicated the process of patient selection for transplantation. This discussion will review the current status of clinical cardiac transplantation, describe the diagnostic algorithms of the acute decompensated heart failure patient that determine appropriate patient selection for cardiac transplantation, and identify the major perioperative risk factors for acute allograft loss and the clinical strategies designed to attenuate these risks.

CARDIAC TRANSPLANTATION: CURRENT STATUS

Registry data from the International Society of Heart and Lung Transplantation demonstrate continued improvement in clinical outcomes with the current expected half life (50% survival) of cardiac allografts at 10 years (2). Conditional half life for patients surviving to 1 year now exceeds 13 years. Indications for transplantation continue to be equally divided between patients with ischemic cardiomyopathy and those with nonischemic dilated cardiomyopathies, and among recent transplant recipients, 40% were receiving inotropic support and 30% were on some form of mechanical circulatory device. However, fewer than half of all patients between 2001 and 2004 were hospitalized at the time of transplant versus a nearly 70% hospitalization rate between 1999 and 2001 (2).

Categoric risk factors for early mortality are essentially unchanged (2). Requirement for dialysis at the time of transplant, female organ recipient, donor with a cerebrovascular accident as cause of death, coronary artery disease as the indication for transplant, and human leukocyte antigen–DR (HLA-DR) mismatches continue to be risk factors for 1-year mortality for patients transplanted between January 2001 and June 2004. Continuous variables contributing to 1-year mortality include older donors, older recipients, longer allograft ischemic times, and physiologic markers of progressive decompensated heart failure (elevated bilirubin, creatinine, and diastolic pulmonary artery pressure of the recipient). Important factors that no longer predict 5-year mortality in patients who survive to 1 year include the presence of a ventricular assist device, continuous mechanical ventilation, intravenous inotrope dependency, or hospitalization at the time of transplant.

Late morbidity after transplantation continues to be defined by increasing renal dysfunction, progressive hyperlipidemia, and diabetes, with nearly 10% of all heart recipients having significant renal insufficiency (creatinine >2.5) by 8 years and an additional 5% requiring long-term dialysis (2). Coronary artery vasculopathy (CAV) and malignancy continue to impact late mortality with the incidence of any malignancy approaching 35% at 10 years. By 10 years, only 44% of patients are free of angiographic CAV. Donor hypertension and early infection (within 2 weeks of transplant) are independent categoric risk factors for coronary artery vasculopathy whereas donor age and elevated recipient body mass index are continuous variables contributing to progressive CAV. This is consistent with our institutional bias that the biology of CAV is an inherent characteristic of allograft selection and early inflammatory injury. Skin cancer is the most common malignancy among solid organ transplant recipients and complicates the care in 21% of heart patients by 10 years (2).

PATIENT SELECTION AND ORGAN ALLOCATION

Hemodynamic Markers of Heart Failure

The decision to transplant should be determined by the natural history of underlying disease, the relative efficacy of medical therapy, and the patient's perception of quality of life. Although the objective hemodynamic criteria used to define end stage heart disease have not changed significantly in the past decade, the clinical profile of patients who die from heart failure is radically different (3). Knowing the risk of dying and the prognosis of patients receiving optimal medical therapy is critical to the determination of transplant candidacy and timing. Here we discuss the objective criteria of oxygen consumption (VO_2) and right heart catheterization that define the hemodynamics of transplant candidacy, discuss the evolving concept of the circulatory-renal limit (CRL) in predicting medical efficacy and the timing of transplant, describe the Heart Failure Survival Score (HFSS), and integrate these issues into the current paradigm of organ allocation. This discussion is focused on the ambulatory patient with acute decompensated heart failure.

Cardiopulmonary testing as a measure of oxygen consumption is routinely used to determine candidacy for transplantation (4). The currently accepted indication for transplantation is a peak VO_2 <10 mL/kg per minute in patients with adequate β-blockade who achieved anaerobic threshold. Patients with a VO_2 between 10 and 14 mL/kg per minute are more problematic, and decisions to list for transplantation should be individualized. The use of VO_2 as a discriminatory variable requires experience and attention to detail in testing performance. It is important to note that patients tolerating β-blockade demonstrate improved survival with equivalent VO_2. It is also notable that appropriate patient selection assumes maximal effort to achieve a plateau of performance. In populations with limited functional status a respiratory exchange ratio (RER) >1.05 is generally considered a maximal exercise test. Peak VO_2 also varies with age and gender and is normalized for body weight with heavier patients having a lower VO_2 at comparable levels of performance. In the era prior to widespread use of β-blockers and angiotensin-converting enzyme (ACE) inhibitors, a VO_2 maximum of <50% was shown to be a significant predictor of cardiac death. Nonetheless, isolated peak VO_2 should not be used as the sole criterion for transplant eligibility.

Right heart catheterization provides information on cardiac output, ventricular filling pressures, and pulmonary vascular resistance (PVR) and is an absolute prerequisite to consideration for transplantation (4–6). A pulmonary vascular resistance greater than 5 Wood units, an indexed PVR greater than 6 Wood units or a transpulmonary gradient (TPG) greater than 16 to 20 mm Hg have been considered relative contraindications to transplant (1 Wood Unit = 80 dynes · s/cm^5). Candidacy for transplantation is less dependent on the absolute measures of PVR than on the responsiveness of the pulmonary vascular bed to therapy. Heart failure patients with pulmonary artery (PA) systolic pressures greater than 50 mm Hg and either a PVR >3 Wood units or a TPG >15 mm Hg are routinely challenged with multiple vasodilators to ascertain whether the elevated pulmonary pressures are reactive. Most patients with acute decompensated heart failure have elevated left-sided filling pressures with secondary pulmonary venous hypertension. Pharmacologically unloading the left ventricle with sodium nitroprusside while maintaining a systolic blood pressure (SBP) of >85 mm Hg is generally considered evidence of a reactive vascular bed and does not preclude transplantation.

A significant minority of patients have evidence of fixed pulmonary hypertension. It is our institutional practice to initially evaluate patients who fail provocative vasodilatory testing for an anatomic substrate of pulmonary hypertension including chronic thromboembolic disease, pulmonary parenchymal disease, or history of significant sleep apnea. Patients without evidence of an anatomic substrate are treated with aggressive diuresis and short-term inotropy with the phosphodiesterase inhibitor milrinone. If subsequent provocative testing demonstrates continued nonreactivity, dobutamine is added to the inotropic support for synergy. Such vasodilatory conditioning generally improves pulmonary vascular resistance, but these patients remain at higher risk for acute cardiac death prior to transplant (7) and in our experience remain at significant risk for elevated PA pressures after transplantation. It is important to recognize that the reversibility of PVR in patients with low left ventricular ejection fraction (LVEF) cannot be assessed without unloading the left ventricle. Fixed pulmonary hypertension has been effectively treated with mechanical circulatory support allowing isolated cardiac transplantation in patients initially thought to require a combined heart–lung procedure (8).

Renal dysfunction is among the most significant clinical variables complicating the decision to transplant and one of the most significant morbidities after transplant (2). A serum creatinine >2 mg/dL or a creatinine clearance (CrCl) <50 mL/minute were initially considered evidence of irreversible renal dysfunction and a contraindication to transplant (4). Current practice patterns are variable and institution specific, but efferent arteriolar vasoconstriction mediated by elevated angiotensin II levels with resultant interstitial fibrosis and glomerular scarring is a common feature of progressive heart failure. We do not consider renal dysfunction a contraindication to transplant and have actively pursued combined heart and kidney transplant in patients at high risk for end-stage renal disease in the early postoperative interval. Outcomes for combined transplant are comparable to those of isolated cardiac allografts (9). Regardless of approach, the decision to exclude patient candidacy secondary to significant renal dysfunction or to simultaneously transplant a renal allograft requires careful consideration of the cause of preoperative renal insufficiency, the degree to which renal insufficiency is irreversible, and the probability of progressive renal failure after transplant.

There is little disagreement that a CrCl >80 mL/minute corrected for body surface area and a urine protein <150 mg per 24 hours present no significant risk for transplant. Elevated creatinine is a common manifestation of decompensated heart failure and even mild increases are associated with poor outcome (2). It is our practice to routinely evaluate any potential recipient with an elevated creatinine (>1.5 mg/dL) or questionable CrCl by estimated glomerular filtration rate (eGFR) using the risk stratified database and analysis of the Modification of Diet in Renal Disease (MDRD) study (*http://nephron.com/cgi-bin/mdrd.cgi*). Patients with decreased GFR or marginal GFR in the context of associated proteinuria are referred to transplant nephrology for formal evaluation and consideration as to candidacy for combined organ transplant. Renal ultrasound is routinely used to assess renal parenchymal disease and screen for renovascular disease, and sequential biopsy may be necessary to determine renal transplant candidacy in the context of progressive heart failure (10). The decision to offer combined heart–kidney transplant remains controversial as the heart recipient removes a renal allograft from the kidney donor pool. Alternatively, transplantation in patients with poorly characterized renal dysfunction carries significant morbidity with nearly 20% of heart recipients demonstrating renal insufficiency by 5 years (2).

Neurohormonal Markers of Heart Failure

The natural history of heart failure is characterized by systemic neurohormonal activation in response to the structural and functional remodeling of decreased ejection fraction and progressive volume overload. Optimal medical therapy of heart failure is designed to ameliorate these neurohormonal changes—β-blockade of adrenergic pathways, diuresis to reduce volume overload and natriuretic hormone production, and various inhibitors of the renin–angiotensin system including ACE inhibitors and angiotensin receptor blockade. Although there is as yet no composite score of multiple neurohormonal markers to describe the dynamic changes in heart failure, there are a number of relationships between various markers and cardiac remodeling that allow risk stratification of patients considered for transplant. Analysis of the RESOLVD (Randomized Evaluation of Strategies for Left Ventricular Dysfunction) trial data demonstrated that temporal increases in brain natriuretic (BNP) and N-terminal atrial natriuretic peptide (NT-ANP) during medical therapy were associated with concurrent reductions in ejection fraction and increases in end-diastolic and systolic volume (11). In a multivariate analysis of the same database, NT-ANP and norepinephrine increases over time and beyond baseline were independently predictive of an increased risk for death and heart failure hospitalization. We use BNP as a marker to evaluate the adequacy and response to acute heart failure therapy and consider it a physiologic marker of volume overload. C-reactive protein (CRP), a nonspecific marker of inflammation, is considered a sensitive marker of the neurohormonal milieu in acute heart failure and a more sensitive marker of prognosis. In patients with decompensated heart failure, CRP is most elevated (CRP >15%–18 mg%) and associated with poor outcomes regardless of ejection fraction (12).

Neurohormonal modulation with nonselective β-blockers, ACE inhibitors, angiotensin receptor blockade, and aldosterone antagonists directly influences patient survival and constitutes the basis for contemporary heart failure therapy. However, the survival advantage of effective early therapy and the prevention of sudden death has created a population of patients very different from that of previous decades. The decision to recommend definitive therapy, whether transplant or mechanical ventricular assist, is contingent on the ability to identify which patients can tolerate aggressive therapy. Intolerance to such medical therapy defines a high-risk population of heart failure patients at risk for early death and has led to the important concept of the *circulatory-renal limit* (13).

Systemic blood pressure, renal perfusion, and sodium homeostasis are controlled by the renin–angiotensin–aldosterone system via angiotensin-II–mediated vasoconstriction of the peripheral and efferent renal arterioles. Vasoconstriction potentiates the sympathetic stimulation of the adrenergic pathways, and serum sodium indirectly influences volume status by influencing intravascular oncotic pressure. Symptomatic hypotension, renal dysfunction, and hyperkalemia define the circulatory-renal limit and identify patients unable to tolerate escalating levels of β-blockade and ACE inhibition. Among ACE inhibitor–intolerant patients, mortality is greater than 50% by 6 months, and patients requiring inotropic support to maintain systemic blood pressure and renal perfusion have even poorer prognosis with no survivors by 4 months (13).

Heart Failure Survival Score (HFSS)

The Heart Failure Survival Score (HFSS) is a clinical descriptor derived from a Cox proportional hazards regression model of noninvasively derived measurements describing ambulatory patients with advanced heart failure (14). The prognostic variables include resting heart rate, mean systemic blood pressure, left ventricular ejection fraction, serum sodium, peak oxygen consumption, intraventricular conduction delay defined as a QRS complex >120 ms, and the presence or absence of ischemic cardiomyopathy (Table 91.1). Based on the absolute value of the sum of weighted variables, three risk-stratified groups were identified: high risk (score <7.19, 35% 1-year survival with medical therapy), medium risk (score 7.20–8.09, 60% 1-year survival), and low risk (score >8.10, 88% 1-year survival with medical therapy). These risk strata were derived before the widespread application of β-blockade and resynchronization therapy. However, the HFSS has been validated against peak oxygen consumption (15) and with the addition of effective β-blocker therapy (16). Application of the HFSS to medical decision making is variable among programs, but we consider high-risk stratification (score <7.2) a relative indication for transplantation. Even with effective medical therapy, 2-year event-free survival for high-risk HFSS patients is only 60%, and limited data suggest that the very significant survival advantage of β-blockers in medium-risk patients (85% 1-year survival) is lost by 3 to 4 years (16).

The Seattle Heart Failure Model is a more recent reiteration of a Cox proportional hazards multivariate analysis of mortality in ambulatory heart failure patients (17). New York Heart Association (NYHA) class, ischemic etiology, diuretic dose, ejection fraction, SBP, serum sodium, hemoglobin, percent lymphocytes, uric acid, and cholesterol each had independent predictive value. The model has been prospectively validated and incorporates both medicine and devices to predict associated changes in patient survival (www.SeattleHeartFailureModel.org). However, neither the Seattle nor the HFSS model is designed to address issues of patients in the critical care environment with acute decompensated heart failure. Analysis of the Acute Decompensated Heart

TABLE 91.1

HEART FAILURE SURVIVAL SCORE (HFSS)

Coronary artery disease (yes = 1, no = 0)	(..... × 0.6931) =	+
Intraventricular conduction delay (yes = 1, no = 0)	(..... × 0.6083) =	+
Left ventricular ejection fraction (%)	(..... × 0.0464) =	+
Heart rate (bpm)	(..... × 0.0216) =	+
Na^+ concentration (mmol/L)	(..... × 0.0470) =	+
Mean arterial pressure (mm Hg)	(..... × 0.0255) =	+
Peak VO_2 (mL/kg/min)	(..... × 0.0546) =	+
		HFSS = ...

High risk <7.19 (35% 1-y survival), medium risk 7.20–8.09 (60% 1-y survival), and low risk >8.10 (88% 1-y survival).

From Aaronson KD, Schawartz JS, Chen TM, et al. Development and prospective validation of a clinical index to predict survival in ambulatory patients referred for cardiac transplant evaluation. *Circulation.* 1997;95:2660.

Failure National Registry (ADHERE) demonstrates that blood urea nitrogen (BUN) >43 mg/dL at admission is the best discriminator between hospital survivors and nonsurvivors, followed by a systolic blood pressure <115 mm Hg and a creatinine >2.75 mg/dL. In-hospital mortality for the high-risk group (elevated BUN and creatinine, low SBP) is approximately 23% (18).

It is our institutional bias that the decision to transplant is individualized and directed toward patient-specific quality of life. Hemodynamic and objective measures of cardiac performance are always used to make transplant decisions, but functional status, a history of acute decompensation, neurohormonal markers of compensated heart failure, and intolerance to optimal medical therapy influence the thought process and timing of decisions. We do not question that transplantation improves cardiac function but always question whether "fixing the heart" will significantly improve the patient. While individual physicians advocate for patients, the decision to transplant is collective and represents the balance of interest between responsible use of a shared limited resource and appropriate patient need. Heart transplantation as an operation should not exist outside an integrated heart failure service and an active mechanical circulatory assist program. We do not consider decompensated heart failure an indication for transplantation. Every effort is made to establish a euvolemic state with adequate end organ perfusion before proceeding to transplantation. Patients intolerant of maximal medical therapy are referred for ventricular device placement, and patients with acute cardiogenic shock refractory to medical therapy are stabilized with extracorporeal life support (ECLS) before placement of definitive ventricular assist devices and consideration for transplant. The separation of mechanical ventricular assist technology and transplantation in this discussion is editorial and does not reflect current thinking in the surgical management of end-stage heart disease.

Organ Allocation

The current allocation system for donor hearts is designed to prioritize patients with the most urgent medical need of transplantation—potential recipients with mechanical circulatory assist devices and patients requiring multiple inotropes or a single high-dose inotrope (dobutamine >7.5 μg/kg per minute or milrinone >0.5 μg/kg per minute) are listed as status 1A. Patients requiring a single continuous low-dose inotrope to maintain hemodynamics and end organ perfusion are listed as 1B. Patients with end-stage heart disease who fail to meet either of these criteria are listed as status 2. Because of the increasing efficacy of medical therapy, the survival benefit of transplantation to United Network for Organ Sharing (UNOS) status 2 patients has been questioned (19). As a result, hearts are now offered to local 1A and 1B recipients and subsequently offered to regional 1A and 1B recipients within 500 miles of a donor hospital before returning to the local transplant centers for UNOS status 2 patients. There have been serious suggestions that heart transplantation be subjected to a randomized trial against medical therapy for patients currently listed as UNOS status 2.

One consequence of regional allocation beyond the local organ procurement organization is the logistic difficulty of cross-matching hearts to allosensitized patients. Nearly 20% of potential recipients in our program have significant anti-HLA antibodies or panel reactive antibody (PRA) >10% requiring a prospective cross-match prior to organ acceptance. Because of the logistic difficulty of maintaining potential recipient sera at all possible donor centers, we have come to rely on the virtual cross-match to exclude organs at significant risk for acute immune mediated rejection (20). Currently, all potential recipients are screened for class I and class II anti-HLA IgG antibodies by flow cytometry. If HLA alloantibodies are detected, the specificity of the HLA antibody is determined by single HLA molecule high-definition reagents. A list of exclusive antigens is used to virtually cross-match and exclude organs with potentially cross-reactive allospecific HLAs. Local donors are prospectively cross-matched using cell based, complement-dependent cytotoxicity assays to identify immunoreactive allografts. It is important to recognize that cytotoxicity assays are subjective and open to significant differences in interpretation, particularly at lower levels of reactivity. Infection and transfusion are the most frequent source of alloreactive antibodies in potential organ recipients and as such should be carefully noted in the critical care environment. It is our practice to screen actively listed potential transplant recipients every 30 days for alloreactive antibodies.

ACUTE ALLOGRAFT LOSS

Within 30 days of transplantation, causes of death include graft failure (primary and/or nonspecific) accounting for 40%, multiorgan system failure (14%), and noncytomegalovirus (non-CMV) infection (13%). Here we discuss the cause and management of primary graft loss focusing on the mechanisms of acute right ventricular failure, acute immune injury in the context of current practices of immunosuppression and induction therapy, and the biology of opportunistic infections in the early posttransplant period.

Right Ventricular Dysfunction and Allograft Failure

Whereas acute right ventricular (RV) failure at the time of allograft implantation is an uncommon but highly morbid condition with historical mortalities approaching 30% to 50%, RV dysfunction after allograft implantation is common. Nearly 20% of orthotopic heart transplants demonstrate some degree of RV dysfunction as manifested by tricuspid regurgitation. Tricuspid regurgitation has recently been shown to be a predictor of late survival after cardiac transplantation, suggesting that early RV dysfunction is a marker of poor outcome (21). The etiology of transplant RV dysfunction is poorly understood but clearly multifactorial and includes primary aspects of donor organ biology (e.g., primary right ventricular graft dysfunction), inherent injury secondary to the procurement process (e.g., ischemia–reperfusion injury), and specific characteristics of recipient pathophysiology (e.g., elevated pulmonary vascular resistance).

Heart donors with cerebrovascular accident as the cause of death have consistently demonstrated a significant negative impact on 1-year posttransplant mortality (2), and experimental data have supported the concept that donor brain death contributes to right ventricular dysfunction after cardiac transplantation. Animal studies have demonstrated a significant decrease in right ventricular function after transplantation in hearts retrieved from a brain dead donor whereas right ventricular function is maintained or increased after implantation of normal hearts even in recipients with chronic pulmonary hypertension (22). Furthermore, large animal models assessing the intrinsic myocardial mechanics of transplanted hearts independent of the severe changes in peripheral loading conditions that accompany the catecholamine storm of brain death (elevated peripheral and pulmonary vascular resistance) demonstrate a nearly 40% reduction in RV contractility without a similar decrease in LV contractility (22). This suggests that RV dysfunction is primarily related to the status of the donor heart, and although elevated pulmonary vascular resistance will increase the severity of postoperative RV dysfunction, it is unlikely that elevated PVR independently creates RV dysfunction.

The early biology of transplanted hearts is defined by denervation and diastolic dysfunction. Loss of afferent parasympathetic vagal tone and corresponding lowering of myocardial catecholamine levels in response to sympathetic denervation results in higher resting heart rates and a blunted response to hypovolemia and decreased preload. A poorly understood but useful consequence of denervation is increased presynaptic sensitivity to β-adrenergic stimulation (22). The transplanted heart is also "stiff," and restrictive physiology is expected in the immediate postoperative period. Elevated diastolic ventricular filling pressures generally diminish within weeks of transplant, but persistent diastolic dysfunction may represent donor–recipient size mismatch, myocardial injury from harvest ischemia, intrinsic characteristics of the donor heart (e.g., hypertension), or evidence of rejection.

Because of limited therapies, prophylaxis for acute allograft dysfunction is a preferable clinical strategy. It is our practice to start inhaled nitric oxide (NO) (20 ppm) prior to weaning from cardiopulmonary bypass to lower pulmonary vascular resistance in patients with preoperative PVR >3 Wood units. All patients exit the operative theatre on low- to moderate-dose epinephrine (0.02–0.06 μg/kg per minute) and patients receiving chronic afterload reduction preoperatively (e.g., intravenous milrinone) are simultaneously started on low-dose norepinephrine (0.02–0.04 μg/kg per minute). Patients are atrially paced (92 beats per minute [bpm]), or AV sequentially paced, in the immediate postoperative period. In the absence of significant tricuspid regurgitation and RV dysfunction, NO is weaned in the immediate postoperative period, and patients are generally extubated within 6 hours of exiting the operating room (OR). Caution should be used in weaning NO as rebound pulmonary hypertension has been observed (23). We have not found this to be a significant clinical problem outside the pediatric population. Inotropic support is maintained for the initial 24 hours and weaned off between 24 and 36 hours as determined by clinical exam.

We routinely start milrinone (0.2–0.5 μg/kg per minute) as a selective pulmonary vasodilator and for peripheral afterload reduction between 12 and 24 hours postoperatively as epinephrine/norepinephrine are withdrawn. Patients frequently remain on low-dose milrinone (0.2 μg/kg per minute) for 3 to 5 days after transplant. Approximately half of our patients have right heart catheters postoperatively. We have found clinical exam and echocardiogram effective for evaluating ventricular function, filling pressures, and RV strain, and right heart catheters are generally placed for specific diagnostic questions and rarely guide clinical management. All patients undergo right heart catheterization and biopsy within 7 to 14 days of transplant. For patients with biventricular dysfunction thought secondary to reperfusion injury, we have anecdotally found the combination of epinephrine and low-dose calcium (50–200 mg/hour) efficacious in the postoperative period. This is consistent with theoretical models identifying calcium homeostasis as a significant pathway in ischemia–reperfusion injury (23).

Ischemia–reperfusion Injury

Over the past three decades, studies of ischemia–reperfusion injury have created an enormous amount of descriptive data, a limited amount of information, and a small amount of integrated knowledge. Traditional views hold that the obligatory ischemia of organ procurement induces endothelial dysfunction, lipid peroxidation with loss of membrane integrity, free radical superoxide production, dysregulation of intracellular and mitochondrial calcium flux, and neutrophil activation with allograft infiltration. Reperfusion at the time of allograft implantation is thought to extend the inflammatory injury with subsequent apoptosis and delayed cell death contributing to graft dysfunction. The volume of translational research directed at the cause of ischemia–reperfusion injury and the efforts to design surgical strategies to diminish its impact on the vascular biology of solid organ transplants precludes any significant discussion, and the subject has been recently reviewed (23). However, two conceptual shifts of probable impact on the treatment and understanding of acute cardiac allograft function in the context ischemia–reperfusion injury deserve mention.

First, reintroduction of blood flow to the thoracic allograft in a stuttering fashion has had wide anecdotal application among transplant surgeons. This is based on anecdotal observations that slow and intermittent reperfusion limits clinical reperfusion injury. Similar patterns of postconditioning have recently been demonstrated to reduce reperfusion injury and enhance myocardial function in patients experiencing acute myocardial infarcts (24). The mechanism of postconditioning appears to involve release of endogenous adenosine and opioid receptor ligands (24). A second observation is the increasing appreciation of toll-like receptors in ischemia–reperfusion injury. Toll-like receptors, one class of the pathogen recognition system involved in innate immunity, have been associated with early cytokine release after reperfusion (23). It is likely that antagonists of both systems will eventually find application in modulating the adhesion molecule engagement and proinflammatory cytokine biology of allograft reperfusion injury.

Rejection and Immunosuppression

With the exception of homozygous twins, all allografts are incompatible. This incompatibility is defined by the predominant mechanism of allorecognition—humoral or cellular—and the temporal pattern of allograft rejection. *Hyperacute rejection* occurs within minutes to hours of allograft reperfusion and is a rare form of perioperative graft loss caused by preformed antibodies directed against donor HLA or endothelial antigen. Complement activation results in intravascular thrombosis and ischemic graft dysfunction. There is no medical therapy as graft loss is nearly immediate and salvage requires mechanical circulatory support (ECLS or VAD) and consideration for retransplantation. Diagnosis is mandatory and should be directed at confirming ABO compatibility and identifying the antibody-specific alloantigen. Although the UNOS ethics committee recognizes retransplantation as a therapeutic option, it also notes that "graft failure, particularly early or immediate failure, evokes significant concerns regarding repeat transplantation" and suggests that "the likelihood of long-term survival of a repeat transplant should receive strong consideration" (*www.UNOS.org/bioethics*). Histologic confirmation of humoral injury requires immunostains for complement (C4d), immunoglobulins, and macrophages (CD68) within capillaries.

Acute rejection is historically considered a T-cell–mediated process with perivascular infiltration of lymphocytes and macrophages and variable degrees of myonecrosis. It can occur anytime after transplantation but is most commonly diagnosed within the first 6 months—nearly 60% of heart recipients—and is the most common form of rejection within days to weeks after allograft implantation (25). The diagnosis and management of acute rejection can be problematic. Early ischemic injury can manifest as significant myocyte injury with various degrees of inflammation. Although *mild* acute cellular rejection (grade 1R) with perivascular mononuclear cells and *severe* acute cellular rejection (grade 3R) with diffuse mononuclear cell infiltrates and extensive myonecrosis are easily distinguished from ischemic injury, *moderate* rejection requires interpretation. Perivascular and interstitial mononuclear cells predominate with few (two or more) foci of myocyte injury in moderate acute cellular rejection. A predominance of neutrophils and organ dysfunction may suggest the possibility of a humoral component (26)

Chronic rejection is characterized by circumferential myointimal proliferation and progressive coronary artery vasculopathy. Nearly half of all heart transplants demonstrate angiographically recognizable CAV by year five. Early acute vascular rejection, inadequately treated acute rejection, CMV infection, non-CMV infection, donor age, and donor hypertension are among the factors associated with the biology of chronic rejection, and early CAV (occurring within 1 year) contributes to significant increases in mortality when compared to patients without CAV (27).

The goal of early biopsy is diagnosis, and the subsequent histology must be interpreted within the patient-specific clinical context. This clinical context requires active participation of both surgeon and cardiologist with the reviewing pathologist, and it is our policy to collectively review all biopsy specimens. Interobserver differences in the interpretation of biopsies can be significant, and there is an understandable tendency to "overcall" inflammation and overtreat mild rejection because of the fear of rejection; overimmunosuppression in the acute postoperative phase can result in catastrophic infection whereas failure to adequately treat rejection can result in significant allograft injury. We do not treat mild rejection (grade 1R). Severe rejection (grade 3R) is always treated with pulse steroids and antilymphocyte therapy, and in the context of organ dysfunction, every attempt is made to rule out humoral rejection. If circulating antibody is detected, patients undergo plasmapheresis although this is uncommon in our practice since all recipients undergo retrospective cross-match to guide post-transplant management. Moderate rejection can be confused with ischemic injury, and we routinely treat grade 2R biopsies with pulse steroids and rebiopsy within 7 to 10 days.

Balanced Risk: Immunosuppression and Infection

Coronary artery vasculopathy is a probable complication of underimmunosuppression whereas early infection and late malignancy are probable complications of overimmunosuppression. These opposing problems represent the major failure of contemporary thoracic transplantation. Immunosuppressive therapies remain institution specific. Drug protocols for thoracic transplant are derived largely from the investigational experiences of renal transplant, and monitoring of immunosuppressive drug therapy is based on pharmacology and presumed therapeutic drug levels rather than the analysis of specific measures of general and donor-specific immune responsiveness. Nonetheless, there are shared immunosuppressive strategies for the *induction* of immune tolerance at the time of allograft implantation and for the *maintenance* of chronic immune suppression over time. *Rescue* (antirejection) therapy in response to histologic rejection remains very problematic as there is no direct relationship between microscopic evidence of allograft rejection, allograft dysfunction, and patient survival. Acute rejection, outside the context of patient noncompliance or unappreciated preformed antibody in the sensitized organ recipient, is uncommon and accounts for only 2% of deaths at 1 year (Fig. 91.1).

Induction Therapy and Maintenance Immunosuppression

The goal of induction therapy is clonal deletion of T cells with allograft-specific antigen recognition. The reality of induction therapy is generalized T-cell anergy with effective immunosuppression at the risk of generalized immunodeficiency. Although the efficacy of induction therapy in cardiac transplantation remains controversial and is necessarily balanced against the risk of increased infection, approximately half of all heart transplant patients receive antilymphocyte induction therapy at the time of allograft implantation (2). Collective registry data suggest no significant differences in survival among patients receiving induction therapy. However, the specific risk profiles for various induction therapies—nonspecific polyclonals versus specific monoclonals—are distinct, and the application of various induction therapies is often patient specific.

Polyclonal antilymphocyte antibody preparations are gamma globulin fractions of serum derived from animals immunized with human lymphoid tissue—rabbit-derived antilymphocyte/thymocyte globulin (ALG, *Thymoglobulin*) or horse-derived antithymocyte globulin (ATG). Both preparations bind various cell surface antigens on B and T cells with subsequent complement-mediated cytolysis and eventual opsinization (28). Therapy is nonspecific, and cross-reactivity may induce leukopenia and thrombocytopenia. The current polyclonals are foreign proteins and induce an immune response in the organ recipient; this limits long-term efficacy

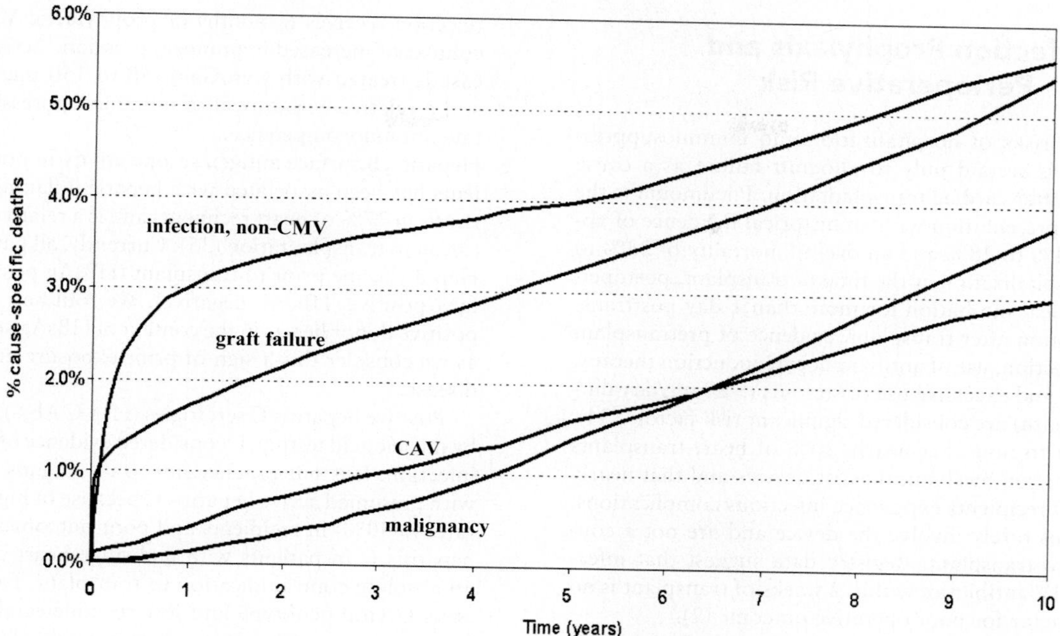

FIGURE 91.1. Causes of specific mortality in heart transplantation. Note the early incidence of infection and graft failure followed by a dose-dependent rise in coronary artery vasculopathy (CAV) and malignancy. CMV, cytomegalovirus. (Adapted from Taylor DO, Edwards LB, Boucek MM, et al. Registry of the International Society of Heart and Lung Transplantation: twenty-third official adult heart transplantation report. *J Heart Lung Transplant.* 2006;25:869.

without recurrent therapy and raises concerns as to the potential for hypersensitivity responses with subsequent exposures. Cytokine release syndrome complicates polyclonal therapy in approximately 20% of patients, and serum sickness has been reported with equine-derived antithymocyte globulin. Nonetheless, while very limited retrospective reviews suggest some efficacy to polyclonal induction therapy (29,30) the practice and experience remains largely institution specific.

Induction therapy with the monoclonal antibody daclizumab (*Zenapax*), directed against the interleukin-2 receptor, is now widespread among cardiac transplant programs. A randomized trial of daclizumab as induction therapy demonstrated a decreased rate of acute cellular rejection (25% vs. 41%) and an increased median time to the primary end points of histologic rejection, allograft dysfunction, retransplantation, or death (31). However, the mortality in the daclizumab group was 6.5% at 6 months versus 3.2% in the nontreatment group with most of the treatment group deaths secondary to infection in patients receiving a second antilymphocyte cytolytic therapy (32). The efficacy of daclizumab may be influenced by the degree of donor–recipient mismatch at the HLA-DR histocompatability locus (33).

It is our institutional practice to use the humanized antiinterleukin-2 receptor monoclonal antibody daclizumab (*Zenapax*) to delay the initiation of calcineurin inhibitor therapy in an attempt to prevent potential nephrotoxicity in the perioperative setting. Patients receive 1 mg/kg intravenously (IV) at the time of transplant with an additional dose given on postoperative day 7 and every 14 days thereafter for a total of three to five cumulative doses. In reality, only 20% of patients receive the full five doses with therapy curtailed in response to leukopenia or two consecutive biopsies with no evidence of rejection in the context of well-tolerated therapeutic levels of calcineurin inhibitor. As an alternative induction therapy, basiliximab (*Simulect*), a chimeric anti-IL-2 receptor monoclonal antibody, is given on induction (20 mg IV) and postoperative day 4 (20 mg IV). We do not use induction therapy with patients on mechanical circulatory devices or in patients who have received any immunosuppressive therapy within 12 weeks of transplant.

Maintenance immunosuppression generally consists of an antiproliferative drug (azathioprine or mycophenolate), a calcineurin inhibitor (tacrolimus or cyclosporine), and steroids. It is our institutional preference to use mycophenolate because of a reported lower rate of death and treated episodes of rejection when compared to azathioprine (32). Tacrolimus is started postoperatively within 72 hours in patients receiving induction therapy or immediately if serum creatinine is <1.8 mg/dL. Heart recipients without induction therapy receive tacrolimus (1 mg via nasogastric tube) in the operative theater and are converted to sublingual therapy in the rare situation of delayed extubation. We do not use IV tacrolimus because of the difficulty in predicting therapeutic levels and our observation of delayed seizures in patients with transient toxic levels of calcineurin inhibitor. Every attempt is made to wean steroids to 5 mg of prednisone or less within 6 months of transplant, and 30% of heart recipients are steroid free by 2 years (2). We have increasingly used the mammalian target of rapamycin (mTOR) inhibitor rapamycin (*Sirolimus*) in conjunction with low-dose calcineurin inhibitors to limit calcineurin-induced nephrotoxicity. Rapamycin is not started until 4 to 6 weeks after transplant because of its significant impact on sternal wound healing.

Infection Prophylaxis and Perioperative Risk

Because of the risks of hospitalization and immunosuppression, infection is second only to allograft failure as a cause of early death after cardiac transplantation. Pneumonia is the most common presentation with an historical incidence of approximately 14% to 28% and an overall mortality of 23% to 31% (34). Hospitalization at the time of transplant, postoperative endotracheal intubation for more than 1 day posttransplant, reintubation after transplant, evidence of pretransplant pulmonary infection, use of antilymphocyte induction therapy, and prolonged and excessive use of steroids (>80 mg/day during the first month) are considered significant risk factors (34). It is important to note that nearly 20% of heart transplants occur in patients on mechanical assist devices and that nearly half of all VAD recipients experience infectious complications. These infections rarely involve the device and are not a contraindication to transplant. Registry data suggest that infection requiring IV antibiotics within 2 weeks of transplant is no longer a risk factor for poor operative outcome (2).

The importance of clinical history and serologic screening of potential organ donors cannot be overemphasized given the potential for disease reactivation. Specific characteristics of the donor population vary widely among geographically distinct transplant centers, and ethnic diversity can influence the prevalence of endemic disease. Nearly half of our thoracic organs derive from donors born in areas of endemic Chagas disease (*Trypanosoma cruzi*), and 20% derive from areas of endemic viral hepatitis B. Geography, not immunosuppression, is also the major risk factor for certain mycoses (e.g., coccidiomycosis, histoplasmosis), and the endemicity of tuberculosis and variable use of immunization can influence the interpretation of donor serologies. The recent deaths of organ recipients receiving allografts from patients with undiagnosed trypanosomal infection (*www.CDC.org*) underscores the increasing globalization of the donor population and the need for increasingly sophisticated screening technologies. Our institutional biases for the prophylaxis and treatment of the common bacterial, viral, and fungal pathogens are listed below:

1. Vancomycin (10–15 mg/kg every 12 h) and piperacillin/tazobactam (3.375 gm IV every 6 h) are empiric bacterial prophylaxis. Therapy is stopped at 72 hours after review of donor cultures.
2. Cytomegalovirus seropositivity is not a contraindication for either donor or recipient. Leukocytes are the source of CMV infection, and seronegative blood products should be used in seronegative patients and patients with seronegative allografts. Primary infection, a seropositive (CMV+) organ into a seronegative (CMV–) recipient, is associated with the greatest risk of CMV disease. These patients receive prophylaxis with CMV immune globulin (CytoGam, CMV-IVIG) at 150 mg/kg IV for 7 days followed by valganciclovir (Valcyte) for 1 year (450 mg twice daily [BID] dosed for renal function). Seropositive patients who receive either CMV-positive or CMV-negative allografts are at moderate to low risk of reactivation disease as are seronegative recipients of CMV-negative transplants. These patients receive prophylactic coverage for 6 months with Valcyte (450 mg orally (PO) BID). Any patient receiving treatment for histologic rejection receives 6 months of prophylactic Valcyte in the context of increased immunosuppression. Active CMV disease is treated with CytoGam (50 to 150 mg/kg IV daily) and a relative withdrawal of immunosuppression to facilitate immunocompetence.
3. Hepatitis B surface antigen seropositivity in potential recipients has been associated with hepatic inflammation or cirrhosis in 37% of heart recipients and is a relative contraindication to transplantation (35). Currently, all patients receive Hep B vaccine prior to transplant (HBsAg positive, HBsAb IgM positive, HBcAb negative). We routinely use HBcAb-positive donor hearts in the context of HBsAg seronegativity as we consider this a sign of prior exposure and not active disease.

   Positive hepatitis C serologies (Hep C Ab+), if confirmed by nucleic acid testing, is considered evidence of active donor infection. It is our practice not to use organs from donors with presumed active hepatitis C because of high conversion rates (>50%) in recipients and poor outcomes (36). Active hepatitis C in patients with end-stage heart disease is not an absolute contraindication to transplant. Favorable hepatitis C viral genotype and low to undetectable viral titre by quantitative polymerase chain reaction (PCR) identifies a group of patients with outcomes comparable to those of thoracic transplant recipients without viral infection. We have also challenged hepatitis C seropositive patients pretransplant with low-dose calcineurin inhibitors (target level of 5–8 ng%) and mycophenolate (1,000 mg BID). Patients without a significant rise in viral titre by quantitative PCR over 3 months have not demonstrated evidence of active viral disease after transplantation.
4. All patients receive trimethoprim/sulfamethoxazole (*Septra*) for *Pneumocystis carinii* prophylaxis. Fluconazole (100 mg PO every week) is given for mucocutaneous candidiasis prophylaxis as long as patients are receiving steroids, and patients with evidence of fungal colonization (e.g., *Aspergillus* spp.) are maintained on voriconazole.

In the absence of allograft dysfunction, the decision to treat moderate histologic (2R) rejection with pulse steroids deserves discussion. There is no compelling data that treatment of mild to moderate rejection significantly influences allograft survival, and there is significant evidence that increased steroids and antilymphocyte therapy increase the incidence of infection. Given the variability of histologic interpretation and the inherent possibility of nonrepresentative biopsy tissue, the decision to treat histologic rejection should be approached with caution as this represents the most significant variable in transplant infections.

CLINICAL PEARLS IN CARDIAC TRANSPLANTATION

1. Neurohormonal markers and the circulatory-renal limit predict the need for transplantation, not isolated hemodynamics.
2. Elevated pulmonary vascular resistance, renal insufficiency, and diabetes mellitus are only *relative* contraindications to transplant.
3. The degree of fixed pulmonary vascular resistance cannot be assessed without unloading the left ventricle.

4. Elevated postoperative PVR exacerbates RV dysfunction.
5. The relationship between histologic rejection and patient outcome remains obscure; microscopic rejection is rarely manifested as graft dysfunction.
6. Balanced risk is the goal of immunosuppression.

References

1. Hunt SA. Taking heart—cardiac transplantation past, present, and future. *N Engl J Med.* 2006;355:231.
2. Taylor DO, Edwards LB, Boucek MM, et al. Registry of the International Society of Heart and Lung Transplantation: twenty-third official heart transplantation report. *J Heart Lung Transplant.* 2006;25:869.
3. Teuteberg, JJ, Lewis EF, Nohria A, et al. Characteristics of patients who die with heart failure and a low ejection fraction in the new millennium. *J Card Fail.* 2006;12:47.
4. Mehra MR, Kobashigawa J, Starling R, et al. Listing criteria for heart transplantation: International Society for Heart and Lung Transplantation guidelines for the care of cardiac transplant candidates—2006. *J Heart Lung Transplant.* 2006;25:1024.
5. Ghio S, Gavazzi A, Campana C, et al. Independent and additive prognostic value of right ventricular systolic function and pulmonary artery pressure in patients with chronic heart failure. *J Am Coll Cardiol.* 2001;37:183.
6. Grigioni F, Poten L, Galie N, et al. Prognostic implications of serial assessments of pulmonary hypertension in severe chronic heart failure. *J Heart Lung Transplant.* 2006;25:1241.
7. Stobierska-Dzierzek B, Awad H, Michler RE. The evolving management of acute right-sided heart failure in cardiac transplant recipients. *J Am Coll Cardiol.* 2001:38:923.
8. Petrofski JA, Hoopes C, Bashore TM, et al. Mechanical ventricular support lowers pulmonary vascular resistance in a patient with congenital heart disease. *Ann Thorac Surg.* 2003;75:1005.
9. Luckraz H, Parameshwar J, Charman SC, et al. Short- and long-term outcomes of combined cardiac and renal transplantation with allografts from a single donor. *J Heart Lung Transplant.* 2003;12:1318.
10. Haas M, Kain R, Mayer G, et al. Heart transplant and combined heart/kidney transplant? Even one renal biopsy may fool you. *Nephrol Dial Transplant.* 1999;14:1014.
11. Yan RT, White M, Yan AT, et al. Usefulness of temporal changes in neurohormones as markers of ventricular remodeling and prognosis in patients with left ventricular systolic dysfunction and heart failure receiving either Candesartan or Enalapril or both. *Am J Cardiol.* 2005;96:698.
12. Mueller C, Laule-Kilan K, Brunner-La Rocca HP, et al. Inflammation and long-term mortality in acute congestive heart failure. *Am Heart J.* 2006;151:845.
13. Kittleso M, Hurwitz S, Shah MR, et al. Development of circulatory-renal limitations to angiotensin-converting enzyme inhibitors identifies patients with severe heart failure and early mortality. *J Am Coll Cardiol.* 2003;41:2029.
14. Aaronson KD, Schawartz JS, Chen TM, et al. Development and prospective validation of a clinical index to predict survival in ambulatory patients referred for cardiac transplant evaluation. *Circulation.* 1997;95:2660.
15. Lund LH, Aaronson KD, Mancini DM. Validation of peak exercise oxygen consumption and the Heart Failure Survival Score for serial risk stratification in advanced heart failure. *Am J Cardiol.* 2005;95:734.
16. Koelling T, Joseph S, Aaronson K. Heart Failure Survival Score continues to predict clinical outcomes in patients with heart failure receiving β-blockers. *J Heart Lung Transplant.* 2004;23:1414.
17. Levy WC, Mozaffarian D, Linker DT. The Seattle Heart Failure Model, prediction of survival in heart failure. *Circulation.* 2006;113:1424.
18. Fonarow GC, Adams KF, Araham WT, et al. Risk stratification for in-hospital mortality in acutely decompensated heart failure. *JAMA.* 2005;293:572.
19. Jimenez J, Edwards LB, Higgins R, et al. Should stable UNOS status 2 patients be transplanted? *J Heart Lung Transplant.* 2005;24:178.
20. Zangwill SD, Ellis TM, Zlotocha J, et al. The virtual crossmatch—a screening tool for sensitized pediatric heart transplant recipients. *Pediatr Transplant.* 2006;10:38.
21. Anderson CA, Shernan SK, MD, Leacche M, et al. Severity of intraoperative tricuspid regurgitation predicts poor late survival following cardiac transplantation. *Ann Thorac Surg.* 2004;78:1635.
22. Bittner HB, Chen EP, Biswas SS, et al. Right ventricular dysfunction after cardiac transplantation: primarily related to status of donor heart. *Ann Thorac Surg.* 1999;68:1605.
23. Land WG. The role of postischemic reperfusion injury and other nonantigen-dependent inflammatory pathways in transplantation. *Transplantation.* 2005;79:505.
24. Gross GJ, Auchampach JA. Reperfusion injury: does it exist? *J Mol Cell Cardiol.* 2006;10:1016.
25. Billingham M, Kobashigawa JA. The revised ISHLT biopsy grading scale. *J Heart Lung Transplant.* 2005;24:1709.
26. Takemoto S, Zeevi A, Feng S, et al. A national conference to assess antibody mediated rejection in solid organ transplantation. *Am J Transplant.* 2004;4:1.
27. Avery RK. Cardiac allograft vasculopathy. *N Engl J Med.* 2003;349:829.
28. Mueller XM. Drug immunosuppression therapy for adult heart transplantation: immune response to allograft and mechanism of action of immunosuppressants. *Ann Thorac Surg.* 2004;77:354.
29. Mueller XM. Drug immunosuppression therapy for adult heart transplantation: clinical application and results. *Ann Thorac Surg.* 2004;77:363.
30. Lindenfield J, Miller GG, Shakar SF, et al. Drug therapy in the heart transplant recipient, 1: cardiac rejection and immunosuppressive drugs. *Circulation.* 2004;110:3734.
31. Hershberger RE, Starling RC, Eisen JH, et al. Daclizumab to prevent rejection after cardiac transplantation. *N Engl J Med.* 2005;352:2705.
32. Hosenpud JD. Immunosuppression in cardiac transplantation. *N Engl J Med.* 2005;352:2749.
33. Lietz K, John R, Beniaminovitz A, et al. Interleukin-2 receptor blockade in cardiac transplantation: influence of HLA-DR locus incompatibility on treatment efficacy. *Transplantation.* 2003;75:781.
34. Montoya JG, Giraldo LF, Efron B, et al. Infectious complications among 620 consecutive heart transplant patients at Stanford University Medical Center. *Clin Infect Dis.* 2001;33:629.
35. Haji SA, Avery RK, Yamani MH, et al. Donor or recipient hepatitis B seropositivity is associated with allograft vasculopathy. *J Heart Lung Transplant.* 2006;25:294.
36. Gasink LB, Blumberg EA, Localio AR, et al. Hepatitis C virus seropositivity in organ donors and survival in heart transplant recipients. *JAMA.* 2006;296:1843.

CHAPTER 92 ■ LUNG TRANSPLANTATION

SEBASTIAN FERNANDEZ-BUSSY • OLUFEMI AKINDIPE • AMY F. ROSENBERG • EDWARD D. STAPLES • MAHER A. BAZ

Lung transplantation has become a therapeutic option for patients with end-stage lung diseases who have severe functional impairment and limited life expectancy. Lung transplantation thus offers the possibility of improving the quality of life and prolonging life in a select population of recipients. It has been applied with success to most advanced lung diseases, with the exception of lung cancers. Nonetheless, complications are frequent, with a median survival of 5 years. The purpose of this chapter is to give the reader a thorough account of lung transplantation, its application, benefits, and potential complications.

PRETRANSPLANT CONSIDERATIONS AND CANDIDATE SELECTION

Waiting Lists, Donor Availability, and Donor Suitability

The number of lung diseases successfully treated by transplantation has increased in the last two decades, resulting in an increase in both the indications for lung transplantation and, as a consequence, in the number of eligible candidates. After many years of stable lung donor supply, it seems that the procurement of lungs from potential donors has slightly increased in the last 1 to 2 years as a result of national collaboration among the transplant centers and the organ procurement organizations (OPO) to improve the medical management of organ donors (Fig. 92.1) (1). This has led to a slight increase in the number of lung transplant operations performed in the last 1 to 2 years. Moreover, it appears that with the implementation of a new lung allocation system (LAS) score on May 4, 2005, the number of deaths on the waiting list is trending downward. The LAS score is based on the principle of maximum benefit from lung transplantation, rather than transplanting the "sickest" patient. A score is calculated based on the probability of surviving 1 year on the waiting list minus the probability of surviving the first year posttransplant. This compound score has resulted in our ability to transplant patients with shorter life expectancy (i.e., pulmonary fibrosis) at a higher rate than the previous system used (2). The previous system was based purely on the waiting time, with seniority on the list going to patients with the most waiting time, regardless of their level of illness or potential benefit from lung transplantation. We are hopeful that in 1 to 2 years, we will be able to unequivocally demonstrate that the new LAS has resulted in a significant decrease in the death rate on the waiting list.

All hospitals are obligated to report all deaths to their local organ procurement organizations (OPO). Each OPO covers several counties—and sometimes a whole state. The OPO reviews and identifies potential organ donors (brain death with consenting families). Once a suitable donor is identified, the OPO offers the lungs first to the transplant centers located within the geographic boundaries of their working area. The local recipient list (Fig. 92.2) is organized first by blood type and height; recipients are usually listed with a height range of ±20%, as height is the primary determinant for lung volumes. Patients on the waiting list with the highest lung allocation system score will be offered the lungs first. The list is then run by compatible blood types if no recipients with identical blood types match in the OPO's region. Lung transplant centers usually prefer to implant taller-donor lungs into recipients with obstructive lung diseases (chronic obstructive pulmonary disease [COPD], cystic fibrosis [CF]) and shorter-donor lungs into recipients with restrictive lung diseases (idiopathic pulmonary fibrosis [IPF]). If the transplant center(s) within the geographic boundaries of the OPO does not accept the lungs, the procurement agency will widen the search to include transplant centers within a radius of 500 miles—as determined by zip codes—with lungs offered to patients with the highest LAS score in those areas. Since lungs can tolerate a 6- to 8-hour period of ischemia, travel time limitations are also a factor for accepting lungs. By way of contrast, livers can tolerate up to 12 hours of ischemia time.

Organ donors are procured from patients declared brain-dead, whose families consent to donation. The most common causes of brain death are from motor vehicle crashes, gunshot wounds, or cerebrovascular accidents. Historically, lung(s) were procured only from about 15% to 20% of potential solid organ donors; in contrast, about 80% of donors have kidneys and livers procured (3–5). Potential lung donors are managed by the OPOs prior to procurement, with the goal of maximizing organ function and suitability. The medical management is ideally geared toward keeping the donor lungs "dry" and minimizing risk of ventilator-associated pneumonia by using aggressive chest percussion and administering intravenous antibacterial therapy to the donor (6,7). With the recent emphasis on optimizing the medical management of donor lungs and the collaboration between OPOs and critical care physicians, some OPOs are now reporting lung procurement rates of 35% to 40%.

Potential lung donors could be considered unsuitable if there is a long history of smoking, evidence of aspiration pneumonia by chest radiograph or bronchoscopy, or evidence of neurogenic pulmonary edema by chest radiographs, especially when there is an associated progressive decline in oxygenation (8) (Table 92.1). Although Table 92.1 has criteria for "ideal" donors, other lungs with less ideal characteristics have been successfully transplanted with reasonable short-term outcomes (9).

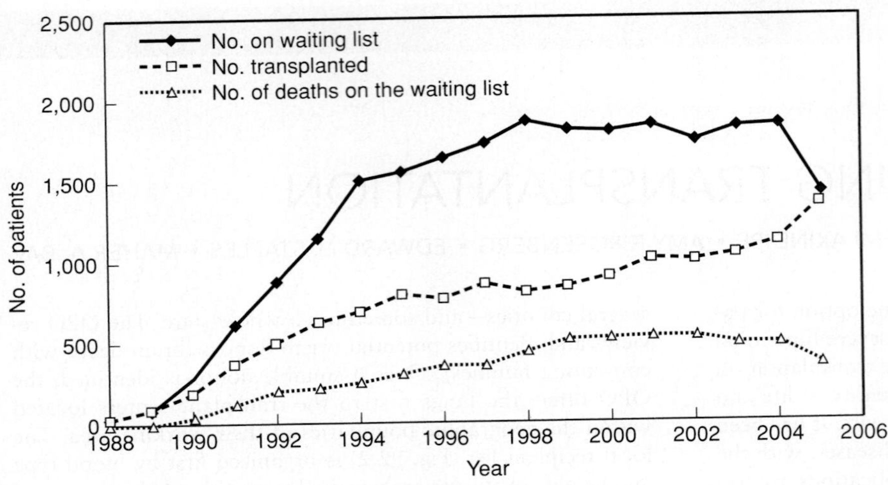

FIGURE 92.1. In the United States: number of lung transplants, number of patients waiting and deaths on the waiting list, 1988 to 2005 (ages 18–64 years). (Adapted from 2005 Annual Report of the U.S. Organ Procurement and Transplantation Network and the Scientific Registry of Transplant Recipients: transplant data 1994–2006.)

Timing of Referrals

Patients should be referred at a point in the course of the disease when death is considered likely in the next few years, especially if the projected 2-year survival is about 50% to 60%. The patient's report of an unacceptable quality of life is an important factor to consider in evaluating his or her candidacy for lung transplantation, but the disease prognosis must be the overriding impetus for referral and listing. An anticipated waiting time of 12 to 24 months, during which the candidate's condition must remain functionally suitable for transplantation, must be integrated into the decision process for referring and listing patients. Disease-specific guidelines for referral are listed in Table 92.2. Between the years of 1995 and 2005, the combination of COPD and alpha-1 antitrypsin deficiency accounted for about 50% of indications for lung transplantation, while IPF and CF accounted for 19% and 16%, respectively (10). However, it appears that there has been a trend toward more transplantation of IPF patients in the last 18 months, possibly due to a higher LAS score at the time of listing in this population since its implementation in May of 2005 (Fig. 92.3).

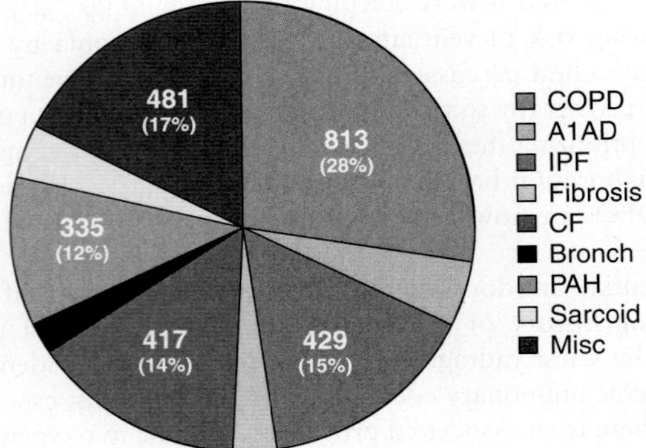

FIGURE 92.2. Adult patients on the waiting list in the United States in 2005, by indication. (Adapted from 2005 Annual Report of the U.S. Organ Procurement and Transplantation Network and the Scientific Registry of Transplant Recipients: transplant data 1994–2006.)

Selection Criteria for Suitable Candidates

Although transplantation has been successful in most lung diseases, not all patients with advanced lung diseases are suitable candidates (11). The patient's medical records are screened carefully prior to the initial clinic visits. Patients are often declined at the initial clinic visit if there is any history of cigarette smoking in the last 6 months or if there is evidence of severe extrapulmonary end organ damage. Patients are also screened for their insurance coverage, as lung transplantation is not an inexpensive endeavor. In most states, Medicaid, Medicare, and private insurance policies cover the costs of lung transplantation and immunosuppressive medications.

After an initial screening of the patient's medical records, the potential lung recipients are seen in the lung transplant clinic. A detailed discussion of lung transplantation, its outcome, and potential complications occurs with the patient if there are no obvious contraindications identified during the clinic visit. If the patient consents to the transplant procedure, he or she is then referred for a more detailed transplant evaluation and testing. Lung transplant evaluation and the guidelines for the selection of recipients are listed in Tables 92.3 and 92.4, respectively. A body mass index (BMI) >30 has recently been identified as an independent predictor of mortality in the first 12 months post transplantation (10,12). BMI >30 is a relative contraindication, as some of these patients have a large muscle volume accounting for their weight. Patients with BMI >30 with a low muscle volume are counseled to lose weight, and usually are not transplanted until they meet the target weight of

TABLE 92.1

CRITERIA FOR "IDEAL" LUNG DONORS

PaO_2 >300 mm Hg on FiO_2 = 1.0 and 5 cm H_2O continuous positive airway pressure (CPAP)
Less than 20 pack-years smoking history
Clear chest radiograph
Minimal secretions on bronchoscopy
Negative viral serology (HIV, hepatitis B and C infections)
Age younger than 55–60 years

TABLE 92.2

DISEASE-SPECIFIC GUIDELINES FOR REFERRAL

Chronic obstructive pulmonary disease (COPD)
FEV_1 (forced expiratory volume in 1 s) <25% of predicted postbronchodilator, especially when associated with mild or moderate pulmonary artery hypertension
Frequent severe exacerbations
BODE index (body-mass index [B], airflow obstruction [O], dyspnea [D], and exercise capacity [E]) of ≥7
Cystic fibrosis (CF)
FEV_1 <30% of predicted
$PaCO_2$ >50 mm Hg
Frequent severe exacerbations
Rapid decline in lung function (especially in females)
Idiopathic pulmonary fibrosis (IPF)
Vital capacity (VC) <65% predicted
10% decline in VC or in diffusion capacity in the last 12 months
Initiation of oxygen therapy
Pulmonary arterial hypertension (PAH)
NYHA (New York Heart Association) functional class III or IV
Cardiac index <2 L/min/m^2
Mean right atrial pressure >12 mm Hg
Failure of medical therapy to improve hemodynamic indexes or functional class
Eisenmenger syndrome
NYHA III or IV despite optimal medical therapy (especially if patients are discontented with their current quality of life)

BMI <30. This is especially important in the COPD population where quality of life is the sole indication for transplantation. Patients who are suitable for lung transplantation are listed with the United Network for Organ Sharing (UNOS).

SURGICAL TECHNIQUES FOR LUNG TRANSPLANTATION

There are four lung transplant surgical procedures: (i) single-lung transplantation (SLT), (ii) bilateral sequential lung transplantation (BLT), (iii) combined heart–lung transplantation (HLT), and (iv) bilateral lobar transplantation from living related donors. Although recipient history of previous talc pleurodesis still gives many transplant centers pause, a history of other chest surgeries is not a contraindication to lung transplantation (13,14).

Historically, SLT used to be the most applied technique, but lately, more centers are adopting BLT as the transplant procedure of choice. The airway anastomosis is performed by telescoping the airways into each other at the mainstem bronchus. The pulmonary venous anastomosis is performed at the level of the donor atrial cuff, and the pulmonary artery anastomosis is performed at the main pulmonary artery branch. The advantages of SLT include a shorter waiting time for the recipient, technical ease, and the fact that lungs from one donor can be potentially used for two recipients. With the exception of suppurative lung diseases, SLT has been applied to all lung diseases (15–17). COPD is the most common indication for lung transplantation in the United States, with most receiving SLT (10,18,19). Most patients with alpha-1 antitrypsin deficiency have recently been receiving BLT (10).

The only absolute indication for BLT is suppurative lung disease such as cystic fibrosis (CF). BLT accounted for about 60% of the lung transplant operations in the United States in the last 1 to 2 years. There is currently debate about whether BLT should be the preferred procedure for all end-stage lung diseases, as BLT has marginal but significant survival advantage after 5 years and because BLT recipients have more lung reserve to buffer complications. Most patients with pulmonary artery hypertension (PAH) receive BLT. This is because PAH patients who have undergone SLT encounter severe hypoxemia with airway injury to the allograft (pneumonia or rejection) due to the resultant severe ventilation/perfusion mismatch (19,20). Recently, there has been a trend to performing more BLT for patients with IPF, especially in the presence of pulmonary vascular disease (10). Most patients with COPD continue to receive SLT at this time.

The only absolute indications for HLT are: pulmonary hypertension with surgically irreparable congenital heart disease (i.e., tetralogy of Fallot, large ventricular septal defect); pulmonary hypertension associated with significant left ventricular systolic dysfunction; or severe end-stage lung disease associated with significant coronary artery disease. In HLT, the airway anastomosis is typically performed at the distal tracheal level. The vascular anastomoses are performed at the right atrium and aorta. Patients with Eisenmenger syndrome secondary to patent ductus arteriosus or atrial septal defect usually undergo BLT with concurrent repair of the congenital heart disease. Right ventricular dysfunction, *per se*, is not an indication for heart–lung transplantation since the recovery of right ventricular function—and the associated tricuspid valve regurgitation—is generally rapid and complete after the restoration of normal pulmonary artery pressures after transplantation (Fig. 92.4) (21–23).

Living related bilateral lobar transplantation is an evolving technique; about 130 transplantations have been performed in the United States since 1991. This technique is generally reserved for patients who meet all the criteria for lung

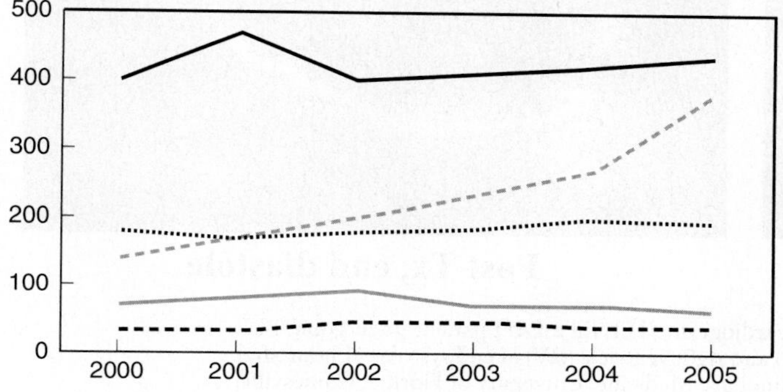

FIGURE 92.3. Indication for lung transplantation in the United States. (Adapted from OPTN data, 2006: http://www.OPTN.org. Accessed September 19, 2007.)

TABLE 92.3

TRANSPLANT EVALUATION TESTING

1. Detailed history and physical exam
2. Chest radiograph, electrocardiogram
3. Computed tomography (CT) scan of chest
4. Pulmonary function tests, arterial blood gas
5. Differential ventilation/perfusion scan
6. Two-dimensional echocardiography
7. Coronary angiography (age older than 45 years or younger than 45 in presence of risk factors)
8. Right heart catheterization (in all candidates)
9. Abdominal ultrasound
10. Bone density (if indicated)
11. Bronchoscopy (rarely indicated)
12. Sputum culture (in patients with suppurative lung disease)
13. Labs: viral serologies (human immunodeficiency virus [HIV], hepatitis B and C, cytomegalovirus [CMV], herpes simplex virus [HSV], Epstein-Barr virus [EBV]), ABO blood typing, human leucocyte antigen [HLA] typing, reactive antibodies panel, complete blood count, liver and chemistry batteries
14. Consults
    a. Physical therapy
       Six-minute walk test
       Musculoskeletal strength assessment
       Rest and exercise oxygen requirements
    b. Social work
    c. Psychology
    d. Nutritional services (when indicated)
    e. Anesthesiology
    f. Transplant thoracic surgeon
    g. Transplant pulmonologist

TABLE 92.4

GENERAL GUIDELINES FOR SELECTION OF RECIPIENTS

INDICATIONS
End-stage lung disease with average life expectancy <2 years
Failed medical and surgical therapy
Severe functional limitation, but ambulatory
Upper age limit has recently been liberalized to include ≤ 69 years

ABSOLUTE CONTRAINDICATIONS
Significant extrapulmonary end organ damage
Acute critical illness
History of cancer in the last 5 years
Active psychosis or history of noncompliance with therapy
Cigarette smoking in the last 6 months
History of substance abuse with risk factors for recidivism
Nonambulatory, with poor rehabilitation potential
Inadequate social support
Systemically active collagen vascular diseases
Extrapulmonary infections (human immunodeficiency virus [HIV], hepatitis B, C active infections)

RELATIVE CONTRAINDICATIONS
Mechanical ventilation
Extensive pleural adhesions from previous surgical procedures (especially talc)
Airway colonization with bacteria panresistant to all antibacterials
Body mass index >30

transplantation but have a minimal chance of surviving the waiting time on the lung transplant waiting list. Most of the recipients have been patients with CF, although a few patients with fibrotic lung diseases or pulmonary hypertension have been transplanted (24). Donors are typically family members who undergo full evaluation for thoracotomy. Because this procedure presents risks to two healthy donors, appropriate recipient and donor selection and timing of transplantation are critical to minimize the morbidity to the donor and maximize the chance of a successful outcome in the recipient. The surgical technique involves explantation of both of the recipient's

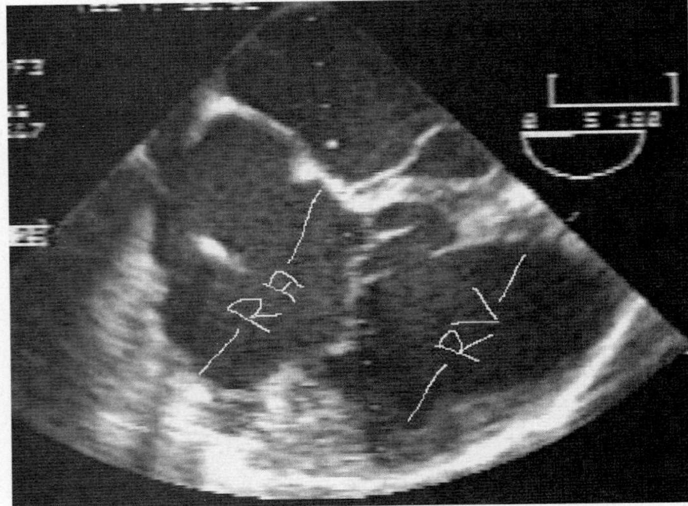

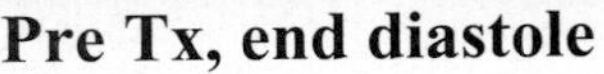

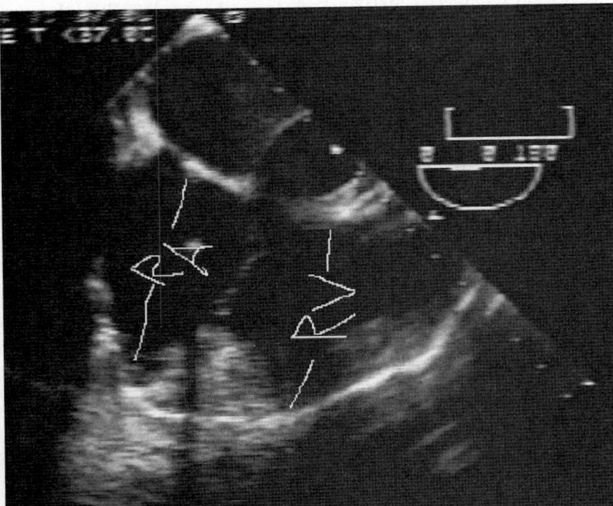

Post Tx, end diastole

FIGURE 92.4. Intraoperative transesophageal echocardiogram (TEE) in a PAH patient undergoing BLT. Note the reduction of the size of the right atrium (RA) and right ventricle (RV) at end systole $\sim$1 hour after reperfusion of the lungs. (Courtesy of Division of Pulmonary Medicine, University of Florida, Gainesville, FL.)

TABLE 92.5

COMMONLY USED IMMUNOSUPPRESSIVE MEDICATIONS

Drug	Dosing and adjustments	Side effects	Drug interactions
Cyclosporine and tacrolimus	Every 12 h	Commonly occur with both: nephrotoxicity, hypertension, neurotoxicity (tremors, headaches, rarely seizures), hyperkalemia, hyperlipidemia, hypomagnesemia Occur only with tacrolimus: myalgias, hyperglycemia Occur only with CyA: hemolytic-uremic syndrome, hirsutism, gingival hyperplasia	Blood levels are increased with all macrolide antibiotics (except azithromycin), azole antifungals, calcium channel blockers (except nifedipine). Blood levels are decreased by anticonvulsants and rifampin.
Sirolimus	Every 24 h	Cytopenias, hyperlipidemia (mainly hypertriglyceridemia)	Same drug interactions as tacrolimus and cyclosporine: Blood levels are increased with all macrolide antibiotics (except azithromycin), azole antifungals (voriconazole contraindicated with sirolimus), calcium channel blockers (except nifedipine). Blood levels are decreased by anticonvulsants and rifampin.
Azathioprine	Every 24 h Decrease dosage in the event of renal or hepatic insufficiency.	Cytopenias, hepatotoxicity, pancreatitis, nausea	Increased bone marrow suppression with allopurinol, ganciclovir, and antithymocyte globulin (ATG).
Mycophenolate mofetil	Every 12 h Decrease dosage in the event of renal or hepatic insufficiency.	Abdominal cramps, diarrhea, vomiting, cytopenias	No significant interactions.
Prednisone	0.3–0.5 mg/kg/d in the first 3 mo, then tapered afterwards.	Hypertension, hyperglycemia, weight gain, myopathy, osteoporosis, cataracts, mood swings, hyperlipidemia	No significant interactions.

lungs, lobectomy—usually lower lobe—from two donors, and implantation of one donor lobe in each thoracic cavity of the recipient. Even though the risk for chronic rejection appears to be lower compared to the cadaveric lung transplantation, the long-term (3–5 years) outcomes of the two techniques are equivalent (25).

Immunosuppression

Immunosuppression initiated intraoperatively is termed *induction immunosuppression* and is continued for the rest of the recipient's life as a maintenance immunosuppressive regimen. An intravenous bolus of 500 to 1,000 mg of methylprednisolone is used for intraoperative induction. Some centers add antilymphocyte antibodies (Thymoglobulin or OKT3) to the induction therapy during the first 72 hours. Cyclosporine A (CyA), or alternatively tacrolimus (Tac), and azathioprine (AZA, 2 mg/kg per day) are also started intraoperatively or in the first 24 hours. Recently, more centers are using interleukin-2 receptor antagonists (basiliximab, daclizumab) as part of the routine induction therapy.

The classic triple maintenance immunosuppressive regimen consists of CyA or Tac, AZA, and prednisone. The steroid dose is rapidly reduced to a maintenance prednisone dose of 0.3 to 0.5 mg/kg per day by the third or fifth day after transplantation, and then patients are gradually weaned over the next 6 to 12 months to about 0.15 to 0.2 mg/kg per day. The CyA dose is adjusted to maintain therapeutic trough serum levels of 250 to 300 ng/mL; the Tac dose is adjusted to maintain trough serum levels of 8 to 12 ng/mL; whereas the AZA dose is adjusted to maintain white blood cell count >3,500 cells/microL. Table 92.5 details the numerous side effects, interactions, and dosing of the immunosuppressive medications.

OUTCOMES FOLLOWING LUNG TRANSPLANTATION

Survival

The median survival after lung transplantation is approximately 5 years. The 1-, 3-, 5-, and 10-year actuarial survivals after lung transplantation are 78%, 61%, 49%, and 25%, respectively (Fig. 92.5). The survival at some transplant centers is higher than the national average, likely because survival is significantly correlated with a center's experience (Fig. 92.6). However, these survival rates lag considerably behind those

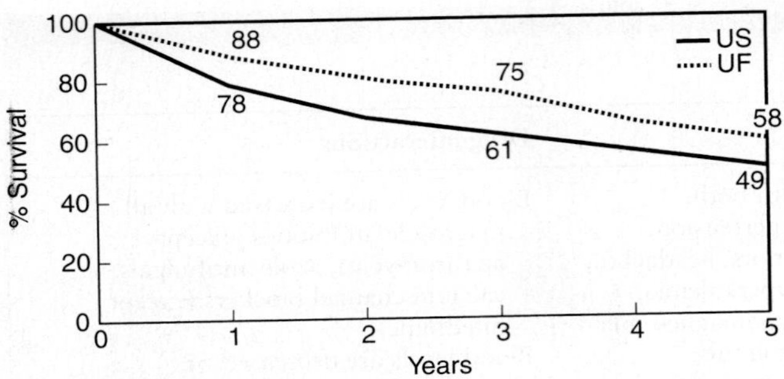

FIGURE 92.5. Five-year actuarial survival after lung transplantation. (From Taylor DO, Edwards LB, Boucek MM, et al. Registry of the International Society for Heart and Lung Transplantation: twenty-third official adult heart transplantation report—2006. *J Heart Lung Transplant*. 2006;25(8):869–879.)

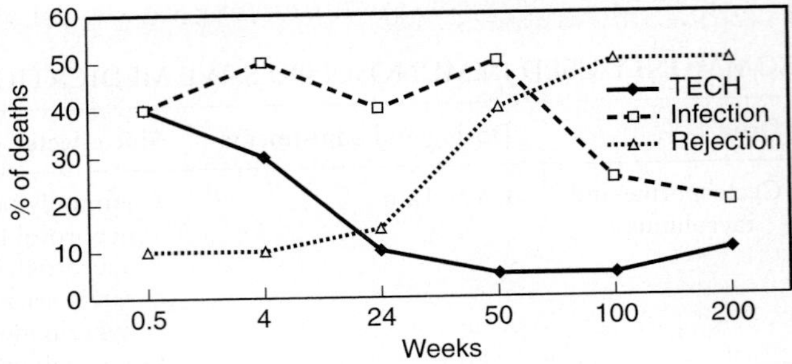

FIGURE 92.7. Causes of death after lung transplantation. (Courtesy of Division of Pulmonary Medicine, University of Florida, Gainesville, FL.)

of liver or kidney transplant recipients, for whom the 5-year actuarial survival approximates 70% to 80%.

In the absence of prospective randomized trials, it is difficult to ascertain whether lung transplantation truly increases survival over the natural history of the lung disease. Hosenpud et al. (26) made a disease-specific comparison of survival after transplantation and found that patients with CF and IPF have higher survival rates. No such advantage has yet been demonstrated for patients with COPD, a disease that typically follows a protracted course with a 5-year survival of 40% to 50% for patients with forced expiratory volume in 1 second (FEV_1) <20% of predicted (27). Thus, the main indication for lung transplantation in patients with COPD is to improve quality of life in patients with FEV_1 in the 15% to 25% range, rather than prolonging survival. Recently, a BODE index (body-mass index [B], airflow obstruction [O], dyspnea [D], and exercise capacity [E]) has been identified that may yet prove to be a predictor of improved survival when transplantation is applied to COPD patients with a high index (28).

The leading causes of death in the first 30 days after transplantation are primary allograft failure and pneumonia (Fig. 92.7) (29). Primary allograft failure manifests in the first 24 hours with severe hypoxemia, a pulmonary edema pattern on chest radiograph, and, often, hypotension. In the first 24 hours, medical management is geared toward establishing adequate systemic perfusion pressure with judicious amount

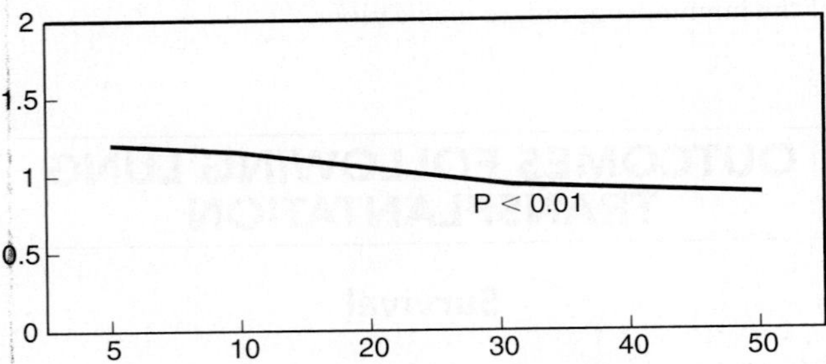

FIGURE 92.6. Impact of center volume on the relative risk (RR) of death within 1 year after lung transplantation. (From Taylor DO, Edwards LB, Boucek MM, et al. Registry of the International Society for Heart and Lung Transplantation: twenty-third official adult heart transplantation report—2006. *J Heart Lung Transplant.* 2006;25(8):869–879.)

of fluids and intravenous pressor support. This approach tends to preserve the kidneys from significant injury, which will later allow the institution of diuresis and extubation. At Shands Hospital at the University of Florida (SUF), our discharge rate post–lung transplantation approximates 95%, with pneumonia being the most common cause of death. Approximately 50% of the patients are liberated from mechanical ventilation within the first 24 hours, and 75% by 48 hours after transplantation.

Pneumonia in the immediate postoperative period is almost always associated with bacterial organisms acquired with the donor lung. Donors are usually on mechanical ventilation for a few days prior to procurement, and they are often colonized with bacteria. Alternatively, the donor aspirates from vomiting at the time of death or during intubation, resulting in pneumonia. These pneumonias can be very subtle, escaping detection at the time of procurement, only to manifest fully 24 hours after implantation. Low found that when donors did not routinely receive antibacterial therapy, 97% of their bronchial washings have potentially pathogenic microbes, with *Staphylococcus* and *Enterobacter* being most common (30). A review of bronchial swab cultures obtained intraoperatively from 50 consecutive non-CF recipients cared for at SUF showed that 32/50 patients had 45 potential bacterial pathogens, with some showing more than one potential pathogen, and 18/50 had "normal oral flora." Twenty-four of the 45 bacterial species were Gram-positive cocci, and 21/45 were Gram-negative rods. Methicillin-sensitive *Staphylococcus aureus* was the most common Gram-positive organism, while *Enterobacter* was the most common Gram-negative organism. The incidence of donor-associated bacterial pneumonia approximated 15% at SUF over the last 18 months. The lower incidence of detecting pathogenic bacteria at our center may result from the routine use of antibacterial therapy 24 to 48 hours prior to organ procurement, or due to the method of collection of the culture specimen as compared to the technique in the study of Low et al. (30)

There have been a few risk factors identified by multivariate analysis that are associated with risk of death 1 year after transplantation: diagnosis of portopulmonary hypertension (PPH) or IPF, ventilator dependence prior to transplantation, and retransplantation (10). However, it is important to remember that those statistics are obtained from multiple centers and reported to the International Society of Heart and Lung Transplantation (ISHLT). Since different centers have different expertise and experience, those risk factors may not be uniform among centers. For example, in carefully selected ventilator-dependent patients who are not critically ill, mechanical ventilation did not influence the 1-year outcome after transplantation at two centers (31,32).

There is a marginal (approximately 8 months) but significant survival advantage of BLT recipients compared to SLT recipients after analysis of survival data in about 6,000 recipients (10). In both groups, the long-term survival is limited by obliterative bronchiolitis (OB). OB, the most common cause of death in patients surviving past the first year after transplantation, is responsible for progressive decline in lung function and, ultimately, respiratory failure. The median survival after the diagnosis of OB is approximately 2 years. This higher survival has caused more and more centers to consider BLT as the procedure of choice, with approximately 60% of lung transplantations being BLT in the United States.

Pulmonary Function and Gas Exchange

Both SLT and BLT patients have significant improvement in pulmonary function tests (PFTs) and in gas exchange post transplantation. The peak improvement in PFTs is achieved at 1 to 3 months after SLT, but after BLT, improvement may not be achieved until 4 to 6 months post transplant. The factors associated with the delay in achieving peak values are reperfusion injury, postoperative pain, altered chest wall mechanics, and respiratory muscle dysfunction after transplant surgery.

After SLT in patients with COPD, the FEV_1 significantly improves to about 45% to 60% of the predicted value and lung volumes approach the normal predicted values (Fig. 92.8) (33). The chest radiograph in COPD recipients of SLT shows hyperinflated native lung with a flat diaphragm and mild herniation across the midline. The transplanted allograft is a normal-sized lung—although it appears small compared to the native lung—with a physiologically domed diaphragm (Fig. 92.9).

After SLT in patients with IPF, the vital capacity improves to about 70% to 80% of the predicted value (Fig. 92.10) (33). Compared to a fibrotic native lung on the contralateral side, the chest radiograph shows a normal-sized lung allograft (Fig. 92.11). After BLT, the chest radiograph and spirometry values approximate predicted values for the recipient size (Figs. 92.12 and 92.13). After lung transplantation, arterial oxygenation rapidly returns to normal, but hypercapnia may take a few days before returning to normal. Supplemental oxygen is unnecessary for most patients at the time of hospital discharge.

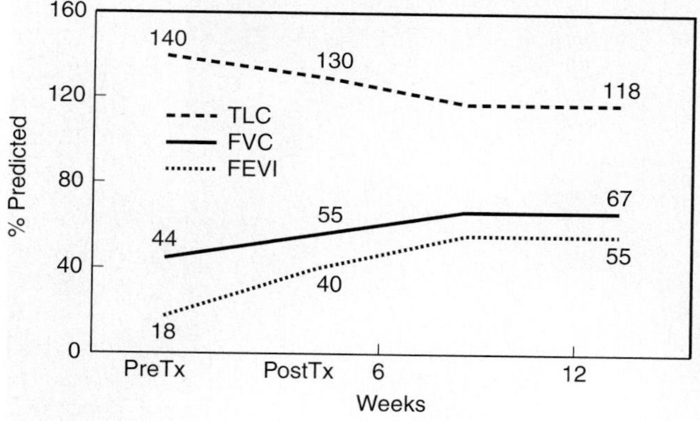

FIGURE 92.8. Lung function in chronic obstructive pulmonary disease (COPD) patients after single lung transplant (SLT) (n = 6). (Courtesy of Division of Pulmonary Medicine, University of Florida, Gainesville, FL.)

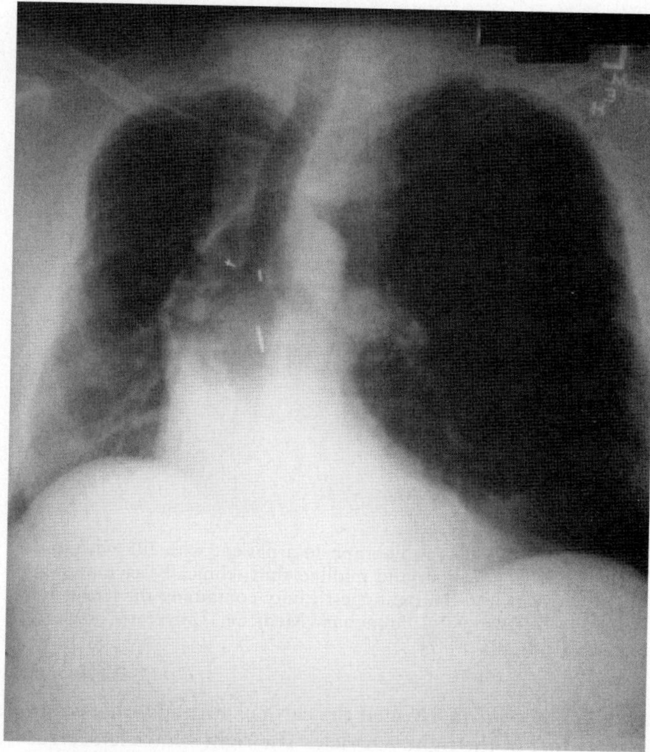

FIGURE 92.9. Chest radiograph after right SLT in a patient with COPD. Note the hyperinflated native lung with (clinically asymptomatic) shift across the midline. (Courtesy of Division of Pulmonary Medicine, University of Florida, Gainesville, FL.)

Hemodynamics

Both SLT and BLT result in immediate and sustained normalization—or near normal in SLT—of pulmonary artery pressures in PPH recipients, barring significant reperfusion injury. This is associated with near total or total resolution of the associated tricuspid valve insufficiency and is accompanied

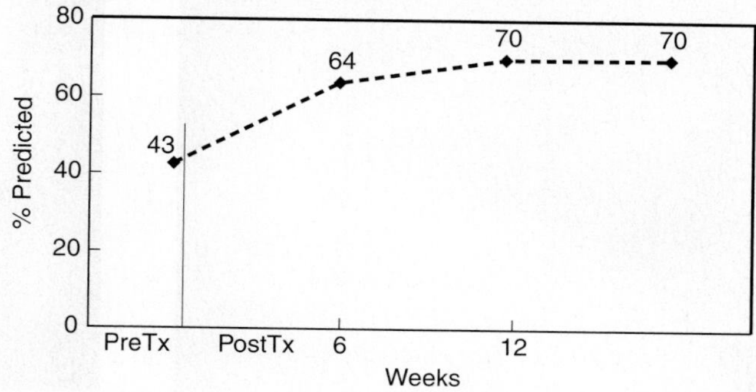

FIGURE 92.10. Vital capacity in idiopathic pulmonary fibrosis (IPF) patients after single lung transplant (SLT) (n = 7). (Courtesy of Division of Pulmonary Medicine, University of Florida, Gainesville, FL.)

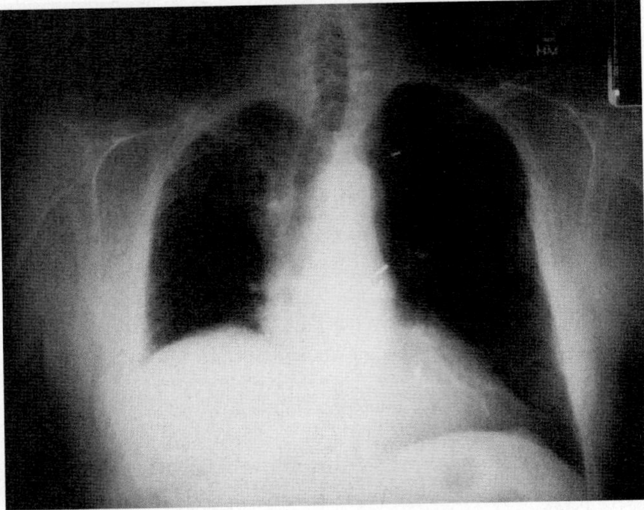

FIGURE 92.11. Chest radiograph in a patient with IPF who underwent left SLT. Note the mild midline shift (clinically asymptomatic) of the allograft into the right chest cavity containing the native lung. (Courtesy of Division of Pulmonary Medicine, University of Florida, Gainesville, FL.)

by an immediate increase of the cardiac output with a gradual remodeling of the right ventricle. The right ventricle decreases in size and regains normal function over the next few days to weeks. This hemodynamic improvement is sustained after successful transplantation. The advantage of BLT over SLT for patients with pulmonary vascular disease is that airway injury is better tolerated in BLT. Due to the resultant severe ventilation/perfusion mismatch, airway injury (caused by pneumonia, or acute or chronic rejection) results in profound hypoxemia in patients with severe pulmonary hypertension who undergo SLT (20).

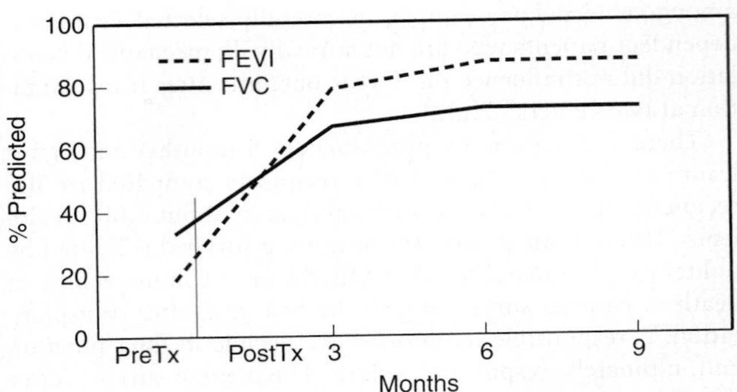

FIGURE 92.12. Spirometry values in cystic fibrosis (CF) patients undergoing bilateral lung transplantation (BLT) ($n = 5$). (Courtesy of Division of Pulmonary Medicine, University of Florida, Gainesville, FL.)

Quality of Life

Several studies show a dramatic, global improvement in all measures of quality of life (physical, social, and psychological) in most recipients as early as 3 months after transplantation. These improvements are maintained for the next 12 to 24 months (34–36). However, because OB causes progressive deterioration of lung function, any newly acquired improvement in the quality of life deteriorates if OB occurs after transplantation (37). Only approximately one third of recipients return to work after transplantation. Factors that may contribute to this relatively low re-employment rate include potential reluctance to hire employees with complex medical conditions, potential loss of income or medical benefits as a result of returning to work, and the change of priorities and goals of recipients after recovering from their previous incapacitating condition (38).

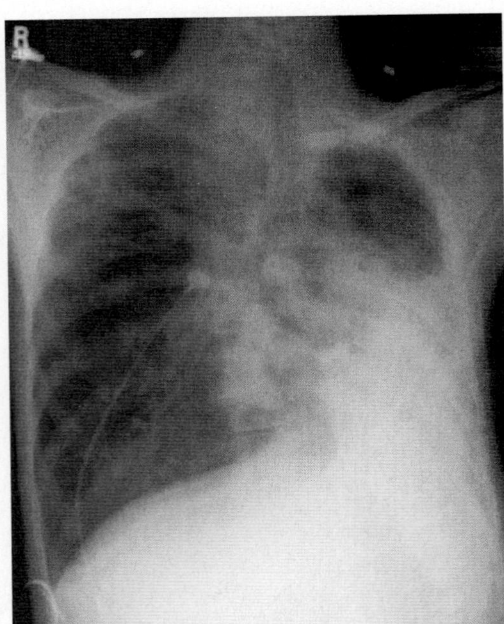

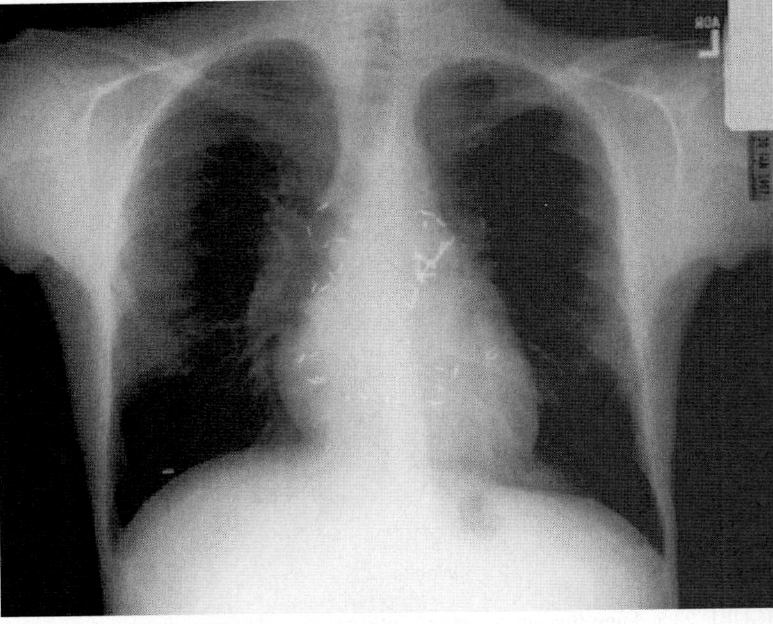

FIGURE 92.13. Pretransplant chest radiograph in a patient with CF showing bilateral bronchiectasis, severe left lower lobe necrosis and volume loss with shift of the heart into the left hemithorax; and 3 month post BLT. (Courtesy of Division of Pulmonary Medicine, University of Florida, Gainesville, FL.)

Exercise Capacity

Peak exercise performance, as measured by cycle ergometry, is characteristically reduced in both SLT and BLT recipients as late as 1 or 2 years after the surgery. These patients have subnormal peak work rate, peak oxygen consumption, and early lactate threshold on incremental exercise testing. Maximal oxygen consumption is significantly increased after lung transplantation, but it typically is 40% to 60% of the maximal predicted value. Interestingly, the limitation to exercise is not cardiac or ventilatory in nature, and, surprisingly, the maximal oxygen consumption attained during exercise testing is similar whether the recipients are of SLT or BLT (39). Reduced mitochondrial oxidative capacity and peripheral oxygen use in the skeletal muscles of lung transplant recipients (40–42) may be secondary to the deconditioning associated with chronic lung diseases or cyclosporine-associated impairment in skeletal muscle mitochondrial respiration (43,44).

COMMON COMPLICATIONS AFTER LUNG TRANSPLANTATION

Primary Graft Dysfunction/Failure

Most allografts have reperfusion lung injury manifesting as pulmonary edema within the first 24 hours after transplantation. The injury is mild to moderate, and the edema is transient in most cases. However, in 5% to 10% of cases, the lung injury is severe enough to cause acute respiratory distress syndrome or severe primary graft failure. Primary graft failure manifests as severe pulmonary edema, severe hypoxemia, high pulmonary artery pressures, high airway pressures, fever, and hypotension. It is presumed to reflect ischemia–reperfusion injury, but hyperacute rejection (caused by preformed antibodies in the recipient) is the cause for the severe injury in a small subset of patients with this complication (45). The chest radiograph and clinical scenario are almost identical in all these etiologic factors, i.e., all have widespread interstitial and alveolar infiltrates in the allograft(s) and severe hypoxemia. The diagnosis of reperfusion injury is established by excluding other causes of graft dysfunction: hyperacute or acute rejection, pneumonia, volume overload, and thrombosis of the pulmonary venous anastomosis. An algorithm for the workup of reperfusion injury is summarized in the article by Zander et al. (29). Inhaled nitric oxide, independent lung ventilation, and extracorporeal membrane oxygenation have been attempted with variable success. The mortality rate reportedly ranges between 40% and 60% in cases of severe hypoxemia. The clinical course in survivors is protracted, but some of the survivors are able to ultimately attain normal allograft function. Variables associated with increased mortality in patients with reperfusion lung injury are age, severity of gas exchange impairment, and severity of hemodynamic failure (46).

Airway Complications

Airway complications requiring intervention occur in 7% to 15% of bronchial anastomosis (47). This reflects both improved surgical techniques that occurred with the advent of bronchial telescoping and relatively lower steroid doses compared to those used with transplantation in the 1970s and early 1980s. Complete dehiscence of the bronchial anastomosis, very rare in the present time, is an emergency situation that requires immediate surgical intervention. Anastomotic stenosis is the most common airway complication, followed by bronchomalacia.

Most airway complications manifest in the first 100 days after transplantation. They may present as wheezing, exertional dyspnea, or decline in FEV_1. As the bronchial arteries are not reconnected at the time of transplantation, the bronchial mucosa distal to the anastomosis could be affected by bronchial artery reperfusion injury. This manifests as bronchial mucosal injury with ischemic mucosal surface. The mucosal injury may heal with minimal sequelae, thereby resulting in airway stricture, or, if the bronchial artery ischemia injures the underlying cartilaginous support of the bronchus, it may cause bronchomalacia. Alternatively, bronchial stenosis may be caused by overgrowth of the scar tissue at the site of the bronchial anastomosis. Thus, airway complications may be at the anastomotic site or a few centimeters distally.

Bronchial mucosal injury has the bronchoscopic appearance of a pseudomembrane, which is sometimes superinfected with fungal organisms (Fig. 92.14). Most airway complications are amenable to correction with stent placement, balloon dilation, or cautery (Fig. 92.15) (47–49).

Infections

The rate of infection among lung transplant recipients is two to three times higher than that for recipients of other solid organs (50). This is most likely related to the exposure of the allograft to the external environment, impaired mucociliary clearance after transplantation, and the denervation of the allograft, which can cause poor cough reflex. Ciliary motility, airway sensation, and lymphatic drainage remain abnormal years after lung transplantation due to bronchial mucosal injury, denervation, and lymphatic resection, respectively. Infection, the most common cause of death in the first 12 months after lung transplantation, is also a common cause of death in patients afflicted with OB (51).

Most recipients will have at least one infection requiring therapy with an antimicrobial agent during the first 12 months after transplantation. At SUF, the rate of freedom from at least one episode of infection is 32% in patients surviving 12 months (Fig. 92.16). Respiratory tract pathogens are the most common source of bacterial infections after transplantation. Microbes from donor lungs cause a significant number of early episodes of bacterial pneumonia, but the incidence has decreased because antibacterial prophylaxis is used at the time of transplantation. *Pseudomonas* and the Enterobacteriaceae cause most bacterial infections after discharge from the transplant hospitalization; infections caused by *Staphylococcus* and *Haemophilus* are also common (52,53). At SUF, the incidence of bacterial pneumonias after lung transplantation in CF patients who are colonized with *Pseudomonas,* sensitive to at least one antibacterial agent prior to transplantation, is comparable to that of non-CF patients. In a single-center study, panresistant *Pseudomonas* was not associated with increased mortality or increased risk of pneumonia after lung transplantation; some

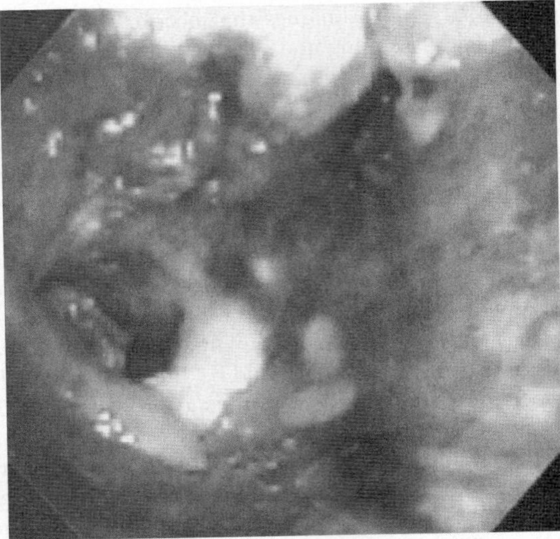

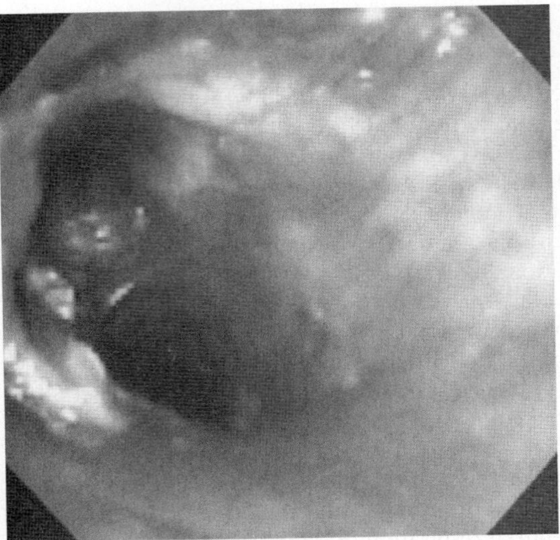

FIGURE 92.14. Bronchial mucosal reperfusion injury and *Aspergillus* superinfection of right upper lobe (RUL) orifice and bronchus intermedius before (**left photo**) and after debridement and suctioning (**right photo**). (Courtesy of Division of Pulmonary Medicine, University of Florida, Gainesville, FL.)

centers, however, continue to consider it as a contraindication to lung transplantation (54). Colonization with *Burkholderia cepacia* is associated with a significantly high incidence of infection and mortality (55).

Viral infections are the second most common cause of infections; cytomegalovirus (CMV) infection is the most common among the viral causes (56). The incidence of CMV infection or reactivation has been reported to be 40% to 75%, which is much higher than for other solid organs. The patients at highest risk of infection and morbidity are CMV-seronegative recipients from a seropositive lung donor. The case fatality rate of CMV infection is reported to be about 5%. Herpes simplex (HSV) and varicella-zoster (VZ) infections are also quite common. HSV and VZ are mostly caused by reactivation of a latent viral infection. Acquired respiratory viral infections are mostly secondary to respiratory syncytial virus (RSV), influenza, and parainfluenza viruses. These viral infections may cause cough, wheezing, or, in extreme cases, acute respiratory distress syndrome. Parvovirus has been reported to cause refractory anemia in recipients of solid organ transplants.

The most common cause of fungal infection is *Candida albicans*, with *Aspergillus* a close second. The lung allograft is a common site of infection; the spectrum of disease ranges from necrotic bronchitis (Fig. 92.10) to invasive fungal pneumonia (57–59). The incidence of *Pneumocystis carinii* pneumonia (PCP), approximately 80% prior to prophylaxis (60), has decreased to between 5% and 10% since the institution of long-term prophylaxis.

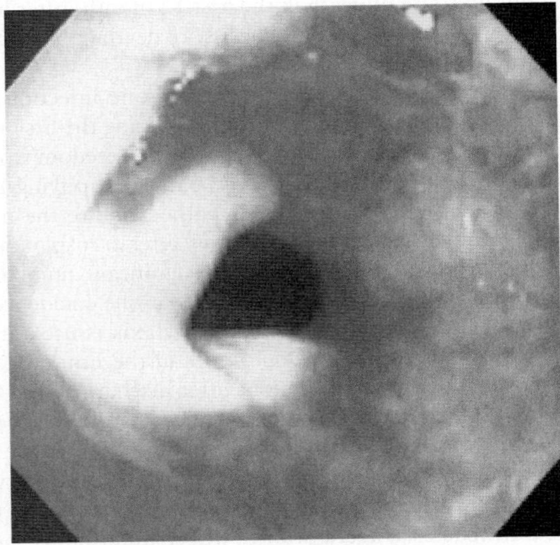

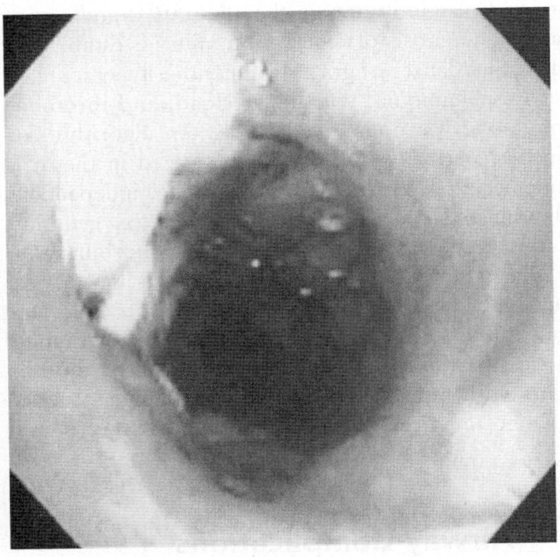

FIGURE 92.15. Bronchus intermedius showing pseudomembrane formation and severe bronchostenosis (**left photo**) prior to stent placement and after 10 mm × 20 mm Ultraflex stent placement (**right photo**). (Courtesy of Division of Pulmonary Medicine, University of Florida, Gainesville, FL.)

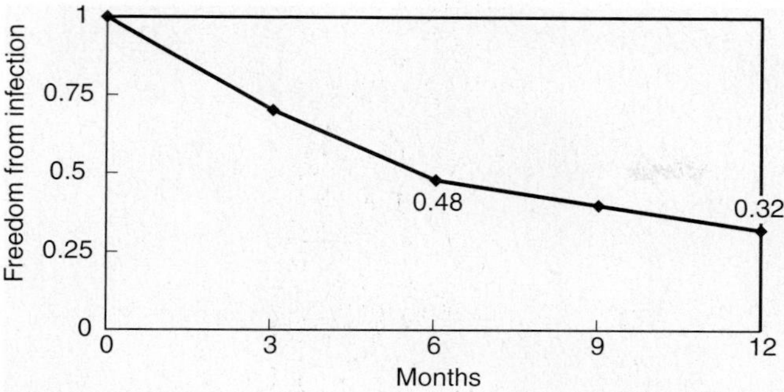

FIGURE 92.16. One-year freedom from any infection at the University of Florida (n = 110). (Courtesy of Division of Pulmonary Medicine, University of Florida, Gainesville, FL.)

Acute Rejection

Acute rejection denotes the infiltration of the allograft by lymphocytes (Fig. 92.17); severity of the rejection is classified by pathologic criteria (61). In a study published in 1996, the incidence of acute lung rejection was highest in the first 30 days after transplantation and plateaued about 3 months after transplantation. A surveillance bronchoscopy program indicated that only 25% of recipients were free from acute rejection at 3 months (Fig. 92.18) (62). In that study, the recipients had induction steroid therapy and subsequent triple maintenance immunosuppression consisting of CyA, prednisone, and AZA. Antilymphocyte therapy and interleukin-2 (IL-2) receptor antagonists were not part of the induction immunosuppression. IL-2 receptor antagonists have recently been shown to decrease the 3-month risk of acute rejection without increasing the risk for infection, but the incidence of acute rejection approached the control arm rate—50% to 70%—by 6 months (63). In a recently completed prospective multicenter, open label randomized study comparing azathioprine (AZA) to mycophenolate mofetil (MMF) with CyA and prednisone, there was no difference in the freedom from acute lung rejection or in the number

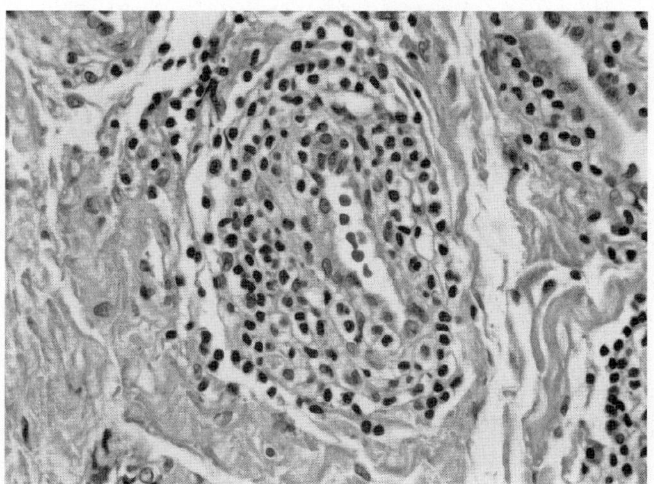

FIGURE 92.17. Perivascular cuffing of a blood vessel (detected by transbronchial biopsy) is diagnostic of acute rejection. (Courtesy of Division of Pulmonary Medicine, University of Florida, Gainesville, FL.)

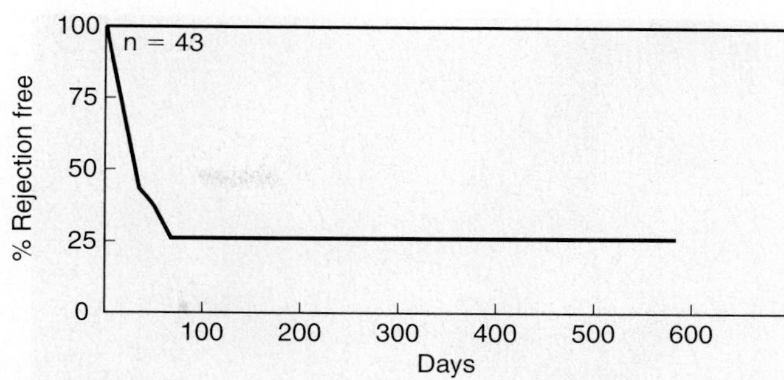

FIGURE 92.18. One-year freedom from acute lung rejection. (From Baz MA, Layish DT, Govert JA, et al. Diagnostic yield of bronchoscopies after isolated lung transplantation. *Chest*. 1996;110(1):84–88.)

of episodes of acute rejection per 100 patient days at 6 months (64).

There have been no large prospective randomized studies showing that tacrolimus is associated with higher freedom from acute rejection when compared to CyA. A prospective study compared a triple immunosuppression maintenance therapy containing CyA to tacrolimus and found that the number of episodes of acute rejection per 100 patient days was lower in the tacrolimus group (65). There have also been uncontrolled studies showing that tacrolimus is as effective as rescue therapy for patients with recurrent acute lung rejection who have switched from CyA to tacrolimus (66).

Acute rejection may present as decline in airflows, cough, oxygen desaturation with exercise, or, rarely, as low-grade temperature elevation. The chest radiograph may be clear and unchanged or may represent a pulmonary edema pattern (Fig. 92.19). While the classic triple maintenance immunosuppressive regimen remains CyA, prednisone, and AZA, acute rejection episodes are treated with a course of pulse steroids consisting of three daily doses of methylprednisolone, dosed at 15 mg/kg per day, followed by oral prednisone taper and optimization of the CyA and AZA doses. Patients resistant to pulse steroid therapy are treated with antilymphocyte antibodies—polyclonal antithymocyte globulin or monoclonal OKT3—and are often switched from CyA to tacrolimus.

Chronic Rejection (Bronchiolitis Obliterans)

Chronic lung rejection is used synonymously with *bronchiolitis obliterans syndrome* (BOS). BOS is a progressive and irreversible decline in airflow, ultimately resulting in respiratory failure. The disease has a variable course: some patients experience a rapid decline in airflow, whereas others experience either slow progressive decline or intermittent decline in airflow punctuated by long periods of stable lung function. BOS is staged by the magnitude of the loss of lung function (Table 92.6). BO is the histologic equivalent of chronic lung rejection, and the histologic diagnosis is difficult because transbronchial biopsy specimens are not sufficiently sensitive for diagnosis.

BO is characterized by initial lymphocytic-mediated cytotoxicity directed at the epithelial cells lining the respiratory bronchioles. The lymphocytes initially infiltrate the submucosa of the airways and migrate through the basement membrane into the epithelial layer. At this site, epithelial cell necrosis occurs, resulting in a secondary cascade of inflammatory

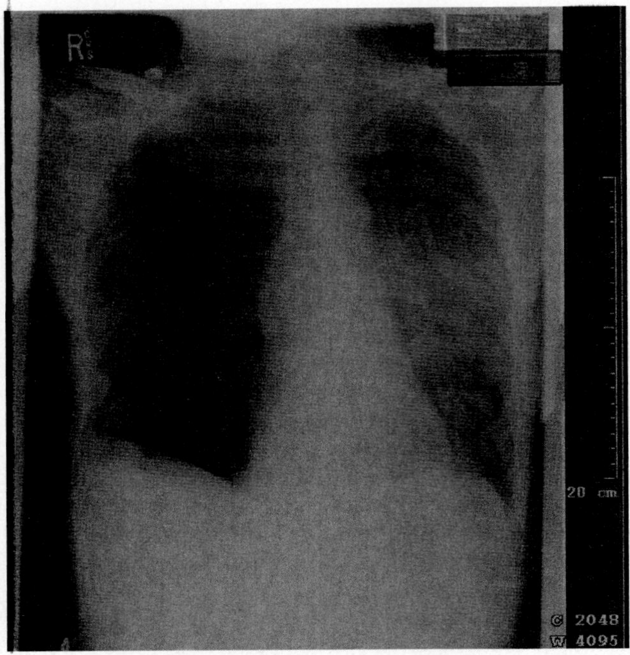

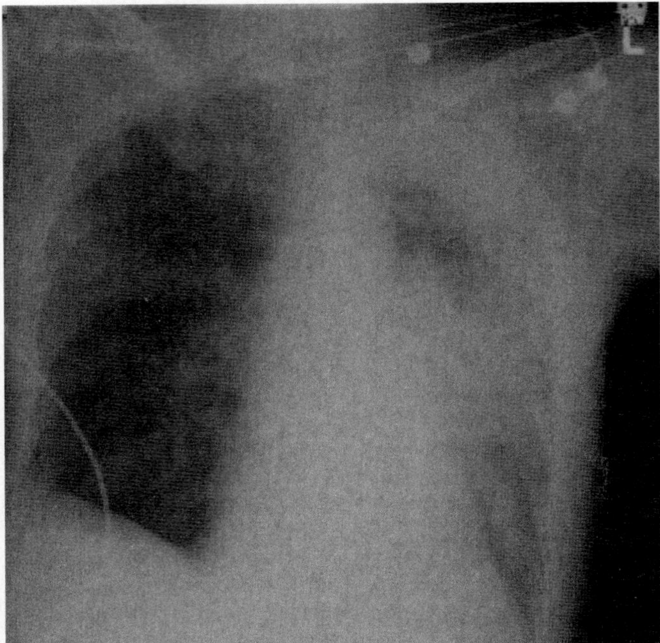

FIGURE 92.19. Steroid-resistant acute rejection. Note the increased perihilar infiltrate 4 weeks post left lung transplantation. The chest Xray and hypoxemia continued to worsen a few days after therapy with pulse steroids. Complete reversal was achieved within a few days after initiation of therapy with anti-lymphocyte antibodies. (Courtesy of Division of Pulmonary Medicine, University of Florida, Gainesville, FL.)

mediators and cytokines attracting neutrophils, fibroblasts, and myofibroblasts. This results in formation of granulation tissue obliterating the bronchiolar lumen, airway obstruction, and proximal bronchiectasis (Fig. 92.20).

After the exclusion of other factors confounding bronchoscopy and transbronchial biopsy, the diagnosis is made by pulmonary function tests. Bronchoscopy is performed to exclude anastomotic complications, infections, acute rejection, or disease recurrence in the allograft. If the decline in FEV_1 is >20% compared to the peak FEV_1 attained after transplantation, and the bronchoscopy—with transbronchial biopsy—excludes confounding factors, the clinical scenario is then diagnostic of BOS (67). Moreover, if the decline in FEV_1 is associated with acute rejection on transbronchial biopsy but does not reverse with augmentation of immunosuppression, it is also consistent with BOS.

BOS occurs in approximately 50% of recipients 5 years after transplantation (Fig. 92.21) (68). It is the most common cause of death in patients surviving >1 year. The median survival after the diagnosis of BOS approximates 2 years. In most patients, BOS is characterized by a relentless decline in airflows, albeit at variable rates in different patients, and ultimately results in respiratory failure. In SLT recipients, BOS is associated with a significantly lower survival when it occurs in IPF patients rather than COPD patients (69). Recurrent episodes of acute lung rejection are a definite risk factor for BOS; CMV pneumonitis is a probable risk factor (70,71). In a retrospective study, mismatching at the HLA-A locus was found to be a risk factor for BOS (72).

TABLE 92.6

STAGING OF BRONCHIOLITIS OBLITERANS SYNDROME (BOS)

BOS-p (potential BOS): 10%–19% decline in forced expiratory volume in 1 s (FEV_1) compared with the peak FEV_1
Stage 1: 20%–33% decline in FEV_1 compared with the peak FEV_1
Stage 2: 33%–50% decline in FEV_1 compared with the peak FEV_1
Stage 3: >50% decline in FEV_1 compared with the peak FEV_1

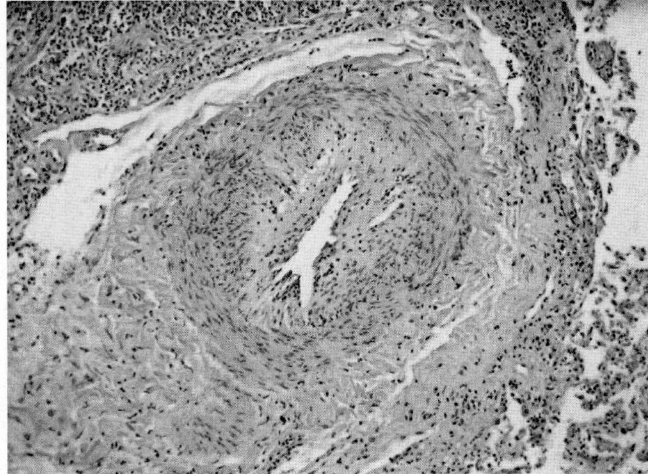

FIGURE 92.20. Open lung biopsy sample showing obliteration of a bronchiolar lumen with granulation tissue, diagnostic of Obliterative Bronchiolitis. (Courtesy of Division of Pulmonary Medicine, University of Florida, Gainesville, FL.)

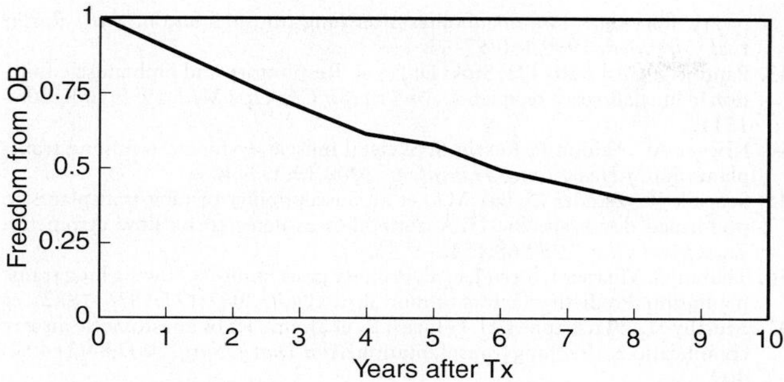

FIGURE 92.21. Freedom from obliterative bronchiolitis (OB). (From Taylor DO, Edwards LB, Boucek MM, et al. Registry of the International Society for Heart and Lung Transplantation: twenty-third official adult heart transplantation report—2006. *J Heart Lung Transplant.* 2006;25(8):869–879.)

BOS presents as cough that later becomes productive, followed by progressive exertional dyspnea. The chest radiograph is clear, but in the advanced stages will show bronchiectasis and interstitial infiltrates. Studies have shown that augmentation of immunosuppression will not reverse the decline in most cases; furthermore, it probably places patients at increased risk of infection, with very little impact on the natural history of the disease. Retransplantation has been attempted for this complication but with variable success.

Posttransplant Lymphoproliferative Disease (PTLD)

The reported incidence of PTLD after lung transplantation varies between 2% and 6%. The presentation and pattern of organ involvement is related to the time of onset. In the first year, intrathoracic involvement is the most common presentation; gastrointestinal tract involvement predominates later (73,74). The incidence of PTLD increases in proportion to the intensity of immunosuppression, especially when antilymphocyte antibodies are used (75).

Most PTLD falls under the spectrum of non-Hodgkin lymphoma, and it is predominantly B-cell lymphocyte in lineage. Epstein-Barr virus (EBV) reactivation or infection results in the unchecked proliferation of infected B lymphocytes caused by the impaired T-lymphocyte response. The EBV-encoded latent membrane protein 1 (LMP1) oncogene represents the major pathogenic factor for enabling the virus to cause PTLD (76). Decreasing the intensity of immunosuppression is the mainstay of therapy, but it carries the risk of allograft rejection. Antiviral therapy, anti-CD20 monoclonal antibody therapy, and radiation therapy have all been used but with variable success; an optimal treatment protocol has, at the time of this writing, not been determined.

Recurrence of Native Lung Diseases

Sarcoidosis, giant cell pneumonitis, lymphangiomyomatosis, and diffuse panbronchiolitis have each been documented to recur in the allograft (77–80). Due to the small number of recipients with these diagnoses, and the relatively short follow-up time, the recurrence rate and its impact on the allograft function is not known with certainty. Furthermore, the transplant community has not developed a bias against transplanting these diseases.

SUMMARY: LUNG TRANSPLANTATION

Lung transplantation has become an acceptable therapeutic option for patients with end-stage lung diseases who have failed all possible medical and surgical interventions. Patients should be referred for transplantation when projected 2-year survival is about 50% and transplantation is expected to increase the probability of survival. The patient's perception of an unacceptable quality of life associated with the end-stage lung disease is an important additional consideration, but the life expectancy must be the overriding impetus for referral. In addition, since the waiting time is between 12 and 24 months, the patient's health must remain stable during this time so that the patient will be able to endure transplantation as well as the pulmonary rehabilitation that follows.

The use of relatively stringent criteria is important in identifying candidates for whom transplantation is likely to be successful. It is important to avoid selecting poor candidates simply because of the desperate nature of their situation. Patients should be functionally disabled but ambulatory. They should also be free of clinically significant cardiac, renal, or hepatic impairment. Lung transplantation has been proven to prolong the 2- and 4-year survival in advanced stage IPF and CF patients, but not in patients with COPD. In COPD patients, we generally wait until the patient has a projected 2-year survival—with or without transplantation—before performing transplantation, with improvement in the quality of life being the most important factor to consider as the justification.

References

1. 2006 Annual Report of the U.S/ Scientific Registry for Transplant Recipients and the Organ Procurement and Transplantation Network—transplant data: 1988–2005. http://www.OPTN.org/data. Accessed September 19, 2007.
2. Egan TM, Murray S, Bustami RT, et al. Development of the new lung allocation system in the United States. *Am J Transplant.* 2006;6(5 Pt 2):1212–1227.
3. Razek T, Olthoff K, Reilly PM. Issues in potential organ donor management. *Surg Clin North Am.* 2000;80:1021–1032.
4. Jenkins DH, Reilly PM, Schwab CW. Improving the approach to organ donation: a review. *World J Surg.* 1999;23:644–649.
5. Hauptman PJ, O'Connor KJ. Procurement and allocation of solid organs for transplantation. *N Engl J Med.* 1997;336:422–431.
6. de Perrot M, Weder W, Patterson GA, et al. Strategies to increase limited donor resources. *Eur Respir J.* 2004;23(3):477–482.
7. Pilcher DV, Scheinkestel CD, Snell GI, et al. High central venous pressure is associated with prolonged mechanical ventilation and increased mortality after lung transplantation. *J Thorac Cardiovasc Surg.* 2005;129:912–918.
8. Orens JB, Boehler A, de Perrot M, et al. A review of lung transplant donor acceptability criteria. *J Heart Lung Transplant.* 2003;22(11):1182–1200.
9. Bhorade SM, Vigneswaran W, McCabe MA, et al. Liberalization of donor criteria may expand the donor pool without adverse consequence in lung transplantation. *J Heart Lung Transplant.* 2000;19(12):1199–1204.
10. Trulock EP, Edwards LB, Taylor DO, et al. Registry of the International Society for Heart and Lung Transplantation: twenty-third official adult lung and heart-lung transplantation report—2006. *J Heart Lung Transplant.* 2006;25(8):880–892.
11. Orens JB, Estenne M, Arcasoy S, et al. International guidelines for the selection of lung transplant candidates: 2006 update. *J Heart Lung Transplant.* 2006;25:745–755.
12. Kanasky WF, Anton SD, Rodrigue JR, et al. Impact of body weight on long-term survival after lung transplantation. *Chest.* 2002;121:401–406.

13. Detterbeck FC, Egan TM, Mill MR. Lung transplantation after previous thoracic surgical procedures. *Ann Thorac Surg.* 1995;60:139–143.
14. Dusmet M, Wilton TL, Kesten S, et al. Previous intrapleural procedures do not adversely affect lung transplantation. *J Heart Lung Transplant.* 1996;15:249–254.
15. Pigula FA, Griffith BP, Zenati MA, et al. Lung transplantation for respiratory failure resulting from systemic disease. *Ann Thorac Surg.* 1997;64:1630–1634.
16. Yeatman M, McNeil K, Smith JA, et al. Lung transplantation in patients with systemic diseases: an eleven-year experience at Papworth Hospital. *J Heart Lung Transplant.* 1996;15:144–149.
17. Sundaresan RS, Shiraishi Y, Trulock EP, et al. Single or bilateral lung transplantation for emphysema? *J Thorac Cardiovasc Surg.* 1996;112:1485–1495.
18. Bavaria JE, Kotloff RM, Palevsky H, et al. Bilateral versus single lung transplantation for chronic obstructive pulmonary disease. *J Thorac Cardiovasc Surg.* 1997;113:520–528.
19. Levine SM, Anzueto A, Peters JI, et al. Single lung transplantation in patients with systemic disease. *Chest.* 1994;105:837–841.
20. Levine SM, Jenkinson SG, Bryan CL, et al. Ventilation-perfusion inequalities during graft rejection in patients undergoing single lung transplantation for primary pulmonary hypertension. *Chest.* 1992;101:401–405.
21. Ritchie M, Waggoner AD, Davila-Roman VG, et al. Echocardiographic characterization of the improvement in right ventricular function in patients with severe pulmonary hypertension after single lung transplantation. *J Am Coll Cardiol.* 1993;22:1170–1174.
22. Kramer MR, Valantine HA, Marshall SE, et al. Recovery of the right ventricle after single-lung transplantation in pulmonary hypertension. *Am J Cardiol.* 1994;73:494–500.
23. Curran WD, Akindipe O, Staples ED, et al. Lung transplantation for primary pulmonary hypertension and Eisenmenger's syndrome. *J Cardiovasc Nurs.* 2005;20(2):124–132.
24. Barr ML, Baker CJ, Schenkel FA, et al. Living donor lung transplantation: selection, technique, and outcome. *Transplant Proc.* 2001;33(7–8):3527–3532.
25. Starnes VA, Bowdish ME, Woo MS, et al. A decade of living lobar lung transplantation: recipient outcomes. *J Thorac Cardiovasc Surg.* 2004;127(1):114–122.
26. Hosenpud JD, Bennett LE, Ked BM, et al. Effect of diagnosis on survival benefit of lung transplantation for end-stage lung disease. *Lancet.* 1998;351:24–27.
27. Anthonisen N. Prognosis in COPD: results from multicenter clinical trials. *Am Rev Respir Dis.* 1989;140:S95–S99.
28. Celli BR, Cote CG, Marin JM, et al. The body-mass index, airflow obstruction, dyspnea, and exercise capacity index in chronic obstructive pulmonary disease. *N Engl J Med.* 2004;350(10):1005–1012.
29. Zander DS, Baz MA, Visner GA, et al. Analysis of early deaths after isolated lung transplantation. *Chest.* 2001;120:225–232.
30. Low DE, Kaiser LR, Haydock DA, et al. The donor lung: infectious and pathologic factors affecting outcome in lung transplantation. *J Thorac Cardiovasc Surg.* 1993;106:614–621.
31. Baz MA, Palmer SM, Staples ED, et al. Lung transplantation after long-term mechanical ventilation: results and 1 year follow up. *Chest.* 2001;119:224–227.
32. Meyers BF, Lynch JP, Battafarano RJ, et al. Lung transplantation is warranted for stable, ventilator-dependent recipients. *Ann Thorac Surg.* 2000;70:1675–1678.
33. Chacon RA, Corris PA, Dark JH, et al. Comparison of the functional results of single lung transplantation for pulmonary fibrosis and chronic airway obstruction. *Thorax.* 1998;53:43–49.
34. TenVergert EM, Vermeulen KM, Geertsma A, et al. Quality of life before and after lung transplantation in patients with emphysema versus other indications. *Psychol Rep.* 2001;89:707–717.
35. Lanuza DM, Lefaiver C, McCabe M, et al. Prospective study of functional status and quality of life before and after lung transplantation. *Chest.* 2000;118:115–122.
36. Rodrigue JR, Kanasky WF, Baz MA, et al. Does lung transplantation improve health-related quality of life? The University of Florida experience. *J Heart Lung Transplant.* 2005;24(6):755–763.
37. van den Berg JW, Geertsma A, van der Bij W, et al. Bronchiolitis obliterans syndrome after lung transplantation and health-related quality of life. *Am J Respir Crit Care Med.* 2000;161:1937–1941.
38. Paris W, Diercks M, Bright J, et al. Return to work after lung transplantation. *J Heart Lung Transplant.* 1998;17:430–436.
39. Schwaiblmair M, Reichenspurner H, Muller C, et al. Cardiopulmonary exercise testing before and after lung and heart-lung transplantation. *Am J Respir Crit Care Med.* 1999;159:1277–1283.
40. Tirdel GB, Girgis R, Fishman RS, et al. Metabolic myopathy as a cause of the exercise limitation in lung transplant recipients. *J Heart Lung Transplant.* 1998;17:1231–1237.
41. Lands LC, Smountas AA, Mesiano G, et al. Maximal exercise capacity and peripheral skeletal muscle function following lung transplantation. *J Heart Lung Transplant.* 1999;18:113–120.
42. Wang XN, Williams TJ, McKenna MJ, et al. Skeletal muscle oxidative capacity, fiber type, and metabolites after lung transplantation. *Am J Respir Crit Care Med.* 1999;160:57–63.
43. Pantoja JG, Andrade FH, Stoki DS, et al. Respiratory and limb muscle function in lung allograft recipients. *Am J Respir Crit Care Med.* 1999;160:1205–1211.
44. Krieger AC, Szidon P, Kesten S. Skeletal muscle dysfunction in lung transplantation. *J Heart Lung Transplant.* 2000;19:392–400.
45. Scornik JC, Zander D, Baz MA, et al. Susceptibility of lung transplants to preformed donor-specific HLA antibodies as detected by flow cytometry. *Transplantation.* 1999;68:1542–1546.
46. Thabut G, Vinatier I, Stern J, et al. Primary graft failure following lung transplantation. Predictive factors of mortality. *Chest.* 2002;121:1876–1882.
47. Murthy SC, Blackstone EH, Gildea TR, et al. Impact of anastomotic airway complications after lung transplantation. *Ann Thorac Surg.* 2007;84(2):401–409.
48. Chhajed PN, Malouf MA, Tamm M, et al. Interventional bronchoscopy for the management of airway complications following lung transplantation. *Chest.* 2001;120(6):1894–1899.
49. Herrera JM, McNeil KD, Higgins RS, et al. Airway complications after lung transplantation: treatment and long-term outcome. *Ann Thorac Surg.* 2001;71:989–993.
50. Speich R, van der Bij W. Epidemiology and management of infections after lung transplantation. *Clin Infect Dis.* 2001;33:S58–S65.
51. Boehler A, Kesten S, Weder W, et al. Bronchiolitis obliterans after lung transplantation: a review. *Chest.* 1998;114:1411–1426.
52. Maurer JR, Tullis DE, Grossman RF, et al. Infectious complications following isolated lung transplantation. *Chest.* 1992;101:1056–1059.
53. Paradis IL, Williams P. Infection after lung transplantation. *Semin Respir Infect.* 1993;8:207–215.
54. Aris RM, Gilligan PH, Neuringer IP, et al. The effect of panresistant bacteria in cystic fibrosis patients on lung transplant outcome. *Am J Respir Crit Care Med.* 1997;155:1699–1704.
55. Snell G, de Hoyos A, Krajden M, et al. Pseudomonas cepacia in lung transplantation recipients with cystic fibrosis. *Chest.* 1993;103:466–471.
56. Snydman DR. Epidemiology of infections after solid organ transplantation. *Clin Infect Dis.* 2001;33:S5–S8.
57. Kanj SH, Welty-Wolf K, Madden J, et al. Fungal infections in lung and heart-lung recipients: report of nine cases and review of the literature. *Medicine.* 1996;75:142–156.
58. Gordon SM, Avery RK. Aspergillosis in lung transplantation: incidence, risk factors, and prophylactic strategies. *Transpl Infect Dis.* 2001;3:161–167.
59. Paradowski LJ. Saprophytic fungal infections and lung transplantation-revisited. *J Heart Lung Transplant.* 1997;16:524–531.
60. Gryzan S, Paradis IL, Zeevi A, et al. Unexpectedly high incidence of *Pneumocystis carinii* infection after lung-heart transplantation. Implications for lung defense and allograft survival. *Am Rev Respir Dis.* 1988;137:1268–1274.
61. Yousem SA, Berry GJ, Cagle PT, et al. Revision of the 1990 working formulation for the classification of pulmonary allograft rejection: Lung Rejection Study Group. *J Heart Lung Transplant.* 1996;15:1–15.
62. Baz MA, Latish DT, Govern JA, et al. Diagnostic yield of bronchoscopies after isolated lung transplantation. *Chest.* 1996;110(1): 84–88.
63. Garrity ER, Villanueva J, Bhorade SM, et al. Low rate of acute lung allograft rejection after the use of daclizumab, an interleukin 2 receptor antibody. *Transplantation.* 2001;71:773–777.
64. Palmer SM, Baz MA, Sanders L, et al. Results of a randomized, prospective, multicenter trial of mycophenolate mofetil versus azathioprine in the prevention of acute lung allograft rejection. *Transplantation.* 2001;71:1772–1776.
65. Treede H, Klepetko W, Reichenspurner H, et al; Munich and Vienna Lung Transplant Group. Tacrolimus versus cyclosporine after lung transplantation: a prospective, open, randomized two-center trial comparing two different immunosuppressive protocols. *J Heart Lung Transplant.* 2001;20:511–517.
66. Vitulo P, Oggionni T, Cascina A, et al. Efficacy of tacrolimus rescue therapy in refractory acute rejection after lung transplantation. *J Heart Lung Transplant.* 2002;21:435–439.
67. Estenne M, Maurer JR, Boehler A, et al. Bronchiolitis obliterans syndrome 2001: an update of the diagnostic criteria. *J Heart Lung Transplant.* 2002;21:297–310.
68. Arcasoy SM, Kotloff RM. Lung transplantation. *N Engl J Med.* 1999;340:1081–1091.
69. Haider Y, Yonan N, Mogulkoc N, et al. Bronchiolitis obliterans syndrome in single lung transplant recipients-patients with emphysema versus patients with idiopathic pulmonary fibrosis. *J Heart Lung Transplant.* 2002;21:327–333.
70. Sharples LD, McNeil K, Stewart S, et al. Risk factors for bronchiolitis obliterans: a systematic review of recent publications. *J Heart Lung Transplant.* 2002;21:271–281.
71. Bando K, Paradis IL, Similo S, et al. Obliterative bronchiolitis after lung and heart-lung transplantation. An analysis of risk factors and management. *J Thorac Cardiovasc Surg.* 1995;110:4–13.
72. Schulman LL, Weinberg AD, McGregor CC, et al. Influence of donor and recipient HLA locus mismatching on development of obliterative bronchiolitis after lung transplantation. *Am J Respir Crit Care Med.* 2001;163:437–442.

73. Parajothi S, Yusen RD, Kraus MD, et al. Lymphoproliferative disease after lung transplantation: comparison of presentation and outcome of early and late cases. *J Heart Lung Transplant.* 2001;20:1054–1063.
74. Ramalingham P, Rybicki I, Smith MD, et al. Posttransplant lymphoproliferative disorders in lung transplant patients: the Cleveland Clinic experience. *Mod Pathol.* 2002;15:647–656.
75. Swinnen LJ, Costanzo-Nordin MR, Fisher SG, et al. Increased incidence of lymphoproliferative disorder after immunosuppression with the monoclonal antibody OKT3 in cardiac transplant recipients. *N Engl J Med.* 1990;323:1723–1728.
76. Knecht H, Berger C, Rothenberger S, et al. The role of EBV in neoplastic transformation. *Oncology.* 2001;60:289–302.
77. Johnson BA, Duncan SR, Ohori NP, et al. Recurrence of sarcoidosis in pulmonary allograft recipients. *Is Rev Respir Dis.* 1993;148:1373–1377.
78. Frost AE, Keller CA, Brown RW, et al. Giant cell interstitial pneumonitis. Disease recurrence in the transplanted lung. *Am Rev Respir Crit Care Med.* 1993;148:1401–1404.
79. O'Brien JD, Lium JH, Parosa JF, et al. Lymphangiomyomatosis recurrence in the allograft after single-lung transplantation. *Am J Respir Crit Care Med.* 1995;151:2033–2036.
80. Baz MA, Kussin PS, Van Trigt P, et al. Recurrence of diffuse panbronchiolitis after lung transplantation. *Am J Respir Crit Care Med.* 1995;151:895–897.

CHAPTER 93 ■ LIVER TRANSPLANT

GIUDITTA ANGELINI • ZOLTAN G. HEVESI • DOUGLAS B. COURSIN

Liver failure or end-stage liver disease (ESLD) is the fourth leading cause of death in the United States in patients 45 to 54 years of age and 12th among all age groups (1). Liver transplantation is the only definitive cure for irreversible liver failure. The etiology of liver failure is well reviewed elsewhere in this textbook. The first several liver transplants performed in the 1960s and 1970s resulted in a 75% mortality within 1 year (2). The intervention that improved survival dramatically was the clinical introduction of cyclosporine in the late 1970s. Since then, many innovations have further improved the prognosis after liver transplantation. Depending on the degree of liver failure, survival is now 73% to 81% at 1 year (3). Several developments have occurred during the intervening time period due to an improved understanding of the physiology of liver failure and management during the perioperative period. Currently in the United States, there are 127 liver transplant centers (4) and about 17,000 patients on the liver transplant waiting list (5). It is important for intensive care unit physicians to understand the process of liver transplantation including preoperative assessment, intraoperative management, and postoperative priorities to optimize their ability to positively affect the outcome of these often complex patients.

KEY POINTS

1. The model for end-stage liver disease (MELD) is a system recently developed and extensively studied to accurately predict short- and intermediate-term mortality. It is based on the parameters of bilirubin, international standardized ratio, and creatinine. It is the new method on which allocation of transplant organs is based.
2. Patients with liver failure can have alterations in their cardiovascular, pulmonary, and renal physiology that can impact their prognosis after liver transplantation.
3. Blood product use during the management of the liver transplant patient should be judicious despite significant coagulation defects. This will also help to avoid hypervolemia, as both of these can significantly impact prognosis after liver transplantation.
4. Patients undergoing liver transplantation need constant surveillance of their fluid and electrolyte status to avoid complications.
5. Although most patients will experience a mild increase in aminotransferases after transplantation, there are several complications that can significantly increase the degree or duration of this rise and require evaluation.

PRESURGICAL PROCESS

The appropriate assignment and prioritization of scarce resources such as solid organs remains a challenge with organizations such as the United Network of Organ Sharing (UNOS), which strives to achieve optimal and fair distribution for transplantation. Since 2001, the MELD scoring system has been the accepted method of prioritizing liver allocation for an individual patient (6). It is calculated as shown in Table 93.1 using logarithmic numbers of the following serum indices: bilirubin, international standardized ratio (INR) for prothrombin time, and creatinine. Any patient who is on dialysis receives an automatic 4 mg/dL for his or her creatinine score. The only exception to the MELD scoring system for listing transplant candidates are status 1 patients who have acute fulminant liver failure (6). Initial research on the MELD score included a fourth number reflecting the cause of liver failure, which is no longer used. However, it is replaced by adding 0.643 for all patients to make the literature comparable despite the change. A calculator for the MELD score can be found at the UNOS Web site (*www.unos.org/resources/meldPeldCalculator.asp*).

The MELD score has been shown to be a better predictor of short- and intermediate-term morbidity and mortality among patients with liver failure than the previously used Child-Pugh Score (7,8) as well as other less well known scoring systems. In addition, once the score rises above 21, it also outperforms composite indicators such as persistent ascites or encephalopathy. There is a subset of patients at higher risk for mortality than calculated by the MELD score; the increased mortality is based on persistent ascites and hyponatremia, factors likely related to the potential for developing renal failure (9).

Patients with hepatocellular cancer (HCC) can have an excellent prognosis if liver transplantation occurs early, but their disease progression is not well represented by MELD. Therefore, the HCC patients are assigned a MELD score based on their stage according to the Milan criteria, which evaluate the number and size of liver tumors present on a CT scan or MRI. This "MELD exception" score attempts to predict the chance of progression to inoperability within 90 days. Periodically, the system is adjusted to make the allocation fair for all patients with ESLD as well as HCC. UNOS continuously monitors waiting list dropout and reviews patient scores to maintain impartiality (10). Other patients may be considered on a case-by-case basis for exception as published by the MELD exception study group (11). Potential candidates include those suffering from hepatopulmonary syndrome, primary hyperoxaluria, familial

TABLE 93.1

MODEL FOR END-STAGE LIVER DISEASE

0.378 × $\log_e$ (bilirubin) [mg/dL]   +   1.120 × $\log_e$ (INR)   +   0.957 × $\log_e$ (creatinine) [mg/dL]   +   0.643   *Add the above 4 numbers and multiply by 10. Round to the nearest integer.*
INR, international normalized ratio. From United Network for Organ Sharing. MELD/PELD calculator documentation. www.unos.org/resources, with permission. Accessed October 12, 2007.

amyloid polyneuropathy, cystic fibrosis, and small-for-size syndrome.

Cardiovascular Issues

The cardiac physiology of liver failure is characterized as a hyperdynamic profile with a high cardiac output. If there is any degree of dysfunction, it has been assumed in the past that the patient suffered from alcohol chronic toxicity, which is responsible for 30% of dilated cardiomyopathies (12). However, it is becoming evident that a significant amount of systolic dysfunction and even more diastolic dysfunction is present in patients with ESLD of all causes including nonalcoholic (13). In addition, the potential for coronary artery disease has been underappreciated previously in the potential liver transplant patient. Current studies suggest that the prevalence of coronary artery disease in patients with ESLD is at least as common and probably more so than in the general population. Patients may also be less symptomatic despite moderate to severe coronary heart disease (14). At least 50% of patients with coronary artery disease will suffer significant morbidity and mortality while undergoing a liver transplantation (1).

Patients with liver failure demonstrate blunted cardiac response to stimuli such as hemorrhage, hypovolemia, and administration of inotropic drugs (15). In ESLD patients, there are several elevated levels of circulating vasodilators such as nitric oxide, tumor necrosis factor-alpha (TNF-α), and prostaglandins, so patients are often autotreated for cardiac failure by their evolving pathophysiology (13). However, when challenged with a dramatic increase in preload from shunted mesenteric venous blood, as occurs in the transjugular intrahepatic portosystemic shunt (TIPS) procedure, cirrhotic patients have a 12% risk of heart failure (16). The risk of mortality secondary to heart failure from liver transplantation is at least 7% (17).

The prevalence of cirrhotic cardiomyopathy is difficult to assess since no firm diagnostic criteria exist, and its presence only becomes evident under stress. The prognosis correlates with the degree of liver failure and does improve over time after transplantation. The presence of cirrhotic cardiomyopathy can potentiate the occurrence of hepatorenal syndrome (13). β-Adrenergic receptor desensitization occurs so the normal inotropic and chronotropic responses to isoproterenol and dobutamine are attenuated (18,19).

The high pressure present in the hepatic sinusoids and hypoalbuminemia associated with ESLD increases Starling forces in the direction to translocate fluid to the abdominal cavity, which results in total body volume overload secondary to resultant ascites but with intravascular depletion (20). Adding the vasodilatory state associated with liver failure results in decreased end organ perfusion and predisposes to complications such as the hepatorenal syndrome discussed below. Every attempt to maintain intravascular repletion and euvolemia should be exercised. At least part of fluid resuscitation in ESLD patients should include albumin, as it has been shown to improve patient survival after the onset of ascites in long-term management of liver failure (21).

Pulmonary Disorders in Liver Failure

There are several reasons for pulmonary disease to develop in patients with liver failure. Some are related to the cause of liver failure such as emphysema with alpha-1 antitrypsin deficiency and fibrosing alveolitis associated with primary biliary cirrhosis. Additionally, complications of portal hypertension can affect lung function due to overwhelming ascites, which can decrease functional residual capacity and cause hepatic hydrothorax. However, the pulmonary issues that receive the most attention include the vascular abnormalities of hepatopulmonary syndrome and portopulmonary hypertension (22).

Approximately 40% of cirrhotic patients have hepatopulmonary syndrome, with approximately 8% to 15% developing impaired oxygenation. Essentially, the patient develops pulmonary arteriovenous dilations due to the increased presence of vasodilators. The gold standard in diagnosis is a contrast echocardiogram demonstrating intrapulmonary shunting. There is no effective treatment for this disease, but transplantation results in an 85% resolution or significant improvement (22). The duration of time until that improvement occurs can be quite variable, anywhere between a few days to 14 months postoperatively. Unfortunately, there are no good indicators to predict reversibility (23). Baseline room air arterial oxygenation of ≤50 mm Hg has been shown to worsen survival despite liver transplantation (24).

Conversely, portopulmonary hypertension is essentially pulmonary hypertension, which occurs in 2% to 5% of cirrhotic patients (25). It does not correlate with the degree of portal hypertension or liver failure. Using a cutoff of 40 mm Hg for right ventricular systolic pressure, the sensitivity of echocardiogram is 80% and the specificity is 96% (26).

The treatment of portopulmonary hypertension is not at all the same as for other types of pulmonary artery hypertension (PAH). At the present time, diuretics and epoprostenol have been the best studied and the most likely to provide benefit. Recommended therapies for PAH such as anticoagulation, calcium channel blockers, beta blockers, and endothelin receptor antagonists can have adverse effects either on the prognosis of portopulmonary hypertension or on liver failure in general. TIPS is contraindicated in this setting. Sildenafil may have some benefit, but it does increase the production of endogenous nitric oxide and can further exacerbate systemic hypotension (25).

When the mean pulmonary artery pressure is >50 mm Hg, liver transplantation is contraindicated, as the mortality has been documented to be 100% (27). It is considered a contraindication due to the fact that transplantation will decrease the amount of circulating prostaglandins and result in worsening of the disease. Below a mean pulmonary artery pressure of 35 mm Hg, proceeding with liver transplantation can occur without delay. Between 35 and 50 mm Hg, optimizing the patient's status with diuretics and epoprostenol is indicated prior to liver transplantation (25).

Hepatorenal Syndrome

Hepatorenal syndrome (HRS) is a functional type of renal impairment that occurs in 11.4% of patients with liver failure within 5 years of the first episode of significant ascites (28). There are two types, which are both potentially reversible with liver transplantation. HRS 1 is rapidly progressive, with a doubling of initial creatinine to above 2.5 mg/dL or 50% reduction of creatinine clearance to less than 20 mL/minute, which occurs in less than 2 weeks. The mortality rate is nearly 100% within 10 weeks of development. HRS 2 is associated with a more moderate, steady decline in renal function (29). The 1-year probability of survival is 38.5% with HRS 2, but the mean survival of HRS 1 is only 7 ± 2 days (28). A more complete discussion of this topic is found in the chapter on liver failure. Therefore, the focus here will be regarding the goals of therapy during liver transplantation in patients with HRS.

The most successful management to prevent further injury during surgery is to alter the physiology that led to the development of HRS. The effect of peripheral and splanchnic vasodilation from cytokines and nitric oxide, as well as the intrarenal vasoconstriction that occurs in response to intravascular depletion are both aspects of liver failure that combine to produce this syndrome (29). Obviously, euvolemia is a primary goal, and in most studies looking at prevention and improvement of HRS, albumin is used as an adjuvant therapy.

Vasopressin analogues administered with albumin to patients with both types of HRS have been shown to improve glomerular filtration rate and creatinine levels (29). Pretransplant normalization of kidney function with terlipressin has been shown to provide similar outcomes after liver transplantation similar to patients with normal renal function (30). There is also a survival advantage while waiting for transplantation if terlipressin is administered, but only if the transplant occurs within 3 months. The major risk associated with vasopressin analogues is the potential for ischemia, which has been shown to be clinically significant with only ornipressin. Terlipressin is not currently available in the United States, however (29).

The combination of octreotide and midodrine has been shown to have some beneficial effects on renal function and mortality in HRS; however, patients treated with vasopressin had improved survival rates and were more likely to receive a liver transplant (31). There is no literature that has investigated the combined effects of all three agents. In a very small study, norepinephrine had comparable efficacy to vasopressin without any adverse side effects (32). In patients with liver failure who develop hypotension, norepinephrine and vasopressin are agents that should be considered first line with less concern regarding renal side effects. Patients who do not respond to the above therapies will likely require some form of renal replacement therapy. Continuous venovenous hemodialysis (CVVHD) is the treatment of choice since it causes less hypotension, with a decreased potential to create ongoing injury compared to hemodialysis performed 3 times a week. However, once a patient has received any type of dialysis for HRS lasting longer than 12 weeks, there is a risk that renal dysfunction will either continue after transplantation or will recur within a few years. For patients who develop renal failure within 13 years of their liver transplant, survival is only 28% compared to 55% for those who do not; yet, it is not clear which patients will definitely develop ongoing renal compromise. Therefore, the selection of which patients will receive a combined liver/kidney transplant remains in evolution (33).

Fulminant Hepatic Failure

The abrupt onset of liver failure within 8 weeks in a previously healthy patient has been the traditional definition of fulminant failure, but modern discussion centers on potentially decreasing the time period to 2 weeks to correlate with the prognosis. There are several potential causes, but acetaminophen is by far the most common. The mortality rate is 80% without liver transplantation (34).

Table 93.2 summarizes the King's College criteria for liver transplantation (35). The MELD score has a higher sensitivity and negative predictive value, but a very high false-positive rate so it may be better to use it in conjunction with King's College criteria to avoid transplantation in patients who may recover spontaneously (36). One of the main components of both scores is the prothrombin time and/or INR. Therefore, it is imperative to give blood products only if bleeding occurs or a procedure is planned. Infection occurs in 80% of patients

TABLE 93.2

KING'S COLLEGE CRITERIA FOR LIVER TRANSPLANTATION IN FULMINANT HEPATIC FAILURE

ACETOMINOPHEN
- pH <7.3 (irrespective of encephalopathy)

Or all three of the following:
- Grade III or IV encephalopathy
- PT >100 sec or INR >6.5
- Serum creatinine >3.4 mg/dL

ALL OTHER CAUSES
- PT >100 s or INR >6.5 (irrespective of encephalopathy)

Or any three of the following:
- Age <10 or >40 years
- Cause: non–A, non–B hepatitis; halothane; idiosyncratic drug reaction; Wilson disease
- Length of time from jaundice to encephalopathy >7 days
- PT >50 seconds or INR >3.5
- Serum bilirubin >17.5 mg/dL

PT, prothrombin time; INR, international normalized ratio.
From O'Grady JG, Alexander GJ, Hayllar KM, et al. Early indications of prognosis in fulminant hepatic failure. *Gastroenterology.* 1989;97:439–445, with permission.

TABLE 93.3

HEPATIC ENCEPHALOPATHY IN FULMINANT HEPATIC FAILURE

Stage	Mental status	EEG
I	Confusion, slow mentation and affect, slurred speech, disordered sleep	Normal
II	Accentuation of stage I, drowsy, inappropriate, loss of sphincter control	Slowing
III	Marked confusion, sleeps mostly but arousable, incoherent	Abnormal
IV	Not arousable; may or may not respond to painful stimuli	Abnormal

EEG, electroencephalograph.
From Sass DA, Shakil AO. Fulminant hepatic failure. *Liver Transplant.* 2005;11(6):594–605, with permission.

with fulminant hepatic failure (FHF), and thus a high index of suspicion and regular surveillance are important. Some centers use prophylactic antibiotics, but this increases the risk of fungal infections, which occur in 30% of patients with FHF. Hemodynamically, FHF is associated with a high cardiac output and vasodilation similar to sepsis, making infection difficult to discern. Optimizing intravascular volume is the main goal in management, but vasopressors may be necessary. Fluid management may be complicated by renal failure since this occurs in 40% to 50% of patients (34).

Encephalopathy inversely correlates with prognosis. Table 93.3 summarizes the four stages of encephalopathy that are seen in FHF (34). Cerebral edema occurs in most cases that progress to stage 4. Typical symptoms of cerebral edema are the Cushing reflex, decerebrate rigidity, dysconjugate eye movements, and a loss of pupillary reflexes. Intracranial pressure (ICP) monitoring should be considered if the patient develops stage 3 or 4 encephalopathy due to the development of increased ICP in the setting of systemic hypotension (34). Cerebral perfusion pressure (CPP) of >60 mm Hg is necessary to maintain intact neurologic function. Liver transplantation in the setting of CPP <40 mm Hg for 2 hours or more is contraindicated (37). Concern for intracranial bleeding associated with the placement of an ICP monitor has precluded use in most liver transplant centers. Recently, factor VIIa has been shown to be effective in transiently correcting coagulopathy to allow for safer placement of this monitor (38). Patients with elevated ICP are candidates for mannitol, mild hyperventilation, and barbiturate or propofol infusions while maintaining systemic blood pressure in an attempt to optimize CPP.

ANESTHETIC AND SURGICAL ISSUES

Anesthetic Drugs

Increasingly, numerous transplant centers demonstrate successful extubation at the end of surgery in over 50% of patients (39). Therefore, careful dosing of anesthetic drugs is warranted to ensure the possibility that patients are awake enough to extubate. Low doses of midazolam based on previous history of exposure to benzodiazepines and alcohol and less than 20 μg/kg of fentanyl will facilitate avoidance of postoperative mechanical ventilation in suitable patients who are able to maintain oxygenation and normocarbia. Maximizing the use of inhaled agents will decrease the need for other sedative agents. Isoflurane is probably the volatile anesthetic of choice to preserve splanchnic flow, as it produces vasodilator effects on the hepatic circulation (1). Cisatracurium is the muscle relaxant of choice since it is degraded by serum esterases. Some reports suggest that a recovery time of more than 150 minutes from rocuronium is predictive of primary graft dysfunction (40).

Blood Product Use

Patients with liver failure have a decrease in all factors except von Willebrand. Platelets are also reduced secondary to hypersplenism, bone marrow suppression, and decreased thrombopoietin production in ESLD (41). Attempts to correct coagulation defects in patients undergoing liver transplantation result in a hypervolemic state, which can lead to an increase in blood transfusion. Restricting the transfusion of products to situations in which clinical bleeding requires control or to treat severe anemia can lead to fewer or no red blood cell transfusions during liver transplantation. This has been shown to improve 1-year survival after transplantation (42). Table 93.4 is a transfusion algorithm based on the thromboelastogram and has been applied successfully in cardiac surgical patients to decrease transfusion (43). Some minor changes make it amenable to liver transplantation patients. Thromboelastography is used because most serum component markers of coagulation do not reflect the intricate dynamics of whole blood clotting to guide transfusion.

Aprotinin use in liver transplantation has been shown to decrease red blood cell transfusion in several randomized trials (44,45). During the anhepatic phase of surgery, the suprahepatic and infrahepatic vena cava may be cross-clamped. This is a stage during which there is rapid increase in tissue-type plasminogen activator in the absence of α-2-antiplasmin and plasminogen activator inhibitor. Therefore, plasmin activity increases, and fibrinolysis can ensue (46). Aprotinin acts to inhibit plasmin. The concern regarding the use of aprotinin on

TABLE 93.4

A THROMBOELASTOGRAM-BASED ALGORITHM IN LIVER TRANSPLANTATION

Platelet administration if platelet count is less than 50,000 or MA is less than 45 mm
Fresh frozen plasma administration if heparinase R time is more than 20 mm
Cryoprecipitate if fibrinogen is less than 100 mg/dL
Protamine if heparinase R time is less than one half nonheparinase R time
Antifibrinolytic therapy if LY 30 is more than 7.5%

R, recombinant.
From Shore-Lesserson L, Manspeizer HE, DePerio M, et al. Thromboelastography-guided transfusion algorithm reduces transfusions in complex cardiac surgery. *Anesth Analg.* 1999;88(2):312–319, with permission.

a prophylactic basis is due to scattered case reports of thrombotic episodes such as clots on pulmonary artery catheters and an increased rate of vein graft occlusions in cardiac surgery (47).

Stagnation of blood flow can lead to clot formation in the vena cava. On reperfusion of the transplanted liver, echocardiographic evidence of embolization has been documented, even in the absence of aprotinin (48). Nonetheless, it is concerning that there are several case reports of massive pulmonary embolism and death during liver transplantation when aprotinin was used (49,50). Given the crude understanding of coagulation in the presence of liver disease, potential aprotinin administration should be reserved for documented fibrinolysis during the reperfusion stage. The lowest effective dose documented in the literature is 500,000 kallikrein inactivation units (KIU) as a bolus, with 150,000 KIU/hour, with equal efficacy to higher doses in limiting the number of blood products transfused (51). If pulmonary embolism occurs, supportive care and thrombolysis may lead to better outcomes compared to embolectomy (50).

The benefit of aprotinin outside of blood conservation includes potential anti-inflammatory activity. Aprotinin has been shown to decrease some of the cytokines that inappropriately vasodilate patients with ESLD such as TNF and nitric oxide (52). This can produce less cardiovascular instability and vasopressor use, and result in improved graft function (46). However, there are several adverse effects with increasing documentation in the cardiac surgery literature. Recent evidence suggests a dose-dependent increase in death, renal failure, and cardiovascular events when aprotinin was used. This information makes routine or even occasional use of aprotinin questionable for reasons other than thromboembolic complications (53).

Aminocaproic acid and tranexamic acid have both been used in liver transplantation but are less studied than aprotinin. There are fewer randomized controlled trials to confirm efficacy. Furthermore, neither agent has the benefit of the anti-inflammatory activity, which is seen with aprotinin. These agents exert their effect by inhibiting the conversion of plasminogen into plasmin (46). In studies with aminocaproic acid, fatal thromboembolism has occurred if the standard dose in cardiac surgery is given with a 5-g bolus and then 1 g per hour. However, it has been safely used without reports of many thromboembolic complications if administered in lower doses, ranging from 0.25 to 1 g as a bolus only. Success was variable in controlling significant bleeding (46). Studies with tranexamic acid have shown a dose-related effect. Low dose (2mg/kg/hour) has minimal effect on transfusion requirements, but high dose (10–40 mg/kg/hour) has been shown to significantly reduce intraoperative bleeding. An optimal dose has not been established (46). Tranexamic acid has not been associated with thromboembolic phenomena, but it is much less frequently used than either aprotinin or Amicar to treat fibrinolysis during liver transplantation.

Factor VIIa is a novel way to increase the thrombin burst and acutely improve coagulation on a short-term basis secondary to rapid factor consumption. Theoretically, it requires an activated platelet so coagulation occurs at the site of bleeding and not systemically (54). It has been studied in cirrhotic patients in trials for gastrointestinal bleeding and liver transplantation (55–57). Neither showed any difference in the degree of bleeding or required transfusions. However, cirrhotic patients are likely to be factor VII deficient. There has been no dose-ranging study to look at efficacy related to the degree of serum levels achieved.

Fluids and Electrolytes

Along the lines of avoiding hypervolemia, minimizing fluid use is the goal during liver transplantation. There is no particular type of fluid that conclusively shows benefit. ESLD patients have a decreased ability to metabolize lactate and are prone to lactic acidosis, especially during the required interruption of blood flow for performing the vascular anastomosis of the liver transplant (58). The exclusive use of lactate-containing solution is likely unwise. In addition, patients may require a small amount of bicarbonate administration to offset ongoing acid production, with attention to the fact that large amounts will result in metabolic alkalosis after surgery (58). Placing 150 mEq of sodium bicarbonate in 1 L of D_5W achieves an isotonic fluid with a modest degree of bicarbonate. Using this fluid during the anhepatic phase of surgery may have the added benefit of aiding renal preservation. ESLD patients experience renal vasoconstriction that may be similar pathophysiologically to what occurs with intravenous dye administration (59).

Hyponatremia at $\leq$127 mEq/L occurs in 3.5% of liver transplant candidates. A change in serum sodium approaching 20 mEq/L is much more likely to produce central pontine myelinolysis (CPM) than a change closer to 7 mEq/L (60). CPM is a source of mortality after liver transplantation (61). Normal saline solutions are actually somewhat hypernatremic and hyperchloremic to serum, and excessive use will lead to hyperchloremic acidosis. Albumin administration has shown benefit during paracentesis and in the long-term management of patients with ESLD. However, there is no conclusive evidence for risks or benefits during liver transplantation, and it is a source of sodium as well. Although a transfusion algorithm will minimize administration, fresh frozen plasma may be required in some amount and also presents a salt load. Potentially, a mixture of crystalloid and colloid provides the best approach.

Attempting to maintain euvolemia in patients who are total body-volume overloaded leads into a discussion of diuretic administration. Intravascular volume depletion chronically present in ESLD complicates the use of furosemide unless there has been significant volume overload requiring removal such as a stable patient who required several different blood products to control bleeding. However, mannitol has many characteristics that make it advantageous to use during liver transplantation. Patients with ESLD may have edema of the abdominal organs due to congestion of blood flow through the fibrosed liver and the hypoalbuminemic state. The osmotic activity of mannitol can aid in removing free water within these organs, particularly in the setting of hepatorenal syndrome, and thus prevent hepatic distention once the transplanted liver is reperfused. It may also provide some renal protection during hypoperfusion of the anhepatic stage while simultaneously increasing portal blood flow. Finally, the patient benefits from the potential of mannitol to provide free radical scavenging (62). Optimal dosing of mannitol is 0.5 to 1 g/kg just prior to cross-clamping or while anhepatic.

In addition to acid-base homeostasis, there are a number of other electrolyte issues of concern during liver transplantation. Due to the presence of cirrhosis-induced insulin resistance, the increase in stress hormones during surgery, and the use of steroid and glucose-containing solutions, patients may become quite hyperglycemic even if there are no glucose control issues prior to surgery (58). Since these patients are going to the intensive care unit, they may benefit from some degree of control with an insulin infusion, with the goal of maintaining the blood sugar >80 mg/dL and <150 mg/dL. With the use of diuretics and the presence of malnutrition, magnesium deficiency is also common in liver failure (58). This places the patient at risk for arrhythmias, which can be resistant to treatment without magnesium replacement (63). In addition, in some patients a hypocoagulable tracing on a thromboelastogram (TEG) has been shown to normalize solely from magnesium supplementation (64). Patients can be hyperkalemic or hypokalemic prior to liver transplantation also based on the degree of diuretic use; hyperkalemia can be exacerbated during surgery, especially since spironolactone has such a long half-life. Transfused blood products are a source of additional potassium during surgery. Depending on the type of preservation solution, revascularization can be a time of excessive hyperkalemia, which can result in cardiac arrest (65). This concern is increased with livers obtained through donation after cardiac death, with resultant warm ischemia and increased cell death.

Patients with significant renal dysfunction and/or those undergoing dialysis at the time of transplantation will most likely require CVVHD during liver transplantation. Although this is helpful to manage electrolyte abnormalities, it is not quick. This is particularly the case with metabolic acidosis in which patients often require the addition of a dilute bicarbonate infusion, which may be faster and safer (66). However, CVVHD can be used to both remove and administer fluid expeditiously. A heating system should be used during CVVHD since serum is exchanged at about the rate of 22 to 30 L in 24 hours, and patients can become hypothermic, which can exacerbate baseline coagulopathy. To prevent the system from developing clots, citrate is often used, as opposed to heparin, in patients with significant coagulopathy. Between this condition and the amount of citrate that may be administered from blood products, calcium supplementation is often required (58).

Surgical Considerations

In the past, venovenous bypass was required for the anhepatic phase of liver transplantation due to the patient's inability to tolerate complete occlusion of the portal vein and inferior vena cava. However, this intervention is not without the potential for complications such as nerve damage and lymphatic disruption, as well as fatal pulmonary embolus (2). The piggyback technique (Fig. 93.1), in which outflow of the donor liver is anastomosed to a vessel formed from combined hepatic veins, results in a shorter anhepatic phase and avoidance of completely cross-clamping the inferior vena cava. The advantages in addition to avoiding venovenous bypass include less bleeding, protection of renal venous outflow, less adrenal injury, and potentially more hemodynamic stability (2).

Cardiopulmonary Management

Intraoperative transesophageal echocardiography (TEE) has increasingly been used as part of an anesthetic in situations that traditionally have been managed with a pulmonary artery catheter. There are no randomized controlled trials demonstrating the efficacy of this technology in liver transplantation. However, it would seem helpful at the time of reperfusion given that cardiac output alone is not as reliable in patients with liver failure and the potential presence of cirrhotic cardiomyopathy. It would also document evidence of thromboembolism during that stage of the surgery. The obvious concern about the use of TEE is the risk of bleeding from varices. No case reports have documented this as an actual risk, and there are some

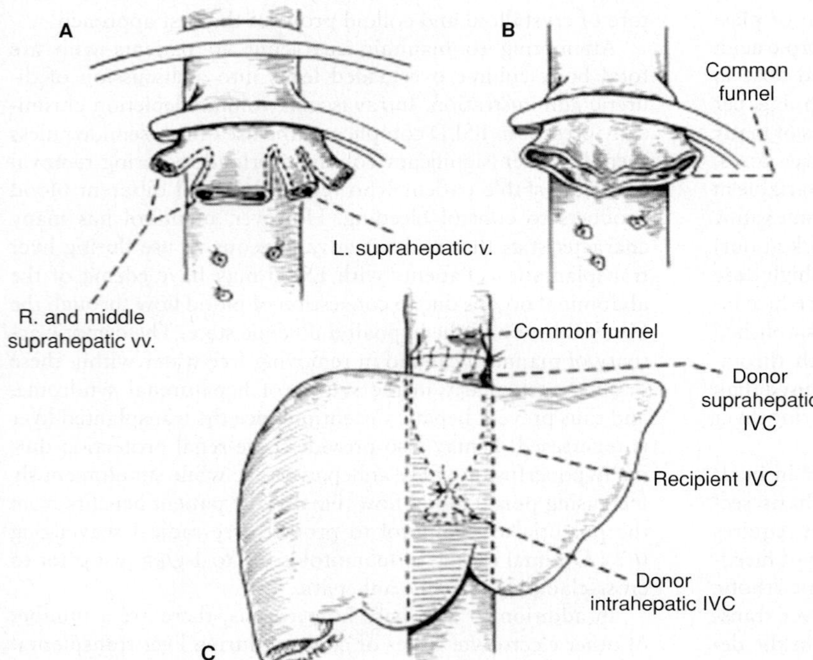

FIGURE 93.1. Piggyback technique. (From Eghtesad B, Kadry Z, Fung J. Technical considerations in liver transplantation: what a hepatologist needs to know (and every surgeon should practice). *Liver Transpl.* 2005;11[8]:861–871, with permission.)

centers that use TEE on a regular basis. Theoretically, varices may deflate after celiotomy, with resultant decrease in abdominal pressure. It would seem prudent to evaluate the use of the technology on a case-by-case basis and maybe restrict its use to an unstable patient (67).

Minimizing intrathoracic pressure will be helpful to improve hepatic outflow. Setting lower tidal volumes (6–8 mL/kg) and avoidance of positive end-expiratory pressure may contribute to maintaining euvolemia in minimizing preload, and therefore decrease the risk for bleeding. Nitric oxide has been shown to improve oxygenation and decrease severe intraoperative pulmonary hypertension (68) as a bridge to more definitive treatment. However, the most commonly used medication for intraoperative therapy of pulmonary hypertension is epoprostenol.

Patients frequently require the use of vasopressor agents. As already discussed above, vasopressin and norepinephrine are considered the best choices due to their potential to improve intra-abdominal vascular stability and enhance renal perfusion without inducing mesenteric ischemia. Since the phenomenon of cirrhotic cardiomyopathy is difficult to demonstrate, there are no studies on the beneficial effects of dobutamine or milrinone.

POSTTRANSPLANT COMPLICATIONS

The postoperative goals in a liver transplant recipient are similar to intraoperative priorities. Therefore, this section will discuss unique and specific postoperative entities. Infections in the immunodepressed posttransplant period are thoroughly discussed in other sections of the textbook.

Primary Nonfunction

Ischemia reperfusion injury of the transplanted organ can result in some degree of graft dysfunction, which can be compensated by the significant regenerative capacity of the liver. However, some patients may develop primary graft nonfunction, with a reported incidence of 7% (69). There is no clear definition or uniform diagnostic criteria for this diagnosis, but generally it includes patients who die or require retransplantation within 1 week without a definite technical or immunologic cause. Patients appear to rapidly go back into hepatic failure with high levels of aminotransferases, prolonged prothrombin time, hepatic encephalopathy, hypoglycemia, and lactic acidosis (70).

Reactive oxygen intermediates and issues in organ preservation represent targets to potentially modulate primary nonfunction, but there are currently no definitive preventative strategies or treatments. Donor age older than 50 years and macrovesicular steatosis of >60% are possible risk factors, but these have not been shown to be consistently so (70).

Vascular Occlusion

Studies concerning the incidence of portal vein thrombosis (PVT) at the time of liver transplant show that it occurs in about 12% of patients. The presence of a pre-existing thrombosis makes surgery more challenging and increases the risk of rethrombosis after transplantation, but it has not been shown to alter mortality (71). The incidence of PVT presenting after transplantation is less than 1%. In addition to a prior history of PVT, the risk factors include a hypercoagulable state, perioperative hypotension, and allograft cirrhosis. Acutely, it can lead to hepatic failure, but chronically there is a more insidious presentation involving portal hypertension with ascites and varices (70). Hepatic vein thrombosis is very unusual except in patients who have undergone transplantation for Budd-Chiari syndrome with subtherapeutic anticoagulation, and it typically takes months to years to develop (70).

The most common vascular complication is hepatic artery thrombosis (HAT), which occurs somewhere between 3% and 9% (72). In addition, mortality is common without retransplantation, with an incidence of about 30% (70). If HAT is tolerated by the liver surviving solely on portal flow, then complications occur usually after 1 month with the development of bile duct strictures since virtually all biliary perfusion comes from the hepatic artery. For patients who cannot be supported solely on portal flow, their presentation is much more acute with severe graft dysfunction or primary nonfunction (70).

Risk factors for HAT include small caliber or complex arterial structure of both the donor and recipient. Increased donor age and a recipient/donor ratio greater than 1.25 can put the recipient at risk for HAT. Medical issues that may predispose to HAT include cytomegalovirus infection, rejection, tobacco use, and hypercoagulable states. Urgent revascularization can be attempted for early presentation of HAT-associated graft dysfunction (70). This can be accomplished angiographically or surgically. However, about 50% of patients in this scenario will require retransplantation. Patients who do receive some type of intravascular therapy have difficulty maintaining long-term hepatic artery patency (72).

Rejection

Not only is rejection less common in liver transplantation than in other solid organ transplants, but less rejection occurs in the latter group when performed in the setting of a concurrent or previous liver transplant (73). In addition, rejection that occurs early after the liver is transplanted does not necessarily affect overall graft survival (74). This effect is not due to antigenic indifference, but instead to an active immune system process in which there are several theoretical causes. Microchimerism is one such hypothesis where donor hematopoietic cells persist in the recipient, producing tolerance through a balance of graft versus host and host versus graft reactions (73).

Nonetheless, transplantation tolerance is not attainable consistently. It has been shown that patients can be weaned off corticosteroid immune suppression 3 to 4 months after transplantation, but complete cessation of immune suppression is associated with about a 30% incidence of rejection (74). The commonly used immune suppressives in liver transplantation with their side effects are listed in Table 93.5 (75). Side effects can result in the alteration of which medications are used, and the development of a lymphoproliferative disorder can be grounds for complete cessation of therapy (73).

Acute rejection occurs within the first 5 to 15 days after transplantation. It is manifested by fever, graft enlargement, tenderness, leukocytosis with increased eosinophils, and

TABLE 93.5

IMMUNE SUPPRESSIVE MEDICATION IN LIVER TRANSPLANT

Medication	Side effects
Steroids	Acne, obesity, hypertension, bone loss, hyperglycemia, bone disease, cataracts, adrenal suppression, muscle wasting
Calcineurin inhibitor (cyclosporine, tacrolimus)	Neurotoxicity, nephrotoxicity, hypertension, hyperglycemia, lipid abnormalities
Mycophenolate	Nausea, diarrhea, leucopenia, thrombocytopenia, anemia
Azathioprine	Gastrointestinal ulceration, myelosuppression
MTOR inhibitor (sirolimus, everolimus)	Increased cholesterol and triglycerides, proteinuria, potentially nephrotoxic[a]
Murine monoclonal antibody (OKT3)	Fever, rigor, headache, dyspnea, nausea, diarrhea, flash pulmonary edema
Rabbit polyclonal antibody (Thymoglobulin)	Similar to OKT3, leukopenia, thrombocytopenia, serum sickness
Anti-interleukin-2 receptor (basiliximab)	Minimal to none

[a]Patients on sirolimus and a calcineurin inhibitor in combination may have more nephrotoxicity than seen with the latter drug alone.
From Hirose R, Vincenti F. Immunosuppression: today, tomorrow and withdrawal. *Semin Liver Dis*, 2006;26(3):201–210, with permission.

reduced bile production. Biopsies are done only when symptoms are present because the morphologic features consistent with acute rejection can be present in a significant percentage of patients in the early posttransplant period (76). Treatment for acute rejection is 3 to 5 days of 500 to 1,000 mg of methylprednisolone daily, with about 75% resolution. A second course is sufficient for treatment in an additional 10%. The rest require some type of antilymphocyte therapy, with a rare case requiring retransplantation (77). Patients who develop rejection in the setting of complete immune suppressive cessation have been shown to have an increased risk of steroid-resistant rejection (74).

Biliary Dysfunction

Posttransplant complications in the biliary tract are relatively common. The reported incidence is somewhere between 9% and 15% (78). A very rare syndrome of diffuse biliary necrosis may require retransplantation. In this scenario, patients present with a combination of sepsis, cholestasis, and bile leakage in which temporizing measures are useless. However, most cases of biliary dysfunction are not a cause for retransplantation or mortality (78).

Early complications of the biliary tract are leaks and strictures. Anastomotic leaks and strictures are the most serious and are usually related to ischemic necrosis of the donor distal bile duct. These can be managed with endoscopic or percutaneous stenting and require surgery only if a major leak is present. The vast majority of these problems present within the first 2 months after transplantation (78).

Live Donor or Living Related Liver Transplantation

For the most part, the recipient receives essentially the same measures. However, there is an increased risk of vascular and biliary problems postoperatively. Unique to this type of transplantation is small-for-size syndrome. Essentially, the patient has poor bile production, delayed synthetic function, prolonged cholestasis, and intractable ascites. These patients are at risk for sepsis and have an increased mortality (79). A similar situation may affect patients who receive a split liver as well.

SUMMARY

The patient undergoing liver transplantation has a significantly altered physiology and undergoes specific management to ensure optimal outcome. Coordinated care from the perioperative physician, surgeon, and anesthesiologist can minimize the risks from this procedure so the intensivist is in the position to effect a prognosis.

References

1. Steadman RH. Anesthesia for liver transplant surgery. *Anesthesiol Clin North Am.* 2004;22:687–711.
2. Eghtesad B, Kadry Z, Fung J. Technical considerations in liver transplantation: what a hepatologist needs to know (and every surgeon should practice). *Liver Transpl.* 2005;11(8):861–871.
3. The Organ Procurement and Transplantation Network. Liver graft survival rates for transplants performed: 1997–2004. www.optn.org/latestData/rptStrat.asp. Accessed November 5, 2007.
4. United Network of Organ Sharing. Transplant Centers. www.unos.org/shoWe Are/transplantCenters.asp. Accessed November 5, 2007.
5. United Network of Organ Sharing. Waiting list by organ. www.optn.org/latestData/rptData.asp. Accessed November 5, 2007.
6. United Network for Organ Sharing. MELD/PELD calculator documentation. www.unos.org/resources. Accessed October 12, 2007.
7. Kamath PS, Wiesner RH, Malinchoc M, et al. A model to predict survival in patients with end-stage liver disease. *Hepatology.* 2001;33(2):464–470.
8. Said A, Williams J, Holden J, et al. Model for end stage liver disease score predicts mortality across a broad spectrum of liver disease. *J Hepatol.* 2004;40:897–903.
9. Heuman DM, Abou-Assi SG, Habib A, et al. Persistent ascites and low serum sodium identify patients with cirrhosis and low MELD scores who are at high risk for early death. *Hepatology.* 2004;40(4):802–810.

10. Hevesi ZG. Member of UNOS Liver and Intestinal Organ Transplantation Committee. Personal communication. October 20, 2007.
11. Freeman RB, Gish RG, Harper A, et al. Model for end-stage liver disease (MELD) exception guidelines: results and recommendations from the MELD Exception Study Group and Conference (MESSAGE) for the approval of patients who need liver transplantation with diseases not considered by the standard MELD formula. *Liver Transpl.* 2006;12(12,S3):S128–S136.
12. Lee WK, Regan TJ. Alcoholic cardiomyopathy: is it dose dependent? *Congest Heart Fail.* 2002;8(6):303–306.
13. Baik SK, Fouad TR, Lee SS. Cirrhotic cardiomyopathy. *Orphanet J Rare Dis.* 2007;2:15–22.
14. Keeffe BG, Valantine H, Keeffe EB. Detection and treatment of coronary artery disease in liver transplant candidates. *Liver Transpl.* 2001;7(9):755–761.
15. Pozzi M, Carugo S, Pecci BG, et al. Evidence of functional and structural cardiac abnormalities in cirrhotic patients with and without ascites. *Hepatolog.* 1997;26:1131–1137.
16. Gines P, Uriz J, Calahorra B, et al. Transjugular intrahepatic portosystemic shunting versus paracentesis plus albumin for refractory ascites in cirrhosis. *Gastroenterology.* 2002;123:1839–1847.
17. Myers RP, Lee SS. Cirrhotic cardiomyopathy and liver transplantation. *Liver Transpl.* 2000;6(4S1):S44–S52.
18. Ramond MJ, Comoy E, Lebrec D. Alterations in isoprenaline sensitivity in patients with cirrhosis: evidence of abnormality of the sympathetic nervous system. *Br J Clin Pharmacol.* 1986;21:191–196.
19. Mikulic E, Munoz C, Puntoni LE, et al. Hemodynamic effects of dobutamine in patients with alcoholic cirrhosis, *Clin Pharmacol Ther.* 1983;34:56–59.
20. Arroyo V, Colmenero J. Ascites and hepatorenal syndrome in cirrhosis: pathophysiological basis of therapy and current management. *J Hepatol.* 2003;38(S1):S69–S89.
21. Romanelli RG, La Villa G, Barletta G, et al. Long-term albumin infusion improves survival in patients with cirrhosis and ascites: an unblended randomized trial. *World J Gastroenterol.* 2006;12(9):1403–1407.
22. Fallon MB, Abrams GA. Pulmonary dysfunction in chronic liver disease. *Hepatology.* 2000;32(4):859–865.
23. Lange PA, Stoller JK. The hepatopulmonary syndrome. *Clin Chest Med.* 1996;17(1):115–123.
24. Swanson KL, Wiesner RH, Krowka MJ. Natural history of hepatopulmonary syndrome: impact of liver transplantation. *Hepatology.* 2005;41(5):1122–1129.
25. Golbin JM, Krowka MJ. Portopulmonary hypertension. *Clin Chest Med.* 2007;28:203–218.
26. Colle IO, Moreau R, Godinho E, et al. Diagnosis of portopulmonary hypertension in candidates for liver transplantation: a prospective study. *Hepatology.* 2003;37(2):401–409.
27. Tam NL, He X. Clinical management of portopulmonary hypertension. *Hepatobiliary Pancreat Dis Int.* 2007;6:464–469.
28. Planas R, Montoliu S, Balleste B, et al. Natural history of patients hospitalized for management of cirrhotic ascites. *Clin Gastroenterol Hepatol.* 2006;4(11):1385–1394.
29. Wadei HM, Mai ML, Ahsan N, et al. Hepatorenal syndrome: pathophysiology and management. *Clin J Am Soc Nephrol.* 2006;1:1066–1079.
30. Restuccia T, Ortega R, Guevara M, et al. Effects of treatment of hepatorenal syndrome before transplantation on posttransplantation outcome. A case-control study. *J Hepatol.* 2004;40:149–146.
31. Kiser TH, Fish DN, Obritsch MD, et al. Vasopressin, not octreotide, may be beneficial in the treatment of hepatorenal syndrome: a retrospective study. *Nephrol Dial Transplant.* 2005;20:1813–1820.
32. Alessandria C, Ottobrelli A, Debernardi-Venon W, et al. Noradrenalin vs terlipressin in patients with hepatorenal syndrome: a prospective, randomized, unblended pilot study. *J Hepatol.* 2007;47:499–505.
33. Davis CL, Gonwa TA, Wilkinson AH. Identification of patients best suited for combined liver-kidney transplantation, II. *Liver Transpl.* 2002;8(3):193–211.
34. Sass DA, Shakil AO. Fulminant hepatic failure. *Liver Transpl.* 2005;11(6):594–605.
35. O'Grady JG, Alexander GJ, Hayllar KM, et al. Early indications of prognosis in fulminant hepatic failure. *Gastroenterology.* 1989;97:439–445.
36. Zaman MB, Hoti E, Qasim A, et al. MELD score as a prognostic model for listing acute liver failure patients for liver transplantation. *Transplant Proc.* 2006;38(7):2097–2098.
37. Hoofnagle JH, Carithers RLJ, Shapiro C, Ascher N. Fulminant hepatic failure: summary of a workshop. *Hepatology.* 1995;21:240–252.
38. Shami VM, Caldwell SH, Hespenheide EE, et al. Recombinant activated factor VII for coagulopathy in fulminant hepatic failure compared with conventional therapy. *Liver Transpl.* 2003;9:138–143.
39. Biancofiore G, Bindi ML, Romanelli AM, et al. Fast track in liver transplantation: 5 years' experience. *Eur J Anesthesiol.* 2005;22:584–590.
40. Marcel RJ, Ramsay MA, Hein HA, et al. Duration of rocuronium-induced neuromuscular block during liver transplantation: a predictor of primary allograft function. *Anesth Analg.* 1997;84(4):870–874.
41. Wiklund RA. Preoperative preparation of patients with advanced liver disease. *Crit Care Med.* 2004;32(S4):S106–S115.
42. Massicotte L, Lenis S, Thibeault L, et al. Effect of low central venous pressure and phlebotomy on blood product transfusion requirements during liver transplantation. *Liver Transpl.* 2006;12:117–123.
43. Shore-Lesserson L, Manspeizer HE, DePerio M, et al. Thromboelastography-guided transfusion algorithm reduces transfusions in complex cardiac surgery. *Anesth Analg.* 1999;88(2):312–319.
44. Findlay JY, Rettke SR, Ereth MH, et al. Aprotinin reduces red blood cell transfusion in orthotopic liver transplantation: a prospective, randomized, double blind study. *Liver Transpl.* 2001;7(9):802–807.
45. Porte RJ, Molenaar IQ, Begliomini B, et al., for the ESMALT Study Group. Aprotinin and transfusion requirements in orthotopic liver transplantation: a multicentre randomized double-blind study. *Lancet.* 2000;355(9212):1303–1309.
46. Groenland THN, Porte RJ. Antifibrinolytics in liver transplantation. *Int Anesthesiol Clin.* 2006;44(3):83–97.
47. Heindel SW, Mill M, Freid EB, et al. Fatal thrombosis associated with a hemi-Fontan procedure, heparin-protamine reversal and aprotinin. *Anesthesiology.* 2001;94(2):369–371.
48. Ellis JE, Lichtor JL, Feinstein SB, et al. Right heart dysfunction, pulmonary embolism, and paradoxical embolization during liver transplantation. A transesophageal two-dimensional echocardiographic study. *Anesth Analg.* 1989;68(6):777–782.
49. Fitzsimmons MG, Peterfreund RA, Raines DE. Aprotinin administration and pulmonary thromboembolism during orthotopic liver transplantation: report of two cases. *Anesth Analg.* 2001;92:1418–1421.
50. O'Connor CJ, Roozeboom D, Brown R, et al. Pulmonary thromboembolism during liver transplantation: possible association with antifibrinolytic drugs and novel treatment options. *Anesth Analg.* 2000;91:296–299.
51. Soilleux H, Gillon MC, Mirand A, et al. Comparative effects of small and large dose aprotinin doses on bleeding during orthotopic liver transplantation. *Anesth Analg.* 1995;80:349–352.
52. Mahdy AM, Webster NR. Perioperative systemic haemostatic agents. *Br J Anaesth.* 2004;93(6):842–858.
53. Mangano DT, Tudor IC, Dietzel C. The risk associated with aprotinin in cardiac surgery. *N Engl J Med.* 2006;354(4):353–365.
54. Martinowitz U. The use of rFVIIa as adjunct treatment for hemorrhage control in trauma and surgery. *Bloodline Rev.* 2001;1:9–11.
55. Bosch J, Thabut D, Bendtsen F, et al. Recombinant factor VIIa for upper gastrointestinal bleeding in patients with cirrhosis: a randomized, double blind trial. *Gastroenterology.* 2004;127:1123–1130.
56. Lodge JPA, Jonas S, Jones RM, et al. Efficacy and safety of repeated perioperative doses of recombinant factor VIIa in liver transplantation. *Liver Transpl.* 2005;11(8):973–979.
57. Planinsic RM, van der Meer J, Testa G, et al. Safety and efficacy of a single bolus administration of recombinant factor VIIa in liver transplantation due to chronic liver disease. *Liver Transpl.* 2005;11(8):895–900.
58. Shangraw RE. Metabolic issues in liver transplantation. *Int Anesthesiol Clin.* 2006;44(3):1–20.
59. Merten GJ, Burgess WP, Gray LV, et al. Prevention of contrast-induced nephropathy with sodium bicarbonate. *JAMA.* 2005;291(19):2328–2334.
60. Abbasoglu O, Goldstein RM, Vodapally MS, et al. Liver transplantation in hyponatremic patients with emphasis on central pontine myelinolysis. *Clin Transplant.* 1998;12:263–269.
61. Lampl C, Yazdi K. Central pontine myelinolysis. *Eur Neurol.* 2002;47:3–10.
62. Vater Y, Levy A, Martay K, et al. Adjuvant drugs for end-stage liver failure and transplantation. *Med Sci Monit.* 2004;10(4):RA77–RA88.
63. Ranasinghe DN, Mallett SV. Hypomagnesaemia, cardiac arrhythmias, and orthotopic liver transplantation. *Anaesthesia.* 1994;49(5):403–405.
64. Choi JH, Lee J, Park CM. Magnesium therapy improves thromboelastographic findings before liver transplantation: a preliminary study. *Can J Anesth.* 2005;52(2):156–159.
65. Shi X, Xu Z, Xu H, et al. Cardiac arrest after graft reperfusion during liver transplantation. *Hepatobiliary Pancreat Dis Int.* 2006;5(2):185–189.
66. Heering P, Ivens K, Thumer O, et al. Acid-base balance and substitution fluid during continuous hemofiltration. *Kidney Int.* 1999;56(S72):S37–S40.
67. Burtenshaw AJ, Isaac JL. The role of trans-oesophageal echocardiography for perioperative cardiovascular monitoring during orthotopic liver transplantation. *Liver Transpl.* 2006;12:1577–1583.
68. Vater Y, Martay K, et al. Intraoperative epoprostenol and nitric oxide for severe pulmonary hypertension during orthotopic liver transplantation: a case report and review of the literature. *Med Sci Monit.* 2006;12(12):CS115–CS118.
69. Bzeizi KI, Jalan R, Plevris JN, et al. Primary graft dysfunction after liver transplantation: from pathogenesis to prevention. *Liver Transplant Surg.* 1997;3(2):137–148.
70. Burton JR, Rosen HR. Diagnosis and management of allograft failure. *Clin Liver Dis.* 2006;10:407–435.
71. Llado L, Fabregat J, Castellote J, et al. Management of portal vein thrombosis in liver transplantation: influence on morbidity and mortality. *Clin Transplant.* 2007;21(6):716–721.
72. Stange BJ, Glanemann M, Nuessler NC, et al. Hepatic artery thrombosis after adult liver transplantation. *Liver Transplant.* 2003;9(6):612–620.
73. Benseler V, McCaughan GW, Schlitt HJ, et al. The liver: a special case in transplantation tolerance. *Semin Liver Dis.* 2007;27(2):194–213.

74. Wiesner RH, Rakela J, Ishtani MB, et al. Recent advance in liver transplantation. *Mayo Clin Proc.* 2003;78:197–210.
75. Hirose R, Vincenti F. Immunosuppression: today, tomorrow and withdrawal. *Semin Liver Dis.* 2006;26(3):201–210.
76. Gornicka B, Ziarkiewicz-Wroblewska M, Bogdanska U, et al. Pathomorphological features of acute rejection in patients after orthotopic liver transplantation: own experience. *Transplant Proc.* 2006;38:221–225.
77. Encke J, Waldemar U, Stremmel W, et al. Immunosuppression and modulation in liver transplantation. *Nephrol Dial Transplant.* 2004;19(S4):iv22–iv25.
78. Moser MAJ, Wall WJ. Management of biliary problems after liver transplantation. *Liver Transpl.* 2001;11(S1):S46–S52.
79. Tanaka K, Ogura Y. "Small-for-size graft" and "small-for-size syndrome" in living donor liver transplantation. *Yonsei Med J.* 2004:45(6):1089–1094.

CHAPTER 94 ■ PANCREATIC TRANSPLANTATION

RAJA KANDASWAMY • DAVID E. R. SUTHERLAND

The treatment options for insulin-dependent diabetes mellitus are (a) exogenous insulin administration or (b) β-cell replacement by pancreas or islet transplantation. Exogenous insulin administration is burdensome to the patient and gives imperfect glycemic control, predisposing to secondary complications of the eyes, nerves, kidneys, and other systems. On the other hand, β-cell replacement, when successful, establishes a constant euglycemic state but requires major surgery (a pancreas transplant) and immunosuppression to prevent rejection, predisposing to complications, often compounded by comorbidities from pre-existing diabetes.

The Diabetes Control and Complications Trial (1) showed that intensive insulin therapy (multiple injections per day with dose adjusted by frequent blood sugar determinations) decreased (although rarely normalized) glycosylated hemoglobin levels and reduced the rate of secondary complications (2). The threshold for totally eliminating the risks of secondary diabetic complications was perfect glycemic control, an objective that cannot be achieved by even the most sophisticated exogenous insulin delivery devices available today. This may change in the future with real-time glucose monitoring systems combined with insulin pumps (3,4). Pancreas transplantation induces insulin independence in diabetic recipients without the risk of hypoglycemia and can ameliorate secondary complications. With major advances in the management of pancreas transplantation, the success rate of pancreas transplants has progressively increased during the past two decades (5). Today's recipients have a high probability of being insulin independent for years, if not indefinitely.

Historically, islet transplants have been less successful for a variety of reasons (6). In the late 1990s at the University of Alberta, insulin independence was achieved in several consecutive recipients by sequential grafting of islets from multiple donors and the use of a steroid-free nondiabetogenic immunosuppressive regimen (7). In another series from the University of Minnesota with a similar regimen, single-donor islet transplants induced insulin independence (8). In the Minnesota series, the donors had a high body mass index and the recipients had a low body mass index. Thus, the net number of islets transplanted per unit weight was similar in the Alberta and Minnesota series. Islet transplants can succeed with stringent donor and recipient selections, but is not yet able to supersede pancreas transplants as the mainstay of β-cell replacement. Until islet transplants can consistently succeed from a single donor, regardless of size or recipient insulin requirements, an integrated approach is likely. Large donors will be used for islet transplants to recipients with low insulin requirements and the remaining donors (the majority) for pancreas transplants to recipients with average or high insulin requirements. This strategy will maximize the number of recipients of allogenic β-cells and eliminate surgical complications for a subset of patients.

Although short-term islet graft survival appears promising (even with single donors) (9), long-term graft function after islet transplants (even with multiple donors) continues to be a major impediment to rapid progress. In the University of Alberta series, only 10% of islet transplant recipients were insulin independent at 5 years posttransplant (10).

The main tradeoff for recipients of β-cell allografts is the need for immunosuppression. A successful graft makes the recipient euglycemic and normalizes glycosylated hemoglobin levels (11,12), but the combined risks of immunosuppression and pancreas transplant surgery must be weighed against the long-term risks of imperfect glycemic control and of development of secondary complications with exogenous insulin. A randomized prospective trial has not been done to weigh these risks. The burden of day-to-day management of diabetes with need for multiple needlesticks to inject insulin and monitor blood sugar levels tilts the balance in favor of a transplant for many diabetic patients. Furthermore, antirejection strategies are continually being developed to decrease the side effects of immunosuppression. Nevertheless, only a few institutions perform pancreas transplants soon after the onset of the disease (13).

The main indications for a pancreas transplant in patients with normal kidney function has been labile diabetes with frequent insulin reactions and hypoglycemic unawareness, a syndrome that may emerge years after the onset of diabetes, particularly in patients with autonomic neuropathy (14). However, even for nonlabile diabetic patients who attempt tight control by intensive glucose monitoring, literature shows a high rate of secondary complications that are just as morbid as (15), if not more so than, chronic immunosuppressive complications in organ allograft recipients (16,17). Thus, for a patient who wishes to avoid a lifetime of insulin injections and glucose monitoring and who prefers the risks of immunosuppressive complications to the secondary complications of diabetes, a pancreas transplant can be performed with good results (18). This also applies to type 2 diabetics who are obligatory insulin dependent. About 5% of pancreas transplants are performed in selected type 2 diabetics (19).

In the past, most pancreas transplant candidates had advanced diabetic nephropathy and required a kidney transplant also. The risks of immunosuppression are about to be assumed because of the kidney transplant, so a simultaneous or sequential pancreas transplant does not pose any additional risks other than surgery (13). Indeed, pancreas transplants have been done in renal allograft recipients who meet the criteria for type 2 diabetes with elimination of the need for exogenous insulin (20).

RECIPIENT CATEGORIES

Diabetic pancreas transplant candidates are divided into three categories: uremic (need a kidney transplant), posturemic (have a functioning kidney transplant), and nonuremic (do not need a kidney transplant). For candidates who are uremic, the options are to receive kidney and pancreas transplants either simultaneously in one operation or sequentially in separate operations. The decision as to which option to take is usually based on the availability and suitability of living and cadaveric donors for one or both organs.

Accordingly, there are three broad categories of recipients: simultaneous pancreas–kidney (SPK), pancreas after kidney (PAK), and pancreas transplants alone (PTA).

1. SPK transplants: Most SPK transplants have been done with both organs coming from the same cadaveric donor. Because a large number of patients are waiting for a kidney, unless priority is given to SPK candidates, waiting times tend to be long (years). Thus, to avoid two operations and a long wait, a simultaneous kidney and segmental pancreas transplant from a living donor can be done (20–22). Only a few centers offer this option (23,24). There has been a report from Japan of a successful islet transplantation from a live donor (25). Therefore, a simultaneous living-donor islet kidney transplant may become a viable option in the future (26,27). If a living donor is suitable for or only willing to give a kidney, another option is a simultaneous living-donor kidney and cadaveric pancreas transplant (23,24). For these options, the living kidney donor usually must be available on a moment's notice (the same as for the recipient), as the cadaveric pancreas must be transplanted soon after procurement. Alternatively, a recipient of a scheduled living-donor kidney transplant could also receive a cadaveric pancreas simultaneously if one became available fortuitously. If not, and only a kidney is transplanted, the recipient becomes a PAK candidate.
2. PAK transplants: For nephropathic diabetic patients who have already undergone a kidney transplant from a living or a cadaveric donor, a PAK transplant can be performed. Most PAK transplants today are done in patients who previously received a living-donor kidney because suitable uremic diabetic patients without a living donor will undergo a cadaveric pancreas transplant. Although a PAK means a uremic diabetic patient requires two operations to achieve both a dialysis-free and insulin-independent state, the two transplants done separately are smaller procedures than a combined transplant. The interval between the living-donor kidney and cadaveric pancreas transplant depends on several factors, including recipient recovery from the kidney transplant and donor availability, but the outcome is similar for all intervals more than 1 month. PAK is the largest pancreas transplant category at the University of Minnesota (28–30).
3. PTA: For recipients with adequate kidney function, a solitary pancreas transplant can be performed from either a living or a cadaveric donor. Because the waiting time for a cadaveric pancreas is relatively short at the present time, living-donor pancreas transplants are done infrequently, but are particularly indicated if a candidate has a high panel-reactive antibody and a negative cross-match to a living donor. Most PTA candidates have problems with glycemic control, hypoglycemic unawareness, and frequent insulin reactions. A successful PTA not only obviates these problems, but also improves the quality of life, and may ameliorate secondary complications, thus increasing the applicability of PTA (28–31).

EVOLUTION AND IMPROVEMENTS

The first clinical pancreas transplant was performed at the University of Minnesota in 1966 (32). The number of transplants remained low during the 1970s, but progressively increased in the 1980s, following the introduction of cyclosporine. By the end of 2000, more than 15,000 pancreas transplants had been performed at more than 1,000 centers worldwide (Figs. 94.1 and 94.2), including more than 11,000 in the United States (33). By the mid-1990s, more than 1,000 pancreas transplants were being done annually in the United States (5).

The history of pancreas transplants involves many different techniques and eras (34). The first series of pancreas transplants at the University of Minnesota used enteric drainage (ED) (32). Urinary drainage was first done into the ureter by Gliedman in the early 1970s (33,34), then via duct injection by Dubernard et al. (35) in 1974, and then via direct bladder drainage (BD) by Sollinger et al. (36) in 1982. During the 1980s, BD became the predominant technique (Fig. 94.3) with good results (37). ED was still used (38), although sparingly, but in the 1990s it became more frequent (Fig. 94.4), especially in SPK transplants.

Venous drainage of the pancreas has also evolved over the years. Portal drainage was used with segmental grafts in the 1980s (39–42). For whole-organ pancreas transplants, systemic drainage was the norm until the 1990s, when portal drainage gained popularity, especially with ED (43,44), as opposed to BD (45). Between 1996 and 2000, about one fifth of all SPKs used portal drainage, by anastomosis either to the recipient splenic vein (40) or, more commonly, to the superior mesenteric vein (46) (Fig. 94.5).

Before techniques were developed to procure both liver and pancreas grafts with intact blood supply (47,48), segmental pancreas grafts were commonly used. Currently, whole-organ pancreaticoduodenal grafts predominate (49), although segmental grafts are still used for living-donor pancreas

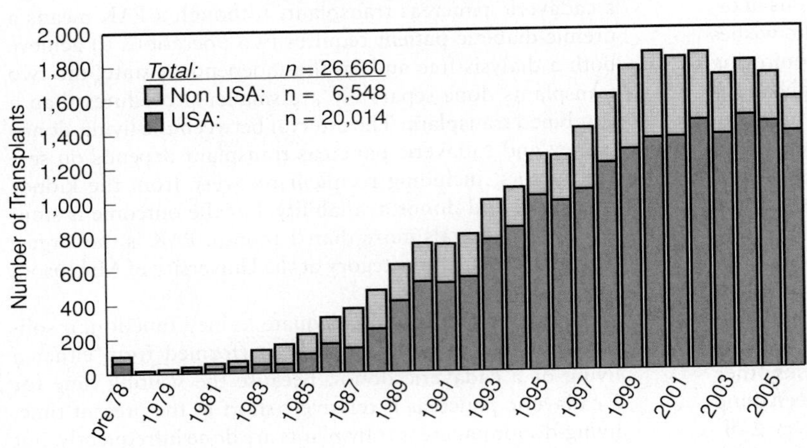

FIGURE 94.1. Number of pancreas transplants worldwide tabulated by the International Pancreas Transplant Registry from 1966 to 2005.

transplants (28). The first living-donor pancreas transplant was performed at the University of Minnesota in 1979 (50). The early series of living-donor pancreas transplants consisted of solitary pancreases because the rejection rate of cadaveric pancreases was high (23). In the 1990s, living-donor pancreas transplants were predominantly performed in combination with a kidney from the same donor (Fig. 94.6) (22,51–53). Recently, living-donor segmental pancreatectomy has been performed laparoscopically (54). Another approach, as previously mentioned, is to perform a living-donor kidney transplant simultaneously with a cadaveric pancreas transplant (24).

Immunosuppressive regimens have made great strides over the years. Today, there are more than 100 pancreas transplant centers in the United States (55). Some centers have reported extensive experience. For example, more than 500 SPK transplants have been performed at the University of Wisconsin (56), and more than 1,000 pancreas transplants of all categories have been performed at the University of Minnesota (28). The International Pancreas Transplant Registry, formed in 1980, collects data from all centers in the world (57) and is the best resource for outcome analysis.

RESULTS

Outcomes after pancreas transplants have consistently improved over the years (5). The latest report from the International Pancreas Transplant Registry (5) outlined recent results, focusing on U.S. transplants from 2000 through 2004, including more than 3,800 SPK, more than 600 PAK, and 290 PTA cases. Patient survival rates for all three categories was more than 95% at 1 year posttransplant (Fig. 94.7). Primary pancreas graft survival rates at 1 year posttransplant were higher for SPK (85%) than for PAK (78%) and PTA (76%) recipients (Fig. 94.8). Graft loss from rejection was low at 1 year in all three categories (2% SPK, 8% PAK, 10% PTA). In the majority of all transplants, ED was used for duct management, and of the ED transplants, portal venous drainage was used in about 25% of cases. Although overall graft function did not vary with ED or BD, the PTA group had a higher immunologic graft loss rate in ED versus BD cases. BD may result in earlier diagnosis of rejection because of the ability to monitor for a decline in urine amylase activity as a marker (28). Nevertheless, the late rejection rate is higher in the PTA than in other categories.

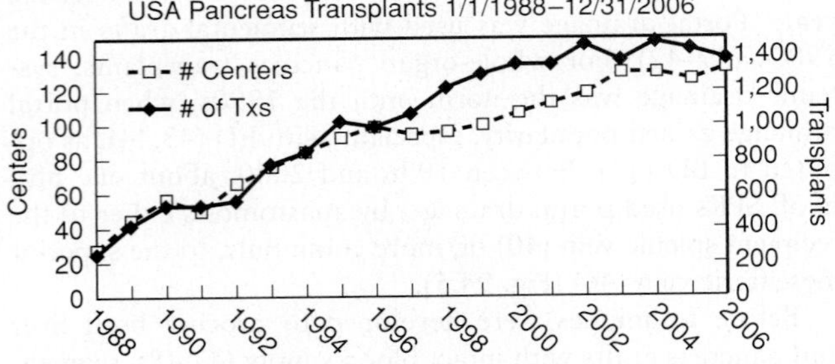

FIGURE 94.2. Number of transplant centers worldwide tabulated by the International Pancreas Transplant Registry from 1966 to 2006. Tx, transplant.

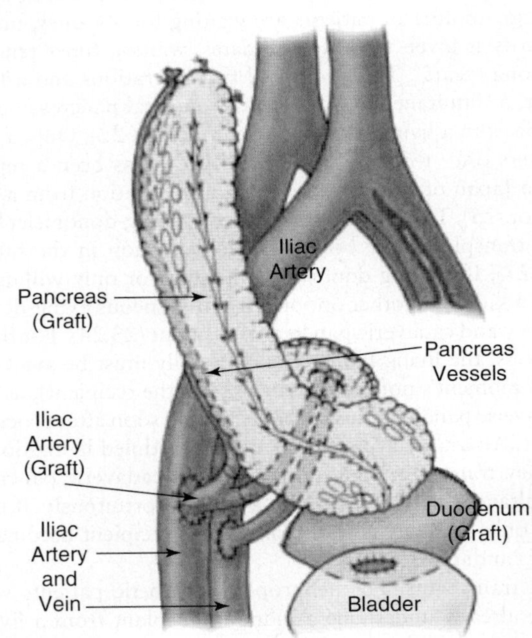

FIGURE 94.3. Bladder-drained (BD) pancreaticoduodenal transplant alone (PTA) from a cadaver donor.

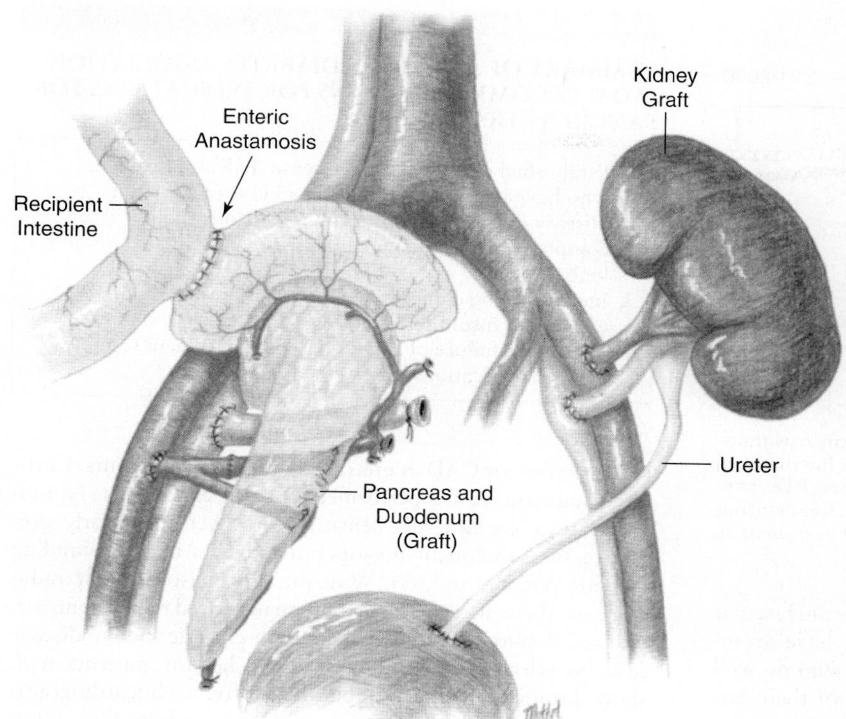

FIGURE 94.4. Enteric-drained (ED) simultaneous pancreas and kidney (SPK) transplant from a cadaver donor with systemic venous drainage.

INDICATIONS AND CONTRAINDICATIONS

The indications for a pancreas transplant have evolved and expanded over the years as the results have improved. The position statement of the American Diabetes Association (58) on indications for a pancreas transplant (Table 94.1) is conservative. A pancreas transplant is also indicated for patients who have developed secondary complications of diabetes. The progression of complications is halted by a functioning pancreas graft. In fact, even an improvement in neuropathy has been documented (22,34,59,60). In addition to improvement in glomerular architecture, a recent study shows that interstitial expansion is reversible, and atrophic tubules can be reabsorbed (61). Advanced retinopathy and vascular disease, however, are unaffected (62). Atherosclerotic risk factors decrease and endothelial function improves posttransplant (63). A pancreas transplant should be offered early, before the onset of complications of diabetes, to interested patients who understand the risk of immunosuppression versus the benefit of insulin independence and freedom from diabetic complications.

Contraindications include those for any other transplant, such as malignancy, active infections, noncompliance,

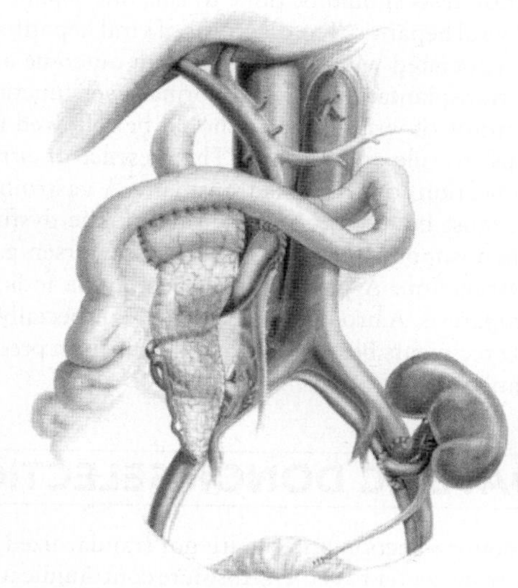

FIGURE 94.5. Enteric drainage (ED) simultaneous pancreas and kidney (SPK) transplants with portal venous drainage of the pancreas graft via the superior mesenteric vein.

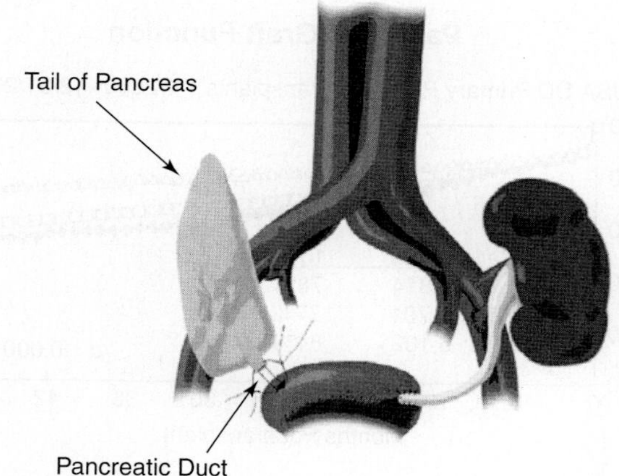

FIGURE 94.6. Simultaneous segmental pancreas and kidney transplant from a living donor (LD). Either bladder drainage (BD) or enteric drainage (ED) can be used, but the BD technique has a lower complication rate and is illustrated.

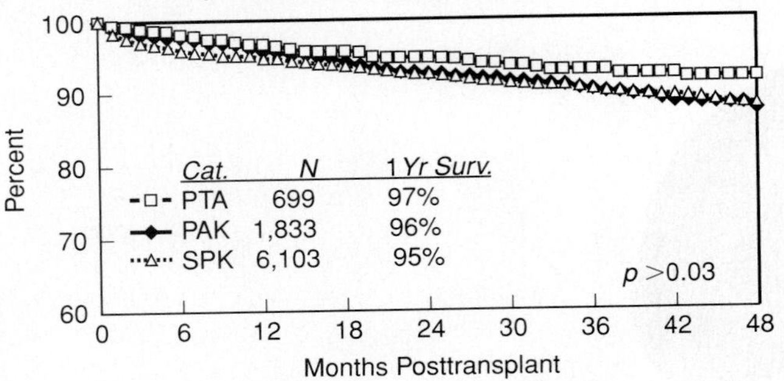

FIGURE 94.7. Patient survival after primary cadaver pancreas transplants in the United States from 1997 to 2006 by the International Pancreas Transplant Registry (IPTR). DD, deceased donor; PTA, pancreas transplant alone; PAK, pancreas after kidney; SPK, simultaneous pancreas–kidney; Cat, category; N, numbers; 1 Yr Surv, 1 year survival.

serious psychosocial problems, and prohibitive cardiovascular risk. Candidates with advanced vascular disease have an increased risk of surgical complications, yet those who do well posttransplant greatly benefit from stabilization of their cardiovascular risk.

Although it was clear that insulin-dependent recipients with renal failure benefited from a pancreas transplant in addition to the kidney, the survival benefit for pancreas transplant in patients with preserved renal function was questioned by at least one study (64). However, a more comprehensive reanalysis revealed that there was no increased mortality for solitary pancreas transplant recipients over wait-listed patients (65,66).

PRETRANSPLANT EVALUATION

The pretransplant workup should include a detailed medical and psychosocial evaluation. Cardiac risk assessment is mandatory because diabetes is a major risk factor for coronary artery disease (CAD). Cardiologists vary on the type of

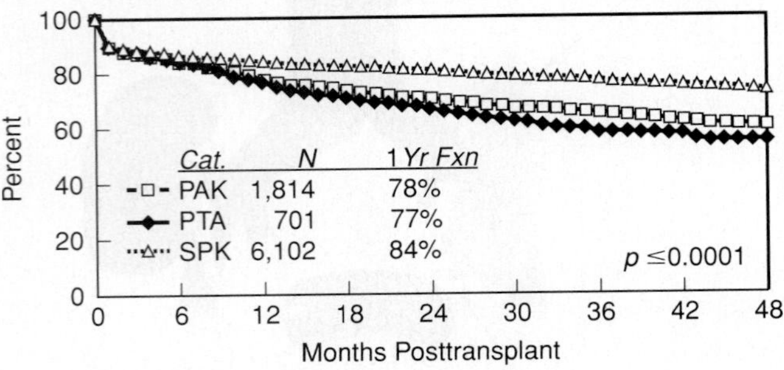

FIGURE 94.8. Pancreas graft survival after primary cadaver pancreas transplants in the United States from 1997 to 2006 by International Pancreas Transplant Registry. DD, deceased donor; PTA, pancreas transplant alone; PAK, pancreas after kidney; SPK, simultaneous pancreas–kidney; Cat, category; N, numbers; 1 Yr Fxn, 1 year function.

TABLE 94.1

SUMMARY OF AMERICAN DIABETES ASSOCIATION (ADA) RECOMMENDATIONS FOR INDICATIONS FOR PANCREAS TRANSPLANTS

1. Established end-stage renal disease (ESRD) in patients who have had, or plan to have, a kidney transplant
2. History of frequent, acute, and severe metabolic complications (e.g., hypoglycemia, hyperglycemia, ketoacidosis)
3. Incapacitating clinical and emotional problems with exogenous insulin prescription
4. Consistent failure of insulin-based management to prevent acute complications

test to screen for CAD in pretransplant diabetic patients. Coronary angiograms are performed in most candidates. Noninvasive tests are not very sensitive for CAD and poorly predictive for subsequent postoperative events in long-standing diabetic patients (67,68). With the use of iso-osmolar radio contrast, there does not seem to be an increased risk of contrast-induced nephropathy in patients with chronic kidney disease (69). In selected patients (i.e., young, healthy patients with short-duration diabetes), dobutamine stress echocardiograms are used for cardiac evaluation with good results (70). Once significant CAD is detected, aggressive treatment by revascularization, angioplasty, or stenting is recommended. In one study, revascularized transplant candidates had significantly fewer postoperative cardiac events, as compared with those who received medical therapy alone (71).

A detailed vascular examination must be done to rule out significant vascular insufficiency. If such insufficiency is found, it may need correction pretransplant because the transplant surgery, involving an anastomosis to the iliac artery, may further diminish lower-extremity blood flow.

Pulmonary function tests are indicated in chronic smokers and patients with a history of chronic pulmonary disease. Postoperative intensive care unit monitoring and perioperative bronchodilator therapy may be indicated in some patients. Liver function tests should be done to rule out hepatic insufficiency and viral hepatitis. The diagnosis of viral hepatitis (either B or C) is associated with worse long-term outcome after extrahepatic transplantation (72). Abnormal liver function tests or the diagnosis of viral hepatitis should be followed up with a liver biopsy to rule out cirrhosis. The presence of cirrhosis is a contraindication for pancreas transplant. A gastrointestinal evaluation must be done to rule out autonomic dysfunction. Some immunosuppressive medications may worsen gastrointestinal dysfunction. A prokinetic agent may be indicated to treat gastroparesis. A urologic examination is especially important for BD recipients because bladder dysfunction predisposes to graft pancreatitis.

CADAVERIC DONOR SELECTION

Pancreas donor selection criteria are not standardized, but instead vary from center to center. Absolute contraindications are the obvious ones applied to most solid organs: active hepatitis B, C, and non A–non B; human immunodeficiency virus; non–central nervous system (CNS) malignancy; surgical or traumatic damage to the pancreas; history of diabetes mellitus; pancreatitis; and extremes of age (younger than 10 or older than 60 years). Prolonged intensive care unit stay and duration of brain death have been associated with an increased risk of graft failure (73). Other studies have shown that donor age is important. Even middle-aged donors (older than 40 years) are associated with increased complications and graft failure (73–75). However, so-called marginal donor organs are associated with good outcome if the pancreas, on inspection, is found to be "healthy" in appearance (76,77).

Donors after cardiac death are being used increasingly to expand the donor pool. However, there may be a higher rate of early organ dysfunction with these donors (78). A recent survey showed equivalent patient and graft survival at 1, 3, and 5 years in SPK transplant recipients from donors after cardiac death compared with donors after brain death (78).

PANCREAS PRESERVATION

University of Wisconsin (UW) solution was first used for pancreas preservation in a preclinical model in 1987 (79). As with most solid organs, *in vivo* flush followed by simple storage in cold University of Wisconsin solution is the standard for pancreas preservation. In the original model, pancreases were preserved for up to 96 hours (80). In clinical transplantation, pancreas cold preservation exceeding 24 hours has been associated with increased graft dysfunction (81). Even less than 24 hours, it has been shown that the longer the cold ischemia time, the greater the technical complication rate (82). Therefore, every effort should be made to minimize the cold ischemia time in order to optimize graft function and to lower complication rates. Recent data suggest a new method of preservation that may be advantageous: the two-layer method using University of Wisconsin solution and perfluorochemical (83). This method allows for longer preservation time while providing a mechanism for repair of ischemic damage due to cold storage (84–86). More clinical trials are needed before the two-layer method becomes routine.

Recently, histidine-tryptophan ketoglutarate solution has been increasingly used in pancreas transplantation (87). Advantages include lower viscosity, less potassium, and lower cost. Early outcome studies do not show inferiority compared to the more expensive UW solution (88,89).

HUMAN LEUKOCYTE ANTIGEN MATCHING

The impact of human leukocyte antigen (HLA) matching on outcome varies. It is generally accepted that HLA matching has little effect on graft outcome for the SPK category (90,91), although higher rejection rates have been reported with poor matches (92–94). For solitary pancreas transplants (PAK and PTA), the data are mixed, ranging from studies showing no impact (95) to registry data showing that HLA A and B matches have a significant impact (91). At the University of Minnesota, SPKs are done regardless of HLA match; for PAKs, generally at least one antigen in the B locus matches, and for PTAs, at least one antigen in each of the A, B, and DR loci.

ANESTHETIC CONSIDERATIONS

A patient with brittle diabetes and secondary complications (e.g., CAD, autonomic neuropathy) can pose special problems for the anesthesiologist. Dysautonomic response to drugs or hypoxia can lead to significant morbidity (96) and even death (97). It has also been documented that long-standing diabetes poses a challenge to the anesthesiologist during intubation (98). Awareness of these risks and employment of an experienced anesthesiology team might help decrease the risks or morbidity. A major operation such as a pancreas transplant or combined kidney–pancreas transplant is often prolonged and can be associated with significant blood loss. Prompt replacement with blood or colloids should be instituted to avoid hypoperfusion after significant blood loss. Before and after revascularization of the pancreas, careful blood glucose monitoring, along with continuous intravenous (IV) insulin therapy to maintain tight control of blood glucose levels, is essential. Perioperative β-blockade should be considered for long-standing diabetic patients with a cardiac history.

BACK-TABLE PREPARATION OF THE DONOR PANCREAS

Once the donor pancreas has been opened in the recipient operating room, some back-table work is necessary to prepare it for the transplant, including these steps:

1. Donor splenectomy (taking care to avoid injury to the pancreatic tail)
2. Trimming down of the donor duodenum to the shortest length without damage to the main or accessory duct (especially important with BD to minimize bicarbonate loss)
3. Oversewing or individual vessel ligation of the mesocolic and mesenteric stumps on the anterior aspect of the pancreas
4. Excision of lymphatic and ganglionic tissue in the periportal area
5. Reconstruction of the splenic and superior mesenteric arteries with a Y graft of the donor iliac A bifurcation (to provide for a single arterial anastomosis in the recipient)

RECIPIENT OPERATION

Several techniques have been described for the recipient operation (99). The techniques vary based on whether a solitary pancreas transplant (PTA, PAK) or a combined transplant (SPK) is done.

Solitary Pancreas Transplant

The major surgical considerations for solitary pancreas transplants include:

1. Choice of exocrine secretion of the pancreas, drainage of bowel or bladder: Currently, for pancreas transplants in the United States, 67% of PAK, 56% of PTA, and 81% of SPK transplants are drained enterically (5). ED is more physiologic and does away with the complications of BD (e.g., acidosis, pancreatitis, urinary infections, hematuria). Between

10% and 20% of BD recipients are ultimately converted to ED because of such complications once they are 6 to 12 months posttransplant and their rejection risk is lower. BD, however, allows for direct measurement of urinary amylase as a marker of exocrine function. A decrease in urine amylase is sensitive, but not very specific, for acute rejection of the pancreas (100). Hyperglycemia is a late event in the rejection, and a decrease in urine amylase occurs early. Thus, rejection episodes are detected early with BD, and the rejection loss rate is lower with BD than with other techniques (55).

In clinical practice, the choice of exocrine drainage varies. Some groups always use ED (101,102), while some always use BD (101). Others base it on the individual recipient's immunologic risk versus the risk of urologic complications (28). The surgical risks and short-term outcome with both techniques are comparable (74,103). ED is likely to predominate as the major technique in the future as immunologic strategies to eliminate rejection are developed (102).

2. Choice of venous drainage, portal or systemic: Currently in the United States, of all ED transplants, 20% of SPK, 23% of PAK, and 35% of PTA cases are drained to the portal vein (5). Portal drainage is more physiologic than systemic drainage (104,105). Theoretically, portal drainage preserves the first-pass metabolism of insulin in the liver. Therefore, portally drained recipients will have lower systemic insulin levels (106). However, there is no evidence of any detrimental effect on lipid levels (107) or on risk of vascular disease (62) as seen in *de novo* hyperinsulinemia (syndrome X).

   Portal venous drainage is difficult to perform with exocrine BD (45). However, portal drainage is likely to increase in popularity, given some reports that rejection rates are lower in this category (103,108). Recent modifications include a retroperitoneal portal-enteric drainage technique (109).
3. Whether to transplant the whole organ or a segment: Almost all cadaveric pancreas transplants performed today use whole-organ grafts. Segmental grafts have little role to play in this group, except when a rare anatomic abnormality is noted such that the head of the pancreas cannot be used. A rare instance of a split cadaveric pancreas transplanted into two different recipients has been described (110). All living-donor pancreas transplants use segmental grafts (body and tail); doing so maintains normoglycemia in the recipient (12).

Simultaneous Pancreas–Kidney

SPK transplants have a lower rejection rate than do solitary pancreases. Further, rejection episodes are rarely isolated to the pancreas alone. Most pancreas rejection episodes can be indirectly detected by monitoring serum creatinine as a marker for kidney rejection. Therefore, most SPK transplants are done using ED, as advocated by the Stockholm group (111) (Fig. 94.4). With ED, the risk of acute technical complications is slightly higher, but the chronic complication rate is lower (112). Choice of venous drainage varies by center. Because ED is the choice for exocrine drainage, there is no impediment to performing portal venous drainage (Fig. 94.4).

POSTOPERATIVE CARE

After an uncomplicated pancreas transplant, the recipient is transferred to the postanesthesia care unit or the surgical intensive care unit. Centers that have a specialized monitored transplant unit (with central venous and arterial monitoring capabilities) transition the postoperative recipients through the postanesthesia care unit to the transplant unit. Others transfer directly to the surgical intensive care unit for the first 24 to 48 hours. Care during the first few hours posttransplant is similar to care after any major operative procedure. Careful monitoring of vital signs, central venous pressure, oxygen saturation, and hematologic and laboratory parameters is crucial. The following factors are unique to pancreas recipients and should be attended to:

1. Blood glucose levels: Any sudden, unexplained increase in glucose levels should raise the suspicion of graft thrombosis. An immediate ultrasound examination must be done to assess blood flow to the graft. Maintenance of tight glucose control (less than 150 mg/dL) using an IV insulin drip is important to "rest" the pancreas in the early postoperative period.
2. Intravascular volume: Because the pancreas is a "low-flow" organ, intravascular volume must be maintained to provide adequate perfusion to the graft. Central venous pressure monitoring is used to monitor intravascular volume status. In some cases, such as patients with depressed cardiac function, pulmonary artery catheter monitoring may be required during the first 24 to 48 hours. If the hypovolemia is associated with low hemoglobin levels, then washed packed red blood cell transfusions should be given. Otherwise, colloid or crystalloid replacement can be used.
3. Maintenance IV fluid therapy: The choice of IV fluid is usually 5% dextrose in half normal saline. The use of dextrose is not contraindicated and may be of benefit, as long as IV insulin is used to maintain good blood glucose control. In SPK recipients, whose IV rate is based on urine output, dextrose should be eliminated if the urine output is high (more than 500 mL/hour). Maintenance solution for BD recipients should include 10 mEq of HCO_3 added to each liter to account for the excess HCO_3 loss (113,114). Sodium lactate can be used as an alternative (115).
4. Antibiotic therapy: Broad-spectrum antibiotic therapy (with strong Gram-negative coverage) and antifungal therapy are instituted before the incision is made in the operating room, then continued for 3 days (for antibiotics) and 7 days (for antifungal). At the University of Minnesota, since the introduction of this protocol, we have noted a decrease in postoperative abdominal infections (74). Cytomegalovirus (CMV) and antiviral prophylaxis is similar to that for other solid organs.
5. Octreotide: The use of octreotide in pancreas recipients helps reduce the incidence of technical complications (116). This benefit should be weighed against evidence, in rat studies, that shows decreased pancreatic islet blood flow with octreotide use (117), although clinically no detrimental effects of octreotide use have been documented. A dose of 100 to 150 μg IV or subcutaneously three times a day is administered for 5 days posttransplant. Dose adjustments may be made for nausea, which is the predominant side effect.

6. Anticoagulation: The use of low-dose heparin in the early postoperative period (days 0–5) decreases the risk of graft thrombosis (118). An intraoperative dose of 70 units/kg is given, followed by an IV infusion of 3 units/kg started at 4 hours postoperatively and gradually increased up to 7 units/kg (depending on hemodynamic stability and hemoglobin levels). Enteric-coated aspirin (8 mg) is started on day 1 and continued for 6 months. At the University of Minnesota, this protocol decreased the thrombosis rate from about 12% to 6%, but increased the relaparotomy rate due to bleeding from 4% to 6%. Segmental pancreas transplants (as in living-donor transplants) have a higher thrombosis risk and therefore therapeutic heparinization (with a target partial thromboplastin time of 50) for 5 days and Coumadin therapy (with a target international normalized ratio of 2–2.5) are recommended for 6 months. The higher risk of thrombosis is due to the smaller vessels in a segmental graft (119,120).

IMMUNOSUPPRESSION

Immunosuppression is essential to thwart rejection in all allotransplant recipients (17). Before the advent of cyclosporine in the early 1980s (121), azathioprine and prednisone were the mainstays of immunosuppression. From the early 1980s to the mid-1990s, cyclosporine was added to the mix and resulted in significant improvement in immunologic outcomes (122). Since the mid-1990s, tacrolimus and mycophenolate mofetil have replaced cyclosporine and azathioprine as the main drugs, resulting in even better pancreas graft survival rates (122–124). In addition, steroids have been successfully withdrawn from some pancreas recipients (125) and, in some cases, avoided (126). With a recently introduced drug, rapamycin, used in combination with tacrolimus, steroids have been successfully avoided in some pancreas recipients (127,128).

Anti–T-cell therapy has always remained a part of the induction protocol for pancreas recipients. With the recent emphasis on steroid withdrawal or avoidance, anti–T-cell therapy has taken on added importance to avoid rejection. Anti-CD25 antibodies are also used frequently as induction therapy (129). Avoidance of calcineurin inhibitors has been attempted in pancreas transplantation. When combined with steroid avoidance, this required prolonged anti–T-cell therapy, which increases the risk of infection without adequately controlling rejection (130). Table 94.2 presents the immunosuppressive protocol for pancreas transplant recipients at the University of Minnesota.

For PTA recipients, whose rejection rates are the highest of all categories, pretransplant immunosuppression has decreased rejection rates and graft loss from rejection (31). Heavy use of

TABLE 94.2

UNIVERSITY OF MINNESOTA STANDARD IMMUNOSUPPRESSION PANCREAS PROGRAM

SPK	PAK & SPLK	PTA	Rejection
Antithymocyte globulin (1.25 mg/kg)* 5 doses First dose intraoperative Give methylprednisolone 500 mg, 250 mg, and 100 mg before first, second, and third doses, respectively **Tacrolimus** 2 mg PO bid Start when creatinine <3 mg/dL or postoperative day #5, whichever is later If tacrolimus is delayed continue TMG until tacrolimus levels are therapeutic Levels 8–10 ng/mL for 3 mo, then 5–8 ng/mL **Mycophenolate** Start postoperative 1 g PO bid	**Antithymocyte globulin** (1.25 mg/kg)* 7 doses First dose intraoperative Give methylprednisolone 500 mg, 250 mg, and 100 mg before first, second, and third doses, respectively **Tacrolimus** 2 mg PO bid Start postoperative If tacrolimus is delayed continue TMG until tacrolimus levels are therapeutic Levels 8–10 ng/mL for 3 mo, then 5–8 ng/mL **Mycophenolate** Start postoperative 1 g PO bid	**Antithymocyte globulin** (1.25 mg/kg)* 7–10 doses First dose intraoperative Give methylprednisolone 500 mg, 250 mg, and 100 mg before first, second, and third doses, respectively **Tacrolimus** 2 mg PO bid Start postoperative If tacrolimus is delayed continue TMG until tacrolimus levels are therapeutic Levels 8–10 ng/mL for 3 mo, then 5–8 ng/mL **Mycophenolate** Start postoperative 1 g PO bid	**Methylprednisolone** Day #0: 500 mg IV Day #1: 250 mg IV Day #2: 125 mg IV **Antithymocyte globulin** 1.25 mg/kg IV* × 5–7 d Give premedication Monitor ALC *Resistant rejection* **OKT3** qd × 5–7 doses First dose = 5 mg IV Subsequent doses = 2.5 mg IV Give premedication Monitor CD3 **Note:** Kidney rejections on the kidney steroid avoidance study should be treated with Thymoglobulin (mild) or OKT3 (moderate/severe or vascular).

SPK, simultaneous pancreas kidney; PAK, pancreas after kidney; SPLK, simultaneous cadaver pancreas living-donor kidney; TMG, antithymocyte globulin; ALC, absolute lymphocyte count; mo, month.
**Round up antithymocyte globulin dose to the nearest 25.*
ALC levels: If zero, hold antithymocyte globulin; if 0.1 give half-dose antithymocyte globulin; if 0.2 or above give full dose.
CD3 levels (if using OKT3): Monitor effectiveness of antibody therapy. Absolute CD3 level should drop to <100 mm^3. Antithymocyte globulin and OKT3 require "premedication."

immunosuppression may increase the infection rate, but effective antimicrobial prophylaxis has helped ameliorate this problem (131,132).

INTRAVENOUS IMMUNOGLOBULIN AND PLASMAPHERESIS

IV immunoglobulin has many applications in transplantation. It has been used successfully to decrease anti-HLA antibodies in transplant recipients on the waiting list and to shorten their waiting times (133,134). It can also be used to control acute humoral rejection in kidney and heart allograft recipients (135). Plasmapheresis has been used to decrease humoral antibody titers in ABO-incompatible liver and kidney recipients (136,137). It has also been used to control hyperacute and accelerated acute rejection in positive cross-match kidney recipients (138,139) and lung (140) recipients. At the University of Minnesota, for ABO-incompatible (A_2 to O, B, or AB) or positive cross-match (T-cell) pancreas recipients, the treatment protocol consists of intraoperative IV immunoglobulin (0.5 mg/kg) followed by a course of 5 to 7 days in combination with daily plasmapheresis. For B-cell positive cross-match recipients, IV immunoglobulin may be used without plasmapheresis.

SURGICAL COMPLICATIONS

1. Bleeding: Postoperative bleeding is a frequent reason for early relaparotomy in pancreas recipients. The incidence ranges from 6% to 8% (74,141). This risk is increased by the use of anticoagulation in the immediate postoperative period. Frequent physical examinations and monitoring of hemoglobin help detect bleeding early. Heparin may be temporarily suspended to stabilize the patient. If bleeding continues, early operative intervention is indicated. If bleeding stops or slows down, heparin should be restarted at a lower rate and judiciously increased as tolerated.
2. Thrombosis: The incidence of thrombosis posttransplant ranges from 5% to 13% (118,141). The risk is increased after segmental pancreas transplants because of the small caliber of vessels (51). Most thromboses are due to technical reasons. A short portal vein (requiring an extension graft) or atherosclerotic arteries in the pancreas graft increases the risk for thrombosis. In the recipient, a narrow pelvic inlet with a deeply placed iliac vein, atherosclerotic disease of the iliac artery, a technically difficult vascular anastomosis, kinking of the vein by the pancreas graft, significant hematoma formation around the vascular anastomosis, and a hypercoagulable state are some of the factors that increase the risk for thrombosis. The most common form of hypercoagulable state is factor V Leiden mutation in the Western population. The incidence ranges from 2% to 5% but may be as high as 50% to 60% in patients with a history (self or family) of thrombosis (142). Other causes of hypercoagulable state include antithrombin deficiency, protein C or S deficiency, activated protein C resistance, and anticardiolipin antibodies (143).
3. Duodenal leaks: The incidence of duodenal leaks ranges from 4% to 6% (74,141). A leak from the anastomosis of the duodenum to the bowel almost always leads to a relaparotomy. Gross peritoneal contamination due to an enteric leak necessitates a graft pancreatectomy. The diagnosis is made by elevated pancreatic enzymes associated with acute abdomen. The differential diagnosis is pancreatitis, abdominal infection, or acute severe rejection. A Roux-en-Y anastomosis to the pancreatic duodenum may be preferred if the risk of leak is thought to be increased during intraoperative inspection of the pancreas. Other novel techniques such as a venting jejunostomy (Roux-en-Y) have been used in selected recipients (144).

   Duodenal leaks in BD recipients are usually managed nonoperatively with prolonged catheter decompression of the urinary bladder. The diagnosis is made using plain or computed tomography (CT) cystography. The size and extent of the leak cannot always be assessed by the imaging studies. Large leaks may require operative intervention, such as a repair or enteric conversion (145).
4. Major intra-abdominal infections: The incidence of intra-abdominal infections requiring reoperation ranges from 4% to 10% (74,141). Opening the duodenal segment intraoperatively, with associated contamination, predisposes to this high rate. Fungal and Gram-negative infections predominate. With the advent of advanced interventional radiologic procedures to drain intra-abdominal abscesses, the incidence of reoperations is fast decreasing. If the infection is uncontrolled or widespread, then graft pancreatectomy followed by frequent washouts may be necessary.
5. Renal pedicle torsion: Torsion of the kidney has been reported after the SPK transplants (146,147). The intraperitoneal location of the kidney (allowing for more mobility) predisposes to this complication. Additional risk factors are a long renal pedicle (more than 5 cm) and a marked discrepancy between the length of artery and vein. Prophylactic nephropexy to the anterior or lateral abdominal wall is recommended in intraperitoneal transplants to avoid this problem.
6. Others: Other surgical complications that may require laparotomy also decreased from 9% to 1%. Improved anti-infective prophylaxis, surgical techniques, immunosuppression, and advances in interventional radiology have all contributed to this disease (74).

NONSURGICAL COMPLICATIONS

1. Pancreatitis: The incidence of posttransplant pancreatitis varies based on the type of exocrine drainage. BD recipients with abnormal bladder function are at increased risk secondary to incomplete bladder emptying or urine retention causing resistance to the flow of pancreatic exocrine secretions. Other causes of pancreatitis include drugs (corticosteroids, azathioprine, cyclosporine), hypercalcemia, viral infections (CMV or hepatitis C), and reperfusion injury after prolonged ischemia. Pancreatitis is usually manifested by an increase in serum amylase and lipase with or without local signs of inflammation. The treatment usually consists of catheter decompression of the bladder for a period of 2 to 6 weeks, depending on the severity. In addition, octreotide therapy may be used to decrease pancreatic secretions. The

underlying urologic problem, if any, should be treated. If repeated episodes of pancreatitis occur, an enteric conversion of exocrine drainage may be indicated (148–150).

2. Rejection: The incidence of rejection is discussed in the Results section earlier in this chapter. The diagnosis is usually based on an increase in serum amylase and lipase and a decrease in urine amylase in BD recipients. A sustained significant drop in urinary amylase from baseline should prompt a pancreas biopsy to rule out rejection (151). In ED recipients, one has to rely on serum amylase and lipase only. A rise in serum lipase has recently shown to correlate well with acute pancreas rejection (149). Other signs and symptoms include tenderness over the graft, unexplained fever, and hyperglycemia (usually a late finding). Diagnosis can be confirmed by a percutaneous pancreas biopsy (153,154). In cases in which percutaneous biopsy is not possible due to technical reasons, empiric therapy may be started. Rarely, open biopsy is indicated. Transcystoscopic biopsy, which was used in the past, has been largely abandoned.
3. Others: Other findings include infectious complications such as CMV, hepatitis C, extra-abdominal bacterial or fungal infections, posttransplant malignancy such as posttransplant lymphoproliferative disorder, and other rare complications such as graft versus host disease that occur in pancreas transplantation. The diagnosis and management of these complications is similar to those of other solid-organ transplants.

RADIOLOGIC STUDIES

1. Ultrasonography: This is the most frequent study used in pancreas recipients. Noninvasive, portable, and relatively inexpensive, it provides prompt information regarding blood flow to the pancreas; the presence of arterial or venous occlusion, thrombi, pseudoaneurysms, or arteriovenous (AV) fistulas; resistance to blood flow within the pancreas (suggestive of either rejection or pancreatitis); and peripancreatic fluid collections.
2. CT scan: A CT scan provides more detail of pancreatic and surrounding anatomy. Use of oral, IV, and bladder contrast (in BD recipients) is recommended. Thus, a CT cystogram can be combined with an abdominal CT scan. A CT scan is frequently used as a guide in pancreas biopsies or in placement of directed intra-abdominal drains.
3. Fluoroscopy: A contrast cystogram can be performed under fluoroscopy and can be used instead of, or in addition to, a CT cystogram to look for bladder leak. The combination of the tests increases the sensitivity for detecting leaks.
4. Magnetic resonance angiogram (MRA): An MRA is done if vascular abnormalities are suspected on the ultrasound and if the patient's kidney function is inadequate to perform standard angiography with contrast. MRA provides resolution comparable to a CT angiogram, without the risk of contrast nephropathy, but it is inferior to standard angiography in providing fine vascular detail.
5. Angiography: This is the gold standard test for evaluating details of arterial anatomy in and around the pancreas. However, it is rarely employed, except in cases in which angiographic intervention (such as angioplasty, stenting of a stenotic segment, or coiling of an AV fistula or pseudoaneurysm) is planned. Contrast nephropathy is feared in a diabetic kidney, and reasonable alternatives (such as ultrasound and MRA) are available.

FUTURE DIRECTIONS

In diabetic patients with kidney dysfunction, SPK or PAK transplant is the standard of care. A PTA, however, is less common because the long-term risks of diabetes are pitted against the long-term risks of immunosuppression. A successful transplant can improve existing neuropathy (62) in diabetic recipients, and the survival after a solitary pancreas transplant is better than remaining on the waiting list (65). As the risks of immunosuppression decrease with novel methods of tolerance and immunomodulation (102), the balance will tilt in favor of an early transplant. The limiting factor will then be the organ shortage, which could be alleviated if xenotransplantation is able to overcome its current barrier of hyperacute rejection (155).

The application of islet transplants is rapidly growing. Recent successes (7,8) suggest that islet transplants can provide all the benefits of pancreas transplants without the risks of major surgery. Xenotransplantation of islets may be more readily achievable using encapsulation (156) than with other organs. Prolonged diabetes reversal after intraportal xenotransplant in primates has been documented (157) and may pave the way for human xenotransplant trials. Also, stem cells that are manipulated to differentiate into islets may provide a rich supply for transplantation (158). Islet transplants can be combined with immunomodulation and tolerogenic strategies to minimize or avoid immunosuppression (159). This combination would provide for minimally invasive cellular (islet) transplants for all type 1 diabetic patients without the need for long-term immunosuppression.

References

1. The effect of intensive treatment of diabetes on the development and progression of long-term complications in insulin-dependent diabetes mellitus. The Diabetes Control and Complications Trial Research Group. *N Engl J Med.* 1993;329:977–986.
2. DCCT Research Group Lifetime benefits and costs of intensive therapy as practiced in the diabetes control and complications trial. *JAMA.* 1997; 277:372.
3. Diabetes Research in Children Network (DirecNet) Study Group, Buckingham B, Beck RW et al. Continuous glucose monitoring in children with type 1 diabetes. *J Pediatr.* 2007;151:388–393.
4. Cobry E, Chase HP, Burdick P, et al. Use of CoZmonitor in youth with type 1 diabetes. *Pediatr Diabetes.* 2008;9:148–151.
5. Gruessner AC, Sutherland DE. Pancreas transplant outcomes for United States (US) and non-US cases as reported to the United Network for Organ Sharing (UNOS) and the International Pancreas Transplant Registry (IPTR) as of June 2004. *Clin Transplant.* 2005;19:433–455.
6. Hering BJ, Ricordi C. Islet transplantation for patients with type I diabetes results, research priorities and reasons for optimism. *Graft.* 1999;2:12–27.
7. Shapiro AM, Lakey JR, Ryan EA, et al. Islet transplantation in seven patients with type 1 diabetes mellitus using a glucocorticoid-free immunosuppressive regimen. *N Engl J Med.* 2000;343:230–238.
8. Hering BJ, Kandaswamy R, Harmon J. Insulin independence after single-donor islet transplantation in type I diabetes with hOKT3–1 (ala-ala), sirolimus, and tacrolimus therapy. *Am J Transplant.* 2001;1:180.
9. Hering BJ, Kandaswamy R, Ansite JD et al. Single-donor, marginal-dose islet transplantation in patients with type 1 diabetes. *JAMA.* 2005;293:830–835.
10. Ryan EA, Paty BW, Senior PA et al. Five-year follow-up after clinical islet transplantation. *Diabetes.* 2005;54:2060–2069.
11. Morel P, Goetz FC, Moudry-Munns K, et al. Long-term glucose control in patients with pancreatic transplants. *Ann Intern Med.* 1991;115:694–699.
12. Robertson RP, Sutherland DE, Lanz KJ. Normoglycemia and preserved insulin secretory reserve in diabetic patients 10–18 years after pancreas transplantation. *Diabetes.* 1999;48:1737–1740.

13. Sutherland DER, Stratta R, Gruessner A. Pancreas transplant outcome by recipient category: single pancreas versus combined kidney-pancreas. *Curr Opin Organ Transplant.* 1998;3:231–241.
14. Gruessner RWG, Sutherland DER, Najarian JS, et al. Solitary pancreas transplantation for nonuremic patients with labile insulin-dependent diabetes mellitus. *Transplantation.* 1997;64:1572–1577.
15. Krolewski AS, Warram JH, Freire MB. Epidemiology of late diabetic complications. A basis for the development and evaluation of preventive programs. *Endocrinol Metab Clin North Am.* 1996;25:217–242.
16. Syndman DR. Infection in solid organ transplantation. *Transplant Infect Dis.* 1999;1:21–28.
17. First MR. Immunosuppressive [correction of immunosupressive] agents and their actions. *Transplant Proc.* 2002;34:1369–1371.
18. Gruessner RW, Sutherland DE, Kandaswamy R, et al. Over 500 solitary pancreas transplants in nonuremic patients with brittle diabetes mellitus. *Transplantation.* 2008;85:42–47.
19. Nath DS, Gruessner AC, Kandaswamy R, et al. Outcomes of pancreas transplants for patients with type 2 diabetes mellitus. *Clin Transplant.* 2005;19:792–797.
20. Light JA, Sasaki TM, Currier CB, et al. Successful long-term kidney-pancreas transplants regardless of C-peptide status or race. *Transplantation.* 2001;71:152–154.
21. Benedetti E, Dunn T, Massad MG, et al. Successful living related simultaneous pancreas-kidney transplant between identical twins. *Transplantation.* 1999;67:915–918.
22. Gruessner RW, Kendall DM, Drangstveit MB, et al. Simultaneous pancreas-kidney transplantation from live donors. *Ann Surg.* 1997;226:471–480.
23. Sutherland DE, Gores PF, Farney AC, et al. Evolution of kidney, pancreas, and islet transplantation for patients with diabetes at the University of Minnesota. *Am J Surg.* 1993;166:456–491.
24. Farney AC, Cho E, Schweitzer EJ, et al. Simultaneous cadaver pancreas living-donor kidney transplantation: a new approach for the type 1 diabetic uremic patient. *Ann Surg.* 2000;232:696–703.
25. Matsumoto S, Okitsu T, Iwanaga Y, et al. Insulin independence after living-donor distal pancreatectomy and islet allotransplantation. *Lancet.* 2005;365:1642–1644.
26. Matsumoto S, Okitsu T, Iwanaga Y, et al. Follow-up study of the first successful living donor islet transplantation. *Transplantation.* 2006;82:1629–1633.
27. Iwanaga Y, Matsumoto S, Okitsu T, et al. Living donor islet transplantation, the alternative approach to overcome the obstacles limiting transplant. *Ann N Y Acad Sci.* 2006;1079:335–339.
28. Sutherland DE, Gruessner RW, Dunn DL, et al. Lessons learned from more than 1,000 pancreas transplants at a single institution. *Ann Surg.* 2001;233:463–501.
29. Gruessner AC, Sutherland DE, Dunn DL, et al. Pancreas after kidney transplants in posturemic patients with type I diabetes mellitus. *J Am Soc Nephrol.* 2001;12:2490–2499.
30. Humar A, Ramcharan T, Kandaswamy R, et al. Pancreas after kidney transplants. *Am J Surg.* 2001;182:155–161.
31. Sutherland DE, Gruessner RG, Humar A, et al. Pretransplant immunosuppression for pancreas transplants alone in nonuremic diabetic recipients. *Transplant Proc.* 2001;33:1656–1658.
32. Kelly WD, Lillehei RC, Merkel FK, et al. Allotransplantation of the pancreas and duodenum along with the kidney in diabetic nephropathy. *Surgery.* 1967;61:827–837.
33. Gold M, Whittaker JR, Veith FJ, et al. Evaluation of ureteral drainage for pancreatic exocrine secretion. *Surg Forum.* 1972;23:375–377.
34. Gliedman ML, Natale DL, Riflan H, et al. Clinical segmental pancreatic transplantation with ureter-to-pancreatic duct anastomosis for exocrine drainage. *Bull Soc Int Chir.* 1975;34:15–20.
35. Dubernard JM, Traeger J, Neyra P, et al. A new method of preparation of segmental pancreatic grafts for transplantation: trials in dogs and in man. *Surgery.* 1978;84:633–639.
36. Sollinger HW, Cook K, Kamps D, et al. Clinical and experimental experience with pancreaticocystostomy for exocrine pancreatic drainage in pancreas transplantation. *Transplant Proc.* 1984;16:749–751.
37. Nghiem DD, Corry RJ. Technique of simultaneous renal pancreatoduodenal transplantation with urinary drainage of pancreatic secretion. *Am J Surg.* 1987;153:405–406.
38. Groth CG, Collste H, Lundgren G, et al. Successful outcome of segmental human pancreatic transplantation with enteric exocrine diversion after modifications in technique. *Lancet.* 1982;2:522–524.
39. Calne RY. Paratopic segmental pancreas grafting: a technique with portal venous drainage. *Lancet.* 1984;1:595–597.
40. Gil-Vernet JM, Fernandez-Cruz L, Caralps A, et al. Whole organ and pancreaticoureterostomy in clinical pancreas transplantation. *Transplant Proc.* 1985;17:2019–2022.
41. Sutherland DE, Goetz FC, Moudry KC, et al. Use of recipient mesenteric vessels for revascularization of segmental pancreas grafts: technical and metabolic considerations. *Transplant Proc.* 1987;19:2300–2304.
42. Tyden G, Lundgren G, Ostman J. Grafted pancreas with portal venous drainage. *Lancet.* 1984;1:964–965.
43. Rosenlof LK, Earnhardt RC, Pruett TL, et al. Pancreas transplantation. An initial experience with systemic and portal drainage of pancreatic allografts. *Ann Surg.* 1992;215:586–595.
44. Shokouh-Amiri MH, Gaber AO, Gaber LW, et al. Pancreas transplantation with portal venous drainage and enteric exocrine diversion: a new technique. *Transplant Proc.* 1992;24:776–777.
45. Muhlbacher F, Gnant MF, Auinger M, et al. Pancreatic venous drainage to the portal vein: a new method in human pancreas transplantation. *Transplant Proc.* 1990;22:636–637.
46. Gaber AO, Shokouh-Amiri MH, Hathaway DK, et al. Results of pancreas transplantation with portal venous and enteric drainage. *Ann Surg.* 1995;221:613–622.
47. Marsh CL, Perkins JD, Sutherland DE, et al. Combined hepatic and pancreaticoduodenal procurement for transplantation. *Surg Gynecol Obstet.* 1989;168:254–258.
48. Delmonico FL, Jenkins RL, Auchincloss H Jr, et al. Procurement of a whole pancreas and liver from the same cadaveric donor. *Surgery.* 1989;105:718–723.
49. Stratta RJ, Taylor RJ, Gill IS. Pancreas transplantation: a managed cure approach to diabetes. *Curr Probl Surg.* 1996;33:709–808.
50. Sutherland DE, Goetz FC, Najarian JS. Living-related donor segmental pancreatectomy for transplantation. *Transplant Proc.* 1980;12: 19–25.
51. Gruessner RW, Sutherland DE. Simultaneous kidney and segmental pancreas transplants from living related donors—the first two successful cases. *Transplantation.* 1996;61:1265–1268.
52. Sutherland DE, Najarian JS, Gruessner R. Living versus cadaver donor pancreas transplants. *Transplant Proc.* 1998;30:2264–2266.
53. Gruessner RW, Sutherland DE, Drangstveit MB, et al. Pancreas transplants from living donors: short- and long-term outcome. *Transplant Proc.* 2001;33:819–820.
54. Gruessner RW, Kandaswamy R, Denny R. Laparoscopic simultaneous nephrectomy and distal pancreatectomy from a live donor. *J Am Coll Surg.* 2001;193:333–337.
55. Gruessner AC, Sutherland DER. Pancreas transplant outcomes for United States (US) and non-US cases as reported to the United Network for Organ Sharing (UNOS) and the International Pancreas Transplant Registry (IPTR) as of October 2002. In: Cecka JM, Terasaki PI, eds. *Clinical Transplants 2002.* Los Angeles: UCLA Immunogenetics Center; 2003.
56. Sollinger HW, Odorico JS, Knechtle SJ, et al. Experience with 500 simultaneous pancreas-kidney transplants. *Ann Surg.* 1998;228:284–296.
57. Sutherland DE. International human pancreas and islet transplant registry. *Transplant Proc.* 1980;12:229–236.
58. American Diabetes Association. Pancreas transplantation for patients with type 1 diabetes. *Diabetes Care.* 2000;23:117.
59. Kennedy WR, Navarro X, Goetz FC, et al. Effects of pancreatic transplantation on diabetic neuropathy. *N Engl J Med.* 1990;322:1031–1037.
60. Solders G, Tyden G, Persson A, et al. Improvement of nerve conduction in diabetic neuropathy. A follow-up study 4 yr after combined pancreatic and renal transplantation. *Diabetes.* 1992;41:946–951.
61. Fioretto P, Sutherland DE, Najafian B, et al. Remodeling of renal interstitial and tubular lesions in pancreas transplant recipients. *Kidney Int.* 2006;69:907–912.
62. Stratta R. Impact of pancreas transplantation on complications of diabetes. *Curr Opin Organ Transplant.* 1998;3:258.
63. Fiorina P, La RE, Venturini M, et al. Effects of kidney-pancreas transplantation on atherosclerotic risk factors and endothelial function in patients with uremia and type 1 diabetes. *Diabetes.* 2001;50:496–501.
64. Venstrom JM, McBride MA, Rother KI, et al. Survival after pancreas transplantation in patients with diabetes and preserved kidney function. *JAMA.* 2003;290:2817–2823.
65. Gruessner RW, Sutherland DE, Gruessner AC. Mortality assessment for pancreas transplants. *Am J Transplant.* 2004;4:2018–2026.
66. Gruessner RW, Sutherland DE, Gruessner AC. Survival after pancreas transplantation. *JAMA.* 2005;293:675–676.
67. Vandenberg BF, Rossen JD, Grover-McKay M, et al. Evaluation of diabetic patients for renal and pancreas transplantation: noninvasive screening for coronary artery disease using radionuclide methods. *Transplantation.* 1996;62:1230–1235.
68. Herzog CA, Marwick TH, Pheley AM, et al. Dobutamine stress echocardiography for the detection of significant coronary artery disease in renal transplant candidates. *Am J Kidney Dis.* 1999;33:1080–1090.
69. Tadros GM, Malik JA, Manske CL, et al. Iso-osmolar radio contrast iodixanol in patients with chronic kidney disease. *J Invasive Cardiol.* 2005; 17:211–215.
70. Bates JR, Sawada SG, Segar DS, et al. Evaluation using dobutamine stress echocardiography in patients with insulin-dependent diabetes mellitus before kidney and/or pancreas transplantation. *Am J Cardiol.* 1996;77:175–179.
71. Manske CL, Wang Y, Rector T, et al. Coronary revascularisation in insulin-dependent diabetic patients with chronic renal failure. *Lancet.* 1992;340: 998–1002.
72. Legendre C, Garrigue V, Le BC, et al. Harmful long-term impact of hepatitis C virus infection in kidney transplant recipients. *Transplantation.* 1998; 65:667–670.

73. Douzdjian V, Gugliuzza KG, Fish JC. Multivariate analysis of donor risk factors for pancreas allograft failure after simultaneous pancreas-kidney transplantation. *Surgery.* 1995;118:73–81.
74. Humar A, Kandaswamy R, Granger D, et al. Decreased surgical risks of pancreas transplantation in the modern era. *Ann Surg.* 2000;231:269–275.
75. Humar A, Harmon J, Gruessner A, et al. Surgical complications requiring early relaparotomy after pancreas transplantation: comparison of the cyclosporine and FK 506 eras. *Transplant Proc.* 1999;31:606–607.
76. Kapur S, Bonham CA, Dodson SF, et al. Strategies to expand the donor pool for pancreas transplantation. *Transplantation.* 1999;67:284–290.
77. Bonham CA, Kapur S, Dodson SF, et al. Potential use of marginal donors for pancreas transplantation. *Transplant Proc.* 1999;31:612–613.
78. Salvalaggio PR, Davies DB, Fernandez LA, et al. Outcomes of pancreas transplantation in the United States using cardiac-death donors. *Am J Transplant.* 2006;6:1059–1065.
79. Wahlberg JA, Love R, Landegaard L, et al. 72-hour preservation of the canine pancreas. *Transplantation.* 1987;43:5–8.
80. Kin S, Stephanian E, Gores P, et al. Successful 96-Hr cold-storage preservation of canine pancreas with UW solution containing the thromboxane A2 synthesis inhibitor OKY046. *J Surg Res.* 1992;52:577–582.
81. D'Alessandro AM, Kalayoglu M, Sollinger HW, et al. Current status of organ preservation with University of Wisconsin solution. *Arch Pathol Lab Med.* 1991;115:306–310.
82. Humar A, Kandaswamy R, Drangstveit MB, et al. Surgical risks and outcome of pancreas retransplants. *Surgery.* 2000;127:634–640.
83. Matsumoto S, Kandaswamy R, Sutherland DE, et al. Clinical application of the two-layer (University of Wisconsin solution/perfluorochemical plus O2) method of pancreas preservation before transplantation. *Transplantation.* 2000;70:771–774.
84. Kuroda Y, Kawamura T, Suzuki Y, et al. A new, simple method for cold storage of the pancreas using perfluorochemical. *Transplantation.* 1988; 46:457–460.
85. Fujita H, Kuroda Y, Saitoh Y. The mechanism of action of the two-layer cold storage method in canine pancreas preservation–protection of pancreatic microvascular endothelium. *Kobe J Med Sci.* 1995;41:47–61.
86. Tanioka Y, Kuroda Y, Saitoh Y. Amelioration of rewarming ischemic injury of the pancreas graft during vascular anastomosis by increasing tissue ATP contents during preservation by the two-layer cold storage method. *Kobe J Med Sci.* 1994;40:175–189.
87. Agarwal A, Murdock P, Pescovitz MD, et al. Follow-up experience using histidine-tryptophan ketoglutarate solution in clinical pancreas transplantation. *Transplant Proc.* 2005;37:3523–3526.
88. Englesbe MJ, Moyer A, Kim DY, et al. Early pancreas transplant outcomes with histidine-tryptophan-ketoglutarate preservation: a multicenter study. *Transplantation.* 2006;82:136–139.
89. Becker T, Ringe B, Nyibata M, et al. Pancreas transplantation with histidine-tryptophan-ketoglutarate (HTK) solution and University of Wisconsin (UW) solution: is there a difference? *JOP.* 2007;8:304–311.
90. Mancini MJ, Connors AF Jr, Wang XQ, et al. HLA matching for simultaneous pancreas-kidney transplantation in the United States: a multivariable analysis of the UNOS data. *Clin Nephrol.* 2002;57:27–37.
91. Gruessner AC, Sutherland DE, Gruessner RW. Matching in pancreas transplantation—a registry analysis. *Transplant Proc.* 2001;33:1665–1666.
92. Malaise J, Berney T, Morel P, et al. Effect of HLA matching in simultaneous pancreas-kidney transplantation. *Transplant Proc.* 2005;37:2846–2847.
93. Lo A, Stratta RJ, Alloway RR, et al. A multicenter analysis of the significance of HLA matching on outcomes after kidney-pancreas transplantation. *Transplant Proc.* 2005;37:1289–1290.
94. Berney T, Malaise J, Morel P, et al. Impact of HLA matching on the outcome of simultaneous pancreas-kidney transplantation. *Nephrol Dial Transplant.* 2005;20(Suppl 2):ii48–53, ii62.
95. Gruber SA, Katz S, Kaplan B, et al. Initial results of solitary pancreas transplants performed without regard to donor/recipient HLA mismatching. *Transplantation.* 2000;70:388–391.
96. Burgos LG, Ebert TJ, Asiddao C, et al. Increased intraoperative cardiovascular morbidity in diabetics with autonomic neuropathy. *Anesthesiology.* 1989;70:591–597.
97. Page MM, Watkins PJ. Cardiorespiratory arrest and diabetic autonomic neuropathy. *Lancet.* 1978;1:14–16.
98. Hogan K, Rusy D, Springman SR. Difficult laryngoscopy and diabetes mellitus. *Anesth Analg.* 1988;67:1162–1165.
99. Krishnamurthi V, Philosophe B, Bartlett ST. Pancreas transplantation: contemporary surgical techniques. *Urol Clin North Am.* 2001;28:833–838.
100. Benedetti E, Najarian JS, Gruessner AC, et al. Correlation between cystoscopic biopsy results and hypoamylasuria in bladder-drained pancreas transplants. *Surgery.* 1995;118:864–872.
101. Elkhammas EA, Demirag A, Henry ML. Simultaneous pancreas-kidney transplantation at the Ohio State University Medical Center. *Clin Transpl.* 1999;211–215.
102. Kirk AD. Immunosuppression without immunosuppression? How to be a tolerant individual in a dangerous world. *Transplant Infect Dis.* 1999;1:65.
103. Stratta RJ, Shokouh-Amiri MH, Egidi MF, et al. A prospective comparison of simultaneous kidney-pancreas transplantation with systemic-enteric versus portal-enteric drainage. *Ann Surg.* 2001;233:740–751.
104. Bagdade JD, Ritter MC, Kitabchi AE, et al. Differing effects of pancreas-kidney transplantation with systemic versus portal venous drainage on cholesteryl ester transfer in IDDM subjects. *Diabetes Care.* 1996;19:1108–1112.
105. Carpentier A, Patterson BW, Uffelman KD, et al. The effect of systemic versus portal insulin delivery in pancreas transplantation on insulin action and VLDL metabolism. *Diabetes.* 2001;50:1402–1413.
106. Diem P, Abid M, Redmon JB, et al. Systemic venous drainage of pancreas allografts as independent cause of hyperinsulinemia in type I diabetic recipients. *Diabetes.* 1990;39:534–540.
107. Konigsrainer A, Foger BH, Miesenbock G, et al. Pancreas transplantation with systemic endocrine drainage leads to improvement in lipid metabolism. *Transplant Proc.* 1994;26:501–502.
108. Philosophe B, Farney AC, Schweitzer EJ, et al. Superiority of portal venous drainage over systemic venous drainage in pancreas transplantation: a retrospective study. *Ann Surg.* 2001;234:689–696.
109. Boggi U, Vistoli F, Signori S, et al. A technique for retroperitoneal pancreas transplantation with portal-enteric drainage. *Transplantation.* 2005; 79:1137–1142.
110. Sutherland DE, Morel P, Gruessner RW. Transplantation of two diabetic patients with one divided cadaver donor pancreas. *Transplant Proc.* 1990;22:585.
111. Tyden G, Tibell A, Sandberg J. Improved results with a simplified technique for pancreaticoduodenal transplantation with enteric exocrine drainage. *Clin Transplant.* 1996;10:306.
112. Becker YT, Collins BH, Sollinger HW. Technical complications of pancreas transplantation. *Curr Opin Organ Transplant.* 1998;3:253.
113. Elkhammas EA, Henry ML, Tesi RJ, et al. Control of metabolic acidosis after pancreas transplantation using acetazolamide. *Transplant Proc.* 1991;23:1623–1624.
114. Schang T, Timmermann W, Thiede A, et al. Detrimental effects of fluid and electrolyte loss from duodenum in bladder-drained pancreas transplants. *Transplant Proc.* 1991;23:1617–1618.
115. Peltenburg HG, Mutsaerts KJ, Hardy EL, et al. Sodium lactate as an alternative to sodium bicarbonate in the management of metabolic acidosis after pancreas transplantation. *Transplantation.* 1992;53:225–226.
116. Benedetti E, Coady NT, Asolati M, et al. A prospective randomized clinical trial of perioperative treatment with octreotide in pancreas transplantation. *Am J Surg.* 1998;175:14–17.
117. Carlsson PO, Jansson L. The long-acting somatostatin analogue octreotide decreases pancreatic islet blood flow in rats. *Pancreas.* 1994;9:361–364.
118. Kandaswamy R, Humar A, Gruessner AC, et al. Vascular graft thrombosis after pancreas transplantation: comparison of the FK 506 and cyclosporine eras. *Transplant Proc.* 1999;31:602–603.
119. Humar A, Gruessner RW, Sutherland DE. Living related donor pancreas and pancreas-kidney transplantation. *Br Med Bull.* 1997;53:879–891.
120. Benedetti E, Rastellini C, Sileri P, et al. Successful simultaneous pancreas-kidney transplantation from well-matched living-related donors. *Transplant Proc.* 2001;33:1689.
121. Calne RY, Rolles K, White DJ, et al. Cyclosporin A initially as the only immunosuppressant in 34 recipients of cadaveric organs: 32 kidneys, 2 pancreases, and 2 livers. *Lancet.* 1979;2:1033–1036.
122. Stratta RJ. Simultaneous use of tacrolimus and mycophenolate mofetil in combined pancreas-kidney transplant recipients: a multi-center report. The FK/MMF Multi-Center Study Group. *Transplant Proc.* 1997;29:654–655.
123. Gruessner AC, Sutherland DE. Analysis of United States (US) and non-US pancreas transplants as reported to the International Pancreas Transplant Registry (IPTR) and to the United Network for Organ Sharing (UNOS). *Clin Transpl.* 1998;53–73.
124. Gruessner RW, Sutherland DE, Drangstveit MB, et al. Mycophenolate mofetil and tacrolimus for induction and maintenance therapy after pancreas transplantation. *Transplant Proc.* 1998;30:518–520.
125. Gruessner RW, Sutherland DE, Parr E, et al. A prospective, randomized, open-label study of steroid withdrawal in pancreas transplantation-a preliminary report with 6-month follow-up. *Transplant Proc.* 2001;33:1663–1664.
126. Kaufman DB, Leventhal JR, Gallon LG. Pancreas transplantation in the prednisone-free era. *Am J Transplant.* 2003;3:322.
127. Salazar A, McAlister VC, Kiberd BA, et al. Sirolimus-tacrolimus combination for combined kidney-pancreas transplantation: effect on renal function. *Transplant Proc.* 2001;33:1038–1039.
128. Kaufman DB, Leventhal JR, Koffron AJ, et al. A prospective study of rapid corticosteroid elimination in simultaneous pancreas-kidney transplantation: comparison of two maintenance immunosuppression protocols: tacrolimus/mycophenolate mofetil versus tacrolimus/sirolimus. *Transplantation.* 2002;73:169–177.
129. Stratta RJ, Alloway RR, Lo A, et al. A multicenter trial of two daclizumab dosing strategies versus no antibody induction in simultaneous kidney-pancreas transplantation: interim analysis. *Transplant Proc.* 2001; 33:1692–1693.
130. Gruessner RW, Kandaswamy R, Humar A, et al. Calcineurin inhibitor- and steroid-free immunosuppression in pancreas-kidney and solitary pancreas transplantation. *Transplantation.* 2005;79:1184–1189.

131. Rubin RH. A new beginning. *Transplant Infect Dis.* 1999;1:1.
132. Villacian JS, Paya CV. Prevention of infections in solid organ transplant recipients. *Transplant Infect Dis.* 1999;1:50.
133. Tyan DB, Li VA, Czer L, et al. Intravenous immunoglobulin suppression of HLA alloantibody in highly sensitized transplant candidates and transplantation with a histoincompatible organ. *Transplantation.* 1994;57:553–562.
134. Glotz D, Haymann JP, Niaudet P, et al. Successful kidney transplantation of immunized patients after desensitization with normal human polyclonal immunoglobulins. *Transplant Proc.* 1995;27:1038–1039.
135. Jordan SC, Quartel AW, Czer LS, et al. Posttransplant therapy using high-dose human immunoglobulin (intravenous gammaglobulin) to control acute humoral rejection in renal and cardiac allograft recipients and potential mechanism of action. *Transplantation.* 1998;66:800–805.
136. Watanabe H, Misu K, Kobayashi T, et al. ABO-incompatible auxiliary partial orthotopic liver transplant for late-onset familial amyloid polyneuropathy. *J Neurol Sci.* 2002;195:63–66.
137. Shishido S, Asanuma H, Tajima E, et al. ABO-incompatible living-donor kidney transplantation in children. *Transplantation.* 2001;72:1037–1042.
138. Montgomery RA, Zachary AA, Racusen LC, et al. Plasmapheresis and intravenous immune globulin provides effective rescue therapy for refractory humoral rejection and allows kidneys to be successfully transplanted into cross-match-positive recipients. *Transplantation.* 2000;70:887–895.
139. Takeda A, Uchida K, Haba T, et al. Acute humoral rejection of kidney allografts in patients with a positive flow cytometry crossmatch (FCXM). *Clin Transplant.* 2000;14(Suppl 3):15–20.
140. Bittner HB, Dunitz J, Hertz M, et al. Hyperacute rejection in single lung transplantation–case report of successful management by means of plasmapheresis and antithymocyte globulin treatment. *Transplantation.* 2001;71:649–651.
141. Reddy KS, Stratta RJ, Shokouh-Amiri MH, et al. Surgical complications after pancreas transplantation with portal-enteric drainage. *J Am Coll Surg.* 1999;189:305–313.
142. Wuthrich RP. Factor V Leiden mutation: potential thrombogenic role in renal vein, dialysis graft and transplant vascular thrombosis. *Curr Opin Nephrol Hypertens.* 2001;10:409–414.
143. Friedman GS, Meier-Kriesche HU, Kaplan B, et al. Hypercoagulable states in renal transplant candidates: impact of anticoagulation upon incidence of renal allograft thrombosis. *Transplantation.* 2001;72:1073–1078.
144. Zibari GB, Aultman DF, Abreo KD, et al. Roux-en-Y venting jejunostomy in pancreatic transplantation: a novel approach to monitor rejection and prevent anastomotic leak. *Clin Transplant.* 2000;14:380–385.
145. Eckhoff DE, Ploeg RJ, Wilson MA, et al. Efficacy of 99mTc voiding cystourethrogram for detection of duodenal leaks after pancreas transplantation. *Transplant Proc.* 1994;26:462–463.
146. Roza AM, Johnson CP, Adams M. Acute torsion of the renal transplant after combined kidney-pancreas transplant. *Transplantation.* 1999;67:486–488.
147. West MS, Stevens RB, Metrakos P, et al. Renal pedicle torsion after simultaneous kidney-pancreas transplantation. *J Am Coll Surg.* 1998;187: 80–87.
148. Del Pizzo JJ, Jacobs SC, Bartlett ST, et al. Urological complications of bladder-drained pancreatic allografts. *Br J Urol.* 1998;81:543–547.
149. Kaplan AJ, Valente JF, First MR, et al. Early operative intervention for urologic complications of kidney-pancreas transplantation. *World J Surg.* 1998;22:890–894.
150. Troppmann C, Gruessner AC, Dunn DL, et al. Surgical complications requiring early relaparotomy after pancreas transplantation: a multivariate risk factor and economic impact analysis of the cyclosporine era. *Ann Surg.* 1998;227:255–268.
151. Kuo PC, Johnson LB, Schweitzer EJ, et al. Solitary pancreas allografts. The role of percutaneous biopsy and standardized histologic grading of rejection. *Arch Surg.* 1997;132:52–57.
152. Papadimitriou JC, Drachenberg CB, Wiland A, et al. Histologic grading of acute allograft rejection in pancreas needle biopsy: correlation to serum enzymes, glycemia, and response to immunosuppressive treatment. *Transplantation.* 1998;66:1741–1745.
153. Klassen DK, Weir MR, Cangro CB, et al. Pancreas allograft biopsy: safety of percutaneous biopsy-results of a large experience. *Transplantation.* 2002; 73:553–555.
154. Malek SK, Potdar S, Martin JA, et al. Percutaneous ultrasound-guided pancreas allograft biopsy: a single-center experience. *Transplant Proc.* 2005;37:4436–4437.
155. Auchincloss H Jr, Sachs DH. Xenogeneic transplantation. *Ann Rev Immunol.* 1998;16:433–470.
156. Lanza RP, Chick WL. Transplantation of encapsulated cells and tissues. *Surgery.* 1997;121:1–9.
157. Hering BJ, Wijkstrom M, Graham ML, et al. Prolonged diabetes reversal after intraportal xenotransplantation of wild-type porcine islets in immunosuppressed nonhuman primates. *Nat Med.* 2006;12:301–303.
158. Shapiro AM, Lakey JR. Future trends in islet cell transplantation. *Diabetes Technol Ther.* 2000;2:449–452.
159. Cooke A, Phillips JM, Parish NM. Tolerogenic strategies to halt or prevent type 1 diabetes. *Nat Immunol.* 2001;2:810–815.

CHAPTER 95 ■ RENAL TRANSPLANTATION

LINDA L. WONG • KIMI R. UEDA • V. RAM PEDDI

Because of advances in critical care and medical treatment, many more patients are living with end-stage renal disease (ESRD). In 2003, more than 324,000 patients in the United States received some form of renal replacement therapy for ESRD. The economic burden of ESRD is staggering, with $27.3 billion spent in the United States in public and private funds in 2003 (1). Renal transplantation is clearly the most cost-effective treatment option for ESRD when compared to all other forms of renal replacement therapy (2,3). The improvement in outcome after renal transplantation has resulted in a more liberal selection of patients. Unfortunately, the demand for kidney transplants far exceeds the supply of available organs. While nearly 70,000 patients currently await renal transplantation in the United States, only 16,477 renal transplant procedures were performed in 2005 (4). As a result, patients on the deceased donor organ transplant waiting list wait prolonged periods and suffer the consequences of chronic disease and associated comorbidities before finally undergoing transplantation. This serious shortage of donor kidneys has prompted many institutions to expand their donor criteria. In an attempt to increase the utilization of suboptimal kidneys, transplantation of both marginal kidneys, a "dual transplant," into a single recipient has been performed at some centers with good short-term results (5). Furthermore, there has been a renewed interest in the use of "non–heart-beating donors," also with good short-term results (6,7). Because of these reasons, which may lead to an increase in the incidence of delayed graft function or slow graft function, the critical care management of these patients has become increasingly important. Furthermore, advances in transplant management now allow for long-term survival after transplant. There are now over 100,000 patients living on chronic immunosuppression after renal transplant in the United States, some of whom may present to the critical care unit for unique problems and complications long after they have undergone transplant surgery (8).

EVALUATION OF POTENTIAL TRANSPLANT CANDIDATE

Before undergoing renal transplantation, each patient must undergo thorough evaluation, as not all ESRD patients are appropriate candidates for transplantation. Each center has a specific protocol for candidate evaluation, but the main purpose of any evaluation is to identify major contraindications to transplantation including active malignancy, advanced cardiopulmonary disease, active infection, substance abuse, and noncompliance with medical therapy. With most malignancies, a waiting period before transplantation is recommended (time period varies with the type of malignancy) and patients should be thoroughly evaluated for any recurrence or metastasis, which would contraindicate transplantation. There is no completely reliable algorithm for evaluating patients for cardiac disease for renal transplant surgery. General recommendations include noninvasive cardiac stress testing for the following population: diabetics, males older than 45 years, females older than 55 years, family history of premature cardiac disease (myocardial infarction [MI] or sudden death in first-degree male relative younger than 55 or first-degree female relative younger than 65), current cigarette smoking, hypertension, total cholesterol >200 mg/dL, and high-density-lipoprotein cholesterol <35 mg/dL. For those with positive stress testing, coronary angiography would be indicated. Some centers routinely advocate coronary angiography for all diabetics as the incidence of ischemic heart disease is high in this population (9).

Patients undergoing evaluation should be screened for viral hepatitis B and C and HIV, and any active infection should be treated. While viral hepatitis B and C and HIV positivity are not absolute contraindications, patients with advanced forms of these infections are generally not candidates for transplantation.

Other potential relative contraindications to transplantation include obesity, severe peripheral vascular/cerebrovascular disease, and advanced age. Although obesity is not an absolute contraindication, U.S. data on over 27,000 patients have indicated that those with morbid obesity (body mass index [BMI] >35) have a higher rate of delayed graft function, acute rejection, and overall survival, as well as longer hospitalizations (10). Thrombophilia, prostatic disease, high immunologic sensitization, psychosocial problems, and renal diseases with a high recurrence rate such as focal and segmental glomerulosclerosis should be identified during this transplant evaluation. Potential anatomic abnormalities such as severe iliac arterial disease and genitourinary anomalies should also be delineated before transplantation.

Candidates on the deceased donor waiting list should be reassessed periodically for any changes in the status of their medical and psychosocial problems. Potential recipients with diabetes mellitus should be evaluated annually as they often have associated ischemic heart disease. As patients wait longer for deceased organ donors, they will need to be monitored carefully as significant changes in their medical status may occur during the waiting period.

TYPES OF DONORS

Kidneys are transplanted from deceased donors after brain death or cardiac death, and from living donors. Brain death is defined by the Uniform Determination of Death Act of 1981 as follows: "an individual is dead if there is irreversible cessation of circulatory and respiratory functions or if there is irreversible cessation of all brain functions of the entire brain, including the brainstem." A brain-dead donor has suffered head trauma, cerebrovascular accident, cerebral anoxia, or a nonmetastasizing brain tumor. Physicians caring for the patient can diagnose brain death with the assistance of physical exam findings, an apnea test, a nuclear brain flow scan, and an electroencephalogram, though none of these tests is specifically required. It is the responsibility of all health professionals and especially critical care medicine physicians to report all patients with brain death and impending brain death to the local organ procurement organization (OPO). Once family members have accepted that their relative is brain dead, the trained donation coordinator may approach the family to discuss organ donation.

Because of the disparity between organ demand and supply, kidneys that traditionally would not have been used are now being considered. These deceased donors have been defined by the United Network for Organ Sharing (UNOS), the national organization that coordinates organ allocation, as "expanded donors." Expanded criteria donors (ECDs) include all kidneys procured from donors of age older than 60 or age between 50 and 59 years and at least two of the following: hypertension, serum creatinine >1.5 mg/dL, or death due to a cerebrovascular accident. Some studies have shown that recipients of kidneys with expanded donor criteria have slightly diminished graft function, but comparable long-term graft and patient survival (11). Use of ECD kidneys may offer survival advantages to those on dialysis and should be offered principally to recipients older than 60 years or perhaps allocated to OPOs with longer waiting times (12). This is a controversial area and some centers advocate ECD kidneys to all diabetics older than age 40 if waiting time is long.

In donation after cardiac death (DCD), death is determined by the usual cardiopulmonary criteria to prove the absence of circulation and can be used in clinical scenarios in which the donor does not meet brain death criteria. Conditions that may warrant consideration of DCD include irreversible brain injury, end-stage musculoskeletal disease, and high spinal cord injury. Early reports suggest that the time between extubation of the donor and the initiation of cold perfusion of the organs (warm ischemia) should be less than 60 minutes for successful kidney removal and function, though this does vary somewhat between centers (13).

Living donors are people who have been evaluated extensively both medically and psychosocially for possible donor nephrectomy. Medical evaluation should include thorough history and physical examination, laboratory studies (chemistry panel, complete blood count, hepatitis B and C and HIV testing, ABO typing, tissue typing, cross-match testing), 24-hour urine for creatinine clearance and protein, chest radiograph, computed tomography (CT), or magnetic resonance imaging (MRI) to evaluate both kidneys. Psychosocial evaluation is done to determine the emotional relation of the donor to the potential recipient and to ensure that the donor truly desires to donate and for altruistic reasons (not financial or other gain). An individual should be considered as a potential living donor only if the following basic requirements have been fulfilled:

1. Donor and recipient are ABO blood group compatible.
2. The warm T-lymphocyte cross-match is negative.
3. The person is in excellent physical condition, emotionally stable, and well motivated.
4. The individual is willing to undergo donor nephrectomy, is fully informed about the procedure, and is not under pressure from family members to donate a kidney.

The cytotoxic T-cell cross-match must be negative immediately before transplantation in order to proceed with surgery. A positive high-titer B-cell cross-match is also a contraindication to transplantation; however, transplantation may proceed in the presence of a low-titer B-cell cross-match, provided that the T-cell cross-match and the flow cytometry cross-match are negative (14).

IMMEDIATE PREOPERATIVE MANAGEMENT

Appropriate recipients are selected based on a list that is generated by UNOS. This list takes into account the following factors: ABO blood type, human leukocyte antigen (HLA) matching, antibody testing, and waiting time. Although potential recipients are familiar to the transplant center physicians, they are carefully evaluated for recent infection or illness with blood tests, chest radiograph, and electrocardiogram (ECG). Because waiting lists are long and patients may have been waiting for several years, other illnesses may have developed in the interim that may contraindicate transplant surgery. Patients may require a treatment of hemodialysis or peritoneal dialysis prior to transplant surgery if there is evidence of hyperkalemia or fluid overload.

IMMEDIATE POSTTRANSPLANT MANAGEMENT

Renal transplantation is carried out in the standard fashion through an incision that exposes the iliac fossa. The donor renal vessels are sutured in an end-to-side fashion to the external iliac artery and vein and a ureteroneocystostomy is created. Patients are monitored with continuous ECG and central venous pressure in the immediate postoperative period. Blood pressures are carefully monitored, as most patients have underlying hypertension and administration of immunosuppressive medications such as corticosteroids can affect blood pressure control. In addition, pain, catecholamine release, and fluid status may contribute to difficulties with blood pressure control. While adequate blood pressure control is important for the integrity of the renal arterial anastomosis, it is equally important to avoid hypotension and therefore prevent renal hypoperfusion and graft thrombosis.

Urine output is carefully monitored on an hourly basis via an indwelling urinary catheter. This urinary catheter also serves to protect the ureteroneocystostomy during the early postoperative period. Any increase in intravesical pressure due to incomplete emptying of the bladder could compromise the newly created anastomosis between the ureter and bladder. Hematuria occurring early posttransplant may be due to bleeding at the ureteral anastomosis, in the bladder, or along the urethra. This can be managed with gentle flushing of the urinary catheter with 20 to 30 mL of sterile saline. Changing the urinary catheter to one of a larger caliber may also help remove clots. Three-way urinary catheters are also used to facilitate

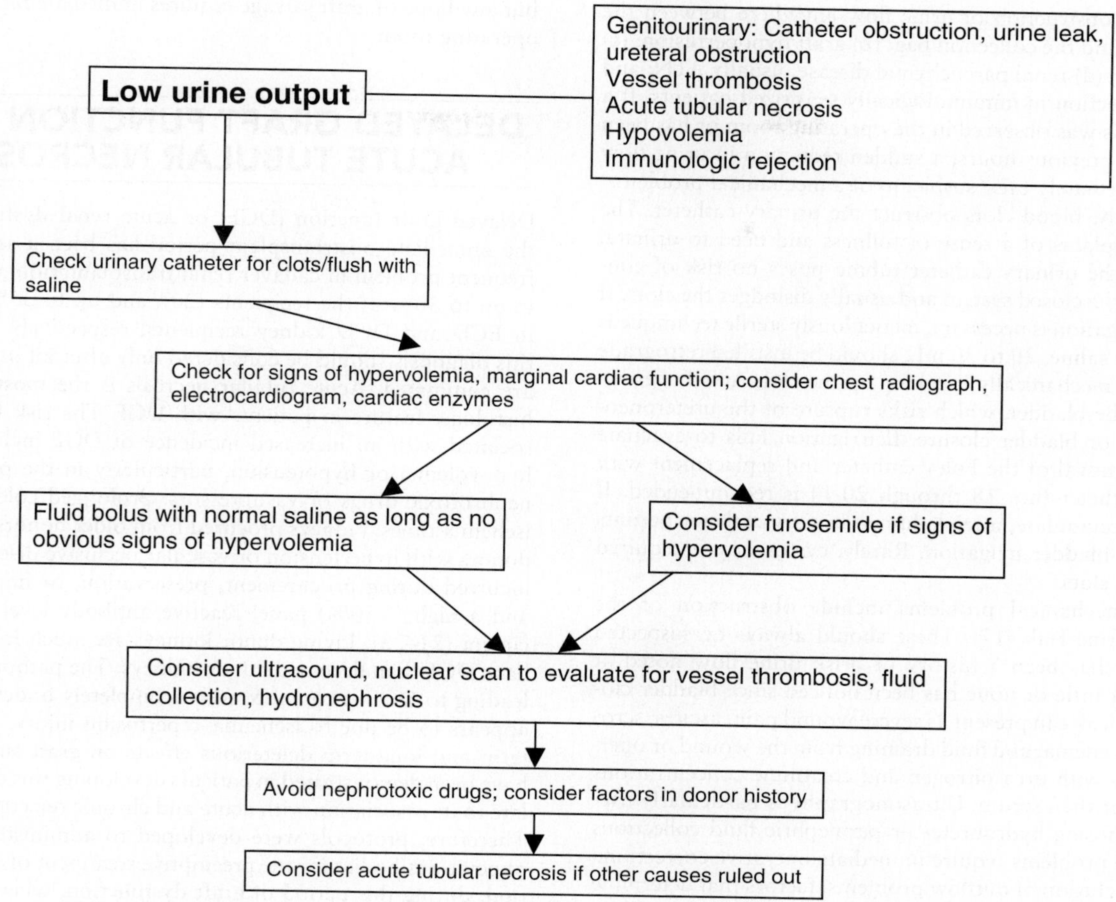

FIGURE 95.1. Algorithm for management of low urine output following renal transplant.

continuous bladder irrigation should other measures fail to treat the hematuria.

Blood glucose monitoring is also done on a regular basis. Many transplant recipients have underlying diabetes mellitus and all patients may have hyperglycemia exacerbation related to administration of steroids and other immunosuppressive agents. Use of continuous insulin infusion and frequent blood glucose monitoring may be necessary to maintain good glycemic control. Optimal control of hyperglycemia in the postoperative period and in critically ill patients has been shown to decrease morbidity and mortality (15,16).

Particular attention should be paid to the volume and electrolyte status as the urine output in the immediate posttransplant period can vary from oliguria (frequently due to delayed graft function) to several liters as a result of generous fluid replacement during the surgery and also due to solute-induced osmotic diuresis. Living donor allografts typically have excellent immediate function and may have prompt and marked diuresis. Most transplant centers utilize a center-specific protocol with a fixed-rate maintenance of intravenous fluids usually with 0.9% normal saline at 50 mL/hour or 100 mL/hr together with replacement fluid at two thirds or one half of previous hour urine output. Some recipients may need hourly fluid replacement on a milliliter-for-milliliter basis in order to keep up with fluid losses. Kidneys from expanded donors or donation after cardiac death or with longer cold ischemia times may not have immediate function due to acute tubular necrosis (ATN). These recipients should be kept on a maintenance volume of intravenous fluids and the central venous pressure can be used to guide fluid status (Fig. 95.1). Other factors to consider would include the timing of the last dialysis and the amount of urine produced by the patient before transplant. Hemodialysis treatment shortly before the transplant surgery may render a recipient relatively hypovolemic during the perioperative period. Patients who have not yet been started on renal replacement therapy or who make a normal amount of urine may not have issues with hypovolemia.

Postoperative evaluation of electrolytes should include monitoring of serum sodium, potassium, bicarbonate, calcium, magnesium, and phosphorous. While some patients require bicarbonate supplements, potassium supplements are usually not necessary. However, supplementation may be required in patients with large-volume posttransplant diuresis.

Prophylaxis with subcutaneous heparin to prevent deep venous thrombosis and H_2 receptor blockers or proton pump inhibitors to prevent gastric and/or duodenal ulcers are often administered. Patients should be evaluated for the need for dialysis based on their electrolyte, metabolic, and volume status.

EARLY COMPLICATIONS

The most common complication early posttransplant is an inappropriately low urine output. The differential diagnosis includes (a) obstruction of urine flow anywhere between the renal pelvis and the collection bag; (b) graft hypoperfusion; (c) urinary leak; (d) renal parenchymal disease, usually ATN; and (e) acute rejection in immunologically sensitized patients. If a brisk diuresis was observed in the operating room or has been recorded in previous hours, a sudden reduction in urine flow should immediately raise suspicion of a mechanical problem.

Frequently, blood clots obstruct the urinary catheter. The patient complains of a sense of fullness and need to urinate. "Milking" the urinary catheter tubing poses no risk of contaminating the closed system and usually dislodges the clots. If catheter irrigation is necessary, meticulously sterile technique is used. Sterile saline, 20 to 30 mL, should be instilled retrograde to facilitate mechanically breaking up the clot. Avoid overdistention of the bladder, which risks rupture of the ureteroneocystostomy or bladder closure. If irrigation fails to evacuate the clot, removal of the Foley catheter and replacement with a larger catheter (no. 18 through 20 F) is recommended. If clots still accumulate, a triple-lumen urinary catheter permits continuous bladder irrigation. Rarely, cystoscopy is required to evacuate clots.

Other mechanical problems include obstruction of the ureter or urine leak (17). These should always be suspected when there has been a history of brisk urine flow noted at surgery, but little or none has been noticed since bladder closure. Urine leak can present as severe wound pain, ascites, scrotal or labial edema, and fluid draining from the wound or operative drains with urea nitrogen and creatinine concentrations much higher than serum. Ultrasonography is particularly useful in diagnosing hydroureter or perinephric fluid collections (18). These problems require immediate operative correction.

After exclusion of outflow problems, factors that determine allograft perfusion should be addressed. Norms for "adequate" blood pressure are higher after transplantation, especially in children receiving adult kidneys and patients with limited cardiac contractility. To some degree, all transplanted kidneys have sustained predonation procurement and reperfusion injuries (19). There is an increase in interstitial edema and increased venocapillary resistance, endothelial swelling and denuding, and activation of vasoactive mediators. The resistance of the renal vascular bed is increased. Renal plasma flow requires a higher mean arterial pressure in this setting. The renal transplant recipient usually requires a blood pressure greater than 120/80 mm Hg. The patient's history of average pretransplant pressures is valuable in targeting perfusion pressure.

Unless there is clear evidence of intravascular volume overload, fluid boluses with normal saline are usually required. A transient response may justify further volume expansion. Most dialysis-dependent patients have total-body fluid overload. Their "dry weight," used to calculate an end point on dialysis, is always in excess of the dry weight they reach with normal renal function. Several centers use low-dose dopamine (2.5 μg/kg/minute) in an attempt to improve renal perfusion. In rare circumstances, the intrarenal vascular resistance may be excessively high, and adequate perfusion pressures do not produce sufficient intrarenal blood flow. This problem dramatically increases the risk of further ischemic injury or even thrombosis. Grafts from pediatric donors, especially those younger than 4 years of age, are prone to thrombosis. As an additional safeguard, in recipients of pediatric en bloc kidneys, low-dose aspirin therapy immediately after surgery to minimize the risk of thrombosis should be considered. Graft thrombosis is rare, but any hope of graft salvage requires immediate return to the operating room.

DELAYED GRAFT FUNCTION AND ACUTE TUBULAR NECROSIS

Delayed graft function (DGF) or acute renal dysfunction in the immediate posttransplant period has been a serious and frequent problem in cadaver renal transplantation and occurs in up to 30% of the recipients (20), and up to 35% to 40% in ECD and DCD kidney recipients, respectively. However, this diagnosis should be considered only after all other causes are eliminated. Acute tubular necrosis is the most common histologic feature in patients with DGF. The risk factors associated with an increased incidence of DGF include donor hypovolemia or hypotension, particularly in the presence of nephrotoxic drugs or vasopressors; prolonged cold or warm ischemia times; kidneys procured from older donors and from donors with hypertension or vascular occlusive disease; injury incurred during procurement, preservation, or implantation; and a high (>50%) panel reactive antibody level in the recipient (21–23). Living donor kidneys are much less likely to have DGF than deceased donor kidneys. The pathophysiology leading to DGF is complex and incompletely understood and appears to be due to ischemia–reperfusion injury. The short-term and long-term deleterious effects on graft survival that have been demonstrated in patients developing this disorder relate to its association with acute and chronic rejection (23,24). Therefore, protocols were developed to administer antilymphocyte antibodies for the preemptive treatment of acute rejection, during this period of graft dysfunction, when a diagnosis of rejection could be difficult. This led to the development of protocols termed sequential quadruple immunosuppressive therapy, where patients receive antibody induction followed by maintenance immunosuppression, usually with three agents.

IMMUNOLOGIC CAUSES OF EARLY GRAFT DYSFUNCTION

Hyperacute rejection is a rare and largely preventable cause of immediate graft failure. It is caused by preformed antibodies present in the recipients' serum at the time of transplantation against donor antigens. These antibodies are the consequence of previous exposure to donor antigens due to blood transfusions, prior transplantation, or pregnancy. It also occurs when transplantation is attempted across ABO-incompatible barriers. The events that lead to hyperacute rejection may occur with such rapidity that the kidney becomes visibly ischemic while the patient is still on the operating table. It always occurs within 24 hours of transplantation. Renal histology shows fibrin thrombi occluding the glomerular capillaries and small vessels with extensive tissue necrosis. Although plasmapheresis and anticoagulation have been advocated, there is no established effective treatment and interventions are seldom successful. A kidney with hyperacute rejection should always be removed promptly. The current cross-match techniques, because of their increased sensitivity, have greatly diminished the incidence of hyperacute rejection. *Antibody-mediated (CD4 positive) acute rejection* is another form of early rejection that can occur in previously sensitized patients but with an initial negative cross-match. This form of acute rejection is potentially reversible if diagnosed early and treated aggressively with plasmapheresis and intravenous immunoglobulin (25).

IMMUNOSUPPRESSION

The different phases of immunosuppressive therapy after transplantation are (a) induction immunosuppression in the immediate posttransplantation period when potent therapy is required to prevent rejection; (b) maintenance immunosuppression for long-term therapy to prevent allograft rejection, but at the same time preserving host defense mechanisms against infections; and (c) intensification of the immunosuppressive therapy for the treatment of an acute rejection episode.

Antilymphocyte antibodies are ideally suited for use as induction immunosuppressive agents and some for the treatment of acute rejection. They have been available for use as immunosuppressive agents since the late 1960s. All early forms of antilymphocyte antibodies were polyclonal, which are made by injecting human lymphocytes into horses, goats, rabbits, or sheep. In contrast to polyclonal antibodies, a monoclonal antibody is highly specific, and recognizes a single antigen epitope. They have a greater potency at lower doses, and have a more predictable and consistent effect. Monoclonal antibodies that are currently approved for use in transplantation are directed either at cell surface receptors such as the CD3/T-cell receptor (TCR) complex (OKT3), or the interleukin-2 (IL-2) receptor (IL-2R; daclizumab and basiliximab). Current maintenance immunosuppression protocols often use the combination of a calcineurin inhibitor, an antimetabolite, and corticosteroids. However, the principles of the different regimens are similar: more intense immunosuppression in the induction phase with gradual reduction in immunosuppression in the maintenance phase. The immunosuppression protocol an institution implements should provide a balance between preventing rejection and avoiding the consequences of overimmunosuppression such as infection and malignancy.

POLYCLONAL ANTIBODIES

Polyclonal antilymphocyte antibodies are produced by the immunization of rabbits (Thymoglobulin) or horses (Atgam) with human thymocytes. Several mechanisms of action have been proposed to explain the immunosuppressive effect of polyclonal antibodies. These include (a) complement-mediated cell lysis, (b) clearance of lymphocytes by opsonization and subsequent phagocytosis by macrophages, and (c) antibody-dependent cell-mediated cytolysis (26).

Polyclonal antibody treatment induces marked lymphocyte depletion that persists during the entire treatment period. The number of circulating T cells will gradually increase after the cessation of treatment and reach pretreatment levels in several weeks, with significant variability among patients. Each polyclonal antilymphocyte preparation varies in its constituent antibodies. Due to this unpredictable antibody mixture and batch-to-batch variability, treatment responses and side effects are variable between the different preparations (27).

There are two formulations of antithymocyte globulin available in the United States: Atgam, an equine polyclonal antithymocyte globulin, and Thymoglobulin, a rabbit polyclonal antithymocyte globulin. Thymoglobulin consists of antibodies specific for T-cell epitopes, including CD2, CD3, CD4, CD8, CD11a, CD18, CD25, HLA-DR, and HLA class I. Comparative studies have demonstrated superior efficacy of Thymoglobulin when compared to Atgam (28,29) and therefore the use of Thymoglobulin has largely superseded that of Atgam.

The most common side effect of polyclonal antibody treatment is the cytokine release syndrome, which usually occurs after the administration of the first few doses. However, these symptoms are not as severe as with OKT3. More severe reactions include the development of skin rashes, hypotension, acute respiratory distress, and anaphylaxis. Polyclonal antibodies often cross-react with antigens on unrelated cells, resulting in such side effects as granulocytopenia, thrombocytopenia, arthralgia, serum sickness, phlebitis, and immune complex glomerulonephritis. Because these agents severely impair the cell-mediated immunity, patients are prone to develop opportunistic infections and posttransplantation malignancies, especially posttransplantation lymphoproliferative disorders (PTLDs).

Thymoglobulin is dosed at 1.5 mg/kg/day, whereas Atgam is dosed at 10 to 15 mg/kg/day. Both antibody preparations are administered as an IV infusion over a period of about 6 hours. Premedication is recommended using high-dose methylprednisolone, an antihistamine, and acetaminophen 1 hour prior to the administration of these antibodies.

MONOCLONAL ANTIBODIES

OKT3 (Muromonab)

OKT3 is a murine monoclonal antibody directed against CD3, a molecule closely associated with the TCR on the surface of human T cells (30). Antigen recognition by the TCR results in signal transduction via the CD3 molecule and subsequent T-cell proliferation and activation. OKT3 inhibits the CD3/TCR complex, thereby inactivating T lymphocytes. OKT3 is used for induction or for the treatment of acute rejection. The standard dose of OKT3 is 5 mg/day administered intravenously through a central or peripheral line.

The most common side effect of OKT3 is the cytokine release syndrome that typically begins 30 to 60 minutes after the administration of the first few doses and may last for several hours. This syndrome is characterized by fever, chills, tremor, nausea, vomiting, diarrhea, headache, myalgia, chest pain and tightness, and wheezing. This syndrome is believed to be mediated by a massive systemic release of cytokines by activated T cells. The cytokine release syndrome may cause severe pulmonary edema in patients who are fluid overloaded. It is therefore essential to assess the volume status of the patient prior to initiating OKT3 treatment and to induce diureses or dialyze as indicated (31). Cytokine nephropathy, a reversible renal dysfunction, has also been reported. In order to minimize or avoid the cytokine release syndrome, premedication is recommended using high-dose corticosteroids, an antihistamine, and acetaminophen 1 hour prior to the administration of OKT3 (32). Another drawback of OKT3 therapy is the production of human antimouse antibodies by the kidney transplant

TABLE 95.1

COMPARISON OF BASILIXIMAB AND DACLIZUMAB

	Basiliximab (Simulect)	Daclizumab (Zenapax)
Nature	Chimeric (mouse variable region with human constant region)	Humanized (murine hypervariable regions, rest of the molecule [90%] is human)
Mechanism of action	Blocks the binding of IL-2 to its receptor	Blocks the IL-2 pathway by binding to the Tac-subunit of the IL-2 receptor
Half-life	7.2 days	20 days
Saturation	36 days	120 days
Affinity	More (9×10^9 mol/L)	Less (3×10^9 mol/L)
Recommended adult dosing schedule	20 mg within 2 h prior to and 20 mg 4 d after transplantation	Five doses of 1 mg/kg. First dose given within 24 h prior to transplantation and four remaining doses at intervals of 14 days
Adverse reactions	Similar to placebo	Similar to placebo
Results[a]		
Biopsy-confirmed acute rejection	29.8% vs. 44% with placebo ($p = 0.012$)	22% vs. 35% with placebo ($p = 0.03$)
Graft survival	87.9% vs. 86.6% with placebo ($p = 0.591$)	95% vs. 90% with placebo ($p = 0.08$)
Patient survival	95.3% vs. 97.3% with placebo ($p = 0.293$)	98% vs. 96% with placebo ($p = 0.51$)

IL, interleukin.
[a] Data from published studies.
From Vincenti F, Kirkman R, Light S, et al., for the Daclizumab Triple Therapy Study Group. Interleukin-2-receptor blockade with daclizumab to prevent acute rejection in renal transplantation. *N Engl J Med.* 1998;338:161; and Nashan B, Moore R, Amlot P, et al., for the CH1B 201 International Study Group. Randomized trial of basiliximab versus placebo for control of acute cellular rejection in renal allograft recipients. *Lancet.* 1997;350:1193.

recipients' immune system. These antibodies may neutralize the efficacy of OKT3 treatment, thus limiting repeated use.

Immunologic monitoring using flow cytometric determination of the lymphocyte subsets to monitor depletion of CD3+ lymphocytes from the peripheral blood plays an essential role in the treatment of patients receiving OKT3 or antithymocyte globulin preparations. The absolute number of CD3+ cells should remain depressed throughout treatment. The guidelines for the number of CD3+ cells varies from fewer than 10/mm^3 to more than 50/mm^3 in different studies (33).

Anti-interleukin-2α Receptor Antibodies

IL-2 is a cytokine responsible for the growth and proliferation of activated T cells. During an immune response, IL-2 exerts its effects by binding to the IL-2R on the surface of the antigen-activated T cell. Anti-interleukin-2α receptor antibodies are monoclonal antibodies directed against the IL-2R on activated T cells. These antibodies are used as induction agents for prophylaxis against acute rejection in renal transplant recipients (34,35).

Basiliximab (Simulect) is a chimeric (human and mouse) $IgG_{1\kappa}$ monoclonal antibody that is administered as an IV infusion of two doses of 20 mg each. The first dose is given within 2 hours prior to transplantation and the second dose is given 4 days after transplantation. Daclizumab (Zenapax) is a humanized IgG_1 monoclonal antibody that is administered as an IV infusion of five doses of 1 mg/kg body weight each. The first dose of 1 mg/kg is given prior to transplantation. Subsequent doses are administered every 2 weeks posttransplantation for a total of five doses. Adverse effects of the IL-2R antibodies are minimal and equivalent to placebo in controlled trials. Hypersensitivity reactions have been reported with both antibodies. The two IL-2R antibodies are compared in Table 95.1.

Alemtuzumab (Campath-1H)

Alemtuzumab (Campath-1H) is a humanized monoclonal antibody directed against the CD52 antigen (36,37) found on approximately 5% of the lymphocyte surface, making it the highest-density cell-surface marker on lymphocytes. Targeting of CD52 with antibody has shown to be exceptionally lytic of lymphocytes. The mechanism of action of alemtuzumab includes complement-mediated lysis, cell-mediated killing (antibody dependent cellular cytotoxicity [ADCC]), and induction of apoptosis of targeted cells. Alemtuzumab is a relatively low-affinity antibody, requiring 20 to 50 μg/mL to saturate its receptors (38). Because of the humanization of alemtuzumab, the first-dose effect is relatively mild. There is an associated tumor necrosis factor (TNF)-α and interferon-γ release that can be reduced with steroids. First infusion reactions such as fever, rash, nausea, vomiting, headache, and rigors due to a cytokine release syndrome have been reported with alemtuzumab treatment; however, these effects have been of a low-grade nature and limited with steroid pretreatment (38). Alemtuzumab effectively depletes immune cells, namely T and B lymphocytes; some natural killer (NK) cells; and some monocyte/macrophage lineage. Currently, alemtuzumab is approved for treatment of patients with B-cell chronic lymphocytic leukemia (39) and is not Food and Drug Administration (FDA) approved for use in transplant recipients in the United States. However, since the introduction of this agent for leukemic patients, a number of single-center trials have taken place in renal transplantation with good results (40,41). Results from a recently completed multicenter trial comparing alemtuzumab induction with that of basiliximab in low-immunologic-risk recipients and with Thymoglobulin for high-immunologic-risk recipients are pending.

Rituximab

Rituximab (Rituxan) antibody is a genetically engineered chimeric (human and mouse) monoclonal antibody directed against the CD20 antigen found on the surface of normal and malignant B lymphocytes (42). Rituximab is approved for the treatment of patients with relapsed or refractory, low-grade or follicular, CD20-positive, B-cell, non-Hodgkin lymphoma (43,44). Because of its effects on the B lymphocytes, rituximab is believed to be effective in the treatment of patients with antibody-mediated (humoral) acute rejection and is also thought to have a role in decreasing the panel reactive antibody (PRA) level in sensitized patients. However, it is not FDA approved for the latter indications and has not gained widespread support for use in transplant recipients, except for treatment in patients with PTLD (45).

CALCINEURIN INHIBITORS

Calcineurin inhibitors are currently considered to be the mainstay of immunosuppression regimens following transplantation. They are potent immunosuppressants that inhibit T-cell activation by inhibiting calcineurin phosphatase, a key step in the regulation of cytokine expression. The introduction of calcineurin inhibitors in the mid-1980s has revolutionized the field of transplantation by dramatically reducing acute rejection rates and improving short-term allograft survival (46).

Cyclosporine

Cyclosporine A (CsA), the first calcineurin inhibitor approved for use in transplant recipients for maintenance immunosuppression, binds to cyclophilin in the T cell. The CsA/cyclophilin complex, in turn, inhibits calcineurin phosphatase, which is responsible for the transcription of IL-2. CsA is highly lipophilic and water insoluble. Early formulations (Sandimmune) were administered orally as an oil-based solution. In this form, bioavailability was erratic and highly variable and bile dependant for its absorption. This erratic absorption profile led to the development of a microemulsion formulation (modified cyclosporine, Neoral) that demonstrated a more reliable and predictable absorption. These two formulations are not bioequivalent and are thus not interchangeable. CsA is available in an IV formulation, as an oral solution, and in a capsule form. The IV formulation should be administered as a continuous infusion and should be limited to patients unable to take CsA orally, and the patient should be monitored closely during the infusion process. The dosage should be titrated based on whole blood concentration. The recommended starting dose of oral solution or capsules is 10 to 14 mg/kg/day for the nonmodified CsA and 6 to 12 mg/kg/day of the modified CsA administered 12 hours apart in divided doses. Various generic formulations of CsA are available. In the United States use of CsA has been superseded by that of tacrolimus in the majority of kidney transplant recipients and in almost all pancreas transplant recipients.

Tacrolimus

Tacrolimus (Prograf, FK-506) is a macrolide agent that inhibits IL-2 production in a similar fashion as CsA in the T lymphocyte. However, instead of binding to cyclophilin, tacrolimus binds to the FK binding protein 12 (FKBP-12) and the resulting complex inhibits calcineurin phosphatase. Tacrolimus is available in IV injection and oral capsule dosage forms. The IV form of tacrolimus is also administered as a continuous infusion and because of the risk of neurotoxicity should be limited to select patients unable to take tacrolimus orally. Tacrolimus is readily absorbed in the stomach and should be given orally or through nasogastric tube whenever feasible. The recommended starting dose of oral tacrolimus is 0.2 mg/kg/day administered 12 hours apart in divided doses.

Adverse Effects of the Calcineurin Inhibitors

Both calcineurin inhibitors have a narrow therapeutic window, multiple side effects, and drug interactions. Both drugs are metabolized by the cytochrome P450–3A4 enzyme system; their blood concentrations are affected by drugs that block or induce the cytochrome P450–3A4 enzyme system. Both drugs interact with some of the commonly used antibiotics, antifungal agents, and antihypertensive agents. Their interactions with other commonly used drugs are listed in Table 95.2. Both drugs cause acute and chronic nephrotoxicity. The acute nephrotoxicity is due in part to hemodynamic changes secondary to their vasoconstrictor effects on the afferent arteriole of the glomerulus. This results in a reduction in the glomerular filtration rate, manifested by an increase in the serum creatinine concentration. This acute change is dose related and reversible. However, the lesions associated with calcineurin inhibitor–induced chronic nephropathy may lead to end-stage renal failure. These lesions, which consist of tubulointerstitial striped fibrosis, tubular atrophy, afferent arteriolopathy, and global or focal glomerular

TABLE 95.2

COMMON DRUG INTERACTIONS WITH CYCLOSPORINE AND TACROLIMUS

Decreased blood concentrations	Increased blood concentrations	
Phenytoin	Diltiazem	Cimetidine
Carbamazepine	Nicardipine	Metoclopramide
Phenobarbital	Nifedipine	Oral contraceptives
Rifampin	Verapamil	Prednisone
Rifabutin	Ketoconazole	Protease inhibitors
St. John's wort	Fluconazole	Grapefruit juice
	Itraconazole	Amiodarone
	Clarithromycin	
	Erythromycin	

TABLE 95.3

ADVERSE-EFFECT PROFILE OF CYCLOSPORINE A AND TACROLIMUS

Adverse event	Cyclosporine A (%)	Tacrolimus (%)	*p*
Hypertension	52.2	49.8	
Hyperlipidemia	38.2	30.7	
Nephrotoxicity	41.5	45.4	
Hyperglycemia	4.0	19.9	<0.001
Headache	37.7	43.9	
Tremors	33.8	54.1	<0.001
Alopecia	1.0	10.7	<0.001
Hirsutism	8.7	0.5	<0.001
Gingival hyperplasia	5.3	0.5	0.004
Gingivitis	8.7	1.5	<0.001

From Pirsch JD, Miller J, Deierhoi MH, et al., for the FK506 kidney transplant study group. A comparison of tacrolimus (FK506) and cyclosporine for immunosuppression after cadaveric renal transplantation. *Transplantation.* 1997;63:977.

sclerosis or collapse, have been well demonstrated in patients with autoimmune diseases treated with cyclosporine, as well as in the various organ transplant recipients: heart, liver, renal, and bone marrow (47,48). The other reported adverse effects of CsA and tacrolimus include hypertension, hyperkalemia, hyperlipidemia, and headache. Adverse effects unique to CsA include hirsutism and gingival hyperplasia, whereas those unique to tacrolimus include alopecia, fine tremor, and hyperglycemia. The adverse-effect profile of both CsA and tacrolimus is compared in Table 95.3.

Dose modifications of both CsA and tacrolimus are based on whole blood trough concentrations. Monitoring of the respective drug concentrations is an essential aid in the management of a transplant recipient for the evaluation of rejection, toxicity, dose adjustments, drug interactions, and compliance. Two methods for monitoring CsA levels in whole blood include high-pressure liquid chromatography (HPLC) and radioimmunoassay, or TDx. For tacrolimus, a microparticle enzyme immunoassay (MEIA) or an enzyme-linked immunosorbent assay (ELISA)-based IMx assay are utilized. Target levels of either drug vary based on the type of assay used, the type of monitoring (trough vs. C2 [drug level 2 hours postdose] vs. AUC [area under the curve]), transplant center standards, time posttransplantation, and the recipients' risk for acute rejection.

ANTIMETABOLITES

Mycophenolic Acid

Mycophenolate mofetil (MMF) (CellCept) and enteric-coated mycophenolate sodium (MPS) (Myfortic) contain the active moiety mycophenolic acid (MPA), a reversible inhibitor of inosine monophosphate dehydrogenase (IMPDH), a key, rate-limiting step in the *de novo* pathway of guanosine nucleotide synthesis. Depletion of the guanosine nucleotides inhibits T- and B-cell proliferation as they are dependent on the *de novo* pathway of purine synthesis rather than salvage pathways.

The recommended dose of MMF is 1,000 mg orally or IV twice daily divided 12 hours apart. MMF is the prodrug of MPA and allows for increased oral bioavailability. Some centers monitor MPA drug levels for dose adjustments. The MPS equivalent is 720 mg orally twice daily 12 hours apart, although due to differences in absorption, these two formulations are not interchangeable. MPS is not available for IV infusion and the enteric-coated tablets should not be cut, crushed, or chewed.

Adverse effects of MPA include gastrointestinal effects (dyspepsia, nausea, vomiting, diarrhea, and constipation) and bone marrow suppression (leukopenia and thrombocytopenia). Diarrhea, leukopenia, and thrombocytopenia are often dose limiting requiring dose reduction to ameliorate the toxic effects. These patients, however, should be monitored closely, as a relation exists between an increased incidence of acute rejection and decreased MPA doses (49,50).

Azathioprine

Azathioprine (Imuran) is an imidazole derivative of 6-mercaptopurine. It is a purine analog that inhibits DNA and RNA production in the T cell. The initial recommended dose of azathioprine is 3 to 5 mg/kg/day administered orally or IV once daily. Adverse effects of azathioprine include hematologic toxicities (pancytopenia, macrocytic anemia, thrombocytopenia, and leukopenia), alopecia, pancreatitis, and hepatotoxicity. Dose reductions may be required for myelosuppressive toxicities. A potent drug interaction may be seen with the coadministration of azathioprine and allopurinol (a xanthine oxidase inhibitor). Although it is recommended that the dose of azathioprine should be reduced by 75% when coadministered with allopurinol, it is more prudent to avoid the use of these two agents together.

mTOR INHIBITORS

Sirolimus (Rapamune) is a macrolide antibiotic produced by *Streptomyces hygroscopicus* and is structurally similar to tacrolimus. Like tacrolimus, sirolimus also binds to FKBP-12. However, unlike tacrolimus, this complex binds to and inhibits the activation of the mammalian target of rapamycin (mTOR). This interferes with biochemical signal transductions from the cell membrane to the nucleus by inhibiting the stimulation of T cells by IL-2, -4, and -6 and by blocking the CD28 costimulatory signal. Sirolimus is available in oral tablets and oral solution. The recommended initial dose of sirolimus is approximately 6 mg (5–10 mg) loading dose, followed by 2 mg once daily maintenance dose. Dose adjustments are made based on weekly or biweekly trough level monitoring ($t_{1/2}$ = 62 hours).

Adverse effects of sirolimus include anemia, leukopenia, thrombocytopenia, hyperlipidemia, prolongation of delayed graft function, impaired wound healing, pneumonitis, arthralgia, aphthous mouth ulcers, lymphocele, and diarrhea.

The advantage of sirolimus is due to its lack of nephrotoxicity (51,52). However, when coadministered with CsA, the nephrotoxic effect of CsA can be potentiated (53). Sirolimus is metabolized by the cytochrome P450–3A4 enzyme system and has a similar drug interaction profile as that of the calcineurin inhibitors.

CORTICOSTEROIDS

Corticosteroids exert their immunosuppressive effects through multiple pathways, the most important of which is through their ability to inhibit cytokine and cytokine receptor transcription. Corticosteroids inhibit the expression of various cytokines responsible for the activation of T cells including IL-1, IL-2, IL-3, IL-6, TNF-α, and interferon-γ (IFN-γ). Corticosteroids function as both induction and maintenance immunosuppressive agents as well as for the treatment of acute rejection episodes. Typical induction protocols call for high-dose methylprednisolone, the first dose administered intraoperatively prior to organ perfusion with tapering doses for the first few days posttransplantation. This is followed by oral prednisone with continued tapering to a baseline maintenance dose. Corticosteroids are typically administered once a day in the morning concurrent with intrinsic cortisol release.

Adverse effects of corticosteroids are numerous and include cosmetic changes, avascular necrosis, cataracts, osteoporosis, impaired wound healing, glucose intolerance, hypertension, hyperlipidemia, increased appetite, hypothalamic–adrenal axis (HPA) suppression, and mood swings.

Corticosteroids were the first used immunosuppressant when renal transplants were done in the 1960s. Because of numerous adverse effects, steroid withdrawal has been attempted, but only with moderate success because of increased acute rejection. However, with the advent of newer and more effective immunosuppressive therapy, there has been a renewed interest in early withdrawal or complete elimination of corticosteroids. Short-term success has been achieved in several small single-center trials and a few larger multicenter trials. Early corticosteroid withdrawal has also been associated with a more favorable cardiovascular risk profile, as evidenced by less hypertension, posttransplant diabetes mellitus (PTDM), and hyperlipidemia (54).

MINIMIZING OPPORTUNISTIC INFECTIONS IN THE TRANSPLANT RECIPIENT

Within the first month following transplantation, surgical wound-related and nosocomial infections are the most common infections observed in renal allograft recipients. As a result, bacterial infections involving the urinary tract, the respiratory tract, the surgical wound, and/or intravenous lines are the ones frequently encountered. In a few instances, infections may be due to reactivation of pre-existing infection in the recipient such as subclinical bacterial infections, especially urinary tract infections and tuberculosis, or transmission of infections from the donor to the recipient.

Infections in the 1-month to 6-month period after transplantation are due to opportunistic organisms, most notably viruses belonging to the herpes group, especially cytomegalovirus (CMV), and due to *Candida* species and *Pneumocystis carinii*. Antimicrobial prophylaxis specific to these opportunistic organisms should be given to all renal allograft recipients early posttransplantation. Prophylaxis protocols differ among centers in antimicrobial selection and duration of therapy. Prophylaxis with antifungals such as clotrimazole, nystatin, or fluconazole may be used against *Candida* infections of the mouth and throat (thrush). Prophylaxis against *P. carinii* pneumonia (PCP) includes cotrimoxazole; or for those patients with a sulfa allergy, monthly inhaled pentamidine or oral dapsone will provide adequate prophylaxis against PCP. Drug and dose selection of antiviral prophylaxis against CMV infection can be stratified by infection risk based on previous CMV exposure, or the presence of anti-CMV antibodies in the recipient (Table 95.4). Valganciclovir is currently the drug of choice for antiviral prophylaxis against CMV.

Several antimicrobial agents adversely interact with cyclosporine and tacrolimus, and careful consideration should be given to the choice of the antimicrobial agent.

TABLE 95.4

CYTOMEGALOVIRUS (CMV) RISK STRATIFICATION AND TREATMENT OPTIONS

Risk status	Donor CMV IgG serostatus	Recipient CMV IgG serostatus	Usual drug of choice	Dose	Duration
High	Positive	Negative	Valganciclovir	450 mg qd	90–180 days
Moderate	Positive	Positive	Valganciclovir	450 mg qd	90 days
	Negative	Positive	Valganciclovir	450 mg qd	90 days
Low	Negative	Negative	Valacyclovir	500 mg bid or tid	30 days

"STABLE" ALLOGRAFT RECIPIENTS READMITTED TO THE INTENSIVE CARE UNIT

Successful transplantation restores patients to an active and functional life, but it does not prevent subsequent occurrence of atherosclerotic cardiovascular disease, cancer, trauma, infections, and other major problems. Furthermore, the care of transplant patients with other diseases demands an awareness of the long-term problems that are unique to this patient population, and these are also discussed below.

INFECTIONS

Viral Infections

Cytomegalovirus is the most important viral infection affecting transplant recipients. CMV infection risk is highest in patients who are CMV IgG seronegative and received an allograft from a CMV-seropositive donor (Table 95.4) or who have received CMV-positive blood transfusion. CMV infection often presents clinically with fever after cessation of anti-CMV prophylaxis and in some instances may present as disseminated or tissue invasive CMV disease affecting the gastrointestinal tract, liver, kidney, or lungs (pneumonitis) and with organ-specific symptoms. CMV is diagnosed by identification and quantification of the viral DNA in the blood by polymerase chain reaction (PCR). Tissue-invasive disease may be diagnosed by the identification of the characteristic *owl-eye* inclusions on tissue biopsy (55). Treatment of CMV viremia and tissue-invasive CMV disease should be initiated promptly with oral valganciclovir or intravenous ganciclovir. Concomitant treatment with CMV immune globulin may be required in some patients with severe tissue disease. Duration of treatment depends on the extent of the disease and continued positivity of the CMV-DNA by PCR.

Other viral infections that may occur in the immunosuppressed renal allograft recipient include Epstein-Barr virus (EBV), which may lead to the development of EBV-positive lymphomas; herpes simplex virus (types I and II); hepatitis B virus; hepatitis C virus; varicella-zoster virus; and the influenza virus. Treatment of viral infections depends on the type of virus and the extent of the disease. All transplant recipients should receive an annual influenza immunization.

Fungal Infections

Fungal infections are a major concern in the immunosuppressed renal allograft recipient. As with the general population, *Candida albicans* infections resulting from endogenous flora are common. However, with immunosuppression, these infections can rapidly develop into more serious infections. Other fungal pathogens seen in transplant recipients include nocardiosis, aspergillosis, *Cryptococcus*, histoplasmosis, coccidiomycosis, blastomycosis, and mucormycosis. Treatment of fungal infections include the use of antifungals specific to the organism, surgical excision (especially in the case of mucormycosis), and reduction in the overall immunosuppression. Careful consideration should be given to the choice of the antimicrobial agent because of drug interactions (azole antifungals) or additive nephrotoxicity (amphotericin B). Invasive fungal infections in transplant recipients are associated with a high risk of graft loss and mortality. Early diagnosis and aggressive treatment can preserve organ function and can be life saving.

Other Opportunistic Infections

Urinary tract infections (UTIs) are a frequent complication of renal transplantation. Although UTIs are frequently asymptomatic, they constitute the major source of bacteremia in this patient population. Therefore, all urinary tract infections, even asymptomatic ones, should be treated appropriately. Fortunately, renal dysfunction is an uncommon complication of urinary tract infections in the transplant recipient. It usually occurs with severe pyelonephritis involving the allograft, usually in the setting of ureteric obstruction or vesicoureteral reflux. Chronic urinary tract infections may require daily prophylactic antibiotic administration.

Renal allograft recipients, especially patients with poor allograft function with a background of intensive acute and chronic immunosuppressive therapy for recurrent rejection episodes, are susceptible to a large range of infections. Empiric treatment should be initiated at the first sign of infection as infections can be aggressive and worsen rapidly.

GASTROINTESTINAL COMPLICATIONS

A wide variety of gastrointestinal complications may occur after transplantation due to infections with organisms such as CMV, *Candida* sp., and *Clostridium difficile*; adverse effects associated with immunosuppressive agents; posttransplantation complications of pre-existing conditions such as diverticulitis; and other complications such as acute appendicitis, gastrointestinal bleeding, colonic or small bowel perforations, pancreatitis, and ischemic colitis. Diarrhea is a common problem in transplant recipients and may be related to the immunosuppressive drugs, due to opportunistic infections, or due to pre-existing autonomic dysfunction often related to diabetes mellitus.

Peptic Ulcer Disease

Gastroduodenal ulcers account for most of the gastrointestinal complications posttransplantation and often occur soon after renal transplantation or acute rejection therapy. Gastroduodenal ulcers presenting posttransplantation can be attributed to a variety of causes including pre-existing ulcer history, viral pathogens (CMV in 15%, herpes simplex in 2%), and immunosuppressive agents, mainly corticosteroids (56–59). The treatment of posttransplantation gastroduodenal ulcers is the same as with the general population. Proton pump inhibitors and H_2-receptor blocking agents may be used for both therapy and prophylaxis. Intermittent therapy with calcium, aluminum, or magnesium salts can provide immediate relief;

however, coadministration of these agents with MMF (CellCept) may inhibit absorption of the active moiety of this drug in the intestinal tract. All kidney transplant recipients diagnosed with gastroduodenal ulcers should be evaluated for *Helicobacter pylori* and CMV infection. Clarithromycin (Biaxin), commonly used for the treatment of *H. pylori*, interacts with CsA and tacrolimus (Table 95.2), and therefore ideally, an alternate antibiotic regimen should be used. For CMV-related gastrointestinal lesions, ganciclovir or valganciclovir treatment should be initiated promptly.

Bowel Perforations

Colonic perforation should be suspected in the presence of one or more of the following: abdominal pain, fever, increased white blood cell count, tenderness, and pneumoperitoneum. These clinical criteria may be blunted in the presence of poor renal function, use of high-dose corticosteroids, or the overall state of immunosuppression. A plain abdominal radiograph, CT scan, or colonoscopy may help in the diagnosis. Mortality rates after colonic perforation can be reduced with minimal delay to perform surgery, broad-spectrum antibiotic therapy, and reduction of immunosuppression. Operative intervention has been shown to improve patient survival significantly (60). Screening for colonic diverticula before transplantation should be applied to all patients older than age 50 years, and a segmental colectomy may be required in patients who have experienced clinical symptoms of diverticulitis (56,60).

Acute Pancreatitis

Acute pancreatitis is an infrequent but severe complication following renal transplantation. A review of the literature has documented an incidence of 2.3% with a mortality rate of 61.3% in 3,253 renal transplant recipients (61). Several etiologic factors have been considered. Azathioprine has been reported to cause pancreatitis with rapid improvement after cessation and with recurrence of symptoms with reinstitution (62). Corticosteroids and cyclosporine have also been reported to cause pancreatitis; however, this association is not as convincing. Other causes of pancreatitis include hyperparathyroidism, CMV infection, biliary tract disease, alcoholism, and hyperlipidemia (63). Although the diagnosis of pancreatitis depends largely on an increase in the serum amylase and/or serum lipase levels, ultrasonography and CT scan may be useful. Intensive medical management with particular attention to volume replacement, electrolyte balance, and nutrition is essential.

Severe diarrhea with ensuing dehydration and acidosis, gastrointestinal bleeding, cholecystitis, and diverticulitis are other commonly encountered gastrointestinal problems in the transplant recipient. Advances in the management of peptic ulcer disease, prophylaxis against CMV disease, and better preparation of recipients prior to transplantation have reduced the overall morbidity and mortality. Several of the gastrointestinal problems may be related to the side effects of the immunosuppressive drugs or due to the net state of overimmunosuppression. Careful consideration should be given to the change in the immunosuppressive agent and to decrease in the dosages of these medications.

Hematologic Complications

Neutropenia is a frequent complication posttransplantation, often as a result of the adverse effects of immunosuppressive medications. Antithymocyte globulin can cause transient decreases in neutrophils that often rebound after cessation of therapy. Maintenance immunosuppression with mycophenolic acid, sirolimus, and prophylaxis with ganciclovir and cotrimoxazole contribute to the development of neutropenia due to their myelosuppressive effects. Careful dose reduction of these agents and/or use of granulocyte-stimulating factors are often required for persistent neutropenia. Of particular importance is that neutropenia can be a sign of CMV infection, and therefore this should always be excluded in transplant recipients with persistent neutropenia.

Anemia is a frequent occurrence in the early posttransplantation period as a result of pre-existing anemia of end-stage renal disease, surgical blood loss, and immunosuppressive medications. Patients with slow or delayed graft function may have a more pronounced and prolonged anemia. Anemia in the late posttransplantation phase can be attributed to a combination of immunosuppressive medications, renal allograft dysfunction, use of angiotensin-converting enzyme (ACE) inhibitors or angiotensin II receptor blockers, and/or iron deficiency (64). As cardiovascular disease is the leading cause of morbidity and mortality in kidney transplant recipients, it is important to manage anemia aggressively in this patient population with the use of erythropoietin. Furthermore, given the high incidence of coexisting cardiovascular disease in this patient population, blood transfusions should not be withheld for acute indications.

Thrombocytopenia is also a frequent occurrence in renal allograft recipients and often is caused by the immunosuppressive medications. Antithymocyte globulin, valganciclovir, and dapsone can cause transient decreases in platelets. Withholding doses or dose adjustments of the responsible agent may be required for thrombocytopenia. Platelet recovery is rapid, often returning to baseline within days. In rare circumstances, thrombocytopenia may be due to hemolytic uremic syndrome (HUS) that is caused by immunosuppressive drugs (calcineurin inhibitors, sirolimus, OKT3), severe acute vascular rejection, transmission from donor, recurrence of previous HUS, or causes similar to those in nontransplant recipients.

CARDIAC AND VASCULAR DISEASES

Coronary Artery Disease

Atherosclerotic vascular disease is the major cause of late morbidity and mortality in transplant recipients, and coronary artery disease is the principal cause of death (65–69). In transplant recipients, risk factors for posttransplantation coronary artery disease include increased age, male gender, history of diabetes mellitus, hypercholesterolemia, smoking history, acute renal allograft rejection episodes, and greater cumulative dose of steroids (70). The key to the early detection of significant coronary artery disease in renal transplant recipients without coronary symptoms is repeated evaluation for the known risk factors. The management of transplant patients with coronary artery disease is similar to that of other patients and should include noninvasive exercise or resting diagnostic testing, coronary arteriography, or both. However, some noninvasive screening tests have been shown to be less useful, especially in the presence of diabetes, uremia, and left ventricular hypertrophy (71). With the increasing number of transplantations performed in the elderly and in patients with diabetes mellitus, cardiovascular disease will continue to be a major cause of posttransplantation morbidity. Of particular note, during cardiac catheterization, femoral arterial puncture on the ipsilateral side to the renal transplant should be avoided whenever feasible to reduce the risks of mechanical injury and atheroembolization to the renal allograft.

Cerebrovascular and Peripheral Vascular Disease

Cerebrovascular disease occurs in 1% to 3% of all renal allograft recipients (65,72). There is also an increased risk of peripheral vascular disease (65,68,73,74). A thorough history to elicit symptoms associated with cerebrovascular and peripheral vascular disease and examination of the carotid arteries and peripheral circulation should be performed annually and the presence of a carotid bruit should be further investigated with duplex ultrasonography and magnetic resonance angiography (MRA). In the presence of more than 60% stenosis of the carotid artery, the patient should be referred to the neurovascular surgeon for further evaluation (75).

Successful transplantation does not reduce the rate of atherosclerosis initiated in renal failure. Factors contributing to the high incidence of vascular disease include hypertension, hyperlipidemia, obesity, cigarette smoking, and the presence of pre-existing diabetes mellitus or the development of posttransplantation diabetes mellitus (65). The mortality rate from coronary artery disease was increased 25-fold to that of age-matched and gender-matched controls in an Australian study (76), was increased 10-fold in a study from Stockholm (77), and was increased three- to fourfold in a Minneapolis study (70). By actuarial analysis, 15% of patients who survived with a functioning allograft for 15 years developed peripheral vascular disease (73).

HYPERTENSION

Hypertension is a common complication of renal transplantation and remains an important risk factor for mortality from cardiovascular disease. Posttransplantation hypertension is a major risk factor for graft survival. It is unclear, however, whether this is because of the deleterious effects of hypertension on the structure and function of the renal allograft or whether hypertension is a marker of underlying renal disease (78,79). The causes of hypertension in renal transplant recipients include acute and/or chronic allograft rejection; recurrent or *de novo* transplant glomerulonephritis; transplant renal artery stenosis; high renin output state from diseased native kidneys; immunosuppressive agents such as steroids, cyclosporine, and tacrolimus; obesity; hypercalcemia; and new-onset essential hypertension (80).

HYPERLIPIDEMIA

As discussed earlier, cardiovascular disease is the most common cause of posttransplantation morbidity and mortality among long-term renal transplant survivors. As in the general population, posttransplantation lipoprotein abnormalities contribute to the development of cardiovascular and peripheral vascular disease in renal transplant recipients (67,73,81,82). The prevalence of posttransplantation hyperlipidemia ranges from 16% to 78% of recipients (65), depending at which time point posttransplantation serum lipid levels were obtained. Elevations in triglycerides, low-density lipoproteins (LDLs), apolipoprotein B, and total cholesterol levels are common (83–91). The pathogenesis of hyperlipidemia in renal transplant recipients is poorly understood and appears to be multifactorial. The numerous factors that have been shown to be associated with hyperlipidemia after renal transplantation are age, body weight, gender, pretransplantation lipid levels, renal dysfunction, proteinuria, concomitant use of diuretics or β-blockers, diabetes, steroid use, and cyclosporine and sirolimus use (81,83–89,92,93).

NEW-ONSET DIABETES AFTER TRANSPLANTATION

New-onset diabetes after transplantation (NODAT) has been reported in 3% to 40% of transplant recipients with an even higher incidence occurring in African Americans, Hispanics, and patients with a family history of diabetes mellitus, increasing with recipient age and weight (65,66,69,72,94–96). NODAT has been attributed to the use of immunosuppressive agents, especially with tacrolimus and corticosteroids; however, cyclosporine has also been implicated (96–99). Patients with NODAT have a poor outcome in terms of patient and graft survival, with increased mortality resulting from cardiovascular and possibly infectious complications (95,100).

Insulin treatment may be required in patients with NODAT who do not respond to lifestyle modification and oral hypoglycemic agents. About half of patients in whom NODAT develops require insulin. Aggressive treatment with either intravenous or subcutaneous insulin may also be indicated during periods of intercurrent illness and stress.

GRAFT DYSFUNCTION AND GRAFT FAILURE

The differential diagnosis of acute allograft dysfunction can be divided into (a) early, occurring <90 days posttransplantation, and (b) late, occurring >90 days after transplantation. It can be further differentiated into medical and surgical problems as outlined in Table 95.5. Some of the more common medical and surgical problems are discussed below.

Acute Rejection

Although acute allograft rejection is the most common cause of graft dysfunction both in the early and late periods, it most commonly occurs during the first 90 days posttransplantation.

TABLE 95.5

CAUSES OF GRAFT DYSFUNCTION AND FAILURE

	Early (0–90 days posttransplantation)	Late (>90 days posttransplantation)
Medical	Hyperacute rejection Delayed graft function Acute rejection Acute calcineurin inhibitor nephrotoxicity Dehydration Other drug toxicities Infection *De novo*/recurrent disease	Acute rejection Calcineurin inhibitor toxicity Chronic rejection Dehydration Other drug toxicities Infection BK virus nephropathy *De novo*/recurrent disease
Mechanical	Lymphocele Ureteric obstruction Urine leak Vascular thrombosis	Renal artery stenosis Ureteric obstruction Urine leak Vascular thrombosis

Recipients of transplants from living donors have a significantly lower incidence of rejection episodes. Factors significantly associated with the development of acute rejection are HLA mismatch, anti-HLA antibodies reactive to greater than 50% of a lymphocyte panel, retransplantation, African American race, and recipient age under 16 (101,102). The classic clinical features associated with acute rejection are fever, oliguria, weight gain, edema, hypertension, and the presence of an enlarged, tender graft. However, these features are frequently absent, and the most common presentation may be an asymptomatic rise in serum creatinine. An increase in serum creatinine greater than 20% is often the cardinal feature of rejection. Percutaneous needle biopsy of the allograft is the most reliable method of diagnosis of acute rejection. Acute rejection is classified histologically using the Banff 97 classification of renal allograft pathology depending on the severity of lymphocytic infiltration of tubules (tubulitis), arterioles (arteritis), and the renal interstitium (103).

The principles and the management of acute rejection include rapid diagnosis, accurate classification, and prompt administration of antirejection therapy. Currently, corticosteroids and antilymphocyte antibodies represent the main components of antirejection treatment protocols. The decision on treatment of acute rejection is based on histologic severity. One approach is to treat mild acute cellular rejection with a course of 250 to 500 mg of intravenous methylprednisolone administered daily for 3 or 4 days, and moderate and severe acute cellular rejection and acute vascular rejection are treated with a 4- to 7-day course of an antilymphocyte antibody, currently either Thymoglobulin or OKT3.

Chronic Rejection

Chronic rejection is characterized clinically by a progressive decline in renal function, persistent proteinuria, and hypertension. The course of chronic rejection is slow and insidious. Chronic rejection often occurs in conjunction with other histologic causes of allograft dysfunction, namely, acute rejection, calcineurin inhibitor nephrotoxicity, and recurrent or *de novo* glomerular diseases. The diagnosis of chronic rejection should therefore be based on morphologic characteristics of allograft histology and the clinical observation of a gradual decline in renal allograft function. The pathophysiology of chronic rejection is not completely understood, but most likely involves both immune and nonimmune factors. Risk factors for the development of chronic rejection include delayed graft function, ischemia–reperfusion injury, degree of HLA mismatching, histoincompatibility, acute rejection episodes, inadequate renal mass, hypertension, hyperlipidemia, and cytomegalovirus infection (104). There is no treatment for chronic rejection at the present time.

Urologic Complications

Urologic problems have been reported in between 2% and 20% of all renal transplants (105–109). These complications can include urinary retention, urine leak, and ureteral stenosis. Urinary retention can occur because of a neurogenic bladder (related to diabetes or a congenital neurologic disorder) or perhaps an undetected prostatic hypertrophy. These can be managed with an initially longer period of urinary catheterization and use of α-antagonists (tamsulosin, terazosin, prazosin) to improve bladder emptying. More extreme cases may require long-term intermittent self-catheterization or surgical urinary diversion. Urine leak or stenosis can occur both early and later after renal transplant and will be manifested by a rising serum creatinine. Urine leaks may also result in increased fluid through an operative drain or fluid leakage through the wound. This fluid can be sent for creatinine level to confirm the presence of a urine leak. Ultrasound studies may demonstrate a fluid collection around the allograft or hydronephrosis in the case of ureteral stenosis. Nuclear medicine scans can also be obtained to confirm the presence of a ureteral stenosis or urine leak. Mild cases of ureteral stenosis/leakage can be managed with percutaneous methods including insertion of ureteral stents and transluminal balloon dilation. Many of these stenoses/leaks will require operative management to reimplant the ureter or a more complex urologic procedure using the recipient's native ureter or bladder (105–109).

Vascular Complications

Vascular complications including vessel thrombosis or stenosis have been reported in 2% to 12% of all renal transplants. Vascular complications in general are significantly associated with ATN and graft loss. Early graft dysfunction should be evaluated for vascular complications with ultrasound with Doppler (110). Patients with underlying thrombophilia are at a higher risk for early allograft loss without appropriate anticoagulation. Screening for thrombophilia in those ESRD patients with a history of a thromboembolic event may be appropriate to prevent this. Those patients with graft loss due to vascular thrombosis in the absence of an obvious technical problem should undergo a thrombophilia evaluation before retransplant (111).

Lymphocele

A lymphocele is a collection of lymphatic fluid around the allografted kidney that can occur due to leakage of small lymphatic channels around the iliac vessels at the time of the transplant. The incidence of lymphoceles has been reported from 0.02% up to 26% following renal transplant (112–114). Consequences of lymphoceles can include distention due to the fluid collection as well as venous or ureteral obstruction and graft compromise. Treatment of lymphoceles can include percutaneous techniques with drainage and sclerosis of the cavity or may include operative marsupialization via the laparoscopic or open technique. Laparoscopic techniques are less invasive, have less morbidity, and are generally the first line of therapy (114).

Stones

Urinary calculi are a relatively uncommon complication of renal transplantation. Calculi may have been present in the donor kidney or may develop after transplantation. Predisposing factors include obstruction, recurrent urinary tract infection, hypercalciuria, hyperoxaluria, internal stents, and nonabsorbable suture material (115). Open removal of a calculus from the transplanted kidney is rarely necessary. Complete stone removal is usually possible by standard urologic techniques.

POSTTRANSPLANT MALIGNANCIES

Prolonged and intensive immunosuppression impairs the ability of the body to cope with cancers caused by carcinogens such as sunlight or oncogenic viruses and may lead to the development of an unusual assortment of malignancies (116,117). Infections with potentially oncogenic viruses are common in immunosuppressed patients, including EBV-related B-cell PTLD, human papillomavirus, hepatitis B and hepatitis C virus–related hepatocellular carcinoma, and the human herpes virus-8 (Kaposi sarcoma) (117). Malignancies that occur in transplant recipients have a pattern that is very different from that of the general population. The frequency of the cancers that are common in the general population, such as carcinomas of the lung, prostate, breast, and colon and invasive carcinomas of the uterine cervix, are not increased among transplant recipients (116). Most patients who develop malignancies posttransplant have received multiple immunosuppressive drugs and no single agent can be implicated. The natural history of tumors associated with immunosuppression used for renal transplantation may be more aggressive than would be expected in patients without immunosuppression or transplantation. Cancers of the lip and skin are the most common malignancies. In contrast to the general population, squamous cell carcinoma outnumbers basal cell carcinoma and occurs at a much younger age.

PTLDs are the second most common malignancies found in renal transplant recipients, with the bulk being non-Hodgkin lymphomas. The EBV genome has been isolated from many lymphomas in transplant recipients and causes a variety of lesions that range from benign polyclonal B-cell hyperplasia to frank monoclonal B-cell lymphomas (116,118). Risk factors for PTLD include the overall extent of immunosuppression of the patient. Use of monoclonal/polyclonal antibodies for induction and repeated treatments for acute rejection will significantly increase the risk for PTLD (116,119). The clinical symptoms of PTLD may be extremely variable, and a high index of suspicion is required for accurate diagnosis. PTLD may present in the lymph nodes or extranodally. There are two basic clinical patterns with some overlap. The first, occurring in the early (usually <90 days) posttransplantation period, usually manifests with widespread lesions in an EBV-susceptible patient. The second pattern occurs in patients who received long-term immunosuppression and may present several years after transplantation, with lesions confined to a single organ (120,121).

Treatment of PTLD consists of partial or complete withdrawal of immunosuppression. Such treatment carries the risk of allograft rejection and return of the renal allograft recipient to dialysis. Treatment with prednisone may be continued, however, because it is an important component of many cancer chemotherapy protocols. If EBV infection is suspected, treatment with acyclovir, ganciclovir, or valacyclovir should be initiated pending documentation of EBV infection. Other treatment options include interferon-γ therapy to enhance the immune attack on the lymphoma cells; surgical excision or local radiotherapy to localized tumors; and in advanced cases, chemotherapy. Rituximab (Rituxan; Genentech), a monoclonal antibody directed against the CD20 antigen, has been used successfully to treat CD20-positive tumors (122–124).

References

1. Kidney and Urologic Diseases Information Clearinghouse. A service of the National Institute of Diabetes and Digestive Diseases and Kidney Diseases, National Institutes of Health. Available at: http://kidney.niddk.nih.gov/kudiseases/pubs/kustats/index.htm. Accessed October 15, 2006.
2. Winkelmayer WC, Weinstein MC, Mittelman MA, et al. Health economic evaluations: the special case of end-stage renal disease treatment. *Med Decis Making.* 2002;22:417.
3. Loubeau PR, Loubeau JM, Jantzen R. The economics of kidney transplantation vs hemodialysis. *Prog Transplant.* 2001;11:291.
4. National transplant statistics, 2005. United Network for Organ Sharing. Available at: www.unos.org. Accessed October 15, 2006.
5. Remuzzi G, Grinyo J, Ruggenenti P, et al. Early experience with dual kidney transplantation in adults using expanded donor criteria. Double Kidney Transplant Group (DKG). *J Am Soc Nephrol.* 1999;10:2591.
6. Gok MA, Buckley PE, Shenton BK, et al. Long-term renal function in kidneys from non-heart beating donors: a single-center experience. *Transplantation.* 2002;74:664.
7. Sanchez-Fructuoso A, Sanchez DP, Vidas MM, et al. Non-heart beating donors. *Nephrol Dial Transplant.* 2004;19(Suppl 3):iii26.

8. U.S. Organ Procurement and Transplantation Network/Scientific Registry of Transplant Recipients, Annual Report 2005.
9. Kasiske BL, Cangro CB, Hariharan S, et al. The evaluation of renal transplant candidates: clinical practice guidelines. *Am J Transplantation.* 2001;2(Suppl 1):5–95.
10. Gore JL, Pham PT, Danovitch GM, et al. Obesity and outcome following renal transplant. *Am J Transplantation.* 2006;6:357.
11. Stratta RJ, Rohr MS, Sundberg AK et al. Intermediate-term outcomes with expanded criteria deceased donors in kidney transplantation: a spectrum or specter of quality. *Ann Surg.* 2006;243:594.
12. Merion RM, Ashby VB, Wolfe RA, et al. Decreased-donor characteristics and the survival benefit of kidney transplantation. *JAMA.* 2005;294:2726.
13. Bernat JL, D'Alessandro AM, Port FK, et al. Report of a national conference on donation after cardiac death. *Am J Transplant.* 2006;6:281.
14. Ting A, Welsh K. HLA matching and crossmatching in renal transplantation. In: Morris PJ, ed. *Kidney Transplantation: Principles and Practice.* 4th ed. Philadelphia: WB Saunders; 1994:109.
15. Furnary AP, Wu Y, Bookin SO. Effect of hyperglycemia and continuous intravenous insulin infusions on outcomes of cardiac surgical procedures: the Portland Diabetic Project. *Endocr Pract.* 2004;10:21.
16. Finney SJ, Zekveld C, Elia A, et al. Glucose control and mortality in critically ill patients. *JAMA.* 2003;290:2041.
17. Starzl TE, Broth CG, Putnam CW, et al. Urologic complications in 216 human recipients of renal transplants. *Ann Surg.* 1973;172:609.
18. Petrek J, Tilney NL, Smith EH, et al. Ultrasound in renal transplantation. *Ann Surg.* 1977;185:441.
19. Maley HT, Bulkley GB, Williams GM. Ablation of free radical-medicated reperfusion injury for the salvage of kidneys taken from non-heartbeating donors. *Transplantation.* 1988;45:284.
20. Sola R, Alarcon A, Jimenez C, et al. The influence of delayed graft function. *Nephrol Dial Transplant.* 2004;19(Suppl 3):iii32.
21. Boom H, Mallat MJ, deFijter JW, et al. Delayed graft function influences renal function, but not survival. *Kidney Int.* 2000;58:859.
22. Irish WD, McCollum DA, Tesi RJ, et al. Nomogram for predicting the likelihood of delayed graft function in adult cadaveric renal transplant recipients. *J Am Soc Nephrol.* 2003;14:2967.
23. Shoskes DA, Halloran PF. Delayed graft function in renal transplantation: etiology, management and long-term significance. *J Urol.* 1996;155:1831.
24. Ojo AO, Wolfe RA, Held PJ, et al. Delayed graft function: risk factors, and implications for renal allograft survival. *Transplantation.* 1997;63:968.
25. Rocha PN, Butterly DW, Greenberg A, et al. Beneficial effect of plasmapheresis and intravenous immunoglobulin on renal allograft survival of patients with acute humoral rejection. *Transplantation.* 2003;75:1490.
26. Bonnefoy-Berard N, Revillard JP. Mechanisms of immunosuppression induced by antithymocyte globulins and OKT3. *J Heart Lung Transplant.* 1996;15:435.
27. Rossi SJ, Schroeder TJ, Hariharan S, et al. Prevention and management of the adverse effects associated with immunosuppressive therapy. *Drug Saf.* 1993;9:104.
28. Gaber AO, First MR, Tesi RJ, et al. Results of the double-blind, randomized, multicenter, phase-III clinical trial of Thymoglobulin versus Atgam in the treatment of acute graft rejection episodes after renal transplantation. *Transplantation.* 1998;66:29.
29. Brennan DC, Flavin K, Lowell JA, et al. A randomized, double-blinded comparison of Thymoglobulin versus Atgam for induction immunosuppressive therapy in adult renal transplant recipients. *Transplantation.* 1999;67:1011.
30. Ortho Multicenter Transplant Study Group. A randomized clinical trial of OKT3 monoclonal antibody for acute rejection of cadaveric renal transplants. *N Engl J Med.* 1985;313:337.
31. First MR, Schroeder TJ, Hariharan S. OKT3-induced cytokine release syndrome: renal effects (cytokine nephropathy). *Transplant Proc.* 1993;25:25.
32. Chatenoud L, Legendre C, Ferran C, et al. Corticosteroid inhibition of the OKT3-induced cytokine release syndrome: dosage and kinetics prerequisites. *Transplantation.* 1991;51:334.
33. Peddi VR, Bryant M, Roy-Chaudhury P, et al. Thymoglobulin induction therapy in cadaveric renal allograft recipients: intermittent dosing with CD3+ lymphocyte count monitoring [Abstract]. *Transplantation.* 2000;69:S160.
34. Vincenti F, Kirkman R, Light S, et al., for the Daclizumab Triple Therapy Study Group. Interleukin-2- receptor blockade with daclizumab to prevent acute rejection in renal transplantation. *N Engl J Med.* 1998;338:161.
35. Nashan B, Moore R, Amlot P, et al., for the CH1B 201 International Study Group. Randomized trial of basiliximab versus placebo for control of acute cellular rejection in renal allograft recipients. *Lancet.* 1997;350:1193.
36. Riechmann L, Clark M, Waldmann H. Reshaping human antibodies for therapy. *Nature.* 1988;332:323.
37. Hale G, Xia MQ, Tighe MJS, et al. The Campath-1H antigen (CDw52). *Tissue Antigens.* 1990;35:118.
38. Hale G. CD52 antigen as a target for immunotherapy. *Transpl Rev.* 2003;17:S8.
39. Waldmann H. Development and clinical use of Campath 1H. *Transpl Rev.* 2003;17:S5.
40. Kaufman DB, Leventhal JR, Axelrod D, et al. Alemtuzumab induction and prednisolone-free maintenance immunotherapy in kidney transplantation: comparison with basiliximab induction. Long-term results. *Am J Transpl.* 2005;78:426.
41. Shapiro R, Basu A, Tan H, et al. Kidney transplantation under minimal immunosuppression after pretransplant lymphoid depletion with Thymoglobulin or Campath. *J Am Coll Surg.* 2005;200:505.
42. Nadler LM, Ritz J, Hardy R, et al. A unique cell surface antigen identifying lymphoid malignancies of B-cell origin. *J Clin Invest.* 1981;67:134.
43. Maloney D, Liles T, Czerwinski D, et al. Phase I clinical trial using escalating single dose infusion of chimeric anti-CD 20 monoclonal antibody in patients with recurrent B-cell lymphoma. *Blood.* 1994;84:2457.
44. Coiffier B, Haioun C, Ketterer N, et al. Rituximab for the treatment of patients with relapsing or refractory aggressive lymphoma: a multicenter phase II study. *Blood.* 1998;92:1927.
45. Blaes AH, Peterson BA, Bartlett N, et al. Rituximab therapy is effective for post transplant lymphoproliferative disorders after solid organ transplantation: results of a phase II trial. *Cancer.* 2005;104:1661.
46. Rosenthal JT, Hakala TR, Iwatsuki S, et al. Cadaveric renal transplantation under cyclosporine-steroid therapy. *Surg Gynecol Obstet.* 1983;157:309.
47. Myers BD, Newton L, Oyer P. The case against the indefinite use of cyclosporine. *Transplant Proc.* 1991;23:41.
48. Bennett WM, DeMattos A, Meyer MM, et al. Chronic cyclosporine nephropathy: the Achilles' heel of immunosuppressive therapy. *Kidney Int.* 1996;50:1089.
49. Hardinger KL, Brennan DC, Mutinga N, et al. Long-term outcome and cost of gastrointestinal complications in renal transplant patients treated with mycophenolate mofetil (MMF). Presented at American Society of Transplantation, May 30–June 4, 2003; Washington DC. Poster #1595.
50. Knoll GA, MacDonald I, Khan A. Mycophenolate mofetil dose reduction and the risk of acute rejection after renal transplantation. *J Am Soc Nephrol.* 2003;14:2381.
51. Morales JM, Wramner L, Kreis H, et al. Sirolimus does not exhibit nephrotoxicity compared to cyclosporine in renal transplant recipients. *Am J Transplant.* 2002;2:436.
52. Reitamo S, Spuls P, Sassolas B, et al. Efficacy of sirolimus (rapamycin) administered concomitantly with a subtherapeutic dose of cyclosporine in the treatment of severe psoriasis: a randomized controlled trial. *Br J Dermatol.* 2001;145:438.
53. Shihab FS, Bennett WM, Yi H, et al. Sirolimus increases transforming growth factor- beta1 expression and potentiates chronic cyclosporine nephrotoxicity. *Kidney Int.* 2004;65:1262.
54. Matas AJ, Kandaswamy R, Humar A, et al. Long-term immunosuppression, without maintenance prednisone, after kidney transplantation. *Ann Surg.* 2004;240:510.
55. Ulrich W, Schlederer MP, Buxbaum P, et al. The histopathologic identification of CMV infected cells in biopsies of human renal allografts. An evaluation of 100 transplant biopsies by *in situ* hybridization. *Pathol Res Pract.* 1986;1981:739.
56. Benoit G, Moukarzel M, Verdelli G, et al. Gastrointestinal complications in renal transplantation. *Transplant Int.* 1993;6:45.
57. Troppmann C, Papalois BE, Chiou A, et al. Incidence, complications, treatment, and outcome of ulcers of the upper gastrointestinal tract after renal transplantation during the cyclosporine era. *J Am Coll Surg.* 1995;180:433.
58. Gianello P, Squifflet JP, Pirson Y, et al. Gastroduodenal complications after transplantation. *Clin Transplant.* 1988;2:221.
59. Hadjiyannakis EJ, Evans DB, Smellie WAB, et al. Gastrointestinal complications after renal transplantation. *Lancet.* 1971;2:781.
60. Carson SD, Krom RAF, Uchida K, et al. Colon perforation after kidney transplantation. *Ann Surg.* 1978;188:109.
61. Fernandez-Cruz L, Targarona EM, Cugat E, et al. Acute pancreatitis after renal transplantation. *Br J Surg.* 1989;76:1132.
62. Kawanishi H, Rudolph E, Bull FE. Azathioprine-induced acute pancreatitis. *N Engl J Med.* 1973;289:357.
63. Fernandez-Cruz L, Targarona EM, Cugat E, et al. Acute pancreatitis after renal transplantation. *Br J Surg.* 1989;76:1132.
64. Vanrenterghem Y, Ponticelli C, Morales JM, et al. Prevalence and management of anemia in renal transplant recipients: a European survey. *Am J Transplant.* 2003;3:835.
65. First MR. Long-term complications after transplantation. *Am J Kidney Dis.* 1993;22:477.
66. Kirkman RL, Strom TB, Weir MR, et al. Late mortality and morbidity in recipients of long-term renal allografts. *Transplantation.* 1982;34:347.
67. Hill MN, Grossman RA, Feldman HI, et al. Changes in causes of death after renal transplantation, 1966 to 1987. *Am J Kidney Dis.* 1991;5:512.
68. Rao KV, Andersen RC. Long-term results and complications in renal transplant recipients: observations in the second decade. *Transplantation.* 1988;45:45.
69. Braun WE. Long-term complications of renal transplantation. *Kidney Int.* 1990;37:1363.
70. Kasiske BL. Risk factors for accelerated atherosclerosis in renal transplant recipients. *Am J Med.* 1988;84:985.
71. Braun WE, Marwick TH. Coronary artery disease in renal transplant recipients. *Cleve Clin J Med.* 1994;61:370.
72. Keown PA, Shackleton CR, Ferguson BM. Long-term mortality, morbidity, and rehabilitation in organ transplant recipients. In: Paul LC, Solez K, eds.

Organ Transplantation: Long-Term Results. New York: Marcel Dekker; 1992:57.

73. Kasiske BL, Buijjaro C, Massy ZA, et al. Cardiovascular disease after renal transplantation. *J Am Soc Nephrol.* 1996;7:158.
74. Vanrenterghem Y, Roels L, Lerut T, et al. Long-term prognosis after cadaveric kidney transplantation. *Transplant Proc.* 1987;19:3762.
75. Brott T, Toole JF. Medical compared with surgical treatment of asymptomatic carotid artery stenosis. *Ann Intern Med.* 1995;123:720.
76. Ibels LS, Stewart JH, Mahony JF, et al. Deaths from occlusive arterial disease in renal allograft recipients. *BMJ.* 1974;3:552.
77. Gunnarsson R, Lofmark R, Nondlander R, et al. Acute myocardial infarction in renal transplant recipients: incidence and prognosis. *Eur Heart J.* 1984;5:218.
78. Held PJ, Port FK, Blagg CR, et al. Survival and mortality. Excerpts from United States Renal Data System 1990 Annual Report. *Am J Kidney Dis.* 1990;16(Suppl 2):44.
79. Luke RG. Pathophysiology and treatment of posttransplant hypertension. *J Am Soc Nephrol.* 1991;2(Suppl 1):S37.
80. Luke RG. Hypertension in renal transplant recipients. *Kidney Int.* 1987;31:1024.
81. Abdulmassih Z, Chevalier A, Bader C, et al. Role of lipid disturbances in the atherosclerosis of renal transplant patients. *Clin Transplant.* 1992;6:106.
82. Summary of the second report of the National Cholesterol Education Program (NCEP) expert panel on detection, evaluation, and treatment of high blood cholesterol in adults (adult treatment panel II). *JAMA.* 1993;269:3015.
83. Cattran DC, Steiner G, Wilson DR, et al. Hyperlipidemia after renal transplantation: natural history and pathophysiology. *Ann Intern Med.* 1979;91:554.
84. Vathsala A, Weinberg RB, Schoenberg L, et al. Lipid abnormalities in cyclosporine-prednisone-treated renal transplant recipients. *Transplantation.* 1989;48:37.
85. Kasiske BL, Umen AJ. Persistent hyperlipidemia in renal transplant recipients. *Medicine.* 1987;66:309.
86. Divaker D, Bailey RR, Frampton CM, et al. Hyperlipidemia in stable renal transplant recipients. *Nephron.* 1991;59:423.
87. Massy ZA, Kasiske BL. Post-transplant hyperlipidemia: mechanisms and management. *J Am Soc Nephrol.* 1996;7:971.
88. Duerke TB, Abdulmassih Z, Lacour B, et al. Atherosclerosis and lipid disorders after renal transplantation. *Kidney Int.* 1991;39:S24.
89. Raine AEG, Carter R, Mann JI, et al. Adverse effect of cyclosporin on plasma cholesterol in renal transplant recipients. *Nephrol Dial Transplant.* 1988;3:458.
90. Jung K, Neumann R, Scholz D, et al. Abnormalities in the composition of serum high density lipoprotein in renal transplant recipients. *Clin Nephrol.* 1982;17:191.
91. Averna MR, Barbagallo CM, Sparacino V, et al. Follow-up of lipid and apoprotein levels in renal transplant level in renal transplant recipients. *Nephron.* 1991;58:255.
92. Kasiske BL, Tortorice KL, Heim-Duthoy KL, et al. The adverse impact of cyclosporine on serum lipids in renal transplant recipients. *Am J Kidney Dis.* 1991;17:700.
93. Bittar AE, Ratcliffe PJ, Richardson AJ, et al. The prevalence of hyperlipidemia in renal transplant recipients associations with immunosuppressive and antihypertensive therapy. *Transplantation.* 1990;50:987.
94. Roth D, Milgrom M, Esquenazi V, et al. Posttransplant hyperglycemia increased incidence in cyclosporine-treated renal allograft recipients. *Transplantation.* 1989;47:278.
95. Sumrani NB, Delaney V, Ding Z, et al. Diabetes mellitus after renal transplantation in the cyclosporine era—an analysis of risk factors. *Transplantation.* 1991;51:343.
96. Jindal RM. Posttransplant diabetes mellitus—a review. *Transplantation.* 1994;58:1289.
97. Pirsch JD, Miller J, Deierhoi MH, et al., for the FK506 kidney transplant study group. A comparison of tacrolimus (FK506) and cyclosporine for immunosuppression after cadaveric renal transplantation. *Transplantation.* 1997;63:977.
98. US multicenter FK506 Liver Study Group. A comparison of tacrolimus (FK506) and cyclosporine for immunosuppression in liver transplantation. *N Engl J Med.* 1994;331:1110.
99. European FK506 Multicentre Liver Study Group. Randomised trial comparing tacrolimus (FK506) and cyclosporin in prevention of liver allograft rejection. *Lancet.* 1994;344:423.
100. Sumrani N, Delaney V, Ding Z, et al. Posttransplant diabetes mellitus in cyclosporine-treated renal transplant recipients. *Transplant Proc.* 1991;23:1249.
101. Koyama H, Cecka JM. Rejection episodes. *Clin Transpl.* 1992;391.
102. Peddi VR, First MR. Early posttransplant care of renal transplant recipients. *Semin Dial.* 1999;12:320.
103. Racusen LC, Solez K, Colvin RB, et al. The Banff 97 working classification of renal allograft pathology. *Kidney Int.* 1999;55:713–723.
104. Monaco AP, Burke JF Jr, Ferguson RM. Current thinking on chronic renal allograft rejection: issues, concerns, and recommendations from a 1997 round table discussion. *Am J Kidney Dis.* 1999;33:150.
105. Hernandez D, Rufino M, Armas S, et al. Retrospective analysis of surgical complications following cadaveric kidney transplantation in the modern transplant era. *Nephrol Dial Transplant.* 2006;10:2908.
106. Dalgic A, Boyvat F, Karakayali H, et al. Urologic complications in 1523 renal transplantations: the Baskent University experience. *Transplant Proc.* 2006;38:543.
107. Juaneda B, Alcaraz A, Buhons A, et al. Endourological management is better in early-onset ureteral stenosis in kidney transplant. *Transplant Proc.* 2005;37:3825.
108. Pisani F, Iaria G, D'Angelo M, et al. Urologic complications in kidney transplantation. *Transplant Proc.* 2005;37:2521.
109. Praz V, Leeisinger HJ, Pascual M, et al. Urological complications in renal transplantation from cadaveric donor grafts: a retrospective analysis of 20 years. *Urol Int.* 2005;75:144.
110. Osman Y, Shokeir A, Ali-el Dein B, et al. Vascular complications after live donor renal transplantation: study of risk factors and effects of graft and patient survival. *J Urol.* 2003;169:859.
111. Morrissey PE, Ramirez PJ, Gohh RY, et al. Management of thrombophilia in renal transplant patients. *Am J Transplant.* 2002;2:872.
112. Smyth GP, Beitz G, Eng MP, et al. Long-term outcome of cadaveric renal transplant after treatment of symptomatic lymphocele. *J Urol.* 2006;176:1069.
113. Atray NK, Moore F, Zaman F, et al. Post-transplant lymphocele: a single centre experience. *Clin Transplant.* 2004;18:46.
114. Bailey SH, Mone MC, Holman JM, et al. Laparoscopic treatment of post renal transplant lymphoceles. *Surg Endosc.* 2003;17:1896.
115. Yigit B, Aydin C, Titiz I, et al. Stone disease in kidney transplantation. *Transplant Proc.* 2004;36:187.
116. Penn I. Cancers complicating organ transplantation. *N Engl J Med.* 1990;323:1767.
117. Penn I. Tumors in the transplant. In: Jacobson HR, Striker GF, Klahr S, eds. *The Principles and Practice of Nephrology.* Philadelphia: Mosby; 1995:833.
118. Hanto DW. Polyclonal and monoclonal posttransplant lymphoproliferative diseases (PTLD). *Clin Transpl.* 1992;6:227.
119. Penn I. The changing pattern of posttransplant malignancies. *Transplant Proc.* 1991;23:1101.
120. Renoult E, Aymard B, Gregoire MJ, et al. Epstein-Barr virus lymphoproliferative disease of donor origin after kidney transplantation: a case report. *Am J Kidney Dis.* 1995;26:84.
121. Alfrey EJ, Friedman AL, Grossman RA, et al. Two distinct patterns of posttransplantation lymphoproliferative disorder (PTLD): early and late onset. *Clin Transpl.* 1992;6:246.
122. Penn I. Immunosuppression—a contributory factor in lymphoma formation. *Clin Transpl.* 1992;6:214.
123. Milpied N, Vasseur B, Parquet N, et al. Humanized anti-CD20 monoclonal antibody (rituximab) in post transplant lymphoproliferative disorder: a retrospective analysis on 32 patients. *Ann Oncol.* 2000;1(Suppl 1):113.
124. Faye A, Van Den Abeele T, Peuchmaur M, et al. Anti-CD20 monoclonal antibody for post-transplant lymphoproliferative disorders. *Lancet.* 1998;352:1285.

CHAPTER 96 ■ CRITICAL CARE ASPECTS OF STEM CELL TRANSPLANTATION

ROBERT PETER GALE • AMIN RAHEMTULLA

Bone marrow and blood cell transplants are widely used to treat aplastic anemia, leukemias, lymphomas, myeloma, and immune deficiency disorders. Transplants are also increasingly used to treat other bone marrow disorders such as sickle cell disease and thalassemia. Morbidity and mortality associated with transplants usually result from regimen-related toxicity, such as adverse effects of drugs and radiation given pretransplant, complications of graft versus host disease (GVHD), as well as infections resulting from bone marrow failure. Morbidity and mortality of transplants has steadily decreased over the past four decades because of better supportive care. Recently, there has also been an increased use of reduced intensity-conditioning transplants, with less attendant regimen-related toxicity, and an increase in transplants from unrelated donors with increased regimen-related toxicity because of more intensive pretransplant therapy.

Pretransplant evaluation of recipients typically includes the following (1–6):

1. Measurement of the left ventricular ejection fraction (LVEF), which should be at least 40%
2. Pulmonary function tests, including diffusing capacity (DL_{CO}), and forced vital capacity (FVC), which should be more than 50% of predicted
3. Hepatic transaminases, which should be less than twice normal
4. Creatinine clearance, which should be more than 50 mL/minute
5. A pretransplant performance score consistent with an independent life

Because the risk of GVHD increases with age, allotransplants are typically done in subjects younger than 55 years of age (7). By way of contrast, autotransplant recipients may be as old as 70 years (8). The risk of infection is minimized by various preventative or isolation procedures (see below). Transplants are typically delayed in subjects with active infections until the infection resolves (9,10). The 100-day transplant-related mortality after autotransplants is 2% to 5%; after related allotransplants, it is 15% to 20%; and after alternative (unrelated) allotransplants, it is about 30% (9,10).

IMMEDIATE CONCERNS—THE FIRST 30 DAYS

Pretransplant Conditioning Regimens

In the setting of allotransplants, the pretransplant conditioning regimen needs to moderate or eliminate recipient immunity to prevent graft rejection (11,12). When the allotransplant recipient has cancer, the pretransplant conditioning regimen must also eradicate it. Most allotransplant conditioning regimens contain cyclophosphamide and busulphan, or total-body radiation (13,14). Antilymphocyte antibodies, such as antilymphocyte globulin (ALG), antithymocyte globulin (ATG), or alemtuzumab (anti-CD52), are often used in reduced-intensity conditioning regimens or in alternative donor transplants. In immune deficiency disorders—for example, severe combined immune deficiency (SCID), pretransplant conditioning is not necessary, as the host is already immune deficient.

For autotransplants, the choice of pretransplant conditioning regimen is based on anticancer effect, a steep dose–response curve, lack of cross-resistance with other drugs, and low non–bone marrow dose-limiting toxicities. In general, these regimens contain alkylating drugs, such as melphalan or cyclophosphamide, combined with two or three other drugs. Immune suppression is unnecessary and an unwanted side effect of therapy. Radiation is not used in autotransplants, as the effective anticancer doses exceed nonbone marrow dose-limiting toxicity.

Pretransplant conditioning regimens are typically empirically determined, with few large randomized trials. Consequently, it is difficult to determine which regimen, if any, is best (15). The choice of a pretransplant conditioning regimen depends not only on effectiveness of the regimen in a specific disease and the need for immune suppression needed for engraftment, but also on avoiding toxicity from prior therapy or current organ dysfunction. For example, prior mantle radiation or exposures to radiosensitizers, such as bleomycin or carmustine (BCNU), increase the pulmonary toxicity of total body irradiation (TBI), whereas prior therapy of subjects with testicular cancer with cisplatin increases kidney toxicity of platinum-based conditioning regimens. The nonbone marrow, dose-limiting toxicities of drugs in commonly used pretransplant conditioning regimens are listed in Table 96.1.

Bone Marrow and Blood Cell Collection

Cells used for transplants are most often collected from the blood but may also be collected from the bone marrow or umbilical cord blood (16–21). Collection of blood cells is an outpatient procedure accomplished with an apheresis device such as the Cobe Spectra. In the context of autotransplants, recipients often receive chemotherapy and/or hematopoietic growth factors to increase the number of blood cells collected. Normal allotransplant donors often receive only hematopoietic growth factors. The timing of apheresis correlates with the method used to increase the number of cells collected: apheresis is

TABLE 96.1

TOXICITY OF CONDITIONING REGIMEN DRUGS

Drug/dose	Extramedullary dose-limiting toxicity	Other toxicities
BCNU	Interstitial pneumonitis	Renal insufficiency, encephalopathy, nausea, vomiting, veno-occlusive disease (VOD).
Busulphan	Mucositis, VOD	Seizures, rash, hyperpigmentation, nausea, vomiting, pneumonitis
CCNU (lomustine)	Interstitial pneumonitis	Renal insufficiency, encephalopathy, nausea, vomiting, VOD
Cyclophosphamide	Heart failure	Hemorrhagic cystitis, syndrome of inappropriate antidiuretic hormone (SIADH), nausea, vomiting, pulmonary edema, interstitial pneumonitis
Cytarabine	Mucositis, cerebellar ataxia	Pulmonary edema, conjunctivitis, rash, fever, hepatitis, toxic epidermal necrolysis
Cisplatin	Renal insufficiency, peripheral neuropathy	Nausea, vomiting, renal tubular acidosis, hypomagnesemia
Carboplatin	Ototoxicity, hepatitis	Renal insufficiency, hypomagnesemia, peripheral neuropathy
Etoposide	Mucositis	Nausea, vomiting, hemorrhagic cystitis, pneumonia, hepatitis
Ifosfamide	Encephalopathy, renal insufficiency	Hemorrhagic cystitis, renal tubular acidosis
Melphalan	Mucositis	Nausea, vomiting, hepatitis, SIADH, pneumonitis, renal insufficiency
Mitoxantrone	Cardiotoxicity	Mucositis
Paclitaxel	Mucositis	Peripheral neuropathy, bradycardia, anaphylaxis
Thiotepa	Mucositis	Intertriginous rash, hyperpigmentation, nausea, vomiting

usually done for 1 to 3 days, starting 4 days after beginning hematopoietic growth factor therapy. In contrast, when chemotherapy is used, apheresis is usually done for 1 to 3 days when neutrophils are present at a level of greater than or equal to 1×10^9 cells/L; this is usually 10 to 16 days after beginning chemotherapy. The advantages of collecting blood rather than bone marrow cells include no need for anesthesia; utility in subjects with hypocellular, fibrotic, or cancer-infiltrated bone marrow; and a more rapid bone marrow recovery post transplant. A disadvantage of using blood as opposed to bone marrow cells is an increased incidence and severity of chronic GVHD. This is probably because blood contains tenfold more T cells, the cells causing chronic GVHD (20). The cost of blood cell collection is similar to collecting bone marrow cells. The complications of blood cell collection are rare, but include infection, anaphylaxis, and hypocalcemia.

Bone marrow cells are collected in the operating room under general, epidural, spinal, or caudal anesthesia. The donor may be admitted on the day of the harvest and discharged the next day. Sometimes, an autologous red blood cell (RBC) unit is collected 3 to 4 weeks before the procedure for autotransfusion. Complications of bone marrow collection are rare but include the risks of anesthesia: hypotension, nausea, vomiting, cardiac arrest, pulmonary emboli, pain, hemorrhage, and infection.

Cord blood cells are obtained from the umbilical cord and placental blood at the time of birth. The target is to collect 2 to 4×10^7 nucleated cells/kg donor weight. This is more than tenfold less than the 2 to 4×10^8 nucleated cells/kg recipient weight collected from the bone marrow. Cord blood cell transplants are often limited to children because of the small number of cells collected. The potential advantages of cord blood are a higher proportion of progenitor cells compared to bone marrow and possibly less GVHD from fewer T cells.

Bone Marrow and Blood Cell Infusion

Bone marrow and blood cells may be frozen in dimethyl sulfoxide (DMSO) for later use (22,23). The intracellular contents of cells destroyed in the freezing and thawing processes—and DMSO itself—may cause hypotension, anaphylaxis, or dysrhythmias, including transient heart block (24). To avoid complications, subjects are premedicated with diphenhydramine hydrochloride (Benadryl) and methylprednisolone sodium succinate (Solu-Medrol). Intubation equipment and epinephrine should be available at the bedside when cells are infused. If hypotension occurs, the infusion is slowed or temporarily interrupted until the blood pressure stabilizes. If the bone marrow or blood cells have not been frozen, the risk of anaphylaxis is similar to a standard blood transfusion, and premedication is unnecessary.

Bone marrow and blood cell collections are routinely analyzed for quality control at various times during collection, processing, storage, and infusion. Approximately 1.2% of cultures obtained during these processes are found to contain bacteria (25). Most cultures show coagulase-negative *Staphylococcus sp.*, which colonize the skin; pathogenic Gram-negative bacteria are occasionally present. Bone marrow and blood cell collections inconvenience the donor and cost approximately $16,000. Thus, despite positive culture results, most centers reinfuse the stem cells after appropriate antibiotic coverage. Although controversial, this approach has generally been without adverse effects.

Fluids and Hypotension

High-dose chemotherapy and radiation damage vascular endothelial cells, resulting in extravascular leakage of fluids. Furthermore, GVHD and cytokines such as tumor necrosis factor (TNF), interleukin 2 (IL-2), and interferon-gamma (IFN-γ) contribute to a post transplant capillary leak syndrome (26–29). In addition, subjects often receive large volumes of intravenous (IV) fluids from drug dilutions, parenteral nutrition, and prophylaxis for hemorrhagic cystitis. Consequently, all transplant recipients gain weight, and diuretics are frequently given to maintain baseline weight and prevent fluid retention. If hypotension develops, emphasis should be placed on early invasive cardiovascular monitoring, inotropic support, and irradiated packed red blood cell transfusion to maintain intravascular oncotic pressure. Aggressive hydration may precipitate pulmonary and peripheral edema, even with normal pulmonary artery wedge pressure and right atrial pressure.

Electrolyte Balance

Electrolyte abnormalities are common in transplant recipients, resulting from the underlying disease, prophylactic hydration for hemorrhagic cystitis, diarrhea, parenteral nutrition, renal insufficiency, diuretics, and other medications. Ifosfamide, especially combined with carboplatin, causes a Fanconi syndrome–like renal tubular acidosis 3 to 7 days after the pretransplant conditioning regimen (30,31). The resulting normal anion gap acidosis may be treated with sodium bicarbonate. Other drugs associated with renal tubular wasting of electrolytes are amphotericin, foscarnet, and aminoglycosides. The syndrome of inappropriate secretion of antidiuretic hormone (SIADH) may result from high-dose cyclophosphamide and/or ifosfamide. Cyclosporine may cause hypomagnesemia and hypokalemia or hyperkalemia. Hypomagnesemia increases the risk of cyclosporine-associated seizures. Tumor lysis syndrome is rare, as most transplant recipients have relatively few cancer cells and receive intensive hydration. Finally, uric acid, a major blood antioxidant, is markedly decreased soon after a transplant, independent of allopurinol which is often given (32).

Blood Product Transfusions

Subjects receiving transplants are immune compromised and at risk for transfusion-associated GVHD. All cellular blood products contain white blood cells (WBC), including immune-competent T cells, and should be irradiated (25 Gy) (33).

Cytomegalovirus (CMV) infection is another risk. Allotransplant recipients should receive CMV-negative blood product transfusions, especially when the recipient is CMV seronegative (34–37). If CMV seronegative blood is unavailable, removal of contaminating WBC with an in-line microfilter is an alternative (38,39). When an allotransplant recipient is CMV seropositive, no special CMV-related precautions are needed. Because autotransplant recipients do not develop GVHD or receive post transplant immune suppression, the risk of CMV-related infection is low (40), and no special CMV-related precautions are needed.

In the allotransplant setting, special consideration is needed regarding ABO compatibility between recipient and donor (41–43). As donor bone marrow engraftment occurs, there is a switch to the ABO type of the donor. However, there is a transition period when RBCs with both recipient and donor ABO types are present. When there is A and/or B incompatibility between recipient and donor, there is the possibility that residual anti-A or -B recipient antibodies may react against donor RBC, or that B cells in the graft may produce anti-A or -B antibodies against residual recipient RBC. This complexity of blood product transfusion support should be viewed in terms of whether there is a major or minor ABO incompatibility between the recipient and donor (Table 96.2). A major ABO incompatibility occurs when the recipient has antibodies to the donor RBC phenotype, for example, recipient group O, donor group A. To prevent RBC destruction, red blood cells should be removed from the graft. Post transplant, the recipient should receive recipient ABO-type RBC transfusions or O-type RBC transfusions from which plasma and platelets are removed. With a minor ABO incompatibility, the donor has anti-A and/or -B antibodies to the recipient's RBC ABO type, for example, donor O type, and recipient A or B type. Donor anti-A and/or B antibodies should be removed from the graft. Post transplant, the recipient should receive O-type RBC transfusions and recipient ABO-type plasma and platelets. When recipient and donor have anti-A and/or -B antibodies to each other's ABO type, for example, recipient A type and donor B type, there is a combined major/minor ABO incompatibility. In this instance, RBC and plasma should be removed from the graft. Post transplant, the recipient should receive O-type RBC transfusions and AB-type platelets and plasma.

Despite using ABO-compatible platelets, many subjects fail to respond to platelet transfusions early post transplant. Causes include fever, hepatic veno-occlusive disease (VOD), drugs, infection, disseminated intravascular coagulation (DIC), and microangiopathic hemolytic anemia related to cyclosporine and/or GVHD (44).

Infection Prevention

Tactics to prevent bacterial, viral, and fungal infections vary considerably between centers (45–47). This reflects the fact that there are few definitive studies and frequent availability of new drugs. The types of infections occurring in transplant recipients correlated with the post transplant interval. Tactics to prevent bacterial infections early post transplant are based on two considerations: most infections arise from endogenous microorganisms; and in studies of neutropenic animals, the oral

TABLE 96.2a

DONOR-RECIPIENT ABO INCOMPATIBILITY

Major ABO incompatibility	Minor ABO incompatibility	Major and minor ABO incompatibility
Recipient has antibody to donor	Donor has antibody to recipient	Recipient has antibody to donor and donor has antibody to recipient
IMMEDIATE HEMOLYSIS		
Prevent by RBC depletion of marrow	Prevent by plasma depletion of marrow	Prevent by RBC and plasma depletion of marrow
DELAYED HEMOLYSIS		
Occurs 2 to 4 weeks after SCT	Occurs Day 9 to Day 16 after SCT	+ Direct antiglobulin test
+ Direct antiglobulin test Risk increased with high recipient isohemagglutinin titer	+ Direct antiglobulin test Risk increased with T-cell depleted marrow	
DELAYED ERYTHROPOESIS		
Plasma exchange, erythropoietin, steroids		Plasma exchange, erythropoietin, steroids

RBC, red blood cell; SCT, stem cell transplantation; +, positive.

inoculum of Gram-negative bacteria required to cause death is increased by colonization of the gastrointestinal tract with anaerobes. This has led to selective aerobic gastrointestinal decontamination, first, with nonabsorbable antibiotics such as gentamicin, Vancomycin, and nystatin, and later, with absorbable antimicrobials selective for aerobes like oral quinolones (48–50).

TABLE 96.2b

ABO TYPE OF BLOOD COMPONENTS USED IN PATIENTS WHO HAVE RECEIVED AN ABO-INCOMPATIBLE TRANSPLANT

Donor	Recipient	Red cells	Platelets*	FFP
MAJOR ABO INCOMPATIBILITY				
A	O	O	A	A
B	O	O	B	B
AB	O	O	A	AB
AB	A	A	A	AB
AB	B	B	B	AB
MINOR ABO INCOMPATIBILITY				
O	A	O	A	A
O	B	O	B	B
O	AB	O	A	AB
A	AB	A	A	AB
B	AB	B	B	AB
MAJOR AND MINOR ABO INCOMPATIBILITY				
A	B	O	B	AB
B	A	O	A	AB

*Occasionally, due to nonavailability of platelets of the requested group, group O platelets (labelled as "low titre," i.e., low titre of anti-A and anti-B) may be used for patients of any group. When full ABO conversion has taken place, all patients receive products of their new ABO group.

Standards for prevention of infection vary from strict isolation in laminar airflow (LAF) rooms to none. In LAF rooms, the subject is in a sterile environment; anyone who enters must be gloved and gowned, and the patient's food is sterilized or has a low microbial content secondary to autoclave or microwave treatment (51–54). Prophylactic oral antibiotics are given to destroy enteric pathogens, which not only are reservoirs for infection, but also may function as superantigens that increase the severity of GVHD (55). The minimal standards to prevent bacterial infections include the following:

1. A transplant unit set aside from general hospital, patients, and visitor traffic
2. High-efficiency particulate air (HEPA) filtration to prevent iatrogenic *Aspergillus* species infection (56,57)
3. Careful hand-washing before entering a patient's room
4. A diet without fresh salads, vegetables, or fruits, as these may be contaminated with Gram-negative bacteria, or without pepper, as this may be contaminated with an *Aspergillus* species (58)

Other measures, such as donning shoe covers, gloves, masks, and gowns and low microbial diets and anterooms are also commonly used, but their cost-effectiveness is debatable. Bacterial prophylactic measures are generally discontinued when the neutrophil count is greater than 0.5×10^9 cells/L.

Tactics to prevent fungal infections include the use of oral triazoles such as itraconazole or fluconazole, given orally or intravenously for the first month post transplant (59). The azole antifungals are effective against most *Candida* species, but in transplant recipients, fluconazole is ineffective and itraconazole is more effective against *Aspergillus* species. Most *Aspergillus* species infections are iatrogenic and preventable by HEPA filtration of rooms. Subjects with prior aspergillus infection are at high risk of recurrence (60), especially when there is

1. Prolonged neutropenia post transplant
2. A more advanced cancer state
3. Less than or equal to a 6-week interval from beginning systemic antiaspergillus therapy to the transplant
4. Severe acute GVHD

Persons with prior aspergillosis should receive amphotericin, voriconazole, or caspofungin early post transplant (61).

Herpes simplex reactivation is usually prevented by using intravenous or oral acyclovir for the first month post transplant (62,63). Treatment thereafter results in frequent acyclovir resistance and delays the development of natural immunity.

Fever and Neutropenia

Transplant recipients are immune compromised from neutropenia, breakdown in mucosal barriers (e.g., mucositis), invasive therapies (e.g., Foley catheter or central venous lines), immune suppressive drugs (e.g., cyclosporine, corticosteroids, and methotrexate), and GVHD. Lymphocyte function is also affected by thymic involution, weak proliferative responses to T- or B-cell mitogens, and inverted $CD4^{+}/CD8^{+}$ ratios for 6 months after autotransplants and more than 1 year after allotransplants (64,65). When an allotransplant is complicated by chronic GVHD, normal lymphocyte function may never return (66). The risk of infection depends on the genetic link between donor and recipient, graft type, and post transplant immune suppression.

In transplant recipients with fever—temperature greater than or equal to 38°C—and a neutrophil count less than 0.5×10^9 cells/L (67), one should try to identify an infection source using a chest radiograph, blood and urine cultures, and physical examination with emphasis on line sites and perineal, oropharyngeal, and sinus regions. Usually no focal source is found, and broad-spectrum antibiotics are begun. The choice of antibiotics may include an antipseudomonal penicillin, aminoglycoside, and vancomycin or a third-generation antipseudomonal cephalosporin. Transplant recipients commonly receive loop diuretics such as furosemide. The ototoxicity of this drug is increased by aminoglycosides and vancomycin. Allotransplant recipients receive cyclosporine, whose nephrotoxicity is increased by aminoglycosides. Recurrent or persistent fever for 3 to 5 days without source in a person with granulocytes less than 0.5×10^9 cells/L is an indication for empiric antifungal therapy with amphotericin. The kidney toxicity of amphotericin is enhanced by cyclosporine and aminoglycosides.

Mucositis

The severity of mucositis depends on the components of the preconditioning regimen. The nonbone marrow dose-limiting toxicity of etoposide, busulfan, cytarabine, thiotepa, and paclitaxel is mucositis. Radiation also contributes to mucositis. Not surprisingly, conditioning regimens containing these drugs and/or radiation are associated with severe mucositis. Other risk factors include post transplant methotrexate and pretransplant interferon-gamma. Methotrexate should be withheld if severe mucositis develops, whereas interferon-gamma should be discontinued at least 2 to 4 weeks before giving radiation.

Management of mucositis includes good oral hygiene, using, for example, saline, chlorhexidine, and nystatin rinses, and topical analgesics (68,69). Opioids are often needed, and should be given intravenously by schedule or using patient-controlled analgesia (PCA). Severe mucositis may require prophylactic intubation for airway protection. Ultimately, the resolution of mucositis generally correlates with recovery of the neutrophil count bone marrow. New drugs, such as palifermin (recombinant human keratinocyte growth factor-1) reduce the incidence and severity of oral mucositis (70).

Diarrhea

Diarrhea in transplant recipients may be caused by high-dose chemoradiotherapy, other drugs such as antibiotics, and bacterial or viral infections, as well as GVHD (71–73). The pretransplant conditioning regimen is the most common cause of diarrhea within 2 to 3 weeks post transplant. Nevertheless, an infection cause should always be considered. including *Clostridium difficile* and *Escherichia coli* (0157:H7), CMV, herpes simplex, adenoviruses, rotaviruses, echoviruses, astroviruses, Norwalk virus, Coxsackie virus, *Strongyloides* species, *Giardia* species, and *Cryptosporidium* species. GVHD also causes diarrhea; the diagnosis can be confirmed by intestinal biopsy showing loss of crypts, vacuolization of crypt epithelium, karyorrhectic apoptotic debris, microabscesses, and, in severe cases, ulceration and denudation of the epithelium. Therapy is directed toward appropriate antibiotics for infections and immune suppression for GVHD. Conditioning regimen- and GVHD-associated diarrhea may respond to octreotide, a somatostatin analogue whose mechanism of action is partly through the inhibition of secretory hormones (74). Some viral infections—for example, CMV—respond to ganciclovir, foscarnet, or cidofovir (75).

Hemorrhagic Cystitis

Hemorrhagic cystitis, occurring 2 to 3 weeks post transplant, usually results from drugs in the pretransplant conditioning regimen, such as cyclophosphamide, ifosfamide, or etoposide (76–78). Prophylaxis for hemorrhagic cystitis includes hydration and diuretics to maintain urine output at 0.2 mL/kg per hour (79,80). Sodium mercaptoethane sulphate (Mesna) is often used, especially with high-dose cyclophosphamide or ifosfamide (81). Mesna is inert in plasma but is hydrolyzed in the urine to reactive monomers that conjugate alkylating drugs. It has a short half-life, and is therefore given by continuous intravenous infusion. Complications of hemorrhagic cystitis are uncontrolled bleeding and clotting of the ureters or urethra, resulting in acute kidney failure. Obstruction of the ureters by clots may be asymptomatic or cause kidney colic from ureteral spasm. Severe pain may occur in the back or flank and radiate into the groin or genitals.

Therapy of hemorrhagic cystitis consists of using a Foley catheter to irrigate the bladder with normal saline at 250 mL/hour to prevent intravesicular clotting. Platelets should be maintained at more than 50×10^9 cells/L with platelet transfusions, and RBC transfusion should be given to replace blood loss. Discomfort from local bladder spasm can be treated with antispasmodic agents such as oxybutynin chloride (Ditropan). In severe cases, arterial embolization or cystectomy may be necessary.

Hemorrhagic cystitis seen more than 2 weeks post transplant can result from pretransplant conditioning or viral infection due to, for example, adenovirus, CMV, JC or BK viruses of the bladder epithelium (82–84). Except for CMV, there are no effective antiviral drugs.

Veno-occlusive Disease of the Liver

Veno-occlusive disease of the liver (VOD) is caused by drugs and/or radiation in the pretransplant conditioning regimen within 1 to 3 months post transplant (85). Unlike the Budd-Chiari syndrome with thrombosis of the large hepatic veins, VOD arises from thrombosis of the central venule. High-dose therapy damages endothelial cells throughout the body. However, metabolism or activation of drugs by hepatocytes results in a high local concentration. Histologically, the central venule is occluded by concentric fibrosis best shown by a trichrome Masson stain. Lesions are composed initially of von Willebrand factor, soon replaced by collagen (86). Obliteration of the central venule results in intrahepatic hypertension, diminished or reversal of portal blood flow, and ascites.

VOD, with a reported incidence of 1% to 56%, is a clinical diagnosis suggested by elevated bilirubin, weight gain, ascites, and tender hepatomegaly (87–89) (Table 96.3). The incidence variability results partly from different pretransplant conditioning regimens and the clinical criteria used to diagnose VOD. For instance, although diagnostic criteria from Johns Hopkins and Seattle seem similar, a retrospective comparison showed VOD incidence rates of 32% versus 8% (90). Risk factors for VOD include increased pretransplant transaminases, conditioning regimen intensity, prolonged fever, and age (88). A positive hepatitis viral serology does not increase the risk of VOD if pretransplant transaminases are normal. Altered drug metabolism is probably responsible for the decreased incidence of VOD in children and increased risk for VOD in persons with abnormal pretransplant transaminases. Cytokines that cause fever also damage endothelial cells and probably cause the increased risk of VOD in persons with prolonged fever. In general, VOD incidence is not significantly different in recipients of allotransplants versus autotransplants.

Clinical symptoms of VOD are also associated with many common but unrelated transplant complications. For instance, jaundice may result from hemolysis—for example, ABO incompatibility, bacterial sepsis, hepatic candidiasis, parenteral nutrition, drugs such as cyclosporine and methotrexate, or GVHD. Initial evaluation for VOD should include ultrasound of the liver, with Doppler measurement of portal vein blood flow. Reversal or diminished portal flow is consistent with intrahepatic obstruction of blood flow secondary to VOD (91). Ultrasonographic findings are generally present only in overt clinical disease (92). Although uncertain cases may require liver biopsy, a percutaneous biopsy is contraindicated because of ascites, coagulopathy, and low platelets. Transjugular biopsy may, in general, be performed safely and provides an opportunity to measure the hepatic venous pressure gradient, which, if greater than 10 mm Hg, is consistent with VOD (93).

Therapy for VOD is predominantly supportive. Emphasis should be on avoiding hepatotoxic drugs that will further damage the liver. Persons with severe VOD may develop the hepatorenal syndrome, marked by kidney insufficiency and a low fractional sodium excretion. Therapy includes diuretics to maintain baseline weight and oral ursodeoxycholic acid to lower the bilirubin and prevent further liver injury from free radicals generated by bile acids (94). Some centers attempt to maintain intravascular volume and kidney perfusion with RBC transfusions, aiming for a hemoglobin of 12 to 15 g/dL. Early studies of defibrotide, a single-stranded polydeoxyribonucleotide with fibrinolytic, antithrombotic, and anti-ischemic properties, in severe VOD suggested activity with complete response rates of 36% to 55% (95–97). No severe hemorrhage or other serious toxicity related to defibrotide was reported.

The prognosis of VOD is poor when bilirubin is more than 15 to 20 mg/dL. Thrombolytic therapy with tissue plasminogen activator and heparin has been used successfully but may be complicated by severe bleeding (98,99). Once the thrombus is replaced by fibrin and collagen, thrombolytic therapy is probably ineffective. However, in late VOD, another option is a transjugular, intrahepatic portal shunt to decompress the portal vein (100–102). If there is engraftment without severe GVHD or recurrence of the underlying disorder prompting the transplant, consideration should also be given to a liver transplant (103–105).

TABLE 96.3

CLINICAL CRITERIA FOR VENO-OCCLUSIVE DISEASE OF THE LIVER

McDonald criteria—Seattle	Jones criteria—Johns Hopkins
Before day 30: Any two of the following	*Before day 21: Any two of the following*
Bilirubin >27 μmol/L = 1.7 mg/dL	Bilirubin >34 μmol/L = 2.0 mg/dL
Hepatomegaly	Hepatomegaly
Ascites or weight gain	Ascites
	Weight gain

Respiratory Failure

Transplant recipients who develop respiratory failure and require mechanical ventilation have a poor prognosis (106,107). Once intubated, 80% of recipients are never extubated and, at 6 months, only 3% of subjects who required intubation survive. Except for procedures performed as a prelude to surgery, the reason for intubation is not correlated with a likelihood of survival, but age younger than 40 years and intubation more than 100 days post transplant correlated with better survival.

Respiratory failure within the first 30 days is usually caused by pretransplant conditioning, regimen-related epithelial cell damage, and/or infection (108–111). Early post transplant radiotherapy and chemotherapy releases free radicals and cytokines, resulting in damage to pulmonary epithelial cells. This leads to blebs in the cell membranes, separation of junctions between cells, and necrosis. The end result is pulmonary edema, occasionally with focal or diffuse pulmonary alveolar hemorrhage (112). This may occur without an increase in pulmonary artery occlusion pressure (PAOP). Median time to onset of alveolar hemorrhage post transplant is about 4 months, but it may occur as late as 1 to 2 years. Symptoms are nonspecific and include dyspnea, hypoxia, and diffuse infiltrates. Although hemoptysis is rare, bronchoalveolar lavage often shows intrapulmonary hemorrhage. Early in the course of respiratory distress, efforts should be directed to preventing intubation. Although not evaluated in prospective studies, and therefore of unproven benefit, management may include early invasive hemodynamic monitoring, RBC transfusions to maintain hemoglobin more than 12 g/dL, ultrafiltration to decrease intravascular volume, and anticytokine monoclonal antibodies or cytokine receptor antagonists. Use of high-dose corticosteroids is controversial but, in theory, inhibits generation of free radicals, decreases cytokine release, and decreases inflammation.

The repair process after high-dose chemotherapy and radiation may further interfere with gas exchange by causing interstitial fibrosis. Further, infection aggravates parenchymal inflammation and protracts the repair of the interstitium. Transplant recipients are especially susceptible to pulmonary infections because of bone marrow failure, immune suppressive drugs, mucositis, aspiration, and bronchial epithelial cell damage with impaired ciliary motility. Gram-negative and -positive pneumonias are common in the first 30 days post transplant. Fungal infections of the lung also occur early post transplant, and isolation of *Aspergillus* species in a nasal or sputum culture should prompt intial therapy with amphotericin, voriconazole, or caspofungin. Risk factors for aspergillosis are long-term duration of impaired immunity pretransplant, for example, aplastic anemia or severe combined immune deficiency (SCID); centers without HEPA filters to prevent inhalation of aerosolized spores; and prior invasive aspergillosis. Viral pneumonia is rare early post transplant; the most common etiologic agent when this does occur is herpes simplex.

Heart Failure

Heart failure may result from volume overload or impairment of left ventricular function from sepsis or toxicity from pretransplant conditioning regimen drugs such as cyclophosphamide, ifosfamide, and/or anthracyclines (113–117). Pretransplant risk factors for cardiac failure are a prior history of heart failure or a low resting left ventricular ejection fraction of less than 40% (3). Prior mediastinal radiation or a high cumulative anthracycline dose are not independent risk factors, provided the ejection fraction is normal. High-dose cyclophosphamide causes hemorrhagic myocarditis. Transient ST-segment depression and T-wave inversions are common during cyclophosphamide infusion but are not a reason to alter therapy. Cyclophosphamide damages cardiac capillary endothelial cells, leading to hemorrhage between, and separation of, myocytes. The end result is loss of voltage, heart failure, and/or pericardial effusion. Unlike anthracycline-related heart damage arising from myocyte damage, even severe cyclophosphamide-induced left ventricular dysfunction is reversible after an interval of weeks to months.

Kidney Failure

Renal insufficiency is usually a multifactorial process whose cause includes the underlying disease—for example, cast nephropathy in myeloma, a prerenal decrease in glomerular filtration, intrinsic renal dysfunction, or postrenal obstruction. The most common reason for renal insufficiency early in the post transplant period is drug related, especially with use of aminoglycosides, cyclosporine, and amphotericin (118,119). Mortality in persons requiring dialysis is about 85% (120). Prerenal causes of azotemia include hepatic VOD, diarrhea, diuretics, third-spacing from sepsis, hypoalbuminemia, and a capillary leak syndrome from high-dose drugs and radiation. Hepatic VOD, like other causes of prerenal azotemia, is marked by decreased fractional excretion of sodium ($FeNa^+$) in the urine.

Azotemia from intrinsic renal failure may result from acute tubular necrosis (ATN), glomerulonephritis, interstitial nephritis, or renal vascular damage. Causes of ATN in transplant recipients include sepsis, hypovolemia, and drugs such as aminoglycosides, amphotericin, platinums, foscarnet, and cyclosporine. In ATN, the $FeNa^+$ is high, and the urine has muddy hyaline casts. Renal insufficiency secondary to glomerulonephritis usually results from streptococcal or staphylococcal bacteremia. In glomerulonephritis, the $FeNa^+$ is low, and the urine sediment contains RBC casts and increased protein. Interstitial nephritis arising in the early stem cell transplantation (SCT) period is usually drug induced. Causes of allergic interstitial nephritis are penicillins, cephalosporins, sulphamethoxazole-trimethoprim, and fluoroquinolones. In allergic interstitial nephritis, the urine $FeNa^+$ is high, and urine sediment contains white blood cells (WBCs), WBC casts, and eosinophils. Renal insufficiency from renovascular damage is usually caused by drugs such as cyclosporine or from hemolytic-uremic syndrome (HUS), which is marked by schistocytes, thrombocytopenia, and azotemia. HUS arises from endothelial cell damage, which may be related to cyclosporine, GVHD, or high-dose drugs and radiation.

Postrenal kidney failure in transplant recipients may result from hemorrhagic cystitis with ureteral or urethral obstruction due to blood clots, retroperitoneal hemorrhage, urate nephropathy, or drugs that undergo intratubular crystallization and obstruction such as acyclovir, ciprofloxacin, and triamterene. Regardless of the cause, post transplant renal insufficiency may require a dose reduction of prophylactic immune suppressive drugs such as cyclosporine or methotrexate; this may increase GVHD.

Engraftment

Definition of graft failure is controversial. After a bone marrow graft, there is usually a rise in the WBC by 3 weeks. After a peripheral blood stem cell transplant, the WBC usually rises by about 2 weeks. Platelet recovery, defined as more than 20×10^9 platelets/L without transfusion, typically occurs 2 to 3 weeks later. Occasionally, recipients require platelet transfusions for months post transplant. Generally, graft failure is defined as a neutrophil count less than or equal to 0.5×10^9 cells/L by day 28. Causes of graft failure include too few normal hematopoietic cells, damage to the bone marrow microenvironment, immune-mediated graft rejection, or drug- or viral-related immune suppression (121,122).

The minimal number of bone marrow or blood cells needed for sustained engraftment is unknown. There are several reasons for this:

TABLE 96.4a

GRAFT VERSUS HOST DISEASE, GRAFT FAILURE, AND DISEASE-FREE SURVIVAL FOR TRANSPLANTS WITH SIBLING-MATCHED OR UNRELATED DONORS

Degree of HLA match	Acute GVHD grade III or IV (%)	Chronic GVHD (%)	Graft failure (%)	DFS-AML or all in remission (%)	DFS-CML in chronic phase (%)	DFS-AML or ALL in relapse (%)	DFS-CML in transformation (%)	DFS-AA (%)
Sibling 6/6	7–15	30–35	<2	50–60	60–80	20	10–35	78–90
Related 5/6	25–30	50	7–9	40–60	60–80	20	10–35	25–40
Related 4/6	45–50	50	21	10–40	—	10	10–30	—
Haplo-identical	50–100	>50	20	10–40	—	10	10–30	—
Unrelated 6/6	45–50	55	6	45	40	20	20	30–40

GVHD, graft versus host disease; DFS, disease-free survival; AML, acute myelogenous leukemia; CML, chronic myelogenous leukemia; ALL, acute lymphoblastic leukemia; AA, aplastic anemia.

1. It is not known what hematopoietic cell(s) are responsible for sustained engraftment.
2. Different hematopoietic cells may operate under different circumstances and in different persons.
3. After autotransplants, there is no need for sustained engraftment in the context of autologous bone marrow recovery.
4. There is no validated method to identify the hematopoietic cell(s) responsible for sustained engraftment (123,124).

Because of these limitations, surrogate markers are used to assess the hematopoietic-restoring functionality of grafts. For instance, CD34 is a surface membrane marker of immature hematopoietic cells. In animals and humans, retrovirus-transduced $CD34^+$ cells contribute to long-term engraftment (but may not be necessary) (125). To ensure sustained engraftment in humans, most data suggest a threshold of 2 to 4 $\times$ 10^8 mononuclear cells or 2 $\times$ 10^6 $CD34^+$ cells/kg of recipient body weight. Autotransplant recipients receiving extensive prior chemotherapy and/or radiation frequently have fewer $CD34^+$ cells. It may be difficult to obtain large numbers of $CD34^+$ cells from these persons, and recipients generally recover bone marrow function later than after grafts from normal or less extensively treated donors. This may reflect decreased numbers and/or function of $CD34^+$ cells and/or damage to the bone marrow microenvironment.

Immune-mediated graft failure is theoretically impossible after autotransplants, but it is the most common cause of graft failure for allotransplants. Risk of immune-mediated graft failure correlates with the degree of HLA disparity between donor and recipient. Graft failure occurs in less than 1% after HLA-identical sibling allotransplants, 6% to 8% after unrelated HLA-phenotype matched allotransplants, and in up to 20% after HLA-haplotype mismatched allotransplants (126–128) (Table 96.4). Immunity to non-HLA antigens, such as H-Y and KIR, also operates to increase risk of immune-mediated graft failure. Other variables influencing the risk of immune-mediated graft failure are transfusion-induced sensitization to HLA and non-HLA antigens, intensity of the pretransplant conditioning regimen, and quantity of T cells in the graft. In persons with aplastic anemia, the volume of pretransplant RBC or platelet transfusions correlates with a higher rate of graft failure. This is presumed to result from sensitization of the recipient to disparate HLA and non-HLA antigens. These observations were made before microfilters were available to deplete WBC from transfused blood products; whether this risk still operates is unknown. However, because of these considerations, potential allotransplant recipients should avoid unnecessary transfusions or receive microfiltered blood products. Removal of donor T cells from the bone marrow graft to prevent GVHD also increases the risk of graft failure; compensation may be possible by more intensive pretransplant immune suppression (129,130). Graft failure risk is also increased after male grafts to parous and/or transfused female recipients. Here, the recipient is presumed to be sensitized to H-Y antigens (131,132).

Several bone marrow suppressive drugs commonly used post transplant may delay and/or reverse engraftment, for example, methotrexate and sulphamethoxazole-trimethoprim. Viruses, especially herpes simplex, parvovirus, HHV-6, parvovirus-B19, and CMV, cause bone marrow suppression, possibly because they infect bone marrow stroma cells. A decline in the WBC and/or platelets after recovery post transplant should prompt a search for a drug- or virus-related cause. Declines are also temporarily associated with tapering immune suppression; whether these are related phenomena is unclear. The effect, if any, of acute GVHD on bone marrow function is poorly understood. However, there is a clear association of decreased bone marrow function and chronic

TABLE 96.4b

INCIDENCE OF GRADES III–IV ACUTE GRAFT VERSUS HOST DISEASE IN CML ACCORDING TO THE NUMBER OF MISMATCHED CLASS I AND CLASS II ALLELES

	0 Class I (%)	1 Class I (%)	≥2 Class I (%)	Total (%)
0 Class II	32	29	36	32
1 Class II	45	31	55	45
≥2 Class II	67	67	86	74
Total	34	30	44	35

There were 467 chronic myeloid leukemia unrelated donor–recipient pairs.

GVHD (see below). The response of chronic GVHD to immune suppression is often correlated with improved bone marrow function.

Treatment for graft failure includes using molecularly cloned hematopoietic growth factors (G- or GM-CSF), a second graft, and/or increased immune suppression. Subjects with primary graft failure (that is, no engraftment) have a poor prognosis, whereas those with secondary graft failure (unsustained engraftment) do better. When graft failure is associated with re-emergence of host T cells, repeat pretransplant conditioning is usually given before the second graft based on the assumption that graft failure is immune mediated; this may not be correct in all instances.

Acute Graft versus Host Disease (GVHD)

The principle manifestations of acute GVHD are rash, diarrhea, and jaundice, present individually or in combination (133,134). Histologically, there is involvement of the basal cell layer of the skin, biliary ductules of the liver, and crypts of the distal gastrointestinal tract. Symptoms occur close to the time of engraftment but may occur earlier or at any time within the first 100 days post transplant. Acute GVHD is an allogeneic response mediated by donor T cells, which recognizes recipient tissues as foreign. The incidence and severity of acute GVHD increase with increasing recipient age and HLA and non-HLA disparity between the recipient and donor (135,136) (Table 96.4).

The major HLA genes are inherited from both paternal and maternal chromosome 6. The classic HLA class-1 genes are A, B, and C, and more HLA molecules are being characterized. The classical HLA class-1 molecules are present on the surface of all cells and function to present small intracellular peptides to T cells. HLA class 2 molecules are DR, DP, and DQ. These surface molecules present extracellular peptides that result from endocytosis of extracellular protein and degradation of these proteins into smaller peptides (137,138). Even after an HLA genotypically matched allotransplant, acute GVHD invariably develops when—usually inadvertently—no post transplant immune suppression is given. This likely arises because of recognition of host-derived peptides presented by HLA molecules and recognized as foreign by donor T cells (139).

Skin involvement in acute GVHD results in a maculopapular, erythematous rash, often beginning on the palms and soles and which may become systemic. In severe cases, acute GVHD with skin involvement may be pruritic with bullae. The skin involvement in acute GVHD may be precipitated by exposure to sunlight and/or drugs. Histologically, one can see the dermal-epidermal border disrupted by vacuolar degeneration of epithelial cells, dyskaryotic bodies, acantholysis (that is, separation of cell–cell contact), epidermolysis (separation of the epidermal and dermal layers), and lymphocytic infiltration. These clinical and histologic findings are not unique to acute GVHD and may occur from drug allergy or the effects of the high-dose chemotherapy and radiation used in the pretransplant conditioning regimen.

Gastrointestinal involvement with acute GVHD results in diarrhea, often accompanied by cramping abdominal pain. In severe cases, the diarrhea may be bloody or associated with a paralytic ileus. Histologically, lymphocytes and apoptotic cells are present and intestinal crypts are lost, which leads to epithelial denudation. Evaluation of gastrointestinal tract signs and symptoms should include stool cultures for bacteria, fungi, and viruses, especially CMV. Sigmoidoscopy with biopsy may be helpful if the diagnosis is in doubt and platelet levels are sufficient. Acute GVHD with hepatic involvement presents as jaundice and an elevated alkaline phosphatase with or without elevated transaminases. The differential diagnosis includes VOD or infections with CMV or *Candida* species and may require a transjugular liver biopsy for acurate diagnosis. In acute GVHD, the liver biopsy may show T-cell infiltration of the portal triad, with apoptosis of epithelial cells lining the biliary tree.

Acute GVHD and infections from immune suppression are major causes of early death after allotransplant. Consequently, acute GVHD prophylaxis is needed for all allotransplant recipients. One effective method to prevent acute GVHD is a 2- to 3-log depletion of T cells from the graft (140–142). However, benefits from preventing acute GVHD are offset by increased graft failure and leukemia relapse. Increased graft failure is presumed to result from immune-mediated graft rejection but may also reflect loss of the interaction of donor T cells and hematopoietic cells. Increased leukemia relapse is presumed to result from decreased T-cell–mediated antileukemia effects, sometimes referred to as *graft versus leukemia* or GvL. Experimental approaches to retain GvL while decreasing acute GVHD include selective T-cell depletion or adding back subsets of T cells or natural killer (NK) cells to the graft, use of cytokines, and modulation of costimulatory T-cell or chemokine pathways (143).

Pharmacologic approaches to preventing acute GVHD are technically simpler and more widely used than T-cell depletion. Cyclosporine and methotrexate given on days 1, 3, 6, and 11 post transplant are the most common preventative regimen (144). Other regimens include cyclosporine and prednisolone or cyclosporine, methotrexate, and methylprednisolone (145). In HLA-identical sibling transplants, weekly intravenous immunoglobulin (IVIG) until day 100 results in a lower incidence of acute GVHD (146). GVHD is associated with a lower leukemia relapse rate, and, therefore, the aim should not be to completely eliminate acute GVHD, but rather to balance the risk of acute GVHD against the risk of a leukemia relapse. Thus, more intensive immune suppressive regimens are used when GVHD risk is high, for instance, in HLA-mismatched transplants, and when the leukemia relapse risk is least, whereas less intensive regimens are used when the leukemia relapse risk is highest such as in advanced leukemia and when acute GVHD risk is least. Convincing data supporting these approaches are lacking.

Clinical staging of acute GVHD considers individual tissue/organ involvement scores, which are combined for an overall grade (Table 96.5). Grade 1 acute GVHD is not clinically important and requires no specific therapy. Grades 2 through 4 acute GVHD are typically treated with corticosteroids such as methylprednisolone, 1 to 2 mg/kg per day, with or without cyclosporine. Acute GVHD unresponsive to this approach has a poor prognosis. Further therapies include monoclonal or polyclonal antibodies to T cells, such as antithymocyte globulin (ATG) or alemtuzumab (anti-CD52), or cytokines such as dacluzimab or infliximab. Dacluzimab binds to the high-affinity IL-2 receptor found on activated T cells, whereas infliximab binds to TNF-α, a cytokine involved in acute GVHD (147). Several reports suggest that giving IVIG—typically used for

TABLE 96.5a

GRADING OF ACUTE GRAFT VERSUS HOST DISEASE

SEVERITY OF INDIVIDUAL ORGAN INVOLVEMENT		
Organ	Grade	Description
Skin	+1	A maculopapular eruption involving less than 25% of the body surface
	+2	A maculopapular eruption involving 25%–50% of the body surface
	+3	Generalized erythroderma
	+4	Generalized erythroderma with bullous formation and often with desquamation
Liver	+1	Moderate increase of AST (150–750 IU) and bilirubin (2.0–3.0 mg/dL)
	+2	Bilirubin rise (3.1–6.0 mg/dL) with or without an increase in AST
	+3	Bilirubin rise (6.1–15 mg/dL) with or without an increase in AST
	+4	Bilirubin rise (greater than 15 mg/dL) with or without an increase in AST
Gut		Diarrhea, nausea, and vomiting graded +1 to +4 in severity. The severity of gut involvement is assigned to the most severe involvement noted.
	+1	Diarrhea more than 500 mL/day
	+2	Diarrhea more than 1,000 mL/day
	+3	Diarrhea more than 1,500 mL/day
	+4	Diarrhea more than 2,000 mL/day; or severe abdominal pain with or without ileus

AST, aspartate transaminase.

CMV-infection prevention (see below)—is associated with less acute GVHD, but these data are inconsistent.

INTERMEDIATE CONCERNS (DAYS 30 TO 100)

CMV Prophylaxis

Prophylaxis for CMV infection after autotransplants is unnecessary. In allotransplants, ganciclovir is often given when a surveillance blood culture or bronchoalveolar lavage (BAL) is CMV-positive by quantitative polymerase chain reaction (PCR). Subjects with CMV viremia and $CD4^+$ T cells less than 0.1×10^9 cells/L are at greatest risk of developing CMV disease (148). Surveillance CMV-PCR is started 2 weeks before transplantation and continued until day 100 post procedure. A positive CMV-PCR usually prompts giving full-dose ganciclovir for 2 weeks or until the CMV-PCR becomes negative, and then for another 2 weeks at one-half dose (149–152). Valaciclovir is then given as prophylaxis until day 100. G-CSF may be given if there is bone marrow suppression, or therapy may be changed to foscarnet, which is associated with less bone marrow suppression.

Pneumonitis

Between 30% and 50% of early post transplant deaths are associated with respiratory failure (153,154). Although bacterial and fungal pulmonary infections can occur, the two most common causes are idiopathic and CMV-related interstitial pneumonia.

Interstitial pneumonia is more common after allotransplantation (40%) as compared to autotransplantation (10%). Risk factors include a radiation-based pretransplant conditioning regimen, severe GVHD, older age, and post transplant use of methotrexate. The median time to onset of interstitial pneumonia is about 50 days post transplant, with only rare cases developing after 6 months. Affected persons are hypoxic and/or hypocapnic; physical examination often shows basilar crackles; and the chest roentgenogram shows an interstitial

TABLE 96.5b

OVERALL GRADE OF GRAFT VERSUS HOST DISEASE*

Grade	Skin	Gut		Liver	ECOG performance
I	+1 to +2	0		0	0
II	+1 to +3	+1 to +2	and/or	+1 to +2	0 to 1
III	+2 to +4	+2 to +4	and/or	+2 to +4	2 to 3
IV	+2 to +4	+2 to +4	and/or	+2 to +4	3 to 4

ECOG, Eastern Cooperative Oncology Group. AST, aspartate transaminase
*If no skin disease, the overall grade is the higher single organ grade.
Adapted from Glucksberg H, Storb R, Fefer A, et al. Clinical manifestations of graft versus host disease in human recipients of marrow from HL-A-matched sibling donors. *Transplantation*. 1974;18:295–304.

reticular-nodular infiltrate. Between 40% and 65% of cases of interstitial pneumonia are CMV related. Diagnosis is usually accomplished by bronchoscopy with BAL. Early intervention with combined IVIG and ganciclovir has a reduced mortality of CMV pneumonia to about 50% (155,156). It is very rare for a subject to develop CMV pneumonia when routine screening for CMV activation by PCR is carried out and appropriate interventions taken. Adoptive immunotherapy, giving CMV-specific cytotoxic T cells has also been used to treat CMV pneumonia (157). Other opportunistic infections causing interstitial pneumonia, such as *Chlamydia trachomatis* and *Legionella pneumophilia*, are less common. Prophylaxis for *Pneumocystis carinii* pneumonia with sulphomethaxozole-trimethoprim (Bactrim) is usually begun after engraftment and continued for 1 year.

The cause(s) of 30% to 50% of post transplant interstitial pneumonias are unknown (158–160). Etiologies are complex and poorly understood; likely contributors include the toxicity of the pretransplant conditioning regimen, chronic GVHD, and unidentified infectious organisms such as human herpes virus 6 (HHV-6) and respiratory syncytial virus (RSV) (161). Carmustine (BCNU)-related interstitial pneumonia may respond to corticosteroids, but most cases of idiopathic pneumonia syndrome do not.

Epstein-Barr Virus Lymphoproliferative Disease

Infection of B cells by Epstein-Barr virus (EBV) results in B-cell proliferation. In a normal person, infection-induced, EBV-specific cytotoxic T cells prevent uncontrolled B-cell proliferation. In immune-deficient allotransplant recipients, failure of immune surveillance by EBV-specific cytotoxic T cells results in a polyclonal or, less often, monoclonal B-cell proliferation of donor or recipient origin (162). EBV-lymphoproliferative syndrome (EBV-LPS) occurs in about 0.5% of allotransplant recipients. Risk factors include T-cell–depleted grafts and the use of ATG or anti-CD3 antibodies post transplant to prevent acute GVHD. EBV-LPS typically develops 45 days to 1.5 years post transplant; the median time to onset is 70 to 80 days. Presenting features of early-onset EBV-LPS include fever and extranodal involvement; the course is typically unfavorable. Later-onset EBV-LPS generally has a more indolent course, manifested by fever and lymph node enlargement. Antiviral therapy of EBV-LPS is generally ineffective. Rituximab (anti-CD20 monoclonal antibody) has been used and is sometimes effective (163). Giving donor EBV-specific cytotoxic T cells sometimes results in prompt remission of polyclonal and monoclonal EBV-LPS (164).

LATE CONCERNS (BEYOND DAY 100)

Chronic GVHD

Chronic GVHD usually occurs after day 100 post transplant. Chronic disease may seemingly develop *de novo* without prior clinically diagnosed acute GVHD, after a quiescent interval following resolution of acute GVHD. Most often, acute GVHD evolves into the chronic process (165,166). The most important risk factors for developing chronic GVHD are older recipient age and severity of acute GVHD. Whereas acute GVHD is predominately an alloimmune disorder, chronic GVHD has features of alloimmunity and autoimmunity.

Skin involvement in chronic GVHD involves scleroderma-like changes with hypopigmentation and hyperpigmentation, loss of hair follicles, thickened skin, and joint contractures. Mucosal involvement manifests by dryness, pain, ulceration, and lacy white buccal mucosal membranes. Occular features include sicca conjunctivitis, ectropion, and, in severe cases, corneal ulceration. In contrast to acute GVHD of the gastrointestinal tract, which is marked by watery or bloody diarrhea, chronic gastrointestinal GVHD manifests as nausea, anorexia, malabsorption, dysphagia, and weight loss. Ulcerations, strictures, and narrowing may occur at any site along the gastrointestinal tract. Hepatic involvement in chronic GVHD presents similarly to acute GVHD with predominance of cholestasis—that is, increased bilirubin and alkaline phosphatase.

Chronic GVHD may have various autoimmune features, including antibodies to DNA, mitochondria, smooth muscle, or connective tissue. Autoimmune syndromes associated with chronic GVHD include polymyositis, myasthenia gravis, systemic lupus erythematosis, rheumatoid arthritis, primary biliary cirrhosis, and thyroiditis. Chronic GVHD of the lung presents with cough and dyspnea caused by progressive obstructive small airway disease with hyperinflated lungs and reduced midexpiratory flows; histologically, the process resembles bronchiolitis obliterans. Chronic GVHD results from underlying immune dysregulation, which also causes immune deficiency that predisposes to infection independent of the immune suppressive drugs used to treat GVHD.

Chronic GVHD may be limited or extensive (Table 96.6). Limited-stage chronic GVHD has a favorable prognosis and requires no therapy. Extensive-stage chronic GVHD has a poor prognosis; therapy is needed (167). Adverse prognostic variables in persons with extensive-stage GVHD include thrombocytopenia (less than 100×10^9 cells/L) and poor performance status. Standard therapy of extensive-stage chronic GVHD is alternate day corticosteroids. Other options include thalidomide, extracorporeal photophoresis, psoralen and ultraviolet irradiation (PUVA) for chronic cutaneous GVHD, and ursodeoxycholic acid for chronic hepatic GVHD (168). Clinical trials with thalidomide analogues, such as lenalidomide and

TABLE 96.6

CHRONIC GRAFT VERSUS HOST DISEASE GRADES

Limited	Disease localized only to skin involvement or hepatic involvement
Extensive	1. Generalized skin involvement 2. Limited skin involvement or hepatic involvement and a. Liver histologic features showing chronic progressive hepatitis, bridging necrosis, or cirrhosis b. Eye involvement (Schirmer's test with less than 5 mm wetting) c. Involvement of minor salivary glands or oral mucosa d. Involvement of any other organ

pomalidomide, are beginning. The natural history of chronic GVHD is to "burn out" or for subjects to die from an opportunistic infection. The therapy paradox here is that one is forced to use immune suppression to treat a disease that kills subjects because of intrinsic immune suppression.

Herpes Zoster

Varicella zoster occurs in 20% of autotransplant (169) and 20% to 50% of allotransplant recipients, usually 100 days to 1 year post transplant (170,171). Infection may present with cutaneous or visceral involvement. Persons with visceral involvement may present with severe acute abdominal pain from virus reactivation in the celiac plexus, which spreads to the pancreas and small bowel. If cutaneous or visceral *Herpes varicella zoster* is suspected, the subject should be hospitalized, placed in isolation, and given IV acyclovir.

Second Cancers

Transplant recipients are at increased risk to develop a second cancer (172–174). Autotransplants are associated with increased clonal cytogenetic changes in bone marrow cells post transplant. Some of these abnormalities are typical of therapy-related myelodysplastic syndrome (MDS), including monosomy 5 or 7 (del[5] and del[7]), and translocations involving 11q23. These abnormalities are reported in up to 9% of recipients at 3 years post transplant and are likely related to the effects of exposing the bone marrow to drugs and radiation as part of disease therapy and as part of pretransplant conditioning. Allotransplant recipients have a fourfold to sixfold age-adjusted risk of developing a cancer. Risk factors include pretransplant conditioning with radiation and acute GVHD equal to or greater than grade 2. The 10-year cumulative incidence of solid cancers after allotransplants is about 3%, while the 15-year probability of a second cancer is about 6% for persons not receiving radiation versus 20% for persons receiving radiation.

Relapse

Relapse of disease after autotransplants or allotransplants may be treated with a second autotransplant or allotransplant (175–178). If the first pretransplant conditioning regimen included radiation, it should not be used prior to the second transplant; if, however, the first pretransplant conditioning regimen lacked radiation, it should be considered for the second transplant if this is disease appropriate. If the first transplant was an autotransplant, it is unlikely that a second autotransplant will succeed, and thus, an allotransplant is preferred.

Subjects relapsing less than 1 year after autotransplant or allotransplant are often not reasonable candidates for a second transplant because of substantial transplant-related morbidity and mortality and a low likelihood of leukemia control. Subjects retransplanted less than 6 months after a first transplant have done particularly poorly. Sometimes leukemia relapse can be reversed by discontinuing post transplant immune suppression or by giving donor lymphocytes, or both (179–181). Donor lymphocyte infusions (DLI) are effective in many subjects with recurrent chronic phase chronic myelogenous leukemia (CML) provided DLI is done in early relapse (182). In acute myelogenous leukemia (AML), about 30% of subjects with relapse respond; the interval to remission after DLI is 1 to 3 months. Complications of DLI include bone marrow failure and worsening of acute GVHD. Mixed chimeras have a lower risk of bone marrow failure than persons with only recipient hematopoeisis. The risk of acute GVHD after DLI is about 80%, with a tendency to cause hepatic acute GVHD. Attempts to modulate precipitating acute GVHD by genetically engineering donor lymphocytes to express herpes simplex virus thymidine kinase (HSVTK) and treating with ganciclovir if acute GVHD develops are reported (183).

Hypothyroidism

For the first 3 to 6 months, post transplant recipients may have a "euthyroid sick syndrome" with decreased tri-iodothyronine (T3), decreased thyroxine (T4), and low thyroid-stimulating hormone (TSH) (184,185). As in other nonthyroid diseases associated with a euthyroid sick syndrome, these abnormalities are reversible and probably are normal physiologic responses to decreased protein catabolism. Hormone replacement therapy is unnecessary.

Primary hypothyroidism post transplant is caused by high-dose radiation in the pretransplant conditioning regimen (186–188). Primary hypothyroidism—elevated TSH and low T4—occurs in less than 2% of recipients not receiving radiation (189) but in about 10% of radiation recipients. A greater proportion of subjects have compensated primary hypothyroidism with increased TSH but normal T4. The time interval to onset of primary hypothyroidism is 6 to 41 months post transplant, with a median of 13 months. The risk of primary hypothyroidism is greater after single-dose than fractionated radiation. Whereas overt hypothyroidism is treated with hormone replacement, compensated disease may be treated with close follow-up or hormone replacement.

Growth and Development

Child and adolescent transplant recipients have delayed or interrupted growth and development; the composition of the pretransplant conditioning regimen is a major determinant (187,190). Other risk factors for growth retardation are central nervous system (CNS) radiation, single-dose radiation pretransplant, chronic GVHD, corticosteroid use, and age. Children receiving only high-dose cyclophosphamide do not, in general, have growth retardation. Radiation regimens, on the other hand, adversely affect the rate of height and growth. Radiation may also inhibit normal dental and facial skeletal development, especially in children younger than 6 years of age. Although chemotherapy regimens were originally not thought to alter growth, combined busulfan and cyclophosphamide pretransplant conditioning causes growth retardation comparable to that of cyclophosphamide combined with fractionated radiation (191). How pretransplant conditioning regimens cause growth retardation is incompletely understood but includes direct injury to the growth plates, decreased pituitary and hypothalamic growth hormone production, and primary gonadal failure with decreased estrogens and testosterone, as well as elevated luteinizing hormone and follicle-stimulating hormone. In premenopausal transplant recipients, secondary sexual characteristics and menarche are usually delayed. Growth hormone therapy may improve final height in children younger than 10 years of age at transplant but has no impact on older children (192).

Fertility

Primary gonadal failure, for example, hypergonadotropic hypogonadism, is common post transplant (187,190,193,194). Recovery of gonadal function depends on recipient age and pretransplant conditioning regimen. In postmenopausal women receiving cyclophosphamide only, gonadal dysfunction is usually transitory. Gonadal failure occurs in about one half of recipients of busulphan and cyclophosphamide (194), whereas almost all recipients of radiation-containing pretransplant conditioning regimens develop gonadal failure. The return of menstruation within 10 years after radiation occurs in more than 90% of recipients who were younger than 18 years of age at the time of transplant and in 10% to 15% of recipients older than 18 years of age at the time of transplant. Post transplant gonadal failure is often associated with symptoms of estrogen deficiency, including hot flashes, dyspareunia, dysuria, and vaginal dryness, which may be helped by hormone replacement therapy (195). Cases have been reported of cryopreservation and orthotopic transplantation of ovarian tissue that has resulted in recovery of ovarian function and subsequent pregnancy (196,197).

Cataracts

Corticosteroid therapy and radiation-containing pretransplant conditioning regimens cause cataracts within a median of 2.5 to 5 years post transplant (198–201). The incidence of cataracts, both subclinical and clinical, is 85% to 100% for unfractionated radiation recipients, 30% to 50% for fractionated radiation recipients, and 5% to 20% for recipients not receiving radiation. The probability of requiring cataract removal within 10 years post transplant is 100% for single-dose radiation and 20% for fractionated radiation. Eye shielding decreases the cataract risk but is not generally done because of the concern of increasing leukemia relapse, as blood cells in the eye would escape irradiation.

Late Renal Effects

Reversible renal dysfunction is common early post transplant, with causes that are multifactorial including, but not limited to, drugs and infections (202,203). Although long-term complications are rare, there are occasional reports of late-onset renal dysfunction consistent with radiation nephropathy occurring after multidrug and radiation-containing pretransplant conditioning regimens. Onset is typically 3 to 7 months post transplant and is characterized by hypertension, edema, uremia, and occasionally hemolytic uremic syndrome (HUS). Cyclosporine may cause a similar picture of hypertension, renal insufficiency, and HUS that can be confused with or complicate transplant-related renal failure.

Late Pulmonary Effects

Late-onset noninfectious pulmonary complications (LONIPC) occur in 10% to 25% of subjects (204–206). These are further classified as bronchiolitis obliterans, bronchiolitis obliterans with organizing pneumonia, interstitial pneumonia, and diffuse alveolar disease. These abnormalities are thought to result from the pretransplant conditioning regimen, especially radiation. Chronic GVHD and pretransplant pulmonary function are the main determinants predicting worsening pulmonary function in long-term survivors post transplant (206). Bronchiolitis obliterans presents as cough and wheezing. Studies typically show severe obstructive lung disease with hyperinflated diaphragms resulting from obliteration of small bronchioles. This typically occurs 3 months to 2 years post transplant. Although usually associated with allotransplants complicated by chronic GVHD, bronchiolitis obliterans occurs rarely after autotransplants. Corticosteroids are usually used to treat bronchiolitis obliterans, but the results are poor at best. Lymphocytic interstitial pneumonia is characterized by a lymphocytic interstitial infiltrate that may progress to fibrosis. The cause is not clear but is thought to be immune-mediated, and is also treated with corticosteroids. Survival of persons with LONIPC is poor; death usually results from respiratory failure and/or infections.

IMMUNE SUPPRESSIVE DRUGS

Antiproliferative Drugs

Mycophenolate mofetil (MPA), used to modify GVHD in allotransplants, is metabolized to mycophenolic acid, a potent, reversible noncompetitive inhibitor of inosine monophosphate dehydrogenase (IMPDH). IMPDH is the first of two enzymes that convert inosine monophosphate (IMP) to guanosine monophosphate (GMP). GMP is normally converted to GDP, GTP, and dGTP. IMPDH is not involved in the salvage pathway of purine biosynthesis. MPA treatment decreases GTP and dGTP in lymphocytes that inhibit DNA synthesis and GTP-dependent metabolic events resulting in immune suppression (207).

Cyclophosphamide is a common component of pretransplant conditioning. It is a cyclic phosphamide ester of mechlorethamine inactive in its native form. Cyclophosphamide is converted in the liver to active alkylating metabolites, acrolein, and phosphoramide mustard, which prevent cell division by cross-linking DNA strands. High-dose cyclophosphamide, if given without mesna, results in hemorrhagic cystitis via acrolein formation. Prior pelvic radiation also increases the risk of cyclophosphamide-related hemorrhagic cystitis.

Corticosteroids and Other Immune Suppressive Drugs

Prednisone is widely used in oncology for anticancer and immune suppression effect. The agent is highly active in acute lymphoblastic leukemia (ALL) and lymphomas. Prednisone is also used to palliate symptomatic advanced cancers where it enhances appetite and produces a sense of well-being.

Corticosteroids are also powerful immune suppressive drugs used to prevent and/or treat GVHD. The relatively high mineralocorticoid activity of cortisone and hydrocortisone with resultant fluid retention makes them unsuitable for long-term immune suppression. Prednisone has predominantly glucocorticoid activity, and is the corticosteroid most commonly used for long-term immune suppression in chronic GVHD. The maintenance dose of prednisone in this setting should be kept as low as possible to minimize adverse effects, including peptic ulcers, proximal myopathy, osteoporosis, kidney suppression, hirsuitism, weight gain, susceptibility to infections, euphoria, depression, cataracts, impaired healing, and others.

Cyclosporine, a calcineurin inhibitor, is a potent immune suppressive drug that adversely affects the kidney but not the bone marrow. Cyclosporine is widely used to prevent and/or treat GVHD.

Tacrolimus is also a calcineurin inhibitor. Although tacrolimus is not chemically related to cyclosporine, it has a similar mode of action and side-effect profile. The incidences of neural and renal toxicity are greater with tacrolimus than cyclosporine. Additionally, cardiomyopathy and glucose intolerance are reported. Hypertrichosis is less a problem with tacrolimus than cyclosporine. Tacrolimus is not commonly used in bone marrow and blood cell allotransplants.

Interleukin-2 (IL-2) and its receptor (IL-2R) are important in T-cell–mediated immunity. Monoclonal antibodies to these moieties, basiliximab and dacluzimab, are used to treat corticosteroid-resistant GVHD (208). Rare side effects include hypersensitivity reactions. Infliximab is also used in the treatment of corticosteroid-refractory GVHD (147,209).

Thalidomide, a member of a class of immune modulating compounds, termed ImiDs, has been used to prevent and/or treat chronic GVHD (210). It is also used, combined with other drugs, to treat multiple myeloma. Thalidomide causes drowsiness, constipation, thrombosis, and neuropathy. Because of its teratogenic effects, it should not be given to sexually active persons without proper precautions. Lenalidomide, a thalidomide analogue, is also used to treat bone marrow disorders, including myelodysplastic syndrome (MDS) and multiple myeloma. Clinical trials of lenalidomide and pomalidomide, a third ImiD, in chronic GVHD are beginning.

Alemtuzumab (Campath-1H) directed at the CD52 molecule on the surface of all lymphocytes is sometimes used to remove T cells from allografts. Alemtuzumab is also sometimes used to treat corticosteroid-resistant, acute GVHD (211). Infusion-related adverse effects may occur, including fever, chills, nausea and vomiting, and allergic reactions. There is also increased susceptibility to infections, particularly with fungi, viruses, and protozoa.

References

1. Ghalie R, Szidon JP, Thompson L, et al. Evaluation of pulmonary complications after bone marrow transplantation: the role of pretransplant pulmonary function tests. *Bone Marrow Transplant.* 1992;10:359–365.
2. Milburn HJ, Prentice HG, du Bois RM. Can lung function measurements be used to predict which patients will be at risk of developing interstitial pneumonitis after bone marrow transplantation? *Thorax.* 1992;47:421–425.
3. Hertenstein B, Stefanic M, Schmeiser T, et al. Cardiac toxicity of bone marrow transplantation: predictive value of cardiologic evaluation before transplant. *J Clin Oncol.* 1994;12:998–1004.
4. Chien JW, Madtes DK, Clark JG. Pulmonary function testing prior to hematopoietic stem cell transplantation. *Bone Marrow Transplant.* 2005; 35:429–435.
5. Parimon T, Au DH, Martin PJ, et al. A risk score for mortality after allogeneic hematopoietic cell transplantation. *Ann Intern Med.* 2006;144:407–414.
6. Singh AK, Karimpour SE, Savani BN, et al. Pretransplant pulmonary function tests predict risk of mortality following fractionated total body irradiation and allogeneic peripheral blood stem cell transplant. *Int J Radiat Oncol Biol Phys.* 2006;66:520–527.
7. Ditschkowski M, Elmaagacli AH, Trenschel R, et al. Myeloablative allogeneic hematopoietic stem cell transplantation in elderly patients. *Clin Transplant.* 2006;20:127–131.
8. Klepin HD, Hurd DD. Autologous transplantation in elderly patients with multiple myeloma: are we asking the right questions? *Bone Marrow Transplant.* 2006;38:585–592.
9. Klingemann HG, Shepherd JD, Reece DE, et al. Regimen-related acute toxicities: pathophysiology, risk factors, clinical evaluation and preventive strategies. *Bone Marrow Transplant.* 1994;14(Suppl 4):S14–18.
10. Reece DE, Bredeson C, Perez WS, et al. Autologous stem cell transplantation in multiple myeloma patients <60 vs ≥60 years of age. *Bone Marrow Transplant.* 2003;32:1135–1143.
11. Barrett AJ. Immunosuppressive therapy in bone marrow transplantation. *Immunol Lett.* 1991;29:81–87.
12. Storb R, Yu C, Deeg HJ, et al. Current and future preparative regimens for bone marrow transplantation in thalassemia. *Ann N Y Acad Sci.* 1998;850: 276–287.
13. Thomas ED, Buckner CD, Banaji M, et al. One hundred patients with acute leukemia treated by chemotherapy, total body irradiation, and allogeneic marrow transplantation. *Blood.* 1977;49:511–533.
14. Santos GW, Tutschka PJ, Brookmeyer R, et al. Marrow transplantation for acute nonlymphocytic leukemia after treatment with busulfan and cyclophosphamide. *N Engl J Med.* 1983;309:1347–1353.
15. Socie G, Clift RA, Blaise D, et al. Busulfan plus cyclophosphamide compared with total-body irradiation plus cyclophosphamide before marrow transplantation for myeloid leukemia: long-term follow-up of 4 randomized studies. *Blood.* 2001;98:3569–3574.
16. Montgomery M, Cottler-Fox M. Mobilization and collection of autologous hematopoietic progenitor/stem cells. *Clin Adv Hematol Oncol.* 2007;5: 127–136.
17. Ikeda K, Kozuka T, Harada M. Factors for PBPC collection efficiency and collection predictors. *Transfus Apher Sci.* 2004;31:245–259.
18. Cesaro S, Marson P, Gazzola MV, et al. The use of cytokine-stimulated healthy donors in allogeneic stem cell transplantation. *Haematologica.* 2002;87:35–41.
19. Siena S, Bregni M, Gianni AM. Mobilization of peripheral blood progenitor cells for autografting: chemotherapy and G-CSF or GM-CSF. *Baillieres Best Pract Res Clin Haematol.* 1999;12:27–39.
20. Group SCTC. Allogeneic peripheral blood stem-cell compared with bone marrow transplantation in the management of hematologic malignancies: an individual patient data meta-analysis of nine randomized trials. *J Clin Oncol.* 2005;23:5074–5087.
21. Weber-Nordt RM, Schott E, Finke J, et al. Umbilical cord blood: an alternative to the transplantation of bone marrow stem cells. *Cancer Treat Rev.* 1996;22:381–391.
22. Berz D, McCormack EM, Winer ES, et al. Cryopreservation of hematopoietic stem cells. *Am J Hematol.* 2007;2(6):463–472.
23. Rowley SD. Hematopoietic stem cell cryopreservation: a review of current techniques. *J Hematother.* 1992;1:233–250.
24. Alessandrino P, Bernasconi P, Caldera D, et al. Adverse events occurring during bone marrow or peripheral blood progenitor cell infusion: analysis of 126 cases. *Bone Marrow Transplant.* 1999;23:533–537.
25. Klein MA, Kadidlo D, McCullough J, et al. Microbial contamination of hematopoietic stem cell products: incidence and clinical sequelae. *Biol Blood Marrow Transplant.* 2006;12:1142–1149.
26. Mackie FE, Umetsu D, Salvatierra O, et al. Pulmonary capillary leak syndrome with intravenous cyclosporin A in pediatric kidney transplantation. *Pediatr Transplant.* 2000;4:35–38.
27. Woywodt A, Haubitz M, Buchholz S, et al. Counting the cost: markers of endothelial damage in hematopoietic stem cell transplantation. *Bone Marrow Transplant.* 2004;34:1015–1023.
28. Schots R, Kaufman L, Van Riet I, et al. Proinflammatory cytokines and their role in the development of major transplant-related complications in the early phase after allogeneic bone marrow transplantation. *Leukemia.* 2003;17:1150–1156.
29. Al-Homaidhi A, Prince HM, Al-Zahrani H, et al. Granulocyte-macrophage colony-stimulating factor-associated histiocytosis and capillary-leak syndrome following autologous bone marrow transplantation: two case reports and a review of the literature. *Bone Marrow Transplant.* 1998;21: 209–214.
30. Rossi R, Pleyer J, Schafers P, et al. Development of ifosfamide-induced nephrotoxicity: prospective follow-up in 75 patients. *Med Pediatr Oncol.* 1999;32:177–182.
31. Skinner R. Chronic ifosfamide nephrotoxicity in children. *Med Pediatr Oncol.* 2003;41:190–197.

32. Durken M, Agbenu J, Finckh B, et al. Deteriorating free radical-trapping capacity and antioxidant status in plasma during bone marrow transplantation. *Bone Marrow Transplant.* 1995;15:757–762.
33. Przepiorka D, LeParc GF, Stovall MA, et al. Use of irradiated blood components: practice parameter. *Am J Clin Pathol.* 1996;106:6–11.
34. Ljungman P, Perez-Bercoff L, Jonsson J, et al. Risk factors for the development of cytomegalovirus disease after allogeneic stem cell transplantation. *Haematologica.* 2006;91:78–83.
35. Takami A, Mochizuki K, Asakura H, et al. High incidence of cytomegalovirus reactivation in adult recipients of an unrelated cord blood transplant. *Haematologica.* 2005;90:1290–1292.
36. Boeckh M, Fries B, Nichols WG. Recent advances in the prevention of CMV infection and disease after hematopoietic stem cell transplantation. *Pediatr Transplant.* 2004;8(Suppl 5):19–27.
37. Gentile G, Picardi A, Capobianchi A, et al. A prospective study comparing quantitative Cytomegalovirus (CMV) polymerase chain reaction in plasma and pp65 antigenemia assay in monitoring patients after allogeneic stem cell transplantation. *BMC Infect Dis.* 2006;6:167.
38. Blajchman MA. The clinical benefits of the leukoreduction of blood products. *J Trauma.* 2006;60:S83–90.
39. van Prooijen HC, Visser JJ, van Oostendorp WR, et al. Prevention of primary transfusion-associated cytomegalovirus infection in bone marrow transplant recipients by the removal of white cells from blood components with high-affinity filters. *Br J Haematol.* 1994;87:144–147.
40. Rossini F, Terruzzi E, Cammarota S, et al. Cytomegalovirus infection after autologous stem cell transplantation: incidence and outcome in a group of patients undergoing a surveillance program. *Transpl Infect Dis.* 2005;7: 122–125.
41. Heal JM, Liesveld JL, Phillips GL, et al. What would Karl Landsteiner do? The ABO blood group and stem cell transplantation. *Bone Marrow Transplant.* 2005;36:747–755.
42. Seebach JD, Stussi G, Passweg JR, et al. ABO blood group barrier in allogeneic bone marrow transplantation revisited. *Biol Blood Marrow Transplant.* 2005;11:1006–1013.
43. Stussi G, Muntwyler J, Passweg JR, et al. Consequences of ABO incompatibility in allogeneic hematopoietic stem cell transplantation. *Bone Marrow Transplant.* 2002;30:87–93.
44. Benson K, Fields K, Hiemenz J, et al. The platelet-refractory bone marrow transplant patient: prophylaxis and treatment of bleeding. *Semin Oncol.* 1993;20:102–109.
45. Trifilio S, Verma A, Mehta J. Antimicrobial prophylaxis in hematopoietic stem cell transplant recipients: heterogeneity of current clinical practice. *Bone Marrow Transplant.* 2004;33:735–739.
46. Nichols WG. Combating infections in hematopoietic stem cell transplant recipients. *Expert Rev Anti Infect Ther.* 2003;1:57–73.
47. Kruger WH, Bohlius J, Cornely OA, et al. Antimicrobial prophylaxis in allogeneic bone marrow transplantation. Guidelines of the infectious diseases working party (AGIHO) of the German society of haematology and oncology. *Ann Oncol.* 2005;16:1381–1390.
48. Patrick CC. Use of fluoroquinolones as prophylactic agents in patients with neutropenia. *Pediatr Infect Dis J.* 1997;16:135–139; discussion 160–132.
49. Reuter S, Kern WV, Sigge A, et al. Impact of fluoroquinolone prophylaxis on reduced infection-related mortality among patients with neutropenia and hematologic malignancies. *Clin Infect Dis.* 2005;40:1087–1093.
50. Gafter-Gvili A, Paul M, Fraser A, et al. Effect of quinolone prophylaxis in afebrile neutropenic patients on microbial resistance: systematic review and meta-analysis. *J Antimicrob Chemother.* 2007;59:5–22.
51. Buckner CD, Clift RA, Sanders JE, et al. Protective environment for marrow transplant recipients: a prospective study. *Ann Intern Med.* 1978;89:893–901.
52. Fenelon LE. Protective isolation: who needs it? *J Hosp Infect.* 1995;30 (Suppl):218–222.
53. Passweg JR, Rowlings PA, Atkinson KA, et al. Influence of protective isolation on outcome of allogeneic bone marrow transplantation for leukemia. *Bone Marrow Transplant.* 1998;21:1231–1238.
54. Russell JA, Poon MC, Jones AR, et al. Allogeneic bone-marrow transplantation without protective isolation in adults with malignant disease. *Lancet.* 1992;339:38–40.
55. Beelen DW, Elmaagacli A, Muller KD, et al. Influence of intestinal bacterial decontamination using metronidazole and ciprofloxacin or ciprofloxacin alone on the development of acute graft-versus-host disease after marrow transplantation in patients with hematologic malignancies: final results and long-term follow-up of an open-label prospective randomized trial. *Blood.* 1999;93:3267–3275.
56. Cornet M, Levy V, Fleury L, et al. Efficacy of prevention by high-efficiency particulate air filtration or laminar airflow against Aspergillus airborne contamination during hospital renovation. *Infect Control Hosp Epidemiol.* 1999;20:508–513.
57. Sherertz RJ, Belani A, Kramer BS, et al. Impact of air filtration on nosocomial Aspergillus infections. Unique risk of bone marrow transplant recipients. *Am J Med.* 1987;83:709–718.
58. Moody K, Charlson ME, Finlay J. The neutropenic diet: what's the evidence? *J Pediatr Hematol Oncol.* 2002;24:717–721.
59. Marr KA, Crippa F, Leisenring W, et al. Itraconazole versus fluconazole for prevention of fungal infections in patients receiving allogeneic stem cell transplants. *Blood.* 2004;103:1527–1533.
60. Martino R, Parody R, Fukuda T, et al. Impact of the intensity of the pretransplantation conditioning regimen in patients with prior invasive aspergillosis undergoing allogeneic hematopoietic stem cell transplantation: A retrospective survey of the Infectious Diseases Working Party of the European Group for Blood and Marrow Transplantation. *Blood.* 2006;108:2928–2936.
61. Richard C, Romon I, Baro J, et al. Invasive pulmonary aspergillosis prior to BMT in acute leukemia patients does not predict a poor outcome. *Bone Marrow Transplant.* 1993;12:237–241.
62. Hann IM, Prentice HG, Blacklock HA, et al. Acyclovir prophylaxis against herpes virus infections in severely immunocompromised patients: randomised double blind trial. *Br Med J (Clin Res Ed).* 1983;287:384–388.
63. Saral R, Burns WH, Laskin OL, et al. Acyclovir prophylaxis of herpes-simplex-virus infections. *N Engl J Med.* 1981;305:63–67.
64. Atkinson K. Reconstruction of the haemopoietic and immune systems after marrow transplantation. *Bone Marrow Transplant.* 1990;5:209–226.
65. Storek J, Saxon A. Reconstitution of B cell immunity following bone marrow transplantation. *Bone Marrow Transplant.* 1992;9:395–408.
66. Friedrich W, O'Reilly RJ, Koziner B, et al. T-lymphocyte reconstitution in recipients of bone marrow transplants with and without GVHD: imbalances of T-cell subpopulations having unique regulatory and cognitive functions. *Blood.* 1982;59:696–701.
67. Glasmacher A, von Lilienfeld-Toal M. An evidence based review of the available antibiotic treatment options for neutropaenic patients and a recommendation for treatment guidelines. *Int J Infect Dis.* 2006;10(Suppl 2): S9–S16.
68. Scully C, Sonis S, Diz PD. Oral mucositis. *Oral Dis.* 2006;12:229–241.
69. Silverman S, Jr. Diagnosis and management of oral mucositis. *J Support Oncol.* 2007;5:13–21.
70. Spielberger R, Stiff P, Bensinger W, et al. Palifermin for oral mucositis after intensive therapy for hematologic cancers. *N Engl J Med.* 2004;351:2590–2598.
71. Cox GJ, Matsui SM, Lo RS, et al. Etiology and outcome of diarrhea after marrow transplantation: a prospective study. *Gastroenterology.* 1994;107:1398–1407.
72. Schiller GJ, Gale RP. A critical reappraisal of gastrointestinal complications of allogeneic bone marrow transplantation. *Cell Transplant.* 1992;1:265–269.
73. Schulenburg A, Turetschek K, Wrba F, et al. Early and late gastrointestinal complications after myeloablative and nonmyeloablative allogeneic stem cell transplantation. *Ann Hematol.* 2004;83:101–106.
74. Ippoliti C, Champlin R, Bugazia N, et al. Use of octreotide in the symptomatic management of diarrhea induced by graft-versus-host disease in patients with hematologic malignancies. *J Clin Oncol.* 1997;15:3350–3354.
75. Meijer E, Boland GJ, Verdonck LF. Prevention of cytomegalovirus disease in recipients of allogeneic stem cell transplants. *Clin Microbiol Rev.* 2003;16:647–657.
76. Cheuk DK, Lee TL, Chiang AK, et al. Risk factors and treatment of hemorrhagic cystitis in children who underwent hematopoietic stem cell transplantation. *Transpl Int.* 2007;20:73–81.
77. Giraud G, Bogdanovic G, Priftakis P, et al. The incidence of hemorrhagic cystitis and BK-viruria in allogeneic hematopoietic stem cell recipients according to intensity of the conditioning regimen. *Haematologica.* 2006;91:401–404.
78. Hale GA, Rochester RJ, Heslop HE, et al. Hemorrhagic cystitis after allogeneic bone marrow transplantation in children: clinical characteristics and outcome. *Biol Blood Marrow Transplant.* 2003;9:698–705.
79. Meisenberg B, Lassiter M, Hussein A, et al. Prevention of hemorrhagic cystitis after high-dose alkylating agent chemotherapy and autologous bone marrow support. *Bone Marrow Transplant.* 1994;14:287–291.
80. Turkeri LN, Lum LG, Uberti JP, et al. Prevention of hemorrhagic cystitis following allogeneic bone marrow transplant preparative regimens with cyclophosphamide and busulfan: role of continuous bladder irrigation. *J Urol.* 1995;153:637–640.
81. Hows JM, Mehta A, Ward L, et al. Comparison of mesna with forced diuresis to prevent cyclophosphamide induced haemorrhagic cystitis in marrow transplantation: a prospective randomised study. *Br J Cancer.* 1984;50:753–756.
82. Spach DH, Bauwens JE, Myerson D, et al. Cytomegalovirus-induced hemorrhagic cystitis following bone marrow transplantation. *Clin Infect Dis.* 1993;16:142–144.
83. Hale GA, Heslop HE, Krance RA, et al. Adenovirus infection after pediatric bone marrow transplantation. *Bone Marrow Transplant.* 1999;23:277–282.
84. Erard V, Storer B, Corey L, et al. BK virus infection in hematopoietic stem cell transplant recipients: frequency, risk factors, and association with postengraftment hemorrhagic cystitis. *Clin Infect Dis.* 2004;39:1861–1865.
85. Bearman SI. The syndrome of hepatic veno-occlusive disease after marrow transplantation. *Blood.* 1995;85:3005–3020.
86. McDonald GB, Hinds MS, Fisher LD, et al. Veno-occlusive disease of the liver and multiorgan failure after bone marrow transplantation: a cohort study of 355 patients. *Ann Intern Med.* 1993;118:255–267.

87. Shulman HM, Gown AM, Nugent DJ. Hepatic veno-occlusive disease after bone marrow transplantation. Immunohistochemical identification of the material within occluded central venules. *Am J Pathol.* 1987;127:549–558.
88. McDonald GB, Sharma P, Matthews DE, et al. Venocclusive disease of the liver after bone marrow transplantation: diagnosis, incidence, and predisposing factors. *Hepatology.* 1984;4:116–122.
89. Jones RJ, Lee KS, Beschorner WE, et al. Venoocclusive disease of the liver following bone marrow transplantation. *Transplantation.* 1987;44:778–783.
90. Blostein MD, Paltiel OB, Thibault A, et al. A comparison of clinical criteria for the diagnosis of veno-occlusive disease of the liver after bone marrow transplantation. *Bone Marrow Transplant.* 1992;10:439–443.
91. Herbetko J, Grigg AP, Buckley AR, et al. Venoocclusive liver disease after bone marrow transplantation: findings at duplex sonography. *AJR Am J Roentgenol.* 1992;158:1001–1005.
92. Hommeyer SC, Teefey SA, Jacobson AF, et al. Venocclusive disease of the liver: prospective study of US evaluation. *Radiology.* 1992;184:683–686.
93. Shulman HM, Gooley T, Dudley MD, et al. Utility of transvenous liver biopsies and wedged hepatic venous pressure measurements in sixty marrow transplant recipients. *Transplantation.* 1995;59:1015–1022.
94. Essell JH, Schroeder MT, Harman GS, et al. Ursodiol prophylaxis against hepatic complications of allogeneic bone marrow transplantation. A randomized, double-blind, placebo-controlled trial. *Ann Intern Med.* 1998;128:975–981.
95. Chopra R, Eaton JD, Grassi A, et al. Defibrotide for the treatment of hepatic veno-occlusive disease: results of the European compassionate-use study. *Br J Haematol.* 2000;111:1122–1129.
96. Kornblum N, Ayyanar K, Benimetskaya L, et al. Defibrotide, a polydisperse mixture of single-stranded phosphodiester oligonucleotides with lifesaving activity in severe hepatic veno-occlusive disease: clinical outcomes and potential mechanisms of action. *Oligonucleotides.* 2006;16:105–114.
97. Richardson PG, Murakami C, Jin Z, et al. Multi-institutional use of defibrotide in 88 patients after stem cell transplantation with severe veno-occlusive disease and multisystem organ failure: response without significant toxicity in a high-risk population and factors predictive of outcome. *Blood.* 2002;100:4337–4343.
98. Bearman SI, Lee JL, Baron AE, et al. Treatment of hepatic venocclusive disease with recombinant human tissue plasminogen activator and heparin in 42 marrow transplant patients. *Blood.* 1997;89:1501–1506.
99. Schriber J, Milk B, Shaw D, et al. Tissue plasminogen activator (tPA) as therapy for hepatotoxicity following bone marrow transplantation. *Bone Marrow Transplant.* 1999;24:1311–1314.
100. Fried MW, Connaghan DG, Sharma S, et al. Transjugular intrahepatic portosystemic shunt for the management of severe venoocclusive disease following bone marrow transplantation. *Hepatology.* 1996;24:588–591.
101. Azoulay D, Castaing D, Lemoine A, et al. Transjugular intrahepatic portosystemic shunt (TIPS) for severe veno-occlusive disease of the liver following bone marrow transplantation. *Bone Marrow Transplant.* 2000;25:987–992.
102. Zenz T, Rossle M, Bertz H, et al. Severe veno-occlusive disease after allogeneic bone marrow or peripheral stem cell transplantation–role of transjugular intrahepatic portosystemic shunt (TIPS). *Liver.* 2001;21:31–36.
103. Hagglund H, Ringden O, Ericzon BG, et al. Treatment of hepatic venoocclusive disease with recombinant human tissue plasminogen activator or orthotopic liver transplantation after allogeneic bone marrow transplantation. *Transplantation.* 1996;62:1076–1080.
104. Nimer SD, Milewicz AL, Champlin RE, et al. Successful treatment of hepatic venoocclusive disease in a bone marrow transplant patient with orthotopic liver transplantation. *Transplantation.* 1990;49:819–821.
105. Rapoport AP, Doyle HR, Starzl T, et al. Orthotopic liver transplantation for life-threatening veno-occlusive disease of the liver after allogeneic bone marrow transplant. *Bone Marrow Transplant.* 1991;8:421–424.
106. Price KJ, Thall PF, Kish SK, et al. Prognostic indicators for blood and marrow transplant patients admitted to an intensive care unit. *Am J Respir Crit Care Med.* 1998;158:876–884.
107. Martin PL. To stop or not to stop: how much support should be provided to mechanically ventilated pediatric bone marrow and stem cell transplant patients? *Respir Care Clin North Am.* 2006;12:403–419.
108. Ho VT, Weller E, Lee SJ, et al. Prognostic factors for early severe pulmonary complications after hematopoietic stem cell transplantation. *Biol Blood Marrow Transplant.* 2001;7:223–229.
109. Khurshid I, Anderson LC. Non-infectious pulmonary complications after bone marrow transplantation. *Postgrad Med J.* 2002;78:257–262.
110. Sharma S, Nadrous HF, Peters SG, et al. Pulmonary complications in adult blood and marrow transplant recipients: autopsy findings. *Chest.* 2005;128:1385–1392.
111. Yen KT, Lee AS, Krowka MJ, et al. Pulmonary complications in bone marrow transplantation: a practical approach to diagnosis and treatment. *Clin Chest Med.* 2004;25:189–201.
112. Afessa B, Tefferi A, Litzow MR, et al. Diffuse alveolar hemorrhage in hematopoietic stem cell transplant recipients. *Am J Respir Crit Care Med.* 2002;166:641–645.
113. Gottdiener JS, Appelbaum FR, Ferrans VJ, et al. Cardiotoxicity associated with high-dose cyclophosphamide therapy. *Arch Intern Med.* 1981;141:758–763.
114. Hochster H, Wasserheit C, Speyer J. Cardiotoxicity and cardioprotection during chemotherapy. *Curr Opin Oncol.* 1995;7:304–309.
115. Murdych T, Weisdorf DJ. Serious cardiac complications during bone marrow transplantation at the University of Minnesota, 1977–1997. *Bone Marrow Transplant.* 2001;28:283–287.
116. Tang WH, Thomas S, Kalaycio M, et al. Clinical outcomes of patients with impaired left ventricular ejection fraction undergoing autologous bone marrow transplantation: can we safely transplant patients with impaired ejection fraction? *Bone Marrow Transplant.* 2004;34:603–607.
117. Morandi P, Ruffini PA, Benvenuto GM, et al. Cardiac toxicity of high-dose chemotherapy. *Bone Marrow Transplant.* 2005;35:323–334.
118. Parikh CR, Coca SG. Acute kidney failure in hematopoietic cell transplantation. *Kidney Int.* 2006;69:430–435.
119. Kersting S, Koomans HA, Hene RJ, et al. Acute kidney failure after allogeneic myeloablative stem cell transplantation: retrospective analysis of incidence, risk factors and survival. *Bone Marrow Transplant.* 2007;39:359–365.
120. Lane PH, Mauer SM, Blazar BR, et al. Outcome of dialysis for acute kidney failure in pediatric bone marrow transplant patients. *Bone Marrow Transplant.* 1994;13:613–617.
121. Woolfrey A, Anasetti C. Allogeneic hematopoietic stem-cell engraftment and graft failure. *Pediatr Transplant.* 1999;3(Suppl 1):35–40.
122. Woodard P, Tong X, Richardson S, et al. Etiology and outcome of graft failure in pediatric hematopoietic stem cell transplant recipients. *J Pediatr Hematol Oncol.* 2003;25:955–959.
123. Shizuru JA, Negrin RS, Weissman IL. Hematopoietic stem and progenitor cells: clinical and preclinical regeneration of the hematolymphoid system. *Annu Rev Med.* 2005;56:509–538.
124. van Os R, Kamminga LM, de Haan G. Stem cell assays: something old, something new, something borrowed. *Stem Cells.* 2004;22:1181–1190.
125. Engelhardt M, Lubbert M, Guo Y. CD34(+) or CD34(−): which is the more primitive? *Leukemia.* 2002;16:1603–1608.
126. Petersdorf EW. HLA matching in allogeneic stem cell transplantation. *Curr Opin Hematol.* 2004;11:386–391.
127. Davies SM, Ramsay NK, Haake RJ, et al. Comparison of engraftment in recipients of matched sibling of unrelated donor marrow allografts. *Bone Marrow Transplant.* 1994;13:51–57.
128. Bearman SI, Mori M, Beatty PG, et al. Comparison of morbidity and mortality after marrow transplantation from HLA-genotypically identical siblings and HLA-phenotypically identical unrelated donors. *Bone Marrow Transplant.* 1994;13:31–35.
129. Holler E. Risk assessment in haematopoietic stem cell transplantation: GvHD prevention and treatment. *Best Pract Res Clin Haematol.* 2007;20:281–294.
130. Champlin R, Giralt S, Gajewski J. T cells, graft-versus-host disease and graft-versus-leukemia: innovative approaches for blood and marrow transplantation. *Acta Haematol.* 1996;95:157–163.
131. Goulmy E, Termijtelen A, Bradley BA, et al. Y-antigen killing by T cells of women is restricted by HLA. *Nature.* 1977;266:544–545.
132. Gahrton G. Risk assessment in haematopoietic stem cell transplantation: impact of donor-recipient sex combination in allogeneic transplantation. *Best Pract Res Clin Haematol.* 2007;20:219–229.
133. Deeg HJ, Antin JH. The clinical spectrum of acute graft-versus-host disease. *Semin Hematol.* 2006;43:24–31.
134. Ferrara JL. Novel strategies for the treatment and diagnosis of graft-versus-host-disease. *Best Pract Res Clin Haematol.* 2007;20:91–97.
135. Hansen JA, Petersdorf E, Martin PJ, et al. Hematopoietic stem cell transplants from unrelated donors. *Immunol Rev.* 1997;157:141–151.
136. Petersdorf EW, Anasetti C, Martin PJ, et al. Tissue typing in support of unrelated hematopoietic cell transplantation. *Tissue Antigens.* 2003;61:1–11.
137. Shastri N, Cardinaud S, Schwab SR, et al. All the peptides that fit: the beginning, the middle, and the end of the MHC class I antigen-processing pathway. *Immunol Rev.* 2005;207:31–41.
138. Villadangos JA, Schnorrer P, Wilson NS. Control of MHC class II antigen presentation in dendritic cells: a balance between creative and destructive forces. *Immunol Rev.* 2005;207:191–205.
139. Ferrara JL, Reddy P. Pathophysiology of graft-versus-host disease. *Semin Hematol.* 2006;43:3–10.
140. Ringden O, Pihlstedt P, Markling L, et al. Prevention of graft-versus-host disease with T cell depletion or cyclosporin and methotrexate. A randomized trial in adult leukemic marrow recipients. *Bone Marrow Transplant.* 1991;7:221–226.
141. Chao NJ, Chen BJ. Prophylaxis and treatment of acute graft-versus-host disease. *Semin Hematol.* 2006;43:32–41.
142. Bacigalupo A, Palandri F. Management of acute graft versus host disease (GvHD). *Hematol J.* 2004;5:189–196.
143. Fowler DH. Shared biology of GVHD and GVT effects: potential methods of separation. *Crit Rev Oncol Hematol.* 2006;57:225–244.
144. Storb R, Deeg HJ, Whitehead J, et al. Methotrexate and cyclosporine compared with cyclosporine alone for prophylaxis of acute graft versus host disease after marrow transplantation for leukemia. *N Engl J Med.* 1986;314:729–735.
145. Leelasiri A, Greer JP, Stein RS, et al. Graft-versus-host-disease prophylaxis for matched unrelated donor bone marrow transplantation:

comparison between cyclosporine-methotrexate and cyclosporine-methotrexate-methylprednisolone. *Bone Marrow Transplant.* 1995;15:401–405.
146. Sullivan KM, Kopecky KJ, Jocom J, et al. Immunomodulatory and antimicrobial efficacy of intravenous immunoglobulin in bone marrow transplantation. *N Engl J Med.* 1990;323:705–712.
147. Jacobsohn DA, Vogelsang GB. Anti-cytokine therapy for the treatment of graft-versus-host disease. *Curr Pharm Des.* 2004;10:1195–1205.
148. Einsele H, Ehninger G, Steidle M, et al. Lymphocytopenia as an unfavorable prognostic factor in patients with cytomegalovirus infection after bone marrow transplantation. *Blood.* 1993;82:1672–1678.
149. Mori T, Okamoto S, Matsuoka S, et al. Risk-adapted pre-emptive therapy for cytomegalovirus disease in patients undergoing allogeneic bone marrow transplantation. *Bone Marrow Transplant.* 2000;25:765–769.
150. Matthes-Martin S, Lion T, Aberle SW, et al. Pre-emptive treatment of CMV DNAemia in paediatric stem cell transplantation: the impact of recipient and donor CMV serostatus on the incidence of CMV disease and CMV-related mortality. *Bone Marrow Transplant.* 2003;31:803–808.
151. Ng AP, Worth L, Chen L, et al. Cytomegalovirus DNAemia and disease: incidence, natural history and management in settings other than allogeneic stem cell transplantation. *Haematologica.* 2005;90:1672–1679.
152. Razonable RR, Emery VC. Management of CMV infection and disease in transplant patients. 27–29 February 2004. *Herpes.* 2004;11:77–86.
153. Scaglione S, Hofmeister CC, Stiff P. Evaluation of pulmonary infiltrates in patients after stem cell transplantation. *Hematology.* 2005;10:469–481.
154. Clark JG, Hansen JA, Hertz MI, et al. NHLBI workshop summary. Idiopathic pneumonia syndrome after bone marrow transplantation. *Am Rev Respir Dis.* 1993;147:1601–1606.
155. Stocchi R, Ward KN, Fanin R, et al. Management of human cytomegalovirus infection and disease after allogeneic bone marrow transplantation. *Haematologica.* 1999;84:71–79.
156. Ljungman P. Cytomegalovirus pneumonia: presentation, diagnosis, and treatment. *Semin Respir Infect.* 1995;10:209–215.
157. Einsele H, Hebart H. CMV-specific immunotherapy. *Hum Immunol.* 2004; 65:558–564.
158. Bilgrami SF, Metersky ML, McNally D, et al. Idiopathic pneumonia syndrome following myeloablative chemotherapy and autologous transplantation. *Ann Pharmacother.* 2001;35:196–201.
159. Keates-Baleeiro J, Moore P, Koyama T, et al. Incidence and outcome of idiopathic pneumonia syndrome in pediatric stem cell transplant recipients. *Bone Marrow Transplant.* 2006;38:285–289.
160. Wong R, Rondon G, Saliba RM, et al. Idiopathic pneumonia syndrome after high-dose chemotherapy and autologous hematopoietic stem cell transplantation for high-risk breast cancer. *Bone Marrow Transplant.* 2003;31:1157–1163.
161. Taplitz RA, Jordan MC. Pneumonia caused by herpesviruses in recipients of hematopoietic cell transplants. *Semin Respir Infect.* 2002;17:121–129.
162. Aguilar LK, Rooney CM, Heslop HE. Lymphoproliferative disorders involving Epstein-Barr virus after hemopoietic stem cell transplantation. *Curr Opin Oncol.* 1999;11:96–101.
163. Ganne V, Siddiqi N, Kamaplath B, et al. Humanized anti-CD20 monoclonal antibody (Rituximab) treatment for post-transplant lymphoproliferative disorder. *Clin Transplant.* 2003;17:417–422.
164. Swinnen LJ. Immune-cell treatment of Epstein–Barr-virus-associated lymphoproliferative disorders. *Best Pract Res Clin Haematol.* 2006;19:839–847.
165. Cutler C, Antin JH. Chronic graft-versus-host disease. *Curr Opin Oncol.* 2006;18:126–131.
166. Baird K, Pavletic SZ. Chronic graft versus host disease. *Curr Opin Hematol.* 2006;13:426–435.
167. Martin PJ, Carpenter PA, Sanders JE, et al. Diagnosis and clinical management of chronic graft-versus-host disease. *Int J Hematol.* 2004;79:221–228.
168. Saksena S, Tandon RK. Ursodeoxycholic acid in the treatment of liver diseases. *Postgrad Med J.* 1997;73:75–80.
169. Offidani M, Corvatta L, Olivieri A, et al. A predictive model of varicella-zoster virus infection after autologous peripheral blood progenitor cell transplantation. *Clin Infect Dis.* 2001;32:1414–1422.
170. Leung TF, Chik KW, Li CK, et al. Incidence, risk factors and outcome of varicella-zoster virus infection in children after haematopoietic stem cell transplantation. *Bone Marrow Transplant.* 2000;25:167–172.
171. Koc Y, Miller KB, Schenkein DP, et al. Varicella zoster virus infections following allogeneic bone marrow transplantation: frequency, risk factors, and clinical outcome. *Biol Blood Marrow Transplant.* 2000;6:44–49.
172. Gallagher G, Forrest DL. Second solid cancers after allogeneic hematopoietic stem cell transplantation. *Cancer.* 2007;109:84–92.
173. Forrest DL, Nevill TJ, Naiman SC, et al. Second malignancy following high-dose therapy and autologous stem cell transplantation: incidence and risk factor analysis. *Bone Marrow Transplant.* 2003;32:915–923.
174. Lenz G, Dreyling M, Schiegnitz E, et al. Moderate increase of secondary hematologic malignancies after myeloablative radiochemotherapy and autologous stem-cell transplantation in patients with indolent lymphoma: results of a prospective randomized trial of the German Low Grade Lymphoma Study Group. *J Clin Oncol.* 2004;22:4926–4933.
175. Meshinchi S, Leisenring WM, Carpenter PA, et al. Survival after second hematopoietic stem cell transplantation for recurrent pediatric acute myeloid leukemia. *Biol Blood Marrow Transplant.* 2003;9:706–713.
176. Eapen M, Giralt SA, Horowitz MM, et al. Second transplant for acute and chronic leukemia relapsing after first HLA-identical sibling transplant. *Bone Marrow Transplant.* 2004;34:721–727.
177. Qazilbash MH, Saliba R, De Lima M, et al. Second autologous or allogeneic transplantation after the failure of first autograft in patients with multiple myeloma. *Cancer.* 2006;106:1084–1089.
178. Yoshimi A, Mohamed M, Bierings M, et al. Second allogeneic hematopoietic stem cell transplantation (HSCT) results in outcome similar to that of first HSCT for patients with juvenile myelomonocytic leukemia. *Leukemia.* 2007;21:556–560.
179. Dazzi F, Goldman J. Donor lymphocyte infusions. *Curr Opin Hematol.* 1999;6:394–399.
180. Loren AW, Porter DL. Donor leukocyte infusions after unrelated donor hematopoietic stem cell transplantation. *Curr Opin Oncol.* 2006;18:107–114.
181. Slavin S, Morecki S, Weiss L, et al. Immunotherapy of hematologic malignancies and metastatic solid tumors in experimental animals and man. *Crit Rev Oncol Hematol.* 2003;46:139–163.
182. Dazzi F, Szydlo RM, Goldman JM. Donor lymphocyte infusions for relapse of chronic myeloid leukemia after allogeneic stem cell transplant: where we now stand. *Exp Hematol.* 1999;27:1477–1486.
183. Ciceri F, Bonini C, Gallo-Stampino C, et al. Modulation of GvHD by suicide-gene transduced donor T lymphocytes: clinical applications in mismatched transplantation. *Cytotherapy.* 2005;7:144–149.
184. Toubert ME, Socie G, Gluckman E, et al. Short- and long-term follow-up of thyroid dysfunction after allogeneic bone marrow transplantation without the use of preparative total body irradiation. *Br J Haematol.* 1997;98:453–457.
185. Vexiau P, Perez-Castiglioni P, Socie G, et al. The 'euthyroid sick syndrome': incidence, risk factors and prognostic value soon after allogeneic bone marrow transplantation. *Br J Haematol.* 1993;85:778–782.
186. Sklar CA, Kim TH, Ramsay NK. Thyroid dysfunction among long-term survivors of bone marrow transplantation. *Am J Med.* 1982;73:688–694.
187. Shalitin S, Phillip M, Stein J, et al. Endocrine dysfunction and parameters of the metabolic syndrome after bone marrow transplantation during childhood and adolescence. *Bone Marrow Transplant.* 2006;37:1109–1117.
188. Faraci M, Barra S, Cohen A, et al. Very late nonfatal consequences of fractionated TBI in children undergoing bone marrow transplant. *Int J Radiat Oncol Biol Phys.* 2005;63:1568–1575.
189. Slatter MA, Gennery AR, Cheetham TD, et al. Thyroid dysfunction after bone marrow transplantation for primary immunodeficiency without the use of total body irradiation in conditioning. *Bone Marrow Transplant.* 2004;33:949–953.
190. Sanders JE. Endocrine complications of high-dose therapy with stem cell transplantation. *Pediatr Transplant.* 2004;8(Suppl 5):39–50.
191. Wingard JR, Plotnick LP, Freemer CS, et al. Growth in children after bone marrow transplantation: busulfan plus cyclophosphamide versus cyclophosphamide plus total body irradiation. *Blood.* 1992;79:1068–1073.
192. Sanders JE, Guthrie KA, Hoffmeister PA, et al. Final adult height of patients who received hematopoietic cell transplantation in childhood. *Blood.* 2005;105:1348–1354.
193. Tauchmanova L, Selleri C, Rosa GD, et al. High prevalence of endocrine dysfunction in long-term survivors after allogeneic bone marrow transplantation for hematologic diseases. *Cancer.* 2002;95:1076–1084.
194. Bakker B, Oostdijk W, Bresters D, et al. Disturbances of growth and endocrine function after busulphan-based conditioning for haematopoietic stem cell transplantation during infancy and childhood. *Bone Marrow Transplant.* 2004;33:1049–1056.
195. Chiodi S, Spinelli S, Cohen A, et al. Cyclic sex hormone replacement therapy in women undergoing allogeneic bone marrow transplantation: aims and results. *Bone Marrow Transplant.* 1991;8(Suppl 1):47–49.
196. Demeestere I, Simon P, Buxant F, et al. Ovarian function and spontaneous pregnancy after combined heterotopic and orthotopic cryopreserved ovarian tissue transplantation in a patient previously treated with bone marrow transplantation: case report. *Hum Reprod.* 2006;21:2010–2014.
197. Donnez J, Dolmans MM, Demylle D, et al. Restoration of ovarian function after orthotopic (intraovarian and periovarian) transplantation of cryopreserved ovarian tissue in a woman treated by bone marrow transplantation for sickle cell anaemia: case report. *Hum Reprod.* 2006;21:183–188.
198. Tichelli A, Gratwohl A, Egger T, et al. Cataract formation after bone marrow transplantation. *Ann Intern Med.* 1993;119:1175–1180.
199. Benyunes MC, Sullivan KM, Deeg HJ, et al. Cataracts after bone marrow transplantation: long-term follow-up of adults treated with fractionated total body irradiation. *Int J Radiat Oncol Biol Phys.* 1995;32:661–670.
200. van Kempen-Harteveld ML, Struikmans H, Kal HB, van der Tweel I, et al. Cataract after total body irradiation and bone marrow transplantation: degree of visual impairment. *Int J Radiat Oncol Biol Phys.* 2002;52: 1375–1380.
201. Zierhut D, Lohr F, Schraube P, et al. Cataract incidence after total-body irradiation. *Int J Radiat Oncol Biol Phys.* 2000;46:131–135.
202. Miralbell R, Bieri S, Mermillod B, et al. Kidney toxicity after allogeneic bone marrow transplantation: the combined effects of total-body irradiation and graft-versus-host disease. *J Clin Oncol.* 1996;14:579–585.
203. Tarbell NJ, Guinan EC, Niemeyer C, et al. Late onset of kidney dysfunction

in survivors of bone marrow transplantation. *Int J Radiat Oncol Biol Phys.* 1988;15:99–104.

204. Sakaida E, Nakaseko C, Harima A, et al. Late-onset noninfectious pulmonary complications after allogeneic stem cell transplantation are significantly associated with chronic graft-versus-host disease and with the graft-versus-leukemia effect. *Blood.* 2003;102:4236–4242.
205. Palmas A, Tefferi A, Myers JL, et al. Late-onset noninfectious pulmonary complications after allogeneic bone marrow transplantation. *Br J Haematol.* 1998;100:680–687.
206. Savani BN, Montero A, Srinivasan R, et al. Chronic GVHD and pretransplantation abnormalities in pulmonary function are the main determinants predicting worsening pulmonary function in long-term survivors after stem cell transplantation. *Biol Blood Marrow Transplant.* 2006;12:1261–1269.
207. Ransom JT. Mechanism of action of mycophenolate mofetil. *Ther Drug Monit.* 1995;17:681–684.
208. Bordigoni P, Dimicoli S, Clement L, et al. Daclizumab, an efficient treatment for steroid-refractory acute graft-versus-host disease. *Br J Haematol.* 2006;135:382–385.
209. Bruner RJ, Farag SS. Monoclonal antibodies for the prevention and treatment of graft-versus-host disease. *Semin Oncol.* 2003;30:509–519.
210. Flowers ME, Martin PJ. Evaluation of thalidomide for treatment or prevention of chronic graft-versus-host disease. *Leuk Lymphoma.* 2003;44:1141–1146.
211. Chakrabarti S, Hale G, Waldmann H. Alemtuzumab (Campath-1H) in allogeneic stem cell transplantation: where do we go from here? *Transplant Proc.* 2004;36:1225–1227.

CHAPTER 97 ■ THE OBSTETRIC PATIENT: GENERAL

MICHAEL A. FRÖLICH • MALI MATHRU

Major scientific advances have occurred in virtually all areas of patient care. One of the major changes in obstetrics has been the recognition of the specialty nature of medical complications related to pregnancy. The physiologic alterations that accompany pregnancy may have profound effects on a variety of pathologic conditions. In addition, maternal disease or its therapy may adversely affect the fetus, which makes these considerations unique to the obstetric patient.

The intensivist must be knowledgeable of the considerations specific to pregnant patients and should also understand the pathophysiologic alterations associated with high-risk conditions such as preeclampsia. Obstetricians have done a remarkably good job in managing common diseases such as diabetes, asthma, and chronic hypertension with great sophistication. Nevertheless, life-threatening emergencies during pregnancy challenge the knowledge and skills of anyone who works with this group of patients. Clinicians have acquired considerable information about the management of critically ill obstetric patients; however, this information is not geared toward the critical care provider in most textbooks. This chapter is intended to fill this gap and provide the essential information about the most severe critical conditions that might arise during pregnancy.

An extensive review of all maternal high-risk conditions would go beyond the scope of this chapter. Therefore, we will limit our review to the discussion of physiologic changes of pregnancy that clearly have to be recognized when managing the critically ill pregnant patient. This review is focused mainly on the most life-threatening pathophysiologic processes, including thrombosis and thromboembolism, hypertensive disease of pregnancy, hemorrhage, and amniotic fluid embolism (Tables 97.1 and 97.2), but is inclusive of other more common pregnancy-related problems that come to the attention of the intensivist, such as peripartum cardiomyopathy and pulmonary edema.

PHYSIOLOGIC CHANGES ASSOCIATED WITH PREGNANCY

Several physiologic changes are associated with normal pregnancy. These adaptations are necessary to meet the demands of the growing fetus, and have to be considered when evaluating and managing pregnant patients.

Body Constitution

Optimal weight gain in pregnancy is currently a matter of debate (1–3). In general, an approximate weight gain of 6 kg is attributed to the fetus, placenta, and uterus, and the remainder of the weight gain to an increase in maternal blood, interstitial fluid volume, and fat. A gestational weight gain of more than 12 kg in women of normal pre-pregnant weight is related to the lowest risk for complications during delivery. Thorsdottir et al. (4) studied the relationship between gestational weight gain and complications during pregnancy, comparing pregnant women with normal weight gain with other higher gestational weight gain. They found that women who exceeded 18 kg of weight gain during pregnancy are considered at greater risk for maternal (pre-eclampsia, gestational diabetes) and fetal (increased incidence of operative delivery) complications.

Changes in maternal physiology occur normally during pregnancy, and have the potential to alter the absorption, distribution, and elimination of drugs used therapeutically in pregnant women (5).

Metabolisms and Respiration

Key physiologic changes of respiration that occur in pregnancy are an increased minute ventilation, which is caused by increased respiratory center sensitivity and drive; a compensated respiratory alkalosis; and a low expiratory reserve volume (6). The vital capacity and measures of forced expiration are well preserved. Patients who have severe lung diseases tolerate pregnancy well, with the exception of those with pulmonary hypertension or chronic respiratory insufficiency from parenchymal or neuromuscular disease.

Lung volumes have been measured in several case series of pregnant women and compared to nonpregnant women or those in the postpartum state (7), with body plethysmography being the preferred technique of measurement (8), and were found well preserved in the majority of cases. The residual volume tends to decrease slightly, which leads to a small increase or stability of the vital capacity (7,9–12). The most consistent change in static lung volumes with pregnancy is the reduction in the functional residual capacity (FRC) and expiratory reserve volume. As the uterus enlarges, FRC decreases by 10% to 25% of the previous value, starting about the 12th week of pregnancy (7). The normal reduction in FRC is accentuated

TABLE 97.1

DIRECT MATERNAL DEATHS, 2000–2002[a]

Cause of death	1985–87	1988–90	1991–93	1994–96	1997–99	2000–02
Thrombosis and thromboembolism	32	33	35	48	35	30
Hypertensive disease of pregnancy	27	27	20	20	15	14
Hemorrhage	10	22	15	12	7	17
Amniotic fluid embolism	9	11	10	17	8	5
Deaths in early pregnancy total	22	24	18	15	17	15
Ectopic	16	15	8	12	13	11
Spontaneous miscarriage	5	6	3	2	2	1
Legal termination	1	3	5	1	2	3
Other	0	0	2	0	0	0
Genital tract sepsis	6[b]	7[b]	9[b]	14[c]	14[c]	11[c]
Other direct total	27	17	14	7	7	8
Genital tract trauma	6	3	4	5	2	1
Fatty liver	6	5	2	2	4	3
Other	15	9	8	0	1	4
Anaesthetic	6	4	8	1	3	6
Total number of deaths	139	145	128	134	106	106

[a]Deaths reported to the Enquiry only and excluding other deaths identified by ONS.
[b]Excluding early pregnancy deaths due to sepsis.
[c]Including early pregnancy deaths due to sepsis.
From Confidential Enquiry into Maternal and Child Health (CEMACH), Chiltern Court (Lower ground floor), 188 Baker Street, London NW1 5SD, Tel: 020 7486 1191; Fax: 020 7486 6543; E-mail: info@cemach.org.uk. Publication 2004: Why Mothers Die 2000–2002.

further in the supine position (13). The reduction in FRC is due to a decrease in chest wall compliance, up to 35% to 40% (14). The lung compliance remains normal during pregnancy, whereas expiratory muscle strength is in the low-normal range (9). The decreased chest wall compliance is the result of the enlarging uterus increasing the abdominal pressure, which leads to a reduction of the FRC (15). The diaphragm elevates about 4 cm, and the circumference of the lower rib cage increases about 5 cm (16). The lower end-expiratory lung volume leads to an increased area of apposition of the diaphragm to the chest wall, which improves the coupling of the diaphragm and chest wall. Thus, the increased tidal volume of pregnancy is achieved without an increase in the respiratory excursions of the diaphragm.

The rib cage undergoes structural changes during pregnancy (17). Progressive relaxation of the ligamentous attachments of the ribs causes the subcostal angle of the rib cage to increase early in pregnancy. This change persists for months into the postpartum period. The increased elasticity of the rib cage is mediated by the polypeptide hormone, relaxin, which is increased during pregnancy and is responsible for the softening of the cervix and relaxation of the pelvic ligaments (18,19). Changes in pulmonary function during pregnancy are summarized in Figure 97.1.

Changes in Arterial Blood Gases

The hormonal changes of pregnancy lead to remarkable respiratory changes throughout its course. The resulting changes of arterial blood gas values have been measured by Templeton et al. (20,21), who obtained serial measurements of maternal blood gases during pregnancy. The same investigators also measured serial alveolar-to-arterial oxygen tension differences (PAO_2-PaO_2), and calculated the pulmonary venous admixture (physiologic shunt), dead space-to-tidal volume ratio (V_D/V_T),

TABLE 97.2

INDIRECT MATERNAL DEATHS, 2000–2002[a]

Causes of indirect deaths	1985–87	1988–90	1991–93	1994–96	1997–99	2000–02
Cardiac	22	18	37	39	35	44
Psychiatric	N/A	N/A	N/A	9	15	16
Other indirect	62	75	63	86	75	90
Indirect malignancies	N/A	N/A	N/A	N/A	11	5
Total number of indirect deaths	84	93	100	134	136	155

[a]Deaths reported to the Enquiry only and excluding other deaths identified by ONS.
From Confidential Enquiry into Maternal and Child Health (CEMACH), Chiltern Court (Lower ground floor), 188 Baker Street, London NW1 5SD, Tel: 020 7486 1191; Fax: 020 7486 6543; E-mail: info@cemach.org.uk. Publication 2004: Why Mothers Die 2000–2002.

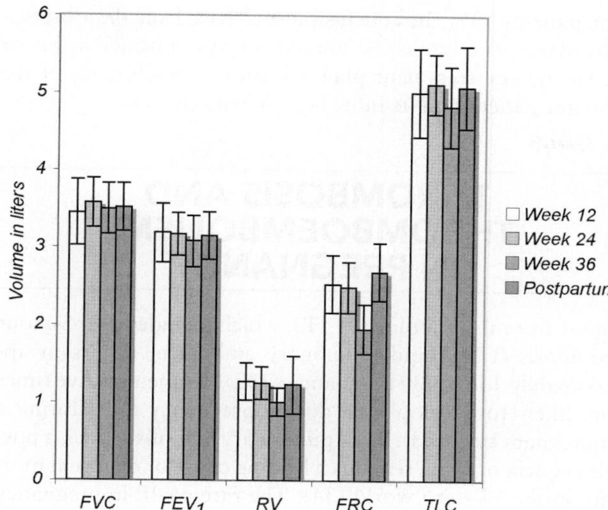

FIGURE 97.1. Pregnancy—pulmonary changes. FVC, forced vital capacity; FEV_1, forced expiratory volume in 1 second; RV, plethysmographic residual volume; FRC, plethysmographic functional residual capacity; TLC, plethysmographic total lung capacity. (Data from Garcia-Rio F, Pino-Garcia JM, Serrano S, et al. Comparison of helium dilution and plethysmographic lung volumes in pregnant women. *Eur Respir J.* 1997;10:2371–2375.)

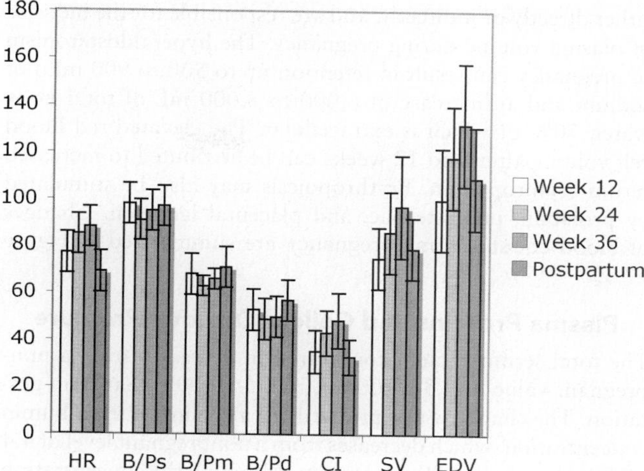

FIGURE 97.2. Pregnancy—cardiovascular changes. HR, heart rate (bpm); B/Ps, systolic blood pressure (mm Hg); B/Pm, mean blood pressure (mm Hg); B/Pd, diastolic blood pressure (mm Hg); CI, cardiac index (L/min/m^2); SV, stroke volume (mL); EDV, end-diastolic volume (mL). (Data from *Circulation.* 1978;58:434–441.)

and respiratory minute volume (Table 97.3). The mean arterial PO_2 during pregnancy was found to be consistently greater than 100 mm Hg throughout pregnancy, with no alterations of dead space-to-tidal volume ratio (V_D/V_T) and shunt.

Cardiovascular System

Management of pregnancy, especially for women with heart disease, requires an understanding of the hemodynamic stress that occurs during gestation. The most important hemodynamic change in the maternal circulation during pregnancy is an increase in the cardiac index of 30% to 40% (22), which can be primarily attributed to an increase in stroke volume, while heart rate and blood pressure do not change significantly (Fig. 97.2).

This alteration has several unique features: (a) the augmentation occurs relatively early in pregnancy (20–24 weeks), (b) it cannot be explained entirely on the basis of fetal needs, and (c) fluctuations in cardiac output occur with changes in body position as the gravid uterus impinges in varying degrees on the inferior vena cava, thus altering systemic venous return (23).

TABLE 97.3

BLOOD GAS ANALYSIS IN LATE PREGNANCY[a]

pH	7.44	HCO_3^- (mval/L)	20
PaO_2 (mm Hg)	103	BE (mval/L)	2.5
$PaCO_2$ (mm Hg)	30		

[a] Averages.
Data from Templeton A, Kelman GR. Maternal blood-gases, PAo2–Pao2), physiological shunt and V_D/V_T in normal pregnancy. *Br J Anaesth.* 1976;48:1001.

Red Blood Cell, Plasma, and Blood Volume

An increase of plasma volume is evident by the sixth week of gestation, reaching a value by the end of the first trimester of 15% above nonpregnant women. There is subsequently a steep increase of this parameter until 28 to 30 weeks of gestation, followed by a more gradual rise, to a final volume at term of 55% above the nonpregnant level (24). Red blood cell mass decreases during the first 8 weeks of gestation, but increases to nearly 30% above the nonpregnant level at term. These physiologic changes result in a 45% increase of total blood volume and a reduction of the hemoglobin concentration and hematocrit to values of approximately 11.6 g/100 mL and 35.5 volume %, respectively (Fig. 97.3). Estrogens, progesterone, and placental lactogen elevate aldosterone production

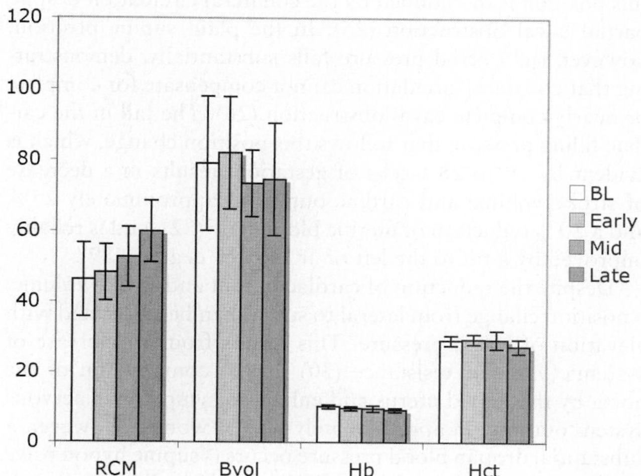

FIGURE 97.3. Changes of blood count during pregnancy. RCM, red cell mass in mL/10; Bvol, blood volume in mL/kg; Hb, hemoglobin in g/100 mL; Hct, hematocrit in %; BL, pre-pregnant data; early, 8th week of pregnancy; mid, 14th week of pregnancy; late, 20th week of pregnancy. (Data from Metcalfe J, Ueland K. A study of pregnancy in Pygmy goats. *Prog Cardiovasc Dis.* 1974;16:363.)

either directly or indirectly, and are responsible for the increase of plasma volume during pregnancy. The hyperaldosteronism of pregnancy can result in retention up to 500 to 900 mEq of sodium and an increase of 6,000 to 8,000 mL of total body water, 70% of which is extracellular. The elevated red blood cell volume after 8 to 12 weeks can be attributed to increased serum erythropoietin. Erythropoiesis may also be stimulated by prolactin, progesterone, and placental lactogen. Changes of blood counts during pregnancy are summarized in Figure 97.3.

Plasma Proteins and Colloid Osmotic Pressure

The total serum protein concentration decreases from a nonpregnant value of 7.3 g/100 mL to 6.5 g/100 mL at term gestation. The change is due primarily to a decline of the albumin concentration, which decreases from a nonpregnant level of 4.4 g/100 mL to 3.4 g/100 mL at term. Although the concentration of globulins declines by 10% during the first trimester, the level rises subsequently to a value at term that is 5% to 10% above the nonpregnant level. These changes result in a progressive decrease in the albumin-to-globulin ratio from approximately 1.5 during pregnancy to 1.1 at term gestation. Maternal colloid osmotic pressure decreases in parallel with the decline in serum albumin concentration from nonpregnant values of 25 to 26 mm Hg to approximately 22 mm Hg at term.

Aortocaval Compression

Angiographic studies show that the aorta and inferior vena cava can be significantly compressed by the gravid uterus in the supine position. In fact, Kerr et al. (25) observed a complete obstruction of the inferior vena cava at the level of the bifurcation in 80% of patients in late pregnancy. Partial obstruction of the aorta at the level of the lumbar lordosis (L3–L5) has also been demonstrated in patients between the 27th week of pregnancy and term gestation (26,27).

The pregnant subject at term, when placed in the lateral decubitus position, exhibits a right ventricular filling pressure (central venous pressure) similar to that of a nonpregnant woman (28). This observation suggests that venous return in this position is maintained by the collateral circulation despite partial caval obstruction (25). In the plain supine position, however, right atrial pressure falls substantially, demonstrating that collateral circulation cannot compensate for complete or nearly complete caval obstruction (26). The fall in the cardiac filling pressure that follows this position change, which is evident by 20 to 28 weeks of gestation, results in a decrease of stroke volume and cardiac output of approximately 25% and a 20% reduction of uterine blood flow (22), and is reliably improved by a tilt to the left of at least 25 degrees (29).

Despite the reduction of cardiac output and stroke volume, a position change from lateral to supine can be associated with elevation of blood pressure. This results from an increase of systemic vascular resistance (30) due to compression of the aorta by the gravid uterus and enhanced sympathetic nervous system outflow. In approximately 5% of women, however, a substantial drop in blood pressure occurs ("supine hypotensive syndrome"), which is associated with bradycardia (usually following a transient tachycardia) and maternal symptoms, low systemic perfusion such as of pallor and sweating, possibly followed by cardiocirculatory collapse. This occasional but profound drop of venous return may be exacerbated by neuraxial block, the preferred method of providing anesthesia in pregnant patients (31). In conclusion and based on the observations above, the intensivist should always consider in his or her emergency treatment plan the proper positioning of the pregnant patient and its influence on hemodynamics.

THROMBOSIS AND THROMBOEMBOLISM IN PREGNANCY

Venous thromboembolism (VTE), which includes deep venous thrombosis (DVT) and pulmonary embolism, occurs in approximately 1 in 1,000 pregnancies (32). Women are five times more likely to develop VTE during pregnancy than during a nonpregnant state (33). Fatal pulmonary embolism (PE), a possible sequela of VTE, remains a leading cause of maternal mortality in the Western world (34). The rate of PE in pregnancy is five times greater than that for nonpregnant women of the same age, and is about 1 in 100 deliveries; the risks are even higher in the puerperium.

Risk Factors and Predisposition to Venous Thrombosis

Compared to nonpregnant females, pregnant women have a 10-fold risk of a thrombotic episode. Risk factors for VTE other than pregnancy are increased maternal age (>35 years), previous cesarean delivery, obesity, multiparity, and a history of DVT (Table 97.4).

Pregnancy is associated with an increased clotting potential, decreased anticoagulant properties, and decreased fibrinolysis. Pregnancy is accompanied by a two- to threefold increased concentration of fibrinogen and a 20% to 1,000% increase in factors VII, VIII, IX, X, and XII, all of which peak at term (35). Levels of von Willebrand factor (vWF) increase up to 400% by term (35). Free protein S levels decline significantly (up to 55%) during pregnancy due to increased circulating levels of its carrier molecular, complement 4 binding protein (35). As a consequence, pregnancy is associated with an increase in resistance to activated protein C (35,36). Levels of plasminogen activation inhibitor-1 increase three- to fourfold during pregnancy, while plasma plasminogen activation inhibitor-2 values, which are negligible before pregnancy, reach concentrations of 160 mg/L at delivery (30).

TABLE 97.4

RISK FACTORS FOR VENOUS THROMBOEMBOLISM (VTE) DURING PREGNANCY

- Cesarean delivery
- History of prior VTE
- Family history of VTE
- Inherited or acquired thrombophilia
- Obesity
- Older maternal age
- Higher parity
- Prolonged immobilization

Pregnancy is also associated with venous stasis in the lower extremities due to compression of the inferior vena cava and pelvic veins by the enlarging uterus and hormone-mediated increases in deep vein capacitance secondary to increased circulating levels of estrogen and local production of prostacyclin and nitric oxide.

Important hereditary risk factors that can increase DVT risk are antithrombin III deficiency, protein S and C deficiency, a G1691A mutation of the factor V gene (37), and a G20210A mutation of the factor II gene (38).

Diagnosis of Venous Thromboembolism during Pregnancy

Bates and Ginsberg have recently addressed the diagnosis of VTE during pregnancy in detail (39). In pregnant women presenting with lower extremity edema, back pain, and/or chest pain, the prevalence of VTE is less than in the general population because of the high frequency of these complaints in the pregnant woman. D-dimer assays, which can be used to exclude VTE in healthy nonpregnant individuals, usually become positive late in pregnancy, which decreases the utility of this assay in pregnancy (40). Radiologic studies used to diagnose VTE in the nonpregnant individual have not been validated in pregnancy, and potential risks to the fetus, particularly in terms of ionizing radiation exposure, need to be considered (41). Compression ultrasonography (CUS) of the proximal veins has been recommended as the initial test for suspected DVT during pregnancy (39). When results are equivocal or an iliac vein thrombosis is suspected, magnetic resonance venography (MRV) can be used. MRV does not carry the radiation risk of contrast venography, and is becoming increasingly available in the United States. The approach to the diagnosis of PE is similar in the pregnant and nonpregnant individual. Ventilation/perfusion (V/Q) scanning confers relatively low radiation exposure to the fetus, a risk less than that of missing a diagnosis of PE in the mother. However, when a V/Q study is indeterminate in a pregnant patient without demonstrated lower extremity thrombosis, it is usually followed by angiography. A brachial approach carries less radiation exposure to the fetus than spiral computed tomography (CT).

Prevention of Thrombosis during Pregnancy

The optimal anticoagulation regimen has not been established. Low-molecular-weight heparins (LMWHs) have become the anticoagulant of choice because, like unfractionated heparin (UFH), they do not cross the placenta, have better bioavailability, and carry less risk of osteoporosis and heparin-induced thrombocytopenia than UFH (42). A recent review of published data on the use of LMWHs in pregnancy supports their use as safe alternatives to UFH as anticoagulants during pregnancy (43).

A more recent practice trend, especially in the United States, has been to switch patients to the longer-acting, subcutaneous UFH a few weeks before delivery to allow the use of activated partial thromboplastin time (aPTT) as a diagnostic test to assess anticoagulation pre- and post labor. (44)

Another means of providing VTE prophylaxis is with elastic compression stockings, which may be used for the entire pregnancy period. Elastic stockings are appropriate for in-hospital patients at increased risk of VTE, and may be combined with the use of LMWH. Vena cava filter placement represents a potentially important but poorly evaluated therapeutic modality in the prevention of pulmonary emboli. Randomized trials to establish the appropriate role of vena cava filters in the treatment of venous thromboembolic disease are lacking (45).

Thrombolytic Therapy for Pulmonary Embolism

The indications for thrombolytic therapy for PE remain controversial. The incidence of intracranial hemorrhage may be as high as 2% to 3% with systemic thrombolytic therapy (46), although rates were lower in a recent trial (47). Fatality rates in patients with PE presenting in cardiogenic shock may be as high as 30% (46); thrombolytic therapy should be considered in this circumstance, although evidence for this subgroup is limited (48). Approximately 10% of symptomatic pulmonary emboli are rapidly fatal (49,50). The International Cooperative Pulmonary Embolism Registry, established to ascertain PE mortality, reported that 2% of patients were first diagnosed with PE at autopsy (51). Of patients diagnosed with PE before death, 5% to 10% have shock at presentation, which is associated with a mortality of 25% to 50% (51–53). Echocardiographic evidence of right ventricular dysfunction at presentation also has been suggested as an indication for thrombolytic therapy (47); however, a recent randomized trial failed to demonstrate a survival benefit with thrombolysis in patients with this finding (47), and mortality rates with conventional therapy are conflicting (46). At the time of this writing, routine thrombolysis cannot be justified in all patients.

HEMORRHAGE

Peripartum hemorrhage remains a significant cause of maternal and fetal morbidity and mortality. In the United States and other industrialized nations, massive obstetric hemorrhage has generally ranked among the top three causes of maternal death despite modern improvements in obstetric practice and transfusion services.

Peripartum hemorrhage includes a wide range of pathophysiologic events. Antepartum bleeding occurs in nearly 4% of pregnant women (54). The causes of serious antepartum bleeding are abnormal implantation (placenta previa, accreta), placental abruption, or uterine rupture. The latter is often caused by a dehiscence of a pre-existing uterine scar. The main reason for postpartum bleeding is uterine atony when myometrial contraction is inadequate. It is not surprising that uterine bleeding may be fatal when considering the massive amount of blood flow perfusing the uterus at term (up to 600 mL/minute).

Patients with hemodynamic instability or massive hemorrhage require prompt resuscitative measures, including the administration of supplemental oxygen, placement of two intravenous lines, intravenous hydration, and blood typing and cross-matching for the replacement of packed red blood cells (Table 97.5). A delay in the correction of hypovolemia, diagnosis and treatment of impaired coagulation, and surgical

TABLE 97.5

MANAGEMENT OF SEVERE POSTPARTUM HEMORRHAGE

CONSERVATIVE MANAGEMENT

General Measures
- Administration of supplemental oxygen
- Placement of adequate intravenous access lines
- Intravenous hydration
- Blood typing and cross-matching
- Placement of arterial line for repeated blood sampling

Pharmacologic Measures
- Oxytocin
- Methylergonovine
- 15-Methyl prostaglandin F_2-α

SURGICAL MANAGEMENT

Vascular Ligation
- Uterine artery
- Hypogastric artery
- Ovarian artery

Hysterectomy
- Supracervical
- Total

control of bleeding are the avoidable factors in most maternal mortality cases caused by hemorrhage. If a transfusion must be given before full cross-matching is finished, type-specific uncross-matched blood can be used (55).

If the placenta has not been delivered when hemorrhage begins, it should be removed, if necessary by manual exploration of the uterine cavity. Placenta accreta is diagnosed if the placental cleavage plane is indistinct. In this situation, the patient should be prepared by the intensivist or the anesthesiologist for probable urgent hysterectomy. Firm bimanual compression of the uterus (with one hand in the posterior vaginal fornix and the other on the abdomen) can limit hemorrhage until help can be obtained. Hemorrhage after placental delivery should prompt vigorous fundal massage while the patient is rapidly given 10 to 30 units of oxytocin in 1 L of intravenous crystalloids. Uterotonic agents such as oxytocin are routinely used in the management of uterine atony (56). This synthetic nonpeptide is a first-line therapeutic agent because of the paucity of side effects and the absence of contraindications. If the fundus does not become firm, uterine atony is the presumed (and most common) diagnosis. While fundal massage continues, the patient may be then given 0.2 mg of methylergonovine (Methergine) intramuscularly, with this dose to be repeated at 2- to 4-hour intervals if necessary. Methylergonovine, an ergot alkaloid, is used as a second-line uterotonic agent in the setting of massive obstetric hemorrhage due to uterine atony. It may cause undesirable adverse effects such as cramping, headache, and dizziness. Coexisting severe hypertension is an absolute contraindication to its use. Injectable prostaglandins may also be used when oxytocin fails. Both prostaglandin E and prostaglandin F_2 stimulate myometrial contractions, and have been used intramuscularly or intravenously for refractory hemorrhage due to uterine atony.

In particular, carboprost (Hemabate), 15-methyl prostaglandin F_2-α, may be administered intramuscularly or intramyometrially in a dosage of 250 μg every 15 to 90 minutes, up to a maximum dosage of 2 mg. Sixty-eight percent of patients respond to a single carboprost injection; 86% respond to a second dose (57). Since oxygen desaturation has been reported with the use of carboprost (58), patients should be monitored by pulse oximetry.

The use of a hydrostatic balloon has been advocated as an alternative to uterine packing for controlling hemorrhage due to uterine atony (59). The inflated Rusch balloon can conform to the contour of the uterine cavity and provides an effective tamponade. Life-threatening hemorrhage can also be treated by arterial embolization by interventional radiology (60). Finally, in cases of continuing hemorrhage, a variety of surgical techniques can be used to avoid a hysterectomy, such as bilateral uterine artery ligation or internal iliac artery ligation (61).

AMNIOTIC FLUID EMBOLISM

Morgan published the first major review on amniotic fluid embolism in 1979 (62), although the entry of amniotic fluid into the maternal circulation was already recognized in 1926 (63). He reviewed 272 cases reported in the English literature up to date. While the true incidence of this disease entity is not known, most authors estimate it to be between 1 in 8,000 and 1 in 80,000 pregnancies.

Clinical Presentation

The classic presentation of amniotic fluid embolism is described as a sudden, profound, and unexpected cardiovascular collapse followed, in many cases, by irreversible shock and death (64). The only known predisposing factor to this life-threatening complication appears to be multiparity, which accounts for 88% of the cases (62). In a smaller percentage of cases (51%), the presenting symptom was respiratory related. Hypotension is present in 27% of surviving cases, with coagulopathy comprising 12% and seizures 10%. Fetal bradycardia (17%) and hypotension (13%) are the next most common presenting features (Table 97.6).

Etiology and Pathophysiology

It has been a common misperception in the literature that the entry of amniotic fluid into maternal circulation is a routine event. This belief arises from the recognized presence of squamous cells in the pulmonary vasculature as a marker signaling the entry of amniotic fluid into the maternal circulation.

TABLE 97.6

CLINICAL PRESENTATION OF AMNIOTIC FLUID EMBOLISM

- Acute cardiorespiratory collapse
- Acute respiratory distress
- Hypotension
- Hemorrhage/coagulopathy
- Seizures
- Fetal distress

TABLE 97.7

DIFFERENTIAL DIAGNOSIS OF AMNIOTIC FLUID EMBOLUS: EXCLUSION CRITERIA

- Thrombosis
- Air embolus
- Septic shock
- Acute myocardial infarction
- Peripartum cardiomyopathy
- Anaphylaxis
- Aspiration
- Placental abruption
- Transfusion reaction
- Local anesthetic toxicity

Studies have now shown that squamous cells can appear in the pulmonary blood of heterogenous populations of both pregnant and nonpregnant patients who have undergone pulmonary artery (PA) catheterization (65–69). The presence of these cells is probably the result of contamination by epithelial cells derived from the cutaneous entry site of the PA catheter (65,66). Since it is difficult to differentiate adult from fetal epithelial cells, the isolated finding of squamous cells in the pulmonary circulation of pregnant patients, with or without coexisting thrombotic pulmonary embolism, should be seen as a contaminant and not indicative of maternal exposure to amniotic fluid (70–72).

Recently, it has been hypothesized that amniotic fluid could act as a direct myocardial depressant. *In vitro* observation documented that amniotic fluid can cause a decrease in myometrial contractility (73). Other humoral factors, including proteolytic enzymes, histamine, serotonin, prostaglandins, and leukotrienes, may contribute to the hemodynamic changes and consumptive coagulopathy associated with amniotic fluid embolus, with a pathophysiologic mechanism similar to distributive or anaphylactic shock (73,74).

Diagnosis and Management

Amniotic fluid embolus syndrome is a diagnosis of exclusion (Table 97.7), and the treatment is essentially supportive. Hemodynamic instability should be treated with optimization of preload by rapid volume infusion. An α-receptor agonist such as phenylephrine may be useful to maintain adequate aortic perfusion pressure (90 mm Hg systolic) while volume is infused. Coagulopathy associated with amniotic fluid embolus should be treated with aggressive administration of blood component therapy. If maternal cardiopulmonary resuscitation (CPR) must be initiated, and the fetus is sufficiently mature and is undelivered at the time of the cardiac arrest, a perimortem cesarean section should be immediately instituted (74,75).

PERIPARTUM CARDIOMYOPATHY

Peripartum cardiomyopathy is a rare disease of unknown cause that strikes women in the childbearing years, and is associated with a high mortality rate.

Definition

Peripartum cardiomyopathy (PPCM) is defined by the development of left ventricular or biventricular failure in the last month of pregnancy or within 5 months of delivery in the absence of other identifiable cause (76). Peripartum cardiomyopathy in the United States can affect women of various ethnic backgrounds at any age, but is more common in women 30 years of age. The strong association of PPCM with gestational hypertension and twin pregnancy should raise the level of suspicion for this condition in pregnant patients who develop symptoms of congestive heart failure (77).

Etiology and Diagnosis

A number of possible causes have been proposed for PPCM, including myocarditis (78), abnormal immune response to pregnancy, maladaptive response to the hemodynamic stresses of pregnancy (79), stress-activated cytokines, and prolonged tocolysis. A genetic tract is probable, as there have been reported few cases of familial PPCM. The diagnosis of PPCM requires the exclusion of more common causes of cardiomyopathy, and should be confirmed by standard echocardiographic assessment of the left ventricular systolic dysfunction, including depressed fractional shortening and ejection fraction documentation.

Treatment and Prognosis

Therapy should be initiated using standard clinical protocols for heart failure. However, angiotensin-converting enzyme inhibitors should be avoided prenatally.

Long-term clinical prognosis is usually defined within 6 months after delivery. In one study, approximately half of 27 women studied had persistent left ventricular dysfunction beyond 6 months, with a cardiac mortality rate of 85% over 5 years, as compared with the group in whom cardiac size returned to normal by the same time interval, with no mortality (76). The identification of the underlying cause of heart failure in the pregnant patient is another important factor that influences long-term survival (80).

HYPERTENSIVE DISEASE OF PREGNANCY

Diagnosis

Hypertensive disorders of pregnancy include chronic hypertension, preeclampsia/eclampsia, preeclampsia superimposed on chronic hypertension, and gestational hypertension (81). Preeclampsia is a pregnancy-specific, multisystem disorder that is characterized by the development of hypertension and proteinuria after 20 weeks of gestation. The disorder complicates approximately 5% to 7% of pregnancies (82), with an incidence of 23.6 cases per 1,000 deliveries in the United States (83). Chronic hypertension is defined by elevated blood pressure that predates the pregnancy, and is documented before 20 weeks of gestation or is present 12 weeks after delivery. Eclampsia,

TABLE 97.8

PHYSICAL EXAMINATION OF THE SEVERELY PREECLAMPTIC PATIENT

- **Funduscopic**
  - Arteriolar spasm (focal or diffuse)
  - Retinal edema
  - Retinal hemorrhages (superficial and flame shaped, or deep and punctate)
  - Retinal exudates (hard or "cotton wool")
  - Papilledema
- **Cardiovascular**
  - Heart failure (rales, elevated jugular venous pressure, S_3) or aortic dissection
  - New or increased murmur of mitral regurgitation
  - Bruits
- **Neurologic**
  - Hypertensive encephalopathy: Disorientation
  - Depressed consciousness (Glasgow coma scale <13)
  - Focal deficits, generalized or focal seizures
- **Abdominal**
  - Palpation for liver tenderness or increase in size
- **Fetal**
  - Assessment of fetal well-being (fetal heart rate strip, biophysical profile)

a severe complication of preeclampsia, is a new onset of seizures in a woman with preeclampsia.

Diagnostic criteria for preeclampsia include new onset of elevated blood pressure and proteinuria after 20 weeks of gestation. Severe preeclampsia is indicated by more substantial blood pressure elevations and a greater degree of proteinuria. Other features of severe preeclampsia include oliguria, cerebral or visual disturbances, and pulmonary edema or cyanosis (81,84) (Table 97.8).

Therapy

Initial therapeutic goals during labor are focused on preventing seizures and controlling hypertension (84). Magnesium sulfate is the medication of choice to prevent eclamptic seizures for either preeclampsia or eclamptic seizures (85). Magnesium sulfate has been shown to be superior to phenytoin (Dilantin) and diazepam (Valium) for the treatment of eclamptic seizures, although they do not prevent the progression of the disorder (86,87). Women with systolic blood pressures of 160–180 mm Hg or higher diastolic blood pressures of 105–110 mm Hg should receive immediate antihypertensive therapy. The treatment goal is to lower systolic pressure to 140–150 mm Hg and diastolic pressure to 90–100 mm Hg. Hydralazine (Apresoline) and labetalol (Normodyne, Trandate) are the antihypertensive drugs most commonly used. Nifedipine (Procardia) and sodium nitroprusside (Nitropress) are potential alternatives, but their use is associated with significant adverse effects and risk of overdose. Similarly, labetalol should not be used in women with asthma or congestive heart failure. Angiotensin-converting enzyme inhibitors are also contraindicated in this group of patients. In women with preeclampsia, blood pressure usually normalizes within a few hours after delivery but may remain elevated for 2 to 4 weeks (88).

TABLE 97.9

ANTIHYPERTENSIVE THERAPY IN PRE-ECLAMPSIA

- **Labetalol (Normodyne, Trandate)**
  IV bolus, 20–40 mg IV. May repeat in 10 min. Usual effective dose is 50–200 mg, or continuous infusion of 2 mg/min (this regimen avoids reflex tachycardia).
- **Nitroglycerin**
  Start at 10 μg/min (6 mL/hr). Titrate by 10–20 μg/min to 400 μg/min until desired effect.
- **Hydralazine (Apresoline)**
  Initial dose: 5 mg IV. Maintenance: 5–10 mg IV q20–30 min.
- **Other Antihypertensive Options**
  Nicardipine, nitroprusside, phentolamine, fenoldopam, diazoxide

Care and Management of the Hypertensive Parturient

Some patients with severe preeclampsia will require admission in the intensive care setting for invasive monitoring and close supervision. Typical indications include (a) a severe increase in blood pressure, with diastolic blood pressures greater than 115 to 120 mg/dL or a systolic blood pressure greater than 200 mm Hg refractory to initial antihypertensive therapy; (b) oliguria refractory to repeated fluid challenges; (c) eclamptic seizures; or (d) respiratory insufficiency with pulmonary edema. The initial physical examination should include a neurologic assessment, funduscopic examination, auscultation of the heart and lungs, and palpation of the abdomen (Table 97.8). If magnesium sulphate is given, it should be continued for 24 hours following delivery or at least 24 hours after the last seizure. Regular assessment of urine output, maternal reflexes, respiratory rate, and oxygen saturation is paramount while magnesium is infused. A loading dose of 4 g should be given by infusion pump over 5 to 10 minutes, followed by a further infusion of 1 g/hour maintained for 24 hours after the last seizure. Gradual antihypertensive therapy can be accomplished with a 25% reduction of mean arterial pressure within minutes to 2 hours, to 160/100 mm Hg (89) (Table 97.9).

Most patients satisfying the criteria for intensive care unit admission should be monitored with central venous access and an arterial catheter. The use of invasive monitoring facilitates the therapeutic goals and can clarify the suspected diagnosis. Occasionally, the use of a pulmonary artery catheter facilitates cardiovascular management by monitoring cardiac output and systemic oxygen delivery while gradually reducing systemic vascular resistance and restoring preload. Other indications for placement of a pulmonary artery catheter include underlying or complicating cardiac diseases with suspected pulmonary hypertension or the progression of respiratory failure to acute lung injury or acute respiratory distress syndrome.

FETAL MONITORING IN THE INTENSIVE CARE SETTING

Electronic fetal monitoring (EFM) is used in the management of labor and delivery in nearly three of four pregnancies in the United States. The apparent contradiction between the widespread use of EFM and expert recommendations to limit its routine use indicates that a reassessment of this practice is warranted (90). Even more difficult is the question of whether fetal monitoring is of any substantial use in the critically ill mother or the mother undergoing surgery. Continuous cardiotocography (CTG) during labor is associated with a reduction in neonatal seizures, but no significant differences in cerebral palsy, infant mortality, or other standard measures of neonatal well-being. On the contrary, this monitoring technique was associated with an increase in cesarean sections and instrumental vaginal births. When considering the use of EFM, the intensivist should consider the effects of many sedative, hypnotic, or analgesic drugs routinely used in the critical care setting on fetal heart rate variability (91–93). At this time, no systematic studies have been performed concerning the value of CTG during general anesthesia for nonobstetric surgery; it is assumed that uneventful sedation and analgesia provide adequate oxygenation and circulatory stability without having any influence on the fetus (91–93).

PULMONARY EDEMA IN PREGNANCY

Pulmonary edema is a rare but well-documented complication of tocolytic therapy in pregnant patients (94–96). The incidence of pulmonary edema related to β-mimetic tocolysis is estimated to be 0.15% (97). The etiology of the pulmonary edema is unclear, but is likely multifactorial (98). Both cardiogenic and noncardiogenic mechanisms have been proposed. Possible cardiogenic causes include fluid overload, catecholamine-related myocardial necrosis, cardiac failure secondary to reduced diastolic compliance, and down-regulation of β-receptors (97–101).

Treatment

Immediate recognition and appropriate therapy can ameliorate the course of respiratory insufficiency in patients who develop pulmonary edema during tocolytic treatment. Therapy involves discontinuing the medication, ensuring adequate ventilation and oxygenation, correcting fluid imbalance and hypotension, and maintaining adequate cardiac output. Continuous assessment of the fetus' well-being is necessary.

Tocolytic Therapy

The development of pulmonary edema during the course of β-adrenergic agonist treatment for preterm labor is an indication for discontinuing the treatment and either switching to a different type of labor-inhibiting drug or terminating all efforts to prevent preterm delivery. Magnesium sulfate, calcium channel blockers, or oxytocin antagonists are the most frequently used alternatives.

Ventilatory Support

This topic is reviewed extensively in other sections of the book. Mechanical ventilation principles are not different for the pregnant patient, and are being standardized by evidence-based medicine and consensus conferences (101–103).

Fetal Considerations

In particular, fetal well-being must be interpreted within the context of maternal respiratory failure. At minimum, intermitted fetal monitoring is indicated. If refractory maternal hypoxemia and acidosis presents, and results in fetal distress, cesarean delivery to salvage the fetus should be considered.

CARDIOPULMONARY RESUSCITATION IN PREGNANCY

The major causes of maternal cardiac arrest are trauma, cardiac arrest, and embolism. Other causes are sepsis, magnesium overdose, complications of eclampsia, or the result of an unanticipated difficult intubation. The general treatment of the pregnant patient in cardiac arrest is no different than any other patient, including drug dosages and defibrillation settings. Chest compressions and ventilations should be performed with the recommended sequence. Because a slight left tilt of the pregnant patient during CPR enhances venous return after 24 weeks of gestation, this position is recommended. Because of the reduced pulmonary reserve, pregnant women do not tolerate hypoxia well. IV fluid should be running wide open on pressure bags, and blood products should be considered if hemorrhage is suspected. Once the age of the fetus is determined, a decision can be made whether to proceed with a perimortem cesarean section. The fetus can tolerate hypoxia longer than normal, but the decision to proceed with a cesarean delivery should be made within 4 minutes (102). In a recent retrospective review on cardiopulmonary resuscitation with perimortem cesarean section, authors found 35 reports with 20 potentially resuscitable causes, of which 13 women survived (103). While this recent review fell short of proving that perimortem cesarean delivery within 4 minutes of maternal cardiac arrest improves maternal and neonatal outcomes, it provided additional support for this procedure. An extensive review of this topic is also available on the American Society of Anesthesiologists (ASA) website.

Anesthesiologists have recognized that the management of the airway in the obstetric patient may be especially challenging. According to a closed claims analysis of the ASA, the main mechanisms for airway problems are inadequate ventilation, esophageal intubation, and difficult intubation (104). If the anesthesiologist encounters an unanticipated difficult airway, alternative airway management attempts may include the laryngeal mask airway or the Combitube. If cricothyrotomy becomes necessary, this maneuver should be initiated in a timely fashion to minimize the chance of maternal hypoxic brain damage.

SUMMARY

The obstetric patient poses exceptional challenges in the intensive care unit. Knowledge of the physiologic changes of pregnancy and specific pregnancy-related disorders is necessary for optimal management. The critically ill obstetric patient is unique in terms of medical management and often requires the input of several specialties. These patients require specialized nursing care and aggressive monitoring of both mother and fetus, and often include invasive monitoring of the mother. Intensive care unit diagnoses may include preeclampsia, including the HELLP syndrome, pulmonary embolic disease, amniotic fluid embolism, status asthmaticus, respiratory infection, acute respiratory distress syndrome, and sepsis. There is little doubt that intensivists in an intensive care unit can best treat these patients. The management of mechanical ventilation is based on modern principles of avoiding lung injury, while hypercapnia may be tolerated even during the pregnancy. The maternal–fetal medicine physician should be included in the treatment team. Care must include the consideration of pregnancy-induced physiologic changes, normal laboratory alterations, and continued fetal well-being if antepartum. Ultimately, the goal of this interdisciplinary approach is to ensure cohesive coordinated care for the pregnant patient. The following chapter will review some of the topics discussed above in more detail.

References

1. Lederman SA. Pregnancy weight gain and postpartum loss: avoiding obesity while optimizing the growth and development of the fetus. *J Am Med Womens Assoc.* 2001;56(2):53–58.
2. Abrams B, Altman SL, Pickett KE. Pregnancy weight gain: still controversial. *Am J Clin Nutr.* 2000;71(5 Suppl):1233S–1241S.
3. Feig DS, Naylor CD. Eating for two: are guidelines for weight gain during pregnancy too liberal? *Lancet.* 1998;351(9108):1054–1055.
4. Thorsdottir I, Torfadottir JE, Birgisdottir BE, et al. Weight gain in women of normal weight before pregnancy: complications in pregnancy or delivery and birth outcome. *Obstet Gynecol.* 2002;99(5 Pt 1):799–806.
5. Frederiksen MC. Physiologic changes in pregnancy and their effect on drug disposition. *Semin Perinatol.* 2001;25(3):120–123.
6. Wise RA, Polito AJ, Krishnan V. Respiratory physiologic changes in pregnancy. *Immunol Allergy Clin North Am.* 2006;26(1):1–12.
7. Cugell DW, Frank NR, Gaensler EA, et al. Pulmonary function in pregnancy. I. Serial observations in normal women. *Am Rev Tuberc.* 1953;67(5): 568–597.
8. Garcia-Rio F, Pino-Garcia JM, Serrano S, et al. Comparison of helium dilution and plethysmographic lung volumes in pregnant women. *Eur Respir J.* 1997;10(10):2371–2375.
9. Gee JB, Packer BS, Millen JE, et al. Pulmonary mechanics during pregnancy. *J Clin Invest.* 1967;46(6):945–952.
10. Gazioglu K, Kaltreider NL, Rosen M, et al. Pulmonary function during pregnancy in normal women and in patients with cardiopulmonary disease. *Thorax.* 1970;25(4):445–450.
11. Baldwin GR, Moorthi DS, Whelton JA, et al. New lung functions and pregnancy. *Am J Obstet Gynecol.* 1977;127(3):235–239.
12. Alaily AB, Carrol KB. Pulmonary ventilation in pregnancy. *Br J Obstet Gynaecol.* 1978;85(7):518–524.
13. Blair E, Hickam JB. The effect of change in body position on lung volume and intrapulmonary gas mixing in normal subjects. *J Clin Invest.* 1955;34(3):383–389.
14. Marx GF, Murthy PK, Orkin LR. Static compliance before and after vaginal delivery. *Br J Anaesth.* 1970;42(12):1100–1104.
15. Contreras G, Gutierrez M, Beroiza T, et al. Ventilatory drive and respiratory muscle function in pregnancy. *Am Rev Respir Dis.* 1991;144(4):837–841.
16. Field SK, Bell SG, Cenaiko DF, et al. Relationship between inspiratory effort and breathlessness in pregnancy. *J Appl Physiol.* 1991;71(5):1897–1902.
17. Oddoy A, Merker G. Lung mechanics and blood gases in pregnant guinea pigs. *Acta Physiol Hung.* 1987;70(2–3):311–315.
18. Sherwood OD, Downing SJ, Guico-Lamm ML, et al. The physiological effects of relaxin during pregnancy: studies in rats and pigs. *Oxf Rev Reprod Biol.* 1993;15:143–189.
19. Goldsmith LT, Weiss G, Steinetz BG. Relaxin and its role in pregnancy. *Endocrinol Metab Clin North Am.* 1995;24(1):171–186.
20. Sheldon CP. Studies on the physiology of respiration in pregnancy. Effects of barbiturates administered during labor. *J Clin Invest.* 1939;18(1):157–164.
21. Templeton A, Kelman GR. Maternal blood-gases, PAo2–Pao2), physiological shunt and VD/VT in normal pregnancy. *Br J Anaesth.* 1976;48(10): 1001–1004.
22. Ueland K, Novy MJ, Peterson EN, et al. Maternal cardiovascular dynamics. IV. The influence of gestational age on the maternal cardiovascular response to posture and exercise. *Am J Obstet Gynecol.* 1969;104(6):856–864.
23. Chesley LC, Duffus GM. Posture and apparent plasma volume in late pregnancy. *J Obstet Gynaecol Br Commonw.* 1971;78(5):406–412.
24. Metcalfe J, Ueland K. Maternal cardiovascular adjustments to pregnancy. *Prog Cardiovasc Dis.* 1974;16(4):363–374.
25. Kerr MG, Scott DB, Samuel E. Studies of the inferior vena cava in late pregnancy. *BMJ.* 1964;1(5382):532–533.
26. Abitbol MM. Aortic compression by pregnant uterus. *N Y State J Med.* 1976;76(9):1470–1475.
27. Bieniarz J, Branda LA, Maqueda E, et al. Aortocaval compression by the uterus in late pregnancy. 3. Unreliability of the sphygmomanometric method in estimating uterine artery pressure. *Am J Obstet Gynecol.* 1968;102(8):1106–1115.
28. Clark SL, Cotton DB, Lee W, et al. Central hemodynamic assessment of normal term pregnancy. *Am J Obstet Gynecol.* 1989;161(6 Pt 1):1439–1442.
29. Newman B, Derrington C, Dore C. Cardiac output and the recumbent position in late pregnancy. *Anaesthesia.* 1983;38(4):332–335.
30. Milsom I, Forssman L. Factors influencing aortocaval compression in late pregnancy. *Am J Obstet Gynecol.* 1984;148(6):764–771.
31. Mendonca C, Griffiths J, Ateleanu B, et al. Hypotension following combined spinal-epidural anaesthesia for Caesarean section. Left lateral position vs. tilted supine position. *Anaesthesia.* 2003;58(5):428–431.
32. Phillips OP. Venous thromboembolism in the pregnant woman. *J Reprod Med.* 2003;48(11 Suppl):921–929.
33. Prevention of venous thrombosis and pulmonary embolism. NIH Consensus Development. *JAMA.* 1986;256(6):744–749.
34. Confidential Enquiry into Maternal and Child Health. Why Mothers Die 2000–2002: The Sixth Report of the Confidential Enquiry into Maternal Death in the United Kingdom. 2004.
35. Bremme KA. Haemostatic changes in pregnancy. *Best Pract Res Clin Haematol.* 2003;16(2):153–168.
36. Ku DH, Arkel YS, Paidas MP, et al. Circulating levels of inflammatory cytokines (IL-1 beta and TNF-alpha), resistance to activated protein C, thrombin and fibrin generation in uncomplicated pregnancies. *Thromb Haemost.* 2003;90(6):1074–1079.
37. Bertina RM, Koeleman BP, Koster T, et al. Mutation in blood coagulation factor V associated with resistance to activated protein C. *Nature.* 1994; 369(6475):64–67.
38. Poort SR, Rosendaal FR, Reitsma PH, et al. A common genetic variation in the 3′-untranslated region of the prothrombin gene is associated with elevated plasma prothrombin levels and an increase in venous thrombosis. *Blood.* 1996;88(10):3698–3703.
39. Hart RG, Halperin JL. Atrial fibrillation and thromboembolism: a decade of progress in stroke prevention. *Ann Intern Med.* 1999;131(9):688–695.
40. Albers GW, Dalen JE, Laupacis A, et al. Antithrombotic therapy in atrial fibrillation. *Chest.* 2001;119(1 Suppl):194S–206S.
41. Mok CK, Boey J, Wang R, et al. Warfarin versus dipyridamole-aspirin and pentoxifylline-aspirin for the prevention of prosthetic heart valve thromboembolism: a prospective randomized clinical trial. *Circulation.* 1985;72(5):1059–1063.
42. Bates SM, Ginsberg JS. How we manage venous thromboembolism during pregnancy. *Blood.* 2002;100(10):3470–3478.
43. Sanson BJ, Lensing AW, Prins MH, et al. Safety of low-molecular-weight heparin in pregnancy: a systematic review. *Thromb Haemost.* 1999;81(5): 668–672.
44. Anderson DR, Ginsberg JS, Burrows R, et al. Subcutaneous heparin therapy during pregnancy: a need for concern at the time of delivery. *Thromb Haemost.* 1991;65(3):248–250.
45. Streiff MB. Vena caval filters: a comprehensive review. *Blood.* 2000;95(12): 3669–3677.
46. Dalen JE. The uncertain role of thrombolytic therapy in the treatment of pulmonary embolism. *Arch Intern Med.* 2002;162(22):2521–2523.
47. Konstantinides S, Geibel A, Heusel G, et al. Heparin plus alteplase compared with heparin alone in patients with submassive pulmonary embolism. *N Engl J Med.* 2002;347(15):1143–1150.
48. Jerjes-Sanchez C, Ramirez-Rivera A, de Lourdes Garcia M, et al. Streptokinase and heparin versus heparin alone in massive pulmonary embolism: a randomized controlled trial. *J Thromb Thrombolysis.* 1995;2(3):227–229.
49. Stein PD, Henry JW. Prevalence of acute pulmonary embolism among patients in a general hospital and at autopsy. *Chest.* 1995;108(4):978–981.
50. Bell WR, Simon TL. Current status of pulmonary thromboembolic disease: pathophysiology, diagnosis, prevention, and treatment. *Am Heart J.* 1982;103(2):239–262.
51. Goldhaber SZ, Visani L, De Rosa M. Acute pulmonary embolism: clinical outcomes in the International Cooperative Pulmonary Embolism Registry (ICOPER). *Lancet.* 1999;353(9162):1386–1389.
52. Grifoni S, Olivotto I, Cecchini P, et al. Short-term clinical outcome of patients with acute pulmonary embolism, normal blood pressure, and echocardiographic right ventricular dysfunction. *Circulation.* 2000;101(24):2817–2822.
53. Goldhaber SZ, Haire WD, Feldstein ML, et al. Alteplase versus heparin in acute pulmonary embolism: randomised trial assessing right-ventricular function and pulmonary perfusion. *Lancet.* 1993;341(8844):507–511.
54. Fong J, Gadalla F, Pierri MK, et al. Are Doppler-detected venous emboli during cesarean section air emboli? *Anesth Analg.* 1990;71(3):254–257.
55. Gervin AS, Fischer RP. Resuscitation of trauma patients with type-specific uncrossmatched blood. *J Trauma.* 1984;24(4):327–331.
56. Dildy GA 3rd. Postpartum hemorrhage: new management options. *Clin Obstet Gynecol.* 2002;45(2):330–344.

57. Hayashi RH, Castillo MS, Noah ML. Management of severe postpartum hemorrhage with a prostaglandin F2 alpha analogue. *Obstet Gynecol.* 1984;63(6):806–808.
58. Hankins GD, Berryman GK, Scott RT Jr, et al. Maternal arterial desaturation with 15-methyl prostaglandin F2 alpha for uterine atony. *Obstet Gynecol.* 1988;72(3 Pt 1):367–370.
59. Johanson R, Kumar M, Obhrai M, et al. Management of massive postpartum haemorrhage: use of a hydrostatic balloon catheter to avoid laparotomy. *BJOG.* 2001;108(4):420–422.
60. Pelage JP, Le Dref O, Mateo J, et al. Life-threatening primary postpartum hemorrhage: treatment with emergency selective arterial embolization. *Radiology.* 1998;208(2):359–362.
61. B-Lynch C, Coker A, Lawal AH, et al. The B-Lynch surgical technique for the control of massive postpartum haemorrhage: an alternative to hysterectomy? Five cases reported. *Br J Obstet Gynaecol.* 1997;104(3):372–375.
62. Morgan M. Amniotic fluid embolism. *Anaesthesia.* 1979;34(1):20–32.
63. Masson RG. Amniotic fluid embolism. *Clin Chest Med.* 1992;13(4):657–665.
64. Steiner PE, Lushbaugh CC. Landmark article, Oct. 1941: Maternal pulmonary embolism by amniotic fluid as a cause of obstetric shock and unexpected deaths in obstetrics. *JAMA.* 1986;255(16):2187–2203.
65. Clark SL, Pavlova Z, Greenspoon J, et al. Squamous cells in the maternal pulmonary circulation. *Am J Obstet Gynecol.* 1986;154(1):104–106.
66. Giampaolo C, Schneider V, Kowalski BH, et al. The cytologic diagnosis of amniotic fluid embolism: a critical reappraisal. *Diagn Cytopathol.* 1987;3(2):126–128.
67. Lee W, Ginsburg KA, Cotton DB, et al. Squamous and trophoblastic cells in the maternal pulmonary circulation identified by invasive hemodynamic monitoring during the peripartum period. *Am J Obstet Gynecol.* 1986;155(5):999–1001.
68. Masson RG, Ruggieri J. Pulmonary microvascular cytology. A new diagnostic application of the pulmonary artery catheter. *Chest.* 1985;88(6):908–914.
69. Lee KR, Catalano PM, Ortiz-Giroux S. Cytologic diagnosis of amniotic fluid embolism. Report of a case with a unique cytologic feature and emphasis on the difficulty of eliminating squamous contamination. *Acta Cytol.* 1986;30(2):177–182.
70. Dib N, Bajwa T. Amniotic fluid embolism causing severe left ventricular dysfunction and death: case report and review of the literature. *Cathet Cardiovasc Diagn.* 1996;39(2):177–180.
71. Clark SL, Cotton DB, Gonik B, et al. Central hemodynamic alterations in amniotic fluid embolism. *Am J Obstet Gynecol.* 1988;158(5):1124–1126.
72. Vanmaele L, Noppen M, Vincken W, et al. Transient left heart failure in amniotic fluid embolism. *Intensive Care Med.* 1990;16(4):269–271.
73. Clark SL. New concepts of amniotic fluid embolism: a review. *Obstet Gynecol Surv.* 1990;45(6):360–368.
74. Dudney TM, Elliott CG. Pulmonary embolism from amniotic fluid, fat, and air. *Prog Cardiovasc Dis.* 1994;36(6):447–474.
75. Clark SL, Hankins GD, Dudley DA, et al. Amniotic fluid embolism: analysis of the national registry. *Am J Obstet Gynecol.* 1995;172(4 Pt 1):1158–1167; discussion 1167–1169.
76. Demakis JG, Rahimtoola SH. Peripartum cardiomyopathy. *Circulation.* 1971;44(5):964–968.
77. Elkayam U, Akhter MW, Singh H, et al. Pregnancy-associated cardiomyopathy: clinical characteristics and a comparison between early and late presentation. *Circulation.* 2005;111(16):2050–2055.
78. Midei MG, DeMent SH, Feldman AM, et al. Peripartum myocarditis and cardiomyopathy. *Circulation.* 1990;81(3):922–928.
79. Mone SM, Sanders SP, Colan SD. Control mechanisms for physiological hypertrophy of pregnancy. *Circulation.* 1996;94(4):667–672.
80. Felker GM, Thompson RE, Hare JM, et al. Underlying causes and long-term survival in patients with initially unexplained cardiomyopathy. *N Engl J Med.* 2000;342(15):1077–1084.
81. Report of the National High Blood Pressure Education Program Working Group on High Blood Pressure in Pregnancy. *Am J Obstet Gynecol.* 2000;183(1):S1–S22.
82. Witlin AG, Sibai BM. Magnesium sulfate therapy in preeclampsia and eclampsia. *Obstet Gynecol.* 1998;92(5):883–889.
83. Samadi AR, Mayberry RM, Zaidi AA, et al. Maternal hypertension and associated pregnancy complications among African-American and other women in the United States. *Obstet Gynecol.* 1996;87(4):557–563.
84. ACOG practice bulletin. Diagnosis and management of preeclampsia and eclampsia. Number 33, January 2002. *Obstet Gynecol.* 2002;99(1):159–167.
85. Altman D, Carroli G, Duley L, et al. Do women with pre-eclampsia, and their babies, benefit from magnesium sulphate? The Magpie Trial: a randomised placebo-controlled trial. *Lancet.* 2002;359(9321):1877–1890.
86. Scott JR. Magnesium sulfate for mild preeclampsia. *Obstet Gynecol.* 2003;101(2):213.
87. Sibai BM. Diagnosis and management of gestational hypertension and preeclampsia. *Obstet Gynecol.* 2003;102(1):181–192.
88. Ferrazzani S, De Carolis S, Pomini F, et al. The duration of hypertension in the puerperium of preeclamptic women: relationship with renal impairment and week of delivery. *Am J Obstet Gynecol.* 1994;171(2):506–512.
89. Chobanian AV, Bakris GL, Black HR, et al. Seventh report of the Joint National Committee on Prevention, Detection, Evaluation, and Treatment of High Blood Pressure. *Hypertension.* 2003;42(6):1206–1252.
90. Alfirevic Z, Devane D, Gyte GM. Continuous cardiotocography (CTG) as a form of electronic fetal monitoring (EFM) for fetal assessment during labour. *Cochrane Database Syst Rev.* 2006;3:CD006066.
91. Liu PL, Warren TM, Ostheimer GW, et al. Foetal monitoring in parturients undergoing surgery unrelated to pregnancy. *Can Anaesth Soc J.* 1985;32(5):525–532.
92. Katz JD, Hook R, Barash PG. Fetal heart rate monitoring in pregnant patients undergoing surgery. *Am J Obstet Gynecol.* 1976;125(2):267–269.
93. Caforio L, Draisci G, Ciampelli M, et al. Rectal cancer in pregnancy: a new management based on blended anesthesia and monitoring of fetal well being. *Eur J Obstet Gynecol Reprod Biol.* 2000;88(1):71–74.
94. Karaman S, Ozcan O, Akercan F, et al. Pulmonary edema after ritodrine therapy during pregnancy and subsequent cesarean section with epidural anesthesia. *Clin Exp Obstet Gynecol.* 2004;31(1):67–69.
95. Kayacan N, Dosemeci L, Arici G, et al. Pulmonary edema due to ritodrine. *Int J Clin Pharmacol Ther.* 2004;42(6):350–351.
96. Paternoster DM, Manganelli F, Fantinato S, et al. Maternal complications from tocolytic treatment with ritodrine. Three cases of pulmonary edema. *Minerva Ginecol.* 2004;56(5):491–492.
97. Gyetvai K, Hannah ME, Hodnett ED, et al. Tocolytics for preterm labor: a systematic review. *Obstet Gynecol.* 1999;94(5 Pt 2):869–877.
98. Lamont RF. The pathophysiology of pulmonary oedema with the use of beta-agonists. *BJOG.* 2000;107(4):439–444.
99. Kleinman G, Nuwayhid B, Rudelstorfer R, et al. Circulatory and renal effects of beta-adrenergic-receptor stimulation in pregnant sheep. *Am J Obstet Gynecol.* 1984;149(8):865–874.
100. Senzaki H, Fetics B, Chen CH, et al. Comparison of ventricular pressure relaxation assessments in human heart failure: quantitative influence on load and drug sensitivity analysis. *J Am Coll Cardiol.* 1999;34(5):1529–1536.
101. Tatara T, Morisaki H, Shimada M, et al. Pulmonary edema after long-term beta-adrenergic therapy and cesarean section. *Anesth Analg.* 1995;81(2):417–418.
102. Katz VL, Dotters DJ, Droegemueller W. Perimortem cesarean delivery. *Obstet Gynecol.* 1986;68(4):571–576.
103. Atta E, Gardner M. Cardiopulmonary resuscitation in pregnancy. *Obstet Gynecol Clin North Am.* 2007;34(3):585–597, xiii.
104. Cheney FW. The American Society of Anesthesiologists Closed Claims Project: what have we learned, how has it affected practice, and how will it affect practice in the future? *Anesthesiology.* 1999;91(2):552–556.

CHAPTER 98 ■ CARDIAC DISEASE AND HYPERTENSIVE DISORDERS IN PREGNANCY

RAYMOND O. POWRIE

PART I: HYPERTENSIVE DISORDERS OF PREGNANCY

Hypertension during pregnancy has been classified by the American College of Obstetricians and Gynecologists into four distinct categories: (a) pre-eclampsia and eclampsia, (b) chronic hypertension (hypertension that was present before pregnancy), (c) chronic hypertension with superimposed pre-eclampsia or eclampsia, and (d) latent or transient hypertension of the third trimester (1). Most chronic hypertensive pregnant patients have essential hypertension, which has no appreciable effect during pregnancy unless end-organ damage is present. Chronic hypertension is seen in a critical care unit typically only when a patient has a hypertensive urgency/emergency unrelated to pregnancy, or if the patient has a secondary cause of hypertension that represents a short-term risk to maternal health. Similarly, latent or transient hypertension is also relatively benign, occurring in the last trimester or the immediate postpartum period, with a return of normotension by the first 3 weeks after delivery. It is pre-eclampsia and eclampsia (whether occurring *de novo* or superimposed upon pre-existing hypertension) that is most likely to require critical care support, and therefore will be the focus of this section.

Pre-eclampsia/Eclampsia

Pre-eclampsia is a multisystem disorder unique to human pregnancies. Its pathophysiology is not well understood, and its cause is unknown. It is associated with an increased risk of fetal loss, intrauterine growth restriction, and preterm birth, and remains a leading cause of maternal death worldwide. Eclampsia refers to pre-eclampsia that is complicated by seizures, but it is our present understanding that the underlying condition is the same (2).

Although much of the care of the pre-eclamptic patient will fall into the domain of the obstetrician, familiarity with the manifestations and management of pre-eclampsia is important for any critical care physician for two reasons. First, pre-eclampsia is far more common among women with medical problems such as chronic hypertension, thrombophilia, renal disease, diabetes, and collagen vascular disease, which are precisely the women that intensivists are most likely to care for during a pregnancy. Second, intensivists are often called to assist with the maternal medical manifestations of severe pre-eclampsia, and the help they provide will be greatly enhanced by an understanding of the underlying condition.

Risk Factors for Pre-eclampsia

Five percent of pregnancies are complicated by pre-eclampsia. It typically occurs in the final weeks prior to the due date, and is very rare prior to 20 weeks of gestation. The risk factors for pre-eclampsia are listed in Table 98.1. The diverse nature of the risk factors suggests that pre-eclampsia may be a common end point for a variety of processes related to placental dysfunction (3).

Etiology/Pathophysiology

Pre-eclampsia is believed to be an abnormal vascular response to the formation of the placenta. It is associated with endothelial cell dysfunction, activation of the coagulation system, enhanced platelet aggregation, and increased systemic vascular resistance. The maternal effects of these changes are manifest in the cardiovascular system, kidneys, lungs, and brain. Pathologic examination of affected maternal organs reveals areas of edema, endothelial swelling, microinfarctions, and microhemorrhages. The cardiovascular features of pre-eclampsia include decreased plasma volume (despite an increase in total body water and salt retention) and colloid osmotic pressure (largely due to a drop in serum albumin) (4,5). Generalized arteriolar vasospasm accounts for the hypertension in pre-eclampsia, which is often very labile.

The etiology of pre-eclampsia is one of medicine's greatest mysteries. Our present understanding suggests that the condition begins early in pregnancy and that there are three distinct, sequential phases that are necessary for its evolution (6,7). The first phase is incomplete invasion of the trophoblast into the endometrium, perhaps due to a maladaptive immune response in the mother, followed by inadequate "placentation" (formation of the placenta), which leads to the second phase in which decreases in the levels of angiogenic growth factors and increased placental debris are found in the maternal circulation. This stage of the development of pre-eclampsia is not associated with any clinical symptoms or signs. However, decreases in placental growth factor (PlGF) and elevations of fms-like tyrosine kinase 1 (sFlt) and endoglin can be detected (8–10). These changes incite a maternal inflammatory response. The third phase that leads to the maternal pre-eclamptic syndrome, as detected clinically, is the response of the maternal endothelium and cardiovascular system to these stressors, which is modulated by the woman's own level of metabolic and cardiovascular health. Although this response is manifested predominantly as hypertension and proteinuria, it is typically the less common cardiac, pulmonary, hematologic, neurologic, and hepatic effects of pre-eclampsia that present to intensivists. The importance of this model for the etiology of pre-eclampsia is the

TABLE 98.1

RISK FACTORS FOR PRE-ECLAMPSIA

Maternal	Fetal
■ First pregnancy ■ New partners ■ Age younger than 18 or older than 35 y ■ Chronic hypertension ■ Prior history of pre-eclampsia ■ Family history of pre-eclampsia ■ Pregestational diabetes ■ Obesity ■ Thrombophilias ■ Systemic erythematosus ■ Renal disease	■ Multiple gestations ■ Molar pregnancies (can cause pre-eclampsia at <20 wk gestation) ■ Fetal hydrops ■ Triploidy

underlying concept that pre-eclampsia is evolving long before it becomes clinically apparent in the maternal syndrome.

Clinical Features

Pre-eclampsia can manifest both as a fetal syndrome (abnormal fetal oxygenation, reduced amniotic fluid, and fetal growth restriction) and a maternal syndrome (proteinuria and hypertension with or without other multisystem abnormalities). In most patients, both the fetal and maternal syndrome will be apparent, but one or the other will often predominate in an individual case. This chapter will focus on the maternal manifestations.

Pre-eclampsia is defined by the maternal manifestations of hypertension and proteinuria occurring in the second half of pregnancy. The presentation and diagnostic features of this condition are reviewed in Tables 98.2A and 98.2B (11–16). Although hypertension >140/90 mm Hg and proteinuria >300 mg/24 hour are required for the diagnosis of pre-eclampsia,

TABLE 98.2A

CLINICAL FEATURES OF PRE-ECLAMPSIA

SYMPTOMS	Headache	The headache that characterizes pre-eclampsia is typically frontal in location, throbbing in character, persistent, and not responsive to mild analgesia.
	Visual phenomena	The visual disturbances that characterize pre-eclampsia are presumed to be due to cerebral vasospasm and are typically scintillations or scotomas. Longer-lasting visual field deficits and rarely transient blindness can result from edema, posterior reversible encephalopathic syndrome, and even infarction in the occipital region of the brain. Serous retinal detachments can also occur in pre-eclampsia and are related to retinal edema. Magnesium, which is commonly used to prevent seizures in pre-eclamptic women, can cause mild visual blurring or double vision, but should not cause scotomas, scintillations, or visual loss.
	Epigastric pain	The epigastric or right upper quadrant discomfort that occurs in pre-eclampsia can be marked, and may be out of proportion to the degree of liver enzyme abnormalities. It is believed to be caused by edema in the liver that stretches the hepatic capsule. In rare cases, it may be caused by hepatic infarction or rupture.
	Edema	Edema is present in more than 30% of normal pregnancies, and is thus not a reliable sign of pre-eclampsia. Rapid weight gain (more than 1 pound per week in the third trimester) or edema in the hands or facial area (nondependent edema) is best viewed as a sign that should lead the clinician to evaluate the patient for other, more specific, evidence of pre-eclampsia.
SIGNS	Hypertension >140/90	Hypertension in pre-eclampsia is due to vasospasm and can be very labile. Ideally, blood pressure should be measured in the sitting position with a manual cuff, with the brachial artery at the level of the heart. There is a literature suggesting that some automated blood pressure cuffs may be less reliable in pre-eclampsia and that either a manual cuff or arterial line should be used to verify blood pressure in pre-eclamptic patients with severe hypertension (12). Although a rise in systolic/diastolic blood pressure of 30/15 mm Hg was once considered a criterion for diagnosing pre-eclampsia, it is now recognized that this definition lacks both sensitivity and specificity.
	Epigastric or right upper quadrant tenderness	Abdominal pain in pre-eclampsia is attributed to hepatic capsular stretching from edema. The degree of tenderness is often out of proportion to the degree of elevation of liver function tests. Epigastric tenderness is suggestive of severe pre-eclampsia, and is associated with an increased risk of both maternal and fetal adverse outcomes.
	Hyperreflexia	Clonus is an important sign of pre-eclampsia but should be distinguished from the very brisk reflexes commonly seen in normal pregnancies.
	Retinal artery vasospasm on funduscopy	Retinal vasospasm, retinal edema (in the form of soft exudates), hemorrhage, and exudative retinal detachment are uncommon findings in pre-eclampsia. Papilledema is rare.

TABLE 98.2B

LABORATORY FEATURES OF PRE-ECLAMPSIA

Complete blood count with elevated hemoglobin and/or thrombocytopenia	The "elevation of hemoglobin" seen with pre-eclampsia (which may manifest as a hemoglobin of 12 g/dL at 37 wk when it would be expected to be closer to 10 g/dL because of the physiologic dilutional anemia that is seen in pregnancy) is due to hemoconcentration. Much less commonly, hemoglobin may fall with pre-eclampsia due to a microangiopathic hemolytic anemia. Platelet consumption in pre-eclampsia can cause an increased mean platelet volume and thrombocytopenia, and is an important manifestation of severe disease (13). In severe cases of pre-eclampsia or HELLP (a subset of pre-eclampsia), schistocytes (fragmented red cells) may be seen on peripheral smear and can lead to a mild drop in hemoglobin. Brisk hemolysis is rare, however, and should lead to the consideration of HUS or TTP.
Elevated serum creatinine	Typically serum creatinine is <0.8 mg/dL (70 μmol/L) in pregnancy and values greater than this are considered abnormal. Renal function impairment is caused by decreased renal blood flow and glomerular filtration rate secondary to swelling of intracapillary glomerular cells, fibrin deposition along the basement membranes, and afferent arteriolar spasm.
Elevated serum uric acid	Typically, serum uric acid is <5.0 mg/dL (280 μmol/L) in pregnancy. Uric acid is the most sensitive test for identifying pre-eclampsia but it is still only elevated in approximately 80% of cases of pre-eclampsia. Uric acid rises in this setting due to impaired excretion of uric acid in the renal tubules that is caused by pre-eclampsia-related changes in the renal microcirculation (14). Although an important sign of pre-eclampsia, the elevated uric acid level is distinct from an elevated creatinine, AST, or decreased platelet count in that the uric acid level is not generally believed to have any direct clinical consequences and should not be used as a marker of disease severity.
Elevated liver enzymes	Mild elevations of AST, typically less than 100 U/L, suggest hepatic involvement. Greater levels may be due to severe pre-eclampsia, HELLP syndrome, hepatic infarction, hepatic rupture, or superimposed acute fatty liver of pregnancy.
Proteinuria	Proteinuria is an essential diagnostic feature of pre-eclampsia. Urine dipsticks are routinely used to screen for proteinuria in asymptomatic patients. However, dipsticks lack the needed sensitivity and specificity to make them a reliable test for proteinuria in patients in whom the diagnosis of pre-eclampsia is suspected because of the presence of other features of this disease. When pre-eclampsia is suspected, a 24-hour urine test for proteinuria with creatinine and creatinine clearance should be obtained. Proteinuria is present if there is more than 300 mg of protein excreted over 24 hours. Total urinary creatinine should be measured to assess the adequacy of urine collection. The creatinine clearance can be used in conjunction with the serum creatinine as a measure of renal function. The use of a random spot urinary protein-to-creatinine ratio to diagnose proteinuria in pregnancy has had many advocates, but it remains unclear at this time whether this test can replace the 24-hour urine in pregnant patients with suspected pre-eclampsia (15,16).
DIC screen	Severe pre-eclampsia can rarely cause DIC, but it is almost always seen in association with thrombocytopenia. Checking INR, PTT, and fibrinogen degradation products is usually only done if the patient with pre-eclampsia has thrombocytopenia or is undergoing an invasive procedure.

HUS, hemolytic uremic syndrome; TTP, thrombotic thrombocytopenic purpura; AST, aspartate aminotransferase; DIC, dissemination intravascular coagulation; INR, international normalized ratio; PTT, partial thromboplastin time.

some cases may present initially without these features, or may present—as in the case of postpartum eclampsia—after some of these features have already resolved.

Severe pre-eclampsia is defined by one or more of the following: systolic blood pressure greater than 160 mm Hg; diastolic blood pressure greater than 110 mm Hg; mean arterial pressure greater than 120 mm Hg; proteinuria greater than 5 g/24 hours; oliguria less than 500 mL/24 hours; and headaches, visual disturbances, epigastric pain, pulmonary edema, or cyanosis. Eclampsia results when seizures occur that are not related to other underlying disorders. These features describe a group of patients with an increased risk of fetal and maternal morbidity for whom delivery should be strongly considered. Pre-eclamptic patients who lack any of the features of severe pre-eclampsia may have to be observed without moving toward delivery if the fetus is significantly premature and the mother remains under close observation; however, such patients are rarely seen in intensive care settings.

Life-threatening maternal complications of pre-eclampsia include severe hypertension, seizure, cerebral hemorrhage, pulmonary edema, disseminated intravascular coagulopathy (DIC), acute renal failure (ARF), and hepatic failure and/or rupture. Although these complications occur in the minority of cases of pre-eclampsia, they are reviewed here, as it is these complications that are most likely to require the care of a critical care physician.

Severe Hypertension. Although most clinicians would agree that the treatment goal for chronic hypertension in pregnancy is to keep the blood pressure below at least 160/100, the level at which elevated blood pressure should be treated in the setting of confirmed pre-eclampsia is controversial. All experts would agree that blood pressures greater than 180 mm Hg (systolic) and 110 mm Hg (diastolic) should be treated urgently, and that in the setting of obvious hypertensive end-organ damage (retinal hemorrhage, papilledema, pulmonary edema, severe headache, or renal failure), the blood pressure should be kept under 160/100 mm Hg. Beyond this consensus, opinions vary considerably.

Although no evidence suggests that treating blood pressures between 160/100 and 180/110 mm Hg in the setting of pre-eclampsia improves maternal or fetal outcomes, many experts believe that the risks for seizure, placental abruption, and cerebral hemorrhage are decreased by bringing blood pressures down into the normal or mildly hypertensive range. Other experts believe that because pre-eclampsia is a dynamic vasospastic disorder with associated target-organ ischemia, the safest approach is to let blood pressures run in a moderately severe range to avoid worsening ischemia in areas of regional vasospasm. This is a particularly important consideration if one believes that part of the reason for maternal hypertension in pre-eclampsia may be to improve placental perfusion. In the absence of direct evidence of end–target-organ damage from severe hypertension, it is our practice to treat all blood pressures over 160/105 mm Hg. However, although we treat these blood pressures urgently, we are careful to avoid any severe, sudden decreases in maternal blood pressure that may adversely affect uteroplacental and cerebral perfusion.

If urgent blood pressure reduction is required, intravenous labetalol or intravenous hydralazine can be used. Increasing evidence indicates that labetalol may be the better choice of the two; it is our preferred agent, although both agents are still acceptable (17). Hydralazine has been associated with an increased risk of an emergency cesarean in women who receive it while still pregnant and with lower Apgar scores in the infants of mothers who have been given this agent prior to delivery. Short-acting oral nifedipine is also used at some centers as an alternative to labetalol or hydralazine for the acute treatment of severe hypertension. Although its use in medical patients is now discouraged, its use for control of blood pressure in young pregnant or postpartum women without coronary artery disease remains an acceptable practice. Previous concerns about a drug interaction between magnesium and calcium channel blockers appear to be ill-founded (18). Diuretics should not be used in this setting unless pulmonary edema is present because, despite the edema that is so common in pre-eclamptic patients, most hemodynamic studies of pre-eclamptic women suggest that they are actually intravascularly volume depleted.

Once the patient has delivered, any antihypertensive agent can be used for blood pressure control. At that point, nitroprusside and nitroglycerin are excellent choices because of their very short half-lives.

Seizures. Seizures are the most well-known severe manifestation of pre-eclampsia. The risk of an eclamptic seizure in a patient with untreated pre-eclampsia is estimated to be about 1 in 200. Because of early identification of pre-eclampsia and the widespread use of magnesium prophylaxis, the incidence of eclampsia in the United States ranges from 1 in 1,000 to 1 in 20,000 deliveries. When it does occur, eclampsia is associated with a maternal mortality rate of 5% and a perinatal mortality rate between 13% and 30%.

Eclamptic seizures are typically of the grand mal variety, with clonic-tonic muscular activity followed by a postictal period. However, focal, jacksonian-type and absence seizures have been described. Most eclamptic seizures occur in the setting of established pre-eclampsia with hypertension and proteinuria. Classically, they are preceded by evidence of neuromuscular irritability such as tremulousness, agitation, nausea, vomiting, and/or clonus. However, some patients will present with seizure as their first manifestation of pre-eclampsia, usually occurring in the absence of hypertension or proteinuria.

The onset of eclamptic convulsions can be antepartum (38%–53%), intrapartum (18%–36%), or postpartum (11%–44%). Postpartum eclamptic seizures generally occur in the first 48 hours after delivery, but it is not unusual to see them occur anytime in the first week after delivery. Eclamptic seizures have been reported as late as 23 days postpartum.

The underlying pathophysiology of the eclamptic seizure is unclear. They cannot be attributed simply to severe hypertension, because eclampsia can be seen in patients with only mild elevations in blood pressure. Electroencephalograms may show epileptiform abnormalities, but usually show only a nonspecific diffuse slowing that may persist for weeks after delivery. Computed tomography (CT) and magnetic resonance imaging (MRI) of the eclamptic patient can be normal, or may show findings ranging from diffuse edema to focal areas of hemorrhage or infarction in the subcortical white matter and adjacent gray matter of the parieto-occipital lobes. The MRI is more sensitive in detecting abnormalities in eclamptic patients, but both CT and MRI of the brain can be normal, particularly if done in the first 24 hours after the seizure. When radiologic changes are present, some—but not all—of these changes usually resolve with time (19).

Management of eclamptic seizures. While moving toward delivery, a pre-eclamptic woman should receive an anticonvulsant to prevent eclamptic seizures. Magnesium sulfate is the drug of choice for this purpose (20). It halves the risk of eclampsia in patients with pre-eclampsia and lowers the risk of recurrent seizures and maternal death in women with eclampsia. It is superior to phenytoin and benzodiazepines in preventing further seizures. Magnesium is typically given as an intravenous bolus of 4 to 6 g, followed by a continuous intravenous infusion of 1 to 4 g/hour. Some clinicians will monitor plasma concentrations (which should run between 4 and 7 mmol/L), but others will simply administer the magnesium and monitor the patient for symptoms and signs of toxicity (hypotension, muscular weakness, and respiratory depression). Carefully monitoring for toxicity is important, particularly in patients with worsening renal function. Severe respiratory depression in a patient on magnesium should be treated with intravenous calcium. The only role of magnesium in pre-eclampsia is that of an anticonvulsant. Despite the possibility of a transient decrease in blood pressure with its initial administration, magnesium has no significant sustained effect on blood pressure. Its mechanism of action remains unclear, but it does not seem to have any intrinsic anticonvulsant effect, and may actually prevent seizures through its action as a cerebral vasodilator.

If the woman does have an acute eclamptic seizure, intravenous benzodiazepine is indicated to acutely stop the seizure, and magnesium should then be initiated if this has not already occurred. If an eclamptic convulsion occurs while a patient is receiving magnesium, most clinicians will add phenytoin to the regimen. Continued seizures should warrant the involvement of neurology and consideration of the use of phenobarbital or other hypnotic agents. Anticonvulsant therapy can generally be stopped once postpartum diuresis has begun and the manifestations of pre-eclampsia have started to improve.

Most patients with eclamptic seizures should have their head imaged with CT or MRI to rule out an intracerebral hemorrhage; the timing of these neuroimaging tests should be determined by the level of clinical suspicion for this diagnosis, and should not substantially delay delivery.

Cerebrovascular Accidents. Cerebrovascular accidents are three to seven times more common in pregnancy. Pre-eclampsia accounts for over a third of the strokes that do occur during pregnancy. At least half of the deaths from pre-eclampsia in the developed world are due to stroke. Most of the strokes in patients with pre-eclampsia will be related to intracerebral hemorrhage, but can also occur due to vasospastic ischemia (21). Pre-eclampsia-related stroke is often, but not always, associated with severe hypertension and/or eclamptic convulsions. Sudden onset or worsening of a headache, a change in mental status, or any focal neurologic complaint occurring in the context of pre-eclampsia should lead to consideration of this diagnosis and urgent neuroimaging.

Pulmonary Edema. Pulmonary edema occurs in about 3% of cases of pre-eclampsia, and can cause significant maternal morbidity (22,23). It occurs as a result of the interplay of pre-eclampsia-related pulmonary endothelial damage and the low plasma oncotic pressure seen in all pregnancies. Excessive intravenous fluid is also typically a contributing factor. It is often seen in the postpartum period after a patient has received a substantial amount of intravenous fluid in labor (or with cesarean delivery) and when mobilization of fluid from the involuting uterus begins. Pulmonary edema in this setting is often amenable to gentle diuresis but may be severe enough to warrant mechanical ventilation.

Echocardiographic studies demonstrate that transient systolic or diastolic ventricular dysfunction is present in up to one third of pre-eclampsia cases associated with pulmonary edema. This pre-eclampsia-related myocardial dysfunction is believed to be a manifestation of vasospastic coronary ischemia, and usually resolves rapidly with resolution of the pre-eclampsia. The author considers this to be a distinct entity from peripartum cardiomyopathy and does not believe there is a substantial recurrence risk of cardiac disease for these patients in a subsequent pregnancy.

Prevention and treatment of pulmonary edema. It is important to avoid excessive fluid administration to patients with pre-eclampsia because of their propensity for pulmonary edema. Ideally, one individual should be designated to approve and monitor all fluid administration in these patients. Regular auscultation of the lungs and use of transcutaneous pulse oximetry in patients with severe pre-eclampsia will help identify cases of pulmonary edema as they evolve. This careful observation should be continued in the postpartum period because pulmonary edema often occurs as late as 2 to 3 days after delivery. Acute treatment of pulmonary edema should involve supplemental oxygen, low-dose furosemide, and, if needed, morphine (23,24). Blood pressure control may help treat pulmonary edema by decreasing afterload. An echocardiogram should be obtained to look for an underlying cardiac contribution. Intubation and mechanical ventilation may become necessary if the above measures do not improve the patient's oxygenation.

Disseminated Intravascular Coagulation. Disseminated intravascular coagulation (DIC) can occur as a late and severe complication of pre-eclampsia or eclampsia (25). Because most patients with pre-eclampsia-related DIC have low platelet counts or elevated transaminase levels, DIC screening in the absence of these abnormalities is generally not necessary (26). However, a DIC screen should be ordered in all pre-eclamptic patients with rising liver enzymes, dropping platelet counts, and/or any abnormal bleeding. This is particularly important if there is a possibility of an operative delivery.

Acute Renal Failure. Pre-eclampsia is often associated with a mild degree of renal impairment manifesting as a slightly elevated creatinine or a decreased urine output. This is due to a combination of intravascular volume depletion, renovascular vasospasm, and a pre-eclampsia-related glomerular lesion known as glomerular endotheliosis. This mild renal impairment usually resolves rapidly after delivery.

Acute renal failure in pre-eclampsia is not common. If it does occur, acute tubular necrosis (ATN) and partial or total cortical necrosis are the most likely underlying lesions, and are thought to be caused by pre-eclampsia-related, vasospasm-induced renal ischemia. A history of transient hypotension is also typically present in these cases. The differential diagnosis includes ATN from sepsis or hemorrhage, an entity known as postpartum renal failure, or renal failure from causes unassociated with pregnancy such as hemolytic uremic syndrome, medication effects, or acute glomerulonephritis.

Most renal failure in the setting of pre-eclampsia is rapidly reversible, but if significant hypotension has occurred (as may happen with placental abruption or DIC-related hemorrhage), ATN or renal cortical necrosis may result and necessitate dialysis. In persons with sustained oliguria in the setting of pre-eclampsia, fluid challenges should be given cautiously because of the risk of pulmonary edema. Poor outcomes in pre-eclampsia are far more commonly related to pulmonary edema than they are to decreased urine output. Diuretics to improve urine output should be avoided in the absence of pulmonary edema because of the intravascular volume depletion present in most patients with pre-eclampsia.

If the patient is unresponsive to small fluid boluses, the use of central venous pressure monitoring may be a helpful, if not completely reliable, guide. The role of the pulmonary artery catheter in this context is unproven, and should only be used by nurses and physicians who are trained and experienced in its use. Increasing data from randomized control trials have shown that pulmonary artery catheters are of less benefit than previously believed in nonpregnant patients, and there is little reason to believe this tool has a uniquely beneficial role in the pregnant population.

Sustained oliguria in pre-eclampsia is unusual, and therefore significant and rapid peripartum renal deterioration should also lead to consideration of differential diagnoses that include the hemolytic uremic syndrome (HUS), thrombotic thrombocytopenic purpura, and an entity known as postpartum renal failure. It is therefore advisable to perform careful microscopic examination of urinary sediment and a peripheral smear in all pregnant or postpartum patients with oliguria (27).

HELLP Syndrome. A distinct clustering of the manifestations of pre-eclampsia is the HELLP syndrome (*h*emolysis, *e*levated *l*iver enzymes, and *l*ow *p*latelet counts). This constellation of findings represents a particularly severe form of pre-eclampsia with significant risk for maternal illness and fetal injury or death (28,29). HELLP occurs in up to 20% of cases of severe pre-eclampsia. The hemolysis is microangiopathic, and therefore schistocytes (fragmented erythrocytes) are seen on peripheral smears of the blood. Lactate dehydrogenase levels are usually increased. The liver enzymes may run into the hundreds. The thrombocytopenia can be precipitous and severe. High-dose dexamethasone is often given to treat patients with HELLP, but it is not clear that this intervention has clinically significant effects on outcomes, and the treatment remains supportive care coupled with delivery (30,31).

Hepatic Rupture or Hemorrhage. Epigastric or right upper quadrant pain and elevation of hepatic enzymes due to pre-eclampsia are common. When these factors are present, it suggests severe disease and pre-eclampsia-related hepatic edema and ischemia. It generally is associated with no more than a two- to fourfold increase in aspartate aminotransferase (AST) or alanine aminotransferase (ALT). When pain is severe and/or hepatic enzymes rise above this level, pre-eclampsia-related hepatic infarction, hemorrhage, and rupture should be considered and investigated with a hepatic ultrasound or CT (32). Acute fatty liver of pregnancy (AFLP) is also part of the differential diagnoses in these cases.

Diabetes Insipidus. Diabetes insipidus is a rare complication of pre-eclampsia with significant hepatic involvement. It can also be seen with acute fatty liver of pregnancy. It has been hypothesized that the acute liver dysfunction in these patients reduces the degradation of vasopressinase (an enzyme which itself degrades vasopressin), and results in a state of relative vasopressin deficiency (33). The course of the condition follows that of the underlying disorder and can be treated with additional vasopressin until it resolves.

The Role of Arterial Lines, Central Venous Pressure Monitors, and Pulmonary Artery Catheters in Pre-eclamptic Patients

Most severe pre-eclamptic patients have normal or hyperdynamic left ventricular function with normal pulmonary artery pressure. Thus, a central venous pressure (CVP) monitor usually is adequate to assess volume status and left ventricular function. However, severely pre-eclamptic patients may develop cardiac failure, progressive and marked oliguria, or pulmonary edema. In such cases, some authors suggest that a pulmonary artery (PA) catheter may be helpful for proper diagnosis and treatment, because right and left ventricular pressures may not correlate (34,35). Given that evidence has evolved that the routine use of pulmonary artery catheters may not be as beneficial in the care of nonobstetric patients as once believed, the rather limited literature about their use in obstetric populations cannot help but be questioned (36,37). No clear consensus exists as to their role in the management of pre-eclampsia (38). We rarely employ them in any obstetric patients, as the risks—especially on labor and delivery units where the personnel have less experience in their placement and interpretation—seem to outweigh the evidence justifying their use. When questions arise as to whether cardiac dysfunction is contributing to a pre-eclamptic patient's pulmonary edema and/or renal failure, we obtain an urgent bedside echocardiogram to guide our care and, in the absence of a significant cardiac cause, manage these patients clinically.

An intra-arterial catheter monitor may be indicated for protracted severe hypertension during therapy with potent antihypertensive agents or when there is a significant disparity between automated and manual cuff measurements of blood pressure.

PART II: CARDIAC DISEASE

Cardiac disease during pregnancy has an incidence rate of 0.4% to 4%, and is associated with a maternal mortality of 0.4% to 6%, depending on the cardiac lesion being discussed (39). It, therefore, remains one of the leading causes of maternal mortality, and may actually be increasing as a cause of maternal mortality in the developed world. While rheumatic heart disease is far less of a concern in the West than it was several decades ago, it remains a problem, along with peripartum cardiomyopathy, pulmonary hypertension, adult congenital heart disease, and myocardial ischemia. These conditions will be the focus of this section. While many of the patients with cardiac disease who end up under the care of a critical care physician will have cardiac disease that was identified prior to pregnancy, a significant portion of patients will also have their cardiac disease present for the first time during pregnancy. The physiologic changes of pregnancy may exacerbate, and thereby unmask, previously undiagnosed cardiac disease, and pregnancy can predispose patients to the onset of certain cardiac diseases such as peripartum cardiomyopathy or ischemic heart disease. Some of the physiologic changes associated with pregnancy are reviewed below and are summarized in Table 98.3.

Physiologic Changes

1. Maternal blood volume gradually increases during pregnancy to 150% of nonpregnant levels (40). The increase in plasma volume (45%–55%) is greater than the increase in red blood cell volume (20%–30%), resulting in a relative anemia of pregnancy. This increase in blood volume is associated with an increase in cardiac output, which begins early in gestation and peaks at levels 30% to 40% over nonpregnant values between 20 and 30 weeks (40). The increase then plateaus until term.
2. The increase in cardiac output with gestation is dependent on heart rate and stroke volume. Heart rate gradually increases throughout pregnancy, starting as early as 4 weeks' gestation, with a 10% to 15% increase by term. Stroke volume, in contrast, peaks during the second trimester, with a 20% to 40% increase over the nonpregnant state.
3. During labor, cardiac output rises another 15% to 45% above prelabor values with an additional increase of 10% to 25% during uterine contractions. The increase in cardiac output in labor during contractions versus that seen

TABLE 98.3

HEMODYNAMIC CHANGES IN PREGNANCY

	% Change[a]		
	Pregnancy	**Labor and delivery**	**Postpartum**
Cardiac output	+30–50	+50–65[b]	+60–80
Heart rate	+10–15	+10–30[b]	−10–15
Stroke volume	+20–30	+40–70	+60–80
Blood volume	+20–80	—	+0–10
Plasma volume	+44–55	—	+0–30
Red cell volume	+20–30	—	−10
Oxygen consumption	+20	+40–100[b]	−10–15
Systemic vascular resistance	−10–25		—
Systemic blood pressure			
Systolic	−5	+10–30[b]	+10
Diastolic	−10	+10–30[b]	+10
Pulmonary vascular resistance	−30	—	—
Pulmonary artery occlusion pressure (PAOP)	0	—	—
Colloid oncotic pressure (COP)	−10	—	—
COP–PAOP	−25	—	—

[a]Percent change from nonpregnant state.
[b]Percent change without regional anesthesia (local anesthetic).

between contractions is greater late in the first stage (34%) versus early in the first stage (16%) (41).

4. Oxygen consumption increases 20% during pregnancy, and may increase as much as 40% to 100% during active labor. In the immediate postpartum period, cardiac output increases 30% to 40% over the labor period or 60% to 80% over the nonpregnant state, with the increased blood volume shifting to the central circulation from the contracted uterus, as well as alleviation of aortocaval compression and a slight decrease in total peripheral resistance.
5. Cardiac output and other hemodynamic parameters are thought to return to their baseline prepregnant state by 6 weeks after delivery. However, cardiac output may remain elevated for up to 12 weeks (42).
6. Systemic arterial pressure decreases by 10 to 15 mm Hg over the first two trimesters and then gradually returns to baseline by term. Systemic vascular resistance decreases 10% to 20% during pregnancy. Moreover, systemic vascular resistance may remain decreased for at least 12 weeks post partum.
7. Venous pressure in the lower extremities increases and peaks near term as the gravid uterus compresses the inferior vena cava—especially when the patient is supine—while central venous pressure remains unchanged. Total body water increases by about 2 kg throughout pregnancy.
8. Invasive PA catheterization in low-risk, near-term pregnant patients (36–38 weeks) reveals a significant decrease in pulmonary vascular resistance, colloid oncotic pressure (COP), and COP–pulmonary artery occlusion pressure (PAOP) gradient, with no change in PAOP or left ventricular stroke work index (43).
9. With a significant increase in oxygen consumption, especially during labor, along with a decrease in functional residual capacity, the importance of adequate preoxygenation before rapid sequence induction of anesthesia cannot be overemphasized. Morbidity and mortality statistics from England and Wales reveal that anesthetic-related maternal mortality is predominantly caused by the inability to intubate the trachea or by pulmonary aspiration during general anesthesia (44). Thus, an awake orotracheal intubation should be considered when airway patency is suspect. The most experienced person available should typically be the individual who intubates pregnant women on a regular basis.
10. Despite an average 200- to 500-mL blood loss for routine, uncomplicated vaginal deliveries and an 800- to 1,000-mL blood loss for cesarean section deliveries, blood transfusions are seldom necessary because of the increased blood volume and the autotransfusion of approximately 500 mL of blood from the contracted uterus in the postpartum period. Although this increase in blood volume protects against blood loss at delivery, pulmonary congestion and cardiac failure can result in patients with underlying cardiac dysfunction.
11. Pregnant women have a predisposition to pulmonary edema. Physiologic changes in pregnancy that favor the development of pulmonary edema include an increase in intravascular volume, decreased blood viscosity ("physiologic anemia of pregnancy"), decreased COP, and fluid shifts, especially in the immediate postpartum period.
12. Patients with minimal cardiac reserve may tolerate early pregnancy, and subsequently decompensate from

increasing blood volume and cardiac output in the late second trimester and early third trimester. Patients with moderate cardiac reserve may tolerate pregnancy well until labor and delivery or the puerperium. Thus, cardiac patients should continue to be closely monitored in the postpartum period because cardiac decompensation most frequently occurs during this time; the prepregnant baseline state may not be reached for as long as 12 weeks after delivery.

13. The enlarging uterus in the third trimester predisposes to aortocaval compression and decreased cardiac output in supine patients. Inferior vena cava compression occurs in up to 90% of near-term parturients in the supine position. However, only about 10% to 15% of patients manifest the supine hypotensive syndrome because of shunting of venous blood away from the caval system to the azygous system by the intervertebral plexus of veins. Patients most susceptible to supine hypotension are those with polyhydramnios and multiple gestation. However, in most patients in the lateral position, cardiac output is maintained. Turning from the supine to the lateral decubitus position increases cardiac output from 8% at 20 to 24 weeks to as much as 30% near term (45). Therefore, to avoid aortocaval compression, measures such as uterine displacement by maternal position (lateral decubitus), bed position (left lateral tilt), or uterine displacement devices are imperative, especially in the last trimester. Moreover, maternal hypotension and placental hypoperfusion from aortocaval compression can be compounded by regional anesthesia that interferes with compensatory sympathetic nervous system mechanisms (46).
14. As a consequence of these cardiovascular changes, normal symptoms of pregnancy can include fatigue, dyspnea, decreased exercise capacity, and light-headedness. Cardiac signs that may be seen in normal pregnancies include distended neck veins, peripheral edema, loud first heart sound, loud third heart sound, systolic ejection murmurs, and continuous murmurs (cervical venous hums and mammary souffle). Fourth heart sounds and diastolic murmurs occur rarely in normal pregnancy and should be considered pathologic unless proven otherwise. These changes are reviewed in Table 98.4. Therefore, the normal signs and symptoms of pregnancy may simulate pathologic disease states, thereby rendering the diagnosis of heart disease difficult.
15. Normal chest radiographic findings demonstrate increased lung markings (prominent pulmonary vasculature partly due to both increased blood volume and increased breast shadow). Electrocardiographic (ECG) changes may include a left QRS axis deviation and nonspecific ST-segment and T-wave changes.

TABLE 98.4

NORMAL CARDIAC SYMPTOMS AND SIGNS IN PREGNANCY

SYMPTOMS
Fatigue
Dyspnea
Decreased exercise tolerance
Light-headedness
Syncope
SIGNS
General
Distended neck veins
Peripheral edema
Hyperventilation
Heart
Loud S_1; increased split S_1
Loud S_3
Systolic ejection murmur
Continuous murmurs (venous hum, mammary souffle)
Chest radiograph
Increased pulmonary vasculature
Horizontal position of heart
Electrocardiogram
Left axis deviation
Nonspecific ST-T–wave changes
Mild sinus tachycardia

Who is Most at Risk, and When is That Risk Greatest?

Table 98.5 classifies the risk of various cardiac lesions in pregnancy. When we speak about "risk" for these patients, we refer to congestive heart failure, arrhythmias, stroke, and death. Overall, about 13% of cardiac patients will suffer one of these outcomes in pregnancy. The presence of pulmonary hypertension is always associated with an increased risk, and this risk is commensurate to its degree of severity. Other factors associated with an increased risk of cardiac complications in pregnancy include the following (47):

1. *New York Heart Association (NYHA) functional class.* This is perhaps the most important predictor of pregnancy outcome. Patients with NYHA class I and II cardiac disease generally have a good prognosis during pregnancy. Patients with NYHA class III and IV are more likely to experience complications and may require special management around the time of delivery.
2. *Left-sided obstructive cardiac lesions.* Patients with lesions such as aortic stenosis may have difficulty accommodating the increased blood volume and cardiac output seen in pregnancy, and become increasingly symptomatic. Interestingly, patients with regurgitant valvular lesions may have less difficulty in pregnancy, as cardiac output in these cases may benefit from the decrease in systemic vascular resistance seen in pregnancy.
3. *Cyanosis*
4. *Left ventricular systolic dysfunction*
5. *Prior cardiac events or previous arrhythmia*

Although pregnant women with cardiac disease may experience complications at any point during pregnancy, there are three periods of particular risk:

1. At the end of the second trimester when cardiac output has increased to its peak
2. At the time of labor and delivery when cardiac work may be increased dramatically by both pain and the autotransfusion of blood from the placenta and uterus with each contraction
3. In the first 72 hours following delivery when the uterine involution and resolution of pregnancy-related edema leads to mobilization of large amounts of fluid.

TABLE 98.5

PERIPARTUM RISK OF VARIOUS CARDIAC LESIONS

Risk category	Lesion
Lower-risk lesion	Mitral valve prolapse Mitral valve prolapse with regurgitation Atrial septal defect Ventricular septal defect with normal pulmonary pressures Trace to mild valvular regurgitation NYHA class I History of SVT with recent good control Pacer
Intermediate-risk lesion	Stable ischemic heart disease Mild to moderate pulmonary hypertension Moderate to severe valvular insufficiency NYHA class II Cardiomyopathy with ejection fraction 30%–50% Poorly controlled SVT
High-risk lesion	Unstable ischemic heart disease Moderate to severe left ventricular obstruction (e.g., aortic <1.5 cm^2 or mitral valvular stenosis <2 cm^2, peak gradient IV outflow tract of >30 mm Hg) NYHA class III Cardiomyopathy with ejection fraction $<30\%$ Dilated aortic root/Marfan/Ehlers-Danlos Moderate pulmonary hypertension History of ventricular tachycardia with or without AICD Mechanical prosthetic heart valve History of TIA or CVA
Highest-risk lesion	Pulmonary hypertension >80 mm Hg Eisenmenger syndrome NYHA class IV Cyanosis

NYHA, New York Heart Association; SVT, supraventricular tachycardia; AICD, automated implantable cardioverter-defibrillator; TIA, transient ischemic attack; CVA, cerebrovascular accident.
Items above can be used to calculate a risk index with 1 point being assigned for each and 0, 1, and >1 points being associated with a risk of some cardiac event during the entire pregnancy of 5%, 27%, and 75%, respectively. (Risk calculation adapted from Siu S, Sermer M, Colman JM, et al. Prospective multicenter study of pregnancy outcomes in women with heart disease. *Circulation*. 2001;104:515.)

General Management of Cardiac Patients During Pregnancy

Management of patients with cardiac disease in pregnancy in general should include good preconception counseling to assess and inform the patient of the risks associated with a pregnancy. Although no woman should be told that she "should never get pregnant," a clear discussion of the risk is essential. With cases such as severe pulmonary hypertension or Eisenmenger syndrome, the patient should be strongly cautioned against pursuing a pregnancy. Women with congenital heart disease need also be informed that they are at increased risk of giving birth to a child with congenital heart disease.

If a woman with cardiac disease decides to pursue a pregnancy after a clear discussion of risk, the cardiologist should ensure that her cardiac status is clearly delineated and optimized. Ideally, any necessary investigations or interventions should be carried out prior to conception.

Once a woman is pregnant, regular visits with a medical specialist and an obstetrician trained in the care of high-risk pregnancies to watch for evidence of heart failure and arrhythmias are essential. Consultation with an obstetric anesthesiologist prior to delivery is also prudent.

As stated earlier, most cardiac medications can be used in pregnancy when indicated. Table 98.7 lists many common cardiac medications, and classifies them as to which drugs we know the most about regarding their safe use during pregnancy and which drugs we know the least. However, it should be emphasized that among the more commonly used cardiac medications, only angiotensin-converting enzyme inhibitors, angiotensin receptor blockers, and warfarin are known or strongly suspected to be human teratogens. Amiodarone has had mixed data with respect to its safety in pregnancy, with some reports of congenital hypothyroidism, goiter, prematurity, hypotonia, and bradycardia (48,49). While use in an acute setting is appropriate, it is not a first-line agent for maintenance therapy in pregnancy. Angiotensin-converting enzymes and angiotensin receptor blockers both have been associated with fetal anomalies, fetal loss, oligohydramnios, cranial ossification abnormalities, and neonatal renal failure. Although their use in the first trimester was once supported, recent evidence suggests

TABLE 98.6

REVIEWS OF DRUG SAFETY DATA FOR PREGNANCY AND LACTATION

Publication title	Format	Details
Drugs in Pregnancy and Lactation	Hardcover	Authors: Briggs GS, Freeman R, Yaffe S. Published by Lippincott Williams & Wilkins; ISBN: 9780781778763; 8th edition (April 2008)
Shepard's Catalog of Teratogenic Agents	Hardcover reference text	Authors: Shepard T, Lemire RS. Published by Johns Hopkins University Press; ISBN: 9780801887420; 12th edition (November 2007)
Handbook for Prescribing Medications in Pregnancy	Paperback	Authors: Coustan D, Michizuki T. Published by Lippincott Williams & Wilkins; ISBN: 0316158267; 3rd edition (January 15, 1998)
Teratogenic Effects of Drugs: A Resource for Clinicians	Hardcover	Authors: Friedman JM, Polifka JE Published by Johns Hopkins University Press; ISBN: 9780801863875; 2nd edition (July 2000)
Reprotox	Online subscription or diskette PDA version available	www.REPROTOX.org; distributed in Micromedix, Inc.'s, TOMES Reprorisk module
TERIS	Online subscription or diskette	http://depts.washington.edu/~terisweb/teris/; distributed in Micromedix, Inc.'s, TOMES Reprorisk module
Medications & Mothers' Milk: A Manual of Lactational Pharmacology	Softcover	Author: Thomas Hale Published by Pharmasoft Medical Pub; ISBN: 9780981525723; 13th edition (July 2008) Associated website at http://neonatal.ttuhsc.edu/lact/

they should not be used at any time in gestation (50). Warfarin is associated with a high risk of miscarriage and anomalies of the eyes, hands, neck, and central nervous system (51). Again, the guiding principle of managing critical illness in pregnancy should be that because fetal well-being is dependent upon maternal well-being, medications that are of benefit to maternal health should also be considered to be in the fetus' best interest. Useful references for reviewing the available safety data for medications during pregnancy and with breastfeeding are listed in Table 98.6.

For any structural cardiac lesion, we typically will obtain an echocardiogram as a baseline early in pregnancy, in the third trimester, and with any change in clinical status. Additional investigations and interventions should be dictated by the patient's clinical status, and no needed test or procedure should be withheld during gestation. In particular, pregnancy should not limit necessary diagnostic testing (52). Ultrasound has a long history of safe use in pregnancy. The radiation exposure associated with plain film radiographs, nuclear medicine scans, angiography, and CT scans are all well below what is deemed acceptable during pregnancy. Contrast agents appear to be well tolerated by the fetus. Magnetic resonance imaging has not been associated with any ill effects in human pregnancies. Because fetal well-being is dependent on maternal well-being, more harm will generally be caused to a mother and her fetus by withholding necessary investigations than by obtaining them.

Women with congenital heart disease should undergo a detailed fetal ultrasound in the early second trimester to allow early diagnosis of congenital heart disease in the fetus. This will allow informed decision making by the mother, and will prepare the neonatology team should a problem be present.

Labor and delivery and the first 72 hours post partum warrant special consideration with respect to assembling the appropriate team and determining what monitoring will be needed. For most cardiac patients, a multidisciplinary patient care conference should be assembled well in advance of the anticipated time of delivery and a written care plan developed for the peripartum management of the patient. This team should generally include representation from critical care, nursing, anesthesia, obstetrics, and cardiology. The plans that are developed should be explicit and detailed and recognize that the labor and delivery room is a place where cardiac care is not commonly provided. Even the best-trained obstetricians and obstetric nurses will lack the volume of experience in the management of cardiac cases that is common among cardiac and critical care providers. It is our conviction that joint nursing of such patients by obstetric and cardiac-trained nurses during labor and delivery, followed by postpartum care in a cardiac or critical care unit, seems the ideal approach when possible. Table 98.8 offers a check list of parameters to be considered and addressed in a patient care conference dedicated to developing a delivery plan for a cardiac patient.

The mode of delivery should not generally be determined by medical concerns. The need for cesarean deliveries is generally dictated by obstetric concerns, and vaginal deliveries should generally be viewed as the safest and best option for cardiac patients. The choice between spontaneous labor and elective induction of labor should be made both on the likelihood of successful induction and the availability of medical expertise and resources should a cardiac patient go spontaneously into labor during the off hours and weekends.

Most patients should be kept in neutral fluid balance over the course of their delivery period, and careful monitoring of both input and output will be essential. Early and good anesthesia is important to decrease the cardiac work of delivery, and most patients should receive regional anesthesia in a manner that will minimize the need for the fluid

TABLE 98.7

COMMONLY USED CARDIAC MEDICATIONS AND THEIR SAFETY IN PREGNANCY

	Use generally justifiable for this indication in pregnancy	Use justifiable in special circumstances for this indication in pregnancy	Use almost never justifiable for this indication in pregnancy
Arrhythmia	Digoxin β-Blockers (all probably safe but most avoid propanolol and atenolol, which may cause intrauterine growth restriction) Calcium channel blockers, especially verapamil and diltiazem (less known about amlodipine) Adenosine Quinidine Procainamide Lidocaine	Amiodarone Disopyramide, mexiletine, and flecainide (less is known about these agents in pregnancy but there is no evidence at this point of human teratogenesis; they should generally be considered second-line agents in pregnancy)	
Ischemia	Nitrates Low-dose (<100 mg) ASA β-Blockers Heparin (unfractionated or low molecular weight) Tissue plasminogen activator Streptokinase	HMG-coA reductase inhibitors ("statins") have concerning animal pregnancy data, but very limited reported human experiences thus far have been encouraging; should only be used in pregnancy when short-term benefits are clear Abciximab (and other glycoprotein IIb/IIIa inhibitors) dipyridamole, ticlopidine, and clopidogrel lack published human data; they are probably safe but should only be used in pregnancy when short-term benefits are clear	Warfarin
Heart failure	Furosemide Digoxin Hydralazine β-Blockers Dopamine Dobutamine	Nitroprusside (fetal cyanide toxicity possible at high doses)	ACE inhibitors Angiotensin II receptor blockers
Hypertension	Labetalol β-Blockers Nifedipine Hydralazine Methyldopa	Thiazide diuretics (in this category for the treatment of hypertension because of effects of blood volume in pregnancy) Clonidine, prazosin, verapamil, diltiazem, and amlodipine (in this category for the treatment of hypertension because of limited data on safety and the availability of many good alternatives with more data) Nitroprusside (fetal cyanide toxicity possible at high doses)	ACE inhibitors Angiotensin II receptor blockers

ASA, acetylsalicylic acid; ACE, angiotensin-converting enzyme.

boluses typically given to decrease the hypotension associated with establishing regional anesthesia. It is also important to consider that certain lesions, such as an aortic stenosis, may be highly volume dependent and require this additional fluid support.

Intra-arterial lines are advisable for cardiac lesions for which moment-to-moment monitoring of blood pressure might be desirable, such as severe aortic stenosis. The role of the pulmonary artery catheter in the laboring patient remains unclear and, in the absence of clear benefit, it is this author's opinion that their use during delivery should be limited to the most severe cardiac cases, if it is used at all.

Bacterial endocarditis prophylaxis is no longer recommended by the American Heart Association for vaginal or cesarean deliveries because the bacteremia associated with delivery is unlikely to cause endocarditis (53). If done at all, endocarditis prophylaxis should be reserved for patients with prosthetic heart valves, a prior history of subacute bacterial endocarditis, complex cyanotic congenital heart disease, or surgically constructed systemic pulmonary shunts or conduits, and an agent active against enterococci such as penicillin, ampicillin, or vancomycin should be utilized.

It is critical that all team members recognize that the cardiac patient remains at risk for at least 72 hours postpartum, so

(*text continues on page 1456*)

TABLE 98.8

CARDIAC PATIENT DELIVERY PLAN CHECK LIST

PRIOR TO HOSPITALIZATION	
Is additional testing needed to assess risk or guide therapy peripartum? ☐ Baseline ECG done in third trimester ☐ Echocardiogram at any time in the past for lowest-risk lesions, in this pregnancy for moderate-risk lesions, and in the third trimester for high- and highest-risk lesions ☐ Stress testing (exercise echo or dobutamine echo in past year for patients with known or suspected ischemic heart disease or more recently if they are symptomatic) ☐ EP testing for life-threatening arrhythmia investigation (often deferred until postpartum but can be done in pregnancy if warranted)	Consider for all levels of risk.
Has the patient's cardiac status been optimized? ☐ Is medical therapy optimized and have appropriate dose adjustments been made for the changes of pharmacokinetics in pregnancy? ☐ Are there interventions that would be done if the woman was not pregnant that should be done while she is pregnant to optimize patient's status for delivery (e.g., diagnostic or therapeutic cardiac catheterization [angioplasty, stent], valvuloplasty, valve replacement, diagnostic or therapeutic EP studies, AICD or pacemaker placement or adjustment)?	Consider for all levels of risk.
☐ Multidisciplinary team meeting needed and arranged (generally should have occurred by 34 wk). Team should include: ● Nursing (LDR and postpartum care RN +/- ICU/CCU nursing)________ ● Maternal fetal medicine________ ● Anesthesia (ideally obstetric anesthesia, also consider cardiac anesthesia for high- and highest-risk cases) ________ ● Cardiology________ ● ICU/CCU doctor________	Consider having meeting of RN/MFM/Anesthesia for moderate-risk patients and all of the listed providers for high- and highest-risk patients.
☐ Written delivery plan should be generated and distributed and made available to all relevant parties including nursing (should include **who to call and how to do so** when the patient comes in)	Consider for all levels of risk
☐ Case-specific nursing education should occur in advance of delivery.	Consider for all levels of risk. For lowest-risk lesions it may be adequate to have a standardized nursing care plan or the written delivery plan.
INTRAPARTUM	
Determine mode and timing of delivery: ☐ Planned induction at what gestation/cervical status ☐ Planned cesarean delivery at what gestation ☐ Spontaneous delivery	Decision to be made on the basis of obstetric factors and the need to ensure availability of necessary members of the care team. Planned delivery may be advisable for high- and highest-risk patients.
Delivery location: ☐ Standard LDR ☐ Specialized LDR ☐ Obstetric ICU ☐ MICU ☐ CCU	Decision to be made on the basis of local facilities and expertise. In general, care during delivery is best provided in LDR and afterwards in medical setting.

(continued)

TABLE 98.8

(CONTINUED)

Delivery personnel who should be notified of admission (make sure needed parties available on day of any planned delivery) Medical Attendants: ☐ Obstetrician ☐ Cardiologist ☐ Anesthesia (ideally obstetric anesthesia; also consider cardiac anesthesia for high- and highest-risk cases) ☐ Intensivist	Consider having both LDR nurse and critical care nurse for high- and highest-risk patients.
Nursing (Consider need for team approach of ICU/CCU/RR/ER nurse with LDR nurse. Define necessary nurse-to-patient ratio): ☐ LDR nurse ☐ LDR nurse with ACLS training ☐ LDR nurse with ACLS and special critical care training ☐ Critical care nurse (ICU/CCU/RR/ER) nurse	Consider required response time of ACLS trained personnel if nursing team caring for patient is not ACLS certified/experienced This question is particularly important for free-standing obstetric centers.
EDUCATION ☐ Verify written care plan is available to all team members ☐ Is a "recap" in-service for care team advisable on day of delivery?	Consider summary in-service on day of delivery for high- and highest-risk patients and any patient for whom medications may be required urgently that are not routinely used on obstetric floors.
MONITORING Cardiac monitor options (choose one) ☐ Not necessary ☐ To be in room but does not need to be on if patient asymptomatic ☐ To be on patient at all times but not continuously observed ☐ To be on patient at all times and should be continually observed by ACLS-trained individual ☐ To be on patient at all times and should be observed at all times by critical care nurse/MD/PA/RNP	Most cardiac patients aside from the highest-risk patients or those with a history of life-threatening hemodynamically unstable arrhythmias will not need continuous monitoring by ACLS-trained personnel. Low-risk lesions may warrant one of the first two approaches. Moderate- and high-risk lesions may warrant only option 3.
Pulse oximeter (choose one) ☐ Not necessary ☐ Readily available but use only with symptoms ☐ In room and check hourly ☐ In room and on continuously	Pulse oximeter may provide evidence of CHF but should always be interpreted in view of strength of pulse signal. Option 2 is probably adequate for most cardiac patients aside from those with cyanotic heart disease or those in CHF, who probably warrant option 4.
Fetal monitoring	Obtain explicit plan from obstetric team including who will read the fetal monitoring strips and the plan of action should they be concerning.
Defibrillator ☐ On the unit with ready access to defibrillator pads ☐ Defibrillator and defibrillator pads in the room ☐ Defibrillator pads on patient but machine not hooked up ☐ Patient to be monitored using defibrillator with defibrillator pads	Option 1 is generally adequate. Consider other options in highest-risk patients.
IV access ☐ No IV necessary ☐ Single peripheral IV lines needed ☐ Two peripheral IV lines needed ☐ Central line ☐ Central line with CVP ☐ Central line with pulmonary artery catheter	Option 2 is enough for most patients. Consider central line in highest-risk lesions.
Fluid balance	
All patients need strict ins and outs measured throughout hospitalization. Most cardiac patients we will want to keep in a neutral fluid balance during hospitalization. Fluid to be run: _______ Rate: _________	Make sure to add in all fluids given with medications and for regional anesthesia.

(continued)

TABLE 98.8

(CONTINUED)

Arterial line ☐ No arterial line needed ☐ Arterial line warranted	Arterial line advisable when hemodynamics make moment-to-moment monitoring of blood pressure useful (e.g., aortic stenosis)
MEDICATIONS ☐ Need for SBE prophylaxis (SBE prophylaxis for high-risk lesions only and even then not absolutely necessary) ☐ Special issues related to interactions with commonly used obstetric medications ☐ Possibly necessary cardiac medications not routinely used on obstetric units______ ● Need for RN/MD education regarding these medications ● Need for written instructions with respect to preparation and administration of this medication ● Need for medication to be at bedside ● Pharmacy notified in advance of request (especially if free-standing obstetrics hospital)	May be given for prosthetic heart valves, prior SBE, complex cyanotic congenital heart disease, surgically constructed systemic pulmonary shunts or conduits but not necessary for the rest ☐ Standard dosing: Ampicillin 2 g IV plus gentamicin 1.5 mg/kg within 30 min of delivery; ampicillin 1 g IV 6 h after delivery ☐ Penicillin allergy: Vancomycin 1 g IV over 1–2 h plus gentamicin 1.5 mg/kg IV within 30 min of delivery
Anesthetic concerns ☐ Special issues related to anesthesia ☐ Special issues with respect to cautery for cesarean delivery	Anesthesia will determine preferred modality of anesthesia timing and precautions in technique. Implanted defibrillators may need to be turned off prior to surgery because of interference from cautery.
Thromboprophylaxis ☐ Intermittent compression stockings ☐ Heparin 5,000 units SQ q12h ☐ Heparin 5,000 units SQ q8h ☐ Enoxaparin 40 units SQ daily ☐ Enoxaparin 30 units SQ q12h ☐ Full anticoagulation necessary in peripartum period (please see peripartum anticoagulation protocol)	Options 1 and 2 compatible with epidural anesthesia. Options 3–6 should only be done after the epidural catheter is removed. Consider option 1 or 2 antepartum and option 2, 3, 4, or 5 for most patients postpartum while in hospital.
POSTPARTUM How long postpartum will patient require special observation? ☐ Usual period of postpartum observation ☐ 6 h ☐ 12 h ☐ 24 h ☐ 48 h ☐ 72 h ☐ 96 h	Low-risk patients probably only warrant the usual period of observation given all patients. Moderate-risk patients warrant 6 h. High-risk patients warrant between 6 and 48 h and highest-risk patients 72–96 h.
Location of special postpartum observation ☐ Room on regular postpartum floor ☐ Room on high-risk antenatal floor ☐ Standard LDR/postop CS area ☐ Specialized LDR/postop CS area ☐ Obstetric ICU ☐ MICU ☐ CCU ☐ Other________	Option 1, 2, or 3 for low-risk; 2, 3, or 4 for moderate-risk; and 4, 5, 6, or 7 for high- and highest-risk patients

(continued)

TABLE 98.8

(CONTINUED)

MONITORING Cardiac monitor options (choose one) ☐ Not necessary ☐ To be in room but does not need to be on if patient asymptomatic ☐ To be on patient at all times but not continuously observed ☐ To be on patient at all times and should be continually observed by ACLS-trained individual ☐ To be on patient at all times and should be observed at all times by critical care nurse/MD/PA/RNP	Option 1 or 2 for low-risk; 2 or 3 for moderate-risk; 3 for high-risk; and 3, 4 or 5 for highest-risk patients
Postpartum monitoring/interventions recommended and for how long ☐ Peripheral IV________ ☐ Central line________ ☐ CVP________ ☐ Arterial line________ ☐ Pulmonary artery catheter________	No special monitoring or interventions for low-risk patients; 1 for 24 h for moderate-risk patients; and 1 or 2 for 48–72 h for high- and highest-risk patients
All patients need strict ins and outs measured throughout hospitalization. Most cardiac patients we will want to keep in a neutral fluid balance during hospitalization. Fluid to be run: ________ Rate: ________	Make sure to add in all fluids given with medications and for regional anesthesia.
Pulse oximeter in room and checked how often ☐ Not necessary ☐ In room but use only with symptoms ☐ In room and check hourly ☐ In room and on continuously	Pulse oximeter may provide evidence of CHF but should always be interpreted in view of strength of pulse signal. Option 2 probably adequate for most cardiac patients aside from those with cyanotic heart disease and those in CHF, who probably warrant option 4.
Availability of ACLS trained physician/PA/RNP: ☐ Special availability not necessary ☐ Special availability necessary with what maximum response time	
Postpartum care team: Identify the care team and circle who will be the initial contact should medical problems arise. Make sure the person's name and contact number are clearly documented in the chart. Medical Attendants: ☐ Obstetrician ☐ Cardiologist ☐ Anesthesia (ideally obstetric anesthesia; also consider cardiac anesthesia for high- and highest-risk cases) ☐ General internist ☐ ICU team ☐ CCU team ☐ Medical ICU vs. LDR with cardiac nursing (consider need for team approach and necessary nurse-to-patient ratio) ☐ LDR nurse ☐ LDR nurse with ACLS training ☐ LDR nurse with ACLS and special critical care training ☐ Critical care (ICU/CCU/RR/ER) nurse	Consider required response time of ACLS-trained personnel if not present

(continued)

TABLE 98.8

(CONTINUED)

Defibrillator □ On the floor □ In the room □ Pads on patient □ Patient to be monitored with defibrillator pads on □ Special issues related to interactions with commonly used obstetric medications	Option 1 is generally adequate. Consider other options in highest-risk patients.
Thromboprophylaxis START___________ DURATION___________ □ Intermittent compression stockings □ Heparin 5,000 units SQ q 2h □ Heparin 5,000 units SQ q8h □ Enoxaparin 40 units SQ daily □ Enoxaparin 30 units SQ q12h □ Full anticoagulation will be needed postpartum: See peripartum anticoagulation protocol □ Possibly necessary cardiac medications not routinely used on obstetric units___________ ● Need for RN/MD education regarding these medications ● Need for written instructions with respect to preparation and administration of this medication ● Need for medication to be at bedside ● Pharmacy notified in advance of request (especially if free-standing obstetric hospital)	
DISCHARGE PLANNING Will there be any adjustments to medication necessary postpartum (e.g., resumption/replacing of medications stopped/started because of pregnancy OR dosing adjustments necessary in postpartum period because of increases made during pregnancy)? Who will follow the patient after discharge and when will patient need to be seen (letter or phone call should be sent/made to receiving MD): □ Cardiology___________ □ Primary care doctor___________ □ Obstetrics___________	

ECG, electrocardiogram; EP, electrophysiologic; AICD, automatic implantable cardioverter-defibrillator; LDR, labor and delivery room; RN, registered nurse; ICU, intensive care unit; CCU, critical care unit; MFM, maternal–fetal medicine; MICU, medical intensive care unit; RR, recovery room; ER, emergency room; ACLS, Advanced Cardiac Life Support; MD, doctor; PA, physician assistant; RNP, registered nurse practitioner; CHF, congestive heart failure; CVP, central venous pressure; SBE, subacute bacterial endocarditis; CS, cesarean section.

despite the sense of completion that comes with a successful delivery, caregivers need to remain vigilant for early signs of deterioration in the days following the birth.

Specific Lesions

Mitral Stenosis. Rheumatic heart disease remains a common form of heart disease in pregnancy despite its declining incidence in the developed world. Mitral stenosis (MS) accounts for approximately 90% of the rheumatic valvular lesions in pregnancy. It often presents for the first time in pregnancy; risk factors include atrial fibrillation, pulmonary edema, and thromboembolic stroke. Most patients will experience some worsening of symptoms during pregnancy (54). Complication rates were found in one study to be 38% in moderately severe MS and 67% in severe cases (55). Avoidance of tachycardia, increased PA pressure, decreased systemic vascular resistance, and increased central blood volume are essential to patient management. For this reason, many patients will benefit from β-blockade to improve filling time during pregnancy (56). Echocardiograms in these patients should be done once every trimester and with any change in status in these patients. Careful attention should be paid to pulmonary pressures (although echocardiography may provide a less reliable estimate of pulmonary pressures in pregnancy). Pulmonary edema should be treated with diuretics and β-blockade. If symptoms persist despite optimal medical management, percutaneous mitral balloon valvuloplasty, commissurotomy, or even valve replacement may be warranted; all have been successfully performed in pregnancy (57–59). Open procedures may be associated with a higher risk of miscarriage, fetal loss, and preterm labor, and thus balloon valvuloplasty may be preferable at centers experienced with this procedure. Although surgery can be performed at any point in the pregnancy, the risk to the fetus is lowest in the second trimester.

If atrial fibrillation occurs, it should be treated promptly to decrease tachycardia and the associated risk of a low cardiac output state or degeneration into more malignant dysrhythmias. Rate control, full anticoagulation with heparin, and consideration of either medical or electrical cardioversion remain the core management principles in pregnant women with atrial fibrillation as they are for nonpregnant women.

For labor, vaginal delivery or cesarean, excellent pain control is important and is best achieved with early establishment of regional anesthesia. Control of pain will limit the undesirable effects of labor on heart rate and blood pressure. A conservatively dosed lumbar epidural anesthetic with special attention to fluid status, left uterine displacement, and careful use of α-adrenergic agents to treat hypotension is often helpful. These patients are dependent on high left ventricular filling pressures for their cardiac output (60,61). Obstetricians will generally try to limit the second stage of delivery (the "pushing" stage) and assist a prolonged second stage through the use of vacuum extractors or forceps to decrease maternal work. The role of pulmonary artery catheters and intra-arterial lines for cardiac patients in labor was discussed previously and remains unclear. If there is a group who benefits from these interventions, it will likely be those patients with severe obstructive lesions or very poor ejection fractions. If the pulmonary artery catheter is used for patients with mitral stenosis, it will be important to remember that the PAOP may overestimate left ventricular end-diastolic pressure.

Aortic Stenosis. Aortic stenosis is a valvular lesion rarely seen during pregnancy, and can be of rheumatic or congenital origin. Although bicuspid aortic valves are common, they are unlikely to be associated with significant stenosis in the childbearing years. They are, however, associated with an increased risk of both coarctation and dissection. While mild to moderate aortic stenosis is generally well tolerated in pregnancy, severe stenosis (defined as <1.0 cm^2) carries a significant fetal and maternal risk. The rate of complication varies from 10% to 31% (62,63). Ideally, symptomatic aortic stenosis should be repaired prior to pregnancy. If the patient is classified as NYHA functional class III or IV while pregnant, consideration should be given to percutaneous valvuloplasty, surgical repair, or valve replacement. Ideally, such procedures are best done in the middle of the pregnancy but, if necessary, can be done at any time. When severe disease is identified after the first trimester, it is important to be aware that both labor and delivery and a late termination are associated with significant risks. Due to the fixed outflow obstruction, these patients will not tolerate sudden drops in volume or preload, and their peripartum period should be managed in such a way as to minimize the risk of such events and ensure the ability to respond rapidly if and when they do occur. Arterial lines are strongly advised, and the use of pulmonary artery catheters, while not proven, may be of benefit.

In the past, with severe stenotic lesions of the aorta, regional anesthesia has been avoided because of the resulting local anesthetic–induced sympathectomy, which can lead to bradycardia and decreased venous return. However, good results have been obtained in patients with severe aortic stenosis managed during labor with a carefully titrated epidural anesthetic (64,65).

Mitral and Aortic Insufficiency. Mitral insufficiency is the second most common valvular lesion seen in pregnancy, and is typically due to rheumatic heart disease (65). Aortic insufficiency is less common, and may be due to rheumatic, infectious, or rheumatologic conditions. These lesions, when found in isolation, tend to do well in pregnancy unless there is associated ventricular decompensation. Treatments when symptomatic may include diuretics, digoxin, or calcium channel blockers, but angiotensin receptor blockers should not be used despite the benefits of afterload reduction. Increases in systemic vascular resistance, decreased heart rate, atrial arrhythmias, and myocardial depressants may be poorly tolerated. Perhaps the most important peripartum issue for these patients is early regional anesthesia to prevent pain-associated increases in systemic vascular resistance.

Congenital Heart Disease

Approximately 25% of heart disease in pregnancy is congenital. It can be categorized as left-to-right shunt, right-to-left shunt, and aortic lesions.

Left-to-right Shunt. The most common congenital heart lesions are atrial septal defects (ASDs) and ventricular septal defects (VSDs), which are usually well tolerated in pregnancy. The risk of cardiac complications is greatest in patients with large defects. Congestive heart failure (due to increased blood volume in pregnancy leading to cardiac decompensation), atrial arrhythmias, shunt reversal (occurring due to sudden systemic hypotension), and thromboembolic disease are all possible complications seen with ASD and VSD in pregnancy. Ideally, hemodynamically significant septal defects should be repaired prior to pregnancy. However, when symptomatic septal defects present in pregnancy, the principles of management include (a) acetylsalicylic acid (ASA) 81 mg daily to prevent thromboembolism, (b) use of diuretics and digoxin to treat heart failure, (c) avoidance of hypotension with epidural administration or postpartum blood loss, and (d) rapid rate control with any arrhythmia.

Right-to-left Shunt and Pulmonary Hypertension. The high-risk congenital disorders in pregnancy include right-to-left shunts, as seen in Eisenmenger syndrome (any congenital heart lesion with a bidirectional or right-to-left shunt at the atrial, ventricular, or aortic level), and any other lesions associated with significant pulmonary hypertension. Patients with uncorrected cyanotic heart disease have increased spontaneous abortion rates, pulmonary embolization, congestive heart failure, and incidence for congenital heart defects in the fetus. A high hematocrit ($\geq$65%) is not only an indication of the severity of the cardiac disease, but also in itself has a poorer prognosis secondary to complications from hyperviscosity (decreased cardiac output, organ hypoperfusion, and thrombosis).

During pregnancy, right-to-left shunting is increased because of decreased systemic vascular resistance, resulting in decreased pulmonary artery perfusion and hypoxia. A review on maternal and fetal outcome in patients with Eisenmenger syndrome reveals maternal mortality rates of 25% to 52% and fetal loss as high as 44% (66–69). Because of the grim prognosis for these pregnancies, these women should be strongly warned about the dangers of pursuing a pregnancy and, if they do become pregnant, should be offered the opportunity for an early termination. If they continue with the pregnancy, they may warrant hospitalization from 20 weeks onward. Oxygen should be administered for dyspnea, and prophylactic heparin should be considered throughout pregnancy and for 6 weeks postpartum. The mode of delivery should be determined on the basis of obstetric indications. Pulmonary artery catheterization can carry additional risks in patients with significant pulmonary hypertension, and should probably be avoided in these patients. Active efforts should be made to avoid sudden decreases in systemic vascular resistance, blood volume, and venous return. Increased pulmonary vascular resistance promotes right-to-left shunting; therefore, hypercapnia and hypoxia are to be avoided. How best to provide peripartum anesthesia to these patients is not clear, and discussion of this matter is beyond the scope of this chapter. What *is* clear is that if regional anesthesia is used, care must be taken to prevent precipitous drops in venous return. Patients with pulmonary hypertension and/or Eisenmenger syndrome should be observed for 72 hours postpartum in a cardiac setting, as many of the maternal deaths associated with these conditions will occur during this period.

Aortic Disease. Coarctation of the aorta and aortic manifestations of Marfan syndrome pose significant problems in pregnancy (70,71). The physiologic changes during pregnancy, including increased blood volume and increased blood pressure during labor and delivery, may promote aortic dissection in either of these conditions. Patients with coarctation of the aorta may also suffer from worsening hypertension or congestive heart failure in pregnancy.

Marfan syndrome is often associated with aortic dilation, aortic valve regurgitation, and mitral valve disease. Aortic dissection occurs in about 10% of patients with Marfan syndrome who undergo a pregnancy, and is most likely to occur if the aortic root measures beyond 4.5 cm in diameter (72,73). Ideally, women with this severity of aortic root dilation should have their aorta repaired prior to pregnancy. However, if they have not, serial echocardiography during pregnancy to watch for worsening dilation should be performed. If the root is increasing in size, aortic repair should be considered. The activity of patients with significant aortic dilation in pregnancy should be limited, and they should be placed on β-blockers to decrease shear stresses upon the vessel wall (74,75). Although we generally teach that the indications for cesarean delivery are obstetric and not medical, it is common practice to deliver women with aortic roots dilated beyond 4.0 cm by cesarean to avoid additional stressors on the aorta associated with the pain and pushing of a vaginal delivery. However, it is worth noting that the majority of aortic dissections in these patients occur prior to the onset of labor.

Aortic coarctation in pregnancy is associated with an increased risk of worsening hypertension and, less commonly, congestive heart failure or pre-eclampsia (76,77). It is much less likely to be associated with aortic dissection than Marfan syndrome, but dissection can and does occur. Blood pressure should be kept less than 160/100 mm Hg in these patients but not brought below 120/70 mm Hg, as there may be a significant gradient between blood pressure measurement in the arm and the estimated blood pressure of the placenta circulation that is distal to the aortic narrowing. β-Blockers are the preferred antihypertensives for these patients. Patients with coarctation can undergo a vaginal delivery but should have a limited second stage (i.e., prolonged pushing should be avoided by the use of vacuum extractor or forceps).

Tetralogy of Fallot

Tetralogy of Fallot is the most common cyanotic congenital heart disease. It consists of a ventricular septal defect, an overriding aorta, infundibular pulmonary stenosis, and secondary right ventricular hypertrophy. Patients with uncorrected tetralogy have significant complications in pregnancy including biventricular failure, arrhythmias, stroke, and risk of shunt reversal with worsening cyanosis. Preconception surgical repair should be undertaken if at all possible. If these patients do proceed with a pregnancy unrepaired, they should be managed in a manner similar to patients with Eisenmenger syndrome.

Patients with a surgically corrected tetralogy of Fallot who enter a pregnancy with a good functional status generally tolerate pregnancy well. The main risks are right-sided heart failure and arrhythmias. Their volume status should be watched throughout pregnancy and complaints of palpitations or syncope investigated with an event monitor. Delivery should include cardiac monitoring (78–81).

Other Repaired Congenital Heart Conditions

An increasing number of women with congenital heart problems that were repaired in childhood are reaching adulthood and undergoing pregnancy. In general, these patients' course in pregnancy is readily predictable by the parameters outlined earlier in this chapter. The majority will have a good pregnancy outcome for both themselves and their offspring if they enter the pregnancy with a good functional status.

Peripartum Cardiomyopathy

The National Heart, Lung, and Blood Institute (NHLBI) defines peripartum cardiomyopathy (PPCM) as the new onset of systolic dysfunction occurring in the absence of other plausible causes anytime between the final month of pregnancy up to 5 months postpartum. The incidence is between 1 in 3,000 and 1 in 15,000 pregnancies, and may be increasing (82,83). It is most commonly found in women who have twins, women who have pre-eclampsia/eclampsia, and older multiparous women. It is not clear if race is an independent risk factor for PPCM, but it is clear that African American women are more likely to die of PPCM than Caucasian women when it does occur. It is generally quoted that one third of these patients have complete resolution in the year following delivery, one third are left with residual cardiac dysfunction, and one third have progressive cardiac decompensation. The mortality rate is between 9% and 56%, and is highest in the subset of patients with persistent cardiomegaly beyond 6 months. Mortality can be due to end-stage heart failure, arrhythmia, or thromboembolism.

Pathologic findings include four-chamber enlargement with normal coronary arteries and valves. Light microscopic findings include myocardial hypertrophy and fibrosis with scattered mononuclear infiltrates. Clinical signs include symptoms of ventricular failure with possible associated arrhythmias and/or pulmonary emboli. Treatment includes bed rest, sodium restriction, diuresis, and preload/afterload reduction with a calcium channel blocker and hydralazine while pregnant and an angiotensin-converting enzyme inhibitor post partum. Patients with an ejection fraction less than 35% should be considered for anticoagulation with low-molecular-weight heparin while pregnant and warfarin post partum. Antidysrhythmics should be utilized in a manner similar to what would be done for any patient with an idiopathic cardiomyopathy. Although the exact risk remains unclear, there is evidence that peripartum cardiomyopathy may recur or worsen with subsequent pregnancies (84).

Hypertrophic Cardiomyopathy

During pregnancy, the course of hypertrophic cardiomyopathy (HCM) is variable because while the normal increase of blood volume is beneficial, the decrease in systemic vascular resistance and the increase in heart rate may be detrimental. Several large case series have highlighted the risks for these patients during pregnancy (85–87). Complications are not common but include congestive heart failure, chest pain, supraventricular tachycardias, ventricular tachycardia, and sudden death. Complications can occur at any point in the pregnancy or during labor as a result of stress, pain, and increased circulating catecholamines. Moreover, the immediate postpartum period can increase risk due to blood loss and decrease in systemic vascular resistance. Atrial fibrillation and supraventricular tachycardias are a common feature of this cardiac anomaly; thus, cardioselective β-blockers and verapamil are usually administered to these patients. Tocolytics, sympathomimetic agents, and digoxin should be avoided in these patients, as they may increase the risk of arrhythmia. The peripartum period should include cardiac monitoring and use of forceps or vacuum extractor so that the mother has to do little or no pushing. If regional anesthesia is employed, it should be done incrementally and with agents that minimize the risk of a sudden drop in preload.

Ischemic Heart Disease in Pregnancy

Although myocardial infarction in pregnancy is uncommon, with an incidence estimated at between 1 in 10,000 and 1 in 35,700, it does appear to be increasing. Risk factors include advancing age, pre-eclampsia, multiparity, chronic hypertension, and diabetes. Myocardial infarctions associated with pregnancy can occur at any time during gestation, with one report finding that 38% occurred antepartum, 21% intrapartum, and 41% in the first 6 weeks postpartum. Maternal mortality rate ranges from 7% to 35%, with a disproportionate number of deaths occurring among the antenatal cases (88–90). A large portion of pregnancy-associated myocardial infarctions are not due to atherosclerotic heart disease but instead due to coronary artery *in situ* thrombus formation, dissection, or spasm.

Diagnosis of ischemic heart disease in pregnancy does require considering it as part of the differential diagnosis, even in the absence of traditional risk factors. Clinicians should also be aware that creatine phosphokinase (CPK) and creatine kinase-MB (CK-MB) can be mildly elevated following a cesarean delivery and that troponin is a more specific marker of cardiac disease in the peripartum period. All forms of stress testing can be safely carried out in pregnancy, including nuclear imaging, although many centers prefer exercise echocardiography for this population. Diagnostic coronary angiography can and should be performed on pregnant women for the same indications as for nonpregnant patients.

Treatment of coronary artery disease remains largely unchanged in pregnancy. None of the medications commonly used to treat ischemic heart disease has been shown to cause adverse effects in the fetus. There is broad experience with low-dose aspirin, nitrates, β-blockers, and heparins in pregnancy. The paucity of data regarding the use of clopidogrel and the platelet glycoprotein IIb/IIIa inhibitors should limit their use in pregnancy to clinical scenarios with proven benefits. Coronary angiography, angioplasty and stenting, and thrombolysis have been and can be carried out safely throughout pregnancy (91–94).

The management of laboring patients with ischemic heart disease should be the same for other cardiac patients as discussed in the section above on general principles of management of cardiac disease at the time of delivery, and has strong parallels with the management of the cardiac patient undergoing general surgery.

Cardiac Arrhythmias in Pregnancy

Arrhythmias during gestation, and especially labor and delivery, appear to be more common than in the nonpregnant population (95). Hormonal changes, stress, and anxiety are contributing factors; however, most arrhythmias are not serious unless they are associated with organic heart disease.

Atrial Fibrillation

Atrial fibrillation occurring in pregnancy is usually associated with underlying disease such as mitral stenosis, peripartum cardiomyopathy, hypertensive heart disease, thyroid disease, or atrial septal defects. Patients with acute atrial fibrillation and significant hemodynamic changes require direct current cardioversion. Cardioversion appears to have no adverse effects on the fetus. Most patients, however, will require only medical management with rate-controlling or rhythm-restoring antidysrhythmics. β-Adrenergic blockers such as metoprolol, calcium channel blockers such as diltiazem or verapamil, and agents such as procainamide or digoxin can all be used safely during pregnancy. Amiodarone would not be considered a first-line agent for hemodynamically stable atrial fibrillation because of its possible effects on the fetal thyroid, but its use in pregnancy is not absolutely contraindicated. Anticoagulation for atrial fibrillation in pregnancy has the same indications as in nonpregnant patients, but the agent that must be used is heparin (usually in the form of subcutaneous low-molecular-weight heparin) because warfarin is associated with adverse fetal effects throughout gestation.

Supraventricular Tachycardia

Supraventricular tachycardias (SVTs) during pregnancy can occur with or without organic heart disease. Four percent of women with SVT report that their condition was first identified in pregnancy, and up to 22% state that pregnancy exacerbated their condition (96). In the absence of underlying cardiac disease, these tachycardias are not usually associated with increased morbidity. However, in patients with underlying structural cardiac disease or cardiomyopathy, SVT can lead to heart failure and death. Treatment protocols for supraventricular tachycardia remain unchanged in pregnancy and include carotid sinus massage, adenosine (97), calcium channel blockers, β-blockers, and direct current cardioversion (98,99).

Ventricular Arrhythmias

Ventricular arrhythmia during pregnancy may be associated with cocaine use, peripartum or any other form of cardiomyopathy, ischemic heart disease, and digitalis toxicity. Antiarrhythmic agents for which we have the most pregnancy data are lidocaine, β-blockers, and procainamide. Amiodarone is associated with an increased risk of fetal thyroid disease and, although its use in pregnancy is permissible, it should not be considered a first-line agent. Implantable defibrillators can and should be used when indicated in pregnancy, although they will need to be turned off during surgical procedures that require the use of cautery.

Bradycardia

Bradyarrhythmias during pregnancy are rare and may result from Lyme disease, hypothyroidism, myocarditis, and drug-induced, or congenital or acquired heart blocks. Permanent pacemakers are indicated for hemodynamically significant bradycardia. Patients with pre-existing pacemakers may need to have their baseline rate increased during pregnancy to mimic the normal physiologic changes of pregnancy.

Antiarrhythmic Drugs

Table 98.7 classifies the commonly used antiarrhythmic agents on the basis of what is known about their safety in pregnancy. Although there are obviously agents that we know more about than others, it is important to re-emphasize here that both mother and fetus benefit from the use of the best agent to control cardiac symptoms in pregnancy, and treatment should never be withheld from a pregnant woman based on theoretic fears of fetal harm.

Cardiac Surgery During Pregnancy

As in other semi-elective nonobstetric surgery during pregnancy, if nonurgent cardiac surgery is necessary, it should ideally take place during the second trimester. Deferring when possible until after the first trimester avoids the period of organogenesis and the risk of miscarriage. Third-trimester surgery carries the risk of precipitating preterm labor. However, surgery that is important to a patient's short-term well-being and survival should be done at any point in gestation as required. Coronary artery bypass grafts, valvuloplasties, valvular replacements, and aortic root replacements have all been done in pregnancy with good outcomes for mother and baby. When medical management can ameliorate the disease process, surgery may be postponed until the patient has recovered at least 4 to 6 weeks post partum; however, such decisions should be based on the best plan of action for the mother's safety rather than a cultural discomfort related to performing surgery in pregnancy.

Special intraoperative considerations in pregnant patients include (a) fetal monitoring during and after surgery, (b) maintenance of high flow and systemic mean arterial pressure (during cardiopulmonary bypass), and (c) uterine displacement devices if the patient is in the supine position for a median sternotomy. Although the pregnant patient has fared well with open heart procedures, fetal mortality rate can be high. Generally, better results are seen in closed heart procedures. Postoperatively, fetal monitoring should be continued and maternal analgesia maintained to avoid precipitating labor from accelerated postoperative pain.

Pregnancy after Prosthetic Valve Surgery

Patients with mechanical heart valve prostheses pose a significant risk during pregnancy as a result of their coagulation status. Fewer maternal and fetal complications occur with bioprosthetic valves but the need for reoperation on these valves for degenerative changes means they are not commonly used in women of reproductive age.

Heparin, typically low-molecular-weight heparin (LMWH), is the anticoagulant agent of choice during pregnancy because its molecular weight prevents placental crossover, and it is not teratogenic. It is now well established as the anticoagulant of choice in pregnancy for all indications except for mechanical heart valves. Questions still remain as to whether LMWH provides the same level of protection against mechanical valve thrombosis as warfarin. Although warfarin and its derivatives are associated with an increased risk of central nervous system anomalies and warfarin embryopathy, it may be that the risk is worth taking to prevent the catastrophic consequences of valve thrombosis (100–102). Some experts therefore recommend that women with mechanical heart valves use LMWH during the period of organogenesis, switch to warfarin for the majority of the pregnancy, and then switch back to LMWH close to term to avoid both fetal and maternal bleeding associated with delivery. Other experts would use LMWH but carry out frequent testing of the peak and trough heparin levels (also known as anti-Xa levels) to ensure that the patient is adequately anticoagulated.

Cardiac Transplant Patients

With the increasing number and survival of heart transplant recipients, increasing numbers of women who have undergone this procedure have become pregnant (40,41). The pregnancy experience with solid tissue transplant patients in general has found a 25% risk of maternal complications (with over half of these complications being hypertension), a 29% risk of miscarriage, and a 41% risk of prematurity (103). The best data specific to cardiac transplantation describes 32 U.S. pregnancies in women who had undergone cardiac transplantation, and found a 44% rate of hypertension, a 22% risk of rejection, and a 13% risk of worsening renal function. Neonatal complications were similar to the data described above for all solid tissue transplants (104). In light of these data, women who have undergone cardiac transplantation are warned of the possible risks of a pregnancy, and are encouraged to wait 2 years after transplantation before becoming pregnant to ensure that the transplant has been a success. Drugs used to prevent rejection should be continued during pregnancy; evidence of their safety is accumulating. If antirejection treatment is continued, pregnancy does not appear to increase the risk of rejection (104,105). The peripartum management should be dictated by the quality of left ventricular function in a manner similar to that discussed previously in this chapter.

Cardiopulmonary Resuscitation

Pregnancy poses some unique problems during cardiopulmonary resuscitation (CPR). In the third trimester and particularly near term, the gravid uterus impairs venous return. Thus, during CPR, the uterus should be displaced (i.e., left uterine tilt). Moreover, if defibrillation is required, the left breast needs to be displaced because of marked enlargement during pregnancy. The unlikely but theoretical possibility that there may be electrical arcing between a defibrillator and any fetal monitoring devices means that fetal monitoring devices should be removed prior to defibrillation. Otherwise, the Advanced Cardiac Life Support (ACLS) protocols, including medications and the use of the defibrillator, should be followed as done in a nonpregnant patient. Some experts would suggest that the use of amiodarone should be deferred in cardiac resuscitation until alternative appropriate agents have failed. However, in the context of a cardiac arrest, this author would support the use of any recommended ACLS medication, as the one-time use of any of these agents is very unlikely to be of any harm, and may be of great benefit to both mother and fetus.

Data about the risk and benefits of an emergency cesarean delivery in the context of maternal resuscitation are very limited. The present-day view is that if the fetus has reached a point in the pregnancy where survival after delivery is possible (typically more than 24 weeks' gestation), emergency cesarean should be considered a part of the resuscitative efforts. Evacuation of the gravid uterus, with the concomitant release of pressure on the inferior vena cava and removal of the low-resistance circulatory unit that is the placenta, may improve the efficacy of chest compressions and improve the outcome for both mother and baby. Present recommendations are for consideration of cesarean delivery in pregnant women greater than 24 weeks' gestation who have had a cardiac arrest and failed to respond to 5 minutes of aggressive and appropriate resuscitative efforts (106).

An extensive review of this topic is available on the American Society of Anesthesiology website.

References

1. National High Blood Pressure Education Program Working Group report on high blood pressure in pregnancy. *Am J Obstet Gynecol.* 1990;163:1689.
2. Powrie RO. A 30-year-old woman with chronic hypertension trying to conceive. *JAMA.* 2007;298(13):1548.
3. Sibai B, Dekker G, Kupferminc M. Pre-eclampsia. *Lancet.* 2005;365(9461):785.
4. Bletka M, Hlavatj V, Tenkova M, et al. Volume of whole blood and absolute amount of serum proteins in the early stages of late toxemia of pregnancy. *Am J Obstet Gynecol.* 1970;106:10.
5. Bletka M, Hlavatj V, Tenkova M, et al. Volume of whole blood and absolute amount of serum proteins in the early stages of late toxemia of pregnancy. *Am J Obstet Gynecol.* 1970;106:10.
6. Redman CW, Sargent IL. Latest advances in understanding pre-eclampsia. *Science.* 2005;308(5728):1592.
7. Sibai B, Dekker G, Kupferminc M. Pre-eclampsia. *Lancet.* 2005;365(9461):785–799.
8. Levine RJ, Lam C, Qian C, Yu KF, et al. Soluble endoglin and other circulating anti-angiogenic factors in pre-eclampsia. *N Engl J Med.* 2006;355(10):992.
9. Levine RJ, Maynard SE, Qian C, et al. Circulating angiogenic factors and the risk of pre-eclampsia. *N Engl J Med.* 2004;350(7):672.
10. Levine RJ, Thadhani R, Qian C, et al. Urinary placental growth factor and risk of pre-eclampsia. *JAMA.* 2005;293(1):77.
11. Powrie RO, Miller MA. Hypertension in pregnancy. In: Rosene-Montella K, Lee R, Keely EJ, et al., eds. *Medical Care of the Pregnant Patient.* Philadelphia: American College of Physicians; 2007:153–162.
12. Natarajan P, Shennan AH, Penny J, et al. Comparison of auscultatory and oscillometric automated blood pressure monitors in the setting of pre-eclampsia. *Am J Obstet Gynecol.* 1999;181(5 Pt 1):1203.
13. von Dadelszen P, Magee LA, Devarakonda RM, et al. The prediction of adverse maternal outcomes in pre-eclampsia. *J Obstet Gynaecol Can.* 2004;26(10):871.
14. Lam C, Lim KH, Kang DH, et al. Uric acid and pre-eclampsia. *Semin Nephrol.* 2005;25(1):56.
15. Rodriguez-Thompson D, Lieberman ES. Use of a random urinary protein-to-creatinine ratio for the diagnosis of significant proteinuria during pregnancy. *Am J Obstet Gynecol.* 2001;185(4):808.
16. Durwald C, Mercer B. A prospective comparison of total protein/creatinine ratio versus 24-hour urine protein in women with suspected pre-eclampsia. *Am J Obstet Gynecol.* 2003;189(3):848.
17. Magee LA, Cham C, Waterman EJ, et al. Hydralazine for treatment of severe hypertension in pregnancy: meta-analysis. *BMJ.* 2003;327(7421):955.
18. Magee LA, Miremadi S, Li J, et al. Therapy with both magnesium sulfate and nifedipine does not increase the risk of serious magnesium-related maternal side effects in women with pre-eclampsia. *Am J Obstet Gynecol.* 2005;193(1):153.
19. Sibai BM. Diagnosis, prevention, and management of eclampsia. *Obstet Gynecol.* 2005;105(2):402.
20. Duley L. Evidence and practice: the magnesium sulphate story. *Best Pract Res Clin Obstet Gynaecol.* 2005;19(1):57.
21. Jeng JS, Tang SC, Yip PK. Stroke in women of reproductive age: comparison between stroke related and unrelated to pregnancy. *J Neurol Sci.* 2004;221(1–2):25.
22. Sibai BM, Mabie BC, Harvey CJ, et al. Pulmonary edema in severe pre-eclampsia-eclampsia: analysis of thirty-seven consecutive cases. *Am J Obstet Gynecol.* 1987;156(5):1174.
23. Bandi VD, Munnur U, Matthay MA. Acute lung injury and acute respiratory distress syndrome in pregnancy. *Crit Care Clin.* 2004;20(4):577.
24. Powrie RO, Levy M. Pulmonary edema in pregnancy. In: Rosene-Montella K, Lee R, Keely EJ, et al., eds. *Medical Care of the Pregnant Patient.* Philadelphia: American College of Physicians; 2007:383–394.
25. Letsky EA. Disseminated intravascular coagulation. *Best Pract Res Clin Obstet Gynaecol.* 2001;15(4):623.
26. Kramer RL, Izquierdo LA, Gilson GJ, et al. Pre-eclamptic labs for evaluating hypertension in pregnancy. *J Reprod Med.* 1997;42:223.
27. Gammil HS, Jeyabalan A. Acute renal failure in pregnancy. *Crit Care Med.* 2005;33(10 Suppl):S372.
28. Dotsch J, Hohmann M, Kuhl PG. Neonatal morbidity and mortality associated with maternal hemolysis elevated liver enzymes and low platelets syndrome. *Eur J Pediatr.* 1997;156:389.
29. Baxter JK, Weinstein L. HELLP syndrome: the state of the art. *Obstet Gynecol Surv.* 2004;59(12):838.
30. van Runnard Heimel PJ, Franx A, Schobben AF, Corticosteroids, pregnancy, and HELLP syndrome a review. *Obstet Gynecol Surv.* 2005;60(1):57.
31. Katz L, de Amorim MM, Figueiroa JN, et al. Postpartum dexamethasone for women with hemolysis, elevated liver enzymes, and low platelets (HELLP) syndrome: a double-blind, placebo-controlled, randomized clinical trial. *Am J Obstet Gynecol.* 2008;198(3):283.
32. Sheikh RA, Yasmeen S, Pauly MP, et al. Spontaneous intrahepatic hemorrhage and hepatic rupture in the HELLP syndrome: four cases and a review. *J Clin Gastroenterol.* 1999;28(4):323.
33. Kalelioglu I, Kubat Uzum A, Yildirim A, et al. Transient gestational diabetes insipidus diagnosed in successive pregnancies: review of pathophysiology, diagnosis, treatment, and management of delivery. *Pituitary.* 2007;10(1):87.
34. Strauss RG, Keefer JR, Burke T, et al. Hemodynamic monitoring of cardiogenic pulmonary edema complicating toxemia of pregnancy. *Obstet Gynecol.* 1980;55:170.
35. Benedetti TJ, Cotton DB, Read JC, et al. Hemodynamic observations in severe pre-eclampsia with a flow-directed pulmonary artery catheter. *Am J Obstet Gynecol.* 1980;136:465.
36. Young P, Johanson R. Haemodynamic, invasive and echocardiographic monitoring in the hypertensive parturient. *Best Pract Res Clin Obstet Gynaecol.* 2001;15(4):605.
37. Fujitani S, Baldisseri MR. Hemodynamic assessment in a pregnant and peripartum patient. *Crit Care Med.* 2005t;33(10 Suppl):S354.
38. Young PF, Leighton NA, Jones PW, et al. Fluid management in severe pre-eclampsia (VESPA): survey of members of ISSHP. *Hypertens Pregnancy.* 2000;19(3):249–259.
39. Elkayam U, Gleicher N. *Cardiac Problems in Pregnancy: Diagnosis and Management of Maternal and Fetal Heart Disease.* New York City: Wiley Liss; 1998.
40. James CF, Banner T, Levelle JP, et al. Noninvasive determination of cardiac output throughout pregnancy. *Anesthesiology.* 1985;63(Suppl 3 A):A434.
41. Robson SC, Dunlop W, Boys RJ, et al. Cardiac output during labour. *BMJ.* 1987;295:1169.
42. Capeless EL, Clapp JF. When do cardiovascular parameters return to their preconception values? *Am J Obstet Gynecol.* 1991;165:883.

43. Clark SL, Cotton DG, Lee W, et al. Central hemodynamic assessment. *Am J Obstet Gynecol.* 1989;161:1439.
44. Munnur U, de Boisblanc B, Suresh MS. Airway problems in pregnancy. *Crit Care Med.* 2005;33(10 Suppl):S259.
45. Ueland K, Hansen JM. Maternal cardiovascular dynamics. II, Posture and uterine contractions. *Am J Obstet Gynecol.* 1969;103.
46. Gogarten W. Spinal anaesthesia for obstetrics. *Best Pract Res Clin Anaesthesiol.* 2003;17(3):377.
47. Siu SC, Sermer M, Colman JM, et al. Prospective multicenter study of pregnancy outcomes in women with heart disease. *Circulation.* 2001;104:515.
48. Pradhan M, Manisha M, Singh R, et al. Amiodarone in treatment of fetal supraventricular tachycardia. A case report and review of literature. *Fetal Diagn Ther.* 2006;21(1):72.
49. Lomenick JP, Jackson WA, Backeljauw PF. Amiodarone-induced neonatal hypothyroidism: a unique form of transient early-onset hypothyroidism. *J Perinatol.* 2004;24(6):397.
50. Cooper WO, Hernandez-Diaz S, Arbogast PG, et al. Major congenital malformations after first-trimester exposure to ACE inhibitors. *N Engl J Med.* 2006;354(23):2443.
51. Schaefer C, Hannemann D, Meister R, et al. Vitamin K antagonists and pregnancy outcome. A multi-centre prospective study. *Thromb Haemost.* 2006;95(6):940.
52. Patel SJ, Reede DL, Katz DS, Subramaniam R, et al. Imaging the pregnant patient for nonobstetric conditions: algorithms and radiation dose considerations. *Radiographics.* 2007;27(6):1705.
53. Wilson W, Taubert KA, Gewitz M, et al. Prevention of infective endocarditis: guidelines from the American Heart Association. *Circulation.* 2007;116:1736.
54. Hameed A, Karaalp IS, Tummala PP, et al. The effect of valvular heart disease on maternal and fetal outcome of pregnancy. *J Am Coll Cardiol.* 2001; 37:893.
55. Silversides CK, Colman JM, Sermer M, et al. Cardiac risk in pregnant women with rheumatic mitral stenosis. *Am J Cardiol.* 2003;91:1382.
56. al Kasab SM, Sabag T, al Zaibag M, et al. Beta-adrenergic receptor blockade in the management of pregnant women with mitral stenosis. *Am J Obstet Gynecol.* 1990;163:37.
57. Esteves CA, Ramos AL, Braga SL. Effectiveness of percutaneous balloon mitral valvotomy during pregnancy. *Am J Cardiol.* 1991;68:930.
58. de Souza JAM, Martinez EE, Ambrose JA, et al. Percutaneous balloon mitral valvuloplasty in comparison with open mitral valve commissurotomy for mitral stenosis during pregnancy. *J Am Coll Cardiol.* 2001;37:900.
59. Sullivan HJ. Valvular heart surgery during pregnancy. *Surg Clin North Am.* 1995;75:59.
60. Oakley C, Child A, Jung B. Expert consensus document on management of cardiovascular disease during pregnancy. *Eur Heart J.* 2003;24:761.
61. Elkayam U, Bitar F. Valvular heart disease and pregnancy. *J Am Coll Cardiol.* 2005;46:223.
62. Silversides CK, Colman JM, Sermer M, et al. Early and intermediate-term outcomes of pregnancy with congenital aortic stenosis. *Am J Cardiol.* 2003;91(11):1386.
63. Singh H, Bolton PJ, Oakley CM. Pregnancy after surgical correction of tetralogy of Fallot. *BMJ.* 1982;285:168.
64. Easterling TR, Chadwick HS, Otto CM, et al. Aortic stenosis in pregnancy. *Obstet Gynecol.* 1988;72:113.
65. Graham TP. Ventricular performance in adults after operation for congenital heart disease. *Am J Cardiol.* 1982;50:612.
66. Gleicher N, Midwall J, Hochberger D, et al. Eisenmenger's syndrome and pregnancy. *Obstet Gynecol Surv.* 1979;34:721.
67. Avila WS, Grinberg M, Snitcowsky R, et al. Maternal and fetal outcome in pregnant women with Eisenmenger's syndrome. *Eur Heart J.* 1995;16:460.
68. Yentis SM, Steer PJ, Plaat F. Eisenmenger's syndrome in pregnancy; maternal and fetal mortality in the 1990s. *Br J Obstet Gynaecol.* 1998;105:921.
69. Elkayam U, Ostzega A, Shotan A, et al. Cardiovascular problems in pregnant women with the Marfan syndrome. *Ann Intern Med.* 1995;123:117.
70. Lipscomb KJ, Smith JC, Clarke B, et al. Outcome of pregnancy in women with Marfan's syndrome. *BJOG.* 1997;104:201.
71. Lind J, Wallenburg HC. The Marfan syndrome and pregnancy: a retrospective study in a Dutch population. *Eur J Obstet Gynecol Reprod Biol.* 2001;98:28.
72. Rossiter JP, Repke JT, Morales AJ, et al. A prospective longitudinal evaluation of pregnancy in the Marfan syndrome. *Am J Obstet Gynecol.* 1995;173:1599.
73. Oakley C, Child A, Jung B. Expert consensus document on management of cardiovascular disease during pregnancy. *Eur Heart J.* 2003;24: 761–781.
74. Carabello BA, Chatterjee K, de Leon AC, et al. ACC/AHA 2006 guidelines for the management of patients with valvular heart disease. *J Am Coll Cardiol.* 2006;48:1.
75. Beauchesne LM, Connolly HM, Ammash NM, et al. Coarctation of the aorta; outcome of pregnancy. *J Am Coll Cardiol.* 2001;38(6):1728.
76. Vriend JW, Drenthen W, Pieper PG, et al. Outcome in pregnancy in patients after repair of aortic coarctation. *Eur Heart J.* 2005;26(20):2173.
77. Fishburne JI Jr, Dormer KJ, Payne GG, et al. Effects of amrinone and dopamine on uterine blood flow and vascular responses in the gravid baboon. *Am J Obstet Gynecol.* 1988;158:829.
78. Meijer JM, Pieper PG, Drenthen W, et al. Pregnancy, fertility and recurrence risk in corrected tetralogy of Fallot. *Heart.* 2005;91:801.
79. Presbitero P, Somerville J, Stone S, et al. Pregnancy in cyanotic congenital heart disease: outcome of mother and fetus. *Circulation.* 1994;89:2673.
80. Patton DE, Lee W, Cotton DB, et al. Cyanotic maternal heart disease in pregnancy. *Obstet Gynecol Surv.* 1990;45:594–600.
81. Bernstein PS, Magriples U. Cardiomyopathy in pregnancy: a retrospective study. *Am J Perinatol.* 2001;18:163.
82. Avila WS, de Carvalho ME, Tschaen CK, et al. Pregnancy and peripartum cardiomyopathy. A comparative and prospective study. *Arq Bras Cardiol.* 2002;79:484.
83. Sliwa K, Fett J, Elkayam U. Peripartum cardiomyopathy. *Lancet.* 2006; 368(9536):687.
84. Autore C, Conte MR, Piccininno M, et al. Risk associated with pregnancy in hypertrophic cardiomyopathy. *J Am Coll Cardiol.* 2002;40:1864.
85. Thaman R, Varnava A, Hamid MS, et al. Pregnancy related complications in women with hypertrophic cardiomyopathy. *Heart.* 2003;89:752.
86. Wigle ED, Rakowski H, Kimball BP, et al. Hypertrophic cardiomyopathy: clinical spectrum and treatment. *Circulation.* 1995;92:1680.
87. James AH, Jamison MG, Biswas MS, et al. Acute myocardial infarction in pregnancy: a United States population-based study. *Circulation.* 2006;113: 1564.
88. Badin E, Enciso R. Acute myocardial infarction during pregnancy and puerperium: a review. *Angiology.* 1996;47:739.
89. Ladner HE, Danielsen B, Gilbert WM. Acute myocardial infarction in pregnancy and the puerperium: a population-based study. *Obstet Gynecol.* 2005;105:480.
90. Turrentine MA, Braems G, Ramirez MM. Use of thrombolytics for the treatment of thromboembolic disease during pregnancy. *Obstet Gynecol Surv.* 1995;50:534.
91. Cowan NC, deBelder MA, Rothman MT. Coronary angioplasty in pregnancy. *Br Heart J.* 1988;59:588.
92. Giudici MC, Artis AK, Webel RR, et al. Postpartum myocardial infarction treated with balloon coronary angioplasty. *Am Heart J.* 1989;118:614.
93. Saxena R, Nolan TE, von Dohlen T, et al. Postpartum myocardial infarction treated by balloon coronary angioplasty. *Obstet Gynecol.* 1992;79:810.
94. Shotan A, Ostrzega E, Mehra A, et al. Incidence of arrhythmias in normal pregnancy and relation to palpitations, dizziness, and syncope. *Am J Cardiol.* 1997;79:1061.
95. Lee SH, Chen SA, Chiang CE, et al. Effects of pregnancy on first onset and symptoms of paroxysmal supraventricular tachycardia. *Am J Cardiol.* 1995;76:675.
96. Nunley WC, Kolp LA, Dabinett LN, et al. Subsequent fertility in women who undergo cardiac surgery. *Am J Obstet Gynecol.* 1989;161:573.
97. Tawan M, Levine J, Mendelson M, et al. Effect of pregnancy on paroxysmal supraventricular tachycardia. *Am J Cardiol.* 1993;72:838.
98. Silversides CK, Harris L, Haberer K, et al. Recurrence rates of arrhythmias during pregnancy in women with previous tachyarrhythmia and impact on fetal and neonatal outcomes. *Am J Cardiol.* 2006;97:1206.
99. Chan WS, Anand S, Ginsberg JS. Anticoagulation of pregnant women with mechanical heart valves: a systematic review of the literature. *Arch Intern Med.* 2000;160:191.
100. Maxwell CV, Poppas A, Dunn E, et al. Pregnancy, mechanical heart valves and anticoagulation: navigating the complexities of management during gestation. In: Rosene-Montella K, Keely EJ, Lee RV, et al., eds. *Medical Care of the Pregnant Patient.* 2nd ed. Philadelphia: American College of Physicians; 2007:344–355.
101. Bonow RO, Carabello BA, Chatterjee K, et al. ACC/AHA 2006 guidelines for the management of patients with valvular heart disease: a report of the American College of Cardiology/American Heart Association Task Force on Practice Guidelines. (Writing Committee to revise the 1998 Guidelines for the Management of Patients With Valvular Heart Disease): developed in collaboration with the Society of Cardiovascular Anesthesiologists: endorsed by the Society for Cardiovascular Angiography and Interventions and the Society of Thoracic Surgeons. *Circulation.* 2006;114:e84.
102. Miniero R, Tardivo I, Curtoni ES, et al. Outcome of pregnancy after organ transplantation: a retrospective survey in Italy. *Transplant Int.* 2005; 17:724.
103. Wagoner L, Taylor D, Olson S, et al. Immunosuppressive therapy, management and outcomes of heart transplant recipients during pregnancy. *J Heart Lung Transplant.* 1993;12:993.
104. Branch KR, Wagoner LE, McGrory CH, et al. Risk of subsequent pregnancies on mother and newborn in female heart transplant recipients. *J Heart Lung Transplant.* 1998;17:698.
105. Wagoner L, Taylor D, Olson S, et al. Immunosuppressive therapy, management and outcomes of heart transplant recipients during pregnancy. *J Heart Lung Transplant.* 1993;12:993.
106. Mallampalli A, Guy E. Cardiac arrest in pregnancy and somatic support after brain death. *Crit Care Med.* 2005;33(10 Suppl):S325.

CHAPTER 99 ■ HEMORRHAGIC AND LIVER DISORDERS OF PREGNANCY

KAREN BORDSON • CARL P. WEINER

IMMEDIATE CONCERNS

Major Problems

Maternal mortality is defined as deaths occurring during pregnancy or within 6 weeks postpartum, with the cause of death identified as complications related to pregnancy, delivery, or the puerperium (International Classification of Diseases, 9th Revision, codes 630–676). It has decreased significantly over the past century, falling from 850 deaths per 100,000 deliveries in 1900 to 7.5 deaths per 100,000 in 1982 (1). This rate has remained stable at approximately 7.5 per 100,000 deliveries between 1982 and 1996. Hemorrhage and hypertensive disorders are the major contributors to maternal death rates (2). Hemorrhagic disorders can become life threatening and quickly challenge the obstetrician. Appropriate care requires an efficient plan with the understanding of the special complications associated with pregnancy and the gravid uterus. There are two main subtopics in this chapter that the reader needs to consider; these include placental complications (abruption and previa) and the HELLP syndrome (hemolysis, elevated liver enzymes, and low platelets)/disseminated intravascular coagulation (DIC).

As hepatic disorders in pregnancy can be devastating to both fetus and the pregnant patient, this chapter will address liver disorders related to pregnancy, specifically hyperemesis gravidarum, intrahepatic cholestasis of pregnancy, and acute fatty liver of pregnancy.

Stress Points

1. The physician must be aware of the potential hemorrhagic complications to which pregnancy predisposes the patient and fetus, and the physiologic and pathologic risk factors. Rapid diagnosis and treatment are critical to patient safety.
2. Liver disorders can vary from irritating and relatively minor, to life threatening with significant morbidity and mortality.

HEMORRHAGIC CONCERNS

Significant bleeding in pregnancy can be quantified by total amount, or by amount and time period over which the bleeding occurred (3,4). Generally, postpartum hemorrhage—defined by the total estimated blood loss—is established when there is greater than 500 mL for vaginal deliveries and more than 1 L for cesarean deliveries; additionally, clinical symptoms and signs with respect to the blood loss are considered in the management.

Coagulation Changes

In pregnancy, if factors are measured, one will note an increase in factors I (fibrinogen), VII, VIII, IX, and X. Functional tests, such as the prothrombin time (PT), partial thromboplastin time (PTT), and bleeding times (BT) should not change in a normal pregnancy.

The reader is asked to refer to Chapter 49 for more detailed description of essential physiologic concerns related to coagulation and Chapter 170 for coagulation disorders.

PLACENTAL COMPLICATIONS

Placental Abruption

Placental abruption (abruptio placentae) is a condition in which the placenta separates from the implantation site of the uterus prior to the delivery of the fetus. The area of hemorrhage along the decidua basalis expands as the bleeding progresses. This hematoma may be concealed or present clinically with vaginal bleeding. The underlying mechanism may be related to vascular damage caused by preeclampsia, trauma, cocaine/alcohol use, or chorioamnionitis. Risk factors for abruption include either maternal or paternal (secondhand) smoking, multiparity, prior caesarean delivery, and African American ethnicity (5,6). The incidence ranges between 0.4% and 0.8%, and there is a 15% recurrence rate for a subsequent pregnancy and a 20% recurrence rate for two previous episodes (7). Morbidity and mortality of both the mother and fetus can be significant with this process if the hemorrhage is significant.

Classic clinical manifestations include vaginal bleeding, abdominal pain/uterine irritability, and fetal heart rate abnormalities or fetal distress; of note, however, is that none or all of these symptoms may be present. Ultrasound has limited usefulness as it reveals a retroplacental blood clot in only 15% of cases, thus giving a high false-negative rate (5).

Treatment with fluid resuscitation, adequate oxygenation, and close fetal monitoring is critical. With evidence of significant hemorrhage or fetal distress, delivery must be expedited. It is critical to anticipate additional postpartum complications, such as uterine atony, to limit further hemorrhage.

Placenta Previa

Placental previa occurs with improper implantation of the placenta such that it overlies the internal os of the cervix during the third trimester. Traditionally, placenta previa was referenced

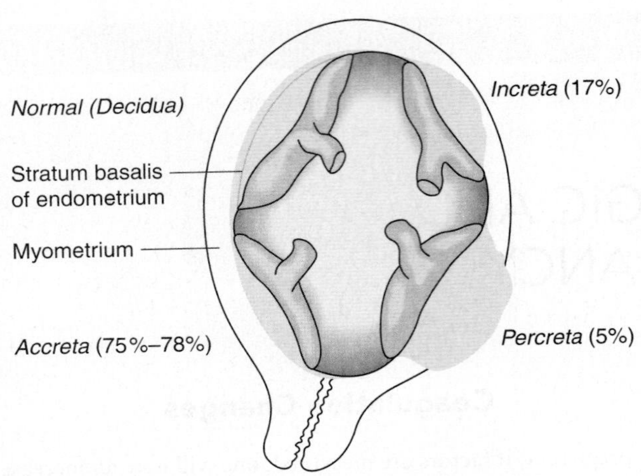

FIGURE 99.1. Placental implantation abnormalities (public domain image per http://en.wikipedia.org/wiki/Image:Placenta_accreta.png).

with different classifications of previa and low-lying placentas. However, with current ultrasound capabilities, this classification scheme has limited utility.

The incidence of placenta previa is noted to be approximately 0.5% (8); however, with the increased rates of cesarean deliveries and advancing maternal age, there is concern regarding an increase in that incidence in the future (9). Risk factors include prior placenta previa, a history of cesarean delivery, a history of suction curettage, maternal age older than 35 years, African American or non-Caucasian ethnicity, and cigarette smoking.

Clinical symptoms include painless vaginal bleeding beginning in the second or third trimester. Ultrasound is then performed to confirm or rule out the diagnosis. Management is expectant unless maternal bleeding or fetal heart rate abnormalities/fetal distress necessitates imminent delivery via cesarean section. If the patient is stable—meaning no bleeding—and the fetal surveillance is reassuring, the patient is closely monitored on pelvic rest (nothing per vagina, no vaginal exam, no intercourse) until fetal lung maturity or 37 weeks' gestation, at which time a cesarean delivery is performed. Risks of placenta previa include other placental implantation abnormalities, such as placenta accreta, placenta increta, and placenta percreta (Fig. 99.1). The physician must be aware of these risks at the time of delivery and be prepared for a possible cesarean hysterectomy (hysterectomy performed at the time of the cesarean delivery) if necessary.

HEMOLYSIS, ELEVATED LIVER ENZYMES, AND LOW PLATELETS (HELLP) SYNDROME AND DISSEMINATED INTRAVASCULAR COAGULATION (DIC)

The topic of preeclampsia/eclampsia is discussed in Chapter 98, Cardiac Disease and Hypertensive Disorders in Pregnancy.

The acronym, HELLP, for the syndrome consisting of hemolysis, elevated liver enzymes, and low platelets, was first used by Weinstein in 1982 (10). The clinical entity was first noted by Pritchard et al. in 1954 (11). It is currently thought to be a distinct variant, rather than a progression, of the preeclampsia/eclampsia continuum. The incidence is rare, with Bhattacharya and Campbell (12) noting 13 cases of HELLP in a population of 4,188 patients with preeclampsia (310 per 100,000 patients). Although much speculated, the true cause is unclear. Older theories dealt with long-chain 3-hydroxyacyl-CoA (LCHAD) and other fatty acid oxidation defects. However, these have not been proven to be major risk factors in HELLP (13,14). Current research has found associations with genetic mutations of the Fas gene and regulation of the immune system (15,16). There are also studies regarding the prognostic values of hyaluronic acid (17) and serotonin (18) to evaluate liver function and platelet activation, respectively. Risk factors have been shown to include African Americans (19) and a history of prior pregnancy with HELLP. The recurrence rate has been reported as 14% (20).

HELLP is a disease with significant morbidity and mortality, both maternal and perinatal. In a prospective study of 442 pregnancies with HELLP, the risk of maternal death was found to be 1.1% (21). Significant maternal morbidity included DIC (21%), placental abruption (16%), acute renal failure (7.7%), pulmonary edema (6%), and rare occurrences of subcapsular liver hematoma and retinal detachment (22). Additionally, case reports of hepatic rupture (23–26) have been documented. Fetal outcome is typically related to the necessity to proceed with preterm delivery. Neonatal outcomes include risk of intensive care requirements, mechanical ventilation, sepsis, and intraventricular hemorrhage (27).

The clinical features and laboratory evaluation of HELLP have not been firmly defined. Generally, the findings reflect the disease process on the vascular supply of the maternal liver. The hemolysis can be noted by an abnormal peripheral smear, elevated serum bilirubin, low serum haptoglobin levels, elevated lactate dehydrogenase (LDH) of subtypes LDH1/LDH2, or a fall in the hemoglobin (22). Elevated liver enzymes, generally aspartate transaminases (AST), alanine transferase (ALT) and/or bilirubin, are present; however, there is no strict definition of the degree of elevation. There is also great variability in establishing the criteria for low platelets, varying from 150,000 to less than 50,000 cells/μL. Patients with HELLP also have altered vascular reactivity (28), and methods of prediction of HELLP by Doppler ultrasound have been examined, revealing a decrease in dual hepatic blood supply preceding the onset of HELLP (29,30). Objective parameters for DIC include prolonged prothrombin time (PT) and activated partial thromboplastin time (aPTT), elevated fibrinogen degradation products, and elevated D-dimers; as fibrinogen is increased in a normal pregnancy, the value in DIC may decrease to "normal" (nonpregnant) values, so it is not used as an objective parameter.

Treatment of HELLP includes supportive care in a facility suited for such high-level care. Prompt delivery of the fetus is indicated if the patient is beyond 34 gestational weeks, or sooner if the disease has progressed to multiorgan dysfunction, DIC, liver infarction or hemorrhage, renal failure, suspected placental abruption, or a nonreassuring fetal status (22).

There is more controversy regarding the recommendations if the pregnancy is less than 34 weeks' gestation and there are only mild to moderate laboratory abnormalities. Generally, expectant management and corticosteroids for fetal lung maturity are given with delivery after completion of the course of steroids. There is significant debate over use of steroids for *treatment* of the laboratory abnormalities of HELLP. Some studies have shown clinical benefit (31,32), whereas others, including a Cochrane Database review (33), find insufficient evidence of beneficial effect. This topic, among others, was specifically discussed at the 2004 Annual Meeting of the Society for Maternal-Fetal Medicine (34), with the conclusion that insufficient evidence of beneficial effect exists and there is a need for further studies. Additionally, the benefit of plasma exchange therapy has been shown to improve treatment outcome (35). Heparin therapy, however, is associated with further bleeding complications (36). Management of DIC must address the underlying cause (37); transfusion of both packed red cells and component therapy as indicated, as well as fluid replacement and oxygenation, are critical. There are investigations examining the role of solvent-detergent plasma (38) and aprotinin (39) in HELLP, the results of which appear safe and improve laboratory indices of coagulopathy.

LIVER CONCERNS

Physiologic Changes Associated with Pregnancy

Pregnancy-related hormones and fetal enzymes significantly affect the maternal liver. Known changes in the liver profile reveal a decrease in serum albumin secondary to the dilutional effect of a 50% increase in maternal plasma volume. There is also an increase in serum alkaline phosphatase due to placental/fetal production. Markers of liver injury, such as aspartate aminotransferase, alanine aminotransferase, and lactate dehydrogenase, will not change in normal pregnancy. Bilirubin and gamma-glutamyl transpeptidase are both significantly lowered (40).

One of the main hormones causing alterations in hepatic physiology is estrogen. Estrogen produces an increase in the hepatic rough endoplasmic reticulum, which increases the production of proteins. The approximate sevenfold increase in estradiol—related to multiple factors, from changes in the binding hormones to changes in metabolism and production—in the first trimester and a further fivefold increase by term stimulates an approximate sixfold increase in the production of the sex hormone–binding globulin (41). Estrogen also has an inverse relationship with bile salt production and bile flow. There is a change in both composition of the bile and in the rate of cholesterol and phospholipid production; these changes produce an increased lithogenicity (42).

Progesterone, another hormone known to cause significant hepatic changes, mainly effects an increase of smooth endoplasmic reticulum and an increase in cytochrome P-450. Additionally, there is notable smooth muscle relaxation of the gallbladder and biliary ductal system. Progesterone can also produce slow wave dysrhythmia in the gastrointestinal tract (43).

It is now thought that there are genetic influences specifically related to MDR3 gene mutations in liver diseases in pregnancy. Refer to Chapter 48 for more detailed description of essential physiologic concerns related to the liver.

Hyperemesis Gravidarum

Hyperemesis gravidarum (HG) is a condition characterized by serious and persistent vomiting that limits fluid intake and adequate nutrition. Clinical manifestations include weight loss greater than 5% of prepregnancy weight, weakness, dehydration, ketosis, and muscle wasting. HG occurs in approximately 0.3% to 2.0% of pregnancies, seems to affect a diverse population with multiple risk factors, and can be associated with a range of outcomes. Studies have associated HG to various hormone levels, including those of human chorionic gonadotropin, estrogen (44), prolactin (45), thyroxine (46), androgens (46), cortisol (47), and maternal prostaglandins (48). Other factors identified included prior history of HG with previous pregnancies (49), female fetal gender (50,51), maternal age, maternal weight (52), and smoking (53). *Helicobacter pylori* may (54–56) or may not (57) have a role. Chronic medical conditions such as history of gastritis, allergies, and gallbladder disease (58) contribute to the risk. Additionally, the interpregnancy interval and paternity (50) have been examined; although the cause cannot be established, the relationship is being studied.

A complete differential diagnosis includes multiple systems; obstetric and gynecologic conditions such as a molar pregnancy, degenerating uterine leiomyoma, or ovarian torsion should be considered. Gastrointestinal causes could include gastroenteritis, gastroparesis, achalasia, biliary tract disease, hepatitis, intestinal obstruction, peptic ulcer disease, pancreatitis, and appendicitis. The patient needs to be evaluated for urinary tract conditions, including pyelonephritis, uremia, and kidney stones. Metabolic diseases, including hyperthyroidism, diabetic ketoacidosis, porphyria, and Addison disease, should be ruled out. Neurologic disorders, drug reactions, and psychiatric conditions are other considerations.

Some studies have found HG to be protective against adverse outcomes (59), whereas more recent studies have failed to prove this relationship (60). Current research shows a relationship between HG and low birth weight that is mostly attributed to poor maternal weight gain (61–63). In addition to potentially compromised fetal outcomes, a worsened maternal morbidity and mortality are also noted. Cases of Wernicke encephalopathy (64–67), central pontine myelinolysis (68–70), severe liver injury (71), splenic avulsion (72), pneumomediastinum following esophageal rupture (73), and acute renal failure (74) have been reported.

Treatment for HG is primarily supportive, with antiemetics, fluid therapy, and electrolyte replacement. Natural remedies such as pyridoxine (vitamin B6) and ginger (75) have been shown to be effective. Additionally, behavior modification with avoidance of strong odors/scents and adjustment of diet may be tried. However, if these measures are inadequate, hospitalization and treatment with steroids (76–78) and parenteral nutrition may be necessary.

Intrahepatic Cholestasis of Pregnancy

Intrahepatic cholestasis of pregnancy (ICP) is the most frequent of the pregnancy-related liver diseases (79), occurring in approximately 1% of pregnancies (80). It is a condition characterized by the progressive pruritus of cholestasis, with elevated fasting bile salts—specifically chenodeoxycholic acid, deoxycholic acid, and cholic acid elevations more than 10 μmol/L—and elevated aminotransferases (81). Clinical manifestations begin in the late second or third trimester and most often will resolve spontaneously within 2 to 3 weeks postpartum. Although the direct cause is unknown, research has shown a strong familial component. Nonetheless, ICP affects specific populations at different rates. For example, ICP occurs in less than 0.2% of pregnancies in women of North American and Central/Western European descent, whereas Scandinavian and Baltic populations show a rate of 1% to 2%, and Chilean and Bolivian populations have shown rates of 5% to 15% (80). The severe form of ICP—bile acid levels more than 40 μmol/L—in the Swedish population is associated with a frame shift mutation in the gene coding for the ATP binding cassette transporter, specifically the ABCB4_5 gene variant (formerly known as multidrug resistance gene 3, MDR3) (82–84). Mutations in the bile salt export pump (BSEP) can also predispose a patient to ICP (85). Other possible causes relate to "leaky gut" theories (86). This theory is based on the increased absorption of bacterial endotoxins and the enterohepatic circulation of cholestatic metabolites of sex hormones and bile salts. Research has also shown an association with low maternal serum estrogen (87,88).

Fetal complication rates are directly related to maternal serum bile acids (89). Bile acid levels greater than 40 μmol/L are associated with preterm delivery, fetal asphyxial events, and meconium staining (90). Additionally, case reports of neonatal respiratory distress syndrome (90) and fetal death (91) are noted; on the other hand, maternal morbidity and mortality are low.

Supportive measures for pruritus with antihistamine is inadequate, as it has limited effectiveness and fails to address the bile acid elevation and fetal concerns. Cholestyramine, S-adenosylmethionine, and dexamethasone were the treatments of choice (92). However, newer research is advocating the use of ursodeoxycholic acid (UDCA), which is a tertiary bile acid. Initial use of UDCA was with bear bile in traditional Chinese medicine for the treatment of liver disease (93). Recent research has shown UDCA to be more effective in reducing bile acids and bilirubin (94–97). Fetal risks are decreased, but not eliminated. Because of this, careful fetal monitoring and delivery at fetal lung maturity should be considered (92). Ondansetron is also being evaluated as a treatment for pruritus; however, no data are noted on fetal benefits of that antiemetic (98).

Acute Fatty Liver Disease of Pregnancy

Acute fatty liver disease of pregnancy (AFLP) is a rare but potentially fatal disease that occurs in the third trimester. Mean gestational ages vary between 34.5 weeks' (99,100) and 37 weeks' gestation (101). Incidence has been documented as 1 in 6,659 births (102) to 1 in 15,900 births (102). It is characterized by significant malaise, nausea/vomiting, anorexia, abdominal pain, and jaundice (103). Clinical signs include hypertension, jaundice, elevated serum transaminases, coagulopathies, thrombocytopenia, and hypoglycemia. A high index of suspicion should be maintained if evidence of these signs and symptoms are noted (104). Imaging studies are often performed but have limited usefulness in making the diagnosis; ultrasound may show nonspecific changes (104). Computerized tomography (CT) has a high false-negative rate (100). Liver biopsy is the gold standard in confirming the diagnosis; however, it is rarely necessary and carries significant maternal risk in the setting of disseminated intravascular coagulation (DIC).

This disease is noted to have significant risks with respect to morbidity and mortality. Older research reported maternal and perinatal mortality rates as high as 75% and 85%, respectively (104). Although the maternal mortality rate has fallen significantly, fetal mortality has remained as high as 66% (101). Maternal morbidity includes coagulopathies (specifically DIC) (105), hepatic encephalopathy (100), respiratory compromise (pulmonary edema or respiratory arrest) (100), and renal insufficiency (102). Current research has found an associated genetic component with mitochondrial trifunctional protein mutations (106,107).

Treatment of this disease is supportive, with management in a higher-level setting, specifically an ICU. Delivery is recommended as efficiently as possible. Debates regarding prolonged inductions and surgical risks of cesarean are common. The decision should be individualized, and should include the patient and her family. Hypoglycemia should be treated with dextrose-containing solutions. Elevated ammonia levels can be decreased with neomycin. Blood transfusions and replacement of clotting factors should be considered as appropriate. AFLP generally resolves within 2 to 3 days postpartum; however, cases of fulminant hepatic failure requiring liver transplantation have been reported (108).

References

1. Chang J, Elam-Evan LD, Berg CJ, et al. Pregnancy-related mortality surveillance—United States, 1991–1999. *MMWR Surveill Summ.* 2003; 52:1–8.
2. Kahn KS, Wojdyla D, Say L, et al. WHO analysis of causes of maternal death: a systematic review. *Lancet.* 2006;367:1066–1074.
3. Sobieszczyk K, Breborowicz G. Management recommendations for postpartum hemorrhage. *Arch Perinat Med.* 2004;10:1–4.
4. Macphail S, Talks K. Massive post-partum haemorrhage and management of disseminated intravascular coagulation. *Curr Obst Gynaecol.* 2004;14:123–131.
5. Tikkanen M, Nuutila M, Hiilesmaa V, et al. Clinical presentation and risk factors of placental abruption. *Acta Obstet Gynecol Scand.* 2006;85:700–705.
6. Getahun D, Oyelese Y, Salihu HM, et al. Previous cesarean delivery and risks of placenta previa and placental abruption. *Obstet Gynecol.* 2006;107:771–778.
7. Rasmussen S, Irgens LM, Dalaker K. The effect on the likelihood of further pregnancy of placental abruption and the rate of its recurrence. *Br J Obstet Gynaecol.* 1997;104:1292–1295.
8. Iyasu S, Saftlas AK, Rowley DL, et al. The epidemiology of placenta previa in the United States, 1979 through 1987. *Am J Obstet Gynecol.* 1993;168: 1424–1429.
9. Oyelese Y, Smulian JC. Placenta previa, placenta accreta, and vasa previa. *Obstet Gynecol.* 2006;107:927–941.
10. Weinstein L. Syndrome of hemolysis, elevated liver enzymes, and low platelet count: a severe consequence of hypertension in pregnancy. *Am. J Obstet. Gynecol.* 1982;142(2):159–167.
11. Pritchard JA, Weisman R Jr, Ratnoff OD, et al. Intravascular hemolysis, thrombocytopenia, and other hematologic abnormalities associated with severe toxemia of pregnancy. *N Engl J Med.* 1954;250:89–98.
12. Bhattacharya S, Campbell DM. The incidence of severe complications of preeclmpsia. *Hypertens Pregnancy.* 2005;24:181–190.
13. Holub M, Bodamer OA, Item C, et al. Lack of correlation between fatty acid oxidation disorders and haemolysis, elevated liver enzymes, low platelets (HELLP) syndrome? *Acta Paediatr.* 2005;94:48–52.
14. den Boer ME, Iilist L, Wiiburg FA, et al. Heterozygosity for the common LCHAD mutation (1528g>C) is not a major cause of HELLP syndrome and the prevalence of the mutation in the Dutch population is low. *Pediatr Res.* 2000;48:151–154.
15. Sziller I, Hupuczi P, Normand N, et al. Fas (TNFRSF6) gene polymorphism in pregnant women with hemolysis, elevated liver enzymes and low platelets and in their neonates. *Obstet Gynecol.* 2006;107:582–587.

16. Harirah H, Donia S, Hsu CD. Serum soluble Fas in the syndrome of hemolysis, elevated liver enzymes and low platelets. *Obstet Gynecol.* 2001;98:295–298.
17. Osmers RG, Schutz E, Diedrich F, et al. Increased serum levels of hyaluronic acid in pregnancies complicated by preeclampsia or hemolysis, elevated liver enzymes and low platelets syndrome. *Am J Obstet Gynecol.* 1998;178:341–3345.
18. Backe J, Bussen S, Steck T. Significant decrease of maternal serum serotonin levels in singleton pregnancies complicated by the HELLP syndrome. *Gynecol Endocrinol.* 1997;11:405–409.
19. Haddad B, Barton JR, Livingston JC, et al. Risk factors for adverse maternal outcomes among women with HELLP (hemolysis, elevated liver enzymes, and low platelet count) syndrome. *Am J Obstet Gynecol.* 2000;183:444–448.
20. Hupuczi P, Rigo B, Sziller I, et al. Follow-up analysis of pregnancies complicated by HELLP syndrome. *Fetal Diagn Ther.* 2006;21:519–522.
21. Sibai BM. Diagnosis, controversies and management of the syndrome of hemolysis, elevated liver enzymes and low platelet count. *Obstet Gynecol.* 2004;103:981–991.
22. Sibai BM, Ramadan MK, Usta I, et al. Maternal morbidity and mortality in 442 pregnancies with hemolysis, elevated liver enzymes and low platelets (HELLP syndrome). *Am J Obstet Gynecol.* 1993;169:1000–1006.
23. Hafeez M, Hameed S. HELLP syndrome and subcapsular liver haematoma. *J Coll Physicians Surg Pak.* 2005;15:733–735.
24. Herring CS, Heywood SG, Hatjis CG. The multiple challenges in the management of a patient with HELLP syndrome, liver rupture and eclampsia. *W V Med J.* 2005;101:261–262.
25. Shrivastava VK, Imagawa D, Wing DA. Argon beam coagulator for treatment of hepatic rupture with hemolysis, elevated liver enzymes, low platelets (HELLP) syndrome. *Obstet Gynecol.* 2006;107:525–526.
26. Araujo AC, Leao MD, Nobrega MH, et al. Characteristics and treatment of hepatic rupture caused by HELLP syndrome. *Am J Obstet Gynecol.* 2006; 195:129–133.
27. Kim HY, Sohn YS, Lim JH, et al. Neonatal outcome after preterm delivery in HELLP syndrome. *Yonsei Med J.* 2006;47:393–398.
28. Fischer T, Schneider MP, Schobel HP, et al. Vascular reactivity in patients with preeclampsia and HELLP (hemolysis, elevated liver enzymes and low platelet count) syndrome. *Am J Obstet Gynecol.* 2000;183:1489–1494.
29. Oosterhof H, Voorhoeve PG, Aarnoudse JG. Enhancement of hepatic artery resistance to blood flow in preeclampsia in presence or absence of HELLP syndrome (hemolysis, elevated liver enzymes, and low platelets). *Am J Obstet Gynecol.* 1994;171:526–530.
30. Kawabata I, Nakai A, Takeshita T. Prediction of HELLP syndrome with assessment of maternal dual hepatic blood supply by using Doppler ultrasound. *Arch Gynecol .Obstet.* 2006;274:303–309.
31. van Runnard Heimel PJ, Huisjes AJ, Franx A, et al. A randomized placebo-controlled trial of prolonged prednisolone administration to patients with HELLP syndrome remote from term. *Eur J Obstet Gynecol Reprod Biol.* 2006;128:187–193.
32. Rose CH, Tigpen BD, Bofill JA, et al. Obstetric implications of antepartum corticosteroid therapy for HELLP syndrome. *Obstet Gynecol.* 2004;104: 10011–10014.
33. Matchaba P, Moodley J. Corticosteroids for HELLP syndrome in pregnancy. *Cochrane Database Syst Rev.* 2004;(1):CD002076.
34. Norwitz ER, Bahtiyar MO, Sibai BM. Defining standards of care in maternal-fetal medicine. *Am J Obstet Gynecol.* 2004;191:1491–1496.
35. Eser B, Guven M, Unal A, et al. The role of plasma exchange in HELLP syndrome. *Clin Appl Thromb Hemost.* 2005;11:211–217.
36. Detti L, Mecacci F, Piccioli A, et al. Postpartum heparin therapy for patients with the syndrome of hemolysis, elevated liver enzymes and low platelets (HELLP) is associated with significant hemorrhagic complications. *J Perinatol.* 2005;25:236–240.
37. Labelle CA, Kitchens CS. Disseminated intravascular coagulation: treat the cause, not the lab values. *Cleve Clin J Med.* 2005;72:377–378.
38. Chekrizova V, Murphy WG. Solvent-detergent plasma: use in neonatal patients, in adults and paedriatric patients with liver disease and in obstetric and gynaecological emergencies. *Transfus Med.* 2006;16:85–91.
39. Stroup J, Haraway D, Beal JM. Aprotinin in the management of coagulopathy associated with amniotic fluid embolus. *Pharmacotherapy.* 2006;26: 689–693.
40. Bacq Y, Zarka O, Brechot J, et al. Liver function tests in normal pregnancy: a prospective study of 103 pregnant women and 103 matched controls. *Hepatology.* 1996;23:1030–1034.
41. O'Leary P, Boyne P, Flett P, et al. Longitudinal assessment of changes in reproductive hormones during Nnormal pregnancy. *Clin Chem.* 1991;37: 667–672.
42. Lynn J, Williams L, O'Brien J, et al. Effects of estrogen upon bile: implications with respect to gallstone formation. *Ann Surg.* 1973;178:514–522.
43. Walsh JW, Hasler WL, Nugent CE, et al. Progesterone and estrogen are potential mediators of gastric slow-wave dysrhythmias in nausea of pregnancy. *Am J Physiol.* 1996;270:506–514.
44. Lagiou P, Tamimi R, Mucci L, et al. Nausea and vomiting in pregnancy in relation to prolactin, estrogens and progesterone: a prospective study. *Obstet Gynecol.* 2003;101:639–644.
45. Panesar NS, Li CY, Rogers MS. Are thyroid hormones or hCG responsible for hyperemesis gravidarum? A matched paired study in pregnant Chinese women. *Acta Obstet Gynecol Scand.* 2001;80:519–524.
46. Carlsen SM, Vanky E, Jacobsen G. Nausea and vomiting associated with increasing maternal androgen levels in otherwise uncomplicated pregnancies. *Acta Obstet Gynecol Scand.* 2003;82:225–228.
47. Jarnfelt-Samsio A. Nausea and vomiting in pregnancy: a review. *Obstet Gynecol Surv.* 1987;42:422–427.
48. Gadsby R, Barnie-Adshead A, Grammatoppoulos D, et al. Nausea and vomiting in pregnancy: an association between symptoms and maternal prostaglandin E2. *Gynecol Obstet Invest.* 2000;50:149–152.
49. Trogstad LI, Stoltenberg C, Magnus P, et al. Recurrent risk in hyperemesis gravidarum. *BJOG.* 2005;112:1641–1645.
50. del Mar Melero-Montes M, Jick H. Hyperemesis gravidarum and the sex of offspring. *Epidemiology.* 2001;12:123–124.
51. Schiff MA, Reed SD, Daling JR. The sex ratio of pregnancies complicated by hospitalization for hyperemesis gravidarum. *BJOG.* 2004;111:27–30.
52. Depue RH, Bernstein L, Ross RK, et al. Hyperemesis gravidarum in relation to estradiol levels, pregnancy outcomes and other maternal factors: a seroepidemiologic study. *Am J Obstet Gynecol.* 1987;156:1137–1141.
53. Zhang J, Cai WW. Severe vomiting during pregnancy: antenatal correlated and fetal outcomes. *Epidemiology.* 1991;2:454–457.
54. Kuscu NK, Koyuncu F. Hyperemesis gravidarum: current concepts and management. *Postgrad Med J.* 2002;78:76–79.
55. Lee RH, Pan VL, Wing DA. The prevalence of *Helicobacter pylori* in the Hispanic population affected by hyperemesis gravidarum. *Am J Obstet Gynecol.* 2005;193:1024–1027.
56. Verberg MF, Gillott D, Al-Fardan N, et al. Hyperemesis gravidarum, a literature review. *Hum Reprod Update.* 2005;11:527–539.
57. Jacobson GF, Autry AM, Somer-Shely TL, et al. *Helicobacter pylori* seropositivity and hyperemesis gravidarum. *J Reprod Med.* 2003;48:578–582.
58. Jarnfelt-Samsioe A, Samsioe G, Velinder GM. Nausea and vomiting in pregnancy—a contribution to epidemiology. *Gynecol Obstet Invest.* 1983; 16:221–229.
59. Weigel RM, Weigel MM. Nausea and vomiting of early pregnancy and pregnancy outcome: a meta-analytical review. *Br J Obstet Gynaecol.* 1989; 96:1312–1318.
60. Weigel MM, Reyes M, Caiza ME, et al. Is the nausea and vomiting of early pregnancy really feto-protective? *J Perinat Med.* 2006;34:115–122.
61. Bailit JL. Hyperemesis gravidarum: epidemiologic finding from a large cohort. *Am J Obstet Gynecol.* 2005;193:811–814.
62. Dodds L, Fell D, Joseph KS, et al. Outcomes of pregnancies complicated by hyperemesis gravidarum. *Obstet Gynecol.* 2006;107:285–292.
63. Fell DB, Dodds L, Joseph KS, et al. Risk factors for hyperemesis gravidarum requiring hospital admission during pregnancy. *Obstet Gynecol.* 2006;107:2477–1384.
64. Chiossi G, Neri I, Cavazzuti M, et al. Hyperemesis gravidarum complicated by Wernicke encephalopathy: background, case report, and review of the literature. *Obstet Gynecol Surv.* 2006;61:255–268.
65. Rastenvte D, Obelieniene D, Kondrackiene J, et al. Wernicke's encephalopathy induced by hyperemesis gravidarum (case report). *Meicina (Kaunas).* 2003;39:56–61.
66. Indraccolo U, Gentile G, Pomili G, et al. Thiamine deficiency and beriberi features in a patient with hyperemesis gravidarum. *Nutrition.* 2005;21: 967–968.
67. Togay-Isikay C, Yigit A, Mutluer N. Wernicke's encephalopathy due to hyperemesis gravidarum—an under-recognized condition. *Aust N Z J Obstet Gynaecol.* 2001;41:453–456.
68. Tonelli J, Zurru MC, Castillo J, et al. Central pontine myelinolysis induced by hyperemesis gravidarum. *Medicina (B Aires).* 1999;59:176–178.
69. Burneo J, Vizcarra D, Miranda H. Central pontine myelinolysis and pregnancy: a case report and review of literature. *Rev Neurol.* 2000;30:1036–1040.
70. Valiulis B, Kelley RE, Hardiasudarma M, et al. Magnetic resonance imaging detection of a lesion compatible with central pontine myelinolysis in a pregnant patient with recurrent vomiting and confusion. *J Neuroimaging.* 2001;11:441–443.
71. Vitoratos N, Bottsis D, Detsis G, et al. Severe liver injury due to hyperemesis gravidarum. *J Obstet Gynaecol.* 2006;26:172–173.
72. Nguyen N, Deitel M, Lacy E. Splenic avulsion in a pregnant patient with vomiting. *Can J Surg.* 1995;38:464–465.
73. Liang SG, Ooka F, Santo A, et al. Pneumomediastinum following esophageal rupture associated with hyperemesis gravidarum. *J Obstet Gynaecol Res.* 2002;28:172–175.
74. Hill JB, Yost NP, Wendel GD Jr. Acute renal failure in association with severe hyperemesis gravidarum. *Obstet Gynecol.* 2002;100:1119–1121.
75. Jewell D, Young G. Interventions for nausea and vomiting in early pregnancy. *Cochrane Database Syst Rev.* 2003;(4):CD 000145.
76. Moran P, Taylor R. Management of hyperemesis gravidarum: the importance of weight loss as a criterion for steroid therapy. *Q J Med.* 2002;95: 153–158.
77. Nelson-Piercy C, Fayers P, de Swiet M. Randomised, double blind, placebo-controlled trial of corticosteroids for the treatment of hyperemesis gravidarum. *BJOG.* 2001;108:9–15.

78. Bondok RS, El Sharnouby NM, Eid HE, et al. Pulsed steroid therapy is an effective treatment for intractable hyperemesis gravidarum. *Crit Care Med.* 2006;34:2781–2783.
79. Lammert F, Marschall H, Glantz A, et al. Intrahepatic cholestasis of pregnancy: molecular pathogenesis, diagnosis and management. *J Hepatol.* 2000;33:1012–1021.
80. Ropponen A, Sund F, Riikonen S, et al. Intrahepatic cholestasis of pregnancy as an indicator of liver and biliary diseases: a population-based study. *Hepatology.* 2006;43:723–728.
81. Beuers U, Pusl T. Intrahepatic cholestasis of pregnancy—a heterogeneous group of pregnancy-related disorders? *Hepatology.* 2006;43:647–649.
82. Dixon PH, Weerasekera N, Linton KJ, et al. Heterozygous MDR3 missense mutation associated with intrahepatic cholestasis of pregnancy: evidence for a defect in protein trafficking. *Hum Mol Genet.* 2000;9:1209–1217.
83. Floreani A, Carderi I, Paternoster D, et al. Intrahepatic cholestasis of pregnancy: three novel MDR3 gene mutations. *Aliment Pharmacol Ther.* 2006;23:1649–1653.
84. Wasmuth H, Glantz A, Keppeler H, et al. Intrahepatic cholestasis of pregnancy: the severe form is associated with common variants of the hepatobiliary phospholipids transporter gene ABCB4. *Gut.* 2007;56(2):265–279. Epub 2006 Aug 4.
85. Kubitz R, Keitel V, Scheuring S, et al. Benign recurrent intrahepatic cholestasis associated with mutations of the bile salt export pump. *J Clin Gastroenterol.* 2006;40:81–85.
86. Reyes H, Zapata R, Hernandez I, et al. Is a leaky gut involved in the pathogenesis of intrahepatic cholestasis of pregnancy? *Hepatology.* 2006;43:715–722.
87. Reyes H, Simon FR. Intrahepatic cholestasis of pregnancy: an estrogen-related disease. *Semin Liver Dis.* 1993;13:289–301.
88. Leslie K, Reznikov L, Simon F, et al. Estrogens in intrahepatic cholestasis of pregnancy. *Obstet Gynecol.* 2000;95:372–376.
89. Glantz A, Marschall HU, Mattsson LA. Intrahepatic cholestasis of pregnancy: relationships between bile acid levels and fetal complication rates. *Hepatology.* 2004;40:467–474.
90. Zeeca E, De Luca D, Marras M, et al. Intrahepatic cholestasis of pregnancy and neonatal respiratory distress syndrome. *Pediatrics.* 2006;117:1669–1672.
91. Sentilhes L, Verspyck E, Pia P, et al. Fetal death in a patient with intrahepatic cholestasis of pregnancy. *Obstet Gynecol.* 2006;107:458–460.
92. Lammert F, Marschall HU, Matern S. Intrahepatic cholestasis of pregnancy. *Curr Treat Options Gastroenterol.* 2003;6:123–132.
93. Hagey L, Crombie D, Espinosa E, et al. Ursodeoxycholic acid in the Ursidae: biliary bile acid of bears, pandas, and related carnivores. *J Lipid Res.* 1993;34:1911–1917.
94. Brites D. Intrahepatic cholestasis of pregnancy: changes in maternal-fetal bile acid balance and improvement by ursodeoxycholic acid. *Ann Hepatol.* 2002;1:20–28.
95. Copaci I, Micu L, Iliescu L, et al. New therapeutical indications of ursodeoxycholic acid. *Rom J Gastroent.* 2005;14:259–266.
96. Glantz A, Marschall H, Lammert F, et al. Intrahepatic cholestasis of pregnancy: a randomized controlled trial comparing dexamethasone and ursodeoxycholic acid. *Hepatology.* 2005;42:1399–1405.
97. Zapata R, Sandoval L, Palma J, et al. Ursodeoxycholic acid in the treatment of intrahepatic cholestasis of pregnancy. A 12-year experience. *Liver Int.* 2005;25:548–554.
98. Schumann R, Hudcova J. Cholestasis of pregnancy, pruritus and 5-hydroxytryptamine 3 receptor antagonist. *Acta Obstet Gynecol Scand.* 2004;83:861–862.
99. Usta IM, Barton JR, Amon EA, et al. Acute fatty liver of pregnancy: an experience in the diagnosis and management of fourteen cases. *Am J Obstet Gnecol.* 1994;171:1342–1347.
100. Mjahed K, Charra B, Hamoudi D, et al. Acute fatty liver of pregnancy. *Arch Gynecol Obstet.* 2006;274(6):349–353. Epub 2006 Jul 26.
101. Castro MA, Fassett MJ, Reynolds TB, et al. Reversible peripartum liver failure: a new perspective on the diagnosis, treatment and cause of acute fatty liver of pregnancy, based on 28 consecutive cases. *Am J Obstet Gynecol.* 1999;181:389–395.
102. Reyes H, Sandoval L, Wainstein A, et al. Acute fatty liver of pregnancy: a clinical study of 12 episodes in 11 patients. *Gut.* 1994;35:101–106.
103. Bacq Y. Acute fatty liver of pregnancy. *Semin Perinatol.* 1998;22:134–140.
104. Kaplan MM. Acute fatty liver of pregnancy. *N Engl J Med.* 1985;313:367–370.
105. Yucesoy G, Ozkan SO, Bodur H, et al. Acute fatty liver of pregnancy complicated with disseminated intravascular coagulation and haemorrhage: a case report. *Int J Clin Pract Suppl.* 2005;147:82–84.
106. Isaaca J, Sims H, Powell C, et al. Maternal acute fatty liver of pregnancy associated with fetal trifunctional protein deficiency: molecular characterization of a novel maternal mutant allele. *Ped Res.* 1996;40:393–398.
107. Blish KR, Ibdah JA. Maternal heterozygosity for a mitochondrial trifunctional protein mutation as a cause for liver disease in pregnancy. *Med Hypotheses.* 2005;64:96–100.
108. Ockner SA, Brunt EM, Cohn SM, et al. Fulminant hepatic failure caused by acute fatty liver of pregnancy treated by orthotopic liver transplant. *Hepatology.* 1990;11:59–64.

CHAPTER 100 ■ ACUTE ABDOMEN AND TRAUMA DURING PREGNANCY

IRA M. BERNSTEIN • CATHLEEN HARRIS

IMMEDIATE CONCERNS

The evaluation of pregnant patients with surgical disorders and trauma is complex, owing to the fact that the woman and her fetus are both regarded as patients. The well-being of the fetus depends entirely on the stability of the physiologic processes of the pregnant woman. Knowledge of normal physiologic changes of pregnancy is essential, as increased morbidity and mortality for mother or baby can result from delays in diagnosis and treatment. This chapter will summarize the approach to the gravid patient with surgical disease, including clinical assessment, diagnostic studies, interpretation of laboratory values, and specific considerations for various clinical conditions.

Approximately 1 in 500 (0.2%) of pregnant women require surgery for nonobstetric conditions (1). Appendectomy, cholecystectomy, and adnexal procedures constitute the most common surgeries during pregnancy. Although pregnancy outcomes after surgery are often good, fetal loss rates can be as high as 2% to 20%, depending on the condition (1). This fact highlights the importance of thoughtful management in these cases. Trauma is an additional important cause for surgical intervention during pregnancy. Most series report the incidence of trauma to be approximately 8%, or 1 in 12 pregnancies (2). Trauma is the leading cause of nonobstetric maternal death, and fetal losses can be significant. One should always consider the possibility of pregnancy in any female between 12 and 44 years of age presenting with abdominal pain or trauma.

TABLE 100.1

KEY POINTS IN THE ABCs OF THE RESUSCITATION OF PREGNANT WOMEN

Airway	Weight gain Breast enlargement Short time to establish airway before desaturation Edema of airway Difficulty in positioning neck Delayed gastric emptying—aspiration risk
Breathing	Elevated diaphragm Decreased fetal heart rate—rapid desaturation Respiratory alkalosis Limited chest wall expansion Limited accessory muscle use Normal large and small airway function
Circulation	Aortocaval compression at >20 weeks gravid Increased cardiac output Increased resting heart rate Decreased peripheral vascular resistance Decreased systolic and diastolic blood pressure Large shunt due to placental blood flow Hypercoagulable state

As in nonpregnant individuals, the first task is to ensure that airway, breathing, and circulation (ABCs) are adequate. It is important to give first priority to these basic elements, because adequate maternal oxygenation and uteroplacental perfusion are the means by which the fetus is also resuscitated. Attention should always be paid to achieving hemodynamic stability in the mother first, before evaluation and treatment of pregnancy issues. Physiologic adaptations of pregnancy affect the clinician's ability to address the ABCs, and key points that should be considered in the pregnant trama victim are summarized in Table 100.1.

Once assured that the patient is hemodynamically stable, attention is turned to a more detailed secondary assessment. This is centered on evaluation of specific injuries or organ systems, as well as the pregnancy itself. A focused patient history is central to the evaluation of abdominal pain or trauma during pregnancy. Abdominal symptoms can be nonspecific during pregnancy, so it is especially valuable to clarify the location, intensity, and quality of pain, including associated symptoms and aggravating or alleviating factors. Any obstetric symptoms, such as contractions, cramps, bleeding, or fluid leakage, should be noted. In the case of trauma, important details of the incident should be elicited, including vehicle speed, position seated in the vehicle, use of restraints, airbag deployment, and injuries to the head, abdomen, or extremities.

Understanding normal physical changes and common complaints associated with pregnancy will help the clinician to determine which symptoms are benign and pregnancy-related versus pathologic. Many patients report nausea and vomiting in early pregnancy, but these symptoms are not typical in the latter two trimesters. Pyrosis due to acid reflux is reported by many gravidas, but is often easily relieved with antacids. Constipation is a common complaint, due to the increased transit time of the gastrointestinal tract. Transient discomfort or intermittent contractions are not rare, but persistent, rhythmic, or severe abdominal pain merits evaluation. In all trimesters, right lower quadrant pain may signal appendicitis. Colicky right upper quadrant pain is suggestive of cholelithiasis, and the symptom profile for biliary tract disease in pregnant women is similar to that of their nonpregnant counterparts.

In the third trimester, it is important to evaluate and exclude the possibility of obstetric complications such as preterm labor (PTL), premature rupture of membranes, placental abruption, and intrauterine infection. A basic obstetric (OB) triage evaluation includes external fetal heart rate monitoring, assessment of contractions, palpation of the uterine fundus, speculum examination for pooling, Nitrazine and fern tests, and digital cervical examination.

A suggested approach to the initial evaluation of the pregnant patient with surgical diseases or trauma is shown in Table 100.2.

TABLE 100.2

KEY STEPS IN THE APPROACH TO THE PREGNANT PATIENT WITH SURGICAL DISEASES OR TRAUMA

1. Consider pregnancy in any woman of reproductive age presenting after trauma or with abdominal complaints—check urine or serum HCG
2. Perform a primary assessment of airway/breathing/circulation (ABCs)
   a. Use a 15-degree left lateral tilt
   b. IV hydration with isotonic crystalloid solution
   c. Supplemental oxygen as necessary
3. Primary assessment of maternal status should be done prior to evaluation and treatment of fetal issues—should be focused and brief
4. Perform a secondary assessment once patient is hemodynamically stable
   a. Investigate specific injuries or organ systems
   b. Evaluate pregnancy viability and gestational age
   c. Assess for pregnancy complications such as preterm labor (PTL), intrauterine infection, placental abruption, or fetomaternal hemorrhage
   d. Perform cardiotocography for patients over 24 weeks' gestation
5. Do not withhold necessary diagnostic procedures
   a. Consider using modalities that do not use ionizing radiation when possible
   b. Limit ionizing radiation exposure to less than a total dose of 5 rad, as doses less than this amount are not associated with fetal loss or anomalies
6. Obstetric consult for all cases of severe abdominal pain or injury in pregnant patients
   a. Determine if intervention for fetal indications is appropriate
   b. Manage pregnancy complications as necessary
   c. Develop contingency plans for route and timing of delivery where appropriate
   d. Consider neonatal, anesthesiology consultations
   e. Ensure equipment and staff available to effect emergency delivery if indicated

HCG, human chorionic gonadotropin; IV, intravenous.

DIAGNOSTIC STUDIES

Laboratory Values

When common laboratory tests are evaluated during pregnancy, results can be misinterpreted or confusing unless pregnancy-specific norms are considered. Physiologic changes of pregnancy, including increased blood and plasma volumes, hormone production, and altered metabolic clearance, cause changes in the plasma concentration of many analytes. Selected laboratory values of interest are displayed in Table 100.3 (3).

OB Tests of Interest

Fetal Fibronectin

Fetal fibronectin (fFN) is a protein produced by fetal membranes involved in adhesion of the placenta and membranes to maternal tissues. Between 24 and 34 weeks, fFN is not normally detectable in cervicovaginal secretions. The presence of fFN may indicate a disruption of the membranes and decidua, due to inflammation or other causes. Numerous studies have shown success in using fFN to predict preterm birth. The clinical utility of the test rests in its high negative predictive value. In a symptomatic patient, a negative test is associated with greater than 95% likelihood of not delivering within 14 days. This information is useful in the management of patients with preterm contractions, not uncommon in the setting of surgical diseases complicating pregnancy (4).

Amniocentesis

In selected cases, evaluation of amniotic fluid may be important to exclude intrauterine infection as a cause of abdominal pain. Abnormal findings in amniotic fluid suggestive of bacterial infection include bacteria seen on Gram stain and/or positive culture. Low glucose, typically less than 15 mg/dL, and a high white cell count are also highly suspicious. In addition, inflammatory markers such as high granulocyte colony-stimulating factor (G-CSF), tumor necrosis factor (TNF)-α, interleukin (IL)-1, and IL-6 are strongly suggestive of amnionitis. Because there is a risk of preterm contractions, premature rupture of the membranes, or fetal loss due to the procedure, amniocentesis should be done on a selective basis. However, these data can be extremely useful when the clinical picture is unclear (5).

TABLE 100.3

NORMAL LABORATORY VALUES DURING PREGNANCY

WBC	Increased	5,000–15,000 cells/mm^3
Hemoglobin	Decreased	10.5–13.5 g/dL
Hematocrit	Decreased	30.5%–39%
Platelet	Decreased	150–380 × $10^3/\mu$L
Fibrinogen	Increased	265–615 mg/dL
D-Dimer	Frequently positive	—
HCO_3–	Mild acidosis	19–25 mEq/L
BUN	Decreased	3–4 mg/dL
Creatinine	Decreased	0.4–0.7 mg/dL
Albumin	Decreased	2.7–3.7 g/dL
AST, ALT	Unchanged	12–38 U/L
Bilirubin	Unchanged	0.2–0.6 mg/dL
Alkaline phosphatase	Increased	60–140 IU/L

ALT, alanine aminotransferase; AST, aspartate aminotransferase; BUN, blood urea nitrogen; HCO_3^-, bicarbonate; WBC, white blood cell count.
From Lockitch G. The effect of normal pregnancy on common biochemistry and hematology tests. In: Barron WM, Lindheimer MD, eds. *Medical Disorders during Pregnancy*. 3rd ed. St. Louis, MO: Mosby; 2000.

Diagnostic Imaging Studies

Several modalities are available for diagnostic imaging to aid in the evaluation of surgical diseases of pregnancy. Medically necessary diagnostic tests should not be withheld solely on the basis of pregnancy, but one should contemplate the potential advantages and disadvantages when selecting a particular testing method.

Ultrasonography uses sound waves and thus does not expose the patient to ionizing radiation. There are no known adverse fetal outcomes associated with the use of prenatal diagnostic ultrasound under current clinical guidelines for energy exposure. Magnetic resonance imaging (MRI) makes use of the altered energy state of protons to enhance imaging. Its chief clinical uses have been to evaluate placental abnormalities and characterize fetal central nervous system (CNS) malformations; however, increasing experience in the acute setting suggests MRI may also be a valuable tool for assessing for intra-abdominal pathology. To date, MRI has been used safely during pregnancy and is consistent with American College of Radiology guidelines, as discussed below. X-ray studies and computed tomography (CT) involve ionizing radiation, and for this reason need to be used judiciously in gravid patients (6).

Obstetric Ultrasound

Obstetric ultrasound serves to confirm fetal viability and offers the opportunity to assess fetal size, anatomy, amniotic fluid volume, and placental location (6). This information provides the basis for decision making in pregnant patients. A basic study can be completed quickly at the bedside and can be done at the time of sonographic evaluation for other indications, such as right upper quadrant ultrasound.

Sonography for Trauma

In the setting of trauma, surgeon-performed focused assessment with sonography for trauma (FAST [focused assessment with sonography for trauma]-US [ultrasound]) is a useful screening tool. At one institution, FAST-US was used not only for trauma evaluation, but as a screen for pregnancy, and 18 of 144 (11%) of patients were newly diagnosed with pregnancy using this procedure. Because of this, FAST-US contributed to a significant decrease in radiation exposure when compared to other trauma patients diagnosed with pregnancy based on serum human chorionic gonadotropin (HCG) screening (7).

FAST-US done to detect intra-abdominal bleeding after trauma has a similar sensitivity and specificity among pregnant and nonpregnant patients. In one study of 127 pregnant trauma patients, ultrasound examination identified intraperitoneal fluid in 5 of 6 patients and was negative in 117 of 120 patients without intra-abdominal injury. Patients with false-positive scans had serous fluid (8). In reproductive-age women with blunt abdominal trauma, free fluid in the cul de sac has been associated with a higher injury rate compared to no free fluid in both pregnant and nonpregnant women. Thus, free fluid is not necessarily a normal or physiologic finding (9).

Ultrasonography is of limited value in the diagnosis of placental abruption after trauma. In fact, ultrasound may miss up to 50% to 58% of cases. The echotexture may be very similar to that of placental tissue, so identification of retroplacental bleeding is not always possible (10,11).

Appendicitis. Graded compression ultrasonography is the initial test of choice in the assessment of appendicitis during pregnancy. Imaging is focused on the self-reported area of maximal pain. The overall accuracy of this technique in diagnosing appendicitis is 86%. However, accuracy may be limited in the setting of a retrocecal appendix or perforated appendicitis, both of which are more common in the gravid patient. Color Doppler sonography can be used as an adjunct for improving the sensitivity of the test. In a series of 42 women with suspected appendicitis during pregnancy, ultrasound was found to be 100% sensitive, 96% specific, and 98% accurate in diagnosing appendicitis (12).

Biliary Tract Disease. The diagnosis of cholelithiasis during pregnancy is similar to that in the nonpregnant patient. Visualization of stones in the gallbladder is reported to be as high as 95% using sonography. Although detection of gallstones in a patient with right upper quadrant pain is suggestive of acute cholelithiasis, other features should be considered, such as gallbladder wall edema or thickening >4 to 5 mm. The Murphy sign can also be elicited, as the patient experiences pain from pressing the transducer over the gallbladder (13).

Computed Tomography

Computed tomography (CT) may be considered for evaluation of the abdomen if the initial examination or other studies are equivocal. The most common indication for CT is blunt abdominal trauma after motor vehicle crashes (13). Other common indications include appendicitis and renal colic. One study of helical CT revealed good success in detecting injuries after trauma during pregnancy. In this cohort, 17 women (35%) had normal evaluations, 11 patients (23%) had abnormal placental enhancement, and 1 uterine rupture occurred. Fifteen women (31%) had nonuterine injuries, and 27% had both uterine and other maternal injuries. The estimated radiation exposure due to helical CT was estimated to be 8.7 to 17.5 mGy, depending on technique (14). Although there are limited data regarding the accuracy of CT for the diagnosis of appendicitis during pregnancy, one series of seven patients correctly identified all cases (15). Depending on the protocol, pelvic CT can deliver a dose of radiation to the fetus as high as 2 to 5 rad. Although the threshold for teratogenesis may not be reached with this level of radiation exposure, the relative risk of childhood cancer may be increased. The odds of dying of childhood cancer increase from a baseline of 1 in 2,000 to approximately 2 in 2,000 after exposure of 5 rads (15,16). The potential risks and benefits of CT during pregnancy should be discussed with patients. CT contrast seems safe to use in pregnancy and should be administered in the usual fashion (6).

Magnetic Resonance Imaging

In recent years, magnetic resonance imaging (MRI) has been used as a tool to identify the cause of abdominal pain during pregnancy. MRI studies confirm that the appendix and cecum are superiorly displaced as pregnancy advances (17). In one series, MRI was able to correctly identify the appendix in 10 of 12 cases where sonography was uninformative (18). In another study, 29 pregnant women were evaluated with MRI for abdominal or pelvic pain, and correct prospective diagnoses were made in all but one patient (19). More recently, a series of 51 patients were evaluated for abdominal pain with both sonography and MRI. Four cases with appendicitis were found, with three inconclusive results. Ultrasound revealed appendicitis in only two of the confirmed cases. MRI compared favorably with sonography—the overall sensitivity was 100%, specificity 93.5%, and accuracy 94% for detecting appendicitis (20).

According to American College of Radiology guidelines, "Pregnant patients may be approved to undergo MR studies at any stage of pregnancy, so long as the attending radiologist determines the risk–benefit ratio warrants that the study be done" (21). After conferring with the referring provider, the radiologist should document the following:

1. The information from the MR will obtain information not obtainable from nonionizing means
2. The data are needed to affect care given to the patient or fetus during the pregnancy
3. The referring physician does not feel it is prudent to wait to obtain the data until after the patient is no longer pregnant (21).

Gadolinium contrast is not recommended for use in pregnancy. Gadolinium crosses the placenta and enters the fetal circulation. It enters the amniotic fluid, where it is swallowed by the fetus and absorbed (22). It is a pregnancy category C drug, since animal studies have revealed adverse effects but no controlled studies have been performed in humans.

Decisions about contrast use should be made on a case-by-case basis after considering the risks and benefits. Written informed consent for MRI during pregnancy is suggested (21). MRI is not recommended for acute evaluation of severely ill persons, because examinations can be lengthy and there is limited access to patients.

SPECIFIC MANAGEMENT

Specific Conditions: Trauma

Trauma complicates 1 in 12 pregnancies. Two thirds of trauma cases in pregnant women are due to motor vehicle crashes, and other common causes are falls, burns, and penetrating wounds. Blunt abdominal trauma is the most frequent mechanism of injury. One percent to 20% of gravidas experience domestic abuse, and up to 60% of women affected report two or more assaults during pregnancy. At one center, nearly 3% of all trauma patients were pregnant, and 11% of these pregnancies were diagnosed during the trauma evaluation (1,23).

Fortunately, severe trauma requiring admission to the ICU is infrequent (3 in 1,000 pregnancies). Maternal death due to trauma is estimated to be 1.9 per 100,000 live births, representing the leading cause of nonobstetric maternal death. It is estimated that 1,300 to 3,900 pregnancies are lost due to maternal trauma each year (24). Mild maternal injuries carry a 1% to 5% fetal loss rate, whereas life-threatening trauma is associated with loss rates up to 40% to 50%. Because mild trauma is more prevalent, most fetal loss is due to minor maternal injury (24). Population-based data indicate that motor vehicle crashes account for 82% of fetal deaths after trauma, with an overall rate of 3.7 per 100,000 live births. The highest rate of fetal death due to trauma is seen in patients between 15 and 19 years of age (25,26).

One study of 271 pregnant women observed after blunt abdominal trauma showed that fetal death was associated with ejection from vehicle, motorcycle crash, pedestrian collision, maternal death, maternal tachycardia, abnormal fetal heart rate (FHR), lack of restraints, and an injury severity score (ISS) greater than 9. Preterm labor was associated with gestational age over 35 weeks, assault, and pedestrian collisions (10). As many as 20% of injured pregnant patients test positive for drugs or alcohol, and one in three do not report using seat belts (27). The worst outcomes take place among those who deliver during their hospital stay for trauma. In this group of patients, the odds ratios (OR) are strikingly high for maternal death (OR 69), fetal death (OR 4.7), uterine rupture (OR 43), and abruption (OR 9.2), compared to women who deliver later or had no trauma (28). Interestingly, fetal survival was 78% among fetuses born to mothers with a high injury severity score (less than 25), whereas maternal survival was only 44%. In contrast, for women with an ISS less than 16, maternal survival was 100% but the fetal survival was only 73%, giving support to the concept that even minor maternal injury places fetuses at risk (29).

Besides fetal death, complications such as abruptio placentae, preterm labor, and fetomaternal hemorrhage can contribute to morbidity and mortality among survivors. The diagnosis of abruption is based on signs and symptoms. One of the best indicators of placental abruption is cardiotocography. In patients with a normal study, the risk of abruption after trauma is approximately 1% to 5%. In patients with more than six contractions per hour or abnormal fetal heart rate patterns, the risk of abruption can be 20% or higher.

All women over 24 weeks' gestation should undergo an initial evaluation with cardiotocographic monitoring for 4 to 6 hours after trauma. Four to 6 hours of observation is sufficient for patients who have experienced minor trauma, and who are hemodynamically stable, with a negative primary evaluation, FAST-US, and reassuring cardiotocography (29). An extended period of observation for 24 hours or more is indicated for women with six or more contractions per hour, nonreassuring FHR patterns, vaginal bleeding, uterine pain or tenderness, premature rupture of membrane (PROM), or serious maternal injury. Consideration for prolonged monitoring is advised if laboratory data are abnormal, such as decreased fibrinogen or a positive Kleihauer-Betke (KB) test. Patients with these characteristics are more likely to experience abruption or other complications (30).

Kleihauer-Betke testing to detect fetomaternal hemorrhage should be considered for patients beyond the first trimester, especially those with Rh-negative status. RhIG 300 μg IM should be administered to all pregnant women with an Rh-negative blood type. Should the KB test be positive, the amount of fetal bleeding can be quantified and additional RhIG administered as necessary. A positive KB test may also be an indicator for adverse pregnancy outcome after trauma. One study reviewed 166 pregnant trauma cases. In 71 of these cases, a KB test was done. The likelihood ratio for preterm labor was 20.8-fold if the KB was positive, whereas clinical assessment did not predict preterm birth accurately (31).

Pregnant women occasionally present with other types of injuries due to trauma to the head, pelvis, or chest. Pelvic fractures, especially those involving the acetabulum, are associated with high maternal and fetal mortality rates. The mechanism of injury and severity influence mortality more than the classification type or trimester of pregnancy (32). Specific management can be complex and requires the coordination of a multidisciplinary team. Penetrating injury is less common during pregnancy than other forms of trauma. In general, the severity of maternal abdominal or vascular injuries may be less than that of nongravid women, but rate of placental injury and fetal loss tends to be high. Management is similar to that of nonpregnant persons, with careful and prompt evaluation of the placenta and fetus.

Specific Conditions: Appendicitis

Acute appendicitis complicates approximately 1 in 1,500 pregnancies, making it the most common indication for nonobstetric surgery during pregnancy. Overall, appendicitis may occur less frequently in gravid patients than in nonpregnant individuals (33).

Although appendicitis occurs in all trimesters, the second trimester is most typical. More than 80% of patients with appendicitis report right lower quadrant pain, irrespective of the trimester (34). Appendicitis can be difficult to diagnose during pregnancy because signs and symptoms can be easily confused with physiologic changes of pregnancy. Nausea and vomiting are common during pregnancy, but not typically associated with pain. Constipation and bowel irregularity, frequent bothersome symptoms of gestation, can be difficult to interpret. Mild leukocytosis is a normal laboratory finding in pregnant women, rendering it of limited value in making the diagnosis of appendicitis. The white blood cell (WBC) count ranges from 5,000 to 15,000 cells/mm^3 in the first two trimesters and can be as high as 20,000 cells/mm^3 in labor (35,36). The classic triad of obturator, psoas, and Rovsing signs is present in less than one in three pregnant patients (37). Imaging plays an important role in the diagnosis of appendicitis during pregnancy and is discussed above.

Complications may be increased when appendicitis occurs during pregnancy. A delay in diagnosis and treatment over 24 hours was associated with perforation in 14% to 43% of cases in one report (38). In another study, the perforation rate for appendicitis occurring in the first and second trimesters was 31%, but rose to 69% in the third trimester (39). Fetal loss rates as high as 33% and preterm delivery rates of 14% have also been reported in women undergoing appendectomy (40). This underscores the importance of a high index of suspicion in evaluating women with right lower quadrant pain during pregnancy.

When appendicitis is strongly suspected, surgery should be performed as per usual clinical indications. An incision over the point of maximal tenderness is most often recommended. Laparoscopy may be considered as an alternative in patients under 24 weeks' gestation. For patients under 24 weeks' gestation, the uterine size and location of the appendix may reduce access for laparoscopic procedures.

Specific Conditions: Gallstones

Cholelithiasis is common among pregnant women, seen in 3% to 4% of OB ultrasounds. Symptomatic gallstones occur less frequently, in approximately 1 in 1,000 cases. Half or more of patients experience recurrent bouts of biliary colic, making management a challenge. Traditional management consists of intravenous hydration, nothing by mouth or a low-fat diet, analgesics, and antibiotics. Cholecystectomy is required in 1 to 6 per 10,000 pregnancies. Typical indications for surgery include acute cholecystitis (38%), gallstone pancreatitis (28%), common bile duct stone (20%), and refractory pain (18%) (41). Laparoscopy has been used successfully during pregnancy for this indication, as discussed below. Traditional management emphasized deferring surgery for symptomatic cholelithiasis until after delivery. More recent data suggest that relapse of symptoms is common, seen in 38%, and labor induction due to refractory symptoms results in preterm delivery in some cases (42).

Specific Conditions: Adnexal Surgery

The true incidence of adnexal masses during pregnancy is unclear, but it is estimated to be approximately 1 in 200. Simple ovarian cysts compose the vast majority of cases, and most do not require intervention. Adnexal surgery is necessary in 1 in 1,300 pregnancies, typically due to masses greater than 6–8 cm, complex masses, and ovarian torsion. Malignancy is uncommon, seen in less than 10% of cases (43). Care should be taken to avoid removal of the corpus luteum in the first trimester prior to 10 weeks' gestation, as this can result in disruption of the ongoing pregnancy unless progesterone supplementation is provided.

Historically, about half of surgeries performed were due to ovarian torsion (1). With improvements in the diagnosis of ovarian masses, surgery during pregnancy for asymptomatic patients with adnexal pathology has become more common. In one series of 44 cases of benign ovarian masses, most surgeries were performed successfully using laparoscopy in the middle trimester, and the most common diagnosis was benign cystic teratoma (44). Outcomes after adnexal surgery during pregnancy have been shown to be excellent, so long as surgery is performed after the 7th week of gestation (45).

FETAL ASSESSMENT

Risk of Fetal Loss and Recommended Fetal Assessment

A review of 55 papers regarding surgery during pregnancy, including 12,452 patients reported in the literature, confirms that the total fetal loss rate is low, at 2.5%. Birth defects after first trimester surgeries occurred in 3.9%, and the miscarriage rate was 5.8%, likely not increased above background rates, but not proven due to lack of controls for comparison. Premature labor after nonobstetric surgery was seen in 3.5%, and the overall rate of preterm birth was 8.2%. The highest risk for preterm birth and fetal loss was seen with appendectomy. In this setting, the preterm delivery rate was 4.6%, and losses occurred in 10.9% of cases (46).

There is no consensus on optimal fetal monitoring in the perioperative period. During the first trimester, no specific fetal evaluation is necessary. Documentation of a live intrauterine pregnancy prior to surgery is prudent in those patients who present with abdominal complaints, primarily to exclude the possibility of ectopic pregnancy or nonviable gestation. From 14 weeks to 24 weeks, assessment of fetal heart tones is advised preoperatively and postoperatively. Perioperative assessment of contractions may be considered after 20 to 24 weeks.

At 24 weeks or beyond, cardiotocography should be performed before and after completion of surgery. In special circumstances, intraoperative monitoring may be chosen. It is important to remember that anesthetic drugs may be associated with decreased fetal heart rate variability, and misinterpretation has led to unnecessary emergency cesarean deliveries (47). In general, if the mother is normotensive and normoxemic, the fetus is well maintained. In the setting of trauma, an initial evaluation consisting of 4 to 6 hours of cardiotocography is warranted, as discussed above.

Decisions about the timing, duration, and methods of fetal monitoring are dependent on the clinical scenario and procedure planned. Such decisions should be made in consultation with an obstetrician and with input from an anesthesiologist.

PRETERM LABOR AND TOCOLYSIS

Preterm labor is a frequent event, due to either the underlying condition or the surgical intervention. In one series of 77 patients undergoing nonobstetric surgery, preterm labor was seen in 26% of patients in the second trimester and in 82% of those in the third trimester. Preterm labor was commonest after appendicitis and adnexal surgery. Actual preterm birth was seen in 16%. Only in 5%, however, was a clear link to the surgical procedure established (1). Another study of 62 pregnant subjects with nonobstetric abdominal surgery during pregnancy revealed 18% delivered preterm, similar to that institution's preterm delivery rate but higher than the national average (48,49).

Most women with preterm labor will not deliver prematurely. Tocolytic medications are given to reduce uterine contractions in many cases, because it is difficult to predict accurately which women will go on to deliver prematurely. There is not a single drug of choice to manage preterm labor. The most commonly used tocolytic agents include nifedipine, magnesium sulfate, and indomethacin. The selection of a tocolytic drug should be based on gestational age, maternal health conditions, and possible side effects. Because tocolytic drugs prolong pregnancy for only 2 to 7 days, their chief utility is to allow for administration of steroids to improve fetal lung maturity (50).

In the postoperative patient, discomfort most often represents typical postsurgical pain, but care should be taken to evaluate for preterm labor or signs of intrauterine infection.

Clinical assessment includes physical examination with palpation of the fundus, cervical examination, and cardiotocography. Adjunctive tests to aid in predicting preterm birth include cervical length measurement, fetal fibronectin testing, and possibly amniocentesis. Tocolysis should be undertaken with caution in the surgical patient, and obstetric consultation is recommended in the event of preterm contractions after surgery.

Corticosteroids for Fetal Lung Maturity Enhancement

All pregnant women between 24 and 34 weeks of gestation who are at risk of preterm delivery within 7 days should be given a single course of corticosteroids for fetal lung maturity enhancement (51).

Recommended regimens for this indication include the following:

Betamethasone, 12 mg intramuscularly every 24 hours for two doses

or

Dexamethasone, 6 mg intramuscularly every 12 hours for four doses

These corticosteroids have been shown to cross the placenta and still retain their biologic effects. They have minimal mineralocorticoid activity and cause little immune suppression. Overall, antenatal corticosteroid use has proved to be one of the most beneficial interventions in the treatment of preterm labor. Corticosteroids for fetal lung maturity enhancement reduce the incidence and severity of respiratory distress syndrome in preterm infants, and betamethasone has been shown to decrease neonatal mortality (52). In addition, intraventricular hemorrhage and necrotizing enterocolitis are decreased with steroid use (52,53). Consideration should be given as to whether a patient may benefit from corticosteroid administration, and decisions individualized. Consultation with an obstetrician regarding this issue is recommended.

Venous Thromboembolism Prevention

Pregnancy is a prothrombotic state, and the risk of venous thromboembolism (VTE) is increased among women who undergo cesarean delivery as compared with vaginal birth (53). However, there are few data regarding the risk for VTE after nonobstetric surgery. There are no clear guidelines or recommendations to address prevention of thromboembolism in the setting of trauma or abdominal surgery during pregnancy. Nonpregnant trauma patients with at least one risk factor for VTE (including estrogen exposure) are recommended to receive thromboprophylaxis (54,55). In the gravid patient, mechanical prophylaxis, such as pneumatic compression, is reasonable, and low-molecular-weight heparin (LMWH) prophylaxis can be considered on a case-by-case basis. For patients with additional risk factors for thromboembolism beyond pregnancy itself, pharmacologic methods should be combined with use of mechanical approaches.

Consultation

Obstetrics

Obstetric consultation should be considered for any patient requiring surgery during pregnancy. Because there are few data to guide clinical management, the American College of Obstetricians and Gynecologists states that "it is important for non-obstetric physicians to obtain obstetric consultation before performing non-obstetric surgery. The decision to use fetal monitoring should be individualized, and each case warrants a team approach to ensure optimal safety for the woman and her baby" (48).

Anesthesia

Prior to delivering anesthesia care, the anesthesiologist is responsible for reviewing the medical record, interviewing and performing a focused examination on the patient, ordering and reviewing appropriate medical tests, ordering appropriate medications, ensuring consent for anesthesia is obtained, and documenting the above in the patient medical record. Preoperative anesthesia consultation should be considered in most cases of nonobstetric surgery during pregnancy, as obstetric complications that may lead to operative delivery are possible (56,57).

Neonatology

In the scenario of surgical diseases affecting third trimester pregnancy, decisions must be made about obstetric and neonatal management. This is especially critical for cases at the threshold of viability. Parents should participate along with physicians in decisions regarding management, including the selection of facility for perinatal care, the type of fetal surveillance planned, and whether or not to perform cesarean birth for fetal indications.

Although the overall prognosis for premature infants has steadily improved, the morbidity and mortality for extremely low-birth-weight infants remains high. The mean survival rates for infants born between 23 and 25 weeks increase from 30%, to 52%, to 76% with each additional week of development. Likewise, the survival for infants weighing 401–800 g ranges from 11% in those under 500 g to 74% in those over 701 g. Severe disability is common among survivors in this group of vulnerable infants.

Neonatal consultation is extremely important for those patients at risk for preterm birth, particularly in the "periviable" period. Parents should be informed about the prospects for infant survival, the likelihood of various outcomes related to prematurity, and the potential risks and benefits of treatments for preterm infants. Decisions regarding the planned level of intervention for the neonate should be documented in the medical record. Noninitiation of resuscitation for newborns less than 23 weeks or 400-g birth weight is appropriate (58).

PERIOPERATIVE MANAGEMENT

Anesthesia

The goals of anesthesia for nonobstetric surgery are different than those of the labor patient. Instead of attempting to preserve uterine tone and minimize fetal sedation, the objective is to provide effective surgical anesthesia while avoiding stimulating uterine contractions. There is little concern for the effects of fetal respiratory depression, but instead a focus on uteroplacental exchange.

In general, regional or local anesthetics are thought to be safer than general anesthesia. Regional anesthesia for abdominal surgery has the advantage of minimal fetal local anesthetic drug exposure and is less likely to be associated with airway complications. Local anesthetics are not known to be teratogenic when used in this clinical setting.

Due to the risk of aspiration from gastroesophageal (GE) reflux and delayed gastric emptying, it is customary to administer a nonparticulate antacid or H2 blocker as well as medication to improve GE sphincter tone preoperatively. If general anesthesia is planned, preoxygenation and rapid-sequence intubation are typically performed. Care should be taken to avoid hyperventilation, as uterine blood flow is impaired. Inhalational agents, such as isoflurane and others, decrease uterine tone and effectively inhibit labor during surgery.

In general, agents used for general anesthesia during pregnancy, including a single dose of benzodiazepines, nitrous oxide, and inhalational agents, have not been shown to be teratogenic. Fetal loss, low birth weight, and perinatal mortality increases after nonobstetric surgery appear not to be influenced by the choice of anesthetic in one study of 5,405 operations in pregnant women (59).

Laparoscopy during Pregnancy

Various conditions are suitable for treatment via laparoscopic surgery. In general, laparoscopy has had a good record of safety during pregnancy. Special considerations for laparoscopy during pregnancy might include use of an open technique to gain access to the abdominal cavity, direct visualization for trocar placement, and lower insufflation pressures. Laparoscopy is of limited utility in late pregnancy, when the size of the uterus obscures views and reduces access to abdominal structures.

Rates of fetal loss in the first trimester have been reported to be about 10% to 15%, similar to persons with no surgery (60). The effects of CO_2 on the fetus are unclear. Insufflation with carbon dioxide has been reported to cause metabolic acidosis in animal studies but is not known to cause harmful sequelae in human cases (60,61).

The largest experience with laparoscopy has been reported by the Swedish Health Registry (2,233 laparoscopies and 2,491 open laparotomies). In both groups, there was an increase in low birthweight (<2,500 g) due to fetal growth restriction and also associated with delivery before 37 weeks. There were no significant differences between the groups with respect to any other obstetric outcomes (62). It would seem reasonable to assess fetal growth periodically among patients who have undergone nonobstetric surgery. Guidelines for laparoscopic surgery during pregnancy are displayed in Table 100.4 (63).

Delivery Considerations

Optimal maternal and infant outcome depends on planning for contingencies. Action items that might impact care when managing pregnant trauma or surgery patients are listed below:

1. Admit the mother to a facility able to provide appropriate specialty care, including neonatology and neonatal intensive care unit (NICU) care.
2. Provide level I trauma center care for any gravid trauma patient whenever possible.
3. Ensure immediate availability of equipment for emergency delivery, in the emergency room (ER), main operating room (OR), intensive care unit (ICU), or surgical unit, where appropriate. This includes all items for infant resuscitation, such as warmer bed, oxygen, endotracheal tubes, suction, other supplies, and emergency medications.
4. Plan for adequate staff to address obstetric issues, including fetal monitoring and/or emergency delivery.
5. Plan for adequate nursing care for perioperative needs on labor and delivery ward.
6. Ensure that clear instructions designate which providers or specialty services are responsible for various aspects of patient care.
7. Display contact information for the various providers prominently in patient medical record, in case emergency evaluation and treatment is necessary.
8. Encourage impeccable communication between specialists, including general surgery, trauma surgery, obstetrics, anesthesiology, neonatology, or others.
9. Obtain consultations early, and document recommendations or treatment plans.
10. Clearly indicate what the plans are for fetal assessment and whether or not intervention is planned for indications, such as emergent cesarean in the event of nonreassuring fetal heart rate patterns.
11. Delivery timing and route may be individualized. In general, delivery at full term (≥37 weeks) is the goal. Cesarean is reserved for usual clinical indications, with the notable exception of the perimortem patient (Table 100.5).
12. A typical trauma care team for a gravid patient includes the following:
    a. ER physician
    b. ER nurse
    c. Trauma surgeon
    d. Obstetrician
    e. OB nurse
    f. Anesthesiology

TABLE 100.4

SOCIETY FOR AMERICAN GASTROINTESTINAL ENDOSCOPIC SURGEONS GUIDELINES FOR LAPAROSCOPIC SURGERY DURING PREGNANCY (2000)

1. Preoperative obstetric consultation
2. If possible, defer operation until second trimester, when fetal risk is lowest.
3. Use pneumatic compression devices whenever possible, as pneumoperitoneum enhances lower extremity venous stasis and pregnancy induced a hypercoagulable state.
4. Monitor fetal and uterine status, and use maternal end-tidal CO_2 and/or arterial blood gas (ABG).
5. Protect uterus with a lead shield if intraoperative cholangiography is possible. Use fluoroscopy selectively.
6. Attain abdominal access using an open technique, as the gravid uterus is enlarged.
7. Shift the uterus off the inferior vena cava by using dependent positioning/lateral tilt.
8. Minimize pneumoperitoneum pressures (8–12 mm Hg) and do not exceed 15 mm Hg.

From Lu E, Curet M, El-Sayed Y, et al. Medical versus surgical management of biliary tract disease in pregnancy. *Am J Surg*. 2004;188:755–759, with permission.

TABLE 100.5

IINDICATIONS FOR EMERGENT CESAREAN

Emergent cesarean may be warranted in the following circumstances:
Fetal heart tones are present (there is a living fetus)
The fetus is at a viable gestational age (≥23 to 24 weeks)
Adequate equipment and personnel are available to perform cesarean
Adequate equipment and personnel are available for neonatal resuscitation
Lack of response to maternal cardiopulmonary resuscitation (CPR) within 4 minutes (discussed in text)
Persistent nonreassuring fetal heart rate (FHR) pattern is present—examples include fetal bradycardia, prolonged decelerations, or repetitive late decelerations
Deteriorating maternal condition—cardiovascular instability
Direct uterine or fetal injury

g. Pediatrician available
h. NICU or nursery nurse available
i. OR team on standby

Maternal CPR or Death

Rarely, a pregnant woman is sufficiently unstable to require cardiopulmonary resuscitation (CPR) or advanced cardiac life support (ACLS) procedures. To be most effective with CPR, it is important to recall the physical changes of pregnancy that affect the efficiency of compressions. Aortocaval compression by the gravid uterus decreases cardiac output by 25%, and hypotension in supine position is not uncommon.

The American Heart Association suggests key components for the resuscitation of the pregnant woman in cardiac arrest, itemized below (64):

1. left lateral position
2. 100% oxygen
3. IV access and fluid bolus
4. Identification of the cause of cardiac arrest, and consideration of other medical conditions that could complicate efforts to revive the patient

Chest compressions should be done higher on the sternum, slightly above the center, because of the elevated diaphragm and abdominal contents. Vasopressors should be used when necessary, but be aware that epinephrine, vasopressin, and dopamine can decrease uterine blood flow. Maintaining maternal circulation is still the most important means of supporting the fetus, even in the event of maternal CPR. Medication doses and defibrillation protocols do not change. If fetal or uterine monitors are in place, these should be removed before delivering shocks. No other changes from the ACLS protocol are advised. Pregnancy-specific complications that providers should consider during their resuscitation efforts include magnesium toxicity, eclampsia, and amniotic fluid embolism (64).

Perimortem Cesarean

Intact survival of a fetus is most likely when cesarean delivery is accomplished within 5 minutes of cardiac arrest in a pregnant patient (65). A recent report of outcomes after 38 cases of perimortem cesarean indicated that there were 34 surviving infants. Of those infants, time of delivery was available for 25 cases. Twelve of 25 (48%) were delivered within 5 minutes, and 9 of these 12 infants had no neurologic deficits on follow-up. Of the remaining cases, four were delivered between 6 and 10 minutes, two between 11 and 15 minutes, and seven delivered more than 15 minutes from cardiac arrest. Neurologic sequelae were present in at least one of the survivors in each of these groups. Interestingly, of 20 perimortem cesareans with resuscitable causes, 13 mothers were revived and discharged from the hospital in good condition (65). Clearly there is a role for this life-saving procedure for both mother and baby.

Maternal Brain Death

On rare occasions maternal brain death is identified in a pregnant woman while somatic support has been maintained and the fetus remains alive. Under these circumstances, a determination must be made as to whether to deliver the fetus immediately, to initiate supportive care to allow further fetal maturation, or to allow the fetus to die as the mother is removed from mechanical ventilation. Immediate delivery when gestational age is consistent with neonatal survival is always preferred. However, if the mother's condition permits, it is possible to support the mother and previable fetus until fetal maturation allows for neonatal survival. This somatic support can be provided for extended periods with no apparent neonatal or pediatric sequelae with 2-year follow-up reported (66,67).

Ethical Decision Making

There is a potential for conflicts in decision making between the clinician and the pregnant woman. Patients may be asked to consent to procedures that carry some risk to the fetus. Alternatively, interventions proposed for fetal benefit may present a risk to maternal health. Principle-based ethics, based on the concepts of autonomy, beneficence, and justice, have been used to aid choices. Providers also need to take into account the social and cultural context within which the patient is making her choices. According to the ACOG Ethical Guidelines, "Every reasonable effort should be made to protect the fetus, but the pregnant woman's autonomy should be respected . . . Intervention against the wishes of a pregnant woman is rarely if ever acceptable" (68).

In the case of a patient who is incapacitated, state laws vary with respect to who may serve as a surrogate decision maker. The designees should base their decisions on the values and wishes of the patient, which may or may not have previously been stated in writing. Clinicians should try to anticipate such scenarios and attempt to adhere to the woman's wishes regarding treatment for herself and/or her fetus. If there is not consensus about who should be designated, the advice of an ethics committee should be considered.

INJURY PREVENTION/REDUCTION

Lack of seat belt use has been shown to contribute to the severity of maternal and fetal injuries. Knowledge of proper seat belt use is low among some patients, especially teens and those with low education levels. In one survey of 450 pregnant women, only 72.5% reported using the seat belt in the proper location. Women who always wore restraints were more likely to report correct placement. 60% of respondents thought restraints would protect their baby, whereas 11.6% thought restraints caused injury to the baby, and 37% were unsure. The most common reasons for lack of use were lack of comfort (52.8%) and forgetting (42.5%). However, only 36.9% of women reported receiving information about seat belt use during that pregnancy (69). Another survey of 807 women revealed that although 79% of women used safety restraints, only 52% of them did so correctly, and only 21% were educated on proper use during pregnancy (70). Educational interventions during prenatal care can improve the proper use of seat belts significantly. At one institution, the proportion of women reporting correct seat belt placement improved from 70.8% to 83% after instruction during prenatal care (71).

There are case reports of complications due to seat belts and air bags, including uterine rupture (72). However, the evidence to date suggests that correct use of seat belts reduces the likelihood of fetal loss. One statewide study reviewed the experience of 8,928 women (2.8% of the overall pregnant population) with a history of motor vehicle crashes during pregnancy. Unbelted women were 2.8 times more likely to experience a fetal death after the incident (73). Prenatal care visits and emergency room encounters provide an opportunity for providers to give health messages to their patients regarding the importance of proper seat belt use.

Domestic Violence Awareness

Studies indicate that women who experience physical violence are at higher risk for pregnancy loss and low-birth-weight infants (74). A recent prospective study of pregnant women indicated that among 949 surveyed, low birth weight was increased in those reporting verbal abuse (7.6% vs. 5.1%). Also, neonatal deaths were more common among those with physical abuse (1.5% vs. 0.2%). Unexpectedly, 94 women who declined interview had higher rates of low-birth-weight infants (12.8%), preterm birth (5.3% vs. 1.2%), abruption (7.4% vs. 2.2%), and NICU admission (7.4% vs. 2.2%) than those reporting no abuse (75).

Women generally feel that a provider asking them about domestic violence in a confidential, private setting is helpful. Universal screening for domestic violence is recommended by several professional organizations, such as American Medical Association (AMA), American College of Obstetricians and Gynecologists (ACOG), and American Academy of Family Physicians (AAFP). Behavioral cues that domestic violence may be an issue include late entry to prenatal care or sporadic attendance at prenatal visits, changes in appointment patterns, overprotective or threatening partner, or multiple visits for somatic complaints. Battered women are commonly reported to seek medical services at eight times the rate of other women, but they are rarely identified or referred for services. Indeed, battered women account for up to a quarter of all women seeking emergency medical services and/or prenatal care. Emergency visits for abdominal complaints or trauma may serve to prompt the clinician to consider domestic violence as an underlying cause of symptoms. Should a patient indicate that domestic violence is a concern, assistance is available from the National Domestic Violence Hotline, 1-800-799-SAFE. This 24-hour, toll-free hotline provides information and referrals from anywhere in the United States.

References

1. Visser BC, Glasgow RE, Mulvihill KK, et al. Safety and timing of nonobstetric abdominal surgery in pregnancy. *Dig Surg.* 2001;18:409–417.
2. Pearlman MD, Tintinalli JE, Lorenz RP. A prospective controlled study of outcome after trauma during pregnancy. *Am J Obstet Gynecol.* 1990;162:1502–1510.
3. Lockitch G, The effect of normal pregnancy on common biochemistry and hematology tests. In: Barron WM, Lindheimer MD, eds. *Medical Disorders during Pregnancy.* 3rd edn. St. Louis, MO: Mosby; 2000.
4. American College of Obstetricians and Gynecologists. Assessment of risk factors for preterm birth. *ACOG Practice Bulletin.* October 2001, Number 31.
5. Goldenberg RL, Hauth JC, Andrews WW. Intrauterine infection and preterm delivery. *N Engl J Med.* 2000;342:1500–1507.
6. American College of Obstetricians and Gynecologists. Guidelines for diagnostic imaging during pregnancy. *ACOG Committee Opinion.* September 2004, Number 299.
7. Bochicchio GV, Haan, JM, Scalea TM. Surgeon-performed focused assessment with sonography for trauma as an early screening tool for pregnancy after trauma. *J Trauma.* 2002;52(6):1125–1128.
8. Goodwin H, Holmes JF, Wisner DH. Abdominal ultrasound examination in pregnant blunt trauma patients. *J Trauma.* 2001;50(4):689–693.
9. Ormsby EL, Geng J, McGahan JP, et al. Pelvic free fluid: clinical importance for reproductive age women with blunt abdominal trauma. *Ultrasound Obstet Gynecol.* 2005;26(3):271–278.
10. Curet MJ, Schermer CR, Demarest GB, et al. Predictors of outcome in trauma during pregnancy: identification of patients who can be monitored for less than 6 hours. *J Trauma.* 2000;49(1):18–24.
11. Reis PM, Sander CM, Pearlman MD. Abruptio placentae after auto accidents. A case-control study. *J Reprod Med.* 2000;45:6–10.
12. Lim HK, Bae SH, Seo GS. Diagnosis of acute appendicitis in pregnant women: value of sonography. *Am J Roentgenol.* 1992;159:539–542.
13. Stauffer RA, Adams A, Wygal J, et al. Gallbladder disease in pregnancy. *Am J Obstet Gynecol.* 1982;144:661–664.
14. Lowdermilk C, Gavant ML, Qaisi W, et al. Screening helical CT for evaluation of blunt traumatic injury in the pregnant patient. *Radiographics.* 1999;19:S243–S255.
15. Castro A, Shipp TD, Castro EE, et al. The use of helical computed tomography in pregnancy for the diagnosis of acute appendicitis. *Am J Obstet Gynecol.* 2001;184:954–957.
16. Damilakis J, Perisinakis K, Voloudaki A, et al. Estimation of fetal radiation dose from computed tomography scanning in late pregnancy: depth-dose data from routine examinations. *Invest Radiol.* 2000;35:527–533.
17. Oto A, Srinivasan PN, Ernst RD, et al. Revisiting MRI for appendix location during pregnancy. *Am J Roentgenol.* 2006;186:883–887.
18. Cobben LP, Groot I, Haans L, et al. MRI for clinically suspected appendicitis during pregnancy. *Am J Roentgenol.* 2004;183:671–675.
19. Birchard KR, Brown MA, Hyslop WB, et al. MRI of acute abdominal and pelvic pain in pregnant patients. *Am J Roentgenol.* 2005;184:452–458.
20. Pedrosa I, Levine D, Eyvazzade AD, et al. MR imaging evaluation of acute appendicitis in pregnancy. *Radiology.* 2006;238:891–899.
21. Kanal E, Borgstede JP, Barkovich AJ, et al. American College of Radiology White Paper on MR Safety. *AJR Am J Roentgenol.* 2002;178:1335–1347.
22. Kanal E, Borgstede JP, Barkovich AJ, et al. American College of Radiology White Paper on MR Safety: 2004 update and revisions. *Am J Roentgenol.* 2004;182:1111–1114.
23. Bochicchio GV, Napolitano LM, Haan J, et al. Incidental pregnancy in trauma patients. *J Am Coll Surg.* 2001;192(5):566–569.
24. American College of Obstetricians and Gynecologists. Obstetric aspects of trauma management. *ACOG Educational Bulletin.* September 1998, Number 251.
25. Horon IL, Cheng D. Enhanced surveillance for pregnancy-associated mortality—Maryland 1993–1998. *JAMA.* 2001;285:1455–1459.
26. Weiss HB, Songer TS, Fabio A. Fetal deaths related to maternal injury. *JAMA.* 2001;286:1863–1868.
27. Ikossi DG, Lazar A, Morabito D, et al. Profile of mothers at risk: an analysis of injury and pregnancy loss in 1,195 trauma patients. *J Am Coll Surg.* 2005;200(1):49–56.
28. El-Kady D, Gilbert W, Anderson J, et al. Trauma during pregnancy: an analysis of maternal and fetal outcomes in a large population. *Am J Obstet Gynecol.* 2004;190(6):1661–1668.

29. Curet MJ, Schermer CR, Demarest GB, et al. Predictors of outcome in trauma during pregnancy: identification of patients who can be monitored for less than 6 hours. *J Trauma.* 2000;49:18–25.
30. Goodwin TM, Breen MT. Pregnancy outcome and fetomaternal hemorrhage after noncatastrophic trauma. *Am J Obstet Gynecol.* 1990;162:665–671.
31. Muench MV, Baschat AA, Reddy UM, et al. Kleihauer-Betke testing is important in all cases of maternal trauma. *J Trauma.* 2004;57(5):1094–1098.
32. Leggon RE, Wood GC, Indeck MC. Pelvic fractures in pregnancy: factors influencing maternal and fetal outcomes. *J Trauma.* 2002;53(4):796–804.
33. Andersson REB, Lambe M. Incidence of appendicitis during pregnancy. *Int J Epidemiol.* 2001;30:1281–1285.
34. Mourad J, Elliott JP, Erickson L, Lisboa L. Appendicitis in pregnancy: new information that contradicts long-held clinical beliefs. *Am J Obstet Gynecol.* 2000;182:1027–1029.
35. Martin C, Varner MW. Physiologic changes in pregnancy: surgical implications. *Clin Obstet Gynecol.* 1994;37:241–255.
36. Delgado I, Neubert R, Dudenhausen JW. Changes in white blood cells during parturition in mothers and newborns. *Gynecol Obstet Invest.* 1994;338:227–235.
37. Tamir IL, Bongard FS, Klein SR. Acute appendicitis in the pregnant patient. *Am J Surg.* 1990;160:571–575.
38. Bickell NA, Siu AL. Why do delays in treatment occur? Lessons learned from ruptured appendicitis. *Health Serv Res.* 2001;36:1–5.
39. Weingold AB. Appendicitis in pregnancy. *Clin Obstet Gynecol.* 1983;26:801–809.
40. Andersen B, Nielsen TF. Appendicitis in pregnancy: diagnosis, management, and complications. *Acta Obstet Gynecol Scan.* 1999;78:758.
41. Cosenza CA, Saffari B, Jabbour N, et al. Surgical management of biliary gallstone disease during pregnancy. *Am J Surg.* 1999;178:545–548.
42. Lu E, Curet M, El-Sayed Y, et al. Medical versus surgical management of biliary tract disease in pregnancy. *Am J Surg.* 2004;188:755–759.
43. Kort B, Katz VL, Watson WJ. The effect of nonobstetric operation during pregnancy. *Surg Gynecol Obstet.* 1993;177:371–376.
44. Ishihara Y, Inoue H, Kohata Y, et al. Delivery outcomes following laparoscopic ovarian cystectomy during pregnancy. *Gynecol Endosc.* 2002;11:417–421.
45. Wang PH, Chao HT, Yuan CC, et al. Ovarian tumors complicating pregnancy. Emergency and elective surgery. *J Reprod Med.* 1999;44:279–287.
46. Cohen-Kerem R, Railton C, Oren D, et al. Pregnancy outcome following non-obstetric surgical intervention. *Am J Surg.* 2005;190:467–473.
47. Immer-Bansi A, Immer FF, Henle S, et al. Unnecessary emergency cesarean section due to silent CTG during anesthesia? *Br J Anaesth.* 2001;87:791–793.
48. American College of Obstetricians and Gynecologists. Nonobstetric surgery during pregnancy. *ACOG Committee Opinion.* August 2003 Number 284.
49. Gerstenfeld TS, Chang DT, Pliego AR, et al. Nonobstetrical abdominal surgery during pregnancy in Women's Hospital. *J Matern Fet Med.* 2002;9:170–172.
50. American College of Obstetricians and Gynecologists. Management of preterm labor. *ACOG Practice Bulletin.* May 2003, Number 43.
51. American College of Obstetricians and Gynecologists. Antenatal corticosteroid therapy for fetal maturation. *ACOG Committee Opinion.* May 2002, Number 273.
52. Roberts D, Dalziel S. Antenatal corticosteroids for accelerating fetal lung maturation for women at risk of preterm birth. *Cochrane Database Syst Rev.* 2006 Jul 19;3: CD004454.
53. Ballard PL, Ballard RA. Scientific basis and therapeutic regimens for use of antenatal corticosteroids. *Am J Obstet Gynecol.* 1995;173:254–262.
54. Greer IA. Thrombosis in pregnancy: maternal and fetal issues. *Lancet.* 1999;353:1258–1265.
55. Geerts WH, Pineo GF, Heit JA, et al. Prevention of venous thromboembolism: the Seventh ACCP Conference on Antithrombotic and Thrombolytic Therapy. *Chest.* 2004;126:338S–400S.
56. Basic standards for preanesthesia care. American Society of Anesthesiologists, 2005.
57. American College of Obstetricians and Gynecologists. Obstetric analgesia and anesthesia. *ACOG Practice Bulletin.* July 2002, Number 36.
58. MacDonald H. American Academy of Pediatrics, Committee on Fetus and Newborn. Perinatal care at the threshold of viability. *Pediatrics.* 2002;110:1024–1027.
59. Maze RI, Kallen B. Reproductive outcome after anesthesia and operation during pregnancy: a registry study of 5405 cases. *Am J Obstet Gynecol.* 1989;161:1178–1185.
60. Rizzo AG. Laparoscopic surgery in pregnancy: long-term follow-up. *J Laparoendosc Adv Surg Tech.* 2003;13(1):11–15.
61. Hunter JG, Swanstrom L, Thornburg K. Carbon dioxide pneumoperitoneum induces fetal acidosis in a pregnant ewe model. *Surg Endosc.* 1995;9:272–279.
62. Reedy MB, Kallen B, Kuehl TJ. Laparoscopy during pregnancy: a study of five fetal outcome parameters with the use of the Swedish Health Registry. *Am J Obstet Gynecol.* 1997;177:673–679.
63. SAGES publication 0023, 2000. SAGES guidelines for laparoscopic surgery during pregnancy. www.sages.org/sagespublication.php?doc=23. Accessed October 22, 2006.
64. American Heart Association. Cardiac arrest associated with pregnancy. *Circulation.* 2005;112:IV-150–IV-153.
65. Katz V, Balderston K, DeFreest M. Perimortem cesarean delivery: were our assumptions correct? *Am J Obstet Gynecol.* 2005;192:1916–1921.
66. Powner DR, Bernstein IM. Extended somatic support for pregnant women after brain death. *Crit Care Med.* 2003;31:1241–1248.
67. Bernstein IM, Watson M, Simmons GM, et al. Maternal brain death and prolonged fetal survival. *Obstet Gynecol.* 1989;74:434–437.
68. American College of Obstetricians and Gynecologists. Patient choice in the maternal-fetal relationship. *Ethics in Obstetrics and Gynecology.* 2nd ed. www.acog.org. Accessed October 22, 2006.
69. McGwin G, Russell SR, Rux RL, et al. Knowledge, beliefs, and practices concerning seat belt use during pregnancy. *J Trauma.* 2004 Mar;56(3):670–675: beliefs and practices. *J Trauma.* 1999 Feb;46(2):241–245.
70. McGwin G Jr, Willey P, Ware A, et al. A focused educational intervention can promote the proper application of seat belts during pregnancy. *J Trauma.* 2004;56(5):1016–1021.
71. Astarita DC, Feldman B. Seat belt placement resulting in uterine rupture. *J Trauma.* 1997;42:738–740.
72. Hyde LK, Cook LJ, Olson LM, et al. Effect of motor vehicle crashes on adverse fetal outcomes. *Obstet Gynecol.* 2003;102(2):279–286.
73. Murphy CC, Schei B, Myhr T, et al. Abuse: a risk factor for low birth weight? A systematic review and meta-analysis. *Can Med Assoc J.* 2001;164:1567–1572.
74. Yost NP, Bloom SL, McIntire DD, et al. A prospective observational study of domestic violence during pregnancy. *Obstet Gynecol.* 2005;106:61–65.

CHAPTER 101 ■ FETAL MONITORING CONCERNS

KERI A. BAACKE • RODNEY K. EDWARDS

The care of a pregnant woman poses a special set of challenges. These challenges are due primarily to the fact that one really is caring for two separate patients: the woman and her fetus. To further complicate matters, one of these patients, the fetus, cannot be assessed directly. The needs of one often are congruent with the needs of the other. However, this may not always be the case. There are times when interventions undertaken on behalf of either the pregnant woman or her fetus may be detrimental to the other. At all times, the needs of each of these patients must be considered when caring for a pregnant woman.

IMMEDIATE CONCERNS

Immediate issues that need to be evaluated when caring for a pregnant woman include viability of the fetus, the gestational age of the fetus, and assessment of the fetal condition. Determination of fetal viability is the first priority in the initial assessment of a pregnant patient—a diagnosis of fetal demise eliminates the fetus as a confounding factor in decisions regarding maternal treatment. In contrast, confirmation of a live fetus indicates a need to avoid teratogenic agents and optimize oxygen delivery to the placenta. In either case, one should consider the physiologic changes that occur during pregnancy when formulating a plan of care.

Estimation of gestational age is an important factor to establish as early into the treatment as is possible. If the pregnancy is near term and nonobstetric surgical treatment is indicated, delivery of the fetus prior to such treatment may be warranted. The earliest gestational age at which neonatal survival may occur is around 23 weeks. However, survival, particularly without significant morbidity, becomes more likely at later gestational ages. Even prior to the time when *ex utero* survival is possible, some treatments may better be avoided for the sake of the fetus, but as the gestational age advances, discussion regarding delivery of the fetus may be appropriate to maximize treatment to the woman without placing the fetus at unnecessary risk.

Finally, fetal assessment is dependent on the current gestational age. At early gestational ages, assessment includes only documentation of fetal cardiac activity. At later gestational ages, the goal of fetal assessment and monitoring is the determination of the adequacy of fetal oxygenation, and, when necessary, alerting the physician to potential hypoxia and/or fetal compromise. These indirect assessments of the fetal condition (discussed later in this chapter) allow for intervention, with the aim of improving fetal oxygenation or delivery if improvement does not occur.

SPECIAL CONSIDERATIONS

When instituting therapies for a pregnant patient, the effect of such therapy on the fetus must be considered. Many treatments provided to pregnant women are also considered to be in the best interest of the fetus. Optimal maternal oxygenation, blood pressure, temperature, and electrolyte balance benefit both the mother and the fetus. Some therapies, however, may be detrimental to the fetus, such as certain radiologic procedures and the administration of some medications. Similar to the blood–brain barrier, not all medications are transported across the placenta. This fact allows the use of some treatments without undue risk to the fetus. However, there are instances when short-term use of some medications may be acceptable or when alternate therapies may provide similar benefit without excessive risk to the fetus. Certainly, all of these factors need to be considered before beginning a course of treatment. Consultation with a maternal-fetal medicine specialist will provide appropriate recommendations regarding the effects of the physiologic changes of pregnancy on the planned treatment and which medications to avoid.

FETAL OXYGENATION

The placenta develops from trophoblastic cells called the syncytiotrophoblast. As these cells proliferate, the intervillous space is created. This space is where maternal blood bathes the fetal chorionic villi and where fetal-maternal and maternal-fetal exchange occurs (1). Although the intervillous space is an area characterized by low pressure, a pressure differential does exist and ensures adequate circulation. The maternal arteriolar pressure exceeds the pressure in the intervillous space, which exceeds the pressure in the maternal veins. The placenta itself is a low-resistance organ, and, accordingly, the pressure differential across the intervillous space is small. Therefore, the vascular resistance of the maternal arteries governs the rate of flow into and across the intervillous space. During uterine contractions, venous pressure increases. This increased venous pressure causes cessation of flow into the intervillous space. However, the villous space becomes somewhat dilated during a contraction, allowing for continued contact with maternal blood and continued gas exchange, although with reduced efficiency.

The placenta has a high rate of oxygen consumption. It serves as the main organ of gas and nutrient exchange for the fetus (2). However, oxygen extracted at the fetal-maternal interface serves not only the fetus, but the placenta as well. This highly metabolic organ uses as much, and possibly more, of the total oxygen and nutrients as the fetus to maintain its own growth and metabolism (3).

Oxygen consumption remains constant over a wide range of changes in oxygen delivery and will decrease only when extraction is maximal and delivery is further reduced (4). A 50% reduction in uterine blood flow is compensated by an increase in umbilical blood flow and an increase in oxygen extraction to maintain oxygen delivery with no change in fetal oxygen consumption (5). This compensatory mechanism remains adequate only with short-term reductions in uterine blood flow. A critical point exists below which oxygen uptake becomes dependent on oxygen delivery (6). Long-term reductions result in decreased consumption secondary to the decrease in delivery. Below this threshold, tissue hypoxia occurs, there is an inability to maintain oxidative metabolism, and fetal acidemia results (7). A chronic decrease in oxygen consumption also will lead to decreases in both fetal growth and fetal activity in an effort to conserve oxygen for cellular homeostasis (8).

Evidence in sheep indicate that low oxygen-diffusing capacity may be the limiting factor in equilibration of maternal and fetal PO_2 across the placenta, particularly in the setting of fetal growth restriction (9). At high altitudes, the diffusion capacity for oxygen increases in an effort to compensate for the low maternal PO_2 (10). The administration of maternal oxygen has no effect on uterine or umbilical blood flow but does, however, increase the fetal venous PO_2. In situations where fetal oxygen consumption is normal, no increase in fetal oxygen consumption occurs (11). In situations in which fetal oxygen consumption is decreased, maternal administration of oxygen will increase fetal oxygen consumption to near-normal range (12).

The placenta carries oxygenated blood to the fetus via the umbilical vein, while deoxygenated blood is carried back to the placenta via the two umbilical arteries. The human fetal umbilical venous PO_2 is low compared to postnatal standards—around 30 mm Hg. Despite this low PO_2, adequate amounts of oxygen can be delivered to the fetal tissues. This delivery is facilitated by the high fetal cardiac output, relative to its body size, and the affinity of fetal hemoglobin for oxygen (13). This situation highlights the importance of the high affinity that fetal hemoglobin has for oxygen. Fetal hemoglobin's high affinity for oxygen ensures that virtually all of the fetal hemoglobin is maximally saturated, even at the low PO_2 of the fetal umbilical venous blood. This affinity can be altered by factors such as acidosis and temperature. An increase in pH or a decrease in temperature causes a shift of the hemoglobin oxygen dissociation curve to the left, indicating a higher oxygen affinity.

The transfer of carbon dioxide across the placenta is limited by the diffusion capacity. The placenta is highly permeable to carbon dioxide, and transfer across the chorionic villi is accomplished faster than the transfer of oxygen. Also favoring the transfer of carbon dioxide is the higher affinity that maternal blood has for carbon dioxide compared to fetal blood. Finally, the mild respiratory alkalosis that is normally present in the pregnant woman results in a lower PCO_2, further enhancing the transfer of carbon dioxide from the fetus to the maternal blood. These physiologic changes also can work to alter the fetal acid-base balance. Alterations in maternal PCO_2 content can lead to disturbances in the fetal PCO_2 content. If maternal PCO_2 is abnormally elevated, fetal transfer is hindered and will result in elevations of fetal PCO_2 and fetal acidosis.

Glucose is a major energy source for the fetus. The fetus primarily obtains glucose from maternal blood, but this may be supplemented by its own glycogenolysis. Fetal glucose deprivation does not alter the weight-specific glucose utilization by the fetus. Instead, this utilization causes fetal hypoglycemia, which results in an increase in the maternal-fetal glucose gradient, and thus increased glucose transport across the placenta. Glucose transport is limited by the availability of transport proteins in the placenta as well as maternal blood glucose levels (2). This facilitated transport differs from that of oxygen and carbon dioxide, which is dependent solely on simple diffusion. Severe glucose deprivation and the resultant decrease in placental uptake may result in fetal growth abnormalities due to the decrease in available substrate (3). Chronic glucose deprivation will decrease glucose utilization and increase glycogenolysis and gluconeogenesis by the breakdown of fetal protein. This net protein loss results in fetal growth disturbances and ultimately may lead to growth restriction.

Transport of waste includes lactate. With a drop in oxygen supply and a change to anaerobic metabolism, the fetus begins to produce large amounts of lactate. In this situation, the placenta becomes a major source of lactate clearance from the fetal circulation (14). The placenta, in response to decreased glucose supply, will decrease its consumption of glucose and increase its consumption of lactate to account for the glucose deficit (15).

FETAL MONITORING

Electronic fetal monitoring, introduced in the 1960s, has become ubiquitous in labor and delivery units in developed countries. This type of fetal monitoring typically is used at any gestational age at which *ex utero* survival is possible. It requires very little in preparation or maintenance but does require an experienced interpreter. This technique results in a continuous tracing of the fetal heart rate, coupled with a tracing of uterine activity.

Regulation of the fetal heart rate is governed by a complex interplay of the sympathetic and parasympathetic nervous systems (16). The sympathetic nervous system exerts influence through the release of norepinephrine, which accelerates the heart rate and increases inotropy. The parasympathetic nervous system influences the fetal heart through the vagus nerve. Stimulation of the vagus nerve leads to a decrease in the heart rate. The fetal heart rate variability results from the constant "push-pull" of these two systems. Gestational age has some effect on the fetal heart rate, with a general decrease in the baseline heart rate occurring with advancing gestation. Finally, fetal heart rate tracing reactivity is defined by the presence of fetal heart rate accelerations. These transient increases in baseline fetal heart rate are due to fetal movement. The presence of reactivity is associated with central nervous system maturation and virtually always is present in a normal fetus after 32 weeks gestational age (17). The absence of fetal heart rate variability for periods of more than 1 hour, and especially in the presence of fetal heart rate decelerations, is associated with fetal acidemia (18).

Decelerations occur when the fetal heart rate falls below the baseline heart rate and are classified according to their location in relation to uterine contractions and their appearance. Different types of decelerations are caused by different mechanisms.

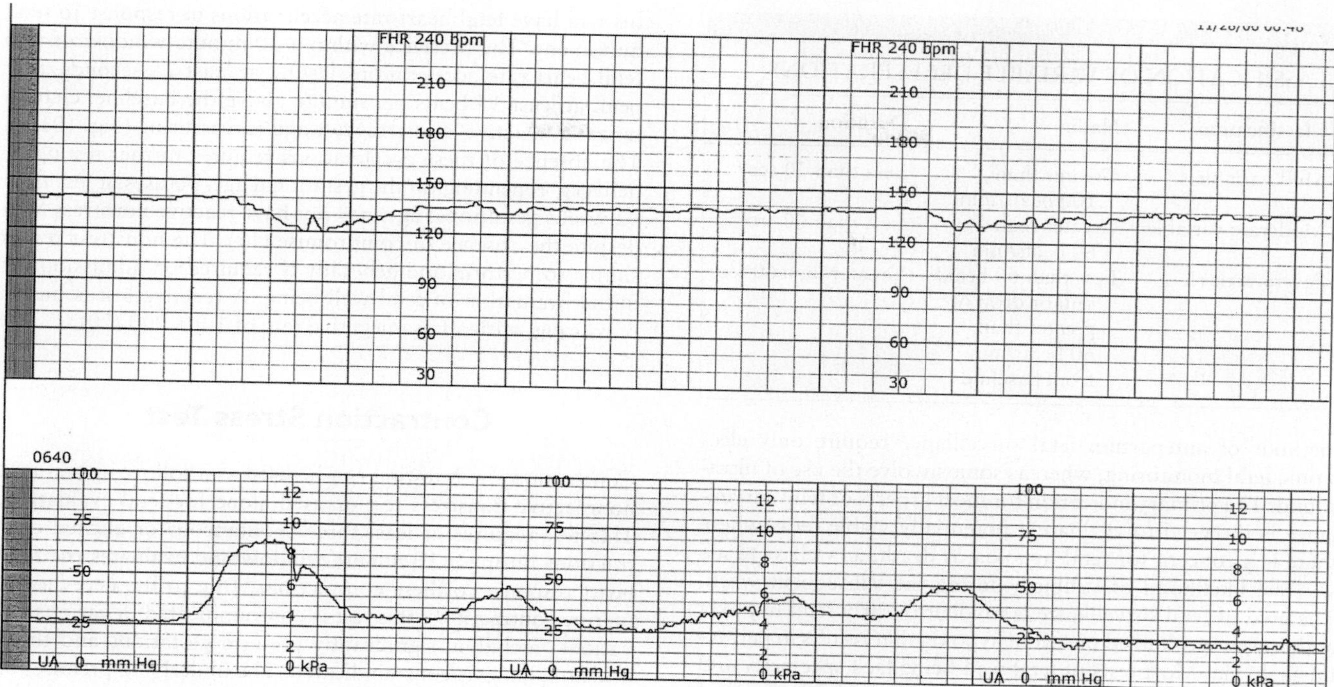

FIGURE 101.1. Early decelerations. Early decelerations mirror the contraction and are not associated with fetal compromise.

Therefore, each type of deceleration has different implications for fetal well-being.

- **Early decelerations:** Early decelerations begin at the onset of uterine contractions and appear to mirror the contraction (Fig. 101.1). They are believed to be caused by pressure on the fetal head. This pressure results in an alteration in cerebral blood flow and stimulation of the vagal center, with a subsequent decrease in the fetal heart rate. Early decelerations generally are not associated with other ominous findings and are not associated with fetal hypoxia, acidosis, or low Apgar scores.
- **Variable decelerations:** Variable decelerations are caused by intermittent umbilical cord compression. Although they occur most often during uterine contractions, they may occur at variable times in relation to uterine contractions and may occur even in the absence of contractions (Fig. 101.2). The physiologic basis for these decelerations results from either a chemoreceptor or a baroreceptor response. On initial cord occlusion, there is an increase in fetal peripheral resistance caused by the interruption of the low resistance placental circulation. This results in fetal hypertension and stimulation of the baroreceptors. The baroreceptor response activates the vagus nerve, resulting in fetal heart rate deceleration. Along with the rise in pressure, there is a fall in fetal PO_2 with umbilical cord compression. This decrease in arterial oxygen content leads to chemoreceptor activation and stimulation of vagal activity. Frequently, "shoulders" can be seen both preceding and following these variable decelerations. These transient increases in fetal heart rate are a result of venous occlusion and a decrease in blood return to the fetal heart. This decreased cardiac output leads to a compensatory rise in heart rate. Mild or isolated variable decelerations are benign. However, repetitive moderate or severe variable decelerations may indicate fetal compromise (Table 101.1).
- **Late decelerations:** Late decelerations occur late in relation to the uterine contraction. Their onset begins after the contraction begins, and they resolve after the resolution of the contraction (Fig. 101.3). These decelerations occur as a result of decreased uteroplacental oxygen delivery to the fetus. This intermittent hypoxia, which may or may not be associated with fetal acidemia, also results in fetal hypertension, leading to both a chemoreceptor and baroreceptor response. In the presence of fetal acidemia, this response may also be mediated by direct myocardial depression (17). There are many clinical causes of late decelerations, primarily those that result in maternal hypotension or decreased uterine blood flow. Persistence of late decelerations, especially in the absence of fetal variability, is an ominous sign of fetal compromise.

Other fetal heart rate patterns may be seen in the presence of fetal central nervous system dysfunction. Although the normal fetus may have episodes of decreased heart rate variability of 30 to 40 minutes due to sleep, fetuses with central nervous system dysfunction may exhibit persistently diminished variability. Unstable, or wandering, baseline heart rates also may be seen. Sinusoidal patterns also can be seen in the presence of fetal central nervous system dysfunction. These patterns resemble a sine wave, with a frequency of 3 to 5 cycles per minute and an absence of fetal heart rate variability. Severe fetal anemia is another potential cause of a sinusoidal fetal heart rate tracing (17).

ANTENATAL TESTING

In addition to fetal heart rate monitoring during labor, certain situations may indicate periodic assessments of fetal well-being during the antepartum period. Several of these

TABLE 101.1

CLASSIFICATION OF VARIABLE DECELERATIONS

Classification	Nadir	Duration
Mild variable	Greater than 100 beats/min	Less than 30 sec
Moderate variable	Greater than 60 beats/min	Less than 60 sec
Severe variable	Less than 60 beats/min or drop of greater than 60 beats/min from baseline	Greater than 60 sec

methods of antepartum fetal surveillance require only electronic fetal monitoring, whereas some involve the use of ultrasound. The primary indication for most aspects of fetal surveillance is the need to evaluate a potentially viable fetus where there is a concern for fetal hypoxia or death, as well as to assess the likelihood of stillbirth during the subsequent week. The goal of fetal surveillance is to identify early fetal hypoxia and prevent prolonged or severe hypoxia that results in perinatal asphyxia. Most tests of fetal well-being lack specificity and have a low positive-predictive value but are used because of their high negative-predictive value. They are frequently used in high-risk obstetric patients but are of limited value when the maternal condition is changing rapidly.

Nonstress Test

Nonstress testing involves fetal heart rate monitoring for a period of 20 to 40 minutes. The underlying premise for this test relates to the fact that a nonacidotic, neurologically intact fetus will have fetal heart rate accelerations in response to fetal movement. The presence within a 20-minute window of two fetal heart rate accelerations lasting at least 15 seconds, that peak at least 15 beats per minute above the baseline, characterizes a 'reactive' nonstress test and is reassuring (Fig. 101.4). The absence of these accelerations requires further testing or delivery, depending on the gestational age. Fetuses at less than 32 weeks gestational age may not have reactive nonstress tests despite the absence of compromise (19). The nonstress test is simple to perform and generally is required on admission for initial evaluation of fetal well-being. A reactive test is highly reassuring, with a false-negative rate of 1.9/1,000 (20).

Contraction Stress Test

Contraction stress testing can be used as a follow-up test to a nonreactive nonstress test or used alone for fetal evaluation. This test requires at least three spontaneous or elicited contractions during a 10-minute window and evaluates the fetal heart response to these contractions. Due to the necessity of uterine contractions, this test is contraindicated in various situations, including significantly preterm gestations and those in whom labor is contraindicated. The underlying premise for this test involves the idea that fetal oxygenation will transiently worsen in the presence of uterine contractions. In the already compromised fetus, this will result in late decelerations. The contraction stress test is interpreted based on the presence or absence of late decelerations. A positive contraction stress test is one in which late decelerations occur with at least 50% of contractions and generally indicates that delivery is warranted. A negative test result with no late decelerations is highly reassuring, with a false-negative rate of only 0.3/1,000 (Fig. 101.5) (20).

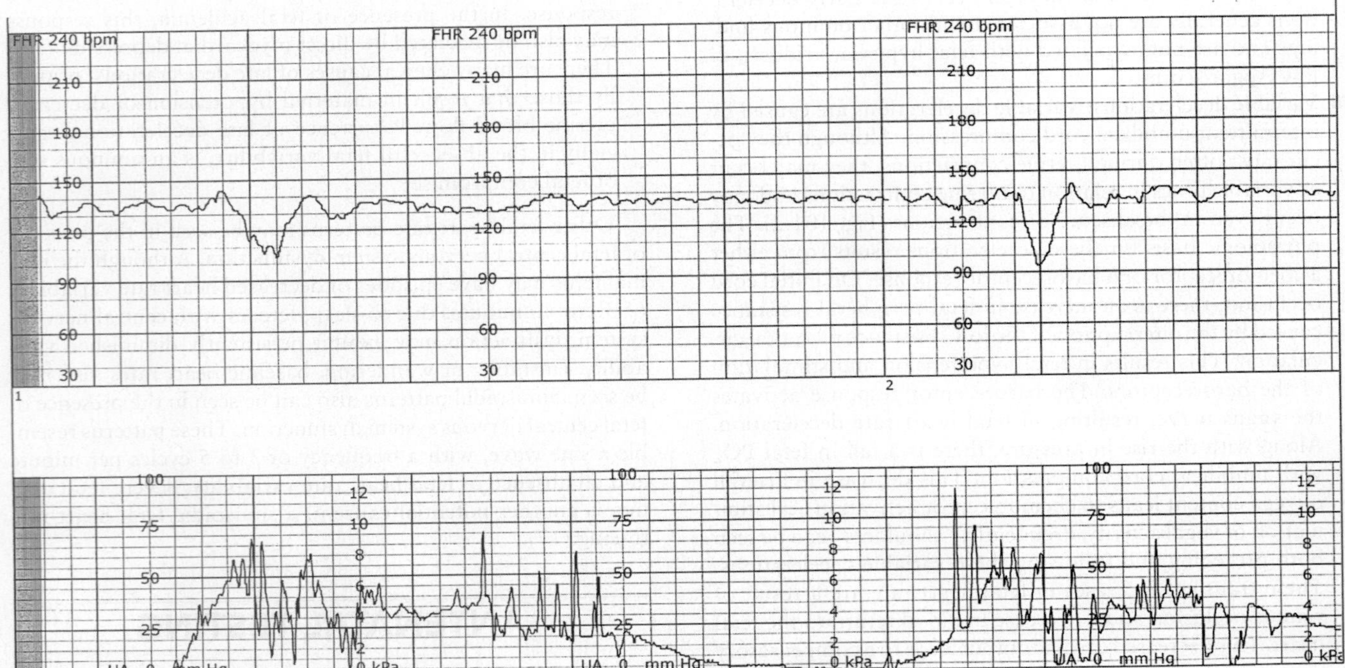

FIGURE 101.2. Variable decelerations. Variable decelerations occur at various times in relation to the contraction and are a result of transient umbilical cord compression.

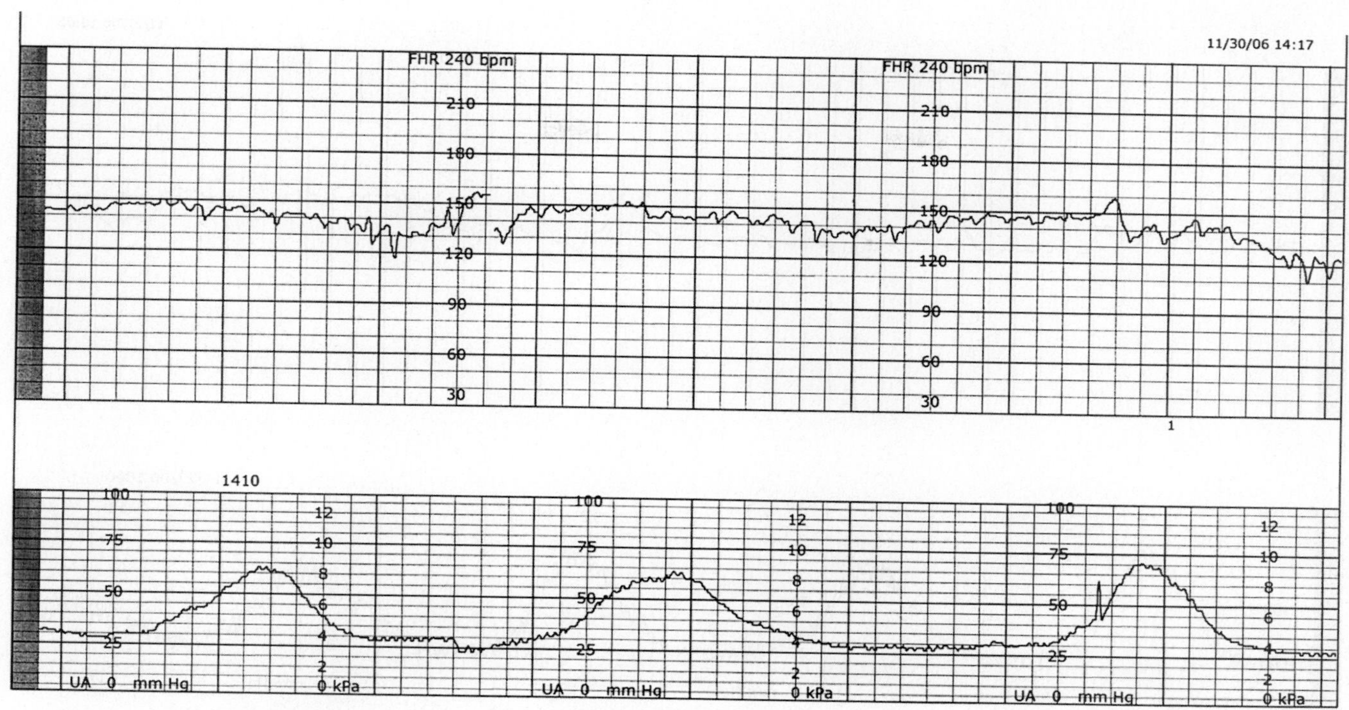

FIGURE 101.3. Late decelerations. Late decelerations occur late in relation to the contraction and may be a sign of fetal compromise.

Biophysical Profile

The biophysical profile consists of a nonstress test and an ultrasound evaluation of several parameters. This test can be performed as a follow-up test to a nonreactive, nonstress test or can be used as a form of surveillance on its own. The biophysical profile attempts to evaluate the fetus in terms of acute and chronic compromise. The nonstress test is one of the parameters used for evaluation. In addition, an ultrasound examination seeks to evaluate the amount of amniotic fluid, fetal tone, gross body movements, and fetal breathing movements

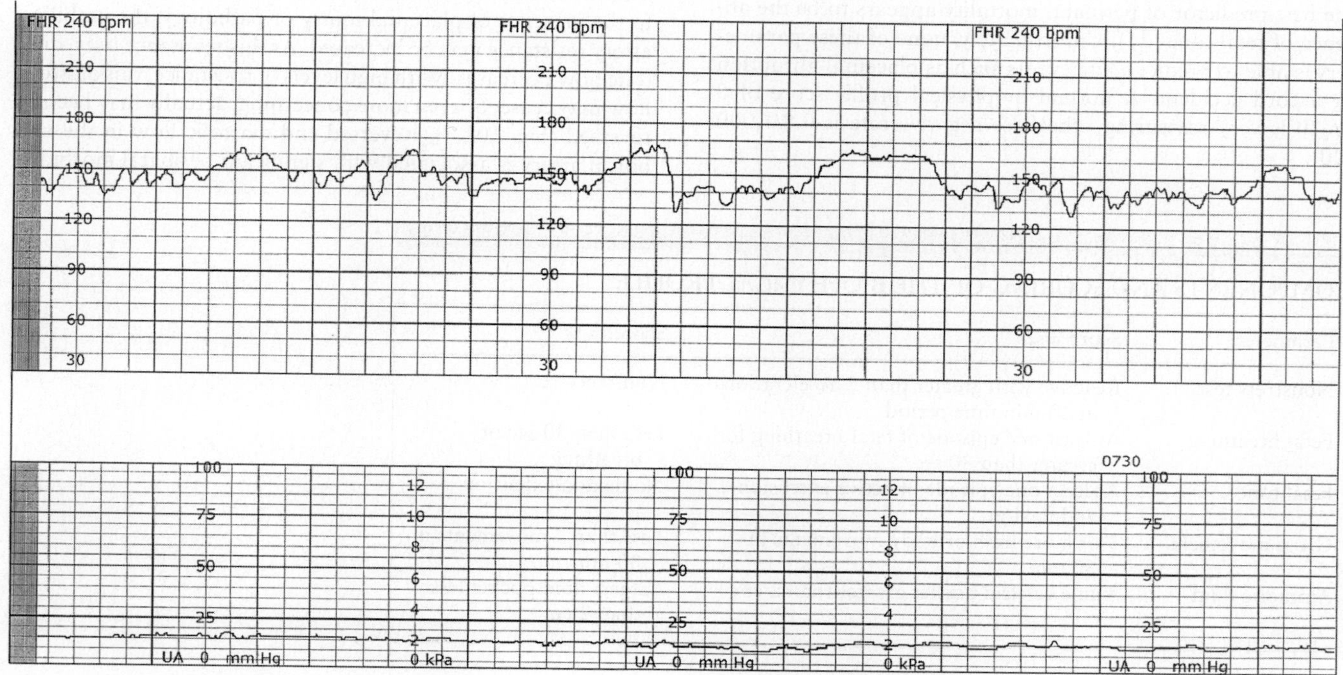

FIGURE 101.4. Reactive nonstress test. This nonstress test is reassuring, indicating fetal well-being.

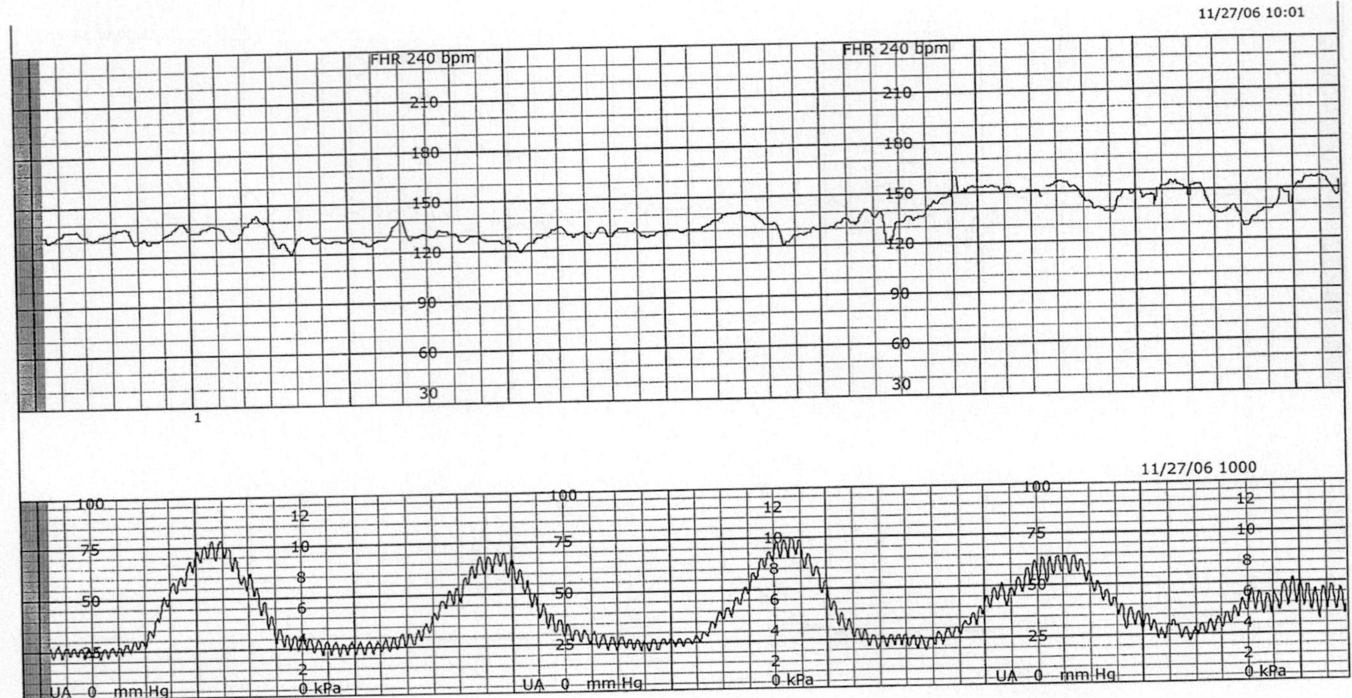

FIGURE 101.5. Negative contraction stress test. This contraction stress test is negative, indicating good fetal reserve.

(Table 101.2). The final score is derived from these various assessments, and intervention is based on both the score and gestational age. There are no contraindications to its use, and the entire evaluation takes less than an hour to complete. Many factors may alter the results of the biophysical profile, including maternal sedation, drug use, or hypoglycemia. There is a high correlation with low scores and fetal compromise, and the best predictor of perinatal mortality appears to be the absence of fetal tone (21). Unfortunately, none of these parameters is able to predict acute events such as placental abruption or a cord accident. A normal biophysical profile score of 8 or 10 is very reassuring—the false-negative rate is 0.8/1,000 (20).

Doppler Velocimetry

Doppler assessment can be accomplished with the use of color Doppler during an ultrasound examination. The umbilical artery is the most widely interrogated vessel for fetal surveillance. In normal fetuses, the umbilical artery has a high diastolic velocity due to low placental resistance (Fig. 101.6). In the presence of placental injury or pathology, the umbilical artery resistance may be increased. As this resistance rises, diastolic flow decreases. With high levels of resistance, this diastolic flow may cease, or even more concerning, actually may become reversed (Fig. 101.7). Reversed end diastolic flow in the umbilical artery is associated with significant perinatal morbidity

TABLE 101.2

COMPONENTS AND SCORING OF THE BIOPHYSICAL PROFILE[a]

Parameter	Score = 2	Score = 0
Nonstress test	Reactive with greater than 2 accelerations in 20-min time period	Non-reactive
Fetal breathing	At least one episode of fetal breathing for greater than 30 sec	Less than 30 sec of breathing
Fetal tone	At least one episode of active extension and flexion	No flexion/extension
Gross movement	3 or more limb or body movements in 30 min	Less than 3 movements in 30 min
Amniotic fluid	Single vertical pocket greater than 2 cm	Largest fluid pocket less than 2 cm

[a]Score is 2 or 0 for each parameter.

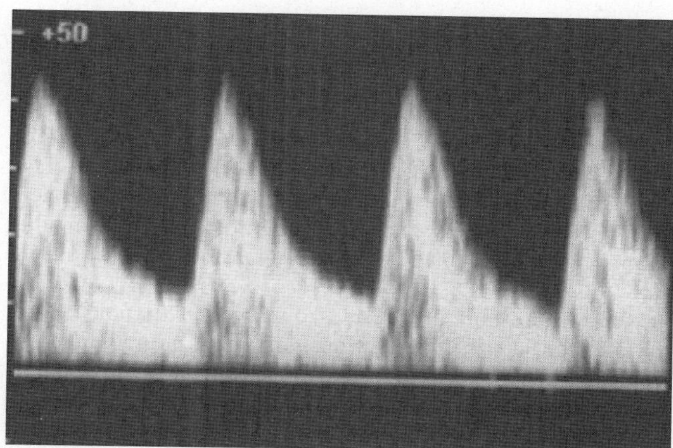

FIGURE 101.6. Doppler velocimetry. Normal umbilical artery Doppler waveform.

and mortality. Although large-scale studies have not been performed using umbilical artery Doppler as the main method of surveillance, small randomized controlled trials have indicated that it is a highly effective means of monitoring, with a negative-predictive value approaching 100% (22). A recent meta-analysis confirms the utility of Doppler assessment in the setting of growth restriction and notes a reduction in the number of perinatal deaths with the use of this technology (23). Doppler assessment has not been shown to be of value in the general obstetric population as a form of fetal surveillance in the absence of fetal growth restriction (24).

Doppler interrogation of the middle cerebral artery also has been shown to be of benefit in certain situations. In the setting of significant fetal anemia, the blood is "thinner" and the cardiac ejection fraction increases. This increase forces an increase in the velocity of blood through the middle cerebral artery. Periodic middle cerebral artery interrogation is replacing the assessment of amniotic fluid for monitoring fetuses at risk of anemia (25). The use of Doppler measurements from the umbilical artery or middle cerebral artery outside of the clinical settings described or the use of measurements from other vessels currently is investigational.

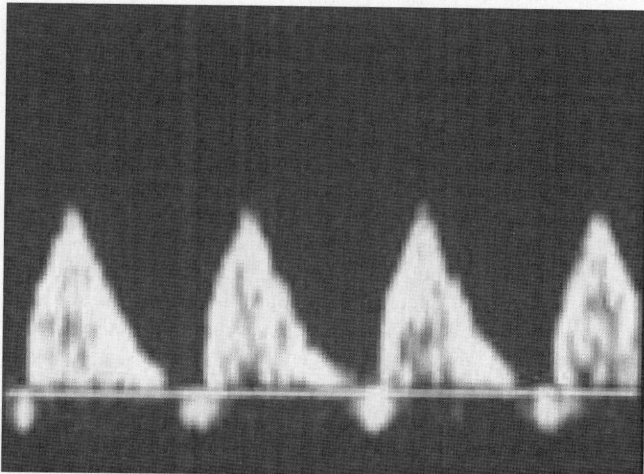

FIGURE 101.7. Abnormal Doppler velocimetry. This umbilical artery Doppler waveform shows reversed end diastolic flow, indicating increased placental resistance.

ADJUNCTS TO INTRAPARTUM FETAL HEART RATE MONITORING

Fetal Scalp Sampling

As mentioned previously, decelerations can occur in the absence of fetal hypoxia or acidemia. In an effort to delineate fetuses with decelerations and acidemia from those with normal pH, fetal scalp sampling may be performed. This is accomplished by taking a blood sample from the fetal scalp. The normal fetal scalp pH is 7.25 to 7.35, with values below 7.20 considered acidotic (17). This direct evaluation of fetal pH has limitations, in that this test can be performed only in the presence of labor with ruptured membranes. Therefore, this technique is not available for evaluating the preterm fetus, or even the term fetus when the membranes are intact, which limits its use to the intrapartum course. However, in the appropriate setting, this test can be an invaluable tool in the assessment of fetal acidosis. This metabolic acidosis can be treated with an adequate supply of oxygen. If the hypoxic insult is reversible, intrauterine resuscitation is preferred to immediate delivery. This can be accomplished with various techniques to improve maternal, and thus fetal, oxygenation, including the administration of supplemental oxygen and maternal position changes.

Many studies have evaluated fetal scalp stimulation and its relation to fetal pH. Fetuses with a fetal heart rate acceleration in response to digital stimulation of the scalp reliably have a pH of greater than 7.20. However, of fetuses without accelerations, 50% have a normal pH, whereas the remaining 50% are noted to be acidotic (26). Because digital stimulation of the fetal scalp can be performed when the membranes are intact, it requires only a cervix that is dilated. Therefore, this more simple evaluation of fetal pH can be used without ruptured membranes, although its use is still confined to evaluation of the fetus during labor.

Fetal Pulse Oximetry

Fetal pulse oximetry, introduced in the 1980s, initially held promise as a method to further assess the fetal oxygen status in the presence of a nonreassuring fetal heart rate tracing (27). As mentioned previously, the presence of late decelerations does not always indicate a state of persistent hypoxia or acidemia. The ability to directly monitor the fetal arterial oxygen saturation was thought to be an advancement in the ability to accurately predict those fetuses in need of more rapid delivery. A large randomized controlled trial was performed to assess the clinical utility of fetal pulse oximetry in the setting of a nonreassuring fetal heart rate tracing. Unfortunately, the results revealed no benefit in terms of overall cesarean delivery rate, with increased cost in the group using pulse oximetry (28). In response to this study, fetal pulse oximetry is not recommended for routine use and should be used only in the setting of a specific research protocol.

ST Segment Analysis

One of the newest advancements in the field of fetal assessment and electronic fetal monitoring is the ability to combine standard fetal heart rate assessment with an automated analysis of the fetal electrocardiogram, ST waveform analysis. Abnormalities in fetal heart rate tracings, as mentioned previously, have a low predictive value for neonatal acidemia. Fetal ST segment analysis is based on the observation that fetal hypoxia results in characteristic changes in the ST segment as well as the T wave on the fetal electrocardiogram. These changes are thought to be caused by anaerobic metabolism resulting from fetal hypoxia (29). A large Swedish trial comparing electronic fetal monitoring alone with electronic fetal monitoring and ST segment analysis showed a reduction in neonates born with metabolic acidosis when using ST segment analysis (30). Although this technology is not currently used in the United States, trials in this country currently are ongoing and should be reported in the very near future. If future trials support this improved sensitivity in the detection of fetuses with acidosis, ST segment analysis will provide more objective data to allow better identification of those fetuses at risk. ST segment analysis is limited by the need to have a fetal scalp electrode in place. Therefore, it is invasive and can be employed only during labor after the membranes have been ruptured.

HYPOXIA

Acute Adaptations

To understand fetal oxygenation, it is necessary to first understand the relationship of maternal to fetal oxygen delivery. As we know from the oxygen dissociation curve, at high partial pressures of oxygen, more oxygen can be bound to hemoglobin. As the hemoglobin protein binds each oxygen molecule, its affinity for oxygen is increased. The opposite also is true, in that, as the oxygen is unloaded at the tissue level, the affinity decreases, allowing for easier uncoupling and supply to the tissue. Various other factors, including pH, temperature, and organic phosphates, can alter that binding. An increase in temperature or decrease in pH causes a decrease in hemoglobin's affinity for oxygen, whereas a decrease in temperature or an increase in pH increases the affinity.

Carbon dioxide in the fetal circulation is exchanged for oxygen from the maternal circulation at the placental interface. The partial pressure of oxygen in the fetal circulation is much lower than that in the maternal circulation. It is this gradient that allows for oxygen transport to the fetus. Fetal hemoglobin is structurally different from adult hemoglobin, consisting of alpha and gamma chains rather than alpha and beta chains. Fetal hemoglobin has an increased affinity for oxygen compared to maternal hemoglobin. This difference in oxygen affinity allows for placental uptake of oxygen even at low partial pressures of oxygen, as is typical in the fetal circulation. At this lower partial pressure of oxygen, the maternal hemoglobin readily is able to unload oxygen, while the fetal hemoglobin readily attracts it. Due to these factors and other adaptations, including a high fetal cardiac output, the fetus normally is able to supply an adequate amount of oxygen to its tissues.

Fetal hypoxia results from either a reduction in placental blood flow or a reduction in oxygen delivery. The process begins with hypoxemia, a reduction in the amount of oxygen carried in the blood as a result of decreased PO_2. Although there are attempts at compensation, if these compensatory mechanisms fail, tissue hypoxia results. Energy requirements then are met using anaerobic mechanisms. However, when anaerobic metabolism is insufficient for continued energy demand, permanent tissue damage, organ failure, and asphyxia result (31).

Acute hypoxemia may result from several situations. Cord compression, uterine contractions, and maternal hypotension are frequent causes. Several defense mechanisms allow the fetus to adapt to acute hypoxemia. The fetal brain has a proportionally higher rate of oxygen consumption and therefore requires a high rate of oxygen delivery. To maintain adequate oxygenation, even during times of hypoxemia, the brain is perfused preferentially over other organ systems (32). To shunt blood to the brain, vasoconstriction occurs in the gastrointestinal tract, the skin, and other less essential organ systems. This redistribution of cardiac output via selective peripheral vasoconstriction is mediated by carotid artery chemoreceptor activation. What results is both a decrease in blood flow and oxygen delivery to the peripheral tissues. The accompanying vasodilation that occurs in the brain is most pronounced in the fetal brainstem. Consequently, it has been noted that the fetal brainstem is more resistant to hypoxic damage than are other areas of the brain (33). Tissue mediators, most importantly adenosine, mediate this cerebral vasodilation in response to acute hypoxemia. Adenosine is felt to be neuroprotective in the presence of hypoxemia by controlling oxygen consumption in the brain (34). Certainly, other mediators also influence the vasodilatory effect in the fetal brain; there are suggestions regarding the roles of nitric oxide and opioids. To what degree these other mediators affect the cerebral response to hypoxemia still is under investigation (35).

Along with circulatory centralization mediated by chemoreceptors, metabolic centralization also occurs. *Metabolic centralization* refers to the fetus's ability to reduce oxygen consumption in the setting of hypoxemia. This process allows the fetus to decrease oxygen delivery to peripheral tissues and allows for increased oxygen delivery to more vital organs. Therefore, when oxygen is in short supply, oxygen delivery still can be maintained to organs such as the brain, heart, and adrenals for continued oxidative metabolism (4). These changes in fetal metabolism contribute to compensatory adaptations to acute hypoxemia. A decrease in oxygen delivery can be compensated for a time. However, once oxygen delivery falls below a critical level, oxygen consumption also falls. Anaerobic metabolism of glycogen allows for maintenance of organ functions in the presence of continued hypoxemia. This anaerobic metabolism, however, leads to the production of lactate and a resulting metabolic acidosis. Lactate accumulates in the fetal tissue and leads to metabolic acidemia. Thus, assessment of fetal pH gives an indirect measure of fetal oxygenation.

Hypoxemia results in decreases in fetal breathing movements, rapid eye movements, general muscle tone and activity, and baseline heart rate (36). These changes minimize the fetus's consumption of oxygen and allow a greater proportion of the cardiac output to be used for maintaining the oxygen supply to the brain (37). Resumption of these activities will occur after several hours, even in the presence of continued hypoxia, as the fetus begins to adapt to a chronic hypoxic condition (38).

Hypoxia affects the fetal heart with a resulting drop in fetal heart rate and ventricular output. There is an elevation in blood pressure but only a small increase in stroke volume (4). To meet the oxygen requirements of the heart, coronary and myocardial blood flow is increased. If hypoxia progresses to acidemia, direct myocardial depression occurs, possibly related to depletion of cardiac glycogen stores. This myocardial depression, in turn, may cause late decelerations seen on fetal heart rate monitoring.

The fetal kidney also is affected by hypoxia. With increasing hypoxia, renal blood flow is decreased, and renal vascular resistance is increased in keeping with the redistribution of cardiac output to the brain, heart, and adrenal glands described previously (39). Prolonged hypoxia will result in a fall in the glomerular filtration rate and a decrease in urine output. The result will be a decrease in the amniotic fluid volume. Studies in sheep show that during recovery from hypoxia, the glomerular filtration rate and urine production actually will increase over control values (40).

Chronic Adaptations

Much of our understanding of the fetal response to chronic oxygen deprivation is a result of animal studies. Prolonged periods of umbilical cord occlusion and reductions in uterine blood flow result in chronic hypoxia for the fetus. The response to chronic hypoxia is different from the response to an acute hypoxic event. In an effort to continue to supply adequate amounts of oxygen to the peripheral tissues, plasma hemoglobin concentrations rise. Vascular endothelial growth factor and erythropoietin are part of the endocrine response to chronic hypoxia. These factors have neuroprotective effects through both direct action on the neuron and stimulation of angiogenesis and thus act to reduce neuronal injury in the presence of hypoxia (41). Blood flow, previously centralized to the brain, begins to normalize. Although cardiac output is depressed by continued hypoxia, the cerebral vasodilation and cerebral blood flow is maintained. Some studies have shown that under chronic hypoxic conditions, an increase in the synthesis of adrenomedullin, a vasodilator in the fetal cerebral cortex, may allow adequate oxygen delivery, even under low oxygen conditions (42). The increased cerebral blood flow to the brainstem that occurred acutely continues as the hypoxia becomes chronic.

Vascular resistance is increased in the setting of chronic hypoxia. This elevated resistance continues to allow the shunting of blood and oxygen preferentially to the brain. Maintenance of brain growth continues to be a priority even in the presence of continued hypoxia. Other organ systems grow at a disproportionately slower rate, and overall fetal weight is slowed. Meanwhile, the increased resistance in vascular beds, such as the gastrointestinal tract, may set the stage for neonatal complications such as necrotizing enterocolitis. This increase in vascular resistance is evident in Doppler studies of the umbilical arteries.

Some evidence points to changes in the venous circulation with chronic hypoxia. It has been noted that ductus venosus flow is increased in the fetus during periods of hypoxia (43). The increase in ductus venosus flow results in a decrease in flow through the liver, and the fall in hepatic perfusion may impair the liver's ability to synthesize and store glycogen. This situation leads to a decreased substrate available for continued fetal growth. The increase in ductus venosus flow is maintained, even in the presence of severe growth restriction. Some studies have associated a finding of decreased or absent flow in the ductus venosus during atrial systole as a late finding in the fetus's response to hypoxia. This finding has been further implicated in poor perinatal outcome (44).

Deep inspiratory efforts and fetal gasping occur with severe hypoxia/asphyxia. Although this inspiratory-like reflex is not effective in the fetus, it has been reported as a preterminal event in animal studies. With normalization of fetal oxygenation, even after prolonged periods of hypoxia, fetal breathing movements and fetal movements can return to normal. These events may occur, however, even in the presence of significant brain damage, including reduced myelination and periventricular necrosis (45). Therefore, fetal heart rate monitoring is limited in its ability to predict poor outcome in cases when significant hypoxic episodes occurred prior to the monitoring period. Prolonged periods of hypoxia have an effect on fetal heart rate—similar to the effect on fetal movements. Initially, bradycardia may be noted, followed by a reflex tachycardia. However, in the absence of acidemia, fetal heart rate will return to normal baseline after 12 to 16 hours (46).

SUMMARY

The presence of the fetus and the physiologic changes that occur during pregnancy significantly complicate the care of the pregnant woman. The ability to accurately evaluate the status of the fetus is limited by current technology. Although most tests of fetal surveillance can reassure the clinician that the fetus is in good condition, the positive-predictive value of nonreassuring results is low, and testing may lead to intervention when the fetus actually is not in jeopardy. As newer methods of evaluating the fetal response to stress and hypoxia are developed, our ability to accurately identify fetuses truly at risk will improve. Despite the limitations of the current methods, frequent monitoring of fetal status in the pregnant critically ill patient is used to guide treatment. Consultation either with maternal-fetal medicine specialists or general obstetrician-gynecologists will improve the ongoing care of pregnant patients, as these physicians are more familiar with the physiologic changes that occur in pregnancy and the methods used to evaluate the fetus.

PEARLS

- Determination of fetal viability is the first priority in the initial assessment of a pregnant patient.
- Fetal hemoglobin's high affinity for oxygen ensures maximal saturation of fetal hemoglobin.
- The primary indication for most aspects of fetal surveillance is the need to evaluate a potentially viable fetus when there is a concern for fetal hypoxia or death.
- The goal of fetal surveillance is to identify early fetal hypoxia and prevent prolonged or severe hypoxia resulting in perinatal asphyxia.

- Persistence of late decelerations, especially in the absence of fetal heart rate variability, is an ominous sign of fetal compromise.
- Antenatal fetal assessment includes the use of a nonstress test, biophysical profiles, and Doppler velocimetry.
- To maintain adequate oxygenation, even during times of hypoxemia, the brain is perfused preferentially over other organ systems.
- When oxygen is in short supply, oxygen delivery still can be maintained to organs such as the brain, heart, and adrenals for continued oxidative metabolism.
- Although the negative-predictive values are high, the positive-predictive values of all tests of fetal well-being are low.
- Consultation either with maternal-fetal medicine specialists or general obstetrician-gynecologists is recommended.

References

1. Ramsey EM, Martin CB Jr, Donner MW. Fetal and maternal placental circulation. *Am J Obstet Gynecol.* 1967;98:419.
2. Hay WW Jr. Placental transport of nutrients to the fetus. *Horm Res.* 1994;42:215.
3. Bell AW, Hay WW Jr, Ehrhardt RA. Placental transport of nutrients and its implications for fetal growth. *J Reprod Fertil Suppl.* 1999;54:401.
4. Jensen A, Garnier Y, Berger R. Dynamics of fetal circulation responses to hypoxia and asphyxia. *Eur J Obstet Gynecol Reprod Biol.* 1999;84:155.
5. Anderson DF, Parks CM, Faber JJ. Fetal O_2consumption in fetal sheep during controlled long term reduction in umbilical blood flow. *Am J Physiol.* 1986;250:H1037.
6. Carter AM. Factors affecting gas transfer across the placenta and the oxygen supply to the fetus. *J Dev Physiol.* 1989;12:305.
7. Carter AM. Placental oxygen consumption, I: in vivo studies—a review. *Placenta.* 2000;21:S31.
8. Peebles DM. Fetal consequence of chronic substrate deprivation. *Semin Fetal Neonatal Med.* 2004;9:379.
9. Wilkening RB, Meschia G. Current topic: comparative physiology of placental oxygen transport. *Placenta.* 1992;13:1.
10. Reshetnikova OS, Burton GJ, Milovanov AP. Effects of hypobaric hypoxia on the fetoplacental unit: the morphometric diffusing capacity of the villous membrane at high altitude. *Am J Obstet Gynecol.* 1994;171:1560.
11. Battaglia C, Artini PG, B'Ambrogi G, et al. Maternal hyperoxygenation in the treatment of intrauterine growth retardation. *Am J Obstet Gynecol.* 1992;167:430.
12. Battaglia FC, Meschia G, Makowski EL, et al. The effect of maternal oxygen inhalation upon fetal oxygenation. *J Clin Inves.* 1968;47:548.
13. Hellegers AE, Schruefer JJ. Nomograms and empirical equations relating oxygen tension, percentage saturation, and pH in maternal and fetal blood. *Am J Obstet Gynecol.* 1961;81:377.
14. Hooper SB, Walker DW, Harding R. Oxygen, glucose and lactate uptake by the fetus and placenta during prolonged hypoxemia. *Am J Physiol.* 1995;268:R303.
15. Gu W, Jones CT, Parer JT. Metabolic and cardiovascular effects on fetal sheep of sustained reduction of uterine blood flow. *J Physiol.* 1985;368:109.
16. Dalton KJ, Dawes GS, Patrick JE. The autonomic nervous system and fetal heart rate variability. *Am J Obstet Gynecol.* 1983;146:456.
17. Freeman RK, Garite TJ, Nageotte MP. Physiologic basis of fetal monitoring. In: *Fetal Heart Rate Monitoring.* 2nd ed. Baltimore, MD: Williams & Wilkins; 1991.
18. Williams KP, Galerneau F. Intrapartum fetal heart rate patterns in the prediction of neonatal academia. *Am J Obstet Gynecol.* 2002;188:820.
19. Smith CV, Phelan JP, Paul RH. A prospective analysis of the influence of gestational age on the baseline fetal heart rate activity and reactivity in a low-risk population. *Am J Obstet Gynecol.* 1985;153:780–782.
20. American College of Obstetrics and Gynecology Practice Bulletin No. 9. Antepartum fetal surveillance. October 1999.
21. Vintzileos AM, Gaffney SE, Salinger LM, et al. The relationship among the fetal biophysical profile, umbilical cord pH, and Apgar scores. *Am J Obstet Gynecol.* 1987;157:627.
22. Almstrom H, Axelsson O, Cnattingius S, et al. Comparison of umbilical artery velocimetry and cardiotocography for surveillance of small-for-gestational age fetuses. *Lancet.* 1992;340:936.
23. Westergaard HB, Langhoff-Roos J, Lingman G, et al. A critical appraisal of the use of umbilical artery Doppler ultrasound in high-risk pregnancies: use of meta-analyses in evidence-based obstetrics. *Ultrasound Obstet Gyneco.* 2001;17:466.
24. Mason GC, Lindow S, Ramsden C, et al. Randomized comparison of routine versus highly selective use of Doppler ultrasound in low risk pregnancies. *Br J Obstet Gynecol.* 1993;100:130.
25. Mari G, Deter RL, Carpenter RL, et al. Noninvasive diagnosis by Doppler ultrasonography of fetal anemia due to maternal red-cell alloimmunization. Collaborative Group for Doppler Assessment of the Blood Velocity in Anemic Fetuses. *N Engl J Med.* 2000;342:9.
26. Clark SL, Gimovsky ML, Miller FC. The scalp stimulation test: a clinical alternative to fetal scalp blood sampling. *Am J Obstet Gynecol.* 1984;148:274.
27. Dildy GA. Fetal pulse oximetry: a critical appraisal. *Best Pract Res Clin Obstet Gynecol.* 2004;18:477.
28. Garite TJ, Dildy GA, McNamara H, et al. A multicenter controlled trial of fetal pulse oximetry in the intrapartum management of nonreassuring fetal heart rate patterns. *Am J Obstet Gynecol.* 2000;183:1049.
29. Westgate J, Harris M, Curnow JSH, Greene KR. Plymouth randomized trial of cardiotocogram for intrapartum monitoring in 2400 cases. *Am J Obstet Gynecol.* 1993;169:1151.
30. Hagberg H, Goteborg I, Amer-Wahlin I, et al. Intrapartum fetal monitoring: cardiotocography versus cardiotocography plus fetal ECG ST waveform analysis. A Swedish randomized controlled trial. *Am J Obstet Gynecol.* 2001;184:S19.
31. Clerici G, Luzietti R, Di Renzo GC. Monitoring of antepartum and intrapartum fetal hypoxemia: Pathophysiological basis and available techniques. *Biol Neonate.* 2001;79:246.
32. Sheldon RE, Peeters LLH, Jones MD Jr, et al. Redistribution of cardiac output and oxygen delivery in the hypoxemic fetal lamb. *Am J Obstet Gynecol.* 1979;135:1071.
33. Tolcos M, Harding R, Loeliger M, et al. The fetal brainstem is relatively spared from injury following intrauterine hypoxia. *Brain Res Dev Brain Res.* 2003;143:73.
34. Koos BJ, Mason BA, Punla O, et al. Hypoxic inhibition of breathing in fetal sheep: relationship to brain adenosine concentrations. *J Appl Physiol.* 1994;77:2734.
35. Pearce W. Hypoxic regulation of the fetal cerebral circulation. *J Appl Physiol.* 2006;100:731.
36. Natale R, Clewlow F, Dawes GS. Measurement of fetal forelimb movements in the lamb in utero. *Am J Obstet Gynecol.* 1981;140:545.
37. Giussani DA, Spencer JAD, Hanson MA. Fetal cardiovascular reflex responses to hypoxaemia. *Fetal Maternal Med Rev.* 1994;6:17.
38. Bocking AD, Gagnon R, Milne KM, et al. Behavioral activity during prolonged hypoxemia in fetal sheep. *J Appl Physiol.* 1988;65:2420.
39. Weismann DN, Robillard JE. Renal hemodynamic response to hypoxemia during development: relationship to circulating vasoactive substances. *Pediatr Res.* 1988;23:155.
40. Wlodek ME, Challis JRG, Richardson B, et al. The effects of hypoxaemia with progressive acidaemia on fetal renal function in sheep. *J Dev Physiol.* 1989;12:323.
41. Marti HH. Erythropoietin and the hypoxic brain. *J Exp Biol.* 2004;207:3233.
42. Jensen RI, Carter AM, Skott O, Jensen BL. Adrenomedullin expression during hypoxia in fetal sheep. *Acta Physiol Scand.* 2005;183:219.
43. Tchirikov M, Rybakowski C, Hunecke B, et al. Blood flow through the ductus venosus in singleton and multifetal pregnancies and in fetuses with intrauterine growth retardation. *Am J Obstet Gynecol.* 1998;178:943.
44. Baschat AA, Gembruch U, Weiner CP, et al. Qualitative venous Doppler wavefrom analysis improve prediction of critical perinatal outcomes in premature growth-restricted fetuses. *Ultrasound Obstet Gynecol.* 2003;22:240.
45. Bocking AD. Assessment of fetal heart rate and fetal movements in detecting oxygen deprivation in-utero. *Eur J Obstet Gynecol Reprod Biol.* 2003;110:S108.
46. Bocking AD, White S, Gagnon R, et al. Effect of prolonged hypoxemia on fetal heart rate accelerations and decelerations in sheep. *Am J Obstet Gynecol.* 1989;161:722.

CHAPTER 102 ■ THE OBESE SURGICAL PATIENT IN THE CRITICAL CARE UNIT

ADRIAN ALVAREZ • JUAN C. CENDAN

Throughout the economically developed world, the incidence of obesity is rising at epidemic proportions. University medical centers are reporting that 25% of routine surgical patients are obese, and at least 10% of all patients are morbidly obese. Given the increasing prevalence of obesity in the general population, it is not surprising that many morbidly obese patients undergoing surgery are treated in intensive care units (ICU). Nevertheless, the real prevalence of critically ill morbidly obese patients, even in the United States, is not known. A retrospective study has allowed researchers to estimate that the incidence rate of morbidly obese patients requiring nonsurgical intensive care treatment approaches 14 cases per 1,000 ICU admissions annually. Bariatric surgical procedures alone have increased in the United States from 37,000 cases in 2000 up to 200,000 in 2006 as reported by the American Society for Bariatric Surgery (1).

The critically ill morbidly obese surgical patient presents the critical care team with many unique problems (2). As a result, every health care provider eventually involved in surgical procedures must be familiar with the management of morbidly obese patients, not only for bariatric procedures, but also for all types of surgery (3,4). Morbidly obese patients have an eightfold higher mortality rate after blunt trauma than nonobese patients presenting with the same diagnosis (5). Retrospective reviews of morbidly obese patients—hospitalized with or without ICU requirements—have shown significant increases in length of ICU stay, mortality, and duration of mechanical ventilation (6–9).

The pathophysiologic consequences of obesity involve all major organ systems (10). Conditions such as diabetes mellitus and hyperlipidemia are associated with obesity and contribute to chronic morbidity in the obese. However, the main concerns for the intensivist, anesthesiologist, and surgeon have been the same for over three decades: the derangements of the cardiopulmonary system (11,12).

The perioperative care of these patients must be understood as a continuous, indivisible, and dynamic process that requires multidisciplinary involvement from surgeons, anesthesiologists, internists, and intensivists. Collaborative and coordinated activity within the surgical team is vital in these scenarios involving the morbidly obese (13). In this chapter, we will discuss cardiac and respiratory diseases in the morbidly obese patient undergoing a surgical procedure, following the above-mentioned focus, from preoperative assessment to postoperative care.

SPECIFIC SURGICAL ISSUES

Obese patients undergoing emergency general surgery are particularly challenging for the team managing the patient before and after surgery. These patients occasionally present with more advanced disease than otherwise might be expected due to the obesity causing delays in diagnosis.

The first decision to be made is whether or not the procedure can be performed laparoscopically, or if an open procedure is required. Where possible, it has been our practice to perform emergency surgery laparoscopically in obese patients; there is evidence to support this approach for laparoscopic appendectomy and cholecystectomy. However, these patients require an additional level of expertise in the operating theater, not only from the surgeon and anesthesiologist, but also from the equipment handlers and the assistants. Colon cases and other cases involving more complicated visceral dissection may be detrimental if performed laparoscopically.

Obese patients are at higher risk for wound infection. The worst-case scenario develops when an obese patient eviscerates in the postoperative period. Emergent management will require closure, but this may not be technically feasible. These patients may require leaving the abdomen "open" with packing, and the patient will generally be intubated and paralyzed until the abdominal contents can be reduced or sufficient granulation develops that allows the construct to stabilize.

CARDIOVASCULAR CONSIDERATIONS IN THE MORBIDLY OBESE

Cardiovascular diseases are common in obese individuals, and manifest as ischemic heart disease, hypertension, and cardiac failure. Cardiovascular disease is reported in 37% of adults with a body mass index (BMI) greater than 30 kg/m^2, 21% with a BMI of 25 to 30 kg/m^2, and only 10% in those with a BMI less than 25 kg/m^2. *Obesity*—defined as a BMI of greater than or equal to 30 kg/m^2—has been observed to be an independent risk factor for the development of hypertension. The Framingham Heart Study suggests that 65% of the risk for hypertension in women and 78% of the risk in men can be related to obesity (14). Interestingly, mortality rates were reported to be 3.9 times greater in the overweight group versus the normal-weight group participating in the Framingham study (15).

The relationship between the increase in blood pressure and the risk of cardiovascular disease is considered to be independent of other risk factors. The chances of myocardial infarction, heart failure, stroke, and kidney disease are all greater as a patient's blood pressure increases (16). Obesity is also well recognized as a risk factor for ischemic heart disease. Many obese individuals also suffer from "metabolic syndrome," which has a strong association as being a precursor in the development of diabetes, cardiovascular disease, and increased mortality rates from cardiovascular disorders. There is also a 5% increased risk of heart failure for men and 7% for women associated with each unit of increase in body mass (15).

Preoperative Considerations

Pathophysiology

In morbidly obese patients, blood volume, cardiac output, systemic and pulmonary artery pressures, and left and right ventricular pressures are all elevated (17,18). These changes manifest clinically as arterial hypertension and, with advancing age, one may note ischemic heart disease and right–left heart failure (19). The incidence of pre-existing, often severe, cardiovascular disease in morbidly obese patients scheduled for elective bariatric surgery is reported to be as great as 20% (20,21). It is the complex interaction of hypertension, ischemic heart disease, and pulmonary hypertension that contribute to the development of global cardiac dysfunction and exacerbates congestive heart failure. This clinical situation is referred to as "obesity cardiomyopathy."

Arterial Hypertension

The pathogenesis of obesity-related hypertension is complex. There is a continuous relationship between body mass index and systolic/diastolic blood pressures (22,23). Blood pressure is normally regulated by a series of feedback loops (baroreceptors) and by the secretion of vasoactive hormones—renin, angiotensin, aldosterone, and catecholamines. A derangement in any of these feedback loops may lead to hypertension.

Many factors act together to promote vasoconstriction, sodium retention, and volume overload in obesity, and are noted in Table 102.1 (24–28). In the long term, these changes cause glomerular injury, ultimately leading to glomerulosclerosis. A review of 7,000 renal biopsies between the years 1990 and 2000 showed a 10-fold increase in obesity-related glomerulopathy (glomerulomegaly and glomerulosclerosis). Prolonged obesity may lead to a gradual loss of nephron function that worsens with time and exacerbates hypertension (29). Hypertension contributes to a pressure overload of the heart, as well as an expansion of extracellular and blood volume combining to create a volume overload.

Other variables that may also lead to hypertension in obese patients include leptin, free fatty acids, and insulin, which stimulate sympathetic activity and vasoconstriction (24). Furthermore, obesity-induced insulin resistance and endothelial dysfunction may act as amplifiers of the vasoconstrictor response. Obstructive sleep apnea (OSA), which also is more prevalent in obese patients, leads to periods of apnea and hypoxia, triggering a chemoreceptor response, which causes sympathetic activation (24,30,31).

TABLE 102.1

FACTORS THAT ACT TOGETHER TO PROMOTE VASOCONSTRICTION, SODIUM RETENTION, AND VOLUME OVERLOAD IN THE OBESE PATIENT

- Elevated glomerular filtration rate, an elevated renal blood flow, and exhibiting delayed urinary sodium excretion in response to the saline load[a]
- Increased renal sympathetic nervous activity, which directly promotes tubular reabsorption of sodium at the proximal and distal tubules[b]
- The renin-angiotensin-aldosterone system is activated, which contributes to sodium retention and an increase in extracellular volume, despite an elevated blood pressure[c]
- Natriuretic peptide levels are low, both at basal levels and also in response to salt loading[d]
- Hyperinsulinemia directly promotes the tubular absorption of sodium.[e] *Compensatory mechanisms in the obese for overcoming increased sodium reabsorption include renal vasodilation, an increased glomerular filtration rate, and a higher blood pressure.*

Data from:
[a] Montani JP, Antic V, Yang Z, et al. Pathways from obesity to hypertension: from the perspective of a vicious triangle. *Int J Obes Relat Metab Disord.* 2002;26(Suppl 2):S28–38.
[b] DiBona GF, Kopp UC. Neural control of renal function. *Physiol Rev.* 1997;77:75–197.
[c] Engeli S, Sharma AM. The renin-angiotensin system and natriuretic peptides in obesity-associated hypertension. *J Mol Med.* 2001;79:21–29.
[d] Dessi-Fulgheri P, Sarzani R, Tamburrini P, et al. Plasma atrial natriuretic peptide and natriuretic peptide receptor gene expression in adipose tissue of normotensive and hypertensive obese patients. *J Hypertens.* 1997;15:1695–1699.
[e] Endre T, Mattiasson I, Berglund G, et al. Insulin and renal sodium retention in hypertension-prone men. *Hypertension.* 1994;23:313–319.

Ischemic Heart Disease

Obesity is a recognized risk factor for ischemic heart disease (19,32). The risk is proportional to the duration of obesity and distribution of fat. A habitually overweight individual is less likely to be at risk than individuals who exhibit continuous weight gain, and individuals with a central distribution of fat are more at risk than individuals with a peripheral distribution. Additionally, hypertension, diabetes, hypercholesterolemia, and increased levels of low-density lipoproteins (LDLs), which are common in obese patients, further increase the risk of coronary stenosis. Nevertheless, more than 40% of obese patients with angina do not have significant coronary artery disease (30,33,34). Angina would then be attributable to the oxygen supply/demand imbalance due to cardiac hypertrophy and other factors. In the morbidly obese, myocardial oxygen consumption is higher than in normal-weight adults. The ventricular cavity dimension is enlarged due to a chronically augmented preload. An enhanced sympathetic activity and subsequent arterial hypertension and/or increased heart rate promote higher wall tension and ventricular systolic stress. In addition, the ventricular wall is commonly hypertrophic (35–39). Patients suffering chronic hypoxemia (pickwickian syndrome, obesity hypoventilation syndrome, and obstructive sleep apnea syndrome) frequently develop secondary polycythemia and, subsequently, elevated blood viscosity. In these patients, due to the higher blood viscosity, the contractility is augmented, which consequently increases myocardial oxygen requirements (40).

It may be assumed that morbidly obese patients are at a higher risk of myocardial ischemia. In these subjects, reducing myocardial oxygen consumption and ensuring the maximum possible oxygen delivery to the heart must be a major therapeutic target.

Cardiac Failure

There is an increased risk of heart failure of 5% for men and 7% for women per each unit of increase in body mass (15). There is a linear relationship between body weight and cardiac weight gain attributed to concentric and eccentric hypertrophy. This event is secondary to pressure overload, which is due to arterial hypertension and possibly increased blood viscosity. In obese patients, circulating blood volume, plasma volume, and cardiac output increase proportionately with rising weight. For a patient with a fat mass of 50 kg, blood flow to this fat mass accounts for an extra cardiac output of 1.5 to 2.0 L/minute, resulting in both ventricular enlargement and an increase in stroke volume. The hypertrophy that ensues subsequently contributes to a reduction in cardiac compliance and left ventricular diastolic function, which leads to increased left ventricular end-diastolic pressure and possible pulmonary edema (41).

In long-standing obesity, systolic function might be reduced if hypertrophy is unable to keep pace with the increasing demand. A decrease in midwall fiber shortening and a decrease in ejection fraction may thus become evident in developing "obesity cardiomyopathy." The right ventricle can also exhibit hypertrophy secondary to pulmonary hypertension due to obstructive sleep apnea and subsequent chronic hypoxemia and hypercapnia.

Preoperative Evaluation and Optimization for Surgery

A significant percentage of obese patients who present for intermediate- to high-risk noncardiac surgery is likely to have cardiovascular disease. It is imperative to know if any related impairment actually exists. If so, assessment of its severity, decisions on whether or not any therapeutic measures can be taken prior to surgery, and consideration of any extra intraoperative or postoperative monitoring are of utmost importance for effective treatment of the obese patient.

Arterial Hypertension

The preoperative assessment, optimization, and treatment of arterial hypertension in the obese patient are guided by the same principles as in the nonobese patient. Urgent and emergent surgeries should be evaluated on a case-by-case basis, and aggressive control of blood pressure in the perioperative period is vital.

Acute hypertensive episodes and hypertensive emergencies should also be approached as they would be in the nonobese, but with the strong recommendation for meticulous and adequate monitoring. Careful drug titration is required due to the particular hemodynamic liability of this population, coupled with the fact that for obvious reasons, pharmacokinetics and dynamics might be altered.

In current clinical practice, measurement of blood pressure may be difficult, even to the point of deciding where to make the measurement. Obese individuals—especially women—tend to have a conical shape of the upper arm, termed *gynoid obesity*, and accurate measurement of blood pressure is difficult with conventional cuffs. As an alternative, the cuff can be placed around the forearm for more predictable cuff pressures. An increasing arm circumference is associated with miscalculation of blood pressure if standard-length cuffs are used. An appropriate-sized cuff that encompasses at least 80% of the arm should be used to ensure accurate measurement of blood pressure in an obese patient (42). If these maneuvers fail to result in adequate and reliable measurements, invasive blood pressure monitoring should then be considered as an alternative.

Ischemic Heart Disease and Cardiac Failure

To date, no specific cardiac risk index has been proposed for obese patients. Preoperative cardiac assessment of obese patients follows the same sequence as for lean patients, and for that reason, the American College of Cardiology/American Heart Association (ACC/AHA) guidelines are thought to be valid for this population (43). However, the guidelines do not take into account the presence of multiple, intermediate, or minor risk factors that are frequently observed in the obese. The presence of multiple cardiac risk factors has been shown to increase the incidence of perioperative cardiac morbidity (44). In addition, surgical risk categories may be modified based on institutional expertise, which is highly dependent on clinical experience, surgical skills, anesthetic care, and nursing quality (45,46). In this regard, there is evidence to suggest significant differences between care and outcomes at different institutions for the same surgical procedure (46–49). In addition to careful appraisal of arterial hypertension and its consequences, a comprehensive cardiac evaluation in obese patients should focus on assessing both cardiac function and the presence and severity of ischemic heart disease. Evaluation of cardiac function by clinical signs can be extremely difficult in the obese and, for that reason, objective evaluation of ejection fraction and cardiac function by echocardiography and/or left ventriculography is usually necessary.

The ACC/AHA recommendation for preoperative noninvasive evaluation of left ventricular function includes patients with current or poorly controlled heart failure, patients with a history of heart failure, and patients with dyspnea of unknown origin—an extremely frequent finding within this population.

Despite the fact that no randomized study has been performed in obese patients to determine the utility of routine evaluation of right and left ventricular function, it is very probable that such evaluation, guided by symptoms prior to intermediate- and high-risk surgery, will be helpful in guiding intraoperative and postoperative management of obese patients.

Evaluation for ischemic heart disease requires stress testing, although there is no consensus on which type of stress test is optimal. The choice among the various noninvasive tests must be made based on local preferences. The patient's weight must be taken into account not only for logistical reasons—as many diagnostic devices have significant weight limitations—but also because the effect of the patient's body habitus has long been recognized as a factor that may reduce the accuracy of myocardial perfusion studies (50,51).

The first decision to be made is whether or not patients can exercise sufficiently to obtain 85% of predicted maximal heart rate. If they cannot, then a pharmacologic stress test is better indicated (e.g., stress echocardiography after dobutamine or atropine administration [DSE] or a dipyridamole thallium nuclear imaging study [DTS]) (52). Patients who have positive stress test results will require coronary angiography.

If cardiac catheterization is indicated, patient weight has to be taken into account because some tables used to perform this study have weight limits as low as 300 lb. Despite the concerns raised by the size of the patients, cardiac catheterization is considered safe in these patients. Fifty-five percent of the time, cardiac catheterization results in negative findings; when positive, medical management, interventional cardiology therapy, or even cardiac bypass surgery may be indicated (52).

Once ischemic heart disease has been identified and its severity quantified in the morbidly obese patient, three therapeutic options are available prior to elective noncardiac surgery:

- Revascularization by surgery (coronary artery bypass grafting [CABG])
- Revascularization by percutaneous coronary intervention (PCI)
- Optimized medical management (typically with β-blockers or α_2-agonists)

There is no irrefutable evidence that indications for preoperative cardiac revascularization are any different for obese patients than for nonobese patients.

Coronary Artery Bypass Grafting. Still a controversial topic, some studies suggest that moderately and morbidly obese patients have a higher rate of deep sternal wound infection, renal failure, prolonged postoperative hospital stay, and operative mortality after coronary artery bypass surgery (53–55).

Coronary revascularization is guided by the patient's cardiac condition—that is, is there unstable angina, left main coronary artery disease (CAD), three-vessel disease, decreased left ventricular (LV) function, and/or left anterior descending artery disease?—as well as by the added risk of the coronary intervention and the potential consequences of delaying the noncardiac surgery for recovery after the cardiac intervention (56). It has been demonstrated that when indicated, patients undergoing coronary revascularization prior to major-risk noncardiac surgery did better postoperatively. Comparing this population of preoperatively revascularized patients with those medically managed suggests that the latter patient group had a mortality rate two times higher than the former (57,58).

Percutaneous Coronary Intervention. Evidence suggests that patients who underwent angioplasty prior to elective noncardiac surgery had better outcomes (59–62). However, angioplasty is now often accompanied by stenting, with postprocedure antiplatelet therapy to prevent acute coronary thrombosis and maintain long-term patency of the intervened vessel. It is strongly suggested that elective noncardiac surgery should be delayed for 4 to 6 weeks after PCI with stenting to allow for complete endothelialization of the stent and completion of aggressive antiplatelet therapy with glycoprotein (GP) IIb/IIIa inhibitors (63).

The introduction of drug-eluting stents may obviate the need for such prolonged systemic anticoagulation, thus allowing patients to undergo noncardiac surgery sooner. The complication rate of PCI in obese patients has not been reported to be different than in nonobese individuals, and similar precautions should also be taken in morbidly obese patients (64).

Medical Management. Perioperative use of β-blockers has been shown to be efficacious in reducing perioperative morbidity and mortality (65–68). The ACC/AHA guidelines recommend initiating β-blockers as early as possible prior to high-risk surgery and titrating the patient's heart rate to 60 bpm (43). Perioperative β-blocker use is recommended for patients with one or more Revised Cardiac Index risk factors despite a negative stress test and for patients with two minor risk factors, even with a good functional status and/or a negative noninvasive stress test (43,67).

Many morbidly obese patients are already receiving β-blocker therapy when they present for their preoperative assessment. β-Blockers have been used intraoperatively to control hemodynamics, intraoperative ischemia, and cardiac arrhythmias (65). Some studies investigating their prophylactic role have demonstrated decreased intraoperative ischemia (69).

The general consensus appears to be that if β-blockers are indicated perioperatively, they should be given not only intraoperatively but, more appropriately, they should be initiated during the preoperative period and—except in the presence of significant contraindications—should be continued through the postoperative period. The pharmacokinetics of β-blockers are affected by obesity, and there exists significant pharmacodynamic variability. The dosage of β-blockers should be initiated based on lean body mass and then titrated until the desired clinical effect is achieved (70,71).

Intraoperative Considerations

Mechanics

Surgical beds are now available that accommodate patients weighing as much as 500 kg. However, these patients require tremendous preparation on behalf of the operative staff. Even with appropriate beds, the obese patient can be at high risk for falling during sudden motion. This situation can be extremely dangerous to the patient and the supporting staff alike. Institution of a lift team and the availability of both "bean" bags and bed extensions in order to keep the folds of pannus stable are of the utmost importance to the surgical team, and have already become widely used in accredited surgical facilities. Finally, institutional investments in lifting equipment such as ceiling-mounted lifts and beds that oscillate and/or transform into chairs may be necessary to fully deploy the necessary mechanical advantage to care for the obese patient.

Rhabdomyolysis

Rhabdomyolysis is often described in the obese patient. This scenario generally follows prolonged operations and presents as dark urine, representing muscle necrosis from groups on the flanks or buttock. Also termed *pressure-induced myoglobinuria*, this is more commonly noted among patients with diabetes mellitus (72,73). It is generally attributed to lying on a hard surface, and has been frequently associated with an

TABLE 102.2

MOST FREQUENT AND PROMINENT RISKS OF THE MORBIDLY OBESE PATIENT UNDERGOING SURGERY

- Pulmonary aspiration of gastric contents
- Difficult mask ventilation and tracheal intubation
- Rapid development of hypoxemia after apnea
- Pulmonary atelectasis
- Hemodynamic instability
- Decreased ability to deal with the physiologic responses to stressful situations (i.e., hyperglycemia, hypertension, cardiac failure, arrhythmias, and myocardial ischemia)
- Delayed recovery
- Postoperative respiratory dysfunction
- Deep venous thrombosis

exaggerated lithotomy position in the operating theater (74). To handle this situation, attending staff should initiate aggressive hydration and monitor creatine phosphokinase (CPK). If CPK exceeds 5,000 IU/L, staff must initiate diuresis with mannitol and alkalinize the urine with sodium bicarbonate (75,76). Acute renal failure may develop, but recovery of renal function is generally expected.

Anesthetic Technique

No randomized, controlled trial provides unquestionable evidence that one or another anesthetic technique is best for the morbidly obese. Total intravenous anesthesia (TIVA) and inhalational, regional, and combined general/epidural or general/spinal anesthetics have been used safely in these individuals (77–81). Selecting one technique over another will depend upon:

- Patient's clinical status
- Type of surgery the patient requires
- Expertise of the senior anesthesiologist
- Availability of institutional resources
- Patient's verbal and/or written requests and consent

What must be absolutely clear are the pathophysiologic alterations and subsequent risks presented in each individual case. This should guide the physician to define the intraoperative goals. Considering only the potential impairments of the cardiovascular and respiratory systems, we must highlight the potential risks and recommended anesthetic goals.

The classic, most frequent and prominent risks of the morbidly obese patient undergoing surgery are listed in Table 102.2. Accordingly, the basic anesthetic goals should be (77):

- Hemodynamically smooth and rapid induction
- Rapid access and securing of the airway
- Prominent attention paid to hemodynamic stability
- A high level of analgesia to avoid increments in catecholamine activity
- Rapid recovery and early ambulation

Postoperative Considerations

Logistic and Technical Issues

The main diagnostic and therapeutic principles related to cardiovascular diseases and/or complications commonly observed in the ICU setting—such as arrhythmias, cardiac failure, hypertensive or ischemic episodes, and so forth—do not differ significantly when comparing the morbidly obese with lean patients. Therefore, a detailed discussion is not warranted. Nevertheless, we will highlight the few—but in our eyes important—differences to consider when presented with a morbidly obese surgical patient in the ICU setting.

Pathophysiologic Principles for a Rational Therapeutic Approach

Obesity has been likened to "exercise," that is, a *constant* state of "exercise." The morbidly obese patient's cardiovascular system is continuously overdemanded, even at rest, mainly because of chronic intravascular volume overload, blood hyperviscosity, and sympathetic hyperactivity. These are components of a "dysfunctional compensating mechanism," which tries to satisfy the increased metabolic rate imposed by the excessive adipose tissue. The resulting eccentric left ventricular hypertrophy (LVH) is associated with a reduced LV compliance, causing elevation of LV filling pressure in many morbidly obese persons (18,82).

The additional increase in cardiac output promoted by any perioperative stress may markedly increase LV filling pressure, often exceeding the threshold for pulmonary edema. Respiratory disease, especially obstructive sleep apnea syndrome (OSAS) and the obesity hypoventilation syndrome (OHS), acting on the pulmonary circulation may affect the right heart cavities as well. The heart of a morbidly obese patient may have less tolerance to any kind of cardiovascular stress—hypovolemia, hypervolemia, hypertension, hypotension, and so forth—and is at a higher risk of organ failure. Consequently, the appropriate diagnostic and therapeutic measures should be applied as soon and as accurately as possible to avoid systemic hypoperfusion and inadequate oxygen delivery, which may predispose to multiple organ system failure.

Importance of Coupled Cardiorespiratory Function

It is vital to maintain the best possible ventilation/perfusion (V/Q) balance, since V/Q mismatch is a prominent mechanism that can trigger respiratory and subsequent cardiac dysfunction in the morbidly obese surgical patient. In mechanically ventilated, morbidly obese patients, airway pressure may be elevated. Additionally, morbid obesity is associated with volume and pressure overload. Volume load conditions may fluctuate according to patient positioning. For example, changing position from the "physiologically ideal" reverse Trendelenburg to the supine position can significantly increase venous blood return to the heart and, as a result, augment cardiac output, pulmonary capillary wedge pressure, and mean pulmonary artery pressure, potentially increasing the risk of acute heart failure (83); one would expect this maneuver to increase airway pressure as well due to the increased weight of the chest.

Compression of the inferior vena cava may reduce venous return to the heart, and is thus a possible mechanism of hypotension. This can be avoided by tilting the operating room table or ICU bed by placing a wedge under the patient. These maneuvers are similar to those performed during caesarean section to reduce the pressure of the gravid uterus on the inferior vena cava (84). Considering that the reverse Trendelenburg position significantly improves cardiac and respiratory performance, it should be maintained during the entire perioperative period unless there is a particular contraindication.

Drug Dosing

The distribution, metabolism, protein binding, and clearance of many drugs are altered by the physiologic changes associated with obesity (85–87). In addition, the patient's underlying disease may substantially influence the pharmacokinetic properties of a drug (88). The net pharmacologic alteration in any patient is, therefore, often uncertain, especially in those suffering from morbid obesity. Nevertheless, for a number of drugs used in the ICU—most notably digoxin, aminophylline, aminoglycosides, and cyclosporine—drug toxicity may occur if the patients are dosed based on their actual, rather than ideal or adjusted, body weight (70,85,87,89–91). For drug dosing, with few exceptions, it is advisable to base drug calculations on ideal body weight (IBW) rather than real weight, and then adjust doses through meticulous monitoring (92).

RESPIRATORY CONSIDERATIONS IN THE MORBIDLY OBESE

The higher morbidity and mortality of hospitalized obese patients may be related to the increased pulmonary complications with which morbidly obese patients present (93). In the postoperative state, obese individuals are at increased risk of developing atelectasis, aspiration, ventilatory failure, and pulmonary embolism (93).

Clinicians caring for morbidly obese patients must be aware of the significant physiologic changes associated with their obesity, such as reduced lung volumes, increased work of breathing, and alterations in control of breathing and gas exchange. Many factors are involved including, but not limited to, BMI, patient's age, duration of obesity, fat distribution (central or peripheral), and the strong association of certain disorders such as OSAS, OHS, and pickwickian syndrome. In addition, obesity itself has a major detrimental impact on the respiratory system (94).

Preoperative Considerations

Respiratory Disorders

Obstructive Sleep Apnea Syndrome. Morbid obesity is the most common and major risk factor for OSAS (95). While its prevalence in the general U.S. population is 2% to 4%, this increases to 40% to 78% in the morbidly obese (95–99). Notwithstanding these facts, it is thought that 80% to 90% of American sleep apnea sufferers are undiagnosed (100,101).

The detection of OSAS among obese surgical patients is vital for several reasons:

- Obese patients are more sensitive to the depressant effects of hypnotics and opioids (102). Perioperative administration may lead to life-threatening respiratory complications (103,104), especially in face of pre-existing OSAS.
- OSAS is associated with difficult laryngoscopy and mask ventilation (104–107).
- Obese patients have, in general, a diminished expiratory reserve volume (ERV) with, consequently, reduced oxygen stores; this promotes faster development of desaturation after apnea (108).

If OSAS is present, these effects become exaggerated. The combination of these factors sets the stage for an airway catastrophe, not only during induction of general anesthesia, but also during tracheal extubation, and especially if an emergent intubation becomes necessary in the ICU or during intra- or interhospital transfer.

Obesity Hypoventilation Syndrome. Some obese patients suffer from a disorder characterized by chronic daytime hypoventilation, also known as obesity hypoventilation syndrome (109). These individuals are typically extremely obese, with a BMI greater than 40 kg/m^2, and the likelihood of OHS increases as the BMI increases. OHS is associated with chronic daytime hypoxemia—with a PaO_2 less than 65 mm Hg—and hypercapnia (107,108,110). It is essential to find out if the obese patient suffers from chronic daytime hypoxemia, as this is a better predictor of pulmonary hypertension and cor pulmonale than the presence and/or severity of OSAS (111–113).

Pickwickian Syndrome. Patients suffering OHS who additionally have signs and symptoms of cor pulmonale are termed *pickwickian*—from the Charles Dickens novel, *The Pickwick Papers*—and they have an increased perioperative morbidity and mortality (93).

Respiratory Insufficiency. Obesity *per se* is not a common cause for chronic respiratory insufficiency (109). Significant respiratory dysfunction is more common when chronic obstructive pulmonary disease (COPD) and obesity coexist. When respiratory insufficiency is present, impairment of gas exchange is greater than expected from a simple summation of the alterations caused by each pathophysiologic process (114).

Simple Obesity

Obese patients with minimal or no coexisting pulmonary conditions are classified as "simple" obesity patients. The pathophysiology of simple obesity consists of alterations in daytime gas exchange and pulmonary function, and may result from compression and restriction of the chest wall and diaphragm by excess adipose tissue (115). The ERV and functional residual capacity (FRC) are particularly affected, being reduced to 60% to 80% of normal, respectively.

If ERV decreases below the alveolar closing volume, then airway closure occurs during normal tidal breathing, and dependent alveoli are relatively or completely underventilated. As a consequence, V/Q mismatch, pulmonary shunt, and daytime hypoxemia results. One may see, in formerly obese patients after massive weight loss, a marked improvement in the PaO_2 and alveolar–arterial oxygen gradient; thus, this improvement is directly proportional to the increase in the ERV (116,117).

Other mechanisms may further impair respiratory function. Sleep apnea in the obese is usually obstructive, secondary to airway narrowing from abundant peripharyngeal adipose tissue, and an abnormal decrease of upper airway muscle tone during rapid eye movement (REM) sleep (95). Hypopneic and apneic events lead to arousal from REM sleep, oxyhemoglobin desaturation, and sympathetic nervous system activation in response to hypoxemia. This may explain the strong association between OSA and systemic hypertension (118). The precise pathophysiologic mechanism of OHS is unclear (93,109).

Of most importance is that vital capacity, reduced to 90% of normal in simple obesity, decreases to 60% of normal in

OHS. This reflects a profound and important decrement in lung volumes in OHS, as compared with simple obesity patients. Thus, one may see:

- A marked increase in distal airway resistance
- A more profound abnormality in V/Q matching
- A more significant impact on the PaO_2
- A larger A–a gradient in patients with OHS

Supine positioning further reduces lung volume and, as a result, increases the magnitude of all these alterations (107,115,119).

Diaphragmatic function is also affected due to overstretching and cephalad displacement resulting from increased intra-abdominal pressure. All of these factors combined may lead to chronic respiratory muscle fatigue and the chronic hypoventilation characteristic of OHS (93).

Venous Thromboembolism

Perioperative venous thromboembolism (VTE) occurs in 0.2% to 2.4% of bariatric patients receiving thromboprophylaxis (120). According to the *Chest* Consensus Statement, obese patients in the ICU will generally fall into either the high or highest risk categories in which, if left untreated, the risk of deep venous thrombosis (DVT) ranges from 20% to 80%. The risk of clinical pulmonary embolus (PE) ranges from 2% to 10%, and fatal PE occurs in 0.4% to 5% of patients (121).

The obese population in the surgical ICU requires thromboprophylaxis; however, the best regimen is not clear. Multiple variables are worthy of mention in regard to this matter. Venous stasis ulcers are more common in the obese, and in turn, are associated with DVT. Prophylactic inferior vena cava filters can be considered, but may also be technically difficult in the heaviest patients. Sequential compression devices (SCDs) are generally recognized as a useful adjunct but, again, may be limited by the patient size. The adequacy of pedal pumps is not clear. Unfractionated or low-molecular-weight heparins are both viable options, though precise dosing regimens and duration of dosage have emerged largely from uncontrolled trials. There are reports in the bariatric literature that 40 mg of enoxaparin every 12 hours may provide better thromboprophylaxis than 30 mg every 12 hours; however, this recommendation came from a retrospective report that coincided with significant changes in patient mobilization and improvements in overall hospital length of stay. It is not clear if it was these improvements in overall patient mobility or the change in medication administered that led to the improved VTE rates (122).

Evaluation and Optimization for Surgery

In simple obesity, preoperative assessment of respiratory function should be similar to that indicated in the assessment of lean and healthy patients. More extensive pulmonary function tests and preoperative treatment may be necessary for the obese patient who smokes or has pulmonary symptoms.

Elements of the history and physical examination can be as important—indeed, more important—as preoperative testing. Obese patients who habitually snore and report daytime somnolence and/or have suffered breath interruptions during sleep should be evaluated with polysomnography, since it is the definitive diagnostic test for OSAS (95). However, morbid obesity and symptoms of OSA are not, *per se*, indications for preoperative pulmonary function testing and room air arterial blood gas (ABG) analyses. These tests have failed to demonstrate predictive values and/or lead to the optimization of postoperative management or outcomes of bariatric surgery patients, and are not routinely indicated (103,123–125). Room air pulse oximetry in both the upright and supine positions may be a useful, noninvasive method for screening patients for daytime hypoxemia. A supine room air SpO_2 less than 96% may merit further investigation. An elevated hematocrit may also be a clue of chronic hypoxemia.

If clinical evidence of OHS is present, ABG analyses are indicated because of chronic daytime hypoxemia—PaO_2 less than 65 mm Hg, but especially sustained hypercapnia—a $PaCO_2$ greater than 45 mm Hg—in the morbidly obese patient without significant obstructive pulmonary disease is diagnostic for this syndrome.

One must differentiate whether morbid obesity coexists with either OHS *or* COPD. These combinations often result in chronic daytime hypoxemia and increase the chances for pulmonary hypertension, right ventricular hypertrophy, and/or right ventricular failure. Assessment of these pickwickian patients may require extensive testing to guide preoperative medical optimization and postoperative management, given that their morbidity and mortality rate is increased (93,102,126).

It is unclear if it is appropriate to delay bariatric surgery for aggressive optimization of airway status and oxygenation with continuous positive airway pressure (CPAP) or bilevel positive airway pressure (BiPAP) therapy. Rennotte et al. observed no major postoperative respiratory complications in 14 patients treated with nasal CPAP for up to 3 weeks prior to surgery (127). Two to three weeks may be necessary not only to maximize medical benefits, but also to allow sufficient time for patients unfamiliar with CPAP or BiPAP therapy to acclimate to the nocturnal use of the device. Three weeks of nightly CPAP treatment prior to bariatric surgery improved left ventricular ejection fraction and afterload in obese patients with coexisting heart failure (128). Eight weeks of preoperative nasal CPAP therapy may be required to treat hypertension secondary to OSA (129).

Intraoperative Considerations

Airway Management

It is still a debatable issue whether or not morbid obesity should be considered a risk factor for difficult airway management. Brodsky et al. observed that neither absolute obesity nor BMI was associated with problematic intubation in morbidly obese patients. They also concluded that only a large neck circumference and a Mallampati score of 3 or more were significantly correlated with a high probability of problematic intubation (130). In our opinion, preoperative airway assessments should be similar in both morbidly obese and lean patients.

Whether or not morbid obesity is considered a risk factor for intubation, issues related specifically to the patient's BMI that impact airway management include:

- Preoxygenation
- Positioning
- Immediate availability to adequate resources, both technical and human (technical: special laryngoscopes, blades, tracheal tubes, oro- and nasopharyngeal cannulae, intubating laryngeal airway [ILA], LMA Fastrach, Combitube, etc.; human: personnel sufficient in both number and expertise)

In the perioperative setting, one never knows when an emergent tracheal intubation or reintubation may be necessary, or when an unpredicted difficult mask ventilation and difficult tracheal intubation combination may appear. Indeed, the latter is a common situation in morbidly obese patients suffering from OSAS or OHS. The presence of any of these urgent/emergent events—taking into account the reduced time to hypoxemia after apnea and possible increased risk for gastric aspiration in morbidly obese individuals—will likely result in a life-threatening, although preventable/treatable, respiratory misadventure.

In our opinion, the same American Society of Anesthesiologists algorithm for difficult airway management and indications for conscious tracheal intubation should be considered for both obese and lean patients. If conscious intubation is indicated, it must be remembered that most episodes of gastroesophageal reflux, and the greatest potential for pulmonary aspiration of gastric contents, occur from and during "bucking" on an endotracheal tube; consequently, appropriate preparation of the patient is crucial (131,132).

Meticulous patient explanation, a low infusion rate of remifentanil (0.05 μg/kg IBW/minute) to avoid loss of response to verbally required active ventilation, and/or local anesthesia—such as bilateral blockade of the internal branch of the glossopharyngeal nerve—have shown to be the most effective and safest induction alternative (77). Finally, although somewhat controversial, it is prudent to treat morbidly obese patients with prophylactic measures against gastric aspiration, such as cimetidine, ranitidine, Bicitra, and/or metoclopramide (133); the timing of administration of these agents is, of course, of great significance.

Preoxygenation and Position

Hypoxemia during induction of general anesthesia in obese individuals is, and must be, a real concern for the anesthesiologist and/or intensivist. These patients may experience rapid arterial oxygen desaturation after apnea (134). Compared with supine-positioned obese patients, preoxygenation in the 25- to 30-degree head-up position with 100% oxygen for 3 minutes achieves higher oxygen tensions—in other words, more time and better oxygenation for intubation and airway control, given that as the BMI increases, it has been shown that the amount of time for desaturation in the patient decreases (135). Preoxygenation in the 30-degree reverse-Trendelenburg position provides a longer, safer apnea period than the 30-degree semi-Fowler and supine positions. Consequently, the Trendelenburg position has been recommended as the optimal position for induction of general anesthesia in obese patients (136). The head-up position results in an unloading of the intra-abdominal contents from the diaphragm; thus, pulmonary compliance and FRC increase, and oxygenation returns toward baseline values, as compared to the same patients who were placed in the supine position (137).

Prior to induction of general anesthesia in any setting—whether the operating room, the ICU, or on the hospital floor—the obese patient should be positioned with pillows under the shoulders, with the head and upper body elevated in a semirecumbent or reverse Trendelenburg position. This "ramped" position is strongly recommended in the morbidly obese, as it improves pulmonary function, oxygenation, cardiovascular function, conditions for mask ventilation, laryngoscopic view, and tracheal intubation (130). Extremely obese patients should never be allowed to lie completely flat. Their upper body should be constantly elevated at 25 to 30 degrees in the perioperative period.

Atelectasis

In the perioperative setting, reduction of chest wall and diaphragmatic muscle tone following the induction of general anesthesia and skeletal muscle relaxation impairs oxygenation. In simple obesity, the net effect may reduce ERV and FRC to less than 50% of preinduction values, excluding even more alveoli from effective gas exchange (115). As reduction of ERV and FRC increases exponentially with increasing BMI, the combination of these factors predisposes the morbidly obese patient to suffer atelectasis not only during anesthesia and surgery, but also in the postoperative period. The importance of this topic will be developed in the postoperative section.

Mechanical Ventilation: Invasive Positive Pressure Ventilation

Respiratory physiology must be taken into account when considering mechanical ventilation. Oxygen consumption and carbon dioxide production increase due to a higher metabolic rate promoted by excessive fat and an augmented workload on supportive tissues (138). Normocapnia is maintained by increased minute ventilation. Regarding mechanics, total compliance of the respiratory system declines exponentially with increasing BMI, as do FRC, ERV, and total lung capacity (139). Clinical correlates of these changes are increased work of breathing, small airway closure, ventilation/perfusion mismatch, pulmonary shunt, and hypoxemia. Sedation, anesthesia, and positioning supine further reduce FRC in the obese as compared to nonobese subjects, and consequently worsen respiratory performance (140).

Considering these factors, the initial tidal volume should be based on ideal body weight rather than actual body weight, and adjustments made according to airway pressures and appropriate respiratory monitoring (141). As lung volumes are reduced and airway resistance is increased, a tidal volume based on the patients' actual body weight would probably result in high airway pressures, alveolar overdistention, and barotrauma. Some data suggest, as a lung-protective strategy, the use of smaller tidal volumes and adequate positive end-expiratory pressure (PEEP)/CPAP (142) to prevent airway closure (143). Although this technique may result in decreased cardiac output, fluid loading will correct the problem. Additionally, in an attempt to improve ventilator–patient synchrony and reduce airway pressure, the patient's spontaneous respiratory effort should be maintained and assisted with pressure support ventilation as needed (144).

Tracheal Extubation and Intrahospital Transfer

As a result of the increased work of breathing and impaired respiratory mechanics, morbid obesity has been associated with prolonged mechanical ventilation, extended weaning periods, and longer ICU and hospital lengths of stay (6). Strategies suggested for facilitating the weaning process include positioning of the patient in a 45-degree reverse Trendelenburg position—thus optimizing lung mechanics, increasing tidal volume, and reducing respiratory rate (145)—and BiPAP post extubation (146).

If hemodynamic stability has been achieved, the trachea should be extubated with the patient's upper body elevated between 30 and 45 degrees. The patient should be transferred from the operating room while in a semirecumbent or tilted reverse Trendelenburg position (147). As obese patients have greater reduction in lung volumes than normal-weight counterparts following abdominal surgery (115), it comes as no surprise that the recovering patient should be kept in a head-up position in order to minimize intrapulmonary shunting (148). On days 1 and 2 postoperatively, a change from the semirecumbent to the supine position may result in significant decreases in PaO_2. Consequently, obese patients should convalesce in the semirecumbent position while receiving supplemental oxygen (148), if at all possible. Intrahospital transfer of a morbidly obese patient is best and most safely accomplished if the patient remains in his or her own hospital bed.

Ideal FiO_2 (Supplemental Oxygen)

It should go without saying that one uses the highest concentration of oxygen necessary to maintain life. Nonetheless, high oxygen concentrations have often been associated with atelectasis formation and recurrence (149). In order to avoid this consequence, using as low an oxygen concentration as possible has been recommended. When 100% oxygen is delivered, shunt increases significantly due to atelectasis development, while with 30% oxygen delivery, shunt and atelectasis are minimal (150). Finally, without any preoxygenation, no atelectasis develops after induction (151,152), although there may be other problems unrelated to atelectasis.

Nevertheless, supplemental oxygen carries clear benefits for patients, especially the morbidly obese. There is evidence that suggests that an FiO_2 of 0.8 ensures appropriate oxygenation without increasing the risk of absorptive atelectasis, reduces the incidence of postoperative nausea and vomiting (PONV) in patients with an increased risk of gastric aspiration, and improves the host's defense mechanisms against infection. The improvement can be seen not only in the wound site, but also in the respiratory system (153–156). Although not proven in morbidly obese surgical patients, this possible benefit should not be ignored. Ideal FiO_2 should, then, result from a balance between a supplemental quantity of oxygen that is sufficient enough to avoid hypoxemia, reduce postoperative infections, and reduce PONV, but not so high as to facilitate the development and maintenance of atelectasis.

Our recommendation is to deliver 100% oxygen before induction of anesthesia to retard the development of hypoxemia after apnea and, once tracheal intubation is confirmed, reduce the FiO_2 to 0.8, if possible, according to respiratory monitoring.

Monitoring

FRC is reduced in the morbidly obese patient; if it drops below closing capacity (CC), the dependent small airways will collapse, promoting:

- Ventilation/perfusion mismatch
- Gas exchange deterioration
- An increase in the shunt fraction
- An increase in the alveolar–arterial oxygen gradient

Consequently, the more obese the patient—the greater will be the alveolar–arterial gas difference, in other words, the less the expiratory gas measurements will correlate with arterial blood gas analysis.

A morbidly obese patient will not be able to reach the same PaO_2/FiO_2 ratio as the normal-weight patient, even if higher inspiratory oxygen concentrations are delivered. Morbid obesity decreases the arterial oxygenation index even further, yet leaves $PaCO_2$ values unaffected if the patient does not suffer from either OHS or pickwickian syndrome (115); this effect is mainly due to intrapulmonary shunts in the atelectatic-dependent lung areas. In this scenario, arterial blood gas analysis becomes increasingly important because blood gases reflect the respiratory status more accurately than expiratory gas measurements. This does not mean that morbidly obese patients routinely require invasive or special monitoring of respiration (157), but morbid obesity, the presence of comorbidities, and the type of surgery, among other factors, should influence the decision of which monitoring devices need be used. Routine noninvasive monitoring will be sufficient in simple obesity cases, while the presence of OSAS, OHS, pickwickian syndrome, daytime hypoxemia, and/or associated COPD should alert the anesthesiologist or intensivist to modify not only the intra- and postoperative respiratory monitoring, but also narcotic use (158). It is a good practice to obtain pulse oximetry or even arterial blood gas analysis values in the awake obese patient prior to any anesthetic premedication in order to obtain a reference reading, and thereby allow a comparison of preoperative values with intra- and postoperative values.

Anesthesia and controlled mechanical ventilation will almost always have a negative impact on oxygenation and alveolar ventilation. In surgeries where large fluid shifts occur, long intraoperative hypotensive episodes are possible, and satisfactory tissue oxygenation cannot be assessed by pulse oximetry or PaO_2 alone. In these cases, decreasing pH values or increasing anionic gap or lactate values may be indicative of inadequate oxygen delivery (159). Inadequate oxygen delivery may be reflected in increased, and sometimes "unexplained," postoperative complications. The degree and duration of postoperative surveillance depend on the surgical intervention, the course of anesthesia, and the patient's condition. Monitoring should at least include pulse oximetry, respiratory rate, cardiac rhythm monitoring, and blood pressure measurement in the immediate postoperative period. In patients with decreasing oxygen saturations, ABG analysis and chest radiographs may be useful in sorting out the differential diagnosis. Sudden onset of respiratory distress, chest pain, and dyspnea may be indicative not only of a cardiac event, but also of pulmonary embolism; most mortality in the 30-day postoperative period after bariatric surgery is due to pulmonary embolism (160).

Obese patients have increased risk of respiratory-related complications in the postoperative period. In one study, the overall rate of critical respiratory events in obese patients was 3% (8). Interestingly, however, another study showed no significant increase of adverse perioperative events, even in patients with confirmed OSAS when the levels of wakefulness were carefully maintained (161). This reflects the importance of the anesthetic and analgesic management on the speed and quality of recovery of central nervous system (CNS) function. It is of utmost importance to take this into account when considering the anesthetic/analgesic strategy. Combined thoracic epidural/general anesthesia techniques may be quite suitable in these major cases.

Patients with confirmed or suspected OSAS, OHS, and pickwickian syndrome require more stringent observation. In the postoperative period, this may warrant prolonged surveillance in the postanesthesia care unit or even admission to the ICU in selected cases, especially in those with surgery lasting for more than 4 hours and in patients with critical comorbidities. The main reasons for ICU admission in morbidly obese patients are disturbances in pulmonary gas exchange, which can be prevented by more prolonged one-on-one surveillance combined with meticulous medical care (162).

Postoperative Considerations

Hypoxemia and Associated Postoperative Respiratory Disorders

Following major open abdominal surgery without postoperative oxygen supplementation, even normal patients experience hypoxemia (SpO_2 less than 90%) (163). On the first postoperative day following open bariatric surgery, 75% of morbidly obese patients had a PaO_2 less than 60 mm Hg, which usually persisted and worsened in the following days (12). Many clinical processes may be suggested to explain this phenomenon. The most frequently observed is atelectasis, but pulmonary aspiration of oral or gastric secretions, pneumonia, acute lung injury, and acute respiratory distress syndrome (ARDS) should also be considered as possible and relatively common respiratory complications of postsurgical morbidly obese patients.

Finally, it is important to remember tracheal tube displacement as a mechanism of perioperative hypoxemia. Abdominal insufflation, as well as changes in operating room table position—usually to the Trendelenburg position—can cause cephalad movement of the diaphragm, and can lead to migration of an initially correctly positioned endotracheal tube (164,165). This phenomenon in morbidly obese patients undergoing laparoscopy can result in right endobronchial intubation and intraoperative hypoxemia. This mechanism should be considered in the intubated ICU patient because of the frequent, necessary changes in the patient's position during care (166).

Atelectasis

General anesthesia may impair pulmonary gas exchange, and consequently decrease oxygenation in the general population; atelectasis is a major cause of this kind of impairment (167–170). Alterations in respiratory mechanics induced by general anesthesia, such as decreased chest wall and lung compliance, and a reduction in functional residual capacity promote atelectasis in nonobese patients. Conscious morbidly obese patients already have prominent alterations of their respiratory mechanics (171), and these patients are, in fact, particularly prone to intra- and postoperative atelectasis. During general anesthesia, as well as during the immediate postoperative period, morbidly obese patients are more likely to have significant impairment of pulmonary gas exchange and respiratory mechanics (115,172,173). Thus, it has been noted, even before the induction of anesthesia, that morbidly obese patients had more atelectasis, expressed in the percentage of the total lung area, than nonobese patients. After tracheal decannulation, atelectasis increased in both groups, but remained significantly more severe in the morbidly obese. Finally, 24 hours postoperatively, a complete re-expansion of the lung parenchyma occurred in nonobese patients, while the amount of atelectasis remained unchanged in the morbidly obese (94).

TABLE 102.3

VITAL MEASURES TO PREVENT OR REDUCE THE SEVERITY AND DURATION OF ATELECTASIS IN THE OBESE PATIENT

- Place patients in the semirecumbent position and, if possible, out of bed in a chair as tolerated, as this maneuver may increase functional residual capacity.
- Provide effective analgesia, which will allow early and effective mobilization, cough, and excellent tolerance to physiotherapy.
- Institute aggressive incentive spirometry.
- During the first 3 postoperative days, deliver humidified "supplemental oxygen," but avoid inspired fractions higher than 0.8. Supplemental humidified oxygen will not reduce atelectasis, but will facilitate respiratory secretion clearance, and will prevent hypoxemic episodes in efforts to improve the host's defenses against bacterial infections.
- During surgery or postoperatively in intubated patients, instituting positive end-expiratory pressure is probably effective in increasing functional residual capacity via recruitment of atelectatic regions of the lung. Applying vital capacity maneuvers (also known as recruitment maneuvers) may also reduce the incidence and/or severity of atelectasis while improving the quality and effective time of alveoli recruitment.[a]
- Noninvasive positive pressure ventilation can be used to avoid intubation in selected patients.

[a] From Magnusson L, Spahn DR. New concepts of atelectasis during general anaesthesia. *Br J Anaesth*. 2003;91:61–72.

The increased atelectasis found in morbidly obese patients explains, at least partially, postoperative pulmonary complications. Various mechanisms have been suggested for the development of atelectasis in the morbidly obese, such as lung parenchyma compression, absorption of alveolar gas in completely or partially collapsed airways, and alterations in surfactant production, function, and/or distribution (174). Our conclusion is that all possible measures to prevent or reduce the severity and duration of atelectasis in this patient population are vital and are listed in Table 102.3.

While some bariatric groups use noninvasive positive pressure ventilation (NIPPV) routinely in the postoperative care of morbidly obese patients immediately after extubation, others are reluctant because of the fear of anastomotic disruption; there are no data to support this concern. Commonly, morbidly obese patients use some form of NIPPV (CPAP or BiPAP) chronically for the treatment of OSA. Postoperatively, morbidly obese patients are at risk for prolonged depressant effects of the drugs administered during surgery. This situation may promote airway collapse not only in those morbidly obese patients with diagnosed OSAS and already under preoperative treatment, but also in previously undiagnosed morbidly obese patients (175,176). Airway collapse is most frequent during REM sleep, which is brief in the initial postoperative period, but significantly longer on the third to fifth postoperative nights. The risk for airway collapse increases even days after surgery. This means that oximetric monitoring and supplementary oxygen must continue to be administered during this dangerous period (177).

A prospective study of 1,067 bariatric patients evaluated the risk of developing anastomotic leaks and pulmonary complications after gastric bypass. Of the 1,067 patients, 420 had OSAS and 159 were dependent on CPAP. There were 15 major anastomotic leaks, two of which occurred in CPAP-treated patients. No correlation between CPAP utilization and incidence of major anastomotic leakage was demonstrated. No episodes of pneumonia were diagnosed in either group. Based on this study, the conclusion was that CPAP is a useful modality for treating hypoventilation after gastric bypass surgery without increasing the risk of developing postoperative anastomotic leaks (178).

Regarding BiPAP, it appears that when used prophylactically during the first 24 hours postoperatively, it significantly reduces pulmonary dysfunction after gastroplasty in morbidly obese patients and accelerates the re-establishment of preoperative pulmonary function (146).

Pulmonary Aspiration

Even though many mechanisms were classically associated with an increased risk of gastric content aspiration in the morbidly obese, this topic remains controversial. While it is still recommended to take precautions against acid aspiration, massive pulmonary aspiration in morbidly obese patients is a rare event in current anesthesia practice, and the occurrence of unwitnessed "microaspirations" in the postoperative period is difficult to assess because of the diagnostic problems observed within this population (144). While massive aspiration is uncommon, the following cautionary list should be carefully noted:

- While in bed, the patient must be adequately positioned in a semirecumbent or reverse Trendelenburg position at all times.
- The care team must be ready for bag-valve-mask ventilation and tracheal intubation in a ramped position, as well as have technical and adequate human resources.
- Drug dosing must be meticulously titrated according to monitoring parameters and clinical response, and based on the IBW.
- Consider the importance of a sufficient and safe analgesic strategy. It will improve the tolerance and cooperation of the patient with the therapeutic measures required for an expeditious recovery.

Radiographic Evaluation and Complications

Radiographic evaluation of the surgically obese patient is complicated and made difficult by the weight limitations of modern scanners and the patient's inability to cooperate with the transfer. Several radiographic tests, including the upper gastrointestinal series, may require the patient to stand for extended periods of time. Although tomographic tables now routinely handle patients weighing 400 lb. (182 kg), these weight limits vary by institutional device. Surgeons and caregivers that are in a position to affect patient selection should consider this when planning operative interventions for obese patients. Further consideration for tables that handle heavier patients should be entertained when new equipment is being purchased. In the absence of excellent radiographic capabilities, these patients may require surgical exploration, and both patients and surgical team members must assume those additional risks.

Venous, Arterial, and Nutritional Access

Venous access is difficult in this population. When peripheral access is inadequate, the point of choice may be the jugular vein. Gilbert et al. found this location to have fewer complications and to require fewer conversions to different locations (179). Arterial access is generally recommended as noninvasive blood pressure cuffs can give inaccurate measurements in this patient population. Nutritional access in critically ill obese patients is imperative; despite their weight, these patients can be relatively malnourished. There is evidence from the trauma literature that obese patients preferentially mobilize protein instead of fats as compared to lean patients (180). As a result of this mobilization, the obese patient will need additional nutrition. Optimally, if the patient requires reoperative interventions, a feeding gastrostomy or jejunostomy can be placed. Although not impossible, achieving percutaneous gastric access can be extremely difficult, especially in a patient following a gastric bypass procedure. In these circumstances, it is a good time to reiterate the importance of communication between the surgical and critical care physicians and staff.

Analgesia

Overview. Acute pain can result in reduced tidal volume, vital capacity, functional residual capacity, and alveolar ventilation (181,182). These factors contribute to atelectasis, V/Q mismatch, hypoxemia, and hypercapnia. Pain-related muscle splinting interferes with the patient's ability to cough, clear secretions, and efficiently participate in chest physiotherapy, all of which increase the chances for pulmonary complications (182).

A major component of segmental and suprasegmental reflex responses is enhanced general sympathetic tones (183). Results of this tone are increased peripheral resistance, stroke volume, and heart rate, which lead to an increase in cardiac output. High blood pressure results in increased myocardial work and myocardial oxygen consumption (181). The rise in heart rate causes decreased diastolic filling time, possibly resulting in reduced oxygen delivery to the myocardium, with a risk of ischemia (181). All of these alterations could result in devastating respiratory and/or cardiovascular complications in at-risk individuals such as the morbidly obese, who commonly are at a higher risk of suffering variable degrees of impaired function affecting both systems.

Every health care provider knows that the efficacy of analgesia must be measured by the ability to cough and move without pain or discomfort, and not only by the absence of pain while in a resting state. All the potential consequences of poor pain control are serious problems in a general population, but they are of outstanding importance in the morbidly obese surgical patient. Early mobilization without discomfort should be considered a major anesthetic target in this population due to the fact that deep vein thrombosis and pulmonary embolism are some of the most frequent causes of mortality during the first 30 postoperative days. In addition, sufficient and safe postoperative pain control would result in a more effective and tolerable respiratory physiotherapy—a critical maneuver in this context—which would certainly reduce the possibilities for other respiratory complications such as atelectasis. Nevertheless, most morbidly obese patients with surgical pain do not receive adequate pain relief (184).

Analgesic Strategies (Intravenous, Thoracic Epidural, Multimodal Approach). Unfortunately, uncertainty remains as to the superiority of one pain treatment modality versus another (185). Open versus laparoscopic surgical techniques, personal skills, and experience may influence the patient's and anesthesiologist's choice of pain treatment. Pain management strategies may offer specific advantages for specific patient outcomes, such as a reduced rate of pulmonary complications after abdominal surgery and superior pain control with thoracic epidural analgesia (TEA) (185–188). Postoperative epidural analgesia, using either local anesthetics or opioids, may be the route of choice for postoperative analgesia in morbidly obese patients, as it allows a more vigorous cough and chest physiotherapy, better diaphragmatic function, more powerful leg exercise, and earlier ambulation and discharge from hospital (11,189,190). These advantages may lead to a more benign postoperative course, as previously noted in other populations who had earlier walking, earlier feeding, a lower incidence of pulmonary alveolar collapse, and fewer thromboembolic complications (11,189,190). TEA can be improved by adding opioids and possibly epinephrine to the epidural solution (191,192).

Thoracic epidural anesthesia/analgesia may be particularly beneficial in the pathophysiologic context observed in morbid obesity. For example, left ventricular work conditions (both preload and afterload) may be improved by the sympathetic blockade, thus reducing the chances for developing heart failure (193,194). Myocardial oxygen balance may be improved as well due to a decrease in oxygen demand and augmented myocardial perfusion induced by coronary vasodilatation, both secondary to sympathetic block, thereby reducing the risk of ischemia (195–202). TEA does not affect chest wall compliance in the postsurgical state, and allows for better diaphragmatic function when compared with general anesthesia alone (190,203–209). Alterations in chest wall compliance and diaphragmatic performance can be considered major determinants of postoperative respiratory dysfunction in most patients, but especially in the morbidly obese after upper open abdominal procedures (182,210–219).

Regarding intravenous analgesia, improved efficacy and safety have been shown when patient-controlled anesthesia management includes adjunct analgesics such as nonsteroidal anti-inflammatory medications and local anesthetic wound infiltration in a multimodal approach (220,221). It must be remembered in the most emphatic way that a continuous and efficient analgesic scheme would certainly improve patient satisfaction and comfort, and very probably—even though still not proven in the morbidly obese—would reduce morbidity and mortality.

References

1. James PT, Leach R, Kalamara E, et al. The worldwide obesity epidemic. *Obes Res.* 2001;9(Suppl 4):228S–233S.
2. Marik FB. Management of the obese critically ill patient in intensive care unit. In: Alvarez A, ed. *Morbid Obesity Peri-operative Management.* Cambridge, UK: Cambridge University Press; 2004:363–368.
3. Dindo D, Muller MK, Weber M, et al. Obesity in general elective surgery. *Lancet.* 2003;361:2032–2035.
4. McTigue KM, Harris R, Hemphill B, et al. Screening and interventions for obesity in adults: summary of the evidence for the U.S. Preventive Services Task Force. *Ann Intern Med.* 2003;139:933–949.
5. Choban PS, Weireter LJ Jr, Maynes C. Obesity and increased mortality in blunt trauma. *J Trauma.* 1991;31:1253–1257.
6. El-Solh A, Sikka P, Bozkanat E, et al. Morbid obesity in the medical ICU. *Chest.* 2001;120:1989–1997.
7. Goldhaber SZ, Grodstein F, Stampfer MJ, et al. A prospective study of risk factors for pulmonary embolism in women. *JAMA.* 1997;277:642–645.
8. Rose DK, Cohen MM, Wigglesworth DF, et al. Critical respiratory events in the postanesthesia care unit. Patient, surgical, and anesthetic factors. *Anesthesiology.* 1994;81:410–418.
9. Yaegashi M, Jean R, Zuriqat M, et al. Outcome of morbid obesity in the intensive care unit. *J Intensive Care Med.* 2005;20:147–154.
10. Fontaine KR, Redden DT, Wang C, et al. Years of life lost due to obesity. *JAMA.* 2003;289:187–193.
11. Fox GS, Whalley DG, Bevan DR. Anaesthesia for the morbidly obese. Experience with 110 patients. *Br J Anaesth.* 1981;53:811–816.
12. Taylor RR, Kelly TM, Elliott CG, et al. Hypoxemia after gastric bypass surgery for morbid obesity. *Arch Surg.* 1985;120:1298–1302.
13. Friederich JA, Heyneker TJ, Berman JM. Anesthetic management of a massively morbidly obese patient. *Reg Anesth.* 1995;20:538–542.
14. Garrison RJ, Kannel WB, Stokes J III, et al. Incidence and precursors of hypertension in young adults: the Framingham Offspring Study. *Prev Med.* 1987;16:235–251.
15. Kenchaiah S, Evans JC, Levy D, et al. Obesity and the risk of heart failure. *N Engl J Med.* 2002;347:305–313.
16. Chobanian AV, Bakris GL, Black HR, et al. The Seventh Report of the Joint National Committee on Prevention, Detection, Evaluation, and Treatment of High Blood Pressure: the JNC 7 report. *JAMA.* 2003;289:2560–2572.
17. Whyte HM. Blood pressure and obesity. *Circulation.* 1959;19:511–516.
18. Alexander J. Obesity and cardiac performance. *Am J Cardiol.* 1964;14:860–865.
19. Kannel WB, LeBauer EJ, Dawber TR, et al. Relation of body weight to development of coronary heart disease. The Framingham study. *Circulation.* 1967;35:734–744.
20. Buckley FP, Robinson NB, Simonowitz DA, et al. Anaesthesia in the morbidly obese. A comparison of anaesthetic and analgesic regimens for upper abdominal surgery. *Anaesthesia.* 1983;38:840–851.
21. Dominguez-Cherit G, Gonzalez R, Borunda D, et al. Anesthesia for morbidly obese patients. *World J Surg.* 1998;22:969–973.
22. Jones DW, Kim JS, Andrew ME, et al. Body mass index and blood pressure in Korean men and women: the Korean National Blood Pressure Survey. *J Hypertens.* 1994;12:1433–1437.
23. Jones DW. Body weight and blood pressure. Effects of weight reduction on hypertension. *Am J Hypertens.* 1996;9:50s–54s.
24. Montani JP, Antic V, Yang Z, et al. Pathways from obesity to hypertension: from the perspective of a vicious triangle. *Int J Obes Relat Metab Disord.* 2002;26(Suppl 2):S28–38.
25. DiBona GF, Kopp UC. Neural control of renal function. *Physiol Rev.* 1997;77:75–197.
26. Engeli S, Sharma AM. The renin-angiotensin system and natriuretic peptides in obesity-associated hypertension. *J Mol Med.* 2001;79:21–29.
27. Dessi-Fulgheri P, Sarzani R, Tamburrini P, et al. Plasma atrial natriuretic peptide and natriuretic peptide receptor gene expression in adipose tissue of normotensive and hypertensive obese patients. *J Hypertens.* 1997;15:1695–1699.
28. Endre T, Mattiasson I, Berglund G, et al. Insulin and renal sodium retention in hypertension-prone men. *Hypertension.* 1994;23:313–319.
29. Hall JE. Mechanisms of abnormal renal sodium handling in obesity hypertension. *Am J Hypertens.* 1997;10:49S–55S.
30. Adams JP, Murphy PG. Obesity in anaesthesia and intensive care. *Br J Anaesth.* 2000;85:91–108.
31. Shamsuzzaman AS, Gersh BJ, Somers VK. Obstructive sleep apnea: implications for cardiac and vascular disease. *JAMA.* 2003;290:1906–1914.
32. Hubert HB, Feinleib M, McNamara PM, et al. Obesity as an independent risk factor for cardiovascular disease: a 26-year follow-up of participants in the Framingham Heart Study. *Circulation.* 1983;67:968–977.
33. McNulty PH, Ettinger SM, Field JM, et al. Cardiac catheterization in morbidly obese patients. *Catheter Cardiovasc Interv.* 2002;56:174–177.
34. Bahadori B, Neuer E, Schumacher M, et al. Prevalence of coronary artery disease in obese versus lean men with angina pectoris and positive exercise stress test. *Am J Cardiol.* 1996;77:1000–1001.
35. Alpert MA, Terry BE, Kelly DL. Effect of weight loss on cardiac chamber size, wall thickness and left ventricular function in morbid obesity. *Am J Cardiol.* 1985;55:783–786.
36. Kasper EK, Hruban RH, Baughman KL. Cardiomyopathy of obesity: a clinicopathologic evaluation of 43 obese patients with heart failure. *Am J Cardiol.* 1992;70:921–924.
37. Merlino G, Scaglione R, Paterna S, et al. Lymphocyte beta-adrenergic receptors in young subjects with peripheral or central obesity: relationship with central haemodynamics and left ventricular function. *Eur Heart J.* 1994;15:786–792.
38. Warnes CA, Roberts WC. The heart in massive (more than 300 pounds or 136 kilograms) obesity: analysis of 12 patients studied at necropsy. *Am J Cardiol.* 1984;54:1087–1091.
39. Alexander JK, Pettigrove JR. Obesity and congestive heart failure. *Geriatrics.* 1967;22:101–108.

40. Avellone G, Di G, V, Cordova R, et al. Coagulation, fibrinolysis and haemorheology in premenopausal obese women with different body fat distribution. *Thromb Res.* 1994;75:223–231.
41. Herrera MF, Oseguera J, Gamino R, et al. Cardiac abnormalities associated with morbid obesity. *World J Surg.* 1998;22:993–997.
42. Iyriboz Y, Hearon CM, Edwards K. Agreement between large and small cuffs in sphygmomanometry: a quantitative assessment. *J Clin Monit.* 1994; 10:127–133.
43. Eagle KA, Brundage BH, Chaitman BR, et al. Guidelines for perioperative cardiovascular evaluation for noncardiac surgery. Report of the American College of Cardiology/American Heart Association Task Force on Practice Guidelines (Committee on Perioperative Cardiovascular Evaluation for Noncardiac Surgery). *J Am Coll Cardiol.* 1996;27:910–948.
44. Lee TH, Marcantonio ER, Mangione CM, et al. Derivation and prospective validation of a simple index for prediction of cardiac risk of major noncardiac surgery. *Circulation.* 1999;100:1043–1049.
45. Pronovost PJ, Jenckes MW, Dorman T, et al. Organizational characteristics of intensive care units related to outcomes of abdominal aortic surgery. *JAMA.* 1999;281:1310–1317.
46. Dimick JB, Pronovost PJ, Cowan JA Jr, et al. Postoperative complication rates after hepatic resection in Maryland hospitals. *Arch Surg.* 2003;138:41–46.
47. Begg CB, Cramer LD, Hoskins WJ, et al. Impact of hospital volume on operative mortality for major cancer surgery. *JAMA.* 1998;280:1747–1751.
48. Hannan EL, O'Donnell JF, Kilburn H Jr, et al. Investigation of the relationship between volume and mortality for surgical procedures performed in New York State hospitals. *JAMA.* 1989;262:503–510.
49. Hannan EL. The relation between volume and outcome in health care. *N Engl J Med.* 1999;340:1677–1679.
50. Dunn RF, Wolff L, Wagner S, et al. The inconsistent pattern of thallium defects: a clue to the false positive perfusion scintigram. *Am J Cardiol.* 1981;48:224–232.
51. Goodgold HM, Rehder JG, Samuels LD, et al. Improved interpretation of exercise Tl-201 myocardial perfusion scintigraphy in women: characterization of breast attenuation artifacts. *Radiology.* 1987;165:361–366.
52. Brusco L Jr. Peri-operative risks and frequent complications. In: Alvarez A, ed. *Morbid Obesity Peri-operative Management.* Cambridge, UK: Cambridge University Press; 2004:13–23.
53. Kuduvalli M, Grayson AD, Oo AY, et al. Risk of morbidity and in-hospital mortality in obese patients undergoing coronary artery bypass surgery. *Eur J Cardiothorac Surg.* 2002;22:787–793.
54. Reeves BC, Ascione R, Chamberlain MH, et al. Effect of body mass index on early outcomes in patients undergoing coronary artery bypass surgery. *J Am Coll Cardiol.* 2003;42:668–676.
55. Prabhakar G, Haan CK, Peterson ED, et al. The risks of moderate and extreme obesity for coronary artery bypass grafting outcomes: a study from the Society of Thoracic Surgeons' database. *Ann Thorac Surg.* 2002;74: 1125–1130.
56. Eagle KA, Berger PB, Calkins H, et al. ACC/AHA Guideline Update for Perioperative Cardiovascular Evaluation for Noncardiac Surgery–Executive Summary. A report of the American College of Cardiology/American Heart Association Task Force on Practice Guidelines (Committee to Update the 1996 Guidelines on Perioperative Cardiovascular Evaluation for Noncardiac Surgery). *Anesth Analg.* 2002;94:1052–1064.
57. Eagle KA, Rihal CS, Mickel MC, et al. Cardiac risk of noncardiac surgery: influence of coronary disease and type of surgery in 3368 operations. CASS Investigators and University of Michigan Heart Care Program. Coronary Artery Surgery Study. *Circulation.* 1997;96:1882–1887.
58. Hassan SA, Hlatky MA, Boothroyd DB, et al. Outcomes of noncardiac surgery after coronary bypass surgery or coronary angioplasty in the Bypass Angioplasty Revascularization Investigation (BARI). *Am J Med.* 2001;110: 260–266.
59. Allen JR, Helling TS, Hartzler GO. Operative procedures not involving the heart after percutaneous transluminal coronary angioplasty. *Surg Gynecol Obstet.* 1991;173:285–288.
60. Posner KL, Van Norman GA, Chan V. Adverse cardiac outcomes after noncardiac surgery in patients with prior percutaneous transluminal coronary angioplasty. *Anesth Analg.* 1999;89:553–560.
61. Elmore JR, Hallett JW Jr, Gibbons RJ, et al. Myocardial revascularization before abdominal aortic aneurysmorrhaphy: effect of coronary angioplasty. *Mayo Clin Proc.* 1993;68:637–641.
62. Gottlieb A, Banoub M, Sprung J, et al. Perioperative cardiovascular morbidity in patients with coronary artery disease undergoing vascular surgery after percutaneous transluminal coronary angioplasty. *J Cardiothorac Vasc Anesth.* 1998;12:501–506.
63. Wilson SH, Fasseas P, Orford JL, et al. Clinical outcome of patients undergoing non-cardiac surgery in the two months following coronary stenting. *J Am Coll Cardiol.* 2003;42:234–240.
64. Powell BD, Lennon RJ, Lerman A, et al. Association of body mass index with outcome after percutaneous coronary intervention. *Am J Cardiol.* 2003;91:472–476.
65. Akhtar S, Barash PG. Perioperative use of beta-blockers: past, present, and future. *Int Anesthesiol Clin.* 2002;40:133–157.
66. Zaugg M, Schaub MC, Pasch T, et al. Modulation of beta-adrenergic receptor subtype activities in perioperative medicine: mechanisms and sites of action. *Br J Anaesth.* 2002;88:101–123.
67. Auerbach AD, Goldman L. beta-Blockers and reduction of cardiac events in noncardiac surgery: clinical applications. *JAMA.* 2002;287:1445–1447.
68. Stevens RD, Burri H, Tramer MR. Pharmacologic myocardial protection in patients undergoing noncardiac surgery: a quantitative systematic review. *Anesth Analg.* 2003;97:623–633.
69. Wallace A, Layug B, Tateo I, et al. Prophylactic atenolol reduces postoperative myocardial ischemia. McSPI Research Group. *Anesthesiology.* 1998;88:7–17.
70. Cheymol G, Poirier JM, Carrupt PA, et al. Pharmacokinetics of beta-adrenoceptor blockers in obese and normal volunteers. *Br J Clin Pharmacol.* 1997;43:563–570.
71. Cheymol G. Effects of obesity on pharmacokinetics implications for drug therapy. *Clin Pharmacokinet.* 2000;39:215–231.
72. Bostanjian D, Anthone GJ, Hamoui N, et al. Rhabdomyolysis of gluteal muscles leading to renal failure: a potentially fatal complication of surgery in the morbidly obese. *Obes Surg.* 2003;13:302–305.
73. Torres-Villalobos G, Kimura E, Mosqueda JL, et al. Pressure-induced rhabdomyolysis after bariatric surgery. *Obes Surg.* 2003;13:297–301.
74. Guzzi LM, Mills LM, Greenman P. Rhabdomyolysis, acute renal failure, and the exaggerated lithotomy position. *Anesth Analg.* 1993;77:635–637.
75. Zager RA, Foerder C, Bredl C. The influence of mannitol on myoglobinuric acute renal failure: functional, biochemical, and morphological assessments. *J Am Soc Nephrol.* 1991;2:848–855.
76. Abassi ZA, Hoffman A, Better OS. Acute renal failure complicating muscle crush injury. *Semin Nephrol.* 1998;18:558–565.
77. Alvarez AO, Cascardo A, Albarracin MS, et al. Total intravenous anesthesia with midazolam, remifentanil, propofol and cisatracurium in morbid obesity. *Obes Surg.* 2000;10:353–360.
78. Pizzirani E, Pigato P, Favretti F, et al. The Post-anaesthetic Recovery in Obesity Surgery: comparison between two anaesthetic techniques. *Obes Surg.* 1992;2:91–94.
79. Shenkman Z, Shir Y, Brodsky JB. Perioperative management of the obese patient. *Br J Anaesth.* 1993;70:349–359.
80. von Ungern-Sternberg BS, Regli A, Reber A, et al. Effect of obesity and thoracic epidural analgesia on perioperative spirometry. *Br J Anaesth.* 2005;94:121–127.
81. Michaloudis D, Fraidakis O, Petrou A, et al. Continuous spinal anesthesia/analgesia for perioperative management of morbidly obese patients undergoing laparotomy for gastroplastic surgery. *Obes Surg.* 2000;10:220–229.
82. Backman L, Freyschuss U, Hallberg D, et al. Cardiovascular function in extreme obesity. *Acta Med Scand.* 1973;193:437–446.
83. Paul DR, Hoyt JL, Boutros AR. Cardiovascular and respiratory changes in response to change of posture in the very obese. *Anesthesiology.* 1976; 45:73–78.
84. Brodsky JB. Positioning the morbid obese patient for surgery. In: Alvarez A, ed. *Morbid Obesity Peri-Operative Management.* Cambridge, UK: Cambridge University Press; 2004:274–283.
85. Abernethy DR, Greenblatt DJ. Drug disposition in obese humans. An update. *Clin Pharmacokinet.* 1986;11:199–213.
86. Cheymol G. Clinical pharmacokinetics of drugs in obesity. An update. *Clin Pharmacokinet.* 1993;25:103–114.
87. Blouin RA, Kolpek JH, Mann HJ. Influence of obesity on drug disposition. *Clin Pharm.* 1987;6:706–714.
88. Li L, Miles MV, Lakkis H, et al. Vancomycin-binding characteristics in patients with serious infections. *Pharmacotherapy.* 1996;16:1024–1029.
89. Zahorska-Markiewicz B, Waluga M, Zielinski M, et al. Pharmacokinetics of theophylline in obesity. *Int J Clin Pharmacol Ther.* 1996;34:393–395.
90. Flechner SM, Kolbeinsson ME, Tam J, et al. The impact of body weight on cyclosporine pharmacokinetics in renal transplant recipients. *Transplantation.* 1989;47:806–810.
91. Traynor AM, Nafziger AN, Bertino JS Jr. Aminoglycoside dosing weight correction factors for patients of various body sizes. *Antimicrob Agents Chemother.* 1995;39:545–548.
92. Luc EC De Baerdemaeker M, Mortier EP, et al. Pharmacokinetics and pharmacodynamics. Essential guide for anesthetic drugs administration. In: Alvarez A, ed. *Morbid Obesity Peri-operative Management.* Cambridge, UK: Cambridge University Press; 2004:211–220.
93. Koenig SM. Pulmonary complications of obesity. *Am J Med Sci.* 2001;321: 249–279.
94. Eichenberger A, Proietti S, Wicky S, et al. Morbid obesity and postoperative pulmonary atelectasis: an underestimated problem. *Anesth Analg.* 2002;95:1788–1792, table.
95. Strollo PJ Jr, Rogers RM. Obstructive sleep apnea. *N Engl J Med.* 1996;334: 99–104.
96. Rajala R, Partinen M, Sane T, et al. Obstructive sleep apnoea syndrome in morbidly obese patients. *J Intern Med.* 1991;230:125–129.
97. Ferretti A, Giampiccolo P, Cavalli A, et al. Expiratory flow limitation and orthopnea in massively obese subjects. *Chest.* 2001;119:1401–1408.
98. Resta O, Foschino-Barbaro MP, Legari G, et al. Sleep-related breathing disorders, loud snoring and excessive daytime sleepiness in obese subjects. *Int J Obes Relat Metab Disord.* 2001;25:669–675.

99. Vgontzas AN, Bixler EO, Chrousos GP. Obesity-related sleepiness and fatigue: the role of the stress system and cytokines. *Ann N Y Acad Sci.* 2006;1083:329–344.
100. Young T, Palta M, Dempsey J, et al. The occurrence of sleep-disordered breathing among middle-aged adults. *N Engl J Med.* 1993;328:1230–1235.
101. Silverberg DS, Iaina A, Oksenberg A. Treating obstructive sleep apnea improves essential hypertension and quality of life. *Am Fam Physician.* 2002;65:229–236.
102. Dhonneur G, Combes X, Leroux B, et al. Postoperative obstructive apnea. *Anesth Analg.* 1999;89:762–767.
103. Boushra NN. Anaesthetic management of patients with sleep apnoea syndrome. *Can J Anaesth.* 1996;43:599–616.
104. Ostermeier AM, Roizen MF, Hautkappe M, et al. Three sudden postoperative respiratory arrests associated with epidural opioids in patients with sleep apnea. *Anesth Analg.* 1997;85:452–460.
105. Hiremath AS, Hillman DR, James AL, et al. Relationship between difficult tracheal intubation and obstructive sleep apnoea. *Br J Anaesth.* 1998; 80:606–611.
106. Siyam MA, Benhamou D. Difficult endotracheal intubation in patients with sleep apnea syndrome. *Anesth Analg.* 2002;95:1098–1102, table.
107. Biring MS, Lewis MI, Liu JT, et al. Pulmonary physiologic changes of morbid obesity. *Am J Med Sci.* 1999;318:293–297.
108. Langeron O, Masso E, Huraux C, et al. Prediction of difficult mask ventilation. *Anesthesiology.* 2000;92:1229–1236.
109. Kessler R, Chaouat A, Schinkewitch P, et al. The obesity-hypoventilation syndrome revisited: a prospective study of 34 consecutive cases. *Chest.* 2001;120:369–376.
110. Akashiba T, Kawahara S, Kosaka N, et al. Determinants of chronic hypercapnia in Japanese men with obstructive sleep apnea syndrome. *Chest.* 2002;121:415–421.
111. Blankfield RP, Hudgel DW, Tapolyai AA, et al. Bilateral leg edema, obesity, pulmonary hypertension, and obstructive sleep apnea. *Arch Intern Med.* 2000;160:2357–2362.
112. Bradley TD, Rutherford R, Grossman RF, et al. Role of daytime hypoxemia in the pathogenesis of right heart failure in the obstructive sleep apnea syndrome. *Am Rev Respir Dis.* 1985;131:835–839.
113. Al-Mobeireek AF, Al-Kassimi FA, Al-Majed SA, et al. Clinical profile of sleep apnea syndrome. A study at a university hospital. *Saudi Med J.* 2000;21:180–183.
114. Chaouat A, Weitzenblum E, Krieger J, et al. Association of chronic obstructive pulmonary disease and sleep apnea syndrome. *Am J Respir Crit Care Med.* 1995;151:82–86.
115. Pelosi P, Croci M, Ravagnan I, et al. Respiratory system mechanics in sedated, paralyzed, morbidly obese patients. *J Appl Physiol.* 1997;82:811–818.
116. Vaughan RW, Cork RC, Hollander D. The effect of massive weight loss on arterial oxygenation and pulmonary function tests. *Anesthesiology.* 1981;54:325–328.
117. Hakala K, Maasilta P, Sovijarvi AR. Upright body position and weight loss improve respiratory mechanics and daytime oxygenation in obese patients with obstructive sleep apnoea. *Clin Physiol.* 2000;20:50–55.
118. Peppard PE, Young T, Palta M, et al. Prospective study of the association between sleep-disordered breathing and hypertension. *N Engl J Med.* 2000;342:1378–1384.
119. Rochester DF. Obesity and pulmonary function. In: Alpert MA, Alexander JK, eds. *The Heart and Lung in Obesity.* Armonk, NY: Futura Publishing Company; 1998:108–132.
120. Eriksson S, Backman L, Ljungstrom KG. The incidence of clinical postoperative thrombosis after gastric surgery for obesity during 16 years. *Obes Surg.* 1997;7:332–335.
121. Geerts W, Selby R. Prevention of venous thromboembolism in the ICU. *Chest.* 2003;124:357S–363S.
122. Scholten DJ, Hoedema RM, Scholten SE. A comparison of two different prophylactic dose regimens of low molecular weight heparin in bariatric surgery. *Obes Surg.* 2002;12:19–24.
123. Hnatiuk OW, Dillard TA, Torrington KG. Adherence to established guidelines for preoperative pulmonary function testing. *Chest.* 1995;107:1294–1297.
124. Roche N, Herer B, Roig C, et al. Prospective testing of two models based on clinical and oximetric variables for prediction of obstructive sleep apnea. *Chest.* 2002;121:747–752.
125. Crapo RO, Kelly TM, Elliott CG, et al. Spirometry as a preoperative screening test in morbidly obese patients. *Surgery.* 1986;99:763–768.
126. Tung A, Rock P. Perioperative concerns in sleep apnea. *Curr Opin Anaesthesiol.* 2001;14:671–678.
127. Rennotte MT, Baele P, Aubert G, et al. Nasal continuous positive airway pressure in the perioperative management of patients with obstructive sleep apnea submitted to surgery. *Chest.* 1995;107:367–374.
128. Tkacova R, Rankin F, Fitzgerald FS, et al. Effects of continuous positive airway pressure on obstructive sleep apnea and left ventricular afterload in patients with heart failure. *Circulation.* 1998;98:2269–2275.
129. Wilcox I, Grunstein RR, Hedner JA, et al. Effect of nasal continuous positive airway pressure during sleep on 24-hour blood pressure in obstructive sleep apnea. *Sleep.* 1993;16:539–544.
130. Brodsky JB, Lemmens HJ, Brock-Utne JG, et al. Morbid obesity and tracheal intubation. *Anesth Analg.* 2002;94:732–736.
131. Illing L, Duncan PG, Yip R. Gastroesophageal reflux during anaesthesia. *Can J Anaesth.* 1992;39:466–470.
132. Hardy JF, Lepage Y, Bonneville-Chouinard N. Occurrence of gastroesophageal reflux on induction of anaesthesia does not correlate with the volume of gastric contents. *Can J Anaesth.* 1990;37:502–508.
133. Beers RA, Roizen MF. Pre-operative evaluation of the patient for bariatric surgery. In: Alvarez A, ed. *Morbid Obesity Peri-operative Management.* Cambridge, UK: Cambridge University Press; 2004:113–125.
134. Berthoud MC, Peacock JE, Reilly CS. Effectiveness of preoxygenation in morbidly obese patients. *Br J Anaesth.* 1991;67:464–466.
135. Dixon BJ, Dixon JB, Carden JR, et al. Preoxygenation is more effective in the 25 degrees head-up position than in the supine position in severely obese patients: a randomized controlled study. *Anesthesiology.* 2005;102:1110–1115.
136. Boyce JR, Ness T, Castroman P, et al. A preliminary study of the optimal anesthesia positioning for the morbidly obese patient. *Obes Surg.* 2003; 13:4–9.
137. Perilli V, Sollazzi L, Bozza P, et al. The effects of the reverse Trendelenburg position on respiratory mechanics and blood gases in morbidly obese patients during bariatric surgery. *Anesth Analg.* 2000;91:1520–1525.
138. Luce JM. Respiratory complications of obesity. *Chest.* 1980;78:626–631.
139. Pelosi P, Croci M, Ravagnan I, et al. The effects of body mass on lung volumes, respiratory mechanics, and gas exchange during general anesthesia. *Anesth Analg.* 1998;87:654–660.
140. Damia G, Mascheroni D, Croci M, et al. Perioperative changes in functional residual capacity in morbidly obese patients. *Br J Anaesth.* 1988;60:574–578.
141. Marik P, Varon J. The obese patient in the ICU. *Chest.* 1998;113:492–498.
142. The ARDS Network. Ventilation with lower tidal volumes as compared with traditional tidal volumes for acute lung injury and the acute respiratory distress syndrome. The Acute Respiratory Distress Syndrome Network. *N Engl J Med.* 2000;342:1301–1308.
143. Pelosi P, Ravagnan I, Giurati G, et al. Positive end-expiratory pressure improves respiratory function in obese but not in normal subjects during anesthesia and paralysis. *Anesthesiology.* 1999;91:1221–1231.
144. Marko P, Gabrielli A, Caruso LJ, et al. Digestive physiology and gastric aspiration. In: Alvarez A, ed. *Morbid Obesity Peri-operative Management.* Cambridge, UK: Cambridge University Press; 2004:89–106.
145. Burns SM, Egloff MB, Ryan B, et al. Effect of body position on spontaneous respiratory rate and tidal volume in patients with obesity, abdominal distension and ascites. *Am J Crit Care.* 1994;3:102–106.
146. Joris JL, Sottiaux TM, Chiche JD, et al. Effect of bi-level positive airway pressure (BiPAP) nasal ventilation on the postoperative pulmonary restrictive syndrome in obese patients undergoing gastroplasty. *Chest.* 1997; 111:665–670.
147. Brodsky JB. Morbid obesity. *Curr Anaesth Crit Care.* 1998;9:249–254.
148. Vaughan RW, Bauer S, Wise L. Effect of position (semirecumbent versus supine) on postoperative oxygenation in markedly obese subjects. *Anesth Analg.* 1976;55:37–41.
149. Rothen HU, Sporre B, Engberg G, et al. Reexpansion of atelectasis during general anaesthesia may have a prolonged effect. *Acta Anaesthesiol Scand.* 1995;39:118–125.
150. Rothen HU, Sporre B, Engberg G, et al. Influence of gas composition on recurrence of atelectasis after a reexpansion maneuver during general anesthesia. *Anesthesiology.* 1995;82:832–842.
151. Reber A, Engberg G, Wegenius G, et al. Lung aeration. The effect of preoxygenation and hyperoxygenation during total intravenous anaesthesia. *Anaesthesia.* 1996;51:733–737.
152. Rothen HU, Sporre B, Engberg G, et al. Prevention of atelectasis during general anaesthesia. *Lancet.* 1995;345:1387–1391.
153. Goll V, Akca O, Greif R, et al. Ondansetron is no more effective than supplemental intraoperative oxygen for prevention of postoperative nausea and vomiting. *Anesth Analg.* 2001;92:112–117.
154. Greif R, Laciny S, Rapf B, et al. Supplemental oxygen reduces the incidence of postoperative nausea and vomiting. *Anesthesiology.* 1999;91:1246–1252.
155. Greif R, Akca O, Horn EP, et al. Supplemental perioperative oxygen to reduce the incidence of surgical-wound infection. Outcomes Research Group. *N Engl J Med.* 2000;342:161–167.
156. Kotani N, Hashimoto H, Sessler DI, et al. Supplemental intraoperative oxygen augments antimicrobial and proinflammatory responses of alveolar macrophages. *Anesthesiology.* 2000;93:15–25.
157. Capella JF, Capella RF. Is routine invasive monitoring indicated in surgery for the morbidly obese? *Obes Surg.* 1996;6:50–53.
158. Esclamado RM, Glenn MG, McCulloch TM, et al. Perioperative complications and risk factors in the surgical treatment of obstructive sleep apnea syndrome. *Laryngoscope.* 1989;99:1125–1129.
159. Tucci M, Bansal V, Camporesi EM. Respiratory monitoring. In: Alvarez A, ed. *Morbid Obesity Peri-operative Management.* Cambridge, UK: Cambridge University Press; 2004:89–106.
160. Sapala JA, Wood MH, Schuhknecht MP, et al. Fatal pulmonary embolism

after bariatric operations for morbid obesity: a 24-year retrospective analysis. *Obes Surg.* 2003;13:819–825.

161. Sabers C, Plevak DJ, Schroeder DR, et al. The diagnosis of obstructive sleep apnea as a risk factor for unanticipated admissions in outpatient surgery. *Anesth Analg.* 2003;96:1328–1335, table.
162. Schroder T, Nolte M, Kox WJ, et al. [Anesthesia in extreme obesity]. *Herz.* 2001;26:222–228.
163. Rosenberg J, Ullstad T, Rasmussen J, et al. Time course of postoperative hypoxaemia. *Eur J Surg.* 1994;160:137–143.
164. Yap SJ, Morris RW, Pybus DA. Alterations in endotracheal tube position during general anaesthesia. *Anaesth Intensive Care.* 1994;22:586–588.
165. Lobato EB, Paige GB, Brown MM, et al. Pneumoperitoneum as a risk factor for endobronchial intubation during laparoscopic gynecologic surgery. *Anesth Analg.* 1998;86:301–303.
166. Ezri T, Hazin V, Warters D, et al. The endotracheal tube moves more often in obese patients undergoing laparoscopy compared with open abdominal surgery. *Anesth Analg.* 2003;96:278–282, table.
167. Hedenstierna G, Tokics L, Strandberg A, et al. Correlation of gas exchange impairment to development of atelectasis during anaesthesia and muscle paralysis. *Acta Anaesthesiol Scand.* 1986;30:183–191.
168. Moller JT, Johannessen NW, Berg H, et al. Hypoxaemia during anaesthesia—an observer study. *Br J Anaesth.* 1991;66:437–444.
169. Bendixen HH, Hedley-Whyte J, Laver MB. Impaired oxygenation in surgical patients during general anesthesia with controlled ventilation. A concept of atelectasis. *N Engl J Med.* 1963;269:991–996.
170. Brismar B, Hedenstierna G, Lundquist H, et al. Pulmonary densities during anesthesia with muscular relaxation-a proposal of atelectasis. *Anesthesiology.* 1985;62:422–428.
171. Zerah F, Harf A, Perlemuter L, et al. Effects of obesity on respiratory resistance. *Chest.* 1993;103:1470–1476.
172. Pelosi P, Croci M, Ravagnan I, et al. Total respiratory system, lung, and chest wall mechanics in sedated-paralyzed postoperative morbidly obese patients. *Chest.* 1996;109:144–151.
173. Tweed WA, Phua WT, Chong KY, et al. Tidal volume, lung hyperinflation and arterial oxygenation during general anaesthesia. *Anaesth Intensive Care.* 1993;21:806–810.
174. Magnusson L, Spahn DR. New concepts of atelectasis during general anaesthesia. *Br J Anaesth.* 2003;91:61–72.
175. Millman RP, Meyer TJ, Eveloff SE. Sleep apnea in the morbidly obese. *R I Med.* 1992;75:483–486.
176. Douglas NJ, Polo O. Pathogenesis of obstructive sleep apnoea/hypopnoea syndrome. *Lancet.* 1994;344:653–655.
177. Murphy PG. Obesity. In: Hemmings HC, Hopkins PM, eds. *Foundation of Anaesthesia. Basic Clinical Sciences.* Philadelphia: Mosby; 2000:703–711.
178. Huerta S, DeShields S, Shpiner R, et al. Safety and efficacy of postoperative continuous positive airway pressure to prevent pulmonary complications after Roux-en-Y gastric bypass. *J Gastrointest Surg.* 2002;6:354–358.
179. Gilbert TB, Seneff MG, Becker RB. Facilitation of internal jugular venous cannulation using an audio-guided Doppler ultrasound vascular access device: results from a prospective, dual-center, randomized, crossover clinical study. *Crit Care Med.* 1995;23:60–65.
180. Jeevanandam M, Young DH, Schiller WR. Obesity and the metabolic response to severe multiple trauma in man. *J Clin Invest.* 1991;87:262–269.
181. Cousins M, Power I. Acute and postoperative pain. In: Wall PD, Melzack R, eds. *Textbook of Pain.* Philadelphia: Elsevier;1999:447–491.
182. Craig DB. Postoperative recovery of pulmonary function. *Anesth Analg.* 1981;60:46–52.
183. Fine PC, Ashburn MA. Functional neuroanatomy and nociception. In: Ashburn MA, Rice LJ, eds. *The Management of Pain.* Philadelphia: Churchill Livingstone; 1998:1–16.
184. Rawal N. 10 years of acute pain services–achievements and challenges. *Reg Anesth Pain Med.* 1999;24:68–73.
185. Provenzano D, Grass J. Is epidural analgesia superior to IV-PCA? In: Fleisher L, ed. *Evidence-Based Practice of Anesthesiology.* Philadelphia: Saunders, Elsevier Inc.; 2004:441–448.
186. Rigg JR, Jamrozik K, Myles PS, et al. Epidural anaesthesia and analgesia and outcome of major surgery: a randomised trial. *Lancet.* 2002;359:1276–1282.
187. Block BM, Liu SS, Rowlingson AJ, et al. Efficacy of postoperative epidural analgesia: a meta-analysis. *JAMA.* 2003;290:2455–2463.
188. Schumann R, Shikora S, Weiss JM, et al. A comparison of multimodal perioperative analgesia to epidural pain management after gastric bypass surgery. *Anesth Analg.* 2003;96:469–474, table.
189. Brodsky JB, Merrell RC. Epidural administration of morphine postoperatively for morbidly obese patients. *West J Med.* 1984;140:750–753.
190. Rawal N, Sjostrand U, Christoffersson E, et al. Comparison of intramuscular and epidural morphine for postoperative analgesia in the grossly obese: influence on postoperative ambulation and pulmonary function. *Anesth Analg.* 1984;63:583–592.
191. Niemi G, Breivik H. Epidural fentanyl markedly improves thoracic epidural analgesia in a low-dose infusion of bupivacaine, adrenaline and fentanyl. A randomized, double-blind crossover study with and without fentanyl. *Acta Anaesthesiol Scand.* 2001;45:221–232.
192. Niemi G, Breivik H. The minimally effective concentration of adrenaline in a low-concentration thoracic epidural analgesic infusion of bupivacaine, fentanyl and adrenaline after major surgery. A randomized, double-blind, dose-finding study. *Acta Anaesthesiol Scand.* 2003;47:439–450.
193. Blomberg S, Emanuelsson H, Ricksten SE. Thoracic epidural anesthesia and central hemodynamics in patients with unstable angina pectoris. *Anesth Analg.* 1989;69:558–562.
194. Saada M, Catoire P, Bonnet F, et al. Effect of thoracic epidural anesthesia combined with general anesthesia on segmental wall motion assessed by transesophageal echocardiography. *Anesth Analg.* 1992;75:329–335.
195. Tevelenok I. [Peridural anesthesia in the acute period of myocardial infarct]. *Anesteziol Reanimatol.* 1977;36–39.
196. Toft P, Jorgensen A. Continuous thoracic epidural analgesia for the control of pain in myocardial infarction. *Intensive Care Med.* 1987;13:388–389.
197. Blomberg SG. Long-term home self-treatment with high thoracic epidural anesthesia in patients with severe coronary artery disease. *Anesth Analg.* 1994;79:413–421.
198. Kataja J. Thoracolumbar epidural anaesthesia and isoflurane to prevent hypertension and tachycardia in patients undergoing abdominal aortic surgery. *Eur J Anaesthesiol.* 1991;8:427–436.
199. Baron JF, Coriat P, Mundler O, et al. Left ventricular global and regional function during lumbar epidural anesthesia in patients with and without angina pectoris. Influence of volume loading. *Anesthesiology.* 1987;66:621–627.
200. Diebel LN, Lange MP, Schneider F, et al. Cardiopulmonary complications after major surgery: a role for epidural analgesia? *Surgery.* 1987;102:660–666.
201. Yeager MP, Glass DD, Neff RK, et al. Epidural anesthesia and analgesia in high-risk surgical patients. *Anesthesiology.* 1987;66:729–736.
202. Her C, Kizelshteyn G, Walker V, et al. Combined epidural and general anesthesia for abdominal aortic surgery. *J Cardiothorac Anesth.* 1990;4:552–557.
203. Meyers JR, Lembeck L, O'Kane H, et al. Changes in functional residual capacity of the lung after operation. *Arch Surg.* 1975;110:576–583.
204. Spence AA, Smith G. Postoperative analgesia and lung function: a comparison of morphine with extradural block. *Br J Anaesth.* 1971;43:144–148.
205. Brown D, Neal J. Chronic obstructive pulmonary disease and perioperative analgesia. In: Brown DL, ed. *Problems in Anesthesia.* Philadelphia: JB Lippincott; 1988:422–434.
206. Hickey RF, Visick WD, Fairley HB, et al. Effects of halothane anesthesia on functional residual capacity and alveolar-arterial oxygen tension difference. *Anesthesiology.* 1973;38:20–24.
207. Garibaldi RA, Britt MR, Coleman ML, et al. Risk factors for postoperative pneumonia. *Am J Med.* 1981;70:677–680.
208. Hendolin H, Lahtinen J, Lansimies E, et al. The effect of thoracic epidural analgesia on respiratory function after cholecystectomy. *Acta Anaesthesiol Scand.* 1987;31:645–651.
209. Cuschieri RJ, Morran CG, Howie JC, et al. Postoperative pain and pulmonary complications: comparison of three analgesic regimens. *Br J Surg.* 1985;72:495–498.
210. Pansard JL, Mankikian B, Bertrand M, et al. Effects of thoracic extradural block on diaphragmatic electrical activity and contractility after upper abdominal surgery. *Anesthesiology.* 1993;78:63–71.
211. Duggan J, Drummond GB. Activity of lower intercostal and abdominal muscle after upper abdominal surgery. *Anesth Analg.* 1987;66:852–855.
212. Ali J, Weisel RD, Layug AB, et al. Consequences of postoperative alterations in respiratory mechanics. *Am J Surg.* 1974;128:376–382.
213. Tarhan S, Moffitt EA, Sessler AD, et al. Risk of anesthesia and surgery in patients with chronic bronchitis and chronic obstructive pulmonary disease. *Surgery.* 1973;74:720–726.
214. Rademaker BM, Ringers J, Odoom JA, et al. Pulmonary function and stress response after laparoscopic cholecystectomy: comparison with subcostal incision and influence of thoracic epidural analgesia. *Anesth Analg.* 1992;75:381–385.
215. Sydow FW. The influence of anesthesia and postoperative analgesic management of lung function. *Acta Chir Scand Suppl.* 1989;550:159–165; discussion 165–168
216. Nunn JF. Effects of anaesthesia on respiration. *Br J Anaesth.* 1990;65:54–62.
217. Weller R, Rosenblum M, Conard P, et al. Comparison of epidural and patient-controlled intravenous morphine following joint replacement surgery. *Can J Anaesth.* 1991;38:582–586.
218. McCarthy GS. The effect of thoracic extradural analgesia on pulmonary gas distribution, functional residual capacity and airway closure. *Br J Anaesth.* 1976;48:243–248.
219. Groeben H. Effects of high thoracic epidural anesthesia and local anesthetics on bronchial hyperreactivity. *J Clin Monit Comput.* 2000;16:457–463.
220. Ballantyne J, Carwood C. Optimal postoperative analgesia. In: Fleisher L, ed. *Evidence-Based Practice of Anesthesiology.* Philadelphia: Saunders, Elsevier Inc.; 2004:449–458.
221. Meyer R. Rofecoxib reduces perioperative morphine consumption for abdominal hysterectomy and laparoscopic gastric banding. *Anaesth Intensive Care.* 2002;30:389–390.

CHAPTER 103 ■ THE GERIATRIC PATIENT

CARL W. PETERS • REBECCA J. BEYTH • MIHO K. BAUTISTA

The elderly population in the United States is growing at a remarkable rate, with considerable implications for delivery of intensive care to those in the later years of life. The numbers tell the story: in the 2000 U.S. census, those 62 years of age and older represented 14.7% of the population. At that time, those 85 years of age and older numbered 4,239,587, or 1.5% of the American population, an increase of 1.2 million more than found within the similar population range 10 years earlier (1). As of 2000, the life expectancy beyond the age of 65 years was nearly 19 years for a woman and 16 years for a man. Similar predictions for those 85 years old were 7 and 6 years, respectively (2). At the dawn of the 20th century, the elderly population of the United States was a small percentage of its total, 4%, or 3.1 million people; presently, the corresponding value is 35 million people. Based on revolutionary advances in public health and the development of medications and techniques of acute medical care provided to those born in the 20 years after World War II, 70,000,000 individuals will find themselves in the population subgroup known as "elderly" by 2030 (3). At that time, those 65 years and older are forecast to compose 26% of the population of Florida, which is projected to have become the third most populous of the 50 states (4). By virtue of the diseases and natural organ aging and deterioration that accompany 65—and more—years of living and working, those who advance into this age range become increasingly voracious consumers of medical care resources, including the specialized capabilities of the intensive care unit. In 2005, spending by Medicare for those older than 65 years totaled $342 billion, representing 17.1% of the total of $2 trillion spent nationwide for health care (5). Intensive care consumes 4% of national health care expenditures (6). During the last 6 months of their lives, 11% of Medicare recipients spend 8 or more days in the ICU; various studies documenting ICU occupancy by those older than 65 years old note that this ranges from one quarter to one half of the available beds (7,8). The magnitude of these statistics portend the profound financial burden that must be borne to provide a medically sound and appropriate depth of care, a significant portion of which will be provided in the ICU. Because of the magnitude of these expenditures, which are projected to continue their slow but exponential growth, the argument has been made that, in the context of *increasing* demand for *limited* health care resources—an economically unsustainable situation—blanket cost-cutting actions such as limiting scarce ICU availability to those who would "most benefit" society and themselves in later life should be instituted. The geriatric population, in some minds, does not qualify for this category of expenditure, given their diminished physical functionality and limited life span—and therefore, less payoff in return for resource use compared to a younger population. This "logic," however, belies reality. Although levels of functionality diminish with advancing age, albeit with a very wide bell curve contour, many individuals continue to perform both complex physical and intellectual tasks well into their eighth or ninth decades of life, bringing to bear resources of experience and problem solving not yet acquired by their descendents. Additionally, while flirting with the tactic of cost savings through measures that "cut out the expensive waste" in the ICU care of the elderly may fascinate some, thoughtful analyses argue persuasively that such a superficially derived position is misleading and inaccurate (9–11). Furthermore, at least in the United States, while increasingly alarmed by the financial implications of medical care costs associated with an aging population, we continue to postpone in-depth reckoning with the consequences and management of this information. Until we are ready to deal with this issue, one must maximize use of the resources available, while being mindful of the individual patient's expectations and likelihood of recovery. In the management of geriatric medical issues, recognition of the unique pathophysiology of the elderly patient may lead to streamlining of what might otherwise be a prolonged and painful ICU admission, either by recognition of the futility of the care or by amending the clinical strategy based on assessment of the distinctive clinical features, thereby extending the availability of scarce resources.

The response of the human body to physiologic insult evolves with age. A parallel with outdoor activity is useful in understanding this evolution. Imagine that a man is placed on a long ridgetop that is quite wide and smooth, and that man is told to walk down the middle of the ridge with his eyes closed. Unknown to him, as he walks, the ridge slowly becomes strewn with larger and larger rocks, and narrows inexorably as he approaches the end. Initially, the man walks quickly, with little risk of tripping or nearing the edge. As he advances farther, however, his drifting excursions off the centerline each take him closer to the treacherous rocky edge, increasing the risk of a fall. If he is careful and walks slowly, he hears the wind blowing near the cliff and is able to redirect himself away from the danger. Eventually, however, the narrowed ridgetop is completely covered with loose rocks to the very edges, and no step is possible without catastrophe. By analogy, one can think of the human body as possessing a certain amount of physiologic reserve that sustains it through times of stress brought on by disease or injury, with the maximum amount of reserve being present in young adulthood. With age, baseline organ function declines at a generally predictable rate, leaving the aging person with progressively less and less capacity to respond fully and expeditiously to stressful demands. Furthermore, there is the accumulation of permanent detrimental consequences of lifestyle decisions, such as tobacco use and lack of exercise, and of only partially controllable genetic influences, such as familial hypercholesterolemia or essential hypertension, with which the aging individual must contend, thereby increasing the likelihood of succumbing to a stressful physiologic insult. The progressive impairment of physiologic vigor is exemplified by the *exponential* increase in the death rate from sepsis with age, although the incidence of sepsis increases only *linearly* (12).

CARDIOVASCULAR DISEASE IN THE ELDERLY

Cardiovascular (CV) disease is pervasive in the elderly. Approximately 35% of all deaths in the United States are attributable to one of several manifestations of this pathophysiology, namely coronary artery disease and other conditions that involve the myocardium, hypertension, and arteriosclerosis of the central and peripheral arterial tree and cerebral vascular system, with three fourths of these deaths directly attributable to a cardiac cause (13). This proportion is higher in the more aged population, with CV disease manifesting itself as a complicating cofactor in the management of *any* older person's serious illness. For example, although only 6% of the U.S. population is 75 years of age or older, such individuals account for 30% of all myocardial infarctions and 60% of the infarction-related deaths (14).

Aging and the CV System

Studying the effect of the natural aging process on cardiovascular physiology is quite complex. From the epidemiologic standpoint, it is difficult to differentiate the basis of decline in cardiovascular function of the well-conditioned octogenarian who exercises aggressively from that of his sedentary twin who has led a life of excess, because some features and consequences of natural aging resemble those seen with disease. Although degenerative cardiovascular processes are most often looked on as what happens as you grow old, these have been demonstrated not to be the obligatory sequence of events in human aging (15,16). For all intents and purposes, the common causative elements within modern civilized existence, such as diet, minimal demands for aerobic exercise, and recurrent and ubiquitous emotional and physical stress are so intimately associated with mere existence that they may be looked on as inevitable and unchangeable. The clinical consequences to these presently unalterable processes may be perceived by the clinician or investigator as the natural process of cardiovascular aging, but the accuracy of this statement is difficult to determine. The steepness of the downward slope of this decline is increased by both a sedentary lifestyle and by the cardiovascular disease processes that are epidemic in western society's geriatric populations. Some features of cardiovascular physiology in the elderly are identical to those of younger individuals, primarily those measured in the resting state, but are affected by processes that are presently characterized as immutable in the aging process.

A degenerative process that occurs in most elderly individuals is that of stiffening of the *central* arterial tree with advancing age. Although the consequences of this process do not manifest in acute ways within the direct purview of the intensivist, they induce chronic progressive conditions that complicate critical illness in the elderly, warranting discussion. Oxygen- and nutrient-bearing blood is carried to organs via the conduit of the vascular arterial tree. In doing so, distensible large arteries perform transport and cushioning functions, transforming pulsatile flow into a steady stream of blood to the periphery (17). Release of the potential energy stored with each heartbeat within the stretched arterial wall elastin fibers propels the column of blood smoothly toward the muscular arterioles and capillary bed (17). With age—and likely related to both replacement of deteriorating, nonregenerating structural elastin fibers with nondistensible collagen, and to the progressive calcification of wall structural components (18)—vascular remodeling causes the progressive slow dilation and stiffening of the arterial wall, transforming the robust, pliant central vasculature typical of youth to that commonly seen in the elderly, more akin to a thick-walled, stiff, nondistensible garden hose (19,20). Augmented tensile and shear stresses related to the nonlaminar flow characteristic of fluid flow through vessels with impaired compliance contribute to progressive occlusive disease (21) that is typically found at turbulent areas of narrowing, bending, and bifurcation (22). The prominent manifestation of this progressive central arterial stiffening is that of the so-called *systolic hypertension syndrome*—the gradual increase in systolic blood pressure with simultaneous diastolic decline or maintenance at the same level (23). In years past, the transmission velocity of the cardiac-generated pressure impulse was discovered to change with patient age and to vary as a function of central arterial stiffness (24–27). With increased central arterial elastance—in other words, stiffness—comes an increased velocity of impulse transmission in both the forward and backward (i.e., reflected) directions. In the young, with distensible central arteries, the arrival of the reflected wave coincides with diastole, thereby augmenting coronary perfusion and modulating the magnitude of the disease-inducing tensile shear forces on the vasculature. Youthful vessels have little disease, and thus seldom display the wide pulse pressure that is the hallmark of central thickening. Aging, stiff central arteries transmit the cardiac impulse outward more rapidly and turbulently such that its reflected return arrives at the end or even the height of systole (27). In those with such vessels—the elderly—is seen isolated *systolic* hypertension, the term seeming to imply a benign connotation consistent with the previous generalized opinion that sustained *diastolic* pressure elevation was the lethal culprit (28). More recently, the insidiously destructive nature of the *augmentation index*—the reflected augmentation of systolic pressure at the expense of diastolic coronary perfusion, yielding an easily observed increased pulse pressure (29)—has been recognized as the true contribution of central vascular stiffness to the morbidity and mortality among the elderly. Indeed, the speed with which the cardiac impulse is propelled outward, known as pulse wave velocity (PWV), and pulse pressure (PP) are recognized as factors strongly associated with all forms of cardiovascular disease:

$$PP = SBP - DBP$$

where SBP is systolic blood pressure and DBP is diastolic blood pressure. These measurements, when elevated over time, strongly predict mortality and are indicative of vascular and cardiac pathology, even if the patient's blood pressure measurements and examination findings at a given moment, such as at the time of the initial evaluation of a geriatric patient on ICU arrival, appear benign (21,28,30,31).

Other specific processes within the cardiovascular system change with age, seen even in the most healthy and intact geriatric physiology. With myocardial aging, there is a predictable loss of myocytes, possibly from apoptosis (32,33). Since cardiac myocytes are unable to regenerate, functional "replacement" of these contractile cells occurs by hypertrophy of the remaining myocytes, with only slight overall loss of myocardial mass. With preservation of cardiac fibroblast synthetic function despite myocyte loss, cardiac tissue becomes infiltrated with an increasing proportion of noncompliant connective tissue, causing the gradual thickening and stiffening of the ventricular wall and impairment of left ventricular diastolic relaxation and filling. This appears similar to the fibrosis seen in pathologic left ventricular hypertrophy leading to congestive heart failure (34). Diastolic relaxation is an energy-requiring process, consuming ATP to recover calcium back into the sarcoplasmic reticulum after its release during systole (35). Malfunction of the calcium-sequestering mechanism, involving a dysfunctional SERCA (smooth endoplasmic reticulum calcium) pump, is felt to be at least partially responsible for the increased percentage of geriatric heart failure patients who display lusitropic dysfunction (36). As a consequence, the filling process is delayed, with a smoother—though steeper, as depicted on the left ventricular pressure–volume loop—slope of passive diastolic ventricular filling (37) into a more slowly relaxing ventricle that ends diastole with lower volume. The ventricle thereby becomes more dependent on the contribution of atrial contraction to ventricular filling for optimum systolic function. In other words, as the aging ventricle becomes progressively more and more lusitropically impaired, it fills progressively less well by virtue of thickening from age-related myocyte depletion and incomplete relaxation from SERCA pump dysfunction. The resulting dependence on volume repletion, control of heart rate, and the robust synchronous atrial contribution to ventricle filling assume increasing importance in managing geriatric cardiac issues. In the critically ill elderly patient in whom there is a very high chance of harboring occult diastolic dysfunction, if not overt congestive heart failure, the strictest attention must be paid to maintenance of both sinus rhythm and volume repletion within a narrow range. Furthermore, the reassurance of a preserved ejection fraction viewed on echocardiogram may be deceptive, since systolic function is preserved in the normal healthy geriatric heart (38) and can be maintained at greater than 50% in a very high proportion of those whose cardiac status has deteriorated to the point of being symptomatic from lusitropically deficient congestive heart failure (39,40).

Equally important is recognition of the progressive decrease in the responsiveness of myocardial and vascular tissue to adrenergic stimulation (41–43). This phenomenon manifests itself as an age-associated lowering of exercise-induced maximal heart rate, with a gradual shift to augmented ventricular filling to meet exercise-related demands. The stressed or exercising younger adult musters additional cardiac output by increasing contractility and heart rate and by vasodilation in the areas of maximum demand—in the case of exercise, the skeletal muscles—in response to increased levels of norepinephrine and epinephrine, with unchanged or reduced end systolic volume as output is ejected into a dilated vascular tree. The elderly, by comparison, with reduced myocardial and vasodilatory responsiveness to exercise-induced beta-1 and beta-2 stimulus (43), have increased reliance on *ventricular filling* (the Frank-Starling mechanism) to achieve augmented cardiac output (44,45).

Optimal care requires clinical awareness of age-related cardiovascular differences such as diastolic dysfunction. Currently, there are no medications that restore the vigor with which calcium is resequestered within the SER during diastole, nor avert the obligate loss of myocardial cells, nor restore the responsiveness of the elderly cardiovascular system to endogenous catecholamines, although supplements can be supplied via a continual infusion in the ICU setting. Meanwhile, the clinician must contend with the challenge of managing the stiff, hypertrophied ventricle perfusing a nondistensible vascular tree. With the fraction of elderly patients who harbor cardiovascular disease being as large as it is in western society, clinical manifestations of this condition may complicate the management of virtually every older patient. In those not displaying the "usual, common" symptoms of heart failure traditionally taught in medical school, one *must* maintain a level of suspicion to recognize the more subtle presentations of age-related lusitropic pathophysiology.

Acute Coronary Syndrome in the Elderly

Acute coronary syndrome (ACS) presents a particular challenge from the standpoints of recognition and management. Optimal management of myocardial ischemia and infarction in the elderly population is less well defined than in younger populations, since those older than 75 years are less commonly included in ischemia-related studies (46). The elderly mortality rate exceeds that found in younger individuals (47), but the elderly stand to benefit most in mortality reduction from intervention (48). In the young, acute ischemic processes are often associated with onset of classic angina or one of its common equivalents; in the elderly, symptoms may be much more subtle and nondistinguishing, but the condition is more likely to be fatal (49). Therefore, proper identification of myocardial ischemia and infarction must occur in a timely manner, as aggressive management is warranted. The diagnostic picture can be further complicated by the postoperative sedated state, when hypotension or arrhythmias may easily be attributed to hydration or electrolyte disturbances rather than to coronary insufficiency. ICU patients often have contraindications to intervention, and the risks of reperfusion therapy must be weighed thoughtfully against the benefits. While evaluating the need for intervention with the cardiologist, the patient, and family members, the intensivist must remember that only a small percentage of elderly patients warranting reperfusion therapy actually receive it (50), even when no absolute contraindication exists. This is attributable to two misperceptions: the magnitude of risk to the geriatric patient, and the likelihood of benefit (48). The cardiology literature contains studies covering enormous numbers of patients evaluating the strategies of treatment to optimize the restoration of coronary blood flow, and in-depth discussion is beyond the scope of this chapter. Nonetheless, a few generalities focusing on the management of the elderly patient can be made.

One relevant observation is the paucity of elderly individuals who have been included in many of the large trials (51), especially considering the prevalence of coronary disease in this group; for this reason, optimal management strategies may not be as well defined as those that address ACS within a younger population. ACS must be identified correctly, nonetheless, since treatment strategies of the patient subgroups within this very large category differ (52). One of the underpinnings of any strategy is that of expeditious implementation, in that the more quickly the intervention is begun, the greater the mass of myocardial tissue preserved and the greater number of lives saved (53). Rapid restoration of coronary blood flow is the major goal of treatment for STEMI (ST-segment elevation myocardial infarction). A decrease in mortality of 25% with reperfusion therapy has been demonstrated (54). From identification of STEMI, it is recommended that the infusion of thrombolytics begin within 30 minutes, or that the dilating balloon be inflated within 90 minutes (55). In general, percutaneous coronary intervention (PCI) is the preferred mode of treatment for STEMI, as long as the time constraints are met (56). Extrapolation of this analysis to the elderly population is done only with trepidation, since only small numbers of elderly patients were included in the studies covered by this meta-analysis. By examining the subgroup data, nevertheless, it appears that elderly patients in this urgent situation of evolving myocardial infarction, in which the risk of death is particularly high by virtue of the risk factors associated with advanced age (57) and by the emergent nature of the situation, are best served by PCI (47,58). PCI yielded lower mortality in the elderly population than did thrombolysis, with more benefit found as age progressively advanced, although possibly at the risk of a slightly increased rate of major bleeding events. In the management of non–ST-segment elevation MI (N-STEMI), early invasive strategy with catheterization and revascularization (when warranted) significantly benefits those older than 65 years of age (59). The early invasive strategy, however, led to a significant increase in in-hospital major bleeding (16.6% vs. 6.5%; $p = 0.009$) and blood transfusion (20.9% vs. 7.9%; $p = 0.002$) in the patients older than 75 years of age. There were no significant increases in minor bleeding or stroke in any study group. The potential benefits of PCI in the elderly patient in the elective and emergent arenas must be weighed closely against the risks incurred by this group of individuals in the form of increased bleeding and vascular complications (60).

Cardiomyopathy

Decompensated heart failure (HF) is frequently encountered in the management of the critically ill elderly. In the United States, 5,000,000 persons suffer from heart failure, with more than 50,000 new cases diagnosed yearly; over 80% of the individuals with heart failure are older than 65 years of age (61–63). Symptomatic heart failure *by itself* carries a dismal prognosis, with a median survival of 1.7 years for men and 3.2 years for women (64). Critical illness superimposed on decompensated HF is challenging for even the most adept clinical wizard. Common causes for HF in the elderly include coronary artery disease and hypertension, followed by diabetes mellitus, valvular disease (especially aortic stenosis and mitral regurgitation) and cardiomyopathies other than ischemic (65). The incidence of heart failure increases with age; Framingham Study data reveal a doubling in incidence with each decade after 45 to 54 years of age (66). Factors abound in the critical care arena that may precipitate HF decompensation, suddenly destabilizing an already tenuous orchestration of treatment modalities. These include ischemia and infarction, which is more often "silent" and subtly manifested in the elderly (67), dysrhythmias and extremes of heart rate, fever and infection, medication side effects, and rapid fluid shifts such as with bleeding and aggressive fluid resuscitation. Suspicion of cardiovascular decompensation warrants aggressive timely investigation. Marginal coronary reserve should be presumed and investigated with measurement of cardiac enzymes and documentation of electrocardiogram patterns. An echocardiogram is usually available relatively quickly and may be useful in separating those suffering from lusitropic dysfunction from those with inotropic insufficiency. Particular points of interest to be investigated include systolic ejection fraction, lusitropic state (i.e., diastolic "relaxability" between contractions, reflecting preload), valvular integrity, and wall motion abnormalities. The wary intensivist should maintain a low threshold in the use of invasive monitoring to clarify an uncertain hemodynamic state and guide infusion of vasoactive medications. In the elderly patient with heart failure, an eroded reserve may not allow more than a trivial aberration beyond the margins of physiologic compensation.

Dysrhythmias

Dysrhythmias are frequent in the elderly patient (68,69), including those who manifest no other overt cardiovascular abnormalities—for example, the so-called *lone atrial fibrillation*. With advancing age, sinus node and conduction system integrity deteriorate, with gradual replacement of cardiac pacemaker cells by collagen and elastic tissue (70–74). Such triggering events as autonomic tone disruption (75,76), ischemia or infarction (which portends worse outcome) (77,78), anatomic alterations such as fluid overload or cardiac surgery (79,80), and a host of other cardiac conditions (81) may initiate potentially injurious tachyarrhythmic events, the most common of which is atrial fibrillation.

The occurrence of atrial fibrillation (AF) increases with age (82), carrying an increased risk of stroke and death (83) in those older than 60 years, even in the absence of other cardiac abnormalities. Several issues remain unsettled in the optimal management of AF (84). Of these, the two that receive the most attention are rate control versus rhythm control, and management of anticoagulation. The AFFIRM investigators (85) found no clear survival advantage to either rate or rhythm control in AF, but the rate control strategy did appear to manifest some advantages in the area of medication side effects. All choices for chemical control of rate and rhythm in the elderly population must be made within the skewed context of the high percentage of these patients who harbor comorbid conditions, especially heart failure. Choices for immediate rate control include beta-blockers and calcium channel blockers, remaining mindful of their impact on the state of heart failure compensation. Amiodarone or digoxin may be used in those with heart failure in the absence of an accessory pathway. Digoxin is not recommended in such patients, as it may precipitate *profound* tachycardia via the accessory pathway, with heart rate nearing 300 beats per minute (bpm), leading to rapid cardiovascular collapse. In the case of acute hemodynamic instability, recovery of sinus rhythm with biphasic DC cardioversion after sedation is appropriate. Digoxin or amiodarone can provide rate control, but the former is *not* recommended for chemical cardioversion, and several medications primarily used by cardiologists surpass the latter in class of recommendation for this purpose (86).

There is no "one size fits all" solution to the question of anticoagulation, although it has been well demonstrated (87) to reduce the incidence of stroke related to AF. Equally well demonstrated (88,89) is the extent to which anticoagulation is *under*used in the elderly, presumably because of concern for bleeding risk in this accident- and fall-prone population, and inadequate awareness of the extent to which AF warrants anticoagulation to minimize the risk of AF-associated stroke. Although use of direct thrombin inhibitors in AF is under investigation, at present for the long-term patient, anticoagulation is best accomplished by using vitamin K antagonists for those at highest risk of severe stroke (>75 years), and aspirin for those elderly (<65) with less stroke risk; in the 65 to 75 age range, either will suffice. Target international normalized ratio (INR) of 2.0 to 3.0 is recommended for those receiving vitamin K antagonists (90). Clearly, maintenance of long-term anticoagulant regimens have limited applicability to the patient who suffers a critical injury or illness, and rapid normalization of INR may be warranted. Quickly reversible heparin may be a better choice in such a situation, if continued anticoagulation is warranted at all. AF that persists beyond 48 hours mandates anticoagulation for 2 weeks (86,90) or transesophageal echocardiogram evaluation by a cardiologist—with particular attention to the left atrium and its appendage—for the presence of clot prior to conversion to sinus rhythm. The most complete and recent American College of Cardiology/American Heart Association/European Society of Cardiology (ACC/AHA/ESC) guidelines for management of all issues relating to atrial fibrillation appear in the references to this chapter (86).

Complex ventricular dysrhythmias and ventricular tachycardia (VT) present a difficult management problem in the elderly. Sudden cardiac death is, to a large extent, a product of untreated VT degenerating into ventricular fibrillation (VF), followed by asystole (91,92). In the elderly population as a whole, ambulatory monitoring reveals a very high instance of ventricular arrhythmias, including VT (93,94). Therefore, there is a high likelihood that any given elderly ICU patient will have worrisome ventricular ectopy, with a significant number displaying VT (95–97). Despite the high prevalence of ventricular ectopy in this population, only those patients with underlying heart disease have a poorer long-term prognosis by virtue of the ectopy (98). Underlying heart failure and left ventricular hypertrophy (99) associated with increased ectopy are prognostic of an increased likelihood of subsequent adverse cardiac events, including myocardial infarction and sudden death (100). Pulseless cardiac arrest due to VF or VT warrants management following current advanced cardiac life support (ACLS) guidelines, using cardiopulmonary resuscitation with chest compressions and immediate defibrillation (101). The timely recognition of these lethal arrhythmias and initiation of most recent ACLS protocols is *crucial* for patient welfare, since survival is a direct function of the immediacy of electrical resynchronization therapy (102). Defibrillation for VF provides the optimal chance of survival if provided within 3 minutes (103). The frequency of ventricular ectopy is increased in the geriatric ICU population where several factors, including ischemia, sepsis, extremes of heart rate, hypoxia, electrolyte imbalance, and autonomic disruption associated with recent surgery, can aggravate cardiac irritability and induce lethal arrhythmias in a marginally compensated individual. These inciting factors should be readily recognized and reversed in the constantly vigilant ICU environment. Empiric treatment of ventricular ectopy *per se*, however, has been demonstrated to be more proarrhythmic than beneficial (104,105), often increasing mortality and/or inducing drug-related side effects. Nonetheless, certain medications warrant closer attention. Beta-blockers after myocardial infarction have been demonstrated to reduce subsequent total mortality and sudden cardiac death (SCD) (106). After initial enthusiasm, amiodarone has not, in a recent study of cardiomyopathy patients, proven to be beneficial in reducing SCD when given prophylactically to patients with ejection fraction ≤35% and New York Heart Association (NYHA) class II or III heart failure, as compared to that achieved with a single-lead automatic implantable cardiac defibrillator (AICD) (107). With the emergence of AICD technology, there has been a gradual reduction in mortality from SCD in elderly patients, in whom there is a higher incidence than in the general population of coronary artery disease. In this situation, the AICD appears superior to medications in preventing SCD (108). Elderly individuals accrue an equal or greater benefit from AICD placement compared to younger individuals, with minimal risk involved in the actual placement of the device (109). The indications for AICD placement continue to evolve (110–112). Clearly, the expertise of a cardiac electrophysiologist is indicated when medications or AICD placement are considered in the management of a patient at risk for or who has survived SCD.

With advancing age comes a parallel increase in conduction system disease, often mandating permanent pacemaker (PPM) placement. In 1990, the implantation rate for cardiac pacemakers was 329 devices per million patients; by 2002, the rate had risen to 612 per million (113). The mean age of implanted patients was 75.1 years (113). Such statistics make it likely that an elderly person with a PPM will at some time arrive in the intensive care unit for a noncardiac ailment. Furthermore, advances in engineering and microcircuitry have allowed the development of single devices that incorporate PPM and AICD capability. Although management of issues directly referable to these increasingly complex machines is more within the purview of the cardiologist, certain data can be gathered quickly that will expedite investigation of such a device's performance, as is well detailed in the recent literature (114–116). Considerable guidance can be formulated based on information found on the manufacturer's card carried by the patient, and on a chest radiograph, showing lead position and integrity, and an electrocardiogram with rhythm strip. Details of electrical patterns should be apparent from the rhythm strip and interrogation findings. Any ICD discharge should be investigated with interrogation.

In the instance of withdrawal or termination of unwanted medical care from a terminally ill patient, the intervention of a normally functioning ICD or PPM is directly contrary to the natural process of dying, analogous to instituting cardiopulmonary resuscitation (CPR) when "Do Not Resuscitate" orders exist. In such an instance, deactivation is indicated (117).

PULMONARY DISEASE

Human pulmonary function deteriorates with age, occurring on the microscopic level with resulting functional changes and on the macroscopic level from alterations of chest wall anatomy. Quantification of this age-induced deterioration is quite difficult. Measurement solely of the effects of aging on the respiratory system would require exclusion of all factors that influence respiratory function other than those relating directly to breathing and gas exchange, namely (A) chest wall mechanics, (B) lung histologic structure, and (C) neural/muscular respiratory control. The list of such influencing factors includes environmental pollution and tobacco smoke exposure, occult disease, and effects of previous nutritional deficiencies. Furthermore, these factors complicate contemporaneous comparison between different generations because of the variability of their impacts on these generations. The alternative is the longitudinal study of a rigorously screened cohort of subjects, which has been performed in a few cases (118,119). Analytic difficulties notwithstanding, it is possible, in some instances, to identify the predictable alterations in respiratory physiology that occur with age, so as to prepare the intensivist to contend with a common form of critical illness pathophysiology in the elderly—that of profound respiratory insufficiency.

Microscopic examination of tissue samples from young and older individuals reveals the basis of age-related changes in pulmonary physiology. One sees alveoli from older patients to be less fully surrounded by the elastin/collagen network (120,121), each less robustly tethered open from without, yielding an increasingly compliant lung with compromised recoil (122). Loss of cartilaginous supporting tissue in the small airways further contributes to loss of lung elasticity. The concepts of first, airway collapse, worsened in the patient with advanced emphysema, and second, the progressive stiffening of the chest wall with age allow one to forecast and better understand the evolution of geriatric respiratory function: alterations in lung volume due to gas trapping at higher residual volumes and deterioration of gas exchange. In addition, neural factors alter responsiveness to changes in $PaCO_2$ and PaO_2 (123,124). The magnitude of these changes varies from person to person.

Geriatric flow–volume curves reveal "scooping" of the expiratory limb, implying early closure of airways, and increased residual volume as seen in obstruction from airway collapse in emphysema, a similar phenomenon (125,126). Furthermore, chest wall compliance decreases from calcification of the cartilaginous rib and thoracic spine joints, with kyphotic changes stiffening the thoracic spine itself (127). Compromised compliance results in a substantial increase in the work of breathing, to be provided by deconditioned, aging muscles, likely in the face of low cardiac output and poor nutrition. Such factors yield the respiratory pattern displayed by a significant percentage of the elderly: rapid, shallow breathing at rest, with little exertional reserve. A diagram of lung volumes versus age reveals a slight increase in functional residual capacity (FRC) and residual volume, with a steep rise in *closing capacity*, the volume at which airway collapse takes place in the dependent airways. Thus, airway closure occurs in the upright person *without pulmonary disease* at a lung volume that exceeds FRC (128). In other words, airway collapse can take place in the upright healthy elderly lung even during quiet resting tidal volume during spontaneous breathing, with ventilation/perfusion (V/Q) mismatch increasing shunt fraction and alveolar-arterial partial pressure of oxygen (PO_2) gradient, with relative hypoxemia for a given inspired fraction of oxygen (FiO_2). Subjecting the supine elderly patient with compromised FRC to controlled positive pressure ventilation demands that meticulous attention must be paid to ventilator management to correct V/Q mismatch. The complex details of mechanical ventilation are addressed elsewhere. (Chapter 130). In general, one must use PEEP (positive end-expiratory pressure) while administering the lowest FiO_2 possible, avoiding overdistention of the better aerated (more superior, nondependent) alveoli, and providing sufficient expiratory time to avoid auto-PEEP and breath stacking, as well as sufficient tidal volume into the restricted thoracic cage without exceeding peak pressure limits.

It is commonly held that healthy elderly individuals have a significantly lower PaO_2 for a given FiO_2, compared to equally healthy younger counterparts. Traditional teaching has proposed the following formulae (129,130):

$$PaO_2\,(\text{mm Hg}) = 104.2 - (0.27 \times \text{age})$$
$$PaO_2 = 100.1 - 0.325 \times \text{age (years)}$$
$$PaO_2 = 109 - 0.43\,(\text{age})$$

More recent studies have yielded varying results (131,132), certainly not confirmatory of a pronounced "predestined" decline in oxygenation with age, and questioning the hypothesis that progressive disruption of the matching of ventilation and perfusion in the elderly is actually the cause of whatever decline actually occurs (133). The related questions of rise in (A–a) gradient with age, and "normal" age-related decline in PaO_2 are, similarly, quantified by different investigators (129,130, 134,135).

NUTRITIONAL ISSUES

Malnutrition, also known as undernutrition, is a common companion of elderly individuals and frequently a complicating factor in the efficient and successful management of an elderly ICU patient. The natural decline in energy expenditure with age begins at about age 30 and accompanies the age-related increase in body fat–to–protein ratio (136–138). The evolution of nutritional intake with age is one of decline that exceeds the decrease in energy expenditure (139,140) for various reasons. Thus, even the healthy individual will eat less and lose weight with time, and will be at risk for malnutrition if illness occurs or social support wanes. For example, in elderly nursing home patients, a population in whom initially minor medical problems can quickly blossom into life-threatening conditions, the incidence of undernutrition can approach 85% (141,142). Malnutrition at the onset of critical illness portends poor outcome, as does insufficient nutritional support during the course of the illness (143,144). Mortality is considerably higher in the malnourished elderly patient, compared to those who are nutritionally replete (143). Undernutrition has several common causes: (i) functional decline and social isolation from family and other support systems, (ii) anorexia associated with older age—the so-called *anorexia of aging*—or chronic illness, (iii) anatomic or gustatory impediments to mastication or swallowing, (iv) abuse or neglect, and (v) insufficient financial resources (145–148). Therefore, the prevalence of undernutrition in hospitalized, geriatric patients is relatively high (149,150) and is often unrecognized unless sought specifically (151). Identification of malnutrition in the elderly patient (151) may be facilitated by the routine employment of easily used physical examination and laboratory screening tools as part of an organized, proactive nutrition screening program (152). There is little literature addressing nutrition in the geriatric intensive care unit patient *per se*, and the principles set forth below are generally applicable to any ill elderly patient.

Undernutrition imposes a considerable burden on the marginally compensated geriatric patient. The conditions known as protein-energy malnutrition (PEM) and micronutrient deficiency complicate the treatment of several conditions seen in the ICU. These include the contribution of gastrointestinal tract nonintegrity to multiorgan system failure (153,154) and other common cardiovascular (155,156), pulmonary (157–159), and infectious issues (160). Wound healing is impeded by a poor nutritional state (161–163); in particular, development of decubitus ulcers is more common in malnourished elderly individuals, and successful management is decidedly more difficult (164). Patients with PEM are at increased risk for serious complications while in the hospital (165), with slower recovery (166), poorer functional status at discharge, and higher rates of mortality after discharge (167,168).

Malnutrition is a disorder of body composition in which macronutrient and/or micronutrient deficiencies occur when nutrient intake is insufficient, resulting in reduced organ function, abnormal blood chemistry studies, and suboptimal clinical outcomes (169). Nutritional deficiency is found in 35% to 65% of elderly hospitalized patients (170). Of the available screening techniques reflective of nutritional status, one of the most revealing is the dietary and weight loss history, as found in such structured nutritional questionnaires as the Mini Nutritional Assessment (MNA) tool and others (171,172). While probably more applicable to the long-term outpatient setting, certain pieces of information gathered from the patient or family via the MNA are helpful in providing a "snapshot" of the patient's nutritional status. Obtaining the patient's weight *immediately on admission* is an obvious step in assessing nutritional condition. Because of the various types of body habitus found in ICU patients, a calculation of the Quetelet body-mass index (BMI) is helpful to standardize weight to height, providing a relatively standardized estimate of body fat (173):

$$\text{BMI} = \text{weight (in kg) divided by height (in m}^2\text{)}.$$

The Department of Health and Human Services defines normal BMI as being within the range of 18 to 24.9, with those with BMIs less than 18 being underweight, the overweight range being 25 to 29.5, and those displaying a BMI above 30 being obese (174). These data, however, cover—in the United States—the adult population as a whole. The picture in a unique subset such as the elderly is more complex. In the geriatric population, BMI less than 20 is predictive of nearly 50% 1-year mortality (175), a stronger predictor of mortality than is diagnosis. Similar results were found among critically ill adults with a BMI less than or equal to the 15th percentile (176). Such data lead researchers to suggest that the optimal BMI lies higher in the elderly than in the general population (177); this supposition has been supported by a large study demonstrating that the detrimental effect on mortality of excess body weight declines with age (178). Furthermore, the BMI calculation does not differentiate between differences in body morphology; obese, malnourished individuals whose BMIs fall within the normal range may go unidentified using this formula (179). Since an age-associated loss of height can be significant in the geriatric population, especially in kyphotic individuals, substitution of arm span as the denominator of the BMI calculation has been suggested to give a more accurate comparison of an individual patient's BMI to the standards that were originally established in younger persons (180,181). Arm span is identical to height in younger years; although height may decline with age, arm span remains unchanged, providing more accuracy within the previously determined younger age frame of BMI reference. Knee height, as measured from plantar surface to top of patella with the ankle at 90 degrees, is another measurement (182) that can be substituted in corrected BMI calculations in those with diminished stature who are unsuitable for arm span measurement. Triceps skin fold thickness and midarm circumference can also provide an idea of body fat content (183).

In general, however, use of the BMI in the elderly is suspect, regardless of the height measurement used, as there are few normal BMI data that specifically describe those older than 65 years. The ages of geriatric patients included in nutrition studies vary, anthropometric characteristics vary in different advanced decades, and incidence of weight-changing diseases and conditions—such as cancer or the anorexia of aging—increases with age (184). These factors make the formulation of accurate statements and recommendations addressing ideal weight and BMI in the elderly difficult to formulate (137). Although the percentage of older Americans falling into the definition of obese continues to climb (185), one should not make the assumption of nutritional integrity. Age-related redistribution of caloric stores may disguise the overweight elderly patient with severe PEM (179) as one who is obese in the mind of the unwary clinician who is not familiar with the metabolism of geriatric patients, and the pathophysiologic implications of these changes (186). Misguided hypocaloric feeding, directed at mobilizing excess fat stores in the obese, but malnourished, elderly patient may worsen the situation by leaving the ongoing catabolic protein breakdown associated with critical illness uncorrected (187).

Several easily measured laboratory parameters are reflective of nutritional status on admission, and some can be followed periodically to assess the success of nutritional support. Albumin is a product of hepatic metabolism, synthesized ultimately from ingested or infused nitrogenous precursors in the presence of adequate caloric support. Although it is held that the serum albumin level is reflective of the nutritional state, various factors influencing serum albumin levels make it only vaguely reflective of overall nutritional status (188), with a ROC (receiver operating characteristic) curve rating of 0.58 compared to the clinical subjective global assessment tool. Serum albumin level does decline somewhat with age—0.8 g/L per decade for individuals older than 60 years of age—but generally remains within the numerical normal range. Significantly reduced albumin concentration, therefore, should be attributed to disease processes (189,190) and be aggressively investigated. A substantial decline in serum albumin concentration is accurately predictive of mortality and worse outcome among the elderly, both in the setting of apparent health and illness (191–195), possibly reflective of the presence of chronic disease- or inflammation-induced mediators that simultaneously suppress albumin gene expression (196). The half-life of albumin, 18 to 19 days (197–199), makes its use less than optimal in monitoring metabolic and synthetic functions, in which rapid change is significant. Alternatives include prealbumin and retinol binding protein. The former has a half-time of 2 days and is not affected by age but is elevated with steroid use. The latter has a half-time of 12 hours, decreases slightly with age, and is elevated in the setting of acute liver injury. The serum level of renally excreted retinol binding protein is artificially elevated in renal failure, which may suggest nutritional integrity (199).

As critical illness induces substantial catabolism (199–201), resting energy expenditure (REE) rises during the first 2 weeks of this state, with mobilization of nitrogen stores as a component of the associated inflammatory response to physiologic insult. Total energy expenditure (TEE) may rise to as high as 40 to 50 kcal/kg/day in critically ill, septic, or trauma patients, repletion of which is most difficult without correcting the underlying inciting process (202,203). In the elderly individual with marginal nutritional reserve at the onset of critical illness, early provision of caloric and protein support is warranted. The farther behind the patient starts, the more difficult is the recovery of positive nitrogen balance. Catabolic processes characteristic of critical illness are not reversible by nutrient supplementation alone; they are incited by inflammatory mediators rather than by pre-existing deficiency or inadequate repletion and are thus not forestalled by aggressive nutritional support. Traditional guidance recommends 25 kcal/kg/day of nutritional support, with an additional protein supply of 1.2 to 1.5 grams/kg/day (169), based on *usual* body weight. Obese individuals, defined as above (204,205), warrant feeding based on *ideal*, rather than usual, body weight:

$$\textbf{Men:}\ \text{IBW (kg)} = 50 + 2.3\ \text{kg per inch over 5 ft}$$
$$\textbf{Women:}\ \text{IBW (kg)} = 45.5 + 2.3\ \text{kg per inch over 5 ft}$$

Where IBW is ideal body weight.

Greater accuracy can be achieved using the Harris-Benedict equations to determine the estimated resting energy expenditure (REE) as a guide to calculation of nutritional needs (206):

$$\begin{aligned}\textbf{Men:}\ \text{REE} &= 66.5 + (13.75 \times \text{weight in kg}) \\ &\quad + (5.003 \times \text{height in cm}) \\ &\quad - (6.775 \times \text{age in years}) \\ \textbf{Women:}\ \text{REE} &= 655.1 + (9.563 \times \text{weight in kg}) \\ &\quad + (1.850 \times \text{height in cm}) \\ &\quad - (4.676 \times \text{age in years})\end{aligned}$$

This may be insufficient in the critically ill geriatric patient in the throes of the inflammatory response, unless the higher stress and activity factor is used (207). Resting metabolic rate may be nearly double in the critically ill or injured individual (202) compared to the healthy noninjured person. Protein supplementation at a rate of 2 g/kg is recommended for the most critically ill, catabolic patients although, in the initial stages of such a condition, the rate of catabolism may just not be ameliorable despite aggressive support in appropriate quantities (208). Initial empiric dosages should subsequently be adjusted based on indirect calorimetry and nitrogen balance studies if there is suspicion of inadequate nutritional support as revealed by following the previously noted markers of protein synthesis as surrogates of metabolic recovery (209). Enthusiastic overprovision of macronutrients in a misguided and vain attempt to thwart and correct inflammatory catabolism, on the other hand, leads to a host of complications and considerable morbidity (210) for which the geriatric patient may be unable to compensate. Furthermore, the confounding factor of obesity sometimes seen in the nutritionally deficient geriatric patient makes the recipe that provides optimal nutritional support frustratingly difficult to determine. In such situations, measurements of energy expenditure performed at frequent intervals are even more strongly advisable, since energy requirements fluctuate with time and medical condition, and vary significantly from those of younger patients, on whose metabolism nutritional recommendations are often based. In general, most, although not all, studies show that enteral nutrition is preferred because of the purported preservative effects on intestinal mucosal integrity, cost issues, and a lesser degree of risk exposure to the patient, both infectious and mechanical, associated with placement of flexible nasointestinal feeding tube versus central line for parenteral nutrition (169,211–215). This statement, however, is the source of endless controversy and the basis of considerable investigation and an inordinate number of publications (216–218). The risks and benefits of the common routes of nutritional support were recently reviewed in exquisite detail (219).

RENAL CONSIDERATIONS

Deterioration of renal function in a critically ill patient has a dramatic impact on survival. Acute renal failure (ARF) carries a mortality of nearly 30% in a general ICU population; a decline of renal function of even lesser severity also impacts mortality significantly (220) and more so in the geriatric population. An elderly patient with compromised renal function will often succumb to the added insult of renal failure after a complex surgical intervention or traumatic injury. The chance for at least partial renal functional recovery after critical illness-related ARF is greater than 90% among those alive a year after their illness (221). Presently, there is little treatment for renal insufficiency or failure other than optimization of hemodynamics, prevention of further damage, and aggressive treatment of the complications. The intensivist holds a pivotal position in the understanding of renal physiology and principles of renal protection to minimize the impact of critical illness on renal function and its influence on outcome.

As in all physiologic systems in the elderly, there is a gradual deterioration of renal function, beginning at age 30 years (222,223). When the sixth decade is reached, this deterioration *generally* continues, although with a very wide bell curve of distribution (224). It is well described (225) that renal blood flow declines after the fourth decade (226). There is loss of renal—primarily cortical—mass (227) and the onset of glomerular sclerosis and involution, causing a decrease in the number of functional glomeruli (228), in turn causing a decrease in glomerular filtration rate (GFR) of 30% to 40% by age 80 (222,229). Deterioration of tubular function parallels that of the glomerulus (230). In the elderly patient, factors other than age-related deterioration may complicate renal function, including pre-existing renovascular disease, hypertensive nephrosclerosis, or hypotension associated with trauma or neglect. Clearly, accurate assessment of GFR is fundamental to the prudent management of the elderly patient's medication dosages and fluid and electrolyte status. Laboratory measurement of serum blood urea nitrogen (BUN) and creatinine (S_{cr}), used individually or in a ratio, act as surrogates of renal function. They are, however, less accurately reflective of renal function in the elderly than in a younger person. BUN rises slightly with age over 60 years, paralleling the gradual decline in renal function. S_{cr} reflects muscle mass and, while completely filtered (and only minimally secreted) into the tubule and therefore generally reflective of GFR, may not climb as expected despite age-related falling renal filtration (231). Age-related diminished muscle mass, often paralleling the deterioration of renal function, generates less creatine (and thus, creatinine), leading to what may erroneously be looked upon as a normal (i.e., lower than expected S_{cr} for given GFR that is diminished from the effects of age and its associated diseases) baseline S_{cr}.

The wary clinician will individualize each assessment of GFR by using the Cockcroft-Gault formula (232) to generate a more accurate estimate of function based on weight, age, and serum creatinine:

$$\text{Creatinine clearance} = [(140 - \text{age})(\text{weight in kg})]/(72 \times S_{cr})$$
$$(\text{arithmetic result} \times 0.85 = \text{clearance for female patients})$$

This formula provides a "snapshot" of function at a given time and is most useful if calculated on ICU arrival and daily thereafter. Recall that S_{cr} may be affected (i.e., increased) by excessive muscle breakdown due to rhabdomyolysis, critical illness, or medications. Other laboratory surrogates of GFR have been devised, such as the measurement of cystatin C (233–235) and MDRD (modification of diet in renal disease) equations (236), but the ease with which the Cockcroft-Gault calculation is performed makes its routine replacement unlikely. If CFR remains uncertain, urine collection for measurement of creatinine clearance can be done with fair accuracy using at least an 8-hour urine collection period (237,238). However, 24-hour collection is preferred in critically ill patients and is easily done in patients with indwelling urinary catheters.

There are alterations of fluid and electrolyte handling by the aging kidney of which the intensivist must be aware, related to tubular dysfunction proportional to the decline in GFR. Although baseline electrolyte values and fluid status are likely within normal ranges in the previously healthy geriatric patient, age-related tubular dysfunction narrows the limits of correction of water and sodium aberrations that the patient can readily accomplish. Sodium excretion and reabsorption declines in efficiency, with those older than 60 years requiring considerably more time to achieve homeostasis in the face of sodium overload or deprivation (239). Similarly, the range of specific gravity and osmolarity achievable in the face of water excess or deficit is narrowed in comparison to that of a younger individual (240). Rectification of acid-base perturbations is similarly deficient (241). The stresses of critical illness or injury typical of the elderly ICU patient intensify the effects of these functional deficiencies, and must be foreseen and addressed aggressively to forestall the profound effects of deterioration of renal function on morbidity and mortality. These stresses include volume depletion from gastrointestinal (GI) bleeding, severe dehydration, diarrhea, aggressive diuresis, insensible losses in burn patients or those with drainage from wounds or fistulas, and disruption of renal blood flow from sepsis, shock, or surgical causes such as complex renovascular surgery.

Management of deteriorating renal function requires accurate diagnosis of the inciting cause, while addressing complicating or resultant metabolic derangements and preventing further insult. The details of the diagnosis of renal pathology are not specific to the geriatric patient and are addressed elsewhere in this text (Chapter 163). It is important to recognize that acute kidney injury occurs in as many as 67% of ICU admissions (220), as identified by RIFLE (risk, injury, failure, loss, end-stage) criteria (242), and that the effect of renal deterioration is quite detrimental to the elderly individual. Initial evaluation must include such fundamental steps as performance of a physical examination that may reveal an occluded urinary catheter causing an enlarged bladder. Hypovolemia, both absolute, as in severe dehydration, and relative, as in sepsis, must be aggressively corrected with appropriate fluid and blood products; invasive monitoring is warranted in this population of patients with compromised reserve. Dosage adjustment of potentially nephrotoxic medications is mandatory, using assessment of GFR as a guide. Antimicrobials such as cephalosporins and aminoglycosides, nonsteroidal anti-inflammatory medications, certain chemotherapeutic medications, and angiotensin-converting enzyme inhibitors are common offenders (243). Loop diuretics, mannitol, and natriuretic peptides have largely been demonstrated to be of no use in preventing incipient acute renal failure that may seem to be starting (244). The role of N-acetylcysteine and bicarbonate to minimize the deleterious effect of radiocontrast medium on renal function in critically ill individuals remains controversial, but it should generally be used in any elderly patient receiving contrast (245–247). Beyond awareness of medications that impact renal function, there is the effect of age-related diminished renal function on drug metabolism and excretion (248). Recall that common indicators of renal function, BUN and S_{cr}, although appearing normal in the elderly, may mask a compromised GFR, risking medication-induced complications if this fact is overlooked. Early nephrology consultation is encouraged when RIFLE criteria suggest compromised renal function; similarly, a critical care pharmacologist can assist in clarifying renal-active medication issues in these complex patients.

ASSESSMENT AND MANAGEMENT OF TRAUMATIC INJURIES

Elderly individuals suffer a significant number of severe and often lethal traumatic injuries, the analysis and management of which can be frustratingly complex (249). In the 55 to 64 age group, unintentional injury was the sixth leading cause of death in 2003; in those older than 65 years, nearly 35,000 deaths were attributed to trauma (250). Most serious injuries are caused by falls, the occurrence rising dramatically as age advances into the 60s and beyond (251). Falls from a standing or even sitting position, imparting an apparently trivial amount of kinetic energy to frail tissue, may result in fatal injury, disproportionately accounting for half the trauma-related deaths when compared to those of younger people (252). Most remaining significant traumatic injuries to the elderly involve motor vehicles, either as vehicle occupants or as pedestrians (253), while there is a small but persistent incidence of injury and death from penetrating trauma in the geriatric population, declining to less than 1% in those older than 75 years (254,255). Evaluation and management of the injured elderly require familiarity with characteristic injury patterns and knowledge of comorbid diseases and particulars of geriatric physiology that impact treatment (256). Practice management guidelines for geriatric trauma (257) are helpful in this situation.

Immediate assessment of the resuscitation status of any patient arriving in the ICU, whether from the operating room, the emergency department, or elsewhere in the hospital, is imperative. The paucity of overt physical findings of intravascular fluid deficiency that may be seen in the elderly patient adds additional urgency to its accurate analysis. The lusitropic compromise that typifies the geriatric patient demands avoidance of overgenerous fluid repletion. Although standard protocols may serve as a guide to ensure that all systems are evaluated, one must remain mindful that standard and acceptable initial hemodynamic measurements may actually conceal unsuspected injury or bleeding in the confused elderly trauma patient who may be taking medications that affect vital signs. Airway management in the elderly carries its own set of difficulties. Age-associated arthritic spinal, mandibular, and arytenoid deformities; an increased incidence of occult cervical spinal injuries (258–260); marginal respiratory drive; and compromised airway reflexes may warrant securing the airway preemptively, avoiding a later "crash" difficult airway emergency. A thorough and detailed physical examination is fundamental. Timely sequential measurement of routine hematology tests, even in the stable geriatric patient, may reveal unsuspected hemorrhage. Arterial blood gas analysis is a convenient tool since it is quickly performed and allows frequent measurement of hemoglobin, base deficit, and lactate. The latter two values are powerful indicators of resuscitation status and, when elevated, predict increased mortality in the elderly population (261,262). In one study of elderly trauma patients, mortality was decreased from 54% to 34% ($p < 0.003$) by institution of a protocol of trauma team activation and early noninvasive and subsequently invasive monitoring for resuscitation of all patients older than age 70 years with an injury severity score (ISS) greater than 15, even for those with nonworrisome initial vital signs and fairly minor injuries (263). This supports the precept that achieving adequate tissue perfusion *early*, while often difficult to accomplish, is fundamental to successful trauma management. One must be mindful, furthermore, that while invasive monitoring carries its own risks, judicious use of these tools can improve outcome and survival in the elderly trauma patient (263–265).

Certain patterns of injury are found in geriatric patients. Traumatic brain injury (TBI) afflicts the elderly with extraordinary severity. High mortality leaves fewer survivors, most of whom suffer debilitating sequelae (266). In 2003, there were 90,000 emergency department visits involving TBI in those older than 65 years, of whom 38.4% died (267). Some series document mortality rates for severe TBI in those older than 55 years of age as high as 80% (268). Initial neurologic examination of an elder with significant intracranial injury may be deceptively normal (269). Suspicion of an occult central nervous system (CNS) injury must be maintained if such individuals arrive in the ICU without radiologic evaluation having been performed, warranting frequent, sequential neurologic evaluations by the same examiner and a conservative approach to ordering a cranial CT scan. Those elderly whose cause of TBI is a fall—nearly 50%, from 1988 to 1998—are likely to have three or more significant comorbid conditions complicating ICU management (270,271). Outcome after TBI is optimized by using meticulous clinical assessment, timely radiologic reevaluation, and aggressive invasive monitoring to facilitate immediate recognition of worsening status, such as that due to recurrent intracranial hemorrhage, while minimizing secondary injury.

Secondary injury may occur when even transient episodes of hypoxia or hypotension affect cerebral perfusion pressure (CPP) (272) and, in the setting of elevated intracranial pressure (273), hyperglycemia (274), hyperthermia (275), or aggressive hyperventilation (276,277). Infusion of hypertonic saline (278) may supplement the management of elevated intracranial pressure that resists control by the usual initial measures. The cornerstone of TBI treatment is the maintenance of cerebral oxygenation by ensuring adequate oxygen content and CPP, guided by data derived via invasive intracranial monitoring devices that are inserted based on specific indications (279). Little, however, has been written specifically addressing geriatric CPP requirements. Although a CPP of 70 mm Hg is considered the standard (279), this has not been rigorously tested specifically in the elderly as it affects outcome. Cerebral autoregulation in the elderly is subject to the same influences as those that affect the younger individual. In this population, the abundance of comorbidities, such as untreated hypertension, may have acclimated the cerebral vasculature to a new baseline, making invasive cerebral monitoring even more critical in ensuring adequate perfusion for the aging brain. The profound influence of even mild TBI (280–282) on short- and long-term outcome in the elderly patient mandates aggressive monitoring and optimization of cerebral perfusion parameters.

Cervical spine injury is not uncommon in the geriatric trauma patient (283); plain radiographs (258,284) may be unrevealing of fracture or difficult to interpret because of age-related boney changes obscuring acute pathology (259). Fracture of the upper cervical spine is more common in the elderly than in younger individuals, especially in those who have fallen (260) and are more likely to be unstable (285). Helical CT is superior to plain radiographs to identify cervical spine injury in this population (284,285–287). Cervical spine pathology may exist in totally asymptomatic individuals with unremarkable examination findings, only to be discovered by a diligent clinician who takes extra steps to search for such an injury (288,289). In the cervically injured geriatric patient, the likelihood of coincident painful injury—a distracting injury in which the pain from another injury distracts the patient's attention from the perception of neck pain or a condition, such as altered mental status—that would affect the examiner's decision to forgo radiographic evaluation is so high as to make such an evaluation imperative in nearly all cases. One must be mindful of the greater likelihood that cervical injuries in the elderly often occur in the arthritis-prone superior vertebrae, which are notoriously difficult to depict on plain films (290), and consider CT evaluation of virtually all geriatric trauma patients in whom even subtle symptoms, history, or mechanism of injury suggest cervical injury, regardless of the initial examination findings or any comforting results of a protocol-based decision-assisting algorithm that suggest the safety of less aggressive investigation.

Traumatic rib fractures impose substantial morbidity. Those older than 45 years of age with more than four fractures are particularly affected (291). In a study of patients traditionally defined as *elderly*—those older than 64 years—rib fractures profoundly affected morbidity and mortality, with longer length of stay in the ICU, more frequent pneumonia, and overall mortality rate of 22% versus 10% ($p < 0.001$) in those less seriously affected (292). Of note in this study was that rates of mortality and pneumonia both increased with each additional rib fracture. Epidural analgesia would appear to be the ideal technique to alleviate the pain associated with rib fractures to optimize pulmonary status and, indeed, has been found to be successful in nongeriatric adults (293,294). In one recent study, however, the opposite has been demonstrated in an elderly population when compared to parenteral analgesia (295).

The management of abdominal trauma follows pathways similar to those for younger patients, with certain caveats. As in other body systems in the elderly, findings on physical examination indicating serious abdominal pathology can be subtle, especially when complicated by distracting orthopedic or mild head injury. Liberal use of CT scanning is strongly recommended if mechanism of injury, external abdominal findings such as a seat belt mark, or laboratory evidence of hypoperfusion (elevated base deficit or serum lactate) suggest visceral injury. Nonoperative management of certain radiologically well-characterized injuries of solid organs—namely the spleen, the liver, and the pancreas—in the hemodynamically stable elderly patient is becoming increasingly accepted as evidence of the success of this approach accumulates (296–298).

Serious orthopedic injuries frequently befall older victims of polytrauma. Decrease in bone mineral density (BMD) with age older than about 30 years heightens the risk of fracture in general; this phenomenon is observed in varying degrees in both genders and all races, but is particularly severe in post-menopausal Caucasian women (299,300). Pelvic fracture in the aged is associated with a greater likelihood of significant blood volume transfusion and mortality ($p < 0.005$) (301). Open pelvic fracture often has substantial associated bleeding, which is seldom treatable, with the exception of arterial bleeding, in any way other than with early stabilization, aggressive transfusion, and correction of coagulopathy in hopes of eventual tamponade of the retroperitoneal bleeding source. Arterial bleeding from lacerated pelvic vessels warrants embolization (302). The more typical scenario, however, is that of diffuse venous oozing, which, nonetheless, may render the elderly patient hemodynamically unstable, requiring large-volume transfusion of blood products as a temporizing measure until anatomic stabilization can be achieved (302,303). The presence of an open pelvic fracture, with frequent associated visceral injuries (304,305), further worsens outcome (301). Hemodynamic consequences of large-volume transfusion and frequent septic complications can drive the mortality in both younger and older adults to nearly 80% (306). Long-bone fractures, in general, warrant early immobilization and stabilization to minimize ongoing hemorrhage and generation of fat emboli; such fixation improves mortality significantly (307). Optimal timing of surgical stabilization of these quite morbid fractures, however, is a complex issue to resolve when they occur in the larger setting of the patient with severe head, chest, or abdominal injuries (308). Although postponing the operative stabilization of a femur or complex pelvic fracture to allow time to achieve hemodynamic stability in a traumatized patient is not without benefits, it is also not without risks (309,310). Prolonged immobilization of the elderly patient with such a fracture prior to stabilization forgoes the profound respiratory benefits of early mobilization, more likely exposing the patient to extended intubation, pulmonary thromboembolus, and infection.

Studies of elderly trauma patients have consistently documented the higher mortality expected in this population (254,264,310,311). The mortality rate begins to climb for those in their sixth decade, even for less severe injuries (312), when compared to younger individuals; for moderate injuries, the mortality curves diverge beginning in the fifth decade, with a steeper turn in the seventh. With advancing age, trauma-related mortality rates for those in the seventh decade and above range as high as 47% for those with an injury severity score (ISS) more than 30, compared to those 45 years old or younger (20.1%) (313). Within the context to which allusion was earlier made—that of future payoff in return for resource use—the complexity and enormity of the issue grows as health care costs rise, and as the percentage of the population represented by the elderly increases. As these rising numbers of individuals cease working, and, thereby, are no longer able to generate an income that can be taxed to finance public health care funding programs such as Medicare, or be used to pay for personal private health insurance to cover costs of traumatic injuries, the costs of providing that trauma—and, indeed, all—care will have to be borne by a source other than the patients themselves. Based on the size of these costs and the likelihood of marginally or poorly acceptable outcomes among a substantial minority of geriatric trauma patients (3,313–316), investigations have been performed that have tried to answer two important trauma outcome-related questions. These are as follows: Is it possible to identify an elderly trauma patient who will certainly die later, even if the patient survives the initial period of resuscitation, surgery, and further stabilization; and to what level of functioning will the elderly survivor of trauma-related intensive care return on discharge? To many elderly individuals, the prospect of lingering in the netherworld of prolonged posttrauma multiorgan system failure with the certainty of death pushed back "only as long as the machines keep me running," or existing debilitated in a nonhome environment where even bowel function and bathing are at the behest of another, is worse than death itself, not really living at all, and is the basis of much concern among the elderly.

There are, however, grounds for hope. In one study of victims of penetrating trauma more than 60 years old, 91% were discharged home, most without assistance (255). The postdischarge level of functioning in elderly patients surviving blunt trauma varies widely, as would be expected in a population whose baseline physiologic attributes are so diverse. Clearly, even the healthiest octogenarian is not the physiologic equal of a two-sets-of-tennis 65-year-old and will have a significantly decreased likelihood of returning to premorbid functionality, although both individuals may be described as elderly. Nonetheless, even after significant traumatic injuries, a substantial percentage of recovering geriatric patients, even the very old, will be able to live relatively independently, albeit for some patients, in a protected environment with assistance. Many will be able to return home with or without periodic professional assistance (314,317–319). In one retrospective study of 38,707 elderly trauma patients with a mean ISS of 11.7 ± 0.05 (standard error of mean), in which 10.3% died in hospital, 52.2% of the survivors went home. The percentage of patients returning home after serious traumatic injuries, many requiring prolonged intensive care, varied considerably with age, from 66.7% of those 65 to 74 years to 30.5% of those 85 years of age or older (320). With aggressive rehabilitation, improvement in function and independence can continue for substantial periods of time after discharge, including in those who have suffered TBI (321). In another study, recovery of elderly trauma patients was improved by early involvement of physicians from a geriatric trauma consult service, who assisted in recognition and treatment of medical issues, and in advanced care and disposition planning (322). The likelihood of leaving the hospital after a trauma-related ICU admission can be improved from the outset, as noted earlier, by aggressive attention to adequate resuscitation to rectify suboptimal perfusion, by attention to maintenance of acceptable CPP in TBI, and by recognition and treatment of the early subtle signs of cardiac and respiratory decompensation. Finally, trauma care outcome must be scrutinized within the context of profound personal and social issues, beyond those solely of medical success, that are integral to ICU care in patients in this age group.

OUTCOME AFTER A CRITICAL ILLNESS IN THE GERIATRIC POPULATION

Most people die after the age of 65 years. Although life expectancy is greater at any given age now than it was even 15 years ago, with an increasing percentage of patients falling within the age range when death within a few years is a real possibility even in the most healthy of individuals, objective evaluation must be made of the appropriateness—and likelihood of successful outcome—of aggressive critical care medical services that are provided to those in this age group. At present, geriatric patients represent between 25% and 50% of all ICU admissions (8,9). In 2000, ICU costs represented 13.3% of hospital costs, 4.2% of health care expenditures, and 0.56% of the U.S. gross domestic product (323). The enormous expense associated with ICU care has prompted some analysts to raise the subject of limits on expenditures for the elderly (324,325), since, for example, an 80-year-old who is supported through a 3-week bout of sepsis is not likely to return to the revenue-generating work force for an additional 30 years as would a similarly afflicted 35-year-old. Indeed, the literature dealing with geriatric medical issues is liberally populated with articles addressing ageism in the context of delivery of services to the elderly (326–328), raising the concept of providing less aggressive or intensive levels of acute care to an elderly person solely on the basis of age. Meaningful discussions addressing the more philosophical issues of critical care such as the correct level of aggressiveness of care and appropriateness of withdrawal of care, to say nothing of the financial issues, simply cannot be addressed in any rational way without an accurate picture of what critical care accomplishes in these elderly patients.

A successful ICU admission is certainly defined within cultural and social, as well as personal, contexts. Although the family member's "do *everything* for Granddad" dictum is familiar, it often represents an unrealistic appraisal of the possible benefit from certain modalities of care that can be done, but possibly should not be done. Although the ICU is designed as a temporary environment that allows support of body functions during recovery, the complicated technology and meticulous attention to detail that characterize that environment is not the basis for such "magical" accomplishments as saving the life of a patient who has a lethal condition, despite the expectations and exhortations of some. Nonetheless, death can often skillfully be forestalled with polished and professional ICU care to such a degree that it may occur immediately after a de-escalation of such care, or later while the patient is on the general ward, in a step-down unit or rehabilitation facility, or after returning home (either early or late) to a life with varying similarity to that prior to the original serious medical occurrence (329). Meaningful discussions with elderly patients and their families, whether prior to complex morbid surgical procedures or as an ICU stay extends past the first few days, *must* include accurate outcome data, so as to facilitate informed decisions regarding the specifics and suitability of continued care. Studies addressing outcome in the critically ill geriatric population have produced various results that vary with the metric employed, the duration over which the outcome is monitored, and broad intrapopulation patient variability. The latter category highlights differences in age, premorbid physical status, statements of preference regarding aggressiveness of long-term medical care, and patient and family declarations addressing such subjective concepts as posthospitalization quality of life.

The term *geriatric population* encompasses a quite heterogeneous group of individuals from the standpoint of age, premorbid general medical health as a reflection of functional status, severity of the event that justifies ICU admission, and cultural mores as they impact interaction with the modern health care structure of the country in question. Studies assessing the results of care delivered to the elderly may or may not reflect this diversity (330), making interpretation of individual study conclusions and their application to individual clinical situations suspect. Furthermore, the term *outcome* must be specifically defined as to the depth of support required by the post-ICU elder and its correspondence with that autonomous person's preferences, which, again, may vary widely based on cultural, religious, national, and other parameters. Although many elders prefer a less aggressive care regimen designed around end-of-life comfort at the expense of duration of remaining life, many desire life extension in the face of critical illness by use of complex technology despite a vanishingly small or nonexistent expectation of recovery (8,331,332). Furthermore, the clinician's perceptions of the patient's desires may not be accurate, and thus may lead to withdrawal of care or withholding of a modality of treatment in a manner that would not be considered in the care of a younger patient (331). It is important to remember that while age may be associated with worse outcome from critical illness, numerous investigations have demonstrated that age, in and of itself, is less a factor than is the severity of the specific condition that warrants intensive care or the general medical condition of the patient prior to the institution of intensive care (333–335). Despite being subjected to procedures that are potentially morbid, the otherwise healthy patient may fare quite as well as a younger individual (335,336). In one study of outcome after intensive care in octogenarians, postdischarge survival was more accurately forecast by care dependency at the time of discharge, as a reflection of premorbid condition and severity of illness, rather than solely by length of stay (337). Quality of life (QOL) in the post-ICU elder is not necessarily inferior to that of younger individuals (338); indeed, overall QOL has been demonstrated to be similarly good across age groups ranging from middle-aged to very old (above 80 years) (339,340). It must be remembered, however, when evaluating outcome data in elderly ICU patients, that while ICU survival is less a function of age than of premorbid condition or severity of illness (30,337,338,341,342), when the aggressive ICU support is de-escalated with recovery, physiologic reserve may no longer suffice to forestall death in the few months after discharge, and thus may not be reflected in ICU outcome statistics. With the wide variability of desires for aggressiveness of care displayed by the elderly and the inaccuracy with which they are analyzed by many physicians (343), the most important function of the geriatric intensivist may be that of conducting a thorough discussion at the outset of care with the patient and involved family members so as to tailor intensiveness of care to the patient's educated and informed preferences.

DRUG DOSING IN THE ELDERLY

As more patients live longer and consume a larger proportion of medications, it is necessary for health care providers to understand the risks, benefits, and consequences of drug

TABLE 103.1

AGE-RELATED CHANGES RELEVANT TO DRUG PHARMACOLOGY

Pharmacologic process	Physiologic change	Clinical significance
Absorption	Decreased absorptive surface Decreased splanchnic blood flow Increased gastric pH Altered gastrointestinal motility	Little change in absorption with age
Distribution	Decreased total body water Decreased lean body mass Increased body fat Decreased serum albumin Altered protein binding	Higher concentration of drugs that distribute in body fluids; increased distribution and often prolonged elimination half-life of fat-soluble drugs Increased free fraction in plasma of some highly protein-bound acidic drugs
Metabolism	Reduced hepatic mass Reduced hepatic blood flow Decreased phase I metabolism	Often decreased first-pass metabolism and decreased rate of biotransformation of some drugs
Elimination	Reduced renal plasma flow Reduced glomerular filtration rate Decreased tubular secretion function	Decreased renal elimination of drugs and metabolites; marked interindividual variation
Tissue sensitivity	Alterations in receptor number Alterations in receptor affinity Alterations in second-messenger function Alteration in cellular and nuclear responses	Patients are more sensitive or less sensitive to an agent

therapy in older patients. Several important pharmacologic and nonpharmacologic issues influence the safety and effectiveness of drug therapy in this population. *Pharmacokinetics*, the study of the action of a drug in the body over a period of time, changes with age. The physiologic changes accompanying aging affect the pharmacologic processes of absorption, distribution, metabolism, and excretion (Table 103.1). The effects of these age-related changes are variable and difficult to predict. Some changes are related solely to aging, whereas others most likely are due to the combined effects of age, disease, and the environment. Although increasing age is often accompanied by decreased physiologic reserve in many organ systems, independent of the effects of disease, this change is not uniform. There is substantial variation from individual to individual, making some older patients more vulnerable than others. The alterations in pharmacokinetics and pharmacodynamics that occur with increasing age suggest a pharmacologic basis for concern about the vulnerability of the elderly to the effects of medications. Unfortunately, the results of epidemiologic studies that explore these relationships are unclear, in part due to the small number of older people included in premarketing studies relative to the patient population most likely to be exposed to the drug. The oldest—those aged 80 years or older—have not generally been included in clinical trials of investigational drugs, and those older subjects who do participate in such trials tend to be healthy "young-old" people. Thus, the results of these trials and the side effects reported often have limited application to the older patient with multiple illnesses, taking several medications. In general, consideration of the individual patient, his or her physiologic status—hydration, nutrition, and cardiac output, and how this status affects the pharmacology of a particular drug are more important in prescribing that drug than any specific age-related changes.

Absorption of drugs, which occurs mainly by passive diffusion, changes little with advancing age. The changes listed in Table 105.1 could potentially affect drug absorption. More important changes result from concurrent administration of several medications. For example, antacids decrease the oral absorption of cimetidine, and alcohol accelerates the absorption of chloral hydrate.

Unlike absorption, drug distribution is affected by age in clinically meaningful ways. In older persons, the relative increase in body fat and the decrease in lean body mass alter drug distribution so that fat-soluble drugs are distributed more widely and water-soluble drugs less so (344) (Table 103.2). The increased distribution of fat-soluble drugs can delay elimination and may result in prolonged duration of action of a single dose. This effect is especially important for drugs such as hypnotics and analgesics, which may be given in single doses on an intermittent basis. For example, the volume of distribution

TABLE 103.2

VOLUME OF DISTRIBUTION OF COMMONLY PRESCRIBED DRUGS

Increased volume	Decreased volume[a]
Acetaminophen	Cimetidine
Chlordiazepoxide	Digoxin
Diazepam	Ethanol
Oxazepam	Gentamicin
Prazosin	Meperidine
Salicylates	Phenytoin
Thiopental	Quinine
Tolbutamide	Theophylline

[a]If the volume of distribution is decreased, drug levels tend to be higher.

of diazepam is increased almost twofold in older patients, and the elimination half-life is prolonged from 24 hours in young patients to approximately 90 hours in the elderly. In contrast, the volume of distribution of water-soluble compounds, such as digoxin, is decreased in older patients, and thus the dose required to reach a target plasma concentration is decreased. Likewise, due to the decreased volume of distribution, the loading dose of aminoglycosides is less in older patients.

For drugs that bind to serum proteins, equilibrium exists between the bound or ineffective portion and the unbound (free), or effective, portion. For acidic drugs that are highly bound to albumin, the free plasma concentration may correlate best with pharmacologic effect. Although albumin levels decrease only slightly with age, they tend to decrease during periods of illnesses. This can result in elevated levels of unbound acidic drugs in older persons during episodes of illnesses, and thus in an increased potential for toxicity. These changes can be significant for drugs such as thyroid hormone, digoxin, warfarin, and phenytoin. On the other hand, some basic drugs, such as lidocaine and propranolol, bind mainly to alpha-1 acid glycoprotein, an acute phase-reactant protein. The concentration of this protein tends to rise as a person ages and is elevated following myocardial infarction and in chronic inflammatory diseases and malignant conditions (345). The plasma binding of these drugs is increased in older patients, but because these age-related changes are not great, their exact clinical relevance is uncertain.

Overall, changes in protein binding are an important consideration initially when a drug is being started, when the dosage is changed, when serum protein levels change, or when a newly administered drug displaces another protein-bound agent. Because the free portion of the drug is generally smaller than the bound portion, the normal mechanisms of metabolism and excretion ultimately eliminate the free drug. If either hepatic or renal function is impaired due to age or disease, this elimination may be slowed.

Although *in vitro* studies of drug-metabolizing enzyme activity from human liver biopsy samples have not demonstrated any changes with aging, some investigators speculate that the decline in liver size with age may result in decreased metabolic capacity. A significant decline in hepatic blood flow occurs with age, reductions of 25% to 47% being reported in persons between the ages of 25 and 90 years. This decrease in hepatic blood flow is clinically important because hepatic metabolism is the rate-limiting step that determines the clearance of most metabolized drugs. This change is especially relevant for drugs that undergo rapid hepatic metabolism (e.g., propranolol). Also, drugs that undergo extensive first-pass metabolism are likely to reach higher blood levels if hepatic blood flow is decreased.

The liver metabolizes drugs through two distinct systems: phase I metabolism, involving drug oxidation, reduction and hydrolysis; and phase II metabolism, involving glucuronidation, sulfation, acetylation, and methylation. Phase I metabolism is catalyzed primarily by the cytochrome P-450 system in the smooth endoplasmic reticulum of hepatocytes. Cytochrome P-450 enzymes are a superfamily of microsomal drug-metabolizing enzymes important in the biosynthesis and degradation of endogenous compounds such as steroids, lipids, and vitamins, as well as the metabolism of most commonly used drugs (346). Phase I metabolism activity decreases substantially with age. Drugs that are metabolized through phase I enzymatic activity have prolonged half-lives. Examples of some drugs whose metabolism is slowed because of these age-related changes in hepatic metabolism include meperidine, phenytoin, diazepam, propranolol, theophylline, labetalol, lidocaine, and quinidine. Age-related changes in phase I metabolism, coupled with the use of multiple medications, place older patients at increased risk for adverse drug reactions. Adverse drug reactions occur due either to inhibition or induction of cytochrome P-450 enzymes, especially CYP3A, which is thought to be involved in the metabolism of more than half of the currently prescribed drugs (347). Clinical outcomes are determined by the potency of the CYP3A inhibitor (moderate versus potent), the availability of alternative pathways, and the seriousness of the symptoms. A drug is considered a potent CYP3A inhibitor if it causes more than a fivefold increase in the plasma concentration of another drug that is primarily dependent on CYP3A for its metabolism (348). Thus, clinicians should be cognizant of potential drug interactions when they prescribe drugs from classes that include potent or moderate inhibitors of CYP3A. If a potent CYP3A inhibitor or inducer and substrate must be taken together, dosage adjustment and close clinical monitoring are warranted to avoid adverse reactions.

Phase II hepatic metabolism involves the conjugation of drugs or their metabolites to organic substrates. The elimination of drugs that undergo phase II metabolism by conjugation is generally altered less with age. Thus, drugs that require only phase II metabolism for excretion (e.g., triazolam) do not have a prolonged half-life in older people. These drugs contrast with agents such as diazepam that undergo both phases of metabolism and have active intermediate metabolites. Although the effect of aging on hepatic drug metabolism is variable, phase I metabolism is the process that is most likely to decrease in older persons. The apparent variable effect of age on drug metabolism is probably due to the fact that age is only one of many factors that affect drug metabolism. For example, cigarette smoking, alcohol intake, dietary modification, drugs, viral illness, caffeine intake, and other unknown factors also affect the rate of drug metabolism. Induction of drug metabolism can occur in older persons. The rate of elimination of theophylline is increased by smoking and by phenytoin in both young and older persons (349). Not all metabolizing isoenzymes are induced equally in the young and the old. For example, antipyrine elimination is increased after pretreatment with dichloralphenazone in younger patients but not in older patients.

An important pharmacokinetic change that occurs in persons of advanced age is that of reduced renal drug elimination. This change results from the age-related decline in both glomerular filtration rate and tubular function. Drugs that depend on glomerular function (e.g., gentamicin) and/or on tubular secretion (e.g., penicillin) for elimination both exhibit reduced excretion in older patients. Because drug elimination is correlated with creatinine clearance, measurement of creatinine clearance is helpful in determining the maintenance dose. As noted earlier, the average creatinine clearance declines by 50% from age 25 to age 85 despite a serum creatinine level that remains unchanged at approximately 1.0 mg/dL. The Cockroft-Gault formula (see earlier discussion) is useful in the accurate assessment of renal function when planning administration of renally excreted drugs. Although helpful in adjusting for age, weight, and the measured serum creatinine level, it does not account for individual variation.

Altered renal clearance leads to two clinically relevant consequences: the half-lives of renally excreted drugs are prolonged, and the serum levels of these drugs are increased. For drugs with large therapeutic indices (e.g., penicillin), this is of little clinical importance, but for drugs with a narrower therapeutic index (e.g., digoxin, cimetidine, aminoglycosides), side effects may occur in older patients if dose reductions are not made. Thus, it is not surprising that digoxin is the drug that most often causes side effects in the elderly, especially if the dose exceeds 0.125 mg daily (350). To define dose requirements further, therapeutic drug monitoring should be performed for drugs with a low therapeutic index.

In addition to the factors that determine the drug concentration at the site of action—the *pharmacokinetics*—the effect of a drug also depends on the sensitivity of the target organ to the drug. The biochemical and physiologic effects of drugs and their mechanisms of action—*pharmacodynamics*—and the effects of aging are not clearly known. Pharmacodynamics has been even less extensively studied in older patients than has been pharmacokinetics. Generalizations are not straightforward, and the effect of age on sensitivity to drugs varies with the drug studied and the response measured. These differences in sensitivity occur in the absence of marked reductions in the metabolism of the drug and its related compounds. Thus, sensitivity to drug effects may either increase or decrease with increasing age. For example, older patients seem to be more sensitive to the sedative effects of given blood levels of benzodiazepine drugs (e.g., diazepam) but less sensitive to the effects of drugs mediated by beta-adrenergic receptors (e.g., isoproterenol, propranolol). Although an age-related decline in hormone receptor affinity or number (e.g., in beta-adrenergic receptors) is suspected, definitive data demonstrating such an alteration are sparse. Other possible explanations offered for these differences are alterations in second-messenger function and alterations in cellular and nuclear responses.

Since the response of older patients to any given medication is variable and cannot be foreseen, all drugs should be used appropriately, but judiciously, in older patients. The physician should resist the temptation to apply protocol medicine. In general, knowledge of the pharmacology of the drugs prescribed, limits on the number used, determination of the preparation and dosage based on the patient's general condition and ability to handle the drug, combined with downward adjustment of the dose in the presence of known hepatic or renal impairment, in concert with surveillance for untoward effects, will minimize the risks of medication use in the elderly.

SPECIAL PROBLEMS OF THE ELDERLY

As has been briefly addressed above, more people are living longer with chronic diseases, thus increasingly older patients are being admitted to the ICU. Over one half of all ICU admissions are patients older than 65 years of age, and they account for almost 60% of all ICU days (7,341,351,352). Unfortunately, many of these older patients' final days before death are spent in the ICU; 40% of Medicare patients who die are admitted to an ICU during their terminal illness, accounting for 25% of all Medicare expenditures (353,354). Additionally, of those who survive, many are discharged to a subacute facility with persistent organ failure where they eventually die. Dardaine et al. (355) reported a 6-month post-ICU survival of 53% in 116 patients over 70 years of age who had required mechanical ventilation for more than 24 hours. Compared to their younger counterparts, octogenarians have a higher ICU mortality rate (10% vs. 6%, $p < 0.01$) and higher discharge rate to a subacute care facility (35% vs. 18%, $p < 0.01$) (337). Furthermore, those discharged to a subacute care facility had a higher mortality rate compared to those discharged home (31% vs. 17%). Preadmission comorbidities and severity of illness were independent predictors of discharge to a subacute care facility. Degenerative brain disease, cerebrovascular disease, chronic heart failure, chronic pulmonary disease, diabetes mellitus, and malnutrition were more commonly associated with care dependency. Thus, the decision to admit an elderly patient to an ICU should be based not only on their comorbidities, acuity of illness, prehospital functional status, including quality of life, but also on their preference for the use of life-sustaining treatments if it is known. The underlying disease process is not altered despite the use of invasive procedures in terminally ill patients (356,357), and potential harm or discomfort can occur if invasive procedures are used inappropriately. To avoid such unintended consequences and enhance optimal end-of-life decision making, health care providers need to identify, explain, and negotiate consensus therapeutic goals (358).

Neurologic Disorders

Neurologic problems common among older adults in the critical care setting are delirium, stroke, and sleep disorders.

Delirium

Background and Risk Factors. Delirium is an acute mental disorder common among elderly patients. Fourteen percent to 56% of the hospitalized elderly develop delirium (359), increasing the 6-month mortality rate among these patients to 10% to 26% (360,361). Recognition is difficult, with only 25% of cases being diagnosed using standard screening tools (362,363). Delirium-associated morbidity complicates the hospitalization of 2.3 million older people annually, adding 17.5 million inpatient days and $4 billion to Medicare expenditures to cover increased lengths of stay and greater need for post-discharge institutionalization, rehabilitation, and home care (364–367). Older adults with multiple comorbidities, particularly pre-existing cognitive deficits, are predisposed (368–370), with a prevalence rate surpassing 50% during intensive care. Symptoms persist in nearly that number after ICU departure (371). Particularly at risk are those with a history of hypertension, smoking, elevated bilirubin level, recent epidural analgesia, and recent administration of morphine (369,370,372). Other predictors of delirium include respiratory disease, infection, fever, hypotension, hypocalcemia, and hyperamylasemia (373). Invasive devices, sensory alteration, and inadequate or overaggressive pain control likely aggravate delirium-inducing medication effects in the critically ill patient (369,372,374).

Pathophysiology. Specific pathophysiologic mechanisms are not well understood. The phenomenon can be viewed as a final pathway of various causes of acute brain dysfunction. These include the following: (a) direct brain injury from trauma, cerebrovascular disease, or central nervous system infection; (b) systemic disturbances such as hypoxemia, hypotension, renal failure, hepatic failure, sepsis, and endocrine dysfunction; (c) effects of toxic or pharmacologic agents such as anticholinergics, narcotics, and sedative-hypnotics; and (d) the consequences of withdrawal of substances to which the brain has developed tolerance (e.g., alcohol or benzodiazepines). Delirium is more likely to occur when these factors coexist in patients with pre-existing comorbidities (375–388). Current theory proposes alteration of central nervous system neurotransmitter levels and metabolism by age, medication, or illness as paramount in producing the mental status that characterizes delirium, particularly acetylcholine and dopamine pathways, and serotonin, GABA, histamine, glutamine, and norepinephrine systems (389–392).

Diagnosis. Criteria defining delirium are detailed in the *Diagnostic and Statistical Manual of Mental Disorders* (DSM-IV) of the American Psychiatric Association, specifically (a) a disturbance of consciousness with impaired ability to focus, sustain, or shift attention; (b) a change in cognitive function (in terms of memory, orientation, and language) or a perceptual disturbance that is not better explained by pre-existing or evolving dementia; (c) disturbance development over a short period of time in hours or days, fluctuating through the day; and (d) history, physical examination, or laboratory data suggestive of the abnormalities caused by a general medical condition (393). Additional features include alteration of sleep/awake cycle and psychomotor activities. Various instruments have been developed that allow accurate and timely diagnosis using these criteria (370,394–396) when the diagnosis is specifically sought. Patterns of psychomotor symptoms are termed hyperactive and hypoactive (397–399). *Hyperactive* patients are agitated and combative, with loud, inappropriately boisterous outbursts and motor activity that can be harmful to self or a caregiver. Those termed *hypoactive* alternate between calm, appropriate behavior and a minimally interactive, withdrawn state, making this variant easy to overlook. Delirium may erroneously be attributed to such conditions as dementia or depression (indeed, the three may coexist) or simply not be recognized (400), delaying the diagnosis. Delays may be explained by the following: (a) the fluctuating nature of the signs and symptoms, (b) inadequate or insufficiently detailed scheduled neurologic and cognitive assessments of patients at risk for delirium, (c) avoidance of interactions with patients displaying altered mental status, or (d) misperception of mental status changes "expected" in critically ill patients (401,402). Altered mental status in any patient suggests delirium; an organized approach to its investigation (403) that focuses on known risk factors is paramount to avoid overlooking the condition.

Of particular interest to the intensivist who manages elderly patients are alterations of mental status temporally related to surgical procedure, specifically delerium developing within the immediate (minutes to days) postoperative time, and the more indolent neurocognitive decline that may appear days to weeks to months later, termed *postoperative cognitive dysfunction* (POCD). The uniqueness of these conditions lies in their association with the postoperative period. Emergence delirium, the transitory restlessness and disorientation often apparent in the postanesthesia care unit or an ICU that receives patients directly from the operating room, is familiar to all anesthesiologists and often resolves within a brief period of time. More worrisome is interval delirium, appearing 2 to 7 days after operation, the patient manifesting disorientation and agitation and being at risk for suboptimal outcome by virtue of its appearance. Risk factors for postoperative delirium are additive to those menacing the nonoperated elderly patient, including perioperative hypoxemia and hypotension, exposure to medications that are used in the operating room—anticholinergics such as atropine, volatile inhalational anesthetics, neuromuscular blocking agents, and potent opioids—and high-volume blood transfusion and rapid fluid shifts associated with surgery. Procedures using cardiopulmonary bypass raise the possibility of microscopic atheromatous or air emboli as contributors. The incidence of postoperative delirium ranges from 0 to 74%, varying with age group, type of surgery, variability of diagnostic criteria, and preoperative and postoperative cognitive status (404). POCD was first identified in 1955 (405), characterized by the appearance weeks to months after a surgical procedure of impairment of memory, concentration, comprehension of language, and social integration (406). Although the intensivist is seldom charged with management of POCD, she or he is instrumental in its prevention, in that delirium in the early postoperative period may forecast its later appearance (407). One well-designed investigation of elderly patients undergoing noncardiac surgery reported the incidence of delirium to be 25% at 1 week after operation, with symptoms of POCD being present in 9.9% of patients at 3 months, significantly worse than controls at both intervals (406), and revealing advancing age as the only factor significantly predictive of POCD. Similarly, abundant literature (408–410) exists addressing this syndrome in cardiac surgery patients following both on- and off-pump procedures, most of whom were older than 60 years of age. Although most cardiac surgery patients suffer various concurrent confounding medical conditions that make the specific effects solely of cardiac surgery on subsequent mental status difficult to isolate, meticulous attention to statistical and study control issues allows identification of a substantial incidence (53%) of coronary artery bypass graft (CABG) patients (average age, 60.9 years ± 10.6 years) showing cognitive deterioration consistent with POCD at time of discharge, and 42% at 5 years (411), with age being a univariate predictor of decline. The specific cause of POCD is obscure. Suggested causes are those noted above as well as more abstract considerations such as brain inflammation, genetic factors, cerebral edema, and blood–brain barrier dysfunction (412–414).

Timely recognition of the onset of delirium is required for optimal treatment, facilitating rapid identification of reversible precipitating factors. Beyond that, treatment is supportive, with aggressive treatment of symptoms and protection of the patient from the sequelae of his or her delirious state. Prevention is central, requiring a multicomponent approach that includes modification of environmental factors and provision of supportive measures, as demonstrated in a prospective, although nonrandomized, study of 852 patients over 70 years old admitted to a general medicine service in which a multicomponent delirium prevention strategy achieved a one-third reduction in the incidence of delirium, compared to those who received standard care (364). Although this study included patients in a general ward, one may extrapolate the findings to profoundly at-risk ICU patients. Symptomatic treatment uses both pharmacologic and nonpharmacologic strategies. Instrumental are the use of repeated reorientation, cognitive stimulating activities, promotion of adequate sleep on a normal sleep/wake cycle, physical therapy and mobilization, early removal of catheters and physical restraints, and provision of eyeglasses and hearing aids, combined with the judicious use of medications particularly targeted at calming agitation. All potentially neuroactive medications such as benzodiazepines, opioids, or those with anticholinergic effects that are not absolutely fundamental to the patient's treatment plan and improvement should be discontinued (370,372,373). Butyrophenone haloperidol is often used in the management of delirium-induced agitation, having few active metabolites and minimal anticholinergic, sedative, and hypotensive effects (415). A recent retrospective analysis suggested that haloperidol use was independently associated with lower mortality in 989 critically ill patients (416). For POCD, there is no management other than prevention; no therapy has been identified that is curative once the syndrome had developed. In all cases, contributing problems must be identified and corrected and the patient protected. Support must also be provided to family members, who likely will be affected by their loved one's distressing symptoms and by the prospect of additional responsibilities for caring for that person.

Stroke

Incidence and Risk Factors. Stroke is the third leading cause of death and the *leading cause of disability* in the elderly. Approximately 500,000 individuals in this age group suffer strokes annually in the United States, corresponding to one event every 45 seconds and leading to one death every 3 minutes. Among those 55 years and older, the incidence of stroke doubles with each additional decade of life (417), despite a decline in the United States, Canada, and Western Europe through the later part of the 20th century to the present, attributable to improved management of modifiable risk factors. Among these factors, hypertension is by far the most powerful; aggressive blood pressure control can reduce the risk of stroke by 40% (417). Coronary atherosclerosis, left ventricular hypertrophy, and atrial fibrillation contribute to stroke risk. Diabetes mellitus may increase likelihood of stroke by a factor of two to four; tight glucose control significantly reduces this risk, and may postpone such vascular complications as retinopathy and nephropathy (418,419). Modifiable factors also include cigarette smoking, hyperlipidemia, and excessive alcohol consumption.

Classification. Stroke classification can be based on location, cause, and time course. Prior to routine availability of CT, history and clinical findings provided the sole method of neurologic lesion identification. Today, rapid CT localization supplemented by the time-sensitive history and clinical examination findings allow much more rapid formulation of a treatment plan. Although the details of stroke syndromes are addressed elsewhere in this textbook (see Chapter 84), discussion of some issues as they affect the elderly is warranted.

Location. The most common location in which a stroke occurs, representing approximately two thirds of ischemic strokes (420), is in the distribution of the middle cerebral artery (MCA). Findings include contralateral hemiplegia and hemianesthesia. Proximal MCA occlusion produces profound symptoms: homonymous hemianopsia, or deviation of the head and eyes toward the side of the lesion. Involvement of the dominant MCA distribution may cause aphasia, expressive or receptive. Dominant hemisphere MCA lesions may induce depression in the elderly, whereas those in the nondominant hemisphere produce visuospatial deficits, unilateral neglect, and emotional lability that can mimic depression, sometimes delaying correct diagnosis. Anterior cerebral artery (ACA) stroke, the least common variety, accounting for about 2% of ischemic infarcts (420), most profoundly affects the contralateral leg and foot, generally with lesser impact on the arm and little involvement of the face. Very proximal ACA occlusion, however, may affect the entire contralateral side. Abundant collateral flow in ACA territory yields various symptoms associated with anterior circulation stroke. One may observe frontal lobe features such as emotional lability, mood impairment, personality changes, and intellectual deficits; aphasia is uncommon. Stroke-related paraplegia and incontinence may leave the elderly victim wheelchair-bound and unable to control critical body functions, greatly complicating rehabilitation and subsequent independent living. Strokes in the distribution of the posterior cerebral artery (PCA) manifest a diversity of findings due to the variability of anatomic origin, namely partial or complete origin from the basilar artery or internal carotid arteries. Neurologic consequences of PCA stroke include contralateral hemianesthesia and hemianopsia with sparing of central macular vision, difficulty with reading and calculations, and hemiballismus from subthalamic involvement (420). With vertebrobasilar atherothrombotic disease, cerebellar dysfunction predominates. Common symptoms include vomiting, dizziness, ataxia, nystagmus, and double vision. Vertigo can be profound, causing an already tenuously balanced elderly person to sustain a fatal fall. Other symptoms include weakness of the face and the opposite side of the body, with dysarthria or dysphasia. Facial numbness may occur. Brain stem involvement may be revealed by altered mental status or quadriplegia (420). Lacunar strokes—small occlusions of the penetrating and subcortical arteries—tend to occur in the basal ganglia, internal capsule, thalamus, or pons. Depending on the specific sites of lesions, a wide variety of presentation may occur, including pure motor or sensory findings, symptoms that appear parkinsonian, or a mixture of presenting abnormalities.

Cause. Strokes are either ischemic or hemorrhagic. Those that are ischemic, about 85% of the total, involve occlusion of the cerebral vessel by embolus or thrombosis; the remaining 15% include hemorrhage into the brain parenchyma or its surrounding spaces (420). Rapid identification of the specific cause of the stroke is fundamental to its management, since modalities of treatment vary with cause. Embolic phenomena most often originate from the heart, commonly associated with atrial fibrillation, which is frequent in the elderly population. Atherosclerotic disease of the aortic arch is emerging as an increasingly important and recognized risk factor for recurrent stroke when the wall thickness exceeds 4 mm (421). Atheroma-associated clot formation may produce neurologic syndromes known as thrombotic stroke. Subintimal vascular disease is the ultimate inciting event, inducing arterial narrowing with ulcerated plaque formation in areas of more turbulent flow, such as the carotid bifurcation, leading ultimately to symptoms ranging from a temporary deficit (i.e., a transient ischemic attack, or TIA) to complete arterial occlusion caused by clot formation.

Time Course. Stroke phases are termed acute, subacute, and chronic, each with its unique needs and goals of care. Time spans are generally said to extend from symptom onset to 48 hours, 48 hours to 3 months, and past 3 months, respectively.

The intensivist is little involved in direct management of stroke-related symptoms after the first few days, although elderly patients who fall within the later stages of recovery may certainly require intensive care for recurrent stroke, a stroke-related complication, or other critical illness.

Acute phase of stroke (admission to 48 hours). Management of the acute phase involves, first and foremost, ensuring airway and hemodynamic stability. Thereafter, the goals of care are (i) identification of the stroke as ischemic or hemorrhagic, (ii) initiation of thrombolytic therapy when indicated, and (iii) recognition and therapy of medical or neurologic complications. The first goal is most easily achieved by obtaining a noncontrast-enhanced CT scan of the brain as quickly as possible when stroke is suspected. Hemorrhage is usually obvious on this scan, although early in the course of ischemic stroke there may be no visible abnormality. Early CT may reveal one of the many mimics of stroke: subarachnoid hemorrhage, subdural hematoma, neoplasm, or hydrocephalus. Contrast enhancement may improve yield if tumor or infection are likely. Recall that comorbid conditions abound in the elderly; cardiac arrhythmias or infarction may provoke or result from a cerebrovascular event, mandating 12-lead electrocardiogram (ECG) and continuous cardiac monitoring in all stroke patients. Questions of the numerous other causes of altered mental status in the geriatric patient must be investigated and settled quickly. For those in whom, with the assistance of expert consultation, it is decided that ischemic stroke is present, the risks and benefits of thrombolytic therapy must be weighed. Current recommendations for management include initiation of intravenous thrombolytic therapy with recombinant tissue plasminogen activator (rt-PA) as soon as possible, within 180 minutes of onset of stroke, in the absence of contraindications (422,423). Intra-arterial thrombolysis is an option for those with occlusion of the middle cerebral artery. Of note is that rt-PA is approved by the Food and Drug Administration (FDA) for intravenous administration, but not for intra-arterial use. Use of rt-PA appears to improve outcome from stroke at 3 months. There is a relative paucity of data documenting treatment of older patients, similar to those studies addressing thrombolysis for myocardial infarction. It does appear, however, that while there may be poorer outcome from stroke in the elderly population, there is no increased likelihood of rt-PA–induced severe intracranial hemorrhage (424,425). A number of stroke scales, including the National Institutes of Health Stroke Scale (NIHSS), have been devised to assist in quantification of severity of stroke-related symptoms, as a guide to optimal management. Important issues such as blood pressure management and anticoagulation are best addressed in concert with expert consultation (426).

Subacute and chronic phases of stroke management. The acute events and aggressive treatment related to stroke often stabilize a patient's condition within 48 hours. Thereafter, close attention to complications or neurologic decompensation is warranted. Early extubation is advisable, with meticulous attention to the return of intact airway reflexes and sufficient recovery of mental status. Otherwise, tracheostomy for airway protection allows withdrawal of sedation, early mobilization, and more robust participation in physical and occupational therapy, with the long-term goal of rehabilitation to maximal recovery. The common companions of those with compromised mental status, namely pulmonary aspiration, skin breakdown, infections, and limitation of extremity range of movement, can be ameliorated by aggressive rehabilitation efforts. Early nutritional support via feeding tube is sometimes overlooked in the flurry of initial management activity but must be initiated as early as possible. Formal rehabilitation programs may be organized in the setting of the acute inpatient rehabilitation unit, or in long-term rehabilitation hospitals, skilled nursing facilities, outpatient rehabilitation centers, or home. Optimal programs incorporate comprehensive assessment and treatment by a multidisciplinary team that includes physical, occupational, and speech therapists, and a geriatrician, physiatrist, psychologist, nurse, and social worker during this first few months during which most neurologic recovery occurs. A pre-existing state of debilitation, however, may limit the 3-hour period of active participation traditional to inpatient environments, mandating alternate plans. General goals of rehabilitation include restoration of motor and sensory function, and strengthening of intact functions to facilitate compensation for residual deficits. Beyond the first few months, while neurologic function likely plateaus, functional recovery continues when encouraged and supported by family presence, social interaction, and adequate nutrition. The stroke recurrence rate of 30% within 10 years warrants continued attention to chronic medical conditions. Framingham Study data documents survival in stroke victims of 50% in 5 years (427–429). Preservation of functional gains, avoidance of complications, and aggressive management of contributing comorbid conditions may well forestall the decline that often follows a stroke in an elderly patient.

Sleep Disorders

Background. Insomnia plagues the elderly, afflicting nearly 50% of older adults (430); the genders are generally equally affected, although sleepless men predominate after 85 years of age. Prevalence increases in the elderly with the number of coincident medical conditions (431,432). Common sleep complaints among the community-dwelling elderly are difficulty in initiation of sleep, and nighttime and early morning awakening (433). Sequelae of insomnia include physical and mental fatigue, anxiety, and irritability, which worsen as bedtime approaches and personal worries re-emerge without the protective diversion of normal daytime activities (434). Chronic dysfunctional sleep induces a state of endless fatigue, affecting memory and concentration (431,435). The elderly are particularly affected, with steepened cognitive decline and risk of falls, with associated morbidity and mortality (436–438). Hospitalization amplifies the morbidity of sleep disturbances; ICU admission likely subverts any semblance of a normal sleep pattern. Sedation to facilitate mechanical ventilation subdues consciousness but disrupts normal variation in sleep stages, preventing rest. Circadian rhythms are disrupted, with dyssynchrony with anticipated light/dark time cycles and adequate daily morning exposure to sufficient bright light (439). Many elderly patients become disoriented at night, exhausted and confused by constant alarms, noises, dressing changes, unscheduled diagnostic procedures, and the impact of acute severe illness, producing delirium in nearly two thirds of elderly ICU patients (372). Dementia contributes to this phenomenon.

Identification and Management of Sleep Disorders. The sleep/wake cycle is regulated by a complex neurochemical interaction subserved by the brainstem, hypothalamus, pons, and preoptic areas of the brain (440). Aberrations of sleep patterns produce dysfunctional sleep (441), disrupting daytime functioning. Sleep architecture is determined for an individual by performance of a sleep study displayed on a hypnogram. Normal sleep architecture displays three segments: light sleep (stages one and two); deep (delta or slow wave) sleep (stages three and four), which is the most restorative segment; and rapid eye movement, or REM, sleep (stages one and four) (442). In nonelderly adults, typical cycle time between REM and non-REM sleep is 90 to 120 minutes (442). Advanced age alters sleep by shortening sleep latency and total sleep time, preserving REM sleep, decreasing the delta segment, and advancing the natural onset of sleepiness to an earlier time in the evening (433). Nocturnal sleep fragmentation worsens, with daytime somnolence and frequent napping being commonplace, sometimes causing reversal of the sleep/wake cycle. Acute insomnia in the geriatric patient may be precipitated by a host of issues, including the critical illness itself. Metabolic derangements related to sepsis or trauma, recent exposure to potent anesthetic agents, and the unfamiliar ICU environment filled with off-schedule and frequent disruptions effectively prevent restful sleep. Although not generally within the purview of the intensivist, investigation of the cause of insomnia may be initiated for the ICU patient by meticulous history gathering, discussion with family members, use of sleep-related questionnaires such as the Multiple Sleep Latency Test (441) and the Epworth sleepiness scale screening tool (443), and observation of the patient for evidence of any of the primary sleep disorders that respond to specific treatment modalities. These include a spectrum of conditions collectively termed sleep-disordered breathing (SDB), periodic limb movements in sleep/restless legs syndrome, and REM sleep behavior disorder. Some causes of SDB (obstructive sleep apnea, specifically) respond to continuous positive airway pressure (CPAP) (444), and the latter two respond to medications (445,446). Secondary causes are legion, including medications, sleep-disruptive behavioral habits (such as prolonged daytime naps, sedentary lifestyle, overindulgence in tobacco or alcohol, late evening meals), numerous medical conditions (heart failure with orthopnea, incomplete bladder emptying with nocturia, gastric reflux, dementia), or environmental deficiencies (insufficient daytime sunlight exposure, inadequate climate control) (442).

Effective treatment obviously requires an accurate diagnosis. Evidence of primary causes should be relayed to the patient, family members, and the physician responsible for long-term management of the patient after transfer. All possible accommodations should be made to minimize interruption of the older patient's restful nighttime sleep periods, minimizing noise, procedures, and cycling of lights on and off. Daily exposure to bright sunlight through nearby windows is beneficial (447,448). Pharmacologic treatments are best addressed on an individual basis, and within certain guidelines (449). Various medications are available (442); each, however, may provoke delirium in elderly patients. In-depth guidelines for the evaluation and treatment of sleep disorders are available (435,450–455).

REHABILITATION AFTER ACUTE ILLNESS

The impact of critical illness on the lives of elderly patients is profound. Beyond the associated death rates, level of functioning is compromised in a substantial percentage of survivors (456). Increasing vulnerability to long-term dependence increases with age (457). Medical intervention in the critically ill or injured patient has evolved to a level of sophistication and capability that allows a previously unsalvageable patient to survive. Thoughtful and comprehensive discharge planning, initiated at the time of admission, can shorten length of stay (LOS) (458) and provide the springboard for return to a reasonable, though often compromised, level of functional autonomy (459). Many of these elderly individuals, after considerable improvement, may nevertheless linger for a prolonged period, requiring a single isolated critical intervention such as mechanical ventilation, further risking the decline of inactivity. The deleterious effects of such a prolonged hospital confinement can be ameliorated by early use of the expertise of rehabilitation professionals. Furthermore, optimal recovery from certain common medical occurrences and conditions simply is not possible without active patient participation, which can be assisted and promoted by the physical medicine team. It is being increasingly recognized that *early* institution of rehabilitation planning and execution by such a team of specialists can reduce health care costs, length of stay, and severity of disability after discharge (460). Shortening of hospitalization decreases the exposure of the marginally compensated patient to its debilitating risks (461). Avoidance of postillness disability is of paramount importance in that it is associated with higher mortality and greater dependence on family and other caregivers (462,463).

Rehabilitation, as a general concept, encompasses several basic tenets that meld smoothly with the critical care frame of reference (464). Fundamental to any rehabilitation plan is stabilization of the primary inciting disorder; such a precept is the essence of the practice of critical care medicine, and thus is accomplished by virtue of the administration of ICU care. The unique jeopardy in which the elderly exist by virtue of their frailty and vulnerability to complications warrants the most meticulous attention to routine ICU precautions, which must be recognized by the intensivist (465). These include frequent turning, early nutrition, appropriate deep venous thrombosis (DVT) prophylaxis, semirecumbent positioning, and maintenance of day–night cycle of auditory and visual stimulation. Early evaluation by a multidisciplinary team of specialists facilitates identification of evolving and anticipated functional deficits that are amenable to treatment, whether preventive or corrective. Integrated rehabilitation treatment and planning should occur in both the immediate and long-term settings by involvement of the physiatry team. Admission of a frail elder to a specialized unit designed around and attentive to specific features of geriatric pathophysiology has been demonstrated to improve functional outcomes (466).

The fundamental tool available to the geriatrician with which to organize the management and treatment of medical issues, including problems warranting formal rehabilitation, is the comprehensive geriatric assessment (CGA) (467). The integrated, patient-centered concept of treatment implicit in CGA is often accomplished in specialized hospital units or within the framework of treatment considerations peculiar to the elderly, managed by a devoted multidisciplinary team. Such units include the geriatric evaluation and management (GEM) unit, as found in some Veterans Administration hospitals (468), or a specifically formulated management plan termed Acute Care for Elders (ACE) (469), or a construct of aggressive hospital-wide screening and treatment for at-risk patients by specialists and volunteers in an organization such as the Hospital

Elder Life Program (HELP) (470). An alternative for the intensivist, whose patients are clearly unavailable for transfer to such a location remote from the ICU, is consultation by an in-patient geriatric consultation service team including individuals knowledgeable in rehabilitation issues (471). To date, the success of CGA in improving functionality and decreasing disability in the elderly after discharge seems clear, although improvement in mortality with this approach, as documented by several studies, seems less so (466,468,472–474).

Several specific medical issues mandating ICU admission require active rehabilitation activities to achieve successful treatment. These include cardiac events related both to ACS and cardiac surgery, stroke, serious injury, various debilitating musculoskeletal conditions, and such morbid orthopedic procedures as lower extremity amputation and hip fracture repair.

Although large studies and reviews (475) document the success of aggressive rehabilitation in reducing cardiac mortality, its success specifically in the elderly appears mostly in small, nonrandomized, or uncontrolled studies. Nevertheless, it appears that an aggressive program of cardiac rehabilitation conducted for elderly patients, although often limited by arthritis or coexistent peripheral vascular or pulmonary disease, is safe, able to improve aerobic capacity, and favorably affects body fat percentage, lipid profiles, and physical function scores (476–478). Less enthusiastic referral habits by physicians may explain lower participation among elderly cardiac patients, especially women, compared to younger people (479–481).

Recovery from acute stroke presents a complex challenge to victim and physician alike. Whereas the cardiac patient may see improvement after surgery that continues during rehabilitation, the stroke patient often must endure compromised mental status and motor/sensory capabilities from the initial insult, yielding a debilitated individual with little motivational reserve with which to sustain himself or herself during recovery. Survival beyond the first few days likely mandates prolonged assistance that may be required for months to achieve optimal improvement. The extent of this improvement hinges on several issues. These include age (482), the nature and severity of the initial deficit (483,484), presence of intracranial hemorrhage-related rather than infarction-related stroke—a patient with the former improves more than one with the latter for a given initial severity (485)—and early initiation of the rehabilitation activities, preferably within 7 days (486). The plasticity of injured and unaffected normal brain tissue allows gradual improvement over the subsequent several months (487). Specific stroke-related rehabilitation issues include the following: (a) optimal location for therapy, (b) speech and swallowing, (c) recovery of upper extremity function, (d) balance and walking, and (e) strengthening exercises (483). Evaluation tools such as the Barthel Index and the Stroke Impact Scale (488) are used to quantify a stroke patient's recovery, which may continue for as long as six months of recovery in the absence of another complication (489,490). Success of recovery from stroke varies over a large population (491) based on aforementioned variables and, to some extent, social status (492).

Rehabilitation of an injured elderly patient often involves continued long-term supportive therapy of conditions from which a younger individual may well recover quickly, namely mild traumatic brain injury and extremity fracture. Indeed, continuity of specialized geriatrician involvement may facilitate continued attention to several issues during a prolonged trauma-ICU admission: comorbid problems, functional abilities and family support, formulation and continuous assessment of an itemized management plan toward realistic goals, and early initiation of planning for discharge and follow-up care (493,494). Of particular concern to intensivists managing elderly patients is hip fracture, of which more than 250,000 occur annually (495), with most patients being older than 50 years of age. Such fractures increase mortality—compared to that of similar patients without fracture—in those older than 65 years of age by 12% to 36% (496), as well as the likelihood of subsequent institutionalization (497) and functional dependence (498). Those whose course is complicated by pre-existing cognitive dysfunction or delirium fare more poorly (497,499). Successful management requires identification and correction/stabilization of comorbid conditions, appropriate surgical treatment, and early initiation of important precepts of rehabilitation (495,500). These include early mobilization, initially to chair followed by standing and walking with weight bearing; prolonged bed rest fosters deconditioning and is to be avoided. The intensivist who manages a particularly ill elder must address the potential for thromboembolic complications by encouraging early mobilization to minimize venous stasis, and by using prophylactic anticoagulant medication; regimens differ according to the exact situation (501–504). Functionality can be profoundly affected after hip fracture (505,506) and is further impacted by a high level of comorbidity (507). Although more men than women die initially after hip fracture, those who survive after the first year experience comparable functional recovery regardless of gender (508). Very advanced age is not necessarily a contraindication to hip fracture surgery in the absence of a prohibitive comorbidity; those older than 90 years often do quite well, returning, with aggressive rehabilitation and social support, to independent living (509).

About 50,000 amputations are performed annually in the United States, most on patients who are older than 60 years (510). Rates of lower extremity amputation declined from the 1980s to the mid 1990s, paralleling the improvement in arterial bypass and angioplasty techniques and the heightened attention to control of risk factors for vascular disease. Rates since then seem to have stabilized (511). Eighty percent of amputations are performed as a result of arteriosclerotic occlusive disease and complications of diabetes mellitus (512), coincident with common comorbidities that may direct an elderly patient to the ICU. Nearly half of lower extremity amputees die within 2 years (513); a substantial percentage of survivors go on to lose the other leg (514) within a few years. Despite the attention paid to morbid consequences of amputation during the immediate postoperative period, this procedure profoundly impacts the patient's entire remaining life span. Optimal therapy for the amputee is achievable only with the early involvement and assistance of a rehabilitation team of physicians, technologists, and therapists skilled specifically in management of amputation-related issues and familiar with prosthetic devices. Level of amputation varies with severity of lower extremity involvement; although medically sound judgement is the pre-eminent guide in this decision, it is important to note that the more joints and muscles are replaced by a prosthesis, the greater the associated forfeiture of mobility and increase in energy cost of ambulation. The transmetatarsal amputee requires fairly trivial energy supplement to return to ambulation; the similar requirement for a transfemoral amputation patient can balloon by nearly 100% (512–515). Such cardiovascular and energy demands are considerable, even in an otherwise healthy amputee (515,516), and may not be achievable in the debilitated geriatric vascular or traumatized patient without risk of further decompensation. Nonetheless, early mobilization is to be encouraged. Prolonged bed rest further compromises balance and endurance, inviting the onset of contractures and loss of strength in compensatory muscle groups during prosthesis introduction. In the past, elderly amputees were seldom offered prosthesis; this picture has reversed with the more modern approach to elderly amputee care (517), in which such an offering is made to nearly 90% of elderly. An early visit from the physiatrist to the amputee's bedside facilitates initiation of an organized rehabilitation care plan to formulate future prosthetic, physical therapy, wound care, and emotional support needs. Parts of these recovery plan components may be initiated by the intensivist while the patient is still critically ill and more fully conducted on a regular hospital ward, a specialty rehabilitation facility, or even at home. Follow-up must be long term; medical, emotional, and physical needs continue long after the amputee's surgical stump has completely healed (518,519).

SUMMARY

The health care needs of the elderly members of the community represent enormous challenges to all members of the medical profession. The aspirations and personal convictions of such individuals are as fundamental to the well-being and fruitfulness of their lives as are those of any other segment of the population. While years of living bring elderly patients with the most complex illnesses and comorbid conditions to the door of the hospital and intensive care unit, it is to be remembered that the elderly often recover fully, or almost so, from profoundly serious illness despite numerous worrisome impediments that would discourage all but the most optimistic clinician. In general, vigilance and dispatch in investigations and treatment of critically ill geriatric patients, using the guidelines listed in this chapter, will facilitate recognition of the subtleties of such conditions. Although a substantial percentage of the elderly cannot be brought back to an independent level of functioning, every effort should be expended to achieve accurate diagnosis and expeditious treatment, providing full intensive support to conditions that are correctable and recognition when reasonable limits have been reached.

References

1. United States Census 2000. www.census.gov/main/www/cen2000.html. Accessed April 1, 2007.
2. CDC National Vital Statistics Report, Vol 54; No. 14, April 19, 2006, Report revised as of 28 March, 2007. www.cdc.gov/nchs/data/nvsr/nvsr54/nvsr54_14.pdf. Accessed April 1, 2007.
3. Rice DP, Fineman N. Economic implications of increased longevity in the United States. *Annu Rev Public Health.* 2004;25:457–473.
4. Office of Demographic and Economic Research; The Florida Legislature. http://edr.state.fl.us/population.htm. AccessedApril 1, 2007.
5. U.S. Department of Health & Human Services: Centers for Medicare & Medicaid Services. www.cms.hhs.gov/NationalHealthExpendData. Accessed April 1, 2007.
6. Alsarraf AA, Fowler R. Health, economic evaluation, and critical care. *J Crit Care.* 2005;20:194–197.
7. Angus DC, Kelley MA, Schmitz RJ, et al. Committee on Manpower for Pulmonary and Critical Care Societies (COMPACCS). Caring for the critically ill patient. Current and projected workforce requirements for care of the critically ill and patients with pulmonary disease: can we meet the requirements of an aging population? *JAMA.* 2000;284:2762–2770.
8. Rockwood K, Noseworthy TW, Gibney RT, et al. One-year outcome of elderly and young patients admitted to intensive care units. *Crit Care Med.* 1993;21:687–691.
9. Luce JM, Rubenfeld GD. Can health care costs be reduced by limiting intensive care at the end of life? *Am J Respir Crit Care Med.* 2002;165:750–754.
10. Fries JF, Koop CE, Beadle CE, et al. Reducing health care costs by reducing the need and demand for medical services. The Health Project Consortium. *N Engl J Med.* 1993;329:321–325.
11. Emanuel EJ, Emanuel LL. The economics of dying. The illusion of cost savings at the end of life. *N Engl J Med.* 1994;330:540–544.
12. Martin GS, Mannino DM, Moss M. The effect of age on the development and outcome of adult sepsis. *Crit Care Med.* 2006;34:15–21.
13. CDC/National Center for Health Statistic. Cardiovascular disease in the elderly. www.cdc.gov/nchs/. Accessed April 1, 2007.
14. Crispell KA. Common cardiovascular issues encountered in geriatric critical care. *Crit Care Clin.* 2003;19:677–691.
15. Timio M. Blood pressure trend and psychosocial factors: the case of the nuns in a secluded order. *Acta Physiol Scand Suppl.* 1997;640:137–139.
16. Poulter NR, Khaw KT, Mugambi M, et al. Blood pressure patterns in relation to age, weight and urinary electrolytes in three Kenyan communities. *Trans R Soc Trop Med Hyg.* 1985;79:389–392.
17. Nichols WW, O'Rourke MF. *McDonald's Blood Flow in Arteries.* London, England: Edward Arnold Publishers; 1990.
18. Greenwald SE; Ageing of the conduit arteries. *J Pathol.* 2007;211:157–172.
19. London GM, Marchais SJ, Guerin AP, et al. Arterial stiffness: pathophysiology and clinical impact. *Clin Exp Hypertens.* 2004;26:689–699.
20. Dao HH, Essalihi R, Bouvet C, et al. Evolution and modulation of age-related medial elastocalcinosis: impact on large artery stiffness and isolated systolic hypertension. *Cardiovasc Res.* 2005;66:307–317.
21. Avolio A, Jones D, Tafazzoli-Shadpour M. Quantification of alterations in structure and function of elastin in the arterial media. *Hypertension.* 1998; 32:170–175.
22. O'Rourke M. Mechanical principles in arterial disease. *Hypertension.* 1995;26:2–9.
23. Izzo JL Jr. Arterial stiffness and the systolic hypertension syndrome. *Curr Opin Cardiol.* 2004;19:341–352.
24. Bramwell JC, Hill AV. Velocity of tansmission of the Pulse Wave. *Lancet.* 1922;1:891–892.
25. O'Rourke MF, Blazek JV, Morreels CL Jr, et al. Pressure wave transmission along the human aorta. Changes with age and in arterial degenerative disease. *Circ Res.* 1968;23:567–579.
26. Nichols WW, O'Rourke MF, Avolio AP, et al. Effects of age on ventricular-vascular coupling. *Am J Cardiol.* 1985;55:1179–1184.
27. Nichols WW, Edwards DG. Arterial elastance and wave reflection augmentation of systolic blood pressure: deleterious effects and implications for therapy. *J Cardiovasc Pharmacol Ther.* 2001;6:5–21.
28. Strandberg TE, Pitkala K. What is the most important component of blood pressure: systolic, diastolic or pulse pressure? *Curr Opin Nephrol Hypertens.* 2003;12:293–297.
29. Nichols WW, Singh BM. Augmentation index as a measure of peripheral vascular disease state. *Curr Opin Cardiol.* 2002;17:543–551.
30. Safar ME. Systolic blood pressure, pulse pressure and arterial stiffness as cardiovascular risk factors. *Curr Opin Nephrol Hypertens.* 2001;10:257–261.
31. Franklin SS, Gustin W 4th, Wong ND, et al. Hemodynamic patterns of age-related changes in blood pressure. The Framingham Heart Study. *Circulation.* 1997;96:308–315.
32. Olivetti G, Melissari M, Capasso JM, et al. Cardiomyopathy of the aging human heart. Myocyte loss and reactive cellular hypertrophy. *Circ Res.* 1991;68:1560–1568.
33. Wei JY. Age and the cardiovascular system. *N Engl J Med.* 1992;327:1735–1739.
34. Weber KT, Brilla CG. Structural basis for pathologic left ventricular hypertrophy. *Clin Cardiol.* 1993;16(5 Suppl 2):II10–II14.
35. Kass DA, Bronzwaer JG, Paulus WJ. What mechanisms underlie diastolic dysfunction in heart failure? *Circ Res.* 2004;94:1533–1542.
36. Periasamy M, Kalyanasundaram A. SERCA pump isoforms: their role in calcium transport and disease. *Muscle Nerve.* 2007;35:430–442.
37. Aurigemma GP, Gaasch WH. Clinical practice. Diastolic heart failure. *N Engl J Med.* 2004;351:1097–1105.
38. Mandinov L, Eberli FR, Seiler C, et al. Diastolic heart failure. *Cardiovasc Res.* 2000;45:813–825.
39. Kitzman DW, Gardin JM, Gottdiener JS, et al.; Cardiovascular Health Study Research Group. Importance of heart failure with preserved systolic function in patients > or = 65 years of age. CHS Research Group. Cardiovascular Health Study. *Am J Cardiol.* 2001;87:413–419.
40. Brucks S, Little WC, Chao T, et al. Contribution of left ventricular diastolic dysfunction to heart failure regardless of ejection fraction. *Am J Cardiol.* 2005;95:603–606.
41. Lakatta EG. Diminished beta-adrenergic modulation of cardiovascular function in advanced age. *Cardiol Clin.* 1986;4:185–200.

42. Lakatta EG, Sollott SJ. Perspectives on mammalian cardiovascular aging: humans to molecules. *Comp Biochem Physiol A Mol Integr Physiol.* 2002;132:699–721.
43. Lakatta EG. Catecholamines and cardiovascular function in aging. *Endocrinol Metab Clin North Am.* 1987;16:877–891.
44. Rodeheffer RJ, Gerstenblith G, Becker LC, et al. Exercise cardiac output is maintained with advancing age in healthy human subjects: cardiac dilatation and increased stroke volume compensate for a diminished heart rate. *Circulation.* 1984;69:203–213.
45. Stratton JR, Levy WC, Cerqueira MD, et al. Cardiovascular responses to exercise. Effects of aging and exercise training in healthy men. *Circulation.* 1994;89:1648–1655.
46. Mehta RH, Granger CB, Alexander KP, et al. Reperfusion strategies for acute myocardial infarction in the elderly: benefits and risks. *J Am Coll Cardiol.* 2005;45:471–478.
47. Goldberg RJ, McCormick D, Gurwitz JH, et al. Age-related trends in short- and long-term survival after acute myocardial infarction: a 20-year population-based perspective (1975–1995). *Am J Cardiol.* 1998;82:1311–1317.
48. Angeja BG, Gibson CM, Chin R, et al. Use of reperfusion therapies in elderly patients with acute myocardial infarction. *Drugs Aging.* 2001;18:587–596.
49. Canto JG, Shlipak MG, Rogers WJ, et al. Prevalence, clinical characteristics, and mortality among patients with myocardial infarction presenting without chest pain. *JAMA.* 2000;283:3223–3229.
50. Giugliano RP, Camargo CA Jr, Lloyd-Jones DM, et al. Elderly patients receive less aggressive medical and invasive management of unstable angina: potential impact of practice guidelines. *Arch Intern Med.* 1998;158:1113–1120.
51. Lee PY, Alexander KP, Hammill BG, et al. Representation of elderly persons and women in published randomized trials of acute coronary syndromes. *JAMA.* 2001;286(6):708–713.
52. Antman EM, Braunwald E. Acute myocardial infarction. In: Braunwald EB, ed. *Heart Disease: A Textbook of Cardiovascular Medicine.* Philadelphia, PA: WB Saunders; 1997
53. Gersh BJ, Anderson JL. Thrombolysis and myocardial salvage. Results of clinical trials and the animal paradigm—paradoxic or predictable? *Circulation.* 1993;88(1):296–306.
54. Indications for fibrinolytic therapy in suspected acute myocardial infarction: collaborative overview of early mortality and major morbidity results from all randomised trials of more than 1000 patients. Fibrinolytic Therapy Trialists' (FTT) Collaborative Group. *Lancet.* 1994;343(8893):311–322.
55. Antman EM, Anbe DT, Armstrong PW, et al. American College of Cardiology/American Heart Association Task Force on Practice Guidelines (Writing Committee to Revise the 1999 Guidelines for the Management of Patients With Acute Myocardial Infarction). ACC/AHA guidelines for the management of patients with ST-elevation myocardial infarction–executive summary: a report of the American College of Cardiology/American Heart Association Task Force on Practice Guidelines (Writing Committee to Revise the 1999 Guidelines for the Management of Patients With Acute Myocardial Infarction). *Circulation.* 2004;110(5):588–636.
56. Keeley EC, Boura JA, Grines CL. Primary angioplasty versus intravenous thrombolytic therapy for acute myocardial infarction: a quantitative review of 23 randomised trials. *Lancet.* 2003;361(9351):13–20.
57. Guagliumi G, Stone GW, Cox DA, et al. Outcome in elderly patients undergoing primary coronary intervention for acute myocardial infarction: results from the Controlled Abciximab and Device Investigation to Lower Late Angioplasty Complications (CADILLAC) trial. *Circulation.* 2004;110(12):1598–1604.
58. Zahn R, Schiele R, Schneider S, et al. Primary angioplasty versus intravenous thrombolysis in acute myocardial infarction: can we define subgroups of patients benefiting most from primary angioplasty? Results from the pooled data of the Maximal Individual Therapy in Acute Myocardial Infarction Registry and the Myocardial Infarction Registry. *J Am Coll Cardiol.* 2001;37(7):1827–1835.
59. Bach RG, Cannon CP, Weintraub WS, et al. The effect of routine, early invasive management on outcome for elderly patients with non-ST-segment elevation acute coronary syndromes. *Ann Intern Med.* 2004;141(3):186–195.
60. Assali AR, Moustapha A, Sdringola S, et al. The dilemma of success: percutaneous coronary interventions in patients > or = 75 years of age-successful but associated with higher vascular complications and cardiac mortality. *Catheter Cardiovasc Interv.* 2003;59(2):195–199.
61. Hunt SA, Abraham WT, Chin MH, et al. American College of Cardiology; American Heart Association Task Force on Practice Guidelines; American College of Chest Physicians; International Society for Heart and Lung Transplantation; Heart Rhythm Society. ACC/AHA 2005 Guideline Update for the Diagnosis and Management of Chronic Heart Failure in the Adult: a report of the American College of Cardiology/American Heart Association Task Force on Practice Guidelines (Writing Committee to Update the 2001 Guidelines for the Evaluation and Management of Heart Failure): developed in collaboration with the American College of Chest Physicians and the International Society for Heart and Lung Transplantation: endorsed by the Heart Rhythm Society. *Circulation.* 2005;112(12):e154–235. Epub 2005 Sep 13.
62. Masoudi FA, Havranek EP, Krumholz HM. The burden of chronic congestive heart failure in older persons: magnitude and implications for policy and research. *Heart Fail Rev.* 2002;7(1):9–16.
63. Kannel WB, Belanger AJ. Epidemiology of heart failure. *Am Heart J.* 1991;121(3 Pt 1):951–957.
64. Kannel WB, Ho K, Thom T. Changing epidemiological features of cardiac failure. *Br Heart J.* 1994;72(2 Suppl):S3–9.
65. Aronow WS. Epidemiology, pathophysiology, prognosis, and treatment of systolic and diastolic heart failure in elderly patients. *Heart Dis.* 2003;5(4):279–294.
66. Kannel WB. Incidence and epidemiology of heart failure. *Heart Fail Rev.* 2000;5(2):167–173.
67. Aronow WS, Tresch DD. Management of the older patient with acute myocardial infarction: difference in clinical presentations between older and younger patients. *J Am Geriatr Soc.* 1998; 46(9):1157–1162.
68. Marinchak RA, Friehling TD, Kowey PR. Diagnosis and treatment of cardiac rhythm disorders in the elderly. *Clin Geriatr Med.* 1988;4(1):83–110.
69. Rials SJ, Marinchak RA, Kowey PR. Arrhythmias in the elderly. *Cardiovasc Clin.* 1992;22(2):139–157.
70. Falk RH. Etiology and complications of atrial fibrillation: insights from pathology studies. *Am J Cardiol.* 1998;82(8A):10N–17N.
71. Fujino M, Okada R, Arakawa K. The relationship of aging to histological changes in the conduction system of the normal human heart. *Jpn Heart J.* 1983;24(1):13–20.
72. Lev M. Aging changes in the human sinoatrial node. *J Gerontol.* 1954; 9(1):1–9.
73. Roberts WC. The aging heart. *Mayo Clin Proc.* 1988;63(2):205–206.
74. Thery C, Gosselin B, Lekieffre J, et al. Pathology of sinoatrial node. Correlations with electrocardiographic findings in 111 patients. *Am Heart J.* 1977;93(6):735–740.
75. Tai CT, Chiou CW, Chen SA. Interaction between the autonomic nervous system and atrial tachyarrhythmias. *J Cardiovasc Electrophysiol.* 2002; 13(1):83–87.
76. Coumel P. Autonomic influences in atrial tachyarrhythmias. *J Cardiovasc Electrophysiol.* 1996;7(10):999–1007.
77. Wong CK, White HD, Wilcox RG, et al. Significance of atrial fibrillation during acute myocardial infarction, and its current management: insights from the GUSTO-3 trial. *Card Electrophysiol Rev.* 2003;7(3):201–207.
78. Wong CK, White HD, Wilcox RG, et al. New atrial fibrillation after acute myocardial infarction independently predicts death: the GUSTO-III experience. *Am Heart J.* 2000;140(6):878–885.
79. Kailasam R, Palin CA, Hogue CW Jr. Atrial fibrillation after cardiac surgery: an evidence-based approach to prevention. *Semin Cardiothorac Vasc Anesth.* 2005;9(1):77–85.
80. McMurry SA, Hogue CW Jr. Atrial fibrillation and cardiac surgery. *Curr Opin Anaesthesiol.* 2004;17(1):63–70.
81. Chatap G, Giraud K, Vincent JP. Atrial fibrillation in the elderly: facts and management. *Drugs Aging.* 2002;19(11):819–846.
82. Hersi A, Wyse DG. Management of atrial fibrillation. *Curr Probl Cardiol.* 2005;30(4):175–233.
83. Kopecky SL, Gersh BJ, McGoon MD, et al. Lone atrial fibrillation in elderly persons: a marker for cardiovascular risk. *Arch Intern Med.* 1999;159(10): 1118–1122.
84. Nattel S, Opie LH. Controversies in atrial fibrillation. *Lancet.* 2006;367 (9506):262–272.
85. Wyse DG, Waldo AL, DiMarco JP, et al. Atrial Fibrillation Follow-up Investigation of Rhythm Management (AFFIRM) Investigators. A comparison of rate control and rhythm control in patients with atrial fibrillation. *N Engl J Med.* 2002;347(23):1825–1833.
86. Fuster V, Ryden LE, Cannom DS, et al: American College of Cardiology; American Heart Association Task Force; European Society of Cardiology Committee for Practice Guidelines; European Heart Rhythm Association; Heart Rhythm Society. ACC/AHA/ESC 2006 guidelines for the management of patients with atrial fibrillation: full text: a report of the American College of Cardiology/American Heart Association Task Force on practice guidelines and the European Society of Cardiology Committee for Practice Guidelines (Writing Committee to Revise the 2001 guidelines for the management of patients with atrial fibrillation) developed in collaboration with the European Heart Rhythm Association and the Heart Rhythm Society. *Europace.* 2006;8(9):651–745.
87. Snow V, Weiss KB, LeFevre M, et al. AAFP Panel on Atrial Fibrillation; ACP Panel on Atrial Fibrillation. Management of newly detected atrial fibrillation: a clinical practice guideline from the American Academy of Family Physicians and the American College of Physicians. *Ann Intern Med.* 2003;139(12):1009–1017.
88. Monette J, Gurwitz JH, Rochon PA, et al. Physician attitudes concerning warfarin for stroke prevention in atrial fibrillation: results of a survey of long-term care practitioners. *J Am Geriatr Soc.* 1997;45(9):1060–1065.
89. Vasishta S, Toor F, Johansen A, et al. Stroke prevention in atrial fibrillation: physicians' attitudes to anticoagulation in older people. *Arch Gerontol Geriatr.* 2001;33(3):219–226.
90. Singer DE, Albers GW, Dalen JE, et al. Antithrombotic therapy in atrial fibrillation: the Seventh ACCP Conference on Antithrombotic and Thrombolytic Therapy. *Chest.* 2004;126(3 Suppl):429S–456S.

91. Zipes DP, Wellens HJ. Sudden cardiac death. *Circulation.* 1998;98(21):2334–2351.
92. Bayes de Luna A, Coumel P, Leclercq JF. Ambulatory sudden cardiac death: mechanisms of production of fatal arrhythmia on the basis of data from 157 cases. *Am Heart J.* 1989;117(1):151–159.
93. Fleg JL, Kennedy HL. Cardiac arrhythmias in a healthy elderly population: detection by 24-hour ambulatory electrocardiography. *Chest.* 1982; 81(3):302–307.
94. Fleg JL, Kennedy HL. Long-term prognostic significance of ambulatory electrocardiographic findings in apparently healthy subjects greater than or equal to 60 years of age. *Am J Cardiol.* 1992;70(7):748–751.
95. Sajadieh A, Nielsen OW, Rasmussen V, et al. Ventricular arrhythmias and risk of death and acute myocardial infarction in apparently healthy subjects of age >or =55 years. *Am J Cardiol.* 2006;97(9):1351–1357.
96. Manolio TA, Furberg CD, Rautaharju PM, et al. Cardiac arrhythmias on 24-h ambulatory electrocardiography in older women and men: the Cardiovascular Health Study. *J Am Coll Cardiol.* 1994;23(4):916–925.
97. Hedblad B, Janzon L, Johansson BW, et al. Survival and incidence of myocardial infarction in men with ambulatory ECG-detected frequent and complex ventricular arrhythmias. 10-year follow-up of the 'Men born 1914' study in Malmo, Sweden. *Eur Heart J.* 1997;18(11):1787–1795.
98. Kennedy HL, Whitlock JA, Sprague MK, et al. Long-term follow-up of asymptomatic healthy subjects with frequent and complex ventricular ectopy. *N Engl J Med.* 1985;312(4):193–197.
99. Kahan T, Bergfeldt L. Left ventricular hypertrophy in hypertension: its arrhythmogenic potential. *Heart.* 2005;91(2):250–256.
100. Aronow WS, Epstein S, Koenigsberg M, et al. Usefulness of echocardiographic left ventricular hypertrophy, ventricular tachycardia and complex ventricular arrhythmias in predicting ventricular fibrillation or sudden cardiac death in elderly patients. *Am J Cardiol.* 1988;62(16):1124–1125.
101. ECC Committee, Subcommittees and Task Forces of the American Heart Association. 2005 American Heart Association Guidelines for Cardiopulmonary Resuscitation and Emergency Cardiovascular Care. *Circulation.* 2005;112(24 Suppl):IV1–203.
102. Valenzuela TD, Roe DJ, Nichol G, et al. Outcomes of rapid defibrillation by security officers after cardiac arrest in casinos. *N Engl J Med.* 2000; 343(17):1206–1209.
103. Eisenberg MS, Mengert TJ. Cardiac resuscitation. *N Engl J Med.* 2001; 344(17):1304–1313.
104. Teo KK, Yusuf S, Furberg CD. Effects of prophylactic antiarrhythmic drug therapy in acute myocardial infarction. An overview of results from randomized controlled trials. *JAMA.* 1993;270(13):1589–1595.
105. Aronow WS, Mercando AD, Epstein S, et al. Effect of quinidine or procainamide versus no antiarrhythmic drug on sudden cardiac death, total cardiac death, and total death in elderly patients with heart disease and complex ventricular arrhythmias. *Am J Cardiol.* 1990;66(4):423–428.
106. Hilleman DE, Bauman AL. Role of antiarrhythmic therapy in patients at risk for sudden cardiac death: an evidence-based review. *Pharmacotherapy.* 2001;21(5):556–575.
107. Bardy GH, Lee KL, Mark DB, et al. Sudden Cardiac Death in Heart Failure Trial (SCD-HeFT) Investigators. Amiodarone or an implantable cardioverter-defibrillator for congestive heart failure. *N Engl J Med.* 2005; 352(3):225–237.
108. Siddiqui A, Kowey PR. Sudden death secondary to cardiac arrhythmias: mechanisms and treatment strategies. *Curr Opin Cardiol.* 2006;21(5):517–525.
109. Tresch DD, Troup PJ, Thakur RK, et al. Comparison of efficacy of automatic implantable cardioverter defibrillator in patients older and younger than 65 years of age. *Am J Med.* 1991;90(6):717–724.
110. Goldberger Z, Lampert R. Implantable cardioverter-defibrillators: expanding indications and technologies. *JAMA.* 2006;295(7):809–818.
111. Gregoratos G, Abrams J, Epstein AE, et al. ACC/AHA/NASPE 2002 Guideline Update for Implantation of Cardiac Pacemakers and Antiarrhythmia Devices–summary article: a report of the American College of Cardiology/American Heart Association Task Force on Practice Guidelines (ACC/AHA/NASPE Committee to Update the 1998 Pacemaker Guidelines). *J Am Coll Cardiol.* 2002;40(9):1703–1719.
112. Prystowsky EN. Prevention of sudden cardiac death. *Clin Cardiol.* 2005;28(11 Suppl 1):I12–I18.
113. Birnie D, Williams K, Guo A, et al. Reasons for escalating pacemaker implants. *Am J Cardiol.* 2006;98(1):93–97.
114. McPherson CA, Manthous C. Permanent pacemakers and implantable defibrillators: considerations for intensivists. *Am J Respir Crit Care Med.* 2004;170(9):933–940.
115. Stone KR, McPherson CA. Assessment and management of patients with pacemakers and implantable cardioverter defibrillators. *Crit Care Med.* 2004;32(4 Suppl):S155–165.
116. Trohman RG, Kim MH, Pinski SL. Cardiac pacing: the state of the art. *Lancet.* 2004;364(9446):1701–1719.
117. Mueller PS, Hook CC, Hayes DL. Ethical analysis of withdrawal of pacemaker or implantable cardioverter-defibrillator support at the end of life. *Mayo Clin Proc.* 2003;78(8):959–963.
118. Ware JH, Dockery DW, Louis TA, et al. Longitudinal and cross-sectional estimates of pulmonary function decline in never-smoking adults. *Am J Epidemiol.* 1990;132(4):685–700.
119. van Pelt W, Borsboom GJ, Rijcken B, et al. Discrepancies between longitudinal and cross-sectional change in ventilatory function in 12 years of follow-up. *Am J Respir Crit Care Med.* 1994;149(5):1218–1826.
120. Lang MR, Fiaux GW, Gillooly M, et al. Collagen content of alveolar wall tissue in emphysematous and non-emphysematous lungs. *Thorax.* 1994; 49(4):319–326.
121. Andreotti L, Bussotti A, Cammelli D, et al. Connective tissue in aging lung. *Gerontology.* 1983;29(6):377–387.
122. Turner JM, Mead J, Wohl ME. Elasticity of human lungs in relation to age. *J Appl Physiol.* 1968;25(6):664–671.
123. Kronenberg RS, Drage CW. Attenuation of the ventilatory and heart rate responses to hypoxia and hypercapnia with aging in normal men. *J Clin Invest.* 1973;52(8):1812–1819.
124. Brischetto MJ, Millman RP, Peterson DD, et al. Effect of aging on ventilatory response to exercise and CO2. *J Appl Physiol.* 1984;56(5):1143–1150.
125. Babb TG, Rodarte JR. Mechanism of reduced maximal expiratory flow with aging. *J Appl Physiol.* 2000;89(2):505–511.
126. Fowler RW, Pluck RA, Hetzel MR. Maximal expiratory flow-volume curves in Londoners aged 60 years and over. *Thorax.* 1987;42(3):173–182.
127. Mittman C, Edelman NH, Norris AH, et al. Relationship between chest wall and pulmonary compliance and age. *J Appl Physiol.* 1965; 20:1211–1216.
128. Levitzky MG. Effects of aging on the respiratory system. *Physiologist.* 1984;27(2):102–107.
129. Mellemgaard K. The alveolar-arterial oxygen difference: its size and components in normal man. *Acta Physiol Scand.* 1966;67(1):10–20.
130. Sorbini CA, Grassi V, Solinas E, et al. Arterial oxygen tension in relation to age in healthy subjects. *Respiration.* 1968;25(1):3–13.
131. Cardus J, Burgos F, Diaz O, et al. Increase in pulmonary ventilation-perfusion inequality with age in healthy individuals. *Am J Respir Crit Care Med.* 1997;156(2 Pt 1):648–653.
132. Delclaux B, Orcel B, Housset B, et al. Arterial blood gases in elderly persons with chronic obstructive pulmonary disease (COPD). *Eur Respir J.* 1994;7(5):856–861.
133. Janssens JP. Aging of the respiratory system: impact on pulmonary function tests and adaptation to exertion. *Clin Chest Med.* 2005;26(3):469–484, vi–vii.
134. Knudson RJ. How aging affects the normal lung. *J Respir Dis.* 1981;2:74–84.
135. Skorodin MS. Respiratory disease and A-a gradient measurement. *JAMA.* 1984;252:1344. (letter).
136. Prentice AM, Jebb SA. Beyond body mass index. *Obes Rev.* 2001;2(3):141–147.
137. Ritz P. Factors affecting energy and macronutrient requirements in elderly people. *Public Health Nutr.* 2001;4(2B):561–568.
138. Steen B. Body composition and aging. *Nutr Rev.* 1988;46(2):45–51.
139. Wurtman JJ, Lieberman H, Tsay R, et al. Calorie and nutrient intakes of elderly and young subjects measured under identical conditions. *J Gerontol.* 1988;43(6):B174–B180.
140. Rolls BJ, Dimeo KA, Shide DJ. Age-related impairments in the regulation of food intake. *Am J Clin Nutr.* 1995;62(5):923–931.
141. Mowe M, Bohmer T. The prevalence of undiagnosed protein-calorie undernutrition in a population of hospitalized elderly patients. *J Am Geriatr Soc.* 1991;39(11):1089–1092.
142. Visvanathan R. Under-nutrition in older people: a serious and growing global problem! *J Postgrad Med.* 2003;49(4):352–360.
143. Cederholm T, Jagren C, Hellstrom K. Outcome of protein-energy malnutrition in elderly medical patients. *Am J Med.* 1995;98(1):67–74.
144. Constans T, Bacq Y, Brechot JF, Guilmot JL, et al. Protein-energy malnutrition in elderly medical patients. *J Am Geriatr Soc.* 1992;40(3):263–268.
145. Brownie S. Why are elderly individuals at risk of nutritional deficiency? *Int J Nurs Pract.* 2006;12(2):110–118.
146. Deschamps V, Astier X, Ferry M, et al. Nutritional status of healthy elderly persons living in Dordogne, France, and relation with mortality and cognitive or functional decline. *Eur J Clin Nutr.* 2002;56(4):305–312.
147. Pearson JM, Schlettwein-Gsell D, Brzozowska A, et al. Life style characteristics associated with nutritional risk in elderly subjects aged 80-85 years. *J Nutr Health Aging.* 2001;5(4):278–283.
148. Hays NP, Roberts SB. The anorexia of aging in humans. *Physiol Behav.* 2006;88(3):257–266.
149. Omran ML, Morley JE. Assessment of protein energy malnutrition in older persons, part I: history, examination, body composition, and screening tools. *Nutrition.* 2000;16(1):50–63.
150. Omran ML, Morley JE. Assessment of protein energy malnutrition in older persons, Part II: laboratory evaluation. *Nutrition.* 2000;16(2):131–140.
151. van Bokhorst-de van der Schueren MA, Klinkenberg M, Thijs A. Profile of the malnourished patient. *Eur J Clin Nutr.* 2005;59(10):1129–1135.
152. Harris D, Haboubi N. Malnutrition screening in the elderly population. *J R Soc Med.* 2005;98(9):411–414.
153. Schmidt H, Martindale R. The gastrointestinal tract in critical illness. *Curr Opin Clin Nutr Metab Care.* 2001;4(6):547–551.

154. Nieuwenhuijzen GA, Deitch EA, Goris RJ. Infection, the gut and the development of the multiple organ dysfunction syndrome. *Eur J Surg.* 1996;162(4):259–273.
155. Witte KK, Nikitin NP, Parker AC, et al. The effect of micronutrient supplementation on quality-of-life and left ventricular function in elderly patients with chronic heart failure. *Eur Heart J.* 2005;26(21):2238–2244.
156. Webb JG, Kiess MC, Chan-Yan CC. Malnutrition and the heart. *CMAJ.* 1986;135(7):753–758.
157. Creutzberg EC, Wouters EF, Mostert R, et al. Efficacy of nutritional supplementation therapy in depleted patients with chronic obstructive pulmonary disease. *Nutrition.* 2003;19(2):120–127.
158. Schols AM. Nutrition in chronic obstructive pulmonary disease. *Curr Opin Pulm Med.* 2000;6(2):110–115.
159. Schols AM. Pulmonary cachexia. *Int J Cardiol.* 2002;85(1):101–110.
160. Lesourd B. Nutrition: a major factor influencing immunity in the elderly. *J Nutr Health Aging.* 2004;8(1):28–37.
161. Hollington P, Mawdsley J, Lim W, et al. An 11-year experience of enterocutaneous fistula. *Br J Surg.* 2004;91(12):1646–1651.
162. Demling RH. The incidence and impact of pre-existing protein energy malnutrition on outcome in the elderly burn patient population. *J Burn Care Rehabil.* 2005;26(1):94–100.
163. Witte MB, Barbul A. Repair of full-thickness bowel injury. *Crit Care Med.* 2003;31(8 Suppl):S538–S546.
164. Mathus-Vliegen EM. Old age, malnutrition, and pressure sores: an ill-fated alliance. *J Gerontol A Biol Sci Med Sci.* 2004;59(4):355–360.
165. Sullivan DH, Bopp MM, Roberson PK. Protein-energy undernutrition and life-threatening complications among the hospitalized elderly. *J Gen Intern Med.* 2002;17(12):923–932.
166. Johansen N, Kondrup J, Plum LM, et al. Effect of nutritional support on clinical outcome in patients at nutritional risk. *Clin Nutr.* 2004;23(4):539–550.
167. Covinsky KE, Martin GE, Beyth RJ, et al. The relationship between clinical assessments of nutritional status and adverse outcomes in older hospitalized medical patients. *J Am Geriatr Soc.* 1999;47(5):532–538.
168. Giner M, Laviano A, Meguid MM, et al. In 1995 a correlation between malnutrition and poor outcome in critically ill patients still exists. *Nutrition.* 1996;12(1):23–29.
169. Cerra FB, Benitez MR, Blackburn GL, et al. Applied nutrition in ICU patients. A consensus statement of the American College of Chest Physicians. *Chest.* 1997;111(3):769–778.
170. Sullivan DH, Sun S, Walls RC. Protein-energy undernutrition among elderly hospitalized patients: a prospective study. *JAMA.* 1999;281(21):2013–2019.
171. Guigoz Y, Vellas B, Garry PJ. Assessing the nutritional status of the elderly: the Mini Nutritional Assessment as part of the geriatric evaluation. *Nutr Rev.* 1996;54(1 Pt 2):S59–S65.
172. Omran ML, Salem P. Diagnosing undernutrition. *Clin Geriatr Med.* 2002;18(4):719–736.
173. Garrow JS, Webster J. Quetelet's index (W/H2) as a measure of fatness. *Int J Obes.* 1985;9(2):147–153.
174. US Department of Health and Human Services; National Institutes of Health: http://www.nhlbi.nih.gov/health/public/heart/obesity/lose_wt/risk.htm (last accessed on 20 April 2007)
175. Flodin L, Svensson S, Cederholm T. Body mass index as a predictor of 1 year mortality in geriatric patients. *Clin Nutr.* 2000;19(2):121–125.
176. Galanos AN, Pieper CF, Kussin PS, et al. Relationship of body mass index to subsequent mortality among seriously ill hospitalized patients. SUPPORT Investigators. The Study to Understand Prognoses and Preferences for Outcome and Risks of Treatments. *Crit Care Med.* 1997;25(12):1962–1968.
177. Beck AM, Ovesen L. At which body mass index and degree of weight loss should hospitalized elderly patients be considered at nutritional risk? *Clin Nutr.* 1998;17(5):195–198.
178. Stevens J, Cai J, Pamuk ER, et al. The effect of age on the association between body-mass index and mortality. *N Engl J Med.* 1998;338(1):1–7.
179. Davidson I, Smith S. Nutritional screening: pitfalls of nutritional screening in the injured obese patient. *Proc Nutr Soc.* 2004;63(3):421–425.
180. Kalliomaki JL, Siltavuori L, Virtama P. Stature and aging. *J Am Geriatr Soc.* 1973;21(11):504–506.
181. Dequeker JV, Baeyens JP, Claessens J. The significance of stature as a clinical measurement of aging. *J Am Geriatr Soc.* 1969;17(2):169–179.
182. Han TS, Lean ME. Lower leg length as an index of stature in adults. *Int J Obes Relat Metab Disord.* 1996;20(1):21–27.
183. Noppa H, Andersson M, Bengtsson C, et al. Body composition in middle-aged women with special reference to the correlation between body fat mass and anthropometric data. *Am J Clin Nutr.* 1979;32(7):1388–1395.
184. Rossner S. Obesity in the elderly—a future matter of concern? *Obes Rev.* 2001;2(3):183–188.
185. Villareal DT, Apovian CM, Kushner RF, et al: NAASO, The Obesity Society. Obesity in older adults: technical review and position statement of the American Society for Nutrition and NAASO, The Obesity Society. *Am J Clin Nutr.* 2005;82(5):923–934.
186. Zamboni M, Mazzali G, Zoico E, et al. Health consequences of obesity in the elderly: a review of four unresolved questions. *Int J Obes* (Lond). 2005;29(9):1011–1029.
187. Liu KJ, Cho MJ, Atten MJ, et al. Hypocaloric parenteral nutrition support in elderly obese patients. *Am Surg.* 2000;66(4):394–399.
188. Covinsky KE, Covinsky MH, Palmer RM, et al. Serum albumin concentration and clinical assessments of nutritional status in hospitalized older people: different sides of different coins? *J Am Geriatr Soc.* 2002;50(4):631–637.
189. Campion EW, deLabry LO, Glynn RJ. The effect of age on serum albumin in healthy males: report from the Normative Aging Study. *J Gerontol.* 1988;43(1):M18–M20.
190. Cooper JK, Gardner C. Effect of aging on serum albumin. *J Am Geriatr Soc.* 1989;37(11):1039–1042.
191. Fuhrman MP, Charney P, Mueller CM. Hepatic proteins and nutrition assessment. *J Am Diet Assoc.* 2004;104(8):1258–1264.
192. Goldwasser P, Feldman J. Association of serum albumin and mortality risk. *J Clin Epidemiol.* 1997;50(6):693–703.
193. Don BR, Kaysen G. Serum albumin: relationship to inflammation and nutrition. *Semin Dial.* 2004;17(6):432–437.
194. Sung J, Bochicchio GV, Joshi M, et al. Admission serum albumin is predicitve of outcome in critically ill trauma patients. *Am Surg.* 2004;70 (12):1099–1102.
195. Corti MC, Guralnik JM, Salive ME, et al. Serum albumin level and physical disability as predictors of mortality in older persons. *JAMA.* 1994;272(13):1036–1042.
196. Chojkier M. Inhibition of albumin synthesis in chronic diseases: molecular mechanisms. *J Clin Gastroenterol.* 2005;39(4 Suppl 2):S143–S146.
197. Nicholson JP, Wolmarans MR, Park GR. The role of albumin in critical illness. *Br J Anaesth.* 2000;85(4):599–610.
198. Rothschild MA, Oratz M, Schreiber SS. Albumin synthesis. 1. *N Engl J Med.* 1972;286(14):748–757.
199. Rothschild MA, Oratz M, Schreiber SS. Albumin synthesis (second of two parts). *N Engl J Med.* 1972;286(15):816–821.
200. Cerra FB. Hypermetabolism, organ failure, and metabolic support. *Surgery.* 1987;101(1):1–14.
201. Wernerman J, Hammarqvist F, Gamrin L, et al. Protein metabolism in critical illness. *Baillieres Clin Endocrinol Metab.* 1996;10(4):603–615.
202. Plank LD, Hill GL. Energy balance in critical illness. *Proc Nutr Soc.* 2003; 62(2):545–552.
203. Uehara M, Plank LD, Hill GL. Components of energy expenditure in patients with severe sepsis and major trauma: a basis for clinical care. *Crit Care Med.* 1999;27(7):1295–1302.
204. Heiat A, Vaccarino V, Krumholz HM. An evidence-based assessment of federal guidelines for overweight and obesity as they apply to elderly persons. *Arch Intern Med.* 2001;161(9):1194–1203.
205. Executive summary of the clinical guidelines on the identification, evaluation, and treatment of overweight and obesity in adults. *Arch Intern Med.* 1998;158(17):1855–1867.
206. Harris J, Benedict F. A biometric study of basal metabolism in man. Washington D.C. Carnegie Institute of Washington. 1919.
207. Cheng CH, Chen CH, Wong Y, et al. Measured versus estimated energy expenditure in mechanically ventilated critically ill patients. *Clin Nutr.* 2002;21(2):165–172.
208. Frankenfield DC, Smith JS, Cooney RN. Accelerated nitrogen loss after traumatic injury is not attenuated by achievement of energy balance. *JPEN J Parenter Enteral Nutr.* 1997;21(6):324–329.
209. Long CL, Schaffel N, Geiger JW, et al. Metabolic response to injury and illness: estimation of energy and protein needs from indirect calorimetry and nitrogen balance. *JPEN J Parenter Enteral Nutr.* 1979;3(6):452–456.
210. Klein CJ, Stanek GS, Wiles CE 3rd. Overfeeding macronutrients to critically ill adults: metabolic complications. *J Am Diet Assoc.* 1998;98(7):795–806.
211. Heyland DK, Dhaliwal R, Drover JW, et al: Canadian Critical Care Clinical Practice Guidelines Committee. Canadian clinical practice guidelines for nutrition support in mechanically ventilated, critically ill adult patients. *JPEN J Parenter Enteral Nutr.* 2003;27(5):355–373.
212. Woodcock NP, Zeigler D, Palmer MD, et al. Enteral versus parenteral nutrition: a pragmatic study. *Nutrition.* 2001;17(1):1–12.
213. Heyland DK, Dhaliwal R, Day A, et al. Validation of the Canadian clinical practice guidelines for nutrition support in mechanically ventilated, critically ill adult patients: results of a prospective observational study. *Crit Care Med.* 2004;32(11):2260–2266.
214. Wernerman J. Guidelines for nutritional support in intensive care unit patients: a critical analysis. *Curr Opin Clin Nutr Metab Care.* 2005;8(2):171–175.
215. Kreymann KG, Berger MM, Deutz NE, et al; ESPEN (European Society for Parenteral and Enteral Nutrition). ESPEN Guidelines on Enteral Nutrition: intensive care. *Clin Nutr.* 2006;25(2):210–223. Epub 2006 May 11.
216. Bistrian BR, McCowen KC. Nutritional and metabolic support in the adult intensive care unit: key controversies. *Crit Care Med.* 2006;34(5):1525–1531.
217. Griffiths RD, Bongers T. Nutrition support for patients in the intensive care unit. *Postgrad Med J.* 2005;81(960):629–636.
218. Griffiths RD. Is parenteral nutrition really that risky in the intensive care unit? *Curr Opin Clin Nutr Metab Care.* 2004;7(2):175–181.
219. Debaveye Y, Van den Berghe G. Risks and benefits of nutritional support during critical illness. *Annu Rev Nutr.* 2006;26:513–538.

220. Hoste EA, Clermont G, Kersten A, et al. RIFLE criteria for acute kidney injury are associated with hospital mortality in critically ill patients: a cohort analysis. *Crit Care.* 2006;10(3):R73. Epub 2006 May 12.
221. Schiffl H. Renal recovery from acute tubular necrosis requiring renal replacement therapy: a prospective study in critically ill patients. *Nephrol Dial Transplant.* 2006;21(5):1248–1252. Epub 2006 Jan 31.
222. Lindeman RD. Overview: renal physiology and pathophysiology of aging. *Am J Kidney Dis.* 1990;16(4):275–282.
223. Epstein M. Aging and the kidney. *J Am Soc Nephrol.* 1996;7(8):1106–1122.
224. Lindeman RD, Tobin J, Shock NW. Longitudinal studies on the rate of decline in renal function with age. *J Am Geriatr Soc.* 1985;33(4):278–285.
225. Lindeman RD, Goldman R. Anatomic and physiologic age changes in the kidney. *Exp Gerontol.* 1986;21(4-5):379–406.
226. Davies DF, Shock NW. Age changes in glomerular filtration rate, effective renal plasma flow, and tubular excretory capacity in adult males. *J Clin Invest.* 1950;29(5):496–507.
227. Hollenberg NK, Adams DF, Solomon HS, et al. Senescence and the renal vasculature in normal man. *Circ Res.* 1974;34(3):309–316.
228. Cortes P, Zhao X, Dumler F, et al. Age-related changes in glomerular volume and hydroxyproline content in rat and human. *J Am Soc Nephrol.* 1992;2(12):1716–1725.
229. Meyer BR. Renal function in aging. *J Am Geriatr Soc.* 1989;37(8):791–800.
230. Wharton WW 3rd, Sondeen JL, McBiles M, et al. Measurement of glomerular filtration rate in ICU patients using 99mTc-DTPA and inulin. *Kidney Int.* 1992;42(1):174–178.
231. Tietz NW, Shuey DF, Wekstein DR. Laboratory values in fit aging individuals—sexagenarians through centenarians. *Clin Chem.* 1992;38(6):1167–1185.
232. Cockcroft DW, Gault MH. Prediction of creatinine clearance from serum creatinine. *Nephron.* 1976;16(1):31–41.
233. Burkhardt H, Bojarsky G, Gretz N, et al. Creatinine clearance, Cockcroft-Gault formula and cystatin C: estimators of true glomerular filtration rate in the elderly? *Gerontology.* 2002;48(3):140–146.
234. Hoek FJ, Kemperman FA, Krediet RT. A comparison between cystatin C, plasma creatinine and the Cockcroft and Gault formula for the estimation of glomerular filtration rate. *Nephrol Dial Transplant.* 2003;18(10):2024–2031.
235. Dharnidharka VR, Kwon C, Stevens G. Serum cystatin C is superior to serum creatinine as a marker of kidney function: a meta-analysis. *Am J Kidney Dis.* 2002;40(2):221–226.
236. Kuan Y, Hossain M, Surman J, et al. GFR prediction using the MDRD and Cockcroft and Gault equations in patients with end-stage renal disease. *Nephrol Dial Transplant.* 2005;20(11):2394–2401. Epub 2005 Aug 22.
237. O'Connell MB, Wong MO, Bannick-Mohrland SD, et al. Accuracy of 2- and 8-hour urine collections for measuring creatinine clearance in the hospitalized elderly. *Pharmacotherapy.* 1993;13(2):135–142.
238. Baumann TJ, Staddon JE, Horst HM, et al. Minimum urine collection periods for accurate determination of creatinine clearance in critically ill patients. *Clin Pharm.* 1987;6(5):393–398.
239. Luft FC, Weinberger MH, Fineberg NS, et al. Effects of age on renal sodium homeostasis and its relevance to sodium sensitivity. *Am J Med.* 1987;82(1B):9–15.
240. Rowe JW, Shock NW, DeFronzo RA. The influence of age on the renal response to water deprivation in man. *Nephron.* 1976;17(4):270–278.
241. Agarwal BN, Cabebe FG. Renal acidification in elderly subjects. *Nephron.* 1980;26(6):291–295.
242. Bellomo R, Ronco C, Kellum JA, et al: Acute Dialysis Quality Initiative workgroup. Acute renal failure—definition, outcome measures, animal models, fluid therapy and information technology needs: the Second International Consensus Conference of the Acute Dialysis Quality Initiative (ADQI) Group. *Crit Care.* 2004;8(4):R204–R212.
243. Taber SS, Mueller BA. Drug-associated renal dysfunction. *Crit Care Clin.* 2006;22(2):357–374, viii.
244. Leblanc M, Kellum JA, Gibney RT, et al. Risk factors for acute renal failure: inherent and modifiable risks. *Curr Opin Crit Care.* 2005;11(6):533–536.
245. van den Berk G, Tonino S, de Fijter C, et al. Bench-to-bedside review: preventive measures for contrast-induced nephropathy in critically ill patients. *Crit Care.* 2005;9(4):361–370. Epub 2005 Jan 7.
246. Meschi M, Detrenis S, Musini S, et al. Facts and fallacies concerning the prevention of contrast medium-induced nephropathy. *Crit Care Med.* 2006;34(8):2060–2068.
247. Bagshaw SM, McAlister FA, Manns BJ, et al. Acetylcysteine in the prevention of contrast-induced nephropathy: a case study of the pitfalls in the evolution of evidence. *Arch Intern Med.* 2006;166(2):161–166.
248. Muhlberg W, Platt D. Age-dependent changes of the kidneys: pharmacological implications. *Gerontology.* 1999;45(5):243–253.
249. Lonner JH, Koval KJ. Polytrauma in the elderly. *Clin Orthop Relat Res.* 1995;(318):136–143.
250. Center for Disease Control: National Center for Injury Control and Prevention: http://www.cdc.gov/ncipc/fact_book/factbook.htm (Last accessed on 20 April, 2007)
251. Hogue CC. Injury in late life: part I. Epidemiology. *J Am Geriatr Soc.* 1982;30(3):183–190.
252. Mosenthal AC, Livingston DH, Elcavage J, et al. Falls: epidemiology and strategies for prevention. *J Trauma.* 1995;38(5):753–756.
253. Spaite DW, Criss EA, Valenzuela TD, et al. Geriatric injury: an analysis of prehospital demographics, mechanisms, and patterns. *Ann Emerg Med.* 1990;19(12):1418–1421.
254. Hannan EL, Waller CH, Farrell LS, et al. Elderly trauma inpatients in New York state: 1994–1998. *J Trauma.* 2004;56(6):1297–1304.
255. Nagy KK, Smith RF, Roberts RR, et al. Prognosis of penetrating trauma in elderly patients: a comparison with younger patients. *J Trauma.* 2000;49(2):190–193; discussion 193–194.
256. McMahon DJ, Shapiro MB, et al. The injured elderly in the trauma intensive care unit. *Surg Clin North Am.* 2000;80(3):1005–1019.
257. Jacobs DG, Plaisier BR, Barie PS, et al. EAST Practice Management Guidelines Work Group. Practice management guidelines for geriatric trauma: the EAST Practice Management Guidelines Work Group. *J Trauma.* 2003;54(2):391–416.
258. Mann FA, Kubal WS, Blackmore CC. Improving the imaging diagnosis of cervical spine injury in the very elderly: implications of the epidemiology of injury. *Emergency Radiol.* 2000; 7(1):36–41.
259. Ehara S, Shimamura T. Cervical spine injury in the elderly: imaging features. *Skeletal Radiol.* 2001;30(1):1–7.
260. Prasad VS, Schwartz A, Bhutani R, et al. Characteristics of injuries to the cervical spine and spinal cord in polytrauma patient population: experience from a regional trauma unit. *Spinal Cord.* 1999;37(8):560–568.
261. MacLeod J, Lynn M, McKenney MG, et al. Predictors of mortality in trauma patients. *Am Surg.* 2004;70(9):805–810.
262. Davis JW, Kaups KL. Base deficit in the elderly: a marker of severe injury and death. *J Trauma.* 1998;45(5):873–877.
263. Demetriades D, Karaiskakis M, Velmahos G, et al. Effect on outcome of early intensive management of geriatric trauma patients. *Br J Surg.* 2002;89(10):1319–1322.
264. McKinley BA, Marvin RG, Cocanour CS, et al. Blunt trauma resuscitation: the old can respond. *Arch Surg.* 2000;135(6):688–693; discussion 694–695.
265. Scalea TM, Simon HM, Duncan AO, et al. Geriatric blunt multiple trauma: improved survival with early invasive monitoring. *J Trauma.* 1990;30(2):129–34; discussion 134–136.
266. Flanagan SR, Hibbard MR, Riordan B, et al. Traumatic brain injury in the elderly: diagnostic and treatment challenges. *Clin Geriatr Med.* 2006;22(2):449–468; x.
267. Rutland-Brown W, Langlois JA, Thomas KE, et al. Incidence of traumatic brain injury in the United States, 2003. *J Head Trauma Rehabil.* 2006;21(6):544–548.
268. Thompson HJ, McCormick WC, Kagan SH. Traumatic brain injury in older adults: epidemiology, outcomes, and future implications. *J Am Geriatr Soc.* 2006;54(10):1590–1595.
269. Rathlev NK, Medzon R, Lowery D, et al. Intracranial pathology in elders with blunt head trauma. *Acad Emerg Med.* 2006;13(3):302–307.
270. Adekoya N, Thurman DJ, White DD, et al. Surveillance for traumatic brain injury deaths—United States, 1989–1998. *MMWR Surveill Summ.* 2002;51(10):1–14.
271. Coronado VG, Thomas KE, Sattin RW, et al. The CDC traumatic brain injury surveillance system: characteristics of persons aged 65 years and older hospitalized with a TBI. *J Head Trauma Rehabil.* 2005;20(3):215–228.
272. Stocchetti N, Furlan A, Volta F. Hypoxemia and arterial hypotension at the accident scene in head injury. *J Trauma.* 1996;40(5):764–767.
273. Eisenberg HM, Frankowski RF, Contant CF, et al. High-dose barbiturate control of elevated intracranial pressure in patients with severe head injury. *J Neurosurg.* 1988;69(1):15–23.
274. Jeremitsky E, Omert LA, Dunham CM, et al. The impact of hyperglycemia on patients with severe brain injury. *J Trauma.* 2005;58(1):47–50.
275. Cairns CJ, Andrews PJ. Management of hyperthermia in traumatic brain injury. *Curr Opin Crit Care.* 2002;8(2):106–110.
276. Coles JP, Fryer TD, Coleman MR, et al. Hyperventilation following head injury: effect on ischemic burden and cerebral oxidative metabolism. *Crit Care Med.* 2007;35(2):568–578.
277. Muizelaar JP, Marmarou A, Ward JD, et al. Adverse effects of prolonged hyperventilation in patients with severe head injury: a randomized clinical trial. *J Neurosurg.* 1991;75(5):731–739.
278. Doyle JA, Davis DP, Hoyt DB. The use of hypertonic saline in the treatment of traumatic brain injury. *J Trauma.* 2001;50(2):367–383.
279. Bullock R, Chesnut RM, Clifton G, et al. Guidelines for the management of severe head injury. Brain Trauma Foundation. *Eur J Emerg Med.* 1996;3(2):109–127.
280. Mosenthal AC, Lavery RF, Addis M, et al. Isolated traumatic brain injury: age is an independent predictor of mortality and early outcome. *J Trauma.* 2002;52(5):907–911.
281. LeBlanc J, de Guise E, Gosselin N, et al. Comparison of functional outcome following acute care in young, middle-aged and elderly patients with traumatic brain injury. *Brain Inj.* 2006;20(8):779–790.
282. Hukkelhoven CW, Steyerberg EW, Rampen AJ, et al. Patient age and outcome following severe traumatic brain injury: an analysis of 5,600 patients. *J Neurosurg.* 2003;99(4):666–673.

283. Hu R, Mustard CA, Burns C. Epidemiology of incident spinal fracture in a complete population. *Spine.* 1996;21(4):492–499.
284. Gale SC, Gracias VH, Reilly PM, et al. The inefficiency of plain radiography to evaluate the cervical spine after blunt trauma. *J Trauma.* 2005;59(5):1121–1125.
285. Lomoschitz FM, Blackmore CC, Mirza SK, et al. Cervical spine injuries in patients 65 years old and older: epidemiologic analysis regarding the effects of age and injury mechanism on distribution, type, and stability of injuries. *AJR Am J Roentgenol.* 2002;178(3):573–577.
286. Widder S, Doig C, Burrowes P, et al. Prospective evaluation of computed tomographic scanning for the spinal clearance of obtunded trauma patients: preliminary results. *J Trauma.* 2004;56(6):1179–1184.
287. Schenarts PJ, Diaz J, Kaiser C, et al. Prospective comparison of admission computed tomographic scan and plain films of the upper cervical spine in trauma patients with altered mental status. *J Trauma.* 2001;51(4):663–668.
288. Mace SE. The unstable occult cervical spine fracture: a review. *Am J Emerg Med.* 1992;10(2):136–142.
289. Barry TB, McNamara RM. Clinical decision rules and cervical spine injury in an elderly patient: a word of caution. *J Emerg Med.* 2005;29(4):433–436.
290. Heffernan DS, Schermer CR, Lu SW. What defines a distracting injury in cervical spine assessment? *J Trauma.* 2005;59(6):1396–1399.
291. Holcomb JB, McMullin NR, Kozar RA, et al. Morbidity from rib fractures increases after age 45. *J Am Coll Surg.* 2003;196(4):549–555.
292. Bulger EM, Arneson MA, Mock CN, et al. Rib fractures in the elderly. *J Trauma.* 2000;48(6):1040–1046.
293. Karmakar MK, Critchley LA, Ho AM, et al. Continuous thoracic paravertebral infusion of bupivacaine for pain management in patients with multiple fractured ribs. *Chest.* 2003;123(2):424–431.
294. Bulger EM, Edwards T, Klotz P, et al. Epidural analgesia improves outcome after multiple rib fractures. *Surgery.* 2004;136(2):426–430.
295. Kieninger AN, Bair HA, Bendick PJ, et al. Epidural versus intravenous pain control in elderly patients with rib fractures. *Am J Surg.* 2005;189(3):327–330.
296. Falimirski ME, Provost D. Nonsurgical management of solid abdominal organ injury in patients over 55 years of age. *Am Surg.* 2000;66(7):631–635.
297. Krause KR, Howells GA, Bair HA, et al. Nonoperative management of blunt splenic injury in adults 55 years and older: a twenty-year experience. *Am Surg.* 2000;66(7):636–640.
298. Franklin GA, Casos SR. Current advances in the surgical approach to abdominal trauma. *Injury.* 2006;37(12):1143–1156. Epub 2006 Nov 7.
299. Looker AC, Johnston CC Jr, Wahner HW, et al. Prevalence of low femoral bone density in older U.S. women from NHANES III. *J Bone Miner Res.* 1995;10(5):796–802.
300. Wehren LE. The epidemiology of osteoporosis and fractures in geriatric medicine. *Clin Geriatr Med.* 2003;19(2):245–258.
301. Henry SM, Pollak AN, Jones AL, et al. Pelvic fracture in geriatric patients: a distinct clinical entity. *J Trauma.* 2002;53(1):15–20.
302. Dyer GS, Vrahas MS. Review of the pathophysiology and acute management of haemorrhage in pelvic fracture. *Injury.* 2006;37(7):602–613.
303. Pohlemann T, Bosch U, Gansslen A, et al. The Hannover experience in management of pelvic fractures. *Clin Orthop Relat Res.* 1994;(305):69–80.
304. Perry JF Jr. Pelvic open fractures. *Clin Orthop Relat Res.* 1980;(151):41–45.
305. Hanson PB, Milne JC, Chapman MW. Open fractures of the pelvis. Review of 43 cases. *J Bone Joint Surg Br.* 1991;73(2):325–329.
306. Dente CJ, Feliciano DV, Rozycki GS, et al. The outcome of open pelvic fractures in the modern era. *Am J Surg.* 2005;190(6):830–835.
307. Bone LB, McNamara K, Shine B, et al. Mortality in multiple trauma patients with fractures. *J Trauma.* 1994;37(2):262–264; discussion 264–265.
308. Dunham CM, Bosse MJ, Clancy TV, et al. EAST Practice Management Guidelines Work Group. Practice management guidelines for the optimal timing of long-bone fracture stabilization in polytrauma patients: the EAST Practice Management Guidelines Work Group. *J Trauma.* 2001;50(5):958–967.
309. Crowl AC, Young JS, Kahler DM, et al. Occult hypoperfusion is associated with increased morbidity in patients undergoing early femur fracture fixation. *J Trauma.* 2000;48(2):260–267.
310. Grossman MD, Miller D, Scaff DW, et al. When is an elder old? Effect of preexisting conditions on mortality in geriatric trauma. *J Trauma.* 2002;52(2):242–246.
311. Perdue PW, Watts DD, Kaufmann CR, et al. Differences in mortality between elderly and younger adult trauma patients: geriatric status increases risk of delayed death. *J Trauma.* 1998;45(4):805–810.
312. Morris JA Jr, MacKenzie EJ, Damiano AM, et al. Mortality in trauma patients: the interaction between host factors and severity. *J Trauma.* 1990;30(12):1476–1482.
313. Taylor MD, Tracy JK, Meyer W, et al. Trauma in the elderly: intensive care unit resource use and outcome. *J Trauma.* 2002;53(3):407–414.
314. McKevitt EC, Calvert E, Ng A, et al. Geriatric trauma: resource use and patient outcomes. *Can J Surg.* 2003;46(3):211–215.
315. Ross N, Timberlake GA, Rubino LJ, et al. High cost of trauma care in the elderly. *South Med J.* 1989;82(7):857–859.
316. Young JS, Cephas GA, Blow O. Outcome and cost of trauma among the elderly: a real-life model of a single-payer reimbursement system. *J Trauma.* 1998;45(4):800–804.
317. Grossman M, Scaff DW, Miller D, et al. Functional outcomes in octogenarian trauma. *J Trauma.* 2003;55(1):26–32.
318. van Aalst JA, Morris JA Jr, Yates HK, et al. Severely injured geriatric patients return to independent living: a study of factors influencing function and independence. *J Trauma.* 1991;31(8):1096–1101.
319. Carrillo EH, Richardson JD, Malias MA, et al. Long term outcome of blunt trauma care in the elderly. *Surg Gynecol Obstet.* 1993;176(6):559–564.
320. Richmond TS, Kauder D, Strumpf N, et al. Characteristics and outcomes of serious traumatic injury in older adults. *J Am Geriatr Soc.* 2002;50(2):215–222.
321. Mosenthal AC, Livingston DH, Lavery RF, et al. The effect of age on functional outcome in mild traumatic brain injury: 6-month report of a prospective multicenter trial. *J Trauma.* 2004;56(5):1042–1048.
322. Fallon WF Jr, Rader E, Zyzanski S, et al. Geriatric outcomes are improved by a geriatric trauma consultation service. *J Trauma.* 2006;61(5):1040–1046.
323. Halpern NA, Pastores SM, Greenstein RJ. Critical care medicine in the United States 1985–2000: an analysis of bed numbers, use, and costs. *Crit Care Med.* 2004;32(6):1254–1259.
324. Callahan D. Old age and new policy. *JAMA.* 1989;261(6):905–906.
325. Levinsky NG. Age as a criterion for rationing health care. *N Engl J Med.* 1990;322(25):1813–1816.
326. Hubbard RE, Lyons RA, Woodhouse KW, et al. Absence of ageism in access to critical care: a cross-sectional study. *Age Ageing.* 2003;32(4):382–387.
327. Nuckton TJ, List ND. Age as a factor in critical care unit admissions. *Arch Intern Med.* 1995;155(10):1087–1092.
328. Attitudes of critical care medicine professionals concerning distribution of intensive care resources. The Society of Critical Care Medicine Ethics Committee. *Crit Care Med.* 1994;22(2):358–362.
329. Somme D, Maillet JM, Gisselbrecht M, et al. Critically ill old and the oldest-old patients in intensive care: short- and long-term outcomes. *Intensive Care Med.* 2003;29(12):2137–2143. Epub 2003 Nov 12.
330. Hennessy D, Juzwishin K, Yergens D, et al. Outcomes of elderly survivors of intensive care: a review of the literature. *Chest.* 2005;127(5):1764–1774.
331. Hamel MB, Teno JM, Goldman L, Lynn J, et al. Patient age and decisions to withhold life-sustaining treatments from seriously ill, hospitalized adults. SUPPORT Investigators. Study to Understand Prognoses and Preferences for Outcomes and Risks of Treatment. *Ann Intern Med.* 1999;130(2):116–125.
332. Somogyi-Zalud E, Zhong Z, Hamel MB, et al. The use of life-sustaining treatments in hospitalized persons aged 80 and older. *J Am Geriatr Soc.* 2002;50(5):930–934.
333. Hamel MB, Davis RB, Teno JM, et al. Older age, aggressiveness of care, and survival for seriously ill, hospitalized adults. SUPPORT Investigators. Study to Understand Prognoses and Preferences for Outcomes and Risks of Treatments. *Ann Intern Med.* 1999;131(10):721–728.
334. Kleinpell RM. Exploring outcomes after critical illness in the elderly. *Outcomes Manag.* 2003;7(4):159–169.
335. Layon AJ, George BE, Hamby B, et al. Do elderly patients overutilize healthcare resources and benefit less from them than younger patients? A study of patients who underwent craniotomy for treatment of neoplasm. *Crit Care Med.* 1995;23(5):829–834.
336. Blair SL, Schwarz RE. Advanced age does not contribute to increased risks or poor outcome after major abdominal operations. *Am Surg.* 2001;67(12):1123–1127.
337. Rady MY, Johnson DJ. Hospital discharge to care facility: a patient-centered outcome for the evaluation of intensive care for octogenarians. *Chest.* 2004;126(5):1583–1591.
338. Wehler M, Geise A, Hadzionerovic D, et al. Health-related quality of life of patients with multiple organ dysfunction: individual changes and comparison with normative population. *Crit Care Med.* 2003;31(4):1094–1101.
339. Kleinpell RM, Ferrans CE. Quality of life of elderly patients after treatment in the ICU. *Res Nurs Health.* 2002;25(3):212–221.
340. Eddleston JM, White P, Guthrie E. Survival, morbidity, and quality of life after discharge from intensive care. *Crit Care Med.* 2000;28(7):2293–2299.
341. Chelluri L, Pinsky MR, Donahoe MP, et al. Long-term outcome of critically ill elderly patients requiring intensive care. *JAMA.* 1993;269(24):3119–3123.
342. Wu AW, Rubin HR, Rosen MJ. Are elderly people less responsive to intensive care? *J Am Geriatr Soc.* 1990;38(6):621–627.
343. Teno JM, Fisher E, Hamel MB, et al. Decision-making and outcomes of prolonged ICU stays in seriously ill patients. *J Am Geriatr Soc.* 2000; 48(5 Suppl):S70–S74.
344. Vestal RE, Norris AH, Tobin JD, et al. Antipyrine metabolism in man: influence of age, alcohol, caffeine, and smoking. *Clin Pharmacol Ther.* 1975;18(4):425–432.
345. Abernethy DR, Kerzner L. Age effects on alpha-1-acid glycoprotein concentration and imipramine plasma protein binding. *J Am Geriatr Soc.* 1984;32(10):705–708.
346. Wilkinson GR. Drug metabolism and variability among patients in drug response. *N Engl J Med.* 2005;352(21):2211–2221.

347. Nebert DW, Russell DW. Clinical importance of the cytochromes P450. *Lancet.* 2002;360(9340):1155–1162.
348. CYP3A and Drug Interactions. *The Medical Letter* 2005;47(1212):54–55.
349. Crowley JJ, Cusack BJ, Jue SG, et al. Aging and drug interactions. II. Effect of phenytoin and smoking on the oxidation of theophylline and cortisol in healthy men. *J Pharmacol Exp Ther.* 1988;245(2):513–523.
350. Nolan L, O'Malley K. Prescribing for the elderly. Part I: Sensitivity of the elderly to adverse drug reactions. *J Am Geriatr Soc.* 1988;36(2):142–149.
351. Knaus WA, Wagner DP, Draper EA, et al. The APACHE III prognostic system. Risk prediction of hospital mortality for critically ill hospitalized adults. *Chest.* 1991;100(6):1619–1636.
352. Suresh R, Kupfer YY, Tessler S. The graying of the intensive care unit: demographic changes 1988–1998. *Crit Care Med* 1999:27(Suppl):A27.
353. Barnato AE, McClellan MB, Kagay CR, et al. Trends in inpatient treatment intensity among Medicare beneficiaries at the end of life. *Health Serv Res.* 2004;39(2):363–375.
354. Lubitz JD, Riley GF. Trends in Medicare payments in the last year of life. *N Engl J Med.* 1993;328(15):1092–1096.
355. Dardaine V, Dequin PF, Ripault H, et al. Outcome of older patients requiring ventilatory support in intensive care: impact of nutritional status. *J Am Geriatr Soc.* 2001;49(5):564–570.
356. Baker R, Wu AW, Teno JM, et al. Family satisfaction with end-of-life care in seriously ill hospitalized adults. *J Am Geriatr Soc.* 2000;48(5 Suppl):S61–S69.
357. Borum ML, Lynn J, Zhong Z. The effects of patient race on outcomes in seriously ill patients in SUPPORT: an overview of economic impact, medical intervention, and end-of-life decisions. Study to Understand Prognoses and Preferences for Outcomes and Risks of Treatments. *J Am Geriatr Soc.* 2000;48(5 Suppl):S194–S198.
358. Braun UK, Beyth RJ, Ford ME, et al. Defining limits in care of terminally ill patients. *BMJ.* 2007;334(7587):239–241.
359. Fick DM, Agostini JV, Inouye SK. Delirium superimposed on dementia: a systematic review. *J Am Geriatr Soc.* 2002;50(10):1723–1732.
360. Kakuma R, du Fort GG, Arsenault L, et al. Delirium in older emergency department patients discharged home: effect on survival. *J Am Geriatr Soc.* 2003;51(4):443–450.
361. O'Keeffe S, Lavan J. The prognostic significance of delirium in older hospital patients. *J Am Geriatr Soc.* 1997;45(2):174–178.
362. Cameron DJ, Thomas RI, Mulvihill M, et al. Delirium: a test of the Diagnostic and Statistical Manual III criteria on medical inpatients. *J Am Geriatr Soc.* 1987;35(11):1007–1010.
363. Foreman MD, Wakefield B, Culp K, et al. Delirium in elderly patients: an overview of the state of the Science. *J Gerontol Nurs.* 2001;27(4):12–20.
364. Inouye SK, Bogardus ST Jr, Charpentier PA, et al. A multicomponent intervention to prevent delirium in hospitalized older patients. *N Engl J Med.* 1999;340(9):669–676.
365. Inouye SK, Viscoli CM, Horwitz RI, et al. A predictive model for delirium in hospitalized elderly medical patients based on admission characteristics. *Ann Intern Med.* 1993;119(6):474–481.
366. McCusker J, Cole MG, Dendukuri N, et al. Does delirium increase hospital stay? *J Am Geriatr Soc.* 2003;51(11):1539–1546.
367. Cole MG, Primeau FJ. Prognosis of delirium in elderly hospital patients. *CMAJ.* 1993;149(1):41–46.
368. Cole MG. Delirium in elderly patients. *Am J Geriatr Psychiatry.* 2004; 12(1):7–21.
369. Cole MG, Primeau FJ, Elie LM. Delirium: prevention, treatment, and outcome studies. *J Geriatr Psychiatry Neurol.* 1998;11(3):126–137.
370. Ely EW, Shintani A, Truman B, et al. Delirium as a predictor of mortality in mechanically ventilated patients in the intensive care unit. *JAMA.* 2004; 291(14):1753–1762.
371. McNicoll L, Pisani MA, Zhang Y, et al. Delirium in the intensive care unit: occurrence and clinical course in older patients. *J Am Geriatr Soc.* 2003;51(5):591–598.
372. Dubois MJ, Bergeron N, Dumont M, et al. Delirium in an intensive care unit: a study of risk factors. *Intensive Care Med.* 2001;27(8):1297–1304.
373. Aldemir M, Ozen S, Kara IH, et al. Predisposing factors for delirium in the surgical intensive care unit. *Crit Care.* 2001;5(5):265–270.
374. Morrison RS, Magaziner J, Gilbert M, et al. Relationship between pain and opioid analgesics on the development of delirium following hip fracture. *J Gerontol A Biol Sci Med Sci.* 2003;58(1):76–81.
375. Mesulam MM, Waxman SG, Geschwind N, et al. Acute confusional states with right middle cerebral artery infarctions. *J Neurol Neurosurg Psychiatry.* 1976;39(1):84–89.
376. Teasdale E, Cardoso E, Galbraith S, et al. CT scan in severe diffuse head injury: physiological and clinical correlations. *J Neurol Neurosurg Psychiatry.* 1984;47(6):600–603.
377. Noldy NE, Carlen PL. Acute, withdrawal, and chronic alcohol effects in man: event-related potential and quantitative EEG techniques. *Ann Med.* 1990;22(5):333–339.
378. van Sweden B, Mellerio F. Toxic ictal delirium. *Biol Psychiatry.* 1989;25(4): 449–458.
379. Trzepacz PT, Sclabassi RJ, Van Thiel DH. Delirium: a subcortical phenomenon? *J Neuropsychiatry Clin Neurosci.* 1989;1(3):283–290.
380. Woods JC, Mion LC, Connor JT, et al. Agitation among ventilated medical intensive care unit patients: frequency, characteristics and outcomes. *Intensive Care Med.* 2004;30(6):1066–1072.
381. Konsman JP, Parnet P, Dantzer R. Cytokine-induced sickness behaviour: mechanisms and implications. *Trends Neurosci.* 2002;25(3):154–159.
382. Allan SM. The role of pro- and antiinflammatory cytokines in neurodegeneration. *Ann N Y Acad Sci.* 2000;917:84–93.
383. Young GB, Bolton CF, Austin TW, et al. The encephalopathy associated with septic illness. *Clin Invest Med.* 1990;13(6):297–304.
384. Sprung CL, Peduzzi PN, Shatney CH, et al. Impact of encephalopathy on mortality in the sepsis syndrome. The Veterans Administration Systemic Sepsis Cooperative Study Group. *Crit Care Med.* 1990;18(8):801–806.
385. Moller K, Strauss GI, Qvist J, et al. Cerebral blood flow and oxidative metabolism during human endotoxemia. *J Cereb Blood Flow Metab.* 2002;22(10):1262–1270.
386. Wong ML, Bongiorno PB, Rettori V, et al. Interleukin (IL) 1beta, IL-1 receptor antagonist, IL-10, and IL-13 gene expression in the central nervous system and anterior pituitary during systemic inflammation: pathophysiological implications. *Proc Natl Acad Sci U S A.* 1997;94(1):227–232.
387. Sharshar T, Gray F, Poron F, et al. Multifocal necrotizing leukoencephalopathy in septic shock. *Crit Care Med.* 2002;30(10):2371–2375.
388. Sharshar T, Annane D, de la Grandmaison GL, et al. The neuropathology of septic shock. *Brain Pathol.* 2004;14(1):21–33.
389. van der Mast RC, Fekkes D. Serotonin and amino acids: partners in delirium pathophysiology? *Semin Clin Neuropsychiatry.* 2000;5(2):125–131.
390. Mussi C, Ferrari R, Ascari S, et al. Importance of serum anticholinergic activity in the assessment of elderly patients with delirium. *J Geriatr Psychiatry Neurol.* 1999;12(2):82–86.
391. Tune LE, Egeli S. Acetylcholine and delirium. *Dement Geriatr Cogn Disord.* 1999;10(5):342–344.
392. Roche V. Southwestern Internal Medicine Conference. Etiology and management of delirium. *Am J Med Sci.* 2003;325(1):20–30.
393. American Psychiatric Association. Task Force on DSM-IV. *Diagnostic and Statistical Manual of Mental Disorders: DSM-IV-TR.* 4th ed. Washington DC: 2000.
394. Trzepacz PT, Mittal D, Torres R, et al. Validation of the Delirium Rating Scale-revised-98: comparison with the delirium rating scale and the cognitive test for delirium. *J Neuropsychiatry Clin Neurosci.* 2001;13(2):229–242.
395. Bergeron N, Dubois MJ, Dumont M, et al. Intensive Care Delirium Screening Checklist: evaluation of a new screening tool. *Intensive Care Med.* 2001;27(5):859–864.
396. Inouye SK, van Dyck CH, Alessi CA, et al. Clarifying confusion: the confusion assessment method. A new method for detection of delirium. *Ann Intern Med.* 1990;113(12):941–948.
397. Meagher DJ, O'Hanlon D, O'Mahony E, et al. Relationship between symptoms and motoric subtype of delirium. *J Neuropsychiatry Clin Neurosci.* 2000;12(1):51–56.
398. Lipowski ZJ. Delirium in the elderly patient. *N Engl J Med.* 1989;320 (9):578–582.
399. Ross CA, Peyser CE, Shapiro I, et al. Delirium: phenomenologic and etiologic subtypes. *Int Psychogeriatr.* 1991;3(2):135–147.
400. Francis J, Martin D, Kapoor WN. A prospective study of delirium in hospitalized elderly. *JAMA.* 1990;263(8):1097–1101.
401. Ely EW, Siegel MD, Inouye SK. Delirium in the intensive care unit: an under-recognized syndrome of organ dysfunction. *Semin Respir Crit Care Med.* 2001;22(2):115–126.
402. Ely EW, Stephens RK, Jackson JC, et al. Current opinions regarding the importance, diagnosis, and management of delirium in the intensive care unit: a survey of 912 healthcare professionals. *Crit Care Med.* 2004;32(1):106–112.
403. Inouye SK. Delirium in older persons. *N Engl J Med.* 2006;354(11):1157–1165.
404. Dyer CB, Ashton CM, Teasdale TA. Postoperative delirium. A review of 80 primary data-collection studies. *Arch Intern Med.* 1995;155(5):461–465.
405. Bedford PD. Adverse cerebral effects of anaesthesia on old people. *Lancet.* 1955;269(6884):259–263.
406. Moller JT. Cerebral dysfunction after anaesthesia. *Acta Anaesthesiol Scand Suppl.* 1997;110:13–16.
407. Rogers MP, Liang MH, Daltroy LH, et al. Delirium after elective orthopedic surgery: risk factors and natural history. *Int J Psychiatry Med.* 1989;19(2):109–121.
408. Selnes OA, Goldsborough MA, Borowicz LM Jr, et al. Determinants of cognitive change after coronary artery bypass surgery: a multifactorial problem. *Ann Thorac Surg.* 1999;67(6):1669–1676.
409. Selnes OA, Royall RM, Grega MA, et al. Cognitive changes 5 years after coronary artery bypass grafting: is there evidence of late decline? *Arch Neurol.* 2001;58(4):598–604.
410. Stroobant N, Van Nooten G, Van Belleghem Y, et al. Relation between neurocognitive impairment, embolic load, and cerebrovascular reactivity following on- and off-pump coronary artery bypass grafting. *Chest.* 2005;127(6):1967–1976.
411. Newman MF, Kirchner JL, Phillips-Bute B, et al: Neurological Outcome Research Group and the Cardiothoracic Anesthesiology Research Endeavors Investigators. Longitudinal assessment of neurocognitive function

after coronary-artery bypass surgery. *N Engl J Med.* 2001;344(6):395–402.
412. Dodds C, Allison J. Postoperative cognitive deficit in the elderly surgical patient. *Br J Anaesth.* 1998;81(3):449–462.
413. Bryson GL, Wyand A. Evidence-based clinical update: general anesthesia and the risk of delirium and postoperative cognitive dysfunction. *Can J Anaesth.* 2006;53(7):669–677.
414. Bekker AY, Weeks EJ. Cognitive function after anaesthesia in the elderly. *Best Pract Res Clin Anaesthesiol.* 2003;17(2):259–272.
415. Jacobi J, Fraser GL, Coursin DB, et al. Task Force of the American College of Critical Care Medicine (ACCM) of the Society of Critical Care Medicine (SCCM), American Society of Health-System Pharmacists (ASHP), American College of Chest Physicians. Clinical practice guidelines for the sustained use of sedatives and analgesics in the critically ill adult. *Crit Care Med.* 2002;30(1):119–141.
416. Milbrandt EB, Kersten A, Kong L, et al. Haloperidol use is associated with lower hospital mortality in mechanically ventilated patients. *Crit Care Med.* 2005;33(1):226–229.
417. Thom T, Haase N, Rosamond W, et al. American Heart Association Statistics Committee and Stroke Statistics Subcommittee. Heart disease and stroke statistics—2006 update: a report from the American Heart Association Statistics Committee and Stroke Statistics Subcommittee. *Circulation.* 2006;113(6):e85–e151.
418. Sacco RL. Risk factors, outcomes, and stroke subtypes for ischemic stroke. *Neurology.* 1997; 49(5 Suppl 4):S39–S44.
419. Sacco RL. Reducing the risk of stroke in diabetes: what have we learned that is new? *Diabetes Obes Metab.* 2002;4 Suppl 1:S27–S34.
420. Zivin JA. Approach to cerebrovascular diseases. In: Goldman L, Ausiello D, eds. *Cecil Textbook of Medicine.* Philadelphia, PA: WB Saunders, 2004.
421. Atherosclerotic disease of the aortic arch as a risk factor for recurrent ischemic stroke. The French Study of Aortic Plaques in Stroke Group. *N Engl J Med.* 1996;334(19):1216–1221.
422. Adams HP Jr, Adams RJ, Brott T, et al. Stroke Council of the American Stroke Association. Guidelines for the early management of patients with ischemic stroke: A Scientific statement from the Stroke Council of the American Stroke Association. *Stroke.* 2003;34(4):1056–1083.
423. Adams H, Adams R, Del Zoppo G, et al. Stroke Council of the American Heart Association; American Stroke Association. Guidelines for the early management of patients with ischemic stroke: 2005 guidelines update a Scientific statement from the Stroke Council of the American Heart Association/American Stroke Association. *Stroke.* 2005;36(4):916–923.
424. Berrouschot J, Rother J, Glahn J, et al. Outcome and severe hemorrhagic complications of intravenous thrombolysis with tissue plasminogen activator in very old (> or =80 years) stroke patients. *Stroke.* 2005; 36(11):2421–2425.
425. Tissue plasminogen activator for acute ischemic stroke. The National Institute of Neurological Disorders and Stroke rt-PA Stroke Study Group. *N Engl J Med.* 1995;333(24):1581–1587.
426. Kasner SE. Clinical interpretation and use of stroke scales. *Lancet Neurol.* 2006;5(7):603–612.
427. Gresham GE, Fitzpatrick TE, Wolf PA, et al. Residual disability in survivors of stroke–the Framingham study. *N Engl J Med.* 1975;293(19):954–956.
428. Kelly-Hayes M, Wolf PA, Kannel WB, et al. Factors influencing survival and need for institutionalization following stroke: The Framingham Study. *Arch Phys Med Rehabil.* 1988;69(6):415–418.
429. Sacco RL, Wolf PA, Kannel WB, et al. Survival and recurrence following stroke. The Framingham study. *Stroke.* 1982;13(3):290–295.
430. Cooke JR, Ancoli-Israel S. Sleep and its disorders in older adults. *Psychiatr Clin North Am.* 2006;29(4):1077–1093.
431. Foley DJ, Monjan A, Simonsick EM, et al. Incidence and remission of insomnia among elderly adults: an epidemiologic study of 6,800 persons over three years. *Sleep.* 1999;22 Suppl 2:S366–S372.
432. Foley D, Ancoli-Israel S, Britz P, et al. Sleep disturbances and chronic disease in older adults: results of the 2003 National Sleep Foundation Sleep in America Survey. *J Psychosom Res.* 2004;56(5):497–502.
433. Neubauer DN. Sleep problems in the elderly. *Am Fam Physician.* 1999; 59(9):2551–2558, 2559–2560.
434. Vgontzas AN, Kales A. Sleep and its disorders. *Annu Rev Med.* 1999;50: 387–400.
435. Schubert CR, Cruickshanks KJ, Dalton DS, et al. Prevalence of sleep problems and quality of life in an older population. *Sleep.* 2002;25(8):889–893.
436. Brassington GS, King AC, Bliwise DL. Sleep problems as a risk factor for falls in a sample of community-dwelling adults aged 64–99 years. *J Am Geriatr Soc.* 2000;48(10):1234–1240.
437. Cricco M, Simonsick EM, Foley DJ. The impact of insomnia on cognitive functioning in older adults. *J Am Geriatr Soc.* 2001;49(9):1185–1189.
438. Manabe K, Matsui T, Yamaya M, et al. Sleep patterns and mortality among elderly patients in a geriatric hospital. *Gerontology.* 2000;46(6):318–322.
439. Shochat T, Martin J, Marler M, et al. Illumination levels in nursing home patients: effects on sleep and activity rhythms. *J Sleep Res.* 2000;9(4):373–379.
440. Espana RA, Scammell TE. Sleep neurobiology for the clinician. *Sleep.* 2004; 27(4):811–820.
441. Feinsilver SH. Sleep in the elderly. What is normal? *Clin Geriatr Med.* 2003; 19(1):177–188, viii.
442. Kamel NS, Gammack JK. Insomnia in the elderly: cause, approach, and treatment. *Am J Med.* 2006;119(6):463–469.
443. Johns MW. A new method for measuring daytime sleepiness: the Epworth sleepiness scale. *Sleep.* 1991;14(6):540–545.
444. Shochat T, Pillar G. Sleep apnoea in the older adult: pathophysiology, epidemiology, consequences and management. *Drugs Aging.* 2003;20(8):551–560.
445. Olson EJ, Boeve BF, Silber MH. Rapid eye movement sleep behaviour disorder: demographic, clinical and laboratory findings in 93 cases. *Brain.* 2000;123 (Pt 2):331–339.
446. Littner MR, Kushida C, Anderson WM, et al. Standards of Practice Committee of the American Academy of Sleep Medicine. Practice parameters for the dopaminergic treatment of restless legs syndrome and periodic limb movement disorder. *Sleep.* 2004;27(3):557–559.
447. Kobayashi R, Kohsaka M, Fukuda N, et al. Effects of morning bright light on sleep in healthy elderly women. *Psychiatry Clin Neurosci.* 1999;53(2): 237–238.
448. Fetveit A, Skjerve A, Bjorvatn B. Bright light treatment improves sleep in institutionalised elderly—an open trial. *Int J Geriatr Psychiatry.* 2003;18(6): 520–526.
449. Kupfer DJ, Reynolds CF 3rd. Management of insomnia. *N Engl J Med.* 1997;336(5):341–346.
450. Chesson A Jr, Hartse K, Anderson WM, et al. Practice parameters for the evaluation of chronic insomnia. An American Academy of Sleep Medicine report. Standards of Practice Committee of the American Academy of Sleep Medicine. *Sleep.* 2000;23(2):237–241.
451. Howes JB, Ryan J, Fairbrother G, et al. Benzodiazepine prescribing in a Sydney teaching hospital. *Med J Aust.* 1996;165(6):305–308.
452. Kripke DF. Chronic hypnotic use: deadly risks, doubtful benefit. REVIEW ARTICLE. *Sleep Med Rev.* 2000;4(1):5–20.
453. Morin CM, Colecchi C, Stone J, et al. Behavioral and pharmacological therapies for late-life insomnia: a randomized controlled trial. *JAMA.* 1999;281(11):991–999.
454. Obermeyer WH, Benca RM. Effects of drugs on sleep. *Neurol Clin.* 1996;14(4):827–840.
455. Smith MT, Perlis ML, Park A, et al. Comparative meta-analysis of pharmacotherapy and behavior therapy for persistent insomnia. *Am J Psychiatry.* 2002;159(1):5–11.
456. Sager MA, Franke T, Inouye SK, et al. Functional outcomes of acute medical illness and hospitalization in older persons. *Arch Intern Med.* 1996;156(6):645–652.
457. Covinsky KE, Palmer RM, Fortinsky RH, et al. Loss of independence in activities of daily living in older adults hospitalized with medical illnesses: increased vulnerability with age. *J Am Geriatr Soc.* 2003;51(4):451–458.
458. Nasraway SA, Button GJ, Rand WM, et al. Survivors of catastrophic illness: outcome after direct transfer from intensive care to extended care facilities. *Crit Care Med.* 2000;28(1):19–25.
459. Montuclard L, Garrouste-Orgeas M, Timsit JF, et al. Outcome, functional autonomy, and quality of life of elderly patients with a long-term intensive care unit stay. *Crit Care Med.* 2000;28(10):3389–3395.
460. Stucki G, Stier-Jarmer M, Grill E, et al. Rationale and principles of early rehabilitation care after an acute injury or illness. *Disabil Rehabil.* 2005;27(7-8):353–359.
461. Creditor MC. Hazards of hospitalization of the elderly. *Ann Intern Med.* 1993;118(3):219–223.
462. Manton KG. A longitudinal study of functional change and mortality in the United States. *J Gerontol.* 1988;43(5):S153–S161.
463. Gill TM, Allore HG, Holford TR, et al. Hospitalization, restricted activity, and the development of disability among older persons. *JAMA.* 2004;292(17):2115–2124.
464. Brummel-Smith K. Rehabilitation. In: Cassel CK, Leipzig RM, Cohen HJ, Larson EB, Meier DE, ed. *Geriatric Medicine: An evidence based approach.* New York, New York: Springer-Verlag, 2003
465. Hoenig H, Nusbaum N, Brummel-Smith K. Geriatric rehabilitation: state of the art. *J Am Geriatr Soc.* 1997;45(11):1371–1381.
466. Landefeld CS, Palmer RM, Kresevic DM, et al. A randomized trial of care in a hospital medical unit especially designed to improve the functional outcomes of acutely ill older patients. *N Engl J Med.* 1995;332(20):1338–1344.
467. Ellis G, Langhorne P. Comprehensive geriatric assessment for older hospital patients. *Br Med Bull.* 2005;71:45–59.
468. Cohen HJ, Feussner JR, Weinberger M, et al. A controlled trial of inpatient and outpatient geriatric evaluation and management. *N Engl J Med.* 2002;346(12):905–912.
469. Counsell SR, Holder CM, Liebenauer LL, et al. Effects of a multicomponent intervention on functional outcomes and process of care in hospitalized older patients: a randomized controlled trial of Acute Care for Elders (ACE) in a community hospital. *J Am Geriatr Soc.* 2000;48(12):1572–1581.
470. Inouye SK, Bogardus ST Jr, Baker DI, et al. The Hospital Elder Life Program: a model of care to prevent cognitive and functional decline in older hospitalized patients. Hospital Elder Life Program. *J Am Geriatr Soc.* 2000;48(12):1697–1706.

471. Winograd CH. Inpatient geriatric consultation. *Clin Geriatr Med.* 1987; 3(1):193–202.
472. Stuck AE, Siu AL, Wieland GD, et al. Comprehensive geriatric assessment: a meta-analysis of controlled trials. *Lancet.* 1993;342(8878):1032–1036.
473. Miller DK. Effectiveness of acute rehabilitation services in geriatric evaluation and management units. *Clin Geriatr Med.* 2000;16(4):775–782.
474. Reuben DB, Borok GM, Wolde-Tsadik G, et al. A randomized trial of comprehensive geriatric assessment in the care of hospitalized patients. *N Engl J Med.* 1995;332(20):1345–1350.
475. Jolliffe JA, Rees K, Taylor RS, et al. Exercise-based rehabilitation for coronary heart disease. *Cochrane Database Syst Rev.* 2000;(4):CD001800.
476. Pasquali SK, Alexander KP, Peterson ED. Cardiac rehabilitation in the elderly. *Am Heart J.* 2001;142(5):748–755.
477. Lavie CJ, Milani RV, Littman AB. Benefits of cardiac rehabilitation and exercise training in secondary coronary prevention in the elderly. *J Am Coll Cardiol.* 1993;22(3):678–683.
478. Kreizman IJ, Allen D. Aging with cardiopulmonary disease: the rehab perspective. *Phys Med Rehabil Clin N Am.* 2005;16(1):251–265, x.
479. Lavie CJ, Milani RV. Effects of cardiac rehabilitation programs on exercise capacity, coronary risk factors, behavioral characteristics, and quality of life in a large elderly cohort. *Am J Cardiol.* 1995;76(3):177–179.
480. Ades PA, Waldmann ML, Polk DM, et al. Referral patterns and exercise response in the rehabilitation of female coronary patients aged greater than or equal to 62 years. *Am J Cardiol.* 1992;69(17):1422–1425.
481. Cottin Y, Cambou JP, Casillas JM, et al. Specific profile and referral bias of rehabilitated patients after an acute coronary syndrome. *J Cardiopulm Rehabil.* 2004;24(1):38–44.
482. Arboix A, Garcia-Eroles L, Massons J, et al. Acute stroke in very old people: clinical features and predictors of in-hospital mortality. *J Am Geriatr Soc.* 2000;48(1):36–41.
483. Dobkin BH. Clinical practice. Rehabilitation after stroke. *N Engl J Med.* 2005;352(16):1677–1684.
484. Macciocchi SN, Diamond PT, Alves WM, et al. Ischemic stroke: relation of age, lesion location, and initial neurologic deficit to functional outcome. *Arch Phys Med Rehabil.* 1998;79(10):1255–1257.
485. Kelly PJ, Furie KL, Shafqat S, et al. Functional recovery following rehabilitation after hemorrhagic and ischemic stroke. *Arch Phys Med Rehabil.* 2003;84(7):968–972.
486. Musicco M, Emberti L, Nappi G, et al: Italian Multicenter Study on Outcomes of Rehabilitation of Neurological Patients. Early and long-term outcome of rehabilitation in stroke patients: the role of patient characteristics, time of initiation, and duration of interventions. *Arch Phys Med Rehabil.* 2003;84(4):551–558.
487. Hallett M. Plasticity of the human motor cortex and recovery from stroke. *Brain Res Brain Res Rev.* 2001;36(2–3):169–174.
488. Duncan PW, Wallace D, Lai SM, et al. The Stroke Impact Scale version 2.0. Evaluation of reliability, validity, and sensitivity to change. *Stroke.* 1999;30(10):2131–2140.
489. Lai SM, Studenski S, Duncan PW, et al. Persisting consequences of stroke measured by the Stroke Impact Scale. *Stroke.* 2002;33(7):1840–1844.
490. Jorgensen HS, Nakayama H, Raaschou HO, et al. Outcome and time course of recovery in stroke. Part II: time course of recovery. The Copenhagen Stroke Study. *Arch Phys Med Rehabil.* 1995;76(5):406–412.
491. Jorgensen HS, Nakayama H, Raaschou HO, et al. Outcome and time course of recovery in stroke. Part I: outcome. The Copenhagen Stroke Study. *Arch Phys Med Rehabil.* 1995;76(5):399–405.
492. Weir NU, Gunkel A, McDowall M, et al. Study of the relationship between social deprivation and outcome after stroke. *Stroke.* 2005;36(4):815–819.
493. Barnes MP. Rehabilitation after traumatic brain injury. *Br Med Bull.* 1999;55(4):927–943.
494. Horan MA, Clague JE. Injury in the aging: recovery and rehabilitation. *Br Med Bull.* 1999;55(4):895–909.
495. Zuckerman JD. Hip fracture. *N Engl J Med.* 1996;334(23):1519–1525.
496. Richmond J, Aharonoff GB, Zuckerman JD, et al. Mortality risk after hip fracture. *J Orthop Trauma.* 2003;17(1):53–56.
497. Cree M, Soskolne CL, Belseck E, et al. Mortality and institutionalization following hip fracture. *J Am Geriatr Soc.* 2000;48(3):283–288.
498. Cree M, Carriere KC, Soskolne CL, et al. Functional dependence after hip fracture. *Am J Phys Med Rehabil.* 2001;80(10):736–743.
499. Marcantonio ER, Flacker JM, Michaels M, et al. Delirium is independently associated with poor functional recovery after hip fracture. *J Am Geriatr Soc.* 2000;48(6):618–624.
500. Koval KJ, Sala DA, Kummer FJ, et al. Postoperative weight-bearing after a fracture of the femoral neck or an intertrochanteric fracture. *J Bone Joint Surg Am.* 1998;80(3):352–356.
501. Handoll HH, Farrar MJ, McBirnie J, et al. Heparin, low molecular weight heparin and physical methods for preventing deep vein thrombosis and pulmonary embolism following surgery for hip fractures. *Cochrane Database Syst Rev.* 2002;(4):CD000305.
502. Bergqvist D, Benoni G, Bjorgell O, et al. Low-molecular-weight heparin (enoxaparin) as prophylaxis against venous thromboembolism after total hip replacement. *N Engl J Med.* 1996;335(10):696–700.
503. Dahl OE, Bergqvist D. Current controversies in deep vein thrombosis prophylaxis after orthopaedic surgery. *Curr Opin Pulm Med.* 2002;8(5):394–397.
504. Freedman KB, Brookenthal KR, Fitzgerald RH Jr, et al. A meta-analysis of thromboembolic prophylaxis following elective total hip arthroplasty. *J Bone Joint Surg Am.* 2000;82-A(7):929–938.
505. Rosell PA, Parker MJ. Functional outcome after hip fracture. A 1-year prospective outcome study of 275 patients. *Injury.* 2003;34(7):529–532.
506. Lin PC, Chang SY. Functional recovery among elderly people one year after hip fracture surgery. *J Nurs Res.* 2004;12(1):72–82.
507. Press Y, Grinshpun Y, Berzak A, et al. The effect of co-morbidity on the rehabilitation process in elderly patients after hip fracture. *Arch Gerontol Geriatr.* 2007; [Epub ahead of print]
508. Hawkes WG, Wehren L, Orwig D, et al. Gender differences in functioning after hip fracture. *J Gerontol A Biol Sci Med Sci.* 2006;61(5):495–499.
509. Shah MR, Aharonoff GB, Wolinsky P, et al. Outcome after hip fracture in individuals ninety years of age and older. *J Orthop Trauma.* 2001;15(1):34–39.
510. Cutson TM, Bongiorni DR. Rehabilitation of the older lower limb amputee: a brief review. *J Am Geriatr Soc.* 1996;44(11):1388–1393.
511. Feinglass J, Brown JL, LoSasso A, et al. Rates of lower-extremity amputation and arterial reconstruction in the United States, 1979 to 1996. *Am J Public Health.* 1999;89(8):1222–1227.
512. Esquenazi A. Geriatric amputee rehabilitation. *Clin Geriatr Med.* 1993; 9(4):731–743.
513. Cruz CP, Eidt JF, Capps C, et al. Major lower extremity amputations at a Veterans Affairs hospital. *Am J Surg.* 2003;186(5):449–454.
514. Waters RL, Perry J, Antonelli D, et al. Energy cost of walking of amputees: the influence of level of amputation. *J Bone Joint Surg Am.* 1976;58(1):42–46.
515. Fisher SV, Gullickson G Jr. Energy cost of ambulation in health and disability: a literature review. *Arch Phys Med Rehabil.* 1978;59(3):124–133.
516. Pagliarulo MA, Waters R, Hislop HJ. Energy cost of walking of below-knee amputees having no vascular disease. *Phys Ther.* 1979;59(5):538–543.
517. Harris KA, van Schie L, Carroll SE, et al. Rehabilitation potential of elderly patients with major amputations. *J Cardiovasc Surg (Torino).* 1991; 32(4):463–467.
518. Legro MW, Reiber G, del Aguila M, et al. Issues of importance reported by persons with lower limb amputations and prostheses. *J Rehabil Res Dev.* 1999;36(3):155–163.
519. Esquenazi A, DiGiacomo R. Rehabilitation after amputation. *J Am Podiatr Med Assoc.* 2001;91(1):13–22.

CHAPTER 104 ■ THE ROLE OF ANTIBIOTICS IN THE MANAGEMENT OF SERIOUS HOSPITAL-ACQUIRED INFECTIONS

MARIN H. KOLLEF • SCOTT T. MICEK • LEE P. SKRUPKY

Antimicrobial resistance has emerged as an important variable influencing patient mortality and overall resource use in the hospital setting (1). Intensive care units (ICUs) worldwide are faced with increasingly rapid emergence and spread of antibiotic-resistant bacteria. Both antibiotic-resistant Gram-negative and Gram-positive bacteria are reported as important causes of hospital-acquired infections. In many circumstances, particularly with methicillin-resistant *Staphylococcus aureus* and *Enterococcus faecium* and Gram-negative bacteria producing extended-spectrum β-lactamases with resistance to multiple other antibiotics, few antimicrobial agents remain for the effective treatment of seriously ill patients (1,2). Within hospitals, ICUs are an important area for the emergence of antimicrobial resistance due to the following (1–6):

- The frequent use of broad spectrum agents
- The physical crowding of patients with high-acuity diseases within relatively small specialized areas
- Reductions in nursing and other support staff due to economic pressures, which increase the likelihood of person-to-person transmission of micro-organisms
- The presence of more chronically and acutely ill patients who require prolonged hospitalizations and often harbor antibiotic-resistant bacteria.

For the reasons listed above, hospitals—and particularly ICUs—are at the center of the problem of escalating bacterial resistance. The antibiotic treatment strategies described in this chapter attempt to balance the need to provide appropriate initial antimicrobial treatment to patients with serious infections while minimizing further development of antibiotic resistance. Many of these strategies—developed in the ICU setting—also have application in non-ICU areas of the hospital. The strategies described in this review adhere to the Centers for Disease Control and Prevention 12-step program for the prevention of antimicrobial resistance (http://www.cdc.gov/drugresistance/healthcare/). One of the key elements in this strategy is to consult experts in the field of antimicrobial resistance (e.g., infectious disease experts, infection control practitioners, microbiologists) when designing interventions aimed at optimizing the treatment of infected patients and minimizing the emergence of antimicrobial resistance.

The primary treatment strategy described in this chapter will be the approach of antibiotic de-escalation (7). De-escalation is a treatment strategy that attempts to provide appropriate initial antimicrobial therapy to optimize patient outcomes while avoiding the consequences of excessive or unnecessary antibiotic administration (Figs. 104.1 and 104.2).

KEY POINTS

1. Efforts should be made to rapidly identify the source and site of infection and to obtain specimens for culture, antimicrobial susceptibility testing, and rapid diagnostic tests. Obtaining these specimens should not delay initial empiric therapy in a critically ill patient.
2. Initial treatment with an appropriate antibiotic regimen is one of the most important factors influencing the outcome of critically ill patients with infection.
3. Infection with antibiotic-resistant micro-organisms increases the likelihood that inappropriate initial antibiotic therapy will be prescribed to critically ill patients.
4. Host factors influence the likelihood that a patient will be infected with antibiotic-resistant pathogens (e.g., prior hospitalization or antibiotic treatment, admission from a nursing home or other high-risk environment).
5. Avoidance of unnecessary antibiotic exposure in the ICU setting is important to reduce the emergence of and subsequent infection with antibiotic-resistant micro-organisms.

ESSENTIAL DIAGNOSTIC TESTS AND PROCEDURES

1. For patients with septic shock, establish adequate intravenous access and assess intravascular volume status (e.g., measure central venous pressure).
2. Perform a directed medical history and physical examination to identify potential sources and sites of infection.
3. Obtain specimens for microbiologic testing including blood, urine, and lower respiratory tract secretions. Other specimens should be directed by the initial history/physical examination (e.g., ascites, pleural fluid, cerebral spinal fluid).
4. Perform radiographic evaluation to identify infection sites requiring expeditious surgical or percutaneous drainage (intra-abdominal abscess, thoracic empyema, necrotizing skin, or visceral infection).

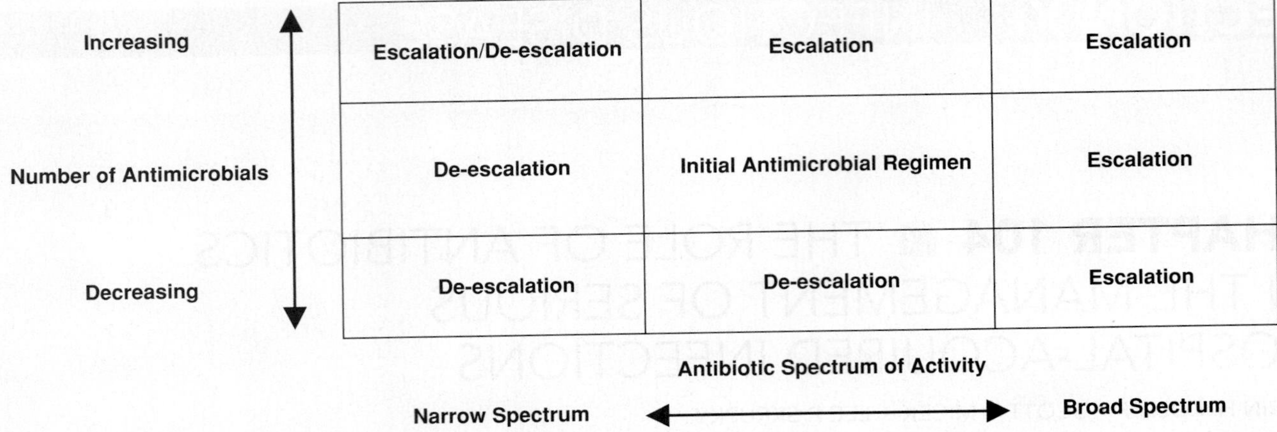

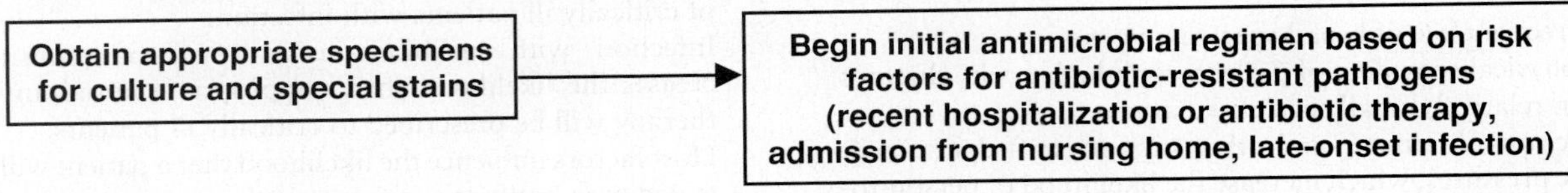

FIGURE 104.1. Antimicrobial de-escalation promotes initial administration of broad-spectrum antibiotics to patients at risk for infection with multidrug-resistant pathogens, followed by the reduction of the number of antimicrobials used and/or their spectrum of activity based on subsequent pathogen identification and antimicrobial susceptibility testing.

INITIAL THERAPY

1. Administer intravenous fluids to the patient with septic shock to achieve predetermined goals (e.g., central venous pressure >8 mm Hg, oxygen saturation of central venous blood [$S_{svc}O_2$] >70%).
2. An initial appropriate antibiotic regimen should be prescribed with adequate activity against all pathogens likely to be responsible for the infection.
3. Initial antibiotic dosing and interval of administration should be pharmacokinetically based to ensure that drug concentrations at the site of infection are adequate to achieve therapeutic drug levels.

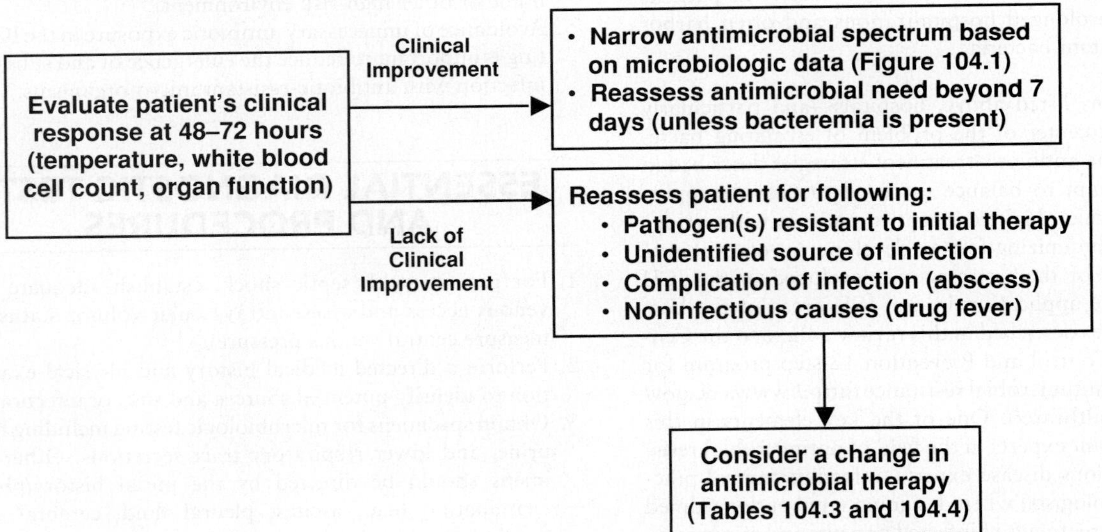

FIGURE 104.2. Clinical algorithm for the de-escalation approach to antibiotic treatment of serious infections in patients with risk factors for multidrug-resistant pathogens. Optimally, de-escalation of antimicrobial treatment would always occur once the pathogen causing infection and its antimicrobial susceptibility are known.

4. Drainage of amenable infection sites should occur once the patient has received adequate intravascular fluid replacement and appropriate initial antibiotic therapy.
5. Antibiotic treatment should be reassessed as soon as microbiologic test results become available.
6. Failure of initial antimicrobial therapy should prompt a thorough re-evaluation to identify the reason for failure (e.g., inadequate fluid resuscitation, inappropriate initial antimicrobial therapy, unidentified collection of infected fluid needing drainage).

ANTIMICROBIAL RESISTANCE: RISK FACTORS AND INFLUENCE ON OUTCOME

Antimicrobial use is the key driver for the emergence of antibiotic resistance. Therefore, antibiotic treatment strategies in the ICU need to take this into account to optimize clinical outcomes, both efficacy and the prevention of subsequent resistance to these drugs. Several investigators have demonstrated a close association between the prior use of antibiotics and the emergence of subsequent antibiotic resistance in both Gram-negative and Gram-positive bacteria (6,8,9). Other factors promoting antimicrobial resistance include prolonged hospitalization, the presence of invasive devices such as endotracheal tubes and intravascular catheters (possibly due to the formation of biofilms on the surfaces of these devices), residence in long-term treatment facilities, and inadequate infection control practices (6). The emergence of new strains of existing pathogens within the community setting has created additional stressors favoring the entry of resistant micro-organisms into the hospital setting. This has most recently been demonstrated by the identification and spread of community-associated, methicillin-resistant *Staphylococcus aureus* (MRSA) (10). However, the prolonged administration of antimicrobial regimens appears to be the most important factor promoting the emergence of antibiotic resistance that is potentially amenable to intervention (9,11,12).

Many clinical investigations have shown that antimicrobial regimens that lack action against identified micro-organisms that cause serious infections (i.e., inappropriate initial antimicrobial therapy) are associated with greater hospital mortality (13–18). Unfortunately, changing antibiotic therapy to an appropriate regimen after antimicrobial susceptibility data become available has not been demonstrated to improve clinical outcomes (19). These studies suggest that the increasing prevalence of antimicrobial resistance has led to greater overall hospital mortality, in part, through the administration of less effective antibiotic agents. The recent Infectious Disease Society of America/American Thoracic Society (IDSA/ATS) guidelines for the treatment of nosocomial pneumonia emphasize the importance of inappropriate initial antimicrobial therapy as a determinant of hospital mortality (20). This guideline also stresses the importance of maintaining local, frequently updated antibiograms within individual hospitals and ICUs to ensure the appropriateness of antibiotic coverage and the use of proper drug doses to optimize tissue concentrations of antibiotics. In addition to increased hospital mortality, antimicrobial resistance is associated with excess costs. Most of this cost is simply associated with the acquisition of a nosocomial infection, much of which is due to potentially antibiotic-resistant bacteria (9,21). However, the presence of antibiotic resistance may also confer added morbidity and costs (22).

CLINICAL FACTORS THAT AFFECT INITIAL ANTIMICROBIAL SELECTION

To provide an empirical antimicrobial regimen with an appropriate spectrum of activity, one must appreciate (a) the likely pathogens causing various infections, (b) local pathogen distribution and resistance patterns, and (c) patient-specific risk factors for resistance. Ideally, administration of appropriately broad-spectrum empiric antimicrobial therapy is based on consideration of all of these factors, and each will be examined in the following section.

Data from the National Nosocomial Infections Surveillance (NNIS) outlines the most frequent infections in participating acute care general hospitals in the United States. This surveillance network was established in 1970 and initially reported only hospital-wide infection rates; however, since 1986, the network has reported ICU infection rates as well. In the 2000 report, device-related infection predominated; 83% of nosocomial pneumonia episodes were associated with mechanical ventilation, 97% of urinary tract infections occurred in catheterized patients, and 87% of primary bloodstream infections occurred in patients with a central catheter (23). A more recent publication of the NNIS data reported pathogen distribution by site of infection and compared data from 1975 and 2003 as demonstrated in Table 104.1 (24). In general, the occurrence of hospital-acquired infections attributed to potentially antibiotic-resistant bacteria (e.g., *Staphylococcus aureus, Pseudomonas aeruginosa*) is increasing (23,24).

The NNIS data outline the changing spectrum of bacterial infection among patients with hospital-acquired pneumonia where Gram-negative aerobes remain the most frequently reported pathogen associated with pneumonia (65.9%); however *Staphylococcus aureus* (27.8%) was the most frequently reported *single* species (23,24). In patients with primary bloodstream infections, coagulase-negative staphylococci (42.9%) has remained the most common pathogen reported and *Staphylococcus aureus* (14.3%) was reported as frequently as enterococci (14.5%). In patients with urinary tract infections, *Escherichia coli* (26%) was the most frequently reported isolate; however, *Pseudomonas aeruginosa* constituted 16.3% of reported isolates, increasing from 10.6% in the 1989 to 1998 data. In surgical site infections, the proportion of isolates that were Gram-negative decreased significantly during the past two decades. Gram-positive pathogens are now more commonly associated with both bloodstream infections and skin and skin structure infections, whereas Gram-negative aerobes predominate in pneumonia and urinary tract infections (23–25).

One of the most concerning trends reported in the NNIS data is the increasing isolation of *Acinetobacter* species in urinary tract infections, pneumonia, and surgical site infections (23–25). Although overall numbers of isolates of *Acinetobacter* are still relatively small (approximately 2.0%), the percentage increase is significant. Even more concerning is the recent report of community-acquired pneumonia now

TABLE 104.1

RELATIVE PERCENTAGE BY SITE OF INFECTION OF PATHOGENS ASSOCIATED WITH NOSOCOMIAL INFECTION

Pathogen	PNEU			BSI			SSI			UTI		
Year	1975	1989–1998	2003	1975	1989–1998	2003	1975	1989–1998	2003	1975	1989–1998	2003
Number	4,018	65,056	4,365	1,054	50,091	2,351	7,848	22,043	2,984	16,434	47,502	4,109
Staphylococcus aureus	13.4	16.8	27.8	16.5	10.7	14.3	18.5	12.6	22.5	1.9	1.6	3.6
Pseudomonas aeruginosa	9.6	16.1	18.1	4.8	3	3.4	4.7	9.2	9.5	9.3	10.6	16.3
Enterococcus subspecies	3	1.9	1.3	8.1	10.3	14.5	11.9	14.5	13.9	14.2	13.8	17.4
Enterobacter subspecies	9.6	10.7	10	6	4.2	4.4	4.6	8.8	9	4.7	5.7	6.9
Escherichia coli	11.8	4.4	5	15	2.9	3.3	17.6	7.1	6.5	33.5	18.2	26
Klebsiella pneumoniae	8.4	6.5	7.2	4.5	2.9	4.2	2.7	3.5	3	4.6	6.1	9.8
Serratia marcescens	2.2	—	4.7	2.6	—	2.3	0.5	—	2	1.4	—	1.6
Acinetobacter species	1.5	—	6.9	1.8	—	2.4	0.5	—	2.1	0.6	—	1.6

PNEU, pneumonia; BSI, blood stream infection; SSI, surgical site infection; UTI, urinary tract infection; —, not reported.
From: Gaynes R, Edwards JR; National Nosocomial Infections Surveillance System. Overview of nosocomial infections caused by Gram-negative bacilli. *Clin Infect Dis.* 2005;41:848–854.

attributed to *Acinetobacter* species, suggesting that this pathogen is extending its area of influence outside of the health care setting (26).

Also disconcerting is the observation made by the NNIS report that for each of the antibiotic-pathogen combinations tested, there was a significant increase in resistance between study periods. Most impressive were trends in carbapenem- and cephalosporin-resistant *Pseudomonas aeruginosa* and *Acinetobacter* species (23,24). Rates of imipenem- and amikacin-resistant *Acinetobacter* isolates are approaching 20% and have been steadily increasing since 1990. The intrinsically multidrug-resistant (MDR) nature of this organism makes these trends particularly worrisome, as many isolates lack effective treatment options and represent a serious public health concern. Last, 2003 rates of third-generation cephalosporin-resistance in *Escherichia coli* (6.4%) and *Klebsiella pneumoniae* (14.2%) provide estimates of the presence of extended-spectrum β-lactamase (ESBL) producing often MDR bacteria, again with very limited treatment options in hospitals in the United States (24,27).

The prevalence of MDR pathogens varies by patient population, hospital, and type of floor or unit in which the patient resides, which underscores the need for local surveillance data. MDR pathogens are more commonly isolated from patients with severe, chronic underlying disease—for example, those with risk factors for health care–associated infection (Table 104.2) and patients with late-onset hospital-acquired infections. The importance of these risk factors was demonstrated by Trouillet et al. (9) for potentially antibiotic-resistant ventilator-associated pneumonia (VAP) in 135 mechanically ventilated patients. The duration of ventilation before the onset of VAP and prior antibiotic use (within 15 days prior to developing VAP) were both significant risk factors associated with VAP caused by antibiotic-resistant pathogens. Late-onset VAP (≥5 days), in patients who had previously received antibiotics was generally caused by MDR pathogens such as *Pseudomonas aeruginosa, Acinetobacter baumannii, Stenotrophomonas maltophilia*, or MRSA. The authors concluded that this study provided evidence for the need of a more rational approach to selecting initial empiric antibiotic therapy before culture results were available in patients with VAP to provide an appropriate initial regimen.

A study by Namias et al. (28) examined how variable MDR pathogen distribution can occur among ICUs even from a single hospital. These investigators found highly variable rates of susceptibility to several problem pathogens in their trauma,

TABLE 104.2

DEFINITIONS OF INFECTION CATEGORIES (WITH FOCUS ON BACTERIAL PATHOGENS)

Infection category	Definition
Community-acquired infection	Patients with a first positive bacterial culture obtained within 48 hours of hospital admission lacking risk factors for health care–associated infection
Hospital-acquired infection	Patients with a first positive bacterial culture >48 hours after hospital admission
Health care–associated infection	Patients with a first positive bacterial culture within 48 hours of admission and any of the following: ■ Admission source indicates a transfer from another health care facility (e.g., hospital, nursing home) ■ Receiving hemodialysis, wound, or infusion therapy as an outpatient ■ Prior hospitalization for ≥3 days within 90 days ■ Immunocompromised state due to underlying disease or therapy (human immunodeficiency virus, chemotherapy)

surgical, and medical ICUs and found that while *Acinetobacter* susceptibility rates to imipenem were low in the surgical ICU, susceptibility was very good in the trauma ICU. Similar variations in infection rates with MDR pathogens have been reported between different cities and countries (29,30). These data suggest that consensus guidelines for antimicrobial therapy will need to be modified at the local level (for example, according to county, city, hospital, and ICU) to take into account local patterns of antimicrobial resistance. In addition, it is helpful for clinicians to appreciate local specific resistance rates of certain Gram-negative pathogens such as ESBL-producing *Klebsiella pneumonia* or *Escherichia coli*, fluoroquinolone-resistant *Pseudomonas aeruginosa*, or carbapenem-resistant *Acinetobacter baumannii.* When risk of these pathogens is identified, empirical therapy must be tailored accordingly.

In addition to local or regional variance, numerous patient-specific factors affect the risk of isolation of a resistant pathogen. Therefore, the choice of empirical antibiotic agents should be based on local patterns of antimicrobial susceptibility and must also take into account patient-specific characteristics that may influence the risk of infection with a resistant pathogen. Patients of particular concern are those at risk for hospital-acquired infections caused by *Staphylococcus aureus*, *Pseudomonas aeruginosa,* and *Acinetobacter species* due to the high frequency with which they cause infection, their resistance to numerous antibiotics, and their associated high mortality rates. Infections with these potentially antibiotic-resistant bacteria have occurred primarily among hospitalized patients and/or among patients with an extensive hospitalization history and other predisposing risk factors like indwelling catheters, past antimicrobial use, decubitus ulcers, postoperative surgical wound infections, or treatment with enteral feedings or dialysis.

DIFFERENTIATING HEALTH CARE–ASSOCIATED INFECTIONS FROM COMMUNITY-ACQUIRED INFECTIONS

Health care–associated bacteremia (HCAB) and health care–associated pneumonia (HCAP) have recently been described as infections developing in patients admitted to the hospital from high-risk environments (20,31–33). These high-risk environments include nursing homes and extended care facilities, or patients' homes if they are receiving chronic dialysis, home infusion therapy, or home wound therapy, or have had a recent hospitalization (Table 104.2) (34). These risk factors increase the likelihood of infection with MDR bacteria that are more commonly seen in nosocomial infections as compared with community-acquired infections.

Health care services, such as dialysis, chemotherapy, and same-day surgery, are increasingly provided in the outpatient environment (34). At present, pneumonia and bloodstream infections related to these health care–associated interventions often are classified as community-acquired infections and are initially treated as such. However, given the frequent transfer of patients and health care workers between these facilities and hospitals, an outpatient facility is likely to be distinct from the true community setting and may more closely resemble the nosocomial setting in terms of the pathogens it might house. For example, MRSA strains isolated from patients infected in health care–associated settings are distinct from those that are truly community-acquired and have different susceptibility to antibiotics (10).

In addition to the complexity introduced by evolving health care practices, the causative pathogens associated with community-acquired infections have also changed in prevalence in recent years. Although *Streptococcus pneumoniae* remains the most common causative pathogen for community-acquired pneumonia, other potential pathogens (e.g., *Chlamydia pneumoniae*, *Mycoplasma pneumoniae*, *Acinetobacter* species, MRSA, and *Legionella* spp) exist and their prevalence changes over time and varies by geographic location (26,35). Furthermore, the emerging antimicrobial resistance of community-acquired pathogens has complicated the management of these infections. These changes necessitate an evolving treatment strategy based on the most recent findings regarding microbiology and epidemiology (10,20,35).

A DE-ESCALATION APPROACH FOR THE ANTIBIOTIC TREATMENT OF SERIOUS INFECTION IN THE HOSPITALIZED PATIENT

Above all, it is imperative to provide an initial antibiotic regimen that is active against the pathogen(s) causing the underlying infection in a seriously ill patient to optimize clinical outcomes (36). Additionally, the prescribed antibiotics must be dosed adequately according to their pharmacodynamic characteristics, given at the proper interval, and monitored for toxicities to achieve tissue levels that will kill the pathogens (6). After an initial appropriately broad-spectrum antibiotic regimen is prescribed, modification of the regimen using a de-escalation strategy should occur based on the results of the patient's clinical response and microbiologic testing (Fig. 104.2). Based on the de-escalation strategy, modification of the initial antibiotic regimen should include decreasing the number and/or spectrum of antibiotics, if possible based on culture and sensitivity results, shortening the duration of therapy in patients with uncomplicated infections who are demonstrating signs of clinical improvement, or discontinuing antibiotics altogether in patients who have a noninfectious cause identified accounting for the patient's signs and symptoms. The following sections describe individual antibiotic classes as well as methods for implementing a de-escalation approach at the local hospital level. These methods should be used, in combination, according to local preferences to achieve the desired balance between prescribing appropriate initial antibiotic treatment to patients with a serious infection and minimizing the emergence of antimicrobial resistance.

ANTIBIOTICS, THEIR MODE OF ACTION, CLINICAL INDICATIONS FOR THEIR USE, AND ASSOCIATED TOXICITIES

Most antimicrobial agents used for the treatment of infections may be categorized according to their principal mechanism of action. For antibacterial agents, the major modes of action include the following (37):

1. Interference with cell wall synthesis
2. Disruption of the bacterial cell membrane
3. Inhibition of protein synthesis
4. Interference with nucleic acid synthesis
5. Inhibition of a metabolic pathway

Tables 104.3, 104.4, and 104.5 review the major pathogens, the antimicrobials of choice by pathogen, and the major toxicities of specific agents, respectively.

Cell Wall Active Antibiotics

Antibacterial drugs that work by inhibiting bacterial cell wall synthesis include the β-lactams—such as the penicillins, cephalosporins, carbapenems, and monobactams—and the glycopeptides, including vancomycin and teicoplanin. β-Lactam agents inhibit the synthesis of the bacterial cell wall by interfering with the enzymes required for the synthesis of the peptidoglycan layer. Vancomycin and teicoplanin also interfere with cell wall synthesis by preventing the cross-linking steps required for stable cell wall synthesis.

Disruption of Bacterial Cell Membrane

Disruption of the bacterial membrane is a less well characterized mechanism of action. Polymyxin antibiotics appear to exert their inhibitory effects by increasing bacterial membrane permeability, causing leakage of bacterial contents. The cyclic lipopeptide, daptomycin, appears to insert its lipid tail into the bacterial cell membrane, causing membrane depolarization and eventual death of the bacterium.

Inhibition of Bacterial Protein Synthesis

Macrolides, aminoglycosides, tetracyclines, chloramphenicol, streptogramins, and oxazolidinones produce their antibacterial effects by inhibiting protein synthesis. Bacterial ribosomes differ in structure from their counterparts in eukaryotic cells. Antibacterial agents take advantage of these differences to selectively inhibit bacterial growth. Macrolides, aminoglycosides, and tetracyclines bind to the 30S subunit of the ribosome, whereas chloramphenicol binds to the 50S subunit. Linezolid is a Gram-positive antibacterial oxazolidinone that binds to the 50S subunit of the ribosome on a site that has not been shown to interact with other classes of antibiotics.

Inhibition of Nucleic Acid Synthesis

Fluoroquinolones exert their antibacterial effects by disrupting DNA synthesis and causing lethal double-strand DNA breaks during DNA replication.

Inhibition of a Metabolic Pathway

Sulfonamides and trimethoprim block the pathway for folic acid synthesis, which ultimately inhibits DNA synthesis. The common antibacterial drug combination of trimethoprim, a folic acid analogue, plus sulfamethoxazole (a sulfonamide) inhibits two steps in the enzymatic pathway for bacterial folate synthesis.

Mechanisms of Resistance to Antibacterial Agents

Most antimicrobial agents exert their effect by influencing a single step in bacterial reproduction or bacterial cell function. Therefore, resistance can emerge with a single point mutation aimed at bypassing or eliminating the action of the antibiotic. Some species of bacteria are innately resistant to at least one class of antimicrobial agents, with resulting resistance to all the members of those antibacterial classes. However, the emergence and spread of acquired resistance due to the selective pressure to use specific antimicrobial agents is of greater concern due to the spread of such resistance. Several mechanisms of antimicrobial resistance are readily transferred to various bacteria. First, the organism may acquire genes encoding enzymes, such as β-lactamases, that destroy the antibacterial agent before it can have an effect. Second, bacteria may acquire efflux pumps that extrude the antibacterial agent from the cell before it can reach its target site and exert its effect. Third, bacteria may acquire several genes for a metabolic pathway that ultimately produces altered bacterial cell walls that no longer contain the binding site of the antimicrobial agent, or bacteria may acquire mutations that limit access of antimicrobial agents to the intracellular target site via down-regulation of porin genes. Susceptible bacteria can also acquire resistance to an antimicrobial agent via new mutations such as are noted above.

STRATEGIES THAT OPTIMIZE THE EFFICACY OF ANTIBIOTICS WHILE MINIMIZING ANTIBIOTIC RESISTANCE

Formal Protocols and Guidelines

Antibiotic practice guidelines or protocols have emerged as a potentially effective means of both avoiding unnecessary antibiotic administration and increasing the effectiveness of prescribed antibiotics. Automated antimicrobial utilization guidelines have been successfully used to identify and minimize the occurrence of adverse drug effects due to antibiotic administration and to improve antibiotic selection (6). Their use has also been associated with stable antibiotic susceptibility patterns for both Gram-positive and Gram-negative bacteria, possibly as a result of promoting antimicrobial heterogeneity and specific end points for antibiotic discontinuation. Automated and nonautomated antimicrobial guidelines have also been employed to reduce the overall use of antibiotics and limit the use of inappropriate antimicrobial treatment, both of which could affect the development of antibiotic resistance (38). One way these guidelines limit the unnecessary use of antimicrobial agents is by recommending that therapy be modified when initial empiric broad-spectrum antibiotics are prescribed and the

TABLE 104.3

MOST COMMON PATHOGENS ASSOCIATED WITH SITES OF SERIOUS INFECTION COMMONLY SEEN IN THE ADULT INTENSIVE CARE UNIT SETTING

Infection site	Pathogens
I. Pneumonia	
1. Community-acquired pneumonia (non-immunocompromised host)	*Streptococcus pneumoniae* *Haemophilus influenzae* *Moraxella catarrhalis* *Mycoplasma pneumoniae* *Legionella pneumophilia* *Chlamydia pneumoniae* Methicillin-resistant *Staphylococcus aureus* (MRSA) Influenza virus
2. Health care–associated pneumonia	MRSA *Pseudomonas aeruginosa* *Klebsiella pneumoniae* *Acinetobacter* species *Stenotrophomonas* species *Legionella pneumophilia*
3. Pneumonia (immunocompromised host)	
a. Neutropenia	Any pathogen listed above *Aspergillus* species *Candida* species
b. Human immunodeficiency virus	Any pathogen listed above *Pneumocystis carinii* *Mycobacterium tuberculosis* *Histoplasma capsulatum* Other fungi Cytomegalovirus
c. Solid organ transplant or bone marrow transplant	Any pathogen listed above (Can vary depending on timing of infection to transplant)
d. Cystic fibrosis	*Haemophilus influenzae* (early) *Staphylococcus aureus* *Pseudomonas aeruginosa* *Burkholderia cepacia*
4. Lung abscess	*Bacteroides* species *Peptostreptococcus* species *Fusobacterium* species *Nocardia* (in immunocompromised patients) Amebic (when suggestive by exposure)
5. Empyema	*Staphylococcus aureus*, *Streptococcus pneumoniae*, Group A *Streptococci*, *Haemophilus influenzae* } Usually acute Anaerobic bacteria, *Enterobacteriaceae*, *Mycobacterium tuberculosis* } Usually subacute or chronic
II. Meningitis	*Streptococcus pneumoniae* *Neisseria meningitidis* *Listeria monocytogenes* *Haemophilus influenzae* *Escherichia coli*, Group B streptococci } Neonates *Staphylococcus aureus*, *Enterobacteriaceae*, *Pseudomonas aeruginosa* } Post-surgical or Post-trauma

(*continued*)

TABLE 104.3

(CONTINUED)

Infection site	Pathogens	
III. Brain abscess	Streptococci *Bacteroides* species	
	Enterobacteriaceae *Staphylococcus aureus*	}Post-surgical or Post-trauma
	Nocardia *Toxoplasma gondii*	}Immunocompromised or HIV infected
IV. Encephalitis	West Nile Herpes simplex Arbovirus Rabies Catscratch disease	
V. Endocarditis	*Streptococcus viridans* *Enterococcus* species *Staphylococcus aureus* *Streptococcus bovis*	
	MRSA	Intravenous drug user, prosthetic value
	Candida species	Prosthetic value
VI. Catheter-associated bacteremia	*Candida* species *Staphylococcus aureus* *Enterococcus* species *Enterobacteriaceae* *Pseudomonas aeruginosa*	
VII. Pyelonephritis	*Enterobacteriaceae* *Escherichia coli* *Enterococcus* species	
	Pseudomonas aeruginosa *Acinetobacter* species	}Catheter-associated, post-surgical
VIII. Peritonitis 1. Primary or spontaneous	*Enterobacteriaceae* *Streptococcus pneumoniae* *Enterococcus* species Anaerobic bacteria (rare)	
2. Secondary (bowel perforation)	*Enterobacteriaceae* *Bacteroides* species *Enterococcus* species *Pseudomonas aeruginosa* (uncommon)	
3. Tertiary (bowel surgery, hospitalized on antibiotics)	*Pseudomonas aeruginosa* MRSA *Acinetobacter* species *Candida* species	
IX. Skin structure infections 1. Cellulitis	Group A streptococci *Staphylococcus aureus*	
	Enterobacteriaceae	Diabetics
2. Decubitus ulcer	Polymicrobial *Streptococcus pyogenes* *Enterococcus* species *Enterobacteriaceae* Anaerobic streptococci *Pseudomonas aeruginosa* *Staphylococcus aureus* *Bacteroides* species	

(*continued*)

TABLE 104.3

(CONTINUED)

Infection site	Pathogens
3. Necrotizing fasciitis	*Streptococcus* species *Clostridia* species Mixed aerobic/anaerobic bacteria
X. Muscle infection	
1. Myonecrosis (gas gangrene)	*Clostridium perfringens* Other *Clostridia* species
2. Pyomyositis	*Staphylococcus aureus* Group A streptococci Anaerobic bacteria Gram-negative bacteria (rare)
XI. Septic shock	
1. Community-acquired	*Streptococcus pneumoniae* *Neisseria meningitidis* *Haemophilus influenzae* *Escherichia coli* *Capnocytophaga* (DF-2 with splenectomy)
2. Health care–associated	MRSA *Pseudomonas aeruginosa* *Acinetobacter* species *Candida* species
3. Toxic shock syndrome	*Staphylococcus aureus* Streptococci species
4. Regional illness or special circumstances	Rickettsial species Ehrlichiosis Babesiosis Catscratch disease (immunocompromised hosts) *Yersinia pestis* *Francisella tularensis* *Leptospira* *Salmonella enteritidis* *Salmonella typhi*

culture results reveal that narrow-spectrum antibiotics can be used.

Hospital Formulary Restrictions

Restricted use of specific antibiotics or antibiotic classes from the hospital formulary has been used as a strategy to reduce the occurrence of antibiotic resistance and antimicrobial costs. Such an approach has been shown to achieve reductions in pharmacy expenses and adverse drug reactions from the restricted drugs. However, not all experiences have been uniformly successful, and the homogenous use of a single limited number of drug classes may actually promote the emergence of resistance (6). Restricted use of specific antibiotics has generally been applied to those drugs with a broad spectrum of action (e.g., carbapenems), rapid emergence of antibiotic resistance (e.g., cephalosporins), and readily identified toxicity (e.g., aminoglycosides). To date, it has been difficult to demonstrate that restricted hospital formularies are effective in curbing the overall emergence of antibiotic resistance among bacterial species. This may be due in large part to methodologic problems. However, their use has been successful in specific outbreaks of infection with antibiotic-resistant bacteria, particularly in conjunction with infection control practices and antibiotic educational activities.

Use of Narrow-Spectrum Antibiotics

Another proposed strategy to curtail the development of antimicrobial resistance, in addition to the judicious overall use of antibiotics, is to use drugs with a narrow antimicrobial spectrum. Several investigations have suggested that infections such as community-acquired pneumonia can usually be successfully treated with narrow spectrum antibiotic agents, especially if the infections are not life threatening. Similarly, the avoidance of broad-spectrum antibiotics, especially those associated with rapid emergence of resistance (cephalosporins, quinolones), and the reintroduction of narrow-spectrum agents (penicillin, trimethoprim, gentamicin), along with infection control practices have been successful in reducing the occurrence of specific infections in the hospital setting (6). Unfortunately, ICU patients often have already received prior antimicrobial treatment, making it more likely that they will be infected with an antibiotic-resistant pathogen (9). Therefore, initial empiric treatment with broad-spectrum agents is often initially necessary for hospitalized patients to avoid inappropriate treatment

TABLE 104.4

DRUGS OF CHOICE IN SERIOUS INFECTIONS[a]

Organism	Drug of choice	Alternative drugs
GRAM-POSITIVE COCCI		
Staphylococcus aureus[b] or *Staphylococcus epidermidis*		
Penicillin-sensitive	Penicillin G	Cephalosporin vancomycin, or clindamycin[c]
Penicillinase-producing[d]	Oxacillin or nafcillin	Cephalosporir vancomycin, or clindamycin
Methicillin-resistant[e]	Vancomycin (linezolid for pneumonia)	Quinolone, T/IP/SMX, minocycline, clindamyci
Nonenterococcal streptococci	Penicillin G	Cephalospori, vancomycin, or clindamycin
Enterococcus	Penicillin or ampicillin + gentamicin	Vancomycin+ gentamicin
Streptococcus pneumoniae[f]	Penicillin G	Cephalospoin, vancomycin, macrolide, or clindamyin
GRAM-POSITIVE BACILLI		
Actinomyces israelii	Penicillin G	Tetracyclie
Bacillus anthracis	Penicillin G	Tetracyclie, macrolide
Clostridium difficile	Metronidazole	Oral vanomycin
Clostridium perfringens	Penicillin[g]	Clindamcin, metronidazole, tetracycline, imipeem
Clostridium tetani	Penicillin[h]	Tetracyine
Corynebacterium diphtheriae	Macrolide[g]	Penicil
Corynebacterium JK	Vancomycin	Penicih G + gentamicin, erythromycin
Listeria monocytogenes	Ampicillin gentamicin	TMP/MX
Nocardia asteroides	TMP/SMX	carbaenem + amikacin
Proprionobacterium sp.	Penicillin	Clinmycin, erythromycin
GRAM-NEGATIVE COCCI		
Moraxella catarrhalis	TMP/SMX	Amicillin-clavulanic acid, ceftriaxone, crolide, tetracycline
Neisseria gonorrhea	Ceftriaxone	Pecillin G, quinolone
Neisseria meningitidis	Penicillin G	Criaxone
ENTERIC GRAM-NEGATIVE BACILLI		
Bacteroides		
Oral source	Penicillin	indamycin, cefoxitin, metronidazole, cefotetan
Bowel source	Metronidazole	efoxitin, cefotetan, imipenem, ampicillin-sulbactam ticar-clavulanate, pip-tazobactam, clindamycin
Citrobacter	Cefepime or imipenem/meropenem	Aminoglycoside, quinolone, piperacillin, aztreonam
Enterobacter sp.[i]	Cefepime or imipenem/meropenem	Ciprofloxacin, aminoglycoside, aztreonam
Escherichia coli[j]	3rd-generation cephalosporin	Aminoglycoside, carbapenem, cefepime, β-lactam/β-lactamase inhibitor, ciprofloxacin, TMP/SMX
Klebsiella[j]	3rd-generation cephalosporin	As for *E. coli*
Proteus mirabilis	Ampicillin	Aminoglycoside, quinolone, cephalosporin, piperacillin, ticarcillin, TMP/SMX
Proteus, nonmirabilis	3rd-generation cephalosporin	Aminoglycoside, quinolone, piperacillin, aztreonam, imipenem
Providencia	2nd- or 3rd-generation cephalospo	Gentamicin, amikacin, piperacillin, aztreonam, imipenem, ticarcillin, mezlocillin, TMP/SMX
Salmonella typhi	Ceftriaxone or quinolone lone	Ampicillin, TMP/SMX
Salmonella, nontyphi[k]	Cefotaxime, ceftriaxone, or qu m	Ampicillin, TMP/SMX
Serratia	Cefepime or imipenem/meror	Aminoglycoside, aztreonam piperacillin, TMP/SMX, quinolone
Shigella	Quinolone	Ampicillin, TMP/SMX, ceftriaxone, cefixime
Yersinia enterocolitica	TMP/SMX	Aminoglycoside, tetracycline, 3rd-generation cephalosporin, quinolone

(continued)

TABLE 104.4

(CONTINUED)

Organism	Drug of choice	Alternative drugs
OTHER GRAM-NEGATIVE BACILLI		
Acinetobacter	Imipenem	Cefepime, aminoglycoside, TMP/SMX, colistin, sulbactam
Eikenella corrodens	Ampicillin	Penicillin G, erythromycin, tetracycline, ceftriaxone
Francisella tularensis	Streptomycin, gentamicin	Tetracycline
Fusobacterium	Penicillin	Clindamycin, metronidazole, cefoxitin
Haemophilus influenzae	3rd-generation cephalosporin	Ampicillin, imipenem, quinolone, cefuroxime[l],
Legionella	Erythromycin (1 g q6h) + rifampin	quinolone, macrolide, TMP/SMX
Pasteurella multocida	Penicillin G	Tetracycline, cephalosporin, amps-sulbactam
Pseudomonas aeruginosa	Antipseudomonal penicillin[m] + aminoglycoside	Aztreonam, cefepime, imipenem, quinolone
Pseudomonas cepacia	TMP/SMX	Ceftazidime
Spirillum minus	Penicillin G	Tetracycline, streptomycin
Streptobacillus moniliforms	Penicillin G	Tetracycline, streptomycin
Vibrio cholerae[n]	Tetracycline	TMP/SMX, quinolone
Vibrio vulnificus	Tetracycline	Cefotaxime
Xanthomonas maltophilia	TMP/SMX	Quinolone, minocycline, ceftazidime
Yersinia pestis	Streptomycin	Tetracycline, gentamicin
CHLAMYDIAE		
Chlamydia pneumoniae (TWAR)	Macrolide	Tetracycline
Chlamydia psittaci	Tetracycline	Chloramphenicol
Chlamydia trachomatis	Macrolide	Sulfonamide, tetracycline
***MYCOPLASMA* sp.**	Macrolide	Tetracycline
	Tetracycline	Quinolone
SPIROCHETES		
Borrelia burgdorferi	Doxycycline, amoxicillin	Penicillin G, macrolide, cefuroxime, ceftriaxone, cefotaxime
Borrelia sp.	Tetracycline	Penicillin G
Treponema pallidum	Penicillin	Tetracycline, ceftriaxone
VIRUSES		
Cytomegalovirus	Ganciclovir[o]	Foscarnet, cidofovir
Herpes simplex	Acyclovir	Foscarnet, ganciclovir
HIV	See Centers for Disease Control Web site	
Influenza	Amantadine	Rimantadine, oseltamivir, zanamivir
Respiratory syncytial	Ribavirin	
Varicella zoster	Acyclovir	Famciclovir[p]
FUNGI		
Aspergillus	Voriconazole	Amphotericin B, echinocandin, Itraconazole
Blastomyces	Amphotericin B or itraconazole	Ketoconazole
Candida[q]		
Mucosal	Fluconazole, echinocandin[s]	Ketoconazole, itraconazole
Systemic	Fluconazole, echinocandin	Amphotericin B
Coccidioides	Amphotericin B or fluconazole	Itraconazole, ketoconazole
Cryptococcus	Amphotericin	Fluconazole, itraconazole
Histoplasma	Itraconazole or Amphotericin B	
Pseudallescheria	Ketoconazole or itraconazole	
Zygomycosis ("mucor")	Amphotericin B	Posaconazole

[a]This table does not consider minor infections that may be treated with oral agents, single-agent therapy, or less toxic drugs. Sensitivity testing must be done on bacterial isolates to confirm the sensitivity pattern.
[b]Some authorities recommend clindamycin as the first choice for susceptible toxin-producing staphylococci, streptococci, or clostridia.
[c]First-generation cephalosporins are most active. If endocarditis is suspected, do not use clindamycin. Some authorities recommend the addition of gentamicin for endocarditis caused by nonenterococcal streptococci or tolerant staphylococci.
[d]Penicillinase-producing staphylococci are also resistant to ampicillin, amoxicillin, carbenicillin, ticarcillin, mezlocillin, and piperacillin

(*continued*)

TABLE 104.4
(CONTINUED)

(*Footnote continued from previous page*).
[e]Methicillin-resistant staphylococci should be assumed to be resistant to all cephalosporins and penicillins, even if disk testing suggests sensitivity. Tigecycline, ceftobiprole, daptomycin, telavancin, and dalbavancin may be alternatives for specific types of methicillin-resistant infection pending future studies and indications.
[f]Some stains show intermediate- or high-level penicillin resistance. Highly resistant strains are treated with vancomycin, or rifampin, or both. In regions with high prevalence of resistant pneumococcus, ceftriaxone or vancomycin should be considered until sensitivity is known.
[g]Use as an adjunct to debridement of infected tissues.
[h]Use as an adjunct to active and passive immunization.
[i]Because of rapid development of resistance, cephalosporins not recommended even if initial tests indicate susceptibility.
[j]*Klebsiella sp.* and *E. coli* producing extended-spectrum beta-lactamase (ESBL) should be preferentially managed with a carbapenem.
[k]Uncomplicated *Salmonella* enteritis should not be treated with antibiotics.
[l]Should not be used in meningitis because of poor CNS penetration.
[m]Antipseudomonal penicillins include ticarcillin, mezlocillin, and piperacillin.
[n]Primary therapy is fluid and electrolyte repletion.
[o]Oral form should be used only in maintenance therapy of retinal cytomegalovirus.
[p]Approved only for mild herpes zoster in immunocompetent hosts.
[q]*Candida kruseii* and *Torulopsis glabrata* may be resistant to azole therapy, *Candida parapsilosis* may be resistant to echinocandins.
[r]In multidrug combinations.
[s]Echinocandins include caspofungin, micafungin, and anidulafungin.

until culture results become available and de-escalation can occur (Fig. 104.2) (14).

Quantitative Cultures and Assessment of Infection Risk

Pneumonia is the most common hospital-acquired infection among mechanically ventilated patients. A recent meta-analysis of four randomized trials demonstrated that the use of quantitative bacterial cultures obtained from the lower respiratory tract may, in theory, facilitate de-escalation of empiric broad-spectrum antibiotics and reduce drug-specific antibiotic days of treatment (39). Another recent study found that patients with a clinical suspicion for VAP and culture-negative bronchoalveolar lavage (BAL) results for a major pathogen could have antimicrobial therapy safely discontinued within 72 hours (40). Interestingly, the mean modified clinical pulmonary infection scores of these patients was approximately six, suggesting that this quantitative clinical assessment of the risk for VAP could have been used to discontinue antibiotics as previously suggested (41). Regardless of whether quantitative culture methods are used, the results of microbiologic testing should be used to routinely modify or discontinue antibiotic treatment in the appropriate clinical setting.

Combination Antibiotic Therapy

Several recent meta-analyses recommend the use of monotherapy with a β-lactam antibiotic, as opposed to combination therapy including an aminoglycoside, for the definitive treatment of severe sepsis once antimicrobial susceptibilities are known (42,43). Additionally, there is no definitive evidence that the emergence of antibiotic resistance is reduced by the use of combination antimicrobial therapy. However, empiric combination therapy directed against high-risk pathogens such as *Pseudomonas aeruginosa* should be encouraged until the results of antimicrobial susceptibility become available. Such an approach to empiric treatment can increase the likelihood of providing appropriate initial antimicrobial therapy with improved outcomes (15).

Antibiotic Cycling and Scheduled Antibiotic Changes

The concept of antibiotic class cycling has been suggested as a potential strategy for reducing the emergence of antimicrobial resistance (6). In theory, a class of antibiotics or a specific antibiotic drug is withdrawn from use for a defined time period and reintroduced at a later time in an attempt to limit bacterial resistance to the cycled antimicrobial agents. Unfortunately, mathematical modeling suggests that the use of antibiotic cycling will be inferior to "mixing" of antibiotics as a strategy to reduce the emergence of antimicrobial resistance (44). Nevertheless, several earlier studies of antimicrobial cycling have found beneficial outcomes in terms of antibiotic resistance, with benefits extending outside of the ICU setting. More recent rigorous studies of antimicrobial cycling have failed to confirm these findings (45,46). Although antimicrobial heterogeneity or mixing seems to be a logical policy, simple cycling of antibiotics combined with prolonged treatment exposures seems to be a strategy that will only promote further antibiotic resistance.

Antimicrobial Decolonization Strategies

The prophylactic administration of parenteral antibiotics has been shown to reduce the occurrence of nosocomial infections in specific high-risk patient populations requiring intensive care (47). Similarly, topical antibiotic administration (i.e., selective digestive decontamination), with or without concomitant parenteral antibiotics, has also been shown to be effective at reducing nosocomial infections (48). However, the routine use of selective digestive decontamination has also been linked to the emergence of antimicrobial resistance. Additionally, the mixed results of recent negative trials for VAP prevention using iseganan and chlorhexidine, an antimicrobial peptide and

TABLE 104.5

TOXICITIES ASSOCIATED WITH ANTIMICROBIALS

Antimicrobial	Serious toxicities, uncommon	Common toxicities[a]
Penicillins Ampicillin Penicillin	Anaphylaxis, seizures, hemolytic anemia, neutropenia, thrombocytopenia, drug fever	Diarrhea, nausea, vomiting, rash
Antistaphylococcal penicillins Nafcillin Oxacillin	Anaphylaxis, neutropenia, thrombocytopenia, acute interstitial nephritis, hepatotoxicity	Diarrhea, nausea, vomiting, rash
***B*-lactam/*B*-lactamase inhibitors** Amoxicillin/clavulanate Ampicillin/sulbactam Piperacillin/tazolbactam* Ticarcillin/clavulanate	Anaphylaxis, seizures, hemolytic anemia, neutropenia, thrombocytopenia *C. difficile* colitis, cholestatic jaundice,* drug fever	Diarrhea, nausea, vomiting, rash
Cephalosporins	Anaphylaxis, seizures, neutropenia, thrombocytopenia, drug fever	Diarrhea, nausea, vomiting, rash
Carbapenems Imipenem Meropenem Ertapenem	Anaphylaxis, seizures (imipenem > meropenem, ertapenem) *C. difficile* colitis, drug fever	Diarrhea, nausea, vomiting
Glycopeptides Vancomycin	Ototoxicity, nephrotoxicity (unlikely without concomitant nephrotoxins), thrombocytopenia	Red-man syndrome
Oxazolidinones Linezolid	*More common with long-term use:* Peripheral and optic neuropathy, myelosuppression *Possible with short-term use:* Lactic acidosis, myopathy anemia	Diarrhea
Lipopeptides Daptomycin		Diarrhea, constipation, vomiting
Streptogramin Quinupristin/dalfopristin		Arthralgia, myalgia, inflammation, pain, edema at infusion site, hyperbilirubinemia
Aminoglycosides Amikacin Gentamicin Tobramycin		Nephrotoxicity, ototoxicity
Fluoroquinolones 2nd generation Ciprofloxacin 3rd generation Levofloxacin 4th generation Gatifloxacin* Moxifloxacin Gemifloxacin	Anaphylaxis, dysglycemia* QTc prolongation, joint toxicity in children, tendon rupture	Nausea, vomiting, diarrhea, photosensitivity, rash CNS stimulation, dizziness, somnolence
Macrolides Erythromycin* Azithromycin Clarithromycin	QTc prolongation (erythromycin > clarithromycin > azithromycin), cholestasis*	Nausea, vomiting, diarrhea, abnormal taste
Ketolides Telithromycin	Acute hepatic failure QTc prolongation	Nausea, vomiting, diarrhea
Clindamycin	*C. difficile* colitis	Nausea, vomiting, diarrhea, abdominal pain, rash
Tetracyclines Tetracycline* Doxycycline Minocycline[†]	Tooth discoloration and retardation of bone growth (in children), renal tubular necrosis,* dizziness,[†] vertigo,[†] pseudotumor cerebri	Photosensitivity, diarrhea
Glycylcyclines Tigecycline		Nausea, vomiting, diarrhea
Trimethoprim/sulfamethoxazole	Myelosuppression Stevens-Johnson syndrome, hyperkalemia, aseptic meningitis, hepatic necrosis	Rash, nausea, vomiting, diarrhea
Metronidazole	Seizures, peripheral neuropathy	Nausea, vomiting, metallic taste, disulfiramlike reaction
Nitrofurantoin	Pulmonary toxicity, peripheral neuropathy	Urine discoloration, photosensitivity

(continued)

TABLE 104.5

(CONTINUED)

Antimicrobial	Serious toxicities, uncommon	Common toxicities[a]
Antifungal Agents		
Azoles	Hepatic failure, increased AST/ALT, cardiovascular toxicity,* hypertension,* edema*	Nausea, vomiting, diarrhea, rash, visual disturbances,† phototoxicity†
Fluconazole		
Itraconazole*		
Voriconazole†		
Amphotericin B products	Acute liver failure, myelosuppression	Nephrotoxicity (less common with lipid formulations), acute infusion-related reactions, hypokalemia, hypomagnesemia
Amphotericin B deoxycholate		
ABLC		
ABCD		
Liposomal amphotericin B		
Echinocandins	Hepatotoxicity, infusion-related rash, flushing, itching	
Caspofungin		
Micafungin		
Anidulafungin		
Flucytosine	Myelosuppression, hepatotoxicity, confusion, hallucinations, sedation	Nausea, vomiting, diarrhea, rash
Antiviral Agents		
Nucleoside analogues	Nephrotoxicity, rash, encephalopathy, inflammation at injection site, phlebitis	Bone marrow suppression,† headache, nausea, vomiting, diarrhea (with oral forms)
Acyclovir		
Valacyclovir		
Ganciclovir†		
Valganciclovir†		
Amantadine	CNS disturbances (amantadine > rimantadine)	Nausea, vomiting, anorexia, xerostomia
Rimantadine		
Neuraminidase inhibitors	Anaphylaxis,* bronchospasm†	Nausea, vomiting,* cough,† local discomfort†
Oseltamivir*		
Zanamivir†		
Cidofovir	Anemia, neutropenia, fever, rash	Nephrotoxicity, uveitis/iritis, nausea, vomiting
Foscarnet	Seizures, anemia, fever	Nephrotoxicity, electrolyte abnormalities (hypocalcemia, hypomagnesemia, hypokalemia, hypophosphatemia), nausea, vomiting, diarrhea, headache

[a]Toxicities were classified as "common" relative to the other toxicities that agent is known to cause. Because toxicities are classified as "common" does not imply they are not serious.

antiseptic, respectively, to decontaminate the oropharynx in mechanically ventilated patients sheds doubt on the overall utility of this practice (49–51). Based on these studies, antimicrobial and nonantimicrobial agents should be considered for oral decontamination only in *appropriate high-risk ICU* patients or to assist in the containment of outbreaks of MDR bacterial infections in conjunction with established infection control practices.

Shorter Courses of Antibiotic Treatment

Prolonged administration of antibiotics to hospitalized patients has been shown to be an important risk factor for the emergence of colonization and infection with antibiotic-resistant bacteria (9,12). Therefore, recent attempts have been made to reduce the duration of antibiotic treatment for specific bacterial infections. Several clinical trials have found that 7 to 8 days of antibiotic treatment is acceptable for most *nonbacteremic* patients with VAP (11,41). Similarly, shorter courses of antibiotic treatment have been successfully used in patients at low risk for VAP (38,40,41) with pyelonephritis (52) and for community-acquired pneumonia (53). In general, the shorter-course treatment regimens have been associated with a significantly lower risk for the emergence of antimicrobial resistance compared to more traditional durations of antibiotic treatment ranging from 14 to 21 days. In the future, more specific markers for the presence of bacterial infection (e.g., procalcitonin, soluble triggering receptor on myeloid cells [sTREM1]) may allow shorter courses of empiric antibiotic administration in patients without identified bacterial infection. Several recently published guidelines for the antibiotic management of nosocomial pneumonia and severe sepsis currently recommend the discontinuation of empiric antibiotic therapy after 48 to 72 hours if cultures are negative or the signs of infection have resolved (2,20).

Optimizing Pharmacokinetic/Pharmacodynamic (Pk/Pd) Principles

Antibiotic concentrations that are sublethal can promote the emergence of resistant pathogens. Optimization of antibiotic

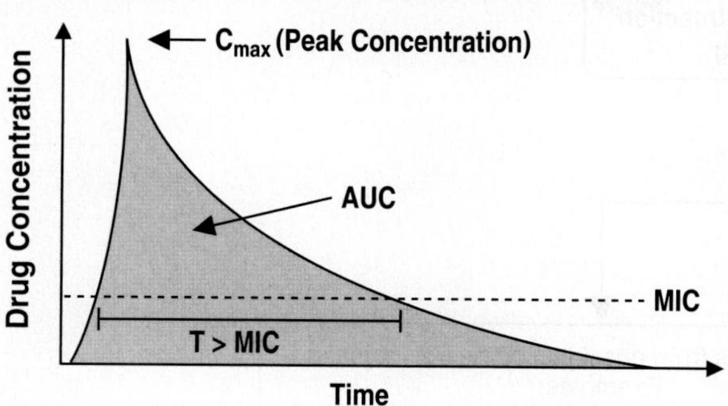

FIGURE 104.3. Pharmacodynamic parameters found to be important for the efficacy of antimicrobial agents. AUC, area under the concentration–time curve; C_{max}, maximum concentration; MIC, minimum inhibitory concentration; T, time.

regimens on the basis of pharmacokinetic/pharmacodynamic principles could play a role in the reduction of antibiotic resistance (8). The duration of time the serum drug concentration remains above the minimum inhibitory concentration of the antibiotic (T > MIC) enhances bacterial eradication with β-lactams, carbapenems, monobactams, glycopeptides, and oxazolidinones (Fig. 104.3). Frequent dosing, prolonged infusion times, or continuous infusions can increase the T > MIC and improve clinical and microbiologic cure rates. To maximize the bactericidal effects of aminoglycosides, clinicians must optimize the maximum drug concentration (C_{max})-to-MIC ratio. A C_{max}:MIC ratio of $\geq$10:1 using once-daily aminoglycoside dosing (5–7 mg/kg) has been associated with preventing the emergence of resistant organisms, improving clinical response to treatment, and avoiding toxicity. The 24-hour area under the antibiotic concentration curve-to-MIC ratio (AUIC) is correlated with fluoroquinolone efficacy and prevention of resistance development. An AUIC value of >100 has been associated with a significant reduction in the risk of resistance development while on therapy. As a general rule, clinicians should use the *maximum approved dose* of an antibiotic for a potentially life-threatening infection to optimize tissue concentrations of the drug and killing of pathogens.

New Antimicrobial Agents

Most new antibiotics have been developed for the treatment of Gram-positive bacteria. Given the increasing prevalence of resistance in Gram-negative bacteria, new agents for these pathogens are urgently needed as well. Until recently, the glycopeptides, vancomycin and teicoplanin, were the only antibacterial compounds available to which MRSA strains remained uniformly susceptible. In 1996, the first clinical isolate of *Staphylococcus aureus* with reduced susceptibility to vancomycin (vancomycin-intermediate *Staphylococcus aureus,* or VISA) was reported in Japan and, since then, similar cases have been reported around the world. Only a few years later, clinical isolates of *Staphylococcus aureus* that were fully resistant to vancomycin were reported in South Africa and Michigan, USA. The emergence of MRSA strains with reduced vancomycin susceptibility has limited the treatment options and increased the incidence of treatment failure (54); infection with one of these strains may be an independent predictor of mortality (55). More concerning are the observations that upward drift in the minimum inhibitory concentrations for vancomycin in MRSA are associated with an increased risk of clinical treatment failures (56). As a result of this upsurge in MRSA resistance, most of the recent advances in the development of new antibiotic agents have predominantly occurred for Gram-positive bacteria. Unfortunately, Gram-negative antibiotic development has lagged behind.

Linezolid

Linezolid is the first licensed member of a new class of antibiotics, the oxazolidinones, that binds to the ribosome and inhibits microbial protein synthesis. This novel mechanism of action provides an antimicrobial activity that is independent of the resistance status toward other antibiotics. Some studies suggest that linezolid may be associated with improved survival and clinical cure rates compared to vancomycin in patients with nosocomial pneumonia. Linezolid is a suitable alternative to vancomycin in nosocomial infections caused by MRSA, particularly in pneumonia. Although a general agreement on the superiority of linezolid to vancomycin and teicoplanin is lacking, it does not require adjustment for renal function at a dosage of 600 mg every 12 hours. Close monitoring of the blood cell count should be done in case of pre-existing myelosuppression and during prolonged treatment.

Daptomycin

Daptomycin is a cyclic lipopeptide active only against Gram-positive organisms, and has been recently approved for the treatment of complicated skin and soft tissue infections, with activity against resistant and susceptible isolates of *Staphylococcus aureus*. Its once-daily dosing (4 mg/kg IV) and safety profile (except for some concerns for rhabdomyolysis) make daptomycin an attractive option for the treatment of staphylococcal infections. Unfortunately, daptomycin may not be a useful agent for deep-seated tissue infections. A recent trial of 740 patients with pneumonia had to be terminated early due to a lower level of efficacy compared to ceftriaxone. This may be related to the molecular size of this drug, its protein-binding characteristics, and inhibition by pulmonary surfactant. Therefore, the current use of daptomycin should be limited to skin infections and bacteremia and/or endocarditis.

Quinupristin-Dalfopristin

Quinupristin-dalfopristin is a semisynthetic, parenteral streptogramin with activity against most of the Gram-positive pathogens. A multicenter study compared quinupristin-dalfopristin and vancomycin in the treatment of nosocomial pneumonia by Gram-positive pathogens. Similar clinical success rates were observed, including in the MRSA subgroup, although very low rates were seen (30.9% in the quinupristin-dalfopristin group versus 44.4% in the vancomycin group) in the bacteriologically evaluable population. These data suggest that quinupristin-dalfopristin is probably not a better option than vancomycin, with both agents seemingly having limited activity against MRSA pneumonia in this study. Although antimicrobial resistance has not been an overriding concern, the side effect profile of quinupristin-dalfopristin (myalgia, arthralgia, and thrombophlebitis) and its lack of proven efficacy over vancomycin have limited its overall use.

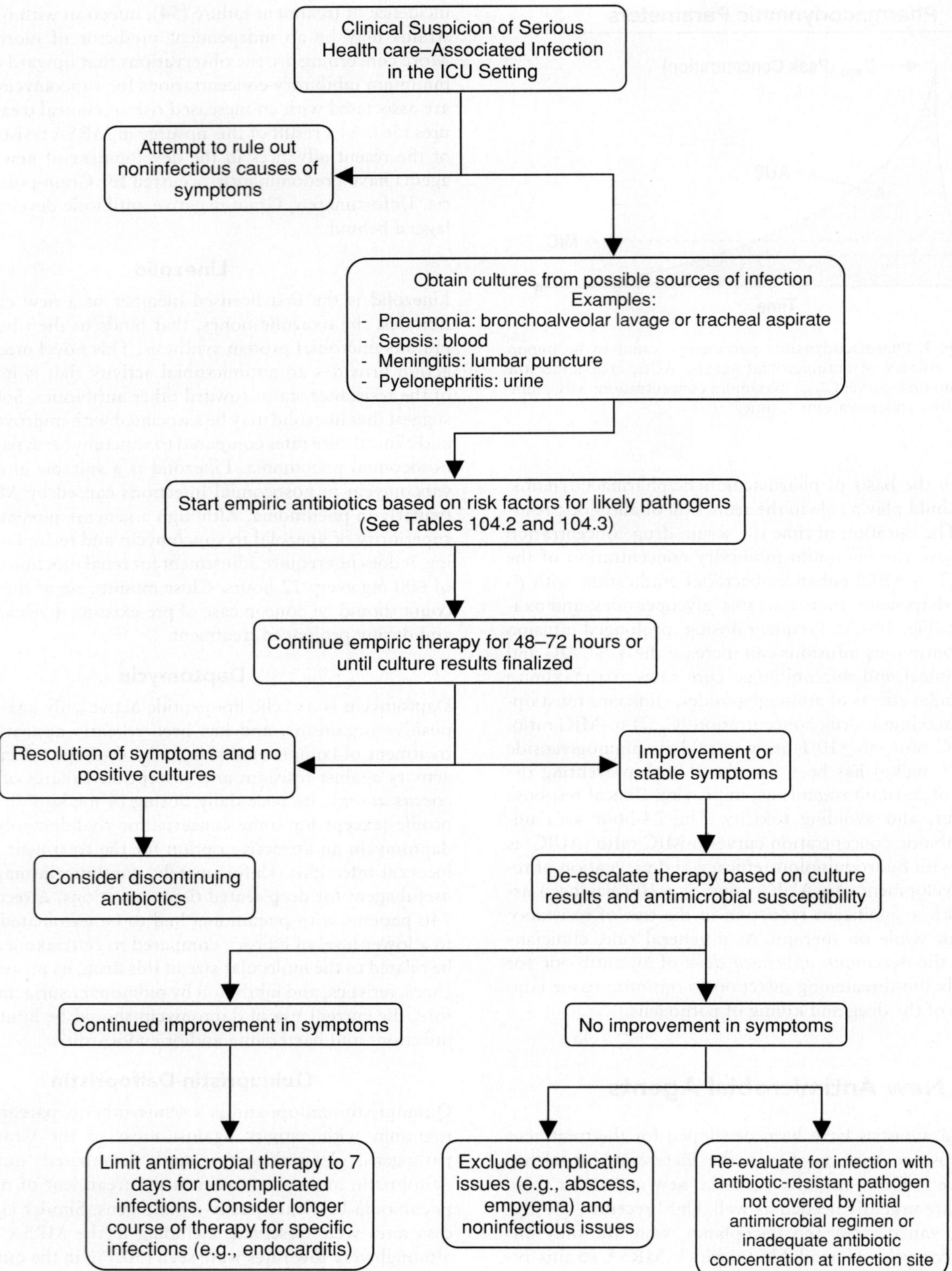

FIGURE 104.4. A step-by-step approach to the antibiotic management of serious or life-threatening health care–associated infections. ICU, intensive care unit.

Tigecycline

Tigecycline is the first glycylcycline to be launched and is one of the very few antimicrobials with activity against Gram-negative bacteria and MRSA. In contrast to classic tetracyclines, tigecycline can be administered only parenterally, and its major side effect appears to be dose-related nausea and emesis. The dosing regimen for tigecycline has been validated in clinical trials that involved a 100-mg loading dose, followed by 50 mg twice daily in patients with complicated infections of the skin and skin structure, as well as intra-abdominal infections. It evades acquired efflux and target-mediated resistance to classical tetracyclines but not chromosomal efflux. The C_{max} is low, but tissue penetration is excellent and, in clinical trials, the compound has shown equivalence to imipenem/cilastatin in intra-abdominal infection and to vancomycin plus aztreonam in skin and skin structure infection. Tigecycline may prove particularly useful for the treatment of surgical wound infections, where both Gram-negative bacteria and MRSA are likely pathogens. Tigecycline may also have a role in the treatment of infections due to multiresistant pathogens, including *Acinetobacter* species and extended-spectrum β-lactamase producing Gram-negatives. Future studies are needed to differentiate the role of tigecycline from other newly available agents including new glycopeptides, linezolid, daptomycin, and ceftobiprole.

Ceftobiprole

Ceftobiprole (BAL5788) is the water-soluble prodrug of BAL9141, a novel broad-spectrum cephalosporin with potent bactericidal activities against MRSA and penicillin-resistant *Streptococcus pneumoniae*. Until recently, efforts to develop β-lactam antibiotics active against MRSA have largely been unsuccessful. One exception is BAL9141, a novel pyrrolidinone-3-ylidenemethyl cephalosporin specifically designed to have strong affinity for penicillin-binding protein (PBP) 2a known to confer resistance in staphylococci and pneumococci. BAL9141 also binds strongly to the relevant PBPs of most Gram-positive and Gram-negative pathogens and is resistant to many β-lactamases. Ceftobiprole is currently being investigated in patients with pneumonia and complicated skin infections.

Dalbavancin

Dalbavancin is a lipoglycopeptide antimicrobial that has been studied in phase two trials for complicated skin and skin structure infections and catheter-related bloodstream infection. Dalbavancin is a bactericidal agent whose long terminal plasma half-life (9–12 days) allows for the unique dosing of 1,000 mg given on day 1 and 500 mg given on day 8. The long half-life may turn out to be the strength of the drug, allowing for more convenient treatment options in patients requiring prolonged antibiotic therapy (e.g., right-sided infective endocarditis or osteomyelitis). However, the impact of this prolonged half-life on adverse reactions also needs further evaluation.

Telavancin

Telavancin is another lipoglycopeptide in development. Telavancin exerts concentration-dependent bactericidal activity against Gram-positive bacteria, including MRSA. This agent's rapid bactericidal activity arises from two mechanisms: inhibition of peptidoglycan synthesis and interaction with the bacterial membrane. In a recent double-blind randomized control trial, it proved effective for the treatment of complicated skin and skin structure infections given as a once-daily dosing. Telavancin's once daily dosing is appealing, and perhaps the dual mechanism of action will eventually slow the development of resistance to this agent. Additional studies are ongoing to determine the efficacy of this agent in other infections including pneumonia.

Doripenem

Doripenem is a novel broad-spectrum parenteral carbapenem antimicrobial. The chemical formula for doripenem confers β-lactamase stability and resistance to inactivation by renal dehydropeptidases. Information from presented *in vitro* studies indicates that doripenem has a spectrum and potency against Gram-positive cocci most similar to imipenem or ertapenem and a Gram-negative activity most like meropenem (twofold or fourfold superiority to imipenem).

SUMMARY

Antimicrobial resistance is a common variable influencing antibiotic prescription decisions and clinical outcomes. Increasingly, clinicians must be able to balance the need to provide appropriate antimicrobial treatment to patients while minimizing the further development of resistance. The practice of antimicrobial de-escalation (Figs. 104.1 and 104.2) should be used to accomplish this difficult but important balance. Moreover, for patients with serious or life-threatening infections, treatment algorithms should be used to ensure that early appropriate therapy is administered to all patients (Fig. 104.4).

References

1. Carlet J, Ben Ali A, Chalfine A. Epidemiology and control of antibiotic resistance in the intensive care unit. *Curr Opin Infect Dis.* 2004;17:309–316.
2. Dellinger RP, Carlet JM, Masur H, et al. Surviving Sepsis Campaign Management Guidelines Committee. Surviving Sepsis Campaign guidelines for management of severe sepsis and septic shock. *Crit Care Med.* 2004;32:858–873.
3. Neuhauser MM, Weinstein RA, Rydman R, et al. Antibiotic resistance among Gram-negative bacilli in US intensive care units: implications for fluoroquinolone use. *JAMA.* 2003;289:885–888.
4. Naiemi NA, Duim B, Savelkoul PH, et al. Widespread transfer of resistance genes between bacterial species in an intensive care unit: implications for hospital epidemiology. *J Clin Microbiol.* 2005;43:4862–4864.
5. Cartolano GL, Cheron M, Benabid D, et al. Association of Hospital Bacteriologists, Virologists and Hygiene Professionals. Methicillin-resistant *Staphylococcus aureus* (MRSA) with reduced susceptibility to glycopeptides (GISA) in 63 French general hospitals. *Clin Microbiol Infect.* 2004;10:448–451.
6. Kollef MH, Fraser VJ. Antibiotic resistance in the intensive care unit. *Ann Intern Med.* 2001;134:298–314.
7. Kollef MH. Gram-negative bacterial resistance: evolving patterns and treatment paradigms. *Clin Infect Dis.* 2005;40:S85–S88.
8. Kollef MH, Micek ST. Strategies to prevent antimicrobial resistance in the intensive care unit. *Crit Care Med.* 2005;33:1845–1853.
9. Trouillet JL, Chastre J, Vuagnat A, et al. Ventilator-associated pneumonia caused by potentially drug-resistant bacteria. *Am J Respir Crit Care Med.* 1998;157:531–539.
10. Kollef MH, Micek ST. Methicillin-resistant Staphylococcus aureus: a new community-acquired pathogen. *Curr Opin Infect Dis.* 2006;19:161–168.
11. Chastre J, Wolff M, Fagon JY, et al. Comparison of 15 vs. 8 days of antibiotic therapy for ventilator-associated pneumonia in adults: a randomized trial. *JAMA.* 2003;290:2588–2598.
12. Dennesen PJW, van der Ven AJ, Kessels AGH, et al. Resolution of infectious parameters after antimicrobial therapy in patients with ventilator-associated pneumonia. *Am J Respir Crit Care Med.* 2001;163:1371–1375.
13. Ibrahim EH, Sherman G, Ward S, et al. The influence of inadequate antimicrobial treatment of bloodstream infections on patient outcomes in the ICU setting. *Chest.* 2000;118:146–155.

14. Kollef MH. Inadequate antimicrobial treatment: an important determinant of outcome for hospitalized patients. *Clin Infect Dis.* 2000;31:S131–S138.
15. Micek ST, Lloyd AE, Ritchie DJ, et al. *Pseudomonas aeruginosa* bloodstream infection: importance of appropriate initial antimicrobial treatment. *Antimicrob Agents Chemother.* 2005;49:1306–1311.
16. Dhainaut JF, Laterre PF, LaRosa S, et al. The clinical evaluation committee in a large multicenter phase 3 trial of drotrecogin alfa (activated) in patients with severe sepsis (PROWESS): role, methodology, and results. *Crit Care Med.* 2003;31:2291–2301.
17. Harbarth S, Garbino JK, Pugin J, et al. Inappropriate initial antimicrobial therapy and its effects on survival in a clinical trial of immunomodulating therapy for severe sepsis. *Am J Med.* 2003;115:529–535.
18. Garnacho-Montero J, Garcia-Garmendia JL, Barrero-Almodovar A, et al. Impact of adequate empirical antibiotic therapy on the outcome of patients admitted to the intensive care unit with sepsis. *Crit Care Med.* 2003;31:2742–2751.
19. Kollef MH, Ward S. The influence of mini-BAL cultures on patient outcomes: implications for the antibiotic management of ventilator-associated pneumonia. *Chest.* 1998;113:412–420.
20. American Thoracic Society. Guidelines for the management of adults with hospital-acquired, ventilator-associated, and healthcare-associated pneumonia. *Am J Resp Crit Care Med.* 2005;171:388–416.
21. Rello J, Ollendorf DA, Oster G, et al. Epidemiology and outcomes of ventilator-associated pneumonia in a large US database. *Chest.* 2002;122: 2115–2121.
22. Shorr AF, Combes A, Kollef MH, et al. Methicillin-resistant *Staphylococcus aureus* prolongs intensive care unit length of stay in ventilator-associated pneumonia – despite initially appropriate antibiotic therapy. *Crit Care Med.* 2006;34:700–706.
23. National Nosocomial Infections Surveillance (NNIS) system report, data summary from January 1992-April 2000, issued June 2000. *Am J Infect Control.* 2000;28:429–448.
24. Gaynes R, EdwardsJR; National Nosocomial Infections Surveillance System. Overview of nosocomial infections caused by gram-negative bacilli. *Clin Infect Dis.* 2005;41:848–854.
25. Richards MJ, Edwards JR, Culver DH, et al. Nosocomial infections in combined medical-surgical intensive care units in the United States, 1. *Infect Control Hosp Epidemiol.* 2000;21:510–515.
26. Leung WS, Chu CM, Tsang KY, et al. Fulminant community-acquired *Acinetobacter baumannii* pneumonia as a distinct clinical syndrome. *Chest.* 2006;129:102–109.
27. Paterson DL, Bonomo RA. Extended-spectrum beta-lactamases: a clinical update. *Clin Micro Rev.* 2005;18:657–686.
28. Namias N, Samiian L, Nino D, et al. Incidence and susceptibility of pathogenic bacteria vary between intensive care units within a single hospital: implications for empiric antibiotic strategies. *J Trauma.* 2000;49:638–645.
29. Rello J, Sa-Borges M, Correa H, et al. Variations in etiology of ventilator-associated pneumonia across four treatment sites. *Am J Respir Crit Care Med.* 1999;160:608–613.
30. Masterton RG, Kuti JL, Turner PJ, et al. The OPTIMA programme: utilizing MYSTIC (2002) to predict critical pharmacodynamic target attainment against nosocomial pathogens in Europe. *J Antimicrob Chemother.* 2005;55:71–77.
31. Tacconelli E, Venkataraman L, De Girolami PC, et al. Methicillin-resistant *Staphylococcus aureus* bacteraemia diagnosed at hospital admission: distinguishing between community-acquired versus healthcare-associated strains. *J Antimicrob Chemother.* 2004;53(3):474–479.
32. Friedman ND, Kaye KS, Stout JE, et al. Health care-associated bloodstream infections in adults: a reason to change the accepted definition of community-acquired infections. *Ann Intern Med.* 2002;137:791–797.
33. Kollef MH, Shorr A, Tabak YP, et al. Epidemiology and outcomes of healthcare-associated pneumonia: results from a large US database of culture-positive pneumonia. *Chest.* 2005;128:3854–3862.
34. Gaynes R. Health-care associated bloodstream infections: a change in thinking. *Ann Intern Med.* 2002;137:850–851.
35. Wilkinson M, Woodhead MA. Guidelines for community-acquired pneumonia in the ICU. *Curr Opin Crit Care.* 2004;10:59–64.
36. Micek ST, Heuring TJ, Hollands JM, et al. Optimizing antibiotic treatment for ventilator-associated pneumonia. *Pharmacotherapy.* 2006;26:204–213.
37. Tenover FC. Mechanisms of antimicrobial resistance in bacteria. *Am J Med.* 2006;119:s3–s10.
38. Micek ST, Ward S, Fraser VJ, et al. A randomized controlled trial of an antibiotic discontinuation policy for clinically suspected ventilator-associated pneumonia. *Chest.* 2004;125:1791–1799.
39. Shorr AF, Sherner JH, Jackson WL, et al. Invasive approaches to the diagnosis of ventilator-associated pneumonia: a meta-analysis. *Crit Care Med.* 2005;33:46–53.
40. Kollef MH, Kollef KE. Antibiotic utilization and outcomes for patients with clinically suspected ventilator-associated pneumonia and negative quantitative BAL culture results. *Chest.* 2005;128:2706–2713.
41. Singh N, Rogers P, Atwood CW, et al. Short-course empiric antibiotic therapy for patients with pulmonary infiltrates in the intensive care unit. A proposed solution for indiscriminate antibiotic prescription. *Am J Respir Crit Care Med.* 2000;162:505–511.
42. Paul M, Benuri-Silbiger I, Soares-Weiser K, et al. Beta-lactam monotherapy versus beta-lactam-aminoglycoside combination therapy for sepsis in immunocompetent patients: systematic review and meta-analysis of randomized trials. *BMJ.* 2004;328:668.
43. Safdar N, Handelsman J, Maki DG. Does combination antimicrobial therapy reduce mortality in Gram-negative bacteraemia? A meta-analysis. *Lancet Infect Dis.* 2004;4:519–527.
44. Bergstrom CT, Lo M, Lipsitch M. Ecological theory suggests that antimicrobial cycling will not reduce antimicrobial resistance in hospitals. *Proc Natl Acad Sci U S A.* 2004;101:13285–13290.
45. Warren DK, Hill HA, Merz LR, et al. Cycling empirical antimicrobial agents to prevent emergence of antimicrobial-resistant Gram-negative bacteria among intensive care unit patients. *Crit Care Med.* 2004;32:2450–2456.
46. van Loon HJ, Vriens MR, Fluit Ac, et al. Antibiotic rotation and development of Gram-negative antibiotic resistance. *Am J Respir Crit Care Med.* 2005;171:480–487.
47. Sirvent JM, Torres A, El-Ebiary M, et al. A protective effect of intravenously administered cefuroxime against nosocomial pneumonia in patients with structural coma. *Am J Respir Crit Care Med.* 1997;155:1729–1734.
48. Krueger WA, Lenhart FP, Neeser G, et al. Influence of combined intravenous and topical antibiotic prophylaxis on the incidence of infections, organ dysfunctions, and mortality in critically ill surgical patients: a prospective, stratified, randomized, double-blind, placebo-controlled clinical trial. *Am J Respir Crit Care Med.* 2002;166:1029–1037.
49. Kollef MH, Pittet D, Sánchez García M, et al. A randomized, double-blind, placebo-controlled, multinational phase III trial of iseganan in prevention of ventilator-associated pneumonia. *Am J Respir Crit Care Med.* 2006;173:91–97.
50. Fourrier F, Dubois D, Pronnier P, et al. Effect of gingival and dental plaque antiseptic decontamination on nosocomial infections acquired in the intensive care unit: a double-blind placebo-controlled multicenter study. *Crit Care Med.* 2005;33:1728–1735.
51. Koeman M, van der Van A, Hak E, et al. Oral decontamination with chlorhexidine reduces the incidence of ventilator-associated pneumonia. *Am J Respir Crit Care Med.* 2006;173:1348–1355.
52. Talan DA, Stamm WE, Hooton TM, et al. Comparison of ciprofloxacin (7 days) and trimethoprim-sulfamethoxazole (14 days) for acute uncomplicated pyelonephritis in women: a randomized trial. *JAMA.* 2000;283:1583–1590.
53. Dunbar LM, Wunderink RG, Habib MP, et al. High-dose, short-course levofloxacin for community-acquired pneumonia: a new treatment paradigm. *Clin Infect Dis.* 2003;37:752–760.
54. Howden BP, Ward PB, Charles PGP, et al. Treatment outcomes for serious infections caused by methicillin-resistant *Staphylococcus aureus* with reduced vancomycin susceptibility. *Clin Infect Dis.* 2004;38:521–528.
55. Fridkin SK, Hageman J, McDougal LK, et al. Epidemiological and microbiological characterization of infections caused by *Staphylococcus aureus* with reduced susceptibility to vancomycin, United States, 1997–2001. *Clin Infect Dis.* 2003;36:429–439.
56. Sakoulas G, Moellering RC, Eliopoulos GM. Adaptation of methicillin-resistant *Staphylococcus aureus* in the face of vancomycin therapy. *Clin Infect Dis.* 2006;42:S40–S50.

CHAPTER 105 ■ AN APPROACH TO THE FEBRILE ICU PATIENT

NEIL A. MUSHLIN • PAUL E. MARIK

Fever is a common problem in the intensive care unit (ICU), with approximately 70% of patients developing a fever at some point during their ICU stay. Infectious and noninfectious etiologies contribute almost equally to the causation of febrile episodes (1). The discovery of fever in an ICU patient has a significant impact on health care costs due to the blood cultures, radiologic imaging, and antibiotics that routinely follow. It is therefore important to have a good understanding of the mechanisms and etiology of fever in ICU patients, how and when to initiate a diagnostic workup, and when initiation of antibiotics is indicated.

The Society of Critical Care Medicine and the Infectious Disease Society of America consider a temperature of 38.3°C or greater (101°F) in an ICU patient a fever that warrants further evaluation (2). This does not necessarily imply that a temperature below 38.3°C (101°F) does not require further investigation, as many variables determine a patient's febrile response to an insult. In addition, it should be recognized that there is a daily fluctuation of temperature by 0.5°C to 1.0°C, with women having wider variations in temperature than men (3). Furthermore, with aging, the maximal febrile response decreases by about 0.15°C per decade (4).

Accurate and reproducible measurement of body temperature is important in detecting disease and in monitoring patients with an elevated temperature. A variety of methods are used to measure body temperature by combining different sites, instruments, and techniques. The mixed venous blood in the pulmonary artery is considered the optimal site for core temperature measurement. However, this method requires placement of a pulmonary artery catheter. Infrared ear thermometry has been demonstrated to provide values that are a few tenths of a degree below temperatures in the pulmonary artery and brain (5–9). Rectal temperatures obtained with a mercury thermometer or electronic probe are often a few tenths of a degree higher than core temperatures (10–12). However, patients perceive having rectal temperatures taken as unpleasant and intrusive. Furthermore, access to the rectum may be limited by patient position, with an associated risk of rectal trauma. Oral measurements are influenced by events such as eating and drinking and the presence of respiratory devices delivering warmed gases (13). Many tachypneic patients are unable to keep their mouth closed to obtain an accurate oral temperature. Axillary measurements substantially underestimate core temperature and lack reproducibility. Body temperature is therefore most accurately measured with an intravascular thermistor; however, measurement by infrared ear thermometry or with an electronic probe in the rectum is an acceptable alternative (2).

PATHOGENESIS OF FEVER

Cytokines released by monocytic cells play a central role in the genesis of fever. The cytokines primarily involved in the development of fever include interleukin-1 (IL-1), interleukin-6 (IL-6), and tumor necrosis factor-α (TNF-α) (14–23). The interaction between these cytokines is complex, with each being able to up-regulate and down-regulate their own expression as well as that of the other cytokines. These cytokines bind to their own specific receptors located in close proximity to the preoptic region of the anterior hypothalamus (14,15). Here, the cytokine receptor interaction activates phospholipase A_2, resulting in the liberation of plasma membrane arachidonic acid as substrate for the cyclo-oxygenase pathway. Some cytokines appear to increase cyclo-oxygenase expression directly, leading to the liberation of prostaglandin E_2 (PGE_2).

Fever appears to be a preserved evolutionary response within the animal kingdom (24,25). With few exceptions, reptiles, amphibians, fish, and several invertebrate species have been shown to manifest fever in response to challenge with microorganisms. Increased body temperature has been shown to enhance the resistance of animals to infection (24,25). Although fever has some harmful effects, it appears to be an adaptive response that has evolved to help rid the host of invading pathogens. Temperature elevation has been shown to enhance several parameters of immune function including antibody production, T-cell activation, production of cytokines, and enhanced neutrophil and macrophage function (26–29). Furthermore, some pathogens such as *Streptococcus pneumoniae* are inhibited by febrile temperatures (30).

Schulman et al. investigated whether it was beneficial to treat the fever of hospitalized patients admitted to a trauma ICU (31). Patients were randomized to an active treatment group, in which acetaminophen and cooling blankets were used to aggressively cool this subgroup, as compared to a permissive group, in which fever was only treated once it reached 40°C. In this study, there was a strong trend toward increased mortality in the active treatment group. It should, however, be noted that all the patients who died in the aggressive treatment group had an infectious etiology as the cause of the fever. Doran et al. demonstrated that children with varicella who were treated with acetaminophen had a more prolonged illness (32). Weinstein et al. reported that patients with spontaneous bacterial peritonitis had improved survival if they had a temperature greater than 38°C (33). These data suggest that fever from an infectious cause should not be treated unless the patient has limited cardiorespiratory reserve.

In contrast to patients with infectious disorders, patients with cerebral ischemia or head trauma have worse outcomes with increased temperature. For these patients, the current recommendation is to maintain the patient's temperature in the normothermic range (34). Antipyresis must always include an antipyretic agent, as external cooling alone increases heat generations and catecholamine production (35). Furthermore, acute hepatitis may occur in ICU patients with reduced glutathione reserves (alcoholics, malnourished, etc.) who have received regular therapeutic doses of acetaminophen.

FEVER PATTERNS

Attempts to derive reliable and consistent clues from evaluation of a patient's fever pattern are fraught with uncertainty and are not likely to be helpful diagnostically (14,36,37). Most patients have remittent or intermittent fever, which, when due to infection, usually follows a diurnal variation (36). Sustained fevers have been reported in patients with Gram-negative pneumonia or central nervous system (CNS) damage (36). The appearance of fever at different time points in the course of a patient's illness may, however, provide some diagnostic clues. Fevers that arise more than 48 hours after the institution of mechanical ventilation may be secondary to a developing pneumonia. Fevers that arise 5 to 7 days postoperatively may be related to abscess formation (38). Fevers that arise 10 to 14 days after institution of antibiotics for intra-abdominal abscess may be due to fungal infections (39–41).

CAUSES OF FEVER IN THE INTENSIVE CARE UNIT

Any disease process that results in the release of the proinflammatory cytokines IL-1, IL-6, and TNF-α will result in the development of fever. While infections are common causes of fever in ICU patients, many noninfectious inflammatory conditions cause the release of the proinflammatory cytokines and induce a febrile response. Similarly, it is important to appreciate that not all patients with infections are febrile. Approximately 10% of septic patients are hypothermic and 35% normothermic at presentation. Septic patients who fail to develop a fever have a significantly higher mortality than febrile septic patients (42–44). The reason that patients with established infections fail to develop a febrile response is unclear; however, preliminary evidence suggests that this aberrant response is not due to diminished cytokine production (45).

The presence of fever in an ICU patient frequently triggers a battery of diagnostic tests that are costly, expose the patient to unnecessary risks, and often produce misleading or inconclusive results. It is therefore important that fever in ICU patients be evaluated in a systematic, prudent, clinically appropriate, and cost-effective manner.

Infectious Causes of Fever in the Intensive Care Unit

The prevalence of nosocomial infection in ICUs has been reported to vary from 3% to 31% (13, 46–49). In a point prevalence study conducted in 1992, the European Prevalence of Infection in Intensive Care (EPIC) study investigators reported on the prevalence of nosocomial infections in 10,038 patients hospitalized in 1,417 European ICUs (50). In this study, 20.6% of patients had an ICU-acquired infection, with pneumonia being most common (46.9%), followed by urinary tract infection (17.6%) and bloodstream infection (12%). The most common infectious causes of fever in ICU patients are listed in Table 105.1.

TABLE 105.1

MOST COMMON INFECTIOUS CAUSES OF FEVER IN THE INTENSIVE CARE UNIT

Catheter-related bloodstream infection
Ventilator-associated pneumonia
Primary septicemia
Sinusitis
Surgical site/wound infection
Clostridia difficile colitis
Cellulitis/infected decubitus ulcer
Urinary tract infection
Suppurative thrombophlebitis
Endocarditis
Diverticulitis
Septic arthritis
Abscess/empyema

Catheter-related Blood Stream Infection

Intravascular catheters are a major source of infection in the ICU. According to the National Nosocomial Infections Surveillance (NNIS) system, the mean incidence of catheter-related bloodstream infection (CRBI) in the United States is 5.3 per 1,000 catheter-days. Coagulase-negative staphylococci account for up to 40% of cases (51). Other common causes of CRBI include enterococci, *Staphylococcus aureus*, *Candida* species, and aerobic Gram-negative bacilli. Methicillin-resistant *S. aureus* (MRSA) and vancomycin-resistant enterococci are now becoming important causes of CRBI. A number of different mechanisms likely lead to CRBI. Skin pathogens can infect the catheter exit site and then migrate down the tract along the external catheter surface. Pathogens can also contaminate the catheter hub, leading to intraluminal catheter colonization and infection. Hematogenous seeding of the external surface of the catheter may also occur (52). In addition, despite rigorous skin disinfection, viable micro-organisms can be impacted during insertion of the distal tip of the catheter, causing infection (53). A number of factors have been identified as increasing the risk of CRBI, including the number of lumens in the central venous catheter, the number of stopcocks, transfusion of blood and blood products, parenteral nutrition, and an open infusion system (54–57). Catheter-related thrombosis is associated with an increased risk of catheter infection, while thrombocytopenia has been suggested to be protective against CRBI (55,58). The acquired immunodeficiency syndrome (AIDS) and hematologic malignancies have been found to be independent risk factors for CRBI (57).

The site of central venous catheter placement and the length of time it can be left indwelling has been a controversial topic for decades. Many studies have been published reporting conflicting data. Generally, however, subclavian catheters have been found to have a lower risk of infection than femoral catheters (59). It has also been suggested that placement of subclavian catheters may result in fewer catheter-related infections than internal jugular placement (60–62). However, a recent study found no difference in the risk of CRBI between subclavian, internal jugular, and femoral catheter placement (63). In this study, the vascular catheters were placed by experienced operators using strict aseptic techniques. While the risk of CRBI increases with the time the catheter remains *in situ*, changing catheters at regularly scheduled intervals has not been shown to reduce the risk of CRBI (64).

The diagnosis of CRBI can be challenging. Routine culture of blood withdrawn from the catheter is not recommended. However, the catheter exit site should be inspected daily for evidence of erythema or pus. The absence of local infection, unfortunately, does not exclude CRBI. In a patient with an indwelling central venous catheter who develops a fever, two sets of blood cultures should be drawn: one from the catheter and one from a peripheral source. If the patient has systemic signs of infection and no other identifiable source of infection, the catheter should be removed and empiric antibiotics commenced pending culture results. In patients with limited venous access, the central catheter may be replaced with a new catheter over a guidewire. However, both the catheter tip as well as the intracutaneous portion of the catheter should be sent for culture. If catheter culture returns positive (greater than 15 colony-forming units [CFU]), or the blood cultures are consistent with a CRBI, the catheter that was changed over a guidewire must be removed and replaced with a new catheter at a clean site (65,66). Follow-up blood cultures should be obtained in patients with CRBI. If blood cultures remain positive, a thorough investigation for septic thrombosis, infective endocarditis, and other metastatic infections should be pursued (67).

The usual approach to patients with suspected CRBI involves removal of the catheter. However, this subjects patients with negative cultures to the added risk of catheter placement. To avoid this problem, a number of methods have been investigated for the diagnosis of CRBI that do not require removal of the central venous catheter. Comparison of blood cultured from the central catheter with that from a peripheral venous site is currently the most useful technique. In patients with CRBI, quantitative culture counts are greater and time to positivity shorter with blood withdrawn from the catheter as opposed to the peripheral site (65). Acridine-orange leukocyte cytospin testing, available in some countries, is a rapid, inexpensive test that can also be used to prevent unnecessary removal of catheters (68–70). Endoluminal brushing, in which the central venous catheter is sampled within 3 to 5 cm of the catheter tip, has also been demonstrated to be useful in the diagnosis of CRBI (71,72). Experience with these alternative methods of diagnosing CRBI is, however, quite limited.

Ventilator-associated Pneumonia

Ventilator-associated pneumonia (VAP) is a common source of fever in the intubated patient. Intubation increases the risk of developing pneumonia from 6- to 21-fold (73). Between 10% and 25% of patients on mechanical ventilation will develop VAP during their ICU stay (74,75). VAP is associated with significant costs and has an attributable mortality of about 25% (76). The risk of acquiring VAP is highest in the first week, at 3% a day, thereafter decreasing to 2% a day in the second week, and down to 1% a day in the third and subsequent weeks (77). The risk of VAP is higher in trauma, burn, and neurosurgical units as compared to medical ICUs.

VAP is usually categorized as either early (occurring less than 48 hours after intubation) or late onset (occurring after 5 to 7 days of intubation) (78). The distinction between these two phases of VAP is vitally important, as they are associated with different pathogens. Early-onset VAP is associated with bacteria that are normally sensitive to antibiotics (methicillin-sensitive *S. aureus, Haemophilus influenzae*, and *Streptococcus pneumoniae*). Late onset is typically associated with antibiotic-resistant bacteria (MRSA, *Pseudomonas aeruginosa, Acinetobacter* species, and *Enterobacter* species) (76,79,80).

The major risk factors for VAP include (74,81,82):

- Age over 60 years
- Male gender
- Chronic lung disease
- Acute respiratory distress syndrome
- Aspiration
- Sinusitis
- Nasogastric tube
- Transport in and out of the ICU
- Failure to elevate the head of the bed
- Endotracheal cuff pressures less than 20 cm of H_2O
- Increased severity of illness
- Delayed extubation
- Continuous sedation
- Cardiopulmonary resuscitation
- Medications including H_2 blockers and paralytic agents

The diagnosis of VAP is challenging. VAP should be suspected when a patient on mechanical ventilation develops a new infiltrate on a chest radiograph along with leukocytosis, fever, and purulent tracheobronchial secretions (83). The presence of a new infiltrate on chest radiograph, together with two of the above-cited clinical findings, has a sensitivity of 69% with a specificity of 75% for the diagnosis of VAP (84). The decision to treat a suspected VAP on clinical grounds alone will frequently overdiagnose the condition and lead to treatment that fails to cover the correct pathogen in patients with true VAP (85). Quantitative cultures of secretions obtained from the lower respiratory tract can facilitate making the diagnosis of VAP. The two most common techniques include protected specimen brush (PSB) sampling and bronchoalveolar lavage (BAL). These techniques can be performed bronchoscopically or blindly. Blind bronchial suctioning and mini-bronchoalveolar lavage are gaining popularity in intensive care units, and have been shown to be as effective as a protected specimen brush (86). These are generally safe, inexpensive tests that can be performed by respiratory therapists without a physician present. A threshold of 1,000 CFU/mL for PSB and 10,000 CFU/mL for BAL is currently recommended. However, we suggest a threshold of 500 and 5,000 CFU/mL, respectively, as this increases the sensitivity of the tests (87). Microscopic examination of the BAL fluid has also been used to facilitate the diagnosis of VAP; if there is less than 50% neutrophils, pneumonia can be excluded (88). The role of quantitative culture of tracheal aspirates (as opposed to lower respiratory tract sampling) is unclear at this time. The effect of quantitative culture techniques on patient outcome is unclear; however, these techniques result in a significant reduction in the use of antibiotics (89–92).

Urinary Tract Infection

Most ICU patients require an indwelling urinary catheter for monitoring fluid balance and renal function. Urinary tract infections (UTIs), according to some studies, are the third most common infection found in the intensive care unit. In a study of 4,465 patients who were admitted to the ICU for at least 48 hours, 6.5% developed a UTI, with an overall incidence of 9.6 cases per 1,000 ICU days (93). However, the incidence of bacteremia and fungemia was only 0.1 case per 1,000 catheter-days. Interestingly, UTIs are reported to be more common in medical ICU patients and least likely in cardiothoracic patients. Reported risk factors for UTIs include (94,95):

- Female gender
- Age over 60 years
- Antimicrobial therapy use
- Severity of illness
- Duration of urinary catheterization

The presence of a urinary catheter for longer than 4 to 5 days significantly increases the risk of UTI (96). Gram-negative bacteria, especially *Escherichia coli* and *Pseudomonas aeruginosa*, account for more than half of the pathogens. Gram-positive organisms, especially *Enterococcus* and *Candida*, account for the remaining cases. Risk factors for funguria include immunosuppression, diabetes, renal failure, structural or functional abnormalities of the urinary tract, recent surgery, chronic illness, and broad-spectrum antibiotics (97). Examination of the urine with "dipsticks" for leukocyte esterase and nitrate is insensitive and should not be substituted for quantitative culture (98).

The significance of UTIs in catheterized ICU patients is unclear, and they appear unlikely to lead to increased morbidity or mortality (99). It is probable that most patients have "asymptomatic bacteriuria" rather than true infections of the urinary tract. The treatment of patients with "asymptomatic bacteriuria" is based on a single study performed in the early 1980s that may not be applicable today (100). Platt et al. demonstrated that in hospitalized patients, bacteriuria with greater than or equal to 10^5 CFU of bacteria per milliliter of urine during bladder catheterization was associated with a 2.8-fold increase in mortality (100). Based on this study, thousands of ICU patients with urinary tract colonization have been, and continue to be, treated with antibiotics. However, recent studies suggest that this approach may not be optimal.

In patients with indwelling urinary catheters, colonic flora rapidly colonizes the urinary tract (101). Stark and Maki have demonstrated that in catheterized patients, bacteria rapidly proliferate in the urinary system to exceed 10^5 CFU/mL over a short period of time (102). Bacteriuria, defined as a quantitative culture of greater than or equal to 10^5 CFU/mL, has been reported in up to 30% of catheterized hospitalized patients (102). The terms *bacteriuria* and *UTI* are generally—although incorrectly—used as synonyms. Indeed, most studies in ICU patients have used bacteriuria to diagnose a UTI. Bacteriuria implies colonization of the urinary tract without bacterial invasion and an acute inflammatory response, while urinary tract infection implies an infection of the urinary tract (103). Criteria have not been developed for differentiating asymptomatic colonization of the urinary tract from symptomatic infection. Furthermore, the presence of white cells in the urine is not useful for differentiating colonization from infection, as most catheter-associated bacteriurias have accompanying pyuria (104). It is therefore unclear how many catheterized patients with greater than or equal to 10^5 CFU/mL actually have urinary tract infections.

While catheter-associated bacteruria is common in ICU patients, data from the early 1980s indicate that less than 3% of catheter-associated bacteriuric patients will develop bacteremia caused by organisms in the urine (105). Therefore, the surveillance for, and treatment of, isolated bacteruria in most ICU patients is currently not recommended (106). Bacteriuria should, however, be treated following urinary tract manipulation or surgery in patients with kidney stones, and in those with urinary tract obstruction. In a patient with systemic signs of infection together with bacteruria and no other obvious source of infection, it would probably be prudent to treat this patient with a short course of antibiotics. Moreover, ultrasonography to exclude urinary tract obstruction and repeat urine culture is recommended. Treatment is clearly indicated in those patients with bacteruria who develop bloodstream infection. Isolated *Candida* lower urinary tract infection is exceedingly uncommon; when this diagnosis is entertained, *Candida* infection of the kidney should be excluded.

Sinusitis

Sinusitis is an underappreciated cause of fever in the ICU and, as a result, the diagnosis is usually not considered or made until other, more common infectious causes of fever have been excluded. Sinusitis, if not diagnosed and treated in a timely fashion, can lead to nosocomial pneumonia and severe sepsis (107–109). Nasal colonization with enteric Gram-negative rods, nasoenteric tubes, and a Glasgow Coma Scale score of less than 7 are all risk factors of acquiring nosocomial sinusitis. Patients who are orally intubated are less prone to develop sinusitis than those who are nasotracheally intubated (110). Indeed, up to 85% of nasally intubated patients will develop sinusitis within a week.

In patients with radiologic evidence of sinusitis, aspiration of the sinuses is required to confirm the diagnosis and to identify the causative pathogen (111). Several radiologic tests have been employed to identify this problem. While a computed tomography (CT) scan of the sinuses is considered the gold-standard study, if a patient is too ill to be transported out of the ICU, plain films of the sinuses may be obtained. In order to maximize the chances of making the diagnosis, multiple views of the sinuses are required (111). Bedside ultrasound has been gaining popularity in European countries over the last decade, and there are data to suggest that it is at least equivalent to CT scanning (108,112–114).

Once sinusitis is diagnosed, all nasal tubes should immediately be removed, with early sinus drainage (115). Broad-spectrum antibiotics should be commenced with coverage that includes *Pseudomonas* and MRSA. The antibiotics should then be de-escalated once culture data are available (116). Topical decongestants and vasoconstrictors, alone or combined with systemic decongestants and antihistamines, are also recommended (111).

Clostridium difficile Colitis

In patients who develop fever with concurrent diarrhea, *Clostridium difficile* must be considered. It is crucial to diagnose this disease early, as it can lead to severe sepsis, multiorgan system failure, and death. Patients with *C. difficile* often present with a leukemoid reaction, with white blood cell counts that may reach greater than 35,000 cells/μL. A leukemoid reaction or unexplained leukocytosis may be the presenting sign of *C. difficile,* even in the absence of diarrheal symptoms (117–119). Interestingly, *C. difficile* presenting with a leukemoid reaction is associated with a worse prognosis and higher mortality rate (120).

Concurrent or prior antibiotic use is a strong risk factor for developing *C. difficile* colitis. Clindamycin, β-lactams (especially cephalosporins), and, more recently, quinolones have been the antibiotics most frequently associated with this form of colitis (121,122). Most patients in the ICU receive stress ulcer prophylaxis, with many receiving proton pump inhibitors (PPIs). PPIs have recently been associated with a higher risk of *C. difficile* infection (123–125); indeed, the number of cases of *C. difficile* colitis has doubled in university hospitals over the past 6 years (126). Recently, epidemics of an extremely virulent strain of *C. difficile* have been reported in the United States and Canada (127–132); it is suggested that the increasing use of fluoroquinolones has played a role. This strain is associated with higher morbidity and mortality, as it produces significantly more toxins than do the other strains.

The diagnosis of *C. difficile* colitis is usually made by immunoassays of stool against both toxin A and toxin B. The presence of *C. difficile* antigen in the absence of the toxin suggests colonization, rather than infection, with *C. difficile*. Due to the low sensitivity of the toxin assay, two stool specimens should be examined. The cytotoxic assay is more sensitive and specific than the immunoassay; however, this test is not readily available and takes longer to perform. In patients where the diagnosis is still in doubt, colonoscopy may be performed to look for pseudomembranes. CT scan may also be helpful, as 50% of patients will have changes that can be seen on imaging. Positive CT scans are associated with leukocytosis, abdominal pain, and diarrhea (133). If *C. difficile* colitis is suspected, empiric treatment should be started until the diagnosis is excluded. It is important to note that alcohol-based hand hygiene, which has rapidly gained popularity in many hospitals, does not kill spore-forming organisms such as *C. difficile* and should not replace handwashing with soap when one is exposed to these patients.

Skin Infections

Skin infections, especially infected pressure ulcers, may be a source of infection in ICU patients. Several factors increase the risk of ICU patients developing pressure ulcers, including (134–136):

- Emergent admissions
- Severity of illness
- Extended ICU length of stay
- Malnutrition
- Age
- Diabetes
- Infusion of vasopressor agents
- Anemia
- Fecal incontinence

Protocols for the prevention of pressure ulcers should be routinely instituted in the ICU. In addition, physicians and nurses should routinely examine their patient's skin, particularly high-pressure areas such as the sacrum and heels, to detect early signs of skin breakdown.

Other Infections

Nosocomial meningitis is exceedingly uncommon in hospitalized patients who have not undergone a neurosurgical procedure (137,138). Lumbar puncture, therefore, does not need to be performed routinely in nonneurosurgical ICU patients who develop a fever, unless they have meningeal signs or contiguous infection (137,138). In patients who have undergone abdominal surgery and develop a fever, intra-abdominal infection must always be excluded, usually with an evaluation that includes CT scanning of the abdomen. Similarly, in patients who have undergone other operative procedures, wound infection must be excluded.

Noninfectious Causes of Fever in the Intensive Care Unit

A large number of noninfectious conditions result in tissue injury with inflammation and a febrile reaction. Those noninfectious disorders that should be considered in ICU patients are listed in Table 105.2. For reasons that are not entirely clear, most noninfectious disorders usually do not lead to a fever in excess of 38.9°C (102°F); therefore, if the temperature increases above this threshold, the patient should be considered to have an infectious etiology as the cause of the fever (139). However, patients with drug fever may have a temperature greater than 102°F. Similarly, fever secondary to blood transfusion may exceed 102°F. In patients with a temperature above 40°C (104°F), neuroleptic malignant syndrome, malignant hyperthermia, the "serotonin syndrome," and subarachnoid hemorrhage must always be considered. Most of those clinical conditions listed in Table 105.2 are clinically obvious and do not require additional diagnostic tests to confirm their presence. However, a few of these disorders require special consideration.

Drug-induced Fever

Most ICU patients receive numerous medications, and all drugs have side effects, including fever. It is estimated that about 10% of inpatients develop drug fever during their hospital stay (140). Patients with human immunodeficiency virus (HIV) appear to be at a particularly high risk of developing a drug fever (141–143). The diagnosis of drug fever in ICU patients is challenging, as the onset of fever can occur immediately after administration of the drug or it can occur days, weeks, months, or even years after the patient has been on the offending medication (140). Furthermore, once the implicated medication is discontinued, the fever can take up to 3 to 4 days to resolve. Associated rashes and leukocytosis occur in less than 20% of cases (144). Penicillins, cephalosporins, anticonvulsants, heparin, and H_2 blockers are commonly used medications in the ICU that are associated with drug fevers (145–148).

Five mechanisms have been described that give rise to drug fevers. First, and the most common mechanism, patients can have a hypersensitivity reaction to the drug. Second, medications can cause fever by disrupting the normal thermoregulatory mechanisms of the body. Third, drugs can cause fever directly related to administration of the drug (e.g., from contamination of the solution with endotoxin or other exogenous pyrogens). The drug can also cause a chemical phlebitis or inflammation at the site of injection. The fourth mechanism

TABLE 105.2

NONINFECTIOUS CAUSES OF FEVER IN THE INTENSIVE CARE UNIT

Drug-related
Drug fever
Neuroleptic malignant syndrome
Malignant hyperthermia
Serotonin syndrome
Drug withdrawal (including alcohol and recreational drugs)
IV contrast reaction
Posttransfusion Fever
Neurologic
Intracranial hemorrhage
Cerebral infarction
Subarachnoid hemorrhage
Seizures
Endocrine
Hyperthyroidism
Pheochromocytoma
Adrenal insufficiency
Rheumatologic
Crystal arthropathies
Vasculitis
Collagen vascular diseases
Hematologic
Phlebitis
Hematoma
Gastrointestinal/Hepatic
Acalculous cholecystitis
Ischemic bowel
Cirrhosis
Hepatitis
Gastrointestinal bleed
Pancreatitis
Pulmonary
Aspiration pneumonitis
Acute respiratory distress syndrome
Thromboembolic disease
Fat embolism syndrome
Cardiac
Myocardial infarction
Dressler syndrome
Pericarditis
Oncologic
Neoplastic syndromes

is due to the direct extension of the pharmacologic action of the drug. This can be seen in chemotherapy with cell necrosis, lysis, and the release of various pyrogenic substances. This can also be seen with antimicrobial therapy with the release of bacterial products into the circulation, known as the Jarisch-Herxheimer reaction. Finally, patients can have idiosyncratic reactions, which include syndromes such as malignant hyperthermia, neuroleptic malignant syndrome, serotonin syndrome, and glucose-6-phosphate dehydrogenase deficiency (140,148–151).

Malignant Hyperthermia. This is a rare genetic disorder of the muscle membrane causing an increase of calcium ions in the muscle cells. This can cause a variety of clinical problems, most commonly a dangerous hypermetabolic state after the use of agents such as succinylcholine and the potent inhaled anesthetic agents (152). This reaction typically occurs within 1 hour of anesthesia but can be delayed for up to 10 hours (153,154). Patients present with continually increasing fevers, muscle stiffness, and tachycardia. They can rapidly develop hemodynamic instability with progression to multiorgan failure. Since the introduction of dantrolene, the mortality of malignant hyperthermia has decreased from 80% in the 1960s to less than 10% today (155).

Neuroleptic Malignant Syndrome. This syndrome is characterized by high fevers, a change in mental status, muscle rigidity, extrapyramidal symptoms, autonomic nervous system disturbances, and altered levels of consciousness (156,157); symptoms usually begin within days to weeks of starting the offending drug. Patients typically have very high creatinine kinase levels (158). Neuroleptic malignant syndrome is caused by excessive dopaminergic blockade causing a dopamine deficiency in the central nervous system (156). Agents most commonly implicated include neuroleptic medications and certain antiemetics. Withdrawal of certain medications, which will be discussed later in this chapter, can cause this syndrome as well. Treatment includes discontinuing the offending drug, aggressive supportive care, and close hemodynamic monitoring. Drug treatment of neuroleptic malignant syndrome is controversial. A case control analysis and a retrospective analysis of published cases suggested that dantrolene, bromocriptine, and amantadine may be beneficial (159,160).

Serotonin Syndrome. Serotonin syndrome shares many of the clinical features found in neuroleptic malignant syndrome. Patients with serotonin syndrome typically have lower fevers than those with neuroleptic malignant syndrome, but have more gastrointestinal dysfunction. Their neuromuscular findings are more consistent with hyperreactivity, and can include tremors, clonus, and muscular hypertonicity (161). The presentation is much more rapid than that of neuroleptic malignant syndrome. In one report, 74.3% of patients presented within 24 hours of medication initiation, overdose, or change in dosage, and 61.5% presented within the first 6 hours (162). The Hunter Serotonin Toxicity Criteria are commonly used to evaluate the likelihood that a patient has the serotonin syndrome. The criteria include the following features in a patient recently administered a serotonergic agent: spontaneous clonus, inducible clonus, ocular clonus, agitation or diaphoresis, tremor and hyperreflexia, hypertonicity, and fever greater than 38°C (163). Benzodiazepines should be used for control of agitation, and physical restraints should be avoided (164–167). Cyproheptadine, an H_1-receptor antagonist with nonspecific 5-HT1A and 5-HT2A antagonistic properties, has been used in patients who respond poorly to benzodiazepines alone (168). Paralysis with nondepolarizing agents, endotracheal intubation, and mechanical ventilation may be needed in severely agitated and hyperthermic patients (164).

Alcohol and Drug Withdrawal

Withdrawal from alcohol and medications is a common cause of noninfectious fever in hospitalized patients, and usually presents within the first few days of hospital admission. Drug withdrawal can present in a variety of ways including fever alone, neuroleptic malignant–like syndromes, and fever with hemodynamic instability. Patients admitted to the ICU are often unable to provide histories and, thus, it is important to get an accurate list of their current medications at the time of admission. Drug withdrawal syndromes have been described with the use of baclofen, selective serotonin reuptake inhibitors (SSRI antidepressants), levodopa, narcotics, certain street drugs, and herbal remedies (169–173).

Crystal-associated Arthritis

Patients in the ICU are at increased risk of developing gout or pseudogout (174). A thorough physical exam focusing on the joints and an arthrocentesis to examine the synovial fluid are essential in making this diagnosis. Gout will typically present as a monoarthritis (174). Patients with increased body mass index, hypertension, alcohol consumption, and renal disease are at an increased risk for gout (175–179). Trauma, surgery, and severe infection are associated with an abrupt drop in uric acid level, which can trigger acute gout (180). Loop diuretics, iodinated contrast dye, and total parenteral nutrition may also precipitate gout (181,182). Calcium pyrophosphate dehydrate crystal deposition disease, also known as pseudogout, most commonly affects the knee. Pseudogout can be triggered by trauma, surgery, or severe medical illness (181–183). Electrolyte disorders such as hypomagnesemia and hypophosphatemia increase the risk for pseudogout. Pseudogout is also associated with endocrine and metabolic disorders such as hyperparathyroidism, hemochromatosis, Wilson disease, and hypothyroidism (174,184–186).

Acalculous Cholecystitis

Acute acalculous cholecystitis is a condition of inflammation of the gallbladder in the absence of calculi. It is a disease with significant morbidity and mortality, as it can lead to empyema, gallbladder gangrene, and gallbladder perforation. A high index of suspicion is required as this can be a difficult diagnosis to make, especially in the intubated and sedated patient. Initially patients present with very few symptoms. Clinical features include fever, leukocytosis, abnormal liver function tests, a palpable right upper quadrant mass, vague abdominal discomfort, and jaundice. Untreated, bacterial superinfection may occur, which can progress to empyema, peritonitis, and septic shock.

The pathophysiology of acalculous cholecystitis is complex and involves hypoperfusion and biliary stasis. Risk factors include everything one expects to see in an ICU patient: trauma, surgery, intermittent positive pressure ventilation, coronary heart disease, cholesterol emboli, fasting, total parental nutrition, immunosuppression, transfusions of blood products, hypotension, multiorgan dysfunction, sedation, opiates, diabetes, infections, childbirth, and renal failure (187–196).

Ultrasound is usually the first diagnostic test performed, as it may be performed at the bedside. In addition, a bedside ultrasound can readily image other abdominal organs. Ultrasound for acute acalculous cholecystitis, however, has been found to be inferior to morphine cholescintigraphy and CT. One study showed ultrasound to have a sensitivity of 50% compared to 67% for morphine cholescintigraphy with a specificity of 94% and 100%, respectively (197). Another study reported a sensitivity of 90% for cholescintigraphy, 67% for CT, and only 29% for ultrasound (198). An abnormal ultrasound can be seen in 50% of ICU patients, even if they are not suspected of having acalculous cholecystitis (199). As soon as the diagnosis is suspected, blood cultures should be drawn, broad-spectrum antibiotics initiated, and a surgical consult requested. In unstable patients, percutaneous drainage may be preferable to surgical intervention.

Postoperative Fever

Surgery alone can cause fever, which is self-limited. In the early postoperative period, a patient's temperature may increase up to 1.4°C, with the peak occurring approximately 11 hours after surgery. Fifty percent of postoperative patients will develop a fever greater than or equal to 38°C, with 25% reaching 38.5°C or higher (200); the fever typically lasts for 2 to 3 days (200–202). Postoperative fever is believed to be caused by tissue injury and inflammation with associated cytokine release (203–205). The invasiveness of the procedure, as well as genetic factors, influences the degree of cytokine release and the febrile response (201,206,207). A good physical examination and history of the timing and sequence of events are crucial to help differentiate this from other causes of infectious and noninfectious fever. Reactions to medications, especially anesthesia; blood products; and infections that might have existed prior to the surgery should be considered during a patient's early postoperative course. Nosocomial and surgical site infections usually develop 3 to 5 days postoperatively.

Atelectasis

While atelectasis is commonly implicated as a cause of fever (38,208), even in standard ICU texts, they provide no primary reference source to support this assertion (38,208). Indeed, a major surgery text states that "... fever is almost always present [in patients with atelectasis] ... " (38). During rounds, many medical students and house-staff have been taught that atelectasis is one of the "five" main causes of postoperative fever. However, there are very little data to support this widely held belief.

Engoren studied 100 postoperative cardiac surgery patients and was unable to demonstrate a relationship between atelectasis and fever (209). Furthermore, when atelectasis is induced in experimental animals by ligation of a mainstem bronchus, fever does not occur (210,211). However, Kisala et al. demonstrated that IL-1 and TNF-α levels in macrophage cultures from atelectatic lungs were significantly increased compared with control lungs (212). While the role of atelectasis as a cause of fever is unclear, atelectasis probably does not cause fever in the absence of pulmonary infection.

Blood Transfusions

A large number of patients in the ICU will receive transfusions of blood products. One study composed of 4,892 ICU patients demonstrated that 44% received a blood transfusion (213). In another study, 85% of patients in the ICU for longer than 1 week were reported to receive a blood transfusion (214). Febrile, nonhemolytic transfusion reactions are exceedingly common following transfusion of blood and blood products. This is likely mediated by the transfusion of cytokines such as IL-1, IL-6, IL-8, and TNF-α, which accumulate with increasing length of blood storage (215–218).

Febrile, nonhemolytic reactions normally manifest within the first 6 hours after transfusion, and are self-limiting. They can present with chills and rigors in addition to fever. It is crucial to differentiate these from febrile acute hemolytic transfusion reactions, which can be life threatening.

Leukoreduction has been shown to reduce the risk of febrile nonhemolytic transfusion reactions (219–221).

Thromboembolic Disease

Fever has been reported in 14% to 18% of patients with thromboembolic disease, and is generally an uncommon cause of fever in hospitalized patients (222–224). If present, the fever is typically low grade (37.5°C–38°C) (225).

AN APPROACH TO THE CRITICALLY ILL PATIENT WITH FEVER

From the foregoing information, the following approach is suggested in ICU patients who develop a fever (see Fig. 107.1). Due to the frequency and excess morbidity and mortality associated with bacteremia, blood cultures are recommended in all ICU patients who develop a fever. A comprehensive physical examination and review of the chest radiograph is essential. Noninfectious causes of fever should be excluded. In patients with an obvious focus of infection—purulent nasal discharge, abdominal tenderness, profuse green diarrhea—a focused diagnostic workup is required. If there is no clinically obvious source of infection, and unless the patient is clinically deteriorating—falling blood pressure, decreased urine output, increasing confusion, rising serum lactate concentration, falling platelet count, or worsening coagulopathy—or the temperature is in excess of 39°C (102°F), it may be prudent to perform blood cultures and then observe the patient before embarking on the further diagnostic tests and commencing empiric antibiotics. However, *all neutropenic* patients with fever, as well as patients with severe—as outlined above—or progressive signs of sepsis should be started on broad-spectrum antimicrobial therapy immediately after obtaining appropriate cultures.

In patients whose clinical picture is consistent with infection and in whom no clinically obvious source has been documented, removal of all central catheters that are more than 48 hours old—with semiquantitative or quantitative cultures performed on the intracutaneous segments—is recommended, as is stool culture for *C. difficile* toxin in those patients with loose stools and CT scan of sinuses with removal of all nasal tubes. Urine culture is indicated only in patients with abnormalities of the renal system or following urinary tract manipulation. If the patient is at risk of abdominal sepsis or has any abdominal signs—tenderness, distention, inability to tolerate enteral feeds—a CT scan of the abdomen is indicated. Patients with right upper quadrant tenderness require an abdominal ultrasound or CT examination.

Reevaluation of the patients' status after 48 hours, using all available results and the evolution of the patients' clinical condition, is essential. If fever persists despite empiric antibiotics and no source of infection has been identified, empiric antifungal therapy may be indicated in patients with risk factors for

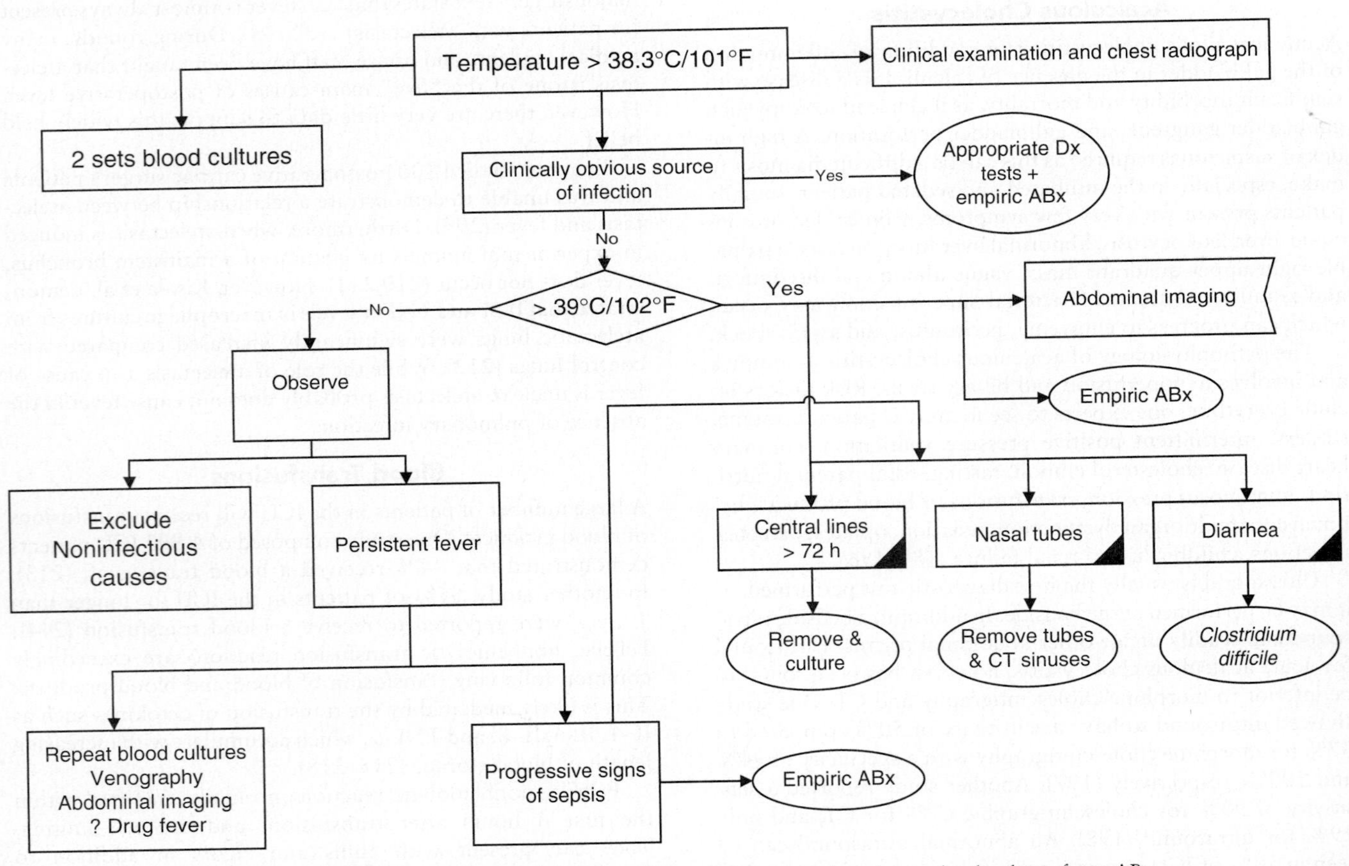

FIGURE 105.1. Suggested diagnostic algorithm for intensive care unit patients who develop a fever. ABx, antibiotics; CT, computed tomography; Dx, diagnostic.

Candida infection. Additional diagnostic tests may be appropriate at this time, including venography, a differential blood count for eosinophils to assist in the diagnosis of drug fever, and abdominal imaging.

SUMMARY

Intensive care physicians are presented with patients who develop a fever on a daily basis. The clinician should be aware of the common infectious and noninfectious causes of fever in ICU patients. A comprehensive history and physical examination as well as a review of the patient's hospital course and medications are essential in formulating a diagnostic and therapeutic plan. Antibiotics are only recommended in patients with a high likelihood of having an infectious cause of fever. The empiric antibiotics should be based on the presumed site of infection as well as the likely pathogens. De-escalation of the antibiotic regimen is important once culture data are available. As a general rule, patients with an infective cause of fever should not be treated with antipyretic agents.

References

1. Circiumaru B, Baldock G, Cohen J. A prospective study of fever in the intensive care unit. *Intensive Care Med.* 1999;25:668–673.
2. O'Grady NP, Barie PS, Bartlett J, et al. Practice parameters for evaluating new fever in critically ill adult patients. *Crit Care Med.* 1998;26:392–408.
3. Sund-Levander M, Forsberg C, Wahren LK. Normal oral, rectal, tympanic and axillary body temperature in adult men and women: a systematic literature review. *Scand J Care Sci.* 2002;16:122–128.
4. Roghmann MC, Warner J, Mackowiak PA. The relationship between age and fever magnitude. *Am J Med Sci.* 2001;322:68–70.
5. Teasell RW, McRae M, Marchuk Y, et al. Pneumonia associated with aspiration following stroke. *Arch Phys Med Rehabil.* 1996;77:707–709.
6. Hayward JS, Eckerson JD, Kemna D. Thermal and cardiovascular changes during three methods of resuscitation from mild hypothermia. *Resuscitation.* 1984;11:21–33.
7. Shiraki K, Konda N, Sagawa S. Esophageal and tympanic temperature responses to core blood temperature changes during hyperthermia. *J Appl Physiol.* 1986;61:98–102.
8. Shiraki K, Sagawa S, Tajima F, et al. Independence of brain and tympanic temperatures in an unanesthetized human. *J Appl Physiol.* 1988;65:482–486.
9. Amoateng-Adjepong Y, Del Mundo J, Manthous CA. Accuracy of an infrared tympanic thermometer. *Chest.* 1999;115:1002–1005.
10. Schmitz T, Bair N, Falk M, et al. A comparison of five methods of temperature measurement in febrile intensive care patients. *Am J Crit Care.* 1995;4:286–292.
11. Milewski A, Ferguson KL, Terndrup TE. Comparison of pulmonary artery, rectal, and tympanic membrane temperatures in adult intensive care unit patients. *Clin Pediatr.* 1991;30:13–16.
12. Nierman DM. Core temperature measurement in the intensive care unit. *Crit Care Med.* 1991;19:818–823.
13. Erickson RS, Kirklin SK. Comparison of ear-based, bladder, oral, and axillary methods for core temperature measurement. *Crit Care Med.* 1993;21:1528–1534.
14. Mackowiak PA. Concepts of fever. *Arch Intern Med.* 1998;158:1870–1881.
15. Saper CB, Breder CD. The neurologic basis of fever. *N Engl J Med.* 1994;330:1880–1886.
16. Dinarello CA, Cannon JG, Mier JW, et al. Multiple biological activities of human recombinant interleukin 1. *J Clin Invest.* 1986;77:1734–1739.
17. Dinarello CA. Interleukin-1 and the pathogenesis of the acute-phase response. *N Engl J Med.* 1984;311:1413–1418.
18. Fontana A, Weber E, Dayer JM. Synthesis of interleukin 1/endogenous pyrogen in the brain of endotoxin-treated mice: a step in fever induction? *J Immunol.* 1984;133:1696–1698.
19. Gourine AV, Rudolph K, Tesfaigzi J, et al. Role of hypothalamic interleukin-1beta in fever induced by cecal ligation and puncture in rats. *Am J Physiol.* 1998;275:R754–R761.
20. Leon LR, White AA, Kluger MJ. Role of IL-6 and TNF in thermoregulation and survival during sepsis in mice. *Am J Physiol.* 1998;275:R269–R277.
21. Kluger MJ, Kozak W, Leon LR, et al. The use of knockout mice to understand the role of cytokines in fever. *Clin Exp Pharmacol Physiol.* 1998;25:141–144.
22. Klir JJ, McClellan JL, Kluger MJ. Interleukin-1 beta causes the increase in anterior hypothalamic interleukin-6 during LPS-induced fever in rats. *Am J Physiol.* 1994;266:R1845–R1848.
23. Klir JJ, Roth J, Szelenyi Z, et al. Role of hypothalamic interleukin-6 and tumor necrosis factor-alpha in LPS fever in rat. *Am J Physiol.* 1993;265:R512–R517.
24. Kluger MJ, Ringler DH, Anver MR. Fever and survival. *Science.* 1975;188:166–168.
25. Kluger MJ, Kozak W, Conn CA, et al. The adaptive value of fever. *Infect Dis Clin North Am.* 1996;10:1–20.
26. Jampel HD, Duff GW, Gershon RK, et al. Fever and immunoregulation. III. Hyperthermia augments the primary in vitro humoral immune response. *J Exp Med.* 1983;157:1229–1238.
27. van Oss CJ, Absolom DR, Moore LL, et al. Effect of temperature on the chemotaxis, phagocytic engulfment, digestion and O2 consumption of human polymorphonuclear leukocytes. *J Reticuloendothelial Soc.* 1980;27:561–565.
28. Biggar WD, Bohn DJ, Kent G, et al. Neutrophil migration in vitro and in vivo during hypothermia. *Infect Immun.* 1984;46:857–859.
29. Azocar J, Yunis EJ, Essex M. Sensitivity of human natural killer cells to hyperthermia. *Lancet.* 1982;1:16–17.
30. Styrt B, Sugarman B. Antipyresis and fever. *Arch Intern Med.* 1990;150:1589–1597.
31. Schulman CI, Namias N, Doherty J, et al. The effect of antipyretic therapy upon outcomes in critically ill patients: a randomized, prospective study. *Surg Infect.* 2005;6:369–375.
32. Doran TF, De AC, Baumgardner RA, et al. Acetaminophen: more harm than good for chickenpox? *J Pediatr.* 1989;114:1045–1048.
33. Weinstein MP, Lannini PB, Stratton CW, et al. Spontaneous bacterial peritonitis. A review of 28 cases with emphasis on improved survival and factors influencing prognosis. *Am J Med.* 1978;64:592–598.
34. Ginsberg MD, Busto R. Combating hyperthermia in acute stroke: a significant clinical concern. *Stroke.* 1998;29:529–534.
35. Lenhardt R, Negishi C, Sessler DI, et al. The effects of physical treatment on induced fever in humans. *Am J Med.* 1999;106:550–555.
36. Musher DM, Fainstein V, Young EJ, et al. Fever patterns. Their lack of clinical significance. *Arch Intern Med.* 1979;139:1225–1228.
37. Mackowiak PA, Bartlett JG, Borden EC, et al. Concepts of fever: recent advances and lingering dogma. *Clin Infect Dis.* 1997;25:119–138.
38. Hiyama DT, Zinner MJ. Surgical complications. In: Schwartz SI, Shires GT, Sencer FC, et al., eds. *Principles of Surgery.* 6th ed. New York: McGraw-Hill; 1994:455–487.
39. Calandra T, Bille J, Schneider R, et al. Clinical significance of Candida isolated from peritoneum in surgical patients. *Lancet.* 1989;2:1437–1440.
40. Petri MG, Konig J, Moecke HP, et al. Epidemiology of invasive mycosis in ICU patients: a prospective multicenter study in 435 non-neutropenic patients. Paul-Ehrlich Society for Chemotherapy, Divisions of Mycology and Pneumonia Research. *Intensive Care Med.* 1997;23:317–325.
41. Nolla-Salas J, Sitges-Serra A, Leon-Gil C, et al. Candidemia in non-neutropenic critically ill patients: analysis of prognostic factors and assessment of systemic antifungal therapy. Study Group of Fungal Infection in the ICU. *Intens Care Med.* 1997;23:23–30.
42. Clemmer TP, Fisher CJ Jr, Bone RC, et al. Hypothermia in the sepsis syndrome and clinical outcome. The Methylprednisolone Severe Sepsis Study Group. *Crit Care Med.* 1992;20:1395–1401.
43. Sprung CL, Peduzzi PN, Shatney CH, et al. Impact of encephalopathy on mortality in the sepsis syndrome. The Veterans Administration Systemic Sepsis Cooperative Study Group. *Crit Care Med.* 1990;18:801–806.
44. Arons MM, Wheeler AP, Bernard GR, et al. Effects of ibuprofen on the physiology and survival of hypothermic sepsis. *Crit Care Med.* 1999;27:699–707.
45. Marik PE, Zaloga GP. Hypothermia and cytokines in septic shock. *Intensive Care Med.* 1999;26:716–721.
46. Jarvis WR, Edwards JR, Culver DH, et al. Nosocomial infection rates in adult and pediatric intensive care units in the United States. National Nosocomial Infections Surveillance System. *Am J Med.* 1991;91:185S–191S.
47. Brown RB, Hosmer D, Chen HC, et al. A comparison of infections in different ICUs within the same hospital. *Crit Care Med.* 1985;13:472–476.
48. Bueno-Cavanillas A, Delgado-Rodriguez M, Lopez-Luque A, et al. Influence of nosocomial infection on mortality rate in an intensive care unit. *Crit Care Med.* 1994;22:55–60.
49. Potgieter PD, Linton DM, Oliver S, et al. Nosocomial infections in a respiratory intensive care unit. *Crit Care Med.* 1987;15:495–498.
50. Vincent JL, Bihari DJ, Suter PM, et al. The prevalence of nosocomial infection in intensive care units in Europe. Results of the European Prevalence of Infection in Intensive Care (EPIC) Study. EPIC International Advisory Committee. *JAMA.* 1995;274:639–644.
51. Richards MJ, Edwards JR, Culver DH, et al. Nosocomial infections in medical intensive care units in the United States. National Nosocomial Infections Surveillance System. *Crit Care Med.* 1999;27:887–892.
52. McGee DC, Gould MK. Preventing complications of central venous catheterization. *N Engl J Med.* 2003;348:1123–1133.
53. Elliott TS, Moss HA, Tebbs SE, et al. Novel approach to investigate a source of microbial contamination of central venous catheters. *Eur J Clin Microbiol Infect Dis.* 1997;16:210–213.

54. Rosenthal VD, Maki DG. Prospective study of the impact of open and closed infusion systems on rates of central venous catheter-associated bacteremia. *Am J Infect Control.* 2004;32:135–141.
55. Hanna HA, Raad I. Blood products: a significant risk factor for long-term catheter-related bloodstream infections in cancer patients. *Infect Control Hosp Epidemiol.* 2001;22:165–166.
56. Beghetto MG, Victorino J, Teixeira L, et al. Parenteral nutrition as a risk factor for central venous catheter-related infection. *JPEN J Parenter Enteral Nutr.* 2005;29:367–373.
57. Tacconelli E, Tumbarello M, Pittiruti M, et al. Central venous catheter-related sepsis in a cohort of 366 hospitalised patients. *Eur J Clin Microbiol Infect Dis.* 1997;16:203–209.
58. Raad II, Luna M, Khalil SA, et al. The relationship between the thrombotic and infectious complications of central venous catheters. *JAMA.* 1994; 271:1014–1016.
59. Merrer J, De JB, Golliot F, et al. Complications of femoral and subclavian venous catheterization in critically ill patients: a randomized controlled trial (see comment). *JAMA.* 2001;286:700–707.
60. Raad I, Darouiche R, Dupuis J, et al. Central venous catheters coated with minocycline and rifampin for the prevention of catheter-related colonization and bloodstream infections. A randomized, double-blind trial. The Texas Medical Center Catheter Study Group. *Ann Intern Med.* 1997;127:267–274.
61. Heard SO, Wagle M, Vijayakumar E, et al. Influence of triple-lumen central venous catheters coated with chlorhexidine and silver sulfadiazine on the incidence of catheter-related bacteremia. *Arch Intern Med.* 1998;158:81–87.
62. McKinley S, Mackenzie A, Finfer S, et al. Incidence and predictors of central venous catheter related infection in intensive care patients. *Anaesth Inten Care.* 1999;27:164–169.
63. Deshpande KS, Hatem C, Ulrich HL, et al. The incidence of infectious complications of central venous catheters at the subclavian, internal jugular, and femoral sites in an intensive care unit population. *Crit Care Med.* 2005;33:13–20.
64. McLaws ML, Berry G. Nonuniform risk of bloodstream infection with increasing central venous catheter-days. *Infect Control Hosp Epidemiol.* 2005;26:715–719.
65. Blot F, Schmidt E, Nitenberg G, et al. Earlier positivity of central-venous versus peripheral-blood cultures is highly predictive of catheter-related sepsis. *J Clin Microbiol.* 1998;36:105–109.
66. Blot F, Nitenberg G, Chachaty E, et al. Diagnosis of catheter-related bacteraemia: a prospective comparison of the time to positivity of hub-blood versus peripheral-blood cultures. *Lancet.* 1999; 354:1071–77.
67. Pettigrew RA, Lang SD, Haydock DA, et al. Catheter-related sepsis in patients on intravenous nutrition: a prospective study of quantitative catheter cultures and guidewire changes for suspected sepsis. *Br J Surg.* 1985;72:52–55.
68. Bong JJ, Kite P, Ammori BJ, et al. The use of a rapid in situ test in the detection of central venous catheter-related bloodstream infection: a prospective study. *JPEN J Parenter Enteral Nutr.* 2003;27:146–150.
69. Kite P, Dobbins BM, Wilcox MH, et al. Rapid diagnosis of central-venous-catheter-related bloodstream infection without catheter removal. *Lancet.* 1999;354:1504–1507.
70. Rushforth JA, Hoy CM, Kite P, et al. Rapid diagnosis of central venous catheter sepsis. *Lancet.* 1993;342:402–403.
71. Catton JA, Dobbins BM, Kite P, et al. In situ diagnosis of intravascular catheter-related bloodstream infection: a comparison of quantitative culture, differential time to positivity, and endoluminal brushing. *Crit Care Med.* 2005;33:787–791.
72. Dobbins BM, Kite P, Catton JA, et al. In situ endoluminal brushing: a safe technique for the diagnosis of catheter-related bloodstream infection. *J Hosp Infect.* 2004;58:233–237.
73. Guideline for prevention of nosocomial pneumonia. Centers for Disease Control and Prevention. *Resp Care.* 1994;39:1191–1236.
74. Rello J, Ollendorf DA, Oster G, et al. Epidemiology and outcomes of ventilator-associated pneumonia in a large US database. *Chest.* 2002;122: 2115–2121.
75. Craven DE, Steger KA. Nosocomial pneumonia in mechanically ventilated adult patients: epidemiology and prevention in 1996. *Semin Resp Infect.* 1996;11:32–53.
76. Kollef MH, Silver P, Murphy DM, et al. The effect of late-onset ventilator-associated pneumonia in determining patient mortality. *Chest.* 1995;108:1655–1662.
77. Cook DJ, Walter SD, Cook RJ, et al. Incidence of and risk factors for ventilator-associated pneumonia in critically ill patients. *Ann Intern Med.* 1998;129:433–440.
78. Pingleton SK, Fagon JY, Leeper KV Jr. Patient selection for clinical investigation of ventilator-associated pneumonia. Criteria for evaluating diagnostic techniques. *Chest.* 1992;102:553S–556S.
79. Niederman MS, Craven DE, Fein AM, et al. Pneumonia in the critically ill hospitalized patient. *Chest.* 1990;97:170–181.
80. Rello J, Ausina V, Ricart M, et al. Impact of previous antimicrobial therapy on the etiology and outcome of ventilator-associated pneumonia. *Chest.* 1993;104:1230–1235.
81. Kollef MH. The prevention of ventilator-associated pneumonia. *N Engl J Med.* 1999;340:627–634.
82. Kollef MH, Von HB, Prentice D, et al. Patient transport from intensive care increases the risk of developing ventilator-associated pneumonia. *Chest.* 1997;112:765–773.
83. Meduri GU. Diagnosis and differential diagnosis of ventilator-associated pneumonia. *Clin Chest Med.* 1995;16:61–93.
84. Fabregas N, Ewig S, Torres A, et al. Clinical diagnosis of ventilator associated pneumonia revisited: comparative validation using immediate post-mortem lung biopsies. *Thorax.* 1999;54:867–873.
85. Fagon JY, Chastre J, Hance AJ, et al. Evaluation of clinical judgment in the identification and treatment of nosocomial pneumonia in ventilated patients. *Chest.* 1993;103:547–553.
86. Pham LH, Brun-Buisson C, Legrand P, et al. Diagnosis of nosocomial pneumonia in mechanically ventilated patients. Comparison of a plugged telescoping catheter with the protected specimen brush. *Am Rev Respir Dis.* 1991;143:1055–1061.
87. Timsit JF, Misset B, Goldstein FW, et al. Reappraisal of distal diagnostic testing in the diagnosis of ICU-acquired pneumonia. *Chest.* 1995;108: 1632–1639.
88. Kirtland SH, Corley DE, Winterbauer RH, et al. The diagnosis of ventilator-associated pneumonia: a comparison of histologic, microbiologic, and clinical criteria. *Chest.* 1997;112:445–457.
89. Sanchez-Nieto JM, Torres A, Garcia-Cordoba F, et al. Impact of invasive and noninvasive quantitative culture sampling on outcome of ventilator-associated pneumonia: a pilot study. *Am J Respir Crit Care Med.* 1998;157:371–376.
90. Fagon JY, Chastre J, Wolff M, et al. Invasive and noninvasive strategies for management of suspected ventilator-associated pneumonia. A randomized trial. *Ann Intern Med.* 2000;132:621–630.
91. Shorr AF, Sherner JH, Jackson WL, et al. Invasive approaches to the diagnosis of ventilator-associated pneumonia: a meta-analysis. *Crit Care Med.* 2005;33:46–53.
92. Rello J, Vidaur L, Sandiumenge A, et al. De-escalation therapy in ventilator-associated pneumonia. *Crit Care Med.* 2004;32:2183–2190.
93. Laupland KB, Bagshaw SM, Gregson DB, et al. Intensive care unit-acquired urinary tract infections in a regional critical care system. *Crit Care.* 2005;9:R60–R65.
94. Leone M, Albanese J, Garnier F, et al. Risk factors of nosocomial catheter-associated urinary tract infection in a polyvalent intensive care unit. *Intensive Care Med.* 2003;29:1077–1080.
95. Rosser CJ, Bare RL, Meredith JW. Urinary tract infections in the critically ill patient with a urinary catheter. *Am J Surg.* 1999;177:287–290.
96. Huang WC, Wann SR, Lin SL, et al. Catheter-associated urinary tract infections in intensive care units can be reduced by prompting physicians to remove unnecessary catheters. *Infect Control Hosp Epidemiol.* 2004;25:974–978.
97. Krcmery S, Dubrava M, Krcmery V Jr. Fungal urinary tract infections in patients at risk. *Int J Antimicrob Agents.* 1999;11:289–291.
98. Mimoz O, Bouchet E, Edouard A, et al. Limited usefulness of urinary dipsticks to screen out catheter-associated bacteriuria in ICU patients. *Anaesth Inten Care.* 1995;23:706–707.
99. Laupland KB, Zygun DA, Davies HD, et al. Incidence and risk factors for acquiring nosocomial urinary tract infection in the critically ill. *J Crit Care.* 2002;17:50–57.
100. Platt R, Polk BF, Murdock B, et al. Mortality associated with nosocomial urinary tract infection. *N Engl J Med.* 1982;307:637–642.
101. Daifuku R, Stamm W. Association of rectal and urethral colonization with urinary tract infection in patients with indwelling catheters. *JAMA.* 1984;252:2028–2030.
102. Stark RP, Maki DG. Bacteriuria in the catheterized patient. What quantitative level of bacteriuria is relevant? *N Engl J Med.* 1984;311:560–564.
103. Paradisi F, Corti G, Mangani V. Urosepsis in the critical care unit. *Crit Care Clin.* 1998;114:165–180.
104. Warren JW. Catheter-associated urinary tract infections. *Infect Dis Clin North Am.* 1997;11:609–619.
105. Krieger JN, Kaiser DL, Wenzel RP. Urinary tract etiology of bloodstream infections in hospitalized patients. *J Infect Dis.* 1983;148:57–62.
106. Garibaldi RA, Mooney BR, Epstein BJ, et al. An evaluation of daily bacteriologic monitoring to identify preventable episodes of catheter-associated urinary tract infection. *Infect Control.* 1982;3:466–470.
107. Rouby JJ, Laurent P, Gosnach M, et al. Risk factors and clinical relevance of nosocomial maxillary sinusitis in the critically ill. *Am J Respir Crit Care Med.* 1994;150:776–783.
108. Lichtenstein D, Biderman P, Meziere G, et al. The "sinusogram," a real-time ultrasound sign of maxillary sinusitis. *Intensive Care Med.* 1998;24:1057–1061.
109. Bert F, Lambert-Zechovsky N. Microbiology of nosocomial sinusitis in intensive care unit patients. *J Infect.* 1995;31:5–8.
110. George DL, Falk PS, Umberto MG, et al. Nosocomial sinusitis in patients in the medical intensive care unit: a prospective epidemiological study. *Clin Infect Dis.* 1998;27:463–470.
111. Holzapfel L, Chevret S, Madinier G, et al. Influence of long-term oro- or nasotracheal intubation on nosocomial maxillary sinusitis and pneumonia:

results of a prospective, randomized, clinical trial. *Crit Care Med.* 1993;21: 1132–1138.
112. Hilbert G, Vargas F, Valentino R, et al. Comparison of B-mode ultrasound and computed tomography in the diagnosis of maxillary sinusitis in mechanically ventilated patients. *Crit Care Med.* 2001;29:1337–1342.
113. Puidupin M, Guiavarch M, Paris A, et al. B-mode ultrasound in the diagnosis of maxillary sinusitis in intensive care unit. *Intensive Care Med.* 1997;23:1174–1175.
114. Westergren V, Berg S, Lundgren J. Ultrasonographic bedside evaluation of maxillary sinus disease in mechanically ventilated patients. *Intensive Care Med.* 1997;23:393–398.
115. Mevio E, Benazzo M, Quaglieri S, et al. Sinus infection in intensive care patients. *Rhinology.* 1996;34:232–236.
116. Ramadan HH, Owens RM, Tiu C, et al. Role of antral puncture in the treatment of sinusitis in the intensive care unit. *Otolaryngol Head Neck Surg.* 1998;119:381–384.
117. Wanahita A, Goldsmith EA, Marino BJ, et al. Clostridium difficile infection in patients with unexplained leukocytosis. *Am J Med.* 2003;115:543–546.
118. Wanahita A, Goldsmith EA, Musher DM. Conditions associated with leukocytosis in a tertiary care hospital, with particular attention to the role of infection caused by Clostridium difficile. *Clin Infect Dis.* 2002;34:1585–1592.
119. Bulusu M, Narayan S, Shetler K, et al. Leukocytosis as a harbinger and surrogate marker of Clostridium difficile infection in hospitalized patients with diarrhea. *Am J Gastroenterol.* 2000;95:3137–3141.
120. Marinella MA, Burdette SD, Bedimo R, et al. Leukemoid reactions complicating colitis due to Clostridium difficile. *South Med J.* 2004;97:959–963.
121. Starr JM, Martin H, McCoubrey J, et al. Risk factors for Clostridium difficile colonisation and toxin production. *Age Ageing.* 2003;32:657–660.
122. McCusker ME, Harris AD, Perencevich E, et al. Fluoroquinolone use and Clostridium difficile-associated diarrhea. *Emerg Infect Dis.* 2003;9:730–733.
123. Al-Tureihi FI, Hassoun A, Wolf-Klein G, et al. Albumin, length of stay, and proton pump inhibitors: key factors in Clostridium difficile-associated disease in nursing home patients. *J Am Med Dir Assoc.* 2005;6:105–108.
124. Dial S, Alrasadi K, Manoukian C, et al. Risk of Clostridium difficile diarrhea among hospital inpatients prescribed proton pump inhibitors: cohort and case-control studies. *CMAJ.* 2004;171:33–38.
125. Cunningham R, Dale B, Undy B, et al. Proton pump inhibitors as a risk factor for Clostridium difficile diarrhoea. *J Hosp Infect.* 2003;54:243–245.
126. Polk RE, Oinonen M, Pakyz A. Epidemic Clostridium difficile. *N Engl J Med.* 2006;354:1199–1203.
127. Todd B. Clostridium difficile: familiar pathogen, changing epidemiology: a virulent strain has been appearing more often, even in patients not taking antibiotics. *Am J Nurs.* 2006;106:33–36.
128. Muto CA, Pokrywka M, Shutt K, et al. A large outbreak of Clostridium difficile-associated disease with an unexpected proportion of deaths and colectomies at a teaching hospital following increased fluoroquinolone use. *Infect Control Hosp Epidemiol.* 2005;26:273–280.
129. Loo VG, Poirier L, Miller MA, et al. A predominantly clonal multi-institutional outbreak of Clostridium difficile-associated diarrhea with high morbidity and mortality. *N Engl J Med.* 2005;353:2442–2449.
130. Pepin J, Valiquette L, Cossette B. Mortality attributable to nosocomial Clostridium difficile-associated disease during an epidemic caused by a hypervirulent strain in Quebec. *CMAJ.* 2005;173:1037–1042.
131. Sunenshine RH, McDonald LC, Sunenshine RH, et al. Clostridium difficile-associated disease: new challenges from an established pathogen. *Cleveland Clinic J Med.* 2006;73:187–197.
132. McDonald LC, Killgore GE, Thompson A, et al. An epidemic, toxin gene-variant strain of Clostridium difficile. *N Engl J Med.* 2005;353:2433–2441.
133. Ash L, Baker ME, O'Malley CM Jr, et al. Colonic abnormalities on CT in adult hospitalized patients with Clostridium difficile colitis: prevalence and significance of findings. *AJR Am J Roentgenol.* 2006;186:1393–1400.
134. Bours GJ, De Laat E, Halfens RJ, et al. Prevalence, risk factors and prevention of pressure ulcers in Dutch intensive care units. Results of a cross-sectional survey. *Intensive Care Med.* 2001;27:1599–1605.
135. Eachempati SR, Hydo LJ, Barie PS. Factors influencing the development of decubitus ulcers in critically ill surgical patients. *Crit Care Med.* 2001;29:1678–1682.
136. Theaker C, Mannan M, Ives N, et al. Risk factors for pressure sores in the critically ill. *Anaesthesia.* 2000;55:221–224.
137. Metersky ML, Williams A, Rafanan AL. Retrospective analysis: are fever and mental status indications for lumbar puncture in a hospitalized patient who has not undergone neurosurgery. *Clin Infect Dis.* 1997;25:285–288.
138. Adelson-Mitty J, Fink MP, Lisbon A. The value of lumbar puncture in the evaluation of critically ill, non-immunosuppressed, surgical patients: a retrospective analysis of 70 cases. *Intensive Care Med.* 1997;23:749–752.
139. Marik PE. Fever in the ICU. *Chest.* 2000;117:855–869.
140. Johnson DH, Cunha BA. Drug fever. *Infect Dis Clin North Am.* 1996;10:85–91.
141. Bayard PJ, Berger TG, Jacobson MA. Drug hypersensitivity reactions and human immunodeficiency virus disease. *J Acquir Immune Defic Syndr.* 1992;5:1237–1257.
142. Ryan C, Madalon M, Wortham DW, et al. Sulfa hypersensitivity in patients with HIV infection: onset, treatment, critical review of the literature. *WMJ.* 1998;97:23–27.
143. Mijch AM, Hoy JF. Unexplained fever and drug reactions as clues to HIV infection. *Med J Aust.* 1993;158:188–189.
144. Mackowiak PA, LeMaistre CF. Drug fever: a critical appraisal of conventional concepts. An analysis of 51 episodes in two Dallas hospitals and 97 episodes reported in the English literature. *Ann Intern Med.* 1987;106:728–733.
145. De Vriese AS, Philippe J, Van Renterghem DM, et al. Carbamazepine hypersensitivity syndrome: report of 4 cases and review of the literature. *Medicine.* 1995;74:144–151.
146. Vittorio CC, Muglia JJ, Vittorio CC, et al. Anticonvulsant hypersensitivity syndrome. *Arch Intern Med.* 1995;155:2285–2290.
147. Hosoda N, Sunaoshi W, Shirai H, et al. Anticarbamazepine antibody induced by carbamazepine in a patient with severe serum sickness. *Arch Dis Child.* 1991;66:722–723.
148. Tabor PA. Drug-induced fever. *Drug Intell Clin Pharm.* 1986;20:413–420.
149. Roush MK, Nelson KM. Understanding drug-induced febrile reactions. *Am Pharm.* 1993;NS33:39–42.
150. Hanson MA. Drug fever. Remember to consider it in diagnosis. *Postgrad Med.* 1991;89:167–170.
151. Beutler B, Munford RS. Tumor necrosis factor and the Jarisch-Herxheimer reaction. *N Engl J Med.* 1996;335:347–348.
152. Denborough M. Malignant hyperthermia. *Lancet.* 1998;352:1131–1136.
153. Hadad E, Weinbroum AA, Ben-Abraham R. Drug-induced hyperthermia and muscle rigidity: a practical approach. *Eur J Emerg Med.* 2003;10:149–154.
154. Simon HB. Hyperthermia. *N Engl J Med.* 1993;329:483–487.
155. Krause T, Gerbershagen MU, Fiege M, et al. Dantrolene—a review of its pharmacology, therapeutic use and new developments. *Anaesthesia.* 2004;59:364–373.
156. Waldorf S. AANA journal course. Update for nurse anesthetists. Neuroleptic malignant syndrome. *AANA J.* 2003;71:389–394.
157. Velamoor VR. Neuroleptic malignant syndrome. Recognition, prevention and management. *Drug Saf.* 1998;19:73–82.
158. Levenson JL. Neuroleptic malignant syndrome. *Am J Psychiatry.* 1985;142:1137–1145.
159. Sakkas P, Davis JM, Janicak PG, et al. Drug treatment of the neuroleptic malignant syndrome. *Psychopharmacol Bull.* 1991;27:381–384.
160. Rosenberg MR, Green M. Neuroleptic malignant syndrome. Review of response to therapy. *Arch Intern Med.* 1989;149:1927–1931.
161. Carbone JR. The neuroleptic malignant and serotonin syndromes. *Emerg Med Clin N Am.* 2000;18:317–325.
162. Mason PJ, Morris VA, Balcezak TJ. Serotonin syndrome. Presentation of 2 cases and review of the literature. *Medicine.* 2000;79:201–209.
163. Dunkley EJ, Isbister GK, Sibbritt D, et al. The Hunter Serotonin Toxicity Criteria: simple and accurate diagnostic decision rules for serotonin toxicity. *Q J Med.* 2003;96:635–642.
164. Boyer EW, Shannon M. The serotonin syndrome. *N Engl J Med.* 2005;352:1112–1120.
165. Nisijima K, Shioda K, Yoshino T, et al. Diazepam and chlormethiazole attenuate the development of hyperthermia in an animal model of the serotonin syndrome. *Neurochem Int.* 2003;43:155–164.
166. Gillman PK. The serotonin syndrome and its treatment. *J Psychopharmacol.* 1999;13:100–109.
167. Hick JL, Smith SW, Lynch MT. Metabolic acidosis in restraint-associated cardiac arrest: a case series. *Acad Emerg Med.* 1999;6:239–243.
168. Graudins A, Stearman A, Chan B. Treatment of the serotonin syndrome with cyproheptadine. *J Emerg Med.* 1998;16:615–619.
169. Hashimoto T, Tokuda T, Hanyu N, et al. Withdrawal of levodopa and other risk factors for malignant syndrome in Parkinson's disease. *Parkinson Relat Disord.* 2003;9(Suppl 1):S25–S30.
170. Reutens DC, Harrison WB, Goldswain PR. Neuroleptic malignant syndrome complicating levodopa withdrawal. *Med J Aust.* 1991;155:53–54.
171. Keyser DL, Rodnitzky RL. Neuroleptic malignant syndrome in Parkinson's disease after withdrawal or alteration of dopaminergic therapy. *Arch Intern Med.* 1991;151:794–796.
172. Rainer C, Scheinost NA, Lefeber EJ. Neuroleptic malignant syndrome. When levodopa withdrawal is the cause. *Postgrad Med.* 1991;89:175–178.
173. Toru M, Matsuda O, Makiguchi K, et al. Neuroleptic malignant syndrome-like state following a withdrawal of antiparkinsonian drugs. *J Nerv Ment Dis.* 1981;169:324–327.
174. Raj JM, Sudhakar S, Sems K, et al. Arthritis in the intensive care unit. *Crit Care Clin.* 2002;18:767–780.
175. Becker MA. Clinical aspects of monosodium urate monohydrate crystal deposition disease (gout). *Rheum Dis Clin N Am.* 1988;14:377–394.
176. Grahame R, Scott JT. Clinical survey of 354 patients with gout. *Ann Rheum Dis.* 1970;29:461–468.
177. Saag KG, Choi H. Epidemiology, risk factors, and lifestyle modifications for gout. *Arthritis Res Ther.* 2006;8(Suppl 1):S2.
178. Choi HK, Atkinson K, Karlson EW, et al. Obesity, weight change, hypertension, diuretic use, and risk of gout in men: the health professionals follow-up study. *Arch Intern Med.* 2005;165:742–748.

179. Choi HK, Atkinson K, Karlson EW, et al. Alcohol intake and risk of incident gout in men: a prospective study. *Lancet.* 2004;363:1277–1281.
180. Diamond HS. Control of crystal-induced arthropathies. *Rheum Dis Clin N Am.* 1989;15:557–567.
181. Agudelo CA, Wise CM. Crystal-associated arthritis in the elderly. *Rheum Dis Clin N Am.* 2000;26:527–546.
182. Michet CJ Jr, Evans JM, Fleming KC, et al. Common rheumatologic diseases in elderly patients. *Mayo Clin Proc.* 1995;70:1205–1214.
183. Ho G Jr, DeNuccio M. Gout and pseudogout in hospitalized patients. *Arch Intern Med.* 1993;153:2787–2790.
184. Doherty M, Dieppe P. Clinical aspects of calcium pyrophosphate dihydrate crystal deposition. *Rheum Dis Clin N Am.* 1988;14:395–414.
185. Jones AC, Chuck AJ, Arie EA, et al. Diseases associated with calcium pyrophosphate deposition disease. *Semin Arthritis Rheum.* 1992;22:188–202.
186. Halverson PB, McCarty DJ. Clinical aspects of basic calcium phosphate crystal deposition. *Rheum Dis Clin North Am.* 1988;14:427–439.
187. Kes P, Vucicevic Z, Sefer S, et al. Acute acalculous cholecystitis in patients with surgical acute renal failure. *Acta Med Croatica.* 2000;54:15–20.
188. Molenat F, Boussuges A, Valantin V, et al. Gallbladder abnormalities in medical ICU patients: an ultrasonographic study. *Intensive Care Med.* 1996;22:356–358.
189. Stevens PE, Harrison NA, Rainford DJ. Acute acalculous cholecystitis in acute renal failure. *Intensive Care Med.* 1988;14:411–416.
190. McChesney JA, Northup PG, Bickston SJ. Acute acalculous cholecystitis associated with systemic sepsis and visceral arterial hypoperfusion: a case series and review of pathophysiology. *Dig Dis Sci.* 2003;48:1960–1967.
191. Wiboltt KS, Jeffrey RB Jr. Acalculous cholecystitis in patients undergoing bone marrow transplantation. *Eur J Surg.* 1997;163:519–524.
192. Nash JA, Cohen SA, Nash JA, et al. Gallbladder and biliary tract disease in AIDS. *Gastroenterol Clin North Am.* 1997;26:323–335.
193. Romero Ganuza FJ, La BG, Montalvo R, et al. Acute acalculous cholecystitis in patients with acute traumatic spinal cord injury. *Spinal Cord.* 1997;35:124–128.
194. Gofrit O, Eid A, Pikarsky A, et al. Cholesterol embolisation causing chronic acalculous cholecystitis. *Eur J Surg.* 1996;162:243–245.
195. Schwesinger WH, Diehl AK. Changing indications for laparoscopic cholecystectomy. Stones without symptoms and symptoms without stones. *Surg Clin N Am.* 1996;76:493–504.
196. Shapiro MJ, Luchtefeld WB, Kurzweil S, et al. Acute acalculous cholecystitis in the critically ill. *Am Surg.* 1994;60:335–339.
197. Mariat G, Mahul P, Prevt N, et al. Contribution of ultrasonography and cholescintigraphy to the diagnosis of acute acalculous cholecystitis in intensive care unit patients. *Intensive Care Med.* 2000;26:1658–1663.
198. Kalliafas S, Ziegler DW, Flancbaum L, et al. Acute acalculous cholecystitis: incidence, risk factors, diagnosis, and outcome. *Am Surg.* 1998;64:471–475.
199. Boland G, Lee MJ, Mueller PR. Acute cholecystitis in the intensive care unit. *New Horiz.* 1993;1:246–260.
200. Frank SM, Kluger MJ, Kunkel SL. Elevated thermostatic setpoint in postoperative patients. *Anesthesiology.* 2000;93:1426–1431.
201. Dauleh MI, Rahman S, Townell NH. Open versus laparoscopic cholecystectomy: a comparison of postoperative temperature. *J Royal Coll Surg Edin.* 1995;40:116–118.
202. Sazbon L, Groswasser Z. Outcome in 134 patients with prolonged posttraumatic unawareness. Part 1: parameters determining late recovery of consciousness. *J Neurosurg.* 1990;72:75–80.
203. Guinn S, Castro FP Jr, Garcia R, et al. Fever following total knee arthroplasty. *Am J Knee Surg.* 1999;12:161–164.
204. Hobar PC, Masson JA, Herrera R, et al. Fever after craniofacial surgery in the infant under 24 months of age. *Plastic Reconstr Surg.* 1998;102:32–36.
205. Livelli FD Jr, Johnson RA, McEnany MT, et al. Unexplained in-hospital fever following cardiac surgery. Natural history, relationship to postpericardiotomy syndrome, and a prospective study of therapy with indomethacin versus placebo. *Circulation.* 1978;57:968–975.
206. Clark JA, Bar-Yosef S, Anderson A, et al. Postoperative hyperthermia following off-pump versus on-pump coronary artery bypass surgery. *J Cardio Vasc Anesth.* 2005;19:426–429.
207. Ghert M, Allen B, Davids J, et al. Increased postoperative febrile response in children with osteogenesis imperfecta. *J Pediatr Ortho.* 2003;23:261–264.
208. Fry DE. Postoperative fever. In: Mackowiak PA, ed. *Fever: Basic Mechanisms and Management.* New York: Raven Press; 1991:243–254.
209. Engoren M. Lack of association between atelectasis and fever. *Chest.* 1995;107:81–84.
210. Shields RT. Pathogenesis of postoperative pulmonary atelectasis an experimental study. *Arch Surg.* 1949;48:489–503.
211. Lansing AM. Mechanism of fever in pulmonary atelectasis. *Arch Surg.* 1963;87:168–174.
212. Kisala JM, Ayala A, Stephan RN, et al. A model of pulmonary atelectasis in rats: activation of alveolar macrophage and cytokine release. *Am J Physiol.* 1993;264:R610–R614.
213. Corwin HL, Gettinger A, Pearl RG, et al. The CRIT study: anemia and blood transfusion in the critically ill–current clinical practice in the United States. *Crit Care Med.* 2004;32:39–52.
214. Corwin HL, Parsonnet KC, Gettinger A. RBC transfusion in the ICU. Is there a reason? *Chest.* 1995;108:767–771.
215. Snyder EL, Snyder EL. The role of cytokines and adhesive molecules in febrile non-hemolytic transfusion reactions. *Immunol Invest.* 1995;24:333–339.
216. Shanwell A, Kristiansson M, Remberger M, et al. Generation of cytokines in red cell concentrates during storage is prevented by prestorage white cell reduction. *Transfusion.* 1997;37:678–684.
217. Stack G, Snyder EL. Cytokine generation in stored platelet concentrates. *Transfusion.* 1994;34:20–25.
218. Heddle NM, Klama LN, Griffith L, et al. A prospective study to identify the risk factors associated with acute reactions to platelet and red cell transfusions. *Transfusion.* 1993;33:794–797.
219. King KE, Shirey RS, Thoman SK, et al. Universal leukoreduction decreases the incidence of febrile nonhemolytic transfusion reactions to RBCs. *Transfusion.* 2004;44:25–29.
220. Paglino JC, Pomper GJ, Fisch GS, et al. Reduction of febrile but not allergic reactions to RBCs and platelets after conversion to universal prestorage leukoreduction. *Transfusion.* 2004;44:16–24.
221. Yazer MH, Podlosky L, Clarke G, et al. The effect of prestorage WBC reduction on the rates of febrile nonhemolytic transfusion reactions to platelet concentrates and RBC. *Transfusion.* 2004;44:10–15.
222. Stein PD, Afzal A, Henry JW, et al. Fever in acute pulmonary embolism. *Chest.* 2000;117:39–42.
223. Calvo-Romero JM, Lima-Rodriguez EM, Perez-Miranda M, et al. Low-grade and high-grade fever at presentation of acute pulmonary embolism. *Blood Coag Fibrinol.* 2004;15:331–333.
224. Mourad O, Palda V, Detsky AS. A comprehensive evidence-based approach to fever of unknown origin. *Arch Intern Med.* 2003;163:545–551.
225. Murray HW, Ellis GC, Blumenthal DS, et al. Fever and pulmonary thromboembolism. *Am J Med.* 1979;67:232–235.

CHAPTER 106 ■ SURGICAL INFECTIONS

PHILIP S. BARIE • FREDERIC M. PIERACCI • SOUMITRA R. EACHEMPATI

Infection is morbid and costly, but also preventable to some degree; therefore, it behooves every practitioner to do the utmost to prevent infection. An ensemble of prevention methods is required, because no single method is universally effective. Infection control is paramount, but often underemphasized. Surgical incisions and traumatic wounds must be handled gently, inspected daily, and dressed if necessary using aseptic technique. Drains and catheters must be avoided if possible, and removed as soon as practicable. Prophylactic and therapeutic antibiotics should be used sparingly so as to minimize antibiotic selection pressure on the development of multidrug-resistant (MDR) pathogens.

Surgical patients are at particular risk of infection for many reasons. Surgery is inherently invasive, which creates portals of entry in natural epithelial barriers for pathogens to invade the host. Surgical illness is immunosuppressive (e.g., trauma, burns, malignant tumors), as is therapeutic immunosuppression following solid organ transplantation. General anesthesia almost always means a period of mechanical ventilation and a period of reduced consciousness during emergence from anesthesia that poses a risk of pulmonary aspiration of gastric contents, all of which increase the risk of pneumonia. Nosocomial pneumonia occurs more frequently among surgical patients than comparably ill medical patients. Surgical patients are also uniquely afflicted by infections of incisions. Considering that the development of a postoperative infection has a negative impact on surgical outcomes, recognizing risk, minimizing it, and taking an aggressive approach to the diagnosis and treatment of such infections is crucial to improve surgical outcomes.

Surgical infections are traditionally considered to be infections that require surgical therapy (e.g., complicated intra-abdominal and soft tissue infections). However, the recognition that surgical patients are especially vulnerable to nosocomial infection has led to an expansive definition to include any infection that affects surgical patients. Intra-abdominal and soft tissue infections are considered in detail elsewhere in this textbook. The emphasis of this chapter is on the epidemiology, prevention, and management of postoperative and posttraumatic infections.

RISK FACTORS FOR POSTOPERATIVE INFECTION

The general principles of surgical care, critical care, and infection control cannot be overemphasized. Resuscitation must be rapid, yet precise. Pathology must be identified and treated as soon as possible. Infection control is sometimes sacrificed under the often chaotic conditions of resuscitation, but it must not be (see below). Central venous catheters inserted under suboptimal barrier precautions (i.e., lack of cap, mask, sterile gown, and sterile gloves for the operator and a full-bed drape for the patient) must be removed and replaced (if necessary) by a new puncture at a new site as soon as the patient's condition permits. Detailed evidence-based guidelines for the general prevention of infection (1,2) and the prevention of ventilator-associated pneumonia have been published (3,4). All who provide critical care must be familiar with the guidelines and adhere to them insofar as possible.

CONTROL OF BLOOD SUGAR

Hyperglycemia is deleterious to host immune function, and may also reflect the catabolism and insulin resistance associated with the surgical stress response. Poor perioperative control of blood glucose increases the risk of infection and worsens outcome from sepsis. Diabetic patients undergoing cardiopulmonary bypass surgery have a higher risk of infection of both the sternal incision and the vein harvest incisions on the lower extremities (5). Moderate hyperglycemia (>200 mg/dL) at any time on the first postoperative day increases the risk of surgical site infection (SSI) fourfold after cardiac (6) and noncardiac surgery (7). Insulin infusion to keep blood glucose concentrations <110 mg/dL was associated with a 40% decrease in mortality among critically ill postoperative patients, and also fewer nosocomial infections and less organ dysfunction (8). Meta-analysis of 35 trials of control of blood glucose indicates that the risk of mortality is decreased significantly (risk ratio [RR] 0.85, 95% confidence interval [CI] 0.75–0.97) by tight glucose control, especially so for critically ill surgical patients (RR 0.58, 95% CI 0.22–0.62), regardless of whether the patients had diabetes mellitus (RR 0.71, 95% CI 0.54–0.93) or stress-induced hyperglycemia (RR 0.73, 95% CI 0.58–0.90) (9).

Nutritional support is crucial, considering that surgical stress causes catabolism and that restoration of anabolism requires the provision of calories and nitrogen far in excess of basal requirements of 25 to 30 kcal and 1 g nitrogen/kg/day. In the midst of the stress response, it is challenging to provide adequate calories and protein while avoiding hyperglycemia. Parenteral nutrition appears to convey no advantage over not feeding the patient at all (10), perhaps because of the inherent morbidity of central intravenous feeding (i.e., the risk of catheter-related bloodstream infection [CR-BSI] and hyperglycemia). In contrast, early enteral feeding (within the first 48 hours, perhaps immediately if the gut is functional) is clearly beneficial, with the possible exception of pneumonia prevention (see below). The risk of infection was reduced by 55% (odds ratio [OR] 0.45, 95% CI 0.30–0.66) in a meta-analysis of 15 randomized trials of early enteral feeding following surgery, trauma, or burns (11).

Blood Transfusion

Blood transfusion can be life saving after trauma or hemorrhage, but an increased risk of infection is the consequence. Transfusions exert immunosuppressive effects through presentation of leukocyte antigens and the induction of a shift to the T-helper 2 (immunosuppressive) phenotype, although the mechanism remains somewhat controversial because transfusion of leukocyte-depleted red blood cell concentrates does not reduce the risk of infection (12). Claridge et al. identified an exponential relationship between transfusion risk and infection risk among trauma patients, detectable with even 1 unit of transfusion and becoming a virtual certainty after more than 15 units of transfused blood (RR 1.084, 95% CI 1.028–1.142) (13). Hill et al. has estimated by meta-analysis the risk of infection related to blood transfusion to be increased for trauma patients by more than fivefold (OR 5.26, 95% CI 5.03–5.43), and for surgical patients by more than threefold (14). This increased risk for infection by transfusion has also been identified for critically ill patients in general (15), and for CR-BSI (16) and ventilator-associated pneumonia (VAP) (17) specifically.

Banked blood is affected by a "storage lesion" characterized by loss of membrane 2-3-diphosphoglycerate and adenosine triphosphate, leading to loss of membrane deformability (18). As a result, erythrocytes cannot deform as they must to transit the microcirculation, causing disruption of nutrient blood flow and impaired oxygen offloading. Consequently, blood transfusion does not increase oxygen consumption for critically ill patients with sepsis (19), and may actually increase the risk of organ dysfunction. The storage lesion becomes fully manifest after about 14 days of storage; transfusion of older blood is an independent risk factor for the development of infection (20). It is safe to be conservative in the administration of red blood cell concentrates to stable patients in the intensive care unit (ICU) (21).

INFECTION CONTROL

Infection control is an individual and a collective responsibility of the critical care team and unit. Hand hygiene is the most effective means known to reduce the spread of infection, yet whenever studied it is invariably underutilized. Hand cleansing with soap and water requires a minimum of 30 to 45 seconds to be effective. Alcohol gel hand cleansers are equally effective (except against the spores of *Clostridium difficile*), compliance with use is higher, and when used, the prevalence of MDR bacteria is reduced (22). Universal precautions (i.e., cap, mask, gown, gloves, and protective eyewear) must be observed whenever there is a risk of splashing of body fluids.

The source of most bacterial pathogens is the patient's endogenous flora. Skin surfaces, artificial airways, gut lumen, wounds, catheters, and inanimate surfaces (e.g., bed rails, computer terminals) may become colonized. Any break in natural epithelial barriers (e.g., incisions, percutaneous catheters, airway or urinary catheters) creates a portal of entry for invasion of pathogens. The fecal-oral route is the most common manner by which pathogens reach the portal, but health care workers definitely facilitate the transmission of pathogens around a unit. Many organisms that cause infection following surgery are inherently avirulent (e.g., *Candida, Enterococcus, Pseudomonas*). Whether infection develops is determined by complex interactions among host defenses, pathogen, and therapy.

Contact isolation is an important part of infection control, and should be used selectively to prevent the spread of pathogens such as methicillin-resistant *Staphylococcus aureus* (MRSA) and vancomycin-resistant enterococci (VRE), or MDR Gram-negative bacilli. However, contact isolation may decrease the amount of direct patient contact. An appropriate balance must be struck, because reduced nurse staffing of ICUs has been independently associated with an increased risk of a number of nosocomial infections (23).

CATHETER CARE

Optimal catheter care includes avoidance of use when unnecessary, appropriate skin cleansing and barrier protection during insertion, proper catheter selection, proper dressing of indwelling catheters, and removal as soon as possible when no longer needed, or after insertion under less than ideal circumstances (e.g., trauma bay, cardiac resuscitation).

The benefit of the information gained by catheterization must always be weighed against the risk of infection. Almost all indwelling catheters carry a risk of infection, but nontunneled central venous catheters (and pulmonary artery catheters) pose the highest risk, including local site infections and CR-BSIs (see below). Other catheters that pose increased infection risk include intercostal thoracostomy catheters (if inserted as an emergency), ventriculostomy catheters for intracranial pressure monitoring, and urinary bladder catheters. Each day of endotracheal intubation and mechanical ventilation increases the risk of pneumonia by 1% to 3%; it is controversial whether tracheostomy decreases that risk.

Chlorhexidine (which is bactericidal, viricidal, and fungicidal) should be used preferentially for skin preparation for vascular catheter insertion, having been shown to be superior to povidone-iodine solution (24). If povidone-iodine solution is used (of which use is discouraged), it must be allowed to dry, as it is not bactericidal when wet. Full barrier precautions are mandatory for all bedside catheterization procedures (2) except arterial and urinary bladder catheterization, for which sterile gloves and a sterile field suffice. Whenever a central venous catheter is inserted under suboptimal conditions it must be removed (and replaced at a different site if still needed) as soon as permitted by the patient's hemodynamic status, but no more than 24 hours after insertion. A single dose of a first-generation cephalosporin (e.g., cefazolin), but no more, may prevent some infections following emergency tube thoracostomy or ventriculostomy, but is not indicated for vascular or bladder catheterizations. Topical antiseptics placed postprocedure at the insertion site are of no benefit for any type of indwelling catheter, and may actually increase the risk of infection.

Dressings must be maintained carefully (25). Maintaining the integrity of dressings is challenging if the patient is agitated or the body surface is irregular (e.g., the neck [internal jugular vein catheterization] as opposed to the chest wall [subclavian vein catheterization]), but its importance is crucial. Marking the dressing clearly with the date and time of each change is a simple and effective way to manage dressing changes. Dressing carts or similar apparatus should not be brought from patient to patient; rather, sufficient supplies should be kept in each patient's room. The possibility for inanimate objects (e.g., scissors) to be transmission vectors if not cleansed thoroughly after contact with each patient must be borne in mind. Dedicated catheter care teams reduce the risk of CR-BSI substantially (26).

The choice of catheter may play a role in decreasing the risk of infection related to endotracheal tubes, central venous catheters, and urinary catheters. Continuous aspiration of subglottic secretions (CASS), via an endotracheal tube with an extra lumen that opens to the airway just above the balloon, facilitates the removal of secretions that accumulate below the vocal cords but above the endotracheal tube balloon, an area that cannot be reached by routine suctioning. The incidence of VAP is decreased by one half by CASS (26). Silver-impregnated endotracheal tubes are effective in reducing airway colonization, but whether the incidence of VAP is reduced is not yet known (27). Antibiotic- (e.g., minocycline/rifampin) or antiseptic-coated central venous catheters (e.g., chlorhexidine/silver sulfadiazine) can reduce the incidence of CR-BSI (28), especially in high-prevalence units; minocycline/rifampin-coated catheters may be more effective. Urinary bladder catheters coated with ionic silver reduce the incidence of catheter-related bacterial cystitis by a similar amount (29).

Ventilator weaning by protocol, combined with daily sedation holidays and spontaneous breathing trials, allows earlier endotracheal extubation and decreases the risk of VAP (see below) (30). An even better strategy may be avoidance of endotracheal intubation entirely. Respiratory failure can sometimes be managed with noninvasive positive pressure ventilation delivered by mask (e.g., continuous positive airway pressure [CPAP]) (31). Improved resuscitation techniques and noninvasive monitoring techniques have decreased the utilization of pulmonary artery catheters, which pose a particularly high risk of infection (32). Most drains do not decrease the risk of infection; in fact, the risk is probably increased (33) because the catheters hold open a portal for invasion by bacteria.

RISK FACTORS FOR SURGICAL SITE INFECTION

The spectrum of bacterial contamination of the surgical site is well described (34). Clean surgical procedures affect only integumentary and musculoskeletal soft tissues. Clean-contaminated procedures open a hollow viscus (e.g., alimentary, biliary, genitourinary, respiratory tract) under controlled circumstances (e.g., elective colon surgery). Contaminated procedures involve extensive introduction of bacteria into a normally sterile body cavity, but too briefly to allow infection to become established during surgery (e.g., penetrating abdominal trauma, enterotomy during adhesiolysis for mechanical bowel obstruction). Dirty procedures are performed to control established infection (e.g., colon resection for perforated diverticulitis).

Numerous factors determine whether a patient will develop an SSI, including factors related to the patient, the environment, and the therapy (Table 106.1) (33). As incorporated in the National Nosocomial Infections Surveillance System (NNIS) (34,35), the most recognized factors are the wound classification, American Society of Anesthesiologists class ≥3 (class 3: Chronic active medical illness), and prolonged operative time, where time is longer than the 75th percentile for each such procedure. According to the NNIS, the risk of SSI increases with an increasing number of risk factors present, irrespective of the type of operation (35). Laparoscopic surgery decreases the incidence of SSI under most circumstances (36). The reasons that laparoscopic surgery decreases the risk of SSI are possibly several, including decreased wound size, limited use of cautery in the abdominal wall, or a diminished stress response to tissue injury.

TABLE 106.1

RATES OF HEALTH CARE-ASSOCIATED PNEUMONIA AND CATHETER-RELATED BLOODSTREAM INFECTION AMONG VARIOUS INTENSIVE CARE UNIT (ICU) TYPES

ICU type	CVC use	CR-BSI rate Mean/median	TT use	VAP rate Mean/median
Medical	0.52	5.0/3.9	0.46	4.9/3.7
Pediatric	0.46	6.6/5.2	0.39	2.9/2.3
Surgical	0.61	4.6/3.4	0.44	9.3/8.3
Cardiovascular	0.79	2.7/1.8	0.43	7.2/6.3
Neurosurgical	0.48	4.6/3.1	0.39	11.2/6.2
Trauma	0.61	7.4/5.2	0.56	15.2/11.4

CVC use, number of days of catheter placement per 1,000 patient-days in ICU; CR-BSI, catheter-related bloodstream infection; TT use, number of days of indwelling endotracheal tube or tracheostomy per 1,000 patient-days in ICU; VAP, ventilator-associated pneumonia. Infection rates are indexed per 1,000 patient-days.
From the National Nosocomial Infection Surveillance System, U.S. Centers for Disease Control and Prevention.
From Reference 6. Data available at www.cdc.gov, and are in the public domain.

Host-derived factors contribute importantly to the risk of SSI, including increased age (36), obesity, malnutrition, diabetes mellitus (5,7), hypocholesterolemia (38), and numerous other factors that are not accounted for specifically by the NNIS system (Table 106.1). In one 6-year study of 5,031 patients undergoing noncardiac surgery, the overall incidence of SSI was 3.2%. Independent risk factors for the development of SSI included ascites, diabetes mellitus, postoperative anemia, and recent weight loss, but not chronic obstructive pulmonary disorder, tobacco use, or corticosteroid use (39). In another prospective study of 9,016 patients, 12.5% of patients developed an infection of some type within 28 days after surgery (40). Multivariable analysis revealed that decreased serum albumin concentration, increased age, tracheostomy, and amputations were associated with an increased probability of an early infection, whereas factors associated with readmission due to infection included a dialysis shunt, vascular repair, and an early infection. Factors associated with 28-day mortality included increased age, low serum albumin concentration, increased serum creatinine concentration, and an early infection (40).

Lapses in the modern operating room can result in increased rates of SSI. Proper sterilization, ventilation, and skin preparation techniques require continuous vigilance. The operating team must be attentive to personal hygiene (e.g., hand scrubbing, hair). Recent data indicate that a brief rinse with soap and water followed by use of an alcohol gel hand rub is equivalent to the prolonged (and ritualized) session at the scrub sink (41).

Hypothermia during surgery is common if patients are not warmed actively, owing to evaporative water losses, administration of room temperature fluids, and other factors (42). Maintenance of normal core body temperature is unequivocally important for decreasing the incidence of SSI. Mild intraoperative hypothermia is associated with an increased rate of SSI following elective colon surgery (43) and diverse operations (44).

It is intuitive that oxygen administration in the postoperative period would be beneficial for wound healing (45,46). The ischemic milieu of the fresh surgical incision is vulnerable to bacterial invasion. Moreover, oxygen has been postulated to have a direct antibacterial effect (46). However, clinical trials have had conflicting results (47,48). Supplemental oxygenation administration specifically to reduce the incidence of SSI remains plausible, and further studies are needed.

Closure of a contaminated or dirty incision is widely believed to increase the risk of SSI, but few good studies exist to help sort out the multiplicity of wound closure techniques available to surgeons. "Open abdomen" techniques of temporary abdominal closure for management of trauma or severe peritonitis are utilized increasingly. Retrospective studies indicate that antibiotics are not indicated for prophylaxis of the open abdomen (49), but infection of the abdominal wall, should it occur, is highly morbid. Inability to achieve primary abdominal closure is associated with several infectious complications (pneumonia, bloodstream infection, and SSI). Infectious complications, in turn, significantly increased costs from prolonged length of stay, but not mortality (50).

Drains placed in incisions probably cause more infections than they prevent. Epithelialization of the wound is prevented and the drain becomes a conduit, holding open a portal for invasion by pathogens colonizing the skin. Several studies of drains placed into clean or clean-contaminated incisions show that the rate of SSI is not reduced (51,52); in fact, the rate is increased (53–56). Considering that drains pose a risk and accomplish little of what is expected of them, they should be used as little as possible and removed as soon as possible (57). Under no circumstances should prolonged antibiotic prophylaxis be administered to "cover" indwelling drains.

Wound irrigation is a controversial means to reduce the risk of SSI. Routine low-pressure saline irrigation of an incision does not reduce the risk of SSI (58), but high pressure (i.e., pulse irrigation) may be beneficial (59). An increasing body of knowledge suggests that intraoperative topical antibiotics can minimize the risk of SSI (60–62), but the use of antiseptics rather than antibiotics might minimize the possibility of the development of resistance.

Risk Factors for Pneumonia

Surgical patients are susceptible to pneumonia, particularly if they require mechanical ventilation. Ventilator-associated pneumonia, defined as pneumonia occurring 48 to 72 hours after endotracheal intubation, is the most common ICU infection among surgical and trauma patients. Unfortunately, VAP is partially iatrogenic. Nonspecific diagnostic criteria, indiscriminate antibiotic use, and unclear therapeutic end points have all contributed to increased episodes of VAP caused by MDR pathogens. In turn, MDR pathogens increase the likelihood of inadequate initial antimicrobial therapy, which exerts further selection pressure for these pathogens, and results in higher mortality.

Distinction is sometimes made between early-onset VAP (occurring <5 days after intubation) and late-onset VAP (occurring ≥5 days after intubation). Early-onset VAP, to which trauma patients are particularly prone, is often a result of aspiration of gastric contents, and is usually caused by antibiotic-sensitive bacteria such as methicillin-sensitive *S. aureus, Streptococcus pneumoniae*, and *Haemophilus influenzae* (4,63,64). Conversely, patients with late-onset VAP are at increased risk for infection with MDR pathogens (e.g., MRSA, *Pseudomonas aeruginosa*, or *Acinetobacter* spp.).

The incidence of VAP depends upon the diagnostic criteria utilized, and thus varies in published reports. Clinical criteria alone overestimate the incidence of VAP as compared with either microbiologic or histologic data (65,66). A systematic review of 89 studies of VAP among mechanically ventilated patients (67) reported a pooled incidence of VAP of 22.8% (95% CI 18.8–26.9). The NNIS system reported recently that VAP occurred at a rate of 4.9 cases per 1,000 ventilator-days in medical ICUs and 9.3 per 1,000 ventilator-days in surgical ICUs (36) (Table 106.2). The risk for trauma patients, especially those with traumatic brain injury, is especially high. The incidence of VAP increases with the duration of mechanical ventilation at a rate of 3% per day during the first 5 days, 2% per day during days 5 to 10, and 1% per day after that (68).

Risk factors for VAP are summarized in Table 106.3 (27). Perhaps most important is airway intubation itself. The risk of VAP increases six- to 20-fold in mechanically ventilated patients (69,70); VAP is also especially common in patients with acute respiratory distress syndrome (ARDS), owing to prolonged mechanical ventilation and devastated local airway host defenses (71–73).

TABLE 106.2

RISK FACTORS FOR THE DEVELOPMENT OF SURGICAL SITE INFECTIONS

PATIENT FACTORS
Ascites (for abdominal surgery)
Chronic inflammation
Corticosteroid therapy (controversial)
Obesity
Diabetes
Extremes of age
Hypocholesterolemia
Hypoxemia
Peripheral vascular disease (for lower extremity surgery)
Postoperative anemia
Prior site irradiation
Recent operation
Remote infection
Skin carriage of staphylococci
Skin disease in the area of infection (e.g., psoriasis)
Undernutrition
ENVIRONMENTAL FACTORS
Contaminated medications
Inadequate disinfection/sterilization
Inadequate skin antisepsis
Inadequate ventilation
TREATMENT FACTORS
Drains
Emergency procedure
Hypothermia
Inadequate antibiotic prophylaxis
Oxygenation (controversial)
Prolonged preoperative hospitalization
Prolonged operative time

Several evidence-based strategies can prevent VAP, but to be used effectively a thorough understanding of modifiable risk factors is required (Table 106.4). Prevention of VAP begins with minimization of endotracheal intubation and the duration of mechanical ventilation. Noninvasive positive pressure ventilation (NIPPV) should be considered in lieu of intubation, as management of respiratory failure with NIPPV leads

TABLE 106.3

RISK FACTORS FOR VENTILATOR-ASSOCIATED PNEUMONIA

Age ≥60 y
Acute respiratory distress syndrome
Chronic obstructive pulmonary disease or other underlying pulmonary disease
Coma or impaired consciousness
Serum albumin <2.2 g/dL
Burns, trauma
Blood transfusion
Organ failure
Supine position
Large-volume gastric aspiration
Sinusitis
Immunosuppression

TABLE 106.4

STRATEGIES TO PREVENT VENTILATOR-ASSOCIATED PNEUMONIA

Strategy	Recommended	Insufficient evidence
Universal infection control precautions	+	
Orotracheal intubation	+	
Maintenance of endotracheal cuff pressure >20 cm H_2O	+	
Continuous aspiration of subglottic secretions	+	
Semirecumbent positioning	+	
Postpyloric feeding		+
Postponement of enteral feeding for at least 48 h following intubation	+	
Selective decontamination of the digestive tract		+
Topical chlorhexidine	+	
Transfusion restriction	+	
Antibiotic cycling		+

to a lower incidence of VAP (74). If endotracheal intubation is required, the orotracheal route is preferred to nasotracheal intubation to decrease the risk of VAP by as much as one half (75), by decreasing the risk of nosocomial sinusitis (76), which often precedes and is caused by the same pathogen as that which caused VAP subsequently. Evidence-based strategies to decrease the duration of mechanical ventilation include daily interruption of sedation (77), standardized weaning protocols, and adequate ICU staffing (78).

After intubation, most VAP preventive measures aim to decrease the risk of aspiration. Both maintenance of endotracheal cuff pressure >20 cm H_2O (51) and CASS reduce the incidence of VAP significantly (26).

Semirecumbent positioning (30- to 45-degree head-up) is also protective as compared to supine positioning, especially during enteral feeding (79–81). Compared to postpyloric feeding, intragastric feeding increases both gastroesophageal reflux and aspiration (82). A meta-analysis of 11 randomized trials reported a RR of 0.77 (95% CI 0.60–1.00, $p = 0.05$) for VAP with postpyloric as compared to gastric feedings (83). Promotility agents such as erythromycin may facilitate safe intragastric feeding, should this route be used (84). However, early enteral feedings may increase the risk of VAP. Shorr et al. reported that enteral nutrition begun ≤48 hours after the initiation of mechanical ventilation was independently associated with the development of VAP (OR 2.65, 95% CI 1.93–3.63, $p < 0.0001$) (17).

Pharmacologic strategies to minimize the risk of aspiration include minimization of stress ulcer prophylaxis, and selective decontamination of the digestive tract (SDD) with either topical or systemic antibiotics or antiseptics. Myriad clinical trials have reported a significant decrease in the incidence of VAP, but the literature is limited by questionable study methodology (85), study in ICUs in which MDR pathogens were rare, and an increased number of infections caused by MDR bacteria observed in the SDD groups (86–88). For these reasons, use of SDD is currently not recommended for the routine prevention of VAP. However, meta-analysis of studies of oropharyngeal decontamination with topical chlorhexidine provides sufficient evidence to recommend the practice (89), especially for cardiac surgical patients.

Stress ulcer prophylaxis is a known risk factor for VAP (90); its use should be reserved for patients at high risk for gastrointestinal mucosal hemorrhage (e.g., mechanical ventilation >2 days, intracranial hemorrhage, coagulopathy, glucocorticoid therapy). Results of randomized trials comparing histamine type 2 antagonists, sucralfate, and antacids are conflicting for prevention of VAP (91,92).

Ample data document the relationship between blood transfusion and infection risk in surgical, trauma, and critically ill patients. Shorr et al. found red blood cell transfusion to be an independent risk factor for VAP (OR 1.89, 95% CI 1.33–2.68, $p = 0.0004$) (17). Earley et al. documented a 90% decreased incidence of VAP in a surgical ICU following implementation of an anemia management protocol that resulted in fewer blood transfusions (93).

Risk Factors for Catheter-related Bloodstream Infection

Critically ill patients often require reliable large-bore central venous access (e.g., femoral, internal jugular, or subclavian vein), but the catheters are highly prone to infection. Strict adherence to infection control and proper insertion technique is crucial for prevention (94), because surgical and especially trauma patients are at high risk (Table 106.1). When placed under elective (controlled) circumstances, optimal insertion technique includes chlorhexidine skin preparation (not povidone-iodine) (24), draping the entire bed into the sterile field, and donning a cap, a mask, and sterile gown and gloves (2). If technique is breached, the risk of infection increases exponentially, and the catheter should be removed and replaced (if still needed) at a different site using strict asepsis and antisepsis as soon as the patient's condition permits, but certainly within 24 hours. Infection risk for femoral vein catheters is highest, and is lowest for catheters placed via the subclavian route (49). Peripheral vein catheters, peripherally inserted central catheters (PICCs), and tunneled central venous catheters (e.g., Hickman, Broviac) pose less risk of infection than percutaneous central venous catheters (25). Information campaigns, educational initiatives (95), and strict adherence to insertion protocols are all effective to decrease the risk of CR-BSI. Antibiotic- and antiseptic-coated catheters are controversial, but may help decrease the risk of infection in units that have a high rate of infection (96).

Risk Factors for Sinusitis

In the ICU, nosocomial sinusitis is an uncommon closed-space infection that may be clinically occult but can have serious consequences (97). Whereas sinusitis is often part of the differential diagnosis of fever, the incidence is low in comparison to other nosocomial infections in the ICU, and the diagnosis can be difficult to document convincingly. The likely pathogenesis of sinusitis is anatomic obstruction of the ostia draining the facial sinuses, especially the maxillary sinuses. Transnasal endotracheal intubation is the leading risk factor, with an incidence of sinusitis estimated to be one third after 7 days of intubation. Maxillofacial trauma, with obstruction of drainage by retained blood clots, is another clear risk factor. Nasogastric intubation, nasal packing for epistaxis, and corticosteroid therapy have also been implicated, but the evidence is less convincing.

ANTIBIOTIC PROPHYLAXIS

Prophylactic antibiotics are used most often to prevent infection of a surgical incision. Antibiotic prophylaxis of surgery does not prevent postoperative nosocomial infections, which actually occur at an increased rate after prolonged prophylaxis (98), selecting for more resistant pathogens when infection does develop (99).

Preoperative antibiotic prophylaxis is proved to reduce the risk of postoperative SSI in many circumstances. However, only the incision itself is protected, and only while it is open and thus vulnerable to inoculation. Therefore, antibiotics are not a panacea. If not administered properly, antibiotic prophylaxis is ineffective and may be harmful.

Antibiotic prophylaxis is indicated for most clean-contaminated and contaminated (or potentially contaminated) operations. An example of a clean-contaminated operation where antibiotic prophylaxis is usually not indicated is elective laparoscopic cholecystectomy (100); meta-analysis of five trials including 899 patients revealed no benefit compared with placebo for prevention of SSI (OR 0.68, 95% CI 0.24–1.91), "major infection," or "distant infection." Antibiotic prophylaxis is indicated for high-risk biliary surgery; high-risk is conferred by age older than 70 years, diabetes mellitus, or a recently instrumented biliary tract (e.g., biliary stent).

Elective colon surgery is a clean-contaminated procedure where preparatory practices are in evolution (101,102), although the evidence of benefit of systemic antibiotic prophylaxis is unequivocal. Antibiotic bowel preparation, standardized in the 1970s by the oral administration of nonabsorbable neomycin and erythromycin base in addition to mechanical cleansing, reduced the risk of SSI to its present rate of approximately 4% to 8% (101). However, mechanical bowel preparation and preoperative oral antibiotics are omitted increasingly out of the belief that there is no additive benefit beyond parenteral antibiotic prophylaxis. Current Surgical Care Improvement Project (SCIP) guidelines for antibiotic prophylaxis of elective colon surgery give equal weighting to oral prophylaxis alone, parenteral prophylaxis alone, or the combination (102) (Table 106.5), despite the fact that two meta-analyses (that asked different questions) are in conflict as to the efficacy of oral prophylaxis for colorectal surgery. Song and Glenny (103) examined oral antibiotics alone compared with oral/systemic antibiotic prophylaxis (five trials), and found a higher SSI rate with oral prophylaxis alone (OR 3.34, 95% CI 1.66–6.72). Lewis performed a meta-analysis of 13 randomized trials of systemic versus combined oral and systemic prophylaxis, and showed significant benefit for the combined approach (RR 0.51, 95% CI 0.24–0.78) (101).

Antibiotic prophylaxis of clean surgery is controversial. Where bone is incised (e.g., craniotomy, sternotomy) or a prosthesis is inserted, antibiotic prophylaxis is generally indicated. Some controversy persists with clean surgery of soft tissues (e.g., breast, hernia). Meta-analysis of randomized controlled trials shows some benefit of antibiotic prophylaxis of breast cancer surgery without immediate reconstruction (104,105), but no decrease of SSI rate for groin hernia surgery (106, 107), even when a nonabsorbable mesh prosthesis is implanted.

Arterial reconstruction with prosthetic graft material is an example of clean surgery where the susceptibility to infection is high, owing to the presence of ischemic tissue and the infrainguinal location of many such operations. A recent meta-analysis (108) identified 23 randomized, controlled trials of prophylactic systemic antibiotics for peripheral arterial reconstruction (Table 106.6). Prophylactic systemic antibiotics

TABLE 106.5

SURGICAL CARE IMPROVEMENT PROGRAM: APPROVED ANTIBIOTIC PROPHYLACTIC REGIMENS FOR ELECTIVE SURGERY

Type of operation	Antibiotic(s)
Cardiac (including CABG)[a], vascular[b]	Cefazolin, cefuroxime, or vancomycin[f]
Hip/knee arthroplasty[b]	Cefazolin, cefuroxime, or vancomycin[f]
Colon[c,d]	Oral: Neomycin sulfate plus either erythromycin base or metronidazole, administered for 18 h before surgery Parenteral: Cefoxitin, cefotetan, or cefazolin plus metronidazole or ampicillin-sulbactam or ertapenem
Hysterectomy[e]	Cefazolin, cefoxitin, cefotetan, cefuroxime, or ampicillin-sulbactam

[a]Prophylaxis may be administered for up to 48 h for cardiac surgery; for all other cases, the limit is 24 h.
[b]For β-lactam allergy, clindamycin or vancomycin is an acceptable substitute for cardiac, vascular, and orthopedic surgery.
[c]For β-lactam allergy, clindamycin plus gentamicin, a fluoroquinolone, or aztreonam; or metronidazole plus gentamicin or a fluoroquinolone is an acceptable choice.
[d]For colon surgery, either oral or parenteral prophylaxis alone, or both combined, is acceptable.
[e]For β-lactam allergy, clindamycin plus gentamicin, a fluoroquinolone, or aztreonam; or metronidazole plus gentamicin or a fluoroquinolone or clindamycin monotherapy is an acceptable choice.
[f]Vancomycin is acceptable with a physician-documented justification for use in the patient's medical record.

TABLE 106.6

META-ANALYSIS OF MEASURES TO PREVENT INFECTION FOLLOWING ARTERIAL RECONSTRUCTION

Intervention	No. of trials	Odds ratio	95% CI
Systemic antibiotic prophylaxis			
Surgical site infection	10	0.25	0.17–0.38
>24 h prophylaxis	3	1.28	0.82–1.98
Early graft infection	5	0.31	0.11–0.85
Rifampicin bonding of polyester grafts			
Graft infection—1 mo	3	0.63	0.27–1.49
Graft infection—2 y	2	1.05	0.46–2.40
Suction wound drainage—groin	2		
Surgical site infection		0.96	0.50–1.86
Preoperative antiseptic bath	3		
Surgical site infection		0.97	0.70–1.36
In situ surgical technique	2		
Surgical site infection		0.48	0.31–0.74

Data from Stewart A, Evers PS, Earnshaw JJ. Prevention of infection in arterial reconstruction. *Cochrane Database Syst Rev.* 2006;3: CD003073.

reduced the risk of SSI by approximately 75%, and early graft infection by about 69%. There was no benefit to prophylaxis for more than 24 hours, antibiotic bonding to the graft material itself, or preoperative bathing with an antiseptic agent compared with unmedicated bathing.

Four principles guide the administration of antimicrobial agents for prophylaxis: safety, an appropriate narrow spectrum of coverage of relevant pathogens, little or no reliance upon the agent for therapy of infection (owing to the possible induction of resistance with heavy usage), and administration within 1 hour before surgery and for a defined, brief period of time thereafter (no more than 24 hours [48 hours for cardiac surgery]; ideally, a single dose) (109). According to these principles, quinolones or carbapenems are undesirable agents for surgical prophylaxis, although ertapenem and quinolone prophylaxes have been endorsed by the SCIP for prophylaxis of colon surgery (the latter with metronidazole for penicillin-allergic patients) (Table 106.5).

Most SSIs are caused by Gram-positive cocci; therefore, prophylaxis should be directed primarily against staphylococci for clean cases and high-risk clean-contaminated elective biliary and gastric surgery. A first-generation cephalosporin is preferred in almost all circumstances (Table 106.7), with clindamycin used for penicillin-allergic patients (109). If Gram-negative or anaerobic coverage is required, a second-generation cephalosporin or the combination of a first-generation agent plus metronidazole is most experts' regimens of first choice. Vancomycin prophylaxis is generally appropriate only in institutions where the incidence of MRSA infection is high (>20% of all SSIs caused by MRSA).

The optimal time to give parenteral antibiotic prophylaxis is within 1 hour prior to incision (110). Antibiotics given sooner are ineffective, as are agents given after the incision is closed. A 2001 audit of prescribing practices in the United States indicated that only 56% of patients who received prophylactic antibiotics did so within 1 hour prior to the skin incision (111); timeliness was documented in only 76% of cases in a 2005 audit in U.S. Department of Veterans Affairs hospitals (112). Most inappropriately timed first doses of prophylactic antibiotic occur too early (111,112); changing institutional processes to administer the drug in the operating room can improve compliance with best practices (112). Antibiotics with short half-lives (<2 hours, e.g., cefazolin or cefoxitin) should be redosed every 3 to 4 hours during surgery if the operation is prolonged or bloody (113). Even though the SCIP specifies a 24-hour limit for prophylaxis, single-dose prophylaxis (with intraoperative redosing, if indicated) is equivalent to multiple doses for the prevention of SSI (114). Unfortunately, excessively prolonged antibiotic prophylaxis is both pervasive and potentially harmful. Recent U.S. data show that only 40% of patients who receive antibiotic prophylaxis do so for less than 24 hours (111). As a result of ischemia caused by surgical hemostasis, antibiotic penetration into the incision immediately after surgery is questionable until neovascularization occurs (24–48 hours). Antibiotics should not be given to "cover" indwelling drains or catheters, in lavage or irrigation fluid, or as a substitute for poor surgical technique. That prophylaxis is prolonged excessively is demonstrated by antibiotic utilization data for U.S. surgical ICUs (Table 106.8); high usage of first-generation cephalosporins in ICUs cannot be explained by therapeutic use.

Prolongation of antibiotic prophylaxis beyond 24 hours is not only nonbeneficial, but also may be harmful. *Clostridium difficile*–associated disease (CDAD) follows disruption of the normal balance of gut flora, resulting in overgrowth of the enterotoxin-producing *C. difficile* (115). Although virtually any antibiotic may cause CDAD (even a single dose), prolonged antibiotic prophylaxis increases the risk. Prolonged prophylaxis also increases the risk of nosocomial infections unrelated to the surgical site, and the emergence of MDR pathogens. Both pneumonia and vascular catheter–related infections have been associated with prolonged prophylaxis (116,117), as has the emergence of SSI caused by MRSA (99).

EVALUATION OF POSSIBLE POSTOPERATIVE INFECTION

A new temperature elevation usually triggers an automatic evaluation that includes many costly tests of limited utility, based on suspicion of a nosocomial infection. During the evaluation, the patient may be exposed to unneeded radiation, require transport outside the controlled environment of the ICU, or experience considerable blood loss due to this testing, which is often repetitive. With utilization of resources under intensive scrutiny, it is appropriate to assess such fevers in a prudent and cost-effective manner.

However, some infected patients do not become febrile, and may even become hypothermic. A hypothermic or euthermic patient may have a life-threatening infection (118,119). Such patients include elderly patients, those with open abdominal wounds or large burns, patients on extracorporeal support (e.g., continuous renal replacement therapy) (120), patients with end-stage liver disease or chronic renal failure, and patients taking anti-inflammatory or antipyretic drugs. Absent a

TABLE 106.7

APPROPRIATE CEPHALOSPORIN PROPHYLAXIS FOR SELECTED OPERATIONS[a]

Operation	Alternative prophylaxis in serious penicillin allergy
First-generation cephalosporin (i.e., cefazolin, cefuroxime)	
Cardiovascular and thoracic	Clindamycin (for all cases herein except amputation)[b]
Median sternotomy	Vancomycin
Pacemaker insertion	
Vascular reconstruction involving the abdominal aorta, insertion of a prosthesis, or a groin incision (except carotid endarterectomy, which requires no prophylaxis)	
Implantable defibrillator	
Pulmonary resection	
Lower limb amputation	Gentamicin and metronidazole
General	
Cholecystectomy (High risk only)	Gentamicin
Gastrectomy (High risk only: Not uncomplicated chronic duodenal ulcer)	Gentamicin and metronidazole
Hepatobiliary	Gentamicin and metronidazole
Major debridement of traumatic wound	Gentamicin
Genitourinary (Ampicillin plus gentamicin is a reasonable alternative)	Ciprofloxacin
Gynecologic	
Cesarean section (stat)	Metronidazole (after cord clamping)
Hysterectomy (cefoxitin is a reasonable alternative)	Doxycycline
Head and neck/oral cavity	
Major procedures entering oral cavity or pharynx	Gentamicin and clindamycin or metronidazole
Neurosurgery	
Craniotomy	Clindamycin, vancomycin
Orthopedics	
Major joint arthroplasty	Vancomycin[b]
Open reduction of closed fracture	Vancomycin[b]
Appendectomy	Metronidazole with or without gentamicin (for all cases herein) Second generation (i.e., cefoxitin)[c]
Colon surgery	
Surgery for penetrating abdominal trauma	

[a]Should be given as a single intravenous dose just before the operation. Consider an additional dose if the operation is prolonged longer than 3–4 h.
[b]Primary prophylaxis with vancomycin (i.e., for the non–penicillin-allergic patient) may be appropriate for cardiac valve replacement, placement of a nontissue peripheral vascular prosthesis, or total joint replacement in institutions where a high rate of infections with methicillin-resistant *Staphylococcus aureus* or *Staphylococcus epidermidis* has occurred. The precise definition of "high rate" is debated. A single dose administered immediately before surgery is sufficient unless operation lasts for more than 6 h, in which case the dose should be repeated. Prophylaxis should be discontinued after a maximum of two doses, but may be continued for up to 48 h.
[c]An intraoperative dose should be given if cefoxitin is used and the duration of surgery exceeds 3–4 h, because of the short half-life of the drug. A postoperative dose is not necessary, but is permissible for up to 24 h.

fever, any of hypotension, tachycardia, tachypnea, confusion, rigors, skin lesions, respiratory manifestations, oliguria, lactic acidosis, leukocytosis, leukopenia, immature neutrophils (i.e., bands >10%), or thrombocytopenia may indicate a workup for infection and immediate empiric therapy.

The definition of fever is arbitrary, and depends on how and when temperature was measured. In addition to host biology, a variety of environmental forces in an ICU can also alter body temperature, such as specialized mattresses, lighting, heating or air conditioning, peritoneal lavage, and renal

TABLE 106.8

COMPARISON OF ANTIBIOTIC UTILIZATION (MEDIAN DEFINED DAILY DOSES) FOR SURGICAL INTENSIVE CARE UNITS (SICUs) AND INPATIENT UNITS, 1998–2002

Agent	Inpatient	SICU
First-generation cephalosporins	76	168
Third-generation cephalosporins	81	142
Vancomycin		104
Fluoroquinolones	62	87
Ampicillins	63	83
Second-generation cephalosporins	34	NR

NR, not reported.
From the National Nosocomial Infections Surveillance System, U.S. Centers for Disease Control and Prevention. Data abstracted from www.cdc.gov. Data are in the public domain.

replacement therapy (121–123). Thermoregulatory mechanisms can be disrupted by drugs or by injury to the central nervous systems. Thus, it is often difficult to determine if an abnormal temperature is a reflection of a physiologic process, a drug, or an environmental influence. Moreover, in surgical patients, the substantial possibility (~50%) that a fever is due to a noninfectious cause must be considered (Fig. 106.1) (124).

Many ICUs consider any patient with a core temperature ≥38.3°C (≥101°F) to be febrile and to warrant evaluation to determine if infection is present. However, a lower threshold may be decided upon for immunocompromised patients. However, laboratory tests or imaging studies to search for infection should be performed only after a clinical assessment (history and physical examination) indicates that infection might be present.

Blood Cultures

Blood cultures should be obtained from patients with a new fever when clinical evaluation does not strongly suggest a noninfectious cause. The site of venipuncture should be cleaned with either 2% chlorhexidine gluconate in 70% isopropyl alcohol or 1% to 2% tincture of iodine. Povidone-iodine (10%), while acceptable, is not bactericidal until dry; some false-positive blood cultures may be due to premature specimen collection (125,126). One blood culture is defined as a 20- to 30-mL sample of blood drawn at a single time from a single site, regardless of how many bottles or tubes are filled for processing. The sensitivity of blood culturing for detection of true bacteremia or fungemia is related to many factors, most importantly the volume of blood drawn and obtaining the cultures before initiation of anti-infective therapy (127,128).

Recent data suggest that the cumulative yield of pathogens is optimized when three blood cultures with adequate volume (20- to 30-mL each) are drawn (127). Each culture should ideally be drawn by separate venipuncture or through a separate intravascular device, but not through multiple ports of the same intravascular catheter (129). There is no evidence that the yield of cultures drawn from an artery or vein is different. Drawing two to three blood cultures with appropriate volume from separate sites of access at the onset of fever is the most effective way to discern whether an organism found in blood culture represents a true pathogen (multiple cultures are often positive), a contaminant (only one of multiple blood cultures is positive for an organism commonly found on skin and clinical

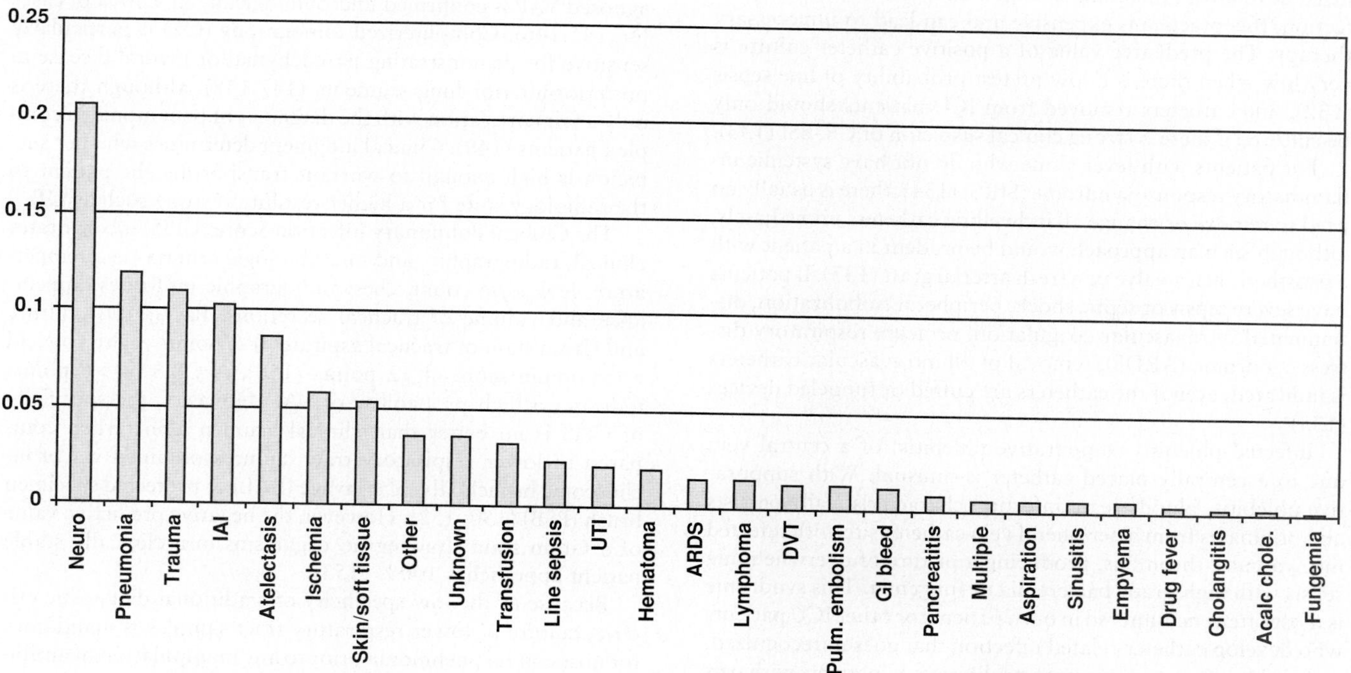

FIGURE 106.1. Causes of fever (%) among more than 600 consecutive surgical intensive care unit patients. IAI, intra-abdominal; UTI, urinary tract infection; ARDS, acute respiratory distress syndrome; DVT, deep venous thrombosis; pulm., pulmonary; GI, gastrointestinal; chole., cholecystitis.

correlation does not support infection), or a bacteremia/fungemia from an infected catheter (one culture from the source catheter is positive, often with a positive catheter tip, and other cultures are not) (130).

Intravascular Devices

All intravascular devices and insertion sites must be assessed daily as part of a comprehensive physical examination to determine if they are still needed and whether signs of infection are present locally (e.g., inflammation or purulence at the exit site or along the tunnel) or systemically. Contaminated catheter hubs are common portals of entry for organisms colonizing the endoluminal surface of the catheter (131). Additionally, infusate (parenteral fluid, blood products, or intravenous medications) can become contaminated and produce bacteremia or fungemia, which is especially likely to result in septic shock. Abrupt onset of signs and symptoms of sepsis or shock in patients with an indwelling vascular catheter should prompt suspicion of infection of an intravascular device. Recovery of certain micro-organisms in multiple blood cultures, such as staphylococci or *Candida* spp., strongly suggests infection of an intravascular device.

Removal and culture of the catheter has historically been the gold standard for the diagnosis of CR-BSI, particularly with short-term catheters. Studies have demonstrated the reliability of semiquantitative or quantitative catheter tip culture methods for the diagnosis of CR-BSI (132), which is confirmed when a colonized catheter is associated with concomitant bloodstream infection with the identical organism, with no other plausible source. Some ICU clinicians culture central venous catheters routinely on removal, regardless of whether infection is suspected. Because ~20% of central venous catheters are colonized at removal, most unassociated with local or systemic infection, this practice is expensive and can lead to unnecessary therapy. The predictive value of a positive catheter culture is very low when there is a low pretest probability of line sepsis (132), and catheters removed from ICU patients should only be cultured if there is strong clinical suspicion of CR-BSI (133).

For patients with fever alone who do not have systemic inflammatory response syndrome (SIRS) (134), there is usually no need to remove or change all indwelling catheters immediately, although such an approach would be prudent in a patient with a prosthetic heart valve or a fresh arterial graft (133). If patients have severe sepsis or septic shock, peripheral embolization, disseminated intravascular coagulation, or acute respiratory distress syndrome (ARDS), removal of all intravascular catheters is indicated, even if the catheters are cuffed or tunneled devices (135).

Infected phlebitis (suppurative phlebitis) of a central vein due to a centrally placed catheter is unusual. With suppurative phlebitis, bloodstream infection characteristically persists and originates from a peripheral vein catheter site with infected intravascular thrombus, producing a picture of overwhelming sepsis with high-grade bacteremia or fungemia. This syndrome is most often encountered in burn patients or other ICU patients who develop catheter-related infection that goes unrecognized, permitting micro-organisms to proliferate. In patients with persistent *S. aureus* bacteremia or fungemia, echocardiography is appropriate to assess for endocarditis and guide further therapy (133).

Intensive Care Unit–acquired Pneumonia

Pneumonia is the second most common cause of ICU-acquired infection and a ubiquitous cause of fever, with the majority of cases occurring in mechanically ventilated patients (65,136). The diagnosis of VAP is especially challenging, as patients commonly also have other, noninfectious processes producing abnormal chest radiographs and gas exchange (e.g., congestive heart failure, atelectasis, ARDS). Intubated, sedated patients cannot cough, or otherwise mobilize abnormal secretions without assistance. In addition, immunocompromised patients such as solid organ transplant recipients may have pneumonia without fever, cough, sputum production, or leukocytosis (137–138).

The diagnosis of VAP requires determination if the patient has pneumonia, and the etiologic pathogen. Poor specificity is problematic because it not only exposes patients to unnecessary risk from overtreatment with antibiotics, but also increases selection pressure and thus the emergence of MDR bacteria (139,140). Conversely, inadequate initial therapy in patients with VAP (poor sensitivity) is associated with increased mortality that cannot be reduced by subsequent changes in antibiotics (141).

Historically, the diagnosis of VAP requires one or more of the following: fever, leukocytosis or leukopenia, purulent sputum, hypoxemia, or a new or evolving chest radiographic infiltrate. However, several noninfectious processes may mimic these nonspecific signs, such as congestive heart failure, atelectasis, pulmonary thromboembolism, pulmonary hemorrhage, and ARDS, making clinical criteria alone unreliable. A new chest radiographic infiltrate, along with two of the three aforementioned criteria, was only 69% sensitive and 75% specific for VAP as compared to postmortem histology (142). Several subsequent reports have confirmed the low specificity of clinical acumen in the diagnosis of VAP (143–144); clinically diagnosed VAP is confirmed microbiologically in <50% of cases (66,145,146). Computerized tomography (CT) is particularly sensitive for demonstrating parenchymal or pleural disease in posterior-inferior lung segments (147,148), although there is only a fair correlation with the diagnosis of pneumonia in complex patients (149). Clinical judgment determines whether suspicion is high enough to warrant transporting the patient to the radiology suite for a higher-resolution study such as CT.

The Clinical Pulmonary Infection Score (CPIS) incorporates clinical, radiographic, and microbiologic criteria (i.e., temperature, leukocyte count, chest radiographic infiltrates, appearance and volume of tracheal secretions, PaO_2:FIO_2, culture and Gram stain of tracheal aspirate [0–2 points each]) to yield a maximum score of 12 points (150). A CPIS of >6 points indicates a high probability of VAP. However, the specificity of CPIS is no better than clinical acumen alone when compared to lower respiratory tract cultures obtained via bronchoscopic bronchoalveolar lavage (BAL) or protected specimen brush (PSB) (150–152). However, the negative predictive value of a Gram stain showing no organisms in a clinically stable patient approaches 100% (153).

Because of the low specificity of traditional diagnostic criteria, culture of lower respiratory tract samples is mandatory for nosocomial pneumonia prior to any manipulation of antibiotics in order to minimize false-negative results. The method of specimen collection (invasive vs. noninvasive) and the method of specimen analysis (semiquantitative vs. quantitative) are debated. Noninvasive techniques include endotracheal suction aspiration (EA), blinded plugged telescoping catheter, blinded PSB, and mini-BAL. Endotracheal aspirates are less specific due to an increased likelihood of contamination by oropharyngeal flora reflecting colonization rather than infection.

Invasive techniques (BAL or PSB) collect samples using fiberoptic bronchoscopy, and also allow direct inspection of the airways, but are more expensive and resource intensive than noninvasive techniques. Furthermore, arterial desaturation may persist for up to 24 hours postbronchoscopy, possibly due to alveolar flooding caused by residual lavage fluid. However, this desaturation has not been correlated with poorer outcomes (154).

Respiratory tract cultures may be reported either semiquantitatively or quantitatively. The crucial issue is distinction of colonization from infection (155). Whereas semiquantitative microbiology reports growth in terms of ordinal categories (e.g., light, moderate, or heavy), quantitative microbiology reports growth in terms of colony forming units (CFU)/mL of aliquot; a threshold value is assigned to distinguish colonization from infection. Commonly used thresholds are 10^3 CFU/mL for PSB, 10^4 CFU/mL for BAL, and 10^5 CFU/mL for EA. Any threshold should be lowered by one order of magnitude if antibiotics have been changed recently or started prior to sample acquisition (156). Clinical interpretation of quantitative cultures is likely to be hampered by prior antibiotic administration, which may lower the observed quantitative inoculum after 24 hours of ongoing antibiotic therapy, and for up to 72 hours after cessation of antibiotics (157,158). The diagnostic threshold is usually lowered by one order of magnitude in the presence of antibiotics or recently discontinued therapy.

Endotracheal aspirates have lower specificity compared to either blinded plugged telescoping catheter (159) or bronchoscopic BAL or PSB (160–163). Two systematic reviews, one of bronchoscopic BAL (154) and one of blinded invasive techniques (163), reported similar test characteristics for the two techniques, but methodologic variability is rampant. Bronchoscopic techniques are more specific than blinded techniques, and both techniques are superior to EAs.

Shorr et al. performed a meta-analysis of randomized trials that compare outcomes of patients with VAP managed with invasive versus noninvasive sampling when both samples were cultured quantitatively (164). Although the pooled OR suggested a survival advantage to the invasive approach (OR = 0.62), the result was not significant. However, patients in the invasive group were significantly more likely to undergo changes in antimicrobial regimen.

Pulmonary secretions for culture should be transported to the laboratory and processed within 2 hours so that fastidious organisms such as *S. pneumoniae* remain viable. For any expectorated specimen, it is important for the laboratory to perform direct microscopy on the specimen to determine if squamous epithelial cells are present, which invalidates the specimen.

Organisms that may be pathogens in VAP or contaminants when recovered from the airway include *P. aeruginosa, Enterobacteriaceae, S. pneumoniae, S. aureus*, and *H. influenzae.* Conversely, isolation of enterococci, viridans streptococci, coagulase-negative staphylococci, and *Candida* spp. (165,166) should rarely be considered the cause of respiratory dysfunction, if ever. Although febrile postoperative patients in an ICU often have small pleural effusions due to fluid overload, hypoalbuminemia, or postoperative processes, it is not necessary to sample such fluid from every febrile patient. Thoracentesis is appropriate if there is sufficient fluid to aspirate safely using ultrasound (US) guidance and there is either an adjacent pulmonary infiltrate or possible contamination of the pleural space by surgery, trauma, or a fistula.

Evaluation for *Clostridium difficile* Infection

Many ICU patients have diarrhea, often due to enteral feedings or drugs. By far the most common enteric cause of fever in the ICU is *C. difficile*, which should be suspected in any patient with diarrhea and fever or leukocytosis who has received an antibacterial agent or antineoplastic chemotherapy within 60 days prior to the onset of diarrhea (167,168). *C. difficile* accounts for 10% to 25% of all cases of antibiotic-associated diarrhea and virtually all of the cases of antibiotic-associated colitis (169). However, some patients, especially those who are postoperative, may present with ileus or toxic megacolon, or leukocytosis without diarrhea, as the manifestation of CDAD. In these patients, the diagnosis is difficult to establish because stool specimens are not accessible (170). *C. difficile*–associated diarrhea may occur with any antibacterial agent, but the most common causes are clindamycin, cephalosporins, and fluoroquinolones (171).

Although less accurate than expensive tissue culture assays, most laboratories now use immunoassays for *C. difficile* toxins, which provide results within hours and are easy to perform. Lower sensitivity may require repeat tests to document disease in seriously ill patients (172). Most strains of *C. difficile* produce toxin A, but 2% to 3% of stains produce only toxin B so an assay that detects both toxins A and B is preferred (173). Cultures for *C. difficile* are technically demanding, and are not specific in distinguishing toxin-positive strains, toxin-negative strains, and asymptomatic carriage (172,174). Cultures may be useful in the setting of nosocomial outbreaks to identify isolates for epidemiologic purposes (168). The North American pulse-field gel electrophoresis type 1 (NAP1) strain, now epidemic in many hospitals in the United States, Canada, and Europe, is associated with serious complications (toxic megacolon, leukemoid reactions, septic shock, and death) (175,176).

Direct visualization of pseudomembranes is nearly diagnostic of CDAD, but only about 70% of seriously ill patients and 25% of patients with mild disease have pseudomembranes by direct visualization (177), diminishing the role of endoscopy for routine diagnostic use. However, a role for direct visualization may exist if false-negative *C. difficile* toxin assays are suspected (168).

Urinary Tract Infection

Catheter-associated bacteriuria or candiduria usually represents colonization, is rarely symptomatic, and is an unlikely cause of fever or secondary bloodstream infection (178), even in immunocompromised patients (179), unless there is urinary tract obstruction; there is a history of recent urologic manipulation, injury, or surgery; or the patient is neutropenic (180,181). Traditional signs and symptoms (dysuria, urgency, pelvic or flank pain, fever or chills) that correlate well with bacteriuria in noncatheterized patients are rarely reported in ICU patients with documented catheter-associated bacteriuria or candiduria (>10^5 CFU/mL) (180,181). In the ICU, the majority of urinary tract infections are related to urinary catheters and are caused by multiresistant nosocomial Gram-negative bacilli other than *Escherichia coli, Enterococcus* spp., and yeasts (178,182,183).

When clinical evaluation suggests the urinary tract as a possible source of fever, a urine specimen should be evaluated by direct microscopy, Gram stain, and quantitative culture. The specimen should be aspirated from the catheter sampling port, not collected from the drainage bag. Health care personnel should wear clean gloves whenever manipulating a urinary device and should scrupulously clean the port with 70% to 90% alcohol prior to specimen collection. For patients without a catheter, a conventional midstream clean-catch urine specimen should be obtained. Urine collected for culture should reach the laboratory promptly to prevent multiplication of bacteria within the receptacle, which might lead to the misdiagnosis of infection; any delay should prompt refrigeration of the specimen.

In contrast to community-acquired urinary tract infections, where pyuria is highly predictive of important bacteriuria, pyuria may be absent with catheter-associated urinary tract infections. Even if present, pyuria is not a reliable predictor of urinary tract infection in the presence of a catheter (178). The concentration of urinary bacteria or yeast needed to cause symptomatic urinary tract infection or fever is unclear. Whereas it is clear that counts >10^3 CFU/mL represent true bacteriuria or candiduria in catheterized patients (184), there are no data to show that higher counts are more likely to represent symptomatic infection. Gram stain of a centrifuged urine specimen, however, will show micro-organisms most of the time if infection is present (185).

Whereas it is appropriate to collect urine specimens in the investigation of fever, routine monitoring or "surveillance" cultures of urine contribute little to patient management. Rapid dipstick tests, which detect leukocyte esterase and nitrite, are unreliable in the setting of catheter-related UTI. The leukocyte esterase test correlates with the degree of pyuria, which may or may not be present in a catheter-related UTI. The nitrite test reflects *Enterobacteriaceae*, which convert nitrate to nitrite, and is therefore unreliable to screen for *Enterococcus* spp., *Candida* spp., and *Staphylococcus* spp. (186,187).

SINUSITIS

The paranasal sinuses are normally sterile, but bacterial overgrowth occurs when drainage is impeded. The etiologic agents responsible for most cases of nosocomial sinusitis are those that colonize the naso-oropharynx (76,188), which occurs at high frequency among critically ill patients. Gram-negative bacilli (particularly *P. aeruginosa*) constitute 60% of bacteria isolated from nosocomial sinusitis, whereas Gram-positive cocci (typically *S. aureus* and coagulase-negative staphylococci) comprise one third of isolates, and fungi the remaining 5% to 10% (76,189,190). Infections are often polymicrobial.

The diagnosis of sinusitis in critically ill, intubated patients is difficult to make. Complaints of facial pain or headache may be impossible to elicit, and purulent nasal discharge is present in only 25% of proved cases of sinusitis. In the ICU, acute sinusitis is diagnosed most efficiently by CT of the facial bones (191), followed by sampling using antiseptic technique if mucosal thickening or sinus fluid is documented. Microbial analysis of fluid obtained by minimally invasive sinus puncture and aspiration under antiseptic conditions is definitive for the diagnosis. Although less well studied, endoscopic-guided middle meatal tissue culture is a safe alternative for patients who are not candidates for antral puncture (e.g., coagulopathy) (192). Pathogen identification and susceptibility testing permit focused, narrow-spectrum antimicrobial therapy. However, specimen collection is susceptible to contamination by bacteria colonizing the overlying mucosa if rigorous antisepsis is not practiced when obtaining the specimen.

INTRACRANIAL DEVICE–RELATED FEVER

When a patient with an intracranial device such as an extraventricular drain (EVD) (ventriculostomy catheter) or a ventriculoperitoneal shunt becomes febrile, cerebrospinal fluid (CSF) should almost always be analyzed. Access to CSF in the patient with an EVD is straightforward. The patient with a shunt or Ommaya reservoir should have the reservoir aspirated. Patients with EVDs who develop stupor or signs of meningitis should have the catheter removed and the tip cultured.

Basic tests of CSF for suspected central nervous system (CNS) infection include cell counts and differential, glucose and protein concentrations, Gram stain, and bacterial cultures. Patients with bacterial meningitis typically have a CSF glucose concentration <35 mg/dL, a CSF:blood glucose ratio <0.23, a CSF protein concentration >220 mg/dL, >2,000 total white blood cells/μL, or >1,180 neutrophils/μL (193). Conversely, the presence of a normal opening pressure, <5 white blood cells/μL, and a normal CSF protein concentration essentially exclude meningitis (193). Measurement of CSF lactate concentration may be useful in neurosurgical patients to distinguish infection from postoperative aseptic meningitis (194,195).

NONINFECTIOUS CAUSES OF FEVER IN THE INTENSIVE CARE UNIT

Postoperative Fever

Fever is common during the initial 72 hours following surgery, and is usually noninfectious in origin (196), presuming that unusual breaks in sterile technique or pulmonary aspiration did not occur. Considerable effort and money can be wasted in overzealous evaluation of early postoperative fever. However, once a patient is more than 96 hours postoperative, fever is more likely to represent infection.

A chest radiograph is not mandatory for evaluation of postoperative fever unless respiratory rate, auscultation, abnormal blood gases, or pulmonary secretions suggest a high yield. Atelectasis is often considered to be a cause of postoperative fever. The clinician must be alert to the possibility that the patient could have aspirated during the perioperative period, or the uncommon event that the patient was incubating a community-acquired pneumonia prior to the operation caused, for example, by pneumococci or influenza A.

Urinary tract infection is common postoperatively in nontrauma patients because of the use of urinary drainage catheters (197). The duration of catheterization increases the risk of bacteriuria by about 5% per day, which in turn increases the risk of nosocomial cystitis or pyelonephritis. A urinalysis or culture is not mandatory to evaluate fever during the initial 3 days postoperatively unless there is reason by history or examination to suspect an infection at this site. After trauma, urinary tract infection is common only after injury to the urinary tract.

Fever can be related to hematoma or infection of the surgical field. Surgical site infection is rare in the first few days after operation, except for group A streptococcal infections and clostridial infections, which can develop within hours to 1 to 3 days after surgery. These causes should be suspected on the basis of inspection of the incision.

Many emergency abdominal operations are performed for control of an infection (e.g., perforated diverticulitis). Even under optimal circumstances (definitive surgical source control and timely administration of appropriate broad-spectrum antibiotics), it may take ≥72 hours for such patients to defervesce. New or persistent fever more than 4 days after surgery should raise suspicion of persistent pathology or a new complication. Thus, it is mandatory to remove the surgical dressing to inspect the incision. Swabbing an open wound or collecting fluid from drains (if present) for culture is rarely helpful because the likelihood of colonization is high. Muscle compression injury (either direct trauma or as a result of compartment syndrome) and tetanus are two rare complications of traumatic wounds that may cause fever. Toxic shock may accompany infection with group A streptococci or *S. aureus*. Other potentially serious noninfectious causes of postoperative fever include deep venous thrombosis, tissue ischemia or necrosis, pulmonary embolism, adrenal insufficiency, drug-induced fever, anesthesia-induced malignant hyperthermia, and acute allograft rejection.

Drug-related Fever

Any drug can cause fever due to hypersensitivity (198), but "drug fever" is decidedly unusual in surgical patients, and must be considered a diagnosis of exclusion. In addition, some drugs cause fever by producing local inflammation at the site of administration (phlebitis, sterile abscesses, or soft tissue reaction), such as amphotericin B, erythromycin, and potassium chloride. Drugs or their delivery systems (diluent, intravenous fluid, or intravascular delivery devices) may also contain pyrogens or, rarely, microbial contaminants (199). Some drugs may also stimulate heat production (e.g., thyroxine), limit heat dissipation (e.g., atropine or epinephrine), or alter thermoregulation (e.g., butyrophenone tranquilizers, phenothiazines, antihistamines, or antiparkinson drugs). Among drug categories, drug fever in surgical ICUs is most often attributed to antimicrobial agents (e.g., vancomycin, β-lactams) and anticonvulsants (especially phenytoin).

Two important syndromes, malignant hyperthermia and neuroleptic malignant syndrome, deserve consideration when fever is especially high because the results can be devastating if left untreated (200). Malignant hyperthermia is more often identified in the operating room than in the ICU, but onset can be delayed for as long as 24 hours, especially if the patient is on steroids. Malignant hyperthermia is believed to be a genetically determined response mediated by a dysregulation of cytoplasmic calcium flux in skeletal muscle, resulting in intense muscle contraction, fever, and increased creatinine phosphokinase concentration. It can be caused by succinylcholine and inhalational anesthetics.

TABLE 106.9

CAUSES OF FEVER RELATED TO NONINFECTIOUS STATES

Acalculous cholecystitis
Acute myocardial infarction
Acute respiratory distress syndrome (fibroproliferative phase)
Adrenal insufficiency
Cytokine release syndrome
Fat embolism
Gout
Hematoma
Heterotopic ossification
Immune reconstitution inflammatory syndrome (IRIS)
Intracranial hemorrhage
Pancreatitis
Pericarditis
Pulmonary infarction
Thyroid storm
Transfusion of blood or blood products
Transplant rejection
Tumor lysis syndrome
Venous thromboembolic disease
Withdrawal syndromes (drug, alcohol)

The neuroleptic malignant syndrome is slightly more common, and more often identified in the ICU than malignant hyperthermia. It has been strongly associated with the neuroleptic medications phenothiazines, thioxanthenes, and butyrophenones (200,201), most frequently haloperidol in the ICU. It also manifests as muscle rigidity, fever, and increasing creatinine phosphokinase concentration. However, unlike malignant hyperthermia, the initiator of muscle contraction is central, the syndrome is often less intense, and mortality is less.

Drug withdrawal syndromes may be associated with fever, tachycardia, diaphoresis, and hyperreflexia, including from alcohol, opioids, barbiturates, and benzodiazepines. It is important to recognize that a history of use of these drugs may not be available when the patient is admitted to the ICU. Withdrawal and related fever may therefore occur several hours or days after admission. Other noninfectious causes of fever are listed in Table 106.9.

CLINICAL INFECTION SYNDROMES

Biliary Tract Infections

Infections of the biliary tree are similar to those found elsewhere in the body in that therapy consists of antibiotics directed at the causative pathogens and source control, typically in the form of drainage. Biliary tract infections remain an important cause of critical illness. They are difficult to diagnose in critically ill patients, owing to their relative rarity and the nonspecificity of symptoms that noncommunicative patients may manifest. Unless diagnosed and treated aggressively, organ dysfunction and death may ensue rapidly. Signs and symptoms of hepatobiliary infection commonly include abdominal pain, fever, nausea, and vomiting; the clinical presentation may range in severity from the appearance of a chronic disease state to overt septic shock. Leukocytosis is common to all but the patterns of liver enzyme abnormalities overlap to such a degree that it may be difficult to make a definitive diagnosis based on history, physical examination, and laboratory values alone. Furthermore, in the critically ill patient, it may be difficult to distinguish liver dysfunction caused by primary infection from that caused by multiple organ dysfunction syndrome. Imaging of the biliary tree is often of paramount importance in the diagnosis and treatment of biliary tract infections, but ultimately a thorough working knowledge of the differential diagnosis and treatment of biliary tract infections is the key to successful management.

Acute Cholecystitis

Among outpatients, acute cholecystitis usually occurs when gallstones migrate into the cystic duct, causing outflow obstruction. This obstruction causes sterile inflammation and edema of the gallbladder wall initially, followed by bacterial superinfection (202). Acute calculous cholecystitis presents with fever, right upper quadrant pain, nausea, and vomiting. Physical examination may range from arrest of inspiration due to tenderness on palpation in the right upper quadrant (Murphy sign) to signs of peritonitis in advanced cases. Concomitant jaundice suggests the presence of choledocholithiasis. Ultrasound is a highly sensitive and specific test (95% and 97%, respectively) for acute cholecystitis and is the initial test of choice. Diagnostic findings include the presence of stones in the gallbladder, thickening of the gallbladder wall (>3.5 mm), pericholecystic fluid, and tenderness with application of the US probe (sonographic Murphy sign) (203). Most cases (~80%) of acute calculous cholecystitis resolve with bowel rest, fluid resuscitation, and intravenous antibiotics, and are treated ultimately by cholecystectomy. Patients who become ill enough to require ICU care generally have gallbladder gangrene that progresses to perforation, resulting in either subhepatic abscess or free perforation with bile peritonitis. Gangrene of the gallbladder is associated with a 30% mortality rate and tends to occur in older patients (204). Emphysematous cholecystitis, a severe manifestation of acute cholecystitis that occurs with a predilection for elderly patients and patients with diabetes mellitus, is defined by the presence of gas in the gallbladder wall as visualized on US or CT and is characterized by polymicrobial infection including *Clostriduim* spp., *E. coli, Klebsiella* spp., and *Streptococcus* spp. Roughly one half of all cases of emphysematous cholecystitis are acalculous (see below); the reported mortality ranges from 15% to 25% (205,206).

Acalculous cholecystitis has been reported in all age groups, but most often occurs in the setting of severe illness or injury. It may also occur in the postoperative setting, particularly in males after emergency surgery complicated by large-volume blood loss. One review of 31,710 cases of cardiac surgery found a 0.05% incidence of acalculous cholecystitis (207); after open abdominal aortic aneurysm repair, the incidence has been reported to be between 0.7% and 0.9% (208). Acute acalculous cholecystitis is a grave condition of insidious onset in patients who are often already critically ill, and the mortality approaches 30% (209). Therefore, the diagnosis of acalculous cholecystitis must always be entertained in a patient with sepsis for whom no clear source of infection can be determined.

The pathogenesis of acalculous cholecystitis is most likely splanchnic ischemia–reperfusion injury. Critically ill patients probably have this pathophysiology even in the presence of gallstones. Alternatively, bile stasis associated with critical illness may lead to distention of the gallbladder, which in combination with hypoperfusion may cause ischemia and ultimately necrosis. Factors such as mechanical ventilation, total parenteral nutrition, cytokine activation, and endotoxemia have also been implicated (210).

The diagnosis of acalculous cholecystitis can be difficult to make in the ICU. Patients who are able to communicate may report abdominal pain localizing to the right upper quadrant or diffuse pain in the case of peritonitis. Fever is usually present. Physical examination may reveal signs ranging from localized tenderness in the right upper quadrant to frank peritonitis. A right upper quadrant abdominal phlegmon may be palpable. All too often, the altered mental status that often accompanies critical illness may obscure any useful information that might be obtained from the history and physical examination. Laboratory values are nonspecific but usually include leukocytosis and elevated liver enzymes, particularly of bilirubin, transaminases, and alkaline phosphatase. Hyperbilirubinemia, perhaps representative of the cholestasis of sepsis, is typical and occurs more often in acalculous than calculous cholecystitis.

Ultrasound is perhaps the ideal radiologic study to investigate the diagnosis of acalculous cholecystitis in the ICU. Ultrasound may reveal hydrops of the gallbladder, pericholecystic fluid, or gallbladder wall thickening. At a gallbladder wall thickness ≥3.5 mm, US is 98.5% sensitive and 80% specific for the diagnosis of acalculous cholecystitis (211). Ultrasound conveniently can be diagnostic at the bedside of patients too ill to be transported to the radiology suite, and followed immediately by percutaneous drainage of the gallbladder under US guidance. Computed tomography is equally accurate in the diagnosis of acalculous cholecystitis (212), but requires a patient stable enough to be transported. The primary advantage of CT scan over US is in its ability to evaluate other potential sources of intra-abdominal infection. Interpretation of radionuclide biliary scans can be confounded in critically ill patients by false-positive scans due to fasting, liver disease, or parenteral nutrition, which are sufficiently common to diminish its utility in this population.

Upon making the diagnosis of acalculous cholecystitis, a decision about the method of source control must be made and empiric antibiotic therapy must be started. Even though up to one half of cases of acute acalculous cholecystitis are associated with culture-negative bile (at least initially, considering that ischemia–reperfusion is paramount and superinfection is a secondary phenomenon), empiric antibiotics are needed because distinguishing sterile from infected cases can be clinically impossible owing to the massive inflammatory response. The organisms most frequently cultured from the bile in acalculous cholecystitis are *E. coli, Klebsiella,* and *Enterococcus faecalis* (211).

Source control for cholecystitis, whether calculous or acalculous, has traditionally been by cholecystectomy. However, patients with acalculous cholecystitis are often critically ill and thus poor surgical candidates. Percutaneous cholecystostomy tube placement is a minimally invasive alternative to cholecystectomy that is favored increasingly. In this technique, the gallbladder is punctured through an anterior transhepatic approach under US guidance and a drainage catheter is placed using the Seldinger technique. A tube study may be performed at the time of catheter placement to discern whether the cystic duct is patent. If not, and concomitant cholangitis is suspected, further drainage of the biliary tree must be performed with endoscopic retrograde cholangiopancreatography (ERCP) or percutaneous transhepatic cholangiopancreatography (PTC). Complications of percutaneous cholecystostomy include bacteremia, hemorrhage, bile peritonitis, and tube dislodgement. Patients with uncomplicated cholecystitis should improve rapidly after gallbladder decompression; failure to improve should raise suspicions of an incorrect diagnosis or inadequate source control. Under such conditions, surgical exploration is mandated. Upon resolution of acalculous cholecystitis, patients treated with percutaneous cholecystostomy may have their tubes removed once sepsis has resolved, the patient has recovered from the precipitating illness, and the cystic duct is demonstrated to be patent. Percutaneous cholecystostomy is the definitive treatment in this group.

Cholangitis

Cholangitis is an acute infection of the main biliary ductal system. The pathogenesis of cholangitis requires both obstruction and bacterial superinfection. The most common cause of intrinsic obstruction in the Western world is choledocholithiasis (213). Both primary and metastatic malignant disease of the abdominal viscera may cause extrinsic obstruction, among other causes. Obstruction from calculi is more likely to cause cholangitis than malignant obstruction (214). Cholangitis may also occur in the postoperative setting, particularly after a biliary-enteric anastomosis.

Bile is sterile in the normal biliary tree. Bile is naturally bacteriostatic, and antegrade flow of bile from liver to duodenum serves as a flushing mechanism. The sphincter of Oddi is an anatomic barrier, preventing reflux of enteric flora. Bile salts serve to absorb intraluminal endotoxins and may also exhibit a trophic effect on small bowel mucosa, thus helping to prevent bacterial and endotoxin translocation. In the absence of bile flow, normal bacterial ecology is perturbed, leading to bacterial overgrowth and degradation of mucosal defenses. The hepatic reticuloendothelial system serves to filter translocated bacteria and endotoxin and is impaired when the biliary tree is obstructed, further increasing the risk of infection (215). Bacteria may gain access to the biliary tree either via the portal vein or by ascending directly from the duodenum. In addition, pathogens may be introduced iatrogenically during surgical, endoscopic, or percutaneous biliary interventions.

The Charcot triad of fever, right upper quadrant pain, and jaundice is observed in 50% to 70% of patients who present with cholangitis, with fever present most consistently (90%). Hypotension and altered mental status (i.e., severe sepsis or septic shock) in addition constitute the Reynolds pentad. Patients with cholangitis typically have leukocytosis, direct hyperbilirubinemia (88%–100%), and elevated alkaline phosphatase (80%) (216); transaminitis is usually mild.

Common duct bile cultures are positive 80% to 100% of the time in cholangitis, with positive blood cultures found in up to two thirds of patients. The concordance rate between bile and blood cultures is 33% to 84%, with bile cultures being polymicrobial in roughly one half of cases. The typical florae are *Klebsiella, E. coli,* and *Enterococcus* (217).

Imaging of patients with cholangitis is possible using US, CT, or magnetic resonance imaging (MRI). Ultrasound detects cholelithiasis and bile duct dilation reliably, but is only 50% sensitive for detecting choledocholithiasis. Computed tomography detects ductal dilation with 98% accuracy and is superior to US in defining the level of obstruction, but may fail to visualize the 85% of biliary calculi that are radiolucent. Stones can be visualized on MRI; therefore, magnetic resonance cholangiopancreatography (MRCP) provides the most complete imaging as to the etiology of biliary obstruction. However, MRCP is expensive, time consuming, and cumbersome for ICU patients, and does not allow for therapeutic intervention. By contrast, ERCP and PTC are both 90% to 100% sensitive for defining the site and nature of biliary obstruction (218). Either can be used diagnostically or therapeutically to decompress the biliary tree. Both ERCP and PTC have rare potential complications (e.g., bile leak, bleeding) that may precipitate ICU admission. In the hemodynamically stable patient with cholangitis, US is the investigation of first choice, followed by further imaging as needed with CT or MRCP. Because of the potential for intervention, ERCP should be considered strongly for unstable patients and other cases where intervention is likely to be necessary. Hemodynamic instability in the setting of suspected or confirmed bacterial cholangitis is a true emergency that requires immediate biliary decompression.

Treatment of cholangitis consists of immediate fluid resuscitation and broad-spectrum antibiotics, followed by urgent or emergent biliary decompression. Numerous antibiotic regimens have been successful historically, but many authorities prefer a single broad-spectrum agent such as piperacillin/tazobactam (219) or a carbapenem. The majority of patients respond to initial medical therapy followed by biliary decompression, but 10% to 15% will require emergent decompression (220). ERCP is the safest and most efficacious treatment for acute cholangitis with a success rate of 90% and a mortality rate of 10%, considerably lower than that of emergency surgical decompression of the common bile duct. Through ERCP, a sphincterotomy can be performed to facilitate drainage and removal of calculi, or a temporizing stent or nasobiliary tube may be placed. Other complications of ERCP include pancreatitis, perforation, aspiration, systemic sepsis, and failure to decompress the bile duct.

Percutaneous transhepatic biliary drainage carries 30% morbidity from complications such as hemorrhage, pneumothorax, subphrenic abscess, and bile peritonitis. The mortality for PTC is estimated to be between 5% and 10%, similar to that seen with ERCP (221). Although the risk is higher, PTC may be used preferentially for intrahepatic choledocholithiasis, for cholangitis from proximal bile duct stricture or neoplasm, or when ERCP is impossible secondary to surgically altered upper gastrointestinal tract anatomy (e.g., after Roux-en-Y reconstruction) or anatomic anomalies (e.g., ampulla of Vater located within a duodenal diverticulum).

Surgery is now infrequent in the primary management of acute cholangitis. In situations that require surgery (e.g., resectable malignant obstruction), patients may be temporized by ERCP or PTC, converting an emergency operation into an elective procedure that can be performed at lower risk. Surgery is also indicated in patients who fail less invasive treatment methods. Standard emergency surgical therapy includes cholecystectomy, choledochotomy, and T-tube placement.

Liver Abscess

The most common cause (50% to 65% of liver abscesses) is now ascending biliary tract infection (222) (e.g., cholangitis, direct extension of acute suppurative cholecystitis). Seeding from the portal vein accounts for 10% to 25% of abscesses and is typically a result of intra-abdominal sources of infection such as diverticulitis. Systemic seeding via the hepatic artery occurs in 1% to 10% of cases from processes such as bacterial endocarditis, dental abscesses, or interventions such as hepatic artery chemoembolization, intraoperative cryoablation, or radiofrequency ablation (221). Liver abscess complicates fewer than 1% of blunt liver injuries managed nonoperatively, and is more common in patients requiring damage-control laparotomy and perihepatic packing to control hemorrhage (222).

Patients with pyogenic hepatic abscess usually present with fever and chills, abdominal pain, and weight loss. Nonspecific abdominal complaints and constitutional symptoms are common, and presentation can range from the appearance of a chronic disease state to overt septic shock. The laboratory workup demonstrates leukocytosis in most patients, with liver enzymes being moderately abnormal as well.

Due to the protean manifestations of liver abscess and the mimicry of a number of disease processes, radiographic imaging is crucial in confirming the diagnosis. Ultrasound and CT both have greater than 95% sensitivity for the diagnosis. One half of patients will present with more than one abscess, and approximately 75% of all liver abscesses will be found in the right lobe of the liver (223).

Pyogenic liver abscesses are equally likely to be polymicrobial as monomicrobial, and approximately 5% to 27% show no growth in culture. In many cases, failure to speciate bacteria in culture may reflect prior antibiotic treatment. The flora found in liver abscesses reflects the underlying source of the infection, but overall the most common Gram-negative aerobes found in pyogenic liver abscesses are *E. coli* and *Klebsiella* spp., whereas the most common Gram-positive aerobes are *Enterococcus* spp., viridans streptococci, and *S. aureus*. Among cultured anaerobes, *Bacteroides* spp. predominate (224).

Historically, medical management of pyogenic liver abscess carried a mortality rate of 60% to 100% (225). Several recent case series demonstrate success rates for antibiotics alone of up to 80% when multiple (military) abscesses are too small or too numerous for percutaneous drainage. Although antibiotics are a necessary adjunct to the treatment of hepatic abscess, most authorities agree that this approach is not sufficient except in the case of very small abscesses or in patients in whom intervention poses a prohibitive risk. The preferred method of treatment is broad-spectrum antibiotics in conjunction with drainage of all abscesses. Most hepatic abscesses can be drained successfully by image-guided percutaneous techniques, with a success rate of 70% to 93%. Surgical drainage is indicated in patients who fail percutaneous drainage, who require surgical management of the underlying problem (e.g., diverticulitis), or who have abscesses that are not amenable to minimally invasive techniques because of their location. Surgical options include simple drainage, debridement, and formal resection. Liver resection should be considered in those patients with extensive tissue loss or with intrahepatic stones, which may serve as a nidus for recurrent infection.

Most contemporary series quote a mortality rate for hepatic abscess between 6% and 31% (221). Factors associated with a worse prognosis include an underlying diagnosis of malignant disease, multiple abscesses, and a high presenting APACHE II score (226).

Postoperative Infections after Biliary Tract Operations

Perihepatic infections may occur as a result of commonly performed hepatobiliary surgical procedures. Postoperative bile leaks may occur after any operation in which a bile duct is opened (such as hepatectomy, hepaticoenterostomy, hepatic transplant, or cholecystectomy). Leaking bile may induce chemical peritonitis, or cause infection with microbial flora present in or introduced into tissue at the time of operation, or by translocation from the gut, leading to an infected intrahepatic or perihepatic collection known as a biloma.

After cholecystectomy, bile leaks occur in up to 1% of patients regardless of the technique used. Bile leakage may occur from the transected cystic duct, the hepatic bed of the gallbladder, or incidental injury to other portions of the biliary tree during dissection. Patients with postoperative bile collections may present with right upper quadrant pain, fever, nausea, vomiting, or jaundice. Discrimination between sterile bile peritonitis and infection may be difficult without culture of the collection.

Postoperative fluid collections may be imaged with US, CT, or nuclear scintigraphy. The diagnosis of bile leak can also be made by image-guided aspiration of the collection. Nuclear scintigraphy is an excellent screening test for the diagnosis of bile leak, but it is not useful in determining the precise anatomy of the leak. For this reason ERCP is used to determine the anatomy once leakage is documented, with some leaks being amenable to concomitant endoscopic therapy by stent placement.

Treatment of postoperative bile leakage hinges first upon drainage and then definitive treatment of the underlying problem. If the leak originates from the bed of the gallbladder, percutaneous drainage alone is indicated. Extravasation from the cystic duct is best managed endoscopically by stent placement with or without sphincterotomy to allow bile to drain preferentially through the ampulla of Vater (227). Major duct injuries discovered at ERCP generally require surgical management.

Perihepatic or intra-abdominal abscess complicates 8% to 30% of major liver resections, and is associated with preoperative biliary stenting, hepaticoenterostomy, increased operative time, greater extent of resection, and the need for blood transfusion (222). Preoperative hyperbilirubinemia as a result of biliary obstruction occurs frequently in patients with malignant biliary tract obstruction; such patients are at increased risk for complications of surgical resection (228). However, recent data demonstrate clearly that preoperative stent placement to alleviate biliary obstruction leads to increased rates of postoperative infectious complications (229).

Resection of hepatic parenchyma leaves dead space in the abdomen that collects bile and blood and is in proximity to ischemic tissue at the resection margin. Bacterial superinfection may occur, leading to the formation of an abscess. Infected bilomas are heralded by fever, right upper quadrant pain, leukocytosis, and elevated liver enzymes. Imaging modalities for posthepatectomy abscesses include CT, US, and MRI as discussed in the prior section on pyogenic hepatic abscess. Cultures reveal that 50% to 75% of postoperative perihepatic abscesses are polymicrobial, with bacteria of enteric origin (e.g., *E. coli*,

Enterococcus) predominating (215). Image-guided percutaneous drainage is the treatment of choice where feasible, with reoperation reserved for those patients in whom percutaneous drainage is not possible or unsuccessful.

Despite recent advances in surgical technique and perioperative management, liver transplantation is plagued by complication rates ranging from 24% to 64%. The incidence of bile leak after orthotopic liver transplantation is between 10% and 40%, with the leaks arising most commonly from hepatic resection lines, T-tube sites, and biliary anastomoses (230). Patients may present up to 6 months after transplantation. Computed tomography is used to image the collection, which may be intrahepatic in up to two thirds of cases. Endoscopic retrograde cholangiopancreatography, PTC, or cholangiogram through a pre-existing T tube may be used to delineate the origin of the leak. Most collections can be drained percutaneously, and in the event of direct communication with the biliary tree, ERCP can be used to re-establish preferential enteric drainage. Because the blood supply to the biliary tree is provided by the hepatic artery, anastomotic leaks after liver transplantation may occur as a result of ischemia from hepatic artery thrombosis. Therefore, assessment of the patency of the graft hepatic artery must be determined. Whereas some cases of biloma associated with hepatic artery thrombosis may respond to conservative measures, up to two thirds will require retransplantation (231).

SURGICAL SITE INFECTION

Surgical site infections are among the most frequently encountered complications in surgical patients regardless of specialty. Local surgical control of the infection remains the crucial aspect of therapy, oftentimes by simply opening and draining the incision in cases of superficial incisional SSI. Infections extending below the superficial fascia (deep incisional SSIs) invariably require formal surgical debridement and open wound care to resolve the infection. Vacuum-assisted closure (VAC) and antimicrobial therapy also improved outcomes, but MDR pathogens may complicate resolution of ostensibly simple infections in the postoperative period (232), especially among patients hospitalized for a period before surgery, particularly if they required antimicrobial therapy.

Surgical site infection remains a clinical diagnosis. Presenting signs and symptoms depend on the depth of infection, typically as early as postoperative day 4 or 5. Clinical signs range from local induration only to the hallmarks of infection (e.g., erythema, edema, tenderness, warm skin, and pain-related immobility), which may manifest before wound drainage. In cases of deep incisional SSIs, tenderness may extend beyond the margin of erythema, and crepitus, cutaneous vesicles, or bullae may be present (233). With ongoing infection, signs of SIRS herald the development of sepsis. If infection involves an intracavitary space (organ/space), symptoms specific to that organ system will usually predominate, such as prolonged postoperative ileus, persistent respiratory distress, or altered neurologic status.

Cultures are not mandatory for management of superficial incisional SSIs, particularly if drainage and wound care alone will suffice without antibiotics. In cases of deeper infection or infection that has arisen in the hospital, exudates or drainage specimens should be sent for analysis. Culturing the surgically opened wound (as opposed to the already opened wound, which becomes colonized) by the swab method has been shown experimentally to be reliable. Computed tomography and MRI are more sensitive in detecting small amounts of gas in soft tissues than plain radiographs, and CT-guided aspiration or drainage often facilitates treatment, and may serve as definitive source control for an organ/space SSI.

More severe SSIs, especially the dangerous forms of necrotizing soft tissue infection (NSTI), are true emergencies that need immediate surgical attention. Even modest delays can increase patient mortality substantially. Freischlag et al. showed that mortality increased from 32% to 70% when therapy was delayed more than 24 hours (234). With an established diagnosis of NSTI, immediate and widespread operative debridement is indicated without waiting for precise determination of the causative pathogen or the identification of a specific clinical symptom. These patients often require planned, sequential, repetitive surgical debridement sessions to control the infection.

When faced with a potential SSI, the first steps in management are to remove the appropriate sutures, open and examine the suspicious portion of the incision, and decide about further surgical treatment (235). If the infection is not confined to the skin and superficial underlying subcutaneous tissue, urgent surgical exploration and debridement is essential to obtain local control of the infection, remove necrotic tissue, and restore aerobic conditions to prevent further spread of the infection. Surgical site infection must also be considered the cause of delayed or failed wound healing and prompt the same decisions as described above (235).

Superficial SSIs, which functionally are subcutaneous abscesses, rarely lead to systemic infection and usually do not make patients seriously ill. Antibiotic therapy is not indicated for patients who do not have systemic signs of infection. Formal surgical intervention is limited to complications such as loculated abscesses or necrosis of the skin or underlying tissue. In contrast, deep incisional SSIs typically present with extensive discomfort in more seriously ill patients. These infections extend to superficial fascia or beneath, and may cause extensive tissue necrosis and liquefaction beyond the obvious limits of the cutaneous signs, making it necessary to explore the wound formally in the operating room. The clinician must be alert to the possibility that necrotizing is present. Broad-spectrum antimicrobial therapy should be given empirically to cover likely pathogens, and reassessed following receipt of the microbiology report.

Organ/space SSIs occur within a body cavity, are directly related to a surgical procedure, and may manifest as intra-abdominal, intrapleural, or intracranial infections. They also may remain occult or present with few symptoms, mimicking incisional SSIs and leading to inadequate initial treatment, becoming apparent only when a major complication ensues. The diagnosis of organ/space SSI usually requires some form of imaging to confirm the site and extent of infection. Adequate source control requires a drainage procedure, whether open or percutaneous.

Experimentally, the value of vacuum-assisted wound closure was first appraised by Morykwas et al. in a swine model in 1997 (236). VAC optimizes blood flow, decreases tissue edema, and removes fluid from the wound bed, thereby facilitating the removal of bacteria from the wound. Mechanical deformation of the wound promotes tissue expansion to cover the defect, and subatmospheric pressure in the milieu may trigger a cascade of intracellular signals that increases the rate of cell division and formation of granulation tissue (237). The clinical value of VAC systems has been described only in small case series and cohort studies, mostly for sternal infections following cardiac surgery, abdominal wall dehiscence, and the management of complex perineal wounds, or as a method to secure skin grafts (238,239). A lack of well-designed randomized, controlled trials precludes more specific recommendations.

PNEUMONIA

The decision to treat pneumonia with an antibiotic is based on clinical suspicion and microscopic examination of Gram-stained sputum, as culture data will not become available for 48 to 72 hours. Choice of agent is based on both individual patient risk factors for infection with MDR organisms and institution-specific susceptibility data. Antimicrobial therapy may be withheld safely if the Gram stain reveals no organisms and the patient has no signs of sepsis (164). Clinical signs of infection with a negative sputum Gram stain suggest either an extrapulmonary source of infection or sterile inflammation.

Patients with micro-organisms on Gram stain or clinical instability should receive empiric therapy for VAP pending the results of cultures. The primary concern is the administration of "adequate therapy," being collectively at least one antimicrobial agent to which the pathogen is sensitive, in the correct dose, via the correct route of administration, and in a timely manner. Treated patients must be re-evaluated serially so that therapy is de-escalated to treat only the specific etiologic pathogen, an end point of therapy may be identified prospectively and adhered to, or therapy may be discontinued if cultures are negative and the patient remains stable.

Choice of initial antimicrobial therapy depends not only on patient risk factors, but also on local (ideally, unit-specific) microbiologic data, which increases the likelihood that appropriate empiric therapy will be prescribed (240). In general, a regimen for patients at risk for infection with an MDR organism should provide coverage against MRSA, *P. aeruginosa*, *Acinetobacter* spp., and extended-spectrum β-lactamase (ESBL)-producing *Klebsiella* spp. At least two drugs are usually required, one effective against MRSA (e.g., vancomycin, linezolid) and one effective against MDR Gram-negative bacilli, particularly *P. aeruginosa* (e.g., piperacillin-tazobactam, meropenem).

Increased mortality is associated with inadequate initial antimicrobial therapy of VAP (241), due to clinical failure and the emergence of MDR bacteria. Appropriate initial dosing is paramount to achieving adequate therapy, for example, of vancomycin (15 mg/kg q12h), aminoglycosides (gentamicin, tobramycin 7 mg/kg daily; amikacin 20 mg/kg daily), and fluoroquinolones (levofloxacin 750 mg daily; ciprofloxacin 400 mg q8h) (all doses assume normal renal function). Abundant data now document an association between fluoroquinolone use and the emergence of VAP caused by MDR pathogens, particularly *Pseudomonas* (242–244) and MRSA (245). Fluoroquinolone use should be judicious, based on current unit-specific susceptibility data.

Whereas multidrug empiric therapy is necessary to treat patients with suspected VAP until culture results become available, combination therapy of a specific pathogen (e.g., "double-coverage" of *Pseudomonas*) is unlikely to provide benefit and may worsen outcomes. Neither *in vitro* nor *in vivo* synergy of such combination therapy has been demonstrated consistently. A meta-analysis of β-lactam monotherapy versus β-lactam–aminoglycoside combination therapy for immunocompetent patients with sepsis (64 trials, 7,586 patients) found no difference in either mortality (RR 0.90, 95% CI 0.77–1.06) or the development of resistance (246). In fact, clinical failure was more common with combination therapy.

Following initiation of therapy for suspected VAP, lower respiratory tract cultures may reveal either (a) no growth or growth below the predetermined threshold value, (b) significant (above threshold) growth of a "sensitive" pathogen, or (c) significant growth of an MDR pathogen. Under the first scenario, antimicrobial therapy may be discontinued if the patient has not deteriorated (164,247). Under the second scenario, therapy is de-escalated to a narrow-spectrum agent active against the pathogen. In the last scenario, the initial broad-spectrum agent active against the pathogen is continued.

Once pathogen-specific therapy has been initiated, its duration must be determined with the goal of avoiding prolonged and unnecessary administration. Resolution of clinical and radiographic parameters typically lags the eradication of infection (248). Vidaur et al. found that improved oxygenation and normothermia occurred within 3 days in VAP patients without ARDS (156). Dennesen et al. observed a clinical response to therapy (e.g., normalization of temperature, white blood cell count, arterial oxygen saturation, and decreased bacterial count in sputum) within 6 days of therapy of VAP (249). A randomized, multicenter trial of 401 patients (VAP proved by bronchoscopy and quantitative microbiology) (250) showed an 8-day course (vs. 15 days) of initially appropriate antimicrobial therapy to be effective, provided that the patient is stable and the pathogen is not a nonfermenting Gram-negative bacillus. In select patients (i.e., those unlikely to have VAP based on a CPIS $\leq$6), a 3-day course of therapy may be effective for therapy of VAP (251).

Nonresponders to therapy for VAP pose a dilemma (247). Inadequate therapy, misdiagnosis, or a pneumonia-related complication (e.g., empyema, lung abscess) must be considered. The diagnostic evaluation should be repeated, including quantitative sputum cultures (using a lower diagnostic threshold when interpreting quantitative microbiology given recent antibiotic exposure). Broadened antibiotic coverage should be considered until new data become available.

CATHETER-RELATED BLOODSTREAM INFECTION

The pathogens of CR-BSI are predominantly Gram-positive cocci, most commonly methicillin-related *Staphylococcus epidermidis* (MRSE), MRSA, and enterococci. Unfortunately, MRSE is both the most common cause of CR-BSI and the most common cause of false-positive blood cultures because of contamination during the collection process. Most authorities consider the isolation of MRSE from a single blood culture to be a contaminant and do not treat, especially if the patient has no indwelling hardware that might become infected secondarily (e.g., prosthetic joint or heart valve). Gram-negative bacillary pathogens are less common (but seldom are contaminants), and fungal CR-BSIs are less common in surgical patients than medical patients.

Treatment is by catheter removal (for peripheral or percutaneous central venous catheters) and parenteral antibiotics, at least initially. It is unclear whether a positive catheter culture requires therapy beyond catheter removal, absent local signs of infection or a true-positive blood culture. Catheter-related bloodstream infections caused by *S. aureus* probably require at least 2 weeks of therapy, although some authorities argue for a longer course (4–6 weeks) because of the risk of metastatic infection (e.g., pneumonia, endocarditis). Vancomycin or linezolid may be chosen for MRSA CR-BSI (or MRSE when treatment is indicated), with daptomycin as an alternative. Therapy for enterococcal or Gram-negative CR-BSI is dictated by bacterial susceptibility, with no clear consensus as to duration of therapy. Beyond removal of the catheter, treatment of fungal CR-BSI is controversial; some authorities recommend at least 2 weeks of systemic antifungal therapy.

PERITONITIS

Only about 15% of patients with secondary peritonitis are ill enough to require ICU care. Severe secondary peritonitis may follow penetrating intestinal injury that is not recognized or treated promptly (>12-hour delay). Other causes include dehiscence of a bowel anastomosis with leakage and development of an intra-abdominal abscess. Secondary peritonitis is polymicrobial, with anaerobic Gram-negative bacilli (e.g., *Bacteroides fragilis*) predominating, and *E. coli* and *Klebsiella* spp. isolated commonly from community-onset infections. Any of a number of antibiotic regimens of appropriate spectrum may be prescribed. Enterococci, *Pseudomonas*, and other bacteria may be isolated, but do not require specific therapy if the patient is otherwise healthy (e.g., not immunocompromised) and responding to therapy as prescribed.

When secondary peritonitis develops in a hospitalized patient as a complication of disease or therapy, the flora are more likely to reflect MDR pathogens encountered in the hospital (252–254), and outcomes are worsened if empiric therapy is not appropriate. For example, enterococci, *Enterobacter*, and *Pseudomonas* are more prevalent, whereas *E. coli* and *Klebsiella* are less common (Fig. 106.2) (254,255). Antibiotic therapy must be adjusted accordingly, and surgical source control must be achieved. Failure of two source control procedures with persistent intra-abdominal collections is referred to as tertiary peritonitis. Tertiary peritonitis is also characterized by complete failure of intra-abdominal host defenses (256). There is controversy whether tertiary peritonitis is a true invasive infection, or rather peritoneal colonization with incompetent local host defenses, and thus, whether antibiotics should be prescribed and if so, for how long. Bacteria isolated in tertiary peritonitis are avirulent opportunists such as MRSE, enterococci, *Pseudomonas*, and *Candida albicans*, supporting the incompetent host defense hypothesis. Some authorities recommend management with an open-abdomen technique, so that

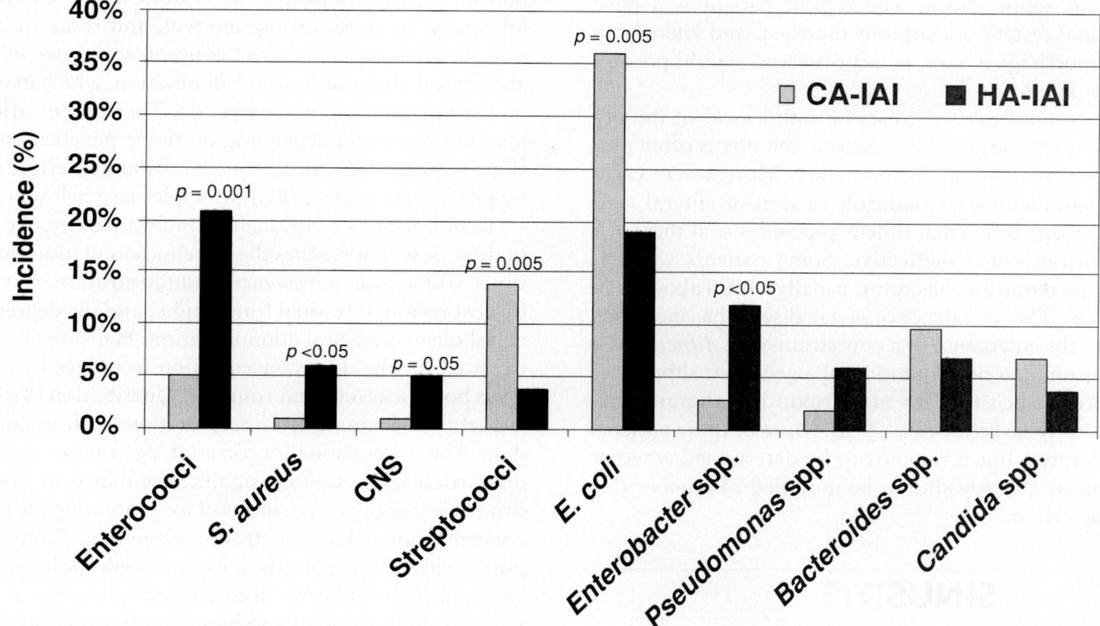

FIGURE 106.2. Microbiology of community-acquired versus health care-acquired intra-abdominal infections. Results from a study in which peritoneal isolates from 67 patients with postoperative peritonitis were compared to those of 68 patients with community-acquired peritonitis. As a consequence of prior antimicrobial use, the florae of the peritoneum are altered. Whereas pathogens such as *Escherichia coli* and streptococci are more commonly isolated in cases of community-acquired intra-abdominal infection (CA-IAI), enterococci and *Staphylococcus aureus* are more prevalent in health care-acquired intra-abdominal infection (HA-IAI). CNS, central nervous system. (Adapted with permission from Nicolau DP, Freeman CD, Belliveau PP, et al. Experience with a once-daily aminoglycoside program administered to 2,184 adult patients. *Antimicrob Agents Chemother.* 1995;39:650–655.)

peritoneal toilet can be provided manually (at the bedside in some cases) under sedation or anesthesia, until local host defenses recover. There may be no alternative to open-abdomen management if the infection extends to involve the abdominal wall and extensive debridement is required.

CLOSTRIDIUM DIFFICILE–ASSOCIATED DISEASE

C. difficile–associated disease, formerly pseudomembranous colitis, develops because antibiotic therapy disrupts the balance of colonic flora, allowing the overgrowth of *C. difficile*, which is present in the fecal flora of about 3% of normal hosts. Any antibiotic can induce this selection pressure, even when given appropriately as surgical prophylaxis, although clindamycin, third-generation cephalosporins, and fluoroquinolones have a predilection (174). Paradoxically, even antibiotics used to treat CDAD (e.g., metronidazole) have been associated with CDAD.

C. difficile–associated disease is unquestionably a nosocomial infection. Spores can persist on inanimate surfaces for prolonged periods, and pathogens can be transmitted from patient to patient by contaminated equipment (e.g., bedpans, rectal thermometers) or on the hands of health care workers. The alcohol gel that is used increasingly for hand disinfection is not active against spores of *C. difficile*; therefore, hand washing with soap and water is necessary when caring for an infected patient, or generally during outbreaks.

The clinical spectrum of CDAD is wide, ranging from asymptomatic (8% of affected patients do not have diarrhea) to life-threatening transmural pancolitis with perforation and severe sepsis or septic shock. The typical patient will have fever, abdominal distention, copious diarrhea, and leukocytosis. Colon hemorrhage is rare, and if observed should prompt an alternative diagnosis.

Treatment of mild cases consists of withdrawal of the putative offending antibiotic; oral antibiotic therapy is often prescribed but may or may not be necessary. More severe cases may require parenteral metronidazole or oral or enteral vancomycin (by gavage or enema, if ileus precludes oral therapy); parenteral vancomycin is ineffective. Some patients with severe disease may require a colectomy, usually a total abdominal colectomy (176). The prevalence of severe disease has increased markedly with the emergence of a new strain of *C. difficile*. The new strain has undergone a mutation of a gene that suppresses toxin production, such that far more toxin is elaborated, resulting in clinically severe disease (175). More of these patients will require surgery, but it remains to be determined whether or how antibiotic therapy should be modified to combat this dangerous bacterium.

SINUSITIS

Nosocomial sinusitis is a dangerous, closed-space infection that is increasing in incidence, but is difficult to diagnose and therefore controversial as to its actual incidence and importance (257).

Sinusitis should be suspected in any patient with sepsis, particularly if initial cultures (e.g., blood, sputum, urine, indwelling vascular catheters) are unrevealing. If sinusitis is suspected, the diagnosis is confirmed by maxillary antral tap, lavage, and culture using aseptic technique. Gram-positive cocci, Gram-negative bacilli (including *P. aeruginosa*), and fungi (incidence, 8%) are possible pathogens, so initial therapy should be based on local susceptibility patterns. Most antibiotics achieve adequate tissue penetration. The optimal duration of therapy is unknown, so it is based on the patient's clinical response. Refractory cases may require repetitive lavage of the sinus, or a formal drainage procedure.

Sinusitis is a predisposing factor for VAP, and may be a source of lower respiratory tract pathogens. There is 85% concordance between pathogens of sinusitis and pneumonia in patients who develop VAP subsequently, lending credence to the hypothesis that purulent sinus drainage inoculates the lower airway.

PRINCIPLES OF ANTIBIOTIC THERAPY

Antimicrobial therapy is a mainstay of the treatment of infections, but widespread overuse and misuse of antibiotics have led to an alarming increase in MDR pathogens. New agents may allow shorter courses of therapy and prophylaxis, which are desirable for cost savings and control of microbial flora. To provide effective therapy with no toxicity requires an understanding of the principles of pharmacokinetics (PK).

Pharmacokinetic Principles

Pharmacokinetics is the principles of drug absorption, distribution, and metabolism (258). Dose-response relationships are influenced by dose, dosing interval, and route of administration. Plasma and tissue drug concentrations are influenced by absorption, distribution, and elimination, which in turn depend on drug metabolism and excretion. The concentrations may or may not correlate, depending on tissue penetration. Relationships between local drug concentration and effect are defined by pharmacodynamic (PD) principles (see below) (258).

Basic concepts of PK include bioavailability, the percentage of drug dose that reaches the systemic circulation. Bioavailability is 100% after intravenous administration, but is affected by absorption, intestinal transit time, and the degree of hepatic metabolism after oral administration. Half-life ($T_{1/2}$), the time required for the drug concentration to reduce by one half, reflects both clearance and volume of distribution (V_D) (258), and is useful to estimate for interpretation of drug concentration data. The proportionality constant V_D, a derived parameter of no particular physiologic significance that is independent of a drug's clearance or $T_{1/2}$, is useful for estimating the plasma drug concentration achievable from a given dose. Volume of distribution varies substantially due to pathophysiology; reduced V_D causes a higher plasma drug concentration for a given dose, whereas fluid overload and hypoalbuminemia (which decrease drug binding) increase V_D, making dosing more complex.

Clearance refers to the volume of liquid from which drug is eliminated completely per unit of time, whether by tissue distribution, metabolism, or elimination; knowledge of drug clearance is important for determining the dose of drug necessary to maintain a steady-state concentration. Drug elimination may be by metabolism, excretion, or dialysis. Most drugs are metabolized by the liver to polar compounds for eventual renal excretion, which may occur by filtration or either active or passive transport. The degree of filtration is determined by molecular size and charge and by the number of functional nephrons. In general, if ≥40% of administered drug or its active metabolites is eliminated unchanged in the urine, decreased renal function will require a dosage adjustment.

Pharmacodynamic Principles

Pharmacodynamics (PD) is unique for antibiotic therapy, because drug–patient, drug–microbe, and microbe–patient interactions must be accounted for (258). In contrast to most drug treatments, the key drug interaction is not with the host, but with the microbe. Microbial physiology, inoculum size, microbial growth phase, mechanisms of resistance, the microenvironment (e.g., local pH), and the host's response are important factors. Because of microbial resistance, mere administration of drug may not be microbicidal.

Antibiotic PD parameters determined by laboratory analysis include the minimal inhibitory concentration (MIC), the lowest serum drug concentration that inhibits bacterial growth (MIC_{90} refers to 90% inhibition). However, some antibiotics may suppress bacterial growth at subinhibitory concentrations (postantibiotic effect [PAE]). Appreciable PAE can be observed with aminoglycosides and fluoroquinolones for Gram-negative bacteria, and with some β-lactam drugs (notably carbapenems) against *S. aureus*. However, MIC testing may not detect resistant bacterial subpopulations within the inoculum (e.g., "heteroresistance" of *S. aureus*) (259, 260). Moreover, *in vitro* results may be irrelevant if bacteria are inhibited only by drug concentrations that cannot be achieved clinically.

Sophisticated analytic strategies utilize both PK and PD, for example, by determination of the peak serum concentration:MIC ratio, the duration of time that plasma concentration remains above the MIC, and the area of the plasma concentration-time curve above the MIC (the *area under the curve* [AUC]) (261). Accordingly, aminoglycosides exhibit concentration-dependent killing (262,263), whereas β-lactam agents exhibit efficacy determined by time above the MIC (264). For β-lactam antibiotics with short $T_{1/2}$, it may be efficacious to administer by continuous infusion (265,266). Some agents (e.g., fluoroquinolones) exhibit both properties; bacterial killing increases as drug concentration increases up to a saturation point, after which the effect becomes concentration independent.

Empiric Antibiotic Therapy

Empiric antibiotic therapy must be administered carefully. Injudicious therapy could result in undertreatment of established infection, or unnecessary therapy when the patient has only inflammation or bacterial colonization; either may be deleterious. Inappropriate therapy (e.g., delay, therapy misdirected against usual pathogens, failure to treat MDR pathogens) leads unequivocally to increased mortality (141,241,267,268).

Strategies have been promulgated to optimize antibiotic administration, including reliance upon physician prescribing patterns, computerized decision support (269), administration by protocol (140,270–275), and formulary restriction programs. Owing to the increasing prevalence of MDR pathogens, it is crucial for initial empiric antibiotic therapy to be targeted appropriately, administered in sufficient dosage to ensure bacterial killing, narrowed in spectrum (*de-escalation*) (276) as soon as possible based on microbiology data and clinical response, and continued only as long as necessary. Appropriate antibiotic prescribing not only optimizes patient care, but also supports infection control practice and preserves microbial ecology (276).

Choice of Antibiotic

Antibiotic choice is based on several interrelated factors (Table 106.10). Paramount is activity against identified or likely (for empiric therapy) pathogens, presuming infecting and colonizing organisms can be distinguished, and that narrow-spectrum coverage is always desired. Estimation of likely pathogens depends on the disease process believed responsible; whether the infection is community, health care, or hospital acquired; and whether MDR organisms are present. Local knowledge of antimicrobial resistance patterns is essential, even at the unit-specific level. Patient-specific factors of importance include age, debility, immunosuppression, intrinsic organ function, prior allergy or other adverse reaction, and recent antibiotic therapy. Institutional factors of importance include guidelines that may specify a particular therapy, formulary availability of specific agents, outbreaks of infections caused by MDR pathogens, and antibiotic control programs.

Numerous agents are available for therapy (Table 106.11) (277–279). Agents may be chosen based on spectrum, whether broad or targeted (e.g., antipseudomonal, antianaerobic), in addition to the above factors. If a nosocomial Gram-positive pathogen is suspected (e.g., wound or surgical site infection, CR-BSI, pneumonia) or MRSA is endemic, empiric vancomycin (or linezolid) is appropriate. Some authorities recommend dual-agent therapy for serious *Pseudomonas* infections (i.e., an antipseudomonal β-lactam drug plus an aminoglycoside), but evidence of efficacy is lacking (247). It is important to use at least two antibiotics for empiric therapy of any infection that may be caused by either a Gram-positive or Gram-negative infection (e.g., nosocomial pneumonia) (248).

Antifungal Prophylaxis and Therapy

The incidence of invasive fungal infections is increasing among critically ill surgical patients. Several conditions are

TABLE 106.10

FACTORS INFLUENCING ANTIBIOTIC CHOICE

Factors
Activity against known/suspected pathogens
Disease believed responsible
Distinguish infection from colonization
Narrow-spectrum coverage most desirable
Antimicrobial resistance patterns
Patient-specific factors
Severity of illness
Age
Immunosuppression
Organ dysfunction
Allergy
Institutional guidelines/restrictions

TABLE 106.11

ANTIBACTERIAL AGENTS FOR EMPIRIC USE

ANTIPSEUDOMONAL
Piperacillin-tazobactam
Cefepime, ceftazidime
Imipenem, meropenem
? Ciprofloxacin, levofloxacin (depending on local susceptibility patterns)
Aminoglycoside
TARGETED SPECTRUM
Gram positive
Glycopeptide
Lipopeptide (not for known/suspected pneumonia)
Oxazolidinone
Gram negative
Third-generation cephalosporin (not ceftriaxone)
Monobactam
Antianaerobic
Metronidazole
BROAD SPECTRUM
Piperacillin-tazobactam
Carbapenems
Fluoroquinolones
Tigecycline (plus an antipseudomonal agent)
ANTIANAEROBIC
Metronidazole
Carbapenems
β-Lactam/β-lactamase combination agents
Tigecycline

predictors for invasive fungal infection complicating critical illness, including intensive care unit length of stay, altered immune responsiveness, and the number of medical devices placed. Neutropenia, diabetes mellitus, new-onset hemodialysis, total parenteral nutrition, broad-spectrum antibiotic administration, bladder catheterization, azotemia, diarrhea, and corticosteroid therapy are also associated with invasive fungal infection (122,154).

Duration of Therapy

The end point of therapy is largely undefined, in part because quality data are few (140,249,280). If cultures are negative, empiric antibiotic therapy should be stopped in most cases. Unnecessary antibiotic therapy in the absence of infection clearly increases the risk of MDR infection; therefore, therapy beyond 48 to 72 hours with negative cultures usually is unjustifiable. The morbidity of antibiotic therapy includes allergic reactions, development of nosocomial superinfections (e.g., fungal, enterococcal, and *C. difficile*–related infections), organ toxicity, promotion of antibiotic resistance, reduced yield from subsequent cultures, and induced vitamin K deficiency with coagulopathy or accentuation of warfarin effect.

If bona fide evidence of infection is evident, then treatment is continued as indicated clinically. Some infections can be treated with therapy lasting 5 days or less. Every decision to start antibiotics must be accompanied by a decision regarding the duration of therapy (66). A reason to continue therapy beyond the predetermined end point must be compelling. Bacterial killing is rapid in response to effective agents, but the host response may not subside immediately. Therefore, the clinical response of the patient should not be the sole determinant for continuation of therapy. If a patient still has SIRS at the predetermined end of therapy, it is more useful to stop therapy and obtain new cultures to look for persistent or new infection, resistant pathogens, and noninfectious causes of SIRS. Seldom should antibacterial therapy continue for more than 7 to 10 days. Examples of bacterial infections that require more than 14 days of therapy include tuberculosis of any site, endocarditis, osteomyelitis, and selected cases of brain abscess, liver abscess, lung abscess, postoperative meningitis, and endophthalmitis.

References

1. Mangram AJ, Horan TC, Pearson ML, et al. Guideline for prevention of surgical site infection, 1999. Hospital Infection Control Practices Advisory Committee. *Infect Control Hosp Epidemiol.* 1999;20:250–278.
2. O'Grady NP, Alexander M, Dellinger EP, et al. Guidelines for the prevention of intravascular catheter-related infections. Centers for Disease Control and Prevention. *MMWR Recomm Rep.* 2002;51(RR-10):1–29.
3. Minei JP, Nathens AB, West M, et al. Inflammation and the host response to injury large scale collaborative research program investigators. Inflammation and the host response to injury, a large-scale collaborative project: patient-oriented research core-standard operating procedures for clinical care. II. Guidelines for prevention, diagnosis and treatment of ventilator-associated pneumonia (VAP) in the trauma patient. *J Trauma.* 2006;60:1106–1113.
4. Guidelines for the management of adults with hospital-acquired, ventilator-associated, and healthcare-associated pneumonia. *Am J Respir Crit Care Med.* 2005;171:388–416.
5. Latham R, Lancaster AD, Covington JF, et al. The association of diabetes and glucose control with surgical-site infections among cardiothoracic surgery patients. *Infect Control Hosp Epidemiol.* 2001;22:607–612.
6. Zerr KJ, Furnary AP, Grunkemeier GL, et al. Glucose control lowers the risk of wound infection in diabetics after open heart operations. *Ann Thorac Surg.* 1997;63:356–361.
7. Pomposelli JJ, Baxter JK 3rd, Babineau TJ, et al. Early postoperative glucose control predicts nosocomial infection rate in diabetic patients. *JPEN J Parenter Enteral Nutr.* 1998;22:77–81.
8. van den Berghe G, Wouters P, Weekers F, et al. Intensive insulin therapy in the critically ill patients. *N Engl J Med.* 2001;345:1359–1367.
9. Pittas AG, Siegel RD, Lau J. Insulin therapy for critically ill hospitalized patients: a meta-analysis of randomized controlled trials. *Arch Intern Med.* 2004;164(18):2005–2011.
10. Heyland DK, MacDonald S, Keefe L, et al. Total parenteral nutrition in the critically ill patient: a meta-analysis. *JAMA.* 1998;280:2013–2019.
11. Marik PE, Zaloga GP. Early enteral nutrition in acutely ill patients: a systematic review. *Crit Care Med.* 2001;29:2264–2270.
12. Nathens AB, Nester TA, Rubenfeld GA, et al. The effects of leukoreduced blood transfusion on infection risk following injury: a randomized controlled trial. *Shock.* 2006;26:342–347.
13. Claridge JA, Sawyer RG, Schulman AM, et al. Blood transfusions correlate with infections in trauma patients in a dose-dependent manner. *Am Surg.* 2002;68:566–572.
14. Hill GE, Frawley WH, Griffith KE, et al. Allogeneic blood transfusion increases the risk of postoperative blood infection: a meta-analysis. *J Trauma.* 2003;54:908–914.
15. Taylor RW, O'Brien J, Trottier SJ, et al. Red blood cell transfusions and nosocomial infections in critically ill patients. *Crit Care Med.* 2006;34:2302–2308.
16. Shorr AF, Jackson WL, Kelly KM, et al. Transfusion practice and blood stream infections in critically ill patients. *Chest.* 2005;127:1722–1728.
17. Shorr AF, Duh MS, Kelly KM, et al., CRIT Study Group. Red blood cell transfusion and ventilator-associated pneumonia: a potential link? *Crit Care Med.* 2004;32:666–674.
18. Fernandes CJ Jr, Akamine N, De Marco FV, et al. Red blood cell transfusion does not increase oxygen consumption in critically ill septic patients. *Crit Care.* 2001;5:362–367.
19. Moore FA, Moore EE, Sauaia A. Blood transfusion. An independent risk factor for postinjury multiple organ failure. *Arch Surg.* 1997;132:620–624.
20. Offner PJ, Moore EE, Biffl WL, et al. Increased rate of infection associated with transfusion of old blood after severe injury. *Arch Surg.* 2002;137:711–716.
21. Hebert PC, Wells G, Blajchman MA, et al. A multicenter, randomized,

controlled clinical trial of transfusion requirements in critical care. Transfusion Requirements in Critical Care Investigators, Canadian Critical Care Trials Group. *N Engl J Med.* 1999;340:409–417.
22. Trick WE, Vernon MG, Welbel SF, et al. Chicago Antimicrobial Resistance Project. Multicenter intervention program to increase adherence to hand hygiene recommendations and glove use and to reduce the incidence of antimicrobial resistance. *Infect Control Hosp Epidemiol.* 2007;28:42–49.
23. Dancer SJ, Coyne M, Speekenbrink A, et al. MRSA acquisition in an intensive care unit. *Am J Infect Control.* 2006;34:10–17.
24. Chaiyakunapruk N, Veenstra DL, Lipsky BA, Saint S. Chlorhexidine compared with povidone-iodine solution for vascular catheter-site care: a meta-analysis. *Ann Intern Med* 2002;136:792–801.
25. McGee DC, Gould MK. Preventing complications of central venous catheterization. *N Engl J Med.* 2003; 348:1123–1133.
26. Wenzel RP, Edmond MB. Team-based prevention of catheter-related infections. *N Engl J Med.* 2006;355:2781–2783.
27. Rello J, Kollef M, Diaz E, et al. Reduced burden of bacterial airway colonization with a novel silver-coated endotracheal tube in a randomized multiple-center feasibility study. *Crit Care Med.* 2006;34:2766–2772.
28. Hanna HA, Raad II, Hackett B, et al. M.D. Anderson Catheter Study Group. Antibiotic-impregnated catheters associated with significant decrease in nosocomial and multidrug-resistant bacteremias in critically ill patients. *Chest.* 2003;124:1030–1038.
29. Johnson JR, Kuskowski MA, Wilt TJ. Systematic review: antimicrobial urinary catheters to prevent catheter-associated urinary tract infection in hospitalized patients. *Ann Intern Med.* 2006;144:116–126.
30. Ely EW, Baker AM, Dunagan DP, et al. Effect on the duration of mechanical ventilation of identifying patients capable of breathing spontaneously. *N Engl J Med.* 1996;335:1864–1869.
31. Esteban A, Frutos-Vivar F, Ferguson ND, et al. Noninvasive positive-pressure ventilation for respiratory failure after extubation. *N Engl J Med.* 2004;350:2452–2460.
32. Shah MR, Hasselblad V, Stevenson LW, et al. Impact of the pulmonary artery catheter in critically ill patients: meta-analysis of randomized controlled trials. *JAMA.* 2005;294:1664–1670.
33. Barie PS. Surgical site infections: epidemiology and prevention. *Surg Infect.* 2002;3(Suppl 1):S9–21.
34. National Nosocomial Infections Surveillance System (NNIS) System Report: data summary from January 1992-June 2001, issued August 2001. *Am J Infect Control.* 2001;29:404–421.
35. National Nosocomial Infections Surveillance (NNIS) System Report, data summary from January 1992 to June 2004, issued October 2004. *Am J Infect Control.* 2004;32:470–485.
36. Garibaldi RA, Cushing D, Lerer T. Risk factors for post-operative infection. *Am J Med.* 1991;91(Suppl 3B):158S–163S.
37. Raymond DP, Pelletier SJ, Crabtree TD, et al. Surgical infection and the ageing population. *Am Surg.* 2001;67:827–832.
38. Delgado-Rodriguez M, Medina-Cuadros M, Martinez-Gallego G, et al. Total cholesterol, HDL cholesterol, and risk of nosocomial infection: a prospective study in surgical patients. *Infect Control Hosp Epidemiol.* 1997;18:9–18.
39. Malone DL, Genuit T, Tracy JK, et al. Surgical site infections: reanalysis of risk factors. *J Surg Res.* 2002;103:89–95.
40. Scott JD, Forrest A, Feuerstein S, et al. Factors associated with postoperative infection. *Infect Control Hosp Epidemiol.* 2001;22:347–351.
41. Parienti JJ, Thibon P, Heller R, et al. Hand-rubbing with an aqueous alcoholic vs. traditional surgical hand-scrubbing and 30-day surgical site infection rates: a randomized equivalence study. *JAMA.* 2002;288:722–727.
42. Hedrick TL, Heckman JA, Smith RL, et al. Efficacy of protocol implementation on incidence of wound infection in colorectal operations. *J MA Coll Surg.* 2007;205:432–438.
43. Kurz A, Sessler DI, Lenhardt R. Perioperative normothermia to reduce the incidence of surgical-wound infection and shorten hospitalization, Study of Wound Infection and Temperature Group. *N Engl J Med.* 1996;334:1209–1215.
44. Flores-Maldonado A, Medina-Escobedo CE, Rios-Rodriguez HM, et al. Mild hypothermia and the risk of wound infection. *Arch Med Res.* 2001; 32:227–231.
45. Gottrupp F. Oxygen in wound healing and infection. *World J Surg.* 2004; 28:312–315.
46. Knighton DR, Halliday B, Hunt TK. Oxygen as an antibiotic. A comparison of the effects of inspired oxygen concentration and antibiotic administration on in vivo bacterial clearance. *Arch Surg.* 1986;121:191–195.
47. Greif R, Akca O, Horn EP, et al. Supplemental perioperative oxygen to reduce the incidence of surgical-wound infection. Outcomes Research Group. *N Engl J Med.* 2000;342:161–167.
48. Pryor KO, Fahey TJ 3rd, Lien CA, et al. Surgical site infection and the routine use of perioperative hyperoxia in a general surgical population: a randomized controlled trial. *JAMA.* 2004;291:79–87.
49. Miller RS, Morris JA Jr, Diaz JJ Jr, et al. Complications after 344 damage-control open celiotomies. *J Trauma.* 2005;59:1365–137.
50. Vogel TR, Diaz JJ, Miller RS, et al. The open abdomen in trauma: do infectious complications affect primary abdominal closure? *Surg Infect.* 2006;7:433–441.
51. Al-Inany H, Youssef G, Abd ElMaguid A, et al. Value of subcutaneous drainage system in obese females undergoing cesarean section using Pfannenstiel incision. *Gynecol Obstet Invest.* 2002;53:75–78.
52. Magann EF, Chauhan SP, Rodts-Palenik D, et al. Subcutaneous stitch closure versus subcutaneous drain to prevent wound disruption after cesarean delivery: a randomized clinical trial. *Am J Obstet Gynecol.* 2002;186:1119–1123.
53. Siegman-Igra Y, Rozin R, Simchen E. Determinants of wound infection in gastrointestinal operations, the Israeli study of surgical infections. *J Clin Epidemiol.* 1993;46:133–140.
54. Noyes LD, Doyle DJ, McSwain NE. Septic complications associated with the use of peritoneal drains in liver trauma. *J Trauma.* 1998;28:337–346.
55. Magee C, Rodeheaver GT, Golden GT, et al. Potentiation of wound infection by surgical drains. *Am J Surg.* 1976;131;28:14–20.
56. Vilar-Compote D, Mohar A, Sandoval S, et al. Surgical site infections at the National Cancer Institute in Mexico: a case-control study. *Am J Infect Control.* 2002;28:14–20.
57. Barie PS. Are we draining the life from our patients? *Surg Infect.* 2002;3: 159–160.
58. Platell C, Papadimitriou JM, Hall JC. The influence of lavage on peritonitis. *J Am Coll Surg.* 2000;191:672–680.
59. Cervantes-Sanchez CR, Gutierrez-Vega R, Vasquez-Carpizio JA, et al. Syringe pressure irritation of subdermic tissue after appendectomy to decrease the incidence of postoperative wound infection. *World J Surg.* 2000;24:38–41.
60. Andersen B, Bendtsen A, Holbraad L, et al. Wound infections after appendectomy. I. A controlled trial on the prophylactic efficacy of topical ampicillin in non-perforated appendicitis. *Acta Chir Scand.* 1972;138:531–536.
61. Yoshii S, Hosaka S, Suzuki S, et al. Prevention of surgical site infection by antibiotic spraying in the operating field during cardiac surgery. *Jpn J Thorac Cardiovasc Surg.* 2001;49:279–281.
62. O'Connor LT Jr, Goldstein M. Topical perioperative antibiotic prophylaxis for minor clean inguinal surgery. *J Am Coll Surg.* 2002;194:407–410.
63. Kollef MH, Shorr A, Tabak YP, et al. Epidemiology and outcomes of health-care-associated pneumonia. *Chest.* 2005;128:3854–3862.
64. Vincent JL, Bihari DJ, Suter PM, et al. The prevalence of nosocomial infection in intensive care units in Europe: results of the European Prevalence of Infection in Intensive Care (EPIC) study. *JAMA.* 1995;274:639–644.
65. Rello J, Ollendorf DA, Oster G, et al. Epidemiology and outcomes of ventilator-associated pneumonia in a large US database. *Chest.* 2002;122: 2115–2121.
66. Fagon JY, Chastre J, Wolff M, et al. Invasive and noninvasive strategies for management of suspected ventilator-associated pneumonia. A randomized trial. *Ann Intern Med.* 2000;132:621–630.
67. Safdar N, Dezfulian C, Collard HR, et al. Clinical and economic consequences of ventilator-associated pneumonia: a systematic review. *Crit Care Med.* 2005;33:2184–2193.
68. Cook DJ, Walter SD, Cook RJ, et al. Incidence and risk factors for ventilator-associated pneumonia in critically ill patients. *Ann Intern Med.* 1998;129:433–440.
69. Celis R, Torres A, Gatell JM, et al. Nosocomial pneumonia: a multivariate analysis of risk and prognosis. *Chest.* 1988;93:318–324.
70. Torres A, Aznar R, Gatell JM, et al. Incidence, risk, and prognosis factors of nosocomial pneumonia in mechanically ventilated patients. *Am Rev Respir Dis.* 1990;142:523–528.
71. Chastre J, Trouillet JL, Vuagnat A, et al. Nosocomial pneumonia in patients with acute respiratory distress syndrome. *Am J Respir Crit Care Med.* 1998;157:1165–1172.
72. Delclaux C, Roupie E, Blot F, et al. Lower respiratory tract colonization and infection during severe acute respiratory distress syndrome: incidence and diagnosis. *Am J Respir Crit Care Med.* 1997;156:1092–1098.
73. Markowicz P, Wolff M, Djedaini K, et al. Multicenter prospective study of ventilator-associated pneumonia during acute respiratory distress syndrome. Incidence, prognosis, and risk factors. ARDS Study Group. *Am J Respir Crit Care Med.* 2000;161:1942–1948.
74. Antonelli M, Conti G, Rocco M, et al. A comparison of noninvasive positive pressure ventilation and conventional mechanical ventilation in patients with acute respiratory failure. *N Engl J Med.* 1998;339:429–435.
75. Holzapfel L, Chevret S, Madinier G, et al. Influence of long-term oro- or nasotracheal intubation on nosocomial maxillary sinusitis and pneumonia: Results of a prospective, randomized trial. *Crit Care Med.* 1993;21:1132–1138.
76. Rouby JJ, Laurent P, Gosnach M, et al. Risk factors and clinical relevance of nosocomial maxillary sinusitis in the critically ill. *Am J Respir Crit Care Med.* 1994;150:776–783.
77. Kress J, Pohlman A, O'Connor M, et al. Daily interruption of sedative infusions in critically ill patients undergoing mechanical ventilation. *New Engl J Med.* 2000;342:1471–1477.
78. Marelich GP, Murin S, Battistella F, et al. Protocol weaning of mechanical ventilation in medical and surgical patients by respiratory care practitioners and nurses: effect on weaning time and incidence of ventilator-associated pneumonia. *Chest.* 2000;118:459–467.
79. Torres A, Serra-Batlles J, Ros E, et al. Pulmonary aspiration of gastric contents in patients receiving mechanical ventilation: the effect of body position. *Ann Intern Med.* 1992;116:540–543.

80. Orozco-Levi M, Torres A, Ferrer M, et al. Semirecumbent position protects from pulmonary aspiration but not completely from gastroesophageal reflux in mechanically ventilated patients. *Am J Respir Crit Care Med.* 1995;152:1387–1390.
81. Drakulovic MB, Torres A, Bauer TT, et al. Supine body position as a risk factor for nosocomial pneumonia in mechanically ventilated patients: a randomised trial. *Lancet.* 1999; 354:1851–1858.
82. Heyland DK, Drover J, MacDonald S, et al. Effect of postpyloric feeding on gastroesophageal regurgitation and pulmonary microaspiration: results of a randomized controlled trial. *Crit Care Med.* 2001;29:1495–1501.
83. Heyland DK, Dhaliwal R, Drover JW, et al. Canadian clinical practice guidelines for nutrition support in mechanically ventilated, critically ill adult patients. *JPEN J Parenter Enteral Nutr.* 2003;27:355–373.
84. Berne JD, Norwood SH, McAuley CE, et al. Erythromycin reduces delayed gastric emptying in critically ill trauma patients: a randomized, controlled trial. *J Trauma.* 2002;53:422–425.
85. van Nieuwenhoven CA, Buskens E, van Tiel FH, et al. Relationship between methodological trial quality and the effects of selective digestive decontamination on pneumonia and mortality in critically ill patients. *JAMA.* 2001;286:335–340.
86. Verwaest C, Verhaegen J, Ferdinande P, et al. Randomized, controlled trial of selective digestive decontamination in 600 mechanically ventilated patients in a multidisciplinary intensive care unit. *Crit Care Med.* 1997;25:63–71.
87. Misset B, Kitzis MD, Conscience G, et al. Mechanisms of failure to decontaminate the gut with polymixin E, gentamycin and amphotericin B in patients in intensive care. *Eur J Clin Microbiol Infect Dis.* 1994;13:165–170.
88. Lingnau W, Berger J, Javorsky F, et al. Changing bacterial ecology during a five-year period of selective intestinal decontamination. *J Hosp Infect.* 1998;39:195–206.
89. Chlebicki MP, Safdar N. Topical chlorhexidine for prevention of ventilator-associated pneumonia: a meta-analysis. *Crit Care Med.* 2007;35:595–602.
90. Bonten MJ, Gaillard CA, de Leeuw PW, et al. Role of colonization of the upper intestinal tract in the pathogenesis of ventilator-associated pneumonia. *Clin Infect Dis.* 1997;24:309–319.
91. Prod'hom G, Leuenberger P, Koerfer J, et al. Nosocomial pneumonia in mechanically ventilated patients receiving antacid, ranitidine or sucralfate as prophylaxis for stress ulcer: a randomized controlled trial. *Ann Intern Med.* 1994;120:653–662.
92. Cook D, Guyatt G, Marshall J, et al. A comparison of sucralfate and ranitidine for the prevention of upper gastrointestinal bleeding in patients requiring mechanical ventilation. *N Engl J Med.* 1998;338:791–797.
93. Earley AS, Gracias VH, Haut E, et al. Anemia management program reduces transfusion volumes, incidence of ventilator-associated pneumonia, and cost in trauma patients. *J Trauma.* 2006;61:1–7.
94. Rizzo M. Striving to eliminate catheter-related bloodstream infections: a literature review of evidence-based strategies. *Semin Anesth.* 2005;24:214–225.
95. Coopersmith CM, Rebmann TL, Zack JE, et al. Effect of an education campaign on decreasing catheter-related bloodstream infections in the surgical intensive care unit. *Crit Care Med.* 2002;30:59–64.
96. Byrnes MC, Coopersmith CM. Prevention of catheter-related blood stream infection. *Curr Opin Crit Care.* 2007;13:411–415.
97. Stein M, Caplan ES. Nosocomial sinusitis: a unique subset of sinusitis. *Curr Opin Infect Dis.* 2005;18:147–150.
98. Velmahos GC, Toutouzas KG, Sarkisyan G, et al. Severe trauma is not an excuse for prolonged antibiotic prophylaxis. *Arch Surg.* 2002;137:537–541.
99. Manian FA, Meyer PL, Setzer J, et al. Surgical site infections associated with methicillin-resistant Staphylococcus aureus: do postoperative factors play a role? *Clin Infect Dis.* 2003;36:863–868.
100. Al-Ghnaniem R, Benjamin IS, Patel AG. Meta-analysis suggests antibiotic prophylaxis is not warranted in low-risk patients undergoing laparoscopic cholecystectomy. *Br J Surg.* 2003;90:365–366.
101. Lewis RT. Oral versus systemic antibiotic prophylaxis in elective colon surgery: a randomized study and meta-analysis send a message from the 1990s. *Can J Surg.* 2002;45:173–180.
102. http://www.cms.hhs.gov/HospitalQualityInits/Downloads/HospitalSDPS MemoRandum.pdf. Accessed September 1, 2007.
103. Song F, Glenny A-M. Antimicrobial prophylaxis in colorectal surgery: a systematic review of randomized controlled trials. *Br J Surg.* 1998;85:1232–1241.
104. Tejirian T, DiFrtonzo LA, Haigh PI. Antibiotic prophylaxis for preventing wound infection after breast surgery: a systematic review and metaanalysis. *J Am Coll Surg.* 2006;203:729–734.
105. Cunningham M, Bunn F, Handscomb K. Prophylactic antibiotics to prevent surgical site infection after breast cancer surgery (review). *Cochrane Database Syst Rev.* 2006;2:CD005360.
106. Aufenacker TJ, Koelemay JW, Gouma DJ, et al. Systematic review and meta-analysis if the effectiveness of antibiotic prophylaxis in prevention of wound infection after mesh repair of abdominal wall hernia. *Br J Surg.* 2006;93:5–10.
107. Sanchez-Manuel FJ, Seco-Gil JL. Antibiotic prophylaxis for hernia repair. *Cochrane Database Syst Rev.* 2004;4:CD003769.
108. Stewart A, Evers PS, Earnshaw JJ. Prevention of infection in arterial reconstruction. *Cochrane Database Syst Rev.* 2006;3:CD003073.
109. Bratzler DW, Houck PM, Surgical Infection Prevention Guideline Writers Workgroup. Antimicrobial prophylaxis for surgery: an advisory statement from the National Surgical Infection Prevention Project. *Am J Surg.* 2005;189:395–404.
110. Classen DC, Evans RS, Pestotnik SL, et al. The timing of prophylactic administration of antibiotics and the risk of surgical-wound infection. *N Engl J Med.* 1992;326:281–286.
111. Bratzler DW, Houck PM, Richards C, et al. Use of antimicrobial prophylaxis for major surgery. Baseline results from the national surgical infection prevention project. *Arch Surg.* 2005;140:174–182.
112. Hawn MT, Gray SH, Vick CC, et al. Timely administration of prophylactic antibiotics for major surgical procedures. *J Am Coll Surg.* 2006;203:803–811.
113. Zaneti G, Giardina R, Platt R. Intraoperative redosing of cefazolin and risk for surgical site infection in cardiac surgery. *Emerg Infect Dis.* 2001;7:828–831.
114. McDonald M, Grabsch E, Marshall C, et al. Single- versus multiple-dose antimicrobial prophylaxis for major surgery: a systematic review. *Aust N Z J Surg.* 1998;68:388–396.
115. Morris AM, Jobe BA, Stoney M, et al. *Clostridium difficile* colitis: an increasingly aggressive iatrogenic disease? *Arch Surg.* 2002;137:1096–1100.
116. Namias N, Harvill S, Ball S, et al. Cost and morbidity associated with antibiotic prophylaxis in the ICU. *J Am Coll Surg.* 1999;188:225–230.
117. Fukatsu K, Saito H, Matsuda T, et al. Influences of type and duration of antimicrobial prophylaxis on an outbreak of methicillin-resistant *Staphylococcus aureus* and on the incidence of wound infection. *Arch Surg.* 1997; 132:1320–1325.
118. Crabtree TD, Pelletier SJ, Antevil JL, et al. Cohort study of fever and leukocytosis as diagnostic and prognostic indicators in infected surgical patients. *World J Surg.* 2001;25:739–744.
119. Swenson BR, Hedrick TL, Popovsky K, et al. Is fever protective in surgical patients with bloodstream infection? *J Am Coll Surg.* 2007;204:815–821.
120. Le Blanc L, Lesur O, Valiquette L, et al. Role of routine blood cultures in detecting unapparent infections during continuous renal replacement therapy. *Intensive Care Med.* 2006;32:1802–1807.
121. Insler SR, Sessler DI. Perioperative thermoregulation and temperature monitoring. *Anesthesiol Clin.* 2006;24:823–837.
122. van der Sande FM, Kooman JP, Leunissen KM. Haemodialysis and thermoregulation. *Nephrol Dial Transplant.* 2006;21:1450–1451.
123. van der Sande FM, Rosales LM, Brener Z, et al. Effect of ultrafiltration on thermal variables, skin temperature, skin blood flow, and energy expenditure during ultrapure hemodialysis. *J Am Soc Nephrol.* 2005;16:1824–1831.
124. Barie PS, Hydo LJ, Eachempati SR. Causes and consequences of fever complicating critical surgical illness. *Surg Infect.* 2004;5:145–159.
125. Trautner BW, Clarridge JE, Darouiche RO. Skin antisepsis kits containing alcohol and chlorhexidine gluconate or tincture of iodine are associated with low rates of blood culture contamination. *Infect Control Hosp Epidemiol.* 2002;23:397–401.
126. Mimoz O, Karim A, Mercat A, et al. Chlorhexidine compared with povidone-iodine as skin preparation before blood culture. A randomized, controlled trial. *Ann Intern Med.* 1999;131:834–837.
127. Cockerill FR 3rd, Wilson JW, Vetter EA, et al. Optimal testing parameters for blood cultures. *Clin Infect Dis.* 2004;38:1724–1730.
128. Mermel LA, Maki DG. Detection of bacteremia in adults: consequences of culturing an inadequate volume of blood. *Ann Intern Med.* 1993;119:270–272.
129. Bates DW, Goldman L, Lee TH. Contaminant blood cultures and resource utilization. The true consequences of false-positive results. *JAMA.* 1991;265:365–369.
130. Clinical and Laboratory Standards Institute. *Principles and Procedures for Blood Cultures; Proposed Guideline.* Wayne, PA: Clinical and Laboratory Standards Institute, CLSI Document M47-P 2006.
131. Leon C, Alvarez-Lerma F, Ruiz-Santana S, et al. Antiseptic chamber-containing hub reduces central venous catheter-related infection: a prospective, randomized study. *Crit Care Med.* 2003;31:1318–1324.
132. Safdar N, Fine JP, Maki DG. Meta-analysis: methods for diagnosing intravascular device-related bloodstream infection. *Ann Intern Med.* 2005; 142:451–466.
133. Mermel LA, Farr BM, Sherertz RJ, et al. Guidelines for the management of intravascular catheter-related infections. *Clin Infect Dis.* 2001;32:1249–1272.
134. Bone RC, Balk RA, Cerra FB, et al. Definitions for sepsis and organ failure and guidelines for the use of innovative therapies in sepsis. The ACCP/SCCM Consensus Conference Committee. American College of Chest Physicians/Society of Critical Care Medicine. *Chest.* 1992;101:1644–1655.
135. Mayhall CG. Diagnosis and management of infections of implantable devices used for prolonged venous access. *Curr Clin Top Infect Dis.* 1992; 12:83–110.
136. Chastre J, Fagon JY. Ventilator-associated pneumonia. *Am J Respir Crit Care Med.* 2002;165:867–903.
137. Sawyer RG, Crabtree TD, Gleason TG, et al. Impact of solid organ

transplantation and immunosuppression on fever, leukocytosis, and physiologic response during bacterial and fungal infections. *Clin Transplant.* 1999;13(3):260–265.
138. Pelletier SJ, Crabtree TD, Gleason TG, et al. Characteristics of infectious complications associated with mortality after solid organ transplantation. *Clin Transplant.* 2000;14(4 Pt 2):401–408.
139. Neuhauser MM, Weinstein RA, Rydman R, et al. Antibiotic resistance among gram-negative bacilli in US intensive care units: implications for fluoroquinolone use. *JAMA.* 2003;289:885–888.
140. Niederman MS. Appropriate use of antimicrobial agents: challenges and strategies for improvement. *Crit Care Med.* 2003;31:608–616.
141. Alvarez-Lerma F. Modification of empiric antibiotic treatment in patients with pneumonia acquired in the intensive care unit: ICU-Acquired Pneumonia Study Group. *Intensive Care Med.* 1996;22:387–394.
142. Fabregas N, Ewig S, Torres A, et al. Clinical diagnosis of ventilatory associated pneumonia revisited: comparative value using immediate post-mortem lung biopsies. *Thorax.* 1999;54:867–873.
143. Fagon JY, Chastre J, Hance AJ, et al. Evaluation of clinical judgment in the identification and treatment of nosocomial pneumonia in ventilated patients. *Chest.* 1993;103:547–555.
144. Mabie M, Wunderink RG. Use and limitations of clinical and radiologic diagnosis of pneumonia. *Semin Respir Infect.* 2003;18:72–79.
145. Fagon JY, Chastre J, Domart Y, et al. Nosocomial pneumonia in patients receiving continuous mechanical ventilation. Prospective analysis of 52 episodes with use of a protected specimen brush and quantitative culture techniques. *Am Rev Respir Dis.* 1989;139:877–884.
146. Rodriguez de Castro F, Sole-Violan J, Aranda Leon A, et al. Do quantitative cultures of protected brush specimens modify the initial empirical therapy in ventilated patients with suspected pneumonia? *Eur Respir J.* 1996;9:37–41.
147. Winer-Muram HT, Steiner RM, Gurney JW, et al. Ventilator-associated pneumonia in patients with adult respiratory distress syndrome: CT evaluation. *Radiology.* 1998;208:193–199.
148. Franquet T. High-resolution computed tomography (HRCT) of lung infections in non-AIDS immunocompromised patients. *Eur Radiol.* 2006;16:707–718.
149. Hiorns MP, Screaton NJ, Muller NL. Acute lung disease in the immunocompromised host. *Radiol Clin North Am.* 2001;39:1137–1151.
150. Luyt CE, Chastre J, Fagon J, et al. Value of the clinical pulmonary infection score for the identification and management of ventilator-associated pneumonia. *Intensive Care Med.* 2004;30:844–852.
151. Fartoukh M, Maitre B, Honore S, et al. Diagnosing pneumonia during mechanical ventilation: the clinical pulmonary infection score revisited. *Am J Respir Crit Care Med.* 2003;168:173–179.
152. Veinstein A, Brun-Buisson C, Derrode N, et al. Validation of an algorithm based on direct examination of specimens in suspected ventilator-associated pneumonia. *Intensive Care Med.* 2006;32:676–683.
153. Blot FB, Raynard B, Chachaty E, et al. Value of gram stain examination of lower respiratory tract secretions for early diagnosis of nosocomial pneumonia. *Am J Respir Crit Care Med.* 2000;162:1731–1737.
154. Torres A, Mustafa E. Bronchoscopic BAL in the diagnosis of ventilator-associated pneumonia. *Chest.* 2000;117:198–202.
155. Niederman MS. Gram-negative colonization of the respiratory tract: Pathogenesis and clinical consequences. *Semin Respir Infect.* 1990;5:173–184.
156. Vidaur L, Gualis B, Rodriquez A, et al. Clinical resolution in patients with suspicion of VAP: a cohort study comparing patients with and without ARDS. *Crit Care Med.* 2005;33:1248–1253.
157. Souweine B, Veber B, Bedos JP, et al. Diagnostic accuracy of protected specimen brush and bronchioalveolar lavage in nosocomial pneumonia: impact of previous antimicrobial treatment. *Crit Care Med.* 1998;26:236–244.
158. Heyland D, Dodek P, Muscedere J, et al. A randomized trial of diagnostic techniques for ventilator-associated pneumonia. *N Engl J Med.* 2006; 355:2619–2630.
159. Elatrous S, Boukef R, Besbes LO, et al. Diagnosis of ventilator-associated pneumonia: agreement between quantitative cultures of endotracheal aspiration and plugged telescoping catheter. *Intensive Care Med.* 2004;30:853–858.
160. Wu CL, Yang DI, Wang NY, et al. Quantitative culture of endotracheal aspirates in the diagnosis of ventilator associated pneumonia in patients with treatment failure. *Chest.* 2002;122:662–668.
161. Brun-Buisson C, Fartoukh M, Lechapt E, et al. Contribution of blinded, protected quantitative specimens to the diagnostic and therapeutic management of ventilator-associated pneumonia. *Chest.* 2005;128:533–544.
162. Sanchez-Nieto JM, Torres A, Garcia-Cordoba F, et al. Impact of invasive and noninvasive quantitative culture sampling on outcome of ventilator-associated pneumonia. *Am J Respir Crit Care Med.* 1998;157:371–376.
163. Campbell GD. Blinded invasive diagnostic procedures in ventilator-associated pneumonia. *Chest.* 2000;117:207S–211S.
164. Shorr AF, Sherner JH, Jackson WL, et al. Invasive approaches to the diagnosis of ventilator-associated pneumonia: a meta-analysis. *Crit Care Med.* 2005;33:46–53.
165. Rello J, Esandi ME, Diaz E, et al. The role of Candida spp. isolated from bronchoscopic samples in nonneutropenic patients. *Chest.* 1998;114:146–149.
166. el-Ebiary M, Torres A, Fabregas N, et al. Significance of the isolation of Candida species from respiratory samples in critically ill, non-neutropenic patients. An immediate postmortem histologic study. *Am J Respir Crit Care Med.* 1997;156(2 Pt 1):583–590.
167. Fekety R. Guidelines for the diagnosis and management of Clostridium difficile-associated diarrhea and colitis. American College of Gastroenterology, Practice Parameters Committee. *Am J Gastroenterol.* 1997;92:739–750.
168. DeMaio J, Bartlett JG. Update on diagnosis of *Clostridium difficile*-associated diarrhea. *Curr Clin Top Infect Dis.* 1995;15:97–114.
169. Bartlett JG. Clostridium difficile: history of its role as an enteric pathogen and the current state of knowledge about the organism. *Clin Infect Dis.* 1994;18(Suppl 4):S265–S272.
170. Fekety R, Shah AB. Diagnosis and treatment of Clostridium difficile colitis. *JAMA.* 1993;269:71–75.
171. Pepin J, Saheb N, Coulombe MA, et al. Emergence of fluoroquinolones as the predominant risk factor for Clostridium difficile-associated diarrhea: a cohort study during an epidemic in Quebec. *Clin Infect Dis.* 2005;41:1254–1260.
172. Manabe YC, Vinetz JM, Moore RD, et al. Clostridium difficile colitis: an efficient clinical approach to diagnosis. *Ann Intern Med.* 1995;123:835–840.
173. Johnson S, Kent SA, O'Leary KJ, et al. Fatal pseudomembranous colitis associated with a variant clostridium difficile strain not detected by toxin A immunoassay. *Ann Intern Med.* 2001;135:434–438.
174. Walker RC, Ruane PJ, Rosenblatt JE, et al. Comparison of culture, cytotoxicity assays, and enzyme-linked immunosorbent assay for toxin A and toxin B in the diagnosis of Clostridium difficile-related enteric disease. *Diagn Microbiol Infect Dis.* 1986;5:61–69.
175. McDonald LC, Killgore GE, Thompson A, et al. An epidemic, toxin gene-variant strain of Clostridium difficile. *N Engl J Med.* 2005;353:2433–2441.
176. Lamontagne F, Labbe AC, Haeck O, et al. Impact of emergency colectomy on survival of patients with fulminant Clostridium difficile colitis during an epidemic caused by a hypervirulent strain. *Ann Surg.* 2007;245:267–272.
177. Talbot RW, Walker RC, Beart RW Jr. Changing epidemiology, diagnosis, and treatment of Clostridium difficile toxin-associated colitis. *Br J Surg.* 1986;73:457–460.
178. Tambyah PA, Maki DG. Catheter-associated urinary tract infection is rarely symptomatic: a prospective study of 1,497 catheterized patients. *Arch Intern Med.* 2000;160:678–682.
179. Safdar N, Slattery WR, Knasinski V, et al. Predictors and outcomes of candiduria in renal transplant recipients. *Clin Infect Dis.* 2005;40:1413–1421.
180. Bryan CS, Reynolds KL. Hospital-acquired bacteremic urinary tract infection: epidemiology and outcome. *J Urol.* 1984;132:494–498.
181. Quintiliani R, Klimek J, Cunha BA, et al. Bacteraemia after manipulation of the urinary tract. The importance of pre-existing urinary tract disease and compromised host defences. *Postgrad Med J.* 1978;54:668–671.
182. Laupland KB, Zygun DA, Davies HD, et al. Incidence and risk factors for acquiring nosocomial urinary tract infection in the critically ill. *J Crit Care.* 2002;17:50–57.
183. Laupland KB, Bagshaw SM, Gregson DB, et al. Intensive care unit-acquired urinary tract infections in a regional critical care system. *Crit Care.* 2005;9:R60–R65.
184. Stark RP, Maki DG. Bacteriuria in the catheterized patient. What quantitative level of bacteriuria is relevant? *N Engl J Med.* 1984;311:560–564.
185. Cornia PB, Takahashi TA, Lipsky BA. The microbiology of bacteriuria in men: a 5-year study at a Veterans' Affairs hospital. *Diagn Microbiol Infect Dis.* 2006;56:25–30.
186. Schwartz DS, Barone JE. Correlation of urinalysis and dipstick results with catheter-associated urinary tract infections in surgical ICU patients. *Intensive Care Med.* 2006;32:1797–1801.
187. Schiotz HA. The value of leukocyte stix results in predicting bacteriuria and urinary tract infection after gynaecological surgery. *J Obstet Gynaecol.* 1999;19:396–398.
188. Westergren V, Forsum U, Lundgren J. Possible errors in diagnosis of bacterial sinusitis in tracheal intubated patients. *Acta Anaesthesiol Scand.* 1994; 3:699–703.
189. Grindlinger GA, Niehoff J, Hughes SL, et al. Acute paranasal sinusitis related to nasotracheal intubation of head-injured patients. *Crit Care Med.* 1987;15:21421–21427.
190. Aebert H, Hunefeld G, Regel G. Paranasal sinusitis and sepsis in ICU patients with nasotracheal intubation. *Intensive Care Med.* 1988;15:27–30.
191. Vargas F, Bui HN, Boyer A, et al. Transnasal puncture based on echographic sinusitis evidence in mechanically ventilated patients with suspicion of nosocomial maxillary sinusitis. *Intensive Care Med.* 2006;32:858–866.
192. Kountakis SE, Skoulas IG. Middle meatal vs antral lavage cultures in intensive care unit patients. *Otolaryngol Head Neck Surg.* 2002;126:377–381.
193. Hayward RA, Shapiro MF, Oye RK. Laboratory testing on cerebrospinal fluid. A reappraisal. *Lancet.* 1987;1:1–4.
194. Leib SL, Boscacci R, Gratzl O, et al. Predictive value of cerebrospinal fluid (CSF) lactate level versus CSF/blood glucose ratio for the diagnosis of bacterial meningitis following neurosurgery. *Clin Infect Dis.* 1999;29:69–74.
195. Tunkel AR, Hartman BJ, Kaplan SL, et al. Practice guidelines for the management of bacterial meningitis. *Clin Infect Dis.* 2004;39:1267–1284.

196. Garibaldi RA, Brodine S, Matsumiya S, et al. Evidence for the non-infectious etiology of early postoperative fever. *Infect Control.* 1985;6:273–277.
197. Cheadle WG. Current perspectives on antibiotic use in the treatment of surgical infections. *Am J Surg.* 1992;164(4A Suppl):44S–47S.
198. Mackowiak PA. Drug fever: mechanisms, maxims and misconceptions. *Am J Med Sci.* 1987;294:275–286.
199. Mermel LA. Bacteriology, safety and prevention of infection associated with continuous intravenous infusions. *Blood Coagul Fibrinolysis.* 1996;7(Suppl 1):S45–S51.
200. Heiman-Patterson TD. Neuroleptic malignant syndrome and malignant hyperthermia. Important issues for the medical consultant. *Med Clin North Am.* 1993;77:477–492.
201. Caroff SN, Mann SC. Neuroleptic malignant syndrome and malignant hyperthermia. *Anaesth Intensive Care.* 1993;21:477–478.
202. Den-Hoed PT, Boelhouwer RU, Veen HF, et al. Infections and bacteriological data after laparoscopic and open gallbladder surgery. *J Hosp Infect.* 1998;39:27–37.
203. Shea JA, Berlin JA, Escarce JJ, et al. Revised estimates of diagnostic test sensitivity and specificity in suspected biliary tract disease. *Arch Intern Med.* 1994;154:2573–2577.
204. Roelofsen H, Van Der Veere CN, Ottenhoff R, et al. Decreased bilirubin transport in the perfused liver of endotoxemic rats. *Gastroenterology.* 1994;107:1075–1080.
205. Mentzer RM, Golden GT, Chandler JG, et al. A comparative appraisal of emphysematous cholecystitis. *Am J Surg.* 1975;129:10–14.
206. Garcia-Sancho Tellez L, Rodriguez-Montes JA, Fernandez de Lis S, et al. Acute emphysematous cholecystitis; report of twenty cases. *Hepatogastroenterology.* 1999;46:2144–2150.
207. Barie PS. Acalculous and postoperative cholecystitis In: Barie PS, Shires GT, eds. *Surgical Intensive Care.* Boston: Little, Brown; 1993:837–849.
208. Hagino RT. Acalculous cholecystitis after aortic reconstruction. *J Am Coll Surg.* 1997;184:245–250.
209. Wang AJ, Wang TE, Lin CC, et al. Clinical predictors of severe gallbladder complications in acute acalculous cholecystitis. *World J Gastroenterol.* 2003;9:2821–2825.
210. Barie PS, Eachempati SR. Acute acalculous cholecystitis. *Curr Gastroenterol Rep.* 2003;5:302–308.
211. Deitch EA. Acute acalculous cholecystitis: ultrasonic diagnosis. *Am J Surg.* 1981;142:290–292.
212. Mirvis SE. CT diagnosis of acalculous cholecystitis. *J Comput Assist Tomogr.* 1987;11:83–88.
213. Kadakia SC. Biliary tract emergencies: acute cholecystitis, acute cholangitis, and acute pancreatitis. *Med Clin North Am.* 1993;77:1015–1019.
214. Lanier AP, Trujillo DE, Schantz PM, et al. Comparison of serologic tests for the diagnosis and follow-up of alveolar hydatid disease. *Am J Trop Med Hyg.* 1987;37:609–613.
215. Krige JEJ, Bornman PC. Infections in hepatic, biliary and pancreatic surgery. In: Blumgart L, Fong Y, eds. *Surgery of the Liver and Biliary Tract.* London: Elsevier; 2002:151–165.
216. Pessa ME, Hawkins IF, Vogel SB. The treatment of acute cholangitis: percutaneous transhepatic biliary drainage before definitive therapy. *Ann Surg.* 1987;205:389–394.
217. Shimada K, Noro T, Inamatsu T, et al. Bacteriology of acute obstructive suppurative cholangitis of the aged. *J Clin Microbiol.* 1989;14:522–526.
218. Yusoff IF. Diagnosis and management of cholecystitis and cholangitis. *Gastroenterol Clin North Am.* 2003;32:1145–1150.
219. Thompson JE Jr, Pitt HA, Doty JE, et al. Broad spectrum penicillin as an adequate therapy for acute cholangitis. *Surg Gynecol Obstet.* 1990;171:275–279.
220. Hanau LH, Stiegbigel NH. Acute (ascending) cholangitis. *Infect Dis Clin North Am.* 2000;14:521–531.
221. Huang C, Pitt HA, Lipsett PA, et al. Pyogenic hepatic abscess. Changing trends over 42 years. *Ann Surg.* 1996;223:600–606.
222. Garwood RA, Sawyer RG, Thompson L, et al. Infectious complications after hepatic resection. *Am Surg.* 2004;70:787–791.
223. Rahimian J, Wilson T, Oram V, et al. Pyogenic liver abscess: recent trends in etiology and mortality. *Clin Infect Dis.* 2004;39:1654–1660.
224. Johannsen EC. Pyogenic liver abscesses. *Infect Dis Clin North Am.* 2000; 14:547–557.
225. Roelofsen H, Shoemaker B, Bakker C, et al. Impaired hepatocanalicular organic anion transport in endotoxemic rats. *Am J Physiol.* 1995;269:427–433.
226. Perez JAA, Gonzalez JJ, Baldonedo RF, et al. Clinical course, treatment, and multivariate analysis of risk factors for pyogenic liver abscess. *Am J Surg.* 2001;181:177–182.
227. Cuschieri A. Cholecystitis. In: Blumgart LH, Fong Y, eds. *Surgery of the Liver and Biliary Tract.* London: Elsevier; 2002:665–675.
228. Cherqui D, Benoist S, Benoit M, et al. Major liver resection for carcinoma in jaundiced patients without preoperative biliary drainage. *Arch Surg.* 2000;135:302–307.
229. Hochwald SN, Burke EC, Jarnagin WR, et al. Association of preoperative biliary stenting with increased postoperative infectious complications in proximal cholangiocarcinoma. *Arch Surg.* 1999;134:261–266.
230. Federle MP, Kapoor V. Complications of liver transplantation: imaging and intervention. *Radiol Clin North Am.* 2003;41:1289–1299.
231. Said A, Safdar N, Lucey MR, et al. Infected bilomas in liver transplant recipients, incidence, risk factors, and implications for prevention. *Am J Transplant.* 2004;23:574–580.
232. Raghavan M, Linden PK. Newer treatment options for skin and soft tissue infections. *Drugs.* 2004;64:1621–1642.
233. Lewis RT. Soft tissue infections. *World J Surg.* 1998;22:146–151.
234. Freischlag JA, Ajalat G, Busuttil RW. Treatment of necrotizing soft tissue infections. The need for a new approach. *Am J Surg.* 1985;149:751–755.
235. Turina M, Cheadle WG. Management of established surgical site infections. *Surg Infect.* 2006;7(Suppl 3):S33–S41.
236. Morykwas MJ, Argenta LC, Shelton-Brown EI, et al. Vacuum-assisted closure: a new method for wound control and treatment: animal studies and basic foundation. *Ann Plast Surg.* 1997;38:553–562.
237. Venturi ML, Attinger CE, Mesbahi AN, et al. Mechanisms and clinical applications of the vacuum-assisted closure (VAC) device: a review. *Am J Clin Dermatol.* 2005;6:185–194.
238. Heller L, Levin SL, Butler CE. Management of abdominal wound dehiscence using vacuum assisted closure in patients with compromised healing. *Am J Surg.* 2006;191:165–172.
239. Schaffzin DM, Douglas JM, Stahl TJ, et al. Vacuum-assisted closure of complex perineal wounds. *Dis Colon Rectum.* 2004;47:1745–1748.
240. Rello J, Sa-Borges M, Correa H, et al. Variations in etiology of ventilator-associated pneumonia across four treatment Sites. Implications for antimicrobial prescribing practices. *Am J Respir Crit Care Med.* 1999;160:608–613.
241. Iregui M, Ward S, Sherman G, et al. Clinical importance of delays in the initiation of appropriate antibiotic treatment for ventilator-associated pneumonia. *Chest.* 2002;122:262–268.
242. Nsier S, Pompeo C, Soubrier S, et al. First-generation fluoroquinolone use and subsequent emergence of multiple drug-resistant bacteria in the intensive care unit. *Crit Care Med.* 2005;33:283–289.
243. Trouillet J, Vuagnat A, Combes A, et al. Pseudomonas aeruginosa ventilator-associated pneumonia: comparison of episodes due to piperacillin-resistant versus piperacillin-susceptible organisms. *Clin Infect Dis.* 2002;34:1047–1054.
244. Daniel F, Sahm D, Critchley I, et al. Evaluation of current activities of fluoroquinolones against gram-negative bacilli using centralized in vitro testing and electronic surveillance. *Antimicrob Agents Chemother.* 2001;45:267–274.
245. McDougall C, Powell JP, Johnson CK, et al. Hospital and community fluoroquinolones use and resistance in Staphylococcus aureus and Escherichia coli in 17 US hospitals. *Clin Infect Dis.* 2005;41:435–440.
246. Paul M, Benuri-Silbiger I, Soares-Weiser K, et al. Beta-lactam monotherapy versus beta-lactam-aminoglycoside combination therapy for sepsis in immunocompetent patients: systematic review and meta-analysis of randomized trials. *BMJ.* 2004;328:668–672.
247. Kollef MH, Kollef KE. Antibiotic utilization and outcomes for patients with clinically suspected VAP and negative quantitative BAL cultures results. *Chest.* 2005;128:2706–2713.
248. American Thoracic Society. Guidelines for the management of adults with hospital-acquired, ventilator-associated, and healthcare-associated pneumonia. *Am J Resp Crit Care Med.* 2005;171:388–410.
249. Dennesen PJ, van der Ven AJ, Kessels AG, et al. Resolution of infectious parameters after antimicrobial therapy in patients with ventilator-associated pneumonia. *Am J Respir Crit Care Med.* 2001;163:1371–1375.
250. Chastre J, Wolff M, Fagon JY, et al. Comparison of 15 vs. 8 days of antibiotic therapy for ventilator-associated pneumonia in adults: a randomized trial. *JAMA.* 2003;290:2588–2598.
251. Singh N, Rogers P, Atwood CW, et al. Short-course empiric antibiotic therapy for patients with pulmonary infiltrates in the intensive care unit. *Am J Respir Crit Care Med.* 2000;162:505–511.
252. Montravers P, Gauzit R, Muller C, et al. Emergence of antibiotic-resistant bacteria in cases of peritonitis after intraabdominal surgery affects the efficacy of empirical antimicrobial therapy. *Clin Infect Dis.* 1996;23:486–494.
253. Sitges-Serra A, Lopez MJ, Girvent M, et al. Postoperative enterococcl infection after treatment of complicated intra-abdominal sepsis. *Br J Surg.* 2002: 361–367.
254. Roehrborn A, Thomas L, Potreck O, et al. The microbiology of postoperative peritonitis. *Clin Infect Dis.* 2001;33:1513–1519.
255. Pieracci FM, Barie PS. Intra-abdominal infections. *Curr Opin Crit Care.* 2007;13:440–449.
256. Bujik SE, Bruining HA. Future directions in the management of tertiary peritonitis. *Intensive Care Med.* 2002;28:1024–1029.
257. Talmor M, Li P, Barie PS. Acute paranasal sinusitis: guidelines for prevention, diagnosis, and treatment. *Clin Infect Dis.* 1997;25:1441–1446.
258. DiPiro JT, Edmiston CE, Bohnen JMA. Pharmacodynamics of antimicrobial therapy in surgery. *Am J Surg.* 1996;171:615–622.
259. Naimi TS, LeDell KH, Como-Sabetti K, et al. Comparison of community- and health care-associated methicillin-resistant Staphylococcus aureus infection. *JAMA.* 2004;290:2976–2984.

260. Anstead GM, Owens AD. Recent advances in the treatment of infections due to resistant Staphylococcus aureus. *Curr Opin Infect Dis.* 2004;17:549–555.
261. Schentag JJ, Gilliland KK, Paladino JA. What have we learned from pharmacokinetic and pharmacodynamic theories? *Clin Infect Dis.* 2001;32:S39–S46.
262. Nicolau DP, Freeman CD, Belliveau PP, et al. Experience with a once-daily aminoglycoside program administered to 2,184 adult patients. *Antimicrob Agents Chemother.* 1995;39:650–655.
263. Kashuba AD, Bertino JS Jr, Nafziger AN. Dosing of aminoglycosides to rapidly attain pharmacodynamic goals and hasten therapeutic response by using individualized pharmacokinetic monitoring of patients with pneumonia caused by gram-negative organisms. *Antimicrob Agents Chemother.* 1998;42:1842–1844.
264. Thomas JK, Forrest A, Bhavnani SM, et al. Pharmacodynamic evaluation of factors associated with the development of bacterial resistance in acutely ill patients during therapy. *Antimicrob Agents Chemother.* 1998;42:521–527.
265. Benko AS, Cappelletty DM, Kruse JA, et al. Continuous infusion versus intermittent administration of ceftazidime in critically ill patients with suspected Gram-negative infections. *Antimicrob Agents Chemother.* 1996;40:691–695.
266. Lau WK, Mercer D, Itani KM, et al. Randomized, open-label, comparative study of piperacillin-tazobactam administered by continuous infusion versus intermittent infusion for treatment of hospitalized patients with complicated intra-abdominal infection. *Antimicrob Agents Chemother.* 2006;50:3556–3561.
267. Kollef MH, Ward S, Sherman G, et al. Inadequate treatment of nosocomial infections is associated with certain empiric antibiotic choices. *Crit Care Med.* 2000;28:3456–3464.
268. Garnacho-Montero J, Garcia-Garmendia JL, Barrero-Almodovar A, et al. Impact of adequate empirical antibiotic therapy on the outcome of patients admitted to the intensive care unit with sepsis. *Crit Care Med.* 2003;31:2742–2751.
269. Evans RS, Pestotnik SL, Classen DC, et al. A computer-assisted management program for antibiotics and other antiinfective agents. *N Engl J Med.* 1998;338:232–238.
270. Kollef MH, Vlasnik J, Sharpless L, et al. Scheduled rotation of antibiotic classes: a strategy to decrease the incidence of ventilator-associated pneumonia due to antibiotic-resistant gram-negative bacteria. *Am J Respir Crit Care Med.* 1997;156:1040–1048.
271. Gruson D, Hilbert G, Vargas F, et al. Strategy of antibiotic rotation: long term effect on incidence and susceptibilities of gram-negative bacilli responsible for ventilator-associated pneumonia. *Crit Care Med.* 2003;31:1908–1914.
272. Raymond DP, Pelletier SJ, Crabtree TD, et al. Impact of a rotating empiric antibiotic schedule on infectious mortality in an intensive care unit. *Crit Care Med.* 2001;29:1101–1108.
273. van Loon HJ, Vriens MR, Fluit AC, et al. Antibiotic rotation and development of gram-negative antibiotic resistance. *Am J Respir Crit Care Med.* 2005;171:480–487.
274. Kollef MH. Is antibiotic cycling the answer to preventing the mergence of bacterial resistance in the intensive care unit? *Clin Infect Dis.* 2006;43:S82–S88.
275. Aarts MA, Granton J, Cook DJ, et al. Empiric antibiotic therapy in critical illness. Results of a Surgical Infection Society survey. *Surg Infect.* 2007;8:329–336.
276. Kollef MH, Micek ST. Strategies to prevent antimicrobial resistance in the intensive care unit. *Crit Care Med.* 2005;33:1845–1853.
277. Giamarellou H. Treatment options for multidrug-resistant bacteria. *Expert Rev Antiinfect Ther.* 2006;4:601–618.
278. Bosso JA. The antimicrobial armamentarium: evaluating current and future treatment options. *Pharmacotherapy.* 2005;25:55S–62S.
279. Padmanabhan RA, Larosa SP, Tomecki KJ. What's new in antibiotics? *Dermatol Clin.* 2005;23:301–312.
280. Dellinger EP. Duration of antibiotic treatment in surgical infections of the abdomen. Undesired effects of antibiotics and future studies. *Eur J Surg.* 1996;576(Suppl):29–31.

APPENDIX A. ABBREVIATIONS

ARDS	Acute respiratory distress syndrome
AUC	Area under curve
BAL	Bronchoalveolar lavage
CASS	Continuous aspiration of subglottic secretions
CI	Confidence interval
CDAD	*Clostridium difficile*–associated disease
CFU	Colony forming units
CNS	Central nervous system
CPAP	Continuous positive airway pressure
CPIS	Clinical pulmonary infection score
CR-BSI	Catheter-related bloodstream infection
CSF	Cerebrospinal fluid
CT	Computerized tomography
CXR	Chest radiograph
EA	Endotracheal suction aspiration
ERCP	Endoscopic retrograde cholangiopancreatography
ESBL	Extended-spectrum β-lactamase
EVD	Extraventricular drain
ICU	Intensive care unit
MDR	Multidrug resistant
MIC	Minimal inhibitory concentration
MIC_{90}	90% inhibition
MRCP	Magnetic resonance cholangiopancreatography
MRI	Magnetic resonance imaging
MRSA	Methicillin-resistant *Staphylococcus aureus*
MRSE	Methicillin-related *S. epidermis*
NAP1	North American pulse-field gel electrophoresis type 1
NIPPV	Noninvasive positive pressure ventilation
NNIS	National Nosocomial Infections Surveillance System
NSTI	Necrotizing soft tissue infection
OR	Odds ratio
PAE	Postantibiotic effect
PD	Pharmacodynamic
PICC	Peripherally inserted central catheters
PK	Pharmacokinetic
PSB	Protected specimen brush
PTC	Plugged telescoping catheter
PTC	Percutaneous transhepatic cholangiopancreatography
RR	Relative risk
SCIP	Surgical care improvement project
SDD	Self-decontamination of the digestive tract
SIRS	Systemic inflammatory response syndrome
SSI	Surgical site infections
$T_{1/2}$	Half-life
US	Ultrasound
UTI	Urinary tract infection
VAP	Ventilator-associated pneumonia
V_D	Volume of distribution
VRE	Vancomycin-resistant enterococci
VAC	Vacuum-assisted closure
WBC	White blood count

CHAPTER 107 ■ SKIN WOUNDS AND MUSCULOSKELETAL INFECTION

MARC J. SHAPIRO • STEVEN SANDOVAL

WOUND CLASSIFICATION

Surgical Site Infections

In the United States alone, an estimated 27 million surgical procedures are performed annually (1). Surgical site infections (SSIs) are the third most common nosocomial infection in most hospitalized patients accounting for 14% to 16% (Fig. 107.1). Among surgical patients, SSIs were the most common nosocomial infection, accounting for 38% of infections. Whereas 66% of the SSIs remained confined to the incision site, the remainder involved organs or spaces accessed during the surgical procedure. In 1980 it was estimated that a SSI increased hospital stay by 10 days and cost an additional $2,000 per patient (2). By 1992 that number had decreased to 7.5 days' increased stay; however, the cost had increased to $3,152 per patient. All told, the contribution to the cost of health care in the United States is calculated at 130 to 180 million dollars per year (3). The effects of SSIs are not only felt locally, such as tissue destruction, pain, scar formation, septic thrombophlebitis, but also extend systemically to septicemia, shock, organ dysfunction, and death.

Center for Disease Control (CDC) Classification of Surgical Site Infections

Superficial Incisional SSIs. Infection occurs within 30 days of surgery and involves only skin or subcutaneous tissue with the following:

1. Purulent drainage
2. Presence of organisms in drainage
3. Pain or tenderness, swelling, redness

Deep Incisional SSIs. Infection within 30 days of surgery, or within 1 year if implant is present. Infection involves deep soft tissues with the following:

1. Purulence from deep incision, not the organ space of operation
2. Dehiscence of deep incision or opened wound by surgeon due to symptoms of fever, pain, tenderness
3. Abscess found on direct exam or reoperation

Organ/Space SSIs. Infection within 30 days of surgery, or within 1 year if implant is present. Infection involves any part of the anatomy other than the incision opened during operation with the following:

1. Purulence from a surgically placed drain in the organ space
2. Positive cultures from that organ space
3. Abscess found on direct exam or reoperation

Purulence alone is not a hallmark of an infected wound. If purulence is present, however, a wound can be considered infected, even if confirmatory cultures are negative. The absence of confirmatory pathogens can be as a result of inadequate techniques of culture, the patient's current antimicrobial therapy, or a particularly fastidious organism. Patients with immunologic dysfunction or those who are granulocytopenic may not always produce purulent material.

Surgical wounds are grouped into four classes, each with its infection risk (Table 107.1):

Class I (clean): An uninfected operative wound in which no inflammation is encountered and the respiratory, alimentary, genital, or uninfected urinary tract is not entered. In addition, clean wounds are primarily closed and, if necessary, drained with closed drainage. Operative incisional wounds that follow nonpenetrating (blunt) trauma should be included in this category if they meet the criteria.

Class II (clean to contaminated): An operative wound in which the respiratory, alimentary, genital, or urinary tracts are entered under controlled conditions and without unusual contamination. Specifically, operations involving the biliary tract, appendix, vagina, and oropharynx are included in this category, provided no evidence of infection or major break in technique is encountered.

Class III (contaminated): These include open, fresh, accidental wounds. In addition, operations with major breaks in sterile techniques (e.g., open cardiac massage) or gross spillage from the gastrointestinal tract, and incisions in which acute nonpurulent inflammation is encountered.

Class IV (dirty to infected): Old traumatic wounds with retained devitalized tissue and those that involve existing clinical infection or perforated viscera. The organisms causing postoperative infection were present in the operative field before the operation.

Risk Factors

All surgical wounds are at risk for infection. It is important to be aware of the risk factors and if possible to take as many preventative measures as possible that will have a positive impact. The National Nosocomial Infection Surveillance (NNIS) system was developed in the early 1970s to monitor the incidence of health care–associated infections (HAIs) and their associated risk factors and pathogens. NNIS has identified wound infection risk factors as the following:

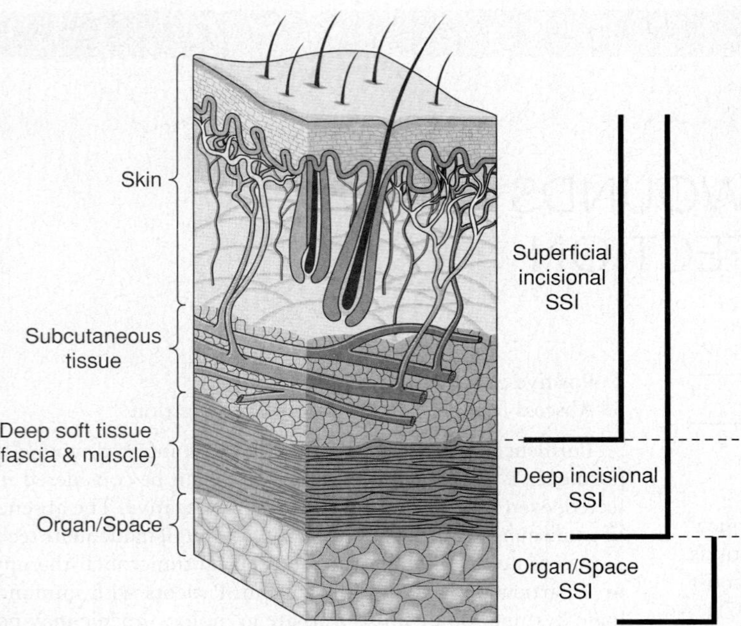

FIGURE 107.1. Surgical site infections (SSI) categorized by depth of involvement.

a. Wound classified as contaminated or dirty
b. A patient with an ASA (American Society of Anesthesiologists) score of 3, 4, or 5 prior to operation
c. A procedure lasting longer than T hours, where T represents the 75th percentile of duration of time expected for that surgery

To identify a patient's risk index category (RIC), each factor, if present, receives a score of 1, with a range between 0 and 3. SSI rates by operative procedure category and risk index are published in NNIS source documents.

The NNIS also publishes recommendations for reducing the risk of SSIs. The weight of these recommendations are based on the scientific evidence used to support the conclusions:

1. Category IA: Strongly recommended for implementation and supported by well-designed experimental, clinical, or epidemiologic studies
2. Category IB: Strongly recommended for implementation and supported by some experimental, clinical, or epidemiologic studies and strong theoretical rationale
3. Category II: Suggested for implementation and supported by suggestive clinical or epidemiologic or theoretical rationale
4. No recommendation or unresolved issue: Practice for which insufficient evidence or no consensus regarding efficacy exists

TABLE 107.1

SURGICAL WOUND CLASSIFICATION AND RISK OF INFECTION (IF NO ANTIBIOTICS USED)

Classification	Description	Infection risk (%)
Class I	Clean	<2
Class II	Clean to Contaminated	<10
Class III	Contaminated	20
Class IV	Dirty	40

Category IA recommendations for SSI prevention:

- Treat remote infection before performing an elective operation.
- Do not remove hair from operative sites unless it interferes with surgery and then only use electric clippers just prior to surgery.
- Select an agent with efficacy against the suspected organism, making sure the therapeutic serum levels exist from the beginning of the operation. Mechanical preparation of the colon with enemas and cathartics before elective colorectal operations and the use of nonabsorbable oral antimicrobials the day before operation have been beneficial.

Category IB recommendations for SSI prevention:

- Control serum glucose prior to operation.
- Cease tobacco use 30 days prior to operation.
- Shower night before surgery.
- Prepare operative site with an antiseptic skin agent.
- Do not routinely use vancomycin for antimicrobial prophylaxis.
- The operative team should keep nails short and not wear artificial nails.
- A 2- to 5-minute preoperative surgical scrub for the surgical team should occur.

Category II recommendations for SSI prevention:

- Prepare skin in concentric circles from the incision site outwards.
- Keep preoperative stay in the hospital as short as possible.
- Clean underneath each fingernail prior to performing first scrub of the day.
- Do not wear hand or arm jewelry.
- Limit the number of personnel entering the operating room.

No recommendation or unresolved issue: Restriction of scrub suits to the operating suite, or coverage of scrub suits outside of theater.

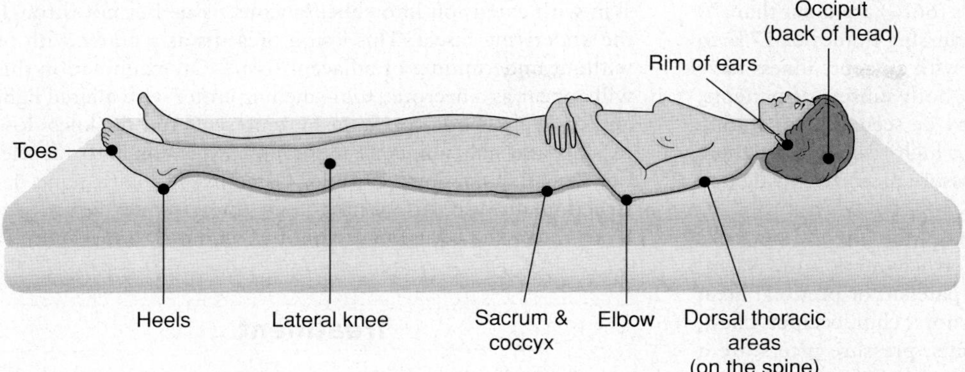

FIGURE 107.2. Pressure points in supine position.

Pressure/Decubitus Ulcers

From the Latin *decumbere*, "to lie down," the term *decubitus* has been applied to any area that develops an ulcer secondary to prolonged pressure between a bony prominence and an unyielding surface. Thus the term *pressure ulcer* is a more accurate description. Although an issue of long duration, it appears to be first addressed in scientific writing in the 19th century.

To overcome arterial and capillary hydrostatic pressure and develop subsequent tissue necrosis with ulceration, an individual must be subjected to 32 mm Hg pressure at the level of the ischium, sacrum, or heels for a prolonged period of time, usually exceeding 2 hours as reported by Lindan et al. (4). The points of greatest pressure with a supine patient are seen over the sacrum, heel, and occiput at 40 to 60 mm Hg (Fig. 107.2).

With the body in a prone position, the chest and knees absorb the greatest pressure, which may be 50 mm Hg. When the patient is sitting, the ischial tuberosities are under the most pressure, measured at near 100 mm Hg (Fig. 107.3).

If sensation is intact, ulceration usually will not occur as the incipient pain would lead to a change in position by the patient. This occurs during the sleep cycle.

The risk factors associated with pressure ulcer development can be divided into external and internal causes. Externally, the patient might be subjected to a constant pressure for a period of time, or friction exists between exposed skin and a surface that remains static, or a region remains moist and may have desquamation, leading to a loss of the epithelial protective mechanism (Fig. 107.4). The placement of splints can also alter a patient's ability to change position in response to pressure-related pain or in itself may cause pressure necrosis. The administration of sedatives or paralytics can also remove the normal feedback pathways that exist to prevent pressure ulcer formation. Internally, factors responsible for pressure ulceration include malnutrition (serum albumin levels less than 3.0 g/dL preoperatively), anemia, and/or endothelial dysfunction. Diabetes, peripheral vascular disease, and episodes of hypotension also increase the risk as do sensory deficits in patients with plegia or paresis. Patients with dementia may also not be sensitive to the importance of changing position frequently and may also be more prone to pressure ulceration.

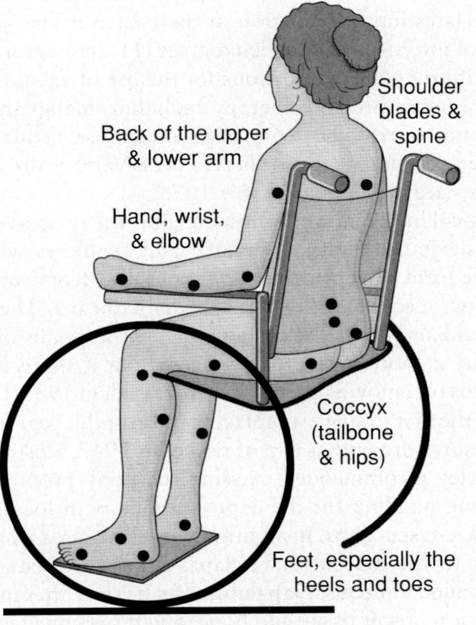

FIGURE 107.3. Pressure points in sitting position.

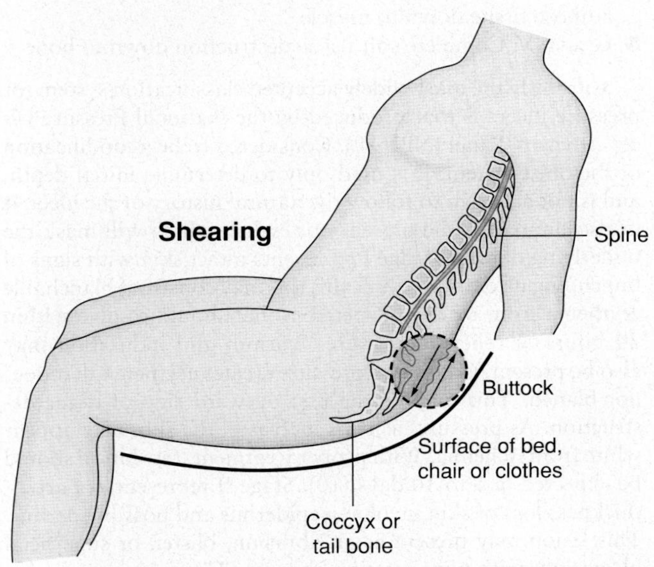

FIGURE 107.4. Shearing effect.

Most patients with pressure ulcers (66%) are older than 70 years old, with a prevalence rate in nursing homes of 17% to 28%. In contrast, patients admitted with an acute illness have an incidence rate of 3% to 11%. In both subsets of patients, recurrence rates as high as 90% may be seen. The operating room, where patients are immobile is a high-risk area, and there is a report that up to 25% of all pressure ulcers are instigated there (5).

Anatomic sites affected are primarily the hip and buttocks (67% of the cases involve ischial, trochanteric, and sacral tuberosity); 25% in malleolar, heel, patellar, or pretibial area; with the remainder occurring on the nose, chin, occiput, chest, back, or elbow. In paraplegic patients, pressure ulcers are a leading cause of death, responsible for an 8% mortality rate (6). Overall an estimated 60,000 people die each year from a pressure ulcer complication. The health care cost in the United States alone per year is in excess of $1 billion (7).

Several scoring systems are used to grade the risk for ulceration. The Braden scale is a summation rating scale made up of six subscores consisting of sensory perception, moisture, activity, mobility, nutrition, and friction/shear, each ranging from 1 to 3 or 4 points, with total scores ranging from 6 to 23. The subscores measure the functional capabilities of the patient that contribute to either higher intensity and duration of pressure or lower tissue tolerance for pressure. A lower Braden score indicates lower levels of functioning with a higher risk for pressure ulcer development

The Daniels classification looks at muscle and subcutaneous tissue breakdown, which occurs before dermal and epidermal changes are observed. Epidermal necrosis occurs later because epidermal cells are able to better withstand prolonged absence of oxygen than cells in the deeper tissues both *in vivo* and *in vitro* (8). Once skin damage is visible, irreversible internal damage may have already occurred (9).

Shea staging describes ulcers that start superficially and progress to deeper structures:

- Grade I: limited to superficial epidermis and dermis
- Grade II: Involving the epidermis and dermis and extending to the adipose tissue
- Grade III: Extending through the superficial structures and adipose tissue down to muscle
- Grade IV: Complete soft tissue destruction down to bone

Currently the most widely accepted classification system for pressure ulcers is that produced by the National Pressure Ulcer Advisory Panel (NPUAP). Considered to be a modification of the Shea system, it is used only to determine initial depth, and is not a system to follow the natural history of the ulcer. It is also limited by the presence of eschar, which will mask the underlying damage. Stage I represents intact skin with signs of impending ulceration. Clinically, this may consist of blanchable erythema from reactive hyperemia that should resolve within 24 hours of relief of pressure. Warmth and induration may also be present. Continued pressure creates erythema that does not blanch. This may be the first outward sign of tissue destruction. As pressure necrosis increases, the skin may appear white from ischemia. With proper treatment, resolution should be expected in 5 to 10 days (10). Stage II represents a partial-thickness loss of skin involving epidermis and possibly dermis. This lesion may present as an abrasion, blister, or superficial ulceration, with pigmentation changes. These too represent a reversible condition. Stage III represents a full-thickness loss of skin with extension into subcutaneous tissue but not through the underlying fascia. This lesion presents as a crater with or without undermining of adjacent tissue. On examination this will appear as a necrotic, foul-smelling crater with altered light and dark pigmentation. Stage IV represents full-thickness loss of skin and subcutaneous tissue and extension into muscle, bone, tendon, or joint capsule. Osteomyelitis with bone destruction, dislocations, or pathologic fractures may be present. Sinus tracts and severe undermining commonly are present.

Treatment

All modalities of care for pressure ulcers fall along four paths:

1. Pressure reduction: Frequent turning and repositioning the patient at least every 2 hours. Historically, this was adopted because of nursing issues (it took 2 hours for the nurse to rotate all ward patients). Currently, there is debate in the literature as to this being an adequate amount of time. In addition to positioning, mattresses that reduce pressure, such as low-air-loss and air-fluidized beds should be used for patients with stage III and IV ulcers, whereas for stage I and II ulcers, the use of static mattresses such as air, foam, or water overlays are the most beneficial.
2. Wound management: Once an ulcer has developed, removal of dead tissue and debris, drainage, and protecting the surrounding healthy tissue are the goals. The pressure needed to clean wounds with no necrotic material is 2 to 5 pounds per square inch (psi). If necrotic debris is present, the pressure required increases by a factor of 2 to 3. The old wound dictum—if it is dry, wet it; if it is wet, dry it—has some validity here. A draining wound needs either a hydrocolloid or alginate, whereas a wound without drainage will respond to simple moist gauze; the surrounding skin of both need to be kept lubricated, but not wet, to reduce friction. Negative pressure therapy enhances wound healing by reducing edema, increasing the rate of granulation tissue formation, and stimulating circulation. Increased blood flow translates into a reduction in the bacterial load and delivery of infection-fighting leukocytes (11). However, there are significant contraindications for the use of vacuum-assisted or negative pressure therapy including malignancy of the wound, untreated osteomyelitis, nonenteric fistulas, and exposed vessels, organs, or nerves (12). Various dressing categories are presented in Table 107.2.
3. Surgical intervention: Debridement is the process of removing devitalized tissue. Stage III and IV ulcers will require some form of debridement, whether it is from surgical, autolytic, mechanical, or via enzymatic means. The patient's wound and overall status will dictate the means of debridement, a more stable patient receiving a more aggressive means of removing the necrotic material. In 1938, Davis (13) was the first to suggest replacing the unstable scar of a healed pressure sore with a flap of tissue. In 1947, Kostrubala and Greeley recommended excising the bony prominence and adding padding for the exposed bone with local fascia or muscle-fascia flaps. In addition, larger wounds may respond only to the placement of flaps, either fasciocutaneous or musculocutaneous. Flap failure can be seen after insufficient excision of soft tissue and bone, and if systemic factors such as nutritional status are suboptimal.

TABLE 107.2

DRESSING CATEGORIES

Category	Properties/Uses
Alginates	Absorption of drainage, dead space obliteration, autolysis of necrotic material
Foams	Absorption of drainage, dead space obliteration, mechanical debridement, moisture retention
Gauzes	Absorption of drainage, dead space obliteration, mechanical debridement, moisture retention
Hydrocolloids	Dead space obliteration, autolysis of necrotic material, moisture retention
Vacuum-assisted closure	Dead space obliteration, induction of granulation
Ostomy appliances	Drainage diversion

4. Nutritional support: Malnourished patients have a higher susceptibility for ulcer formation. Once formed these patients also have a diminished ability to heal or to prevent further ulcer formation in other sites. Patients with serum albumin levels less than 3 mg/dL may be candidates for supplemental feedings via enteral or parenteral routes

PRIMARY BACTERIOLOGIC INFECTIONS

Skin and soft tissue infections are usually easily treated but have the potential of being lethal. Any break in the usual protection of the integument such as occurs with a cut, scrape, insect bite, splinter, or traumatic injury allows bacteria to enter underlying tissues. Although a scrape or a cut will not usually result in a cellulitis, a tender, firm, painful, and rapidly expanding area of redness on the skin surrounding violation of the skin barrier should be a cause for concern. Red streaks between lymph node–bearing areas may be visible, and this is indicative of a potentially spreading infection. Certain areas are more prone in becoming infected depending on the age group, such as facial cellulitis occurring more commonly in adults older than 50 years and in children 6 months to 3 years of age.

Most common causative organisms in skin infections are group A β-hemolytic streptococci and *Staphylococcus aureus*. Depending on the source of contamination and whether the patient is immunocompromised, Gram-negative rods and fungus can be seen. If the insult occurs during exposure to fresh water, the causative organism may be *Aeromonas*, a Gram-negative rod.

Predisposing states in which a minor break in the skin barrier leads to a significant infection include those patients with diabetes, immunodeficiency, varicella; venous, arterial or lymphatic insufficiency, such as that seen after lymphatic removal during mastectomy; or vein stripping for varicosities.

Treatment of uncomplicated cellulitis begins with removing the nidus of infection, cleansing the wound with an antiseptic agent, dressing the wound with an antiseptic ointment if indicated, and considering a course of oral antibiotics, such as dicloxacillin, 500 mg PO (orally) four times a day for 7 days, or cephalexin, 500 mg PO four times a day for 7 days. For patients with a suspected or known penicillin allergy, clindamycin, 400 mg, is given PO four times a day (14).

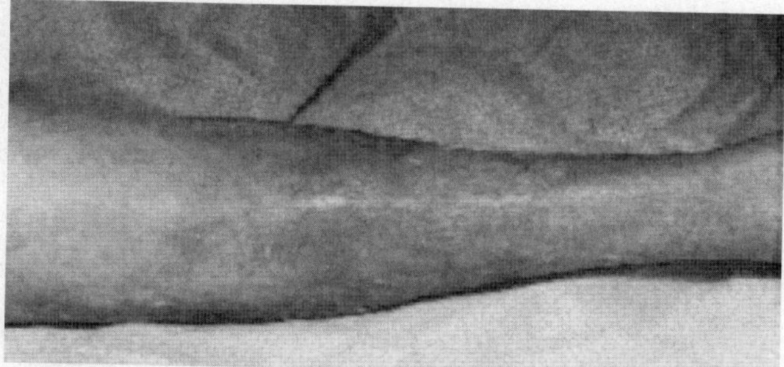

FIGURE 107.5. Erysipelas.

Erysipelas

Erysipelas (Fig. 107.5) is a form of cellulitis that affects the epidermis primarily extending into the cutaneous lymphatics. During the Middle Ages, it was referred to as St. Anthony's fire, named after the Egyptian healer who was successful in treating this condition. It shares the same underlying cause as cellulitis with bacterial inoculation into an area of skin violation. It is more commonly seen in children and the elderly. Erysipelas differs from cellulitis in that the inflamed area is distinct from the surrounding skin, being raised and demarcated. Erysipelas is often found on the face; however, it can also develop on the arms and legs. Sometimes the skin will have what is called a *peau d'orange*, or orange peel, look to it. As with cellulitis, streptococcus is the primary organism identified with its toxin responsible for the brisk inflammation associated with this condition.

Treatment consists of elevation of the affected extremity, penicillin, 250 to 500 mg PO or 0.6 to 1.2 million Units intramuscularly, given every 4 to 6 hours for a 10- to 20-day course. In cases of penicillin allergy, a macrolide or cephalosporin usually suffices. If the area affected becomes ulcerated, saline dressings changed every 12 hours will assist with wound closure.

Impetigo

Also known as pyoderma, impetigo (Fig. 107.6) is the most common bacterial infection of the skin seen. It is contagious and can happen at any age but is more common in young children. Patients report skin lesions, often with associated adenopathy, with minimal systemic signs and symptoms. Impetigo may present in two forms: small vesicles with a honey-colored crust known as *impetigo contagiosa*, or purulent-appearing bullae, known as *bullous impetigo*. Most commonly caused by *S. aureus*, group A beta-hemolytic strep is also commonly seen in the over-2-year-old population. Warm temperatures, humidity, poor hygiene, and crowded living conditions can exacerbate the spread of impetigo. When associated with lymphadenitis in deeper infections, the term *ecthyma* is given. Topical mupirocin (Bactroban) applied three times a day for 5 days is successful in treating >90% of cases and is more

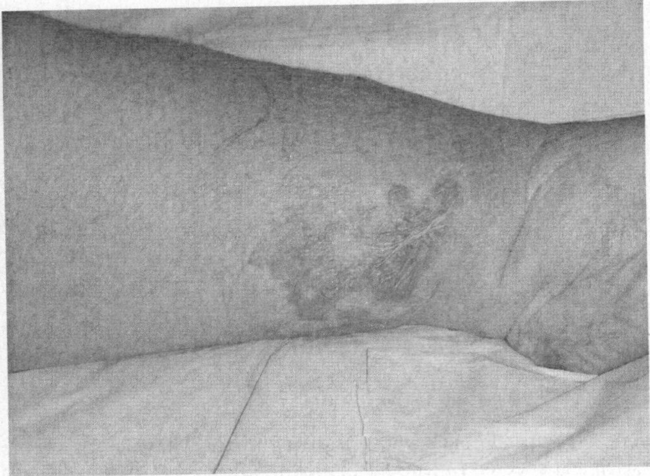

FIGURE 107.6. Impetigo due to *Staphylococcus aureus* in a 68-year-old diabetic who fell onto concrete while walking and developed this lesion after 6 days. This resolved with conservative care and antibiotics.

effective than oral erythromycin (2). Lesions usually resolve completely within 7 to 10 days.

CUTANEOUS FUNGAL INFECTIONS

The most common important fungal infections that occur in the ICU setting are for the most part due to *Candida*, especially *albicans*, *glabrata*, and *tropicalis* (2). In immunocompromised or morbidly obese patients, this usually manifests itself as cutaneous moniliasis and can be treated with topical powders or ointments. Vaginitis, of course, should be treated with suppositories, and funguria is addressed by removing or replacing the urinary catheter, which will be successful in about one third of patients.

MUSCULOSKELETAL INFECTIONS

First described in 1848, deep soft tissue infection remained a disease of unknown cause until 1920 when Meleney identified 20 patients in China in whom a hemolytic streptococcus was identified in the wounds. In Meleney gangrene, there is extensive necrosis of the skin and subcutaneous tissue caused by synergistic infection between microaerobic staphlococcal and hemolytic streptococcal infection.

Break in skin integrity
↓
Wound contamination with anaerobic and/or aerobic necrotizing bacteria
↓
Edema
↓
Tissue hypoxia
↓
Release of exotoxins
↓
Necrosis of fat, subcutaneous tissue, and muscle
Production of hydrogen sulfide and carbon dioxide as a result.
↓ ↑
Decreased blood flow Causing further tissue hypoxia → Liquefactive necrosis of tissues due to enzymes from anaerobic bacteria.

FIGURE 107.7. Pathophysiology of necrotizing fasciitis.

The term *necrotizing fasciitis* (NF) was first coined in 1952 by Wilson (15) and involves the underlying fascia and subcutaneous tissue and spares the muscle. Myositis results in muscle involvement, which becomes exquisitely tender and indurated. The muscle involvement leads to elevation of the creatine phosphokinase and can spread over several hours to contiguous muscle groups, thus heightening the need for early diagnosis and treatment. Fournier's gangrene is listed here as a separate entity due to its predilection for the perineum.

All of these subgroups have in common pathogenicity with the organisms spreading from subcutaneous tissues to both superficial and deep fascial planes (Figs. 107.1 and 107.7). The local effect is vascular occlusion, ischemia, and necrosis. The systemic effect is sepsis, end organ dysfunction with a mortality rate as high as 75% with Fournier's gangrene (16) and up to 100% in patients with multiple organ failure. Mortality rate varies with age and extent of involvement (17) with survivors being younger. The male:female ratio of affliction ranges 2 to 3:1.

Types of Necrotizing Fasciitis

Table 107.3 presents types of necrotizing fasciitis. Further details are discussed in the paragraphs that follow.

TABLE 107.3

SUBTYPES OF NECROTIZING FASCIITIS (NF)

Subtype	Organisms present	Treatment	Mortality
Type I	Gram-negative, gram-positive, aerobes and anaerobes	Antibiotics, penicillin, clindamycin, debridement	Without organ dysfunction, 25%; with organ dysfunction, 75%; dependent on age
Type II	Streptococcus	Antibiotic, cessation of NSAID use, debridement	Same as above
Type III	*Clostridium perfringens*, *Clostridium septicum*	Wide local debridement, hyperbaric oxygen, immunoglobulin, antibiotics	75%
Fournier's	Polymicrobial, same as type III	Wide local debridement, hyperbaric oxygen, antibiotics	75%

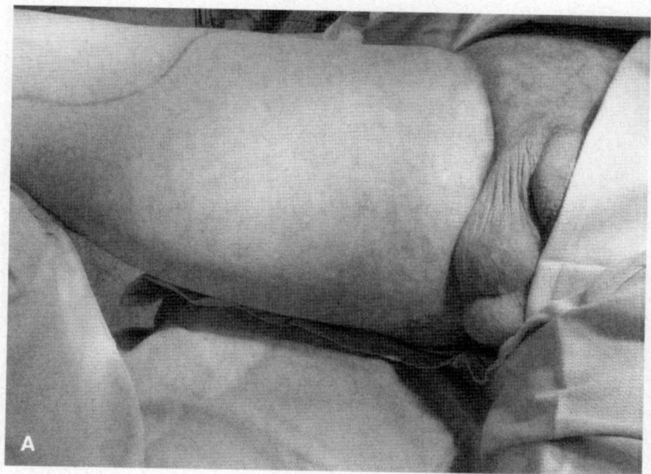

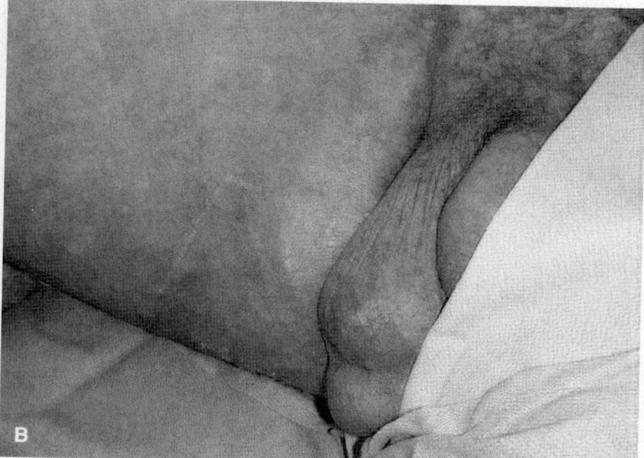

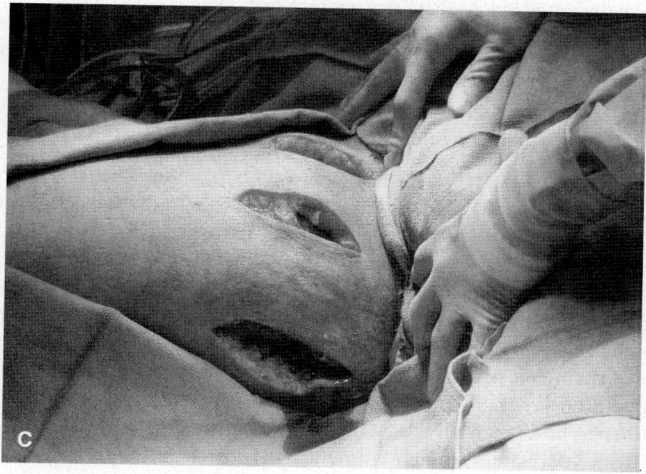

FIGURE 107.8. A–C: Meleney's synergistic gangrene in a 45-year-old pipe layer who noticed initially a wheal and subsequently required incision and drainage for beta-hemolytic streptococcus.

a. Type I (polymicrobial): Usually occurring after injury or surgery, it can be misdiagnosed as a simple cellulitis; however, as tissue necrosis and hypoxia continue, pain and systemic symptoms of fever, chills, and malaise increase as the underlying tissue liquefies while the overlying skin may show minimal changes. In the late stages, extension into the muscle itself occurs. Over 2 to 3 days erythema increases, with occasional bullae formation. Cultures may reveal a combination of aerobic and anaerobic organisms. Deep soft tissue infection of the perineum is termed *Fournier's gangrene* (15). Many of these patients have predisposing systemic issues such as diabetes or the presence of immunosuppressed states. Histologically, thrombosis of blood vessels and abundant bacteria with many polymorphonuclear cells are typically seen.
b. Type II (group A streptococcal) (Figs. 107.8A–C and 107.9A,B): Also known familiarly as 'flesh-eating bacteria' or as Meleney's synergistic gangrene. As with type I, a nearly normal appearing overlying skin may result in a delay in diagnosing the underlying ongoing necrosis. A simple incision into the region affected can demonstrate drainage or even gas in advanced cases. Other predisposing factors include varicella infection and the use of nonsteroidal anti-inflammatory drugs (NSAIDs) (18). NSAID use is seen as an immunomodulator, which may predispose to this condition. With type II there is an association with the streptococcal toxic shock syndrome, similar to its staphylococcal counterpart except for the presence of necrosis as the precipitant event.
c. Type III (gas gangrene/clostridial myonecrosis): A rapidly progressive infection coined necrotizing fasciitis, it is most commonly caused by *C. perfringens* and less frequently by *C. septicum*. Most cases arise in the setting of recent surgery or trauma, being less commonly spontaneous as in types I and II. *C. perfringens* (formally *C. welchii*) is an anaerobic Gram-positive spore-forming organism that produces at least ten distinct exotoxins. The most important exotoxin leading to human pathogenesis is the alpha-toxin, which hemolyzes red blood cells, hydrolyzes cell membranes, and exerts a direct cardiodepressive effect. Within 12 to 24 hours, crepitation (Fig. 107.10) of the soft tissues may be detected by palpation (19,20). A variant of type III, known as anaerobic streptococcal myonecrosis, has a slower progression and less gas production. *Aeromonas hydrophilia*, a facultatively anaerobic, Gram-negative bacillus most commonly encountered in freshwater, can also yield a type III-like syndrome.
d. Fournier's gangrene (idiopathic gangrene of the penis and scrotum) (21): Although first described in 1764 by Baurienne, this entity received its name from a French venereologist, Jean-Alfred Fournier. In 1883 he presented a case

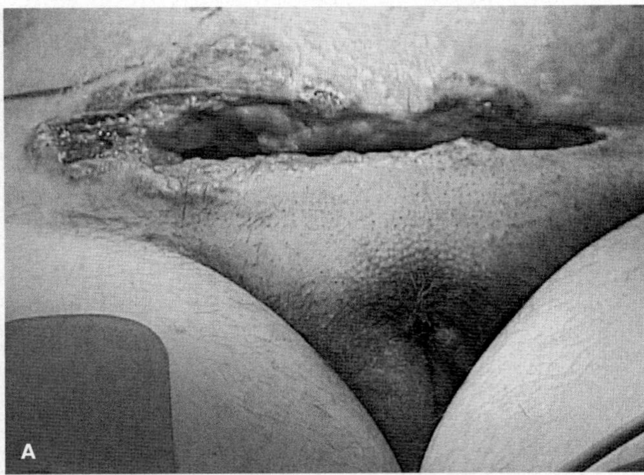

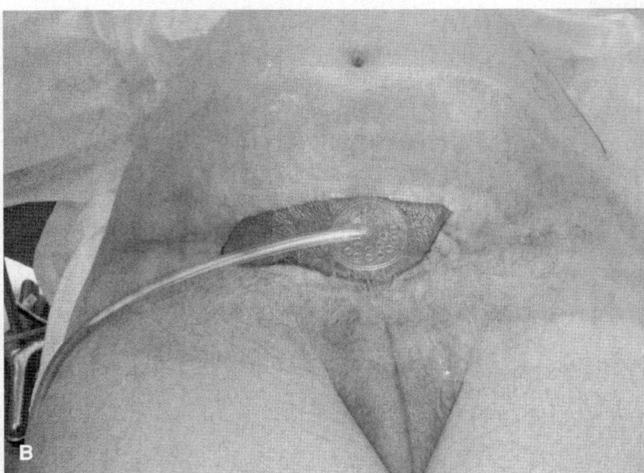

FIGURE 107.9. A,B: A 25-year-old female who had a c-section 1 week prior for placenta previa and accreta who 48 hours later developed these purplish minimally raised lesions that grew out beta-hemolytic streptococcus.

of gangrene of the perineum in an otherwise healthy young man. In 95% of cases, an identifiable cause can be found, with the disease process originating from the anorectum, the urogenital tract, or the skin of the genitalia. Anorectum causes include malignancy, diverticulitis, or appendicitis. Urethral injury, urethral stricture, urogenital manipulation, or infection can initiate Fournier's gangrene, whereas cutaneous conditions like hidradenitis suppurativa or trauma can be precursors. In addition to local predisposing conditions, systemic factors such as leukemia, systemic lupus erythematosus, Crohn's disease, HIV, or other conditions of immunodeficiency may predispose one. Other predisposing comorbidities associated with Fournier's include obesity, cirrhosis, vasculitides of the perineum, steroid use, and diabetes. On exam the typical Fournier's patient will be an elderly male in his sixth or seventh decade of life with one or more of the above comorbidities. Clinically, this patient may have a history of fever and lethargy for approximately 1 week. Pain, tenderness, and erythema of the genitalia and overlying skin will progress to a dusky appearance, ultimately with purulent-appearing drainage.

FIGURE 107.10. Necrotizing fasciitis on chest radiograph with soft tissue air in right shoulder.

There are no predictive tests as to when a superficial infection will develop into a deep infection nor is there a chemistry test for identifying a soft tissue infection. Investigation has focused on polymerase chain reaction tests specific for streptococcal pyrogenic exotoxin (SPE) genes, variants A, B, and C along with streptococcal superantigens. These superantigens cause the release of cytokines through binding to a specific segment of the T-cell receptor, resulting in an overwhelming production of TNF-α, IL-1, and IL-6 with subsequent systemic effects of sepsis and septic shock. Work has also centered on the filamentous M-protein, which is anchored to the cell membrane and has antiphagocytic properties (Fig. 107.11).

Imaging Studies for Necrotizing Fasciitis

A summary of different imaging studies is presented in Table 107.4.

Imaging studies, in particular computerized tomography, have shown with great sensitivity the presence and extent of gas or subcutaneous air. MRI T2-weighted images (Fig. 107.12) can show well-defined areas of high signal intensity significant for tissue necrosis, and absence of gadolinium contrast enhancement on T1 images reliably detects fascial necrosis in those who might require operative debridement. Ultrasound, although able to detect fluid or gas within soft tissues, requires the probe to be applied directly on the involved tissues. Many patients with NF, especially those with Fournier's, may not tolerate this, plus there may be a limitation of the anatomic site causing difficulty in visualizing deep tissues. Yen et al. (22) found ultrasound to have a sensitivity of 88% and a specificity of 93% (positive predictive value of 83%). Their diagnostic criteria included diffuse thickening of the subcutaneous tissue accompanied by fluid accumulation more than 4 mm in depth along the fascial layer.

In addition, the diagnosis can be made with culture and biopsy of the affected tissue; a Gram stain to identify single or multiple organisms would be helpful in distinguishing type I

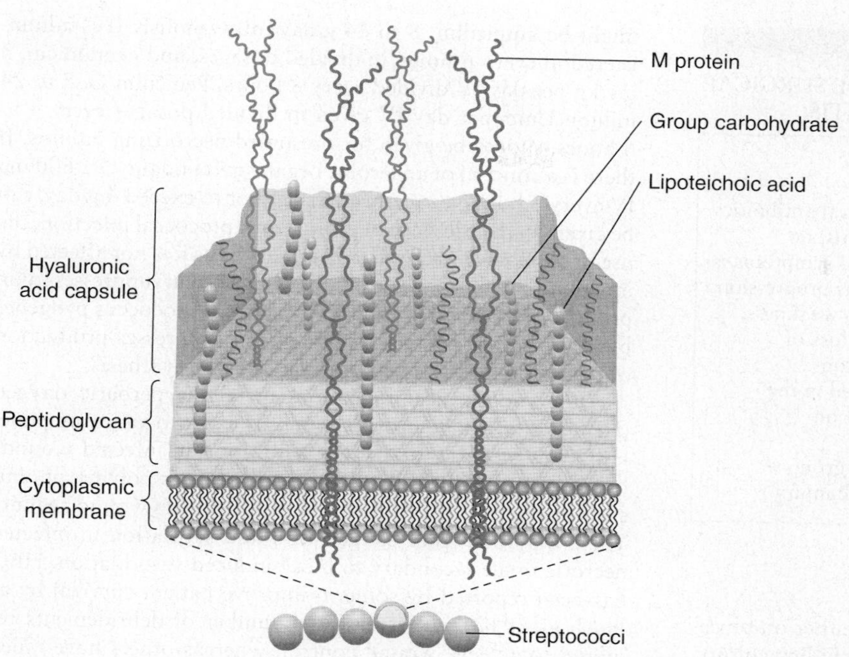

FIGURE 107.11. Action of streptococci.

TABLE 107.4

IMAGING STUDIES

Type	Role of study	Limitations	Advantages
Ultrasound	Detection of fluid and gas within soft tissues	Requires direct contact, painful	Fast, reproducible, portable to bedside
Magnetic resonance imaging (Fig. 107.12)	T2-weighted images. T1-weighted images	Unstable patients unable to tolerate time required for study	High sensitivity for extent of involvement
Plain radiographs (Fig. 107.10)	Identification of air in subcutaneous location	Seen in <50% of cases	Fast, reproducible
Computerized tomography	Detection of extent of fluid/gas in soft tissues	Requires transport, dye is nephrotoxic	High sensitivity for extent of involvement

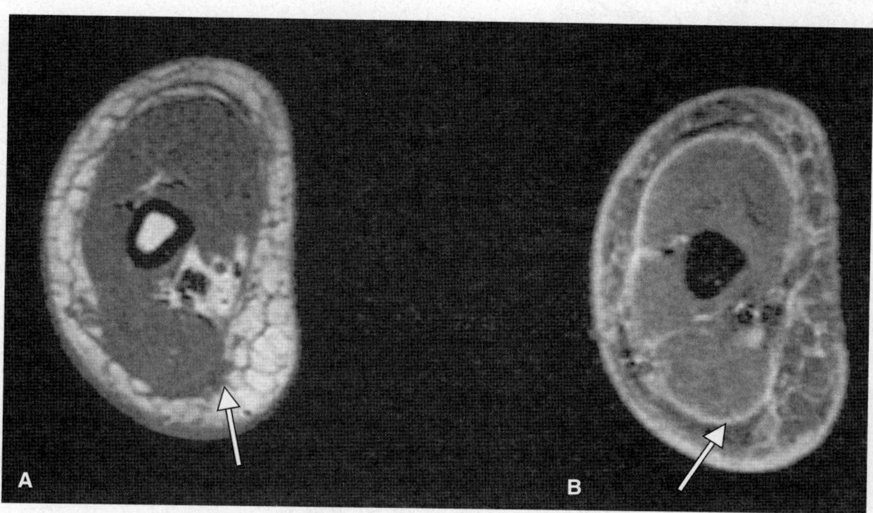

FIGURE 107.12. T1-weighted and T2-weighted magnetic resonance (MR) image of the lower extremity showing fascial thickening and fluid accumulation between the subcutaneous tissues (A) and fascial layer (B), respectively, in this patient with necrotizing fasciitis.

TABLE 107.5

CLINICAL INDICATORS PROMPTING WIDE SURGICAL INTERVENTION IN NECROTIZING FASCIITIS

Indicator	Remarks
Failure of improvement	After hours of parenteral antibiotics for presumed cellulitis, no decrease in signs and symptoms is detected or if there is progression
Profound toxic effects occurring at the onset of infection	These include malaise, weakness, generalized aching, loss of appetite/concentration
Extensive necrosis	Necrosis or gas is noted in the wound or is evident on radiographs
Compartment syndrome suspected	Edema within muscle group resulting in ischemic injury

from type II NF. Once the diagnosis is made, either on physical exam or through other diagnostic means including culture, biopsy, or excision, multimodality therapy should be used early due to the rapidity of progression.

Therapy

Until the organism is identified, broad-spectrum antibiotics should be administered. For aerobic organisms, one regimen might be ampicillin, 8 to 14 g/day intravenously (IV) administered in every-6-hours in divided dosages, and gentamicin, 3 mg/kg per day IV divided every 8 hours. Penicillin G, 8 to 24 million Units per day IV given in divided dosages every 4 to 6 hours, should be given for presumed necrotizing fasciitis. If there is a concern of anaerobic organisms clindamycin, 600 mg IV every 6 hours, or metronidazole, not to exceed 4 g/day, can be given. In the presence of group A streptococcal infection, the use of clindamycin may be advantageous as it is not affected by inoculum size or stage of growth. Clindamycin suppresses toxin production, facilitates phagocytosis of streptococcus pyogenes by inhibiting M-protein synthesis, and suppresses production of regulatory elements controlling cell wall synthesis.

Other nonsurgical modalities include hyperbaric oxygen (HBO), although no prospective study exists to justify its value. HBO can increase the oxygen saturation in infected wounds by a thousandfold, is bacteriocidal, improves polymorphonuclear leukocytes (PMN) function, and enhances wound healing. There may be higher oxygenation and saturation in infected necrotic tissue secondary to HBO-induced vasodilation. HBO has been reported by some to improve patient survival by as much as 50% and decrease the number of debridements required to achieve wound control, whereas others have failed to show any beneficial effect (23). A typical treatment protocol involves HBO given aggressively after the first surgical debridement.

Three treatment sessions, in a multiplace chamber at 3 atmospheres absolute (ATA) at 100% oxygen for 90 minutes each, can be given in the first 24 hours; in a monoplace chamber, 2.5 to 2.8 ATA, 100% oxygen for 90 minutes per session can be given. Beginning with the second day, twice-daily treatments

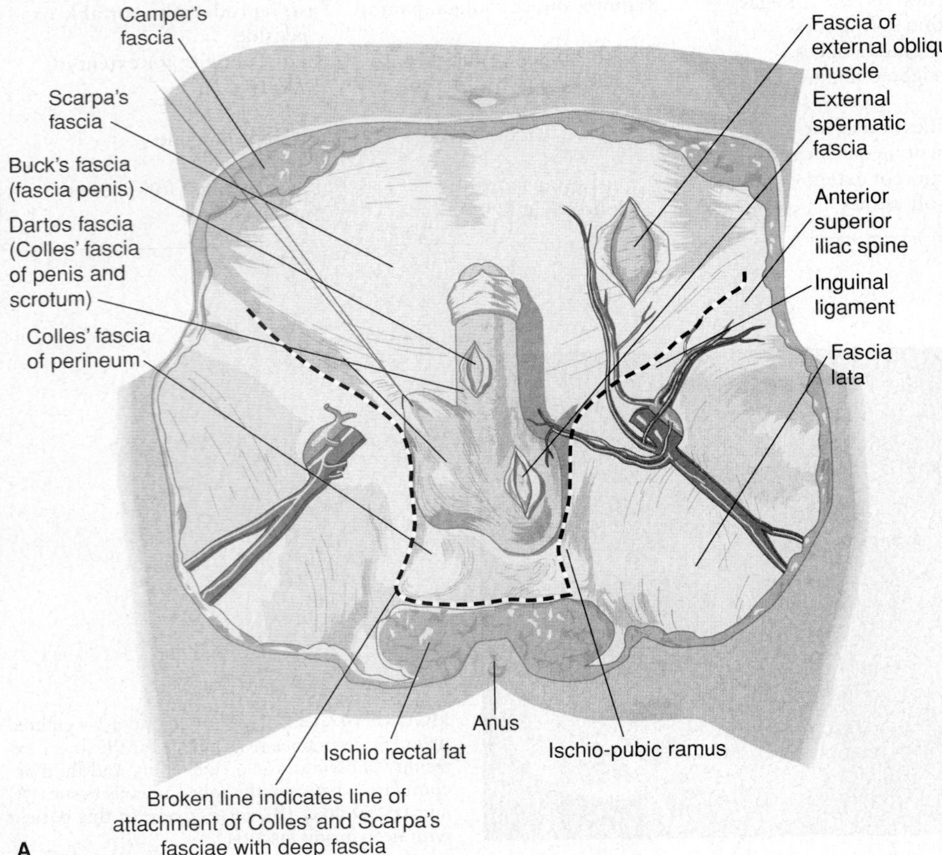

FIGURE 107.13. A-C: Fournier's gangrene involving the perineum but sparing the penis and testicles. Wide debridement has been performed. *(continued)*

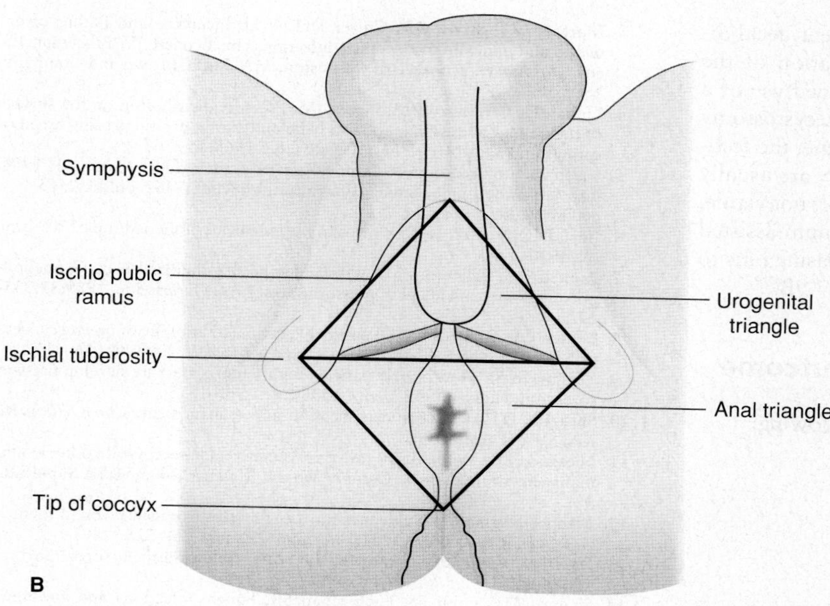

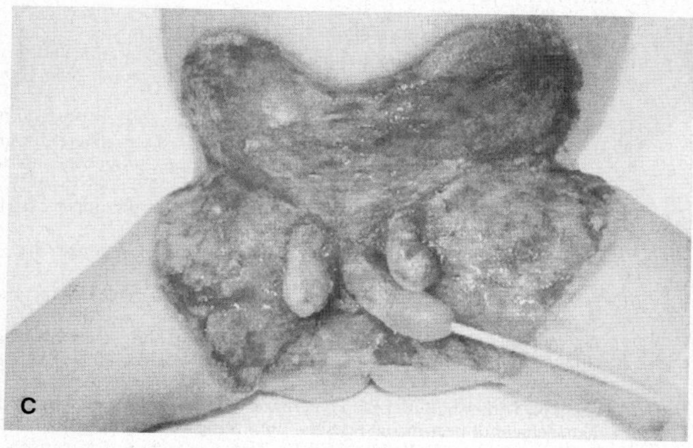

FIGURE 107.13. (continued)

are given until granulation tissue is seen, usually requiring a total of 10 to 15 treatments (24). Since clostridial myonecrosis is a monobacterial anaerobic infection, hyperbaric therapy has a greater logistic role in inhibiting clostridial growth and alpha toxin production.

Intravenous immunoglobulins (IVIG) has also been used with necrotizing soft tissue infections although there are no prospective randomized trials to support its use. Case reports indicate that IVIG inhibits activation of T cells by superantigens and thereby decreases the production of TNF-α and IL-6 by T cells, providing a beneficial effect. The Canadian Streptococcal Study Group in 1998 compared 21 consecutive patients with group A streptococcal toxic shock syndrome who were administered IVIG and had a survival benefit rate of 33% (25). Several adverse side effects occurred in $<5\%$ of patients, which can mimic a worsening course of NF. Adverse effects include pallor, flushing, fever, muscle aches, hypotension, anaphylaxis, erythema multiforme, and blood-borne pathogen transmission.

Although wide local debridement may be the classical therapy for cases of necrotizing soft tissue infections (Table 107.5), initially, diagnostic surgical exploration can be limited (26,27). A series of small incisions under local anesthesia can be performed to delineate the extent and presence of muscle or facial necrosis. In addition, frozen sections of tissue specimens obtained can establish the diagnosis. However, once the diagnosis is confirmed, there exists no role for conservative debridement or incision and drainage. In the case of Fournier's gangrene, an understanding of the anatomic relationship between the perineum and abdominal wall is important. Below the area of the inguinal ligament, Scarpa's fascia blends into the Colles's fascia, which is contiguous with the dartos fascia of the penis and scrotum (Fig. 107.13A–C). This allows a potential space to exist between the Scarpa's fascia and abdominal oblique musculature, contributing to a potential spread from the perineum to the anterior abdominal wall. Due to Buck's fascia, a deep fascia that covers the corpora and anterior urethra, and due to the retroperitoneal blood supply to the testis, the penis and testicles may be spared.

The two most common pitfalls with a necrotizing soft tissue infection are diagnostic delay and inadequate debridement. Excision of nonviable areas should be early and aggressive, with repeat debridements performed until the local process has been controlled. The use of electrocautery will aid in reducing the considerable operative blood loss if the area of involvement is extensive. With perineal involvement, fecal diversion via colostomy allows for less contamination of the wound site. With urogenital involvement, continued use of a urethral catheter is safe; occasionally suprapubic cystostomy will be necessary. In the case of Fournier's gangrene, the testicles are usually spared. To prevent dessication they are usually placed in a surgically made subcutaneous pocket. If not viable, orchiectomy is performed. In all cases of NF, vacuum-assisted closure devices have shown great promise in decreasing time to grafting and closure of the debrided area (Fig. 107.9B).

Factors Associated with Poor Outcome

Factors associated with poor outcome are the following:

Older age
Female sex
Elevated creatinine and lactate
Extent of tissue involved
Inadequate debridement
Advanced age
Truncal involvement
Chest wall involvement (28)
Presence of diabetes when in conjunction with renal dysfunction or peripheral vascular disease (29)

SUMMARY

The major points to remember with all soft tissue and musculocutaneous infections is that aggressive and early therapy in general yields the best results. This includes local care, surgical debridement, and the use of appropriate antibiotics, which can be guided by the cultures obtained. There are many new topical products coming out on the market place which can further assist in the management of these conditions and allow for improved outcome.

References

1. Centers for Disease Control and Prevention, National Center for Health Statistics. Vital and health statistics, detailed diagnoses and procedures, national hospital discharge survey, 1994. Vol. 127. Hyattsville, MD: DHHS Publication; 1997.
2. Cruse PJ, Foord R. The epidemiology of wound infections: a 10-year prospective study of 62,939 wounds. *Surg Clin North Am.* 1980;60(1):27–40.
3. Martone WJ, Jarvis WR, Culver DH, et al. Incidence and nature of endemic and epidemic nosocomial infections. In: Bennett JV, Brachman PS, eds. *Hospital Infections.* 3rd ed. Boston, MA: Little, Brown and Company; 1992:577–596.
4. Lindan O, Greenway RM, Piazza JM. Pressure distribution on the surface of the human body. Evaluation in lying and sitting positions using a bed of springs and nails. *Arch Phys Med Rehabil.* 1965;46:378.
5. Up to 25% of bedsores begin in surgery: Doctor's guide. March 11, 1998. http://www.docguide.com/dg.nsf/printprint/68cbdfa3462eofdd852565c4005496d9. Accessed
6. Revis DR. Decubitus ulcers. http://www.emedicine.com/med/topic2709.htm. Accessed
7. Bennett RG, Bellantoni MF, Ouslander JG. Air-fluidized bed treatment of nursing home patients with pressure sores. *J Am Geriatr Soc.* 1989;37:235–242.
8. Bouten CV, Oomens CW, Baaijens FP, et al. The etiology of pressure ulcers: skin deep or muscle bound? *Arch Phys Med Rehab.* 2003;84:616–619.
9. Versluysen M. How elderly patients with femoral fracture develop pressure sores in the hospital. *Br Med J.* 1986;292:1311–1313.
10. Shea JD. Pressure sores: classification and management. *Clin Orthop Rel Res.* 1975;112:89–100.
11. Niezgoda JA. Combining negative pressure wound therapy with other wound management modalities. *Ostomy Wound Manage.* 2005;51(2A Suppl):36–38.
12. Mendez-Eastman S. Guidelines for using negative pressure wound therapy. *Adv Skin Wound Care.* 2001;14(6):314–22; quiz 324–325.
13. Davis JS. Operative treatment of scars following bed sores. *Surgery.* 1938;3:1.
14. Shapiro MJ, Smith ES, Eachempati SR. Fungal infections and antifungal therapy in the surgical intensive care unit. In: Asensio J, Trunkey D, eds. *Current Therapy of Trauma and Surgical Critical Care.* Philadelphia, PA: Mosby/Elsevier; 2008:702–710.
15. Wilson B. Nectrotizing Fasciitis. *Am Surg.* 1952;18:416.
16. Clayton MD, Fowler JE Jr, Sharifi R, et al. Causes, presentation and survival of 57 patients with necrotizing fasciitis of the male genitalia. *Surg Gynecol Obstet.* 1990;170:49–55.
17. Trent JT, Kirsner RS. Necrotizing fasciitis. *Wounds.* 2002;14(8):284–292.
18. Kaul R, McGeer A, Low DE, et al. Population-based surveillance for group A streptococcal necrotizing fasciitis: clinical features, prognostic indicators and microbiologic analysis of 77 cases. *Am J Med.* 1997;103:18–24.
19. Gonzalez MH. Necrotizing fasciitis and gangrene of the upper extremity. *Hand Clin.* 1998;14:635–645.
20. Kramer LM. Necrotizing fasciitis: a case of clostridial myonecrosis. *Am J Crit Care.* 2001;10(3):181–187.
21. Yanar H, Taviloglu K, Ertekin C, et al. Fournier's gangrene: risk factors and strategies for management. *World J Surg.* 2006;30:1750–1754.
22. Yen ZS, Wang HP, Ma HM, et al. Ultrasonographic screening of clinically suspected necrotizing fasciitis. *Acad Emerg Med.* 2002;9(12):1448–1451.
23. Jallali N, Withey S, Butler PE. Hyperbaric oxygen as adjuvant therapy in the management of necrotizing fasciitis. *Am J Surg.* 2005;189(4):462–468.
24. Korhonen K, Kuttila K, Niinikoski J. Tissue gas tensions in patients with necrotising fasciitis and healthy controls during treatment with hyperbaric oxygen: a clinical study. *Eur J Surg.* 2000;166(7):530–534.
25. Kaul R, McGeer A, Norrby-Teglund A. Intravenous immunoglobulin therapy for toxic shock syndrome. *Clin Infect Dis.* 1998;28:800–807.
26. Yong JM. Rationale for the use of intravenous immunoglobulin in streptococcal necrotizing fasciitis. *Clin Immunother.* 1995;4(1):61–71.
27. Urschel JD. Necrotizing soft tissue infections. *Postgrad Med J.* 1999;75:645–649.
28. Hammainen P, Kostiainen S. Postoperative necrotizing chest wall infections. *Scand Cardiovasc J.* 1998;32:243–245.
29. Elliot DC, Kufera JA, Myers RA. Necrotizing soft tissue infections: risk factors for mortality and strategies for management. *Ann Surg.* 1996;224:672–683.

CHAPTER 108 ■ NEUROLOGIC INFECTIONS

WENDY I. SLIGL • STEPHEN D. SHAFRAN

Infections of the central nervous system (CNS) are often rapidly progressive and can be fatal if left undiagnosed and/or treatment is delayed. Prompt diagnosis and treatment are, therefore, crucial to decreasing morbidity and mortality. Patients with CNS infections commonly require intensive care unit (ICU) support, particularly for airway protection and mechanical ventilation in the presence of an altered mental status. Similarly, patients with undiagnosed CNS infections may be admitted to the ICU, offering intensivists the opportunity to make challenging diagnoses and alter patient outcomes with early and effective therapy.

Identifying the presence or absence of focal neurologic findings is the most important distinction to be made in patients with suspected neurologic infections. This distinction helps to focus the differential diagnosis and identifies patients in whom lumbar puncture may be contraindicated—at least until neuroimaging is completed. The major neurologic infections encountered in the critically ill include acute bacterial meningitis, encephalitis, brain abscess, subdural empyema, epidural abscess, and suppurative intracranial thrombophlebitis. Neurologic findings may also be the result of primary nonneurologic syndromes such as bacterial endocarditis and are covered in other chapters. Neurologic infections in advanced HIV/AIDS are also covered separately elsewhere.

The central nervous system is normally protected by various host defenses, the most important of which is the blood–brain barrier. Once micro-organisms gain entry, however, they are able to proliferate rapidly due to the low concentration of immunoglobulins and leukocytes in the CNS. Central nervous system infections can be caused by viral, bacterial, mycobacterial, fungal, or parasitic agents. Patient age, underlying host factors, and epidemiologic exposures including travel, animal or vector exposures, and contacts with infectious cases are important risk factors for acquiring specific types of infections or pathogens. Prompt physical examination to identify patients in need of urgent interventions—including endotracheal intubation—should be performed, followed by lumbar puncture and/or imaging studies. New techniques in the areas of molecular diagnostics and neuroimaging have revolutionized the approach to the diagnosis and management of patients with central nervous system infections. New therapeutic options, as well as improvements in intensive care support, have also enhanced outcomes in these patients.

The remainder of this chapter will specifically address the epidemiology, clinical presentation, diagnosis, management, and prevention of neurologic infections in the critically ill.

MENINGITIS

Key Points

- Untreated acute bacterial meningitis is universally fatal; early recognition, rapid diagnostic testing, and emergent administration of antimicrobials are crucial.
- The classic triad of fever, nuchal rigidity, and change in mental status occurs in less than 66% of patients with bacterial meningitis; however, the absence of all three of these findings effectively excludes the diagnosis with 99% to 100% sensitivity.
- Lumbar puncture should be performed urgently in all patients with suspected meningitis.
- Neuroimaging with computed tomography (CT) or magnetic resonance imaging (MRI) to rule out mass lesions should precede lumbar puncture in those with an abnormal level of consciousness, focal neurologic deficits, papilledema, a history of CNS disease, immune compromise, or seizure within 1 week of presentation.
- Empiric antimicrobial agents should be administered as soon as possible after blood cultures are collected if neuroimaging is to be performed prior to lumbar puncture or immediately following cerebrospinal fluid (CSF) collection.
- The specific microbiology and choice of empiric therapy in bacterial meningitis depend on patient risk factors, especially age, underlying host immune status, and history of preceding infections or neurosurgical procedures.
- Dexamethasone has been shown to decrease mortality in adults with *Streptococcus pneumoniae* meningitis and children with *Haemophilus influenzae*, and should therefore be administered before or concomitant with the first dose of antimicrobial in all cases pending Gram stain and culture results.
- Neurologic complications of bacterial meningitis include seizure, cerebral edema, cerebral infarction, cranial nerve involvement, venous sinus thrombosis, brain abscess, subdural empyema, and coma. Intracranial pressure monitoring and/or other surgical interventions may be required.
- Chemoprophylaxis and/or immunoprophylaxis are available for *Neisseria meningitidis*, *Haemophilus influenzae*, and infections in specific circumstances.
- In suspected meningococcal or *Haemophilus influenzae* meningitis, droplet isolation should be strictly enforced until 24 hours of effective antimicrobial therapy has been completed or an alternate diagnosis is reached. Isolation in other

cases of meningitis, including pneumococcal meningitis, is not required.

- Aseptic meningitis refers to inflammation of the meninges not attributed to bacterial infection. CSF analysis usually reveals a normal glucose, elevated protein, elevated white blood cell count with lymphocytic predominance, and negative Gram stain and bacterial cultures.
- Viral, mycobacterial, syphilitic, fungal, amoebic, and parameningeal infections should be considered in the differential diagnosis of aseptic meningitis.

Meningitis, or inflammation of the meninges, may be caused by a wide variety of micro-organisms (Table 108.1). Infectious agents gain entry to the CSF via hematogenous, transdural, or transparenchymal routes. It is important to consider noninfectious syndromes in the differential diagnosis of meningitis. Such examples include meningeal carcinomatosis, vasculitic syndromes, or drug effect (e.g., nonsteroidal anti-inflammatories, antimicrobials, immunosuppressants, anticonvulsants). Identification of such noninfectious conditions is essential, as their therapies differ from those used in the treatment of infectious syndromes; specifically, high dose corticosteroid therapy may be indicated in some of these cases. Aseptic meningitis refers to inflammation of the meninges not attributed to bacterial infection. Critically ill patients, however, present much more commonly with bacterial meningitis by virtue of the more rapid and fulminant presentation of bacterial as opposed to aseptic meningitis.

TABLE 108.1

CAUSES OF ACUTE MENINGITIS

	Common	Uncommon
Viruses	Enteroviruses non-polio Human immunodeficiency virus (HIV) Arboviruses (including West Nile virus, St. Louis encephalitis virus) Herpes simplex virus types 1 and 2 (HSV-2)	Influenza Parainfluenza Lymphocytic choriomeningitis virus (LCM) Varicella-zoster virus (VZV) Polio Mumps Cytomegalovirus (CMV) Epstein-Barr virus (EBV) Adenovirus
Bacteria	*Streptococcus pneumoniae* *Neisseria meningitidis* *Haemophilus influenzae* *Listeria monocytogenes* Enterobacteriaceae *Staphylococcus aureus* *Mycobacterium tuberculosis* *Borrelia burgdorferi* (Lyme disease) *Streptococcus agalactiae*	*Treponema pallidum* (syphilis) *Rickettsiae* *Mycoplasma* *Brucella* *Chlamydia* *Leptospira*
Fungi	*Cryptococcus neoformans* *Histoplasma capsulatum* *Coccidioides immitis*	*Candida* *Aspergillus* *Blastomyces dermatitidis* *Sporothrix schenckii*
Parasites		*Toxoplasma gondii* *Naegleria fowleri* (free-living amoeba) *Angiostrongylus cantonensis* (eosinophilic meningitis) *Strongyloides stercoralis* (hyperinfection syndrome)
Other infectious syndromes	Parameningeal focus (brain abscess, subdural empyema, epidural abscess) Infective endocarditis	
Noninfectious causes	Medications Intracranial tumor Stroke Lymphoma/leukemia Meningeal carcinomatosis Post procedure (neurosurgery) Seizure	Autoimmune diseases (SLE, sarcoid, Behçet) Migraine syndromes

SLE, systemic lupus erythematosus.

TABLE 108.2

PREDISPOSING HOST FACTORS TO SPECIFIC ETIOLOGIC AGENTS OF MENINGITIS

Immunoglobulin deficiency	*S. pneumoniae*
Asplenia	*S. pneumoniae*
Complement deficiency	*N. meningitidis*
Corticosteroid excess	*L. monocytogenes, Cryptococcus*
HIV infection	*Cryptococcus, L. monocytogenes, S. pneumoniae*
Bacteremia	*S. aureus,* Enterobacteriaceae
Fracture of cribiform plate	*S. pneumoniae*
Basal skull fracture	*S. pneumoniae, H. influenzae, S. pyogenes*
Neurotrauma, postneurosurgery	*S. aureus, S. epidermidis,* Gram-negative bacilli including *P. aeruginosa*

HIV, human immunodeficiency virus.

Bacterial Meningitis

Acute bacterial meningitis accounts for approximately 1.2 million cases annually worldwide (1). Because untreated bacterial meningitis is universally fatal, early recognition, rapid diagnostic testing, and emergent administration of antimicrobial and adjunctive agents are crucial. The most common meningeal pathogens include *Streptococcus pneumoniae* and *Neisseria meningitidis*, although specific etiologic agents and their frequencies vary with underlying host factors such as age, immune status, and route of acquisition. The case fatality rate for adults with bacterial meningitis is approximately 25%, with transient or permanent neurologic sequelae in 21% to 28% of survivors (2,3).

Bacterial meningitis develops as a result of several mechanisms (4). Certain micro-organisms that colonize the nasopharynx may invade local tissues and subsequently spread to the bloodstream and CNS. Bacteremia and subsequent CNS invasion may also develop from localized sources such as pneumonia or urinary tract infection. Last, direct entry from contiguous infection (such as via the sinuses or mastoids), trauma, neurosurgery, or prosthetic devices such as CSF shunts or cochlear implants also occurs. Host factors including functional or anatomic asplenia, complement deficiency, and congenital or acquired immunodeficiency predispose to bacterial meningitis (Table 108.2). Other risk factors for the development of meningitis include recent exposure to a patient with acute bacterial meningitis, recent travel to areas with endemic meningococcal disease, injection drug use, recent neurotrauma or CSF leak, and otorrhea.

The median duration of symptoms prior to admission in bacterial meningitis is impressively short, averaging approximately 24 hours (5). The classic triad of fever, nuchal rigidity, and change in mental status occurs in less than 66% of cases; however, almost all patients have at least one of these findings (6). It bears reiterating that the absence of any of these findings effectively excludes the diagnosis with 99% to 100% sensitivity.

Nuchal rigidity can be detected with passive or active flexion of the neck. Tests, such as the Kernig and Brudzinski signs, are well-described physical examination techniques but are neither sensitive nor specific (7). In addition to severe headache, patients often note photophobia, and seizures, focal neurologic deficits, and papilledema may be seen on physical examination. Some patients may not manifest the classic signs and symptoms of bacterial meningitis, particularly neonates and those with underlying immunosuppressive conditions including diabetes, chronic organ failure, neutropenia, chronic corticosteroid use, transplantation, and HIV infection.

Certain micro-organisms may present with specific physical findings. Meningococcal meningitis may present with characteristic skin manifestations consisting of diffuse petechiae and purpura on the distal extremities. Skin findings occur in approximately one fourth of bacterial meningitis cases, over 90% of which are due to *Neisseria meningitidis* infection (8).

As a result of the widespread use of conjugate vaccine for *H. influenzae* type b in infants, *Streptococcus pneumoniae* has become the most frequently observed cause of bacterial meningitis, accounting for 47% of total cases (9). *S. pneumoniae* serotypes causing bacteremic disease are also those commonly responsible for meningitis. Focal infection is common with contiguous or distant sites, including sinusitis, mastoiditis, pneumonia, otitis media, and endocarditis. The major risk factors for pneumococcal meningitis include asplenia, hypogammaglobulinemia, alcoholism, chronic renal or hepatic disease, malignancy, diabetes mellitus, basal skull fracture with CSF leak, and the presence of a cochlear implant. Mortality rate range from 19% to 30% (9–13).

Neisseria meningitidis commonly causes meningitis in children and young adults. Serogroups B, C, and Y are responsible for most endemic disease in North America, accounting for 32%, 35%, and 26% of cases, respectively (14). Epidemic disease is most commonly caused by serogroup C, with fewer outbreaks due to serogroup A. In 2000, epidemic W-135 was associated with the Hajj pilgrimage to Mecca in Saudi Arabia (15). Subsequently, meningococcal vaccination has become legally required prior to undertaking this activity. Risk factors for invasive meningococcal disease include nasopharyngeal carriage, terminal complement deficiency, and properdin deficiency (16,17). Although a characteristic rapidly evolving petechial or purpuric rash strongly suggests *N. meningitidis*, a similar rash may be seen in splenectomized patients with overwhelming *S. pneumoniae* or *H. influenzae* type b infection.

Haemophilus influenzae previously accounted for a large proportion of cases of bacterial meningitis; however, widespread vaccination against *H. influenzae* type b has now markedly decreased its incidence (Table 108.3). Isolation of *H. influenzae* type b in adults suggests the presence of an

TABLE 108.3

INCIDENCE BY CAUSE OF BACTERIAL MENINGITIS IN THE UNITED STATES, 1995

Micro-organism	Rate per 100,000
Streptococcus pneumoniae	1.1
Neisseria meningitidis	0.6
Streptococcus agalactiae (group B streptococcus)	0.3
Listeria monocytogenes	0.2
Haemophilus influenzae type b	0.2

From Schuchat A, et al. Bacterial meningitis in the United States in 1995. Active Surveillance Team. *N Engl J Med.* 1997;337(14): 970–976, with permission.

underlying condition such as sinusitis, otitis media, pneumonia, diabetes mellitus, alcoholism, CSF leak, asplenia, or immune deficiency.

Listeria monocytogenes meningitis carries a mortality rate of 15% to 29% (9,12). It occurs in neonates, adults older than 50 years of age, and in those with risk factors including alcoholism, malignancy, pregnancy, and immune suppression secondary to corticosteroid therapy or transplantation. It is interesting that this infection is seen infrequently in HIV-infected patients for unknown reasons. Pregnant women may be asymptomatic carriers and transmit infection to their infants. *L. monocytogenes* commonly makes up part of the fecal flora of farm animals and can be isolated from soil, water, or contaminated vegetables. Outbreaks have been associated with unpasteurized dairy products such as milk and cheeses, vegetables, and processed meats (18–20).

Aerobic Gram-negative bacilli can cause meningitis in specific groups of patients. Predisposing risk factors include neurosurgical procedures, neonatal status, advanced age, immune suppression, Gram-negative bacteremia, and disseminated *Strongyloides stercoralis* infection with hyperinfection syndrome. *Escherichia coli* is a common cause of meningitis in neonates.

Staphylococcus aureus or *Staphylococcus epidermidis* can both cause meningitis but are, however, less common than the previously described micro-organisms. Both staphylococcal species exist as part of the normal skin flora, predominantly causing infections following neurosurgery or neurotrauma, or when prosthetic material is present, particularly external ventricular drains or ventriculoperitoneal shunts. Some patients with staphylococcal bacterial meningitis have underlying infective endocarditis, paraspinal or epidural infection, sinusitis, osteomyelitis, or pneumonia.

Other less common causes of bacterial meningitis include enterococci, viridans group streptococci, beta-hemolytic streptococci, diphtheroids and *Propionibacterium acnes*—generally only in the setting of prosthetic material—and anaerobic species.

Viral Meningitis

Viruses are the most commonly isolated pathogens in aseptic meningitis. The nonpolio enteroviruses, especially Coxsackie viruses A and B, and echoviruses are common, accounting for 85% to 95% of all cases of aseptic meningitis with an identified pathogen (21). Enteroviruses occur worldwide, are transmitted by fecal-oral or respiratory droplet spread, and exhibit summer and fall seasonality in temperate climates. Infants, children, and young adults are commonly affected. Clinical manifestations depend on host age and immune status but generally include abrupt onset of severe headache, fever, nausea, vomiting, photophobia, nuchal rigidity, and malaise. Rash and upper respiratory symptoms are common. Only rarely is illness severe enough to require critical care.

Arboviruses more commonly cause encephalitis but have also been isolated in cases of aseptic meningitis. Arboviruses endemic to North America include the flaviviruses—such as St. Louis encephalitis virus, Colorado tick fever, Japanese encephalitis virus, and West Nile virus—and California encephalitis viruses. Arboviruses occur predominantly in the summer and early fall when vector exposure is most likely. St. Louis encephalitis virus is mosquito borne and causes epidemic disease in the Mississippi River area. Japanese encephalitis virus less commonly causes meningitis, is endemic in Asia, and requires prolonged stays in rural settings for acquisition so is uncommon even in returned travelers.

West Nile virus (WNV) came to widespread attention in 1999 when the first North American cases were identified. Since then, the virus has spread extensively across North America and should be considered in all patients with meningitis, particularly in late summer or early fall. WNV infection is asymptomatic in 80% of cases. The remaining patients present with West Nile nonneurologic syndrome (approximately 20%; formerly named West Nile fever) or West Nile neurologic syndrome (WNNS; less than 1%). West Nile nonneurologic syndrome is a self-limited febrile illness characterized by fever, headache, malaise, myalgias, and often a rash (50%). WNNS may present as encephalitis, meningitis, or flaccid paralysis. Meningitis, however, is the least common presentation of WNNS.

Lymphocytic choriomeningitis (LCM) virus is a zoonotic disease, transmitted by contact with infected rodents—such as house mice, rats, hamsters—or their feces. Though now rare, LCM virus was one of the first viruses to be associated with aseptic meningitis (4). Infection is more common in the winter months. Presenting manifestations include an influenza-like syndrome and meningismus, with occasional rash, orchitis, arthritis, myopericarditis, and transient alopecia.

Six of the eight recognized human herpesviruses can cause meningitis. Herpes simplex viruses (HSV) are most commonly associated with aseptic meningitis during primary genital infection, affecting 36% of women and 13% of men with primary genital herpes (22). HSV-2 infection is responsible for most infections; nonetheless, HSV-1 genital infection and concomitant meningitis can also occur. Meningitis is much less likely in the setting of genital herpes recurrences. Headache, photophobia, and meningismus are common presenting symptoms. Genital lesions are present in 85% of patients with primary HSV-2 meningitis and generally precede meningeal symptoms by several days.

Herpes zoster aseptic meningitis, with or without typical skin lesions, has also been reported, particularly in older patients. Cytomegalovirus (CMV), Epstein-Barr virus (EBV), and human herpes virus 6 (HHV-6) are all capable of causing aseptic meningitis but occur very rarely, predominantly in immune-suppressed populations.

HIV-associated aseptic meningitis can occur with primary infection in approximately 5% to 10% of patients (22). Cranial neuropathies may be present along with headache, fever, and meningismus. Symptoms are usually self-limited.

Mumps, now rare as a result of universal vaccination programs, was once a relatively common cause of aseptic meningitis. The clinical manifestations include fever, vomiting, headache, and parotitis in approximately 50% of patients. Meningismus, lethargy, and abdominal pain may also be present.

Other Less Common Infectious Causes

Spirochetal meningitis may be caused by *Treponema pallidum* or *Borrelia burgdorferi*. *T. pallidum*, the etiologic agent of syphilis, is acquired by sexual contact, placental transfer, or direct contact with active lesions; these include condyloma lata, mucous patches, or the rash of secondary syphilis. Syphilitic meningitis usually occurs during primary or secondary infection, complicating 0.3% to 2.4% of untreated infections during the first 2 years (4). *B. burgdorferi* is transmitted by the *Ixodes* tick and causes Lyme disease. It is the most common vector-borne disease in the United States. Meningitis can occur during the first stage of disease, concurrently with erythema migrans at the tick bite site. Dissemination of the microorganism in the second stage of disease, 2 to 10 weeks following exposure, may also result in aseptic meningitis. Late or chronic disease may include subacute encephalopathy but not meningitis.

Mycobacterium tuberculosis may cause a subacute or chronic form of meningitis. Infection of the meninges results from rupture of a tuberculous focus into the subarachnoid space. In very young patients, concomitant disseminated systemic infection is common. Epidemiologic risk factors include a known prior history of tuberculosis (TB) exposure, residence in an endemic area, contact with an active case, incarceration, homelessness, and HIV infection. Tuberculin skin testing is negative in over half of patients with tuberculous meningitis (23,24). A negative skin test, therefore, cannot be used to exclude tuberculous meningitis, as is also the case with other active tuberculous infections. Newer tests, such as the QuantiFERON-TB Gold test, may be available in some centers (25).

Fungal meningitis, although uncommon, should be considered, particularly given the high mortality associated with untreated infection. *Cryptococcus neoformans* predominantly affects immunocompromised hosts but can also infect the immunocompetent. The encapsulated yeast is distributed worldwide but prefers wet forested regions with decaying wood and is found in particularly high concentrations in pigeon guano. Risk factors for cryptococcal infection include HIV/AIDS, prolonged corticosteroid therapy, immunosuppression post-transplantation, malignancy, and sarcoidosis. Clinical presentation is typically indolent, occurring over 1 to 2 weeks, and is characterized by fever, malaise, and headache. Meningismus, photophobia, and vomiting occur in less than 33% of patients. *Cryptococcus gattii*, a serotype usually restricted to tropical climates, emerged on Vancouver Island, British Columbia (BC), Canada in 1999 and has since been responsible for numerous cases of CNS infection in predominantly immunocompetent hosts in BC and the U.S. Pacific Northwest.

Coccidioides immitis, a dimorphic fungus, is found in soil in the dry desert regions of the southwest United States, Mexico, and Central and South America. Infection results after inhalation of arthroconidia, usually following a dust storm or during building construction. Infection is usually confined to the respiratory system in those with competent immune systems. However, extrapulmonary dissemination to the meninges can occur in patients with immune compromise or during pregnancy. Patients present with headache, vomiting, and altered level of consciousness. Risk factors for the development of disease include travel to or residence in an endemic region and immune deficiency. Coccidioidal meningitis is universally fatal if untreated.

Less common fungal causes of meningitis include *Blastomyces dermatitidis*, *Histoplasma capsulatum*, *Sporothrix schenckii*, and rarely, *Candida* species. *B. dermatitis*, *H. capsulatum*, and *S. schenckii* are all dimorphic fungi with similar presentations to coccidioidal meningitis. Primary infection occurs via inhalation, and disseminated infection occurs predominantly in immune compromised populations. *B. dermatitidis* and *H. capsulatum* are endemic in the Mississippi and Ohio River Valleys. *S. schenckii* has been reported worldwide, with most cases in the tropical regions of the Americas.

Candida exists only in yeast form and is part of the normal flora of skin and gastrointestinal tract. CNS involvement is most commonly due to candidemia with subsequent meningeal seeding. Predisposing risk factors for candidemia include the use of broad-spectrum antibiotics, the presence of indwelling devices such as vascular or urinary catheters, parenteral nutrition, intensive care unit admission, prolonged hospital stay, and immune compromise. Specific risk factors for *Candida* CNS infection include ventricular shunts, trauma, neurosurgery, or lumbar puncture (26,27). *C. albicans* is the most commonly isolated species; however, nonalbicans species are becoming more prevalent, particularly in ICU populations (28–30).

Meningitis caused by protozoa or helminths is extremely rare. The free-living amoebas *Acanthamoeba*, *Balamuthia*, and *Naegleria fowleri* are associated with fresh water exposure. They are usually acquired by individuals diving into contaminated lakes or swimming pools. CNS invasion occurs via penetration of the nasal mucosa and cribriform plate. *N. fowleri* can cause a primary amoebic meningoencephalitis. *Acanthamoeba* and *Balamuthia* rarely cause meningitis; they commonly present as encephalitis.

Angiostrongylus cantonensis, the rat lungworm, is the classic infectious cause of eosinophilic meningitis (>10% eosinophils in the CSF) (Table 108.4). Humans are incidental hosts and develop neurologic symptoms as a result of larval migration through the CNS. *A. cantonensis* is endemic in Southeast Asia and the Pacific Islands and is acquired by ingesting raw mollusks such as snails or slugs. *Gnathostoma spinigerum*, acquired by ingestion of raw and undercooked fish and poultry, is not primarily neurotropic like *A. cantonensis* but may also cause eosinophilic meningitis as a result of migration of larvae up the nerve tracts to the CNS. Gnathostomiasis is endemic in Asia, especially Thailand and Japan, and more recently in Mexico. *Baylisascaris procyonis*, a roundworm infection of raccoons, rarely causes human eosinophilic meningoencephalitis following accidental ingestion of ova from raccoon feces in contaminated water, soil, or foods.

Diagnosis

Lumbar puncture (LP) should be performed emergently in all patients suspected of having bacterial meningitis unless

TABLE 108.4

CEREBROSPINAL FLUID TESTS IN SUSPECTED CNS INFECTION

Routine tests	Further testing
Cell count and differential	Lactate Viral studies: Viral culture PCR for Enteroviruses, HSV, WNV, VZV, influenza
Protein	AFB stain and Mycobacterial culture
Glucose (preferably with simultaneous serum glucose)	Cryptococcal antigen test (can send serum as well, sensitivity comparable to CSF)
Gram stain	Fungal culture
Bacterial culture and sensitivity	VDRL, FTA-Abs, *T. pallidum* PCR[a] Cytology Cytospin and flow cytometry if available Wet mount if PAM suspected Lyme-specific Ab and PCR[a]

CNS, central nervous system; PCR, polymerase chain reaction; HSV, herpes simplex virus; WNV, West Nile virus; VZV, varicella-zoster virus; AFB, acid-fast bacillus; CSF, cerebrospinal fluid; VDRL, Venereal Diseases Research Laboratory; FTA-Abs, fluorescent treponemal antibody absorption; PAM, primary amoebic meningoencephalitis.
[a]Experimental, available only in research laboratories

contraindicated, although it is commonly unnecessarily delayed while neuroimaging is performed to exclude mass lesions. Complications associated with lumbar puncture are uncommon; however, the incidence of life-threatening brain herniation has been reported to range from less than 1% to 6% (31,32). A recent study evaluating the clinical features at baseline associated with abnormal findings on CT scan, and thus, increased risk of brain herniation, identified: age greater than or equal to 60 years; a history of CNS disease such as a mass lesion, stroke, and focal infection; immune compromise such as HIV or immunosuppressive therapy; a history of seizure less than or equal to 1 week before presentation; and specific abnormal neurologic findings (33). Based on these findings, guidelines for which adult patients should undergo CT prior to LP have been recommended (Table 108.5) (34).

TABLE 108.5

INDICATIONS FOR IMAGING PRIOR TO LUMBAR PUNCTURE IN ADULTS WITH SUSPECTED BACTERIAL MENINGITIS

Indications
Immunocompromised state (HIV/AIDS, immunosuppressive therapy)
History of CNS disease (mass lesion, stroke, or focal infection)
New-onset seizure (less than or equal to 1 week of presentation)
Papilledema
Abnormal level of consciousness
Focal neurologic deficit (dilated nonreactive pupil, abnormalities of ocular motility, abnormal visual fields, arm or leg drift)

HIV, human immunodeficiency virus; AIDS, acquired immunodeficiency syndrome; CNS, central nervous system.

Nosocomial meningitis is rare in nonneurosurgical patients; nevertheless, lumbar punctures are often performed in hospitalized patients with unexplained fever and/or decreased level of consciousness. The yield of performing an LP in the nonneurosurgical population is extremely low and of questionable utility (35).

CSF analysis is extremely important in the diagnosis of meningitis. Basic laboratory analyses, including cell count and differential, protein, glucose, Gram stain, and bacterial cultures, are most useful in distinguishing between viral, bacterial, tuberculous, and fungal infection (Table 108.3).

Bacterial Meningitis

Bacterial meningitis usually presents with an elevated systemic white blood cell (WBC) count and left shift (immature forms such as bands and myeloids). Leukopenia is occasionally present in severe infection. Thrombocytopenia may be the result of sepsis, disseminated intravascular coagulation, or meningococcemia alone. Renal and hepatic dysfunction may occur as part of multiorgan failure in severe disease. Blood cultures are often positive and should always be drawn prior to the administration of antimicrobials, particularly if the LP cannot be performed immediately. Approximately 66% of patients with bacterial meningitis have positive blood cultures (8).

CSF analysis in bacterial meningitis classically reveals a neutrophilic pleocytosis with hundreds to thousands of cells and greater than 80% neutrophils. In fact, a low CSF WBC count is usually a marker of poor prognosis in this setting. The CSF glucose concentration is usually low and should always be compared with a simultaneous serum glucose measurement. An abnormal CSF-to–serum glucose ratio (less than 0.5) is common in bacterial meningitis—and it is often much lower than 0.5. Acute illness in diabetics may increase serum glucose levels markedly, making the CSF-to–serum glucose ratio inaccurate. In the postoperative neurosurgical patient, elevated CSF

TABLE 108.6

TYPICAL CSF PARAMETERS IN PATIENTS WITH MENINGITIS

Etiology	WBC Count (cells/mm^3)	Predominant cell type	Protein (mg/dL)	Glucose (mg/dL)	Opening Pressure (cm H_2O)
Normal	0–5	Lymphocyte	15–40	50–75	8–20
Viral	10–500	Lymphocyte[a]	Normal	Normal	9–20
Bacterial	100–5,000	Neutrophil	>100	<40	20–30
Tuberculous	50–300	Lymphocyte	>100	<40	18–30
Cryptococcal	20–500	Lymphocyte	50–200	<40	18–30

CSF, cerebrospinal fluid.
[a]Neutrophils may predominate in the first 24 hours.

lactate concentrations (greater than or equal to 4.0 mMol/L) have been shown to be superior to CSF-to–blood glucose ratios (36), and initiation of empirical antimicrobial therapy in this setting should be considered pending the results of additional studies (34). CSF protein and opening pressure are usually elevated in bacterial meningitis (Table 108.6).

Gram staining permits rapid identification of bacterial species and is positive in approximately 50% to 60% of patients with bacterial meningitis. The presence of bacteria is virtually 100% specific, but sensitivity is variable. The Gram stain is more likely to be positive in patients with high bacterial loads. Gram-positive diplococci suggest *S. pneumoniae* infection, Gram-negative diplococci suggest *N. meningitidis* infection, Gram-positive rods suggest *L. monocytogenes* infection, and small pleomorphic coccobacilli suggest *H. influenzae* infection.

CSF bacterial cultures are positive in approximately 70% to 85% of cases. The yield decreases significantly in patients treated with antimicrobials prior to CSF collection. Antigen assays (latex agglutination tests) have been used in these cases, but due to their low sensitivity are no longer routinely offered by many laboratories. Broad-based polymerase chain reaction (PCR) may be useful for excluding the diagnosis of bacterial meningitis (34) but is unavailable in many centers.

Viral Meningitis

In acute viral meningitis, the CSF cell count is usually in the low hundreds with lymphocytic predominance. A predominance of neutrophils may be seen in the first 24 hours of disease, occasionally confusing the diagnosis. The CSF glucose concentration is usually within normal range. CSF protein is usually mildly elevated, and the opening pressure is usually normal.

Viral cultures and nucleic acid amplification tests are most commonly used in the diagnosis of viral meningitis. Enteroviruses may be cultured from CSF, throat, or rectal swabs, with a sensitivity of 65% to 70%, or identified by nucleic acid amplification testing. Enteroviral PCR is both sensitive and specific. PCR for HSV is also widely available, and in studies of HSV-1 encephalitis, HSV PCR demonstrated a specificity of approximately 100% and sensitivity of 75% to 98% (37,38). False negatives occur mostly within the first 72 hours of infection. The diagnosis of WNV can be made by detection of serum IgM or a fourfold rise in IgG between acute and convalescent titers. WNV PCR of serum and CSF are also available; however, the sensitivity is higher in CSF specimens due to the short-lived viremia in humans.

Other Less Common Causes

CSF analysis in syphilitic meningitis is characterized by a mild lymphocytic pleocytosis, decreased glucose, and elevated protein. *T. pallidum* cannot be cultured, so diagnosis must be made using alternate methods, predominantly serology. Direct visualization by darkfield microscopy or direct fluorescent antibody testing may be possible if a primary chancre or skin lesion of secondary syphilis—condyloma latum or mucous patch—is present. Serologic testing should include nontreponemal (RPR, rapid plasma reagin; VDRL, Venereal Diseases Research Laboratory) and treponemal (TPPA, *Treponema pallidum* particle agglutination; FTA-Abs, fluorescent treponemal antibody absorption) tests for the diagnosis of active syphilis infection. *Treponema*-specific enzyme immunoassays (EIA) for IgM and IgG are replacing the above traditional serologic tests as the initial laboratory diagnostic test in some centers. CSF VDRL may be used in the diagnosis of syphilitic meningitis. The specificity is high, but false positives occur in bloody specimens. The major limitation of CSF VDRL is its low sensitivity (30% to 70%), so a negative result should not be used to rule out infection in the setting of high clinical suspicion. CSF FTA-Abs is more sensitive; however, false positives are common due to serum antibody leak into the CSF. Last, PCR has been recently used to detect *T. pallidum* DNA in the CSF. Further studies are needed to ascertain the sensitivity and specificity of this test.

Lyme meningitis is characterized by a mild lymphocytic pleocytosis, low glucose, and an elevated protein. The CSF concentration of *B. burgdorferi* antibody, compared to serum levels, is a sensitive and specific diagnostic method. PCR is currently available only in research laboratories, although it will likely become the diagnostic test of choice in the near future. CSF oligoclonal bands and *B. burgdorferi* culture are also available, but neither is sensitive or specific.

The CSF analysis in tuberculosis meningitis demonstrates a lymphocytic pleocytosis, low glucose, and markedly elevated protein and opening pressure. The elevation in protein is particularly marked in the setting of CSF block. Acid-fast bacillus (AFB) smears are very low yield; only 10% to 22% of cases will be positive (24,39,40). Mycobacterial cultures, although slow growing—taking several weeks—become positive in up to 88% of cases (4). DNA probes and nucleic acid amplification techniques (mainly PCR) have recently become available with great improvements in sensitivity and specificity. Meningeal biopsy is rarely performed but may show caseating granulomata. Skin testing and QuantiFERON-TB Gold testing have been discussed in the previous section. Sputum and urine AFB, as well as mycobacterial blood cultures, should also be included as part of the TB workup in these patients.

Cryptococcal meningitis is characterized by a lymphocytic pleocytosis, decreased glucose, and elevated protein. Opening pressures may be markedly elevated. Culture of *C. neoformans* or *C. gattii* from the CSF is diagnostic; however, other simpler tests are now available. Detection of serum or CSF cryptococcal antigen (CrAg) is highly sensitive (greater than 90%). India ink was previously regarded as the standard diagnostic test, but due to its low sensitivity (50%), it has been largely replaced by antigen testing. Fungal blood cultures may also be useful, as cryptococcal meningitis occasionally occurs in the setting of disseminated cryptococcal infection with cryptococcemia, especially in HIV-infected patients.

Other fungal meningitides are similarly characterized by a lymphocytic pleocytosis, low to normal glucose, and an elevated protein. Coccidioidal meningitis may present with an eosinophilic pleocytosis and peripheral eosinophilia. Fungal cultures are diagnostic and are most useful in *Candida* or *Aspergillus* infection. Dimorphic fungal infection may be diagnosed serologically, as isolating these organisms from the CSF is challenging and of low yield. Detection of complement-fixing (CF) IgG antibodies or immunodiffusion tests for IgM and IgG in CSF are currently the standard diagnostic tests. Low-titer false positives may occur in the setting of parameningeal foci. As well, false negatives may occur in early disease.

Primary amoebic meningoencephalitis due to *N. fowleri* results in a neutrophilic pleocytosis, increased red blood cells, low glucose, and an elevated protein. Demonstration of motile trophozoites on a wet mount of CSF or biopsy specimens is diagnostic. The diagnosis of *A. cantonensis, G. spinigerum*, or *B. procyonis* requires an appropriate epidemiologic exposure, peripheral blood eosinophilia, and a characteristic eosinophilic pleocytosis. Serologic tests are helpful but performed only in reference laboratories.

Treatment

The initial management of the patient with suspected meningitis is primarily guided by epidemiologic risk factors and lumbar puncture results. The CSF cell count, glucose, and Gram stain are crucial in guiding empiric therapy. If the LP is delayed for any reason, empiric antimicrobial therapy should not be withheld (Table 108.7), as delays in therapy have been associated with adverse clinical outcomes and increased mortality (41,42). The administration of antimicrobials should immediately follow blood culture collection and should not be delayed by neuroimaging or other tests performed prior to LP.

Bacterial Meningitis

As noted above, lumbar puncture should be performed urgently in those with suspected meningitis. A protocol for the management of bacterial meningitis is presented in Figure 108.1. Imaging should be performed prior to LP in specific populations (Table 108.5) but should not result in a delay in the initiation of antimicrobial therapy. Empiric therapy should be based on

TABLE 108.7

EMPIRIC THERAPY OF BACTERIAL MENINGITIS BASED ON AGE AND HOST FACTORS

	Most common causes	Recommended therapy
Age: Preterm to less than 1 month	*Streptococcus agalactiae* *Escherichia coli* *Listeria monocytogenes*	Ampicillin + cefotaxime or ceftriaxone
Age: 1 month to 50 years	*Streptococcus pneumoniae* *Neisseria meningitidis* *Haemophilus influenzae*	Cefotaxime or ceftriaxone + vancomycin[a] + dexamethasone[b]
Age: greater than 50 years or alcoholism or other debilitating diseases or impaired cellular immunity	*Streptococcus pneumoniae* *Listeria monocytogenes* Coliform Gram-negative bacilli	Ampicillin + cefotaxime or ceftriaxone + vancomycin[a] + dexamethasone[b]
Post neurosurgery, neurotrauma, or cochlear implant	*Streptococcus pneumoniae* *Staphylococcus aureus* Coliform Gram-negative bacilli *Pseudomonas aeruginosa*	Vancomycin + ceftazidime or meropenem
Ventriculitis/meningitis due to infected shunt	*Staphylococcus epidermidis* *Staphylococcus aureus* Coliform Gram-negative bacilli Diphtheroids *Propionibacterium acnes*	Vancomycin + ceftazidime or meropenem

[a]Vancomycin should be added in centers where *S. pneumoniae* may be resistant to third-generation cephalosporins
[b]Dexamethasone is efficacious in children with *H. influenzae* and in adults with *S. pneumoniae*. The first dose is to be given 15 to 20 minutes prior to or concomitant with first dose of antibiotic. Dose, 0.15 mg/kg IV every 6 hours for 2 to 4 days; discontinue if micro-organism isolated other than listed above.

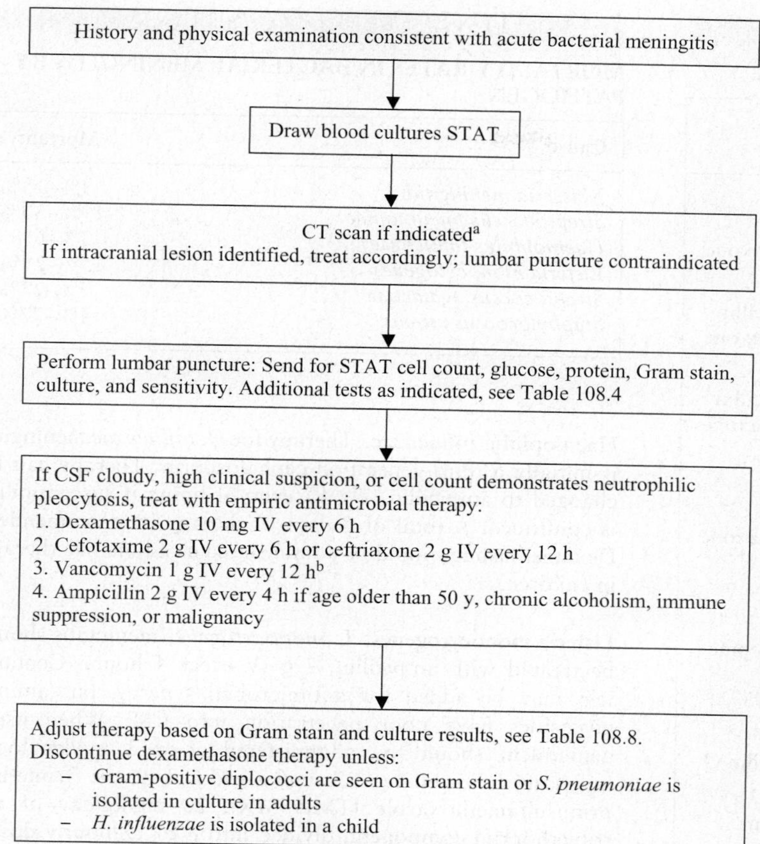

History and physical examination consistent with acute bacterial meningitis
Draw blood cultures STAT
CT scan if indicated[a]
If intracranial lesion identified, treat accordingly; lumbar puncture contraindicated
Perform lumbar puncture: Send for STAT cell count, glucose, protein, Gram stain, culture, and sensitivity. Additional tests as indicated, see Table 108.4
If CSF cloudy, high clinical suspicion, or cell count demonstrates neutrophilic pleocytosis, treat with empiric antimicrobial therapy:
1. Dexamethasone 10 mg IV every 6 h
2 Cefotaxime 2 g IV every 6 h or ceftriaxone 2 g IV every 12 h
3. Vancomycin 1 g IV every 12 h[b]
4. Ampicillin 2 g IV every 4 h if age older than 50 y, chronic alcoholism, immune suppression, or malignancy
Adjust therapy based on Gram stain and culture results, see Table 108.8.
Discontinue dexamethasone therapy unless:
– Gram-positive diplococci are seen on Gram stain or S. pneumoniae is isolated in culture in adults
– H. influenzae is isolated in a child
[a]Indications: Decreased mental status, focal neurologic deficits, history of recent head trauma or intracranial malignancy, immune suppression (HIV, transplantation, chronic corticosteroid use).
[b]Vancomycin is recommended if third-generation cephalosporin–resistant S. pneumoniae isolates have been documented locally

FIGURE 108.1. Bacterial Meningitis Protocol

age, underlying host factors, and initial CSF Gram stain results (Table 108.7).

The choice of antimicrobial therapy in bacterial meningitis is influenced by blood–CSF barrier penetration, effect of meningeal inflammation on penetration, and the bactericidal efficacy. In general, CSF penetration is enhanced in the setting of meningeal inflammation due to increased permeability. Additionally, high lipid solubility, low molecular weight, and low protein binding increase CSF drug levels. Bactericidal efficacy may be decreased in purulent CSF, particularly with aminoglycosides, due to the low pH. Penicillins, third-generation cephalosporins, carbapenems, fluoroquinolones, and rifampin achieve high CSF levels and are all bactericidal. Antimicrobials should be adjusted based on renal and hepatic function. Therapeutic drug monitoring may be required to ensure adequate levels and prevent toxicity (e.g., vancomycin, aminoglycosides). Antimicrobial therapy should be adjusted based on culture and susceptibility results as soon as possible (Table 108.8). In suspected meningococcal or *H. influenzae* meningitis, droplet isolation (single room, gowns, gloves, surgical masks, and dedicated patient care equipment) should be strictly enforced until 24 hours of effective antimicrobial therapy have been completed or an alternate diagnosis is reached. Isolation in other cases of meningitis, including pneumococcal meningitis, is not required (Table 108.9).

Streptococcus pneumoniae. Empiric therapy guidelines for pneumococcal meningitis have been recently modified due to the increasing incidence of penicillin resistance. *S. pneumoniae* organisms were once uniformly susceptible to penicillin; however, mutations in penicillin-binding proteins have resulted in varying levels of resistance. Empiric therapy therefore consists of a third-generation cephalosporin until susceptibility results become available. Once the minimum inhibitory concentrations (MIC) are available, therapy should be adjusted accordingly. For isolates with penicillin MIC less than 0.1 μg/mL, penicillin G (4 million units IV every 4 hours) or ampicillin (2 g IV every 4 hours) should be used. For isolates with a MIC greater than or equal to 0.1 μg/mL, treatment with a third-generation cephalosporin should be continued; either cefotaxime (2 g IV every 6 hours) or ceftriaxone (2 g IV every 12 hours). For isolates with a ceftriaxone MIC greater than or equal to 1 μg/mL, vancomycin and a third-generation cephalosporin are the recommended therapy; some clinicians administer very high doses of third-generation cephalosporins in these cases. Vancomycin should be dosed 1 g IV every 12 hours, or 500 to 750 mg IV every 6 hours, to a maximum of 2 to 3 g/day, and adjusted based on therapeutic drug monitoring to maintain a trough serum concentration of between 15 and 20 μg/mL. Meropenem is a reasonable alternative to the above agents and does not carry the theoretical risk of decreasing

TABLE 108.8

SPECIFIC THERAPY OF BACTERIAL MENINGITIS

Bacterium	Recommended therapy
Haemophilus influenzae	
Ampicillin susceptible	Ampicillin
Ampicillin resistant	Cefotaxime or ceftriaxone
Neisseria meningitidis	
Penicillin MIC <0.1 μg/mL	Penicillin G or ampicillin
Penicillin MIC 0.1–1.0 μg/mL	Cefotaxime or ceftriaxone
Streptococcus pneumoniae	
Penicillin MIC <0.1 μg/mL	Penicillin G or ampicillin
Penicillin MIC ≥0.1 μg/mL	Cefotaxime or ceftriaxone
Ceftriaxone MIC ≥1.0 μg/mL	Vancomycin plus cefotaxime or ceftriaxone
Enterobacteriaceae	Cefotaxime or ceftriaxone unless member of SPICEM group[a]
Pseudomonas aeruginosa	Meropenem or ceftazidime or cefepine or aztreonam or ciprofloxacin PLUS tobramycin
Listeria monocytogenes	Ampicillin or penicillin G
Staphylococcus aureus	
Methicillin susceptible	Nafcillin or oxacillin
Methicillin resistant	Vancomycin
Prosthesis associated	Consider adding rifampin to above choices
Staphylococcus epidermidis	Vancomycin
Prosthesis associated	Consider adding rifampin
Streptococcus agalactiae	Ampicillin or penicillin G

MIC, minimum inhibitory concentration.
[a]SPICEM group: includes *Serratia marcescens*, *Providencia*, indole-positive *Proteus* (*P. vulgaris*), *Citrobacter freundii* group, *Enterobacter* spp., and *Morganella morganii*). These micro-organisms carry chromosomal, inducible ß-lactamases (ampC), which are capable of inactivating third-generation cephalosporin even if reported to be susceptible. Carbapenems (meropenem has greatest cerebrospinal fluid penetration), fluoroquinolones, or trimethoprim/sulfamethoxazole may be used to treat these micro-organisms, if susceptible.

seizure threshold as is seen with imipenem. The efficacy of newer antimicrobials, such as linezolid and daptomycin, have not been established. Dexamethasone should be administered prior to or with the first dose of antimicrobial (see Adjunctive Therapy). Treatment duration is 10–14 days.

Neisseria meningitidis. The initial treatment of meningococcal meningitis is with a third-generation cephalosporin—for example, cefotaxime (2 g IV every 6 hours) or ceftriaxone (2 g IV every 12 hours); however, therapy should be stepped down to penicillin if susceptibility is confirmed. The duration of treatment is 7 days. Chloramphenicol (25 mg/kg, to a maximum of 1 g IV every 6 hours) is a reasonable alternative in the beta-lactam–allergic patient. Meropenem (2 g IV every 8 hours) is another alternative, although there is a high degree of cross-reaction in penicillin-allergic patients. Dexamethasone is not indicated in confirmed meningococcal meningitis.

TABLE 108.9

MORTALITY RATES IN BACTERIAL MENINGITIS BY PATHOGEN

Cause	Mortality
Neisseria meningitidis	3%–13%
Streptococcus pneumoniae	19%–30%
Haemophilus influenzae	3%–6%
Listeria monocytogenes	15%–29%
Streptococcus agalactiae	7%–27%
Staphylococcus aureus	14%–77%

Haemophilus influenzae. Therapy for *H. influenzae* meningitis is initially a third-generation cephalosporin. Therapy can be changed to ampicillin, 2 g IV every 4 hours if susceptibility is confirmed. A total of 7 days of therapy is recommended. Dexamethasone should be administered as adjunctive therapy in children.

Listeria monocytogenes. *L. monocytogenes* meningitis should be treated with ampicillin, 2 g IV every 4 hours. Gentamicin may be added for antimicrobial synergy, but aminoglycosides have poor penetration into CSF. When used, gentamicin should be administered as a 2 mg/kg loading dose, followed by 1.7 mg/kg every 8 hours. Trimethoprim/sulfamethoxazole (TMP/SMX), 20 mg/kg/day of the trimethoprim component, divided into 6 to 12 hourly doses, can be used in penicillin-allergic patients. Alternate therapies include meropenem and, potentially, linezolid and rifampin. Third-generation cephalosporins have no activity against *L. monocytogenes* and should not be used. Treatment duration is 14 to 21 days.

Aerobic Gram-negative bacilli. Aerobic Gram-negative bacilli should be treated empirically with a third-generation cephalosporin or meropenem. Susceptibility results should be obtained as soon as possible to guide therapy in consultation with an infectious diseases specialist. For *Pseudomonas aeruginosa* infections, ceftazidime or cefepime, 2 g IV every 8 hours, or meropenem, 2 g IV every 8 hours, with tobramycin 2 mg/kg IV every 8 hours, should be used. Cefotaxime and ceftriaxone should not be used as they do not have antipseudomonal activity. Ciprofloxacin or aztreonam are acceptable alternatives if the isolate is susceptible. The duration of therapy is prolonged, generally 21 days.

Staphylococcus. Staphylococcal meningitis therapy depends on methicillin susceptibility. Methicillin-susceptible strains should be treated with nafcillin or oxacillin, 2 g IV every 4 hours, whereas methicillin-resistant strains should be treated with vancomycin, 1 g IV every 12 hours or 500 to 750 mg IV every 6 hours, to a maximum of 2 to 3 g/day, with therapeutic drug monitoring to ensure adequate serum levels—15 to 20 μg/mL—are achieved. Vancomycin is recommended in patients with penicillin allergy. Infected prosthetic material should be removed if possible and antimicrobial therapy continued for 10 to 14 days after removal. If removal is not possible, rifampin may be added; however, cure rates are poor with hardware retention. Linezolid and daptomycin may become alternate therapies, but data on efficacy are currently lacking.

Adjunctive therapies in bacterial meningitis include corticosteroids, procedures to reduce intracranial pressure, and surgery. Corticosteroid therapy aims to decrease the inflammatory response while allowing antimicrobial therapy to eradicate infection. Although corticosteroid administration may decrease CSF penetration and bactericidal activity of antimicrobials, recent randomized controlled trials suggest benefit with its use. In children, the administration of dexamethasone has demonstrated a reduction in the incidence of hearing impairment and severe neurologic complications in *H. influenzae* meningitis (43). Adjunctive corticosteroid therapy has also been evaluated in adults, showing a mortality benefit in patients with pneumococcal meningitis (5). Based on these results, treatment recommendations suggest dexamethasone, 0.15 mg/kg, be given 10 to 20 minutes before, or at least concomitant with, the first dose of antimicrobial therapy and continued every 6 hours. Dexamethasone should therefore be administered to all patients with suspected meningitis until Gram stain or culture results are available. Dexamethasone should be continued for 2 to 4 days only if the Gram stain or cultures demonstrate *H. influenzae* in children or *S. pneumoniae* in adults. The potential disadvantage of decreased CSF penetration by non–beta-lactam antimicrobials with concomitant dexamethasone administration has yet to be thoroughly studied. Treatment with adjunctive dexamethasone has not been associated with an increased risk for long-term cognitive impairment (44).

Placement of an intracranial pressure monitoring device may be beneficial for patients with bacterial meningitis and elevated intracranial pressure. Admission to an ICU with expertise in this type of monitoring is most appropriate. Surgical intervention may be required in some patients, for example, those with basal skull fractures with persistent CSF leaks or dural defects.

Complications of bacterial meningitis can be divided into neurologic and nonneurologic complications. Neurologic complications include seizures, cerebral edema, cerebral infarction, cranial nerve palsies, venous sinus thrombosis, brain abscess, subdural empyema, and coma. Late complications include hearing impairment, obstructive hydrocephalus, learning disabilities, sensory and motor deficits, mental retardation, cortical blindness, and seizures. Nonneurologic complications include septic shock, coagulopathy, and the syndrome of inappropriate antidiuretic hormone secretion (SIADH).

Viral Meningitis

In general, the treatment for viral meningitis is supportive given its benign and self-limited course. Pleconaril has been evaluated for enteroviral meningitis with modest benefit but remains experimental (45,46). Intravenous immunoglobin has been used in agammaglobulinemic patients with chronic enteroviral meningitis. No specific therapy exists for arboviruses, mumps, or LCM. HIV-associated meningitis should be treated with combination antiretroviral therapy.

It is not clear whether antiviral treatment alters the course of HSV meningitis; nevertheless, primary episodes of genital herpes should be treated as per guidelines. Some physicians extend therapy to 14 days with concomitant meningitis. Intravenous acyclovir, dosed at 5 mg/kg every 8 hours, has been used in severe disease. Ganciclovir is the treatment of choice for CMV meningitis in immunocompromised hosts.

Other Less Common Causes

Syphilitic meningitis does not respond to benzathine penicillin, which is used to treat most forms of syphilis; it requires a 2-week course of high-dose IV penicillin G (4 million units every 4 hours). RPR titers should be monitored after therapy, and repeat CSF examination should be performed if titers do not decline fourfold 6 months after therapy. All HIV patients with syphilitic meningitis should have a lumbar puncture repeated 6 months following therapy. Patients with penicillin allergy should undergo desensitization, as there are no proven effective alternative therapies for syphilitic meningitis.

The treatment of Lyme meningitis is achieved with ceftriaxone, 2 g daily, or cefotaxime, 2 g IV every 8 hours for 14 to 28 days. Alternate therapy is penicillin (4 million units every 4 hours) for 14 to 28 days.

The treatment of tuberculous meningitis depends largely on the resistance pattern in the community and results of susceptibility testing; consultation with an infectious diseases specialist is recommended. In general, standard combination therapy includes isoniazid (INH), rifampin (RIF), ethambutol (ETB), and pyrazinamide (PZA). ETB may be discontinued once INH and RIF susceptibilities are confirmed. Treatment should be continued for a minimum of 12 months and up to 24 months. Adjunctive therapy with dexamethasone for the first month has been shown to decrease complications and is recommended. Pyridoxine, 25 to 50 mg daily, should also be administered to prevent INH-related neuropathy.

Therapy for fungal meningitis is complicated by the lack of standardized susceptibility testing and interpretation for many fungi. The area of antifungal therapy, however, is an evolving area with an increasing number of antifungal agents from which to choose.

Cryptococcal meningitis should be treated with a 14-day induction phase of amphotericin B, 0.7 to 1 mg/kg/day IV, with or without flucytosine, 100 mg/kg/day PO dosed every 6 hours. Consolidation therapy with fluconazole, 400 mg daily, should be continued for 8 weeks following induction. Maintenance (or suppressive) therapy with fluconazole, 200 mg per day, should be continued in patients with HIV/AIDS until immune reconstitution is achieved. Cryptococcal meningitis may require daily therapeutic lumbar punctures, an external ventricular drain, or a ventriculoperitoneal shunt to relieve increased intracranial pressure. Therapy is identical in non-HIV/AIDS patients, with the exception that consolidation therapy is continued for 10 weeks; further prolongation may be required in transplant patients. Echinocandins, such as caspofungin and micafungin, are not active in cryptococcosis.

The treatment for coccidioidal meningitis is oral fluconazole, 400 mg daily. Some clinicians initiate therapy with a higher dose of 800 mg per day or may add intrathecal amphotericin B. Treatment must be continued lifelong, as relapses are frequently lethal. Therapy for *H. capsulatum* meningitis consists of amphotericin B, 0.7 to 1 mg/kg/day to complete a total dose of 35 mg/kg. Fluconazole, 800 mg per day, for an additional 9 to 12 months, may be used to prevent relapse. If relapse does occur, long-term therapy with fluconazole or intraventricular amphotericin B is recommended. Itraconazole should be avoided due to poor CSF penetration. Although very rare, *S. schenckii* meningitis is treated with amphotericin B. Itraconazole, despite its poor CSF penetration, may be tried after initial therapy for lifelong suppression.

For candidal meningitis, the preferred initial therapy is amphotericin B, 0.7 mg/kg/d, with flucytosine, 25 mg/kg dosed every 6 hrs and adjusted to maintain serum levels of 40 to 60 μg/mL. Fluconazole therapy, in susceptible species, may be used for follow-up or suppressive therapy. The duration of therapy should continue for at least 4 weeks after resolution of symptoms. All prosthetic material must be removed to achieve cure.

Primary amoebic meningoencephalitis caused by *N. fowleri* is usually fatal. A few cases have been successfully treated with early diagnosis and treatment with high-dose intravenous and intrathecal amphotericin B or miconazole and rifampin. Eosinophilic meningitis caused by *A. cantonensis* and *G. spinigerum* are treated supportively. Corticosteroids are recommended to decrease the inflammatory response to intracranial larvae. Antihelminthic therapy is relatively contraindicated, as clinical deterioration and death may occur following severe inflammatory reactions to dying larvae.

Prevention

Chemoprophylaxis (medications) and immunoprophylaxis (vaccines) are available to prevent infection in contacts of cases or in times of epidemic spread. Temporary nasopharyngeal carriage with *H. influenzae*, *N. meningitidis*, and *S. pneumoniae* may occur following exposure to an index case and is a risk factor for the development of invasive disease. Chemoprophylaxis is recommended to eliminate nasopharyngeal carriage in some individuals at risk.

Prophylaxis is indicated in household contacts—those residing with the index case or with greater than 4 hours of close contact—and day care contacts—same day care as index case for 5 to 7 days before onset of disease—of cases of *H. influenzae* type b. If there is an unvaccinated contact less than or equal to 4 years of age in the household, chemoprophylaxis is recommended for all household contacts except pregnant women. Rifampin, 20 mg/kg, with a usual adult dose of 600 mg daily, for four doses, is the recommended therapy.

Prophylaxis for *N. meningitidis* is recommended for close contacts of cases. This includes intimate contacts (e.g., kissing) and close contacts with greater than or equal to 4 hours contact 1 week prior to the onset of illness. Most close contacts include house mates, day care center contacts, cellmates, and/or military recruits. Medical personnel exposed to oropharyngeal secretions during intubation, nasotracheal suctioning, or mouth-to-mouth resuscitation should also receive chemoprophylaxis. Rifampin, 600 mg orally every 12 hours for a total of four doses, or single doses of ciprofloxacin (500 mg orally) or ceftriaxone (250 mg intramuscularly) are all efficacious. It is recommended that ciprofloxacin be avoided in children younger than 16 years of age and in pregnant women, based on joint cartilage injury demonstrated in animal studies. Chemoprophylaxis is not indicated in *S. pneumoniae* infection.

Vaccination is available for the prevention of *H. influenzae*, *N. meningitidis*, and *S. pneumoniae* (47,48). Vaccination against *H. influenzae* type b is part of routine childhood immunization. Unvaccinated children less than or equal to 2 years of age exposed to an index case should receive chemoprophylaxis and vaccination.

S. pneumoniae vaccination is available in two preparations: the 23-valent polysaccharide vaccine and the 7-valent conjugate vaccine. The conjugate vaccine is recommended routinely in all children less than or equal to 23 months of age and in those at high risk of invasive disease—sickle cell disease and other hemoglobinopathies, functional or anatomic asplenia, HIV infection, immunocompromising conditions, and chronic medical conditions—who are greater than 23 months of age. The polysaccharide vaccine is recommended for all individuals greater than 65 years old and in those greater than 5 years old with the above high-risk conditions, but is of limited immunogenicity and efficacy. Studies of conjugate pneumococcal vaccine in adults are ongoing. *S. pneumoniae* vaccination is not an indicated as postexposure prophylaxis.

N. meningitidis vaccine is also available in two forms: conjugate and polysaccharide vaccines. Available conjugate vaccines include a quadrivalent (MCV4) vaccine, as well as the monovalent serogroup C (Men-C) vaccine. Available polysaccharide vaccines include a quadrivalent vaccine containing A, C, Y, and W-135 and a bivalent vaccine with serogroups A and C. *N. meningitidis* vaccination is indicated in high-risk populations, including those with specific immune deficiencies (Table 108.2), those traveling to endemic and epidemic regions, laboratory workers routinely exposed to *N. meningitidis*, first-year college students living in dormitories, and military recruits. Vaccination during outbreaks of meningococcal disease due to a serogroup contained in a vaccine should be performed in consultation with public health authorities.

ENCEPHALITIS

Key Points

- In distinguishing encephalitis from meningitis, the most useful finding is altered mental status.
- Encephalitis is most commonly viral or postinfectious in etiology.
- Herpes simplex encephalitis is the most common cause of sporadic encephalitis in Western countries, accounting for 10% to 20% of cases. Temporal lobe involvement on MRI and electroencephalogram (EEG) are characteristic. PCR is 75% to 98% sensitive, with false negatives occurring predominantly during the first 72 hours of illness. Mortality approaches 70% without therapy but can be significantly reduced with early antiviral therapy.

Encephalitis is defined as inflammation of the brain parenchyma. Although encephalitis and meningitis may present with similar clinical findings, the two syndromes are pathophysiologically distinct. The major distinguishing feature is the presence or absence of normal brain function. Patients with meningitis may be drowsy or lethargic but should have normal cerebral function, whereas those with encephalitis generally have altered mental status. Occasionally patients may present with a combination of findings in an overlap syndrome of meningoencephalitis. It is important to distinguish between the two syndromes, as the etiologic agents and treatments may differ.

Encephalitis is most commonly viral or postinfectious (Table 108.10). Viral encephalitis is caused by direct viral invasion of the CNS whereas postinfectious encephalitis is an immune-mediated process. Unfortunately it may be difficult to differentiate between the two; however, encephalitis with resolving infectious symptoms suggests a postviral cause. The most common viruses causing postinfectious encephalitis

TABLE 108.10

MOST COMMON VIRAL CAUSES OF ENCEPHALITIS, THEIR VECTORS OR ANIMAL HOSTS, AND GEOGRAPHIC DISTRIBUTIONS

Viral cause	Vector or animal host	Geographic distribution
Alpha viruses	Mosquitoes	
Eastern equine (EEE)	*Culiseta melanura*	New England
Western equine (WEE)	*Culex tarsalis*	West of Mississippi River
Venezuelan equine (VEE)	*Culex spp.*	South and Central America
Flaviviruses	Mosquitoes or ticks	
St. Louis	*Culex* spp.	Throughout the United States
West Nile (WNV)	*Culex pipiens* and *tarsalis*	Americas, Africa, Asia, Middle East, Europe
Japanese	*Culex tritaeniorhyunchus*	Asia and SE Asia
Murray Valley	*Culex* and *Aedes spp.*	Western Australia
Tick-borne	*Ixodes ricinus* and *persulcatus* ticks	Russia, Central Europe, China, North America, British Isles
Powassan virus		
Louping ill virus		
Herpes viruses	N/A	Worldwide
Herpes simplex virus (HSV-1)		
Varicella-zoster virus (VZV)		
Cytomegalovirus (CMV)		
Epstein-Barr virus (EBV)		
Human herpesviruses 6, 7		
Enteroviruses	N/A	Worldwide
Polioviruses		
Coxsackieviruses		
Echoviruses		
Adenoviruses	N/A	Worldwide
Human immunodeficiency virus (HIV)	N/A	Worldwide; particularly high prevalence in sub-Saharan Africa, Central and Southeast Asia, Eastern Europe
Rabies	Dogs, cats, raccoons, wolves, foxes, bats	Worldwide
Colorado tick fever	*Dermacentor andersoni* tick	Western United States and Canada
Mumps	N/A	Unvaccinated populations worldwide
Measles	N/A	Unvaccinated populations worldwide

N/A, not applicable.

include mumps, measles, varicella-zoster virus, rubella, and influenza.

Access to the CNS is highly virus-specific and occurs via hematogenous or neuronal routes. In hematogenous invasion, viral infection is acquired at an initial site of entry, with primary site replication, transient viremia, and CNS seeding. Retrograde transport within motor and sensory axons to the CNS occurs in the neuronal route of entry. After CNS entry, viruses enter neural cells, causing inflammation and cell dysfunction. Clinical manifestations are the result of specific cell-type invasion. Oligodendroglial cell invasion causes demyelination, whereas cortical invasion results in altered mental status, and neuronal invasion may result in focal or generalized seizures. Thus, focal pathology is the result of specific neural tropism.

Arboviruses are acquired via vector exposure, mainly mosquitoes and ticks. These include eastern equine encephalitis (EEE), western equine encephalitis (WEE), St. Louis encephalitis, Venezuelan equine encephalitis (VEE), California encephalitis (caused by La Crosse virus), Japanese encephalitis, yellow fever, and West Nile virus (WNV). Arbovirus-related encephalitides are most prevalent during the summer and early fall months when mosquitoes and ticks are most active.

EEE has a high mortality rate and occurs in the New England area, whereas WEE is a much milder illness, occurring west of the Mississippi River. VEE occurs from Florida to South America, whereas St. Louis encephalitis virus is found throughout much of the United States. The California encephalitis viruses mainly affect children in the Midwest and Eastern states. West Nile virus, identified in North America in 1999, causes West Nile neurologic syndrome (WNNS) in less than 1% of exposed individuals. WNNS most commonly manifests as encephalitis and occurs in those with diabetes mellitus, alcoholism, and of older age (49). Muscle weakness and flaccid paralysis may present concurrently in patients with encephalitis. Japanese virus encephalitis, occurring principally in Southeast Asia, China, India, and Japan, is the most common viral encephalitis outside of the United States.

Colorado tick fever is prevalent in the western United States, and most affected individuals have a history of camping and hiking in wooded endemic areas. Malaria, in those with an appropriate travel history, should also be considered in the differential diagnosis of encephalitis.

Rabies, a zoonotic disease that requires contact with infected animals, should be considered in all cases of encephalitis. Once CNS infection is established, however, the mortality is essentially 100%. Rabies can be acquired from many sources including dogs, cats, raccoons, bats, and foxes. The history of an animal bite, although useful if present, is absent in most cases of rabies.

Herpes viruses cause disease by primary infection or reactivation. Herpes simplex encephalitis (HSE) is the most common cause of sporadic encephalitis in Western countries, accounting for 10% to 20% of cases (50). HSE is caused by type 1 virus in greater than 90% of cases, occurs year-round, and affects all age groups. Two thirds of cases are due to reactivation of the virus in the trigeminal ganglion, with retrograde transport along the olfactory tract to the orbitofrontal and mediotemporal lobes. Untreated HSE has a mortality rate of 50% to 75%, and all survivors suffer neurologic sequelae. Outcomes correlate strongly with the severity of disease at presentation, as well as the time to initiation of antiviral therapy. Varicella-zoster encephalitis generally affects immune-compromised patients and may occur with or without concomitant cutaneous lesions.

Nonviral causes of encephalitis include bacterial, rickettsial, fungal, and parasitic infections. Bacterial causes include *Mycoplasma*, *Listeria monocytogenes*, *Borrelia burgdorferi* (Lyme disease), *Leptospira* spp., *Brucella*, *Legionella*, *Nocardia*, *Treponema pallidum* (syphilis), *Salmonella typhi*, and mycobacterial species, *Coxiella burnetii* (Q-fever), and Ehrlichiae. The most common rickettsial species include *R. rickettsii* (Rocky Mountain spotted fever) and *R. typhi* (endemic typhus). Fungal causes include *Cryptococcus* spp., *Aspergillus* spp., *Candida*, *Coccidioides immitis*, *Histoplasma capsulatum*, and *Blastomyces dermatitidis*. Last, *Trypanosoma brucei* complex (African sleeping sickness), malaria, *Toxoplasma gondii*, *Echinococcus granulosus*, and *Schistosoma* species can cause encephalitis but require epidemiologic exposures or specific risk factors. For example, toxoplasma encephalitis is most common in advanced HIV.

Clinical findings of encephalitis include the classic triad of fever, headache, and altered mental status. The onset of symptoms may be acute, subacute, or chronic; the acuity and severity of symptoms at presentation correlate with prognosis. Encephalitic symptoms may be preceded by a viral prodrome consisting of fever, headache, nausea, vomiting, lethargy, and myalgias.

Disorientation, amnesia, behavioral and speech changes, movement disorders, and focal or diffuse neurologic abnormalities such as hemiparesis, cranial nerve palsies, or seizures are common presenting; neck stiffness and photophobia may also be noted. VZV, EBV, CMV, measles, and mumps may present with rash, lymphadenopathy, and hepatosplenomegaly. HSE incidence is unrelated to a history of oral or genital lesions.

Laboratory findings may include peripheral leukocytosis or leukopenia. CSF examination usually reveals a pleocytosis with lymphocytic predominance; neutrophilic predominance may be present early in infection. Red blood cells, in the absence of a traumatic tap, are suggestive of HSV but may be seen in other necrotizing viral encephalitides. Protein levels are usually elevated, and glucose may be normal or slightly decreased. Because viral cultures are rarely positive, molecular methods have become the diagnostic tests of choice. Demonstration of HSV DNA in the CSF by PCR is both sensitive and specific (75%–98% and 100%, respectively) but may miss cases in the first 72 hours of illness. PCR testing is available for WNV, VZV, enteroviruses, adenoviruses, rabies, CMV, EBV, HHV-6, and HHV-7 in most reference laboratories. Serology may be diagnostic if IgM is detected or a fourfold rise in acute and convalescent IgG titers is demonstrated. Corneal or neck (posterior, at the hairline) biopsies and saliva PCR can be diagnostic for rabies. Brain biopsy may be considered in patients with encephalitis if all other tests are nondiagnostic.

Other investigations that may aid in diagnosis include EEG, CT, or MRI. EEG is particularly helpful in HSE, showing characteristic focal changes (spiked and slow wave patterns) from the temporal regions in 80% of patients. MRI is the most sensitive imaging modality at detecting early viral encephalitis and may show virus-specific changes. CT scans are more available on an urgent basis and are useful in ruling out space-occupying lesions; however, they are rarely able to visualize encephalitic changes.

It is most unfortunate that there are few specific therapies for viral encephalitis. Treatment of HSE with acyclovir, 10 mg/kg IV every 8 hours, is the main exception. Treatment should be initiated as soon as possible, as delays in therapy correlate with mortality. Therapy should be started empirically in all patients with encephalitis until confirmatory testing is available, given the dramatic effect on outcome. Acyclovir should also be considered in VZV encephalitis even though data regarding efficacy in this form of VZV disease are only anecdotal. Supportive therapy, including ICU admission with intubation and mechanical ventilation, may be required. Ganciclovir or foscarnet for ganciclovir-resistant strains is used to treat CMV encephalitis. The role of antivirals for EBV and HHV-6 encephalitides is unproven, but the International Herpes Management Forum has recommended the use of ganciclovir or foscarnet for HHV-6 encephalitis.*

Outcomes are related to multiple factors including host age and immune response, organism virulence, and time to effective therapy. Poor outcomes are more common in younger (less than 1 year of age) and older (greater than 55 years of age) populations. HSE, Japanese encephalitis, and EEE have the highest mortality rates. HSE mortality approaches 70% without therapy but can be reduced to 28% with early antiviral treatment. Most patients with HSE (62%) recover with significant neurologic deficits (paresis, seizures, cognitive and memory deficits).

BRAIN ABSCESS

Key Points

- Brain abscess results from focal infection, trauma, or surgery.
- A solitary abscess is usually the result of contiguous infection from otitis, mastoiditis, sinusitis, or dental infection.

*Data on CMV encephalitis come from several papers related to HIV patients, including International Herpes Management Forum (IHMF) recommendations (*Herpes*. 2004;11(Suppl 2):95A–104A). Data on HHV-6 are more limited, but antivirals are still suggested by the IHMF (*Herpes*. 2004;11(Suppl 2):105A–111A).

- Multiple abscesses commonly result from hematogenous spread from chronic pulmonary, endocardial, skin, intra-abdominal, or pelvic infections.
- The microbiology of brain abscess depends on the primary site of infection, patient age, and underlying host factors. Infections are commonly polymicrobial, and empiric therapy should include targeted anaerobic activity.
- Clinical manifestations are nonspecific and depend on the size and location of the abscess. Headache is the most common presenting feature.
- MRI is more sensitive than CT scanning and is the neuroimaging test of choice.
- Blood and abscess culture results should be used to tailor antimicrobial therapy, which is generally prolonged (6 to 8 weeks) and guided by serial imaging.
- Surgical excision may be indicated in patients with traumatic brain abscesses, fungal abscesses, and multiloculated or large (greater than 2.5 cm) abscesses.

Brain abscess is an uncommon but potentially life-threatening infection. Characterized by localized intracranial suppurative collections, brain abscesses are usually the result of extension of focal infection (45%), trauma (10%), or surgery. Bacteria may also gain entry to the CNS by hematogenous seeding in 25% of cases. Mortality rates with treatment range from 4.5% to 13%, even with new imaging techniques, antimicrobials, and surgical therapies (51–53). Infection begins as a localized area of cerebritis, with subsequent central necrosis, suppuration, and fibrous capsule formation (Table 108.11).

Solitary abscesses are usually the result of contiguous infection including otitis, mastoiditis, frontal or ethmoid sinusitis, or dental infection. Bullet fragments or other foreign bodies may serve as a nidus of infection and develop into abscesses even years after initial injury. Postneurosurgical brain abscesses may also present in a delayed fashion.

Multiple abscesses are more commonly the result of hematogenous seeding from chronic pulmonary, endocardial, skin, intra-abdominal, or pelvic infections. For example, patients with hereditary hemorrhagic telangiectasia (Osler-Weber-Rendu syndrome) and children with congenital cyanotic heart disease are predisposed to brain abscesses. A primary site or underlying condition cannot be identified in approximately 20% to 40% of patients with brain abscess.

The location of the brain abscess may be suggestive of the source. Temporal lobe or cerebellar abscesses commonly result

TABLE 108.11

RISK FACTORS FOR BRAIN ABSCESS

Otic infection (otitis media, mastoiditis)
Sinusitis (frontal, ethmoid, sphenoid)
Dental infection
Neurosurgical intervention or neurotrauma
Bacterial endocarditis
Neutropenia
Immune compromise (HIV infection, immunosuppressive therapy)
Chronic lung infection (abscess, bronchiectasis, empyema)
Congenital heart disease

HIV, human immunodeficiency virus.

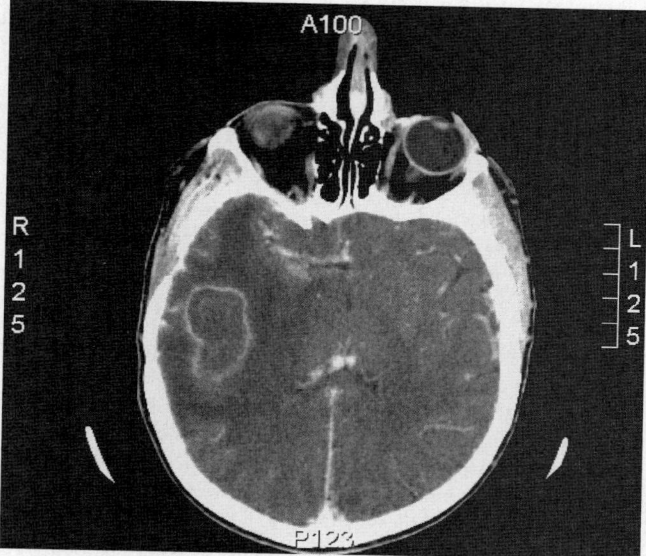

FIGURE 108.2. Axial contrast CT scan of a right temporal lobe abscess. This 36-year-old patient with cyanotic heart disease underwent a previous right craniotomy for subdural hematoma evacuation. Due to the presence of a pacemaker an MRI could not be performed. The image shows a 3.8 cm × 2.4 cm abscess in the posterior right temporal lobe underlying the previously noted right craniotomy. Decreased central attenuation of the lesion and surrounding vasogenic edema with uncal and subfalcine herniation are noted. There is no hydrocephalus. Abscess cultures grew *Streptococcus anginosus* group.

from otic infections, frontal lobe abscesses from sinusitis or dental infection, and abscesses in the distribution of the middle cerebral artery from hematogenous seeding.

The microbiology of brain abscesses is diverse and depends on the primary site of infection, age of the patient, and underlying host factors. Common aerobic species include streptococci (viridans, anginosus group, and microaerophilic species), which are isolated in up to 70% of cases (54). Aerobic Gram-negative bacilli—commonly *Klebsiella pneumoniae*, *Pseudomonas* spp., *Escherichia coli*, and *Proteus* spp.—and *S. aureus* are common pathogens with contiguous infection (55,56). Less common pathogens, such as *Rhodococcus*, *Listeria*, *Nocardia*, mycobacteria, and fungi—including *Candida*, *Cryptococcus*, *Aspergillus*, agents of zygomycosis, *Pseudallescheria boydii*, and the dimorphic fungi such as *Histoplasma*, *Coccidioides*, and *Blastomyces*—cause disease in immunocompromised hosts. Postsurgical and posttraumatic abscesses are usually due to *S. aureus* and aerobic Gram-negative bacilli. HIV-infected patients with advanced disease commonly present with *Toxoplasma gondii* infection.

Anaerobes are present in 40% to 100% of brain abscesses (55), although anaerobic cultures may not be routinely performed in all laboratories and, even if performed, may be falsely negative. Anaerobic species identified may originate from the oropharynx with contiguous head and neck infections, or from the abdomen or pelvis when infection is due to hematogenous seeding. Commonly isolated anaerobes include *Peptococcus*, *Peptostreptococcus*, *Bacteroides* spp, *Prevotella* spp., *Propionibacterium*, *Fusobacterium*, *Eubacterium*, *Veillonella*, and *Actinomyces*.

Helminths may occasionally cause localized brain infection in immigrant populations. Neurocysticercosis, intracranial

TABLE 108.12

COMMON PRESENTING FEATURES IN BRAIN ABSCESS

Headache
Mental status changes
Fever
Focal neurologic deficits
Neck stiffness
Papilledema, nausea, or vomiting with increased intracranial pressure
Seizures

infection with the larval cyst of *T. solium* or pork tapeworm, is most common and results from the ingestion of *T. solium* ova. *Entamoeba histolytica*, *Schistosoma japonicum* and *mekongi* species, *Paragonimus,* and *Toxocara* have also been described as causes of brain abscess.

The clinical manifestations of brain abscess are relatively nonspecific, resulting in delays in presentation and diagnosis (Table 108.12). The onset may be acute or chronic, and most of the presenting features are related to the size and location of the abscess. Systemic toxicity is uncommon. Headache is the most common presenting symptom and is usually localized to the side of the abscess. Sudden worsening of headache may be due to rupture of the abscess into the ventricular space. Fever is present in only half of patients and thus is not a reliable sign; seizure is, however, a common presenting feature. Focal neurologic findings are relatively uncommon. Neck stiffness occurs in 15% of patients and is most commonly seen with occipital abscesses. Altered mental status and vomiting are late signs, indicating the development of elevated intracranial pressure.

Specific presenting features correlate with abscess location. Patients with frontal lobe abscesses often present with changes in personality or mental status, hemiparesis, motor speech difficulties, and seizures. Temporal lobe abscesses may cause visual field defects or dysphasia if located in the dominant hemisphere. Patients with cerebellar abscesses may present with ataxia, nystagmus, and dysmetria. Brainstem abscesses usually extend longitudinally, with minimal compressive effect, and therefore present with few classic features. Papilledema occurs late with increased intracranial pressure.

Imaging of the brain parenchyma is the diagnostic test of choice. Lumbar puncture is contraindicated in patients with focal findings or papilledema and should be avoided in patients with suspected brain abscess. Computed tomography (CT) scanning or magnetic resonance imaging (MRI) should be performed, with the choice of test depending on the stability of the patient and availability of the imaging technique. CT scanning with contrast is not as sensitive as MRI but is generally more easily obtained on an urgent basis. MRI with gadolinium enhancement is more sensitive than CT in detecting early cerebritis and can more accurately estimate the extent of central necrosis, ring enhancement, and cerebral edema. MRI is also better able to visualize the brainstem, cerebellum, and spinal cord and can detect lesions 1.5 cm or smaller, which the CT scan may miss.

Blood cultures should be drawn in all patients with suspected or confirmed brain abscess. Abscess specimens should be obtained by stereotactic CT-guided aspiration or surgery to confirm the diagnosis and guide antimicrobial therapy. Bacterial, mycobacterial, and fungal cultures should be requested. Serology may be helpful for specific causes, such as *Toxoplasma gondii* and neurocysticercosis. In toxoplasma brain abscesses, IgG should be positive, as most infections are due to

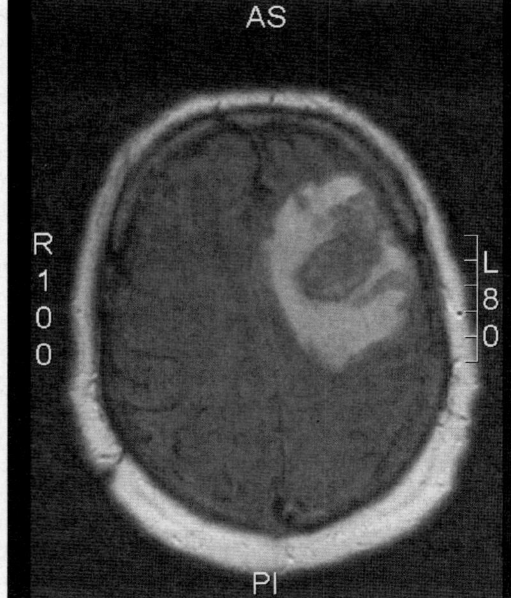

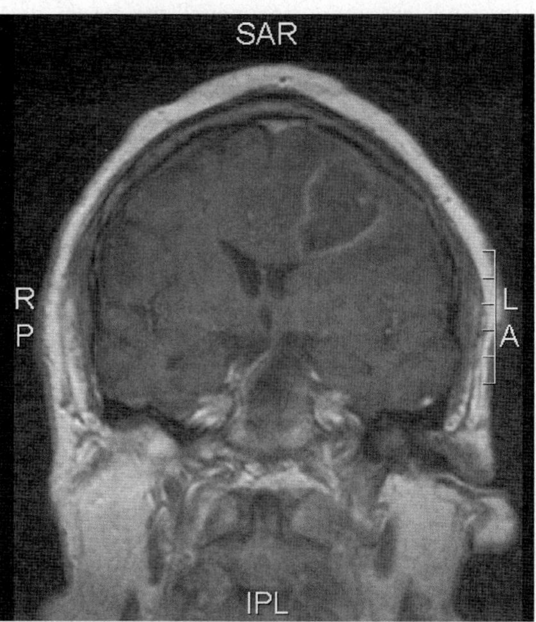

FIGURE 108.3. Axial and coronal MRI images of a frontal brain abscess. This 59-year-old diabetic male presented with a 10-day history of confusion, headache, right upper extremity weakness, as well as a generalized tonic-clonic seizure. Axial T2 FLAIR and coronal T1 post-gadolinium MRI images are shown above demonstrating a 3.4 cm × 3.4 cm × 4.3 cm intra-axial frontal lobe abscess with surrounding edema and mass effect. An urgent craniotomy was performed when the patient's level of consciousness decreased abruptly. Approximately 8 mL of pus were drained; cultures grew *Streptococcus anginosus*. Blood cultures were negative and the primary source of abscess was never identified.

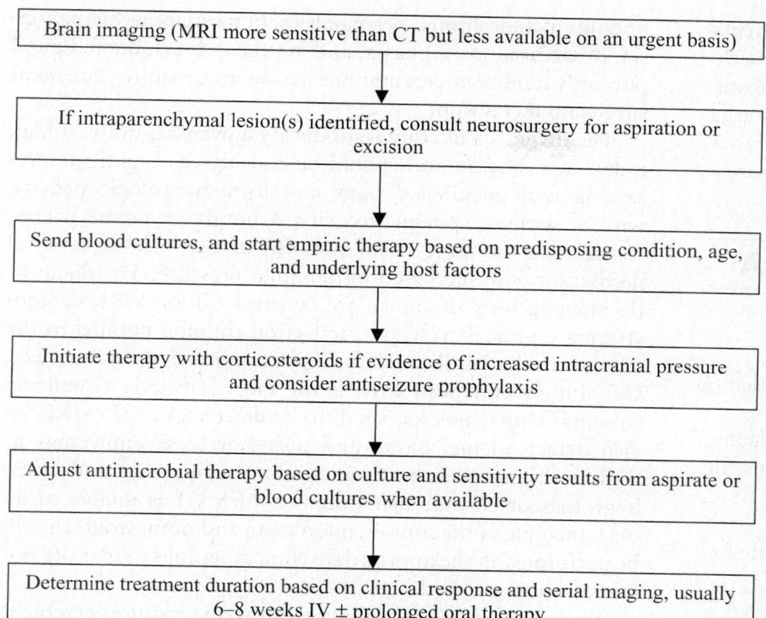

Brain imaging (MRI more sensitive than CT but less available on an urgent basis)
If intraparenchymal lesion(s) identified, consult neurosurgery for aspiration or excision
Send blood cultures, and start empiric therapy based on predisposing condition, age, and underlying host factors
Initiate therapy with corticosteroids if evidence of increased intracranial pressure and consider antiseizure prophylaxis
Adjust antimicrobial therapy based on culture and sensitivity results from aspirate or blood cultures when available
Determine treatment duration based on clinical response and serial imaging, usually 6–8 weeks IV ± prolonged oral therapy

FIGURE 108.4. Management of Brain Abscess

reactivation and not primary infection. A positive IgG antibody, however, does not prove *T. gondii* is the cause of a brain abscess. Brain biopsy may establish the diagnosis but is not routinely recommended given the risks involved and availability of less invasive diagnostic methods. Empiric therapy without aspiration for microbiologic samples is not generally advised except in specific situations where there is a high likelihood of a specific pathogen. For example, empiric treatment for toxoplasma infection may be warranted in a patient with advanced HIV (CD4 count less than 100 cells/μL) not receiving prophylaxis, with multiple lesions and positive IgG *T. gondii* serology. If clinical and radiologic responses are not evident within 7 and 14 days respectively, a microbiologic specimen should be obtained.

The therapy for brain abscess (Fig. 108.4) requires combination medical and surgical therapy for cure, as antimicrobial therapy alone is rarely effective. Empiric therapy should be initiated after imaging confirms the presence of an intraparenchymal lesion, pending aspiration for definitive diagnosis. Empiric therapy should be directed by the most likely source and respective pathogens.

For patients with presumed otic, mastoid, sinus, or dental sources, or temporal or cerebellar abscesses, treatment with a third-generation cephalosporin (cefotaxime, 2 g IV every 4 hours, or ceftriaxone, 2 g IV every 12 hours) and metronidazole (15 mg/kg IV load, followed by 7.5 mg/kg IV every 8 hours) is appropriate.

For patients with suspected hematogenous spread, an antimicrobial with activity against *S. aureus* should be used. Nafcillin or oxacillin, 2 g IV every 4 hours, is appropriate in settings with a low prevalence of methicillin resistance. Vancomycin, 15 mg/kg IV every 12 hours—adjusted for renal function and monitored with therapeutic drug levels—should be used where methicillin resistance is common or in penicillin-allergic patients. Vancomycin penetrates the CNS poorly and should be used only when indicated; a trough level of 15 to 20 μg/mL should be achieved. Metronidazole and/or a third-generation cephalosporin may be added, depending on the clinical setting.

For postneurosurgical or posttrauma patients with brain abscess, nafcillin, oxacillin, or vancomycin plus meropenem, a third-generation cephalosporin, preferably one with antipseudomonal activity such as ceftazidime, should be used.

Antimicrobial therapy should be adjusted once pathogen identification and susceptibility results are available and continued intravenously for 6 to 8 weeks, guided by clinical response and serial imaging. Prolonged oral antimicrobial therapy (2–6 months) is often administered if an appropriate regimen is available, although the efficacy of this approach has not been established. Therapy should be continued until there is complete resolution of symptoms and CT/MRI findings.

Antifungal therapy must be guided by fungal cultures and used in combination with surgical therapy. Candidal brain abscesses should be treated with amphotericin B and flucytosine. The efficacy of fluconazole has not been sufficiently evaluated in this clinical setting to recommend its use. Aspergillus brain abscesses have been historically treated with amphotericin B. However, due to recent data, voriconazole has become the treatment of choice (57), and combination antifungal therapy with voriconazole, plus either an echinocandin or an amphotericin B formulation, is increasingly used. Cerebral zygomycosis is almost invariably fatal, although amphotericin B is the treatment of choice. Posaconazole may be an alternative for zygomycoses, but voriconazole is inactive in these cases. *P. boydii* demonstrates *in vitro* resistance to amphotericin B, and, due to the lack of alternative agents, voriconazole is recommended as the antifungal of choice in these cases.

Neurosurgical consultation should be sought at the time of diagnosis. Aspiration through a burr hole or complete excision following craniotomy are both appropriate treatment options, although aspiration is generally preferred. Therapeutic aspiration may also be performed with CT or MRI guidance. Surgical excision is indicated in patients with traumatic brain abscesses, fungal abscesses, and large (greater than 2.5 cm) or multiloculated abscesses. If there is no clinical improvement within 1 week of initiation of treatment and aspiration, mental status declines, or intracranial pressure or abscess size increases despite therapy, surgical excision is also indicated. Antibiotic therapy may be shortened to 2 to 4 weeks following surgical excision.

Therapy with dexamethasone should be initiated in patients with significant edema and mass effect. Prophylactic antiseizure medications are also frequently administered. Poor prognostic factors in brain abscess include rapid progression, mental status or neurologic impairment on presentation, and rupture into a ventricle (51). Neurologic sequelae, most commonly seizures, occur in 30% to 60% of patients (51).

CRANIAL SUBDURAL EMPYEMA

Key Points

- Cranial subdural empyema and brain abscess share epidemiologic risk factors and microbiology.
- Presenting symptoms include high fever, unilateral headache, and a recent history of contiguous otic, mastoid, sinus, or meningeal infection.
- MRI is the diagnostic test of choice.
- Therapy should include prolonged antimicrobials and surgical drainage for cure.

Cranial subdural empyema is an intracranial collection of pus in the subdural space, the area between the dura and arachnoid. It is a potentially life-threatening condition, accounts for 15% to 20% of all intracranial infections (58–60,61), and was universally fatal prior to antimicrobial therapy. Recent data indicate that mortality with combined medical and surgical therapy now approximates 12% (61,62) with usually complete recovery in survivors.

Spread of infection to the subdural space occurs via the emissary veins or by direct extension of cranial osteomyelitis with accompanying epidural abscess. The subdural space lacks septations, so infection may spread rapidly and progressively. Most cranial subdural empyemas involve the frontal lobe, but the area of involvement is generally related to contiguous infection. Cerebral edema and hydrocephalus may develop when blood or cerebrospinal flow is disrupted by increased intracranial pressure. Cerebral infarction may also result from septic venous thrombosis.

Common predisposing infections include otic and sinus infections in up to 50% to 80% of cases (63). In patients with chronic otitis media, the middle ear and mastoids are commonly the predisposing sites of infection. Other predisposing conditions include traumatic brain injury with skull fracture, neurosurgical procedures, infection of a pre-existing hematoma, chronic pulmonary infection, or preceding meningitis.

Cranial subdural empyema is invariably polymicrobial, including streptococci, staphylococci, aerobic Gram-negative bacilli, and anaerobes. *S. aureus*, Enterobacteriaceae, and *Pseudomonas* are more common following neurosurgical procedures or neurotrauma.

The clinical presentation of cranial subdural empyema can be rapidly progressive so early diagnosis and treatment are crucial. Presenting symptoms generally include high fever and unilateral headache. A recent history of sinusitis, otitis media, mastoiditis, meningitis, cranial surgery or trauma, sinus surgery, or pulmonary infection within 2 weeks is common. Altered mental status, present in approximately 50% of patients on admission, is initially characterized by confusion and drowsiness and progresses to coma in most untreated cases. Focal neurologic signs most commonly include hemiparesis or hemiplegia, and seizures develop in up to 50% of patients (61). Other focal findings include cranial nerve palsies, homonymous hemianopsia, dysarthria or dysphasia, and ataxia. A fixed, dilated pupil portends imminent cerebral herniation and requires emergent surgical intervention.

The diagnosis of cranial subdural empyema requires a high index of suspicion and should be considered in patients presenting with meningeal signs and focal neurologic deficits, with or without systemic toxicity. A lumbar puncture is contraindicated in these cases because of the risk of cerebral herniation with increased intracranial pressure. The diagnostic imaging tests of choice are contrast CT or MRI, demonstrating a typical crescentic collection running parallel to the cranial vault. Midline shift implies significant mass effect. Gadolinium-enhanced MRI is the most sensitive, visualizing subdural empyemas too small to be detected by CT. MRI can also detect falcine, basal, and posterior fossa empyemas as well as differentiate between subdural empyemas and cystic hygromas or chronic hematomas, which CT is unable to do (61). Imaging of the sinuses, middle ear, and/or mastoids should be performed in the appropriate clinical settings to identify potential sources.

Treatment of cranial subdural empyema requires emergent combined medical and surgical therapy. Surgical drainage is mandatory, as antimicrobials alone cannot effectively cure empyemas. Cultures are, of course, required to guide antimicrobial therapy. Antiseizure treatment and/or prophylaxis may be warranted, and standard therapy for increased intracranial pressure should be instituted.

Empiric antimicrobial therapy should be initiated as soon as aspiration of the empyema is performed, or immediately on admission in unstable patients. Empiric therapy should be guided by the most likely source of primary infection. Recommended therapy includes a third-generation cephalosporin (cefotaxime, 2 g IV every 4 hours, or ceftriaxone, 2 g IV every 12 hours) or meropenem, 2g IV every 8 hours with metronidazole (15 mg/kg IV load, followed by 7.5 mg/kg IV every 12 hours). If *S. aureus* is suspected, nafcillin or oxacillin (2 g IV every 4 hours) should be used. Vancomycin, 1 g IV every 12 hours or 500 to 750 mg IV every 6 hours, to a maximum of 2 to 3 g/day, should be used in patients with penicillin allergy or in regions with high prevalence of methicillin resistance. Vancomycin dosing requires adjustment in patients with renal dysfunction, and serum levels should be monitored; a trough level of 15 to 20 μg/mL is desired. If *Pseudomonas aeruginosa* infection is suspected, ceftazidime, cefepime, or meropenem should be used in place of other third-generation cephalosporins. Intravenous antimicrobial therapy should be administered for 3 to 6 weeks, depending on clinical response and serial imaging. Prolonged therapy (6–8 weeks) may be warranted if contiguous osteomyelitis or mastoiditis is present.

Surgical therapy of cranial subdural empyema includes either burr hole drainage or craniotomy. Debridement of necrotic bone and surgical correction of sinus and otic infections are important adjuvant surgical therapies.

EPIDURAL ABSCESS

Key Points

- Epidural abscesses may be cranial (between the dura and skull) or spinal (overlying the vertebral column).

- Spinal epidural abscesses are nine times more common than cranial epidural abscesses, and result most commonly from hematogenous seeding of the intervertebral disk or vertebral body. They can also occur as a complication of spinal surgery or spinal/epidural anesthesia.
- Risk factors for spinal epidural abscess include injection drug use, diabetes mellitus, bacteremia, infective endocarditis, chronic indwelling catheters, decubitus ulcers, back surgery or procedures, and trauma.
- *S. aureus* is the most common pathogen.
- Consider tuberculosis in those at epidemiologic risk.
- Common presenting features of spinal epidural abscess include fever, back pain, and neurologic deficits.
- MRI is the diagnostic test of choice.
- Management includes prolonged antimicrobial therapy and early surgical decompression. Surgical intervention is preferred when symptoms have been present for less than 24 hours.

An epidural abscess is a localized collection of pus between the dura and overlying skull (cranial epidural abscess) or vertebral column (spinal epidural abscess). Because severe symptoms may result due to compression of the brain or spinal cord, prompt diagnosis and treatment are crucial.

Cranial epidural abscess is commonly accompanied by subdural empyema, as emissary veins may translocate infection across the cranial dura. The microbiology is therefore identical to that of cranial subdural empyema (see previous section).

Spinal epidural abscess is nine times more common than cranial epidural abscess. The epidural space is a potential space extending from the foramen magnum down the length of the spinal canal. The space is larger in the lumbar area and is predominantly posterior, and thus most spinal epidural abscesses occur in this area. Spinal epidural abscesses most commonly originate when the intervertebral disk (diskitis) or vertebral body (osteomyelitis) become infected via hematogenous seeding. As the abscess extends, it may track longitudinally in the epidural space causing damage via direct compression of the spinal cord or local vascular damage (thrombosis, thrombophlebitis, vasculitis). Most spinal epidural abscesses extend approximately three to five vertebral spaces but can extend the entire length of the spinal canal in some cases.

Risk factors for the development of spinal epidural abscess include injection drug use, diabetes mellitus, bacteremia, infective endocarditis, chronic indwelling venous catheterization, epidural catheterization, decubitus ulcers, chronic skin conditions, paraspinal abscess, back surgery, lumbar puncture, CT-guided needle biopsies, and blunt or penetrating spinal trauma. Secondary hematogenous spread occurs in 25% to 50% of cases.

S. aureus is the most common pathogen isolated from spinal epidural abscesses, accounting for approximately 65% of cases (64). Other implicated micro-organisms include streptococci; aerobic Gram-negative bacilli, particularly *Escherichia coli* and *Pseudomonas aeruginosa;* coagulase-negative staphylococci, usually with previous spinal instrumentation; and anaerobes. Less common pathogens include *Actinomyces*, *Nocardia,* and fungi, predominantly *Candida*. Infections are polymicrobial in 5% to 10% of cases. *Mycobacterium tuberculosis* makes up approximately 25% of spinal epidural abscess and should be suspected in patients with a previous history of tuberculosis, residence in a TB-endemic region, or other TB risk factors.

Clinical manifestations in patients with cranial epidural abscess are usually insidious. Headache is the most common presenting feature. Once infection spreads to involve the meninges, subdural space, and brain perenchyma, focal neurologic signs and symptoms may develop. If the abscess is located near the petrous bone, osteomyelitis of the petrous ridge may result in Gradenigo syndrome–cranial nerve V and VI palsies with unilateral pain or otalgia.

Spinal epidural abscess presents classically with fever, back pain, and neurologic deficits. However, all three symptoms are present in only 13% of patients (65). Back pain is usually the first symptom, with paresthesias, motor weakness, and sensory changes occurring in the affected nerve roots. Bladder and bowel dysfunction, as well as paralysis, are late signs and should prompt urgent surgical consultation.

The diagnosis of epidural abscess begins with the identification of risk factors and clinical suspicion. Routine blood work may demonstrate a peripheral leukocytosis or elevated erythrocyte sedimentation rate (ESR) or C-reactive protein (CRP). MRI with gadolinium enhancement is the imaging modality of choice for both cranial and spinal epidural abscesses. CT scanning cannot visualize the spinal cord adequately and is less sensitive at identifying contiguous diskitis or osteomyelitis. Blood cultures should be collected in all patients, as they are positive in 62% of patients (64). Lumbar puncture is relatively contraindicated in the setting of epidural abscess; however, studies have shown that CSF analysis is routinely Gram stain–negative, but cultures are positive in 19% of cases. The highest-yield (90%) culture comes from the abscess itself. Ultrasound- or CT-guided drainage should be performed as soon as possible. Bacterial, mycobacterial, and fungal cultures should be requested. Additional studies to diagnose active tuberculosis should be performed—for example, sputum AFB smears and cultures, urine AFB culture, and tuberculin skin testing or QuantiFERON-TB Gold testing—in patients with suspected spinal TB.

The management of epidural abscess requires a combination of medical and surgical therapy. Empiric antimicrobial therapy for cranial epidural abscess should include a third-generation cephalosporin or meropenem plus metronidazole. Nafcillin, oxacillin, or vancomycin may be added if *S. aureus* is strongly suspected. Surgical drainage is crucial for cure.

The management of spinal epidural abscess similarly requires empiric antimicrobial therapy and surgical decompression, drainage, and debridement. Because of the predominance of *S. aureus* infection, empiric therapy is fairly targeted; vancomycin if methicillin-resistant *S. aureus* is likely or if the patient is penicillin-allergic; and nafcillin or oxacillin if the local prevalence of methicillin resistance is low. Early surgical intervention, specifically within the first 24 hours of presentation, results in improved outcomes (66,67). Medical therapy alone may be successful when blood or abscess aspirate cultures are available to guide therapy and there are no neurologic deficits on presentation (68,69). Serial imaging is required in these cases to confirm improvement in abscess size. Surgery should be pursued if neurologic deterioration occurs at any time, or if resolution of the abscess is not evident with medical therapy alone.

Therapy with antimicrobials is prolonged, usually 4 to 8 weeks, and should be guided by serial imaging to ensure complete resolution of the abscess. Repeat imaging should occur at approximately 4-week intervals or at any time if neurologic deterioration occurs. Although the prognosis is fair, 37% of patients experience residual neurologic deficits. The degree of residual deficit is affected by the duration of neurologic deficit prior to surgery and diagnostic delays of greater than 24 hours (65).

SUPPURATIVE INTRACRANIAL THROMBOPHLEBITIS

Key Points

- Suppurative intracranial thrombophlebitis is a complication of otic, sinus, mastoid, oropharyngeal, facial, or neurologic (bacterial meningitis, epidural abscess, or subdural abscess) infections.
- Staphylococci, streptococci, aerobic Gram-negative bacilli, and anaerobic bacteria are the most common pathogens.
- Symptoms depend on the location of septic intracranial thrombosis.
- MRI is the diagnostic test of choice.
- Management includes antimicrobials, surgical therapy, and anticoagulation.

Suppurative intracranial thrombophlebitis is septic venous thrombosis of the cortical veins. It may occur as a complication of sinus, middle ear, mastoid, oropharyngeal, or facial infections. Bacterial meningitis, epidural abscess, or subdural abscess may also result in intracranial suppurative thrombophlebitis. The absence of valves in the cerebral veins and venous sinuses aids the spread of infection from proximal sites.

Anatomically, the location of intracranial infection depends on the original source of infection. In bacterial meningitis, infection is spread via drainage of the meningeal veins into the superior sagittal sinus. The superior sagittal sinus may also be involved following facial, scalp, subdural, and epidural space infections. Otitis media and mastoiditis are the usual causes of lateral sinus and petrosal sinus thromboses. Paranasal sinus, facial, or oropharyngeal infections may result in cavernous sinus thrombosis. Risk factors for cerebral venous stasis include hypercoagulable states—specifically antiphospholipid antibody syndrome—volume depletion, polycythemia, pregnancy, the use of oral contraceptives, malignancy, sickle cell disease, and traumatic brain injury (63).

The bacterial pathogens involved in intracranial suppurative thrombophlebitis depend on the originating source of infection. *S. aureus* is commonly involved following facial infection; otherwise, sinusitis and otitis media pathogens cause most infections; these include staphylococci, streptococci, aerobic Gram-negative bacilli, and anaerobes such as *Fusobacterium* and *Bacteroides*. *Aspergillus* and the agents of zygomycosis rarely cause suppurative intracranial thrombophlebitis and are most often seen in patients with diabetes mellitus or immune deficiencies.

The clinical manifestations of suppurative intracranial thrombophlebitis depend on the anatomic site(s) involved. Septic thrombosis of the superior sagittal sinus presents with fever, headache, confusion, nausea, vomiting, and seizures. Mental status depression and progression to coma may occur rapidly. Upper motor neuron lower extremity weakness or hemiparesis may be present. When septic thrombosis is a complication of bacterial meningitis, nuchal rigidity may also be present.

Cranial nerve palsies may result from compression due to increased pressure in the cavernous sinus. Cranial nerves III, IV, V-1, V-2, and VI, as well as the internal carotid artery, travel through the cavernous sinus. Classic symptoms of septic cavernous sinus thrombosis include fever, headache, diplopia, and retro-orbital pain. Depending on the specific nerves involved, ptosis, proptosis, chemosis, hyperesthesia, and decreased corneal reflexes may be present. Venous engorgement of the retinal veins and papilledema are commonly present.

Septic transverse sinus thrombosis presents with headache and otitis. Intracranial suppurative thrombophlebitis may also be a complication of Gradenigo syndrome with spread of infection around the carotid sheath and surrounding venous plexus; patients with sigmoid sinus and internal jugular vein thrombosis may present with neck pain.

The diagnosis of suppurative intracranial thrombophlebitis is made by MRI, demonstrating absence of flow within the affected veins and venous sinuses. MR venography or angiography can be used to confirm the diagnosis, and sinus imaging should be concomitantly performed. Compared to CT scanning, MRI offers the additional benefits of detecting cerebritis, intracranial abscess, cerebral infarction, hemorrhage, or edema. Despite its lower sensitivity, CT scanning is commonly performed before MRI, as it is more easily obtained on an urgent basis.

The treatment of suppurative intracranial thrombophlebitis includes antimicrobials, surgical therapy, and anticoagulation. The choice of antimicrobial therapy depends on risk factors, the most probable source of infection, and culture results, if available. In antecedent sinusitis, empiric therapy with cefotaxime or ceftriaxone, and metronidazole is a reasonable choice. In cavernous sinus thrombosis, an agent active against *S. aureus* should be included. Antimicrobial therapy should be continued for 6 weeks or until radiographic resolution of thrombosis.

If antimicrobial therapy is ineffective, surgical therapy may be required for drainage of infected sinuses, ligation of the internal jugular vein, or for source control (e.g., oropharyngeal or dental infections). Anticoagulation with heparin is beneficial in cavernous sinus thrombosis, particularly if used early, and should be strongly considered (70). Intracerebral hemorrhage, if small, is not an absolute contraindication to heparin therapy; however, this form of therapy must be individualized. The efficacy of thrombolysis in septic intracranial thrombosis has not been adequately evaluated to suggest its use.

References

1. Scheld WM, Koedel U, Nathan B, et al. Pathophysiology of bacterial meningitis: mechanism(s) of neuronal injury. *J Infect Dis.* 2002;186(Suppl 2):S225–233.
2. Durand ML, Calderwood SB, Weber DJ, et al. Acute bacterial meningitis in adults. A review of 493 episodes. *N Engl J Med.* 1993;328(1):21–28.
3. Aronin SI, Peduzzi P, Quagliarello VJ. Community-acquired bacterial meningitis: risk stratification for adverse clinical outcome and effect of antibiotic timing. *Ann Intern Med.* 1998;129(11):862–869.
4. Tunkel AR, Scheld WM. Acute meningitis. In: Mandell GL, Bennett JE, Dolin R, eds. *Mandell, Douglas, and Bennett's Principles and Practice of Infectious Diseases.* 6th ed. Philadelphia, PA: Elsevier; 2005.
5. de Gans J, van de Beek D. Dexamethasone in adults with bacterial meningitis. *N Engl J Med.* 2002;347(20):1549–1556.
6. Attia J, Hatala R, Cook DJ, et al. The rational clinical examination. Does this adult patient have acute meningitis? *JAMA.* 1999;282(2):175–181.
7. Thomas KE, Hasburn R, Jekel J, et al. The diagnostic accuracy of Kernig's sign, Brudzinski's sign, and nuchal rigidity in adults with suspected meningitis. *Clin Infect Dis.* 2002;35(1):46–52.

8. van de Beek D, de Gans J, Spanjaard L, et al. Clinical features and prognostic factors in adults with bacterial meningitis. *N Engl J Med.* 2004;351(18):1849–1859.
9. Schuchat A, Robinson K, Wenger JD, et al. Bacterial meningitis in the United States in 1995. Active Surveillance Team. *N Engl J Med.* 1997;337(14):970–976.
10. Weisfelt M, van de Beek D, Spanjaard L, et al. Clinical features, complications, and outcome in adults with pneumococcal meningitis: a prospective case series. *Lancet Neurol.* 2006;5(2):123–129.
11. Schlech WF 3rd, Ward JI, Band JD, et al. Bacterial meningitis in the United States, 1978 through 1981. The National Bacterial Meningitis Surveillance Study. *JAMA.* 1985;253(12):1749–1754.
12. Wenger JD, Hightower AW, Facklam RR, et al. Bacterial meningitis in the United States, 1986: report of a multistate surveillance study. The Bacterial Meningitis Study Group. *J Infect Dis.* 1990;162(6):1316–1323.
13. Sigurdardottir B, Björnsson OM, Jónsdóttir KE, et al. Acute bacterial meningitis in adults. A 20-year overview. *Arch Intern Med.* 1997;157(4):425–430.
14. Rosenstein NE, Perkins BA, Stephens DS, et al. The changing epidemiology of meningococcal disease in the United States, 1992–1996. *J Infect Dis.* 1999;180(6):1894–1901.
15. Wilder-Smith A, Goh KT, Barkham T, et al. Hajj-associated outbreak strain of *Neisseria meningitidis* serogroup W135: estimates of the attack rate in a defined population and the risk of invasive disease developing in carriers. *Clin Infect Dis.* 2003;36(6):679–683.
16. Fijen CA, Kuijper EJ, Tjia HG, et al. Complement deficiency predisposes for meningitis due to nongroupable meningococci and *Neisseria*-related bacteria. *Clin Infect Dis.* 1994;18(5):780–784.
17. Sjoholm AG, Kuijper EJ, Tijssen CC, et al. Dysfunctional properdin in a Dutch family with meningococcal disease. *N Engl J Med.* 1988;319(1):33–37.
18. Lorber B. Listeriosis. *Clin Infect Dis.* 1997;24(1):1–9.
19. Linnan MJ, Mascola L, Lou XD, et al. Epidemic listeriosis associated with Mexican-style cheese. *N Engl J Med.* 1988;319(13):823–828.
20. Bula CJ, Bille J, Glauser MP. An epidemic of food-borne listeriosis in western Switzerland: description of 57 cases involving adults. *Clin Infect Dis.* 1995;20(1):66–72.
21. Connolly KJ, Hammer SM. The acute aseptic meningitis syndrome. *Infect Dis Clin North Am.* 1990;4(4):599–622.
22. Corey L, Adams HG, Brown ZA, et al. Genital herpes simplex virus infections: clinical manifestations, course, and complications. *Ann Intern Med.* 1983;98(6):958–972.
23. Kent SJ, Crowe SM, Yung A, et al. Tuberculous meningitis: a 30-year review. *Clin Infect Dis.* 1993;17(6):987–994.
24. Klein NC, Damsker B, Hirschman SZ. Mycobacterial meningitis. Retrospective analysis from 1970 to 1983. *Am J Med.* 1985;79(1):29–34.
25. Mazurek GH, Jereb J, Lobue P, et al. Guidelines for using the QuantiFERON-TB Gold test for detecting *Mycobacterium tuberculosis* infection, United States. *MMWR Recomm Rep.* 2005;54(RR-15):49–55.
26. Montero A, Romero J, Vargas JA, et al. *Candida* infection of cerebrospinal fluid shunt devices: report of two cases and review of the literature. *Acta Neurochir (Wien)* 2000;142(1):67–74.
27. Nguyen MH, Yu VL. Meningitis caused by *Candida* species: an emerging problem in neurosurgical patients. *Clin Infect Dis.* 1995;21(2):323–327.
28. Bassetti M, Righi E, Costa A, et al. Epidemiological trends in nosocomial candidemia in intensive care. *BMC Infect Dis.* 2006;6:21.
29. Sobel JD, Vazquez J. Candidiasis in the intensive care unit. *Semin Respir Crit Care Med.* 2003;24(1):99–112.
30. Tortorano AM, Caspani L, Rigoni AL, et al. Candidosis in the intensive care unit: a 20-year survey. *J Hosp Infect.* 2004;57(1):8–13.
31. Korein J, Cravioto H, Leicach M. Reevaluation of lumbar puncture; a study of 129 patients with papilledema or intracranial hypertension. *Neurology.* 1959;9(4):290–297.
32. Horwitz SJ, Boxerbaum B, O'Bell J. Cerebral herniation in bacterial meningitis in childhood. *Ann Neurol.* 1980;7(6):524–528.
33. Hasbun R, Abrahams J, Jekel J, et al. Computed tomography of the head before lumbar puncture in adults with suspected meningitis. *N Engl J Med.* 2001;345(24):1727–1733.
34. Tunkel AR, Hartman BJ, Kaplan SL, et al. Practice guidelines for the management of bacterial meningitis. *Clin Infect Dis.* 2004;39(9):1267–1284.
35. Metersky ML, Williams A, Rafanan AL. Retrospective analysis: are fever and altered mental status indications for lumbar puncture in a hospitalized patient who has not undergone neurosurgery? *Clin Infect Dis.* 1997;25(2):285–288.
36. Leib SL, Boscacci R, Gratzl O, et al. Predictive value of cerebrospinal fluid (CSF) lactate level versus CSF/blood glucose ratio for the diagnosis of bacterial meningitis following neurosurgery. *Clin Infect Dis.* 1999;29(1):69–74.
37. Koskiniemi M, Piiparinen H, Mannonen L, et al. Herpes encephalitis is a disease of middle aged and elderly people: polymerase chain reaction for detection of herpes simplex virus in the CSF of 516 patients with encephalitis. The Study Group. *J Neurol Neurosurg Psychiatry.* 1996;60(2):174–178.
38. Tyler KL. Update on herpes simplex encephalitis. *Rev Neurol Dis.* 2004;1(4):169–178.
39. Stockstill MT, Kauffman CA. Comparison of cryptococcal and tuberculous meningitis. *Arch Neurol.* 1983;40(2):81–85.
40. Verdon R, Chevret S, Laissy JP, et al. Tuberculous meningitis in adults: review of 48 cases. *Clin Infect Dis.* 1996;22(6):982–988.
41. Miner JR, Heegaard W, Mapes A, et al. Presentation, time to antibiotics, and mortality of patients with bacterial meningitis at an urban county medical center. *J Emerg Med.* 2001;21(4):387–392.
42. Lu CH, Huang CR, Chang WN, et al. Community-acquired bacterial meningitis in adults: the epidemiology, timing of appropriate antimicrobial therapy, and prognostic factors. *Clin Neurol. Neurosurg.* 2002;104(4):352–358.
43. McIntyre PB, Berkey CS, King SM, et al. Dexamethasone as adjunctive therapy in bacterial meningitis. A meta-analysis of randomized clinical trials since 1988. *JAMA.* 1997;278(11):925–931.
44. Weisfelt M, Hoogman M, van de Beek D, et al. Dexamethasone and long-term outcome in adults with bacterial meningitis. *Ann Neurol.* 2006;60(4):456–468.
45. Desmond RA, Accortt NA, Talley L, et al. Enteroviral meningitis: natural history and outcome of pleconaril therapy. *Antimicrob Agents Chemother.* 2006;50(7):2409–2414.
46. Steiner I, Budka H, Chaudhuri A, et al. Viral encephalitis: a review of diagnostic methods and guidelines for management. *Eur J Neurol.* 2005;12(5):331–343.
47. Centers for Disease Control and Prevention. Recommended childhood and adolescent immunization schedule-United States, 2006. *MMWR Morb Mortal Wkly Rep.* 2005;54 (51,52):Q1–Q4.
48. Centers for Disease Control and Prevention. Recommended adult immunization schedule(United States, October 2005–September 2006. *MMWR Morb Mortal Wkly Rep.* 2005;54:Q1–Q4.
49. Bode AV, Sejvar JJ, Pape WJ, et al. West Nile virus disease: a descriptive study of 228 patients hospitalized in a 4-county region of Colorado in 2003. *Clin Infect Dis.* 2006;42(9):1234–1240.
50. Levitz RE. Herpes simplex encephalitis: a review. *Heart Lung.* 1998;27(3):209–212.
51. Seydoux C, Francioli P. Bacterial brain abscesses: factors influencing mortality and sequelae. *Clin Infect Dis.* 1992;15(3):394–401.
52. Tattevin P, Bruneel F, Clair B, et al. Bacterial brain abscesses: a retrospective study of 94 patients admitted to an intensive care unit (1980 to 1999). *Am J Med.* 2003;115(2):143–146.
53. Yang SY, Zhao CS. Review of 140 patients with brain abscess. *Surg Neurol.* 1993;39(4):290–296.
54. Wispelwey B, Scheld WM. Brain abscess. In: Scheld WM, Whitley RJ, Durack DT, eds. *Infections of the Central Nervous System.* 2nd ed. Philadelphia, PA: Lippincott-Raven Publishers, 1997:463–493.
55. de Louvois J, Gortavai P, Hurley R. Bacteriology of abscesses of the central nervous system: a multicentre prospective study. *Br Med J.* 1977;2(6093):981–984.
56. Mandell GL, Bennett JE, Dolin R, eds. *Mandell, Douglas, and Bennett's Principles and Practice of Infectious Diseases.* 6th ed. Philadelphia, PA: Elsevier Churchill Livingstone; 2005.
57. Johnson LB, Kauffman CA. Voriconazole: a new triazole antifungal agent. *Clin Infect Dis.* 2003;36(5):630–637.
58. Silverberg AL, DiNubile MJ. Subdural empyema and cranial epidural abscess. *Med Clin North Am.* 1985;69(2):361–374.
59. Coonrod JD, Dans PE. Subdural empyema. *Am J Med.* 1972;53(1):85–91.
60. Kaufman DM, Miller MH, Steigbigel NH. Subdural empyema: analysis of 17 recent cases and review of the literature. *Medicine (Baltimore).* 1975;54(6):485–498.
61. Tunkel AR. Subdural empyema, epidural abscess, and suppurative intracranial thrombophlebitis. In: Mandell GL, Bennett JE, Dolin R, eds. *Mandell, Douglas, and Bennett's Principles and Practice of Infectious Diseases.* 6th ed. Elsevier; 2005.
62. Nathoo N, Nadvi SS, van Dellen JR, et al. Intracranial subdural empyemas in the era of computed tomography: a review of 699 cases. *Neurosurgery.* 1999;44(3):529–535; discussion 535–536
63. Kaufman DM, Litman N, Miller MH. Sinusitis: induced subdural empyema. *Neurology.* 1983;33(2):123–132.
64. Darouiche RO, Hamill RJ, Greenberg SB, et al. Bacterial spinal epidural abscess. Review of 43 cases and literature survey. *Medicine (Baltimore).* 1992;71(6):369–385.
65. Davis DP, Wold RM, Patel RJ, et al. The clinical presentation and impact of diagnostic delays on emergency department patients with spinal epidural abscess. *J Emerg Med.* 2004;26(3):285–291.
66. Rigamonti D, Liem L, Wolf Al, et al. Epidural abscess in the cervical spine. *Mt Sinai J Med.* 1994;61(4):357–362.
67. Liem LK, Rigamonti D, Wolf AL, et al. Thoracic epidural abscess. *J Spinal Disord.* 1994;7(5):449–454.
68. Wheeler D, Keiser P, Rigamonti D, et al. Medical management of spinal epidural abscesses: case report and review. *Clin Infect Dis.* 1992;15(1):22–27.
69. Siddiq F, Chowfin A, Tight R, et al. Medical vs surgical management of spinal epidural abscess. *Arch Intern Med.* 2004;164(22):2409–2412.
70. Levine SR, Twyman RE, Gilman S. The role of anticoagulation in cavernous sinus thrombosis. *Neurology.* 1988;38(4):517–522.

CHAPTER 109 ■ INFECTIONS OF THE HEAD AND NECK

MARIA SUURNA • ALLEN M. SEIDEN

OTOLOGIC INFECTIONS

Otitis Externa

Acute otitis externa (AOE) is defined as a diffuse inflammation of the external ear canal, which may also involve the pinna or tympanic membrane (1). This condition is also known as "swimmer's ear" or "tropical ear" due to a higher prevalence in individuals with prolonged water exposure during swimming or who live in warm and humid climates (2). The annual incidence of AOE is about 1:100 to 1:250 within the general population (3).

The external ear comprises the auricle and external ear canal. The medial 60% of the external auditory canal is osseous and contains thin skin densely adherent to the underlying periosteum (Fig. 109.1). The lateral 40% of the external auditory canal is cartilaginous and contains a thin layer of subcutaneous tissue between the skin and cartilage. This subcutaneous layer contains hair follicles and sebaceous and apocrine glands. The skin of the auditory canal has a property of migrating from the tympanic membrane outward, resulting in self-cleansing. Cerumen is formed by glandular secretions and sloughed epithelium and provides both a chemical and mechanical protective barrier to infection. Cerumen is slightly acidic, maintaining a canal pH of 5 to 6.5, which helps inhibit bacterial and fungal growth. The lipid content of cerumen prevents maceration and breakdown of the epithelium. It is the breakdown in this natural defense mechanism that allows for opportunistic infections, giving rise to otitis externa (4).

The risk factors for acute otitis externa are prolonged exposure to water from swimming; dermatologic conditions such as seborrhea, psoriasis, eczema; trauma from ear cleaning, and foreign objects; use of assistive devices such as earplugs or hearing aids; anatomic abnormalities such as exostoses and narrow ear canals; immunocompromising systemic conditions such as diabetes, HIV; concomitant ear diseases such as cholesteatoma, suppurative otitis media; and a history of cancer radiotherapy (1,5).

Symptoms and signs of ear canal inflammation usually have rapid onset. Some of the presenting symptoms may be otalgia, itching, aural fullness, decreased hearing, and pain with chewing. Patients with AOE will often have disproportionately severe pain and will have significant tenderness when pushed on the tragus, or with manipulation of the pinna. Otoscopic exam usually reveals ear canal cellulitis and edema. Depending on the severity of the ear canal swelling, the tympanic membrane may or may not be visualized. The ear canal is often filled with purulent discharge and debris. Inflammation may spread to involve the entire auricle and adjacent skin. Regional lymphadenopathy may be present on the exam (1).

Most cases of AOE are bacterial. *Pseudomonas aeruginosa* and *Staphylococcus* species have been found to be the most common pathogens (6). Fungal involvement is uncommon in primary AOE. It is more often seen in chronic otitis externa or as secondary overgrowth following the treatment of bacterial infection.

Initial treatment of otitis externa involves removal of debris from the external ear canal, pain control, use of topical medications, acidification of the ear canal, and control of predisposing factors. Debridement of the external ear canal removes infectious material and allows for better penetration of topical medications. Topical medications can usually be administered directly into the ear canal. However, in many cases marked edema of the ear canal will prevent proper penetration of the medicated drop down into the canal. In this situation, placement of a cotton wick directly into the ear canal for several days will facilitate delivery of the medication (1).

Currently recommended topical preparations consist of antibiotics and steroid combinations. Quinolone antibiotic preparations may have broader microbial coverage and a low risk of contact dermatitis. Caution should be used when treating with neomycin-containing topical preparations due to a potential for neomycin to cause contact sensitivity and in turn lead to worsening of symptoms. Neomycin-containing preparations also have a low risk of causing permanent sensorineural hearing loss and should be used with caution in patients with perforated tympanic membranes. Acetic acid, boric acid, aluminum acetate, and silver nitrate have also been found to be effective. When treating immunocompromised patients, or if otitis externa infection has spread beyond the ear canal, consideration should be given to the use of systemic antibiotics as well. The choice of antibiotics should be based on their antipseudomonal and antistaphylococcal properties (1).

Chronic Otitis Externa

Chronic otitis externa (COE) is a persistent inflammatory disorder of the ear canal usually caused by repeated mechanical debridement or water exposure. Other potential causes are allergic, contact dermatitis, or dermatologic disorders. Chronic inflammation may lead to development of granulation. The treatment of COE involves debridement, avoidance of ear canal manipulation, elimination of the offending agent, and topical corticosteroids. Regular flushing of the ear canal with a mild acidic solution, such as acetic acid or vinegar and distilled water, can help to eradicate infection and keep the canal free of debris (7,8).

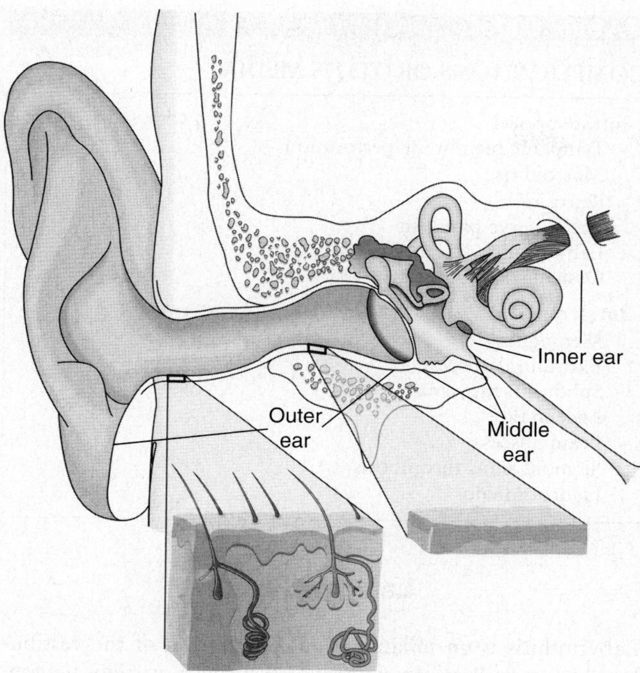

FIGURE 109.1. Anatomic depiction of the external, middle, and inner ear.

Otomycosis

Otomycosis is a fungal infection of the external ear canal. It constitutes roughly 10% of all cases of otitis externa and is more common in geographic locations with a warm and humid climate, in patients following long-term topical antibiotic therapy, and in patients with diabetes, HIV, or other immunocompromising condition (9). The ear canal will often have cellulitis and edema on otoscopic examination. The canal debris may have a cheeselike or grayish appearance with visualized fungal hyphae. *Aspergillus* species and *Candida* species are the most common pathogens (10). Treatment consists of debridement, acidification, and drying of the ear canal. For candidal infections, topical antifungal therapy may also be effective.

Necrotizing Otitis Externa

Malignant or necrotizing otitis externa (MOE) is an aggressive infection that begins as otitis externa but spreads through surrounding tissues toward the skull base. It is seen predominantly in the elderly, diabetic, or immunocompromised patient. *Pseudomonas aeruginosa* is the most common causative pathogen; however, staphylococcal species are also known to cause the infection (11,12). Fungal causes of MOE are less common, with *Aspergillus* species the predominating pathogen (13).

MOE initially presents with symptoms and signs of AOE. Subsequently it may progress to temporal bone osteomyelitis and affect adjacent cranial nerves (VII–XII), blood vessels, and soft tissue. If not treated aggressively, the infection can expand intracranially, leading to neurologic symptoms. On otoscopic exam, granulation tissue is classically seen at the bony-cartilaginous junction (11–14). A raised erythrocyte sedimentation rate and abnormal computed tomography (CT) or magnetic resonance imaging (MRI) scan help to confirm the clinical diagnosis. Other imaging techniques that assist in diagnosis include gallium scan, indium-labeled leukocyte scan, technetium bone scan, and single photon emission tomographs (12,15). Patients will require treatment with systemic antibiotics that cover pseudomonal and staphylococcal infection, including methicillin-resistant *Staphylococcus aureus* (11,12).

Furunculosis (Ear Canal Abscess)

Furunculosis is a localized infection of the ear canal that is usually caused by an infected hair follicle. It may present with otalgia, otorrhea, and localized tenderness. A tender, often fluctuant nodule within the lateral ear canal can be identified on the exam. The most common pathogen is *S. aureus*. The treatment includes application of heat, incision and drainage of the infected area, and systemic antibiotic treatment with staphylococcal coverage (16).

Acute Otitis Media

Acute otitis media is an inflammation of the middle ear that is generally characterized by the rapid onset of otalgia, aural fullness, and occasionally fever. In the pediatric patient, more common signs are irritability, sleeplessness, and pulling at the affected ear. On pneumatic otoscopy, the tympanic membrane will have a red, opaque, and bulging appearance with decreased mobility due to the accumulation of purulent fluid in the middle ear space. Erythema of the tympanic membrane may be noted, and if the tympanic membrane is ruptured, patients will present with otorrhea (17,18).

Predominant pathogens in AOM are *Streptococcus pneumoniae*, *Haemophilus influenzae*, and *Moraxella catarrhalis* (19). Observation for 24 to 48 hours in the case of a nonsevere illness in an otherwise healthy individual older than 6 months of age is an initial option. If symptoms persist, antimicrobial therapy should be initiated. Amoxicillin is recommended for initial treatment of acute otitis media, at a recommended dose of 80 to 90 mg/kg per day. In the case of penicillin allergy, azithromycin, clarithromycin, erythromycin-sulfisoxazole or trimethoprim-sulfamethoxazole could be used. Due to the increased incidence of beta-lactamase–producing organisms, the bacterial coverage should be expanded if there is no improvement within 48 to 72 hours. In very rare cases, if pain or fever is excessive, immediate tympanocentesis or myringotomy may be required (18,19).

Otitis media with effusion is the presence of fluid in the middle ear without signs or symptoms of acute ear infection and should be distinguished from acute otitis media. Otitis media with effusion often occurs as a result of eustachian tube dysfunction, or middle ear inflammation following acute infection. It is most common in the pediatric population between the ages of 6 months and 4 years, although it may occur at any age. On pneumatic otoscopy, the tympanic membrane is usually retracted, will have decreased mobility, and an air–fluid level or bubbles are often visualized. Patients often report a decrease in hearing. Otitis media with effusion is often self-limited and is likely to resolve spontaneously within 3 months. If it persists, hearing testing is recommended, particularly in children with language delay, learning problems, or suspicion of significant hearing loss (17,20). In individuals with persistent middle ear effusion leading to hearing loss or structural damage, surgical intervention, such as myringotomy with tympanostomy tube insertion, should be considered. Medical treatment, such as decongestants, has not been shown to be effective in the treatment of middle ear effusion. In an adult presenting with a unilateral middle ear effusion, an examination of the nasopharynx should be performed to rule out the possibility of a nasopharyngeal mass causing obstruction of the eustachian tube.

Chronic Otitis Media

Chronic otitis media is diagnosed when infection persists for more than 1 to 3 months. It may present as chronic suppurative otitis media (CSOM), which is characterized by persistent bacterial infection and drainage from the ear, or as chronic otitis media with effusion (COME), which results from unresolving inflammation of the middle ear and persistent middle ear secretions with an intact tympanic membrane. Chronic otitis media may be associated with cholesteatoma, which is a keratin cyst that forms from an accumulation of squamous debris in the middle ear with potential for growth and erosion of surrounding structures (21).

Patients with CSOM will present with hearing loss, painless purulent otorrhea, and a chronic tympanic membrane perforation. Evaluation includes visual exam, bacterial culture, and radiographic imaging. Gram-negative and anaerobic organisms are usually seen on cultures with *Pseudomonas aeruginosa* being a predominant organism. Temporal bone CT scan allows evaluation of the extent of disease and reveals potential complications. Medical treatment of CSOM consists of topical debridement, along with topical and systemic antibiotics. Topical drops often consist of antibiotic and steroid combinations. Ciprofloxacin is recommended for systemic use; however, it cannot be given to children younger than 17 years of age. Surgical treatment is performed for eradication of the infection and reconstruction of the middle ear (21,22).

COME is characterized by persistent hearing loss and a middle ear space filled with thick mucus. Chronic inflammation of the middle ear often begins with obstruction of the eustachian tube. The resulting negative pressure in the middle ear leads to collection of transudate. Secondary to chronic inflammation, the middle ear lining becomes hyperplastic and produces further mucus. On exam the tympanic membrane is intact and has a thickened, opaque appearance. On pneumatic otoscopy, the tympanic membrane does not move. As the disease progresses, the tympanic membrane starts to retract and drape over the ossicles. Nasal obstruction and sinus disease may contribute to eustachian tube insufficiency and lead to middle ear fluid accumulation. Treatment of COME consists of fluid drainage, which is accomplished by myringotomy with ventilation tube insertion. Treating sinus disease and relieving nasal obstruction may improve eustachian tube function (21).

Acute or chronic forms of otitis media, if left untreated, may lead to extracranial or intracranial complications (Table 109.1). Hearing loss, tympanic membrane perforation, atelectasis of the middle ear, mastoiditis, apical petrositis, facial nerve paralysis, labyrinthitis, and ossicular discontinuity are some of the possible intratemporal sequelae of otitis media. Meningitis, extradural abscess, subdural empyema, encephalitis, brain abscess, sigmoid sinus thrombosis, and hydrocephalus are potential intracranial complications. Intracranial complications should be suspected in individuals presenting with changes in mental status (17,23–25).

TABLE 109.1

COMPLICATIONS OF OTITIS MEDIA

Intratemporal
Tympanic membrane perforation
Mastoiditis
Petrositis
Facial nerve paralysis
Labyrinthitis
Ossicular discontinuity
Intracranial
Meningitis
Extradural abscess
Subdural empyema
Encephalitis
Brain abscess
Sigmoid sinus thrombosis
Hydrocephalus

Labyrinthitis

Labyrinthitis is an inflammation or infection of the vestibular apparatus. Patients typically present with vertigo, nausea, vomiting, and malaise. The cause is most often viral or traumatic but can be bacterial. Bacterial labyrinthitis most often arises as a spread of infection from meningitis or otitis media. It can be serous or suppurative. Viral infections such as mumps, measles, Lassa fever, varicella-zoster, and herpes simplex have been associated with labyrinthitis. Labyrinthitis may or may not be associated with a sensorineural hearing loss, which can be temporary or permanent depending on the cause, patient's age, and severity of the loss (26).

Bell's Palsy

Bell's palsy is defined as an acute unilateral peripheral facial nerve weakness. Diagnosis is made when other causes of facial nerve paralysis such as systemic diseases, infection, trauma, central nervous system disorders, and neoplasm are ruled out. Patients will usually present with abrupt onset of unilateral facial weakness. Other symptoms may include numbness or pain around the ear, decreased taste, and increased sensitivity to sounds (27). Herpes simplex virus is thought to be an etiologic factor for this disease (28). Bell's palsy most commonly occurs in individuals between 10 to 40 years of age. Pregnant women and individuals with diabetes mellitus are at a higher risk of developing Bell's palsy. Most cases spontaneously improve within 6 months. Residual facial nerve weakness may persist in about 15% of affected individuals (27). Recommended treatment consists of the early administration of high-dose prednisone and acyclovir (29). Patients should be educated about using artificial tears and protecting the eye during sleep to prevent corneal abrasion and eye infection. Preferably, treatment should be initiated within 72 hours of the onset of symptoms (27).

Ramsay Hunt Syndrome

Ramsay Hunt syndrome is caused by reactivation of varicella-zoster virus (VZV) in the geniculate ganglion and is associated with eruption of an auricular or oropharyngeal vesicular rash, facial paralysis, and otalgia (30,31). In addition tinnitus, hearing loss, nausea, vomiting, vertigo, and nystagmus can be accompanying symptoms (32). Patients with Ramsay Hunt syndrome present more severe symptoms and have a worse prognosis for recovery of facial nerve function relative to patients with Bell's palsy. The timing between onset of facial paralysis and vesicular eruption may vary. Some patients present with facial paralysis, have a rise in VZV antibody, but never develop cutaneous manifestations. Such cases are termed *Ramsay Hunt sine herpete* and often are labeled as Bell's palsy (30). Initiation of early treatment with prednisone and acyclovir is currently recommended (33).

Chondritis/Perichondritis

Chondritis/perichondritis of the ear is an infection of auricular cartilage/perichondrium. It is often caused by penetrating injury to the ear, particularly piercing of the pinna. Blunt trauma with auricular hematoma can also lead to infection. Cartilage involvement can also be seen in spreading otitis externa. Due to its relative avascularity, cartilage is more susceptible to infection. Infections are more often reported during warm weather, after exposure to water in pools, lakes, or hot tubs. Patients present with a very tender, erythematous, and indurated auricle. It is generally doughy on palpation and is rarely fluctuant. *Pseudomonas aeruginosa* has been identified as the most likely cause of the infection (34,35). Treatment consists of removing any foreign body, and drainage of any abscess or hematoma. Patients should be treated aggressively with antibiotics that provide coverage for *Pseudomonas*. Cartilage necrosis or subperichondrial fibrosis leading to auricular deformity may be seen following the infectious process (34). Recurrent auricular chondritis should raise suspicion for the diagnosis of relapsing polychondritis (36).

NASAL INFECTIONS

Septal Abscess

Septal abscess is rare and is defined as a collection of pus between the cartilaginous or bony nasal septum and overlying mucoperichondrium or mucoperiosteum (37). The leading cause is trauma that leads to a septal hematoma. It has also been shown to occur in association with influenza, sinusitis, nasal furuncle, and dental infection. Immunocompromised patients are at a higher risk of dangerous complications. Patients complain of nasal congestion, nasal pain, fever, and headache. On exam there is evidence of an anterior intranasal mass, as the septum will appear swollen and fluctuant. Most common causative organisms are *S. aureus* and group A beta-hemolytic streptococcus; however, *Staphylococcus epidermidis, S. pneumoniae, H. influenzae*, and anaerobes are also possible pathogens. Treatment involves antibiotics and surgical drainage. Ischemic necrosis of the septal cartilage may lead to saddle nose deformity or septal perforation. Other complications may involve intracranial infections such as meningitis, brain abscess, and subarachnoid empyema (37,38).

Rhinoscleroma

Rhinoscleroma is a chronic infectious granulomatous disease that originates in the nose but can involve any part of the respiratory tract. It is more common in the Middle East, parts of Latin America, and Eastern Europe, and is often diagnosed in young adults. Three clinical stages are recognized: (i) the catarrhal-atrophic stage, which consists of mucosal congestion and suppurative discharge; (ii) the granulomatous stage, which may present with epistaxis and nasal deformity and is associated with granulomatous nodules and infiltration; and (iii) the sclerotic stage in which fibrosis and stenosis develop (39). Typically patients present with crusting and nodular thickening of the nasal mucosa. Biopsy and culture of the diseased area provides a diagnosis. The presence of *Klebsiella rhinoscleromatis* is diagnostic of rhinoscleroma. Diagnosis is usually made in the proliferation stage. Biopsy shows an abundance of Mikulicz cells (40). Surgical debridement and prolonged antibiotic therapy is effective against the disease. Streptomycin, tetracycline, rifampin, second- or third-generation cephalosporins, and fluoroquinolones have been found to be effective against *Klebsiella rhinoscleromatis*. Treatment requires months to years, and relapses are common. Patients require long-term follow-up with repeat cultures and biopsies (39).

Rhinosinusitis

Acute Bacterial Rhinosinusitis

Acute bacterial rhinosinusitis most often develops following a viral upper respiratory infection. Some of the presenting diagnostic symptoms include purulent nasal discharge; nasal congestion; maxillary, tooth, or facial pain; and worsening of symptoms following initial improvement. Other symptoms include general malaise and a more generalized headache, although fever is unusual. Predisposing physiologic factors include obstruction of sinus ostia, reduction in number or function of sinus cilia, and a change in the quality of secretions (41). The most common pathogens are *S. pneumoniae, H. influenzae, Moraxella catarrhalis*, and *S. aureus*. In immunocompromised patients, in patients with cystic fibrosis, and in patients with sinusitis of nosocomial origin (on mechanical ventilation, with nasal tubing), *P. aeruginosa* and other aerobic Gram-negative rods are common causative pathogens (42). Anaerobic bacteria are usually associated with sinusitis of dental origin (43). It is often difficult to distinguish between viral and bacterial sinusitis. The diagnosis is usually based on medical history and clinical findings. With bacterial sinusitis symptoms are usually present for >7 days. Sinus puncture with aspiration of sinus contents is the most accurate diagnostic technique; however, since it is invasive, it is not commonly used. Radiographic imaging may help confirm the presence of sinus disease. Plain films can be difficult to interpret and are rarely ordered. CT findings will include thickened mucosa, sinus opacification, or air–fluid levels, and CT is the preferred exam although these findings are nonspecific (Fig. 109.2). A CT is rarely ordered to confirm acute infection unless there is concern about possible complications, such as in the case of frontal or sphenoid sinus infection. Nasal endoscopy will often demonstrate swelling within the middle meatus or sphenoethmoidal recess, with purulent discharge. Antimicrobial treatment of acute sinusitis includes amoxicillin,

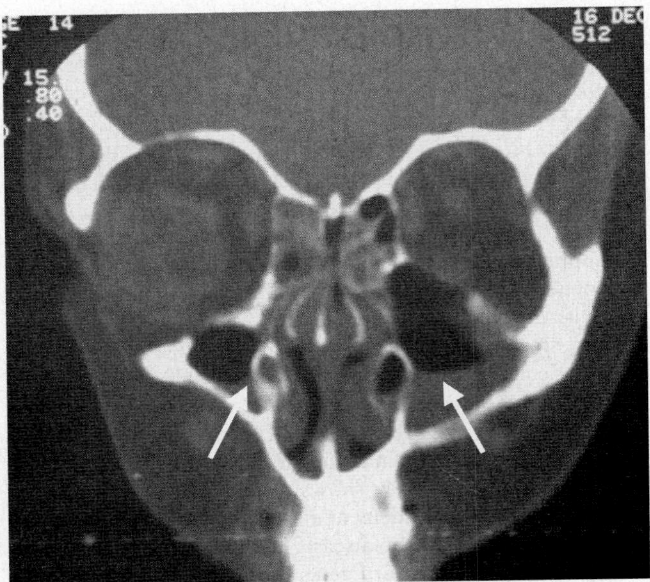

FIGURE 109.2. A coronal computed tomography (CT) image depicting inflammatory sinus disease. A coronal CT without contrast is the preferred radiographic study to evaluate for the presence and extent of sinus infections.

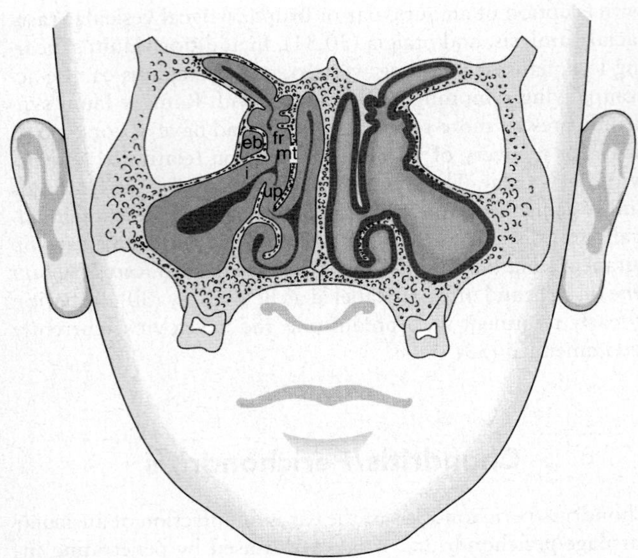

FIGURE 109.3. The ostiomeatal complex, referring to the anterior ethmoid sinus, and the ostia of the maxillary and frontal sinus as they drain into the middle meatus. Most sinus infections begin and persist because of obstruction in this area. The *right* side depicts these areas swollen; the *left* demonstrates the postsurgical appearance after the ostiomeatal complex has been opened. Eb, ethmoidal bulla; fr, frontal recess; i, infundibulum; mt, middle turbinate; up, uncinate process.

amoxicillin-clavulanic acid, cephalosporins, trimethoprim-sulfamethoxazole, macrolides, doxycycline, and quinolones. Treatment can be supplemented with nasal saline irrigation, antihistamines, decongestants, and intranasal steroids (41). If not treated, acute bacterial sinusitis may be complicated by development of several orbital and intracranial complications, particularly when the infection involves the ethmoid, frontal, or sphenoid sinuses (44,45) (Table 109.2).

Chronic Bacterial Rhinosinusitis

Chronic bacterial rhinosinusitis is diagnosed when symptoms are present for at least 12 weeks. Symptoms are similar to an acute infection, with nasal congestion and purulent discharge predominating, sometimes associated with facial pressure, aural fullness, and anosmia. Nasal endoscopy may reveal nasal polyps, edema, or purulent discharge (46,47). CT findings may reveal mucosal thickening, sinus opacification, polyps, or air–fluid levels (47). Predisposing factors include smoking, inhalant allergies, obstruction of the ostiomeatal complex (Fig. 109.3), immune deficiency, and genetic factors (48). Pathogens are similar to those found in acute infections, with a greater predominance of staphylococcus, *Pseudomonas*, and possibly anaerobes. The most common anaerobic bacteria include *Peptostreptococcus* species, *Fusobacterium* species, *Prevotella* and *Porphyromonas* species. In cases of *P. aeruginosa*, aminoglycosides, fourth-generation cephalosporins, or fluoroquinolones are used (42). A more prolonged course of antibiotic therapy may be required, ranging from 3 to 6 weeks. Adjunctive therapy including decongestants, mucolytics, and steroids may be helpful. If patients do not respond to medical therapy, surgical drainage should be considered (47).

TABLE 109.2

POTENTIAL COMPLICATIONS OF SINUSITIS

- Acute sinusitis
  - Orbital
    - Periorbital cellulitis
    - Orbital cellulitis
    - Subperiosteal abscess
    - Orbital abscess
    - Optic neuritis
    - Cavernous sinus thrombosis
  - Intracranial
    - Meningitis
    - Epidural abscess
    - Subdural empyema
    - Brain abscess
- Chronic sinusitis
  - Mucocele
  - Osteitis/osteomyelitis

Viral Rhinosinusitis

Viral rhinosinusitis is more common than bacterial. The most common pathogens are rhinovirus, influenza viruses, adenoviruses, parainfluenza viruses, and respiratory syncytial virus (RSV). Inflammatory symptoms of viral rhinosinusitis are thought to be due to the host response to the virus. Patients may present with symptoms of the common cold such as nasal congestion, nasal discharge, sneezing, cough, fever, malaise, and muscle ache. Viral rhinosinusitis is usually self-limited. Antiviral therapy may be used for specific viruses. Nasal saline irrigation and various anti-inflammatory medications may aid with symptomatic relief (49).

Fungal Rhinosinusitis

Acute Necrotizing Fungal Rhinosinusitis. Acute necrotizing fungal rhinosinusitis is a fulminant invasive fungal infection that is often life threatening. It usually affects

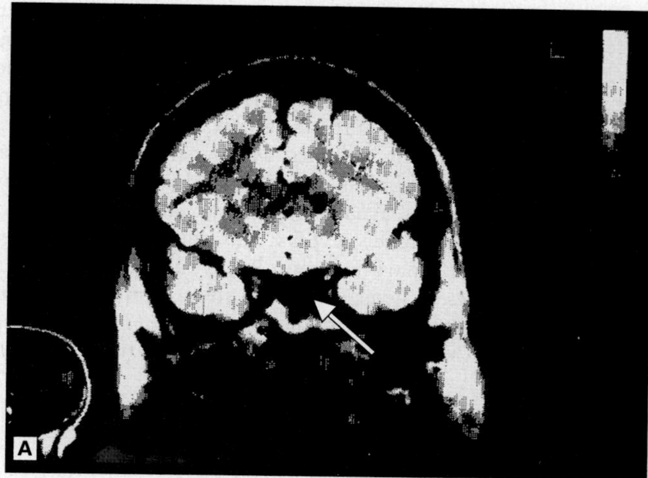

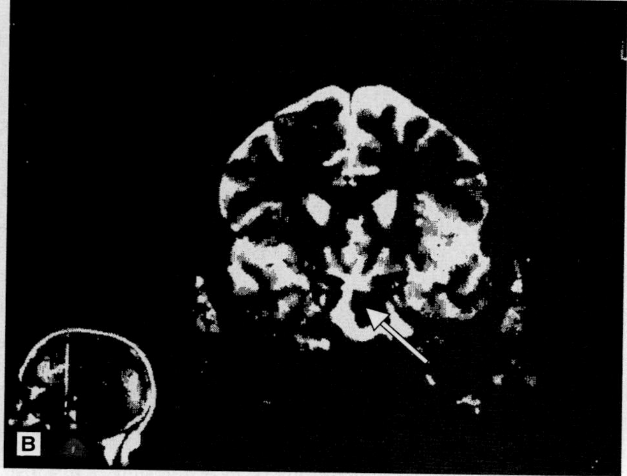

FIGURE 109.4. Magnetic resonance imaging (MRI) of a mycetoma or fungal ball within the sphenoid sinus, demonstrating isodense opacification on T1 images (A), with a ring of enhancement and central attenuation on T2 (B).

immunocompromised patients, such as diabetics, patients with immunodeficiency disorders, patients undergoing chemotherapy, or patients requiring prolonged stays in the intensive care unit. Patients often present with acute onset of fever, headache, cough, mucosal ulcerations, and epistaxis. On exam, nasal eschar spreading through mucosa, soft tissue, and bone is seen. Histopathologic evaluation of involved tissue reveals necrosis and inflammatory infiltrate with giant cells, lymphocytes, and neutrophils. Gomori methenamine silver or periodic acid-Schiff histologic fungal stains demonstrate tissue and vascular invasion by fungal hyphae. Most common pathogens are *Aspergillus, Rhizopus*, and *Mucor* species. Treatment involves emergent surgical debridement, intravenous antifungal drugs such as amphotericin B, and treatment of the underlying immunocompromising disorder. If the disease is not treated, it may lead to rapid dissemination and death (50,51).

Chronic Invasive Fungal Rhinosinusitis. Chronic invasive fungal rhinosinusitis is a chronic, more indolent, and slowly invasive fungal infection. It too usually affects immunocompromised patients, particularly diabetics and patients requiring prolonged corticosteroid treatment, but has also been reported in otherwise healthy individuals. Patients may present with orbital apex syndrome due to the extension of the infection into the orbit. This will result in decreased vision, ocular immobility, and proptosis. Erosion may also occur into the infratemporal fossa, the anterior cranial fossa, or the premaxillary region. Histopathology reveals a dense accumulation of hyphae, with a chronic inflammatory infiltrate of lymphocytes, giant cells, and necrotizing granulomas. If left untreated, the disease may invade cerebral blood vessels leading to ischemic injury or directly invade the brain. Treatment involves repeated surgical debridement and antifungal drugs (50).

Mycetoma

Mycetoma, also described as a fungal ball, is an accumulation of degenerating fungal hyphae within a sinus cavity. It usually involves one sinus, most often the maxillary sinus. Patients are generally immunocompetent and will present with symptoms of nasal obstruction, postnasal drainage, and localized facial pain. Risk factors include previous sinus surgery, oral-sinus fistula, and chemotherapy treatment. The presence of chronic mucosal inflammation may be noted on nasal endoscopy, along with green-black concretions within the middle meatus. A CT study will reveal sinus opacification, often with areas of calcification. Magnetic resonance imaging (MRI) may be definitive, demonstrating isodense opacification on T1 images, with a ring of enhancement and central attenuation on T2 (Fig. 109.4). This result is from ferromagnetic deposits related to the fungal infection. *Aspergillus* is the most common organism, although fungal cultures are often found to be negative. Treatment involves surgical removal of the fungal ball with adequate drainage of the affected sinus (51,52).

Allergic Fungal Sinusitis

Allergic fungal sinusitis (AFS) is a form of chronic hypertrophic sinus disease and not really a true infection. The cause of AFS is thought to be in part an allergic response to the presence of noninvasive fungi in the sinus cavity and has been likened to allergic bronchopulmonary aspergillosis (51). Patients will commonly present with hypertrophic sinus disease and nasal polyps. Symptoms of headache, paranasal fullness, and nasal discharge are often reported. Sinus CT often reveals the presence of chronic sinusitis with hyperattenuation present in the opacified sinus, creating an inhomogeneous appearance often with areas of calcification (Fig. 109.5). Serum IgE levels are often elevated. Histologic evaluation reveals the presence of allergic mucin, containing fungal hyphae and elevated eosinophils. There is no evidence of mucosal invasion. Intraorbital and intracranial expansion may occur secondary to pressure resorption of surrounding bone. The most common causative agents are *Bipolaris spicifera* and *Curvularia lunata*. Other causative agents are *Exserohilum rostratum*, *Alternaria* species, and *Aspergillus* species. Treatment consists of sinus surgery to remove the diseased mucosa and allergic mucin, although recurrence is common. Once AFS is diagnosed, if there are no contraindications, treatment with corticosteroids should be initiated (52,53).

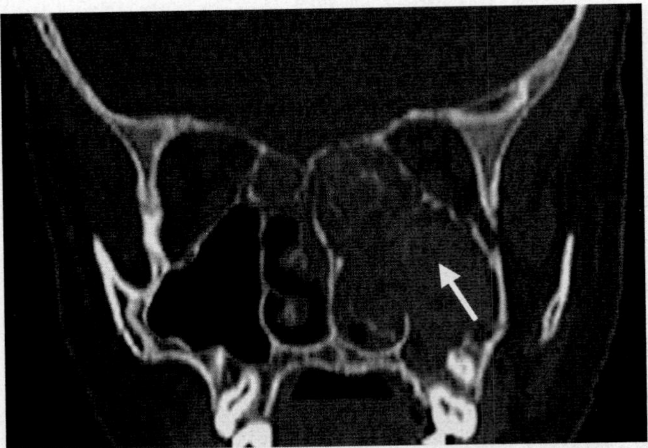

FIGURE 109.5. Computed tomography (CT) of the sinuses in a patient with allergic fungal sinusitis, demonstrating an inhomogeneous appearance with areas of calcification.

ORAL CAVITY

Gingivitis

Gingivitis affects 50% to 90% of the adult population. It has an infectious etiology caused by oral microflora in the accumulating dental plaque and usually contains both aerobic and anaerobic bacteria. Gingivitis is a reversible disease. Chronic gingivitis often leads to bleeding of the gums during tooth brushing (54). Gingivitis may progress to periodontitis, which involves inflammation of deeper tissues leading to the loss of supporting connective tissue and alveolar bone. This disease is nonreversible and may lead to loss of involved teeth (55,56). Treatment involves primarily good oral hygiene along with the mechanical removal of plaque and calculus (55).

Acute Necrotizing Ulcerative Gingivitis (Trench Mouth)

Acute necrotizing ulcerative gingivitis (trench mouth, Vincent stomatitis) is a rare periodontal disease characterized by gingival necrosis, ulceration, pain, and bleeding (57). Disease is most commonly seen in young adults. Patients will often present with sudden onset of gingival inflammation. Gingival lacerations covered with gray membranes and gingival bleeding are noted on the exam. The causative organisms are fusospirochetal bacteria, which become pathogenic during periods of compromised immune system function. *Bacteroides* and *Selenomonas* species have also been implicated in the disease (57). Diagnosis is based on clinical findings. Risk factors include dental crowding, physical fatigue, increased stress, low socioeconomic status, immunosuppression, smoking, and poor oral hygiene (58). Treatment includes eliminating precipitating factors, treatment of underlying immunosuppression, oral hygiene, mechanical debridement of affected areas, and antibiotics. Penicillin or metronidazole is recommended for antibiotic treatment (57).

Herpetic Gingival Stomatitis

Herpetic gingivostomatitis is an infection due to herpes simplex virus. Primary infection most commonly manifests in children between the ages of 2 and 5 years. Patients may present with fever and irritability. Oropharyngeal pain, mucosal edema and erythema are often present. Vesicular lesions appear on mobile or nonkeratinized mucosal surfaces (buccal, labial) and attached or keratinized surfaces (gingiva, hard palate). These usually rupture within 24 hours, leaving small ulcers with an elevated margin. Diagnosis is confirmed by viral studies and biopsy. Treatment is usually supportive, although acyclovir may help to shorten the severity and duration of the infection. Once the primary infection resolves, infection remains dormant, the reservoir usually being the trigeminal ganglion. Periodic reactivation of infection may occur. In most cases, individuals must have an active lesion to be able to transmit the virus (59,60).

Herpangina

Herpangina is a disease that commonly occurs in children (61). Coxsackie A virus is the most common causative organism (62). Patients will present with fever, malaise, and sore throat. On exam patients are noted to have oropharyngeal erythema. Vesicles and small ulcers are present on the posterior pharynx, often on the uvula and soft palate. The course is usually self-limiting (61).

Candidiasis

Candidiasis is caused by overgrowth of *Candida albicans*. Often the patient is predisposed, with a history of immunosuppression, radiation, or altered microflora following long-term broad-spectrum antibiotic use. In the pseudomembranous form, yellow-white plaques are present that have been likened to milk curds (Fig. 109.6A), whereas in the erythematous form, these plaques have disappeared (Fig. 109.6B). Clinical diagnosis may be confirmed with potassium hydroxide staining revealing fungal hyphae. Initial therapy usually consists of oral hygiene and topical treatment. Some of the available agents include oral nystatin preparations, amphotericin lozenges, and clotrimazole troches. Ketoconazole, fluconazole, and itraconazole can be used for systemic treatment if indicated (63).

Odontogenic Infections

Odontogenic infections often originate from infected pulp and may spread to the fascial spaces of the head and neck where an abscess may form (Fig. 109.7). The potential spaces are found around the face—masticator, buccal, canine, and parotid; in the suprahyoid area—submandibular, sublingual, and parapharyngeal; and in the infrahyoid area—retropharyngeal and paratracheal. The most common causative organisms are *S. aureus*, group A streptococci, and anaerobic bacteria. Treatment with broad-spectrum antibiotics is recommended (64,65).

Ludwig's Angina

Ludwig's angina is an infection that involves the left and right sublingual and submandibular spaces, generally spreading rapidly through fascial planes. It occurs most often in adults with poor dentition, usually from an infection involving the second or third molar. Other sources may include inflammation of the tongue or floor of mouth, and lingual tonsillitis (65,66).

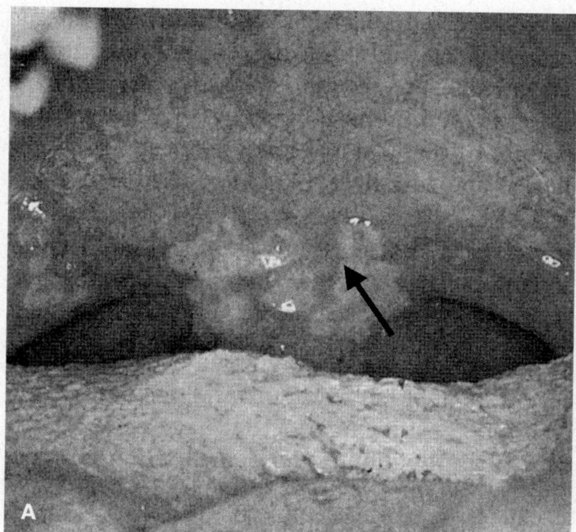

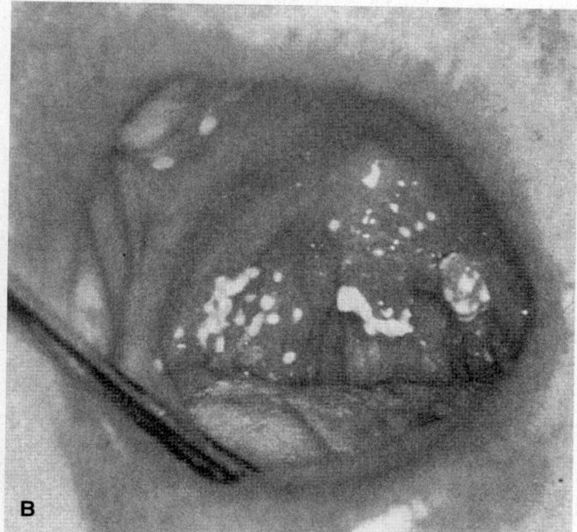

FIGURE 109.6. Oropharyngeal infection by *Candida albicans* (thrush). These photos demonstrate the pseudomembranous form (**A**) associated with yellow-white plaques, and the erythematous form (**B**). (From Walner DL, Shott SR. Infectious and inflammatory disorders. In: Seiden AM, Tami TA, Pensak ML, et al., eds. *Otolaryngology: The Essentials*. New York, NY: Thieme Medical Publishers; 2001:188, with permission.)

Patients will often present with submandibular swelling but not fluctuance, and swelling of the floor of the mouth that pushes the tongue upward and backward toward the palate. In the case of advanced disease, patients may present in acute distress with fever, difficulty handling secretions, and dyspnea that favors a seated and head forward position. Infection can be rapidly progressive, leading to airway compromise. Anaerobic organisms and streptococci are the most common cause of Ludwig angina. Treatment requires close airway monitoring with prophylactic tracheotomy in most cases for airway protection, administration of antibiotics, and surgical drainage (66,67).

PHARYNX

Tonsillitis/Pharyngitis

Tonsillopharyngitis is a common disease characterized by infection of the nasopharynx and oropharynx and associated lymphoid tissue. Acute tonsillopharyngitis may be caused by viral or bacterial infection, a virus being most common. It is often difficult to distinguish between a bacterial and viral cause based on clinical exam. Patients present with fever, malaise, odynophagia, and lymphadenitis. On exam tonsillar enlargement, erythema, and exudate may be present. Upper respiratory viruses such as rhinovirus, coronavirus, and adenovirus are the most common causes of viral infection (68). The most common cause of bacterial tonsillopharyngitis is a group A beta-hemolytic streptococci (GABHS). It can be diagnosed by performing a group A *Streptococcus* test. Other pathogens have also been associated with the disease such as *M. catarrhalis*, *H. influenzae*, *S. aureus*, and *S. pneumoniae* (69). Diphtheria and gonococcal infections should also be considered. If GABHS infection is suspected, antibiotic treatment should be initiated. Penicillin, amoxicillin, erythromycin, and first-generation cephalosporins are recommended for treatment. It is recommended to perform a group A *Streptococcus* test prior to initiation of antibiotic treatment (68,70). If not treated, bacterial tonsillopharyngitis may lead to complications that can be suppurative and nonsuppurative. The nonsuppurative complications include scarlet fever, acute rheumatic fever, and post-streptococcal glomerulonephritis. Suppurative complications include peritonsillar, parapharyngeal, and retropharyngeal cellulites and/or abscess (71). In cases of recurrent streptococcal tonsillopharyngitis or infections unresponsive to antimicrobial therapy, tonsillectomy might be indicated (72).

Peritonsillar Abscess

Peritonsillar abscess is the most common deep infection of the head and neck. It usually occurs as a complication of bacterial tonsillitis or less frequently in cases of infectious mononucleosis. Infection may spread through the tonsillar capsule into the space between the tonsil and superior constrictor muscle and sequentially develop into an abscess. Peritonsillar abscess is most commonly diagnosed in adults or adolescents. Patients will present with increasing pharyngeal pain, dysphagia, trismus, dysarthria, drooling, and a muffled voice. The clinical exam reveals trismus, peritonsillar bulging that displaces the soft palate medially, and uvular deviation toward the opposite side. Patients will often have tonsillar exudates and tender cervical lymphadenopathy (65). A peritonsillar abscess is usually polymicrobial, with Group A streptococci and anaerobes the most common pathogens (73). The diagnosis is usually made on physical exam. A CT scan may help if the diagnosis is uncertain. Treatment involves aspiration or incision and drainage of the abscess along with antibiotic therapy (74). If the peritonsillar abscess becomes recurrent, a tonsillectomy would be indicated (75). A peritonsillar space infection has the potential for spreading to the parapharyngeal space, the manifestations of which may be delayed (65).

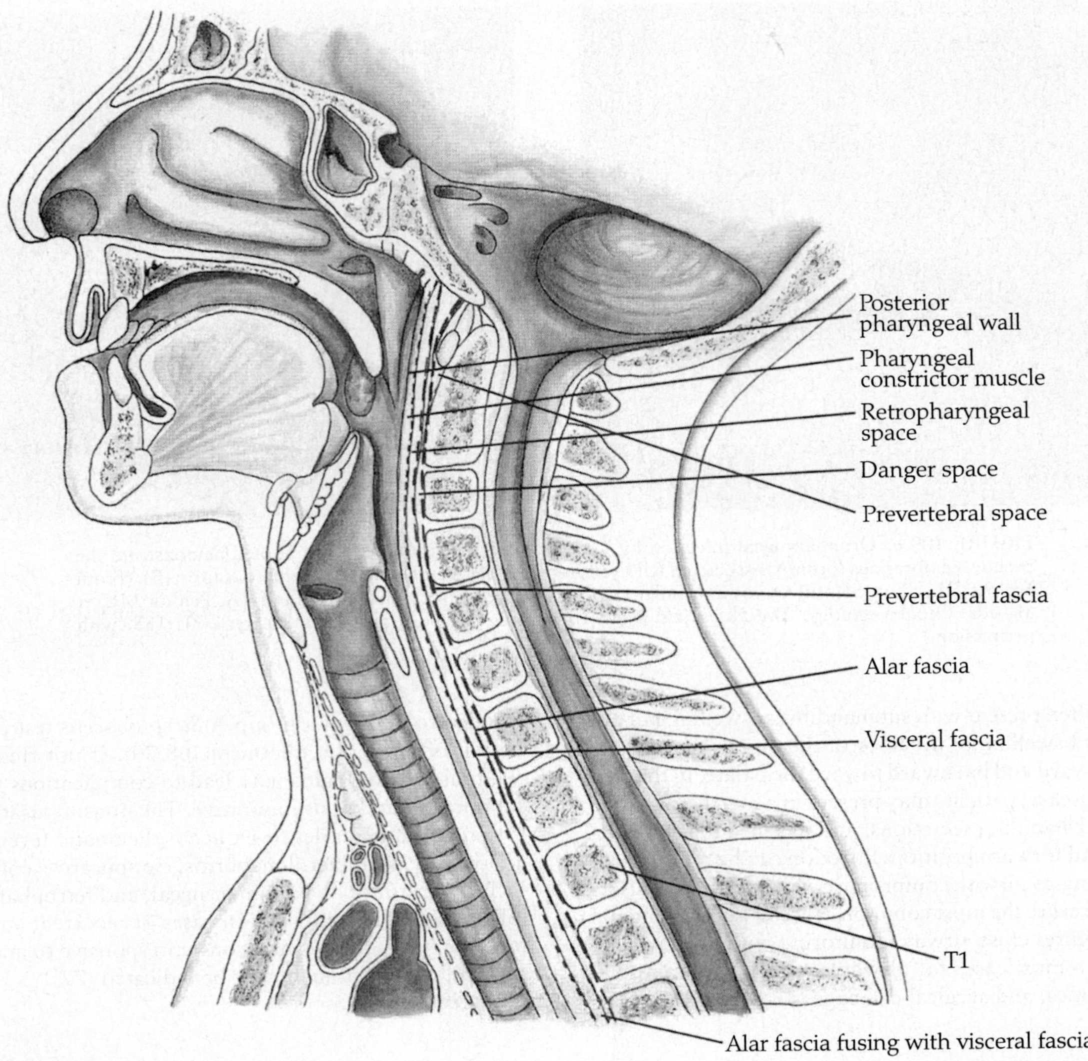

FIGURE 109.7. Schematic representation of the deep fascial spaces of the head and neck. (From Portugal LG, Padhya TA, Gluckman JL. Anatomy and Physiology. In: Seiden AM, Tami TA, Pensak ML, et al., eds. *Otolaryngology: The Essentials*. New York, NY: Thieme Medical Publishers; 2001:477, with permission.)

Lemierre Syndrome

Lemierre syndrome is described as the presence of oropharyngeal infection, sepsis, internal jugular vein thrombosis, and septic emboli caused by *Fusobacterium necrophorum* (76). This is a Gram-negative anaerobic organism that can be part of the normal human oropharyngeal, gastrointestinal, or genitourinary flora. In the present time disease is rather uncommon due to the availability of antibiotics. Most often Lemierre syndrome affects young adults with a recent history of oropharyngeal, tonsillar, or peritonsillar infection. Patients will often present with tenderness and swelling of the lateral neck, secondary to thrombophlebitis of the internal jugular vein. Septic emboli may spread and affect other organs, especially the lungs. The disease requires immediate antibiotic treatment with agents such as clindamycin, metronidazole, ampicillin-sulbactam, or ticarcillin-clavulanate for a period of at least 6 weeks (76,77). In the case of abscess formation, surgical drainage might be required. In rare cases of refractory disease, ligation or excision of the jugular vein might be indicated (77,78).

Infectious Mononucleosis

Infectious mononucleosis is a systemic disease caused by Epstein-Barr virus (EBV). It most commonly occurs in teenagers and young adults. The virus is transmitted through saliva. Patients will present with fever, fatigue, malaise, sore throat, and generalized nontender lymphadenopathy. On exam patients will have inflamed tonsils with exudate. Hepatosplenomegaly may also be present. Diagnosis is confirmed by the presence of atypical lymphocytes on peripheral smear, a positive monospot test, and positive EBV titers. Treatment of mononucleosis is supportive (79,80). Corticosteroids are used to decrease inflammation, particularly in cases where airway obstruction is a concern due to marked tonsillar enlargement. In severe cases of airway obstruction, establishing a secure airway might be indicated. Patients will develop a rash if treated with amoxicillin for presumed bacterial tonsillitis; thus administration of amoxicillin should be avoided (79).

LARYNX/AIRWAY

Supraglottitis/Epiglottitis

Epiglottitis is an infectious disease of the epiglottis and supraglottis, most commonly bacterial in origin. It usually has a sudden onset, with patients developing high fever, pain with swallowing, drooling due to difficulty handling secretions, and respiratory distress. On presentation the patient is often found sitting in a hunched-forward position with an extended neck and open mouth (sniffing position) (81). On a lateral neck film, edema of the epiglottis and a ballooning of the hypopharynx (thumb sign) will be noted (Fig. 109.8). On direct visualization the epiglottis will appear erythematous (cherry-red) and swollen. Care should be taken with airway manipulation as it may quickly precipitate complete airway obstruction. *H. influenzae* type b used to be the most common causative agent; however, with the introduction of the vaccine the incidence of *H. influenzae*–related epiglottitis has significantly decreased (82). Currently *S. pneumoniae* group A beta-hemolytic streptococci are the most common causative agents (82,83). Epiglottitis is considered an emergency as it has a potential for rapid complete airway obstruction, particularly in children. When epiglottitis is diagnosed, in most cases a secure airway should be established via endotracheal intubation or tracheostomy. The decision to extubate or decannulate is based on clinical improvement. Treatment with intravenous antibiotics (ceftriaxone or ampicillin/sulbactam) and steroids is initiated (81,82). Adults may sometimes present with supraglottitis where the epiglottis is not involved. In these cases, the airway can often be managed more conservatively, although close in-hospital observation is required.

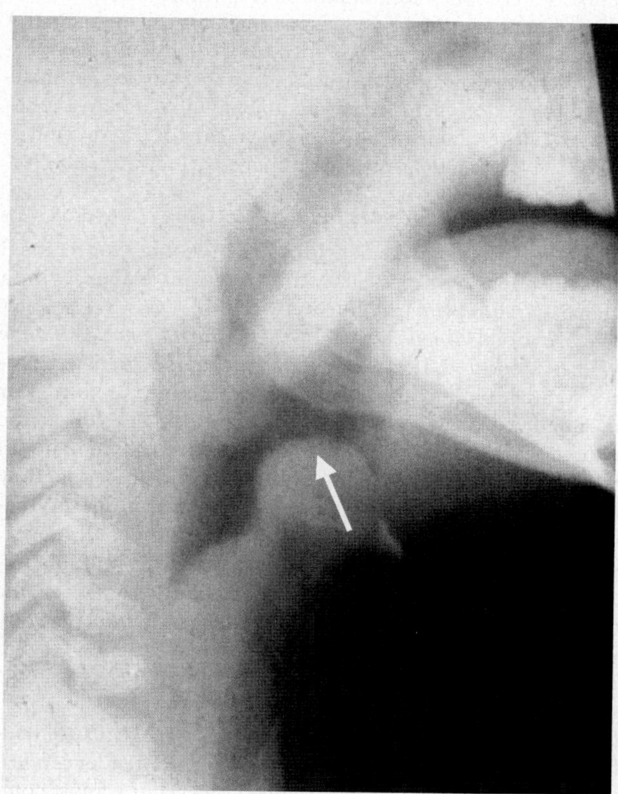

FIGURE 109.8. Lateral plain neck radiograph demonstrating edema of the epiglottis associated with epiglottitis.

Laryngitis

Acute laryngitis most often occurs as part of an upper respiratory infection and therefore is usually caused by rhinovirus (84). Laryngoscopy reveals diffuse laryngeal erythema and edema, often producing a cough and hoarseness. The treatment is often supportive, including voice rest, humidification, and occasionally anti-inflammatory medications.

Croup

Croup is an inflammatory disease of the subglottic airway. Almost always it is associated with a viral infection, most commonly caused by parainfluenza and influenza viruses. It most commonly occurs in the pediatric population between the ages of 1 and 3 years. Patients usually present with fever, tachypnea, inspiratory stridor, hoarseness, and a barking cough. The history often includes a preceding upper respiratory infection. Radiographic studies reveal subglottic narrowing, the so-called steeple sign (Fig. 109.9). Depending on the severity of the symptoms, patients might require close observation and establishment of a secure airway. Administration of glucocorticoids is recommended to decrease airway inflammation, and racemic

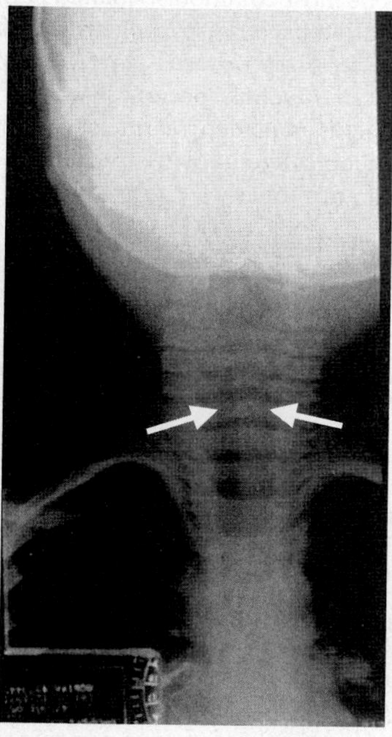

FIGURE 109.9. Subglottic edema causing narrowing and the so-called steeple sign associated with croup. (From Stern Y, Myer CM. Infectious and inflammatory disorders. In: Seiden AM, Tami TA, Pensak ML, et al., eds. *Otolaryngology: The Essentials*. New York, NY: Thieme Medical Publisher; 2001:304, with permission.)

epinephrine treatments are often helpful. When croup is recurrent, an airway evaluation with laryngoscopy and bronchoscopy is recommended to assess for anatomic abnormalities (85).

Diphtheria

Diphtheria is an infectious disease of the upper airway. It is caused by *Corynebacterium diphtheriae* and is rather rare due to widespread immunization. Patients will present with fever and malaise. Bloody nasal discharge and pseudomembranes in the nose, oropharynx, and larynx may be noted on exam. The presence of membranes may lead to airway obstruction and respiratory failure. Exotoxins produced by the bacteria may affect the heart, liver, kidney, and brain. Clinical diagnosis is confirmed by bacterial smear and cultures on Löffler or tellurite media. The treatment consists of ensuring a secure airway, administration of antitoxin, and antibiotics. Penicillin or erythromycin is recommended for treatment (68,86).

Bacterial Tracheitis

Bacterial tracheitis is a rare, potentially life-threatening respiratory infection. It is characterized by the presence of thick membranous tracheal secretions that do not readily clear with coughing and may lead to occlusion of the airway. Patients will present with fever, cough, stridor, and generalized malaise. Patients do not respond to racemic epinephrine treatment. Radiographic findings often reveal irregular tracheal margins with a normal-appearing epiglottis. Diagnosis is made with direct visualization of thick membranous tracheal secretions or the presence of purulent tracheal secretions in the glottis and subglottis (87,88). The most commonly isolated pathogen is *S. aureus*. Other causative bacterial pathogens include *H. influenzae, S. pneumoniae, Streptococcus pyogenes, M. catarrhalis, Klebsiella,* and *Pseudomonas* species (87–89). If the diagnosis of bacterial tracheitis is made, treatment consists of securing the airway, endoscopically removing tracheal membranes, and administration of antibiotics (87).

NECK

Salivary Gland Infections

Viral Infections

Mumps. Mumps is a viral infection caused by paramyxovirus and is the most common viral infection that involves the salivary glands. Infected patients display signs of fever and malaise. Painful parotid swelling occurs within 24 hours and is often bilateral. Ten percent of patients have submandibular gland involvement. Patients may experience pain with salivation. Twenty-five percent of affected adolescent or adult males will develop orchitis, and 5% of females may present with oophoritis. Mastitis, pancreatitis, and central nervous system involvement may also occur in affected individuals. Mumps infection can also lead to sensorineural hearing loss. The treatment is usually supportive. In children the disease has a less severe course than in adults (90).

Other potential viruses that may infect the salivary glands include coxsackie A, echovirus, choriomeningitis, parainfluenza type 1 and 3, and cytomegalovirus (90,91).

Bacterial Infections

Bacterial infections of the salivary glands often develop following salivary stasis, secondary to ductal obstruction by a stone or mass, or a decrease of salivary flow secondary to dehydration. Any sort of intraoral trauma, such as extensive dental work, may also cause an inflammatory obstruction of the duct. The most common causative pathogens are *S. aureus* and *Streptococcus viridans*. The parotid gland is affected more often, likely due to lower bacteriostatic activity of saliva from this gland as compared to the submandibular or sublingual glands. Patients will present with pain, swelling, and erythema in the region of the salivary gland, exacerbated by eating. Patients may also have fever, malaise, and an elevated white count. Treatment involves hydration to increase salivary flow, massaging of the affected gland, sialogogues, and administration of antistaphylococcal antibiotics. In cases of chronic or recurrent sialadenitis, removal of the obstructing stone or excision of the gland might be recommended (91,92).

Lymphadenitis

Lymphadenitis is an inflammatory process involving lymph nodes. The pediatric group is more commonly affected. Upper respiratory viral infections are the most common cause of cervical lymphadenopathy. This condition is self-limited and usually does not require treatment. Bacterial lymphadenitis usually occurs as a complication of skin or respiratory infection. The most common causative organisms are *S. aureus* and group A streptococci. Patients may present with tender lymphadenopathy, which may progress to formation of an abscess. If bacterial lymphadenitis is suspected, treatment with beta-lactamase–resistant antibiotics is recommended. In case of progression to abscess formation, incision and drainage are indicated (93,94).

Catscratch Disease

This disease usually presents with subacute solitary or regional lymphadenopathy in patients with a previous contact with a kitten or cat. It is primarily caused by *Bartonella henselae*; however, cases of *Bartonella clarridgeiae* and *Bartonella elizabethae* have been reported. Lymphadenopathy occurs 1 to 3 weeks after a scratch, bite, or other contact with an infected kitten or cat. Small red-brown nontender papules may develop at the site of inoculation 3 to 30 days after contact. The lymph nodes draining the affected site gradually enlarge and are moderately tender, with the overlying skin appearing warm and erythematous. Up to 10% of lesions may require surgical drainage. Histologic examination reveals granulomas with multiple microabscesses. The indirect fluorescent antibody test and enzyme immunoassay are used for detection of specific serum antibody to *B. henselae* (95).

Mycobacterium

Nontuberculous mycobacterial infection is a rare cause of lymphadenitis. It presents as a slowly enlarging, nontender cervical mass. The infection can affect adults; however, it is most commonly found in children younger than 5 years of age. It is often diagnosed after failure to respond to treatment with antibiotics.

The most common causative pathogen is *Mycobacterium avium-intracellulare*. Other reported pathogens are *M. scrofulaceum, M. kanasasaii, M. fortuitum*, and *M. malmoense* (96). Nontuberculous mycobacteria are found ubiquitously in the environment—in soil, food, water, animals, and so on. It is usually acquired from the environment, and there is no evidence of person-to-person transmission. An intradermal PPD test (purified protein derivative of tuberculin) aids in the diagnosis of nontuberculous lymphadenitis. However, positive cultures will be more definitive (97). Complete surgical resection of infected tissues has been the gold standard for the treatment of nontuberculous mycobacterial infections. Treatment with antituberculous medications, such as macrolides (clarithromycin), has also been shown to be effective in some cases. Recent studies have suggested an antibiotic therapeutic trial prior to surgical excision or as an adjunct to surgical excision (98).

Actinomycosis

Actinomycosis is an infection caused by *Actinomyces israelii*, a Gram-positive anaerobic bacterium. The disease has multiple presentations and is often misdiagnosed. Most of these infections occur in the head and neck region (>50%), most often entering the tissue through an area of prior trauma. As the infection develops, patients will be noted to have a woody induration that eventually leads to central abscess formation. This abscess will generally track to a mucosal surface or externally to the skin, forming a sinus or fistulous tract. The suppurative drainage will contain so-called sulfur granules, yellow flecks containing the bacterial colonies. The diagnosis is best made by culture, but as anaerobic cultures can be unreliable, diagnosis may have to rely on the clinical picture and histology. The organisms stain best with Gram and Gomori methenamine silver stains. Treatment consists of drainage and debridement of the infected area with administration of penicillin (99).

Deep Neck Space Infections

Retropharyngeal Space Abscess

The retropharyngeal space is defined by the prevertebral fascia posteriorly, the posterior layer of the deep cervical fascia anteriorly, the skull base superiorly, and the posterior mediastinum inferiorly (Fig. 109.7). Infection usually develops from infected retropharyngeal lymph nodes, which receive lymphatic drainage from the paranasal sinuses, nasopharynx, and middle ear, and are more common in children. Trauma is another common cause. Patients commonly present with fever, pain with swallowing, decreased oral intake, drooling, malaise, and torticollis. Trismus and neck swelling are often present. The most common causative organisms are *S. pyogenes* and anaerobic bacteria (73). Lateral radiographic images of the neck in extension reveal thickened prevertebral soft tissue. Computed tomography aids in determining the presence of an abscess. Therapy involves the administration of intravenous antibiotics and drainage of the abscess. Transoral drainage is recommended unless there is extension lateral to the great vessels, i.e., the carotid artery (100). If left untreated, spontaneous rupture of the abscess may lead to aspiration of infectious material. Infection may spread to the parapharyngeal and prevertebral spaces, and lead to mediastinitis, or involve the great vessels (65).

Parapharyngeal Space Abscess

The parapharyngeal space is a potential space that extends from the skull base to the greater cornu of the hyoid bone (Fig. 109.7). The pharynx and superior constrictor muscle are the medial boundaries; the internal pterygoid muscle, parotid gland, and mandible are lateral structures; the prevertebral fascia lies posteriorly; and the pterygomandibular ligament is an anterior structure that surrounds the parapharyngeal space. The styloid process divides the space into an anterior and posterior division. Pharyngeal infections, molar tooth infections, gingivitis, and even mastoiditis may spread to the parapharyngeal space. If untreated, infection has the potential to spread to the retropharyngeal space, to the mediastinum, and to involve the great vessels causing internal jugular thrombosis and erosion of the internal carotid artery. Airway compromise may occur. Patients typically present with a prior history of a sore throat or tooth infection. Initial symptoms are fever and pain with swallowing. Tender, erythematous swelling at the angle of the mandible and parotid is typically found on clinical exam, but it will not appear fluctuant even if an abscess is present. Examination of the pharyngeal will often reveal medial displacement of the ipsilateral tonsil. Trismus may develop secondary to inflammation of the medial pterygoid muscle. Torticollis toward the opposite side often results from inflammation of lymph nodes under the sternocleidomastoid muscle. Patients may also complain of otalgia (65,101,102). The most common causative pathogens are *S. aureus, S. pyogenes*, and anaerobic bacteria (73). Computed tomography aids in evaluation of the site and the extent of infection, distinguishing between cellulitis and abscess (Fig. 109.10). Parapharyngeal space infections require immediate treatment with intravenous antibiotics and surgical drainage if an abscess is present. This is usually done

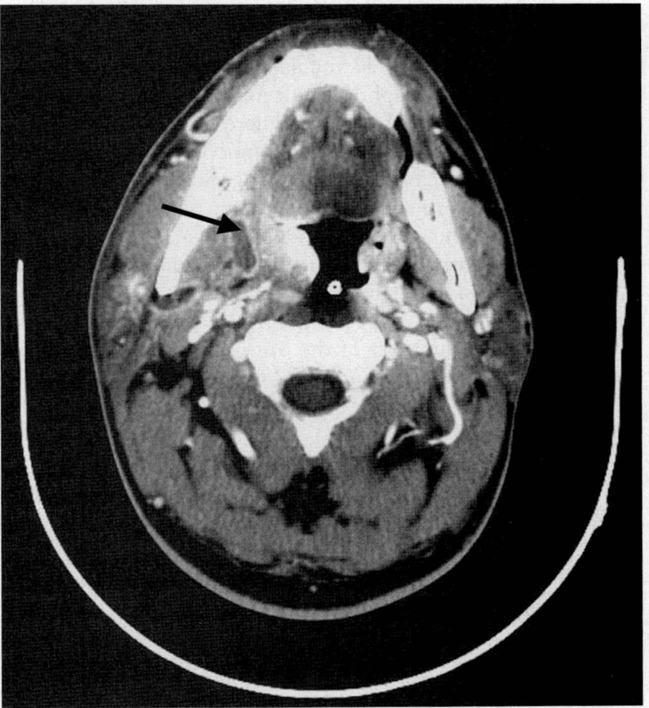

FIGURE 109.10. Computed tomography (CT) of the neck demonstrating a parapharyngeal space abscess.

through an external approach. Transoral drainage is not recommended (65,102).

TIPS AND PEARLS

Infections of the head and neck may be an occult source of sepsis in critically ill patients, especially since nasopharyngeal and oropharyngeal tubes may cause obstruction and mucosal breakdown.

- In a patient presenting with an ear infection, pushing on the tragus will elicit pain if it is an outer or external ear infection, but not if it is a middle ear infection.
- Oral antibiotics are rarely helpful in the treatment of external otitis, a condition that is more effectively treated with topical preparations.
- Otomycosis caused by *aspergillus* usually presents with grayish black or yellow dots (fungal conidiophores) surrounded by a cottonlike material (fungal hyphae) that is easily visible when examining the ear canal.
- Otitis externa with granulation tissue in a diabetic patient should be considered diagnostic of necrotizing otitis externa and treated aggressively.
- In an adult presenting with a unilateral middle ear effusion, it is essential to evaluate the nasopharynx to rule out the presence of a nasopharyngeal mass obstructing the eustachian tube.
- Auricular perichondritis should be treated early and aggressively to prevent the sequela of auricular deformity.
- The presence of a nasal septal hematoma or abscess requires immediate drainage to prevent secondary necrosis of the septal cartilage and the subsequent development of a saddle nose deformity.
- A bacterial rather than viral sinus infection should be suspected when symptoms have been present for >7 to 10 days or symptoms are worsening after 5 days.
- Primary herpes can be distinguished from aphthous ulceration by the fact that aphthous ulcers appear only on mobile or unattached mucosal surfaces, whereas herpetic lesions appear on both mobile and attached mucosa.
- Ludwig's angina can be rapidly progressive and should be considered an airway emergency, with a prophylactic tracheotomy recommended in most cases.
- Due to its potential for rapid airway compromise, epiglottitis should be considered an airway emergency.
- Due to its deep location, a parapharyngeal space abscess will cause tender induration of the upper neck, but not fluctuance.

References

1. Rosenfeld RM, Brown L, Cannon CR, et al. American Academy of Otolaryngology–Head and Neck Surgery Foundation. Clinical practice guideline: acute otitis externa. *Otolaryngol Head Neck Surg.* 2006;134(4 Suppl):S4–23.
2. Russell JD, Donnelly M, McShane DP, et al. What causes acute otitis externa? *J Laryngol Otol.* 1993;107:898–901.
3. Guthrie RM. Diagnosis and treatment of acute otitis externa: an interdisciplinary update. *Ann Otol Rhinol Laryngol.* 1999;17:2–23.
4. Kelly KE, Mohs DC. The external auditory canal. Anatomy and physiology. *Otolaryngol Clin North Am.* 1996;29:725–739.
5. Rutka J. Acute otitis externa: treatment perspectives. *Ear Nose Throat J.* 2004;83(9 Suppl 4):20–21.
6. Clark WB, Brook I, Bianki D, et al. Microbiology of otitis externa. *Otolaryngol Head Neck Surg.* 1997;116:23–25.
7. Osguthorpe JD, Nielsen DR. Otitis externa: review and clinical update. *Am Fam Physician.* 2006;74(9):1510–1516.
8. Schapowal A. Otitis externa: a clinical overview. *Ear Nose Throat J.* 2002; 81(8 suppl 1):21–22.
9. Kaur R, Mittal N, Kakkar M, et al. Otomycosis: a clinicomycologic study. *Ear Nose Throat J.* 2000;79:606–609.
10. Lucente FE. Fungal infections of external ear. *Otolaryngol Clin North Am.* 1993;26:995–1006.
11. Amorosa L, Modugno GC, Pirodda A. Malignant external otitis: review and personal experience. *Acta Otolaryngol Suppl.* 1996;521:3–16.
12. Slattery WH, Brackmann DE. Skull base osteomyelitis: malignant external otitis. *Otolaryngol Clin North Am.* 1996;29:795–806.
13. Kountakis SE, Kemper JV, Chang CYJ, et al. Osteomyelitis of the base of the skull secondary to Aspergillus. *Am J Otolaryngol.* 1997;18:19–22.
14. Chandler JR. Malignant external otitis. *Laryngoscope.* 1968;78:1257–1294
15. Okpala NC, Siraj QH, Nilssen E, et al. Radiological and radionuclide investigation of malignant otitis externa. *J Laryngol Otol.* 2005;119(1):71–75.
16. Bojarb DI, Bruderly T, Abdulrazzak Y. Otitis externa. *Otolaryngol Clin North Am.* 1996;29:761–782.
17. Bluestone CD, Gates GA, Klein JO, et al. Definitions, terminology, and classification of otitis media. *Ann Otol Rhinol Laryngol.* 2002;111: 8–18.
18. Lieberthal AS, Ganiats TG, Cox EO, et al. American Academy of Pediatrics Subcommittee on Management of Acute Otitis Media. Diagnosis and management of acute otitis media. *Pediatrics.* 2004;113(5):1451–1465.
19. Hoberman A, Marchant CD, Kaplan SL, et al. Treatment of acute otitis media consensus recommendations. *Clin Pediatr.* 2002;41:373–390.
20. Rosenfeld RM, Culpepper L, Doyle KJ, et al. American Academy of Pediatrics Subcommittee on Otitis Media with Effusion; American Academy of Family Physicians; American Academy of Otolaryngology—Head and Neck Surgery. Clinical practice guideline: Otitis media with effusion. *Otolaryngol Head Neck Surg.* 2004;130(5 Suppl):S95–118.
21. Jahn AF. Chronic otitis media: diagnosis and treatment. *Med Clin North Am.* 1991;75(6):1277–1291
22. Kenna MA. Treatment of chronic suppurative otitis media. *Otolaryngol Clin North Am.* 1994;27(3):457–472.
23. Leskinen K, Jero J. Acute complications of otitis media in adults. *Clin Otolaryngol.* 2005;30:511–516.
24. Penido NO, Borin A, Iha L, et al. Intracranial complications of otitis media: 15 years of experience in 33 patients. *Otolaryngol Head Neck Surg.* 2005; 132:37–42.
25. Osma U, Cureoglu S, Hosoglu S. The complications of chronic otitis media: report of 93 cases. *J Laryngol Otol.* 2000;114:97–100.
26. Hyden D, Akerlind B, Peebo M. Inner ear and facial nerve complications of acute otitis media with focus on bacteriology and virology. *Acta Otolaryngol.* 2006;126(5):460–466.
27. Ahmed A. When is facial paralysis Bell palsy? Current diagnosis and treatment. *Cleve Clin J Med.* 2005;72(5):398–401, 405.
28. Jackler RK, Furuta Y. Reactivation of herpes simplex virus type 1 in patients with Bell's palsy. *Am J Otol.* 1998;19:236–245.
29. Abour KK, Ruboylanes JM, Von Doersten PG, et al. Bell's palsy treatment with acyclovir and prednisone compared with prednisone alone: a double blind, randomized, controlled trial. *Ann Otol Rhinol Laryngol.* 1996; 105:307–378.
30. Sweeney CJ, Cilden DH. Ramsay Hunt syndrome. *J Neurol Neurosurg Psychiatry.* 2001;71:149–154.
31. Murakami S, Nakashiro Y, Mizobuchi M, et al. Varicella-zoster virus distribution in Ramsay Hunt syndrome revealed by polymerase chain reaction. *Acta Otolaryngol.* 1998;118:145–149.
32. Kuhweide R, Van de Steene V, Vlaminck S, et al. Ramsay Hunt syndrome: pathophysiology of cochleovestibular symptoms. *J Laryngol Otol.* 2002;116(10):844–848
33. Murakami S, Hato N, Horiuch J, et al. Treatment of Ramsay Hunt syndrome with acyclovir-prednisone: significance of early diagnosis and treatment. *Ann Neurol.* 1997;41:353–357.
34. More DR, Seidel JS, Beyan PA. Ear-piercing techniques as a cause of auricular chondritis. *Pediatr Emerg Care.* 1999;15:189–192
35. Keene WE, Markum AC, Samadpour M. Outbreak of *Pseudomonas aeruginosa* infections caused by commercial piercing of upper ear cartilage. *JAMA.* 2004;291(8):981–985.
36. Bachor E, Blevins NH, Karmody C, et al. Otologic manifestations of relapsing polychondritis. Review of literature and report of nine cases. *Auris Nasus Larynx.* 2006;33(2):135–141.
37. Ambrus PS, Eavey RD, Baker AS, et al. Management of nasal septal abscess. *Laryngoscope.* 1981;91:575–582.
38. Canty PA, Berkowitz RG. Hematoma and abscess of the nasal septum in children. *Arch Otolaryngol Head Neck Surg.* 1996;122:1373–1376.
39. Andraca R, Edson RS, Kern EB. Rhinoscleroma: a growing concern in the United States? Mayo Clinic experience. *Mayo Clin Proc.* 1993;68(12): 1151–1157.
40. Stiernberg CM, Clark WD. Rhinoscleroma—a diagnostic challenge. *Laryngoscope.* 1983;93(7):866–870.

41. Marple BF, Brunton S, Ferguson BJ. Acute bacterial rhinosinusitis: a review of U.S. treatment guidelines. *Otolaryngol Head Neck Surg.* 2006;135(3): 341–348.
42. Brook I. Microbiology and antimicrobial management of sinusitis. *Otolaryngol Clin North Am.* 2004;37(2):253–266.
43. Brook I. Sinusitis of odontogenic origin. *Otolaryngol Head Neck Surg.* 2006;135(3):349–355.
44. Younis RT, Lazar RH, Anand VK. Intracranial complications of sinusitis: a 15-year review of 39 cases. *Ear Nose Throat J.* 2002;81(9):636-8, 640-2, 644.
45. Jackson LL, Kountakis SE. Classification and management of rhinosinusitis and its complications. *Otolaryngol Clin North Am.* 2005;38(6):1143–1153.
46. Benninger MS, Ferguson BJ, Hadley JA, et al. Adult chronic rhinosinusitis: definitions, diagnosis, epidemiology, and pathophysiology. *Otolaryngol Head Neck Surg.* 2003;129(3 Suppl):S1–32.
47. Devaiah AK. Adult chronic rhinosinusitis: diagnosis and dilemmas. *Otolaryngol Clin North Am.* 2004;37(2):243–252.
48. Kennedy DW. Pathogenesis of chronic rhinosinusitis. *Ann Otol Rhinol Laryngol Suppl.* 2004;193:6–9.
49. Winther B, Gwaltney JM Jr, Mygind N, et al. Viral-induced rhinitis. *Am J Rhinol.* 1998;12(1):17–20.
50. DeShazo RD, Chapin K, Swain RE. Fungal sinusitis. *N Engl J Med.* 1997; 337:254–259.
51. DeShazo RD, Swain RE. Diagnostic criteria for allergic fungal sinusitis. *J Allergy Clin Immunol.* 1995;96:24–35.
52. Schubert MS. Allergic fungal sinusitis. *Otolaryngol Clin North Am.* 2004; 37(2):301–326.
53. DeShazo RD, O'Brien M, Chapin K, et al. Criteria for the diagnosis of sinus mycetoma. *J Allergy Clin Immunol.* 1997;99475–99485.
54. Pihlstrom BL, Michalowicz BS, Johnson NW. Periodontal diseases. *Lancet.* 2005;306:1809–1820.
55. Preshaw PM, Seymour RA, Heasman PA. Current concepts in periodontal pathogenesis. *Dent Update.* 2004;31:570–578.
56. Tatakis DN, Kumar PS. Etiology and pathogenesis of periodontal diseases. *Dent Clin North Am.* 2005;49:491–516.
57. Johnson BD, Engel D. Acute necrotizing ulcerative gingivitis. A review of diagnosis, etiology and treatment. *J Periodontol.* 1986;57(3):141–150.
58. Rowland RW. Necrotizing ulcerative gingivitis. *Ann Periodontol.* 1999; 4:65–73.
59. Amir J. Clinical aspects and antiviral therapy in primary herpetic gingivostomatitis. *Paediatr Drugs.* 2001;3(8):593–597.
60. Ajar AH, Chauvin PJ. Acute herpetic gingivostomatitis in adults: a review of 13 cases, including diagnosis and management. *J Can Dent Assoc.* 2002; 68(4):247–251.
61. Cherry JD, Jahn CL. Herpangina: the etiologic spectrum. *Pediatrics.* 1965; 36(4):632–634.
62. Zavate O, Avram G, Pavlov E. Coxsackie A virus-associated herpetiform angina. *Virologie.* 1984;35(1):49–53.
63. Greenspan D, Greenspan JS. HIV-related oral disease. *Lancet.* 1996;348 (9029):729–733.
64. Flynn TR. The swollen face. Severe odontogenic infections. *Emerg Med Clin North Am.* 2000;18(3):481–519.
65. Baker AS, Montgomery WW. Oropharyngeal space infections. *Curr Clin Top Infect Dis.* 1987;8:227–265.
66. Busch RF, Shah D. Ludwig's angina: improved treatment. *Otolaryngol Head Neck Surg.* 1997;117:5172–5175.
67. Baqain ZH, Newman L, Hyde N. How serious are oral infections? *J Laryngol Otol.* 2004;118:561–565.
68. Bisno AL. Acute pharyngitis. *N Engl J Med.* 2001;344(3):205–211.
69. Brook I, Gober AE. Increased recovery of *Moraxella catarrhalis* and *Haemophilus influenzae* in association with group A beta-haemolytic streptococci in healthy children and those with pharyngo-tonsillitis. *J Med Microbiol.* 2006;55(Pt 8):989–992.
70. Rufener JB, Yaremchuk KL, Payne SC. Evaluation of culture and antibiotic use in patients with pharyngitis. *Laryngoscope.* 2006;116:1727–1729.
71. Tewfik TL, Al Garni M. Tonsillopharyngitis: clinical highlights. *J Otolaryngol.* 2005;34(Suppl 1):S45–49.
72. Darrow DH, Siemens C. Indications for tonsillectomy and adenoidectomy. *Laryngoscope.* 2002;112:6–10.
73. Brook I. Microbiology and management of peritonsillar, retropharyngeal, and parapharyngeal abscess. *J Oral Maxillofac Surg.* 2004;62:1545–1550.
74. Herbild O, Bonding P. Peritonsillar abscess. *Arch Otolaryngol.* 1981; 107(9):540–542.
75. Kronenberg J, Wolf M, Leventon G. Peritonsillar abscess: recurrence rate and the indication for tonsillectomy. *Am J Otolaryngol.* 1987 Mar–Apr; 8(2):82–84.
76. Moreno S, Garcia Altozano J, Pinilla B, et al. Lemierre's disease: postanginal bacteremia and pulmonary involvement caused by *Fusobacterium necrophorum. Rev Infect Dis.* 1989;11:319–324.
77. Brook I. Microbiology and management of deep facial infections and Lemierre syndrome. *ORL J Otorhinolaryngol Related Spec.* 2003;65:117–120.
78. Nadkarni MD, Verchick J, O'Neill JC. Lemierre syndrome. *J Emerg Med.* 2005;28:297–299.
79. Ebell MH. Epstein-Barr virus infectious mononucleosis. *Am Fam Physician.* 2004;70(7):1279–1287.
80. Rea TD, Russo JE, Katon W, et al. Prospective study of the natural history of infectious mononucleosis caused by Epstein-Barr virus. *J Am Board Fam Pract.* 2001;14(4):234–242.
81. Carey MJ. Epiglottitis in adults. *Am J Emerg Med.* 1996;14(4):421–424.
82. Shah RK, Roberson DW, Jones DT. Epiglottitis in the *Haemophilus influenzae* type B vaccine era: changing trends. *Laryngoscope.* 2004;114:557–560.
83. Trollfors B, Nylen O, Carenfelt C, et al. Aetiology of acute epiglottitis in adults. *Scand J Infect Dis.* 1998;30(1):49–51.
84. Monto AS. Epidemiology of viral respiratory infections. *Am J Med.* 2002;112(Suppl 6A):4S–12S.
85. Stroud RH, Friedman NR. An update on inflammatory disorders of the pediatric airway: epiglottitis, croup, and tracheitis. *Am J Otolaryngol.* 2001; 22(4):268–275.
86. Hadfield TL, McEvoy P, Polotsky Y, et al. The pathology of diphtheria. *J Infect Dis.* 2000;181(Suppl 1):S116–120.
87. Friedman EM, Jorgensen K, Healy GB, et al. Bacterial tracheitis–two-year experience. *Laryngoscope.* 1985;95(1):9–11.
88. Mahajan A, Alvear D, Chang C, et al. Bacterial tracheitis, diagnosis and treatment. *Int J Pediatr Otorhinolaryngol.* 1985;10(3):271–7.
89. Salamone FN, Bobbitt DB, Myer CM, et al. Bacterial tracheitis reexamined: is there a less severe manifestation? *Otolaryngol Head Neck Surg.* 2004; 131(6):871–876.
90. Johnson A. Inflammatory conditions of the major salivary glands. *Ear Nose Throat J.* 1989;68(2):94–102.
91. Blitzer A. Inflammatory and obstructive disorders of salivary glands. *J Dent Res.* 1987;66:675–679.
92. Travis LW, Hecht DW. Acute and chronic inflammatory diseases of the salivary glands: diagnosis and management. *Otolaryngol Clin North Am.* 1977;10:329–38
93. Gosche JR, Vick L. Acute, subacute, and chronic cervical lymphadenitis in children. *Semin Pediatr Surg.* 2006;15(2):99–106.
94. Leung AK, Robson WL. Childhood cervical lymphadenopathy. *J Pediatr Health Care.* 2004;18:3–7.
95. Massei F, Gori L, Macchia P, et al. The expanded spectrum of bartonellosis in children. *Infect Dis Clin North Am.* 2005;19:691–711.
96. Flint D, Mahadevan M, Barber C, et al. Cervical lymphadenitis due to non-tuberculous mycobacteria: surgical treatment and review. *Int J Pediatr Otorhinolaryngol.* 2000;53(3):187–194.
97. Danielides V, Patrikakos G, Moerman M, et al. Diagnosis, management and surgical treatment of non-tuberculous mycobacterial head and neck infection in children. *ORL J Otorhinolaryngol Related Spec.* 2002;64:284–289.
98. Luong A, McClay JE, Jafri HS, et al. Antibiotic therapy for nontuberculous mycobacterial cervicofacial lymphadenitis. *Laryngoscope.* 2005;115: 1746–1751.
99. Richtsmeier WJ, Johns ME. Actinomycosis of the head and neck. *CRC Crit Rev Clin Lab Sci.* 1979;11(2):175–202.
100. Kirse DJ, Roberson DW. Surgical management of retropharyngeal space infections in children. *Laryngoscope.* 2001;111:1413–1422.
101. Sethi DS, Stanley RE. Parapharyngeal abscesses. *J Laryngol Otol.* 1991; 105(12):1025–1030.
102. Boscolo-Rizzo P, Marchiori C, Zanetti F, et al. Conservative management of deep neck abscesses in adults: the importance of CECT findings. *Otolaryngol Head Neck Surg.* 2006;135(6):894–899.

CHAPTER 110 ■ CATHETER-RELATED BLOODSTREAM INFECTIONS

DANY E. GHANNAM • ISSAM I. RAAD

Central venous catheter (CVC) use now permeates every sector of medicine, spanning the spectrum of both the inpatient and outpatient clinical settings. Their use is primarily directed at securing vascular access for fluids, medications, blood products, total parenteral nutrition (TPN), and hemodialysis (1). However, these intravascular devices are becoming a ready conduit for bacterial and fungal invasion, resulting in catheter-related bloodstream infection (CRBSI) (Table 110.1) that ultimately can be complicated by septic thrombophlebitis, infective endocarditis, and other metastatic infections, such as lung abscess, brain abscess, and endophthalmitis.

CRBSIs are the most common cause of hospital-acquired infections in the critically ill (2). More than 80,000 CRBSIs are estimated to occur annually in intensive care units (ICUs) in the United States, with an attributable mortality ranging from 12% to 25% (3). Therefore, 9,600 to 20,000 patients die from CRBSI in ICUs annually. The added cost ranges from $28,690 to $56,167 per each individual episode in ICU patients (4). Non-ICU patients, especially the immunocompromised hosts with CVCs in place, are also at significant risk. These infections are often difficult to diagnose, treat, and prevent. This chapter will concentrate on the latter aspects of CRBSI.

PATHOGENESIS

Diagnosis, treatment, and prevention of CRBSIs are based on our understanding of the pathogenesis of these infections. The first step in primary infection is the colonization of the CVC. For short-term, nontunneled, noncuffed, multilumen catheters—which make up 90% of CRBSIs—the skin insertion site is the source of the colonization; organisms migrate along the external surface of the catheter and through the subcutaneous layers and infect the catheter tip (5,6).

For long-term catheters—the cuffed, tunneled, silicone catheters, Hickman or Broviac—or implantable devices, the lumen of the hub or belt of the port is the primary source of entry (7,8). Micro-organisms are introduced via the hands of medical personnel while manipulating the hub during, for example, flushing and drawing of blood (7–9). Of note is that colonization is universal after insertion of a CVC, can occur as early as 1 day after insertion, and is quantitatively independent of a catheter-related infection (7).

These sources explain the prevalence of *Staphylococcus aureus*, coagulase-negative *Staphylococcus* (CNS), enterococci, nonenteric hospital-acquired Gram-negative bacilli (*Stenotrophomonas maltophilia*, *Pseudomonas aeruginosa*, *Acinetobacter* spp.), mycobacteria, and *Candida* spp. as primary organisms of CRBSI (10). Secondary seeding of the CVC, whereby organisms become blood-borne and colonize the catheter, has been suggested (11,12) to the point of recommending treatment of urinary tract infections *prior* to CVC insertion to prevent a potential CRBSI (13). However, its role in CRBSI has not been documented (13).

Contamination of the infusate or additives, such as contaminated heparin flush, are rare causes of colonization and infection of the vascular devices (14–16). The nationwide outbreaks of *Enterobacter agglomerans* and *Enterobacter cloacae* in 1971 led to widespread changes and surveillance at industry, hospital, and state and federal levels. The nutritional components present in the TPN promote the growth of certain fungi such as *Candida parapsilosis* and *Malassezia furfur,* as well as bacteria such as *Klebsiella pneumoniae* and *E. cloacae* (17–19).

The second step in the pathogenesis of CRBSI is the ability of some microbes to form a biofilm of extracellular, polysaccharide-rich, slimy material (20,21), promoting the adhesiveness of the bacteria to the surface of the CVC. Biofilms form on the external surface of short-term catheters and the internal surface of long-term catheters—that is, those with a dwell time of at least 30 days. This biofilm enables bacteria not only to adhere to the surface of the catheter, but also to resist antibiotics, such that "chronic" biofilm eradication becomes a difficult task (22). Another factor promoting adherence is the thrombin layer that covers both surfaces of a catheter during its insertion; the rich composition of the host's own blood components enables *S. aureus*, for example, to adhere to fibrinogen, CNS to fibronectin, and *Candida* spp. to fibrin (23–27).

Finally, other factors could also potentiate the risk for a CRBSI, including femoral catheterization, which was associated with a higher rate of infections and thrombotic complications when compared to subclavian catheterization in a prospective randomized, controlled trial involving intensive care unit patients (28). Another prospective controlled trial demonstrated that a transparent occlusive dressing was associated with significantly increased rates of insertion site colonization ($p < 0.001$) in patients having CVCs for more than 3 days when compared to gauze dressing (29). This difference was explained by the warm atmosphere created by occlusive dressings, which promoted microbial growth.

CLINICAL MANIFESTATIONS

Clinical manifestations of CRBSIs can be divided into two categories: local and systemic. Local manifestations include erythema, edema, tenderness, and purulent discharge. These signs and symptoms are neither sensitive nor specific, and cannot be relied on to identify catheter colonization or CVC-related

TABLE 110.1

DEFINITIONS OF CATHETER-RELATED BLOODSTREAM INFECTIONS (CRBSIs)

PROBABLE CRBSI

- Clinical manifestations of infection (fever >38°C, chills/rigors, or hypotension)
- No apparent source of the sepsis/bloodstream infection other than the catheter
- Common skin organisms (e.g., coagulase-negative staphylococci) isolated from two blood cultures from patients with intravascular device or a known pathogen (*Staphylococcus aureus* or *Candida*) isolated from a single blood culture

DEFINITE CRBSI

Probable CRBSI criteria outlined above with any of the following:

- Differential quantitative blood cultures with 5:1 ratio of the same organism isolated from blood drawn simultaneously from the central venous catheter (CVC) and peripheral vein

OR

- Differential positivity time (positive result of culture from a CVC is obtained at least 2 h earlier than positive result of culture from peripheral blood)

OR

- Positive quantitative skin culture whereby the organism isolated from an infected insertion site is identical to that isolated from blood

OR

- Isolation of the same organisms from the peripheral blood and from a quantitative or semiquantitative culture of a catheter segment or tip

bloodstream infection. On one hand, they could be completely absent, especially in immunocompromised and neutropenic patients. On the other hand, peripherally inserted central catheters (PICCs) (inserted in the basilic or cephalic veins) are associated with a 26% rate of sterile local exit site inflammation secondary to irritation of small veins (i.e., cephalic vein) by insertion of a large catheter (30); to this must be added the finding that coagulase-negative staphylococci, the most frequent pathogen involved, incites little local or systemic inflammation (31).

The Centers for Disease Control and Prevention (CDC) suggested the following definitions:

1. ***Exit-site infection***: Purulent drainage from the catheter exit site, or erythema, tenderness, and swelling within 2 cm of the catheter exit site, and colonization of the catheter if removed
2. ***Port-pocket infection***: Erythema and/or necrosis of the skin or subcutaneous tissues either over or around the reservoir of an implanted catheter, and colonization of the catheter if removed
3. ***Tunnel infection:*** Erythema, tenderness, and induration of the tissues above the catheter and more than 2 cm from the exit site, and colonization of the catheter if removed

The systemic features of CRBSIs are generally indistinguishable from those of secondary bloodstream infections arising from other foci of infection, and include fever and chills, which may be accompanied by hypotension, hyperventilation, altered mental status, and nonspecific gastrointestinal manifestations such as nausea, vomiting, abdominal pain, and diarrhea. Deep-seated infections such as endocarditis, osteomyelitis, retinitis, and organ abscess may complicate CRBSIs caused by some virulent organisms such as *S. aureus*, *P. aeruginosa*, and *Candida albicans*.

DIAGNOSIS

A clinical diagnosis of CRBSI is frequently inaccurate, as outlined before. Removal of the CVC had previously been mandatory to prove the CRBSI. Microbiologic methods requiring removal of the CVC were studied with the semiquantitative roll plate catheter cultures developed by Maki et al. in 1977 and considered the gold standard. However, the majority of the catheters were removed unnecessarily (32), exposing the patient to the complications related to reinsertion of a new central catheter and adding to the cost as well. To prevent that, techniques allowing accurate diagnosis without removing the line have been elaborated. In the following section, we will review different methods used for the microbiologic diagnosis of CRBSI (Table 110.2).

Catheter-sparing Diagnostic Methods

Simultaneous Quantitative Blood Cultures

This method consists of obtaining paired quantitative blood cultures (QBCs) simultaneously from the CVC and a peripheral vein. The target is to have both samples drawn <10 minutes apart with the same volume of blood. The hypothesis is that the higher load of organisms on the internal lumen of the CVC signifying CRBSI would translate into a colony count

TABLE 110.2

SENSITIVITY AND SPECIFICITY OF TESTS USED IN THE DIAGNOSIS OF CRBSI[a]

Diagnostic tests	Sensitivity	Specificity
Paired quantitative blood cultures	75%–93%	97%–100%
Differential time to positivity		
Short-term CVCs	89%	87%
Long-term CVCs	90%	72%
Acridine orange leukocyte cytospin technique	87%	94%
Semiquantitative culture of catheter tip (roll-plate technique)		
Short-term CVCs	84%	85%
Long-term CVCs	45%	75%
Quantitative catheter culture		
Short-term CVCs	82%	89%
Long-term CVCs	83%	97%

CRBSI, catheter-related bloodstream infection; CVC, central venous catheter.

[a]The data on the sensitivities and specificities are based on a meta-analysis of diagnostic methods by Safdar et al. (Safdar N, Fine JP, Maki DG. Meta-analysis: methods for diagnosing intravascular device-related bloodstream infection. *Ann Intern Med.* 2005;142[6]: 451–466).

from the CVC greater by manyfold than the peripheral stick. A CVC/peripheral ratio of CFU/mL of 5:1 has been chosen by the Infectious Diseases Society of America to represent true infection. However, multiple cutoffs have been used, including 2:1 (33), 3:1 (34), 4:1 (35, 36), 5:1 (37), and 10:1 (38).

A recent meta-analysis found that quantitative blood culture is the most accurate, with a pooled sensitivity of 75% to 93% and specificity of 97% to 100% (39). That same study recommended not culturing all catheter tips, but rather culturing *only* if CRBSI is suspected clinically. Keutgen et al. found that a 3:1 ratio has a sensitivity and specificity very close to the 5:1 ratio, and concluded that the latter might be missing true CRBSI episodes (40). This method is limited by the fact that it is expensive and labor intensive, in addition to the difficulty in obtaining samples through the catheter in some cases (41).

Differential Time to Positivity

The differential time to positivity (DTP) of qualitative paired CVC and peripheral blood culture has been a more practical test for centers that lack the logistics for QBCs, especially with the introduction of automated radiometric blood culture systems that record the time at which a culture turns positive. The hypothesis suggests that time to positivity of a culture is closely related to the inoculum size of micro-organisms. The technique involves measuring the difference between the time required for culture positivity in simultaneously drawn samples of catheter blood and peripheral blood. In a single center trial of CRBSI, a DTP of 120 minutes was associated with 81% sensitivity and 92% specificity for short-term catheters and 93% sensitivity and 75% specificity for long-term catheters (42). A meta-analysis showed that the DTP of 120 minutes predicts CRBSI, with a pooled sensitivity and specificity of 89% and 87% for short-term catheters and 90% and 72% for long-term catheters, respectively (39). This technique also demands a simultaneous blood draw (within 10 minutes) from the line and the peripheral vein with the same amount of blood. One limitation of this study is that its sensitivity could be compromised when antibiotics are given intraluminally at the time of drawing the blood cultures through the catheters (42).

Acridine Orange Cytospin Technique

This test involves 1 mL of ethylenediaminetetraacetic acid (EDTA) blood aspirated through the CVC. The sample is added to 10% formalin saline solution for 2 minutes. The sample is then centrifuged, the supernatant decanted, and the cellular deposit homogenized and cytocentrifuged. A monolayer is stained with 1 in 10,000 acridine orange staining and viewed by ultraviolet light. A positive test is indicated by the presence of any bacteria (43). This method is expensive but takes 30 minutes, with a sensitivity of 87% and specificity of 94% (44). It should be noted that this technique has only been tested by a small group of investigators and is not easy to perform correctly in order to reproduce the Kite method (45).

Catheter-drawn Quantitative Blood Culture

This method includes a single quantitative blood culture drawn through the CVC. The cutoff of 100 CFU/mL establishes the diagnosis with a pooled sensitivity of 81% to 86% and pooled specificity of 85% to 96% (39). In a retrospective study in a pediatric cancer population (46), this technique showed a sensitivity of 75%, specificity of 69%, positive predictive value of 79%, and likelihood ratio of 2.44—that is, the odds of having a true CRBSI with the >100 CFU/mL cutoff increase by 2.44 when compared to <100 CFU/ mL. One major drawback to this technique is that it cannot distinguish between CRBSI and high-grade bacteremia, especially in immunocompromized patients.

Diagnostic Methods Requiring Catheter Removal

Semiquantitative Roll-plate Catheter Culture

This method was described by Maki et al. in 1977 and remains the international reference diagnostic method (47). It consists of rolling a 3- to 5-cm section of the distal tip of the CVC at least four times back and forth over an agar plate surface and leaving it to incubate overnight. A cutoff of ≥15 CFU defines catheter colonization; if at the same time a peripheral culture grows with the same organism, then a CRBSI is diagnosed. However, this method does not sample the internal lumen of a CVC that is the source of the infection in long-term catheters. Nevertheless, pooled sensitivity and specificity in 14 trials involving short-term catheters was 84% and 85%, respectively (39); this number decreased to 45% and 75%, respectively, with long-term CVCs (i.e., those with more than 30 days of dwell time) (6,48).

Quantitative Catheter Cultures

This type of culture involves flushing or sonicating a catheter segment in broth with the target of retrieving organisms from both surfaces of the line. A threshold of ≥1,000 CFU correlated best with colonization; CRBSI would be defined by the same cutoff accompanied by a high clinical suspicion and absence of evidence of other sites of infection. As would be expected, the sonication method had a higher sensitivity than the roll-plate method for long-term CVCs (6); however, both sonication and vortexing had the same sensitivity and specificity of the roll-plate method for short-term CVCs (49). A recent meta-analysis revealed a pooled sensitivity and specificity of 82% and 89% for short-term catheters and 83% and 97% for long-term catheters, respectively (39).

Stain and Microscopy Rapid Diagnostic Techniques

This method suggests staining of the removed catheter segments and subsequent microscopy testing. The cutoff value of 1 organism per 20 oil immersion fields indicates that the catheter is colonized. Cooper and Hopkins (50) reported 100% sensitivity, 97% specificity, a positive predictive value of 84%, and a negative predictive value of 100%, but the results were not reproduced in another study (51). In a similar technique, acridine orange staining has been used for diagnosis, in which fluorescence is indicative of positivity (52). In addition to achieving a sensitivity of 84% and a specificity of 99%, acridine orange staining perhaps may be more easily performed than Gram staining, though microscopic techniques as a whole are labor intensive.

PREVENTIVE STRATEGIES

It should go without saying—but obviously does not—that CVCs should only be used when medically necessary, and

TABLE 110.3

PREVENTIVE MEASURES TO DECREASE THE RISK OF COLONIZATION OF CENTRAL VENOUS CATHETERS

- Hand hygiene
- Avoiding femoral site insertion if possible
- Removing unnecessary catheters
- Cutaneous antiseptic agents (2% chlorhexidine-based preparation)
- Maximal sterile barrier (handwashing, sterile gloves, large drape, and sterile gown, mask, and cap)
- Antimicrobial catheter lock solutions (a combination of an anticoagulant like heparin or ethylenediaminetetraacetic acid plus an antimicrobial agent, such as vancomycin, minocycline, or ciprofloxacin)
- Antimicrobial coating of catheter (with minocycline/rifampin or chlorhexidine/silver sulfadiazine)

should be removed as soon as possible to prevent potential complications. In a large study that included 1,981 ICU months of data, collective antiseptic measures consisting of handwashing, maximal sterile barriers during insertion, cutaneous antisepsis with chlorhexidine, avoidance of femoral site, and removal of CVCs determined to be unnecessary were associated with a significant decrease in CRBSI rate—from 7.7 per 1,000 catheter-days to 1.4 per 1,000 catheter-days ($p < 0.001$) over 18 months of follow-up (53). In 1992, Cobb et al., in an attempt to reduce catheter-related infection, conducted a controlled study whereby CVCs or pulmonary artery catheters were changed or exchanged over guidewire every 3 days. The former procedure resulted actually in an increase in the risk of mechanical complications, whereas the latter technique increased the risk of bloodstream infection (9). Table 110.3 provides a listing of preventive strategies to decrease the risk of colonization of central venous catheters. We review below the novel strategies implemented by the Healthcare Infection Control Practices Advisory Committee (HICPAC) and other professional organizations, including the Infectious Diseases Society of America (IDSA), Society for Healthcare Epidemiology of America (SHEA), and American Society of Critical Care Anesthesiologists (ASCCA) aiming at controlling all factors that could lead to colonization of the CVC, and hence decreasing the rate of CRBSI.

Cutaneous Antiseptics

The HICPAC/CDC guidelines recommend with level 1A evidence—data derived from multiple randomized clinical trials proving general agreement on its effectiveness—the usage of 2% chlorhexidine (CHX)-based preparation (54). Maki et al. prospectively randomized 68 ICU patients to 10% povidone-iodine, 70% alcohol, or 2% aqueous chlorhexidine to disinfect the site before insertion of CVCs and for site care every other day thereafter, and demonstrated that 2% aqueous chlorhexidine preparation tended to decrease the rate of CRBSI substantially (55). Using lower concentrations of CHX decreased the effectiveness of this method. Tincture of chlorhexidine gluconate 0.5% is no more effective in preventing CRBSI or CVC colonization than 10% povidone-iodine, as demonstrated by a prospective, randomized study in adults (56). A meta-analysis of eight randomized trials found an overall reduction of 49% in catheter-associated bloodstream infections when a disinfectant containing chlorhexidine was used (57).

Maximal Sterile Barrier

This involves wearing a sterile gown, gloves, and a cap and using a large drape similar to those used in the operating room during the insertion of catheters as opposed to the regular precautions consisting of sterile gloves and a small drape only. The HICPAC/CDC guidelines recommend this technique while inserting CVCs, PICC lines, and pulmonary artery catheters (54) (category 1A) based on a number of studies (58–60).

A prospective study conducted by Raad et al. with long-term, nontunneled silicone CVCs and PICC lines in a cancer patient population demonstrated not only a reduction of CRBSIs ($p = 0.03$), but also that this practice was cost effective (58). Mermel et al., in another prospective study with Swan-Ganz pulmonary artery (PA) catheters, found that less stringent barrier precautions were associated with a significantly increased risk of catheter-related infection (relative risk = 2.1, $p = 0.03$) (59). Of note is that this technique failed to reduce the colonization of CRBSIs associated with arterial catheters (60).

Antimicrobial Catheter Lock Solutions

Antimicrobial catheter lock involves flushing the catheter lumen and then filling it with 2 to 3 mL of a combination of an anticoagulant plus an antimicrobial agent. The dwell (lock) time varies between clinicians, but 20 to 24 hours is the most preferred. However, this might not be possible if the catheter has to be used (61). This intervention has often been used in long-term CVCs that remain in place longer than 30 days. Henrickson et al. showed that a combination of vancomycin and heparin, with or without ciprofloxacin, was equivalent, but each was superior to heparin alone (62). Heparin prevents the formation of the fibrin sheath on the inner surface of the line. Of six studies, four revealed a significant reduction in CRBSI with the above lock solution (63–65), and two demonstrated no benefit (66,67). Vancomycin-heparin lock solutions did not promote vancomycin resistance (66), but the risk of superinfection with Gram-negative bacilli and *Candida* is present since the vancomycin spectrum is limited to Gram-positive bacteria. A recent meta-analysis concluded that the use of a vancomycin lock solution in high-risk patient populations being treated with long-term central intravascular devices (IVDs) reduces the risk of bloodstream infection with a risk ratio of 0.34 (95% confidence interval [CI], 0.12–0.98; $p = 0.04$) (68).

Minocycline and EDTA (M-EDTA), another lock solution, was reported in a prospective randomized trial to significantly reduce the risk of catheter colonization and infection when compared with heparin in long-term hemodialysis CVCs (69). This solution was superior in an *in vitro* biofilm model and in an animal model to vancomycin-heparin lock solution (70,71). A clinical study of pediatric cancer populations showed that M-EDTA significantly reduces the risk of catheter infection and colonization when compared to heparin (72).

In a prospective nonrandomized study of tunneled CVCs in a pediatric cancer population, ethanol as a lock solution reduced the risk of relapse of CRBSI and was well tolerated (73). However, symptoms of fatigue, nausea, dizziness, and headache were reported. The study involved filling the catheter lumen with 2.3 mL of a 74% ethanol solution for 20 to 24 hours. The solution was then flushed through to prevent clotting inside the catheter. Each port was alternately blocked for 3 days, allowing the unblocked port to be used. In a recent study by Raad et al. (74), M-EDTA in 25% ethanol was found to be highly effective in eradicating organisms embedded in biofilm, even after a short exposure of 15 to 60 minutes. Hence, the addition of a low concentration of ethanol (25%) to M-EDTA could expedite its activity and decrease the necessary dwell time. A prolonged dwell time of more than 8 hours is often required for nonalcohol based antibiotic lock solutions, which makes their use limited, particularly in critically ill patients or patients requiring TPN.

Antimicrobial Impregnation of Catheters

This technique consists of the impregnation of the external and/or internal surface of the catheter with antiseptic or antibiotics; the slow release of antimicrobials would prevent initial bacterial adherence and biofilm formation, with virtually undetectable serum levels. The HICPAC/CDC, with a category 1B, recommends use of the coated CVCs described herein. The first-generation catheters were impregnated on the external surface with CHX and silver sulfadiazine (CHX/SSD) (Arrow Gard and Arrow Gard Plus, Arrow International, Inc.). That technique lowered the rate of CRBSI from 7.6 cases per 1,000 catheter-days to 1.6 cases per 1,000 catheter-days ($p = 0.03$), with a decrease in the rate of colonization (relative risk, 0.56 [95% CI, 0.36–0.89]; $p = 0.005$) (75); the estimated cost savings per CVC insertion was $196 (76). However, three subsequent studies failed to show that difference (77–79). This was explained by the fact that short-term catheter infection is due to external colonization, whereas long-term CRBSIs due to internal colonization are not prevented by external coating. Moreover, Mermel showed that these catheters do not protect if the CVC dwell time is more than 3 weeks, secondary to wearing off of the antimicrobial activity (3). The second-generation CHX/SSD-coated catheters were impregnated on both surfaces. In a multicenter, randomized double-blind prospective study from 14 French ICUs, second-generation catheters failed to decrease the rate of CRBSI (80,81) when compared to noncoated catheters, although they significantly decreased the rate of colonization (11/1,000 catheter-days to 3.6/1,000 catheter-days, $p = 0.01$).

In 1997, Raad et al. launched the polyurethane catheter impregnated on both surfaces with minocycline-rifampin (M/R). In a prospective randomized, double-blind trial, M/R CVCs showed more efficacy when compared to noncoated catheters (81). Another prospective trial comparing M/R catheters with first-generation CHX/SSD-impregnated catheters found that the former were three times less likely to be colonized ($p < 0.001$), and CRBSI was 12-fold more likely to occur in the CHX/SSD catheters ($p < 0.002$) (82). The use of antibiotic-impregnated CVCs in medical and surgical units was associated with a significant decrease in nosocomial bloodstream infections, including vancomycin-resistant enterococci (VRE) bacteremia, catheter-related infections, and length of hospital and ICU stay (83). Furthermore, the MR-coated catheters saved $9,600 per each CRBSI and $81 per each catheter placed when compared to first-generation CHX/SSD (84).

The concern for the emergence of antibiotic-resistant organisms was raised with the catheters coated with minocycline and rifampin. Four prospective studies evaluated the skin at the catheter insertion site before and after the insertion of antibiotic-coated catheters and failed to detect any emergence of resistance (81,82,85,86). A retrospective review of the M/R-coated CVC experience in bone marrow transplant patients also detected no emergence of resistance of staphylococci to either component (87). Through prospective randomized studies, the M/R-coated CVCs were shown to bring the risk of CRBSI to a level ≤ 0.3 per 1,000 catheter-days in nontunneled, noncuffed CVCs (81,82,86), which is lower than the 1.4 per 1,000 catheter-days achieved with multiple other aseptic measures applied collectively (such as the maximal sterile barrier, chlorhexidine cutaneous antisepsis, and hand hygiene).

Silver-impregnated Catheters

Other catheters incorporate silver, platinum, and carbon (SPC) into the polyurethane, allowing topical silver ion release (Vantex CVC with oligan, Edwards Life Sciences, Irvine, CA). A recent prospective randomized study compared these catheters to the M/R-coated type; the latter was more efficacious in reducing, to a significant degree, CVC colonization with Gram-positive and Gram-negative bacteria ($p = 0.039$). However, the CRBSI rates were low and similar between the two groups (88). In another prospective, randomized, controlled, open-label, multicenter clinical trial, the SPC CVCs failed to show any benefit in reducing CRBSI or colonization (89). Management of CRBSI is based on the organisms causing such an infection, and is detailed below.

MANAGEMENT

The management of CRBSIs involves confirming the source of infection, determining the choice of antimicrobials, determining the duration of therapy, and deciding whether to remove the catheters.

Confirmation of the infection is dependent on the diagnostic measures outlined above. The duration of therapy depends on whether the infection is complicated (i.e., by a septic phlebitis or endocarditis) or uncomplicated.

Coagulase-negative Staphylococcus (CNS)

Coagulase-negative staphylococci are the primary organisms involved in CRBSIs because they are the most common skin organisms. However, and for the same reason, they are the most frequent blood contaminants. A recent study indicated that QBC collected through CVC, with a cutoff point of 15 CFU/mL, could be a useful laboratory criterion, together with positive clinical findings for differentiating true bacteremia from false-positive contaminated blood cultures, with a sensitivity of 96%, specificity of 94%, positive predictive value of 86%, and negative predictive value of 98% (90). The IDSA guidelines recommend removing the CVC and treating for

5 to 7 days. Otherwise, if the CVC is to be retained, duration of treatment should be 10 to 14 days, and antibiotic lock therapy should be considered (91). Leaving the CVC in place carries a risk of recurrence of 20% (92).

Lock solutions used included vancomycin plus heparin. The limited activity of vancomycin against *Staphylococcus* embedded in biofilms (66,68,93) led investigators to consider other alternatives. Minocycline and EDTA, ethanol, or the triple combination (94,95) was used as an alternative. Systemically, vancomycin has been the most frequently used glycopeptide. Dalbavancin, a new, long-acting glycopeptide that is dosed weekly, was noted to be superior to vancomycin for adult patients with CRBSIs caused by CNS and *S. aureus*, including methicillin-resistant *S. aureus* (MRSA) in a phase 2, open-label, randomized, multicenter study; the side effect profile was comparable (96). Linezolid and daptomycin were also used successfully (97,98).

Staphylococcus aureus

S. aureus CRBSI is associated with high rates of deep-seated infection such as osteomyelitis, septic phlebitis, and endocarditis (99). In addition, Fowler et al. showed that patients whose intravascular device was not removed were 6.5 times more likely to relapse or die of their infection than were those whose device was removed (99). IDSA guidelines recommend removing the CVC, as this results in a more rapid response and lower relapse rate but, at the same time, gives the option of keeping it and initiating systemic and lock solutions in case of thrombocytopenia or lack of other vascular access (91). Capdevila et al. used the antibiotic lock technique in addition to standard parenteral therapy for patients with a hemodialysis catheter–related infection. All 40 CRBSIs—including all 12 cases reported to involve *S. aureus*—were cured and the catheter salvaged (100). The lock solutions most frequently used *in vivo* and *in vitro* are vancomycin plus heparin, or minocycline plus EDTA (64,95). However, the former combination—with or without ceftazidime, depending on the organism—was associated with a 60% failure rate in hemodialysis MRSA catheter infections (101). Ethanol is another very appealing component for use in combination lock solutions. Raad et al. found that the combination of minocycline–EDTA in 25% ethanol was highly efficacious in eradicating *S. aureus* in biofilm within 60 minutes of dwell time (74).

For methicillin-sensitive *S. aureus*, nafcillin or first-generation cephalosporins are the first-choice agents (91). Vancomycin, linezolid, daptomycin, and dalbavancin (96–98) are all appropriate options for MRSA. Duration of therapy usually consists of 10 to 14 days of intravenous therapy if the CVC is removed, with no deep-seated infection present (91). If fever or bacteremia persists for more than 72 hours after catheter removal, transesophageal echocardiography should be considered to rule out infectious endocarditis, with the intravenous therapy duration expanded to at least 4 weeks (91,102).

Gram-negative Bacilli

Gram-negative bacilli (GNB) bacteremia is rarely due to a CVC; rather, it generally arises from a visceral source of infection such as the genitourinary, pulmonary, or gastrointestinal tracts. However, CRBSIs caused by such organisms as *K. pneumoniae*, *Enterobacter* spp., *P. aeruginosa* spp., *Acinetobacter* spp., and *Stenotrophomonas maltophilia* have been reported (103,104). Elting and Bodey reported a 15-year experience of 149 episodes of septicemia caused by *Xanthamonas maltophilia* and *Pseudomonas* spp. in cancer patients where the CVC was the most common source (103). Hanna et al. demonstrated that catheter removal within 72 hours of the onset of the catheter-related GNB was the only independent protective factor against the relapse of infection (odds ratio, 0.13; 95% confidence interval, 0.02–0.75; $p = 0.02$) (104). IDSA guidelines (91) recommend removing nontunneled CVCs and treating for 10 to 14 days; there are no data to guide the use of intravenous versus oral antibiotics. It is considered appropriate to attempt to salvage the CVC in certain situations (e.g., when unable to access other vascular sites due to anatomic challenges or if there is a high risk of hemorrhagic complications because of thrombocytopenia or elevated prothrombin time) using systemic and lock solution therapies. However, lock therapy for GNB CRBSIs is anecdotal; successful cases were salvaged using gentamicin, amikacin, or ceftazidime (91,101).

Candida

Five large prospective studies proved that catheter retention was associated with increased mortality and an increase in the mean duration of candidemia in cases of *Candida* CRBSI (105–109). Hung et al. investigated the predisposing factors and prognostic determinants of candidemia in a Taiwan hospital, and concluded that higher severity scores, nonremoval of the catheter, persistent candidemia, and lack of antifungal therapy adversely affect the outcome (107). Raad et al., in a retrospective study of 404 patients with candidemia and an indwelling CVC, using a multivariate analysis, demonstrated that catheter removal 72 hours or sooner after onset of candidemia improved the response to antifungal therapy exclusively in patients with catheter-related candidemia ($p = 0.04$) (110). IDSA guidelines recommend removing the CVC and treating for 14 days after the last positive blood culture in uncomplicated cases. Endophthalmitis merits 6 weeks of therapy (91). Further studies are needed to define the role of antifungal lock solution in these cases. Fluconazole and caspofungin were equivalent to amphotericin B in candidemia, but with a better safety profile (109, 110); therefore, fluconazole or caspofungin should be considered in documented cases of catheter-related candidemia. If the rates of fluconazole-resistant *Candida glabrata* and *Candida krusei* in the hospital are high, an echinocandin (caspofungin, micafungin, or anidulafungin) would be the best alternative to amphotericin B.

SUMMARY

Central venous catheters are as much a part of modern ICU practice as are mechanical ventilators and antibiotics. When CVCs are placed with the appropriate technique, accessed, and cared for, it is possible to use these devices while approximating a zero incidence of infection. As is true in the majority of the practice of critical care medicine, it is in the details that the battle is won or lost.

References

1. Maki DG, Mermel LA. Infections due to infusion therapy. In: Bennett JV, Brachman PS, eds. *Hospital Infections.* 4th ed. Philadelphia: Lippincott-Raven; 1998:689–724.
2. Fletcher SJ. Central venous catheter related infection. *Anaesth Intensive Care.* 1999;27(4):425.
3. Mermel LA. Prevention of intravascular catheter-related infections. *Ann Intern Med.* 2000;132:391–402.
4. Dimick JB, Pelz RK, Consunji R, et al. Increased resource use associated with catheter-related bloodstream infection in the surgical intensive care unit. *Arch Surg.* 2001;136:229–234.
5. Maki DG, Stolz SM, Wheeler S, et al. Prevention of central venous catheter-related bloodstream infection by use of an antiseptic impregnated catheter: a randomized controlled trial. *Ann Intern Med.* 1997;127:257–266.
6. Safdar N, Maki DG. The pathogenesis of catheter-related bloodstream infection with noncuffed short-term central venous catheters. *Intensive Care Med.* 2004;30(1):62–67.
7. Raad I, Costerton W, Sabharwal U, et al. Ultrastructural analysis of indwelling vascular catheters: a quantitative relationship between luminal colonization and duration of placement. *J Infect Dis.* 1993;168:400–407.
8. Sitges-Serra A, Puig P, Linares J, et al. Hub colonization as the initial step in an outbreak of catheter-related sepsis due to coagulase negative staphylococci during parenteral nutrition. *J Parenter Enteral Nutr.* 1984;8:668–672.
9. Cobb DK, High KP, Sawyer RG, et al. A controlled trial of scheduled replacement of central venous and pulmonary artery catheters. *N Engl J Med.* 1991;327:1062–1068.
10. Raad II, Hanna HA. Intravascular catheter-related infections: new horizons and recent advances. *Arch Intern Med.* 2002;162(8):871–878.
11. Kovacevich DS, Faubion WC, Bender JM, et al. Association of parenteral nutrition catheter sepsis with urinary tract infections. *J Parenter Enter Nutr.* 1986;10:639–641.
12. Pettigrew RA, Lang DSR, Haycock DA, et al. Catheter-related sepsis in patients on intravenous nutrition: a prospective study of quantitative catheter cultures and guideline changes for suspected sepsis. *Br J Surg.* 1985;72:52–55.
13. Anaissie E, Samonis G, Kontoyiannis D, et al. Role of catheter colonization and infrequent hematogenous seeding in catheter-related-infections. *Eur J Clin Microbiol Infect Dis.* 1995;14(2):134–137.
14. Centers for Disease Control. Nosocomial bacteremia associated with intravenous fluid therapy. *MMWR.* 1971;20(Suppl 9):S1–S2.
15. Maki DG, Rhame FS, Mackel DC, et al. Nation-wide epidemic of septicemia caused by contaminated intravenous products. *Am J Med.* 1976;60:471–485.
16. Kimura AC, Calvet H, Higa JI, et al. Outbreak of *Ralstonia pickettii* bacteremia in a neonatal intensive care unit. *Pediatr Infect Dis J.* 2005; 24(12):1099–1103.
17. Jarvis WR, Highsmith AK. Bacterial growth and endotoxin production in lipid emulsion. *J Clin Microbiol.* 1984;19:17–20.
18. Danker WM, Spector SA, Fierer J. Malassezia fungemia in neonates and adults: complication of hyperalimentation. *Rev Infect Dis.* 1987;9:743–837.
19. Plouffe JF, Brown DG, Silva J, et al. Nosocomial outbreak of *Candida parapsilosis* fungemia related to intravenous infusions. *Arch Intern Med.* 1977;137:1686–1699.
20. Christensen GD, Simpson WA, Bisno AL, et al. Adherence of slime producing strains of *Staphylococcus epidermidis* to smooth surfaces. *Infect Immun.* 1982;17:318–326.
21. Costerton JW, Irvin RT, Cheng KJ. The bacterial glycocalyx in nature and disease. *Annu Rev Microbiol.* 1981;35:299–324.
22. Anwar H, Strap JL, Chen K, et al. Dynamic interactions of biofilms of mucoid *Pseudomonas aeruginosa* with tobramycin and piperacillin. *Antimicrob Agents Chemother.* 1992;36(6):1208–1214.
23. Hawiger J, Timmons S, Strong DD, et al. Identification of a region of human fibrinogen interacting with staphylococcal clumping factor. *Biochemistry.* 1982;21:1407–1413.
24. Kuusela P. Fibronectin binds to *Staphylococcus aureus*. *Nature.* 1978;276: 718–720.
25. Lopes JD, Dos Reis M, Brentani RR. Presence of laminin receptors in *Staphylococcus aureus*. *Science.* 1985;229:275–277.
26. Vaudaux P, Pittet D, Haeberli A, et al. Host factors selectively increase staphylococcal adherence on inserted catheters: a role for fibronectin and fibrinogen or fibrin. *J Infect Dis.* 1989;160:865–875.
27. Bouali A, Robert R, Tronchin G, et al. Characterization of binding of human fibrinogen to the surface of germ-tubes and mycelium of *Candida albicans*. *J Gen Microbiol.* 1987;133(3):545–551.
28. Merrer J, De Jonghe B, Grolliot F, et al. Complications of femoral and subclavian venous catheterization in critically ill patients: a randomized controlled trial. *JAMA.* 2001;286(6):700–707.
29. Conly JM, Grieves K, Peters B. A prospective, randomized study comparing transparent and dry gauze dressings for central venous catheters. *J Infect Dis.* 1989;159(2):310–319.
30. Raad I, Davis S, Becker M, et al. Low infection rate and long durability of nontunneled silastic catheters: a safe and cost-effective alternative for long-term venous access. *Arch Intern Med.* 1993;153:1791–1796.
31. Safdar N, Maki DG. Inflammation at the insertion site is not predictive of catheter-related bloodstream infection with short-term, noncuffed central venous catheters. *Crit Care Med.* 2002;30(12):2632–2635.
32. Ryan JA Jr, Abel RM, Abbott WM, et al. Catheter complications in total parenteral nutrition. A prospective study of 200 consecutive patients. *N Engl J Med.* 1974;290(14):757–761.
33. Chatzinikolaou I, Hanna H, Hachem R, et al. Differential quantitative blood cultures for the diagnosis of catheter-related bloodstream infections associated with short- and long-term catheters: a prospective study. *Diagn Microbiol Infect Dis.* 2004;50(3):167–172.
34. Douard MC, Clementi E, Arlet G, et al. Negative catheter-tip culture and diagnosis of catheter-related bacteremia. *Nutrition.* 1994;10(5):397–404.
35. Capdevila JA, Planes AM, Palomar M, et al. Value of differential quantitative blood cultures in the diagnosis of catheter-related sepsis. *Eur J Clin Microbiol Infect Dis.* 1992;11(5):403–407.
36. Douard MC, Arlet G, Longuet P, et al. Diagnosis of venous access port-related infections. *Clin Infect Dis.* 1999;29(5):1197–1202.
37. Flynn PM, Shenep JL, Barrett FF. Differential quantitation with a commercial blood culture tube for diagnosis of catheter-related infection. *J Clin Microbiol.* 1988;26:1045–1046.
38. Raucher HS, Hyatt AC, Barzilai A, et al. Quantitative blood cultures in the evaluation of septicemia in children with Broviac catheters. *J Pediatr.* 1984;104:29–33.
39. Safdar N, Fine JP, Maki DG. Meta-analysis: methods for diagnosing intravascular device-related bloodstream infection. *Ann Intern Med.* 2005;142(6):451–466.
40. Keutgen X, Ghannam D, Hackett B, et al. Differential quantitative blood cultures (QBC) for the diagnosis of catheter-related bloodstream infection: what is the cutoff ratio? [Abstract D0472]. In: Programs and abstracts of the 46th Interscience Conference on Antimicrobial Agents and Chemotherapy, September 27–30, 2006, San Francisco, CA.
41. Catton JA, Dobbins BM, Kite P, et al. In situ diagnosis of intravascular catheter-related bloodstream infection: a comparison of quantitative culture, differential time to positivity, and endoluminal brushing. *Crit Care Med.* 2005;33(4):787–791.
42. Raad I, Hanna HA, Alakech B, et al. Differential time to positivity: a useful method for diagnosing catheter-related bloodstream infections. *Ann Intern Med.* 2004;140(1):18–25.
43. Kite P, Dobbins BM, Wilcox MH, et al. Rapid diagnosis of central-venous-catheter-related bloodstream infection without catheter removal. *Lancet.* 1999;354:1504–1507.
44. Rushforth JA, Hoy CM, Kite P, et al. Rapid diagnosis of central venous catheter sepsis. *Lancet.* 1993;342(8868):402–403.
45. Farina C, Bonanomi E, Benetti G, et al. Acridine orange leukocyte cytospin test for central venous catheter-related bloodstream infection: a pediatric experience. *Diagn Microbiol Infect Dis.* 2005;52(4):337–339.
46. Franklin JA, Gaur AH, Shenep JL, et al. In situ diagnosis of central venous catheter-related bloodstream infection without peripheral blood culture. *Pediatr Infect Dis J.* 2004;23(7):614–618.
47. Maki DG, Weise CE, Sarafin HW. A semiquantitative culture method for identifying intravenous-catheter-related infection. *N Engl J Med.* 1977; 296(23):1305–1309.
48. Rello J, Gatell JM, Almirall J, et al. Evaluation of culture techniques for identification of catheter-related infection in hemodialysis patients. *Eur J Clin Microbiol Infect Dis.* 1989;8(7):620–622.
49. Bouza E, Alvarado N, Alcala L, et al. A prospective, randomized and comparative study of three different methods for the diagnosis of intravascular catheter colonization. *Clin Infect Dis.* 2005;40(8):1096–1100.
50. Cooper GL, Hopkins CC. Rapid diagnosis of intravascular catheter-associated infection by direct Gram staining of catheter segments. *N Engl J Med.* 1985;312:1142–1147.
51. Spencer RC, Kristinsson KG. Failure to diagnose intravascular-associated infection by direct Gram staining of catheter segments. *J Hosp Infect.* 1986;7:305–306.
52. Zufferey J, Rime B, Francioli P, et al. Simple method for rapid diagnosis of catheter-associated infection by direct acridine orange staining of catheter tips. *J Clin Microbiol.* 1988:26:175–177.
53. Pronovost P, Needham D, Berenholtz S, et al. An intervention to decrease catheter-related bloodstream infections in the ICU. *N Engl J Med.* 2006;355(26):2725–2732.
54. O'Grady NP, Alexander M, Dellinger EP, et al. Guidelines for the prevention of intravascular catheter-related infections. Centers for Disease Control and Prevention. *MMWR Recomm Rep.* 2002;51(RR-10):1–29.
55. Maki DG, Ringer M, Alvarado CJ. Prospective randomized trial of povidone-iodine, alcohol, and chlorhexidine for prevention of infection associated with central venous and arterial catheters. *Lancet.* 1991; 338(8763):339–343.
56. Humar A, Ostromecki A, Direnfeld J, et al. Prospective randomized trial of 10% povidone-iodine versus 0.5% tincture of chlorhexidine as cutaneous antisepsis for prevention of central venous catheter infection. *Clin Infect Dis.* 2000;31:1001–1007.

57. Chaiyakunapruk N, Veenstra DL, Lipsky BA, et al. Chlorhexidine compared with povidone-iodine solution for vascular catheter-site care: a meta-analysis. *Ann Intern Med.* 2002;136:792–801.
58. Raad II, Hohn DC, Gilbreath B, et al. Prevention of central venous catheter-related infections using maximal sterile barrier precautions during insertion. *Infect Control Hosp Epidemiol.* 1994;15:231–238.
59. Mermel LA, McCormick RD, Springman SR, et al. The pathogenesis and epidemiology of catheter-related infection with pulmonary artery Swan Ganz catheters: a prospective study utilizing molecular subtyping. *Am J Med.* 1991;91(Suppl 3B):197S–205S.
60. Rijnders BJ, Van Wijngaerden E, Wilmer A, et al. Use of full sterile barrier precautions during insertion of arterial catheters: a randomized trial. *Clin Infect Dis.* 2003;36(6):743–748.
61. Segarra-Newnham M, Martin-Cooper EM. Antibiotic lock technique: a review of the literature. *Ann Pharmacother.* 2005;39(2):311–318.
62. Henrickson KJ, Axtell RA, Hoover SM, et al. Prevention of central venous catheter-related infections and thrombotic events in immunocompromised children by the use of vancomycin/ciprofloxacin/heparin flush solution: a randomized, multicenter, double-blind trial. *J Clin Oncol.* 2000;18(6):1269–1278.
63. Schwartz C, Henrickson KJ, Roghmann K, et al. Prevention of bacteremia attributed to luminal colonization of tunneled central venous catheters with vancomycin-susceptible organisms. *J Clin Oncol.* 1990;8(9):1591–1597.
64. Carratala J, Niubo J, Fernandez-Sevilla A, et al. Randomized, double-blind trial of an antibiotic-lock technique for prevention of gram-positive central venous catheter-related infection in neutropenic patients with cancer. *Antimicrob Agents Chemother.* 1999;43(9):2200–2204.
65. Garland JS, Henrickson KJ, Maki DG. A prospective randomized trial of vancomycin-heparin lock for prevention of catheter-related bloodstream infection in an NICU (abstract 1734). In: Program and abstracts of the 2002 Annual Meeting of the Pediatric Academic Societies (Baltimore). Pediatric Academic Societies; 2002:235.
66. Rackoff WR, Weiman M, Jakobowski D, et al. A randomized, controlled trial of the efficacy of a heparin and vancomycin solution in preventing central venous catheter infections in children. *J Pediatr.* 1995;127(1):147–151.
67. Daghistani D, Horn M, Rodriguez Z, et al. Prevention of indwelling central venous catheter sepsis. *Med Pediatr Oncol.* 1996;26(6):405–408.
68. Safdar N, Maki DG. Use of vancomycin-containing lock or flush solutions for prevention of bloodstream infection associated with central venous access devices: a meta-analysis of prospective, randomized trials. *Clin Infect Dis.* 2006;43(4):474–484.
69. Bleyer AJ, Mason L, Russell G, et al. A randomized, controlled trial of a new vascular catheter flush solution (minocycline-EDTA) in temporary hemodialysis access. *Infect Control Hosp Epidemiol.* 2005;26(6):520–524.
70. Raad I, Chatzinikolaou I, Chaiban G, et al. In vitro and ex vivo activities of minocycline and EDTA against microorganisms embedded in biofilm on catheter surfaces. *Antimicrob Agents Chemother.* 2003;47(11):3580–3505.
71. Raad I, Hachem R, Tcholakian RK, et al. Efficacy of minocycline and EDTA lock solution in preventing catheter-related bacteremia, septic phlebitis, and endocarditis in rabbits. *Antimicrob Agents Chemother.* 2002;46(2):327–332.
72. Chatzinikolaou I, Zipf TF, Hanna H, et al. Minocycline-ethylenediaminetetraacetate lock solution for the prevention of implantable port infections in children with cancer. *Clin Infect Dis.* 2003;36(1):116–119.
73. Dannenberg C, Bierbach U, Rothe A, et al. Ethanol-lock technique in the treatment of bloodstream infections in pediatric oncology patients with Broviac catheter. *J Pediatr Hematol Oncol.* 2003;25(8):616–621.
74. Raad I, Hanna H, Dvorak T, et al. Optimal antimicrobial catheter lock solution, using different combinations of minocycline, EDTA and 25% ethanol: rapid eradication of organisms embedded in biofilm. *Antimicrob Agents Chemother.* 2007;51(1):78–83.
75. Maki DG, Stolz SM, Wheeler S, et al. Prevention of central venous catheter-related bloodstream infection by use of an antiseptic-impregnated catheter. A randomized, controlled trial. *Ann Intern Med.* 1997;127(4):257–266.
76. Veenstra DL, Saint S, Sullivan SD. Cost-effectiveness of antiseptic impregnated central venous catheters for the prevention of catheter-related bloodstream infection. *JAMA.* 1999;282(6):554–560.
77. Heard SO, Wagle M, Vijayakumar E, et al. Influence of triple-lumen central venous catheters coated with chlorhexidine and silver sulfadiazine on the incidence of catheter-related bacteremia. *Arch Intern Med.* 1998;158:81–87.
78. Ciresi D, Albrecht RM, Volkers PA, et al. Failure of an antiseptic bonding to prevent central venous catheter-related infection and sepsis. *Ann Surg.* 1996;62:641–646.
79. Pemberton LB, Ross V, Cuddy P, et al. No difference in catheter sepsis between standard and antiseptic central venous catheters: a prospective randomized trial. *Arch Surg.* 1996;131:986–989.
80. Brun-Buisson C, Doyon F, Sollet JP, et al. Prevention of intravascular catheter-related infection with newer chlorhexidine-silver sulfadiazine-coated catheters: a randomized controlled trial. *Intensive Care Med.* 2004;30(5):837–843.
81. Raad I, Darouiche R, Dupuis J, et al. Central venous catheters coated with minocycline and rifampin for the prevention of catheter-related colonization and bloodstream infections: a randomized, double-blind trial. The Texas Medical Center Study Group. *Ann Intern Med.* 1997;127:267–274.
82. Darouiche RO, Raad II, Heard SO, et al. Comparison of two anti-microbial impregnated central venous catheters. *N Engl J Med.* 1999;340:1–8.
83. Hanna HA, Raad II, Hackett B, et al. Anderson Catheter Study Group. Antibiotic-impregnated catheters associated with significant decrease in nosocomial and multidrug resistant bacteremias in critically ill patients. *Chest.* 2003;124(3):1030–1038.
84. Shorr AF, Humphreys CW, Helman DL. New choices for central venous catheters: potential financial implications. *Chest.* 2003;124(1):275–284.
85. Chatzinikolaou I, Finkel K, Hanna H, et al. Antibiotic-coated hemodialysis catheters for the prevention of vascular catheter-related infections: a prospective, randomized study. *Am J Med.* 2003;115(5):352–357.
86. Hanna H, Benjamin R, Chatzinikolaou I, et al. Long-term silicone central venous catheters impregnated with minocycline and rifampin decrease rates of catheter-related bloodstream infection in cancer patients: a prospective randomized clinical trial. *J Clin Oncol.* 2004;22(15):3163–3171.
87. Chatzinikolaou I, Hanna H, Graviss L, et al. Clinical experience with minocycline and rifampin-impregnated central venous catheters in bone marrow transplantation recipients: efficacy and low risk of developing staphylococcal resistance. *Infect Control Hosp Epidemiol.* 2003; 24(12):961–963.
88. Fraenkel D, Rickard C, Thomas P, et al. A prospective, randomized trial of rifampicin-minocycline-coated and silver platinum-carbon-impregnated central venous catheters. *Crit Care Med.* 2006;34(3):668–675.
89. Moretti EW, Ofstead CL, Kristy RM, et al. Impact of central venous catheter type and methods on catheter-related colonization and bacteraemia. *J Hosp Infect.* 2005;61(2):139–145.
90. Chatzinikolaou I, Hanna H, Darouiche R, et al. Prospective study of the value of quantitative culture of organisms from blood collected through central venous catheters in differentiating between contamination and bloodstream infection. *J Clin Microbiol.* 2006;44(5):1834–1835.
91. Mermel LA, Farr BM, Sherertz RJ, et al. Infectious Diseases Society of America; American College of Critical Care Medicine; Society for Healthcare Epidemiology of America. Guidelines for the management of intravascular catheter-related infections. *Clin Infect Dis.* 2001;32(9):1249–1272.
92. Raad I, Davis S, Khan A, et al. Impact of central venous catheter removal on the recurrence of catheter-related coagulase negative staphylococcal bacteremia. *Infect Control Hosp Epidemiol.* 1992;13(4):215–221.
93. Farber BF, Kaplan MH, Clogston AG. *Staphylococcus epidermidis* extracted slime inhibits the antimicrobial action of glycopeptide antibiotics. *J Infect Dis.* 1990;161(1):37–40.
94. Raad I, Buzaid A, Rhyne J, et al. Minocycline and ethylenediaminetetraacetate for the prevention of recurrent vascular catheter infections. *Clin Infect Dis.* 1997;25(1):149–151.
95. Metcalf SC, Chambers ST, Pithie AD. Use of ethanol locks to prevent recurrent central line sepsis. *J Infect.* 2004;49(1):20–22.
96. Raad I, Darouiche R, Vazquez J, et al. Efficacy and safety of weekly dalbavancin therapy for catheter-related bloodstream infection caused by gram-positive pathogens. *Clin Infect Dis.* 2005;40(3):374–380.
97. Birmingham MC, Rayner CR, Meagher AK, et al. Linezolid for the treatment of multidrug-resistant, gram positive infections: experience from a compassionate-use program. *Clin Infect Dis.* 2003;36(2):159–168.
98. Carpenter CF, Chambers HF. Daptomycin: another novel agent for treating infections due to drug-resistant gram-positive pathogens. *Clin Infect Dis.* 2004;38(7):994–1000.
99. Fowler VG Jr, Sanders LL, Sexton DJ, et al. Outcome of *Staphylococcus aureus* bacteremia according to compliance with recommendations of infectious diseases specialists: experience with 244 patients. *Clin Infect Dis.* 1998;2(3):478–486.
100. Capdevila JA, Segarra A, Planes A, et al. Long term follow-up of patients with catheter related sepsis (CRS) treated without catheter removal [abstract J3]. In: Program and abstracts of the 35th Interscience Conference on Antimicrobial Agents and Chemotherapy (San Francisco). Washington, DC: American Society for Microbiology; 1995.
101. Poole CV, Carlton D, Bimbo L, et al. Treatment of catheter-related bacteraemia with an antibiotic lock protocol: effect of bacterial pathogen. *Nephrol Dial Transplant.* 2004;19(5):1237–1244.
102. Raad II, Sabbagh MF. Optimal duration of therapy for catheter-related *Staphylococcus aureus* bacteremia: a study of 55 cases and review. *Clin Infect Dis.* 1992;14(1):75–82.
103. Elting LS, Bodey GP. Septicemia due to *Xanthomonas* species and non *aeruginosa Pseudomonas* species: increasing incidence of catheter-related infections. *Medicine (Baltimore).* 1990;69(5):296–306.
104. Hanna H, Afif C, Alakech B, et al. Central venous catheter-related bacteremia due to gram-negative bacilli: significance of catheter removal in preventing relapse. *Infect Control Hosp Epidemiol.* 2004;25(8):646–649.
105. Nguyen MH, Peacock JE Jr, Tanner DC, et al. Therapeutic approaches in patients with candidemia: evaluation in a multicenter, prospective observational study. *Arch Intern Med.* 1995;155:2429–2435.

106. Nucci M, Colombo AL, Silveira F, et al. Risk factors for death in patients with candidemia. *Infect Control Hosp Epidemiol.* 1998;19:846–850.
107. Hung C-C, Chen Y-C, Chag S-C, et al. Nosocomial candidemia in a university hospital in Taiwan. *J Formasan Med Assoc.* 1996;95:19–28.
108. Rex JH, Bennett JE, Sugar AM, et al. Intravascular catheter-exchange and duration of candidemia. *Clin Infect Dis.* 1995;21:995–996.
109. Karkowicz MG, Hashimoto LN, Kelly RE, et al. Should central venous catheters be removed as soon as candidemia is detected in neonates? *Pediatrics.* 2000;106:E63.
110. Raad I, Hanna H, Boktour M, et al. Management of central venous catheters in patients with cancer and candidemia. *Clin Infect Dis.* 2004; 38(8):1119–1127.

CHAPTER 111 ■ RESPIRATORY INFECTIONS IN THE ICU

OLIVIER Y. LEROY • SERGE ALFANDARI

PNEUMONIA

Traditionally, pneumonia is differentiated as being either community acquired or hospital acquired. For *community-acquired pneumonia*, the infection begins while the patient is in an outpatient setting. Conversely, *hospital-acquired pneumonia* occurs while the patient is in an inpatient setting. Usually, a pneumonia that was apparently not incubating at the time of admission is defined as hospital acquired when it occurs 48 hours or more after admission (1).

It has increasingly become clear that this dichotomous classification scheme cannot be sufficient to characterize all patients suffering from pneumonia. First, among hospital-acquired pneumonias, those occurring during mechanical ventilation must be distinguished from others. One reason for this distinction comes from the fact that a significant number of *ventilator-associated pneumonias* (VAPs) occur within 48 hours of hospital admission. Consequently, the 48-hour threshold used to define the infection as hospital acquired is no longer appropriate for pneumonia acquired during mechanical ventilation (2), although it does remain adequate for hospital-acquired pneumonia occurring apart from mechanical ventilation (3). Second, numerous outpatients benefit from health care services such as dialysis, chemotherapy, or ambulatory surgery. Similarly, in most nursing homes and rehabilitation hospitals, patients can receive intensive and/or invasive medical therapies. Sometimes categorized as community acquired and other times as hospital acquired, a pneumonia developing in such patients is now defined as a *health care–associated pneumonia* (3).

Thus, four classes of pneumonia can be distinguished:

1. Community-acquired pneumonia
2. Ventilator-associated pneumonia
3. Hospital-acquired pneumonia
4. Health care–associated pneumonia

We will discuss each of these below, and will also briefly touch on the topics of tracheobronchitis, pleural infections, and pulmonary abscess.

Severe Community-acquired Pneumonia

Immediate Concerns

Community-acquired pneumonia (CAP) is a common infectious disease affecting about 1 per 1,000 of the adult population per year. An intensive care unit (ICU) admission for severe CAP is required for 2% of patients. The most frequent pathogen is *Streptococcus pneumoniae*. Despite progress in antibiotic therapy and ICU management, the mortality of pneumococcal pneumonia remains elevated. The changing pattern of antimicrobial resistance of pneumonia pathogens complicates therapeutic guidelines.

Diagnosis of Community-acquired Pneumonia

CAP is suspected on the basis of clinical symptoms: cough, dyspnea, sputum production, pleuritic chest pain, and elevated body temperature. These symptoms can be absent or moderated in older patients. However, these signs are not specific of pneumonia; a chest radiograph or computed tomography (CT) scan revealing a new infiltrate is required to document a pneumonia diagnosis (4).

The chest radiograph might offer insights into the etiologic diagnosis, with intracellular pathogens typically presenting with interstitial pneumonia, and *S. pneumoniae* resulting in lobar pneumonia. However, none of these findings is specific, and caution should be exercised in interpreting radiographs, particularly in critically ill patients. The chest radiograph allows for staging of severity according to the localization and number of involved lobes. It is helpful to detect complications (pleural effusion, cavitation, acute respiratory distress syndrome [ARDS], etc.), for which the CT scan can be used to reveal evocative patterns, particularly in immunosuppressed patients (e.g., halo or crescent signs in pulmonary aspergillosis of neutropenic patients, cavitation in tuberculosis).

Definition of Severe Community-acquired Pneumonia and Decision for Admission to the Intensive Care Unit

Although there is no gold standard to define severe CAP, criteria do exist that may be used to assess the severity of CAP and define the need for ICU admission.

According to the original American Thoracic Society (ATS) guidelines (5), CAP was considered severe when any one of the following criteria was present:

- Respiratory frequency greater than 30 breaths per minute on admission
- Severe respiratory failure (PaO_2/FiO_2 <250 mm Hg)
- Requirement for mechanical ventilation
- Bilateral or multilobar or extensive (greater than or equal to 50% within 48 hours of admission) involvement of the chest radiograph
- Shock (systolic blood pressure less than 90 mm Hg or diastolic blood pressure less than 60 mm Hg)
- Requirement for vasopressors for more than 4 hours
- Low urine output (less than 20 mL/hour or less than 80 mL/4 hours) or acute renal failure requiring dialysis

In 1998, Ewig et al. (6) demonstrated that using any one of these factors as the definition of severe CAP had a high sensitivity but a low specificity. They proposed a new definition of severe CAP, which, in 2001, was adopted by the ATS (7). Today, the diagnosis of CAP is considered severe and requiring ICU admission for patients exhibiting either one of two major criteria (need for mechanical ventilation and septic shock) or two of three minor criteria (systolic blood pressure less than or equal to 90 mm Hg, multilobar involvement on chest radiograph, or PaO_2/FiO_2 less than 250 mm Hg) (7). Unfortunately, two recent studies suggest that this revised ATS criteria rule does not discriminate enough to guide individual decision making and underlines the need for additional criteria not presently available that may be identified in future studies (8,9).

In 2001, the British Thoracic Society (BTS) proposed assessing the severity of CAP utilizing three groups of adverse prognostic features: Four "core" factors (**CURB** score: Confusion, blood Urea nitrogen greater than 19 mg/dL [7 mmol/L], Respiratory rate greater than or equal to 30 breaths/minute, and low Blood pressure—systolic less than 90 mm Hg and/or diastolic less than or equal to 60 mm Hg); two "additional" factors (hypoxemia defined by SpO_2 less than 92% or PaO_2 less than 60 mm Hg [8kPa] and bilateral or multilobar involvement on chest radiograph); and two "pre-existing" factors (age 50 years or older and the presence of coexisting disease) (10). CAP was considered and treated as severe in patients having two or more core adverse prognostic features. In patients exhibiting only one of these core factors, the decision, based on clinical judgment, could be assisted by taking into account pre-existing and additional factors (10).

Diagnostic Studies

Evaluation for the etiologic diagnosis is helpful to confirm the infectious origin of the pneumonia and allow adequate antimicrobial therapy (including secondary deescalation therapy). Numerous methods are available for the microbiologic diagnosis of pneumonia:

- Sputum stains and cultures necessitate rigorous interpretation criteria. The presence of more than 25 polymorphonuclear cells and less than 10 squamous epithelial cells per high power field is required to interpret a sample. A single predominant organism on Gram stain suggests the etiology. Other stains can be used according to particular clinical context and may allow for a positive diagnosis without any sample validation (*Mycobacterium tuberculosis*, *Legionella pneumophila*, *Pneumocystis jirovecii*).
- More invasive sampling methods (endotracheal aspiration, protected brush, bronchoalveolar lavage, and transtracheal aspiration) are discussed in the ventilator-associated pneumonia section but can also be used to diagnose CAP.
- Blood cultures, drawn before antibiotic therapy, are rarely positive (6%–20% of cases) and, when positive, are most often for *S. pneumoniae*, *Staphylococcus aureus*, and Gram-negative bacilli.
- Rapid diagnostic tests have recently been introduced. The urinary antigen test is highly sensitive for the diagnosis of *L. pneumophila* type 1. A more recent urinary antigen test has been introduced for the diagnosis of pneumococcal pneumonia; a recent study in ICU patients with severe CAP displayed sensitivity, specificity, and positive and negative predictive values of 72%, 90%, 68%, and 92%, respectively (11). Rapid diagnosis is available for influenza A (12). Available tests can detect influenza viruses in 30 minutes. The types of specimens acceptable for use (i.e., throat, nasopharyngeal, or nasal; and aspirates, swabs, or washes) vary by test. The specificity and, in particular, the sensitivity of rapid tests are lower than for viral culture and vary by test.
- Serologic testing is less useful for rapid diagnosis. The presence of IgM with a titer greater than or equal to 16 generally indicates recent infection. This titer is, however, rarely observed in the initial phase of infection when antibiotic therapy must be chosen. A fourfold rise in antibody titer requiring samples drawn 2 weeks apart indicates, retrospectively, infection. Serologic diagnosis can be useful for some pathogens (e.g., *Mycoplasma pneumoniae*, *Chlamydia pneumoniae*, *Chlamydophila psittaci*, *Legionella* spp., *Coxiella burnetii*, adenovirus, parainfluenza viruses, and influenza A virus).
- Polymerase chain reaction (PCR) testing is a promising future field. To date, it cannot be recommended routinely, as questions concerning sensitivity, specificity, and clinical relevance remain.

Minimal diagnostic testing for patients admitted to the ICU with CAP can be done via endotracheal aspiration, blood cultures, *L. pneumophila* urinary antigen, and thoracentesis if pleural effusion is present. More invasive investigations should be reserved for the most critically ill patients, immunosuppressed patients, and those with failure of a first-line treatment (7).

Etiology of Severe Community-acquired Pneumonia

Despite intensive microbiologic testing, a definitive diagnosis is obtained in only about 50% of cases.

Organisms Causing Community-acquired Pneumonia in Hospitalized Patients Requiring Intensive Care Unit Admission. The epidemiology of CAP patients admitted to the ICU does not appear to be different from other hospitalized individuals with CAP. The most frequent pathogen isolated in ICU-hospitalized CAP patients is *S. pneumoniae* (Table 111.1) (13–15).

Other pathogens responsible for severe CAP, *L. pneumophila* or *S. aureus*, occur with variable frequency, probably reflecting different settings and diagnostic management strategies. *S. aureus* pneumonia is typically a complication of influenza pneumonia. Less frequent pathogens are mostly recovered from immunosuppressed patients and include *Pseudomonas aeruginosa*, *Aspergillus* spp., influenza, and other pathogens.

Drug-resistant Pathogens. One major challenge is the emergence and dissemination of drug-resistant micro-organisms. Resistant pathogens increase regularly. Major concerns are caused by penicillin-resistant pneumococci (PRP) and methicillin-resistant staphylococci.

For *S. pneumoniae*, macrolide resistance is above 20% in the United States and higher than 50% in some European or Asian-Pacific countries (16). Decreased susceptibility or resistance to penicillin is observed in 30% to 50% of strains in some studies. While the prevalence is higher for noninvasive infections, it reached 19% in blood cultures worldwide (17, 18). PRP risk factors include recent previous hospitalization, recent administration of antimicrobial agents, and immunodeficiency. The impact of drug resistance on outcome is

TABLE 111.1

MICROORGANISMS CAUSING SEVERE COMMUNITY-ACQUIRED PNEUMONIA REQUIRING ADMISSION TO AN INTENSIVE CARE UNIT[a]

References	Yoshimoto et al.[b]	Leroy et al.[c]	Shorr et al.[d]
Number of patients	72	308	199
Unknown pathogen	55.6%	45%–45.9%	43.7%
Streptococcus pneumoniae	13.9%	38.7%–41%	44.7%
Haemophilus influenzae	2.8%	15.8%–24.5%	10.6%
Legionella pneumophila	2.8%	3.2%–3.8%	8.9%
Staphylococcus aureus	2.8%	2.8%–7.4%	8.9%
Pseudomonas aeruginosa	8.3%	ND	4.9%
Other Gram-positive	2.8%	17%–17.9%	ND
Enterobacteriaceae	11.1%	7.5%–8.4%	6.5%
Chlamydia spp.	ND	1.9%–3.2%	ND
Mycobacterium tuberculosis	2.8%	ND	2.4%
Other	1.4%	3.2%–3.8%	13%

ND, no data.
[a] Data presented as number or percentage.
[b] Yoshimoto A, Nakamura H, Fujimura M, et al. Severe community-acquired pneumonia in an intensive care unit: risk factors for mortality. *Intern Med.* 2005;44:710.
[c] Leroy O, Saux P, Bedos JP, et al. Comparison of levofloxacin and cefotaxime combined with ofloxacin for ICU patients with community-acquired pneumonia who do not require vasopressors. *Chest.* 2005;128:172.
[d] Shorr AF, Bodi M, Rodriguez A, et al. Impact of antibiotic guideline compliance on duration of mechanical ventilation in critically ill patients with community-acquired pneumonia. *Chest.* 2006;130:93.

controversial, although adverse outcomes have been described (19). A recent Spanish study noted a nonsignificant trend to higher mortality in patients with pneumococcal pneumonia caused by intermediately resistant strains (20). However, the patients did not have a poorer outcome when treated with amoxicillin. Fluoroquinolone resistance is increasing, and fluoroquinolone-prescribing habits may affect resistance rates (21). Resistance to fluoroquinolones reaches 5.6% in Italy, where clonal spreading is thought to be responsible for the rapid dissemination of resistance (22).

Emergence of community-acquired methicillin-resistant *S. aureus* (MRSA) is a new challenge. An MRSA strain carrying Panton-Valentine leukocidin (PVL) genes was recently described in the community. It primarily causes skin and soft tissue infections but can be responsible for rapidly progressing necrotizing pneumonia (23).

P. aeruginosa are naturally resistant to numerous antibiotics and can elevate to a high-level resistance under treatment. Risk of *P. aeruginosa* is increased in patients presenting with a previous chronic pulmonary disease such as chronic obstructive pulmonary disorder (COPD) or cystic fibrosis, recent antibiotic therapy, or a stay in the hospital, especially the ICU (24,25).

Specific Etiologies in Immunosuppressed Patients. Immunosuppressed patients have an increased risk of severe CAP. All patients have more frequent bacterial pneumonia, particularly due to *S. pneumoniae* or *P. aeruginosa*. Moreover, different types of immunodeficiency can also result in different epidemiology.

Human immunodeficiency virus (HIV)-infected patients used to have a 25-fold higher risk of developing bacterial pneumonia (26). In developed countries, this risk has been tremendously decreased with the use of newer antiretroviral drugs. This incidence of bacterial pneumonia in a French cohort was 0.8 per 100 patient-years—very little difference from the general population (27). *P. jirovecii* pneumonia remains a frequent acquired immunodeficiency syndrome (AIDS)-defining diagnosis. Less frequent causes of severe pneumonias include cytomegalovirus (CMV), toxoplasma, and mycobacteria.

Patients with chemotherapy-induced neutropenia, particularly when severe (below 500 neutrophils/μL) and prolonged (greater than 10 days), have an increased risk of invasive pulmonary aspergillosis (28) and severe bacterial pneumonia (29). This risk also exists with targeted monoclonal antibody therapies, which increase the risk of CMV and *P. jirovecii* pneumonia (30). Patients with solid organ transplant have an increased risk of severe CAP. The usual bacterial pathogens, as well as *P. jirovecii* and *Aspergillus*, have been described (31). Patients treated by anti–tumor necrosis factor (TNF)-α monoclonal antibodies have an increased risk of infection, including severe pneumonia (32). Bacterial, viral, and fungal pneumonia have been described.

Treatment of Severe Community-acquired Pneumonia

Antibiotic Therapy

Antimicrobial spectrum. The ideal antibiotic should have a "kill spectrum" to cover all pathogens responsible for severe CAP. Because other factors (e.g., cost effectiveness and selective pressure) need to be assessed, the choice of antimicrobial regimen usually results in a compromise. The most frequent and/or most severe pathogens (*S. pneumoniae, Haemophilus influenzae, L. pneumophila*) should be covered by the initial antimicrobial regimen. Initial coverage of other pathogens (i.e., *S. aureus, P. aeruginosa,* opportunistic agents) should be evaluated on a case-by-case basis according to patient history and clinical presentation.

One should be aware that, compared to drugs used to treat other diseases, antimicrobial agent efficacy should not be considered constant over time and in every location. Drug resistance is a major concern worldwide, and drugs consistently effective 20 years ago may be nearly useless for the next patient admitted to the ICU.

Timing of initial therapy. The most recent Infectious Diseases Society of America (IDSA) guidelines recommend initial antibiotics administration within 4 hours of admission (24). A reduced mortality (adjusted odds ratio, 0.85, 95% confidence interval [CI] 0.76–0.95) was observed in patients with early therapy in a retrospective study of 18,209 Medicare patients (33). However, other studies contradict this finding, suggesting the time to first antibiotic dose to be a marker of disease severity rather than an indicator of prognosis (34,35).

Antimicrobial choices. Drug choice depends on numerous factors: pharmacodynamics/pharmacokinetics, spectrum, dosing schedule, adverse events, costs, and availability.

The antimicrobial should have sufficient diffusion in pulmonary tissues. β-Lactam antibiotics have a good extracellular diffusion, but are ineffective on intracellular organisms. Their concentration in the alveolar lining fluid (ALF) reached 10% to 20% of the serum concentration after a single administration. Macrolides, on the other hand, have a variable intracellular distribution—low for erythromycin and elevated for the newer macrolides (clarithromycin, azithromycin). Fluoroquinolones have an excellent intracellular and ELF diffusion. Newer quinolones have an enhanced activity against *S. pneumoniae*, and levofloxacin is reported to be the most active drug against *Legionella* spp. (36).

Little data are available on the best antimicrobial regimen for CAP. Retrospective studies have suggested that some combination regimens, including a macrolide, might be superior to β-lactam monotherapy for CAP (37,38), particularly for bacteremic pneumococcal pneumonia (39,40). Similar results were reported with a β-lactam–fluoroquinolone combination (41). However, these studies presented with potential biases and confounding factors.

The impact of combination therapy on the prognosis of pneumococcal bacteremia was confirmed in an international, multicenter, prospective observational study (38). Lower mortality was associated with combination therapy for critically ill patients (14-day mortality, 23.4% vs. 55.3%; $p = 0.0015$), but not for all patients receiving combination versus monotherapy (10.4% vs. 11.5%, $p = \text{NS}$). All combinations using a β-lactam had an enhanced response.

Recommendations. Regularly updated guidelines published by North American and European medical societies mostly recommend the utilization of a β-lactam with a macrolide or a fluoroquinolone. The 2007 IDSA/American Thoracic Society (ATS) guidelines are presented in Table 111.2, and take into account new data on antimicrobial susceptibility patterns and newly available antibiotics.

Duration of therapy. Length of treatment is usually based on the pathogen, response to treatment, comorbid illness, and complications (42). Length of treatment for pneumonia caused by *S. pneumoniae* should continue, at least, until the patient has been afebrile for 72 hours. Bacteria causing necrosis of the pulmonary parenchyma (e.g., *S. aureus, P. aeruginosa, Klebsiella,* and anaerobes) should probably be treated for no less

TABLE 111.2

INITIAL EMPIRIC ANTIBIOTIC THERAPY IN PATIENTS ADMITTED TO AN INTENSIVE CARE UNIT FOR SEVERE COMMUNITY-ACQUIRED PNEUMONIA

Clinical characteristics	Recommended antibiotics
No *Pseudomonas* or methicillin-resistant *Staphylococcus aureus* (MRSA) or penicillin allergy	A β-lactam (cefotaxime, ceftriaxone, ampicillin/sulbactam) **plus** azithromycin or a respiratory fluoroquinolone[a]
Patients with penicillin allergy	A respiratory fluoroquinolone, with azithromycin
Suspected *Pseudomonas* infection	An antipseudomonal β-lactam[b] plus ciprofloxacin or levofloxacin[a] or plus an aminoglycoside and an antipneumococcal fluoroquinolone[a]
Suspected community-acquired MRSA	Addition of vancomycin or linezolid

[a] Dosage of levofloxacin should be 750 mg daily.
[b] Antipseudomonal agents include piperacillin-tazobactam, imipenem, meropenem, or cefepime. Azithromycin can be substituted for penicillin allergy.
Adapted from Mandell LA, Wunderink RG, Anzueto A, et al. Infectious Diseases Society of America/American Thoracic Society consensus guidelines on the management of community-acquired pneumonia in adults. *Clin Infect Dis.* 2007;44(Suppl 2):S27.

than 2 weeks. Pneumonia caused by intracellular organisms should probably be treated for at least 2 weeks.

Nonantimicrobial Therapy. Besides antimicrobial therapies, most patients admitted to the ICU for severe CAP need additional treatments. Organ dysfunctions such as respiratory failure, septic shock, or renal failure require supportive, as well as specific, treatments. Similarly, the standard care of acutely ill patients (i.e., nutrition, prevention of ICU-related complications, and treatment of underlying diseases) must be utilized. These points are detailed in other chapters of this textbook. Only two recent aspects of the nonantibiotic treatment of severe CAP will be discussed further.

Activated Protein C. Severe sepsis is associated with a generalized inflammation and procoagulant response to infection. Activated protein C is an important endogenous modulator of this response. The activation of protein C can be impaired during sepsis, and there are reduced levels of activated protein C in most patients with severe sepsis.

Drotrecogin-α activated, a recombinant form of human activated protein C (r-aPC), exhibits profibrinolytic, antithrombotic, and anti-inflammatory characteristics. A large randomized, double-blind, placebo-controlled, multicenter study (PROWESS) composed of 1,690 patients demonstrated that treatment with r-aPC significantly decreased 28-day and hospital discharge mortality rates in patients with severe sepsis (43,44).

A retrospective analysis of these 1,690 patients included in the PROWESS trial identified 602 patients (r-aPC, $n = 324$; placebo, $n = 278$) classified as exhibiting severe CAP (45). Compared with placebo, r-aPC provided a relative risk reduction in a 28-day mortality of 28%. This survival benefit was even more pronounced in patients with severe pneumococcal CAP and in patients with a high risk of death assessed by an Acute Physiology and Chronic Health Evaluation (APACHE) II score of at least 25, or a Pneumonia Severity Index score of 4 or greater.

Conversely, in patients with severe sepsis but a low risk of death defined by an APACHE II score less than 25 or a single organ failure, r-aPC compared with placebo provided no beneficial effect and was associated with an increased incidence of bleeding events (46). Consequently, as recommended by regulatory agencies, the use of r-aPC should be limited in severe CAP, as in other severe infections, to patients at high risk of death. An APACHE II score of 25 or more or multiple organ failure must be present.

Corticosteroids. In a recent preliminary randomized trial, hydrocortisone (200 mg IV bolus followed by infusion at a rate of 10 mg/hour for 7 days) was compared with placebo in 46 patients (47). On day 8, hydrocortisone treatment was associated with a significant improvement in PaO_2/FiO_2 and chest radiograph score, as well as a significant decrease in C-reactive protein levels and Multiple Organ Dysfunction Syndrome score, and a lower incidence of delayed septic shock. Moreover, length of hospital stay and mortality were decreased. These results, suggesting that low doses of hydrocortisone could hasten the resolution of severe CAP and prevent the occurrence of sepsis-related complications, are as yet insufficient to propose the systematic use of hydrocortisone in severe CAP. Future trials are needed before such routine use.

Expected Clinical Course

Evaluation on Day 3. Generally, a decrease in fever and oxygenation requirements is not observed in responding patients prior to day 3 or 4. In the absence of rapid clinical deterioration, initial therapy should not be changed prior to completion of 48 to 72 hours of the initial therapy.

Day 3 usually sees the return of microbiologic exams, including cultures and antimicrobial sensitivity. This can allow for treatment adaptation (de-escalation or treatment for a pathogen not covered by first-line therapy). For example, negative results of urinary antigen test combined with blood cultures positive for *S. pneumoniae* make it possible to simplify therapy to target *S. pneumoniae* with an aminopenicillin.

Complications and failure to improve. A poor clinical response by day 3 is usually a sign of treatment failure. However, in the ICU, other diagnoses such as pulmonary embolism or cardiac failure should be considered. Treatment failure can be due to an organism not covered by the first-line antimicrobial therapy, thus demanding a change or addition to the previous treatment regimen. Other causes of treatment failure can include complications despite adequate antimicrobial therapy. These include lung abscess, necrosis, meningitis, endocarditis, or superinfection.

Prognosis of Severe Community-acquired Pneumonia

Despite advances in antimicrobial therapy and supportive measures, mortality in patients with severe CAP requiring admission to the ICU remains high, ranging in the literature from 18% to 46% (8,48–54). A meta-analysis of 788 evaluable ICU patients found a mean mortality rate of 36.5% (55). In this meta-analysis, Fine et al. identified 11 independent prognostic factors associated with a mortality of CAP (55). They were (a) male gender (odds ratio [OR] = 1.3), (b) pleuritic chest pain (OR = 0.5), (c) hypothermia (OR = 5.0), (d) systolic hypotension (OR = 4.8), (e) tachypnea (OR = 2.9), (f) diabetes mellitus (OR = 1.3), (g) neoplastic disease (OR = 2.8), (h) neurologic disease (OR = 4.6), (i) bacteremia (OR = 2.8), (j) leukopenia (OR = 2.5), and (k) multilobar pulmonary involvement (OR = 3.1). This analysis included 33,148 patients suffering from CAP, although only 788 of them were admitted to an ICU.

Numerous studies have focused on the prognosis of patients admitted to the ICU for severe CAP (48–50,52–54,56–58). Although inclusion criteria were different from one study to another and no meta-analysis was performed, most independent prognostic factors identified in these studies are quite similar. They demonstrate that the prognosis of severe CAP depends on the preadmission health status of the patient, the initial severity of illness, and the evolution during ICU stay (Table 111.3).

Although these findings might suggest that physicians minimally influence the prognosis of severe CAP, since prior health status and initial severity cannot be modified, the following points must be underlined: the initial empiric treatment must be instituted as soon as possible (less than 4 hours after hospital admission) and must be adequate to be as effective as possible. Moreover, nonpneumonia-related complications—such as upper gastrointestinal bleeding, catheter-related infection, deep venous thrombosis, and pulmonary embolism—and complications attributed only to underlying medical conditions must be prevented during the ICU stay.

TABLE 111.3

INDEPENDENT PROGNOSTIC FACTORS ASSOCIATED WITH MORTALITY OF PATIENTS WITH SEVERE COMMUNITY-ACQUIRED PNEUMONIA

PREADMISSION HEALTH STATUS

- Age older than 70 yr
- Immunosuppression
- Comorbidities with anticipated death within 5 yr

INITIAL SEVERITY OF ILLNESS

- Antibiotic administration prior to hospital presentation
- Simplified Acute Physiologic Score (SAPS) I more than 12 or SAPS II more than 45
- Septic shock
- Requirement for mechanical ventilation
- Acute renal failure
- Bilateral or multilobar pulmonary involvement
- *K. pneumonia* or *P. aeruginosa* as etiologic agent
- Bacteremia
- Nonaspiration pneumonia

EVOLUTION DURING INTENSIVE CARE UNIT STAY

- Radiographic spread of pneumonia
- Number of nonpulmonary organs that failed
- Increase in Logistic Organ Dysfunction score from D1 to D3
- Delay in hospital antibiotic administration of more than 4 h
- Ineffective initial antimicrobial therapy
- Occurrence of non–pneumonia-related complications
- Increase of procalcitonin level in serum from D1 to D3

Data from Pachon J, Prados MD, Capote F, et al. Severe community-acquired pneumonia. Etiology, prognosis, and treatment *Am Rev Respir Dis.* 1990;142:369; Almirall J, Mesalles E, Klamburg J, et al. Prognostic factors of pneumonia requiring admission to the intensive care unit. *Chest.* 1995;107:511; Leroy O, Santré C, Beuscart C, et al. A five-year study of severe community-acquired pneumonia with emphasis on prognosis in patients admitted to an intensive care unit. *Intensive Care Med.* 1995;21:24; Paganin F, Lilienthal F, Bourdin A, et al. Severe community-acquired pneumonia: assessment of microbial aetiology as mortality factor. *Eur Respir J.* 2004;24:779; Tejerina E, Frutos-Vivar F, Restrepo MI, et al. Prognosis factors and outcome of community-acquired pneumonia needing mechanical ventilation. *J Crit Care.* 2005;20:230; Boussekey N, Leroy O, Alfandari S, et al. Procalcitonin kinetics in the prognosis of severe community-acquired pneumonia. *Intensive Care Med.* 2006;32:469; Torres A, Serra-Batlles J, Ferrer A, et al. Severe community-acquired pneumonia. Epidemiology and prognostic factors. *Am Rev Respir Dis.* 1991;144:312; Leroy O, Devos P, Guery B, et al. Simplified prediction rule for prognosis of patients with severe community-acquired pneumonia in ICUs. *Chest.* 1999;116:157; Wilson PA, Ferguson J. Severe community-acquired pneumonia: an Australian perspective. *Intern Med J.* 2005;35:699.

Some studies have shown that empiric initial antimicrobial treatment based on an antibiotics combination employing a macrolide or a fluoroquinolone as a second agent could reduce mortality from CAP (37,59,60). Similarly, it was suggested that an antibiotic combination could decrease mortality from bacteremic pneumococcal CAP (39,40,61). Despite the interest of these findings, it must be underlined that most of these studies were retrospective and often even excluded severely ill ICU patients. To the best of our knowledge, only one study compared the survival impact of various antimicrobial regimens for patients admitted to the ICU for severe CAP (38). This study was unable to demonstrate the superiority of any antimicrobial regimen to another, and only suggested that combinations including aminoglycosides could be suboptimal.

Mortality risk scores specific to CAP have been elaborated; Fine et al. derived a prediction rule from data on 14,199 adults hospitalized for CAP, stratifying patients into five classes according to the risk of death within 30 days (62). This rule, validated with data on 38,039 patients, is now entitled the Pneumonia Severity Index (PSI) and stratifies risk using a two-step approach. First, patients with a low risk (class I) are identified by age younger than 50 years and the absence of comorbidities and vital sign abnormalities. For the remaining patients, a score is determined by adding points assigned to age and different variables, taking into account comorbid conditions, physical examination findings, and laboratory and radiographic abnormalities (Table 111.4). According to the value of this score, patients are classified into class II (70 points or less), III (71–90 points), IV (91–130 points), or V (more than 130 points). From class I to class V, mortality rates observed in the validation cohort were 0.1%, 0.6%, 2.8%, 8.2%, and 29.2%, respectively. Despite the major interest of this PSI, it must be emphasized that this score was primarily built to identify patients at low risk who might be safely treated as outpatients. Consequently, the implications of the PSI for the medical care of patients exhibiting severe CAP, requiring admission into an ICU, may be questionable.

A specific prediction rule for mortality of patients with severe CAP admitted to an ICU has been proposed by our group (57). This rule takes into account data on prognostic factors, emphasizing that the prognosis of severe CAP depends on both *initial* baseline characteristics of the patient and *evolution* during the ICU stay, and is based on two successive steps. On ICU admission, an initial risk score based on six independent variables associated with the prognosis is established. These variables and their respective point value are (a) age 40 years or older (+1 point), (b) anticipated death within 5 years (+1 point), (c) nonaspiration pneumonia (+1 point), (d) chest radiograph involvement greater than one lobe (+1 point), (e) acute respiratory failure requiring mechanical ventilation (+1 point), and (f) septic shock (+3 points). The initial risk score, obtained by summing up these points, allows inclusion of each patient into one of the three risk classes of increasing mortality. In class I (0–2 points) mortality risk is low (less than 5%), whereas in class III (6–8 points), mortality risk is high (more than 50%). In class II (3–5 points), mortality risk is intermediate (25%). A risk score based on three independent factors identified during the ICU stay allows a definite evaluation of the final prognosis. These three independent factors and their point scoring are (a) hospital-acquired, lower respiratory tract superinfections (+1 point), (b) nonspecific CAP-related complications (+2 points), and/or (c) sepsis-related complications (+4 points) occurring during the ICU stay. This risk score appears particularly useful for patients in the intermediate-risk class II on ICU admission. Indeed, for these patients, the mortality rate estimated on ICU admission by the initial risk score is quite similar to the mortality rate observed in the overall population of patients admitted into the ICU for severe CAP. According to the occurrence or the nonoccurrence of complications during the ICU stay, the adjusted risk score determined subgroups of patients exhibiting significantly different mortality rates; in the studied cohort, rates ranged from 2% to 86%.

TABLE 111.4

CRITERIA AND POINT SCORING SYSTEM USED IN THE PNEUMONIA SEVERITY INDEX (STEP 2; CLASSES II–V)

Variables	Points	Variables	Points
Age	Age (yr)	**Vital sign abnormality**	
Female gender	−10	Altered mental status	+20
Nursing home resident	+10	Respiratory rate more than 30 breaths/min	+20
		Systolic blood pressure less than 90 mm Hg	+20
		Temperature less than 35°C or greater than or equal to 40°C	+15
		Tachycardia more than 125 breaths/min	+10
Comorbidity		**Laboratory and radiographic data**	
Neoplastic disease	+30	Arterial pH less than 7.35	+30
Liver disease	+20	Blood urea nitrogen greater than or equal to 30 mg/dL	+20
Congestive heart failure	+10	Sodium less than 130 mmol/L	+20
Cerebrovascular disease	+10	Glucose greater than or equal to 250 mg/dL	+10
Renal disease	+10	Hematocrit less than 30%	+10
		PaO_2 less than 60 mm Hg	+10
		Pleural effusion	+10

Adapted from Fine MJ, Auble TE, Yealy DM, et al. A prediction rule to identify low-risk patients with community-acquired pneumonia. *N Engl J Med.* 1997;336:243.

Therefore, this score may help clinicians to reassess severe CAP patients during the ICU stay.

Prevention of Community-acquired Pneumonia

Many of the factors associated with an increase in CAP risk (tobacco use, malnutrition, chronic pulmonary disease, diabetes, liver disease, older age, confinement to a nursing home) are not amenable to prevention. Immunization remains the most significant method of prevention (24).

Two vaccines are available for preventing pneumococcal disease. Pneumococcal polysaccharide vaccine is recommended for persons 65 or more years of age, and for persons 2 or more years of age who are immunocompetent but at an increased risk for illness and death associated with pneumococcal disease because of chronic illness, with functional or anatomic asplenia, who live in environments in which the risk for disease is high, or are immunosuppressed and at high risk for infection (63). The more recent pneumococcal conjugate vaccine is, at the time of this writing, recommended only for children (64–66).

The Advisory Committee on Immunization Practices (ACIP) recommends inactivated influenza A vaccine for all persons older than 50 years of age, those at risk for influenza complications, and household contacts of high-risk persons (including health care workers) (67).

Ventilator-associated Pneumonia

Ventilator-associated pneumonia (VAP) is defined as a pneumonia occurring in intubated or tracheotomized patients undergoing mechanical ventilation. Although usual guidelines suggest a delay of 48 to 72 hours between the beginning of mechanical ventilation and the occurrence of pneumonia to qualify for this diagnosis (68), recent data suggest that a pneumonia acquired earlier than the 48th hour of mechanical ventilation could also be considered a VAP (2,69). VAP represents 80% of pneumonia acquired during hospitalization, and is the most frequent hospital-acquired infection in ICUs.

Immediate Concerns

The major dilemmas regarding VAP at the present time are the following:

- Prevention remains a challenge.
- There is no gold standard for diagnosis.
- The rate of multidrug-resistant causative pathogens has dramatically increased during recent years.
- Prompt initiation of an adequate antibiotic therapy is essential.

Incidence

The exact incidence of VAP is difficult to assess for a number of reasons. Study populations vary greatly from one study to another, the criteria used to diagnose VAP can be quite different (i.e., clinical vs. bacteriologic diagnosis), and, finally, an overlap between VAP and other hospital-acquired lower respiratory tract infections such as nosocomial tracheobronchitis exists. With this in mind, one must carefully analyze the existent studies, which show an incidence varying from 5.6% to 82.4% (Table 111.5) (70–77).

In a large U.S. inpatient database composed of 9,080 patients mechanically ventilated for more than 24 hours, the incidence of VAP was 9.3% (69). The percentages of episodes of VAP occurring during the first 2 days of hospitalization—between days 3 and 6 and after hospital day 6—were 45.2%, 29.1%, and 25.7%, respectively. Most episodes of VAP (63.2%) developed within 48 hours of mechanical ventilation. Thereafter, 16% occurred between 48 hours and 96 hours of mechanical ventilation, and 20.8% after 96 hours of mechanical ventilation.

TABLE 111.5

INCIDENCE OF VENTILATOR-ASSOCIATED PNEUMONIA (VAP) IN THE INTENSIVE CARE UNIT

References	No. of patients	Characteristics of patients	Diagnostic criteria	Incidence of VAP
Torres et al.[a]	322	Medicosurgical patients	Clinical and Rx	24%
Chevret et al.[b]	540	Medicosurgical patients	Clinical and Rx	12.6%
Baker et al.[c]	514	Trauma patients	Clinical, Rx, and Q. bacteriologic cultures	5.6%
Chastre et al.[d]	56	Patients with ARDS	Clinical, Rx, and Q. bacteriologic cultures	55%
Tejada Artigas et al.[e]	103	Trauma patients	Clinical, Rx, and Q. bacteriologic cultures	22.3%
Ibrahim et al.[f]	880	Medicosurgical patients	Clinical and Rx	15%
Bouza et al.[g]	356	Heart surgical patients	Clinical, Rx, and Q. bacteriologic cultures	7.9%
Hilker et al.[h]	17	Patients with acute stroke	Clinical and Rx	82.4%

Rx, radiologic; ARDS, acute respiratory distress syndrome; Q., quantitative.
[a] Torres A, Aznar R, Gatell JM, et al. Incidence, risk, and prognosis factors of nosocomial pneumonia in mechanically ventilated patients. *Am Rev Respir Dis.* 1990;142:523.
[b] Chevret S, Hemmer M, Carlet J, et al. Incidence and risk factors of pneumonia acquired in intensive care units. Results from a multicenter prospective study on 996 patients. European Cooperative Group on Nosocomial Pneumonia. *Intensive Care Med.* 1993;19:256.
[c] Baker AM, Meredith JW, Haponik EF. Pneumonia in intubated trauma patients. Microbiology and outcomes. *Am J Respir Crit Care Med.* 1996;153:343.
[d] Chastre J, Trouillet JL, Vuagnat A, et al. Nosocomial pneumonia in patients with acute respiratory distress syndrome. *Am J Respir Crit Care Med.* 1998;157:1165.
[e] Tejada Artigas A, Bello Dronda S, Chacon Valles E, et al. Risk factors for nosocomial pneumonia in critically ill trauma patients. *Crit Care Med.* 2001;29:304.
[f] Ibrahim EH, Tracy L, Hill C, et al. The occurrence of ventilator-associated pneumonia in a community hospital: risk factors and clinical outcomes. *Chest.* 2001;120:555.
[g] Bouza E, Perez A, Munoz P, et al. Ventilator-associated pneumonia after heart surgery: a prospective analysis and the value of surveillance. *Crit Care Med.* 2003;31:1964.
[h] Hilker R, Poetter C, Findeisen N, et al. Nosocomial pneumonia after acute stroke: implications for neurological intensive care medicine. *Stroke.* 2003;34:975.

In a cohort of 1,014 patients ventilated for 48 hours or more, the overall incidence of VAP was 14.8 cases per 1,000 ventilator-days. The daily risk for developing VAP is highest in the early course of hospital stay. It is estimated to be 3% per day at day 5, 2% at day 10, and 1% at day 15 (78).

Pathogenesis

Pneumonia occurs resultant to the entry of bacteria into the normally sterile lower respiratory tract, leading to colonization and subsequently to infection when bacteria overwhelm host defenses secondary to a large bacterial inoculum, a virulent pathogen, or a defect in the local host defenses (68,80).

Bacteria can reach the lower respiratory tract by four different pathogenic mechanisms: (a) contiguous spread, (b) hematogenous spread, (c) inhalation, and (d) aspiration. The first two mechanisms of invasion are infrequent (79). Inhalation of gastric material or direct inoculation of bacteria into the lower respiratory tract through contaminated "devices" (aerosol, bronchoscopes, ventilator circuit, nebulizer, tracheal suctioning) is rarely associated with VAP. Aspiration of bacteria colonizing the oropharynx is the main route of entry into the lower respiratory tract.

Colonization of the oropharyngeal airways by pathogenic micro-organisms occurs during the first hospital week in most critically ill patients. These micro-organisms that replace the normal microflora of the oropharynx can be either endogenous (enteric Gram-negative bacteria) or exogenous *via* a cross-contamination from other patients in the ICU. The stomach, sinuses, and dental plaque may be potential reservoirs for pathogens colonizing the oropharynx. However, their exact contribution still remains controversial. The endotracheal tube compromises the natural barrier between the oropharynx and lower respiratory tract, and leakage of contaminated secretions around the endotracheal tube cuff allows bacterial entry into the trachea (68,80).

Risk Factors

Many risk factors for VAP are host related and, thus, not accessible to intervention. Patient-related risk factors include male gender, pre-existing pulmonary disease, coma, AIDS, head trauma, age older than 60 years, neurosurgical procedures, and multiorgan system failure (81).

Among accessible risk factors, the most important is the presence of mechanical ventilation, associated with a 3- to 21-fold risk (71). The endotracheal tube limits the draining of secretions that leak around the cuff, favors bacterial multiplication, offers a focus for bacterial adherence and colonization, and impairs ciliary clearance and cough. Furthermore, the mechanically ventilated patient requires other devices such as nebulizers or humidifiers, which can be a source of micro-organisms. The risk of infection is highest during the first 8 to 10 days (82) of mechanical ventilation and increases with the duration of mechanical ventilation (78).

Accidental extubation, rather than reintubation, increases the risk of VAP (83), likely due to preparation for extubation that is—obviously—inadequate to nonexistent. Enteral nutrition administered by a nasogastric, rather than a post-pyloric, tube also increases the risk of VAP (78,81). The nasogastric tube might increase the risk of reflux and subsequent colonization of the airways. The use of H_2 blockers or antacids favors gastric colonization and may contribute to VAP.

Other factors facilitating the inhalation of oropharyngeal secretions favor VAP: supine position, patient transportation out of the ICU (84), sedation (85), failed subglottic aspiration (82), intracuff pressure less than 20 cm H_2O, tracheostomy, and aerosol treatment. Identifying these risk factors will guide the prevention measures of VAP.

Etiology

VAP may be caused by a wide spectrum of bacteria and is often polymicrobial (Table 111.6) (86,87,88). Gram-negative enteric bacilli, *P. aeruginosa,* and *S. aureus* are the leading etiologies. However, micro-organisms responsible for VAP may differ according to patient groups, unit types, hospitals, and countries (88). Moreover, the main epidemiologic patterns—principally the susceptibility patterns of causative pathogens—may also vary in a given unit over the course of time.

Several studies have tried to identify specific risk factors for VAP due to a given causative pathogen. The presence of an altered level of consciousness, admission into a medical ICU, and a high Simplified Acute Physiologic Score are independent factors associated with the development of VAP caused by anaerobes (89). In trauma patients, VAP due to *Stenotrophomonas maltophilia* are independently associated with prior exposure to cefepime and tracheostomy (90). Cytotoxic chemotherapy and use of corticosteroids are independent factors predisposing to the development of nosocomial pneumonia due to *L. pneumophila* (91). Neurosurgery, acute respiratory distress syndrome, head trauma, and large-volume pulmonary aspiration are independent risk factors for VAP due to *Acinetobacter baumannii* (92). Chronic obstructive pulmonary disease, prior use of antibiotics, and duration of mechanical ventilation longer than 8 days are independently associated with VAP due to *P. aeruginosa* (93). Finally, coma is an independent risk factor for VAP caused by *S. aureus* (94). Even if such factors are important to consider, there is major overlap between these different factors and, consequently, they are not sufficiently discriminant to allow focusing the empirical antimicrobial treatment on a specific etiologic agent.

The time of onset of VAP influences the etiology of VAP, making it useful to distinguish early-onset VAP from late-onset VAP. In early-onset VAP, the main causative pathogens are *S. pneumoniae*, methicillin-susceptible *S. aureus*, *H. influenzae*, and susceptible Gram-negative enteric bacilli (95). In late-onset VAP, MRSA, *P. aeruginosa*, *A. baumannii*, and *S. maltophilia* are the main causative organisms. Although this distinction between early- and late-onset VAP is useful, we must emphasize that there is no consensus on the number of days considered that separate these types of VAP. According to the literature, the threshold varies from 3 to 7 days (80). Similarly, it is unclear whether the threshold refers to the number of days in the hospital or to the number of days of mechanical ventilation (95). In the recent ATS/IDSA guidelines (68), duration of hospitalization fewer than, or more than 5 days, respectively, separates early- from late-onset VAP.

TABLE 111.6

MICRO-ORGANISMS CAUSING VENTILATOR-ASSOCIATED PNEUMONIA (VAP)[a]

References	Trouillet et al.[b]	Leroy et al.[c]	Rello et al.[d]
Number of episodes of VAP	135	124	290
Number of bacteria identified	245	154	321
Pseudomonas aeruginosa	39 (15.9%)	48 (31.1%)	102(31.7%)
Acinetobacter baumannii	22 (9%)	9 (5.8%)	38 (11.8%)
Stenotrophomonas maltophilia	6 (2.4%)	8 (5.2%)	8 (2.5%)
Klebsiella species	9 (3.7%)	5 (3.2%)	ND
Escherichia coli	8 (3.3%)	8 (5.2%)	ND
Proteus species	7 (2.9%)	5 (3.2%)	ND
Enterobacter species	5 (2.0%)	7 (4.5%)	ND
Morganella species	4 (1.6%)	—	ND
Serratia species	4 (1.6%)	7 (4.5%)	ND
Haemophilus species	15 (6.1%)	10 (6.5%)	26 (8.1%)
Methicillin-resistant *Staphylococcus aureus*	32 (13.1%)	10 (6.5%)	10 (4.0%)
Methicillin-sensitive *S. aureus*	20 (8.2%)	19 (12.4%)	38 (11.8%)
Streptococcus pneumoniae	3 (1.2%)	9 (5.8%)	25 (7.8%)
Streptococcus species	33 (13.5%)	2 (1.3%)	10 (3.1%)
Enterococcus species	5 (2.0%)	—	ND
Coagulase-negative staphylococcus	4 (1.6%)	1 (0.6%)	ND
Anaerobic pathogens	6 (2.4%)	—	ND

ND, no data.
[a] Data are presented as number and (percentage).
[b] Trouillet JL, Chastre J, Vuagnat A, et al. Ventilator-associated pneumonia caused by potentially drug-resistant bacteria. *Am J Respir Crit Care Med.* 1998;157:531.
[c] Leroy O, Girardie P, Yazdanpanah Y, et al. Hospital-acquired pneumonia: microbiological data and potential adequacy of antimicrobial regimens. *Eur Respir J.* 2002;20:432.
[d] Rello J, Sa-Borges M, Correa H, et al. Variations in etiology of ventilator-associated pneumonia across four treatment sites: implications for antimicrobial prescribing practices. *Am J Respir Crit Care Med.* 1999;160:608.

TABLE 111.7

RISK FACTORS FOR MULTIDRUG-RESISTANT PATHOGENS AS CAUSATIVE ORGANISMS IN VENTILATOR-ASSOCIATED PNEUMONIA (VAP)

- Admission from a nursing home or an extended-care facility
- History of regular visits to an infusion or dialysis center
- Prior antimicrobial treatment in the preceding 90 days
- Prior use of broad-spectrum antibiotics
- Prior hospitalization in the preceding 90 days
- Current hospitalization for greater than or equal to 5 days
- Duration of mechanical ventilation greater than or equal to 7 days
- Immunosuppression
- High level of antibiotic resistance in the community or in local intensive care unit

Data from American Thoracic Society, Infectious Diseases Society of America. Guidelines for the management of adults with hospital-acquired, ventilator-associated, and healthcare-associated pneumonia. *Am J Respir Crit Care Med.* 2005;171:388; Trouillet JL, Chastre J, Vuagnat A, et al. Ventilator-associated pneumonia caused by potentially drug-resistant bacteria. *Am J Respir Crit Care Med.* 1998;157:531; Leroy O, Girardie P, Yazdanpanah Y, et al. Hospital-acquired pneumonia: microbiological data and potential adequacy of antimicrobial regimens. *Eur Respir J.* 2002;20:432; Porzecanski I, Bowton DL. Diagnosis and treatment of ventilator-associated pneumonia. *Chest.* 2006;130:597; Rello J, Torres A, Ricart M, et al. Ventilator-associated pneumonia by *Staphylococcus aureus*. Comparison of methicillin-resistant and methicillin-sensitive episodes. *Am J Respir Crit Care Med.* 1994;150:1545; Trouillet JL, Vuagnat A, Combes A, et al. *Pseudomonas aeruginosa* ventilator-associated pneumonia: comparison of episodes due to piperacillin-resistant versus piperacillin-susceptible organisms. *Clin Infect Dis.* 2002;34:1047; Leroy O, Jaffre S, D'Escrivan, et al. Hospital-acquired pneumonia: risk factors for antimicrobial-resistant causative pathogens in critically ill patients. *Chest.* 2003;123:2034.

Among these potential causative pathogens, the rate of multidrug-resistant pathogens has dramatically increased during recent years. Numerous factors are associated with the emergence of these resistant strains and are summarized in Table 111.7. As demonstrated in numerous studies, duration of hospitalization (and/or mechanical ventilation) and prior exposure to antimicrobial agents are the major risk factors for VAP due to multidrug-resistant pathogens (86,87,96–99). Finally, it must be underlined that VAP due to fungi such as *Candida* species and *Aspergillus* species or to viruses such as influenza, parainfluenza, measles, adenovirus, and respiratory syncytial virus is uncommon in immunocompetent patients (68).

To conclude this section, we must emphasize that the etiologic characteristics of VAP vary widely from one ICU to another. Consequently, every ICU is encouraged to determine the local microbiology of VAP and the antimicrobial susceptibilities of these specific pathogens. Such a determination will assist in choosing adequate initial empiric antimicrobial treatment.

Diagnostic Strategies and Diagnostic Testing

In the ICU, the diagnosis of VAP remains a challenge. Difficulties encountered by physicians are mainly explained by the absence of a gold standard for this diagnosis. Usually, the diagnostic approach is based on two successive steps: (a) the diagnosis of pneumonia must be established and (b) the etiologic pathogen(s) of this pulmonary parenchymal infection must be identified (68).

Pneumonia is suspected when a patient exhibits signs and symptoms suggesting both pulmonary involvement and infection. The most current signs of infection are fever or hypothermia, leukocytosis or leucopenia, and tachycardia. Purulent sputum, a decline in oxygenation, and pulmonary infiltrates on chest radiograph are suggestive of pulmonary involvement. Unfortunately, among these signs and symptoms, none is specific for pneumonia. Most inflammatory processes and nonpulmonary infectious diseases are associated with fever, leukocytosis, or tachycardia. Similarly, cardiogenic and noncardiogenic pulmonary edema, pulmonary embolism, pulmonary contusion, and atelectasis are all associated with radiographic infiltrates. Finally, purulent sputum, even when associated with fever and leukocytosis, may be due only to nosocomial tracheobronchitis (100). To address the high sensitivity of these criteria and avoid too high a number of false-positive diagnoses, current recommendations are to combine them (68). Currently, the presence of a new or progressive radiographic infiltrate associated with at least two of three major clinical findings (fever greater than 38°C, purulent tracheal secretions, and leukocytosis or leucopenia) is considered the most accurate combination (101).

Numerous techniques have been proposed to identify causative organism(s) of VAP. Blood cultures are rarely positive. Moreover, a positive result is far from being specific since it could reflect more a severe extrapulmonary infection than identify the causative agent of VAP (102). A positive pleural effusion culture is generally considered as a specific result. However, the spread of infection to the pleural space is a rare event. Thus, analysis of lower respiratory secretions is the most frequently used technique to identify causative organism(s) of VAP. Numerous sampling methods have been described, with the major ones being endotracheal aspiration and bronchoscopic techniques with protected specimen brush and/or bronchoalveolar lavage. Numerous microbiologic techniques can be applied to these samples: direct examination with Giemsa or Gram staining and qualitative, semiquantitative, and quantitative cultures. Among all described methods of sampling and microbiologic techniques applied to these samples, it is not possible, to date, to identify the best method because the data are controversial.

The advantages and disadvantages of each technique evaluating lower respiratory tract samples have been recently reviewed (68,80). The main points summarizing these data are as follows:

- Microscopy and qualitative culture of expectorated sputum or endotracheal aspirates are associated with a high percentage of false-positive results because of colonization of the upper respiratory tract and/or tracheobronchial tree. However, the initial empiric antimicrobial treatment of VAP could be guided by a reliable tracheal aspirate Gram stain. Quantitative cultures with a threshold of 10^6 colony-forming units (CFU)/mL to differentiate colonization from lung infection provide a diagnostic accuracy nearly similar to that of quantitative cultures from samples obtained by bronchoscopic techniques (103,104). Moreover, when the culture of endotracheal secretions is sterile in a patient with no recent (less than 72 hours) change in antimicrobial therapy, the diagnosis of VAP can be ruled out with a high probability (the negative predictive value is greater than 90%) (105), and an extrapulmonary infectious process must be investigated.

- A protected specimen brush (PSB) allows the collection of uncontaminated specimens from the infected pulmonary area. A threshold set at 10^3 CFU/mL is the most adequate for quantitative cultures (106); false-positive results are infrequent (104). False-negative results may be observed when sampling is performed at an early stage of infection, in a technically incorrect (unaffected pulmonary area) manner, in a patient where a new antimicrobial treatment has been initiated, and/or if the specimens are incorrectly processed. Bronchoalveolar lavage explores a larger lung area than PSB. Quantitative cultures of bronchoalveolar lavage (BAL) fluid, with a threshold set at 10^4 CFU/mL, seem to provide results similar to those obtained by PSB (106). However, a possible microscopic examination of BAL fluid immediately after the procedure is a clear advantage. The detection with Gram or Giemsa staining of BAL cells containing intracellular bacteria allows for a rapid diagnosis and guides the initial antibiotic treatment (107,108). The arguments favoring these bronchoscopic techniques are their ability to confirm the diagnosis of VAP by identifying the causative organism(s) and guide the antimicrobial treatment. Furthermore, when cultures are negative, they can point to an alternative diagnosis. When cultures are positive, a more targeted antimicrobial treatment plan is possible, and the selective pressure for antibiotic resistance may be reduced. Finally, having an accurate microbiologic diagnosis may reduce VAP mortality (109). The major limitations of these bronchoscopic techniques are a questionable accuracy in patients in whom a new antimicrobial treatment has been introduced before sampling, the significant cost, a possible occurrence of complications (i.e., hypoxemia), and, perhaps, a low impact on therapeutic decisions since physicians are often reluctant to modify (or discontinue) an effective treatment.

Over many years, experts have discussed the best means to diagnose VAP. Some have preferred a clinical strategy based on radiologic, clinical, and biologic signs previously described; this approach is now considered overly sensitive. Other experts preferred a bacteriologic strategy based on a positive quantitative culture of lower respiratory tract secretions to define both pneumonia and the causative pathogen(s); this approach is now considered insufficiently sensitive, especially in patients in whom an antimicrobial treatment was recently started or changed. The recent ATS/IDSA guidelines propose a "mixed" diagnostic strategy as follows (68):

- The diagnosis of VAP is suspected in the presence of a new or progressive pulmonary infiltrate associated with at least two of the following three infectious signs: fever greater than 38°C, leukocytosis or leucopenia, and/or purulent secretions. For patients with ARDS, radiographic changes are difficult to analyze; consequently, hemodynamic instability and/or deterioration of blood gases could be considered sufficient to suspect VAP.
- As soon as the diagnosis is suspected, lower respiratory tract samples are obtained for microscopy, and quantitative or semiquantitative cultures and empiric antimicrobial therapy is started unless there is both a low clinical suspicion for VAP and a negative microscopy of the respiratory sample.
- On days 2 and 3, the results of cultures should be available, and the clinical response is assessed. According to whether the clinical picture is improving or worsening and the results of cultures, antimicrobial therapy will be stopped, de-escalated, or adjusted, and an investigation for other pathogens, other diagnoses, other sites of infection, or complications is performed.

The major points and recommendations for diagnostic testing following this diagnostic strategy are the following. All acutely ill, mechanically ventilated patients should have a complete daily investigation including physical examination, an anteroposterior portable chest radiograph, measurement of arterial oxygenation saturation, and determination of necessary laboratory values (complete blood count, serum electrolytes, renal function). When VAP is suspected, each patient should have a complete physical examination to search for another source of infection; arterial blood analysis must be performed; and blood cultures collected. In case of large pleural effusion, a diagnostic thoracentesis must be performed, unless there is a contraindication. Samples of lower respiratory tract secretions must be obtained in all patients. They can include endotracheal aspirate and/or bronchoscopic samples (PSB and/or BAL). Quantitative cultures of respiratory samples appear more accurate than qualitative or semiquantitative cultures for diagnosis of VAP (68).

Antibiotic Treatment

Principles of Initial Empiric Treatment. Prompt initiation of adequate antimicrobial treatment is a cornerstone of therapy for VAP (96). This rule is based on the following data: an inadequate initial antibiotic treatment is associated with a significantly increased mortality due to VAP (110–112). The timing of adequate antibiotic treatment is an important determinant of outcome. Iregui et al. studied 107 patients suffering from VAP (113). Among them, 33 received delayed appropriate antibiotic treatment—defined as a period greater than or equal to 24 hours between the time VAP was suspected and the administration of adequate treatment. These patients exhibited a significantly higher mortality than those receiving nondelayed treatment (69.7% vs. 28.4%; $p < 0.001$). It must be emphasized that patients with delayed treatment received antibiotics, on average, only 16 hours later than patients without delay. Once bacteriologic and susceptibility data become available, it does not reduce the excess mortality induced by the inadequate treatment given initially (111,112).

Combining various definitions in the literature, an adequate antibiotic therapy could be defined as the administration, at an appropriate dose, of at least one antibiotic with good penetration into lung tissues and to which all causative pathogens are susceptible *in vitro*. Although inappropriate doses and/or choice of agents with poor lung penetration could explain the inadequacy of treatment, the most common reason is the resistance of the causative pathogen(s). Consequently, antibiotics must be selected according to the presence or absence of risk factors for multidrug-resistant pathogens (Table 111.7) and the local microbiologic patterns of VAP.

Guidelines for Initial Empiric Antibiotic Therapy. On the basis of the time of onset of VAP and the presence or absence of risks for multidrug-resistant pathogens, the recent ATS/IDSA guidelines propose two different schemes for initial empiric antibiotic therapy (68). In patients with no risk factors for

TABLE 111.8

INITIAL EMPIRIC ANTIBIOTIC THERAPY IN PATIENTS WITH VENTILATOR-ASSOCIATED PNEUMONIA (VAP)

Characteristics of patient	Recommended antibiotics and recommended dosages[a]
Early-onset VAP and no risk factors for multidrug-resistant pathogens	■ Ceftriaxone (1–2 g/24 h) *or* ■ Levofloxacin (750 mg/24 h), moxifloxacin (400 mg/24 h), or ciprofloxacin (400 mg/8 h) *or* ■ Ampicillin (1–2 g) plus sulbactam (0.5–1 g)/6 h *or* ■ Ertapenem (1 g/24 h)
Late-onset VAP or risk factors for multidrug-resistant pathogens	■ Antipseudomonal cephalosporin: Cefepime (1–2 g/8–12 h) or ceftazidime (2 g/8 h) *or* ■ Antipseudomonal carbapenem: Imipenem (500 mg/6 h or 1 g/8 h) or meropenem (1 g/8 h) *or* ■ β-Lactam/β-lactamase inhibitor: Piperacillin-tazobactam (4.5 g/6 h) *plus* ■ Antipseudomonal fluoroquinolone: Levofloxacin (750 mg/24 h) or ciprofloxacin (400 mg/8 h) *or* ■ Aminoglycoside[b]: Gentamicin (7 mg/kg/24 h) or tobramycin (7 mg/kg/24 h) or amikacin (20 mg/kg/24 h) *plus* ■ Vancomycin (15 mg/kg/12 h)[c] *or* ■ Linezolid (600 mg/12 h)

Adapted from American Thoracic Society, Infectious Diseases Society of America. Guidelines for the management of adults with hospital-acquired, ventilator-associated, and health care–associated pneumonia. *Am J Respir Crit Care Med.* 2005;171:388.
[a] Dosages are based on normal hepatic and renal function.
[b] Trough levels for gentamicin and tobramycin should be <1 mg/L and for amikacin should be <4–5 mg/L.
[c] Trough levels for vancomycin should be <15–20 mg/L.

multidrug-resistant pathogens and an early-onset VAP (duration of hospitalization less than 5 days), limited-spectrum antibiotic therapy based on monotherapy seems appropriate (Table 111.8). Conversely, in patients with late-onset VAP (greater than or equal to 5 days) or exhibiting risk factors for multidrug-resistant pathogens, a broad-spectrum antibiotic regimen based on two or three combined antibiotics is usually required (Table 111.8).

Among all proposed antimicrobial agents, the initial choice should take into account patient characteristics (underlying diseases associated with contraindications to specific antibiotic agents or classes), class of antibiotic to which the patient was recently exposed, and local microbiologic data (resistance patterns). A recent exposure to one antibiotic could lead to resistance to the entire class. Consequently, if patients develop VAP shortly after, or during, antibiotic treatment, it is recommended that an antibiotic be chosen from a different antimicrobial class for empiric treatment. Local epidemiologic patterns (predominant pathogens and local antibiotic susceptibility) must lead to the implementation of specific institutional guidelines for the treatment of VAP, which are of particular importance. Ioanas et al. demonstrated that guidelines such as those of the ATS have a good ability to predict the causative pathogens of VAP (114). Conversely, their accuracy in regard to the adequacy of a proposed antimicrobial regimen is lower, mainly due to the resistance patterns of locally identified causative organisms. Consequently, institutional guidelines tailored to local microbiologic data are imperative to increase the rate of adequacy of the initial empiric antibiotic treatment of VAP, as demonstrated by Ibrahim et al. (115).

Finally, it is important to report the results from a recent study from Michel et al. (116). These authors demonstrated that routine quantitative cultures of endotracheal aspirates obtained twice a week in mechanically ventilated patients before the onset of VAP was identified, in 95% of cases, the same micro-organisms as the BAL cultures are obtained when VAP was suspected. Consequently, an antibiotic choice based on the results of the last available quantitative culture of endotracheal aspirate could increase the adequacy of the initial empiric treatment. Although prospective comparative studies are required to validate these results, it is possible to imagine that routine cultures of endotracheal aspirates could also help the clinician to choose the most appropriate antibiotic(s) among all proposed agents.

De-escalation Strategy. Considering the negative prognostic impact of an inadequate initial antibiotic therapy in VAP, a therapeutic strategy based on narrow-spectrum initial therapy, followed by a broadened-spectrum therapy once culture results are available, must be avoided. As previously noted, current recommendations propose an initial therapy for which the antimicrobial spectrum depends on potential causative pathogens and the risk of multidrug-resistant pathogens.

As demonstrated in numerous studies (86,87,114), most patients suffering from VAP exhibited either a late-onset VAP or risk factors for multidrug-resistant pathogens. Consequently, most patients with VAP are treated with a broad-spectrum antibiotic therapy that combines two or three agents. One great concern about the widespread use of broad-spectrum empiric therapy in the ICU is the emergence of multidrug-resistant pathogens. Such an emergence could lead, in the future, to ineffective treatment with broad-spectrum antibiotics. To preempt this vicious circle, a de-escalating strategy has been proposed (117).

Once the results of blood or respiratory tract cultures become available, this strategy recommends the change from a broad- to a narrow-spectrum antibiotic to which the isolated organism is sensitive (i.e., imipenem to ceftriaxone when the enteric Gram-negative bacilli do not exhibit extended-spectrum β-lactamase [ESBL]), as well as removing an antibiotic from an initial combination when the anticipated organism is not recovered (i.e., discontinuation of vancomycin or linezolid when MRSA is not present). Rello et al. demonstrated that de-escalation was possible in 31.4% of the 115 patients included in their study (118). This strategy was applied to 40.7% of patients with early-onset and 12.5% of patients with late-onset VAP. Obviously, a de-escalation strategy is not possible in patients without cultures (118). This emphasizes the importance of an initial diagnostic strategy for all patients as soon as VAP is suspected and before the initiation of empiric antibiotic treatment, which includes blood cultures and samples of lower respiratory tract secretions for culture.

Duration of Therapy. Until recently, the optimal duration of antibiotic therapy for VAP was unknown. Lacking prospective controlled studies devoted to this issue, experts empirically recommended a 14- to 21-day treatment duration (1). This was theoretically justified to avoid relapses with short treatment duration. However, this is now in conflict with our knowledge of the impact of prolonged antibiotic duration on the emergence of resistant strains in the ICU.

A prospective, multicenter, randomized, double-blind trial was performed to determine whether 8 versus 15 days of antibiotic treatment were equally effective. Patients receiving appropriate antimicrobial treatment during 8 days had neither excess mortality nor more recurrent infection than patients treated for 15 days. For patients suffering from VAP due to nonfermenting Gram-negative bacilli (mainly *P. aeruginosa* and *A. baumannii*), although the outcome was similar in the two groups, there was a trend to greater rates of pulmonary infection recurrences (relapses and/or superinfection) in the short duration of treatment group (119). Consequently, recent ATS/IDSA guidelines suggest shortening the duration of therapy to 7 days, providing that the causative pathogen is neither *P. aeruginosa* nor *A. baumannii* and the patient exhibits a good clinical response (68). Whatever the treatment duration, when aminoglycosides are used in combination with other agents, they may be stopped after no more than 5 to 7 days (68).

As previously discussed, prompt initiation of empiric antibiotic therapy is a cornerstone of VAP treatment. Unfortunately, in the absence of a gold standard, the diagnosis of VAP remains difficult and, among all empirically treated patients, some will not have VAP. Recent studies demonstrated that empiric antibiotic therapy could be safely discontinued after 72 hours when a noninfectious etiology for the pulmonary infiltrates is discovered or when signs and symptoms of active infections resolve (120,121). Finally, a sterile culture of lower respiratory tract secretions rules out, in the absence of a new antibiotic in the past 72 hours, the presence of bacterial pneumonia (68). In a case such as this, withholding antibiotics is justified.

Specific Antibiotic Regimens. As previously noted, *P. aeruginosa*, *A. baumannii*, and MRSA are the main causative pathogens of VAP. Some points about their specific antimicrobial treatment must be discussed.

A combination of antibiotics for *P. aeruginosa* VAP is commonly used by most clinicians. The aim of the combination is to achieve antibiotic synergy and prevent the emergence of resistant strains during therapy. Two recent meta-analyses showed that, for septic patients, the combination β-lactam plus aminoglycoside compared with β-lactam monotherapy provides no clinical benefit (122), and has no beneficial effect on the development of antimicrobial resistance among initially antimicrobial-susceptible isolates (123). However, these meta-analyses, like previous ones, suffer from limitations that weaken the interpretation (low number of studies included in the analysis, heterogeneity of those studies, outdated aminoglycoside administration schedules). Consequently, we do not think these results are sufficiently strong to justify discontinuing the use of short-term aminoglycoside–β-lactam combination therapy for *P. aeruginosa* VAP.

Vancomycin remains the accepted standard therapy for treatment of serious infections due to MRSA. Linezolid is a recent agent proposed for treatment of these infections. Two multicenter studies demonstrated the equivalence between linezolid and vancomycin for treatment of hospital-acquired pneumonia due to MRSA (124,125). When the results of these studies were combined, linezolid appeared to provide a better outcome and a lower mortality than vancomycin (126). However, these results appear conflicting, and a prospective validation of the superiority of linezolid is still required. Nevertheless, linezolid may be preferred to vancomycin in patients with or at risk for renal insufficiency (68).

A. baumannii exhibits native resistance to many classes of antimicrobial agents and has seen the emergence of resistance to carbapenems. Despite the reported nephrotoxicity of polymyxins, they may be safely used. Garnacho-Montero et al. demonstrated the safety and the efficacy of intravenous colistin in patients with VAP due to *A. baumannii* resistant to carbapenems (127).

Local Instillation and Aerosolized Antibiotics. Although aminoglycosides and polymyxin B have been used for local instillation or aerosolization to treat VAP due to pathogens that are "resistant" to systemic antimicrobial agents, there is a lack of large or randomized prospective studies evaluating the value of these administration routes. Consequently, the routine use of local instillation or aerosolized antibiotics is not recommended (68).

Response to Therapy

Normal Pattern of Resolution. Improvement usually becomes apparent only after 48 to 72 hours of adequate antibiotic therapy. Thus, unless there is rapid clinical deterioration, antimicrobial therapy should not be changed during this period following the initiation of therapy (68).

Two clinical variables, fever and hypoxemia, appear as the best indicators to monitor the response to treatment. In patients without ARDS, most respond with a resolution of fever to less than 38°C and resolution of hypoxemia with a PaO_2/FiO_2 improving to greater than 250 within the first 72 hours of adequate treatment. For responding patients with ARDS, hypoxemia resolves more slowly and, consequently, this parameter should not be used to define the resolution of VAP. In this subset of patients, although fever takes twice as long to resolve, core temperature appears as the most useful indicator of clinical response (128).

Monitoring of white blood cell count is not accurate to evaluate the response to therapy (128,129). Similarly, chest radiographs are of limited value for defining clinical improvement in VAP; indeed, initial radiograph deterioration is common (68). However, a quick radiographic resolution suggests that the initial diagnosis of VAP could be erroneous (128).

Reasons for Deterioration or Nonresolution. When a patient fails to improve or exhibits rapid deterioration, several causes may be considered (Table 111.9) (68). In these patients, the following therapeutic approach can be proposed:

- When possible, the antimicrobial spectrum should be broadened while waiting for culture results and complementary diagnostic studies. A careful clinical evaluation to rule out diagnostic possibilities based on the differential diagnosis must be performed, and sampling of respiratory tract secretions must be repeated.

TABLE 111.9

CAUSES OF NONRESOLUTION OR DETERIORATION IN PATIENTS WITH VENTILATOR-ASSOCIATED PNEUMONIA (VAP)

Factors	Comments
Wrong initial diagnosis of VAP	Many noninfectious processes can mimic VAP: ■ Pulmonary embolism ■ Congestive heart failure ■ Lung contusion ■ Atelectasis ■ Chemical pneumonitis from aspiration ■ ARDS ■ Pulmonary hemorrhage
Host factors	Despite adequate treatment, many conditions are known to be associated with failure: ■ Underlying fatal condition ■ Age older than 60 yr ■ Prior pneumonia ■ Prior antibiotic treatment ■ Chronic lung diseases
Bacterial factors	■ Infecting bacteria can be resistant and can acquire resistance during treatment (*Pseudomonas aeruginosa*) ■ Infecting pathogen can be a nonbacterial pathogen: □ Mycobacteria □ Virus □ Fungus ■ Some pathogens, even with effective treatment, are difficult to eradicate (*P. aeruginosa*)
Occurrence of complications	■ Complications of initial pneumonia: □ Empyema □ Lung abscess ■ Other sites of infection: □ Urinary tract infection □ Catheter-related infection □ Sinusitis □ Pseudomembranous enterocolitis ■ Drug fever, pulmonary embolism, and sepsis with multiple system organ failure

ARDS, acute respiratory distress syndrome.
Adapted from American Thoracic Society, Infectious Diseases Society of America. Guidelines for the management of adults with hospital-acquired, ventilator-associated, and healthcare-associated pneumonia. *Am J Respir Crit Care Med.* 2005;171:388.

- If cultures reveal a resistant pathogen (inadequate initial empiric choice, development of resistance or superinfection with a resistant strain), an adequate antibiotic therapy must be rapidly instituted, even if such a change has a low prognostic impact.
- If cultures do not yield a resistant pathogen, one must consider a noninfectious process, another site of infection, or occurrence of complications. Vascular catheters must be removed and cultured, and blood and urine samples must be drawn for culture. Radiographic procedures such as CT scanning of the thorax and, possibly, of extrathoracic sites (sinuses, abdomen) may reveal complications (e.g., lung abscess, empyema) or other infectious sites (e.g., sinusitis).

Finally, when the entire workup remains negative—including the microbiologic and radiographic evaluations for VAP, with or without resistant pathogens, noninfectious processes mimicking VAP, VAP complications, or an extrapulmonary site of infection, physicians must consider the following: (a) coverage for unusual pathogens (i.e., mycobacteria, fungi), (b) the need for an open-lung biopsy, and (c) initiation of anti-inflammatory therapy such as corticosteroids.

Ioanas et al., studying 71 patients with ICU-acquired pneumonia, demonstrated that the rate of nonresponding patients was high (62%) (130). The main causes of nonresponsiveness were inappropriate initial treatment (23%), superinfections (14%), another site of infection (27%), and a noninfectious process (16%). In 36% of nonresponding patients, no cause of failure could be identified.

Prognosis of Ventilator-associated Pneumonia

According to the literature, crude mortality rates associated with VAP vary from 24% to 76% (80). These widely diverging crude mortality rates can be explained by differences both in the studied populations and the diagnostic criteria used.

One of the most important concerns about VAP is to know whether it is associated with significant attributable mortality. Case-control studies comparing patients with and without VAP with a matching process including variables such as cause of ICU admission, duration of mechanical ventilation, and severity of underlying diseases provide discordant results. In some studies, VAP was not associated with any significant attributable mortality (69,131). Conversely, in others, VAP was associated with a significant attributable mortality set around 25% (132–134).

Numerous independent prognostic factors associated with hospital mortality of patients suffering from VAP were identified. These reflect the patients' underlying illnesses (malignancy, immunosuppression, anticipated death within 5 years, American Society of Anesthesiology grade 3 or more), age older than 64 years, severity of disease justifying ICU admission (high APACHE II score, Simplify Acute Physiology Score greater than 37), initial severity of VAP (chest radiographic involvement of more than one lobe, platelet count less than 150,000 cells/μL, Logistic Organ Dysfunction score greater than 4, time of onset of VAP greater than 3 days, surgery, or hypotension), and initial therapeutic approach (delayed initial appropriate antibiotic treatment) (111–113,135–138).

Prevention of Ventilator-associated Pneumonia

Basic infection control techniques such as hand washing, glove use, sterile equipment, and adequate staffing are necessary to limit cross-contamination of resistant organisms through health care workers.

Prevention of nosocomial pneumonia has been the subject of two recent reviews (81,139). The primary intervention to reduce VAP is to minimize intubation frequency and duration. Noninvasive positive pressure ventilation using a face mask could be an interesting alternative ventilation mode in ICU patients. It is associated with a relative risk reduction for VAP ranging from 0.67 to 0.87. When intubation is necessary, the orotracheal route is preferred. Strategies to reduce the duration of mechanical ventilation, such as optimized sedation and weaning protocols, are also effective. Continuous aspiration of subglottic secretions is associated with a relative risk reduction for VAP of 0.45. A semirecumbent (45-degree) patient position also reduces VAP, particularly compared to the supine position with enteral nutrition. Stress ulcer prophylaxis has a controversial impact on VAP. The benefit it offers by decreasing risks of gastric hemorrhage might outweigh the increased risk of VAP. Similarly, enteral nutrition is associated with VAP, but the alternative—parenteral nutrition—carries the risk of catheter-related bacteremia. Postpyloric feeding has been reported to reduce VAP. Ventilator circuit management, transfusion practices, and glycemic control are also issues that may be addressed to reduce VAP (140).

The Centers for Disease Control and Prevention (CDC) published 2004 guidelines on the prevention of VAP (141). These graded guidelines offer a comprehensive view on the different interventions useful in reducing VAP. Only four measures are recommended (Table 111.10).

ICU providers caring for immunosuppressed patients with severe neutropenia and/or allogeneic hematopoietic stem cell transplant recipients must take measures to prevent legionellosis or aspergillosis. Legionellosis prevention is based on the control of the hot water system, while aspergillosis prevention necessitates rooms with high-efficiency particulate air filters and the use of high-efficiency respiratory protection devices (e.g., N95 respirators) by patients when they leave their rooms and/or when dust-generating activities are ongoing in the facility.

One last highly controversial issue is the use of selective digestive decontamination (SDD) (81,139,142). This has

TABLE 111.10

MEASURES RECOMMENDED BY THE CENTERS FOR DISEASE CONTROL AND PREVENTION TO REDUCE THE INCIDENCE OF VENTILATOR-ASSOCIATED PNEUMONIA

- Changing the breathing circuits of ventilators only when they malfunction or are visibly contaminated
- Preferential use of orotracheal rather than nasotracheal tubes
- Use of noninvasive ventilation
- Use of an endotracheal tube with a dorsal lumen to allow drainage of respiratory secretions

Data from Tablan OC, Anderson LJ, Besser R, et al. Healthcare Infection Control Practices Advisory Committee, Centers for Disease Control and Prevention. Guidelines for preventing health-care–associated pneumonia, 2003: recommendations of the CDC and the Healthcare Infection Control Practices Advisory Committee. *MMWR Recomm Rep.* 2004;53(RR-3):1.

TABLE 111.11

MICRO-ORGANISMS THAT CAUSE HOSPITAL-ACQUIRED PNEUMONIA (HAP)[a]

References	Valles et al.[b]	Sopena et al.[c]	Kollef et al.[d]
Number of episodes of HAP	96	165	835
Number of bacteria identified	75	60	ND
Pseudomonas aeruginosa	18 (24%)	7 (11.7%)	18.4%
Acinetobacter baumannii	1	5 (8.3%)	2.0%
Stenotrophomonas maltophilia	ND	ND	ND
Enterobacteriaceae	7 (9.3%)	8 (13.3%)	16.1%
Haemophilus species	2	2 (3.3%)	5.6%
Legionella pneumophila	9 (12%)	7 (11.7%)	ND
Methicillin-resistant *Staphylococcus aureus* } Methicillin-sensitive *S. aureus*	9 (12%)	1 (1.6%)	22.9%
Streptococcus pneumoniae	11 (15%)	3 (5%)	26.2%
Streptococcus species	2	16 (26.7%)	3.1%
Enterococcus species	ND	ND	13.9%
Coagulase-negative staphylococcus	ND	ND	ND
Anaerobic pathogens	ND	ND	ND
Aspergillus species	13 (17%)	ND	ND
		7 (11.7%)	ND

ND, no data.
[a] Data are presented as number and/or (percentage).
[b] Valles J, Mesalles E, Mariscal D, et al. A 7-year study of severe hospital-acquired pneumonia requiring ICU admission. *Intensive Care Med.* 2003;29:1981.
[c] Sopena N, Sabria M, Neunos 2000 Study Group. Multicenter study of hospital-acquired pneumonia in non-ICU patients. *Chest.* 2005;127:213.
[d] Kollef MH, Shorr A, Tabak YP, et al. Epidemiology and outcomes of health-care-associated pneumonia: results from a large US database of culture-positive pneumonia. *Chest.* 2005;128:3854.

been the subject of multiple trials using the application and ingestion of topical nonabsorbed antimicrobials (usually combining polymyxin, aminoglycoside, and amphotericin B) with or without the addition of a short-duration systemic broad-spectrum antibiotic. The theory is that topical agents will eradicate potential pathogens (Gram-negative aerobic intestinal bacteria, *S. aureus,* and fungi) but not the anaerobic flora. Impressive results have been recently published, with a 20% decrease in ICU mortality (143). However, methodologic flaws (ward, no patient randomization, and unblinded trials) and an extremely low rate of drug-resistant organisms, including zero MRSA colonization, make the generalization of these results difficult. The preventive effects of SDD for VAP are lower in ICUs with high endemic levels of antibiotic resistance, and, in such cases, SDD increases the selective antibiotic pressure and can increase the incidence of drug-resistant micro-organisms. Thus, to date, the generalized routine use of SDD in ICUs is not recommended; it should be decided according to the patient population studied and the characteristics of ICU.

Hospital-acquired Pneumonia

As recently reported by Kollef et al. (3), a hospital-acquired pneumonia (HAP) may be defined as a pneumonia occurring less than 2 days from hospital admission, but without any criteria defining ventilator-associated pneumonia. Data about HAP acquired outside the ICU, treated outside the ICU, or requiring ICU admission for treatment are scarce. Information from recent studies (3,144,145) suggests that most patients who acquired HAP in medical wards exhibited severe underlying diseases (i.e., chronic pulmonary diseases, immunosuppression) and developed HAP late during the hospital stay. Microbiologic data demonstrate both the major role played by the Enterobacteriaceae, *P. aeruginosa,* and MRSA and variations in local epidemiology (Table 111.11). Mortality rate varies from one study to another between 18.8% and 53%. Resultant from this lack of data about HAP, recent ATS/IDSA guidelines suggest, by extrapolation, that all patients with HAP be managed as if they were VAP cases (68).

Health care–associated Pneumonia and Nursing Home Pneumonia

Health care–associated pneumonia (HCAP) includes any patient who was hospitalized in an acute care hospital for 2 or more days within 90 days of the infection; resides in a nursing home or long-term care facility (LTCF); received recent intravenous antibiotic therapy, chemotherapy, or wound care within 30 days of the current infection; or attends a hospital or hemodialysis clinic. Moreover, most pneumonia occurring in hosts with therapeutic immunodeficiency may now be classified as HCAP.

In nursing homes, pneumonia is a leading cause of mortality, morbidity, and transfers to acute care facilities among residents. Pneumonia is the second most common infection in LTCFs, with an incidence of 0.3 to 4.7 cases per 1,000 resident-days (146). It is an independent risk factor for death in LTCF patients (147). Mortality in these at-risk patients ranges from 5% to 40%, and coincides with mortality seen in community-dwelling patients diagnosed with pneumonia and admitted to an intensive care unit (148). These pneumonias differ in presentation due to the modified host response often seen in the elderly.

In these older individuals, fever and respiratory signs may be minimal, while an altered mental status might be the only evident symptom (149). Pneumonia risk factors in nursing home residents include decreased functional status, diminished ability to clear airways, underlying comorbidities (such as chronic obstructive pulmonary disease and heart disease), swallowing disorders, and use of sedatives.

The etiology of nursing home–acquired pneumonia remains controversial. Studies identified a large proportion of Gram-negative bacilli and *S. aureus* based on sputum culture without assessing the quality of the sample. However, when using strict criteria (150), *S. pneumoniae* and *H. influenzae* are the major pathogens (151), while Gram-negative bacilli account for 0% to 12% of cases.

The ATS/IDSA (68) guidelines recommend that, in the hospital, these patients be managed like those with HAP until an etiologic diagnosis is made. Recommendations are summarized in Tables 111.8 and 111.9.

TRACHEOBRONCHITIS

Acute Exacerbations of Chronic Obstructive Pulmonary Disease

Acute exacerbation of COPD is defined by an impairment in the patient's baseline dyspnea, cough, and/or sputum (152). The need for ICU or special care unit admission is based on the severity of respiratory failure and/or the presence of associated organ dysfunction (i.e., shock, hemodynamic instability, neurologic disturbances) (152). Therapy in the ICU is based on supplemental oxygen, ventilatory support, bronchodilators, corticosteroids, and antibiotics (152). Only the latter point will be further discussed.

Notwithstanding a literature extending years into the past, the role of bacterial infection in acute exacerbation of COPD remains controversial. As explained by Murphy et al. (153), this point is still debated for the following reasons: (a) even in the absence of symptoms of exacerbation, numerous bacteria colonize the lower respiratory tract of COPD patients; (b) bacteria colonizing the lower respiratory tract vary from one patient to another, as COPD patients are heterogeneous; (c) information provided by sputum culture does not really reflect conditions in the distal airways; (d) only half of the episodes of acute exacerbations of COPD are linked to bacterial infection; (e) animal models are limited by the fact that the most often isolated bacteria (*S. pneumoniae*, *H. influenzae*, *Moraxella catarrhalis*) are exclusively human pathogens; and (f) clinical studies addressing the impact of antibiotic therapy during acute exacerbation of COPD suggest that such a treatment provides only a small improvement in the most severely ill patients (154).

Despite these uncertainties, the recent ATS/European Respiratory Society Task Force proposed to institute antibiotic treatment in all patients suffering from a severe acute exacerbation of COPD requiring ICU admission (152). Two studies that focused on the impact of antibiotic treatment in COPD patients admitted in the ICU for severe exacerbation requiring mechanical ventilation reinforce this recommendation. Nouira et al. (155) performed a prospective, randomized, double-blind, placebo-controlled trial assessing the effects of ofloxacin. They showed that antibiotic treatment reduced the mortality rate, the need for additional antibiotics in preventing the occurrence of nosocomial pneumonia, and the duration of mechanical ventilation and hospital stay. Similarly, Ferrer et al. (156) demonstrated that an inadequate initial antibiotic treatment increased hospital mortality and was significantly associated with failure of noninvasive ventilation, leading to secondary intubation and invasive mechanical ventilation. Inadequacy of initial empiric treatment mainly occurred when colonizing pathogens were not the usual community-acquired pathogens (*S. pneumoniae*, *H. influenzae*, *M. catarrhalis*), but were instead nonfermenting (*P. aeruginosa*) or enteric Gram-negative bacilli.

Current recommendations (152) propose an antibiotic therapy based on amoxicillin/clavulanate or respiratory fluoroquinolones (gatifloxacin, levofloxacin, moxifloxacin). If *Pseudomonas* spp. or *Enterobacteriaceae* spp. are suspected, combination therapy should be considered. As in hospital-acquired pneumonia, a wide-spectrum β-lactam combined with an antipseudomonal fluoroquinolone or an aminoglycoside may be of use. Finally, an ongoing study of local microbiology and susceptibility patterns by routine bacteriologic investigation in COPD patients appears as the best means to provide an initial adequate antibiotic treatment for acute exacerbations of COPD (152,157).

Nosocomial Tracheobronchitis

As recently noted, only a few studies have addressed nosocomial tracheobronchitis acquired during mechanical ventilation (158). Most recent data are provided by Nseir et al. (100), with the potentially major limitation that their studies were performed in a single ICU. Consequently, the results may not be applicable to other units.

In a retrospective analysis of 2,128 patients mechanically ventilated more than 48 hours, the incidence of nosocomial tracheobronchitis was 10.6%, without any significant difference between medical (9.9%; 165 of 1,655) and surgical patients (15.3%; 36 of 234) (100). In patients without underlying chronic respiratory insufficiency, the incidence was 8% (159). In most patients, the delay between initiation of mechanical ventilation and occurrence of tracheobronchitis was up to 10 days. In medical patients, nosocomial tracheobronchitis was significantly associated with age younger than 60 years (OR = 1.8), COPD (OR = 1.57) and receiving prior antibiotics within the 2 weeks preceding ICU admission (OR = 1.52). The main pathogens identified in culture of tracheal aspirates were *P. aeruginosa*, *A. baumannii*, and MRSA.

The impact of nosocomial tracheobronchitis on patient outcome remains difficult to assess. Nseir et al. performed two case-control studies comparing patients with and without nosocomial tracheobronchitis (159,160). In both COPD patients and in patients without chronic respiratory insufficiency, nosocomial tracheobronchitis was significantly associated with longer durations of mechanical ventilation and ICU stay. Conversely, the occurrence of tracheobronchitis had no significant influence on mortality rates.

Indications for antibiotic treatment in these patients are still being debated. Some physicians consider that antibiotic treatment is not justified, whereas others consider antibiotics to be useful in patients with tracheobronchitis and weaning difficulties. In Nseir's trial (159), including patients without underlying chronic respiratory insufficiency, only 21% of patients received antibiotics. Despite results suggesting that appropriate antibiotic treatment might reduce the duration of mechanical ventilation (160), only well-designed prospective studies will answer the question of whether or not patients with nosocomial tracheobronchitis should be treated with antibiotics.

LUNG ABSCESS

Lung abscesses can be associated with aspiration pneumonia, poor dental hygiene, alcohol consumption, or chronic lung disease (161). It is relatively uncommon in developed countries, where it occurs mostly in immunosuppressed patients or as a postobstructive complication. Risk factors and underlying diseases from two studies are presented in Table 111.12 (161,162).

Bacteriology of Lung Abscesses

The predominant pathogens are considered to be anaerobes, which account for 60% to 80% of cases (163). Hammond et al., in a study of 34 patients with community-acquired lung abscess, identified 2.3 bacterial species per episode (161); anaerobes were identified in 75% of cases, with infection due to an aerobe observed in only 19% of cases. More recent studies reveal a more mixed pattern. A study of 90 patients with lung abscesses in Taiwan observed polymicrobial infection in only 20% of cases (162). Gram-negative bacilli, mostly *Klebsiella pneumoniae*, were the most frequently isolated microorganisms (47%), while anaerobes were only isolated in 31% (162). Despite limitations (the study excluded nosocomial, nonbacterial, and undocumented infections), it probably describes a change in the epidemiology of lung abscess that could modify the preferred antimicrobial regimen. Main bacteriologic data are reported in Table 111.13.

TABLE 111.12

RISK FACTORS AND UNDERLYING DISEASES OF ADULT PATIENTS WITH COMMUNITY-ACQUIRED LUNG ABSCESS[a]

References	Hammond et al.[b]	Wang et al.[c]
Number of patients	34	90
Characteristic (%)		
Smoking	ND	57%
Chronic lung disease	29%	37%
Diabetes mellitus	ND	31%
Previous aspiration pneumonia	29%	32%
Malignancy	3%	19%
Alcohol abuse	38%	14%
Dental caries	26%	ND
CNS disease	9%	11%
Chronic liver disease	ND	11%
Steroid use/SLE	9%	6%
None	12%	18%

ND, no data; CNS, central nervous system; SLE, systemic lupus erythematosus.
[a] Data are presented as number or percentage.
[b] Hammond JM, Potgieter PD, Hanslo D, et al. Etiology and antimicrobial susceptibility patterns of micro organisms in acute community-acquired lung abscess. *Chest*. 1995;108:937.
[c] Wang JL, Chen KY, Fang CT, et al. Changing bacteriology of adult community-acquired lung abscess in Taiwan: *Klebsiella pneumoniae* versus anaerobes. *Clin Infect Dis*. 2005;40:915.

TABLE 111.13

PATHOGENS ISOLATED FROM ADULT PATIENTS WITH COMMUNITY-ACQUIRED LUNG ABSCESS[a]

References	Hammond et al.[b]	Wang et al.[c]
Number of patients	34	90
Number of bacteria identified	79	118
Anaerobes	59 (75%)	40 (34%)
Microaerophilic streptococci	7 (20%)	11 (12%)
Prevotella	17 (50%)	8 (9%)
Bacteroides	4 (12%)	6 (7%)
Fusobacterium	4 (12%)	3 (3%)
Porphyromonas	7 (20%)	1 (1%)
Gram-negative bacilli	3 (9%)	42 (47%)
Klebsiella pneumoniae	2 (6%)	30 (33%)
Gram-positive cocci	12 (35%)	30 (33%)
Streptococcus milleri	ND	19 (21%)
Staphylococcus aureus	5 (15%)	2 (2%)
Viridans streptococci	7 (20%)	5 (5%)
Other	5 (15%)	5 (5%)

ND, no data.
[a] Data are presented as number and (percentage).
[b] Hammond JM, Potgieter PD, Hanslo D, et al. Etiology and antimicrobial susceptibility patterns of micro organisms in acute community-acquired lung abscess. *Chest*. 1995;108:937.
[c] Wang JL, Chen KY, Fang CT, et al. Changing bacteriology of adult community-acquired lung abscess in Taiwan: *Klebsiella pneumoniae* versus anaerobes. *Clin Infect Dis*. 2005;40:915.

Diagnosis

Blood cultures and sputum examination are rarely positive (161,162). Methods to obtain a specimen uncontaminated with colonizing bacteria from the upper airway are preferred. Percutaneous aspiration, transtracheal aspiration, or thoracocentesis from empyema fluid make isolation of both aerobic and anaerobic bacteria possible.

Treatment

Lung abscess is a severe disease. Historical studies reported death in one third of cases (163) when surgical resection or drainage was the only available tool.

Antimicrobial Therapy

Lung abscesses are generally treated successfully with prolonged systemic antibiotic therapy. The preferred antimicrobial therapy, based on the high frequency of anaerobes, was clindamycin (163). A β-lactamase inhibitor/aminopenicillin is also effective (164). Both regimens obtain cure rates between 60% and 70% with a 3-week course of therapy.

Other Therapies

Lack of improvement may necessitate drainage procedures in 10% to 20% of patients who remain symptomatic and eventually require other therapy.

Percutaneous radiographic-guided drainage is effective in only a selected subgroup of patients. Reported catheter drainage times averaged 9.8 to 20.1 days, with a range of 4 to 59 days (165). This invasive procedure may be difficult in patients with hemostatic abnormalities. Furthermore, there is a risk of soiling the pleural space with abscess contents. Surgical resection of the diseased lung and abscess might be necessary in some cases. Endoscopic drainage is a more recent procedure that could be useful in patients who have an airway connection to the abscess or an endobronchial obstruction preventing drainage (166).

PLEURAL EMPYEMA

Pathophysiology of Pleural Infection

The pleural space is normally sterile. Pleural effusion is favored by an increase in the hydrostatic pressure, a decrease of oncotic pressure, or alterations of pleural permeability. Infection follows colonization of pleural fluid. The formation of an empyema is arbitrarily divided into three phases: (a) an exudative phase with accumulation of pus, (b) a fibropurulent phase with fibrin deposition and loculation of pleural exudate, and (c) an organization phase with fibroblast proliferation leading to scar formation and lung entrapment (167).

In up to half of cases, empyema is a complication of pneumonia. Approximately one fourth of empyemas are due to a traumatic or iatrogenic injury (surgery, thoracocentesis, chest tube placement). In the remaining cases, pleural infection is due to a contiguous infection (i.e., mediastinum, esophagus, subdiaphragmatic areas) extending to the pleura (167).

Bacteriology of Pleural Infection

The bacterial etiology of empyema depends on the underlying mechanism leading to pleural colonization. With three fourths of empyemas developing as a complication of pneumonia or traumatic or iatrogenic injury, most isolated aerobic organisms are *Streptococcus* species, *S. pneumoniae,* and *S. aureus.* The main isolated aerobic Gram-negative organisms are *Klebsiella* species, *P. aeruginosa*, *H. influenzae,* and *Escherichia coli.* These organisms are commonly part of mixed growths with anaerobes. Anaerobic isolates are identified in 12% to 34% of cultures. They can cause empyema without aerobic copathogens in about 15% of cases (167,168).

Management of Patients with Pleural Infection

Identification of Pleural Effusion

In patients suffering from empyema, clinical symptoms may be nonspecific (fever, chills, chest pain, night sweats). Physical examination alterations may be limited to diminished breath sounds, basilar dullness to percussion, and/or a pleural friction rub. In mechanically ventilated patients, these signs and symptoms may be less relevant (167). Chest radiographic study remains the most important clue for diagnosis of pleural effusion. As soon as the volume of pleural fluid exceeds 200 mL, blunting of the posterior costodiaphragmatic sulcus occurs. Moreover, chest radiograph can reveal a pulmonary infiltrate, which suggests the possibility of a parapneumonic collection (168).

Ultrasonography is particularly useful in unstable or critically ill patients, since devices can be transported to the bedside. This investigation is able to precisely locate the fluid collection and allows for a guided diagnostic aspiration. Moreover, according to some ultrasonographic characteristics (i.e., echogenicity, septations), it may help distinguish empyema from transudative pleural effusion and solid mass, and may detect the presence of loculated collections (167).

When diagnosis appears difficult, a contrast-enhanced CT scan is useful to differentiate pleural empyema from a lung abscess, to detect complications of pleural infection, and, finally, to identify an intra- or extrathoracic focus of infection that extends to the pleura.

Indication of Pleural Fluid Sampling

In most cases, management of pleural effusion is guided by biologic characteristics of pleural fluid. Consequently, diagnostic pleural fluid sampling is recommended in all patients exhibiting pleural effusion in association with pneumonia, recent chest surgery or trauma, or an infectious process contiguous to pleura (168).

However, in the ICU, numerous patients develop pleural effusion without any relationship to pleural infection (i.e., hypoalbuminemia, heart failure, and atelectasis). In these patients at low risk of infection, pleural fluid sampling does not appear immediately useful in the absence of sepsis (168).

Gross appearance and chemical, physical, and microscopic characteristics of pleural fluid must be determined. The pH, lactic dehydrogenase (LDH) and glucose levels, and white blood cell count must be measured, and an appropriate microscopic examination of stained smears and cultures of pleural fluid must be performed. Empyema usually has a pH value of less than 7.0, an LDH level greater than 1,000 IU/L, a glucose level less than 40 mg/dL, and positive Gram stain and/or culture (167).

In patients with parapneumonic pleural effusions, gross appearance and biologic characteristics of pleural fluid can differentiate simple parapneumonic effusion from complicated parapneumonic effusion and empyema and, consequently, guide the management (168). In simple parapneumonic effusion, macroscopic appearance reveals a clear fluid, pH is greater than 7.2, LDH level is less than 1,000 IU/L, glucose level is greater than 40 mg/dL, and no organism is identified on Gram stain and culture. In complicated parapneumonic effusion, pleural fluid is clear, cloudy, or turbid; pH is less than 7.2; LDH level is greater than 1,000 IU/L; glucose level is greater than 40 mg/dL; and the Gram stain and/or culture are positive. Finally, in empyema, macroscopic examination reveals frank pus exhibiting the biologic characteristics previously described.

Treatment

Treatment of empyema requires adequate antimicrobial therapy, drainage of pus, and re-expansion of the lung.

Antibiotics. As soon as pleural infection is diagnosed, antibiotic treatment must be started. When pleural fluid cultures are positive, antibiotics must be chosen according to organisms identified and their sensitivities. Both penicillins and cephalosporins exhibit good penetration into the pleural space. They are the drugs of choice for treating empyemas due to *Streptococcus* species and *S. pneumoniae*. Nafcillin is the drug of choice for methicillin-sensitive *S. aureus* infection. Third-generation cephalosporins and carbapenems are preferred choices in case of empyema due to Gram-negative aerobic bacilli. Infections due to MRSA and penicillin- and cephalosporin-resistant *S. pneumoniae* should be treated with vancomycin. Aminoglycosides must be avoided, as their penetration into the pleural space is poor and they lose their activity in acid pleural fluid. When anaerobic organisms are causative pathogens, a β-lactam combined with a β-lactamase inhibitor, imipenem, metronidazole, and clindamycin are the drugs of choice (167,168).

When cultures are negative, antibiotics must be chosen according to the likely causative organisms. Choice depends on the mechanism of empyema, the origin of infection (community acquired vs. hospital acquired), and the local hospital policy. Recent guidelines from the British Thoracic Society (168) suggest the following empirical antibiotic regimens:

- In community-acquired infection, second- and third-generation cephalosporins, amoxicillin, β-lactam–β-lactamase inhibitor combination, meropenem, clindamycin, and benzyl penicillin combined with quinolone may be proposed.
- In hospital-acquired infection, such as empyema following a nosocomial pneumonia or recent chest surgery, antibiotics should cover both Gram-positive and Gram-negative aerobes and anaerobes. Antipseudomonal penicillins (piperacillin-tazobactam, ticarcillin-clavulanic acid), carbapenems, and third-generation cephalosporins combined with vancomycin may be used.

The duration of antibiotic treatment remains controversial since specific clinical trials are absent. Recent BTS guidelines suggest that a duration of 3 weeks is probably appropriate.

Chest Tube Drainage. Prompt chest tube drainage is indicated in patients with frankly purulent or turbid/cloudy pleural fluid on sampling. Similarly, a pleural fluid pH less than 7.2 and the presence of pathogens identified by Gram stain or culture of nonpurulent pleural fluid require prompt chest tube drainage (168). When, despite appropriate antibiotic treatment, clinical improvement is poor or when radiologic investigations demonstrate the presence of a loculated pleural collection, chest tube drainage may be suggested.

There is no consensus about the optimal size of the chest tube or about the efficacy of intrapleural fibrinolytic drugs. A recent randomized, double-blind trial compared intrapleural streptokinase (250,000 IU twice daily for 3 days) to placebo. Among the 427 studied patients, streptokinase did not reduce mortality, need for drainage surgery, or duration of hospital stay, and it did not improve radiographic and spirometric outcomes (169). A recent meta-analysis does not support the routine use of fibrinolytic treatment for patients requiring chest tube drainage for empyema or complicated parapneumonic effusion (170). Further evaluation is needed to define patients that would benefit from this therapy.

Surgical Treatment. Surgical treatment must be considered in all patients exhibiting a persisting sepsis associated with continuous pleural collection despite being appropriately treated with antibiotics and chest tube drainage. Different surgical approaches have been described. The choice between video-assisted thoracoscopic surgery, open thoracic drainage, or thoracotomy with decortication depends on the patient status (age, comorbidity), surgical preferences, and anatomy of pleural effusion assessed by recent thoracic CT scanning (168).

SUMMARY

Pneumonia remains a frequent disease in the community and in ventilated patients. Management of severe pneumonia in the ICU is challenging on many fronts. Diagnosis is difficult, as community-acquired pneumonias are only documented in about 50% of cases, and no consensual gold standard exists for ventilator-associated pneumonia. Preventive strategies such as vaccination have a low impact on community-acquired pneumonia, and the best strategies remain to be determined for ventilator-associated pneumonia.

Despite adequate treatment, the death rate remains elevated, reaching 18% to 46% in community-acquired pneumonia and 24% to 76% in ventilator-associated pneumonia. Adequate antimicrobial therapy is paramount for successful treatment but is increasingly complex. Drug choice depends on numerous factors: pharmacodynamics/pharmacokinetics, spectrum, dosing schedule, adverse events, costs, and availability. The rise of antimicrobial resistance in pneumonia pathogens complicates therapeutic guidelines that need to be regularly adapted to local resistance patterns.

References

1. American Thoracic Society. Hospital-acquired pneumonia in adults: diagnosis, assessment of severity, initial antimicrobial therapy, and preventive strategies. A consensus statement. *Am J Respir Crit Care Med.* 1996;153:1711.
2. Ewig S, Bauer T, Torres A. The pulmonary physician in critical care. Nosocomial pneumonia. *Thorax.* 2002;57:366.
3. Kollef MH, Shorr A, Tabak YP, et al. Epidemiology and outcomes of health-care-associated pneumonia: results from a large US database of culture-positive pneumonia. *Chest.* 2005;128:3854.
4. Bartlett JG, Mundy LM. Community-acquired pneumonia. *N Engl J Med.* 1995;333:1618.
5. Niederman MS, Bass JB Jr, Campbell GD, et al. Guidelines for the initial management of adults with community-acquired pneumonia: diagnosis, assessment of severity, and initial antimicrobial therapy. *Am Rev Respir Dis.* 1993;148:1418.
6. Ewig S, Ruiz M, Mensa J, et al. Severe community-acquired pneumonia. Assessment of severity criteria. *Am J Respir Crit Care Med.* 1998;158:1102.
7. Niederman MS, Mandell LA, Anzueto A, et al. Guidelines for the management of adults with community-acquired pneumonia. Diagnosis, assessment of severity, antimicrobial therapy, and prevention. *Am J Respir Crit Care Med.* 2001;163:1730.
8. Angus DC, Marrie TJ, Obrosky DS, et al. Severe community-acquired pneumonia: use of intensive care services and evaluation of American and British Thoracic Society Diagnostic criteria. *Am J Respir Crit Care Med.* 2002;166:717.
9. Riley PD, Aronsky D, Dean NC. Validation of the 2001 American Thoracic Society criteria for severe community-acquired pneumonia. *Crit Care Med.* 2004;32:2398.
10. British Thoracic Society Standards of Care Committee. BTS Guidelines for the Management of Community Acquired Pneumonia in Adults. *Thorax.* 2001;56(Suppl 4):1.
11. Lasocki S, Scanvic A, Le Turdu F, et al. Evaluation of the Binax NOW *Streptococcus pneumoniae* urinary antigen assay in intensive care patients hospitalized for pneumonia. *Intensive Care Med.* 2006;32:1766.
12. Cox NJ, Subbarao K. Influenza. *Lancet.* 1999;354:1277.
13. Yoshimoto A, Nakamura H, Fujimura M, et al. Severe community-acquired pneumonia in an intensive care unit: risk factors for mortality. *Intern Med.* 2005;44:710.

14. Leroy O, Saux P, Bedos JP, et al. Comparison of levofloxacin and cefotaxime combined with ofloxacin for ICU patients with community-acquired pneumonia who do not require vasopressors. *Chest.* 2005;128:172.
15. Shorr AF, Bodi M, Rodriguez A, et al. Impact of antibiotic guideline compliance on duration of mechanical ventilation in critically ill patients with community-acquired pneumonia. *Chest.* 2006;130:93.
16. Hyde TB, Gay K, Stephens DS, et al. Macrolide resistance among invasive *Streptococcus pneumoniae* isolates. *JAMA.* 2001;286:1857.
17. Hoban DJ, Doern GV, Fluit AC, et al. Worldwide prevalence of antimicrobial resistance in *Streptococcus pneumoniae, Haemophilus influenzae,* and *Moraxella catarrhalis* in the SENTRY Antimicrobial Surveillance Program, 1997–1999. *Clin Infect Dis.* 2001;32(Suppl 2):81.
18. Hoban D, Baquero F, Reed V, et al. Demographic analysis of antimicrobial resistance among *Streptococcus pneumoniae*: worldwide results from PROTEKT 1999–2000. *Int J Infect Dis.* 2005;9:262.
19. Metlay JP, Hofmann J, Cetron MS, et al. Impact of penicillin susceptibility on medical outcomes for adult patients with bacteremic pneumococcal pneumonia. *Clin Infect Dis.* 2000;30:520.
20. Falco V, Almirante B, Jordano Q, et al. Influence of penicillin resistance on outcome in adult patients with invasive pneumococcal pneumonia: is penicillin useful against intermediately resistant strains? *J Antimicrob Chemother.* 2004;54:481.
21. Low DE. Quinolone resistance among pneumococci: therapeutic and diagnostic implications. *Clin Infect Dis.* 2004;38(Suppl 4):357.
22. Deshpande LM, Sader HS, Debbia E, et al., SENTRY Antimicrobial Surveillance Program (2001–2004). Emergence and epidemiology of fluoroquinolone-resistant Streptococcus pneumoniae strains from Italy: report from the SENTRY Antimicrobial Surveillance Program (2001–2004). *Diagn Microbiol Infect Dis.* 2006;54:157.
23. Francis JS, Doherty MC, Lopatin U, et al. Severe community-onset pneumonia in healthy adults caused by methicillin-resistant *Staphylococcus aureus* carrying the Panton-Valentine leukocidin genes. *Clin Infect Dis.* 2005;40:100.
24. Mandell LA, Wunderink RG, Anzueto A, et al. Infectious Diseases Society of America/American Thoracic Society consensus guidelines on the management of community-acquired pneumonia in adults. *Clin Infect Dis.* 2007;44(Suppl 2):S27.
25. Rello J, Rodriguez A, Torres A, et al. Implications of COPD in patients admitted to the intensive care unit by community-acquired pneumonia. *Eur Respir J.* 2006;27:1210.
26. Feikin DR, Feldman C, Schuchat A, et al. Global strategies to prevent bacterial pneumonia in adults with HIV disease. *Lancet Infect Dis.* 2004;4:445.
27. Le Moing V, Rabaud C, Journot V, et al., APROCO Study Group. Incidence and risk factors of bacterial pneumonia requiring hospitalization in HIV-infected patients started on a protease inhibitor-containing regimen. *HIV Med.* 2006;7:261.
28. Pagano L, Caira M, Fianchi L. Pulmonary fungal infection with yeasts and pneumocystis in patients with hematological malignancy. *Ann Med.* 2005;37:259.
29. Rano A, Agusti C, Benito N, et al. Prognostic factors of non-HIV immunocompromised patients with pulmonary infiltrates. *Chest.* 2002;122:253.
30. Martin SI, Marty FM, Fiumara K, et al. Infectious complications associated with alemtuzumab use for lymphoproliferative disorders. *Clin Infect Dis.* 2006;43:16.
31. Cervera C, Agusti C, Angeles Marcos M, et al. Microbiologic features and outcome of pneumonia in transplanted patients. *Diagn Microbiol Infect Dis.* 2006;55:47.
32. Colombel JF, Loftus EV Jr, Tremaine WJ, et al. The safety profile of infliximab in patients with Crohn's disease: the Mayo clinic experience in 500 patients. *Gastroenterology.* 2004;126:19.
33. Houck PM, Bratzler DW, Nsa W, et al. Timing of antibiotic administration and outcomes for Medicare patients hospitalized with community-acquired pneumonia. *Arch Intern Med.* 2004;164:637.
34. Waterer GW, Kessler LA, Wunderink RG. Delayed administration of antibiotics and atypical presentation in community-acquired pneumonia. *Chest.* 2006;130:11–15.
35. Metersky ML, Sweeney TA, Getzow MB, et al. Antibiotic timing and diagnostic uncertainty in Medicare patients with pneumonia: is it reasonable to expect all patients to receive antibiotics within 4 hours? *Chest.* 2006;130:16.
36. Pedro-Botet L, Yu VL. Legionella: macrolides or quinolones? *Clin Microbiol Infect.* 2006;12(Suppl 3):25.
37. Gleason PP, Meehan TP, Fine JM, et al. Associations between initial antimicrobial therapy and medical outcomes for hospitalized elderly patients with pneumonia. *Arch Intern Med.* 1999;159:2562.
38. Rello J, Catalan M, Diaz E, et al. Associations between empirical antimicrobial therapy at the hospital and mortality in patients with severe community-acquired pneumonia. *Intensive Care Med.* 2002;28:1030.
39. Waterer GW, Somes GW, Wunderink RG. Monotherapy may be suboptimal for severe bacteremic pneumococcal pneumonia. *Arch Intern Med.* 2001;161:1837.
40. Martinez JA, Horcajada JP, Almela M, et al. Addition of a macrolide to a beta-lactam-based empirical antibiotic regimen is associated with lower in-hospital mortality for patients with bacteremic pneumococcal pneumonia. *Clin Infect Dis.* 2003;36:389.
41. Mortensen EM, Restrepo MI, Anzueto A, et al. The impact of empiric antimicrobial therapy with a β-lactam and fluoroquinolone on mortality for patients hospitalized with severe pneumonia. *Crit Care.* 2006;10:R8 doi:10.1186/cc3934
42. Bartlett JG, Dowell SF, Mandell LA, et al. Practice guidelines for the management of community-acquired pneumonia in adults. Infectious Diseases Society of America. *Clin Infect Dis.* 2000;31:347.
43. Bernard GR, Vincent JL, Laterre PF, et al. Efficacy and safety of recombinant human activated protein C for severe sepsis. *N Engl J Med.* 2001;344:699.
44. Angus DC, Laterre PF, Helterbrand J, et al. The effect of drotrecogin alfa (activated) on long-term survival after severe sepsis. *Crit Care Med.* 2004;32:2199.
45. Laterre PF, Garber G, Levy H, et al. Severe community-acquired pneumonia as a cause of severe sepsis: data from the PROWESS study. *Crit Care Med.* 2005;33:952.
46. Abraham E, Laterre PF, Garg R, et al. Drotrecogin alfa (activated) for adults with severe sepsis and a low risk of death. *N Engl J Med.* 2005;353:1332.
47. Confalonieri M, Urbino R, Potena A, et al. Hydrocortisone infusion for severe community-acquired pneumonia: a preliminary randomized study. *Am J Respir Crit Care Med.* 2005;171:242.
48. Pachon J, Prados MD, Capote F, et al. Severe community-acquired pneumonia. Etiology, prognosis, and treatment *Am Rev Respir Dis.* 1990;142:369.
49. Almirall J, Mesalles E, Klamburg J, et al. Prognostic factors of pneumonia requiring admission to the intensive care unit. *Chest.* 1995;107:511.
50. Leroy O, Santré C, Beuscart C, et al. A five-year study of severe community-acquired pneumonia with emphasis on prognosis in patients admitted to an intensive care unit. *Intensive Care Med.* 1995;21:24.
51. Pascual FE, Matthay MA, Bacchetti P, et al. Assessment of prognosis in patients with community-acquired pneumonia who require mechanical ventilation. *Chest.* 2000;117:503.
52. Paganin F, Lilienthal F, Bourdin A, et al. Severe community-acquired pneumonia: assessment of microbial aetiology as mortality factor. *Eur Respir J.* 2004;24:779.
53. Tejerina E, Frutos-Vivar F, Restrepo MI, et al. Prognosis factors and outcome of community-acquired pneumonia needing mechanical ventilation. *J Crit Care.* 2005;20:230.
54. Boussekey N, Leroy O, Alfandari S, et al. Procalcitonin kinetics in the prognosis of severe community-acquired pneumonia. *Intensive Care Med.* 2006;32:469.
55. Fine MJ, Smith MA, Carson CA, et al. Prognosis and outcomes of patients with community-acquired pneumonia. A meta-analysis. *JAMA.* 1996;275:134.
56. Torres A, Serra-Batlles J, Ferrer A, et al. Severe community-acquired pneumonia. Epidemiology and prognostic factors. *Am Rev Respir Dis.* 1991;144:312.
57. Leroy O, Devos P, Guery B, et al. Simplified prediction rule for prognosis of patients with severe community-acquired pneumonia in ICUs. *Chest.* 1999;116:157.
58. Wilson PA, Ferguson J. Severe community-acquired pneumonia: an Australian perspective. *Intern Med J.* 2005;35:699.
59. Houck PM, MacLehose RF, Niederman MS, et al. Empiric antibiotic therapy and mortality among medicare pneumonia inpatients in 10 western states: 1993, 1995, and 1997. *Chest.* 2001;119:1420.
60. Brown RB, Iannini P, Gross P, et al. Impact of initial antibiotic choice on clinical outcomes in community-acquired pneumonia: analysis of a hospital claims-made database. *Chest.* 2003;123:1503.
61. Baddour LM, Yu VL, Klugman KP, et al. Combination antibiotic therapy lowers mortality among severely ill patients with pneumococcal bacteremia. *Am J Respir Crit Care Med.* 2004;170:440.
62. Fine MJ, Auble TE, Yealy DM, et al. A prediction rule to identify low-risk patients with community-acquired pneumonia. *N Engl J Med.* 1997;336:243.
63. Recommendations of the Advisory Committee on Immunization Practices (ACIP): prevention of pneumococcal disease. *MMWR.* 1997;46(RR-08):1.
64. Recommendations of the Advisory Committee on Immunization Practices (ACIP): preventing pneumococcal disease among infants and young children. *MMWR.* 2000;49(RR09):1.
65. Whitney CG, Farley MM, Hadler J, et al. Decline in invasive pneumococcal disease after the introduction of protein-polysaccharide conjugate vaccine. *N Engl J Med.* 2003;348:1737.
66. Kyaw MH, Lynfield R, Schaffner W, et al. Active Bacterial Core Surveillance of the Emerging Infections Program Network Effect of introduction of the pneumococcal conjugate vaccine on drug-resistant *Streptococcus pneumoniae. N Engl J Med.* 2006;354:1455.
67. Recommendations of the Advisory Committee on Immunization Practices (ACIP). Prevention and control of influenza. *MMWR.* 2006;55(RR10):1.
68. American Thoracic Society, Infectious Diseases Society of America. Guidelines for the management of adults with hospital-acquired, ventilator-associated, and healthcare-associated pneumonia. *Am J Respir Crit Care Med.* 2005;171:388.
69. Rello J, Ollendorf DA, Oster G, et al. Epidemiology and outcomes of ventilator-associated pneumonia in a large US database. *Chest.* 2002;122:2115.

70. Torres A, Aznar R, Gatell JM, et al. Incidence, risk, and prognosis factors of nosocomial pneumonia in mechanically ventilated patients. *Am Rev Respir Dis.* 1990;142:523.
71. Chevret S, Hemmer M, Carlet J, et al. Incidence and risk factors of pneumonia acquired in intensive care units. Results from a multicenter prospective study on 996 patients. European Cooperative Group on Nosocomial Pneumonia. *Intensive Care Med.* 1993;19:256.
72. Baker AM, Meredith JW, Haponik EF. Pneumonia in intubated trauma patients. Microbiology and outcomes. *Am J Respir Crit Care Med.* 1996;153:343.
73. Chastre J, Trouillet JL, Vuagnat A, et al. Nosocomial pneumonia in patients with acute respiratory distress syndrome. *Am J Respir Crit Care Med.* 1998;157:1165.
74. Tejada Artigas A, Bello Dronda S, Chacon Valles E, et al. Risk factors for nosocomial pneumonia in critically ill trauma patients. *Crit Care Med.* 2001;29:304.
75. Ibrahim EH, Tracy L, Hill C, et al. The occurrence of ventilator-associated pneumonia in a community hospital: risk factors and clinical outcomes. *Chest.* 2001;120:555.
76. Bouza E, Perez A, Munoz P, et al. Ventilator-associated pneumonia after heart surgery: a prospective analysis and the value of surveillance. *Crit Care Med.* 2003;31:1964.
77. Hilker R, Poetter C, Findeisen N, et al. Nosocomial pneumonia after acute stroke: implications for neurological intensive care medicine. *Stroke.* 2003;34:975.
78. Cook DJ, Walter SD, Cook RJ, et al. Incidence of and risk factors for ventilator-associated pneumonia in critically ill patients. *Ann Intern Med.* 1998;129:433.
79. Rello J, Diaz E, Rodriguez A. Advances in the management of pneumonia in the intensive care unit: review of current thinking. *Clin Microbiol Infect.* 2005;11(Suppl 5):30.
80. Chastre J, Fagon JY. Ventilator-associated pneumonia. *Am J Respir Crit Care Med.* 2002;165:867.
81. Bonten MJ, Kollef MH, Hall JB. Risk factors for ventilator-associated pneumonia: from epidemiology to patient management. *Clin Infect Dis.* 2004;38:1141.
82. Rello J, Sonora R, Jubert P, et al. Pneumonia in intubated patients: role of respiratory airway care. *Am J Respir Crit Care Med.* 1996;154:111.
83. de Lassence A, Alberti C, Azoulay E, et al. Impact of unplanned extubation and reintubation after weaning on nosocomial pneumonia risk in the intensive care unit: a prospective multicenter study. *Anesthesiology.* 2002;97:148.
84. Kollef MH, von Harz B, Prentice D, et al. Patient transport from intensive care increases the risk of developing ventilator-associated pneumonia. *Chest.* 1997;112:765–773.
85. Kollef MH. Ventilator-associated pneumonia: a multivariate analysis. *JAMA.* 1993;27:1965–1970.
86. Trouillet JL, Chastre J, Vuagnat A, et al. Ventilator-associated pneumonia caused by potentially drug-resistant bacteria. *Am J Respir Crit Care Med.* 1998;157:531.
87. Leroy O, Girardie P, Yazdanpanah Y, et al. Hospital-acquired pneumonia: microbiological data and potential adequacy of antimicrobial regimens. *Eur Respir J.* 2002;20:432.
88. Rello J, Sa-Borges M, Correa H, et al. Variations in etiology of ventilator-associated pneumonia across four treatment sites: implications for antimicrobial prescribing practices. *Am J Respir Crit Care Med.* 1999;160:608.
89. Dore P, Robert R, Grollier G, et al. Incidence of anaerobes in ventilator-associated pneumonia with use of a protected specimen brush. *Am J Respir Crit Care Med.* 1996;153:1292.
90. Hanes SD, Demirkan K, Tolley E, et al. Risk factors for late-onset nosocomial pneumonia caused by *Stenotrophomonas maltophilia* in critically ill trauma patients. *Clin Infect Dis.* 2002;35:228.
91. Carratala J, Gudiol F, Pallares, et al. Risk factors for nosocomial *Legionella pneumophila* pneumonia. *Am J Respir Crit Care Med.* 1994;149:625.
92. Baraibar J, Correa H, Mariscal D, et al. Risk factors for infection by *Acinetobacter baumannii* in intubated patients with nosocomial pneumonia. *Chest.* 1997;112:1050.
93. Rello J, Ausina V, Ricart M, et al. Risk factors for infection by *Pseudomonas aeruginosa* in patients with ventilator-associated pneumonia. *Intensive Care Med.* 1994;20:193.
94. Rello J, Quintana E, Ausina V, et al. Risk factors for *Staphylococcus aureus* nosocomial pneumonia in critically ill patients. *Am Rev Respir Dis.* 1990;142:1320.
95. Torres A, Carlet J. Ventilator-associated pneumonia. European Task Force on ventilator-associated pneumonia. *Eur Respir J.* 2001;17:1034.
96. Porzecanski I, Bowton DL. Diagnosis and treatment of ventilator-associated pneumonia. *Chest.* 2006;130:597.
97. Rello J, Torres A, Ricart M, et al. Ventilator-associated pneumonia by *Staphylococcus aureus*. Comparison of methicillin-resistant and methicillin-sensitive episodes. *Am J Respir Crit Care Med.* 1994;150:1545.
98. Trouillet JL, Vuagnat A, Combes A, et al. *Pseudomonas aeruginosa* ventilator-associated pneumonia: comparison of episodes due to piperacillin-resistant versus piperacillin-susceptible organisms. *Clin Infect Dis.* 2002;34:1047.
99. Leroy O, Jaffre S, D'Escrivan, et al. Hospital-acquired pneumonia: risk factors for antimicrobial-resistant causative pathogens in critically ill patients. *Chest.* 2003;123:2034.
100. Nseir S, Di Pompeo C, Pronnier P, et al. Nosocomial tracheobronchitis in mechanically ventilated patients: incidence, aetiology and outcome. *Eur Respir J.* 2002;20:1483.
101. Fabregas N, Ewig S, Torres A, et al. Clinical diagnosis of ventilator associated pneumonia revisited: comparative validation using immediate post-mortem lung biopsies. *Thorax.* 1999;54:867.
102. Luna CM, Videla A, Mattera J, et al. Blood cultures have limited value in predicting severity of illness and as a diagnostic tool in ventilator-associated pneumonia. *Chest.* 1999;116:1075.
103. Marquette CH, Copin MC, Wallet F, et al. Diagnostic tests for pneumonia in ventilated patients: prospective evaluation of diagnostic accuracy using histology as a diagnostic gold standard. *Am J Respir Crit Care Med.* 1995;151:1878.
104. Torres A, Martos A, Puig de la Bellacasa J, et al. Specificity of endotracheal aspiration, protected specimen brush, and bronchoalveolar lavage in mechanically ventilated patients. *Am Rev Respir Dis.* 1993;147:952.
105. Blot F, Raynard B, Chachaty E, et al. Value of gram stain examination of lower respiratory tract secretions for early diagnosis of nosocomial pneumonia. *Am J Respir Crit Care Med.* 2000;162:1731.
106. Baselski VS, el-Torky M, Coalson JJ, et al. The standardization of criteria for processing and interpreting laboratory specimens in patients with suspected ventilator-associated pneumonia. *Chest.* 1992;102(Suppl 1):571.
107. Timsit JF, Cheval C, Gachot B, et al. Usefulness of a strategy based on bronchoscopy with direct examination of bronchoalveolar lavage fluid in the initial antibiotic therapy of suspected ventilator-associated pneumonia. *Intensive Care Med.* 2001;27:640.
108. Chastre J, Fagon JY, Bornet-Lecso M, et al. Evaluation of bronchoscopic techniques for the diagnosis of nosocomial pneumonia. *Am J Respir Crit Care Med.* 1995;152:231.
109. Fagon JY, Chastre J, Wolff M, et al. Invasive and noninvasive strategies for management of suspected ventilator-associated pneumonia. A randomized trial. *Ann Intern Med.* 2000;132:621.
110. Alvarez-Lerma F. Modification of empiric antibiotic treatment in patients with pneumonia acquired in the intensive care unit. *Intensive Care Med.* 1996;22:387.
111. Kollef MH, Ward S. The influence of mini-BAL cultures on patient outcomes: implications for the antibiotic management of ventilator-associated pneumonia. *Chest.* 1998;113:412.
112. Luna CM, Vujacich P, Niederman MS, et al. Impact of BAL data on the therapy and outcome of ventilator-associated pneumonia. *Chest.* 1997;111:676.
113. Iregui M, Ward S, Sherman G, et al. Clinical importance of delays in the initiation of appropriate antibiotic treatment for ventilator-associated pneumonia. *Chest.* 2002;122:262.
114. Ioanas M, Cavalcanti M, Ferrer M, et al. Hospital-acquired pneumonia: coverage and treatment adequacy of current guidelines. *Eur Respir J.* 2003;22:876.
115. Ibrahim EH, Ward S, Sherman G, et al. Experience with a clinical guideline for the treatment of ventilator-associated pneumonia. *Crit Care Med.* 2001;29:1109.
116. Michel F, Franceschini B, Berger P, et al. Early antibiotic treatment for BAL-confirmed ventilator-associated pneumonia: a role for routine endotracheal aspirate cultures. *Chest.* 2005;127:589.
117. Hoffken G, Niederman MS. Nosocomial pneumonia: the importance of a de-escalating strategy for antibiotic treatment of pneumonia in the ICU. *Chest.* 2002;122:2183.
118. Rello J, Vidaur L, Sandiumenge A, et al. De-escalation therapy in ventilator-associated pneumonia. *Crit Care Med.* 2004;32:2183.
119. Chastre J, Wolff M, Fagon JY, et al. Comparison of 8 vs 15 days of antibiotic therapy for ventilator-associated pneumonia in adults: a randomized trial. *JAMA.* 2003;290:2588.
120. Micek ST, Ward S, Fraser VJ, et al. A randomized controlled trial of an antibiotic discontinuation policy for clinically suspected ventilator-associated pneumonia. *Chest.* 2004;125:1791.
121. Kollef MH, Kollef KE. Antibiotic utilization and outcomes for patients with clinically suspected ventilator-associated pneumonia and negative quantitative BAL culture results. *Chest.* 2005;128:2706.
122. Paul M, Benuri-Silbiger I, Soares-Weiser K, et al. Beta lactam monotherapy versus beta lactam-aminoglycoside combination therapy for sepsis in immunocompetent patients: systematic review and meta-analysis of randomised trials. *BMJ.* 2004;328:668.
123. Bliziotis IA, Samonis G, Vardakas KZ, et al. Effect of aminoglycoside and beta-lactam combination therapy versus beta-lactam monotherapy on the emergence of antimicrobial resistance: a meta-analysis of randomized, controlled trials. *Clin Infect Dis.* 2005;41:149.
124. Rubinstein E, Cammarata S, Oliphant T, et al. Linezolid (PNU-100766) versus vancomycin in the treatment of hospitalized patients with nosocomial pneumonia: a randomized, double-blind, multicenter study. *Clin Infect Dis.* 2001;32:402.
125. Wunderink RG, Cammarata SK, Oliphant TH, et al. Continuation of a randomized, double-blind, multicenter study of linezolid versus

vancomycin in the treatment of patients with nosocomial pneumonia. *Clin Ther.* 2003;25:980.
126. Wunderink RG, Rello J, Cammarata SK, et al. Linezolid vs vancomycin: analysis of two double-blind studies of patients with methicillin-resistant Staphylococcus aureus nosocomial pneumonia. *Chest.* 2003;124:1789.
127. Garnacho-Montero J, Ortiz-Leyba C, Jimenez-Jimenez FJ, et al. Treatment of multidrug-resistant *Acinetobacter baumannii* ventilator-associated pneumonia (VAP) with intravenous colistin: a comparison with imipenem-susceptible VAP. *Clin Infect Dis.* 2003;36:1111.
128. Vidaur L, Gualis B, Rodriguez A, et al. Clinical resolution in patients with suspicion of ventilator-associated pneumonia: a cohort study comparing patients with and without acute respiratory distress syndrome. *Crit Care Med.* 2005;33:1248.
129. Luna CM, Blanzaco D, Niederman MS, et al. Resolution of ventilator-associated pneumonia: prospective evaluation of the clinical pulmonary infection score as an early clinical predictor of outcome. *Crit Care Med.* 2003;31:676.
130. Ioanas M, Ferrer M, Cavalcanti M, et al. Causes and predictors of nonresponse to treatment of intensive care unit-acquired pneumonia. *Crit Care Med.* 2004;32:938.
131. Papazian L, Bregeon F, Thirion X, et al. Effect of ventilator-associated pneumonia on mortality and morbidity. *Am J Respir Crit Care Med.* 1996;154:91.
132. Nseir S, Di Pompeo C, Soubrier S, et al. Impact of ventilator-associated pneumonia on outcome in patients with COPD. *Chest.* 2005;128:1650.
133. Bercault N, Boulain T. Mortality rate attributable to ventilator-associated nosocomial pneumonia in an adult intensive care unit: a prospective case-control study. *Crit Care Med.* 2001;29:2303.
134. Fagon JY, Chastre J, Hance AJ, et al. Nosocomial pneumonia in ventilated patients: a cohort study evaluating attributable mortality and hospital stay. *Am J Med.* 1993;94:281.
135. Moine P, Timsit JF, De Lassence A, et al. Mortality associated with late-onset pneumonia in the intensive care unit: results of a multi-center cohort study. *Intensive Care Med.* 2002;28:154.
136. Dupont H, Montravers P, Gauzit R, et al. Outcome of postoperative pneumonia in the Eole study. *Intensive Care Med.* 2003;29:179.
137. Leroy O, Meybeck A, d'Escrivan T, et al. Impact of adequacy of initial antimicrobial therapy on the prognosis of patients with ventilator-associated pneumonia. *Intensive Care Med.* 2003;9:2170.
138. Clec'h C, Timsit JF, De Lassence A, et al. Efficacy of adequate early antibiotic therapy in ventilator-associated pneumonia: influence of disease severity. *Intensive Care Med.* 2004;30:1327.
139. Alp E, Voss A. Ventilator associated pneumonia and infection control. *Ann Clin Microbiol Antimicrob.* 2006;5:7.
140. Isakow W, Kollef MH. Preventing ventilator-associated pneumonia: an evidence-based approach of modifiable risk factors. *Semin Respir Crit Care Med.* 2006;27:5.
141. Tablan OC, Anderson LJ, Besser R, et al. Healthcare Infection Control Practices Advisory Committee, Centers for Disease Control and Prevention. Guidelines for preventing health-care–associated pneumonia, 2003: recommendations of the CDC and the Healthcare Infection Control Practices Advisory Committee. *MMWR Recomm Rep.* 2004;53(RR-3):1.
142. van Nieuwenhoven CA, Buskens E, van Tiel FH, et al. Relationship between methodological trial quality and the effects of selective digestive decontamination on pneumonia and mortality in critically ill patients. *JAMA.* 2001;286:335.
143. de Jonge E, Schultz M, Spanjaard L, et al. Effects of selective decontamination of the digestive tract on mortality and acquisition of resistant bacteria in intensive care: a randomized controlled trial. *Lancet.* 2003;362:1011.
144. Valles J, Mesalles E, Mariscal D, et al. A 7-year study of severe hospital-acquired pneumonia requiring ICU admission. *Intensive Care Med.* 2003;29:1981.
145. Sopena N, Sabria M, Neunos 2000 Study Group. Multicenter study of hospital-acquired pneumonia in non-ICU patients. *Chest.* 2005;127:213.
146. Capitano B, Nicolau DP. Evolving epidemiology and cost of resistance to antimicrobial agents in long-term care facilities. *J Am Med Dir Assoc.* 2003;4(3S):90.
147. Mylotte JM, Goodnough S, Tayara A. Antibiotic-resistant organisms among long-term care facility residents on admission to an inpatient geriatrics unit: retrospective and prospective surveillance. *Am J Infect Control.* 2001;29:139.
148. Dosa D. Should I hospitalize my resident with nursing home-acquired pneumonia? *J Am Med Dir Assoc.* 2006;7(Suppl 3):74.
149. Crossley KB, Peterson PK. Infections in the elderly. *Clin Infect Dis.* 1996;22:209.
150. Muder RR. Pneumonia in residents of long-term care facilities: epidemiology, etiology, management, and prevention. *Am J Med.* 1998;105:319.
151. Mylotte JM. Nursing home-acquired pneumonia: update on treatment options. *Drugs Aging.* 2006;23(5):377.
152. Celli BR, MacNee W, ATS/ERS Task Force. Standards for the diagnosis and treatment of patients with COPD: a summary of the ATS/ERS position paper. *Eur Respir J.* 2004;23:932.
153. Murphy TF, Sethi S, Niederman MS. The role of bacteria in exacerbations of COPD. A constructive view. *Chest.* 2000;118:204.
154. Saint S, Bent S, Vittinghoff E, et al. Antibiotics in chronic obstructive pulmonary disease exacerbations. A meta-analysis. *JAMA.* 1995;273:957.
155. Nouira S, Marghli S, Belghith M, et al. Once daily oral ofloxacin in chronic obstructive pulmonary disease exacerbation requiring mechanical ventilation: a randomised placebo-controlled trial. *Lancet.* 2001;358:2020.
156. Ferrer M, Ioanas M, Arancibia F, et al. Microbial airway colonization is associated with noninvasive ventilation failure in exacerbation of chronic obstructive pulmonary disease. *Crit Care Med.* 2005;33:2003.
157. Ewig S, Soler N, Gonzalez J, et al. Evaluation of antimicrobial treatment in mechanically ventilated patients with severe chronic obstructive pulmonary disease exacerbations. *Crit Care Med.* 2000;28:692.
158. Cavalcanti M, Valencia M, Torres A. Respiratory nosocomial infections in the medical intensive care unit. *Microbes Infect.* 2005;7:292.
159. Nseir S, Di Pompeo C, Soubrier S, et al. Effect of ventilator-associated tracheobronchitis on outcome in patients without chronic respiratory failure: a case-control study. *Crit Care.* 2005;9:R238.
160. Nseir S, Di Pompeo C, Soubrier S, et al. Outcomes of ventilated COPD patients with nosocomial tracheobronchitis: a case-control study. *Infection.* 2004;32:210.
161. Hammond JM, Potgieter PD, Hanslo D, et al. Etiology and antimicrobial susceptibility patterns of micro organisms in acute community-acquired lung abscess. *Chest.* 1995;108:937.
162. Wang JL, Chen KY, Fang CT, et al. Changing bacteriology of adult community-acquired lung abscess in Taiwan: *Klebsiella pneumoniae* versus anaerobes. *Clin Infect Dis.* 2005;40:915.
163. Bartlett JG. The role of anaerobic bacteria in lung abscess. *Clin Infect Dis.* 2005;40:923.
164. Allewelt M, Schuler P, Bolcskei PL, et al. Study group on aspiration pneumonia. *Clin Microbiol Infect.* 2004;10:163.
165. Podbielski FJ, Rodriguez HE, Wiesman IM, et al. Pulmonary parenchymal abscess: VATS approach to diagnosis and treatment. *Asian Cardiovasc Thorac Ann.* 2001;9:339.
166. Herth F, Ernst A, Becker HD. Endoscopic drainage of lung abscesses: technique and outcome. *Chest.* 2005;127:1378.
167. Bryant RE, Salmon CJ. Pleural empyema. *Clin Infect Dis.* 1996;22:747.
168. Davies CW, Gleeson FV, Davies RJ, Pleural Diseases Group, Standards of Care Committee, British Thoracic Society. BTS guidelines for the management of pleural infection. *Thorax.* 2003;58(Suppl 2):18.
169. Maskell NA, Davies CW, Nunn AJ, et al. U.K. Controlled trial of intrapleural streptokinase for pleural infection. *N Engl J Med.* 2005;352:865.
170. Tokuda Y, Matsushima D, Stein GH, et al. Intrapleural fibrinolytic agents for empyema and complicated parapneumonic effusions: a meta-analysis. *Chest.* 2006;129:783.

CHAPTER 112 ■ ADULT GASTROINTESTINAL INFECTIONS IN THE ICU

SRIDIVYA JAINI • HERBERT L. DUPONT

Diarrhea occurs in close to one occurrence per person per year in the United States. It varies from a short-lasting mild illness to various more serious enteric syndromes that include watery diarrhea with dehydration, febrile dysentery, and gastroenteritis with sepsis.

Although diarrhea may be acquired directly from an infected person, it is usually acquired by exposure to contaminated food, water, or the environment. Foodborne diseases became particularly important during 2006. The foodborne enteric diseases have been estimated to cause approximately 76 million cases of illness, 325,000 hospitalizations, and 5,000 deaths in the United States each year. Known pathogens account for an estimated 14 million cases of illnesses, 60,000 hospitalizations, and 1,800 deaths (1).

Diarrhea has two important definitions:

1. An increase in the normal frequency of stools associated with a decrease in their form, progressing from formed stools to those showing a watery or loose (soft) consistency.
2. Passage of more than 200 gm per day of unformed stool in an adult person on a standard western diet.

Diarrhea may be divided into three stages based on duration: (i) *acute* (less than or equal to 14 days), (ii) *persistent* (14 days or more), or (iii) *chronic* (30 days or more). The cause of the illness is different in the three groups. Viruses, bacteria, and toxins explain most episodes of acute diarrhea (Table 112.1); parasitic agents are more involved in the persistent cases (Table 112.1); and noninfectious causes are characteristically associated with chronic diarrhea. The severity of diarrhea can be determined according to a functional definition:

1. Mild—requires no change in activities
2. Moderate—requires a change in activities but doesn't disable
3. Severe—disables, usually confining the affected person to bed. It is the severe forms of diarrhea that usually lead to hospitalization.

ETIOLOGY OF ACUTE DIARRHEA IN THE UNITED STATES

Community-acquired, acute infectious diarrhea is caused by various micro-organisms including bacteria, viruses, and parasites (Table 112.1). Bacterial causes include the following: *Shigella, Salmonella, Campylobacter, Clostridium difficile*, and various *Escherichia coli* species—enterotoxigenic (ETEC), enteroaggregative (EAEC), shigatoxin-producing (STEC) including *E. coli* O157:H7, enteropathogenic (EPEC), enteroinvasive (EIEC)—and, less commonly, others that include *Aeromonas, Plesiomonas, Yersinia* species, *Vibrio cholerae*, and other *Vibrios*. Important viral causes include rotavirus in infants and noroviruses in all age groups. Protozoan parasitic causes include *Giardia, Entamoeba histolytica, Cryptosporidium, Isospora, Cyclospora* and *Microsporidia*.

In the community, the most common causes of diarrhea are viral, with noroviruses being the most important. These cases are usually mild and do not require any specific treatment. The cause of diarrhea may vary depending on the season, with more viral cases in spring and winter and more bacterial cases in summer and spring (2).

The etiology of diarrheal cases presenting to a hospital and hospital-acquired diarrhea is different from the community-based diarrhea. In diarrheal cases presenting to the hospital, the disease is more severe compared to community diarrhea, and the causative agent may be a bacterial (most common), parasitic, or viral agent (rarely). Diarrhea acquired in the hospital may be due to bacteria (*Clostridium difficile* or *Salmonella*), viruses (rotavirus, noroviruses), or fungi (*Candida albicans*), or most commonly to noninfectious agents.

EVALUATION OF THE PATIENT WITH SEVERE DIARRHEA

Emergency Department

The first priority is to evaluate vital signs and the hydration status of the patient. Second, electrolyte disturbances need to be sought and corrected. The primary concern is to immediately reverse circulatory or organ failure resulting from loss of fluid and salt. Electrolyte imbalances may vary depending on the cause and also on other comorbid conditions. Diagnostic investigations for identifying the causative agent should be done either simultaneously or after stabilization of the patient. Most of the cases requiring hospitalization are due to bacterial causes rather than viral, which tend to be mild. Epidemiologic history and clinical features may provide clues to the diagnosis. Prior travel to an economically developing country suggests a bacterial cause of the diarrhea. Diarrhea in a person receiving antibacterial or chemotherapeutic drugs suggests *C. difficile* as the etiologic agent. Proctitis in a male with a history of having sex with men suggests sexually transmitted pathogens including *Neisseria gonorrhoeae, Chlamydia trachomatis*, herpes simplex or *Treponema pallidum*. In Figure 112.1, an algorithm is provided to help identify important steps in the workup of patients with acute diarrhea.

TABLE 112.1

POTENTIAL ETIOLOGIC AGENTS IN PATIENTS WITH ACUTE DIARRHEA

Viral	Bacterial	Protozoal
Noroviruses	*Shigella* sp.	*Entamoeba histolytica*
Rotavirus	*Salmonella* sp.	*Giardia lamblia*
Cytomegalovirus	*Vibrio cholerae*	*Cryptosporidium*
	Clostridium difficile	*Cyclospora*
	Campylobacter jejuni	*Isospora*
	Staphylococcus aureus	*Microsporidia*
	Bacillus cereus	
	Shigatoxin-producing *E. coli* (STEC)	
	Enteropathogenic *E. coli* (EPEC)	
	Enteroaggregative *E. coli* (EAEC)	
	Enterotoxigenic *E. coli* (ETEC)	
	Aeromonas	
	Plesiomonas	
	Yersinia sp.	
	Clostridium perfringens	
	Non-cholera *Vibrio*	

The laboratory will help establish the diagnosis. Finding many fecal leukocytes indicates the patient has diffuse colonic inflammation. Finding occult blood in the stool supports an inflammation. Finding occult blood in the stool supports an inflammatory type of diarrhea. Gross blood passed in stool may indicate a dysenteric pathogen including *Shigella*, *Campylobacter*, Shigatoxin-producing *E. coli* (often *E. coli* O157:H7), and *C. difficile*. Stool cultures, parasite examination, or stool toxin test for *C. difficile* may help define the cause of the illness. Some characteristics, when present, that require aggressive and thorough laboratory workup are fever greater than 102°F with systemic findings, suggesting the presence of sepsis; among enteric pathogens, *Salmonella* is an important cause or an extraintestinal focus of infection such as an intra-abdominal abscess. If associated cases of diarrhea are known to be present, local health department authorities should be notified. In the United States and other economically developed nations, the most important etiologic agent to consider in patients suffering from diarrhea after being admitted to the hospital is *C. difficile*. Once disease onset, presentation, and progression of associated symptoms are evaluated and immediate laboratory work has been performed, it may be useful to categorize the diarrhea into one of two physiologic classifications. Diarrhea can be divided into noninflammatory and inflammatory (Table 112.2). A subcategory of inflammatory is hemorrhagic or dysenteric diarrhea. Distinction of the specific type of diarrhea is helpful to focus on appropriate empiric management options.

Hospital-Acquired Diarrhea

Illness occurring after the expected incubation period of an identified enteric pathogen is considered nosocomial or health care-associated. For practical purposes, diarrhea developing 3 days or longer after admission can be considered health care associated. In Figure 112.2, the relative importance of causes of diarrhea in hospitalized patients in one study is provided. Between 10% and 30% of nosocomial diarrhea is due to *C. difficile* (3,4). The other important causes of nosocomial diarrhea include antibiotics, chemotherapeutic agents, proton pump inhibitors, tube feedings, laxatives, other drugs, and various iatrogenic and idiopathic conditions (Fig. 112.2).

It is appropriate in all hospital-associated diarrheas, when a patient is receiving antibacterial treatment, to consider *C. difficile* as the causative agent, and empiric treatment is advisable in the more severe cases while laboratory tests are pending. Rarely, other pathogens can be found in hospital-associated diarrhea, including rotaviruses in pediatric wards, noroviruses, and *Salmonella* spp.

The International Traveler

The incidence of traveler's diarrhea (TD) ranges from 13.6% to 54.6% in the high-risk regions (5) and approximately 4% in low-risk regions. (6) The various parts of the world have been classified into three different groups: low, intermediate, and high risk, based on the frequency of TD in the traveling public (7).

The important causes of TD are ETEC, EAEC, noroviruses, *Campylobacter*, *Shigella*, and *Salmonella* (7–12). Less commonly, the parasitic agents cause TD and should be suspected in persistent illness. The important parasitic pathogens in persistent TD include *Giardia*, *Cryptosporidium*, and *Cyclospora*.

The Immunosuppressed Patient

An immunosuppressed or immune-compromised patient—that is, with congenital or acquired immune deficiency, HIV/AIDS, or receiving immunosuppressive or cancer chemotherapy drugs—will have increased susceptibility to diarrhea. The etiology of diarrheal diseases in immunocompromised hosts is different from that of other populations in that they are at risk of developing infections from various opportunistic organisms in addition to the routine diarrheal pathogens. The use of various chemotherapy drugs or immunomodulators such as cyclosporine, mycophenolate mofetil, tacrolimus, or sirolimus results in drug-induced diarrhea (13). Diarrhea in transplant recipients can also be due to graft versus host disease (GVHD). Various organisms to consider as causes of diarrhea in this group of patients include *Clostridium difficile*, *Salmonella* enterica, noroviruses, *Cryptosporidium*, *Isospora*, *Cyclospora*, cytomegalovirus, and *Mycobacterium avium intracellulare* complex. A thorough and quick evaluation for identifying the causative organism is the key in treating/controlling diarrhea in this patient population. Appropriate rapid diagnostic tests include direct stool examination for ova, cysts, and parasites; stool test for *C. difficile* toxin; polymerase chain reaction (PCR) for cytomegalovirus or herpesvirus; stool cultures; and blood cultures. If the above tests do not provide a specific diagnosis, endoscopy and mucosal biopsy should be pursued to establish an etiologic diagnosis.

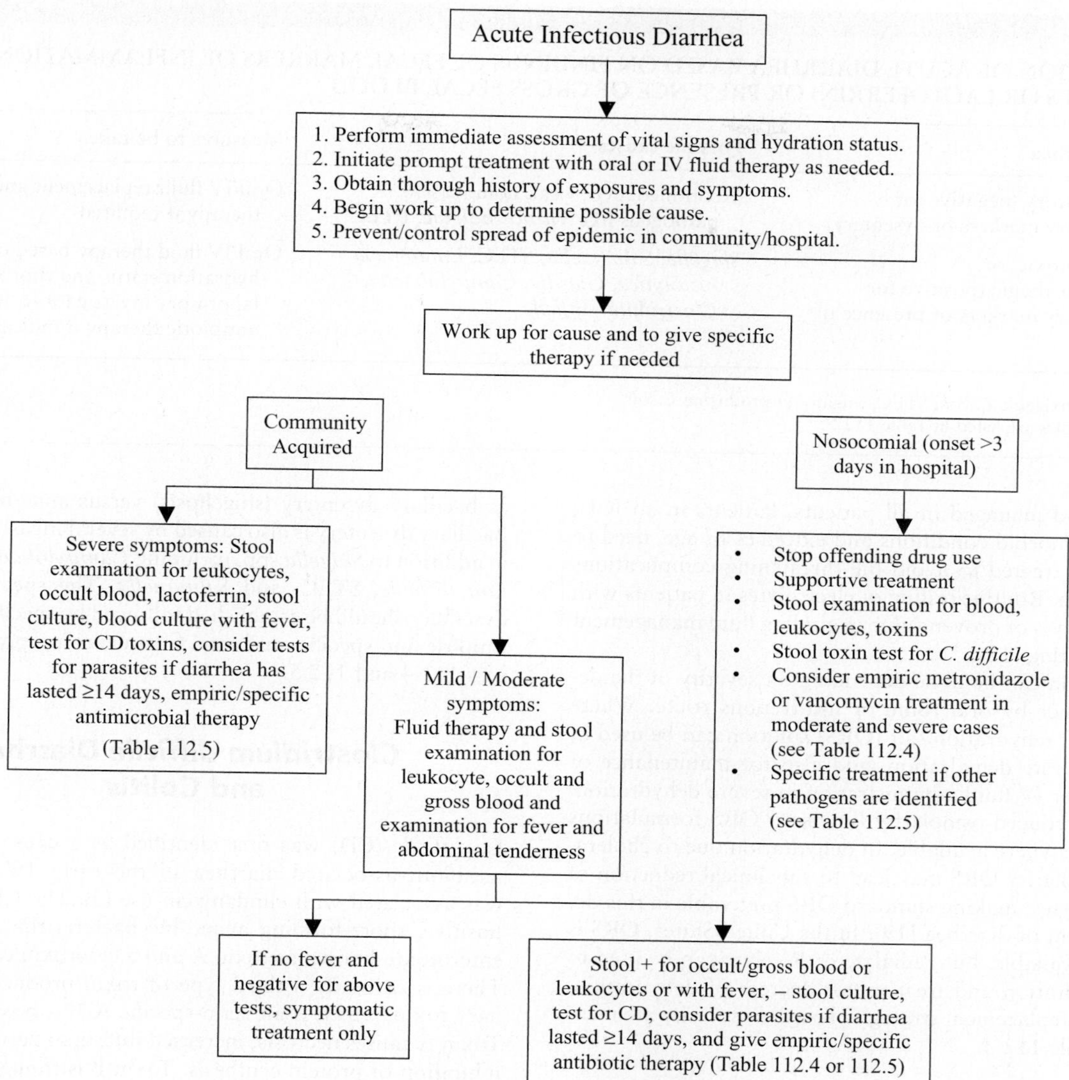

FIGURE 112.1. Flow chart showing approach to a patient with acute infectious diarrhea.

The Patient with Extraintestinal Disease

Diagnostic evaluation of patients with diarrhea and systemic symptoms and signs will often take the clinician's focus away from the gut for the diagnosis. Blood cultures, CT of the abdomen, and serology (for *Entamoeba histolytica*) may help determine the primary cause of the disease. In cases of sepsis, blood cultures and stool studies may provide the diagnosis. Systemic complications are often seen with invasive bacterial and parasitic infections. Systemic complications of enteric infection include hemolytic uremic syndrome (HUS) or thrombotic thrombocytopenic purpura (TTP), Guillain-Barré syndrome, sepsis, infective endocarditis, and abdominal abscesses or localized abscess elsewhere, or pyogenic arthritis (14). In immunocompromised patients with diarrhea, systemic complications can occur with any of the etiologic agents. Antimotility drugs should not be used in inflammatory diarrhea, as they can prolong or complicate the disease (15,16). Amoebiasis, which is uncommon in the United States, shows an extended spectrum of extraintestinal complications including liver abscess and disseminated infection (14,17).

MANAGEMENT OF ACUTE DIARRHEA

Dehydration

Dehydration is defined as excess loss of body fluids resulting in fluid and electrolyte abnormalities. In Table 112.3, the classifications of dehydration are provided. Dry skin and dry mucous membranes, sunken eyes, decreased urine output, loss of skin turgor, dizziness/light-headedness are all manifestations of moderate to severe dehydration. Dehydration is the most common serious complication of diarrhea and should be promptly

TABLE 112.2

CLASSIFICATION OF ACUTE DIARRHEA BASED ON FINDINGS OF FECAL MARKERS OF INFLAMMATION (LEUKOCYTES OR LACTOFERRIN) OR PRESENCE OF GROSS FECAL BLOOD

Types of diarrhea	Possible causes	Measures to be taken
Noninflammatory (negative for inflammatory markers or dysentery)	Toxin-mediated, viral, noninvasive pathogens like *Vibrio cholerae*, ETEC	Oral/IV fluid replacement and empiric therapy if required
Invasive, cytotoxic, or enterohemorrhagic (positive for inflammatory markers or presence of dysentery)	*Shigella, Salmonella,* STEC, *Entamoeba histolytica, Giardia, Campylobacter, Clostridium difficile*	Oral/IV fluid therapy based on hydration status and thorough laboratory investigations with specific antibiotic therapy if indicated[a]

ETEC, enterotoxigenic *E. coli*; STEC, shigatoxin-producing *E.coli*.
[a]Specific therapies are listed in Table 112.5.

recognized and managed in all patients. Patients in an ICU, with other comorbid conditions and extremes of age, need to be vigorously treated to avoid life-threatening complications of dehydration. Routine testing of electrolytes in patients with severe diarrhea is of proven value in guiding fluid management in the ICU setting (18).

Rehydration can be done depending on severity of the dehydration either by oral route or intravenous route. Where available, oral rehydration salt (ORS) solution can be used in mild or moderate dehydration, and also for maintenance of hydration after IV fluid administration in severe dehydration. Standard or reduced osmolarity (low-salt) ORS formulations are preferable where available. In dehydration due to cholera, reduced-osmolarity ORS may lead to subclinical reduction of body electrolytes, making standard ORS preferable in this dehydrating form of diarrhea (19). In the United States, ORS is not readily available, but Pedialyte or Ricelyte can be used to maintain hydration and treat minor degrees of dehydration. Specific fluid replacement strategies based on severity are mentioned in Table 112.3.

Dysentery

Dysentery is the diagnosis when subjects are passing grossly bloody stools. The disease has been historically classified as bacillary dysentery (shigellosis) versus amoebic dysentery. Bacillary dysentery is also caused by several invasive pathogens in addition to *Shigella* spp. including *Campylobacter, Clostridium difficile*, STEC, and *Salmonella*. The specific cause of dysentery should be established followed by specific treatment. Empiric and specific antibiotic treatments are provided in Tables 112.4 and 112.5.

Clostridium difficile Diarrhea and Colitis

C. difficile (CD) was first identified as a causative agent of antibiotic-associated diarrhea in the early 1970s and then was associated with clindamycin use (20,21). CD is a Gram-positive, spore-forming anaerobic bacteria that produces an enterotoxin known as toxin A and a cytotoxin called toxin B. There is currently a third type of toxin produced, called binary toxin, which is an actin-specific ADP ribosylating toxin. Toxin A causes necrosis, increased intestinal permeability, and inhibition of protein synthesis. Toxin B is thought to become effective once the gut wall has been damaged (22,23). There has been an increased virulence of CD strains, which is presumably associated with higher levels of toxin production by a fluoroquinolone-resistant CD strain variably classified as PCR ribotype 027, pulsed-field gel electrophoresis (PFGE) type

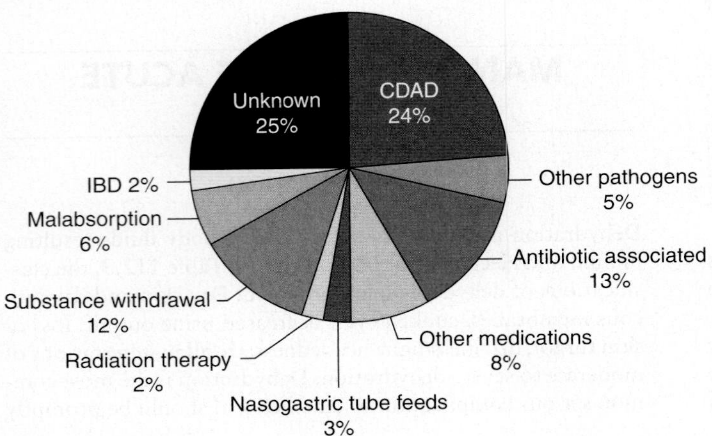

FIGURE 112.2. Relative importance of etiologic agents in hospital-acquired diarrhea. This figure shows the percentage of incidence of each of the common diarrhea-causing bacteria. CDAD, *C. difficile*–associated disease; IBD, inflammatory bowel disease. (Adapted from McFarland LV. Epidemiology of infectious and iatrogenic nosocomial diarrhea in a cohort of general medicine patients. *Am J Infect Control*. 1995;23(5):295–305, with permission.)

TABLE 112.3

CLASSIFICATION OF DEHYDRATION IN A PATIENT WITH ACUTE DIARRHEA

Dehydration		Symptoms	Suggested management
Mild dehydration	3%–5% loss in body weight	Increased thirst and slightly dry mucous membranes	Oral rehydration solution (ORS) 50 mL/kg over first 2–4 h
Moderate dehydration	6%–9% loss in body weight	Loss of skin turgor, dry mucous membranes, tenting of skin	ORS 100 mL/kg over first 2–4 h
Severe dehydration	≥10% loss in body weight	Lethargy, altered consciousness, prolonged skin retraction time, cool extremities, decreased capillary refill	Immediate IV fluid replacement with 20 mL/kg of lactated Ringer solution to restore perfusion and mental status. Continue with 100 mL/kg ORS or IV 5% dextrose and 1/2 normal saline at two times the maintenance rate.

From Duggan C, Santosham M, Glass RI. The management of acute diarrhea in children: oral rehydration, maintenance, and nutritional therapy. Centers for Disease Control and Prevention. *MMWR Recomm Rep*. 1992;41(RR-16):1–20; and King CK, Glass R, Bresee JS, et al. Managing acute gastroenteritis among children: oral rehydration, maintenance, and nutritional therapy. *MMWR Recomm Rep*. 2003;52(RR-16):1–16, with permission.

NAP1, restriction endonuclease analysis (REA) type BI, and toxinotype III (24).

The incidence of CD acute diarrhea (CDAD) has been rising in recent years due to excess use of antibiotics and emergence of resistant and more virulent strains. According to the Centers for Disease Control and Prevention (CDC) national nosocomial infection surveillance systems data, nosocomial CDAD has been increasing both in the intensive care units of large hospitals and hospital-wide in smaller hospitals (25). This rise has nearly doubled from 1996 to 2003 and has disproportionately increased in the elderly population (26). A conservative estimate of the cost of this disease in the United States is $1.1 billion per year, with a 54% increase in individual adjusted hospital costs and an extension of hospital stay by 3.6 days for each affected person (27). In a study done by our group (4), normal hospital surveillance of CDAD identified only half of the affected patients in our institution. Thus, the real burden of CDAD seems to be much more than estimated.

Major risk factors for CDAD include antimicrobial use, age older than 65 years, severity of existing health condition, use of other drugs such as chemotherapeutic agents and proton pump inhibitors, renal insufficiency, and gastrointestinal surgery. Our research team recently identified a genetic factor that allows identification of persons at high risk for CDAD (28). In CDAD, advanced age and comorbidity, plus severity of underlying impairment, predict frequency of infection and outcome (29).

When assessing institutionalized individuals, such as nursing home patients with diarrhea, associated risk factors for CDAD should be considered. Some of the risk factors other than antibiotic use and comorbidity are low albumin level

TABLE 112.4

EMPIRIC ANTIMICROBIAL THERAPY OF ACUTE DIARRHEA

Indication	Recommended therapy	References
Febrile dysentery: Fever (temperature >100.2°F [>38°C]) plus dysentery (passage of grossly bloody stools)	Azithromycin, 500 mg PO daily for 3 days	50–52
Moderate to severe traveler's diarrhea with fever and dysentery	Azithromycin, 500 mg PO daily for 3 days	50–52
Moderate to severe traveler's diarrhea without fever and dysentery	Rifaximin, 200 mg tid for 3 days; ciprofloxacin, 500 mg bid for 3 days; or levofloxacin, 500 mg once a day for 3 days; or azithromycin, 500 mg once a day for 3 days	53–57
Severe hospital-acquired diarrhea in a patient with comorbidity and prior receipt of antibacterial therapy	Oral metronidazole, 500 mg tid for 10 days; or vancomycin, 125–500 mg qid for 10 days	43, 58–60

bid, twice a day; PO, orally; qid, four times a day; tid, three times a day.

TABLE 112.5

SPECIFIC THERAPY FOR PATHOGEN-SPECIFIC DIARRHEA, ONCE ETIOLOGIC DIAGNOSIS IS ESTABLISHED

Identified pathogen	Suggested antimicrobial therapy	References
Clostridium difficile	Oral metronidazole, 500 mg tid for 10 days; or vancomycin, 125 to 500 mg qid for 10 days (newer therapies being evaluated including nitazoxanide, rifaximin, and *Saccharomyces*)	43, 58–60
Salmonella sp. (treat only for suspected sepsis based on presence of high-risk host*)	For high-risk host[a]: Fluoroquinolones: ciprofloxacin, 500 mg bid; or levofloxacin, 500 mg once a day for 7 to 10 days	61–63
Shigella	Fluoroquinolones, dose as in *Salmonella* above, give for 3 days	64–66
Campylobacter	Azithromycin, 500 mg once a day for 3 days; or erythromycin, 500 mg bid for 5 days	52, 67–69
Shigatoxin-producing *E. coli* (STEC)	No antimotility drugs, antibiotic treatment not usually given as they may increase the risk of occurrence of hemolytic uremic syndrome (HUS)	15, 70–73
Enterotoxigenic *E. coli* (ETEC)	Rifaximin, 200 mg tid for 3 days; fluoroquinolone in above dose for 3 days; or azithromycin, 500 mg once a day for 3 days.	53–55, 74
Enteropathogenic *E. coli* (EPEC)	Same as *Shigella*	
Enteroaggregative *E. coli* (EAEC)	Same as ETEC	
Enteroinvasive *E. coli* (EIEC)	Same as *Shigella*	
Vibrio spp. (*Vibrio cholerae* or noncholera *Vibrios*)	Tetracycline, 500 mg qid for 3 days; or 300 mg doxycycline, single 100-mg dose for adults	75, 76
Aeromonas/Plesiomonas	Same as *Shigella*	62, 77–79
Yersinia	Same as *Shigella*	61, 80–82
Entamoeba histolytica	Metronidazole, 750 mg tid for 5–10 days and diloxanide furoate, 500 mg tid for 10 days; or paromomycin, 500 mg tid for 10 days	61
Giardia	Metronidazole, 250–750 mg tid for 7–10 days; tinidazole, 2 g as a single dose	62, 83, 84
Cryptosporidium	Nitazoxanide, 500 mg bid for 3 days; in HIV/AIDS or immunosuppressed patients nitazoxanide, 500/1,000 mg bid for 14 days or more. Paromomycin, 500 mg qid for 7–14 days; or spiramycin, 3 g/day for up to 1 week	85–91
Cyclospora	TMP-SMZ, 160 and 800 mg, respectively, bid for 7 days; in AIDS patients, TMP-SMZ treatment is given for 14 days followed by 3 times weekly for up to 10 weeks	92, 93
Isospora	TMP-SMZ, 160 and 800 mg, respectively, bid for 7 days; in AIDS patients, treatment is followed by thrice weekly TMP-SMZ for up to 10 weeks	93
Microsporidium	Albendazole, 400 mg bid for 7 days and for 4 weeks in immunocompromised patients	94–96
Cytomegalovirus	In immunocompromised patient, ganciclovir, 5 mg/kg bid for 14 days	97, 98

bid, twice a day; ETEC, enterotoxigenic *E. coli*; qid, four times a day; tid, three times a day; TMP-SMZ, trimethoprim-sulfamethoxazole.
[a]High-risk patients for *Salmonella* enterica species (nontyphoid *Salmonella*): Any subject who is toxic with fever greater than 102°F (39°C), age less than 3 months or 65 years of age or greater, and subjects with malignancy or AIDS, on steroids, with inflammatory bowel disease or renal failure, or undergoing hemodialysis, with hemoglobinopathy such as sickle cell disease. Patients with simple gastroenteritis are best not given antibacterial drugs.

(less than 2.5 g/dL), recent admission to a health care institution, and use of proton pump inhibitors (30). In nonhospitalized patients with other predisposing conditions such as cancer, prolonged antibiotic usage—especially with first-generation cephalosporins, fluoroquinolones, or clindamycin—is a recognized risk factor for CDAD (31).

Recurrence is very common in CDAD as, after the first episode, it is estimated that nearly 15% to 30% of patients have recurrent illness after initial treatment (32,33). Recurrences include both re-infections with new strains and relapse of the original infecting strain. In one study, 56% of recurrences were due to re-infection (34). Some of the risk factors for early recurrence of CDAD are renal failure, white blood cell counts greater than 15,000 cells/μL with the initial episode, and community-acquired CDAD with the first episode (35). Failure to mount a serum antibody response to toxin A during an initial episode of CDAD is associated with CD recurrence (36).

Diagnosis of CDAD is based on both clinical and laboratory findings. The customary way to make the diagnosis is to recover a toxigenic strain of CD through microbiologic culture or to detect one or both of the known CD toxins, A and B, in stool samples. The stool toxin studies include a commercial tissue culture cytotoxin assay for toxin B or an enzyme immunoassay

(EIA) for one or both of the toxins. In a highly probable clinical case with severe disease or fragile clinical picture, it is often advisable to initiate prompt empiric treatment before stool test results are back or even in the face of negative laboratory tests for the toxins. Colonoscopy should be considered in patients in whom the diagnosis is not obvious, after initial screening, when there are extraintestinal complications, and in those not responding to empiric treatment (37).

Treatment

Prompt diagnosis and treatment are important to successful management of CDAD (Table 112.5). Cessation of causative antibiotic use if possible and initiation of either oral metronidazole (most consider first-line therapy) or oral vancomycin for 10 days is the standard practice in treating symptomatic patients (38–40). Vancomycin may be slightly more effective than metronidazole but its widespread use could promote the development of vancomycin resistance in the hospital setting, especially among *Enterococcus* spp.

Both metronidazole and vancomycin are used in the treatment of recurrent CD diarrhea. Independent predictors of a second recurrence are age and duration of hospitalization after the first recurrence (41). Strategies for treating recurrent CD diarrhea or colitis include repeating antibiotics either with metronidazole or vancomycin, with tapering of the antibiotic dose after a 10-day standard and administering the drug for 2 months or longer; use of probiotics such as *Saccharomyces boulardii* along with high-dose (500 mg four times a day) vancomycin; and use of intravenous immunoglobulin (IVIG) (42). When *Saccharomyces* was used in one study, the risk of recurrence was reduced by 50% (43).

If more than one recurrence occurs, various drugs may be used for prolonged therapy including vancomycin, rifaximin, and *Saccharomyces*. Other microbiologic approaches that may be useful include the restoration of normal colonic flora by fecal enema or by nasogastric tube administration (42). Surgical management of CDAD is done after failure of medical therapy or if life-threatening complications occur, including colonic perforation, peritonitis, or bowel infarction.

Diarrhea Epidemics in the Hospital

Early identification and controlling the spread of rare hospital epidemics of enteric disease are the keys to successful management. Universal protocols of isolation and personal hygiene measures play an important role. Cohorting subjects by putting infected persons in contiguous areas away from uninfected persons and using dedicated hospital personnel for their care is an important strategy. Judicious use of antibiotics in the hospital and prompt discontinuation of possible inciting drugs also can be helpful. Agents showing potential for epidemics in hospitals are *C. difficile, Salmonella* spp, *Shigella, Campylobacter, Vibrio, Aeromonas, Yersinia,* noroviruses, and rotavirus. Early therapy of treatable enteric pathogens should occur (Table 112.5). Health care worker and patient education regarding various personal hygiene and isolation procedures could help in stopping the spread within the institution.

Prevention of Diarrhea in the Hospital

Appropriate use of antibiotics in hospitalized patients, along with use of the narrowest-spectrum antibiotics safely possible to minimize the disruption of gut flora should prevent cases of CDAD. Additionally, at least in a research setting, *Saccharomyces* has been used to prevent CDAD (44). Enteric isolation practices for patients with known enteric infection in the hospital will help prevent the spread of diarrhea and lower its incidence. Effective and widespread hand washing with soap and water—note that alcohol-based hand cleaners are not effective against *C. difficile*—by patients and health care workers, using disposable thermometers for recording temperature, and meticulous environmental cleaning with chlorine-based bleach products in clinical settings where *C. difficile*-infected patients have been housed are proven to prevent spread of infections in the hospital (45–47).

References

1. Mead PS, Slutsker L, Dietz V, et al. Food-related illness and death in the United States. *Emerg Infect Dis.* 1999;5(5):607–625.
2. Denno DM, Stapp JR, Boster DR, et al. Etiology of diarrhea in pediatric outpatient settings. *Pediatr Infect Dis J.* 2005;24(2):142–148.
3. McFarland LV. Epidemiology of infectious and iatrogenic nosocomial diarrhea in a cohort of general medicine patients. *Am J Infect Control.* 1995;23(5):295–305.
4. Garey KW, Graham G, Gerard L, et al. Prevalence of diarrhea at a university hospital and association with modifiable risk factors. *Ann Pharmacother.* 2006;40(6):1030–1034.
5. Steffen R, Tornieporth N, Clemens SA, et al. Epidemiology of travelers' diarrhea: details of a global survey. *J Travel Med.* 2004;11(4):231–238.
6. Steffen R. Epidemiologic studies of travelers' diarrhea, severe gastrointestinal infections, and cholera. *Rev Infect Dis.* 1986;8(Suppl 2):S122–130.
7. DuPont HL, Ericsson CD. Prevention and treatment of traveler's diarrhea. *N Engl J Med.* 1993;328(25):1821–1827.
8. Ko G, Garcia C, Jiang ZD, et al. Noroviruses as a cause of traveler's diarrhea among students from the United States visiting Mexico. *J Clin Microbiol.* 2005;43(12):6126–6129.
9. Bouckenooghe AR, Jiang ZD, De La Cabada FJ, et al. Enterotoxigenic *Escherichia coli* as cause of diarrhea among Mexican adults and US travelers in Mexico. *J Travel Med.* 2002;9(3):137–140.
10. Adachi JA, Ericsson CD, Jiang ZD, et al. Natural history of enteroaggregative and enterotoxigenic *Escherichia coli* infection among US travelers to Guadalajara, Mexico. *J Infect Dis.* 2002;185(11):1681–1683.
11. Gallardo F, Gascon J, Ruiz J, et al. *Campylobacter jejuni* as a cause of traveler's diarrhea: clinical features and antimicrobial susceptibility. *J Travel Med.* 1998;5(1):23–26.
12. Adachi JA, Jiang ZD, Mathewson JJ, et al. Enteroaggregative *Escherichia coli* as a major etiologic agent in traveler's diarrhea in 3 regions of the world. *Clin Infect Dis.* 2001;32(12):1706–1709.
13. Ginsburg PM, Thuluvath PJ. Diarrhea in liver transplant recipients: etiology and management. *Liver Transpl.* 2005;11(8):881–890.
14. Rees JR, Pannier MA, McNees A, et al. Persistent diarrhea, arthritis, and other complications of enteric infections: a pilot survey based on California FoodNet surveillance, 1998–1999. *Clin Infect Dis.* 2004;38(Suppl 3):S311–317.
15. Cimolai N, Basalyga S, Mah DG, et al. A continuing assessment of risk factors for the development of *Escherichia coli* O157:H7-associated hemolytic uremic syndrome. *Clin Nephrol.* 1994;42(2):85–89.
16. DuPont HL, Hornick RB. Adverse effect of Lomotil therapy in shigellosis. *JAMA.* 1973;226(13):1525–1528.
17. Landzberg BR, Connor BA. Persistent diarrhea in the returning traveler: think beyond persistent infection. *Scand J Gastroenterol.* 2005;40(1):112–114.
18. Wathen JE, MacKenzie T, Bothner JP. Usefulness of the serum electrolyte panel in the management of pediatric dehydration treated with intravenously administered fluids. *Pediatrics.* 2004;114(5):1227–1234.
19. Murphy C, Hahn S, Volmink J. Reduced osmolarity oral rehydration solution for treating cholera. In: Murphy C, Hahn S, Volmink J. Reduced osmolarity oral rehydration solution for treating cholera. *Cochrane Database Syst Rev.* 2004 Oct 18;(4):CD003754.
20. Tedesco FJ, Barton RW, Alpers DH. Clindamycin-associated colitis. A prospective study. *Ann Intern Med.* 1974;81(4):429–433.
21. Bartlett JG, Chang TW, Gurwith M, et al. Antibiotic-associated pseudomembranous colitis due to toxin-producing *Clostridia*. *N Engl J Med.* 1978;298(10):531–534.
22. Poxton IR, McCoubrey J, Blair G. The pathogenicity of *Clostridium difficile*. *Clin Microbiol Infect.* 2001;7(8):421–427.
23. Rupnik M, Grabnar M, Geric B. Binary toxin producing *Clostridium difficile* strains. *Anaerobe.* 2003;9(6):289–294.

24. Kuijper EJ, Coignard B, Tull P, et al. Emergence of *Clostridium difficile*-associated disease in North America and Europe. *Clin Microbiol Infect.* 2006;12(Suppl 6):2–18.
25. Archibald LK, Banerjee SN, Jarvis WR. Secular trends in hospital-acquired *Clostridium difficile* disease in the United States, 1987-2001. *J Infect Dis.* 2004;189(9):1585–1589.
26. McDonald LC, Owings M, Jernigan DB. *Clostridium difficile* infection in patients discharged from US short-stay hospitals, 1996-2003. *Emerg Infect Dis.* 2006;12(3):409–415.
27. Kyne L, Hamel MB, Polavaram R, et al. Health care costs and mortality associated with nosocomial diarrhea due to *Clostridium difficile*. *Clin Infect Dis.* 2002;34(3):346–353.
28. Jiang ZD, DuPont HL, Garey K, et al. A common polymorphism in the interleukin 8 gene promoter is associated with *Clostridium difficile* diarrhea. *Am J Gastroenterol.* 2006;101(5):1112–1116.
29. Andrews CN, Raboud J, Kassen BO, et al. *Clostridium difficile*-associated diarrhea: predictors of severity in patients presenting to the emergency department. *Can J Gastroenterol.* 2003;17(6):369–373.
30. Al-Tureihi FI, Hassoun A, Wolf-Klein G, et al. Albumin, length of stay, and proton pump inhibitors: key factors in *Clostridium difficile*-associated disease in nursing home patients. *J Am Med Dir Assoc.* 2005;6(2):105–108.
31. Palmore TN, Sohn S, Malak SF, et al. Risk factors for acquisition of *Clostridium difficile*-associated diarrhea among outpatients at a cancer hospital. *Infect Control Hosp Epidemiol.* 2005;26(8):680–684.
32. Fekety R, McFarland LV, Surawicz CM, et al. Recurrent *Clostridium difficile* diarrhea: characteristics of and risk factors for patients enrolled in a prospective, randomized, double-blinded trial. *Clin Infect Dis.* 1997;24(3):324–333.
33. McFarland LV, Surawicz CM, Rubin M, et al. Recurrent *Clostridium difficile* disease: epidemiology and clinical characteristics. *Infect Control Hosp Epidemiol.* 1999;20(1):43–50.
34. Wilcox MH, Fawley WN, Settle CD, et al. Recurrence of symptoms in *Clostridium difficile* infection–relapse or reinfection? *J Hosp Infect.* 1998;38(2):93–100.
35. Do AN, Fridkin SK, Yechouron A, et al. Risk factors for early recurrent *Clostridium difficile*-associated diarrhea. *Clin Infect Dis.* 1998;26(4):954–959.
36. Kyne L, Warny M, Qamar A, et al. Association between antibody response to toxin A and protection against recurrent *Clostridium difficile* diarrhoea. *Lancet,* 2001;357(9251):189–193.
37. Bauer TM, Lalvani A, Fehrenbach J, et al. Derivation and validation of guidelines for stool cultures for enteropathogenic bacteria other than *Clostridium difficile* in hospitalized adults. *JAMA.* 2001;285(3):313–319.
38. Aslam S, Musher DM. An update on diagnosis, treatment, and prevention of *Clostridium difficile*-associated disease. *Gastroenterol Clin North Am.* 2006;35(2):315–335.
39. Bergogne-Berezin E. Treatment and prevention of antibiotic associated diarrhea. *Int J Antimicrob Agents.* 2000;16(4):521–526.
40. Bricker E, Garg R, Nelson R, et al. Antibiotic treatment for *Clostridium difficile*-associated diarrhea in adults. *Cochrane Database Syst Rev.* 2005 Jan 25;(1):004610.
41. Pepin J, Routhier S, Gagnon S, et al. Management and outcomes of a first recurrence of *Clostridium difficile*-associated disease in Quebec, Canada. *Clin Infect Dis.* 2006;42(6):758–764.
42. Surawicz CM. Treatment of recurrent *Clostridium difficile*-associated disease. *Nature Clin Practice Gastroenterol Hepatol.* 2004;1(1):32–38.
43. Surawicz CM, McFarland LV, Greenberg RN, et al. The search for a better treatment for recurrent *Clostridium difficile* disease: use of high-dose vancomycin combined with *Saccharomyces boulardii. Clin Infect Dis.* 2000;31(4):1012–1017.
44. McFarland LV. Meta-analysis of probiotics for the prevention of antibiotic associated diarrhea and the treatment of *Clostridium difficile* disease. *Am J Gastroenterol.* 2006;101(4):812–822.
45. Jernigan JA, Siegman-Igra Y, Guerrant RC, et al. A randomized crossover study of disposable thermometers for prevention of *Clostridium difficile* and other nosocomial infections. *Infect Control Hospital Epidemiol.* 1998;19(7):494–499.
46. Worsley MA. Infection control and prevention of *Clostridium difficile* infection. *J Antimicrob Chemother.* 1998;41(Suppl C):59–66.
47. Robinson B. Be alert to an avoidable problem. Management and prevention of antibiotic-acquired diarrhoea. *Prof Nurse.* 1993;8(8):510–512.
48. Duggan C, Santosham M, Glass RI. The management of acute diarrhea in children: oral rehydration, maintenance, and nutritional therapy. Centers for Disease Control and Prevention. *MMWR Recomm Rep.* 1992;41(RR-16):1–20.
49. King CK, Glass R, Bresee JS, et al. Managing acute gastroenteritis among children: oral rehydration, maintenance, and nutritional therapy. *MMWR Recomm Rep.* 2003;52(RR-16):1–16.
50. Adachi JA, Ostrosky-Zeichner L, DuPont HL, et al. Empirical antimicrobial therapy for traveler's diarrhea. *Clin Infect Dis.* 2000;31(4):1079–1083.
51. Adachi JA, Ericsson CD, Jiang ZD, et al. Azithromycin found to be comparable to levofloxacin for the treatment of US travelers with acute diarrhea acquired in Mexico. *Clin Infect Dis.* 2003;37(9):1165–1171.
52. Kuschner RA, Trofa AF, Thomas RJ, et al. Use of azithromycin for the treatment of *Campylobacter* enteritis in travelers to Thailand, an area where ciprofloxacin resistance is prevalent. *Clin Infect Dis.* 1995;21(3):536–541.
53. DuPont HL. Use of quinolones in the treatment of gastrointestinal infections. *Europ J Clin Microbiol Infect Dis.* 1991;10(4):325–329.
54. Salam I, Katelaris P, Leigh-Smith S, et al. Randomised trial of single-dose ciprofloxacin for travellers' diarrhoea. *Lancet.* 1994;344(8936):1537–1539.
55. Ericsson CD, DuPont HL, Mathewson JJ. Optimal dosing of ofloxacin with loperamide in the treatment of non-dysenteric travelers' diarrhea. *J Travel Med.* 2001;8(4):207–209.
56. DuPont HL, Jiang ZD, Ericsson CD, et al. Rifaximin versus ciprofloxacin for the treatment of traveler's diarrhea: a randomized, double-blind clinical trial. *Clin Infect Dis.* 2001;33(11):1807–1815.
57. DuPont HL, Ericsson CD, Mathewson JJ, et al. Rifaximin: a nonabsorbed antimicrobial in the therapy of travelers' diarrhea. *Digestion.* 1998;59(6):708–714.
58. Musher DM, Logan N, Hamill RJ, et al. Nitazoxanide for the treatment of *Clostridium difficile* colitis. *Clin Infect Dis.* 2006;43(4):421–427.
59. Wenisch C, Parschalk B, Hasenhundl M, et al. Comparison of vancomycin, teicoplanin, metronidazole, and fusidic acid for the treatment of *Clostridium difficile*-associated diarrhea. *Clin Infect Dis.* 1996;22(5):813–818.
60. Wullt M, Odenholt I. A double-blind randomized controlled trial of fusidic acid and metronidazole for treatment of an initial episode of *Clostridium difficile*-associated diarrhoea. *J Antimicrob Chemother.* 2004;54(1):211–216.
61. DuPont HL. Guidelines on acute infectious diarrhea in adults. the practice parameters committee of the American College of Gastroenterology. *Am J Gastroenterol.* 1997;92(11):1962–1975.
62. Guerrant RL, Van Gilder T, Steiner TS, et al. Practice guidelines for the management of infectious diarrhea. *Clin Infect Dis.* 2001;32(3):331–351.
63. Soe GB, Overturf GD. Treatment of typhoid fever and other systemic salmonelloses with cefotaxime, ceftriaxone, cefoperazone, and other newer cephalosporins. *Rev Infect Dis.* 1987;9(4):719–736.
64. Khan WA, Seas C, Dhar U, et al. Treatment of shigellosis, V: comparison of azithromycin and ciprofloxacin. A double-blind, randomized, controlled trial. *Ann Intern Med.* 1997;126(9):697–703.
65. Bhattacharya SK, Bhattacharya MK, Dutta P, et al. Randomized clinical trial of norfloxacin for shigellosis. *Am J Trop Med Hyg.* 1991;45(6):683–687.
66. Salam MA, Bennish ML. Antimicrobial therapy for shigellosis. *Rev Infect Dis.* 1991;13(Suppl 4):S332–341.
67. Pai CH, Gillis F, Tuomanen E, et al. Erythromycin in treatment of *Campylobacter* enteritis in children. *Am J Dis Child.* 1983;137(3):286–288.
68. Mandal BK, Ellis ME, Dunbar EM, et al. Double-blind placebo-controlled trial of erythromycin in the treatment of clinical *Campylobacter* infection. *J Antimicrob Chemother.* 1984;13(6):619–23.
69. Endtz HP, Ruijs GJ, van Klingeren B, et al. Quinolone resistance in *Campylobacter* isolated from man and poultry following the introduction of fluoroquinolones in veterinary medicine. *J Antimicrob Chemother.* 1991;27(2):199–208.
70. Wong CS, Jelacic S, Habeeb RL, et al. The risk of the hemolytic-uremic syndrome after antibiotic treatment of *Escherichia coli* O157:H7 infections. *N Engl J Med.* 2000;342(26):1930–1936.
71. O'Ryan M, Prado V. Risk of the hemolytic-uremic syndrome after antibiotic treatment of *Escherichia coli* O157:H7 infections. *N Engl J Med.* 2000;343(17):1271.
72. Aragon T, Fernyak S, Reiter R. Risk of the hemolytic-uremic syndrome after antibiotic treatment of *Escherichia coli* O157:H7 infections. *N Engl J Med.* 2000;343(17):1271–1272.
73. Cimolai N, Carter JE, Morrison BJ, et al. Risk factors for the progression of *Escherichia coli* O157:H7 enteritis to hemolytic-uremic syndrome. *J Pediatr.* 1990;116(4):589–592.
74. DuPont HL, Reves RR, Galindo E, et al. Treatment of travelers' diarrhea with trimethoprim/sulfamethoxazole and with trimethoprim alone. *N Engl J Med.* 1982;307(14):841–844.
75. Hossain MS, Salam MA, Rabbani GH, et al. Tetracycline in the treatment of severe cholera due to *Vibrio cholerae* O139 Bengal. *J Health Popul Nutr.* 2002;20(1):18–25.
76. Alam AN, Alam NH, Ahmed T, et al. Randomised double blind trial of single dose doxycycline for treating cholera in adults. *BMJ.* 1990;300(6740):1619–1621.
77. Holmberg SD, Farmer JJ 3rd. *Aeromonas hydrophila* and *Plesiomonas shigelloides* as causes of intestinal infections. *Rev Infect Dis.* 1984;6(5):633–639.
78. Kain KC, Kelly MT. Clinical features, epidemiology, and treatment of *Plesiomonas shigelloides* diarrhea. *J Clin Microbiol.* 1989;27(5):998–1001.
79. Nathwani D, Laing RB, Harvey G, et al. Treatment of symptomatic enteric *Aeromonas hydrophila* infection with ciprofloxacin. *Scand J Infect Dis.* 1991;23(5):653–654.
80. Abdel-Haq NM, Papadopol R, Asmar BI, et al. Antibiotic susceptibilities of *Yersinia enterocolitica* recovered from children over a 12-year period. *Int J Antimicrob Agents.* 2006;27(5):449–452.
81. Hoogkamp-Korstanje JA, Moesker H, Bruyn GA. Ciprofloxacin vs. placebo for treatment of *Yersinia enterocolitica* triggered reactive arthritis. *Ann Rheum Dis.* 2000;59(11):914–917.
82. Pai CH, Gillis F, Tuomanen E, et al. Placebo-controlled double-blind evaluation of trimethoprim-sulfamethoxazole treatment of *Yersinia enterocolitica* gastroenteritis. *J Pediatr.* 1984;104(2):308–311.

83. Levi GC, de Avila CA, Amato Neto V. Efficacy of various drugs for treatment of giardiasis. A comparative study. *Amer J Trop Med Hyg.* 1977;26(3):564–565.
84. Penggabean M, Norhayati, Oothuman P, et al. Efficacy of albendazole in the treatment of *Trichuris trichiura* and *Giardia intestinalis* infection in rural Malay communities. *Med J Malaysia.* 1998;53(4):408–412.
85. Carr A, Marriott D, Field A, et al. Treatment of HIV-1-associated microsporidiosis and cryptosporidiosis with combination antiretroviral therapy. *Lancet.* 1998;351(9098):256–261.
86. Fichtenbaum CJ, Ritchie DJ, Powderly WG. Use of paromomycin for treatment of cryptosporidiosis in patients with AIDS. *Clin Infect Dis.* 1993;16(2):298–300.
87. Foudraine NA, Weverling GJ, van Gool T, et al. Improvement of chronic diarrhoea in patients with advanced HIV-1 infection during potent antiretroviral therapy. *AIDS.* 1998;12(1):35–41.
88. Portnoy D, Whiteside ME, Buckley E 3rd, et al. Treatment of intestinal cryptosporidiosis with spiramycin. *Ann Intern Med.* 1984;101(2):202–204.
89. Rossignol JF, Ayoub A, Ayers MS. Treatment of diarrhea caused by *Cryptosporidium parvum*: a prospective randomized, double-blind, placebo-controlled study of nitazoxanide. *J Infect Dis.* 2001;184(1):103–106.
90. Rossignol JF, Hidalgo H, Feregrino M, et al. A double-'blind' placebo-controlled study of nitazoxanide in the treatment of cryptosporidial diarrhoea in AIDS patients in Mexico. *Trans R Soc Trop Med Hyg.* 1998;92(6):663–666.
91. Rossignol J. Nitazoxanide in the treatment of acquired immune deficiency syndrome-related cryptosporidiosis: results of the United States compassionate use program in 365 patients. *Aliment Pharmacol Ther.* 2006;24(5):887–894.
92. Hoge CW, Shlim DR, Ghimire M, et al. Placebo-controlled trial of co-trimoxazole for *Cyclospora* infections among travellers and foreign residents in Nepal. *Lancet.* 1995;345(8951):691–693.
93. Verdier RI, Fitzgerald DW, Johnson WD Jr, et al. Trimethoprim-sulfamethoxazole compared with ciprofloxacin for treatment and prophylaxis of *Isospora belli* and *Cyclospora cayetanensis* infection in HIV-infected patients. A randomized, controlled trial. *Ann Intern Med.* 2000;132(11):885–888.
94. Blanshard C, Ellis DS, Tovey DG, et al. Treatment of intestinal microsporidiosis with albendazole in patients with AIDS. *AIDS.* 1992;6(3):311–313.
95. Tremoulet AH, Avila-Aguero ML, París MM, et al. Albendazole therapy for *Microsporidia* diarrhea in immunocompetent Costa Rican children. *Pediatr Infect Dis J.* 2004;23(10):915–918.
96. Farthing MJ. Treatment options for the eradication of intestinal protozoa. *Nature Clin Pract Gastroenterol Hepatol.* 2006;3(8):436–445.
97. Dieterich DT, Kotler DP, Busch DF, et al. Ganciclovir treatment of cytomegalovirus colitis in AIDS: a randomized, double-blind, placebo-controlled multicenter study. *J Infect Dis.* 1993;167(2):278–282.
98. Mayoral JL, Loeffler CM, Fasola CG, et al. Diagnosis and treatment of cytomegalovirus disease in transplant patients based on gastrointestinal tract manifestations. *Arch Surg.* 1991;126(2):202–206.

CHAPTER 113 ■ CATHETER-ASSOCIATED URINARY TRACT INFECTIONS IN THE ICU: IMPLICATIONS FOR CLINICAL PRACTICE

MARC LEONE • CLAUDE MARTIN

OBJECTIVE

Intensive care units (ICUs) represent a meeting point between the most seriously ill patients receiving aggressive therapy and the most resistant pathogens that are selected by the use of broad-spectrum antimicrobial therapy. Most patients who are hospitalized in ICUs receive an indwelling urinary catheter to monitor urine output. Urinary tract infection (UTI) remains a leading cause of nosocomial infections with significant morbidity, mortality, and, hence, additional hospital costs (1).

Although UTI represents 30% to 40% of nosocomial infections (1,2), its prevalence in patients admitted to the ICU is approximately 20% (3). In a large European survey, UTI was the third most common cause of nosocomial infections in the ICU (3). Another study suggests that the incidence of urosepsis, defined as an inflammation of the upper urinary tract that causes sepsis, occurs in approximately 16% of the ICU patient population (4). The aim of this chapter is to focus on the prevention and management of UTI in patients hospitalized in the ICU.

DEFINITIONS

The Centers for Disease Control and Prevention (CDC) definitions of symptomatic UTIs and asymptomatic UTIs are collected in Tables 113.1, 113.2, and 113.3 (5). In the ICU, UTI is the consequence of placement of an indwelling catheter. This results in the concept of *catheter-associated UTI*, the definition of which is restricted to the presence of bacteria in the bladder of a patient with an indwelling catheter. Bacteriuria is defined as the detection of greater than or equal to 10^5 micro-organisms/mL of urine with no more than two species of organisms (5). It is of interest to note that, contrary to non–ICU-acquired urinary tract infections, this definition does not take into account the clinical symptoms.

PATHOPHYSIOLOGY

With the exception of the distal urethra, the urinary tract is normally sterile. Resistance to UTI is influenced by exposure to uropathogenic bacteria, age, hormonal status, and urine flow

TABLE 113.1

DEFINITIONS FOR SYMPTOMATIC URINARY TRACT INFECTIONS

At least one of the following criteria:

CRITERION 1
Patient has at least one of the following signs or symptoms with no other recognized cause : fever (>38°C), urgency, frequency, dysuria, or suprapubic tenderness *and* patient has a positive urine culture with $\geq 10^5$ micro-organisms/mL of urine with no more than two species of micro-organisms.

CRITERION 2
Patient has at least one of the following signs or symptoms with no other recognized cause: fever (>38°C), urgency, frequency, dysuria, or suprapubic tenderness *and at least one of the following*: (a) positive dipstick for leukocyte esterase and/or nitrate; (b) pyuria (urine specimen with 10 white blood cells (WBC)/μL or $\geq$3 WBC/high-power field of unspun urine); (c) organisms seen on Gram stain of unspun urine; (d) at least two urine cultures with repeated isolation of the same uropathogen (Gram-negative bacteria or *Staphylococcus saprophyticus*) with $\geq 10^2$ colonies/mL in nonvoided specimens; (e) $\leq 10^5$ colonies/mL of a single uropathogen (Gram-negative bacteria or *S. saprophyticus*) in a patient being treated with an effective antimicrobial agent for a urinary tract infection; (f) physician diagnosis of a urinary tract infection; or (g) physician institutes appropriate therapy for a urinary tract infection.

CRITERION 3
Patient $\leq$1 year of age with *at least one of the following signs or symptoms with no other recognized cause*: fever (>38°C), hypothermia (<37°C), apnea, bradycardia, dysuria, lethargy, or vomiting *and* positive urine culture with $\geq 10^5$ micro-organisms/mL of urine with no more than two species of micro-organisms.

CRITERION 4
Patient $\leq$1 year of age with *at least one of the following signs or symptoms with no other recognized cause*: fever (>38°C), hypothermia (<37°C), apnea, bradycardia, dysuria, lethargy, or vomiting *and* (a) positive dipstick for leukocyte esterase and/or nitrate; (b) pyuria (urine specimen with 10 WBC/μL or $\geq$3 WBC/high-power field of unspun urine); (c) organisms seen on Gram stain of unspun urine; (d) at least two urine cultures with repeated isolation of the same uropathogen (Gram-negative bacteria or *S. saprophyticus*) with $\geq 10^2$ colonies/mL in nonvoided specimens; (e) $\leq 10^5$ colonies/mL of a single uropathogen (Gram-negative bacteria or *S. saprophyticus*) in a patient being treated with an effective antimicrobial agent for a urinary tract infection; (f) physician diagnosis of a urinary tract infection; or (g) physician institutes appropriate therapy for a urinary tract infection.

From Garner JS, Jarvis WR, Emori TG, et al. CDC definitions for nosocomial infections, 1988. *Am J Infect Control.* 1988;16:128.

(6). Insertion of a catheter allows organisms to gain access to the bladder. The catheter induces an inflammation of the urethra, allowing bacteria to ascend into the bladder in the space between the urethral mucosa and the catheter. Catheter-associated UTI usually follows the formation of biofilm, which consists of adherent micro-organisms, their extracellular products, and host components deposited on both the internal and external catheter surfaces. The biofilm protects the organisms from both antimicrobials and the host immune response (7). The ascending route of infection is predominant in women, owing to their short urethra and contamination with anal flora. An internal route of contamination (i.e., through the lumen of the catheter) is less frequent and related to reflux of pathogens from the drainage system into the bladder. This contamination occurs when the drainage system fails to close or contamination of urine in the collection bag.

TABLE 113.2

DEFINITIONS FOR ASYMPTOMATIC URINARY TRACT INFECTIONS

One of the following criteria:

CRITERION 1
Patient has had an indwelling urinary catheter within 7 d before the culture *and* patient has a positive urine culture with $\geq 10^5$ micro-organisms/mL of urine with no more than two species of micro-organisms and patient has no fever (>38°C), urgency, frequency, dysuria, or suprapubic tenderness.

CRITERION 2
Patient has not had an indwelling urinary catheter within 7 d before the first positive culture and patient has had at least two positive urine cultures with $\geq 10^5$ micro-organisms/mL with repeated isolation of the same micro-organism and no more than two species of micro-organisms and patient has no fever (>38°C), urgency, frequency, dysuria, or suprapubic tenderness.

From Garner JS, Jarvis WR, Emori TG, et al. CDC definitions for nosocomial infections, 1988. *Am J Infect Control.* 1988;16:128.

TABLE 113.3

OTHER URINARY TRACT INFECTIONS

One of the following criteria:

CRITERION 1
Patient has organisms isolated from culture of fluid (other than urine) or tissue from affected site.

CRITERION 2
Patient has an abscess or other evidence of infection seen on direct examination, during surgical operation, or during a histopathologic examination.

CRITERION 3
Patient has at least two of the following signs or symptoms with no other recognized cause: fever (>38°C), localized pain, or tenderness at the involved site *and at least one of the following*: (a) purulent drainage from affected site; (b) organisms cultured from blood that are compatible with suspected site of infection; (c) radiographic evidence of infection (e.g., abnormal ultrasound, computed tomography [CT] scan, magnetic resonance imaging [MRI], or radiolabel scan); (d) physician diagnosis of infection of the kidney, ureter, bladder, urethra, or tissues surrounding the retroperitoneal or perinephric space; or (e) physician institutes appropriate therapy for an infection of the kidney, ureter, bladder, urethra, or tissues surrounding the retroperitoneal or perinephric space.

CRITERION 4
Patient ≤1 year of age with at least one of the following signs or symptoms with no other recognized cause: fever (>38°C), hypothermia (<37°C), apnea, bradycardia, dysuria, lethargy, or vomiting *and at least one of the following*: (a) purulent drainage from affected site; (b) organisms cultured from blood that are compatible with suspected site of infection; (c) radiographic evidence of infection (e.g., abnormal ultrasound, CT scan, MRI, or radiolabel scan); (d) physician diagnosis of infection of the kidney, ureter, bladder, urethra, or tissues surrounding the retroperitoneal or perinephric space; or (e) physician institutes appropriate therapy for an infection of the kidney, ureter, bladder, urethra, or tissues surrounding the retroperitoneal or perinephric space.

From Garner JS, Jarvis WR, Emori TG, et al. CDC definitions for nosocomial infections, 1988. *Am J Infect Control.* 1988;16:128.

MICROBIOLOGY

The isolated pathogens in ICU patients with bacteriuria are essentially relatively few: *Escherichia coli*, *Pseudomonas aeruginosa*, and *Enterococcus* species (Table 113.4) (8–10). Polymicrobial infections represent a relatively small percentage—5% to 12% (2,8,9)—of total infections. In a large report investigating nosocomial infections in ICU patients, Gram-negative bacteria caused 71% of UTIs, with stability over a 17-year period of surveillance (10). Resistance to antimicrobials increased during this period, with rates of resistance to third-generation cephalosporins up to 20% for *E. coli* (10,11). Although its role is demonstrated in a urologic ward, cross-transmission probably plays a much greater role than suggested up to the present (12).

RISK FACTORS

As stated, in ICU patients, UTIs are associated with the presence of indwelling catheters. The first step of prevention is to highlight the risk factors of catheter-associated UTI in this specific population. In a study assessing risk factors for bacteriuria in 553 patients with a urinary catheter for more than 48 hours and hospitalized in an ICU (8), female sex, length of ICU stay, prior use of antibiotics, severity score on admission, and duration of catheterization were independently associated with an increased risk of catheter-associated bacteriuria; these results mirrored those from a previous clinical study (13). Such results emphasize that reducing the duration of catheterization appears to be the most important clinical step that can be identified for prevention. One notable study showed that in 21% of 202 patients, the initial indication for the placement of a urinary catheter was unjustified. In a medical intensive care unit, excessive duration of urinary catheter use for monitoring urine output resulted in 64% of the total of unjustified patient-days (14).

IMPACT OF URINARY TRACT INFECTIONS IN THE INTENSIVE CARE UNIT

Although adverse consequences of asymptomatic UTIs have been described during pregnancy or in nursing home patients (15), the real impact of ICU-acquired UTIs on outcome remains unclear. In a general hospital population, Platt et al. showed that nosocomial UTIs were associated with significant attributable mortality (16). The picture is probably different in a specific ICU population. Indeed, even after controlling for many risk factors, UTIs have a higher incidence in ICUs as compared to other wards (17), although the urinary tract is the source of sepsis in only 10% to 14% of the cases, which is far less than the lung (Table 113.5) (18,19). Development of ICU-acquired UTIs is associated with both an increase in the length of ICU stay and the crude rate of mortality (8,9). However, adequately powered studies demonstrate that UTIs are not dependent factors for mortality (9,17).

Urosepsis is defined as an inflammation of the upper urinary tract that causes seeding of the blood with bacteria, resulting in local and distant destruction of tissue. A retrospective study evaluated 126 trauma patients with a urinary catheter for

TABLE 113.4

PERCENTAGE OF PATHOGENS ASSOCIATED WITH NOSOCOMIAL URINARY TRACT INFECTIONS

	Percentage of isolates		
Pathogens	**Leone et al.[a] (*n* = 53)**	**Laupland et al.[b] (*n* = 290)**	**Gaynes et al.[c] (*n* = 4,109)**
Gram negative			
Escherichia coli	39	23	26
Pseudomonas aeruginosa	22	10	16.3
Enterobacter species	15	3	6.9
Acinetobacter acinus	11	—	1.6
Proteus species	11	5	—
Klebsiella species	11	5	9.8
Citrobacter species	2	1	
Gram positive			
Enterococcus species	4	15	17.4
Staphylococcus aureus	2	1	3.6
Coagulase-negative *Staphylococcus*	2	5	4.9
Yeast			
Candida albicans	2	20	—
Candida non-*albicans*		8	

[a] Leone M, Albanese J, Garnier F, et al. Risk factors of nosocomial catheter-associated urinary tract infection in a polyvalent intensive care unit. *Intensive Care Med.* 2003;29:1077.
[b] Laupland KB, Bagshaw SM, Gregson DB, et al. Intensive care unit-acquired urinary tract infections in a regional critical care system. *Crit Care.* 2005;9:R60.
[c] Gaynes R, Edwards JR, National Nosocomial Infections Surveillance System. Overview of nosocomial infections caused by gram-negative bacilli. *Clin Infect Dis.* 2005;41:848.

sepsis. Twenty (16%) were diagnosed with urosepsis, which was correlated with age older than 60 years, extended length of stay in the ICU and/or hospital, and duration of catheterization. The mortality rates (15%) of the patients without urosepsis and with urosepsis did not differ (4). Similarly, in a prospective study, 6 out of 60 (10%) catheterized patients with asymptomatic bacteriuria developed urosepsis (20). Another prospective, cohort study of 235 catheter-acquired infections among 1,497 patients, 90% of whom were asymptomatic, reported only one (0.42%) secondary bloodstream infection (21).

TABLE 113.5

RATES OF SEPSIS ACCORDING TO EACH SITE

	Percentages of patients	
Sites	**Vincent et al.[a] (*n* = 1,177)**	**Angus et al.[b] (*n* = 192,980)**
Lung	68%	44.0%
Abdomen	22%	8.6%
Blood	20%	17.3%
Urine	14%	9.1%

[a] Vincent JL, Sakr Y, Sprung CL, et al. Sepsis in European intensive care units: results of the SOAP study. *Crit Care Med.* 2006;34:344.
[b] Angus DC, Linde-Zwirble WT, Lidicker J, et al. Epidemiology of severe sepsis in the United States: analysis of incidence, outcome, and associated costs of care. *Crit Care Med.* 2001;29:1303.

Finally, UTIs can incur significant additional cost. An episode of symptomatic nosocomial UTI in a hospitalized patient is expected to result in an average of $676 in additional cost (22). Interestingly, however, a Turkish study calculated the daily antibiotic costs per infected ICU patient. Among the sites of nosocomial infections, urinary tract infections had the lowest daily antibiotic cost per infected patient ($52) (23).

DIAGNOSTIC TOOLS IN THE INTENSIVE CARE UNIT

Urosepsis should be suspected any time a patient has a febrile episode. Because of the prevalence of bacteriuria in patients with urinary catheters, some have advocated daily monitoring of urine in catheterized patients. Routine daily bacteriologic monitoring of the urine from all catheterized patients is not an effective way to decrease the incidence of symptomatic, catheter-associated UTI, and is not recommended (24).

Three clinical trials have assessed the effectiveness of urinary dipsticks (leukocyte esterase and nitrite) for screening patients instead of quantitative urine culture in the ICU (Table 113.6) (25–27). Leukocyte esterase activity is an indicator of pyuria, and urinary nitrite production is an indicator of bacteriuria. In the medical ICU, it has been demonstrated that the urinary dipstick strategy is a rapid and cost-effective test with which to screen asymptomatic catheterized patients. This effectiveness is observed only for a positive quantitative urine culture level of 10^5 micro-organisms/mL. The urinary dipstick

TABLE 113.6

ASSESSING URINARY REAGENT STRIPS IN THE INTENSIVE CARE UNIT

	Tissot et al.[a]	Mimoz et al.[b]	Legras et al.[c]
Prevalence (%)	31	38	42
Sensitivity (%)	87	84	90
Specificity (%)	61	41	65
Positive predictive value (%)	31	46	61
Negative predictive value (%)	96	81	91

[a] Tissot E, Woronoff-Lemsi MC, Cornette C, et al. Cost-effectiveness of urinary dipsticks to screen asymptomatic catheter-associated urinary infections in an intensive care unit. *Intensive Care Med.* 2001;27:1842.
[b] Mimoz O, Bouchet E, Edouard A, et al. Limited usefulness of urinary dipsticks to screen out catheter-associated bacteriuria in ICU patients. *Anaesth Intens Care.* 1995;23:706.
[c] Legras A, Cattier B, Perrotin D. Dépistage des infections urinaires dans un service de rintérêt des bandelettes réactives. *Med Mal Infect.* 1993;23:34.

strategy decreases the cost of diagnosis of nosocomial infection and the daily workload in the microbiology laboratory (25). One limitation of this study is that the incidence of asymptomatic bacteriuria was 31%, as compared with 6% to 9% in other studies (8,9).

In a prior study, analysis of 102 urine samples determined a positive predictive value of 81%. Those authors did not recommend the use of urinary dipsticks (27). Our best sense of these data is that the use of dipsticks—instead of quantitative urine culture—cannot be recommended for symptomatic UTIs in ICU patients. The Infectious Disease Society of America (IDSA) guidelines recommend that asymptomatic bacteriuria or funguria not be screened in patients with an indwelling urethral catheter (28). Hence, in symptomatic patients, quantitative urine culture with Gram stain examination is recommended to obtain rapid identification of the pathogen.

PREVENTION

The best prevention of ICU-acquired UTIs is to simply reduce the use of indwelling urethral catheters. In a medical ICU, an independent observer determined that 64% of the total unjustified patient-days with urethral catheter resulted from its prolonged use for monitoring urine output (14). Hence, each member of the critical care medicine team should attempt to reduce the length of urethral catheterization and, whenever possible, this evaluation should occur during daily rounds. Other measures, described below, can be useful only in units with a restrictive policy of catheterization (Table 113.7).

Urinary Drainage System

In order to prevent infection, the maintenance of a closed sterile drainage system is recommended as the most successful method (29). A closed drainage system was described for the first time in 1928 (30), and its benefit has been subsequently re-enforced (16). A subgroup analysis of a randomized study, in which analyzed patients did not receive antibiotic treatment, showed a reduction in mortality in the group using the closed system (16). Historically, "open systems" were large, uncapped glass bottles. The drainage catheters were inserted into the glass bottles,

TABLE 113.7

COMPARATIVE STUDIES PERFORMED IN THE INTENSIVE CARE UNIT ON THE PREVENTION OF CATHETER-ASSOCIATED URINARY TRACT INFECTION

	Leone et al.[a]	Leone et al.[b]	Thibon et al.[c]	Bologna et al.[d]
Method (number of patients)	Prospective Not randomized (311)	Prospective Randomized (224)	Prospective Randomized Multicenter (199)	Prospective Not randomized Multicenter (108)
Rate of bacteriuria (%)	8	12	11	8.1 vs. 4.9
Study group	Two-chamber simple closed drainage system	Two-chamber simple closed drainage system	Catheter coated with hydrogel and silver salts	Hydrogel latex Foley catheter with silver metal
Control group	Complex closed system	Complex closed system	Standard catheter	Standard catheter
Conclusion	No difference	No difference	No difference	No difference

[a] Leone M, Garnier F, Dubuc M, et al. Prevention of nosocomial urinary tract infection in ICU patients. Comparison of effectiveness of two urinary drainage systems. *Chest.* 2001;120:220.
[b] Leone M, Garnier F, Antonini F, et al. Comparison of effectiveness of two urinary drainage systems in intensive care unit: a prospective, randomized clinical trial. *Intensive Care Med.* 2003;29:410.
[c] Thibon P, Le Coutour X, Leroyer R, et al. Randomized multi-centre trial of the effects of a catheter coated with hydrogel and silver salts on the incidence of hospital-acquired urinary tract infections. *J Hosp Infect.* 2000;45:117.
[d] Bologna RA, Tu LM, Polansky M, et al. Hydrogel/silver ion-coated urinary catheter reduces nosocomial urinary tract infection rates in intensive care unit patients: a multicenter study. *Urology.* 1999;54:982.

often below the level of urine. Urine was stagnant, and bacteria could easily grow and ascend through the drainage catheter. The introduction of closed drainage systems was a major improvement, and their use has greatly reduced the rate of bacteriuria. However, in the modern era, several studies have failed to confirm the benefit of complex closed systems compared with simple devices (31–33).

There are only two studies in the literature specifically focused on ICU patients (34,35) and comparing a two-chamber, open drainage system with a complex closed drainage system. Both of them, which were performed by the same team of investigators, found similar results, although one of these studies was not randomized (34). In the randomized and prospective trial, 311 patients requiring an indwelling urinary catheter for longer than 48 hours were assigned to the two-chamber drainage system group or to the complex closed drainage system group to compare the rates of bacteriuria. The rates of UTIs were 12.1 and 12.8 episodes per 1,000 days of catheterization, respectively (35). The data extracted from the recent literature do not support the use of complex closed drainage systems in ICU patients in view of the increased cost.

Owing to the lack of specific ICU studies, the guidelines for the management of drainage systems should be viewed as recommendations at best.

The following are reasonable suggestions:

1. Only people who know the proper technique of aseptic insertion and maintenance of the catheter should handle catheters.
2. Hospital personnel should be given periodic in-service training stressing the proper techniques and potential complications of urinary catheterization.
3. Hand washing should be performed immediately before and after any manipulation of the catheter site or apparatus.
4. If small volumes of fresh urine are needed for examination, the distal end of the catheter, or preferably the sampling port if present, should be cleansed with a disinfectant, and urine then aspirated with a sterile needle and syringe.
5. Larger volumes of urine for special analyses should be obtained aseptically from the drainage bag.
6. Unobstructed flow should be maintained.
7. In order to achieve free flow of urine, (a) the catheter and collection tube should be kept from kinking; (b) the collection bag should be emptied regularly using a separate collecting container for each patient (the draining spigot and nonsterile collection container should never come into contact); (c) poorly functioning or obstructed catheters should be irrigated or, if necessary, replaced; (d) collection bags should always be kept below the level of the bladder; and (e) indwelling catheters should not be changed at arbitrary fixed intervals (36).

Types of Urethral Catheters

There are a large number of articles in the literature that stress the efficacy of antiseptic-impregnated catheters, including silver oxide or silver alloy, and antibiotic-impregnated catheters in hospitalized patients (37–39). The results of two meta-analyses clarify some points (38,39) related to these devices.

Silver oxide catheters are not associated with a reduction in bacteriuria in short-term catheterized adults, whereas silver alloy catheters reduce the incidence of asymptomatic bacteriuria and the risk of symptomatic UTI in catheterized adults. Further, economic evaluation is required to confirm that the reduction of infection compensates for their increased cost. Catheters coated with a combination of minocycline and rifampin or nitrofurazone may also be beneficial in reducing bacteriuria in hospitalized men catheterized less than 1 week, but this requires further testing (38,39). No trials directly compare nitrofurazone-coated and silver alloy–coated catheters.

In a specific ICU patient population, a randomized, prospective, double-blind multicenter trial compared catheters coated with hydrogel and silver salt with classic urinary tract catheters in 199 patients requiring urethral catheterization for more than 3 days (40). The cumulative incidence of UTIs associated with catheterization was 11.1% overall, 11.9% for the control group, and 10% for the coated catheter group. The odds ratio was 0.82 (95% confidence interval [CI] 0.3–2.2). The differences between the two groups were not significant, although the power of the study was more than 90% (40). A prior trial, which included five hospitals selected to participate in a blinded prospective study, exchanged the standard latex Foley catheter for a hydrogel latex Foley catheter with a monolayer of silver metal applied to the inner and outer surfaces of the device. The adjusted catheter-associated infection rate during the baseline and intervention periods was 8.1 and 4.9 infections per 1,000 catheter-days ($p = 0.13$), respectively (41).

Meatal Care

Twice-daily cleansing of the urethral meatus with povidone-iodine solution and daily cleansing with soap and water have failed to reduce catheter-associated UTIs. Thus, at this time, daily meatal care with either of these two regimens cannot be endorsed.

A randomized, controlled, prospective clinical trial involving 696 patients hospitalized in medical and surgical units was undertaken to determine the effectiveness of 1% silver sulfadiazine cream applied twice daily to the urethral meatus in preventing transurethral catheter-associated bacteriuria. The overall incidence of bacteriuria was approximately 13% in both groups ($p = 0.56$) (42). In the absence of data from an ICU-specific patient population, the current guidelines should be followed.

There are no data available on the level of sterility required to insert a urinary catheter. Experts recommend that catheters should be inserted using an aseptic technique and sterile equipment, including gloves, drapes, and sponges. However, in a prospective study conducted in the operating room, 156 patients underwent preoperative urethral catheterization, randomly allocated to "sterile" or "clean/nonsterile" technique groups. There was no statistical difference between the two groups with respect to the incidence of UTI, but the cost differed considerably between the two groups (43).

Vesical Irrigation and Antiseptic in the Drainage System

The objective of antibiotic irrigation is to clear bacteria from the urinary tract. A randomized study compared 89 patients receiving a neomycin-polymyxin irrigation administered through a closed urinary catheter to 98 patients not so irrigated. Although the number of ICU patients was not specified in this clinical study, 19 of the 98 (18%) patients not irrigated became infected as compared with 14 out of the 89 (16%) of those who were irrigated; the organisms from the irrigated patients were more resistant (44). Another study was conducted in 264 urology patients, evaluating the effect of povidone-iodine bladder irrigation prior to catheter removal on subsequent bacteriuria. Of 264 patients, 138 received irrigation and 126 were controls. Urine cultures were positive in 22% in the control group and 18% in the study group (45). Thus, irrigation methods failed to demonstrate efficacy in surgical patients, and its use is not recommended in ICU patients.

The addition of antimicrobial agents to the drainage device has not been studied in the ICU. The largest reported clinical trial evaluating the effect of H_2O_2 insertion into the drainage device of 353 patients, and comparing this to 315 control patients, failed to show a benefit in the treatment group. It is of interest to note that 68% of these patients required an indwelling catheter for hemodynamic monitoring, with antimicrobial therapy prescribed in 75% of the patients, suggesting that these results may apply to ICU patients (46). Expert opinion recommends that we not use irrigation unless obstruction is anticipated, as might occur with bleeding after prostatic or bladder surgery.

Alternatives to a Urinary Catheter

For selected patients, other methods of urinary drainage, such as condom catheters, suprapubic catheterization, and intermittent urethral catheterization, should be considered as alternatives to indwelling urethral catheterization. There are limited ICU data available to assess these alternative devices. There is evidence, however, that suprapubic catheterization is advantageous, as compared to indwelling catheters, with respect to bacteriuria, recatheterization, and discomfort (47,48). The use of a condom connected to a collection bag has been evaluated in a study comparing 167 patients over two periods of 6 months. The occurrence of bacteriuria was significantly decreased for the period using the condom catheters (26.7 vs. 2.4%) (49). However, this issue merits further study to determine whether or not this alternative method may actually reduce bacteriuria rates. The use of intermittent catheterization is also associated with a lower risk of bacteriuria than indwelling urethral catheter, although such a procedure has never been investigated in ICU patients (48,50,51).

Miscellaneous Measures

While there is a low risk of bacteremia during urinary catheterization (52), the administration of antimicrobial therapy at the time the device is placed leads to a reduction in bacteriuria (53–55). The efficacy of antibiotic treatment has been assessed as optimal for catheterization lasting less than 14 days (54). However, the prophylactic use of antibiotic in the ICU can be detrimental to the bacterial ecology by increasing the pressure for antimicrobial resistance among bacteria. The practice of administration of prophylactic antimicrobials in this manner must be discouraged in our ICUs. It should be noted that in most ICU studies, 75% of the patients with an indwelling catheter require antibiotics for reasons unrelated to the urinary catheter (8). Further, all measures aimed at reducing the burden of nosocomial infections can reduce the rate of UTIs (56–58).

TREATMENT AND MANAGEMENT

The management of catheter-associated UTI has not been evaluated in ICU patients. Several nonspecific measures, including hydration, have been advocated in the therapy of UTI. Adequate hydration would appear to be important, although there is no evidence that it improves the effectiveness of an appropriate antimicrobial therapy (59). The management of complicated UTIs in the ICU may include mechanical intervention. Consequently, appropriate diagnostic tests and urologic consultation should be included in the algorithm of the management of these patients (Fig. 113.1).

Management of Asymptomatic Bacteriuria

According to leaders in our field, asymptomatic catheter-associated UTI does not require treatment (28). However, antimicrobial treatment may be considered for asymptomatic women with a catheter-acquired UTI that persists 48 hours after catheter removal (60). In a specific ICU patient population, 60 patients with an indwelling urethral catheter for longer than 48 hours who developed an asymptomatic positive urine culture were randomized to receive either a 3-day course of antibiotics associated with the replacement of the indwelling urethral catheter 4 hours after the first antibiotic administration or no antibiotics and no catheter replacement. Six patients equally distributed in the two groups developed urosepsis. The profile of bacterial resistance was similar in the two groups. Hence, treating a positive urine culture in an asymptomatic patient with an indwelling urethral catheter does not reduce the occurrence of urosepsis (20).

Management of Symptomatic Urinary Tract Infections

Choice of Antimicrobial Agents

The optimal characteristics of agents to treat urinary tract infection must include activity against the major pathogens involved in these infections, good tissue penetration, and minimal side effects. High urinary levels should be present for an adequate period to eliminate the organisms, since disappearance of bacteriuria correlates with the sensitivity of the pathogen to the concentration of the antimicrobial agent achieved in the urine (61). Inhibitory urinary concentrations are achieved after administration of essentially all commonly used antibiotics. However, an antibiotic that achieves active concentrations in the renal tissue is required for infection of the renal tissue. The antibiotic concentration in the serum or plasma can be used as surrogate markers for the antibiotic concentrations in the renal tissue (62). For drugs with concentration-dependent time-kill activity such as the aminoglycosides or the fluoroquinolones, the peak antibiotic concentration is the most important parameter for the *in vivo* effect. Experimentally, gentamicin and

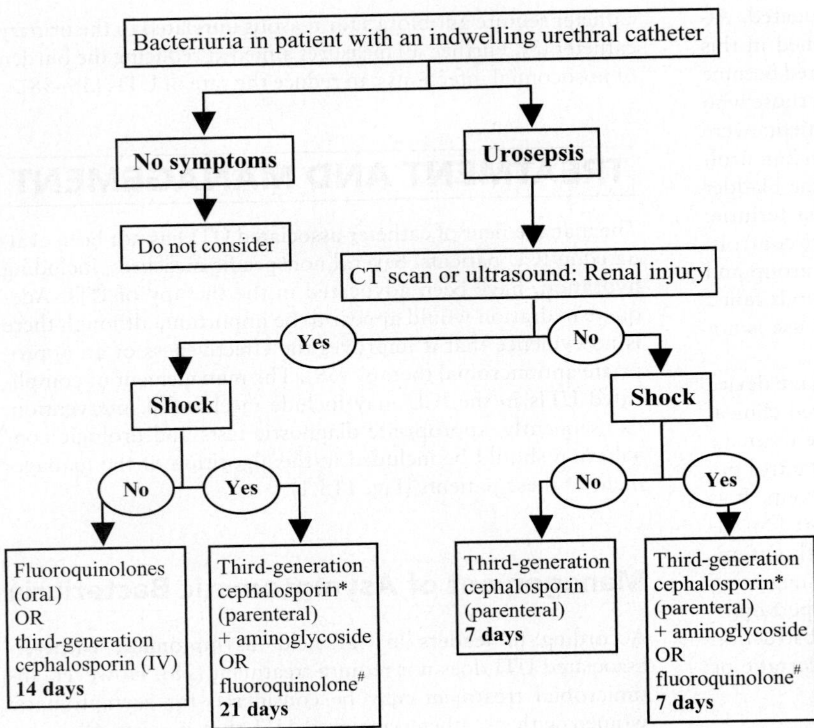

FIGURE 113.1. Suggested algorithm for the management of urinary tract infections related to an indwelling catheter in the intensive care unit. CT, computed tomography. *Discuss the need for antipseudomonal coverage according to the duration of hospitalization, prior medical history, and local ecology. #Discuss if renal failure.

fluoroquinolone treatment are both more effective than the β-lactam antibiotics in rapid bacterial killing (62).

Most clinical studies have shown that the renal concentrations of the cephalosporins remained higher than the minimal inhibitory concentration for the most common bacteria during the time interval between the administration of two doses (63–65). By contrast, β-lactam antibiotics, which have a low pKa and poor lipid solubility, penetrate poorly into the prostate, except for some cephalosporins. Good to excellent penetration into the prostatic tissue has been demonstrated with many antimicrobial agents, such as aminoglycosides, fluoroquinolones, sulfonamides, and nitrofurantoin (66).

In ICU patients, the side effects of treatment should be minimized at both the individual and the community level. Many patients develop renal failure, associated with the inability to concentrate antimicrobial agents in the urine. Additionally, administration of drugs with potential renal toxicity may worsen renal insufficiency. This may be an important limiting factor for using aminoglycosides in patients with renal failure. Otherwise, antimicrobial treatment must produce a minimal effect on the bacterial flora of the community (67). From this standpoint, there is significant literature demonstrating that the use of fluoroquinolone is associated with the emergence of resistant pathogens (68–70). This implies that an indication for antibacterial therapy should be weighed thoroughly and fluoroquinolones should be used in accordance with sensitivity testing (70). Hence, it is of importance to stress that UTI should not be treated before the results of sensitivity testing, except in patients with pyelonephritis and those with severe sepsis or septic shock who require empirical antimicrobial therapy.

Cystitis

As acute uncomplicated cystitis is infrequent in ICU patients, most recommendations focus on the treatment of nonhospitalized women, which makes their relevance in ICU patients questionable; *E. coli* is the evident target pathogen. The 1999 IDSA guidelines recommend treatment with trimethoprim-sulfamethoxazole for 3 days as standard therapy for acute uncomplicated cystitis. Single-dose therapy is less effective in eradicating initial bacteriuria than longer durations of treatment with trimethoprim-sulfamethoxazole, trimethoprim, norfloxacin, ciprofloxacin, fleroxacin, and, as a group, β-lactam antibiotics (71). In contrast, a meta-analysis determined that 3 days of antibiotic therapy is similar to 5 to 10 days in achieving symptomatic cure during uncomplicated UTI treatment, while the longer treatment is more effective in obtaining bacteriologic cure. Consequently, such durations should be considered for treatment of women in whom eradication is critical (72). Quinolones are recommended for acute cystitis in regions where the level of resistance to trimethoprim-sulfamethoxazole is high. There were no significant differences in clinical or microbiologic efficacy between quinolones. The rate of adverse events causing antimicrobial withdrawal tends to be lower with norfloxacin and ciprofloxacin than with other quinolones (73).

Antibiotic treatment of UTI depends on the ability of the antibiotic to inhibit the growth or kill the bacteria present in the urinary tract. This is related to the concentration of antibiotics at the site of infection. Very high concentrations of antibiotics with renal clearance are obtained in urine. Consequently, even in the presence of pathogens exhibiting *in vitro* resistance, the high concentrations of antibiotics in urine inhibit the growth of pathogens, rendering them effective to treat a UTI.

Prostatitis

For outpatients, bacterial prostatitis is a common diagnosis and a frequent indication for antibiotics. Although urethral instrumentation and prostatic surgery are known causes of prostatitis, the incidence of prostatitis among ICU patients has never been assessed, and there is only a weak relation between acute and chronic prostatitis.

Acute prostatitis is an acute infection producing local heat, tenderness, and fever, with the presence of IgA and IgG bacteria-specific immunoglobulins in the prostatic secretions. Few symptoms, usually perineal discomfort, are exhibited with prostatitis. Most patients with chronic prostatitis have no history of positive urine or urethral cultures (74).

In ICU patients, acute bacterial prostatitis is probably a common infection. The patient presents septic, but without an evident source of infection. There may be a history of urine retention due to bladder outlet obstruction. Rectal examination, a crucial step in the diagnosis, reveals a warm, swollen, and tender prostate. The prostatic fluid contains leukocytes and the pathogen responsible for the infection. However, massage of the prostate is proscribed to avoid bacteremia. Fluoroquinolones are the drugs of choice to treat acute prostatitis because of their excellent penetration in the tissue and excretions (75,76). The targeted pathogens are *E. coli*, *Proteus* sp., *Klebsiella* sp., *Enterococcus* sp., *Staphylococcus aureus*, *Neisseria gonorrhoeae*, and *Chlamydia trachomatis*. For acute prostatitis occurring without bacteremia, antimicrobial treatment consists of oral ofloxacin 200 mg twice per day for 28 days; ceftriaxone 2 g/day has good prostatic tissue penetration and represents an alternative to ofloxacin (77). Gentamicin 3 mg/kg/day is added in the presence of positive blood cultures (Table 113.8). Of importance, urethral instrumentation should be discouraged, and if acute retention occurs, suprapubic drainage of urine is required. Treatment of chronic prostatitis is based on the oral administration of ofloxacin 200 mg twice per day, or trimethoprim 160 mg–sulfamethoxazole 800 mg twice per day for at least 28 days. The indications for this treatment should be discussed with specialists.

Acute Pyelonephritis

There are no specific data available in the literature on the management of acute pyelonephritis in the ICU. The urine of all patients with suspicion of complicated pyelonephritis should be cultured and a Gram stain of the spun urine performed. Blood cultures, which are positive in 36% of women not admitted to the ICU, are also required (78). All patients with acute pyelonephritis should have an ultrasound examination or a renal computed tomography scan to evaluate for obstruction and stones.

For uncomplicated acute pyelonephritis, the IDSA, in 1999, derived two conclusions from the analysis of randomized clinical trials. The first is that trimethoprim-sulfamethoxazole is preferred over ampicillin. Indeed, there is a relatively high prevalence of organisms causing acute pyelonephritis that are resistant to ampicillin, and even for susceptible organisms, there is a significantly increased recurrence rate in patients given ampicillin compared with those given trimethoprim-sulfamethiazole. The second conclusion is that 10 to 14 days of therapy appears to be adequate for the majority of women (71). There has been little additional information since the publication of these recommendations. However, 255 outpatients were randomized to oral ciprofloxacin, 500 mg twice per day for 7 days, followed by placebo for 7 days versus trimethoprim-sulfamethoxazole, 160/800 mg twice per day for 14 days. In this study, a 7-day ciprofloxacin regimen was associated with greater bacteriologic and clinical cure rates than a 14-day trimethoprim-sulfamethoxazole regimen (79)

TABLE 113.8

ANTIMICROBIAL TREATMENT OF URINARY TRACT INFECTIONS[a]

Source of infection	Pathogens	Treatment	Duration
Acute prostatitis (without bacteremia)	*Escherichia coli*, *Proteus* sp., *Klebsiella* sp., *Enterococcus* sp., *Staphylococcus aureus*, *Neisseria gonorrhoeae*, *Chlamydia trachomatis*	Ofloxacin 200 mg twice daily (oral)	28 d
Acute prostatitis (with bacteremia)	*E. coli*, *Proteus* sp., *Klebsiella* sp., *Enterococcus* sp., *S. aureus*, *N. gonorrhoeae*, *C. trachomatis*	Ofloxacin 200 mg twice daily (oral) or Ceftriaxone 2 g/d and gentamicin 3 mg/kg/d IV	28 d 3 d
Chronic bacterial prostatitis	*E. coli*, *Proteus* sp., *Klebsiella* sp., *Enterococcus* sp., *S. aureus*, *N. gonorrhoeae*, *C. trachomatis*	Ofloxacin 200 mg twice daily (oral) or Trimethoprim 160 mg/sulfamethoxazole 800 mg twice daily (oral)	28 d
Acute pyelonephritis (uncomplicated)	Enterobacteriaceae, *E. coli*, *Proteus* sp., *Enterococcus* sp.	Ciprofloxacin 500 mg twice daily (oral) If oral route not possible: Ceftriaxone 2 g/d IV	14 d
Acute pyelonephritis (complicated)	Enterobacteriaceae, *E. coli*, *Proteus* sp., *Enterococcus* sp.	Ciprofloxacin 500 mg twice daily (oral) or Ceftriaxone 2 g/d IV AND Gentamicin 3 mg/kg/d	14–21 d 3 d

Each empirical treatment must be adapted to the susceptibility testing results.

(Table 113.8). Gatifloxacin appears to be equivalent to ciprofloxacin for this indication (80).

Patients with complicated acute pyelonephritis should be hospitalized and initial administration of broad-spectrum intravenous antibiotics begun. The targeted bacteria are *Enterobacter* sp., *E. coli*, *Proteus* sp., and *Enterococcus* sp. Ciprofloxacin, 500 mg twice daily, is administered orally for 14 to 21 days. Gentamicin, 3 mg/kg/day intravenously, is added during the first 3 days. Interestingly, oral ciprofloxacin is as effective as the intravenous regimen in the initial empirical management of complicated pyelonephritis (81), and gatifloxacin is as effective as ciprofloxacin (80). If needed, ceftriaxone, 2 g/day intravenously, is an alternative choice to ciprofloxacin. Further, the success rates are similar in patients given ceftriaxone or ertapenem (82).

The drainage of urine must be urgently performed using bladder catheterization, percutaneous nephrostomy drainage, or definitive surgery. Antimicrobial treatment is administered after urine and blood specimen collection. The antibiotic selection is based on the result of the Gram stain of the urine and the knowledge of the local ecology. Antimicrobial treatment should be adapted to the susceptibility testing results as soon as possible, and de-escalation should be performed in favor of a narrow-spectrum antibiotic.

Specificities of Complicated Urinary Tract Infections in the Intensive Care Unit

Although there is little in the literature on the treatment of UTIs in the ICU, one presumes the need for intravenous antibiotics for these patients because of the possibility of bacteremia or sepsis. The guidelines from the Surviving Sepsis Campaign state that (a) antibiotic therapy should be started within the first hour of recognition of severe sepsis, after appropriate cultures have been obtained; (b) initial empirical anti-infective therapy should include one or more drugs that have activity against the likely pathogens and that penetrate the presumed source of sepsis; and (c) monotherapy is as effective as combination therapy with a β-lactam and an aminoglycoside as empiric therapy of patients with severe sepsis or septic shock (83). Hence, empirical antimicrobial therapy should include drugs with good penetration in the urinary tract, and the choice is guided by the susceptibility patterns of micro-organisms in the hospital. For the septic shock patients whose presumed source is urine, we recommend, empirically, a combination of a β-lactam antibiotic with antipseudomonal activity and a fluoroquinolone. This broad-spectrum treatment is narrowed as soon as the results of the susceptibility testing are known. The durations of treatment should be tailored to the source of infection.

Management of Candiduria

Candiduria represents from 3% to 15% of catheter-associated UTI in the ICU (8,9,13). *Candida albicans* and *Candida (Torulopsis) glabrata* are found in 46% and 31% of cases, respectively (84). According to the International Conference for the Development of a Consensus on the Management and Prevention of Severe Candidal Infections, colonized patients without evidence of infection do not require treatment, but the contributing cause should be addressed, such as changing or removing the indwelling catheter and discontinuing inappropriate antibiotic therapy. Fluconazole may be the best option for treating a candiduria (85), but only if the species is *C. albicans*. Voriconazole may be more effective against non-*albicans* species.

Clinician reaction to isolating *Candida* organisms in urine was assessed in a retrospective review of 133 consecutive patients. The average patient age was 68.8 years old, most (78%) had an indwelling catheter, and many (35%) were in the ICU. In response to culture results, clinicians initiated antifungal therapy in 80 instances (60%). Treatment was often based on a single culture result without evidence of infection (66%) and in the absence of risk of invasive disease. Removal of the indwelling catheter was never attempted and antibiotics were rarely discontinued or modified (1.3%). Fluconazole was most frequently utilized (52%), followed by amphotericin B bladder irrigation (32%) and combined fluconazole/amphotericin B bladder irrigation (15%). Therapy was more frequently initiated in ICU cases (77 vs. 56%; $p = 0.02$) (86). These results show the poor adherence to guidelines.

A prospective, randomized trial compared fungal eradication rates among 316 hospitalized patients with candiduria treated with fluconazole (200 mg) or placebo daily for 14 days. Candiduria cleared by day 14 in 50% of the patients receiving fluconazole and 29% of those receiving placebo, with higher eradication rates among patients completing 14 days of therapy. Fluconazole initially produced high eradication rates, but cultures at 2 weeks revealed similar candiduria rates among treated and untreated patients. In 41% of the catheterized subjects, candiduria was resolved as the result of catheter removal only. The outcomes of patients were not provided in the results (87).

Bladder irrigation using amphotericin B has been proposed as an alternative technique to clear *Candida* from the urine. A comparative and randomized study of 109 elderly patients showed that funguria was eradicated in 96% of the patients treated with amphotericin B and 73% of those treated with fluconazole ($p < 0.05$). One month after study enrollment, the mortality rate associated with all causes was greater among patients who were treated with amphotericin B bladder irrigation than among those who received oral fluconazole therapy (41% vs. 22%, respectively; $p < 0.05$). This finding suggests that irrigation therapy could be associated with poorer survival (88).

There has only been one study performed in ICU patients developing candiduria, which reached the same conclusions; unfortunately, methodologic issues restrict the interest of this study. The authors retrospectively compared three means to manage candiduria in ICU patients: successful bladder irrigation with amphotericin B (10 of 27 patients), failure of bladder irrigation requiring the use of parenteral amphotericin B (17 of 27), and patients treated with parenteral fluconazole ($n = 20$). Severity score on admission day was significantly lower in the first group than in the two others. However, the mortality rate was 53% and 5% in patients experiencing a failure of bladder irrigation and in patients receiving fluconazole, respectively (89). These results must be considered with caution because of serious methodologic limitations. However, these data indicate that bladder irrigation of critically ill patients has a negative survival advantage.

SUMMARY

Bacteria in the bladder constitute a reservoir for the development of multiresistant bacterial strains, and the rate of bacteriuria may be used as a marker of the level of care in the

ICU. Prevention of UTIs in the ICU is not improved by the use of expensive devices, but can reflect the level of general unit hygiene. While management of UTIs in the ICU is poorly described in the literature, it is reasonably clear that there is no need to treat asymptomatic bacteriuria. However, although infrequent, severe sepsis with a urine source requires empirical broad-spectrum antimicrobial treatment based on the local bacterial ecology. Treatment is de-escalated after identification of the pathogen and reporting of the susceptibility testing.

References

1. Richards MJ, Edwards JR, Culver DH, et al. Nosocomial infections in medical intensive care units in the United States. National Nosocomial Infections Surveillance System. *Crit Care Med.* 1999;27:887.
2. Bagshaw SM, Laupland KB. Epidemiology of intensive care unit-acquired urinary tract infections. *Curr Opin Infect Dis.* 2006;19:67.
3. Vincent JL, Bihari DJ, Suter PM, et al. The prevalence of nosocomial infection in intensive care units in Europe. Results of the European Prevalence of Infection in Intensive Care (EPIC) Study. EPIC International Advisory Committee. *JAMA.* 1995;274:639.
4. Rosser CJ, Bare RL, Meredith JW. Urinary tract infections in the critical ill patient with a urinary catheter. *Am J Surg.* 1999;177:287.
5. Garner JS, Jarvis WR, Emori TG, et al. CDC definitions for nosocomial infections, 1988. *Am J Infect Control.* 1988;16:128.
6. Agace W, Connell H, Svanborg C. Host resistance to urinary tract infection. In: Mobley HLT, Warren JW, eds. *Urinary Tract Infections. Molecular Pathogenesis and Clinical Management.* Washington, DC: ASM Press; 1996: 221.
7. Trautner BW, Darouiche RO. Role of biofilm in catheter-associated urinary tract infection. *Am J Infect Control.* 2004;32:177.
8. Leone M, Albanese J, Garnier F, et al. Risk factors of nosocomial catheter-associated urinary tract infection in a polyvalent intensive care unit. *Intensive Care Med.* 2003;29:1077.
9. Laupland KB, Bagshaw SM, Gregson DB, et al. Intensive care unit-acquired urinary tract infections in a regional critical care system. *Crit Care.* 2005;9:R60.
10. Gaynes R, Edwards JR, National Nosocomial Infections Surveillance System. Overview of nosocomial infections caused by gram-negative bacilli. *Clin Infect Dis.* 2005;41:848.
11. Wagenlehner FME, Naber KG. Emergence of antibiotic resistance and prudent use of antibiotic therapy in nosocomially acquired urinary tract infection. *Int J Antimicrobial Agents.* 2004;23(Suppl 1):24.
12. Wagenlehner FME, Krcmery S, Held C, et al. Epidemiological analysis of the spread of pathogens from a urological ward using genotypic, phenotypic and clinical parameters. *Int J Antimicrobial Agents.* 2002;19:583.
13. Tissot E, Limat S, Cornette C, et al. Risk factors for catheter-associated bacteriuria in a medical intensive care unit. *Eur J Clin Microbiol Infect Dis.* 2001;20:260.
14. Jain P, Parada JP, David A, et al. Overuse of the indwelling urinary tract catheter in hospitalized medical patients. *Arch Intern Med.* 1995;155:1425.
15. Platt R. Adverse consequences of asymptomatic urinary tract infections in adults. *Am J Med.* 1987;82(Suppl 6B):47.
16. Platt R, Polk BF, Murdock B, et al. Mortality associated with nosocomial urinary-tract infection. *N Engl J Med.* 1982;307:637.
17. Mnatzaganian G, Galai N, Sprung CL, et al. Increased risk of bloodstream and urinary infections in intensive care unit (ICU) patients compared with patients fitting ICU admission criteria treated in regular wards. *J Hosp Infect.* 2005;59:331.
18. Vincent JL, Sakr Y, Sprung CL, et al. Sepsis in European intensive care units: results of the SOAP study. *Crit Care Med.* 2006;34:344.
19. Angus DC, Linde-Zwirble WT, Lidicker J, et al. Epidemiology of severe sepsis in the United States: analysis of incidence, outcome, and associated costs of care. *Crit Care Med.* 2001;29:1303.
20. Leone M, Perrin AS, Granier I, et al. A randomized trial of catheter change and short course of antibiotics for asymptomatic bacteriuria in catheterized ICU patients. *Intensive Care Med.* 2007;33:726.
21. Tambyah PA, Maki DG. Catheter associated urinary tract infection is rarely symptomatic: a prospective study of 1497 catheterized patients. *Arch Intern Med.* 2000;160:678.
22. Saint S. Clinical and economic consequences of nosocomial catheter-related bacteriuria. *Am J Infect Control.* 2000;28:68.
23. Inan D, Saba R, Gunseren F, et al. Daily antibiotic cost of nosocomial infections in a Turkish university hospital. *BMC Infect Dis.* 2005;5:5.
24. Garibaldi RA, Mooney BR, Epstein BJ, et al. An evaluation of daily bacteriologic monitoring to identify preventable episodes of catheter-associated urinary tract infection. *Infect Control.* 1982;3:466.
25. Tissot E, Woronoff-Lemsi MC, Cornette C, et al. Cost-effectiveness of urinary dipsticks to screen asymptomatic catheter-associated urinary infections in an intensive care unit. *Intensive Care Med.* 2001;27:1842.
26. Legras A, Cattier B, Perrotin D. Dépistage des infections urinaires dans un service de réanimation: intéret des bandelettes réactives. *Med Mal Infect.* 1993;23:34.
27. Mimoz O, Bouchet E, Edouard A, et al. Limited usefulness of urinary dipsticks to screen out catheter-associated bacteriuria in ICU patients. *Anaesth Intens Care.* 1995;23:706.
28. Nicolle LE, Bradley S, Colgan R, et al. Infectious diseases society of America guidelines for the diagnosis and treatment of asymptomatic bacteriuria in adults. *Clin Infect Dis.* 2005;40:643.
29. Warren JW. Catheter-associated urinary tract infections. *Int J Antimicrob Agents.* 2001;17:299.
30. Kunin CM, McCormack RC. Prevention of catheter-induced urinary-tract infections by sterile closed drainage. *N Engl J Med.* 1966;274:1155.
31. Huth TS, Burke JP, Larsen LA, et al. Clinical trial of junction seals for the prevention of urinary catheter-associated bacteriuria. *Arch Intern Med.* 1992;152:807.
32. Degroot-Kosolcharoen J, Guse J, Jones JM. Evaluation of a urinary catheter with a preconnected closed drainage bag. *Infect Control Hosp Epidemiol.* 1998;9:72.
33. Wille JC, Blusse Van Oud Alblas A, Thewessen EAPM. Nosocomial catheter-associated bacteriuria: a clinical trial comparing two closed urinary drainage systems. *J Hosp Infect.* 1993;25:191.
34. Leone M, Garnier F, Dubuc M, et al. Prevention of nosocomial urinary tract infection in ICU patients. Comparison of effectiveness of two urinary drainage systems. *Chest.* 2001;120:220.
35. Leone M, Garnier F, Antonini F, et al. Comparison of effectiveness of two urinary drainage systems in intensive care unit: a prospective, randomized clinical trial. *Intensive Care Med.* 2003;29:410.
36. Leone M, Garnier F, Avidan M, et al. Catheter-associated urinary tract infections in intensive care units. *Microbes Infect.* 2004;6:1026.
37. Davenport K, Keeley FX. Evidence for the use of silver-alloy-coated urethral catheters. *J Hosp Infect.* 2005;60:298.
38. Brosnahan J, Jull A, Tracy C. Types of urethral catheters for management of short-term voiding problems in hospitalized adults. *Cochrane Database Syst Rev.* 2004;1:CD004013.
39. Johnson JR, Kuskowski MA, Wilt TJ. Systematic review: antimicrobial urinary catheters to prevent catheter-associated urinary tract infection in hospitalized patients. *Ann Intern Med.* 2006;144:116.
40. Thibon P, Le Coutour X, Leroyer R, et al. Randomized multi-centre trial of the effects of a catheter coated with hydrogel and silver salts on the incidence of hospital-acquired urinary tract infections. *J Hosp Infect.* 2000;45:117.
41. Bologna RA, Tu LM, Polansky M, et al. Hydrogel/silver ion-coated urinary catheter reduces nosocomial urinary tract infection rates in intensive care unit patients: a multicenter study. *Urology.* 1999;54:982.
42. Huth TS, Burke JP, Larsen RA, et al. Randomized trial of meatal care with silver sulfadiazine cream for the prevention of catheter-associated bacteriuria. *J Infect Dis.* 1992;165:14.
43. Carapeti EA, Andrew SM, Bentley PG. Randomised study of sterile versus non-sterile urethral catheterisation. *Ann R Surg Engl.* 1994;76:59.
44. Warren JW, Platt R, Thomas RJ, et al. Antibiotic irrigation and catheter-associated urinary-tract infections. *N Engl J Med.* 1978;299:570.
45. Schneeberger PM, Vreede RW, Bogdanowicz JFTA, et al. A randomized study on the effect of bladder irrigation with povidone-iodine before removal of an indwelling catheter. *J Hosp Infect.* 1992;21:223.
46. Thompson RL, Haley CE, Searcy MA, et al. Catheter associated with bacteriuria. Failure to reduce attacks rates using periodic instillations of a disinfectant into urinary drainage system. *JAMA.* 1984;251:747.
47. Vandoni RE, Lironi A, Tschantz P. Bacteriuria during urinary tract catheterization: suprapubic versus urethral route: a prospective randomized trial. *Acta Chir Belg.* 1994;94:12.
48. Niel-Weise BS, van den Broek PJ. Urinary catheter policies for short-term bladder drainage in adults. *Cochrane Database Syst Rev.* 2005;3: CD004203.
49. Harti A, Bouaggad A, Barrou H, et al. Prévention de l'infection urinaire nosocomiale: sondage vésical versus Pénilex. *Cah Anesthesiol.* 1994;42:31.
50. Tang MW, Kwok TC, Hui E, et al. Intermittent versus indwelling urinary catheterization in older female patients. *Maturitas.* 2006;53:274.
51. Ghalayini IF, Al-Ghazo MA, Pickard RS. A prospective randomized trial comparing transurethral prostatic resection and clean intermittent self-catheterization in men with chronic urinary retention. *BJU Int.* 2005;96: 93.
52. Bregenzer T, Frei R, Widmer AF, et al. Low risk of bacteremia during catheter replacement in patients with long-term urinary catheters. *Arch Intern Med.* 1997;157:521.
53. van der Wall E, Verkooyen RP, Mintjes-de Groot J, et al. Prophylactic ciprofloxacin for catheter-associated urinary-tract infection. *Lancet.* 1992;339:946.
54. Hustinx WNM, Mintjes-de Groot AJ, Verkooyen RP, et al. Impact of concurrent antimicrobial therapy on catheter-associated urinary tract infection. *J Hosp Infect.* 1991;18:45.
55. Niel-Weise BS, van den Broek PJ. Antibiotic policies for short-term catheter bladder drainage in adults. *Cochrane Database Syst Rev.* 2005;3: CD005428.
56. Verwaest C, Verhaegen J, Ferdinande P, et al. Randomized, controlled trial of selective digestive decontamination in 600 mechanically ventilated patients in a multidisciplinary intensive care unit. *Crit Care Med.* 1997;25:63.

57. Senkal M, Mumme A, Eickhoff U, et al. Early postoperative enteral immunonutrition: clinical outcome and cost-comparison analysis in surgical patients. *Crit Care Med.* 2000;28:1255.
58. Nourdine K, Combes P, Carton MJ, et al. Does noninvasive ventilation reduce the ICU nosocomial risk? A prospective clinical survey. *Intensive Care Med.* 1999;25:567.
59. Beetz R. Mild dehydration: a risk factor of urinary tract infection? *Eur J Clin Nutr.* 2003;57(Suppl 2):S52.
60. Harding GKM, Nicolle LE, Ronald AR, et al. How long should catheter-associated urinary tract infection in women be treated. *Ann Intern Med.* 1991;114:713.
61. Stamey TA, Fair WR, Timothy MM, et al. Serum versus urinary antimicrobial concentrations in case of urinary tract infections. *N Engl J Med.* 1974;291:1159.
62. Frimodt-Moller N. Correlation between pharmacokinetic/pharmacodynamic parameters and efficacy for antibiotics in the treatment of urinary tract infection. *Int J Antimicrob Agents.* 2002;19:546.
63. Leone M, Albanese J, Tod M, et al. Ceftriaxone (1 g intravenously) penetration into abdominal tissues when administered as antibiotic prophylaxis during nephrectomy. *J Chemother.* 2003;15:139.
64. Leroy A, Oser B, Grise P, et al. Cefixime penetration in human renal parenchyma. *Antimicrob Agents Chemother.* 1995;39:1240.
65. Saito I, Saiko Y, Tahara T, et al. Penetration of cefpirome into renal and prostatic tissue. *Int J Clin Pharmacol Res.* 1993;13:317.
66. Charalabopoulos K, Karachalios G, Baltogiannis D, et al. Penetration of antimicrobial agents into the prostate. *Chemotherapy.* 2003;49:269.
67. Neu HC. Optimal characteristics of agents to treat uncomplicated urinary tract infections. *Infection.* 1992;20(Suppl 4):S266.
68. Ray GT, Baxter R, DeLorenze GN. Hospital-level rates of fluoroquinolone use and the risk of hospital-acquired infection with ciprofloxacin-nonsusceptible *Pseudomonas aeruginosa*. *Clin Infect Dis.* 2005;41: 441.
69. Lautenbach E, Strom BL, Nachamkin I, et al. Longitudinal trends in fluoroquinolone resistance among Enterobacteriaceae isolates from inpatients and outpatients, 1989–2000: differences in the emergence and epidemiology of resistance across organisms. *Clin Infect Dis.* 2004;38:655.
70. Naber KG, Witte W, Bauernfeind A, et al. Clinical significance and spread of fluoroquinolone resistant uropathogens in hospitalised urological patients. *Infection.* 1994;22(Suppl 2):S122.
71. Warren JW, Abrutyn E, Hebel JR, et al. Guidelines for antimicrobial treatment of uncomplicated acute bacterial cystitis and acute pyelonephritis in women. Infectious Diseases Society of America (IDSA). *Clin Infect Dis.* 1999;29:745.
72. Milo G, Katchman EA, Paul M, et al. Duration of antibacterial treatment for uncomplicated urinary tract infection in women. *Cochrane Database Syst Rev.* 2005;2:CD004682.
73. Rafalsky V, Andreeva I, Rjabkova E. Quinolones for uncomplicated acute cystitis in women. *Cochrane Database Syst Rev.* 2006;3:CD003597.
74. Krieger JN, Riley DE. Prostatitis: what is the role of infection. *Int J Antimicrob Agents.* 2002;19:475.
75. Wagenlehner FME, Naber KG. Current challenges in the treatment of complicated urinary tract infections and prostatitis. *Clin Microbiol Infect.* 2006;12(Suppl 3):67.
76. Sampol-Manos E, Leone M, Karouia D, et al. Prophylaxis with ciprofloxacin for open prostatectomy: comparison of tissue penetration with two oral doses. *J Chemother.* 2006;18:225.
77. Martin C, Viviand X, Cottin A, et al. Concentrations of ceftriaxone (1,000 milligrams intravenously) in abdominal tissues during open prostatectomy. *Antimicrob Agents Chemother.* 1996;40:1311.
78. Smith WR, McClish DK, Poses RM, et al. Bacteremia in young urban women admitted with pyelonephritis. *Am J Med Sci.* 1997;313:50.
79. Talan DA, Stamm WE, Hooton TM, et al. Comparison of ciprofloxacin (7 days) and trimethoprim-sulfamethoxazole (14 days) for acute uncomplicated pyelonephritis in women: a randomized trial. *JAMA.* 2000;283:1583.
80. Naber KG, Bartnicki A, Bischoff W, et al. Gatifloxacin 200 mg or 400 mg once daily is as effective as ciprofloxacin 500 mg twice daily for the treatment of patients with acute pyelonephritis or complicated urinary tract infections. *Int J Antimicrob Agents.* 2004;23(Suppl 1):S41.
80. Mombelli G, Pezzoli R, Pinoja-Lutz G, et al. Oral vs intravenous ciprofloxacin in the initial empirical management of severe pyelonephritis or complicated urinary tract infections: a prospective randomized clinical trial. *Arch Intern Med.* 1999;159:53.
81. Wells WG, Woods GL, Jiang Q, et al. Treatment of complicated urinary tract infection in adults: combined analysis of two randomized, double-blind, multicentre trials comparing ertapenem and ceftriaxone followed by appropriate oral therapy. *J Antimicrob Chemother.* 2004;53(Suppl 2):ii67.
82. Bochud PY, Bonten M, Marchetti O, et al. Antimicrobial therapy for patients with severe sepsis and septic shock: an evidence-based review. *Crit Care Med.* 2004;32(11 Suppl):S495.
83. Leone M, Albanese J, Antonini F, et al. Long-term epidemiological survey of Candida species: comparison of isolates found in an intensive care unit and in conventional wards. *J Hosp Infect.* 2003;55:169.
84. Edwards JE, Bodey GP, Bowden RA, et al. International conference for the development of a consensus on the management and prevention of severe candidal infections. *Clin Infect Dis.* 1997;25:43–59.
85. Ayeni O, Riederer KM, Wilson FM, et al. Clinician's reaction to positive urine culture for candida organisms. *Mycoses.* 1999;42:285.
86. Sobel JD, Kauffman CA, McKinsey D, et al. Candiduria: a randomized, doubleblind study of treatment with fluconazole and placebo. *Clin Infect Dis.* 2000;30:19.
87. Jacobs LG, Skidmore EA, Freeman K, et al. Oral fluconazole compared with amphotericin B for treatment of fungal urinary tract infections in elderly patients. *Clin Infect Dis.* 1996;22:30.
88. Nassoura Z, Ivatury RR, Simon RJ, et al. Candiduria as an early marker of disseminated infection in critically ill surgical patients: the role of fluconazole therapy. *J Trauma.* 1993;35:290.

CHAPTER 114 ■ FUNGAL AND VIRAL INFECTIONS

MINH-LY NGUYEN • MINH-HONG NGUYEN • KEVIN J. FARRELL • CORNELIUS J. CLANCY

FUNGAL INFECTIONS

Fungal Pathogens

Medically relevant fungi are classically considered as one of three types of organism: yeasts, molds, or dimorphic agents. The yeasts grow as smooth colonies on culture plates. Microscopically, they are oval or spherical, and they reproduce by budding. The two most common human yeast pathogens are *Candida* spp. and *Cryptococcus* spp.; the molds appear as fuzzy colonies on agar plates. Microscopically, they have hyphae, which are tubular or filamentous morphologies that grow by branching and longitudinal extension. Hyphae can be septated (i.e., with cross walls perpendicular to hyphal cell wall) or aseptated (no cross walls). The most common human pathogens are *Aspergillus* spp. and *Rhizopus* spp. The term, *dimorphic fungi*, is used to describe the endemic fungi, which are found in distinct geographic locations. These fungi grow as filaments in the environment at ambient temperatures and as yeasts at higher body temperatures. The three most common pathogens are *Histoplasma capsulatum*, *Coccidioides immitis*, and *Blastomyces dermatitidis*. Clinicians should recognize that the term, dimorphic fungi, as commonly used in the medical literature is misleading. *Candida albicans*, although not grouped with the endemic dimorphic fungi, frequently assumes filamentous morphologies in tissue (pseudohyphae and hyphae).

Most fungal pathogens, except for *Candida* spp., are widespread in nature and are acquired by inhalation into the lungs. In immunocompetent hosts, inhaled fungi are generally arrested in the lungs by the host immune system. *Candida* spp., with the exception of *Candida parapsilosis*, are part of the human gastrointestinal flora, and infections with these organisms are usually endogenous in origin.

Due to the widespread environmental distribution of many fungal pathogens and the presence of Candida as human commensals, the diagnosis of infection (i.e., fungal disease) is often difficult to distinguish from colonization. As such, definitive diagnoses generally require either the presence of the organism at sterile sites or histopathology demonstrating tissue-invasive disease. Since many fungi show morphologies that are indistinguishable by histopathology (e.g., *Aspergillus* spp. versus *Fusarium* spp. and other acute-angle branching, septated molds), identification of the organism from culture is the only means to ascertain the etiologic agent.

In intensive care unit (ICU) settings, *Candida* spp. and, to a much lesser extent, *Aspergillus* are the major fungal pathogens. This chapter will concentrate on these fungi.

Infections Caused by *Candida* species (Candidiasis)

Candida spp. cause a wide range of clinical syndromes, from benign cutaneous to fatal deep-seated infections (Table 114.1). *Candida* spp. can affect otherwise healthy patients, as well as those with defective immune systems. In the ICU setting, the most common and serious form of disease is invasive candidiasis, which will be the focus of the rest of this section. Other types of candidiasis are alluded to in Table 114.1.

Invasive candidiasis typically refers to candidemia and deep-organ infections resulting from bloodborne dissemination. Candidemia is not always detected, and deep-seated organ involvement is, not infrequently, the first evidence of candidiasis.

Epidemiology

In the ICU, *Candida* spp. are the third most common cause of blood stream infections (1), accounting for approximately 10% of cases (1,2). The crude mortality rates range from 40% to 75%, and candidemia is associated with excess ICU and hospital stays and increased costs of care (3). Postmortem studies suggest that mortality rates due to invasive candidiasis may be higher than generally realized because of undiagnosed infections.

Risk Factors

The leading predisposing factors for invasive candidiasis include prolonged ICU stay, previous surgery (especially solid organ transplant and gastrointestinal surgery), acute renal failure, receipt of antibacterial agents or hyperalimentation, and the presence of a central venous catheter. In these settings, *Candida* colonization of different body sites and immunosuppression are major risk factors. Solid organ transplant recipients are at highest risk among the surgical patients, particularly small bowel, liver, and pancreas recipients, in whom the prevalence ranges from 9% to 59%. The types of surgical procedure and posttransplant immunosuppression confer additional risk. Although risk factors are well defined, the diversity of factors and underlying diseases associated with invasive candidiasis make it difficult to reliably identify large subgroups of patients within the ICU who might merit particular attention or targeted interventions.

Microbiology

C. albicans is the most common *Candida* species involved in invasive candidiasis, followed by *C. glabrata*, *C. tropicalis*, and *C. parapsilosis*. Other species are less common and often associated with underlying malignancy or chemotherapy. Whereas *C. tropicalis* and *C. glabrata* are found largely in adults, *C. parapsilosis* is the leading pathogen in the neonatal population. In many tertiary care centers, *C glabrata* has surpassed *C. albicans* to become the most common *Candida* sp. in invasive candidiasis, accounting for up to 35% of all candidemias (4,5). Among non-*albicans Candida* species, *C. krusei* and *C. glabrata* are particularly important because of their resistance and decreased susceptibility to fluconazole, respectively.

Clinical Manifestations

Clinical manifestations are often nonspecific. Fever is frequently the first and only sign of invasive candidiasis. Other signs that should raise concern for candidemia are papulopustular or macronodular skin lesions or ocular involvement such as chorioretinitis or endophthalmitis. Deep-seated infections often present, with findings localized to the particular tissue site.

Invasive candidiasis can be divided into four major clinical entities: catheter-related candidemia, acute disseminated candidiasis, chronic disseminated candidiasis, and deep-organ candidiasis (Table 114.2).

Diagnosis

The diagnosis of invasive candidiasis is a challenge due to nonspecific clinical manifestations and the low sensitivity of microbiologic culture techniques. Blood cultures should be routinely obtained in patients who have suggestive signs and symptoms, as well as those at high risk for invasive candidiasis. Although candidemia is the most common manifestation of invasive candidiasis, and whereas the other forms of invasive candidiasis generally originate from bloodborne dissemination, deep-seated candidiasis can occur without a positive blood culture. Indeed, blood cultures are positive in less than 50% of patients, and autopsy data demonstrate that as few as 15% to 40% of patients with invasive candidiasis have an antemortem diagnosis of the disease (6). Diagnosis, therefore, should also rely on histopathology and/or fungal cultures obtained by biopsy of sterile sites. As mentioned earlier, *Candida* spp. are common

TABLE 114.1

MAJOR CLINICAL CANDIDAL SYNDROMES

Type of candidiasis	Specific clinical syndromes	Frequency	Risk factors	Types of hosts	Treatment
Cutaneous: skin, nails		Most common form of candidiasis; Self-limited	Prolonged exposure of skin to moisture	Immunocompetent Immunocompromised	Topical antifungals
Mucocutaneous: Mucous membranes of the mouth, esophagus, vagina	Oropharyngeal	About 25% in patients with solid tumors and 60% in patients with hematologic malignancies and/or following bone marrow transplantation; up to 90% in AIDS	Extremes of age, broad-spectrum antibiotics, inhaled or systemic steroids, radiation to the head and neck	Immunocompetent Immunocompromised, especially patients receiving cytotoxic chemotherapy or systemic immunosuppressive therapy, those with AIDS, malignancy, or chronic mucocutaneous candidiasis	Topical or systemic azole agents
	Esophagitis	15%–20% in AIDS	Broad-spectrum antibiotics, acid-suppressive therapy, prior gastric surgery, mucosal barrier injury, inhaled or systemic steroids, esophageal motility disorders	Mostly immunocompromised, especially patients receiving cytotoxic chemotherapy or systemic immunosuppressive therapy, those with AIDS or malignancy	Systemic antifungal agents: oral azole (preferred treatment), parenteral echinocandin or AmB
	Vaginitis	70%–75% of healthy adult women	Pregnancy, diabetes mellitus, and broad-spectrum antibiotics	Immunocompetent Immunocompromised	Topical or systemic azole agents
Disseminated candidiasis			Colonization with *Candida*, broad-spectrum antibiotics, end-stage renal disease, central venous catheters, critically ill patients, hyperalimentation, GI surgery, burn patients, neonates	Immunocompetent Immunocompromised, especially granulocytopenia, bone marrow or solid organ transplant, chemotherapy, mucositis	Systemic antifungal agents

AIDS, acquired immunodeficiency syndrome; AmB, amphotericin B; GI, gastrointestinal.

colonizers of humans, which often makes it difficult to differentiate between colonization or true infections when organisms are isolated from the urine and nonsterile sites (see below).

Given the potential for antifungal resistance among the non-*albicans Candida* spp., isolates recovered from blood or sterile sites should be identified to the species level. The availability of special fungal media (such as CHROMagar) and rapid *in situ* hybridization techniques have significantly shortened the time to speciation.

Efforts have been devoted to develop nonculture-based diagnostic methods for invasive candidiasis. Antibody-based assays have not been useful. Beta D-glucan assay, an antigen test, has recently been approved for the diagnosis of invasive fungal infections. The assay measures the [1, 3]-beta-D-glucan

TABLE 114.2

FORMS OF INVASIVE CANDIDIASIS

Forms	Portal of entry	Characteristics	Blood cultures	Management
Catheter-related candidemia	Intravascular catheter	Frequently self-limited, but can rarely spread to deep-seated organs	Positive for *Candida* sp.	Systemic antifungal agents and removal of the catheter
Acute disseminated candidiasis	Intravascular catheter or GI tract is most common	Frequently involves deep-seated organ(s)	Can be positive or negative	Systemic antifungal
Chronic disseminated candidiasis (or hepatosplenic candidiasis)	GI tract is the most common portal; intravascular catheter	Almost exclusively seen in neutropenic patients or bone marrow transplant recipients. Typical presentation: Persistent fever, right upper quadrant pain, elevated alkaline phosphatase, lucencies on CT or ultrasound of the liver	Typically negative at the time of the diagnosis	Systemic antifungal
Deep-organ candidiasis	Intravascular catheter or GI tract is most common	Frequently follows an episode of undiagnosed candidemia	Typically negative at the time of the diagnosis	Systemic antifungal

GI, gastrointestinal; CT, computed tomography.

levels released from the cell wall of most fungi. The sensitivity, specificity, and positive and negative predictive values (PPV and NPV) for this test in diagnosing invasive candidiasis are 81%, 84%, 84%, and 75%, respectively (7). Although this test is able to detect various *Candida* spp., a potential drawback is its nonspecificity for *Candida*, as it also detects *Aspergillus*, *Fusarium*, and *Trichosporon*. Other factors that can contribute to false-positive tests results include dialysis filters, gauze, and sponges.

Studies have demonstrated that azole minimum inhibitory concentrations (MICs) correlate with the likelihood of success in treating patients. Nevertheless, antifungal susceptibility testing of *Candida* is currently performed in relatively few clinical laboratories, and it is not considered the standard of care, unlike antibacterial susceptibility testing. In fact, antifungal susceptibility patterns are predictable in most cases based on species and prior exposure to antifungal agents (8). For this reason, identification of isolates to the species level is usually more important than MIC data in the management of individual patients. For example, *C. krusei* is intrinsically resistant to fluconazole and a significant minority of *C. glabrata* strains develop resistance to the drug. For other species, the vast majority of bloodstream isolates remain susceptible to fluconazole, although resistance is a concern in the setting of prior exposure to the drug. Cross-resistance to other azoles is often seen, which limits the utility of this class against fluconazole-resistant isolates.

Reports of resistance to the new echinocandin class of antifungals are beginning to appear, but experience is too limited to know how widespread the phenomenon will be or the extent to which use of these agents will be influenced (9). Of note, MICs of echinocandins against *C. parapsilosis* are generally higher than against other species, and breakthrough infections among patients receiving these agents have been described (10). Since the significance of these observations on the use of echinocandins in the treatment of *C. parapsilosis* infections is unclear, susceptibility testing does not have a role in the management of individual patients as yet. Amphotericin B resistance is difficult to document using current testing methods. Resistance among *C. lusitaniae* and *C. guilliermondii* isolates is well described but not seen with all isolates. Clinicians should probably avoid amphotericin B if elevated MICs are documented. At centers where candidiasis is a particular problem and antifungal use is widespread, it is useful to conduct periodic susceptibility testing to generate an institutional antibiogram. Clinicians should be aware if such reports exist at their institution, as susceptibility patterns against different species can be used to guide empiric antifungal therapy.

Management

Invasive Candidiasis. The major antifungal agents and their activity are summarized in Table 114.3. The current guidelines for management of invasive candidiasis are summarized in Table 114.4 (11–13). Amphotericin B (conventional or lipid formulations) or caspofungin should be the first-line treatment of critically ill patients with invasive candidiasis. Caspofungin, an echinocandin agent, is better tolerated and has fewer side effects than amphotericin B. Fluconazole can also be considered once resistant species such as *C. krusei* are ruled out. Recent data show that anidulafungin and micafungin, two newly approved echinocandin agents, are as effective as caspofungin in management.

All patients with candidemia should have an ophthalmologic exam to rule out retinal involvement. In addition, all vascular catheters should be removed if possible. *Candida* spp. tend to form biofilms on catheters, which can render otherwise susceptible isolates resistant to antifungal agents.

TABLE 114.3

CURRENTLY AVAILABLE SYSTEMIC ANTIFUNGAL AGENTS

Class of antifungal	Mechanisms of actions of specific drugs	Routes of administration and daily doses	Spectrum of activity	Side effects and toxicity
Polyene	Potent antifungal agents that act by binding to ergosterol in the fungal cell membrane, leading to leakage and cell death Amphotericin B (AmB), available in 4 formulations: ■ AmB deoxycholate (dAmB; often called conventional AmB) ■ AmB colloidal dispersion (ABCD) ■ AmB lipid complex (ABLC) ■ Liposomal AmB (L-AmB)	IV for invasive candidiasis Usual daily dosages: dAmB, 0.3–1.5 mg/kg ABCD, 3–6 mg/kg ABLC, 5 mg/kg L-AmB, 3–5 mg/kg	AmB is active (fungicidal) against most pathogenic fungi, except the following: *Trichosporon beigelii*, *Aspergillus terreus*, *Pseudallescheria boydii*, *Malassezia furfur*, *Fusarium* spp. Some *Candida lusitaniae* and *C. guilliermondii* isolates are resistant.	Infusion-related (fever, chills, and myalgia). Nephrotoxicity: Azotemia, electrolyte wasting (potassium, magnesium), renal tubular acidosis. Overall, the lipid formulations of AmB are less nephrotoxic.
Azoles	Inhibition of cytochrome P450 14α-demethylase, an enzyme involved in the sterol biosynthesis pathway Fluconazole	PO and IV Usual daily dosage: 6 mg/kg. Doses of 12 mg/kg are increasingly used to overcome intermediately susceptible (i.e., dose-dependent) organisms.	Fungistatic agent, active against *Candida* spp., *Cryptococcus* spp., and *Coccidioides immitis*. *Candida krusei* is intrinsically resistant, and resistance has been reported among isolates of several other *Candida* spp., especially *C. glabrata*. No activity against molds. Limited activity against *Histoplasma capsulatum*, *Blastomyces dermatitidis*, and *Sporothrix schenckii*.	In general, well-tolerated. Hepatotoxicity is rare.
	Itraconazole	PO and IV Daily dosage: PO: 100–400 mg (at 400 mg/day doses, better levels are achieved with bid dosing) IV: 200 mg bid for 2 days, followed by 200 mg/day	Active against yeasts, molds, and dimorphic fungi. Limited activity against *Fusarium* and Zygomycetes. Resistance has been reported among *Candida* and *Aspergillus* spp.	Generally benign. Hepatotoxicity is rare.
	Voriconazole	PO and IV Daily dosage: PO: 200 mg bid IV: 3–6 mg/kg every 12 h	Active against yeasts, molds and dimorphic fungi. Variable activity against *Fusarium*. Limited activity against Zygomycetes. Resistance has been reported among *Candida* and *Aspergillus* spp.	Dose-related, transient visual disturbances, skin rash, and elevated hepatic enzyme levels have been reported.
	Posaconazole	PO Daily dosage: 600–800 mg/day in divided doses with food	Active against yeasts, molds (including Zygomycetes) and dimorphic fungi. Variable activity against *Fusarium*.	Nausea and headache. Rash, dry skin, nausea, taste disturbance, abdominal pain, dizziness, and flushing can occur. Posaconazole can cause abnormalities in liver function.
Glucan synthesis inhibitors (echinocandins)	Block the synthesis of a major fungal cell wall component, 1-3-beta-D-glucan Caspofungin Anidulafungin Micafungin	IV Caspofungin: 70 mg load, then 50 mg daily Anidulafungin: 200 mg, then 100 mg/day Micafungin: 100 mg/kg	Activity is mainly against *Candida* spp. and *Aspergillus* spp. No activity against *Cryptococcus* or Zygomycetes.	Side-effects are limited Liver toxicity

TABLE 114.4

RECOMMENDED ANTIFUNGAL AGENTS AGAINST INVASIVE CANDIDIASIS

Host	Primary therapy	Alternative therapy	Comments
Nonneutropenic	AmB, 0.6–1 mg/kg/d IV *or* Fluconazole, 400–800 mg/d IV or PO *or* Caspofungin, 70 mg IV once, then 50 mg/d IV *or* Voriconazole, 6 mg/kg IV every 12 h for 2 doses, then 3 mg/kg/d IV every 12 h (can be switched to 200 mg bid PO after 3 days) *or* Anidulafungin, 200 mg IV for 1 dose, then 100 mg/d IV *or* Micafungin, 100 mg/d IV	AmB, 0.7 mg/kg IV plus fluconazole, 800 mg IV or PO for 4 to 7 days, then fluconazole, 800 mg/d	Duration: 14 days after the last positive blood culture and resolution of signs and symptoms Removal of all vascular catheters
Neutropenic	AmB, 0.7–1 mg/kg/d IV *or* Lipid formulations of AmB, 3–5 mg/kg/d IV *or* Caspofungin, 70 mg IV for 1 dose, then 50 mg/d IV	Fluconazole, 6 to 12 mg/kg/d	Duration: 14 days after the last positive blood culture, resolution of signs and symptoms, and of neutropenia Removal of vascular catheters if possible (controversial issue)

Candida **Recovered from Urine or Sputum/Bronchoalveolar Lavage (BAL).** As mentioned above, *Candida* spp. are part of endogenous flora and frequent colonizers of mucosal surfaces. In the ICU setting, urine and sputum are the two most common sites of colonization.

Candida in the Urine. *Candida* spp. are now the most common organisms recovered from the urine of surgical ICU patients. The risk factors include urinary catheters, old age, and receipt of antibacterial agents. Unlike the assessment of bacteriuria, colony counts and urine analysis are not helpful in deciding whether candiduria is of clinical importance (14,15). Many studies have demonstrated that asymptomatic candiduria in the low-risk patient is of little clinical relevance and should not be treated. In a small subset of patients, candiduria is a marker for invasive candidiasis. Treatment is indicated for symptomatic patients and those who are neutropenic, have undergone a urologic manipulation, or received a kidney transplant (9). Treatment entails removal of the urinary catheter and therapy with a systemic antifungal agent (fluconazole or amphotericin B) for 7 to 14 days. In the event that catheter removal is not possible, changing the catheter might be of benefit and should be performed (9).

Candida in the Sputum. Specimens from the airways—sputum, tracheal aspirates, and BAL—are frequently contaminated with oropharyngeal flora, including *Candida* spp. Despite the frequency with which *Candida* spp. are isolated from the respiratory tree of ICU patients, primary *Candida* pneumonia is extremely rare (16,17). Cases are generally encountered among neutropenic hosts. The diagnosis of *Candida* pneumonia requires evidence of parenchymal invasion by hyphae on a biopsy specimen. Antifungal therapy should not be instituted in response to *Candida* isolates recovered from respiratory samples. In fact, strategies of not identifying or reporting *Candida* spp. in respiratory samples decrease length of stay, hospital costs, and unnecessary antifungal therapy, without any negative effects on the accurate diagnosis of *Candida* pneumonia or patient outcome (18).

Prevention

Given the nonspecific clinical manifestations, low yield of blood cultures, and high mortality rates of invasive candidiasis, investigators have studied three treatment strategies in the absence of a definitive diagnosis:

- Prophylactic strategy: Administration of an antifungal agent at a period of high risk to prevent candidiasis
- Preemptive strategy: Administration of an antifungal agent to treat suspected invasive candidiasis based on particular warning signs
- Empiric therapy: Administration of an antifungal agent in persistently febrile patients without a known source or with no response to appropriate antibacterial agents

Prophylactic Strategy. The role of prophylactic antifungal therapy is controversial, as results from several clinical trials are contradictory. The most popular antifungal agent used for prophylaxis is fluconazole, given its benign side effect profile and good absorption. Trials that showed a positive clinical impact of fluconazole prophylaxis are summarized in Table 114.5 (19–22). It should be pointed out that only a small subset of patients is at sufficient risk for invasive candidiasis to justify this strategy. Thus, universal prophylaxis to all ICU patients is not warranted. To date, the specific patient populations that would benefit most are not clearly defined.

Preemptive Strategy. Preemptive antifungal therapy based on specific findings on computed tomography (CT) scan or laboratory markers such as galactomannan is a popular approach in patients undergoing bone marrow transplantation or those with neutropenia from a hematologic malignancy. At this time, however, there are no good indicators for preemptive approaches in nonneutropenic ICU patients.

Empiric Strategy. This practice, although widely used, is not validated by clinical trials. Mathematical models suggest that empiric strategies might be proven effective. A theoretical cost-effectiveness analysis was performed on a target population of

TABLE 114.5

CLINICAL TRIALS DEMONSTRATING A POSITIVE IMPACT OF ANTIFUNGAL PROPHYLAXIS IN NONNEUTROPENIC ICU PATIENTS

Patient population	Intervention	Impact on fungal infections	References
Surgical patients with recurrent gastrointestinal perforations or anastomotic leakage	Randomized prospective double-blind, placebo-controlled study: fluconazole (400 mg IV/day) ($N =$ 25) or placebo ($N = 22$) continued until resolution of the underlying surgical condition	Fluconazole reduced candida colonization by 47% (15% vs. 62%; $p = 0.04$) and *Candida* peritonitis by 31% (4% vs. 35%; $p = 0.02$) No impact on survival	19
Medical and surgical adult ICU patients with mechanical ventilation for at least 48 h	Randomized double-blind, placebo-controlled study: fluconazole, 100 mg daily ($N =$ 103) or placebo ($N = 101$)	Fluconazole reduced *Candida* infections by about 10% (5.8% vs. 16%). No impact on survival (mortality rate 39% vs. 41%)	20
Medical and surgical adult ICU patients in septic shock	Randomized double-blind study: fluconazole, 200 mg IV daily (N $= 32$) or placebo ($N = 39$) during the course of their septic shock	Fluconazole improved 30-day survival by 32% (78% vs. 46%) in patients with intra-abdominal sepsis. No impact on survival in patients with septic shock due to nosocomial pneumonia	21
Surgical ICU patients with a length of ICU stay of at least 3 days	Randomized placebo-controlled study: fluconazole, 400 mg orally or placebo (total $N = 260$)	Fluconazole reduced the risk of fungal infection by 55%. No impact on survival	22

ICU patients with fever, hypothermia, or unexplained hypotension who had not responded to 3 days of antibacterial therapy (23). Assuming that 10% of the target population would have invasive candidiasis, the authors concluded that empiric fluconazole was the most reasonable strategy (cost: $12,593 per discounted life-year saved; one life saved for 71 patients treated). Empiric fluconazole was estimated to decrease mortality from 44% to 30.4% in patients with invasive candidiasis, and from 22.4% to 21.0% in the overall target cohort. The authors calculated that this strategy would be justifiable if the likelihood of invasive candidiasis were at least 2.5%. Until clinical trials validate empiric strategies within well defined at-risk populations, however, they cannot be broadly recommended.

Infections Caused by *Aspergillus* Species (Aspergillosis)

Aspergillus spp. are less common human pathogens in the ICU than *Candida* spp. but cause greater morbidity and mortality. These molds are ubiquitous in the environment. In normal hosts, they are generally saprophytes that colonize the bronchopulmonary tree. The four classical clinical syndromes of pulmonary aspergillosis are presented in Table 114.6. This section will focus on the two syndromes most commonly encountered in ICU setting: chronic necrotizing pulmonary aspergillosis (CNPA) and invasive pulmonary aspergillosis (IPA). In both of these diseases, *Aspergillus* spp. invade tissue and blood vessels, causing necrosis and possibly disseminating to the brain and elsewhere. Of note, entities similar to allergic bronchopulmonary aspergillosis, CNPA, and IPA are also found in the sinuses.

Epidemiology

IPA is estimated to occur in 5% to 13% of patients who have undergone bone marrow transplantation, 5% to 25% of patients who have received heart or lung transplants, and 10% to 20% of patients receiving intensive chemotherapy for leukemia; mortality rates are 50% to 90%. The disease is not as common in patients with less profound immunosuppression and exceedingly uncommon in immunocompetent hosts. In immunocompetent hosts, the rare cases of IPA often follow influenza or other infectious respiratory processes. CNPA is generally a disease of patients with underlying lung disease.

Risk Factors

The major risk factors predisposing to invasive aspergillosis are summarized in Table 114.7. In addition to these, there are increasing reports of disease among debilitated patients in the ICU.

Microbiology

Although there are over 100 species of *Aspergillus*, only a few cause diseases in humans. *A. fumigatus* is most common, followed by *A. flavus*. Less common pathogens include *A. terreus*, *A. niger*, and *A. clavatus*. Antifungal susceptibility testing against molds is not recommended as routine practice. Reproducible testing methodologies have been developed, but interpretive criteria have not been established. Nevertheless, elevated MICs to amphotericin B have been documented against

TABLE 114.6

CLINICAL SPECTRUM OF ASPERGILLOSIS

Clinical syndromes	Description and epidemiology	Predisposing factors	Clinical characteristics	Outcome
Aspergilloma	Fungus ball (a mass of fungal mycelia, inflammatory cells, tissue debris) within a pre-existing lung cavity. Usually, the fungus does not invade the surrounding lung parenchyma or blood vessels. 17% of patients with pre-existing lung cavity have aspergilloma.	Pre-existing lung cavity.	Often asymptomatic. Some develop hemoptysis. Chest radiograph shows a mobile intracavitary mass with an air crescent in the periphery.	Asymptomatic patients: No treatment. Symptomatic patients: Intracavitary AmB or antimold azole agents. Surgical resection: Reserved for patients with massive hemoptysis; carries significant morbidity and mortality.
Allergic bronchopulmonary aspergillosis (ABPA)	Hypersensitivity reaction to *Aspergillus* colonization of the tracheobronchial tree. This can occur by itself or in conjunction with aspergillus sinusitis. 7%–10% of patients with steroid-dependent asthma and 7% of patients with cystic fibrosis have ABPA. The incidence is much less among all patients with asthma (<1%).	Patients with asthma or cystic fibrosis.	Typical presentations: fever and pulmonary infiltrates unresponsive to antibacterial therapy; cough with mucous plugs. Suggestive findings: asthma, eosinophilia, a positive skin test result for *A. fumigatus*, serum IgE level >1,000 IU/dL, fleeting pulmonary infiltrates, central bronchiectasis, mucoid impaction, and positive test results for *Aspergillus* precipitins.	Systemic corticosteroids (inhaled steroids have no effect). For recurrent ABPA, itraconazole in conjunction with systemic steroids speeds the resolution of symptoms and facilitates steroid taper.
Chronic necrotizing aspergillosis	Chronic, indolent destructive process of the lung due to invasion by *Aspergillus*. The rate of disease is not known.	Underlying lung disease. Patients with mild immunosuppression, diabetes, poor nutrition, chronic lung diseases (such as COPD, inactive tuberculosis, previous radiation therapy, pneumoconiosis, cystic fibrosis), lung infarction, sarcoidosis. This syndrome can also follow aspergilloma.	Typical presentations: fever, cough, sputum production, and weight loss for several months. Chest radiographs show an infiltrative process with or without a fungal ball. The diagnosis requires confirmation by demonstration of fungal tissue invasion and the growth of *Aspergillus* species on culture.	Systemic antifungal therapy with voriconazole (or itraconazole) or lipid formulations of AmB. Caspofungin might also be considered. Surgical resection is considered if the disease is focal and refractory to antifungal therapy.
Invasive aspergillosis	Rapidly progressive, often fatal infection. Characterized by fungal invasion of blood vessels. Infection can disseminate to various organs. Epidemiology: refer to discussion in text.	Patients with profound immunosuppression: prolonged neutropenia; recipients of bone marrow transplant or solid organ transplant; advanced AIDS or chronic granulomatous disease; severe burn.	Typical presentations: fever refractory to antibacterial agents, cough, pleuritic chest pain, or hemoptysis. Suggestive chest radiograph findings: pulmonary nodules with or without surrounding halo sign, crescent sign (indicative of cavitation), wedge-shaped or pleural-based nodules or infiltrates.	Systemic antifungal therapy with voriconazole. Itraconazole, lipid formulations of amphotericin B, and caspofungin are alternative treatments.

COPD, chronic obstructive pulmonary disease; AIDS, acquired immunodeficiency syndrome.

TABLE 114.7

PREDISPOSING FACTORS TO INVASIVE ASPERGILLOSIS

Underlying conditions	Notes	Predisposing factors
Allogeneic bone marrow transplant (BMT) recipients	Risk highest for transplantation from an unrelated donor > HLA-mismatched related donor > HLA-matched related donor	Early after BMT: receipt of T-cell-depleted or CD34-selected stem cell products; neutropenia; use of steroids; CMV disease; respiratory viral infections 1–6 mo: defective cellular immunity; use of steroids >6 mo: use of steroids for GVHD; CMV disease
Cord blood transplant	Higher risk of fungal infections than other allograft recipients during the early and late transplant period	Early: slower myeloid engraftment Greater than 6 mo: use of steroids for GVHD
Autologous bone marrow transplant	Lowest risk of infections among the bone marrow transplants	Use of CD34-enriched autografts Use of previous potent immunosuppression for treatment of refractory malignancy
Solid organ transplant	Lung transplant has the highest risk	Immunosuppression to treat allograft rejection
Neutropenia	Highest risk among patients treated with chemotherapy for acute leukemia or aplastic anemia	Intensity (absolute neutrophil count less than 200 cells/μL) and duration of neutropenia (more than 10 days)
Receipt of immunosuppressive therapy	Therapy for autoimmune diseases	Receipt of high-dose steroids (dose equivalent to prednisone more than 20 mg for greater than 3 weeks), antilymphocyte immunoglobulin, anti-TNFα agents, and other immunosuppressive drugs
AIDS	Advanced HIV infection with CD4$^+$ less than 100 cells/μL	

CMV, cytomegalovirus; GVHD, graft versus host disease; TNF, tumor necrosis factor.

a number of *A. terreus* isolates and elevated MICs of itraconazole against a small percentage of *A. fumigatus* isolates.

Clinical Manifestations

Most infections caused by *Aspergillus* spp. originate from the inhalation of fungal spores into the lungs. Cases of direct skin inoculation of *Aspergillus* have been described in association with the insertion of intravenous devices or the taping of arm boards to the extremities. Patients with severe burns can also develop local burn wound infections, especially if they are rolled in the dirt to extinguish flames. Regardless of the portal of entry, any local form of aspergillosis can disseminate to various sites if host immune function is impaired.

Almost any organ may be involved in disseminated aspergillosis, including integument (onychomycosis, cutaneous aspergillosis), ear (otomycosis), respiratory tract (sinusitis, pneumonia, empyema), heart (endocarditis, myocarditis), gastrointestinal (GI, hepatosplenic aspergillosis), central nervous system (cerebral aspergillosis, meningitis), eye (endophthalmitis), bone (osteomyelitis, mediastinitis), and so forth. The lungs and sinuses are the two most common primary sites of aspergillosis. The central nervous system is the most common secondary site.

Diagnosis

The diagnosis of invasive aspergillosis is problematic. Since *Aspergillus* spores are ubiquitous, they are common colonizers of the bronchopulmonary tree. A definitive diagnosis, therefore, requires histologic evidence of tissue invasion by hyphal elements, as well as culture of the organism. It should be noted, however, that the sensitivity of tissue biopsy in diagnosing invasive aspergillosis is low (e.g., 30% for lung biopsies). Moreover, recovery of *Aspergillus* from the blood is extremely rare, with a recovery rate approximating 5% in cases of *Aspergillus*.

In immunocompromised hosts, a positive culture from a respiratory sample (sputum or BAL) is highly associated with invasive pulmonary disease. However, the sensitivity of culture of sputum or BAL is only 50%.

Radiography. In neutropenic patients and bone marrow transplant recipients, high-resolution CT scan of the chest has become an important adjunct to the diagnosis of IPA. One or more nodules surrounded by halo signs (ground glass opacity or haziness) are early findings of angioinvasive mold infections (24); cavitation is a late finding. Although these lesions are highly suggestive of IPA in high-risk patients, it should be emphasized that other infections (other fungi, *Nocardia*, and so forth) can also present with halo signs. In one study, classic CT scan findings led to the earlier diagnosis of IPA, more timely administration of antifungal therapy, and improved outcome (24).

Serologic Detection. A double-sandwich enzyme-linked immunosorbent assay (ELISA) for the detection of galactomannan

(GM) in serum has been used as a marker for aspergillosis. GM is a cell wall polysaccharide of most *Aspergillus* and *Penicillium* species that is released in serum during growth in tissue. The sensitivity of the test in different reports has ranged from 30% to 100%, with the wide range explained in part by various definitions of positive tests (e.g., different cutoff values and number of values above a cutoff) and different patient populations. In adult neutropenic patients, a single serum GM level of 0.8 ng/mL or greater is equivalent to two consecutive serum GM levels of 0.5 ng/mL or greater. The sensitivity, specificity, positive and negative predictive values (PPV and NPV) for these cutoffs are 96.5%, 96.5%, 97.3%, and 98.6%, and 93.3%, 98.6%, 98.6%, and 98.4%, respectively. A major limitation of this assay is false-positive results. Drugs such as piperacillin-tazobactam or cyclophosphamide and certain foods can result in falsely high serum GMs.

In a meta-analysis of 27 studies encompassing about 4,000 patients, the overall sensitivity of the serum ELISA was 61% to 71% with specificity of 89% to 93%, PPV of 26% to 53%, and NPV of 95% to 98% (25). The test performed best among bone marrow transplant recipients and patients with hematologic malignancies; serial testing strategies in these populations are widely accepted. Experience among patients undergoing solid organ transplantation is much more limited. In studies of lung and liver transplant recipients, the sensitivities of the assay were 30% and 56%, respectively (26,27), with specificities of 93% to 95% and 87% to 94%, respectively (26–28). Given the lack of data, it is not clear at present whether serial GM testing of serum plays a useful role in surveillance for IPA among solid organ transplant recipients (26,27). It has been suggested that the moderate sensitivity and relatively low positive predictive value of the serum GM in diagnosing IPA might be improved by applying the assay to bronchoalveolar lavage (BAL) samples (29). Among bone marrow transplant recipients and patients with hematologic malignancies, detection of GM within BAL samples has been reported to add to the sensitivity of both BAL culture and serum GM detection (30–33). Although the specificity of BAL GM detection has generally been good (29,31), high rates of false-positive results were reported in at least one study (34). Moreover, BAL testing is likely to be influenced by the collection techniques of individual bronchoscopists.

Management

Voriconazole should be the first-line therapy against invasive aspergillosis, as it has been proven superior to conventional amphotericin B (35). To date, there have not been head-to-head comparisons of voriconazole versus lipid formulations of amphotericin B. Therapy is generally prolonged for at least 6 weeks or until the primary infection is resolved. The role of other systemic antifungal agents is summarized in Table 114.8 (36–40).

Debridement of the involved sinuses or primary cutaneous aspergillosis should be performed in conjunction with systemic antifungal therapy. Recent data show that combined antifungal therapy and surgical resection of single lesions from the lungs or central nervous system (CNS) might clear the infection faster than antifungal therapy alone, improve outcome, and prevent reactivation during consecutive chemotherapy courses (40–45). The procedures are generally well tolerated and associated with low rates of complications and mortality.

Patients who recover from an episode of invasive aspergillosis are at risk for recurrence of disease during subsequent chemotherapy or transplantation. These patients should be treated with a systemic antifungal agent for at least 6 weeks or until the primary infection resolves, whichever is longer, before further immunosuppressive therapy is considered. In addition, secondary prophylaxis is advised during any subsequent periods of immunosuppression.

TABLE 114.8

RECOMMENDED ANTIFUNGAL AGENTS AGAINST ASPERGILLOSIS

Antifungal agents	Primary therapy	Alternative therapy
Monotherapy		
Voriconazole	More effective and yields better outcome than conventional AmB. There have not been head-to-head comparisons between voriconazole and lipid formulations of AmB.	
Posaconazole	Has not been evaluated as initial monotherapy for invasive aspergillosis.	Yields favorable response (42%) when used as salvage therapy (36)
Caspofungin	Has not been evaluated as initial monotherapy for invasive aspergillosis.	Yields favorable response (45%) when used as salvage therapy. To date only caspofungin has been evaluated for invasive aspergillosis among echinocandins (37)
Lipid formulations of AmB	Have not been evaluated in controlled trials.	Anecdotal reports demonstrating efficacy as salvage therapy
Combination Therapy		
Liposomal formulations of AmB and caspofungin	Have not been evaluated in controlled trials.	Yield favorable outcome in 40%–60% of patients (38,39)
Voriconazole and caspofungin	Has not been evaluated in controlled trials.	Superior to voriconazole alone in salvage therapy of invasive aspergillosis (40)

VIRAL INFECTIONS

Recent years have seen the emergence of unexpected viral diseases with high case fatality rates, including Hantavirus pulmonary syndrome, West Nile virus encephalitis, severe adult respiratory syndrome, and avian influenza. There are several reasons for critical care physicians to be familiar with a range of viral infections and to consider viral causes in their differential diagnosis. First, there is a small window of time to effectively intervene with antiviral agents in many of these diseases. Second, the timely identification of persons with potentially infectious viral diseases has significant public health implications and may reduce the risk of transmission to other persons. Third, in the era of long-distance travel, clinicians must recognize previously unfamiliar diseases. Finally, viruses such as those causing hemorrhagic fevers are possible agents of bioterrorism.

In general, viral infections can be diagnosed by several means (46):

- Serologic tests: The antibody response to viral antigens can be detected in the serum of patients with viral infections. An IgM response usually indicates recent exposure to a virus, whereas the presence of IgG reflects past exposure.
- Culture: Several types of cells are available for growing viruses, and no single cell line is appropriate for all of them. Therefore, it is helpful for the laboratory to know which virus the clinician suspects.
- Pathology: Histologic examination of biopsy and autopsy tissues may demonstrate changes that are typical of certain viruses (e.g., DNA viruses usually produce inclusions in the cytoplasm).
- Detection of viral antigens: Viral antigens can be detected in tissues by direct or indirect immunofluorescence using appropriate antibodies.
- Amplification of viral nucleic acids: Small copy numbers of viral DNA and RNA can be detected by polymerase chain reaction (PCR) and reverse transcription-PCR (RT-PCR), respectively. Real-time amplification methods permit simultaneous detection and quantification of viral nucleic acids.

Table 114.9 lists the leading viruses that might be encountered in the ICU, as of the writing of this chapter. We will review major viral illnesses encountered in critically ill patients, their diagnosis, and treatment. A review of human immunodeficiency virus (HIV) medicine is covered elsewhere (see Chapter 120).

Viral Infections on Admission to the Intensive Care Unit

Viral Pneumonitis

Severe community acquired pneumonia is caused by bacteria in approximately 60% of cases. In a French ICU, bronchoscopy of 41 patients with severe pneumonia revealed that 30% of all BALs and 63% of bacteria-negative BALs were positive for a respiratory virus (47). Influenza A and B are the most common causes of viral pneumonia in immunocompetent adults, whereas CMV and other herpes viruses are more important in immunocompromised patients.

It is frequently difficult to differentiate bacterial from viral pneumonia, but patients who have viral pneumonia often have a less severe illness and may complain of a dry hacking cough. Cultures are often necessary to make a definitive diagnosis. The radiographic findings of viral pneumonia are generally nonspecific, ranging from minimal changes on chest radiograph to hyperinflation or bilateral reticular opacities that are diffuse in distribution. Uncommonly, viral pneumonias can be associated with thickened interlobular septae that result in Kerley B lines. Viral pneumonias are rarely associated with pleural effusions, unless complicated by secondary bacterial pneumonia (48). CT scan of the chest may show poorly defined air space nodules, patchy areas of peribronchial ground glass opacity, and consolidation.

Influenza Virus

In the United States, epidemics of influenza typically occur during the winter. Approximately 66% of patients hospitalized with influenza are older than 64 years of age. Morbidity and mortality are highest among the elderly, children younger than 2 years of age, and persons of any age who have comorbid illnesses such as cardiac, pulmonary, or renal diseases, diabetes mellitus, and/or immunosuppression (49,50).

Microbiology. Human infections are caused by influenza A, B, or C viruses. Wild birds are the natural host for influenza A, and the virus infects humans, birds, pigs, and other animals. Influenza B and C viruses are usually found only in humans. Influenza A and B can cause severe disease and occur in epidemics. Influenza A can also be responsible for pandemics. Influenza C, on the other hand, causes only mild illness in humans and does not result in epidemics or pandemics.

Influenza A viruses are divided into subtypes on the basis of the two main surface glycoproteins, hemagglutinin (HA) and neuraminidase (NA). There are 16 known HA and 9 known NA subtypes of influenza A. New influenza virus variants result from frequent antigenic change, termed *antigenic drift*, resulting from point mutations that occur during viral replication. Influenza B viruses undergo antigenic drift less rapidly than influenza A viruses. In 2006–2007, H5N1 virus (avian influenza) was the circulating virus in Asia and Europe and caused severe respiratory diseases, life-threatening complications, and death (51).

Immunity to the surface antigens, particularly HA, reduces the likelihood of infection and severity of disease. Antibody against one influenza virus type or subtype confers limited or no protection against another type or subtype of influenza. Furthermore, antibody to one antigenic variant of influenza virus might not completely protect against a new antigenic variant of the same type or subtype. Antigenic drift is the basis for seasonal epidemics and the reason for the incorporation of one or more new strains in each year's influenza vaccine. More dramatic antigenic changes, or shifts, occur less frequently and can result in the emergence of a novel influenza virus with the potential to cause a pandemic.

Clinical Manifestations. The classic influenza symptoms in healthy adults include abrupt fever, myalgia, headaches, and upper respiratory symptoms. In the elderly or immunocompromised hosts, these classic symptoms might be absent, and patients might present only with fever and altered mental status.

TABLE 114.9

VIRAL PATHOGENS MOST LIKELY TO BE ENCOUNTERED IN THE ICU

DNA Viruses		
Family	**Viruses**	**Acute critical illness**
Adenoviridae	Adenovirus	Myocarditis
Hepadnaviridae	Hepatitis B	Fulminant liver failure, myocarditis
	Hepatitis delta virus	Fulminant liver failure
Herpesviridae	Herpes simplex	Myocarditis
	Varicella zoster	Pneumonitis
	Cytomegalovirus	Opportunistic infection in immunosuppressed hosts
	EBV	
	HHV8 (Kaposi sarcoma virus)	Fulminant liver failure
		Pulmonary or GI bleeding in HIV
Papovaviridae	JC, BK, other polyomavirus	Renal failure, encephalitis
Parvoviridae	Parvovirus B19	Myocarditis
Poxviridae	Vaccinia	Postvaccinia vaccine complication
RNA Viruses		
Family	**Viruses**	**Acute critical illness**
Arenaviridae	Lymphocytic choriomeningitis virus	Encephalitis
	South American hemorrhagic fever	Hemorrhagic fever
Bunyaviridae	California encephalitis	Encephalitis
	Hantavirus pulmonary syndrome	Pneumonitis
	Bunyavirid hemorrhagic fever	Hemorrhagic fever
Coronaviridae	Coronavirus (including SARS associated)	Pneumonitis
Filoviridae	Marburg	Hemorrhagic fever
	Ebola	Hemorrhagic fever
Flaviviruses	Yellow fever	Encephalitis
	Dengue, dengue hemorrhagic fever	Hemorrhagic fever
	Japanese encephalitis	Encephalitis
	West Nile encephalitis	Encephalitis
	St. Louis encephalitis	Encephalitis
	Tick-borne encephalitis	Encephalitis
	Hepatitis C	Myocarditis
Orthomyxoviridae	Influenza virus	Pneumonitis, myocarditis
	Avian influenza	Pneumonitis
Paramyxoviridae	Parainfluenza	Pneumonitis
	Mumps	Myocarditis
	Respiratory syncytial virus	Pneumonitis in children, IC
	Human meta-pneumovirus	
	Measles virus (rubeola)	Encephalitis, myocarditis
Picornaviridae	Enterovirus	Myocarditis
	Hepatitis A	Fulminant hepatic failure
	Poliovirus	Myocarditis
	Coxsackievirus, echovirus, and newer enteroviruses	Myocarditis
	Rhinovirus	
Retroviridae	Human T-cell lymphotropic virus I and II	Acute adult T cell leukemia
	Human immunodeficiency virus	Refer to Chapter 120
Rhabdoviridae	Vesicular stomatitis virus and related virus	Encephalitis
	Rhabdovirus	
Togaviridae	Rubella virus (German measles)	Myocarditis

EBV, Epstein-Barr virus; HHV8, human herpes virus 8; GI, gastrointestinal; SARS, severe acute respiratory syndrome; IC, intensive care.

Influenza-associated lower respiratory tract infections can be classified into four general forms (52):

1. Influenza without radiographic evidence of pneumonia: Up to 30% of hospitalized patients with influenza have no evidence of pulmonary infiltrates (53).
2. Viral pneumonia followed by bacterial pneumonia: The true incidence is unknown. The most common bacteria are *Staphylococcus aureus* and *Streptococcus pneumoniae*.
3. Rapidly progressive diffuse viral pneumonia: This entity may be decreasing due to the increased rate of influenza vaccination in the elderly.
4. Concomitant viral and bacterial pneumonia: In addition to *S. aureus* and *S. pneumoniae*, the most common bacteria is *Haemophilus influenzae*. These patients are generally more ill than the other groups, with a higher rate of ICU admission and greater morbidity. Poor outcomes result from worsening of underlying heart or lung conditions, secondary bacterial pneumonia, toxic shock syndrome, endotoxemia, myopericarditis, cytokine-induced shock syndrome, encephalitis, and transverse myelitis.

Diagnosis. Several tests can be performed to diagnose influenza. Nasopharyngeal swabs, nasal washes, and aspirates obtained within the first 4 days of illness are preferred respiratory samples.

- *Rapid influenza tests* (54) can provide results within 30 minutes, and some distinguish between influenza A and B. The overall sensitivity is 70% to 75%, with a specificity of 90% to 95%. These tests are useful in the diagnosis of individual patients and in detecting outbreaks.
- *Direct immunofluorescent antibody (DFA) staining* requires 2 to 4 hours for results. It distinguishes influenza A and B and is often performed in a panel that also detects parainfluenza and respiratory syncytial viruses.
- *RT-PCR* detects and distinguishes both influenza A and B in 1 to 2 days.
- *Viral culture* might take up to 10 days. The culture is essential for determining influenza A subtypes and influenza A or B strains, information that can be incorporated into the following year's vaccine.
- *Serology* is used mainly for research or public health investigations, as results are not helpful for clinical decision making.

Treatment. Two classes of antiviral drugs are available for the prevention and treatment of influenza (see Table 114.10 and Fig. 114.1):

1. *Amantadine* and *rimantadine* target the M2 protein of influenza A and are not effective against other influenza viruses. These agents were not recommended in the 2006–2007 season due to the emergence of a high level of resistance (54). Both amantadine and rimantadine are generally well tolerated, but central nervous system (CNS) side effects are more common in the elderly. Dosing modification is based on renal function.
2. *Zanamivir* and *oseltamivir* are neuraminidase inhibitors that are active for prevention and therapy against both influenza A and influenza B. They work best if initiated within 48 hours of clinical symptoms. Although all antiviral medications lessen symptoms and shorten the duration of illness, only oseltamivir has been shown to reduce lower respiratory tract complications requiring antibiotics. Patients with asthma or chronic obstructive pulmonary disease (COPD) are advised to have a fast-acting inhaled bronchodilator available when inhaling zanamivir. Zanamivir should be stopped if patients develop difficulty breathing.

Prevention. Yearly vaccination is the best means to prevent influenza. Vaccination is particularly important in people who are at high-risk of having serious complications, such as those 65 years of age or older, and those with cardiac or pulmonary diseases, diabetes or other metabolic diseases, renal dysfunction, hemoglobinopathies, or immunosuppression, or people (physicians, nurses) caring for those at high risk for serious complications. During influenza outbreaks within an institution or community, public health practice is to combine influenza vaccine and antiviral medications. The vaccine is given to the exposed patients and staff, and the antiviral agent is also given for about 2 weeks until the vaccine takes effect.

Respiratory Syncytial Virus

Respiratory syncytial virus (RSV) causes acute respiratory illness in persons of all ages. The annual frequency of RSV infection in the elderly and high-risk adults is about 5.5% (55). Among patients admitted to a hospital for community-acquired pneumonia, RSV is second to influenza among viral causes. RSV and influenza A result in comparable lengths of stay, admissions to ICUs, and mortality (8% and 7%, respectively).

Transmission. RSV is transmitted person-to-person through close contact or inhalation of large droplets following sneezing or coughing, or by contact with infected fomites. In the United States, RSV outbreaks occur in the winter. In tropical regions, outbreaks occur usually in the rainy season.

Clinical Manifestations. The clinical presentation varies depending on the patient's age and health status. Older children and young adults typically present with upper respiratory symptoms or tracheobronchitis. The elderly and immunocompromised may develop pneumonia. Wheezing occurs in 35% of elderly patients with RSV infection. The presentations can be difficult to differentiate from other causes of viral illnesses, including influenza. In general, however, the upper respiratory infection (URI) symptoms tend to last longer than those caused by other respiratory viruses, and are associated with a bronchitic cough and wheezing (55). Findings on chest radiograph range from focal interstitial or lobar consolidations to diffuse alveolar interstitial infiltrates. Infections are particularly severe in compromised hosts, with a mortality of 30% to 100% in bone marrow transplant recipients (56).

Diagnosis. The diagnosis is made by viral detection (by culture or immunofluorescence) or by detection of viral antigens, RNA, or serology. Cultures are performed on respiratory secretions and require 4 to14 days for results. Rapid assays using *antigen capture technology* can be performed in less than 30 minutes, and sensitivity and specificity approach 90%. Multiplex PCR ELISA is being developed to allow the simultaneous diagnosis of multiple respiratory pathogens (55). In general, the diagnosis is more difficult to establish in adults than in children due to the low titers of viral shedding.

TABLE 114.10

ANTIVIRAL AGENTS (EXCLUDING ANTI-HIV DRUGS)

Drugs	Description	Viral agents	Infection and sites	Dose in patients with normal renal function	Toxicities	Viral resistance	Mechanism of resistance
Acyclovir	Acyclic guanosine nucleoside analogue	HSV1, HSV2, and VZV	Mucocutaneous HSV infection HSV or VZV encephalitis or VZV pneumonitis	400 mg tid PO or 5 mg/kg q8h IV (also available as topical agent) 10 mg/kg q8h IV	Headache, nausea Renal, neurologic toxicities	Less than 1% in immunocompetent hosts 6%–8% in immunocompromised hosts 11%–17% in patients with AIDS and transplant recipients	Most common: no or low production of viral thymidine-kinase (TK) → cross-resistant to penciclovir and ganciclovir Altered TK substrate specificity Altered viral DNA polymerase
Valacyclovir	L-valine ester prodrug of acyclovir	HSV1, HSV2, and VZV	Mucocutaneous HSV Cutaneous HZV	1 g bid PO 1 g tid PO	Similar to acyclovir		Same as acyclovir
Famciclovir	Ester prodrug of penciclovir	HSV1, HSV2, and VZV	Mucocutaneous HSV Cutaneous VZV	125–500 mg bid PO 500–750 mg bid to tid PO	Headache, nausea, and diarrhea		Inactive against TK-deficient strains of HSV and VZV
Ganciclovir	Acyclic guanosine nucleoside analogue	HSV1, HSV2, VZV, CMV, EBV	CMV retinitis, pneumonitis, or other organ disease	5 mg/kg q12h IV	Hematologic	About 8% of isolates in AIDS patients are resistant to ganciclovir after a course of therapy; resistance also documented among transplant recipients	Mutation of UL97 gene or of viral DNA polymerase Some ganciclovir-resistant strains with DNA polymerase mutations are cross-resistant to foscarnet and cidofovir
Valganciclovir	Ester prodrug of ganciclovir	CMV	CMV retinitis	900 mg bid po	Hematologic	Same as ganciclovir	Same as ganciclovir
Foscarnet	Pyrophosphate analogue	HSV1, HSV2, VZV, CMV, HIV	CMV HSV VZV	60 mg/kg q8h IV or 90 mg/kg IV q12h IV 40 mg/kg q8 hours or 60 mg/kg q12 hours IV 60–90 mg/kg q12h IV	Renal (azotemia, acute tubular necrosis) Metabolic and electrolyte imbalance Neurotoxicity (tremor, headache)	Less than 5% of patients on foscarnet therapy	Point mutations in DNA polymerase of HSV and CMV, and reverse transcriptase of HIV. In general, no cross-resistance with ganciclovir or cidofovir, although some ganciclovir-resistant strains with DNA polymerase mutations are cross-resistant to foscarnet and cidofovir

(Continued)

TABLE 114.10

(CONTINUED)

Drugs	Description	Viral agents	Infection and sites	Dose in patients with normal renal function	Toxicities	Viral resistance	Mechanism of resistance
Cidofovir	Nucleotide analogue	HSV1, HSV2, VZV, HHV-6, HHV-8, CMV, EBV, DNA viruses (papilloma, poyloma, pox viruses)	CMV retinitis	5 mg/kg once a week IV	Renal (proximal tubular dysfunction), Ocular (anterior uveitis or ocular hypotony)	Uncommon	Ganciclovir-resistant CMV (due to DNA polymerase mutations plus UL97 mutations) and some foscarnet-resistant CMV strains are cross-resistant to cidofovir
Amantadine Rimantadine	Tricyclic amine	Influenza A	Influenza A within 48 h of symptoms	100 mg bid po	Gastrointestinal complaints and neurologic toxicities (rimantadine has lower neuro effects)	Up to 30% of patients treated shed-resistant viruses by the 5th day	Cross-resistance between amantadine and rimantadine Resistant viruses remain susceptible to neuraminidase inhibitors
Zanamivir	Neuraminidase inhibitor	Influenza A, B	Influenza within 48 h of symptoms	10 mg bid via inhalation	Bronchospasm		
Oseltamivir	Neuraminidase inhibitor	Influenza A, B	Influenza within 48 h of symptoms	75 mg bid po	Neuropsych, nausea		
Ribavirin	Nucleoside analogue	RSV	RSV in infants	6 g/300 mL over 12–18 h/d via aerosol	Teratogenic, embryotoxic Anemia	No viral resistance has been detected (except for Sindbis virus)	
		Hepatitis C	Hepatitis C	500–600 bid po (together with IFN)	Reversible hyperbilirubinemia		
		Lassa fever or Hantavirus		IV, may be obtained from CDC			
Interferon alpha		Hepatitis C virus	Hepatitis C (with ribavirin)	Peg IFN alfa-2a 180 mg SC/week (in combination with ribavirin)	Depression Flulike symptoms Bone marrow toxicity		
		Hepatitis B virus	Hepatitis B	Peg IFN alfa-2a 180 mg SC/week			
Lamivudine	Nucleoside analogue	Hepatitis B HIV	Hepatitis B	100 mg daily po	Benign	16%–31% resistance after 6 mo to 1 y. Rate is higher in transplant recipients	Mutations in HBV DNA polymerase
Entecavir	Nucleoside analogue	Hepatitis B	Hepatitis B	0.5–1 mg PO daily	Headache, Abdominal pain Pharyngitis	Rare in nucleoside-naïve patients (89)	
Adefovir	Nucleotide analogue	Hepatitis B	Hepatitis B	10 mg PO daily		9%, 18%, and 28% resistance after 3, 4, and 5 y, respectively (89)	Mutations in HBV reverse transcriptase domain

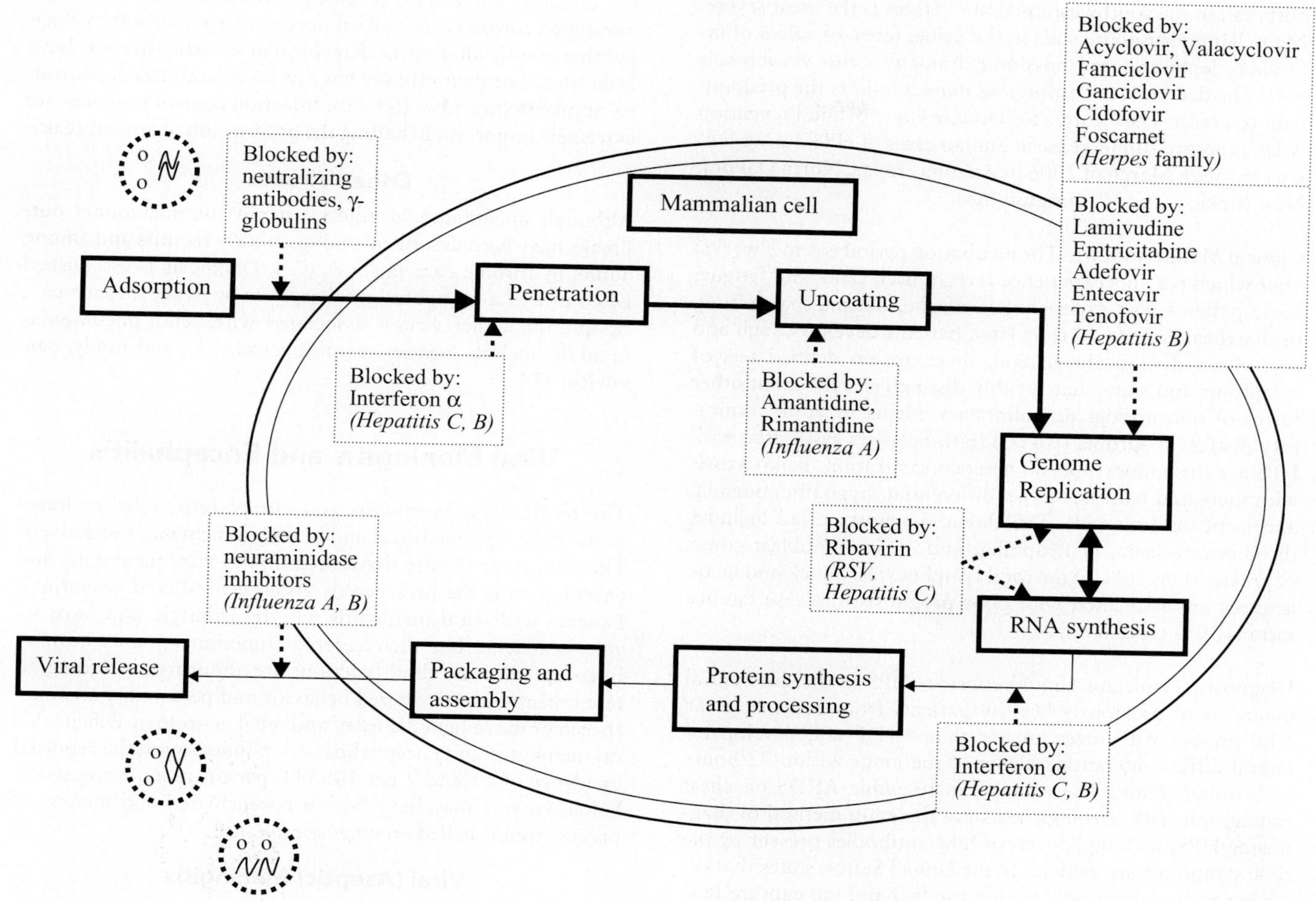

FIGURE 114.1. Sites of action of antiviral agents.

Treatment. Therapy is mainly supportive. Bronchodilators may help to relieve bronchospasm in some patients. Early use of inhaled ribavirin has been shown to reduce morbidity and mortality in adult bone marrow transplant patients who develop RSV infections (56). More aggressive therapy with combined ribavirin, intravenous immunoglobulin with high titers of neutralizing RSV antibody, and/or steroids can be considered in immunosuppressed patients with severe RSV pneumonia (55–57).

Varicella-zoster Virus

Varicella-zoster virus (VZV) causes chickenpox or shingles. Primary infection usually occurs in childhood and is generally a benign self-limited illness in immunocompetent hosts. Although pneumonia is an uncommon complication of varicella in healthy children, it is the most frequent complication in healthy adults. The reported incidence rate is about 2.3 in 400 cases in the United States, and the overall mortality is between 10% and 30% (58,59). In patients with respiratory failure due to varicella pneumonia who require mechanical ventilation, mortality rates approach 50% despite institution of aggressive therapy and supportive measures. Cigarette smoking, pregnancy, immunosuppression, and male sex are risk factors for varicella pneumonia (58,59).

Clinical Manifestations. Varicella pneumonia develops insidiously 1 to 6 days after the onset of the vesicular rash, with symptoms of cough, shortness of breath, fever, and occasionally pleuritic chest pain or hemoptysis. Examination of the chest may reveal rhonchi or wheezes. Chest radiograph typically reveals diffuse or patchy nodular infiltrates with a prominent peribronchial distribution. Reticular markings, pleural effusions, and hilar adenopathy may be seen as well (60).

Treatment. Prompt treatment with intravenous acyclovir at a dose of 10 mg/kg every 8 hours has been associated with clinical improvement and resolution of pneumonia (58,59). The addition of steroids for the treatment of life-threatening varicella pneumonia is controversial and has not been well studied. In one study, patients who received steroids as adjunctive therapy had shorter hospitalizations and ICU stays and no mortality (61,62). Rapid institution of extracorporeal life support has been reported to improve outcome in patients with severe life-threatening varicella pneumonia (63).

Hantavirus Pulmonary Syndrome

Among the agents causing Hantavirus pulmonary syndrome (HPS), the *Sin Nombre* (Spanish for "nameless" or "without a name") virus that caused the 1993 Four Corners outbreak in the southwestern United States is the most severe. Many hantaviruses are shed in the urine, feces, or saliva of infected rodents, and transmission to humans occurs via aerosols (64). The deer mouse *Peromyscus maniculatus* is the predominant reservoir. The Centers for Disease Control and Prevention (CDC) reported an increase in human cases of HPS during January through March of 2006 in Arizona, Texas, North Dakota, New Mexico, and Washington (65).

Clinical Manifestations. The incubation period is 1 to 3 weeks, after which patients experience fever, muscle pain, and fatigue; some patients also experience headache, dizziness, vomiting, or diarrhea. Four to 10 days later, patients develop cough and respiratory distress. In general, there are no defined sets of symptoms and signs that reliably distinguish HPS from other forms of noncardiogenic pulmonary edema or adult respiratory distress syndrome (ARDS) (64). Features associated with HPS are thrombocytopenia, hemoconcentration, leukocytosis with increased band forms on differential, hypoalbuminemia, and lactic acidosis (64). The classic diagnostic triad includes thrombocytopenia, neutrophilia, and an immunoblast count of greater than 10% of the total lymphocytes. Shock and lactic acidosis are associated with poor prognosis; the case fatality ratio is 30% to 40%.

Diagnosis. Clinicians should consider HPS in the differential diagnosis of previously healthy patients from endemic areas who present with fever greater than 101°F and develop bilateral diffuse interstitial edema of the lungs within 72 hours of hospitalization. The edema can resemble ARDS on chest radiograph (64). Serologic tests are the main method of diagnosing HPS, with high levels of IgM antibodies present by the time symptoms are evident. In the United States, states that offer hantavirus diagnostic testing use IgG and mu capture IgM ELISA assays developed and distributed by CDC (64).

Treatment. There is no specific antiviral therapy for HPS, and treatment is mainly supportive, with early initiation of mechanical ventilation to treat respiratory failure. In specialized centers, the use of extracorporeal membrane oxygenation (ECMO) should be considered in patients with a cardiac index of less than 2.5 L/minute/m^2 despite inotropes (66). A placebo-controlled double-blind trial of intravenous ribavirin for the treatment of hantavirus cardiopulmonary syndrome in North America was terminated early due to the drug's probable ineffectiveness (67).

Severe Acute Respiratory Syndrome

Severe acute respiratory syndrome (SARS) is a serious pulmonary illness caused by a coronavirus that jumped species from semidomesticated animals to humans and spread from China to Hong Kong in late 2002 (68–70). The infection is spread by close person-to-person contact via respiratory droplets; incubation period is 2 to 10 days. The patients first experience a high fever associated with chills, headache, and myalgia. Diarrhea is seen in approximately 10% to 20% of patients. Two to 7 days later, patients develop a dry nonproductive cough and hypoxia that progresses to ARDS and multiple organ dysfunction (68–71). Ten percent to 20% of patients require mechanical ventilation. RT-PCR, serology, and cultures of blood, stool, and nasal secretions are possible diagnostic tools but have shortcomings that make routine clinical use difficult. There is no specific treatment against the SARS-associated coronavirus, and supportive care remains the principal therapeutic alternative. Rivabirin and corticosteroids have been used, but their efficacy has not been established. Mortality approximates 11% (68–70). Infection control practices are extremely important in halting the progression of an outbreak.

Other Viruses

Although uncommon in adults, adenovirus pneumonia outbreaks have been described among military recruits and among adults in chronic care facilities (72). Diagnosis is established by culture of a nasopharyngeal aspirate or swab, throat swab, or sputum. Other viruses associated with acute pneumonias in adults include measles, parainfluenza (73), and rarely, parvovirus (74).

Viral Meningitis and Encephalitis

The terms, *viral meningitis* and *encephalitis*, refer to infections of the leptomeninges and brain parenchyma, respectively. The important feature that differentiates viral meningitis and encephalitis is the presence or absence of altered sensorium. Patients with viral meningitis may be lethargic and have severe headache, but their cerebral function remains normal. In encephalitis, cerebral functions are abnormal, including altered mental status, altered behavior and personality changes, speech or movement disorder, and focal neurologic deficits. Viral meningitis and encephalitis are common, with the reported incidence of 11 and 7 per 100,000 person-years, respectively. Some patients may have both a parenchymal and meningeal process that is called *meningoencephalitis*.

Viral (Aseptic) Meningitis

The common causes of viral meningitis are summarized in Table 114.11 (75–77). Other viruses such as Epstein-Barr virus (EBV), cytomegalovirus (CMV), human herpes virus 6 (HHV-6), and herpes zoster (reactivation of VZV infection) are even rarer causes of aseptic meningitis. Arboviruses such as St. Louis encephalitis and California encephalitis (SLE and CE, respectively) more commonly cause encephalitis or meningoencephalitis but can also cause aseptic meningitis.

The clinical presentations of viral meningitis are nonspecific with fever, headache, photophobia, and nuchal rigidity as common symptoms. Helpful clues to the diagnosis include travel to arbovirus endemic areas, exposure history (rodents, ticks), sexual activity (HSV-2), and contact with other people with similar symptoms (enteroviruses). Clinicians should look for pharyngitis and pleurodynia (enteroviruses), rash (zosteriform rash of VZV, vesicular rash of HSV, maculopapular rash measles or enteroviruses), and adenopathy (primary HIV or EBV). Cerebrospinal fluid (CSF) findings include white blood cells (WBC) less than 500 per μL, of which greater than 50% are lymphocytes; protein less than 80 mg/dL; normal glucose; and negative Gram stain. CSF should be sent for bacterial and viral cultures, HSV PCR, and HIV viral load. Other tests that can be sent if indicated include enterovirus PCR and acute/convalescent serologic testing for specific viruses.

If the patient is neither immunocompromised nor toxic appearing, one can observe without giving antibiotic therapy. Treatment for enteroviral meningitis is mostly supportive (pain management and hydration). Pleconaril, which inhibits viral

TABLE 114.11

COMMON CAUSES OF VIRAL MENINGITIS AND ENCEPHALITIS

Types of infection	Viral pathogen	Comments
Viral meningitis	Enterovirus	Most common cause of viral meningitis More than 50 serotypes of enteroviruses Can cause meningitis or meningoencephalitis
	Herpes simplex type 2	Associated with genital herpes infection
	HIV	Generally develops at the time of HIV seroconversion
	Lymphocytic choriomeningitis (LCM)	Sporadic cause of meningitis Can cause meningitis or meningoencephalitis
	Adenovirus	Rare cause of viral meningitis Can cause severe meningoencephalitis in children
Encephalitis	Japanese encephalitis	Most common cause worldwide
	Herpes simplex type 1	Most common cause of sporadic viral encephalitis Associated with focal symptoms
	Arboviruses	Transmitted by mosquitoes or ticks.
	CMV, VZV	Causes disease in immunocompromised patients only

HIV, human immunodeficiency virus; CMV, cytomegalovirus; VZV, varicella-zoster virus.

attachment to host cells and viral uncoating, has shown disappointing results in the treatment of enteroviral meningitis. If the patient is immunosuppressed, elderly, or toxic appearing, or has received antibiotics before presentation, one may consider empiric antibiotics for 48 hours while waiting for culture results.

Viral Encephalitis

In the United States, the most common cause of sporadic encephalitis is HSV-1. Arboviruses account for approximately 5% of viral encephalitis, with SLE virus being the most common. Clues to arboviral infection include the season (arboviruses cause disease when mosquitoes are active, whereas HSV-1 can occur at any time), location (woody or marshy areas would suggest viruses such as the cause of Colorado tick fever or nonviral illness such as Lyme disease or Rocky Mountain spotted fever), geographic region (SLE occurs in the midwest and southern United States, whereas West Nile virus [WNV] occurs in multiple continents), or a history of animal exposure (rabies). Clues on physical exam include parotitis (mumps); flaccid paralysis (WNV); tremors of the eyelids, tongue, lips, and extremities (SLE); or findings of hydrophobia, aerophobia, and hyperactivity (rabies).

The CSF findings can be similar to those of viral meningitis. Depending on clinical suspicion, the CSF can also be sent for PCR for enteroviruses, HSV, or CMV. Acute and convalescent sera against specific viral pathogens such as arboviruses, and lymphocytic choriomeningitis virus (LCMV) might also be useful in determining a cause. CT scan with IV contrast or magnetic resonance imaging (MRI) should be obtained to exclude an intracranial process (cerebritis, abscess, subdural empyema, mass occupying lesions) or to detect findings suggestive of a viral cause. Temporal and basal frontal lobe involvement suggests HSV encephalitis, whereas basal ganglia and thalamic involvement suggest Eastern equine encephalitis.

Until HSV encephalitis is ruled out, acyclovir at 10 mg/dL IV every 8 hours should be considered in patients with suspected viral encephalitis.

HSV Encephalitis. HSV encephalitis is a fulminant hemorrhagic and necrotizing meningoencephalitis that involves primarily the temporal and basal frontal cortices and the limbic system (78). Herpes simplex type 1 (HSV-1) accounts for most fatal cases of sporadic encephalitis in adults. HSV-1 encephalitis can arise either from primary infections or reactivation of a latent infection; there is no difference in outcome from patients suffering encephalitis from a primary or reactivation HSV infection. Herpes simplex virus type 2 (HSV-2) accounts for herpes encephalitis in 80% to 90% of neonates and children.

Clinical Manifestations. The most common early symptoms are fever and headache. Additional symptoms include meningeal irritation, nausea, vomiting, altered consciousness, and generalized seizures. Other changes are referable to the involved areas of the brain and include anosmia, memory loss, abnormal behavior, speech defects, olfactory and gustatory hallucinations, and focal seizures. There can be rapid progression of the disease in some patients with the development of focal paralysis, hemiparesis, and coma.

Diagnosis. The diagnosis of HSV encephalitis can be strongly suggested if the typical clinical presentations are associated with specific findings on electroencephalogram (EEG) and MRI. The typical EEG findings are focal temporal abnormalities, which are found in about 80% of patients; periodic lateralized epileptiform discharges also suggest HSV encephalitis, although they are not as specific. In HSV encephalitis, a normal EEG essentially excludes the diagnosis. The typical MRI appearance is medial temporal abnormalities that do not respect hippocampal borders. CSF findings are similar to other cases of viral meningoencephalitis. Isolation of HSV from the CSF is rare, occurring in less than 5% of cases. A definitive diagnosis is made by detection of HSV DNA in CSF by PCR, which is very sensitive and specific. The availability of PCR has largely obviated the need for brain biopsy, which was the previous gold standard diagnostic test.

Treatment. Morbidity and mortality are reduced by early antiviral therapy. Intravenous acyclovir, 10 mg/kg every 8 hours, is continued for 14 to 21 days. There is a 5% relapse rate after the discontinuation of antiviral therapy.

Rabies. Rabies is caused by neurotropic RNA viruses (79). In addition to the classic rabies virus, at least ten other rabies-related viruses can cause clinically indistinguishable fatal encephalitis (79). Rabies has a worldwide distribution and is found throughout the United States except Hawaii. In developing countries, dogs are the major reservoir. Wild animals remain the most important reservoir in the United States; most reported cases occur in carnivores (raccoons in the northeast, skunks in the south and southwest, and foxes in the southwest and Alaska) or insectivorous bats (79). In the United States, there have been an average of three fatal human cases per year since 1980 (79).

Acquisition of rabies usually occurs after a bite from an infected animal or scratching and licking by a rabid animal. Cases have also been reported after solid organ, cornea, or vascular tissue transplantation from unsuspected rabies-infected individuals (80,81).

Clinical Manifestations. Human rabies assumes two forms: furious (encephalitic) and paralytic (dumb). The furious form (observed in 80% of patients) manifests as hyperactivity, hydrophobia, pharyngeal spasms, and aerophobia. The paralytic presentation can mimic Guillain-Barré syndrome with quadriparesis, sphincter involvement, and late cerebral involvement. Some bat-associated rabies may present atypically with neuropathic pain, sensory or motor deficits, choreiform movements of the bitten limb, focal brainstem signs, myoclonus, and seizures (82). Regardless of presentation, the disease is almost always fatal.

Diagnosis. The diagnosis can be confirmed in several ways: (a) detection of viral RNA in saliva by RT-PCR; (b) biopsy of the nape of the neck for detection of RNA or viral antigen within hair follicles by RT-PCR or immunofluorescence staining, respectively; (c) antibodies in serum and cerebrospinal fluid; (d) the presence of pathognomonic Negri bodies (eosinophilic neuronal cytoplasmic inclusions) in brain biopsy (79).

Treatment. There is no proven effective treatment for rabies after the onset of illness. Only six survivors have been reported, five of whom received postexposure vaccination. The sixth patient survived after induction of coma and treatment with ribavirin and amantadine (83). Clinicians who wish to consider this protocol should contact Dr. Rodney Willoughby at Children's Hospital of Wisconsin (414-266-2000). Rabies vaccination after the onset of illness is not recommended and may be detrimental. After definitive diagnosis, the primary focus is comfort care.

Management of patients with rabies poses no greater risk to health care providers than caring for patients with more common infections. Adherence to standard precautions should be maintained, including gloves, gowns, masks, eye protection, and face shield (particularly during intubation or suctioning). Because of the lack of effective treatment, postexposure prophylaxis should be initiated as soon as possible after exposure to rabid or unknown animals. This includes the administration of human rabies immune globulin (HRIG: Hyper-Rab Tm S/D or Imogam Rabies-HT) and rabies vaccination (purified chick embryo cell vaccine (PCECV; 1-800-244-7668; www.rabavert.com).

West Nile Virus. West Nile virus (WNV) is a single-stranded RNA virus that can infect humans, mosquitoes, and animals such as birds and horses. In temperate climates, WNV is transmitted primarily in the summer or early fall, whereas transmission can occur year round in warmer climates. Most human WNV infections result from mosquito bites. Infection can also be transmitted via transfusion of WNV-infected blood products, transplacental fetal infection, and transplantation of infected organs.

Clinical Manifestations. Patients infected with WNV can be asymptomatic (80%), develop West Nile fever (WNF, 20%) or West Nile neuroinvasive disease (WNND, less than 1%) (84). WNND includes meningitis, encephalitis, and acute flaccid paralysis. WNV encephalitis is more common in the elderly or immunocompromised patients. The incubation period ranges from 3 to 14 days, and symptoms generally last 3 to 6 days. Patients with WNF or WNND present with an abrupt onset of fever, headache, fatigue, anorexia, gastrointestinal complaints, myalgia, lymphadenopathy, and generalized nonpruritic maculopapular rash. Patients with WNND also present with altered mental status (46%–74%), tremor (12%–80% of patients), extrapyramidal features such as rigidity or bradykinesia (67%), and cerebellar abnormalities (11%–57%). Myoclonus, which is present in 33% of cases, is a clue to WN infection since it is rare in other causes of viral encephalitis. Seizures are unusual (1%–16%).

Diagnosis. Diagnosis of WNV infection is based on a high index of suspicion and obtaining specific laboratory tests. An IgM antibody capture ELISA (MAC-ELISA) can detect WNV in nearly all CSF and serum specimens from WNV-infected patients. Because IgM antibody does not cross the blood–brain barrier, IgM antibody in the CSF strongly suggests acute CNS infection. WNV testing of patients with encephalitis, meningitis, or other serious CNS infections can be obtained through local or state health departments.

Treatment. Treatment is supportive, with hospitalization, IV fluids, respiratory support, and prevention of secondary infections for patients with severe disease. Although ribavirin and interferon alpha 2b were found to have some activity against WNV *in vitro*, no controlled studies have been completed. The role of corticosteroids has not been assessed.

Viral Infections Acquired during Intensive Care Unit Stay

Herpes family viruses have been recognized as pathogens in immunosuppressed transplant patients and HIV/AIDS patients. Recently, they have been increasingly reported as pathogens in the nonimmunosuppressed critically ill. A retrospective review demonstrated that at least 14% of chronic critically ill surgical patients had occult CMV or HSV infection/reactivation (85).

CMV Infection

CMV infects about 60% to 70% of people during their lifetimes. Like other members of the herpes family, CMV becomes latent or persistent after primary infection. The infection can reactivate at a later time, especially in the settings of immunodeficiency or significant stress from operations or injuries.

Transmission. CMV can be found in body secretions (such as urine, saliva, sputum, breast milk, semen, and cervical fluid) or in circulating mononuclear and polymorphonuclear cells, vascular endothelium, and renal epithelium. CMV spreads from person to person by contact with body fluids. Transmission is particularly high among toddlers in day care. Day care employees are also at significant risk for CMV exposure and/or infection, as are health care personnel with direct patient contact. Congenital transmission from a mother with acute infection during pregnancy is a significant cause of neurologic abnormalities and deafness in newborns. CMV can also be transmitted by breastfeeding, blood transfusion, or receipt of an organ transplant. The major risk factors for CMV disease in solid organ transplant recipients are CMV mismatch (i.e., transplantation of a CMV-positive organ into a CMV-seronegative recipient) and the degree of immunosuppression.

Clinical Manifestations. Most immunocompetent children and adults who are infected with CMV do not develop symptoms. Some may experience an illness resembling infectious mononucleosis with fever, swollen glands, and mild hepatitis. Rare complications of primary CMV infection include hepatitis, interstitial pneumonia, Guillain-Barré syndrome, meningoencephalitis, pericarditis, myocarditis, thrombocytopenia, and hemolytic anemia. In patients who are immunocompromised, primary CMV infection can be life threatening; myelosuppression, encephalitis, hepatitis, pneumonitis, retinitis, and GI infection are the most common manifestations. Moreover, reactivation of latent CMV also causes disease in immunocompromised hosts, although typically milder than primary infection. In general, the severity of CMV disease is related to the degree of immunosuppression. CMV appears to target allografts in particular. Hepatitis, for example, is common in liver transplant recipients, pancreatitis in pancreatic transplant, and pneumonitis in lung and heart-lung transplant. CMV pneumonia is highest among bone marrow transplant recipients.

In solid organ transplant recipients, CMV infections predispose to other opportunistic infections, especially fungal or *Pneumocystis* infections. CMV infection can also affect graft survival, causing early allograft rejection in renal transplant recipients, chronic allograft rejection in cardiac transplant recipients (allograft atherosclerosis), and vanishing bile duct syndrome in liver transplant recipients.

Diagnosis. Since CMV can be shed in biologic fluids from patients with no evidence of CMV disease, the gold standard for diagnosis remains finding intranuclear inclusion bodies in histologically examined tissue. CMV infection may be confirmed by *in situ* hybridization or direct or indirect staining of intranuclear inclusions using specific antibodies linked to an indicator system. Histopathology is limited by poor sensitivity. Tests that can detect and quantify CMV or its products in blood, leukocytes, or tissues are reviewed in Table 114.12.

CMV excretion in the saliva and urine is common in patients who are immunocompromised and is generally of little consequence. In contrast, viremia in organ transplant patients identifies those at greatest risk for CMV disease. In bone marrow transplant recipients, the sensitivity of viremia as a marker for CMV pneumonia is 60% to 70%; lack of viremia also has a high negative predictive value. In general, detection of CMV or its products in the blood of transplant recipients is a basis for starting antiviral therapy. The value of positive CMV tests in the nontransplant ICU patient is less clear. Studies indicate that asymptomatic CMV infection is common, and low level viremia can be detected in almost a third of patients after 2 weeks in the ICU (85,86). Viremia, therefore, does not necessarily signify CMV disease in ICU patients. Further studies are needed to elucidate the impact of CMV infection/reactivation in critically ill patients and to clarify the effects of CMV treatment on morbidity and mortality.

Management. Ganciclovir, foscarnet, and cidofovir are antiviral agents active against CMV (Table 114.10). To date, the efficacy of anti-CMV therapy has been evaluated primarily in immunocompromised hosts (transplant recipients and AIDS patients). CMV disease in transplant recipients is typically treated with a 3-week course of ganciclovir. Foscarnet is an alternative for patients who cannot tolerate, or fail to respond to, ganciclovir; but experience is more limited, and foscarnet is associated with high rates of nephrotoxicity. CMV retinitis requires a longer course of systemic therapy; intravitreal administration of ganciclovir or fomivirsen, an antisense inhibitor of CMV, is frequently used in addition to systemic therapy. Although long-term maintenance therapy is required for AIDS patients who do not undergo immune reconstitution, this strategy is generally not required for transplant recipients. Recurrence of CMV disease, which can occur in up to 25% of transplant recipients, appears to respond to ganciclovir as well as the initial episode.

HSV Infection

HSV-1 and HSV-2 are closely related, but the epidemiology of infections by the viruses is distinct. HSV-1 is transmitted mainly by contact with infected saliva, and HSV-2 by contact with the genital tract. HSV-1 is acquired more commonly and at an earlier age than HSV-2. By the age of 50 years, over 90% of people have antibodies against HSV-1. Consistent with this, HSV-1 is also more common among ICU patients.

Clinical Manifestations. HSV encephalitis and meningitis are discussed above. HSV-1 can infect virtually any mucocutaneous or visceral site. Typically, primary infections are associated with systemic signs and symptoms, mucosal and extramucosal involvement, longer duration of symptoms and viral shedding, and higher complication rates. Gingivostomatitis and pharyngitis are the most common clinical syndromes of HSV-1

TABLE 114.12

DIAGNOSTIC TESTS FOR CMV INFECTION

Test	Concept	Advantages/disadvantages	Interpretation of positive tests in the immunocompromised host	Interpretation of tests in the immunocompetent host
SEROLOGY				
CMV-specific IgG	Detect IgG seroconversion.	Disadvantage: Need acute and convalescent sera (or known baseline negative IgG).	Documented seroconversion implies primary CMV infection.	Documented seroconversion implies primary CMV infection.
CMV-specific IgM	Acute phase of primary CMV infection should have positive CMV-specific IgM and negative IgG antibodies.	Advantage: Depending on assays used, sensitivity and specificity can be as high as 100% and 98%, respectively. Disadvantage: Interference due to presence of rheumatoid factor and antinuclear antibody.	Primary infection. Since IgM can also be elevated in reactivation, positive IgM alone does not indicate primary CMV infection. In this setting, should interpret in conjunction with CMV-specific IgG. In the immunocompromised host, IgM might persist for a long time after primary infection.	Primary infection. Problems with false-positive and persistent IgM due to reactivation are less than with the immunocompromised hosts.
Detection of virus	Recovery of CMV from the biologic sites signifies either primary infection, reactivation, or asymptomatic shedding without infection.			
Shell-vial assay	Detection and quantitation of viremia.	Disadvantage: 1. Tissue culture is time-consuming. Shell-vial assay can provide results within 24 hours. 2. Low sensitivity. 3. Loss of CMV viability in stored clinical samples.	High risk of developing CMV disease. Marker for initiation of antiviral therapy and monitoring the efficacy of therapy.	Specific for primary CMV infection. Sensitivity of 26.3%, highest within 1 mo of primary infection. Test positivity can last up to 4–6 mo. Low false-positive rate.
Antigenemia	Detection and quantitation of leukocytes that are positive for CMV phosphoprotein pp65.	Advantages: 1. Rapid test with turnover time of a few hours. 2. In transplant recipients, antigenemia becomes positive before viremia detection, but later than DNA-emia at the onset of CMV infection. Disadvantages: 1. Subjective slide reading. 2. Levels of antigenemia might lag behind clinical response to antiviral therapy.	Associated with CMV disease.	Specific for primary CMV infection. Sensitivity of 57.1%, highest within 1 mo of primary infection. Test positivity can last 4–6 mo. Negligible false-positive rate.
CMV DNA in blood (DNA-emia)	Detection and quantitation of CMV DNA in whole blood and leukocytes: PCR and hybridization techniques.	Advantages: 1. Useful for diagnosis of systemic or local CMV infections (CNS, eye, central nervous system, amniotic fluid). 2. Useful for evaluation of efficacy of antiviral therapy	1. Systemic and local site CMV infections.	Marker for primary CMV infection. Leukocyte DNA-emia has sensitivity of 100%, highest within 1 month of primary infection. Test positivity can last 4–6 mo.
Immediate-early and late CMV mRNA (RNA-emia)	Detection of immediate-early and late CMV mRNA transcripts in blood	Advantage: slightly more sensitive than DNA-emia in diagnosing early phase of primary CMV infection. Disadvantage: Slightly less sensitive than DNA-emia in the late phase of primary CMV infection.	1. RNA-emia in blood is a marker of CMV replication 2. Late viral transcripts are markers for active CMV replication and dissemination.	Immediate-early mRNA in the blood is a marker for primary infection.

infection. Lesions are ulcerative with or without exudates, and can be difficult to differentiate from bacterial pharyngitis. HSV-1 also has a predilection for regenerating epithelium. Therefore, healing partial-thickness skin burns, skin donor sites, skin diseases (e.g., eczema, pemphigus, Darier disease), and areas of cutaneous trauma are common sites of infection. HSV-1 keratitis is the most frequent cause of corneal blindness. HSV-1 can also cause chorioretinitis—a sign of disseminated infection—and acute necrotizing retinitis, affecting both immunocompetent and immunocompromised hosts.

In immunocompromised hosts and patients with atopic eczema or burns, severe orofacial HSV lesions can rapidly spread and disseminate infection. Bone marrow and solid organ transplant recipients are at highest risk for HSV reactivation during the pre-engraftment period or within the first month posttransplant. Complications include pneumonitis, tracheobronchitis, esophagitis, hepatitis, and disseminated viral infection.

HSV-1 shedding is observed in immunocompetent but critically ill patients. In one study, HSV-1 was recovered from the mouth swabs or respiratory secretions of 27% of patients requiring mechanical ventilation (87). Although the presence of HSV was associated with a higher APACHE II score and increased mortality (88), it is not clear whether HSV was the cause of the excess deaths or simply a marker for impaired immune function. HSV-1 may predispose to subsequent bacterial or fungal infection (87).

Diagnosis. The diagnosis of HSV-1 infection can be made using a direct immunofluorescence test or by culture of tissue or aspirated fluid. Serology is helpful in diagnosing primary HSV infection. Improved testing methods have led to increased detection of HSV-1 in ICU patients. As with CMV, however, it is often unclear whether HIV-1 is an active pathogen or merely a marker of immune dysfunction. Large randomized trials are needed to determine the impact of CMV and HSV isolation from respiratory specimens of patients in the ICU and the effect of treatment on morbidity and mortality of critically ill patients.

Management. For mucocutaneous and visceral infections, acyclovir or related agents (famciclovir and valacyclovir) are the standard therapy. For disseminated disease or encephalitis due to HSV-1, intravenous acyclovir is recommended. For HSV keratitis, debridement along with topical therapy with idoxuridine or vidarabine is the treatment of choice. Other ophthalmologic disease such as chorioretinitis or retinal necrosis requires systemic antiviral therapy.

SUMMARY

Although the field of antiviral therapy has developed extensively over the last 30 years, many issues remain. Most agents have a similar target of action, which frequently results in cross-resistance among agents. Furthermore, the range of viral infections for which treatment options exist is still limited. A lack of culture systems for many viruses hinders drug development. Moreover, the intracellular parasitism of viruses increases the potential for host toxicity. One needs to keep clinical suspicion for viral illness high since the window of opportunity for treatment is often very narrow. Clearly, there is a critical need for new therapies that expand the rather limited present armamentarium. Until that time, vaccination and other preventive strategies are the best hope for the control of viral infections.

References

1. Wisplinghoff H, Bischoff T, Tallent SM, et al. Nosocomial bloodstream infections in US hospitals: analysis of 24,179 cases from a prospective nationwide surveillance study. *Clin Infect Dis.* 2004;39:309–317.
2. Alberti C, Brun-Buisson C, Burchardi H, et al. Epidemiology of sepsis and infection in ICU patients from an international multicentre cohort study. *Intensive Care Med.* 2002;28:108–121.
3. Gudlaugsson O, Gillespie S, Lee K, et al. Attributable mortality of nosocomial candidemia, revisited. *Clin Infect Dis.* 2003;37:1172–1177
4. Pfaller MA, Diekema DJ, Jones RN, et al. International surveillance of bloodstream infections due to *Candida* species: frequency of occurrence and *in vitro* susceptibilities to fluconazole, ravuconazole, and voriconazole of isolates collected from 1997 through 1999 in the SENTRY antimicrobial surveillance program. *J Clin Microbiol.* 2001;39:3254–3259.
5. Bodey GP, Mardani M, Hanna HA, et al. The epidemiology of *Candida glabrata* and *Candida albicans* fungemia in immunocompromised patients with cancer. *Am J Med.* 2002;112:380–385.
6. Rodriguez LJ, Rex JH, Anaissie EJ. Update on invasive candidiasis. *Adv Pharmacol.* 1997;37:349–400.
7. Ostrosky-Zeichner L, Alexander BD, Kett DH, et al. Multicenter clinical evaluation of the (1->3) beta-D-glucan assay as an aid to diagnosis of fungal infections in humans. *Clin Infect Dis.* 2005;41:654–659.
8. Rex JH, Pfaller MA. Has antifungal susceptibility testing come of age? *Clin Infect Dis.* 2002;35:982–989.
9. Krogh-Madsen M, Arendrup MC, Heslet L, et al. . Amphotericin B and caspofungin resistance in *Candida glabrata* isolates recovered from a critically ill patient. *Clin Infect Dis.* 2006;42:938–944.
10. Mora-Duarte J, Betts R, Rotstein C, et al; Caspofungin Invasive Candidiasis Study Group. Comparison of caspofungin and amphotericin B for invasive candidiasis. *N Engl J Med.* 2002;347:2020–2029.
11. Pappas PG, Rex JH, Sobel JD, et al. Guidelines for treatment of candidiasis. *Clin Infect Dis.* 2004;38:161–189.
12. Bennett JE. Echinocandins for candidemia in adults without neutropenia. *N Engl J Med.* 2006;355:1154–1159.
13. Kullberg BJ, Sobel JD, Ruhnke M, et al. Voriconazole versus a regimen of amphotericin B followed by fluconazole for candidaemia in non-neutropenic patients: a randomised non-inferiority trial. *Lancet.* 2005;366:1435–1442.
14. Kauffman CA. Candiduria. *Clin Infect Dis.* 2005;41(Suppl 6):S371–376.
15. Lundstrom T, Sobel J. Nosocomial candiduria: a review. *Clin Infect Dis.* 2001;32:1602–1607.
16. el-Ebiary M, Torres A, Fabregas N, et al. Significance of the isolation of *Candida* species from respiratory samples in critically ill, non-neutropenic patients. An immediate postmortem histologic study. *Am J Respir Crit Care Med.* 1997;156:583–590.
17. Rello J, Esandi ME, Diaz E, et al. The role of *Candida* sp isolated from bronchoscopic samples in nonneutropenic patients. *Chest.* 1998;114:146–149.
18. Barenfanger J, Arakere P, Cruz RD, et al. Improved outcomes associated with limiting identification of *Candida* spp. In respiratory secretions. *J Clin Microbiol.* 2003;41:5645–5649.
19. Eggimann P, Francioli P, Bille J, et al. Fluconazole prophylaxis prevents intra-abdominal candidiasis in high-risk surgical patients. *Crit Care Med.* 1999;27:1066–1072.
20. Garbino J, Lew DP, Romand JA, et al. Prevention of severe *Candida* infections in nonneutropenic, high-risk, critically ill patients: a randomized, double-blind, placebo-controlled trial in patients treated by selective digestive decontamination. *Intensive Care Med.* 2002;28:1708–1717.
21. Jacobs S, Price Evans DA, et al. Fluconazole improves survival in septic shock: a randomized double-blind prospective study. *Crit Care Med.* 2003;31:1938–1946.
22. Pelz RK, Hendrix CW, Swoboda SM, et al. Double-blind placebo-controlled trial of fluconazole to prevent candidal infections in critically ill surgical patients. *Ann Surg.* 2001;233:542–548.
23. Golan Y, Wolf MP, Pauker SG, et al. Empirical anti-*Candida* therapy among selected patients in the intensive care unit: a cost-effectiveness analysis. *Ann Intern Med.* 2005;143:857–869.
24. Caillot D, Casasnovas O, Bernard A, et al. Improved management of invasive pulmonary aspergillosis in neutropenic patients using early thoracic computed tomographic scan and surgery. *J Clin Oncol.* 1997;15:139–147.
25. Pfeiffer CD, Fine JP, Safdar N. Diagnosis of invasive aspergillosis using a galactomannan assay: a meta-analysis. *Clin Infect Dis.* 2006;42:1417–1427.
26. Husain S, Kwak EJ, Obman A, et al. Prospective assessment of Platelia *Aspergillus* galactomannan antigen for the diagnosis of invasive aspergillosis in lung transplant recipients. *Am J Transplant.* 2004;4:796–802.
27. Kwak EJ, Husain S, Obman A, et al. Efficacy of galactomannan antigen in the Platelia *Aspergillus* enzyme immunoassay for diagnosis of invasive

aspergillosis in liver transplant recipients. *J Clin Microbiol.* 2004;42:435–438.
28. Fortun J, Martin-Davila P, Alvarez ME, et al. *Aspergillus* antigenemia sandwich-enzyme immunoassay test as a serodiagnostic method for invasive aspergillosis in liver transplant recipients. *Transplantation.* 2001;71:145–149.
29. Musher B, Fredricks D, Leisenring W, et al. *Aspergillus* galactomannan enzyme immunoassay and quantitative PCR for diagnosis of invasive aspergillosis with bronchoalveolar lavage fluid. *J Clin Microbiol.* 2004;42:5517–5522.
30. Sanguinetti M, Posteraro B, Pagano L, et al. Comparison of real-time PCR, conventional PCR, and galactomannan antigen detection by enzyme-linked immunosorbent assay using bronchoalveolar lavage fluid samples from hematology patients for diagnosis of invasive pulmonary aspergillosis. *J Clin Microbiol.* 2003;41:3922–3925.
31. Salonen J, Lehtonen OP, Terasjarvi MR, et al. *Aspergillus* antigen in serum, urine and bronchoalveolar lavage specimens of neutropenic patients in relation to clinical outcome. *Scand J Infect Dis.* 2000;32:485–490.
32. Siemann M, Koch-Dorfler M. The Platelia *Aspergillus* ELISA in diagnosis of invasive pulmonary aspergillosis (IPA). *Mycoses.* 2001;44:266–272.
33. Siemann M, Koch-Dorfler M, Gaude M. False-positive results in premature infants with the Platelia *Aspergillus* sandwich enzyme-linked immunosorbent assay. *Mycoses.* 1998;41:373–377.
34. Verweij PE, Erjavec Z, Sluiters W, et al. Detection of antigen in sera of patients with invasive aspergillosis: intra- and interlaboratory reproducibility. The Dutch Interuniversity Working Party for Invasive Mycoses. *J Clin Microbiol.* 1998;36:1612–1616.
35. Herbrecht R, Denning DW, Patterson TF, et al. Voriconazole versus amphotericin B for primary therapy of invasive aspergillosis. *N Engl J Med.* 2002;347:408415.
36. Walsh TJ, Raad I, Patterson TF, et al. Treatment of invasive aspergillosis with posaconazole in patients who are refractory to or intolerant of conventional therapy: an externally controlled trial. *Clin Infect Dis.* 2007;44:2–12.
37. Kartsonis NA, Saah AJ, Joy Lipka C, et al. Salvage therapy with caspofungin for invasive aspergillosis: results from the caspofungin compassionate use study. *J Infect.* 2005;50:196–205.
38. Aliff TB, Maslak PG, Jurcic JG, et al. Refractory *Aspergillus* pneumonia in patients with acute leukemia: successful therapy with combination caspofungin and liposomal amphotericin *Cancer.* 2003;97:1025–1032.
39. Kontoyiannis DP, Hachem R, Lewis RE, et al. Efficacy and toxicity of caspofungin in combination with liposomal amphotericin B as primary or salvage treatment of invasive aspergillosis in patients with hematologic malignancies. *Cancer.* 2003;98:292–299.
40. Marr KA, Boeckh M, Carter RA, et al. Combination antifungal therapy for invasive aspergillosis. *Clin Infect Dis.* 2004;39:797–802.
41. Matt P, Bernet F, Habicht J, et al. Predicting outcome after lung resection for invasive pulmonary aspergillosis in patients with neutropenia. *Chest.* 2004;126:1783–1788.
42. Matt P, Bernet F, Habicht J, et al. Short- and long-term outcome after lung resection for invasive pulmonary aspergillosis. *Thorac Cardiovasc Surg.* 2003;51:221–225.
43. Ali R, Ozkalemkas F, Ozcelik T, et al. Invasive pulmonary aspergillosis: role of early diagnosis and surgical treatment in patients with acute leukemia. *Ann Clin Microbiol Antimicrob.* 2006;5:17.
44. Cesaro S, Cecchetto G, De Corti FD, et al. Results of a multicenter retrospective study of a combined medical and surgical approach to pulmonary aspergillosis in pediatric neutropenic patients. *Pediatr Blood Cancer.* 2007;49(7):909–913.
45. Middelhof CA, Loudon WG, Muhonen MD, et al. Improved survival in central nervous system aspergillosis: a series of immunocompromised children with leukemia undergoing stereotactic resection of aspergillomas. Report of four cases. *J Neurosurg.* 2005;103(4 Suppl):374–378.
46. Janelle JW, Howard RJ. Viral infection. *In:* Souba WW, et al., eds. *ACS Surgery: Principles and Practice.* WebMD Inc; 2007.
47. Legoff J, Guerot E, Ndjoyi-Mbiquino A, et al. High prevalence of respiratory viral infections in patients hospitalized in an intensive care unit for acute respiratory infections as detected by nucleic acid based assays. *J Clin Microbiol.* 2005;431:455–457.
48. Kim EA, Lee KS, Primack SL, et al. Viral pneumonias in adults: radiologic and pathologic findings. *Radiographics.* 2002;22:S137–S149.
49. Centers for Diseases Control and Prevention. Update: influenza activity—United States and worldwide, 2005–2006 season. *MMWR Morb Mortal Wkly Rep.* 2006:55:648–653.
50. de Roux A, Marcos MA, Garcia E, et al. Viral community acquired pneumonia. *Chest.* 2004;125:1343–1351.
51. http://www.who.int/csr/disease/avian_influenza/en.
52. Louria DE, Blumenfeld HL, Ellis JT, et al. Studies on influenza in the pandemic of 1957–1958, II: Pulmonary complications of influenza. *J Clin Invest.* 1959;38:213–265.
53. Oliveira EC, Marik PE, Colice G. Influenza pneumonia: a descriptive study. *Chest.* 2001;119:1717–1723.
54. http://www.cdc.gov/flu. Accessed 2/19/07.
55. Falsey AR, Hennessey PA, Formica MA. The disease burden of respiratory syncytial virus infection in elderly and high risk adults. *N Engl J Med.* 2005;352:1749–1759.
56. McColl MD, Corser RB, Brenner J, et al. Respiratory syncytial virus infection in adult BMT recipients: effective therapy with short duration nebulized ribavirin. *Bone Marrow Transplant.* 1998;21:423–425.
57. Krinzman S, Basgoz N, Kradin R, et al. Respiratory syncytial virus associated infections in adult recipients of solid organ transplants. *J Heart Lung Transplant* 1998;17:202–210.
58. Feldman S. Varicella zoster virus pneumonitis. *Chest.* 1994;106:22S–27S.
59. Gogos CA, Bassaris HP. Varicella pneumonia in adults: a review of pulmonary manifestations, risk factors and treatment. *Respiration.* 1992;59(6):339–343.
60. Schlossberg D, Littman M. Varicella pneumonia. *Arch Intern Med.* 1988;148:1630–1632.
61. Mer M, Richards GA. Corticosteroids in life threatening varicella pneumonia. *Chest.* 1998;114:426–431.
62. Adhami N, Arabi Y, Raees A, et al. Effect of corticosteroids on adult varicella pneumonia: cohort study and literature review. *Respirology.* 2006;11:437–441.
63. Lee WA, Kolla S, Schreiner RJ, et al. Prolonged extracorporeal life support for varicella pneumonia. *Crit Care Med.* 1997;25:977–982.
64. Engelthaler D, Levy C, Mosley DG, et al. Hantavirus pulmonary syndrome: five states, 2006. *MMWR Morb Mortal Wkly Rep.* 2006;55:627–629.
65. Centers for Diseases Control and Prevention. Update: Hantavirus pulmonary syndrome—United States, 1999. *MMWR Morb Mortal Wkly Rep.* 1999;48:521–525.
66. Serna D, Brenner M, Chen JC, et al. Severe Hantavirus pulmonary syndrome: a new indication for extracorporeal life support? *Crit Care Med.* 1998;26:217–218.
67. Mertz GJ, Miedzinski L, Goade D, et al. Placebo controlled, double blind trial of intravenous ribavirin for the treatment of hantavirus cardiopulmonary syndrome in North America. *Clin Infect Dis.* 2004;39:1307–1313.
68. www.cdc.gov/ncidod/sars/. Accessed 2/19/07.
69. Booth CM, Stewart TE. Severe acute respiratory syndrome and critical care medicine: the Toronto experience. *Crit Care Med.* 2005;33(S1):S53–S60.
70. Holmes KV. SARS-associated coronavirus. *N Engl J Med.* 2003;348:1948–1951.
71. Ksiazek TG, Erdman D, Goldsmith CS, et al. A novel coronavirus associated with severe acute respiratory syndrome. *N Engl J Med.* 2003;348:1953–1966.
72. Klinger JR, Sanches MO, Curtin LA, et al. Multiple cases of life-threatening adenovirus pneumonia in a mental health care center. *Am J Respir Crit Care Med.* 1998;157:645–651.
73. Hall CB. Respiratory syncytial virus and parainfluenza virus. *N Engl J Med.* 2001;344:1917–1928.
74. Wardeh A, Marik P. Acute lung injury due to parvovirus pneumonia. *J Intern Med.* 1998;244:257–260.
75. Desmond RA, Accort NA, Talley L, et al. Enteroviral meningitis: natural history and outcome of pleconaril therapy. *Antimicrob Agents Chemother.* 2006;50:2409–2414.
76. Rotbart HA. Viral meningitis. *Semin Neurol.* 2000;20:277–292.
77. Sejvar HH. The evolving epidemiology of viral encephalitis. *Curr Opin Neurol.* 2006;19:350–357.
78. Whitley RJ. Herpes simplex encephalitis: adolescents and adults. *Antiviral Res.* 2006;71:141–148.
79. Hemachudha T, Wacharapluesadee S, Laothamatas J, et al. Rabies. *Curr Neurol Neurosci Rep.* 2006;6:460–468.
80. Burton EC, Burns DK, Opatowsky MJ, et al. Rabies encephalomyelitis: clinical, neuroradiological, and pathological findings in 4 transplant recipients. *Arch Neurol.* 2005;62:873–882.
81. World Health Organization. WHO expert consultation on rabies. *World Health Organ Tech Rep Ser.* 2005;931:1–88.
82. Sellal F, Stoll-Keller F. Rabies: ancient yet contemporary cause of encephalitis. *Lancet.* 2005;365:921–923.
83. Centers for Disease Control and Prevention (CDC). Recovery of a patient from clinical rabies–Wisconsin, 2004. *MMWR Morb Mortal Wkly Rep.* 2004;53:1171–1173.
84. Davis LE, DeBiasi R, Goade DE, et al. West Nile virus neuroinvasive disease. *Ann Neurol.* 2006;60:286–300.
85. Carrat F, Leruez-Ville M, Tonnelier M, et al. A virologic survey of patients admitted to a critical care unit for acute cardiorespiratory failure. *Int Care Med.* 2006;32:156–159.
86. Von Muller L, Klemm A, Weiss M, et al. Active cytomegalovirus infection in patients with septic shock. *Emerg Infect Dis.* 2006;12:1517–1522.
87. Bruynseels P, Jorens PG, Demey HE, et al. Herpes simplex virus in the respiratory tract of critical care patients: a prospective study. *Lancet.* 2003;362:1536–1541.
88. Ong GM, Lowry K, Mahajan S, et al. Herpes simplex type 1 shedding is associated with reduced hospital survival in patients receiving assisted ventilation in a tertiary referral intensive care unit. *J Med Virol.* 2004;72:121–125.
89. Tillmann HL. Antiviral therapy and resistance with hepatitis B infection. *World J Gastroenterol.* 2007;13:125–140.

CHAPTER 115 ■ INFECTIONS IN THE IMMUNOCOMPROMISED HOST

KAREN E. DOUCETTE • JAY A. FISHMAN

The population of immunocompromised patients has multiplied greatly in recent years due to an expansion of indications for immunosuppressive therapies combined with improved survival following organ and bone marrow transplantation, cancer chemotherapy, and other chronic diseases requiring immunosuppressive therapy. Despite advances in prophylactic strategies and antimicrobial therapies, infectious complications remain a leading complication of immunosuppressive therapy. Familiarity with the clinical presentation, differential diagnosis, and management of infectious complications in immunocompromised patients is essential for the practice of critical care medicine. An understanding of the nature of the patient's underlying immune deficits—neutropenia and humoral- or cell-mediated immune deficit—and their epidemiologic exposure—intensity and virulence of offending pathogens—will often define the most likely pathogens responsible for an infectious syndrome.

The following points should be considered when evaluating any immunocompromised patient presenting with a suspected infection.

KEY POINTS

1. Due to the impaired inflammatory response, the classic signs and symptoms of infection may be absent in immunocompromised patients. For example, an organ transplant recipient with a perforated viscus may present with fever but without clinical evidence of peritonitis; a neutropenic patient with pneumonia may have cough but absence of a pulmonary infiltrate on chest radiograph.
2. A thorough, repeated history and physical examination remain vital, and are the basis upon which investigations and management are directed in order to achieve a rapid diagnosis and early appropriate therapy. Subtle signs are often the basis for fruitful investigations.
3. Assessment of the immune deficits based on the underlying condition and immunosuppressive therapies, and other therapeutic interventions—surgery, surgical drains, vascular access, antimicrobial therapies—will suggest the most probable pathogens.
4. An aggressive initial approach to diagnosis is generally warranted given the broad spectrum of pathogens potentially causing disease in this population. Routine noninvasive investigations—cultures of blood, urine, and sputum; chest radiograph; and so forth—should be performed, and invasive procedures such as biopsy and bronchoscopy considered early. A delay in arriving at a diagnosis results in delays of appropriate therapy or exposure to toxicities of unneeded therapies, and will compromise treatment outcomes.
5. When tissue or body fluids are collected, histopathologic and microbiologic specimens must be evaluated for both infectious and noninfectious syndromes, such as malignancy, drug toxicity, rejection, and graft versus host disease. Consultation with the pathology and microbiology departments can help ensure maximal yields from clinical specimens.
6. Initial empiric antimicrobial therapy is often warranted due to the severity of initial presentation and/or potential for rapid clinical deterioration. Microbiologic specimens obtained prior to antimicrobial therapy will facilitate microbiologic diagnosis and directed therapy that will limit toxicities and improve patient outcome.

THE IMMUNOCOMPROMISED HOST WITH SUSPECTED INFECTION

The risk of infection in the immunocompromised host, as for any individual, is determined by the interaction of two factors:

- The epidemiologic exposures of the patient including the timing, intensity, and virulence of the organisms to which the individual is exposed
- The patient's "net state of immunosuppression," a measure of all host factors potentially contributing to the risk for infection (Table 115.1) including anatomic defects, as well as exogenous immunosuppression. Specific immunosuppressive therapies and deficits predispose to specific types of infection (Table 115.2).

Consideration of these factors for each patient allows development of a differential diagnosis for "infectious syndromes" and can also be used to direct preventative strategies, such as prophylaxis and vaccination, appropriate to each individual's degree of risk for specific infections. Additional clues to possible etiologies of infection can be obtained from a careful epidemiologic exposure history including travel, occupation, hobbies, animal contact, exposure to ill contacts, and recent hospitalization.

A thorough physical examination should be completed, with particular focus on organ systems commonly involved with infectious complications in immunocompromised hosts; these include the skin, respiratory tract, central nervous system (CNS), and urinary tract. A careful assessment for cutaneous lesions should be performed, as this may be the earliest manifestation of disseminated infection. Examination of the skin

TABLE 115.1

FACTORS CONTRIBUTING TO THE NET STATE OF IMMUNOSUPPRESSION

IMMUNOSUPPRESSIVE THERAPY
- Type
- Temporal sequence
- Intensity
- Cumulative dose

PRIOR THERAPIES
- Chemotherapy or antimicrobials

MUCOCUTANEOUS BARRIER INTEGRITY
- Surgery
- Catheters
- Lines
- Drains
- Fluid collections

NEUTROPENIA, LYMPHOPENIA
- Often drug induced

UNDERLYING IMMUNE DEFICIENCY
- Hypogammaglobulinemia (e.g., from proteinuria)
- Complement deficiencies
- Autoimmune diseases (e.g., systemic lupus erythematosus)
- Other disease states:
  - Human immunodeficiency virus
  - Lymphoma/leukemia

METABOLIC CONDITIONS
- Uremia
- Malnutrition
- Diabetes mellitus
- Cirrhosis

IMMUNOMODULATORY VIRAL INFECTIONS
- Cytomegalovirus
- Hepatitis B and C
- Respiratory viruses

should include the perirectal area, looking for evidence of erythema or tenderness, as this is a common site of infection, such as a perirectal abscess, and source of fever in neutropenic patients. Examination of the respiratory tract should include the paranasal sinuses in addition to the lungs. Signs and symptoms of infection in immunocompromised hosts are often subtle, and minor complaints may be the only clues to localize infection.

In all immunocompromised patients with fever or suspected infection, routine investigations should include a complete blood count (CBC) with differential, serum creatinine, liver enzymes (alanine aminotransferase [ALT], aspartate aminotransferase [AST], alkaline phosphatase), and liver function tests (bilirubin, international normalized ratio [INR]) in addition to blood cultures. A chest radiograph should be performed, as signs and symptoms of respiratory infection may be absent despite an active pulmonary process. Chest computed tomography (CT) scans will often reveal important abnormalities missed by routine radiographs. Additional investigations should be guided by the history, examination, and results of the initial investigations.

An aggressive approach to making a specific microbiologic diagnosis should be undertaken, because delays in appropriate therapy may compromise outcome. Based upon the clinical stability of the patient, the severity of immune deficits, and the most likely cause of infection, the physician may initiate empiric therapy while awaiting the results of investigations, or therapy may be deferred until these are available. Increasingly, infections in compromised hosts are due to organisms with antimicrobial resistance patterns that make selection of empiric therapy more difficult. Compromised hosts have an increased susceptibility to both community-acquired—methicillin-resistant *Staphylococcus aureus* and multiresistant *Pneumococcus*—and nosocomial—vancomycin-resistant enterococcus, fluconazole-resistant *Candida* species—organisms. Consultation with an infectious diseases specialist may be useful to assist in decisions regarding empiric therapy and for guidance regarding appropriate investigations, specimen collection, and transport.

Whenever tissue or body fluids are collected, appropriate histologic and microbiologic investigations should be performed, and consultation with the pathologist and/or microbiologist is recommended to ensure appropriate testing. Diagnosis of many pathogens that cause disease in immunocompromised hosts requires special stains (e.g., modified acid-fast stain for *Nocardia,* silver stain for *Pneumocystis carinii [jirovecii]*) or culture media (e.g., for *Mycobacteria* species). In addition, given that noninfectious etiologies such as organ rejection, drug toxicity, and graft versus host disease (GVHD) are often in the differential diagnosis, histology is integral to making a definitive diagnosis. The diagnosis of virally driven diseases such as tissue-invasive cytomegalovirus (CMV) disease (1) and Epstein-Barr virus (EBV)-associated posttransplant lymphoproliferative disorder (PTLD) (2) also require histology for diagnosis.

THE NEUTROPENIC PATIENT

Neutropenic patients, generally as a result of cytotoxic chemotherapy for hematologic or solid tumors, are among the most commonly encountered immunocompromised hosts. The relationship between the absolute neutrophil count (ANC) and risk of infection was initially described by Bodey et al., who correlated the risk for infection with the degree and duration of neutropenia, notably in leukemic patients, with neutrophil counts less than 500 cells/μL (3,4). This reduction in ANC impairs the innate host immune response of phagocytosis, thus predisposing the neutropenic patient to an array of bacterial and fungal infections, usually from endogenous colonization.

Presentation, Common Pathogens, and Infectious Disease Syndromes

Fever, defined as a single oral temperature of greater than or equal to 38.3°C (101°F) or a temperature of greater than or equal to 38°C (100.4°F) for an hour or more, is often the only predictor of infection (5). About 50% of neutropenic patients with fever have a documented infection, and about 20% of those with neutrophil counts less than 100 cells/μL have bacteremia (5).

The gastrointestinal tract, including the oropharynx and periodontium where chemotherapeutic agents induce mucosal damage, is the most common source of infection in febrile

TABLE 115.2

INFECTIONS ASSOCIATED WITH SPECIFIC IMMUNE DEFECTS

Defect	Common causes	Associated infections
Granulocytopenia	Leukemia, cytotoxic chemotherapy, acquired immunodeficiency syndrome (AIDS), drug toxicity, Felty syndrome	Enteric Gram negatives, *Pseudomonas*, *Staphylococcus aureus*, *Staphylococcus epidermidis*, streptococci, *Aspergillus*, *Candida*, and other fungi
Neutrophil chemotaxis	Diabetes, alcoholism, uremia, Hodgkin disease, trauma (burns), Lazy leukocyte syndrome, connective tissue disease	*S. aureus*, *Candida*, streptococci
Neutrophil killing	Chronic granulomatous disease, myeloperoxidase deficiency	*S. aureus*, *Escherichia coli*, *Candida*, *Aspergillus*, *Torulopsis*
T-cell defects	AIDS, congenital lymphoma, sarcoidosis, viral infection, connective tissue disease, organ transplants, steroids	Intracellular bacteria (*Legionella*, *Listeria*, *Mycobacteria*), herpes simplex virus, varicella-zoster virus, cytomegalovirus, Epstein-Barr virus, parasites (*Strongyloides*, *Toxoplasma*), fungi (*Candida*, *Cryptococcus*) *Pneumocystis carinii (jirovecii)*
B-cell defects	Congenital/acquired agammaglobulinemia, burns, enteropathies, splenic dysfunction, myeloma, acute lymphocytic leukemia	*Streptococcus pneumoniae*, *Haemophilus influenzae*, *Salmonella* and *Campylobacter* spp., *Giardia lamblia*
Splenectomy	Surgery, sickle cell, cirrhosis	*S. pneumoniae*, *H. influenzae*, *Salmonella* spp., *Capnocytophaga*
Complement	Congenital/acquired defects	*S. aureus*, *Neisseria* spp., *H. influenzae*, *S. pneumoniae*
Anatomic	Vascular/Foley catheters, incisions, anastomotic leaks, mucosal ulceration, vascular insufficiency	Colonizing organisms, resistant nosocomial organisms

neutropenic patients (6). However, this is often difficult to document, making pulmonary infections and bacteremia—especially related to vascular lines—more commonly documented (6). Although historically, Gram-negative organisms such as *Escherichia coli*, *Klebsiella* species, and *Pseudomonas aeruginosa* accounted for most bloodstream infections (4), Gram-positive organisms, particularly *Streptococcus* species and coagulase-negative *Staphylococcus,* are now isolated in almost two thirds of bloodstream infections (6). This shift from Gram-negative to Gram-positive bacteremia is related to the now almost universal placement of central venous catheters (CVCs) in patients undergoing chemotherapy, as well as a reduction in the risk of Gram-negative infections with the use of fluoroquinolone prophylaxis (7). The skin, particularly CVC sites, and the lower respiratory and urinary tracts are other common sites of infection.

The risk of opportunistic fungal infection increases with the duration and severity of neutropenia (8). Up to one third of febrile neutropenic patients who fail to respond to a 1-week course of empiric antibacterial therapy have systemic fungal infections, most commonly (over 80%) due to *Candida* or *Aspergillus* species (9,10). The epidemiology of invasive fungal infections has evolved with the growing "at risk" population and increased use of azole prophylaxis. Over half of the bloodstream isolates at most centers are due to non-*albicans Candida* species with increasing intrinsic (e.g., seen with *Candida krusei*) or acquired (e.g., seen with *Candida glabrata*) fluconazole resistance (11). Similarly, neutropenic patients have been found to become infected with highly resistant non-*Aspergillus* molds in addition to *Aspergillus* species (12,13).

Approach to Diagnosis

Signs and symptoms of inflammation may be minimal or absent in the neutropenic host (14). Cutaneous infection often occurs at former sites of intravenous catheters or drains, and may be tender or edematous, without the usual signs of cellulitis. Urinary tract infection may present without pyuria—often with viral pathogens—and the chest radiograph is often normal despite rapidly progressive pneumonia. Up to 50% of neutropenic patients with a normal chest radiograph and fever lasting 2 days, despite empiric antibiotic therapy, will have findings on chest CT suggestive of pneumonia (15). A daily search for subtle signs and symptoms of infection, particularly pain at the most commonly involved sites—periodontium, oropharynx, perianal, skin, and vascular access sites—should be undertaken.

Basic investigations of the neutropenic patient with possible infection include a CBC with differential, serum creatinine, liver enzymes, and liver function tests in addition to cultures of blood, urine, and sputum. A chest radiograph should be performed. If the chest radiograph is normal but the patient has pulmonary symptoms or no identified source of infection, a CT scan should be performed. Collection of additional specimens is guided by the clinical presentation and preliminary investigations. For example, oral ulcerations should be swabbed for viral (herpes simplex virus [HSV]) studies, skin lesions biopsied for culture and histology, and unexplained pulmonary infiltrates assessed with bronchoscopy and bronchoalveolar lavage and/or transbronchial biopsy, or open lung biopsy, as indicated.

While these investigations are not without risk, it is likely that the patient will become *less* tolerant of invasive studies as infection progresses. In those recovering from neutropenia with persistent fever, liver function tests and chest and abdominal imaging should be performed to look for hepatosplenic candidiasis, typhlitis, or invasive mold infection. Many infections will be asymptomatic during a neutropenic event, only becoming apparent with recovery.

Management

Identification of the best candidates for empiric therapy and avoiding the excessive use of prophylactic antimicrobial agents and the toxicities associated with many therapies are central goals for the care of the sick, neutropenic host. After obtaining appropriate microbiologic studies, empiric antimicrobial therapy is indicated in neutropenic patients at the onset of fever or, in the case of suspected infection, without fever (5). In critically ill neutropenic patients, there is no single empiric regimen appropriate for all patients (5,16,17). The selection of an initial empiric antibiotic regimen should take into consideration the general trend of increasing Gram-positive infections, the local hospital epidemiology, and the susceptibility patterns of isolates from neutropenic patients, in addition to the clinical presentation, epidemiologic exposures, and antimicrobial use history.

Options include monotherapy with (a) a third- or fourth-generation cephalosporin (e.g., ceftazidime or cefepime), (b) a carbapenem such as imipenem or meropenem, or (c) piperacillin-tazobactam. Dual therapy may be used without a glycopeptide, such as an antipseudomonal β-lactam plus an aminoglycoside or fluoroquinolone, or, for inpatients with recent surgery or vascular access catheters, a glycopeptide such as vancomycin can be combined with one- or two-drug therapy.

The empiric addition of vancomycin therapy in febrile neutropenia has not been shown to alter outcomes in those patients without pulmonary infiltrates, septic shock, clinically documented infections likely due to Gram-positive organisms such as central venous catheter or skin and soft tissue infections, or documented Gram-positive infections resistant to the primary empiric therapy (18). Vancomycin use has also been associated with the emergence of vancomycin-resistant enterococci, and thus its use in febrile neutropenic patients should be limited as indicated above.

For those who have a source of infection identified—usually less than half of patients under consideration—antimicrobial therapy can be tailored based on culture results, while those who defervesce on empiric antibacterial therapy should have the antimicrobials continued until neutrophil recovery.

Controversy exists regarding the optimal timing of adding antifungal therapy. In patients who have been in the intensive care unit (ICU) for more than 5 to 7 days and have been hypotensive or otherwise critically ill, anti-*Candida* therapy may be added after cultures are obtained (Table 115.3) (19,20). In others who have failed to defervesce on empiric antibiotic therapy after 5 to 7 days, and in whom no source of infection is identified, there is a high risk of systemic fungal infection, and empiric antifungal therapy should be added (5,8,10). Amphotericin B is the historical gold standard for empiric therapy in this setting; however, lipid products of amphotericin B (e.g., liposomal amphotericin B [AmBisome, Astellas] and amphotericin B lipid complex [Abelcet, Elan]) have similar efficacy with less toxicity (21). Recently, voriconazole (22), caspofungin (23), other echinocandins (e.g., anidulafungin and micafungin), and posaconazole have been demonstrated to be effective in persistently febrile patients with neutropenia. Renal and hepatic function, potential drug interactions, cost, and suspected source of fungal infection are all considerations when choosing an initial empiric antifungal agent.

Adjunctive therapies studied in the setting of febrile neutropenia include granulocyte transfusion and the use of hematopoietic growth factors. The role of neutrophil transfusion has been controversial, limited by technical aspects, and made essentially obsolete with the availability of hematopoietic growth factors (24). Although the use of hematopoietic growth factors such as granulocyte colony-stimulating factor (G-CSF) increase the neutrophil count, they have not been shown to have benefit in the management of febrile neutropenia; hence, their use is not routinely recommended (25,26).

TABLE 115.3

RISK FACTORS FOR CANDIDEMIA IN THE INTENSIVE CARE UNIT SETTING[a]

■ Prolonged length of stay (10 d or more)	■ Immune suppression
■ High acuity of illness	■ Cancer and chemotherapy
■ Acute renal failure	■ Severe acute pancreatitis
■ Hemodialysis	■ Surgery (gastrointestinal)
■ Broad-spectrum antibiotics	■ Transplantation
■ Central venous catheter (3 d or more)	■ Prematurity/low Apgar/congenital malformations
■ Parenteral nutrition	■ Burns
■ *Candida* colonization at multiple sites (longer than about 8 d)	■ Mechanical ventilation
■ Diabetes	

d, days.
[a]Reviewed in Rex JH, Sobel JD. Prophylactic antifungal therapy in the intensive care unit. *Clin Infect Dis.* 2001;32(8):1191; and Ostrosky-Zeichner L, Pappas PG. Invasive candidiasis in the intensive care unit. *Crit Care Med.* 2006;34(3):857.

THE CORTICOSTEROID-TREATED PATIENT

Corticosteroids have been used for the treatment of inflammatory, autoimmune, and lymphoproliferative diseases as well as for the prevention of graft rejection since the 1950s. Corticosteroids have an effect, both negative and positive, on various components of the immune system (27). Treatment with corticosteroids results in reduced proliferation of B and T lymphocytes, inhibition of neutrophil adhesion to endothelial cells, inhibition of macrophage differentiation, and reduced recruitment of mononuclear cells, including monocytes, into sites of immune inflammation (27,28). In addition, these agents suppress cellular (Th1) immunity and promote humoral (Th2) immunity (27).

The risk of infection in corticosteroid-treated patients is related to the dose and duration of therapy (29,30). Those treated with more than 10 to 20 mg/day of prednisone for more than a month are at risk for infectious complications. Although corticosteroids have a broad effect on the immune system, the primary immune deficit is in cell-mediated immunity, thus placing the host at risk for fungal, viral, protozoal, and intracellular bacterial infections. Common pathogens to be considered in corticosteroid-treated patients presenting with a suspected infectious complication include *P. carinii (jirovecii), Listeria monocytogenes, Legionella,* and *Nocardia* species.

Pneumocystis carinii (jirovecii)

The human species of *Pneumocystis* has recently been renamed *P. jirovecii,* although considerable controversy persists regarding the appropriate nomenclature of this protozoan (31). *P. carinii (jirovecii)* has a worldwide distribution and is an important cause of pneumonia in immunocompromised patients, most notably those with human immunodeficiency virus (HIV) infection, but also those immunosuppressed due to malnutrition, organ transplantation, and prolonged corticosteroid use, usually at a dose greater than 15 to 20 mg/day. Those requiring prolonged steroid therapy are appropriate candidates for prophylaxis with trimethoprim-sulfamethoxazole (TMP-SMX) (32).

Presentation

The onset of symptoms is often associated with recent dose reduction or discontinuation of steroids and/or with intensification of the overall immunosuppressive regimen. Although generally presenting as a subacute illness within weeks of progressive dyspnea and nonproductive cough in HIV-infected individuals, non-HIV immunocompromised patients with *Pneumocystis* pneumonia (PCP) tend to have a more acute presentation. Patients with PCP are generally hypoxemic with few physical or radiographic findings. In addition to nonproductive cough and dyspnea, low-grade fever is frequently present. Physical examination findings are nonspecific, but may reveal inspiratory crackles on auscultation, with or without hypoxia or other signs of respiratory distress. The illness may progress to respiratory failure requiring intubation and mechanical ventilation.

Diagnosis

The classic chest radiograph appearance of PCP is bilateral interstitial infiltrates with perihilar predominance. The radiographic appearance can be highly variable, however, including patchy airspace disease and small pulmonary nodules. An elevated lactate dehydrogenase level is a nonspecific finding associated with PCP. Since *P. carinii (jirovecii)* cannot be routinely cultured, a definitive diagnosis relies on the identification of the organism by staining techniques from pulmonary secretions or tissue. The diagnosis may be made by staining secretions obtained through sputum induction with hypertonic saline, which has a 97% negative predictive value (33). If respiratory secretions cannot be obtained by sputum induction, or if this is negative and the diagnosis remains uncertain, bronchoscopy with transbronchial tissue biopsy remains the gold standard for diagnosis of PCP, yielding better results than bronchoalveolar lavage (34). Examination of respiratory secretions may be done quickly by staining with Gomori methenamine silver (GMS) or calcofluor white; however, diagnosis has been improved through the use of immunofluorescent staining with monoclonal antibodies (35).

Treatment

Treatment for PCP is outlined in Table 115.4. First-line therapy for the treatment of PCP is TMP-SMX at a dose of 15 to 20 mg/kg per day of the TMP component, divided every 6 or 8 hours for 21 days (36). In those with severe disease who are allergic to or fail TMP-SMX, alternatives include atovaquone suspension 750 to 1,500 mg orally twice daily, pentamidine 4 mg/kg/day to a maximum of 300 mg, dapsone 100 mg orally plus TMP 15 to 20 mg/kg/day, or clindamycin 600 mg intravenously every 6 hours plus primaquine 15 to 30 mg (as base) per day. Although adjunctive administration of corticosteroids to patients with PCP and HIV has been documented to improve outcomes, this has not been studied in a randomized clinical trial in non-HIV immunocompromised patients with PCP. In practice, a short course of tapering steroids is often beneficial in preventing intubation and in rapidly progressive disease. After completion of therapy, secondary prophylaxis with TMP-SMX should be administered to those who remain at risk due to continued immunosuppression.

Listeria monocytogenes

Listeria monocytogenes is a Gram-positive bacillus capable of intracellular survival after phagocytosis by macrophages (37). Although capable of infecting normal hosts, invasive disease is seen predominantly in those with cell-mediated immune deficits due to such factors as extremes of age (neonates and the elderly), pregnancy, malignancy, organ transplantation, or other immunosuppressive therapy.

Presentation

Though a food-borne pathogen, *L. monocytogenes* infection presents as meningitis or primary bacteremia in 80% to 90% of cases (38–40). Gastrointestinal symptoms are present in only a minority of cases. Onset of symptoms may be acute or subacute, with fever being nearly universal. CNS involvement may present as meningitis with headache and neck stiffness, focal parenchymal involvement with cerebritis and/or abscess, or meningoencephalitis with impaired level of consciousness.

TABLE 115.4

TREATMENT MODALITIES FOR THE COMMONEST INFECTIONS

Infectious agent	Primary therapy	Secondary therapy	Other considerations
Pneumocystis jirovecii (PCP)	Trimethoprim-sulfamethoxazole (TMP-SMX), dosed as 15–20 mg/kg/d of TMP component, divided every 6–8 h × 21 days	■ Atovaquone 750–1,500 mg orally bid ■ Pentamidine 4 mg/kg/d, to max of 300 mg ■ Dapsone 100 mg orally plus TMP as above ■ Clindamycin 600 mg IV every 6 h plus primaquine 15–30 mg/d (as base)	Adjunctive use of corticosteroids common but not evidence based in non-HIV patients
Listeria monocytogenes	*Empiric or confirmed:* Ampicillin 2 g IV every 4 h × 21 d or more *For synergy:* Ampicillin plus TMP-SMX 20 mg/kg/d divided every 6 h	Ampicillin plus gentamicin 2 mg/kg IV load, then 1.7 mg/kg IV every 8 h	
Legionella pneumophila and other species	Levofloxacin 250–750 mg IV every 24 h × 7–14 d	Azithromycin 500 mg daily for 7–14 d	
Nocardia asteroides complex	TMP-SMX, dosed as 15 mg/kg/d of TMP component, divided every 6–12 h, PO or IV	■ Imipenem 500 mg IV every 6 h plus amikacin 7.5 mg/kg IV every 12 h, both × 3–4 wk, then switch to PO regimen ■ Linezolid 300–600 mg orally bid × 3–24 mo	■ Surgical resection of necrotic material often necessary ■ Therapy duration is 6–12 mo; for central nervous system infection 9–12 mo

Diagnosis

The diagnosis of listeriosis is generally made through culture of blood or cerebrospinal fluid (CSF). Approximately 75% of cases of CNS listeriosis are associated with bacteremia, and a positive blood culture for *Listeria* should prompt a CSF examination. CSF parameters are variable, but a common presentation is pleocytosis with neutrophil predominance, elevated protein, and normal glucose. The Gram stain is frequently negative.

Treatment

In patients at risk for *Listeria* who present with meningitis of uncertain etiology, empiric therapy should include ampicillin, 2 g intravenously every 4 hours, as part of the initial regimen. If listeriosis is confirmed, ampicillin is the drug of choice. *In vitro* data suggest bactericidal synergy of the combination of ampicillin and gentamicin (41). *In vitro* synergy has also been demonstrated between ampicillin and TMP-SMX; this combination has been demonstrated to be superior to ampicillin and gentamicin in the treatment of *Listeria* meningoencephalitis (41,42), suggesting that this combination may be indicated in those with severe disease. The minimum duration of therapy recommended is 3 weeks, but this may need to be extended based on the clinical response and radiographic resolution of CNS parenchymal disease if present.

Legionella

Legionella species are small Gram-negative bacilli that are widely distributed in the aqueous environment. Both community and hospital outbreaks have occurred in association with contaminated water sources such as air conditioners, cooling towers, and whirlpools (43). Although capable of causing disease in normal hosts, those with impaired cell-mediated immunity are at highest risk (44).

Presentation

Most commonly, *Legionella* infection presents as pneumonia—termed *Legionnaires disease*—although extrapulmonary disease and a self-limited febrile illness—termed *Pontiac fever*—may occur. The physical and laboratory findings and radiographic appearance of *Legionella* pneumonia are not specific. Fever with pulse–temperature dissociation, diarrhea, hyponatremia, and elevated liver enzymes may occur, but are not distinctive enough for Legionnaires disease to allow a clinical differentiation from other causes of pneumonia. In patients at risk, *Legionella* must be considered in the differential diagnosis of pneumonia, and empiric therapy administered when appropriate.

Diagnosis

Legionella is a fastidious organism, and culture of respiratory secretions for diagnosis is both insensitive and time consuming (45); immunofluorescent microscopy can improve the sensitivity of culture techniques. Serology can be used, but also results in delays in diagnosis, as paired sera must be collected. Newer methods that may allow more rapid diagnosis include a urinary antigen test and nucleic acid detection. Urinary antigen tests have a high sensitivity for the detection of *Legionella pneumophila* serogroup 1, but perform less well in those infected with other serogroups of *L. pneumophila,* or with other

Legionella species. A combination of culture, urinary antigen detection, and serology has been suggested to optimize diagnosis (45).

Treatment

Both macrolides and fluoroquinolones have *in vitro* activity against *Legionella* species. Three observational studies have compared the clinical efficacy of macrolides—not including azithromycin—and quinolones, mainly levofloxacin, in patients with Legionnaires disease. The results suggested that quinolones may be superior to macrolides, with fewer complications and shorter hospital stays in those receiving quinolones (46). There are no studies comparing newer macrolides (e.g., azithromycin) to new quinolones.

Nocardia

Nocardia species are part of the aerobic actinomycetes genus, and are ubiquitous environmental saprophytes. While there are several species, the *Nocardia asteroides* complex—*Nocardia asteroides senso strictu, Nocardia farcinica,* and *Nocardia nova*—are the most common cause of disease (47). Immunosuppression is the major risk factor for nocardial infections, and disease is seen most often in solid organ transplant recipients, patients with advanced HIV infection (i.e., with $CD4^+$ counts of less than 100 cells/μL), patients with lymphoreticular malignancy, and those on chronic corticosteroid therapy.

Presentation

Nocardia predominantly causes pneumonia, and the initial presentation includes respiratory symptoms generally in association with fever (48). Chest radiograph typically demonstrates nodular lesions, which may progress to cavitation; however, diffuse infiltrates or consolidation may also occur. *Nocardia* has a high propensity to disseminate to the CNS, and immunocompromised patients with nocardiosis may present with CNS symptoms with or without concomitant pulmonary symptoms. Although the usual route of infection is inhalational, direct cutaneous inoculation with resultant skin disease—generally subcutaneous nodules—may also be seen.

Diagnosis

Definitive diagnosis of nocardial disease is made through special stain and culture of the organism from the suspected site of infection. Modified acid-fast stain (Kinyoun) demonstrates branching and beading Gram-positive bacilli. *Nocardia* grow on nonselective media; however, the lab should be notified if this diagnosis is suspected, as selective media can be used to avoid overgrowth by other organisms. Whenever a diagnosis of pulmonary nocardiosis is made, further investigations should include neuroimaging to exclude CNS dissemination.

Treatment

Antimicrobial therapy is the foundation of treatment of nocardiosis, although adjunctive surgical resection of necrotic tissue is necessary on occasion. TMP-SMX, dosed as the TMP component at 15 mg/kg/day divided in two or four doses and administered either orally or intravenously, is the preferred agent for treating nocardial infections; this agent achieves high concentrations in lung, brain, skin, and bone (49). Given that some species may be resistant to TMP-SMX, combination therapy may be considered until susceptibilities are available. Other antimicrobial agents with activity against *Nocardia* species include imipenem, amikacin, minocycline, ceftriaxone, linezolid, ciprofloxacin, and amoxicillin/clavulanate. While the duration of therapy should be individualized based on clinical response, pulmonary and cutaneous disease should be treated for at least 6 to 12 months, and CNS disease for at least 9 to 12 months. Immunosuppression should be reduced as much as possible to aid in treatment.

PATIENTS TREATED WITH IMMUNOMODULATORY AGENTS

In recent years, a number of monoclonal antibody therapies have been developed and have revolutionized the treatment of rheumatologic as well as other systemic inflammatory and autoimmune conditions (Table 115.5). Immune modulation using these agents results in selected immune deficits and infectious complications have been recognized in association with several of these agents. As more patients are treated with these therapies, with a longer-term follow-up, our understanding of the risk of infection associated with these biologic compounds will undoubtedly be refined.

Tumor Necrosis Factor-α Antagonists

Three tumor necrosis factor-α (TNF-α) antagonists are currently marketed in the United States: Infliximab (Remicade, Centocor Inc.), etanercept (Enbrel, Amgen and Wyeth Pharmaceuticals), and adalimumab (Humira, Abbott). These agents

TABLE 115.5

SELECTED THERAPEUTIC ANTIBODIES

Antibody	Trade name	Target	Indication
Antithymocyte globulin	Thymoglobulin (others)	T cells (polyclonal rabbit IgG)	Transplant induction, rejection
Muromonab OKT3	Orthoclone OKT3	$CD3^+$	Transplant induction, rejection
Alemtuzumab	Campath-1H	$CD52^+$	B-cell chronic lymphoid leukemia
Daclizumab	Zenapax	Interleukin (IL)-2 receptor a chain ($CD25^+$)	Transplant induction
Basiliximab	Simulect	IL-2 receptor a chain ($CD25^+$)	Transplant induction
Efalizumab	Raptiva	$CD11a^+$	Psoriasis
Natalizumab	Tysabri	α_4-integrin	Multiple sclerosis, Crohn disease

are effective in the treatment of rheumatoid arthritis, active Crohn disease, and ankylosing spondylitis. Blockade of TNF-α, a proinflammatory cytokine, results in improvement in systemic inflammatory conditions; however, TNF-α, along with interferon-γ and other cytokines, is an important component in maintaining cellular immunity.

Tuberculosis has been associated with use of TNF-α antagonists, probably as a result of the resultant cell-mediated immune deficits (50,51). The majority of cases have occurred in patients receiving infliximab; however, cases have also been described in association with etanercept and adalimumab. In general, cases have occurred in those with risk factors for latent tuberculosis infection. As a result, tuberculosis skin testing (TST) is recommended in all patients prior to the initiation of a TNF-α antagonist. Regardless of TST results, tuberculosis should be considered in the differential diagnosis in a patient presenting on a TNF-α antagonist with compatible symptoms.

A number of other infections including histoplasmosis, listeriosis, aspergillosis, coccidiomycosis, and candidiasis have been associated with the use of TNF-α antagonists; however, the magnitude of risk and whether or not a causative association exists are unclear (51).

Rituximab

Rituximab (Rituxan, Genentech Inc. and Biogen Idec) is a chimeric murine/human monoclonal antibody that binds the $CD20^+$ marker, expressed on B lymphocytes. Treatment with rituximab results in rapid depletion of circulating $CD20^+$ B cells. This agent is approved for the treatment of $CD20^+$ B-cell lymphoma, as well as in combination with methotrexate for the treatment of rheumatoid arthritis. In addition to these conditions, rituximab has been used for the treatment of posttransplant lymphoproliferative disease, immune thrombocytopenic purpura, autoimmune hemolytic anemia, systemic lupus erythematosus, multiple sclerosis, graft versus host disease, and treatment of antibody-mediated graft rejection (52).

Following rituximab therapy, antibody production is maintained by plasma cells, which are CD20, negative. Peripheral B-cell recovery takes 3 to 12 months (53). Despite this B-cell deficiency and extensive use of rituximab for the treatment of malignant and autoimmune conditions, there has been no evidence of an increased risk of infection in patients treated.

Natalizumab

Natalizumab (Tysabri, Biogen Idec and Elan Pharmaceuticals) is a recombinant humanized monoclonal antibody that binds to α_4-integrin, thereby inhibiting α_4-integrin–mediated leukocyte adhesion. Disruption of binding prevents the transmigration of leukocytes across the endothelium into inflamed tissue. Natalizumab is indicated as monotherapy for the treatment of patients with relapsing forms of multiple sclerosis and in those with inadequate response to, or who are unable to tolerate, alternate therapies (54). It also increases the rate of remission and improves the quality of life in patients with active Crohn disease (55).

Progressive multifocal leukoencephalopathy (PML), a demyelinating disease of the central nervous system caused by the human polyomavirus JC virus, has been reported in three patients who received natalizumab (56–58). The U.S. Food and Drug Administration (FDA) approved an application for resumed marketing in June of 2006. Given the mechanism of action and inhibition of leukocyte migration, it is possible that further opportunistic infections may be associated with the use of this agent.

THE SOLID ORGAN TRANSPLANT RECIPIENT

With improvements in surgical techniques and immunosuppressive therapy, a growing number of people are living with solid organ transplants. With intensified immune suppression, the incidence of graft rejection has decreased, while infectious complications are an important cause of morbidity and mortality. Although all transplant recipients are at increased risk of infection compared to the general population, the risk of infection in an individual recipient is determined largely by two factors: the degree of exposure to potential pathogens and the overall or "net state of immunosuppression" (Table 115.1) (59). These patients are differentiated from other immunocompromised hosts by the technical aspects (complex surgery) and, in general, the need for lifelong immune suppression to maintain graft function.

In an individual, the net state of immunosuppression is determined not only by the immunosuppressive agents used, but also by their dose, duration, and sequence of use. In addition, factors such as underlying immune deficiency, metabolic derangements, the presence of foreign bodies (e.g., central venous catheters) or fluid collections, and infection with immune-modulating viruses such as CMV or EBV all contribute to overall immunosuppression and the risk of infection (59).

Timeline of Posttransplant Infections

With standardized immunosuppressive regimens, specific infections vary in a predictable pattern depending on the time elapsed since transplantation (Fig. 115.1) (59). This is a reflection of the changing risk factors over time including surgery/hospitalization, immune suppression, acute and chronic rejection, emergence of latent infections, and exposures to novel community infections. The pattern of infection changes with the immunosuppressive regimen (e.g., pulse dose steroids or the intensification for graft rejection), intercurrent viral infections, neutropenia, or significant epidemiologic exposures, such as travel or food. The timeline remains a useful starting point, although it has been altered by the introduction of newer immunosuppressive agents and patterns of use; the reduced use of corticosteroids and calcineurin inhibitors; the increased use of antibody-based induction therapies or sirolimus; routine antimicrobial prophylaxis; improved molecular assays; antimicrobial resistance; transplantation in HIV- and hepatitis C virus (HCV)-infected individuals; and broader epidemiologic exposures, again, such as travel. Figure 115.1 demonstrates three overlapping periods of risk for infection after transplantation, each most often associated with unique groups of pathogens:

- The perioperative period to approximately 4 weeks after transplantation, reflecting surgical and technical complications

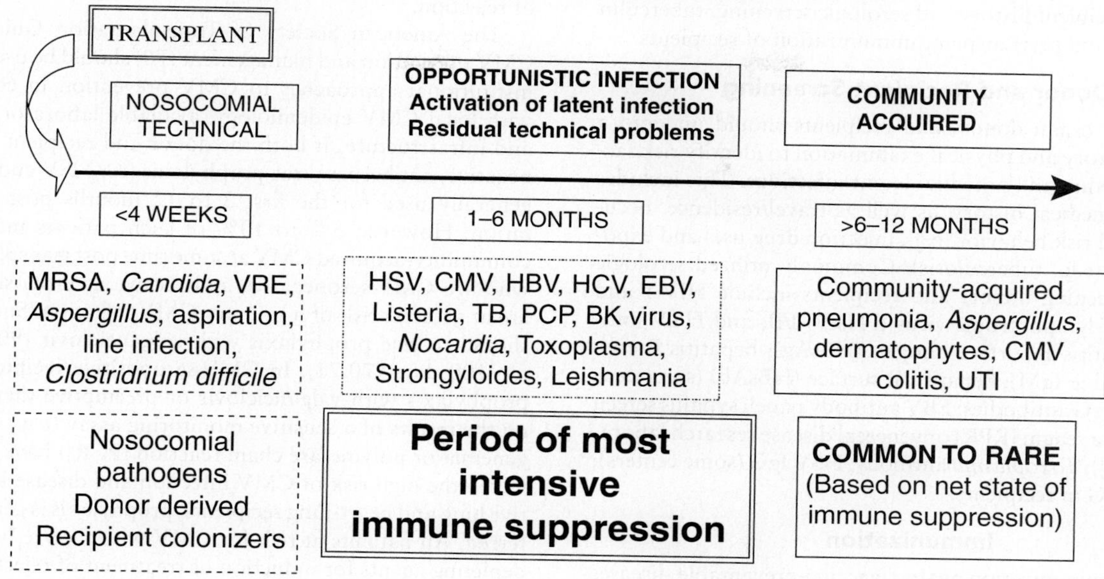

FIGURE 115.1. The timeline of infection after transplantation. MRSA, methicillin-resistant *Staphylococcus aureus*; VRE, vancomycin-resistant enterococcus; HSV, herpes simplex virus; CMV, cytomegalovirus; HBV, hepatitis B virus; EBV, Epstein-Barr virus; TB, tuberculosis; PCP, *Pneumocystic carinii*; UTI, urinary tract infection. (Adapted from Fishman JA, Rubin RH. Infection in organ-transplant recipients. *N Engl J Med.* 1998;338[24]:1741.)

- The period 1 to 6 months after transplantation, depending on the rapidity of tapering immune suppression and the use of antilymphocyte "induction" therapy, reflecting intensive immune suppression with viral activation and opportunistic infections
- The period beyond 6 to 12 months after transplantation, reflecting community-acquired exposures and some unusual pathogens based on the level of maintenance immune suppression

In the first month after transplantation, most infections are related to the surgery, similar to those occurring in the complex general surgical population. These include pneumonia and surgical site, urinary tract, and central venous catheter–associated infections caused by typical bacterial and fungal pathogens such as *Candida*. Exposure to nosocomial pathogens and colonization will alter the use of empiric antimicrobial therapy, including for methicillin-resistant *S. aureus* (MRSA), vancomycin-resistant enterococcus (VRE), fluconazole-resistant *Candida* species, *Clostridium difficile,* and *P. aeruginosa*. Opportunistic infections rarely occur within the first month posttransplant unless there has been pretransplant immunosuppression. In the absence of prophylaxis, however, 24% to 34% of transplant recipients will have HSV disease, with most cases of HSV occurring as orolabial or genital disease due to reactivation of latent infection in the recipient during the first post transplant month (60).

Uncommonly, infections may be transmitted from a bacteremic or fungemic donor with potentially serious complications, including seeding of the vascular suture line. The use of prophylactic antibiotics in the recipient, directed by donor culture results, allows organs from donors with bacteremia and/or meningitis to be safely used without compromising transplant outcomes (61–63).

The first month through the sixth month post transplant is the highest-risk period for opportunistic infections, since the effects of immunosuppression are greatest during this period. These infections may include viral (CMV, varicella-zoster virus [VZV], EBV, and hepatitis B), bacterial (*Nocardia*, *Listeria*, and tuberculosis), fungal (*Aspergillus* and *Cryptococcus*), or parasitic (*Pneumocystis, Toxoplasma* and *Strongyloides*) infections.

Beyond 6 months post transplant, most recipients are on reduced levels of maintenance immunosuppression with good graft function and at low risk for opportunistic infections. Most infectious complications during this time are due to conventional community-acquired pathogens occurring in the general population. These include viral respiratory infections, pneumococcal pneumonia, and gastroenteritis. Intense exposure to an opportunistic pathogen, however, may still result in disease, and transplant recipients should be counseled regarding strategies to avoid high-risk exposures (64). Recipients requiring augmentation of immunosuppression for management of acute chronic rejection, as well as those with chronic or recurrent CMV infection, remain at risk for other opportunistic infections, particularly *P. carinii* (*jirovecii*), invasive fungal infection, and EBV-associated, posttransplant lymphoproliferative disease.

Prevention of Infections

Treatment of infections in transplant recipients may be complicated by rapid progression, precipitation of rejection, and antimicrobial toxicity related to drug interactions or nephrotoxicity. Whenever possible, prevention of infections is therefore a principal goal. Approaches to prevention include donor and recipient history and serologic screening, tuberculin skin testing, and pretransplant immunization of recipients.

Donor and Recipient Screening

All potential organ donors and recipients should undergo a thorough history and physical examination to identify risk factors for infection and potential latent infections. This includes a complete medical history, as well as travel/residence, occupational, and risk behavior (e.g., injection drug use) and exposure history (e.g., tuberculosis). Commonly utilized serologic tests for screening donors and recipients include HIV-1 and -2, human T-lymphotropic virus (HTLV)-I/II, and HCV antibodies; hepatitis B surface antigen (HBsAg); hepatitis B core (HBcAb total ± IgM); hepatitis B surface (HBsAb) (some centers); CMV IgG antibodies; EBV antibody panel; syphilis screen (rapid plasma reagin [RPR] or venereal disease research laboratory [VDRL]); *Toxoplasma* antibody; HSV IgG (some centers); and VZV IgG in recipients.

Immunization

Optimally, immunization against vaccine-preventable diseases should be completed prior to transplantation and as early in the course of the disease as possible. This is based on three principal factors: (a) the response to vaccine declines with progressive end-organ failure; (b) despite this, the response to vaccination may be better before transplantation than after; and (c) live viral vaccines (e.g., mumps, measles, rubella [MMR], varicella) are generally contraindicated post transplant. Attention to the appropriate and timely administration of as many immunizations as possible is of particular importance in pediatric transplant candidates. National immunization guidelines should be followed by consultation with an infectious diseases specialist as needed and, based on vaccine type and urgency of transplant, accelerated vaccination schedules used prior to transplant where appropriate. In addition to routine vaccinations, all transplant candidates should receive a pneumococcal vaccine, yearly influenza vaccine, and hepatitis B vaccine. Hepatitis B vaccination, with a documented serologic response, allows for the safe use of HBcAb-positive donors, thus expanding the donor pool (65). Susceptible individuals should receive varicella vaccine (live vaccine) a minimum of 4 weeks prior to transplantation.

Tuberculosis Screening

There is a 50- to 100-fold increased risk of tuberculosis (TB) following organ transplantation, with an increased risk of dissemination compared to the general population (66,67). Management of TB post transplant is also associated with significant morbidity and mortality, and its therapy is complicated by the multiple drug interactions between antituberculous and antirejection medications (68,69). Transplant candidates should undergo TB screening with TST and risk factor assessment prior to transplantation.

Disease-specific Prevention and Management

Cytomegalovirus. CMV remains a significant cause of morbidity in organ transplant recipients; however, strategies for prevention have decreased the morbidity and mortality from CMV. The risk of CMV disease depends on a number of factors, including the donor and recipient serostatus, as well as the immunosuppression, particularly the use of antilymphocyte antibody (ALA) preparations for induction or treatment of rejection.

The American Society of Transplantation Guidelines on CMV prevention and management (70) should be used to guide institutional approaches to CMV prevention in conjunction with local CMV epidemiology, available laboratory support, and infrastructure. If both the donor and recipient are CMV-negative, antiherpes virus prophylaxis (for HSV and VZV) are generally used for the first 3 to 12 months post transplantation. However, 5% to 10% of such patients may develop community-acquired CMV at some time post transplant. Those who are CMV-seronegative and receive a seropositive organ are at greatest risk of a primary CMV infection. Such patients should receive prophylaxis with valganciclovir (900 mg/day) for 100 days (70,71). In CMV-seropositive recipients, either prophylaxis with valganciclovir or preemptive therapy based on the results of a sensitive monitoring assay (e.g., CMV antigenemia or polymerase chain reaction [PCR]) have been used. Given the high risk of CMV infection and disease in seropositive lung and heart-lung recipients, prophylaxis is generally preferred. All patients at risk for CMV who receive lymphocyte-depleting agents for induction or treatment of rejection should receive antiviral prophylaxis.

CMV disease refers to the presence of symptoms attributable to CMV in the face of viral replication, and can be further divided into (a) "CMV syndrome" and (b) tissue-invasive disease. "CMV syndrome" is defined by the constellation of fever greater than 38°C, neutropenia or thrombocytopenia, and the detection of CMV in the blood by antigenemia, PCR, or shell vial culture. Tissue-invasive disease requires a biopsy for confirmation, except in the case of retinitis, and is defined by the presence of signs or symptoms of organ dysfunction in association with histologic evidence of CMV in the affected tissue (1).

Established CMV syndrome or tissue-invasive disease should be treated with intravenous ganciclovir, 5 mg/kg every 12 hours. Although oral ganciclovir and valganciclovir have been shown to be effective in the prevention of CMV infection, there are, as yet, no data to support their use in the treatment of disease due to CMV. Therapy should be continued for a minimum of 14 days until symptoms have resolved and viremia has cleared (i.e., until the CMV PCR/antigenemia is undetectable) in order to minimize the risk of relapse (72,73).

Ganciclovir-resistant CMV is an emerging problem; risk factors include donor–recipient mismatch, in which the donor is seropositive and the recipient seronegative; prolonged use of ganciclovir; suboptimal ganciclovir levels; intense immunosuppression; and high CMV viral load. Ganciclovir-resistant CMV should be suspected in the setting of a stable, or rising, viral load in patients treated with ganciclovir; no decrease in antigenemia after 7 days of therapy; lack of clinical improvement after 14 days of full-dose intravenous ganciclovir; or CMV infection developing shortly after a prolonged course of low-dose ganciclovir. If ganciclovir resistance is suspected, infectious diseases/microbiology should be consulted for consideration of molecular resistance testing and either alternative (e.g., foscarnet, cidofovir) or adjunctive (CMV-Ig) therapies (74).

Epstein-Barr Virus and Posttransplant Lymphoproliferative Disease. Primary EBV infection after transplantation has been identified as the most important risk factor for PTLD, a complication with mortality reported to range as high as 40% to 60%. This risk is exacerbated by the occurrence of CMV disease and treatment with polyclonal or monoclonal ALA. Studies comparing transplant recipients having received antiviral prophylaxis with either acyclovir or ganciclovir to historical controls suggest some benefit of antiviral prophylaxis (75). Recently, quantitative EBV viral load monitoring has also been shown to decrease the risk of PTLD (76). In those at high risk for PTLD (i.e., EBV donor seropositive/recipient seronegative), preventative strategies with antiviral prophylaxis and/or EBV viral load monitoring may be considered. If EBV viremia is detected, immunosuppression reduction should be considered.

PTLD represents a highly diverse spectrum of disease with variable clinical presentation, from benign B-cell proliferation (mononucleosis) to true monoclonal malignancy. It may be nodal or extranodal and localized or disseminated, and commonly involves the allograft. The diagnosis of PTLD requires histologic confirmation and staging of the disease (2).

Options for the treatment of PTLD depend on the histology and stage of the disease; however, in all cases, attempts should be made to reduce or withdraw immunosuppression. Additional considerations for treatment will depend on the clinical presentation, histology, and stage of disease. A multidisciplinary approach to management is generally indicated with collaboration of the transplant physician with hematology/oncology, infectious diseases, and surgery specialists, depending on the clinical setting. In addition to immunosuppression reduction or withdrawal, potential options for therapy include antiviral agents, intravenous immunoglobulin, surgical resection, and local radiation. The use of rituximab, the anti-CD20 monoclonal antibody, is an attractive second-line option if reduction in immunosuppression alone fails given its low toxicity and response rates, which range from 61% to 76% (77). Cytotoxic chemotherapy is generally considered a third-line option due to a high incidence of toxicity in this population.

Pneumocystis carinii (jirovecii). In the absence of prophylaxis, *P. pneumoniae* occurs in 5% to 15% of solid organ transplant recipients. Prophylaxis with trimethoprim-sulfamethoxazole, one single-strength tablet daily, essentially eliminates this risk and is indicated in all nonallergic transplant recipients for a minimum of 6 months following transplantation. This also acts as prophylaxis for a number of other infections such as *Nocardia*, *Listeria,* and community-acquired pneumonia. In sulfa-allergic patients, dapsone 100 mg daily, aerosolized pentamidine 300 mg monthly, or atovaquone 1,500 mg daily are alternatives (32).

Toxoplasmosis. Toxoplasmosis is of particular concern among cardiac transplant recipients given that the site of latency is the cardiac muscle. Seronegative recipients of a seropositive heart are at risk due to donor transmission and primary infection, and therefore require prophylaxis. TMP-SMX has been used effectively for prophylaxis as one double-strength tablet daily; lifelong prophylaxis is recommended (78).

Diagnosis and Treatment of Infectious Syndromes

The diagnosis and management of infectious complications in transplant recipients can be complex, and thus, consultation with local infectious diseases specialists is recommended. The initial approach to the transplant patient with suspected infection includes a thorough history and physical examination to assess the overall state of immune function and exposure history and localize the potential site of infection. Basic testing should include a complete blood count, creatinine, liver enzyme and function studies, blood cultures, and a chest radiograph. Additional specimens for microbiologic testing should be obtained as directed by the history and physical examination (e.g., urine cultures, stool for bacterial culture, *Clostridium difficile* toxin, ova and parasites, blood for CMV antigenemia, or PCR).

Identification of the etiologic agent of infection is extremely important and, hence, early aggressive testing (e.g., tissue biopsy, bronchoscopy) should be considered. Due to the possibility of unusual pathogens, close coordination with microbiology and pathology is recommended to ensure proper collection and testing of specimens. Because infections may progress rapidly in immunocompromised hosts, empiric therapy directed at likely pathogens may be considered after collection of appropriate diagnostic samples.

Fever and Pulmonary Infiltrate

Transplant recipients are susceptible to both common and unusual respiratory pathogens. In transplant patients presenting with fever and a pulmonary infiltrate, the differential diagnosis is broad and includes both infectious and noninfectious etiologies. However, infection is ultimately identified in 75% to 90% of such cases, and dual or sequential infections are common. Because pneumonia may rapidly progress in immunocompromised hosts with a resultant high mortality, initial empiric therapy directed at the most likely pathogens should be considered following the collection of blood and sputum cultures, viral respiratory studies, a complete blood count, and serum creatinine; consultation with pulmonary and infectious diseases specialists is recommended. Identification of the pathogen is key to directing appropriate therapy, and thus, early invasive diagnostic tests (e.g., bronchoscopy, lung biopsy) should be considered, particularly in those who are critically ill or fail to respond to initial empiric therapy.

Findings on chest radiograph combined with the clinical presentation, rate of progression, exposure history, and assessment of the net state of immunosuppression can help narrow the differential diagnosis. Table 115.6 summarizes the differential diagnosis based on chest radiographic findings and clinical presentation. Chest CT may be useful to delineate the extent of pulmonary disease and guide invasive diagnostic tests.

Central Nervous System Infections

Similar to pulmonary infections, the presentation of CNS infection in transplant patients may differ from the general population due to immunosuppression. Fever may or may not be present, and the presentation can be subtle, with headache or minor changes in mental status. The differential diagnosis in transplant patients presenting with neurologic symptoms—with or without fever—is broad, including both infectious and noninfectious etiologies. Clinical presentations include meningitis—acute or subacute/chronic—encephalitis, seizures, focal neurologic deficits, and progressive cognitive impairment. Among the common causes of infection are *L. monocytogenes* and *Cryptococcus neoformans*, as well as the common community-acquired bacteria pathogens. Metastatic infection due to *Aspergillus* and *Nocardia* species are also common.

TABLE 115.6

DIFFERENTIAL DIAGNOSIS OF FEVER AND PULMONARY INFILTRATE IN ORGAN TRANSPLANT RECIPIENTS

Chest radiograph finding	Acute onset	Subacute/chronic onset
Consolidation	Bacteria Pulmonary embolism Hemorrhage Pulmonary edema	Fungal *Nocardia* Tuberculosis Viral (adenovirus)
Reticulonodular	Pulmonary edema Viral *P. carinii (jirovecii)* Bacterial	*Pneumocystis carinii (jirovecii)* Drug reaction (including sirolimus) Viral
Nodular	Bacterial	Fungal *Nocardia* Tuberculosis Tumor (including PTLD)

PTLD, posttransplant lymphoproliferative disease.

Table 115.7 lists the most common causes of these symptoms. Consultation with infectious diseases/microbiology should be considered to assist in diagnosis and to ensure that appropriate samples are collected for diagnostic testing. Cerebral spinal fluid analysis after neuroimaging with CT and/or magnetic resonance imaging (MRI) should be obtained in all such individuals.

TABLE 115.7

COMMON CENTRAL NERVOUS SYSTEM INFECTIONS IN TRANSPLANT RECIPIENTS

COMMUNITY-ACQUIRED PATHOGENS
- Pneumococcus
- Meningococcus
- *Listeria monocytogenes*
- Herpes simplex virus (HSV)
- *Cryptococcus neoformans*
- Lyme disease

METASTATIC INFECTION
- Bacteremia (endocarditis)
- *Mycobacterium tuberculosis*
- *Aspergillus*
- *Nocardia* species
- *Strongyloides stercoralis* (Gram-negative meningitis)
- Mucoraceae (sinuses)
- Dematiaceae—cerebral phaeohyphomycosis (skin)
- *Histoplasma* and *Pseudoallescheria/Scedosporium, Fusarium*

OTHER CENTRAL NERVOUS SYSTEM PROCESSES
- Cytomegalovirus (nodular angiitis)
- Varicella-zoster virus
- Human herpesvirus 6
- *Toxoplasma gondii*
- JC virus (progressive multifocal leukoencephalopathy)
- West Nile virus, lymphocytic choriomeningitis virus
- Lymphoma (PTLD)
- *Naegleria/Acanthamoeba*

THE HEMATOPOIETIC STEM CELL TRANSPLANT RECIPIENT

A growing number of patients are undergoing allogeneic and autologous hematopoietic stem cell transplantation (HSCT) procedures for both malignant and nonmalignant indications (79). Despite the advances, severe infectious complications are not uncommon, with up to 40% of HSCT recipients requiring ICU admission, and 60% of these needing mechanical ventilation, which is associated with a high mortality rate (80,81). Although traditionally poor, the outcomes of HSCT recipients admitted to the ICU are improving with advances in infection prevention, diagnosis and management, and ICU care (82).

Historically, bone marrow has been relied upon as a source of stem cells, but recent developments now include the use of peripheral blood stem cell (PBSC) and umbilical cord blood (UCB) for transplantation. In an attempt to eliminate malignant cells and decrease the risk of graft versus host disease, positively selected $CD34^+$ progenitor cells may be used for transplantation; however, this results in significant T-lymphocyte and monocyte depletion of the graft, and therefore an increased risk of opportunistic infection (83). In an attempt to extend treatment by allogeneic HSCT to older patients and those with comorbid conditions, reduced-intensity or nonmyeloablative-conditioning regimens have been developed (84). Although the period of neutropenia is shorter, and potent antitumor effects result from this type of transplant, patients remain at high risk for GVHD and require GVHD prophylaxis (85). Thus, despite shorter periods of neutropenia and less severe mucositis, and though the risk of early bacterial infections appears to be decreased, the risk of late viral, fungal, and bacterial infections persists (86).

As a result of pretransplant conditioning chemotherapy, with or without total body irradiation, both humoral- and cell-mediated immunity are diminished. Natural host barrier defenses are also impaired by mucositis and the use of vascular access catheters. The risk of infectious complications in the HSCT recipient is generally divided into three phases: (a) the period from conditioning therapy to engraftment when patients are neutropenic—the pre-engraftment phase—carries a high risk of bacterial and fungal infections; (b) the second phase, from engraftment to day 100—or during the period of treatment for acute GVHD—in which viral and filamentous fungal infections predominate; and (c) beyond day 100—late phase or with chronic GVHD—the incidence of infections is reduced, and is determined by the level of immune suppression needed for chronic GVHD.

Phase 1: Pre-engraftment Infections

The early pre-engraftment, neutropenic phase usually lasts 10 to 15 days in most current nonmyeloablative HSCT patients, and longer with ablative regimens. The predominant infections seen during conditioning chemotherapy to the time of engraftment are similar to those seen in association with neutropenia (see previous section on the neutropenic patient). Similar to other neutropenic hosts, there has been a shift from predominantly Gram-negative to Gram-positive—coagulase-negative *Staphylococci*, *Streptococci*, *Enterococci*—bacterial infections with the use of fluoroquinolone prophylaxis (7). Although azole prophylaxis has reduced the incidence of candidemia, this continues to be an early cause of bloodstream infection with an increase in the risk of azole-resistant *Candida* (87). Herpes simplex virus may also reactivate during this phase but can be prevented with prophylactic acyclovir in seropositive HSCT recipients.

Phase 2: Engraftment to Day 100 (Acute Graft versus Host Disease)

This phase is characterized by deficits in cellular immunity; therefore, the most important infectious complications are viral infections, particularly CMV and invasive mold infections. The most common manifestations of CMV disease in HSCT recipients are pneumonia and gastrointestinal disease (88). The highest risk of disease occurs in seropositive recipients of seronegative transplants (89), and CD34$^+$ selected PBSC transplantation is associated with an increased risk of CMV infection due to T-lymphocyte depletion. The use of ganciclovir for prophylaxis or preemptive therapy has resulted in a decreased risk of CMV infection during this period, with most infections now occurring after ganciclovir has been discontinued.

Interstitial pneumonitis is an important clinical syndrome presenting during the postengraftment phase, and etiologies include CMV, respiratory viruses, *Pneumocystis*, or idiopathic pneumonia syndrome (IPS). The diagnosis of CMV pneumonitis requires histology for definitive diagnosis; however, this is often impractical, and a presumptive diagnosis may be made on the basis of the presence of interstitial pneumonia, detection of CMV antigen or nucleic acid in the peripheral blood, and/or respiratory secretions combined with negative investigations for other etiologies of pneumonitis. Despite treatment with intravenous ganciclovir and CMV hyperimmune globulin or intravenous immunoglobulin, the mortality from CMV pneumonitis remains high at 50% or greater (90).

P. carinii (jirovecii) has essentially been eliminated as a cause of pneumonitis with the use of TMP-SMX prophylaxis. Respiratory viral infections, such as respiratory syncytial virus, parainfluenza virus, and human metpneumovirus, have been increasingly recognized as an etiology of pneumonia in HSCT (91). A number of noninfectious etiologies of pneumonia also exist, including IPS and diffuse alveolar hemorrhage, which must also be considered in the differential diagnosis of HSCT recipients with pneumonitis.

The majority of invasive mold infections occur during the postengraftment phase, and are associated with treatment of acute GVHD (92). Although *Aspergillus* continues to be the predominant pathogen, non-*Aspergillus* molds, including Zygomycetes, are emerging pathogens in this population (93). Invasive mold infections generally present as pulmonary nodules, but invasive sinus disease and disseminated disease including CNS involvement are other common presentations. Given the high mortality associated with invasive mold infections, empiric antifungal therapy should be initiated while a definitive diagnosis is aggressively pursued. Empiric therapy with liposomal amphotericin is preferred to voriconazole in HSCT patients with fever or pulmonary infiltrates, given that it has the broadest spectrum of activity. By contrast, the treatment of choice for documented invasive aspergillosis is voriconazole, which has a survival benefit over amphotericin B deoxycholate therapy and is associated with less toxicity, particularly nephrotoxicity (94). Despite appropriate therapy, the mortality of invasive mold infections remains high in HSCT recipients, particularly in those with disseminated or CNS disease, where the mortality reaches 80% to 100%. Newer antifungal agents, such as posaconazole, and combination therapies have not yet been fully studied for therapy in these populations.

Phase 3: Late Infections beyond 100 Days

Beyond 100 days post transplant, there is gradual recovery of humoral and cellular immune function, but infection risk is driven to a large extent by the additional immunosuppression induced by chronic GVHD and its treatment. Up to 40% of HSCT recipients develop varicella-zoster virus infection, generally as a result of reactivation of latent infection, with most cases occurring during the first year. Disseminated disease is associated with a high mortality rate and should be treated with intravenous acyclovir, 10 mg/kg every 8 hours. Late CMV disease may occur and is associated with a history of early CMV disease and GVHD (95). Late CMV disease is treated the same as that occurring early; the outcome of late disease is poor, particularly for CMV pneumonia. Late invasive mold infections may also occur, particularly in those with GVHD and preceding viral (CMV) infection. As with CMV, the management of late mold infections mimics that of early infections. Every attempt should be made to decrease immunosuppression to assist in the treatment of infection.

About one third of patients with chronic GVHD may develop recurrent infection with encapsulated bacteria (sinopulmonary, bacteremia) (96). The predominant pathogen is *Streptococcus pneumoniae*, with *Haemophilus influenzae* and *S. aureus* also commonly isolated. This risk is related to a deficit in opsonizing antibody (97). Because HSCT recipients respond poorly to pneumococcal vaccine within the first 1 to 2 years post transplant, antibiotic prophylaxis with penicillin or TMP-SMX is recommended in those with chronic GVHD. In patients with chronic GVHD admitted with sepsis, broad-spectrum empiric antibiotic therapy is recommended pending microbiologic identification.

References

1. Ljungman P, Griffiths P, Paya C. Definitions of cytomegalovirus infection and disease in transplant recipients. *Clin Infect Dis.* 2002;34(8):1094.
2. Preiksaitis JK, Keay S. Diagnosis and management of posttransplant lymphoproliferative disorder in solid-organ transplant recipients. *Clin Infect Dis.* 2001;33(Suppl 1):S38.
3. Bodey GP, Buckley M, Sathe YS, et al. Quantitative relationships between circulating leukocytes and infection in patients with acute leukemia. *Ann Intern Med.* 1966;64(2):328.
4. Bodey GP, Rodriguez V, Chang HY, et al. Fever and infection in leukemic patients: a study of 494 consecutive patients. *Cancer.* 1978;41(4):1610.
5. Hughes WT, Armstrong D, Bodey GP, et al. 2002 guidelines for the use of antimicrobial agents in neutropenic patients with cancer. *Clin Infect Dis.* 2002;34(6):730.
6. Peacock JE, Herrington DA, Wade JC, et al. Ciprofloxacin plus piperacillin compared with tobramycin plus piperacillin as empirical therapy in febrile neutropenic patients. A randomized, double-blind trial. *Ann Intern Med.* 2002;137(2):77.
7. Leibovici L, Paul M, Cullen M, et al. Antibiotic prophylaxis in neutropenic patients: new evidence, practical decisions. *Cancer.* 2006;107(8):1743.
8. Gerson SL, Talbot GH, Hurwitz S, et al. Prolonged granulocytopenia: the major risk factor for invasive pulmonary aspergillosis in patients with acute leukemia. *Ann Intern Med.* 1984;100(3):345.
9. Empiric antifungal therapy in febrile granulocytopenic patients. EORTC International Antimicrobial Therapy Cooperative Group. *Am J Med.* 1989; 86(6 Pt 1):668.
10. Pizzo PA, Robichaud KJ, Gill FA, et al. Empiric antibiotic and antifungal therapy for cancer patients with prolonged fever and granulocytopenia. *Am J Med.* 1982;72(1):101.
11. Wisplinghoff H, Bischoff T, Tallent SM, et al. Nosocomial bloodstream infections in US hospitals: analysis of 24,179 cases from a prospective nationwide surveillance study. *Clin Infect Dis.* 2004;39(3):309.
12. Pagano L, Girmenia C, Mele L, et al. Infections caused by filamentous fungi in patients with hematologic malignancies. A report of 391 cases by GIMEMA Infection Program. *Haematologica.* 2001;86(8):862.
13. Richardson MD. Changing patterns and trends in systemic fungal infections. *J Antimicrob Chemother.* 2005;56(Suppl 1):i5.
14. Sickles EA, Greene WH, Wiernik PH. Clinical presentation of infection in granulocytopenic patients. *Arch Intern Med.* 1975;135(5):715.
15. Heussel CP, Kauczor HU, Heussel G, et al. Early detection of pneumonia in febrile neutropenic patients: use of thin-section CT. *AJR Am J Roentgenol.* 1997;169(5):1347.
16. Viscoli C, Cometta A, Kern WV, et al. Piperacillin-tazobactam monotherapy in high-risk febrile and neutropenic cancer patients. *Clin Microbiol Infect.* 2006;12(3):212.
17. Bow EJ, Rotstein C, Noskin GA, et al. A randomized, open-label, multicenter comparative study of the efficacy and safety of piperacillin-tazobactam and cefepime for the empirical treatment of febrile neutropenic episodes in patients with hematologic malignancies. *Clin Infect Dis.* 2006;43(4):447.
18. Cometta A, Kern WV, De Bock R, et al. Vancomycin versus placebo for treating persistent fever in patients with neutropenic cancer receiving piperacillin-tazobactam monotherapy. *Clin Infect Dis.* 2003;37(3):382.
19. Rex JH, Sobel JD. Prophylactic antifungal therapy in the intensive care unit. *Clin Infect Dis.* 2001;32(8):1191.
20. Ostrosky-Zeichner L, Pappas PG. Invasive candidiasis in the intensive care unit. *Crit Care Med.* 2006;34(3):857.
21. Wingard JR, White MH, Anaissie E, et al. A randomized, double-blind comparative trial evaluating the safety of liposomal amphotericin B versus amphotericin B lipid complex in the empirical treatment of febrile neutropenia. L Amph/ABLC Collaborative Study Group. *Clin Infect Dis.* 2000;31(5): 1155.
22. Walsh TJ, Pappas P, Winston DJ, et al. Voriconazole compared with liposomal amphotericin B for empirical antifungal therapy in patients with neutropenia and persistent fever. *N Engl J Med.* 2002;346(4):225.
23. Walsh TJ, Teppler H, Donowitz GR, et al. Caspofungin versus liposomal amphotericin B for empirical antifungal therapy in patients with persistent fever and neutropenia. *N Engl J Med.* 2004;351(14):1391.
24. Schiffer CA. Granulocyte transfusion therapy. *Curr Opin Hematol.* 1999; 6(1):3.
25. Update of recommendations for the use of hematopoietic colony-stimulating factors: evidence-based clinical practice guidelines. American Society of Clinical Oncology. *J Clin Oncol.* 1996;14(6):1957.
26. Berghmans T, Paesmans M, Lafitte JJ, et al. Therapeutic use of granulocyte and granulocyte-macrophage colony-stimulating factors in febrile neutropenic cancer patients. A systematic review of the literature with meta-analysis. *Support Care Cancer.* 2002;10(3):181.
27. Franchimont D. Overview of the actions of glucocorticoids on the immune response: a good model to characterize new pathways of immunosuppression for new treatment strategies. *Ann N Y Acad Sci.* 2004;1024:124.
28. Boumpas DT, Chrousos GP, Wilder RL, et al. Glucocorticoid therapy for immune-mediated diseases: basic and clinical correlates. *Ann Intern Med.* 1993;119(12):1198.
29. Dale DC, Petersdorf RG. Corticosteroids and infectious diseases. *Med Clin North Am.* 1973;57(5):1277.
30. Stuck AE, Minder CE, Frey FJ. Risk of infectious complications in patients taking glucocorticosteroids. *Rev Infect Dis.* 1989;11(6):954.
31. Hughes WT. Pneumocystis carinii versus Pneumocystis jirovecii (jiroveci) Frenkel. *Clin Infect Dis.* 2006;42(8):1211.
32. Fishman JA. Prevention of infection due to Pneumocystis carinii. *Antimicrob Agents Chemother.* 1998;42(5):995.
33. LaRocque RC, Katz JT, Perruzzi P, et al. The utility of sputum induction for diagnosis of Pneumocystis pneumonia in immunocompromised patients without human immunodeficiency virus. *Clin Infect Dis.* 2003;37(10):1380.
34. Stover DE, Zaman MB, Hajdu SI, et al. Bronchoalveolar lavage in the diagnosis of diffuse pulmonary infiltrates in the immunosuppressed host. *Ann Intern Med.* 1984;101(1):1.
35. Kovacs JA, Ng VL, Masur H, et al. Diagnosis of Pneumocystis carinii pneumonia: improved detection in sputum with use of monoclonal antibodies. *N Engl J Med.* 1988;318(10):589.
36. Fishman JA. Treatment of infection due to Pneumocystis carinii. *Antimicrob Agents Chemother.* 1998;42(6):1309.
37. Freitag NE, Jacobs KE. Examination of Listeria monocytogenes intracellular gene expression by using the green fluorescent protein of Aequorea victoria. *Infect Immun.* 1999;67(4):1844.
38. Lorber B. Listeriosis. *Clin Infect Dis.* 1997;24(1):1.
39. Taege AJ. Listeriosis: recognizing it, treating it, preventing it. *Cleve Clin J Med.* 1999;66(6):375.
40. Gellin BG, Broome CV. Listeriosis. *JAMA.* 1989;261(9):1313.
41. MacGowan AP, Holt HA, Bywater MJ, et al. In vitro antimicrobial susceptibility of Listeria monocytogenes isolated in the UK and other Listeria species. *Eur J Clin Microbiol Infect Dis.* 1990;9(10):767.
42. Merle-Melet M, Dossou-Gbete L, Maurer P, et al. Is amoxicillin-cotrimoxazole the most appropriate antibiotic regimen for listeria meningoencephalitis? Review of 22 cases and the literature. *J Infect.* 1996;33(2):79.
43. Roig J, Sabria M, Pedro-Botet ML. Legionella spp.: community acquired and nosocomial infections. *Curr Opin Infect Dis.* 2003;16(2):145.
44. Saravolatz LD, Burch KH, Fisher E, et al. The compromised host and Legionnaires' disease. *Ann Intern Med.* 1979;90(4):533.
45. Den Boer JW, Yzerman EP. Diagnosis of Legionella infection in Legionnaires' disease. *Eur J Clin Microbiol Infect Dis.* 2004;23(12):871.
46. Pedro-Botet L, Yu VL. Legionella: macrolides or quinolones? *Clin Microbiol Infect.* 2006;12(Suppl 3):25.
47. McNeil MM, Brown JM. The medically important aerobic actinomycetes: epidemiology and microbiology. *Clin Microbiol Rev.* 1994;7(3):357.
48. Lerner PI. Nocardiosis. *Clin Infect Dis.* 1996;22(6):891.
49. Smego RA Jr, Moeller MB, Gallis HA. Trimethoprim-sulfamethoxazole therapy for Nocardia infections. *Arch Intern Med.* 1983;143(4):711.
50. Keane J, Gershon S, Wise RP, et al. Tuberculosis associated with infliximab, a tumor necrosis factor alpha-neutralizing agent. *N Engl J Med.* 2001;345(15):1098.
51. Rychly DJ, DiPiro JT. Infections associated with tumor necrosis factor-alpha antagonists. *Pharmacotherapy.* 2005;25(9):1181.
52. Rastetter W, Molina A, White CA. Rituximab: expanding role in therapy for lymphomas and autoimmune diseases. *Annu Rev Med.* 2004;55:477.
53. Maloney DG, Grillo-Lopez AJ, White CA, et al. IDEC-C2B8 (Rituximab) anti-CD20 monoclonal antibody therapy in patients with relapsed low-grade non-Hodgkin's lymphoma. *Blood.* 1997;90(6):2188.
54. Miller DH, Khan OA, Sheremata WA, et al. A controlled trial of natalizumab for relapsing multiple sclerosis. *N Engl J Med.* 2003;348(1):15.
55. Ghosh S, Goldin E, Gordon FH, et al. Natalizumab for active Crohn's disease. *N Engl J Med.* 2003;348(1):24.
56. Langer-Gould A, Atlas SW, Green AJ, et al. Progressive multifocal leukoencephalopathy in a patient treated with natalizumab. *N Engl J Med.* 2005; 353(4):375.
57. Kleinschmidt-DeMasters BK, Tyler KL. Progressive multifocal leukoencephalopathy complicating treatment with natalizumab and interferon beta-1a for multiple sclerosis. *N Engl J Med.* 2005;353(4):369.
58. Van Assche G, Van Ranst M, Sciot R, et al. Progressive multifocal leukoencephalopathy after natalizumab therapy for Crohn's disease. *N Engl J Med.* 2005;353(4):362.
59. Fishman JA, Rubin RH. Infection in organ-transplant recipients. *N Engl J Med.* 1998;338(24):1741.
60. Other herpesviruses: HHV-6, HHV-7, HHV-8, HSV-1 and -2, VZV. *Am J Transplant.* 2004;4(Suppl 10):66.
61. Lopez-Navidad A, Domingo P, Caballero F, et al. Successful transplantation of organs retrieved from donors with bacterial meningitis. *Transplantation.* 1997;64(2):365.
62. Lumbreras C, Sanz F, Gonzalez A, et al. Clinical significance of donor-unrecognized bacteremia in the outcome of solid-organ transplant recipients. *Clin Infect Dis.* 2001;33(5):722.
63. Freeman RB, Giatras I, Falagas ME, et al. Outcome of transplantation of organs procured from bacteremic donors. *Transplantation.* 1999;68(8):1107.
64. Strategies for safe living following solid organ transplantation. *Am J Transplant.* 2004;4(Suppl 10):156.
65. Chung RT, Feng S, Delmonico FL. Approach to the management of allograft recipients following the detection of hepatitis B virus in the prospective organ donor. *Am J Transplant.* 2001;1(2):185.

66. Kotloff RM, Ahya VN, Crawford SW. Pulmonary complications of solid organ and hematopoietic stem cell transplantation. *Am J Respir Crit Care Med.* 2004;170(1):22.
67. Klote MM, Agodoa LY, Abbott K. Mycobacterium tuberculosis infection incidence in hospitalized renal transplant patients in the United States, 1998–2000. *Am J Transplant.* 2004;4(9):1523.
68. Singh N, Paterson DL. Mycobacterium tuberculosis infection in solid-organ transplant recipients: impact and implications for management. *Clin Infect Dis.* 1998;27(5):1266.
69. Mycobacterium tuberculosis. *Am J Transplant.* 2004;4(Suppl 10):37.
70. Cytomegalovirus. *Am J Transplant.* 2004;4(Suppl 10):51.
71. Paya C, Humar A, Dominguez E, et al. Efficacy and safety of valganciclovir vs. oral ganciclovir for prevention of cytomegalovirus disease in solid organ transplant recipients. *Am J Transplant.* 2004;4(4):611.
72. Sia IG, Wilson JA, Groettum CM, et al. Cytomegalovirus (CMV) DNA load predicts relapsing CMV infection after solid organ transplantation. *J Infect Dis.* 2000;181(2):717.
73. Humar A, Kumar D, Boivin G, et al. Cytomegalovirus (CMV) virus load kinetics to predict recurrent disease in solid-organ transplant patients with CMV disease. *J Infect Dis.* 2002;186(6):829.
74. Preiksaitis JK, Brennan DC, Fishman J, et al. Canadian society of transplantation consensus workshop on cytomegalovirus management in solid organ transplantation final report. *Am J Transplant.* 2005;5(2):218.
75. Green M, Reyes J, Webber S, et al. The role of antiviral and immunoglobulin therapy in the prevention of Epstein-Barr virus infection and post-transplant lymphoproliferative disease following solid organ transplantation. *Transpl Infect Dis.* 2001;3(2):97.
76. Lee TC, Savoldo B, Rooney CM, et al. Quantitative EBV viral loads and immunosuppression alterations can decrease PTLD incidence in pediatric liver transplant recipients. *Am J Transplant.* 2005;5(9):2222.
77. Milpied N, Vasseur B, Parquet N, et al. Humanized anti-CD20 monoclonal antibody (Rituximab) in post transplant B-lymphoproliferative disorder: a retrospective analysis on 32 patients. *Ann Oncol.* 2000;11(Suppl 1):113.
78. Parasitic infections. *Am J Transplant.* 2004;4(Suppl 10):142.
79. Ljungman P, Urbano-Ispizua A, Cavazzana-Calvo M, et al. Allogeneic and autologous transplantation for haematological diseases, solid tumours and immune disorders: definitions and current practice in Europe. *Bone Marrow Transplant.* 2006;37(5):439.
80. Soubani AO, Kseibi E, Bander JJ, et al. Outcome and prognostic factors of hematopoietic stem cell transplantation recipients admitted to a medical ICU. *Chest.* 2004;126(5):1604.
81. Afessa B, Tefferi A, Hoagland HC, et al. Outcome of recipients of bone marrow transplants who require intensive-care unit support. *Mayo Clin Proc.* 1992;67(2):117.
82. Soubani AO. Critical care considerations of hematopoietic stem cell transplantation. *Crit Care Med.* 2006;34(9 Suppl):S251.
83. Kawabata Y, Hirokawa M, Komatsuda A, et al. Clinical applications of CD34+ cell-selected peripheral blood stem cells. *Ther Apher Dial.* 2003;7(3):298.
84. Baron F, Storb R. Allogeneic hematopoietic cell transplantation following nonmyeloablative conditioning as treatment for hematologic malignancies and inherited blood disorders. *Mol Ther.* 2006;13(1):26.
85. Sandmaier BM, McSweeney P, Yu C, et al. Nonmyeloablative transplants: preclinical and clinical results. *Semin Oncol.* 2000;27(2 Suppl 5):78.
86. Junghanss C, Marr KA. Infectious risks and outcomes after stem cell transplantation: are nonmyeloablative transplants changing the picture? *Curr Opin Infect Dis.* 2002;15(4):347.
87. Marr KA, Seidel K, White TC, et al. Candidemia in allogeneic blood and marrow transplant recipients: evolution of risk factors after the adoption of prophylactic fluconazole. *J Infect Dis.* 2000;181(1):309.
88. Boeckh M, Bowden R. Cytomegalovirus infection in marrow transplantation. *Cancer Treat Res.* 1995;76:97.
89. Meyers JD, Flournoy N, Thomas ED. Risk factors for cytomegalovirus infection after human marrow transplantation. *J Infect Dis.* 1986;153(3):478.
90. Boeckh M. Current antiviral strategies for controlling cytomegalovirus in hematopoietic stem cell transplant recipients: prevention and therapy. *Transpl Infect Dis.* 1999;1(3):165.
91. Martino R, Porras RP, Rabella N, et al. Prospective study of the incidence, clinical features, and outcome of symptomatic upper and lower respiratory tract infections by respiratory viruses in adult recipients of hematopoietic stem cell transplants for hematologic malignancies. *Biol Blood Marrow Transplant.* 2005;11(10):781.
92. Jantunen E, Ruutu P, Niskanen L, et al. Incidence and risk factors for invasive fungal infections in allogeneic BMT recipients. *Bone Marrow Transplant.* 1997;19(8):801.
93. Walsh TJ, Groll AH. Emerging fungal pathogens: evolving challenges to immunocompromised patients for the twenty-first century. *Transpl Infect Dis.* 1999;1(4):247.
94. Herbrecht R, Denning DW, Patterson TF, et al. Voriconazole versus amphotericin B for primary therapy of invasive aspergillosis. *N Engl J Med.* 2002;347(6):408.
95. Boeckh M, Leisenring W, Riddell SR, et al. Late cytomegalovirus disease and mortality in recipients of allogeneic hematopoietic stem cell transplants: importance of viral load and T-cell immunity. *Blood.* 2003;101(2):407.
96. Atkinson K, Storb R, Prentice RL, et al. Analysis of late infections in 89 long-term survivors of bone marrow transplantation. *Blood.* 1979;53(4):720.
97. Winston DJ, Schiffman G, Wang DC, et al. Pneumococcal infections after human bone-marrow transplantation. *Ann Intern Med.* 1979;91(6):835.

CHAPTER 116 ■ HUMAN IMMUNODEFICIENCY VIRUS IN THE INTENSIVE CARE UNIT

ALISON MORRIS • KRISTINA CROTHERS • LAURENCE HUANG

Human immunodeficiency virus (HIV)-infected patients require critical care for various reasons that may or may not be related to their underlying immunodeficiency. The evaluation of HIV-infected persons admitted to the intensive care unit (ICU) requires consideration of all processes that can occur in HIV-*un*infected persons, as well as those particular to HIV infection, namely opportunistic infections, neoplasms, and HIV-associated comorbidities or toxicities associated with antiretroviral therapy. Management of acute, life-threatening conditions requires institution of similar therapies in HIV-infected persons as in HIV-uninfected persons, with awareness of potential drug toxicities and drug interactions that can occur in those on antiretroviral therapy.

This chapter reviews the critical care of HIV-infected patients, including causes of ICU admission and patient outcomes. Special emphasis is placed on the etiology and management of respiratory failure, particularly that due to *Pneumocystis* pneumonia (PCP), which carries an especially high mortality risk. The potential impact of highly active antiretroviral therapy (HAART) on the critical care of HIV-infected patients is summarized, and issues regarding HIV testing and decreasing transmission of HIV in the health care setting are discussed.

EPIDEMIOLOGY OF HIV-INFECTED PATIENTS IN THE ICU

ICU Admission Rates and Outcomes

The first cases of HIV/AIDS were reported in 1981. Since that time, there have been many developments in the treatment of HIV and its associated diseases, most notably the introduction of HAART in 1996. Rates of ICU admission and mortality related to ICU admission for HIV-infected patients have shifted multiple times during the AIDS epidemic. Reasons for these changing patterns are likely related in part to patient and provider attitudes regarding the utility of intensive care (1). A series of investigations focusing on outcomes of HIV-infected patients requiring intensive care at San Francisco General Hospital illustrates these changes. An analysis of ICU admissions during the early 1980s reported mortality rates of nearly 70% for HIV-infected patients, with most patients admitted for PCP (2). Despite increasing hospital admissions of HIV-infected patients after 1984, the rates of ICU admission declined, likely the result of both the physicians' and patients' views of ICU care as futile (1). Subsequently, in the late 1980s, mortality rates decreased coincident with the introduction of adjunctive corticosteroids to treat PCP (3). However, in the early 1990s, ICU mortality increased in the setting of increased rates of ICU use, possibly because of renewed optimism in outcomes (4). Data from the immediate pre-HAART period of 1992–1995 demonstrated an overall improvement in the mortality rate to 37% compared to the early days of the AIDS epidemic (5).

Studies have suggested a further decline in ICU mortality after the introduction of HAART, although this has not been demonstrated in all reports. In studies from San Francisco General Hospital, ICU mortality decreased significantly from 37% in 1992–1995 to 29% in 1996–1999 (1,6). Likewise, studies comparing the mortality rate between 1991–1992 and 2001 from Beth Israel Medical Center in New York demonstrated a decrease in mortality from 51% to 29% (7). In contrast, analyses of ICU admissions at a hospital in Paris, France, found that ICU mortality was unchanged when comparing admissions before and during the HAART era (8,9). Overall, in recent studies, the average reported in-hospital mortality for HIV-infected patients admitted to the ICU ranged between 25% and 40%, with a median ICU length of stay of 5 to 11 days (5–12) (Table 116.1).

Despite decreasing hospitalization rates for HIV-infected patients, ICU admission rates have not changed substantially in the HAART era (6–9,13). Approximately 5% to 12% of hospital admissions for HIV-infected patients involve ICU care (8,12). Possible reasons why ICU admissions have remained relatively constant include the fact that a large proportion of HIV-infected patients continue to be admitted to the ICU without prior known HIV infection (range 28%–40%) (8,9). In addition, approximately 50% of patients are not on HAART at the time of admission (8,9,12). Thus, these patients may be presenting with critical HIV-associated illnesses, as they have not been receiving care or have not been able to benefit from HAART. Furthermore, as overall survival has improved in HIV-infected patients on HAART, the number of persons living with HIV has increased. Given this improved survival, providers may be more likely to admit patients to the ICU and pursue aggressive life support measures (8,13).

Indications for ICU Admission

Studies of critically ill HIV-infected patients indicate that the spectrum of diseases requiring ICU admission is changing in the setting of HAART. Early in the epidemic, most patients were admitted with an AIDS-associated condition, most often PCP. Increasingly, patients with HIV infection are admitted with a non–AIDS-associated condition. In a study from Beth Israel Medical Center in New York, ICU admissions for non–HIV-related disease increased substantially from 12% of all admissions in 1991–1992 to 67% in 2001 (7). Likewise, in a study from France, the proportion of admissions for non–AIDS-related conditions increased significantly from 42% to 63% when admissions between 1995–1996 and 1997–1999 (9) were compared. Data from San Francisco General Hospital found a similarly high proportion of patients (63%) admitted with non–AIDS-related conditions from 1996 through 1999 (6).

Acute respiratory failure is the most common indication for ICU care, accounting for approximately 25% to 50% of ICU admissions in HIV-infected patients (5,6,9–12,14,15). *Pneumocystis jirovecii* was the responsible pathogen in approximately 25% to 50% of these patients in earlier investigations (5,10,16). Although decreased in some studies (7), it remains a significant cause of respiratory failure in recent studies, accounting for 14% to nearly 50% of cases of respiratory failure (6,7,12,17). Bacterial pneumonia is also a frequent cause of acute respiratory failure and in some studies is now as common (6) or more common (7) than PCP.

Sepsis is an increasingly frequent indication for ICU admission, in one study increasing from 3% to 23% of all admissions for HIV-infected patients during recent years (9). Other commonly reported causes of ICU admission include CNS dysfunction (11%–27%), gastrointestinal bleeding (6%–15%), and cardiovascular disease (8%–13%) (5,6,9,10,15,16). Other reasons for ICU admission unrelated to immunodeficiency include trauma, routine postoperative care, noninfectious pulmonary diseases such as asthma and pulmonary embolism, renal failure, metabolic disturbances, and drug overdose. Given the frequent coinfection with hepatitis C among patients with HIV, liver disease may be increasing as a cause of death (18,19), and complications related to cirrhosis often require ICU admission. In addition, solid organ transplantation (liver, kidney) is currently being studied in HIV-infected patients; thus, these patients may also be encountered in the ICU setting.

Predictors of Mortality during ICU Admission

Mortality in the ICU is clearly related to the reason for ICU admission. The highest mortality rates for HIV-infected patients requiring ICU admission are associated with sepsis and respiratory failure. Mortality rates of approximately 50% (5,15), and as high as 68%, have been reported for sepsis (20). If

TABLE 116.1

MORTALITY ASSOCIATED WITH ICU ADMISSION AMONG HIV-INFECTED PATIENTS IN THE HAART ERA

Setting (reference)	ICU patients (*N*)	Time period	HIV unknown at admission	HAART at admission	HIV or AIDS-related illness	Overall ICU mortality	Independent predictors of ICU or in-hospital mortality[a]
University hospital, Jacksonville, FL, USA (11)	141	1995–1999	—	—	—	30%[b]	Transfer from another hospital ward, APACHE II score
University hospital, Paris, France (9)	230	1997–1999	40%	28%	37%	20%	SAPS II score, mechanical ventilation, Omega score
University hospital, Paris, France (8)	236	1998–2000	28%	50%	50%	25%	PCP with pneumothorax; mechanical ventilation; Kaposi sarcoma; inotropic support; $CD4^+$ count <50 cells; SAPS II score
Urban hospital, New York, NY, USA (12)	259	1997–1999	—	48%	60%	30%	Mechanical ventilation; admission with HIV-related illness
Urban hospital, New York, NY, USA (7)	53	2001	—	52%	33%	29%[b]	No multivariate analysis provided; low albumin associated with increased mortality on univariate analysis
Urban hospital, San Francisco, CA, USA (6)	295	1996–1999	7%	25%	37%	29%[b]	Mechanical ventilation; PCP; APACHE II scores >13; albumin <2.6 g/dL; AIDS-associated diagnosis
Hospital Virgen de la Victoria, Malaga, Spain (17)	49	1997–2003	31%	31%	61%	57%	Not reported

ICU, intensive care unit; HIV, human immunodeficiency virus; HAART, highly active antiretroviral therapy; AIDS, acquired immunodeficiency syndrome; APACHE, Acute Physiology and Chronic Health Evaluation; SAPS, Simplified Acute Physiology Score; PCP, *Pneumocystis* pneumonia.
[a]In order of descending magnitude of association.
[b]Data given as in-hospital rather than ICU mortality.

respiratory failure is due to PCP, mortality remains nearly 50% (6,12) and is increased if complicated by PCP-associated pneumothorax (6,8). For AIDS patients admitted to the ICU for other HIV-related reasons, the reported mortality is generally lower. For example, the reported mortality for CNS dysfunction is 20% to 48% (5,10–12,15), whereas the mortality for gastrointestinal disease is approximately 30% to 35% (5,10,11). However, patients admitted with non–HIV-related conditions may have better outcomes. In a study from San Francisco General Hospital, patients admitted with a non–AIDS-associated diagnosis were significantly more likely to survive than patients admitted with an AIDS-associated condition (odds ratio [OR] 2.9, 95% confidence interval [CI] 1.5–5.8, $p = 0.002$) (6). In a study from New York, ICU admission with an HIV-related illness was independently associated with increased mortality (OR 4.2, 95% CI 2.0–9.0, $p < 0.001$) (12).

Mortality during hospitalization is also related to the severity of the acute illness (Table 116.1). Predictors of increased hospital mortality include the need for mechanical ventilation and disease severity (as assessed by scoring systems such as the Simplified Acute Physiology Score I [SAPS I], and the Acute Physiology and Chronic Health Evaluation II [APACHE II] score) (5,6,9,12,15). ICU mortality has also been related to the preadmission health status of the patient. Patients with a decreased serum albumin level or a history of weight loss may also have a higher mortality (5,6,15). The $CD4^+$ T-cell count and the plasma HIV RNA level have generally not been independent predictors of short-term mortality during the ICU stay (5–7,11,12,16). However, long-term mortality after ICU admission is related to the underlying severity of HIV disease (5,15,16). Compared to pre-HAART, long-term survival following ICU discharge is improved in the HAART era (8,9).

Impact of Antiretroviral Therapy on ICU Mortality

The full impact of HAART on outcome of HIV patients in the ICU remains unclear, as prospective, randomized trials assessing the initiation of HAART on outcome in critically ill patients have not been completed. Two retrospective studies conducted at San Francisco General Hospital suggest that HAART may improve outcomes in critically ill HIV patients. In a review of all HIV-infected patients admitted to the ICU between 1996 and 1999, patients receiving combination HAART at the time of ICU admission were less likely to present with two conditions associated with decreased survival, an AIDS-associated diagnosis and decreased serum albumin, but HAART itself was not independently associated with survival (6). In a study of all HIV-infected patients with PCP who were admitted to the ICU at San Francisco General Hospital between 1996 and mid-2001, patients who were on HAART at the time of ICU admission or started HAART during hospitalization had an improved survival compared to patients not receiving HAART (21). However, in another study from New York City, ICU mortality was not different in patients admitted between 1997 and 1999 when comparing patients receiving HAART versus those not on HAART (12). Furthermore, the prior use of HAART was not associated with differences in overall hospital mortality or length of stay (12). Another study found that although ICU mortality had improved in recent years, this improvement could not be attributed to HAART because none of the patients received this therapy (22). Conclusions regarding the impact of HAART on outcome are limited by the nonrandomized nature of these retrospective studies and by the inability to measure potential bias in the selection of which patients received HAART. In addition, these studies do not address treatment failure, drug resistance, or medication nonadherence prior to or after ICU admission, all of which influence long-term outcome (12).

IMMEDIATE CONCERNS IN MANAGING CRITICALLY ILL HIV-INFECTED PATIENTS

The initial management of critically ill HIV-infected patients includes all the immediate concerns in HIV-uninfected patients such as securing a stable airway and ensuring adequate respiration and circulation. The immediate management of patients with respiratory failure depends on the underlying reason for respiratory compromise, but consideration of opportunistic infections is warranted early in the course of care to ensure prompt diagnostic evaluation and initiation of appropriate antibiotic therapy. Management of patients in shock consists of similar strategies as in HIV-uninfected patients and depends on the cause of shock, with use of volume resuscitation, vasopressors, and/or inotropic agents as appropriate to maintain adequate mean arterial pressures and systemic perfusion. For patients with septic shock, early goal-directed therapy should be instituted (23). Given the increased association of HIV with cardiovascular disease, cardiomyopathy (24), and adrenal insufficiency (25), providers should be alert to the possibility that these conditions may also cause shock in HIV-infected patients.

Certain aspects of the patient's history are important for initiating early appropriate management. The degree of immunosuppression related to HIV infection is a critical determinant of risk for opportunistic infections. In addition, use of and adherence to antiretroviral therapy and prophylactic antibiotics, as well as intravenous drug use and exposures to endemic fungi and mycobacteria, are key components of the patient's history. The evaluation and management of the most common indications for ICU admission among HIV-infected patients are discussed in detail below.

PULMONARY MANIFESTATIONS OF HIV

Spectrum of Respiratory Diseases and Approach to Diagnosis

Although the spectrum of diseases leading to respiratory failure has changed during the HAART era, acute respiratory failure is still the most common cause of ICU admission for HIV-infected patients (5,6,9–12,14,15). Respiratory failure can occur from a multitude of causes including infections, neoplasms, drug overdose, and neurologic conditions that may be both HIV- and non–HIV-related. Rapid diagnosis and initiation of appropriate therapy is crucial, particularly in patients with HIV-associated infections. Although many of the conditions have typical signs and symptoms, many of the presentations can overlap. Therefore, definitive diagnosis should be pursued whenever possible.

Appropriate workup includes chest radiograph and occasionally chest computed tomography (CT). Blood and sputum cultures should be obtained, and bronchoscopy with bronchoalveolar lavage (BAL) should be strongly considered for definitive diagnosis. In some cases, pulmonary disease becomes disseminated, and biopsy of other sites such as lymph nodes or bone marrow can be useful in obtaining a diagnosis. It is important to remember that all the conditions leading to respiratory failure in the non–HIV-infected patient also occur in those with HIV infection. Diagnoses such as pulmonary embolism, asthma, chronic obstructive pulmonary disease, and cardiogenic pulmonary edema also present with respiratory failure, and appropriate testing should be performed.

Pneumocystis Pneumonia

Pneumocystis pneumonia (PCP) has historically been the most common cause of respiratory failure in AIDS patients (5,10,16). PCP is caused by the organism *Pneumocystis jirovecii*, formerly *Pneumocystis carinii*. The numbers of patients admitted to the ICU with PCP has decreased since the introduction of HAART, but it remains an important cause of morbidity and mortality in the HIV-infected ICU patient. In the 1980s, patients with PCP who were admitted to the ICU had a mortality rate as high as 81%, with mortality for those requiring mechanical ventilation approaching 90% (2). The introduction of adjunctive corticosteroids for moderate to severe PCP in the mid-1980s led to an improvement in mortality for PCP-associated respiratory failure to approximately 60% (3,26,27). Since that time, there has been little change in outcomes from severe PCP, with recent studies still reporting a hospital mortality of approximately 60% (5,6). The primary factors that determine mortality in patients with PCP are the need for mechanical ventilation and the development of a pneumothorax. Either of these factors portends a poor prognosis, and the occurrence of both is almost uniformly fatal (6,28). Other factors that have been reported to be associated with mortality in some studies include low serum albumin, admission to the ICU after 3 to 5 days of hospitalization, increased age, and elevated serum lactate dehydrogenase (LDH) (6,22,28–30).

Clinical Presentation. PCP is most frequent in patients with a $CD4^+$ cell count below 200 cells/μL, with the risk of PCP increasing as the $CD4^+$ count decreases below that level (31,32). Although use of PCP prophylaxis decreases the incidence of PCP, patients receiving prophylaxis may still develop PCP, especially if severely immunocompromised (33). However, many patients with PCP do not know that they are HIV-infected, and therefore never receive PCP prophylaxis. Recent studies have reported that 28% to 57% of patients admitted to the ICU are diagnosed with PCP as their first manifestation of HIV; thus clinicians need to consider PCP in *any* patient with a consistent clinical picture if the patient's HIV status is unknown (21,28). HIV-infected patients continue to present with PCP because of a lack of regular medical care, nonadherence to PCP prophylaxis, or failure to have appropriate prophylaxis prescribed (34,35).

Risk factors for PCP other than a low $CD4^+$ cell count, the presence of oropharyngeal candidiasis, and prior PCP are debated. For example, exposure to an infected rodent can result in PCP in immunosuppressed rodents, but whether human exposure increases PCP risk is still unclear (36). Certain activities such as gardening have been associated with increased risk, and there appears to be geographic variation in PCP risk (37,38). The influence of cigarette smoking has also been debated, although some studies have reported an increased risk of PCP in smokers (39,40).

The symptoms of PCP can be nonspecific but include fever, tachypnea, dyspnea, and cough. The cough associated with PCP is most often nonproductive or productive of clear sputum. Patients with purulent sputum are more likely to have bacterial pneumonia. The pace and duration of symptoms is also important in distinguishing PCP from bacterial pneumonia. Unlike in the non–HIV-infected immunosuppressed population, HIV-infected patients with PCP generally report the subacute onset of symptoms over several weeks, with the median duration of symptoms in one study being 28 days (41).

Many patients with PCP have an unremarkable lung examination. They will often manifest hypoxemia and an increased alveolar-arterial oxygen gradient. Laboratory tests can suggest the diagnosis, but are often nonspecific. The white blood cell count can be normal, decreased, or increased. Serum LDH is often elevated in patients with PCP. The test has a sensitivity of 83% to 100%, and a normal LDH does not rule out the diagnosis (42–44). Also, multiple pulmonary and nonpulmonary conditions can result in an elevated LDH, so an elevated LDH does not rule in the diagnosis. In general, the LDH is more useful as a prognostic rather than a diagnostic test. The degree of elevation correlates with outcome and response to therapy, and patients with a rising serum LDH in the face of treatment have a worse prognosis (44). The arterial blood gas in PCP demonstrates hypoxemia and a widened alveolar-arterial gradient, which can be seen in any pulmonary disease but is useful in determining the need for adjunctive corticosteroids and ICU care. A recent study examined the utility of serum procalcitonin measurement in distinguishing PCP from tuberculosis and bacterial pneumonia (45). The authors found that procalcitonin levels were significantly lower in PCP than in either TB or bacterial pneumonia, but this test has not been applied in large-scale clinical studies.

The classic chest radiographic appearance of PCP is a diffuse interstitial, reticular, or granular infiltrate (Fig. 116.1). PCP can

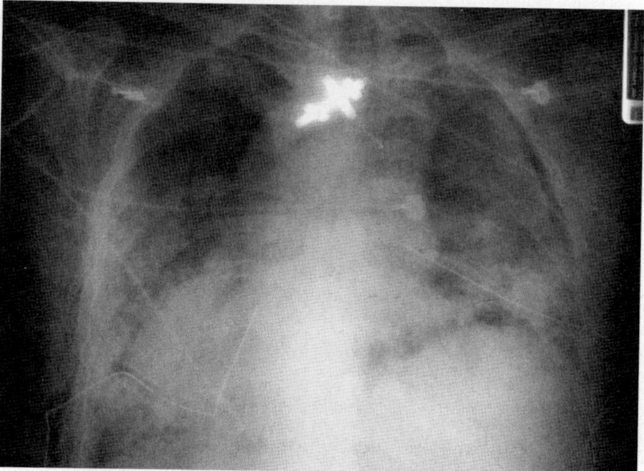

FIGURE 116.1. Portable chest radiograph from a patient with *Pneumocystis* pneumonia demonstrating diffuse bilateral infiltrates and pneumothoraces. (Courtesy of Laurence Huang, M.D., M.A.S., Professor of Medicine, University of California, San Francisco.)

also result in focal airspace consolidation, although this presentation is less common. Infiltrates are occasionally unilateral or asymmetric and, in patients receiving aerosolized pentamidine for prophylaxis, there may be an upper lobe predominance. In general, the pattern (reticular or granular) is more suggestive of the diagnosis than the distribution. Severe PCP is similar to the acute respiratory distress syndrome (ARDS) in causing widespread capillary leak that results in bilateral infiltrates, and these two entities may be indistinguishable radiographically. Cysts or pneumatoceles occur in about 10% to 20% of patients, and these changes can be seen before, during, or after PCP treatment (46,47). Patients with PCP are at risk for developing spontaneous pneumothoraces, and PCP should be high in the differential for any HIV-infected patient presenting with a pneumothorax. Radiographic findings such as pleural effusions or lymphadenopathy are uncommon in PCP, and their presence should lead the clinician to consider alternate or concurrent diagnoses. High-resolution CT scans can be helpful in demonstrating diffuse ground glass opacities typical of PCP, but these findings are not specific.

Diagnosis. Although patients may present with typical signs and symptoms of PCP, a definitive diagnosis is preferred, particularly in patients in the ICU. Many HIV-associated respiratory diseases have overlapping or nonspecific presentations, which makes it difficult for even experienced clinicians to diagnose empirically. Definitive diagnosis allows for the timely administration of appropriate antibiotics and avoids exposure to unnecessary medications. We are currently unable to culture *Pneumocystis*, and thus, the diagnosis relies on visualization of the organism in a respiratory sample from a patient with a compatible clinical presentation.

PCP can be diagnosed either through examination of induced sputum or from samples obtained at bronchoscopy. Spontaneous sputum is generally not acceptable for diagnosis of PCP (48). Rarely, open lung biopsy is used to provide a diagnosis. Induced sputum has a sensitivity ranging from 56% to over 80%, but these numbers were generated by centers experienced in the technique (49–53). The usefulness of this test is often limited because many hospitals lack experience in examining induced sputum, and a negative sputum induction should be followed by a bronchoscopy. A recent study reported that serial sputum samples can improve PCP diagnosis (7). In the ICU, the technique is usually not used because patients are generally not able to tolerate the procedure or are intubated.

Bronchoscopy with BAL should be obtained when sputum induction is negative or cannot be obtained. For patients with HIV infection, BAL has a sensitivity of over 90% for diagnosis of PCP and should be performed as early as possible in undiagnosed patients (54). Transbronchial biopsy does not add significantly to the yield for PCP in an HIV-infected individual and is technically challenging in an intubated patient; however, it may be useful in diagnosing other pulmonary infections that are also in the differential (55). It is reasonable to perform transbronchial biopsy as part of the initial procedure when the probability of PCP is low or as a follow-up test when the initial BAL is nondiagnostic.

Traditional staining methods for PCP include Gomori methenamine silver, toluidine blue O stain, or a modified Wright-Giemsa stain. Immunofluorescent antibody staining can also be used to examine induced sputum or BAL and has a high sensitivity (56,57). Newer methods based on the molecular technique of polymerase chain reaction (PCR) are currently under investigation. A recent study compared PCR of BAL and sputum with traditional methods and found 100% sensitivity for BAL and 85% sensitivity for sputum, with a specificity of 90% to 100% for both (58). Because PCR is quite sensitive, its use might obviate the need to obtain invasive samples. For example, a study of quantitative touch down PCR of oral washes found that the technique had a sensitivity of 88% and a specificity of 85% (59). When a cutoff value was applied to the *Pneumocystis* copy number, specificity improved to 100%. PCR-based diagnosis is not yet widely available for PCP.

Treatment and Corticosteroids. The duration of PCP treatment is 21 days. First-line therapy for moderate to severe PCP is intravenous trimethoprim-sulfamethoxazole (TMP-SMX) (Table 116.2). TMP-SMX is curative in 60% to 86% of patients (60,61). The dosage of TMP-SMX is 15 to 20 mg/kg of trimethoprim and 75 to 100 mg/kg of sulfamethoxazole daily, divided every 6 to 8 hours. TMP-SMX is associated with a high rate of adverse reactions, particularly in those with HIV infection. Approximately one fourth to one half of patients will develop therapy-limiting toxicity (41,60,62–64). Adverse

TABLE 116.2

SUMMARY OF TREATMENT REGIMENS FOR PCP IN THE ICU IN DECREASING ORDER OF PREFERENCE

Agent	Dose	Side effects
Trimethoprim-sulfamethoxazole	15 to 20 mg/kg/d trimethoprim with 75 to 100 mg/kg/d sulfamethoxazole IV, divided every 6 to 8 h	Bone marrow suppression, hyponatremia, hyperkalemia, nausea, nephrotoxicity, rash, transaminitis
Pentamidine isethionate	3 to 4 mg/kg/d IV	Bone marrow suppression, hypoglycemia or hyperglycemia, hypotension, nausea, pancreatitis, nephrotoxicity
Clindamycin-primaquine	900 mg IV every 8 h (clindamycin) 30 mg PO daily (primaquine)	Diarrhea, hemolytic anemia, leukopenia, methemoglobinemia, nausea, rash
Adjunctive therapy: Prednisone if PaO_2 less than 70 mm Hg or A-a gradient more than 35 mm Hg	40 mg PO every 12 h for 5 d, 40 mg PO daily for 5 d, 20 mg PO daily for 11 d	Psychosis, hyperglycemia

PCP, *Pneumocystis* pneumonia; ICU, intensive care unit; IV, intravenously; PO, by mouth; PaO_2, arterial oxygen tension; A-a, alveolar-arterial; d, day; h, hour.

reactions to TMP-SMX include nausea, integumentary rash, elevation of transaminases, hyponatremia, hyperkalemia, renal insufficiency, and bone marrow suppression.

Intravenous pentamidine isethionate is the preferred alternative treatment for patients who cannot tolerate TMP-SMX or have failed treatment. Patients should receive 3 to 4 mg/kg/day of pentamidine. Some studies have found that the efficacy of pentamidine is similar to TMP-SMX, but others have reported a lower survival rate with pentamidine (61% vs. 86% for TMP-SMX) (60,61,65). Pentamidine has several serious adverse effects that can limit therapy and may be seen in as many as 50% of patients. Toxicity from pentamidine includes nausea, hypotension, bone marrow suppression, hepatic transaminitis, and nephrotoxicity. Glucose levels should be monitored in patients receiving pentamidine because it is toxic to pancreatic islet cells and can result in initial hypoglycemia from a surge of insulin release, followed by hyperglycemia from inadequate insulin. Some patients can even progress to chronic diabetes mellitus. Pancreatitis also occurs with pentamidine and may be fatal (66,67). Other side effects that have been reported include myoglobinuria, hyperkalemia, and increases in creatinine kinase. Pentamidine also has cardiac effects with bradycardia, prolonged Q-T intervals, and ventricular arrhythmias (68,69).

When TMP-SMX and pentamidine are either ineffective or toxic, it is possible to use clindamycin and primaquine as another salvage regimen option, but this use may be limited in the ICU because primaquine is administered orally and its absorption may be impaired. Clindamycin should be dosed 600 to 900 mg every 6 to 8 hours intravenously, with primaquine given 15 to 30 mg orally daily. Patients should be tested for G6PD deficiency before starting primaquine. Side effects include rash, diarrhea, and methemoglobinemia.

Adjunctive corticosteroids have been shown to decrease mortality in those patients with moderate to severe PCP (26,27,70,71). A recent meta-analysis of all randomized trials of corticosteroids found that the administration of corticosteroids was associated with a risk ratio of 0.56 for mortality and 0.38 for requiring mechanical ventilation (72,73). Patients with a room air arterial oxygen pressure less than 70 mm Hg or with an alveolar-arterial gradient greater than 35 mm Hg should receive corticosteroids. Corticosteroid therapy should be started within 24 to 72 hours of initiation of PCP treatment, whether the diagnosis is confirmed or only suspected. Corticosteroids act to reduce the inflammatory response seen during the first few days of treatment, thereby preventing respiratory deterioration. The recommended regimen is 40 mg of oral prednisone given twice daily for 5 days, then 40 mg once daily for 5 days, and 20 mg daily for 11 days. If patients are unable to tolerate oral medications, intravenous methylprednisolone or dexamethasone can be substituted.

Treatment Failure. Due to the increased inflammatory response during the initial phase of treatment, clinical deterioration can frequently be seen in the first 3 to 5 days of PCP treatment. Patients may experience worsening hypoxemia and respiratory distress, and radiographic infiltrates may progress. This worsening is likely due to an inflammatory response to dead or dying organisms that results in increased capillary permeability and formation of pulmonary edema. Assessment of treatment failure is challenging given this potential for initial worsening combined with the inability to culture *Pneumocystis* or determine antibiotic sensitivities. In general, treatment should be continued for at least 5 to 10 days before diagnosing treatment failure and switching to another agent. It is important to remember that other diagnoses present at baseline or that have developed since admission can explain the patient's lack of improvement, and these diagnoses must be excluded before concluding that treatment failure is solely to blame. Other diagnoses to consider include nosocomial, community-acquired, or other opportunistic pneumonia, and cardiogenic or noncardiogenic pulmonary edema. Patients who worsen or fail to improve while receiving PCP treatment should undergo diagnostic procedures such as chest CT, sputum cultures, or echocardiography as clinically indicated. Repeat bronchoscopy is useful to identify pathogens other than PCP but is not useful to evaluate treatment failure because *Pneumocystis* can persist in the BAL, even in patients who are successfully treated (74).

It is unknown if treatment failure is more likely in patients with previous exposure to anti-*Pneumocystis* prophylaxis. *Pneumocystis* develops mutations at the dihydropteroate synthase (DHPS) locus with exposure to sulfa- or sulfone-containing medications such as TMP-SMX and dapsone (75–77). In other micro-organisms, mutations at this locus have been shown to produce resistance to TMP-SMX, but the evidence for clinically important resistance in *Pneumocystis* is not clear-cut. Some authors have found an increased mortality and rate of treatment failure in patients with DHPS mutations (78–81), but others have not observed this association (76,82). In general, most patients with previous exposure to TMP-SMX or dapsone respond to treatment with TMP-SMX, and it should still be regarded as first-line therapy for these patients.

Ventilatory Support. Because the physiology of PCP is very similar to that of ARDS, principles of ventilatory management should be the same. Barotrauma is of particular concern in ventilated patients with PCP, as the development of a pneumothorax heralds a poor prognosis. Although patients with PCP were not included in the ARDSnet study, these patients should probably be ventilated in a similar fashion—with tidal volumes of 6 mL/kg and levels of positive end-expiratory pressure as needed to maintain oxygenation according to the ARDSnet guidelines (83). Noninvasive positive pressure ventilation (NIPPV) with continuous positive airway pressure (CPAP) or bilevel positive airway pressure (BiPAP) may be useful in patients with PCP. One study found that use of noninvasive ventilation decreased the rate of intubation, lowered the number of pneumothoraces, and improved survival (84). NIPPV may be tried as a first-line ventilation mode in patients with PCP who are awake, cooperative, and able to protect their airway.

Bacterial Pneumonia

Both the use of TMP-SMX for PCP prophylaxis and HAART have contributed to an overall decline in the numbers of cases of HIV-associated bacterial pneumonia (BP) (85–88). Although absolute numbers of cases of BP have declined since the introduction of HAART, in some series it now accounts for a greater percentage of ICU admissions since the number of PCP cases has also declined (6,11). Clinical risk factors for BP include injection drug use, cigarette smoking, older age, and lower $CD4^+$ cell count, although BP can occur in patients with any $CD4^+$ cell count (87,89–91). There are limited data regarding ICU mortality, but one study found that 83% of HIV-infected patients admitted to the ICU with BP survived (7). $CD4^+$ cell count below 100 cells/μl, shock, and radiographic progression have been associated with mortality from BP in HIV-infected patients (92). Nosocomial pneumonia has also declined since the introduction of HAART but is still common in mechanically ventilated patients (88).

Clinical Presentation. Clinical presentation of BP in the HIV-infected patient is similar to that in the non–HIV-infected population. Patients typically present with an acute onset of fever, cough, shortness of breath, and purulent sputum. Chest radiographs frequently reveal lobar infiltrates that may progress to an ARDS-like picture in severe cases. The most common causes of BP in HIV include *Streptococcus pneumoniae, Haemophilus influenzae, Pseudomonas aeruginosa,* and *Staphylococcus aureus*. Drug resistant *S. pneumoniae* and *S. aureus* are more common in HIV-infected patients (93–95). Atypical pneumonia with *Mycoplasma pneumoniae* is reported in approximately 20% to 30% of HIV-infected patients with community-acquired pneumonia (CAP) but is less commonly a cause of ICU admission (96). HIV-infected patients are more likely to be bacteremic, particularly those with *Streptococcus pneumoniae* infection (97).

Diagnosis and Treatment. Diagnosis and treatment for both CAP and hospital-acquired pneumonia should generally follow published guidelines, although these guidelines do not specifically address pneumonia in HIV-infected patients (98–100). Blood cultures should be obtained. Sputum should be sent for Gram stain and culture, and bronchoscopy should be considered. Treatment should include empiric coverage for the organisms above. Because of the higher incidence of pseudomonal and staphylococcal pneumonia in HIV-infected patients with severe pneumonia, it is important to initiate coverage for these organisms. As methicillin-resistant *Staphylococcus aureus* (MRSA) is common in HIV infection and is associated with decreased survival (88), empiric antibiotics effective against this pathogen are warranted pending results of cultures and antimicrobial sensitivities.

Other Respiratory Diseases

Other respiratory diseases that occur in HIV-infected ICU patients include *Mycobacteria tuberculosis* pneumonia; fungal pneumonias such as *Cryptococcus neoformans, Histoplasma capsulatum, Coccidioides immitis,* and *Aspergillus fumigatus*; cytomegalovirus pneumonia, and *Toxoplasma gondii* pneumonitis. Malignancies such as Kaposi sarcoma and non-Hodgkin lymphoma can also lead to respiratory failure, but they are far less common than infections.

IMMUNE RECONSTITUTION INFLAMMATORY SYNDROME

The immune reconstitution inflammatory syndrome (IRIS) is a life-threatening syndrome occurring in HIV-infected patients who are started on HAART. In the days to months following initiation of HAART, patients experience a paradoxical worsening or new onset of infectious signs or symptoms. The syndrome results from an improvement in the immune system with an increased inflammatory response against infectious agents that can occur before the $CD4^+$ cell count has risen (101). Immune reconstitution is most often seen in infection with *Mycobacterium tuberculosis*, cytomegalovirus (CMV), *Pneumocystis, Mycobacterium avium* complex, and endemic fungi (101–107). Manifestations of IRIS that can result in the need for ICU care include pneumonitis, meningitis, hepatitis, and pericarditis.

Respiratory failure secondary to IRIS is most common in tuberculosis and PCP (105,108–110). Paradoxical worsening in these cases presents with fever, hypoxemia, and new or increased radiographic infiltrates. Care is supportive, and corticosteroids are generally advocated, particularly in cases of PCP. Antiretroviral regimens should be continued whenever possible. Because this syndrome can be difficult to distinguish from acute opportunistic infections or other causes of respiratory deterioration, it is imperative that other causes of respiratory failure are sought before assigning a diagnosis of IRIS.

SEPSIS AND BACTEREMIA

Sepsis is increasingly common among HIV-infected patients admitted to the ICU, and its mortality rate has been reported to be as high as 68% (9,20,111). In the HAART era, more deaths in the HIV population have been attributed to sepsis (112). Care of the HIV-infected patient with sepsis should follow current guidelines (113). Broad-spectrum antibiotics should be based on the patient's $CD4^+$ cell count, the presumed source, and previous use of prophylactic antibiotics that might predispose to resistant bacteria. Clinicians should consider empiric coverage for mycobacterial diseases and endemic fungi as suggested by the patient's presentation. The use of corticosteroids or recombinant-activated protein C has not been extensively studied in the HIV-infected population. Because HIV-infected patients have a high incidence of adrenal insufficiency, it is prudent to evaluate all septic HIV-infected patients and initiate therapy if cortisol levels do not increase appropriately with stimulation. Use of activated protein C can be difficult in this population because it should not be administered to patients with platelet counts below 30,000 cells/μL or to those with a history of a central nervous system (CNS) lesion.

NEUROLOGIC MANIFESTATIONS OF HIV

The spectrum of neurologic disorders requiring critical care for patients with HIV infection includes all the causes commonly seen in the non–HIV-infected population in addition to particular opportunistic infections, neoplasms, and sequelae of HIV. In one series, neurologic diagnoses accounted for 12% of ICU admissions and had a 75% survival in the HAART era (6). An earlier series found that as many as 80% of these conditions required mechanical ventilation (114). A recent study of neurologic causes of ICU admission found that CNS toxoplasmosis and progressive multifocal leukoencephalopathy (PML) had decreased, but the incidence of ischemic stroke, hemorrhagic stroke, and primary CNS lymphoma had increased (115).

CNS toxoplasmosis is one of the most frequent CNS infections seen, although the number of cases has fallen dramatically with the introduction of HAART. Patients typically present with fever, headache, focal neurologic deficits, and a decreased level of consciousness; seizures can also occur. CT scan reveals characteristic ring-enhancing lesions (Fig. 116.2). Similar findings can also be seen with CNS lymphoma. Treatment

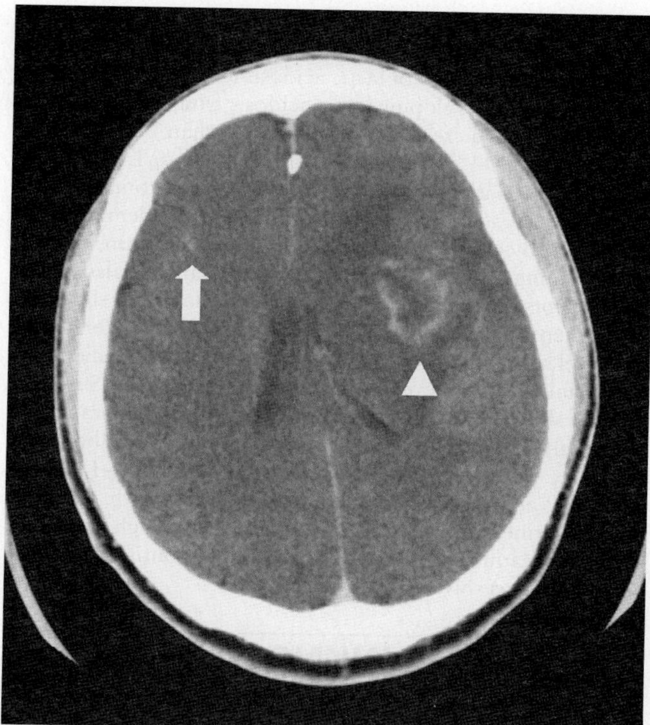

FIGURE 116.2. Contrast-enhanced head computed tomography scan from an AIDS patient with headache, word-finding difficulty, and several seizures showing a left frontoparietal ring-enhancing lesion (*arrowhead*) with mass effect on the lateral ventricle and a subtler focus of enhancement on the right at the gray-white junction (*arrow*). (Courtesy of Cheryl Jay, M.D., Associate Clinical Professor of Neurology, University of California, San Francisco.)

for CNS toxoplasmosis is pyrimethamine given as a 200-mg loading dose, followed by 50 to 75 mg orally every 24 hours, with sulfadiazine at a dose of 1 to 1.5 g every 6 hours orally. Patients should also receive 10 to 20 mg of folic acid daily while receiving pyrimethamine. Other CNS infections that are seen in HIV infection include bacterial and *Cryptococcus neoformans* meningitis. Diagnosis of *C. neoformans* is confirmed by visualization of encapsulated yeast on cerebrospinal fluid (CSF), a positive CSF culture, or a positive CSF cryptococcal antigen. Treatment should be initiated with amphotericin B (0.7 mg/kg/day intravenously) and flucytosine (100 mg/kg/day orally, divided into four doses). Repeated lumbar puncture is often required to normalize CSF pressure. Other CSF infections that occur in HIV include PML, which is a progressive demyelinating disease, CMV, and herpes simplex virus. Any of these diseases can worsen and present with a neurologic immune reconstitution inflammatory syndrome in the setting of introduction of HAART (115).

GASTROINTESTINAL MANIFESTATIONS OF HIV

Gastrointestinal (GI) diseases, in particular liver diseases, have increased as a cause of death in HIV-infected patients (112). These diseases are either the primary cause or a complicating factor in the ICU admission of many HIV-infected patients. As in the non-ICU population, significant GI bleeding often results in ICU admission. Upper GI bleeding is more common than lower GI bleeding, and approximately half of the cases are HIV-related (116). Common HIV-associated diagnoses include infectious esophagitis (e.g., CMV) and ulcers, Kaposi sarcoma, and AIDS-associated lymphoma (116). In cases of lower GI bleeding, approximately 70% are a result of HIV infection (116). CMV colitis and idiopathic colon ulcers are most common, but Kaposi sarcoma, AIDS-associated lymphoma, and infections such as *Mycobacterium avium* complex may also contribute (117). Hemorrhoids and anal fissures can also result in significant bleeding in HIV-infected patients with thrombocytopenia (118). Care of the HIV-infected patient with a GI bleed is the same as for a non–HIV-infected patient and should include immediate resuscitation, source identification, reversal of coagulation defects, and achievement of hemostasis.

Coinfection with HIV and hepatitis C is increasingly common and complicates the management of both diseases. Mortality from hepatitis C has increased in recent years (119–121), and infection in HIV-infected individuals seems to be more severe with a higher mortality and risk of cirrhosis (122–124). There is also an increased risk of renal failure in hospitalized patients coinfected with HIV and hepatitis C (125). Hepatitis B is also common among HIV-infected patients.

Other GI conditions that are common in HIV-infected patients include peritonitis and bowel perforation. The most common cause of life-threatening abdominal pain is small bowel or colon peritonitis from CMV (126). Kaposi sarcoma, AIDS-associated lymphoma, and mycobacterial infection have also been associated with bowel perforation (117). Pancreatitis can also be seen, particularly with exposure to certain antiretroviral medications or pentamidine. AIDS cholangiopathy can result from various infectious and neoplastic processes and can be asymptomatic or present with fulminant biliary sepsis (117). In addition to the usual care of cholangitis with intravenous fluids and broad-spectrum antibiotics, endoscopic retrograde cholangiopancreatography (ERCP) with sphincterotomy may be helpful in patients with common bile duct dilatation (126).

OTHER HIV-ASSOCIATED CONDITIONS

Cardiac Disease

Since the introduction of HAART, there has been growing evidence that HIV-infected patients are developing premature atherosclerosis, and cardiovascular disease is now a primary cause of non–HIV-related deaths in these patients (112,127). Therefore, these patients may be more commonly admitted to the ICU with acute coronary syndromes.

The development of metabolic abnormalities that contribute to atherosclerosis has been associated with the use of nonnucleoside reverse transcriptase inhibitors (NNRTIs) and/or protease inhibitors (PIs). Elevated triglycerides, hypercholesterolemia, decreased high-density lipoproteins, glucose intolerance, and frank diabetes have all been associated with various antiretrovirals (128–131). There may also be direct endothelial effects of PIs or HIV itself that play a role in the development of vascular complications (132). Because of the higher rate of these metabolic abnormalities, combined with a high prevalence of cigarette smoking, it has been postulated that

HIV-infected patients might have advanced cardiac and cerebrovascular disease, but several large-scale studies have had varying results (133–135). Even if the risk of cardiovascular events is elevated compared to non–HIV-infected patients, it is still low, particularly in comparison to the dramatic improvements in morbidity and mortality associated with HAART. There are few data on treatment or outcomes of cardiac disease specifically in the HIV-infected population, but treatment of acute coronary syndromes should be the same as in the non–HIV-infected population. A study of HIV-infected patients undergoing cardiac surgery found that these patients had favorable outcomes and should be referred for coronary artery bypass grafting when appropriate (136).

Renal Disease

HIV-infected patients are at risk of acute and chronic renal failure that can either lead to ICU admission or complicate care in the ICU. Renal function is abnormal in approximately 30% of HIV-infected subjects, and HIV-associated nephropathy is a common cause of end-stage renal disease (137). Renal dysfunction can occur from use of certain antiretroviral medications and other therapies such as pentamidine, TMP-SMX, and amphotericin B. HIV-infected patients who are coinfected with hepatitis C also have an increased risk of renal failure (125). HIV-associated nephropathy is another common cause of renal dysfunction and seems to improve with the administration of HAART (137). The diagnostic workup and treatment of renal dysfunction in HIV-infected patients is similar to that for the non–HIV-infected patient and should include renal ultrasound to rule out obstruction, examination of the urine, discontinuation of nephrotoxic medications, and renal biopsy if indicated. Dialysis should be offered to appropriate patients.

Metabolic Abnormalities

Metabolic abnormalities are common in the HIV-infected ICU patient. As described above, lipid and glucose abnormalities are often seen. Hyperglycemia secondary to drugs such as pentamidine also occurs in this population. It has been noted that hospitalized patients with HIV have high rates of hyponatremia (138–140). Causes of hyponatremia include hypovolemia, adrenal insufficiency, drugs, and the syndrome of inappropriate antidiuretic hormone (SIADH). A high incidence of adrenal abnormalities has been noted on autopsy of HIV-infected patients (141,142). Causes of adrenal pathology include infections such as CMV, tumors such as Kaposi sarcoma, and drugs such as ketoconazole and pentamidine. The clinical significance of the adrenal abnormalities is uncertain, but it seems that HIV-infected patients have a higher likelihood of adrenal dysfunction (25,143). Adrenal insufficiency can present with hyperkalemia, hyponatremia, and hypotension, and patients with these symptoms should be evaluated and treated appropriately. As with non–HIV-infected patients, adrenal insufficiency is likely common in sepsis.

Lactic acidosis is another metabolic abnormality that can occur in HIV-infected patients receiving HAART. This syndrome was first described in the 1990s and can occur with any nucleoside/nucleotide reverse transcriptase inhibitor (NRTI) but is most commonly seen with didanosine and stavudine (144,145). Mitochondrial toxicity secondary to impaired synthesis of adenosine triphosphate (ATP)-generating enzymes is believed to be the cause of lactic acidosis (146). Patients particularly at risk of developing lactic acidosis from these drugs include those with a creatinine clearance less than 70 mL/minute and a nadir CD4$^+$ cell count below 250 cells/μL (147). Although some patients may have only an asymptomatic lactic acidosis, others present with life-threatening acidemia. These patients also commonly complain of abdominal pain, nausea, and vomiting. Hepatic steatosis and transaminitis also occur, and patients can progress to respiratory failure and shock. In any patient presenting with these symptoms, an arterial lactate level should be checked and all antiretroviral medications discontinued if the level is greater than 5 mmol/L. Supportive care should be administered with bicarbonate therapy and hemodialysis if necessary. Based on anecdotal data, riboflavin, thiamine, and L-carnitine may reverse toxicity (148–151). Riboflavin is administered at a dose of 50 mg daily with 50 mg/kg of L-carnitine, and 100 mg of thiamine. Although the exact length of treatment is unknown, it should be continued at least until acidosis resolves.

FEVER OF UNKNOWN ORIGIN

Fever is common in all ICU patients. The differential for fever is broad in the HIV-infected patient and includes infections, neoplasms, medications, and collagen vascular diseases. Several studies have examined the etiology of fevers of unknown origin in those with HIV infection. Most studies have found that infectious causes are responsible for most prolonged fevers in the HIV-infected patient, with mycobacterial diseases diagnosed most commonly. PCP and bacterial infections are also seen (152–155). The most common neoplastic cause of prolonged fever is lymphoma. Patients receiving HAART are less likely to present with a fever of unknown origin than those not receiving HAART (156).

Recurrent fever in an HIV-infected ICU patient should also prompt evaluation of those conditions commonly seen in non–HIV-infected ICU patients. Common infectious causes of fever in the ICU include hospital-acquired pneumonia, catheter-related infections, sinusitis, and pseudomembranous colitis. Noninfectious causes include drug reactions (which are particularly common in those with HIV), pancreatitis, venous thromboembolism, acalculous cholecystitis, adrenal insufficiency, and thyroid storm. Diagnostic workup should include standard evaluation for infections such as blood, sputum, and urine cultures. Bronchoscopy with BAL should be performed in patients who demonstrate a new infiltrate on chest radiograph or have a worsening respiratory status. Testing should be performed for mycobacterial and fungal pathogens. Other testing should be performed as would be done in the non–HIV-infected population.

ANTIRETROVIRAL THERAPY IN THE ICU

Treatment Strategies

HIV-infected patients may be receiving antiretroviral therapy at the time of ICU admission or may have antiretroviral therapy initiated in the ICU. The use of antiretroviral therapy in critically ill patients presents distinct issues related to drug delivery, dosing, drug interactions, and antiretroviral-associated toxicities. The success of HAART in decreasing HIV-associated morbidity and mortality has raised questions regarding the ability of HAART to improve outcome in critically ill HIV-infected patients. It is unclear if the risks associated with HAART outweigh the potential benefits and if patients who are already receiving HAART should continue therapy in the ICU.

There are several factors related to using HAART in the ICU that are important to consider. HAART improves immune function. In chronic HIV infection, improving immune function with HAART significantly reduces the risk of opportunistic infections and neoplasms. This could contribute to reductions in morbidity and mortality in critically ill HIV-infected patients by decreasing the risk of subsequent HIV-associated diseases. HAART is also important in treating conditions such as PML that otherwise lack effective therapy. For these patients, HAART use may be necessary, even in the face of significant risks. For patients already receiving HAART, discontinuing therapy could result in the selection of drug-resistant virus that could limit future therapy. This is especially true if patients are receiving efavirenz or nevirapine, as these antiretroviral medications have longer half-lives than other antiretroviral medications. As a result, levels of these medications may persist as the levels of the other antiretroviral medications decrease, resulting in functional monotherapy.

HAART is also associated with several risks. Drug interactions and HAART-associated toxicities complicate management. In addition to issues regarding antiretroviral drug delivery and absorption, there are uncertainties surrounding dosing in acute and multiple organ system failures. These uncertainties could place patients at risk for subtherapeutic drug levels and drug resistance or, conversely, supratherapeutic levels and toxicity. Immune reconstitution inflammatory syndromes could result in significant clinical worsening of an already critical disease. The potential threat of this syndrome may make physicians reluctant to initiate HAART in the ICU.

There are no randomized clinical trials and no consensus guidelines to assist in decisions regarding HAART use in the ICU. Only a few retrospective studies address some of the clinical issues that clinicians face. Although decisions regarding HAART use in the ICU require a case-by-case basis review, Huang et al. (157) suggested the following framework (Fig. 116.3). Patients receiving HAART prior to ICU admission who have evidence of virologic suppression (plasma HIV RNA below the limit of detection) should continue HAART, if possible. These patients should have no contraindications to continuing HAART such as drug interactions or HAART-associated toxicities. Prompt placement of a feeding tube is especially critical in these patients, as lapses in therapy create the potential for

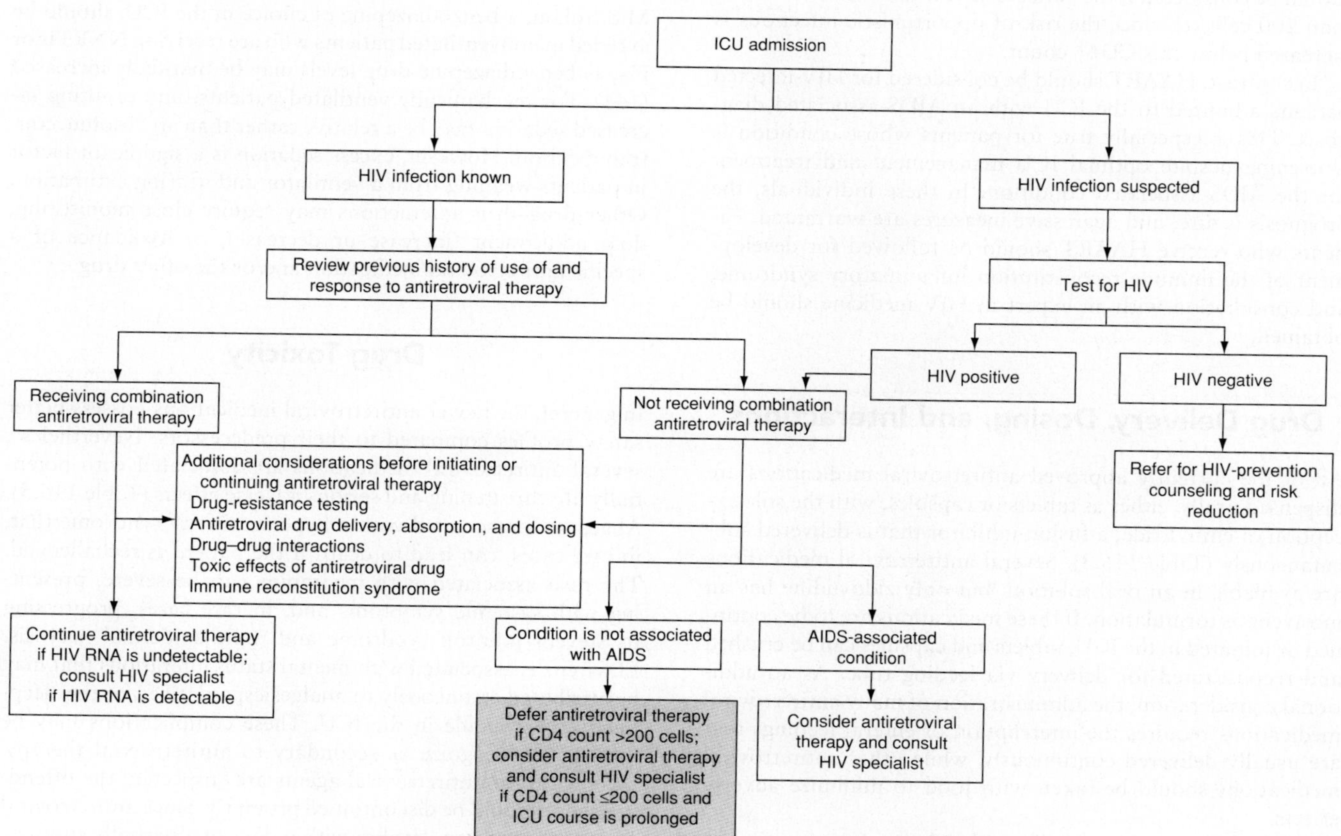

FIGURE 116.3. Treatment strategies for patients with HIV in the ICU. This algorithm provides a framework for making decisions regarding the use of antiretroviral therapy in the ICU. (Reproduced from Huang L, Quartin A, Jones D, et al. Intensive care of patients with HIV infection. *N Engl J Med.* 2006;355:179, with permission.)

subtherapeutic antiretroviral drug levels and the emergence of HIV drug resistance. In patients whose plasma HIV RNA is detectable despite HAART, the risks of continuing HAART may outweigh the benefits of this incomplete HIV viral suppression. However, consultation with an expert in HIV medicine should be obtained prior to any decision to continue, switch, or discontinue HAART.

Patients not receiving HAART prior to ICU admission represent the largest proportion of HIV-infected patients admitted to the ICU (6–9). Two studies from the HAART era suggest that patients admitted with an AIDS-defining diagnosis, especially PCP, have the poorest prognosis and, thus, the greatest theoretical benefit from HAART (6,21). Although one study found that patients receiving or started on HAART during admission for PCP had decreased mortality (25% versus 63%), this study was retrospective and based on a limited number of patients.

Based on the limited available data, HAART initiation should be deferred in HIV-infected patients admitted to the ICU with a non–AIDS-associated condition (Fig. 116.3) (157). The immediate prognosis in these patients is generally better than for an AIDS-associated diagnosis, and the short-term outcome is most likely related to successful treatment of the underlying non-AIDS condition (6). As a result, the risks of HAART initiation in the ICU outweigh the short-term benefits of this therapy. If, however, patients remain in the ICU for a prolonged period, HAART (and opportunistic infection [OI] prophylaxis) should be considered if the patients have a $CD4^+$ cell count less than 200 cells/μL since the risk of opportunistic infections is increased below this $CD4^+$ count.

In contrast, HAART should be considered for HIV-infected patients admitted to the ICU with an AIDS-associated diagnosis. This is especially true for patients whose condition is worsening despite optimal ICU management and treatment for the AIDS-associated condition. In these individuals, the prognosis is dire, and aggressive measures are warranted. Patients who receive HAART should be followed for development of the immune reconstitution inflammatory syndrome, and consultation with an expert in HIV medicine should be obtained.

Drug Delivery, Dosing, and Interactions

All of the currently approved antiretroviral medications are dispensed orally, either as tablets or capsules, with the sole exception of enfuvirtide, a fusion inhibitor that is delivered subcutaneously (Table 116.3). Several antiretroviral medications are available in an oral solution, but only zidovudine has an intravenous formulation. If these medications are to be continued or initiated in the ICU, tablets and capsules can be crushed and reconstituted for delivery via feeding tube. As an additional consideration, the administration of many antiretroviral medications requires the interruption of enteral feedings that are usually delivered continuously, while other antiretroviral medications should be taken with food to minimize adverse effects.

Critical illness may complicate the absorption of antiretroviral medications. Decreased gastric motility (158,159), continuous feeding (160), nasogastric suctioning, and gastric alkalinization recommended for stress ulcer prophylaxis (113) may contribute to variations in the absorption of enterally administered drugs. H_2-blockers and proton pump inhibitors, used for stress ulcer prophylaxis, are contraindicated with certain antiretroviral medications, necessitating the use of alternative prophylaxis agents or antiretroviral medications (Table 116.4) (161). Absorption of subcutaneously injected medications may also be altered (162,163). Furthermore, atypical drug volumes of distribution and compromise of elimination pathways due to acute organ failures may confound the achievement of appropriate drug levels (164).

The impact of acute and multiple organ system failures on the pharmacokinetics of antiretroviral medications, particularly when used in combination, have been largely unstudied. The presence of renal insufficiency or hepatic impairment will affect antiretroviral dosing. Renal insufficiency will reduce the clearance of all NRTIs except abacavir and will require dose adjustment of these NRTIs (Table 116.3). Patients with renal insufficiency cannot use most of the fixed-dose NRTI combinations. Instead, each antiretroviral medication must be used individually and dosed accordingly. Liver impairment will reduce the hepatic metabolism of many PIs and NNRTIs and will require dose adjustment of these medications (Table 116.3). Finally, as the patient's renal and hepatic functions change, the dose of these medications must be readjusted accordingly.

Antiretroviral medications, especially NNRTIs and ritonavir-boosted PI regimens, have several important drug interactions with other medications (Table 116.4). These interactions involve other HIV-associated medications, including those for opportunistic infection treatment or prevention, and common ICU medications, especially benzodiazepines. Midazolam, a benzodiazepine of choice in the ICU, should be avoided in nonventilated patients who are receiving NNRTIs or PIs, as benzodiazepine drug levels may be markedly increased (161). For mechanically ventilated patients, any resulting increased sedation may be a relative rather than an absolute contraindication. However, excess sedation is a significant factor in patients weaning from a ventilator and nearing extubation. Other drug–drug interactions may require close monitoring, dose adjustment (increase or decrease), or avoidance of a specific antiretroviral medication and/or the other drug.

Drug Toxicity

In general, the newer antiretroviral medications possess better safety profiles compared to their predecessors. Nevertheless, several antiretroviral medications are associated with potentially life-threatening and serious adverse effects (Table 116.5). Abacavir is associated with a hypersensitivity syndrome that, in rare cases, can lead to death if the patient is rechallenged. The rash associated with nevirapine can be severe, presenting with systemic symptoms and, in rare cases, progressing to Stevens-Johnson syndrome and toxic epidermal necrosis. Efavirenz is associated with mental status alterations that may be attributed erroneously to analgesics, sedatives, or the sleep-disrupted schedule in the ICU. These complications may be difficult to recognize as secondary to antiretroviral therapy. If toxicities to antiretroviral agents are suspected, the offending agent should be discontinued promptly. Since antiretroviral drug resistance can develop within days of a partially suppressive regimen, all antiretroviral medications should be discontinued or a replacement drug should be substituted for the suspected agent. Consultation with an expert in HIV medicine is

(*text continues on page 1747*)

TABLE 116.3

ANTIRETROVIRAL MEDICATION FORMULATIONS AND DOSING

Medication	Available formulation(s): Tablet/capsule	Available formulation(s): Other	Daily dose	Dosing in renal insufficiency	Dosing in hepatic impairment
Nucleoside/Nucleotide Reverse Transcriptase Inhibitors					
Abacavir, ABC (Ziagen)	300 mg tablets	20 mg/mL oral solution	300 mg BID or 600 mg QD	No dosage adjustment	No dosage recommendation
Didanosine, ddI (Videx EC)[a]	125, 200, 250, 400 mg enteric coated (EC) capsules		More than 60 kg 400 mg QD *With tenofovir* 250 mg QD Less than 60 kg 250 mg QD *With tenofovir* 200 mg QD	(EC capsules) — Dose/d CrCl (mL/min) / >60 kg / <60 kg 30–59 / 200 mg / 125 mg 10–29 / 125 mg / 100 mg <10* / / 125 mg 75 mg *Includes patients receiving CAPD and HD; administer dose after dialysis.	No dosage recommendation
Emtricitabine, FTC (Emtriva)	200 mg hard gelatin capsule	10 mg/mL oral solution	200 mg QD or 240 mg (240 mL) oral solution QD	CrCl (mL/min) / Capsule dose 30–49 / 200 mg q48h 15–29 / 200 mg q72h <15* / 200 mg q96h CrCl (mL/min) / Oral solution dose 30–49 / 120 mg q24h 15–29 / 80 mg q24h <15* / 60 mg q24h *Includes patients receiving HD; administer dose after dialysis.	No dosage recommendation
Lamivudine, 3TC (Epivir)	150, 300 mg tablets	10 mg/mL oral solution	150 mg BID or 300 mg QD	CrCl (mL/min) / Dose 30–49 / 150 mg QD 15–29 / 150 mg once, then 100 mg QD 5–14 / 150 mg once, then 50 mg QD <5* / 50 mg once, then 25 mg QD *Includes patients receiving HD; administer dose after dialysis.	No dosage recommendation
Stavudine, d4T (Zerit)	15, 20, 30, 40 mg capsules	1 mg/mL oral solution	More than 60 kg 40 mg BID Less than 60 kg 30 mg BID	Dose/d CrCl (mL/min) / >60 kg / <60 kg 26–50 / 20 mg q12h / 15 mg q12h 10–25* / 20 mg q24h / 15 mg q24h *Includes patients receiving CAPD and HD; administer dose after dialysis.	No dosage recommendation

(*Continued*)

TABLE 116.3

(*Continued*)

Medication	Available formulation(s)		Daily dose	Dosing in renal insufficiency	Dosing in hepatic impairment
	Tablet/capsule	Other			
Tenofovir disoproxil fumarate, TDF (Viread)	300 mg tablet		300 mg QD	CrCl (mL/min) / Dose: 30–49: 300 mg q48h 10–29: 300 mg twice weekly ESRD*: 300 mg q7d *Includes patients receiving HD; administer dose after dialysis.	No dosage recommendation
Zidovudine, AZT, ZDV (Retrovir)	100 mg capsules 300 mg tablets	10 mg/mL oral solution 10 mg/mL IV solution	300 mg BID 200 mg TID	Severe renal impairment or HD: 100 mg TID	No dosage recommendation
Combination					
Zidovudine + lamivudine (Combivir)	300 + 150 mg tablets		300/150 mg BID	Use individual antiretroviral medications dosed accordingly	No dosage recommendation
Zidovudine + lamivudine + abacavir (Trizivir) 2	300 + 150 + 300 mg tablets		300/150/300 mg BID	Use individual antiretroviral medications dosed accordingly	No dosage recommendation
Abacavir + lamivudine (Epzicom)	600 + 300 mg tablets		600/300 mg QD	Use individual antiretroviral medications dosed accordingly	No dosage recommendation
Tenofovir + emtricitabine (Truvada)	300 + 200 mg tablets		300/200 mg QD	CrCl (mL/min) / Dose: 30–49: 300/200 mg q48h <30: Not recommended	No dosage recommendation
Tenofovir + emtricitabine + efavirenz (Atripla)	300 + 200 + 600 mg tablets		300 + 200 + 600 mg QD	Use individual antiretroviral medications dosed accordingly CrCl <50 mL/min Not recommended	No dosage recommendation
Nonnucleoside Reverse Transcriptase Inhibitors					
Delavirdine, DLV (Rescriptor)[b]	100, 200 mg tablets		400 mg TID	No dosage adjustment	No dosage recommendation; use with caution
Efavirenz, EFV (Sustiva)[a]	50, 100, 200 mg capsules 600 mg tablets		600 mg QD on an empty stomach	No dosage adjustment	No dosage recommendation; use with caution
Nevirapine, NVP (Viramune)	200 mg tablets	50 mg/5 mL oral suspension	200 mg QD for 14 days, then 200 mg BID	No dosage adjustment	No data available; avoid use in patients with moderate to severe impairment

Atazanavir, ATV (Reyataz)[c]	100, 150, 200 mg capsules		400 mg QD *With tenofovir or efavirenz* RTV 100 mg QD must be added to ATV 300 mg QD	No dosage adjustment	C-P Score / Dose 7–9: 300 mg QD >9: Not recommended
Darunavir, DRV Prezista[c,d,f]	300 mg tablet		*With ritonavir* 600 mg BID (RTV 100 mg BID)	No dosage adjustment	No dosage recommendation; use with caution
Fosamprenavir, f-AP (Lexiva)	700 mg tablet		ARV naïve 1,400 mg BID *With ritonavir* 1,400 mg QD (RTV 200 mg QD) or 700 mg BID (RTV 100 mg BID) *With efavirenz* (RTV 100 mg BID must be added to f-APV 700 mg BID or RTV 300 mg QD added to f-APV 1,400 mg QD)	No dosage adjustment	C-P Score / Dose 5–8: 700 mg BID >9: Not recommended RTV boosting should not be used
Indinavir, IDV (Crixivan)[b,d]	200, 333, 400 mg capsules		800 mg q8h[a] *With ritonavir* 800 mg q12h (RTV 100 or 200 mg q12h)	No dosage adjustment	Mild to moderate insufficiency due to cirrhosis: 600 mg q8h
Lopinavir/ritonavir, LPV/r (Kaletra)	200/50 mg capsule	400/100 mg/5 mL oral solution Oral solution contains 42% alcohol	400/100 mg BID or 800/200 mg QD (only if ARV naïve) *With efavirenz or nevirapine* 600/150 mg BID	No dosage adjustment	No dosage recommendation; use with caution
Nelfinavir, NFV (Viracept)[b,c]	250, 625 mg tablets	50 mg/g oral powder	1,250 mg BID or 750 mg TID	No dosage adjustment	No dosage recommendation; use with caution
Ritonavir, RTV (Norvir)[b,e]	100 mg capsules	600 mg/7.5 mL oral solution	600 mg q12h (when used as sole protease inhibitor) 100 to 400 mg daily in 1 to 2 divided doses (when used as pharmacokinetic booster)	No dosage adjustment	No dosage adjustment in mild impairment; no data for moderate to severe impairment, use with caution

(*Continued*)

TABLE 116.3

(*Continued*)

Medication	Available formulation(s): Tablet/capsule	Available formulation(s): Other	Daily dose	Dosing in renal insufficiency	Dosing in hepatic impairment
Saquinavir hard gel capsule, SQV HGC (Invirase)[b,d]	200 mg capsules		*With ritonavir* 1,000 mg BID (RTV 100 mg BID)	No dosage adjustment	No dosage recommendation; use with caution
Tipranavir, TPV (Aptivus)[c,d,f]	250 mg capsules		*With ritonavir* 500 mg BID (RTV 200 mg BID)	No dosage adjustment	No dosage recommendation; use with caution; contraindicated in C-P Class B and C
Enfuvirtide, T20 (Fuzeon)[b,f]		108 mg/1.1 mL sterile H_2O (90 mg/1 mL)	90 mg SQ BID	No dosage adjustment	No dosage recommendation

BID, twice a day; QD, once daily; CAPD, continuous ambulatory peritoneal dialysis; HD, hemodialysis; ESRD, end-stage renal disease; TID, three times a day; C-P, Child-Pugh; SQ, subcutaneously.

[a]Hold enteral nutrition 2 h before and 1 h after administration.

[b]Generally not recommended as initial therapy if alternatives are available due to inferior virologic activity, inconvenient dosing, high pill burden, and/or increased toxicity and adverse events.

[c]Administration with food increases bioavailability. Take with food. For atazanavir, avoid taking with antacids.

[d]Generally not recommended unless accompanied by ritonavir as a pharmacokinetic booster.

[e]Generally not recommended as the sole protease inhibitor, but used in combination with other protease inhibitors as a pharmacokinetic booster.

[f]No clinical trial data in antiretroviral therapy-naïve patients.

Adapted from Guidelines for the Use of Antiretroviral Agents in HIV-1-Infected Adults and Adolescents. These guidelines are updated frequently, and the most recent information is available on the AIDS*info* Web site: http://AIDSinfo.nih.gov. Accessed October 10, 2006.

TABLE 116.4

COMMON ICU MEDICATIONS AND POTENTIALLY SERIOUS LIFE-THREATENING INTERACTIONS WITH ANTIRETROVIRALS

Drug	Antiretroviral	Interaction
NEUROLOGIC AGENTS		
Anticonvulsants Phenytoin, phenobarbital, carbamazepine	Darunavir Delavirdine Efavirenz	May decrease ARV levels May decrease anticonvulsant levels
SEDATIVES/ANALGESICS		
Midazolam/triazolam[a]	Most PIs, NNRTIs	Increased sedative effects
Methadone	Most PIs, NNRTIs, NRTIs	Narcotic withdrawal
Meperidine	Ritonavir	Increased normeperidine levels
ANTIMICROBIALS		
Metronidazole	Amprenavir Ritonavir Tipranavir	Disulfiram-like reaction
Rifampin	Most PIs Delavirdine Efavirenz Nevirapine	Decreased ARV levels Increased hepatotoxicity
Voriconazole	Efavirenz Ritonavir	Decreased voriconazole levels Increased ARV levels
RESPIRATORY AGENTS		
Fluticasone	Most PIs	Increased plasma fluticasone levels and adrenal suppression
CARDIAC AGENTS		
Amiodarone	Most PIs	Increased cardiac effects
Diltiazem	Amprenavir Atazanavir Indinavir	Increased cardiac effects
Nifedipine	Amprenavir Darunavir Delavirdine Lopinavir/ritonavir	Increased cardiac effects
Simvastatin/lovastatin	PIs Delavirdine Efavirenz	Increased statin levels
Sildenafil	Most PIs	Increased sildenafil effects
GASTROINTESTINAL AGENTS		
Proton pump inhibitors/ H_2 blockers	Atazanavir Delavirdine	Decreased ARV levels

ICU, intensive care unit; ARV, antiretroviral; PI, protease inhibitor; NNRTI, nonnucleoside reverse transcriptase inhibitor; NRTI, nucleoside reverse transcriptase inhibitor.
[a]Midazolam can be used with caution as a single dose and given in a monitored situation for procedural sedation.

recommended for patients with suspected antiretroviral-associated toxicities.

HIV TESTING IN THE ICU

In the current era, up to 40% of patients are unaware of their HIV infection at the time of their ICU admission (6–9). For these patients, the first opportunity for HIV testing and diagnosis occurs in an ICU setting. Current guidelines recommend HIV testing whenever HIV infection is suspected (165). However, the prompt recognition of previously undiagnosed HIV infection and HIV testing and disclosure requirements present challenges to critical care physicians.

Most states have specific legislation regarding HIV testing, and significant differences exist between states, requiring health

TABLE 116.5

POTENTIALLY LIFE-THREATENING AND SERIOUS ADVERSE EFFECTS OF ANTIRETROVIRAL AGENTS

Life-threatening and adverse effect	Principal antiretroviral agent	Estimated frequency, onset	Prevention/monitoring and management
Dermatologic- Hypersensitivity reaction (HSR)—fever, diffuse rash; may progress to hypotension, respiratory distress, and vascular collapse	Abacavir (ABC)	Approximately 5%–8% Onset, 9 days (median); approximately 90% within first 6 weeks	■ Discontinue ABC and other ARVs. Most signs and symptoms resolve 48 hrs after discontinuation ■ Rule out other causes of symptoms ■ Discontinue other potential agent(s) ■ Do not rechallenge patients with ABC after suspected HSR
Dermatologic- Stevens-Johnson syndrome/toxic epidermal necrolysis (TEN)	Chiefly NNRTIs: Nevirapine (NVP) more than efavirenz (EFV), delavirdine (DLV)	NVP: 0.3%–1%, EFV and DLV: 0.1%; case reports for other ARVs Onset within first few days to weeks	■ NVP: 2-week lead in period with 200 mg QD dosing, then increase to 200 mg BID. Avoid use of corticosteroids during lead-in period—may increase incidence of rash ■ Discontinue NNRTI and other ARVs ■ Rule out other causes of symptoms ■ Discontinue other potential agent(s) ■ Do not rechallenge patients with NNRTI
Neurologic- Central nervous system (CNS) effects including drowsiness, somnolence, insomnia, hallucination, psychosis, suicidal ideation, exacerbation of psychiatric illness	Efavirenz (EFV)	More than 50% may have some symptoms Onset within first few days; most symptoms subside or diminish after 2–4 weeks	■ Administer at bedtime or 2–3 hrs before bedtime for nonintubated, nonsedated patients ■ Take on an empty stomach to reduce drug concentration and CNS effects ■ Consider discontinuing EFV if symptoms persist and cause significant impairment or exacerbation of psychiatric illness
Gastrointestinal- Hepatotoxicity	All ARVs, especially nevirapine (NVP)	Frequency varies with ARV Onset (NRTIs), months to years; PIs generally weeks to months; NVP, 2/3 within first 12 weeks	■ Monitor liver enzymes ■ Rule out other causes of hepatotoxicity ■ For symptomatic patients, discontinue all ARVs ■ Discontinue other potential agent(s)
Gastrointestinal- Pancreatitis	Didanosine (ddI), also stavudine (d4T) plus ddI	ddI: 1%–7%, d4T plus ddI: increased frequency Onset usually weeks to months	■ ddI should not be used in patients with a history of pancreatitis ■ Avoid concomitant use of ddI with d4T ■ Monitoring of serum amylase/lipase in asymptomatic patients is generally not recommended ■ Discontinue offending agent
Hematologic- Bone marrow suppression	Zidovudine (AZT, ZDV)	Anemia: 1.1%–4%; neutropenia: 1.8%–8% Onset, weeks to months	■ Avoid use in patients at risk ■ Avoid other bone marrow suppressants if possible ■ Monitor CBC with differential ■ Switch to another NRTI if there is an alternative ■ Discontinue concomitant bone marrow suppressants if there are alternatives ■ Identify and treat other causes for anemia and neutropenia ■ Blood transfusion if indicated ■ Consider erythropoietin therapy for anemia ■ Consider filgrastim for neutropenia

(Continued)

TABLE 116.5

(Continued)

Life-threatening and adverse effect	Principal antiretroviral agent	Estimated frequency, onset	Prevention/monitoring and management
Lactic acidosis, hepatic steatosis ± pancreatitis (severe mitochondrial toxicities)	NRTIs, especially stavudine (d4T), didanosine (ddI), and zidovudine (AZT, ZDV)	Rare, but mortality up to 50% in some case series Onset, months	■ Discontinue ARV if this syndrome is highly suspected ■ Routine monitoring of lactic acid is generally not recommended ■ Some patients may require IV bicarbonate infusion, hemodialysis, or hemofiltration ■ Thiamine, riboflavin, and/or L-carnitine resulted in rapid resolution of hyperlactatemia in some case reports
Lactic acidosis, rapidly progressive ascending neuromuscular weakness	Stavudine (d4T), most frequent	Rare Onset, months; then dramatic motor weakness may occur within days to weeks	■ Discontinue ARV. Symptoms may be irreversible ■ Do not rechallenge patients with suspected ARV ■ Plasmapheresis, high dose corticosteroids, intravenous immunoglobulin, carnitine, acetylcarnitine attempted with varying success
Renal- Nephrolithiasis/ urolithiasis/crystalluria	Indinavir (IDV) most frequent	Approximately 12% Onset is any time after beginning of therapy, especially at times of decreased fluid intake	■ Maintain hydration, increase hydration at first sign of darkened urine ■ Monitor serum creatinine, urinalysis ■ Consider switching to alternative agent or therapeutic drug monitoring ■ Stent placement may be required
Renal- Nephrotoxicity	Indinavir (IDV), potentially tenofovir (TDF)	Frequency unknown Onset-(IDV): months; (TDV): weeks to months	■ Avoid use of other nephrotoxic medications ■ IDV: Maintain hydration, increase hydration at first sign of darkened urine ■ Monitor serum creatinine, urinalysis, serum potassium and phosphorus ■ Stop offending agent (generally reversible)

ARV, antiretroviral; NNRTI, nonnucleoside reverse transcriptase inhibitor; QD, daily; BID, twice a day; NRTI, nucleoside reverse transcriptase inhibitor; PI, protease inhibitor; CBC, complete blood count.
This table only lists potential life-threatening and serious adverse effects with an onset starting from initial dose up to months after initiation of therapy. However, there are several important adverse effects including cardiovascular effects, hyperlipidemia, insulin resistance or diabetes mellitus, and osteonecrosis that may result from antiretroviral therapy.
Adapted from Guidelines for the Use of Antiretroviral Agents in HIV-1-Infected Adults and Adolescents. These guidelines are updated frequently, and the most recent information is available on the AIDS*info* Web site: http://AIDSinfo.nih.gov. Accessed October 10, 2006.

care providers to be aware of their state statutes and health codes. In general, HIV testing requires consent from the patient. If a patient is incapacitated, some states permit a surrogate to consent on the patient's behalf. HIV testing cannot be performed if a patient or their surrogate refuses HIV testing. As a result, physicians must weigh the risks and benefits of diagnostic procedures and empiric therapy without a confirmed diagnosis; these decisions may harm patients with and without HIV infection. For example, physicians may decide against pursuing bronchoscopy to diagnose PCP or initiating empiric PCP therapy that could be life-saving in an HIV-infected patient with PCP. Conversely, physicians may perform procedures or initiate therapies based on an incorrect assumption of underlying HIV infection, subjecting a patient without HIV to the resulting complications and toxicities.

In cases where HIV testing cannot be performed, well-intentioned physicians may wish to order plasma HIV RNA assays or CD4$^+$ cell counts to infer HIV status. This practice is ill-advised and may be in violation of legal statutes in some states, which specifically prohibit plasma HIV RNA testing without the appropriate counseling. Although a normal CD4$^+$ cell count argues strongly against the presence of an

HIV-associated opportunistic infection such as PCP, low CD4+ counts characteristic of advanced HIV disease are often seen in critically ill patients without HIV (166–168).

CONTROL OF HIV INFECTION IN THE ICU

Blood-borne Pathogen Precautions

Risks for occupational transmission of HIV depend on the type and severity of exposure. Potentially infectious fluids include blood, any visibly bloody body fluid, semen, vaginal secretions, and cerebrospinal, synovial, pleural, peritoneal, pericardial, and amniotic fluid. Transmission may occur via percutaneous injury or via contact with mucous membranes or nonintact skin with infectious material. The average risk for transmission of HIV following a percutaneous exposure to HIV-infected blood is estimated to be approximately 0.3% (169). Transmission after mucous membrane exposure is estimated to be approximately 0.09% (170).

Primary preventive measures should be used to decrease the risk of exposure to HIV, as well as other infections including hepatitis B and C. Health care workers should use universal precautions for handling blood and body fluids for all patients, regardless of known HIV status. These precautions include the routine use of personal protective equipment such as gloves, face protection, and gown, depending on the nature of the procedure, anticipated contact with blood or bodily fluids, and the potential for splashing or splattering of fluids (171). Additional components of a primary prevention strategy include work practice controls—for example, not recapping needles, announcing all sharps introduced onto or removed from the field, not leaving sharps on the field—and engineering controls—for example, self-retracting needles, needleless systems, and sharps disposal containers (172).

Management of Needle Sticks

In health care workers exposed to potentially infectious body fluids, secondary prevention measures should be used promptly. The first step in postexposure management is the immediate cleaning of the site of injury or skin exposure with soap and water (172). Mucous membranes should be flushed with copious amounts of water (173). Exposures should be reported promptly to the appropriate contact at each facility. If the HIV status of the source patient is unknown, evaluation of the risk factors and HIV testing following proper consent procedures should be performed.

In workers with a potential exposure to HIV, postexposure prophylaxis (PEP) should be offered urgently. Decisions of whether to initiate PEP when exposure occurs from a patient with unknown HIV status depend on the type and severity of exposure, prevalence of HIV in the community, and HIV risk factors of the patient. However, the decision to start prophylaxis will often need to be made prior to establishing the HIV status of the source patient. PEP should be begun within hours of exposure, as data suggest that postexposure prophylaxis is likely to be more effective if started shortly after exposure (170,172).

Selection of the PEP antiretroviral regimen depends on the efficacy of the antiretroviral agents and likelihood that the strain of HIV will be susceptible to different agents, as well as the pill burden, tolerability, and any comorbidities or use of concurrent medications in the health care worker. Basic two- or three-drug antiretroviral regimens are recommended by the Centers for Disease Control and Prevention (CDC), depending on the HIV status of the patient and the severity and type of exposure; specific recommendations are available from the CDC (170). Expert consultation should be considered early, particularly in cases with exposure to documented HIV drug resistance. In an earlier study, use of zidovudine following exposure in health care workers was associated with a decrease in the risk of transmission by an estimated 80% (174). No studies have specifically addressed the additional benefit of combination antiretroviral therapy following occupational exposure, but the risk of transmission is likely to be further decreased with multidrug regimens (170).

Substantial side effects are associated with PEP. A full 4-week course of treatment is recommended, although studies suggest that many are unable to finish a complete course (170). Side effects are reported in as many as 75% of persons on PEP (172). Balancing the risk of toxicity related to a three-drug compared to a two-drug regimen depends on the degree of risk associated with the exposure. Because of toxicity, PEP is not justified in exposures that have a negligible risk for transmission of HIV.

Health care workers with potential exposure to HIV should undergo serial HIV antibody testing. The CDC-recommended schedule is initial testing at the time of exposure, with repeat testing at 6 weeks, 12 weeks, and 6 months after exposure (170). Testing should be extended to 12 months in those with dual exposure to HIV and hepatitis C. Health care workers should also receive counseling at the time of exposure to discuss ways to decrease risk of exposures in the future, measures to decrease the risk of secondary transmission, and side effects of any treatments. Re-evaluation within 72 hours after exposure is warranted, particularly as additional information regarding the source patient may be available, and PEP may be discontinued if HIV testing of the source patient is negative.

Respiratory Isolation

As with HIV-uninfected patients, HIV-infected patients with suspected airborne-spread infections should be placed in respiratory isolation. Airborne precautions in the hospital setting consist of the use of personal protective equipment in the form of respirators and engineering controls such as the use of negative-pressure rooms (175). Diseases requiring airborne isolation precautions include tuberculosis, varicella (chickenpox and herpes zoster), measles, and the severe acute respiratory syndrome (SARS) (175). Because tuberculosis is common in the HIV-infected population and is often difficult to distinguish from other types of pneumonia, most HIV-infected patients with respiratory symptoms and chest radiographic abnormalities should be considered for respiratory isolation. The immune status of staff caring for the patient should also be considered, and limiting the number of staff exposed to the patient may be warranted. Patients with suspected airborne-transmitted diseases should wear a surgical mask during transport. Criteria for removing patients from respiratory isolation vary by disease. For example, patients with tuberculosis can be removed from respiratory isolation when the patient is on effective therapy, is clinically improving, and has three consecutive negative sputum smears for acid-fast bacilli on different days or tuberculosis has been ruled out.

SUMMARY

In summary, the outcome for HIV-infected ICU patients has improved dramatically since the beginning of the AIDS epidemic. The spectrum of admitting diagnoses in the ICU has shifted to include more non–HIV-related conditions and diagnoses related to side effects of HAART. Because many patients are admitted to the ICU as their first manifestation of HIV, clinicians also need to consider a diagnosis of HIV in any patient with a compatible clinical history. Issues regarding continuing or starting HIV therapy are complex, and although HAART seems to have had some impact on the outcomes of critically ill HIV-infected patients, much remains to be discovered about its role in the ICU. Unfortunately, few data exist to guide clinicians in this difficult decision, and until future randomized, controlled studies examine this question, physicians must balance the risks and benefits for individual patients.

PEARLS

- Intensive care survival of HIV-infected patients has improved over the course of the AIDS epidemic with survival rates that justify ICU care for most patients.
- Diagnoses such as bacterial pneumonia, sepsis, and non–AIDS-related conditions have increased in frequency since the introduction of highly active antiretroviral therapy (HAART).
- Definitive diagnosis is highly recommended in patients with HIV. Early bronchoscopy with bronchoalveolar lavage should be performed in patients with pneumonia who do not have an established microbiologic diagnosis.
- Despite decreasing numbers of cases of *Pneumocystis* pneumonia (PCP), PCP is still common in HIV-infected patients. It is associated with a high mortality, particularly in those patients with a pneumothorax while on mechanical ventilation. Many patients admitted with PCP are not aware of their HIV status.
- First-line treatment for PCP is intravenous trimethoprim-sulfamethoxazole, although many patients develop side effects. Corticosteroids should be given to those meeting oxygenation criteria.
- Immune reconstitution inflammatory syndrome can result in pneumonitis, meningitis, hepatitis, and pericarditis. Respiratory failure is most often from tuberculosis and PCP. The syndrome occurs after starting HAART and needs to be distinguished from acute opportunistic infections.
- Patients can develop fatal lactic acidosis as a result of antiretroviral medications. Treatment consists of drug discontinuation. Administration of riboflavin, thiamine, and l-carnitine might be helpful but is unproven.
- Coinfection with HIV and hepatitis C is increasingly common and can complicate ICU care.
- Administration of HAART in the ICU is challenging because of the multiple side effects and drug interactions, difficulty with administration of oral medications, and the possibility of inducing viral resistance; however, use of these medications may be beneficial in certain patients.

References

1. Morris A, Masur H, Huang L. Current issues in critical care of the human immunodeficiency virus-infected patient. *Crit Care Med.* 2006;34:42.
2. Wachter RM, Luce JM, Turner J, et al. Intensive care of patients with the acquired immunodeficiency syndrome. Outcome and changing patterns of utilization. *Am Rev Respir Dis.* 1986;134:891.
3. Wachter RM, Russi MB, Bloch DA, et al. *Pneumocystis carinii* pneumonia and respiratory failure in AIDS. Improved outcomes and increased use of intensive care units. *Am Rev Respir Dis.* 1991;143:251.
4. Wachter RM, Luce JM, Safrin S, et al. Cost and outcome of intensive care for patients with AIDS, *Pneumocystis carinii* pneumonia, and severe respiratory failure. *JAMA.* 1995;273:230.
5. Nickas G, Wachter RM. Outcomes of intensive care for patients with human immunodeficiency virus infection. *Arch Intern Med.* 2000;160:541.
6. Morris A, Creasman J, Turner J, et al. Intensive care of human immunodeficiency virus-infected patients during the era of highly active antiretroviral therapy. *Am J Respir Crit Care Med.* 2002;166:262.
7. Narasimhan M, Posner AJ, DePalo VA, et al. Intensive care in patients with HIV infection in the era of highly active antiretroviral therapy. *Chest.* 2004;125:1800.
8. Vincent B, Timsit JF, Auburtin M, et al. Characteristics and outcomes of HIV-infected patients in the ICU: impact of the highly active antiretroviral treatment era. *Intensive Care Med.* 2004;30:859.
9. Casalino E, Wolff M, Ravaud P, et al. Impact of HAART advent on admission patterns and survival in HIV-infected patients admitted to an intensive care unit. *AIDS.* 2004;18:1429.
10. Rosen MJ, Clayton K, Schneider RF, et al. Intensive care of patients with HIV infection: utilization, critical illnesses, and outcomes. Pulmonary Complications of HIV Infection Study Group. *Am J Respir Crit Care Med.* 1997;155:67.
11. Afessa B, Green B. Clinical course, prognostic factors, and outcome prediction for HIV patients in the ICU. The PIP (Pulmonary complications, ICU support, and Prognostic factors in hospitalized patients with HIV) study. *Chest.* 2000;118:138.
12. Khouli H, Afrasiabi A, Shibli M, et al. Outcome of critically ill human immunodeficiency virus-infected patients in the era of highly active antiretroviral therapy. *J Intensive Care Med.* 2005;20:327.
13. Nuesch R, Geigy N, Schaedler E, et al. Effect of highly active antiretroviral therapy on hospitalization characteristics of HIV-infected patients. *Eur J Clin Microbiol Infect Dis.* 2002;21:684.
14. Gill JK, Greene L, Miller R, et al. ICU admission in patients infected with the human immunodeficiency virus—a multicentre survey. *Anaesthesia.* 1999;54:727.
15. Lazard T, Retel O, Guidet B, et al. AIDS in a medical intensive care unit: immediate prognosis and long-term survival. *JAMA.* 1996;276:1240.
16. Casalino E, Mendoza-Sassi G, Wolff M, et al. Predictors of short- and long-term survival in HIV-infected patients admitted to the ICU. *Chest.* 1998;113:421.
17. Palacios R, Hidalgo A, Reina C, et al. Effect of antiretroviral therapy on admissions of HIV-infected patients to an intensive care unit. *HIV Med.* 2006;7:193.
18. Mocroft A, Brettle R, Kirk O, et al. Changes in the cause of death among HIV positive subjects across Europe: results from the EuroSIDA study. *AIDS.* 2002;16:1663.
19. Smit C, Geskus R, Walker S, et al. Effective therapy has altered the spectrum of cause-specific mortality following HIV seroconversion. *AIDS.* 2006;20:741.
20. Rosenberg AL, Seneff MG, Atiyeh L, et al. The importance of bacterial sepsis in intensive care unit patients with acquired immunodeficiency syndrome: implications for future care in the age of increasing antiretroviral resistance. *Crit Care Med.* 2001;29:548.
21. Morris A, Wachter RM, Luce J, et al. Improved survival with highly active antiretroviral therapy in HIV-infected patients with severe *Pneumocystis carinii* pneumonia. *AIDS.* 2003;17:73.
22. Miller RF, Allen E, Copas A, et al. Improved survival for HIV infected patients with severe *Pneumocystis jirovecii* pneumonia is independent of highly active antiretroviral therapy. *Thorax.* 2006;61:716.
23. Rivers E, Nguyen B, Havstad S, et al. Early goal-directed therapy in the treatment of severe sepsis and septic shock. *N Engl J Med.* 2001;345:1368.
24. Hsue PY, Waters DD. What a cardiologist needs to know about patients with human immunodeficiency virus infection. *Circulation.* 2005;112:3947.
25. Marik PE, Kiminyo K, Zaloga GP. Adrenal insufficiency in critically ill patients with human immunodeficiency virus. *Crit Care Med.* 2002;30:1267.
26. Bozzette SA, Sattler FR, Chiu J, et al. A controlled trial of early adjunctive treatment with corticosteroids for *Pneumocystis carinii* pneumonia in the acquired immunodeficiency syndrome. California Collaborative Treatment Group. *N Engl J Med.* 1990;323:1451.
27. el-Sadr W, Sidhu G, Diamond G, et al. High-dose corticosteroids as adjunct therapy in severe *Pneumocystis carinii* pneumonia. *AIDS Res.* 1986;2:349.
28. Bedos JP, Dumoulin JL, Gachot B, et al. *Pneumocystis carinii* pneumonia

requiring intensive care management: survival and prognostic study in 110 patients with human immunodeficiency virus. *Crit Care Med.* 1999;27:1109.
29. Antinori A, Maiuro G, Pallavicini F, et al. Prognostic factors of early fatal outcome and long-term survival in patients with *Pneumocystis carinii* pneumonia and acquired immunodeficiency syndrome. *Eur J Epidemiol.* 1993;9:183.
30. Forrest DM, Zala C, Djurdjev O, et al. Determinants of short- and long-term outcome in patients with respiratory failure caused by AIDS-related *Pneumocystis carinii* pneumonia. *Arch Intern Med.* 1999;159:741.
31. Phair J, Munoz A, Detels R, et al. The risk of *Pneumocystis carinii* pneumonia among men infected with human immunodeficiency virus type 1. Multicenter AIDS Cohort Study Group. *N Engl J Med.* 1990;322:161.
32. Stansell JD, Osmond DH, Charlebois E, et al. Predictors of *Pneumocystis carinii* pneumonia in HIV-infected persons. Pulmonary Complications of HIV Infection Study Group. *Am J Resp Crit Care Med.* 1997;155:60.
33. Saah AJ, Hoover DR, Peng Y, et al. Predictors for failure of *Pneumocystis carinii* pneumonia prophylaxis. Multicenter AIDS Cohort Study. *JAMA.* 1995;273:1197.
34. Kaplan JE, Hanson D, Dworkin MS, et al. Epidemiology of human immunodeficiency virus-associated opportunistic infections in the United States in the era of highly active antiretroviral therapy. *Clin Infect Dis.* 2000; 30(Suppl 1):S5.
35. Morris A, Lundgren JD, Masur H, et al. Current epidemiology of *Pneumocystis* pneumonia. *Emerg Infect Dis.* 2004;10:1713.
36. Morris A, Beard CB, Huang L. Update on the epidemiology and transmission of *Pneumocystis carinii. Microbes Infect.* 2002;4:95.
37. Dohn MN, White ML, Vigdorth EM, et al. Geographic clustering of *Pneumocystis carinii* pneumonia in patients with HIV infection. *Am J Resp Crit Care Med.* 2000;162:1617.
38. Morris AM, Swanson M, Ha H, et al. Geographic distribution of human immunodeficiency virus-associated *Pneumocystis carinii* pneumonia in San Francisco. *Am J Respir Crit Care Med.* 2000;162:1622.
39. Nieman RB, Fleming J, Coker RJ, et al. The effect of cigarette smoking on the development of AIDS in HIV-1-seropositive individuals. *AIDS.* 1993;7:705.
40. Miguez-Burbano MJ, Ashkin D, Rodriguez A, et al. Increased risk of *Pneumocystis carinii* and community-acquired pneumonia with tobacco use in HIV disease. *Int J Infect Dis.* 2005;9:208.
41. Kovacs JA, Hiemenz JW, Macher AM, et al. *Pneumocystis carinii* pneumonia: a comparison between patients with the acquired immunodeficiency syndrome and patients with other immunodeficiencies. *Ann Intern Med.* 1984;100:663.
42. Kales CP, Murren JR, Torres RA, et al. Early predictors of in-hospital mortality for *Pneumocystis carinii* pneumonia in the acquired immunodeficiency syndrome. *Arch Intern Med.* 1987;147:1413.
43. Zaman MK, White DA. Serum lactate dehydrogenase levels and *Pneumocystis carinii* pneumonia. Diagnostic and prognostic significance. *Am Rev Respir Dis.* 1988;137:796.
44. Garay SM, Greene J. Prognostic indicators in the initial presentation of *Pneumocystis carinii* pneumonia. *Chest.* 1989;95:769.
45. Nyamande K, Lalloo UG. Serum procalcitonin distinguishes CAP due to bacteria, *Mycobacterium tuberculosis* and PJP. *Int J Tuberc Lung Dis.* 2006;10:510.
46. Sandhu JS, Goodman PC. Pulmonary cysts associated with *Pneumocystis carinii* pneumonia in patients with AIDS. *Radiology.* 1989;173:33.
47. Kennedy CA, Goetz MB. Atypical roentgenographic manifestations of *Pneumocystis carinii* pneumonia. *Arch Intern Med.* 1992;152:1390.
48. Metersky ML, Aslenzadeh J, Stelmach P. A comparison of induced and expectorated sputum for the diagnosis of *Pneumocystis carinii* pneumonia. *Chest.* 1998;113:1555.
49. Bigby TD, Margolskee D, Curtis JL, et al. The usefulness of induced sputum in the diagnosis of *Pneumocystis carinii* pneumonia in patients with the acquired immunodeficiency syndrome. *Am Rev Respir Dis.* 1986;133:515.
50. Pitchenik AE, Ganjei P, Torres A, et al. Sputum examination for the diagnosis of *Pneumocystis carinii* pneumonia in the acquired immunodeficiency syndrome. *Am Rev Respir Dis.* 1986; 133:226.
51. Hopewell PC. *Pneumocystis carinii* pneumonia: diagnosis. *J Infect Dis.* 1988;157:1115.
52. Zaman MK, Wooten OJ, Suprahmanya B, et al. Rapid noninvasive diagnosis of *Pneumocystis carinii* from induced liquefied sputum. *Ann Intern Med.* 1988;109:7.
53. Ng VL, Gartner I, Weymouth LA, et al. The use of mucolysed induced sputum for the identification of pulmonary pathogens associated with human immunodeficiency virus infection. *Arch Pathol Lab Med.* 1989;113:488.
54. Golden JA, Hollander H, Stulbarg MS, et al. Bronchoalveolar lavage as the exclusive diagnostic modality for *Pneumocystis carinii* pneumonia. A prospective study among patients with acquired immunodeficiency syndrome. *Chest.* 1986;90:18.
55. Cadranel J, Gillet-Juvin K, Antoine M, et al. Site-directed bronchoalveolar lavage and transbronchial biopsy in HIV-infected patients with pneumonia. *Am J Respir Crit Care Med.* 1995;152:1103.
56. Kovacs JA, Ng VL, Masur H, et al. Diagnosis of *Pneumocystis carinii* pneumonia: improved detection in sputum with use of monoclonal antibodies. *N Engl J Med.* 1988;318:589.
57. Ng VL, Yajko DM, McPhaul LW, et al. Evaluation of an indirect fluorescent-antibody stain for detection of *Pneumocystis carinii* in respiratory specimens. *J Clin Microbiol.* 1990;28:975.
58. Pinlaor S, Mootsikapun P, Pinlaor P, et al. PCR diagnosis of *Pneumocystis carinii* on sputum and bronchoalveolar lavage samples in immunocompromised patients. *Parasitol Res.* 2004;94:213.
59. Larsen HH, Huang L, Kovacs JA, et al. A prospective, blinded study of quantitative touch-down polymerase chain reaction using oral-wash samples for diagnosis of *Pneumocystis* pneumonia in HIV-infected patients. *J Infect Dis.* 2004;189:1679.
60. Sattler FR, Cowan R, Nielsen DM, et al. Trimethoprim-sulfamethoxazole compared with pentamidine for treatment of *Pneumocystis carinii* pneumonia in the acquired immunodeficiency syndrome. A prospective, non-crossover study. *Ann Intern Med.* 1988;109:280.
61. Klein NC, Duncanson FP, Lenox TH, et al. Trimethoprim-sulfamethoxazole versus pentamidine for *Pneumocystis carinii* pneumonia in AIDS patients: results of a large prospective randomized treatment trial. *AIDS.* 1992;6:301.
62. Gordin FM, Simon GL, Wofsy CB, et al. Adverse reactions to trimethoprim-sulfamethoxazole in patients with the acquired immunodeficiency syndrome. *Ann Intern Med.* 1984;100:495.
63. Wofsy CB. Use of trimethoprim-sulfamethoxazole in the treatment of *Pneumocystis carinii* pneumonitis in patients with acquired immunodeficiency syndrome. *Rev Infect Dis.* 1987;9(Suppl 2):S184.
64. Hardy WD, Feinberg J, Finkelstein DM, et al. A controlled trial of trimethoprim-sulfamethoxazole or aerosolized pentamidine for secondary prophylaxis of *Pneumocystis carinii* pneumonia in patients with the acquired immunodeficiency syndrome. AIDS Clinical Trials Group Protocol 021. *N Engl J Med.* 1992;327:1842.
65. Masur H. Prevention and treatment of *Pneumocystis* pneumonia. *N Engl J Med.* 1992;327:1853.
66. Salmeron S, Petitpretz P, Katlama C, et al. Pentamidine and pancreatitis. *Ann Intern Med.* 1986;105:140.
67. Zuger A, Wolf BZ, el-Sadr W, et al. Pentamidine-associated fatal acute pancreatitis. *JAMA.* 1986;256:2383.
68. Gonzalez A, Sager PT, Akil B, et al. Pentamidine-induced torsade de pointes. *Am Heart J.* 1991;122:1489.
69. Quadrel MA, Atkin SH, Jaker MA. Delayed cardiotoxicity during treatment with intravenous pentamidine: two case reports and a review of the literature. *Am Heart J.* 1992;123:1377.
70. MacFadden DK, Edelson JD, Hyland RH, et al. Corticosteroids as adjunctive therapy in treatment of *Pneumocystis carinii* pneumonia in patients with acquired immunodeficiency syndrome. *Lancet.* 1987;1:1477.
71. Walmsley S, Salit IE, Brunton J. The possible role of corticosteroid therapy for *Pneumocystis* pneumonia in the acquired immune deficiency syndrome (AIDS). *J Acquir Immune Defic Syndr.* 1988;1:354.
72. Briel M, Boscacci R, Furrer H, et al. Adjunctive corticosteroids for *Pneumocystis jiroveci* pneumonia in patients with HIV infection: a meta-analysis of randomised controlled trials. *BMC Infect Dis.* 2005;5:101.
73. Briel M, Bucher HC, Boscacci R, et al. Adjunctive corticosteroids for *Pneumocystis jiroveci* pneumonia in patients with HIV-infection. *Cochrane Database Syst Rev.* 2006;3:6150.
74. Shelhamer JH, Ognibene FP, Macher AM, et al. Persistence of *Pneumocystis carinii* in lung tissue of acquired immunodeficiency syndrome patients treated for *Pneumocystis* pneumonia. *Am Rev Resp Dis.* 1984;130: 1161.
75. Lane BR, Ast JC, Hossler PA, et al. Dihydropteroate synthase polymorphisms in *Pneumocystis carinii. J Infect Dis.* 1997;175:482.
76. Ma L, Borio L, Masur H, et al. *Pneumocystis carinii* dihydropteroate synthase but not dihydrofolate reductase gene mutations correlate with prior trimethoprim-sulfamethoxazole or dapsone use. *J Infect Dis.* 1999;180: 1969.
77. Huang L, Crothers K, Atzori C, et al. Dihydropteroate synthase gene mutations in *Pneumocystis* and sulfa resistance. *Emerg Infect Dis.* 2004; 10:1721.
78. Helweg-Larsen J, Benfield TL, Eugen-Olsen J, et al. Effects of mutations in *Pneumocystis carinii* dihydropteroate synthase gene on outcome of AIDS-associated *P. carinii* pneumonia. *Lancet.* 1999;354:1347.
79. Kazanjian P, Armstrong W, Hossler PA, et al. *Pneumocystis carinii* mutations are associated with duration of sulfa or sulfone prophylaxis exposure in AIDS patients. *J Infect Dis.* 2000;182:551.
80. Takahashi T, Hosoya N, Endo T, et al. Relationship between mutations in dihydropteroate synthase of *Pneumocystis carinii* f. sp. *hominis* isolates in Japan and resistance to sulfonamide therapy. *J Clin Microbiol.* 2000; 38:3161.
81. Crothers K, Beard CB, Turner J, et al. Severity and outcome of HIV-associated *Pneumocystis* pneumonia containing *Pneumocystis jirovecii* dihydropteroate synthase gene mutations. *AIDS.* 2005;19:801.
82. Navin TR, Beard CB, Huang L, et al. Effect of mutations in *Pneumocystis carinii* dihydropteroate synthase gene on outcome of *P carinii* pneumonia in patients with HIV-1: a prospective study. *Lancet.* 2001; 358:545.
83. The Acute Respiratory Distress Syndrome Network. Ventilation with lower tidal volumes as compared with traditional tidal volumes for acute lung injury and the acute respiratory distress syndrome. *N Engl J Med.* 2000; 342:1301.

84. Confalonieri M, Calderini E, Terraciano S, et al. Noninvasive ventilation for treating acute respiratory failure in AIDS patients with *Pneumocystis carinii* pneumonia. *Intensive Care Med.* 2002;28:1233.
85. Kohli R, Lo Y, Homel P, et al. Bacterial pneumonia, HIV therapy, and disease progression among HIV-infected women in the HIV epidemiologic research (HER) study. *Clin Infect Dis.* 2006;43:90.
86. Alves C, Nicolas JM, Miro JM, et al. Reappraisal of the aetiology and prognostic factors of severe acute respiratory failure in HIV patients. *Eur Respir J.* 2001;17:87.
87. Puro V, Serraino D, Piselli P, et al. The epidemiology of recurrent bacterial pneumonia in people with AIDS in Europe. *Epidemiol Infect.* 2005; 133:237.
88. Franzetti F, Grassini A, Piazza M, et al. Nosocomial bacterial pneumonia in HIV-infected patients: risk factors for adverse outcome and implications for rational empiric antibiotic therapy. *Infection.* 2006;34:9.
89. Hirschtick RE, Glassroth J, Jordan MC, et al. Bacterial pneumonia in persons infected with the human immunodeficiency virus. Pulmonary Complications of HIV Infection Study Group. *N Engl J Med.* 1995;333:845.
90. Crothers K, Griffith TA, McGinnis KA, et al. The impact of cigarette smoking on mortality, quality of life, and comorbid illness among HIV-positive veterans. *J Gen Intern Med.* 2005;20:1142.
91. Le Moing V, Rabaud C, Journot V, et al. Incidence and risk factors of bacterial pneumonia requiring hospitalization in HIV-infected patients started on a protease inhibitor-containing regimen. *HIV Med.* 2006;7:261.
92. Cordero E, Pachon J, Rivero A, et al. Community-acquired bacterial pneumonia in human immunodeficiency virus-infected patients: validation of severity criteria. The Grupo Andaluz para el Estudio de las Enfermedades Infecciosas. *Am J Resp Crit Care Med.* 2000;162:2063.
93. Bedos JP, Chevret S, Chastang C, et al. Epidemiological features of and risk factors for infection by *Streptococcus pneumoniae* strains with diminished susceptibility to penicillin: findings of a French survey. *Clin Infect Dis.* 1996;22:63.
94. Meynard JL, Barbut F, Blum L, et al. Risk factors for isolation of *Streptococcus pneumoniae* with decreased susceptibility to penicillin G from patients infected with human immunodeficiency virus. *Clin Infect Dis.* 1996;22:437–440.
95. Madhi SA, Petersen K, Madhi A, et al. Increased disease burden and antibiotic resistance of bacteria causing severe community-acquired lower respiratory tract infections in human immunodeficiency virus type 1-infected children. *Clin Infect Dis.* 2000;31:170.
96. Shankar EM, Kumarasamy N, Balakrishnan P, et al. Detection of pulmonary *Mycoplasma pneumoniae* infections in HIV-infected subjects using culture and serology. *Int J Infect Dis.* 2007;11:232.
97. Afessa B, Green B. Bacterial pneumonia in hospitalized patients with HIV infection: the Pulmonary Complications, ICU Support, and Prognostic Factors of Hospitalized Patients with HIV (PIP) Study. *Chest.* 2000;117:1017.
98. Guidelines for the management of adults with community-acquired pneumonia. *Am J Resp Crit Care Med.* 2001;163:1730.
99. Mandell LA, Bartlett JG, Dowell SF, et al. Update of practice guidelines for the management of community-acquired pneumonia in immunocompetent adults. *Clin Infect Dis.* 2003;37:1405.
100. Guidelines for the management of adults with hospital-acquired, ventilator-associated, and healthcare-associated pneumonia. *Am J Resp Crit Care Med.* 2005;171:388.
101. Shelburne SA 3rd, Hamill RJ, Rodriguez-Barradas MC, et al. Immune reconstitution inflammatory syndrome: emergence of a unique syndrome during highly active antiretroviral therapy. *Medicine (Baltimore).* 2002;81:213.
102. Dworkin MS, Fratkin MD. *Mycobacterium avium* complex lymph node abscess after use of highly active antiretroviral therapy in a patient with AIDS. *Arch Intern Med.* 1998;158:1828.
103. Komanduri KV, Viswanathan MN, Wieder ED, et al. Restoration of cytomegalovirus-specific CD4+ T-lymphocyte responses after ganciclovir and highly active antiretroviral therapy in individuals infected with HIV-1. *Nat Med.* 1998;4:953.
104. Narita M, Ashkin D, Hollender ES, et al. Paradoxical worsening of tuberculosis following antiretroviral therapy in patients with AIDS. *Am J Resp Crit Care Med.* 1998;158:157.
105. Barry SM, Lipman MC, Deery AR, et al. Immune reconstitution pneumonitis following *Pneumocystis carinii* pneumonia in HIV-infected subjects. *HIV Med.* 2002;3:207.
106. Chien JW, Johnson JL. Paradoxical reactions in HIV and pulmonary TB. *Chest.* 1998;114:933.
107. Jenny-Avital ER, Abadi M. Immune reconstitution cryptococcosis after initiation of successful highly active antiretroviral therapy. *Clin Infect Dis.* 2002;35:e128.
108. Wislez M, Bergot E, Antoine M, et al. Acute respiratory failure following HAART introduction in patients treated for *Pneumocystis carinii* pneumonia. *Am J Respir Crit Care Med.* 2001;164:847.
109. Dean GL, Williams DI, Churchill DR, et al. Transient clinical deterioration in HIV patients with *Pneumocystis carinii* pneumonia after starting highly active antiretroviral therapy: another case of immune restoration inflammatory syndrome. *Am J Resp Crit Care Med.* 2002;165:1670.
110. Goldsack NR, Allen S, Lipman MC. Adult respiratory distress syndrome as a severe immune reconstitution disease following the commencement of highly active antiretroviral therapy. *Sex Transm Infect.* 2003;79:337.
111. Rosen MJ, Narasimhan M. Critical care of immunocompromised patients: human immunodeficiency virus. *Crit Care Med.* 2006;34:S245.
112. Palella FJ, Jr., Baker RK, Moorman AC, et al. Mortality in the highly active antiretroviral therapy era: changing causes of death and disease in the HIV outpatient study. *J Acquir Immune Defic Syndr.* 2006;43:27.
113. Dellinger RP, Carlet JM, Masur H, et al. Surviving Sepsis Campaign guidelines for management of severe sepsis and septic shock. *Crit Care Med.* 2004;32:858.
114. Bedos JP, Chastang C, Lucet JC, et al. Early predictors of outcome for HIV patients with neurological failure. *JAMA.* 1995;273:35.
115. Subsai K, Kanoksri S, Siwaporn C, et al. Neurological complications in AIDS patients receiving HAART: a 2-year retrospective study. *Eur J Neurol.* 2006;13:233.
116. Chalasani N, Wilcox CM. Gastrointestinal hemorrhage in patients with AIDS. *AIDS Patient Care STDS.* 1999;13:343.
117. Lew E, Dieterich D, Poles M, et al. Gastrointestinal emergencies in the patient with AIDS. *Crit Care Clin.* 1995;11:531.
118. Betz ME, Gebo KA, Barber E, et al. Patterns of diagnoses in hospital admissions in a multistate cohort of HIV-positive adults in 2001. *Med Care.* 2005;43:III3.
119. Bica I, McGovern B, Dhar R, et al. Increasing mortality due to end-stage liver disease in patients with human immunodeficiency virus infection. *Clin Infect Dis.* 2001;32:492.
120. Monga HK, Rodriguez-Barradas MC, Breaux K, et al. Hepatitis C virus infection-related morbidity and mortality among patients with human immunodeficiency virus infection. *Clin Infect Dis.* 2001;33:240.
121. Sulkowski MS, Thomas DL. Hepatitis C in the HIV-infected patient. *Clin Liver Dis.* 2003;7:179.
122. Greub G, Ledergerber B, Battegay M, et al. Clinical progression, survival, and immune recovery during antiretroviral therapy in patients with HIV-1 and hepatitis C virus coinfection: the Swiss HIV Cohort Study. *Lancet.* 2000;356:1800.
123. Sansone GR, Frengley JD. Impact of HAART on causes of death of persons with late-stage AIDS. *J Urban Health.* 2000;77:166.
124. Dodig M, Tavill AS. Hepatitis C and human immunodeficiency virus coinfections. *J Clin Gastroenterol.* 2001;33:367.
125. Wyatt CM, Arons RR, Klotman PE, et al. Acute renal failure in hospitalized patients with HIV: risk factors and impact on in-hospital mortality. *AIDS.* 2006;20:561.
126. Wilcox CM. Serious gastrointestinal disorders associated with human immunodeficiency virus infection. *Crit Care Clin.* 1993;9:73.
127. Sackoff JE, Hanna DB, Pfeiffer MR, et al. Causes of death among persons with AIDS in the era of highly active antiretroviral therapy: New York City. *Ann Intern Med.* 2006;145:397.
128. Grunfeld C, Kotler DP, Hamadeh R, et al. Hypertriglyceridemia in the acquired immunodeficiency syndrome. *Am J Med.* 1989;86:27.
129. Hommes MJ, Romijn JA, Endert E, et al. Insulin sensitivity and insulin clearance in human immunodeficiency virus-infected men. *Metabolism.* 1991;40:651.
130. Carr A, Samaras K, Burton S, et al. A syndrome of peripheral lipodystrophy, hyperlipidaemia and insulin resistance in patients receiving HIV protease inhibitors. *AIDS.* 1998;12:F51.
131. Friis-Moller N, Sabin CA, Weber R, et al. Combination antiretroviral therapy and the risk of myocardial infarction. *N Engl J Med.* 2003;349:1993.
132. de Gaetano Donati K, Rabagliati R, Iacoviello L, et al. HIV infection, HAART, and endothelial adhesion molecules: current perspectives. *Lancet Infect Dis.* 2004;4:213.
133. Bozzette SA, Ake CF, Tam HK, et al. Cardiovascular and cerebrovascular events in patients treated for human immunodeficiency virus infection. *N Engl J Med.* 2003;348:702.
134. Holmberg SD, Moorman AC, Williamson JM, et al. Protease inhibitors and cardiovascular outcomes in patients with HIV-1. *Lancet.* 2002;360:1747.
135. Friis-Moller N, Weber R, Reiss P, et al. Cardiovascular disease risk factors in HIV patients–association with antiretroviral therapy. Results from the DAD study. *AIDS.* 2003;17:1179.
136. Trachiotis GD, Alexander EP, Benator D, et al. Cardiac surgery in patients infected with the human immunodeficiency virus. *Ann Thorac Surg.* 2003;76:1114.
137. Gupta SK, Eustace JA, Winston JA, et al. Guidelines for the management of chronic kidney disease in HIV-infected patients: recommendations of the HIV Medicine Association of the Infectious Diseases Society of America. *Clin Infect Dis.* 2005;40:1559.
138. Agarwal A, Soni A, Ciechanowsky M, et al. Hyponatremia in patients with the acquired immunodeficiency syndrome. *Nephron.* 1989;53:317.
139. Cusano AJ, Thies HL, Siegal FP, et al. Hyponatremia in patients with acquired immune deficiency syndrome. *J Acquir Immune Defic Syndr.* 1990; 3:949.
140. Vitting KE, Gardenswartz MH, Zabetakis PM, et al. Frequency of hyponatremia and nonosmolar vasopressin release in the acquired immunodeficiency syndrome. *JAMA.* 1990;263:973.
141. Guarda LA, Luna MA, Smith JL Jr, et al. Acquired immune deficiency syndrome: postmortem findings. *Am J Clin Pathol.* 1984;81:549.
142. Klatt EC, Shibata D. Cytomegalovirus infection in the acquired immunodeficiency syndrome. Clinical and autopsy findings. *Arch Pathol Lab Med.* 1988;112:540.

143. Grinspoon SK, Bilezikian JP. HIV disease and the endocrine system. *N Engl J Med.* 1992;327:1360.
144. Chattha G, Arieff AI, Cummings C, et al. Lactic acidosis complicating the acquired immunodeficiency syndrome. *Ann Intern Med.* 1993;118:37.
145. Freiman JP, Helfert KE, Hamrell MR, et al. Hepatomegaly with severe steatosis in HIV-seropositive patients. *AIDS.* 1993;7:379.
146. Lonergan JT, Behling C, Pfander H, et al. Hyperlactatemia and hepatic abnormalities in 10 human immunodeficiency virus-infected patients receiving nucleoside analogue combination regimens. *Clin Infect Dis.* 2000;31:162.
147. Bonnet F, Bonarek M, Morlat P, et al. Risk factors for lactic acidosis in HIV-infected patients treated with nucleoside reverse-transcriptase inhibitors: a case-control study. *Clin Infect Dis.* 2003;36:1324.
148. Fouty B, Frerman F, Reves R. Riboflavin to treat nucleoside analogue-induced lactic acidosis. *Lancet.* 1998;352:291.
149. Luzatti R, Del Bravo P, DiPerri G, et al. Riboflavine and severe lactic acidosis. *Lancet.* 1999;353:901.
150. Brinkman K, Vrouenraets S, Kauffmann R, et al. Treatment of nucleoside reverse transcriptase inhibitor-induced lactic acidosis. *AIDS.* 2000;14:2801.
151. Claessens YE, Cariou A, Monchi M, et al. Detecting life-threatening lactic acidosis related to nucleoside-analog treatment of human immunodeficiency virus-infected patients, and treatment with L-carnitine. *Crit Care Med.* 2003;31:1042.
152. Miller RF, Hingorami AD, Foley NM. Pyrexia of undetermined origin in patients with human immunodeficiency virus infection and AIDS. *Int J STD AIDS.* 1996;7:170.
153. Armstrong WS, Katz JT, Kazanjian PH. Human immunodeficiency virus-associated fever of unknown origin: a study of 70 patients in the United States and review. *Clin Infect Dis.* 1999;28:341.
154. Lambertucci JR, Rayes AA, Nunes F, et al. Fever of undetermined origin in patients with the acquired immunodeficiency syndrome in Brazil: report on 55 cases. *Rev Inst Med Trop Sao Paulo.* 1999;41:27.
155. Barbado FJ, Gomez-Cerezo J, Pena JM, et al. Fever of unknown origin: classic and associated with human immunodeficiency virus infection. a comparative study. *J Med.* 2001;32:152.
156. Lozano F, Torre-Cisneros J, Santos J, et al. Impact of highly active antiretroviral therapy on fever of unknown origin in HIV-infected patients. *Eur J Clin Microbiol Infect Dis.* 2002;21:137.
157. Huang L, Quartin A, Jones D, et al. Intensive care of patients with HIV infection. *N Engl J Med.* 2006;355:173.
158. Heyland DK, Tougas G, King D, et al. Impaired gastric emptying in mechanically ventilated, critically ill patients. *Intensive Care Med.* 1996;22:1339.
159. Tarling MM, Toner CC, Withington PS, et al. A model of gastric emptying using paracetamol absorption in intensive care patients. *Intens Care Med.* 1997;23:256.
160. Mimoz O, Binter V, Jacolot A, et al. Pharmacokinetics and absolute bioavailability of ciprofloxacin administered through a nasogastric tube with continuous enteral feeding to critically ill patients. *Intensive Care Med.* 1998;24:1047.
161. Department of Health and Human Services. Guidelines for the use of antiretroviral agents in HIV-1-infected adults and adolescents. http://AIDSinfo.nih.gov. October 6, 2005.
162. Dorffler-Melly J, de Jonge E, Pont AC, et al. Bioavailability of subcutaneous low-molecular-weight heparin to patients on vasopressors. *Lancet.* 2002;359:849.
163. Priglinger U, Delle Karth G, Geppert A, et al. Prophylactic anticoagulation with enoxaparin: is the subcutaneous route appropriate in the critically ill? *Crit Care Med.* 2003;31:1405.
164. Townsend PL, Fink MP, Stein KL, et al. Aminoglycoside pharmacokinetics: dosage requirements and nephrotoxicity in trauma patients. *Crit Care Med.* 1989;17:154.
165. Aberg JA, Gallant JE, Anderson J, et al. Primary care guidelines for the management of persons infected with human immunodeficiency virus: recommendations of the HIV Medicine Association of the Infectious Diseases Society of America. *Clin Infect Dis.* 2004;39:609.
166. Lin RY, Astiz ME, Saxon JC, et al. Altered leukocyte immunophenotypes in septic shock. Studies of HLA-DR, CD11b, CD14, and IL-2R expression. *Chest.* 1993;104:847.
167. Feeney C, Bryzman S, Kong L, et al. T-lymphocyte subsets in acute illness. *Crit Care Med.* 1995;23:1680.
168. Lebedev MJ, Ptitsina JS, Vilkov SA, et al. Membrane and soluble forms of Fas (CD95) in peripheral blood lymphocytes and in serum from burns patients. *Burns.* 2001;27:669.
169. Bell DM. Occupational risk of human immunodeficiency virus infection in healthcare workers: an overview. *Am J Med.* 1997;102:9.
170. Panlilio AL, Cardo DM, Grohskopf LA, et al. Updated U.S. Public Health Service guidelines for the management of occupational exposures to HIV and recommendations for postexposure prophylaxis. *MMWR Recomm Rep.* 2005;54:1.
171. Garner JS. Guideline for isolation precautions in hospitals. The Hospital Infection Control Practices Advisory Committee. *Infect Control Hosp Epidemiol.* 1996;17:53.
172. Calfee DP. Prevention and management of occupational exposures to human immunodeficiency virus (HIV). *Mt Sinai J Med.* 2006;73:852.
173. Updated U.S. Public Health Service Guidelines for the Management of Occupational Exposures to HBV, HCV, and HIV and Recommendations for Postexposure Prophylaxis. *MMWR Recomm Rep.* 2001;50:1.
174. Cardo DM, Culver DH, Ciesielski CA, et al. A case-control study of HIV seroconversion in health care workers after percutaneous exposure. Centers for Disease Control and Prevention Needlestick Surveillance Group. *N Engl J Med.* 1997;337:1485.
175. Rebmann T. Management of patients infected with airborne-spread diseases: an algorithm for infection control professionals. *Am J Infect Control.* 2005;33:571.

CHAPTER 117 ■ UNUSUAL INFECTIONS

SANKAR SWAMINATHAN

This chapter describes the epidemiology, clinical presentation, diagnosis, therapy, and prevention of several relatively unusual infections. Although the incidence of these infections in the United States is low, they have the potential to cause rapidly progressive disease and, in some cases, present unique problems in management and infection control in the critical care setting. Since rapid treatment is critical in many of these infections, prompt diagnosis is likewise essential. Many of the organisms causing these infectious diseases have also gained new relevance as potential biologic warfare agents. The epidemiology, clinical presentation, and management of infections resulting from an intentional release of micro-organisms may differ significantly from disease resulting from traditional modes of spread. In addition to an intentional bioterrorist attack, large social disruptions that affect housing, public hygiene, and mass migration have the potential to allow epidemic transmission of some of these agents. Outbreaks of diseases previously thought to be under control have occurred as a result of natural disasters and human activities, both in the United States and abroad. Finally, globalization, leading to increasing travel of humans, and transport of animals and plant materials all increase the likelihood that, hitherto, unusual infections will become more prevalent in the United States. Recognition of such unusual infections will require familiarity with their epidemiology and clinical presentation and will allow diagnosis and treatment in a timely fashion.

TULAREMIA

Tularemia is a multisystem zoonotic infection caused by a Gram-negative coccobacillus, *Francisella tularensis*. Tularemia, named after Tulare County, California, where the disease was first characterized in ground squirrels (1), has been recognized since the 1800s and is primarily transmitted through contact with infected animals, contaminated food and water, or arthropod bites (2). Tularemia has been listed as a category A bioterrorism agent (3), defined as follows:

High-priority agents include organisms that pose a risk to national security because they

- can be easily disseminated or transmitted from person to person
- result in high mortality rates and have the potential for major public health impact
- might cause public panic and social disruption; and require special action for public health preparedness.

Epidemiology

The incidence of tularemia in the United States has declined since the 1950s and is currently less than 200 per year (4,5). Most cases in the United States occur in the western and southwestern states in small sporadic clusters. Tularemia primarily occurs during the summer months, most likely due to the increased exposure to biting arthropods. Cases also occur during the fall and winter and are linked to hunting and handling infected animals. Perhaps because of a greater likelihood of exposure to animals and arthropods, there is a 3-to-1 preponderance of male-to-female cases. The most recent cases in the United States have been young adults, although a significant percentage of cases occurs among children younger than the age of 14 years (6). Inhalational exposures have occurred in Martha's Vineyard in Massachusetts and were associated with mowing grass and cutting brush (7).

In the United States, ticks and biting flies are the most important arthropod vectors. Major animal reservoirs are lagomorphs (rabbits and hares), as well as rodents including prairie dogs, squirrels, and rats. Mosquitoes were implicated as a primary vector in Scandinavia in one large outbreak (8). Direct contact with infected animals is another significant mode of transmission (9). Hunting, trapping, butchering animal carcasses, and handling meat are all risk factors for tularemia. Contamination of food and water by rodents and other carriers has also been linked to human infection. The organism survives well in cold, moist conditions and can withstand freezing. Finally, cats and other carnivores may transiently carry organisms in their mouths or claws and can thereby transmit infection to humans (10). Pets may also increase the likelihood of tick-borne transmission to humans.

Inhalational exposure may occur in the laboratory or as the consequence of a deliberate release of weaponized *Francisella* cultures. Human-to-human transmission of tularemia is not known to occur.

Clinical Presentation

Tularemia has been classically described as presenting in one of six syndromes: ulceroglandular, oculoglandular, glandular, pharyngeal, typhoidal, and pneumonic (11). However, it is clear that individual patients may have symptoms of several of these types simultaneously. After initial entry into the host—either through cutaneous inoculation, ingestion, or inhalation—*Francisella* organisms multiply at the site of infection (11). A vigorous inflammatory response ensues, leading to subsequent necrosis. The organism multiplies within macrophages and travels to regional lymph nodes, kidney, liver, lung, and spleen (12). The meninges and pericardium are occasionally involved secondarily in untreated tularemia. Inhalation or cutaneous inoculation of 10 to 50 organisms is sufficient for infection (13,14). Symptoms usually begin 3 to 5 days after infection, although longer incubation periods are possible (15).

Differences in clinical presentation may be partly attributable to the type and route of infection. Thus tick-borne infection is more likely to result in skin lesions on the head and neck, trunk, and perineum, whereas animal-associated infections more commonly result in upper extremity lesions (16). Ingestion of contaminated water or food is more likely to cause pharyngeal infection. Inoculation into mucous membranes of the eye results in the oculoglandular syndrome, an ocular lesion with local lymphadenopathy. Inhalation of the organism leads to the pneumonic form of tularemia, although other forms of tularemia can also cause prominent pulmonary involvement through hematogenous dissemination. A typhoidal form of tularemia occurs in less than 30% of cases, in which there are no characteristic localized mucocutaneous or glandular signs or symptoms. The distinction between typhoidal and nontyphoidal infections appears to reflect differences in the host response. In nontyphoidal forms, there is a vigorous inflammatory reaction, and the prognosis is good compared to typhoidal infection, which has a higher mortality and in which pneumonia is more common (16).

In general, the onset of systemic symptoms in tularemia is abrupt and includes fever, headache, myalgia, coryza, cough, malaise, and chest pain or tightness. In mucocutaneous infection, the presenting complaint is usually painful lymphadenopathy, which may precede or follow the skin lesion. In the purely glandular form, there is no apparent skin lesion. Skin lesions usually begin as erythematous painful papules, which progress to necrotic ulcers that are slow to heal. Enlarged lymph nodes are also slow to resolve and may suppurate. In ocular infection, a painful conjunctivitis occurs. Pharyngeal tularemia presents as an exudative pharyngitis with adenopathy that is unresponsive to standard therapy. Tularemic pneumonia is characterized by fever, cough, and pleuritic pain, but sputum production and hemoptysis are unusual. A relative bradycardia, with a normal pulse despite an elevated temperature, is common (40%) in tularemia and may be a useful diagnostic finding (16). Chest radiographic findings include hilar adenopathy, patchy or less commonly lobar infiltrates, and pleural effusions.

Although there has not been a documented biologic attack with weaponized tularemia organisms, several probable aspects of such a scenario are worth noting to allow early recognition and management. If an aerosolized release of organisms were to occur, cases are likely to be pneumonic, although aerosolized tularemia would also likely result in ocular and cutaneous forms (2). Occurrence of tularemia in urban settings and among healthy individuals should also prompt suspicion of a biologic attack. Onset of symptoms is expected to be rapid and, as described above, closely resemble the acute onset of influenza. The differential diagnosis of pneumonia due to an aerosolized biologic weapon attack would include anthrax, plague, and Q fever. Important distinguishing characteristics between these causes would include a more rapid and fulminant course in both anthrax and plague. In addition, pneumonic anthrax would not be expected to cause bronchopneumonia but would result in mediastinal widening. Pneumonic plague results in frankly purulent sputum with hemoptysis and rapid progression. Laboratory testing is important in distinguishing between these various entities (see below), but initial empiric treatment will, by necessity, require diagnosis based primarily on clinical and epidemiologic data.

Diagnosis

Cultures for *Francisella tularensis* require incubation on special supportive media. The laboratory must be notified in advance if tularemia is suspected, both to perform appropriate testing and to institute protective measures to prevent infection of laboratory workers. Cultures of pharyngeal washings, sputum, and fasting gastric aspirates are most likely to yield positive results, whereas blood samples are usually negative (17). Direct fluorescent staining of specimens can be performed by specialized laboratories for a relatively rapid diagnosis. Serology is positive approximately 10 days after infection. Although serology is not helpful for diagnosing acute infection, it is useful for confirmation of suspected cases. It is important to promptly contact the hospital epidemiologist or infection-control practitioner and the local health department in cases of tularemia to aid in management and diagnosis of suspected outbreaks.

Treatment

Treatment regimens for most of the select agents have been devised for either a contained casualty setting or a mass casualty setting (Table 117.1). The recommendations for the latter situation take into account the likelihood that services may be limited and parenteral or inpatient therapy may not be possible. The first-line treatment of tularemia in a contained casualty setting is an aminoglycoside, either streptomycin or gentamicin (2). Alternatives are doxycycline, chloramphenicol, or ciprofloxacin given intravenously. Treatment with aminoglycosides or ciprofloxacin should be given for a minimum of 10 days, and treatment with doxycycline or chloramphenicol for 14 to 21 days. In a mass casualty setting or for postexposure prophylaxis, oral doxycycline or ciprofloxacin for 14 days is recommended. As is the case with other organisms described later in this chapter, several potentially toxic antibiotics that are not routinely given to children or pregnant women are included in the recommended treatment regimens. For example, the use of tetracyclines and quinolones carries the risk of potential side effects in pregnant women and children. Nevertheless, given the high mortality of tularemia, these agents are recommended as acceptable alternatives if aminoglycosides cannot be administered or are not available. The Centers for Disease Control and Prevention (CDC) Web site should be consulted for the most current details regarding the CDC recommendations for treatment as well as more detailed information regarding usage in renal failure and in special situations (18).

PLAGUE

Plague, caused by the Gram-negative bacillus *Yersinia pestis*, is one of the oldest and most feared illnesses known to man. Millions of people were killed by three pandemics occurring in AD 540, the Middle Ages, and in the late 19th century (19,20). Plague has been developed by various groups and nations as a biologic weapon since the 1950s and has been listed as an important potential agent of bioterrorism (3).

Epidemiology

Plague is primarily a rural disease that occurs in all continents except Australia (19). Although most common in rural settings in developing nations, sporadic clusters occur regularly in the United States. For example, 107 cases were reported in the United States between 1990 and 2005, with a median number of seven cases per year (6). However, in 2006, 13 cases were reported in the first 10 months of the year (6). Most cases occur between spring and autumn in the Western states where the disease is enzootic in wild rodents. Humans are infected via bites from infected rodent fleas or by handling infected animals, either domestic pets or wild animals. Worldwide, the most important reservoir is the domestic rat, but as in the United States, sylvatic foci (in wild animals) also exist (21). Human-to-human transmission can occur in pneumonic plague but requires close contact. The last known case acquired in this manner in the United States was reported in 1925 (22).

Clinical Manifestations

The three main types of plague are bubonic, septicemic, and pneumonic. Although there is no current experience with pneumonic plague acquired from a biologic attack, the clinical presentation is expected to differ from that of natural infection and is discussed below.

Bubonic Plague

Bubonic plague is the most common type of plague, occurring in 76% of the cases reported in the United States between 1990 and 2005 (6). Large numbers of bacteria are inoculated at the site of the flea bite and multiply locally, followed by rapid replication in nearby lymph nodes (21). The incubation period is between 2 and 7 days. There is abrupt onset of fever, chills, and headache. The characteristic bubo typically develops as a smooth, firm oval mass which is extremely tender. The overlying skin is warm and erythematous, but suppuration is rare. The primary lesion is often inapparent but can develop into an ulcer. The most common site of the buboes is in the femoral lymph nodes, but they are also seen in inguinal, cervical, and axillary locations depending on the location of the inoculation. Bacteremia occurs in about 25% of case, and in untreated cases, the mortality is approximately 50% (6,21). In untreated cases,

TABLE 117.1

TREATMENT RECOMMENDATIONS FOR TULAREMIA

Contained casualty setting	
Adults	*Preferred choices:* Streptomycin, 1 g IM twice daily Gentamicin, 5 mg/kg IM or IV once daily *Alternative choices:* Doxycycline, 100 mg IV twice daily Chloramphenicol, 15 mg/kg IV 4 times daily Ciprofloxacin, 400 mg IV twice daily
Children	*Preferred choices:* Streptomycin, 15 mg/kg IM twice daily (not to exceed 2 g/d) Gentamicin, 2.5 mg/kg IM or IV 3 times daily *Alternative choices:* Doxycycline If weight 45 kg or more, 100 mg IV twice daily If weight less than 45 kg, 2.2 mg/kg IV twice daily Chloramphenicol, 15 mg/kg IV 4 times daily Ciprofloxacin, 15 mg/kg IV twice daily
Pregnant women	Same as adults above except chloramphenicol is not recommended.
Mass casualty setting	
Adults, including pregnant women	*Preferred choices:* Doxycycline, 100 mg orally twice daily Ciprofloxacin, 500 mg orally twice daily
Children	*Preferred choices:* Doxycycline If 45 kg or more, 100 mg orally twice daily If less than 45 kg, 2.2 mg/kg orally twice daily Ciprofloxacin, 15 mg/kg orally twice daily[a]

For full details and most current treatment recommendations, the reader is referred to the CDC Web site: Centers for Disease Control and Prevention. Consensus statement: tularemia as a biological weapon: medical and public health management. http://www.bt.cdc.gov/agent/tularemia/tularemia-biological-weapon-abstract.asp#4. Accessed February 6, 2007.

[a]Ciprofloxacin dosage should not exceed 1 g/d in children.

deterioration is usually rapid, with progression of typical signs of shock and death occurring as early as 2 to 3 days.

Septicemic Plague

Septicemic plague is defined as plague in the absence of an apparent bubo. As with other systemic infections without clear localization, diagnosis of septicemic plague is often delayed, and the prognosis is thus poorer. In the United States from 1990 to 2005, 18% of reported plague cases were defined as septicemic, although 38% of the cases in 2006 were of this variety (6). A useful clue to the diagnosis of septicemic plague is that gastrointestinal symptoms of nausea and vomiting, diarrhea, and abdominal pain were prominent in several recent cases (6). Disseminated intravascular coagulation may develop rapidly with cutaneous and visceral hemorrhage. Rapidly progressive gangrene may also develop in this setting. Both septicemic plague and pneumonic plague are fatal if untreated. Even with treatment, mortality rates of 33% in septicemic plague were reported from New Mexico in the 1980s (23).

Pneumonic Plague

Pneumonic plague may develop secondary to either bubonic or septicemic plague. The incidence of secondary pulmonary involvement is approximately 12% (19). Recent cases of primary pneumonic plague in the United States have occurred either from laboratory accidents or from exposure to cats (24). Pneumonic plague is similar to other acute pneumonia, with abrupt onset of fever and dyspnea. Watery or purulent, and bloody sputum is produced and is highly infectious. Transmission is via respiratory droplets, and therefore simple respiratory isolation with droplet precautions is sufficient. The chest radiograph usually reveals bronchopneumonia and multilobar consolidation, or cavitation may be seen (25).

Clues to plague arising as the result of a biologic attack include cases outside areas of known enzootic infection; occurrences in an area without associated rodent die-offs, and numerous cases of pneumonia in otherwise healthy patients (25). In general, routine laboratory tests are not markedly different from those seen in other causes of fulminant pneumonia and sepsis. The white blood cell count is often markedly elevated, and fibrin degradation products are detectable in cases where disseminated intravascular coagulation is present (26).

Diagnosis

Specialized laboratory tests to definitively and rapidly identify *Y. pestis* are not widely available. When plague is suspected, coordination with state public health officials and the Centers for Disease Control and Prevention will allow more specialized tests and susceptibility testing to be performed. Blood, sputum, lymph node aspirates, and lesion swabs should be examined by Gram or Wright-Giemsa stain for the presence of bipolar-staining Gram-negative bacilli, which have the appearance of safety pins. The laboratory should be alerted to the possibility of plague so that appropriate biosafety procedures can be followed.

Treatment

The recommendations for therapy of plague provided here are derived from the recommendations of the Working Group on Civilian Biodefense and the CDC (25). Treatment recommendations for plague are complicated by the lack of clinical efficacy trials, lack of experience with widespread pneumonic plague, and potentially unpredictable clinical responses in infections due to a biologic attack. Although some recommendations are not FDA-approved uses of the antibiotics, they are the consensus recommendations for the best alternatives for therapy in various situations and clinical scenarios.

The historically proven, effective antibiotic therapy for plague has been streptomycin. Because of the limited availability of streptomycin, gentamicin—used successfully to treat plague—is the recommended alternative. Both tetracycline and doxycycline are effective against plague and are also recommended. For pregnant women and children, the use of tetracyclines and quinolones carry the risk of potential side effects. Nevertheless, given the high mortality of plague, these agents are recommended as acceptable alternatives if aminoglycosides cannot be administered or are not available. In the setting of a mass casualty, oral regimens are recommended, as these allow treatment of large numbers of people and are also useful in settings where parenteral therapy may not be possible.

The recommended duration of therapy for plague (Table 117.2) is 10 days, and oral therapy should be substituted when the patient's condition improves. Duration of postexposure prophylaxis to prevent plague infection is 7 days. For full details regarding usage in pregnant women and children as well as in special settings including renal failure, please consult the CDC Web site where the most current recommendations may be found (27).

ANTHRAX

Anthrax was an extremely rare disease in the United States until the bioterrorism attacks of 2001. The disease is caused by a Gram-positive, spore-forming bacillus, *Bacillus anthracis*. However, anthrax was tested as a biologic weapon by the United States in the 1960s and by several other countries until at least the 1970s. The technology to produce highly infectious anthrax spores and disseminate them widely as an aerosol exists and is known to have been developed for use as a biologic warfare agent (28). It is therefore important for all physicians to be aware of the manifestations of anthrax and especially of the expected characteristics of an outbreak due to a biologic attack.

Epidemiology

There are three major modes of infection with anthrax: inhalational, cutaneous, and gastrointestinal. *Cutaneous anthrax* is the most common type of anthrax. However, it is still extremely rare in the United States, with 224 cases having been reported in the 50 years from 1944 to 1994 (29). Barring exposure to intentionally produced anthrax, *inhalational anthrax* is even less common and occurs primarily in those with occupational or laboratory exposure. Prior to 2001, there were only 18 cases of inhalational anthrax reported from 1900 to 1978 (30). *Gastrointestinal anthrax* is most commonly reported where improperly cooked meat contaminated with large numbers of anthrax bacilli has been consumed (31).

Clinical Manifestations

The presentation of anthrax due to a biologic attack is still incompletely characterized. Most of the information relevant to inhalational anthrax from anthrax manufactured as a biologic weapon is from the 2001 U.S. attacks and an unintentional release in Sverdlosk, Russia, in 1979 (32). There were 11 cases of inhalational anthrax resulting from the exposures in 2001. Several aspects of the pathophysiology of inhalational anthrax are highly relevant to the clinician. Infection occurs after spores are inhaled and deposited in the alveoli. The spores are phagocytosed by macrophages and transported to regional lymph nodes where they germinate and replicate vegetatively (33). There may be a period of extended latency in the lymph node because of spores that remain dormant. Therefore, although the usual period of incubation is 2 to 6 days, cases have occurred as late as 6 weeks after exposure to aerosolized anthrax (32). When replication does occur, toxin production leads to edema, necrosis, and hemorrhage.

Typical symptoms are fever and chills, chest discomfort and dyspnea, severe fatigue, and vomiting. Two stages may occur, with an initial period of improvement followed by rapid deterioration. The initial finding on chest radiograph is a widened mediastinum due to mediastinal lymph node involvement (34). A hemorrhagic mediastinal lymphadenitis ensues, often accompanied by bloody pleural effusions. Eight of 11 patients in 2001 developed bloody pleural effusions, and 10 of 11 had radiologic evidence of mediastinal adenopathy (35). Although anthrax does not cause a typical bronchopneumonia, pulmonary infiltrates or consolidation were observed in 8 of 11 cases. In addition, in an autopsy series from the Sverdlosk outbreak, primary focal hemorrhagic necrotizing pneumonia was described in 11 of 42 cases (36).

An important point emphasized by Lucey is that while there are three known modes of exposure—inhalational, cutaneous, and gastrointestinal—anthrax may actually present as meningitis, which was the initial presentation of the index case in 2001

TABLE 117.2

RECOMMENDATIONS FOR TREATMENT OF PATIENTS WITH PNEUMONIC PLAGUE IN CONTAINED AND MASS CASUALTY SETTINGS AND FOR POSTEXPOSURE PROPHYLAXIS

	CONTAINED CASUALTY SETTING
Adults	*Preferred choices:* Streptomycin, 1 g IM twice daily Gentamicin, 5 mg/kg IM or IV once daily or 2 mg/kg loading dose followed by 1.7 mg/kg IM or IV three times daily *Alternative choices:* Doxycycline, 100 mg IV twice daily or 200 mg IV once daily Ciprofloxacin, 400 mg IV twice daily Chloramphenicol, 25 mg/kg IV 4 times daily
Children	*Preferred choices:* Streptomycin, 15 mg/kg IM twice daily (maximum daily dose, 2 g) Gentamicin, 2.5 mg/kg IM or IV 3 times daily[†] *Alternative choices:* Doxycycline If 45 kg or more, give adult dosage If less than 45 kg, give 2.2 mg/kg IV twice daily (maximum, 200 mg/d) Ciprofloxacin, 15 mg/kg IV twice daily Chloramphenicol, 25 mg/kg IV 4 times daily In children, ciprofloxacin dose should not exceed 1 g/d, and chloramphenicol should not exceed 4 g/d. Children younger than 2 y should not receive chloramphenicol.
Pregnant Women	Same as adults above except chloramphenicol is not recommended.
	MASS CASUALTY SETTING AND POSTEXPOSURE PROPHYLAXIS
Adults, including pregnant women	*Preferred choices:* Doxycycline, 100 mg orally twice daily Ciprofloxacin, 500 mg orally twice daily Alternative choice: Chloramphenicol, 25 mg/kg orally 4 times daily
Children	*Preferred choices:* Doxycycline If 45 kg or more, give adult dosage If less than 45 kg, give 2.2 mg/kg orally twice daily Ciprofloxacin, 20 mg/kg orally twice daily *Alternative choice:* Chloramphenicol, 25 mg/kg orally 4 times daily (maximum 200 mg/dL)

(28). Furthermore, as many as 50% of inhalational anthrax cases may develop meningitis (36). Anthrax causes a rapidly progressive hemorrhagic meningitis with characteristic large Gram-positive bacilli in the cerebrospinal fluid (CSF). Similarly, although the portal of infection is the lung, hemorrhagic submucosal lesions may develop in the gastrointestinal tract along with mesenteric infection; such lesions were seen in 39 of 42 of the autopsy cases reported in the Sverdlosk outbreak (36) and in one 2001 case. Importantly, this patient presented with primarily gastrointestinal symptoms (37).

The diagnosis of inhalational anthrax may be difficult, especially in the early stages. In addition to the signs and symptoms listed above, tachycardia and severe diaphoresis may be present. Rhinorrhea or sore throat are common in viral respiratory infections but were uncommon in inhalational anthrax (38). A high index of clinical suspicion should be maintained, especially since the risk of exposure may be unknown in the early stages of a biologic attack. Blood cultures are invariably positive if obtained prior to antibiotics.

Cutaneous anthrax is also expected to occur as a result of a biologic anthrax attack. Cutaneous cases occurred up to 12 days after the exposure in the Sverdlovsk outbreak (32). The initial lesion is a papule or macule, leading to ulceration at the site of inoculation within two days, followed by vesiculation. The lesion is painless, although it may be highly pruritic, and the vesicular fluid contains large amounts of bacteria. The characteristic depressed black eschar that subsequently develops is painless. Surrounding edema is often a prominent feature of cutaneous anthrax lesions. In the one case of cutaneous anthrax that developed in a 7-month-old infant in 2001, microangiopathic hemolytic anemia and renal insufficiency occurred (39).

Diagnosis

Blood cultures should be obtained promptly if anthrax is suspected. Blood smears should be examined for the presence of organisms. Chest radiograph and chest CT scans should be obtained to look for evidence of mediastinal widening, pleural effusions, and parenchymal abnormalities. Thoracentesis of any pleural effusions should be performed, and lumbar puncture should be done as indicated. The clinical microbiology laboratory and the state public health department should both be notified of the possibility of anthrax. If indicated, specimens can be sent to specialized laboratories participating in the Laboratory Response Network for specific testing such as immunohistochemical staining or polymerase chain reaction (PCR). Cutaneous lesions, especially vesicle fluid, should be swabbed for stain and culture. Punch biopsy of the periphery of lesions may also be performed and analyzed by immunohistochemistry or PCR if the Gram stain is negative. Nasal swabs are not sensitive indicators of exposure or infection and should not be used to diagnose or rule out infection in individual patients (40). Sputum culture is generally negative in inhalational anthrax.

Treatment

The current recommendations for therapy of anthrax provided here are derived from the Working Group on Civilian Biodefense (41) and the CDC guidelines (Table 117.3). As with recommendations for plague, these are based on expert opinion and a risk–benefit calculation that takes into account the extremely high mortality of inhalational anthrax. As such, the recommendations include therapy with drugs that are not specifically FDA-approved for anthrax and drugs that may have potential side effects in pregnant women and children.

Several factors are important in choosing an empiric regimen for inhalational anthrax. The 60% survival rate in the 2001 cases, which were treated with multidrug regimens, was superior to historical experience. Partly because of these data, the CDC has recommended the use of ciprofloxacin and at least one or two other drugs for the initial treatment of inhalational anthrax. Other factors to be considered are the penetration of drugs into the central nervous system (CNS) in cases where meningitis may be present, as well as the possibility of engineered or primary drug resistance. Although penicillin is FDA-approved for anthrax, the presence of inducible beta-lactamases dictate against the use of penicillin alone. Parenteral therapy is recommended initially. In a mass exposure setting or for postexposure prophylaxis, ciprofloxacin as an oral agent is recommended.

The duration of therapy is an important consideration both in treatment and in postexposure prophylaxis. Although the longest period of latency in the Sverdlovsk episode was reported to be 43 days, viable spores have been demonstrated in the mediastinal lymph nodes of monkeys as late as 100 days after exposure, and disease has occurred 98 days after exposure (42,43). In addition, antibiotic treatment may prevent not only disease, but also the development of an effective immune response; therefore, treatment regimens are recommended for 60 days, with close follow-up after discontinuation of antibiotics. Postexposure vaccination, if available, was also used as an option in addition to antibiotic prophylaxis. Treatment summary guidelines are as follows:

- Recommendations for a mass exposure setting—for both treatment and prophylaxis, where parenteral or multidrug therapy may be problematic—essentially consist of oral ciprofloxacin, 500 mg every 12 hours or 10 to 15 mg/kg twice daily for children.
- For gastrointestinal and oropharyngeal anthrax, use regimens recommended for inhalational anthrax.

TABLE 117.3

INHALATIONAL ANTHRAX TREATMENT PROTOCOL IN THE CONTAINED CASUALTY SETTING

Adults (including pregnant women)	Ciprofloxacin, 400 mg every 12 h *or* Doxycycline[a] 100 mg every 12 h *and* one or two additional antimicrobials[b]	IV treatment initially. Switch to oral antimicrobial therapy when clinically appropriate. Continue for 60 days (IV and PO combined)
Children	Ciprofloxacin[c], 10–15 mg/kg every 12 h *or* Doxycycline[a] Older than 8 y and greater than 45 kg: 100 mg every 12 h Younger than 8 y or 45 kg or less: 2.2 mg/kg every 12 h *and* One or two additional antimicrobials[b]	Same as adult

[a]If meningitis is suspected, doxycycline may be less optimal because of poor central nervous system penetration.
[b]Other agents with *in vitro* activity include rifampin, vancomycin, penicillin, ampicillin, chloramphenicol, imipenem, clindamycin, and clarithromycin. Because of concerns of constitutive and inducible beta-lactamases in *Bacillus anthracis*, penicillin and ampicillin should not be used alone.
[c]The ciprofloxacin dosage in children should not exceed 1 g/d.

- For cutaneous anthrax, the recommendations are ciprofloxacin or doxycycline alone at the same doses as in inhalational anthrax.
- The recommended duration of treatment is a minimum of 60 days after exposure because of the risk of latent spores that may cause reactivation.
- Based on the experience with other bacterial types of meningitis, the use of adjunctive steroids may be considered in anthrax meningitis.
- Initial therapy may be altered based on the clinical course of the patient; one or two first-line antimicrobial agents—ciprofloxacin or doxycycline—may be adequate as the patient improves.

VIRAL HEMORRHAGIC FEVER

The major diseases that will be considered in this section are Marburg, Ebola, and Lassa fevers. Marburg and Ebola viruses are filoviruses, whereas Lassa virus is an arenavirus with different clinical characteristics. Nevertheless, they have the potential to create similar problems in hospital management because of the sometimes dramatic nature of the illness and the potential for human-to-human transmission.

Epidemiology

Since 1976, there have been approximately a dozen outbreaks of Ebola in Africa, with mortality generally ranging from 53% to 88% (44). There have also been eight cases of documented human infection in the United States from contact with imported monkeys from the Philippines. Infections with this Reston strain of Ebola virus have been subclinical. Marburg virus has been associated with six outbreaks since the disease was recognized in 1976 in German and Yugoslav laboratory workers infected by African green monkeys of Ugandan origin (45). Since then, there have been six other clusters of infection in Africa, the most recent in Angola and the Democratic Republic of Congo. Involving more than 400 people, the mortality was 83% and 90%, respectively, in these last two outbreaks.

Both infections are transmitted by exposure to infected primate blood or cell culture (46). Secondary transmission occurs from exposure to blood and body fluids, as well as by intimate contact. Ebola transmission has ranged from 3% to 17% in household contacts (47). Droplet and, possibly, small-particle aerosol transmission is thought to have occurred in the Reston outbreak but has not been documented in human-to-human transmission (46). Nosocomial transmission is associated with percutaneous exposure and mucous membrane or cutaneous exposure to infected body fluids. The skin of patients is also infected and may serve as a source of secondary transmission (46).

Lassa virus causes a chronic infection of rodents, and is endemic throughout West Africa (48). Transmission to humans is through exposure to infected rodents, primarily through contact with urine (49). Person-to-person transmission is thought to be primarily via contact with infected body fluids, although aerosol transmission may also occur. Incubation is between 3 and 16 days. Other arenaviruses are present worldwide in rodent reservoirs and are a potential source of new clinical syndromes (48).

Clinical Manifestations

The clinical pictures of Ebola and Marburg infection are similar (46). The incubation period ranges between 5 and 10 days. Abrupt onset of fever, myalgias, and headache is typical. Nausea and vomiting, abdominal pain, diarrhea, chest pain, and pharyngitis are common. Photophobia, lymph node enlargement, jaundice, and pancreatitis are all manifestations of widespread organ involvement. CNS involvement may manifest as obtundation or coma. A bleeding diathesis is seen in at least 50% of patients. A characteristic maculopapular rash is described by day 5 of the illness. By the second week, there is either a period of defervescence and improvement, or further deterioration with multiorgan system failure. Disseminated intravascular coagulation, as well as hepatic and renal failure may ensue; convalescence is often protracted. Mortality is estimated at 25% for Marburg, 50% for Ebola-Sudan, and 90% for Ebola-Zaire (46). As described above, Ebola-Reston has not led to any known human deaths. There is viremia with infection of all organs, leading to necrosis in areas of viral replication (50). Pathogenesis is thought to be also due to cytokine release, leading to increased vascular permeability and hemodynamic instability (51).

Lassa fever presents with relatively nonspecific signs and symptoms, making recognition of cases in the initial stages difficult (48,52). A combination of fever, retrosternal pain, pharyngitis, and proteinuria has been suggested to be indicative of Lassa fever (52). A diffuse capillary leak syndrome in the second week of illness is a cardinal manifestation of this disorder. Mortality of hospitalized cases ranges from 15% to 25%. Seventh cranial nerve deafness is a common sequela of Lassa infection, occurring in approximately one third of cases (53); persistent vertigo is another reported side effect (54). The pathogenic mechanism of Lassa fever is not well understood, but there is variable necrosis in affected organs, and the systemic manifestations of vascular dysfunction may be due to soluble macrophage-derived factors.

Diagnosis

A history of travel to endemic areas and a clinical syndrome compatible with viral hemorrhagic fever (VHF) are key elements of making a diagnosis. Nevertheless, a cluster of cases with signs and symptoms indicative of VHF may the first clue of a biologic attack. Specialized testing for Marburg and Ebola, including PCR and direct antigen visualization in clinical samples, is available through reference laboratories. Contact with local public health authorities and the CDC will allow testing via mobile laboratory facilities. BSL-4 level containment facilities are required for attempts to isolate virus and BSL-3 facilities for routine testing.

Lassa virus is easily cultured, as the levels of viremia are usually high; reverse transcription-PCR (RT-PCR) may also be used to identify Lassa virus.

Treatment

Treatment of Marburg and Ebola virus is primarily supportive, as there is no effective specific therapy, and interferon is felt not to be useful. Unnecessary movement or manipulation of the patient should be avoided. Contact and respiratory isolation of the patient is necessary, including use of goggles and face shields to prevent exposure to body fluids (55). Thorough disinfection of all materials that have come into patient contact should be performed, and containers of biologic waste should be externally disinfected (55).

In cases of Lassa fever, where the aspartate transaminase levels exceed 150 IU/L, early treatment with intravenous ribavirin has been reported to be beneficial in tapering doses over 12 days (56).

SMALLPOX

Smallpox is caused by infection with variola, a double-stranded DNA orthopoxvirus. Smallpox, one of the most feared and lethal diseases known to man, was virtually eliminated as a natural threat by vaccination (57). By 1980, the World Health Organization declared it to be eradicated worldwide, with the last case known to have occurred naturally in 1977. In the United States, universal childhood vaccination ended in 1972, and thus, most people in the United States today are susceptible to smallpox infection. The anthrax attacks in 2001 again raised the possibility of smallpox being used as a biologic weapon. Smallpox is classified as a category A bioterrorism agent, a high-priority organism that poses a risk to national security (see above under Tularemia for full definition of Category A agents) (3) and should be considered one of the most dangerous agents because of its high infectiousness, capability for rapid spread, lack of effective treatment, and capacity to induce mass social disruption and overburden the public health system.

Epidemiology

Smallpox is spread by direct close contact via large droplet inhalation (58); there are no known animal reservoirs. Spread can also occur by contact with lesions or infected fomites. Household spread has been reported to range from 30% to 80% (59). Smallpox outbreaks were most common during the winter and early spring (60). All ages are susceptible although, historically, vaccination rates and prior infection modulated the attack rates among different groups. Patients are most contagious when they have a rash, although they may be infectious during the symptomatic prodrome prior to the development of skin lesions (see below). Incubation is from 7 to 17 days, during which period the patient is not infectious.

Clinical Manifestations

During the prodromal phase, the patient experiences high fever with back pain and prostration (57). The rash follows within a day or two, with more lesions on the face, oral mucosa, and extremities than on the trunk—termed a *centrifugal pattern*. The lesions begin as macules, progress to vesicles, and become pustules over the first week. Fever is usually persistent throughout the period of rash development. The lesions are deep seated, firm, painful, and—important for the diagnosis—all lesions are at the same stage of development at each phase. All of these characteristics of the rash serve to differentiate it from the rash of chickenpox, which is superficial, appears in crops, is centripetal in distribution, and is associated with a relatively mild prodrome. The extent of the smallpox rash correlates with mortality, which may range from 10% to 75%. In fatal cases, death usually occurs by the second week. The lesions begin to crust over after 7 to 9 days, and the patient is noninfectious only after all scabs have fallen off. Scarring and pitting result in the characteristic pock-marked appearance of survivors. The pathologic damage in smallpox is generally confined to the skin and mucous membranes, although virus is present throughout the internal organs (57). The systemic manifestations and fatalities are attributed to toxinemia and antigenemia.

Vaccine-modified smallpox presents as a milder illness with fewer lesions and mortality less than 10% (57). A hemorrhagic form of smallpox may occur in which there is diffuse erythema, followed by petechial hemorrhages; it is reported to have mortality approaching 100% (61). In malignant or "flat" smallpox, discrete lesions do not develop, but confluent rubbery lesions are present (62). A form of smallpox known as variola minor, with much milder symptoms and mortality less than 10%, is now known to be due to a genetically distinct strain of the virus (63).

Diagnosis

Specimens of vesicular or pustular fluid should be obtained for culture and electron microscopic examination; these are transported in double-sealed, leakproof containers designed for transport of body fluids. Specimens should be handled only in BSL-4 laboratories, and public health authorities should be notified to assist with specimen handling if a case of smallpox is suspected. The diagnosis of orthopoxvirus infection can be made by electron microscopic examination, and speciation can be performed by molecular techniques such as PCR and DNA sequencing.

Treatment and Prevention

Although a full discussion of infection control and vaccination protocols is beyond the scope of this text, the following principles should be followed (64). The patient should be isolated, and contact and airborne precautions should be instituted when a case of smallpox is suspected. All personnel who had face-to-face contact with the patient should be vaccinated, as should all personnel who had contact with the patient while the latter was febrile. Local health authorities should be contacted immediately, and the CDC will provide assistance with prioritizing contacts for vaccination and monitoring. It should also be noted that contraindications to vaccinations do not apply to high-risk exposures. Treatment is primarily supportive and is aimed at maintaining hemodynamic stability and treating secondary infections.

MONKEYPOX

Monkeypox is a disease clinically similar to smallpox that has been sporadically reported in Africa since 1960. Pronounced lymphadenopathy is an additional sign of monkeypox that may help differentiate it from smallpox (65,66). Monkeypox is thought to be endemic in rodents and transmitted to humans via direct animal contact, with occasional human-to-human transmission. In 2003, there was a large cluster of human cases in the United States associated with prairie dogs that had become infected by imported African rodents (67). Although there were no fatalities, several patients required hospitalization. Vaccination against smallpox is thought to ameliorate symptoms and lessen the likelihood of infection. Cidofovir, an antiviral agent, has activity against monkeypox *in vitro* and may be used in severe infection, although there are no clinical data regarding its effectiveness (68).

MALARIA

Malaria, the fourth largest killer of children younger than 5 years of age, causes over 350 million clinical episodes and one million deaths per year. Although a comprehensive discussion of the management of malaria will not be possible here, we will cover the recognition and treatment of severe malaria, which may be encountered in the critical care setting in a nonendemic setting. As such, this chapter will focus on infection with *Plasmodium falciparum*, the strain of the parasite that is most likely to cause high-level parasitemia and severe life-threatening malaria.

Epidemiology

Malaria is endemic throughout much of the world, with the greatest number of cases in Africa and Asia (69). Malaria has been officially eradicated in the United States since 1970, but approximately 1,200 cases are reported annually (70), most in travelers from endemic areas. Other cases are due to local transmission from infected mosquitoes (so-called airport malaria), congenital malaria, and malaria acquired from blood transfusion. Local transmission of malaria in the United States has occurred at least 11 times since 1970, with 20 probable cases (71). In a recent outbreak in Florida, seven cases were verified as being caused by the same strain of *P. vivax* (71). Thus, domestic transmission of malaria is possible, especially in warmer regions of the United States.

In endemic areas, many adults are partially immune to malaria and, although infected, may even be asymptomatic. Children are particularly prone to infection and to developing severe disease. Other high-risk groups include pregnant women, asplenic individuals, and other immunocompromised hosts.

Clinical Manifestations

Malaria typically has an incubation period of 1 to 3 weeks. However, this may be extended by partial immunity or chemoprophylaxis. Therefore, it has been suggested that any traveler returning from an endemic area should be considered at risk for development of malaria for as long as 3 months (72). The clinical presentation is usually nonspecific. Fever and headache are universally present, and myalgia, sweats, and weakness are common. Paroxysmal and cyclical fever, although classically associated with malaria, are not consistently present. Especially in the case of falciparum malaria, the fever is often continuous. Although other infections are common in malaria-endemic areas, malaria should be considered one of the most likely diagnoses in any patient with a consistent clinical picture and travel history. If malaria is suspected, prompt infectious disease consultation is indicated to help with management and assess the likelihood of alternate diagnoses.

The pathogenesis of malaria is complex and related to both the direct effects of the parasite on erythrocytes and the vasculature and indirect effects on cytokine production, tissue oxygen consumption, and other systemic effects (72). Several aspects of the biology of *Plasmodium falciparum* are relevant to the development of severe malaria. *P. falciparum* sequesters itself in the venous microcirculation of virtually all tissues, including the brain. Hypoglycemia is common during *P. falciparum* infection and is thought to be due to oxygen consumption by replicating parasites, as well as a result of increased tissue metabolism. Severe anemia may occur and is due to lysis of infected erythrocytes and the clearance of uninfected erythrocytes and decreased erythrocyte production. Thus, the anemia in severe malaria is often normochromic and normocytic. This combination of factors aggravates tissue hypoxia and leads to metabolic acidosis. A capillary leak syndrome due to parasite sequestration and cytokine production may lead to pulmonary edema. Renal failure in malaria is multifactorial and is more common in adults than children. Hemoglobinuria may be severe enough to cause dark urine, termed, when present, *blackwater fever*.

Diagnosis

The gold standard for diagnosis of malaria remains the microscopic identification of parasites on the blood smear. Examination of thick and thin blood smears should be performed immediately by trained personnel. If the initial examination is negative, smears should be repeated every 12 to 24 hours for a total of 48 to 72 hours (70). When parasites are detected, the percentage of parasitemia can be calculated by counting the number of infected and noninfected red blood cells (RBCs). The number of white blood cells (WBCs) in the microscopic field can also be used as an internal standard to aid in estimated parasite density and percentage when thick smears are examined. Malaria is a nationally notifiable disease, and the state health authorities should be notified when a diagnosis of malaria is made. The Centers for Disease Control and Prevention maintains a 24-hour malaria hotline to assist clinicians with the management of suspected and confirmed malaria cases. The numbers to call are at the time of this publication: 770-488-7788 Monday to Friday, 8:00 a.m. to 4:30 p.m. Off-hours, weekends, and federal holidays, call 770-488-7100 and ask to have the malaria clinician on call to be paged (73).

Treatment

It should be emphasized that patients, particularly those who are nonimmune, may deteriorate rapidly. Thus hospitalization of patients during the initial phase of treatment is prudent. Furthermore, nonimmune patients may have severe illness before manifesting high degrees of parasitemia. Therefore, patients who manifest any of the symptoms or signs of severe malaria and have any degree of parasitemia on blood smear should be

TABLE 117.4

WORLD HEALTH ASSOCIATION CRITERIA FOR SEVERE MALARIA

Criteria for severe malaria requiring parenteral therapy:
■ Impaired consciousness/coma
■ Severe normocytic anemia
■ Renal failure
■ Pulmonary edema
■ Acute respiratory distress syndrome
■ Circulatory shock
■ Disseminated intravascular coagulation
■ Spontaneous bleeding
■ Acidosis
■ Hemoglobinuria
■ Jaundice
■ Repeated generalized convulsions
■ Parasitemia of more than 5%

treated as a case of severe malaria. The World Health Organization (WHO) has promulgated criteria for the diagnosis of severe malaria (Table 117.4) (74).

Cases that meet these criteria should be treated with intravenous therapy. Intravenous quinidine gluconate is currently the only available parenteral drug recommended for severe malaria in the United States. It should be administered as a loading dose of 6.25 mg base/kg (= 10 mg salt/kg), over 1 to 2 hours, followed by a continuous infusion administered at 0.0125 mg base/kg/minute (= 0.02 mg salt/kg/minute). Quinidine levels should be maintained in the range of 3 to 8 mg/L. After 24 hours of intravenous therapy, and if the patient is able to take oral drugs, treatment can be switched to oral quinine (10 mg salt/kg every 8 hours) for a total of 7 days of therapy. All patients with severe malaria should also be treated with intravenous doxycycline (100 mg every 12 hours) or clindamycin (5 mg base/kg every 8 hours) in addition to quinidine until oral therapy is tolerated. If the hospital pharmacy is unable to obtain intravenous quinidine quickly, Eli Lilly may be contacted at 1-800-821-0538. Assistance from the company to arrange a rapid shipment of the drug is available between the hours of 6 a.m. and 6 p.m. The CDC may also be contacted for advice at the malaria hotline (see above).

Two aspects of quinidine therapy in this setting are very important to remember. The first is the possibility of ventricular arrhythmias. Prolongation of the Q-T_C interval is commonly seen during quinidine therapy, and careful monitoring of the electrocardiogram and electrolytes is mandatory. Combination with other drugs that may prolong the Q-T_C interval should be avoided. The second is the propensity of quinidine and quinine to cause hypoglycemia. Given the likelihood of hypoglycemia in severe malaria due to the disease itself, serum glucose must be carefully monitored and supplemented as necessary. Given these considerations, quinidine should be administered in an intensive care unit, with the assistance of a cardiologist as needed.

It is recommended by the CDC that exchange transfusion be considered in cases where parasitemia exceeds 10% or when severe complications are present (75,76). Although the benefits have not been proven in a randomized trial, exchange transfusion has the potential benefit of both reducing the parasite burden and circulating cytokines and toxins. Exchange transfusion is recommended until parasitemia is below 1%.

ROCKY MOUNTAIN SPOTTED FEVER

Rocky Mountain spotted fever (RMSF) is a disease that presents with nonspecific signs and symptoms, for which there is no specific, rapid diagnostic test; when not treated appropriately, RMSF has a high mortality. It is therefore important for the practicing clinician to have a high index of suspicion for RMSF and to be familiar with its epidemiology, clinical manifestations, and treatment.

Epidemiology

RMSF is caused by *Rickettsia rickettsii*, an intracellular bacterium that is transmitted in the United States primarily by the dog tick, *Dermacentor variabilis*, in the Eastern states, and the wood tick *Dermacentor andersoni*, in the Rocky Mountain States; ticks are also the primary reservoir for *R. rickettsii*. Despite the name, most cases of RMSF occur in the southeastern United States, and more than half of all reported cases are from North Carolina, South Carolina, Tennessee, Oklahoma, and Arkansas. However, cases have been reported in all 48 continental states except Vermont and Maine (77). Most cases occur between April and September. Children are at highest risk of RMSF, and the peak incidence is between 5 and 9 years of age (77). Although males are reported to be at higher risk, a recent study of children with RMSF found more cases among girls than boys (78). Most bites are unnoticed, and the tick must be attached for 6 to 10 hours for feeding and infection to take place.

Clinical Manifestations and Pathogenesis

The rickettsial organisms primarily target and infect endothelial cells (79). The primary pathology consists of diffuse cell injury and increased vascular permeability caused by cell-to-cell spread of the organisms after initial hematogenous and lymphatic seeding. Infection occurs in virtually all internal organs, and vascular injury occurs in lung, heart, brain, gastrointestinal tract, and skin as well as other sites.

Symptoms typically begin 2 to 14 days after the tick bite. Virtually all patients experience the classical triad of fever, headache, and rash (78,80,81). However, it should be emphasized that the rash is present in only about 50% of cases within the first 3 days. Rash usually appears by the second to fifth day, but is absent in about 10% of patients. The rash is often faint in the initial stages and may be more difficult to detect in patients with dark skin (81). It begins as a blanching, pink maculopapular exanthem, most commonly beginning at the wrists and ankles, and develops into palpable lesions that spread centrally. The rash often becomes petechial and may involve the palms and soles. Commonly associated symptoms occurring in more than 50% of patients are myalgias, nausea, vomiting, and abdominal pain. The serum AST (aspartate aminotransferase) is often elevated, and thrombocytopenia and hyponatremia occur in up to 50% of cases (81).

CNS abnormalities occur in about 25% and carry a poor prognosis. CSF abnormalities are observed in one third of patients and consist of pleocytosis and elevated protein levels, although the CSF glucose is usually normal. A fulminant form of the disease, with death occurring in the first 5 days, has been described; glucose-6-phosphate dehydrogenase deficiency has been linked to this form of the disease (82). Neurologic deficits and limb loss are the most serious sequelae observed in survivors of RMSF (83).

Diagnosis

Delay in diagnosis and delay in seeking medical attention are associated with poor outcome in RMSF. Factors that are likely to lead to delay in diagnosis include absence of rash or delayed appearance of the rash, no history of tick bite, and presentation early in the course of disease (81,84,85). *R. rickettsii* can be isolated in culture or demonstrated by immunohistochemistry in tissue specimens. However, these methods are not routinely available, and empiric therapy should not await the result of laboratory testing. Serology is likewise useful for confirmation of diagnosis. Diagnosis should therefore be made on the basis of epidemiologic and clinical findings described above.

Treatment

The recommended therapy for RMSF is doxycycline, administered at a dose of 100 mg twice daily (86). Therapy is continued for 7 days and a minimum of 3 days after the patient has defervesced. Treatment of suspected RMSF should be instituted promptly with doxycycline either intravenously or orally. Doxycycline for RMSF is not contraindicated in children (86).

References

1. McCoy G. A plague-like illness of rodents. *Public Health Bull.* 1911;43:53.
2. Dennis DT, Inglesby TV, Henderson DA, et al. Tularemia as a biological weapon: medical and public health management. *JAMA.* 2001;285:2763.
3. Centers for Disease Control and Prevention. Emergency preparedness and response, bioterrorism agents/diseases. http://www.bt.cdc.gov/agent/agentlist-category.asp. Accessed January 9, 2007.
4. Boyce JM. Recent trends in the epidemiology of tularemia in the United States. *J Infect Dis.* 1975; 131:197.
5. Dennis DT. Tularemia. *In:* Wallace RB, ed. *Maxcy-Rosenau-Last Public Health and Preventive Medicine.* 14th ed. Stamford, Ct: Appleton & Lange; 1998:354.
6. Human plague–four states, 2006. *MMWR Morb Mortal Wkly Rep.* 2006; 55:940.
7. Feldman KA, Enscore RE, Lathrop SL, et al. An outbreak of primary pneumonic tularemia on Martha's Vineyard. *N Engl J Med.* 2001;345:1601.
8. Christenson B. An outbreak of tularemia in the northern part of central Sweden. *Scand J Infect Dis.* 1984;16:285.
9. Young LS, Bickness DS, Archer BG, et al. Tularemia epidemia: Vermont, 1968. Forty-seven cases linked to contact with muskrats. *N Engl J Med.* 1969;280:1253.
10. Capellan J, Fong IW. Tularemia from a cat bite: case report and review of feline-associated tularemia. *Clin Infect Dis.* 1993;16:472.
11. Penn RL. Tularemia. In: Mandell GL, Bennett JE, Dolin R, eds. *Principles and Practice of Infectious Diseases.* Vol. 2. Philadelphia, PA: Churchill Livingstone; 2004:2674.
12. Fortier AH, Green SJ, Polsinelli T, et al. Life and death of an intracellular pathogen: *Francisella tularensis* and the macrophage. *Immunol Ser.* 1994;60:349.
13. Saslaw S, Eigelsbach HT, Wilson HE, et al. Tularemia vaccine study, I: intracutaneous challenge. *Arch Intern Med.* 1961;107:689.
14. Saslaw S, Eigelsbach HT, Prior JA, et al. Tularemia vaccine study, II: respiratory challenge. *Arch Intern Med.* 1961;107:702.
15. Sanders CV, Hahn R. Analysis of 106 cases of tularemia. *J La State Med Soc.* 1968;120:391.
16. Evans ME, Gregory DW, Schaffner W, et al. Tularemia: a 30-year experience with 88 cases. *Medicine (Baltimore).* 1985;64:251.
17. Overholt EL, Tigertt WD, Kadull PJ, et al. An analysis of forty-two cases of laboratory-acquired tularemia. Treatment with broad spectrum antibiotics. *Am J Med.* 1961;30:785.
18. Centers for Disease Control and Prevention. Abstract: consensus statement: tularemia as a biological weapon: medical and public health management. http://www.bt.cdc.gov/agent/tularemia/tularemia-biological-weapon-abstract.asp#4. Accessed February, 2007.
19. Perry RD, Fetherston JD. Yersinia pestis–etiologic agent of plague. *Clin Microbiol Rev.* 1997;10:35.
20. Slack P. The black death past and present, 2: some historical problems. *Trans R Soc Trop Med Hyg.* 1989;83:461.
21. Butler T, Dennis DT. Plague. In: Mandell GL, Bennett JE, Dolin R, eds. *Principles and Practice of Infectious Diseases.* Vol. 2. Philadelphia, PA: Churchill Livingstone; 2004:2691.
22. Meyer KF. Pneumonic plague. *Microbiol Mol Biol Rev.* 1961;25:249.
23. Hull HF, Montes JM, Mann JM. Septicemic plague in New Mexico. *J Infect Dis.* 1987;155:113.
24. Gage KL, Dennis DT, Orloski KA, et al. Cases of cat-associated human plague in the Western US, 1977–1998. *Clin Infect Dis.* 2000;30:893.
25. Inglesby TV, Dennis DT, Henderson DA, et al. Plague as a biological weapon: medical and public health management. *JAMA.* 2000;283:2281.
26. Butler T. A clinical study of bubonic plague. Observations of the 1970 Vietnam epidemic with emphasis on coagulation studies, skin histology and electrocardiograms. *Am J Med.* 1972;53:268.
27. Centers for Disease Control and Prevention. Abstract: plague as a biological weapon: medical and public health management. http://www.bt.cdc.gov/Agent/Plague/plague-biological-weapon-abstract.asp#therapy. Accessed November 25, 2007.
28. Lucey D. Anthrax. In: Mandell GL, Bennett JE, Dolin R, eds. *Principles and Practice of Infectious Diseases.* 6th ed. Vol. 2. Philadelphia, PA: Churchill Livingstone; 2004:3618.
29. Summary of notifiable diseases, 1945–1994. *MMWR Morb Mortal Wkly Rep.* 1994;43:70.
30. Brachman PS. Inhalation anthrax. *Ann N Y Acad Sci.* 1980;353:83.
31. Sirisanthana T, Brown AE. Anthrax of the gastrointestinal tract. *Emerg Infect Dis.* 2002;8:649.
32. Meselson M, Guillemin J, Hugh-Jones M, et al. The Sverdlovsk anthrax outbreak of 1979. *Science.* 1994;266:1202.
33. Hanna PC, Ireland JA. Understanding *Bacillus anthracis* pathogenesis. *Trends Microbiol.* 1999;7:180.
34. Jernigan JA, Stephens DS, Ashford DA, et al. Bioterrorism-related inhalational anthrax: the first 10 cases reported in the United States. *Emerg Infect Dis.* 2001;7:933.
35. Bartlett JG, Inglesby TV Jr, Borio L. Management of anthrax. *Clin Infect Dis.* 2002;35:851.
36. Abramova FA, Grinberg LM, Yampolskaya OV, et al. Pathology of inhalational anthrax in 42 cases from the Sverdlovsk outbreak of 1979. *Proc Natl Acad Sci U S A.* 1993;90:2291.
37. Borio L, Frank D, Mani V, et al. Death due to bioterrorism-related inhalational anthrax: report of 2 patients. *JAMA.* 2001;286:2554.
38. Hupert N, Bearman GM, Mushlin AI, et al. Accuracy of screening for inhalational anthrax after a bioterrorist attack. *Ann Intern Med.* 2003;139:337.
39. Freedman A, Afonja O, Chang MW, et al. Cutaneous anthrax associated with microangiopathic hemolytic anemia and coagulopathy in a 7-month-old infant. *JAMA.* 2002;287:869.
40. Kiratisin P, Fukuda CD, Wong A, et al. Large-scale screening of nasal swabs for *Bacillus anthracis*: descriptive summary and discussion of the National Institutes of Health's experience. *J Clin Microbiol.* 2002;40:3012.
41. Inglesby TV, O'Toole T, Henderson DA, et al. Anthrax as a biological weapon, 2002: updated recommendations for management. *JAMA.* 2002;287:2236.
42. Henderson DW, Peacock S, Belton FC. Observations on the prophylaxis of experimental pulmonary anthrax in the monkey. *J Hyg (Lond).* 1956;54:28.
43. Glassman HN. Industrial inhalation anthrax. *Microbiol Mol Biol Rev.* 1966;30:657.
44. Centers for Disease Control and Prevention, Special Pathogens Branch. Ebola hemorrhagic fever. Table showing known cases and outbreaks, in chronological order. 2003. http://www.cdc.gov/ncidod/dvrd/spb/mnpages/dispages/ebotabl.htm. Accessed February 1, 2007.
45. Centers for Disease Control and Prevention, Special Pathogens Branch. Known cases and outbreaks of Marburg hemorrhagic fever, in chronological order, 2005.
46. Peters C. Marburg and Ebola virus hemorrhagic fevers. In: Mandell GL, Bennett JE, Dolin R, eds. *Principles and Practice of Infectious Diseases.* Vol. 2. Philadelphia, PA: Churchill Livingstone; 2004:2057.
47. Baron RC, McCormick JB, Zubeir OA. Ebola virus disease in southern Sudan: hospital dissemination and intrafamilial spread. *Bull World Health Organ.* 1983;61:997.
48. Peters C. Lymphocytic choriomeningitis virus, lassa virus, and the South American hemorrhagic fevers. In: Mandell GL, Bennett JE, Dolin R, eds. *Principles and Practice of Infectious Diseases.* Vol. 2. Philadelphi, PA: Churchill Livingstone; 2004:2090.
49. Keenlyside RA, McCormick JB, Webb PA, et al. Case-control study of *Mastomys natalensis* and humans in Lassa virus-infected households in Sierra Leone. *Am J Trop Med Hyg.* 1983;32:829.

50. Zaki SR, Goldsmith CS. Pathologic features of filovirus infections in humans. *Curr Top Microbiol Immunol.* 1999;235:97.
51. Geisbert TW, Young HA, Jahrling PB, et al. Pathogenesis of Ebola hemorrhagic fever in primate models: evidence that hemorrhage is not a direct effect of virus-induced cytolysis of endothelial cells. *Am J Pathol.* 2003;163:2371.
52. McCormick JB, King IJ, Webb PA, et al. A case-control study of the clinical diagnosis and course of Lassa fever. *J Infect Dis.* 1987;155:445.
53. Cummins D, McCormick JB, Bennett D, et al. Acute sensorineural deafness in Lassa fever. *JAMA.* 1990;264:2093.
54. Rose JR. An outbreak of encephalomyelitis in Sierra Leone. *Lancet.* 1957;273:914.
55. Management of patients with suspected viral hemorrhagic fever. *MMWR Morb Mortal Wkly Rep.* 1988;37(Suppl 3):1.
56. McCormick JB, King IJ, Webb PA, et al. Lassa fever. Effective therapy with ribavirin. *N Engl J Med.* 1986;314:20.
57. Smallpox and its eradication. 1988. http://whqlibdoc.who.int/smallpox/9241561106.pdf. Accessed
58. Wehrle PF, Posch J, Richter KH, et al. An airborne outbreak of smallpox in a German hospital and its significance with respect to other recent outbreaks in Europe. *Bull World Health Organ.* 1970;43:669.
59. Damon I. Orthopoxviruses: vaccinia (smallpox vaccine), variola (smallpox), monkeypox, and cowpox. In: Mandell GL, Bennett JE, Dolin R, eds. *Principles and Practice of Infectious Diseases.* Vol. 2. 6th ed. Philadelphia, PA: Churchill Livingstone; 2004:1742.
60. Joarder A, Tarantola D, Tulloch J. *The Eradication of Smallpox from Bangladesh.* New Delhi, India: World Health Organization South-East Asia Regional Office; 1980.
61. Downie AW, Fedson DS, Saint Vincent L, et al. Haemorrhagic smallpox. *J Hyg (Lond).* 1969;67:619.
62. Rao AR. *Smallpox.* Bombay, India: Kothari Book Depot; 1972.
63. Esposito JJ, Knight JC. Orthopoxvirus DNA: a comparison of restriction profiles and maps. *Virology.* 1985;143:230.
64. Centers for Disease Control and Prevention. The CDC Smallpox Response Plan and Guidelines. http://www.bt.cdc.gov/agent/smallpox/response-plan/index.asp#annex. Accessed November 25, 2007.
65. Nalca A, Rimoin AW, Bavari S, et al. Reemergence of monkeypox: prevalence, diagnostics, and countermeasures. *Clin Infect Dis.* 2005;41:1765.
66. Huhn GD, Bauer AM, Yorita K, et al. Clinical characteristics of human monkeypox, and risk factors for severe disease. *Clin Infect Dis.* 2005; 41:1742.
67. Reed KD, Melski JW, Graham MB, et al. The detection of monkeypox in humans in the Western Hemisphere. *N Engl J Med.* 2004;350:342.
68. Updated interim CDC guidance for use of smallpox vaccine, cidofovir, and vaccinia immune globulin (VIG) for prevention and treatment in the setting of an outbreak of monkeypox infections. 2003. http://www.cdc.gov/ncidod/monkeypox/treatmentguidelines.htm. Accessed January 25, 2007.
69. World Malaria Report 2005. 2005. http://rbm.who.int/wmr2005/. Accessed January 27, 2005.
70. Centers for Disease Control and Prevention. Treatment of malaria, 1: reporting and epidemiology: evaluation and diagnosis. http://www.cdc.gov/malaria/diagnosis_treatment/clinicians1.htm. Accessed
71. *MMWR*, Local Transmission of Plasmodium vivax Malaria—Palm Beach County, Florida, 2003. 2003. http://www.cdc.gov/mmwr/preview/mmwrhtml/mm5238a3.htm. Accessed January 25, 2007.
72. Fairhurst RM, Wellems TE. Plasmodium species (malaria). In: Mandell GL, Bennett JE, Dolin R, eds. *Mandell's Principles and Practice of Infectious Diseases.* Philadelphia, PA: Churchill Livingstone; 2004.
73. Centers for Disease Control and Prevention. Treatment of malaria, 2: treatment: general approach and treatment: uncomplicated malaria. http://www.cdc.gov/malaria/diagnosis_treatment/clinicians2.htm. Accessed January 28, 2007.
74. Severe falciparum malaria. World Health Organization, Communicable Diseases Cluster. *Trans R Soc Trop Med Hyg.* 2000;94(Suppl 1):S1.
75. Zucker JR, Campbell CC. Malaria. Principles of prevention and treatment. *Infect Dis Clin North Am.* 1993;7:547.
76. Powell VI, Grima K. Exchange transfusion for malaria and *Babesia* infection. *Transfus Med Rev.* 2002;16:239.
77. Dalton MJ, Clarke MJ, Holman RC, et al. National surveillance for Rocky Mountain spotted fever, 1981–1992: epidemiologic summary and evaluation of risk factors for fatal outcome. *Am J Trop Med Hyg.* 1995;52:405.
78. Buckingham SC, Marshall GS, Schutze GE, et al. Clinical and laboratory features, hospital course, and outcome of Rocky Mountain spotted fever in children. *J Pediatr.* 2007;150:180.
79. Walker DH, Valbuena GA, Olano JP. Pathogenic mechanisms of diseases caused by *Rickettsia*. *Ann N Y Acad Sci.* 2003;990:1.
80. Kirk JL, Fine DP, Sexton DJ, et al. Rocky Mountain spotted fever. A clinical review based on 48 confirmed cases, 1943–1986. *Medicine (Baltimore).* 1990;69:35.
81. Helmick CG, Bernard KW, D'Angelo LJ. Rocky Mountain spotted fever: clinical, laboratory, and epidemiological features of 262 cases. *J Infect Dis.* 1984;150:480.
82. Walker DH, Hawkins HK, Hudson P. Fulminant Rocky Mountain spotted fever. Its pathologic characteristics associated with glucose-6-phosphate dehydrogenase deficiency. *Arch Pathol Lab Med.* 1983;107:121.
83. Archibald LK, Sexton DJ. Long-term sequelae of Rocky Mountain spotted fever. *Clin Infect Dis.* 1995;20:1122.
84. Kirkland KB, Wilkinson WE, Sexton DJ. Therapeutic delay and mortality in cases of Rocky Mountain spotted fever. *Clin Infect Dis.* 1995;20:1118.
85. Hattwick MA, Retailliau H, O'Brien RJ, et al. Fatal Rocky Mountain spotted fever. *JAMA.* 1978;240:1499.
86. Centers for Disease Control and Prevention. Diagnosis and management of tickborne rickettsial diseases in the United States Rocky Mountain spotted fever, ehrlichioses, and anaplasmosis: a practical guide for physicians and other health care and public health professionals. *MMWR Recomm Rep.* 2006;55(RR-4):1–28.

SECTION XII ■ CARDIOVASCULAR DISEASE AND DYSFUNCTION

CHAPTER 118 ■ EVALUATION OF CHEST PAIN AND ACUTE CORONARY SYNDROME IN THE ICU

GIUSEPPE DE LUCA • SALVATORE CASSESE • PAOLO MARINO

This chapter deals with the clinical presentation and evaluation of chest pain in the intensive care unit (ICU). Please see Chapters 119 and 120 for a full discussion of non–ST-segment elevation myocardial infarction and ST-segment elevation myocardial infarction.

EVALUATION OF CHEST PAIN

Immediate Concerns

Despite insights and innovations over the last decades, acute nontraumatic chest pain still represents one of the most difficult diagnostic challenges in medicine. In fact, it is commonly observed in several life-threatening illnesses, including cardiovascular, pulmonary, and gastrointestinal diseases and, when symptoms are atypical, it may be difficult to interpret (Table 118.1) (1). Algorithms have been proposed to improve the accuracy of diagnosis and the patient's risk stratification via the integrated use of clinical data, biomarkers, and noninvasive diagnostic tests (2,3) (Fig. 118.1).

Main Tips

When confronted with a patient suffering from acute chest pain:

1. First, exclude major life-threatening processes, such as myocardial infarction, pulmonary embolism (PE), or aortic dissection.
2. Obtain a careful history and perform a meticulous physical examination, particularly in patients with atypical chest pain, which is commonly seen in the emergency department (Table 118.2).
3. Use this information to select the most appropriate tests or procedures needed to confirm or reject the suspected diagnosis.

Clinical Evaluation

The evaluation of patients with acute chest pain should include the following.

History

1. *Symptoms and description of the current illness:* The patient should be allowed to describe the character (pressure, sharp, burning, pleuritic), duration (minutes, hours, days), intensity (scale of 0–10), location, radiation, and onset (sudden, gradual) of the pain. Associated symptoms and signs such as nausea, vomiting, diaphoresis, dyspnea, presyncope, and syncope should be noted. Factors that worsen or relieve the symptoms should be obtained (Table 118.2).
2. *Past medical history:* A thorough investigation on history of cardiopulmonary and gastrointestinal disease is mandatory (Table 118.1).
3. *Family history:* A family history of glucose intolerance, coronary artery disease, and sudden or premature death should be investigated.
4. *Social history:* A history of alcohol, cigarette, cocaine, or other drug use should be sought.

Physical Examination

1. *Vital signs:* Changes in heart rate, blood pressure, pulse pressure, pulmonary artery waveforms and pressure, ventilatory parameters, temperature, and urine output should be noted.
2. *Inspection and palpation:* Examination of the head, neck, chest, and abdomen may reveal significant disease. Disrobe the patient and visually inspect for obvious deformities and asymmetry. Significant point tenderness and crepitation should be sought by applying firm pressure to the anterior, lateral, and posterior chest wall. Cardiac impulses may reveal significant underlying disease. Palpate and note the symmetry of all upper and lower extremity pulses. Palpation of the abdomen for tenderness and pulsatile masses is vital in making the diagnosis of thoracic and intra-abdominal disease.
3. *Auscultation:* The neck should be auscultated to evaluate for the presence of significant upper airway obstruction (stridor). Careful auscultation of the chest should assess symmetry of breath sounds. Abnormal sounds (i.e., rales, wheezing, rhonchi, friction rubs) and their location should be noted. Heart sounds should be carefully studied. The cardiac rate and rhythm should be noted. Close attention to findings suggestive of valvular heart disease is important. The abdomen should be auscultated, and the presence and quality of bowel sounds should be noted.

TABLE 118.1

DIFFERENTIAL DIAGNOSIS OF CHEST PAIN

CARDIOVASCULAR
Myocardial infarction
Angina pectoris
Aortic valve disease
Hypertrophic cardiomyopathy
Myocarditis
Pericarditis
Dressler syndrome
Pulmonary embolism
Pulmonary hypertension
Aortic dissection
Thoracic aneurysm
Pericardial effusion
Mitral valve prolapse
PULMONARY
Pulmonary embolism
Pneumothorax
Asthma
Pleuritis
Pneumonia
Chronic obstructive pulmonary disease
Intrathoracic tumor
Tracheitis and tracheobronchitis
GASTROINTESTINAL
Esophageal spasm
Esophageal reflux
Esophagitis
Esophageal rupture
Foreign bodies (food, pills)
Peptic ulcer disease
Nasogastric tube erosions
Gastritis
Colonic distention
Biliary disease
MUSCULOSKELETAL
Costochondritis
Intercostal muscle cramps
Rib fractures
Trauma
OTHER
Herpes zoster
Mediastinitis
Diaphragmatic flutter
Psychoneurosis

Diagnostic Tests for Acute Chest Pain

1. *Electrocardiogram (ECG):* An electrocardiogram should be obtained as soon as possible, particularly in patients with persistent chest discomfort at the time of evaluation. Nondiagnostic ECG changes (i.e., old left bundle branch block) or a *normal* ECG may neither prove nor disprove significant cardiac ischemia. Right axis deviation, right bundle branch block, and inversion of T waves in chest (V-) leads may be observed in acute pulmonary embolism. Diffusely concave ST-segment elevation or inversion of T waves may be observed in patients with pericarditis.
2. *Biomarkers*
   A) Markers of myocardial injury: Several markers are currently available that allow accurate identification of patients with myocardial injury. Cardiac troponin I and T represent a more accurate and sensitive marker of myocardial injury (3,4). It is imperative to consider that a single negative troponin assay at the time of a patient's admission cannot always be relied upon to exclude myocardial infarction. In this setting, it is recommended to repeat the test 6 to 12 hours after admission and after any further episode of chest pain. Myoglobin might be considered between 2 and 6 hours from symptom onset, as compared to creatine kinase (CK)-MB mass and troponin, but the maximal negative predictive value of myoglobin reaches only 89% during this time frame (5). Elevation of troponin may be observed also in patients with acute pulmonary embolism, where it correlates well with the extent of right ventricular dysfunction and prognosis (6–8), and in patients with myocarditis, pericarditis, or acute heart failure (4).

   B) Natriuretic peptides: Cardiac natriuretic peptides are useful diagnostic and prognostic markers for patients with heart failure (8,9). Similar to cardiac troponin, elevations in brain natriuretic peptide (BNP) and in *N*-terminal proBNP (the prohormone) are associated with right ventricular dysfunction in acute pulmonary embolism, and may help to identify a subgroup of hemodynamically stable patients at especially high risk for adverse clinical events (8) (Fig. 118.2).

   C) D-dimer: Fibrin d-dimer (DD) has been proposed as a diagnostic tool in patients with suspected pulmonary thromboembolism (Fig. 118.2) (10). In fact, the dimeric d-domain serves as an indicator of *in vivo* fibrin formation. However, many conditions are associated with fibrin formation:
   - *Nonpathologic:* Cigarette smoking, aging, functional impairment, pregnancy, and postoperative state
   - *Pathologic:* Trauma, pre-eclampsia, malignancy, infection, disseminated intravascular coagulation, arterial or venous thromboembolism, atrial fibrillation, acute coronary syndromes, stroke, and acute upper gastrointestinal hemorrhage

   Because of this low specificity, DD testing may not be helpful in hospitalized patients in whom comorbidities are common. In addition, DD assays (especially qualitative latex agglutination assays) are not 100% sensitive, limiting their utility as a single screening test.
3. ***Imaging techniques:***
   A) Echocardiography: The echocardiogram plays an important role in evaluating chest pain and is frequently used to diagnose regional wall motion abnormalities, aortic stenosis, dissecting aortic aneurysm, pericardial effusion, and cardiac tamponade. Preserved regional wall motion occasionally occurs early in the process of significant cardiac ischemia. Contrast echocardiography may further improve diagnostic accuracy in the evaluation of acute chest pain (11). Transesophageal echocardiography (TEE) has a sensitivity approaching 100% for aortic dissection (12).

   B) Radionuclide myocardial perfusion imaging: Tc-99m–based tracers have been shown to be highly sensitive in the detection of myocardial infarction, although

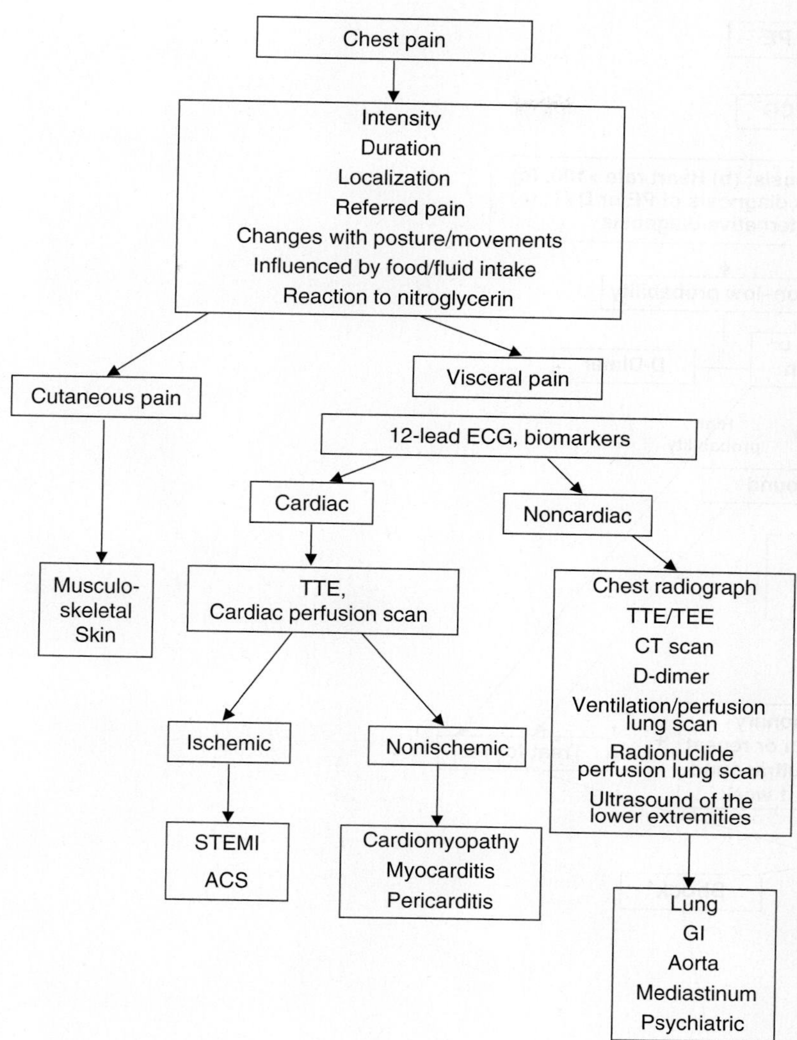

FIGURE 118.1. Diagnostic flow chart in patients with chest pain. ECG, electrocardiogram; TTE, transthoracic echocardiography; TEE, transesophageal echocardiography; CT, computed tomography; STEMI, ST-segment elevation myocardial infarction; ACS, acute coronary syndrome; GI, gastrointestinal.

somewhat less specific. However, data acquisition in a gated mode for additional wall motion score information results in a significant increase in specificity (13). The most suitable population for this method are patients judged at low to intermediate probability of having myocardial ischemia, with an atypical chest pain and a normal or nondiagnostic ECG (14,15).

C) Chest radiography: The chest radiograph may provide important clues regarding the cause of chest pain. The presence or absence of the following radiographic abnormalities should be determined: subcutaneous air, rib fractures, pneumothorax, pulmonary infiltrates, widened mediastinum, pleural effusions, and intraperitoneal free air.

TABLE 118.2

CLINICAL FEATURES OF CHEST PAIN ACCORDING TO THE ETIOLOGY

			RESPONSE TO		
Cause of chest pain	Type of pain	Referred pain	Posture/movement	Food/fluid	Nitroglycerin
Ischemic cardiac pain	Visceral	Yes	No	No	Yes
Nonischemic cardiac pain	Visceral	Yes	No	No	No
Pulmonary disease	Visceral/cutaneous	Usually no	No	No	No
Pneumothorax	Visceral/cutaneous	No	No	No	No
Musculoskeletal	Cutaneous	No	Yes	No	No
Gastrointestinal	Visceral	Sometimes	No	Yes	No
Aortic aneurysm	Visceral	Yes	No	No	No
Psychiatric	Visceral/cutaneous	No	No	No	No

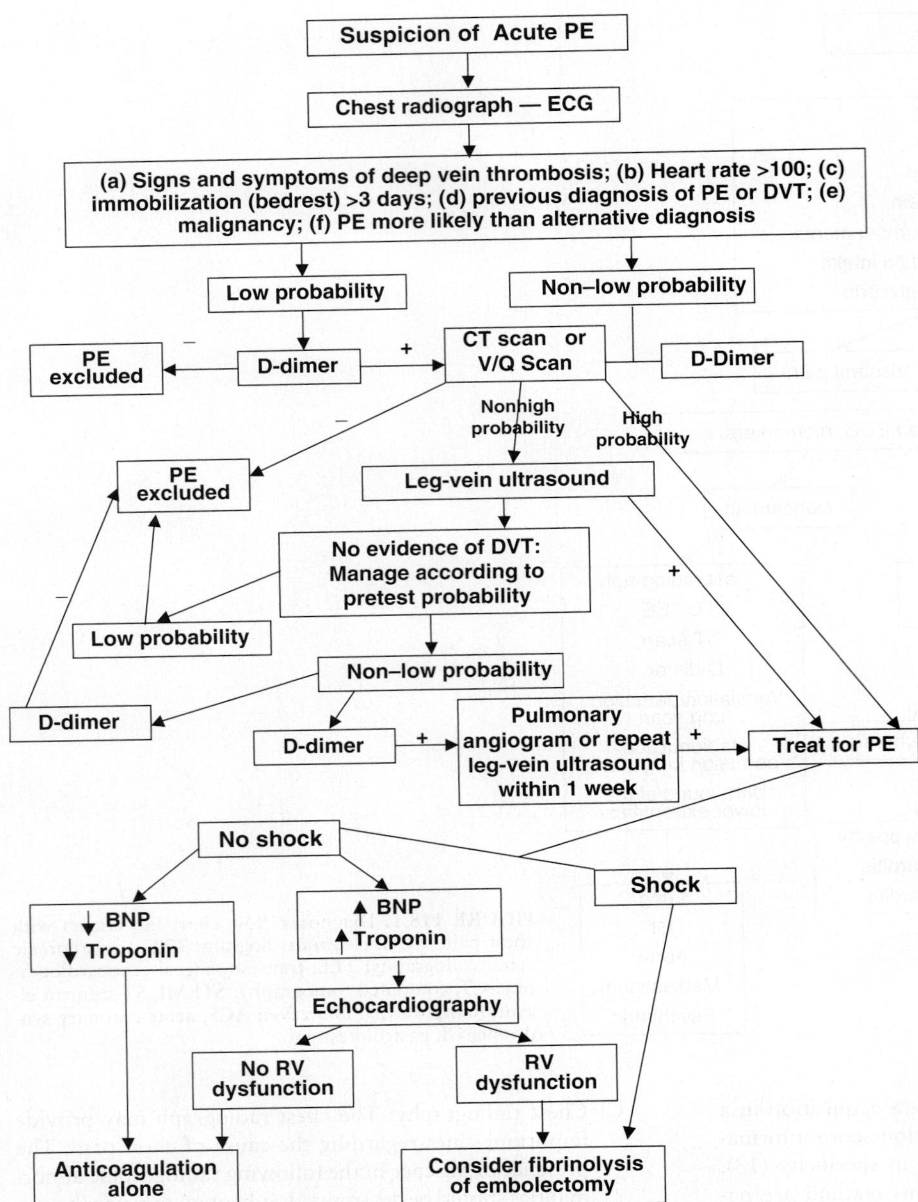

FIGURE 118.2. Algorithm on diagnosis and management of patients with acute pulmonary embolism (PE). ECG, electrocardiogram; DVT, deep vein thrombosis; CT, computed tomography; V/Q, ventilation/perfusion; BNP, brain natriuretic peptide; RV, right ventricle.

D) Radionuclide perfusion lung scan: Intubated patients or patients too ill for transport who are believed to have PE may undergo bedside perfusion lung scanning. Whereas this test is often nondiagnostic, a normal scan result is a sensitive negative predictor for the presence of pulmonary emboli. This test is no longer a principal diagnostic test in PE, being supplanted by computed tomography (CT) scan, unless patients are too unstable for transportation.

E) Radionuclide ventilation/perfusion ($\dot{V}/\dot{Q}$) lung scan: Normal- and high-probability findings on $\dot{V}/\dot{Q}$ scan often are sensitive enough to dictate therapy without further evaluation. Patients with low- and intermediate-probability $\dot{V}/\dot{Q}$ scan results, depending on the level of clinical suspicion, frequently require additional examinations (see Chapter 144). This is no longer a principal diagnostic test in PE, being supplanted by CT scan. It is usually reserved for patients with renal insufficiency, contrast allergy, or pregnancy (because of lower radiation exposure as compared to CT scan).

F) Duplex ultrasound of the lower extremities: Venous ultrasonography is useful if it demonstrates deep venous thrombosis (DVT) in patients with suspected PE. However, the majority of patients with PE have no imaging evidence of DVT. Therefore, if clinical suspicion of PE is high, patients without evidence of DVT should still be investigated for PE.

G) CT scan: It is readily available in most emergency departments, and performed rapidly. It may help in challenging cases when the chest radiograph is not conclusive (e.g., pneumothorax). Furthermore, CT angiography scan may evaluate coronary, aortic, and pulmonary anatomy with great clarity. Several studies have shown that 64-slice computed tomography coronary angiography is very accurate in the diagnosis of coronary artery disease (16). The multidetector CT seems at least as good as stress nuclear imaging for the detection and exclusion of an acute coronary syndrome in low-risk chest pain patients (17). A recent large study has shown that CT scan is effective in the evaluation and management of patients with clinically suspected pulmonary embolism (18). In cases of acute aortic syndromes, in addition to making the initial diagnosis, CT angiography can assess the extent of aortic involvement and depict involvement of visceral and iliac arteries. The average sensitivity exceeds 95%, with specificities of 87% to 100%, and may be more accurate than magnetic resonance imaging (MRI) or TEE in the detection of aortic arch vessel involvement (19).

H) Gadolinium-enhanced magnetic resonance angiography (MRA): Despite the high accuracy for the detection of coronary artery disease, acute aortic dissection, and PE (16,20) and the clear advantages due to the fact that this examination does not require ionizing radiation or use of iodinated contrast agents, MRA is currently used as a second-line diagnostic study when a first imaging study is not adequate or the true diagnosis remains uncertain. The reasons include the limited availability of MRI, especially on an emergency basis, and the issues surrounding patient inconvenience and limited applicability (MRI cannot be performed on patients with claustrophobia, pacemakers, aneurysm clips, or other metal devices).

CHEST PAIN SYNDROMES

Pinpointing the origin of chest pain is often problematic because nociceptors from within the myocardium, aorta, pleura, lungs, and esophagus traverse a common neuronal pathway to the cortex (21). Structures within the thorax that are relatively insensitive to pain include the lung parenchyma and visceral pleura. The parietal pleura, upper airways, musculoskeletal structures of the upper torso, diaphragm, and mediastinal structures respond to trauma and inflammation with pain impulses. Diabetic neuropathy, differing pain thresholds, medications, and varying levels of consciousness all may greatly influence a patient's description of the chest pain.

Classic Chest Pain

Certain disease processes are associated with characteristic pain patterns (Table 118.2). For example, an inflammatory process involving the pleural surfaces of the lungs or heart may produce pleuritic chest pain. This type of pain is described as a sharp, scratchy, or catch-like discomfort. Pneumonia, PE, and pericarditis produce inflammatory processes with this type of pain. Patients who describe their chest discomfort as retrosternal, squeezing, pressure-like, or heavy in nature often are diagnosed with myocardial ischemia (22,23). One of the most dramatic presentations of chest pain is that of acute aortic dissection. Patients frequently describe an excruciating, sharp, knifelike retrosternal pain radiating to the back. The evaluation of patients presenting with classic chest pain syndromes should be directed to specifically confirm or exclude the suspected diagnosis.

Atypical Chest Pain

As shown in Figure 118.1, the approach to patients with chest pain can be systematic and organized. Musculoskeletal or cutaneous causes of atypical chest pain should be excluded. An ECG and cardiac enzymes should thus be obtained. If the index of suspicion for cardiac ischemia is high, irrespective of the ECG and cardiac enzymes, one should proceed with further studies to either confirm or negate the suspected diagnosis. If the index of suspicion for cardiac ischemia is low, causes of chest pain such as PE, aortic dissection, pleural inflammation, pneumothorax, and gastroesophageal disease should be considered. If the ECG reveals new ischemic changes, one may assume that this is the primary cause of the patient's discomfort. Many patients in the adult ICU have significant undiagnosed coronary artery disease. An echocardiogram, unless the result is totally normal, usually is not sensitive enough to exclude acute and significant cardiac ischemia. Stress echocardiography, nuclear medicine studies, angio-CT, and, finally, cardiac catheterization may be necessary under these circumstances. The urgency with which to pursue these tests depends on the acuity of illness.

LIFE-THREATENING CAUSES OF CHEST PAIN

Differential Diagnosis: Pulmonary Causes of Chest Pain

Pulmonary Embolism

Approximately 200,000 patients die yearly from PE. The mortality of untreated PE is five times greater than treated cases (24). The multiple factors that appear to predispose to pulmonary thromboembolism are detailed in Table 118.3. The signs and symptoms of PE have been well described (25). The clinical presentation of acute PE includes the following:

- Abrupt onset of dyspnea
- Chest pain unrelieved with nitroglycerin
- Apprehension
- Tachypnea
- Diaphoresis
- Fever
- Tachycardia
- Increased P2
- Dyspnea at rest
- Thrombophlebitis of the lower extremity
- Decreasing PaO_2

The most common complaint is the sudden onset of pleuritic chest pain; nonpleuritic discomfort occurs less frequently. Approximately 84% of patients complain of dyspnea, and apprehension, cough, and hemoptysis are noted in 50% of patients. Syncope may also be a presenting sign.

On physical examination, most patients have tachycardia and tachypnea. Fever is seen in nearly half of affected patients. Patients with large or multiple emboli often have evidence of

TABLE 118.3

PREDISPOSING FACTORS TO ACUTE AORTIC SYNDROME, PULMONARY EMBOLISM, AND ACUTE CORONARY SYNDROME

Acute aortic syndrome	Pulmonary embolism	Acute coronary syndrome
Long-standing arterial hypertension Connective tissue disorders Hereditary vascular disease - Marfan syndrome - Vascular Ehlers-Danlos syndrome - Bicuspid aortic valve, coarctation of the aorta - Hereditary thoracic aortic aneurysm/dissection Vascular inflammation - Giant cell arteritis - Takayasu arteritis - Behçet's disease - Syphilis Deceleration trauma Iatrogenic factors - Diagnostic catheterization or intervention - Vascular or aortic surgery Advanced age - Atherosclerotic disease	Hereditary - Factor V mutation - Protein C mutation - Protein S deficiency - Antithrombin III deficiency - Plasminogen deficiency - Factor VIII overexpression - Hyperhomocysteinemia Acquired - Antiphospholipid antibody - Orthopedic or pelvic surgery - Obesity - Oral contraceptive/pregnancy - Cancer or chemotherapy - Central venous catheters - Immobilization - Heart failure - Previous deep venous thrombosis - Aging - Hyperhomocysteinemia	Hereditary - Factor V mutation - Protein C mutation - Protein S deficiency - Antithrombin III deficiency - Plasminogen deficiency - Factor VIII overexpression - Hyperhomocysteinemia - Obesity - Advanced age - Antiphospholipid antibody Acquired - Hypertension - Smoking - Diabetes - Dyslipidemia

hypoperfusion. A narrowed pulse pressure, poor peripheral perfusion, hypotension, low urine output, and mental status changes are common signs of hypoperfusion. Once a suspicion of PE is entertained, one should proceed with further diagnostic studies (Fig. 118.2) (26–28) (see Chapter 144).

Pneumothorax

Pneumothorax, a common entity in the ICU setting, is an abnormal collection of air between the parietal and visceral pleurae, which may be, if undiagnosed, rapidly fatal. Pneumothoraces are either spontaneous, traumatic, or iatrogenic. Irrespective of the etiology, a pneumothorax can have a significant impact on oxygenation and hemodynamics. The array of clinical presentations ranges from mild pleuritic chest pain with the sensation of shortness of breath to cardiac arrest. The clinician should look for the following signs and symptoms when pneumothorax is suspected:

- Tachypnea
- Dyspnea at rest
- Dyspnea with exertion
- Localized decrease in breath sounds
- Unilateral hyperresonance to chest percussion
- Dyspnea of abrupt onset
- Increased peak airway pressure
- Sudden hemodynamic instability
- Arterial desaturation

Patients are often apprehensive and demonstrate tachypnea and tachycardia. Auscultation and percussion of the chest often reveal decreased breath sounds and hyperresonance of the affected side. Tracheal deviation, jugular venous distention, hypotension, and shock are indicators of an immediate life-threatening process (tension pneumothorax). A chest radiograph should be obtained in the relatively stable patient believed to have a pneumothorax. Expiratory radiographs increase the likelihood of visualizing a small pneumothorax. Chest radiographs are usually diagnostic when the lung parenchyma is normal. The diagnosis of tension pneumothorax should ideally be made clinically, and the pneumothorax evacuated without waiting for results of a chest radiograph.

Patients who are critically ill and undergoing mechanical ventilation are at risk for a pneumothorax. Such patients may have increased peak airway pressures, arterial desaturation, and increased oxygen extraction. Despite sedation, some patients may become agitated and diaphoretic. Compression of the mediastinal structures with a subsequent decrease in preload may result in a significant decrease in the cardiac output and hemodynamic instability. If a ball-valve mechanism occurs during positive-pressure ventilation, a life-threatening tension pneumothorax may rapidly develop.

A pneumothorax in a patient with severe underlying pulmonary disease may be extremely difficult to diagnose (29,30). Loculated pneumothoraces are frequently missed on portable radiographs of critically ill patients. Once suspected, this diagnosis must be confirmed or negated, as nearly half of all untreated pneumothoraces progress to tension pneumothorax. In these circumstances, a CT scan of the chest often is necessary to make the diagnosis.

Differential Diagnosis: Cardiovascular Causes of Chest Pain

Acute Aortic Syndrome

Acute aortic syndrome is the modern term that includes aortic dissection, intramural hematoma (IMH), and symptomatic aortic ulcer (12). Clinical manifestations, etiology, and treatment can be readily differentiated by using the Stanford or DeBakey

TABLE 118.4

PROPOSED CLASSIFICATIONS OF AORTIC DISSECTION

STANFORD CLASSIFICATION
Type A: Dissection of the ascending and descending aorta
Type B: Dissection of the descending aorta
DEBAKEY CLASSIFICATION
Type 1: Dissection of the entire aorta
Type 2: Dissection of the ascending aorta
Type 3: Dissection of the descending aorta
NEW CLASSIFICATION
Class 1: Classic aortic dissection with an intimal flap between true and false lumen
Class 2: Medial disruption with formation of intramural hematoma/hemorrhage
Class 3: Discrete/subtle dissection without hematoma, eccentric bulge at tear site
Class 4: Plaque rupture leading to aortic ulceration, penetrating aortic atherosclerotic ulcer with surrounding hematoma, usually subadventitial
Class 5: Iatrogenic and traumatic dissection

classification of aortic dissection. Due to new studies demonstrating that intramural hemorrhage, intramural hematoma, and aortic ulcers may be signs of evolving dissections or dissection subtypes, a new system of differentiation has been proposed (Table 118.4).

Among several factors (Table 118.3), the most common risk condition for acute aortic syndromes is hypertension, with chronic exposure of the aorta to high pressures leading to intimal thickening, fibrosis, calcification, and extracellular fatty acid deposition.

Patients complain of the sudden onset of excruciating chest discomfort. This discomfort is sharp and tearing in nature, radiating to the back, abdomen, and extremities. Syncope, diaphoresis, and generalized weakness may occur. Patients may have evidence of shock with mental status changes, cool clammy skin, low urine output, hypertension or hypotension, and lactic acidosis. The clinical presentation of acute aortic syndromes may include the following signs and symptoms:

- Abrupt onset
- Maximal severity at onset
- Knifelike or tearing substernal chest pain
- Severe back pain
- Chest pain unrelieved by nitroglycerin
- Fever
- Tachycardia
- Elevated diastolic blood pressure
- Diaphoresis

Untreated acute aortic dissection is associated with a 50% mortality within the first 48 hours.

Classic Aortic Dissection

Acute aortic dissection is characterized by the rapid development of an intimal flap separating the true and false lumens (12,31). The dissection can spread from the intimal tear in an antegrade or retrograde fashion, often involving side branches and causing malperfusion syndromes, tamponade, or aortic insufficiency (12,32). Once a patient survives to hospital discharge, further prognostic stratification based on clinical and imaging parameters is challenging. Spontaneous false lumen thrombosis (better prognosis), evidence of persistent communication, and/or a patent false channel (worse prognosis) may be used to estimate late risk of expansion (12,33,34).

Type A dissections are most often seen in young patients with Marfan syndrome or cystic medial necrosis. Upper extremity weakness, diminished or loss of upper extremity pulses, asymmetric upper extremity blood pressure, hemiplegia, Horner syndrome, recurrent laryngeal nerve damage, hemopericardium, and cardiac tamponade all are associated with type A dissections. Acute aortic valvular insufficiency and dissection of the coronary artery ostium resulting in an acute myocardial infarction may occur. A prominent diastolic murmur of aortic insufficiency and congestive heart failure may be present. Type B aortic dissections are usually seen in older patients with a history of hypertension and atherosclerosis. Paresthesias, weakness, and pain of the lower extremities may result from compromised blood flow to the spinal arteries, iliac arteries, or both. Diminished or unequal lower extremity pulses and pressures relative to the upper extremities also are suggestive of distal dissection of the aorta. Manifestations of mesenteric and renal ischemia may occur (35).

The radiographic data suggestive of a type A dissection include a widened superior mediastinum and left pleural effusion. Chest radiographs of type B dissections are usually unrevealing. One may, however, see a widened descending aorta relative to the ascending aorta. When a dissection is suspected, immediate surgical consultation is required and a rapid diagnosis is warranted. The CT scan, MRI, and TEE are sensitive and specific (36–38).

Surgery is the preferred approach in case of proximal dissection, whereas medical therapies, including sodium nitroprusside, β-blockers or labetalol, and morphine, may be preferred in distal dissection. However, it is important to monitor the patient vigilantly for any evidence of branch arterial compromise, with the most lethal consequence being mesenteric ischemia.

Intramural Hematoma

Aortic IMH is considered a precursor of dissection, originating from ruptured vasa vasorum in medial wall layers and resulting in an aortic wall infarct that may provoke a secondary tear, causing a classic aortic dissection. It is similar to classic dissection in its natural history in that IMH may extend, progress, regress, or reabsorb. Whereas IMH resorption has been reported in about 10% of cases, resorption of aortic dissection has rarely been so reported (12,39,40). Most IMHs (50%–85%) are located in the descending aorta and are typically associated with hypertension (41,42). Although clinical manifestations of IMH are similar to acute aortic dissection, IMH tends to be a segmental process; therefore, radiation of pain to the head or legs is less common. Chest pain is more common with ascending (type A) IMH; upper or lower back pain is more common with descending (type B) lesions. Nonetheless, the diagnosis of IMH versus acute aortic dissection cannot be made clinically. IMH is a tomographic imaging diagnosis in the appropriate clinical setting. These patients should be managed as those with classic aortic dissection.

Plaque Rupture/Penetrating Atherosclerotic Ulcer

Deep ulceration of atherosclerotic aortic plaques can lead to IMH, aortic dissection, or perforation (43–46). Noninvasive imaging has further elucidated this disease process that often further complicates IMH and appears as an ulcer-like projection into the hematoma. In association with IMH, limited series have reported penetrating atherosclerotic ulcers almost exclusively in patients with type B IMH (46). Symptomatic ulcers with signs of deep erosion are more prone to rupture than others. In these patients, endovascular stent grafting is emerging as an attractive therapeutic modality.

Acute Pericarditis

Acute pericarditis is an inflammatory process of the pericardium caused by a variety of disorders. It is the most common disease of the pericardium. Pericarditis is commonly caused by infection, trauma, autoimmune disease, or neoplasm (see Chapter 127).

The diagnosis of acute pericarditis is established by the presence of chest pain, pericardial friction rub, and ECG abnormalities. A more complete list of the clinical features of acute pericarditis is as follows:

- Chest pain at rest
- Exacerbation of chest pain with breathing
- Chest pain lasting longer than 20 minutes
- Chest pain unrelieved with nitroglycerin
- Fever; sinus tachycardia
- ST-segment elevation without reciprocal depression
- Inverted T waves
- Pericardial friction rub
- Leukocytosis

Pericardial effusions of various sizes are seen by echocardiography (47). The pain of acute pericarditis is pleuritic in nature and often is described as a sharp, retrosternal discomfort radiating to the back and shoulders. This pain is relieved by leaning forward and worsened by recumbency, inspiration, and cough. The chest pain of acute pericarditis may be band-like with radiation to the arms, similar to that of a myocardial infarction.

Pathognomonic for acute pericarditis is a three-component friction rub that is heard best over the left sternal border with the patient sitting upright and leaning forward. It is high pitched and scratching in nature. The rub is often transitory and may be confused with aortic stenosis or mitral regurgitation; careful auscultation of the early diastolic component makes the distinction. In the absence of a large pericardial effusion, subepicardial inflammation often yields a classic triphasic ECG. In the acute stages, one may see diffuse ST-segment elevation with concurrent PR depression in the limb and precordial leads. At 24 to 48 hours, ST and PR segments normalize; however, diffuse T-wave inversion occurs. The T-wave abnormalities subsequently resolve with time. Because there may be elevation of cardiac enzymes, the distinction between myocardial infarction and pericarditis may be difficult initially. Sequential ECGs demonstrating concave morphologic features of the ST segments and absence of Q waves are suggestive of pericarditis. With the development of a large pericardial effusion, reduced QRS voltage, oscillatory voltage pattern, and atrial arrhythmias are sometimes present (48,49).

TABLE 118.5

DIAGNOSTIC TESTS FOR ACUTE PERICARDITIS

Echocardiogram
Pericardiocentesis
Evaluation of pericardial fluid:
The following suggests bacterial pericarditis:
Greater than 2,000 WBCs
Purulent pericardial fluid
Positive Gram stain/culture
CBC with differential
Serum urea and creatinine
Blood cultures
Tuberculin skin test
Antinuclear antibodies
Rheumatoid factor
Serologic tests for Brucella
Salmonella
Toxoplasma
Mycoplasma
Human immunodeficiency virus
Thyrotropin

WBCs, white blood cells; CBC, complete blood cell count.

Most patients who are diagnosed with acute pericarditis have an uneventful recovery with bedrest and anti-inflammatory drug therapy. However, a substantial number of individuals have persistent chest discomfort, fever, leukocytosis, generalized illness, or hemodynamically significant pericardial effusions. In these patients, aggressive diagnostic strategies including pericardiocentesis are warranted (Table 118.5). Despite an aggressive search, a diagnosis is obtained in only approximately 20% of cases (50,51).

Cardiac Ischemia

An imbalance between myocardial oxygen supply and demand is the basic pathophysiologic process for a variety of disease entities. Myocardial infarction, myocardial ischemia, aortic stenosis, hypertrophic cardiomyopathy, right ventricular hypertension, and severe anemia all are associated with the development of such an imbalance. The distinction between these disease processes is made by medical history, symptoms, physical examination, ECG, cardiac enzymes, chest radiographs, and other related studies.

Acute Coronary Syndrome (see below and Chapters 121 and 122)

ST-segment Elevation Myocardial Infarction (see Chapter 122)

Aortic Stenosis

Aortic stenosis is a narrowing of the aortic valve orifice secondary to congenital abnormality, valvular degeneration (calcific), or rheumatic heart disease (see Chapter 125). Discomfort associated with aortic stenosis mimics typical angina pectoris. The clinical presentation of aortic stenosis includes the following:

- Exertional dyspnea
- Chest pain at rest

- Heart gallop
- Forceful localized apical impulse
- Murmur of aortic stenosis
- Decreased aortic component of S_2 or presence of S_4
- Left-axis deviation on ECG
- Left ventricular hypertrophy on ECG

Although the syndrome of chest pain in patients with aortic stenosis is anginal, only 40% of such patients have coronary artery disease. The remaining patients develop ischemia secondary to altered perfusion pressures within a hypertrophied ventricle (52). The diagnosis of aortic stenosis is based on symptoms, with confirmation by echocardiography, coronary angiography, or both; heart catheterization with left ventricular and aortic pressure gradient is also a diagnostic tool. Patients with severe aortic stenosis—less than 1.0 cm^3 valve area—who develop chest pain and hypotension are at a high risk of immediate death and require aggressive management.

Differential Diagnosis: Gastrointestinal Causes of Chest Pain

Unless chest pain is related to obvious life-threatening gastrointestinal disease, many patients initially undergo an evaluation for myocardial ischemia. Most patients with severe gastrointestinal disease have a prior history of gastroesophageal reflux, peptic ulcer disease, caustic ingestion, forceful vomiting, or recent instrumentation.

Esophageal Injury and Rupture

Most causes of esophageal injury are suggested by history. Patients who attempt suicide by ingesting lye or other caustic agents may have obvious injury to the oropharynx. In this circumstance, emergency endoscopy may be warranted. Less obvious causes of chest pain related to esophageal injury include mucosal damage by ingested pills or the presence of pill fragments lodged in the distal esophagus. Occasionally, nasogastric tubes have been found to be the culprit of significant esophageal trauma with resultant chest pain.

Acute increases in intra-abdominal pressure secondary to vomiting, heavy lifting, trauma, or straining during defecation have been associated with esophageal wall tear and rupture. Without a preceding event, making the diagnosis is extremely difficult because this process may easily mimic myocardial infarction, pneumothorax, or esophageal spasm. Undiagnosed esophageal rupture may result in life-threatening mediastinitis. The diagnosis of a nonperforating esophageal injury is frequently obtained by upper endoscopy. The presence of *subcutaneous emphysema, pleural effusion,* or *mediastinal air* on chest radiograph is suggestive of esophageal perforation. This may be confirmed by barium or water-soluble contrast studies of the entire esophagus (see Chapter 160).

Esophageal Spasm

Esophageal spasm is a motility disorder characterized by abnormal lower esophageal sphincter tone. Phasic propulsive contractions cause diffuse spasm of the esophagus. These spasms are associated with substernal chest pain that is squeezing in nature and may occur with exercise, thus making this disorder difficult to distinguish from angina pectoris. Unlike angina pectoris, the discomfort is often induced by very hot or cold liquids. Dysphagia with liquid and solid food may accompany the discomfort.

Once this disease entity is considered, a variety of tests can aid the clinician in establishing the diagnosis. Esophageal scintigraphy, esophageal manometry, and provocative tests all have been used.

NONLIFE-THREATENING CAUSES OF CHEST PAIN

Costochondritis

Inflammation of the costochondral joints frequently results in chest wall pain. This pain is exacerbated by applying pressure over the affected area, by deep breathing, or by coughing. Often, patients can point to the exact area of inflammation.

Herpes Zoster

Reactivation of latent varicella-zoster virus with subsequent posterior root neuronal viral replication and inflammation can result in severe chest pain. This process can be triggered by trauma, surgery, immunosuppression, and a multitude of other immunologic stresses. The distribution of pain is usually along a particular dermatome, with eventual eruption of vesiculopustules on an erythematous base. The Tzanck test demonstrating multinucleated giant epidermal cells is diagnostic.

Asthma and Chronic Obstructive Lung Disease

A well-known association exists between atypical chest pain and obstructive lung disease. Patients describe a variety of symptoms ranging from sharp stabbing discomfort to pressure-like sensations. Bronchodilators may provide relief in some patients.

Psychosomatic Chest Pain

Psychosomatic chest pain is a diagnosis of exclusion. Patients may present with either classic or atypical symptoms. Significant coronary artery disease is frequently excluded by coronary angiography. Many of these patients have clinical depression and need aggressive intervention.

Summary

The evaluation of patients with chest pain should be organized and proceed rapidly in logical sequence. The evaluation should include a review of the patient's past medical history, history of present illness, risk factors, and a detailed physical examination. This initial evaluation should narrow the differential diagnosis and direct the clinician so that appropriate tests or procedures are performed.

EVALUATION OF ACUTE CORONARY SYNDROMES

Immediate Concerns

Acute coronary syndrome (ACS) is a broad term that encompasses a range of acute manifestations of coronary atherosclerosis, including ST-segment elevation myocardial infarction (see Chapter 122), non–ST-segment elevation myocardial infarction (N-STEMI), and unstable angina (UA) (see Chapter 123). The diagnosis and the optimal treatment of these patients may be associated with significant improvement in outcome and survival. We focus on patients with UA/N-STEMI, although, as noted above, there are separate chapters within this textbook that will deal with these topics in detail.

Main Tips

When confronted with a patient suffering from acute coronary syndrome (UA/N-STEMI):

1. Obtain a careful history and perform a meticulous physical examination (Table 118.1), particularly in patients with atypical chest pain, which is commonly seen in the ICU, to exclude:
   - Noncardiac causes of chest pain
   - Nonischemic cardiac disorders (pericarditis, valvular disease)
   - Precipitating extracardiac causes (anemia)
   - Signs of potential hemodynamic instability
2. Monitor ECG and repeat marker of myonecrosis if initially negative (at least 6 hours after initial measurement).
3. Perform echocardiography to identify regional dysfunction and/or nonischemic disorders.
4. After confirmation of the diagnosis, start medical therapy as soon as possible.
5. Risk stratification: high-risk patients may benefit from aggressive antiplatelet therapy and early angiography and revascularization.

Clinical Evaluation

Patients with acute coronary syndromes should undergo rapid and accurate evaluation (see Chapters 120, 121 and 122). Obtaining a careful history and a meticulous physical examination are mandatory as a guide toward a definite diagnosis, which may influence therapeutic strategies.

Unstable angina is defined as angina pectoris (or equivalent type of ischemic discomfort) with at least one of the three features:

1. Occurrence at rest (or with minimal exertion) and lasting more than 20 minutes (if not interrupted by nitroglycerin)
2. Severe new-onset chest pain (i.e., within 1 month)
3. Occurrence with a crescendo pattern (i.e., more severe, prolonged, or frequent than previously) (53,54)

These symptoms may be associated with ECG changes, such as inversion of T waves or ST-segment depression, and elevation of cardiac biomarkers of necrosis (such as CK-MB or troponin T or I, or both); when this is the case, the condition is defined as non–ST-segment elevation myocardial infarction (53,54). Asymptomatic patients with ECG changes and/or elevation of cardiac enzymes are also included in these categories. ST-segment elevation myocardial infarction is defined as prolonged chest pain at rest (greater than 30 minutes), the presence of ST-segment elevation in the 12-lead ECG (more than 0.1 mV in at least two contiguous peripheral leads or more than 0.2 mV in at least two contiguous chest leads), or new-onset left bundle branch block (see Chapter 122).

The discomfort associated with acute coronary syndromes typically radiates to the left shoulder and the left arm, and may be associated with diaphoresis, nausea, and vomiting. Left ventricular failure—manifested by pulmonary edema and shock—may occur. During attacks, increased heart rate, distant heart sounds, and a diffuse apical impulse may develop. Localized papillary muscle dysfunction may cause the late systolic murmur of mitral regurgitation. The tools for diagnosing the problem include ECG changes during attacks, biomarkers, echocardiography, nuclear medicine scan, exercise stress testing, CT scan, and cardiac catheterization.

Risk Stratification

Due to differences in the extent and severity of underlying coronary artery disease, and the different degree of thrombotic risk, identification of high-risk patients is of high clinical relevance in order to prevent, by adequate pharmacologic therapies and mechanical revascularization, the progression and the extent of myocardial infarction and the risk of death (53–55). As previously noted, medical history, clinical examination, ECG, and biomarkers provide key elements for risk assessment (Fig. 118.3).

The characteristics of patients with non–ST-segment elevation ACS at high risk for rapid progression to myocardial infarction or death who should undergo coronary angiography within 48 hours include:

- Recurrent rest pain
- Dynamic ST-segment changes: ST-segment depression of more than or equal to 0.1 mV or transient (less than 30 minutes) ST-segment elevation more than or equal to 0.1 mV
- Elevated troponin-I, troponin-T, or CK-MB levels
- Hemodynamic instability within the observation period
- Major dysrhythmias (ventricular tachycardia, ventricular fibrillation)
- Early postinfarction unstable angina (56–60)

Furthermore, the following markers of severe underlying disease (i.e., a high long-term risk) might also be helpful for risk assessment in non–ST-segment elevation ACS:

- Age older than 65 to 70 years
- History of known coronary artery disease, previous MI, prior percutaneous coronary intervention (PCI), or coronary artery bypass grafting (CABG)
- Congestive heart failure, pulmonary edema, and new mitral regurgitant murmur
- Elevated inflammatory markers (i.e., C-reactive protein [CRP], fibrinogen, interleukin (IL)-6)
- BNP or NT-proBNP in upper quartiles
- Renal insufficiency

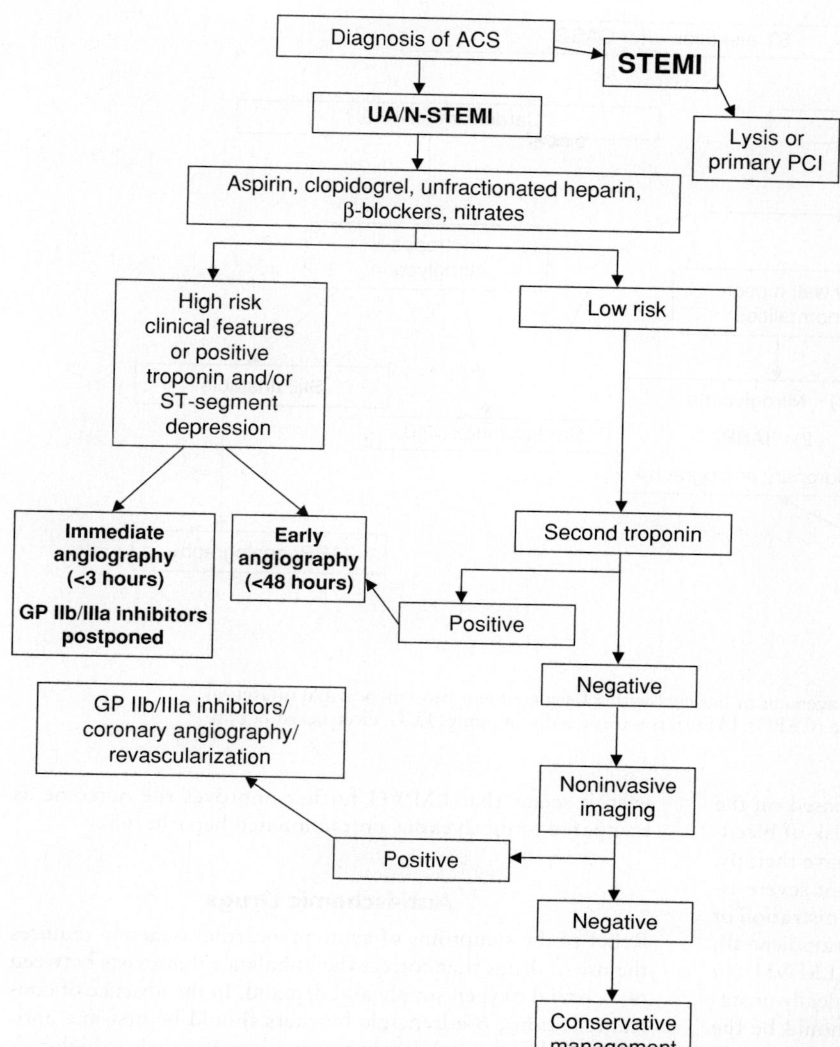

FIGURE 118.3. Algorithm on management of patients with acute coronary syndrome (ACS). STEMI, ST-segment elevation myocardial infarction; UA, unstable angina; N-STEMI, non–ST-segment elevation myocardial infarction; GP, glycoprotein.

The Thrombolysis in Myocardial Infarction (TIMI) risk score has been shown to be an accurate tool for risk stratification that can be easily applied at the bedside of a patient with N-STEMI (61).

Perioperative Management

Cardiac Surgery

Despite improvements in intraoperative myocardial protection, between 5% and 15% of patients undergoing cardiac surgery actually experience a perioperative myocardial infarction due to diffuse atherosclerotic disease of the distal coronary arteries, spasm, embolism, thrombosis of native coronary vessels or bypass graft, technical problems with graft anastomoses, or increased myocardial oxygen need (as in left ventricular hypertrophy).

The diagnosis of postoperative MI is difficult because of the nonspecific ST–T-wave abnormalities frequently present in those patients. In addition, troponins are elevated in almost all patients who undergo CABG. A 12-lead ECG should be obtained upon arrival in the ICU after surgery and every 24 hours, since it represents the most reliable tool to diagnose perioperative MI. CK and CK-MB should be evaluated every 8 hours for the first 36 hours, if postprocedural MI is suspected. Bedside echocardiography, by detecting new regional wall motion abnormalities, represents a major diagnostic tool, particularly when ECG and serum marker measurements are unclear. The appropriate management strategy should be defined according to an integrated evaluation of clinical findings and diagnostic tests (Fig. 118.4).

Major Noncardiac Surgery

Myocardial infarction and ischemia occurring during or after major noncardiac surgery are difficult to diagnose, since they are often silent and because of the confounding effects of analgesics and postoperative surgical pain. The diagnosis is often based on evaluation of cardiac troponins, since CK and CK-MB are less specific and may be elevated during aortic surgery or mesenteric ischemia. Furthermore, most perioperative MIs are non–Q wave, and nonspecific ST changes are common after surgery with or without MI. Echocardiography may certainly help by identifying new wall motion abnormalities.

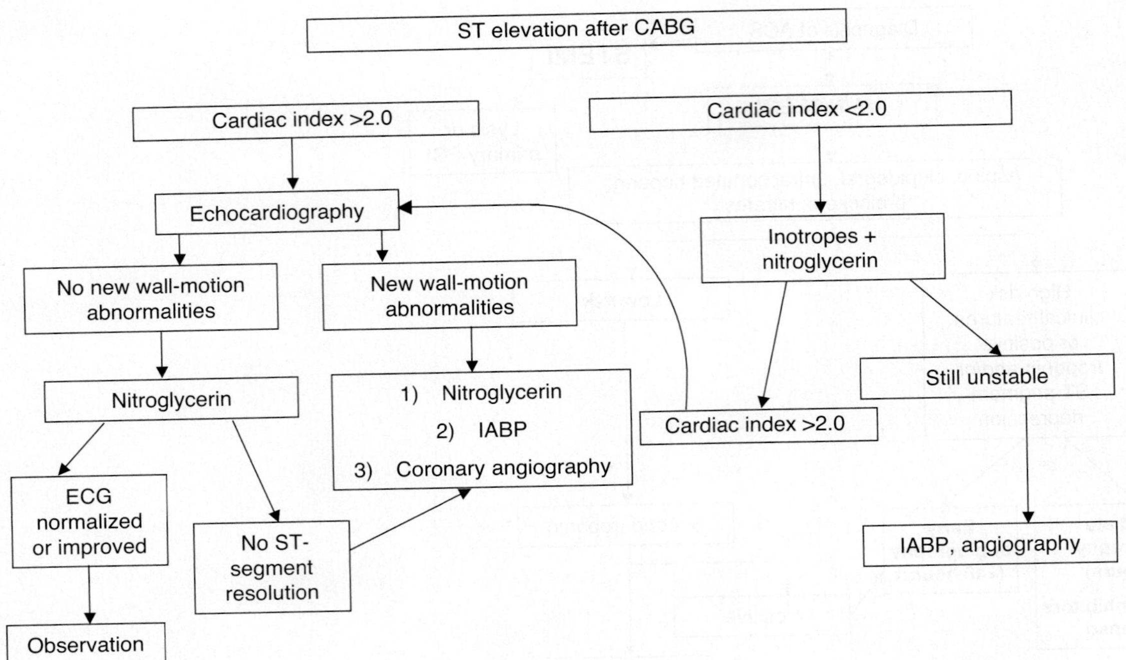

FIGURE 118.4. Algorithm on management of patients with ST-segment elevation myocardial infarction after coronary artery bypass grafting (CABG). IABP, intra-aortic balloon pump; ECG, electrocardiogram.

The management of these patients should be based on the extension and severity of ischemia, weighing the risk of bleeding complications and the benefits from an aggressive therapy. Patients in stable hemodynamic condition, without severe ischemia, may be managed conservatively with administration of acetylsalicylic acid (ASA), β-blockers (if not contraindicated), nitroglycerin, and low-molecular-weight heparin (LMWH). In patients with large STEMI or who are hemodynamically unstable, immediate coronary angiography and PCI should be the preferred strategy.

Drug Therapy

The main objectives of medical therapy in patients with ACS are to stabilize and "cool" the culprit lesion, treat residual ischemia, and prevent long-term complications.

Antiplatelet and Anticoagulation Therapies

Aspirin and clopidogrel, as shown by several large randomized trials (62,63), improve the outcome, and thus represent a cornerstone in the initial treatment of ACS. Glycoprotein IIb/IIIa inhibitors have been shown to reduce mortality. However, the benefits were restricted to patients with positive troponin. A strategy of upstream administration—starting 48 hours before angiography—is currently recommended with eptifibatide or tirofiban. Abciximab may be considered for downstream administration in the cardiac catheterization laboratory in patients with positive troponin undergoing percutaneous revascularization due to the significant benefits shown in a recent randomized trial (64).

Intravenous heparin or LMWH are considered a fundamental therapy for treating ACS and are a class IA therapy when given in conjunction with antiplatelet agents (53–55). However, it seems that LMWH further improves the outcome as compared to intravenous unfractionated heparin (65).

Anti-ischemic Drugs

Relief of the symptoms of acute myocardial ischemia requires the use of drugs that correct the imbalance that exists between myocardial oxygen supply and demand. In the absence of contraindications, β-adrenergic blockers should be first-line anti-ischemic therapy and should be given intravenously in high-risk patients, particularly if ischemia is ongoing. A meta-analysis of three randomized clinical trials comparing β-blockers with placebo in unstable angina showed a significant reduction in rates of progression to acute myocardial infarction, but not death, by active treatment (66).

There are no randomized, placebo-controlled trials investigating the effect of nitrates on symptoms or prognosis in ACS. A number of small, uncontrolled datasets have been published (67,68), but the routine use of this group of drugs is almost entirely based on anecdotal experience of their efficacy in relieving symptoms. It is recommended that sublingual glyceryl trinitrate should be given in all cases where ischemic chest discomfort is present at the time of initial clinical assessment. If symptoms are not relieved rapidly thereafter and after administration of intravenous β-blockers, an intravenous nitrate infusion should be started.

Randomized studies of calcium channel blockers in ACS have shown their efficacy in relieving symptoms (69,70). In addition, diltiazem may have a protective effect (71,72), whereas there is strong evidence that immediate-release nifedipine (a dihydropyridine) increases mortality rate, particularly if given without β-blockers (73,74). Current guidelines recommend reserving the dihydropyridine calcium antagonists for use as second- or third-line therapy after β-blockers and nitrates, whereas the rate-limiting, nondihydropyridine agents (diltiazem and verapamil) may be reasonable alternatives when β-blockers are contraindicated.

Statins represent the main agents for treatment of hypercholesterolemia today. Recent studies have shown that their effects on progression of atherosclerosis may be explained by additional properties beyond lowering cholesterol (75–77). In particular, their antithrombotic and anti-inflammatory properties make statins a therapeutically attractive option in ACS patients. In fact, early statin therapy has been shown to be associated with a significant improvement in clinical outcome (78), and is strongly recommended after ACS (53,54).

SUMMARY

The evaluation of patients with ACS should be organized and proceed rapidly in logical sequence. The evaluation should include a review of the patient's past medical history, history of present illness, risk factors, and a detailed physical examination, to exclude noncardiac or nonischemic disorders and precipitating extracardiac causes. After confirmation of the diagnosis, all patients should be treated with optimal medical therapy. Risk stratification is mandatory, since high-risk patients may benefit from aggressive antiplatelet therapy and early angiography and revascularization, whereas patients at lower risk should undergo early, noninvasive testing for inducible myocardial ischemia, followed by coronary angiography when such testing is positive.

References

1. Lee T, Goldmann L. Evaluation of the patients with acute chest pain. *N Eng J Med.* 2006;342:1187–1195.
2. Puleo PR, Meyer D, Wathen C, et al. Use of a rapid assay of subforms of creatine kinase-MB to diagnose or rule out acute myocardial infarction. *N Engl J Med.* 1994;331:561–566.
3. Newby LK, Goldmann BU, Ohman EM. Troponin: an important prognostic marker and risk-stratification tool in non-ST-segment elevation acute coronary syndromes. *J Am Coll Cardiol.* 2003;41(4 Suppl S):31S–36S.
4. Korff S, Katus HA, Giannitsis E. Differential diagnosis of elevated troponin. *Heart.* 2006;92:987–993.
5. de Winter RJ, Koster RW, Sturk A, et al. Value of myoglobin, troponin T, and CK-MBmass in ruling out an acute myocardial infarction in the emergency room. *Circulation.* 1995;92:3401–3407.
6. Konstantinides S, Geibel A, Olschewski M, et al. Importance of cardiac troponins I and T in risk stratification of patients with acute pulmonary embolism. *Circulation.* 2002;106:1263–1268.
7. Giannitsis E, Muller-Bardorff M, Kurowski V, et al. Independent prognostic value of cardiac troponin T in patients with confirmed pulmonary embolism. *Circulation.* 2000;102:211–217.
8. Kucher N, Goldhaber SZ. Cardiac biomarkers for risk stratification of patients with acute pulmonary embolism. *Circulation.* 2003;108:2191–2194.
9. Panteghini M. Role and importance of biochemical markers in clinical cardiology. *Eur Heat J.* 2004;25:1187–1196.
10. Wakai A, Gleeson A, Winter D. Role of fibrin D-dimer testing in emergency medicine. *Emerg Med J.* 2003;20:319–325.
11. Kang DH, Kang SJ, Song JM, et al. Efficacy of myocardial contrast echocardiography in the diagnosis and risk stratification of acute coronary syndrome. *Am J Cardiol.* 2005;96:1498–1502.
12. Tsai TT, Nienaber CA, Eagle KA. Acute aortic syndromes. *Circulation.* 2005;112:3802–3813.
13. Conti A, Zanobetti M, Grifoni S, et al. Implementation of myocardial perfusion imaging in the early triage of patients with suspected acute coronary syndromes. *Nucl Med Commun.* 2003;24:1055–1060.
14. Wackers FJ, Brown KA, Heller GV, et al. American Society of Nuclear Cardiology position statement on radionuclide imaging in patients with suspected acute ischemic syndromes in the emergency department or chest pain center. *J Nucl Cardiol.* 2002;9:246–250.
15. Bulow H, Schwaiger M. Nuclear cardiology in acute coronary syndromes. *Q J Nucl Med Mol Imaging.* 2005;49:59–71.
16. Schuijf JD, Bax JJ, Shaw LJ, et al. Meta-analysis of comparative diagnostic performance of magnetic resonance imaging and multislice computed tomography for noninvasive coronary angiography. *Am Heart J.* 2006;151:404–411.
17. Gallagher MJ, Ross MA, Raff GL, et al. The diagnostic accuracy of 64-slice computed tomography coronary angiography compared with stress nuclear imaging in emergency department low-risk chest pain patients. *Ann Emerg Med.* 2007;49(2):125–136.
18. van Belle A, Buller HR, Huisman MV, et al. Effectiveness of managing suspected pulmonary embolism using an algorithm combining clinical probability, D-dimer testing, and computed tomography. *JAMA.* 2006;295:172–179.
19. Erbel R, Alfonso F, Boileau C, et al. Task Force on Aortic Dissection, European Society of Cardiology. Diagnosis and management of aortic dissection. *Eur Heart J.* 2001;22:1642–1681.
20. Ohno Y, Higashino T, Takenaka D, et al. MR angiography with sensitivity encoding (SENSE) for suspected pulmonary embolism: comparison with MDCT and ventilation-perfusion scintigraphy. *AJR Am J Roentgenol.* 2004;183:91–98.
21. Richter JE. Overview of diagnostic testing for chest pain of unknown origin. *Am J Med.* 1992;92:41S.
22. Levine HJ. Difficult problems in the diagnosis of chest pain. *Am Heart J.* 1980;100:108.
23. Christie LG Jr, Conti CR. Systematic approach to evaluation of angina-like chest pain: pathophysiology and clinical testing with emphasis on objective documentation of myocardial ischemia. *Am Heart J.* 1981;102:897.
24. Rude RE, Poole VVK, Muller JE, et al. Electrocardiographic and clinical criteria for recognition of acute myocardial infarction based on analysis of 3,697 patients. *Am J Cardiol.* 1983;52:936.
25. Bell WR, Simon TL, DeMets DL. The clinical features of submassive and massive pulmonary emboli. *Am J Med.* 1977;62:355.
26. Piazza G, Goldhaber SZ. Acute pulmonary embolism. Part I: epidemiology and diagnosis. *Circulation.* 2006;114:e28–e32.
27. PIOPED Investigators. Value of ventilation/perfusion scan in acute pulmonary embolism: results of the Prospective Investigation of Pulmonary Embolism Diagnosis (PIOPED). *JAMA.* 1990;263:2753.
28. Goldhaber SZ, Norpurgo M. Diagnosis, treatment and prevention of pulmonary embolism. *JAMA.* 1972;268:1727.
29. Tocino IM, Miller MH, Fairfax WR. Distribution of pneumothorax in the supine and semirecumbent critically ill adult. *AJR Am J Roentgenol.* 1981; 137:699.
30. Ziter FMH, Westcott JL. Supine subpulmonic pneumothorax. *AJR Am J Roentgenol.* 1981;137:699.
31. DeSanctis RW, Doroghazi RM, Austen WG, et al. Aortic dissection. *N Engl J Med.* 1987;317:1060–1067.
32. Suzuki T, Mehta RH, Ince H, et al. Clinical profiles and outcomes of acute type B aortic dissection in the current era: lessons from the International Registry of Aortic Dissection (IRAD). *Circulation.* 2003;108(suppl II):II-312–II-317.
33. Erbel R, Oelert H, Meyer J, et al. Effect of medical and surgical therapy on aortic dissection evaluated by transesophageal echocardiography: implications for prognosis and therapy: the European Cooperative Study Group on Echocardiography. *Circulation.* 1993;87:1604–1615.
34. Glower DD, Speier RH, White WD, et al. Management and long-term outcome of aortic dissection. *Ann Surg.* 1991;214:31–41.
35. Cambria RP, Brewster DC, Gertler J, et al. Vascular complications associated with spontaneous aortic dissection. *J Vasc Surg.* 1988;7:199.
36. Chan K. Impact of transesophageal echocardiography on the treatment of patients with aortic dissection. *Chest.* 1992;101:406.
37. Cigarroa JE, Isselbacher EM, DeSanctis RW, et al. Diagnostic imaging in the evaluation of suspected aortic dissection: old standards and new directions. *N Engl J Med.* 1993;328:35.
38. Nienaber CA, Spielmann RP, von Kodolitsch Y, et al. Diagnosis of thoracic aortic dissection: magnetic resonance imaging versus transesophageal echocardiography. *Circulation.* 1991;85:434.
39. Nienaber CA, von Kodolitsch Y, Petersen B, et al. Intramural hemorrhage of the thoracic aorta: diagnostic and therapeutic implications. *Circulation.* 1995;92:1465–1472.
40. Vilacosta I, San Roman JA, Ferreiros J, et al. Natural history and serial morphology of aortic intramural hematoma: a novel variant of aortic dissection. *Am Heart J.* 1997;134:495–507.
41. Yacoub MH, Gehle P, Chandrasekaran V, et al. Late results of a valve-preserving operation in patients with aneurysms of the ascending aorta and root. *J Thorac Cardiovasc Surg.* 1998;115:1080–1090.
42. Maraj R, Rerkpattanapipat P, Jacobs LE, et al. Meta-analysis of 143 reported cases of aortic intramural hematoma. *Am J Cardiol.* 2000;86:664–668.
43. von Kodolitsch Y, Nienaber CA. Ulcer of the thoracic aorta: diagnosis, therapy and prognosis [in German]. *Z Kardiol.* 1998;87:917–927.
44. Stanson AW, Kazmier FJ, Hollier LH, et al. Penetrating atherosclerotic ulcers of the thoracic aorta: natural history and clinicopathologic correlations. *Ann Vasc Surg.* 1986;1:15–23.
45. Movsowitz HD, Lampert C, Jacobs LE, et al. Penetrating atherosclerotic aortic ulcers. *Am Heart J.* 1994;128:1210–1217.

46. Ganaha F, Miller DC, Sugimoto K, et al. Prognosis of aortic intramural hematoma with and without penetrating atherosclerotic ulcer: a clinical and radiological analysis. *Circulation.* 2002;106:342–348.
47. Horowitz MS, Schults CS, Stinson EB, et al. Sensitivity and specificity of echocardiographic diagnosis of pericardial effusion. *Circulation.* 1974;50:239.
48. Spodick DH. Arrhythmias during acute pericarditis (100) cases. *JAMA.* 1976;235:39.
49. Spodick DH. Diagnostic electrocardiographic sequences in acute pericarditis. *Circulation.* 1973;48:575.
50. Zayas R, Anguita M, Torres F, et al. Incidence of specific etiology and role of methods for specific diagnosis of primary acute pericarditis. *Am J Cardiol.* 1995;75:378.
51. Permanyer-Miralda G, Sagrista-Sauleda J, Soler-Soler J. Primary acute pericardial disease: a prospective series of 231 consecutive patients. *Am J Cardiol.* 1985;56:623.
52. Marcus ML, Doty DB, Hiratzka LF, et al. Decreased coronary reserve: a mechanism for angina pectoris in patients with aortic stenosis and normal coronary arteries. *N Engl J Med.* 1982;307:1362.
53. Bertrand ME, Simoons ML, Fox KA, et al. Task Force on the Management of Acute Coronary Syndromes of the European Society of Cardiology. Management of acute coronary syndromes in patients presenting without persistent ST-segment elevation. *Eur Heart J.* 2002;23(23):1809–1840.
54. Gibler WB, Cannon CP, Blomkalns AL, et al. American Heart Association Council on Clinical Cardiology (Subcommittee on Acute Cardiac Care); Council on Cardiovascular Nursing, and Quality of Care and Outcomes Research Interdisciplinary Working Group; Society of Chest Pain Centers. Practical implementation of the guidelines for unstable angina/non-ST-segment elevation myocardial infarction in the emergency department: a scientific statement from the American Heart Association Council on Clinical Cardiology (Subcommittee on Acute Cardiac Care), Council on Cardiovascular Nursing, and Quality of Care and Outcomes Research Interdisciplinary Working Group, in collaboration with the Society of Chest Pain Centers. *Circulation.* 2005;111:2699–2710.
55. Silber S, Albertsson P, Aviles FF, et al. Task Force for Percutaneous Coronary Interventions of the European Society of Cardiology. Guidelines for percutaneous coronary interventions. The Task Force for Percutaneous Coronary Interventions of the European Society of Cardiology. *Eur Heart J.* 2005; 26:804–847.
56. McKay RG. "Ischemia-guided" versus "early invasive" strategies in the management of acute coronary syndrome/non-ST-segment elevation myocardial infarction: the interventionalist's perspective. *J Am Coll Cardiol.* 2003;41:96S–102S.
57. Antman EM, Cohen M, Bernink PJ, et al. The TIMI risk score for unstable angina/non-ST elevation MI: a method for prognostication and therapeutic decision making. *JAMA.* 2000;284:835–842.
58. Garcia S, Canoniero M, Peter A, et al. Correlation of TIMI risk score with angiographic severity and extent of coronary artery disease in patients with non-ST-elevation acute coronary syndromes. *Am J Cardiol.* 2004;93:813–816.
59. Boersma E, Pieper KS, Steyerberg EW, et al. Predictors of outcome in patients with acute coronary syndromes without persistent ST-segment elevation. Results from an international trial of 9461 patients. The PURSUIT Investigators. *Circulation.* 2000;101:2557–2567.
60. Cannon CP. Evidence-based risk stratification to target therapies in acute coronary syndromes. *Circulation.* 2002;106:1588–1591.
61. Antman EM, Cohen M, Bernink PJ, et al. The TIMI risk score for unstable angina/non-ST elevation MI: a method for prognostication and therapeutic decision making. *JAMA.* 2000;284:835–842.
62. Risk of myocardial infarction and death during treatment with low dose aspirin and intravenous heparin in men with unstable coronary artery disease. The RISC Group. *Lancet.* 1990;336:827–830.
63. Yusuf S, Zhao F, Mehta SR, et al., Clopidogrel in Unstable Angina to Prevent Recurrent Events Trial Investigators. Effects of clopidogrel in addition to aspirin in patients with acute coronary syndromes without ST-segment elevation. *N Engl J Med.* 2001;345:494–502.
64. Kastrati A, Mehilli J, Neumann FJ, et al. Intracoronary Stenting and Antithrombotic: Regimen Rapid Early Action for Coronary Treatment 2 (ISAR-REACT 2) Trial Investigators. Abciximab in patients with acute coronary syndromes undergoing percutaneous coronary intervention after clopidogrel pretreatment: the ISAR-REACT 2 randomized trial. *JAMA.* 2006;295:1531–1538.
65. Petersen JL, Mahaffey KW, Hasselblad V, et al. Efficacy and bleeding complications among patients randomized to enoxaparin or unfractionated heparin for antithrombin therapy in non-ST-segment elevation acute coronary syndromes: a systematic overview. *JAMA.* 2004;292:89–96.
66. Yusuf S, Wittes J, Friedman L. Overview of results of randomized clinical trials in heart disease. II. Unstable angina, heart failure, primary prevention with aspirin, and risk factor modification. *JAMA.* 1988;260:2259–2263.
67. Kaplan K, Davison R, Parker M, et al. Intravenous nitroglycerin for the treatment of angina at rest unresponsive to standard nitrate therapy. *Am J Cardiol.* 1983;51:694–698.
68. Roubin GS, Harris PJ, Eckhardt I, et al. Intravenous nitroglycerine in refractory unstable angina pectoris. *Aust N Z J Med.* 1982;12:598–602.
69. Theroux P, Taeymans Y, Morissette D, et al. A randomized study comparing propranolol and diltiazem in the treatment of unstable angina. *J Am Coll Cardiol.* 1985;5:717–722.
70. Parodi O, Simonetti I, Michelassi C, et al. Comparison of verapamil and propranolol therapy for angina pectoris at rest: a randomized, multiple-crossover, controlled trial in the coronary care unit. *Am Cardiol.* 1986;57:899–906.
71. Gibson RS, Hansen JF, Messerli F, et al. Long-term effects of diltiazem and verapamil on mortality and cardiac events in non-Q-wave acute myocardial infarction without pulmonary congestion: post hoc subset analysis of the multicenter diltiazem postinfarction trial and the second Danish verapamil infarction trial studies. *Am J Cardiol.* 2000;86:275–279.
72. Gibson RS, Young PM, Boden WE, et al. Prognostic significance and beneficial effect of diltiazem on the incidence of early recurrent ischemia after non-Q-wave myocardial infarction: results from the multicenter diltiazem reinfarction study. *Am J Cardiol.* 1987;60:203–209.
73. Yusuf S, Held P, Furberg C. Update of effects of calcium antagonists in myocardial infarction or angina in light of the second Danish verapamil infarction trial (DAVIT-II) and other recent studies. *Am J Cardiol.* 1991;67:1295–1297.
74. Psaty BM, Heckbert SR, Koepsell TD, et al. The risk of myocardial infarction associated with antihypertensive drug therapies. *JAMA.* 1995;274:620–625.
75. Undas A, Brozek J, Musial J. Anti-inflammatory and antithrombotic effects of statins in the management of coronary artery disease. *Clin Lab.* 2002;48:287–296.
76. Thompson PD, Moyna NM, White CM, et al. The effects of hydroxy-methylglutaryl co-enzyme A reductase inhibitors on platelet thrombus formation. *Atherosclerosis.* 2002;161:301–306.
77. Dangas G, Badimon JJ, Smith DA, et al. Pravastatin therapy in hyperlipidemia: effects on thrombus formation and the systemic hemostatic profile. *J Am Coll Cardiol.* 1999;33:1294–1304.
78. Schwartz GG, Olsson AG, Ezekowitz MD, et al. Myocardial Ischemia Reduction with Aggressive Cholesterol Lowering (MIRACL) Study Investigators. Effects of atorvastatin on early recurrent ischemic events in acute coronary syndromes: the MIRACL study: a randomized controlled trial. *JAMA.* 2001;285:1711–1718.

CHAPTER 119 ■ NON ST ELEVATION ACUTE CORONARY SYNDROME: CONTEMPORARY MANAGEMENT STRATEGIES

ACHILLE GASPARDONE • LEONARDO DE LUCA

OVERVIEW

Definition of Terms

The term, *acute coronary syndrome* (ACS), describes a spectrum of clinical conditions ranging from ST-segment elevation myocardial infarction (STEMI) to non–ST-segment elevation MI (N–STEMI) and unstable angina (UA) (Fig. 119.1) (1). These manifestations of acute myocardial ischemia may revert to the presymptomatic state or evolve into a non-Q wave (also termed nontransmural) MI or to Q wave (or transmural) MI (Fig. 119.1).

The boundaries between UA, N-STEMI, and STEMI are not always well defined. Indeed, the three entities should be considered as different and dynamic clinical manifestations of a continuous pathogenetic spectrum; N-STE-ACS are represented by UA and N-STEMI.

Unstable Angina (UA)

Anginal pain is the pivotal symptom for the diagnosis of UA, and its intensity, duration, and exercise-related threshold are usually graded according to the Canadian Cardiovascular Society (CCS) classification (Table 119.1) (2). UA may have three clinical presentations (Table 119.2) (3): (1) *de novo* or new-onset angina of at least CCS III-IV severity in patients without previously diagnosed angina; (2) *crescendo,* or increasing angina in patients with previously diagnosed angina that has become significantly more frequent, more severe in duration, and with a markedly reduced threshold (CCS Class III-IV); (3) postinfarction angina in patients with an MI within 2 weeks in whom biomarkers of myocardial necrosis have returned within normal range.

In all three clinical presentations of UA, pain may occur at rest and, typically, the low threshold for angina (CCS III and IV) represents an essential clinical feature for the diagnosis of UA. In all three clinical manifestations of UA, the presence of angina at rest is associated with a worse prognosis and a higher rate of events (4). In all cases, of course, it is crucial to exclude extracardiac conditions that can intensify or precipitate myocardial ischemia (secondary UA) such as anemia, fever, infection, hypotension, uncontrolled hypertension, hypoxemia, and thyrotoxicosis. The resting ECG may show ST-segment depression and/or T-wave inversion or transient ST-segment elevation or, rarely, may remain normal. The serum markers (troponin I, troponin T, and CK-MB) may remain within their normal biological ranges or fall between the normal range and the level diagnostic of myocardial infarction, the latter being, according to ACC/AHA recommendations, more than twice the upper normal limit (1). In the absence of release of myocardial markers of necrosis, the diagnosis of UA may be made, whereas if markers of myocardial necrosis have been released, the patient with ACS can be considered to have experienced N-STEMI. In the latter condition, ECG ST-segment or T-wave changes may be persistent, whereas in UA, they may or may not occur and, if they are seen, are usually transient.

A peculiar clinical manifestation of UA was described in 1959 by Prinzmetal and associates detailing an atypical ischemic coronary syndrome characterized by sudden onset angina occurring almost exclusively at rest, particularly in the first hours of the day, associated with ST segment elevation on the ECG (1). Because of its peculiar clinical pattern, this acute coronary syndrome was defined as a *variant* form of angina. Prinzmetal and colleagues hypothesized that variant angina is caused by a focal spasm of a coronary artery (5); this initial hypothesis has been convincingly demonstrated by coronary angiography. Variant angina may be associated with acute myocardial infarction, severe cardiac arrhythmias—including ventricular tachycardia and fibrillation, and sudden death. Despite these potentially devastating consequences, long term followup of patients with documented coronary vasospasm is not well documented. In a large population of patients with variant angina—i.e. normal or near normal coronary arteries—and treated with calcium channel blockers, the 7.5-year incidence of sudden death and myocardial infarction were 3.6% and 6.5%, respectively (6). Although the clinical presentation of this variant form of angina is also characterized by instability, with evidence of subendocardial and/or transmural myocardial ischemia, the specific pathogenetic mechanisms—i.e. coronary spasm—is completely different from those leading to N-STE-ACS.

Non-ST-Segment Elevation Myocardial Infarction

N-STEMI may have symptoms and a clinical pattern indistinguishable from UA. While the resting ECG more frequently shows ST-segment depression or T-wave inversion (Fig. 119.2), ST-segment elevation, while sometimes observed, is, by definition, never sustained. There will always be a clear-cut rise in the serum biomarkers to levels that are diagnostic for myocardial infarction. Thus, the essential difference between UA and N-STEMI is mainly related to the amount of biomarkers of myocardial injury.

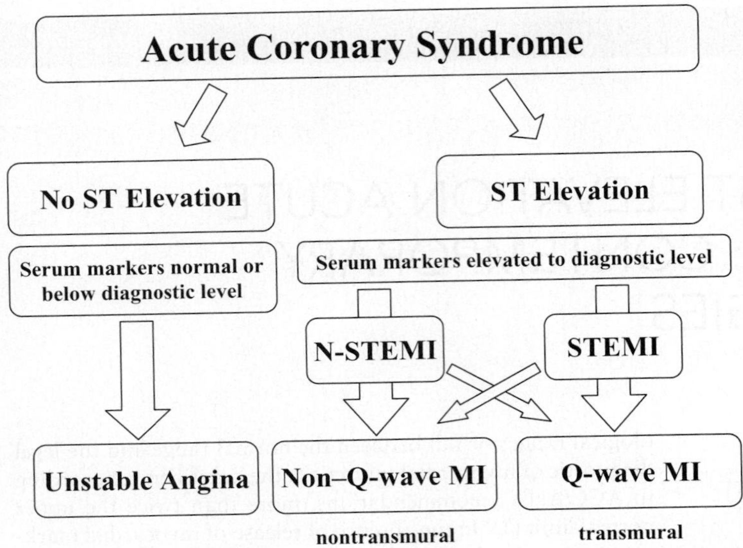

FIGURE 119.1. The interrelationship of the components of ACS on presentation, during evolution and at final outcome [Adapted from Braunwald E, et al. (1)].

Epidemiology of N-STEMI. In the United States, two million patients are admitted annually to cardiac care units with ACS. The number of hospital admissions for patients with UA/N-STEMI is greater than the number with STEMI: 1.4 million and 600,000, respectively (7). The consequences of N-STE-ACS are not benign: among those who reach the hospital alive, approximately 13% of patients will die in the succeeding six months, and 8% will be left with unstable angina (8). The frequency of new stroke ranges between 1.5% and 3%, and rehospitalization for a further episode of ACS ranges between 17% and 20% over the same time interval. Survival data indicate that the risk associated with N-STEMI is greatest during the first 15 to 30 days from symptom presentation.

The Euro Heart Survey–Acute Coronary Syndromes (EHS–ACS) (9) and the Global Registry of Acute Coronary Events (GRACE) studies (8) provided insight into the practice of cardiology in different hospital settings and in different countries. EHS–ACS recorded prospectively 14,271 patients admitted with chest pain, with subsequently documented ACS in 10,484 (73%) of these. GRACE identified, in a prospective or retrospective manner, 11,543 patients with a final diagnosis of myocardial infarction or unstable angina—i.e., an ACS—in 10,709 patients (93%).

In both EHS–ACS and GRACE, about half of all patients underwent diagnostic coronary angiography, and percutaneous revascularization (PCI) was performed in 40% of patients admitted with ST elevation and in about a quarter of patients without initial ST elevation. Inpatient medical therapy included aspirin in over 90% of patients, appropriate use of unfractionated or low molecular weight heparin, but low use of glycoprotein IIb/IIIa receptor blockers when compared to guideline recommendations. Therapy at discharge included aspirin and/or ticlopidine/clopidogrel in over 90% of patients, ACE inhibitors (EHS–ACS 56%, GRACE 55%), β-blockers (EHS–ACS 73%, GRACE 71%), and statins (EHS–ACS 53%, GRACE 47%) (8,9). These findings indicate an increasing awareness of the need for preventive medication in most patients with ACS.

TABLE 119.1

PRINCIPAL PRESENTATIONS OF UNSTABLE ANGINA

New-Onset Angina	New-onset angina of at least CCS Class III severity.
Increasing Angina	Previously diagnosed angina that has become distinctly more frequent, longer in duration, or lower in threshold (i.e., increased by greater than or equal to 1 CCS class to at least CCS Class III severity).
Postinfarction Angina	Patients with recent myocardial infarction (within 2 weeks) in whom biomarkers of myocardial necrosis have returned within normal range.

TABLE 119.2

GRADING OF ANGINA PECTORIS ACCORDING TO THE CANADIAN CARDIOVASCULAR SOCIETY CLASSIFICATION [MODIFIED FROM REFERENCE 1]

I	Ordinary physical activity does not cause angina, such as walking two blocks or climbing stairs. Angina occurs with strenuous, rapid, or prolonged exertion at work or recreation.
II	"Slight limitation of ordinary activity." Angina occurs on walking or climbing stairs rapidly; walking uphill; walking or stair climbing after meals; in cold, in wind, or under emotional stress; or only during the few hours after awakening. Angina occurs on walking more than 2 blocks on level ground and climbing more than 1 flight of ordinary stairs at a normal pace and under normal conditions.
III	"Marked limitations of ordinary physical activity." Angina occurs on walking 1 to 2 blocks on the level and climbing 1 flight of stairs under normal conditions and at a normal pace.
IV	"Inability to carry on any physical activity without discomfort—anginal symptoms may be present at rest."

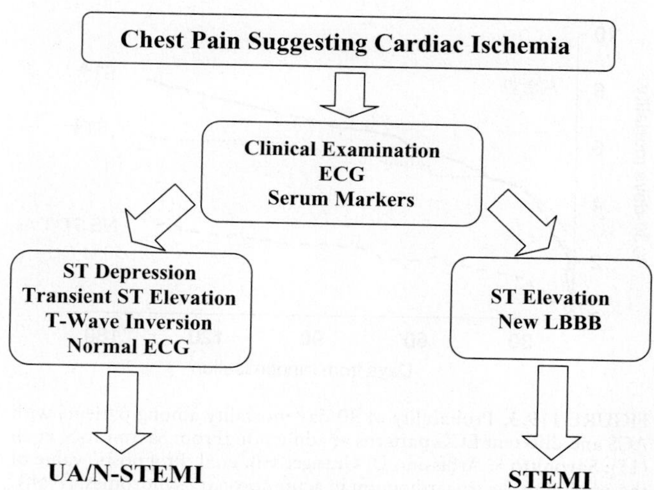

FIGURE 119.2. The differentiation of unstable angina/non–ST-segment elevation myocardial infarction from ST-segment elevation myocardial infarction.

Pathogenesis of N-STE-ACS. N-STE-ACS are usually caused by a sudden reduction of myocardial perfusion resulting from coronary artery narrowing due to a nonocclusive thrombus. The latter, in turn, is a consequence of disruption or erosion of an atherosclerotic coronary artery plaque. Distal microembolization of thrombus and disrupted plaque components may further reduce perfusion of the distal microvasculature. Recent research has focused on the characterization of coronary atherosclerotic plaques more prone to rupture—termed, *vulnerable plaque* (10). The vulnerable plaque is characterized by a necrotic lipid core infiltrated by inflammatory cells—macrophages and lymphocytes, with evidence of intraplaque hemorrhage and abundant generation of *vasa vasorum* on the adventitial site, surrounded by a thin fibrous cap (10). The most convincing hypothesis to explain plaque rupture is based on the critical role of inflammatory mediators driving the expression of proteases and proteolytic inhibitors that progressively weaken the fibrous cap, leading to plaque rupture (11).

The severity of coronary arterial obstruction and the volume of affected myocardium determine the pattern of clinical presentation. Patients with complete occlusion may manifest with a STEMI if the lesion occludes an artery supplying a substantial volume of myocardium, although the same occlusion in the presence of extensive collateralization may manifest as a N-STEMI or UA.

EARLY EVALUATION AND RISK STRATIFICATION

Immediate Concerns

ACS constitutes a clinical emergency. Therefore, early recognition and initiation of treatment is mandatory. Every patient with chest pain should be comprehensively evaluated, including a history and clinical examination of the cardiovascular system, the immediate recording of a resting ECG, and urgent evaluation of the serum markers of myocardial injury. Particular attention must be paid to the factors that influence the patient's risk stratification. These factors are found among the clinical features, the magnitude of ECG change, and the elevation of serum markers of myocardial necrosis. Among those without ST elevation on the ECG, an ACS is diagnosed by the presence of a clinical syndrome of acute ischemia with either pain at rest or a crescendo pattern of ischemic pain with minimal exertion, plus electrocardiographic and/or marker evidence of acute ischemic injury. The predictive accuracy of ST elevation for a final diagnosis of MI is very high, but for non-ST elevation MI, less than 50% are suspected as infarction on initial presentation.

Within the spectrum of ACS, N-STEMI represents the most difficult diagnostic challenge. Separation of N-STEMI from UA is based on the biomarker elevation in the former and the absence of detectable marker release in the latter (repeat assay at 6 to 12 hours after presentation is recommended).

Tools for Risk Stratification

Symptoms and Physical Examination

The features of cardiac ischemic chest pain are usually well recognized. The pain may vary in severity from mild compressive discomfort to sharp, severe pain. It may be located in the anterior chest, particularly substernally, or predominantly involve the mandible, neck, shoulders, either or both arms, the back, or epigastrium. It may be associated with shortness of breath, perspiration, palpitations, nausea or vomiting; however, none of these features predicts the severity of the underlying coronary involvement. The pain is generally of short duration but may last longer than 30 minutes without necessarily resulting in myocardial infarction. In ACS, the chest pain is frequently spontaneous in onset and unrelated to the usual stressors known to precipitate stable angina pectoris. It may occur with no—or less than the usual amount of—provocation, and be more severe or more prolonged. Less frequently, ACS may present with little or no chest pain but, instead, with atypical pain, or it can be accompanied by the features of an acute transient reduction in cardiac output—tachycardia, hypotension, and poor peripheral circulation, pulmonary venous congestion, breathlessness or pulmonary edema or, rarely, a potentially lethal ventricular tachyarrhythmia—a rapid heart rate with a weak or nonpalpable pulse (1).

Male gender, age above 50 years and, in women, early menopause, as well as a history of smoking, dyslipidemia, hypertension, diabetes mellitus, and/or a family history of coronary disease all increase the likelihood of ACS in a given patient with chest pain. Repeated attacks of chest pain or ongoing chest pain before admission, or pain which recurs on treatment, is associated with a worse outcome.

Physical examination often fails to contribute to the diagnosis of ACS. There may be no abnormal findings. However, a fourth heart sound, a mitral regurgitant murmur, or signs of pulmonary congestion are suggestive of transient ischemic myocardial dysfunction (1).

Heart failure (HF) is a frequent complication of ACS (12) and significantly worsens the prognosis of patients with ischemic heart disease (13). In a recent subanalysis of the GRACE Registry, HF on hospital admission was associated with an approximately 3- to 4-fold increase in hospital and 6-month death rates (14). HF was also associated with longer hospital stay and higher readmission rates. As in previous studies, the development of HF during hospital stay—as opposed to HF at admission—was associated with an even worse outcome (13,15). Importantly, there was a reduced frequency of PCI and lower β-blocker usage among patients with HF on admission. Notably, given the high mortality rate of patients with HF and ACS, this group would be expected to derive an even greater benefit from revascularization and, indeed, patients with HF who underwent revascularization had lower cumulative 6-month mortality rates than those who did not, even after adjustment for baseline differences (14).

Electrocardiogram

The presence of ECG changes, especially when occurring at rest and associated with angina, are a powerful indicator of higher risk. ST elevation and ST depression are well recognized electrocardiographic markers of risk. It has been demonstrated that when the other elements of baseline risk have been under control, ST *deviation* conveys the same risk for death whether this deviation is upwards or downwards (16) (Fig. 119.3). New onset T-wave changes—especially T-wave inversion, although less specific—are also important markers of subendocardial ischemia. Clinically, the normalization of ECG alterations and anginal relief are very important within minutes after sublingual nitrate administration; persistence of pain and ECG alterations for more than 20 minutes despite repeated nitrate administration is a marker of increased risk for myocardial infarction (1).

Biochemical Markers

Not all patients presenting with N-STE-ACS have elevated serum markers; at the time of the initial assessment, these markers may be within normal ranges, especially when they have been obtained very shortly after the onset of chest pain. All patients who have normal serum marker results on presentation must have a second assessment 4 to 6 hours later, or 8 to 12 hours after the onset of symptoms, whichever is longer. Elevated levels of creatine kinase (CK), creatine kinase MB iso-enzyme (CK-MB), troponin T or I, and myoglobin are indicators of myocardial injury (Table 119.3).

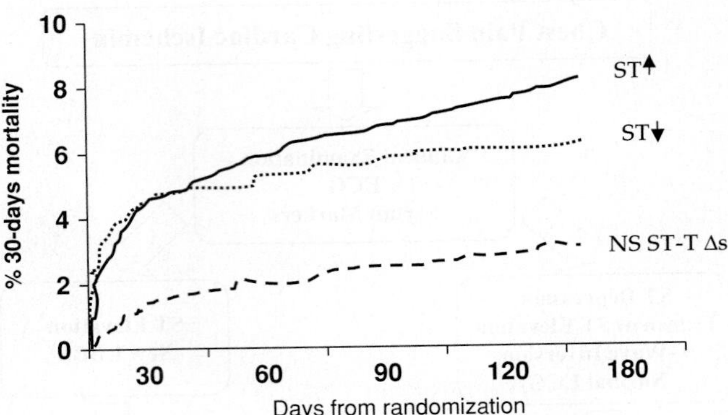

FIGURE 119.3. Probability of 30-day mortality among patients with ACS and different ECG patterns at admission [From Savonitto S, et al. (15): Savonitto S, Ardissino D, Granger CB, et al. Prognostic value of the admission electrocardiogram in acute coronary syndromes. *JAMA.* 1999;281:707–713.]

Myoglobin is the earliest marker of an infarct event to appear in the serum. Although myoglobin is a very sensitive indicator of infarction, its clinical usefulness as the sole marker of myocardial injury/infarction is limited by the high incidence of false-positive results. CK in conjunction with CK-MB, CK-MB alone (17), and the troponins (18) are all sensitive and specific markers of myocardial injury/infarction that appear within the

TABLE 119.3

ADVANTAGES AND DISADVANTAGES OF BIOCHEMICAL CARDIAC MARKERS FOR THE EVALUATION AND MANAGEMENT OF PATIENTS WITH SUSPECTED ACS [MODIFIED FROM BRAUNWALD E, ET AL. (1)].

Marker	Advantages	Disadvantages
CK-MB	1. Rapid, cost-efficient, accurate assays 2. Ability to detect early reinfarction	1. Loss of specificity in setting of skeletal muscle disease or injury, including surgery 2. Low sensitivity during very early MI (less than 6 h after symptom onset) or later after symptom onset (more than 36 h) and for minor myocardial damage (detectable with troponins)
CK-MB Isoforms	1. Early detection of MI	1. Specificity profile similar to that of CK-MB 2. Current assays require special expertise
Myoglobin	1. High sensitivity 2. Useful in early detection of MI 3. Detection of reperfusion 4. Most useful in ruling out MI	1. Very low specificity in setting of skeletal muscle injury or disease 2. Rapid return to normal range limits sensitivity for later presentations
Cardiac Troponins	1. Powerful tool for risk stratification 2. Greater sensitivity and specificity than CK-MB 3. Detection of recent MI up to 2 weeks after onset 4. Useful for selection of therapy 5. Detection of reperfusion	1. Low sensitivity in very early phase of MI (less than 6 h after symptom onset) and requires repeat measurement at 8 to 12 h, if negative 2. Limited ability to detect late minor reinfarction

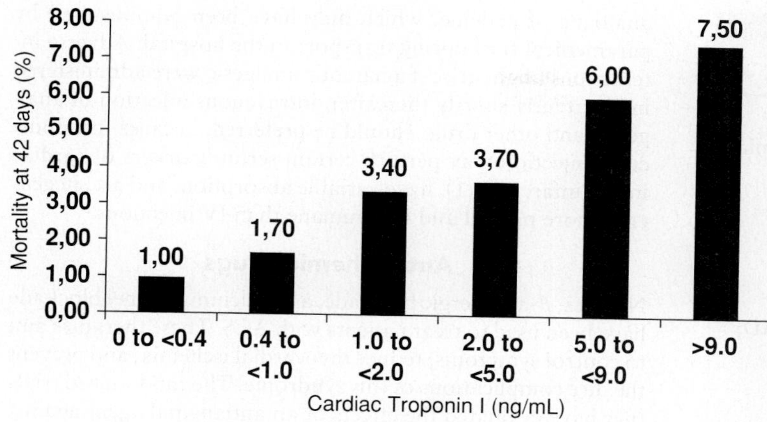

FIGURE 119.4. Relationship between cardiac troponin levels and risk of mortality in patients with ACS. [From Antman EM, et al. (20): Antman EM, Tanasjevic MJ, Thompson B, et al. Cardiac specific troponin I levels to predict the risk of mortality in patients with acute coronary syndromes. *N Engl J Med* 1996;335:1342–1349.]

serum in raised amounts from about 4 hours after the onset of the ischemic event. Whereas CK and CK-MB are cleared from the serum within 2 to 3 days, an elevation of the troponin level may persist for up to 14 days after an event, making the troponins poor markers of early reinfarction.

The bedside use of a "multi-marker strategy" that evaluated CK-MB, troponin I or T, *and* myoglobin in combination proved much superior to any "single-marker" strategy, and was also better than CK-MB and troponin *without* myoglobin in reaching an earlier diagnosis and identifying those at higher risk of death or MI by 30 days (19). Elevated levels of troponin T or I (20–22) or CK-MB (17) on admission indicate a poorer outcome (Fig. 119.4). The later appearance of an elevated troponin level, suggesting ongoing ischemia, is also associated with higher risk (23).

Extensive evidence supports the powerful and independent prediction of thrombotic complications, including MI and death, associated with troponin elevation (21). Furthermore, the evidence from trials of PCI revascularization suggests that troponins can be used as one part of the measures to identify higher risk—although it is not the sole arbiter of risk—and the potential for gain from the interventional procedures (24,25). Newer generation troponin assays have higher sensitivity and diagnostic accuracy. With newer generation assays, very minor increases in troponins are noted when as little as 1 gram of myocardium is necrotic. These minor increases do predict a higher risk of cardiac complications and death. In all instances, the risk predictors should complete, rather than replace, clinical judgment.

Certain biomarkers reflect an upregulation of the inflammatory/thrombotic systems—for example, high sensitivity C reactive protein (hsCRP), interleukin 6 (IL-6), CD40 ligand, and platelet–monocyte complexes. These inflammatory markers may be upregulated before the patient's presentation with ACS, but the acute phase reactant biomarkers are also elevated as a consequence of myocyte injury. Elevation of both hsCRP and troponin signifies a substantially higher risk of death—approximately 14% at one year—than either marker alone. In the absence of both markers, the patient is at very low risk of future cardiac events—less than 2%—based on FRISC 2 data (26). Importantly, whereas troponins predict the hazard of acute events, including acute MI and death, hsCRP on presentation does not independently predict the risk of death during hospitalization but is a powerful predictor of death in the following 1 to 2 years. The extent to which these biomarkers add to the predictive accuracy of established risk models remains to be tested (27). Finally, recent investigations demonstrated the association of a single B-type natriuretic peptide (BNP) measured after presentation with an ACS with short-term and long-term risk of death and HF (28). More recently, changes in BNP over time predicted long-term outcomes, thus providing a tool that could be used to tailor therapy after ACS (29).

Imaging Modalities

Echocardiographic ultrasound evaluation may be extremely useful in early evaluation of left ventricular function and to exclude nonischemic causes of chest pain, ECG alterations, and elevated biomarker levels. With increasing emphasis on early reperfusion and prevention of left ventricular remodeling, echocardiography is also assuming a prominent role in the setting of ACS (30). This imaging modality is noninvasive, cheap, and is an ideal portable imaging technique. Newer modalities, including myocardial contrast echocardiography for the assessment of perfusion, also hold promise (31). Other techniques such as single photon emission computed tomography or magnetic resonance imaging can detect wall motion abnormalities in patients with recent or established infarction, but their role remains to be determined.

After clinical stabilization of low-risk ACS patients, exercise stress testing may be appropriate. Early-onset symptoms during exercise, a short exercise time, a fall in blood pressure during exertion, ST-segment elevation, new postexercise ST-segment depression and/or prolonged ST-segment depression are the characteristics of a strongly positive test. Stress echocardiography and/or myocardial perfusion imaging should be reserved for the patient with a particular clinical problem, when such specialized facilities are available locally. If the functional test demonstrates ischemia, investigation by coronary angiography is advised. The more strongly positive the test, the earlier angiography should be undertaken. Angiography defines the nature and extent of the coronary disease and enables the planning of appropriate revascularization.

ESTIMATION OF THE LEVEL OF RISK AND RISK SCORES

The patient with N-STE-ACS is at risk of major cardiovascular complications and death, and the extent of this risk is

TABLE 119.4

RISK INDICATORS OF A POOR OUTCOME IN ACS

Event-Related	■ Ongoing or recurring chest pain ■ ST-segment depression/new ischemia on ECG ■ Elevated serum biomarkers of cardiac injury/infarction ■ Hemodynamic instability
Preexisting	■ Age over 65 years ■ Three or more risk factors for CAD, especially diabetes mellitus ■ Aspirin use within 7 days ■ Known CAD ■ Prior left ventricular dysfunction

dependent upon acute and preexisting risk factors (Table 119.4). These risk factors not only predict the hazards of early cardiac events, but also of future cerebrovascular and peripheral vascular complications. In such patients, early risk stratification plays a central role, as the benefit of newer, more aggressive, and costly treatment strategies seem to be proportional to the risk of adverse clinical events (32–34) (Figs. 119.5–119.7). Different scores are now available based on initial clinical history, ECG, and laboratory tests that enable early risk stratification on admission (Table 119.5).

The Thrombolysis In Myocardial Infarction (TIMI) (35) and platelet glycoprotein IIb/IIIa in unstable angina: Receptor Suppression Using Integrilin (PURSUIT) (36) scores were developed with the databases from large clinical trials of N-STE-ACS. The more recent Global Registry of Acute Coronary Events (GRACE) score was developed from the registry (27), with a population of patients across the entire spectrum of ACS. All these scores were developed for short-term prognosis: events in-hospital for the GRACE risk score (RS) (37), at 14 days for the TIMI RS, and at 30 days for the PURSUIT RS. Nevertheless, a significant proportion of adverse events in N-STE-ACS patients occur after the first 30 days, and it is not known whether these RSs can also predict their occurrence. On the other hand, it has been demonstrated that an early invasive strategy has a prognostic benefit long term (38). Recently, the GRACE risk model has been demonstrated to have a good predictive accuracy for death or nonfatal MI at 1 year (37).

HOSPITAL CARE AND MANAGEMENT STRATEGIES

Early Pharmacologic Treatment

Control of Pain

While analgesics have no influence on the pathophysiological process, narcotic analgesia with IV morphine sulphate and/or sedation with oral benzodiazepines in standard doses may assist in alleviating the patient's pain and anxiety. As morphine may induce nausea and vomiting, it is advisable to premedicate the patient with IV metoclopramide prior to commencing the IV morphine titration. It is important to be aware of other analgesic treatments such as tramadol, a synthetic analogue of codeine, which may have been administered by paramedical staff during transport to the hospital. Adverse interactions might arise if a narcotic analgesic were administered inadvertently shortly thereafter. Intravenous injection of analgesics and other drugs should be preferred, because intramuscular injection may perturb certain serum markers of cardiac injury/infarction (1), have variable absorption, and are, in general, more painful and less humane than IV injections.

Anti-ischemic Drugs

Nitrates, β-adrenergic blockade, and calcium channel blockade have been used to treat patients with ACS. These therapies aim to control symptoms, reduce myocardial ischemia, and prevent the dire complications of this syndrome. The randomized trials that have evaluated the effects of an antianginal agent against placebo therapy or compared one class of antianginal agent with another in ACS are relatively few and fairly small.

Nitrates. Nitrates act by reducing preload and afterload, promoting coronary vasodilation, relieving coronary vasospasm or vasoconstriction, and by putative effects upon platelet aggregability. These effects combine to improve myocardial blood flow and relieve ischemia. Although nitrates effectively relieve cardiac ischemic pain, they have not been found to improve the outcome in ACS (39). They may be administered sublingually, orally, or intravenously in standard doses (Table 119.6).

Beta-blockers. Beta-blockade reduces myocardial oxygen demand and diminishes ischemia. Although there are large trials that have demonstrated the benefit of β-blockade following acute myocardial infarction, there is limited evaluation of this treatment in N-STE-ACS. The effects of β-blockade upon subsequent myocardial infarction and survival are uncertain. The drugs that have been scrutinized in smaller trials or retrospective subgroup analysis are metoprolol (40), propranolol (41), and esmolol (42). Whichever β-blocker is selected, the dose should be titrated to obtain a resting heart rate of 50 to 60 beats per minute, while maintaining an adequate blood pressure and satisfactory peripheral perfusion.

Calcium Channel Blockers. Calcium channel blockers are a diverse group of compounds that cause smooth muscle relaxation by blocking cellular calcium entry. Their action results in coronary vasodilation and afterload reduction. The dihydropyridine group of calcium channel blockers may increase the resting heart rate, whereas the nondihydropyridine group—diltiazem and verapamil—reduce the resting heart rate, and thus tend to diminish myocardial oxygen demand. The Holland Interuniversity Nifedipine/Metoprolol Trial (40) showed that the short-acting dihydropyridine, nifedipine, was detrimental in comparison with placebo in unstable angina. Calcium channel blockers should be reserved for the control of intractable chest pain or hypertension that cannot be alleviated by other means. Diltiazem is a nondihydropyridine calcium channel blocker that is superior to placebo treatment in reducing reinfarction and postinfarction angina in non-Q wave myocardial infarction (43). Mortality was unaffected in the trial. A trial comparing diltiazem treatment to propranolol found no differences in outcome in groups of patients with unstable angina or Prinzmetal angina (44). In a trial that compared intravenous glyceryl trinitrate with intravenous diltiazem, the combined end point of refractory angina and myocardial infarction

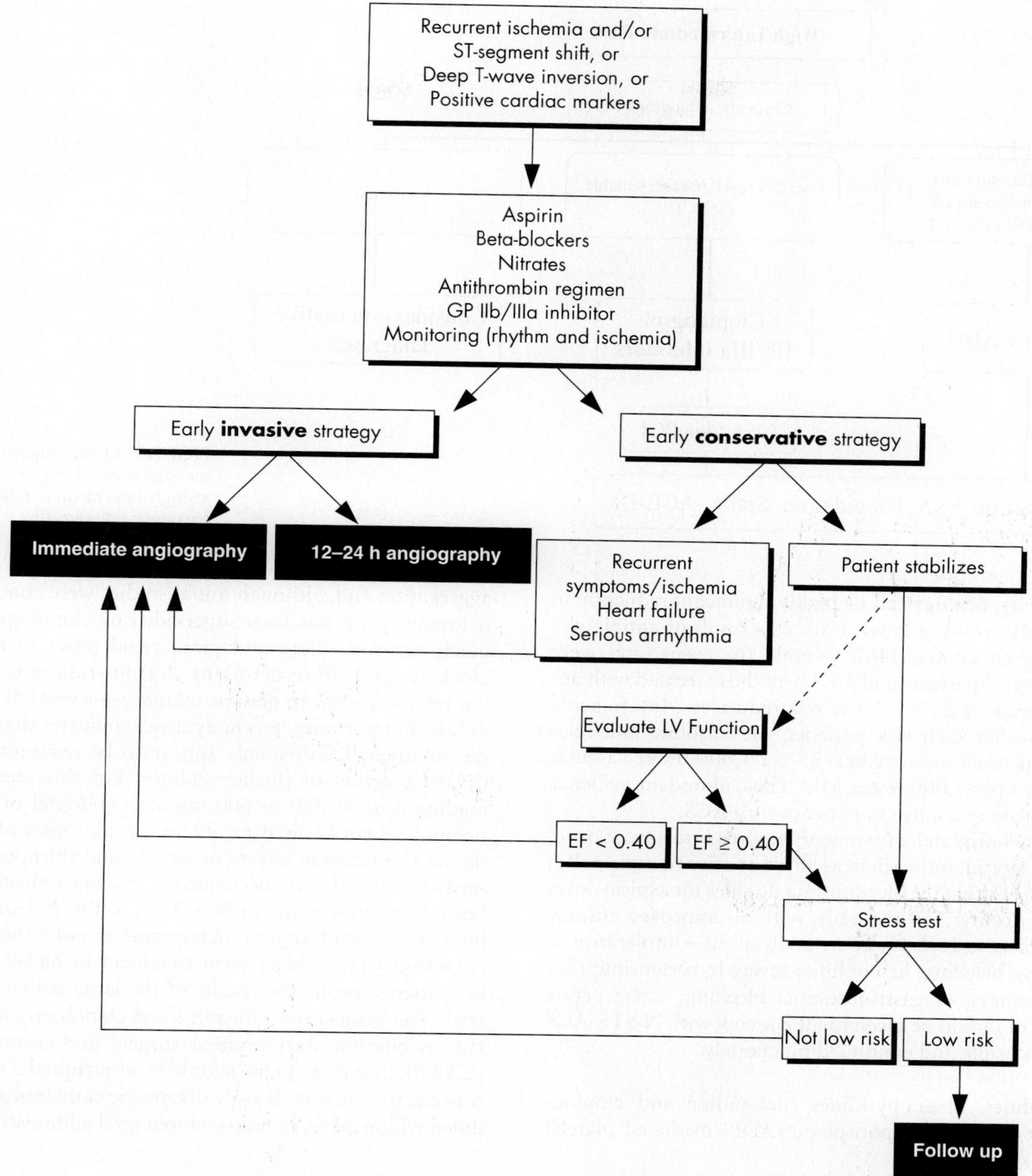

FIGURE 119.5. Acute ischemia pathway [From Braunwald E, et al. (1): Braunwald E, Antman EM, Beasley JW, et al.; American College of Cardiology; American Heart Association. Committee on the Management of Patients With Unstable Angina. ACC/AHA 2002 guideline update for the management of patients with unstable angina and non–ST-segment elevation myocardial infarction–summary article: a report of the American College of Cardiology/American Heart Association task force on practice guidelines (Committee on the Management of Patients With Unstable Angina). *J Am Coll Cardiol.* 2002;40(7):1366–1374.]

was less with diltiazem than with the nitrate (45). Although verapamil has similar effects to diltiazem, its effects in ACS have not been evaluated in any large trial. Dihydropyridines should be used only in combination with β-blockade, as the combination avoids induction of tachycardia. Short-acting dihydropyridine calcium channel blockers should not be used at all. The nondihydropyridine calcium channel blocker, diltiazem, may be used alone as an alternative therapy if it is not possible to use β-blockade. However, β-blockers are preferred in all other patients, as they have marked benefits in those who go on to develop MI. Furthermore, the use of any calcium channel blocker is contraindicated when there is left ventricular dysfunction.

Antiplatelet Therapy (see Table 119.7)

Aspirin. Aspirin irreversibly inhibits cyclooxygenase-1, thus reducing the generation of thromboxane A2, a potent mediator of platelet aggregation. The most recent update of the Antithrombotic Trialists' Collaboration, based upon 287 studies in

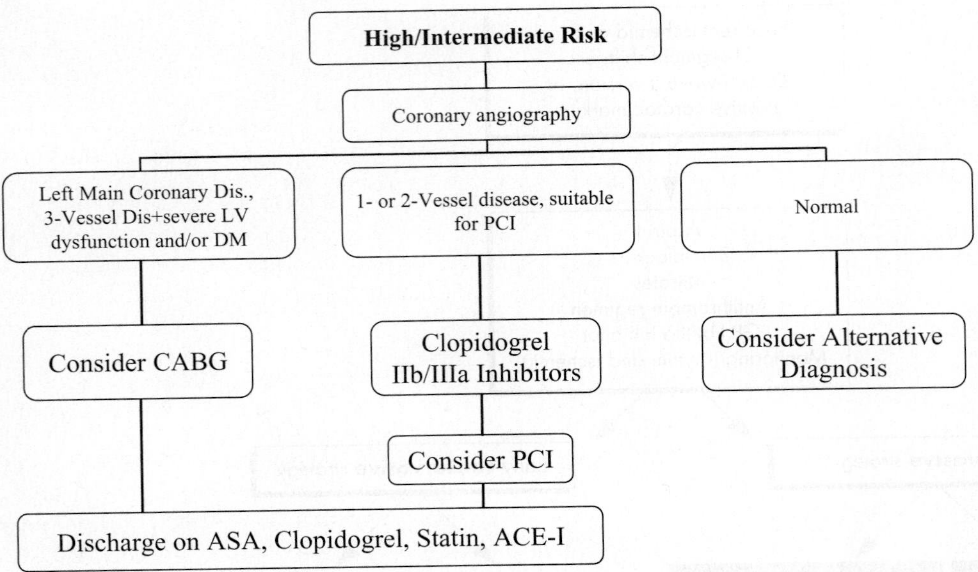

FIGURE 119.6. Algorithm for the management of NSTE-ACS patients at high-intermediate risk undergoing coronary angiography.

13,500 patients, demonstrates a highly significant reduction in the risk of MI/stroke/vascular death as a result of antiplatelet treatment versus control (46). Overall, the event rates were 13.2% in control patients and 10.7% in those treated with antiplatelet therapy, a 22% relative risk reduction (46). In acute MI, and in other high risk patients, the absolute and relative risk reductions were greater: 23 per 1,000 fewer vascular deaths and 13 per 1,000 fewer MIs. Thus, abundant evidence supports the use of aspirin in patients with ACS.

Additional antiplatelet treatment requires evidence of benefit on top of aspirin, rather than as an alternative to aspirin. Recent data suggest that the bleeding risk doubles for aspirin doses above versus below 160 mg daily, with no improved efficacy (1). Unless there are specific contraindications—intolerance or allergy; active bleeding; hemophilia; severe hypertension; retinal, genitourinary, or gastrointestinal bleeding; active peptic ulcer—aspirin should be given to all patients with N-STE-ACS as soon as possible and continued indefinitely.

Thienopyridines. Thienopyridines (ticlopidine and clopidogrel) inhibit adenosine diphosphate (ADP) mediated platelet aggregation and, although initial studies were conducted with ticlopidine, this has been superseded by clopidogrel due to a much superior safety and more rapid onset of action. The blockade of ADP receptors by thienopyridines is irreversible but relatively slow to became manifest—several days for ticlopidine. Furthermore, recent evidence indicates that a substantial number of individuals appear to be resistant to the antiplatelet action of thienopyridines. For this reason, a high loading dose of 300 to 600 mg of clopidogrel or 500 mg of ticlopidine can be used to obtain a rapid onset of action. As the antiaggregation effects of aspirin and thienopyridines are mediated by different mechanisms, an additive benefit by using both drugs may exist. In N-STE-ACS, the AHA/ACC guidelines recommend approximately nine months treatment with clopidogrel (1). Longer term treatment in higher risk vascular patients awaits the results of the large scale CHARISMA trial. The association of aspirin and clopidogrel increases the risk of bleeding during major surgery and coronary surgery (CABG), thus clopidogrel should be interrupted 5 to 7 days before elective surgery. If early diagnostic catheterization is scheduled within 24 to 36 hours, clopidogrel administration can be

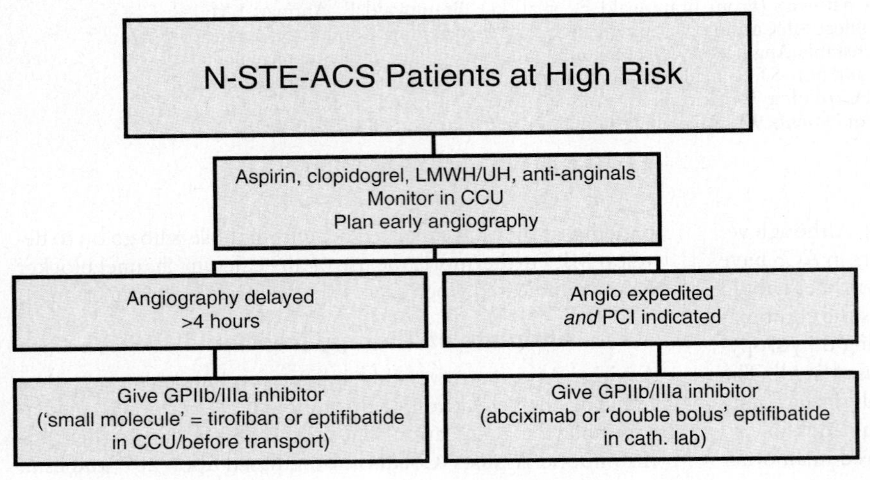

FIGURE 119.7. Algorithm for the treatment of high risk patients with unstable angina/non–ST-segment elevation myocardial infarction.

TABLE 119.5

RISK SCORES FOR N-STE-ACS

TIMI (0–7)	Age 65 years or greater	1
	3 or more risk factors for CAD	1
	Use of ASA (last 7 days)	1
	Known CAD (stenosis 50% or more)	1
	More than 1 episode rest angina in less than 24 h	1
	ST-segment deviation	1
	Elevated cardiac markers	1
PURSUIT (0–18)	Age, separate points for enrollment diagnosis	
	Decade [UA (MI)]	
	50	8 (11)
	60	9 (12)
	70	11 (13)
	80	12 (14)
	Sex	
	Male	1
	Female	0
	Worst CCS-class in previous 6 weeks	
	No angina or CCS I/II	0
	CCS III/IV	2
	Signs of heart failure	2
	ST-depression on presenting ECG	1
GRACE (0–258)	Age (years)	
	less than 40	0
	40–49	18
	50–59	36
	60–69	55
	70–79	73
	80 or older	91
	Heart rate (bpm)	
	less than 70	0
	70–89	7
	90–109	13
	110–149	23
	150–199	36
	200 or more	46
	Systolic BP (mm Hg)	
	less than 80	63
	80–99	58
	100–119	47
	120–139	37
	140–159	26
	160–199	11
	200 or higher	0
	Creatinine (mg/dL)	
	0–0.39	2
	0.4–0.79	5
	0.8–1.19	8
	1.2–1.59	11
	1.6–1.99	14
	2 –3.99	23
	4 or higher	31
	Killip class	
	Class I	0
	Class II	21
	Class III	43
	Class IV	64
	Cardiac arrest at admission	43
	Elevated cardiac markers	15
	ST-segment deviation	30

initiated after coronary angiography when it is clear that CABG will not be undertaken; in the case of immediate percutaneous revascularization, the therapy can be initiated with a loading dose immediately.

Thienopyridines reduce the risk of stent thrombotic occlusion and are now part of standard treatment for at least four weeks in all patients undergoing elective PCI. With drug eluting stents, at least six months and perhaps 12 months of clopidogrel and aspirin are required (1). The CURE trial tested clopidogrel in 12,562 N-STE-ACS patients on top of background treatment and aspirin (47). A 2.1% absolute risk reduction (20% relative risk reduction, $p < 0.0001$) occurred in the frequency of nonfatal MI, stroke, or cardiovascular death (47). The treatment effect was evident within the first 24 hours of starting therapy and, although the absolute benefits were greatest in the first three months of treatment, the relative risk reduction was the same beyond three months. Approximately 1% more patients experienced major bleeding, but there was no significant excess of life-threatening bleeding or hemorrhagic strokes (47). Nevertheless, in view of the irreversible nature of the ADP antagonism, current guidelines suggest that clopidogrel should be withheld for five days before CABG surgery. In candidates for very urgent CABG, a small molecule Gp IIb/IIIa inhibitor—eptifibatide or tirofiban—can be used before surgery.

Three new antiplatelet drugs are in phase III clinical trials, including a potent, fast-acting thienopyridine (prasugrel [48]), a reversible oral PGY12 inhibitor (AZD6140, a cyclopentyltriazolopyridimidine [49]), and a potent, short-acting intravenous PGY12 inhibitor (cangrelor [50]). In patients with N-STE-ACS, preliminary data from the DISPERSE 2 (Safety, Tolerability and Preliminary Efficacy of AZD6140, the First Oral Reversible ADP Receptor Antagonist, Compared with Clopidogrel in Patients with Non-ST-Segment Elevation Acute Coronary Syndrome) trial comparing AZD6140 with placebo demonstrated that AZD6140, 180 mg twice daily, achieved greater and more consistent platelet inhibition, and showed favorable effects on clinical outcomes without an increase in major bleeding (51).

Glycoprotein IIb/IIIa Receptor Antagonists. Platelet aggregation involves the GP IIb/IIIa receptor linked to fibrinogen or von Willebrand factor. Intravenous GP IIb/IIIa receptor antagonists have been extensively tested in patients with ACS and, in a meta-analysis of all the major randomized trials, the absolute risk reduction for death or MI at 30 days was 1% (11.8% control vs. 10.8% with Gp IIb/IIIa) (52). The absolute treatment benefit was largest in high risk patients—in particular, those with evidence of troponin release or those undergoing acute PCI (52). Among those without troponin elevation or PCI, no significant benefits were observed with Gp IIb/IIIa administration.

The CREDO (Clopidogrel for the Reduction of Events During Observation) trial has helped to resolve the question of whether clopidogrel plus GP IIb/IIIa receptor antagonists may be required in patients undergoing PCI (53). Approximately half of the patients received GP IIb/IIIa antagonists (a nonrandomized subset) and two thirds had presented with an ACS. The frequency of MI, stroke, or death at one year was reduced with clopidogrel from 11.5% to 8.5% ($p = 0.02$), with similar risk ratios in the presence or absence of GP IIb/IIIa inhibitors (53). In the ISAR-REACT 2 (Abciximab in Patients with Acute Coronary Syndromes Undergoing Percutaneous Coronary Intervention After Clopidogrel Pre-treatment) trial, abciximab

TABLE 119.6

DOSAGES OF NTG AND NITRATES IN ANGINA [MODIFIED FROM BRAUNWALD ET AL. (1).]

Agent	Route	Dosage
NTG	■ Sublingual tablets ■ Spray ■ Transdermal ■ Intravenous	■ 0.3 to 0.6 mg up to 1.5 mg ■ 0.4 mg as needed ■ 0.2 to 0.8 mg/h every 12 h ■ 5 to 200 mcg/min
Isosorbide dinitrate	■ Oral ■ Oral, slow release	■ 5 to 80 mg, 2 or 3 times daily ■ 40 mg 1 or 2 times daily
Isosorbide mononitrate	■ Oral ■ Oral, slow release	■ 20 mg twice daily ■ 60 to 240 mg once daily
Pentaerythritol tetranitrate	■ Sublingual	■ 10 mg as needed
Erythritol tetranitrate	■ Sublingual ■ Oral	■ 5 to 10 mg as needed ■ 10 to 30 mg 3 times daily

TABLE 119.7

COMMONLY USED ANTIPLATELET AND ANTICOAGULANT AGENTS IN UNSTABLE ANGINA AND N-STEMI—DRUG DOSES AND SPECIAL PRECAUTIONS

Agent	Dose	Precautions
Oral antiplatelet agent		
Aspirin	Initially 300 mg p.o.; then 75 to 150 mg daily	■ GI bleeding ■ Peptic ulceration ■ Aspirin allergy
Clopidogrel (Plavix/Iscover)	Initial loading dose of 300 mg (or 600 mg); then 75 mg daily	■ Increased bleeding risk ■ Antiplatelet therapy contraindicated
Heparins		
Unfractionated heparin	60 U/kg IV bolus to a maximum of 4,000 units; then 12 units/kg/h infusion to a maximum of 1,000 units/h	■ Monitor PTT: keep at 50–70 seconds ■ Any abnormal bleeding ■ Any major surgery <30 days ■ Thrombocytopenia ■ Risk of bleeding
Low-molecular-weight heparin		
Dalteparin (Fragmin)	120 IU/kg subcutaneously every 12 h	
Enoxaparin (Clexane)	1 mg/kg subcutaneously every 12 h	■ As above
Glycoprotein IIb/IIIa inhibitors		
Eptifibatide (Integrilin)	180 μg/kg IV over 1 to 2 min; then 2 μg/kg/min infusion over 72 h or until hospital discharge, whichever occurs first When initiating immediately before PCI, as above but repeat 180 μg/kg IV bolus 10 min after the first bolus	■ Bleeding disorder ■ Thrombocytopenia ■ Surgery <6 weeks ■ Abnormal bleed <30 d ■ Active GI ulceration ■ Puncture of a non-compressible vessel ■ Prior stroke, organic CNS pathology ■ Any systolic BP >180 mm Hg during the acute event ■ As above ■ 1/2 dose in renal insufficiency ■ As above
Tirofiban (Aggrastat)	0.4 μg/kg/min IV over 30 min; then 0.1 μg/kg/min infusion for 48 to 108 h	
Abciximab (ReoPro)	0.25 mg/kg IV bolus 10 to 60 min before PCI, then 10 μg/min IV infusion for 12 h	

reduced the composite of death, MI, or urgent target vessel revascularization within 30 days compared with placebo by 25% among 2,022 patients with N-STE-ACS, all of whom received clopidogrel, 600 mg, at least 2 h before PCI (54). However, the benefit of abciximab was observed only in patients with N-STEMI (54).

The EVEREST (Randomized Comparison of Upstream Tirofiban versus Downstream High Bolus Dose Tirofiban or Abciximab on Tissue-Level Perfusion and Troponin Release in High-Risk Acute Coronary Syndromes Treated with Percutaneous Coronary Interventions) trial of 93 patients with high risk N-STE-ACS compared upstream tirofiban given in the CCU several hours before coronary angiography to downstream (immediately after coronary angiography) high bolus-dose tirofiban and downstream abciximab given 10 min before PCI (55). Upstream tirofiban improved TIMI myocardial perfusion before and after PCI, achieved a higher myocardial contrast echocardiographic score, and resulted in lower rates of postprocedure troponin elevation (55). Results from the open-label ACUITY (Acute Catheterization and Urgent Intervention Triage strategy) timing trial in 9,207 patients randomized to upstream GP IIb/IIIa inhibitors administered, on average, 6 hours before PCI compared with downstream use begun in the catheterization laboratory demonstrated that a downstream strategy was noninferior for a quaternary net clinical benefit end point—death, myocardial infarction, unplanned revascularization for ischemia, major bleeding—but did not satisfy the noninferiority criterion for the triple ischemic end point (56). A cost-effective analysis using data from the TACTICS–TIMI-18 (Prognostic Implications of Elevated Troponin in Patients with Suspected Acute Coronary Syndrome but no Critical Epicardial Coronary Disease–Thrombolysis In Myocardial Infarction-18) trial concluded that the upstream use of tirofiban was superior to selective use and was cost-effective in moderate to high risk patients (57). Taken together, these studies suggest that upstream GPI therapy may be more effective than downstream use in moderate to high risk patients managed with an invasive strategy in whom immediate catheterization is *not* planned. The EARLY ACS (Early Glycoprotein IIb/IIIa Inhibition in Non-ST-Segment Elevation Acute Coronary Syndrome) study (58) is an ongoing randomized, double-blind, clinical trial comparing upstream double-bolus eptifibatide to downstream selective use in high risk patients with N-STE-ACS who are *not* undergoing PCI in the first 12 hours, and should help shed further light on this issue.

Anticoagulation Therapy

Thrombin (Factor IIa) is a highly potent stimulus not only of the generation of fibrin, but also platelet activation. In addition, it leads to monocyte chemotaxis, mitogenesis, increased permeability of the vascular wall, and secretion of cytokines and growth factors from smooth muscle cells. Effective antithrombotic treatment requires the inhibition of both platelet function and thrombin.

Unfractionated heparin has been widely used, but suffers from practical difficulties in maintaining antithrombin activity within the therapeutic range, which are influenced by acute phase proteins and binding to antithrombins. Nevertheless, there is clear evidence that a form of heparin, either unfractionated or low molecular weight heparin (LMWH), is superior to placebo in patients with ACS. The meta-analysis of trials demonstrates a reduction in absolute rates of death or MI from 7.4% to 4.5% (odds ratio 0.53, 95% CI 0.38 to 0.73) (59).

Direct antithrombins may provide significant advantages over the indirect inhibitors (unfractionated and LMWH). Combined analysis of the hirudin studies suggests a relative risk reduction compared to unfractionated heparin. At this point in time, hirudin has only been approved for patients with heparin-induced thrombocytopenia, and none of the hirudins are licensed for ACS. LMWHs partially inhibit factor Xa of the coagulation cascade, but newer specific inhibitors of Xa have been developed—for example, bivaliridin and fondaparinux. Such agents inhibit thrombin generation as distinct from thrombin activity. In the recently published ACUITY trial, 13,819 patients with moderate to high risk N-STE-ACS were randomized to 1 of 3 arms: (1) heparin + GP IIb/IIIa inhibitors (standard), (2) bivalirudin + GP IIb/IIIa inhibitors (combination), or (3) bivalirudin alone (monotherapy) (56). Combination therapy was noninferior to the standard (neither arm was superior), while monotherapy was superior to standard therapy, driven by a reduction in bleeding with bivalirudin monotherapy (56). A common theme among the studies evaluating bivalirudin is the marked reduction in bleeding observed when GP IIb/IIIa inhibitors are *not* routinely administered.

Direct comparisons with LMWH did not show advantages for fondaparinux over enoxaparin in reducing the risk of ischemic events at nine days, but it substantially reduces major bleeding and improves long term mortality and morbidity (60). The results of a randomized, double-blind trial of fondaparinux versus enoxaparin in 20,000 patients with unstable angina or non-STEMI are pending (OASIS 5) (61).

An alternative approach involves an orally administered, direct thrombin antagonist, ximelagatran. It is converted to melagatran in the circulation and directly binds with the active site of the thrombin molecule. Ximelagatran does not require anticoagulation monitoring, and is administered as a fixed dose. In a phase II trial, it reduced the frequency of death, nonfatal MI, and severe recurrent ischemia compared to placebo treatment (hazard ratio 0.76, 95% CI 0.59 to 0.98) (62). Ximelagatran has also been used as an alternative to warfarin in the management of atrial fibrillation (SPORTIF trials), and demonstrates similar efficacy but less bleeding than warfarin. A potential hazard of ximelagatran involves alterations in liver enzymes: 6% to 10% of patients experience a rise in alanine aminotransferase to at least three times the upper limit of normal (62). This appears to resolve with or without cessation of drug treatment. Widespread application of ximelagatran as an alternative to other antithrombins in ACS requires large scale safety and efficacy studies.

HMG-CoA Reductase Inhibitors

In the past year, ancillary analyses from randomized trials of intensive statin therapy and mechanistic studies provided new insights into the role of lowering lipids in patients with ACS. The case for intensive statin therapy after N-STE-ACS was strengthened by a meta-analysis of 6 randomized controlled trials demonstrating that intensive, but not moderate, statin treatment reduces early recurrent ischemic events and stroke (63). A detailed comparison of two trials comparing intensive to moderate statin therapy emphasized the importance of intensive therapy beginning in the early post-ACS phase, and suggested that the early benefit may be associated with a more profound reduction in CRP achieved with earlier intensive therapy (64).

These results have been rapidly reflected in subsequent changes in the particular statin and dose prescribed. A trend-over-time analysis in Ontario, Canada, documented a greater than two-fold increase in the use of atorvastatin, 80 mg, within months after publication of the PROVE IT–TIMI-22 (Pravastatin or Atorvastatin Evaluation and Infection Therapy Thrombolysis In Myocardial Infarction-22) and REVERSAL (Reversing Atherosclerosis With Aggressive Lipid Lowering) studies (65).

The benefit of atorvastatin, 80 mg, compared with pravastatin, 40 mg, occurred within 30 days in the PROVE IT–TIMI-22 trial (28% reduction in the hazard ratio of death, myocardial infarction, or rehospitalization for recurrent ACS) consistent with greater early pleiotropic effects (66). A number of potential early benefits of statins independent of LDL have been postulated and include favorable effects on inflammation, endothelial function, and the coagulation cascade (67). In a secondary analysis from the PROVE IT–TIMI-22 trial, randomization to intensive statin therapy was associated with a lower CRP level, irrespective of the presence of a single or multiple uncontrolled cardiovascular risk factors (68). Endothelium-dependent, flow-mediated dilation increased between one and four months after initiating either atorvastatin, 80 mg, or pravastatin, 40 mg, in the BRAVER (Intensity of Lipid Lowering with Statins and Brachial Artery Vascular Endothelium Reactivity After Acute Coronary Syndromes) trial, independent of reductions in LDL and CRP (69).

Two important observations regarding the safety of statins were reported during the past year. An analysis of 15,693 patients from the GRACE (Global Registry of Acute Coronary Events) registry demonstrated that, in general, patients receiving the combination of clopidogrel and a statin did *not* have an increase in clinical events, thus suggesting no adverse interaction exists between these two therapies. Indeed, even after adjustment for differences in baseline variables and bias in treatment allocation, an analysis of patients administered aspirin with or without clopidogrel and with or without statin revealed that the group taking all 3 drugs had the lowest mortality (70). In an analysis of patients who achieved very low LDL concentrations in the PROVE IT–TIMI-22 trial, there was no adverse safety signal, while clinical efficacy improved as the LDL was lowered to less than 40 mg/dL (71), thus suggesting that downward adjustment of the statin dose is not required in patients who achieve very low LDL concentrations. Despite such favorable results with high intensity statins, only 44% of patients randomized to atorvastatin, 80 mg, with baseline total cholesterol less than 240 mg/dL (average LDL 106 mg/dL) achieved the dual goals of LDL less than 70 mg/dL and CRP less than 2 mg/L (72). Better control of traditional risk factors (68) and even more potent pharmacologic therapy are necessary to achieve these ambitious targets that have been associated with relatively lower rates of death and recurrent ischemic complications (73).

Invasive Strategies

The Role of Coronary Angiography

Presently, coronary angiography represents the only reliable tool for the assessment of coronary anatomy in patients with N-STE-ACS. Patients with high risk coronary lesions—left main disease, three vessel disease, and proximal left anterior descending coronary artery disease—represent about 50% of all patients with N-STE-ACS (74,75) and, despite the use of risk scores and biomarkers of myocardial damage, it is frequently impossible to correctly identify these high risk patients who are most likely to benefit from revascularization both in terms of survival and symptom improvement (Table 119.8). Thus, the concept of *low* and *high* risk patients suggested by the various scores derived by investigational studies and registry is rather relative. According to the TIMI risk score, about 50% of patients with N-STE-ACS are in the low risk subgroup (below score 3); nevertheless about 25% of these patients develop a major event—death, nonfatal MI, or urgent revascularization—within 14 days from hospitalization. Thus, as the predictive accuracy of these risk scores is rather low, all patients with N-STE-ACS should be regarded at risk to develop major coronary events. In this context, the early knowledge of coronary anatomy and the possibility to promptly restore myocardial perfusion appear to have important therapeutic and prognostic implications.

TABLE 119.8

HIGH RISK FEATURES FAVORING AN EARLY INVASIVE STRATEGY

- Recurrent angina/ischemia at rest or with low-level activities despite intensive anti-ischemic therapy
- Elevated troponin level
- New or presumably new ST-segment depression
- Recurrent angina/ischemia with symptoms of heart failure, an S_3 gallop, pulmonary edema, worsening rales, or new or worsening mitral regurgitation
- High risk findings on noninvasive stress testing
- Left ventricular systolic dysfunction (ejection fraction less than 40% on a noninvasive study)
- Hemodynamic instability
- Sustained ventricular tachycardia
- Percutaneous coronary intervention within

Early Conservative versus Invasive Strategies

Studies comparing head-to-head early conservative versus an early invasive strategy are flawed by the substantial rate of crossover patients originally randomized into the conservative arm who were treated invasively because of unstable symptoms. Indeed, when the difference in revascularization rate between the treatment arms is large, the benefit of revascularization strategy is evident. According to a recently published meta-analysis, managing N-STE-ACS by early invasive approach improves long-term survival and reduces late nonfatal myocardial infarction and rehospitalization for symptoms recurrence (76–78). Thus the issue is not *whether* but *when* a patient with N-STE-ACS should undergo coronary angiography and eventually revascularization. Combined data from seven large randomized trials indicate that the goal in patients with N-STE-ACS should be to perform early invasive therapy within 48 hours from hospital admission (76,77) (Fig. 119.8).

Obviously, coronary angiography should be anticipated if clinical instability occurs. This time interval is also supported by the CRUSADE (Can Rapid risk stratification of Unstable

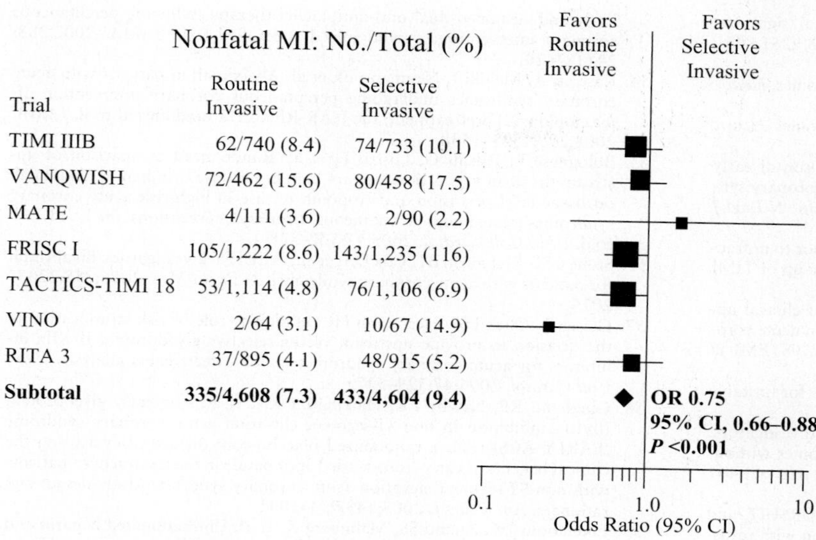

Nonfatal MI: No./Total (%)
Favors Routine Invasive
Favors Selective Invasive
Trial
Routine Invasive
Selective Invasive
TIMI IIIB 62/740 (8.4) 74/733 (10.1)
VANQWISH 72/462 (15.6) 80/458 (17.5)
MATE 4/111 (3.6) 2/90 (2.2)
FRISC I 105/1,222 (8.6) 143/1,235 (116)
TACTICS-TIMI 18 53/1,114 (4.8) 76/1,106 (6.9)
VINO 2/64 (3.1) 10/67 (14.9)
RITA 3 37/895 (4.1) 48/915 (5.2)
Subtotal 335/4,608 (7.3) 433/4,604 (9.4)
OR 0.75
95% CI, 0.66–0.88
P <0.001
0.1
1.0
10
Odds Ratio (95% CI)

FIGURE 119.8. Odds of non-fatal myocardial infarction (MI) from randomization to end of follow-up in a meta-analysis of 7 trials of routine versus selective invasive management of acute coronary syndromes (77). P = 0.51 for heterogeneity across the trials. CI = confidence interval; OR = odds ratio.

angina patients Suppress ADverse outcomes with Early implementation of the ACC/AHA guidelines) registry data, indicating that a delay of 46 hours is not associated with increased adverse events compared with a delay of only 23 hours (79). As clinical stabilization can be obtained pharmacologically in about 90% of patients with N-STE-ACS, this time delay appears reasonably applicable in the majority of cardiology centers. The best revascularization strategy (PCI or CABG) should be evaluated for each case according to coronary anatomy, clinical symptoms, and associated diseases.

References

1. Braunwald E, Antman EM, Beasley JW, et al.; American College of Cardiology; American Heart Association. Committee on the Management of Patients with Unstable Angina. ACC/AHA 2002 guideline update for the management of patients with unstable angina and non–ST-segment elevation myocardial infarction–summary article: a report of the American College of Cardiology/American Heart Association task force on practice guidelines (Committee on the Management of Patients with Unstable Angina). *J Am Coll Cardiol.* 2002;40(7):1366–1374.
2. Myler RK, Shaw RE, Stertzer SH, et al. Unstable angina and coronary angioplasty. *Circulation.* 1990;82(3 Suppl):II88–95.
3. Maseri A, Liuzzo G, Biasucci LM. Pathogenic mechanisms in unstable angina. *Heart.* 1999 Sep;82(Suppl 1):I2–4.
4. Giugliano RP, Braunwald E. The year in non-ST-segment elevation acute coronary syndromes. *J Am Coll Cardiol.* 2006;48(2):386–395.
5. Haywood LJ, Khan AH, de Guzman M. Prinzmetal angina. Normal arteries and multifocal electrocardiographic changes. *JAMA.* 1976;235(1):53–56.
6. Bory M, Pierron F, Panagides D, et al. Coronary artery spasm in patients with normal or near normal coronary arteries. Long-term follow-up of 277 patients. *Eur Heart J.* 1996;17:1015–1021.
7. National Center for Health Statistics. Detailed diagnoses and procedures: national hospital discharge survey, 1996. Hyattsville, MD: National Center for Health Statistics; 1998:13. Data from Vital and Health Statistics.
8. Fox KAA, Goodman SG, Klein W, et al; for the GRACE Investigators. Management of acute coronary syndromes. Variations in practice and outcome; findings from the Global Registry of Acute Coronary Events (GRACE). *Eur Heart J.* 2002;23:1177–1189.
9. Hasdai D, Behar S, Wallentin L, et al. A prospective survey of the characteristics, treatments and outcomes of patients with acute coronary syndromes in Europe and the Mediterranean Basin; the Euro Heart Survey of acute coronary syndromes (Euro Heart Survey ACS). *Eur Heart J.* 2002;23:1190–1201.
10. Virmani R, Burke AP, Farb A, et al. Pathology of the vulnerable plaque. *J Am Coll Cardiol.* 2006;47(Suppl C):C13–18.
11. Libby P. Act local, act global: inflammation and the multiplicity of "vulnerable" coronary plaques. *J Am Coll Cardiol.* 2005;45:1600–1602.
12. Steg PG, Goldberg RJ, Gore JM, et al. Baseline characteristics, management practices, and in-hospital outcomes of patients hospitalized with acute coronary syndromes in the Global Registry of Acute Coronary Events (GRACE). *Am J Cardiol.* 2002;90:358–363.
13. Bart BA, Shaw LK, McCants CB Jr, et al. Clinical determinants of mortality in patients with angiographically diagnosed ischemic or nonischemic cardiomyopathy. *J Am Coll Cardiol.* 1997;30:1002–1008.
14. Steg PG, Dabbous OH, Feldman LJ, et al. Determinants and prognostic impact of heart failure complicating acute coronary syndrome: observations from the Global Registry of Acute Coronary Events (GRACE). *Circulation.* 2004;109:494–499.
15. Spencer FA, Meyer TE, Gore JM, et al. Heterogeneity in the management and outcomes of patients with acute myocardial infarction complicated by heart failure: the National Registry of Myocardial Infarction. *Circulation.* 2002;105:2605–2610.
16. Savonitto S, Ardissino D, Granger CB, et al. Prognostic value of the admission electrocardiogram in acute coronary syndromes. *JAMA.* 1999;281:707–713.
17. Lloyd-Jones DM, Camargo CA, Giugliano RP, et al. Characteristics and prognosis of patients with suspected acute myocardial infarction and elevated MB relative index but normal total creatine kinase. *Am J Cardiol.* 1999;84:957–962.
18. Hamm CW, Goldmann BU, Heeschen C, et al. Emergency room triage of patients with acute chest pain by means of rapid testing for cardiac troponin T or troponin I. *N Engl J Med.* 1997;337:1648–1653.
19. Newby LK, Storrow AB, Gibler WB, et al. Bedside multimarker testing for risk stratification in chest pain units: the Chest Pain Evaluation by Creatine Kinase-MB, Myoglobin and Troponin I (CHECKMATE) Study. *Circulation.* 2001;103:1832–1837.
20. Ohman EM, Armstrong PW, Christenson RH, et al. Cardiac troponin T levels for risk stratification in acute myocardial ischaemia. *N Engl J Med.* 1996;335:1333–1341.
21. Antman EM, Tanasjevic MJ, Thompson B, et al. Cardiac specific troponin I levels to predict the risk of mortality in patients with acute coronary syndromes. *N Engl J Med.* 1996;335:1342–1349.
22. Heeschen C, Goldmann BU, Terres W, et al. Cardiovascular risk and therapeutic benefit of coronary intervention for patients with unstable angina according to the troponin T status. *Eur Heart J.* 2000;21:1159–1166.
23. Newby LK, Christenson RH, Ohman M, et al. Value of serial troponin T measures for early and late risk stratification in patients with acute coronary syndromes. *Circulation.* 1998;98:1853–1859.
24. Wallentin L, Lagerqvist B, Husted S, et al. Outcome at 1 year after an invasive compared with a non-invasive strategy in unstable coronary-artery disease: the FRISC II invasive randomised trial. *Lancet.* 2000;356:9–16.
25. Cannon CP, Weintraub WS, Demopoulos LA, et al. Comparison of early invasive and conservative strategies in patients with unstable coronary syndromes treated with the glycoprotein IIb/IIIa inhibitor tirofiban. *N Engl J Med.* 2001;344:1879–1887.
26. Lindahl B, Toss H, Siegbahn A, et al. Markers of myocardial damage and inflammation in relation to long-term mortality in unstable coronary artery disease. *N Engl J Med.* 2000;343:1139–1147.
27. Granger CB, Goldberg RJ, Dabbous O, for the Global Registry of Acute Coronary Events Investigators, et al. Predictors of hospital mortality in the global registry of acute coronary events. *Arch Intern Med.* 2003;163:2345–2353.
28. Pfeffer MA, Pfeffer JM, Lamas GA. Development and prevention of congestive heart failure following myocardial infarction. *Circulation.* 1993; 87(Suppl IV):IV-120–IV-125.

29. Stevenson LW, Perloff JK. The limited reliability of physical signs for estimating hemodynamics in chronic heart failure. *JAMA*. 1989;261:884–888.
30. Greaves SC. Role of echocardiography in acute coronary syndromes. *Heart*. 2002;88(4):419–425.
31. Greaves SC. Role of echocardiography in acute coronary syndromes. *Heart*. 2002;88(4):419–425.
32. Cannon CP, Weintraub WS, Demopoulos LA, et al. Comparison of early invasive and conservative strategies in patients with unstable coronary syndromes treated with the glycoprotein IIb/IIIa inhibitor tirofiban. *N Engl J Med*. 2001;344:1879–1887.
33. Antman EM, Cohen M, McCabe C, et al. Enoxaparin is superior to unfractionated heparin for preventing clinical events at 1-year follow-up of TIMI 11B and ESSENCE. *Eur Heart J*. 2002;23:308–314.
34. Morrow DA, Antman EM, Snapinn SM, et al. An integrated clinical approach to predicting the benefit of tirofiban in non-ST elevation acute coronary syndromes. Application of the TIMI risk score for UA/NSTEMI in PRISM-PLUS. *Eur Heart J*. 2002;23:223–229.
35. Antman EM, Cohen M, Bernink PJ, et al. The TIMI risk score for unstable angina/non-ST elevation MI. *JAMA*. 2000;284:835–842.
36. Boersma E, Pieper KS, Steyerberg EW, et al., for the PURSUIT Investigators. Predictors of outcome in patients with acute coronary syndromes without persistent ST-segment elevation. Results from an international trial of 9461 patients. *Circulation*. 2000;101:2557–2567.
37. de Araùjo Gonçalves P, Ferreira J, Aguiar C, et al. TIMI, PURSUIT, and GRACE risk scores: sustained prognostic value and interaction with revascularization in NSTE-ACS. *Eur Heart J*. 2005;26:865–872.
38. Fragmin and Fast Revascularization during Instability in Coronary artery disease (FRISC II) Investigators. Invasive compared with non-invasive treatment in unstable coronary artery disease: FRISC II prospective randomised multicentre study. *Lancet*. 1999;354:708–715.
39. Curfman GD, Heinsimer JA, Lozner EC, et al. Intravenous nitroglycerin in the treatment of spontaneous angina pectoris: a prospective randomized trial. *Circulation*. 1983;67:276–282.
40. HINT Group. Early treatment of unstable angina in the coronary care unit: a randomised double-blind, placebo controlled comparison of recurrent ischaemia in patients treated with nifedipine, metoprolol or both. Report of the Holland Interuniversity Nifedipine/Metoprolol Trial (HINT) Research Group. *Br Heart J*. 1986;56:400–413.
41. Gheorghiade M, Schultz L, Tilley B, et al. Effects of propranolol in non-Q wave acute myocardial infarction in the beta blocker heart attack trial. *Am J Cardiol*. 1990;66:129–133.
42. Hohnloser SH, Meinertz T, Kingenheben T, et al. Usefulness of esmolol in unstable angina pectoris. European Esmolol Study Group. *Am J Cardiol*. 1991;67:1319–1323.
43. Gibson RS, Boden WE, Theroux P, et al. Diltiazem and reinfarction in patients with non-Q wave myocardial infarction: results of a double-blind, randomized, multicenter trial. *N Engl J Med*. 1986;315:423–429.
44. Theroux P, Taeymans Y, Morissette D, et al. A randomized trial comparing propanolol and diltiazem in the treatment of unstable angina. *J Am Coll Cardiol*. 1985;5:717–722.
45. Gobel EJAM, Hautvast RWM, van Gilst WH, et al. Randomised, double blind trial of intravenous diltiazem versus glyceryl trinitrate for unstable angina pectoris. *Lancet*. 1995;346:1653–1657.
46. Antithrombotic Trialists' Collaboration. Collaborative meta-analysis of randomised trials of antiplatelet therapy for prevention of death, myocardial infarction, and stroke in high risk patients. *BMJ*. 2002;324:71–86.
47. The Clopidogrel in Unstable Angina to Prevent Recurrent Events Trial Investigators. Effects of clopidogrel in addition to aspirin in patients with acute coronary syndromes without ST-segment elevation. *N Engl J Med*. 2001;345:494–502.
48. Wiviott SD, Antman EM, Gibson CM, et al. Evaluation of prasugrel compared to clopidogrel in patients with acute coronary syndromes: design and rationale for the TRial to assess Improvement in Therapeutic Outcomes by optimizing platelet inhibition with prasugrel (TRITON-TIMI 38). *Am Heart J*. 2006;152:627–635.
49. Husted S, Emanuelsson H, Heptinstall S, et al. Pharmacodynamics, pharmacokinetics, and safety of the oral reversible P2Y12 antagonist AZD6140 with aspirin in patients with atherosclerosis: a double-blind comparison to clopidogrel with aspirin. *Eur Heart J*. 2006;27:1038–1047.
50. Greenbaum AB, Grines CL, Bittl JA, et al. Initial experience with an intravenous P2Y12 platelet receptor antagonist in patients undergoing percutaneous coronary intervention: results from a 2-part, phase II, multicenter, randomized, placebo- and active-controlled trial. *Am Heart J*. 2006;151: e1–689.
51. Cannon CP, Husted S, Storey RF, et al. The DISPERSE 2 trial: safety, tolerability and preliminary efficacy of AZD6140, the first oral reversible ADP receptor antagonist, compared with clopidogrel in patients with non-ST segment elevation acute coronary syndrome [Abstract]. *Circulation*. 2005;112:II615.
52. Boersma E, Harrington RA, Moliterno DJ, et al. Platelet glycoprotein IIb/IIIa inhibitors in acute coronary syndromes: a meta-analysis of all major randomised clinical trials. *Lancet*. 2002;359:189–198.
53. Steinhubl SR, Berger PB, Mann JT 3rd, et al., for the CREDO Investigators. Clopidogrel for the Reduction of Events During Observation. Early and sustained dual oral antiplatelet therapy following percutaneous coronary intervention: a randomized controlled trial. *JAMA*. 2002;288: 2411–2420.
54. Kastrati A, Mehilli J, Neumann FJ, et al. Abciximab in patients with acute coronary syndromes undergoing percutaneous coronary intervention after clopidogrel pretreatment: the ISAR-REACT 2 randomized trial. *JAMA*. 2006;295:1531–1538.
55. Bolognese L, Falsini G, Liistro F, et al. Randomized comparison of upstream tirofiban versus downstream high bolus dose tirofiban or abciximab on tissue-level perfusion and troponin release in high-risk acute coronary syndromes treated with percutaneous coronary interventions: the EVEREST trial. *J Am Coll Cardiol*. 2006;47:522–528.
56. Stone GW, McLaurin BT, Cox DA, et al.; ACUITY Investigators. Bivalirudin for patients with acute coronary syndromes. *N Engl J Med*. 2006;355:2203–2016.
57. Glaser R, Glick HA, Herrmann HC, et al. The role of risk stratification in the decision to provide upstream versus selective glycoprotein IIb/IIIa inhibitors for acute coronary syndromes: a cost-effectiveness analysis. *J Am Coll Cardiol*. 2006;47:529–537.
58. Giugliano RP, Newby LK, Harrington RA, et al. The early glycoprotein IIb/IIIa inhibition in non-ST-segment elevation acute coronary syndrome (EARLY ACS) trial: a randomized placebo-controlled trial evaluating the clinical benefits of early front-loaded eptifibatide in the treatment of patients with non-ST-segment elevation acute coronary syndrome-study design and rationale. *Am Heart J*. 2005;149:994–1002.
59. Eikelboom JW, Anand SS, Malmberg K, et al. Unfractionated heparin and low-molecular-weight heparin in acute coronary syndrome without ST elevation: a meta-analysis. *Lancet*. 2000;355:1936–1942.
60. Fifth Organization to Assess Strategies in Acute Ischemic Syndromes Investigators; Yusuf S, Mehta SR, Chrolavicius S, et al. Comparison of fondaparinux and enoxaparin in acute coronary syndromes. *N Engl J Med*. 2006;354:14641476.
61. MICHELANGELO OASIS 5 Steering Committee. Design and rationale of the MICHELANGELO Organization to Assess Strategies in Acute Ischemic Syndromes (OASIS)-5 trial program evaluating fondaparinux, a synthetic factor Xa inhibitor, in patients with non-ST-segment elevation acute coronary syndromes. *Am Heart J*. 2005;150:1107.
62. Wallentin L, Wilcox RG, Weaver WD, et al. Oral ximelagatran for secondary prophylaxis after myocardial infarction: the ESTEEM randomised controlled trial. *Lancet*. 2003;362:789–797.
63. Schwartz GG, Olsson AG. The case for intensive statin therapy after acute coronary syndromes. *Am J Cardiol*. 2005;96:45F–53F.
64. Wiviott SD, de Lemos JA, Cannon CP, et al. A tale of two trials: a comparison of the post-acute coronary syndrome lipid-lowering trials A to Z and PROVE IT-TIMI 22. *Circulation*. 2006;113:1406–1414.
65. Austin PC, Mamdani MM. Impact of the pravastatin or atorvastatin evaluation and infection therapy-thrombolysis in myocardial infarction 22/Reversal of Atherosclerosis with Aggressive Lipid Lowering trials on trends in intensive versus moderate statin therapy in Ontario, Canada. *Circulation*. 2005;112:1296–1300.
66. Ray KK, Cannon CP, McCabe CH, et al. Early and late benefits of high-dose atorvastatin in patients with acute coronary syndromes: results from the PROVE IT-TIMI 22 trial. *J Am Coll Cardiol*. 2005;46:1405–1410.
67. Ray KK, Cannon CP. The potential relevance of the multiple lipid-independent (pleiotropic) effects of statins in the management of acute coronary syndromes. *J Am Coll Cardiol*. 2005;46:1425–1433.
68. Ray KK, Cannon CP, Cairns R, et al. Relationship between uncontrolled risk factors and C-reactive protein levels in patients receiving standard or intensive statin therapy for acute coronary syndromes in the PROVE IT-TIMI 22 trial. *J Am Coll Cardiol*. 2005;46:1417–1424.
69. Dupuis J, Tardif JC, Rouleau JL, et al. Intensity of lipid lowering with statins and brachial artery vascular endothelium reactivity after acute coronary syndromes (from the BRAVER trial). *Am J Cardiol*. 2005;96:1207–1213.
70. Lim MJ, Spencer FA, Gore JM, et al. Impact of combined pharmacologic treatment with clopidogrel and a statin on outcomes of patients with non-ST-segment elevation acute coronary syndromes: perspectives from a large multinational registry. *Eur Heart J*. 2005;26:1063–1069.
71. Wiviott SD, Cannon CP, Morrow DA, et al. Can low-density lipoprotein be too low? The safety and efficacy of achieving very low low-density lipoprotein with intensive statin therapy: a PROVE IT-TIMI 22 substudy. *J Am Coll Cardiol*. 2005;46:1411–1416.
72. Ridker PM, Morrow DA, Rose LM, et al. Relative efficacy of atorvastatin 80 mg and pravastatin 40 mg in achieving the dual goals of low-density lipoprotein cholesterol <70 mg/dL and C-reactive protein <2 mg/L: an analysis of the PROVE-IT TIMI-22 trial. *J Am Coll Cardiol*. 2005;45:1644–1648.
73. Ridker PM, Cannon CP, Morrow D, et al. C-reactive protein levels and outcomes after statin therapy. *N Engl J Med*. 2005;352:20–28.
74. Fox KA, Anderson FA, Dabbous OH, et al. Intervention in acute coronary syndromes: do patients undergo intervention on the basis of their risk characteristics? The global registry of acute coronary events (GRACE). *Heart*. 2007 Feb;93(2):177–182. Epub 2006 Jun 6.
75. Heras M, Bueno H, Bardaji A, et al; DESCARTES Investigators. Magnitude and consequences of undertreatment of high-risk patients with non-ST segment elevation acute coronary syndromes: insights from the DESCARTES Registry. *Heart*. 2006;92:1571–1576.

76. Mehta SR, Cannon CP, Fox KAA, et al. Routine versus selective invasive strategies in patients with acute coronary syndromes: a collaborative meta-analysis of the randomized trials. *JAMA.* 2005;293:2908–2917.
77. Bavry AA, Kumbhani DJ, Rassi AN, et al. Benefit of early invasive therapy in acute coronary syndromes: a meta-analysis of contemporary randomized clinical trials. *J Am Coll Cardiol.* 2006;48:1319–1325.
78. Bavry AA, Kumbhani DJ, Quiroz R, et al. Invasive therapy along with glycoprotein IIb/IIIa inhibitors and intracoronary stents improves survival in non-ST-segment elevation acute coronary syndromes: a meta-analysis and review of the literature. *Am J Cardiol.* 2004;93:830–835.
79. Ryan JW, Peterson ED, Chen AY, et al.; CRUSADE Investigators. Optimal timing of intervention in non-ST-segment elevation acute coronary syndromes: insights from the CRUSADE (Can Rapid risk stratification of Unstable angina patients Suppress ADverse outcomes with Early implementation of the ACC/AHA guidelines) Registry. *Circulation.* 2005;112:3049–3057.

CHAPTER 120 ■ ST ELEVATION MYOCARDIAL INFARCTION (STEMI) CONTEMPORARY MANAGEMENT STRATEGIES

ACHILLE GASPARDONE • LEONARDO DE LUCA

OVERVIEW OF ST ELEVATION MYOCARDIAL INFARCTION

Definition of Terms

The definition of acute myocardial infarction (MI) may refer to different perspectives related to clinical, electrocardiographic (ECG), biochemical, and pathologic characteristics, all reflecting death of cardiac myocytes caused by prolonged ischemia (1,2). A definition for acute *evolving* myocardial infarction in the presence of clinically appropriate symptoms has been established as:

1. Patients with ST-segment elevation (ST elevation MI [STEMI])—that is, new ST-segment elevation at the J-point with the cutoff points greater than or equal to 0.2 mV in V_1 through V_3 and greater than or equal to 0.1 mV in other leads, or
2. Patients without ST-segment elevation (non–ST elevation MI [N-STEMI])—that is, ST-segment depression or T-wave abnormalities with elevated biomarkers of myocardial damage. ST-segment elevation is usually indicative of transmural MI, while ST-segment depression—whether associated or not with T-wave abnormalities—is more likely indicative of subendocardial MI.

Clinically *established* myocardial infarction may be defined by any Q wave in leads V_1 through V_3, or a Q wave greater than or equal to 0.03 s in leads I, II, aVL, aVF, V_4, V_5, or V_6. In the setting of acute MI, ECG changes are associated with elevation of the biomarkers of myocardial damage. The standard biomarker for myocardial damage is cardiac troponin (I or T), which has an elevated myocardial tissue specificity as well as high sensitivity, and creatine kinin (CK)-MB mass, which is less tissue specific than cardiac troponin but more specific for irreversible injury (1,2). Recently, a Global Task Force composed by several worldwide scientific working groups redefined the ESC/ACC criteria for the diagnosis of MI from various perspectives (2A) (Table 120.1). Clinically, the various types of MI, according to this new definition, can be classified as shown in Table 120.2.

Epidemiology

Acute MI represents a significant public and social health problem in industrialized countries, and is becoming an increasingly significant issue in developing countries (3). Although the exact incidence is difficult to ascertain, using primary listed and secondary hospital discharge data, the incidence has been estimated at 500,000 STEMI events per year in the United States (3). Several registries have reported significant declines in the incidence of STEMI such that ST-elevation MIs are becoming less frequent (4). Accompanying these trends, the overall proportion of admissions for chest pain caused by STEMI is also declining, while several sources have indicated that the incidence of unstable angina and N-STEMI is increasing (4).

Pathogenesis of ST Elevation Myocardial Infarction and Its Complications

ST elevation is conventionally thought of as representing transmural ischemia in response to fissuring or rupture of an atheromatous plaque with total and prolonged occlusion of a major coronary artery. Less frequently vessel occlusion may be caused by a prolonged coronary artery spasm.

After an acute MI, mechanical problems that result from dysfunction or disruption of critical myocardial structures (e.g., loss of contracting muscle causing left ventricular dysfunction,

TABLE 120.1

NEW DEFINITION OF MYOCARDIAL INFARCTION (FROM REF 2A)

Criteria for acute MI

The term MI should be used when there is evidence of myocardial necrosis in a clinical setting consistent with myocardial ischemia. Under these conditions any of the following criteria meets the diagnosis for MI:

- Detection of rise and/or fall of cardiac biomarkers (preferably troponin) with at least one value above the 99th percentile of the URL together with evidence of myocardial ischemia with at least one of the following:
  a. Symptoms of ischemia
  b. ECG changes indicative of new ischemia (new ST-T changes or new LBBB)
  c. Development of pathological Q waves in the ECG
  d. Imaging evidence of new loss of viable myocardium or new regional wall motion abnormality
- Sudden, unexpected cardiac death, involving cardiac arrest, often with symptoms suggestive of myocardial ischemia, and accompanied by presumably new ST elevation, or new LBBB, and/or evidence of fresh thrombus by coronary angiography and/or at autopsy, but death occurring before blood samples could be obtained, or at a time before appearance of cardiac biomarkers in the blood
- For PCI and CABG in patients with normal baseline troponin values, elevation of cardiac biomarkers above the 99th percentile URL are indicative of periprocedural myocardial necrosis. By convention, increases of biomarkers greater than 3 × 99th percentile URL has been designated as defining PCI-related myocardial infarction and elevations of biomarkers greater than 5 × 99th percentile URL plus either new pathological Q waves or new LBBB or angiographically documented new graft or native coronary artery occlusion, or imaging evidence of new loss of viable myocardium have been designated as defining CABG-related myocardial infarction
- Pathological findings of an acute MI

Criteria for prior MI

Any one of the following criteria meets the diagnosis for prior MI:

- Development of new pathological Q waves with or without symptoms
- Imaging evidence of a region of loss of viable myocardium that is thinned and fails to contract, in the absence of a non-ischemic cause.
- Pathological findings of a healed or healing MI

CABG, coronary artery bypass grafting; LBBB, left bundle branch block; MI, myocardial infarction; PCI, percutaneous coronary intervention; URL, upper reference limit.

mitral regurgitation, rupture of the interventricular septum or of the free wall, or ventricular aneurysm formation) may occur and require an immediate combination of pharmacologic, catheter-based, and surgical treatments. This may lead to *ventricular remodeling*, a term that refers to changes in size, shape, and thickness of the left ventricle involving both the infarcted and noninfarcted segments of the left ventricle (1,2,5,6). An extra load is placed on the residual functioning myocardium, which results in compensatory hypertrophy. Additionally, cardiac dysrhythmias may result from electrical instability, pump failure/excessive sympathetic stimulation, and conduction disturbances (1,2,5,6).

TABLE 120.2

CLINICAL CLASSIFICATION OF DIFFERENT TYPES OF MYOCARDIAL INFARCTION (FROM REF 2A)

Type 1
Spontaneous MI related to ischemia due to a primary coronary event such as plaque erosion and/or rupture, fissuring, or dissection

Type 2
MI secondary to ischemia due to either increased oxygen demand or decreased supply, e.g. coronary spasm, coronary embolism, anaemia, arrhythmias, hypertension, or hypotension

Type 3
Sudden unexpected cardiac death, including cardiac arrest, often with symptoms suggestive of myocardial ischemia, accompanied by presumably new ST elevation, or new LBBB, or evidence of fresh thrombus in a coronary artery by angiography and/or autopsy, but death occurring before blood samples could be obtained, or at a time before the appearance of cardiac biomarkers in the blood

Type 4a
MI associated with PCI

Type 4b
MI associated with stent thrombosis as documented by angiography or at autopsy

Type 5
MI associated with CABG

CABG, coronary artery bypass grafting; LBBB, left bundle branch block; MI, myocardial infarction; PCI, percutaneous coronary intervention.

TABLE 120.3

AIMS OF ACUTE MANAGEMENT OF ST ELEVATION MYOCARDIAL INFARCTION

- Rapidly establish a working diagnosis following presentation.
- Treat acute dysrhythmic and hemodynamic complications, including cardiac arrest.
- Provide prompt pain relief and adequate arterial oxygen concentration.
- Initiate reperfusion therapy to limit the extent of infarction and minimize the complications of pump failure and dysrhythmias.
- Treat complications of acute myocardial infarction.
- Provide risk assessment for longer-term management and to initiate secondary prevention.

EARLY EVALUATION

Immediate Concerns and Questions to Be Addressed at the Initial Evaluation

Rapid diagnosis and early risk stratification are essential to identify patients with acute chest pain in whom early revascularization can improve outcomes (Table 120.3). A working diagnosis of acute MI is usually based on the history of severe chest pain lasting for 20 minutes or more, not responding to nitroglycerin (Fig. 120.1). Important clues are a previous history of coronary artery disease (CAD) and radiation of the pain to the neck, lower jaw, or left arm. The pain may not be severe and, particularly in the elderly, other presentations such as fatigue, dyspnea, feeling faint or simply feeling "poorly," or syncope are common. There are no individual physical signs diagnostic of myocardial infarction, but most patients have evidence of autonomic nervous system activation (e.g., pallor and/or sweating) and either hypotension or a narrow pulse pressure. Features may also include irregularities of the pulse, bradycardia or tachycardia, and a third heart sound (7,8). The presence and severity of basal pulmonary rales is an easy, immediate, and pivotal tool for an early risk stratification of STEMI patients (Table 120.4).

An ECG should be obtained as soon as possible. In case of ST-segment elevations, or new or presumed new left bundle branch block, reperfusion therapy should be initiated as soon as possible. However, the ECG is often equivocal in the early hours and, even in proven infarction, it may never demonstrate the classic features of ST-segment elevation and new Q waves. During the early evolution of infarction, the ECG may be abnormal without significant ST elevation. Typical changes may evolve over minutes or hours, and it is critically important to institute continuous ST monitoring or perform repeat ECGs to ensure that such evolution is detected promptly (7,8).

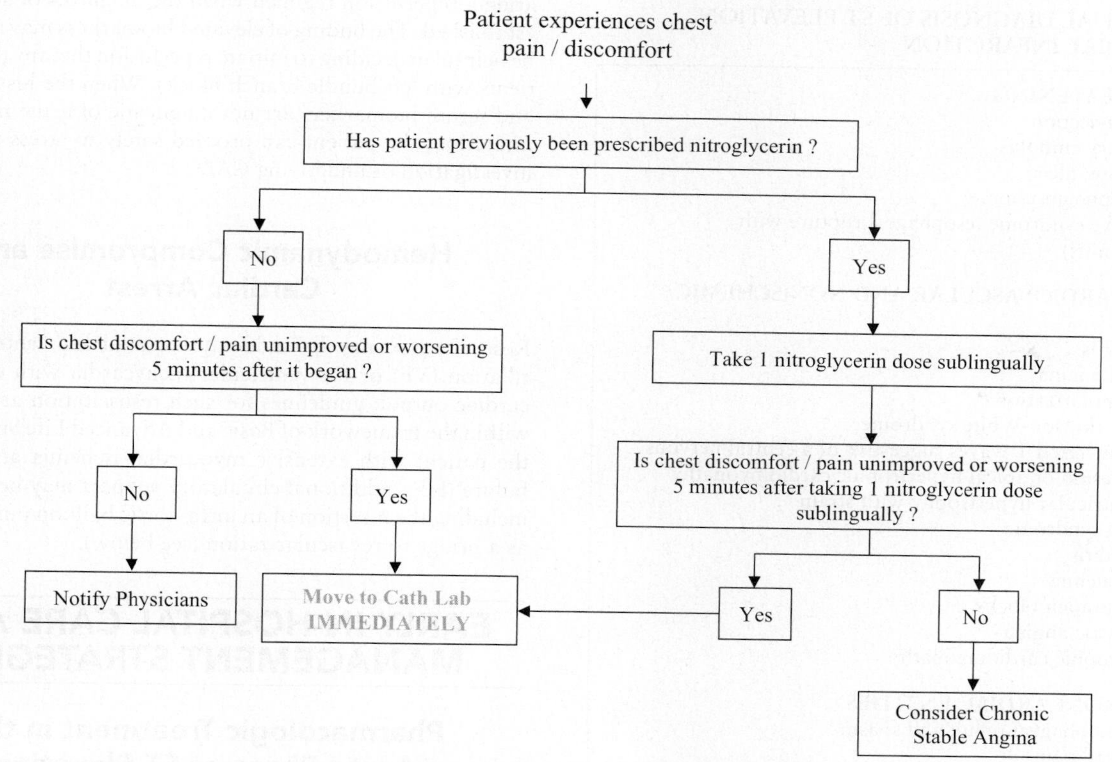

FIGURE 120.1. Patient (advance) instructions for nitroglycerin use and emergency medical service (EMS) contact in the setting of non–trauma-related chest discomfort/pain. (Modified from Antman EM, Anbe DT, Armstrong PW, et al. American College of Cardiology; American Heart Association Task Force on Practice Guidelines; Canadian Cardiovascular Society. ACC/AHA guidelines for the management of patients with ST-elevation myocardial infarction: a report of the American College of Cardiology/American Heart Association Task Force on Practice Guidelines [committee to revise the 1999 Guidelines for the Management of Patients with Acute Myocardial Infarction]. *Circulation*. 2004;110[9]:e82–e292.)

TABLE 120.4

PERCENT MORTALITY BY KILLIP CLASS[a]

Killip class	Killip and Kimball (in-hospital)	Fibrinolytic trials (30 d)			
		GISSI-1		International Study Group: Fibrinolytic	ASSENT-2: Fibrinolytic
		Placebo	Fibrinolytic		
I = no rales	6	7	6	5	5
II = rales less than 50%	17	20	16	18	13
III = pulmonary edema	38	39	33	32	26
IV = cardiogenic shock	81	70	70	72	56[b]

[a]*Values cited are subject to survivor bias.
[b]Highly selected group of patients.

In patients with symptoms suggestive of infarction but without diagnostic ECG changes, alternative diagnoses must be considered, including aortic dissection, gastroesophageal disease, and musculoskeletal and mediastinal conditions (Table 120.5). A normal ECG in the presence of suspected cardiac pain should prompt the search for an alternative diagnosis. Similarly, myocardial perfusion scintigraphy or magnetic resonance imaging (MRI) may be used to detect the presence of ischemia or infarction, and a normal result effectively excludes significant MI. Certain groups of patients, including the elderly and those with diabetes, may present without typical symptoms of MI. They may present with evolving ECG changes of MI or hemodynamic/mechanical complications. Their treatment should be similar to patients with typical painful infarction.

Blood sampling for serum biomarkers is routinely done in the acute phase. Considering that the first blood sample may be negative for elevated biomarkers, even in the presence of acute MI, it is not reasonable to wait for the next results before initiating a reperfusion regimen when the diagnosis of acute MI is established. The finding of elevated biomarkers may sometimes be helpful in deciding to initiate reperfusion therapy (e.g., in patients with left bundle branch block). When the history, ECG, and serum biomarkers are not diagnostic of acute myocardial infarction, the patient can proceed safely to stress testing for investigation of underlying CAD.

TABLE 120.5

DIFFERENTIAL DIAGNOSIS OF ST ELEVATION MYOCARDIAL INFARCTION

LIFE THREATENING
- Aortic dissection
- Pulmonary embolus
- Perforating ulcer
- Tension pneumothorax
- Boerhaave syndrome (esophageal rupture with mediastinitis)

OTHER CARDIOVASCULAR AND NONISCHEMIC ENTITIES
- Pericarditis
- Atypical angina
- Early repolarization
- Wolff-Parkinson-White syndrome
- Deeply inverted T waves suggestive of a central nervous system lesion or apical hypertrophic cardiomyopathy
- Left ventricular hypertrophy with strain
- Brugada syndrome
- Myocarditis
- Hyperkalemia
- Bundle branch blocks
- Vasospastic angina
- Hypertrophic cardiomyopathy

OTHER NONCARDIAC ENTITIES
- Gastroesophageal reflux and spasm
- Chest wall pain
- Pleurisy
- Peptic ulcer disease
- Panic attack
- Biliary or pancreatic pain
- Cervical disc or neuropathic pain
- Somatization and psychogenic pain disorder

Hemodynamic Compromise and Cardiac Arrest

Resuscitation may be suddenly required for ventricular fibrillation (VF) or for ventricular tachycardia with diminished cardiac output; guidelines for such resuscitation are provided within the framework of Basic and Advanced Life Support. For the patient with extensive myocardial ischemia and/or heart failure (HF), additional circulatory support may be necessary, including the insertion of an intra-aortic balloon pump (IABP), as a bridge to revascularization (see below).

EARLY IN-HOSPITAL CARE AND MANAGEMENT STRATEGIES

Pharmacologic Treatment in the Acute Phase of ST Elevation Myocardial Infarction

Pain Control

Pain relief is a key element in the early management of the patient with STEMI. Pain management should be directed toward

TABLE 120.6

CONTRAINDICATIONS TO FIBRINOLYTIC THERAPY

ABSOLUTE CONTRAINDICATIONS
- Hemorrhagic stroke or stroke of unknown origin at any time
- Ischemic stroke in preceding 6 mo
- Central nervous system damage or neoplasms
- Recent major trauma/surgery/head injury (within preceding 3 wk)
- Gastrointestinal bleeding within the last month
- Known bleeding disorder
- Aortic dissection

RELATIVE CONTRAINDICATIONS
- Transient ischemic attack in preceding 6 mo
- Oral anticoagulant therapy
- Pregnancy or within 1 wk postpartum
- Noncompressible punctures
- Traumatic resuscitation
- Refractory hypertension (systolic blood pressure greater than 180 mm Hg)
- Advanced liver disease
- Infective endocarditis
- Active peptic ulcer

acute relief of symptoms of ongoing myocardial ischemia and necrosis, and toward general relief of anxiety and apprehension, the latter of which can heighten pain perception. Morphine sulfate remains the analgesic agent of choice for management of pain associated with STEMI, the exception being documented cases of morphine sensitivity. The dose required for adequate pain relief varies in proportion to age and body size, as well as blood pressure and heart rate. Anxiety reduction secondary to morphine administration reduces the patient's restlessness and the activity of the autonomic nervous system, with a consequent reduction of the heart's metabolic demands. Morphine administration for patients with pulmonary edema is clearly beneficial and may promote peripheral arterial and venous dilation, reducing the work of breathing and slowing the heart rate secondary to a combined decrease in sympathetic tone and augmentation of vagal tone (7,8). Side effects of morphine administration, such as hypotension, can be minimized by keeping the patient supine and elevating the lower extremities if systolic pressure decreases below 100 mm Hg, assuming pulmonary edema is not present.

Fibrinolysis

Prompt and effective reperfusion by pharmacologic therapy is the cornerstone of treatment for STEMI. It is the only widely applicable acute treatment that can diminish infarct size and major cardiac complications (Table 120.6). In trials of fibrinolysis versus control, more than 150,000 patients were randomized and showed that the treatment benefit was approximately 50 lives saved per 1,000 patients treated with the combination of thrombolytic agent and aspirin (9).

Limitations of Fibrinolysis. The major limitation of fibrinolytic drug treatment is that reperfusion is gradual and, in addition, is incomplete or inadequate in a significant proportion of patients. This proportion may range from about 40% showing failure to achieve Thrombolysis in Myocardial Infarction (TIMI) 3 flow within the first 3 hours of reperfusion therapy when streptokinase is used, to 20% to 30% with tissue plasminogen activator (tPA) or tenecteplase (TNK) (Table 120.7).

The principal hazard of fibrinolytic therapy is stroke and intracranial hemorrhage. Overall, about four extra strokes occur per 1,000 patients treated and, of these, two are fatal. The use of accelerated tPA (alteplase) results in ten fewer deaths per 1,000 patients treated, but at the risk of three additional strokes compared with streptokinase treatment (10). Single-bolus agents provide logistic advantages, and both reteplase-PA or weight-adjusted TNK have equivalent efficacy to accelerated tPA. TNK has a lower rate of noncerebral bleeds and a lesser need for blood transfusion. Bolus agents are particularly advantageous in minimizing time delay in the prehospital and emergency room settings (10).

Prehospital Fibrinolysis. In clinical trials, it has been shown that prehospital thrombolysis (PHT) could be used safely in patients presenting with evidence of acute MI (11).

TABLE 120.7

COMPARISON OF APPROVED FIBRINOLYTIC AGENTS

	Streptokinase	Alteplase	Reteplase	Tenecteplase-tPA
Dose	1.5 MU over 30–60 min	Up to 100 mg in 90 min based on weight[a]	10 U × 2 each over 2 min	30–50 mg based on weight[b]
Bolus administration	No	No	Yes	Yes
Antigenic	Yes	No	No	No
Allergic reactions	Yes	No	No	No
Systemic fibrinogen depletion	Marked	Mild	Moderate	Minimal
90-min patency rates, approximate %	50	75	7	75
TIMI grade 3 flow, %	32	54	60	63
Cost per dose (US $)	613	2,974	2,750	2,833 for 50 mg

MU, mega units; TIMI, Thrombolysis in Myocardial Infarction.
[a]Bolus 15 mg, infusion 0.75 mg/kg × 30 min (maximum 50 mg), then 0.5 mg/kg not to exceed 35 mg over the next 60 min to an overall maximum of 100 mg.
[b]Thirty milligrams for weight less than 60 kg; 35 mg for 60–69 kg; 40 mg for 70–79 mg; 45 mg for 80–89 kg; and 50 mg for 90 kg or more.

The efficacy of PHT has initially been demonstrated in the Grampian Region Early Anistreplase Trial (GREAT) (12) in which administration of thrombolysis by the general practitioners before hospital admission resulted in a 50% reduction in 1-year mortality. Recently, a meta-analysis of six trials comparing PHT and in-hospital thrombolysis confirmed this beneficial effect, showing a 17% reduction in in-hospital mortality with the use of PHT (11). The Comparison of Angioplasty and Prehospital Thrombolysis In acute Myocardial infarction (CAPTIM) trial (13), which compared PHT with primary percutaneous coronary intervention (PCI), showed that 1-month mortality was lower in the group that received PHT. These data are concordant with the observation from the meta-analysis of trials of thrombolytic therapy that showed an exponential decrease in the efficacy of thrombolysis in the patients treated more than 3 hours after the onset of chest pain (14).

In this regard, it is now clear that myocardial salvage is highly dependent on the time from the beginning of symptoms to reperfusion, and that very early administration of thrombolytics are likely to result in superior myocardial salvage compared with in-hospital thrombolysis and possibly also primary PCI, for which the time delay observed in the real-world setting is often 1 hour or more (15,16).

Fibrinolysis Combined with Newer Antithrombotic Agents. To improve the rates of patients achieving TIMI 3 flow by pharmacologic reperfusion therapy, glycoprotein (GP) IIb/IIIa antagonists have been combined with fibrinolytic agents to achieve both platelet disaggregation and fibrinolysis (1,2,17). This pharmacologic combination has been tested in seven studies, including two large trials (ASSENT 3 and GUSTO V) involving more than 30,000 patients. There was no overall advantage noted when combining the thrombolytic agent with a GP IIb/IIIa inhibitor. In patients older than 70 years of age, the combination increased the risk of intracranial hemorrhage and extracranial bleeding (10). Similarly, the combination of streptokinase with a specific antithrombin (bivalirudin) failed to improve survival in the HERO 2 trial (18). Two ongoing randomized trials (CARESS and FINESS) are investigating the impact of a combination therapy in the early treatment of STEMI.

Anti-ischemic Drugs

Oxygen. Although oxygen administration to virtually all patients with suspected STEMI has become universal practice, it is still unknown whether this therapy limits myocardial damage or reduces morbidity or mortality. Experimental results indicate that oxygen administration may limit myocardial injury (19), and may reduce ST-segment elevation (20). The rationale for use of oxygen is based on the observation that even with uncomplicated MI, some patients are modestly hypoxemic initially, presumably because of ventilation/perfusion mismatch and excessive lung water (21). For patients without complications, excess administration of oxygen can lead to systemic vasoconstriction, and high flow rates can be harmful to patients with chronic obstructive airway disease. In the absence of compelling evidence for established benefit in uncomplicated cases, and in view of its expense, there appears to be little justification for continuing its routine use beyond 6 hours.

Nitrates. The rationale for using nitrates in the setting of STEMI is that they reduce preload and afterload through peripheral arterial and venous dilation, improve coronary flow by relaxation of epicardial coronary arteries, and dilate collateral vessels, potentially creating a more favorable subendocardial-to-epicardial flow ratio (22,23). Nitrate-induced vasodilatation may also have particular utility in those rare patients with coronary spasm presenting as STEMI.

Clinical trial results have suggested only a modest benefit from nitroglycerin used acutely in STEMI and continued subsequently. A pooled analysis of more than 80,000 patients treated with nitratelike preparations intravenously or orally in 22 trials yielded a mortality rate of 7.7% in the control group, which was reduced to 7.4% in the nitrate group. These data are consistent with a possible small treatment effect of nitrates on mortality, such that three to four fewer deaths would occur for every 1,000 patients treated (24). Nitrates in all forms should be avoided in patients with initial systolic blood pressures less than 90 mm Hg or greater than or equal to 30 mm Hg below baseline, marked bradycardia or tachycardia, or known or suspected right ventricular (RV) infarction.

β-Adrenergic Blockers. The emergency treatment of suspected STEMI with intravenous (IV) β-blocker therapy has also been studied in more than two dozen randomized trials (25–29). Overall, those trials included more than 27,000 patients, but nearly all were done before fibrinolytic and antiplatelet therapy had become routine, and they mainly involved fairly low-risk patients. Collectively, though not separately, their results indicated that this treatment was safe and moderately effective in such low-risk patients (25). However, in the recently published COMMIT trial, 45,852 patients admitted within 24 hours of suspected STEMI onset were randomly allocated metoprolol—up to 15 mg intravenously, followed by 200 mg oral daily—or matching placebo (29). Allocation to early metoprolol was associated with reduced risk of reinfarction and ventricular fibrillation, but increased risk of cardiogenic shock, especially during the first day or so after admission (29). Consequently, it might generally be prudent to consider starting β-blocker therapy in hospital only when the hemodynamic condition after STEMI has been stabilized.

Antiplatelet Therapy

Aspirin. Aspirin should be given to the patient with suspected STEMI as early as possible and continued indefinitely, regardless of the strategy for reperfusion or whether additional antiplatelet agents are administered. Known true aspirin allergy is the only exception to this recommendation. Maintenance aspirin doses for secondary prevention of cardiovascular events in large trials have varied from 75 to 325 mg/day, but no trial has directly compared the efficacy of different doses after STEMI (1,2).

Thienopyridine. A thienopyridine (e.g., ticlopidine or clopidogrel) should be substituted for aspirin in patients with STEMI for whom aspirin is contraindicated because of hypersensitivity or major gastrointestinal intolerance. Clopidogrel is generally preferred to ticlopidine because of fewer side effects, lack of need for laboratory monitoring, and once-daily dosing. On the basis of several randomized trials (30–33), clopidogrel, in combination with low-dose aspirin—75 to 162 mg, to minimize the risk of bleeding—is recommended for all patients after stent implantation (1,2,34). Recently, two randomized trials of 7,000 patients with STEMI showed that adding clopidogrel to aspirin improved the patency of the infarct-related coronary artery after fibrinolytic therapy, and suggested some reduction in clinical events (35,36). In addition, these trials demonstrated that adding clopidogrel 75 mg daily to aspirin and other standard treatments, such as fibrinolytic therapy, in STEMI patients safely reduces mortality and major vascular events in hospital (35,36).

Prasugrel is a new thienopyridine derivative that is about ten times more potent than clopidogrel in preclinical studies (37). It has been evaluated both in healthy individuals and in patients undergoing elective or urgent PCI, in which it was shown to result in low and similar rates of bleeding when compared with clopidogrel (38).

Platelet Glycoprotein IIb/IIIa Receptor Antagonists. It is reasonable to start treatment with GP IIb/IIIa (abciximab, tirofiban, and eptifibatide) as early as possible in patients undergoing primary PCI. Several randomized studies have demonstrated that adjunctive antiplatelet therapy with GP IIb/IIIa blockade reduces the incidence of acute ischemic events by as much as 35% to 50% among the broad population of patients undergoing primary PCI (39).

GP IIb/IIIa inhibitors were also shown to decrease coronary thrombus, improve TIMI flow grade, enhance epicardial reperfusion when combined with thrombolysis, improve 30-day clinical outcomes post-MI (Fig. 120.2), speed resolution of ST-segment elevation, and in one study of elective percutaneous coronary intervention, improve coronary artery flow reserve and myocardial blush grade (40). A recent meta-analysis of all completed, published, randomized trials of abciximab in STEMI showed that, when compared with the control group, adjunctive abciximab was associated with a significant reduction in 30-day and long-term mortality in patients treated with primary PCI, but not in those receiving fibrinolysis (41). The 30-day reinfarction rate was significantly reduced in patients treated with either fibrinolysis or primary PCI. A higher risk of major bleeding complications is observed with abciximab in association with fibrinolysis (41).

Antithrombotic Therapy

Unfractionated Heparin. Despite the use of unfractionated heparin (UFH) (42) in STEMI for over 40 years, there is continued controversy regarding its role. In patients who are treated with fibrinolytic therapy, recommendations for UFH therapy depend on the fibrinolytic agent chosen. The nonspecific fibrinolytic agents—streptokinase, anistreplase, and urokinase—that produce a systemic coagulopathy, including depletion of factors V and VIII, and massive production of fibrinogen degradation products are themselves anticoagulants. From this perspective, the need for adjunctive systemic anticoagulation with these agents is conceptually less compelling. When primary PCI is chosen as the route of reperfusion, weight-adjusted boluses of heparin in the range of 70 to 100 U/kg are recommended. This recommendation does not come specifically from empirical data in the setting of STEMI, but from general observations in the setting of angioplasty that an activated clotting time of at least 250 to 350 seconds is associated with a lower rate of complications than lower activated clotting times (43).

When GP IIb/IIIa antagonists are used, the UFH bolus should be reduced to 50 to 70 U/kg to achieve a target activated clotting time of 200 seconds (34). UFH doses used during PCI for failed fibrinolysis should be similarly reduced and further lowered if used with GP IIb/IIIa antagonists.

Low-molecular-weight Heparin. In the setting of STEMI, low-molecular-weight heparin (LMWH) may be an attractive alternative to UFH, as demonstrated by several clinical trials including those with LMWH as ancillary therapy to fibrinolysis and those that randomized patients not receiving fibrinolysis (44–49). The two LMWHs studied most extensively in patients with STEMI are enoxaparin and dalteparin.

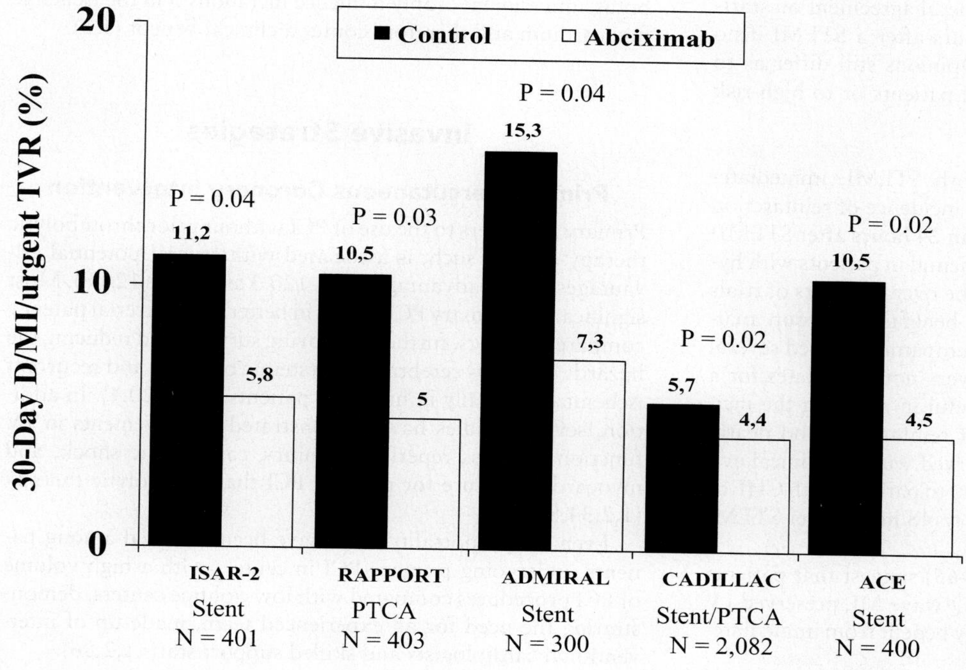

FIGURE 120.2. Randomized trials demonstrating the clinical benefits of abciximab in the setting of ST elevation myocardial infarction (STEMI). D, death; MI, myocardial infarction; TVR, target vessel revascularization; PTCA, percutaneous transluminal coronary angioplasty.

Direct Antithrombin Agents. Selective factor Xa inhibition appears to be a reasonable therapeutic concept in patients presenting with STEMI. A meta-analysis evaluated 11 trials that collectively enrolled more than 35,000 patients, comparing direct thrombin inhibitors with UFH (50). There was an approximate 25% reduction in the incidence of re-MI in patients treated with either hirudin or bivalirudin, but there was less evident efficacy for univalent thrombin inhibitors such as argatroban, efegatran, and inogatran. Other large randomized trials recently completed have confirmed the safety and long-term efficacy of bivalirudin alone compared with heparin or heparin and GP IIb/IIIa in the setting of STEMI (51,52).

Fondaparinux is a synthetic pentasaccharide that is a highly selective inhibitor of factor Xa. It selectively binds antithrombin III, inducing a conformational change that increases the anti-Xa activity of antithrombin III more than 300 times, which results in dose-dependent inhibition of factor Xa (53). In patients with STEMI, particularly those not undergoing primary PCI, fondaparinux seems to reduce mortality and reinfarction without increasing bleeding and strokes (54).

Other Pharmacologic Agents

Angiotensin-converting Enzyme Inhibitors. It is now well established that angiotensin-converting enzyme (ACE) inhibitors should be given to patients who have an impaired left ventricular (LV) ejection fraction or who have experienced congestive heart failure (CHF) in the early phase of an MI. The GISSI-3 (55), ISIS-4 (56), and Chinese study (57) have shown that ACE inhibitors started on the first day after a STEMI reduce mortality in the succeeding 4 to 6 weeks by a small but significant amount. The CONSENSUS II study (58), however, failed to show a benefit of early IV ACE inhibitor administration in STEMI patients. This may have been due to chance, or the fact that treatment was initiated early with an intravenous formulation. However, a systematic overview of trials of ACE inhibition early in acute MI indicated that this therapy is safe, well tolerated, and associated with a small but significant reduction in 30-day mortality, with most of the benefit observed in the first week. Therefore, there is now general agreement on starting ACE inhibitors in the first 24 hours after a STEMI if no contraindications are present (59). Opinions still differ as to whether to give ACE inhibitors to all patients or to high-risk patients only.

Calcium Antagonists. In patients with STEMI, immediate-release nifedipine does not reduce the incidence of reinfarction or mortality when given early (less than 24 hours after STEMI) or late, and may be particularly detrimental in patients with hypotension or tachycardia. Although the overall results of trials with verapamil showed no mortality benefits, subgroup analysis showed that immediate-release verapamil initiated several days after STEMI, in patients who were not candidates for a β-blocking agent, may have been useful in reducing the incidence of the composite end point of reinfarction and death, provided LV function was well preserved with no clinical evidence of CHF. Verapamil is detrimental to patients with CHF or bradyarrhythmias during the first 24 to 48 hours after STEMI (60–65).

Data from randomized trials (60–65) suggest that patients with non–Q-wave MI or those with Q-wave MI, preserved LV function, and no evidence of CHF may benefit from immediate-release diltiazem.

Inodilators. Administration of inodilator agents may be particularly threatening to patients with acute MI and should be avoided, except when severe hypotension occurs. Positive inotropic agents, especially phosphodiesterase inhibitors and adrenergic agonists such as dobutamine, may be associated with increasing myocardial oxygen demand and the potential to induce malignant dysrhythmias and myocardial ischemia, contributing to further cell death or necrosis (66–69).

Levosimendan is a calcium sensitizer that, by virtue of its unique mechanism of action and its negligible effect on myocardial oxygen demand, is the only inodilator that has been associated with favorable short-term outcomes in patients with acute MI, but large mortality studies are warranted (70).

Magnesium. Although a meta-analysis of seven randomized trials suggested a significant mortality benefit of magnesium in acute MI (71,72), subsequently a total of 68,684 patients were studied in a series of 15 randomized trials with controversial findings (73–80). On the basis of the totality of available evidence, in current coronary care practice, there is no indication for the routine administration of intravenous magnesium to patients with acute MI at any level of risk. Magnesium can continue to be administered for repletion of documented electrolyte deficits and life-threatening ventricular arrhythmias such as torsades de pointes (81).

Lidocaine. Although it has been demonstrated that lidocaine can reduce the incidence of ventricular fibrillation in the acute phase of MI (82,83), this drug significantly increases the risk of asystole (83). A meta-analysis of 14 trials showed a nonsignificantly higher mortality in lidocaine-treated patients than in controls (84). The routine prophylactic use of this drug is therefore not justified.

Glucose-Insulin-Potassium. There is experimental and limited clinical evidence that routine administration of glucose-insulin-potassium may favorably influence metabolism in the ischemic myocardium and therefore confer a clinical benefit (1,2).

Invasive Strategies

Primary Percutaneous Coronary Intervention

Primary PCI refers to the use of PCI without prior thrombolytic therapy and, as such, is associated with several potential advantages and disadvantages (Fig. 120.3 and Table 120.8). Most significantly, primary PCI results in better acute arterial patency compared to lytics, further improving survival and reducing the hazards of excess cerebral and systemic bleeding and recurrent ischemia, especially in high-risk patients (Fig. 120.4). In addition, several studies have demonstrated improvements in LV function and less reperfusion injury, cardiogenic shock, and myocardial rupture for primary PCI than fibrinolytic therapy (1,2,34,85).

Even lower mortality rates have been reported among patients undergoing primary PCI in centers with a high volume of PCI procedures compared with low-volume centers, demonstrating the need for an experienced team, made up of interventional cardiologists and skilled support staff (1,2,86).

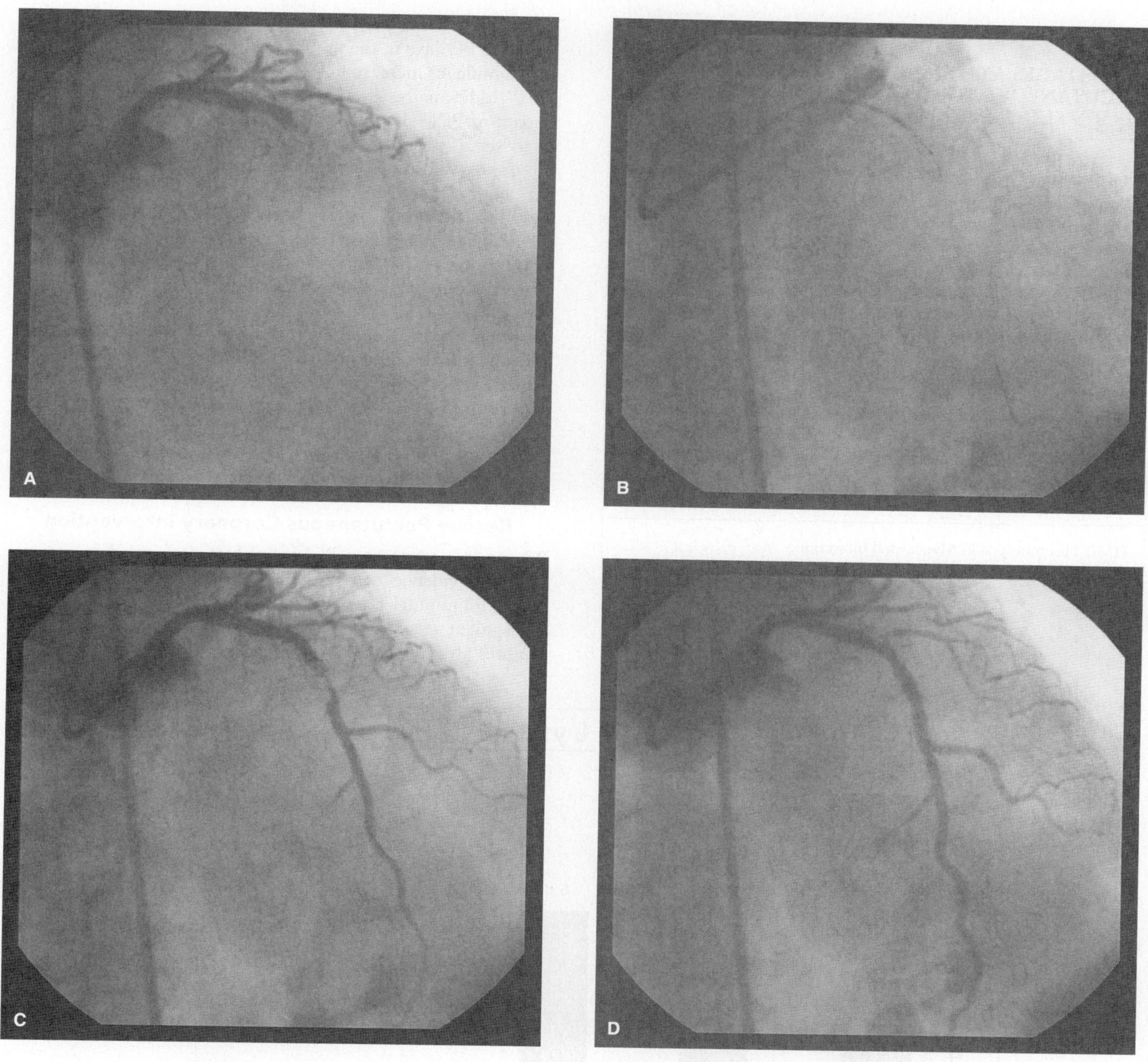

FIGURE 120.3. A case of successful revascularization of anterior ST elevation myocardial infarction (STEMI) by primary percutaneous coronary intervention (PCI). **A:** Total occlusion (TIMI 0) in the middle tract of the left anterior descending (LAD) coronary artery. **B:** Crossing of the guidewire and thrombus removal by a manual thromboaspiration device. **C:** Restoration of a TIMI 3 flow on the LAD. **D:** Final angiographic result after stent placement.

Facilitated Percutaneous Coronary Intervention

Facilitated PCI refers to treatment with low-dose thrombolytic therapy, platelet GP IIb/IIIa inhibitors, or both, before PCI. The rationale is to provide the earliest possible pharmacologic reperfusion before an attempt at definitive mechanical revascularization (87,88). These strategies may offer advantages, but larger-scale trials are still awaited (89).

Recently, the Assessment of the Safety and Efficacy of a New Treatment Strategy for Acute Myocardial Infarction (ASSENT)-4 PCI study was prematurely terminated. The study was intended to be a large, randomized trial in acute MI patients facing very long delays—3 to 4 hours—before receiving therapy, as is typical for patients facing long travel distances or who must be transferred to a hospital with interventional facilities (90). It was an open-label, 1:1 study that randomized patients to either full-dose tenecteplase plus PCI (facilitated PCI) or to primary PCI with unfractionated heparin. GP IIb/IIIa inhibitors were used either in bail-out situations in patients pretreated with fibrinolytic therapy or at the investigator's discretion in the PCI-alone arm. The primary end point—death, cardiogenic shock, or congestive heart failure within 90 days—was significantly lower in the PCI-alone group compared with

TABLE 120.8

ADVANTAGES AND DISADVANTAGES OF PRIMARY PERCUTANEOUS CORONARY INTERVENTION (PCI) VERSUS THROMBOLYSIS

ADVANTAGES OF PRIMARY PCI VERSUS THROMBOLYSIS

- Immediate definition of coronary anatomy
- Early risk stratification
- Superior acute vessel patency and TIMI flow grade
- Less reocclusion, recurrent ischemia, and reinfarction
- Better survival in high-risk patients
- Less reperfusion injury and myocardial rupture
- Lower risk of intracranial hemorrhage
- Useful in thrombolytic ineligible patients
- Shorter length of hospital stay

DISADVANTAGES OF PRIMARY PCI VERSUS THROMBOLYSIS

- Skilled interventional cardiologists and catheterization laboratory must be available
- Logistic delays

TIMI, Thrombolysis in Myocardial Infarction.

the facilitated PCI arm (90). The significantly higher rate of stroke at 90 days in the facilitated PCI group was mainly due to a significant increase in the rate of intracranial hemorrhage (90). Additionally, in the recent BRAVE trial examining the impact of PCI with two boluses of 5 U reteplase plus abciximab versus abciximab alone (12 hours), the infarct size was not improved after PCI with reteplase, and bleeding was more frequent (91).

On the other hand, the recently published CARESS-in-AMI (Combined Abciximab RE-teplase Stent Study in Acute Myocardial Infarction) suggested that immediate transfer for PCI improves outcomes (composite of death, reinfarction, or refractory ischaemia at 30 days) in high-risk patients with STEMI treated at a non-interventional centre with half-dose reteplase and abciximab compared to standard medical therapy with transfer for rescue angioplasty (91A). Based on these findings and waiting for further trial results, organisation of networks to move patients given a thrombolytic drug to institutions with catheterisation laboratories seems a reasonable option, since primary angioplasty cannot be implemented everywhere.

Rescue Percutaneous Coronary Intervention

Rescue PCI refers to a PCI procedure performed in patients without evidence of a response to thrombolytic treatment within 90 minutes after therapy; that is, there is less than 50% ST-segment resolution and/or symptom regression within 90 minutes after treatment.

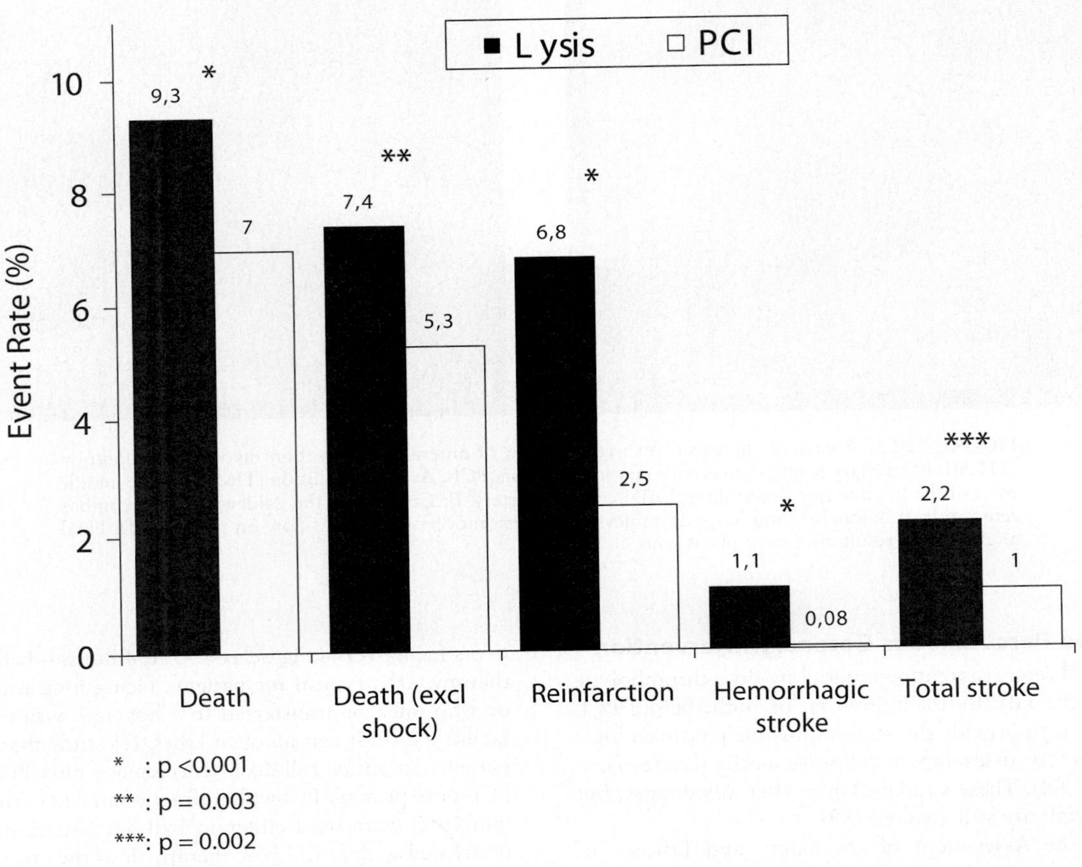

FIGURE 120.4. Meta-analysis of 23 randomized trials of primary percutaneous coronary intervention (PCI) versus thrombolysis. (Modified from Keeley EC, Grines CL. Primary coronary intervention for acute myocardial infarction. *JAMA*. 2004;291[6]:736–739.)

Feasibility studies have demonstrated success of PCI in achieving coronary patency and flow, and current guidelines recommend it only for certain high-risk subgroups of patients (1,2,34).

In the recently published Rescue Angioplasty versus Conservative Treatment or Repeat Thrombolysis (REACT) trial, event-free survival after failed thrombolytic therapy was significantly higher with rescue PCI than with repeated thrombolysis or conservative treatment (92). However, available data are still insufficient to demonstrate whether there is improvement in mortality or further MI with this strategy.

Transport for Primary Percutaneous Coronary Intervention

For hospitals without on-site PCI facilities, careful consideration needs to be given to the potential benefits of PCI following transfer to an intervention center versus fibrinolysis (93). For instance, the DANAMI 2 study suggested that for transfer times of 2 hours or less from a community hospital to the start of PCI, there is a significant reduction in death, reinfarction, and stroke compared with thrombolysis (94). After early reports of feasibility (95), five trials (94,96–99) randomly assigned patients with STEMI in community hospitals without PCI capability to immediate transfer to hospitals that could perform primary PCI or to on-site thrombolytic therapy (Fig. 120.5). Complications were rare during the transfer, with a 0.5% risk for death, a 0.7% to 1.4% risk for ventricular dysrhythmias, and a 2% risk for second- or third-degree heart block (94,96–99). A meta-analysis of these trials (100), which included a trial comparing primary PCI with prehospital thrombolytic therapy (13), compared outcomes of 1,887 patients randomly assigned to emergency transfer for primary PCI and 1,863 patients randomly assigned to on-site or prehospital thrombolytic therapy. The combined end point of death, reinfarction, and stroke at 30 days was reduced by 42% ($p < 0.001$) in the group transferred for primary PCI as compared with the group receiving thrombolytic therapy (100). However, these findings have a limited application in the daily clinical practice. For instance, most patients randomly assigned to transfer for primary PCI were treated in high-volume PCI centers: in the largest trial 96% of patients were transferred in less than 2 hours and the median interval from symptom onset to first balloon inflation was only 224 minutes (94). Accordingly, these data should not be extrapolated to transfer for primary PCI in low-volume centers or to situations in which transfer delays exceed 2 to 3 hours. More importantly, the time from symptom onset to first balloon inflation must be minimized, requiring that the transferred patient is delivered directly to an experienced "ready and waiting" catheterization laboratory (101).

The Crucial Role of Time in Reperfusion Therapies

The shorter the time is from symptom onset to treatment, the greater the survival benefit with either reperfusion therapy (102–107). The choice between therapies should take into account reperfusion treatment times (1,2) (Figs. 120.6 and 120.7). Time delay is critically important, especially within the first 3 to 4 hours following symptom onset (1,2,108). Overall, there is a progressive decrease of about 1.6 deaths per hour of delay per 1,000 patients treated. However, within the first 2 hours, the reduction in mortality is twice as large as beyond 2 hours (Fig. 120.8). Hence, the European guidelines for the management of acute MI recommend that for those patients with clear-cut changes of acute infarction, no more than 20 minutes should elapse between hospital arrival and the administration of thrombolytic therapy (or prehospital administration) or no more than 60 minutes between hospital arrival and balloon inflation for primary PCI (1,2). A second and critically important reason for minimizing prehospital delay is to treat early ventricular fibrillation. At least as many deaths may be saved by prompt resuscitation therapy in early acute MI as are saved by reperfusion therapy.

While the relationship between mortality and time delay from symptom onset to treatment is stringent in patients with STEMI who are receiving thrombolytic therapy (109–111), it is much weaker in patients undergoing primary PCI (108,112,113) (Fig. 120.9). Consequently, favorable results obtained from primary PCI depend less on the time to treatment than does thrombolytic therapy. On the other hand, more recent trials showed that the benefits of primary PCI may diminish with excessive delays in opening the infarct-related artery (106,107,114,115) (Fig. 120.10).

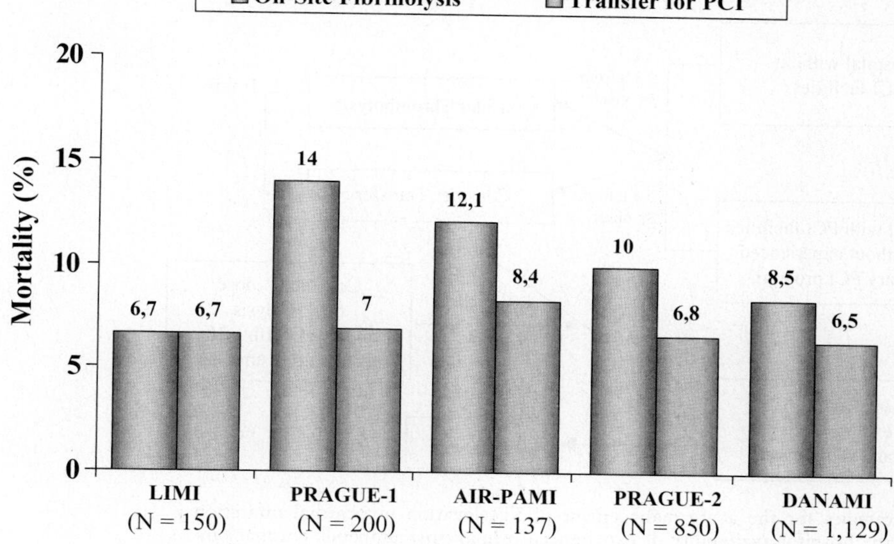

FIGURE 120.5. Randomized trials comparing on-site fibrinolysis and transfer for primary percutaneous coronary intervention (PCI).

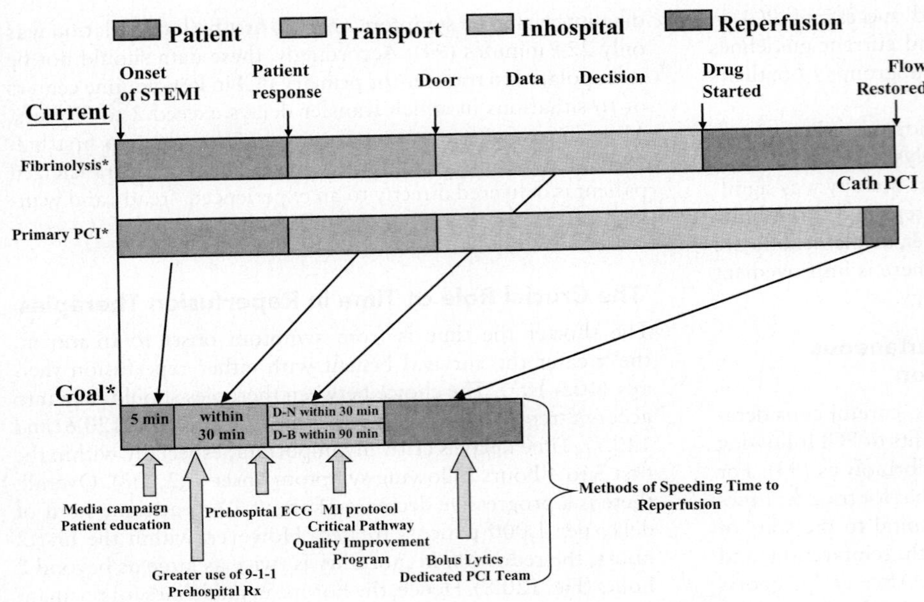

FIGURE 120.6. Major components of time delay between onset of symptoms from ST elevation myocardial infarction (STEMI) and restoration of flow in the infarct related artery. PCI, percutaneous coronary intervention. (Modified from Antman EM, Anbe DT, Armstrong PW, et al. American College of Cardiology; American Heart Association Task Force on Practice Guidelines; Canadian Cardiovascular Society. ACC/AHA guidelines for the management of patients with ST-elevation myocardial infarction: a report of the American College of Cardiology/American Heart Association Task Force on Practice Guidelines [committee to revise the 1999 Guidelines for the Management of Patients with Acute Myocardial Infarction]. *Circulation.* 2004;110[9]:e82–e292.)

Several mechanisms have been proposed to explain this difference in time-to-treatment effect. With thrombolytic therapy, there is an inverse relationship between the rate of achieving normal blood flow and the time-to-treatment interval (116). In addition, patients treated with thrombolytic therapy have an increased risk for mechanical complications, such as myocardial rupture, with progressive increases in time to treatment (116). In patients treated with primary PCI, on the other hand, mechanical complications are rare. Interestingly, thrombolytic therapy is more often complicated by reocclusion of the infarct-related artery, reinfarction, and worse long-term survival as compared with primary PCI (117). Finally, the extent of myocardial salvage is inversely proportional to the time to treatment in patients treated with thrombolytic therapy, but is independent of time to treatment in primary PCI, particularly with adjunctive stenting (118).

Coronary Artery Bypass Surgery

The number of patients who need coronary artery bypass grafting (CABG) in the acute phase of STEMI is quite limited. It may, however, be indicated when PCI has failed, when there has been a sudden occlusion of a coronary artery during catheterization, if PCI is not feasible, in selected patients in cardiogenic shock, or in association with surgery for a ventricular septal defect or mitral regurgitation due to papillary muscle dysfunction and rupture (1,2).

LONG-TERM POST–MYOCARDIAL INFARCTION PHARMACOLOGIC TREATMENT

The results of large randomized clinical trials have formed the basis for the long-term management of acute MI. Evidence from these trials has demonstrated that pharmacologic therapies aimed at limiting risk factors and coronary plaque instability with lipid-lowering therapies, and focused on inhibiting post-MI remodeling with neurohumoral antagonists—namely ACE inhibitors, angiotensin II receptor blockers (ARBs;

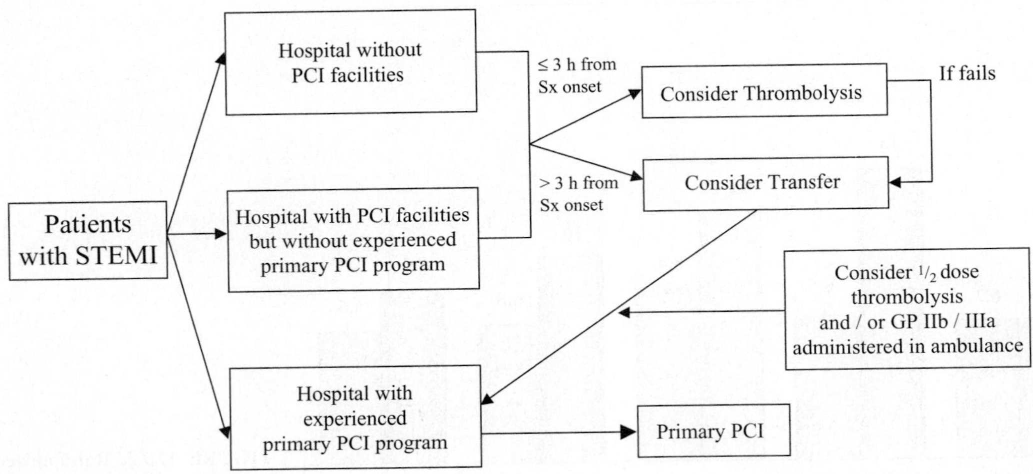

FIGURE 120.7. Possible strategies for the acute management of ST elevation myocardial infarction (STEMI) patients based on the hospital availability of experienced primary percutaneous coronary intervention (PCI) program. GP, glycoprotein.

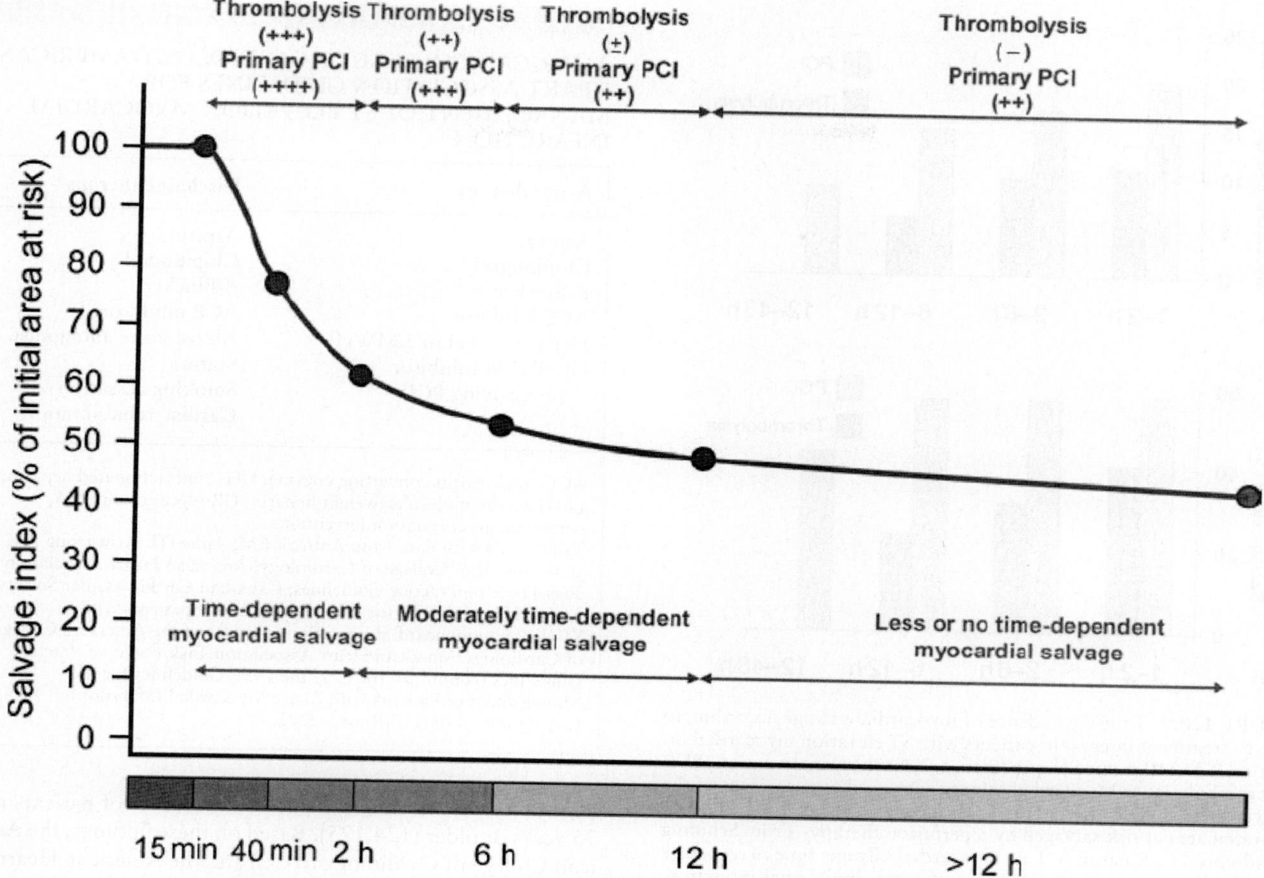

FIGURE 120.8. Time dependency of myocardial salvage expressed as percentage of initial area at risk. The initial parts of the curve up to 2 hours were reconstructed based on the experimental studies. The other parts of the curve showing myocardial salvage from 2 to 12 hours from the symptom onset are reconstructed according to the data of scintigraphic studies. Efficacy of reperfusion is expressed as follows: ++++, very effective; +++, effective; ++, moderately effective; ±, uncertainly effective; −, not effective. PCI, percutaneous coronary intervention. (From Schomig A, Ndrepepa G, Kastrati A. Late myocardial salvage: time to recognize its reality in the reperfusion therapy of acute myocardial infarction. *Eur Heart J*. 2006;27:1900–1907.)

e.g., valsartan), β-blockers (e.g., carvedilol), and, most recently, aldosterone antagonists (e.g., eplerenone)—can significantly improve long-term outcomes including death, reinfarction, and worsening CHF (1,2) (Table 120.9). Clinical trials have also shown the benefits of antiplatelet and anticoagulant therapies, including aspirin and warfarin, as well as newer platelet inhibitors in limiting recurrent myocardial ischemia and its consequences (1,2) (Table 120.10).

SPECIAL ISSUES

Acute Congestive Heart Failure and Cardiogenic Shock

Acute CHF arises from a sudden injury or structural failure and constitutes approximately 10% of CHF admissions. Etiologies include acute coronary syndromes (ACSs), acute valvular dysfunction (e.g., those due to endocarditis, aortic dissection, or papillary muscle rupture), pericardial disease, new arrhythmia (especially atrial fibrillation), myocarditis, and malignant hypertension (119).

Patients who present with ACS accompanied by CHF have considerable mortality and clearly benefit from emergent revascularization (120,121) (Fig. 120.11). Medical management includes the standard therapies for ACS (antiplatelet therapy and anticoagulation), with the exception that β-blockers are contraindicated in the presence of systolic CHF. β-Blockers are not contraindicated, and are probably helpful, in an ACS with diastolic CHF.

For patients with hypotension or hypoperfusion, serious consideration should be given to placement of a pulmonary artery catheter. An IABP is the most physiologic for improving cardiac output in the setting of ACS as it improves coronary perfusion while increasing blood pressure and decreasing afterload (122) (Fig. 120.12). Notably, all currently available inotropes will worsen ischemia and are proarrhythmic.

Cardiogenic shock remains the leading cause of death in patients hospitalized with acute MI (123). The SHOCK randomized trial (124,125) demonstrated that in patients with acute MI complicated by cardiogenic shock, early mechanical revascularization reduced 6- and 12-month mortality compared with initial medical stabilization—including IABP counterpulsation and fibrinolytic therapy—followed by late or no revascularization (Fig. 120.13). There was a significant interaction between treatment and age, with apparent lack of benefit

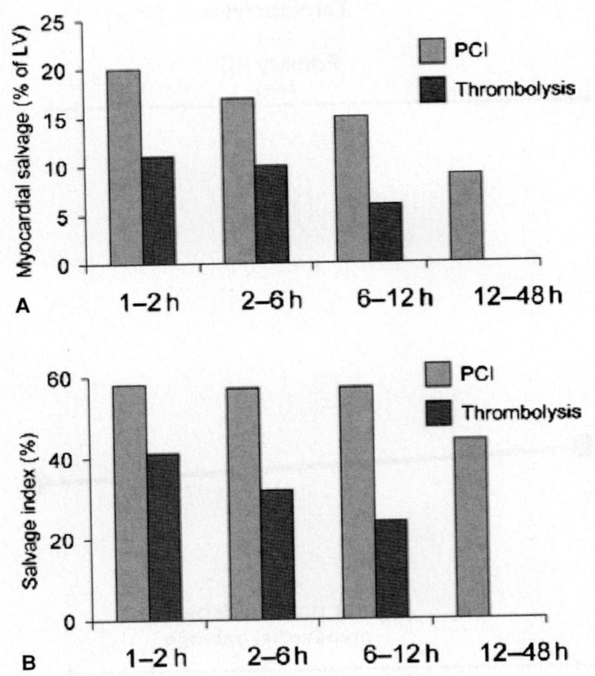

FIGURE 120.9. Time dependence of myocardial salvage according to time-to-treatment interval in patients with ST elevation myocardial infarction (STEMI) treated by percutaneous coronary intervention (PCI) or thrombolysis. A: Myocardial salvage expressed as percentage of the left ventricle (LV). B: Myocardial salvage expressed as proportion of the initial area at risk salvaged by reperfusion therapy. (From Schomig A, Ndrepepa G, Kastrati A. Late myocardial salvage: time to recognize its reality in the reperfusion therapy of acute myocardial infarction. *Eur Heart J.* 2006;27:1900–1907.)

TABLE 120.9

AMERICAN COLLEGE OF CARDIOLOGY/AMERICAN HEART ASSOCIATION GUIDELINES FOR MANAGEMENT OF ST ELEVATION MYOCARDIAL INFARCTION

Acute therapy	Discharge therapy
Aspirin	Aspirin
Clopidogrel	Clopidogrel
β-Blocker	β-Blocker
ACE inhibitor	ACE inhibitor
Heparin (UFH or LMWH)	Aldosterone antagonist
GP IIb/IIIa Inhibitor (if receiving PCI)	Statin
	Smoking cessation
	Cardiac rehabilitation

ACE, angiotensin-converting enzyme; UFH, unfractionated heparin; LMHW, low-molecular-weight heparin; GP, glycoprotein; PCI, percutaneous coronary intervention.
Table made with data from Antman EM, Anbe DT, Armstrong PW, et al. American College of Cardiology; American Heart Association Task Force on Practice Guidelines; Canadian Cardiovascular Society. ACC/AHA guidelines for the management of patients with ST-elevation myocardial infarction: a report of the American College of Cardiology/American Heart Association Task Force on Practice Guidelines (committee to revise the 1999 Guidelines for the Management of Patients with Acute Myocardial Infarction). *Circulation.* 2004;110(9):e82–e292.

of early revascularization for the small subset of patients aged 75 years or older (124,125). Based on these findings, the American College of Cardiology (ACC) and the American Heart Association (AHA) elevated early mechanical revascularization for cardiogenic shock to a class I recommendation for patients

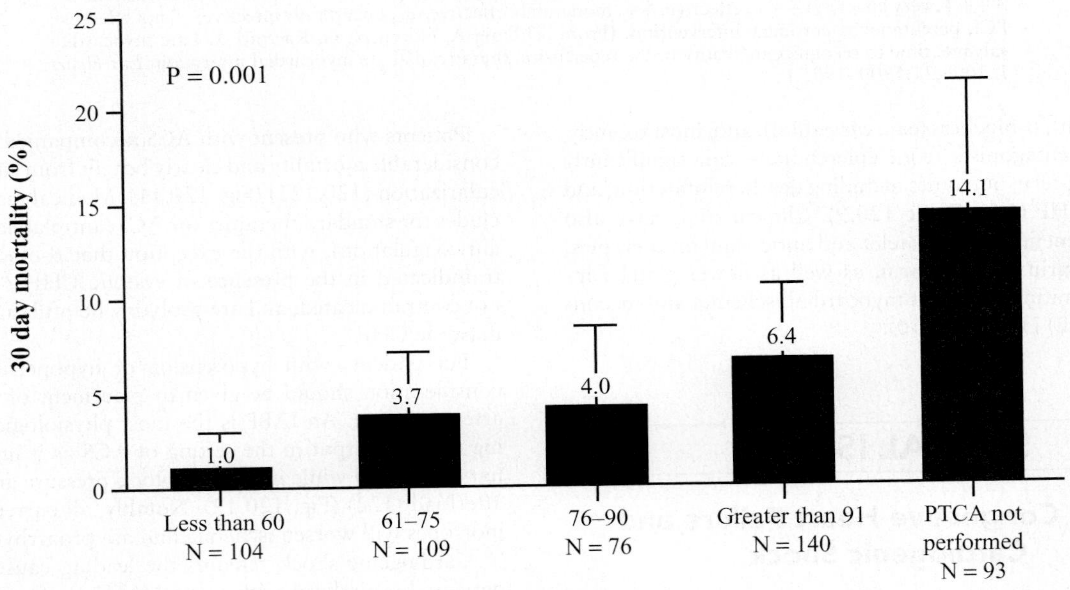

FIGURE 120.10. Relationship between 30-day mortality and time from study enrollment to first balloon inflation. PTCA, percutaneous transluminal coronary angioplasty. (Modified from Berger PB, Ellis SG, Holmes DR Jr, et al. Relationship between delay in performing direct coronary angioplasty and early clinical outcome in patients with acute myocardial infarction: results from the Global Use of Strategies to Open Occluded Arteries in Acute Coronary Syndromes [GUSTO-IIb] trial. *Circulation.* 1999;100:14–20.)

TABLE 120.10

LARGE-SCALE CLINICAL TRIALS OF THERAPY FOR AMI SURVIVORS

Study	Reference	Patient Population (n)	Treatment	Background Therapy	Average Duration	All-cause Mortality Risk Reduction	Reinfarction
Antiplatelet							
ATC	*BMJ.* 1994;308: 81–106	AMI (20,000)	Aspirin	none	4.5 y	25% $p<0.02$	34% $p<0.02$
ACE Inhibitors /ARBs							
SMILE	*N Engl J Med.* 1995;332: 80–85	AMI (1,556)	Zofenopril	Aspirin (53%) β-blockers (18%) CCBs (10%)	6 week	29%[a] $p = 0.01$	37% $p =$ N/A
ISIS-4	*Lancet.* 1995;345: 669–685	AMI (58,050)	Captopril	Nitrates / diuretics	15m	7% at 1 month $p = 0.02$	No difference
GISSI-3	*Lancet.* 1987;2: 871–874	AMI (18,895)	Lisinopril	IV β-blockers (31%), Fibrinolytic therapy (72%), Aspirin (84%), Antiplatelets (4%)	6w	11% $p = 0.03$	No difference
Including patients with LVD or HF							
SAVE	*N Engl J Med.* 1992;327: 669–77	AMI with LVD (2,231)	Captopril	Aspirin (59%) β-blockers (75%) Thrombolytics (32%) PCI (17%) CCBs (42%)	3.5 y	19% $p = 0.019$	25% $p = 0.015$
AIRE	*Lancet.* 1993;342: 821–828	AMI with HF (2,006)	Ramipril	Aspirin (77%) β-blockers (24%) Thrombolytics (59%) CCBs (15%)	15m	27% $p = 0.002$	$p =$ NS
TRACE	*N Engl J Med.* 1995;333: 1670–1676	AMI with LVD (1,749)	Trandolapril	Aspirin (92%) β-blockers (17%) Thrombolytics (45%) CCBs (28%)	2–4 y	22% $p = 0.0001$	14% $p =$ NS
OPTIMAAL	*Lancet.* 2002;360: 752–760	AMI with HF (5,477)	Losartan vs Captopril	Aspirin (96%) β-blockers (79%) Thrombolytics (55%) PCI (17%), CCBs (22%), Statins (31%)	2.7 y	13% Increase in risk $p = 0.07$	3% increase in risk $p =$ NS
VALIANT	*N Engl J Med.* 2003;349: 1893–1906	AMI with HF/LVD (14,703)	Valsartan Vs. Valsartan plus captopril Vs. captopril	Aspirin (91%) β-blockers (70%) ACEIs (40%) Antiplatelet (25%) PCI (20%) Thrombolytics (35%)	24.7 months	No difference $p =$ NS	No difference $p =$ NS
STATINS							
CARE	*N Engl J Med.* 1996;335: 1001–1009	AMI (4,159)	Pravastatin	Aspirin (83%) β-blockers (41%) ACEIs (15%), CCBs (40%)	5y	No difference	24%[b] $p = 0.003$
HPS	*Lancet.* 2002;360: 7–22	History of MI (8,510)	Simvastatin	Aspirin (21%) β-blockers (19.5%) ACEIs (25%)	5y		24%[b]
MIRACL	*JAMA.* 2001;285: 1711–1718	ACS (3,086)	Atorvastatin	Aspirin (91%) β-blockers (78%) ACEIs/ARBs (49%) Antiplatelet (11%) CCBs (48%)	16 weeks	16%[c] $p = 0.048$	10% $p =$ NS
PROVE IT-TIMI	*N Engl J Med.* 2004;3: 1495–1504	ACS (4,162)	Pravastatin or Atorvastatin	Aspirin (93%) β-blockers (85%) ACEIs/ARBs (83%) Antiplatelet (72%) PCI (69%)	2y	28% $p = 0.07$	18% $p = 0.06$

(*Continued*)

TABLE 120.10

(CONTINUED)

Study	Reference	Patient Population (n)	Treatment	Background Therapy	Average Duration	All-cause Mortality Risk Reduction	Reinfarction
A to Z trial	*JAMA.* 2004;292: 1307–1316	ACS (4,497)	Simvastatin 40 mg for 30 days then 80 mg vs. placebo for 4 months then 20 mg	Aspirin (98%) β-blockers (90%) ACEIs/ARBs (71%)	6–24 months	11 %[d] p = NS	4% p = NS
Aldosterone Antagonists							
EPHESUS	*Cardiovasc Drugs Ther.* 2001;15: 79–87	AMI with LYD or HF (6,642)	Eplerenone	Aspirin (88%) β-blockers (75%) ACEIs/ARBs (87%) statin (47%) Thrombolysis or PCI (45%)	16 m	15% $p = 0.008$	N/A
β-Blockers							
Goteborg	*Lancet.* 1981;2: 823–827	AMI (1,395)	Metoprolol tartrate	None	3 m	36% $p = 0.03$	p = NS
MIAMI	*Am J Cardiol.* 1985;56: 15G-22G	AMI (5,778)	Metoprolol tartrate	Antihypertensives (5%) Anticoagulants (2%)	15 days	p = NS	p = NS
ISIS-1	*Lancet.* 1986;2: 57–66	AMI (16,027)	Atenolol	Antiplatelets (5%) Anticoagulants (6%)	1 week	15% $p < 0.04$	p = NS
TIMI II-B	*Circulation.* 1991;83: 422–437	AMI (1,434)	Immediate vs. Late Metoprolol tartrate	N/A	12 m	NS	p = NS
Lopressor Intervention Trial	*Eur Heart J.* 1987;8: 1056–1064	AMI (2,395)	Metoprolol tartrate	None	12m	Increase risk 4% NS	p = NS
Norwegian	*N Engl J Med.* 1985;313: 1055–8	AMI (1,884)	Timolol	None	17 m	39% $p = 0.0003$	28% $p = 0.0006$
BHAT	*JAMA.* 1981;246: 2073–4	AMI (3,837)	Propranolol	Aspirin (21%)	25 m	26% $p < 0.005$	16% p = NS
Including Patients with LVD or HF							
CAPRICORN	*Lancet.* 2001;357: 1385–1390	AMI with LVD (1,959)	Carvedilol	ACEIs (98%), Aspirin (86%), Lipid-lowering (24%), Thrombolytics (36%), PCI (12%)	15 m	23% $p = 0.031$	41% $p = 0.014$

ACEI, angiotensin-converting enzyme inhibitor; ACS, acute coronary syndrome; AMI, acute myocardial infarction; ARB, angiotensin-II receptor blocker; HF, heart failure; IV, intravenous; LVD, left ventricular dysfunction; CCB, calcium channel blockers; PCI, percutaneous coronary intervention.

[a]Risk reduction at one year

[b] Cardiac death or reinfarction

[c] Primary end point event defined as death, nonfatal acute myocardial infarction, cardiac arrest with resuscitation, or recurrent symptomatic myocardial ischemia with objective evidence and requiring emergency rehospitalization.

[d] Composite of cardiovascular death, nonfatal myocardial infarction, readmission for ACS, and stroke

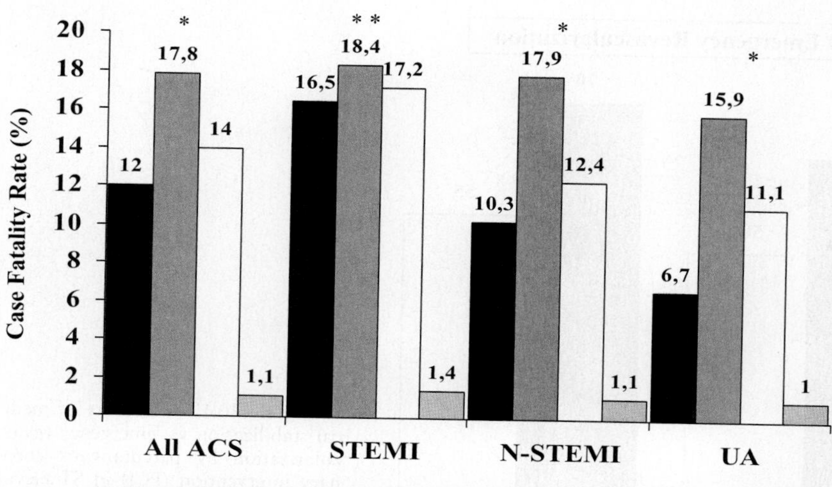

FIGURE 120.11. Impact of presence of heart failure (HF) at admission or development of HF during hospitalization (H) in all patients with acute coronary syndromes (ACSs). STEMI, ST elevation myocardial infarction; N-STEMI, non–ST elevation myocardial infarction; UA, unstable angina. (Modified from Steg PG, Dabbous OH, Feldman LJ, et al.; Global Registry of Acute Coronary Events Investigators. Determinants and prognostic impact of heart failure complicating acute coronary syndromes: observations from the Global Registry of Acute Coronary Events [GRACE]. *Circulation*. 2004;109:494–499.)

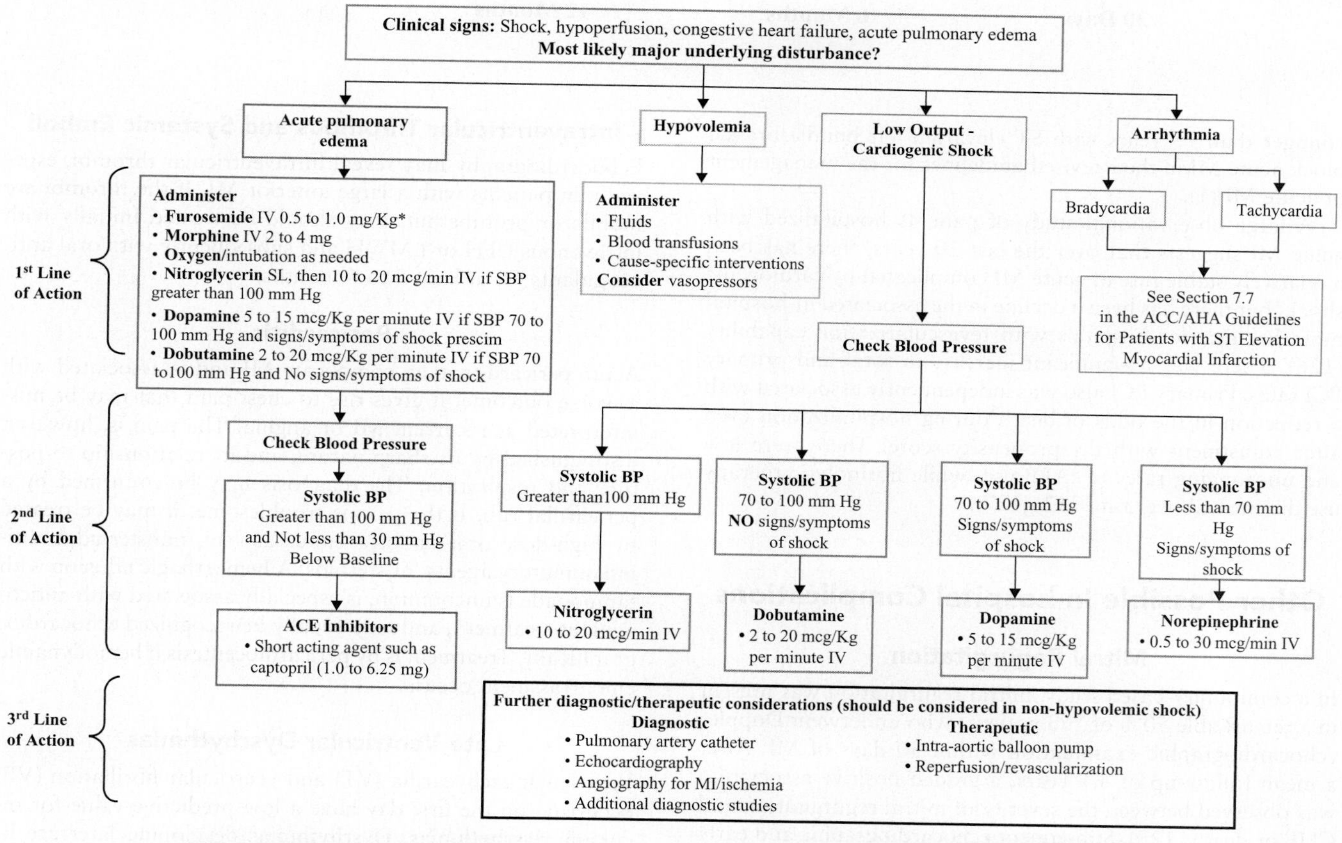

Clinical signs: Shock, hypoperfusion, congestive heart failure, acute pulmonary edema
Most likely major underlying disturbance?

Acute pulmonary edema

1st Line of Action

Administer
- **Furosemide** IV 0.5 to 1.0 mg/Kg*
- **Morphine** IV 2 to 4 mg
- **Oxygen**/intubation as needed
- **Nitroglycerin** SL, then 10 to 20 mcg/min IV if SBP greater than 100 mm Hg
- **Dopamine** 5 to 15 mcg/Kg per minute IV if SBP 70 to 100 mm Hg and signs/symptoms of shock prescim
- **Dobutamine** 2 to 20 mcg/Kg per minute IV if SBP 70 to100 mm Hg and No signs/symptoms of shock

2nd Line of Action

Check Blood Pressure

Systolic BP
Greater than 100 mm Hg and Not less than 30 mm Hg Below Baseline

ACE Inhibitors
- Short acting agent such as captopril (1.0 to 6.25 mg)

Hypovolemia

Administer
- Fluids
- Blood transfusions
- Cause-specific interventions

Consider vasopressors

Low Output - Cardiogenic Shock

Check Blood Pressure

Systolic BP Greater than100 mm Hg → **Nitroglycerin**
- 10 to 20 mcg/min IV

Systolic BP 70 to 100 mm Hg **NO** signs/symptoms of shock → **Dobutamine**
- 2 to 20 mcg/Kg per minute IV

Systolic BP 70 to 100 mm Hg Signs/symptoms of shock → **Dopamine**
- 5 to 15 mcg/Kg per minute IV

Systolic BP Less than 70 mm Hg Signs/symptoms of shock → **Norepinephrine**
- 0.5 to 30 mcg/min IV

Arrhythmia

Bradycardia | Tachycardia

See Section 7.7 in the ACC/AHA Guidelines for Patients with ST Elevation Myocardial Infarction

3rd Line of Action

Further diagnostic/therapeutic considerations (should be considered in non-hypovolemic shock)

Diagnostic
- Pulmonary artery catheter
- Echocardiography
- Angiography for MI/ischemia
- Additional diagnostic studies

Therapeutic
- Intra-aortic balloon pump
- Reperfusion/revascularization

FIGURE 120.12. Emergency management of complicated ST elevation myocardial infarction (STEMI). The emergency management of patients with cardiogenic shock, acute pulmonary edema, or both is outlined. HF, heart failure; IV, intravenous; SL, sublingual; SBP, systolic blood pressure; BP, blood pressure; ACE, angiotensin-converting enzyme; MI, myocardial infarction. (Modified from Antman EM, Anbe DT, Armstrong PW, et al. American College of Cardiology; American Heart Association Task Force on Practice Guidelines; Canadian Cardiovascular Society. ACC/AHA guidelines for the management of patients with ST-elevation myocardial infarction: a report of the American College of Cardiology/American Heart Association Task Force on Practice Guidelines [committee to revise the 1999 Guidelines for the Management of Patients with Acute Myocardial Infarction]. *Circulation*. 2004;110[9]:e82–292.)

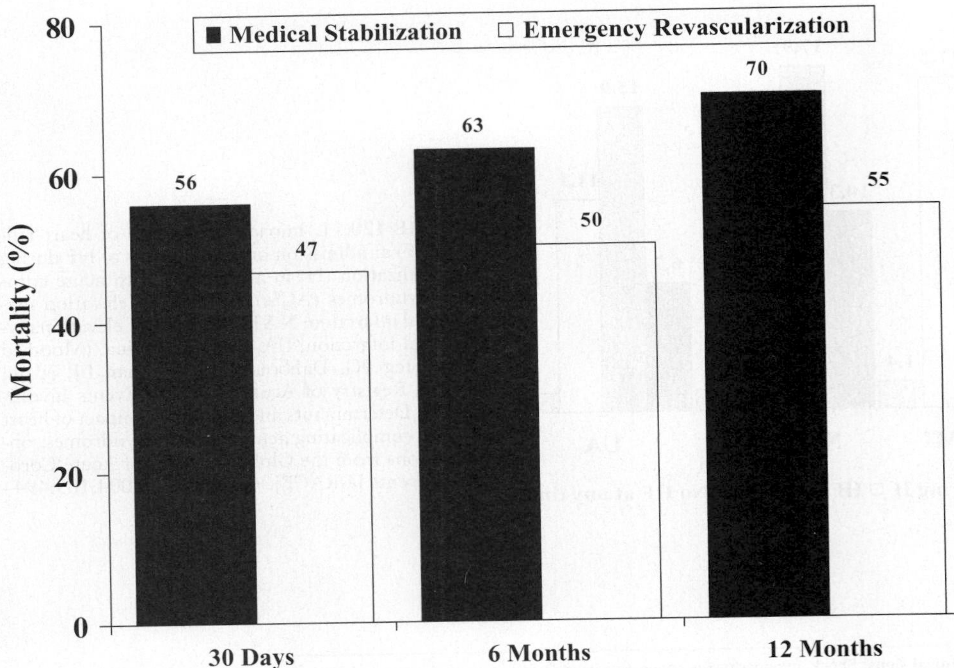

FIGURE 120.13. Mortality of medical stabilization vs. emergency revascularization by percutaneous coronary intervention (PCI) in ST elevation myocardial infarction (STEMI) patients with shock. (Modified from Hochman JS, Sleeper LA, Webb JG, et al.; SHOCK Investigators. Early revascularization in acute myocardial infarction complicated by cardiogenic shock. *N Engl J Med.* 1999;341:625–634.)

younger than 75 years with ST elevation left bundle branch block acute MI in their revised guidelines for the management of acute MI (1).

A large observational study of patients hospitalized with acute MI suggests that over the last 10 years, there has been a relatively stable rate of acute MI complicated by cardiogenic shock, but there has been a decline in the associated in-hospital mortality rate for hospitals with revascularization capability (126). There was a significant increase in total and primary PCI rates. Primary PCI also was independently associated with a reduction in the odds of death during hospitalization even after adjustment with the propensity score. There were low and unchanging rates of IABP use, while fibrinolytic therapy use diminished over time (126,127).

Other Possible In-hospital Complications

Mitral Regurgitation

In a community-based study, mitral regurgitation was present in a remarkable 50% of 773 patients who underwent Doppler echocardiographic examination within 30 days of MI. After a mean follow-up of 4.7 years, a graded positive association was observed between the severity of mitral regurgitation and CHF or death (128). Subsequent echocardiographic and early invasive studies demonstrated the prognostic significance of even mild mitral regurgitation after an acute MI (129).

Deep Vein Thrombosis and Pulmonary Embolism

These complications are now relatively uncommon after MI, except in patients kept in bed for comorbidities or complications of MI. When they occur they should be treated with therapeutic doses of LMWH, followed by oral anticoagulation for 3 to 6 months.

Intraventricular Thrombus and Systemic Emboli

Echocardiography may reveal intraventricular thrombi, especially in patients with a large anterior MI. If the thrombi are mobile or protuberant, they should be treated initially with intravenous UFH or LMWH and subsequently with oral anticoagulants for at least 3 to 6 months.

Pericarditis

Acute pericarditis may complicate MI and is associated with a worse outcome. It gives rise to chest pain that may be misinterpreted as recurrent MI or angina. The pain is, however, distinguished by its sharp nature, and its relationship to posture and respiration. The diagnosis may be confirmed by a pericardial rub. If the pain is troublesome, it may be treated by high-dose oral or intravenous aspirin, nonsteroidal anti-inflammatory agents, or steroids. A hemorrhagic effusion with tamponade is uncommon, is especially associated with anticoagulant treatment, and may usually be recognized echocardiographically. Treatment is by pericardiocentesis if hemodynamic embarrassment occurs.

Late Ventricular Dysrhythmias

Ventricular tachycardia (VT) and ventricular fibrillation (VF) occurring on the first day have a low predictive value for recurring dysrhythmias. Dysrhythmias developing later are liable to recur and are associated with a high risk of death. VT or VF during the first week postinfarction is associated with more extensive myocardial damage; a careful assessment of coronary anatomy and ventricular function should always be undertaken. If it is probable that the arrhythmia is induced by ischemia, revascularization by PCI or surgery should be considered. If this is unlikely, a variety of therapeutic approaches are available, which are, as yet, inadequately researched. These include the use of β-blockers, amiodarone, electrophysiologically guided antidysrhythmic therapy, and/or insertion of an implantable converter defibrillator.

Postinfarction Angina and Ischemia

The routine use of elective PCI following fibrinolytic therapy has been compared with a conservative approach in several randomized trials. It may be concluded that routine PCI in the absence of spontaneous or provocable ischemia does not improve LV function or survival (130,131). In treating angina or recurrent or inducible ischemia, however, whether due to reocclusion or to a residual stenosis, revascularization by PCI or CABG has a definite role (130). It may also be of value in managing dysrhythmias associated with persistent ischemia. CABG surgery may be indicated if symptoms are not controlled by other means or if coronary angiography demonstrates lesions, such as left main stenosis or three-vessel disease with poor LV function, for which surgery improves prognosis.

Right Ventricular Infarction

Right ventricular infarction encompasses a spectrum of disease states ranging from asymptomatic mild RV dysfunction through cardiogenic shock. Most patients demonstrate a return of normal RV function over a period of weeks to months, which suggests that RV stunning, rather than irreversible necrosis, has occurred. In this sense, RV ischemia can be demonstrated in up to half of all inferior STEMIs, although only 10% to 15% of patients show classic hemodynamic abnormalities of clinically significant RV infarction (132,133). Right ventricular infarction with hemodynamic abnormalities accompanying inferior STEMI is associated with a significantly higher mortality (25%–30%) and thus identifies a high-risk subgroup of patients with inferior STEMIs (6%) who should be considered high-priority candidates for reperfusion (132). One group of investigators reported a 31% in-hospital mortality rate in patients with inferior STEMIs complicated by RV infarction compared with 6% in patients who had an inferior STEMI without RV involvement (131). An analysis of patients with predominant RV infarction and cardiogenic shock from the SHOCK trial registry demonstrated an unexpectedly high mortality rate similar to that for patients with LV shock (53.1% vs. 60.8%) (134).

The treatment of patients with RV ischemic dysfunction is different and, in several ways, diametrically opposed to management of LV dysfunction. It includes early maintenance of RV preload, reduction of RV afterload, inotropic support of the dysfunctional RV, and early reperfusion (135). Because of their influence on preload, drugs routinely used in management of LV infarctions, such as nitrates and diuretics, may reduce cardiac output and produce severe hypotension when the RV is ischemic. Indeed, a common clinical presentation is profound hypotension after administration of sublingual nitroglycerin, with the degree of hypotension often out of proportion to the ECG severity of the infarct. Volume loading with normal saline alone often resolves in patients with RV ischemia/infarction (136).

Although volume loading is a critical first step in the management of hypotension associated with RV ischemia/infarction, inotropic support—in particular, with dobutamine—should be initiated promptly if cardiac output fails to improve after 0.5 to 1 L of fluid has been administered. Excessive volume loading may further complicate the right-sided filling pressure increase and RV dilatation, resulting in decreased LV output (136,137) secondary to shift of the interventricular septum toward the LV.

INDICATIONS FOR HEMODYNAMIC MONITORING

It is important to accurately assess the severity of left ventricular dysfunction because maneuvers performed in the coronary care unit may worsen this state. More than half of the patients with a moderate reduction in resting cardiac output and an increase in left ventricular filling pressure have no *clinical* signs of left ventricular dysfunction. Clinical evaluation frequently does not identify patients with low cardiac output who have normal chest radiographs and physical examinations. However, correlation of the chest radiograph and clinical evaluation with hemodynamic measurements have demonstrated that the presence of cardiomegaly, gallop rhythms, and pulmonary edema may help predict which patients with MI will develop shock (138–140).

There is an unfortunate tendency to institute potent therapeutic measures in patients with myocardial infarction before precise hemodynamic indices are known. Intravenous furosemide, for example, may create a decline in pulmonary artery occlusion pressure (PAOP) without compromising the cardiac output if ventricular filling pressures are elevated and there is pulmonary congestion. However, if the clinical diagnosis of CHF is incorrect and the PAOP is normal, diuretic therapy may actually decrease the cardiac output and cause deterioration of an already compromised myocardial flow reserve. This can be particularly detrimental in patients who present with RV infarction.

References

1. Antman EM, Anbe DT, Armstrong PW, et al. American College of Cardiology; American Heart Association Task Force on Practice Guidelines; Canadian Cardiovascular Society. ACC/AHA guidelines for the management of patients with ST-elevation myocardial infarction: a report of the American College of Cardiology/American Heart Association Task Force on Practice Guidelines (committee to revise the 1999 Guidelines for the Management of Patients with Acute Myocardial Infarction). *Circulation.* 2004;110(9):e82–e292.
2. Van de Werf F, Ardissino D, Betriu A, et al. Task Force on the Management of Acute Myocardial Infarction of the European Society of Cardiology. Management of acute myocardial infarction in patients presenting with ST-segment elevation. The Task Force on the Management of Acute Myocardial Infarction of the European Society of Cardiology. *Eur Heart J.* 2003;24(1):28–66.

2a. Thygesen K, Alpert JS, White HD. Joint ESC/ACCF/AHA/WHF Task Force for the Redefinition of Myocardial Infarction. Universal definition of myocardial infarction. *Circulation.* 2007;116:2634–2653.

3. Rogers WJ, Canto JG, Lambrew CT, et al. Temporal trends in the treatment of over 1.5 million patients with myocardial infarction in the US from 1990 through 1999: the National Registry of Myocardial Infarction 1, 2 and 3. *J Am Coll Cardiol.* 2000;36:2056–2063.
4. Kleiman NS, White HD. The declining prevalence of ST elevation myocardial infarction in patients presenting with acute coronary syndromes. *Heart.* 2005;91;1121–1123.
5. Braunwald E, Pfeffer MA. Ventricular enlargement and remodeling following acute myocardial infarction: mechanisms and management. *Am J Cardiol.* 1991;68:1D–6D.
6. Pfeffer MA. Left ventricular remodeling after acute myocardial infarction. *Annu Rev Med.* 1995;46:455–466.
7. Antman EM, Braunwald E. Acute myocardial infarction. In: Braunwald E, Zipes DP, Libby P, eds. *Heart Disease: A Textbook of Cardiovascular Medicine.* 6th ed. Philadelphia: WB Saunders Co Ltd; 2001:1114–1251.

8. Hochman JS, Califf RM. Acute myocardial infarction. In: Smith TW, ed. *Cardiovascular Therapeutics: A Companion to Braunwald's Heart Disease.* 2nd ed. Philadelphia: WB Saunders Co Ltd; 2001:235–291.
9. Collins R, Peto R, Baigent C, et al. Aspirin, heparin, and fibrinolytic therapy in suspected acute myocardial infarction. *N Engl J Med.* 1997;333:847–860.
10. Boersma E, Mercado N, Poldermans D, et al. Acute myocardial infarction. *Lancet.* 2003;361:847–858.
11. Morrison LJ, Verbeek PR, McDonald AC, et al. Mortality and prehospital thrombolysis for acute myocardial infarction: a meta-analysis. *JAMA.* 2000;283:2686–2692.
12. GREAT Group. Feasibility, safety and efficacy of domiciliary thrombolysis by general practitioners. *BMJ.* 1992;305:548–553.
13. Bonnefoy E, Lapostolle F, Leizorovicz A, et al., on behalf of the CAPTIM Study Group. Primary angioplasty versus prehospital fibrinolysis in acute myocardial infarction: a randomised study. *Lancet.* 2002;360:825–829.
14. Boersma E, Maas AC, Deckers JW, et al. Early thrombolytic treatment in acute myocardial infarction: reappraisal of the golden hour. *Lancet.* 1996; 348:771–775.
15. Danchin N, Blanchard D, Steg PG, et al. Impact of prehospital thrombolysis for acute myocardial infarction on 1-year outcome results from the French nationwide USIC 2000 registry. *Circulation.* 2004;110:1909–1915.
16. Stenestrand U, Lindback J, Wallentin L; RIKS-HIA Registry. Long-term outcome of primary percutaneous coronary intervention vs prehospital and in-hospital thrombolysis for patients with ST-elevation myocardial infarction. *JAMA.* 2006;296(14):1749–1756.
17. Gibson CM, Cannon CP, Murphy SA, et al. Relationship of TIMI myocardial perfusion grade to mortality after administration of thrombolytic drugs. *Circulation.* 2000;101:125–130.
18. White H; Hirulog and Early Reperfusion or Occlusion (HERO)-2 Trial Investigators. Thrombin-specific anticoagulation with bivalirudin versus heparin in patients receiving fibrinolytic therapy for acute myocardial infarction: the HERO-2 randomised trial. *Lancet.* 2001;358(9296):1855–1863.
19. Maroko PR, Radvany P, Braunwald E, et al. Reduction of infarct size by oxygen inhalation following acute coronary occlusion. *Circulation.* 1975; 52:360–368.
20. Madias JE, Hood WB. Reduction of precordial ST-segment elevation in patients with anterior myocardial infarction by oxygen breathing. *Circulation.* 1976;53:I198–200.
21. Fillmore SJ, Shapiro M, Killip T. Arterial oxygen tension in acute myocardial infarction: serial analysis of clinical state and blood gas changes. *Am Heart J.* 1970;79:620–629.
22. Abrams J. Hemodynamic effects of nitroglycerin and long-acting nitrates. *Am Heart J.* 1985;110:216–224.
23. Gorman MW, Sparks HV. Nitroglycerin causes vasodilatation within ischaemic myocardium. *Cardiovasc Res.* 1980;14:515–521.
24. ISIS-4 (Fourth International Study of Infarct Survival) Collaborative Group. ISIS-4: a randomised factorial trial assessing early oral captopril, oral mononitrate, and intravenous magnesium sulphate in 58,050 patients with suspected acute myocardial infarction. *Lancet.* 1995;345:669–685.
25. Yusuf S, Peto R, Lewis J, et al. Beta-blockade during and after myocardial infarction: an overview of the randomised trials. *Prog Cardiovasc Dis.* 1985;27:335–371.
26. The MIAMI Trial Research Group. Metoprolol in acute myocardial infarction (MIAMI). A randomised placebo controlled international trial. *Eur Heart J.* 1985;6:199–211.
27. Herlitz J, Waagstein F, Lindqvist J, et al. Effect of metoprolol on the prognosis for patients with suspected acute myocardial infarction and indirect signs of congestive heart failure (a subgroup analysis of the Goteborg Metoprolol Trial). *Am J Cardiol.* 1997;80:40J–44J.
28. ISIS-1 collaborative group. Randomised trial of intravenous atenolol among 16 027 cases of suspected acute myocardial infarction: ISIS-1. *Lancet.* 1986; 2:57–66.
29. COMMIT (ClOpidogrel and Metoprolol in Myocardial Infarction Trial) collaborative group. Early intravenous then oral metoprolol in 45 852 patients with acute myocardial infarction: randomised placebo-controlled trial. *Lancet.* 2005;366:1622–1632
30. Mehta SR, Yusuf S, Peters RJ, et al., for the Clopidogrel in Unstable angina to prevent Recurrent Events trial (CURE) Investigators. Effects of pretreatment with clopidogrel and aspirin followed by long-term therapy in patients undergoing percutaneous coronary intervention: the PCI-CURE study. *Lancet.* 2001;358:527–533.
31. Schömig A, Neumann FJ, Kastrati A, et al. A randomized comparison of antiplatelet and anticoagulant therapy after the placement of coronary-artery stents. *N Engl J Med.* 1996;334:1084–1089.
32. CAPRIE Steering Committee. A randomised, blinded, trial of clopidogrel versus aspirin in patients at risk of ischaemic events (CAPRIE). *Lancet.* 1996;348:1329–1339.
33. Leon MB, Baim DS, Popma JJ, et al., for the Stent Anticoagulation Restenosis Study Investigators. A clinical trial comparing three antithrombotic-drug regimens after coronary-artery stenting. *N Engl J Med.* 1998;339:1665–1671.
34. Smith SC Jr, Dove JT, Jacobs AK, et al. ACC/AHA guidelines for percutaneous coronary intervention (revision of the 1993 PTCA guidelines): a report of the American College of Cardiology/American Heart Association Task Force on Practice Guidelines (committee to revise the 1993 Guidelines for Percutaneous Transluminal Coronary Angioplasty). *Circulation.* 2001;103:3019–3041.
35. Sabatine MS, Cannon CP, Gibson CM, et al. Addition of clopidogrel to aspirin and fibrinolytic therapy for myocardial infarction with ST-segment elevation. *N Engl J Med.* 2005;352:1179–1189.
36. Scirica BM, Sabatine MS, Morrow DA, et al. The role of clopidogrel in early and sustained arterial patency after fibrinolysis for ST-segment elevation myocardial infarction. The ECG CLARITY–TIMI 28 Study. *J Am Coll Cardiol.* 2006;48:37–42.
37. Sugidachi A, Asai F, Ogawa T, et al. The *in vivo* pharmacological profile of CS-747, a novel antiplatelet agent with platelet ADP receptor antagonist properties. *Br J Pharmacol.* 2000;129:1439–1446.
38. Wiviott SD, Antman EM, Winters KJ, et al. A randomised comparison of prasugrel (CS-747), a novel thienopyridine P2Y12 antagonist, to clopidogrel in percutaneous coronary intervention; results of the Joint Utilization of Medications to Block Platelets Optimally (JUMBO)-TIMI 26 Trial. *Circulation.* 2005;111:3366–3373.
39. Lincoff AM, Califf RM, Topol EJ. Platelet glycoprotein IIb/IIIa blockade in coronary artery disease. *J Am Coll Cardiol.* 2000;35:1103–1115.
40. Kloner RA, Dai W. Glycoprotein IIb/IIIa inhibitors and no-reflow. *J Am Coll Cardiol.* 2004;43:284–286.
41. De Luca G, Suryapranata H, Stone GW, et al. Abciximab as adjunctive therapy to reperfusion in acute ST-segment elevation myocardial infarction: a meta-analysis of randomized trials. *JAMA.* 2005;293(14):1759–1765.
42. Antman EM. The search for replacements for unfractionated heparin. *Circulation.* 2001;103:2310–2314.
43. Ogilby JD, Kopelman HA, Klein LW, et al. Adequate heparinization during PTCA: assessment using activated clotting times. *Cathet Cardiovasc Diagn.* 1989;18:206–209.
44. Assessment of the Safety and Efficacy of a New Thrombolytic Regimen (ASSENT)-3 Investigators. Efficacy and safety of tenecteplase in combination with enoxaparin, abciximab, or unfractionated heparin: the ASSENT-3 randomised trial in acute myocardial infarction. *Lancet.* 2001;358:605–613.
45. Wallentin L, Goldstein P, Armstrong PW, et al. Efficacy and safety of tenecteplase in combination with the low-molecular-weight heparin enoxaparin or unfractionated heparin in the prehospital setting: the Assessment of the Safety and Efficacy of a New Thrombolytic Regimen (ASSENT)-3 PLUS randomized trial in acute myocardial infarction. *Circulation.* 2003; 108:135–142.
46. Ross AM, Molhoek P, Lundergan C, et al., for the HART II Investigators. Randomized comparison of enoxaparin, a low-molecular-weight heparin, with unfractionated heparin adjunctive to recombinant tissue plasminogen activator thrombolysis and aspirin: second trial of Heparin and Aspirin Reperfusion Therapy (HART II). *Circulation.* 2001;104:648–652.
47. Baird SH, Menown IB, Mcbride SJ, et al. Randomized comparison of enoxaparin with unfractionated heparin following fibrinolytic therapy for acute myocardial infarction. *Eur Heart J.* 2002;23:627–632.
48. Antman EM, Louwerenburg HW, Baars HF, et al. Enoxaparin as adjunctive antithrombin therapy for ST-elevation myocardial infarction: results of the ENTIRE-Thrombolysis in Myocardial Infarction (TIMI) 23 Trial. *Circulation.* 2002;105:1642–1649.
49. Wallentin L, Bergstrand L, Dellborg M, et al. Low molecular weight heparin (dalteparin) compared to unfractionated heparin as an adjunct to rt-PA (alteplase) for improvement of coronary artery patency in acute myocardial infarction-the ASSENT Plus study. *Eur Heart J.* 2003;24:897–908.
50. Direct thrombin inhibitors in acute coronary syndromes: principal results of a meta-analysis based on individual patients' data. *Lancet.* 2002;359:294–302.
51. Stone GW, McLaurin BT, Cox DA, et al.; ACUITY Investigators. Bivalirudin for patients with acute coronary syndromes. *N Engl J Med.* 2006; 355(21):2203–2216.
52. Exaire JE, Butman SM, Ebrahimi R, et al.; REPLACE-2 Investigators. Provisional glycoprotein IIb/IIIa blockade in a randomized investigation of bivalirudin versus heparin plus planned glycoprotein IIb/IIIa inhibition during percutaneous coronary intervention: predictors and outcome in the Randomized Evaluation in Percutaneous coronary intervention Linking Angiomax to Reduced Clinical Events (REPLACE)-2 trial. *Am Heart J.* 2006;152(1):157–163.
53. Coussement PK, Bassand JP, Convens C, et al., for the PENTALYSE investigators. A synthetic factor-Xa inhibitor (ORG31540/SR9017A) as an adjunct to fibrinolysis in acute myocardial infarction. The PENTALYSE study. *Eur Heart J.* 2001;22:1716–1724.
54. Yusuf S, Mehta SR, Chrolavicius S, et al.; OASIS-6 Trial Group. Effects of fondaparinux on mortality and reinfarction in patients with acute ST-segment elevation myocardial infarction: the OASIS-6 randomized trial. *JAMA.* 2006;295(13):1519–1530.
55. GISSI-3. Effects of lisinopril and transdermal glyceryl trinitrate singly and together on 6-week mortality and ventricular function after acute

myocardial infarction. Gruppo Italiano per lo Studio della Sopravvivenza nell'infarto Miocardico. *Lancet.* 1994;343:1115–1122.

56. ISIS-4. A randomised factorial trial assessing early oral captopril, oral mononitrate, and intravenous magnesium in 58,050 patients with suspected acute myocardial infarction. ISIS-4 (Fourth International Study of Infarct Survival) Collaborative Group. *Lancet.* 1995;345:669–685.
57. Chinese Cardiac Study Collaborative Group. Oral captopril versus placebo among 13,634 patients with suspected myocardial infarction: interim report from the Chinese Cardiac study (CCS-1). *Lancet.* 1995;345:686–687.
58. Swedberg K, Held P, Kjekshus J, et al. Effects of the early administration of enalapril on mortality in patients with acute myocardial infarction: results of the Cooperative New Scandinavian Enalapril Survival Study II (CONSENSUS II). *N Engl J Med.* 1992;327:678–684.
59. Pfeffer MA, Hennekens CH. When a question has an answer: rationale for our early termination of the HEART trial. *Am J Cardiol.* 1995;75:1173–1175.
60. The Danish Study Group on Verapamil in Myocardial Infarction. Verapamil in acute myocardial infarction. *Eur Heart J.* 1984;5:516–528.
61. Held PH, Yusuf S. Effects of beta-blockers and calcium channel blockers in acute myocardial infarction. *Eur Heart J.* 1993;14:18–25.
62. Hilton TC, Miller DD, Kern MJ. Rational therapy to reduce mortality and reinfarction following myocardial infarction. *Am Heart J.* 1991;122:1740–1750.
63. Effect of verapamil on mortality and major events after acute myocardial infarction: the Danish Verapamil Infarction Trial II (DAVIT II). *Am J Cardiol.* 1990;66:779–785.
64. The Multicenter Diltiazem Postinfarction Trial Research Group. The effect of diltiazem on mortality and reinfarction after myocardial infarction. *N Engl J Med.* 1988;319:385–392.
65. Gibson RS, Boden WE, Theroux P, et al. Diltiazem and reinfarction in patients with non–Q-wave myocardial infarction: results of a double-blind, randomized, multicenter trial. *N Engl J Med.* 1986;315:423–429.
66. Caldicott LD, Hawley K, Heppel R, et al. Intravenous enoximone or dobutamine for severe heart failure after acute myocardial infarction: a randomized double-blind trial. *Eur Heart J.* 1993;14:696–700.
67. Karlsberg RP, DeWood MA, DeMaria AN, et al. The milrinone-dobutamine Study Group. Comparative efficacy of short-term intravenous infusions of milrinone and dobutamine in acute congestive heart failure following acute myocardial infarction. *Clin Cardiol.* 1996;19:21–30.
68. Gillespie TA, Ambos HD, Sobel BE, et al. Effects of dobutamine in patients with acute myocardial infarction. *Am J Cardiol.* 1977;39:588–594.
69. Bayram M, De Luca L, Massie BM, et al. Dobutamine, milrinone and dopamine in acute heart failure syndromes: a reassessment. *Am J Cardiol.* 2005;96(6A):47G–58G.
70. De Luca L, Colucci WS, Nieminen MS, et al. Evidence-based use of levosimendan in different clinical settings. *Eur Heart J.* 2006;27(16):1908–1920.
71. Teo KK, Yusuf S, Collins R, et al. Effects of intravenous magnesium in suspected acute myocardial infarction: overview of randomised trials. *BMJ.* 1991;303:1499–1503.
72. Antman EM, Lau J, Kupelnick B, et al. A comparison of results of meta-analyses of randomized control trials and recommendations of clinical experts: treatments for myocardial infarction. *JAMA.* 1992;268:240–248.
73. Magnesium in Coronaries (MAGIC) Trial Investigators. Early administration of intravenous magnesium to high-risk patients with acute myocardial infarction in the Magnesium in Coronaries (MAGIC) Trial: a randomised controlled trial. *Lancet.* 2002;360:1189–1196.
74. Rasmussen HS, McNair P, Norregard P, et al. Intravenous magnesium in acute myocardial infarction. *Lancet.* 1986;1:234–236.
75. Smith LF, Heagerty AM, Bing RF, et al. Intravenous infusion of magnesium sulphate after acute myocardial infarction: effects on arrhythmias and mortality. *Int J Cardiol.* 1986;12:175–183.
76. Abraham AS, Rosenmann D, Kramer M, et al. Magnesium in the prevention of lethal arrhythmias in acute myocardial infarction. *Arch Intern Med.* 1987;147:753–755.
77. Ceremuzynski L, Jurgiel R, Kulakowski P, et al. Threatening arrhythmias in acute myocardial infarction are prevented by intravenous magnesium sulfate. *Am Heart J.* 1989;118:1333–1334.
78. Shechter M, Hod H, Marks N, et al. Beneficial effect of magnesium sulfate in acute myocardial infarction. *Am J Cardiol.* 1990;66:271–274.
79. Feldstedt M, Boesgaard S, Bouchelouche P, et al. Magnesium substitution in acute ischaemic heart syndromes. *Eur Heart J.* 1991;12:1215–1218.
80. Woods KL, Fletcher S, Roffe C, et al. Intravenous magnesium sulphate in suspected acute myocardial infarction: results of the second Leicester Intravenous Magnesium Intervention Trial (LIMIT-2). *Lancet.* 1992;339:1553–1558.
81. Guidelines 2000 for Cardiopulmonary Resuscitation and Emergency Cardiovascular Care: part 6: advanced cardiovascular life support: section 5: pharmacology I: agents for arrhythmias. The American Heart Association in collaboration with the International Liaison Committee on Resuscitation. *Circulation.* 2000;102:I112–128.
82. Lie KJ, Wellens HJ, Van Capelle FJ, et al. Lidocaine in the prevention of primary ventricular fibrillation. A double-blind randomized study of 212 consecutive patients. *N Engl J Med.* 1974;29:1324–1326.
83. Koster RW, Dunning AJ. Intramuscular lidocaine for prevention of lethal arrhythmias in the prehospitalization phase of acute myocardial infarction. *N Engl J Med.* 1985;313:1105–1110.
84. MacMahon S, Collins R, Peto R, et al. Effects of prophylactic lidocaine in suspected acute myocardial infarction. An overview of results from the randomized, controlled trials. *JAMA.* 1988;260:1910–1916.
85. Keeley EC, Grines CL. Primary coronary intervention for acute myocardial infarction. *JAMA.* 2004;291(6):736–739.
86. Magid DJ, Calonge BN, Rumsfeld JS, et al.; National Registry of Myocardial Infarction 2 and 3 Investigators. Relation between hospital primary angioplasty volume and mortality for patients with acute MI treated with primary angioplasty vs thrombolytic therapy. *JAMA.* 2000;284(24):3131–3138.
87. Collet JP, Montalescot G, Le May M, et al. Percutaneous coronary intervention after fibrinolysis: a multiple meta-analyses approach according to the type of strategy. *J Am Coll Cardiol.* 2006;48(7):1326–1335.
88. Gersh BJ, Stone GW, White HD, et al. Pharmacological facilitation of primary percutaneous coronary intervention for acute myocardial infarction: is the slope of the curve the shape of the future? *JAMA.* 2005;293(8):979–986.
89. Borden WB, Faxon DP. Facilitated percutaneous coronary intervention. *J Am Coll Cardiol.* 2006;48(6):1120–1128.
90. Assessment of the Safety and Efficacy of a New Treatment Strategy with Percutaneous Coronary Intervention (ASSENT-4 PCI) investigators. Primary versus tenecteplase-facilitated percutaneous coronary intervention in patients with ST-segment elevation acute myocardial infarction (ASSENT-4 PCI): randomised trial. *Lancet.* 2006;367(9510):569–578.
91. Kastrati A, Mehilli J, Schlotterbeck K, et al.; Bavarian Reperfusion Alternatives Evaluation (BRAVE) Study Investigators. Early administration of reteplase plus abciximab vs abciximab alone in patients with acute myocardial infarction referred for percutaneous coronary intervention: a randomized controlled trial. *JAMA.* 2004;291(8):947–954.

91a. Di Mario C, Dudek D, Piscione F, et al. for the CARESS-in-AMI (Combined Abciximab RE-teplase Stent Study in Acute Myocardial Infarction) investigators. *Lancet.* 2008;371:559–568.

92. Gershlick AH, Stephens-Lloyd A, Hughes S, et al.; REACT Trial Investigators. Rescue angioplasty after failed thrombolytic therapy for acute myocardial infarction. *N Engl J Med.* 2005;353(26):2758–2768.
93. Ting HH, Yang EH, Rihal CS. Reperfusion strategies for ST-segment elevation myocardial infarction. *Ann Intern Med.* 2006;145(8):610–617.
94. Andersen HR, Nielsen TT, Rasmussen K, et al.; DANAMI-2 Investigators. A comparison of coronary angioplasty with fibrinolytic therapy in acute myocardial infarction. *N Engl J Med.* 2003;349(8):733–742.
95. Zijlstra F, van't Hof AW, Liem AL, et al. Transferring patients for primary angioplasty: a retrospective analysis of 104 selected high risk patients with acute myocardial infarction. *Heart.* 1997;78:333–336.
96. Widimsky P, Groch L, Zelízko M, et al. Multicentre randomized trial comparing transport to primary angioplasty vs immediate thrombolysis vs combined strategy for patients with acute myocardial infarction presenting to a community hospital without a catheterization laboratory. The PRAGUE study. *Eur Heart J.* 2000;21:823–831.
97. Widimsky P, Budesinsky T, Vorac D, et al. Long distance transport for primary angioplasty vs immediate thrombolysis in acute myocardial infarction. Final results of the randomized national multicentre trial—PRAGUE-2. *Eur Heart J.* 2003;24:94–104.
98. Vermeer F, Oude Ophuis AJ, vd Berg EJ, et al. Prospective randomised comparison between thrombolysis, rescue PTCA, and primary PTCA in patients with extensive myocardial infarction admitted to a hospital without PTCA facilities: a safety and feasibility study. *Heart.* 1999;82:426–431.
99. Grines CL, Westerhausen DR Jr, Grines LL, et al. A randomized trial of transfer for primary angioplasty versus on-site thrombolysis in patients with high-risk myocardial infarction: the Air Primary Angioplasty in Myocardial Infarction study. *J Am Coll Cardiol.* 2002;39:1713–1719.
100. Dalby M, Bouzamondo A, Lechat P, et al. Transfer for primary angioplasty versus immediate thrombolysis in acute myocardial infarction: a meta-analysis. *Circulation.* 2003;108:1809–1814.
101. Keeley EC, Grines CL. Primary percutaneous coronary intervention for every patient with ST-segment elevation myocardial infarction: what stands in the way? *Ann Intern Med.* 2004;141:298–304.
102. Goldberg RJ, Mooradd M, Gurwitz JH, et al. Impact of time to treatment with tissue plasminogen activator on morbidity and mortality following acute myocardial infarction (the Second National Registry of Myocardial Infarction). *Am J Cardiol.* 1998;82:259–264.
103. Cannon CP, Gibson CM, Lambrew CT, et al. Relationship of symptom-onset-to-balloon time and door-to-balloon time with mortality in patients undergoing angioplasty for acute myocardial infarction. *JAMA.* 2000;283:2941–2947.
104. Berger AK, Radford MJ, Krumholz HM. Factors associated with delay in reperfusion therapy in elderly patients with acute myocardial infarction: analysis of the Cooperative Cardiovascular Project. *Am Heart J.* 2000;139:985–992.

105. Berger PB, Ellis SG, Holmes DR Jr, et al. Relationship between delay in performing direct coronary angioplasty and early clinical outcome in patients with acute myocardial infarction: results from the Global Use of Strategies to Open Occluded Arteries in Acute Coronary Syndromes (GUSTO-IIb) trial. *Circulation.* 1999;100:14–20.
106. De Luca G, Suryapranata H, Ottervanger JP, et al. Time delay to treatment and mortality in primary angioplasty for acute myocardial infarction: every minute of delay counts. *Circulation.* 2004;109:1223–1225.
107. De Luca G, Suryapranata H, Zijlstra F, et al. Symptom-onset-to-balloon time and mortality in patients with acute myocardial infarction treated by primary angioplasty. *J Am Coll Cardiol.* 2003;42:991–997.
108. Schomig A, Ndrepepa G, Kastrati A. Late myocardial salvage: time to recognize its reality in the reperfusion therapy of acute myocardial infarction. *Eur Heart J.* 2006;27:1900–1907.
109. Steg PG, Laperche T, Golmard JL, et al. Efficacy of streptokinase, but not tissue-type plasminogen activator, in achieving 90-minute patency after thrombolysis for acute myocardial infarction decreases with time to treatment. PERM Study Group. Prospective Evaluation of Reperfusion Markers. *J Am Coll Cardiol.* 1998;31:776–779.
110. Zeymer U, Tebbe U, Essen R, et al. Influence of time to treatment on early infarct-related artery patency after different thrombolytic regimens. ALKK-Study Group. *Am Heart J.* 1999;137:34–38.
111. Newby LK, Rutsch WR, Califf RM, et al. Time from symptom onset to treatment and outcomes after thrombolytic therapy. GUSTO-1 Investigators. *J Am Coll Cardiol.* 1996;27:1646–1655.
112. Brodie BR, Stuckey TD, Wall TC, et al. Importance of time to reperfusion for 30-day and late survival and recovery of left ventricular function after primary angioplasty for acute myocardial infarction. *J Am Coll Cardiol.* 1998;32:1312–1319.
113. Antoniucci D, Valenti R, Migliorini A, et al. Relation of time to treatment and mortality in patients with acute myocardial infarction undergoing primary coronary angioplasty. *Am J Cardiol.* 2002;89:1248–1252.
114. Cannon CP, Gibson CM, Lambrew CT, et al. Relationship of symptom-onset-to-balloon time and door-to-balloon time with mortality in patients undergoing angioplasty for acute myocardial infarction. *JAMA.* 2000;283:2941–2947.
115. Nallamothu BK, Bates ER. Percutaneous coronary intervention versus fibrinolytic therapy in acute myocardial infarction: is timing (almost) everything? *Am J Cardiol.* 2003;92:824–826.
116. Kahn JK, O'Keefe HJ Jr, Rutherford BD, et al. Timing and mechanism of in-hospital and late death after primary coronary angioplasty during acute myocardial infarction. *Am J Cardiol.* 1990;66:1045–1048.
117. Gibson CM, Karha J, Murphy SA, et al. Early and long-term clinical outcomes associated with reinfarction following fibrinolytic administration in the Thrombolysis in Myocardial Infarction trials. *J Am Coll Cardiol.* 2003; 42:7–16.
118. Schomig A, Ndrepepa G, Mehilli J, et al. Therapy-dependent influence of time-to-treatment interval on myocardial salvage in patients with acute myocardial infarction treated with coronary artery stenting or thrombolysis. *Circulation.* 2003;108:1084–1088.
119. Gheorghiade M, Zannad F, Sopko G, et al., for the International Working Group on Acute Heart Failure Syndromes. Acute heart failure syndromes: current state and framework for future research. *Circulation.* 2005;112:3958–3968.
120. Gheorghiade M, Sopko G, De Luca L, et al. Navigating the crossroads of coronary artery disease and heart failure *Circulation.* 2006;114:1202–1213.
121. Steg PG, Dabbous OH, Feldman LJ, et al.; Global Registry of Acute Coronary Events Investigators. Determinants and prognostic impact of heart failure complicating acute coronary syndromes: observations from the Global Registry of Acute Coronary Events (GRACE). *Circulation.* 2004;109:494–499.
122. Trost JC, Hillis LD. Intra-aortic balloon counterpulsation. *Am J Cardiol.* 2006;97(9):1391–1398.
123. Becker RC, Gore JM, Lambrew C, et al. A composite view of cardiac rupture in the United States National Registry of Myocardial Infarction. *J Am Coll Cardiol.* 1996;27:1321–1326.
124. Hochman JS, Sleeper LA, Webb JG, et al.; SHOCK Investigators. Early revascularization in acute myocardial infarction complicated by cardiogenic shock. *N Engl J Med.* 1999;341:625–634.
125. Hochman JS, Sleeper LA, White HD, et al.; SHOCK Investigators. One-year survival following early revascularization for cardiogenic shock. *JAMA.* 2001;285:190–192.
126. Babaev A, Frederick PD, Pasta DJ, et al.; NRMI Investigators. Trends in management and outcomes of patients with acute myocardial infarction complicated by cardiogenic shock. *JAMA.* 2005;294(4):448–454.
127. Rogers WJ, Bowlby LJ, Chandra NC, et al.; for the participants in the National Registry of Myocardial Infarction. Treatment of myocardial infarction in the United States (1990 to 1993). *Circulation.* 1994;90:2103–2114.
128. Bursi F, Enriquez-Sarano M, Nkomo VT, et al. Heart failure and death after myocardial infarction in the community: the emerging role of mitral regurgitation. *Circulation.* 2005;111:295–301.
129. Salukhe TV, Henein MY, Sutton R. Ischemic mitral regurgitation and its related risk after myocardial infarction. *Circulation.* 2005;111:254–256.
130. Hochman JS, Lamas GA, Buller CE, et al. Coronary intervention for persistent occlusion after myocardial infarction. *N Engl J Med.* 2006;355:2395–2407.
131. Dzavik V, Buller CE, Lamas GA, et al.; TOSCA-2 Investigators. Randomized trial of percutaneous coronary intervention for subacute infarct-related coronary artery occlusion to achieve long-term patency and improve ventricular function: the Total Occlusion Study of Canada (TOSCA)-2 trial. *Circulation.* 2006;114(23):2449–2457.
132. Zehender M, Kasper W, Kauder E, et al. Right ventricular infarction as an independent predictor of prognosis after acute inferior myocardial infarction. *N Engl J Med.* 1993;328:981–988.
133. Berger PB, Ryan TJ. Inferior myocardial infarction: high-risk subgroups. *Circulation.* 1990;81:401–411.
134. Jacobs AK, Leopold JA, Bates E, et al. Cardiogenic shock caused by right ventricular infarction: a report from the SHOCK registry. *J Am Coll Cardiol.* 2003;41:1273–1279.
135. Kinch JW, Ryan TJ. Right ventricular infarction. *N Engl J Med.* 1994;330:1211–1217.
136. Dell'Italia LJ, Starling MR, Blumhardt R, et al. Comparative effects of volume loading, dobutamine, and nitroprusside in patients with predominant right ventricular infarction. *Circulation.* 1985;72:1327–1335.
137. Love JC, Haffajee CI, Gore JM, et al. Reversibility of hypotension and shock by atrial or atrioventricular sequential pacing in patients with right ventricular infarction. *Am Heart J.* 1984;108:5–13.
138. Cotter G, Berger PB. Cardiogenic shock–beyond the large infarction. *Crit Care Med.* 2006;34(8):2234–2235.
139. Bromet DS, Klein LW. Cardiogenic shock: art and science. *Crit Care Med.* 2004;32(1):293–294.
140. Puri VK. Cardiogenic shock: what has changed? *Chest.* 2003;124(5):1634–1636.

CHAPTER 121 ■ EVALUATION AND MANAGEMENT OF HEART FAILURE

JAMES E. CALVIN, Jr. • STEPHANIE H. DUNLAP

Heart failure is a complex syndrome physiologically characterized as low cardiac output leading to inadequate blood supply of tissues and vital organs. No matter the etiology, damage to the cardiocytes starts a complicated neurohormonal cascade that causes poor renal perfusion, leading to stimulation of the renin–angiotensin–aldosterone system and elevated levels of circulating catecholamines. These compensatory mechanisms lead to sodium and water retention and tachycardia that may cause pulmonary, hepatic, and splenic congestion, as well as peripheral and splanchnic bed constriction. The patient may experience symptoms such as dyspnea on exertion, lower extremity edema, early satiety, paroxysmal nocturnal dyspnea, fatigue, dizziness, and/or syncope.

Heart failure is a serious public health concern in the United States and other industrialized countries. It continues to increase in incidence and prevalence, with a prevalence of 5 million Americans having the syndrome in 2003 and with an incidence 550,000 new persons diagnosed annually (1). These derangements lead to frequent hospitalizations, totaling 1,093,000 hospital discharges (2) and 3.4 million visits to physicians, emergency departments, and hospital outpatient departments annually (3). The mortality rate remains high despite complex and expensive medical regimens, with self-assessment of the patient's quality of life rated as poor. The Framingham Heart Study now has 44 years of follow-up and, based upon these data, heart failure incidence approaches 10 per 1,000 population after age 65 (1). The lifetime risk for development of symptomatic heart failure is one in five for both men and women (4). The lifetime risk for heart failure is doubled for both sexes with blood pressure greater than or equal to 160/100 mm Hg compared to those without hypertension. Thus, given current demographics, cases of heart failure are predicted to continue to rise.

Risk factors for heart failure continue to include hypertension, with 75% of heart failure cases having antecedent hypertension (1). About 22% of male and 46% of female victims of myocardial infarction (MI) will become disabled with heart failure within 6 years of the MI (1). Diabetes mellitus is another significant risk factor for heart failure. In women with coronary heart disease, diabetes mellitus was found to be the strongest risk factor for the development of heart failure. Additionally, in this study, those with an elevated body mass index or depressed creatinine (Cr) clearance in diabetic women were noted to be at highest risk, with annual incidence rates of 7% and 13%, respectively (5). In another study of patients with heart failure, African American women with elevated body mass index and pre-existing hypertension were the cohort with the highest risk for the development of heart failure (6). With regard to mortality, deaths from heart failure based on the International Classification of Disease (Code 428) increased 20.5% from 1993 to 2003. In 2003, the overall death rate for heart failure was 19.1%. Examined by race and gender, death rates were 20.3% for Caucasian males, 22.9% for African American males, 18.3% for Caucasian females, and 19.0% for African American females. Heart failure discharges from hospitals were 1,093,000 in 2003.

Heart failure is a syndrome with diverse etiologies, anatomies, and physiologic presentations. The World Health Organization developed classification nomenclature for the cardiomyopathies. This nomenclature is based on anatomic and physiologic findings: restrictive, hypertrophic, and dilated. This chapter focuses on the dilated cardiomyopathies. The myocardial muscle disease causing dilated cardiomyopathy may be either a primary cardiocyte disorder or secondary to another disease process. Whether primary or secondary, the hallmark findings of dilated cardiomyopathy are a dilated left ventricle and a low left ventricular ejection fraction. The most common etiology of dilated cardiomyopathy (DCM) is secondary to ischemic heart disease. Ischemic cardiomyopathy accounts for nearly half of all cases of DCM in the United States. All the remaining dilated cardiomyopathies are considered primary muscle diseases. Although 75% of patients diagnosed with heart failure have antecedent hypertension, only about 22% of patients with DCM have hypertension as the only identifiable etiology (1). Nearly 25% of patients with dilated cardiomyopathy have no pre-existing risk factors for DCM and are given the diagnosis of idiopathic dilated cardiomyopathy. Nearly 25% of patients with idiopathic dilated cardiomyopathy have a familial component, likely related to abnormalities in cardiac β-adrenergic receptors (7). Once the common etiologies are excluded, a small but important number of other causes remains, including DCM secondary to toxins such as alcohol, anthracyclines, and cocaine. Endocrine diseases such as diabetes mellitus and thyroid disease may also cause heart failure. Other possible etiologies include human immunodeficiency virus (HIV) and Lyme disease infections, sarcoidosis, thiamine deficiency, peripartum cardiomyopathy, hemochromatosis, and underlying collagen vascular diseases.

CELLULAR DETERMINANTS OF MYOCARDIAL CONTRACTION

The Contractile Proteins

The interaction of the proteins actin, myosin, and the troponin complex is responsible for myocardial contraction.

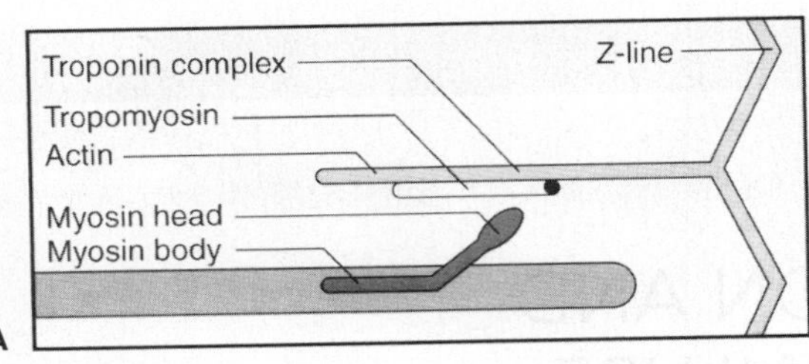

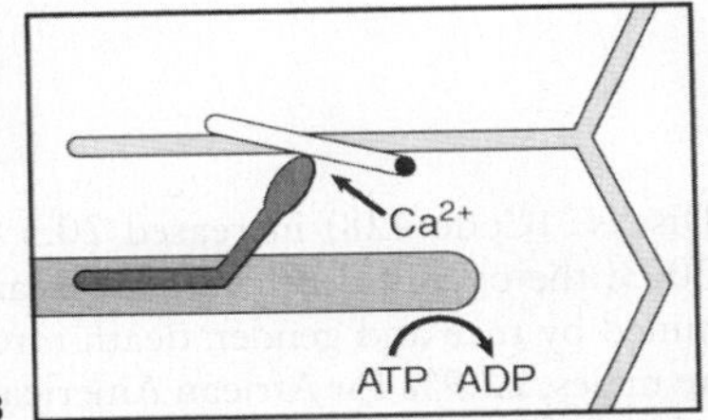

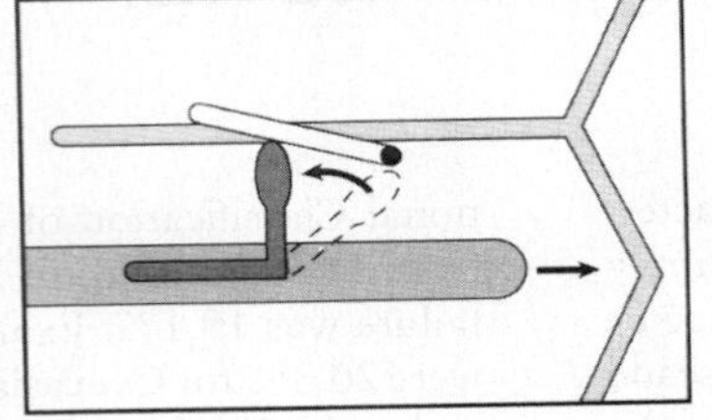

FIGURE 121.1. A schematic representation of tropomyosin, troponin complex, actin, myosin, and calcium during relaxation (A), activation (B), and contraction (C). During relaxation, the myosin is prevented from interacting with actin by tropomyosin. Activation by the interaction of calcium with troponin C confers a configurational change in tropomyosin allowing the interaction of myosin and actin.

Engagement of actin and myosin occurs when calcium (Ca^{2+}) levels in the cytosol increase in the presence of adequate adenosine triphosphate (ATP). This process is regulated by a complex that consists of troponin C and other proteins. Troponin C contains a Ca^{2+}-specific binding site with a variable affinity for Ca^{2+} (8). This binding of Ca^{2+} to troponin C is regulated by troponin I. When Ca^{2+} is bound to troponin C, tropomyosin—a protein, bound to the troponin complex by troponin T, which inhibits actin–myosin interaction in the absence of troponin C—undergoes a conformational change, allowing for actin–myosin interaction and contraction (Fig. 121.1).

Removal of Ca^{2+} from the cytosol results in dissociation from troponin C, with subsequent cessation of actin–myosin cross-linkage. This event signals the end of contractile activity and the start of relaxation—a process known as *inactivation* (9).

Calcium and Cyclic Adenosine Monophosphate

Alterations in the delivery, use, and myofibrillar sensitivity to Ca^{2+} and removal of Ca^{2+} from the myofibril and the myocyte cytosol constitutes the biologic basis for the vast majority, if not all, of the abnormalities in both contractility and relaxation. Entry of Ca^{2+} from extracellular locations occurs through either voltage-dependent, gated "slow channels" activated by membrane depolarization or via sodium–calcium (Na^{+}–Ca^{2+}) exchange across the sarcolemma. In addition, elevated levels of cyclic adenosine monophosphate (cAMP), the major intracellular second messenger, causes increased Ca^{2+} influx by recruitment of additional voltage-dependent channels on the sarcolemma, previously dormant. This is accomplished by cAMP-mediated transfer of phosphates to phospholamban, a protein linked to the voltage-gated channels. This Ca^{2+}, rather than participating directly in activation of contraction, causes release of Ca^{2+} from the sarcoplasmic reticulum (SR) (10), termed *Ca^{2} -dependent Ca^{2+} release*. The Ca^{2+} released from the SR binds to troponin with subsequent contractile activity (Fig. 121.2).

Altered Ca^{2+} kinetics are responsible for the increases in contractility observed in other circumstances. The increased contractility of postextrasystolic beats (11,12), increased heart rate (HR) (13,14), and, during pharmacologic manipulation with cardiac glycosides, phosphodiesterase inhibitors (15), sympathomimetic amines (14), and caffeine (16) are dependent on changes in intracellular Ca^{2+} and/or cAMP levels.

Absolute blood Ca^{2+} levels—by raising cytosolic Ca^{2+} levels (17)—and hormonal changes such as hyperthyroidism increase contractility (18,19) secondary to increased troponin C affinity for Ca^{2+}, increased ATPase activity with concomitant increased cAMP levels, and changes in intracellular Ca^{2+} handling.

Individual muscle units in the failing and hypertrophied ventricle have been found to have depressed function (20). The myocardial depression accompanying anoxia (21), acidosis (22), hypothyroidism (18), barbiturate use, administration of local and general anesthetics, Ca^{2+} antagonists (23), and ischemia (24) all result from abnormalities in the Ca^{2+}-dependent mechanisms described here.

CELLULAR DETERMINANTS OF RELAXATION

Just as abnormalities of contraction have as their cellular basis derangements of Ca^{2+} handling, so too does relaxation. Cessation of the inward Ca^{2+} current—or inactivation—by closure of voltage-limited channels of the sarcolemma begins the period of relaxation, with the rate and extent of Ca^{2+} removal affecting the rate and extent of relaxation. As alluded to earlier, inactivation signals the end of actin–myosin interaction. However, this single term does not adequately describe the interplay of processes that are occurring at the cellular level to facilitate relaxation. The SR Ca^{2+} pump, in the presence of adequate ATP, pumps Ca^{2+} into the SR from the cytosol. Phospholamban, a protein within the SR, when phosphorylated by cAMP-dependent mechanisms, results in increased SR uptake of Ca^{2+} by the reticulum Ca^{2+} ATPase (SERCA) (16,25). This is noted to occur primarily after adrenergic stimuli. In addition, the Na^{+}–Ca^{2+} exchange pump—also requiring ATP—allows

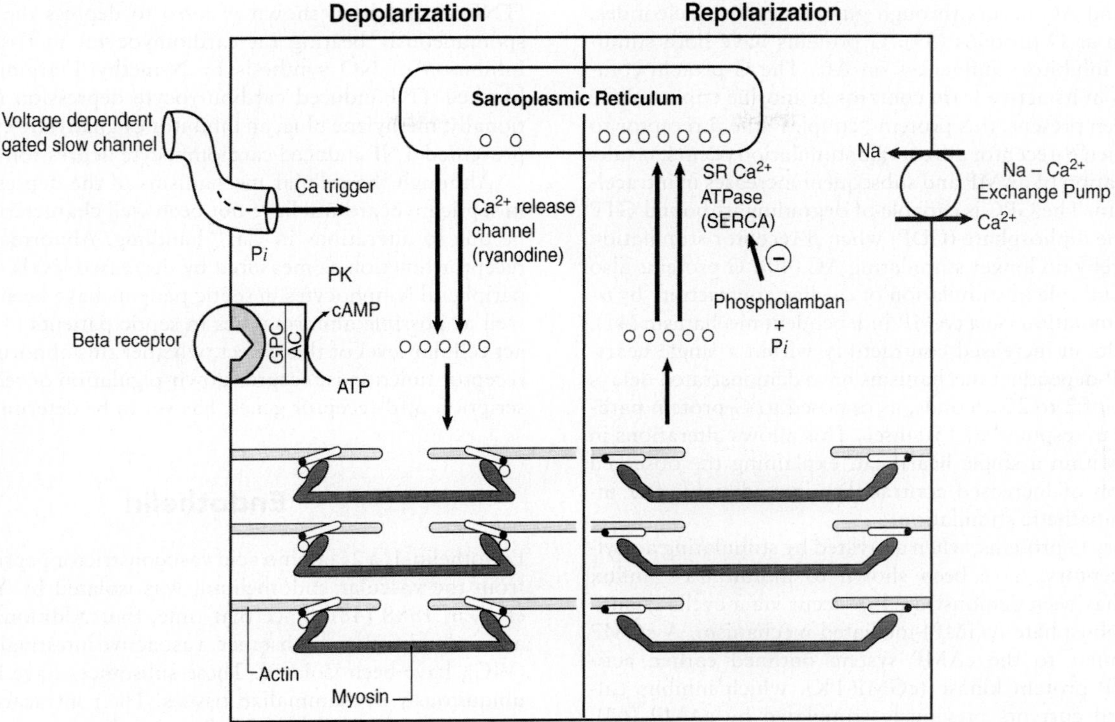

FIGURE 121.2. The role of calcium in excitation and contraction in the human myocyte. During depolarization, Ca^{2+} enters from the extracellular space through the voltage-dependent, gated slow channel, the so-called L-type channel. This entry is facilitated by β-receptor stimulation of a protein receptor, which in turn stimulates adenyl cyclase (AC) producing cyclic adenosine monophosphate (cAMP) and phosphorylation of the calcium channel. However, this intrusion of calcium into the cell does not moderate the interaction of actin and myosin. Rather, it acts as a trigger for the release of calcium from the sarcoplasmic reticulum through the Ca^{2+} release or ryanodine receptor channel. During repolarization, the sarcoplasmic reticulum (SR) Ca^{2+} ATPase (SERCA) mediates the uptake of cytosolic calcium into the SR. cAMP-mediated phosphorylation of phospholamban prevents the inhibition by phospholamban of SERCA activity. The Na–Ca^{2+} exchange pump is the dominant mechanism of Ca^{2+} extrusion out of the cytosol into the extracellular space.

the efflux of Ca^{2+} into the extracellular space from the cytosol (Fig. 121.2). The affinity of myofibrils for Ca^{2+} also affects relaxation. As the myofibril shortens, its affinity for Ca^{2+} decreases, limiting Ca^{2+} effects (26). All of these mechanisms will be facilitated or inhibited by drugs or neurohumoral factors.

The process of relaxation has been extensively studied in DCM, left ventricular (LV) hypertrophy, ischemia, and hypertrophic cardiomyopathy (HCM). Impairment of relaxation in these patients occurs secondary to increased levels of Ca^{2+} within the myocyte in diastole (27,28), owing to diminished function of the SR uptake pump, decreased expression at the genetic level for this pump as evidenced by decreased mRNA levels (29), decreased phospholamban activity (30) and levels of phospholamban mRNA (31), down-regulation or uncoupling of β receptors (32,33), and inhibition of β-receptor function via G-protein inhibition (34).

MEDIATORS OF CONTRACTILITY

Various mediators, acting independently by linking stimulated α, β, or acetylcholine receptors to intracytoplasmic enzyme systems, alter the contractile state of the myocardium. The best characterized of these systems, the guanine nucleotide regulatory proteins (35,36), are coupled to β, α, and acetylcholine receptors, and possibly to receptors for nitric oxide and endothelins.

β Receptors and Guanine Nucleotide Regulatory Proteins

As alluded to earlier, adrenergic stimulation of cardiac myocytes is a very important regulator of both Ca^{2+} influx and cAMP levels within the cell (Fig. 121.2) (37). The predominant (β) receptor of myocytes, when stimulated, increases the manufacture of cAMP. Via the mechanisms previously described, this action, in turn, results in increased Ca^{2+} influx. Ca^{2+} channels that are under the influence of β-receptor–mediated increases in cAMP are known as "receptor-operated channels" (38). Stimulation of β receptors on the cell surface results in activation of adenylate cyclase (AC) and subsequent increases in cAMP levels. This results in increased Ca^{2+} influx, with resultant increases in contractile force. The coupling between β

receptors and AC occurs through guanine cyclic nucleotides, also known as G proteins (39). G proteins have both stimulatory and inhibitory influences on AC. The G-protein complex (GPC) in its active form contains guanosine triphosphate (GTP). When present, this protein "couples" the β receptor to AC, and when β-receptor adrenergic stimulation occurs, results in the formation of cAMP and subsequent increases in intracellular calcium. The GPC is capable of degrading its bound GTP to guanosine diphosphate (GDP) when β-receptor stimulation ceases, thereby no longer stimulating AC (40). G proteins also have a pivotal role in stimulation of cardiac contractility by α-receptor stimulation via a cAMP-independent mechanism (41), which results in increased contractility within a single heartbeat. cAMP-dependent mechanisms have demonstrated delays in response of 2 to 20 seconds, as opposed to G-protein pathway delays in response of 150 msec. This allows alterations in Ca^{2+} flux within a single heartbeat, explaining the observed phenomenon of increased contractility immediately after increased sympathetic stimulation.

Inhibitory G proteins, when activated by stimulating acetylcholine receptors, have been shown to inhibit Ca^{2+} influx (42). This has been demonstrated to occur via a cyclic guanosine monophosphate (cGMP)-mediated mechanism. A cGMP system, similar to the cAMP system outlined earlier, activates cGMP protein kinase (cGMP-PK), which inhibits calcium inward currents previously stimulated by cAMP (43). Additionally, cGMP-mediated inhibition of Ca^{2+} channels has been demonstrated not to be a result of cAMP hydrolysis or a result of inhibition of cAMP-PK, but a direct effect of cGMP-PK.

In addition to changes in receptor function, molecular alterations in β-receptor production in various disease states have been shown to occur. In dilated cardiomyopathies, both β_1-receptor mRNA and absolute receptor levels were found to be depressed (32). At the same time, β-receptor kinase (βARK) levels were elevated. βARK, the molecule responsible for the phosphorylation of β-adrenergic receptors, is elevated when β receptors are dysfunctional (uncoupled). This may provide an explanation for the catecholamine insensitivity observed in failing hearts as well as after cardiopulmonary bypass (44).

Nitric Oxide

Nitric oxide (NO) has been shown to affect cardiac contractility. It has been found in many tissue types, including ventricular myocytes, where its physiologic effects are mediated via cGMP. Cholinergic myocardiac depressant effects, as evidenced by inhibition of the effect of the muscarinic agonist carbachol, were inhibited by antagonists of NO (methylene blue and oxyhemoglobin) as well as by L-arginine (the natural substrate of NO synthesis analogs), which inhibits NO. In addition, the positive inotropic action of the β agonist isoproterenol is enhanced by NO inhibition. These data indicate that the effect of NO is to activate the inhibitory receptor cyclic nucleotide interaction via cGMP mechanisms.

Nitric oxide has been implicated in the myocardial response to sepsis. It has been well documented that myocardial depression in septic shock occurs secondary to a yet undefined substance. One potential substance, tumor necrosis factor-α (TNF-α), has been shown *in vitro* to depress the activity of spontaneously beating rat cardiomyocytes in tissue culture. Inhibition of NO synthesis by N-methyl-L-arginine (NMA) blocked TNF-induced cardiomyocyte depression (45). Additionally, methylene blue, an inhibitor of guanylate cyclase (46), prevented TNF-induced cardiomyocyte depression.

Although the cellular mechanisms of the depression noted in septic myocardium have not been well characterized, it may be due to alterations in Ca^{2+} handling. Abnormalities of β-receptor function as measured by decreased levels of cAMP in peripheral lymphocytes in septic patients have been elicited, as well as possible abnormalities in septic patients (47). The exact cellular level of this defect, whether this abnormality of β-receptor function is receptor down-regulation or reduced transcription of β-receptor genes, has yet to be determined.

Endothelin

Endothelin-1, a 21-amino acid vasoconstrictor peptide released from the vascular endothelium, was isolated by Yanagisawa et al. in 1988 (48). Since that time, four additional isoforms and a closely related substance, vasoactive intestinal contractor (VIC), have been isolated. These substances have been found ubiquitously in mammalian tissues. Their intracardiac site of genesis is unknown, but is believed to be the endothelium of the coronary arteries and microvasculature. Various vasodilator and vasoconstrictor substances released from the vascular endothelium alter blood flow and, in this way, indirectly affect cardiac contractility (49). Of these locally elaborated paracrine substances, the endothelins have been most extensively studied.

High-affinity receptors for endothelins in mammalian atria and ventricles have been isolated. *In vitro*, these substances have been shown to be potent vasoconstrictors and positive inotropes, acting via a yet incompletely defined mechanism. Kelly et al. (50) demonstrated that at constant cytosolic Ca^{2+} levels using the Ca^{2+}-specific intracellular probe Fura-2, endothelins cause marked increases in the contractility of isolated rat ventricular myocytes. This observation suggests that endothelins may sensitize the myofibrils to calcium, although this finding has not been duplicated by others.

As previously discussed, an increase in intracellular pH results in increased myofibrillar sensitivity for Ca^{2+}, thereby increasing contractility. Endothelin causes an increase in intracellular pH, with a subsequent increase in contraction when studied in rat ventricular myocytes. This effect is completely inhibited by pretreatment with amiloride, which inhibits Na^+–H^+ exchange across the sarcolemmal membrane and, hence, prevents increases in intracellular pH (51). Furthermore, the effect of endothelin appears to be mediated via G proteins participating in signal transduction after binding of endothelin to its sarcolemmal receptor.

THE CELLULAR BASIS OF HEART FAILURE

Heart failure, either acute or chronic, results from loss of myocytes or loss of intrinsic contractility within individual myocytes. Several functional abnormalities involving excitation–contraction coupling of contractile proteins within myocytes and myocardial energetics have been identified.

The importance of Ca^{2+} in the regulation of myocardial contraction cannot be overstated. Evidence has mounted about the role of disturbances in calcium handling in heart failure (52–58). Prolonged elevation of Ca^{2+} concentration intracellularly is apparent in heart failure. Furthermore, there is a blunted rise of depolarization, causing slower activation and a slower rate of fall during repolarization. This is likely mediated via the impaired reuptake of calcium into the sarcoplasmic reticulum because Ca^{2+}–adenosine triphosphatase activity (SERCA2) is reduced. The activity of SERCA2 activity is inhibited by phosphorylation of phospholamban through cAMP stimulated by β-adrenergic receptors.

The calcium release channel (CRC) of the sarcoplasmic reticulum mediates release of Ca^{2+} from the SR into the cytosol during contraction and is critical for activation of the contractile elements. It now appears that the CRC is hyperphosphorylated by protein kinase A in heart failure, resulting in a high rate of Ca^{2+} leakage from the SR (59) throughout the cardiac cycle. Other abnormalities identified in heart failure include increased activity in the Na^{+}–Ca^{2+} exchanger, perhaps as a compensation for reduced SERCA2, and decreased mRNA and protein levels of the voltage-dependent Ca^{2+} channel.

Contractile Protein Alteration in the Failure Heart

Considerable data now exist (60,61) demonstrating alterations in contractile proteins in heart failure. Both myosin heavy and light chains have been demonstrated to revert to fetal phenotypes in chronic heart failure. In addition, troponin I and T have also been shown to revert to fetal phenotypes.

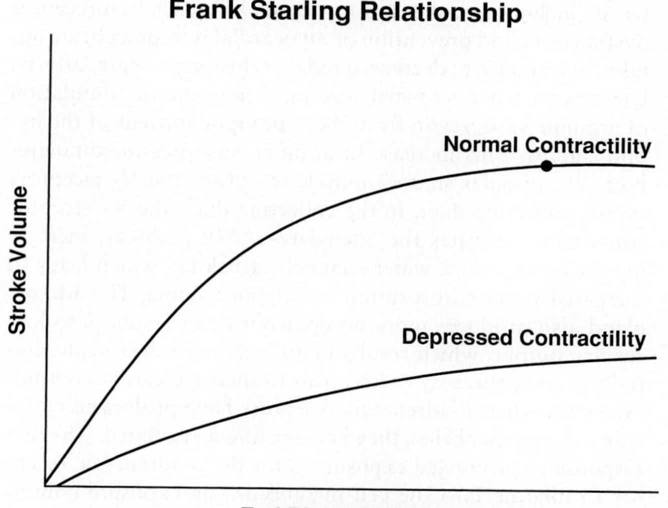

FIGURE 121.3. Typical Frank-Starling curves for normal and depressed myocardium. For a given end-diastolic volume, stroke volume is decreased with depressed contractility.

Regulation of Interstitial Collagen

Collagen provides stents along which myocytes are aligned. The quantity and nature of the collagen in the extracellular matrix (ECM) are determined by the balance between synthesis and degradation. The latter is regulated by matrix metalloproteinases (MMPs) (62,63). In heart failure, there appears to be a maladaptation of collagen stents, perhaps mediated by increased activity of MMPs. Paradoxically, in hypertension and pressure overload, an increase in interstitial collagen has been noted.

Adaptations to Changes in Load or Myocardial Injury

In situations where an excessive load is placed on either ventricle, or where an injury has occurred that depresses myocardial contraction, the ventricle (14) can adapt to maintain cardiac output by doing the following:

1. Increase ventricular preload (so-called *Frank Starling effect*) (Fig. 121.3) (64)
2. Activation of neurohumeral systems such as the renin–angiotensin–aldosterone system (65)
3. The release of norepinephrine (66)
4. Myocardial remodeling via chamber dilatation and augmentation of myocardial mass (67)

The first adaptation increases cardiac output by increasing preload (end-diastolic pressure and volume). The second increases blood volume and blood pressure by increasing peripheral vascular resistance. The third attempts to increase contractility by shifting the Frank-Starling curves upward, and the fourth enhances contractility by restoring the number of contractile units. The next effect of these adaptations is maintenance of cardiac output and blood pressure in the face of increased afterload (peripheral vascular resistance [PVR]) at the expense of increasing ventricular dilatation.

Myocardial remodeling takes longer to develop and there are two distinct patterns (67,68): (a) concentric hypertrophy (increased mass without ventricular dilatation) and (b) eccentric hypertrophy (increased mass and ventricular dilatation) (69). Concentric hypertrophy usually occurs in response to pressure overload, and is characterized by parallel replication of myofibrils and thickening of individual myocytes. Eccentric hypertrophy occurs in response to volume overload, leading to increased diastolic stress with a series replication of sarcomeres, elongation of myocytes, and ventricular dilatation. In both of these cases, wall stress is returned toward normal, at least initially. There appears to be differences in patterns of gene activation for several peptide growth factors.

At the cellular level, there is an increase in the number of mitochondria, an increase in cell size, and an increase in the amount of collagen within the extracellular matrix. When the injury or stress exceeds the ability of these adaptive mechanisms to compensate, myocardial contractility decreases. The transition from a compensated state to failure involves the following processes:

1. Inadequate hypertrophy to maintain contractility
2. Re-expression of fetal genes and decreased expression of adult genes (70)
3. Alteration in proteins involved in excitation–contraction coupling
4. Myocardial death by necrosis or apoptosis (71)
5. Changes in myocardial energetics

Neurohormonal Abnormalities in Heart Failure

When low cardiac output occurs, renal perfusion pressure is decreased. This causes stimulation of renin in the juxtaglomerular apparatus. Renin is then converted in the kidney to angiotensinogen, and then to angiotensin I. Angiotensin I is released into the circulation and is converted in the lung by angiotensin-converting enzyme to angiotensin II, a potent vasoconstrictor. A major breakthrough in therapeutic options for heart failure was the discovery of this enzyme system that then led to pharmaceutical development of angiotensin-converting enzyme inhibitors to interrupt this pathway. Another major breakthrough was the realization that other enzymes, located in the myocardium, could cleave the decapeptide angiotensin I into the octapeptide angiotensin II. These enzymes are chymase, CAGE, and cathepsin G. This discovery cemented the idea that the heart was a neuroendocrine organ. The potent vasoconstrictor effects of angiotensin II were part of the cardiovascular system's compensatory mechanisms: angiotensin II increased renal perfusion pressure.

Elevated levels of aldosterone are also seen in patients with left ventricular systolic dysfunction. Stimulation of renin and angiotensin II leads to increased production of aldosterone by the adrenal gland. Additional mechanisms of increased aldosterone levels are decreased hepatic clearance of the hormone as well as stimulation by sodium-restricted diets. Since elevated aldosterone levels lead to sodium and water retention, plasma volume is increased. Low cardiac output also causes the adrenal gland to produce more norepinephrine. Elevated levels of circulating catecholamines in patients with heart failure have been shown to have prognostic significance, with higher norepinephrine levels predicting higher mortality (72). With increased levels of norepinephrine, heart rate is increased, thus aiding in maintenance of cardiac output since:

$$CO = SV \times HR$$

where CO = cardiac output, SV = stroke volume, and HR = heart rate.

Elevated levels of norepinephrine, angiotensin II, and aldosterone result in maladaptive changes in LV structure. These neurohormones lead to dilatation of the left ventricle as well as changes in cardiocyte architecture, collagen type and content, and β-adrenergic receptor abnormalities. Collectively, these changes in LV architecture are known as remodeling. Complex signaling pathways have been shown to activate cellular responses during hypertrophy of cardiocytes *in vivo*. These include accumulation and assembly of contractile proteins, increase in size of cardiocytes, and expression of embryonic genes resulting in eccentric hypertrophy. Eccentric hypertrophy is found in DCM and is a result of contractile protein units being assembled in series, rather than in parallel, as seen in concentric hypertrophy. Scientific advances that have led to this knowledge were achieved by first identifying mutant genes, such as those that cause familial idiopathic cardiomyopathy, then being able to culture cardiocytes, followed by studying genetically engineered animals. Factors that led to the hypertrophic response include growth factors, peptides, and cytokines, with the most comprehensively studied substances being insulin growth factor I, angiotensin II, endothelin, and those that activate a form of GTP-binding protein (ras) signaling pathways, cytokines including interleukin-6, and heteromeric (G_q) (70).

The presence of these neurohormones in abnormal amounts has been intensively studied. These substances are produced as part of compensatory mechanisms used to alleviate the adverse effects of low cardiac output. The vasoconstrictors include endothelin and angiotensin II. These are the two strongest intrinsic vasoconstrictors discovered in humans, with endothelin being the most potent. Vasoconstrictors aid the failing ventricle by keeping perfusion pressure up. Another compensatory mechanism is stimulation of aldosterone. Increased production of aldosterone results in the kidney retaining sodium—and thus, water—in exchange for increased secretion of potassium, retention of sodium and water, and increased plasma volume. Other adverse effects of this compensatory release of aldosterone include vascular and myocardial fibrosis, baroreceptor dysfunction, and prevention of myocardial norepinephrine uptake. In response to decreased renal perfusion pressure, arterial baroreceptors are activated, leading to nonosmotic stimulation of arginine vasopressin from the supraoptic nucleus of the hypothalamus. This increase in arginine vasopressin stimulates both V_{1a} vascular smooth muscle receptors and V_2 receptors on the collecting duct. In the collecting duct, the V_2 receptor stimulation activates the adenylate–cAMP pathway, increasing the aquaporin-2 water channel trafficking, which leads to increased water reabsorption and hyponatremia. The adrenal gland also produces more norepinephrine in response to low cardiac output, which results in an increase in heart rate, initially a compensatory mechanism to increase cardiac output. However, when β-adrenergic receptors have prolonged exposure to norepinephrine, they become down-regulated. The first response to prolonged exposure is for the β-adrenergic receptor to migrate into the cell membrane. As exposure continues, it is then transported intracellularly and becomes phagocytized (73), as was shown by Bristow et al. by performing endomyocardial biopsies of patients with systolic heart failure. This group noted that there were fewer β-adrenergic receptors in patients with heart failure and that the β receptors that were present were less responsive to isoproterenol, a β-adrenergic agonist (73). Mann et al. found that cultured cardiac myocytes exposed to norepinephrine first began to contract normally and then, after prolonged exposure, became irreversibly hypercontracted and cell viability decreased over time (74). Thus, with low cardiac output, a variety of neurohormones are produced in abnormal amounts, leading to left ventricular remodeling, apoptosis, resting tachycardia, β-receptor down-regulation, arrhythmias, increased systemic vascular resistance (elevated afterload), and edematous states (increased preload).

Another group of neurohormones produced in response to the failing heart has been determined to be beneficial. These include the natriuretic peptides made in response to left ventricular dilatation, especially brain natriuretic peptide (BNP). This hormone has natriuretic and vasodilatory properties that are beneficial in patients with heart failure, their function being an attempt to counteract the deleterious effects of aldosterone and angiotensin II. Levels of BNP are elevated in patients with heart failure, compared to those with normal LV function. Additionally, data suggest that BNP levels are more elevated as the patient becomes more symptomatic—that is, as the New York Heart Association Functional Class increases—and levels may be more elevated when patients present in decompensated heart failure compared to their compensated state. Despite elevated BNP production, the patient may continue to deteriorate, the current explanation being that BNP is rapidly overwhelmed by more potent vasoconstrictor substances present in the heart failure milieu.

Other substances with vasodilatory properties include bradykinin, nitric oxide, and prostaglandins. One mechanism for vasodilatation with angiotensin-converting enzyme (ACE) inhibitors is that degradation of bradykinin is inhibited by ACE inhibitors, since kininase, the enzyme that degrades bradykinin, is also known as angiotensin-converting enzyme. Cytokines are also produced in abnormal amounts, including interleukins and TNF-α. Once LV dysfunction is present, the overexpression of these compounds contributes to the progression of heart failure, promoting LV dilatation and remodeling. Moreover, elevated TNF-α levels are found in patients with advanced heart failure, and a trend toward higher mortality with higher TNF-α levels was found in an analysis of the Studies of Left Ventricular Dysfunction (SOLVD) trial (75,76).

Remodeling

Remodeling is a complex process in response to either acute or chronic injury to cardiocytes. The term encompasses LV dilatation, eccentric hypertrophy, apoptosis (programmed cell death not secondary to ischemia), changes in valvular structure, and arrhythmias. Increases in left ventricular end-diastolic and end-systolic dimensions occur, as well as increased size at the cellular level with cardiocytes developing increased cell volume and eccentric hypertrophy. White et al. (77) found that the most potent predictor of death following acute myocardial infarction was end-systolic volume and, in a multivariable model, was more potent than the extent of coronary artery disease. With the increase in chamber size, LV geometry is also altered, with the left ventricle losing its elliptical shape and developing a more spherical shape. The more spherical LV has been associated with higher end-systolic wall stress and abnormal distribution of fiber shortening (78). Additionally, one small study of patients with idiopathic dilated cardiomyopathy found poorer survival in those that had developed a more spherical ventricle and more uniform distribution of afterload (79).

Mitral regurgitation frequently accompanies LV remodeling. This occurs due to misalignment of papillary muscles and the subvalvular structures, as well as distortion at the mitral annulus secondary to LV enlargement. Left atrial enlargement and pulmonary venous hypertension are frequent sequelae of mitral regurgitation. Electrocardiographic abnormalities and arrhythmias are also common problems in patients with heart failure. These include left bundle branch block, P-R interval prolongation, atrial flutter and atrial fibrillation, and ventricular tachycardia. Development of atrial fibrillation is frequently seen in patients with decompensated heart failure and, in a chicken and egg type phenomenon, may either cause the decompensation or may occur as a result of the decompensation. Syncope, an ominous predictor for sudden cardiac death, may be secondary to ventricular tachycardia or atrial arrhythmias, with rapid ventricular response. Any patient, presenting with syncope should have a thorough investigation for its etiology.

Given that LV remodeling is a harbinger for poor outcomes, attempts to delay or reverse the remodeling process have become therapeutic targets for altering the outcome and improving survival in patients afflicted with heart failure. The Cooperative Northern Scandinavian Enalapril Survival (CONSENSUS) (80) and SOLVD Treatment trials (75,76) determined that therapy with enalapril improved survival in patients with pre-existing mild to moderate and advanced heart failure, most likely by its impact on angiotensin II production. The Survival and Ventricular Enlargement (SAVE) trial (81) revealed that patients surviving myocardial infarction with resultant left ventricular enlargement—but not clinical heart failure—had better survival with the ACE inhibitor, captopril. Additionally, those patients receiving captopril had less morbidity and mortality secondary to cardiovascular events and less recurrent myocardial infarctions. The SOLVD Prevention trial showed that therapy with the ACE inhibitor, enalapril, delayed development of heart failure symptoms and decreased both all-cause hospitalizations and hospitalizations for heart failure, whether for patients with recent myocardial infarcts or those with pre-existing heart failure. Trials with β-adrenergic receptor therapy, in addition to ACE inhibitor therapy, revealed that these agents were capable of decreasing LV size and improving the ejection fraction. Cardiac resynchronization of therapy has also been shown to reverse remodeling the left ventricle.

DIASTOLIC DYSFUNCTION IN HEART FAILURE

Left ventricular diastolic function is dependent on many factors, some *intrinsic* to the heart itself (e.g., the active energy-dependent process of relaxation and material properties of the myocardium) and some *extrinsic* to the LV (e.g., pericardial constraining forces and ventricular interaction). Furthermore, Gilbert and Glantz (82) have suggested that relaxation can be further divided into the *extent of relaxation* (i.e., the completeness of relaxation) and the *rate of relaxation*. Alterations in the extent, rate, or both characterize the abnormalities of relaxation and result in characteristic hemodynamic patterns (82).

Left Ventricular Compliance and the Diastolic Left Ventricular Pressure–Volume Relationship

A nonlinear relationship normally exists between pressure and volume during ventricular diastole. Shifts in this relationship are reflected either by a change in the slope of the relationship of filling pressure and volume—stiffness of the left ventricle—as filling volume increases (83), or by changes in either the slope or intercept of the relationship resulting from various disease states (82).

Extent of Relaxation

The extent of relaxation is the major determinant of end-diastolic volume (EDV) and end-diastolic pressure (EDP), because these are measurements made at the end of the relaxation process. Abnormalities in extent of relaxation affect the end-diastolic pressure–volume (P–V) relationship to the greatest extent. Abnormalities in the rate of relaxation, however, tend to have minimal effect on the end-diastolic P–V relationship, because of the fact that they occur early in diastole and therefore do not alter EDP and EDV to any appreciable extent.

The extent of relaxation, as stated earlier, may be viewed as the compliance properties of the LV at the point where relaxation is complete (i.e., end-diastole). Alterations in the determinants of this relationship, intrinsic to the myocardium, result in shifts of the diastolic P–V curve. LV geometry (i.e., thickness, size, and chamber dimension) in large part determines the LV end-diastolic P–V relationship, as determined by mathematic approximations based on Laplace's law (82). Alterations in the LV end-diastolic P–V relationship may occur secondary to the change in elastic properties as the ventricle stretches during filling. Changes in the diastolic P–V relationship that depend on the rate at which the LV deforms are known as *viscoelasticity*, a property that myocardium shares with most biomaterials (84). This property is manifest when filling rates are highest, occurring during the first half of diastole, or after atrial contraction. *Stress relaxation*—a decrease in the distending pressure of the ventricle over time—or creep, a rightward shift in the diastolic P–V relationship—are two experimental manifestations of viscosity. The clinical importance of viscoelasticity has been disputed, however.

Other dynamic changes in relaxation that occur during ventricular filling are due to alterations in the elastic properties and the rate of relaxation of the myocardium, mediated via changes in the load sensed by the LV during relaxation. These *load-dependent relaxation* phenomena cause instantaneous changes in the LV compliance as well as in the rate of relaxation (9), which are independent of heart rate when LV muscle is abruptly stretched.

An additional determinant of the diastolic P–V relationship previously alluded to is *coronary vascular turgor*. The effect of this condition on the extent of relaxation is primarily through its erectile effect on LV stiffness (85). This decreases LV diastolic compliance by increasing LV *wall* volume, resulting in a higher EDP for a given volume. This effect seems to be independent of pericardial influences and predominates in the late diastolic filling period, thereby influencing the extent of relaxation, albeit to a small degree. In addition, the constraining effect of the pericardium and the degree of ventricular interaction affect the extent of relaxation (discussed later in the text).

LV hypertrophy results in abnormalities of relaxation that are characteristic of the manner in which the hypertrophy developed and of the type of hypertrophy formed (86). Eccentric hypertrophy, as seen with mitral or aortic insufficiency, is characterized by increased ventricular volume but little or no change in elasticity. This results in little increase in pressure at increased volumes. In contrast, concentric hypertrophy, seen with aortic stenosis or chronic untreated hypertension (87), is characterized by increased elastic stiffness and an elevated EDP for a given volume. Geometrically, pressure overload or hypertrophy is characterized by additional myocytes in parallel with existing cells; volume overload (eccentric hypertrophy) results in increased length of existing myocytes. Alterations in Ca^{2+} metabolism, as discussed, result in elevated myocyte diastolic Ca^{2+} levels. These factors account for the elevated EDP seen in chronic pressure overload hypertrophy.

Ischemia affects the extent of relaxation as evidenced by upward shift in the end-diastolic P–V relationship when myocardial oxygen demand outstrips supply (88,89). Pacing-induced ischemia after the creation of a coronary stenosis in dogs results in such a shift in the P–V relationship at end-diastole. These effects are independent of pericardial, right ventricular (RV), or lung interactions, implying a change in the intrinsic myocardial elastic properties. As previously discussed, changes in diastolic properties secondary to changes in myocardial Ca^{2+} handling (90,91), as well as in hydrogen ion accumulation (92) and repeated systolic stretch of the ischemia segment (93), interact to produce the observed changes.

The changes in ventricular compliance seem to be restricted to the region of active ischemia (93). Furthermore, uninvolved areas show evidence of a proportional increase in regional size and pressure—with a resultant constant diastolic P–V relation—to maintain SV by the Frank-Starling mechanism. Hence, during acute ischemia, the remaining normal areas of myocardium appear to utilize the Frank-Starling mechanism to maintain SV in compensation for the effects of abnormal contractility or an upward shift of the regional diastolic P–V relationship within the ischemic areas.

Rate of Relaxation

The rate of relaxation, as stated earlier, results primarily in changes in the rate of diastolic early filling (82). The determinants of relaxation rate are many, and their interactions complicated. Increases in heart rate and inotropy (94) result in increased rates of relaxation. Alterations in end-diastolic loading conditions result in changes in the rate of relaxation during experimental conditions (9,95). Nonuniformity of relaxation (9), which describes a nonuniform distribution of load and electric inactivation during diastole in space and time, results in alterations in the rate of relaxation. Ventricular suction, or the ability of the ventricle to generate pressures below equilibrium diastolic pressures, may alter the rate and extent of LV filling (94). Finally, ischemia can alter the rate as well as the extent of relaxation. Resolution of ischemia results in reversal of these changes.

EXTRINSIC INFLUENCES ON THE DIASTOLIC PRESSURE–VOLUME RELATIONSHIP

External loads can also profoundly influence ventricular compliance properties. Specifically, the RV (96), the pericardium (97), and the lungs (98,99) all may acutely induce shifts of the LV diastolic P–V relationship. While not widely studied in acute decompensated heart failure, it is likely that each of these influences may be exerted when both ventricles are dilated and when the lungs are hyperinflated during ventilator therapy.

The influence of the pericardium in the diastolic P–V relationship is a function of both its stiffness and its ability to constrain the entire heart (100). An increase in size of one ventricle therefore causes an increase in the EDP for a given volume (i.e., a shift upward in the P–V relationship) (Fig. 121.4). The constraining effect of a normal pericardium is dependent on its intrinsic compliance and how it affects LV pressures. Just as dilatation of the RV affects the LV diastolic P–V relation (discussed later), dilatation of the LV (i.e., a high LV filling pressure) amplifies the pericardium's influence. This has been demonstrated by measurement of the diastolic P–V relation before and after removal of the pericardium (97,101). Little normal pericardial effect is observed at normal filling pressures.

In addition, the intact pericardium allows interaction between the atria and the LV as well as between the RV and LV. The effect of left atrial (LA) pressure was approximately one-fourth that of the RV pressure in determining the LV diastolic pressure (102). Studies of the influence of the RV on LV compliance (102–104) have demonstrated that an upward shift of the LV diastolic P–V curve (i.e., reduced compliance) accompanies RV volume increases at end-diastole (Fig. 121.4). Although this effect is present with the pericardium open, the coupling is much stronger when it is closed (97). Ventricular interaction is therefore an important mechanism underlying acute reductions in LV compliance, whether the RV is enlarged as a result of pressure or volume overload. Ventricular interaction may also be responsible for some of the improved LV compliance properties observed with the administration of vasoactive medications that reduce volume return to the RV, such as nitrates (105).

Alterations in LV geometry were also noted with increasing pulmonary hypertension. The LV septal/free wall axis appears disproportionately reduced when compared with either the base-to-apex or the anteroposterior axis (96,98). Acute pulmonary hypertension induced by glass bead embolization confirms that upward shifts in the LV diastolic P–V relationship occur with changes in RV afterload (i.e., a reduction in LV compliance) and that this effect is largely mediated via a reduction in the LV septum to the free wall dimension and an increase in intrapericardial pressure (98).

The Special Case of Acute Right Ventricular Failure

The established mechanisms for acute RV failure are shown in Table 121.1. As mentioned previously, an inverse relationship between the vascular load and stroke output has been previously demonstrated (106). Calvin et al. (98) demonstrated that RV stroke volume was inversely related to the pulmonary input resistance, which is a more precise measurement of vascular load. In another study, it was demonstrated that tripling of the pulmonary artery pressure (PAP) by glass bead embolism is well tolerated by the RV, with cardiac output being maintained by both the heart rate (chronotropic) response and the Frank-Starling mechanism (preload reserve) (107,108). However, further increases in PAP sufficient to decrease the cardiac output by 20% result in a disproportionate increase in end-systolic volume compared with end-diastolic volume (i.e., stroke volume

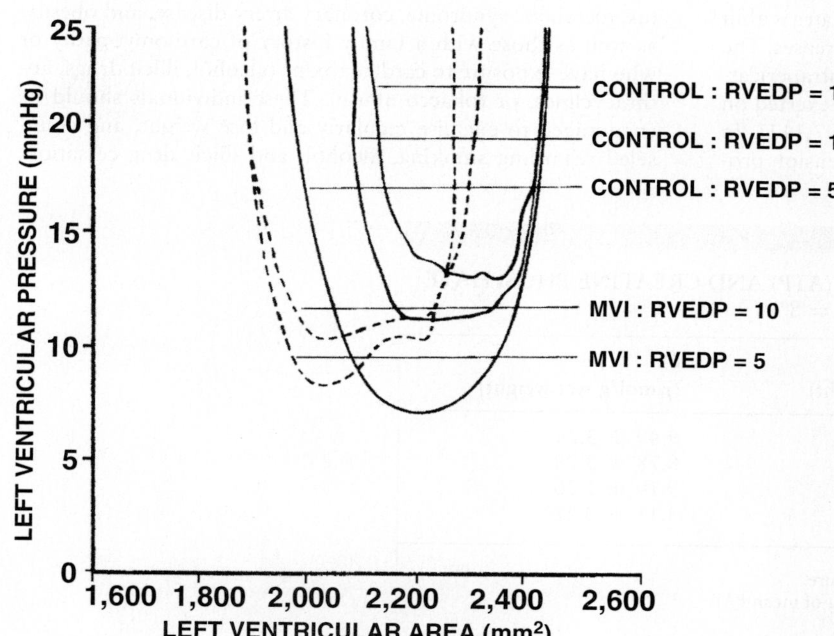

FIGURE 121.4. Diastolic portions of left ventricular pressure–area loops. Representative loops are depicted during both control and a microvascular injury (MVI) of the lungs at different right ventricular preloads or right ventricular end-diastolic pressures of 5, 10, and 15 mm Hg. The loops during both control and MVI are shifted upward by increasing right ventricular end-diastolic pressure (RVEDP), although left ventricular end-diastolic area is reduced at a given RVEDP during MVI.

TABLE 121.1

CAUSES OF RIGHT VENTRICULAR FAILURE

INCREASED PRESSURE LOAD
Pulmonary embolism
Pulmonary disease (hypoxic pulmonary vasoconstriction, destruction of pulmonary vascular bed)
Chronic airflow obstruction (emphysema, chronic bronchitis)
Interstitial lung disease
Neuromuscular chest wall restriction
Primary pulmonary hypertension
Elevated pulmonary venous pressure
Left ventricular failure
Mitral stenosis and insufficiency
Adult respiratory distress syndrome
Positive-pressure ventilation
Pulmonic valve stenosis
INCREASED VOLUME LOAD
Atrial septal defect
Ventricular septal defect
Tricuspid valve insufficiency
DECREASED CONTRACTILITY
Ischemia
Right coronary artery occlusion
Systemic hypotension (poor right coronary perfusion)
Right ventricular contusion (chest trauma)
Mediastinal radiation
β-Blockade

and ejection fraction decrease as a result). At this particular point, the RV is performing largely pressure work and very little flow work. ATP and creatine phosphate levels are normal at this point (Table 121.2). These phenomena represent evidence of an afterload mismatch; further decreases in stroke volume because of RV afterload mismatches are associated with ATP and creatine phosphate depletion (Table 121.2) (109,110).

The pericardium plays a significant role in mediating a direct interaction between the RV and the LV. As the RV dilates within an intact pericardium, RV end-diastolic pressure increases. The first implication of this observation is that the intrapericardial pressure increases and this external pressure is exerted on the LV and affects its distensibility (Fig. 121.4) (97,111). In an experimental model of acute pulmonary hypertension produced by ventricular glass bead embolism, it was determined that the LV diastolic pressure–segment length relationship was shifted upward, indicating decreased distensibility. This effect was found to be independent of any change in heart rate.

The second implication of these events is that the transeptal pressure gradient decreases or, in fact, reverses. Kingma et al., in a model of pulmonary hypertension produced by pulmonary artery banding, demonstrated that the septum shifts leftward, further impairing LV filling (112) as the RV dilates and septal curvature—normally rightward—is flattened. Kingma et al. also clearly demonstrated the inverse relationship between the transeptal pressure gradient and the LV septal–free wall dimension.

EVALUATION AND TREATMENT

With heart failure a growing public health and economic concern, rigorous and expert analysis of therapies and procedures with attention to their risks and benefits have led to publication of guidelines by the Heart Failure Society of America, joint guidelines by the American Heart Association (AHA) and the American College of Cardiology (ACC), with endorsement of the latter by the Heart Rhythm Society (1). The latest documents emphasize recognition of patients at risk to develop heart failure and target interventions to halt its development. Examples include patients with hypertension, diabetes mellitus, or coronary artery disease but without demonstrable abnormalities in cardiac structure or function; these individuals would be termed stage A. Stage B patients are defined as those with similar risk factors that are asymptomatic, but with cardiac abnormalities such as left ventricular hypertrophy (Fig. 121.5). The guidelines also give recommendations for initial evaluation of patients presenting with both systolic and diastolic heart failure, chronic outpatient management for the wide range of NYHA classes, and inpatient management of those presenting with acute decompensated heart failure (ADHF).

Individuals with risk factors for the development of heart failure (stage A) are those with hypertension, diabetes mellitus, metabolic syndrome, coronary artery disease, and obesity, as well as those with a family history of cardiomyopathy or who have exposure to cardiac toxins (alcohol, illicit drugs, anthracyclines, or tobacco abuse). These individuals should be encouraged to exercise regularly and lose weight, and counseled regarding smoking, alcohol, and illicit drug cessation.

TABLE 121.2

MYOCARDIAL ADENOSINE TRIPHOSPHATE (ATP) AND CREATINE PHOSPHATE (CP) IN OPEN PERICARDIA EXPERIMENTS ($n = 8^a$)

	ATP (μmol/g wet weight)	CP (μmol/g wet weight)
Baseline	5.52 ± 1.33	9.49 ± 3.24
Doubling of mean PAP	5.41 ± 1.28	8.78 ± 3.28
Tripling of mean PAP	5.12 ± 0.60	9.19 ± 1.20
RVF	3.63 ± 1.73[b]	3.11 ± 3.22[b]

PAP, pulmonary artery pressure; RVF, right ventricular failure.
[a] $p < .05$, compared with baseline and doubling and tripling of mean PAP.
[b] Values are expressed as mean ± standard deviation.

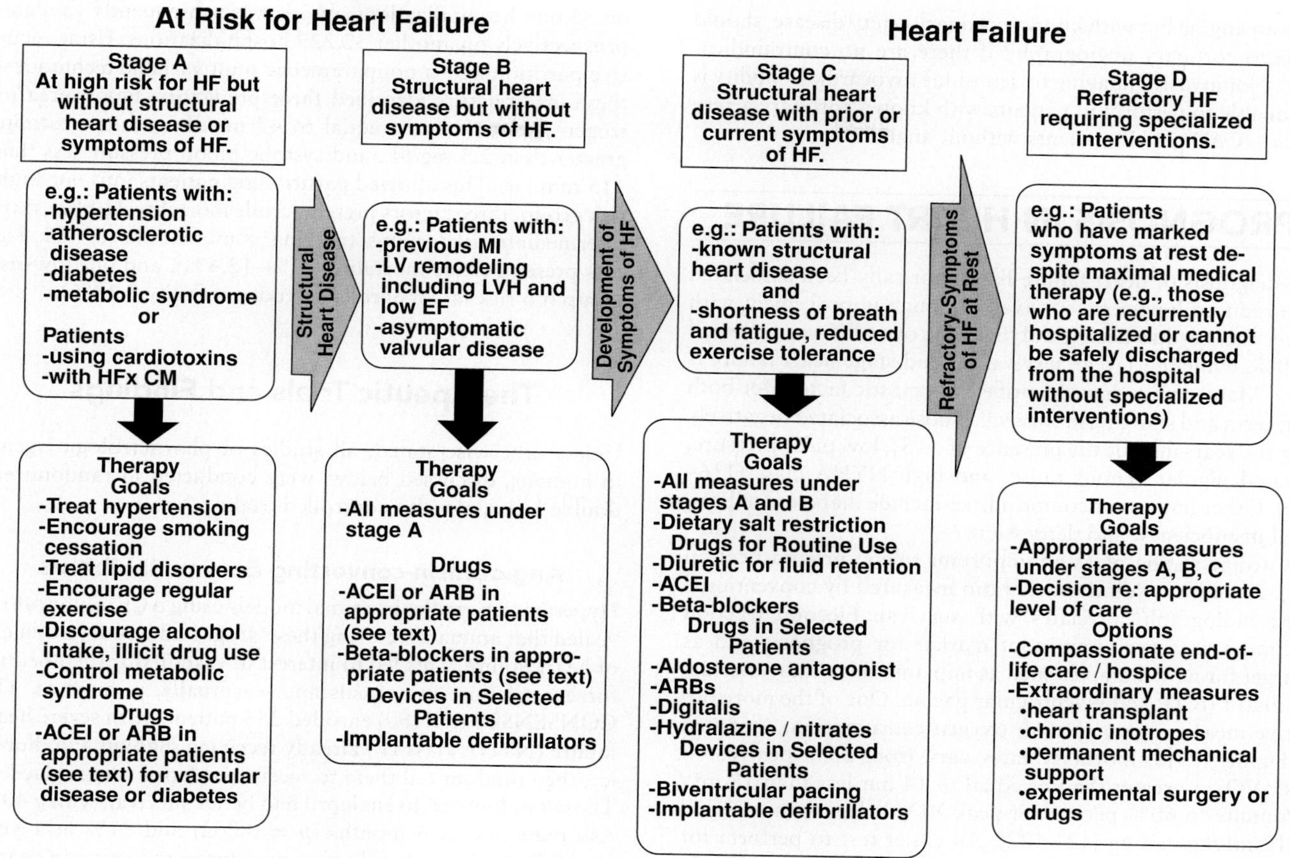

FIGURE 121.5. American College of Cardiology/American Heart Association 2005 guideline update for the diagnosis and management of chronic heart failure in the adult—summary article. A report of the American College of Cardiology Heart Association. Task Force in Practice Guidelines. (Writing Committee to Update the 2001 Guidelines for the Evaluation and Management of Heart Failure. *J Am Coll Cardiol.* 2005;46:1116–1143.)

Additionally, therapy for hypertension, dyslipidemia, and diabetes mellitus should be maximized according to the latest guidelines as published in the seventh report of the Joint National Committee on Prevention, Detection, Evaluation and Treatment of High Blood Pressure (JNC VII) (113); the American Diabetes Association (114); and ACC/AHA (115) joint practice guidelines regarding hypercholesterolemia. Therapeutic options for stage A individuals include appropriate therapy for vascular disease and diabetes mellitus, and ACE inhibitors or angiotensin II receptor blockers (ARBs) as appropriate. Stage B patients remain asymptomatic, but exhibit abnormalities in cardiac structure and function such as LV remodeling, low LV ejection fraction (LVEF), or LV hypertrophy (LVH). These individuals should have all therapeutic measures as those in stage A and should receive ACE inhibitors, ARBs, and β-adrenergic antagonists as appropriate. Additionally, patients in stage B should receive implantable cardioverter defibrillators as appropriate for their LVEF and pre-existing disease. Individuals classified as stage C and D have overt heart failure; their care is subsequently discussed.

Initial Evaluation

Patients presenting with new-onset heart failure should have a thorough history and physical examination, with special attention to risk factors and noncardiac disorders that may aggravate their cardiac condition. Behaviors or therapies that may cause heart failure or exacerbate LV dysfunction should also be sought. Thorough laboratory data, such as a 12-lead electrocardiogram, complete blood count, blood urea nitrogen, creatinine, electrolytes, fasting lipid panel and glucose, hemoglobin A_{1C} in diabetics, and thyroid-stimulating hormone, should be obtained. If suspicion is high that common etiologies of heart failure are not present, patients may be tested for HIV, hemochromatosis, sleep apnea, amyloidosis, pheochromocytoma, and rheumatologic disorders. BNP may be useful to obtain as a baseline. Endomyocardial biopsy should be considered only if the results would influence therapy.

Individuals should also receive posteroanterior (PA) and lateral chest radiographs initially, as well as echocardiography to assess for pulmonary congestion, LV dimensions, LVEF, LVH, and valvular and wall motion abnormalities. Radionuclide ventriculography may also be performed to assess LVEF and LV volumes, and may also be useful to assess right ventricular ejection fraction (RVEF). In patients with angina pectoris or ischemia, coronary angiography should be performed unless contraindicated, since maneuvers to reverse or halt progression of heart failure, such as revascularization, should always be entertained. Additionally, patients with chest pain either consistent or not consistent with cardiac ischemia who have not previously undergone coronary angiography, as well as patients without angina but with known coronary artery disease, should undergo coronary angiography if there are no contraindications. Noninvasive imaging to determine myocardial viability is reasonable to perform in patients with known coronary artery disease (CAD) in HF patients without angina.

PROGNOSIS IN HEART FAILURE

The diagnosis of heart failure has historically been associated with reduced long-term survival, although improvement with newer therapy has been gratifying. The overall 5-year survival is 50%, while the 1-year survival for end-stage heart failure is 75%. Many studies have identified prognostic factors for both long-term and short-term survival. Those associated negatively over the years include the presence of an S_3, low pulse pressure, elevated jugular venous pulse, and high NYHA class (116–120). Other important comorbidities include diabetes mellitus, renal insufficiency, and depression.

Cardiac testing plays an important role in prognostication (72). A simple cardiothoracic ratio measured by conventional chest radiograph correlates with survival. Ejection fraction continues as a very important marker for prognosis and as a target for new therapies such as implantable cardioverter defibrillator (ICD) and biventricular pacing. One of the more objective measurements is peak oxygen consumption. As noted in Figure 121.6, mortality rates vary from 20% per year if peak VO_2 is greater than or equal to 14 but less than 18 mL/kg/minute to 60% per year if peak VO_2 is less than or equal to 10 mL/kg/minute (121,122). An easier test to perform for chronic congestive heart failure is the 6-minute walk (123). In this test, a patient's distance walked after 6 minutes is measured and is predictive of morbidity and mortality (123).

Hemodynamic variables measured at heart catheterization, such as cardiac index, systemic and pulmonary vascular resistances, pulmonary artery pressures, and pulmonary capillary wedge pressures, are important indicators of prognosis as well as aiding in diagnosis. Stroke work index is an especially important predictor, as it incorporates both flow and pressure work.

Inverse relationships exist between survival and plasma norepinephrine, renin, vasopressin, aldosterone, atrial and B-type natriuretic peptides, and endothelin-1 (124–127) (Fig. 121.6). While many of these reflect abnormalities in pathophysiology, only B-type natriuretic peptide has become a routine laboratory test in suspected heart failure patients. Multivariate analyses of heart failure patients randomized in clinical trials have confirmed independent prognostic information from several factors including exercise tolerance parameters, plasma norepinephrine, pro-BNP, and BNP.

Studies of critically ill patients in the past have utilized multivariate models that can be used to assess the severity of acute decompensated heart failure. Teskey et al. (128) looked at the use of the Acute Physiology and Chronic Health Evaluation (APACHE) II score in patients admitted to the coronary care unit and found that it predicted mortality in acute heart failure. Survivors had lower APACHE II scores than nonsurvivors. This score weighs the degree of deviation from normal of selected clinical variables, as well as comorbid conditions. Later, Gracin et al. (129) demonstrated that APACHE II also predicted outcome after ventricular assist device implantation (Fig. 121.7). The Acute Decompensated Heart Failure Registry (ADHERE) has recently published an acuity model for heart failure based on 33,046 hospitalizations, which was subsequently validated prospectively on another 32,229 hospitalizations. Using recursive partitioning—a nonparametric multivariable technique—these investigators identified three predictors: blood urea nitrogen greater than or equal to 43 mg/dL, serum creatinine greater than 2.5 mg/dL, and systolic blood pressure less than 115 mm Hg. This allowed partitioning patients into one high-risk group (three factors present, crude mortality 21.9%), three intermediate-risk groups (varying combinations of risk factors present, crude mortality 5.5%–12.4%), and one low-risk group (no risk factors present, crude mortality 2.14%).

Therapeutic Trials and Findings

Unless otherwise stated, all studies of pharmacologic agents in humans, discussed below, were conducted in randomized, double-blind, placebo-controlled trials.

Angiotensin-converting Enzyme Inhibitors

Hypertension studies in animal models using ACE inhibitors revealed that animals receiving these drugs had less development of heart failure. This led to interest in vasodilator therapeutics for heart failure in animals and, eventually, in humans. The CONSENSUS trial (80) enrolled 253 patients with severe heart failure (NYHA class IV) already receiving digoxin and diuretics, then randomized them to receive enalapril versus placebo. Those randomized to enalapril had better survival, with a 40% risk reduction at 6 months ($p = 0.002$) and 31% at 1 year ($p = 0.001$). The risk reduction was due to reduction in deaths from progressive heart failure. Additionally, the NYHA functional class improved in a significant number of those receiving enalapril. Based on the CONSENSUS trial, and other studies of ACE inhibitors investigating symptoms and hemodynamic indexes, the National Institutes of Health sponsored the SOLVD trials (75,76). The SOLVD treatment trial enrolled 2,569 patients with left ventricular systolic dysfunction (LVEF less than or equal to 35%) and symptoms of heart failure, ranging from NYHA class I through IV, with the majority of enrollees being classes II and III. The primary end point was mortality. Subjects randomized to receive enalapril had better survival than those receiving placebo; risk reduction with enalapril was 16% (95% confidence interval [CI] 5%–26%; $p = 0.0036$). As seen in the CONSENSUS trial, the chief difference in mortality was in deaths due to progressive heart failure, with risk reduction 22% (95% CI 6%–35%; $p < 0.0045$) (79).

The SOLVD prevention trial randomized 4,228 patients with LV systolic dysfunction, but without symptoms, to receive enalapril versus placebo. End points in the SOLVD prevention trial were total mortality and two composite end points: Death or development of heart failure requiring hospitalization, and death in the hospital from heart failure. In these asymptomatic patients, there was no significant decrease in total mortality in those receiving enalapril. However, for those receiving enalapril, the combined end point of death plus development of heart failure was reached less often than those receiving placebo (630 vs. 818; risk reduction 29%; 95% CI 21%–36%; $p < 0.001$). Additionally, those receiving enalapril had fewer hospitalizations for heart failure or death (434 in the enalapril group vs. 518 in the placebo group; risk reduction 20%; 95% CI 9%–30%; $p < 0.001$) (76).

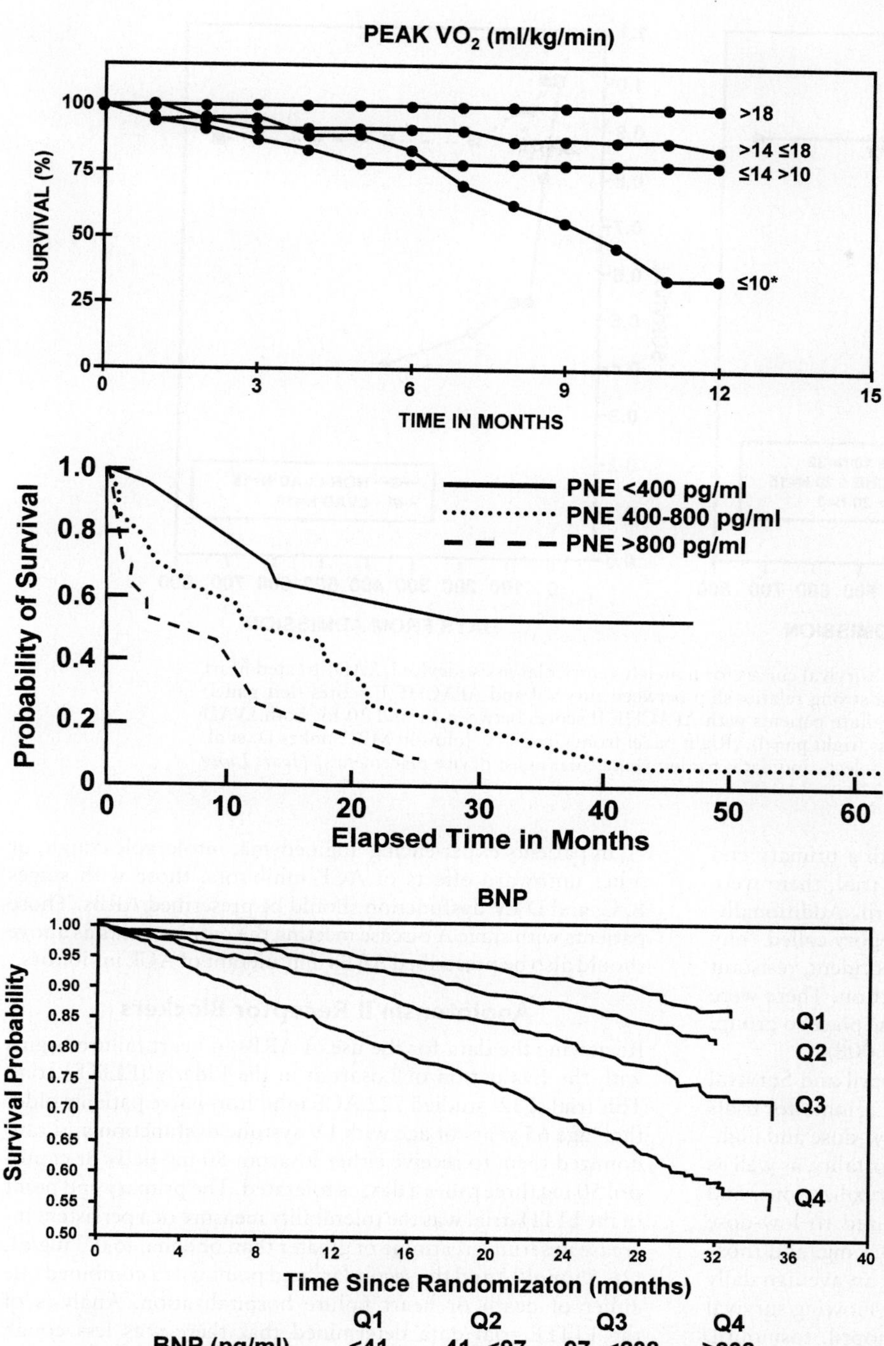

FIGURE 121.6. Survival curves for heart failure patients by peak VO_2 (upper panel), plasma norepinephrine (middle), and brain natriuretic peptide (BNP, lower panel). Survival is best with peak VO_2 greater than 18 mL/kg/minute, plasma norepinephrine less than 400 pg/mL, and BNP less than 100 pg/mL. (Reproduced from Mancin DM, Eisen H, Kausmaul W, et al. *Circulation.* 1991;83:778–786; Cohn JN, Levin B, Olivari MT, et al. *N Engl J Med.* 1984;311:819–823; and Anand IS, Fisher LD, Chiang Y, et al. Changes in brain natriuretic peptide and norepinephrine over time and mortality and morbidity in the Valsartan Heart Failure Trial (Val-HeFT) *Circulation.* 2003;107:1278–1283.)

The SAVE trial enrolled 2,231 patients within 3 to 16 days of an acute myocardial infarction and with LV systolic dysfunction (LVEF less than 40%) to receive the ACE inhibitor captopril versus placebo (81). The primary end point was all-cause mortality. Other SAVE trial end points included cardiovascular deaths, treatment failure requiring open-label ACE inhibitor, and all-cause mortality plus progressive LV systolic dysfunction. All-cause mortality was significantly decreased in the captopril group compared to the placebo group (228 deaths vs. 275 deaths; risk reduction 19%; 95% CI 3%–32%; p = 0.019). The incidence of both fatal and nonfatal major cardiovascular events was less in those receiving captopril. For death from cardiovascular causes, the risk reduction was 21% (95% CI 5%–35%; p = 0.014) and for the development of severe heart failure, the risk reduction for those randomized to captopril was 37% (95% CI 20%–50%; p <0.001). Those receiving captopril also had fewer congestive heart failure end points requiring hospitalization and fewer recurrent myocardial infarctions (130).

The Assessment of Treatment with Lisinopril and Survival (ATLAS) (131) investigators randomized 2,006 patients with an acute myocardial infarction and clinical evidence of heart

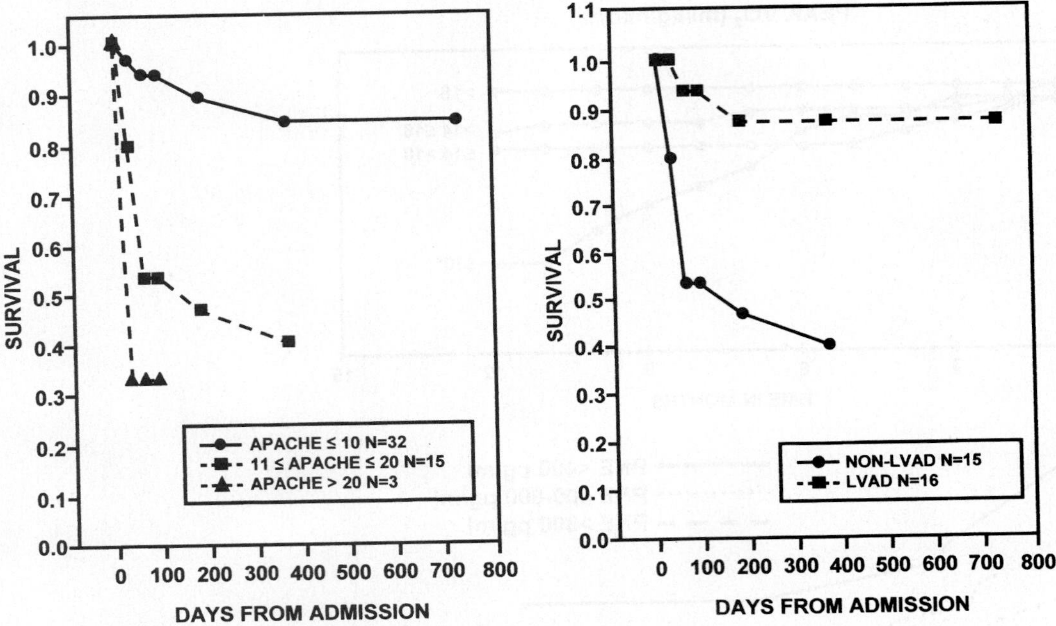

FIGURE 121.7. Kaplan Meier survival curves for non–left ventricular assist device (LVAD)-treated heart failure patients demonstrates a strong relationship between survival and APACHE II scores (**left panel**) and survival curves for heart failure patients with APACHE II scores between 11 and 20 for both LVAD and non–LVAD-treated patients (**right panel**). (Right panel from Gracin N, Johnson MR, Spokes D, et al. The use of Apache II scores to select candidates for left ventricular assist device placement. *J Heart Lung Transplant.* 1998;17:1017–1023.)

failure to receive ramipril versus placebo, with a primary end point of all-cause mortality. As in the SAVE trial, there were fewer deaths in those randomized to ramipril. Additionally, other events examined were grouped in a category called "any event" that included death, cerebrovascular accident, resistant heart failure, and recurrent myocardial infarction. There were fewer events in the ramipril as compared to the placebo group: 28% versus 35% (risk reduction 19%; $p = 0.008$).

The Assessment of Treatment with Lisinopril and Survival (ATLAS) trial (131) differed from the other ACE inhibitor trials since it compared the safety and efficacy of low-dose and high-dose lisinopril on the outcomes of all-cause mortality, as well as cardiovascular mortality, cardiovascular hospitalizations, and combined end points (131). Those randomized to low-dose lisinopril received an average daily dose of 4.5 mg, and those randomized to the high-dose group received an average daily dose of 33.2 mg (129). Other ACE inhibitors showing survival benefit in heart failure patients include lisinopril, fosinopril, and quinapril. Trials of ACE inhibitors in survivors of myocardial infarction showing improved survival with the ACE inhibitors and less development of LV systolic dysfunction now tally approximately 100,000 patients.

Based on the above-cited overwhelming evidence of the impact of this class of drug in patients with symptomatic LV systolic dysfunction and in asymptomatic patients with LV dysfunction, ACE inhibitors are the foundation of therapy for heart failure. Thus, ACE inhibitors should be prescribed for all patients with asymptomatic LV systolic dysfunction and asymptomatic valvular heart disease (stage B), as well as in patients with symptomatic and/or refractory heart failure (stages C and D) unless the patient is intolerant to ACE inhibitors. In stage A patients, ACE inhibitors are indicated for those with diabetes mellitus and LVH.

In patients experiencing angioedema, intolerable cough, or other untoward effects of ACE inhibitors, those with stages B, C, and D LV dysfunction should be prescribed ARBs. Those patients with stage A disease meeting the requirements as above should also be prescribed ARBs if intolerant of ACE inhibitors.

Angiotensin II Receptor Blockers

Reviewing the data for the use of ARBs in heart failure begins with the Evaluation of Losartan in the Elderly (ELITE) trial. This trial (132) studied 722 ACE inhibitor–naïve patients older than age 65 years of age with LV systolic dysfunction and randomized them to receive either losartan 50 mg daily or captopril 50 mg three times a day, as tolerated. The primary end point of the ELITE trial was the tolerability measure of a persistent increase in serum creatinine of greater than or equal to 0.3 mg/dL (26.5 μmol/L) and the secondary end point was a combined one either of death or heart failure hospitalization. Analysis of the ELITE trial data determined that there was less cough in the losartan group, that the increases in serum creatinine were the same in both groups, but that the combined end point was less frequent in those randomized to losartan as compared to captopril, 9.4% vs. 13.2% (risk reduction 32%, 95% CI –4% to +55%, $p = 0.075$). The majority of decreased events in the losartan group were due to a decrease in all-cause mortality: 4.8% versus 8.7% (risk reduction 46%; 95% CI 5%–69%; $p = 0.035$). To confirm the findings found in the ELITE trial, the ELITE II trial (133) was designed as a mortality trial, this time enrolling 3,152 subjects and decreasing the enrollment age to 60 years. Patients were also stratified according to β-blocker use, and were once again randomized to the previous target dosages of losartan and captopril. With a median follow-up of 555 days, there was no difference in all-cause mortality—11.7% versus 10.4% (hazard ratio [HR] 1.13; 95%

CI 0.95–1.35; $p = 0.16$), or in sudden death—9.0% versus 7.3% (HR 1.225; 95% CI 0.98–1.60; $p = 0.08$) between the two treatment groups. The investigators concluded that the differences in the first ELITE trial and ELITE II were likely different secondary to the small number of deaths seen in the original ELITE trial, and that ELITE II had four times as many study subjects and ten times more events. However, losartan was, again, well tolerated.

Valsartan, another ARB, was studied in mortality trials for both chronic heart failure and in heart failure following myocardial infarction. The Valsartan Heart Failure Trial (Val-HeFT) was designed to assess the efficacy of adding valsartan to standard therapy for heart failure (134). Val-HeFT examined 5,010 subjects with LVEFs less than 40% and NYHA class II through IV heart failure judged to be clinically stable by the investigator. Background therapy included ACE inhibitors (93%), diuretics, digoxin, and β-blockers (35%). Subjects were randomized to receive valsartan versus placebo, and randomization was stratified by β-blocker therapy. Thus, most study subjects in the valsartan group were also receiving ACE inhibitor therapy. Mortality was similar in the two treatment groups as was the adjudicated cause of death: 19.7% versus 19.4% (risk reduction 1.02; 95% CI 0.88–1.18; $p = 0.80$). For the combined end point of mortality and morbidity, subjects receiving valsartan had significantly fewer events than those receiving placebo: 28.8% versus 32.1% (0.87; 95% CI 0.77–0.97; $p = 0.009$). This end point was consistent across all prespecified subgroups: men and women, young and old, those with and without diabetes mellitus or coronary artery disease, LVEFs above and below the median, and in the different NYHA classes. The investigators did not find a difference in response to valsartan therapy based on background therapy with neurohormonal inhibitors. They examined four subgroups: those receiving ACE inhibitors or not, and those receiving β-blockers or not. In the three groups (group 1 = neither ACE inhibitor nor β-blockers, group 2 = ACE inhibitor but not β-blockers, group 3 = β-blockers but not ACE inhibitors), there was a favorable effect of valsartan on the combined end point of mortality and morbidity ($p = 0.003$, $p = 0.002$, and $p = 0.037$, respectively). However, in patients receiving both ACE inhibitors and β-blockers, valsartan had an adverse effect on mortality ($p = 0.009$) and was associated with a trend to more events in the combined end point of morbidity and mortality. The investigators were uncertain whether this finding was a chance or true interaction, as other ARB trials in heart failure have not found this same outcome. In a mortality trial of patients with myocardial infarction complicated by heart failure, 14,808 patients were randomized to receive valsartan, captopril, or valsartan plus captopril in addition to conventional therapy (135). In this trial (the VALIANT trial), valsartan was found to be noninferior to captopril with regard to mortality ($p = 0.004$), as well as with regard to the composite end point of fatal plus nonfatal cardiovascular events ($p < 0.001$). The valsartan plus captopril group was found to have the most drug-related adverse events.

The Candesartan in Heart failure Assessment of Reduction in Mortality and morbidity (CHARM) program evaluated the effects of candesartan on mortality and morbidity in a variety of patients with chronic heart failure (136). Unlike the previous heart failure trials, the CHARM-Preserved arm of the program investigated the use of ARBs in heart failure patients with preserved LV systolic dysfunction (e.g., diastolic dysfunction) as well as in patients intolerant to ACE inhibitors. Similar to other trials, the CHARM-Added arm examined the results of adding candesartan to patients still symptomatic despite the presence of ACE inhibitors and other conventional therapy. In the CHARM-Preserved trial, subjects were NYHA class II through IV and baseline LVEF was greater than 40%. The primary outcome of cardiovascular death or admission to hospital for heart failure was not different for those in the candesartan versus the placebo group, although there was a trend toward fewer events in the candesartan group. As could be expected in patients intolerant to ACE inhibitors (CHARM-Alternative), patients receiving candesartan had fewer events than those receiving placebo; 33% of patients receiving candesartan met the combined end point of cardiovascular death or hospitalization for heart failure versus 40% in the placebo group (HR 0.77; 95% CI 0.60–0.81; $p < 0.0001$). In the CHARM-Added trial, patients with LVEF <40% already on ACE inhibitors but still experiencing heart failure symptoms were randomized to candesartan versus placebo. For the primary outcome of cardiovascular death or hospitalization for heart failure, fewer events occurred in the candesartan group versus the placebo group, 38% versus 42%, respectively (HR 0.85; 95% CI 0.75–0.96; $p = 0.010$). The CHARM investigators did not uncover the same untoward effects as did the Val-HeFT investigators with regard to patients receiving ARBs (candesartan) plus ACE inhibitors plus β-blockers. The frequency of new diabetes was lower in the candesartan group than in the placebo group.

β-Adrenergic Receptor Antagonists

Early reports of treating heart failure patients with β-adrenergic receptor antagonists were met with skepticism (137). Then, the initial randomized, double-blind, placebo-controlled trials did not meet the primary end point of decreased mortality but did have some success with decreased need for transplantation in the Metoprolol in Dilated Cardiomyopathy (MDC) trial (138) and improvement in ejection fraction in both the MDC and Cardiac Insufficiency Bisoprolol Study (CIBIS) trials (139). The above trials used different β-adrenergic blockers with different mechanisms of action: metoprolol, a β_1-selective β-blocker in the MDC trial, and bisoprolol, a nonselective β-blocker, in the CIBIS trial. Carvedilol was studied in four efficacy, dosing, and safety trials that were combined into a single report appearing in the literature in 1996. Although mortality was not a primary end point, the trial was not a single trial designed with the power to detect changes in mortality, seven deaths in the open-label run-in period were not included in the analysis, and there were a small number of deaths reported in a short followup time, the results were definitive enough for decreasing hospitalization and improving quality of life that the drug was approved for use in patients with NYHA class II and III heart failure for the end points that the program did have the power to detect. Thus, carvedilol, a nonselective β-blocker as well as an α-blocker, was the first drug approved by the Food and Drug Administration (FDA) for the treatment of heart failure, 21 years after the first report with practolol appeared in the literature.

Carvedilol was further studied in two other trials. The first of these, the Carvedilol Prospective Randomized Cumulative Survival (COPERNICUS) trial studied the outcome of carvedilol on survival in 2,289 patients with severe heart failure already receiving standard heart failure therapy (ACE inhibitors or ARBs plus diuretic) (140). Study subjects had an LVEF of less than 25% and had symptoms of dyspnea or fatigue at rest or on minimal exertion (NYHA class IIIB to IV) for 2 months prior to randomization. Unlike the prior studies with carvedilol, COPERNICUS found that patients randomized to carvedilol had fewer deaths (130) than those randomized to placebo (190). This was a 35% decrease in the risk of death with carvedilol (95% CI 19%–48%; $p = 0.00013$ and $p = 0.00014$ after adjustment for interim analyses). Subjects in the carvedilol group also had significantly fewer events for the combined end point of death or hospitalization, and the results with carvedilol for both the primary end point and the combined end point were the same across all prespecified groups of age, gender, LVEF, heart failure etiology, study center location, and history of prior hospitalization for heart failure within 1 year prior to randomization. Additionally, fewer patients in the carvedilol group required discontinuation of study drug for adverse events than did the placebo group. A second trial with carvedilol following acute myocardial infarction with left ventricular dysfunction Carvediol Post Infarct Survival Control in Left Ventricular Dysfuntion (CAPRICORN) study had reduced all-cause mortality, cardiovascular mortality, and recurrent, nonfatal myocardial infarctions (141). The CIBIS II trial enrolled 2,647 symptomatic heart failure patients to receive bisoprolol versus placebo, in addition to standard therapy with ACE inhibitors, to determine if bisoprolol, a selective β_1 antagonist, could decrease all-cause mortality. After a follow-up of 1.3 years, bisoprolol significantly decreased all-cause mortality as well as sudden death (HR 0.56; 95% CI 0.39–0.80; $p = 0.0011$) (142).

Another selective β_1 antagonist, extended-release metoprolol (Toprol-XL) was examined in the Metoprolol CR/XL Randomized Intervention Trial in Congestive Heart Failure (MERIT-HF) trial (144) for possible benefits to survival in heart failure patients. When randomized to extended-release metoprolol, in addition to optimum standard therapy for heart failure, all-cause mortality and sudden death were once again significantly decreased. However, these data should not be extrapolated to mean that any β-blocker can be used in heart failure patients. The warning bell was sounded with the Beta-blocker Evaluation of Survival Trial (BEST) trial (143), which examined the effects of bucindolol on mortality in a group of patients very similar to the study subjects in the COPERNICUS trial. Bucindolol, a nonselective β-blocker and a weak α-blocker, did not improve survival, unlike carvedilol, bisoprolol, and extended-release metoprolol. Unlike the other β-blockers studied in heart failure patients in the late 1990s, bucindolol has sympatholytic activity, meaning that it is able to decrease norepinephrine levels. Another explanation for the failure of bucindolol to improve survival is that the makeup of its heart failure cohort was designed to enroll more African Americans and women. Not only did bucindolol not improve survival, but it also worsened mortality in African Americans and those with NYHA class IV versus class III heart failure, and, although the hazard ratio for women favored bucindolol, the 95% confidence interval was wide and crossed the line of unity. Another β-blocker trial, the Carvedilol or Metoprolol European Trial (COMET), randomized subjects to receive either carvedilol or short-acting metoprolol. In this trial, carvedilol was found to improve survival and short-acting metoprolol did not. Therefore, short-acting metoprolol has been found ineffective in two trials: the COMET (145) and the MDC trial. Use of β-adrenergic receptor antagonists should be limited to those shown to improve survival in large, randomized clinical trials: carvedilol and extended-release metoprolol in the United States and bisoprolol in Europe.

Aldosterone Receptor Antagonists

Since aldosterone promotes retention of sodium, sympathetic activation, inhibition of the parasympathetic nervous system, myocardial and vascular fibrosis, and loss of magnesium and potassium, it was reasonable to propose that blockade of aldosterone receptors could alter the course of progressive LV dysfunction and, thereby, mortality. Although some may think that ACE inhibitors suppress aldosterone production, there is evidence suggesting that they do it transiently. Thus, investigators postulated that there might be a role for spironolactone, an aldosterone receptor antagonist, in the therapy for heart failure, and the Randomized Aldactone Evaluation Study (RALES) was formed (146). A total of 1,663 patients were randomized to receive spironolactone in addition to standard therapy for heart failure, including ACE inhibitors and diuretics, and sometimes digoxin and other vasodilators. Patients with hyperkalemia (K^+ greater than 5.5 mmol/L) and serum creatinine greater than 2.5 mg/dL were excluded. Spironolactone successfully decreased mortality versus placebo: 35% versus 46%, respectively (relative risk of death 0.70; 95% CI 0.60–0.82; $p < 0.001$).

Other Vasodilators

The combination of hydralazine and oral nitrates for heart failure therapy has been studied in three large randomized clinical trials. The first of these was the Veterans Administration Cooperative Vasodilator Heart Failure Trial (VeHeFT-I) (147), which enrolled 642 patients taking standard heart failure therapy—at the time, digoxin and a diuretic—to three other groups: placebo, prazosin 20 mg/day, or combination of hydralazine (300 mg/day) and isosorbide dinitrate (160 mg/day). This study determined that prazosin was equal to placebo, and that combination vasodilator therapy with hydralazine and isosorbide dinitrate reduced mortality at 2 years with a risk reduction of 34% ($p < 0.028$). Following the publication of the CONSENSUS trial, questions arose about superiority for heart failure therapy: enalapril versus combination hydralazine and isosorbide dinitrate. Study investigators enrolled 804 men—already receiving digoxin and diuretic—in the Veterans Administration Cooperative Vasodilator Heart Failure comparison of enalapril with hydralazine-isosorbide dinitrate Trial (VeHeFT-II) to receive either enalapril 20 mg/day or combination of hydralazine 300 mg/day plus isosorbide dinitrate 160 mg/day. Mortality after 2 years was 18% in the enalapril group and 25% in the hydralazine-isosorbide dinitrate arm (RR 28%; $p = 0.016$) (148). Following retrospective analyses of the combined data sets of VeHeFT-I and -II, interest arose in different treatments based on racial findings in the original trials, with the understanding that race is likely a phenotypic marker of a particular genotype. These analyses showed an absence of treatment effect in Caucasians in VeHeFT-I no matter the assignment arm, but a mortality benefit for African Americans receiving combination therapy. In contrast, Caucasians had survival benefit from enalapril but not combination therapy in VeHeFT-II, whereas mortality was similar in the same trial in the two treatment groups for African Americans. Some clinical investigations found that persons who identify themselves as African American may have a less active renin–angiotensin system (149,150) and lower nitric oxide bioavailability than other racial groups (151,152). This led to the hypothesis that a survival benefit with combination therapy—hydralazine plus isosorbide dinitrate—was possible for NYHA class III and IV African Americans who remained symptomatic with heart failure despite standard therapy, including ACE inhibitors or ARBs in ACE-intolerant patients, β-blockers, digoxin, spironolactone, and diuretics. The African-American Heart Failure Trial (A-HeFT) enrolled 1,050 subjects, at which point randomization stopped, secondary to the independent data and safety monitoring board determining a significantly higher mortality rate in those receiving placebo: 54 patients in the placebo group died versus 32 patients in the combination therapy group. With combination therapy there was a 43% survival improvement (HR 0.57; $p = 0.01$) (153).

Digoxin

Digitalis glycosides have been used for more than 200 years since first described by Sir William Withering in his account of foxglove.[1] Following acceptance of ACE inhibitors for the treatment of heart failure, the efficacy of digoxin became controversial. Two small withdrawal trials in the early 1990s studied the efficacy of digoxin in heart failure patients; in both, patients were already receiving digoxin as part of their heart failure regimen. The Randomized Study assessing the Effect of Digoxin Withdrawal in Patients with Mild to Moderate Chronic Congestive Heart Failure (PROVED) trial withdrew digoxin from 42 subjects receiving diuretic and digoxin and 46 subjects continued with both drugs. In patients withdrawn from digoxin, maximal exercise capacity worsened and patients had more treatment failure with a decreased time-to-treatment failure (154). In the Randomized Assessment of the Effect of Digoxin on Inhibitors of the Angiotensin Converting Enzyme (RADIANCE) trial, digoxin was once again withdrawn, in a randomized fashion, from patients receiving ACE inhibitors and diuretics. Exercise capacity was assessed using treadmill testing and exercise endurance was assessed using the 6-minute walk test. Functional capacity deteriorated in patients withdrawn from digoxin compared with those continuing to receive digoxin ($p = 0.019$ for NYHA class, $p = 0.033$ for maximal exercise tolerance, and $p = 0.01$ for submaximal exercise endurance). Additionally, left ventricular ejection fractions decreased in the placebo group and those in the placebo group also had increases in both weight and heart rate (155). Despite the evidence from the PROVED and RADIANCE trials demonstrating the efficacy of digoxin in the treatment of heart failure, concerns remained regarding the effect of digoxin on survival. The Digitalis Investigation Group trial studied the long-term effect of digoxin on all-cause mortality and heart failure hospitalizations. Study subjects were required to have left ventricular ejection fractions less than 45% and the majority were receiving diuretics and ACE inhibitors at baseline. Patients enrolled into the digoxin arm numbered 3,397, and those randomized to placebo numbered 3,403. There was no difference in mortality between those randomized to digoxin or placebo (34.8% vs. 35.1%; $p = 0.80$), but there were fewer hospitalizations for worsening heart failure in those randomized to digoxin than in those in the placebo group: 910 versus 1,180 (0.72; 95% CI 0.66–0.79; $p < 0.001$). Total hospitalizations were also less frequent in those randomized to the digoxin group, but there were no differences in hospitalizations for ventricular arrhythmias or cardiac arrest between the two groups. Thus, in the era prior to β-blockers, digoxin was shown to be efficacious for treatment of heart failure and to have a neutral effect on mortality.

[1] *An Account of the Foxglove, and Some of its Medical Uses: With Practical Remarks on Dropsy, and Other Disease.* Birmingham, England; M. Sinney; 1785.

ACUTE DECOMPENSATED HEART FAILURE

Although acute decompensated heart failure has a variety of presentations, common symptoms include fatigue, shortness of breath, and congestion of the lungs and abdominal organs. Many disease states may present with all or some of the above symptoms, such as pneumonia, pulmonary embolus, sepsis, and other volume overload states. Patients with preserved systolic function and systemic hypertension comprise the majority of hospitalized patients. The minority are those with poor end-organ perfusion, low ejection fractions, and hypotension. Despite advances in therapeutics, both pharmacologic and devices, risk of death and rehospitalization continues to be high for patients admitted with acute decompensated heart failure. Cost of hospitalization for ADHF remains the bulk of the cost in caring for those afflicted with heart failure. The ability to measure BNP, a neurohormone secreted by the LV in response to volume overload, has become a useful diagnostic test in those presenting with symptoms of ADHF. Normal values range from 0 to 100 pg/mL, and those over 400 have a high probability for heart failure, whether systolic or diastolic in origin (156). The decision to hospitalize patients for ADHF continues to be based on clinical judgment. The Heart Failure Society of America guidelines recommend hospitalization for patients with altered mentation, worsening renal function, hypotension, resting dyspnea, hemodynamically significant arrhythmias, and acute coronary syndromes (157). They further state that hospitalization should be considered when congestion has worsened with evidence of weight gain of greater than or equal to 5 kg, and when there are signs and symptoms of abdominal or pulmonary congestion, even in the absence of weight gain. Other considerations include major electrolyte abnormalities, repeated ICD discharges, and associated comorbid conditions. Recently, the ADHERE collected data for hospitalized patients in community, tertiary, and academic centers in the United States (158,159): 33,046 hospitalization episodes from the ADHERE were analyzed for predictors of in-hospital mortality and were then subjected to a classification and regression tree (CART) analysis to develop the best predictors of in-hospital mortality as well as a risk stratification model (160). Thirty-nine variables were identified and, following the CART method, blood urea nitrogen level greater than 43 mg/dL at hospital admission was identified as the best single discriminator between survivors and nonsurvivors of hospitalization for ADHF. The second best predictor was systolic blood pressure less than 115 mm Hg.

Few trials for those with ADHF admitted to the hospital have been published. To date, only two trials of therapeutics for ADHF have been published: these are the Outcome of a Prospective Trial of Intravenous Milronone for Exacerbations (OPTIME) trial and the Vasodilation in the Management of Acute Congestive Heart Failure (VMAC) trials. Another two trials, the Evaluation Study of Congestive heart Failure

And Pulmonary artery catheterization Effectiveness (ESCAPE) and the Pulmonary Artery Catheters in patient MANagement (PAC-MAN) trials, assess the effectiveness of pulmonary artery catheters in the management of ADHF. A variety of patients were enrolled in the PAC-Man trial (161). Diagnoses at enrollment included multiorgan failure, decompensated heart failure, and respiratory failure; surgical as well as medical patients were enrolled. The investigators noted no differences in hospital mortality in those managed with or without pulmonary artery catheters. Additionally, there were no differences in length of stay in either intensive care unit settings or in hospital. A 10% complication rate was noted in those receiving pulmonary artery catheters, with the most frequent complication being hematoma at the insertion site and arrhythmias requiring treatment within 1 hour of insertion. The ESCAPE trial randomized 433 subjects with decompensated heart failure to receive therapy guided by clinical assessment and a pulmonary artery catheter or by clinical assessment alone. The primary end point of the ESCAPE trial was days alive out of hospital during the first 6 months. Secondary end points included quality of life, exercise, and biochemical and echo changes. Those randomized to pulmonary artery catheters did not impact the primary end point of number of days alive and out of the hospital during 6 months of follow-up, mortality, or the number of days hospitalized. There were no deaths due to use of pulmonary artery catheters, but there were more complications, with the most common being infection (162).

The Vasodilator in the Management of Acute Heart Failure trial randomized 489 patients hospitalized with ADHF to a complicated schema testing nitroglycerin, nesiritide, and standard therapy for the treatment; based on clinical judgment, half of patients received a pulmonary artery catheter. The primary end point of the trial was a change in pulmonary capillary wedge pressure (PCWP) from baseline and change in dyspnea score from baseline at 3 hours (163). Nesiritide lowered pulmonary capillary wedge pressure from baseline by 6.5 mm Hg, and statistically significantly better than placebo ($p < 0.001$) and nitroglycerin ($p = 0.03$).

Based on the paucity of data for treating patients with ADHF admitted to the hospital, current guidelines include identification of precipitating factors and etiology, optimizing volume status, treating with recommended vasodilator therapy, and minimizing side effects. Educating patients about lifestyle changes, including sodium and fluid restriction, as well as self-management techniques are recommended general measures. Precipitating factors include development of arrhythmias, acute infections, and nonadherence with medications and dietary restrictions. Optimization of medical therapy should also be attempted during hospitalization. During hospitalization, the patient should be weighed daily and accurate recordings of intake and output should be kept. Loop diuretics administered intravenously are recommended and, in those not achieving adequate diuresis, continuous intravenous infusion of loop diuretics or addition of other diuretics, such as metolazone, should be considered. In those not responding to the above measures, and without symptomatic hypotension, intravenous nitroglycerin, nitroprusside, or nesiritide may be used in addition to intravenous diuretics. Intravenous inotropes should be reserved for those with advanced heart failure and evidence of end-organ dysfunction and/or decreased peripheral perfusion, especially if systolic blood pressure is <90 mm Hg. Small studies have investigated ultrafiltration (UF) as an alternative to diuretics for volume removal since the procedure does not require central venous access but instead is able to utilize peripheral veins, such as in the antecubital fossa, with a 16-gauge, 35-cm catheter. In one study, after 24 hours 4,650 mL was removed via UF, whereas 2,838 mL was removed in the usual care group, which included diuretics. Those in the ultrafiltration group were also able to receive diuretics after the 8 hours of UF was completed. The authors concluded that UF was feasible and well tolerated (164).

NONPHARMACOLOGIC AND NONSURGICAL THERAPY FOR CHRONIC HEART FAILURE

Electrophysiologic therapy is a new addition to the heart failure management arsenal and is having enormous impact. Defibrillator therapy with an Automatic Implantable Cardioverter Defibrillator (AICD) was first shown to be effective at improving long-term survival in survivors of cardiac arrest (165) and later it was proven beneficial in post-MI patients with low ejection fraction and ventricular dysrhythmia (166). Recent studies have shown its benefits in both ischemic and nonischemic dilated cardiomyopathy (167). Biventricular pacing is a newer electrophysiologic therapy that attempts to improve cardiac efficiency by reducing dyssynchrony in cardiac contraction. It also has been shown to improve NYHA class (168), exercise tolerance (169), and ejection fraction (170); mortality benefits have also been demonstrated. In this section, we will review both defibrillator and biventricular pacing and their role in managing heart failure.

Implantable Cardioverter Defibrillators

Data from the Antiarrhythmic versus Implantable Defibrillator (AVID) trial (165), the Multicenter Automatic Defibrillator Implantation Trial (MADIT) (166), the Multicenter Unstrained Tachycardia Trial (MUSTT) (171), and the Multicenter Automatic Defibrillator Implantation Trial II (172) support the use of ICDs in patients who have survived symptomatic ventricular tachycardia or cardiac arrest, patients with ischemic cardiomyopathy with ejection fraction less than 30%, and patients with asymptomatic ventricular tachycardia that is inducible.

Recently, data from the Sudden Cardiac Death in Heart Failure Trial (SCD-HEFT) (167) and Comparison of Medical Therapy, Pacing and Defibrillation in Chronic Heart Failure (COMPANION) trial (168,173) have broadened the indications to other heart failure patients, including nonischemic cardiomyopathy patients who had QRS duration greater than 120 msec, whose LVEF was less than 35%, and who had an admission for heart failure in the previous year. Patients were randomized to (a) medical therapy, (b) medical therapy and biventricular pacing, and (c) medical therapy, biventricular pacing, and defibrillator implantation. In this study, the addition of the combination therapies reduced mortality by 50% in the nonischemic group and 27% in the ischemic group.

At present, the indications for ICD for primary prevention of sudden cardiac death in heart failure (174) are:

- As primary prevention in patients with prior MI greater than 40 days old, with an ejection fraction between 30% and 40%, and who are NYHA class II or III on optimal therapy
- Patients with prior MI greater than or equal to 40 days previously, or ejection fraction between 30% and 35%

- Patients with nonischemic cardiomyopathy, ejection fraction between 30% and 35%, and NYHA class II or III on optimal medical therapy

Biventricular Pacing

Biventricular pacing is achieved by implantation of a left ventricular lead, generally via the coronary sinus to the great cardiac vein, in addition to a right ventricular lead. This strategy is based on the fact that most patients with intraventricular conduction delay have dyssynchronous left ventricular contraction, which reduces cardiac efficiency (decreased contractile force and impaired myocardial energetics). Studies have shown that biventricular pacing increases dp/dt, ejection fraction, and cardiac index (61,175–178). The COMPANION trial (noted above) demonstrated a significant decrease in mortality (50%) with the combination of biventricular pacing plus ICD compared to biventricular pacing alone (9% mortality reduction).

CARDIAC TRANSPLANTATION AND LEFT VENTRICULAR ASSIST DEVICES

When patients continue to experience advanced heart failure symptoms despite maximization of medical therapy, cardiac transplantation and left ventricular assist devices may be considered. There are currently three left ventricular assist devices available for use in the United States. The Abiomed system is available for temporary use as either right, left, or biventricular assist systems. It is most commonly used after high-risk coronary artery bypass surgery in patients who fail to wean from the cardiopulmonary bypass machine. Cannulae are placed in the atria and the pumps are external to the body. Since the cannulae are implanted in the atria, removal is feasible should the patient recover. Additionally, one ventricular system may be removed at a time; this system requires full anticoagulation. The Thoratec Heart Mate device is approved for use as a bridge to transplantation and as destination therapy in those not considered transplant candidates. The outflow cannula is placed in the proximal ascending aorta, and the inflow cannula is placed in the left ventricular apex. Cannulae are named with respect to the pump that is commonly implanted in the left upper abdominal quadrant preperitoneally. This device does not require anticoagulation, although antiplatelet therapy with aspirin is recommended. The World Heart left ventricular assist device is implanted in a similar fashion to the Heart Mate device and is currently FDA approved as a bridge to transplantation. Currently, a clinical trial is under way for its potential use as destination therapy. The World Heart left ventricular assist device requires full anticoagulation with warfarin, aspirin, and clopidogrel.

There have been 40,192 cardiac transplant procedures between 1988 and August 31, 2006; 2,125 of these procedures were performed in 2005. Kaplan-Meier survival rates for heart transplant procedures performed between 1997 and 2004 ranged from 85.7% to 90.6% at 1 year, 75.2% to 81.8% at 3 years, and 68.8% to 72.6% at 5 years. Ranges are given since the data were based on the United Network of Organ Sharing (UNOS) status at the time of transplantation. Criteria to be considered for transplantation include advanced symptoms despite maximization of medical therapy—including tailoring therapy via hemodynamic monitoring with pulmonary artery catheterization—and a peak oxygen consumption less than 15.0 mL/kg/minute during exercise testing. Exclusion criteria include fixed pulmonary hypertension with greater than 4 Wood units not responsive to vasodilator therapy; tobacco, alcohol, or illicit drug use, or other life-threatening illnesses such as cancer or advanced peripheral arterial disease; noncompliance with physician visits, diet, and medications or psychiatric or personality disorders likely to become exacerbated by, or that would interfere with, posttransplant care; and lack of social support.

THERAPEUTIC GUIDELINES FOR SYMPTOMATIC LEFT VENTRICULAR SYSTOLIC DYSFUNCTION

Polypharmacy has become standard therapy for patients with symptomatic systolic dysfunction. ACE inhibitors are recommended for all patients fitting the above parameters. In those patients with contraindications to ACE inhibitor therapy—or if intolerable side effects develop—treatment should be with ARBs. After the introduction of ACE inhibitor or ARB therapy, a patient should be started on β-adrenergic receptor blockade consisting of either carvedilol or long-acting metoprolol (Toprol XL). β-Blockers should be instituted in patients with euvolemia, starting with low doses and titrating up the dose every 2 weeks as tolerated, to doses achieved in clinical trials; achievement of these doses may take 8 to 12 weeks. For patients being discharged from the hospital with ADHF, low-dose β-blockers may be instituted in-hospital once euvolemia has been achieved. In patients on stable doses of β-blockers who then experience an acute decompensation requiring hospitalization, continuation of β-blocker therapy is recommended. ARBs are recommended for patients intolerant to ACE inhibitors for reasons other than renal insufficiency or hyperkalemia. Hydralazine and oral nitrate combination may be considered in those not tolerating ACE inhibitors or ARBs. Aldosterone antagonists are recommended for patients with NYHA class III or IV symptoms in addition to standard therapy, including diuretics. Aldosterone antagonists are not recommended in patients with creatinine clearance less than 30 mL/minute, serum potassium greater than 5.0 mmol/L, or serum creatinine greater than 2.5 mg/dL. Guidelines recommend frequent monitoring of serum potassium levels following initiation of or change in dose of aldosterone antagonists. The combination of hydralazine and oral nitrates is recommended for African American patients—in addition to ACE inhibitors and β-blockers—who remain NYHA class III or IV despite these drugs. Loop and distal tubule diuretics should be viewed as necessary adjuncts to relieve sodium and water retention. Guidelines recommend that digoxin should be considered for symptomatic patients receiving standard therapy and that the dose should be 0.125 mg in the majority of patients. Serum digoxin level should be less than 1.0 ng/mL. Amiodarone and other antiarrhythmic medications should not be used for primary prevention of sudden death, but amiodarone may be considered in those with ICDs to decrease the frequency of repetitive ICD discharges should this become an issue with the devices. Patients with mild heart failure symptoms (NYHA class II) should restrict their sodium intake to 2 to 3 g daily. Those with more advanced symptoms (NYHA class III to IV) should restrict their sodium intake to 2 g daily. Patients with severe hyponatremia—serum sodium less than 130 mEq/L—should restrict their fluid intake to less than 2 liters per day, as should individuals in whom fluid balance is difficult to maintain despite sodium restriction and high-dose diuretics.

SUMMARY

Heart failure is a complex syndrome characterized by both insufficient cardiac output to meet the body's energy requirements and elevated filling pressures leading to systemic and pulmonary edema. In this chapter, the pathophysiology at a biochemical, cellular, organ, and total body level was reviewed. Evidence-based therapies such as ACE inhibitors, β-blockers, ARBs, and aldosterone antagonists, and the clinical studies supporting their use have been reviewed. Novel therapies such as implantable defibrillators, biventricular pacing, and ventricular assist devices have been presented along with present recommendations for their use.

ACKNOWLEDGMENT

The authors would like to thank Geri Byrd for her patience, expertise, and tireless effort in the preparation of this manuscript. Thanks to Kristen Wienandt Marzejon for preparation of the figures included in the text.

References

1. Thom T, Haase N, Rosamond W, et al. Heart disease and stroke statistics–2006 update: a report from the American Heart Association Statistics Committee and Stroke Statistics Subcommittee. *Circulation.* 2006;113(6):e85–151.
2. National Hospital Discharge Survey CDC/National Center for Health Statistics (NCHS). *Vital Health Stat.* 2005;225 (July 10).
3. National Center for Health Statistics (NCHS). *Vital Health Stat.* 2004; 13:157.
4. Lloyd-Jones DM, Larson MG, Lup EP, et al. Lifetime risk for developing congestive heart failure. The Framingham Heart Study. *Circulation.* 2002;106:3068–3072.
5. Bibbins-Domingo K, Lin F, Vittinghoff E, et al. Predictors of heart failure among women with coronary disease. *Circulation.* 2004;110:1424–1430.
6. Dunlap SH, Sueta CA, Tomasko L, et al. Association of body mass, gender and race with heart failure primarily due to hypertension. *J Am Coll Cardiol.* 1999;34:1602–1608.
7. Liggett SB, Mialet-Perez J, Thaneemit-Chen S, et al. A polymorphism within a conserved beta (1)-adrenergic receptor motif alters cardiac function and beta-blocker response in human heart failure. *Proc Nat Acad Sci USA.* 2006;103(30):11288–11293.
8. Housmans PR, Lee NKM, Blinks JR. Active shortening retards the decline of the intracellular calcium transient in mammalian heart muscle. *Science.* 1983;221:159.
9. Brutsaert DL, Rademakers FE, Sys SU. Triple control of relaxation: implications in cardiac disease. *Circulation.* 1984;69:190.
10. Kohmoto O, Spitzer KW, Movsesian MA, et al. Effects of intracellular acidosis on [Ca2+]i transients, transsarcolemmal C2+ fluxes, and contraction in ventricular myocytes. *Circ Res.* 1990;66:622.
11. Hoffman BF, Bindler E, Suckling EE., et al. Postextrasystolic potentiation of contraction in cardiac muscle. *Am J Physiol.* 1956;185:95.
12. Ross J, Sonnenblick EH, Kaiser GA, et al. Electroaugmentation of ventricular performance and oxygen consumption by repetitive application of paired electrical stimuli. *Circ Res.* 1965;16:332.
13. Higgins CB, Vatner SF, Franklin D, et al. Extent of regulation of the heart's contractile state in the conscious dog by alteration in the frequency of contraction. *J Clin Invest.* 1973;52:1187.
14. Katz AM. Regulation of myocardial contractility 1958–1983: an odyssey. *J Am Coll Cardiol.* 1983;1:42.
15. Colluci WS, Wright RF, Braunwald E. New positive inotropic agents in the treatment of congestive heart failure (second of two parts). *N Engl J Med.* 1986;314:349.
16. Lee HC, Smith N, Mohabir R, et al. Cytosolic calcium transients from the beating mammalian heart. *Physiol Sci.* 1987;84:7793.
17. Lang RM, Fellner SK, Neumann A, et al. LV contractility varies directly with blood ionized calcium. *Ann Intern Med.* 1988;108:524.
18. MacKinnon R, Gwathmey JK, Allen PD, et al. Modulation by the thyroid state of intracellular calcium and contractility in ferret ventricular muscle. *Circ Res.* 1988;63:1080.
19. Morkin E, Flink IL, Goldman S. Biochemical and physiologic effects of thyroid hormone on cardiac performance. *Prog Cardiovasc Dis.* 1983;25:435.
20. Braunwald E, Sommenblick EH, Ross J Jr. Mechanisms of cardiac contraction and relaxation in heart disease. In: Braunwald E, ed. *A Textbook of Cardiovascular Medicine.* 4th ed. Philadelphia: W.B. Saunders Co.; 1992:351.
21. Beierholm EA, Grantham RN, O'Keefe DD, et al. Effects of acid-base changes, hypoxia, and catecholamines on ventricular performance. *Am J Physiol.* 1975;228:1555.
22. Williamson JR, Schaffer SW, Ford C, et al. Contribution of tissue acidosis to ischemic injury in the perfused rat heart. *Circulation.* 1976;53(Suppl 1):3.
23. Braunwald E. Mechanism of action of calcium-channel-blocking agents. *N Engl J Med.* 1982;307:1618.
24. Levine MJ, Harada K, Meuse AJ, et al. Excitation contraction uncoupling during ischemia in the blood perfused dog heart. *Biochem Biophys Res Comm.* 1991;179:502.
25. Hicks MJ, Shigekawa M, Katz AM. Mechanism by which cyclic adenosine 3′:5′-monophosphate-dependent protein kinase stimulates calcium transport in cardiac sarcoplasmic reticulum. *Circ Res.* 1979;44:384.
26. Gwathmey JK, Slawsky MT, Hajjar RJ, et al. Role of intracellular calcium handling in force-interval relationships of human ventricular myocardium. *J Clin Invest.* 1990;85:1599.
27. Gwathmey JK, Copelas L, MacKinnon R, et al. Abnormal intracellular calcium handling in myocardium from patients with end-stage heart failure. *Circ Res.* 1987;61:70.
28. Limas CJ, Olivari M, Goldenberg IF, et al. Calcium uptake by cardiac sarcoplasmic reticulum in human dilated cardiomyopathy. *Cardiovasc Res.* 1987;21:601.
29. Mercadier J, Lompré A, Duc P, et al. Altered sarcoplasmic reticulum CA2+/ATPase gene expression in the human ventricle during end-stage heart failure. *J Clin Invest.* 1990;85:305.
30. Feldman MD, Copelas L, Gwathmey JK, et al. Deficient production of cyclic AMP: pharmacologic evidence of an important cause of contractile dysfunction in patients with end-stage heart failure. *Circulation.* 1987;75:331.
31. Feldman AM, Ray PE, Silan CM, et al. Selective gene expression in failing human heart. *Circulation.* 1991;83:1866.
32. Ungerer M, Bohm M, Elce JS, et al. Altered expression of β-adrenergic receptor kinase and β1-adrenergic receptors in the failing human heart. *Circulation.* 1993;87:454.
33. Bristow MR, Hershberger RE, Port JD, et al. β-adrenergic pathways in nonfailing and failing human ventricular myocardium. *Circulation.* 1990; 82(Suppl 1):12.
34. Feldman AM, Cates AE, Veazey WB, et al. Increase of the 40,000-mol wt pertussis toxin substrate (G protein) in the failing human heart. *J Clin Invest.* 1988;82:189.
35. Gilman AG. G proteins: transducers of receptor-generated signals. *Ann Rev Biochem.* 1987;56:615.
36. Spiegel AM, Gierschik P, Levine MA, et al. Clinical implications of guanine nucleotide-binding proteins as receptor-effector couplers. *N Engl J Med.* 1985;312:26.
37. Katz AM. Cyclic adenosine monophosphate effects on the myocardium: a man who blows hot and cold with one breath. *J Am Coll Cardiol.* 1983; 2:143.
38. Homcy CJ, Graham RM. Molecular characterization of adrenergic receptors. *Circ Res.* 1985;56:635.
39. Neer EJ, Clapham DE. Roles of G protein subunits in transmembrane signaling. *Nature.* 1988;333:129.
40. Colluci WS, Wright RF, Braunwald E. New positive inotropic agents in the treatment of congestive heart failure (first of two parts). *N Engl J Med.* 1986;314:290.
41. Yatani A, Brown AM. Rapid β-adrenergic modulation of cardiac calcium channel currents by a fast G protein pathway. *Science.* 1989;245:71.
42. Mery PF, Lohmann SM, Walter U, et al. Ca^{2+} current is regulated by cyclic GMP-dependent protein kinase in mammalian cardiac myocytes. *Proc Natl Acad Sci.* 1991;88:1197.
43. Nawrath H. Cyclic AMP and cyclic GMP may play opposing roles in influencing force of contraction in mammalian myocardium. *Nature.* 1976;262:509.
44. Schranz D, Droege A, Broede A, et al. Uncoupling of human cardiac β-adrenoceptors during cardiopulmonary bypass with cardioplegic cardiac arrest. *Circulation.* 1993;87:422.
45. Kumar A, Kosuri R, Kandula P, et al. Tumor necrosis factor-induced myocardial cell depression is mediated by nitric oxide and cyclic GMP generation. *Crit Care Med.* 1994;22:A191.

46. Schneider F, Lutun P, Hasselmann M, et al. Methylene blue increases systemic vascular resistance in human septic shock. *Int Care Med.* 1992; 18:309.
47. Silverman HJ, Penaranda R, Orens JB. Impaired β-adrenergic receptor stimulation of cyclic adenosine monophosphate in human septic shock: association with myocardial hyporesponsiveness to catecholamines. *Crit Care Med.* 1993;21:31.
48. Yanagisawa M, Kurihara H, Kimura S, et al. A novel potent vasoconstrictor peptide produced by vascular endothelial cells. *Nature.* 1988;332:411.
49. Kramer BK, Nishida M, Kelly RA, et al. Myocardial actions of a new class of cytokines. *Circulation.* 1992;85:350.
50. Kelly RA, Eid H, Kramer BK, et al. Endothelin enhances the contractile responsiveness of adult rat ventricular myocytes to calcium by a pertussis toxin-sensitive pathway. *J Clin Invest.* 1990;86:1164.
51. Kramer BK, Smith TW, Kelly RA, et al. Endothelin and increased contractility in adult rat ventricular myocytes: role of intracellular alkalosis induced by activation of the protein kinase C-dependent Na^+-H^+. *Circ Res.* 1991;68:269.
52. del Monte F, Hajjar RJ. Targeting calcium cycling proteins in heart failure through gene transfer. *J Physiol.* 2003;546(Pt 1):49–61.
53. Placentino V III, Weber CR, Chen X, et al. Cellular basis of abnormal calcium transients of failing human ventricular myocytes. *Circ Res.* 2003; 92:651.
54. Hasenfuss G, Mulieri LA, Leavitt BJ, et al. Alteration of contractile function and excitation-contraction coupling in dilated cardiomyopathy. *Circ Res.* 1992;70(6):1225–1232.
55. Flesch M, Schwinger RH, Schnabel P, et al. Sarcoplasmic reticulum Ca2+ATPase and phospholamban mRNA and protein levels in end-stage heart failure due to ischemic or dilated cardiomyopathy. *J Mol Med.* 1996;74(6):321–332.
56. Hobai IA, O'Rourke B. Decreased sarcoplasmic reticulum calcium content is responsible for defective excitation-contraction coupling in canine heart failure. *Circulation.* 2001;103(11):1577–1584.
57. Meyer M, Bluhm WF, He H, et al. Phospholamban-to-SERCA2 ratio controls the force-frequency relationship. *Am J Physiol.* 1999;276(3 Pt 2): H779–785.
58. Marks AR, Reiken S, Marx SO. Progression of heart failure: is protein kinase a hyperphosphorylation of the ryanodine receptor a contributing factor? *Circulation.* 2002;105(3):272–275.
59. Shannon TR, Ginsburg KS, Bers DM. Quantitative assessment of the SR Ca^{++} leak load relationship. *Circ Res.* 2002;91:594.
60. Abraham WT, Gilbert EM, Lowes BD, et al. Coordinate changes in Myosin heavy chain isoform gene expression are selectively associated with alterations in dilated cardiomyopathy phenotype. *Mol Med.* 2002;8(11):750–760.
61. Lowes BD, Minobe W, Abraham WT, et al. Changes in gene expression in the intact human heart. Down regulation of alpha myosin heavy chain in hypertrophied failing ventricular myocardium. *J Clin Invest.* 1997;100: 2362.
62. Thomas CV, Coker ML, Zellner JL, et al. Increased matrix metalloproteinase activity and selective up regulation in LV myocardium from patients with end-stage dilated cardiomyopathy. *Circulation.* 1998;97(17):1708–1715.
63. Coker ML, Thomas CV, Clair MJ, et al. Myocardial matrix metalloproteinase activity and abundance with congestive heart failure. *Am J Physiol.* 1998;274:H1516–1523.
64. Meerson, FZ. The myocardium in hyperfunction, hypertrophy, and heart failure. *Circ Res.* 1998;25(Suppl 2):1.
65. Chaudhry PA, Anagnostopouls PV, Mishima T, et al. Acute ventricular reduction with the acorn cardiac support device: effect on progressive left ventricular dysfunction and dilation in dogs with chronic heart failure. *J Card Surg.* 2001;16(2):118–126.
66. Francis GS, Cohn JN, Johnson G, et al. Plasma norepinephrine plasma renin activity and congestive heart failure. Relations to survival and the effects of therapy in V-HeFT II. *Circulation.* 1993;87:VI-400.
67. Cohn JN, Ferrari R, Sharpe N. Cardiac remodeling–concepts and clinical implications: a consensus paper from an international forum on cardiac remodeling. Behalf of an International Forum on Cardiac Remodeling. *J Am Coll Cardiol.* 2000;35(3):569–582.
68. Grossman W, Jones D, McLaurin LP. Wall stress and patterns of hypertrophy in the human left ventricle. *J Clin Invest.* 1975;56(1):56–64.
69. Calderone A, Takahashi N, Izzo NJ, et al. Pressure- and volume-induced left ventricular hypertrophies are associated with distinct myocyte phenotypes and differential induction of peptide growth factor mRNAs. *Circulation.* 1995;92(9):2385–2390.
70. Hunter JJ, Chien K. Signaling pathways for cardiac hypertrophy and failure. *N Engl J Med.* 1999;341(17):1276–1283.
71. Kang PM, Yue P, Izumo S. New insights into the role of apoptosis in cardiovascular disease. *Circ J.* 2002;66(1):1–9.
72. Cohn JN, Levine TB, Olivari MT, et al. Plasma norepinephrine as a guide to prognosis in patients with chronic congestive heart failure. *N Engl J Med.* 1984;311:819–823.
73. Bristow MR, Ginsburg R, Minobe W, et al. Decreased catecholamine sensitivity and beta-adrenergic-receptor density in failing human hearts. *N Engl J Med.* 1982;307(4):205–222.
74. Mann DL, Kent RL, Parsons B, et al. Adrenergic effects on the biology of the adult mammalian cardiocyte. *Circulation.* 1992;85:790–804.
75. The SOLVD Investigators. Effect of enalapril on survival in patients with reduced left ventricular ejection fractions and congestive heart failure. *N Engl J Med.* 1992;325:293–302.
76. The SOLVD Investigators. Effect of enalapril on mortality and the development of heart failure in asymptomatic patients with reduced left ventricular ejection fractions. *N Engl J Med.* 1992;327:685–691.
77. White HD, Norris RM, Brown MA, et al. Left ventricular and end-systolic volume as the major determinant of survival after recovery from myocardial infarction. *Circulation.* 1987;76:44–51.
78. Borow KM, Lang RM, Neumann A, et al. Physiologic mechanisms governing hemodynamic responses to positive inotropic therapy in dilated cardiomyopathy. *Circulation.* 1988;77:625–637.
79. Douglas PS, Morrow R, Ioli A, et al. Left ventricular shape, afterload and survival in idiopathic dilated cardiomyopathy. *J Am Coll Cardiol.* 1989;13: 311–315.
80. The CONSENSUS Trial Study Group. Effects of enalapril on mortality in severe congestive heart failure: results of the Cooperative North Scandinavian Enalapril Survival Study (CONSENSUS). *N Engl J Med.* 1987;316:1429–1435.
81. Pfeffer MA, Braunwald E, Moye LA, et al.; SAVE Investigators. Effect of captopril on mortality and morbidity in patients with left ventricular dysfunction after myocardial infarction: results of the Survival and Ventricular Enlargement Trial. *N Engl J Med.* 1992;327:669–677.
82. Gilbert JC, Glantz SA. Determinants of LV filling and of the diastolic P-V relation. *Circ Res.* 1989;64:827.
83. Gaasch WH, Levine HJ, Quinones MA, et al. LV compliance: mechanisms and clinical implications. *Am J Cardiol.* 1976;38:645.
84. Nikolic SD, Tamura K, Tamura T, et al. Diastolic viscous properties of the intact canine left ventricle. *Circ Res.* 1990;67:352.
85. Momomura S, Ingwall JS, Parker JA, et al. The relationships of high energy phosphates, tissue pH, and regional blood flow to diastolic distensibility in the ischemic dog myocardium. *Circ Res.* 1985;57:822.
86. Lorell BH, Grossman W. Cardiac hypertrophy: the consequences for diastole. *J Am Coll Cardiol.* 1987;9:1189.
87. Cuocolo A, Sax FL, Brush JE, et al. LV hypertrophy and impaired diastolic filling in essential hypertrophy and impaired diastolic filling in essential hypertension. *Circulation.* 1990;81:978.
88. Apstein CS, Grossman W. Opposite initial effects of supply and demand ischemia on LV diastolic compliance: the ischemia-diastolic paradox. *J Mol Cell Cardiol.* 1987;19:119.
89. Paulus WJ, Grossman W, Serizawa T, et al. Different effects of two types of ischemia on myocardial systolic and diastolic function. *Am J Physiol.* 1985;248:H719.
90. Gordon AM, Huxley AF, Julian FJ. The variation in isometric tension with sarcomere length in vertebrate muscle fibres. *J Physiol.* 1966;184:170.
91. Milnor WR. Cardiac dynamics. In: Milnor WR, ed. *Hemodynamics.* Baltimore: Williams & Wilkins Co.; 1982:244.
92. Ikenouchi H, Kohmoto O, McMillan M, et al. Contributions of [Ca2+]i, [Pi], and pHi to altered diastolic myocyte tone during partial metabolic inhibition. *J Clin Invest.* 1991;88:55.
93. Sasayama S, Nonogi H, Miyazaki S, et al. Changes in diastolic properties of the regional myocardium during pacing-induced ischemia in human subjects. *J Am Coll Cardiol.* 1985;5:599.
94. Miyazaki S, Guth BD, Miura T, et al. Changes of LV diastolic function in exercising dogs without and with ischemia. *Circulation.* 1990;81:1058.
95. Nikolic S, Yellin EL, Tamura K, et al. Effect of early diastolic loading on myocardial relaxation in the intact canine left ventricle. *Circ Res.* 1990; 66:1217.
96. Stool EW, Mullins CB, Leshin SJ, et al. Dimensional changes of the left ventricle during acute pulmonary arterial hypertension in dogs. *Am J Cardiol.* 1974;33:868.
97. Glantz SA, Misbach GA, Moores WY, et al. The pericardium substantially affects the LV diastolic P-V relationship in the dog. *Circ Res.* 1978;42: 433.
98. Calvin JE, Baer RW, Glantz SA. Pulmonary injury depresses cardiac systolic function through Starling mechanism. *Am J Physiol.* 1986;251:H722.
99. Cassidy SS, Ramanathan M. Dimensional analysis of the left ventricle during PEEP: relative septal and lateral wall displacements. *Am J Physiol.* 1984;246:H792.
100. Tyson GS, Maier GW, Olsen CO, et al. Pericardial influences on ventricular filling in the conscious dog. *Circ Res.* 1984;54:173.
101. Slinker BK, Glantz SA. End-systolic and end-diastolic ventricular interaction. *Am J Physiol.* 1986;251:H1062.
102. Calvin JE. Optimal RV filling pressures and the role of pericardial constraint in RV infarction in dogs. *Circulation.* 1991;84:852.
103. Calvin JE, Langlois S, Garneys G. Ventricular interaction in a canine model of acute pulmonary hypertension and its modulation by vasoactive drugs. *J Crit Care.* 1988;3:43.
104. Visner MS, Arentzen CE, O'Connor MJ, et al. Alterations in LV three-dimensional dynamic geometry and systolic function during acute RV hypertension in the conscious dog. *Circulation.* 1983;67:353.
105. Ludbrook PA, Byrne JD, McKnight RC. Influence of RV hemodynamics on LV diastolic P-V relations in man. *Circulation.* 1979;59:21.

106. Calvin JE, Baer RW, Glantz SA. Pulmonary artery constriction produces a greater RV dynamic afterload than lung microvascular injury in the open chest dog. *Circ Res.* 1985;56:40.
107. Calvin JE, Quinn B. RV pressure overload during acute lung injury: cardiac mechanics and the pathophysiology of RV systolic dysfunction. *J Crit Care.* 1989;4:251.
108. Calvin JE. RV afterload mismatch during acute pulmonary hypertension and its treatment with dobutamine: a pressure segment length analysis in a canine model. *J Crit Care.* 1989;4:239.
109. Vlahakes GJ, Turley K, Hoffman JIE. The pathophysiology of failure in acute RV hypertension: hemodynamic and biochemical correlations. *Circulation.* 1981;63:87.
110. Gold FL, Bache RJ. Transmural right ventricular blood flow during acute pulmonary artery hypertension in the sedated dog. *Circ Res.* 1982;51:196–204.
111. Taylor R, Covell J, Sonnenblick E, et al. Dependence of ventricular distensibility on filling of the opposite ventricle. *Am J Physiol.* 1967;213:711–718.
112. Kingma I, Tyberg J, Smith E, et al. Effects of diastolic transeptal pressure gradient on ventricular septal position and motion. *Circulation.* 1983;68(6):1304–1314.
113. Chobanian AV, Bakris GL, Black HR, et al. Seventh Report of the Joint National Committee on Prevention, Detection, Evaluation, and Treatment of High Blood Pressure. *Hypertension.* 2003;42:1206–1252.
114. American Diabetes Association. Position Statement: Standards of Medical Care in Diabetes—2006. *Diabetes Care.* 2006;29(Supp 1):S4–S42.
115. Smith SC, Allen J, Blair SN, et al. AHA/ACC Guidelines for Secondary Prevention for Patients with Coronary and Other Atherosclerotic Vascular Disease: 2006 update: endorsed by the National Heart, Lung, and Blood Institute. *Circulation.* 2006;113:2363–2372.
116. Levy D, Kenchaiah S, Larson MG, et al. Long-term trends in the incidence of and survival with heart failure. *N Engl J Med.* 2002;347(18):1397–1402.
117. Ho KK, Anderson KM, Kannel WB, et al. Survival after the onset of congestive heart failure in Framingham Heart Study subjects. *Circulation.* 1993;88(1):107–115.
118. Rector TS, Cohn JN. Prognosis in congestive heart failure. *Ann Rev Med.* 1994;45:341–350.
119. Deedwania PC. The key to unraveling the mystery of mortality in heart failure: an integrated approach. *Circulation.* 2003;107(13):1719–1721.
120. Bart BA, Shaw LK, McCants CB, et al. Clinical determinants of mortality in patients with angiographically diagnosed ischemic or nonischemic cardiomyopathy. *J Am Coll Cardiol.* 1997;30(4):1002–1008.
121. Metra M, Faggiano P, D'Aloia A, et al. Use of cardiopulmonary exercise testing with hemodynamic monitoring in the prognostic assessment of ambulatory patients with chronic heart failure. *J Am Coll Cardiol.* 1999;33(4):943–950.
122. Myers J, Gullestad L, Vagelos R, et al. Clinical, hemodynamic, and cardiopulmonary exercise test determinants of survival in patients referred for evaluation of heart failure. *Ann Intern Med.* 1998;129(4):286–293.
123. Bittner V, Weiner DH, Yusuf S, et al. Prediction of mortality and morbidity with a 6 minute walk test in patients with left ventricular dysfunction. *JAMA.* 1993;270:1702.
124. Francis GS, Cohn JN, Johnson G, et al. Plasma norepinephrine, plasma renin activity, and congestive heart failure. Relations to survival and the effects of therapy in V-HeFT II. The V-HeFT VA Cooperative Studies Group. *Circulation.* 1993;87(6 Suppl):VI40–48.
125. Anand IS, Fisher LD, Chiang YT, et al. Changes in brain natriuretic peptide and norepinephrine over time and mortality and morbidity in the Valsartan Heart Failure Trial (Val-HeFT). *Circulation.* 2003;107(9):1278–1283.
126. Berger R, Stanek B, Frey B, et al. B-type natriuretic peptides (BNP and PRO-BNP) predict long-term survival in patients with advanced heart failure treated with atenolol. *J Heart Lung Transplant.* 2001;20(2):251.
127. Hulsmann M, Stanek B, Frey B, et al. Value of cardiopulmonary exercise testing and big endothelin plasma levels to predict short-term prognosis of patients with chronic heart failure. *J Am Coll Cardiol.* 1998;32(6):1695–1700.
128. Teskey RJ, Calvin JE, McPhail I. Disease severity in the coronary care unit. *Chest.* 1991;100(6):1637–1642.
129. Gracin N, Johnson MR, Spokas D, et al. The use of APACHE II scores to select candidates for left ventricular assist device placement. *J Heart Lung Transplant.* 1998;17:1017–1023.
130. The Acute Infarction Ramipril Efficacy (AIRE) Study Investigators. Effect of ramipril on mortality and morbidity of survivors of acute myocardial infarction with clinical evidence of heart failure. *Lancet.* 1993;342(8875):821–828.
131. Packer M, Poole-Wilson PA, Armstrong PW, et al. Comparative effects of low and high doses of the angiotensin-converting enzyme inhibitor, lisinopril, on morbidity and mortality in chronic heart failure. *Circulation.* 1999;100:2312–2318.
132. Pitt B, Segal R, Martinez FA, et al.; ELITE Study Investigators. Randomized trial of losartan versus captopril in patients over 65 with heart failure (Evaluation of Losartan in the Elderly study, ELITE). *Lancet.* 1997;349:747–752.
133. Pitt B, Poole-Wilson PA, Segal R, et al.; ELITE II Investigators. Effect of losartan compared with captopril on mortality in patients with symptomatic heart failure; randomized trial—the Losartan Heart Failure Survival study ELITE II. *Lancet.* 2000;355:1582–1587.
134. Cohn JN, Tognoni G; Valsartan Heart Failure Trial Investigators. A randomized trial of the angiotensin-receptor blocker valsartan in chronic heart failure. *N Engl J Med.* 2001;345:1667–1675.
135. Pfeffer MA, McMurray JJV, Velazquez EJ, et al. Valsartan, captopril, or both in myocardial infarction complicated by heart failure, left ventricular dysfunction or both. *N Engl J Med.* 2003;349:1893–1906.
136. Pfeffer MA, Swedberg K, Granger CB, et al.; CHARM Investigators and Committees. Effects of candesartan on mortality and morbidity in patients with chronic heart failure: the CHARM-Overall programme. *Lancet.* 2003;362:759–766.
137. Waagstein F, Hjalmarson A, Varnauskas E, et al. Effect of chronic beta-adrenergic receptor blockade in congestive cardiomyopathy. *Br Heart J.* 1975;37:1022–1036.
138. Waagstein F, Bristow MR, Swedberg K, et al. Beneficial effects of metoprolol in idiopathic dilated cardiomyopathy. *Lancet.* 1993;342:1441–1446.
139. CIBIS Investigators and Committees. A randomized trial of beta-blockade in heart failure: the Cardiac Insufficiency Bisoprolol Study (CIBIS). *Circulation.* 1994;90:1765–1773.
140. Packer M, Coats AJS, Fowler MB, et al.; Carvedilol Prospective Randomized Cumulative Survival Study Group. Effect of carvedilol on survival in severe chronic heart failure. *N Engl J Med.* 2001;344:1651–1658.
141. The CAPRICORN Investigators. Effect of carvedilol on outcome after myocardial infarction in patients with left ventricular dysfunction: the CAPRICORN randomised trial. *Lancet.* 2001;357:1385–1390.
142. CIBIS-II Investigators and Committees. The Cardiac Insufficiency Bisoprolol Study II (CIBIS-II) a randomised trial. *Lancet.* 1999;353:9–13.
143. Domanski MJ, Krause-Steinrauff H, Massie BM, et al. A comparative analysis of the results from 4 trials of beta-blocker therapy for heart failure: BEST, CIBIS-II, MERIT-HF, and Copernicus. *J Card Fail.* 2003;9(5):354–363.
144. Goldstein S, Fagerberg B, Hjalmarson A, et al. Metoprolol controlled release/extended release in patients with severe heart failure: analysis of the experience in the MERIT-HF study. *J Am Coll Cardiol.* 2001;38(4):932–938.
145. Poole-Wilson PA, Swedberg K, Cleland JGF, et al., for the COMET Investigators. Comparison of carvedilol and metoprolol on clinical outcomes in patients with chronic heart failure in the Carvedilol or Metoprolol European Trial (COMET): randomised controlled trial. *Lancet.* 2003;362:7–13.
146. Pitt B, Zannad F, Remme WJ, et al.; Randomized Aldactone Evaluation Study Investigators. The effect of spironolactone on morbidity and mortality in patients with severe heart failure. *N Engl J Med.* 1999;341:709–717.
147. Cohn JN, Archibald DG, Ziesche S, et al. Effect of vasodilator therapy on mortality in chronic congestive heart failure. results of a veterans administration cooperative study. *N Engl J Med.* 1986;314:1547–1552.
148. Cohn JN, Johnson G, Ziesche S, et al. A comparison of enalapril with hydralazine-isosorbide dinitrate in the treatment of chronic congestive heart failure. *N Engl J Med.* 1991;325:303–310.
149. Yancy CW. Heart failure in African Americans: a cardiovascular enigma. *J Card Fail.* 2000;6:183–186.
150. Gillum RF. Pathophysiology of hypertension in blacks and whites: a review of the basis of racial blood pressure differences. *Hypertension.* 1979;1:468–475.
151. Hinderliter AL, Sager AR, Sherwood A, et al. Ethnic differences in forearm vasodilator capacity. *Am J Cardiol.* 1996;78:208–211.
152. Stein CM, Lang CC, Nelson R, et al. Vasodilation in black Americans: attenuated nitric oxide-mediated responses. *Clin Pharmacol Ther.* 1997;62:436–443.
153. Taylor AL, Ziesche S, Yancy C, et al.; African-American Heart Failure Trial Investigators. Combination of isosorbide dinitrate and hydralazine in blacks with heart failure. *N Engl J Med.* 2004;351:2049–2057.
154. Uretsky BF, Young JB, Shahidi FE, et al. Randomized study assessing the effect of digoxin withdrawal in patients with mild to moderate chronic congestive heart failure: results of the PROVED trial. *J Am Coll Cardiol.* 1993;22:955–962.
155. Packer M, Gheorghiade M, Young JB, et al.; The RADIANCE Study. Withdrawal of digoxin from patients with chronic heart failure treated with angiotensin-converting–enzyme inhibitors. *N Engl J Med.* 1993;329:1–7.
156. Maisel AS, McCord J, Nowak RM, et al. Bedside B-type natriuretic peptide in the emergency diagnosis of heart failure with reduced or preserved ejection fraction. Results from the breathing not properly multinational study. *J Am Coll Cardiol.* 2003;41:2010–2017.
157. Heart Failure Society of America 2006 comprehensive heart failure practice guideline. *J Card Fail.* 2006;12.
158. Fonarow GC; ADHERE Scientific Advisory Committee. The Acute Decompensated Heart Failure National Registry (ADHERE): opportunities to improve care of patients hospitalized with acute decompensated heart failure. *Rev Cardiovasc Med.* 2003;4(suppl 7):S21–S30.
159. Adams KF, Fonarow GC, Eneman CL, et al. Characteristics and outcomes of patients hospitalized for heart failure in the United States (2001–2003): rationale, design and preliminary observations from the Acute Decompensated Heart Failure National Registry (ADHERE). *Am Heart J.* 2005;149(2):209–216.
160. Fonarow GC, Adams KF, Abraham WT, et al.; ADHERE Scientific Advisory Committee, Study Group, and Investigators. Risk stratification for

in-hospital mortality in acutely decompensated heart failure: classification and regression tree analysis. *JAMA.* 2005;293:572–580.
161. Harvey S, Harrison DA, Singer M, et al.; PAC-Man study collaboration. Assessment of the clinical effectiveness of Pulmonary Artery Catheters in Management of patients in intensive care (PAC-Man); a randomized controlled trial. *Lancet.* 2005;366:472–477.
162. The ESCAPE Investigators and ESCAPE Study Coordinators. Evaluation study of congestive heart failure and pulmonary artery catheterization effectiveness: the ESCAPE trial. *JAMA.* 2005;294:1625–1633.
163. Publication Committee for the JMAC Investigators. Intravenous nesiritide vs. nitroglycerin for treatment of decompensated congestive heart failure: a randomized controlled trial. *JAMA.* 2002;287:1531–1540.
164. Bart BA, Boyle A, Bank AJ, et al. Ultrafiltration versus usual care for hospitalized patients with heart failure: the Relief for Acutely Fluid-overloaded Patients with Decompensated Congestive Heart Failure (RAPID-CHF) trial. *J Am Coll Cardiol.* 2005;46:2043–2046.
165. AVID Investigator. A comparison of antiarrhythmic-drug therapy with implantable defibrillators in patients resuscitated from near-fatal ventricular arrhythmias. The Antiarrhythmics versus Implantable Defibrillators. *N Engl J Med.* 1997;337(22):1576–1583.
166. MADIT Investigator. Improved survival with an implanted defibrillator in patients with coronary artery disease at high risk for ventricular arrhythmia. *N Engl J Med.* 1996;335:1933–1940.
167. Mark DB, Nelson CL, Anstrom KJ, et al. SCD-HeFT Investigators. Cost-effectiveness of defibrillator therapy or a amiodarone in chronic stable heart failure: results from the sudden cardiac death in heart failure trial (SCD-Heft). *Circulation.* 2006;114(2):135–142.
168. Bristow MR, Feldman AM, Saxon LA. Heart failure management using implantable devices for ventricular resynchronization: Comparison of Medical Therapy, Pacing, and Defibrillation in Chronic Heart Failure (COMPANION) trial. COMPANION Steering Committee and COMPANION clinical investigators. *J Card Fail.* 2000;6(3):276–285.
169. Leclercq C, Cazeau S, Le Breton H, et al. Acute hemodynamic effects of biventricular DDD pacing in patients with end-stage heart failure. *J Am Coll Cardiol.* 1998;32(7):1825–1831.
170. Kass DA, Chen CH, Curry C, et al. Improved left ventricular mechanics from acute VDD pacing in patients with dilated cardiomyopathy and ventricular conduction delay. *Circulation.* 1999;99:1567–1573.
171. Buxton AE, Lee KL, Fisher JD, et al. A randomized study of the prevention of sudden death in patients with coronary artery disease. *N Engl J Med.* 1999;341:1882–1890.
172. Moss AJ, Zareba W, Hall WJ, et al. Prophylactic implantation of a defibrillator in patients with myocardial infarction and reduced ejection fraction. *N Engl J Med.* 2002;346(12):877–883.
173. Bristow MR, Saxon LA, Boehmer, et al. Cardiac resynchronization therapy with or without an implantable defibrillator in advanced chronic heart failure: the COMPANION trial. *N Engl J Med.* 2004;350:2140.
174. Zipes, DP, Camm AJ, Borggrefe M, et al.; Writing Committee Members. ACC/AHA/ESC 2006 guidelines for management of patients with ventricular arrhythmias and the prevention of sudden cardiac death—executive summary. *Circulation.* 2006;114:1008–1132.
175. Kerwin WF, Botvinick EH, O'Connell JW. Ventricular contraction abnormalities in dilated cardiomyopathy: effect of biventricular pacing to correct interventricular dyssynchrony. *J Am Coll Cardiol.* 2000;35:1221–1227.
176. Cazeau S, Leclercq C, Lavergne T, et al. Effects of multisite biventricular pacing in patients with heart failure and intraventricular conduction delay. *N Engl J Med.* 2001;344(12):873–880.
177. Saxon LA, De Marco T, Schafer J, et al. Effects of long-term biventricular stimulation for resynchronization on echocardiographic measures of remodeling. *Circulation.* 2002;105(11):1304–1310.
178. St John Sutton MG, Plappert T, Abraham WT, et al. Effect of cardiac resynchronization therapy on left ventricular size and function in chronic heart failure. *Circulation.* 2003;107(15):1985–1990.

CHAPTER 122 ■ CARDIAC MECHANICAL ASSIST DEVICES

CHARLES T. KLODELL

IMMEDIATE GOALS AND PURPOSE OF USE

Cardiac mechanical assist devices are used during periods of hemodynamic instability and persistent low cardiac output in an attempt to restore normal hemodynamic parameters. The primary goal of their use is to normalize inflow and drainage of vital organs so that kidney and liver function return to normal with improved hemostatic potential. The deleterious effects of elevated atrial pressure on many of the major organs are well known, with the lungs being most adversely affected. Increased central venous pressure is also particularly detrimental to the liver and kidneys, causing outflow disorders that compromise organ function. Elevated atrial and central venous pressures, secondary to ventricular dysfunction, are often rapidly normalized by the use of cardiac mechanical assist devices.

There is a stepwise progression of therapy that is followed in the intensive care unit with respect to cardiac assist interventions. Therapy begins with inotropic and vasodilator drugs and, if the sought-after end point is not achieved, typically progresses to the use of an intra-aortic balloon pump. Ultimately, mechanical ventricular assist device placement may be necessary. In this chapter, we will briefly discuss these devices with special emphasis on the indications, contraindications, placement, complications, and potential pitfalls.

INTRA-AORTIC BALLOON PUMP

Indications

- Acute myocardial infarction and shock: 10% to 15% of acute myocardial infarctions may require hemodynamic support with the temporary use of an intra-aortic balloon pump (Fig. 122.1). This may translate into as many as 1.5 million patients annually.
- Unstable angina

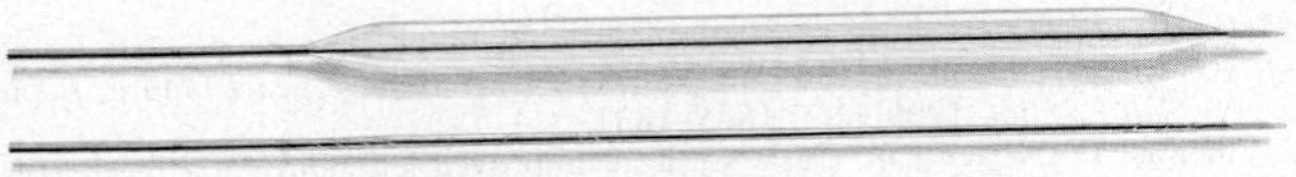

FIGURE 122.1. Intra-aortic balloon pulsation (IABP). Example of standard 7.5 French 40-mL IABP.

- Prophylaxis for high-risk surgery or percutaneous coronary intervention
- Acute mitral insufficiency
- Ventricular septal rupture following an ischemic event (usually several days after ischemic insult)
- Postcardiotomy failure: Inability to separate patient from cardiopulmonary bypass following cardiac surgical procedure
- Traumatic myocardial contusion with low cardiac output

Contraindications

- *Aortic insufficiency:* Leaking of the aortic valve makes the use of an intra-aortic balloon pump potentially detrimental. During periods of diastolic augmentation, enhanced reversal of flow actually exacerbates the aortic insufficiency.
- *Atheromatous aorta:* Patients who are known to have severe atheromatous disease of the aorta are poor candidates for balloon pump therapy. There is the risk of atheroembolization, either distally or retrograde into the cerebral vasculature, during pump use or manipulation.
- *Severe peripheral vascular disease or aortic dissection:* The balloon pump is typically inserted in a retrograde fashion from the groin. This relative contraindication of peripheral vascular disease can be overcome by the use of alternate insertion techniques.

Techniques of Insertion

The most commonly used method of intra-aortic balloon pump insertion is via the retrograde approach from percutaneous access to the femoral artery (Fig. 122.2). This can be performed with or without a vascular sheath. Typically the femoral artery is accessed with a needle. A wire is then passed retrograde into the descending aorta. A sheath may or may not be placed depending on the size of the femoral artery and the circumstances. The balloon pump is then carefully inserted over the wire into the descending aorta to a point immediately distal to the left subclavian artery. When there has already been an incision made to the groin related to coronary artery bypass cannulation or some other intervention, it is possible to insert the balloon pump via direct arterial access.

In special circumstances, there are alternate sites for insertion. This is especially true in patients who either have their balloon pump for an extended period of time or have a need for ambulation during balloon pump use. In these circumstances,

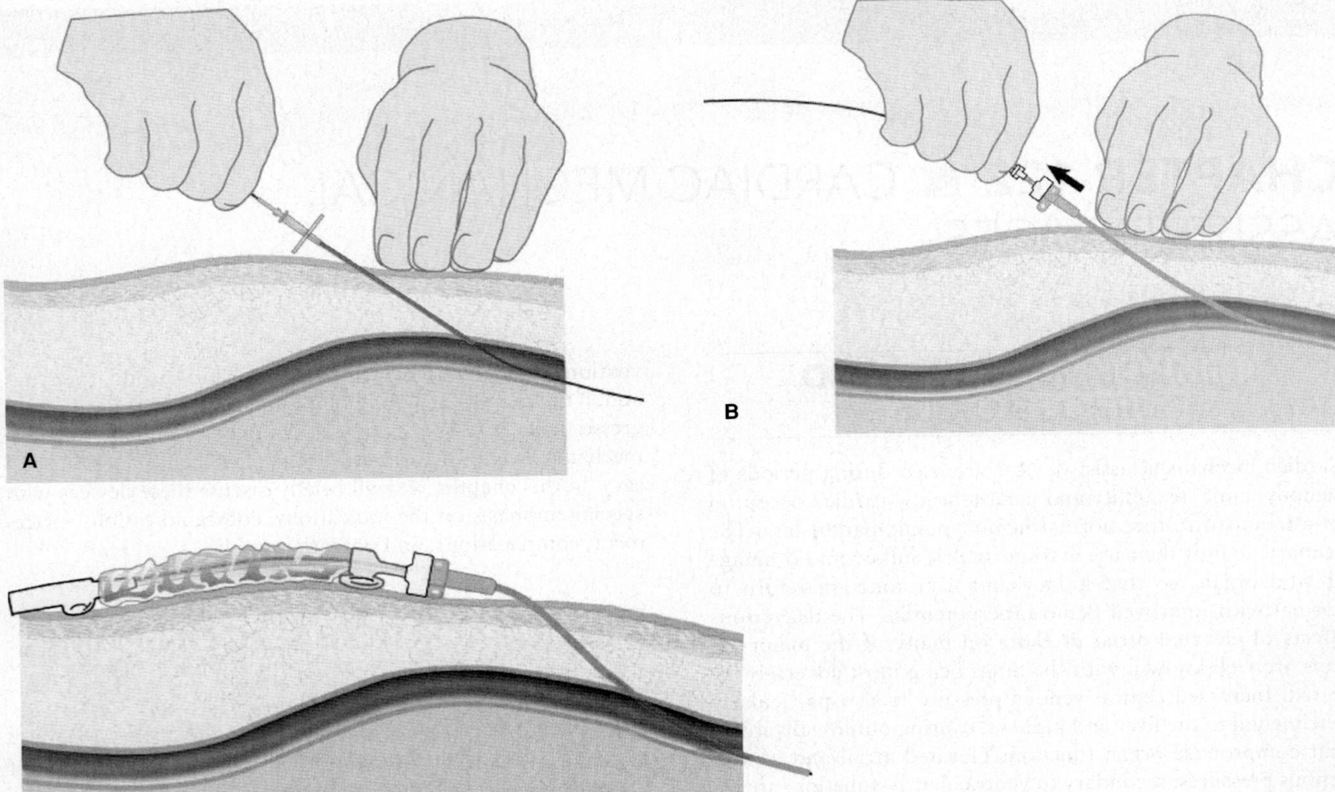

FIGURE 122.2. Intra-aortic balloon pulsation (IABP). Insertion from femoral approach. A: Artery is accessed and wire advanced. B: Sheath inserted over wire. C: IABP advanced over wire and through sheath to appropriate level.

a balloon pump may also be placed directly through the axillary artery (1). When placed via the axillary artery, a sheath is not routinely used for placement. In more extreme circumstances, placement may require an antegrade approach either directly into the arch or through a small graft sewn onto the ascending aorta or arch and tunneled to the chest wall (2,3). This method may be necessary for patients with coexisting peripheral vascular disease and postcardiotomy failure to wean during cardiopulmonary bypass.

Verification of Location

It is important that the appropriate location of the balloon pump be confirmed after insertion. It should be positioned just distal to the left subclavian artery in the descending thoracic aorta (Fig. 122.3). A more proximal placement risks an increased incidence of cerebral atheroembolization or of thromboembolization from microthrombi forming on the balloon pump itself. A more distal placement may cause the pump to impede the visceral arteries. The location of the balloon pump may be verified either by fluoroscopy or a chest roentgenogram. The tip should be high in the left chest in appropriate relation to the aortic arch. Another convenient mechanism to verify location involves using transesophageal echocardiography if performed concurrently with balloon pump insertion.

It is also important to select the appropriate sized balloon pump for the patient. Balloon pumps are manufactured in various sizes, ranging from those appropriate for a small infant to those used in large adults (Fig. 122.4). The standard adult size is 40 mL. The manufacturer's labeling and recommendations and the patient's habitus should be considered in size selection.

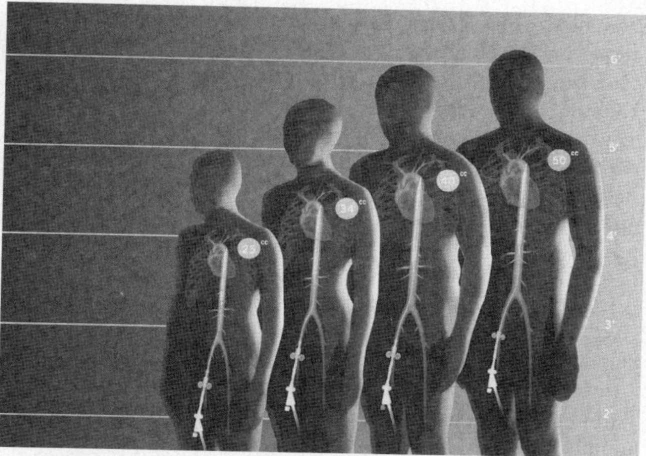

FIGURE 122.4. Different sizes of intra-aortic balloon pulsation (IABP) devices.

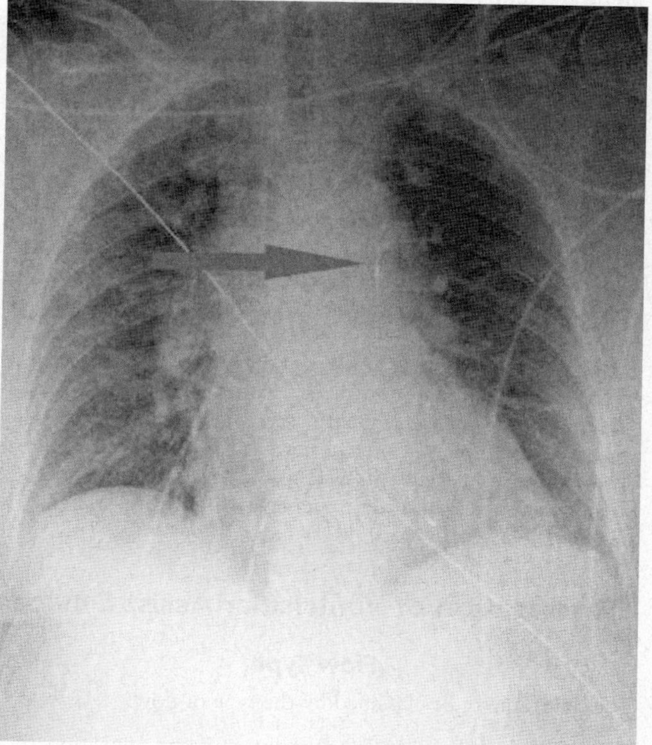

FIGURE 122.3. Chest radiograph showing intra-aortic balloon pulsation (IABP) in place—marked distal tip of IABP.

Mechanism of Action

There are two complimentary effects of an intra-aortic balloon pump. The first is the diastolic augmentation of coronary blood flow. The balloon pump is carefully timed to the cardiac cycle so that the pump inflates during aortic valve closure and thus enhances the diastolic pressure in the proximal aorta. This allows increased coronary blood flow and enhanced myocardial oxygen delivery. The second action involves the afterload reduction at the time of cardiac systole, thereby allowing enhanced runoff for the failing ventricle. The balloon should be properly timed to deflate during aortic valve opening, thereby creating a pocket of reduced afterload and thus enhancing the ability of the heart to eject the blood during systole. This action serves to lower the left ventricular end systolic volume. Both of these mechanisms augment left ventricular function and serve in complementary fashion to help those patients with right ventricular dysfunction. It is a common misperception that a balloon pump is not beneficial, or indicated, for patients with right ventricular dysfunction. In clinical practice, patients with right ventricular dysfunction benefit from the diastolic augmentation of coronary blood flow in the right coronary artery. Additional benefit is derived from the reduced left ventricular end-diastolic pressure and left atrial pressure, thereby allowing increased forward flow and decreased afterload for the failing right ventricle.

Complications

Although complications related to balloon pump insertion and use are relatively infrequent, they can be quite serious. The first potential complication can occur during insertion of the balloon pump and involves direct trauma to the arterial insertion site. It is important that insertion occurs relatively high in the thigh in the femoral artery, near the inferior edge of the inguinal ligament. It is possible for a misplaced balloon to shear off one of the major arterial branches. Misplacing the balloon through a smaller-caliber artery may completely occlude the artery and create an ischemic limb. In arteries that are not particularly calcified, it is relatively easy to use the dilator and place the balloon pump without the use of a vascular sheath. This serves to reduce the maximal diameter of obstruction in the artery, and perhaps reduces the potential for thrombus within the artery.

There is also the potential for mishap in both placement and location of intra-aortic balloon pumps. It is important to remember that when the balloon pump is placed as part of a cardiopulmonary bypass procedure, the blood is equally oxygenated in the arterial and venous vessels because of the bypass oxygenator. Additionally, there is zero pulsatile flow at the time of insertion, making it difficult to differentiate artery from vein. This situation has led some to inadvertently placed balloon pumps via the femoral vein into the right atrium. Additionally, hemodynamic instability at the time of insertion may also lead to suboptimal confirmation of balloon pump location. Improper placement can thus lead to impingement of the arch vessels, causing cerebral ischemia or thromboembolism.

In more chronic management of the balloon pump, ranging from several days to weeks or months, infectious complications become more predominant. In addition to meticulous sterile insertion techniques, balloon pumps also require daily attention from the nursing staff. Like any other percutaneously inserted central catheter, they have the potential to become a source of infection. Attention to the insertion site for signs of erythema or purulence and close monitoring of the patient's temperature is mandatory in all patients using a balloon pump. When a patient's hemodynamic status fails to stabilize with balloon pump therapy, a ventricular assist device is the next course of progressive therapy.

VENTRICULAR ASSIST DEVICES

Preoperative Considerations

Indications for ventricular assist devices include unstable hemodynamic measurements and failure to stabilize measurements with other less invasive therapies previously discussed. Common hemodynamic parameters that are indications for a ventricular assist device placement are listed in Table 122.1.

In the preoperative assessment, it is important to determine the likelihood that right ventricular support will be needed as a course of therapy. There are several scoring systems that are commonly used (4–6). Most of these scoring systems center on the calculation of right ventricular stroke work and other hemodynamic indices. Generally, practitioners should use caution if the central venous pressure is greater than the pulmonary capillary wedge pressure, or if the patient's central venous pressure is greater than 20 mm Hg after optimization. Dependence on the right ventricle to support a left-sided device in such instances may prove to be difficult. It is also important to look at the overall illness of the patient. Patients who are very debilitated at the time of implantation, with organ deterioration caused by right heart dysfunction, are more likely to require right-sided support devices. Thus, it is important to take elevated liver enzymes, abnormal coagulation parameters, and renal dysfunction into consideration.

Finally, it is important to select the device based on the goal of implantation. Devices may be implanted as a *bridge to recovery,* a *bridge to transplantation,* or as a *destination therapy.* The lines between bridge to recovery and bridge to transplantation can sometimes become blurred when the neurologic status of patients cannot be defined prior to implantation. These patients have been termed *bridge to decision,* where a short-term device may be appropriate to stabilize hemodynamics until the neurologic status and overall candidacy for transplantation is better elucidated. Finally, in patients who are not candidates for transplantation because of age or end organ dysfunction, consideration of destination therapy may be appropriate. Destination therapy refers to permanent device implantation, intended to remain in use for the duration of the patient's lifetime.

TABLE 122.1

HEMODYNAMIC PARAMETERS SUGGESTING NEED FOR MECHANICAL SUPPORT

Hemodynamic Parameters	Values
Pulmonary capillary wedge pressure	>20 mm Hg
Central venous pressure	>20 mm Hg
Cardiac index	<2.0 L/m^2
Mean arterial pressure	<60 mm Hg

Preparation of the Patient

Before the operative implantation of the ventricular assist device, it is often useful to have a period of volume optimization, or a preoperative "tune up." This is done to ensure that right ventricular function is as well preserved as possible for placement of a left ventricular assist device. This may include diuretic and inotropic therapy. In some cases, where the decision for biventricular support is difficult, a 24- to 48-hour period of intra-aortic balloon pumping may be a useful prognostic indicator. This helps to demonstrate the response of the right ventricular function to a reduced left ventricular end-diastolic pressure (7). During this period of optimization, it is ideal to use an arterial pressure monitor and a pulmonary artery catheter to allow fine tuning of medications and volume status.

It is essential that attention be given to antimicrobial prophylaxis during the period of preoperative optimization. This usually involves selective skin decontamination with Hibiclens scrub (Regent Medical, London, UK). Additionally, Bactroban (mupirocin) is often used to reduce the number of pathogens in the nasal passages of the patient. It may also be useful to use red cell augmentation in patients who are having semi-elective implants, as frequently there may be a 5- to 7-day delay before implantation, during which time erythropoiesis-stimulating drugs, such as erythropoietin, can be combined with iron supplementation to achieve a significant increase of hematocrit.

Classification of Ventricular Assist Devices

Flow Type

The devices may be classified by the type of flow:

- **Pulsatile:** In these devices, the intermittent relocation of a pusher plate or blood sack emits a pulsatile wave similar to that of the natural heart (Fig. 122.5).

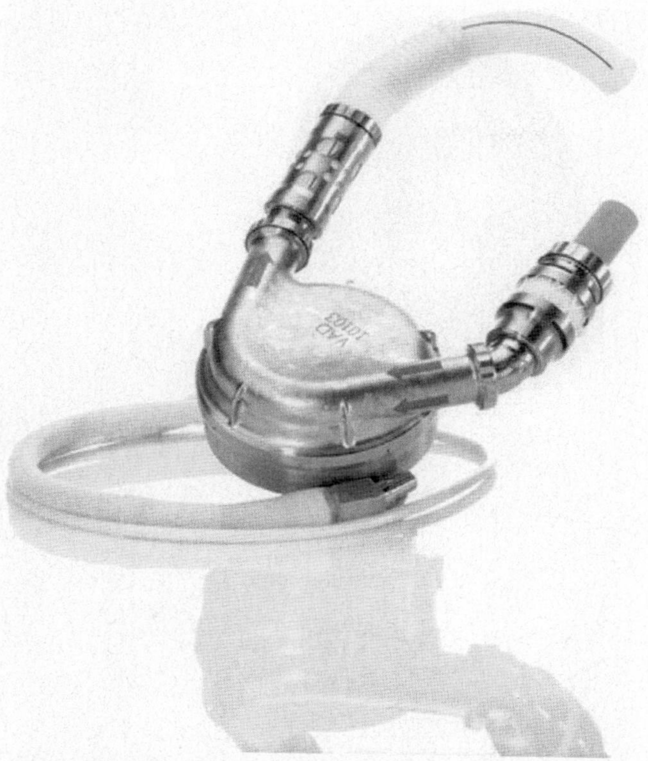

FIGURE 122.5. HeartMate XVE. An example of a pulsatile pusher plate device. (Thoratec Corp, Pleasanton, CA, with permission.)

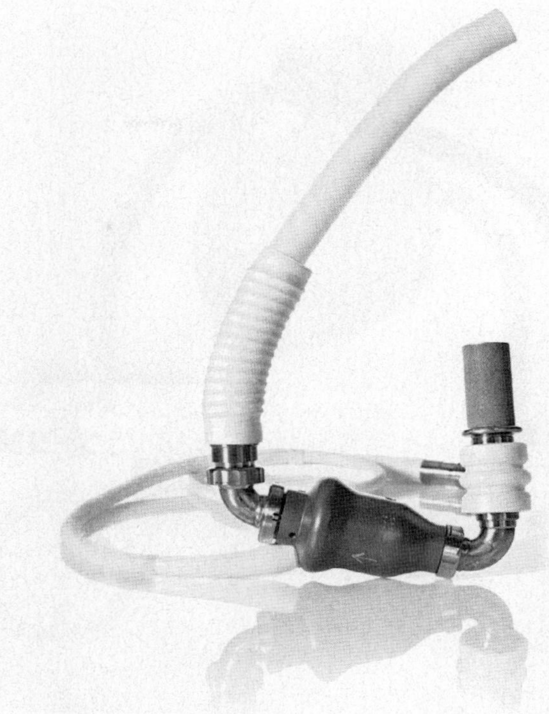

FIGURE 122.6. HeartMate II. An example of an axial flow device. (Thoratec Corp, Pleasanton, CA, with permission.)

- **Axial flow:** The term *nonpulsatile* is frequently applied to these devices, although this is a misnomer. These pumps actually have a central blade that rotates at a rapid rate, similar to a jet engine in an airplane (Fig. 122.6). The native function of the left ventricle does intermittently augment the inflow to the pump, which generates a pulsatile output at appropriate speeds.
- **Centripetal flow:** These pumps have a continuous spinning impeller that generates a flow similar to axial pumps. However, the more advanced pumps, currently in development, may be magnetically levitated to function without bearings (Fig. 122.7).

Mechanism

- **Pneumatic:** These pumps are operated by air, where intermittent external application of compressed gas through a tube to a blood sac emits the pulse of the pump (Fig. 122.8).
- **Electric:** Electric pumps are driven by batteries or AC current via an adapter. They may have the axial flow motor, or the pusher plate-driven motor (Figs. 122.5 and 122.6).

Location

- **Paracorporeal:** These pumps are placed outside of, but in continuity with, the body, usually connected via transcutaneous cannulas that are surgically implanted into the heart (Figs. 122.8 and 122.9).
- **Intracorporeal.** This term typically refers to those pumps that are placed completely within the body with only a drive line exiting the skin (Fig. 122.10). The main pumping mechanism is within the body, rather than external to it.
- **Percutaneous:** *Percutaneous* refers to a small group of pumps that are indicated for extremely short term use and are inserted transcutaneously, either via the femoral vein and then transseptally into the left atrium, or retrograde across the aortic valve (Fig. 122.11).

Potential Duration of Support Based on Device Type

- **Short term:** These devices are placed to resolve immediate hemodynamic instability as either a bridge to recovery, a bridge to decision, or for use during a short-term procedure. Their use is intended for hours to weeks.

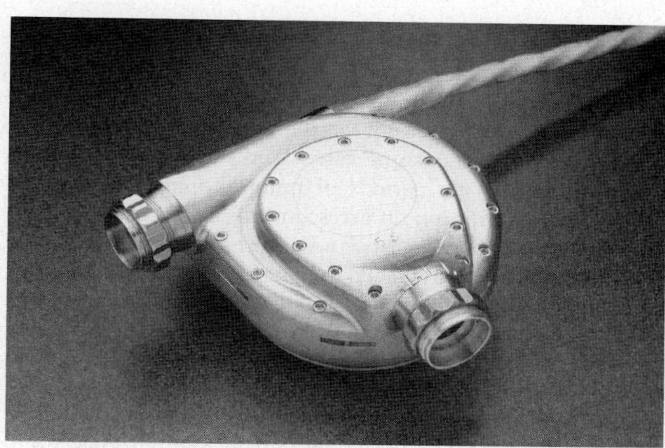

FIGURE 122.7. WorldHeart Levacor. Magnetically levitated, centripetal pump (in development).

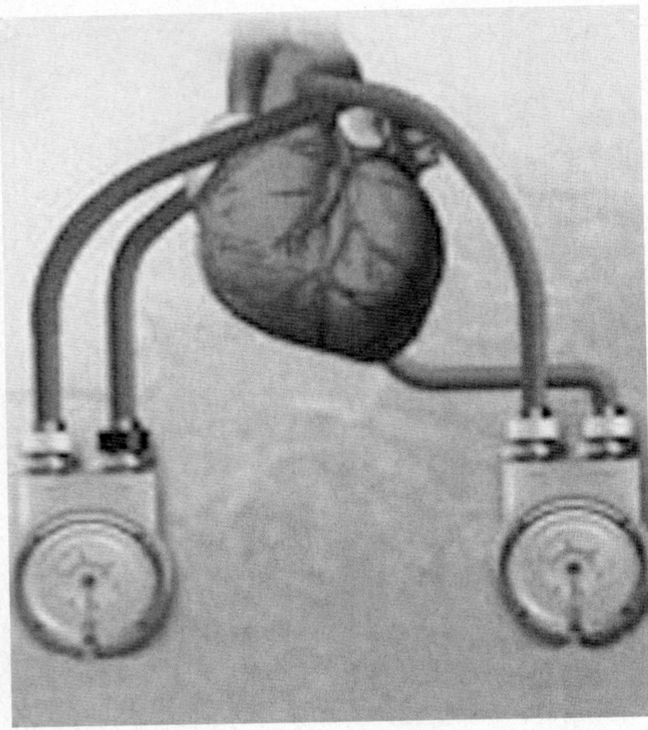

FIGURE 122.8. Thoratec pVAD. An example of pneumatically actuated ventricular assist device as biventricular support.

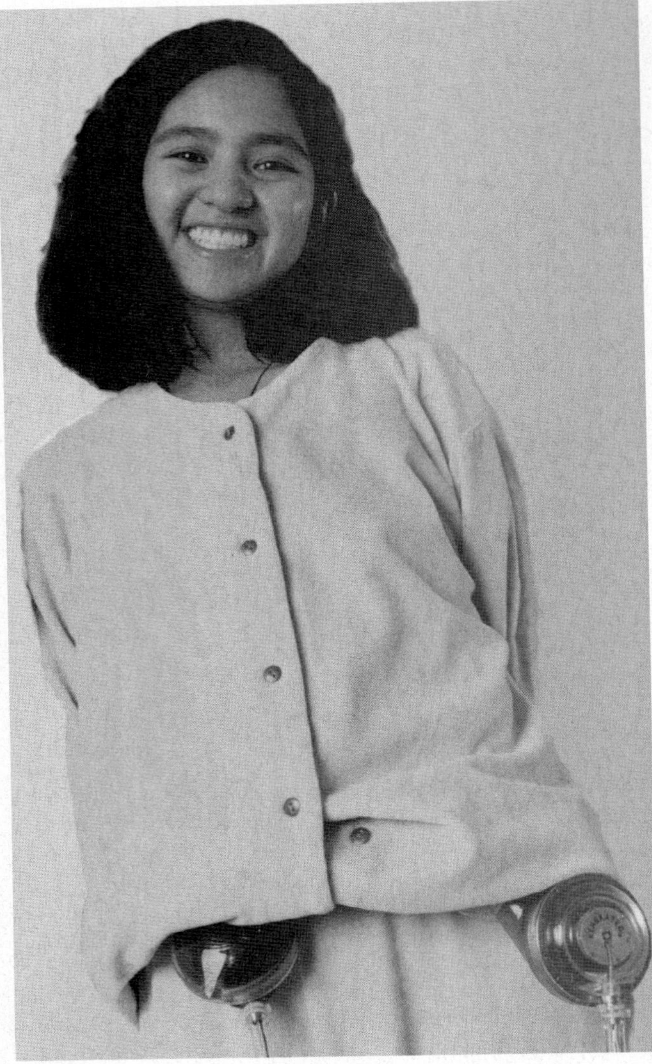

FIGURE 122.9. Picture of Thoratec pVAD. Paracorporeal device.

- **Medium term:** These devices are inserted with the intention of being used to allow recovery of the native heart function, or as a short-term bridge to transplantation. They are indicated for weeks to months.
- **Long term:** These devices are intended to be used for either long-term bridge patients who will require an extended period of time to acquire donor hearts, or for those patients who may potentially have the device as destination therapy.

Important Implications for Potential Emergency Situations while the Patient Is Supported by Ventricular Assist Devices

It is important to understand the physiologic implications of each ventricular assist device, not only while they are in use, but also during periods of unintended pump arrest. One of the critical differentiations between the various types of pumps is the presence or absence of valves and the potential for retrograde flow during periods of pump stoppage. In the devices with valves, a pump arrest merely means that the augmented flow no longer exists, and the presence of valves should prevent retrograde flow. This is a key point to consider during emergency management. The pumps with no valves, such as the axial flow devices, will allow volumes in excess of 1.5 L per minute of retrograde flow during periods of pump arrest. This degree of acute aortic insufficiency will frequently lead to ventricular arrhythmias and cardiovascular collapse. Knowledge of these internal components and working mechanisms leads to proper decision-making during emergencies. Health care providers must know whether the pump can be temporally actuated via an external mechanism (blood sac pumps) by an individual (as opposed to the driver), and whether or not the pump electronics are defibrillation-compatible.

FUTURE DEVICES

Although this chapter is not intended to be comprehensive of all devices currently in development, a few general trends are relevant. Most future generations of these devices are currently being designed to have a longer life span so that they are better suited for destination therapy. Enhanced battery life will allow for greater independence, and a reduced need for transcutaneous attachment to the device, thus reducing infectious complications. Additionally, to extend the life span of these devices, future development will focus on total elimination of bearings and metal-to-metal contact through magnetically levitated bearingless designs. Currently, the primary vulnerabilities of such devices remain issues of anticoagulation and thromboembolic events.

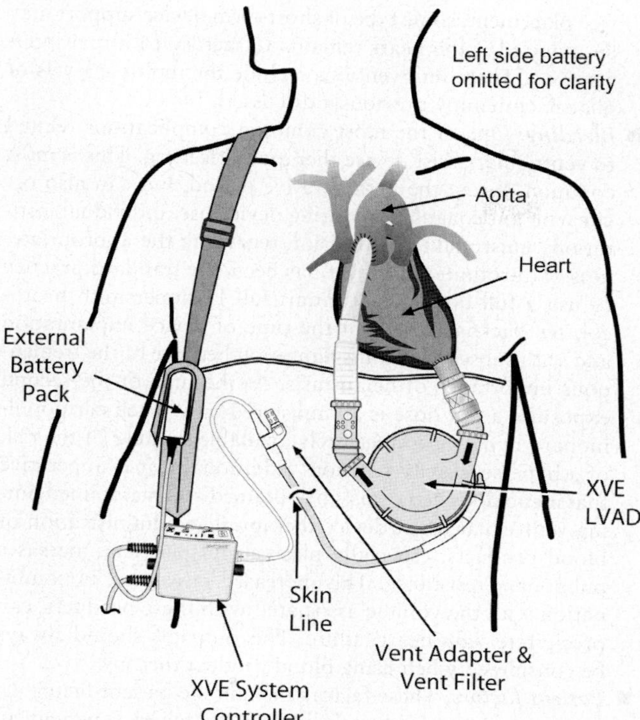

FIGURE 122.10. Picture diagram of HeartMate XVE implanted, an intracorporeal LVAD. (Thoratec Corp, Pleasanton, CA, with permission.)

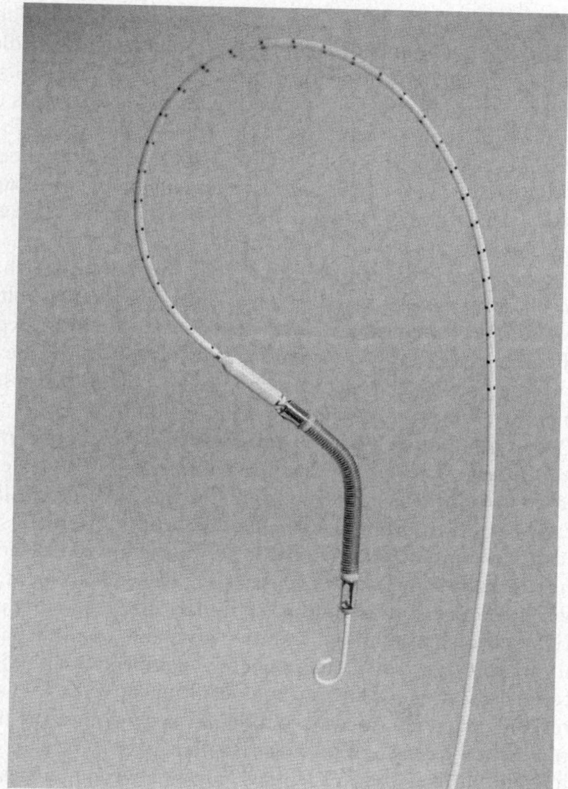

FIGURE 122.11. Impella (Abiomed). Temporary percutaneous ventricular assist device. (Courtesy of Abiomed, Danvers, Mass.)

Management of the Post–Left Ventricular Assist Device Patient

Most ventricular assist device (VAD) centers strive to support patients with left-sided devices only and limit the number of patients who require right ventricular assist devices whenever possible. Patients on single ventricular support are more mobile and more rapidly rehabilitated. Thus, a major focus of post–left ventricular assist device management is the stabilization of right heart function and prevention of right heart failure. To accomplish this goal, the most important factor is the selection of patients who have sustainable right ventricular hemodynamic parameters preoperatively. The previously discussed period of optimization often allows patients with marginal right ventricular function to have significant improvement. This is crucial and ranks just under the requirement that the right heart can support the function of the left ventricular assist device. Additionally, right heart function is frequently supported for some period of time with inotropic therapy. The most commonly used drugs are dobutamine or a phosphodiesterase inhibitor such as milrinone (7). Aggressive attempts are made to lower the pulmonary artery resistance by using nitroso-dilators, such as sodium nitroprusside, nitroglycerin, and inhaled nitric oxide. There is some enthusiasm for the use of inhaled prostacyclin as a less expensive alternative to inhaled nitric oxide (8,9). Other more novel options in evolution include the use of orally available, direct-acting drugs on the pulmonary vasculature, such as the use of sildenafil, a phosphodiesterase type 5 inhibitor (10,11).

After placement of a left ventricular assist device, meticulous care of the drive line site is important to reduce the risk of ascending infection. This typically involves diligent immobilization of the drive line and the use of topical treatments, initially several times a day. In cases where infection is noted at the drive line site despite all efforts, topical treatments can be used with success (12).

Dysfunction and Complications of Left Ventricular Assist Devices

- *Cannula kinking:* In the paracorporeal devices, this is particularly problematic. Shifting of patient position or rolling in the bed can lead to either dislodgement or, more frequently, kinking of the transcutaneous cannula. This will lead to flow alarms and sudden dysfunction of the device, and can usually be addressed by simply removing the kink in the cannula. Often, centers have found it beneficial to keep a folded towel under the device to keep it off the patient's skin and to keep the cannulas straight. With the intracorporeal devices, this problem is usually secondary to device migration, either from chest closure in the operating room or from postoperative ambulation. With intracorporeal devices, this frequently requires reoperation for adjustment of the device.
- *Thrombosis and embolism:* The Achilles heel of all device therapy remains the poorly understood human coagulation system and the effects of foreign bodies in the bloodstream. Depending on the specific device selected and the type of

valves within the device, variable amounts of anticoagulation are recommended by the manufacturer. Regardless of the anticoagulation therapy used, thrombosis, embolism, and bleeding events are a concern with all devices. It is important to treat patients with any new symptom, such as abdominal pain or a cold leg, as if it were a thromboembolic event. With appropriate management of anticoagulation and diligent patient care, these events are relatively infrequent.

- *Mechanical device issues:* The devices themselves may have mechanical issues related to valve dysfunction or problems with either bearings or motor wear. These are addressed in the materials supplied by the manufacturers. All of the devices require some type of ongoing surveillance and assessment for wear and potential mechanical failure.
- *Patent foramen ovale and hypoxemia following left ventricular assist placement:* Patients need to be carefully screened in the operating room with transesophageal echocardiography and provocation maneuvers during a bubble test to identify a patent foramen ovale. With the altered hemodynamics following left ventricular assist device placement, the left atrial pressure is suddenly dramatically lower than the right atrial pressure. This allows even the smallest patent foramen ovale to become clinically significant, with right-to-left shunting occurring and resulting in hypoxemia. A recent report described partial digital occlusion of the main pulmonary artery as a provocative maneuver to be used during the bubble study (13). Such a maneuver enhances the intraoperative detection of patent foramen ovale during device placement. A patent foramen ovale discovered in the operating room prior to placement of the ventricular assist device and those discovered after the device is activated in the operating room should be closed at that time. There are some reports of patients being treated with percutaneous device closure, when discovered as a cause of persistent hypoxemia several hours or days following device placement (14).
- *Right heart failure and the potential need for a right ventricular assist device:* One of the greatest concerns when implanting a left ventricular assist device is the potential need for right ventricular assist device therapy. This risk can be minimized by careful adherence to the post–left ventricular assist device management protocols discussed earlier in the chapter. However, despite best efforts, a small percentage of patients will still develop refractory right heart failure necessitating device therapy. If this occurs in the operating room, it is possible to use temporary support of the right heart while the cardiopulmonary bypass cannulas are still in place. This is done by using a Y off the arterial line and clamping the line to the aorta, thus redirecting blood flow from the pump directly into the pulmonary artery via a separate cannula. This sets up a circuit in which the blood is drawn from the right atrium, oxygenated by the cardiopulmonary bypass circuit, and then returned to the pulmonary artery. The effect of superoxygenated blood on the pulmonary artery may result in a reduction in pulmonary resistance over several minutes and obviate the need for a right ventricular assist device. This is often referred to as a *Berlin bridge* and may be a beneficial intermediate step before placing a right ventricular assist device when right ventricular dysfunction is apparent in the operating room. When right heart dysfunction and failure develop several days after a left ventricular assist device placement, some type of short-term device support may be required if the heart remains refractory to initial interventions. These interventions include the multiple levels of pharmacotherapy previously discussed.
- *Bleeding:* One of the most common complications related to ventricular assist device therapy is bleeding. This is most common during the perioperative period, but can also occur with anticoagulation during device use. Individual institutions must make the decision regarding the appropriateness of aprotinin therapy. It has been our standard practice to use a full dose of aprotinin (full Hammersmith protocol, see package insert) at the time of device implantation and with subsequent transplantation because of the tremendous importance of hemostasis. At the time of the second exposure, a test dose is administered only when cardiopulmonary bypass is immediately available because of the risk of a hypersensitivity reaction. Additionally, it is imperative that meticulous hemostasis be obtained and maintained during ventricular assist device therapy. The administration of blood products, especially plasma and platelets, increases pulmonary resistance. This increased resistance, in combination with the volume associated with these products, can precipitate right heart failure. This outcome should always be considered when using blood product therapy.
- *Patient factors:* These factors include the patient factors of devices such as accidental disconnects, where a patient, in spite of optimal education from physicians and VAD staff, simultaneously disconnects all power sources to their device, resulting in pump stoppage. Additionally, traction injuries are common. Particular attention should be given to entering and exiting vehicles and traversing through narrow doorways, as these seem to be particularly problematic for the drive lines of ventricular assist devices.

TRANSITION FROM ICU TO THE FLOOR AND OUTPATIENT MANAGEMENT

It is beyond the scope of this chapter to discuss personnel management. However, dedicated staff members are essential and must be thoroughly trained to deal with outpatient management of ventricular assist devices. Communication and current knowledge of the device is paramount to the success of the ventricular assist device program. This requires the establishment of community resources and alternate caregiver training so that there is redundancy at every level of the system. Although minor problems with these patients and their devices are not uncommon, most are easily handled if the support staff are prepared and adequately trained. Mechanical assist devices can enhance not only the quantity, but also the quality of life for these patients.

References

1. Marcu CB, Donohue TJ, Ferneini A, et al. Intraaortic balloon pump insertion through the subclavian artery. Subclavian artery insertion of IABP. *Heart Lung Circ.* 2006;15(2):148–150.
2. Kaplan LJ, Weiman DS, Langan N, et al. Safe intraaortic balloon pump placement through the ascending aorta using transesophageal ultrasound. *Ann Thorac Surg.* 1992;54(2):374–375.

3. Meldrum-Hanna WG, Deal CW, Ross DE. Complications of ascending aortic intraaortic balloon pump cannulation. *Ann Thorac Surg.* 1985;40(3):241–244.
4. Fukamachi K, McCarthy PM, Smedira NG, et al. Preoperative risk factors for right ventricular failure after implantable left ventricular assist device insertion. *Ann Thorac Surg.* 1999;68(6):2181–2184.
5. Kavarana MN, Pessin-Minsley MS, Urtecho J, et al. Right ventricular dysfunction and organ failure in left ventricular assist device recipients: a continuing problem. *Ann Thorac Surg.* 2002;73(3):745–750.
6. Ochiai Y, McCarthy PM, Smedira NG, et al. Predictors of severe right ventricular failure after implantable left ventricular assist device insertion: analysis of 245 patients. *Circulation.* 2002;106(12 Suppl 1):I198–1202.
7. Klodell CT, Staples ED, Aranda JM Jr, et al. Managing the post-left ventricular assist device patient. *Congest Heart Fail.* 2006;12(1):41–45.
8. Fattouch K, Sbraga F, Bianco G, et al. Inhaled prostacyclin, nitric oxide, and nitroprusside in pulmonary hypertension after mitral valve replacement. *J Card Surg.* 2005;20(2):171–176.
9. Muzaffar S, Shukla N, Angelini GD, et al. Inhaled prostacyclin is safe, effective, and affordable in patients with pulmonary hypertension, right-heart dysfunction, and refractory hypoxemia after cardiothoracic surgery. *J Thorac Cardiovasc Surg.* 2004;128(6):949–950.
10. Trachte AL, Lobato EB, Urdaneta F, et al. Oral sildenafil reduces pulmonary hypertension after cardiac surgery. *Ann Thorac Surg.* 2005;79(1):194–197; discussion 197.
11. Lobato EB, Beaver T, Muehlschlegel J, et al. Treatment with phosphodiesterase inhibitors type III and V: milrinone and sildenafil is an effective combination during thromboxane-induced acute pulmonary hypertension. *Br J Anaesth.* 2006;96(3):317–322.
12. Baradarian S, Stahovich M, Krause S, et al. Case series: clinical management of persistent mechanical assist device driveline drainage using vacuum-assisted closure therapy. *Asaio J.* 2006;52(3):354–356.
13. Majd RE, Kavarana MN, Bouvette M, et al. Improved technique to diagnose a patent foramen ovale during left ventricular assist device insertion. *Ann Thorac Surg.* 2006;82(5):1917–1918.
14. Kavarana MN, Rahman FA, Recto MR, et al. Transcatheter closure of patent foramen ovale after left ventricular assist device implantation: intraoperative decision making. *J Heart Lung Transplant.* 2005;24(9):1445.

CHAPTER 123 ■ VALVULAR HEART DISEASE

KATHIRVEL SUBRAMANIAM • JEAN-PIERRE YARED

IMMEDIATE CONCERNS

Critically ill patients with valvular heart disease (VHD) presenting to the intensive care unit (ICU) fall into three primary categories: (a) patients who are critically ill as a result of acute onset, newly acquired VHD; (b) patients with exacerbation or complications of pre-existing VHD; or (c) patients with concomitant VHD who are critically ill from other causes. Most patients present with instability secondary to left heart valvular disease, which, if severe, impairs right heart function, but in patients, right heart valvular lesions can be the predominant problem. Hemodynamic consequences of decompensated left-sided valvular lesions include diminished cardiac output with tissue hypoperfusion, and pulmonary venous hypertension with pulmonary edema that, if severe, leads to pulmonary arterial hypertension and right heart failure. Isolated right-sided valvular lesions present with reduced cardiac output and systemic venous congestion. Management is determined by the type of lesion and its hemodynamic consequences, and is modified by coexisting derangements. Noninvasive assessment of the hemodynamic derangement by history, physical exam, chest radiography, or transthoracic echocardiography (TTE) is essential, but useful information may also be derived from invasive measurements such as arterial blood pressure, cardiac filling pressures, cardiac output, mixed venous oxygen saturation, and calculated cardiovascular variables such as left ventricular stroke work index, systemic vascular resistance, and pulmonary vascular resistance. Invasive monitoring is particularly useful for guiding and assessing the results of management.

Patients with life-threatening valvular disease generally present to the critical care unit with one or more manifestations of congestive heart failure that require immediate stabilization. The most common initial interventions are aimed at controlling circulatory shock and respiratory failure. Two levels of diagnosis must then be established. The first level involves defining the type and severity of valvular heart disease. The second level of diagnosis involves determination of acute precipitating events in the patient's deterioration. These can include cardiac problems such as acute changes in the valvular lesion ranging from obstruction to severe insufficiency, endocarditis, myocardial infarction, and cardiac dysrhythmias to systemic problems impacting cardiac performance such as uncontrolled hypertension, noncompliance with diet or medication regimens, infection, pulmonary embolism, endocrine abnormalities—particularly diabetic ketoacidosis or hyperthyroid crisis—and acute renal failure.

Once both levels of diagnosis have been made, an estimate of the reversibility of the hemodynamic defect is possible, and plans for management can be developed. Specific management decisions depend on the lesion, its inherent physiology, and the presence of complicating factors.

CRITICAL ILLNESS CAUSED BY VALVULAR HEART DISEASE

Although valvular disease is often known from the patient's history, detection by physical examination may be made difficult by environmental noise, pulmonary rhonchi, or other factors. Further, with severe aortic or mitral stenosis and a failing left ventricle, cardiac murmurs may be unimpressive or even absent. Electrocardiography frequently reveals the existence of concomitant ischemic heart disease, left ventricular hypertrophy, atrial abnormalities, arrhythmias, or right ventricular hypertrophy. Portable plain film chest radiography can be invaluable in revealing pulmonary venous or arterial hypertension, pulmonary edema, pleural effusions, and lung parenchymal abnormalities, and in allowing evaluation of the cardiac contour. Because of the distortion produced by anteroposterior supine radiographs, every effort should be made to obtain sitting 183-cm (72-inch) posteroanterior radiographs as well as lateral radiographs when the patient's condition allows. Early performance of echocardiography is imperative in patients with unexplained heart failure. If the quality of the transthoracic echocardiogram is not optimal, transesophageal echocardiography should be performed.

CRITICAL ILLNESS IN PATIENTS WITH UNDERLYING VALVULAR HEART DISEASE

Patients with underlying valvular disease may become critically ill from noncardiac causes. The effect of valvular disease on the management plan is determined by the presence of other cardiac abnormalities, the severity of the physiologic derangements, and the resultant hemodynamic burden. Because these patients present with other illnesses, valvular disease is often detected only by the discovery of cardiac murmurs on physical examination, valve calcification or cardiac contour abnormalities on chest radiograph, or unexplained evidence of left ventricular hypertrophy or atrial abnormality on electrocardiogram (ECG). When abnormalities are suspected, echocardiography is the most useful diagnostic tool for defining the type and extent of the valvular abnormality.

Once the valvular abnormality is defined, its impact on the management plan can be determined by consideration of its severity and specific hemodynamic characteristics (see below). All valve lesions share several common considerations. Antibiotic prophylaxis for endocarditis is important since community-acquired, as well as nosocomial, infections are common in critically ill patients, particularly when invasive procedures are undertaken or indwelling catheters are inserted.

Fever and increased work of breathing may increase oxygen demand to a degree not well tolerated, and should be treated vigorously. Sinus tachycardia, atrial fibrillation with rapid ventricular response, and paroxysmal atrial tachycardia reduce left ventricular filling time and may lead to hemodynamic deterioration. They should be aggressively treated, particularly in patients with severely stenotic lesions. Treatment of dysrhythmias includes correction of electrolyte abnormalities, judicious use of digoxin, and intermittent or constant infusion of β-adrenergic blockers, calcium channel blockers, amiodarone, or other antidysrhythmic drugs. Hemodynamically compromised patients who do not promptly respond to the above measures may need urgent cardioversion.

CRITICAL ILLNESSES WITH SPECIFIC VALVULAR ABNORMALITIES

Aortic Stenosis

Etiology

Aortic stenosis (AS) is the most common primary valvular heart disease. Stenosis of the normal tricuspid aortic valve caused by pathology similar to coronary artery disease is the usual cause. A fibrocalcific process may involve the bicuspid aortic valve, though the process is slower. Rheumatic aortic valve disease, though rare in industrialized societies, may be seen along with mitral valve disease.

Hemodynamics

Obstruction to forward blood flow causes compensatory concentric hypertrophy of the left ventricle. Hypertrophy decreases the wall stress, but comes at the price of increased oxygen demand and dependence of ventricular filling on left atrial contractions. As the hypertrophy increases, subendocardial ischemia predisposes these patients to ventricular dysrhythmias. Decrease in forward flow with exercise and associated peripheral vasodilatation can cause syncope. Sudden death has been reported in patients with AS. Later in the course, the ventricles dilate and cardiac function is maintained by Frank-Starling mechanisms. The triad of symptoms—syncope, angina, and dyspnea—indicates severe AS and requires surgical intervention. Clinical signs of common valve lesions are noted in Table 123.1.

Diagnosis

Common features on ECG include left ventricular hypertrophy with strain pattern, left bundle branch block, and left atrial hypertrophy (biphasic P waves in precordial lead V_1). Chest radiography may reveal a boot-shaped heart, calcification of the aortic valve, poststenotic dilatation of the aorta, and pulmonary venous congestion. Echocardiography is the principal modality for confirming the diagnosis of AS (Fig. 123.1); the severity of AS is determined by peak gradients across the aortic valve and calculation of valve area (Table 123.2). It is important to recognize that the gradients will be lower with severe aortic stenosis if the flow across the valve is reduced by hypovolemia or by poor left ventricular function. Echocardiography also provides information about left ventricular function. Patients with AS may have preserved systolic function but with significant diastolic dysfunction. Diastolic dysfunction predisposes these patients to pulmonary edema. Coronary angiography is indicated in patients with aortic stenosis before surgery to rule out associated coronary artery disease (CAD).

Therapeutic Considerations

Patients with AS may require ICU admission because of acute cardiogenic shock, pulmonary edema, severe angina, ventricular dysrhythmias, or, less commonly, atrial fibrillation and systemic embolization.

Drugs

Drugs commonly used to treat these conditions carry significant risks in patients with AS. β-Blockers, calcium channel blockers, and other antidysrhythmics should be used with caution as patients with AS are sensitive to drugs causing myocardial depression. Pulmonary congestion should be relieved by careful administration of diuretics, digitalis, and nitroglycerin. The use of diuretics and nitroglycerin, however, may result in inadequate preload. Digitalis carries the risk of dysrhythmias. Increased left ventricular mass and intracavitary systolic pressure increase oxygen demands, thereby decreasing the patient's tolerance to vasodilatation and tachycardia. Angiotensin-converting enzyme (ACE) inhibitors and other vasodilators such as nitroprusside may precipitate syncope or even sudden death in severe AS, and are relatively contraindicated.

TABLE 123.1

CLINICAL SIGNS IN VALVULAR HEART DISEASE

	Aortic stenosis	Aortic regurgitation	Acute mitral regurgitation	Chronic mitral regurgitation	Mitral stenosis
General signs	Nothing remarkable	Look for Marfan syndrome, ankylosing spondylitis, or seronegative arthropathies	Tachypnea, circulatory shock	Tachypnea	Mitral facies (malar flush), tachypnea, peripheral cyanosis
Pulse	Small volume (parvus) and late peaking (tardus)	Water-hammer pulse, wide pulse pressure	Sinus tachycardia	Irregularly irregular in AF	Reduced or normal volume, irregularly irregular in AF
Neck and JVP	Prominent a wave	Prominent carotid pulsations (Corrigan sign)	Prominent a wave	Absent a wave in AF	Prominent a wave in PHT, absent a wave in AF
Precordium	Sustained, nondisplaced or slightly displaced apical impulse, palpable S_4, systolic thrill at the base and at carotids	Diffuse, hyperdynamic and displaced apical impulse	Nondisplaced hyperdynamic apical impulse, systolic thrill	Hyperdynamic, inferolateral displaced apical impulse, parasternal heave (LAE)	Tapping apical impulse (palpable S_1), palpable P_2 and parasternal heave in PHT, diastolic thrill rarely
AUSCULTATION					
S_1	Soft	Soft in acute AR	Normal/soft	Soft	Loud
S_2	Narrow split or reverse split S_2, absent A_2 in severe AS	P_2 loud in acute AR	Accentuated P_2/wide paradoxical split	Normal P_2/wide paradoxical split	P_2 loud in PHT
S_3/S_4	Prominent S_4	S_3 heard	Present/present	Present/absent	
Clicks and added sounds	Systolic ejection click indicates mobile valve			Mid systolic click in MVP	Opening snap
Murmur	Systolic soft musical murmur, decreasing intensity in advanced disease	High-pitched, long diastolic murmur in chronic versus low-pitched short diastolic murmur in acute AR along left sternal border, diastolic murmur of early mitral diastolic closure	Early systolic loud radiating toward base (anterior directed jet) or axilla (posterior directed jet)	Holosystolic, soft or harsh and radiating toward axilla/back, late systolic murmur in MVP	Mid-diastolic murmur with late diastolic accentuation best heard at apex

AF, Atrial fibrillation; PHT, pulmonary hypertension; LAE, left atrial enlargement; MVP, mitral valve prolapse; AR, aortic regurgitation; AS, aortic stenosis.

Undesirable hemodynamic effects of sedative drugs such as propofol, benzodiazepines, and narcotics should also be considered. Propofol can cause significant vasodilatation and hypotension, and therefore should be avoided in patients with fixed cardiac output. Narcotics can blunt the hypertensive sympathetic responses without significant myocardial depression and are usually the agents of choice.

Fluids

Fluid is administered with extreme caution in patients with AS. Patients with diastolic dysfunction, even when systolic function and ejection fraction are preserved, are extremely sensitive to fluids and can develop pulmonary edema. Filling pressures may need to be monitored with a pulmonary artery catheter (PAC) in such critical situations.

Monitoring

Hemodynamic stabilization with drugs and fluids should be carried out with careful monitoring of arterial pressure and cardiac filling pressures. Normal central venous pressure (CVP) does not ensure adequate filling pressures in patients with a stiff left ventricle. Placement of a PAC, while helpful, is not without risks, as it may precipitate malignant dysrhythmias and sudden deterioration. However, the PAC can provide useful

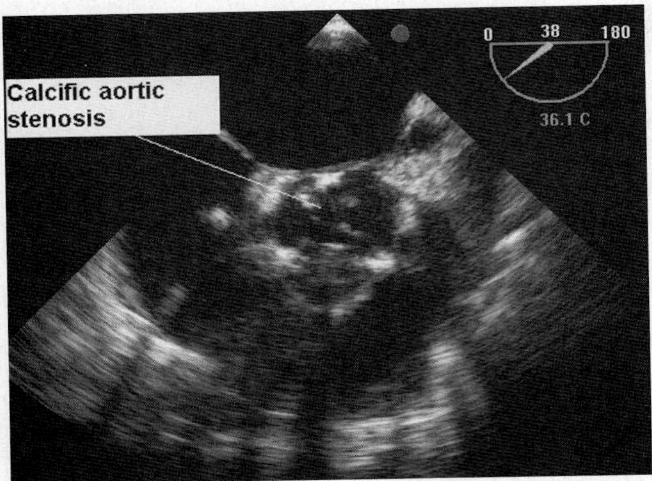

FIGURE 123.1. Transesophageal echocardiographic appearance of severe calcific aortic stenosis.

information about left ventricular filling pressures, cardiac output, and mixed venous oxygenation, and can be used, if needed, for transvenous pacing. It is intuitive that the risks must be weighed against the potential benefits when PAC use is considered. It is important to note that pulmonary capillary wedge pressure (PCWP) can underestimate left ventricular end-diastolic pressure (LVEDP) in patients with markedly reduced ventricular compliance; echocardiography can provide useful information in such situations. Monitoring for ischemia with continuous ECG leads V_5 and II should be carried out in all patients with AS, as they are vulnerable to ischemia. However, the ECG manifestations of left ventricular hypertrophy may make detection of ischemic changes more difficult.

Hemodynamic Goals

Left ventricular hypertrophy renders the atrial contraction—and thus sinus rhythm and preload—more crucial for diastolic filling. Atrial fibrillation should be reversed with prompt cardioversion and initiation of antidysrhythmic therapy with amiodarone and/or β-blocking drugs. Procainamide may also be used, but carries an increased risk of myocardial depression and hypotension. If cardioversion is unsuccessful, pharmacologic control of the ventricular rate is essential. It is imperative to avoid tachycardia, which will decrease the diastolic ventricular filling time and increase the risk of ischemia. Severe bradycardia also should be avoided because severe aortic stenosis results in a fixed stroke volume, therefore potentially reducing cardiac output. Adequate preload should be maintained, and one must recognize that afterload reduction may be hazardous as it can impair coronary perfusion pressure. Severe myocardial dysfunction with low blood pressure and ischemia may require administration of inotropes. Maintenance of adequate coronary perfusion pressure by vasopressors such as phenylephrine may be necessary in patients with optimized volume and myocardial contractile status. Patients who are refractory to medical management may benefit from insertion of an intra-aortic balloon counterpulsation pump (IABP) to improve coronary perfusion pressure.

TABLE 123.2

ECHOCARDIOGRAPHIC ASSESSMENT OF AORTIC STENOSIS (AS)

	Mild AS	Moderate AS	Severe AS
Valve area (cm^2)	More than 1.5	1–1.5	Less than 1
Mean transvalvular gradient (mm Hg)	Less than 25	25–40	Greater than 40
Jet velocity of blood flow across the valve (m/s)	Less than 3	3–4	Greater than 4

Definitive Therapy

Considering the unfavorable natural history of AS, any ICU patient with severe AS who continues to deteriorate despite medical therapy should be seen by a cardiologist and a cardiac surgeon for possible balloon valvotomy or open valve replacement. Balloon valvotomy affords temporary improvement in transvalvular gradient—usually with restenosis in about 6 months—and may relieve symptoms in some patients, thus serving as a bridge to definitive surgery. Balloon valvotomy is often very effective for young adults and adolescents with bicuspid valves, although it carries a mortality of 10% in patients with calcific AS (1).

Aortic Regurgitation

Patients with aortic regurgitation (AR) may present to the critical care physician either because of decompensated chronic AR or due to acute onset of severe regurgitation.

Etiology

Acute AR results from infective endocarditis, with leaflet perforation, vegetations, or perivalvular fistula, and aortic dissection extending into the aortic annulus or aortic root, and from trauma, with avulsions of the annulus and tears of the cusps. Severe, acute hypertension may also cause sudden onset of AR that often reverses after control of hypertension. The causes of chronic AR are diverse; the disease may directly involve the valve or the aortic root. Primary valvular diseases include congenital bicuspid valve, prolapse of aortic cusp, rheumatic heart disease, calcific degenerative disease, connective tissue diseases, and subacute bacterial endocarditis. Diseases associated with aortic root dilatation include systemic hypertension, Marfan disease (Fig. 123.2), Ehlers-Danlos disease, granulomatous diseases of the aorta, senile and cystic medial degeneration, annuloaortic ectasia, and syphilis.

Hemodynamics

In chronic AR, the left ventricle (LV) dilates and hypertrophies when subjected to volume overload. This keeps wall stresses in check and maintains normal forward stroke volume. As the disease progresses and the compensatory limit is reached, the wall stress begins to rise and systolic function deteriorates, with decreasing forward stroke volume as well as increasing LV end-diastolic volume (LVEDV) and LVEDP, resulting in symptoms of heart failure. The presence of symptoms, systolic dysfunction, and an increase in end-systolic dimensions indicate severe

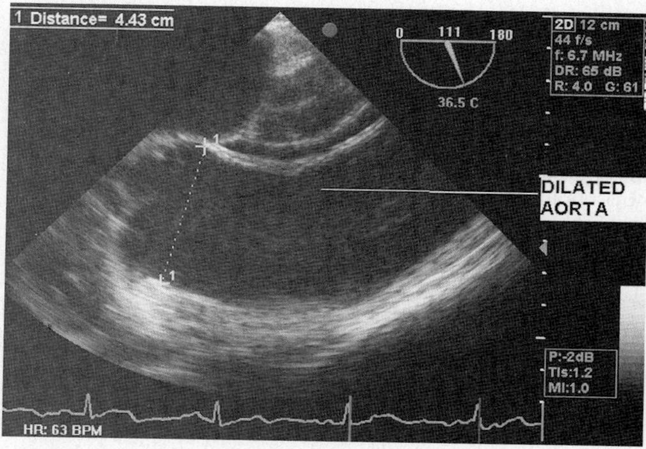

FIGURE 123.2. Dilatation of aortic root and ascending aorta by transesophageal echocardiography in a patient with Marfan disease.

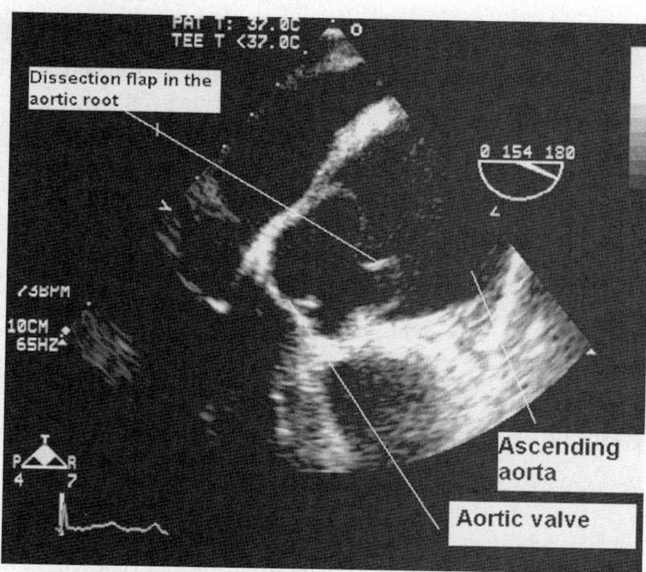

FIGURE 123.3. Aortic dissection intimal flap involving aortic root.

and decompensated AR. During the relatively asymptomatic phase, the patient develops symptoms at a rate of 3.7% per year. In acute AR, the LV is subject to a sudden increase in volume, with no opportunity for a compensatory increase in compliance and eccentric hypertrophy to occur. Without these adaptations, the increase in end-diastolic pressures causes pulmonary venous congestion and pulmonary edema. The severity is dependent on the regurgitant orifice size, duration of diastole—as the degree of AR increases with bradycardia—and the diastolic pressure gradient between aorta and left ventricle. Thus, the patient with acute AR may present with heart failure if the AR is severe, or the initiating event—aortic dissection, trauma, or endocarditis—may dominate if AR is mild.

Diagnosis

An ECG is performed to rule out ischemic heart disease in situations of acute AR. The chest radiograph will reveal cardiomegaly in chronic AR or pulmonary congestion with a normal-sized heart in acute AR. TTE is performed to define the mechanism and severity of AR. Transesophageal echocardiography (TEE) is useful in patients with limited TTE windows. TEE defines the nature of perivalvular pathology (e.g., an abscess) better than TTE. An acute aortic dissection may be diagnosed with high sensitivity and specificity with TEE. Other techniques such as computerized tomographic (CT) scanning, magnetic resonance imaging (MRI), and aortography have been used. Each modality has its own advantages and disadvantages (2). TEE is clearly superior to MRI and CT scanning to characterize the valve pathology in cases of acute dissection, and obviates the need for aortography (Fig. 123.3). Coronary angiography can rule out ischemic heart disease before surgery in chronic AR, but is rarely indicated before emergency surgery in acute AR. Echocardiography may also be helpful to rule out the coronary artery involvement in dissections.

Therapeutic Considerations

Patients with acute AR are generally ill enough to require ICU admission. While medical therapy may allow patients with mild acute AR to reach a chronic compensated state, emergency aortic valve replacement is almost always indicated in a patient with severe acute AR after medical stabilization.

The principle of therapy is to optimize cardiac output and systemic perfusion, reduce pulmonary venous congestion, and initiate therapy for any underlying disorder. Invasive monitoring is initiated and volume is optimized. Tachycardia is beneficial in maintaining cardiac output, and decreases the regurgitant fraction by decreasing the duration of diastole. β-Blockers are avoided in acute severe AR before surgery, as it inhibits compensatory tachycardia and may precipitate circulatory failure. Hypertension and increased afterload are to be avoided; afterload reduction is indicated with vasodilators such as nitroprusside. Inotropic therapy is advised only in patients with depressed systolic function. The hemodynamic response to therapy is an increased cardiac output with reduction of filling pressures. An IABP is absolutely contraindicated in patients with AR, as it will increase the regurgitant fraction.

In contrast to other causes of AR, inotropic therapy is avoided in patients with aortic dissection, as it occurs as a result of long-standing, poorly controlled hypertension or trauma. In both situations, left ventricular contractility is preserved and inotropes are not indicated. β-Adrenergic blockade may be initiated to reduce the velocity of LV ejection and aortic wall stress, therefore preventing extension of the aortic dissection or aortic rupture. In patients with chronic AR who present with an acute decompensation, a search should be made for the precipitating cause, with particular attention to possible infectious endocarditis. Most patients stabilize with medical therapy, but early elective surgery should be considered, as the outlook for medically treated symptomatic patients is poor. Decompensated patients who do not improve with aggressive medical therapy should undergo emergency valve replacement. Mortality with medical therapy alone in this group approaches 100%, while many moribund patients will survive with surgery.

Mitral Regurgitation

The mitral valve apparatus is composed of the valve leaflets, mitral annulus, chorda tendineae, papillary muscles, and adjacent

TABLE 123.3

FUNCTIONAL CLASSIFICATION OF MITRAL REGURGITATION (MR)

Type of MR	Pathology	Disease
Type I	Normal motion of leaflets	Endocarditis (leaflet perforation) or various etiologies causing left ventricular dysfunction (annular dilatation)
Type II	Increased leaflet motion with free edge of the leaflet traveling above the plane of the annulus; this is due to chordal elongation or rupture, papillary muscle rupture	Degenerative myxomatous valve disease
Type IIIA	Restricted leaflet motion during diastole and systole	Rheumatic heart disease
Type IIIB	Restricted leaflet motion during systole, papillary muscle displacement	Ischemic or dilated cardiomyopathy

cardiac chambers, namely the left atrium and left ventricle. Any disruption in the integrity of the mitral valve apparatus may result in regurgitation. One of the major breakthroughs in the management of mitral regurgitation was the functional classification of mitral regurgitation (MR) by Carpentier in early 1980s (3) (Table 123.3).

Etiology

An acute presentation of MR to the critical care physician usually results from infective endocarditis with leaflet perforations, vegetations, and perivalvular leaks; connective tissue or myxomatous disorders (e.g., chordal rupture); and ischemic heart disease—infarction and rupture of papillary muscles, or transient papillary muscle dysfunction due to ischemia. Acute rheumatic mitral valvulitis as the cause of mitral regurgitation is less common today.

Hemodynamics

Chronic MR leads to adaptation of the left ventricle by dilatation and eccentric hypertrophy. Over many years of increasing regurgitant volume, systolic function may fail, resulting in decreased ejection fraction (EF) and pulmonary hypertension. Left atrial (LA) dilatation leads to atrial fibrillation. In the absence of a precipitating event such as an infection or a second hemodynamic abnormality, patients with chronic MR are rarely critically ill on presentation. In acute MR, on the other hand, the regurgitant volume is mainly ejected into the noncompliant left atrium. As a result, left atrial pressure increases, which is transmitted to the pulmonary venous system, resulting in pulmonary edema. Sudden volume overload increases the burden on the LV and it fails. Cardiac output falls and systemic vascular resistance rises, which further increases the regurgitant fraction. Patients may present with acute onset of fatigue, dyspnea, and chest pain, or can be admitted with pulmonary edema and circulatory shock, depending on the etiology. The differences in clinical signs between acute and chronic forms of MR are given in Table 123.1.

Diagnosis

The ECG may show atrial fibrillation, left ventricular hypertrophy, and right ventricular strain, while the chest radiograph may show cardiomegaly, indicating pre-existing heart disease. Pulmonary venous congestion and/or edema with a normal-sized heart indicate acute MR. An ECG may suggest the etiology in cases of ischemic MR.

Echocardiography remains the standard for the diagnosis of mitral regurgitation. TTE is easy, safe, and quick, and can be performed at the bedside. The mechanism and type of MR should be defined. Qualitative and quantitative assessment of MR can be done by color and spectral Doppler methods. Finally, the suitability for repair and left ventricular function should be assessed. TEE may provide better detail because of superior resolution and, further, has a significant advantage in that it allows definition of anatomic details of the mitral valve apparatus and mechanism of MR; the severity of MR is better evaluated by TEE (Fig. 123.4). Indices of left ventricular function such as EF are unreliable in the presence of severe MR. EF in MR is increased when contractility is normal. Normal EF indicates a significant loss of myocardial function; when EF is reduced to 50% or less, advanced myocardial dysfunction is generally present (4). The American Heart Association/American College of Cardiology (AHA/ACC) guidelines recommend medical treatment when EF is less than 30% and

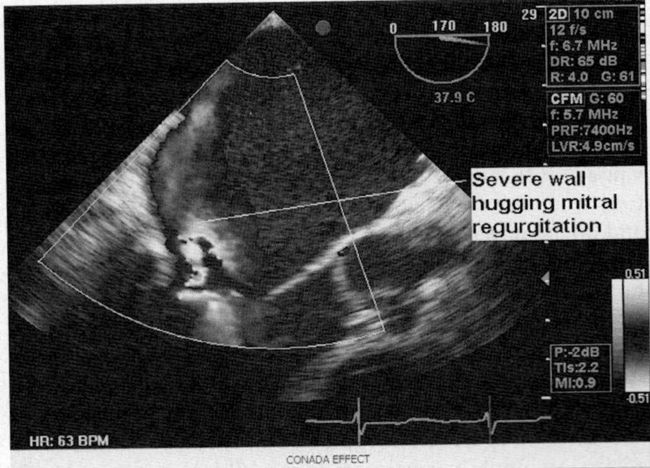

FIGURE 123.4. Transesophageal echocardiographic diagnosis of mitral regurgitation (MR) severity. Left atrial wall hugging eccentric regurgitant jet indicates severe MR.

surgical treatment, even in asymptomatic patients, with EF less than 60% to prevent progression of disease (5). Urgent coronary angiography is indicated if myocardial ischemia or infarction is a real consideration. Coronary angiography may delineate a culprit lesion, which may be amenable to catheter-based interventions. Severe triple-vessel disease should be referred for surgery. In the case of chordal rupture or infective endocarditis without risk factors for CAD, angiography may be deferred.

Therapeutic Considerations

In acute, severe MR, medical therapy has a limited role and is aimed at stabilizing the patient's hemodynamics in preparation for surgical intervention. Early valve surgery is life saving, and therefore should not be delayed. Since acute MR is often a complication of myocardial infarction, therapy should include the need to maintain coronary perfusion pressure and reduce myocardial oxygen consumption. The utilization of a PAC and invasive arterial pressure monitoring are recommended. The pulmonary artery waveform may show typical V waves of mitral regurgitation. Sinus tachycardia maintains the forward flow and, thus, should not be suppressed. Hypertension and the use of vasopressors should be avoided, as the increased afterload will increase the regurgitant fraction. Diuretics may be needed to reduce pulmonary venous congestion. While in the normotensive patient, vasodilators—such as nitroprusside—can be useful in increasing the forward flow and decreasing the regurgitant fraction, the same cannot be said when the patient is hypotensive. In this case, nitroprusside may further impair coronary perfusion pressure and should not be used except in combination with inotropes. When patients fail to respond adequately to medical management, IABP may be life saving, as it increases forward flow and blood pressure while diminishing filling pressures. It is effective in increasing coronary perfusion pressure and reducing oxygen consumption, the key factors in maintaining a favorable balance between myocardial oxygen supply and demand. Thus, IABP can be used to stabilize patients while they are prepared for surgery.

The surgical intervention is determined by the nature of the lesion. Chordal rupture or prolapse of the posterior leaflet can be successfully repaired. Revascularization alone may improve ischemic MR in selected patients with transient papillary muscle ischemia without rupture (6). Revascularization can be done using angioplasty, thrombolysis, or bypass surgery, depending on the anatomic characteristics and the severity of the lesions. However, revascularization alone may leave many of these patients with significant degrees of postoperative MR (7). Current lines of evidence suggest that a combination of complete revascularization with mitral valve repair or replacement with posterior chordal sparing is the standard of care for acute ischemic MR refractory to medical management and nonsurgical revascularization techniques (8). Mitral valve annuloplasty is the best approach for ischemic MR due to annular dilatation, diminished systolic contraction of the annulus, or papillary muscle malalignment. Mitral valve replacement should be considered if the repair is unsatisfactory. Papillary muscle rupture carries a high mortality without surgical intervention; surgery does improve the long-term outcome in functional class in these patients.

Infective endocarditis should be treated with antibiotics. However, if surgery is indicated, it should not be delayed for microbiologic clearance. Indications for surgery include congestive heart failure refractory to medical treatment, uncontrolled infection despite antibiotics, recurrent systemic embolism, perivalvular or pericardial extension of infection, fungal endocarditis, and prosthetic valve endocarditis (5).

Mitral valve prolapse (MVP) deserves special mention because MVP is the most prevalent valvular heart disease and the most common cause of MR. Patients with this condition may present to the ICU because of severe MR, atrial fibrillation with transient ischemic attacks, long QT syndrome and tachyarrhythmias, pulmonary hypertension, cerebral embolism from MVP-related fibrin, infective endocarditis, or even sudden death (9). Medical stabilization and elective surgical repair of the mitral valve are recommended therapies.

Mitral Stenosis

Etiology

Mitral stenosis (MS) is mostly related to rheumatic heart disease. Degenerative calcific stenosis, congenital stenosis, and connective tissue disorders such as systemic lupus erythematosus and Lutembacher syndrome (atrial septal defect with MS) are the other causes for MS. Atrial myxomas and left atrial ball-valve thrombus can present with intermittent obstruction to mitral inflow and mimic MS.

Hemodynamics

In rheumatic MS, inflammation of the connective tissue leads to leaflet thickening and calcification, and commissural and chordal fusion. Ultimately, many patients are left with a funnel-shaped mitral apparatus. As the condition progresses, left atrial pressure and the transmitral gradient increase, thus maintaining flow. However, the subsequent increase in pulmonary venous pressure leads to hydrostatic pulmonary edema. Pulmonary vasoconstriction increases pulmonary arterial pressure and right ventricular afterload. Over the course of rheumatic heart disease, persistently elevated pulmonary arterial pressure leads to structural changes such as intimal hyperplasia and medial hypertrophy. These structural changes are permanent and result in fixed pulmonary hypertension. Right ventricular dilatation and failure result in tricuspid insufficiency and systemic venous congestion, respectively. The impact of MS on cardiac output is initially determined by the severity of the stenosis itself and the limitation to flow across the narrowed mitral orifice. However, as the disease progresses, right ventricular failure may become severe enough to limit cardiac output. Similarly, progression of rheumatic disease with its associated inflammation, fibrosis, and calcium deposition may impair left ventricular function. Although this effect is not a major determinant of cardiac output in patients with MS, it may become important to consider in some patients after surgical repair. In such situations, the increase in transmitral flow may expose the left ventricle to a sudden increase in preload, causing failure.

Presentation

Patients with mitral stenosis often present to the ICU with acute cardiogenic pulmonary edema. Precipitating factors such as infective endocarditis, fever, anxiety, pain, atrial fibrillation, and pregnancy should be identified. Occlusion from an enlarging atrial myxoma should be ruled out. Right-sided heart failure with hepatic dysfunction, acute hemoptysis, systemic embolism, and hoarseness of voice may also be present.

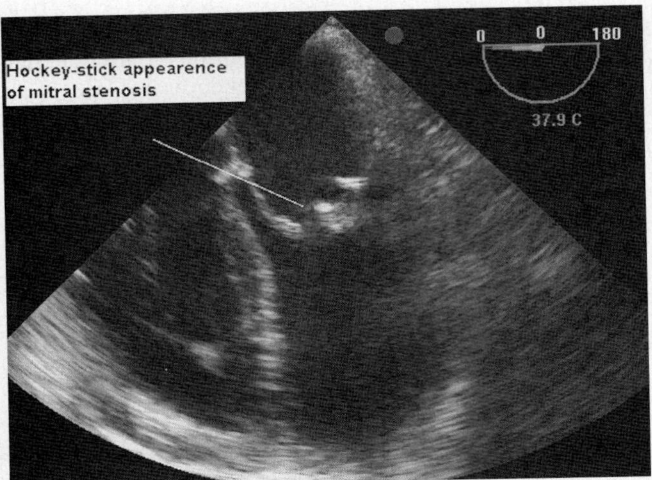

FIGURE 123.5. Typical appearance of rheumatic mitral stenosis.

Diagnosis

The ECG may show left atrial enlargement, right ventricular hypertrophy, and atrial fibrillation in MS. Chest radiography shows straightening of the left heart border, indicating left atrial and pulmonary artery enlargement. Kerley A and B lines indicate pulmonary venous hypertension. TTE findings include doming of the anterior leaflet, decreased leaflet mobility, increased leaflet calcification and thickness, commissural fusion, calcification of the subvalvular apparatus, increased LA size, and the presence of an LA thrombus (Fig. 123.5). Color flow will show associated mitral regurgitation. Doppler echocardiography allows calculation of pressure gradients, mitral valve area, and estimation of pulmonary artery systolic pressure. Cardiac MRI is increasingly being used in the evaluation of stenotic valvular lesions; it measures valve area by planimetry. Its advantage over echocardiography is the lack of dependence upon good echocardiographic windows.

Therapeutic Considerations

New onset atrial fibrillation with hemodynamic instability should be treated with cardioversion. Cardioversion of a patient with atrial fibrillation of unknown duration or that is known to have persisted for more than 48 hours must be preceded by 3 weeks of anticoagulation or by a TEE to exclude the presence of left atrial thrombus. Anticoagulation should be continued for 4 weeks following cardioversion because the enlarged LA remains "stunned" and does not recover a normal contractile state immediately following cardioversion (10). Anticoagulants should also be used in patients with a prior embolic event and left atrial diameter greater than 55 mm by echocardiography (5). Antidysrhythmics, such as amiodarone, may be used to maintain sinus rhythm but should not be expected to provide indefinite success.

Patients admitted with pulmonary edema should be stabilized with oxygen, morphine, anxiolytics, diuretics, and digoxin; the latter is especially useful in patients with atrial dysrhythmias and congestive heart failure. Sympathetic nervous system activity is increased in patients with mitral stenosis, and sympathetic overactivity worsens the symptom complex; β-blockers are very useful in this situation. Intravenous nesiritide, a synthetic human natriuretic peptide, is also used in the critically ill patients with acute decompensated cardiac failure and pulmonary hypertension. Short-term intravenous infusion of nesiritide is associated with hemodynamic and symptomatic improvements in patients with acutely decompensated congestive heart failure (CHF). Nesiritide may offer tolerability and practical advantages over currently used vasodilators, inodilators, and inotropes in this condition; in particular, nesiritide does not appear to have proarrhythmic effects. Nesiritide also appears to be effective and well tolerated in patients receiving concomitant β-blocker therapy and those with renal insufficiency (11, 12). If the patients are hypotensive, inotropes to improve left ventricular function may not be useful, but may worsen tachycardia and pulmonary edema. Inodilators may be useful in improving right ventricular dysfunction and reducing pulmonary hypertension. Systemic blood pressure may need to be supported with vasopressors, with the caveat that they may adversely impact pulmonary vascular resistance. Assessment of volume status is difficult, as the PCWP does not correlate with LVEDP in patients with MS. However, the PCWP gives useful information about the propensity to develop pulmonary edema.

Emergency invasive intervention is rarely required to relieve MS. If the precipitating events are controlled, intervention by surgery or balloon valvotomy can be scheduled electively after medical optimization. Balloon valvotomy is indicated in patients with suitable anatomy: pliable leaflets, no commissural fusion, and minimal subvalvular calcification. LA thrombus and significant (3+ to 4+) MR should be excluded by echocardiography. Patients who are not candidates for balloon intervention should be referred for surgery. Because of extensive calcifications and marked anatomic distortion, mitral valve repair often is not possible in rheumatic mitral disease, and replacement is necessary in those patients.

Tricuspid Stenosis

Etiology

Tricuspid valve obstruction can be due to anatomic disease of the tricuspid valve or functional, causes secondary to right atrial (RA) tumors and thrombus. Anatomic disease is usually related to rheumatic heart disease, and involvement of mitral valve is common. Other anatomic causes are carcinoid syndrome, infective endocarditis, congenital stenosis or atresia, and methysergide toxicity.

Hemodynamics

Obstruction to right ventricular inflow results in systemic venous congestion: elevated jugular venous pulse (JVP), congestive hepatomegaly, and peripheral edema. Diastole is shortened by increasing heart rate, thus causing dramatic increases in transvalvular gradients. Most patients are symptomatic from coexisting mitral stenosis. The presence of systemic venous congestion out of proportion to pulmonary venous congestion should raise the suspicion for involvement of the tricuspid valve.

Clinical Signs

Physical exam will reveal an elevated JVP, a prominent a wave, and distension of veins of the upper arm and dorsum of extended hand. The JVP increases by compression of the liver—*the hepatojugular reflux*. A diastolic thrill may be palpated at the lower left sternal border; the S_1 is increased, and an opening snap and diastolic murmur may be heard at the lower left sternal border. Assigning the murmur to the tricuspid valve is based on its location; the higher, shorter, and softer nature of tricuspid stenosis (TS) in comparison to MS; and the absence of crackles that commonly accompany the murmur of MS. Right-sided murmurs are increased during inspiration.

Diagnosis

The ECG may show evidence of RA enlargement—a P wave exceeding 2.5 mm in lead II and 1.5 mm in V_1. RA enlargement may increase the distance from sinus node to atrioventricular node, causing first-degree heart block; atrial fibrillation may occur in advanced disease. The chest radiograph may show cardiomegaly and RA enlargement, and calcification of the valve may be evident. Typically, echocardiographic visualization shows thickened leaflets, limited mobility, and a dome-shaped structure in diastole. Right ventricular function and the presence of tumor, thrombus, and vegetations can also be assessed. Spectral and color Doppler methods allow calculation of pressure gradients to grade the stenosis—that is, mild less than 5 mm Hg, moderate 5 to 10 mm Hg, and severe greater than 10 mm Hg—and valve area. Catheterization is unnecessary in patients with good echocardiographic windows.

Therapeutic Interventions

Complete obstruction of the tricuspid valve by vegetations, thrombus, and/or tumors is an indication for emergency valve surgery (Fig. 123.6). As seen in other valvular lesions, the disease progresses slowly, becoming symptomatic as obstruction to flow increases. Sodium restriction, careful diuresis, rate control, and anticoagulation are helpful, but surgical correction is required when the transvalvular gradient exceeds 5 mm Hg and the valve area falls below 2 cm^2. Percutaneous valvotomy or, more often, a bioprosthetic valve replacement is necessary. Mechanical valves are avoided because of the very high risk of thromboembolism in this position.

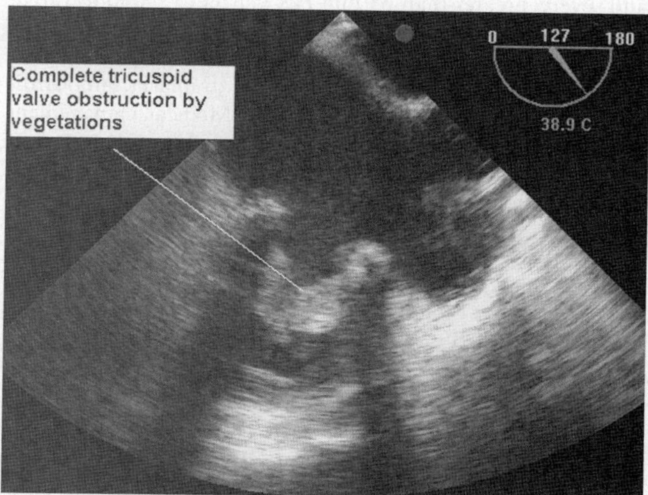

FIGURE 123.6. Complete obstruction of prosthetic tricuspid valve by vegetations requiring emergency surgery.

Tricuspid Regurgitation

Etiology

Tricuspid regurgitation (TR) can be classified as structural or functional. Structural diseases of the valve are caused by rheumatic disease, infective endocarditis, carcinoid syndrome, radiation therapy, Marfan syndrome, congenital heart disease, or tricuspid valve prolapse. Functional TR is usually secondary to left-sided pathology, such as left ventricular failure or mitral or—less frequently—aortic valve disease, but may also result from primary pulmonary hypertension, pulmonic stenosis, right ventricular (RV) infarction, and dilated cardiomyopathy; a small number of cases may not have an etiology identified. While most cases of TR are chronic, an acute presentation may occur following penetrating trauma, RV infarction, infective endocarditis, and, more recently, repeated endomyocardial biopsies to diagnose allograft rejection of heart transplantation.

Hemodynamics

Acutely following the development of TR, elevated RA pressure gives rise to the signs and symptoms of systemic venous congestion. Over time, the RA dilates, with the possible sequelae of atrial fibrillation and thrombus formation. Formation of an RA thrombus may lead to pulmonary and systemic emboli, the latter in patients with patent foramen ovale. RV volume overload leads to eccentric hypertrophy and dilatation. RV systolic dysfunction develops, leading to further decompensation and dilatation, which in turn causes annular dilatation and an increase in the severity of TR. The left heart also suffers from low cardiac output because the RV fails to deliver enough blood to the LV. Ventricular interdependence and paradoxical septal motion also decrease left ventricular output in patients with RV volume overload.

Clinical Symptoms and Signs

Symptoms of low cardiac output and venous congestion present in these patients. Shock and hypotension may develop following acute TR after RV infarction or papillary muscle rupture. Other patients maintain blood pressure but demonstrate signs of right-sided failure. Distended neck veins with a prominent c-v wave, pulsatile hepatomegaly, a precordial bulge, and parasternal heave from RV hypertrophy; soft S_1, prominent P_2, and right-sided S_3 from RV dilatation; pansystolic thrill; and a murmur heard at the left lower sternal border are associated signs. Cases of isolated tricuspid valve endocarditis may disseminate emboli to the lungs, resulting in multiple septic emboli and abscess formation. Peripheral stigmata of infective emboli are usually absent, but may indicate paradoxical embolism or left-sided lesions if present.

Diagnosis

The ECG may show atrial fibrillation, right axis deviation, RV hypertrophy, and a right bundle branch block. Right-sided leads will show ST elevation in RV infarction and may be associated with LV inferior wall infarction. Enlarged RV and cardiomegaly are seen on chest radiography. Echocardiography can yield details about the structural issues with the tricuspid valve—prolapse, vegetations, annular diameter, and rheumatic disease—and helps to rule out thrombus and patent foramen ovale. The diagnosis of a patent foramen ovale is important, since the elevated right atrial pressure frequently exceeds left atrial pressure, causing a right-to-left shunt that may cause refractory hypoxemia. Severity of TR can be assessed by hepatic venous systolic flow reversal and estimation of regurgitant orifice area (greater than 40 mm^2 is severe). Also, pulmonary systolic pressure can be estimated by continuous wave Doppler signal of tricuspid regurgitation. Augmenting ultrasound signal with 10% air, 10% patient's blood, and 80% saline, and estimation of pulmonary artery systolic pressures correlate well with PAC-measured PA systolic pressures (13). Right heart catheterization shows RV pressure greater than 60 mm Hg in functional TR compared to less than 40 mm Hg in structural TR.

Therapeutic Considerations

In general, the hemodynamic impact of acute TR is less severe and can be effectively managed with diuretics and inotropes. In rare instances, acute severe TR may require valvular surgery when the process is refractory to medical therapy. Once stabilized, these patients' long-term prognosis depends on the etiology and severity of the TR. Patients tolerate mild and moderate degrees of chronic TR in the presence of normal LV function. Correction of left-sided heart lesions and treatment of left-sided failure and pulmonary hypertension take priority. If functional TR is severe, surgical intervention may be needed. Ring annuloplasty can improve TR and survival in these patients (14). Cardiac resynchronization therapy with biventricular pacemakers and the Dor procedure (endoventricular circular patch plasty) help patients with functional TR due to systolic heart failure (15).

Rheumatic TR may be treated with open valvotomy or valve replacement. Valves compromised by infective endocarditis can simply be removed after an aggressive course of antibiotics. Valve replacement can be performed later if there is no recurrence of drug abuse in these patients. When acute TR is the result of RV infarction, the usual management of acute coronary insufficiency must be observed, including β-blockers, aspirin, fluids, thrombolysis, coronary angiography, angioplasty, and stenting and, in suitable patients, coronary artery bypass grafting.

Pulmonic Stenosis

Etiology

Pulmonic stenosis (PS) is usually congenital. While valvular PS does occur in isolation, subvalvular and supravalvular stenosis usually comprise part of a larger syndrome. Severe forms, or those associated with other cardiac anomalies, are generally identified and treated in childhood. Acquired forms of pulmonary stenosis include rheumatic, carcinoid disease; infundibular stenosis from pulmonary hypertension; extrinsic compression from aneurysm of the sinus of Valsalva; tumors; and scarring from previous surgery.

Pathophysiology

PS causes obstruction to right ventricular outflow. Right ventricular hypertrophy results, and, if right ventricular failure or tricuspid regurgitation develops, systemic venous hypertension can result. The degree of stenosis, once established, tends to be stable; if decompensation does not occur in childhood, subsequent deterioration is unlikely. Occasionally, patients manifest increasing right ventricular outflow obstruction, perhaps caused by secondary infundibular hypertrophy.

Presentation

Mild PS is often asymptomatic. Patients with more severe stenosis commonly develop fatigue, atypical chest pain, and syncope. When right ventricular failure or tricuspid regurgitation occurs, systemic venous hypertension may be present. Elevated right atrial pressures in the presence of a patent foramen ovale or atrial septal defect can result in a right-to-left shunt at the atrial level.

Physical examination typically reveals a large jugular venous a wave. In the absence of right ventricular failure or tricuspid regurgitation, jugular venous pressure remains normal. A left parasternal systolic lift is common with significant pulmonic stenosis. The murmur is best heard at the left upper sternal border and typically radiates to the left clavicle. A palpable thrill may be present. The intensity of the murmur does not correlate well with severity, but increasing duration and late systolic peaking are indicators of significant stenosis. An ejection click is usually present. As severity increases, P_2 is increasingly delayed; thus, wide splitting of the second sound indicates more severe stenosis.

Diagnostic Studies

The ECG is normal in mild pulmonic stenosis. With increasing severity, right ventricular hypertrophy and right atrial enlargement are common. The chest radiograph may reveal poststenotic dilatation of the main and left pulmonary arteries. Echocardiography is particularly useful in assessing the valve morphology, calculating pressure gradients across the pulmonic valve, grading the severity of stenosis, and evaluating right ventricular function. The presence of other congenital abnormalities, tricuspid regurgitation, and right atrial enlargement can also be ruled out by echocardiography. Cardiac catheterization provides confirmation of pressure gradients, full hemodynamic assessment, and identification of associated pulmonary artery branch stenosis. Pulmonary stenosis is graded based on the peak pressure gradient: mild, with a gradient of 25 to 49 mm Hg; moderate, 50 to 75 mm Hg; and severe, greater than 75 mm Hg. Currently, balloon valvuloplasty is recommended for symptomatic patients and those with a peak gradient greater than 50 mm Hg. Surgical valvuloplasty is reserved for severe calcification, dysplasia, endocarditis, and previous valvuloplasty failure. Medical management includes infective endocarditis prophylaxis, treatment of right heart failure and atrial fibrillation, and anticoagulation to prevent thromboembolic complications.

Pulmonic Insufficiency

Pulmonic insufficiency (PI) generally has a benign course as an isolated abnormality. The natural history is that of the associated lesions.

Etiology

PI may be secondary to pulmonary hypertension or, rarely, to leaflet damage caused by infectious endocarditis, rheumatic fever, or carcinoid syndrome. Occasionally, PI is congenital.

Pathophysiology

In the absence of pulmonary hypertension, volume overload of the right ventricle is well tolerated. Decompensation with resulting right ventricular failure can occur when pulmonary hypertension develops from other causes.

Presentation

PI is usually an incidental auscultatory finding in patients admitted to the ICU for other reasons. Physical findings include the typical decrescendo diastolic murmur along the upper left sternal border. The intensity of the murmur does not correlate well with the severity of regurgitation.

Diagnostic Studies

The ECG is usually normal. The presence of right ventricular hypertrophy suggests pulmonary hypertension. The chest radiograph is normal in mild insufficiency. The pulmonary trunk may be prominent when the insufficiency is moderate to severe. Pulmonary hypertension may be present. Echocardiography with Doppler study can be useful for differentiating pulmonic from aortic insufficiency and for establishing right heart chamber sizes and associated abnormalities.

Therapeutic Considerations

Specific treatment is rarely required. However, therapy should be directed toward control of pulmonary hypertension when present. When the right heart fails, diuretics and sodium restriction are useful, and some clinicians suggest that cardiac glycosides are helpful. Surgical treatment (bioprosthetic valve replacement) is reserved for advanced right heart failure. In patients with a remote repair of tetralogy of Fallot and chronic PI, RV dilatation has been linked to sudden death. This has led some clinician-investigators to pursue valve replacement in early stages of RV dilatation.

Mixed Valve Lesions

Mitral Stenosis with Regurgitation

The combination of pressure and volume overload on LA favors early development of symptoms, atrial fibrillation, and congestive heart failure. Because transvalvular gradients may overestimate the degree of stenosis, Doppler measurement of valve area should be considered. Decision making is complex, and intervention is often required before either of the lesions reaches a severe degree. Moderate MR is a contraindication for balloon valvotomy.

Aortic Stenosis and Regurgitation

This combination causes both pressure and volume overload on the LV. The predominant lesion is indicated by the size of the LV: a normal-sized, but hypertrophied, LV signifies predominant AS; a dilated LV suggests dominant AR. As with combined MS and MR, transvalvular gradients may overestimate AS, so planimetry or the continuity equation method should be considered. The threshold for surgery is lowered as compared to single valve–defect patients. Those with severe AS with accompanying AR should be operated on in higher calculated valve areas or in the presence of mild symptoms. Surgery in patients with predominant AR with accompanying AS can be delayed until symptoms develop or asymptomatic LV dysfunction becomes apparent on echocardiography (enlarged ventricular dimensions).

Mitral Stenosis and Aortic Stenosis

This combination causes serial obstructions resulting in reduced cardiac output and early development of pulmonary venous congestion and hypertension. Low transvalvular gradients characterize this aortic stenosis because of low cardiac output. Mitral valvotomy is done first, followed by aortic valve replacement as indicated.

Mitral Stenosis and Aortic Regurgitation

This combination creates a challenge for the physician attempting to make a diagnosis. MS decreases the volume overload of AR, and AR attenuates antegrade mitral valve flow by increasing LV diastolic pressure, thereby decreasing transmitral gradients. Balloon mitral valvotomy followed by aortic valve replacement (AVR), as indicated, is a reasonable approach.

Mitral Regurgitation and Aortic Stenosis

Aortic stenosis aggravates MR by increasing the afterload. MR, by its pressure release effect, obscures even severe AS. Systolic function remains normal with low transaortic gradients. If both lesions are severe, AVR with mitral valve repair or replacement is necessary. Moderate or mild MR may improve after AVR for AS, especially if there is no anatomic lesion in the mitral valve. Intraoperative TEE plays an important role in this decision.

Mitral Regurgitation and Aortic Regurgitation

These lesions create additive volume loads on the LV; consequently, the sequelae of dyspnea and LV dysfunction appear sooner.

Prosthetic Valve Dysfunction

Prosthetic valves in common use are broadly divided into mechanical, bioprosthetic, and homograft valves. St. Jude bileaflet valves are commonly used mechanical valves which need lifelong anticoagulation. Carpentier-Edwards and Hancock bioprosthetic valves are common tissue valves in use. They do not require long-term anticoagulation, but have a short life span and are prone to degenerative changes and failure. Acute valvular complications may result from infective endocarditis, paravalvular leak, valve ring abscess, thrombosis, pannus formation, degenerative calcification, lipid infiltration, dehiscence of the valve, and strut fracture.

Progressive congestive cardiac failure is a common presentation with stenosis and regurgitation. Acute, complete valvular obstruction may lead to sudden death in the absence of surgical intervention. Embolic phenomenon, hemolytic anemia—indicating a paravalvular leak, and a new atrioventricular block—indicating a valve ring abscess may be other presenting symptoms. Prosthetic valve thrombosis may present with nonspecific cardiac symptoms. Normally functioning prosthetic valves are associated with clicks and murmurs; hence, disappearance of clicks or a new or changing murmur is important in making the diagnosis.

Echocardiography is essential to make a diagnosis in these patients. As previously noted, TEE is more sensitive and specific in the evaluation of prosthetic valve pathologies than TTE; echocardiography has replaced cardiac catheterization in these cases. Fluoroscopy may be needed in some cases to identify the nature of the disease and assess the effects of thrombolysis. Excessive rocking motion of the valve ring or limited motion of the valve components due to thrombus or vegetation; calcification; thickening around the valve due to an abscess; and a pseudoaneurysm can be identified with two-dimensional echocardiography. The color Doppler technique may show a paravalvular leak, pseudoaneurysms, and/or fistula formation. Calculation of transvalvular gradients help in the diagnosis of prosthetic valve stenosis. Gradients depend on the type and size of the valve and dynamic conditions such as cardiac output, blood volume, heart rate, and contractility. Therefore, it is recommended that the measurements be compared to the control values obtained immediately after valve replacement. It has also been suggested that it may be more appropriate to calculate the prosthetic valve area using the continuity equation:

$$\text{Area}_1 \times \text{velocity time integral}_1 = \text{Area}_2 \times \text{velocity time integral}_2$$

Medical therapy is directed toward treatment of congestive heart failure—diuretics, vasodilators, and inotropes; initiation of antibiotics for infective endocarditis after obtaining blood cultures; and thrombolysis for certain cases of prosthetic valve thrombosis. Staphylococcal organisms predominate in early (less than 60 days postplacement) prosthetic valve endocarditis, whereas in late (greater than 60 days postplacement) endocarditis, there are equal percentages of infection caused by streptococcal and staphylococcal organisms (16). Empiric antibiotics are started until culture results and sensitivities are available. Fibrinolytic therapy is recommended for right-sided thrombosis with a large clot burden or New York Heart Association class III to IV symptoms (see http://www.abouthf.org/questions_stages.htm). Fibrinolysis for left-sided lesions is reserved for patients in whom emergency surgery is high risk or contraindicated because this is associated with a 12% to 15% risk of cerebral embolism (17). Ultimately, all prosthetic valve lesions require valve replacement surgery. Reoperative mortality is high in this patient population.

IMPORTANT CONSIDERATIONS IN THE TREATMENT OF RIGHT VENTRICULAR FAILURE SECONDARY TO VALVULAR HEART DISEASE

Chronic RV failure secondary to VHD presents major therapeutic challenges to the intensive care physician. These patients are usually debilitated with low cardiac output and pulmonary, hepatic, and renal dysfunction. Patients develop hepatic failure secondary to congestive hepatic cirrhosis. Ascites, malnutrition, reduced systemic vascular resistance, jaundice, coagulopathy, and renal failure—the hepatorenal syndrome—are the manifestations of hepatic dysfunction. The management of hepatorenal syndrome is challenging and will require invasive monitoring and, often, renal replacement therapy.

Treatment of pulmonary hypertension in the critically ill patient with VHD decreases RV afterload and helps prevent and decrease RV failure. This approach, combined with maintenance of adequate coronary perfusion pressure, forms the mainstay of treatment of acute RV failure. Exacerbating factors of pulmonary hypertension, such as hypoxemia, hypercarbia, acidosis, hypothermia, hypervolemia, and increased intrathoracic pressure, should be corrected aggressively. Recent advances in pharmacology provide intensivists with a wide variety of options for selective pulmonary vasodilatation, with studies favoring the use of inhaled prostaglandins and nitric oxide (18). Inhaled pulmonary vasodilators are preferred over intravenous agents because they do not decrease systemic blood pressure and also do not increase shunt fraction. Many newer drugs—including nitric oxide donors and phosphodiesterase inhibitors—are promising and are under investigation.

References

1. Lieberman EB, Bashore TM, Hermiller JB, et al. Balloon aortic valvuloplasty in adults: failure of procedure to improve long-term survival. *J Am Coll Cardiol.* 1995;26:1522.
2. Shiga T, Wajima Z, Apfel CC, et al. Diagnostic accuracy of transesophageal echocardiography, helical computed tomography, and magnetic resonance imaging for suspected thoracic aortic dissection: systematic review and meta-analysis. *Arch Intern Med.* 2006;166:1350.
3. Carpentier A. Cardiac valve surgery—the 'French correction.' *J Thorac Cardiovasc Surg.* 1983;86:323.
4. Gillam LD, Ford-Mukkamala L. Assessment of ventricular systolic function. In: Mathew JP, Ayoub CM, eds. *Clinical Manual and Review of Transesophageal Echocardiography.* New York: McGraw-Hill; 2005:75.
5. Bonow RO, Carabello B, de Leon AC Jr, et al. ACC/AHA guidelines for management of patients with valvular heart disease. *J Am Coll Cardiol.* 2006;48:598.
6. Durate IG, Shen Y, McDonald MJ, et al. Treatment of mitral regurgitation and coronary disease by coronary bypass alone: late results. *Ann Thorac Surg.* 1999;68:426.
7. Prifti E, Bonacchi M, Frati G, et al. Ischemic mitral valve regurgitation grade II-III: correction in patients with impaired left ventricular function undergoing simultaneous coronary revascularization. *J Heart Valve Dis.* 2001;10:754.
8. Edmunds LHJ. Ischemic mitral regurgitation. In: Edmunds LH Jr, ed. *Cardiac Surgery in the Adult.* New York: McGraw-Hill, Co.; 1997:657
9. Fontana ME, Sparks EA, Boudoulas H, et al. Mitral valve prolapse and the mitral valve prolapse syndrome. *Curr Probl Cardiol.* 1991;16:309.
10. Dabek J, Gasior Z, Monastyrska-Cup B, et al. Cardioversion and atrial stunning. *Pol Merkur Lekarski.* 2007;22:224–228.
11. Maisel AS. Nesiritide; a new therapy for the treatment of heart failure. *Cardiovasc Toxicol.* 2003;3:37.
12. Keating GM, Goa KL. Nesiritide: a review of its use in acute decompensated heart failure. *Drugs.* 2003;63:47.
13. Jeon D, Luo H, Iwami T, et al. The usefulness of a 10% air-10%blood-80% saline mixture for contrast echocardiography: Doppler measurement of pulmonary artery systolic pressure. *J Am Coll Cardiol.* 2002;39:124.
14. Onoda K, Yasuda F, Takao M, et al. Long-term follow-up after Carpentier-Edwards ring annuloplasty for tricuspid regurgitation. *Ann Thorac Surg.* 2000;70:796.
15. Trichon BH, O'Connor CM. Secondary mitral and tricuspid regurgitation accompanying left ventricular systolic dysfunction: is it important and how is it treated?. *Am Heart J.* 2002;144:373.
16. Karchmer AW. Infective endocarditis. In: Braunwald E, Zipes DP, Lippy P, eds. *Heart Disease: A Textbook of Cardiovascular Medicine.* 6th ed. Philadelphia: WB Saunders; 2001:1723.
17. Roudaut R, Labbe T, Lorient-Roudaut MF, et al. Mechanical cardiac valve thrombosis. Is fibrinolysis justified? *Circulation.* 1992;86(Suppl5):II8.
18. Blaise G, Langleben D, Hubert B. Pulmonary arterial hypertension: pathophysiology and anesthetic approach. *Anesthesiology.* 2003;99:1415.

CHAPTER 124 ■ CARDIAC DYSRHYTHMIAS

SHERRY J. SAXONHOUSE • WILLIAM M. MILES • JAMIE B. CONTI

BRADYARRHYTHMIAS

Bradycardia is a common finding in hospitalized patients, especially during sleep. An increase in vagal tone may result in sinus bradycardia, sinus pauses, or atrioventricular (AV) nodal block—all physiologic findings that may have no clinical significance. Bradyarrhythmias can generally be categorized as either sinoatrial (SA) or AV conduction abnormalities.

SA Abnormalities

Sinus pauses may be caused by either sinoatrial conduction block or sinus arrest. SA conduction block occurs when impulses generated by the sinus node are not conducted to the atrial myocardium. Three categories of block are first-, second-, and third-degree SA block. First-degree SA block is not manifested on electrocardiogram, as it is merely the delay between the sinus impulse formation and atrial activation. Second-degree SA block can be type I or type II. Type I (Wenckebach) is manifested by group beating, with progressive shortening of PP intervals until a P wave is absent; this PP interval is usually less than twice the shortest cycle. Type II SA block has fixed PP intervals, followed by a pause without a P wave that is twice the PP interval (Fig. 124.1). Third-degree SA block is not visible on electrocardiogram, as no sinus impulse can escape the SA node. This disorder cannot be differentiated from sinus arrest.

Sinus arrest is the failure of automaticity in which no impulses are generated by the sinus node (Fig. 124.2). *Sick sinus syndrome* is dysfunction of the sinus node or SA conduction in which no adequate escape mechanism is present and the patient becomes symptomatic because of bradycardia. There are intrinsic and extrinsic causes of SA abnormalities. The most prevalent intrinsic cause of sinus node dysfunction is aging, with replacement of the sinus node and the surrounding atrium by fibrotic degeneration. Extrinsic causes of sinus node dysfunction include drugs (Table 124.1), electrolyte abnormalities (hyperkalemia), endocrine disorders (hypothyroidism), neurally mediated conditions (vasovagal syncope), and intracranial hypertension.

Diagnosis and Treatment of SA Abnormalities

1. Record a 12-lead electrocardiogram (ECG).
2. If hypotension, dizziness, and presyncope are absent, no immediate treatment is required. Symptoms dictate the treatment plan. Asymptomatic bradycardia due to sinus node dysfunction is not an emergency!
3. Evaluate the ECG for the following:
   A. Myocardial infarction
   B. Mechanism of bradycardia
      - P-wave regularity (sinus or an atrial rhythm)
      - Abrupt pauses or group beating in the sinus rhythm suggests SA block
      - P waves without QRS complexes suggest AV block
      - QRS axis and width for coexistent bundle branch block
4. In case of sinus bradycardia, give no treatment unless hypotension is present, then give intravenous (IV) atropine, 0.04 mg/kg of body weight.
5. In case of sinoatrial block or sinus arrest, give no treatment unless hypotension is present or the rhythm is digitalis induced (*stop drug*).
6. If sick sinus syndrome, then treatment depends on symptoms such as dizziness, presyncope, congestive heart failure.
7. In case of acute inferoposterior myocardial infarction (MI) with sinoatrial block, coronary reperfusion is indicated.

AV Conduction Abnormalities

AV conduction abnormalities can be categorized as first-, second-, or third-degree AV block. In first-degree AV block, every P wave is conducted to the ventricles but with a prolonged PR interval. Second-degree AV block is characterized by intermittent P waves not conducted to the ventricles and is further broken down into type I (Wenckebach), type II, and two-to-one conduction. Third-degree AV block demonstrates no conduction between the atrium and ventricles. To make the diagnosis of complete or third-degree AV block, the sinus rate must be faster than the ventricular rate.

Noninvasive Methods for Determining Site of AV Block

In AV block, the conduction abnormality may be located within the AV node, the His bundle, or the bundle branches (1). Determining the location of block is important, as this will affect immediate and long-term treatment. A 12-lead ECG and diagnostic maneuvers are helpful in diagnosing the level of block. Baseline intervals on the ECG, including PR interval, QRS duration, and axis, are important. Bedside responses to noninvasive interventions, including IV atropine administration, exercise, or vagal maneuvers, may differentiate between AV nodal and infranodal (below the AV node) block (Table 124.2). Specifically, interventions that slow AV nodal conduction, such as carotid sinus massage, will worsen AV nodal block but, because of sinus slowing, will seem to improve infranodal block. Conversely, interventions that improve AV nodal conduction, such as exercise and atropine, may worsen infranodal conduction because of acceleration of sinus rate.

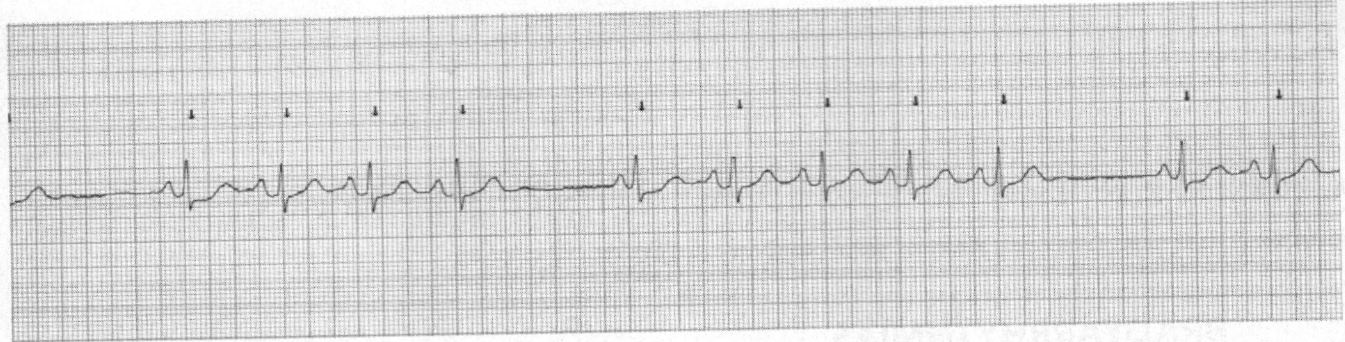

FIGURE 124.1. Lead II rhythm strip. Second-degree type II sinoatrial block. The P-P interval is initially 720 ms and appears to prolong to 1,440 ms.

First-Degree AV block or Prolonged PR Interval

The PR interval is a reflection of AV conduction time and is measured from the onset of the P wave to the beginning of the QRS complex. Conduction delay in the atrium, AV node, bundle of His, or bundle branches all may result in a prolonged PR interval. Prolongation to ≥280 ms usually indicates abnormal AV nodal conduction.

Second-Degree Type I AV Block (AV Wenckebach)

In type I AV block (Wenckebach), there is progressive lengthening of the PR interval before there is a blocked P wave (Fig. 124.3). The QRS duration may be narrow or wide, depending on the presence of bundle branch block. When the QRS is narrow, it is most likely a block occurring at the level of the AV node that will improve with atropine and exercise and worsen with carotid sinus message. It can be seen in young healthy individuals with increased vagal tone. Patients with an acute inferior myocardial infarction can have AV nodal block (≤20%), indicating a proximal right coronary occlusion (2).

Second-Degree Type II AV Block

In type II (Mobitz II) AV block, the PR intervals are normal or slightly prolonged, and are exactly the same length before and after the nonconducted P waves (Fig. 124.4). AV conduction may worsen with sinus acceleration due to atropine and exercise but may improve with carotid massage. Type II AV block is most likely infranodal in the His bundle if there is a narrow QRS duration (rare) or in the bundle branches if there is wide QRS duration (common). These patients are often symptomatic, with shortness of breath, fatigue, and syncope, and sudden progression to complete AV block.

Two-to-One AV Block

In a two-to-one AV block, every other P wave conducts to the ventricle, and the conducted PR interval may be either normal or prolonged (Fig. 124.5). The level of block—AV nodal versus infranodal—cannot be determined with certainty without an electrophysiology study. A narrow QRS duration suggests that the block is in the AV node or the His bundle whereas a wide QRS suggests block in the bundle branches.

Third-Degree AV Block or Complete AV Block

There is no P wave to QRS relationship. Sinus rate (P-to-P intervals) is usually faster than the escape rate. The escape rate is usually <50 beats per minute (bpm), with the exception of a congenital AV block (Fig. 124.6). If the escape rhythm has a narrow QRS complex, then it originates in the AV junction and the site of block is either AV nodal or, less likely, bundle of His. If the QRS is wide, the site of block is likely within the bundle branches.

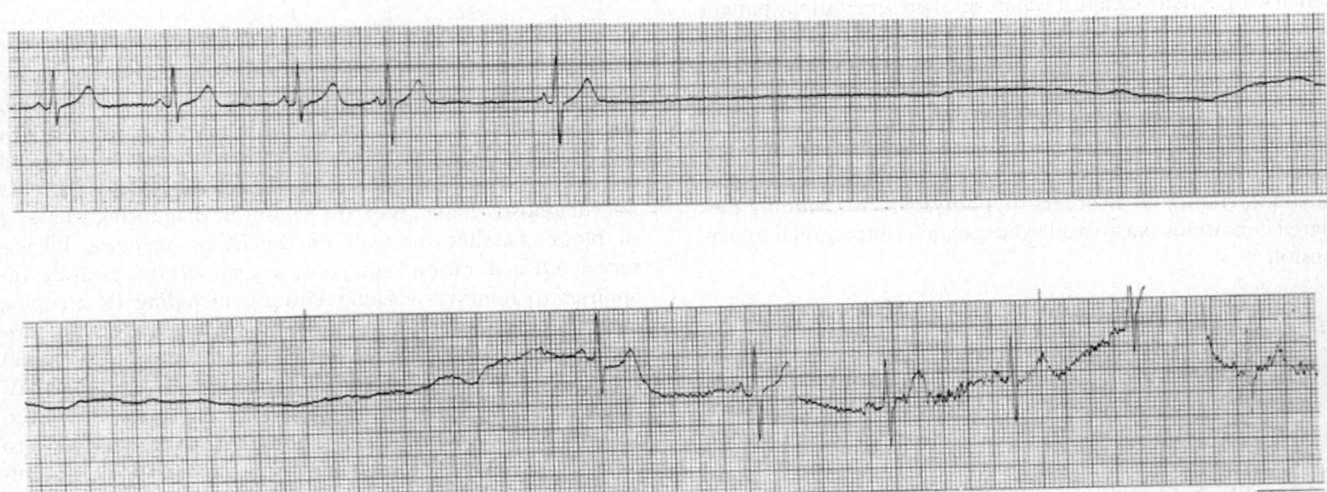

FIGURE 124.2. Lead II rhythm strip. Sinus arrest with no ventricular escape.

TABLE 124.1

DRUGS AFFECTING SINUS NODE FUNCTION

DRUG TYPES	
Antiarrhythmics	Class IA (quinidine, procainamide, disopyramide)
	Class IC (flecainide, propafenone)
	Class III (sotalol, amiodarone)
Beta-blocking agents	
Calcium channel blockers	Verapamil
	Diltiazem
Cardiac glycosides	
Miscellaneous	Lithium
	Cimetidine
	Diphenylhydantoin
	Clonidine and dexmedetomidine

Diagnosis of AV Conduction Abnormalities

1. Record a 12-lead ECG and try to determine site of block by noninvasive methods.
2. In the setting of an acute inferior wall myocardial infarction (MI), the site of block is usually the AV node and is usually transient with successful reperfusion.
   a. Insert a temporary pacemaker if there is cardiogenic shock secondary to heart block.
   b. Use permanent pacing only if there is chronic, symptomatic second- or third-degree AV nodal block.
3. Type II AV block
   a. If there is no PR prolongation prior to block, it is most likely in the His-Purkinje system.
   b. Temporary pacemaker is required when associated with syncope.
   c. Permanent pacemaker can be used in most cases.
4. Two-to-one AV block
   a. PR interval (≤160 ms suggests His bundle or below)
   b. Temporary pacemaker indicated in patients with acute MI, wide QRS, and/or if symptomatic
5. Third-degree AV block
   - Temporary pacemaker required in acute anterior MI, wide QRS, and/or if symptomatic

NARROW QRS TACHYCARDIA

Narrow QRS tachycardia is defined as an arrhythmia with a rate faster than 100 bpm and QRS duration of <120 ms. Patients are usually symptomatic, complaining of palpitations, lightheadedness, shortness of breath, or anxiety. ECG documentation of the tachycardia is extremely important to help determine the mechanism of the tachycardia. The differential diagnosis for narrow QRS tachycardia includes the following: sinus tachycardia, atrial tachycardia, atrial flutter, atrial fibrillation, AV nodal re-entry tachycardia (AVNRT), and AV re-entrant tachycardia (AVRT) using an accessory pathway.

Sinus tachycardia can be differentiated from other narrow QRS tachycardias by the sinus morphology of the P wave on a 12-lead ECG. Atrial fibrillation results in an irregular narrow QRS tachycardia with variable AV conduction, resulting in varying R-to-R intervals. The ventricular response to atrial flutter can be regular or irregular. The three most common causes of regular narrow QRS tachycardia are AVNRT, AVRT, and atrial tachycardia, respectively (3).

Physical examination, 12-lead ECG features during tachycardia and sinus rhythm in the same leads, and tachycardia response to carotid sinus massage will facilitate the correct diagnosis of the tachycardia. Pulsations in the neck may often reveal the mechanism of the tachycardia (Table 124.3) (4).

TABLE 124.2

NONINVASIVE INTERVENTIONS TO DETERMINE SITE OF ATRIOVENTRICULAR (AV) BLOCK

Intervention	AV nodal site of block	Infranodal site of block
Atropine	AV block improves	AV block worsens
Exercise	AV block improves	AV block worsens
Carotid sinus massage	AV block worsens	AV block improves

Atrial Tachycardia

During episodes of atrial tachycardia, an ectopic (nonsinus) P wave precedes the QRS complex. AV block can occur during tachycardia. The atrial rate is regular, with P-to-P intervals ranging between 120 and 250 bpm. The site of origin of the tachycardia within the atria can often be localized using the ECG morphology of the P wave (Fig. 124.7). Atrial tachycardias may be paroxysmal or persistent (incessant). Paroxysmal tachycardias can originate from a focal area of the myocardium or may be due to re-entry within a macrore-entrant circuit. Persistent or incessant atrial tachycardia is rare but important to recognize; patients who are in tachycardia >50% of the time may develop tachycardia-induced dilated cardiomyopathy.

Atrial Flutter

Atrial flutter typically has an atrial rate of 250 to 350 bpm. The most common form of atrial flutter uses a right atrial macrore-entrant circuit, including the cavotricuspid isthmus. Typical atrial flutter has a classic sawtooth pattern of atrial activation in the inferior leads of the ECG (Fig. 124.8). Flutter waves can be better appreciated during rapid tachycardia with slowing of the ventricular response by carotid sinus massage.

Atrial Fibrillation

Atrial fibrillation is the most common supraventricular tachyarrhythmia in the United States (5,6). It is a major cause of cardiovascular morbidity and mortality, with an increased risk of death, congestive heart failure, and stroke. The incidence of atrial fibrillation increases with age, with a lifetime risk of one in four men and women older than the age of 40 y (6). Similarly, the risk of embolic stroke from atrial fibrillation increases with age (>65 years), as well as other risk factors including hypertension, prior history of strokes, heart failure, left ventricular function of ≤35%, mitral stenosis, prosthetic heart valve, and diabetes. Therefore, stroke prevention is the key

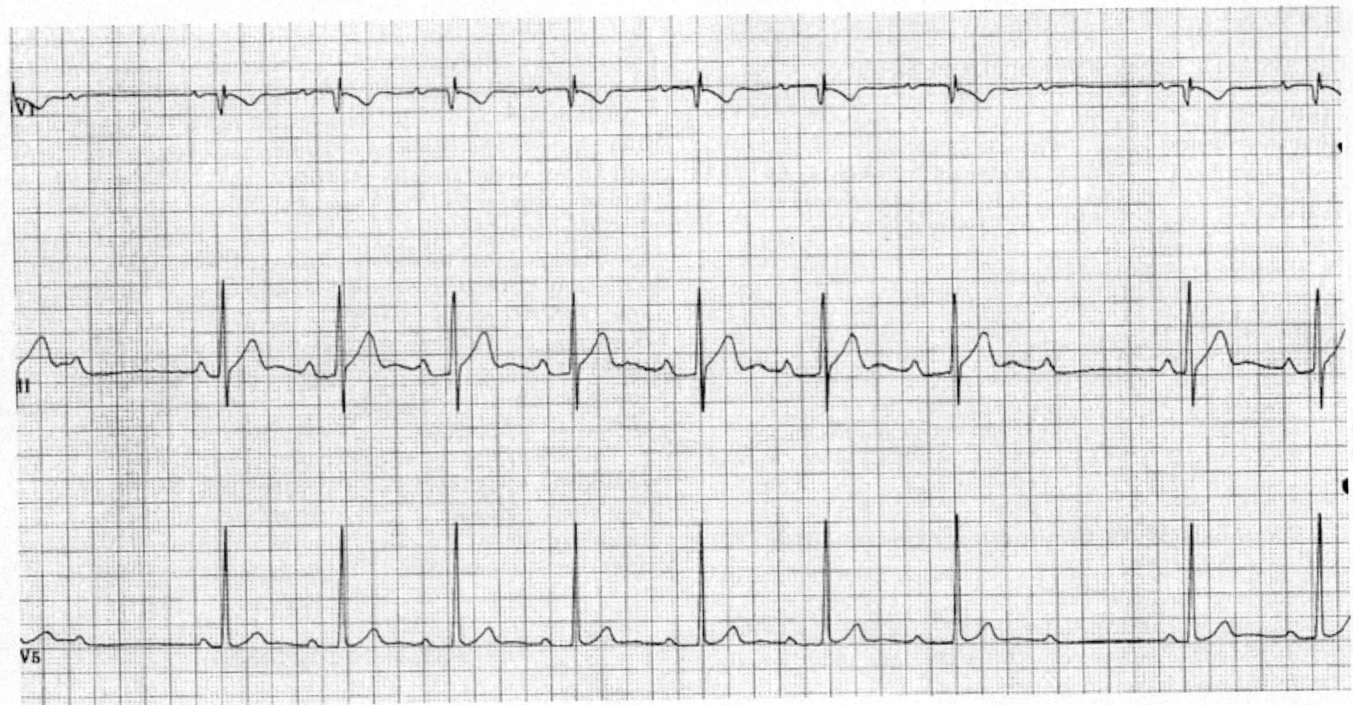

FIGURE 124.3. A 12-lead electrocardiogram. Sinus rhythm with type I second-degree atrioventricular conduction block.

focus in the management of atrial fibrillation. Anticoagulation with warfarin, with an international normalized ratio (INR) between 2.0 and 3.0, is recommended in patients with atrial fibrillation and one or two of the above-mentioned risk factors. Recent practice guidelines have been published by Fuster et al. (7) for the management of patients with atrial fibrillation.

Atrial fibrillation can be divided into four categories: (i) new onset; (ii) paroxysmal (spontaneous termination); (iii) persistent (terminates only by pharmacologic or electrical conversion); and (iv) permanent. The atrial rhythm is irregular, with an atrial rate of 350 to 500 bpm (Fig. 124.9).

AV Nodal Re-entry Tachycardia

AV nodal re-entrant tachycardia (AVNRT) is the most common form of a regular SVT and is due to re-entry within AV nodal and perinodal tissue. The heart rhythm is regular, usually between 130 and 250 bpm. Different forms of AVNRT are classified based on the direction of the circuit and the electrophysiologic properties of the circuit. Typically, there is simultaneous activation of the atria and ventricles, with P waves either hidden or partially visible at the end of the QRS

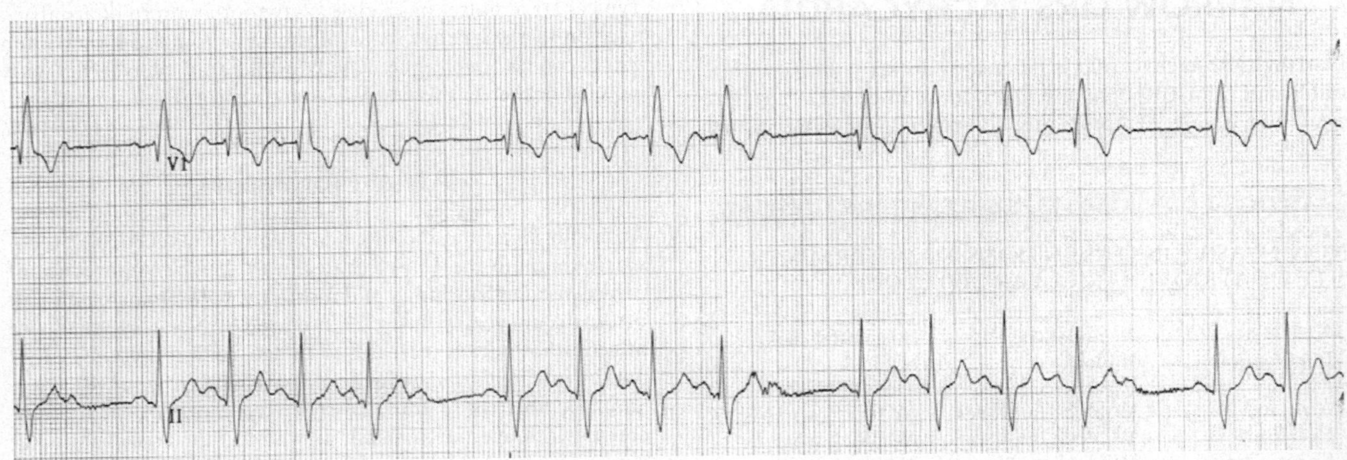

FIGURE 124.4. A 12-lead electrocardiogram. Sinus rhythm with second-degree type II atrioventricular conduction block.

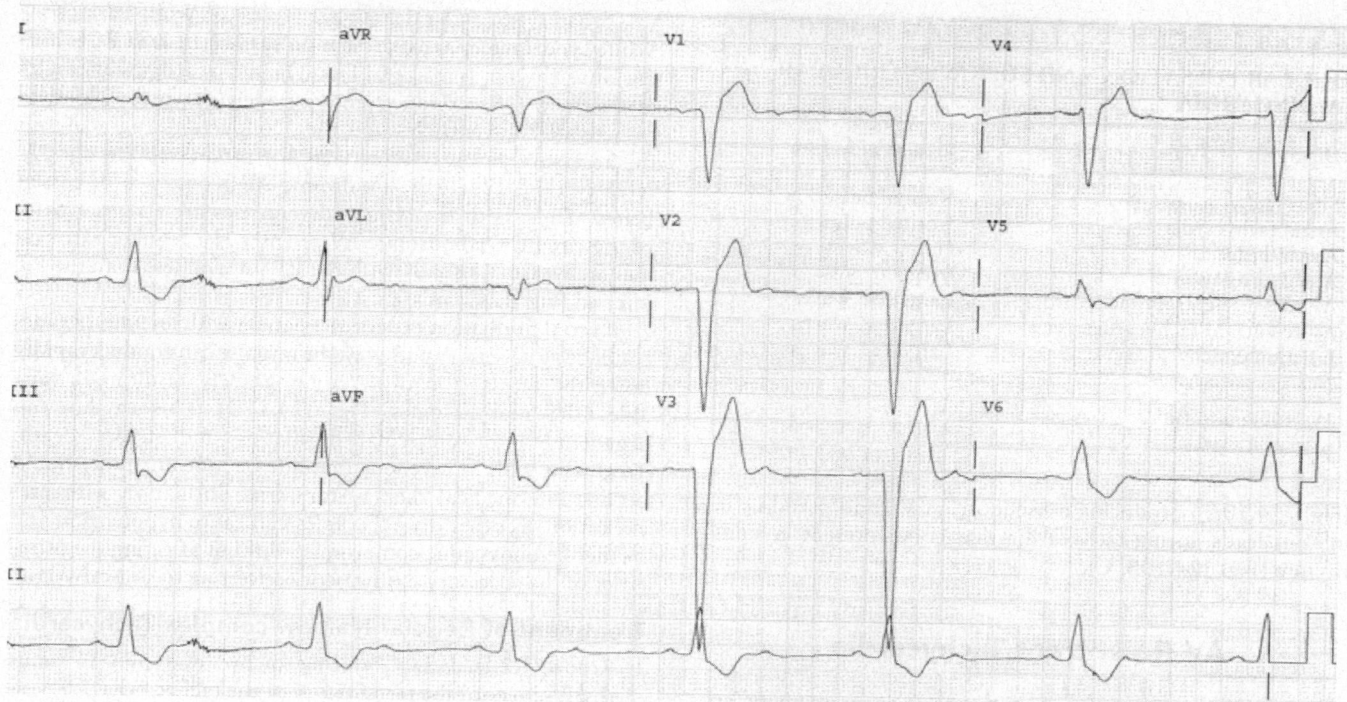

FIGURE 124.5. A 12-lead electrocardiogram. Sinus rhythm with 2:1 atrioventricular conduction block with left bundle branch block suggesting block below the His bundle.

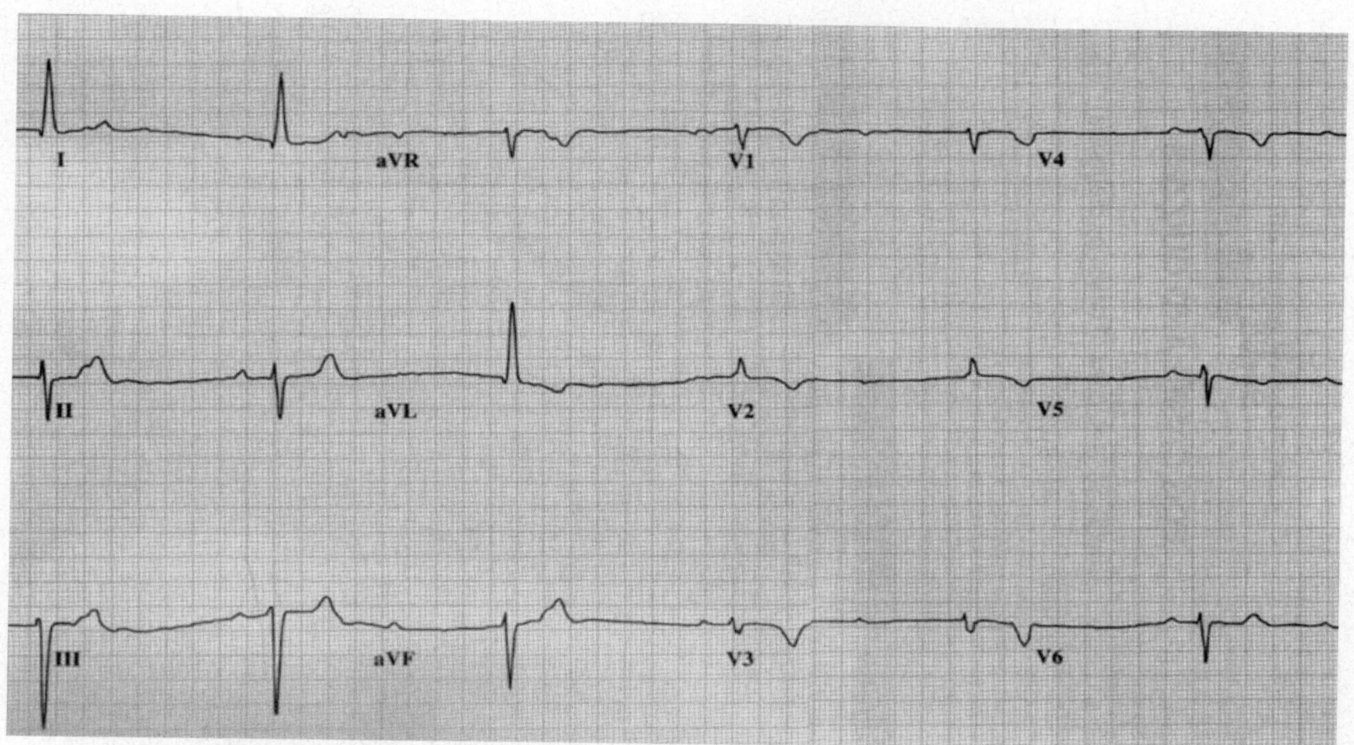

FIGURE 124.6. A 12-lead electrocardiogram. Sinus bradycardia with third degree AV conduction block.

TABLE 124.3

JUGULAR PULSATION AND SUPRAVENTRICULAR TACHYCARDIA

Diagnosis of SVT	Jugular pulsation
Sinus tachycardia	Normal pulsation
Atrial tachycardia	Normal pulsation
Atrial flutter	Flutter waves
Atrial fibrillation	Irregular pulse
AV nodal re-entrant tachycardia	Large "a" waves
AV re-entrant tachycardia	Large "a" waves
Junctional tachycardia	Large "a" waves

AV, atrioventricular.

(Fig. 124.10A), producing a pseudo-r′ in V1 and pseudo-s in inferior leads during tachycardia that is not present in sinus rhythm (Fig. 124.10B, C).

AV Re-entrant Tachycardia

AV re-entrant tachycardia occurs due to re-entry involving an accessory pathway, an abnormal electrical connection between the atria and ventricle (8). If the accessory pathway conducts anterogradely, certain characteristics, such as a short PR interval, broad QRS, and a delta wave typical of Wolff-Parkinson-White syndrome, may be present on surface 12-lead ECG during sinus rhythm (Fig. 124.11A). The tachycardia that results in a narrow QRS conducts anterogradely down the AV node to activate the ventricles and then conducts retrogradely up the accessory pathway to activate the atria (orthodromic AV re-entry (Fig. 124.11B); antidromic AV re-entry is discussed below. Thus, both the atria and ventricles are essential parts of the circuit. Orthodromic AV re-entry is a regular paroxysmal tachycardia, usually with the RP interval less than the PR interval (Fig. 124.11C).

If atrial fibrillation occurs in a patient with an anterograde-conducting accessory pathway, the impulse can conduct rapidly down the accessory pathway anterogradely, resulting in variable QRS morphologies (Fig. 124.11D). This rhythm can degenerate into ventricular fibrillation and sudden death. Treatment with intravenous ibutilide or procainamide should be first-line medical therapy for atrial fibrillation with pre-excitation, as other drug therapies can cause hypotension and further hemodynamic compromise without affecting the properties of the accessory pathway or converting to sinus rhythm.

Treatment of Regular Narrow-complex Tachycardia

1. Record 12-lead ECG during tachycardia and in sinus rhythm; record the termination of the tachycardia
2. Physical examination evaluating jugular pulse
3. Vagal maneuver; if no success, then 6 mg of rapid IV adenosine and repeat with 12 mg of IV adenosine

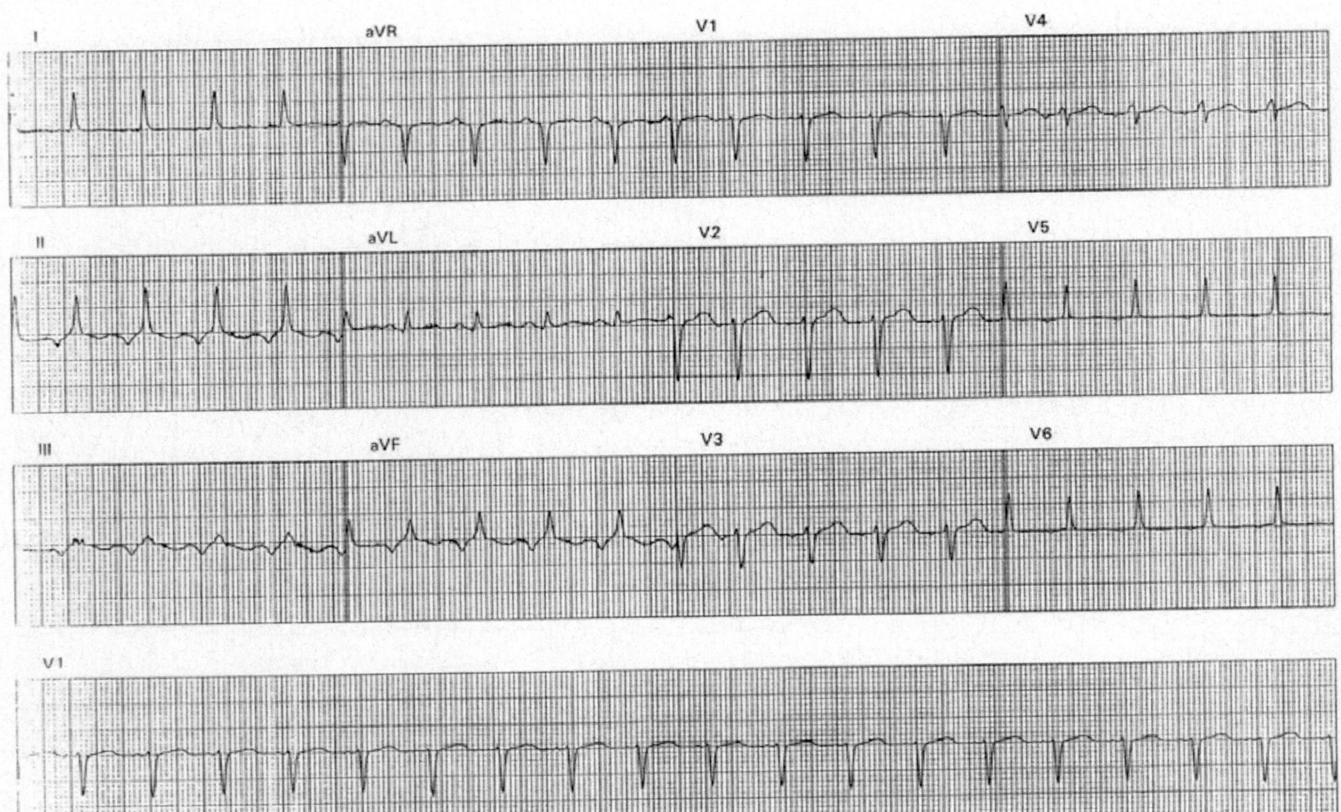

FIGURE 124.7. A 12-lead electrocardiogram. Atrial tachycardia with a p wave preceding each QRS complex. The origin of the p wave is low atrial septal.

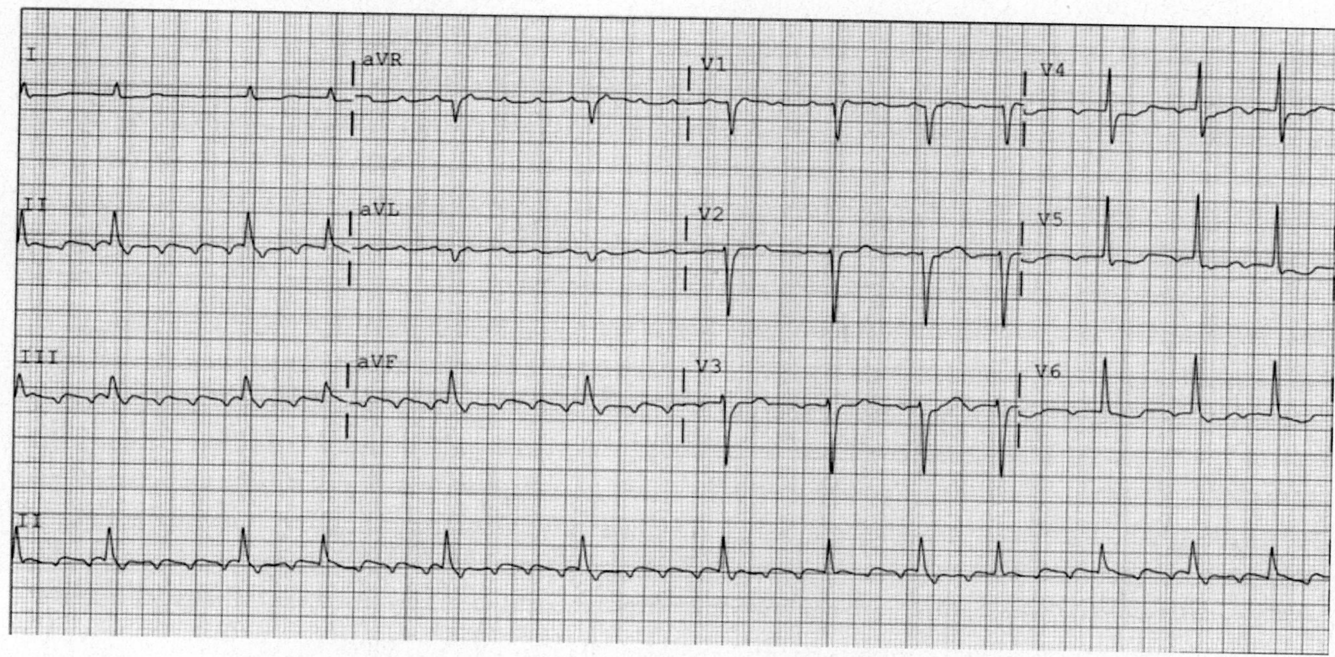

FIGURE 124.8. A 12-lead electrocardiogram. Atrial flutter with variable atrioventricular conduction.

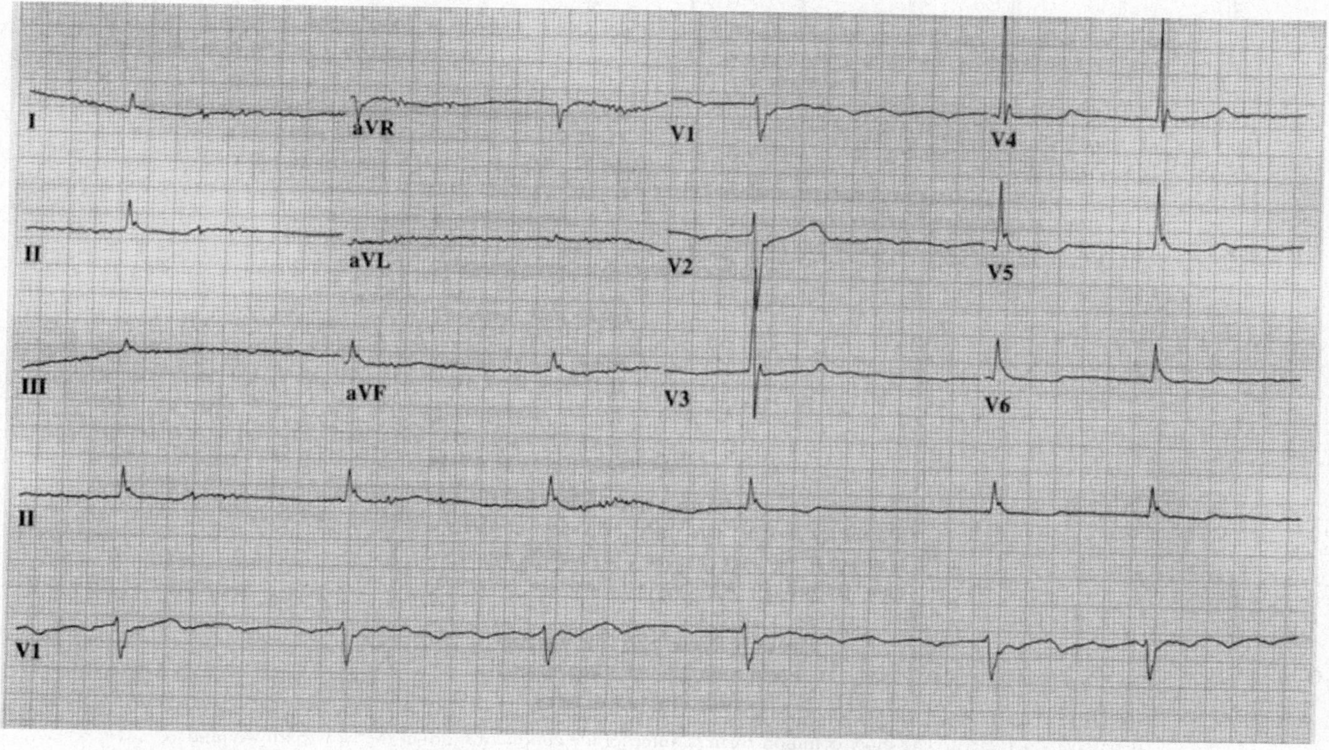

FIGURE 124.9. A 12-lead electrocardiogram. Atrial fibrillation with slow ventricular response. Note that there are no discernible p waves and that the rhythm is irregular.

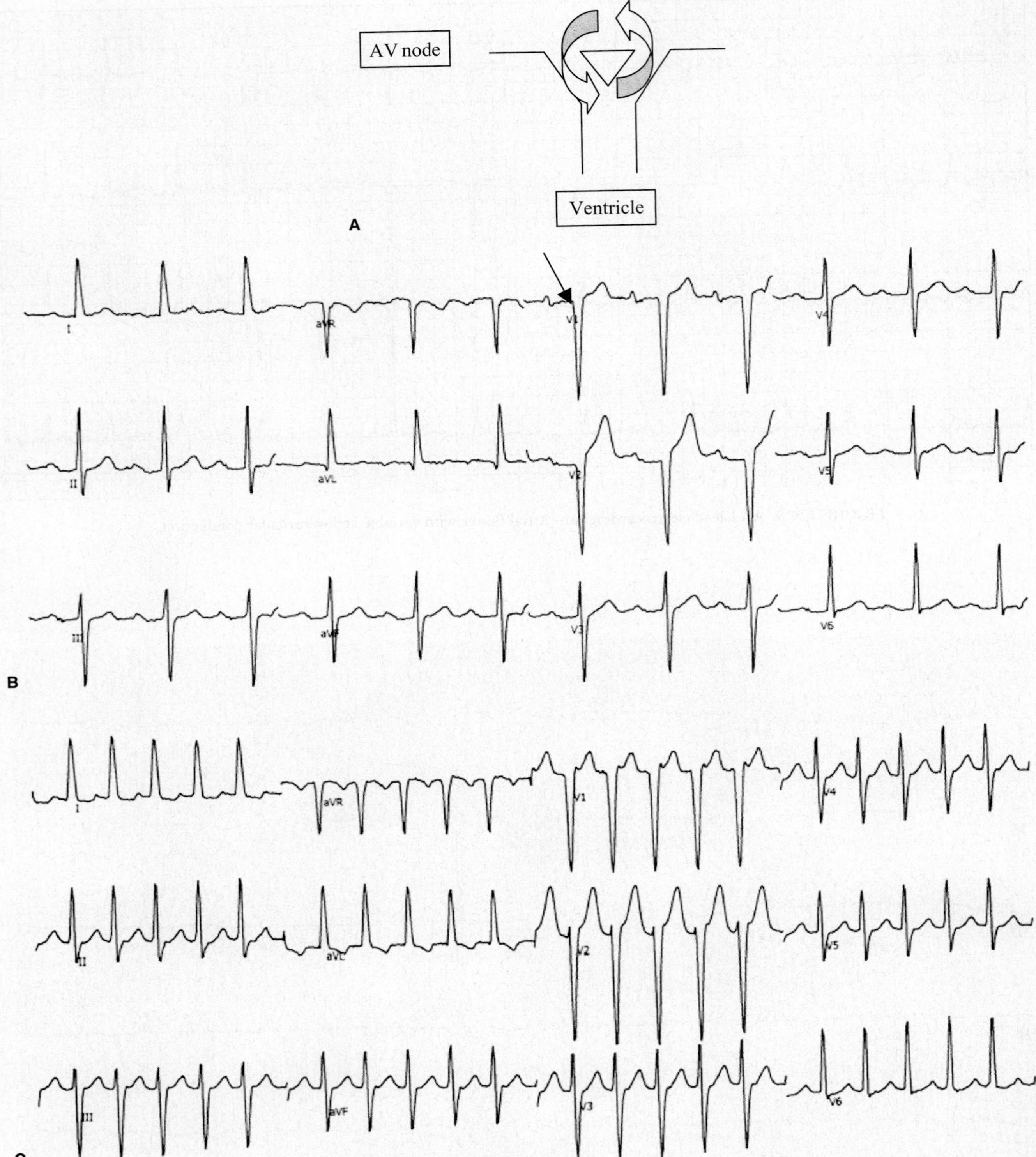

FIGURE 124.10. A: Schematic of atrioventricular (AV) nodal re-entrant tachycardia where the ventricle is passively activated. The most common form is anterograde conduction down the slow pathway and retrograde conduction up the fast pathway. B: A 12-lead electrocardiogram. Sinus rhythm of a patient with AV nodal re-entry tachycardia (AVNRT); there is no r′ in lead V1. C: A 12-lead electrocardiogram. AVNRT with pseudo r′ in lead V1 denoted by the *arrow*.

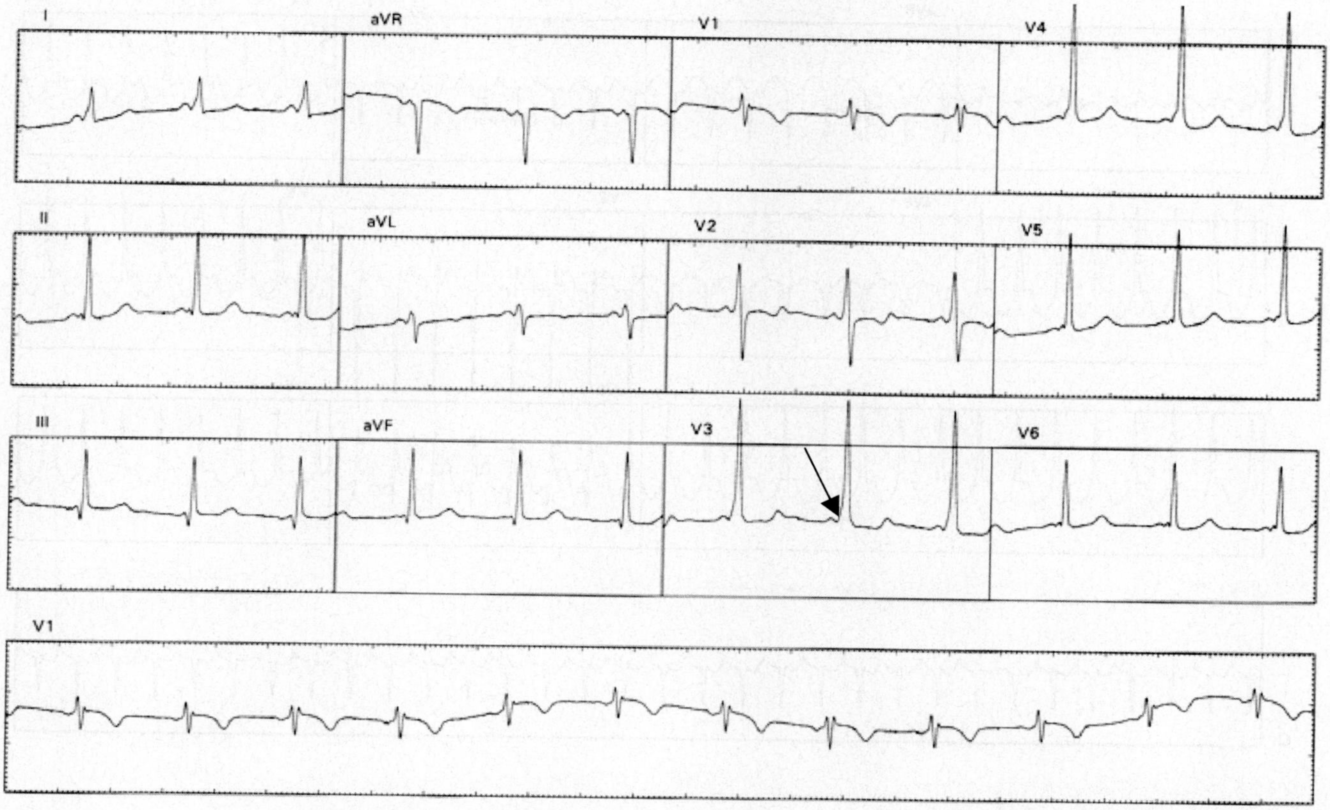

A

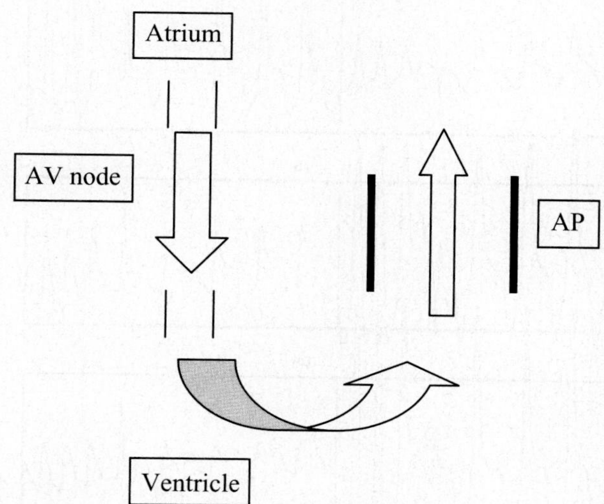

B

FIGURE 124.11. **A:** A 12-lead electrocardiogram. Sinus rhythm with ventricular pre-excitation manifested as a delta wave (*arrow*), consistent with Wolff-Parkinson-White syndrome. **B:** Schematic of orthodromic atrioventricular (AV) re-entrant tachycardia with anterograde ventricular activation from the AV node and retrograde activation through an accessory pathway (AP). Next page. **C:** A 12-lead electrocardiogram. Narrow-complex tachycardia in the same patient was found to be AV re-entrant tachycardia with anterograde conduction down the AV node and retrograde conduction up the accessory pathway. **D:** A 12-lead electrocardiogram. Atrial fibrillation in a patient with anterogradely conducting accessory pathway. There are various QRS width as there is conduction simultaneously down both the AV node and the accessory pathway. This patient is at risk for ventricular fibrillation and sudden cardiac death.

4. If tachycardia continues, then consider beta-blockers, calcium channel blockers (verapamil 5–10 mg IV, if normal left ventricular function), or digoxin
5. If tachycardia persists, use antiarrhythmic medications such as IV amiodarone, IV procainamide (10 mg/kg, no faster than 50 mg/minute), or sotalol
6. If tachycardia persists and/or patient is hemodynamically unstable, cardiovert

Treatment of Atrial Fibrillation

1. Recent onset (<48 hours) without significant heart disease and stable:
   a. Pharmacologic cardioversion with flecainide (300 mg per mouth once), propafenone (600 mg per mouth), procainamide (5–10 mg/kg IV over 20 minutes), ibutilide (1 mg IV over 10 minutes, then repeat), or amiodarone (1,000 mg IV over first 24 hours)

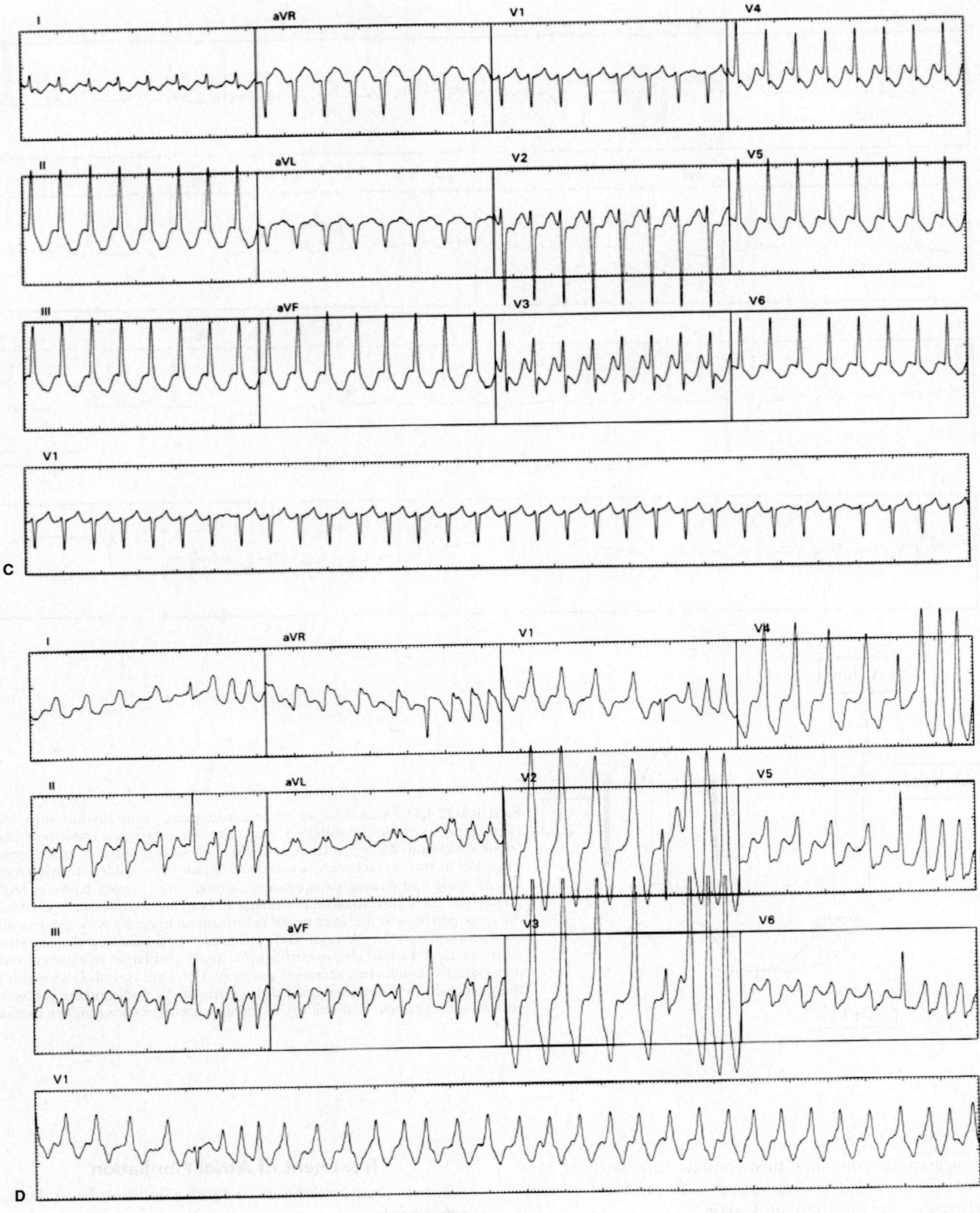

FIGURE 124.11. (*Continued*)

   b. Electrical cardioversion with sedation
2. Recent onset (<48 hours) and unstable: Proceed with immediate cardioversion
3. More than 48 hours and stable:
   a. Control ventricular rate with beta-blockers, calcium channel blockers, and/or digoxin
   b. Aspirin can be used in patients with lone atrial fibrillation (AF) (with no risk factors of heart failure, history of thromboembolism, hypertension, or diabetes)
   c. Patients with risk factors should be on oral anticoagulation with warfarin, with a goal of INR of 2.0 to 3.0
   d. If plan to cardiovert or treat with antiarrhythmic medications, then either anticoagulate for ≥3 weeks prior to cardioversion with therapeutic INR or use transesophageal echocardiography with cardioversion if no thrombus identified, followed by warfarin anticoagulation
4. More than 48 hours and difficulty obtaining adequate rate control: Proceed with transesophageal echocardiogram and cardioversion.
   a. If no thrombus, then cardiovert and anticoagulate
   b. If thrombus is present, then anticoagulate and control rate until thrombus has resolved

WIDE QRS TACHYCARDIA

There are three causes of wide-complex tachycardia: ventricular tachycardia (VT), supraventricular tachycardia (SVT) with aberrant conduction to the ventricles, or a pre-excited tachycardia. A correct and rapid diagnosis is essential, as incorrect treatment may result in hemodynamic decompensation and death (9,10).

Ventricular Tachycardia

Independent atrial and ventricular activity (AV dissociation) is an important electrocardiographic finding that is present in 60% of patients with ventricular tachycardia (Fig. 124.12). Physical examination findings of an irregular jugular pulse, known as cannon "A" waves, varying intensity of the first heart sound, and beat-to-beat changes in systolic blood pressure all are consistent with AV dissociation.

In addition, the presence of supraventricular capture beats (sinus beats that are conducted to the ventricle with a narrow QRS during a wide-complex tachycardia) or fusion beats

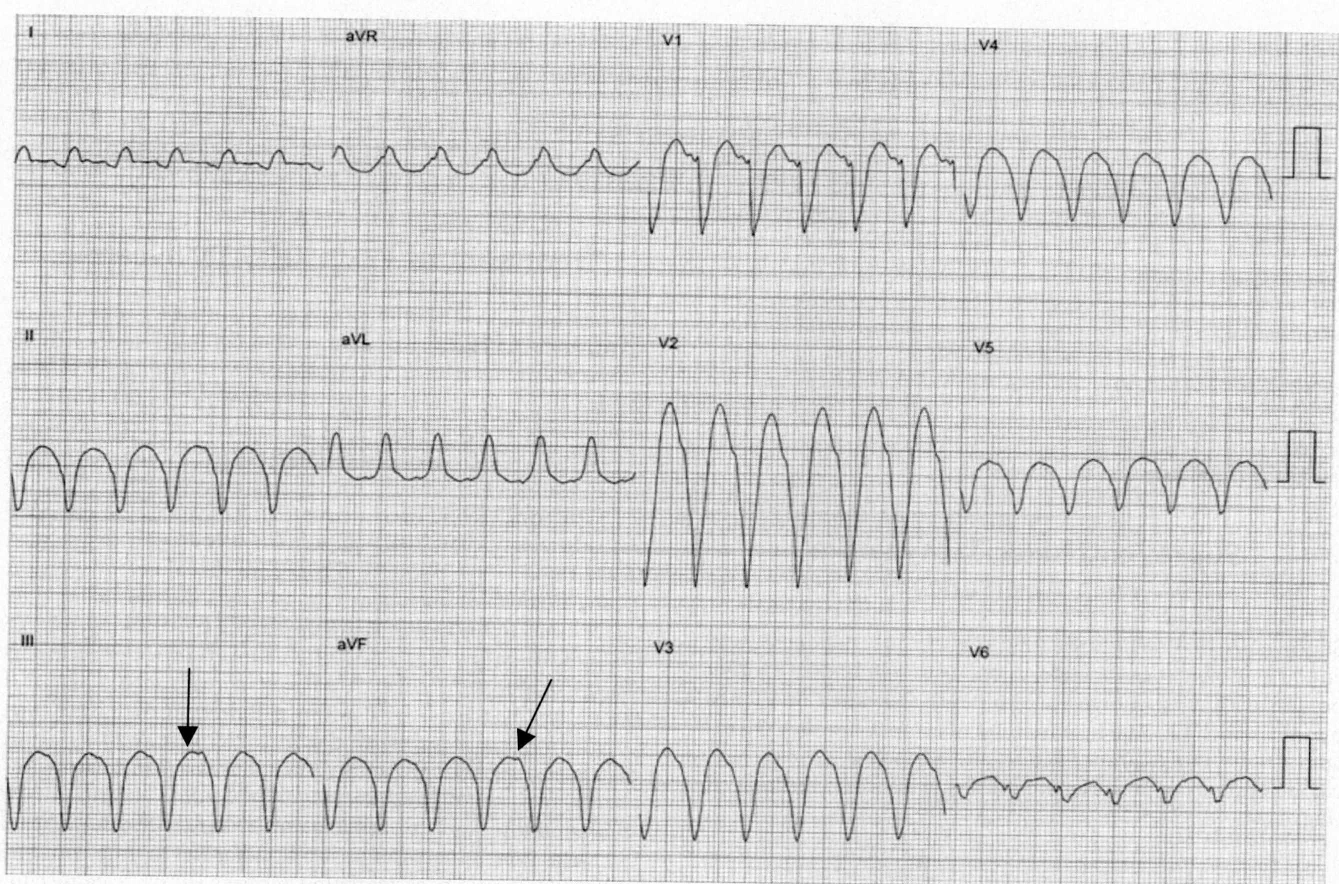

FIGURE 124.12. A 12-lead electrocardiogram. Ventricular tachycardia with atrioventricular dissociation (*arrows* indicate p waves) and negative concordance. There is an atypical left bundle branch block pattern.

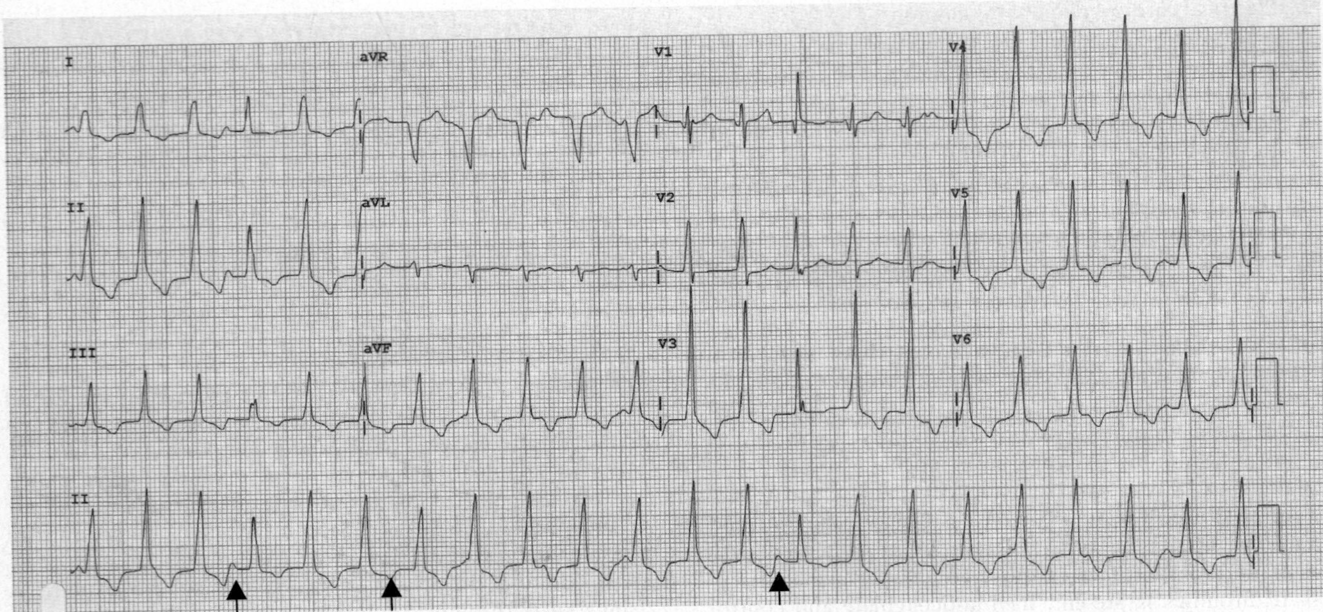

FIGURE 124.13. A 12-lead electrocardiogram. Ventricular tachycardia with AV dissociation and fusion beats (first and second arrow) and supraventricular capture beats (third arrow) confirming the diagnosis of ventricular tachycardia.

(sinus beats that fuse with the wide-complex beat, resulting in a QRS that is narrower than the tachycardia) would be consistent with a diagnosis of ventricular tachycardia (Fig. 124.13). The wide QRS of ventricular tachycardia does not usually mimic a true bundle branch block, since in ventricular tachycardia the impulse is generated in the ventricles; therefore, careful examination of the QRS morphology can usually differentiate ventricular tachycardia from right or left bundle branch block aberrancy. In addition, if all the QRS complexes in the precordial leads V1 to V6 are negative (negative concordance), this is consistent with the diagnosis of ventricular tachycardia (Fig. 124.12). Furthermore, the wider the QRS, the more likely that tachycardia is ventricular in origin. Hemodynamic stability, age of the patient, and ventricular rate or regularity should never be used to distinguish between supraventricular or ventricular tachycardia, as they can be misleading.

Supraventricular Tachycardia with Aberrancy

Supraventricular tachycardia that is aberrantly conducted still conducts down the AV node to the ventricle and can either present with a functional (intermittent) aberrancy or a fixed bundle branch block. The pattern of aberrancy is either typical left or right bundle branch block, and a baseline 12-lead ECG can determine the presence of underlying bundle branch block (Fig. 124.14A, B).

Pre-excited Tachycardia

In patients with AV accessory pathways or Wolff-Parkinson-White syndrome, wide-complex (pre-excited) tachycardias can be seen. In the antidromic AV re-entrant variety, the atrial impulse activates the ventricle anterogradely via the accessory pathway, and retrograde conduction to the atrium is through either the AV node or another accessory pathway (Fig. 124.15). Atrial tachycardias or atrial flutter can conduct via the accessory pathway to produce pre-excited tachycardias.

Treatment of Wide QRS Tachycardia

Monomorphic wide-complex tachycardia that is thought to be ventricular in origin in a stable patient can be treated with intravenous amiodarone (150 mg IV over 10 minutes; repeat as needed to a maximum dose of 2.2 grams IV per 24 hours). If amiodarone is not successful or the patient develops hemodynamic instability or symptoms, then electrical cardioversion is appropriate (11).

If the wide-complex tachycardia is thought to be SVT with aberrancy, then adenosine administration is recommended (6 mg rapid IV push followed by 12 mL of saline. If no effect, 12 mg IV push of adenosine can be tried). Adenosine may be therapeutic (terminating the tachycardia by blocking the AV node) if the patient has a re-entrant supraventricular tachycardia, or diagnostic (causing transient increase in AV block) if the patient has atrial fibrillation or flutter. In the latter case, if patient remains stable, rate-controlling intravenous drugs that have longer-lasting effects, such as beta-blockers or diltiazem, may be administered. Avoid the administration of IV verapamil if the patient has left ventricular dysfunction, heart failure, and/or if there is a possibility that the rhythm could be ventricular in origin, as verapamil has been shown to cause clinical deterioration and death (9). If the patient is hemodynamically unstable, then synchronized cardioversion is appropriate (11).

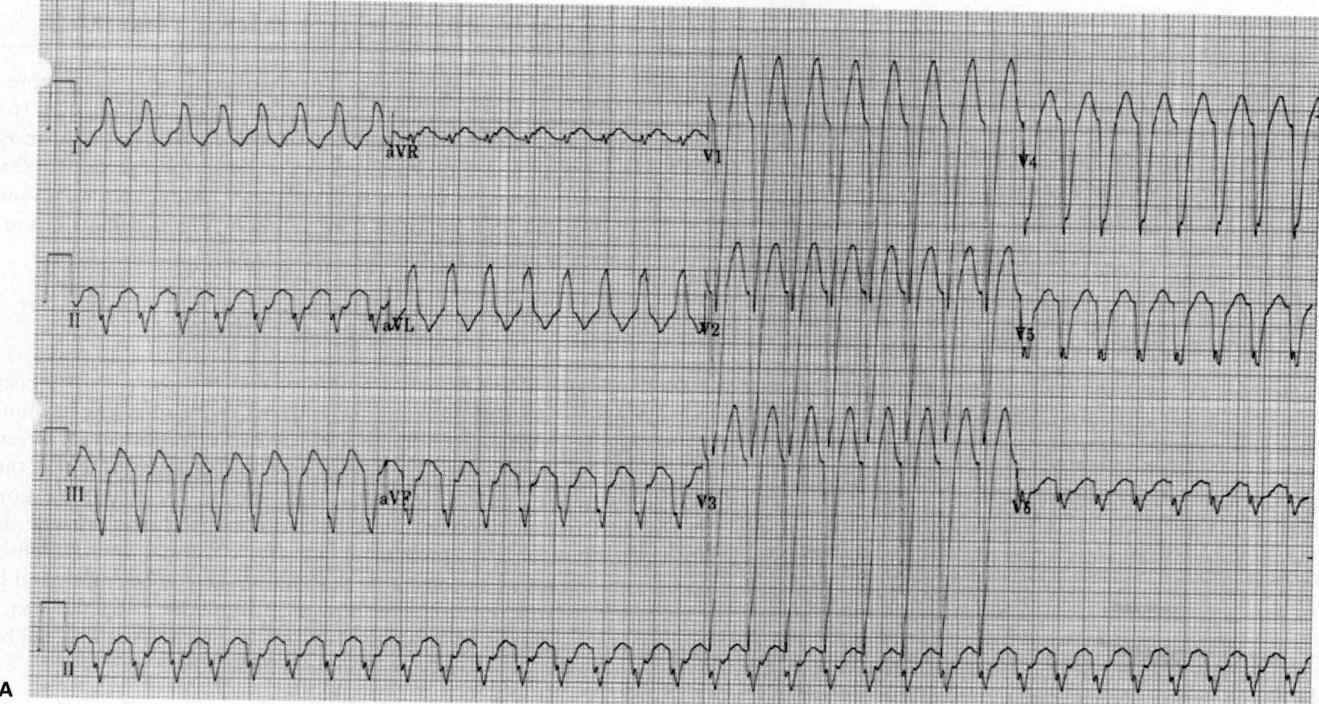

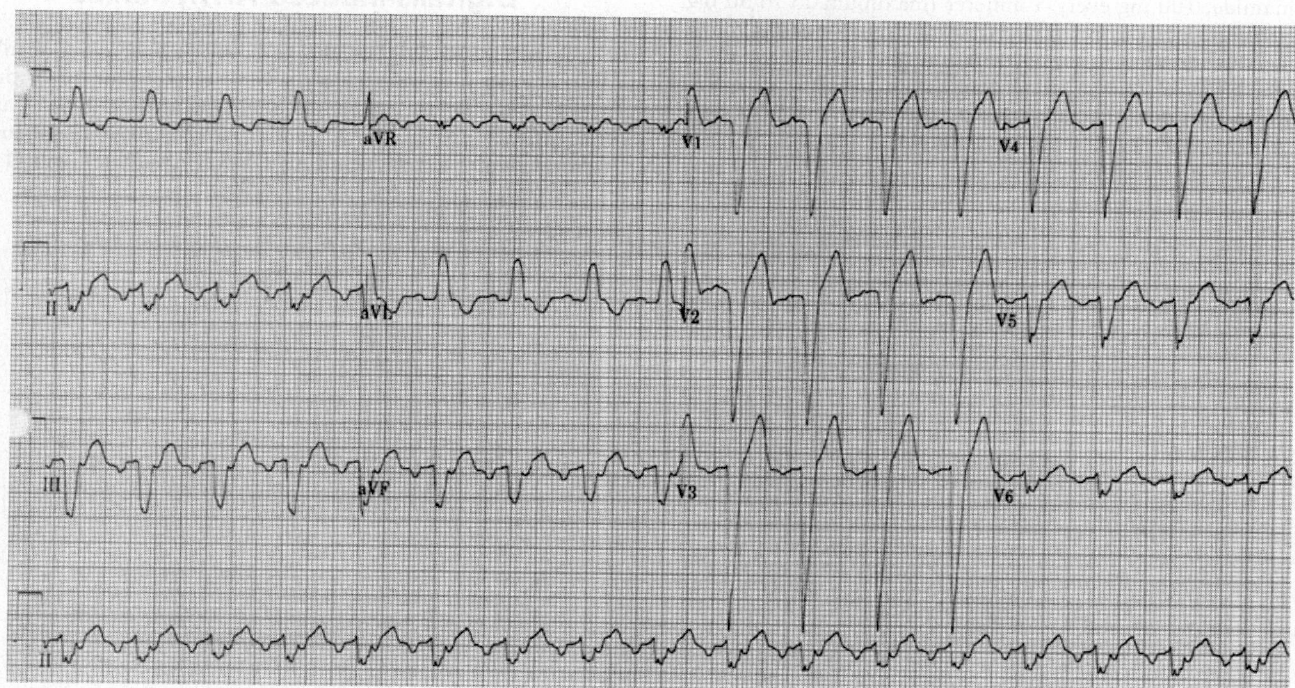

FIGURE 124.14. **A:** A 12-lead electrocardiogram. Atrial flutter with 1:1 conduction and typical left bundle branch block aberrancy. **B:** A 12-lead electrocardiogram. Atrial flutter with 2:1 conduction and typical left bundle branch block aberrancy in the same patient as in Figure 124.12A.

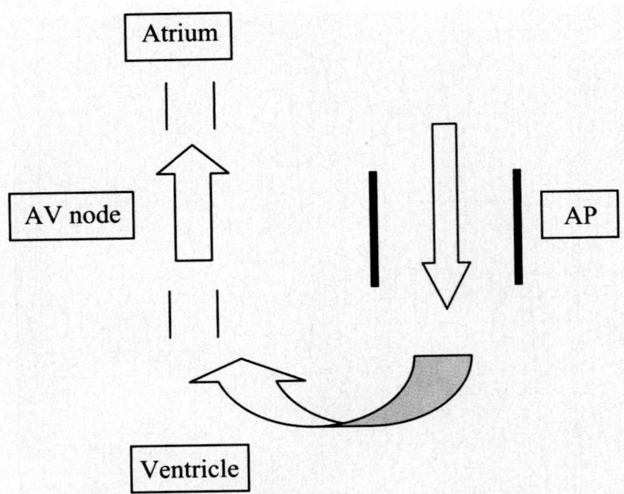

FIGURE 124.15. Schematic of antidromic atrioventricular (AV) reentry, a pre-excited tachycardia with anterograde conduction down the accessory pathway (AP) and retrograde conduction up the AV node.

In a patient with Wolff-Parkinson-White who is in atrial fibrillation with anterograde conduction down the accessory pathway, first-line medical therapy should be intravenous procainamide, 100 mg every 5 minutes (maximum 25 to 50 mg/minute or 17 mg/kg maximum if normal renal function) or intravenous ibutilide, 1 mg over 10 minutes (may be repeated). These drugs block the rapid conduction over the accessory pathway and may also terminate the atrial fibrillation. If there is no effect, then cardiovert. If the patient is unstable, immediate cardioversion is indicated (11).

DRUG-INDUCED ARRYTHMIAS

Many antiarrhythmic agents, noncardiac drugs, and nonprescription medications can cause QT prolongation (Fig. 124.16) and subsequently torsade de pointes (12). The mechanism is thought to be related to reaching the threshold potential for the slow calcium channel, resulting in early after-depolarizations and ectopic impulse formation, triggering re-entrant excitation, which results in torsade de pointes (13,14).

Torsade de Pointes

Torsade de pointes is a polymorphic VT with beat-to-beat changes in the QRS axis (Fig. 124.17); there is QT prolongation, often with a pause or bradycardia-dependent initiation of the arrhythmia. If a drug is responsible for prolonging the QT duration, it should be discontinued. The administration of IV magnesium is effective for the treatment of torsade de pointes, even when serum magnesium is normal. Hypokalemia should also be corrected. Close monitoring is essential, and if bradycardia persists, give atropine or institute temporary pacing. Isoproterenol infusion, between 1 and 4 μg/minute, can be used transiently to increase the heart rate.

Digitalis-induced Arrhythmias

Digitalis, frequently used in heart failure and atrial fibrillation, is a positive inotrope. It slows the ventricular rate during atrial fibrillation, increases vagal tone, causes diuresis, and has vasodilatory effects. Digitalis has a narrow therapeutic window, with women requiring a lower dose than men (15).

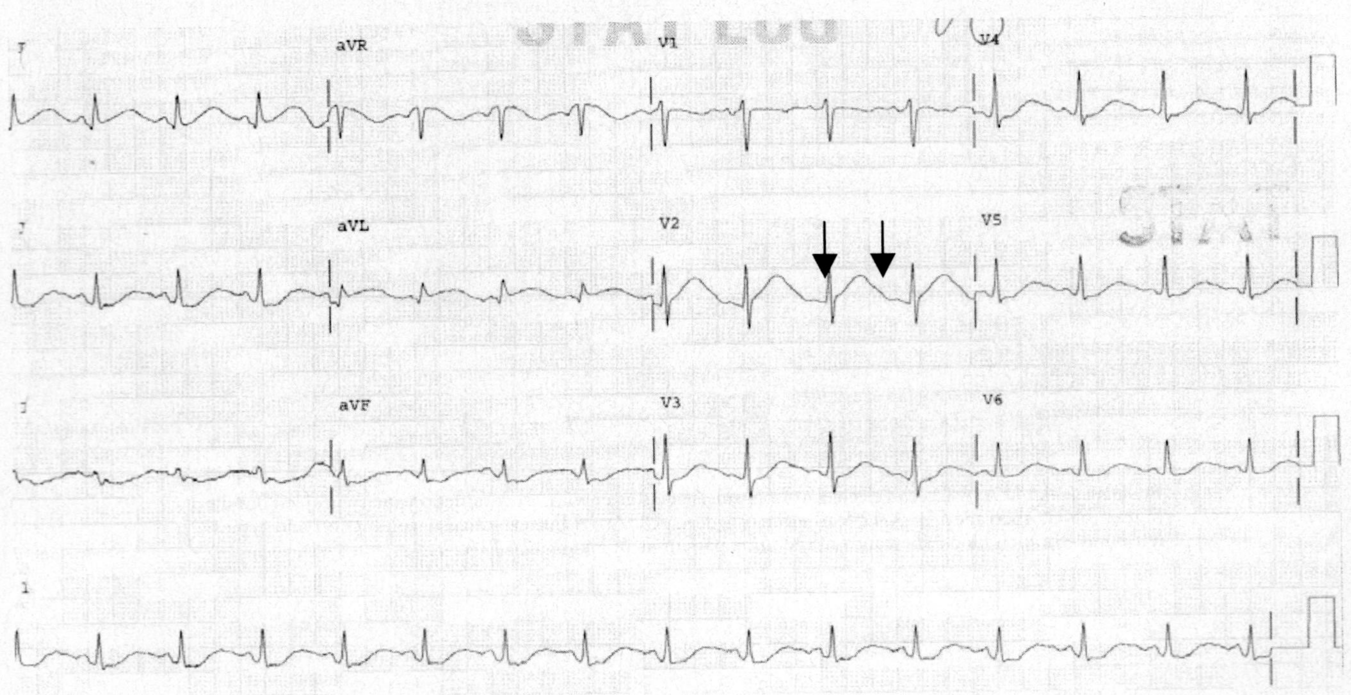

FIGURE 124.16. A 12-lead electrocardiogram. Sinus rhythm with a long QT interval (*arrows* indicate QT measured at approximately 520 ms).

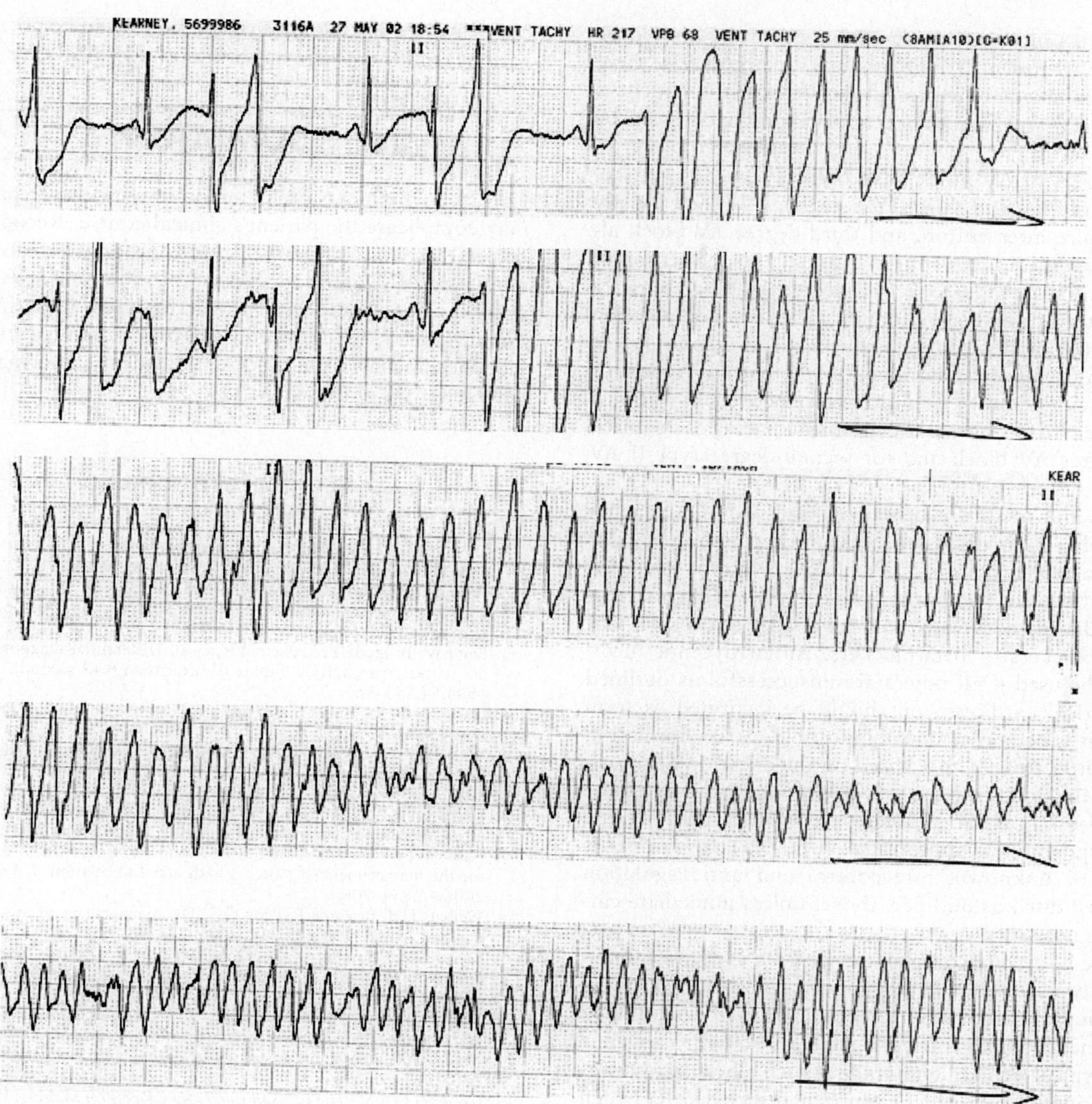

FIGURE 124.17. Lead II rhythm strip. Long QT interval with torsade de pointes.

Unrecognized digitalis intoxication is a common problem and often missed by clinicians (16,17) because the symptoms of digitalis intoxication are nonspecific (gastrointestinal symptoms, visual changes, neuropsychiatric problems, and weakness), and serum drug levels do not correlate well with toxicity. It is important for any health care professional caring for patients who take digitalis to be familiar with ECG findings consistent with digitalis toxicity (17).

Diagnosis and Treatment

Arrhythmias due to digitalis toxicity include atrial tachycardia, junctional tachycardia, ventricular tachycardia, and bradyarrhythmias, including AV block. Many other comorbidities and conditions can potentiate digitalis toxicity, including sympathetic stimulation, hypokalemia, hypercalcemia, hypomagnesemia, diuretics, ischemia and reperfusion, and heart failure. Digitalis toxicity can manifest as four ECG features: (i) bradycardia when the heart rate was previously normal or fast; (ii) tachycardia when the heart rate was previously normal; (iii) unexpected regular rhythm when the patient previously had an irregular rhythm; and (iv) an irregular rhythm that regularly repeats itself (12).

The treatment of digitalis toxicity depends on the clinical condition and not the drug level. The first step when suspecting digitalis toxicity is to discontinue the medication. Rest, continuous ECG monitoring, and correction of electrolyte abnormalities will often help. If the arrhythmia is life threatening, administering digitalis antibodies or phenytoin may be indicated (12). The patient's kidney function must be determined to estimate the severity of the suspected intoxication.

SUMMARY

Cardiac arrhythmias are prevalent in the intensive care setting. Once the mechanism of the arrhythmia is identified, appropriate treatment can be initiated. Bradycardia caused by sinoatrial or AV nodal conduction disorders have been outlined in this chapter. In sinus node dysfunction, symptoms should be used to guide treatment. If patients are asymptomatic, there is no need for immediate treatment; however, if the patient is symptomatic, IV atropine and/or transvenous pacing can be used.

Three degrees of AV block have been reviewed: first, second (types I and II), and third. First-degree AV block usually does not require intervention, and third-degree AV block almost always requires intervention, especially in the setting of an acute MI or heart failure. Second-degree AV block requires immediate intervention if symptomatic. The site of conduction abnormality (AV node versus His-Purkinje) in second-degree AV block can usually be determined by the pattern (type 1 or 2), the QRS width, and by noninvasive maneuvers as outlined in the chapter. In most cases, permanent pacing is required for third-degree AV block and for second-degree type II AV block.

Diagnosis and treatment of narrow and wide QRS tachycardia has also been discussed. The most common regular supraventricular tachycardia is AV nodal re-entrant tachycardia. The treatment of regular narrow-complex supraventricular tachycardia includes vagal maneuvers, IV adenosine, and IV calcium blockers or beta-blockers. Antiarrhythmic medications can be used if all others are unsuccessful as outlined above. Electrical cardioversion should be instituted as soon as the patient is hemodynamically unstable. Atrial fibrillation and atrial flutter treatment is based on the duration of the arrhythmia. If the time from onset is <48 hours, patients can be cardioverted using antiarrhythmics as outlined above, along with anticoagulation as appropriate. If the time from onset is >48 hours or unknown, rate control and anticoagulation should be instituted as outlined above, unless immediate cardioversion is necessary.

The cause of a wide-complex tachycardia should be determined quickly, as it will facilitate appropriate treatment of the patient. Various methods of differentiation have been outlined above. In general, supraventricular tachycardia with aberrancy will have a typical right or left bundle branch block pattern versus a pre-excited tachycardia or ventricular tachycardia which will not have a typical bundle branch block pattern. Differentiation between supraventricular and ventricular tachycardia can be determined with other criteria such as AV dissociation, fusion, or supraventricular capture beats as seen in ventricular tachycardia. With pre-excited tachycardia, there is usually preexcitation (delta wave) present in sinus rhythm and a known history of Wolf-Parkinson-White.

Finally, drug-induced arrhythmias can be seen in the critical care setting. Certain drugs can prolong the QT interval and increase the risk of torsade de pointes, especially if the patient is a female and/or genetically predisposed. Other arrhythmias can be caused by digoxin toxicity, which can be potentiated by various conditions that are common in critical care patients.

SUMMARY

Cardiac arrhythmias are common in critical care patients and may complicate the patient's clinical course. Recognition and correct diagnosis are critical for appropriate treatment to be administered. Careful evaluation of symptoms, electrocardiographic documentation of the arrhythmia, initiating and terminating factors, and response to drug administration all provide the clinician with important diagnostic information in the emergent care of these patients.

References

1. OS N. *Cardiac Arrhythmias: Electrophysiology, Diagnosis, and Management*. Baltimore, MD: Lippincott Williams & Wilkins; 1979.
2. Wellens HJJ, Gorgels APM, Doevendans PA. *The ECG in Acute MI and Unstable Angina: Diagnosis and Risk Stratification*. Boston, MA: Kluwer Academic Publishers; 2003:51.
3. Bar FW, Brugada P, Dassen WR, et al. Differential diagnosis of tachycardia with narrow QRS complex (shorter than 0.12 second). *Am J Cardiol*. 1984;54:555–560.
4. Harvey WP, Ronan JA Jr. Bedside diagnosis of arrhythmias. *Prog Cardiovasc Dis*. 1966;8:419–431.
5. Wolf PA, Abbott RD, Kannel WB. Atrial fibrillation: a major contributor to stroke in the elderly. The Framingham Study. *Arch Intern Med*. 1987;147:1561–1564.
6. Lloyd-Jones DM Wang TJ, Leip EP, et al. Lifetime risk for development of atrial fibrillation: The Framingham Study. *Circulation*. 2004;110:142–146.
7. Fuster V, Ryden LE, Cannom DS, et al. ACC/AHA/ESC 2006 guidelines for the management of patients with atrial fibrillation. *J Am Coll Cardiol*. 2006;48:854–906.
8. Wellens HJJ, Brugada P, Penn OC. The management of pre-excitation syndromes. *JAMA*. 1987;257(17):2325–2333.
9. Buxton AE, Marchlinski FE, Doherty JU, et al. Hazards of intravenous verapamil for sustained ventricular tachycardia. *Am J Cardiol*. 1987;59:1107–1110.
10. Stewart RB, Bardy GH, Greene HL. Wide complex tachycardia: misdiagnosis and outcome after emergent therapy. *Ann Intern Med*. 1986;104:766–771.
11. Management of symptomatic bradycardia and tachycardia. *Circulation*. 2005;112;67–77.
12. Conover HWM. *The ECG in Emergency Decision Making*. Vol. 1. St. Louis, MO: Saunders Elsevier; 2006.
13. Brachmann J, Scherlag BJ, Rosenshtraukh LV, et al. Bradycardia-dependent triggered activity: relevance to drug-induced multiform ventricular tachycardia. *Circulation*. 1983;68:846–856.
14. Roden DM, Hoffman BF. Action potential prolongation and induction of abnormal automaticity by low quinidine concentrations in canine Purkinje fibers. *Relationship to potassium and cycle length. Circ Res*. 1985;56:857–867.
15. Adams KF Jr, Gheorghiade M, Uretsky BF, et al. Clinical benefits of low serum digoxin concentrations in heart failure. *J Am Coll Cardiol*. 2002;39:946–953.
16. Gandhi AJ, Vlasses PH, Morton DJ, et al. Economic impact of digoxin toxicity. *Pharmacoeconomics*. 1997;12:175–181.
17. Williamson KM, Thrasher KA, Fulton KB, et al. Digoxin toxicity: an evaluation in current clinical practice. *Arch Intern Med*. 1998;158:2444–2449.

CHAPTER 125 ■ PERICARDIAL DISEASE

CARSTEN M. SCHMALFUSS

THE NORMAL PERICARDIUM

The normal pericardium forms a sac around the heart and proximal large arteries and veins. It has a thin visceral mesothelial layer that closely adheres to the epicardial surface of the heart. The parietal layer consists of the same thin mesothelium and a thicker (up to 2 mm), fairly nonelastic fibrous layer on the outside. Physiologically, the space between both mesothelial layers contains 20 to 30 mL of fluid.

The fibrous part of the pericardium is attached to the surrounding mediastinal structures and holds the heart in its position within the chest. It limits cardiac dilatation, contributes to the interventricular interaction, and primarily affects diastolic function. The smooth mesothelial surfaces and the pericardial fluid between them reduce friction and act as a barrier to inflammation from surrounding structures. The pericardium is well innervated, and pathologic processes can cause severe episodic or continuous pain.

The intrapericardial pressure is usually negative; it is approximately equal to and varies with the pleural pressure at the same hydrostatic level. Pericardial pressure affects myocardial transmural pressure by the following relationship:

$$\text{Transmural pressure} = \text{cavitary pressure} - \text{adjacent intrapericardial pressure}$$

Because the intrapericardial pressure is normally negative, this usually adds to the normal transmural pressure gradient (1).

The relationship between intrapericardial and pleural pressures causes a simultaneous fall of pressures in both spaces during inspiration and leads to an increased venous return into the right chambers (increased preload), with a subsequent increase in cardiac output. Inspiration influences filling and cardiac output of the left heart only indirectly and very little. The parietal pericardium is very resistant to acute stretching but adapts and expands to great dimension when subjected to a chronic stretching process. The pericardial pressure–volume curve is generally flat as pericardial volume increases, and when further distention is impossible, a sharp rise in the intrapericardial pressure occurs. This exponential curve accounts for the rapid clinical response when even small amounts of fluid are removed in cardiac tamponade (2).

This chapter deals with the most common clinical pericardial problems encountered in critical care medicine. They include acute pericarditis, pericardial effusion, cardiac tamponade, and pericardial constriction.

ACUTE PERICARDITIS

Etiology

Inflammation of the pericardial sac results in acute pericarditis and is either an isolated problem or part of a systemic process. Exudation of inflammatory fluid into the pericardial space can result in pericardial effusion. Depending on the frequency and time course, pericarditis can be acute, recurrent, or chronic. Common causes of acute pericarditis are shown in Table 125.1. Most often, clinically recognizable pericarditis in the adult is idiopathic. In these cases, various viruses are often the suspected causes; an etiologic agent is infrequently demonstrated. The most commonly demonstrated virus is the Coxsackie B group, which causes myopericarditis in children and pleuropericarditis in adults—also called Bornholm disease (3). ECHO, influenza, Epstein-Barr, varicella, hepatitis, mumps, and human immunodeficiency viruses can also cause pericarditis.

Up to one third of patients with end-stage renal disease will develop uremic pericarditis. Most of them have not started dialysis when they present with pericarditis, and the symptoms usually disappear after beginning or increasing the frequency of dialysis (4). There is no direct association with serum blood urea nitrogen level or serum creatinine and the acute illness. However, it is suspected that increased toxin levels from declining renal function cause the inflammatory process. It is important to remember that the uremic patient is susceptible to infections and that the pericarditis may be infectious. Last but not least, the underlying disease process leading to the renal insufficiency (i.e., lupus erythematosus) may also be the cause for the pericardial inflammation.

Acute pericarditis after myocardial injury is thought to be due to direct irritation of the visceral mesothelium. In the past, pericarditis occurred in up to 20% of patients after transmural myocardial infarction; recently, the frequency has decreased due to the increased use of reperfusion therapy—that is, thrombolytic therapy or angioplasty (5). Typically, symptoms occur 1 to 3 days after the myocardial damage and can mimic recurrent angina pectoris. If the patient is receiving anticoagulants, the inflammation can lead to hemorrhagic intrapericardial effusion and possibly cardiac tamponade. Acute pericardial inflammation is also found after open heart surgery, implantation of cardiac pacemakers, percutaneous coronary interventions, or external cardiac trauma, and the presentation is similar to that after transmural infarction.

TABLE 125.1

COMMON CAUSES OF PERICARDITIS

Idiopathic
Viral
Uremic
Neoplastic
Metastatic
Contiguous spread
Primary
Autoimmune
Systemic lupus erythematosus
Postpericardiotomy syndrome (Dressler)
Rheumatoid arthritis
Scleroderma
Postmyocardial infarction
Bacterial
Parasitic
Mycotic
Trauma with contusion of the heart
Aortic dissection or ventricular rupture
Radiation induced
Myxedema
Drug-induced
Procainamide
Hydralazine
Quinidine
Isoniazid
Methysergide
Daunorubicin
Penicillin
Streptomycin
Phenylbutazone
Minoxidil
Sarcoid
Amyloidosis
Acute pancreatitis
Chylopericardium

The postpericardiotomy syndrome was originally described as postmyocardial infarction pericarditis. Later, Engle and Ito (6) noted the same clinical syndrome in children and adults who experienced an opening of the pericardium. The syndrome occurs in 10% to 30% of patients who have undergone pericardiotomy and is thought to be an immune complex reaction to the patient's own pericardium (7). In contrast to pericarditis caused by myocardial injury, these patients usually have symptoms of chest pain and fever beginning several weeks to months after cardiac surgery or other myocardial injury.

Neoplastic pericarditis is most often caused by cancer of the lung, breast, or esophagus as well as lymphoma and melanoma (8). The tumor directly invades the pericardial space or metastasizes through lymphatics or blood vessels; primary pericardial tumors like mesothelioma are rare. The likelihood of finding previously undiagnosed cancer in a patient presenting with pericarditis is about 6% to 7% (9). The cause of pericarditis in patients with known malignancy is neoplastic in only 50% to 60%; idiopathic pericarditis and radiation-induced pericarditis are the most common benign causes (10,11). The prognosis of neoplastic pericarditis and effusion is poor.

Pericarditis is also seen in patients with systemic lupus erythematosus, rheumatoid arthritis, and scleroderma. Inflammation of the pericardium is often the first manifestation of lupus in female patients; this diagnosis should be ruled out during the workup for a first episode of idiopathic pericarditis. Radiation pericarditis often follows a mediastinal dose of 4,000 rad or more and can lead to pericardial effusion and acute cardiac tamponade. The long-term effects of radiation also can lead to constrictive pericarditis.

Pericarditis caused by infectious organisms other than viruses is less frequent now than it was in the preantibiotic era. Pneumonia is still the most common cause; others include sepsis from peritonitis and urinary tract infection, or direct spread of the infectious process from mediastinitis or necrotizing fasciitis of the head or neck. Immunocompromised and elderly patients are more prone to infectious pericarditis than the general population. In adults, *Staphylococcus aureus* is still the most common organism, and there is an apparent decline in infections with *Streptococcus* spp., *Pneumococcus* spp., and *Haemophilus influenzae*.

Tuberculous pericarditis was once a common cause of acute and constrictive pericarditis, but with the overall decline of tuberculosis, it has become a rare entity in the United States (12). More recently, states with a high percentage of immigrants have again reported rising numbers of tuberculous pericarditis (13). One to two percent of patients with pulmonary tuberculosis will develop tuberculous pericarditis (14). Mycobacterial infection must be ruled out in any case of suspected purulent pericarditis.

The most common fungal organism to cause pericarditis is *Histoplasma capsulatum*. Histoplasmosis in the United States is most common in the Mississippi and Ohio River Valleys (15). Diagnosis is usually delayed and made by positive fungal culture of the pericardial fluid and/or a significant rise of serologic antibody titers (greater than 1:32) against *Histoplasma capsulatum*.

Clinical Presentation

The typical patient presenting with pericarditis is young and was previously healthy. Symptoms of acute pericarditis include sharp and, usually, persistent chest pain that is generally increased with respiration and motion. It is worse in the supine position and usually improves sitting up and/or with shallow breathing. The pain can radiate to the neck, and dyspnea may also be present. Other common findings preceding or accompanying pericarditis are fever, myalgia, malaise, and tachycardia. The characteristic and pathognomonic three-component friction rub is best described as coarse, leathery, superficial—like "pulling Velcro". The rub is only intermittently heard during the episode of pericarditis, and therefore, it is important to auscultate frequently. The patient is ideally examined in a quiet setting in an upright position leaning forward; the rub is best heard at the left sternal border or the cardiac apex.

An electrocardiogram (ECG) should be obtained in every patient presenting with chest pain. Four ECG stages, evolving over hours to days and weeks, have been described:

- Stage I includes classic and diffuse ST elevations with a concave ST segment and significant PR-segment depression (Fig. 125.1).
- Stage II is normalization of the ECG.
- Stage III is the development of diffuse T-wave inversion that may persist or normalize.
- Stage IV is final normalization of the ECG (16).

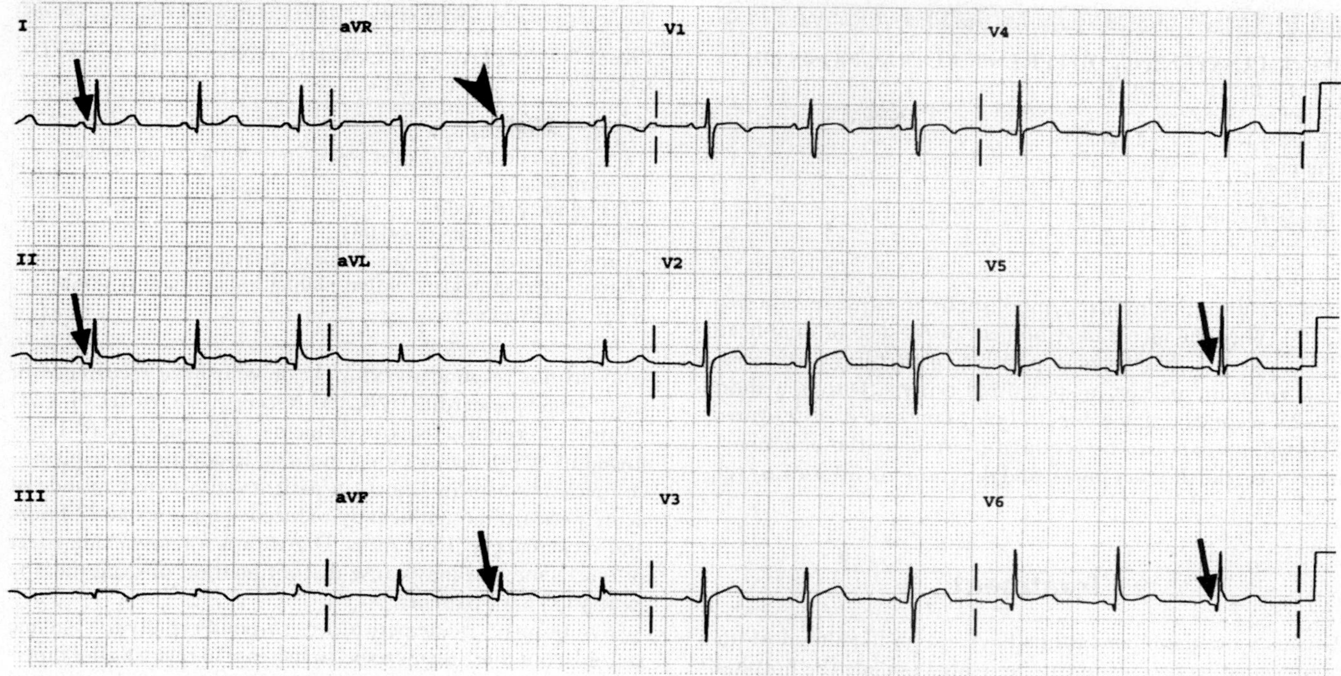

FIGURE 125.1. Electrocardiogram of a patient with acute pericarditis. Note the PR-segment depressions (*arrows*) and convex ST-segment elevations in the inferolateral leads and PR-segment elevation (*arrowhead*) and ST-segment depression in lead aVR consistent with stage I of electrocardiogram findings in acute pericarditis.

The ECG may show all, several, or none of the stages during an episode of acute pericarditis. Atrial arrhythmias are rare but do occur in acute pericarditis (17) and can be the first manifestation of acute pericarditis. However, sustained atrial or ventricular arrhythmias are suggestive of concomitant myocarditis.

The key to an ECG diagnosis of pericarditis is the diffuse nature of the ECG changes, the absence of localization to a particular ECG anatomic area, PR-segment depression, and the absence of ST depression except in lead aVR.

Every patient suspected to have pericarditis should have a chest radiograph taken. It will be normal in most cases of pericarditis; a new finding of an enlarged cardiac silhouette is, however, suggestive of a pericardial effusion (greater than 200 mL) and should be further evaluated.

The laboratory may report positive acute-phase reactants (especially the erythrocyte sedimentation rate) and an elevated white blood cell count; however, these are nonspecific findings. Cardiac troponin T or I and CK-MB isoenzymes are cardiac—but not pericardium—specific and are often found minimally elevated in acute pericarditis. Viral studies may confirm a viral cause of the pericarditis; however, their yield is low, and the result does not change management. In cases of suspected infectious etiology, cultures from blood and pericardial fluid, if available, should be examined for bacterial and mycobacterial pathogens.

Echocardiography should be performed in every patient with the suspected diagnosis of pericarditis to evaluate for and follow pericardial effusion (Fig. 125.2) and to help diagnose cardiac tamponade.

The triad of typical chest pain, pericardial friction rub, and the aforementioned ECG changes confirms the diagnosis of acute pericarditis. However, this diagnosis should be made only after life-threatening conditions with similar presentation (Table 125.2) have been ruled out. Electrocardiographic differential diagnosis also includes variant angina, hypertrophic cardiomyopathy, and the benign finding of early repolarization—all of which can mimic the ECG changes described earlier.

Aside from history and physical exam, ECG, chest radiographs, blood work, and echocardiogram, it may be necessary to evaluate the patient with computed tomography (CT) of the

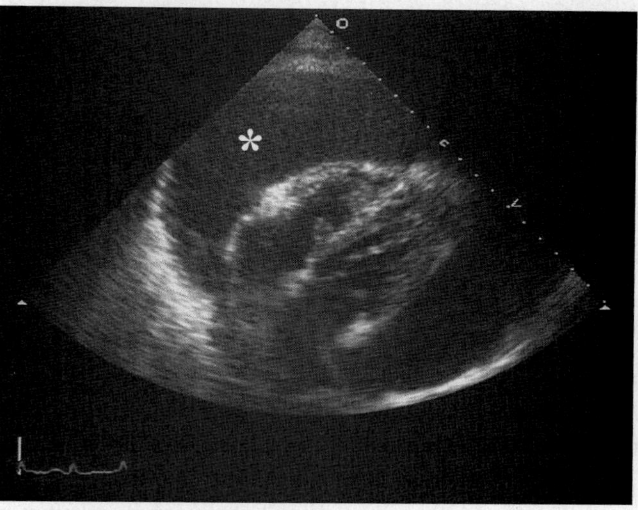

FIGURE 125.2. Subcostal echocardiogram showing a giant pericardial effusion (*asterisk*) in a patient with neoplastic pericarditis.

TABLE 125.2

LIFE-THREATENING DIFFERENTIAL DIAGNOSIS OF ACUTE PERICARDITIS

Acute coronary syndrome
Pulmonary embolism
Aortic dissection
Pericardial tamponade

TABLE 125.3

PRESENTING FACTORS PREDICTING COMPLICATED COURSE

Fever greater than 38° C
Symptoms developing over weeks in immune-compromised patient
Traumatic pericarditis
Patient on oral anticoagulants
Large effusion (more than 20 mm) or tamponade
Failure to respond to nonsteroidal anti-inflammatory drugs

chest to rule out pulmonary embolism or aortic dissection (Fig 125.3). With the recent development of 64-slice or dual-head CT scanners, it has become possible to perform a so-called *triple rule-out*, at least in specialized centers. During a short (20–25 seconds), single breath-hold, contrasted, ECG-gated CT scan, all data can be acquired to evaluate the pulmonary artery tree, the thoracic aorta, and the coronary arteries as well (18).

Treatment

Patients with acute pericarditis have a high likelihood of uncomplicated recovery and can be treated outside the hospital. However, several factors are described as being associated with a complicated course (Table 125.3), and patients with any of these factors should be hospitalized for their initial treatment (19).

Acute idiopathic or viral pericarditis usually responds to nonsteroidal anti-inflammatory drugs (NSAIDs). The drug regimen consists of high-dose aspirin (325–975 mg three to four times daily for 4 weeks), with the addition of a proton pump inhibitor to lessen gastrointestinal effects. Alternatively, indomethacin (25–50 mg four times daily) or ibuprofen (400–600 mg four times daily) can be given. Colchicine has been shown to be effective as a second-line treatment for patients who do not respond to NSAIDs or who have recurrence of their acute pericarditis (20,21). Recently, Imazio et al. (22) found that routine use of colchicine (1–2 mg on day 1 followed by 0.5–1 mg/day for 3 months) in addition to aspirin—compared to aspirin alone—in patients with a first episode of acute pericarditis significantly reduced symptoms at 72 hours and recurrence at 18 months. Diarrhea is a known side effect of colchicine and may cause discontinuation of drug therapy in about 5% of patients.

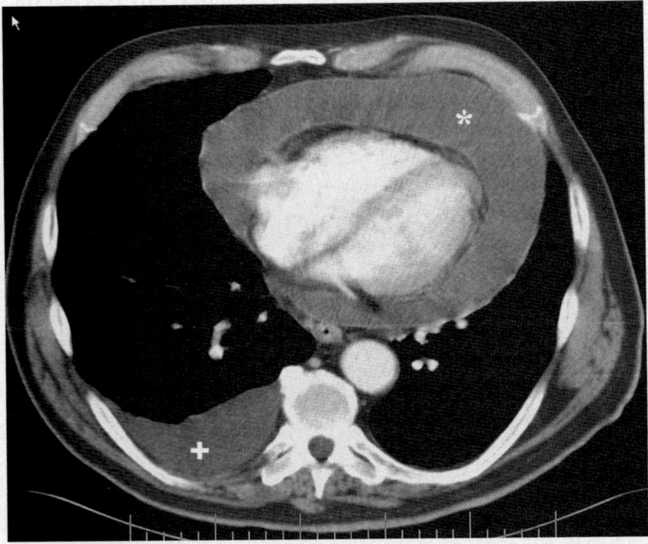

FIGURE 125.3. Computed tomography (CT) of the chest with large pericardial effusion (*asterisk*) and small right-sided pleural effusion (*plus sign*). The dark rim between the pericardial effusion and the right heart represents epicardial fat.

Symptoms of acute pericarditis respond rapidly to systemic steroids, but there seems to be an increase in relapse after tapering (23). Therefore, corticosteroid therapy should be reserved only for patients with recurrent pericarditis not responding to NSAIDs and colchicine. The recommended regimen is 1 to 1.5 mg/kg of prednisone for at least 1 month before slowly tapering the dose by 5 mg/week until the drug is withdrawn (24). The possible side effects of corticosteroid treatment include peptic ulcer disease, sodium retention, hypokalemia, hyperglycemia, Cushing syndrome, and suppression of the adrenal axis. Treatment with corticosteroids also requires the exclusion of infection or an appropriate antibiotic regimen before initiation of therapy.

The treatment of choice for uremic pericarditis consists of intensive, initially daily dialysis therapy. Heparin should be used sparingly during dialysis to reduce the risk of intrapericardial hemorrhage and possible tamponade. The presence of acute pericarditis in acute myocardial infarction also requires caution with the use of intravenous anticoagulants. These drugs are not, however, absolutely contraindicated. Thrombolytic agents have been reported to lead to cardiac tamponade and should be used with caution in the patient with acute myocardial infarction and acute pericarditis.

The postpericardiotomy syndrome is usually self-limited if left untreated; however, the disease may increase the risk of early coronary artery bypass graft closure. Therefore, aggressive treatment has been recommended; NSAIDs often decrease symptoms and speed recovery (25). Refractory cases may occur but usually respond rapidly to systemic corticosteroids as outlined above. Advocates of corticosteroid therapy claim that this treatment reduces the incidence of late constrictive pericarditis.

Nonviral infectious etiology of pericarditis requires prompt evacuation of pus from the pericardium, usually by operative intervention, because of the need to establish a definitive diagnosis, eradicate the infection, and prevent constrictive pericarditis.

Recurrence of acute pericarditis is quite common and often requires long-term drug therapy as noted above. In a few selected cases refractory to medical therapy, radical pericardectomy may need to be considered (23).

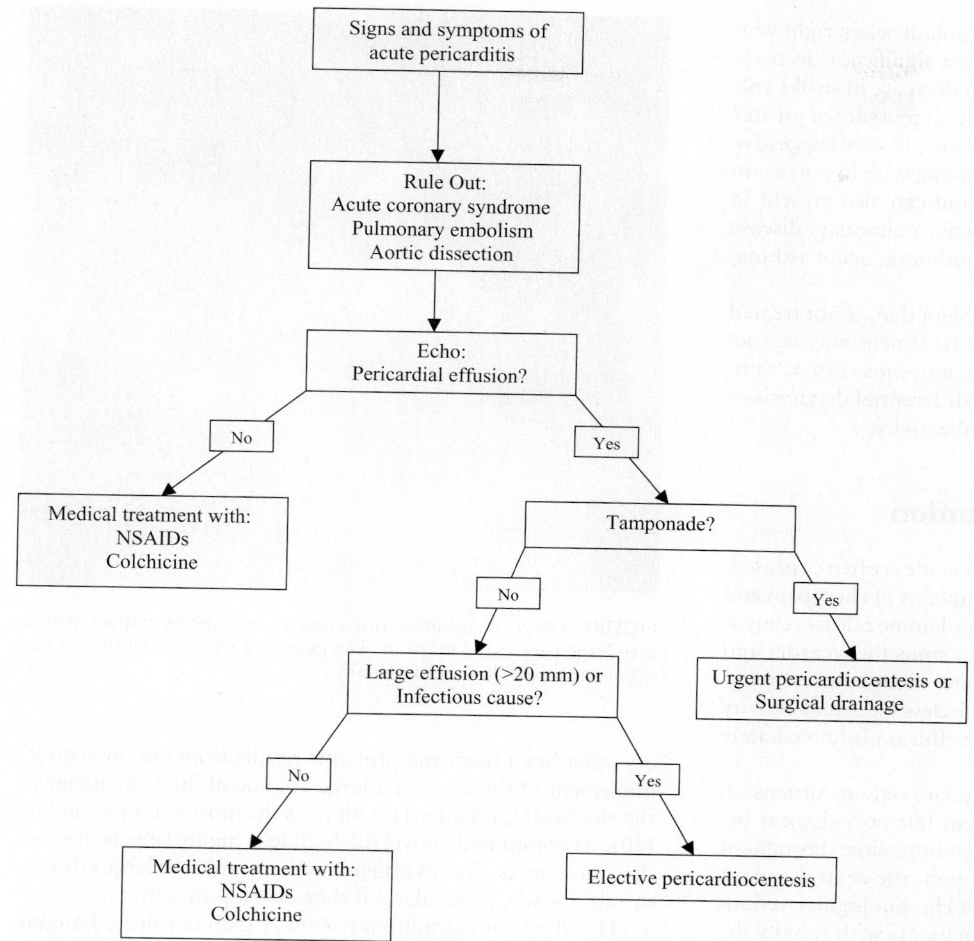

FIGURE 125.4. Diagnostic and treatment algorithm for patients presenting with signs and symptoms of acute pericarditis.

In general, acute pericarditis symptoms subside within several days to weeks. The major immediate complication is cardiac tamponade, which occurs in less than 5% of patients. For diagnostic and treatment approach in patients with suspected acute uncomplicated or complicated pericarditis, see Fig. 125.4.

PERICARDIAL EFFUSION AND CARDIAC TAMPONADE

Etiology

Pericardial effusion often develops with acute pericarditis. It is caused by an inflammatory exudation and an occlusion of the normal drainage through epicardial venous and lymphatic systems by the inflammatory process. The most common causes of tamponade include idiopathic pericarditis, cancer of the lung and breast, lymphoma, renal failure, and tuberculosis (26). Pericardial effusion may also occur in the absence of pericardial inflammation—for example, as a hemorrhagic effusion from internal sources such as a pacemaker, angioplasty, coronary artery bypass grafting (CABG) surgery, aortic dissection, ventricular rupture—or external cardiac trauma. Regardless of their size, pericardial effusions can either be clinically silent or cause hemodynamic compromise. The latter situation is called *cardiac tamponade*. The most important factor contributing to the development of cardiac tamponade is not the total amount of pericardial fluid but the rate at which it accumulates. The pericardium resists sudden stretching but can gradually expand in response to a chronic distending force. A small but rapidly developing effusion—less than 200 mL—in a trauma patient can cause tamponade, because the fibrous pericardial membrane does not have enough time to stretch and accommodate the increased volume. Conversely, a patient with a very large pericardial effusion—1,000 mL—developing over weeks or months may be completely asymptomatic, given that the parietal pericardium has had time to adjust to the increased volume.

It is also important to note that the pressure–volume curve for the stretchable pericardium is curvilinear; a large amount of fluid accumulating over a long time raises the intrapericardial pressure very little. However, at some point, the ability of the pericardium to stretch further is exceeded, and the addition of a very small volume raises the intrapericardial pressure significantly. Once the intrapericardial pressure exceeds the filling pressures of the right atrium and/or the right ventricle, central venous pressure rises, cardiac output drops, and cardiac tamponade—and consequently cardiogenic shock—occur (27,28). Physiologically, the total cardiac volume is limited, and volume in one chamber can increase only if volume in another chamber decreases. This physiologic interdependence of the ventricles is accentuated in cardiac tamponade when right ventricular filling during inspiration causes a significant decrease in left ventricular filling and a significant decrease in stroke volume. This inspiratory drop in systolic blood pressure of greater than 10 mm Hg, termed *pulsus paradoxus*, is very suggestive of cardiac tamponade in a patient presenting with hypotension and tachycardia, but it is not specific and can also present in other conditions such as chronic obstructive pulmonary disease (COPD), pulmonary embolism, pneumothorax, acute asthma, and hypovolemic shock (29).

Cardiac tamponade is a serious problem that, if not treated aggressively and rapidly, may be fatal. Treatment may be successful if diagnosed in a timely fashion, and thus cardiac tamponade needs be included in the initial differential diagnosis of cardiogenic shock or pulseless electrical activity.

Clinical Presentation

The patient with early pericardial tamponade is often confused, agitated, pale, and diaphoretic and complains of chest pain and dyspnea. Initially, compensatory catecholamine release, caused by a decreased cardiac output, leads to sinus tachycardia and often to peripheral vasoconstriction. Later in the course, bradycardia occurs, indicating imminent pulseless electrical activity and cardiorespiratory arrest unless the effusion is immediately decompressed.

Classic clinical signs include jugular venous distension (JVD), demonstrating a rapid x-descent but no y-descent because of right atrial and ventricular compression throughout the entire diastolic cycle. In this situation, the central venous pressure is usually greater than 15 mm Hg, but jugular venous distention may be missing in trauma patients with rapidly developing hemorrhagic tamponade or in patients with uremic pericarditis due to volume depletion from blood loss or dialysis, respectively (*low-pressure tamponade*).

Pulsus paradoxus is often present and can be ascertained through invasive arterial pressure tracing by palpation of an artery or with a sphygmomanometer. The amount of paradox is gauged by measuring the systolic blood pressure and observing the difference in the level at which the Korotkoff sounds are heard only during expiration and the level at which they are heard throughout the respiratory cycle. A paradoxical pulse greater than 10 mm Hg is abnormal; patients with tamponade physiology often drop their systolic blood pressure more than 20 mm Hg with inspiration. Paradoxical pulse is absent in patients with severe aortic insufficiency or atrial septal defect and is difficult to assess in acute cardiac tamponade with hypotension, as the pulse may be unobtainable or disappear completely with inspiration. Other clinical signs of cardiac tamponade are distant and muffled heart sounds and clear lungs. The patient with chronic tamponade may present with a low-output state, right upper quadrant pain caused by swelling of the hepatic capsule, or even ascites and lower extremity edema. The two main differential diagnoses for cardiac tamponade are tension pneumothorax and pulmonary edema; both conditions can present with tachycardia, hypotension, and JVD.

The ECG usually shows signs of acute pericarditis, including sinus tachycardia, PR depression, and abnormal T-wave changes. Electrical alternans of the ECG is almost pathognomonic of pericardial tamponade; it represents a change of direction and amplitude of the P, QRS, and T vectors with every other heart beat, and probably results from the "swinging" movement of the heart in a large volume of fluid. A change of the electrical QRS alternans alone is the most common finding (30). As mentioned above, the finding is highly specific for cardiac tamponade, but its absence does not rule out large effusion or tamponade, particularly if they develop rapidly.

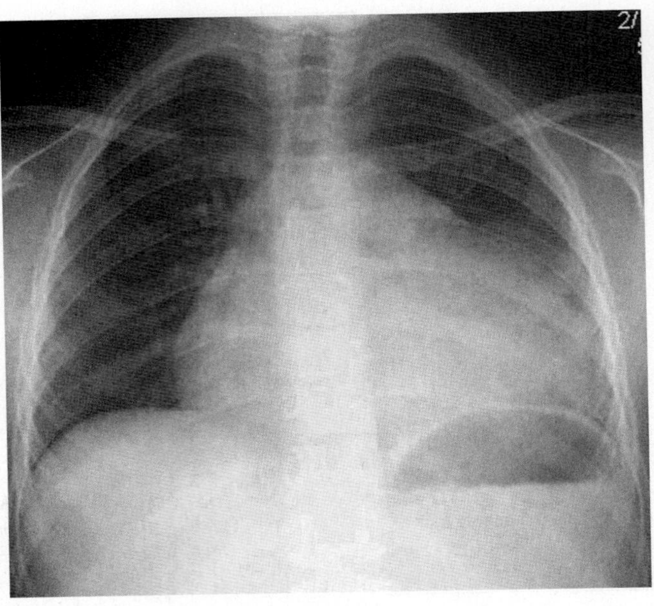

FIGURE 125.5. Anteroposterior chest radiograph in patient with a very large pericardial effusion. The extensive widening of the cardiac silhouette resembles a water bottle.

The chest radiograph may show a globular heart hanging down in the mediastinum—*the water bottle heart* (Fig. 125.5). It is also helpful to rule out diagnoses presenting similarly to tamponade, such as tension pneumothorax and pulmonary edema.

Cardiac tamponade is a clinical diagnosis based on the previously described symptoms and findings. However, the best adjunctive test to assess for pericardial effusion and cardiac tamponade is the echocardiogram (31). Pericardial effusion is seen as an echo-free space surrounding the heart. An echocardiogram can detect even very small amounts of pericardial effusion (less than 20 mL), helps to estimate amount and distribution of the effusion, and visualizes clot or tumor in the fluid if present. Small effusions (less than 1 cm) are seen only inferolaterally and around the right atrium (Fig. 125.6). Effusions causing tamponade are mostly large (greater than 2 cm) and circumferential. Effusions seen with acute tamponade are usually smaller than those seen with chronic tamponade. An echocardiogram can distinguish pericardial from pleural effusion; pericardial effusion tracks between the inferolateral wall and the descending thoracic aorta in the parasternal long axis view and separates both structures (Fig. 125.7), whereas pleural effusion is found only posterior to the aorta in this view.

Once a pericardial effusion begins to compromise the hemodynamics, there are several characteristic echocardiographic findings. There is diastolic collapse, first of the right atrium, and then right ventricle, both of which worsen during expiration when right-sided filling is reduced (32,33). Diastolic collapse lasting more than one third of diastole is considered indicative for tamponade (Fig. 125.8). Reciprocal respiratory variation of

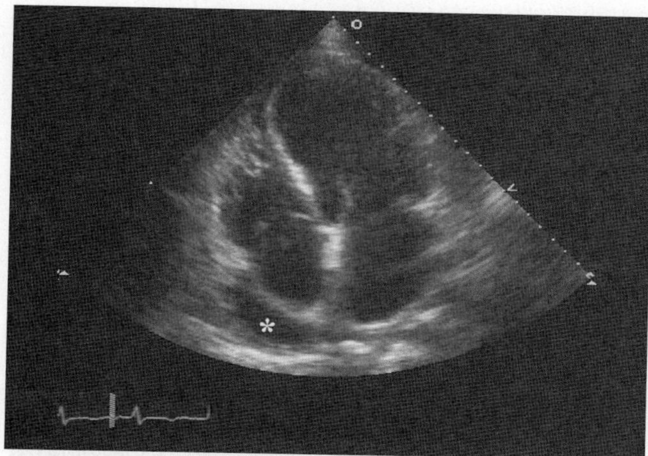

FIGURE 125.6. Apical four-chamber view echocardiogram in patient presenting with acute pericarditis. The very small pericardial effusion is seen only around the right atrial wall (*asterisk*). The right atrium is not compressed by the effusion. This location may be the only one in which an early or small pericardial effusion can be seen in a patient with poor subcostal windows.

greater than 20% to 25% of the peak transmitral and transtricuspid Doppler velocities is another very specific indicator for hemodynamically significant pericardial effusion (Fig. 125.9).

Echocardiography is a very useful tool to assess pericardial effusion and determine its hemodynamic significance. However, life-saving treatments for an unstable or deteriorating patient suffering from cardiac tamponade should not be delayed by waiting for an echocardiogram to be performed.

The invasive hemodynamic profile of acute cardiac tamponade is characteristic and can be assessed by placement of a pulmonary artery catheter. The right-sided cardiac pressures are elevated, and the diastolic pressures equilibrate. The mean right atrial pressure, right ventricular diastolic pressure, pulmonary artery diastolic pressure, and the pulmonary capillary wedge pressure are elevated and are measured within 2 to 3 mm Hg of each other. The pressure contour does not show a dip and plateau sign as seen in constrictive pericarditis. The pressures in chronic congestive heart failure are elevated but do not equilibrate in diastole. These measurements made in the intensive care unit (ICU) setting can confirm the diagnosis of cardiac tamponade.

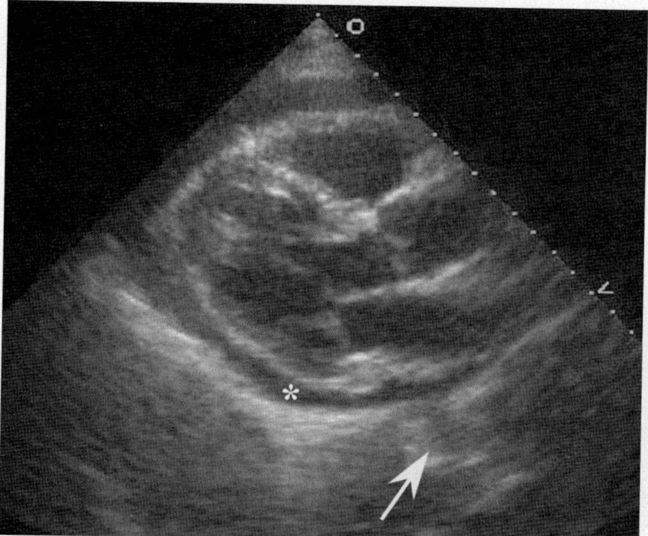

FIGURE 125.7. Parasternal long-axis echocardiographic view in a patient presenting with clinical symptoms of acute pericarditis. There is a small to moderate-sized concentric effusion (*asterisk*). It tracks between the inferolateral wall and the descending thoracic aorta (*arrow*) and thereby confirms the diagnosis of pericardial effusion. A pleural effusion may be seen in the same inferolateral location but would not separate the heart from the aorta.

Treatment

Patients with newly diagnosed pericardial effusion, without tamponade physiology, should be monitored in the hospital for 24 to 48 hours, with at least one repeat echocardiogram prior to discharge. A repeat echocardiogram should be performed in patients with large pericardial effusions 4 to 6 weeks after the initial presentation or with change in symptoms suggestive of beginning hemodynamic significance of the pericardial effusion.

Patients diagnosed with hemodynamically significant cardiac tamponade, defined as systolic blood pressure less than 110 mm Hg or pulsus paradoxus greater than 10 mm Hg, should receive immediate aggressive fluid resuscitation with normal saline to increase right-sided filling pressures to at least temporarily stabilize hemodynamics. Additionally, inotropic support with dobutamine, dopamine, isoproterenol, or norepinephrine may be needed to further stabilize the blood pressure. More definitive treatment with percutaneous pericardiocentesis or surgically created pericardial window should follow promptly. Any patient presenting with traumatic hemopericardium should be treated surgically (34).

Pericardiocentesis should be performed in any patient with acute tamponade and hemodynamic compromise, or when an infectious or malignant cause of the pericardial effusion is suspected. The procedure is usually performed in the cardiac catheterization laboratory, but in an emergency, may be done at the bedside if clinically necessary (34).

The patient should be placed in a supine position at a 45-degree angle. The area between the xiphoid and the left costal arch should be sterilely prepped using a tinted (so clinicians can see where they have prepped) chlorhexidine–alcohol solution and draped in the usual fashion, and anesthetized with a 1% or 2% lidocaine solution. A 7.6-cm (3-inch) aspiratory needle (16–18 gauge) with a short bevel should be directly attached to a three-way stopcock and a 50-mL syringe, and the needle advanced with negative pressure at an angle of 30 to 45 degrees to the abdominal wall and oriented in a posterocephalad direction toward the left shoulder (35). Once it enters the pericardial space, fluid can be easily removed. Removal of a small amount of fluid may provide significant clinical improvement. A temporary catheter is then placed into the pericardial space via Seldinger technique and connected to a bag draining to gravity for several days. This approach provides more complete drainage and reduces the risk for reaccumulation of the effusion.

The first sample of fluid retrieved should be sent for microbiologic studies and several other diagnostic tests (Table 125.4).

Echocardiography can be used to locate the ideal spot for percutaneous puncture (36). It is helpful to determine the

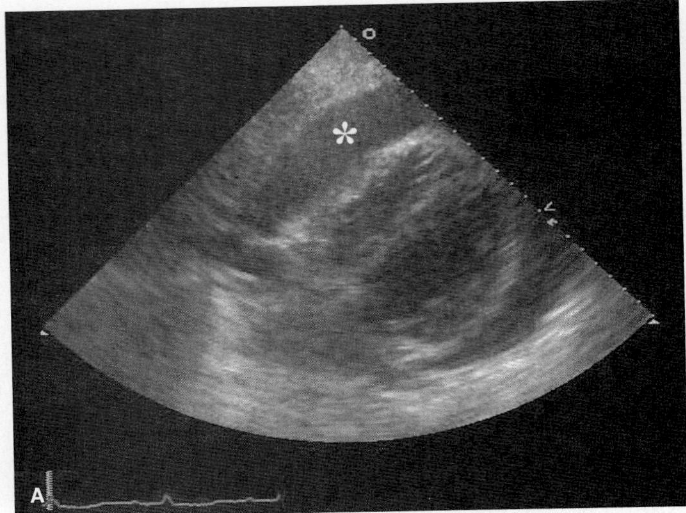

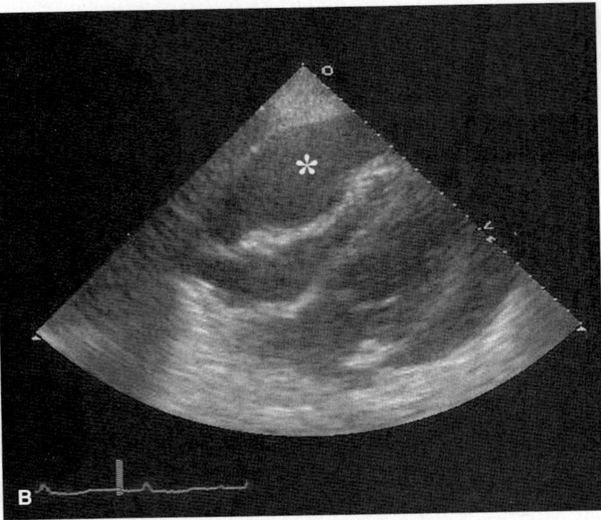

FIGURE 125.8. Subcostal echocardiogram in a patient with cardiogenic shock. Compared to early systole (A), there is significant collapse of the right ventricular free wall until very late into the diastolic filling phase (B), consistent with pericardial tamponade. The treatment of choice is immediate decompression of the effusion (*) by percutaneous or surgical drainage.

distance from the surface to the effusion and demonstrates liver or lung tissue that may be in the projected path of the needle. After the puncture, an echocardiogram confirms the correct position when bubbles generated with sterile, agitated saline injected through the needle are demonstrated within the pericardial effusion. Alternatively, ECG can be used to determine the position of the needle; the needle is connected to a V lead of the ECG via an alligator clamp. If the tip of the needle contacts the epicardium, the ECG will suddenly demonstrate ST-segment elevation. The needle should then be withdrawn until the changes disappear. Complications of this procedure include pneumothorax, myocardial and coronary artery laceration, dysrhythmias, and death. Many authors have pointed out the significant risks associated with this procedure, which should be approached with experience and caution.

If the patient with acute cardiac tamponade can be stabilized by volume expansion and vasopressor support, a safer and equally effective drainage of pericardial fluid can be accomplished by surgical subxiphoid pericardial resection and drainage (34). Subxiphoid resection can be performed in a sterile environment under local anesthesia; pericardial fluid can be removed and pericardial tissue obtained for biopsy and culture (37).

Malignant recurrent pericardial effusions often require surgical creation of a pericardial window to allow fluid to drain into the adjacent pleural space. More recently, percutaneous balloon pericardiotomy has been developed as a nonsurgical approach to create such a window and to drain large pericardial effusions (38).

CONSTRICTIVE PERICARDITIS

Etiology

Constrictive pericarditis occurs when chronic inflammation leads to scarring and, in some cases, calcification of the pericardium. Tuberculosis is the most common cause of constrictive pericarditis worldwide; the leading causes in the United States are idiopathic pericarditis, previous mediastinal radiation, or

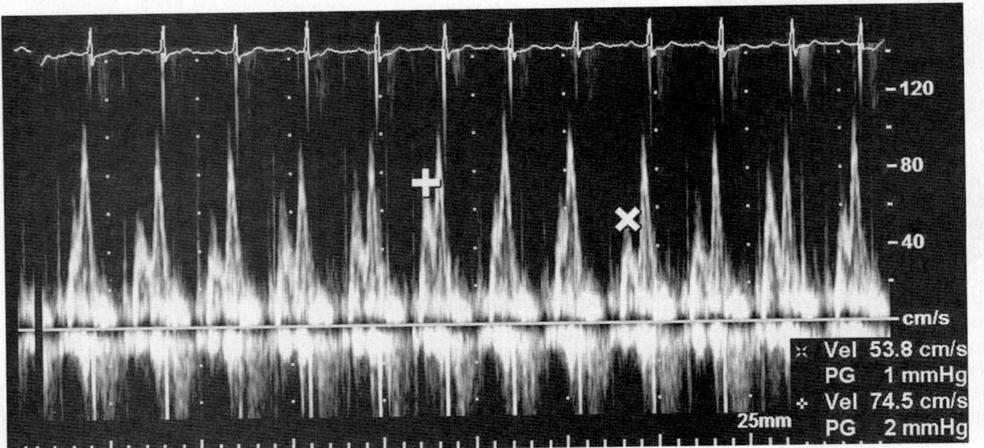

FIGURE 125.9. Transmitral pulse-wave Doppler tracing with significant (greater than 20%) decrease of E-wave velocity during inspiration (x) when compared to velocity during expiration (+). This finding indicates hemodynamic significance if found in conjunction with a pericardial effusion, and immediate drainage of the effusion via percutaneous or surgical route should be considered.

TABLE 125.4

DIAGNOSTIC TESTS ON PERICARDIAL FLUID

- Complete blood count (CBC) and differential
- Microbiology (Gram stain, culture, acid fast bacillus smear)
- Chemistry (glucose, protein, albumin, LDH, amylase)
- Cytology

LDH, lactate dehydrogenase.

cardiac surgery (34). The thickened (greater than 2 to 3 mm) and shrunken pericardium leads to compromise of diastolic filling and elevation and equalization of end-diastolic pressures in all four cardiac chambers (39). Of note is that up to 20% of patients with surgically proven constriction may present without any pericardial thickening (40) (Fig. 125.10). Contrary to pericardial tamponade, the initial diastolic ventricular filling is not inhibited and is very rapid (dip on central pressure tracing). However, once the ventricular volume has reached the limits allowed by the constricted pericardium, filling abruptly ceases (plateau on central pressure tracing). Together, these two findings compose the dip and plateau or square root sign of constrictive pericarditis seen during pulmonary artery catheterization (Fig. 125.11). The signs and symptoms of constrictive pericarditis generally develop over a prolonged period and are similar to those of biventricular congestive heart failure, restrictive cardiomyopathy, cor pulmonale, cirrhosis, and pericardial tamponade. Features of cardiac tamponade and constrictive pericarditis can occur simultaneously, referred to as *effusive-constrictive pericarditis*. This likely represents a transitional state from effusive to constrictive pericarditis, and is commonly seen in patients with thoracic neoplasm who present with malignant pericardial effusion and constrictive pericarditis after radiation to the chest.

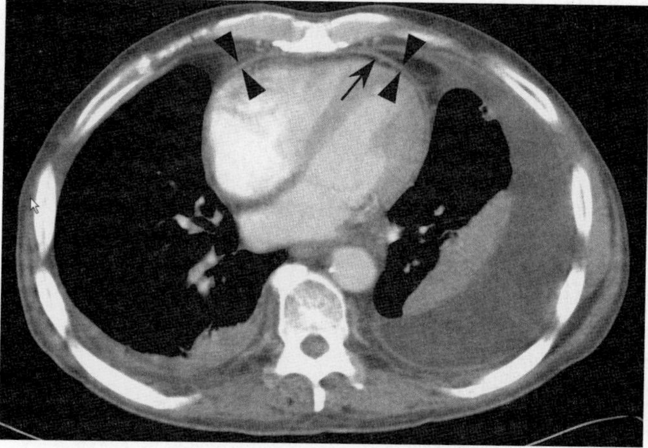

FIGURE 125.10. Axial slice of chest computed tomography in a patient with clinical findings of severe right heart failure. The pericardium is well seen (*arrowheads*) due to the separation from the myocardium by a very small pericardial effusion (*arrow*). Of note is that the pericardium is neither thickened (maximally 3 mm in thickness) nor calcified; however, preoperative cardiac catheterization results and the intraoperative findings during surgical pericardial stripping confirmed the diagnosis of constrictive pericarditis.

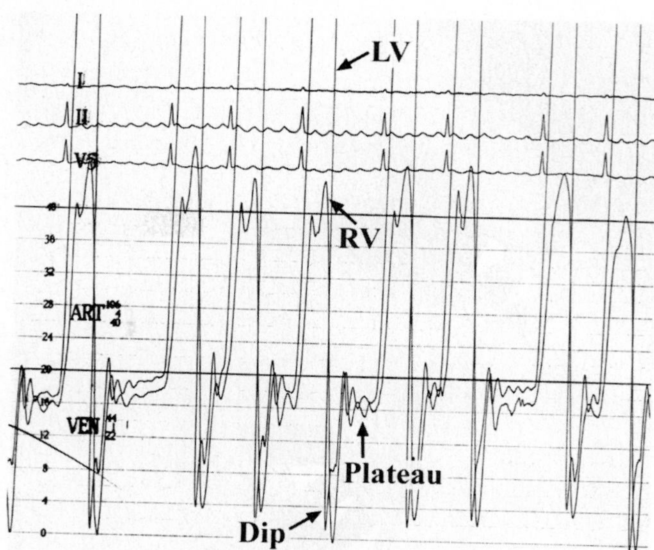

FIGURE 125.11. Right (RV) and left ventricular (LV) pressure tracings in a patient with clinical findings consistent with constrictive pericarditis. The early diastolic dip is followed by plateau, with elevation and equalization of right and left ventricular pressures. Note that contrary to ventricular discordance, the dip and plateau sign is classic but not specific for constrictive pericarditis and can be found in several other medical conditions (see text for details). The ECG tracing shows atrial fibrillation seen often in constrictive pericarditis.

Clinical Presentation

Patients often complain of fatigue, increasing dyspnea on exertion, abdominal discomfort, and abdominal and lower extremity swelling.

Physical findings include increased jugular venous pressure with a prominent x- and y-descent. A loud early diastolic sound, a "pericardial knock," is heard in up to 50% of patients. It is caused by the sudden cessation of ventricular filling and is pathognomonic for pericardial constriction. The lungs remain clear initially, and later in the course, left-sided or bilateral pleural effusions develop. The liver is enlarged secondary to congestion; ascites, splenomegaly, and significant lower extremity edema are also present. Unlike in cardiac tamponade, blood pressure is maintained, and less than 20% of patients have a significant pulsus paradoxus. A lateral chest radiograph may show pericardial calcium in up to 50% (Fig. 125.12).

The ECG findings are nonspecific and include T-wave inversions, low voltage, and atrial fibrillation. Echocardiography is helpful to distinguish right heart failure from pericardial constriction; however echocardiographic findings are not specific for the diagnosis of pericardial constriction. They include paradoxical septal motion, rapid deceleration of the early diastolic mitral inflow velocity (E wave), significant respiratory variation of mitral inflow velocity (more than 25%), and normal mitral valve annular tissue Doppler velocity. In the absence of a pericardial effusion, a thickened pericardium is often hard to distinguish from the myocardium. On the other hand, cardiac CT and cardiac magnetic resonance imaging (MRI) are very useful imaging modalities to precisely determine the pericardial thickness. Cardiac MRI is better suited to image soft tissues and can, in contrast to CT, show normal pericardium,

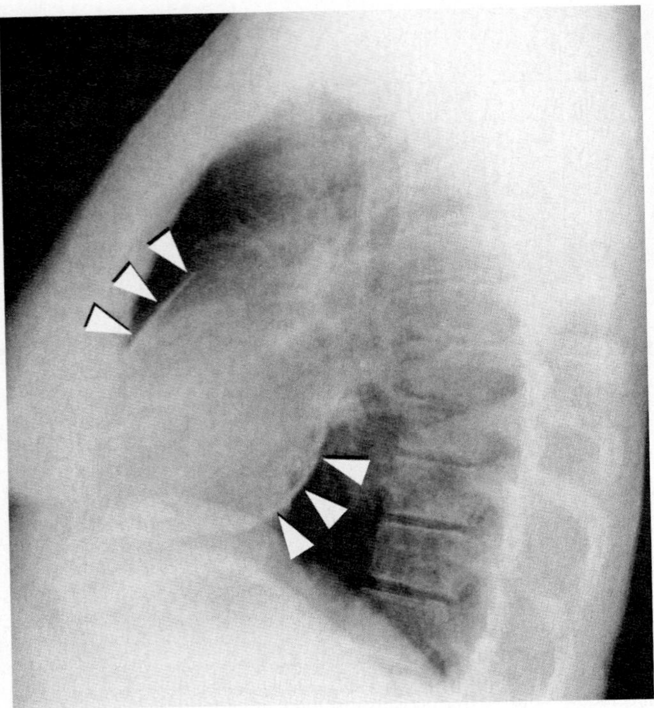

FIGURE 125.12. Lateral chest radiograph showing calcifications of the anterior and inferolateral pericardium in a patient with constrictive pericarditis (*arrowheads*).

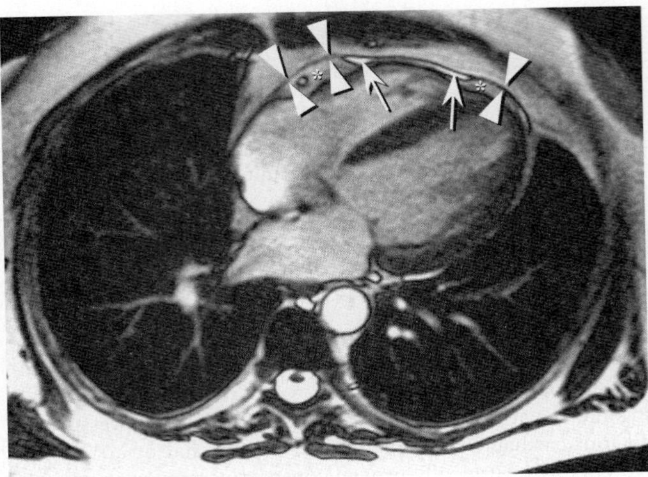

FIGURE 125.13. Four-chamber view of electrocardiogram (ECG)-gated cardiac magnetic resonance imaging (MRI) in a patient with suspected pericardial constriction. The normal-appearing pericardium (*arrowheads*) is very precisely visualized in areas with pericardial effusion (*arrows*) and with pericardial fat (*asterisk*) only. The outstanding soft-tissue imaging capabilities of MRI make it preferable over cardiac computed tomography (CT) to evaluate the pericardium in patients with no or very little pericardial effusion.

even in the absence of pericardial effusion (Fig. 125.13). Furthermore, tagged cine MRI is able to demonstrate adhesions between the pericardium and myocardium (41).

Cardiac catheterization pressure tracings are still the gold standard to diagnose constrictive pericarditis and to differentiate it from restrictive cardiomyopathy. The hemodynamic findings of elevated and equalized diastolic pressures in all four chambers and the dip and plateau sign are classic, although not very specific for constriction. In contrast, respiratory variation of ventricular pressures (right ventricular [RV] pressure rises and left ventricular [LV] pressure falls during inspiration and vice versa during expiration, causing ventricular discordance) has been shown to be highly sensitive and specific for the diagnosis of constrictive pericarditis (42) (Fig. 125.14). Hemodynamically silent constrictive pericarditis can be evaluated by performing volume loading during catheterization; the initially normal right and left heart pressures may elevate and equilibrate in diastole.

Treatment

Patients with acute onset of constrictive symptoms may improve significantly with medical treatment that includes NSAIDs, colchicine, and steroids (43). Chronic constrictive pericarditis can be treated initially with diuretics, and sodium and fluid restriction, if symptoms are mild. Moderate to severe

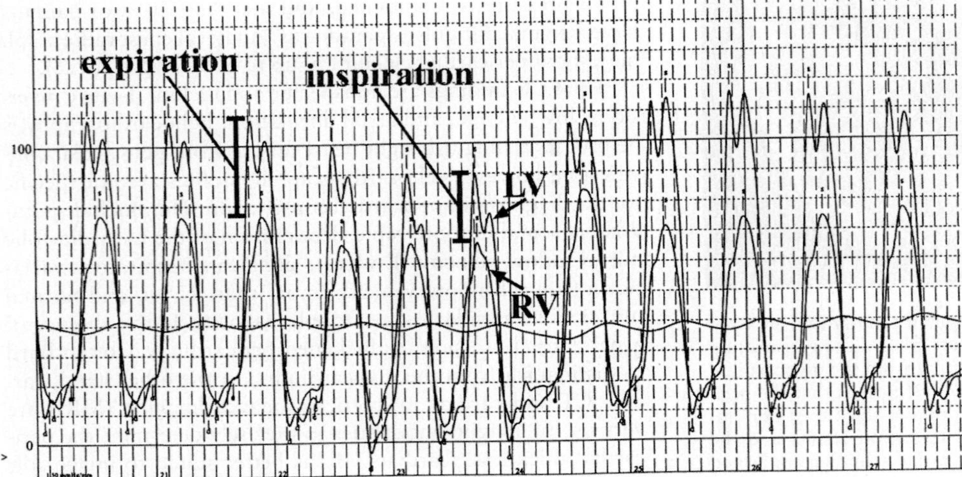

FIGURE 125.14. Simultaneous invasive left (LV) and right ventricular (RV) pressure tracings. Note the ventricular discordance with respiration (RV pressure rises and LV pressure falls during inspiration and vice versa during expiration). This finding is highly sensitive and specific for the diagnosis of constrictive pericarditis; its presence rules out the differential diagnosis of restrictive cardiomyopathy.

disease requires definitive treatment with complete removal of the pericardium by surgical stripping (34). This major procedure is associated with a perioperative mortality of greater than 6%; it can be life-saving and improves symptoms drastically in most patients; however, poor outcome is likely if the constriction is radiation induced.

SUMMARY

Disease processes affecting the pericardium are relatively rare. Inflammation and accumulation of fluid in the pericardial space occur first; in some patients, these conditions can progress to pericardial constriction or tamponade with hemodynamic compromise. The presentation can be acute or chronic; the signs and symptoms are often nonspecific and can mimic other acute conditions as described in the chapter. It is therefore important to include pericardial diseases in the differential diagnosis during the initial workup of a patient presenting with chest symptoms or hemodynamic compromise to avoid inappropriate (i.e., lytic therapy for presumed myocardial infarction in a patient with acute hemorrhagic pericarditis) or delayed treatment (delayed pericardiocentesis in a patient with pericardial tamponade) with possible fatal outcome.

ACKNOWLEDGMENTS

I would like to thank Dr. Ilona Schmalfuss, Radiology and the Medical Media Service, and particularly Mr. John Richardson, both at the Malcom Randall VA Medical Center, for their assistance with the figures for this chapter.

References

1. Morgan BC, Guntheroth WG, Dillard DH, et al. Relationship of pericardial to pleural pressure during quiet respiration and cardiac tamponade. *Cir Res.* 1965;16:493.
2. Shabetai R. Function of the pericardium. In: Fowler NO, ed. *The Pericardium in Health and Disease.* Mount Kisco, NY: Futura Publishing; 1985: 19.
3. Shabetai R. Acute viral and idiopathic pericarditis. In: Shabetai R, ed. *The Pericardium.* New York, NY: Grune & Stratton; 1981:348.
4. Gunukula SR, Spodick DH. Pericardial disease in renal patients. *Semin Nephro.* 2001;21:52.
5. Coreale E, Maggioni AP, Romano S, et al. Comparison of frequency, diagnostic and prognostic significance of pericardial involvement in acute myocardial infarction treated with and without thrombolytics. *Am J Cardiol.* 1993;71:1377.
6. Engle MA, Ito T. The post-pericardiotomy syndrome. *Am J Cardiol* 1961; 7:73.
7. Engle MA, McCabe JC, Ebert PA, et al. The post-pericardiotomy syndrome and antiheart antibodies. *Circulation.* 1974;49:401.
8. Abraham KP, Reddy V, Gattuso P, et al. Neoplasms metastatic to the heart: review of 3314 consecutive autopsies. *Am J Cardiovasc Pathol.* 1990;3: 195.
9. Permanyer-Miralda G, Sagrista-Sauleda J, Soler-Soler J, et al. Primary acute pericardial disease: a prospective series of 231 consecutive patients. *Am J Cardiol.* 1985;56:623.
10. Gornik HL, Gerhard-Herman M, Beckman JA, et al. Abnormal cytology predicts poor prognosis in cancer patients with pericardial effusion. *J Clin Oncol.* 2005;23:5211.
11. Posner MR, Cohen GI, Skarin AT, et al. Pericardial disease in patients with cancer. The differentiation of malignant from idiopathic and radiation-induced pericarditis. *Am J Med.* 1981;71:407.
12. McCaughan BC, Schaff HV, Piehler JM, et al. Early and late results of pericardiectomy for constrictive pericarditis. *J Thorac Cardiovasc Surg.* 1985; 89:340.
13. Trautner BW, Darouiche RO: Tuberculous pericarditis: optimal diagnosis and management. *Clin Infect Dis.* 2001;33:954.
14. Larrieu AJ, Tyers GFO, Williams EH, et al. Recent experience with tuberculous pericarditis. *Ann Thorac Surg.* 1980;29:464.
15. Hammerman KJ, Powell KE, Tosh FE, et al. The incidence of hospitalized cases of systemic mycotic infections. *Sabouraudia.* 1974;12:33.
16. Spodick DH. Diagnostic electrocardiographic sequences in acute pericarditis. *Circulation.* 1973;48:575.
17. Spodick DH. Arrhythmias during acute pericarditis (100 cases). *JAMA.* 1976;235:39.
18. Johnson TR, Nikolaou K, Wintersperger BJ, et al. ECG-gated 64-MDCT angiography in the differential diagnosis of acute chest pain: *AJR Am J Roentgenol.* 2007;188:76.
19. Imazio M, Demichellis B, Parrini I, et al. Day-hospital treatment of acute pericarditis: a management program for outpatient therapy. *J Am Coll Cardiol.* 2004;43:1042.
20. Guindo J, de la Serna AR, Ramio J, et al. Recurrent pericarditis: relief with colchicine. *Circulation.* 1990;82:1117.
21. Adler Y, Finkelstein Y, Guindo J, et al. Colchicine treatment for recurrent pericarditis: a decade of experience. *Circulation.* 1998;97:2183.
22. Imazio M, Bobbio M, Cecchi E, et al. Colchicine in addition to conventional therapy for pericarditis: results of the COlchicine for acute PEricarditis (COPE) Trial. *Circulation.* 2005;112:2012.
23. Shabetai R. Recurrent pericarditis: recent advances and remaining questions. *Circulation.* 2005;112,1921.
24. Maisch B. Recurrent pericarditis: mysterious or not so mysterious? *Eur Heart J.* 2005;26:631.
25. Urschel HC, Razzuk MA, Gardner M, et al. Coronary artery bypass occlusion secondary to postpericardiotomy syndrome. *Ann Thorac Surg.* 1976;22:528.
26. Guberman BA, Fowler NO, Engel PJ, et al. Cardiac tamponade in medical patients. *Circulation.* 1981;64:633.
27. Fowler NO. Physiology of cardiac tamponade and pulsus paradoxus. *Mod Concept Cardiovasc Dis.* 1978;48:115.
28. Shabetai R. Cardiac tamponade. In: Shabetai R, ed. *The Pericardium.* New York, NY: Grune & Stratton; 1981:224.
29. Fowler NO. The paradoxical pulse (pulses paradoxus). In: Fowler NO, ed. *The Pericardium in Health and Disease.* Mount Kisco, NY: Futura Publishing; 1985:235.
30. Spodick DH. Electric alternation of the heart. *Am J Cardiol.* 1962;10:155.
31. Horowitz MS, Schultz CS, Stinson EB, et al. Sensitivity and specificity of echocardiographic diagnosis of pericardial effusion. *Circulation.* 1974;50: 239.
32. Armstrong WF, Schilt BF, Helper DJ, et al. Diastolic collapse of the right ventricle with cardiac tamponade: an echocardiographic study. *Circulation.* 1982;65:1491.
33. Singh S, Wann S, Schuchard GH, et al. Right ventricular and right atrial collapse in patients with cardiac tamponade: a combined echocardiographic and hemodynamic study. *Circulation.* 1984;70:966.
34. Maisch B, Seferovic PM, Ristic AD, et al. Task force on the diagnosis and management of pericardial diseases of the European Society of Cardiology. Guidelines on the diagnosis and management of pericardial disease: executive summary. *Eur Heart J.* 2004;25:587.
35. Lorell BH, Braunwald E. Pericardial disease. In: Braunwald E, ed. *Heart Disease: A Textbook of Cardiovascular Medicine.* Philadelphia, PA: WB Saunders; 1984: 1487.
36. Tsang TS, Enriquez-Sarano M, Freeman WK, et al. Consecutive 1127 therapeutic echocardiographically guided pericardiocenteses: clinical profile, practice patterns, and outcomes spanning 21 years. *Mayo Clin Proc.* 2002;77:429.
37. Santos GH, Frater RW. The subxiphoid approach in the treatment of pericardial effusion. *Ann Thorac Surg.* 1977;23:468.
38. Wang HJ, Hsu KL, Chiang FT, et al. Technical and prognostic outcomes of double-balloon pericardiotomy for large malignancy-related pericardial effusions. *Chest.* 2002;122:893.
39. Shabetai R. Constrictive pericarditis. In: Shabetai R, ed. *The Pericardium.* New York, NY: Grune & Stratton; 1981:154.
40. Talreja DR, Edwards DW, Danielson GK, et al. Constrictive pericarditis in 26 patients with histologically normal pericardial thickness. *Circulation.* 2003;108:1852.
41. Kojima S, Yamada N, Goto Y, et al. Diagnosis of constrictive pericarditis by tagged cine magnetic resonance imaging. *N Engl J Med.* 1999;341:373.
42. Hurrell DG, Nishimura RA, Higano ST, et al. Value of dynamic respiratory changes in left and right ventricular pressures for the diagnosis of constrictive pericarditis. *Circulation.* 1996;93:2007.
43. Haley JH, Tajik J, Danielson GK, et al. transient constrictive pericarditis: causes and natural history. *J Am Coll Cardiol.* 2004;43:271.

CHAPTER 126 ■ ACUTE HYPERTENSION MANAGEMENT IN THE ICU

ANDREAS H. KRAMER • THOMAS P. BLECK

DEFINITIONS

Acute hypertension is a common issue in the intensive care unit (ICU). The settings in which blood pressure elevation occur are highly variable, and optimal care must be tailored to the pathophysiology of the specific circumstances in which it is encountered. The terminology used in the literature to classify this heterogeneous group of disorders has been somewhat inconsistent and confusing (Table 126.1). The terms, *hypertensive emergency* or *hypertensive crisis*, are commonly defined as a marked increase in blood pressure associated with target-organ damage, implying that the blood pressure should be lowered emergently.

Some authors have reserved the definition of hypertensive emergency for the situation where blood pressure elevation itself is directly responsible for causing end-organ damage. However, clinicians more often need to rapidly lower blood pressure in situations where hypertension, although not necessarily directly responsible for causing the condition, may contribute to deterioration. For example, acute hypertension is usually the result of, rather than the immediate cause of, an acute ischemic stroke. If the patient is to be treated with thrombolytics, it becomes imperative to maintain the blood pressure within certain narrow limits to minimize the risk of hemorrhagic transformation while at the same time not compromising cerebral blood flow (CBF). Thus, in this chapter, we define a hypertensive emergency broadly—as any condition in which blood pressure should be lowered immediately. Although the term, *malignant hypertension*, has been discouraged by some, it is still widely used in the literature to describe the syndrome where organ dysfunction is a direct *consequence* of the elevated blood pressure, rather than an epiphenomenon. The presence of papilledema is not necessarily required for this diagnosis to be made (1,2).

In contrast, a *hypertensive urgency* is defined as a condition with severe blood pressure elevation and no target-organ damage, such that the blood pressure can be decreased more gradually over the course of several hours, often with oral medications. It is therefore the presence or absence of organ dysfunction, rather than the absolute degree of blood pressure elevation, that determines whether a patient is classified as having a hypertensive emergency or urgency. It is not always clear how clinicians distinguish between hypertensive urgencies and the situation where a patient simply has severe, poorly controlled, chronic hypertension. The most recent Joint National Committee Guidelines (JNV 7) classify patients with hypertension into stage 1 (systolic blood pressure [SBP] 140–159 mm Hg or diastolic blood pressure [DBP] 90–99 mm Hg) and stage 2 (SBP exceeding 160 mm Hg or DBP exceeding 100 mm Hg). The previously used category of "stage 3 hypertension" (SBP exceeding 180 mm Hg or DBP exceeding 110 mm Hg) has been combined with stage 2 (3).

EPIDEMIOLOGY AND ETIOLOGY

Hypertension is extraordinarily common, with over 1 billion individuals affected worldwide, and only a minority of these having adequate blood pressure control (4). The incidence of hypertensive emergencies and urgencies has not been assessed in population-based studies. Less than 1% of persons with chronic hypertension ever present in this fashion (2). Nevertheless, because hypertension is so common, and because such a wide variety of conditions other than malignant hypertension can be categorized as hypertensive emergencies, acutely elevated blood pressure is still a factor in a substantial number of medical visits to emergency departments and a frequent problem in the ICU (5,6) (Table 126.2).

Malignant Hypertension

The peak incidence of malignant hypertension occurs between the ages of 40 and 50, and risk factors include poor long-term blood pressure control, lack of a primary care physician, noncompliance with antihypertensive medications, male gender, African American ethnicity, illicit drug use, and lower socioeconomic class (7–10). Prior to the availability of effective antihypertensive therapy, the mortality of malignant hypertension was very high, with approximately 80% of patients dying within a year (hence, the term *malignant*) (11).

At least 90% to 95% of patients with chronically elevated blood pressure can be classified as having "essential" hypertension, meaning that the underlying cause is multifactorial and not specifically known. A small proportion of patients have "secondary" hypertension, where there is an identifiable and sometimes treatable condition that is responsible for raising blood pressure (3). In contrast, among patients who present with malignant hypertension, as many as 50% to 80% may have a secondary etiology (12). Other clues that should alert clinicians to the possibility of secondary hypertension include a history of blood pressure that is resistant to medical therapy, sudden worsening in a previously well-controlled patient, and the onset of hypertension at an unusually young or old age (13).

Renovascular disease, the most common cause of secondary hypertension, may be present in as many as 45% of patients with severe or malignant hypertension, although

TABLE 126.1

DEFINITIONS

1. *Hypertensive emergency:* Any condition where hypertension is causing or potentially exacerbating organ dysfunction and should be lowered emergently
2. *Hypertensive urgency:* Severe hypertension that is not associated with acute organ dysfunction and requires gradual reduction in blood pressure over several hours
3. *Malignant hypertension:* A syndrome in which uncontrolled hypertension directly causes organ dysfunction (note that this is a subtype of #1). Although previous definitions have sometimes mandated the presence of retinopathy with papilledema, this is only one of several possible clinical manifestations, and should not necessarily be required.

the proportion is higher in Caucasians than African Americans (14). Features that suggest renovascular hypertension include atherosclerotic vascular disease in other organ systems, systolic-diastolic abdominal bruits, a history of deterioration in renal function with exposure to angiotensin-converting enzyme (ACE) inhibitors or angiotensin II receptor blockers (ARBs), recurrent flash pulmonary edema, and small kidneys (determined by ultrasound or other imaging).

Hypertension is almost universally present in patients with acute or chronic kidney disease, especially when the etiology is a glomerulonephropathy (15). Hypertension is a common manifestation of obstructive sleep apnea, and can be improved by the administration of noninvasive positive airway pressure (16). Various rare endocrine causes, including primary aldosteronism, Cushing syndrome, hypercalcemia, hypothyroidism, and pheochromocytoma, are also responsible for a small proportion of cases. Several illicit drugs can cause malignant hypertension in addition to other hypertensive emergencies. Sympathomimetics, such as cocaine and methamphetamine, have been implicated in causing intracerebral and subarachnoid hemorrhage, ischemic stroke, and aortic dissection (17–19). However, various drugs used in clinical practice have also been reported to cause severe hypertension, or even hypertensive emergencies. The most commonly implicated are erythropoietin and various immunosuppressants, most notably cyclosporine, tacrolimus, interferon, and high-dose corticosteroids, although it is sometimes difficult to separate the hypertension-inducing effects of these drugs from the complications of the diseases they are intended to treat (20,21). A careful history, physical examination, and appropriate diagnostic testing to exclude causes of secondary hypertension are indicated during the hypertensive emergency and after it has resolved (Table 126.3).

TABLE 126.2

TYPES OF HYPERTENSIVE EMERGENCIES

MALIGNANT HYPERTENSION
- Hypertensive encephalopathy/RPLS
- Retinopathy and papilledema
- Acute heart failure
- Myocardial ischemia
- Malignant nephrosclerosis and acute renal failure
- Microangiopathy

NEUROCRITICAL CARE EMERGENCIES
- Acute ischemic stroke requiring thrombolysis
- Acute intracerebral hemorrhage
- Subarachnoid hemorrhage
- Severe hypertension following craniotomy
- Cerebral hyperperfusion syndrome (postendarterectomy or stenting)
- Normal perfusion pressure breakthrough (post-AVM resection)

CARDIOVASCULAR EMERGENCIES
- Acute myocardial infarction
- Acute heart failure
- Aortic dissection
- Severe hypertension following cardiovascular surgery

PRE-ECLAMPSIA/ECLAMPSIA

AVM, arteriovenous malformation; RPLS, reversible posterior leukoencephalopathy syndrome.

TABLE 126.3

ETIOLOGIES OF MALIGNANT HYPERTENSION

Essential hypertension
Secondary hypertension
- Renovascular disease
  - Atherosclerosis, thrombosis
  - Fibromuscular dysplasia
  - Medium and large vessel vasculitis
- Glomerular disease
  - Glomerulonephritis
  - Small vessel vasculitis
  - Microangiopathies
  - Scleroderma
- Renal parenchymal disease
  - Polycystic kidney disease (and others)
  - Renin-producing tumors
- Endocrine causes
  - Pheochromocytoma
  - Primary hyperaldosteronism
  - Cushing syndrome
  - Hypercalcemia
- Aortic coarctation
- Medications (e.g., cyclosporine, tacrolimus, erythropoietin)
- Sympathomimetic drugs (e.g., cocaine, amphetamines)

Neurologic Hypertensive Emergencies

Acute stroke is one of the most common indications for which emergent blood pressure control may be necessary, and often the most frequent form of end-organ damage in a consecutive series of patients with hypertensive emergencies (5). Stroke is the second leading cause of death worldwide, and is also a major reason for long-term disability. Cerebral ischemia is responsible for 70% to 80% of strokes, while intracerebral hemorrhage (ICH) and subarachnoid hemorrhage account for 5% to 20% and 1% to 7%, respectively (22). Overall, more than 80% of patients with ischemic or hemorrhagic strokes are initially hypertensive to some degree (23). Even without treatment, the blood pressure usually declines gradually over the first several hours or days in-hospital. In the well-known National Institute of Neurological Diseases (NINDS) trial evaluating recombinant tissue plasminogen activator (rt-PA) for the management of acute ischemic stroke, 19% of patients had an initial blood pressure of more than 185/110 mm Hg, and 60% had a blood pressure of more than 180/105 mm Hg during the first 24 hours in-hospital (24). Whether or not it is appropriate (see below), more than half of these patients receive antihypertensive medications during the first few days of hospitalization (25). An even larger proportion of patients with intracerebral hemorrhage (ICH) develop, and are treated for, acute hypertension (26). The incidence of hypertension with subarachnoid hemorrhage (SAH) is somewhat lower, but aggressive treatment is sometimes advocated in order to minimize the initial risk of rebleeding from the aneurysm (27).

Perioperative Hypertension

Depending on the patient population, type of surgery, and how hypertension is defined, 3% to 34% of operations are complicated by postoperative hypertension in the recovery room or ICU, with the most important risk factors being inadequately controlled pain and a pre-existing history of hypertension, especially if antihypertensives were withdrawn preoperatively (28,29). Elevations in blood pressure occur most often during the initial 30 to 60 minutes after surgery, may last for several hours, and have been associated with higher rates of postoperative hemorrhage and myocardial ischemia in certain patient populations (30). Hypertension is particularly frequent following neurosurgical and cardiovascular procedures, occurring in approximately 54% to 91% and 30% to 80% of patients undergoing craniotomy and coronary artery bypass grafting, respectively (31,32). A common dilemma faced by anesthetists involves patients who present for surgery with poorly controlled blood pressure. Preoperative hypertension is predictive of intra- and postoperative blood pressure fluctuations, and has been associated with the occurrence of complications and worse outcomes in some studies (33,34). The American Heart Association recommends that nonemergent surgery be deferred if the blood pressure exceeds 180/110 mm Hg (35). However, it remains controversial whether delaying surgery ultimately modifies perioperative risks, with one randomized controlled trial arguing that it does not (36).

Pregnancy-induced Hypertension

Hypertension complicates approximately 12% of pregnancies, and is responsible for 18% of maternal deaths in the United States. When blood pressure elevation occurs prior to 20 weeks' gestation, it is considered chronic hypertension. If it occurs without complication after 20 weeks, it is referred to as gestational hypertension. In contrast, pre-eclampsia is a form of pregnancy-induced hypertension that is associated with vasoconstriction, endothelial dysfunction, platelet aggregation, and increased coagulation. Although it is usually defined by the concomitant presence of hypertension and proteinuria (more than 300 mg of protein per 24 hours), some patients can develop severe symptoms in the absence of proteinuria. Pre-eclampsia occurs in 2% to 10% of pregnancies, with important risk factors including nulliparity, antiphospholipid antibodies, diabetes mellitus, obesity, family history, multiple (twin) pregnancies, maternal age over 40, and a previous history during other pregnancies. Maternal complications can include progression to eclampsia, pulmonary edema, microangiopathy, and renal failure. The most common neonatal complications are prematurity and growth restriction. Eclampsia is defined as the development of severe neurologic manifestations, including seizures and a depressed level of consciousness, in women with pre-eclampsia (37,38).

Cardiovascular Hypertensive Emergencies

Acute heart failure is responsible for 5% to 10% of hospital admissions. Hospital mortality is about 4%, but increases to more than 50% by 1 year. In a large American registry, 73% of patients had a history of chronic hypertension, and 50% were hypertensive at admission (39). In patients presenting with flash pulmonary edema, acute hypertension is particularly common, and is likely to be both a consequence and contributing cause.

A history of chronic hypertension exists in about 40% to 70% of patients with acute coronary syndromes, and about 30% have an elevated blood pressure when initially assessed (40,41). Severe uncontrolled hypertension at admission (greater than 180/110 mm Hg) is a relative contraindication to thrombolysis for ST elevation myocardial infarction (STEMI) (42).

Aortic dissection is a relatively rare condition, with an annual incidence of about 3 to 4 cases per 100,000 persons per year. With modern medical and surgical therapy, the mortality has decreased from as high as 90% to about 20%–35%. More than 70% of patients have a history of chronic hypertension, but blood pressure can be highly variable at presentation. Most patients (70%) with type B dissections (descending aorta) have an admission systolic pressure of more than 150 mm Hg compared with just over a third of those with type A dissections (ascending aorta), of whom approximately 25% actually present with hypertension or in frank shock (43).

PATHOPHYSIOLOGY OF HYPERTENSION-INDUCED END-ORGAN DYSFUNCTION

Blood flow to organs is kept relatively constant despite variations in blood pressure. This process is called *autoregulation*, and its limits are usually between mean arterial pressure (MAP) values of about 60 and 150 mm Hg. Increases in blood pressure induce arteriolar smooth muscle contraction and vasoconstriction, while reductions lead to vasodilatation. Extreme hypertension exceeding the upper range of autoregulation causes edema, hemorrhage, and organ dysfunction, while reductions in blood pressure beyond the lower limits of autoregulation result in tissue hypoperfusion and ischemia (Fig. 126.1). In addition to a widespread, systemic myogenic response, there are also more organ-specific vascular regulatory mechanisms to protect against the effects of acute hypertension. For example, increased delivery of filtrate to the distal nephron stimulates a tubuloglomerular feedback system that promotes afferent arteriolar vasoconstriction (44). The likelihood of end-organ damage increases not only with the absolute degree of blood pressure elevation, but also with the rate at which this occurs (1). With chronic hypertension, there is hypertrophy in the walls of small arteries and arterioles, and the autoregulation curve is shifted toward the right, such that blood flow can be

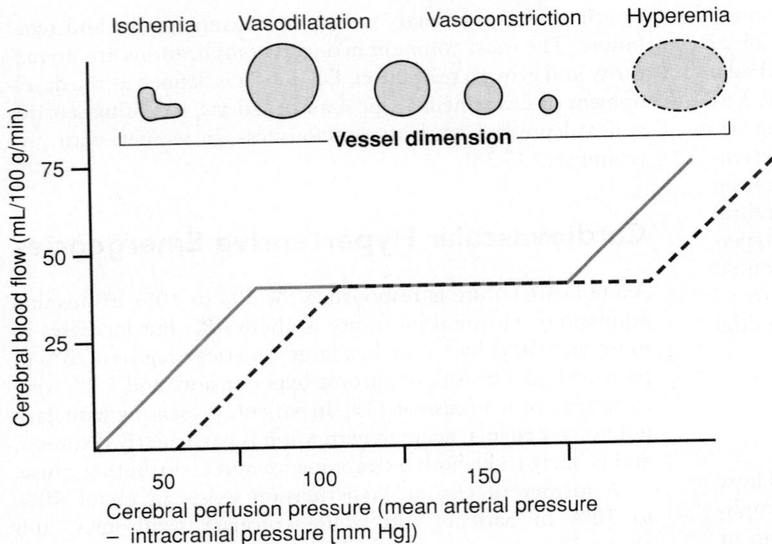

FIGURE 126.1. Cerebral blood flow autoregulation: Effect of changes in cerebral perfusion pressure on cerebral blood flow and vascular caliber in normal and hypertensive patients (*dashed line*).

maintained constant, even at unusually high blood pressures. Conversely, ischemia may occur when blood pressure falls to levels that would otherwise be well tolerated. In the setting of neurologic injury, autoregulation is often impaired, and cerebral blood flow becomes directly dependent on blood pressure (Fig. 126.1).

Normal endothelial function is necessary for the regulation of vascular tone, blood pressure, and regional blood flow. The endothelium is involved in maintaining a delicate balance between vasodilating substances (e.g., nitric oxide, bradykinin, prostacyclin) and vasoconstrictors (e.g., endothelin), as well as between coagulation and fibrinolysis. When blood pressure is elevated, natriuretic peptides are released from the endothelium, which in turn induce sodium and water loss, with decreased intravascular volume (1). Excessive activation of the renin-angiotensin system causes vasoconstriction and inflammation, and has been demonstrated to cause hypertensive emergencies in animal models, an effect that can be inhibited with the use of ACE inhibitors (45). Angiotensin II levels are elevated in most cases of malignant hypertension, particularly when the etiology is a renal condition (46). Increased wall stress and prolonged vasoconstriction in the face of severe hypertension eventually causes endothelial compensatory mechanisms to fail, such that a vicious cycle ensues, with consequent hyperemia, increased permeability, inflammation (endarteritis), platelet aggregation, coagulation, and thrombosis. Transmural necrosis and the entry of blood components into the vessel wall lead to obliteration of the lumen and replacement of smooth muscle with fibrous tissue, a process called *fibrinoid necrosis* (47). Patients with malignant hypertension may therefore paradoxically develop both hyperemia (due to endothelial dysfunction and loss of autoregulation) and ischemia (due to thrombosis and fibrinoid necrosis) (Fig. 126.2).

Manifestations

Hypertensive Encephalopathy/Reversible Posterior Leukoencephalopathy Syndrome

Severe elevations in blood pressure eventually cause a breakdown of the blood–brain barrier, with subsequent development of vasogenic cerebral edema. White matter is less tightly packed than the overlying cerebral cortex, making it more vulnerable to the spread of edema (48). Swelling occurs predominantly, but not exclusively, in the posterior regions of the brain. This is thought to be due to a larger concentration of sympathetic fibers around arterioles in the anterior brain, which results in a greater degree of vasoconstriction and relative protection against the effects of severe hypertension (49). The characteristic clinical features and magnetic resonance imaging (MRI) findings of vasogenic edema in posterior white matter led to the description of a clinical radiologic syndrome, now most commonly termed *reversible posterior leukoencephalopathy syndrome* (RPLS) or *posterior reversible encephalopathy syndrome* (PRES) (50). Although occurring most commonly in association with severe hypertension, there are other conditions that may at least predispose to, if not directly cause, the development of RPLS, perhaps because they induce endothelial toxicity. RPLS has been described in association with certain medications—most notably cyclosporine (21)—and other immunosuppressive agents, as well as in the setting of microangiopathies (51), connective tissue diseases, vasculitis, and pre-eclampsia (52). Although cerebral edema can sometimes be seen on computed tomography (CT) scans, RPLS is best visualized using T2 and fluid-attenuated inversion recovery (FLAIR) MRI sequences. Diffusion-weighted MRI has confirmed that vasogenic edema is much more prominent than cytotoxic edema and, although RPLS is usually "reversible," some patients do develop ischemic strokes (53). Many patients do not adhere perfectly to the typical patterns of RPLS: gray matter involvement of the cerebral cortex and basal ganglia, as well as edema occurring in the frontal lobes, posterior fossa, and brainstem have all been described. It is rare for only one vascular territory to be involved (Fig. 126.3).

The clinical manifestations of RPLS in the setting of acute blood pressure elevation are collectively described by the term, *hypertensive encephalopathy*, which is characterized by the subacute development of neurologic signs and symptoms and may include headache, altered mental status, seizures, and visual disturbances (54,55). Headaches are usually generalized, severe, and poorly responsive to analgesics and improve rapidly with treatment of hypertension (56). Altered mental status can

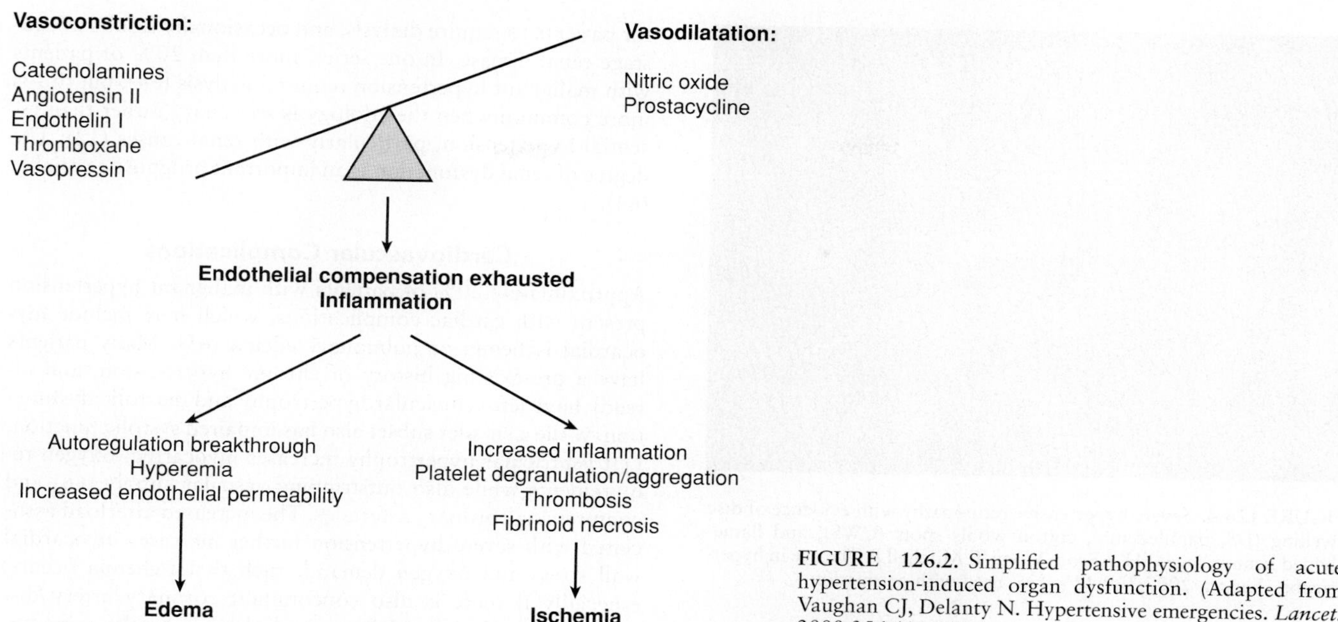

FIGURE 126.2. Simplified pathophysiology of acute hypertension-induced organ dysfunction. (Adapted from Vaughan CJ, Delanty N. Hypertensive emergencies. *Lancet.* 2000;356:411–417.)

range from lethargy and confusion to stupor and coma, although the latter is unusual. The posterior predominance of RPLS is reflected by the frequent occurrence of unilateral or bilateral visual disturbances, including hemianopsia, visual neglect, cortical blindness, Anton syndrome (patient is not aware of blindness), and visual hallucinations. Focal seizures originating in the occipital regions have also been described, although they most often generalize, and may be recurrent (57).

Retinopathy

Endothelial damage and leakage of plasma proteins into the retina lead to edema and the formation of hard exudates (Fig. 126.4). Focal areas of ischemia and infarction within the nerve fiber layer cause white areas, called *cotton-wool spots*, to appear. Breakdown of the blood–retinal barrier results in the emergence of flame-shaped hemorrhages within the retina. The development of papilledema has historically been used to differentiate "accelerated" from "malignant" hypertension. However, the presence or absence of papilledema has little impact on the natural history and prognosis of hypertensive emergencies, nor should it significantly alter management (58). The mechanism of papilledema may include raised intracranial pressure (ICP), which is known to be present in some patients with hypertensive encephalopathy (59), as well as ischemia of the optic nerve head (60). It should be noted that ophthalmoscopic examination for hypertensive retinopathy has relatively high rates of inter- and intraobserver variability, particularly among nonophthalmologists (61).

Nephropathy and Microangiopathy

Certain conditions causing acute renal failure may cause hypertensive emergencies, but severely elevated blood pressure can also cause renal dysfunction, a condition called *malignant nephrosclerosis*. Renal biopsies reveal fibrinoid necrosis, hyperplastic arteriolitis, neutrophilic infiltration, and thrombosis of glomerular capillaries. The histologic appearance can

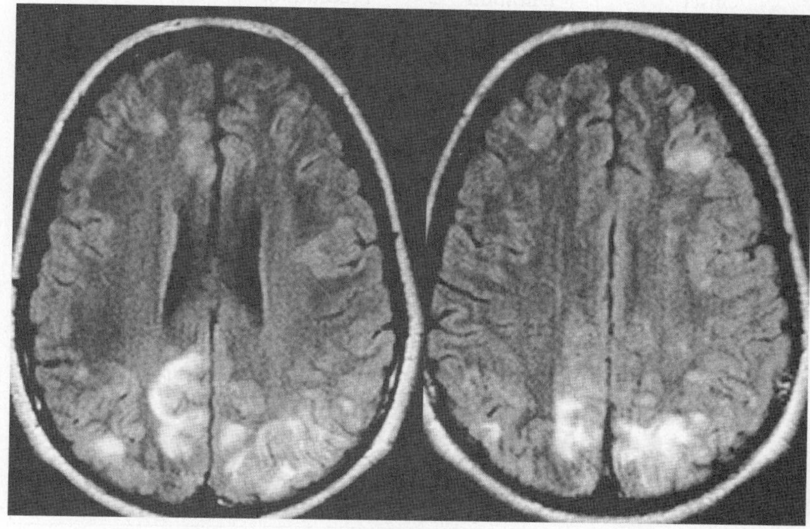

FIGURE 126.3. Fluid-attenuated inversion recovery magnetic resonance imaging sequences of a 15-year-old patient with a history of Wegener granulomatosis presenting with seizures and altered mental status. The findings are consistent with reversible posterior leukoencephalopathy syndrome (RPLS). Although vasogenic edema is seen predominantly posteriorly, anterior changes are also present.

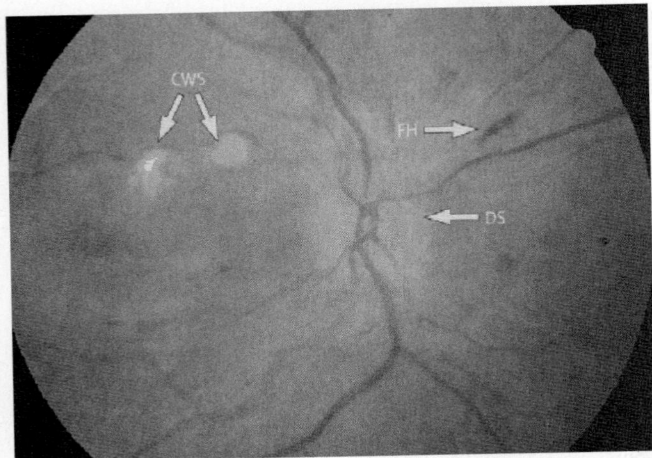

FIGURE 126.4. Severe hypertensive retinopathy with evidence of disc swelling (DS, papilledema), cotton wools spots (CWS), and flame-shaped hemorrhage (FH). (From Wong T, Mitchell P. The eye in hypertension. *Lancet.* 2007;369:425–435, used with permission.)

be difficult to distinguish from other microangiopathies, like hemolytic uremic syndrome and thrombotic thrombocytopenic purpura (62). It is therefore not surprising that more than a quarter of patients with malignant hypertension, especially those with acute renal failure, have typical clinical features of microangiopathy, including thrombocytopenia, elevated lactate dehydrogenase, and schistocytes on blood smear (63). Impaired renal perfusion leads to greater activation of the renin-angiotensin system, which further augments vasoconstriction, fluid retention, and blood pressure elevation. The earliest evidence of renal involvement is the presence of abnormal urine sediment, with proteinuria, hematuria, and the appearance of red and white blood cell casts. This is followed by the development of acute renal failure, which is sometimes severe enough for patients to require dialysis, and occasionally results in end-stage renal disease. In one series, more than 20% of patients with malignant hypertension required dialysis (64), but this is more common when the etiology is secondary rather than essential hypertension, particularly with renal causes (12). The degree of renal dysfunction is an important prognostic variable (64).

Cardiovascular Complications

Approximately 20% of patients with malignant hypertension present with cardiac complications, which may include myocardial ischemia or pulmonary edema (65). Many patients have a pre-existing history of chronic hypertension, and already have left ventricular hypertrophy and diastolic dysfunction, while a smaller subset also has impaired systolic function. Left ventricular hypertrophy increases myocardial oxygen requirements while also outstripping vascular supply (66) and compressing coronary arterioles. The increased afterload associated with severe hypertension further increases myocardial wall stress and oxygen demand, such that ischemia occurs, especially if there is also concomitant coronary artery disease. Increased wall thickness and changes to the extramyocardial collagen network impair myocardial relaxation, and cause pressure within the left ventricle to rise at relatively lower volumes during diastole. As a result, even small increases in intravascular volume and afterload can produce pulmonary edema (67).

Treatment

Pharmacologic Agents

An ideal pharmacologic agent (Table 126.4) for treatment of hypertensive emergencies should have a rapid onset in order to immediately reduce the progression of organ failure, but should also be short-acting and easy to titrate to avoid

TABLE 126.4

INTRAVENOUS PHARMACOLOGIC AGENTS FOR MANAGEMENT OF HYPERTENSIVE EMERGENCIES

Drug	Dose	Onset	Duration	Precautions
Nitroprusside	0.25–10 μg/kg/min (ideally <2 μg/kg/min)	Immediate	1–10 min	Cyanide toxicity with prolonged infusions; coronary steal; ↑ ICP
Nitroglycerin	10–200 μg/min	Immediate	3–10 min	Severe hypotension in hypovolemic patients; ↑ ICP; contraindicated if on PDE-5 inhibitors
Labetalol	10–40-mg boluses 1–4 mg/min infusion	5–15 min	2–4 h	Bradycardia, heart block; LV dysfunction; asthma
Esmolol	0.5 mg/kg load, 50–200 μg/kg/min	5 min	10–30 min	Bradycardia, heart block; LV dysfunction; asthma
Nicardipine	3–15 mg/min	5–15 min	30–60 min	Rebound tachycardia; ICP effects require more study
Fenoldopam	0.1–1.6 μg/kg/min	5–15 min	20–60 min	Glaucoma
Enalaprilat	0.625–2.5-mg bolus, every 6 h	15 min	4–6 h	Renal failure; hyperkalemia
Hydralazine	10–20 mg every 4–6 h	5–20 min	2–6 h	Reflex tachycardia; ischemic heart disease

ICP, intracranial pressure; LV, left ventricular; PDE-5, phosphodiesterase-5.

excessively lowering the blood pressure for long periods of time. The following agents are the most commonly used.

Sodium Nitroprusside. Sodium nitroprusside (NTP) has been used in the management of hypertensive emergencies for over 40 years, and continues to be considered first-line therapy, largely because of its rapid onset, short duration of action, affordability, familiarity, and efficacy (1,68). NTP is a parenterally administered, potent arterial and venous vasodilator, which has an onset within less than 30 seconds and a duration of action of only 2 to 3 minutes, such that cessation of the infusion allows blood pressure to rise back to previous levels within 1 to 10 minutes. Cardiac output is either preserved or increased, and cardiac filling pressures decrease (69,70). The mechanism of action involves the release of nitric oxide into the bloodstream, activation of guanylate cyclase, and subsequent conversion of guanosine triphosphate (GTP) to cyclic guanosine monophosphate (cGMP) in vascular smooth muscle, which in turn inhibits the intracellular movement of calcium. The usual starting dose of NTP is 0.25 to 0.5 μg/kg/minute, and it is increased in increments of 0.5 μg/kg/minute every 5 to 10 minutes until the goal blood pressure is achieved.

NTP has the potential for several serious, life-threatening complications. First, despite lowering preload and afterload, NTP may induce coronary steal, whereby excessive vasodilatation of coronary arterioles shunts blood away from ischemic regions. This effect may help explain the findings of a large clinical trial in which patients with acute myocardial infarction and high left ventricular filling pressures had a worse outcome when treated with nitroprusside within the first 8 hours but improved outcomes thereafter (71).

Second, NTP is often avoided in neurologic emergencies because of the observation in several studies that it vasodilates cerebral vasculature, increases cerebral blood volume, and therefore raises ICP (72). The demonstration of this phenomenon is not entirely consistent in the literature (73), and it may be avoidable with a somewhat slower administration (74).

Third, each nitroprusside molecule has five cyanide moieties, such that cyanide makes up 44% of its molecular weight. Cyanide is metabolized by transulfuration in the liver to thiocyanate, which is 100 times less toxic than cyanide, and is cleared in the urine and stool. When this pathway is overwhelmed, cyanide accumulates and causes toxicity. Patients receiving NTP are particularly vulnerable when treated with prolonged, high-dose infusions, especially if hepatic and renal function are impaired, or if sulfur stores are depleted because of malnutrition (68,75). Cyanide blocks oxidative phosphorylation and essentially causes tissue anoxia and lactic acidosis despite adequate oxygen delivery and high venous oxygen saturation levels. Manifestations of cyanide poisoning include depressed mental status, seizures, and, eventually, bradycardia and hemodynamic collapse. Cyanide levels are not easily monitored, and the development of lactic acidosis is a late finding. The development of tachyphylaxis to nitroprusside, with consequent increasing dose requirements, may be a harbinger of toxicity (68,76).

Treatment of cyanide poisoning consists of discontinuation of nitroprusside, supportive care with the delivery of 100% oxygen, and the administration of sodium nitrite (300 mg IV), followed by sodium thiosulfate (12.5 g IV). The use of sodium nitrite is controversial, as it actually causes the production of methemoglobin, which, although also potentially toxic, binds avidly to cyanide. Sodium thiosulfate acts as a sulfur donor to promote the formation of thiocyanate, and has been used effectively as monotherapy. Hydroxycobalamin combines with cyanide to form cyanocobalamin, and may provide synergy with sodium thiosulfate (77). Both agents have been used prophylactically with infusions of nitroprusside to prevent cyanide accumulation (78,79). Accumulation of thiocyanate, although far less toxic than cyanide, may also cause complications (68,79).

Despite these concerns, NTP has an extensive track record, and many prospective studies have not found evidence of clinical toxicity even after using it for several days. Still, NTP should be administered at as low a dose as possible, and for as short a duration as possible. Newer, alternative agents are increasingly being used as they become available, largely because of concerns about cyanide toxicity with NTP.

Nitroglycerin. Because nitroglycerin produces more venous than arterial vasodilatation, it is usually not used as first-line therapy for hypertensive emergencies, unless there is concurrent pulmonary edema or myocardial ischemia. It is usually started at 5 to 10 μg/minute, and can be titrated up every 5 to 10 minutes to doses as high as 200 to 300 μg/minute. Particular caution must be exercised in the setting of hypovolemia. Patients using drugs for erectile dysfunction should not be given nitroglycerin or nitroprusside, as this may induce profound hypotension (80). As with nitroprusside, there are case reports of nitroglycerin increasing ICP, such that it should be used with caution in brain-injured patients (81).

β-Blockers. Labetalol is the most commonly used intravenous β-blocker for the management of hypertensive emergencies. One of its unique properties is that it blocks both α and β receptors, although the β-blocking effect is more prominent (82). Labetalol is usually administered as 10- to 20-mg boluses, which can be repeated every 15 minutes until the desired effect is achieved. Blood pressure lowering begins within 2 to 5 minutes, with maximal effect after about 10 to 15 minutes. Labetalol can also be delivered as an infusion, beginning at a dose of 1 to 2 mg/minute. It has been demonstrated to be safe and effective in the management of severe hypertension, with advantages including that it does not cause reflex tachycardia, and has little effect on cerebral blood flow or ICP (83). Labetalol does not cross the placenta well, and there is extensive experience using it in pregnancy, making it one of the preferred agents in the management of pre-eclampsia and eclampsia (84).

Esmolol is an extremely short-acting, relatively cardioselective β-blocker, has an onset within less than a minute, and is uniquely metabolized by red blood cell esterases, such that its duration of action is only 10 to 20 minutes. A loading dose of 0.5 mg/kg is administered over 1 minute, followed by an infusion of 50 μg/kg/minute, which can be adjusted as often as every 5 minutes to a maximum dose of 200 μg/kg/minute (85). It is a useful agent when blood pressure is elevated and cardiac output is preserved, especially when there are concerns about myocardial ischemia.

Nicardipine. Nicardipine is a dihydropyridine calcium channel blocker that inhibits calcium influx through L-type channels, thereby preventing smooth muscle contraction, particularly in vascular smooth muscle, rather than cardiac myocytes. Thus, nicardipine causes arterial vasodilatation, with minimal venodilatation or change in cardiac output. It is most often administered as an intravenous infusion, beginning at 3 to 5 mg/hour, to a maximum of 15 mg/hour, but it can also be given as 0.5- to 3-mg boluses. Because of a distribution half-life of less than 3 minutes and an intermediate elimination half-life of less than 45 minutes, nicardipine has a relatively rapid onset and offset (86). It has compared favorably with NTP in clinical trials, with therapeutic targets achieved in a similar amount of time, fewer episodes of severe hypotension, and less frequent dose adjustment (86,87). Nicardipine has been used in a variety of settings, including malignant hypertension, perioperative hypertension, pre-eclampsia, and acute heart failure. It is generally well tolerated, with few adverse effects when used with caution. Given that nicardipine increases cerebral blood flow, one might expect that it would raise ICP. Although this has been reported, it does not appear to be a major concern in most studies (86,88).

Fenoldopam. Fenoldopam is a selective dopamine-1 (DA-1)-receptor agonist, which produces peripheral, renal, splanchnic, and, to a lesser degree, coronary vasodilatation. Stimulation of DA-1 receptors also promotes natriuresis. Unlike dopamine, fenoldopam does not have any effect on DA-2 receptors, nor does it act at the α- or β-adrenergic receptor level. It does not cross the blood–brain barrier, and therefore has little effect on cerebral blood flow and ICP. It is typically administered in doses of 0.025 to 1 μg/kg/minute, and begins to lower blood pressure after as little as 2 minutes, although the maximal effect is not seen for at least 20 to 30 minutes or more. With discontinuation of an infusion, the elimination half-life is less than 10 minutes. Reflex tachycardia, thought to be related to activation of the baroreflex, may occur and can be attenuated with concomitant use of a β-blocker (89). A theoretical advantage of fenoldopam is improved renal blood flow, but despite a slight increase in creatinine clearance, it remains unclear that this will translate into clinically important prevention of renal failure (90). Fenoldopam has been demonstrated to be effective at controlling blood pressure in hypertensive emergencies, with similar efficacy to nitroprusside (91), but has shown no clear improvement in outcomes; it is also considerably more expensive (92). Overall, fenoldopam seems to have few adverse effects. It does raise intraocular pressure, and should therefore probably be avoided in patients with a known history of glaucoma (93).

Treatment for Specific Hypertensive Emergencies

Malignant Hypertension

Because of the shift in the autoregulatory curve that occurs with prolonged hypertension, rapid reductions in blood pressure may cause organ ischemia (94). With hypertensive urgencies, the blood pressure should therefore be reduced carefully and gradually with oral medications over the course of several days. It is not certain how long it takes for the autoregulatory curve to recover and shift back toward the left, such that the initial goal should never be a normal blood pressure.

With hypertensive emergencies, the blood pressure must be reduced immediately, with an initial goal of no more than a 15% reduction. Specific treatment goals should be individualized to ensure that the pressure is reduced sufficiently for organ failure to resolve without compromising perfusion. To facilitate keeping blood pressure within a narrow range, placement of an arterial catheter and careful observation in the ICU are recommended.

Neurologic

Acute Ischemic Stroke. Although acute hypertension is common in patients with ischemic stroke, optimal treatment remains uncertain. The greatest priority in these patients is to preserve as much of the ischemic penumbra as possible. Because autoregulation is usually impaired within the penumbra, pressure reductions may cause blood flow to fall, which in turn may increase infarct size (95). Accordingly, there are several observational studies demonstrating that lowering blood pressure may cause clinical deterioration (96). Preliminary studies have even suggested that transcranial Doppler middle cerebral artery (MCA) flow velocities, cerebral perfusion as determined by MRI, and neurologic examination may improve with supranormal augmentation of blood pressure using a vasopressor (97). The International Stroke Trial of more than 17,000 patients found a U-shaped relationship, where the best outcomes occurred in patients with a presenting systolic blood pressure of about 150 mm Hg (98). The American Stroke Association guidelines currently recommend not treating hypertension unless the systolic pressure exceeds 220 mm Hg or the diastolic pressure exceeds 120 mm Hg (99).

The exception to this rule is if the patient is a candidate for intravenous, or possibly intra-arterial, thrombolysis. Of patients who receive intravenous rt-PA for treatment of acute ischemic stroke, approximately 5% to 6% will develop ICH (100). Whether lowering blood pressure helps to limit this risk is not certain. However, patients in whom systolic and diastolic pressure could not easily be lowered to less than 185 mm Hg and 110 mm Hg, respectively, were excluded from the definitive clinical trial (101). Patients who did receive thrombolysis had a goal blood pressure of less than 180/105 mm Hg. Approximately 10% of patients require intravenous antihypertensive therapy prior to receiving thrombolysis, while 25% to 30% require treatment in the 24 hours after thrombolysis (24).

Intracerebral Hemorrhage. Good neurologic recovery is very uncommon if the volume of ICH exceeds 30 to 60 mL. Hematoma growth is a dynamic process that occurs over several hours, with a significant proportion of patients having detectable expansion even within the first few hours after presentation to the emergency department or ICU (102). Patients with early hematoma enlargement have substantially worse outcomes, and it is likely that therapy that can limit this early growth will improve outcomes. Numerous studies have suggested that patients with higher blood pressure at presentation are more likely to develop hematoma expansion (103) and have a higher mortality (104). However, a randomized controlled trial of lowering blood pressure for acute ICH has not yet been performed. At present, the American Heart Association guidelines are conservative, and recommend the following goals: MAP less than 130 mm Hg, SBP less than 180 mm Hg, and DBP less than 105 mm Hg (105). The main reason for concern has been the observation that there is reduced blood flow around areas of ICH and the belief that this represents an ischemic penumbra that could be compromised with lower blood pressure. However, recent studies using positive emission tomography and MRI have suggested that decreased flow surrounding ICH is appropriate for the corresponding reduction in cerebral metabolic rate (106). Furthermore, CBF autoregulation in this region appears to be preserved, such that lowering blood pressure does not adversely impact regional blood flow (107).

Subarachnoid Hemorrhage. Nontraumatic subarachnoid hemorrhage results from a ruptured intracranial aneurysm in more than 80% of cases (27). The risk of recurrent hemorrhage from the aneurysm is about 4% on the first day, followed by 1% to 2% per day for the next 2 to 3 weeks (108). Although the risk of rebleeding has decreased with the practice of securing aneurysms early, with either surgical clipping or endovascular coil embolization, the incidence of this devastating complication remains approximately 7%, with a mortality of over 50% (109). Many centers attempt to decrease the risk of recurrent hemorrhage by reducing blood pressure prior to the aneurysm being secured, with review articles often citing goal systolic pressures of less than 140 to 180 mm Hg (27). However, the efficacy of this practice remains uncertain, with conflicting results from observational studies. Particular caution should be exercised when treating patients with high-grade SAH who are stuporous or comatose, because these patients may have a raised ICP, and excessive reduction in blood pressure may compromise cerebral perfusion and promote ischemia.

After the aneurysm has been treated, the most concerning complication is the development of cerebral vasospasm and delayed ischemic neurologic deficits, which occur in approximately 20% to 30% of patients, with maximum risk between days 4 and 12 after the event. Hypertension should not routinely be treated during this time, even at relatively high levels, since this practice increases the risk of delayed infarction. If clinical vasospasm develops, first-line therapy actually involves hemodynamic augmentation, using vasopressors to raise blood pressure in order to increase CBF and improve cerebral perfusion.

Perioperative Neurosurgery. Hypertension occurs in the setting of craniotomy more often than with any other type of surgery (31). Neurosurgery results in the release of large amounts of vasoactive substances that raise blood pressure, including catecholamines, endothelin, and renin (110). Importantly, severe hypertension occurring intraoperatively or during the first 12 postoperative hours has been associated with a higher risk of ICH-complicated craniotomy (31).

There are certain neurosurgical procedures where tight postoperative blood pressure control is particularly important. In most patients undergoing carotid stenting or endarterectomy, the sudden resolution of carotid stenosis results in a sudden, asymptomatic, 20% to 40% increase in ipsilateral CBF. However, in some patients, the increase can be much more profound, to the degree that it overcomes the autoregulatory capacity of the corresponding, previously hypoperfused territory. The resulting cerebral hyperperfusion syndrome (CHS) is characterized by the presence of vasogenic edema, which resembles RPLS in that there is a posterior predilection. Patients who are most vulnerable are those with relatively severe carotid stenosis and poor collateral circulation, but postoperative hypertension is also an important risk factor. CHS is treated with tight blood pressure control, but agents that cause cerebral vasodilatation, including nitroprusside and perhaps calcium channel blockers, ideally should be avoided (111).

Mild intraoperative hypotension is sometimes used for vascular neurosurgical procedures, such as microsurgical excision or endovascular obliteration of arteriovenous malformations (AVMs) in order to reduce the risk of hemorrhage. With AVMs, the sudden "repressurization" of previously hypotensive arterioles may contribute to the development of regional hyperemia, edema, and bleeding, a condition sometimes referred to as "normal perfusion pressure breakthrough." Consequently, hypertension should be avoided in the immediate postoperative period. Conversely, the sacrifice of vascular branches during the procedure, or vasospasm from surgical manipulation and retraction, may also create areas of relative underperfusion, such that hypotension would also be deleterious (112).

Cardiovascular Hypertensive Emergencies

Aortic Dissection. The purpose of emergently lowering blood pressure in aortic dissection is to decrease shear stress in the aorta and limit propagation of the intimal tear and false lumen. In order to concomitantly reduce both blood pressure and the force of left ventricular contraction, first-line therapy consists of a β-blocker or, if contraindicated, a calcium channel blocker with negative inotropic and chronotropic properties (e.g., diltiazem or verapamil). Pure vasodilators should not be used in isolation. If possible, the heart rate should be lowered to less than 60 beats per minute, and the blood pressure reduced as much as can be tolerated, ideally below a systolic pressure of 120 mm Hg. Because patients often have substantial chest discomfort, the use of opiates to ameliorate pain may greatly reduce antihypertensive requirements. If the blood pressure remains elevated despite adequate β-blockade, a vasodilator can be added. There is extensive experience with nitroprusside in this setting, although other agents have also been used (86,113).

Acute Pulmonary Edema. Acute hypertension exists in the majority of patients presenting with flash pulmonary edema, and is likely to be both a consequence and contributing cause (39,114). The venodilating properties of nitroglycerin make it an excellent initial choice as an antihypertensive in both normotensive and hypertensive patients, especially if there is failure to improve after administration of a loop diuretic. In titrating the dose of intravenous nitroglycerin, clinicians should be aware that relatively large doses, often in excess of 100 μg/minute, may be required to significantly lower cardiac filling pressures and improve symptoms (115). Patients who benefit from aggressive afterload reduction, such as those with acute aortic or mitral regurgitation (if not hypotensive), may require a more potent arterial vasodilator than nitroglycerin, such as nitroprusside or nicardipine. Although ACE inhibitors are standard care for chronic heart failure, there is little evidence of benefit for acute decompensated heart failure. The only intravenous preparation, enalaprilat, was potentially harmful when routinely administered to patients within the first 24 hours following STEMI, and is therefore not recommended (116). Considerable caution must be exercised when intubating hypertensive patients with acute pulmonary edema, since it is very common for blood pressure to drop precipitously with sedation and positive pressure ventilation. Another agent that has been proposed for use in acute heart failure is nesiritide (recombinant human brain natriuretic peptide). However, it has not been demonstrated to improve clinically important outcomes when compared with standard therapy (117), may worsen renal function (118), and has been linked to a possible increased risk of short-term death (119).

Acute Coronary Syndromes. Although definitive therapy for acute coronary syndromes (ACSs) involves revascularization, tachycardia and hypertension increase myocardial oxygen requirements, and can potentially worsen ischemia and increase infarct size. β-Blockers are recommended for all ACS patients without a contraindication. An intravenous β-blocker is therefore a good initial choice as an antihypertensive (42). Intravenous β-blockers must be used with caution in patients with reduced left ventricular systolic function and in those in whom there is concern about impaired cardiac conduction (e.g.. inferior myocardial infarction). A large clinical trial of early β-blockade in patients with STEMI has demonstrated an increased risk of cardiogenic shock (41). If the blood pressure remains significantly elevated, especially with ongoing chest pain or pulmonary edema, then nitroglycerin should be used. In addition to reducing preload and afterload, nitrates also vasodilate coronary arteries, especially at the site of plaque disruption. If three sublingual tablets (0.4 mg over 5 minutes) are ineffective, then an intravenous infusion should be started and adjusted to alleviate chest pain and reduce blood pressure (10% reduction in normotensive patients, 30% reduction in hypertensive patients) (42).

Pre-eclampsia and Eclampsia

Although hypertensive encephalopathy and eclampsia have largely been considered separate entities, they have a similar pathophysiology and essentially the same MRI findings (RPLS) (120). Definitive treatment for severe pre-eclampsia and eclampsia is delivery, but careful intravenous blood pressure control is frequently also necessary.

Treatment of hypertension in severe pre-eclampsia has not been shown to improve perinatal outcomes, and may actually contribute to a decrease in neonatal birth weight (121). Thus, pharmacologic therapy is not recommended unless the degree of blood pressure elevation is severe (defined as SBP exceeding 160 mm Hg or DBP exceeding 105–110 mm Hg) or there are end-organ complications. Oral medications, with a goal pressure of 140 to 155/90 to 105 mm Hg, may be sufficient in the absence of organ dysfunction, but more rapid and tighter control is necessary for severe pre-eclampsia and eclampsia. Although there has been extensive experience with intravenous hydralazine (5–10 mg every 15–20 minutes to a maximum dose of 30 mg), this agent has a relatively slow onset, has not commonly been used as an infusion, may overshoot blood pressure goals, and has recently been linked to worse outcomes, including more placental abruption, adverse effects on fetal heart rate, lower Apgar scores, and a greater need for cesarean section (122). Other intravenous agents that have been successfully and safely used include labetalol and nicardipine (84,86). In addition to the above, magnesium sulfate should be given to prevent the development of seizures in patients with severe pre-eclampsia (123), and should be used to treat acute seizures when eclampsia occurs (124).

SUMMARY

The occurrence of acute hypertension in critically ill patients is not uncommon and can have serious consequences with regard to outcome. Careful evaluation of the underlying causes is important in selecting the best treatment options. Furthermore, the severity of the condition is determined by the magnitude of the acute increase in blood pressure from baseline more than by the absolute blood pressure level. Thus, in the presence of primarily normotensive baseline values (such as those in pre-eclampsia), a minor increase of blood pressure may lead to a life-threatening condition. Organ manifestations in the course of a hypertensive emergency concern the cardiovascular system and brain, and greatly affect therapeutic options and goals. With few exceptions from the rule (aortic dissection or severe pulmonary edema), the patient's blood pressure should be reduced in a stepwise approach and with precision by intravenous medications rapidly delivered, all the while monitoring the cardiovascular and central nervous systems. The selection of the antihypertensive agent, therefore, depends on the existing organ failure as well as its reliable effectiveness.

References

1. Vaughan CJ, Delanty N. Hypertensive emergencies. *Lancet.* 2000;356:411–417.
2. Calhoun DA, Oparil S. Treatment of hypertensive crisis. *N Engl J Med.* 1990;323:1177–1183.
3. Chobanian AV, Bakris GL, Black HR, et al. The seventh report of the Joint National Committee on prevention, detection, evaluation, and treatment of high blood pressure: the JNC 7 report. *JAMA.* 2003;289:2560–2572.
4. Hajjar I, Kotchen TA. Trends in prevalence, awareness, treatment, and control of hypertension in the United States, 1988–2000. *JAMA.* 2003; 290:199–206.
5. Zampaglione B, Pascale C, Marchisio M, et al. Hypertensive urgencies and emergencies. Prevalence and clinical presentation. *Hypertension.* 1996;27:144–147.
6. Karras DJ, Ufberg JW, Heilpern KL. Elevated blood pressure in urban emergency department patients. *Acad Emerg Med.* 2005;12:835–843.
7. Bennett NM, Shea S. Hypertensive emergency: case criteria, sociodemographic profile, and previous care of 100 cases. *Am J Public Health.* 1988; 78:636–640.
8. Shea S, Misra D, Ehrlich MH, et al. Predisposing factors for severe, uncontrolled hypertension in an inner-city minority population. *N Engl J Med.* 1992;327:776–781.
9. Bender SR, Fong MW, Heitz S, et al. Characteristics and management of patients presenting to the emergency department with hypertensive urgency. *J Clin Hypertens.* 2006;8:12–18.
10. Tisdale JE, Huang MB, Borzak S. Risk factors for hypertensive crisis: importance of out-patient blood pressure control. *Fam Pract.* 2004;2:420–424.
11. Keith NM, Wagener HP, Kernohan JW. The syndrome of malignant hypertension. *Arch Intern Med.* 1928;41:141–188.
12. Scarpelli PT, Livi R, Caselli GM, et al. Accelerated (malignant) hypertension: a study of 121 cases between 1974 and 1996. *J Nephrol.* 1997;10:207–215.
13. Hemmelgran BR, Zarnke KB, Campbell NR, et al. The 2004 Canadian hypertension education program recommendations for the management of hypertension: part I—blood pressure measurement, diagnosis and assessment of risk. *Can J Cardiol.* 2004;20:31–40.
14. Mann SJ, Pickering TG. Detection of renovascular hypertension. State of the art: 1992. *Ann Intern Med.* 1992;117:845–853.
15. Buckalw VM Jr, Berg RL, Wang SR, et al. Prevalence of hypertension in 1795 subjects with chronic renal disease: the modification of diet in renal disease study baseline cohort. Modification of Diet in Renal Disease Study Group. *Am J Kidney Dis.* 1996;28:811–821.
16. Becker HF, Jerrentrup A, Ploch T, et al. Effect of nasal continuous positive airway pressure treatment on blood pressure in patients with obstructive sleep apnea. *Circulation.* 2003;107:68–73.
17. Levine SR, Brust JC, Futrell N, et al. Cerebrovascular complications of the use of the "crack" form of alkaloidal cocaine. *N Engl J Med.* 1990;323:699–704.
18. Green RM, Kell KM, Gabrielsen T, et al. Multiple intracerebral hemorrhages after smoking "crack" cocaine. *Stroke.* 1990;21:957–962.
19. Hsue PY, Salinas CL, Bolger AF, et al. Acute aortic dissection related to crack cocaine. *Circulation.* 2002;105:1592–1595.
20. Novak BL, Force RW, Mumford BT, et al. Erythropoietin-associated hypertensive posterior leukoencephalopathy. *Neurology.* 1997;49:686–689.
21. Schwartz RB, Bravo SM, Klufas RA, et al. Cyclosporine neurotoxicity and its relationship to hypertensive encephalopathy: CT and MR findings in 16 cases. *Am J Roentgenol.* 1995;165:627–631.

22. Feigin VL, Lawes CM, Bennett DA, et al. Stroke epidemiology: a review of population-based studies of incidence, prevalence and case fatality in the late 20th century. *Lancet Neurol.* 2003;2:43–53.
23. Wallace JD, Levy LL. Blood pressure after stroke. *JAMA.* 1981;246:2177–2180.
24. Brott T, Lu M, Kothari R, et al. Hypertension and its treatment in the NINDS rt-PA stroke trial. *Stroke.* 1998;29:1504–1509.
25. Lindenauer PK, Mathew MC, Ntuli TS, et al. Use of antihypertensive agents in the management of patients with acute ischemic stroke. *Neurology.* 2004;63:318–323.
26. Jauch EC, Lindsell CJ, Adeoye O, et al. Lack of evidence for an association between hemodynamic variables and hematoma growth in spontaneous intracerebral hemorrhage. *Stroke* 2006;37:2061–2065.
27. Suarez J, Tarr RW, Selman WR. Aneurysmal subarachnoid hemorrhage. *N Engl J Med.* 2006;354:387–396.
28. Gal TJ, Cooperman LH. Hypertension in the immediate postoperative period. *Br J Anaesth.* 1975;47:70–74.
29. Kutz JD, Cronau LH, Barash PG. Postoperative hypertension hazard of abrupt cessation of antihypertensive medication in preoperative period. *Am Heart J.* 1976;92:79.
30. Towne JB, Bernhard VM. The relationship of postoperative hypertension to complications following carotid endarterectomy. *Surgery.* 1980;88:575–580.
31. Basali A, Mascha EJ, Kalfas I, et al. Relation between perioperative hypertension and intracranial hemorrhage after craniotomy. *Anesthesiology.* 2000;93:48–54.
32. Leslie JB. Incidence and etiology of perioperative hypertension. *Acta Anaesthesiol Scand Suppl.* 1993;99:5–9.
33. Prys-Roberts C, Meloche R, Foex P. Studies of anesthesia in relation to hypertension. I: cardiovascular responses of treated and untreated patents. *Br J Anesth.* 1971;43:122.
34. Aronson S, Boisvert D, Lapp W. Isolated systolic hypertension is associated with adverse outcomes from coronary artery bypass grafting surgery. *Anesth Analg.* 2002;94:1079–1084.
35. Eagle KA, Berger PB, Calkins H, et al. ACC/AHA guideline update for perioperative cardiovascular evaluation for noncardiac surgery—executive summary: A report of the American College of Cardiology/American Heart Association Task Force on practice guidelines (committee to update the 1996 guidelines on perioperative cardiovascular evaluation for noncardiac surgery). *Circulation.* 2002;105:1257–1267.
36. Weksler N, Klein M, Szendro G, et al. The dilemma of immediate preoperative hypertension: to treat and operate, or to postpone surgery? *J Clin Anesth.* 2003;15:179–183.
37. Vidaeff A, Carroll MA, Ramin SM. Acute hypertensive emergencies in pregnancy. *Crit Care Med.* 2005;33:S307–S312.
38. Sibai B, Dekker G, Kupfermink M. Pre-eclampsia. *Lancet.* 2005;365:785–799.
39. Adams Jr KF, Fonarow GC, Emerman CL, et al. Characteristics and outcomes of patients hospitalized for heart failure in the United States: rationale, design, and preliminary observations from the first 100,000 cases in the Acute Decompensated Heart Failure National Registry (ADHERE). *Am Heart J.* 2005;149:209–216.
40. Fifth Organization to Assess Strategies in Acute Ischemic Syndromes Investigators; Yusuf S, Mehta SR, Chrolvaicius S, et al. Comparison of fondaparinux and enoxaparin in acute coronary syndromes. *N Engl J Med.* 2006;354:1464–1476.
41. Chen ZM, Pan HC, Chen YP, et al. Early intravenous then oral metoprolol in 45,852 patients with acute myocardial infarction: a randomised placebo-controlled trial. *Lancet.* 2005;366:1622–1632.
42. Antman EM, Anbe DT, Armstrong PW, et al. ACC/AHA guidelines for the management of patients with ST elevation myocardial infarction: a report of the American College of Cardiology/American Heart Association Task Force on Practice Guidelines. *Circulation.* 2004;110:e82–292.
43. Hagan PG, Nienaber CA, Isselbacher EM, et al. The international registry of acute aortic dissection (IRAD). *JAMA.* 2000;283:897–903.
44. Louzenhiser R, Griffin KA, Bidani AK. Systolic blood pressure as the trigger for the renal myogenic response: protective or autoregulatory? *Curr Opin Nephrol Hypertens.* 2006;15:41–49.
45. Montgomery HE, Kiernan LA, Whitworth CE, et al. Inhibition of tissue angiotensin converting enzyme activity prevents malignant hypertension in TGR(mREN2)27. *J Hypertens.* 1998;16:635–643.
46. Davies DL, Schalekamp MA, Beevers DG, et al. Abnormal relationship between exchangeable sodium and the renin-angiotensin system in malignant hypertension. *Lancet.* 1973;1:683–687.
47. Fleming S. Malignant hypertension—the role of the paracrine renin-angiotensin system. *J Pathol.* 2000;192:135–139.
48. Kalimo H, Fredriksson K, Nordberg C, et al. The spread of brain injury in hypertensive injury. *Med Biol.* 1986;64:133–137.
49. Beausang-Linder M, Bill A. Cerebral circulation in acute arterial hypertension—protective effects of sympathetic nervous activity. *Acta Physiol Scand.* 1981;111:193–199.
50. Hinchey J, Chaves C, Appignani B, et al. A reversible posterior leukoencephalopathy syndrome. *N Engl J Med.* 1996;334:494–500.
51. Bakshi R, Shaikh ZA, Bates VE, et al. Thrombotic thrombocytopenic purpura. Brain CT and MRI findings in 12 patients. *Neurology.* 1999;52:1285–1288.
52. Schwartz RB, Feske SK, Polak JK, et al. Preeclampsia-eclampsia: clinical and neuroradiologic correlates and insights into the pathogenesis of hypertensive encephalopathy. *Radiology.* 2000;217:371–376.
53. Covarrubius DJ, Luetmer PH, Campeau NG. Posterior reversible encephalopathy syndrome: prognostic utility of quantitative diffusion-weighted MR images. *Am J Neuroradiol.* 2002;23:1038–1048.
54. Chester EM, Agamanolis DP, Banker BQ, et al. Hypertensive encephalopathy: a clinicopathologic study of 20 cases. *Neurology.* 1978;28:928–939.
55. Healton EB, Brust JC, Feinfeld DA, et al. Hypertensive encephalopathy and the neurologic manifestations of malignant hypertension. *Neurology.* 1982;32:127–132.
56. Stott VL, Hurrell MA, Anderson TJ. Reversible posterior leukoencephalopathy syndrome: a misnomer reviewed. *Intern Med J.* 2005;35:83–90.
57. Bakshi R, Bates VE, Mechtler LL, et al. Occipital lobe seizures as the major clinical manifestation of reversible posterior leukoencephalopathy syndrome: magnetic resonance imaging findings. *Epilepsia.* 1998;39:295–299.
58. Ahmed ME, Walker JM, Beevers DG, et al. Lack of difference between malignant and accelerated hypertension. *BMJ.* 1986;292:235–237.
59. Griswold WR, Viney J, Mendoza SA, et al. Intracranial pressure monitoring in severe hypertensive encephalopathy. *Crit Care Med.* 1981;9:573–576.
60. Hammond S, Wells JR, Marcus DM, et al. Ophthalmoscopic findings in malignant hypertension. *J Clin Hypertens (Greenwich).* 2005;8:222–223.
61. Dimmitt SB, West JN, Eames SM, et al. Usefulness of ophthalmoscopy in mild to moderate hypertension. *Lancet.* 1989;1:1103–1106.
62. Alpers CE. The kidney. In: Kumar V, Fausto N, Abbas A, eds. *Robbins and Cotran: Pathological Basis of Disease.* 7th ed. Philadelphia: Saunders; 2005.
63. van den Born BJH, Honnebier UPF, Koopmans RP, et al. Microangiopathy hemolysis and renal failure in malignant hypertension. *Hypertension.* 2004;45:246.
64. James SH, Meyers AM, Milne FJ, et al. Partial recovery of renal function in black patients with apparent end-stage renal failure due to primary malignant hypertension. *Nephron.* 1995;71:29–34.
65. Lip GY, Beevers M, Beevers G. The failure of malignant hypertension to decline: a survey of 24 years' experience in a multiracial population in England. *J Hypertens.* 1994;12:1297–1305.
66. Nixenberg A, Antony I. Epicardial coronary arteries are not adequately sized in hypertensive patients. *J Am Coll Cardiol.* 1996;27:1115–1123.
67. Aurigemma GP, Gaasch WH. Diastolic heart failure. *N Engl J Med.* 2005; 351:1097–1105.
68. Friederich JA, Butterworth JF. Sodium nitroprusside: twenty years and counting. *Anesth Analg.* 1995;81:152–162.
69. Armstrong PW, Walker DC, Burton JR, et al. Vasodilator therapy in acute myocardial infarction. A comparison of sodium nitroprusside and nitroglycerin. *Circulation.* 1975;52:1118–1122.
70. Campbell CS, Wallwork J, Taylor KM, et al. The hemodynamic effects of sodium nitroprusside following cardiopulmonary bypass: a clinical study. *J Cardiovasc Surg.* 1982;23:41–48.
71. Cohn JN, Franciosa JA, Francis GS, et al. Effect of short-term infusion of sodium nitroprusside on mortality rate in cute myocardial infarction complicated by left ventricular failure: results of a Veterans Administration cooperative study. *N Engl J Med.* 1982;306:1129–1135.
72. Davis RF, Douglas ME, Heenan TJ, et al. Brain tissue pressure measurement during sodium nitroprusside infusion. *Crit Care Med.* 1981;9:17–21.
73. Ekhart E, Bayer H, Auer L, et al. Sodium nitroprusside in neurosurgery and intensive care of neurosurgical patients. *Aneaesthetist.* 1978;27:527–532.
74. Marsh ML, Aidinis SJ, Naughton KV, et al. The technique of nitroprusside administration modifies the intracranial pressure response. *Anesthesiology.* 1979;51:538–541.
75. Ivankovich AD, Miletich DJ, Tinker JH. Sodium nitroprusside: metabolism and general considerations. *Int Anesthesiol Clin.* 1978;16:1–29.
76. Robin ED, McCauley R. Nitroprusside-related cyanide poisoning. Time (long past due) for urgent, effective interventions [special report]. *Chest.* 1992;102:1842–1845.
77. Hall AH, Rumack BH. Hydroxocobalamin/sodium thiosulfate as a cyanide antidote. *J Emerg Med.* 1987;5:115–121.
78. Cottrell JE, Casthely P, Brodie JD, et al. Prevention of nitroprusside-induced cyanide toxicity with hydroxocobalamin. *N Engl J Med.* 1978;15:809–811.
79. Hall VA, Guest JM. Sodium nitroprusside-induced cyanide intoxication and prevention with sodium thiosulfate prophylaxis. *Am J Crit Care.* 1992;1: 19–27.
80. Ishikura F, Beppu S, Hamada T, et al. Effects of sildenafil citrate (Viagra) combined with nitrate on the heart. *Circulation.* 2000;102:2516–2521.
81. Ghani GA, Sung YF, Weinstein MS, et al. Effects of intravenous nitroglycerin on the intracranial pressure and volume pressure response. *J Neurosurg.* 1983;58:562–565.
82. Lund-Johansen P. Pharmacology of combined alpha-beta blockade. II. Hemodynamic effects of labetalol. *Drugs.* 1984;Suppl 2:35–50.

83. Orlowski JP, Shiesley D, Vidt DG, et al. Labetalol to control blood pressure after cerebrovascular surgery. *Crit Care Med.* 1988;16:765–768.
84. Mabie WC, Gonzalez AR, Sibai BM, et al. A comparative trial of labetalol and hydralazine in the acute management of severe hypertension complication pregnancy. *Obstet Gynceol.* 1987;70:328–333.
85. Gray RJ. Managing critically ill patients with esmolol. An ultra short-acting beta blocker. *Chest.* 1988;93:398–403.
86. Curran MP, Robinson DM, Keating GM. Intravenous nicardipine: its use in the short-term treatment of hypertension and various other indications. *Drugs.* 2006;66:1755–1782.
87. Neutel JM, Smith DH, Wallin D, et al. A comparison of intravenous nicardipine and sodium nitroprusside in the immediate treatment of severe hypertension. *Am J Hypertens.* 1994;7:623–628.
88. Nishiyama T, Omote K, Namiki A, et al. The effects of nicardipine on cerebrospinal fluid pressure in humans. *Anesth Analg.* 1986;65:507–510.
89. Murphy MB, Murray C, Shorten GD. Fenoldopam: a selective peripheral dopamine-receptor agonist for the treatment of severe hypertension. *N Engl J Med.* 2001;345:1548–1557.
90. Elliott WJ, Weber RR, Nelson KS, et al. Renal and hemodynamic effects of intravenous fenoldopam versus nitroprusside in severe hypertension. *Circulation.* 1990;81:970–977.
91. Panacek EA, Bednarczyk EM, Dunbar LM, et al. Randomized, prospective trial of fenoldopam vs sodium nitroprusside in the treatment of acute severe hypertension. Fenoldopam Study Group. *Acad Emerg Med.* 1995;2:959–965.
92. Devlin JW, Seta ML, Kanji S, et al. Fenoldopam versus nitroprusside for the treatment of hypertensive emergency. *Ann Pharmacother.* 2004;38:755–759.
93. Elliott WJ, Karnezis TA, Silverman RA, et al. Intraocular pressure increases with fenoldopam, but not nitroprusside, in hypertensive humans. *Clin Pharacmol Ther.* 1991;49:285–293.
94. Reed WG, Anderson RJ. Effects of rapid blood pressure reduction on cerebral blood flow. *Am Heart J.* 1986;111:226–222.
95. Powers WJ. Acute hypertension after stroke: the scientific basis for treatment decisions. *Neurology.* 1993;43:461–467.
96. Oliveira-Filho J, Silva SC, Trabuco CC, et al. Detrimental effect of blood pressure reduction in the first 24 hours of acute stroke onset. *Neurology.* 2003;61:1047–1051.
97. Rordorf G, Koroshetz WJ, Ezzeddine MA, et al. A pilot study of drug-induced hypertension for treatment of acute stroke. *Neurology.* 2001; 56:1210–1213.
98. Leonardi-Bee J, Bath PM, Phillips SJ, et al. Blood pressure and clinical outcomes in the International Stroke Trial. *Stroke.* 2002;33:1315–1320.
99. Adams HP Jr, Adams RJ, Brott T, et al. Guidelines for the early management of patients with ischemic stroke: a scientific statement from the stroke council of the American Stroke Association. *Stroke.* 2003;34:1056–1083.
100. Hill MD, Buchan AM. Thrombolysis for acute ischemic stroke: results of the Canadian Alteplase for Stroke Effectiveness Study. *CMAJ.* 2005;172:1307–1312.
101. The National Institute of Neurological Disorders and Stroke rt-PA Stroke Study Group. Tissue plasminogen activator for acute ischemic stroke. *N Engl J Med.* 1995;333:1581–1587.
102. Brott T, Broderick J, Kothari R, et al. Early hemorrhage growth in patients with intracerebral hemorrhage. *Stroke.* 1997;28:1–5.
103. Willmot M, Leonardi-Bee J, Bath PM. High blood pressure in acute stroke and subsequent outcome: a systematic review. *Hypertension.* 2004;43:18–24.
104. Leira R, Davalos A, Silva Y. Early neurologic deterioration in intracerebral hemorrhage: predictors and associated factors. *Neurology.* 2004;63:461–467.
105. Broderick JP, Adams HP Hr, Barsan W, et al. Guidelines for the management of spontaneous intracerebral hemorrhage: a statement for healthcare professionals from a special writing group of the Stroke Council, American Heart Association. *Stroke.* 1999;30:905–915.
106. Zazulia AR, Diringer MN, Videen TO, et al. Hypoperfusion without ischemia surrounding acute intracerebral hemorrhage. *J Cereb Blood Flow Metab.* 2001;21:804–810.
107. Powers WJ, Zazulia AR, Videen TO, et al. Autoregulation of cerebral blood flow surrounding acute (6 to 22 hours) intracerebral hemorrhage. *Neurology.* 2001;57:18–24.
108. Mayberg MR, Batjer HH, Dacey R, et al. Guidelines for the management of aneurysmal subarachnoid hemorrhage: a statement for healthcare professionals from a special writing group of the Stroke Council, American Heart Association. *Circulation.* 1994;90:2592–2605.
109. Naidech AM, Janjua N, Kreiter KT, et al. Predictors and impact of aneurysm rebleeding after subarachnoid hemorrhage. *Arch Neurol.* 2005; 62:410–416.
110. Olsen K, Pedersen CB, Madsen JB, et al. Vasoactive modulators during and after craniotomy: relation to postoperative hypertension. *J Neurosurg Anesthesiol.* 2002;14:171–179.
111. van Mook W, Rennenberg R, Schurink GW, et al. Cerebral hyperperfusion syndrome. *Lancet Neurol.* 2005;4:877–888.
112. Hashimoto T, Young WL. Anesthesia-related considerations for cerebral arteriovenous malformations. *Neurosurg Focus.* 2001;11:1–6.
113. Tsai TT, Nienaber CA, Eagle KA. Acute aortic syndromes. *Circulation.* 2005;112:3802–3813.
114. Kramer K, Kirkman P, Kitzman D, et al. Flash pulmonary edema: association with hypertension and reoccurrence despite coronary revascularization. *Am Heart J.* 2000;140:451–455.
115. Elkayam U, Akhter MW, Singe H, et al. Comparison of effects on left ventricular filling pressure of intravenous nesiritide and high-dose nitroglycerin in patients with decompensated heart failure. *Am J Cardiol.* 2004;93:237–240.
116. Sigurdsson A, Swedberg K. Left ventricular remodelling, neurohormonal activation and early treatment with enalapril (CONSENSUS II) following myocardial infarction. *Eur Heart J.* 1994;15:14–19.
117. Publication Committee for VMAC Investigators. Intravenous nesiritide vs nitroglycerin for treatment of decompensated congestive heart failure: a randomized controlled trial. *JAMA.* 2002;287:1531–1540.
118. Sackner-Bernstein JD, Skopicki HA, Aaronson KD. Risk of worsening renal function with nesiritide in patients with acutely decompensated heart failure. *Circulation.* 2005;111:1487–1491.
119. Sackner-Bernstein JD, Kowalski M, Fox M, et al. Short-term risk of death after treatment with nesiritide for decompensated heart failure: a pooled analysis of randomized controlled trials. *JAMA.* 2005;293:1900–1905.
120. Zeeman GC, Hatab MR, Twickler DM. Increased cerebral blood flow in preeclampsia with magnetic resonance imaging. *Am J Obstet Gynec.* 2004; 191:1425–1429.
121. von Dadelszen P, Magee LA. Fall in mean arterial pressure and fetal growth restriction in pregnancy hypertension: an updated metaregression analysis. *J Obstet Gynaec Can.* 2002;24:941–945.
122. Magee LA, Cham C, Waterman EJ, et al. Hydralazine for treatment of severe hypertension in pregnancy: a meta-analysis. *BMJ.* 2003;327:955–960.
123. Altman D, Carroli G, Duley L, et al. Do women with pre-eclampsia, and their babies, benefit from magnesium sulphate? The Magpie Trial: a randomised placebo-controlled trial. *Lancet.* 2002;359:1877–1890.
124. Lucas MJ, Leveno KJ, Cunningham FG. A comparison of magnesium sulphate with phenytoin for the prevention of eclampsia. *N Engl J Med.* 1995; 333:201–205.
125. Wong T, Mitchell P. The eye in hypertension. *Lancet.* 2007;369:425–435.

CHAPTER 127 ■ HEART–LUNG INTERACTIONS

MICHAEL R. PINSKY

This work was supported in part by the NIH grants HL67181, HL07820, and HL073198.

KEY POINTS

1. Spontaneous ventilation is exercise.
   a. Failure to wean may connote cardiovascular insufficiency.
   b. Weaning is a cardiovascular stress test.
   c. Breathing loads both the heart and lungs.
2. Changes in lung volume alter autonomic tone, pulmonary vascular resistance, and at high lung volumes compress the heart in the cardiac fossa in a fashion analogous to cardiac tamponade.
   a. Low lung volumes increase pulmonary vasomotor tone by stimulating hypoxic pulmonary vasoconstriction.
   b. High lung volumes increase pulmonary vascular resistance by increasing transpulmonary pressure.
3. Spontaneous inspiration and spontaneous inspiratory efforts decrease intrathoracic pressure.
   a. Increasing venous return
   b. Increasing left ventricular afterload
4. Positive pressure ventilation increases intrathoracic pressure.
   a. Decreasing venous return
   b. The decrease in venous return is mitigated by the associated increase in intra-abdominal pressure
   c. Decreasing left ventricular afterload
   d. Abolishing negative swings in intrathoracic pressure selectively reduces left ventricular (LV) afterload without reducing venous return.

OVERVIEW

Perhaps the most obvious and least understood aspect of cardiopulmonary disease is the profound and intimate relation between cardiac and pulmonary dysfunction. Heart–lung interactions go in both directions. They include the effect of the circulation on ventilation wherein acute ventricular failure causes hypoxemia and ischemic respiratory failure; and the effect of ventilation on circulation where hyperinflation can induce tamponade and spontaneous inspiration acute heart failure. Although most references to heart–lung interactions usually refer to the effect of ventilation on the circulation, the opposite interactions also exist and are relevant to the bedside clinician.

Heart–lung interactions can be grouped into interactions that involve three basic concepts that usually coexist (1,2). First, spontaneous ventilation is exercise, requiring O_2 and blood flow, thus placing demands on cardiac output, and producing CO_2, adding additional ventilatory stress on CO_2 excretion. Second, inspiration increases lung volume above resting end-expiratory volume. Thus, some of the hemodynamic effects of ventilation are due to changes in lung volume and chest wall expansion. Third, spontaneous inspiration decreases intrathoracic pressure (ITP) whereas positive pressure ventilation increases ITP. Thus the differences between spontaneous ventilation and positive pressure ventilation primarily reflect the differences in ITP swings and the energy necessary to produce them.

THE EFFECTS OF CARDIOVASCULAR DYSFUNCTION ON VENTILATION

Cardiogenic shock can induce hydrostatic pulmonary edema, impairing acute hypoxic respiratory failure. Circulatory shock, by limiting blood flow to the respiratory muscles, can induce respiratory muscle failure and respiratory arrest. These points underscore a fundamental aspect of ventilation, namely that it is exercise, and like any form of exercise, it must place a certain metabolic demand on the cardiovascular system (3). If cardiovascular reserve is limited, this metabolic demand may exceed the heart's ability to deliver O_2 to meet the increased metabolic activity associated with spontaneous ventilation. Thus, ventilator-dependent patients with cardiovascular insufficiency may not be able to wean from mechanical ventilation because the metabolic demand of spontaneous ventilation is too great. Since this increased stress occurs only during the weaning trial, such insufficiency may not be apparent prior to weaning attempts.

Under normal conditions, respiratory muscle blood flow is not the limiting factor determining maximal ventilatory effort even with marked respiratory efforts. Although ventilation normally requires less than 5% of total O_2 consumption (3), if the work of breathing is increased, such as in pulmonary edema, pulmonary fibrosis, or bronchospasm, the work cost of breathing can increase to 25% of total O_2 consumption (3–6). If cardiac output is limited, then blood flow to all organs including the respiratory muscles may be compromised, inducing both tissue hypoperfusion and lactic acidosis (7–10). Under these severe heart failure conditions respiratory muscle failure may develop despite high central neuronal drive (11). Supporting spontaneous ventilation by the use of mechanical ventilation will reduce O_2 consumption increasing SvO_2 for a constant cardiac output and arterial O_2 content. Thus, intubation and mechanical ventilation in patients in severe heart failure will not only decrease the work of breathing but increase the available O_2 delivery to other vital organs, decreasing serum lactate levels. These cardiovascular benefits are not limited to intubated patients but can also be seen with the noninvasive continuous positive airway pressure (CPAP) ventilation mask (12).

Ventilator-dependent patients who fail to wean during spontaneous breathing trials often have impaired baseline cardiovascular performance that may not be apparent when they are on at least partial ventilatory support (13). However, such at-risk patients can develop overt signs of heart failure only during spontaneous breathing trials. The spontaneous ventilation-induced heart failure can present abruptly with the development of acute pulmonary edema (13,14), myocardial ischemia (15–18), tachycardia, and gut ischemia (19). Since breathing is exercise, all subjects will increase their cardiac outputs in response to a spontaneous breathing trial. However, those who subsequently fail to wean demonstrate a reduction in mixed venous O_2, consistent with a failing cardiovascular response to an increased metabolic demand (20). Importantly, the increased work of breathing may come from the endotracheal tube flow resistance (21). Thus, some subjects who fail a spontaneous breathing trial may actually be able to breathe on their own if extubated. Weaning from mechanical ventilatory support is a cardiovascular stress test. In fact, numerous studies have documented weaning-associated ischemic electrocardiogram (ECG) changes and thallium cardiac blood flow ventilation-related signs of ischemia in both subjects with known coronary artery disease (15) and those with normal coronaries (17,18). Using this same logic in reverse, placing patients with severe heart failure and/or ischemia on mechanical ventilatory support by either intubation and ventilation (22) or noninvasive continuous positive airway pressure (23) often reverses myocardial ischemia.

HEMODYNAMIC EFFECTS OF VENTILATION AND VENTILATORY MANEUVERS

Ventilation can profoundly alter cardiovascular function. The specific response will be dependent on myocardial contractile and preload reserve, circulating blood volume, blood flow distribution, autonomic tone, endocrinologic responses, lung volume, intrathoracic pressure (ITP), and the surrounding pressures for the remainder of the circulation (24,25).

To understand this issue better one must understand, at least in part, the relation between airway pressure (Paw) and ITP: the transpulmonary pressure. Paw is relatively easy to measure (26,27), whereas ITP is not. Positive pressure ventilation–induced increases in Paw do not necessarily equate to proportional increases in ITP. The primary determinants of the hemodynamic responses to ventilation are due to changes in ITP and lung volume (28), not Paw. The relation between Paw, ITP, pericardial pressure (Ppc) and lung volume varies with spontaneous ventilatory effort, as well as lung and chest wall compliance. Lung expansion during positive pressure inspiration pushes on the surrounding structures, distorting them and causing their surface pressures to increase, increasing both Ppl and Ppc (29). Only lung and thoracic compliance determine the relation between end-expiratory Paw and lung volume in the sedated and paralyzed patient. However, if a ventilated patient actively resists lung inflation or sustains expiratory muscle activity at end-inspiration, then end-inspiratory Paw will exceed resting Paw for that lung volume. Similarly, if the patient activity prevents full exhalation by expiratory breaking, then for the same end-expiratory Paw, lung volume may be higher than predicted from end-expiratory Paw values. At end-expiration, if the respiratory system is at rest, Paw equals alveolar pressure and lung volume is at functional residual capacity. If incomplete exhalation occurs, then alveolar pressure will exceed Paw. The difference between measured Paw and alveolar pressure is called intrinsic *positive end-expiratory pressure* (PEEP). Finally, if chest wall compliance decreases, as may occur with increased abdominal pressure, both Paw and ITP will increase for the same tidal breath.

Since the heart is fixed within a cardiac fossa and cannot be displaced in any direction, juxtacardiac Ppl will increase more than lateral chest wall or diaphragmatic Ppl during inspiration. Ppc is the outside pressure to LV intraluminal ventricular pressure determining LV filling. Ppc and ITP may not be similar nor increase by similar amounts with the application of positive Paw, if the pericardium acts as a limiting membrane (30,31). With pericardial restraint, as in tamponade, Ppc exceeds juxtacardiac Ppl (32). With progressive increases in PEEP, juxtacardiac Ppl will increase toward Ppc levels, whereas Ppc will initially remain constant. Once these two pressures equalize, further increases in PEEP by increasing lung volume will increase both juxtacardiac Ppl and Ppc in parallel. Thus, if pericardial volume restraint exists, as may occur with acute cor pulmonale or tamponade, then juxtacardiac Ppl will underestimate Ppc.

The presence of lung parenchymal disease, airflow obstruction, and extrapulmonary processes that directly alter chest wall-diaphragmatic contraction or intra-abdominal pressure may also alter these interactions. Static lung expansion occurs as Paw increases because the transpulmonary pressure (Paw relative to ITP) increases. If lung injury induces alveolar flooding or increased pulmonary parenchyma stiffness, then greater increases in Paw will be required to distend the lungs to a constant end-inspiratory volume (9,29,33). Thus, the primary determinants of the increase in Ppl and Ppc during positive pressure ventilation are lung volume change and chest wall compliance, not Paw change (34). Since acute lung injury (ALI) is often nonhomogeneous, with aerated areas of the lung displaying normal specific compliance, increases in Paw above approximately 30 cm H_2O will overdistend these aerated lung units (35). Vascular structures that are distended will have a greater increase in their surrounding pressure than collapsible structures that do not distend (36). Despite this nonhomogeneous alveolar distention, if tidal volume is kept constant, then Ppl increases equally, independent of the mechanical properties of the lung (33,37,38). Thus, under constant tidal volume conditions, changes in peak and mean Paw will reflect changes in the mechanical properties of the lungs and patient coordination, but may not reflect changes in ITP. Thus, one cannot predict the amount of change in ITP or Ppc that will occur in a given patient as PEEP is varied. Accordingly, assuming some constant fraction of Paw transmission to the pleural surface as a means of calculating the effect of increasing Paw on ITP is inaccurate and potentially dangerous if used to assess transmural intrathoracic vascular pressures. However, if the patient has a pulmonary artery catheter *in situ*, then one can estimate end-expiratory ITP. *The clinician has* the ability to measure on-PEEP intrathoracic vascular pressures by calculating the airway pressure transmission index to the pleural space (39) or by briefly removing PEEP while these pressures are directly measured (38). The ratio of end-inspiratory to end-expiratory pulmonary artery diastolic pressure (reflecting ITP changes) to Paw (reflecting alveolar pressure changes) defines the pulmonary transmission index. If one assumes that lung compliance is linear over the given tidal volume, then the product of this transmission index and PEEP represents the end-expiratory ITP.

HEMODYNAMIC EFFECTS OF CHANGES IN LUNG VOLUME

Changing lung volume alters autonomic tone, pulmonary vascular resistance, and at high lung volumes, compresses the heart in the cardiac fossa, limiting absolute cardiac volumes analogous to cardiac tamponade. However, unlike tamponade where Ppc selectively increases in excess of Ppl, with hyperinflation both juxtacardiac Ppl and Ppc increase together.

Autonomic Tone

Cyclic changes in lung volume induce cyclic changes in autonomic inflow. The lungs are richly enervated with integrated somatic and autonomic fibers that originate, traverse through, and end in the thorax. These neuronal pathways mediate many homeostatic processes through the autonomic nervous system that alter both instantaneous cardiovascular function and steady-state cardiovascular status (40,41). Lung inflation to normal tidal volumes ($<$10 mL/kg) induces parasympathetic withdrawal, increasing heart rate. This inspiration-induced cardioacceleration is referred to as *respiratory sinus arrhythmia* (42). The presence of respiratory sinus arrhythmia connotes normal autonomic control (43) and is used in diabetics with peripheral neuropathy to assess peripheral dysautonomia (44). Inflation to larger tidal volumes ($>$15 mL/kg) decreases heart rate by a combination of both increased vagal tone (45) and sympathetic withdrawal. The sympathetic withdrawal also creates arterial vasodilation (40,46–50). This inflation–vasodilatation response induces expiration-associated reductions in LV contractility in healthy volunteers (51), and in ventilator-dependent patients with the initiation of high-frequency ventilation (40) or hyperinflation (48). Humeral factors, including compounds blocked by cyclooxygenase inhibition (52), released from pulmonary endothelial cells during lung inflation may also induce this depressor response (53–55). However, these interactions do not appear to grossly alter cardiovascular status (56). Although overdistention of aerated lung units in patients with acute lung injury (ALI) may induce such cardiovascular depression, unilateral lung hyperinflation (unilateral PEEP) does not appear to influence systemic hemodynamics (57). Thus, these cardiovascular effects are of uncertain clinical significance.

Ventilation also compresses the right atrium and through this mechanical effect alters control of intravascular fluid balance. Both positive pressure ventilation and sustained hyperinflation decrease right atrial stretch stimulating endocrinologic responses that induce fluid retention. Plasma norepinephrine, plasma renin activity (58,59), and atrial naturietic peptide (60) increase during positive pressure ventilation owing to right atrial collapse. Potentially, one of the benefits of the use of nasal CPAP in patients with congestive heart failure (CHF) is to decrease plasma atrial naturietic peptide activity in parallel with improvements in blood flow (61,62). Thus, some of the observed benefit of CPAP therapy in heart failure patients may be mediated through humoral mechanisms.

Pulmonary Vascular Resistance

Ventilation alters pulmonary vascular resistance, and thus pulmonary arterial pressure. Right ventricular (RV) ejection performance is markedly limited by increases in RV ejection pressure because the right ventricle has thin walls that cannot distribute increased wall stress. Sudden increases in pulmonary arterial pressure can induce cardiovascular collapse. This is the common cause of cardiovascular collapse, for example, with massive pulmonary embolism. The mechanisms inducing changes in pulmonary vascular resistance with changing lung volume are often complex, often conflicting, and include both humoral and mechanical interactions. Increasing lung volume occurs because transpulmonary pressure increases. For example, although obstructive inspiratory efforts, as occur during obstructive sleep apnea, are usually associated with increased RV afterload, the increased afterload is due primarily to either increased vasomotor tone (hypoxic pulmonary vasoconstriction) or backward LV failure and not lung volume–induced changes in pulmonary vascular resistance (63,64). RV afterload, like LV afterload, can be defined as the maximal RV systolic wall stress during contraction (65). Thus, it is a function of the maximal product of the RV free wall radius of curvature (a function of end-diastolic volume) and transmural pressure (a function of systolic RV pressure) during ejection (66). Systolic RV pressure equals transmural pulmonary artery pressure. Increases in transmural Ppa impede RV ejection (67), decreasing RV stroke volume (68) and inducing RV dilation, and passively impede venous return (52,54). If not relieved quickly, acute cor pulmonale rapidly develops (69). Furthermore, if RV dilation and RV pressure overload persist, RV free wall ischemia and infarction can develop (70). Importantly, rapid fluid challenges in the setting of acute cor pulmonale can precipitate profound cardiovascular collapse due to excessive RV dilation, RV ischemia, and compromised LV filling.

The pulmonary vasculature constricts if alveolar PO_2 (P_AO_2) decreases to below 60 mm Hg (71). This process of hypoxic pulmonary vasoconstriction is mediated, in part, by variations in the synthesis and release of nitric oxide by endothelial nitric oxide synthase localized on pulmonary vascular endothelial cells and in part by an NAD/NADH voltage-dependent calcium channel in the pulmonary vasculature. Hypoxic pulmonary vasoconstriction, by reducing pulmonary blood flow to hypoxic lung regions, minimizes shunt blood flow. However, if generalized alveolar hypoxia occurs, then pulmonary vasomotor tone increases, increasing pulmonary vascular resistance and impeding RV ejection (65). Importantly, at low lung volumes, alveoli spontaneously collapse as a result of loss of interstitial traction and closure of the terminal airways. This collapse causes both absorption atelectasis and alveolar hypoxia. Patients with acute hypoxemic respiratory failure have small lung volumes and are prone to spontaneous alveolar collapse (72,73). Therefore, pulmonary vascular resistance is often increased in patients with acute hypoxemic respiratory failure due to small lung volumes and atelectasis (e.g., ALI).

Mechanical ventilation may reduce pulmonary vasomotor tone, reducing pulmonary artery pressure and RV afterload by any one of many related processes. First, hypoxic pulmonary vasoconstriction can be inhibited if O_2-enriched inspired gas increases PaO_2 (74–77) or if the mechanical breaths and PEEP, by recruiting collapsed alveolar units, increases PaO_2 in those local alveoli (28,78–80). Second, mechanical ventilation often reverses respiratory acidosis by increasing alveolar ventilation, which itself stimulates pulmonary vasoconstriction (77). Finally, decreasing central sympathetic output by sedation during mechanical ventilation will also reduce vasomotor tone (81–83).

Increases in lung volume directly increase pulmonary vascular resistance by compressing the alveolar vessels (72,79,80). The actual mechanisms by which this occurs have not been completely resolved, but appear to reflect differential extraluminal pressure gradient–induced vascular compression. The pulmonary circulation can be conceptually viewed as existing in two distinct compartments based on the pressure outside the blood vessels, which will be either alveolar pressure (alveolar vessels) or extra-alveolar or ITP (extra-alveolar vessels) (79). The small pulmonary arterioles, venules, and alveolar capillaries sense alveolar pressure as their surrounding pressure while the large pulmonary arteries and veins, as well as the heart and intrathoracic great vessels of the systemic circulation, sense interstitial pressure or ITP as their surrounding pressure. Since alveolar pressure minus ITP is the transpulmonary pressure, and increasing lung volume requires transpulmonary pressure to rise, increases in lung volume augments the extraluminal pressure gradient from extra-alveolar vessels to alveolar vessels. Increases in lung volume progressively raise alveolar vessel resistance, becoming most noticeable above functional residual capacity (FRC) (75,84) (Fig. 127.1). Since the intraluminal pressure in the pulmonary arteries is generated by RV ejection relative to ITP, but the outside pressure of the alveolar vessels is alveolar pressure, if transpulmonary pressure exceeds intraluminal pulmonary arterial pressure, then the pulmonary vasculature will collapse where extra-alveolar vessels pass into alveolar loci, reducing the vasculature cross-sectional area and increasing pulmonary vascular resistance. Hyperinflation can create significant pulmonary hypertension and may precipitate acute RV failure (acute cor pulmonale) (85) and RV ischemia (70), especially in patients prone to hyperinflation (e.g., chronic obstructive pulmonary disease [COPD]). Thus, PEEP may increase pulmonary vascular resistance if it induces lung overdistention (86). Similarly, if lung volumes are reduced, increasing lung volume back to baseline levels by the use of PEEP decreases pulmonary vascular resistance by reversing hypoxic pulmonary vasoconstriction (87).

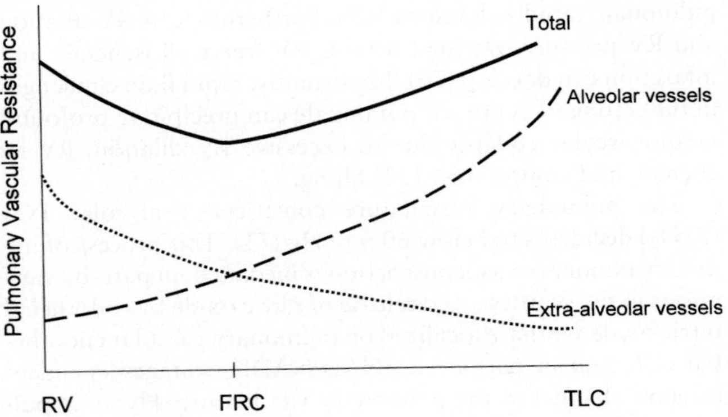

FIGURE 127.1. Schematic diagram of the relation between changes in lung volume and pulmonary vascular resistance, where the extra-alveolar and alveolar vascular components are separated. Note that pulmonary vascular resistance is minimal at resting lung volume or functional residual capacity (FRC). As lung volume increases toward total lung capacity (TLC) or decreases toward residual volume (RV), pulmonary vascular resistance also increases. However, the increase in resistance with hyperinflation is due to increased alveolar vascular resistance, whereas the increase in resistance with lung collapse is due to increased extra-alveolar vessel tone.

Ventricular Interdependence

Although LV preload must eventually be altered by changes in RV output because the two ventricles are in series, changes in RV end-diastolic volume can also alter LV preload by altering LV diastolic compliance by the mechanism of ventricular interdependence (88). Ventricular interdependence functions through two separate processes. First, increasing RV end-diastolic volume will induce an intraventricular septal shift into the LV, decreasing LV diastolic compliance (89). Thus, for the same LV filling pressure, RV dilation will decrease LV end-diastolic volume and, therefore, cardiac output. Second, if pericardial restraint limits absolute biventricular filling, then RV dilation will increase Ppc without septal shift (2,90). This ventricular interaction is believed to be the major determinant of the phasic changes in arterial pulse pressure and stroke volume seen in tamponade, and is referred to as *pulsus paradoxus*. Pulsus paradoxus can be demonstrated during loaded spontaneous inspiration in normal subjects as an inspiration-associated decrease in pulse pressure. Pulse pressure is defined as systolic minus the diastolic blood pressure. If the pulse pressure change is greater than 10 mm Hg or 10% of the mean pulse pressure, then it is referred to as pulsus paradoxus (2). Maintaining a constant rate of venous return, either by volume resuscitation (91) or vasopressor infusion (27), will minimize hyperinflation-induced cardiac compression.

Hyperinflation-induced Cardiac Compression

As lung volume increases, the heart is compressed between the expanding lungs (92), raising juxtacardiac ITP. This compressive effect of the inflated lungs can be seen with either spontaneous (93) or positive pressure–induced hyperinflation (5,38,94–96). As described above, both Ppc and ITP are increased and no pericardial restraint exists. This decrease in apparent LV diastolic compliance (91) was previously misinterpreted as impaired LV contractility, because LV stroke work for a given LV end-diastolic pressure or pulmonary artery occlusion pressure is decreased (97,98). However, when such patients are fluid resuscitated to return LV end-diastolic volume to its original level, both LV stroke work and cardiac output also returned to their original levels (91,99) despite the continued application of PEEP (100).

HEMODYNAMIC EFFECTS OF CHANGES IN INTRATHORACIC PRESSURE

The heart within the thorax is a pressure chamber within a pressure chamber. Therefore, changes in ITP must affect the pressure gradients for both systemic venous return to the RV and systemic outflow from the LV, independent of the heart itself. Increases in ITP, by increasing right atrial pressure and decreasing transmural LV systolic pressure, will reduce the pressure gradients for venous return and LV ejection, decreasing intrathoracic blood volume. Conversely, decreases in ITP will augment venous return and impede LV ejection, increasing intrathoracic blood volume. Everything else below follows from these two simple truths.

Venous Return

Blood flows back from the systemic venous reservoirs into the right atrium through low-pressure, low-resistance venous conduits (101). Right atrial pressure is the back pressure for venous return. Ventilation alters both right atrial pressure and venous reservoir pressure. It is these changes in right atrial and venous capacitance vessel pressure that induce most of the observed cardiovascular effects of ventilation. Pressure in the upstream venous reservoirs is called *mean systemic pressure*, and is, itself, a function of blood volume, peripheral vasomotor tone, and the distribution of blood within the vasculature (102). Usually mean systemic pressure does not change rapidly during positive pressure ventilation, whereas right atrial pressure does owing to concomitant changes in ITP. Thus, variations in right atrial pressure represent the major factor determining the fluctuation in pressure gradient for systemic venous return during ventilation (103,104). The positive pressure inspiration increases in right atrial pressure decrease the pressure gradient for venous return, decreasing RV filling (68) and RV stroke volume (68,103,105–113). During normal spontaneous inspiration, the opposite occurs (2,27,68,69,107,110,114,115). The detrimental effect of positive pressure ventilation on cardiac output can be minimized by either fluid resuscitation to increase mean systemic pressure (27,105,116,117) or by keeping both mean ITP and swings in lung volume as low as possible. Accordingly, prolonging expiratory time, decreasing tidal volume, and avoiding PEEP all minimize this decrease in systemic venous return to the RV (4,24,103,107–111,118).

However, if positive pressure ventilation–induced increases in right atrial pressure always proportionally decreased venous return, then most mechanically ventilated patients would display profound cardiovascular insufficiency, especially at higher levels of PEEP. Fortunately, when lung volumes increase the diaphragm descend, compressing the abdominal compartment and increasing intra-abdominal pressure (119,120). Since a large proportion of venous blood exists in intra-abdominal vasculature, this venous blood is pressurized as well, increasing mean systemic pressure. Accordingly, the pressure gradient for venous return is often not reduced by PEEP (116). Inspiration-induced abdominal pressurization by diaphragmatic descent is probably the primary mechanism by which the decrease in venous return is minimized during positive pressure ventilation (121–125). However, laparotomy, by abolishing the inspiration-associated increases in intra-abdominal pressure, makes surgery patients especially sensitive to mechanical ventilation, requiring increased fluid resuscitation to sustain a constant cardiac output. This is one of the reasons why abdominal surgery patients often leave the operating room many liters positive.

Spontaneous inspiratory efforts usually increase venous return because of the combined decrease in right atrial pressure (2,26,108–110) and increase in intra-abdominal pressure (119,120). However, this augmentation of venous return is limited (126–128) because as ITP decreases below atmospheric pressure, central venous pressure also becomes subatmospheric, collapsing the great veins as they enter the thorax and creating a flow-limiting segment (101).

Ventricular Interdependence

Changes in RV volume induce reciprocal changes in LV diastolic compliance. Although decreasing RV volume during positive pressure inspiration increases LV diastolic compliance by decreasing RV filling, the hemodynamic impact of this effect is usually minimal (88,127–132) (Fig. 127.2).

However, with spontaneous inspiration RV volumes increase, causing an immediate reduction in LV diastolic compliance. This process is the primary cause for the inspiration-associated decrease in LV stroke volume and pulse pressure (87,89,132,133). If the pulse pressure change is greater than 10 mm Hg or 10% of the mean pulse pressure, then it is referred to as pulsus paradoxus (2). Since spontaneous inspiratory

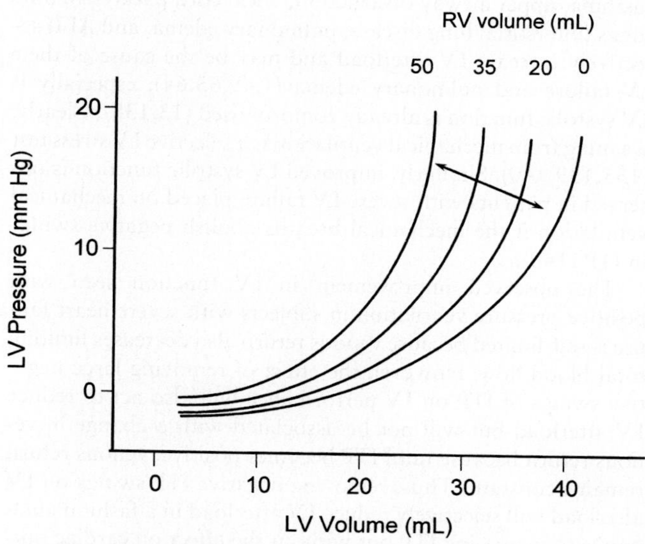

FIGURE 127.2. Schematic diagram of the effect of increasing right ventricular (RV) volumes on the left ventricular (LV) diastolic pressure–volume (filling) relationship. Note that increasing RV volumes decrease LV diastolic compliance, such that a higher filling pressure is required to generate a constant end-diastolic volume. (Adapted from Taylor RR, Corell JW, Sonnenblick EH, et al. Dependence of ventricular distensibility on filling the opposite ventricle. *Am J Physiol.* 1967;213:711–718.)

efforts can also occur during positive pressure ventilation, the use of ventilation-associated pulse pressure variation during positive pressure ventilation can reflect ventricular interdependence. Presently, positive pressure–induced changes in pulse pressure and LV stroke volume have been advocated to be a useful parameter of preload responsiveness (134). However, to assess volume responsiveness using pulse pressure variation, it is essential that no spontaneous inspiratory efforts be present.

LV Afterload

Changes in ITP can directly and indirectly alter LV afterload by altering both LV end-diastolic volume and ejection pressure. LV ejection pressure can be estimated as arterial pressure relative to ITP. Since baroreceptor mechanisms located in the extrathoracic carotid body maintain arterial pressure constant relative to atmosphere, if arterial pressure were to remain constant as ITP increased, then transmural LV pressure and thus LV afterload would decrease. Similarly, if transmural arterial pressure were to remain constant as ITP decreased, then LV wall tension would increase (135). Thus, under steady-state conditions increases in ITP decrease LV afterload and decreases in ITP increase LV afterload (136,137). The spontaneous inspiration–associated decrease in ITP-induced increase in LV afterload is one of the major mechanisms thought to be operative in the wean-induced LV ischemia described in the first part of this chapter since increased LV afterload must increase myocardial O_2 consumption (MVO_2). Thus, spontaneous ventilation not only increases global O_2 demand by its exercise component (3–5), but also increases MVO_2.

Profoundly negative swings in ITP commonly occur during forced spontaneous inspiratory efforts in patients with bronchospasm and obstructive breathing. This condition may rapidly deteriorate into acute heart failure and pulmonary edema (63) as has been described for airway obstruction (asthma, upper airway obstruction, vocal cord paralysis). Stiff lungs (interstitial lung disease, pulmonary edema, and ALI) selectively increase LV afterload and may be the cause of their LV failure and pulmonary edema (1,49,63,64), especially if LV systolic function is already compromised (13,138). Clearly, weaning from mechanical ventilation is a selective LV stress test (135,139,140). Similarly, improved LV systolic function is observed in patients with severe LV failure placed on mechanical ventilation if the mechanical breaths abolish negative swings in ITP (140).

The observed improvement in LV function seen with positive-pressure ventilation in subjects with severe heart failure is self-limited because venous return also decreases limiting total blood flow. However, the effect of removing large negative swings of ITP on LV performance will also act to reduce LV afterload but will not be associated with a change in venous return because until ITP becomes positive, venous return remains constant. Thus, removing negative ITP swings on LV afterload will selectively reduce LV afterload in a fashion analogous to increasing ITP but without the effect on cardiac output (27,101,141–144). This concept has been validated to be a very important clinical approach for patients with obstructive sleep apnea. For example, the cardiovascular benefits of positive airway pressure in nonintubated patients can be seen with CPAP therapy (145,146). Even low levels of CPAP, if they inhibit airway obstruction, will be beneficial (147–149). Prolonged nighttime nasal CPAP can selectively improve respiratory muscle strength, as well as LV contractile function if the patients had pre-existent heart failure (150,151). These benefits are associated with reductions of serum catecholamine levels (152).

Using Heart–Lung Interactions to Diagnose Cardiovascular Insufficiency

Since the cardiovascular response to positive pressure breathing is determined by the baseline cardiovascular state, ventilation-associated changes in arterial pulse pressure and stroke volume should monitor dynamic changes in venous return and the responsiveness of the heart to these transient and cyclic changes in preload (153). Systolic pressure variations during positive pressure ventilation nicely describe both preload responsiveness if the systolic pressure decreases below an apneic baseline value and also predict heart failure with volume overload if the systolic pressure increases above apneic baseline values (154–157). However, it is often difficult to assess if the variation in systolic arterial pressure is primarily up or down in clinical settings. A more physiologic approach is to measure arterial pulse pressure and assess pulse pressure variation (134,158). This technique can be modified to assess stroke volume variation (159) and has profound clinical potential as newer monitoring devices allow for the bedside display of both pulse pressure and stroke volume variation. In subjects on controlled mechanical ventilation, a pulse pressure variation of $>13\%$ or a stroke volume variation of $>10\%$ accurately predict preload responsiveness. This novel and exciting application of heart–lung interactions has been validated in many studies and is presently being assessed in prospective clinical trials, Assuming that this practical application of heart–lung interactions becomes commonplace, then a basic understanding of the principals described in this chapter will be an essential part of the training of acute care physicians.

References

1. Bromberger-Barnea B. Mechanical effects of inspiration on heart functions: a review. *Fed Proc.* 1981;40:2172–2177.
2. Wise RA, Robotham JL, Summer WR. Effects of spontaneous ventilation on the circulation. *Lung.* 1981;159:175–192.
3. Roussos C, Macklem PT. The respiratory muscles. *N Engl J Med.* 1982;307:786–797.
4. Grenvik A. Respiratory, circulatory and metabolic effects of respiratory treatment. A clinical study in postoperative thoracic surgical patients. *Acta Anaesth Scand.* 1966;(19 Suppl):1–122.
5. Shuey CB, Pierce AK, Johnson RL. An evaluation of exercise tests in chronic obstructive lung disease. *J Appl Physiol.* 1969;27:256–261.
6. Stock MC, David DW, Manning JW, et al. Lung mechanics and oxygen consumption during spontaneous ventilation and severe heart failure. *Chest.* 1992;102:279–283.
7. Kawagoe Y, Permutt S, Fessler HE. Hyperinflation with intrinsic PEEP and respiratory muscle blood flow. *J Appl Physiol.* 1994;77:2440–2448.
8. Aubier M, Vires N, Sillye G, et al. Respiratory muscle contribution to lactic acidosis in low cardiac output. *Am Rev Respir Dis.* 1982;126:648–652.
9. Frazier SK, Stone KS, Schertel ER, et al. A comparison of hemodynamic changes during the transition from mechanical ventilation to T-piece, pressure support, and continuous positive airway pressure in canines. *Biol Res Nurs.* 2000;1:253–264.
10. Magder S, Erian R, Roussos C. Respiratory muscle blood flow in oleic acid-induced pulmonary edema. *J Appl Physol.* 1986;60:1849–1856.
11. Vires N, Sillye G, Rassidakis A, et al. Effect of mechanical ventilation on respiratory muscle blood flow during shock. *Physiologist.* 1980;23:1–8.

12. Baratz DM, Westbrook PR, Shah K, et al. Effects of nasal continuous positive airway pressure on cardiac output and oxygen delivery in patients with congestive heart failure. *Chest.* 1992;102:1397–1401.
13. Lemaire F, Teboul JL, Cinoti L, et al. Acute left ventricular dysfunction during unsuccessful weaning from mechanical ventilation. *Anesthesiology.* 1988;69:171–179.
14. Richard C, Teboul JL, Archambaud F, et al. Left ventricular dysfunction during weaning in patients with chronic obstructive pulmonary disease. *Intensive Care Med.* 1994;20:171–172.
15. Hurford WE, Lynch KE, Strauss HW, et al. Myocardial perfusion as assessed by thallium-201 scintigraphy during the discontinuation of mechanical ventilation in ventilator-dependent patients. *Anesthesiology.* 1991;74:1007–1016.
16. Abalos A, Leibowitz AB, Distefano D, et al. Myocardial ischemia during the weaning period. *Am J Crit Care.* 1992;1:32–36.
17. Chatila W, Ani S, Guaglianone D, et al. Cardiac ischemia during weaning from mechanical ventilation. *Chest.* 1996;109:1421–1422.
18. Srivastava S, Chatila W, Amoateng-Adjepong Y, et al. Myocardial ischemia and weaning failure in patients with coronary disease: an update. *Crit Care Med.* 1999;27:2109–2112.
19. Mohsenifar Z, Hay A, Hay J, et al. Gastric intramural pH as a predictor of success or failure in weaning patients from mechanical ventilation. *Ann Intern Med.* 1993;119:794–798.
20. Jabran A, Mathru M, Dries D, et al. Continuous recordings of mixed venous oxygen saturation during weaning from mechanical ventilation and the ramifications thereof. *Am J Respir Crit Care Med.* 1998;158:1763–1769.
21. Straus C, Lewis B, Isebey D, et al. Contribution of the endotracheal tube and the upper airway to breathing workload. *Am J Respir Crit Care Med.* 1998;157:23–30.
22. Rasanen J, Nikki P, Heikkila J. Acute myocardial infarction complicated by respiratory failure. The effects of mechanical ventilation. *Chest.* 1984;85:21–28.
23. Rasanen J, Vaisanen IT, Heikkila J, et al. Acute myocardial infarction complicated by left ventricular dysfunction and respiratory failure. The effects of continuous positive airway pressure. *Chest.* 1985;87:156–162.
24. Cournaud A, Motley HL, Werko L, et al. Physiologic studies of the effect of intermittent positive pressure breathing on cardiac output in man. *Am J Physiol.* 1948;152:162–174.
25. Tyberg JV, Grant DA, Kingma I, et al. Effects of positive intrathoracic pressure on pulmonary and systemic hemodynamics. *Repsir Physiol.* 2000; 119:171–179.
26. Milic-Emili J, Mead J, Turner JM. Improved method for assessing the validity of the esophageal balloon technique. *J Appl Physiol.* 1964;19:207–211.
27. Braunwald E, Binion JT, Morgan WL, et al. Alterations in central blood volume and cardiac output induced by positive pressure breathing and counteracted by metaraminol (Aramine). *Circ Res.* 1957;5:670–675.
28. Whittenberger JL, McGregor M, Berglund E, et al. Influence of state of inflation of the lung on pulmonary vascular resistance. *J Appl Physiol.* 1960;15:878–882.
29. Novak RA, Matuschak GM, Pinsky MR. Effect of ventilatory frequency on regional pleural pressure. *J Appl Physiol.* 1988;65:1314–1323.43. Taha BH, Simon PM, Dempsey JA, et al.
30. Kingma I, Smiseth OA, Frais MA, et al. Left ventricular external constraint: relationship between pericardial, pleural and esophageal pressures during positive end-expiratory pressure and volume loading in dogs. *Ann Biomed Eng.* 1987;15:331–346.
31. Tsitlik JE, Halperin HR, Guerci AD, et al. Augmentation of pressure in a vessel indenting the surface of the lung. *Ann Biomed Eng.* 1987;15:259–284.
32. Pinsky MR, Guimond JG. The effects of positive end-expiratory pressure on heart-lung interactions. *J Crit Care.* 1991;6:1–11.
33. Romand JA, Shi W, Pinsky MR. Cardiopulmonary effects of positive pressure ventilation during acute lung injury. *Chest.* 1995;108:1041–1048.
34. O'Quinn RJ, Marini JJ, Culver BH, et al. Transmission of airway pressure to pleural pressure during lung edema and chest wall restriction. *J Appl Physiol.* 1985;59:1171–1177.
35. Gattinoni L, Mascheroni D, Torresin A, et al. Morphological response to positive end-expiratory pressure in acute respiratory failure. *Intensive Care Med.* 1986;12:137–142.
36. Globits S, Burghuber OC, Koller J, et al. Effect of lung transplantation on right and left ventricular volumes and function measured by magnetic resonance imaging. *Am J Respir Crit Care Med.* 1994;149:1000–1004.
37. Scharf SM, Ingram RH Jr. Effects of decreasing lung compliance with oleic acid on the cardiovascular response to PEEP. *Am J Physiol.* 1977; 233:H635–H641.
38. Pinsky MR, Vincent JL, DeSmet JM. Estimating left ventricular filling pressure during positive end-expiratory pressure in humans. *Am Rev Respir Dis.* 1991;143:25–31.
39. Teboul JL, Pinsky MR, Mercat A, et al. Estimating cardiac filling pressure in mechanically ventilated patients with hyperinflation. *Crit Care Med.* 2000;28:3631–3636.
40. Glick G, Wechsler AS, Epstein DE. Reflex cardiovascular depression produced by stimulation of pulmonary stretch receptors in the dog. *J Clin Invest.* 1969;48:467–472.
41. Painal AS. Vagal sensory receptors and their reflex effects. *Physiol Rev.* 1973;53:59–88.
42. Anrep GV, Pascual W, Rossler R. Respiratory variations in the heart rate, I: the reflex mechanism of the respiratory arrhythmia. *Proc R Soc Lond B Biol Sci.* 1936;119:191–217.
43. Respiratory sinus arrhythmia in humans: an obligatory role for vagal feedback from the lungs. *J Appl Physiol.* 1995;78:638–645.
44. Bernardi L, Calciati A, Gratarola A, et al. Heart rate-respiration relationship: computerized method for early detection of cardiac autonomic damage in diabetic patients. *Acta Cardiol.* 1986;41:197–206.
45. Persson MG, Lonnqvist PA, Gustafsson LE. Positive end-expiratory pressure ventilation elicits increases in endogenously formed nitric oxide as detected in air exhaled by rabbits. *Anesthesiology.* 1995;82:969–974.
46. Cassidy SS, Eschenbacher WI, Johnson RL Jr. Reflex cardiovascular depression during unilateral lung hyperinflation in the dog. *J Clin Invest.* 1979;64:620–626.
47. Daly MB, Hazzledine JL, Ungar A. The reflex effects of alterations in lung volume on systemic vascular resistance in the dog. *J Physiol (London).* 1967;188:331–351.
48. Shepherd JT. The lungs as receptor sites for cardiovascular regulation. *Circulation.* 1981;63:1–10.
49. Stalcup SA, Mellins RB. Mechanical forces producing pulmonary edema in acute asthma. *N Engl J Med.* 1977;297:592–596.
50. Vatner SF, Rutherford JD. Control of the myocardial contractile state by carotid chemo- and baroreceptor and pulmonary inflation reflexes in conscious dogs. *J Clin Invest.* 1978;63:1593–1601.
51. Karlocai K, Jokkel G, Kollai M. Changes in left ventricular contractility with the phase of respiration. *J Auton Nerv Syst.* 1998;73:86–92.
52. Said SI, Kitamura S, Vreim C. Prostaglandins: release from the lung during mechanical ventilation at large tidal ventilation. *J Clin Invest.* 1972;51:83a.
53. Bedetti C, Del Basso P, Argiolas C, Carpi A. Arachidonic acid and pulmonary function in a heart-lung preparation of guinea-pig. Modulation by PCO_2. *Arch Int Pharmacodyn Ther.* 1987;285:98–116.
54. Berend N, Christopher KL, Voelkel NF. Effect of positive end-expiratory pressure on functional residual capacity: role of prostaglandin production. *Am Rev Respir Dis.* 1982;126:641–647.
55. Pattern MY, Liebman PR, Hetchman HG. Humorally mediated decreases in cardiac output associated with positive end-expiratory pressure. *Microvasc Res.* 1977;13:137–144.
56. Berglund JE, Halden E, Jakobson S, et al. PEEP ventilation does not cause humorally mediated cardiac output depression in pigs. *Intensive Care Med.* 1994;20:360–364.
57. Fuhrman BP, Everitt J, Lock JE. Cardiopulmonary effects of unilateral airway pressure changes in intact infant lambs. *J Appl Physiol.* 1984;56:1439–1448.
58. Payen DM, Brun-Buisson CJL, Carli PA, et al. Hemodynamic, gas exchange, and hormonal consequences of LBPP during PEEP ventilation. *J Appl Physiol.* 1987;62:61–70.
59. Frage D, de la Coussaye JE, Beloucif S, et al. Interactions between hormonal modifications during PEEP-induced antidiuresis and antinatriuresis. *Chest.* 1995;107:1095–1100.
60. Frass M, Watschinger B, Traindl O, et al. Atrial natriuretic peptide release in response to different positive end-expiratory pressure levels. *Crit Care Med.* 1993;21:343–347.
61. Wilkins MA, Su XL, Palayew MD, et al. The effects of posture change and continuous positive airway pressure on cardiac natriuretic peptides in congestive heart failure. *Chest.* 1995;107:909–915.
62. Shirakami G, Magaribuchi T, Shingu K, et al. Positive end-expiratory pressure ventilation decreases plasma atrial and brain natriuretic peptide levels in humans. *Anesth Analg.* 1993;77:1116–1121.
63. Fletcher EC, Proctor M, Yu J, et al. Pulmonary edema develops after recurrent obstructive apneas. *Am J Respir Crit Care Med.* 1999;160:1688–1696.
64. Chen L, Shi Q, Scharf SM. Hemodynamic effects of periodic obstructive apneas in sedated pigs with congestive heart failure. *J Appl Physiol.* 2000; 88:1051–1060.
65. Maughan WL, Shoukas AA, Sagawa K, et al. Instantaneous pressure-volume relationships of the canine right ventricle. *Circ Res.* 1979;44:309–315.
66. Sibbald WJ, Driedger AA. Right ventricular function in disease states: pathophysiologic considerations. *Crit Care Med.* 1983;11:339.
67. Piene H, Sund T. Does pulmonary impedance constitute the optimal load for the right ventricle? *Am J Physiol.* 1982;242:H154–H160.
68. Pinsky MR. Determinants of pulmonary arterial flow variation during respiration. *J Appl Physiol.* 1984;56:1237–1245.
69. Theres H, Binkau J, Laule M, et al. Phase-related changes in right ventricular cardiac output under volume-controlled mechanical ventilation with positive end-expiratory pressure. *Crit Care Med.* 1999;27:953–8.
70. Johnston WE, Vinten-Johansen J, Shugart HE, et al. Positive end-expiratory pressure potentates the severity of canine right ventricular ischemia-reperfusion injury. *Am J Physiol.* 1992;262:H168–H176.
71. Madden JA, Dawson CA, Harder DR. Hypoxia-induced activation in small isolated pulmonary arteries from the cat. *J Appl Physiol.* 1985;59:113–118.
72. Hakim TS, Michel RP, Chang HK. Effect of lung inflation on pulmonary vascular resistance by arterial and venous occlusion. *J Appl Physiol.* 1982;53:1110–1115.

73. Quebbeman EJ, Dawson CA. Influence of inflation and atelectasis on the hypoxic pressure response in isolated dog lung lobes. *Cardiovas Res.* 1976;10:672–677.
74. Brower RG, Gottlieb J, Wise RA, et al. Locus of hypoxic vasoconstriction in isolated ferret lungs. *J Appl Physiol.* 1987;63:58–65.
75. Hakim TS, Michel RP, Minami H, et al. Site of pulmonary hypoxic vasoconstriction studied with arterial and venous occlusion. *J Appl Physiol.* 1983;54:1278–1302.
76. Marshall BE, Marshall C. A model for hypoxic constriction of the pulmonary circulation. *J Appl Physiol.* 1988;64:68–77.
77. Marshall BE, Marshall C. Continuity of response to hypoxic pulmonary vasoconstriction. *J Appl Physiol.* 1980;49:189–196.
78. Dawson CA, Grimm DJ, Linehan JH. Lung inflation and longitudinal distribution of pulmonary vascular resistance during hypoxia. *J Appl Physiol.* 1979;47:532–536.
79. Howell JBL, Permutt S, Proctor DF, et al. Effect of inflation of the lung on different parts of the pulmonary vascular bed. *J Appl Physiol.* 1961;16:71–76.
80. West JB, Dollery CT, Naimark A. Distribution of blood flow in isolated lung; relation to vascular and alveolar pressures. *J Appl Physiol.* 1964;19:713–724.
81. Fuhrman BP, Everitt J, Lock JE. Cardiopulmonary effects of unilateral airway pressure changes in intact infant lambs. *J Appl Physiol.* 1984;56:1439–1448.
82. Fuhrman BP, Smith-Wright DL, Kulik TJ, et al. Effects of static and fluctuating airway pressure on the intact, immature pulmonary circulation. *J Appl Physiol.* 1986;60:114–122.
83. Thorvalson J, Ilebekk A, Kiil F. Determinants of pulmonary blood volume. Effects of acute changes in airway pressure. *Acta Physiol Scand.* 1985;125:471–479.
84. Lopez-Muniz R, Stephens NL, Bromberger-Barnea B, et al. Critical closure of pulmonary vessels analyzed in terms of Starling resistor model. *J Appl Physiol.* 1968;24:625–635.
85. Block AJ, Boyson PG, Wynne JW. The origins of cor pulmonale, a hypothesis. *Chest.* 1979;75:109–114.
86. Vieillard-Baron A, Loubieres Y, Schmitt JM, et al. Cyclic changes in right ventricular output impedance during mechanical ventilation. *J Appl Physiol.* 1999;87:1644–1650.
87. Canada E, Benumnof JL, Tousdale FR. Pulmonary vascular resistance correlated in intact normal and abnormal canine lungs. *Crit Care Med.* 1982;10:719–723.
88. Taylor RR, Corell JW, Sonnenblick EH, et al. Dependence of ventricular distensibility on filling the opposite ventricle. *Am J Physiol.* 1967;213:711–718.
89. Brinker JA, Weiss I, Lappe DL, et al. Leftward septal displacement during right ventricular loading in man. *Circulation.* 1980;61:626–633.
90. Takata M, Harasawa Y, Beloucif S, et al. Coupled vs. uncoupled pericardial restraint: effects on cardiac chamber interactions. *J Appl Physiol.* 1997;83:1799–1813.
91. Marini JJ, Culver BN, Butler J. Mechanical effect of lung distention with positive pressure on cardiac function. *Am Rev Respir Dis.* 1980;124:382–386.
92. Butler J. The heart is in good hands. *Circulation.* 1983;67:1163–1168.
93. Cassidy SS, Wead WB, Seibert GB, et al. Changes in left ventricular geometry during spontaneous breathing. *J Appl Physiol.* 1987;63:803–811.
94. Hoffman EA, Ritman EL. Heart-lung interaction: effect on regional lung air content and total heart volume. *Ann Biomed Eng.* 1987;15:241–257.
95. Olson LE, Hoffman EA. Heart-lung interactions determined by electron beam X-ray CT in laterally recumbent rabbits. *J Appl Physiol.* 1995;78:417–427.
96. Jayaweera AR, Ehrlich W. Changes of phasic pleural pressure in awake dogs during exercise: potential effects on cardiac output. *Ann Biomed Eng.* 1987;15:311–318.
97. Cassidy SS, Robertson CH, Pierce AK, et al. Cardiovascular effects of positive end-expiratory pressure in dogs. *J Appl Physiol.* 1978;4:743–749.
98. Conway CM. Hemodynamic effects of pulmonary ventilation. *Br J Anaesth.* 1975;47:761–766.
99. Jardin F, Farcot JC, Boisante L. Influence of positive end-expiratory pressure on left ventricular performance. *N Engl J Med.* 1981;304:387–392.
100. Berglund JE, Halden E, Jakobson S, et al. Echocardiographic analysis of cardiac function during high PEEP ventilation. *Intensive Care Med.* 1994;20:174–180.
101. Guyton AC, Lindsey AW, Abernathy B, et al. Venous return at various right atrial pressures and the normal venous return curve. *Am J Physiol.* 1957;189:609–615.
102. Goldberg HS, Rabson J. Control of cardiac output by systemic vessels: circulatory adjustments of acute and chronic respiratory failure and the effects of therapeutic interventions. *Am J Cardiol.* 1981;47:696.
103. Pinsky MR. Instantaneous venous return curves in an intact canine preparation. *J Appl Physiol.* 1984;56:765–771.
104. Kilburn KH. Cardiorespiratory effects of large pneumothorax in conscious and anesthetized dogs. *J Appl Physiol.* 1963;18:279–283.
105. Chevalier PA, Weber KC, Engle JC, et al. Direct measurement of right and left heart outputs in Valsalva-like maneuver in dogs. *Proc Soc Exper Biol Med.* 1972;139:1429–1437.
106. Guntheroth WC, Gould R, Butler J, et al. Pulsatile flow in pulmonary artery, capillary and vein in the dog. *Cardiovascular Res.* 1974;8:330–337.
107. Guntheroth WG, Morgan BC, Mullins GL. Effect of respiration on venous return and stroke volume in cardiac tamponade. Mechanism of pulsus paradoxus. *Circ Res.* 1967;20:381–390.
108. Guyton AC. Effect of cardiac output by respiration, opening the chest, and cardiac tamponade. In: *Circulatory Physiology: Cardiac Output and Its Regulation.* Philadelphia, PA: WB Saunders; 1963:378–386.
109. Holt JP. The effect of positive and negative intrathoracic pressure on cardiac output and venous return in the dog. *Am J Physiol.* 1944;142:594–603.
110. Morgan BC, Abel FL, Mullins GL, et al. Flow patterns in cavae, pulmonary artery, pulmonary vein and aorta in intact dogs. *Am J Physiol.* 1966;210:903–909.
111. Morgan BC, Martin WE, Hornbein TF, et al. Hemodynamic effects of intermittent positive pressure respiration. *Anesthesiology.* 1960;27:584–590.
112. Scharf SM, Brown R, Saunders N, et al. Hemodynamic effects of positive pressure inflation. *J Appl Physiol.* 1980;49:124–131.
113. Jardin F, Vieillard-Baron A. Right ventricular function and positive-pressure ventilation in clinical practice: from hemodynamic subsets to respirator settings. *Intensive Care Med.* 2003;29:1426–1434.
114. Scharf SM, Brown R, Saunders N, et al. Effects of normal and loaded spontaneous inspiration on cardiovascular function. *J Appl Physiol.* 1979;47:582–590.
115. Groeneveld AB, Berendsen RR, Schneider AJ, et al. Effect of the mechanical ventilatory cycle on thermodilution right ventricular volumes and cardiac output. *J Appl Physiol.* 2000;89:89–96.
116. Van den Berg P, Jansen JRC, Pinsky MR. The effect of positive-pressure inspiration on venous return in volume loaded post-operative cardiac surgical patients. *J Appl Physiol.* 2002;92:1223–1231.
117. Magder S, Georgiadis G, Cheong T. Respiratory variation in right atrial pressure predict the response to fluid challenge. *J Crit Care.* 1992;7:76–85.
118. Harken AH, Brennan MF, Smith N, et al. The hemodynamic response to positive end-expiratory ventilation in hypovolemic patients. *Surgery.* 1974;76:786–793.
119. Fessler HE, Brower RD, Wise RA, et al. Effects of positive end-expiratory pressure on the canine venous return curve. *Am Rev Respir Dis.* 1992;146:4–10.
120. Takata M, Robotham JL. Effects of inspiratory diaphragmatic descent on inferior vena caval venous return. *J Appl Physiol.* 1992;72:597–607.
121. Matuschak GM, Pinsky MR, Rogers RM. Effects of positive end-expiratory pressure on hepatic blood flow and hepatic performance. *J Appl Physiol.* 1987;62:1377–1383.
122. Chihara E, Hasimoto S, Kinoshita T, et al. Elevated mean systemic filling pressure due to intermittent positive-pressure ventilation. *Am J Physiol.* 1992;262:H1116–H1121.
123. Takata M, Wise RA, Robotham JL. Effects of abdominal pressure on venous return: abdominal vascular zone conditions. *J Appl Physiol.* 1990;69:1961–1972.
124. Barnes GE, Laine GA, Giam PY, et al. Cardiovascular responses to elevation of intra-abdominal hydrostatic pressure. *Am J Physiol.* 1985;248:R208–R213.
125. Lichtwarck-Aschoff M, Zeravik J, Pfeiffer UJ. Intrathoracic blood volume accurately reflects circulatory volume status in critically ill patients with mechanical ventilation. *Intensive Care Med.* 1992;18:142–145.
126. Brecher GA, Hubay CA. Pulmonary blood flow and venous return during spontaneous respiration. *Circ Res.* 1955;3:210–214.
127. Terada N, Takeuchi T. Postural changes in venous pressure gradients in anesthetized monkeys. *Am J Physiol.* 1993;264:H21–H25.
128. Scharf S, Tow DE, Miller MJ, et al. Influence of posture and abdominal pressure on the hemodynamic effects of Mueller's maneuver. *J Crit Care.* 1989;4:26–34.
129. Rankin JS, Olsen CO, Arentzen CE, et al. The effects of airway pressure on cardiac function in intact dogs and man. *Circulation.* 1982;66:108–120.
130. Robotham JL, Rabson J, Permutt S, et al. Left ventricular hemodynamics during respiration. *J Appl Physiol.* 1979;47:1275–1303.
131. Ruskin J, Bache RJ, Rembert JC, et al. Pressure-flow studies in man: effect of respiration on left ventricular stroke volume. *Circulation.* 1973;48:79–85.
132. Olsen CO, Tyson GS, Maier GW, et al. Dynamic ventricular interaction in the conscious dog. *Circ Res.* 1983;52:85–104.
133. Janicki JS, Weber KT. The pericardium and ventricular interaction, distensibility and function. *Am J Physiol.* 1980;238:H494–H503.
134. Michard F, Boussat S, Chemla D, et al. Relation between respiratory changes in arterial pulse pressure and fluid responsiveness in septic patients with acute circulatory failure. *Am J Respir Crit Care Med.* 2000;162:134–138.
135. Beyar R, Goldstein Y. Model studies of the effects of the thoracic pressure on the circulation. *Ann Biomed Eng.* 1987;15:373–383.
136. Buda AJ, Pinsky MR, Ingels NB, et al. Effect of intrathoracic pressure on left ventricular performance. *N Engl J Med.* 1979;301:453–459.
137. Pinsky MR, Summer WR, Wise RA, et al. Augmentation of cardiac function by elevation of intrathoracic pressure. *J Appl Physiol.* 1983;54:950–955.
138. Beach T, Millen E, Grenvik A. Hemodynamic response to discontinuance of mechanical ventilation. *Crit Care Med.* 1973;1:85–90.

139. Cassidy SA, Wead WB, Seibert GB, et al. Geometric left-ventricular responses to interactions between the lung and left ventricle: positive pressure breathing. *Ann Biomed Eng.* 1987;15:285–295.
140. Scharf SM, Brown R, Warner KG, et al. Intrathoracic pressure and left ventricular configuration with respiratory maneuvers. *J Appl Physiol.* 1989;66:481–491.
141. Sharpey-Schaffer EP. Effects of Valsalva maneuver on the normal and failing circulation. *Br Med J.* 1955;1:693–699.
142. Khilnani S, Graver LM, Balaban K, et al. Effects of inspiratory loading on left ventricular myocardial blood flow and metabolism. *J Appl Physiol.* 1992;72:1488–1492.
143. Garpestad E, Parker JA, Katayzama H, et al. Decrease in ventricular stroke volume at apnea termination is independent of oxygen desaturation. *J Appl Physiol.* 1994;77:1602–1608.
144. Sibbald WH, Calvin J, Driedger AA. Right and left ventricular preload, and diastolic ventricular compliance: implications of therapy in critically ill patients. In: *Critical Care State of the Art.* Fullerton, CA: Society of Critical Care; 1982:Vol. 3.
145. De Hoyos A, Liu PP, Benard DC, et al. Haemodynamic effects of continuous positive airway pressure in humans with normal and impaired left ventricular function. *Clin Sci (Lond).* 1995;88:173–178.
146. Naughton MT, Rahman MA, Hara K, et al. Effect of continuous positive airway pressure on intrathoracic and left ventricular transmural pressures in patients with congestive heart failure. *Circulation.* 1995;91:1725–1731.
147. Joet-Philip FF, Paganelli FF, Dutau HL, et al. Hemodynamic effects of bi-level nasal positive airway pressure ventilation in patients with heart failure. *Respiration.* 1999;66:136–143.
148. Lin M, Yang Y-F, Chiang H-T, et al. Reappraisal of continuous positive airway pressure therapy in acute cardiogenic pulmonary edema. *Chest.* 1995;107:1379–1386.
149. Buckle P, Millar T, Kryger M. The effect of short-term nasal CPAP on Cheyne-Stokes respiration in congestive heart failure. *Chest.* 1992;102:31–35.
150. Granton JT, Naughton MT, Benard DC, et al. CPAP improves inspiratory muscle strength in patients with heart failure and central sleep apnea. *Am J Respir Crit Care Med.* 1996;153:277–282.
151. Kaneko Y, Floras JS, Usui K, et al. Cardiovascular effects of continuous positive airway pressure in patients with heart failure and obstructive sleep apnea. *N Engl J Med.* 2003;348:1233–1241.
152. Naughton MT, Benard DC, Liu PP, et al. Effects of nasal CPAP on sympathetic activity in patients with heart failure and central sleep apnea. *Am J Respir Crit Care Med.* 1995;152:473–479.
153. Denault AY, Gasior TA, Gorcsan J 3rd, et al. Determinants of aortic pressure variation during positive-pressure ventilation in man. *Chest.* 1999;116:176–86.
154. Abel JG, Salerno TA, Panos A, et al. Cardiovascular effects of positive pressure ventilation in humans. *Ann Thorac Surg.* 1987;43:36–43.
155. Baeaussier M, Coriat P, Perel A, et al. Determinants of systolic pressure variation in patients ventilated after vascular surgery. *J Cardiothorac Vasc Anesth.* 1995;9:547–551.
156. Coriat P, Vrillon M, Perel A, et al. A comparison of systolic blood pressure variations and echocardiographic estimates of end-diastolic left ventricular size in patients after aortic surgery. *Anesth Analg.* 1994;78:46–53.
157. Szold A, Pizov R, Segal E, Perel A. The effect of tidal volume and intravascular volume state on systolic pressure variation in ventilated dogs. *Intensive Care Med.* 1989;15:368–371.
158. Michard F, Boussat S, Chemla D, et al. Relation between respiratory changes in arterial pulse pressure and fluid responsiveness in septic patients with acute circulatory failure. *Am J Respir Crit Care Med.* 2000;162(1):134–138.
159. Monnet X, Rienzo M, Osman D, et al. Esophageal Doppler monitoring predicts fluid responsiveness in critically ill ventilated patients. *Intensive Care Med.* 2005;31(9):1195–1201.

CHAPTER 128 ■ ANATOMY OF MECHANICAL VENTILATION

PAUL B. BLANCH

IMMEDIATE CONCERNS

Ventilation/Perfusion (V_A/Q) in the Normal Lung

The lung's primary function is to add oxygen (O_2) to, and remove carbon dioxide (CO_2) from, blood passing through the pulmonary capillary beds. For this to occur, the gas we breathe must be matched to the blood flowing through our lungs. Average minute alveolar ventilation (V_A) for a healthy adult is 4 liters (L) per minute, while resting cardiac output (Q) is 5 L/minute; therefore that optimal ventilation/perfusion matching (V_A/Q ratio) is 4 L/minute divided by 5 L/minute or 0.8. Perfect V_A/Q matching is unlikely because the distribution of gas and blood flow varies across the lung fields for several reasons. Both gases and blood have mass and are therefore gravity dependent (Fig. 128.1); as a result, both increase as we progress from the apex to the base of the lung. Gravity's effect on blood flow is, however, predominant; it has been estimated that in an upright subject, six times as much blood passes through each lung base compared to its apex, whereas only 2½ times as much air reaches each lung base. These different gradients dictate that the V_A/Q ratio rises progressively from the bottom to the top of the lungs.

Furthermore, the lungs are composed of millions of alveoli, connected to each other and eventually to the trachea by a labyrinth of pathways and interconnections (pores of Kohn). Few connections are consistent in either length or diameter; this effect conspires to further disrupt the distribution of inhaled gases. Even the healthiest athletes exhibit areas of shunt and dead space (Fig. 128.2). About 30% of the air a healthy adult breathes each minute is wasted as dead space ventilation (V_D), and 3% to 5% of the cardiac output passes through the lungs without undergoing gas exchange (shunt). Any pathophysiologic stimulus that acutely increases or decreases ventilation or cardiac output is likely to have a pronounced impact on V_A/Q ratios and in turn, on oxygenation and CO_2 removal.

Positive Pressure Breathing

Positive pressure mechanical ventilation, unlike normal breathing, increases transpulmonary pressure, reduces venous return,

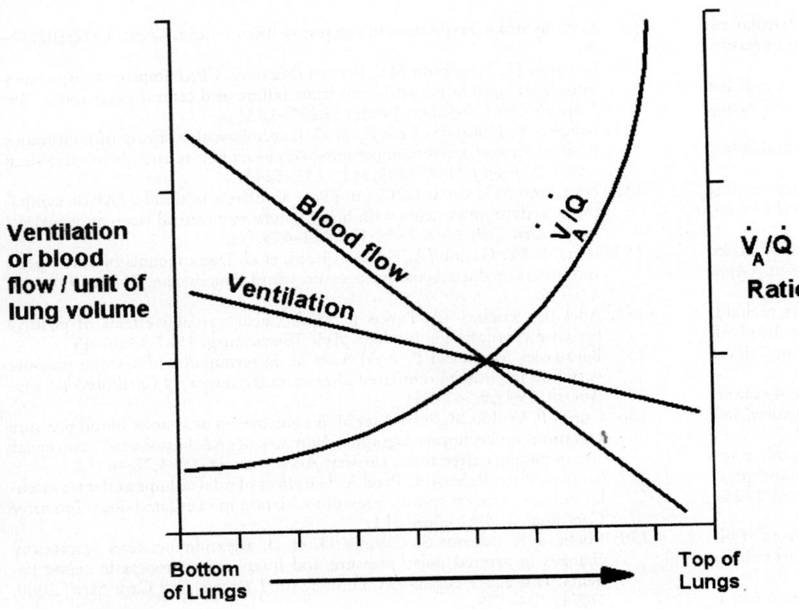

FIGURE 128.1. The effects of gravity on ventilation (V_A)/perfusion (Q) ratio (V_A/Q). In the upright subject, gravity affects V_A, Q, and concomitantly, the V_A/Q ratio. Gravitational forces pull on both the gases we breathe and pulmonary blood flow; as a result, V_A and Q increase from a lung's apex to its base. Due to blood's greater mass, gravity's effect on Q predominates; it is estimated that Q at a lung's base is six times as great as at its apex, compared to only 2½ times as much V_A at the lung's base versus its apex. The resultant V_A/Q ratio is therefore greater at the lung apices than the bases.

and ultimately lowers cardiac output. Positive pressure breathing also preferentially forces gas into areas of the lung with the lowest airway resistance (R_{aw}) and highest compliance (C_{RS}). It is not uncommon for ventilated patients to require airway pressures (P_{aw}) of 30 cm H_2O or more; yet, normal systolic pulmonary arterial pressures seldom exceed 20 to 25 mm Hg. It follows that during positive pressure inflations, if intraluminal alveolar pressure exceeds the hydrostatic pressure, blood flow and gas exchange cease—until alveolar pressure falls below hydrostatic levels again during exhalation. Given these factors, it is easy to understand how mechanical ventilation often disrupts V_A/Q, and why up to 60% or more of each positive pressure breath is wasted as V_D. Allowing patients to breathe spontaneously between mechanical breaths significantly reduces mean transpulmonary and transluminal pressures and improves venous return and cardiac output, which in turn improves V_A/Q.

V_A/Q Inequalities in Respiratory Failure

It is not necessary that alveoli be completely deprived of V_A or Q for life-threatening symptoms to exist. When significant areas of a patient's lungs receive too much or too little V_A or Q, these regions exhibit abnormally high or low V_A/Q ratios, referred to as *relative shunt* and *relative dead space* (Fig. 128.3). Relative shunt and V_D are extremely common in the intensive care unit (ICU) setting, and disrupt CO_2 removal and oxygenation just as quickly as comparable but smaller areas of absolute V_D or shunt.

Conditions Affecting Lung Structure

Along with conditions that affect only V_A or Q, several disorders actually damage lung structure. Furthermore, failure to properly manage the ventilator, in some situations, may play a role in determining the ultimate severity and progression of the lung disease (1–7). Critical care personnel called on to manage ventilators for these patients, whether in a primary or consulting role, must possess a thorough understanding of the pathophysiology and treatment of acute respiratory failure.

Reductions in the arterial partial pressure of oxygen (PaO_2) and carbon dioxide ($PaCO_2$) are characteristic of the early stages of acute respiratory distress syndrome (ARDS).

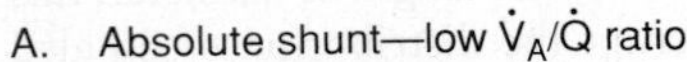

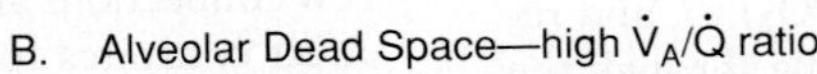

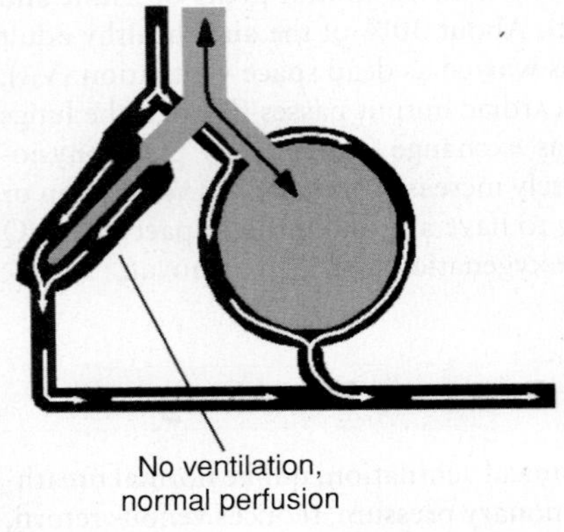

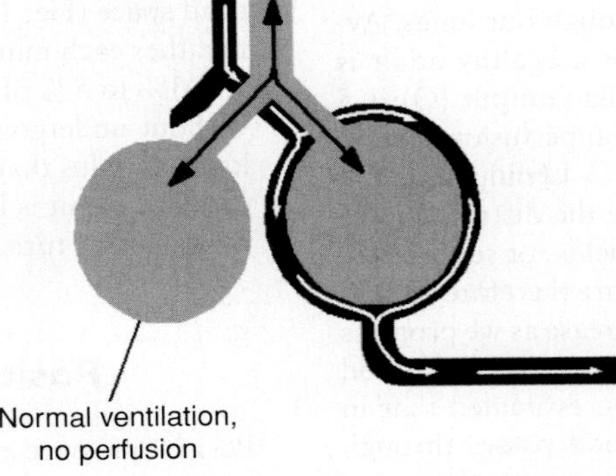

FIGURE 128.2. Ventilation (V_A)/perfusion (Q) (V_A/Q) abnormalities. **A:** *Absolute shunt—low V_A/Q ratio.* An intrapulmonary, or absolute, shunt occurs when blood continues to perfuse collapsed or otherwise unventilated alveoli; blood literally shunts past or bypasses the lung, without participating in gas exchange. **B:** *Alveolar dead space—high V_A/Q ratio.* Dead space or wasted ventilation exists when alveoli receive ventilation but no blood flow.

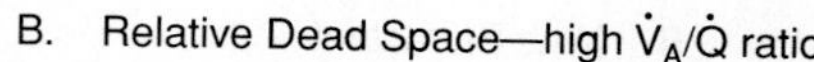

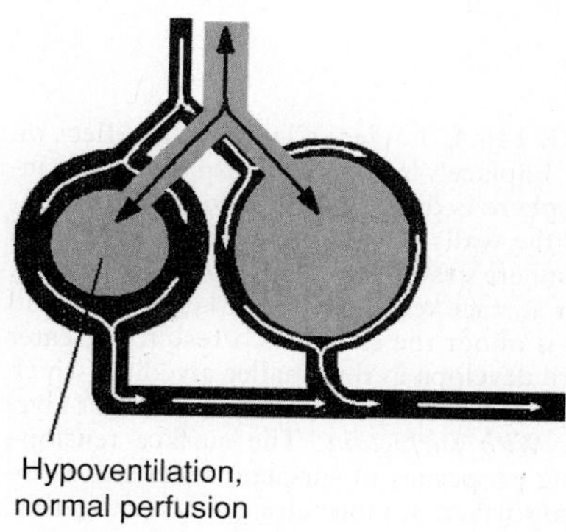

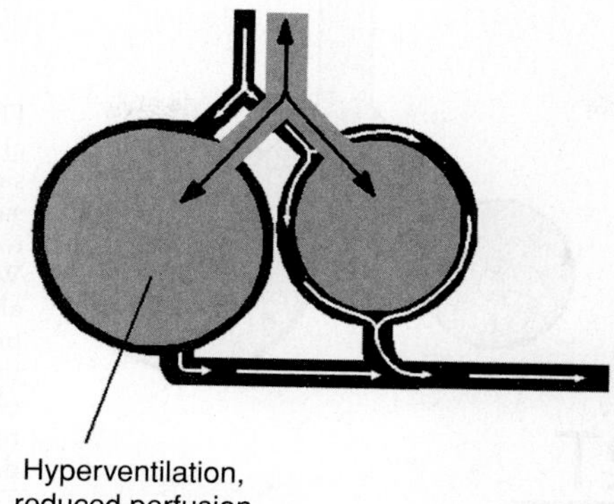

FIGURE 128.3. Relative ventilation (V_A)/perfusion (Q) (V_A/Q) abnormalities. **A:** *Relative shunt—low V_A/Q ratio.* A relative shunt occurs when an alveolus receives too much Q in relation to V_A. **B:** *Relative dead space—high V_A/Q ratio.* Relative dead space exists when an alveolus receives too much V_A relative to its Q.

Widespread, but not uniform, alveolar destabilization and collapse (atelectasis) are hallmarks of ARDS. If ARDS is not aggressively managed in its early stages, pulmonary consolidation (secondary to atelectasis) develops and may lead to a fibro-prolific phase; the chances for recovery are significantly reduced if the disease progresses to this point (8). Hypoxemia results from both relative and absolute shunting caused by complete or partial alveolar collapse and the continued perfusion of these lung regions.

Ventilator Therapy

With respect to therapy, a shifting emphasis in the role of mechanical ventilation has occurred. Positive pressure ventilation was clearly responsible for the decrease in mortality following the poliomyelitis epidemic. Yet, a similar reduction in mortality has been slow to respond following the widespread application of mechanical ventilatory support to ARDS or to acute exacerbations of chronic obstructive pulmonary disease (COPD). Although this is in part due to the multisystem dysfunction that frequently accompanies such problems, it now appears that the inappropriate use of mechanical ventilation has played a significant role.

Poliomyelitis, Guillain-Barré syndrome, and other neuromuscular disease states produce respiratory insufficiency because of mechanical and neural failure to control diaphragmatic driven ventilation. In the absence of complications such as aspiration of gastric contents, pulmonary parenchymal function remains intact. By contrast, ARDS represents a failure of gas exchange that is related almost entirely to parenchymal involvement. Furthermore, neuromuscular and musculoskeletal function generally remain unimpaired during ARDS, although there are exceptions such as flail chest associated with underlying pulmonary contusion after trauma. Even in this situation, however, the musculoskeletal abnormality is of secondary importance compared with the underlying lung contusion.

Even the simplest ventilator provides a satisfactory means for sustaining V_A when neuromuscular and musculoskeletal problems predominate. Yet, it would be very surprising if a simple ventilator performed equally well in the therapy of ARDS, in which an entirely different spectrum of pathophysiologic changes occur. Thus, when a decrease in residual alveolar volume is present—whether caused by surfactant depletion, partial airway obstruction, interstitial and alveolar pulmonary edema, or a combination of these factors—a simple mechanical ventilator can have salutary effects only while it restores alveolar volume and improves oxygen exchange during the inhalation phase, provided, of course, that ventilatory pressures do not approach or exceed pulmonary hydrostatic pressures. During exhalation, the beneficial effects of inflation quickly dissipate, especially if alveolar volume is allowed to return to its starting point.

In fact, opening alveoli during inhalation and allowing them to close again during exhalation may exacerbate the problem. It seems that when alveoli collapse, surfactant activity is lost. There are two putative theories to explain this: first, surfactant molecules are forced into close proximity during collapse; ultimately they collide and clump together (9,10); and/or second, surfactant is forced up into the airways during alveolar collapse (11)—once in the airways, surfactant is either damaged or removed by ciliary action.

Positive End-expiratory Pressure (PEEP)

Reduced levels of surfactant, such as occur during ARDS, lead to widespread atelectasis and hypoxemia; these conditions respond poorly to mechanical ventilation alone. The law of Laplace states that pressure inside a spherical structure is directly proportional to tension in that structure's wall and inversely proportional to its radius. Normally, alveolar surface forces, at alveolar-capillary membranes, are essentially identical. Laplace's law dictates that a loss of surfactant means a greater pressure is required to keep smaller alveoli open (Fig. 128.4). When this occurs, smaller alveoli empty into larger ones, eventually collapsing. A plot of the lung's pressure–volume relationship during ARDS helps to better visualize this phenomenon (Fig. 128.5). Without adequate surfactant, significant portions of the lungs collapse at end-exhalation. During inhalation, as pressure is applied to the airways (x-axis, Fig. 128.5), nothing initially happens. However, when the applied pressure reaches sufficient magnitude, in this instance 14 cm H_2O, some of the collapsed alveoli start to open and gas begins entering the lungs. This "opening" pressure is commonly referred to as the *lower inflection point* (Fig. 128.5) and provides the theoretical underpinnings for the use of PEEP; that is, an ARDS-related surfactant deficiency predisposes to alveolar collapse unless counteracted by force. Clinically, the easiest way to accomplish this goal is by maintaining PEEP,

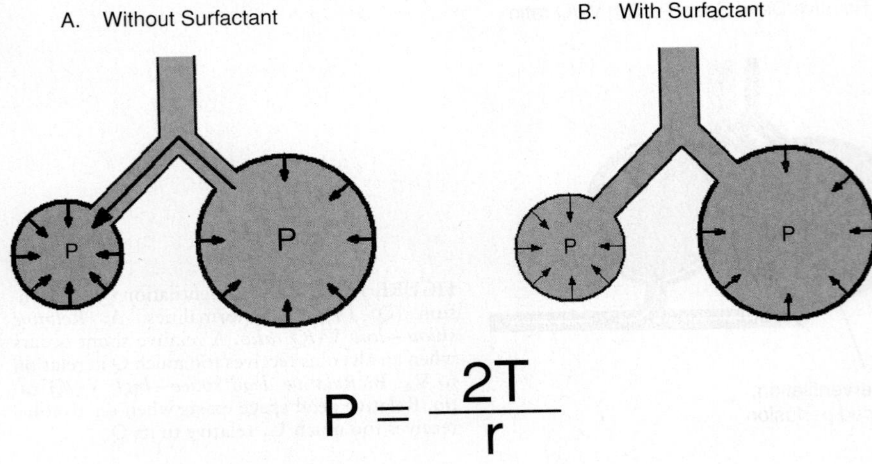

FIGURE 128.4. Laplace's law and its effect on alveoli. Laplace's law states that pressure (P) inside a sphere is directly proportional to the tension in the walls (T) and inversely proportional to the sphere's radius (r). **A:** *Without surfactant.* Wall or surface tension in both large and small alveoli is about the same. As a result, a greater pressure develops in the smaller alveolus, which then proceeds to empty into adjacent larger alveoli. **B:** *With surfactant.* The surface tension–reducing properties of surfactant increase as individual surfactant molecules get closer together. This property counteracts Laplace's law and reduces the tendency for small alveoli to empty into nearby larger alveoli.

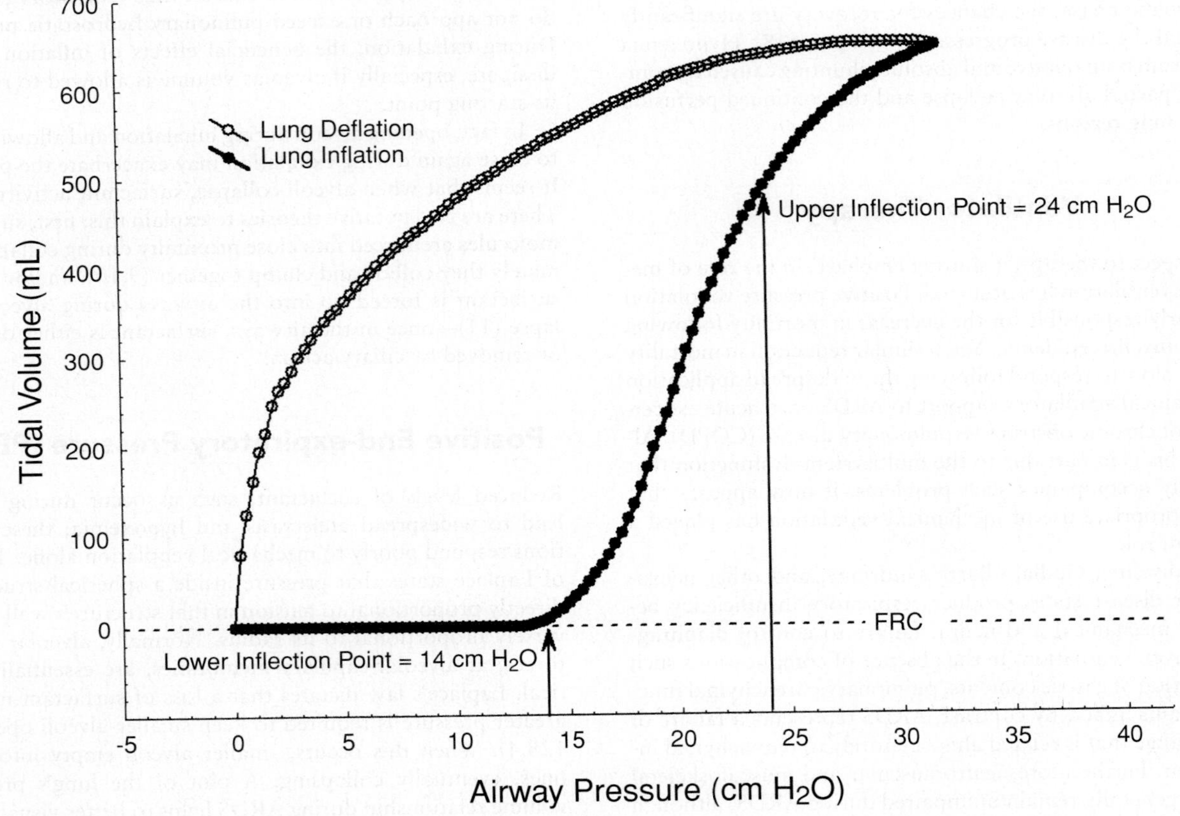

FIGURE 128.5. Inflation and deflation characteristics in the surfactant-deficient lung. Surfactant-deficient alveoli generally remain open throughout exhalation (*open circles*); at end-exhalation, unstable alveoli empty into adjacent larger alveoli and collapse, significantly reducing functional residual capacity (FRC). Furthermore, once collapsed, alveoli tend to stay collapsed until a relatively high pressure is applied. In this idealized example, airway pressure is steadily increased to inflate the lungs (*solid circles*). Note that airway pressure reaches 14 cm H_2O before any measurable volume enters the lungs; at this point (lower inflection point), collapsed alveoli begin to open, the lungs begin to accept volume, and the pressure–volume curve changes slope upward. Alveoli continue to open, those already open expand, and airway pressure continues to rise until the average patent alveoli begin to approach their maximum volume. At this point, the pressure–volume curve flattens; in other words, from this point on, larger changes in pressure will be required to produce a complementary change in volume. This slope change is referred to as the upper inflection point. Although the pressure–volume curve may be difficult to measure at the bedside, avoiding ventilator-induced lung injury likely requires that all mechanical ventilation occur between the upper and lower inflection points; that is, patient airway pressure should not be allowed above the upper inflection point or below the lower inflection point.

preferably somewhat above the lower inflection point (12). Since the therapeutic objective is to prevent alveolar collapse—that is, to keep the alveoli open—the approach is often referred to as the *open lung* approach (13,14).

Combining mechanical ventilation and PEEP usually decreases shunt and improves oxygenation (15–18), often significantly; nevertheless, ARDS mortality rates have to improve. The reasons for this are complex, but theories for these failures are starting to emerge (19). It now appears that, to reduce ARDS-associated morbidity and mortality, we must avoid the risks associated with both low-volume (4–7) and high-volume (1–3) lung injury. To this end, all tidal ventilation must occur between the lower and upper inflection points (19). It sounds easy, but bedside determination of inflection points is difficult; nevertheless, it is worth the effort.

To date, a universally agreed on ventilatory approach, or mode, for managing critically ill patients has failed to emerge. Considering the wide variety of conditions ameliorated by mechanical ventilation, and the extreme range of severity between patients with the same problem, a single, always best approach may not exist. Clinicians, therefore, must understand and recognize the potential and limitations of their favored approaches.

VENTILATOR CLASSIFICATION

Positive versus Negative Pressure

Today, virtually all ventilators function by providing some variant of positive pressure. Yet, during the polio epidemic, "iron lungs" or negative pressure ventilators were in common use. Negative pressure devices require that the patient's body be tightly enclosed within a tube or box while the head remains outside. Once the patient is sealed inside, a pump or bellows evacuates gas from inside the box; this creates a negative pressure around the patient's thorax, making atmospheric pressure positive in relation to alveolar pressure. As a result, gas flows from the mouth to alveoli, trying to equalize the pressure difference. Since this process is nearly identical to normal breathing, negative pressure ventilators tend to provide better V_A/Q ratios (20) and produce less interference with cardiac output (21) than positive pressure counterparts. Nevertheless, these devices quickly lost favor for several compelling reasons: (a) iron lungs are very large and difficult to move; (b) maintaining an airtight seal around the patient's neck, *without irritation*, is nearly impossible; (c) personnel responsible for providing patient monitoring and routine care could not easily access important areas of their patient's body.

Controlled versus Assisted Breaths

Although modern ICU ventilators offer many different operational modes, from the patient's standpoint, only two breath types remain: controlled (mechanical or mandated) and assisted-spontaneous. Controlled breaths, used during controlled mechanical ventilation (CMV), are completely defined by the attending clinician. Controlled breaths are always delivered on schedule and without regard for the patient. For this reason, clinicians favoring CMV must hyperventilate (to suppress respiration), heavily sedate, or even paralyze their patients to avoid patient–ventilator interface complications. From another perspective, CMV strategies should replace 100% of a patient's work of breathing (WOB). Patients allowed to breathe spontaneously during CMV frequently end up out of phase with the ventilator—that is, attempting to breathe when the ventilator is not in the inspiratory phase. Also known as *dyssynchrony,* out of phase breathing during CMV produces very high patient WOB (22). Assisted-spontaneous breathing strategies involve a work-sharing approach between patient and ventilator (23). Theoretically speaking, a work-sharing approach makes perfect sense; ideally, the ventilator functions to "unload" the WOB the patient cannot tolerate. Critically ill patients face an above-normal workload, primarily from their pulmonary disease process, and secondarily, from their artificial breathing apparatus, including the endotracheal tube (ET), breathing circuits, humidifiers, and the ventilator (24,25). Unfortunately, there is a fatal flaw in the ventilator–patient work-sharing concept: until recently (26) we have not been able to find a reliable, readily available, easy-to-perform, and noninvasive methodology for determining just how much WOB our patients can actually tolerate (27–29), and this determination is absolutely crucial. If the ventilator off-loads too much work, the patient's respiratory muscles are predisposed to atrophy. If the ventilator provides insufficient support, fatigue is likely. Either scenario can add unnecessary days, or even weeks, to the period of time patients require ventilatory support. Fatigued or weak patients make poor candidates for weaning and attempts at liberation from the ventilator; moreover, the risk for developing ventilator-associated pneumonia (VAP) correlates directly to the time spent on ventilatory support (30). For some, these concepts imply that hyperventilation, sedation, and paralysis predispose to atrophy, and that CMV should be used with extreme caution. Research suggests that the diaphragm, which evolved to contract without interruption from birth until death, begins to loose contractility shortly after initiating CMV (31); the loss of contractility is time dependent and continues to worsen as mechanical ventilation is prolonged (31).

Ventilator Breaths—Defining Characteristics

The idea of trying to classify each ventilator type, to better understand how specific ventilators interact with and affect physiology, remains as common a goal today as ever. Yet, today's ventilators include so many modes and options, they are nearly impossible to classify. For a time, some tried to classify ventilator modes (32), but even this strategy is no longer reliable because many ventilators now incorporate dual-mode capabilities—the ability to switch modes *within* an individual ventilator breath.

Instead of trying to classify ventilators, modes, or even submodes, it may be easier to develop and use a standardized set of terms and describe the breath types in use. This is possible since, regardless of ventilator or breath type, all ventilator breaths are delivered in four distinct phases or variables (Fig. 128.6).

Phase or Control Variables

Each ventilator breath must begin for some reason and at some specific moment in time. The physical change that initiates a breath is known as the *trigger variable* (labeled A, Fig. 128.6). Once a breath is triggered "on," the ventilator must somehow

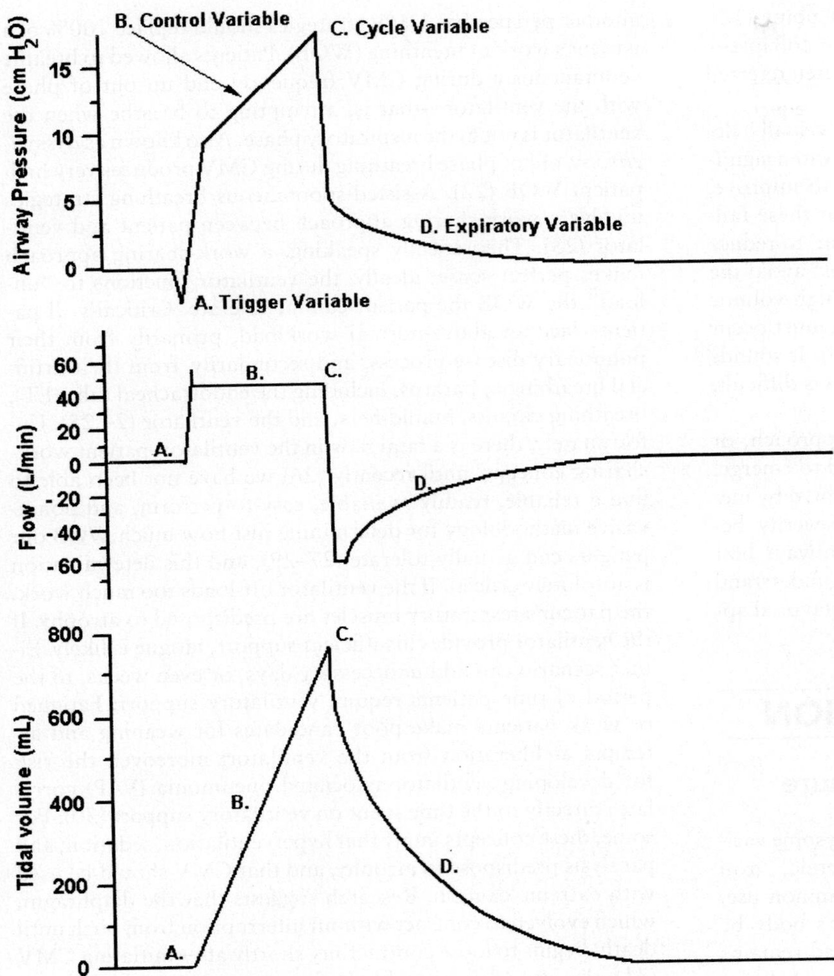

FIGURE 128.6. Pressure, flow, and volume curves for a mechanical ventilator breath. (*A*) The *trigger variable* is the physical characteristic used by the ventilator to initiate a mechanical inflation of the lungs. In this case, pressure falls before the breath starts; the represented ventilator breath is likely pressure triggered. (*B*) *Control variable*. For patient safety, the ventilator must precisely control an important aspect involved with inflating the patient's lungs. For this breath, flow is held constant; the ventilator is described as flow controlled. (*C*) *Cycle variable*. Each mechanical breath must end such that the lungs are properly filled and then allow the patient to exhale. The physical characteristic that determines appropriate lung filling is the cycle variable. This example shows that the breath ending after the control variable (flow) has continued for a specific interval of time; this ventilator is time cycled. (*D*) *Expiratory variable*. Modern ventilators either control pressure during exhalation or they do not. In this example, pressure returns to ambient (0 cm H_2O), so this ventilator has no operative expiratory variable.

precisely manage how gas is forced into the patient's lungs; the physical characteristic managed during lung inflation is the *control variable* (labeled B, Fig. 128.6). After delivering the prescribed volume or pressure, inflation must end. This physical change responsible for ending inflation is called the *cycle variable*, or cycling (labeled C, Fig. 128.6). Immediately following inhalation is exhalation, or the *exhalation variable* (labeled D, Fig. 128.6). Unlike the previous three variables, use of an exhalation variable is optional.

In early attempts at ventilator classification, author(s) often used the term "cycling" for both breath initiation and termination. Do *not* confuse the breath initiation, triggering, with breath termination, cycling; the ambiguous use of the term cycling continues to produce confusion.

All ventilators systematically change the pressure, flow, and volume with respect to time (Fig. 128.6). Thus, when characterizing any of the four phase variables, pressure, flow, volume, or time are the only possible physical characteristics a ventilator could change or control during any phase of the respiratory cycle (Table 128.1). It is also important to note that although some of these characteristics correlate and may change jointly, in direction and magnitude, they do not always do so. The practical side of this translates into an important tenet: ventilators can control only one characteristic at a time. This does not, however, preclude using multiple characteristics, provided they are used in a logical sequence, and one at a time.

Trigger Variable

Ventilators are triggered "on" by time, pressure, flow, or volume. Today's ventilators, however, often depend on multiple trigger variables used sequentially. For example, with a trigger sensitivity set for 2 (actually, −2 cm H_2O), breath rate set to ten breaths per minute (bpm) and in the CMV mode, this ventilator has at least two trigger variables. First, breaths may be pressure-triggered when the ventilator is in the expiratory phase and baseline airway pressure is reduced by 2 cm H_2O or more. If, however, the patient makes no attempt to breathe, the CMV rate timer count reaches zero and a time-triggered breath results—exactly 6 seconds (s) after the last ventilator breath. This mode is known as *assist-control* (A/C), because patients can assist as often as they like, but if they stop breathing (assisting), the ventilator reverts to the predefined CMV rate. Another way ventilators employ multiple trigger variables is by using two sensors, for instance pressure and flow; triggering occurs in response to the variable's threshold (pressure or flow) that is breached first.

Control Variable

Once a breath is triggered "on," patient safety cannot be ensured unless the delivery of gas into the lungs is precisely controlled. Of the four potential physical changes (Table 128.1), only pressure and *flow* are used to any extent. Flow is emphasized to underscore an engineering issue: volume-controlled

TABLE 128.1

VENTILATOR BREATH CLASSIFICATION

Breath variable	Variable characteristics	Frequency of use and examples
Trigger	Time	Common, IMV, CMV, PCV, APRV
	Pressure	Common, SIMV, ACV, PSV, CPAP
	Flow	Common, SIMV, ACV, PSV, CPAP
	Volume	Infrequent, SIMV (some neovents)
Inspiratory control	Time	Never
	Pressure	Common, all pressure-based breaths
	Flow	Common, most volume-based breaths
	Volume	Infrequent, some piston ventilators
Cycle	Time	Common, PCV, APRV
	Pressure	Common, IPPB
	Flow	Common, PSV
	Volume	Common, all volume-targeted modes
Expiratory	Time	Never
	Pressure	Common, CPAP, PEEP, NEEP
	Flow	Infrequent, retard
	Volume	Never

IMV, intermittent mandatory ventilation; CMV, controlled mechanical ventilation; PCV, pressure controlled ventilation; APRV, airway pressure release ventilation; SIMV, synchronized IMV; ACV, assist controlled ventilation; PSV, pressure support ventilation; CPAP, continuous positive airway pressure; IPPV, intermittent positive pressure ventilation; PEEP, positive end-expiratory pressure; NEEP, negative end-expiratory pressure.

ventilators are actually flow controlled. There are several reasons: First, the integral of flow, with respect to time, is volume. Therefore, precisely controlling inspiratory flow (V_I) for a preset inspiratory time (T_I) produces an exact tidal volume (V_T) based on the following equation:

$$V_I \times T_I = V_T \quad [1]$$

Algebraically speaking, the operator can preset only two of these variables, in this case V_I and T_I; the third variable (V_T) cannot be preset because it is a consequence of V_I and T_I. Given a choice, however, most clinicians prefer to preset the V_I and V_T; in this situation, T_I becomes the consequential or resultant variable. In an effort to obviate this preference, most of today's ventilators use an algebraic variant of equation 1:

$$V_T/V_I = T_I \quad [2]$$

This design allows operators to preset V_T and V_I. Furthermore, since the operator actually predefines V_T—referring to the ventilator as a volume controller, or as volume-controlled ventilation (VCV)—this is perfectly acceptable; this nomenclature will be used henceforth.

Volume-controlled strategies differ markedly from pressure-controlled ventilation (PCV). When we opt for VCV, our priorities are clear: we wish to prescribe (preset) V_T, V_I, and flow pattern. If we want these parameters reliably delivered, then airway pressure (P_{aw}) must not be restricted. When P_{aw} is allowed to vary, V_T, V_I, and flow pattern are delivered, regardless of the patient's pulmonary mechanics (Fig. 128.7). High peak inflation pressures (PIP) are a concern, so ventilators allow clinicians to preset a maximum safe level of P_{aw}; this setting, referred to as a *high-pressure limit*, functions as a cycle variable—that is, ending inspiration (or diverting gas flow) the moment P_{aw} violates the established threshold. Keep in mind, though, cycling *via* a high-pressure limit truncates breath delivery, negates volume control, and reduces V_T.

Pressure-controlled strategies allow us to preset a desired P_{aw} and T_I; conversely, V_T, V_I, and flow waveform cannot be predetermined. Pressure-controlled breaths always generate an exponentially decelerating flow pattern; the individual's C_{RS} and R_{aw} determine the magnitude of V_I and V_T (Fig. 128.8) (33,34). Inasmuch as PCV does not control V_T, and preset pressure never varies, clinicians must ensure that PCV is carefully monitored; always carefully set low/high V_T alarms (if available), as well as low/high minute ventilation alarms.

Cycle Variable

All four physical changes are commonly used for cycling ventilator breaths. Pressure cycling is common during intermittent positive pressure breathing (IPPB); flow cycling predominates during pressure support ventilation (PSV); and either time or volume is common during VCV. Without question, time is the most commonly used cycle variable, particularly if one remembers that with today's VCVs, cycling occurs when T_I lapses, not in response to volume.

Expiratory Variable

The expiratory phase is the least varied of the four; attempts at manipulating the expiratory phase variable have met with little success. Varying flow resistance (retard), negative end-expiratory pressure (NEEP), and PEEP have all been thoroughly tried and discarded. Compelling evidence, however, substantiates using continuous positive airway pressure (CPAP) and PEEP to restore or increase functional residual capacity (FRC) (35–37), reduce shunt and improve oxygenation (15–18), and reduce WOB (38).

Classifying Breaths

The four phase variables provide us with a method for classifying ventilator breaths that is easy to use and understand.

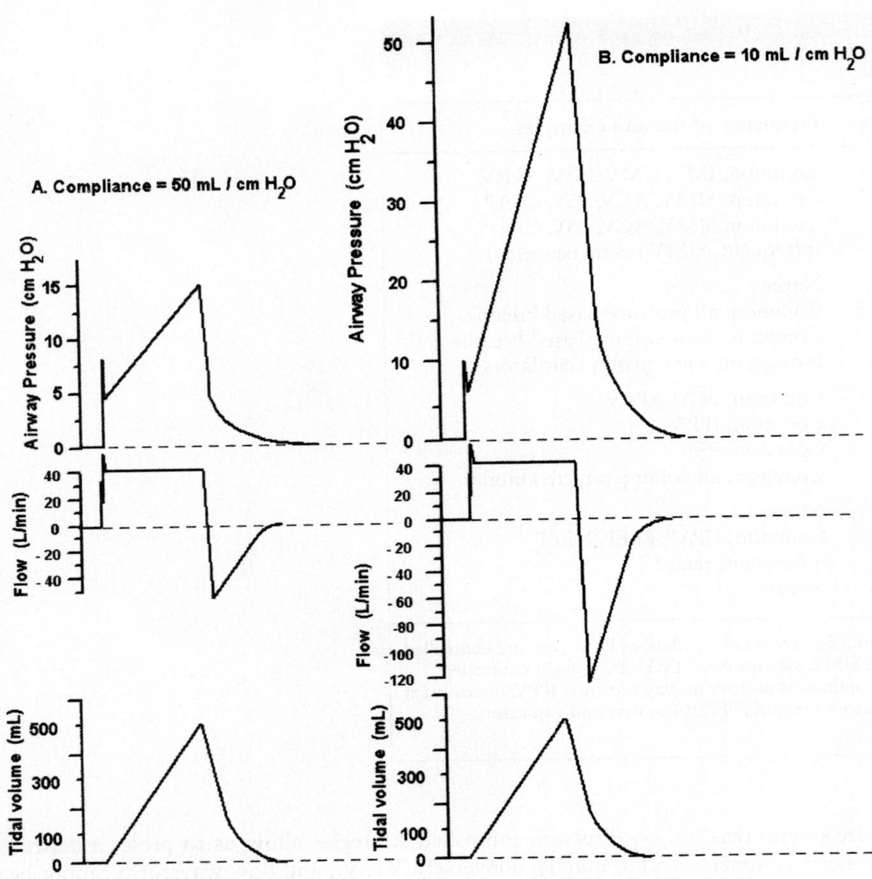

FIGURE 128.7. Response of volume-controlled ventilation (VCV) to a sudden change in respiratory system compliance (C_{RS}). **A:** Compliance = 50 mL/cm H_2O. An airway pressure, flow, and tidal volume curve for a patient with this C_{RS} and receiving VCV. **B:** Compliance = 10 mL/cm H_2O. An airway pressure, flow, and tidal volume curve for the same patient as shown in **A** except that the patient's C_{RS} is acutely reduced. Note that volume and flow are essentially unaffected, but airway pressure is dramatically elevated as the ventilator required far more pressure to provide the same flow and volume into the much stiffer lungs.

It makes sense to classify by breath behavior because today's ventilators offer so many breath types. For instance, the breath depicted in Figure 128.6 is pressure-triggered, volume-controlled, and time or volume cycled; there is no exhalation phase variable. In Figures 128.7 and 128.8, the breaths are time triggered, volume controlled, and time or volume cycled; and time triggered, pressure controlled, and time cycled, respectively. Some ventilator modes like intermittent mandatory ventilation (IMV) or synchronized IMV (SIMV) allow two different breath types. Mandated breaths might be time triggered, volume controlled, and time cycled, whereas between scheduled breaths, spontaneous breaths might be pressure triggered, pressure controlled, and pressure cycled.

VENTILATOR DESIGN

Modern ICU ventilators are expensive and seemingly complex; yet, although the electronics may be complicated, the basic ventilator component configuration is simple and has changed very little over the last 20 years. In its simplest form, a mechanical ventilator requires only a few essential components (Fig. 128.9).

Power Sources

Pneumatics

Ventilators must have power. Most patients require at least some oxygen; this makes the energy stored within compressed oxygen a reliable and convenient power source. Gas-powered ventilators are called *pneumatic*. The powering gas source can be oxygen or compressed air, as long as the gas source is free of contaminants and debris and is dry. Hospital oxygen supplies virtually never pose contamination or water concerns; whether in bulk form or in cylinders, oxygen is certified clean and pure (99.99%). Compressed air sources are, however, a completely different matter. Compressors aspirate air from the environment; if aspirated air is contaminated, so too will be the compressed air. There have been instances of hospitals locating compressor intakes too close to parking lots and, on occasion, compressing exhaust gases along with air. Also, environmental air contains water vapor, some of which condenses and becomes liquid during the compression process; any and all water must be removed or it can cause serious damage to ventilators and other pneumatic equipment. Finally, most compressors use rapidly moving pistons or rotors to compress the air; operating at such high speed requires lubrication. Compressed air, for human consumption, should never involve using an oil-lubricated device. Small oil particles are compressed along with the air and can cause serious lung injury if inhaled.

Despite potential drawbacks associated with using compressed air sources, pneumatic ventilators offer several advantages, particularly when used for transport. For instance, pneumatic ventilators are always ready to go; they never require time-consuming recharging as battery-powered units do. Moreover, pneumatic ventilators use no expensive batteries, power supplies, or electric cables that can fail or must be periodically replaced. Furthermore, batteries often contain

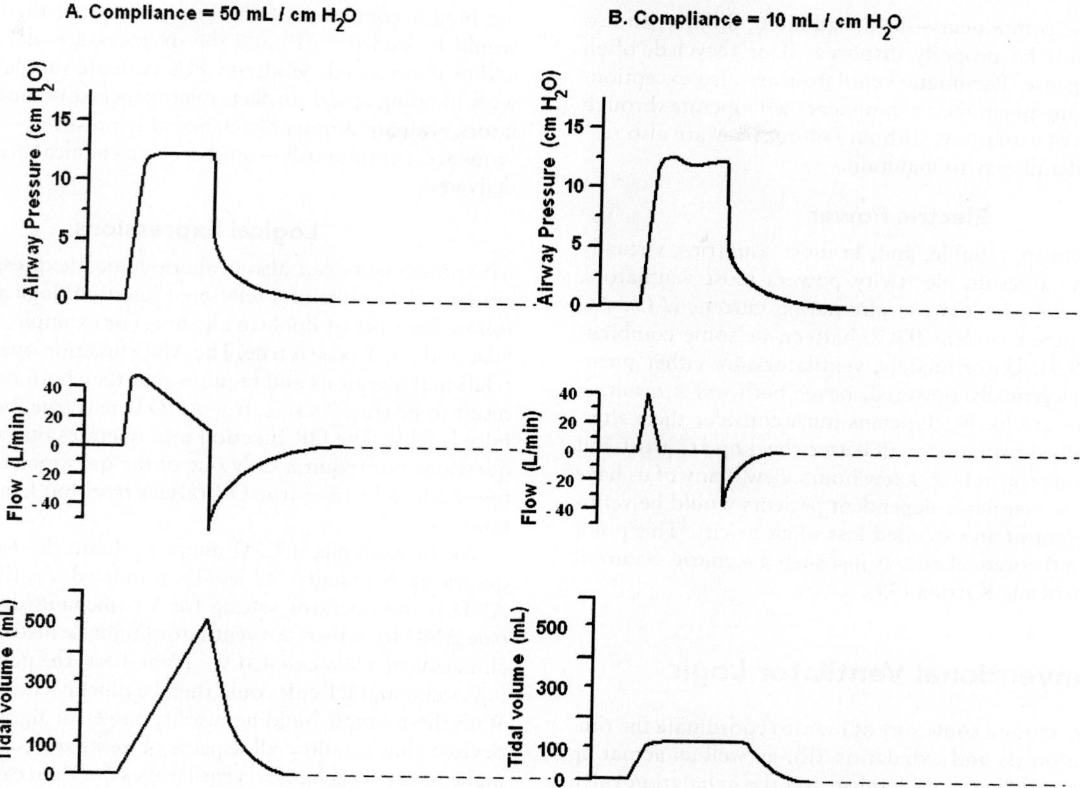

FIGURE 128.8. Response of pressure-controlled ventilation (PCV) to a sudden change in respiratory system compliance (C_{RS}). A: *Compliance* = *50 mL/cm* H_2O. An airway pressure, flow, and tidal volume curve for a patient with this C_{RS} and receiving PCV. B: *Compliance* = *10 mL/cm* H_2O. An airway pressure, flow, and tidal volume curve for the same patient as shown in panel A, except the patient's C_{RS} is acutely reduced. Note pressure is essentially unaffected, but flow and volume are dramatically reduced as the far stiffer lungs respond to the same airway pressure with less flow and volume.

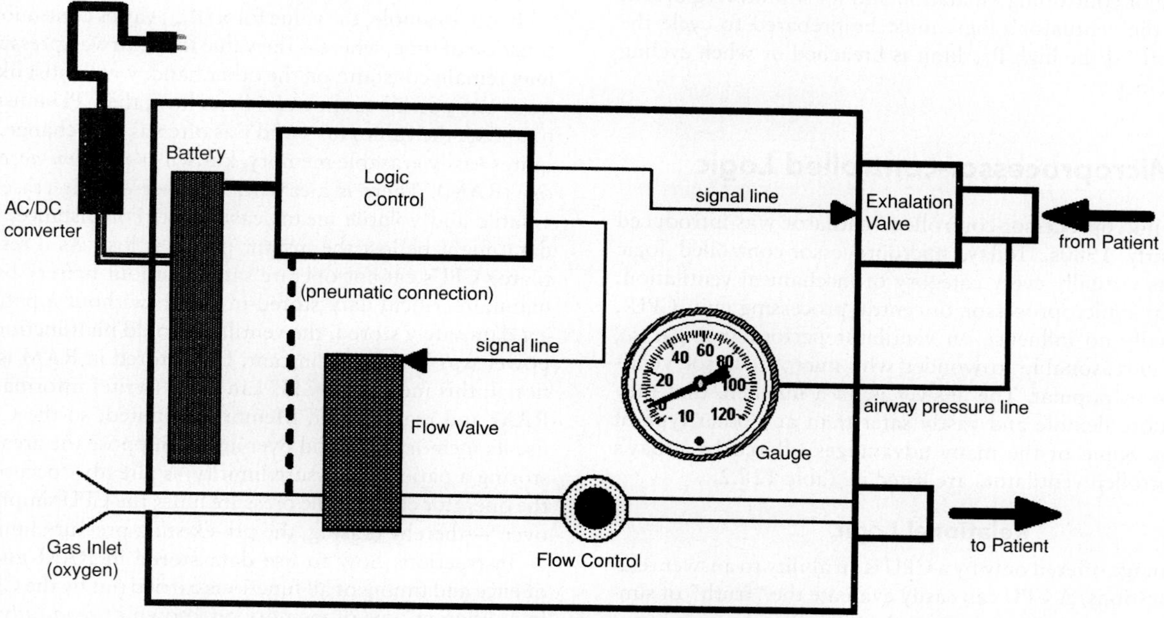

FIGURE 128.9. Schema of a basic ventilator. This schematic includes all of the major components necessary for ventilator operation. The logic component provides timing signals responsible for the inspiratory and expiratory phases. Ventilator logic must also synchronize the onset of each breath by the closing of the exhalation valve. Ventilator logic may be provided by fluidics, analog electronics, digital electronics (microprocessors), or pneumatics. All ventilators, regardless of simplicity, are either electrically powered (with or without battery backup) or pneumatically powered. None so far are powered by both modes.

extremely toxic components—lead, cadmium, lithium, and so forth—and must be properly disposed of or recycled, often at hospital expense. Pneumatic ventilators are also exceptionally robust; many pneumatic components will operate through many millions of actuations without failure. They are also reasonably priced and easy to maintain.

Electric Power

Electricity is cheap, reliable, and, in most countries, virtually ubiquitous. As a result, electricity powers most ventilators. Electrically powered units use alternating current (AC), AC converted to direct current (DC), battery, or some combination (Fig. 128.9). Unfortunately, ventilators are either pneumatically or electrically powered, never both. As a result, if power outages are likely, clinicians must consider their alternatives carefully; ventilators with battery backup are great, but will only operate for, at best, a few hours. Few if any of us have considered how ventilator-dependent patients would be ventilated in the event of an extended loss of electricity. This point is not simply a theoretical one, as just such a scenario occurred following Hurricane Katrina (39).

Conventional Ventilator Logic

All ventilators require some sort of logic to coordinate the timing of inhalation (I) and exhalation (E), as well as actuating the flow/volume delivery mechanism and the exhalation valve (Fig. 128.9).

Traditionally, ventilator logic involved pneumatics, standard electronics, fluidics, or some combination of these. To initiate and maintain inhalation, logic signals simultaneously activate both the flow/volume delivery system and the exhalation valve. At the same time, ventilator logic is responsible for timing or controlling inhalation and for monitoring breath delivery; the ventilator's logic must be prepared to cycle the breath "off" if the high P_{aw} limit is breached or when cycling criteria is met.

Microprocessor-controlled Logic

The first microprocessor-controlled ventilator was introduced in the early 1980s. Today, microprocessor-controlled logic dominates virtually every category of mechanical ventilation. Given that a microprocessor, or central processing unit (CPU), has virtually no influence on ventilator performance *per se*, it is not unreasonable to wonder why microprocessor ventilators are so popular. The answer is, in a nutshell, that they are far more flexible and vastly safer than any other type of ventilator. Some of the many advantages offered by today's CPU-controlled ventilators are listed in Table 128.2.

Relational Logic

An advantage offered only by a CPU is an ability to answer relational questions. A CPU can easily evaluate the "truth" of simple relational expressions such as the following: Is $x < y$?, $x = y$?, or is $x > y$?. A relational question can either be *true* or *false*. For instance, x might be the patient's P_{aw} and y the operator-selected high-pressure limit. During each breath, the CPU could be instructed to evaluate, every few milliseconds, the relational expression Is $x > y$? If the answer is false, then the ventilator breath continues; if the answer is true, then the breath would be cycled "off" and the overpressure alarms sounded and/or illuminated. Modern CPUs evaluate simple expressions with blinding speed. In fact, microprocessor-controlled ventilators evaluate dozens of relational expressions—in a specific sequence, continuously—until each mechanical breath is safely delivered.

Logical Expressions

Microprocessors can also evaluate logical expressions or operate on the results of a relational question; logical operations follow the rules of Boolean algebra. For example, NOT true is false and NOT false is true. The AND function operates on two relational questions and requires that they both be true for the result to be true. That is, true AND true is true, but true AND false is false. The OR function also operates on two relational questions but requires only one of the questions to be true for the result to be true; true OR false is true, but false OR false is false.

As an example, a CPU might evaluate the following two questions: Is exhaled V_T less than inhaled V_T, divided by 2?, AND is the operator setting for V_T unchanged? If answered true AND true, then the ventilator might be instructed to warn clinicians of a low exhaled V_T; from there, the patient's breathing circuit and ET cuff could then be quickly checked for leaks. With these simple building blocks, powerful algorithms can be devised that monitor all aspects of ventilator operations and make today's mechanical ventilators safer than ever before.

Computer Memory

A CPU, no matter how powerful or fast, cannot function without memory. How could a CPU answer the relational question, Is x (P_{aw}) greater than y (airway pressure limit)? if it couldn't remember the value of y? Additionally, how would a CPU know when, or how often, to answer relational questions?

In our example, the value for x (P_{aw}) varies continuously as a function of time, whereas the value for y (airway pressure limit) may remain constant; on the other hand, y will most likely vary from one patient to the next. Somehow, the CPU must be able to update the values for x and y as often as they change. This requires easily erasable memory, known as *random-access memory* (RAM). There is a caveat, however—easily erased means volatile and volatile means easily lost. For instance, valuable data might be lost the instant power is lost. As a result, ventilator CPUs cannot operate safely without battery backup to maintain critical data stored in RAM; without a patient's *exact* data safely stored, the ventilator could malfunction, even if power was lost for an instant. Data stored in RAM is bidirectional; this means the CPU can store (write) information into RAM and read it later. Memory is limited, so the CPU must use its memory over and over again. Suppose the area used for storing a patient's pressure limit (y) is already "occupied" and the operator changes the pressure limit; the CPU simply "writes over"—thereby erasing, the pre-existing pressure limit value.

Instructions how to use data stored in RAM and the sequence and timing of all functions carried out by the CPU reside in a different type of memory on known as *read-only memory* (ROM). This form of memory is nonvolatile and not easily altered. It is this memory that cues the CPU as to how often and when to evaluate the relational and logical operations. In fact, the entire sequence, or code, responsible for every conceivable ventilator function is stored in ROM. The use of ROM comes

TABLE 128.2

ADVANTAGES OF MICROPROCESSOR-CONTROLLED VENTILATORS

GENERAL VERSATILITY

- Can provide virtually any desired mode of positive-pressure ventilation
- Can provide a wide variety of inspiratory flow waveforms
- Offers choice of cycling or trigger variable in many modes
- Can be easily reprogrammed to meet changing trends in mechanical ventilation
- Can ventilate adults, pediatric, and neonatal patients
- Can provide adaptive modes of ventilation such as volume-targeted, pressure ventilation or proportional assist ventilation (PAV)

MONITORING

- Provides real-time monitoring and alarms for various ventilatory parameters
- Can measure and display lung-thorax compliance (C_{LT}), airway resistance (R_{aw}), plateau pressure, minute exhaled ventilation, auto-PEEP
- Provides on-board computer memory that saves, for later retrieval, ventilation data for trend analysis

COMPUTER CORRECTION AND SAFETY

- Can automatically correct for many internal variations that might affect prescribed tidal volume (V_T) or target pressure
- Can automatically maintain the set inspiratory flow rate, waveform, and V_T, even when the patient's impedance (C_{LT}, R_{aw}) decreases or increases
- Measures and displays tidal and minute volumes corrected to BTPS
- Measures compliance/compression of the specific breathing circuit and humidifier in use and compensates for the lost volume on a breath-by-breath basis
- Monitors all critical computer and patient parameters; declares an inoperative condition, terminates ventilation, opens the safety valve (to allow spontaneous breathing from the room), or begins a backup mode of ventilation any time a dangerous situation is detected
- Saves and stores, for later retrieval and analysis, all errors, including patient alarms or other important issues detected during operation

DISPLAY AND COMMUNICATIONS CAPABILITY

- Can process and display any monitored data and important patient ventilation parameters
- Can communicate and interface with remote monitors
- Can communicate with separate microcomputers (personal computers) for monitoring and storage of data

REPAIRS AND MAINTENANCE

- Provides troubleshooting programs or extensive testing programs that pinpoint problems, facilitate repairs, and minimize downtime
- Contains few moving parts; maintenance may involve only routine filter changes
- Provides modular design and easily removable printed circuit boards that facilitate repair

PEEP, positive end-expiratory pressure; BTPS, body temperature and pressure saturated.

with a caveat too: ROM is nonvolatile, but it is not impervious. Even the slightest change in a critical instruction could harm a patient. As a result, ventilator CPUs *must* have powerful "watchdog" systems that constantly evaluate every aspect of their behavior. Watchdogs always err on the side of safety—should they detect anything out of the ordinary, they immediately terminate CPU operation, protect the patient, and alert the operator of the malfunction—often referred to as a *vent-inop*. Once a bizarre or unusual behavior has been detected, manufacturers ensure that CPU integrity is verified *before* the ventilator will function again. Unfortunately, too often vent-inop conditions require technical assistance from a biomedical engineer or factory representative. To obviate such problems, engineers have tried two, or even three, CPUs, which are programmed to constantly evaluate each other. This strategy eliminates the need for watchdogs but, in the case of only two CPUs, does not eliminate the problem; when one CPU detects a problem, who decides which CPU is still functioning properly? With a three-CPU design, there is always a "referee"; the aberrant CPU, once detected, can be shut off leaving two CPUs to continue safely operating the ventilator until it can be safely replaced.

Ventilator Control Systems

Open Loop Control

Open loop ventilator designs (Fig. 128.10) are economical and straightforward but functionally limited. Ventilators using open loops offer VCV or PCV; they seldom provide both. Open loop systems are also not fault tolerant. For instance, suppose over time and with prolonged usage, a ventilator's flow valve

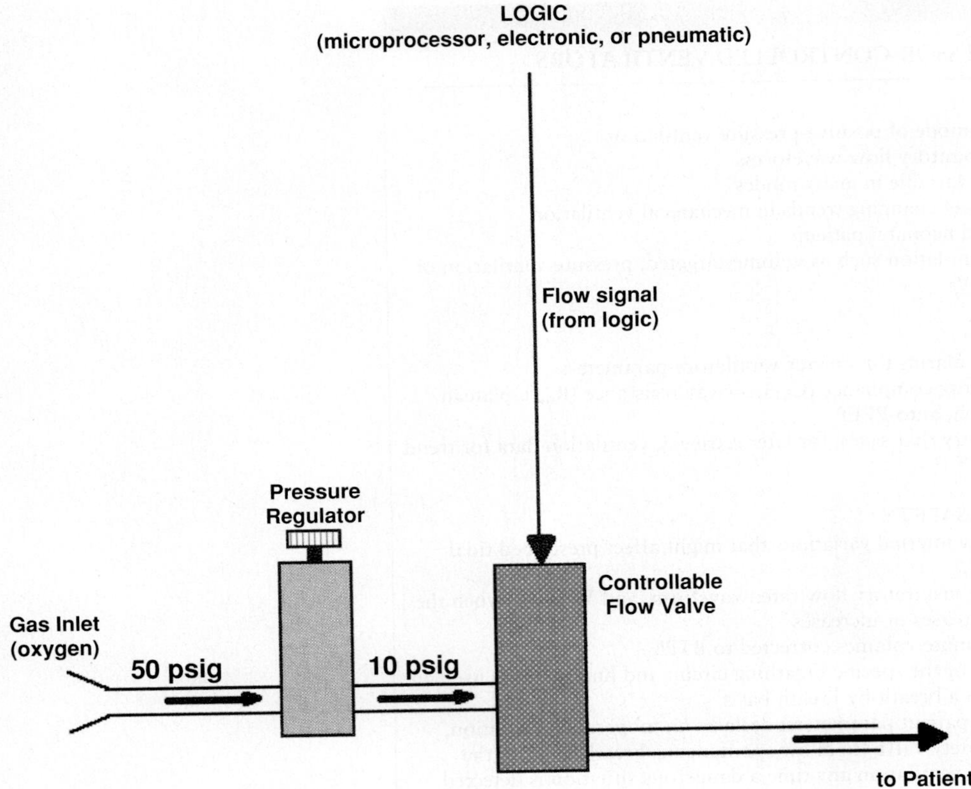

FIGURE 128.10. Schema of open loop ventilator control. Virtually all positive pressure ventilators control flow (shown) or pressure during each mechanical breath. The simplest control system involves a properly synchronized signal from the logic element that produces the output (flow); the ventilator does not verify accuracy, so the operator must do so.

gradually drifts out of calibration. Now, consider that the signal designed to produce 0.75 L/s yields only 0.60 L/s, and V_T is preset to 0.75 L. This patient will receive a V_T no greater than 0.6 L, and the ventilator, even if CPU controlled, would have no way of detecting this problem.

Closed Loop Control

Closed loop, or feedback, designs (Fig. 128.11) are far more complex and expensive than open loop designs. In return, they deliver exceptional accuracy and automatically correct for many common failures and variances. Using the same preset V_T of 0.75 L and V_I of 0.75 L/s, a closed loop ventilator delivers the requested V_T even if the flow valve is no longer calibrated, thereby protecting the patient. Given the example above, ventilator logic opens the flow valve, expecting 0.75 L/s; yet, a flow sensor, located just downstream from the flow valve, measures the actual flow (0.6 L/s) and sends an electric signal—proportional to measured flow—to the comparator (Fig. 128.11). The comparator functions to analyze (electrically) the difference between the measured flow and actuating signals; if the signals are identical, nothing happens; if the signals vary, the comparator provides an output signal proportional in magnitude to the difference. The comparator's output adds to, or removes from, the existing signal actuating the valve—in this case, the combined signals open the valve to produce a higher flow. Comparators function nearly instantaneously, so the flow valve's output can be corrected repeatedly, as often as the valve's response time and the programmed T_I allow. A response time of 10 ms allows 100 corrections in a T_I of 1 second, if necessary.

Closed loop feedback also corrects the ventilator outputs when affected by changing pulmonary impedance, different breathing circuits, and high-resistance humidifiers. Closed loop designs that incorporate flow and pressure sensors do not require separate valves for VCV and PCV. In this instance, a flow valve is either opened and a prescribed V_T delivered, or the valve is opened to provide an initial high flow, and a closed loop pressure algorithm maintains any desired target pressure by manipulating the valve's output flow based on the target pressure.

Closed loop designs require accurate onboard flow and pressure sensors as well as sophisticated control algorithms; these are relatively costly and can be damaged by rough handling. For these reasons, transport ventilators often incorporate open loop designs.

Microprocessors and Closed Loop Control

The first CPU-powered ventilators were too slow to perform all of the tasks involved in operating the ventilator and provide the corrected signals required for closed loop control. To maintain accuracy and speed, the first generation of CPU-powered ventilators combined digital logic with analog, closed loop control systems. In contrast, today's CPUs perform billions of operations per second, leaving adequate time for the CPU to provide "corrected" signals necessary for closed loop control (Fig. 128.12).

Microprocessors operate using digital (D) signals, but most of our real-world hardware (valves, sensors, transducers) require analog (A) signals. It follows that for a CPU to actuate a valve, a digital signal from the CPU must first be converted to analog; this takes place in a D-to-A signal processing chip (Fig. 128.12). Analog information, such as measured flow signals, must be similarly converted A to D before the CPU can

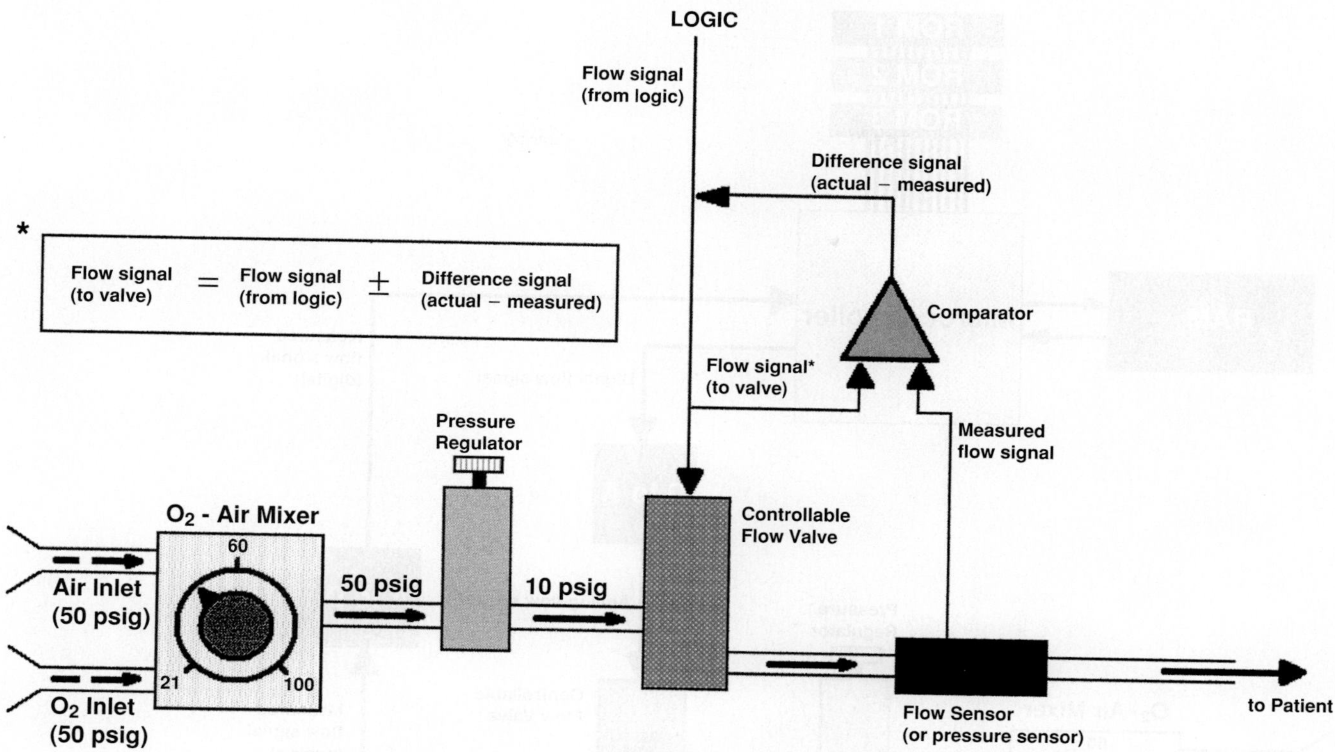

FIGURE 128.11. Schema of closed loop ventilator control. Ventilator reliability and accuracy is vastly improved by measuring the actual output (flow), comparing the measured to desired, and correcting the actuating signal by the difference. At the onset of each breath, a signal from the ventilator's logic actuates (opens) the output valve. The resultant output (flow) is measured immediately by a flow sensor positioned downstream. The flow sensor converts measured gas flow into an analog electric signal, which is routed to one side of an electronic comparator. The actuating signal (actual) from the logic element is fed into the other side of the comparator, where it is compared to the measured signal. If the two signals differ, the comparator adds (or subtracts) an amount of electricity proportional to the signal difference to (or from) the actuating signal. The entire loop requires only about 10 msec to complete; that means the actual signal could theoretically be corrected as many as 100 times in a typical mechanical breath lasting just 1 sec. Normally, however, it requires only a few iterations before the measured and desired signals are identical.

use them. During closed loop control, once a measured signal is converted A to D and reaches the CPU, it is compared to the current actuating signal. Based on the difference, the CPU computes a new actuating signal; its digital representation is sent to the D to A, and from there, it proceeds to replace the existing signal. As each of these transformations take time, it is easy to see why early CPUs did not have sufficient speed to provide closed loop corrections. The state-of-the-art CPUs are so fast, digital control rivals that of analog comparators for controlling closed loop systems.

CONVENTIONAL MECHANICAL VENTILATORY TECHNIQUES

Compliance and Resistance—The End-inspiratory Plateau

Operational Principles

The terms *postinflation hold*, *end-inspiratory pause*, and *end-inspiratory plateau* (EIP) all refer to the same ventilator routine; the instant V_T delivery is complete, the ventilator stops gas flow but does not allow the patient to exhale until a specified period of time, the EIP, elapses (Fig. 128.13). The EIP is considered part of T_I because the V_T volume remains in the lungs and the patient does not exhale until the EIP is complete; ventilators often allow plateaus as long as 2 seconds. Although this may not seem excessive, when combined with the existing T_I, EIPs are often long enough to adversely impact hemodynamics and are poorly tolerated by spontaneously breathing patients.

Clinical Applications

An end-inspiratory plateau has been advocated as a method to improve the distribution of inhaled gases, thereby decreasing V_D/V_T and $PaCO_2$ (40). Theoretically, this makes sense; if inhalation was long enough, gas redistribution into slow-filling spaces would improve overall distribution (41). Gas redistribution during EIP is thought to result secondary to collateral ventilation and Pendelluft flow.

Collateral ventilation occurs when gas enters the alveoli from adjacent alveoli through channels in the alveolar walls (pores of Kohn) or through cross-communications between bronchioles (Lambert canals). Pendelluft flow occurs when, during EIP, volume from fast-filling spaces redistributes into

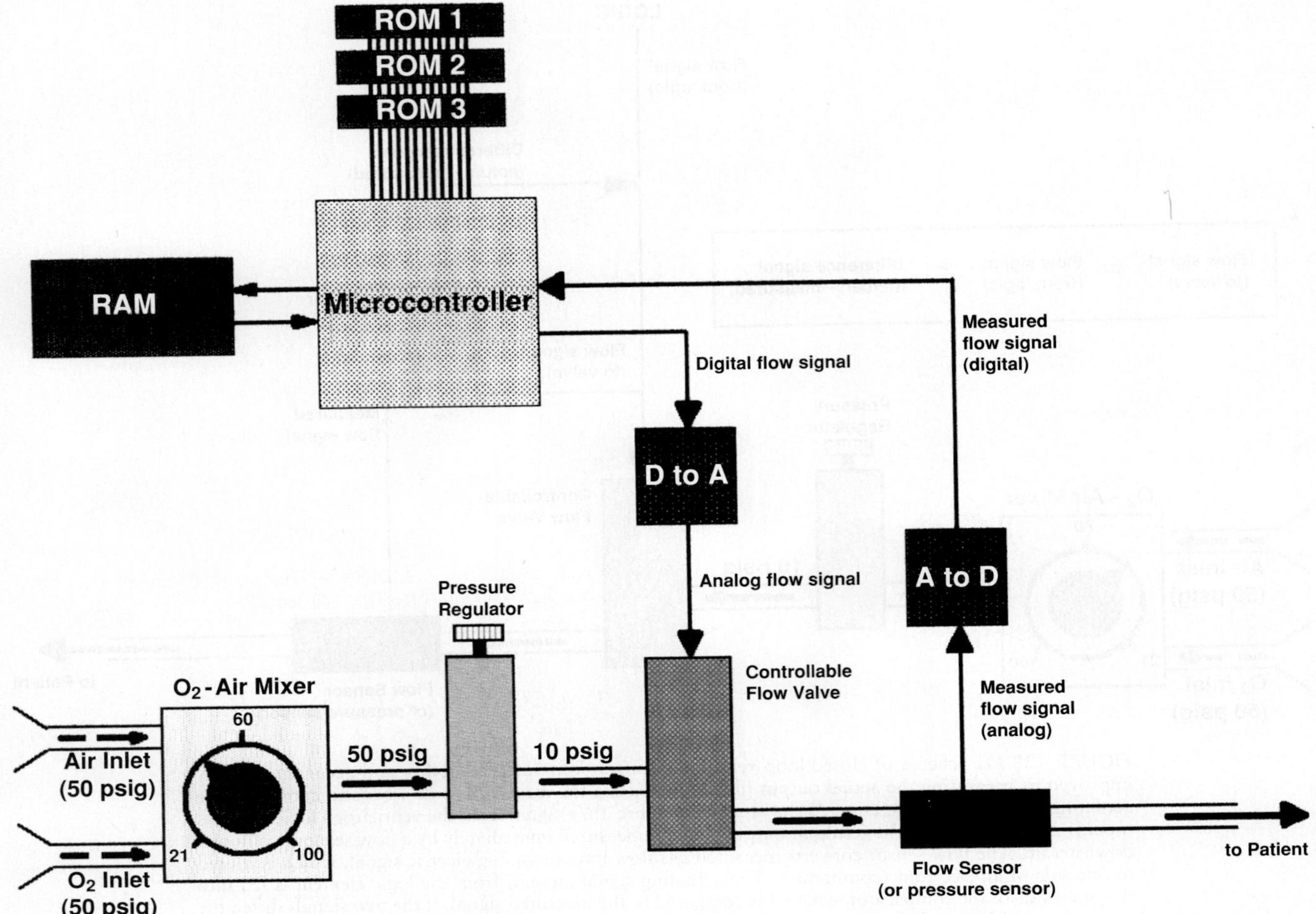

FIGURE 128.12. Schema of a microprocessor-controlled closed loop control system. First-generation microprocessor-controlled ventilators combined digital (D) signals converted to analog (A) with an analog closed loop system. This approach was necessary because digital control of closed loop feedback added several time-consuming steps: corrected signals had to be converted D to A before they could operate ventilator valves, and the measured signal had to be converted A to D before the microprocessor could compare it to desired and determine an appropriate correction. Unfortunately, microprocessors available at the time were simply not fast enough to adequately monitor lung inflation and provide corrected closed loop signals. Today's microprocessors easily perform billions of operations per second, and most second- or third-generation microprocessor-controlled ventilators provide closed loop control using only digital signal processing.

slow-filling spaces. Such gas flow is caused by regional pressure gradients that arise as a consequence of maldistribution secondary to positive pressure inflation.

The EIP is seldom used to improve distribution, but rather to determine C_{RS} and R_{aw}. During the plateau time, as gas flow ceases, the flow-resistive component of PIP disappears. The remaining pressure—the plateau pressure—also reflects the static elastic recoil pressure (ERP) of the lungs. Exhaled V_T, PIP, and ERP are used in determining the patient's C_{RS} and R_{aw} (Table 128.3). These measurements are often performed routinely to assess the patient's progress or to gauge the response to bronchodilators.

Inspiratory Flow Waveforms

Before the advent of microprocessor-powered ventilators, different ventilator brands delivered gas flow using a wide variety of methodologies: pistons, injectors, bellows, solenoids, and so forth. Each flow-generating technique produced a different inspiratory flow pattern: square or constant (Fig. 128.14A), sinusoidal, decelerating (Fig. 128.14B), accelerating. Clinicians immediately began to wonder which waveform was best, or, could matching specific waveforms with specific pulmonary conditions make a difference? To this day, these questions remain essentially unresolved. Some tried various waveforms and found little or no difference in the distribution of ventilation (42). Other studies, modeling multiple lung compartments with different R_{aw}, showed improved distribution with the decelerating waveform compared to others (43,44). Clinical reports confirmed the utility of a decelerating pattern (45–47). In one investigation, V_T, T_I, I:E ratio, and ventilator rate were held constant. Compared to the constant-flow pattern, the decelerating waveform significantly reduced patient PIP, $PaCO_2$, V_D/V_T ratio, and alveolar-to-arterial oxygen pressure gradient

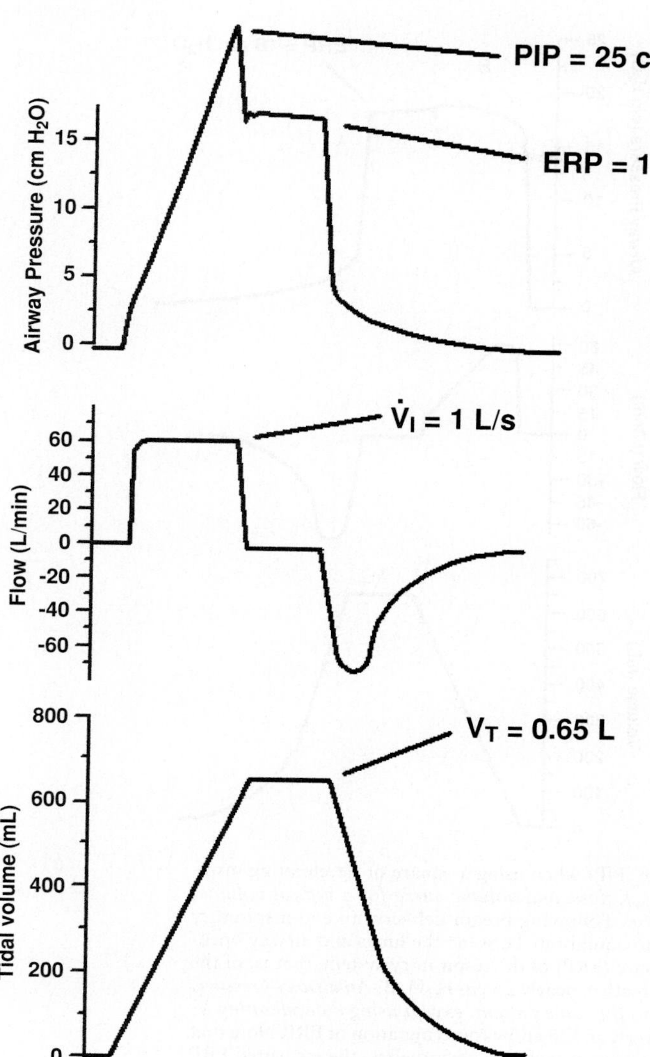

FIGURE 128.13. Compliance and resistance determination in the ventilator patient. Respiratory system compliance (C_{RS}) and airway resistance (R_{aw}) determination by end-inspiratory plateau (EIP) requires volume-controlled mode, square flow pattern, inspiratory flow rate (V_I) of exactly 1 liter (L)/second (s) (or 60 L/minute), and an EIP of $\geq$0.25 second. In this example, the peak inflation pressure (PIP) reaches 25 cm H_2O the instant flow ceases. After the preset tidal volume (V_T) is delivered, the EIP begins, that is, gas flow from the ventilator ceases and the patient is not permitted to exhale. During the EIP, pressure equilibrates between the lungs and breathing circuit and elastic recoil pressure (ERP) of the lungs can be measured at the airway opening. The greater the difference between a patient's PIP and ERP, the greater the R_{aw}. Compliance is computed by dividing V_T (0.65 L) by measured ERP minus the baseline pressure (0 cm H_2O), and is given in units of L/cm H_2O or mL/cm H_2O. Resistance is computed as PIP minus ERP divided by V_I (must be 1 L/s) and is stated in units of cm H_2O/L/s. In this example, C_{RS} is 0.038 L/cm H_2O and R_{aw} is 8 cm H_2O/L/s.

TABLE 128.3

MEASUREMENT OF COMPLIANCE AND AIRWAY RESISTANCE

Definition:

End-inspiratory pause may be used to differentiate dynamic (C_{RS}) (L/cm H_2O) from static lung–thorax compliance (C_{RS}) (L/cm H_2O) and to determine airway resistance (R_{aw}) (cm H_2O/L/s).

1. Dynamic $C_{RS} = V_T/(\text{PIP} - \text{baseline airway pressure})$
   Where: V_T = exhaled tidal volume (L)
   PIP = peak inflation pressure (cm H_2O)
   Baseline airway pressure = atmospheric pressure, continuous positive airway pressure (CPAP) (cm H_2O), or positive end-expiratory pressure (PEEP) (cm H_2O)
   e.g., $C_{RS} = 0.65\ L/(25\ cm\ H_2O - 0\ cm\ H_2O) = 0.026\ L/cm\ H_2O$
2. Static $C_{RS} = V_T/(\text{ERP} - \text{baseline airway pressure})$
   Where: ERP = static elastic recoil pressure of the respiratory system (cm H_2O)
   e.g., $C_{RS} = 0.65\ L/(17\ cm\ H_2O - 0\ cm\ H_2O) = 0.038\ L/cm\ H_2O$
3. $R_{aw} = (\text{PIP} - \text{ERP}) \times V_I$
   Where: V_I = inspiratory flow rate[a] (L/s)
   e.g., $R_{aw} = (25\ cm\ H_2O - 17\ cm\ H_2O) \times 1\ L/s = 8\ cm\ H_2O/L/s$

[a] The selected inspiratory flow pattern must be constant (square).

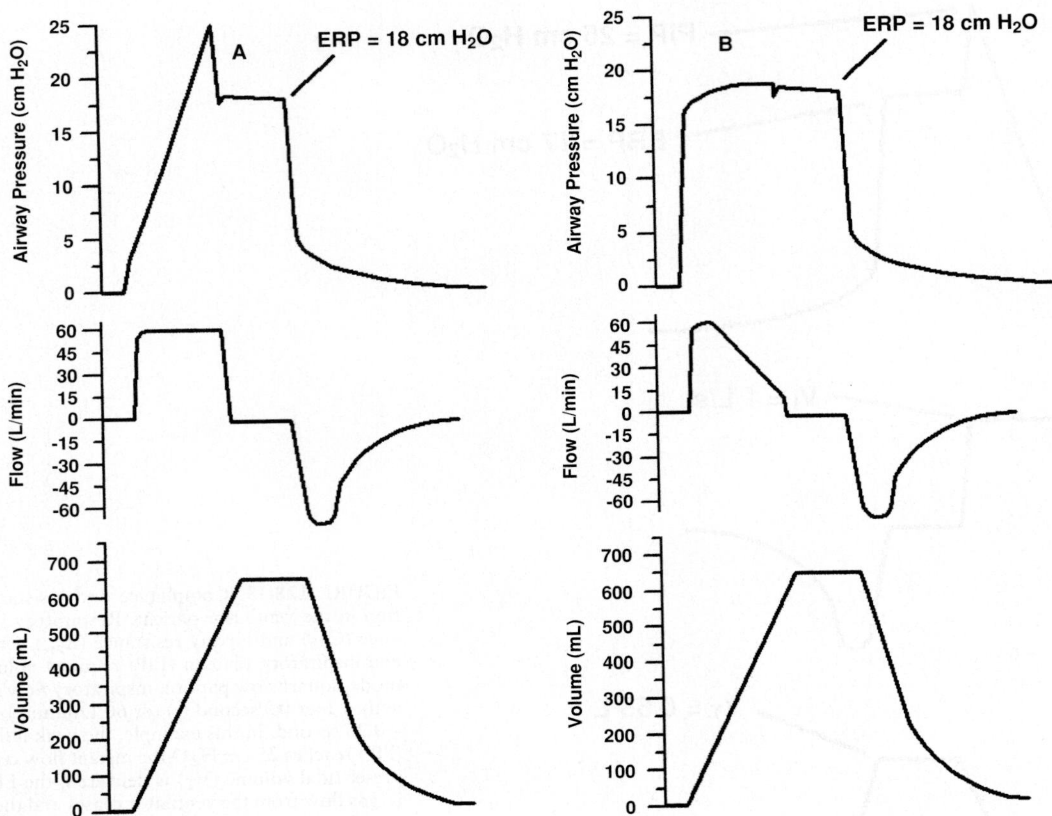

FIGURE 128.14. Differences in peak inflation pressure (PIP) when using a square or decelerating inspiratory flow (V_I) waveform. **A:** *An airway pressure (P_{aw}), flow, and volume curve for a typical volume-controlled breath delivered using a square V_I waveform.* Following breath delivery, an end-inspiratory plateau (EIP) terminates gas flow and allows pressure to equilibrate between the lungs and airway opening; at equilibration, P_{aw} reflects the elastic recoil pressure (ERP) of the respiratory system; that is, of the lungs and thorax combined. Note that the PIP of this breath is nearly 25 cm H_2O. **B:** *An airway pressure, flow, and volume curve for the same breath, delivered to the same patient, except using a decelerating V_I waveform in this instance.* Again, following breath delivery, an EIP allows determination of ERP. Note that the PIP of this breath is 8 cm H_2O lower than for the square waveform; nevertheless, the measured ERP (18 cm H_2O) is exactly the same as that using the square flow pattern. This occurs because a decelerating flow pattern reduces gas flow to near zero (as during an EIP) *before* the breath cycles "off" and the EIP begins.

$P(_{A-a})O_2$ (46). However, mean P_{aw} was significantly greater, predisposing to adverse hemodynamic effects.

In addition to the potential to improve distribution, decelerating waveforms significantly reduce PIP, especially when contrasted to square (Fig. 128.14) or accelerating patterns. Some clinicians opt for a decelerating pattern, believing the lower PIPs may help protect their patients from ventilator-induced lung injury (VILI). This logic is flawed; the pulmonary edema and lung injury, often seen during mechanical ventilation, are now believed to be the consequence of excessive volume (volutrauma) rather than excessive pressure (barotrauma) (48,49). Furthermore, the main determinant of volutrauma appears to be end-inspiratory lung volume (the overall lung distention) rather than the FRC (which depends on PEEP) (19,37). Based on this information, reducing PIP by waveform selection offers no advantage; patients supported with VCV receive the same V_T, and therefore overall lung expansion, regardless of waveform (Fig. 128.14).

Inspiratory flow waveforms impact yet another aspect of mechanical ventilation: patient–ventilator synchrony. During any form of patient-triggered mechanical ventilation, the spontaneous inspiratory effort may extend well into mechanical inflation. If, at any point, spontaneous flow demand exceeds the preset V_I, flow starvation results. Flow starvation distorts pressure patterns and exaggerates WOB. Decelerating flow patterns often provide initial V_I spontaneous sufficient to meet patient demand; if at any point, however, V_I is reduced below that the patient is demanding, flow starvation follows. Often, flow starvation of this nature can be managed by simply switching from a decelerating to a constant waveform to maintain a higher V_I throughout the breath (Fig. 128.15).

Controlled Ventilation

Operational Principles

Mechanical ventilation is indicated when spontaneous ventilation is inadequate or absent. Physiologically, this means the patient is incapable of maintaining acceptable $PaCO_2$ and arterial pH levels. CMV delivers an operator-selected breathing rate, V_T, peak V_I, and flow pattern; CMV operates completely independent of patient efforts to breathe (Fig. 128.16A). When patients attempt to breathe during CMV, the result can be

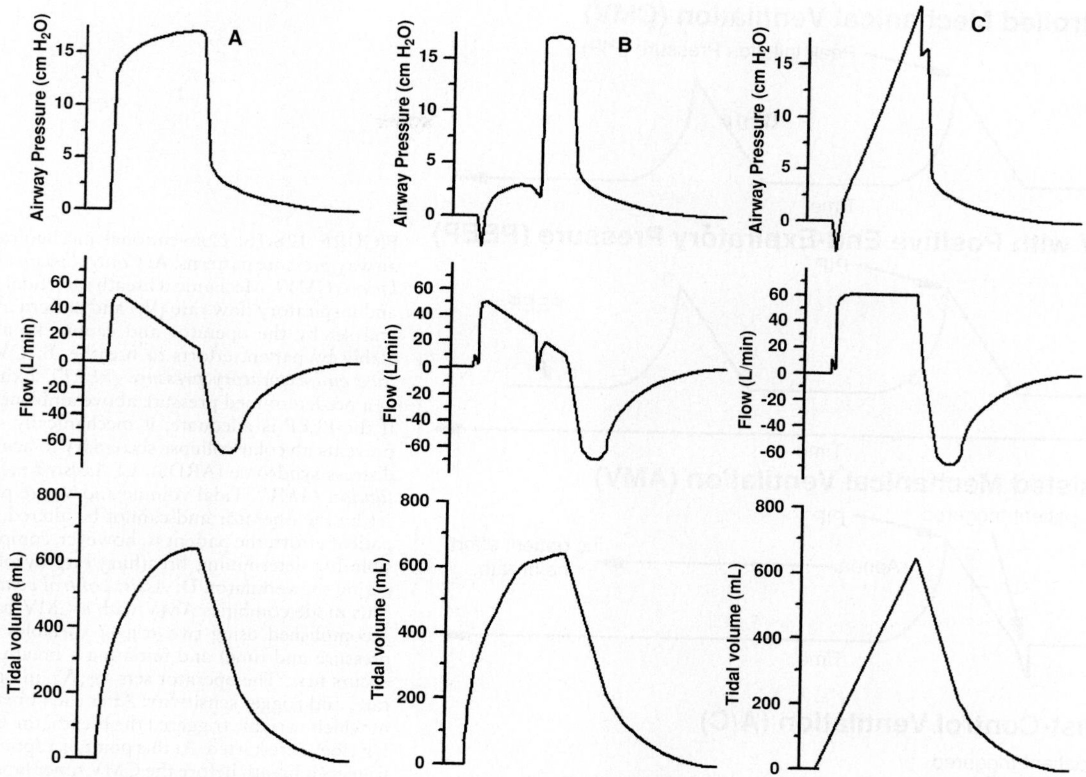

FIGURE 128.15. Improving patient–ventilator synchrony using a square instead of decelerating flow waveform, during volume-controlled ventilation (VCV). **A:** *An airway pressure (P_{aw}), flow, and tidal volume (V_T) curve for a heavily sedated or very relaxed patient receiving VCV.* **B:** *An airway pressure, flow, and V_T curve for the same patient, except the patient is awake, alert, and "fighting the ventilator,"*; that is, attempting to breathe spontaneously during machine breaths. Note that both the P_{aw} pressure pattern and V_I pattern are distorted by the patient's effort. Distortions are often exacerbated by the selected flow pattern, particularly the decelerating pattern, which progressively reduces V_I while patient flow demands may remain high. In situations where the patient flow demand exceeds V_I from the ventilator, a tremendous additional workload is imposed on the patient; this predisposes to fatigue and makes managing the patient difficult. **C:** *An airway pressure, flow, and V_T curve for the same patient, making the same effort to breathe spontaneously, except the selected V_I pattern is switched from decelerating to square.* Note that peak V_I is nearly identical in each case; yet, by maintaining a high flow longer, a square flow pattern better meets the patient flow demand.

violent patient–ventilator dyssynchrony. Consequently, patients supported by CMV often require hyperventilation to blunt the normal stimulus to breathe, heavy sedation, or even pharmacologic paralysis.

Clinical Applications

Indications for CMV and CMV with PEEP (Fig. 128.16B) include apnea, ARDS, central nervous system depression, drug overdose, or neuromuscular dysfunction. For this subset of patients, an accidental disconnection from the ventilator or a ventilator failure is life threatening. Thus, CMV requires vigilant monitoring and carefully set disconnect and failure-to-cycle alarms.

Patient-triggered Ventilation

Operational Principles

There are two basic forms of patient-triggered breaths: mechanical and spontaneous. Patient-triggered mechanical breaths (Fig. 128.16C) are nearly identical to CMV breaths in that the V_T, peak V_I, and flow pattern are all operator selected; the only difference is assisted mechanical ventilation (AMV) which requires that the patient trigger each and every breath. Thus, when supported by AMV, patients must not experience an acute apneic episode; otherwise, all ventilation ceases. Concern for this possibility explains why so few physicians opted to use AMV before ventilators came equipped with backup ventilator modes. For AMV, a backup mode might allow the operator to select desired CMV settings which the ventilator defaults to and uses in the event of apnea.

Clinical Applications

Patient-triggered ventilation is considered a vital link between CMV and extubation. In theory, it allows the patient to breathe spontaneously in preparation for removal of the ventilator. Spontaneous breathing is never consistent, however, meaning AMV is extraordinarily difficult to optimize to a patient's efforts. If the preset V_I, V_T, or both are too high, patient WOB falls to essentially zero; if they are insufficient or the patient becomes dyssynchronous, WOB skyrockets.

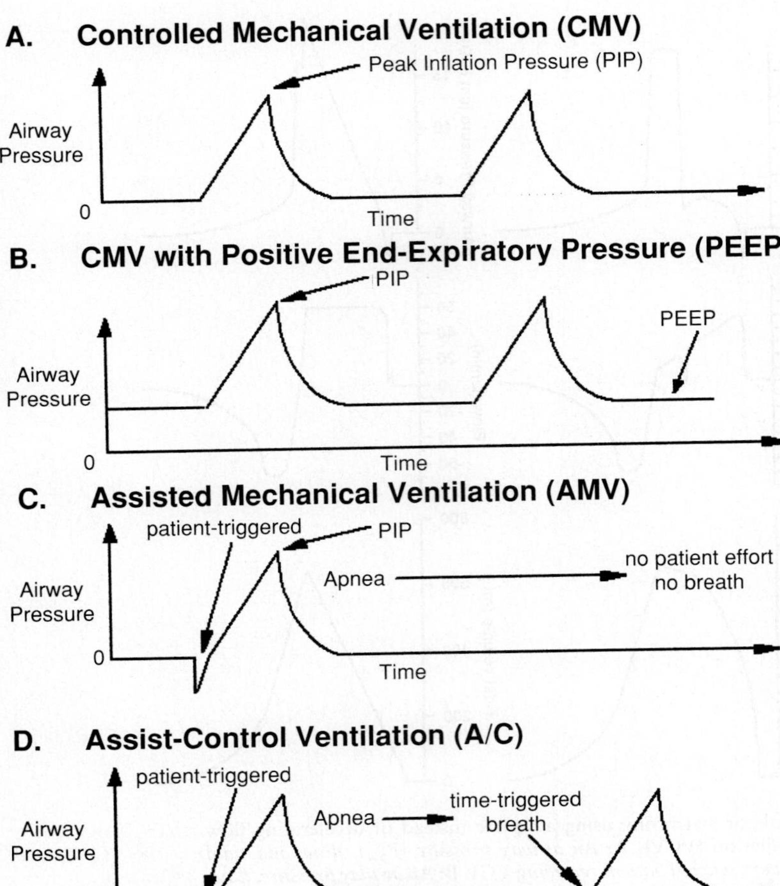

FIGURE 128.16. Conventional mechanical ventilatory airway pressure patterns. **A:** *Controlled mechanical ventilation (CMV)*. Mechanical breath rate, tidal volume (V_T), and inspiratory flow rate (V_I) and pattern are all selected and set by the operator and cannot be altered appreciably by patient efforts to breathe. **B:** *CMV with positive end-expiratory pressure (PEEP)*. Exhalation stops at a predetermined pressure above ambient (PEEP level). If the PEEP is adequate, it mechanically stabilizes and prevents alveolar collapse secondary to acute respiratory distress syndrome (ARDS). **C:** *Assisted mechanical ventilation (AMV)*. Tidal volume and V_I are prescribed and set by the operator and cannot be altered, regardless of patient effort; the patient is, however, completely responsible for determining breathing rate by physically triggering the ventilator. **D:** *Assist-control ventilation (A/C)*. This mode combines AMV with a CMV backup. This is accomplished using two trigger variables (for instance, pressure and time) and initiating a breath to whichever occurs first. The operator sets V_T, V_I and pattern, CMV rate, and trigger sensitivity. After each breath, regardless of which variable triggered the breath, the CMV rate timing clock is restarted. At this point, if a spontaneous effort triggers a breath before the CMV timer lapses, the breath is pressure triggered and the CMV clock restarted. If the patient fails to breathe or cannot spontaneously trigger, the CMV clock will run down and the next breath will be time triggered. Using the A/C strategy, patients may breathe as rapidly as they desire, but never at a rate lower than the CMV mechanical rate setting.

CMV Backup

The use of dual-trigger variables allowed clinicians to safely use AMV well before the incorporation of backup modes. Patient-triggered support with a time-triggered CMV backup was coined *assist/controlled ventilation* (A/C) (Fig. 128.16D). When using A/C, the operator sets a minimum acceptable breathing rate using the CMV rate control, and adjusts trigger sensitivity (usually pressure). As with AMV, the patient triggers breaths, as often as desired, by breaching the trigger threshold. If the patient stops breathing, however, or the spontaneous breathing rate drops below the preset minimum, time-triggered CMV intercedes until a clinician investigates or adequate breathing activity resumes.

Potential Problems

Assisted mechanical ventilation and CMV, used alone or in conjunction, predispose to hyperventilation, ventilator-induced V_A/Q abnormalities, and excessive WOB. These untoward effects are related to anxiety-driven ventilator–patient dyssynchrony and maldistribution of ventilation, respectively. A disproportionate amount of the V_T is delivered anteriorly to nondependent lung regions with decreased perfusion when patients are in the supine position (50). Conversely, spontaneous breathing tends to promote better V_A/Q distribution. Some studies have demonstrated that V_D increases during CMV and AMV, with or without PEEP (51,52) Downs and Mitchell (51) reported that increases in V_D were related to the rate of mechanical breathing, regardless of the ventilatory pattern, mode, and whether or not PEEP was used.

As mentioned, ventilator-patient dyssynchrony is very common during CMV, AMV, and A/C modes of ventilation. These modes all require preset V_I and flow waveforms while patient breathing patterns frequently vary. When patient flow demand exceeds that provided by the ventilator, the WOB imposed on the patient may become excessive (22). Recent trends toward smaller mechanical V_Ts have exacerbated the issue (53). Patients allowed to breathe spontaneously while receiving low-V_T lung-protective ventilation will likely suffer from both flow and volume starvation (Fig. 128.17); the additional WOB can be enormous. Clinicians facing this situation are left with few palatable options: increasing V_T and V_I predispose to ventilator-induced lung injury; yet, continued sedation or paralysis will undoubtedly complicate or prolong the weaning process.

Intermittent Mandatory Ventilation

Operational Principles

With spontaneous breathing rates often >100 breaths per minute, infants with hyaline membrane disease confounded even the best early efforts at patient–ventilator synchronization. The simple concept of providing a continuous flow, from which these babies could breathe spontaneously between

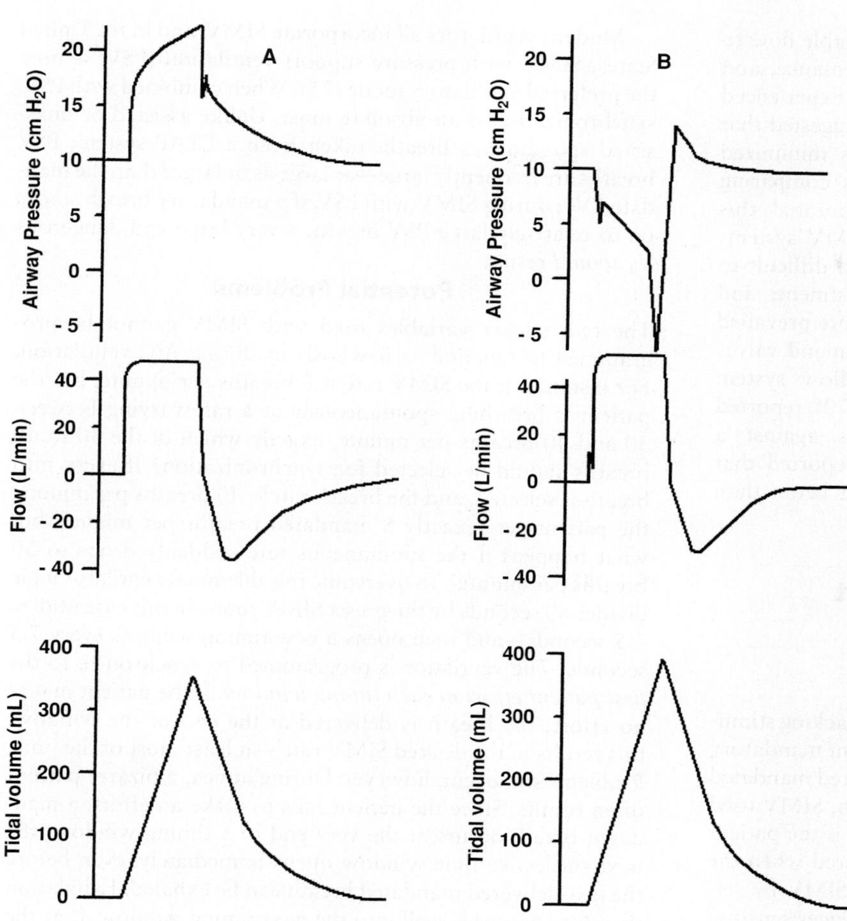

FIGURE 128.17. Flow and volume starvation during low tidal volume (V_T) ventilation. **A:** *An airway pressure (P_{aw}), flow, and tidal volume (V_T) curve for a heavily sedated or very relaxed patient receiving lung-protective low-V_T ventilation.* **B:** *An airway pressure, flow, and V_T curve for the same patient who is now awake, alert, and "fighting the ventilator."* Note that because both flow and V_T are insufficient, P_{aw} remains below baseline pressure throughout the entire inspiratory phase of the mechanical breath; distortions of this magnitude are frequently encountered if patients are allowed to breathe spontaneously when using lung-protective low-V_T ventilation.

mandated mechanical breaths (54–56), resulted in a new ventilatory mode referred to as *intermittent mandatory ventilation* (IMV). After proving its utility on neonates, IMV was later advocated for adults, especially those difficult to wean from mechanical ventilation (57). Neonatal IMV systems provided a continuous flow of gas throughout the respiratory cycle; tidal ventilation was accomplished by simply closing the exhalation valve and diverting flow into the lungs (54,55).

When applying IMV, the operator preselects the desired ventilator rate, V_T, V_I, and flow pattern; in this aspect, it does not differ from CMV. With IMV, however, the patient breathes as often as desired between sequential positive pressure breaths. In theory, a designed and adjusted IMV system provides an unrestricted gas flow equal to or greater than the patient's peak V_I demand; these conditions minimize WOB. Early IMV systems were "homemade" (58,59), leading some to opine that reported failures due to poor system design, not were to IMV, *per se* (60).

Clinical Applications

Most clinicians set an IMV rate sufficient to complement the patient's own spontaneous breathing and still maintain an acceptable alveolar ventilation, $PaCO_2$, and pH. Mandated breathing rates of 4 to 6 breaths per minute were popular because they provided an adequate V_A in the event of apnea. When patients with pre-existing COPD were managed with IMV and compared to others managed with patient-triggered ventilation, IMV offered better control of $PaCO_2$ and pH (61,62). When IMV is combined with CPAP, the cardiopulmonary effects are improved compared to CMV or A/C modes of ventilation; as a result, IMV makes it possible to maintain higher mean expiratory positive pressures with fewer deleterious effects on venous return and cardiac output (63,64).

Potential Problems

IMV and CMV share many similarities, such as preset V_T, V_I, and flow waveform. Furthermore, with both modes, all mandated breaths are time triggered, unresponsive to any patient effort. During IMV, however, the patient breathes freely, as desired. It follows that, occasionally, a time-triggered breath might be delivered at or near end-inhalation for a spontaneous breath (breath-stacking); if the stacked volumes were large enough, they would predispose to elevated PIP, mean P_{aw}, and cardiovascular embarrassment; without any compelling evidence validating this hypothesis, many clinicians nevertheless completely avoided IMV.

The concept of providing an unimpeded continuous gas flow equal to or exceeding the patient's peak V_I introduced an unexpected consequence to developing safe and effective IMV systems: finding a humidifier capable of the task. Poulton and Downs (65) studied the issue and reported that with the exception of the Bird humidifier, the others tested either imposed significant flow resistance—which would certainly affect patient WOB—or failed to provide sufficient humidity at the high flow rates IMV often required.

Breathing spontaneously requires patient WOB; the amount of work required, however, depends on a number of physiologic and external apparatus variables such as C_{RS}, R_{aw}, effort required to trigger breaths (if needed), available flow to that demanded, ET size, exhalation valve performance, and the magnitude and duration of the pressure drop experienced during inhalation. Downs (60) and others (66) suggested that properly adjusted continuous-flow IMV systems minimized the apparatus portion of WOB; several studies comparing continuous-flow to demand-flow valves corroborated this theory (67–69). Nevertheless, continuous-flow IMV systems were never popular—they were bulky, noisy, and difficult to adequately humidify; required frequent readjustment; and wasted massive amounts of gas. Clinicians therefore prevailed on manufacturers to refine and improve their demand valves or demand-flow systems. Gradually, demand-flow system performance improved; by 1985, Katz et al. (70) reported comparing seven demand-flow CPAP systems against a continuous-flow system (at 60 L/minute) and reported that some demand-flow systems performed as well or better than the continuous-flow system.

Synchronized Intermittent Mandatory Ventilation

Operational Principles

Clinical concerns about the potential for breath-stacking stimulated the development of synchronized intermittent mandatory ventilation (SIMV), which allowed patient-triggered mandated breaths. That is, like the A/C mode of ventilation, SIMV used two trigger variables, usually pressure and time; if the patient failed to trigger, an IMV breath was time triggered when the rate clock reached zero. Operators established SIMV by setting patient rate, V_T, V_I, flow waveform, and trigger sensitivity. Otherwise, as with IMV, the patient was free to breathe spontaneously as desired.

Clinical Applications

Proponents believed SIMV would eliminate breath-stacking, promote patient–ventilator synchrony, and minimize cardiovascular effects. These benefits were not all easily substantiated. Shapiro et al. (71) reported that mean intrapleural pressure was substantially lower with SIMV than with IMV in normal volunteers. Hasten et al. (72) compared SIMV and IMV in 25 critically ill patients; they found that although PIP was higher, blood pressure, cardiac output, stroke index, central venous pressure, and pulmonary artery pressure did not differ significantly. In a similar study, Heenan et al. (73) studied anesthetized, near-drowned dogs ventilated with IMV or SIMV. Again, no differences were noted with respect to cardiac output, stroke volume, intrapleural pressure, and intrapulmonary shunt. Mean airway pressure and PIP were significantly elevated with IMV, and some breath-stacking occurred, but the authors noted no adverse effects from these differences. Based on these data, SIMV seems to offer little clinical advantage compared to IMV with CPAP. There is a logical explanation for these findings, however: spontaneously breathing critically ill patients seldom inspire large spontaneous V_T from CPAP systems. In fact, the high-rate/low-V_T breathing pattern is extremely common; indeed, a high breathing frequency (f) to V_T or f/V_T ratios correlates well with extubation success (74). So, IMV breath-stacking, when it does occur, is unlikely to result in dangerously high spontaneous V_T, PIP, or cardiovascular interference.

Modern ventilators all incorporate SIMV, and in the United States, SIMV with pressure support ventilation (PSV) is now the preferred ventilatory mode (75). When combined with PSV, synchronization is an absolute must. Unlike assisted or unassisted spontaneous breaths taken from a CPAP system, PSV breaths are frequently large—as large as or larger than the mandated V_T; during SIMV with PSV, if a mandatory breath stacks on to relatively large PSV breath, a very large and dangerous V_T *would* result.

Potential Problems

The two trigger variables used with SIMV cannot be programmed to function as flawlessly as during A/C ventilation. For instance, if the SIMV rate is 8 breaths per minute, but the patient is breathing spontaneously at a rate varying between 30 and 40 breaths per minute, exactly which of the 30 to 40 breaths should be selected for synchronization? If every fifth breath is selected, and the breath rate is 40 breaths per minute, the patient gets exactly 8 mandated breaths per minute; but what happens if the spontaneous rate suddenly drops to 30 breaths per minute? To overcome this dilemma, ventilator logic divides 60 seconds by the preset SIMV rate—in this case $60/8 = 7.5$ seconds—and then opens a new timing window every 7.5 seconds. The ventilator is programmed to synchronize to the *first patient effort in each timing window*. If the patient makes no effort, the breath is delivered at the end of the window; this results in the desired SIMV rate—at least most of the time. Problems still occur, however. During apnea, a bizarre pattern often results. Since the patient fails to make an effort, a mandated breath occurs at the very end of a timing window; the next successive time window opens immediately, even before the just-delivered mandated breath can be exhaled. Exhalation therefore proceeds well into the next timing window. If at the end of this exhalation, P_{aw} falls a few cm H_2O below baseline pressure, as often happens, the ventilator often mistakes this pressure drop for the first patient effort in the timing window and—delivers a second successive SIMV breath, a phenomenon often referred to as *autotriggering*. The strange behavior does not end there. Since the ventilator has already "synchronized" to the first breath in the present timing window, and because the patient is apneic, it will not trigger again until the next successive timing window expires. A breathing pattern consisting of two consecutive mandated breaths, followed by 15 seconds without a mandated breath, followed by two consecutive mandated breaths repeats over and over (Fig. 128.18). Despite the bizarre appearance, the patient actually receives the eight mandated breaths per minute, just not in the pattern expected. Autotriggering is easily rectified by increasing trigger sensitivity to a point just below the pressure drop noted at end-exhalation. There is a caveat to this solution, however. Increasing trigger sensitivity makes triggering more difficult. Therefore, the operator must be sure to readjust the sensitivity as soon as spontaneous breathing activity resumes.

Pressure Support Ventilation

Operational Principles

Pressure support ventilation likely developed as a method to counteract the additional WOB imposed by early, poorly designed demand valves and demand-flow systems (28).

As demand systems improved, the WOB imposed by the breathing apparatus approached zero; still, patients often

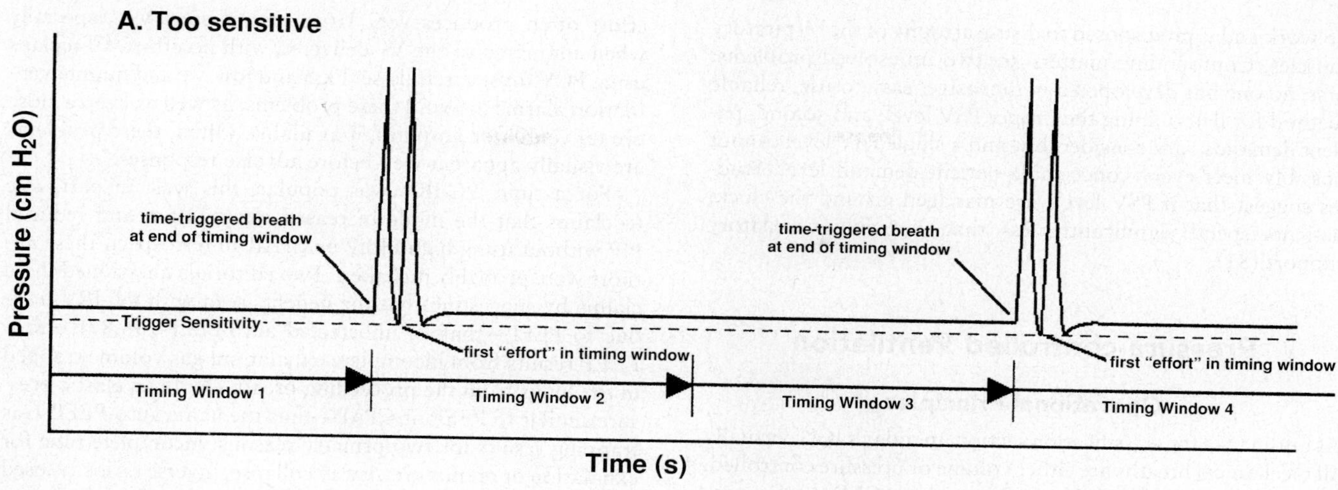

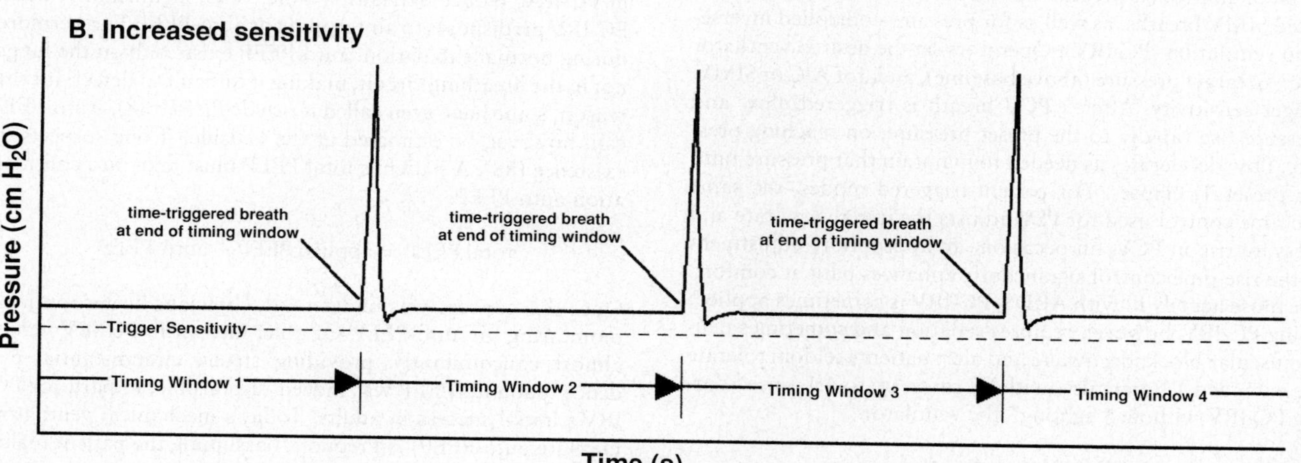

FIGURE 128.18. Synchronized intermittent mandatory ventilation (SIMV) and autotriggering during apnea. A: *Too sensitive*. An airway pressure curve demonstrating how trigger sensitivity set for normal breathing may be too sensitive during apnea. SIMV modes are programmed to synchronize to the first patient effort in each timing window. When no effort occurs, as during apnea, the ventilator must time trigger at the end of the timing window. If sensitivity is set too low (1–2 cm H_2O), exhalation from the previous breath may appear as the first effort in the next timing window and autotrigger a breath. This scenario results in a bizarre breathing pattern: two breaths in succession, followed by a very long pause and two breaths in succession; the pattern then repeats. Interestingly, this pattern delivers the preset breathing rate, but not in the sequence expected. B: *Increased sensitivity*. An airway pressure curve of the same apneic patient, except that trigger sensitivity is increased to a pressure lower than that occurring during exhalation; this eliminates autotriggering and results in a more uniform pattern of ventilation.

struggled to overcome the WOB imposed by the ET (29,30). Furthermore, increased R_{aw} and/or reduced C_{RS} increased patient physiologic WOB, often significantly (76). There were plenty of reasons to continue using PSV.

Pressure support is an assisted spontaneous breathing mode; it can be used alone or in conjunction with SIMV. It is patient triggered, pressure controlled, and is generally flow cycled (at 25%–50% of peak V_I). Patients receiving PSV control their own breathing rate and exert some control over V_T, peak V_I, and T_I. Originally, operators preset only the desired PSV level in cm H_2O above the baseline pressure. PSV, however, generates very high initial V_I; on occasion, the flow was too high for patient comfort (77). This shortcoming was corrected in the latest generation of ventilators by adding a "rise time" control. Clinicians use this control to adjust peak V_I up or down to meet patient needs.

Clinical Application

Pressure support has replaced CPAP as the spontaneous breathing mode used during SIMV. PSV helps to reduce WOB by partially unloading the respiratory muscles. Approaches to the use of PSV vary; some advocate just enough PSV to zero-out any additional WOB imposed by the breathing apparatus and ET (25,27,29,78), whereas others try to neutralize both the imposed WOB and some of the physiologic WOB—enough to provide comfort and avoid fatigue. With backup modes for safety, some use PSV as a stand-alone (79,80).

Potential Problems

Despite its promise, PSV may have created more problems than it solved. If set too low, the patient continues to struggle and may fatigue; set too high, the patient does essentially no work and is predisposed to disuse atrophy of the respiratory muscles. Confounding matters are two unresolved problems: first, no one has developed a noninvasive, easy-to-use, reliable method for determining the proper PSV level; and second, patient demands vary considerably, and a single PSV level cannot possibly meet every conceivable patient demand level. Studies suggest that if PSV levels are managed around the clock, patients spend significantly less time receiving ventilatory support (81).

Pressure-controlled Ventilation

Operational Principles

As outlined in the classification section, in today's ICU, virtually all mechanical breaths are either volume or pressure controlled. Pressure-controlled breaths can be used for CMV, A/C, mandated SIMV breaths, as well as for pressure-controlled inverse-ratio ventilation (PC-IRV). Operators set the desired ventilator rate, T_I, target pressure (above baseline), and, for A/C or SIMV, trigger sensitivity. After a PCV breath is triggered, flow and pressure rise rapidly to the preset pressure; on reaching pressure, flow decelerates as needed to maintain that pressure until the preset T_I elapses. For patient-triggered modes, the same rise time control used for PSV adjusts the initial flow rate and pressure rise in PCV; on occasion, an appropriate adjustment of the rise time control significantly enhances patient comfort. For those acutely ill with ARDS, PC-IRV is sometimes applied. Using PC-IRV, however, requires sedation and sometimes neuromuscular blockade; awake and alert patients seldom tolerate the extended T_I intervals—with I:E ratios up to 4:1—used during PC-IRV without "fighting" the ventilator.

Clinical Applications

Clinicians opt for PCV instead of VCV for three reasons or some combination thereof: (i) to provide higher initial and average V_I for patients breathing spontaneously during mechanical breaths; (ii) to control PIP and limit the possibility of VILI; and/or (iii) to use PC-IRV. Although several studies report improvements in oxygenation at lower PIP using PC-IRV with infants (82,83), its use in adults (84,85) remains limited. Clearly, PC-IRV elevates mean P_{aw}, which in turn raises FRC. Proponents of PC-IRV, however, claimed similar improvements in oxygenation to those seen using VCV but at much lower CPAP or PEEP levels. Using PCV as a method to control PIP and minimize the risk of VILI is an interesting approach. However, if the culprit in VILI is the end-inspiratory lung volume and not the PIP, then the approach is terribly flawed. That is, during PCV, the patient is free to interact with the ventilator. If the patient inhales deeply during any pressure-controlled breath, the resultant spontaneous V_T may be quite large. Thus, while PCV may control P_{aw} precisely, it fails to limit V_T to a safe level. Along the same lines, using PCV to provide higher peak and average V_I makes sense only if the attending clinician is comfortable with the potential for a large range in spontaneous V_T.

Potential Problems

The defining characteristics of PCV are high peak V_I, decelerating flow waveform, and no control over V_T. At one extreme, PCV continues to control pressure even if the ET occludes and V_T drops to zero; at the other extreme, a vigorous patient effort often produces very large spontaneous V_T, especially when compared to the V_T delivered with no effort. Clinicians using PCV must carefully set high and low V_T and minute ventilation alarms to avoid these problems, as well as keep a close eye on ventilator graphics, if available. Often, these problems are visually apparent well before adverse responses.

For a time, PC-IRV was popular; this was, in part, due to claims that the mode increased oxygenation and reduced PIP without using high PEEP or CPAP. In retrospect, these authors were probably mistaken. Two editorials questioned these claims by suggesting that the benefits seen with PC-IRV *were* due to PEEP—that is, undetected auto-PEEP (86,87). *Auto-PEEP* results from incomplete exhalation; gas volume trapped in the lungs from the proceeding breath exerts an elastic pressure similar to PEEP or CPAP—thus the name auto-PEEP. Gas trapping results for two primary reasons: incomplete time for exhalation or premature airway collapse. Inverse ratios, as used in PC-IRV, reduce exhalation time, often significantly; hence PC-IRV predisposes to air trapping or auto-PEEP. Furthermore. during normal exhalation, auto-PEEP exists only in the lungs, not in the breathing circuit, making it difficult to detect; for this reason, some have even called it *occult-PEEP* (88). Auto-PEEP can, however, be estimated at the bedside, if one suspects its existence (88). A patient's total PEEP must take into consideration auto-PEEP:

$$\text{total PEEP} = \text{applied PEEP} + \text{auto-PEEP} \qquad [3]$$

Once this concept was understood, clinicians began routinely monitoring for auto-PEEP. Of note, interest in PC-IRV waned almost concomitantly, providing strong circumstantial evidence that auto-PEEP was indeed responsible, in part, for PC-IRV's initial success in adults. Today's mechanical ventilators measure auto-PEEP "on request," assuming the patient makes no effort to breathe during the measurement.

SPONTANEOUS BREATHING

CPAP and Spontaneous PEEP

Operational Principles

Given the improvements in oxygenation, V_A/Q, C_{RS}, and WOB attributed to using PEEP or CPAP during mechanical ventilation (14–16,68,89), it seems logical to use them as stand-alone modes. With CPAP, both inspiratory and expiratory pressures remain positive. As a practical matter, the inspiratory pressures are lower than expiratory during CPAP. This occurs for three reasons: (i) during inspiration, the removal of gas from the continuous flow by the patient causes pressure to fall; (ii) triggering a demand CPAP system generally requires that pressure fall; (iii) the CPAP system cannot meet the patient's inspiratory flow demands. By definition, spontaneous PEEP requires that the patient reduce P_{aw} to zero or less during the inspiratory phase; P_{aw} returns to the PEEP level during exhalation. Spontaneous PEEP differs from CPAP in that the large pressure fluctuations during inspiration impose a significantly greater WOB on the patient (90) (Fig. 128.19). When tolerated, however, the same large pressure swings improve venous return and cardiac output (91). Conversely, CPAP reduces patient WOB, but at the expense of cardiac output.

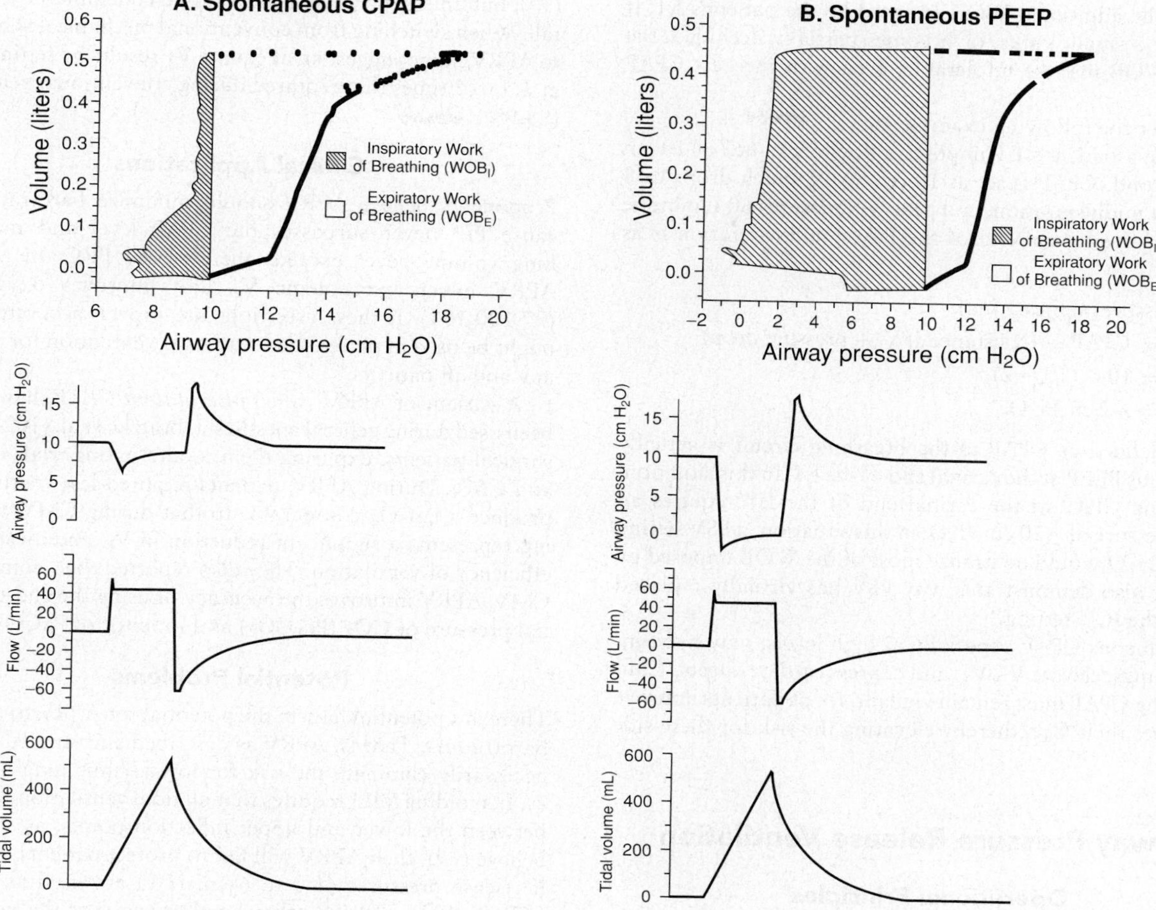

FIGURE 128.19. Work imposed by spontaneous continuous positive airway pressure (CPAP) or positive end-expiratory pressure (PEEP) breathing systems. The inspiratory work of breathing (WOB_I) encountered by patients breathing spontaneously is affected by the type of breathing system. Additional workloads imposed on spontaneously breathing patients are determined by measuring the area under the curve obtained by plotting airway pressure (P_{aw}) versus volume (V_T) loops taken at the proximal airway (i.e., at the endotracheal tube opening). End-expiratory pressure is 10 cm H_2O, while the simulated patient effort is identical for both systems. The additional WOB_I (*cross-hatched areas*) is computed from the area within the P_{aw}/V_T loop while P_{aw} remains below the starting point (10 cm H_2O). With the CPAP system, P_{aw} initially falls to 7 cm H_2O (during triggering) but quickly returns to 9 cm H_2O for the remainder of inspiration; with the spontaneous PEEP system, the same patient effort initially reduces P_{aw} to −2 cm H_2O, but it quickly returns to 0 cm H_2O. The computed WOB_I for the CPAP system is approximately 0.1 joules (J) and for the PEEP system 0.48 J, an increase of 480%. The expiratory work of breathing (WOB_E) is generally a nonfactor; the energy required to exhale is provided by the energy released as patients' highly elastic lungs, which were stretched during inflation, recoil to their resting position (like releasing a just-inflated party balloon).

Years ago, most CPAP and PEEP devices were "homemade"—there were no commercially available systems. Modern ventilators easily provide either spontaneous PEEP or CPAP and have obviated the need for homemade systems, particularly in the ICU setting. Using a ventilator to provide spontaneous PEEP or CPAP has distinct advantages; if the patient deteriorates, the ventilator is already on hand. Furthermore, modern ventilators often incorporate backup modes that automatically begin ventilating patients following any predefined. For example, a 15- to 60-second period of apnea.

The optimum level of PEEP or CPAP can be difficult to determine. For this reason, clinicians often start with a conservative level and then titrate based upon quantitative criteria such as serial blood gases (92,93), oximetry (94), computers (95), or even conjunctival oximetry (96).

Clinical Applications

The rationale for applying spontaneous PEEP or CPAP is the same, of whether they are used with or without mechanical ventilation: both techniques improve oxygenation, V_A/Q, C_{RS}, FRC, and WOB. Furthermore, CPAP/PEEP prevents airway collapse during exhalation and reduces the potential for low-volume lung injury.

Potential Problems

Both spontaneous PEEP and CPAP impose an additional workload on the patient's respiratory muscles. Of the two, there is no argument that spontaneous PEEP imposes a far greater workload. However, even a "perfect" CPAP system—one that allows little or no pressure deflection during inhalation—still does not eliminate the additional WOB imposed by the patient's ET. If an ET is too small, kinks, or becomes partially occluded, the patient's WOB may be intolerable, even with the best CPAP system.

Consider the following example:

Suppose a patient's ET imposes a flow resistance of 10 cm H_2O/L/second, CPAP is set at 10 cm H_2O, which drops to 8 cm H_2O at midinspiration, and peak V_I measures 60 L/minute; pressure at the carinal end of the ET at midinspiration is as follows:

$$\begin{aligned}&\text{pressure (at the carina)}\\&= \text{CPAP} - (\text{resistance at } V_I + \text{pressure drop})\\&= 10 - (10 + 2)\\&= -2\,\text{cm}\,H_2O\end{aligned}$$

What is defined as CPAP in the breathing circuit is actually spontaneous PEEP at the carinal end of the ET. In this situation, maintaining CPAP at the carinal end of the ET requires an airway pressure of $\geq$20 cm H_2O; in this situation, a PSV setting of 10 cm H_2O would neutralize most of the WOB imposed by the ET. It also demonstrates why PSV has virtually replaced CPAP in the ICU setting.

Spontaneous CPAP, especially at high levels, may hyperinflate the lungs, elevate V_D/V_T, and depress cardiac output. Clinicians using CPAP must remain vigilant, for as patients improve so too does their C_{RS}, thereby elevating the risk for these side effects.

Airway Pressure Release Ventilation

Operational Principles

Unlike conventional mechanical ventilation, airway pressure release ventilation (APRV) establishes an elevated baseline pressure—or CPAP level—ostensibly to restore FRC; tidal ventilation occurs by decreasing, or releasing, the CPAP. APRV allows unrestricted spontaneous breathing at all times, even during releases. Interestingly, with conventional ventilation, a higher breathing rate means a higher mean P_{aw}, which, in turn, reduces venous return and cardiac output; with APRV, however, a higher breathing rate actually lowers the mean P_{aw}. As a result, APRV has far less influence on cardiovascular parameters than a comparable level of CPAP.

During the process of initiating APRV, the operator presets the desired CPAP level, number of releases/minute (or breath rate), release time, and release pressure. Although it is possible to set V_T during APRV, it is a difficult trial-and-error process. V_T is limited by the CPAP level, release pressure, release time, and patient C_{RS}. For example, suppose a patient's CPAP level is set at 10 cm H_2O, C_{RS} is 50 mL/cm H_2O, and the release pressure is set to 0 cm H_2O. The maximum V_T for this patient is (assuming complete exhalation) as follows:

$$\begin{aligned}V_T &= \text{change in pressure} \times C_{RS}\\&= (10 - 0)\,\text{cm}\,H_2O \times 50\,\text{mL/cm}\,H_2O\\&= 500\,\text{mL}\end{aligned} \qquad [4]$$

Release volume or V_T also varies with release time; we get the maximum V_T only if release time is long enough for the lungs to completely empty. On many occasions, however, oxygenation deteriorates when using a release pressure of zero. When this happens, raising the release pressure will restore oxygenation (97), but unless the CPAP level is raised concomitantly, V_T will fall. When switching from conventional mechanical ventilation to APRV, some suggest an adequate V_T results by setting CPAP at 1.5 to 2 times that required during conventional ventilation (98,99).

Clinical Applications

Proponents believe APRV should minimize barotrauma because PIP never surpasses the CPAP level and maximum lung volume never exceeds the restored FRC. In addition, APRV lowers physiologic V_D and improves oxygenation (97,100,101). If these assertions are proven accurate, APRV might be used in place of conventional ventilation for virtually any and all patients.

A variant of APRV, called *intermittent CPAP*, has recently been used during general anesthesia. Bratzke et al. (102) studied surgical patients, exposing them to alternating trials of APRV and CMV. During APRV, patients required less ventilation to produce a $PaCO_2$ comparable to that during CMV; this finding represents a significant reduction in V_D and an improved efficiency of ventilation. They also reported that, compared to CMV, APRV improves the accuracy of using the end-tidal partial pressure of CO_2 ($P_{ET}CO_2$) as a monitor of $PaCO_2$.

Potential Problems

There is a potential flaw in the potential for APRV to minimize barotrauma. That is, APRV as described and studied does not necessarily eliminate the risk for low-volume lung injury (4–7). If avoiding VILI requires that all tidal ventilation take place between the lower and upper inflection points, as some now believe (19), then APRV will fail to protect patients, especially if release pressures of 0 to 6 cm H_2O are used as reported (97,100,101). On the other hand, given that the volumetric distance between the lower and upper inflection point is often small and that APRV maintains the same $PaCO_2$ levels as CMV with less ventilation, APRV may well offer the best lung-protective ventilatory strategy available. This assumes, of course, that the CPAP level is set to a pressure below the upper inflection point and the release level to a pressure above the lower inflection point (19).

SPECIAL TECHNIQUES

Pressure-targeted Volume Ventilation

Operational Principles

For years, the Food and Drug Administration (FDA) resisted approving any sort of "smart" ventilator setting. Pressure-targeted volume ventilation, pressure-regulated volume control (PRVC), or volume ventilation plus represent a distinct departure from that stance; this mode is far more automated than any before it. To initiate the mode, the operator presets a ventilator rate, V_T, T_I, and trigger sensitivity (if patient triggering is desired). On connecting the patient, the ventilator performs up to three test breaths. Test breaths are, as a rule, square flow pattern, volume-controlled breaths with a short end-inspiratory pause. Assuming one of the test breaths is not disturbed by patient attempts to breathe, the ventilator determines the patient's C_{RS} (Fig. 128.13 and Table 128.3). Once V_T and C_{RS} are known, the ventilator rearranges and solves equation 4:

$$\text{Pressure change (target)} = V_T/C_{RS}$$

Having determined the target pressure, the ventilator switches from the test breath protocol into what amounts to a smart PCV. For safety reasons, the ventilator begins PRVC using a pressure substantially below that calculated (above). The ventilator "watches" the exhaled V_T and gradually, over the next five to ten mechanical breaths, ramps up its pressure until the exhaled V_T equals that requested. At this point, the operator must thoughtfully set the ventilator's high P_{aw} limit based on the current target pressure and the maximum P_{aw} deemed safe for the patient. This setting is crucial because PRVC is not limited to the initial or starting target pressure. In fact, PRVC changes target pressure as often as required, within limits, to maintain an exhaled V_T equal to that requested. If, for instance, patient C_{RS} suddenly deteriorates, V_T also falls in direct proportion and concomitantly. The ventilator immediately detects the reduced exhaled V_T and increases target pressure at a rate of 2 or 3 cm H_2O per breath. Target pressure continues to increase with each breath until either exhaled V_T is restored or target pressure reaches a value no greater than the high P_{aw} limit minus 2 to 3 cm H_2O. The same but opposite response occurs should C_{RS} improve and V_T increase; that is, target pressure is reduced by 2 or 3 cm H_2O until the exhaled V_T is re-established, but target pressure can go no lower than baseline pressure (PEEP or CPAP level, if applicable) plus 3 cm H_2O.

Clinical Applications

In theory, PRVC combines the best aspects of both VCV and PCV: consistent V_T, delivered at lower PIP with high initial peak V_I. Some clinicians will consider using this mode for its ability to deliver the same V_T at lower PIP. There is no doubt this strategy works to lower PIP, but the same V_T produces the same ERP, regardless of how that volume is forced into the lungs (Fig. 128.14). This explains why, in two carefully controlled studies comparing PRVC to VCV, the researchers found significantly lower PIPs but were unable to detect any difference in outcome (103,104).

Others might consider using PRVC for its ability to provide high initial peak V_I, reduce WOB, and better synchronize with spontaneously active patients. Kallet et al. (53) looked at this issue during lung-protective ventilation, and concluded that PCV and PRVC offer no advantage in reducing WOB when compared to VCV with a high preset V_I.

Potential Problems

Conceptually, PRVC appears inherently safer than traditional PCV because it automatically maintains the preset V_T. Nevertheless, if the operator does not carefully set the high P_{aw} limit, PRVC may produce unexpected and dangerous changes. For instance, imagine a patient supported by PRVC with a V_T of 500 mL and a target pressure of 25 cm H_2O; the operator sets a high P_{aw} limit of 50 cm H_2O. Suppose this patient develops an acute tension pneumothorax and the affected lung collapses. The patient's apparent C_{RS} would suddenly be reduced by one half or more. If the mode were traditional PCV, V_T would be reduced to the same extent, thereby leaving the contralateral lung inflated by essentially the same V_T as prior to the pneumothorax. In contrast, V_T would also be initially reduced with PRVC, but almost immediately, PRVC would begin increasing the target pressure at 3 cm H_2O per breath in an effort to re-establish the preset exhaled volume. If the desired V_T was re-established by 47 cm H_2O (high P_{aw} limit minus 3 cm H_2O), then the entire initial V_T for both lungs is forced into the remaining good lung, risking hyperinflation and damage to this lung as well.

Proportional Assist Ventilation (PAV)

Operational Principles

As explained, PSV unloads potentially fatiguing workloads from spontaneously breathing patients. Unfortunately, it is difficult to determine the needed level of PSV, and PCV does not accommodate changes in patient breathing pattern. As a consequence, PSV either oversupports or undersupports the patient most of the time. Ideally, we need a variable support mode that automatically raises or lowers its response to maintain the same level of support, regardless of patient effort. Younes proposed such a mode, which he named *proportional assist ventilation* (PAV) (105,106). This mode relies on what is referred to as the equation of motion of the respiratory system, which states:

$$P_{aw} = V_T/C_{RS} + V_I \times R_{aw} \quad [5]$$

If C_{RS} and R_{aw} are known and the ventilator measures V_T and V_I instantaneously, as it provides them, the work required—measured as pressure—can easily be computed, regardless of effort level; recall that work is defined as the integral of P_{aw} with respect to time. If the ventilator also knows the ET size and flow resistance, stored in ROM, the ventilator can compute nearly the total WOB, although this approach cannot determine the work needed to inflate the chest wall. Estimating patient WOB in real time, throughout each and every breath, allows the ventilator to unload any quantifiable amount or percentage of that WOB; in fact, most PAV systems are preset to unload a specific percentage of the total WOB provided by the ventilator. For instance, if PAV was preset for 50%, the ventilator would measure the work being performed and provide exactly half of it. By measuring V_I and V_T, many times within each breath, PAV provides 50% of the work generated, regardless of how much or little effort the patient expends.

Assuming PAV works as theorized, it should meet a patient's varying needs by proportionally altering its response, a feature PSV cannot match. Nevertheless, PAV brings us no closer to a quantifiable and reliable method for determining an appropriate level of support; that is, we do not know what percentage of the total WOB the patient can tolerate. Manufacturers recommend starting PAV at a high percentage and gradually tapering down as the patient improves; the statement simply states the obvious and applies equally well to PSV.

Clinical Applications

If PAV proves effective, clinicians should use it in any instance when they would previously have used PSV. So far, PAV remains unproven and controversial. Giannouli et al. (107) compared different levels of PSV and PAV; they reported that PAV seemed more synchronous, but the differences had no effect on gas exchange or spontaneous breathing rate. Hart et al. (108) compared PAV to PSV in patients with neuromuscular and chest wall deformity and concluded that both modes produced similar improvements. Finally, Passam et al. (109) compared different levels of PSV and PAV on breathing pattern, WOB, and gas exchange in mechanically ventilated, hypercapnic COPD patients. They concluded that in COPD, although both PAV and PSV produced similar improvements in blood gases, higher levels of PSV often resulted in spontaneous efforts that failed to trigger breaths, whereas under similar circumstances, PAV developed the "runaway" phenomenon. Runaway occurs when, during PAV, the ventilator begins to trigger on and cycle off at rates much higher than the patient's actual spontaneous breathing frequency. Finally, another group reported that PAV was not superior to PSV in unloading the respiratory muscles following artificially increased ventilatory demand (110). These failures have caused some to question whether PAV represents any improvement over PSV (111,112).

Potential Problems

Based on existing research, patients respond very differently PAV than PSV; yet, the end results so far appear similar. To date, we have over 20 years of clinical experience using PSV. It makes little sense switching to PAV without a compelling reason to do so, especially if PAV is going to affect patients differently and in ways we may not yet understand. One of those differences involves the previously mentioned runaway, which results when the pressure provided by PAV exceeds the patient's elastance (inverse of C_{RS}) and R_{aw}, and persists into the exhalation phase. The physiologic problems that might result during runaway PAV remain to be thoroughly understood and unexplained.

TRANSPORT VENTILATION

Automatic or Manual Ventilation

Ventilation during transport is still often supported using a self-inflating bag (e.g., the Ambu device), a flow-inflating (Mapleson) system, or oxygen-powered breathing devices (Elder demand valve or similar device). This is indeed surprising in an era dominated by evidence-based medicine. The use of bags and valves, even in the most skilled hands, results in significant breath-to-breath differences in V_T, respiratory rate, minute ventilation, PIP and, in some cases, inspired fraction of oxygen (F_IO_2). These differences, acting alone or in combination, may disrupt arterial blood gases at the end of even a short intrahospital transport (113–116). Furthermore, bags and valves may not deliver an effective level of PEEP/CPAP and can make spontaneous breathing difficult. A portable ventilator with the proper capabilities is clearly a better choice.

Important Features for Transport Ventilation

Typical ICU-type mechanical ventilators are too large, cumbersome, and fragile to use for transports. Repairing a $30,000 ICU ventilator unintentionally tipped over or dropped during a rushed transport could easily cost as much or more than the purchase price of a new transport ventilator. Ruggedness is one of the more important, but often overlooked, characteristics desired in a transport ventilator (Table 128.4). Most practitioners opt for units that are electrically powered, with battery backup; nevertheless, an ideal unit would also work when powered only by compressed air or oxygen. Several hospitals in Hurricane Katrina's wake lost electric power for days following the storm. Absolutely nothing electric worked and batteries were all dead in a few hours; yet they had plenty of oxygen. Without properly equipped, pneumatically powered ventilators, however, these physicians and nurses simply could not adequately ventilate their sickest patients (39). Unfortunately, there are no currently manufactured transport or

TABLE 128.4

DESIRABLE CHARACTERISTICS FOR TRANSPORT VENTILATORS

Adult/pediatric use (>5 kg or 11 lb)
Transportable, rugged (<15 lb) and easily stored
Power source (pneumatic/electric with battery backup)
Battery life a minimum of 3 hrs
Nonproprietary, single use, universal breathing circuit
NBC filter–compliant (for use in nuclear, biologic, or chemically hazardous environments)
V_T (50–3,000 mL)
Rate (spontaneous—100 breaths/min)
F_IO_2 (adjustable at least between 0.6 and 1.0, preferably between 0.21 and 1.0)
PEEP/CPAP (0–20 cm H_2O)
Trigger sensitivity (<5 cm H_2O, regardless of CPAP level)
Inspiratory time (adjustable to 3.0 sec)
Breath types: Volume control (VC) and/or pressure control (PC), spontaneous continuous positive airway pressure (CPAP)
Alarms (audible and visual) should include:
- Low pressure/disconnect
- High pressure (3–75 cm H_2O)
- Loss of power (pneumatic or electric)
- Battery low (if applicable)
- Vent-inop
- Alarm silence (≥60 sec)

PEEP, positive end-expiratory pressure.

emergency ventilators that are powered either electrically or pneumatically. It seems only reasonable that disaster preparedness teams consider having at least a few pneumatic transport ventilators available; at present, with certain exceptions, this does not seem to be the case.

Spontaneous Breathing during Transport

Disaster preparedness for mass casualty scenarios or avian flu outbreaks has taken the country by storm. To meet the demand, many companies are either modifying existing ventilators for emergency use or are bringing new products to market. Currently, dozens of brands of transport and emergency ventilators are available; this makes the selection process truly difficult at best.

Perhaps a transport ventilator's spontaneous breathing capabilities provide us with a useful metric. Clearly, the act of spontaneous breathing reduces V_D (51,52,117,118). True spontaneous breathing, however, dramatically improves virtually every parameter associated with V_A/Q matching. Putensen et al. (117) compared APRV, which allows unrestricted spontaneous breathing, to PSV, which provides pressure assistance during each spontaneous breath. The APRV group demonstrated improved V_A/Q matching, venous return, right ventricular end-diastolic filling, stroke index, PaO_2, O_2 delivery, and mixed venous oxygen content when compared to PSV. In addition, APRV reduced V_D, intrapulmonary shunting, pulmonary vascular resistance, and O_2 extraction when compared to PSV (117). Given the compelling strength of the data, it is surprising so few clinicians consider the idea of spontaneous breathing during transport. Perhaps this oversight developed because so few transport ventilators allow effortless spontaneous breathing. Some might argue that patients do not really need to breathe spontaneously during a 10-minute transport. On the other hand, heavy sedation, paralysis, and CMV really do not appear to be in the best interest of potential avian flu victims.

The vast majority of true emergency or transport ventilators simply do not facilitate spontaneous breathing. Making matters worse, many use optional PEEP valves that attach to the exhalation valve, and demand valves that trigger at subambient pressure; these greatly magnify patient WOB as compared to CPAP, often requiring a herculean effort to trigger and maintain flow during spontaneous breaths (Fig. 128.19). To circumvent these issues, clinicians take one of several approaches: heavily sedate or even paralyze patients they plan to transport, thus allowing the use of CMV; or moderately sedate patients, allowing them to use the A/C mode of ventilation with minimal patient interaction.

For those wishing to avoid sedatives and paralytic agents, the transport ventilator needed is one that allows unimpeded, extremely low WOB spontaneous breathing. The pNeuton ventilator (Airon Corporation) is pneumatic and claims spontaneous WOB comparable to that of an ICU ventilator; unfortunately, this claim has not been scientifically validated. Without scientific data, testing ventilators with actual breathing will often expose a system's strengths and weaknesses in terms of its spontaneous breathing claims. Considering the potential benefit to patients allowed to spontaneously breathe during transport, it is surprising there are so few scientific studies thoroughly examining WOB as it applies to transport ventilators. Furthermore, the studies done so far are now dated; that is, they do not include many of today's newer and more popular models. For example, one study found the LTV 1000 (Pulmonetics) consistently produced WOB values comparable to those of critical care ventilators (117). The LTV 1000 has two distinct drawbacks as a transport ventilator. First, it will not tolerate the many "crash landings" most transport ventilators must endure. Second, the LTV 1000 uses a very precise, high-speed turbine compressor. When used in a dehumidified, heated, and air-conditioned environment like a hospital, the LTV 1000 will likely work for many hours without incident. On the other hand, if the LTV 1000 is even briefly exposed to the heat and humidity often found outdoors and is then moved back indoors, a potential exists for condensation to develop on the turbine's bearings. If this occurs, the lifespan of the turbine can be dramatically shortened.

SIDE EFFECTS AND COMPLICATIONS

Spontaneous Breathing

An understanding of the effects of any form of positive airway pressure requires a working knowledge of the physiology that drives spontaneous breathing. Normal spontaneous inspiration at ambient pressure involves contraction of the diaphragm. As the diaphragm contracts, a pressure gradient develops between the pleural space and the mouth; in response, air rushes from the mouth into the lungs. During expiration, the diaphragm relaxes, the gradient reverses, and the gas leaves the lungs.

Hemodynamics

Return of venous blood to the heart is dependent on the pressure gradient between the peripheral vasculature and the right atrium. If mean pressure rises or right atrial pressure (RAP) falls, venous return increases. Conversely, a fall in mean pressure or a rise in RAP decreases venous return. Because output of the right ventricle is dependent on the venous return factors that alter mean pressure and RAP also affect cardiac output (119).

Intrapleural Pressure Changes

A decrease in intrapleural pressure during inhalation is associated with a similar decrease in RAP which enhances venous return. During exhalation, intrapleural pressure increases and venous return falls; these fluctuations are familiar to anyone who has viewed a recording of central venous pressure in a spontaneously breathing patient.

Ventricular Interdependence

Because the right and left ventricles are surrounded by the pericardium, volume changes in one chamber affect the other. An increase in right ventricular volume during inspiration pushes the interventricular septum toward the left (posteriorly), thereby increasing left ventricular pressure; this in turn reduces left ventricular filling and changes the spatial configuration and compliance of the left ventricle.

Left Ventricular Afterload

The decrease in intrapleural pressure is also transmitted to the left ventricle. At the peak of spontaneous inspiration (lowest intrapleural pressure), the left ventricular end-diastolic pressure is reduced correspondingly. In contrast, the pressure that must be developed by the ventricle to perfuse the systemic vessels outside the thoracic cavity remains the same. Because the ventricle is initiating contraction from a lower baseline pressure, however, the gradient of pressure that must be generated is increased.

The increment in necessary wall tension represents an increase of the left ventricular afterload and may be tolerated poorly by patients with ischemic heart disease and compromised ventricular function. Spontaneous breathing with PEEP, which requires greater decrements in airway pressure and pleural pressures for gas to flow, predisposes to this chain of events. Conversely, a properly functioning CPAP system, which requires minimal deflections in airway and intrapleural pressures, minimizes such changes.

Pulmonary Vascular Changes

Expansion of the lungs also affects hemodynamic function. Alveolar vessels are compressed and elongated while pressure and alveolar volume increase. Extra-alveolar vessels, however, are opened by traction of lung inflation, with a consequent decrease in their resistance. When the alveolar vessels are engorged, inspiration decreases net pulmonary blood volume, and pulmonary venous return to the left ventricle may rise. Conversely, when alveolar vessels contain less blood, spontaneous inspiration changes alveolar blood volume very little, but a net increase in pulmonary blood volume and a concomitant decrease in pulmonary venous flow to the left ventricle occurs.

Spontaneous PEEP and CPAP

Common hemodynamic alterations seen during spontaneous PEEP or CPAP involve five major areas:

1. *Decreased venous return*: Most studies confirm increased intrapleural pressures, secondary to the increased mean airway pressures used by these modalities. This reduces the mean pressure/RAP gradient, which in turn reduces venous return. The heart has less blood to pump and output falls.
2. *Decreased right ventricular function*: Acute respiratory failure and PEEP/CPAP may, in some circumstances, increase pulmonary vascular resistance. Conceivably, the right ventricle might fail under these conditions; yet, this is probably not a major direct cause of positive pressure–induced cardiovascular insufficiency.
3. *Decreased left ventricular function*: Left ventricular dysfunction can result from increased mean airway pressures, but the changes are most likely the result of right ventricular dilatation and encroachment. Some investigators question this hypothesis, however. Prewitt and Wood (120) suggest that in selected instances (for example, high PEEP), 50% of the reduction in cardiac output results from left ventricular failure. Clearly, the mechanisms are complex and incompletely understood.
4. *Neural and humoral depression*: In canine cross-circulation studies, PEEP applied to one dog's lungs resulted in a reduction in cardiac output in both animals (121). The nature and composition of the depressant substance or substances is unknown.
5. *Reduction of endocardial blood flow*: It has been suggested that an increased mean airway pressure may act to impede coronary arterial blood flow (122). Such a decrease has been demonstrated experimentally during the use of PEEP.

Most studies show that spontaneous PEEP does not affect circulatory function adversely, as long as patients are not hypovolemic. These observations, oddly, are diametrically opposed to those expected during normal breathing. This phenomenon is best explained by the fact that PEEP is not generally used on *normal* lungs; when it is, FRC is raised above normal, often significantly. With more volume in the lungs, even during exhalation, venous return may be compromised. When either PEEP or CPAP is used therapeutically, however, patients invariably have reduced compliance and a significantly reduced FRC. Collapsed and underventilated alveoli produce hypoxic vasoconstriction in the affected areas; this often markedly increases pulmonary vascular resistance and abnormal loading of the right ventricle. As end-expiratory pressure is raised, FRC increases back toward normal, and underventilated alveoli reexpand; this releases some of the hypoxic vasoconstriction, and unloading of the right ventricle may occur.

Sturgeon et al. (91) reported the effects of 15 cm H_2O spontaneous CPAP, 15 cm H_2O spontaneous PEEP, and zero pressure on a group of patients following coronary artery bypass grafting. When receiving spontaneous PEEP, this group's cardiac output was 1 L/minute more when compared to spontaneous PEEP or zero pressure. The authors suggested that the very large intrapleural pressure drops of >15 cm H_2O—required to breathe from 15 cm H_2O PEEP—resulted in a substantially greater venous return. Also, as pleural pressure increased back to the 15 cm H_2O baseline during exhalation, the associated and likely pericardial compression may have aided ventricular ejection.

Large intrapleural pressure fluctuations are not always beneficial, and could easily overfill the right ventricle, resulting in an elevated left ventricular afterload. It is quite possible a worst case scenario could involve a patient with severe coronary artery disease and left ventricular failure, managed using a high level of spontaneous PEEP. The resultant increase in the left ventricular afterload on an already failing myocardium would predispose to a dramatic and potentially dangerous fall in systemic cardiac output, as well as acute pulmonary edema. Substituting a properly functioning spontaneous CPAP system with a minimal trigger sensitivity would, all other things being equal, unload the left ventricle by decreasing the preloading of the right ventricle.

Mechanical Ventilation

Hemodynamics

Falling Pressures. As a rule, any form of positive pressure breathing will reduce venous return and decrease right ventricular preload; with normal lungs, the effect is pronounced. Even modest increases in airway pressure will elevate the FRC well above normal; an increased intrapleural pressure from the overexpanded lungs presses the pericardium and compresses the heart. These conditions make interpreting filling pressures a challenge, as the central venous pressure (CVP) and pulmonary artery occlusion pressure may be elevated while ventricular stroke volumes are actually decreased.

Ventricular Function. As stated, the elevated airway pressures associated with positive pressure breathing increase the right ventricular afterload and, in turn, decrease venous inflow to the right heart. At the same time, transmural aortic pressure, left ventricular afterload, and end-systolic left ventricular volume fall. The reduced output volume is easily restored by intravascular volume expansion—enough to counteract some or all of airway pressure on venous return. If, after re-expansion of intravascular volume, the source of elevated airway pressure—i.e., ventilator or PEEP/CPAP system—is suddenly removed, a venous return surge that may be well beyond the initial baseline predisposes the patient to acute pulmonary edema (123); this complication is especially likely if the patient's left ventricle is compromised.

Robotham et al. (124) summarized the known and postulated effects of positive pressure inflation of the lungs on cardiopulmonary function; most of these have already been reviewed. They concluded that mechanical ventilation may act as a (relatively) noninvasive cardiac assist device and deserves further evaluation as such.

IMV/SIMV/CPAP. The hemodynamic effects of spontaneous breathing, with or without CPAP, and those secondary to positive pressure ventilation become complicated when combined, as during IMV/SIMV with CPAP. The cumulative effect likely depends on the relative contributions of spontaneous versus mandated breaths, as well as the absolute values of the inspiratory and expiratory pressures, V_T, baseline cardiovascular status, intravascular volume, and so forth. Ventilator performance also plays an important role, especially during spontaneous breathing.

A difficult-to-trigger CPAP system, or a poorly designed and slow-to-respond demand-flow valve, often requires major inspiratory efforts by the patient. These factors were the primary reason many early trials of IMV failed; that is, patients were simply fatigued to the point of failure by work imposed by the system—not by the technique.

Barotrauma and Ventilator-Induced Lung Injury

For many years, the concept of pulmonary barotrauma was limited to extra-alveolar air leaks. It is now abundantly clear that human lungs can be damaged internally by the ventilator with or without air leaks; this type of damage is known as *ventilator-associated lung injury* (VALI) and is reviewed in depth elsewhere (see Chapter 138).

Extra-alveolar Air Leaks. All forms of mechanical ventilation, whether by virtue of positive or negative pressure, rhythmically drive air in and out of the lungs. As outlined, mechanical ventilation disrupts normal hemodynamics, alters V_A/Q ratios, and occasionally damages the lungs. Pulmonary barotrauma (PBT) represents the classic form of VILI. Pulmonary barotrauma includes pneumothorax, pneumomediastinum, pneumopericardium, pneumoperitoneum, pneumoretroperitoneum, subcutaneous air, and air embolization—either venous or arterial. Interestingly, none of these conditions actually describe lung injury. Rather, each of these represents a form of extra-alveolar air; each occurs after the lung fabric is torn and an air leak follows. Air leaks occur following a tear in the fabric of lung parenchyma. If the tear involves the visceral pleura, a pneumothorax often results as the air quickly moves into the pleural space, which the pressure is negative relative to alveolar pressure most of the time. Tension pneumothorax is the most threatening variety of this problem and can obliterate cardiac output if not immediately decompressed. When an air leak occurs away from the pleura, the repeated stretching associated with positive pressure ventilation facilitates the dissection of air along the perivascular sheaths that parallel the airways. Eventually, the dissecting air reaches the pulmonary hilum, where it may invade the subcutaneous tissues of the neck or enter the mediastinum and beyond. Rarely, the rent exposes a vessel large enough for air to enter, and with sufficient air pressure changes (positive or negative), air may enter the circulation. Scuba divers who ascend too rapidly or hold their breath while surfacing can easily rupture their lungs. Because divers normally surface with their heads up, the air bubbles rise and may reach the brain. Cerebral air emboli can be fatal, particularly when the diver cannot be quickly recompressed in a hyperbaric chamber.

A common misconception—that PEEP and CPAP increase the incidence of barotrauma—persists even today. Yet, no increase in the incidence of barotrauma occurs when positive pressure ventilation and CPAP are compared with positive pressure alone (125,126).

SUMMARY

Mechanical ventilators continue to evolve rapidly in complexity, design, and function. It is quite likely this brisk pace will persist for many years. As outlined, it also seems likely that controversies regarding how and when to use ventilators safely and effectively will not be conclusively resolved anytime soon. This set of circumstances means that those of us responsible for prescribing, operating, monitoring, or repairing ventilators must rise to the challenge of maintaining an up-to-date knowledge base. This is no easy task but one that will result in significant benefits for all parties involved.

References

1. Kolobow T, Moretti MP, Famagalli R, et al. Severe impairment of lung function induced by high peak airway pressure during mechanical ventilation. *Am Rev Respir Dis.* 1987;135:312.
2. Tsuno K, Prato P, Kolobow T. Acute lung injury from mechanical ventilation at moderately high airway pressures. *J Appl Physiol.* 1990;69:956.
3. Bowton DL, Kong DL. High tidal volume ventilation increases lung water in oleic acid-injured rabbit lungs. *Crit Care Med.* 1989;17:908.
4. Hernandez LA, Cohen PJ, May AL, et al. Mechanical ventilation increases microvascular permeability in oleic injured lungs. *J Appl Physiol.* 1990;69:2057.
5. Taskar V, Evander JJE, Robertson B, et al. Surfactant dysfunction makes lungs vulnerable to repetitive collapse and reexpansion. *Am J Respir Crit Care Med.* 1997;155:313.
6. Argiras EP, Blakeley CR, Dunnill MS, et al. High PEEP decreases hyaline membrane formation in surfactant deficient lungs. *Br J Anaesth.* 1987; 59:1278.

7. Muscedere JG, Mullen JBM, Gan K, et al. Tidal ventilation at low airway pressures can augment lung injury. *Am J Respir Crit Care Med.* 1994; 149:1327.
8. Martin C, Papazian L, Payan MJ, et al. Pulmonary fibrosis correlates with adult respiratory distress syndrome: a study in mechanically ventilated patients. *Chest.* 1995;107:196.
9. Fariday EE, Permutt S, Riley RL. Effect of ventilation on surface forces in excised dogs' lungs. *J Appl Physiol.* 1966;21:1453.
10. Brown ES, Johnson RP, Clements JA. Pulmonary surface tension. *J Appl Physiol.* 1959;14:717.
11. Fariday EE. Effect of ventilation on movement of surfactant in the airways. *Respir Physiol.* 1976;27:323.
12. Dreyfuss D, Saumon G. Should the lungs be rested or recruited? The Charybdis and Scylla of ventilator management. *Am J Respir Crit Care Med.* 1994;149:1066.
13. Lachmann B. Open up the lung and keep the lung open. *Intensive Care Med.* 1992;18:319.
14. va Kaam AH, Haitsma JJ, DeJaegere, et al. Open lung ventilation improves gas exchange and attenuates secondary lung injury in a piglet model of meconium aspiration. *Crit Care Med.* 2004;32(2):443.
15. Falke KJ, Pontoppidan H, Kumar A, et al. Ventilation with end-expiratory pressure in acute lung disease. *J Clin Invest.* 1972;51:2315.
16. Suter PM, Fairley HB, Isenberg MD. Optimum end-expiratory pressure in patients with acute pulmonary failure. *N Engl J Med.* 1975;292:284.
17. Matamis D, Lemaire F, Harf A, et al. Total respiratory pressure-volume curves in the adult respiratory distress syndrome. *Chest.* 1984;86:58.
18. Benito S, Lemaire F. Pulmonary pressure-volume relationship in acute respiratory distress syndrome in adults: role of positive end-expiratory pressure. *J Crit Care.* 1990;5:27.
19. Dreyfuss D, Saumon G. Ventilator-induced lung injury: lessons from experimental studies. *Am J Resp Crit Care Med.* 1998;157:294.
20. Fernandez E, Weiner P, Meltzer E, et al. Sustained improvement in gas exchange after negative pressure ventilation for 8 hours per day on 2 successive days in chronic airflow limitation. *Am Rev Respir Dis.* 1991;144(2):390.
21. Skarburkis M, Rivero A, Fitchett D, et al. Hemodynamic effects of continuous negative chest pressure ventilation in heart failure. *Am Rev Respir Dis.* 1990;141:938.
22. Marini JJ, Capps JS, Culver BH. The inspiratory work of breathing during assisted mechanical ventilation. *Chest.* 1985;87(5):612.
23. Banner MJ, Kirby RR, Gabrielli A, et al. Partially and totally unloading the respiratory muscles based upon real-time measurements of work of breathing. A clinical approach. *Chest.* 1994:106(6):1835.
24. French CJ, Bellomo R, Buckmaster J. Effect of ventilation equipment on imposed work of breathing. *Crit Care Resuscitation.* 2001;3(3):148.
25. Bersten AD, Rutten AJ, Verdig AE, et al. Additional work of breathing imposed by endotracheal tubes, breathing circuits, and intensive care ventilators. *Crit Care Med.* 1989;17(7):671.
26. Banner MJ, Euliano NR, Brennan V, et al. Power of breathing determined non-invasively using an artificial neural network in patients with respiratory failure. *Crit Care Med.* 2006;34:1052–1059.
27. Banner MJ, Kirby RR, Blanch PB, et al. Decreasing imposed work of breathing apparatus to zero using pressure support ventilation. *Crit Care Med.* 1993;21(9):1333.
28. Kacmarek RM. The role of pressure support ventilation in reducing work of breathing. *Respir Care.* 1988;33(2):99.
29. Fiastro JF, Habib MP, Quan SF. Pressure support compensation for inspiratory work due to endotracheal tubes and demand continuous positive airway pressure. *Chest.* 1988;93(3):499.
30. Myny D, Depuydt P, Colardyn F, et al. Ventilator-associated pneumonia in a tertiary care ICU: analysis of risk factors for acquisition and mortality. *Acta Clin Belg.* 2005;60(3):114.
31. Jubran A. Critical illness and mechanical ventilation: effects on the diaphragm. *Respir Care.* 2006;51(9):1054.
32. Branson RD, Chatburn RL. Technical description and classification of modes of ventilator operation. *Respir Care.* 1992;37(9):1026.
33. Blanch PB, Jones MR, Layon AJ, et al. Pressure-preset ventilation, I: physiologic and mechanical considerations. *Chest.* 1993;104(2):590.
34. Blanch PB, Jones MR, Layon AJ, et al. Pressure-preset ventilation, II: mechanics and safety. *Chest.* 1993;104(3):904.
35. Hopewell PC, Murray JF. Effects of continuous positive pressure ventilation in experimental pulmonary edema. *J Appl Physio.* 1976;40:568.
36. Luce JM, Huang TW, Robertson HT, et al. The effects of prophylactic expiratory positive airway pressure on the resolution of oleic acid-induced injury in dogs. *Ann Surg.* 1983;197:327.
37. Dreyfuss D, Saumon G. The role of tidal volume, FRC and end-inspiratory volume in the development of pulmonary edema following mechanical ventilation. *Am Rev Respir Dis.* 1993;148:1194.
38. Smith TC, Marini JJ. Impact of PEEP on lung mechanics and work of breathing in severe airflow obstruction. *J Appl Physiol.* 1988;65(4):1488.
39. de Boisblanc BP. Black Hawk, please come down: reflections on a hospital's struggle to survive in the wake of Hurricane Katrina. *Am Rev Respir Crit Care Med.* 2005;172(10):1239.
40. Fuleihan SF, Wilson RS, Pontoppidan H. Effect of mechanical ventilation with end-expiratory pause on blood gas exchange. *Anesth Anal.* 1976; 55:122.
41. Banner MJ, Lampotang S. Clinical use of inspiratory and expiratory waveforms. In: Kacmarek RM, Stoller JK, eds. *Current Respiratory Care.* Philadelphia, PA: BC Decker; 1988:139.
42. Dammann JF, McAslan TC. Optimal flow pattern for mechanical ventilation of the lungs. *Crit Care Med.* 1977;5:128.
43. Hedenstierna G, Johansson H. Different flow patterns and their effect on gas distribution in a lung model. *Acta Anaesthesiol Scand.* 1973;17:190.
44. Jansson L, Jonson B. A theoretical study of flow patterns of ventilators. *Scand J Respir Dis.* 1972;55:237.
45. Al-Saady N, Bennett ED. Decelerating inspiratory flow waveform improves lung mechanics and gas exchange in patients on intermittent positive-pressure ventilation. *Intensive Care Med.* 1985;11:68.
46. Baker AB, Colliss JE, Cowie RW. Effects of varying inspiratory flow waveforms and time in intermittent positive-pressure ventilation, II: various physiologic variables. *Br J Anaesth.* 1977;49:1221.
47. Johansson H, Lofstrom JB. Effects on breathing mechanics and gas exchange of different inspiratory gas flow patterns during anesthesia. *Acta Anaesthesiol Scand.* 1975;19:8.
48. Dreyfuss D, Soler G, Basset C, et al. High inflation pressure pulmonary edema: respective effects of high airway pressure, high tidal volume, and positive end-expiratory pressure. *Am Rev Respir Dis.* 1988;137:1159.
49. Dreyfuss D, Saumon G. Barotrauma is volutrauma, but which volume is the one responsible? *Intensive Care Med.* 1992;18:139.
50. Froese AB, Bryan AC. Effects of anesthesia and paralysis on diaphragmatic mechanics in man. *Anesthesiology.* 1974;41:242.
51. Downs JB, Mitchell LA. Pulmonary effects of ventilatory pattern following cardiopulmonary bypass. *Crit Care Med.* 1976;4:295.
52. Murphy EJ, Downs JB. Ventilator induced ventilation-perfusion mismatching. *Anesthesiology.* 1976;45:A345.
53. Kallet RH, Campbell AR, Dicker RA, et al. Work of breathing during lung-protective ventilation in patients with acute lung injury and acute respiratory distress syndrome: a comparison between volume and pressure-regulated breathing modes. *Respir Care.* 2005;50(12):1623.
54. Kirby RR, Robison E, Schultz J. Continuous flow ventilation as an alternative to assisted or controlled ventilation in infants. *Anesth Analg.* 1972;51:871.
55. Kirby RR, Robison E, Shultz J. A new pediatric volume ventilator. *Anesth Analg.* 1971;50:533.
56. Munson ES, Eger EI 2nd. Controlled ventilation in the newborn. *Anesthesiology.* 1963;24:871.
57. Downs JB, Klein EF, Desautels D. Intermittent mandatory ventilation: a new approach to weaning patients from mechanical ventilators. *Chest.* 1973;64:331.
58. Desautels DA. PEEP and open IMV systems. *Respir Care.* 1977;22(11): 1230.
59. Bruining HA. Two simple assemblies for the application of intermittent mandatory ventilation with positive end expiratory pressure. *Intensive Care Med.* 1984;10(1):33.
60. Downs JB. Inappropriate applications of IMV. *Chest.* 1980;78(6):897.
61. Groeger JS, Levinson MR, Carlon GC. Assist control versus synchronized intermittent mandatory ventilation during acute respiratory failure. *Crit Care Med.* 1989;17:607.
62. Kirby RR. Synchronized intermittent mandatory ventilation versus assist control: just the facts ma'am. *Crit Care Med.* 1989;17:706.
63. Kirby RR, Perry JC, Calderwood HW. Cardiorespiratory effects of high end-expiratory pressure. *Anesthesiology.* 1975;43:533.
64. Kirby RR, Downs JB, Civetta JM. High level positive end-expiratory pressure (PEEP) in acute respiratory insufficiency. *Chest.* 1975;67:156.
65. Poulton TJ, Downs JB. Humidification of rapidly flowing gas. *Crit Care Med.* 1981;9:59.
66. Op't Holt TB. Work of breathing and other aspects of patient interaction with PEEP devices and systems. *Respir Care.* 1988;33(6):444.
67. Op't Holt TB, Hall MW, Bass JB, et al. Comparisons of changes in airway pressure during continuous positive airway pressure (CPAP) between demand valve and continuous flow devices. *Respir Care.* 1982;27(10):1200.
68. Gibney RT, Wilson RS, Pontoppidan H. Comparison of work of breathing on high gas flow and demand valve continuous positive airway pressure systems. *Chest.* 1982;82(6):692.
69. Henry WC, West GA, Wilson RA. A comparison of the oxygen cost of breathing between a continuous-flow CPAP system and a demand-flow system. *Respir Care.* 1983;28(10):1273.
70. Katz JA, Kraemer RW, Gjerde GE. Inspiratory work and airway pressure with continuous positive airway pressure delivery systems. *Chest.* 1985;88(4):519.
71. Shapiro BA, Harrison RA, Walton JR. Intermittent demand ventilation (IDV): a new technique for supporting ventilation in critically ill patients. *Respir Care.* 1976;21:521.
72. Hasten RW, Downs JB, Heenan TJ. A comparison of synchronized and nonsynchronized intermittent mandatory ventilation. *Respir Care.* 1980; 25:554.
73. Heenan TJ, Downs JB, Douglas ME. Intermittent mandatory ventilation: is synchronization important? *Chest.* 1980;77:598.
74. Yang KL, Tobin MJ. A prospective study of indexes predicting the outcome of trials of weaning from mechanical ventilation. *N Eng J Med.* 1991; 324(21):1445.

75. Esteban A, Anzueto A, Alia I, et al. How is mechanical ventilation employed in the intensive care unit? An international utilization review. *Am J Respir Crit Care Med.* 2000;161:1450.
76. Brochard L, Harf A, Lorino H, et al. Inspiratory pressure support prevents diaphragmatic fatigue during weaning from mechanical ventilation. *Am Rev Resp Dis.* 1989;33:99.
77. MacIntyre NR, Ho L-I. Effects of initial flow rate and breath termination criteria on pressure support ventilation. *Chest.* 1991;99:134.
78. Bolder PM, Healy EJ, Bolder AR, et al. The extra work of breathing through adult endotracheal tubes. *Anesth Analg.* 1986;65:853.
79. MacIntyre NR. Weaning from mechanical ventilatory support: volume-assisting intermittent breaths versus pressure-assisting every breath. *Respir Care.* 1988;33:121.
80. MacIntyre NR. Pressure support ventilation. *Prob Crit Care.* 1990;4:225.
81. Kirton OC, DeHaven B, Hudson-Civetta J, et al. Re-engineering ventilatory support to decrease days and improve resource utilization. *Ann Surg.* 1996;224(3):396.
82. Reynolds EOR. Effect of alterations in mechanical ventilator settings on pulmonary gas exchange in hyaline membrane disease. *Arch Dis Child.* 1971;46:159.
83. Spahr RC, Klein AM, Brown DR, et al. Hyaline membrane disease: a controlled study of inspiratory to expiratory ratio and its management by ventilator. *Am J Dis Child.* 1980;134:373.
84. Tharatt RS, Allen RP, Albertson TE. Pressure controlled inverse ratio ventilation in severe adult respiratory failure. *Chest.* 1988;94:755.
85. Gurevitch MJ, Van Dyke J, Young ES, et al. Improved oxygenation and lower peak airway pressure in severe adult respiratory syndrome: treatment with inverse ratio ventilation. *Chest.* 1986;89:211.
86. Duncan SR, Rizk NW, Raffin TA. Inverse ratio ventilation. PEEP in disguise [Editorial]? *Chest.* 1989;92:390.
87. Kacmarek RM, Hess D. Pressure-controlled inverse-ratio ventilation: panacea or auto-PEEP [Editorial]? *Respir Care.* 1990;35(10):945.
88. Pepe P, Marini JJ. Occult positive end-expiratory pressure in mechanically ventilated patients with airflow obstruction: the auto-PEEP effect. *Am Rev Respir Dis.* 1982;126(1):166.
89. Katz JA, Marks JD. Inspiratory work with and without continuous positive airway pressure in patients with acute respiratory failure. *Anesthesiology.* 1985;63:598.
90. Gherini S, Peters RM, Virgilio RW. Mechanical work on the lung and work of breathing with positive end expiratory pressure and continuous positive airway pressure. *Chest.* 1979;76:251.
91. Sturgeon CL, Douglas ME, Downs JB, et al. PEEP and CPAP: cardiopulmonary effects during spontaneous ventilation. *Anesth Analg.* 1977;56:633.
92. Kirby RR, Downs JB, Civetta JM, et al. High level positive end-expiratory pressure (PEEP) in acute respiratory failure. *Chest.* 1975;67(2):156.
93. Civetta JM, Kirby RR. Criteria for optimum PEEP. *Respir Care.* 1977;22(11):1171.
94. Rasanen J, Downs JB, DeHaven B. Titration of continuous positive airway pressure by real-time oximetry. *Chest.* 1987;92(5):853.
95. Mrochen H. Optimum PEEP selection using a desk top computer. *Int J Biomed Comput.* 1982;13(4):303.
96. Kram HB, Appel PL, Fleming AW, et al. Determination of optimum positive end-expiratory pressure by means of conjunctival oximetry. *Surgery.* 1987;101(3):329.
97. Rasanen J, Cane R, Downs JB, et al. Airway pressure release ventilation in severe acute respiratory failure. *Crit Care Me.* 1989;17:S32.
98. Banner MJ, Kirby RR, Banner TE. Airway pressure release ventilation in patients with acute respiratory failure. *Crit Care Med.* 1989;17(4):S32.
99. Florete O, Banner MJ, Banner TE, et al. Airway pressure release ventilation in a patient with acute pulmonary injury. *Chest.* 1989;96:679.
100. Stock MC, Downs JB, Frolicher DA. Airway pressure release ventilation. *Crit Care Med.* 1987;15:462.
101. Garner W, Downs JB, Stock MC, et al. Airway pressure release ventilation: a human trial. *Chest.* 1988;94:779.
102. Bratzke E, Downs JB, Smith RA. Intermittent CPAP: a new mode of ventilation during general anesthesia. *Anesthesiology.* 1998;89:334.
103. D'Angio CT, Chess PR, Kovacs SJ, et al. Pressure-regulated volume control vs synchronized intermittent mandatory ventilation for very low birth weight infants: a randomized controlled trial. *Acrh Pediatr Adolesc Med.* 2005;159(9):868.
104. Guldager H, Nielsen SL, Carl P, et al. A comparison of volume control and pressure-regulated volume control in acute respiratory failure. *Crit Care.* 1997;1(2):75.
105. Younes M. Proportional assist ventilation, a new approach to ventilatory support. Theory. *Am Rev Respir Dis.* 1992;145(1):114.
106. Younes M, Puddy A, Roberts D, et al. Proportional assist ventilation. Results of an initial clinical trial. *Am Rev Respir Dis.* 1992;145(1):121.
107. Giannouli E, Webster K, Roberts D, et al. Response of ventilator-dependent patients to different levels of pressure support and proportional assist. *Am J Respir Crit Care Med.* 1999;159(6):1716.
108. Hart N, Hunt A, Polkey MI, et al. Comparison of proportional assist ventilation and pressure support ventilation in chronic respiratory failure due to neuromuscular and chest wall deformity. *Thorax.* 2002;57(11):979.
109. Passam F, Hoing S, Prinianakis G, et al. Effect of different levels of pressure support and proportional assist ventilation on breathing pattern, work of breathing, and gas exchange in mechanically ventilated hypercapnic COPD patients with acute respiratory failure. *Respiration.* 2003;70(4):355.
110. Varelmann D, Wrigge H, Zinserling J, et al. Proportional assist versus pressure support ventilation in patients with acute respiratory failure: cardiorespiratory responses to artificially increased ventilatory demand. *Crit Care Med.* 2005;33(9):2125.
111. Vitacca M. New things are not always better: proportional assist ventilation vs pressure support ventilation. *Intensive Care Med.* 2003;29(7):1038.
112. Appendini L. Proportional assist ventilation: back to the future? *Respiration.* 2003;70(4):345.
113. Gervais HW, Eberle B, Konietzke D, et al. Comparison of blood gases of ventilated patients during transport. *Crit Care Med.* 1987;15(8):761.
114. Braman SS, Dunn SM, Amico CA, et al. Complications of intrahospital transport in critically ill patients. *Ann Int Med.* 1987;107(4):469.
115. Hurst JM, Davis JR, Branson RD, et al. Comparison of blood gases during transport using two methods of ventilatory support. *J Trauma.* 1989;29(12):1637.
116. Nakamura T, Fujino Y, Uchiyama A, et al. Intrahospital transport of critically ill patients using ventilator with patient-triggering function. *Chest.* 2003;123(1):159.
117. Putensen C, Mutz NJ, Putensen-Himmer G, et al. Spontaneous breathing during ventilatory support improves ventilation-perfusion distribution in patients with acute respiratory distress syndrome. *Am J Respir Crit Care Med.* 1999;159(4):1241.
118. Austin PN, Campbell RS, Johannigman JA, et al. Work of breathing of seven portable ventilators. *Resuscitation.* 2001;49(2):159.
119. Pinsky MR. Cardiovascular effects of ventilatory support and withdrawal. *Anesth Analg.* 1994;79:567.
120. Prewitt RM, Wood LH. Effects of positive end-expiratory pressure on ventricular function in dogs. *Am J Physiol.* 1972;236:H534.
121. Patten MT, Liebman PR, Hechtman HB. Humorally medicated decrease in cardiac output associated with positive end-expiratory pressure. *J Microvasc Res.* 1977;13:137.
122. Laver MB. The pulmonary response to trauma and mechanical ventilation: its consequences on hemodynamic function. *World J Surg.* 1983;7:31.
123. Beach T, Millen E, Grenvik A. Hemodynamic response to discontinuation of mechanical ventilation. *Crit Care Med.* 1973;1:85.
124. Robotham JL, Cherry D, Mitzner W, et al. A reevaluation of the hemodynamic consequences of intermittent positive pressure ventilation. *Crit Care Med.* 1983;11:783.
125. Kumar A, Pontoppidan H, Falke KJ, et al. Pulmonary barotrauma during mechanical ventilation. *Crit Care Med.* 1973:1:181.
126. Kirby RR. Best PEEP: issues and choices in the selection and monitoring of PEEP levels. *Respir Care.* 1988;33:569.

CHAPTER 129 ■ NONINVASIVE VENTILATORY SUPPORT MODES

MASSIMO ANTONELLI • GIORGIO CONTI • GIUSEPPE BELLO

Noninvasive ventilation (NIV) refers to the provision of ventilatory assistance using techniques that do not bypass the upper airway. The theoretical advantages of NIV include avoiding the complications associated with endotracheal intubation, improving patient comfort, and preserving airway defense mechanisms. NIV may be delivered through various devices including negative and positive pressure ventilators. During the first half of the 20th century, negative pressure ventilation was the main means of providing mechanical ventilatory assistance outside the anesthesia suite. Because of several disadvantages relative to negative pressure ventilation, including patient discomfort, restrictions on positioning, lack of airway protection, problems with correct fitting, time-consuming application, and lack of portability, negative pressure ventilators have seen diminishing use in favor of positive pressure assistance modes since the early 1960s. Therefore, only positive pressure support modes are discussed here.

The following sections deal with the history and epidemiology of NIV, as well as currently available equipment and techniques, practical applications, appropriate indications, and possible adverse effects. In this chapter, continuous positive airway pressure delivered noninvasively is referred to as CPAP, and NIV using intermittent positive pressure ventilation (IPPV) with or without positive end-expiratory pressure (PEEP) is referred to as NPPV (noninvasive positive-pressure ventilation). The term NIV is considered to include either CPAP or NPPV.

BACKGROUND

The first noninvasive report of positive pressure dates back to 1912, when Bunnell (1) used a face mask to maintain lung expansion during thoracic surgery. In 1936, Poulton and Oxon (2) used a vacuum cleaner to generate gas flow and a spring-loaded valve to oppose expiration to treat a patient with cardiogenic pulmonary edema (CPE). A number of studies conducted by Barach et al. (3–5) over the 1930s showed that CPAP delivered through a face mask could be useful in the treatment of CPE and other forms of respiratory failure. Noninvasive IPPV administered through a mouthpiece was first described by Motley (6) in the 1940s and was used widely until the early 1980s, either for aerosol delivery in patients with chronic obstructive pulmonary disease (COPD) and asthma, or as a means of ventilatory assistance. The use of noninvasive IPPV declined sharply after the demonstration of lack of benefit in comparison to simple nebulizing treatments (7).

The proliferation of NIV occurred during the 1980s, after the introduction of nasal mask ventilation in the management of obstructive sleep apnea (8). Despite a lack of randomized controlled trials, NIV became the ventilatory mode of first choice for patients with neuromuscular diseases and chest wall deformities (9–12). In the early 1990s, the encouraging results obtained in the treatment of acute respiratory failure (ARF) by using NPPV (13–15) stimulated investigation on various applications in the acute care setting. The desire of avoiding complications of endotracheal intubation (16–19), potentially lowering morbidity and mortality rates in selected patients with ARF (20–23), has been the major driving force of the increasing use of NPPV in the acute care setting over the past decade.

In their 28-day international study on patients admitted to 361 ICUs who received mechanical ventilation for more than 12 hours, Esteban et al. (24) found that NPPV through a facial mask was used in 4.9% of overall patients and in 16.9% of patients ventilated because of an exacerbation of COPD. In a prospective 3-week survey of 70 French ICUs performed in 2002, Demoule et al. (25) showed that 23% of patients requiring ventilatory assistance received NPPV as a first-line treatment, a significant increase compared to 1997 (16%) (26); the incidence of NIV for patients admitted to the ICU without intubation was also significantly increased compared to 1997 (52% vs. 35%); furthermore, 3% of patients in 2002 received NPPV before ICU admission compared to none in 1997 (25,26).

EQUIPMENT AND TECHNIQUES

The following paragraphs will discuss various interfaces and ventilatory modes available for administration of NIV. Cough-enhancing techniques will also be described.

Interfaces

Interfaces are devices that connect ventilator tubing to the face, allowing the delivery of pressurized gas into the airway during NIV. Currently available interfaces include nasal and oronasal masks, helmets, and mouthpieces. Selection of a comfortable interface that fits properly is a key issue for the success of NIV.

Nasal Masks

The standard nasal mask is a triangular or cone-shaped clear plastic device that fits over the nose and uses a soft cushion or flange to seal over the skin (Fig. 129.1). Because of the pressure exerted over the bridge of the nose, the mask may cause skin irritation and redness, and occasionally ulceration (Fig. 129.2). For occasional patients who cannot tolerate

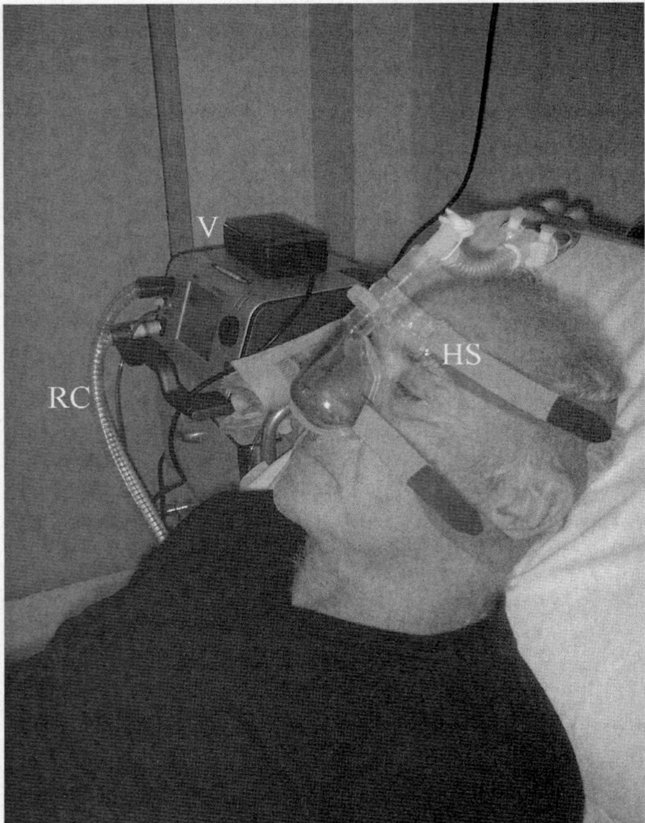

FIGURE 129.1. Noninvasive ventilation delivered through a nasal mask. HS, head straps; RC, respiratory circuit; V, ventilator. (Photograph printed with the permission of the patient.)

commercially available masks, custom-molded, individualized masks that conform to facial contours of the patient can be constructed. Several types of strap systems have been used to hold the mask in place. Depending on the interface, straps attach at two or as many as five points on the mask and may be provided with Velcro fasteners. The nasal mask is generally

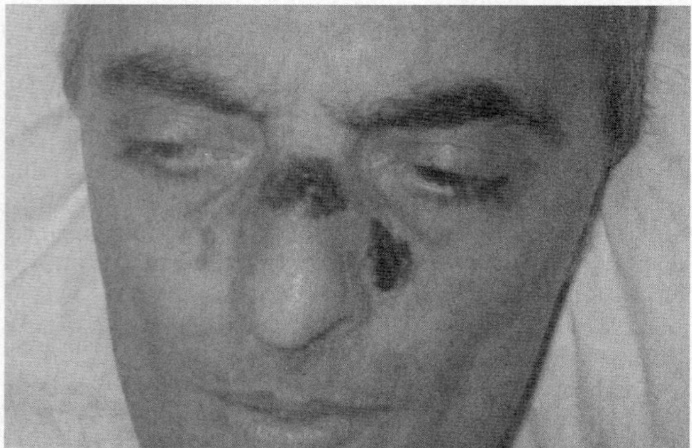

FIGURE 129.2. Skin lesions caused by a mask. Please note that the point at major risk to develop a skin necrosis is the bridge of the nose. (Photograph printed with the permission of the patient.)

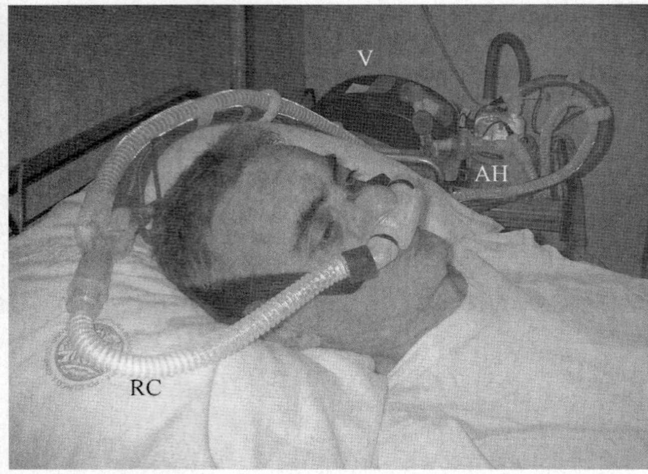

FIGURE 129.3. Noninvasive ventilation delivered through nasal pillows. AH, active humidifier; RC, respiratory circuit; V, ventilator. (Photograph printed with the permission of the patient.)

preferred for chronic administration of NIV. In patients with a nasogastric tube, a seal connector in the dome of the mask may be used to avoid air leakage.

Nasal Pillows

Nasal pillows or seals consist of soft rubber or silicone plugs that are inserted directly into the nostrils (Fig. 129.3). As they exert no pressure over the bridge of the nose, nasal pillows may be useful in patients who develop irritation or ulceration on the nasal bridge while using nasal or oronasal masks.

Oronasal Masks

Oronasal or face masks cover both the nose and the mouth (Fig. 129.4). The oronasal mask is largely used in patients with copious air leaking through the mouth during nasal mask ventilation. Interference with speech, eating, and expectoration, and the likelihood of claustrophobic reactions, are greater with oronasal than with nasal masks. In the acute setting, however, oronasal masks are preferable to nasal masks because dyspneic patients are mouth breathers, predisposing to greater air leakage during nasal mask ventilation. The oronasal masks, like the nasal mask, may cause skin necrosis over the nasal bridge (27). When the opening pressure of the upper esophageal sphincter (25–30 cm H_2O) is overcome, the positioning of a nasogastric tube may protect from gastric distension, even though this is not a common event.

A type of oronasal mask is the "total" face mask (28), which is made of clear plastic and uses a soft silicone flange that seals around the perimeter of the face like a hockey goalie's mask, avoiding direct pressure on facial structures.

Helmet

The helmet (Fig. 129.5) is made of transparent latex-free polyvinyl chloride and is secured by two armpit braces at two hooks (one anterior and the other posterior) of the plastic ring that joins the helmet with a seal connection soft collar adherent to the neck (29,30). The pressure increase during ventilation makes the soft collar sealing comfortable to the neck and shoulders, avoiding air leakage (29). The whole apparatus is

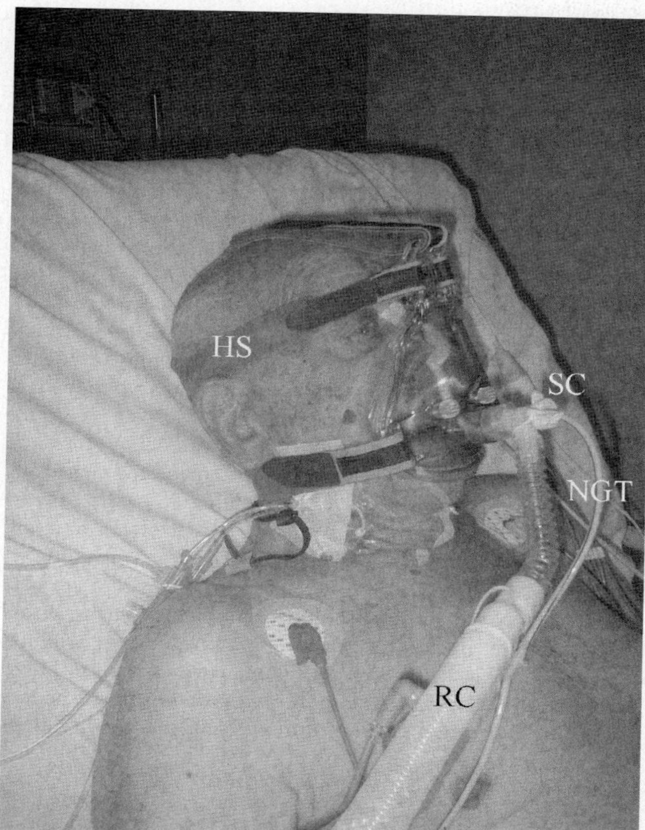

FIGURE 129.4. Noninvasive ventilation delivered through an oronasal mask. HS, head straps; NGT, nasogastric tube; RC, respiratory circuit; SC, seal connection. (Photograph printed with the permission of the patient.)

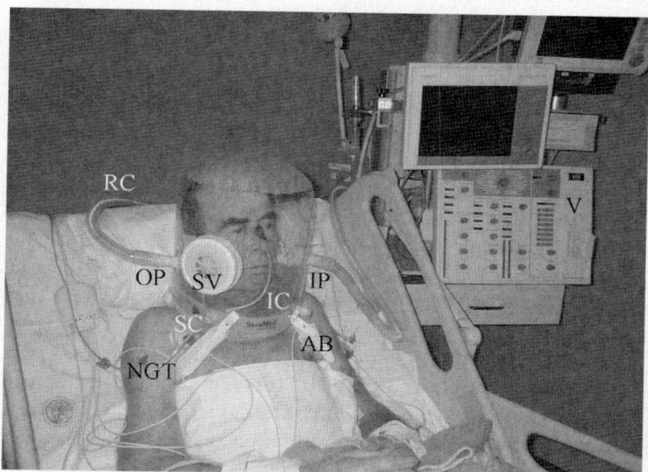

FIGURE 129.5. Noninvasive ventilation delivered through a helmet. AB, armpit braces; IC, inflated cushion; IP, inlet port; NGT, nasogastric tube; OP, outlet port; RC, respiratory circuit; SC, seal connection; SV, security valve; V, ventilator. (Photograph printed with the permission of the patient.)

connected to an ICU ventilator by a standard respiratory circuit. The two ports of the helmet act as inlet and outlet for inspiratory and expiratory gas flows. The inspiratory and expiratory valves are those of the mechanical ventilator. A specific connector placed in the plastic ring can be used to allow the passage of a nasogastric tube, thus reducing air leaks. The patient is allowed to drink through a straw or to be fed a liquid diet. A new version of the helmet, recently developed, has an antiasphyxia device and two inner inflatable cushions to increase comfort and reduce the internal volume. The main advantages of the helmet include a good tolerability in both adult and pediatric populations (31), with a satisfactory interaction of the patients with the environment; a lower risk of dermal lesions; and, compared with the mask, easier applicability to any patient regardless of the face contour.

Mouthpieces

Mouthpieces are simple and inexpensive devices used to provide NPPV for as long as 24 hours a day to patients with chronic respiratory failure (Fig. 129.6). If nasal air leaking reduces efficacy, ventilator tidal volume may be increased or cotton plugs or nose clips may be used for occluding the nostrils. NPPV via mouthpieces has proved to be a valid alternative to tracheostomy in some patients with chronic respiratory muscle insufficiency (32).

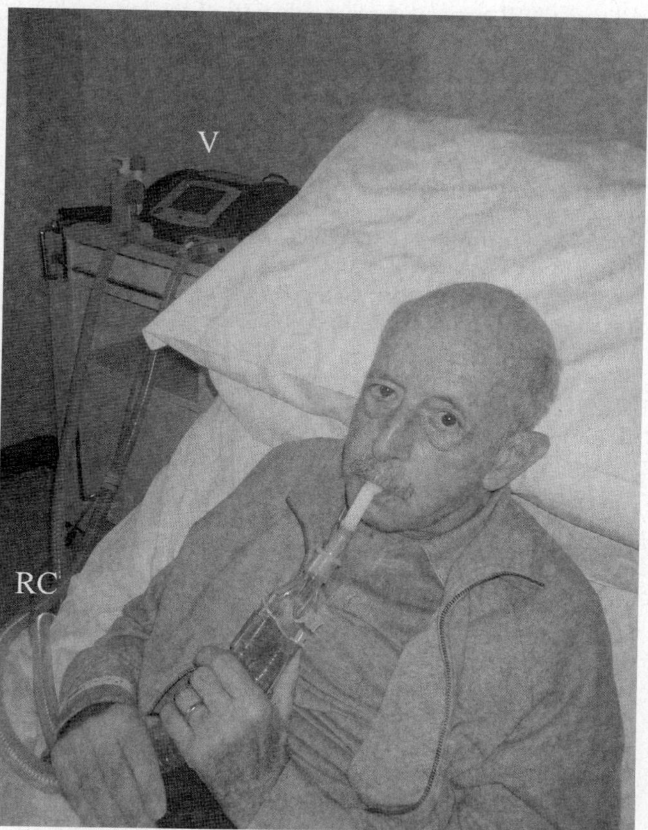

FIGURE 129.6. Noninvasive ventilation delivered through a mouthpiece. RC, respiratory circuit; V, ventilator. (Photograph printed with the permission of the patient.)

Physiologic Aspects and Patient–Ventilator Interaction during NPPV Delivered by Different Types of Interfaces

The choice of an appropriate interface is one of the crucial issues affecting NIV outcome. Data obtained from physiologic evaluations of NPPV delivered by different types of interfaces have been useful to improve devices and patient–ventilator synchrony.

The study of mask mechanics and air leak dynamics during NPPV may guide mask fit and inspiratory pressure (33). The pressure that fits the mask's cushion against the patient's face is represented by the pressure inside the cushion and is measured by connecting a pressure transducer to the cushion's inflation valve. The mask occlusion pressure is obtained by calculating the gradient between the mask fit pressure and airway pressure.

In a controlled study of a group of stable hypercapnic patients (34), the nasal mask used for delivering NPPV was better tolerated than either nasal pillows or an oronasal mask but was less effective at lowering $PaCO_2$. In another controlled trial of 70 patients with acute respiratory failure (ARF) who randomly received either nasal mask or oronasal NPPV (35), both masks performed similarly with regard to improving vital signs and gas exchange and avoiding intubation, but the nasal mask was significantly less well tolerated than the oronasal mask.

In contrast to NIV via nasal or oronasal masks, with helmet-delivered NIV, patients receive only part of the large volumes administered by the ventilator after inspiratory trigger activation. The rest of the volume is compressed around the head, pressurizing the helmet. It is therefore impossible to measure patient tidal volumes and flows with conventional bedside monitoring. The internal volume surrounding the head varies between 6 and 8 L, but this usually does not represent a problem for rebreathing, provided that sufficient levels of pressure support are delivered (29). When measuring partial pressure of inspired CO_2 and end-tidal CO_2 in healthy volunteers at 10 cm H_2O pressure support, CO_2 rebreathing with the helmet is less than 1.5% and is similar to that detected with the oronasal mask (30).

In a physiologic study of eight healthy subjects randomized to receive either face mask or helmet CPAP, Patroniti et al. (36) showed that helmet CPAP is as effective as face mask CPAP in increasing end-expiratory lung volume and in minimizing respiratory airway pressure oscillations, without the need of a reservoir bag. In addition, the authors suggested that high gas flow rates should always be considered during helmet-delivered CPAP, to improve CO_2 washout and decrease CO_2 rebreathing, given the elevated dead space. In a physiologic evaluation of different levels of pressure support ventilation (PSV) during helmet-delivered NPPV (37), the helmet was effective in reducing the inspiratory effort and was efficient in providing ventilation to eight healthy volunteers, without relevant CO_2 rebreathing. Furthermore, a low level of PSV (5–10 cm H_2O) allowed optimal comfort even at high PEEP (10 cm H_2O), whereas a significant discomfort was observed with PSV at 15 cm H_2O.

During NPPV, the ventilator must first pressurize the interface and then the respiratory system (38). Some physiologic studies on healthy subjects (38,39) showed that the use of the helmet to deliver PSV increased inspiratory muscle effort and required a longer time to reach the selected level of airway pressure compared with the standard face mask, thus worsening patient–ventilator asynchrony. More recently, Moerer et al. (40) reported a bench study of ventilatory performance by using an *in vitro* lung model capable of stimulating spontaneous breathing, and compared a helmet and face mask during NPPV at different levels of PSV and PEEP. Measurements included the time delay to activate the ventilatory trigger, the time between the initiation of an inspiratory effort until the preset PEEP level is reached, and the inspiratory pressure–time product (which reflects the inspiratory muscle effort) during these two periods. The helmet, although presenting a significantly longer time delay, caused a lower pressure–time product compared to the face mask. In addition, by increasing the level of PSV or PEEP, the helmet furthermore significantly reduced the delay times and pressure–time product. The investigators suggested that using a minimum PEEP of 6 cm H_2O and adding PSV may shorten the delay times and reduce inspiratory muscle effort, and will hardly promote the occurrence of wasted efforts. The longer delay times observed during helmet-delivered NPPV are presumably a consequence of the high compliance of the actual design of the helmet, which needs higher inspiratory volumes than the face mask to reach the same airway pressure. However, the patient can use the large air reservoir within the helmet at the beginning of an inspiration, thus reducing the initial inspiratory muscle effort.

Ventilatory Modes

Continuous Positive Airway Pressure

Continuous positive airway pressure (CPAP) delivers a constant pressure throughout spontaneous inspiration and exhalation *without* assisting inspiration. Because spontaneous breathing is not assisted, this technique requires an intact respiratory drive and adequate alveolar ventilation. CPAP increases functional residual capacity and opens underventilated alveoli, thus decreasing right-to-left intrapulmonary shunt and improving oxygenation and lung mechanics (41). Moreover, CPAP may reduce the work of breathing and dyspnea in COPD patients by counterbalancing the inspiratory threshold load imposed by intrinsic PEEP (42). Effects on hemodynamics during CPAP have been widely described. By lowering left ventricular transmural pressure in patients with left congestive heart failure, CPAP may reduce left ventricular afterload without compromising cardiac index (43,44). For several years, it was hypothesized that positive airway pressure, by increasing right atrial pressure (45), reduced venous return by decreasing the pressure gradient between mean systemic filling pressure and right atrial pressure (46). However, as demonstrated in experimental (47,48) and human (49) studies, positive airway pressure does not affect the gradient for venous return, because pleural pressure is transmitted to the same extent to both the mean systemic and right atrial pressures. CPAP can be applied by various devices including low flow generators with an inspiratory reservoir, high-flow jet venturi circuits (Fig. 129.7) (both of them with an expiratory mechanical or water valve), and bilevel and critical care ventilators. Continuous positive pressure may be administered using the demand flow (DF) or the gold standard continuous flow (CF) system. With DF CPAP, the patient has to trigger a preset pressure to open the

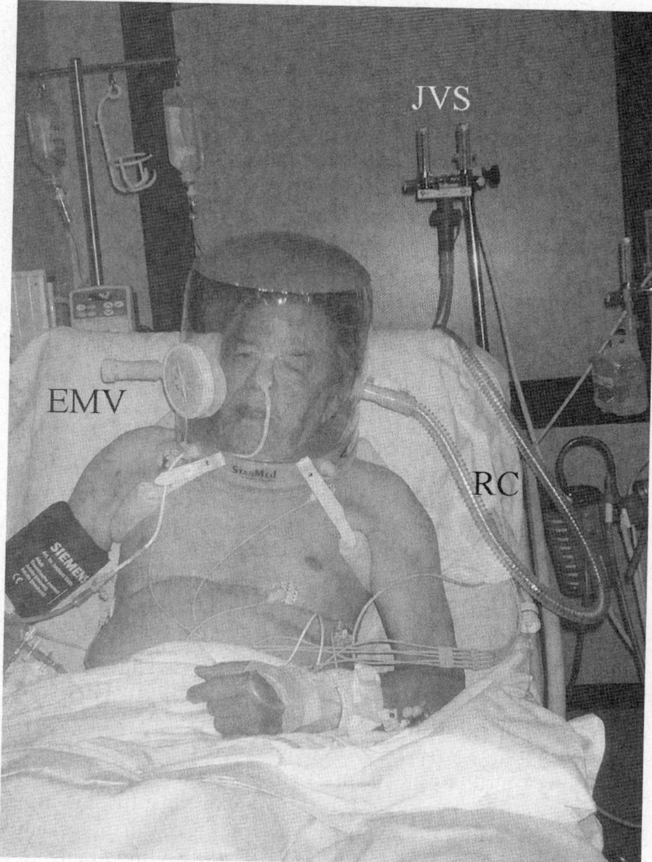

FIGURE 129.7. Helmet continuous positive airway pressure (CPAP) delivered by a high-flow jet venturi system. EMV, expiratory mechanical valve; JVS, jet venturi system; RC, respiratory circuit. (Photograph printed with the permission of the patient.)

demand valve, whereas with CF CPAP, no valves are present. The work of breathing is significantly greater with the DF system than with the CF one (50–52). It is crucial to provide an adequate air flow rate for maintaining a continuous positive pressure, especially in dyspneic patients who breathe at high flow rates.

Pressure Support Ventilation

Pressure support ventilation (PSV) is a pressure-triggered, pressure-targeted, flow-cycled mode of ventilation. It delivers a preset inspiratory pressure to assist spontaneous breathing, augmenting spontaneous breaths and offsetting the work imposed by the breathing apparatus. A sensitive patient-initiated trigger causes the delivery of inspiratory pressure support that is maintained throughout inspiration, and a reduction in inspiratory flow drives the ventilator to cycle into expiration. Therefore, the patient can control either inspiratory duration or breathing rate. Typical starting pressures are a PEEP of 3 to 5 cm H_2O and an inspiratory airway pressure of 8 to 12 cm H_2O (Table 129.1).

Bilevel Positive Airway Ventilation

In bilevel positive airway pressure (BiPAP), a valve sets two pressure levels, the expiratory positive airway pressure (EPAP) level, and the inspiratory positive airway pressure (IPAP) level,

TABLE 129.1

PROPOSED VENTILATOR SETTINGS FOR PRESSURE SUPPORT VENTILATION MODE

	Initial setting	Treatment setting
PEEP	3–5 cm H_2O	Slowly increased to up to 8–12 cm H_2O in hypoxemic patients
PSV	8–12 cm H_2O	Increased as tolerated to 20 cm H_2O to obtain an exhaled tidal volume of about 7 mL/kg and respiratory rate <25 breaths/min
FiO$_2$	Titrated to achieve an arterial saturation >90% or 85%–90% in patients at risk of worsening hypercapnia	Titrated to achieve an arterial saturation >90% or 85%–90% in patients at risk of worsening hypercapnia

even in the presence of rapidly changing flows. With this technique, ventilation is produced by the cyclic delta pressure between IPAP and EPAP. EPAP also recruits underventilated lung and offsets eventual intrinsic PEEP.

Controlled Mechanical Ventilation

In the mandatory controlled mechanical ventilation (CMV) mode, no patient effort is required, as full ventilatory support is provided. In this mode, ventilator settings include inflation pressure or tidal volume, frequency, and the timing of each breath.

Pressure control ventilation (PCV) delivers time-cycled preset inspiratory and expiratory pressures with adjustable inspiratory-to-expiratory ratios at a controlled rate. The resulting tidal volume is determined by the compliance of the lungs and chest wall, and the resistance to flow of ventilator tubing.

In volume control ventilation (VCV), tidal volume is set and the resulting pressure depends on the thoracic and circuit compliance. VCV can be preferred for those patients with severe chest wall deformity or obesity who may need higher inflation pressures.

Assist/Control Ventilation

In assist/control (A/C) ventilation, the ventilator delivers a breath either when triggered by the patient's inspiratory effort (assist) or independently, if such an effort does not occur within a preselected period (control). When triggering occurs, the ventilator delivers an identical breath to mandatory breaths. Volume-cycled and pressure-limited or pressure-targeted modes are available.

Proportional Assist Ventilation

Proportional assist ventilation (PAV) is an alternative technique in which both flow and volume are independently adjusted. In this technique, the ventilator generates volume and pressure in proportion to the patient's effort, increasing comfort and so improving success and compliance with NPPV (53). Despite the promising concept, there is a substantial lack of large clinical studies.

Ventilatory Mode Selection

All ventilatory modes of NPPV have been used to achieve physiologic or clinical benefit, with theoretical advantages and limitations. Spontaneously breathing patients with respiratory failure of various causes may benefit from CPAP to correct hypoxemia. In acute CPE, mask CPAP can result in early physiologic improvement and reduce the need for intubation (54). In one study (55), BiPAP improved ventilation and vital signs more rapidly in patients with CPE, but it was associated with a higher rate of myocardial infarction compared with CPAP. Conversely, a more recent study (56) found no difference in the risk for developing myocardial infarction during NIV delivered by CPAP or BiPAP modes.

VCV can be useful in patients with changing respiratory impedance. In the presence of elevated peak inspiratory airway pressure, however, this technique is susceptible to air leaks, gastric distention, skin irritation and, consequently, poor patient tolerance.

Pressure-targeted modes maintain delivered tidal volume in patients with air leaking better than volume-targeted modes. Therefore, pressure-targeted ventilators are preferred over volume-targeted ventilators to deliver NPPV in the presence of substantial leaks (57). To best compensate for air leaks, pressure-targeted ventilators should have high and sustained maximal inspiratory flow capabilities (>3 L/second), adjustable I:E ratios and other mechanisms to limit inspiratory duration so that inversion of the I:E ratio is avoided, and adjustable trigger sensitivities or algorithms to prevent autocycling (57). Ventilatory systems for air leak detection, calculation, and compensation are now largely available.

When PSV is used as a noninvasive ventilatory assistance mode, some forms of patient–ventilator asynchrony might be intensified, causing breathing discomfort. During PSV, indeed, brief rapid inhalations may not permit adequate time for the ventilator to cycle into expiration, so that the patient's expiratory effort begins while the unit is still delivering inspiratory pressure (58). Also, eventual air leaks during noninvasive PSV may prevent adequate reduction in inspiratory flow required to open the expiratory valve, thereby prolonging inspiratory flow despite expiratory efforts. When this occurs, a time-cycled expiratory trigger provides a better patient–machine interaction than flow-cycled expiratory trigger (59).

In acute hypercapnic exacerbations of COPD, NPPV performed by different ventilatory modes including PSV, ACV, and PAV is able to provide respiratory muscle rest and improve respiratory physiologic parameters (60–62). No difference in clinical outcome or arterial blood gas tensions between patients ventilated in ACV and PSV modes has been found, even though PSV has seemed to be more acceptable to patients and associated with fewer side effects in comparison with ACV (63). As in the intubated mechanically ventilated COPD patients, application of external PEEP is effective in counterbalancing the effects of auto-PEEP and dynamic hyperinflation. The use of noninvasive ventilatory modes in patients with hypoxemic ARF of various causes can improve arterial blood gases, respiratory rate, and dyspnea, and unload the accessory muscles of respiration (20,21,64).

Triggering systems are critical to the success of NPPV in both assist and control modes. During assisted ventilation, flow triggering reduces breathing effort more effectively as compared with pressure triggering, obtaining a better patient–ventilator interaction (65–67).

In the absence of evidence favoring a specific ventilatory mode, the choice should be dictated by personal experience, as well as cause and severity of the pathologic process responsible for ARF (68). However, assisted modes (and particularly PSV) are usually best tolerated and can be safely and effectively performed. A modality that provides a backup rate is needed for patients with inadequate ventilatory drive.

Techniques to Assist Cough

The cough mechanism may be severely impaired in neuromuscular diseases when weak expiratory muscles are combined with a markedly reduced vital capacity. An effective cough depends on the ability to generate adequate expiratory airflow, estimated at >160 L/minute (69), which is determined by lung and chest wall elasticity, airway conductance, and expiratory muscle force. Also, an intact glottic function is needed for yielding high peak expiratory cough flows. Manually assisted coughing consists of quick thrusts applied to the abdomen using the palms of the hands, timed to coincide with the patient's cough effort. The maneuver should be applied cautiously after meals and with the patient positioned semiupright to reduce the risk of aspiration of gastric contents.

Manually assisted coughing may enhance expiratory force, but it does not increase inspired volume, so that patients with severely restricted volumes may still achieve insufficient cough flows. Such a limitation may be overcome by using the mechanical insufflator–exsufflator (Fig. 129.8), which delivers a positive inspiratory pressure of 30 to 40 cm H_2O via a face mask and then rapidly switches to an equal negative pressure (70). The positive pressure produces an adequate tidal volume, whereas the negative pressure stimulates the high peak expiratory cough flows. Insufflator–exsufflator may be combined with manually assisted coughing to further augment cough effectiveness. Any technique used to assist cough can be performed effectively and frequently by skilled caregivers, with minimal discomfort to the patient.

PRACTICAL APPLICATION

NIV should be considered early when patients first develop signs of incipient respiratory failure needing ventilatory assistance. It is crucial that caregivers can identify patients who are likely to benefit from NIV and exclude those for whom NIV would be unsafe. Once the decision to institute NIV has been taken, an interface and ventilatory mode must be chosen, and a close monitoring in an appropriate hospital location must be provided. The initial approach should consist in fitting the interface and familiarizing the patient with the apparatus, explaining the purpose of each piece of equipment. Patients should be motivated and reassured by the clinician, instructed to coordinate their breathing with the ventilator, and encouraged to communicate any discomfort or fears. Collaboration among medical practitioners including physicians, respiratory therapists, and nurses is critical to the success of NIV during the early phase of milder respiratory failure and after an initial period to 20 minutes interruption. For patients with more severe failure, NIV application has to be continuous for at least

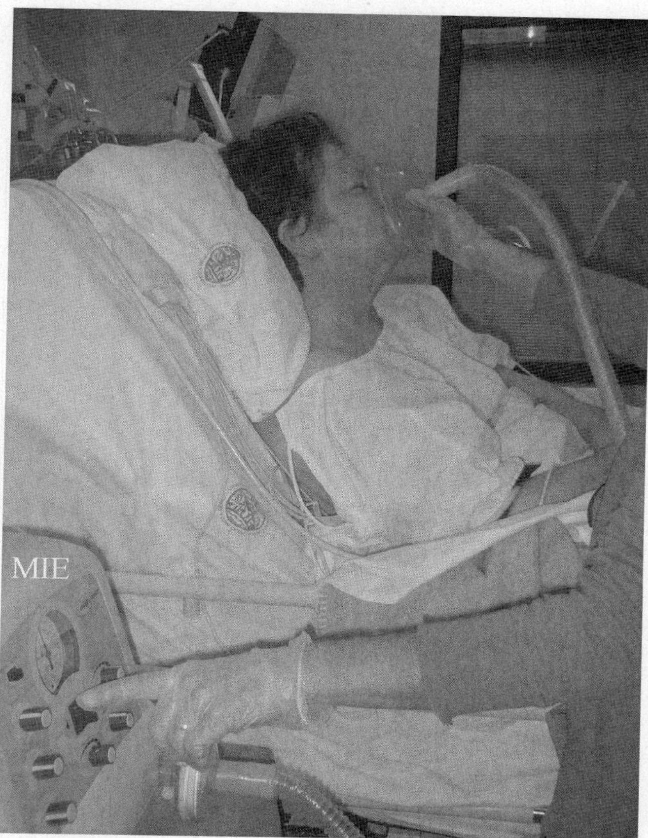

FIGURE 129.8. Mechanical insufflator–exsufflator (MIE). (Photograph printed with the permission of the patient.)

12 to 24 hours (20), and discontinuation is allowed for short periods only when the clinical situation improves. Aggressive physiotherapy is crucial during the periods of NIV discontinuation. Endotracheal intubation must be rapidly accessible, when indicated (Table 129.2).

Patient Selection

The criteria for selecting appropriate patients to receive NIV for ARF include clinical indicators of acute respiratory distress, such as moderate to severe dyspnea, tachypnea, accessory muscle use and paradoxical abdominal breathing, and gas exchange deterioration. Blood gas parameters aid in identifying patients

TABLE 129.2

CRITERIA FOR NONINVASIVE VENTILATION DISCONTINUATION AND ENDOTRACHEAL INTUBATION

Technique intolerance (pain, discomfort, or claustrophobia)
Inability to improve gas exchanges and/or dyspnea
Hemodynamic instability or evidence of shock, cardiac ischemia, or ventricular dysrhythmia
Inability to improve mental status within 30 min after the application of NIV in hypercapnic, lethargic COPD patients or agitated hypoxemic patients

TABLE 129.3

CONTRAINDICATIONS TO NONINVASIVE VENTILATION

Unconsciousness or mental obtundation (chronic obstructive pulmonary disease [COPD] patient may be an exception)
Inability to protect the airway
Inability to clear respiratory secretions
Severe upper gastrointestinal bleeding
Life-threatening hypoxemia
Unstable hemodynamic conditions (blood pressure or rhythm instability)
Recent gastroesophageal surgery
Fixed obstruction of the upper airway
Vomiting
Recent facial surgery, trauma, burns, or deformity
Undrained pneumothorax

with acute or acute superimposed on chronic CO_2 retention. A conscious and cooperative patient is crucial for initiating NIV (Table 129.3), although hypercapnic patients with narcosis who are otherwise good candidates for NIV may represent an exception (71,72).

During NIV, patients can achieve a level of control and independence totally different from when intubated, and sedation is infrequently required. If benzodiazepines or opiates are administered, caution is advised to prevent undue hypoventilation. NIV should be avoided in patients with hemodynamic instability and in those who are unable to protect the airways (coma, impaired swallowing, and so on) (Table 129.3). Patients with severe hypoxemia (PaO_2/FiO_2 <100) or morbid obesity (>200% of ideal body weight) should be closely managed only by experienced personnel and with a low threshold for intubation (20,21,73). In the presence of a pneumothorax, NIV can be initiated provided an intercostal drain is inserted. Criteria for NIV discontinuation and endotracheal intubation must be thoroughly considered to avoid dangerous delays (Table 129.2).

Identification of predictors of success or failure may help in recognizing patients who are appropriate candidates for NIV and those in whom NIV is not likely to be effective, thereby avoiding its application and unnecessary delays before invasive ventilation is given. The severity of acidosis at baseline is a logical starting point for identifying patients who might benefit from NPPV. In a retrospective review aimed at identifying patients with COPD who could be treated successfully with NPPV, Ambrosino et al. (74) found that patients in whom NPPV treatment failed were significantly more acidemic at baseline than those successfully treated (mean pH 7.22 versus 7.28). Similarly, Brochard et al. (75), using *a priori* criteria for the need for intubation, found that success was less likely with a lower starting pH. Also the tolerance of NPPV and the change in arterial blood gas tensions and respiratory rate in the early hours are reasonable predictors of the subsequent outcome in ARF patients with or without hypercapnia (64,74–79). NPPV is less likely to be successful if there are associated complications or if the patient's premorbid condition is poor (78,79). Late failure, considered as occurring after 48 hours of successful NPPV, is recognized, with rates reported at 0 to 20%, and has been associated with poor outcomes (78). Patients affected by acute respiratory distress syndrome (ARDS) with a

Simplified Acute Physiology Score (SAPS) II >34, and whose PaO_2/FiO_2 does not improve over 175 after 1 hour of NPPV should be carefully treated, under strict monitoring within the ICU where endotracheal intubation and invasive ventilation are promptly available (64). It is still unclear if the higher mortality observed in patients who failed NPPV and are eventually intubated might be due to a delayed intubation (64).

Machine Settings

Pressures commonly used to administer CPAP in patients with ARF range from 5 to 12 cm H_2O. For pressure-cycled ventilation, it is suggested to start at low pressures to facilitate patient tolerance (appropriate initial pressures are a CPAP of 3 to 5 cm H_2O and an inspiratory pressure of 8 to 12 cm H_2O) and, if necessary, gradually increase pressure settings as tolerated to obtain alleviation of dyspnea, decreased respiratory rate, adequate exhaled tidal volume, and good patient–ventilator interaction (Table 129.1). In the presence of air leaks, adequate inspiratory flows and durations should be set, triggering sensitivity should be adjusted to prevent autocycling, and a mechanism to limit inspiratory time and avoid I:E ratio inversion should be considered when available (57). A backup rate should be applied in patients with inadequate triggering. When VCV is used to deliver NPPV, tidal volume is usually set higher (10–15 mL/kg) to compensate for air leaking. In any case, excessive inflation can cause activation of expiratory muscles during inspiration with consequent patient–ventilator asynchrony. Oxygen supplementation should be provided as needed to keep oxygen saturation above 90% or between 85% and 90% in patients at risk of worsening hypercapnia. When the duration of NIV is expected to be more than a few hours, a heated humidifier may help oronasal dryness and patient's comfort.

Monitoring

In the acute setting, patients can initiate NIV anywhere, at the onset of the acute respiratory distress, but after initiation, they should be transferred to an ICU or a step-down unit for continuous monitoring until they are sufficiently stable to be moved to a medical ward. During transfers, NIV and monitoring should not be discontinued. The early use of NIV for less acutely ill patients with COPD on a medical ward seems to be effective, but if pH is lower than 7.30, admission to an environment with intensive care monitoring is highly recommended (80).

Monitoring of patients undergoing NIV is aimed at determining whether the initial goals are being achieved, including relief of symptoms, reduced work of breathing, improved or stable gas exchange, good patient–ventilator synchrony, and patient comfort (Table 129.4). Gas exchanges are monitored by continuous oximetry and arterial blood gases at baseline, after 1 to 2 hours, and as clinically indicated; physiologic responses are evaluated by continuous electrocardiography, respiratory rate, blood pressure and heart rates; finally, dyspnea, as well as tolerance of the technique, symptoms of impaired sleep, patient–ventilatory asynchrony, and air leaking can be easily assessed through patient queries, bedside observation, and flow, volume, and pressure waveform analysis. If a poor response to NIV occurs and the specific measures used to correct the situation fail to address an adequate improvement within a few hours, NIV should be considered a failure, and invasive ventilation should be promptly considered.

TABLE 129.4

MONITORING OF PATIENTS RECEIVING NONINVASIVE VENTILATION IN THE ACUTE CARE SETTING

BEDSIDE OBSERVATION
- Conscious level
- Comfort
- Chest wall motion
- Accessory muscle recruitment
- Patient–ventilator synchrony

VITAL SIGNS
- Respiratory rate
- Exhaled tidal volume (and flow, volume, and pressure waveform for poor synchrony problems)
- Heart rate
- Blood pressure
- Continuous electrocardiography

GAS EXCHANGE
- Continuous oximetry
- Arterial blood gas at baseline, after 1–2 h, and as clinically indicated

INDICATIONS

The following sections will review the available evidence on the efficacy of NIV for various applications in the acute care setting.

Acute Exacerbations of Chronic Obstructive Pulmonary Disease

In patients with ARF resulting from acute exacerbations of COPD, the use of NPPV has been proven to be effective in ameliorating dyspnea (77), improving vital signs and gas exchange (75,77,80–82), preventing endotracheal intubation (75,77,80,81), and improving hospital survival (75,80,81). Consequently, there is a general agreement concerning the early use of NPPV in such patients (68,83).

In COPD patients with acute respiratory decompensations, the increased flow resistance and the impossibility to complete the expiration before inspiration determine high levels of dynamic hyperinflation, and substantial shortening of the diaphragm and the inspiratory intercostals and accessory muscles, thereby reducing their mechanical efficiency and endurance. The need to overcome the inspiratory threshold load due to auto-PEEP and to drive the tidal volume against airway resistances increases the respiratory muscle fatigue. During NPPV, the combination of external PEEP and PSV offsets the auto-PEEP level and reduces the work of breathing that the inspiratory muscles must generate to produce the tidal volume (60).

In an early study on the use of face mask NPPV in patients with ARF, Meduri et al. (13) obtained improvements of gas exchanges and avoided endotracheal intubation in a group of

COPD patients. Soon thereafter, Brochard et al. (14) described the short-term (45-minute) physiologic effects of inspiratory assistance with a face mask on gas exchange and respiratory-muscle work in 11 patients with COPD and evaluated the therapeutic use of the technique in 13 patients with COPD exacerbations, comparing the results in the latter group with the results of conventional treatment in 13 matched historical-control patients. In the physiologic study, arterial pH rose from 7.31 to 7.38 ($p < 0.01$), $PaCO_2$ fell from 68 to 55 mm Hg ($p < 0.01$) PaO_2 rose from 52 to 69 mm Hg ($p < 0.05$), and respiratory rate reduced from 31 to 21 breaths per minute ($p < 0.01$) (14). Only 1 of 13 patients treated with NPPV needed intubation, as compared with 11 of the 13 historical controls ($p < 0.001$). In addition, the NPPV-treated patients were weaned from the ventilator faster and spent less time in the ICU than did the control subjects (14). Subsequently, numerous randomized controlled trials using NPPV in ARF caused by COPD have been published (Table 129.5).

In the first randomized, prospective study on 60 COPD patients, Bott et al. (77) compared NPPV delivered through nasal mask with conventional therapy as a treatment of ARF. Patients receiving NPPV had a significant reduction of $PaCO_2$ and dyspnea score, and 30-day mortality (10% vs. 30%). A multicenter European trial (75) on the efficacy of NPPV in acute exacerbation of COPD randomized 85 COPD patients to receive face mask PSV or conventional treatment (oxygen therapy plus drugs). After 1 hour of NPPV, respiratory rate but not $PaCO_2$ showed a significant decrease. The group of patients treated with NPPV had a significantly lower intubation rate, a lower complication rate (14% vs. 45%), length of hospital stay, and mortality rate. In another randomized study on 23 COPD patients that compared NPPV with conventional treatment, the investigators reported a reduction of intubation rate, with a significant improvement in PaO_2, heart rate, and respiratory rate in the NPPV group, even though $PaCO_2$ did not significantly decrease (81). A randomized study on 30 COPD patients with ARF (82) confirmed that early application of NPPV facilitates gas exchange improvement, reduces the need for invasive mechanical ventilation, and decreases the duration of hospitalization. In a randomized trial on 50 COPD patients with acute exacerbation, NPPV reduced weaning time, shortened the length of stay in the ICU, decreased the incidence of nosocomial pneumonia, and improved 60-day survival rates (88). Other and more recent prospective randomized controlled studies on patients with ARF due to COPD exacerbations (89,90) have confirmed the benefit of applying NPPV in improving clinical status and blood gases.

A randomized prospective study by Conti et al. (91) has compared the short- and long-term response to face mask NPPV versus invasive conventional ventilation in COPD patients with ARF failing to sustain the initial improvement with conventional medical therapy in the emergency ward and needing ventilatory assistance. In this study, the intubation rate of 52% in the NPPV group was higher than in other randomized controlled trials, which is not surprising given the higher severity of illness of these patients, as evidenced by the mean pH of 7.2, compared with 7.27 in the study of Brochard et al. (75) and 7.32 in the study of Plant et al. (80). Although the patients who received NPPV were sicker than those reported in previous studies, they showed a trend toward a lower incidence of nosocomial pneumonia during the ICU stay and a better outcome at a 1-year follow-up, as well as no significant differences in ICU and hospital mortality, overall complications, duration of mechanical ventilation and ICU. These findings support early use of NPPV during the course of acute exacerbation of COPD patients. However, also if NPPV is started later, after the failure of medical treatment, it is comparable to invasive mechanical ventilation in terms of survival.

In a matched case-control study conducted in ICU, 64 COPD patients with advanced ARF (pH $\leq$7.25, $PaCO_2$ $\geq$70 torr, and respiratory rate $\geq$35 breaths/minute) prospectively received NPPV and their outcomes were compared with those of a control group of 64 COPD patients (92). NPPV had a high rate of failure (40/64), although mortality rate, duration of mechanical ventilation, and lengths of ICU and post-ICU stay were not different between the two groups, and the NPPV group had fewer complications. In this study, patients who failed NPPV were not harmed by the delayed institution of invasive ventilation, and those who avoided endotracheal intubation had a clear-cut benefit. Based on these results, the authors suggested that in COPD patients with advanced ARF, it might be worthwhile to attempt a trial of NPPV prior to a shift to invasive ventilation with endotracheal intubation.

In summary, NPPV should be considered the first-line therapeutic option to prevent endotracheal intubation and improve outcome in patients with exacerbations of COPD who have no contraindication to NPPV (Table 129.3).

Asthma

NPPV is considered an option in asthmatic patients at risk for endotracheal intubation. However, mechanical ventilation may be dangerous in patients with asthma, first, by worsening lung hyperinflation with the risk of causing barotrauma, and second, by inducing hemodynamic deterioration by increased intrathoracic pressure. To date, guidelines for NPPV in severe asthma are not supported by strong data. In one study (93), only two of 17 severe asthmatic patients (average initial pH of 7.25 and $PaCO_2$ of 65 mm Hg) required intubation after starting therapy with face mask PSV, and the use of NPPV was associated with a rapid correction of gas exchange abnormalities and improvement in dyspnea. In a retrospective analysis of 33 asthmatic patients treated with NPPV or invasive mechanical ventilation (94), although the NPPV patients were less hypercapnic than the other group, gas exchange and vital signs improved rapidly in the NPPV group, and only three patients eventually required endotracheal intubation. A prospective, randomized, placebo controlled study compared 15 patients with acute asthma who received NPPV plus conventional therapy versus conventional therapy alone, and found an improvement in lung function and decreased hospital admission rate in the NPPV group (95). In contrast, another randomized trial found no significant advantages of NPPV in patients with acute asthma (96), and medical therapy alone can be highly effective in the management of asthmatic patients (97). Therefore, in the absence of clear evidence, no conclusions can be drawn regarding the relative effectiveness of NPPV versus conventional therapy in acute exacerbations of asthma.

Hypoxemic Respiratory Failure

Trials of NPPV in patients with hypoxemic respiratory failure, defined as those with ARF not related to COPD, have yielded

TABLE 129.5

RANDOMIZED CONTROLLED STUDIES USING NONINVASIVE VENTILATION IN CHRONIC OBSTRUCTIVE PULMONARY DISEASE

Author, year (reference)	Population	Site	Intervention (NIV/control)	Sample size (NIV/control)	Need for ETI (NIV/control, %)	ICU LOS (NIV/control, days)	Hospital LOS (NIV/control, days)	Survival (NIV/control, %)
Bott et al., 1993 (77)	COPD	Ward	ACV/UMC	30/30	0.0/6.6	NA/NA	9/9	90[a]/70
Brochard et al., 1995 (75)	COPD	ICU	PSV/UMC	43/42	25.6[a]/73.8	7 ± 3[a]/19 ± 13	23 ± 17[a]/35 ± 33	90.7[a]/71.4
Kramer et al., 1995 (81)	Varied	ICU	Bi PAP/UMC	11/8[b]	9.1[a]/66.6[b]	NA/NA	14.9 ± 3.3/17.3 ± 3.0[b]	NA/NA
Barbé et al., 1996 (84)	COPD	Ward	Bi PAP/UMC	10/10	0/0	NA/NA	10.6 ± 0.9/11.3 ± 1.3	100/100
Angus et al., 1996 (85)	COPD	IRCU	PSV/UMC	9/8	NA/NA	NA/NA	NA/NA	100/62.5
Celikel et al., 1998 (82)	COPD	ICU	PSV/UMC	15/15	6.7[a]/40.0	NA/NA	11.7 ± 3.5[a]/14.6 ± 4.7	100/93.3
Nava et al., 1998 (88)	Weaning	ICU	PSV/PSV (invasive)	25/25	NA/NA	15.1 ± 5.4[a]/24 ± 13.7	NA/NA	92[a]/72
Confalonieri et al., 1999 (86)	CAP	IRCU	PSV/UMC	12/11[b]	0.0[a]/54.6[b]	0.25 ± 2.1[a]/7.6 ± 2.2[b]	14.9 ± 3.4/22.5 ± 3.5[b]	91.7/81.8[b]
Plant et al., 2000 (80)	COPD	Ward	Bi PAP/UMC	118/118	15[a]/27	NA/NA	NA/NA	90[a]/80
Martin et al., 2000 (87)	Varied	ICU	Bi PAP/UMC	12/11[b]	25/45[b]	NA/NA	NA/NA	92/91[b]
Conti et al., 2002 (91)	COPD	ED	PSV/ACV, PSV(invasive)	23/26	52/NA	22 ± 1 /21 ± 20	NA/NA	74/54

NIV, noninvasive ventilation; ETI, endotracheal intubation; ICU; intensive care unit; LOS, length of stay; COPD, chronic obstructive pulmonary disease; ACV, assist control ventilation; UMC, usual medical care; NA, not applicable; BiPAP, bilevel positive airway pressure; IRCU, intermediate respiratory care unit; PSV, pressure support ventilation; Weaning, patients in whom NIV was used to facilitate weaning from mechanical ventilation; CAP, community-acquired pneumonia.

[a]Significant difference.

[b]Subset analysis.

conflicting results. In hypoxemic ARF patients, NPPV has been adopted to decrease the amount of work of breathing, correct the rapid shallow breathing, and prevent respiratory muscle fatigue and endotracheal intubation. The studies reviewed in these sections have been conducted on heterogeneous groups of patients with hypoxemic respiratory failure, whereas the analyses of homogeneous patient populations are discussed under each specific topic. Randomized controlled trials using NPPV in hypoxemic ARF patients are shown in Table 129.6.

Meduri et al. (13) in 1989 reported one of the first clinical applications of NPPV in patients with hypoxemic respiratory failure. Subsequently, Pennock et al. (99) reported a 50% success in a large group of patients with ARF of different causes, and similar good results were achieved using NPPV with nasal mask in a second study (100). Wysocki et al. (101) randomized 41 non-COPD patients with ARF to NPPV delivered by face mask versus conventional medical therapy. NPPV reduced the need of endotracheal intubation, the duration of ICU stay, and mortality rate only in those patients with hypercapnia ($PaCO_2$ >45 mm Hg), while having no significant advantages in the hypoxemic group without concomitant hypercarbia. On the basis of these results, the investigators concluded that NPPV may not be beneficial in all forms of ARF not related to COPD. In a study conducted by Meduri et al. (102) on the use of NPPV to treat respiratory failure of varied origins, 41 of 158 patients were hypoxemic. These patients required endotracheal intubation in only 34% of cases and showed a mortality rate of 22% compared with a predicted mortality (using the APACHE II score) of 40%. In a pilot study on patients with hematologic malignancies complicated by ARF (103), 15 of 16 individuals showed a significant improvement in blood gases and respiratory rate within the first 24 hours of nasal mask NPPV treatment.

Antonelli et al. (20) conducted a prospective, randomized study comparing NPPV via a face mask to endotracheal intubation with conventional mechanical ventilation in 64 patients with hypoxemic ARF who required ventilatory assistance after failure to improve with aggressive medical therapy. After 1 hour of mechanical ventilation, both groups had a significant improvement in oxygenation. Ten (31%) patients treated with NPPV required endotracheal intubation. Patients randomized to conventional ventilation developed significantly more frequent septic complications such as pneumonia or sinusitis (31% vs. 3%). Among survivors, NPPV patients had a lower duration of mechanical ventilation ($p = 0.006$) and a shorter ICU stay ($p = 0.002$). On the basis of these results, this trial suggested that NPPV may lead to more favorable outcomes than conventional ventilation in the management of patients with hypoxemic respiratory failure. Conversely, Wood et al. (104) had a substantially negative evaluation of the use of NPPV when applied to patients with hypoxemic ARF. These investigators randomized 27 patients in the emergency department to receive conventional medical therapy or NPPV for the treatment of hypoxemic respiratory failure. The 16 patients who were randomized to the NPPV group had an intubation rate and duration of ICU stay similar to the 11 patients who received medical treatment alone, but there was a trend toward a greater rate of hospital mortality among the patients in the NPPV group compared to patients in the conventional medical therapy group. Several factors may have influenced these negative results of this study. Among patients requiring endotracheal intubation, those of the NPPV group had a longer delay to intubation (26 vs. 4.8 hours, $p = 0.055$). In addition, it cannot be excluded that a sicker patient population was randomized to NPPV. Indeed, NPPV patients had a lower PaO_2 (60 vs. 71), fewer patients with COPD (12% vs. 36%), and more patients with pneumonia (44% vs. 18%), ARDS (1 vs. 0), and interstitial lung disease (1 vs. 0). Furthermore, they had a higher APACHE II score (18 vs. 16), and more required admission to an ICU (81% vs. 64%).

In a study on 10 hemodynamically stable patients with severe acute lung injury or acute respiratory distress syndrome (ARDS) (105), NPPV had a high success rate (66%) and high hospital survival (70%). Three of the six patients who received NPPV as initial mode of ventilatory assistance were discharged from the ICU within 48 hours. Survival for the 10 patients was 70%, and duration of successful NPPV ranged from 23 to 80 hours. Ferrer et al. (106) have prospectively randomized 105 patients with severe hypoxemic ARF to receive NPPV or high-concentration oxygen. Compared with oxygen therapy, NPPV decreased the need for intubation (13 [25%] vs. 28 [52%]), the incidence of septic shock (6 [12%] vs. 17 [31%]), and the ICU mortality (9 [18%] vs. 21 [39%]), and increased the cumulative 90-day survival (all, $p < 0.05$). Also the improvement of tachypnea and arterial hypoxemia was higher in the NPPV group. In a physiologic study performed by L'Her et al. (107) in patients with acute lung injury, noninvasive PSV combined with PEEP improved dyspnea and gas exchange and lowered neuromuscular drive and inspiratory muscle effort.

In ARDS, transient loss of positive pressure during mechanical ventilation may seriously compromise lung recruitment and gas exchange. For this reason, most NPPV studies have excluded patients with ARDS, and limited data are currently available in the literature. The first application of NIV (via face mask CPAP) in patients with increased permeability pulmonary edema ARDS was reported by Barach et al. in 1938 (4). In 1982, Covelli et al. (108) applied face mask CPAP in 35 patients with ARDS of varied causes, with all patients improving their oxygenation within the first hour of therapy. Only five patients were ultimately intubated, two from mask discomfort and three from a change in mental status and lack of cooperation. In two randomized studies, Antonelli et al. (20,21) reported that among patients with ARDS ($n = 31$), NPPV avoided intubation in 60%, whereas in their trial including a small number of ARDS patients ($n = 7$), Ferrer et al. (106) reported an 86% intubation rate. Two NPPV observational studies involving 98 ARDS patients reported an intubation rate of 50% (79,105), which was similar in patients with ARDS of pulmonary or extrapulmonary origin (79). Antonelli et al. (64) prospectively investigated, under close ICU observation, the application of NPPV as first-line intervention in 147 patients with early ARDS. NPPV improved gas exchange and avoided intubation in 54% of treated patients. Avoidance of intubation was associated with less ventilator-associated pneumonia (2% vs. 20%, $p < 0.001$) and a lower ICU mortality rate (6% vs. 53%, $p < 0.001$). SAPS II >34 and a PaO_2/FIO_2 <175 after 1 hour of NPPV were independently associated with NPPV failure and need for endotracheal intubation.

The above findings are, for the most part, supportive of the use of NPPV to treat hypoxemic patients without hypercapnia. However, an extremely prudent approach is needed, limiting the application of NPPV to hemodynamically stable patients who can be closely monitored in the ICU where endotracheal intubation is promptly available. A decisional flow

TABLE 129.6

RANDOMIZED CONTROLLED STUDIES USING NONINVASIVE VENTILATION I \ IN NONCHRONIC OBSTRUCTIVE PULMONARY DISEASE

Author, year (reference)	Population	Site	Intervention (NIV/control)	Sample size (NIV/control)	Need for ETI (NIV/control, %)	ICU LOS (NIV/ control, days)	Hospital LOS (NIV/control, days)	Survival (NIV/control, %)
Wysocki et al., 1993 (101)	Varied	ICU	PSV + PEEP/UMC	21/20	62/70	17 ± 19/25 ± 23	NA/NA	65/70
Antonelli et al., 1998 (20)	AHRF	ICU	PSV + PEEP/ACV, SIMV	32/32	31.3/NA	9 ± 7[a]/16 ± 17	NA/NA	68.8/50.0
Wood et al., 1998 (104)	Varied	ED	Bi PAP/UMC	16/11	45.5/43.8	5.8 ± 5.5/4.9 ± 3.2	17.4 ± 34.3/9.1 ± 5.7	75/100
Girault et al., 1999 (98)	Weaning	ICU	PSV, ACV/PSV	17/16	NA/NA	12.4 ± 6.8/14.1 ± 7.5	27.7 ± 13.1/27.1 ± 14.3	100/87.5
Confalonieri et al., 1999 (86)	CAP	IRCU	PSV/UMC	16/17[b]	37.5/47.1[b]	2.9 ± 1.8/4.8 ± 1.7[b]	17.9 ± 2.9/15.1 ± 2.8[b]	62.5[ac]/76.5[b]
Antonelli et al., 2000 (21)	IC	ICU	PSV + PEEP/UMC	20/20	20/70[a]	5.5 ± 3/9 ± 4[a]	NA/NA	65/45
Martin et al., 2000 (87)	Varied	ICU	Bi PAP/UMC	16/13[b]	37.5[a]/77.0[b]	NA/NA	NA/NA	75/46[b]
Hilbert et al., 2001 (127)	IC	ICU	PSV + PEEP/UMC	26/26	46/77[a]	7 ± 3/10 ± 4	NA/NA	50/81[a]
Ferrer et al., 2003 (106)	AHRF	ICU	Bi PAP/UCM	51/54	25[a]/52	9.6 ± 12.6/11.3 ± 12.6	20.7 ± 16.6/26.8 ± 19.8	82[a]/61

NIV, noninvasive ventilation; ETI, endotracheal intubation; ICU, intensive care unit; LOS, length of stay; PSV, pressure support ventilation; PEEP, positive end-expiratory pressure; UMC, usual medical care; NA, not applicable; AHRF, acute hypoxemic respiratory failure; ACV, assist control ventilation; SIMV, synchronous mandatory ventilation; ED, emergency department; BiPAP, bilevel positive airway pressure; Weaning, patients in whom NIV was used to facilitate weaning from mechanical ventilation; CAP, community-acquired pneumonia; IRCU, intermediate respiratory care unit; IC, immunocompromised.

[a]Significant difference.

[b]Subset analysis.

[c]Hospital survival (no difference noted in 2-month mortality).

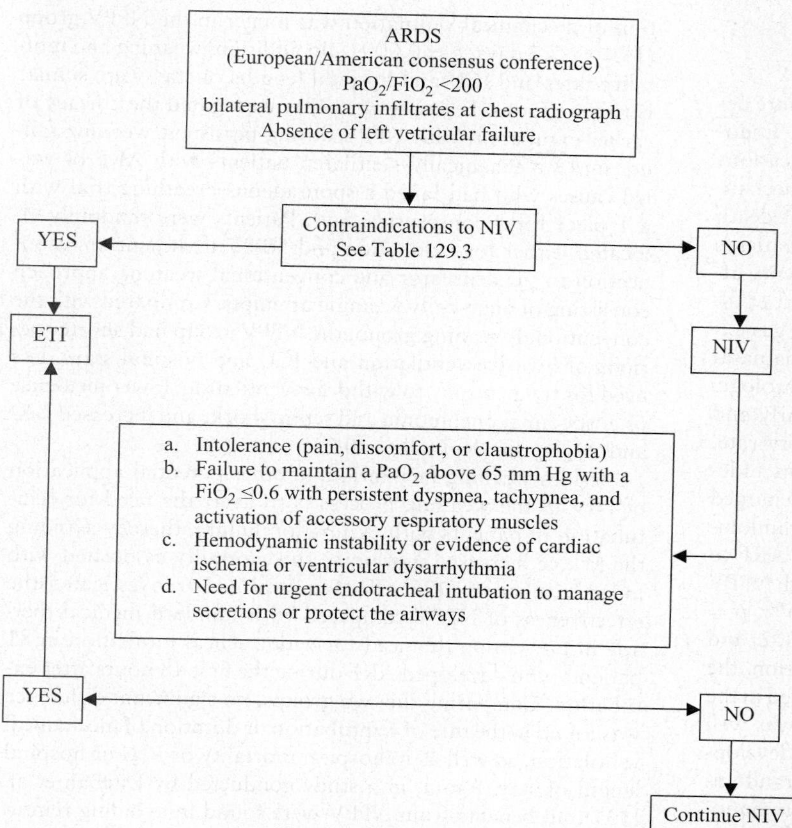

FIGURE 129.9. Decisional flow chart for the application of noninvasive ventilation to acute respiratory distress syndrome (ARDS). ETI, endotracheal intubation; NIV, noninvasive ventilation.

chart may be adopted in applying NPPV to patients with ARDS (Fig. 129.9).

Cardiogenic Pulmonary Edema

Applying positive air pressure has been shown to decrease the work of breathing (41) and left ventricular afterload while maintaining cardiac index (44), thereby benefiting patients with cardiac dysfunction and ARF. The use of mask CPAP in patients with CPE was first described in the 1930s by Poulton and Oxon (2) and Barach et al. (3,4). More recently, several studies have examined responses to NIV of patients with CPE (54–56,109–117).

A systematic review and meta-analysis performed by Collins et al. (118) suggested that early application of NIV in the emergency department can decrease the relative risk of mortality by 39% and the necessity of endotracheal intubation by 57% when compared with standard medical therapy alone. However, in patients with CPE, NIV should not be viewed as the exclusive therapy, but should be accompanied by the aggressive conventional medical treatment.

In the comparison of NIV modalities, BiPAP has the potential advantage over CPAP of assisting the respiratory muscles during inspiration, which would result in faster alleviation of dyspnea and exhaustion (119). Nevertheless, according to all available data, there is no evidence to suggest superiority of either CPAP or BiPAP in terms of intubation or mortality, even in patients with CPE and hypercapnia (118,120,121). The results of one of the earlier studies showed that BiPAP compared with CPAP might increase the risk for new-onset acute myocardial infarction in patients with CPE (55). A recent study specifically examining myocardial infarction rates with BiPAP compared to CPAP (56) showed no significant difference between groups (CPAP, 3/22; BiPAP, 2/24).

In conclusion, NIV should be strongly considered as a first-line treatment in patients with CPE. Future studies are needed to address the NIV modality of choice and to clarify the actual risk of myocardial infarction.

Pneumonia

The application of NIV to treat pneumonia has yielded no definitive conclusions. In a large controlled trial conducted by Ferrer et al. (106) on patients with severe acute hypoxemic failure, NPPV prevented intubation and improved ICU survival in a subgroup of 34 patients with pneumonia compared with high-concentration oxygen. Confalonieri et al. (86) conducted a prospective, randomized study comparing NPPV delivered through a face mask to standard treatment in 56 patients with severe community-acquired pneumonia and ARF. NPPV was associated with a significant reduction in the rate of endotracheal intubation and duration of ICU stay. However, a post hoc analysis showed that the benefits occurred only in patients with underlying COPD. Jolliet et al. (122) used face mask NPPV in non-COPD patients with severe community-acquired pneumonia. Despite initial improvements in arterial oxygenation and respiratory rate in 22 of 24 patients, the intubation rate was high (66%). Thus, NPPV is indicated in COPD patients with community-acquired pneumonia, but caution should be applied in pneumonia patients without COPD, as the benefit of NPPV in such patients is currently unclear.

Immunocompromised Patients

Immunocompromised patients in whom respiratory failure develops often require mechanical ventilatory assistance. Endotracheal intubation is associated with numerous complications (16–19), and in immunosuppressed patients, invasive mechanical ventilation is associated with a significant risk of death (123–125). The use of NPPV in immunosuppressed patients has been reported in several studies. Among 11 patients affected by AIDS and opportunistic pneumonia, Meduri et al. (102) reported a 73% NPPV success rate in improving gas exchange. Conti et al. (103) evaluated NPPV delivered via nasal mask in 16 patients affected by ARF complicating hematologic malignancies. Fifteen of the 16 patients showed an early and significant improvement in blood gases and respiratory rate. Five patients died in the ICU following complications independent of the respiratory failure, whereas 11 were discharged from the ICU in stable condition. Antonelli et al. (21) randomized 40 recipients of solid organ transplantation with ARF to NPPV versus conventional therapy. Patients treated with NPPV more often had increases in oxygenation (60% vs. 25%, $p = 0.03$) and had lower intubation (20% vs. 70%, $p = 0.002$) and ICU mortality rates (20% vs. 50%, $p = 0.05$). In addition, the incidence of fatal complications was significantly reduced in the NPPV group. In another study, NPPV via face mask was well tolerated and avoided intubation in 18 of 21 patients developing ARF after bilateral lung transplantation (126). A randomized trial of 52 ARF patients with pneumonia and immunocompromised state of varied origin (127) showed reductions in the need for intubation (46% vs. 77%, $p = 0.03$) and hospital mortality rate (50% vs. 81%, $p = 0.02$) in NPPV-treated patients compared with conventionally-treated controls. It is reasonable to consider NPPV as a useful tool to avoid intubation and associated infectious complications in selected patients with immunocompromised states.

Facilitation of Weaning and Extubation

NPPV has been used to permit early extubation in patients who fail to meet standard extubation criteria, thus reducing the complications related to endotracheal tube.

Nava et al. (88) conducted a randomized, controlled trial of 50 patients intubated for ARF because of COPD who failed a T-piece weaning trial after 48 hours of invasive mechanical ventilation. Patients were randomized to undergo early extubation followed by face mask PSV or to remain intubated and undergo routine weaning. Patients receiving NPPV had higher overall weaning rates (88% vs. 68%), shorter durations of mechanical ventilation (10.2 vs. 16.6 days), briefer stays in the ICU (15.1 vs. 24 days), and improved 60-day survival rates (92% vs. 72%) (all $p < 0.05$). Furthermore, none of the patients of the NPPV-treated group developed nosocomial pneumonia, compared with seven of the control group. Girault et al. (98) conducted a prospective, randomized controlled study in 33 patients with acute or chronic respiratory failure who failed a 2-hour T-piece weaning trial, although they met simple criteria for weaning. Sixteen patients initiated conventional invasive PSV, and 17 patients received NPPV immediately after extubation. The NPPV group had a shorter duration of endotracheal intubation (4.6 vs. 7.7 days, $p = 0.004$), but the total duration of mechanical ventilation was longer in the NPPV group (16.1 vs. 7.7 days, $p = 0.0001$). In addition, weaning and mortality rates and ICU and hospital lengths of stay were similar between groups. Ferrer et al. (128) investigated the efficacy of earlier extubation with NPPV during persistent weaning failure in 43 mechanically ventilated patients with ARF of varied causes who had failed a spontaneous breathing trial with a T piece for 3 consecutive days. Patients were randomly allocated, either for extubation and NPPV treatment or reconnection to the ventilator and conventional weaning approach consisting of once-daily weaning attempts. Compared with the conventional-weaning group, the NPPV group had shorter periods of invasive ventilation and ICU and hospital stays, less need for tracheotomy to withdraw ventilation, lower incidence of nosocomial pneumonia and septic shock, and increased ICU and 90-day survival (all $p < 0.05$).

Besides weaning facilitation, another potential application of NIV in the weaning process is to avert the need for reintubation in patients with extubation failure, thereby avoiding the risk of increased morbidity and mortality associated with failed extubation (129). Keenan et al. (130) investigated the effectiveness of NPPV compared with standard medical therapy in preventing the need for endotracheal intubation in 81 patients who developed ARF during the first 48 hours after extubation. Comparing the two groups, no significant difference was found in the rate of reintubation or duration of mechanical ventilation, as well as in hospital mortality or ICU or hospital length of stay. Again, in a study conducted by Esteban et al. (131), no benefits from NPPV were found in avoiding reintubation in patients who had developed ARF after extubation, and NPPV was even associated with higher mortality rates as compared with patients treated according to standard treatment. In this study, the time from extubation to reintubation, which is an independent risk factor for increased mortality in reintubated patients (132), was longer in patients who received NPPV. Conversely, positive results were achieved by Ferrer et al. (133) who tested a strategy based on the early use of NPPV to avert reintubation in patients at risk for ARF after extubation. These authors randomized 162 mechanically ventilated patients who tolerated a spontaneous breathing trial but had increased risk for ARF after extubation to receive NPPV for 24 hours versus conventional management with oxygen therapy. In the NPPV group, ARF after extubation was less frequent ($p = 0.029$) and the ICU mortality was lower ($p = 0.015$), whereas 90-day survival did not change significantly between groups. Separate analyses of patients without and with hypercapnia ($PaCO_2$ >45 mm Hg) during the spontaneous breathing trial showed that NPPV significantly improved ICU mortality and 90-day survival in hypercapnic patients only.

In summary, further studies are needed to establish the real efficacy of NPPV either in shortening weaning time or to avoid extubation failure, as well as to better define which patient categories are most likely to benefit from NPPV during the weaning process.

Do-Not-Intubate Orders

Applying NPPV has been described in patients with ARF who are poor candidates for endotracheal intubation or who are reluctant to undergo invasive ventilation. In one study of 30 patients, most elderly and COPD, in whom invasive ventilation was "contraindicated or postponed," 18 patients (60%) were able to be successfully weaned from nasal mask NPPV (134). In a case series of 11 terminally ill patients with ARF who refused endotracheal intubation (135), NPPV delivered via face mask was effective in correcting gas exchange abnormalities in 7 patients, all of whom survived and left the ICU. The authors concluded that even when respiratory failure did not resolve, NPPV offered an effective, comfortable, and dignified method for these patients in providing symptomatic relief of dyspnea and maintaining continuous verbal communication with loved ones. In a trial conducted on 114 patients who declined intubation but accepted NPPV to treat their ARF (136), 49 patients (43%) survived to discharge. Awake patients with congestive heart failure or COPD and those with a more efficient cough mechanism had an increased probability of survival. Another study on 37 COPD patients with do-not-intubate orders who underwent NPPV because of ARF reported a 1-year survival of 30% (137).

A lack of agreement on applying NPPV in do-not-intubate patients does remain, with some authors warning of the potential ethical and economic cost of delaying the inevitable in patients with terminal respiratory failure (138). In patients with the do-not-intubate code, the use of NPPV is justifiable when the acute process responsible for ARF is known to respond well, such as CPE or COPD exacerbation. If NPPV is considered in these terminal patients, the caring clinician should inform the patient or surrogate that NPPV is being used as a form of life support and that it can be stopped at any time if not tolerated.

Postoperative Patients

Thoracic and upper abdominal surgery are associated with a prolonged postoperative gas exchange deterioration and reduction in functional residual capacity, PaO_2, and forced vital capacity (139,140). Mask CPAP was initially used by Bunnell (1) in 1912 to maintain lung expansion in patients undergoing thoracic surgery, and by Boothby (141) et al. in 1940 for treating postoperative hypoxemic ARF. Applying mask CPAP or NPPV improves oxygenation and pulmonary function following upper abdominal surgery (139,142–144) or coronary artery bypass graft (145–147). Squadrone et al. (143) randomized 209 patients who developed severe hypoxemia after major elective abdominal surgery to receive oxygen or oxygen plus CPAP. CPAP-treated patients had a lower intubation rate (1% vs. 10%) and a lower occurrence rate of pneumonia (2% vs. 10%), infection (3% vs. 10%), and sepsis (2% vs. 9%) (all $p < 0.05$) than patients treated with oxygen alone. NPPV improves gas exchange and reduces the need for intubation after lung resection (148,149) or bilateral lung transplantation (126). Thus, accumulating evidence supports the use of NIV to improve gas exchange and avoid reintubation and its attendant complications in selected postoperative patients with respiratory failure.

Obstructive Sleep Apnea

CPAP is recognized to be effective in correcting the respiratory and arousal abnormalities and improving sleep quality in obstructive sleep apnea syndrome (150,151). CPAP is believed to act by pneumatically "splinting" the pharyngeal airway, thus preventing its collapse during sleep (152,153). Also, nasal NPPV has been used in patients with ARF following obstructive sleep apnea syndrome, with improvements in clinical status and arterial blood gas values (154).

Trauma

ARF in trauma patients is generally associated with reduced pulmonary compliance and functional residual capacity, and subsequent restrictive defects (155). In a study of 33 trauma patients with ARF who received face mask CPAP, Hurst et al. (155) found rapid improvements in gas exchange, avoiding intubation in 94% of the cases. In a retrospective survey of 46 trauma patients with ARF who had been given mask NPPV, 33 patients (72%) were successfully weaned to spontaneous breathing (156). In another study (157), NPPV used as first-line treatment in 22 patients with ARF due to blunt chest trauma resulted in rapid improvement in blood gases and respiratory rate, and avoided intubation in 18 patients (82%). In a study of patients with acute hypoxemic respiratory failure needing ventilatory assistance, Antonelli et al. (20) reported that 7 of the 32 patients (22%) randomized to receive NPPV had trauma with pulmonary contusion or atelectasis. NPPV was associated with a rapid improvement in oxygenation, and all seven patients avoided intubation and survived. Despite the favorable results obtained, large randomized studies are needed before definitive recommendations on the use of NIV in posttraumatic ARF can be made.

Restrictive Diseases

NPPV has a role in the treatment of respiratory failure caused by some types of restrictive thoracic diseases. Bach et al. (158) demonstrated that NPPV can prolong survival while decreasing the respiratory morbidity and hospitalization rates in patients with Duchenne muscular dystrophy. Using NPPV prevented intubation in 7 of 11 episodes of ARF in a group of 9 patients with myasthenic crises (159). In ARF due to pulmonary fibrosis, prognosis is poor even when invasive mechanical ventilation is used (160). Aggressive respiratory physiotherapy is crucial in all patients with thoracic restriction.

Bronchoscopy

In nonintubated patients, severe hypoxemia is an accepted contraindication to fiberoptic bronchoscopy (FB). Since PaO_2 routinely decreases after uncomplicated FB, these patients are at high risk for developing ARF or serious cardiac arrhythmias. Antonelli et al. (161,162) proposed a technique to perform FB with bronchoalveolar lavage in hypoxemic, nonintubated patients by means of facial mask NPPV (Fig. 129.10). The fiberoptic bronchoscope was passed through a T adapter and then advanced transnasally. The technique was safe and effective to avoid gas exchange worsening during FB and to allow an early and accurate diagnosis of pneumonia, preventing undesired intubation, in spontaneously breathing, hypoxemic patients. Similar results were achieved by using the helmet to deliver NPPV, allowing a safe diagnostic FB with bronchoalveolar lavage (163). The specific seal connector placed in the plastic

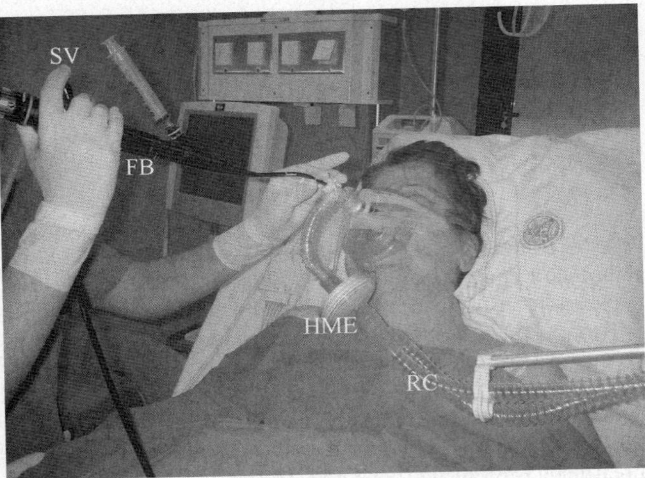

FIGURE 129.10. Fiberoptic bronchoscopy performed during noninvasive ventilation delivered through an oronasal mask. FB, fiberoptic bronchoscope; HME, heat and moisture exchanger; RC, respiratory circuit; SC, seal connection; SV, suction valve. (Photograph printed with the permission of the patient.)

ring of the helmet permitted the passage of the instrument, maintaining assisted ventilation.

ADVERSE EFFECTS AND COMPLICATIONS

Major adverse effects of NIV seldom occur in appropriately selected patients and are minimized when the technique is applied by experienced caregivers (164). The most frequently encountered complications are related to the interface, ventilator airflow or pressure, or patient–ventilator interaction.

The pressure of the mask over the bridge of the nose may induce discomfort, erythema, or ulceration (Fig. 129.2). There are various remedies to ameliorate this complication such as application of a hydrocolloid sheet over the nasal bridge or switching to alternative interfaces.

Air leakage under the mask into the eyes may cause conjunctival irritation, and excessive pressure may be responsible for sinus or ear pain. To minimize these problems, refitting the mask or lowering inspiratory pressure may be useful. Patient–ventilator asynchrony is a common cause of NIV failure and is often related to patient agitation or inability of the ventilator to sense the onset of patient expiration because of excessive air leaking. A judicious use of sedatives may be safe and effective in the treatment of NIV failure due to low tolerance (165), and minimizing air leaks (57,59) may improve patient–ventilator synchrony.

Presumably because of the low inflation pressure used compared with invasive ventilation, NPPV is well tolerated hemodynamically, but it should be avoided in patients with an unstable hemodynamic status, arrhythmias, or uncontrolled ischemia until these problems are stabilized. Gastric insufflation occurs commonly, but it is usually well tolerated. Aspiration pneumonia has been reported in as many as 5% of patients (102). The risk for aspiration is minimized by excluding patients with compromised upper airway function or problems clearing secretions and positioning a nasogastric tube in those with excessive gastric distention, an ileus, or nausea or vomiting. Although pneumothoraces occur very infrequently, inspiratory pressures should be kept at the minimum effective level in patients with bullous lung disease.

SUMMARY

To date, the best-established indication for NIV in the acute care setting is ARF related to exacerbations of COPD. However, evidence has been rapidly accumulating to support application of NIV to treat many other types of ARF in selected patients. Further research should better define indications and patient selection criteria, as well as establish optimal techniques of administration.

PEARLS

- NIV has the potential of avoiding the complications associated with endotracheal intubation, improving patient comfort, and preserving speech and airway defense mechanisms.
- Advances in patient–ventilator interfaces and ventilatory modes have fostered the increasing use of NIV in the acute care setting.
- The choice of ventilatory mode should be dictated by personal experience, as well as the patient's respiratory drive, and etiologic factors and severity of the underlying disease causing respiratory failure.
- It is crucial to identify patients who are likely to benefit from NIV and exclude those for whom NIV would be unsafe.
- Several factors are critical to the success of NIV: properly timed initiation, comfortable and well-fitting interface, patient preparation, careful ventilatory mode selection, and respiratory physiotherapy.
- Patients should receive NIV in an intensive care unit or a step-down unit for continuous monitoring until sufficient stabilization.
- NIV can be used to avoid intubation, *but not to replace it.* Invasive ventilation remains the method of choice for patients with respiratory failure who have contraindications to NIV.
- NIV is indicated as the ventilator mode of first choice in selected patients with COPD exacerbations.
- In acute hypoxemic respiratory failure without hypercapnia, NIV can be used as long as patients are hemodynamically stable and are closely monitored in the intensive care unit to avoid dangerous delays if intubation becomes necessary.
- NIV has a central role in the management of acute respiratory failure of varied causes, improving patient outcome and efficiency of care in the acute setting.

References

1. Bunnel S. The use of nitrous oxide and oxygen to maintain anesthesia and positive pressure for thoracic surgery. *JAMA.* 1912;58:835.
2. Poulton EP, Oxon DM. Left-sided heart failure with pulmonary edema—its treatment with the "pulmonary plus pressure machine." *Lancet.* 1936;231: 981.
3. Barach AL, Martin J, Eckman M: Positive-pressure respiration and its application for the treatment of acute pulmonary edema and respiratory obstruction. *Proc Am Soc Clin Invest.* 1937;16:664.

4. Barach AL, Martin J, Eckman M. Positive-pressure respiration and its application to the treatment of acute pulmonary edema. *Ann Intern Med.* 1938;12:754.
5. Barach AL, Swenson P. Effect of breathing gases under positive pressure on lumens of small and medium sized bronchi. *Arch Intern Med.* 1939;63:946.
6. Motley HL, Lang LP, Gordon B. Use of intermittent positive pressure breathing combined with nebulization in pulmonary disease. *Am J Med.* 1948;5:853.
7. The Intermittent Positive Pressure Breathing Trial Group. Intermittent positive pressure breathing therapy of chronic obstructive pulmonary disease. *Ann Intern Med.* 1983;99:612.
8. Sullivan CE, Issa FG, Berthon-Jones M, et al. Reversal of obstructive sleep apnea by continuous positive airway pressure applied through the nares. *Lancet.* 1981;1:862.
9. Rideau Y, Gatin G, Bach J, et al. Prolongation of life in Duchenne's muscular dystrophy. *Acta Neurol Belg.* 1983;5:118.
10. Kerby GR, Mayer LS, Pingleton SK. Nocturnal positive pressure ventilation via nasal mask. *Am Rev Respir Dis.* 1987;135:738.
11. Ellis ER, Bye PT, Bruderer JW, et al. Treatment of respiratory failure during sleep in patients with neuromuscular disease: positive-pressure ventilation through a nose mask. *Am Rev Respir Dis.* 1987;135:148.
12. Bach JR, Alba AS. Management of chronic alveolar hypoventilation by nasal ventilation. *Chest.* 1990;97:52.
13. Meduri GU, Conoscenti CC, Menashe P, et al. Noninvasive face mask ventilation in patients with acute respiratory failure. *Chest.* 1989;95:865.
14. Brochard L, Isabey D, Piquet J, et al. Reversal of acute exacerbations of chronic obstructive lung disease by inspiratory assistance with a face mask. *N Engl J Med.* 1990;95:865.
15. Elliott MW, Steven MH, Phillips GD, et al. Noninvasive mechanical ventilation for acute respiratory failure. *BMJ.* 1990;300:358.
16. Zwillich CW, Pirson DJ, Creagh CE, et al. Complications of assisted ventilation. *Am J Med.* 1974;57:161.
17. Stauffer JL, Olson DE, Petty TL. Complications and consequences of endotracheal intubation. *Am J Med.* 1981;70:65.
18. Craven DE, Kunches LM, Kilinsky V, et al. Risk factors for pneumonia and fatality in patients receiving continuous mechanical ventilation. *Am Rev Respir Dis.* 1986;113:792.
19. Pingleton SK. Complications of acute respiratory failure. *Am Rev Respir Dis.* 1988;137:1463.
20. Antonelli M, Conti G, Rocco M, et al. A comparison of noninvasive positive-pressure ventilation and conventional mechanical ventilation in patients with acute respiratory failure. *N Engl J Med.* 1998;339:429.
21. Antonelli M, Conti C, Bufi M, et al. Noninvasive ventilation for treatment of acute respiratory failure in patients undergoing solid organ transplantation. *JAMA.* 2000;283:235.
22. Nourdine K, Combes P, Carton MJ, et al. Does noninvasive ventilation reduce the ICU nosocomial infection risk? A prospective clinical survey. *Intensive Care Med.* 1999;25:567.
23. Girou E, Schortgen F, Delclaux C, et al. Association of noninvasive ventilation with nosocomial infections and survival in critically ill patients. *JAMA.* 2000;284:2361.
24. Esteban A, Anzueto A, Frutos F, et al. Characteristics and outcomes in adult patients receiving mechanical ventilation: a 28-day international study. *JAMA.* 2002;287:345.
25. Demoule A, Girou E, Richard JC, et al. Increased use of noninvasive ventilation in French intensive care units. *Intensive Care Med.* 2006;32:1747.
26. Carlucci A, Richard JC, Wysocki M, et al. Noninvasive versus conventional mechanical ventilation. An epidemiologic survey. *Am J Respir Crit Care Med.* 2001;163:874.
27. Antonelli M, Conti G. Noninvasive ventilation in intensive care unit patients. *Curr Opin Crit Care.* 2000;6:11.
28. Criner GJ, Travaline JM, Brennan KJ, et al. Efficacy of a new full face mask for noninvasive positive pressure. *Chest.* 1994;106:1109.
29. Antonelli M, Conti G, Pelosi P, et al. New treatment of acute hypoxemic respiratory failure: noninvasive pressure support ventilation delivered by helmet—a pilot controlled trial. *Crit Care Med.* 2002;30:602.
30. Antonelli M, Pennisi MA, Pelosi P, et al. Noninvasive positive pressure ventilation using a helmet in patients with acute exacerbation of chronic obstructive pulmonary disease: a feasibility study. *Anesthesiology.* 2004;100:16.
31. Piastra M, Antonelli M, Chiaretti M, et al. Treatment of acute respiratory failure by helmet-delivered non-invasive ventilation in children with acute leukemia: a pilot study. *Intensive Care Med.* 2004;30:472.
32. Bach JR, Alba AS, Saporito LR. Intermittent positive pressure ventilation via the mouth as an alternative to tracheostomy for 257 ventilator users. *Chest.* 1993;103:174.
33. Schettino GP, Tucci MR, Sousa R, et al. Mask mechanics and leak dynamics during noninvasive pressure support ventilation: a bench study. *Intensive Care Med.* 2001;27:1887.
34. Navalesi P, Fanfulla F, Frigeiro P, et al. Physiologic evaluation of noninvasive mechanical ventilation delivered with three types of masks in patients with chronic hypercapnic respiratory failure. *Chest.* 2000;28:1785.
35. Kwok H, McCormack J, Cece R, et al. Controlled trial of oronasal versus nasal mask ventilation in the treatment of acute respiratory failure. *Crit Care Med.* 2003;31:468.
36. Patroniti N, Foti G, Manfio A, et al. Head helmet versus face mask for non-invasive continuous positive airway pressure: a physiological study. *Intensive Care Med.* 2003;29:1680.
37. Costa R, Navalesi P, Antonelli M, et al. Physiologic evaluation of different levels of assistance during noninvasive ventilation delivered through a helmet. *Chest.* 2005;128:2984.
38. Chiumello D, Pelosi P, Carlesso E, et al. Noninvasive positive pressure ventilation delivered by helmet vs. standard face mask. *Intensive Care Med.* 2003;29:1671.
39. Racca F, Appendini L, Gregoretti C, et al. Effectiveness of mask and helmet interfaces to deliver noninvasive ventilation in a human model of resistive breathing. *J Appl Physiol.* 2005;99:1262.
40. Moerer O, Fisher S, Quintel M, et al. Influence of two different interfaces for noninvasive ventilation compared to invasive ventilation on the mechanical properties and performance of a respiratory system: a lung model study. *Chest.* 2006;129:1424.
41. Katz JA, Marks JD. Inspiratory work with and without continuous positive airway pressure in patients with acute respiratory failure. *Anesthesiology.* 1985;63:598.
42. Petrof BJ, Legere M, Goldberg P, et al. Continuous positive airway pressure reduced work of breathing and dyspnea during weaning from mechanical ventilation in severe chronic obstructive pulmonary disease. *Am Rev Respir Dis.* 1990;141:281.
43. Rasanen J, Heikkila J, Downs J, et al. Continuous positive airway pressure by face mask in acute cardiogenic pulmonary edema. *Am J Cardiol.* 1985;55:296.
44. Naughton MT, Rahman MA, Hara K, et al. Effect of continuous positive airway pressure on intrathoracic and left ventricular transmural pressures in patients with congestive heart failure. *Circulation.* 1995;91:1725.
45. Scharf SM, Caldini P, Ingram RH. Cardiovascular effects of increasing airway pressure in the dog. *Am J Physiol.* 1977;232:H35.
46. Braunwald E, Binion JT, WL Morgan, et al. Alterations in central blood volume and cardiac output induced by positive pressure breathing counteracted by metaraminol (Aramine). *Circ Res.* 1957;5:670.
47. Fessler H, Brower R, Wise R, et al. Effects of positive end-expiratory pressure on the gradient for venous return. *Am Rev Respir Dis.* 1991;143:19.
48. Nanas S, Magder S. Adaptation of the peripheral circulation to PEEP. *Am Rev Respir Dis.* 1992;146:688.
49. Jellinek H, Krenn H, Oczenski W, et al. Influence of positive airway pressure on the pressure gradient for venous return in humans. *J Appl Physiol.* 2000;88:926.
50. Gibney RT, Wilson RS, Pontoppidan H. Comparison of work of breathing on high gas flow and demand valve continuous positive airway pressure systems. *Chest.* 1982;82:692.
51. Beydon L, Chasse M, Harf A, et al. Inspiratory work of breathing during spontaneous ventilation using demand valves and continuous flow systems. *Am Rev Respir Dis.* 1988;138:300.
52. Sassoon CSH, Lodia R, Rheeman CH, et al. Inspiratory muscle work of breathing during flow-by, demand-flow and continuous-flow systems in patients with chronic obstructive pulmonary disease. *Am Rev Respir Dis.* 1992;145:1219.
53. Younes M, Puddy A, Roberts D, et al. Proportional assist ventilation: results of an initial clinical trial. *Am Rev Respir Dis.* 1992;145:121.
54. Bersten AD, Holt AW, Vedig AE, et al. Treatment of severe cardiogenic pulmonary edema with continuous positive airway pressure delivered by face mask. *N Engl J Med.* 1991;325:1825.
55. Mehta S, Jay GD, Woolard RH, et al. Randomized prospective trial of bilevel versus continuous positive airway pressure in acute pulmonary edema. *Crit Care Med.* 1997;25:620.
56. Bellone A, Monari A, Cortellaro F, et al. Myocardial infarction rate in acute pulmonary edema. *Crit Care Med.* 2004;32:1860.
57. Mehta S, McCool FD, Hill NS. Leak compensation in positive pressure ventilators: a lung model study. *Eur Respir J.* 2001;17:259.
58. Jubran A, Van de Graffe WB, Tobin MJ. Variability of patient–ventilator interaction with pressure support ventilation in patients with chronic obstructive pulmonary disease. *Am J Respir Crit Care Med.* 1995;152:129.
59. Calderini E, Confalonieri M, Puccio PG, et al. Patient–ventilator asynchrony during noninvasive ventilation: the role of expiratory trigger. *Intensive Care Med.* 1999;25:662.
60. Appendini L, Palessio A, Zanaboni S, et al. Physiologic effects of positive end-expiratory pressure and mask pressure support during exacerbations of chronic obstructive pulmonary disease. *Am J Respir Crit Care Med.* 1994;149:1069.
61. Vitacca M, Clini E, Pagani M, et al. Physiologic effects of early administered mask proportional assist ventilation in patients with chronic obstructive pulmonary disease and acute respiratory failure. *Crit Care Med.* 2000;28:1791.
62. Girault C, Richard JC, Chevron V, et al. Comparative physiologic effects of noninvasive assist-control and pressure support ventilation in acute hypercapnic respiratory failure. *Chest.* 1997;111:1639.
63. Vitacca M, Rubini F, Foglio K, et al. Non-invasive modalities of positive pressure ventilation improve the outcome of acute exacerbations in COLD patients. *Intensive Care Med.* 1993;19:450.
64. Antonelli M, Conti G, Esquinas A, et al. A multiple-center survey on the

use in clinical practice of noninvasive ventilation as a first-line intervention for acute respiratory distress sindrome. *Crit Care Med.* 2007;35:18–25.
65. Aslanian P, El Atrous S, Isabey D, et al. Effects of flow triggering on breathing effort during partial ventilatory support. *Am J Respir Crit Care Med.* 1998 Jan;157(1):135.
66. Giuliani R, Mascia L, Recchia F, et al. Patient–ventilator interaction during synchronized intermittent mandatory ventilation. Effects of flow triggering. *Am J Respir Crit Care Med.* 1995;151:1.
67. Nava S, Ambrosino N, Bruschi C, et al. Physiological effects of flow and pressure triggering during non-invasive mechanical ventilation in patients with chronic obstructive pulmonary disease. *Thorax.* 1997;52:249.
68. Organized jointly by the American Thoracic Society, the European Respiratory Society, the European Society of Intensive Care Medicine, and the Societe de Reanimation de Langue Francaise, and approved by ATS Board of Directors, December 2000. International Consensus Conferences in Intensive Care Medicine: noninvasive positive pressure ventilation in acute respiratory failure. *Am J Respir Crit Care Med.* 2001;163:283.
69. Bach JR, Saporito LR. Criteria for extubation and tracheostomy tube removal for patients with ventilatory failure: a different approach to weaning. *Chest.* 1996;110:1566.
70. Bach JR, Mechanical insufflation-exsufflation: comparison of peak expiratory flows and manually assisted and unassisted coughing techniques. *Chest.* 1993;104:1553.
71. Diaz GG, Alcaraz AC, Talavera JC, et al. Noninvasive positive-pressure ventilation to treat hypercapnic coma secondary to respiratory failure. *Chest.* 2005;127:952.
72. Scala R, Naldi M, Archinucci I, et al. Noninvasive positive pressure ventilation in patients with acute exacerbations of COPD and varying levels of consciousness. *Chest.* 2005;128:1657.
73. Pankow W, Hijjeh N, Schuttler F, et al. Influence of noninvasive positive pressure ventilation on inspiratory muscle activity in obese subjects. *Eur Respir J.* 1997;10:2847.
74. Ambrosino N, Foglio K, Rubini F, et al. Non-invasive mechanical ventilation in acute respiratory failure due to chronic obstructive pulmonary disease: correlates for success. *Thorax.* 1995;50:755.
75. Brochard L, Mancebo J, Wysocki M, et al. Noninvasive ventilation for acute exacerbations of chronic obstructive pulmonary disease. *N Engl J Med.* 1995;333:817.
76. Soo Hoo GW, Santiago S, Williams J. Nasal mechanical ventilation for hypercapnic respiratory failure in chronic obstructive pulmonary disease: determinants of success and failure. *Crit Care Med.* 1994;27:417.
77. Bott J, Carroll MP, Conway JH, et al. Randomized controlled trial of nasal ventilation in acute ventilatory failure due to chronic obstructive airways disease. *Lancet.* 1993;341:1555.
78. Moretti M, Cilione C, Tampieri A, et al. Incidence and causes of non-invasive mechanical ventilation failure after initial success. *Thorax.* 2000;55:819.
79. Antonelli M, Conti G, Moro ML, et al. Predictors of failure of noninvasive positive pressure ventilation in patients with acute hypoxemic respiratory failure: a multi-center study. *Intensive Care Med.* 2001;27:1718.
80. Plant PK, Owen JL, Elliott MW. Early use of noninvasive ventilation for acute exacerbations of chronic obstructive pulmonary disease on general respiratory wards: a multicenter randomized controlled trial. *Lancet.* 2000;355:1931.
81. Kramer N, Meyer TJ, Meharg J, et al. Randomized, prospective trial of noninvasive positive pressure ventilation in acute respiratory failure. *Am J Respir Crit Care Med.* 1995;151:1799.
82. Celikel T, Sungur M, Ceyhan B, et al. Comparison of noninvasive positive pressure ventilation with standard medical therapy in hypercapnic acute respiratory failure. *Chest.* 1998;114:1636.
83. Mehta S, Hill NS. Noninvasive ventilation. *Am J Respir Crit Care Med.* 2001;163:540.
84. Barbé F, Togores B, Rubi M, et al. Noninvasive ventilatory support does not facilitate recovery from acute respiratory failure in chronic obstructive pulmonary disease. *Eur Respir J.* 1996;9:1240.
85. Angus RM, Ahmed AA, Fenwick LJ, et al. Comparison of the acute effects on gas exchange of nasal ventilation and doxapram in exacerbations of chronic obstructive pulmonary disease. *Thorax.* 1996;51:1048.
86. Confalonieri M, Potena A, Carbone G, et al. Acute respiratory failure in patients with severe community-acquired pneumonia. A prospective randomized evaluation of noninvasive ventilation. *Am J Respir Crit Care Med.* 1999;160:1585.
87. Martin TJ, Hovis JD, Constantino JP, et al. A randomized prospective evaluation of noninvasive ventilation for acute respiratory failure. *Am J Respir Crit Care Med.* 2000;161:807.
88. Nava S, Ambrosino N, Clini E, et al. Noninvasive mechanical ventilation in the weaning of patients with respiratory failure due to chronic obstructive pulmonary disease. A randomized, controlled trial. *Ann Intern Med.* 1998;128:721.
89. Thys F, Roeseler J, Reynaert M, et al. Noninvasive ventilation for acute respiratory failure: a prospective randomised placebo-controlled trial. *Eur Respir J.* 2002;20:545.
90. Dikensoy O, Ikidag B, Filiz A, et al. Comparison of non-invasive ventilation and standard medical therapy in acute hypercapnic respiratory failure: a randomised controlled study at a tertiary health centre in SE Turkey. *Int J Clin Pract.* 2002;56:85.
91. Conti G, Antonelli M, Navalesi P, et al. Noninvasive vs. conventional mechanical ventilation in patients with chronic obstructive pulmonary disease after failure of medical treatment in the ward: a randomized trial. *Intensive Care Med.* 2002;28:1701.
92. Squadrone E, Frigerio P, Fogliati C, et al. Noninvasive vs. invasive ventilation in COPD patients with severe acute respiratory failure deemed to require ventilatory assistance. *Intensive Care Med.* 2004;30:1303.
93. Meduri GU, Cook TR, Turner RE, et al. Noninvasive positive pressure ventilation in status asthmaticus. *Chest.* 1996;110:767.
94. Fernandez MM, Villagra A, Blanch L, et al. Non-invasive mechanical ventilation in status asthmaticus. *Intensive Care Med.* 2001;27:486.
95. Soroksky A, Stav D, Shpirer I. A pilot prospective, randomized, placebo-controlled trial of bilevel positive airway pressure in acute asthmatic attack. *Chest.* 2003;123:1018.
96. Holley MT, Morrissey TK, Seaberg DC, et al. Ethical dilemmas in a randomized trial of asthma treatment: can Bayesian statistical analysis explain the results? *Acad Emerg Med.* 2001;8:1128.
97. Levy BD, Kitch B, Fanta CH. Medical and ventilatory management of status asthmaticus. *Intensive Care Med.* 1998;24:105.
98. Girault C, Daudenthun I, Chevron V, et al. Noninvasive ventilation as a systematic extubation and weaning technique in acute-on-chronic respiratory failure: a prospective, randomized controlled study. *Am J Respir Crit Care Med.* 1999;160:86.
99. Pennock BE, Crawshaw L, Kaplan PD. Noninvasive nasal mask ventilation for acute respiratory failure. *Chest.* 1994;105:441.
100. Lapinsky SE, Mount DNB, Mackey D, et al. Management of acute respiratory failure due to pulmonary edema with nasal positive pressure support. *Chest.* 1994;105:229.
101. Wysocki M, Tric L, Wolff MA, et al. Noninvasive pressure support ventilation in patients with acute respiratory failure. *Chest.* 1993;103:907.
102. Meduri GU, Turner RE, Abou-Shala N, et al. Noninvasive positive pressure ventilation via face mask. *Chest.* 1996;109:179.
103. Conti G, Marino P, Cogliati A, et al. Noninvasive ventilation for the treatment of acute respiratory failure in patients with hematologic malignancies: a pilot study. *Intensive Care Med.* 1998;24:1283.
104. Wood KA, Lewis L, Von Harz B, et al. The use of noninvasive positive pressure ventilation in the emergency department. *Chest.* 1998;113:1339.
105. Rocker GM, Mackensie M-G, Willilams B, et al. Noninvasive positive pressure ventilation: successful outcome in patients with acute lung injury/ARDS. *Chest.* 1999;115:173.
106. Ferrer M, Esquinas A, Leon M, et al. Noninvasive ventilation in severe hypoxemic respiratory failure: a randomized clinical trial. *Am J Respir Crit Care Med.* 2003;168:1438.
107. L'Her E, Deye N, Lellouche F, et al. Physiologic effects of noninvasive ventilation during acute lung injury. *Am J Respir Crit Care Med.* 2005;172:1112.
108. Covelli HD, Weled BJ, Beekman JF. Efficacy of continuous positive airway pressure administered by face mask. *Chest.* 1982;81:147.
109. Masip J, Betbese AJ, Paez J, et al. Non-invasive pressure support ventilation versus conventional oxygen therapy in acute cardiogenic pulmonary edema: a randomized study. *Lancet.* 2000;356:2126.
110. Levitt MA. A prospective, randomized trial of BIPAP in severe acute congestive heart failure. *J Emerg Med.* 2001;21:363.
111. Kelly CA, Newby DE, McDonagh TA, et al. Randomised controlled trial of continuous positive airway pressure and standard oxygen therapy in acute pulmonary oedema. *Eur Heart J.* 2002;23:1379.
112. Nava S, Carbone G, Dibatista N, et al. Noninvasive ventilation in cardiogenic pulmonary edema. *Am J Respir Crit Care Med.* 2003;168:1432.
113. Cross AM, Cameron P, Kierce M, et al. Non-invasive ventilation in acute respiratory failure. *Emerg Med J.* 2003;20:531.
114. L'Her E, Duquesne F, Girou E, et al. Noninvasive continuous positive airway pressure in elderly cardiogenic pulmonary edema patients. *Intensive Care Med.* 2004;30:882.
115. Park M, Sangean MC, Volpe MC, et al. Randomized, prospective trial of oxygen, continuous positive airway pressure, and bilevel positive airway pressure by face mask in acute cardiogenic pulmonary edema. *Crit Care Med.* 2004;32:2407.
116. Crane SD, Elliott MW, Gilligan P, et al. Randomised controlled comparison of continuous positive airways pressure, bilevel non-invasive ventilation, and standard treatment in emergency department in patients with acute cardiogenic pulmonary oedema. *Emerg Med J.* 2004;21:155.
117. Bellone A, Vettorello M, Monari A, et al. Noninvasive pressure support ventilation vs. continuous positive airway pressure in acute hypercapnic pulmonary edema. *Intensive Care Med.* 2005;31:807.
118. Collins SP, Mielniczuk LM, Whittingham HA, et al The use of noninvasive ventilation in emergency department patients with acute cardiogenic pulmonary edema: a systematic review. *Ann Emerg Med.* 2006;48:260.
119. Wysocki M. Noninvasive ventilation in acute cardiogenic pulmonary edema: better than continuous positive airway pressure? *Intensive Care Med.* 1999;25:1.
120. Masip J, Roque M, Sanchez B, et al. Noninvasive ventilation in acute cardiogenic pulmonary edema: systematic review and meta-analysis. *JAMA.* 2005;294:3124.
121. Ho KM, Wong K. A comparison of continuous and bi-level positive

airway pressure non-invasive ventilation in patients with acute cardiogenic pulmonary oedema: a meta-analysis. *Crit Care.* 2006;10:R49.
122. Jolliet P, Abajo B, Pasquina P, et al. Non-invasive pressure support ventilation in severe community-acquired pneumonia. *Intensive Care Med.* 2001;27:812.
123. Estopa R, Torres-Marti A, Kastanos N, et al. Acute respiratory failure in severe hematologic disorders. *Crit Care Med.* 1984;12:26.
124. Blot F, Guignet M, Nitenberg G, et al. Prognostic factors for neutropenic patients in an intensive care unit: respective roles of underlying malignancies and acute organ failures. *Eur J Cancer.* 1997;33:1031.
125. Ewig S, Torres A, Riquelme R, et al. Pulmonary complications in patients with haematological malignancies treated at a respiratory ICU. *Eur Respir J.* 1998;12:116.
126. Rocco M, Conti G, Antonelli M, et al. Non-invasive pressure support ventilation in patients with acute respiratory failure after bilateral lung transplantation. *Intensive Care Med.* 2001;27:1622.
127. Hilbert G, Gruson D, Vargas F, et al. Noninvasive ventilation in immunosuppressed patients with pulmonary infiltrates, fever, and acute respiratory failure. *N Engl J Med.* 2001;344:481.
128. Ferrer M, Esquinas A, Arancibia F, et al. Noninvasive ventilation during persistent weaning failure: a randomized controlled trial. *Am J Respir Crit Care Med.* 2003;168:70.
129. Epstein SK, Ciubotaru RL, Wong JB. Effect of failed extubation on the outcome of mechanical ventilation. *Chest.* 1997;112:186.
130. Keenan SP, Powers C, McCormack DG, et al. Noninvasive positive-pressure ventilation for postextubation respiratory distress: a randomized controlled trial. *JAMA.* 2002;287:3238.
131. Esteban A, Frutos-Vivar F, Ferguson ND, et al. Noninvasive positive-pressure ventilation for respiratory failure after extubation. *N Engl J Med.* 2004;350:2452.
132. Epstein SK, Ciubotaru RL. Independent effects of etiology of failure and time to reintubation on outcome for patients failing extubation. *Am J Respir Crit Care Med.* 1998;158:489.
133. Ferrer M, Valencia M, Nicolas JM, et al. Early noninvasive ventilation averts extubation failure in patients at risk: a randomized trial. *Am J Respir Crit Care Med.* 2006;173:164.
134. Benhamou D, Girault C, Faure C, et al. Nasal mask ventilation in acute respiratory failure. Experience in elderly patients. *Chest.* 1992;102:912.
135. Meduri GU, Fox RC, Abou-Shala N, et al. Noninvasive mechanical ventilation via face mask in patients with acute respiratory failure who refused endotracheal intubation. *Crit Care Med.* 1994;22:1584.
136. Levy M, Tanios MA, Nelson D, et al. Outcomes of patients with do-not-intubate orders treated with noninvasive ventilation. *Crit Care Med.* 2004;32:2002.
137. Chu CM, Chan VL, Wong IW, et al. Noninvasive ventilation in patients with acute hypercapnic exacerbation of chronic obstructive pulmonary disease who refused endotracheal intubation. *Crit Care Med.* 2004;32:372.
138. Clarke DE, Vaughan L, Raffin TA. Noninvasive positive pressure ventilation for patients with terminal respiratory failure: the ethical and economic costs of delaying the inevitable are too great. *Am J Crit Care.* 1994;3:4.
139. Craig DB. Postoperative recovery of pulmonary function. *Anesth Analg.* 1981;60:46.
140. Linder KH, Lotz P, Ahnefeld FW. Continuous positive airway pressure effect on functional residual capacity, vital capacity and its subdivisions. *Chest.* 1987;92:66.
141. Boothby WM, Mayo Cw, Lovelace WR, II. The use of oxygen and oxygen-helium, with special reference to surgery. *Surg Clin North Am.* 1940; 20:1107.
142. Joris JL, Sottiaux TM, Chiche JD, et al. Effect of bi-level positive airway pressure (BiPAP) nasal ventilation on the postoperative pulmonary restrictive syndrome in obese patients undergoing gastroplasty. *Chest.* 1997; 111:665.
143. Squadrone V, Coha M, Cerutti E, et al. Continuous positive airway pressure for treatment of postoperative hypoxemia: a randomized controlled trial. *JAMA.* 2005;293:589.
144. Jaber S, Chanques G, Sebbane M et al. Non-invasive positive pressure ventilation in patients with respiratory failure due to severe acute pancreatitis. *Respiration.* 2006;73:166.
145. Pinilla J, Oleniuk FH, Tan L, et al. Use of a nasal continuous positive airway pressure mask in the treatment of postoperative atelectasis in aortocoronary bypass surgery. *Crit Care Med.* 1990;18:836.
146. Pennock BE, Kaplan PD, Carlin BW, et al. Pressure support ventilation with a simplified ventilatory support system administered with a nasal mask in patients with respiratory failure. *Chest.* 1991;100:1371.
147. Matte P, Jacquet L, Van Dyck M, et al. Effects of conventional physiotherapy, continuous positive airway pressure and non-invasive ventilatory support with bilevel positive airway pressure after coronary artery bypass grafting. *Acta Anaesthesiol Scand.* 2000;44:75.
148. Aguilo R, Togores B, Pons S, et al. Noninvasive ventilatory support after lung resectional surgery. *Chest.* 1997;112:117.
149. Auriant I, Jallot A, Hervè O, et al. Non-invasive ventilation reduces mortality in acute respiratory failure following lung resection. *Am J Respir Crit Care Med.* 2001;164:1231.
150. Jenkinson C, Davies RJ, Mullins R, et al. Comparison of therapeutic and subtherapeutic nasal continuous positive airway pressure for obstructive sleep apnoea: a randomised prospective parallel trial. *Lancet.* 1999;353: 2100.
151. Loredo JS, Ancoli-Israel S, Kim EJ, et al. Effect of continuous positive airway pressure versus supplemental oxygen on sleep quality in obstructive sleep apnea: a placebo-CPAP-controlled study. *Sleep.* 2006;29: 564.
152. Abbey NC, Block AJ, Green D, et al. Measurement of pharyngeal volume by digitized magnetic resonance imaging. Effect of nasal continuous positive airway pressure. *Am Rev Respir Dis.* 1989;140:717.
153. Schwab RJ, Pack AI, Gupta KB, et al. Upper airway and soft tissue structural changes induced by CPAP in normal subjects. *Am J Respir Crit Care Med.* 1996;154:1106.
154. Sturani C, Galavotti V, Scarduelli C, et al. Acute respiratory failure, due to severe obstructive sleep apnoea syndrome, managed with nasal positive pressure ventilation. *Monaldi Arch Chest Dis.* 1994;49:558.
155. Hurst JM, DeHaven CB, Branson RD. Use of CPAP mask as the sole mode of ventilatory support in trauma patients with mild to moderate respiratory insufficiency. *J Trauma.* 1985;25:1065.
156. Beltrame F, Lucangelo U, Gregori D, et al. Noninvasive positive pressure ventilation in trauma patients with acute respiratory failure. *Monaldi Arch Chest Dis.* 1999;54:109.
157. Xirouchaki N, Kondoudaki E, Anastasaki M, et al. Noninvasive bilevel positive pressure ventilation in patients with blunt thoracic trauma. *Respiration.* 2005;72:517.
158. Bach JR, Ishikawa Y, Kim H. Prevention of pulmonary morbidity for patients with Duchenne muscular dystrophy. *Chest.* 1997;112:1024.
159. Rabinstein A, Wijdicks EF. BiPAP in acute respiratory failure due to myasthenic crisis may prevent intubation. *Neurology.* 2002;59:1647.
160. Fumeaux T, Rothmeier C, Jolliet P. Outcome of mechanical ventilation for acute respiratory failure in patients with pulmonary fibrosis. *Intensive Care Med.* 2001;27:1868.
161. Antonelli M, Conti G, Riccioni L, et al. Noninvasive positive-pressure ventilation via face mask during bronchoscopy with BAL in high-risk hypoxemic patients. *Chest.* 1996;110:724.
162. Antonelli M, Conti G, Rocco M, et al. Noninvasive positive-pressure ventilation vs. conventional oxygen supplementation in hypoxemic patients undergoing diagnostic bronchoscopy. *Chest.* 2002;121:1149.
163. Antonelli M, Pennisi MA, Conti G, et al. Fiberoptic bronchoscopy during noninvasive positive pressure ventilation delivered by helmet. *Intensive Care Med.* 2003;29:126.
164. Hill NS. Complications of noninvasive positive pressure ventilation. *Respir Care.* 1997;42:432.
165. Constantin JM, Schneider E, Cayot-Constantin S, et al. Remifentanil-based sedation to treat noninvasive ventilation failure: a preliminary study. *Intensive Care Med.* 2006;33(1):82–87.

CHAPTER 130 ■ INVASIVE VENTILATORY SUPPORT MODES

CLAUDIA CRIMI • DEAN R. HESS • LUCA M. BIGATELLO

Mechanical ventilation facilitates gas exchange by substituting, in full or in part, for the action of the respiratory muscles. Indications for the institution of mechanical ventilation include hypoxemia, acute respiratory acidosis, excessive ventilatory workload, and acute cardiac failure. Mechanical ventilation can be provided by applying positive pressure to the proximal airway (positive pressure ventilation) or by applying negative pressure to the chest wall (negative pressure ventilation). Moreover, positive pressure ventilation can be delivered through an endotracheal tube or tracheostomy tube (invasive ventilation), or by use of a face mask or other interface applied to the upper airway (noninvasive ventilation). Negative pressure ventilators (iron lung, cuirass) are virtually never used for acute respiratory failure. This chapter focuses on invasive ventilator modes, although many of the principles can be applied to noninvasive mechanical ventilation as well.

PHYSICS OF VENTILATION: THE EQUATION OF MOTION

During spontaneous breathing, air flows into the lungs as the result of the pressure generated by the respiratory muscles. Exhalation normally occurs passively due to the elastic recoil pressure of the respiratory system. The pressure generated by the respiratory muscles during inspiration is opposed by the elastic forces of the lungs and chest wall, and by the resistance to gas flow that occurs in the airways (1,2):

$$P_{MUS} = P_E + P_R$$

where P_{MUS} is the pressure generated by the respiratory muscles, P_E is the pressure required to overcome the elastic properties of the respiratory system, and P_R is the pressure required to overcome the resistive properties of the respiratory system. During positive pressure ventilation, the driving pressure for air to flow is applied by the ventilator and, depending on the mode, the respiratory muscles. Hence:

$$P_{APPL} = P_{MUS} + P_{VENT} = P_E + P_R$$

where P_{APPL} is the pressure applied across the respiratory system to inflate the lungs, and is the combination of contributions from the respiratory muscles (P_{MUS}) and the ventilator (P_{VENT}). P_E is the result of elastance (E) and tidal volume (V_T):

$$P_E = \text{elastance} \times V_T$$

Because elastance is the reciprocal of compliance (C), a more familiar version is

$$P_E = V_T/C$$

P_R is determined by the resistance of the airways:

$$P_R = \dot{V} \times R$$

where $\dot{V}$ is gas flow and R is resistance. These physiologic relationships are described by the equation of motion of the respiratory system for both spontaneous breathing and mechanical ventilation:

$$P_{APPL} = P_{MUS} + P_{VENT} = V_T/C + \dot{V} \times R$$

This states that a pressure applied to the respiratory system—whether it is from the respiratory muscles, the ventilator, or both—generates gas flow through the airways and volume change in the lungs that is opposed by the airways resistance and respiratory system elastance. From the equation of motion, we can derive three important principles to guide the delivery of positive pressure ventilation:

1. The result of any ventilator setting depends not only on what is set on the ventilator, but also on the physiologic characteristics of the patient, namely compliance and resistance, and any active inspiratory effort of the respiratory muscles. Hence, for the appropriate application of mechanical ventilation, we must understand the ventilator operation as well as the patient's respiratory mechanics and the interaction between the ventilator and any active breathing efforts of the patient.
2. For any independent variable set on the ventilator (e.g., P_{VENT}), physiologic variables (compliance and resistance) in the patient, and respiratory muscle pressure generated by the patient (P_{MUS}), there is only one possible result for the dependent variables (e.g., flow and tidal volume). The ventilator typically controls the independent variables of flow (volume-controlled ventilation [VCV]) or pressure (pressure-controlled [PCV] or pressure support ventilation [PSV]). The ventilator cannot regulate both pressure and volume (i.e., flow) during mechanical ventilation.
3. If we know the volume and flow during VCV, we can calculate resistance and compliance from the pressures required. Similarly, if we know the resistance and compliance during PCV, we can calculate the flow and tidal volume. This is relatively straightforward if the patient is being passively ventilated ($P_{MUS} = 0$) but becomes more difficult if the patient is actively breathing. Hence, it is difficult to predict

respiratory mechanics in the actively breathing patient receiving PCV or PSV.

NOMENCLATURE: DESCRIPTION OF A VENTILATOR BREATH

As ventilators become increasingly complex, understanding how each mode of ventilation works is not always simple. As a starting point, it is helpful to describe the way that a breath is delivered. Although the technical detail of this can vary, there are three principal components of ventilator breaths: (i) how inspiration begins (trigger); (ii) what limits the size of the breath (limit); and (iii) how inspiration ends (cycle).

The Trigger

The trigger starts inspiration. Breaths are triggered either by the patient or by the ventilator (3). If the ventilator initiates the breath, the trigger is time, i.e., the operator sets a respiratory rate, and the ventilator will deliver the breath at time intervals to achieve that rate. If the breath is initiated by the patient, inspiration starts when the ventilator detects a pressure or flow change at the airway (pressure trigger and flow trigger).

With a pressure trigger (Fig. 130.1), a decrease of pressure at the airway relative to positive end-expiratory pressure (PEEP) (adjustable sensitivity, but generally set at 0.5–2 cm H_2O) results in closure of the expiratory valve, opening of the inspiratory valve, and delivery of gas to the airway. With a flow trigger (Fig. 130.1), a flow increase at the airway (adjustable sensitivity, but generally set at 1–3 L/minute) results in initiation of the inspiratory phase. Often, but not always, a continuous low flow (bias flow) through the ventilator circuit is used in conjunction with flow triggering. The change in pressure or flow that triggers inspiration is usually caused by the contraction of the respiratory muscles but can result from artifact such as transmission of cardiac oscillations to the proximal airway (4), leaks in the system (e.g., around the airway cuff or through a chest tube), or movement of the circuit (e.g., water condensate in the tubing).

In modern ventilators, both flow triggers and pressure triggers are very sensitive (5). If the trigger sensitivity is set correctly, either flow triggering or pressure triggering is acceptable (6). With either, the sensitivity can be set to insensitive, resulting in missed trigger efforts by the patient, or it can be set too sensitive, resulting in autotriggering with no effort by the patient. Failure to trigger is usually the result of a physiologic problem such as auto-PEEP (7) or respiratory muscle weakness, rather than a problem with the trigger setting on the ventilator. Moreover, in the presence of auto-PEEP, neither flow nor pressure triggering is superior to the other.

The Limit

The limit determines the size of a breath. This is the independent or control variable, i.e., the variable set and controlled by the ventilator. Within limits set by alarms and safety mechanisms, this variable is applied independently of the patient's respiratory mechanics or inspiratory effort. When volume is the preset variable (VCV), flow and volume delivery by the ventilator are limited, but the pressure applied to the airway can vary. When pressure is the preset limit variable (PCV or PSV), the pressure applied at the airway is limited, but the flow and tidal volume are variable.

The Cycle

The cycle is what ends the breath. This can be volume, time, flow, or pressure. In first-generation ventilators, inspiration was volume cycled when the volume was delivered from a bellows (e.g., Puritan-Bennett MA-1) or piston (e.g., Emerson Post-Op). In modern ventilators, time is the cycle criteria with VCV or PCV. Note that for VCV, the ventilator actually controls the flow during inspiration, and inspiration is time cycled. With PSV, the cycle is usually flow; inspiration ends when the flow rate reaches a fraction of the peak flow (adjustable on some ventilators) or a fixed flow. During VCV or PCV, pressure cycle is an alarm condition that avoids application of unsafe high pressure to the airway.

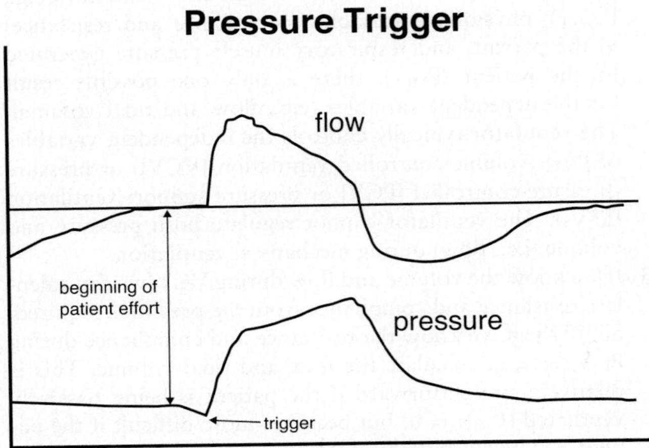

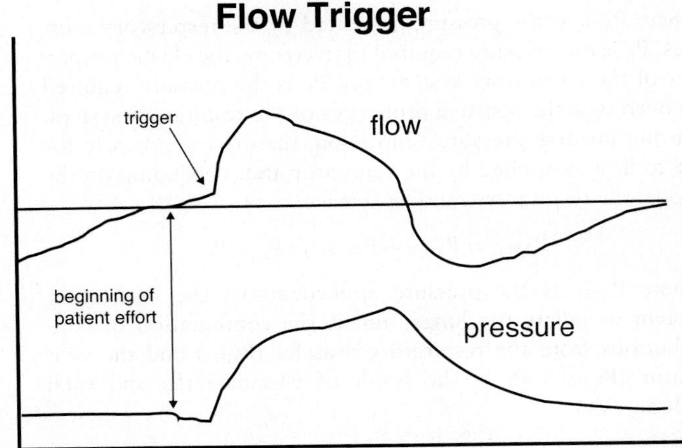

FIGURE 130.1. Pressure triggering and flow triggering. With pressure triggering, the ventilator responds to a decrease in airway pressure. With flow triggering, the ventilator responds to a change in flow.

VENTILATOR MODES

Modern ventilators are equipped to provide various modes. For all modes, the ventilator delivers one of two types of breath: mandatory or spontaneous (Fig. 130.2). A mandatory breath is triggered by the ventilator or the patient and cycled by the ventilator. A set volume (VCV) or pressure (PCV) is delivered regardless of the contribution from the patient and regardless of whether the breath is triggered by the patient or the ventilator. A spontaneous breath is triggered and cycled by the patient.

A ventilator mode describes the pattern of breath delivery from the ventilator. With continuous mandatory ventilation (CMV), also called assist/control ventilation (ACV), every breath is a mandatory breath type. With continuous spontaneous ventilation, every breath is a spontaneous breath type. With synchronized intermittent mandatory ventilation (SIMV), the ventilator delivers a mix of mandatory and spontaneous breaths. With CMV or SIMV, a minimum backup rate is set on the ventilator, but the patient can trigger at a more rapid rate. With continuous spontaneous ventilation, there is no backup rate other than the alarm parameter set on the ventilator. The taxonomy of ventilator modes is shown in Figure 130.2.

Continuous Mandatory Ventilation (CMV)

The main feature of CMV (or assist/control ventilation—ACV) is that it supplies full support of the patient's respiratory muscles, provided that the level of support is set appropriately. Disadvantages of CMV are the possibilities of hyperventilation and/or dyssynchrony. The concern of hyperventilation relates to the fact that the patient will always receive the full volume-controlled or pressure-controlled breath, even when triggering at a high frequency. However, this is uncommon because the minute ventilation is controlled by the patient's $PaCO_2$, which will decrease with hyperventilation, thus blunting the drive to breathe. Hyperventilation during CMV may be no more prevalent than with other modes (8). Dyssynchrony can occur particularly when the level of support is insufficient (8).

Volume-controlled Ventilation (VCV)

With VCV, the ventilator controls the flow and the inspiratory time to deliver the resultant tidal volume. In some cases (e.g., Draeger ventilators), tidal volume, flow, and inspiratory time are each set. In this case, an inspiratory breath hold occurs if the inspiratory time setting is greater than that required to deliver the tidal volume at the flow selected. For example, for a tidal volume of 0.5 L, flow 60 L/minute, and inspiratory time 1 second, a 0.5-second inspiratory breath hold will result. On other ventilators (e.g., Puritan-Bennett 840), an inspiratory hold (pause) is set separately, which prolongs the inspiratory time. For VCV, tidal volume, flow, and inspiratory time are the independent variables. The dependent variable is the inflating pressure applied to the lungs, which is affected by the ventilator settings, the patient's lung mechanics, and the inspiratory effort of the patient, as explained by the *equation of motion* (see above) (9,10). Hence, during VCV, the pressure applied by the ventilator will increase with a higher tidal volume, higher flow, lower compliance, and higher resistance. Also, the pressure applied by the ventilator will decrease if the patient generates a vigorous inspiratory effort (i.e., a higher P_{MUS}). This explains the deformation of the airway pressure waveform during VCV in patients who are generating vigorous inspiratory efforts and are dyssynchronous with the ventilator (9). Inspiratory flow should be set to meet the demand of patients in respiratory failure (11).

On most ventilators, volume-controlled breaths are delivered by a constant inspiratory flow. This is called a square wave or (more precisely) rectangular flow pattern. In some ventilators, the inspiratory flow can also be set to a descending ramp waveform. With such a flow pattern, the preset peak inspiratory flow is reached early during the breath, after which the flow decreases in a linear fashion, reaching a very low level or zero flow at end-inspiration. This affects the shape of the applied

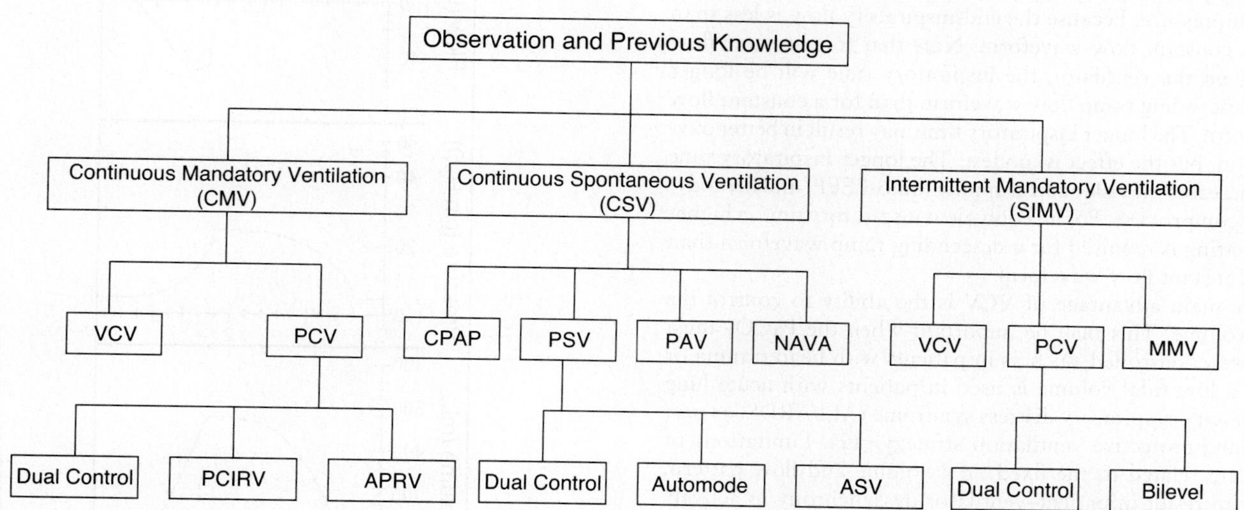

FIGURE 130.2. The taxonomy of ventilator modes. APRV, airway pressure release ventilation; ASV, adaptive support ventilation; CPAP, continuous positive airway pressure; MMV, mandatory minute ventilation; NAVA, neurally adjusted ventilatory assist; PAV, proportional assist ventilation; PCIRV, pressure-controlled inverse ratio ventilation; PCV, pressure-controlled ventilation; PSV, pressure support ventilation; VCV, volume-controlled ventilation.

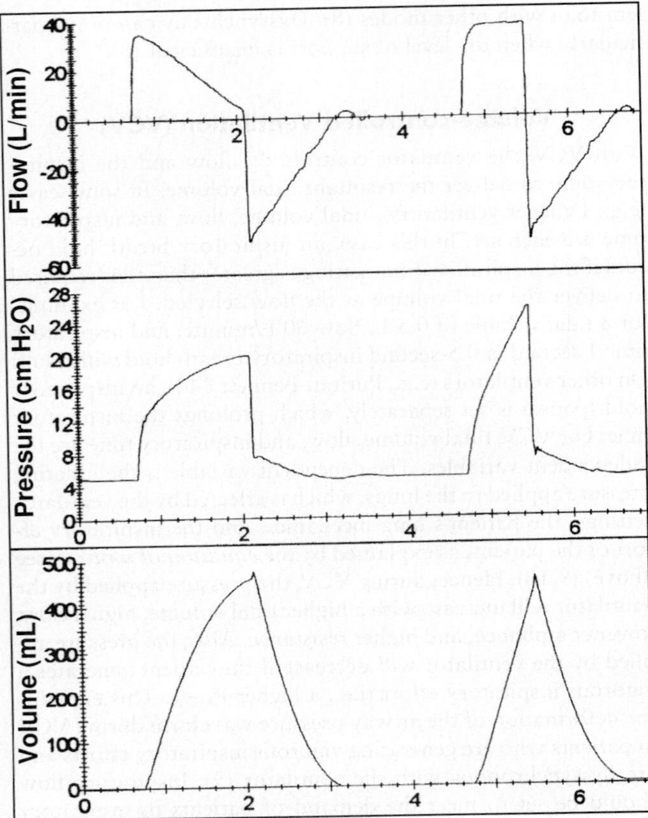

FIGURE 130.3. Waveforms for decelerating and constant flow during volume-controlled ventilation. Note the differences in the shape of the pressure waveform and peak inspiratory pressure.

pressure waveform, in which the pressure increases more rapidly at the beginning of inspiration than near the end of inhalation (Fig. 130.3). Moreover, with a descending ramp waveform, the peak inspiratory pressure is lower and approaches the plateau pressure, because the end-inspiratory flow is less than with a constant flow waveform. Note that for the same flow setting on the ventilator, the inspiratory time will be longer for a descending ramp flow waveform than for a constant flow waveform. The longer inspiratory time may result in better oxygenation, but the effect is modest. The longer inspiratory time also increases the risk or air trapping (auto-PEEP) and hemodynamic compromise. For an equivalent inspiratory time, a higher flow setting is required for a descending ramp waveform than for a constant flow waveform.

The main advantage of VCV is the ability to control the tidal volume. This may be important when the $PaCO_2$ must be closely controlled, such as in patients with head trauma or when a low tidal volume is used in patients with acute lung injury/acute respiratory distress syndrome (ALI/ARDS) as part of a lung-protective ventilation strategy (12). Limitations of VCV are related to the fixed tidal volume and flow pattern. This can result in patient–ventilator dyssynchrony in actively breathing patients if efforts are not made to set the inspiratory flow appropriately or to provide adequate sedation (13). With VCV, a high peak inspiratory pressure may occur with changes in lung mechanics. However, this only increases the risk of lung injury if the high peak inspiratory pressure is associated with an increase in plateau pressure. Accordingly, it is important to monitor plateau pressure on a regular basis when VCV is used.

Pressure-controlled Ventilation (PCV)

With PCV, airway pressure and inspiratory time are set on the ventilator. In some cases (e.g., Draeger ventilators), the inspiratory pressure setting is the peak pressure, but more commonly the pressure control setting is the pressure applied above PEEP. For PCV, pressure and inspiratory time are the independent variables. The dependent variables are flow and volume, which are affected by the ventilator settings, the patient's lung mechanics, and the inspiratory effort of the patient as described by the *equation of motion* (see above) (9,10). Hence, during PCV, the flow and tidal volume will increase with a higher pressure control setting, higher compliance, and lower airways resistance. Also, the flow and tidal volume will increase if the patient generates a vigorous inspiratory effort (i.e., an increase in P_{MUS}). In other words, during PCV, the distending pressure ($P_{VENT} + P_{MUS}$) and tidal volume increase if the patient makes an active inspiratory effort. Compared to VCV, this may improve patient–ventilator synchrony (14), but with an increased risk of overdistention lung injury. An understanding of the equation of motion as it applies to PCV prevents errors when assessing lung mechanics or risk of overdistention when PCV is used.

During PCV, the inspiratory flow waveform is a descending ramp (Fig. 130.4). After triggering the breath (by the patient or the ventilator), the ventilator delivers gas to the airway dependent on the capability of the ventilator, respiratory mechanics, and patient effort. The set pressure is applied to the airway until the set inspiratory time is reached. The slope of the descending portion of the inspiratory flow waveform depends on the lung mechanics (Fig. 130.5). The initial flow is high, the flow descent is rapid, and the tidal volume is small when the compliance is

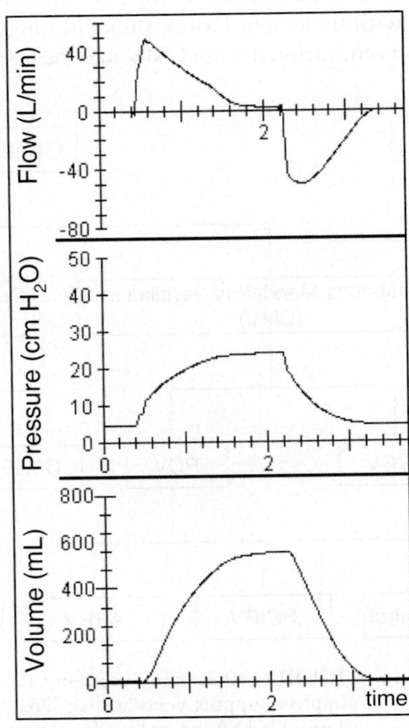

FIGURE 130.4. Flow, pressure, and volume waveforms during pressure-controlled ventilation.

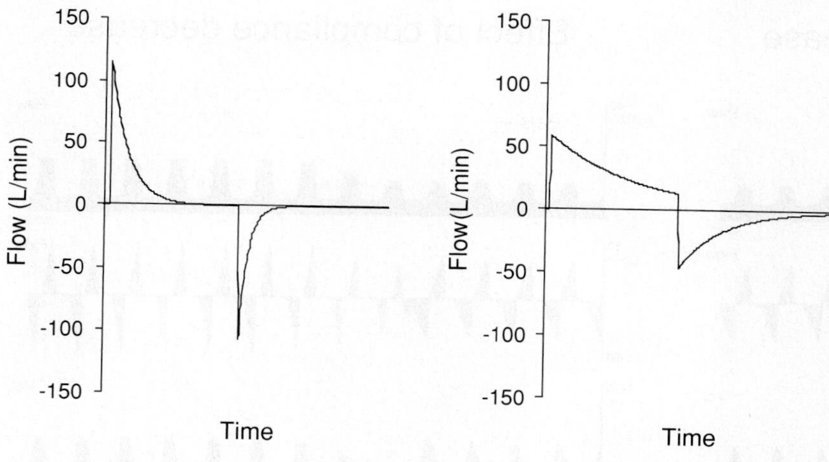

FIGURE 130.5. Effect of changes in respiratory mechanics on gas flow delivery during pressure-controlled ventilation. The **left panel** shows the effect of a significant decrease in compliance; respiratory mechanics were resistance 10 cm H_2O/L/s and compliance 20 mL/cm H_2O; the inspiratory time was 1.5 s, and the resulting tidal volume (the area under the flow curve) 400 mL. The **right panel** shows the effect of a significant increase in airway resistance; resistance was 20 cm H_2O/L/s and compliance 50 mL/cm H_2O; the inspiratory time was 1.5 s, and the resulting tidal volume 775 mL.

low (e.g., ALI/ARDS). On the other hand, the initial flow is low, and the flow descent is slow when the airways resistance is high (e.g., chronic obstructive pulmonary disease [COPD]).

Many current-generation ventilators allow the clinician to adjust the rise time (or pressurization rate), which is the time required for the ventilator to reach the pressure control setting at the onset of inspiration. A fast rise time (one in which the ventilator reaches the target pressure quickly) is associated with a high flow at the onset of inhalation. A slow rise time (one in which the ventilator reaches the target pressure slowly) is associated with a lower flow at the onset of inhalation (Fig. 130.6). Patients with a high respiratory drive should benefit from a fast rise time whereas those with a lower respiratory drive might benefit from a slower rise time (15).

A potential advantage of PCV is that it limits the pressure applied to the alveoli and the risk of ventilator-induced lung injury. However, it is important to note that this benefit occurs only if the patient is making no inspiratory effort, because any inspiratory efforts of the patient will increase the transpulmonary distending pressure during PCV. This theoretical advantage of PCV has not been confirmed by appropriately designed clinical trials. The only randomized controlled trial that compared VCV to PCV reported no difference in patient outcomes attributable to the choice of VCV or PCV (16). The variable inspiratory flow pattern may improve patient–ventilator synchrony during active breathing efforts (14), although this has not been tested in the setting of a low lung volume, lung-protective ventilation strategy.

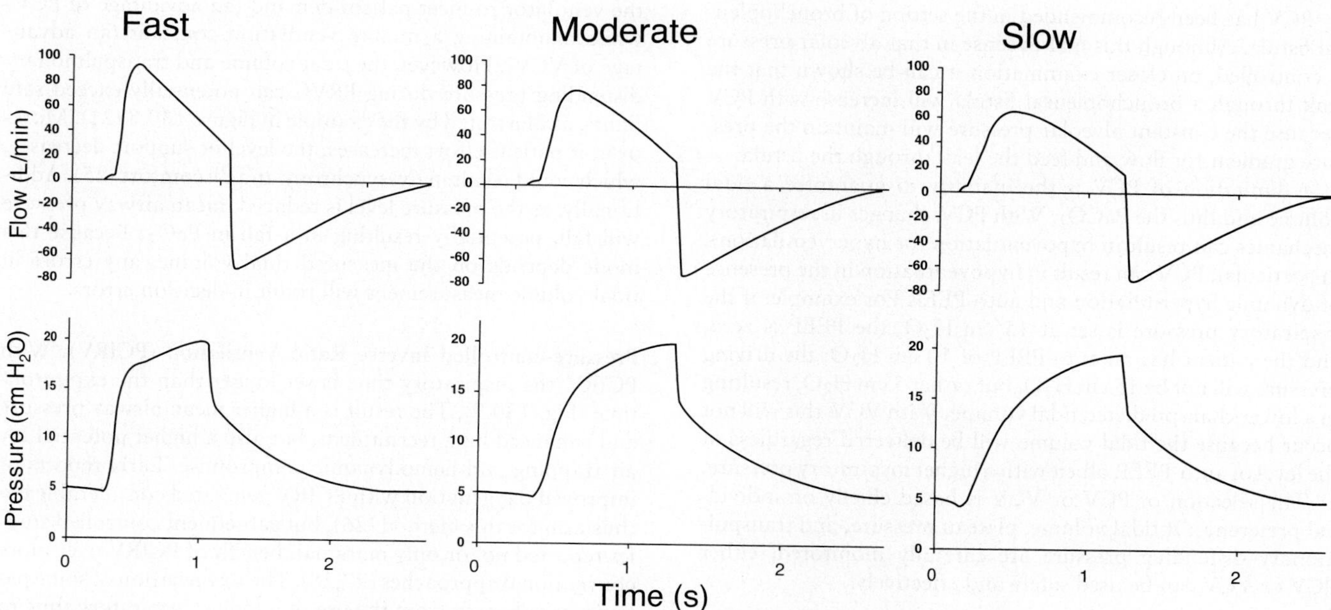

FIGURE 130.6. Flow and pressure waveforms for three rise times (pressurization rates) at a pressure support of 20 cm H_2O. Note the effect of rise time on flow at the initiation of the inspiratory phase. (From Gibbons FK, Hess DR. Mechanical ventilation. In: Bigatello LM, ed. *Critical Care Handbook of the Massachusetts General Hospital*. 4th ed. Philadelphia, PA: Lippincott Williams & Wilkins; 2006, with permission.)

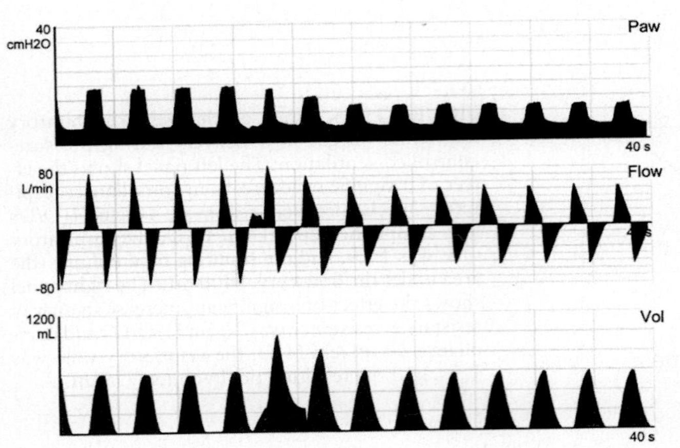

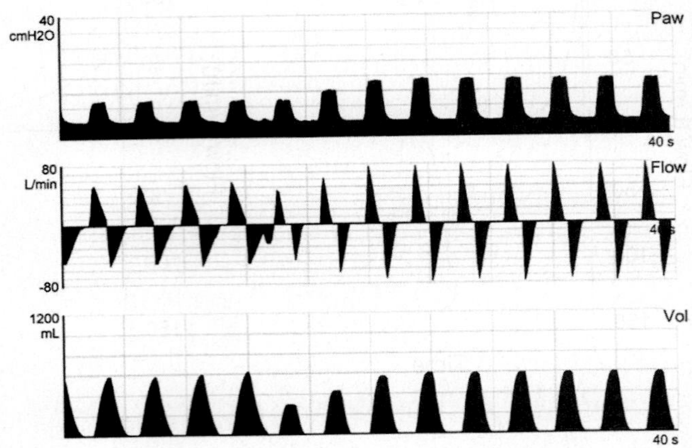

FIGURE 130.7. Left panel: Effects of an increase in lung compliance on airway pressure (Paw), volume, and flow during dual control with a target tidal volume of 600 mL. **Right panel:** Effects of a decrease in lung compliance on airway pressure and flow during dual-control ventilation with a target tidal volume of 600 mL. (From Branson RD, Johannigman JA. The role of ventilator graphics when setting dual-control modes. *Respir Care.* 2005;50:187, with permission.)

The pressure waveform with PCV produces a higher mean airway (and alveolar) pressure than the pressure waveform associated with constant flow volume ventilation. Theoretically, this may produce better alveolar recruitment for the same end-inspiratory airway pressure. However, the same may be achieved using VCV and a descending ramp flow waveform (17). Compared to constant flow VCV, the low end-inspiratory flow with PCV may improve the distribution of ventilation, which may increase PaO_2 and decrease PCO_2, but the effect is usually modest.

PCV has been recommended in the setting of bronchopleural fistula. Although this makes sense in that alveolar pressure is controlled, on closer examination it can be shown that the leak through a bronchopleural fistula will increase with PCV because the constant alveolar pressure will maintain the pressure gradient for flow and feed the leak through the fistula.

A limitation of PCV is the inability to guarantee a tidal volume and thus the $PaCO_2$. With PCV, changes in respiratory mechanics can result in hypoventilation (or hyperventilation). In particular, PCV can result in hypoventilation in the presence of dynamic hyperinflation and auto-PEEP. For example, if the inspiratory pressure is set at 15 cm H_2O, the PEEP is zero, and the patient has an auto-PEEP of 10 cm H_2O; the driving pressure will not be 15 cm H_2O, but rather 5 cm H_2O, resulting in a lower-than-predicted tidal volume. With VCV, this will not occur because the tidal volume will be delivered regardless of the level of auto-PEEP, albeit with a higher inspiratory pressure.

The selection of PCV or VCV is based chiefly on individual preference. If tidal volume, plateau pressure, and transpulmonary distending pressure are carefully monitored, either PCV or VCV can be used safely and effectively.

Dual-controlled Ventilation. Dual-controlled modes allow the ventilator to control pressure or volume based on a feedback loop. At any given time, the ventilator controls either pressure or volume, but cannot do both at the same time. Pressure-regulated volume control (PRVC) provides PCV, and in addition ensures a minimum tidal volume (18–24). PRVC (Servo, Viasys), AutoFlow (Draeger), and VC+ (Puritan-Bennett) are trade names that function in a similar manner. Each mode increases or decreases the pressure breath-to-breath by no more than 3 cm H_2O per breath in an attempt to deliver the desired tidal volume. The pressure limit fluctuates between PEEP and 5 cm H_2O below the upper pressure alarm setting, as illustrated by the example in Figure 130.7. An alarm occurs if the tidal volume and maximum pressure settings are incompatible. The proposed advantage of dual control is the ability of the ventilator to meet patient demand (an advantage of PCV) while maintaining a minute ventilation constant (an advantage of VCV). However, the tidal volume and transpulmonary distending pressure during PRVC can potentially exceed safe limits, as illustrated by the example in Figure 130.8 (21). Moreover, if patient effort increases, the level of support decreases, which could result in dyssynchrony and discomfort (25). Additionally, as the pressure level is reduced, mean airway pressure will fall, potentially resulting in a fall in PaO_2. Because this mode depends on the measured tidal volume, any errors in tidal volume measurement will result in decision errors.

Pressure-controlled Inverse Ratio Ventilation (PCIRV). With PCIRV, the inspiratory time is set longer than the expiratory time (Fig. 130.9). The result is a higher mean airway pressure and enhanced lung recruitment, but also a higher potential for air trapping and hemodynamic compromise. Early reports of improved oxygenation with PCIRV generated considerable enthusiasm for this method (26), but subsequent controlled studies reported no, or only marginal, benefit of PCIRV over more conventional approaches (27,28). The oxygenation of some patients may benefit from the use of a longer inspiratory time to increase mean airway pressure. However, the target variable should be the inspiratory time and not an inverse ratio, *per se*. The likelihood of an improvement in oxygenation using PCIRV is small, and the risk of auto-PEEP and hemodynamic compromise is great. Moreover, the prolonged inspiratory time may

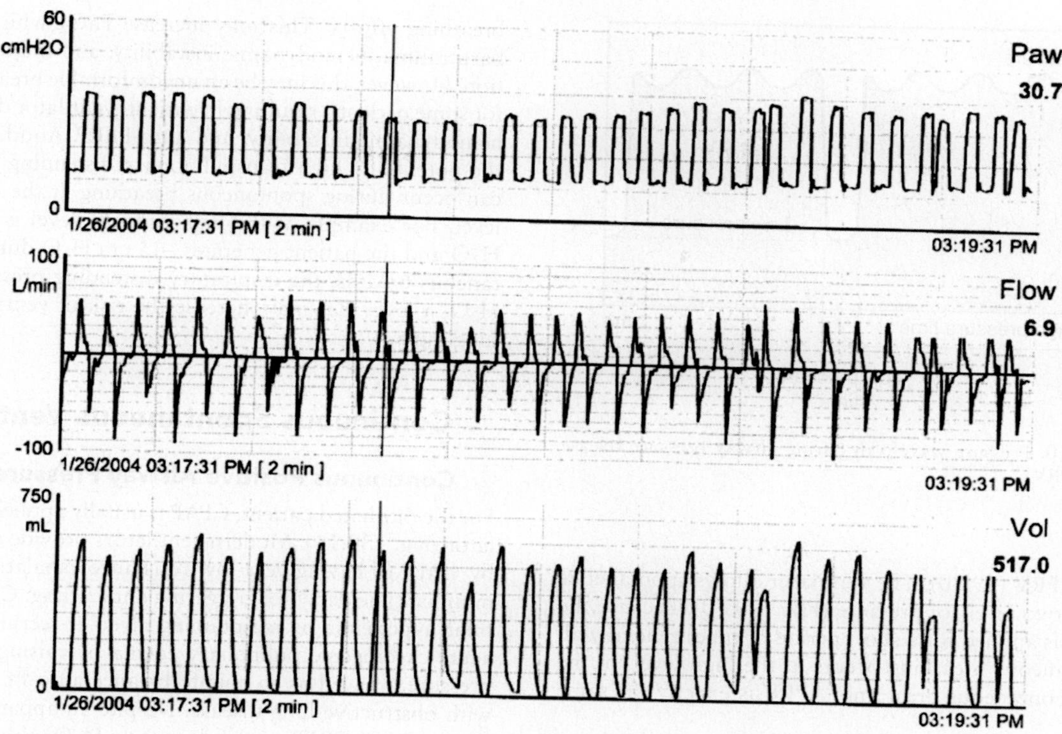

FIGURE 130.8. Airway pressure (Paw), flow, and volume waveforms demonstrating the response of a dual-control algorithm over a 2-minute period with varying patient effort. The tidal volume varies above and below the target (500 mL) by as much as 150 mL. (From Branson RD, Johannigman JA. The role of ventilator graphics when setting dual-control modes. *Respir Care.* 2005;50:187, with permission.)

not be well tolerated and may require high levels of sedation and, in some cases, paralysis.

Airway Pressure Release Ventilation (APRV). Current-generation ventilators use an active exhalation valve; thereby the ventilator controls the inspiratory pressure by allowing the exhalation valve to open if pressure increases and by adding additional flow if the pressure decreases below the pressure control setting. Such a design can also allow spontaneous breathing during the inspiratory phase of the ventilator, which is what

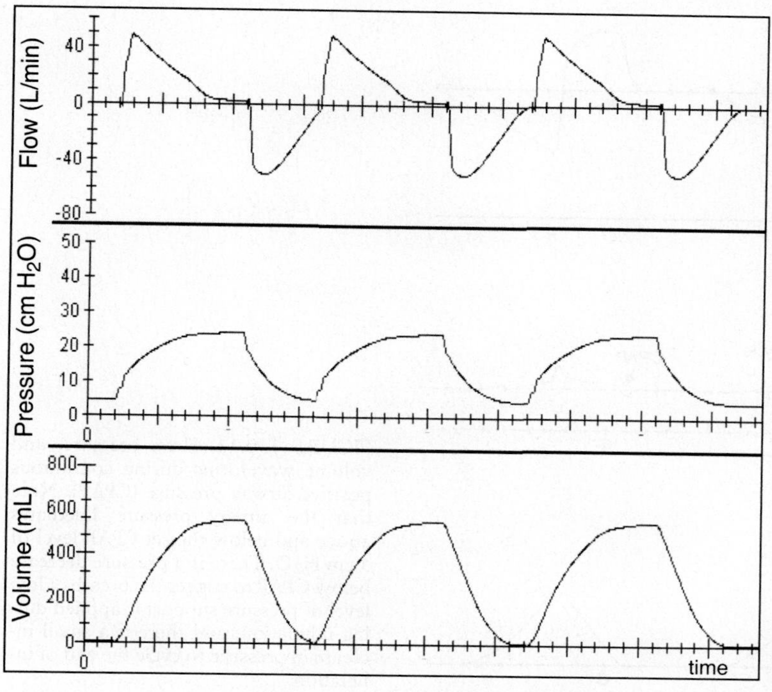

FIGURE 130.9. Flow, pressure, and volume waveforms during pressure-controlled inverse ratio ventilation.

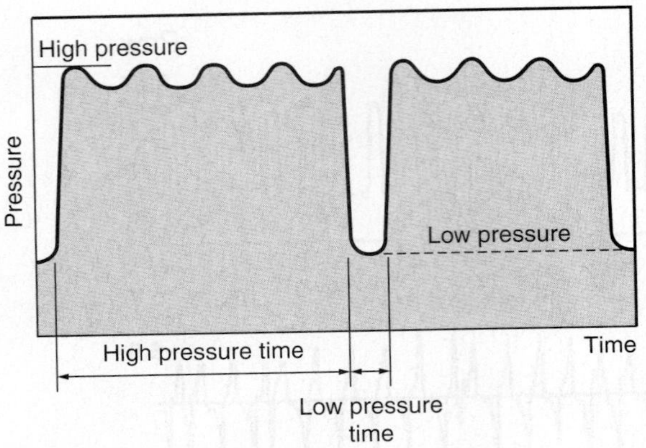

FIGURE 130.10. Pressure waveform during airway pressure release ventilation (APRV).

happens in APRV (29,30). The ventilator allows spontaneous breathing at two levels of pressure (Fig. 130.10). Because the low pressure is applied for a short period of time, generally all of the spontaneous breathing occurs at the high level. In the absence of spontaneous breathing, APRV is exactly the same as PCIRV.

The minute ventilation during APRV results from the amount of spontaneous breathing, the difference between the two pressure levels, and the frequency at which the pressure is released to the lower level. The high pressure level is the main determinant of arterial oxygenation, but the additional spontaneous breaths may further improve gas exchange by preferentially recruiting the dependent lung regions (31,32).

The potential advantage of APRV is to provide lung recruitment at lower airway pressures than with traditional positive pressure ventilation by taking advantage of the spontaneous breathing efforts. This may increase PaO_2 while minimizing barotrauma, hemodynamic instability, and the need for sedation. However, this may be an uncomfortable breathing pattern for some patients, resulting in patient–ventilator dyssynchrony, hemodynamic instability, and auto-PEEP. Another concern is the potentially high transpulmonary distending pressure that can occur during spontaneous breathing at the high pressure level. For example, if the high pressure level is set at 25 cm H_2O and the patient generates −15 cm H_2O during the spontaneous breaths, the inspiratory distending pressure is 40 cm H_2O, a level that may increase the risk of ventilator-induced lung injury.

Continuous Spontaneous Ventilation

Continuous Positive Airway Pressure (CPAP)

For the intubated patient, CPAP is usually applied with a ventilator (Fig. 130.11). Modern ventilators provide efficient CPAP by virtue of having very-low-resistance exhalation valves and minimal time delay for triggering and cycling. CPAP is used to treat hypoxemia by maintaining alveolar recruitment to treat acute cardiogenic pulmonary edema by raising intrathoracic pressure, as well as to counterbalance auto-PEEP in patients with obstructive lung disease. Despite an apparent contradiction in terms, CPAP can be set to 0 cm H_2O (although in reality the ventilator often applies a small level of inspiratory pressure support), and is commonly used as a spontaneous breathing trial to test extubation readiness.

Pressure Support Ventilation (PSV)

With PSV, the ventilator applies a set inspiratory pressure to support each patient-initiated breath (Fig. 130.12) (33). Tidal volume is determined by the level of inspiratory pressure support, respiratory mechanics, and the patient's inspiratory effort.

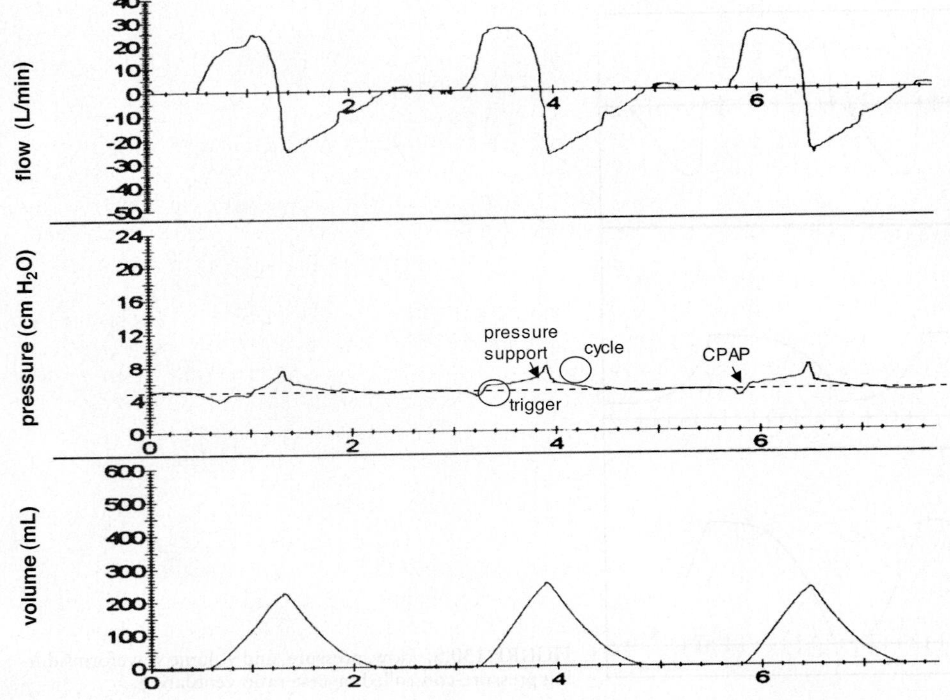

FIGURE 130.11. Flow, pressure, and volume waveforms during continuous positive airway pressure (CPAP). Note that the airway pressure fluctuates above and below the set CPAP level of 5 cm H_2O. There is a pressure decrease below CPAP to trigger the breath, a low level of pressure support is applied during inhalation, and there is a small increase in pressure to cycle the end of inhalation.

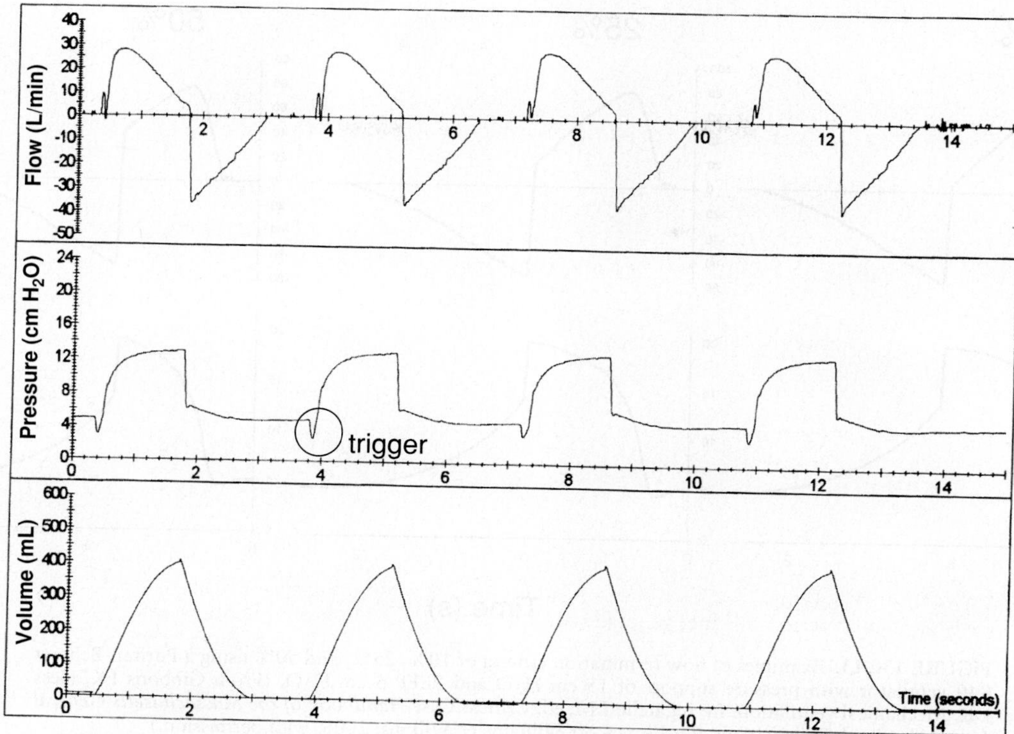

FIGURE 130.12. Flow, pressure, and volume waveforms during pressure support ventilation. (From Gibbons FK, Hess DR. Mechanical ventilation. In: Bigatello LM, ed. *Critical Care Handbook of the Massachusetts General Hospital*. 4th ed. Philadelphia, PA: Lippincott Williams & Wilkins; 2006, with permission.)

The initial part of the breath is delivered in a manner similar to PCV. During inspiration, the flow is delivered at a variable rate. In addition, rise time can be adjusted in a manner similar to that during PCV (34,35). When the set pressure is reached, the flow decreases at a rate determined by lung mechanics and the patient's inspiratory effort.

The inspiratory cycle is what distinguishes PCV from PSV. With PSV, inspiration continues until the inspiratory flow falls to a ventilator preset value—commonly 25% of the peak flow or a fixed flow such as 5 L/minute. In newer-generation ventilators, the flow cycle criteria can be adjusted (expiratory sensitivity, Fig. 130.13) (36–40). Setting a high flow cycle (e.g., 50% of the peak rate) will shorten the duration of the breath, whereas a low flow cycle (e.g., 5% of the peak rate) will increase its duration. A higher flow cycle may be desirable for patients with obstructive lung disease, whereas a lower flow cycle is suitable for patients with restrictive lung disease (i.e., acute lung injury). Time and pressure are secondary criteria that can also cycle the breath during PSV, allowing inspiratory termination if the patient actively exhales (pressure cycle) or if there is a leak (time cycle).

PSV is a commonly used mode of ventilation. In many patients, it effectively assists respiratory muscles during invasive mechanical ventilation (41). However, as with any mode, patient–ventilator dyssynchrony can occur if careful attention is not paid to the level of pressure support, the rise time, and the inspiratory cycle. Because there is no backup rate with PSV, it has also been shown that patients receiving this mode of ventilation are more likely to have apnea and sleep-disordered breathing (42).

SmartCare (Draeger) is a closed-loop knowledge-based weaning system for PSV (43). It adapts the level of pressure support to the patient's ventilatory needs, with the goal of keeping the patient within a comfort zone. Comfort is defined primarily as a respiratory rate that can vary in the range of 15 to 30 breaths/minute, a tidal volume above a minimum threshold, and an end-tidal CO_2 below a maximum threshold. The level of support is periodically adapted by the system in increments of 2 to 4 cm H_2O. The system automatically tries to reduce the pressure level to a minimum value. At this value, a spontaneous breathing trial with a minimal low pressure support level is performed. If successful, a message on the screen recommends removal from the ventilator (i.e., extubation). This mode was shown to reduce the duration of mechanical ventilation as compared with physician-controlled weaning (44).

Dual Control. Dual-controlled ventilation can also be applied during a PSV breath. Volume-assured pressure support (VAPS) combines the high initial flow of PSV with the constant flow delivery of a volume-controlled breath (Fig. 130.14) (18,19). After inspiration is triggered, the ventilator reaches the set airway pressure as occurs with PSV. The ventilator's microprocessor determines the volume that has been delivered and compares this to the set tidal volume. If the set tidal volume is not reached, the ventilator prolongs the inspiratory phase until the set tidal volume is delivered. VAPS is designed to reduce the work of breathing (pressure support) while maintaining a minimum tidal volume (volume control). Choosing the appropriate pressure and flow settings is critical to the success of VAPS. If the pressure is set too high or the tidal volume is set too low,

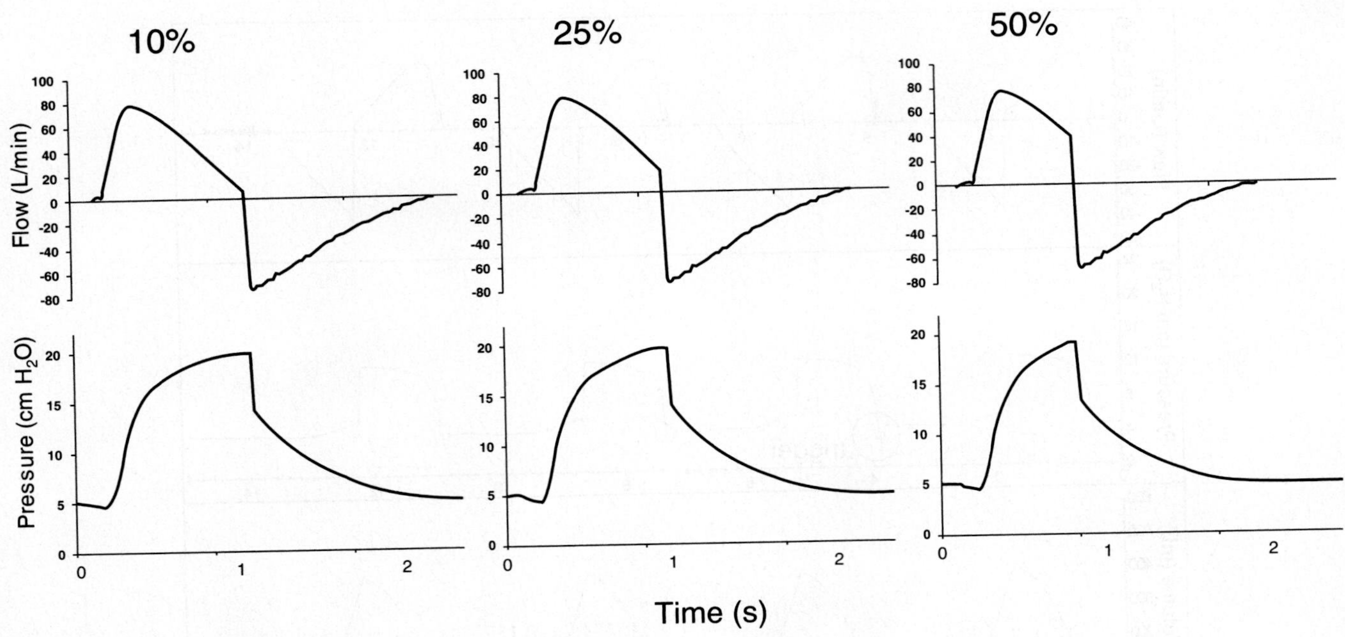

FIGURE 130.13. Examples of flow termination criteria of 10%, 25%, and 50% using a Puritan-Bennett 840 ventilator with pressure support of 15 cm H_2O and PEEP 5 cm H_2O. (From Gibbons FK, Hess DR. Mechanical ventilation. In: Bigatello LM, ed. *Critical Care Handbook of the Massachusetts General Hospital*. 4th ed. Philadelphia, PA: Lippincott Williams & Wilkins; 2006, with permission.)

all breaths will be PSV breaths. If the flow is set too high, all the breaths will be VCV. If the flow is set too low, the switch from pressure support to volume control will occur late in the breath, and inspiratory time may be unnecessarily prolonged.

Volume support (VS) uses PSV in a manner analogous to how PRVC uses PCV (18–23). In other words, the ventilator adjusts the inspiratory pressure according to a set minimum tidal volume. If the patient's effort increases (increased tidal volume for the set level of PSV), the ventilator decreases the support of the next breath. If the compliance or patient effort decreases, the ventilator increases the support to maintain the set volume. This combines the attributes of PSV with the guaranteed minimum tidal volume. A concern with this mode is that the ventilator takes away support if the patient's respiratory demand increases and tidal volume exceeds the set tidal volume. This results in increased work of breathing for the patient (25).

AutoMode

AutoMode is a dual-controlled mode available on the Servo 300 and Servo 300A ventilators (18,19). It provides automated weaning from PCV to PSV, and automated escalation of support if patient effort diminishes. The ventilator provides PRVC if the patient is making no breathing efforts. If the patient triggers two consecutive breaths, the ventilator switches to VS. If the patient becomes apneic, the ventilator switches back to PRVC. AutoMode can also switch between PCV and PSV or VCV and VS.

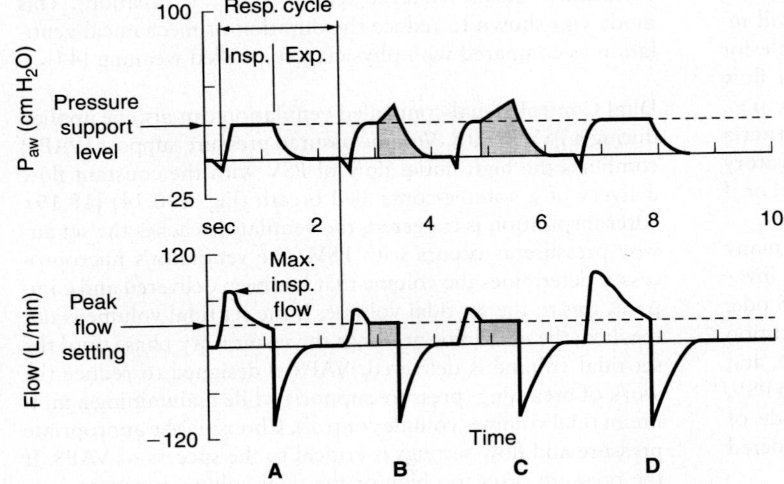

FIGURE 130.14. The possible breath types during volume-assured pressure support ventilation. In breath A, the set tidal volume (V_T) and delivered V_T are equal. This is a pressure support breath (patient triggered, pressure limited, and flow cycled). Breath B represents a reduction in patient effort. As flow decreases, the ventilator determines that delivered V_T will be less than the minimum set volume. At the *shaded* portion of the waveform, the breath changes from a pressure-limited to a volume-limited (constant flow) breath. Breath C demonstrates a worsening of compliance and the possibility of extending inspiratory time to ensure the minimum V_T delivery. Breath D represents a pressure support breath in which the V_T is greater than the set V_T. (From Branson RD, Johannigman JA. The role of ventilator graphics when setting dual-control modes. *Respir Care*. 2005;50:187, with permission.)

Adaptive Support Ventilation (ASV)

Adaptive support ventilation (ASV) is based on the minimal work-of-breathing concept, which suggests that the patient will breathe at a tidal volume and respiratory frequency that minimizes the elastic and resistive loads while maintaining oxygenation and acid-base balance (45). The ventilator attempts to deliver 100 mL/minute/kg of minute ventilation for an adult and 200 mL/minute/kg for children. This can be adjusted by setting the % minute volume control from 20% to 200%, which allows the clinician to provide full ventilatory support or encourage spontaneous breathing and facilitate weaning.

When first connected to the patient, the ventilator delivers a series of test breaths and measures compliance, resistance, and auto-PEEP. The input of body weight allows the ventilator's algorithm to choose a required minute volume. Lung mechanics are measured on a breath-to-breath basis, and ventilator settings are altered to meet the desired targets. If the patient breathes spontaneously, the ventilator will support breaths. Spontaneous and mandatory breaths can be combined to meet the minute ventilation target. The pressure limit of both the mandatory and spontaneous breaths is adjusted continuously. This means that ASV is continuously using dual-control breath-to-breath of mandatory and spontaneous breaths.

The ventilator adjusts the I:E ratio and inspiratory time of mandatory breaths by calculation of the expiratory time constant (compliance × resistance) and maintains sufficient expiratory time to prevent auto-PEEP. If the patient is not triggering, the ventilator determines the respiratory frequency, tidal volume, and pressure limit required to deliver the tidal volume, the inspiratory time, and the I:E ratio. If the patient is triggering, the number of mandatory breaths decreases, and the ventilator chooses a pressure support that maintains a tidal volume sufficient to ensure alveolar ventilation based on a dead space calculation of 2.2 mL/kg. ASV can provide pressure-limited, time-cycled ventilation, add dual control of those breaths on a breath-to-breath basis, allow for mandatory breaths and spontaneous breaths (dual-control SIMV + PSV), and eventually switch to pressure support with dual control breath-to-breath (variable pressure with PSV). During mandatory breath delivery, the ventilator sets the inspiratory time and I:E ratio.

Tube Compensation (TC)

TC is designed to overcome the flow-resistive work of breathing imposed by the endotracheal or tracheostomy tube (46,47). TC uses the known resistive coefficients of the artificial airway (tracheostomy or endotracheal tube) and measurement of instantaneous flow to apply a pressure proportional to resistance throughout the total respiratory cycle. With TC, the ventilator targets the tracheal pressure, rather than proximal airway pressure, increasing the proximal airway pressure necessary to overcome the flow-resistive properties of the artificial airway (Fig. 130.15). The clinician can set the fraction of tube resistance for which compensation is desired (e.g., 50% compensation rather than full compensation). Because *in vivo* tracheal tube resistance tends to be greater than *in vitro* resistance, incomplete compensation for endotracheal tube resistance may occur. Additionally, kinks or bends in the tube as it traverses the upper airway and accumulation of secretions in the inner lumen will change the tube's resistive coefficient and result in incomplete compensation. Available evidence suggests that TC can effectively compensate for resistance through the artificial airway but has not shown improved outcomes with this mode (48,49). On some ventilators, TC can be used with any mode, whereas on others, it can be used only with CPAP.

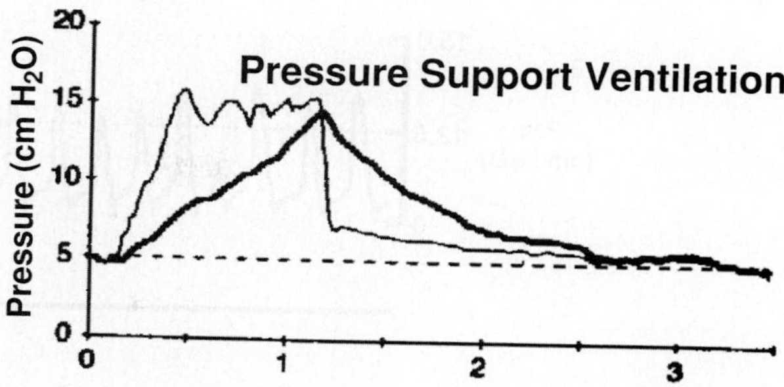

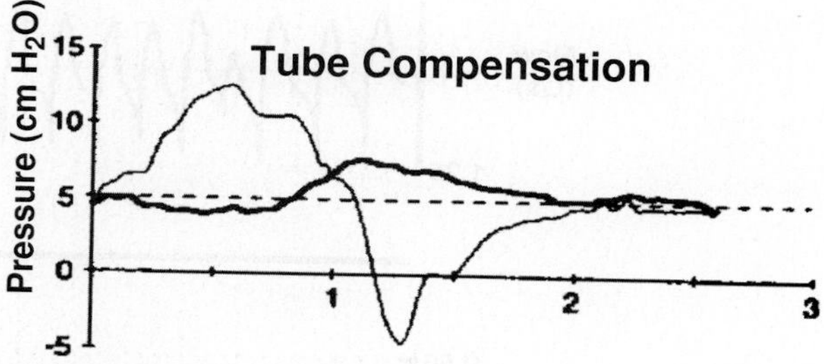

FIGURE 130.15. Tube compensation. Pressure waveforms from the trachea (*heavy lines*) and the proximal airway (*light lines*) during pressure support ventilation and automatic tube compensation. Note that the tracheal pressure fluctuates very little during automatic tube compensation. (From Fabry B, Haberthur C, Zappe D, et al. Breathing pattern and additional work of breathing in spontaneously breathing patients with different ventilatory demands during inspiratory pressure support and automatic tube compensation. *Intensive Care Med.* 1997;23:545, with permission.)

Proportional Assist Ventilation (PAV)

With proportional assist ventilation (PAV) (50,51), the ventilator delivers gas as a positive feedback controller, where respiratory elastance and resistance are the feedback signal gains, defined as K_1 (cm H_2O/L) and K_2 (cm H_2O/L/s), respectively. In such a system, the pressure at the airway opening is adjusted according to the *equation of motion* (see above) (9,10)

$$P = K_1 \times V + K_2 \times \dot{V}$$

where P is the pressure applied at the airway, $\dot{V}$ is the inspiratory flow, and K_1 and K_2 substitute elastance and resistance, respectively. K_1 and K_2 are the volume and flow gains of the proportional assist ventilator. The ventilator measures the patient's instantaneous inspiratory flow rate and provides the set support through a rapid positive feedback loop (Fig. 130.16).

A potential advantage of PAV is that it should provide optimal patient–ventilator synchrony. By following and amplifying the patient's inspiratory flow and volume on a breath-by-breath basis, the ventilator provides support in proportion to patient demand. This differs from PSV, in which the level of support is constant regardless of demand, and VCV, in which the level of support decreases when demand increases. It is important to note that, like other continuous spontaneous breathing modes, PAV requires the presence of an intact ventilatory drive. In addition, if K_1 and K_2 are $\geq$100% of elastance and resistance, "runaway" occurs where the ventilator no longer tracks inspiratory effort. This is similar to the prolonged inspiratory time that can occur during PSV if the pressure is set too high.

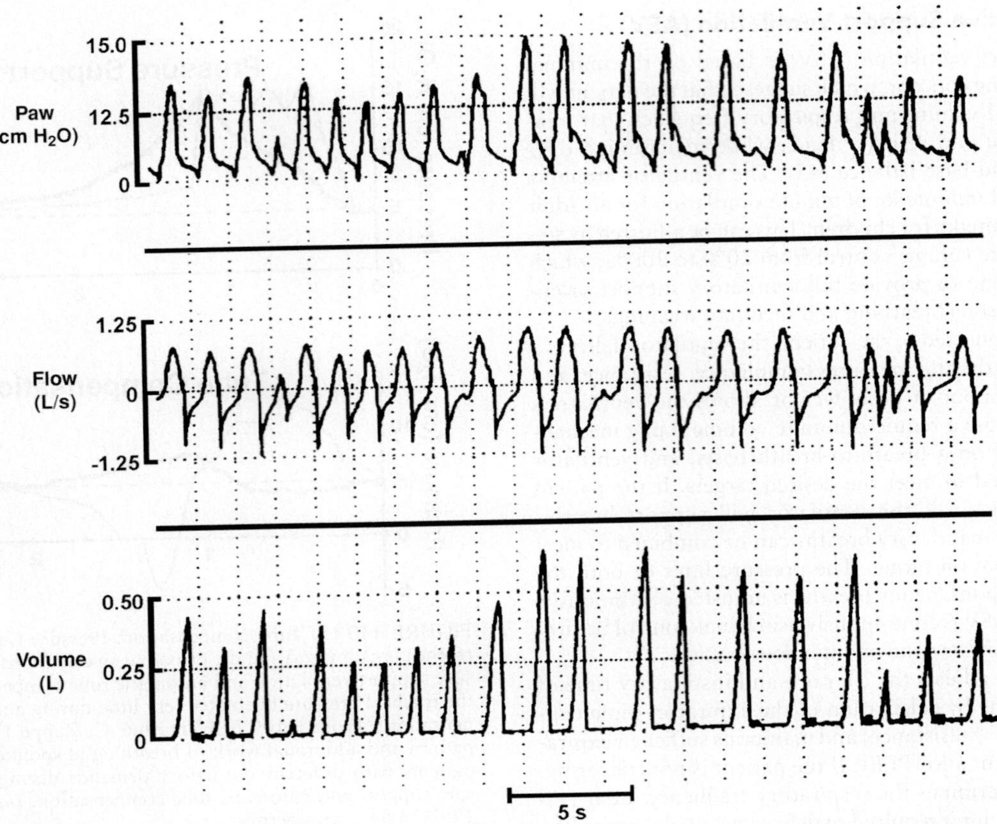

FIGURE 130.16. Airway pressure (Paw), flow, and volume waveforms during proportional assist ventilation. Note that the airway pressure varies with the inspiratory flow and volume demands of the patient. (From Marantz S, Patrick W, Webster K, et al. Response of ventilator-dependent patients to different levels of proportional assist. *J Appl Physiol.* 1996;80:397, with permission.)

A concern with PAV is its dependence on measures of resistance and compliance. These can be difficult to measure during spontaneous breathing, and they change frequently over the course of mechanical ventilation. In its initial application, the clinician measured (or estimated) compliance and resistance and set the proportion of inspiratory support that the ventilator would provide, generally as a percentage of elastic and resistive work, respectively. This has been simplified on the commercially available form of PAV (PAV+, Puritan-Bennett 840). Currently, the ventilator applies end-inspiratory and end-expiratory pause maneuvers periodically to determine resistance, compliance, and auto-PEEP. The clinician sets the trigger, the cycle (3 L/minute default), and the % support. The % support is used to partition the work of breathing between the patient and the ventilator. In other words, for 50% support, half of the work of breathing is performed by the patient and the other half is performed by the ventilator.

Neurally Adjusted Ventilatory Assist (NAVA)

Control of the ventilator through direct measurement of the output of the respiratory center is presently not possible. However, it is possible to transform neural drive into ventilatory output (neuroventilatory coupling) by measuring the electrical activation of the diaphragm. Computer technology and newly developed methods for signal acquisition and processing have made it possible to reliably obtain real-time diaphragmatic electrical activity that is free of artifacts and noise. Diaphragmatic electrical activity can provide a means to give ventilatory assist in proportion to the neural drive, both within a given breath and between breaths (Fig. 130.17). This is called neurally adjusted ventilatory assist (NAVA) (51,52). With NAVA, the magnitude of the support will vary on a moment-by-moment basis according to diaphragmatic electrical activity and the gain factor selected on the ventilator. This allows the patient's respiratory center to be in direct control of the mechanical support provided throughout the course of each breath, provided there is a functioning phrenic nerve and neuromuscular junction, and also that the diaphragm is the primary inspiratory muscle. Through this process, the neural respiratory output is matched to the level of ventilatory assistance. The level of assistance is adjusted in response to changes in neural drive, respiratory system mechanics, inspiratory muscle function, and behavioral influences. Because the trigger is based on diaphragmatic activity rather than pressure or flow measured at the proximal airway, triggering is not adversely affected in patients with flow limitation and auto-PEEP. Although NAVA is clinically attractive, it is not yet commercially available.

Synchronized Intermittent Mandatory Ventilation (SIMV)

With SIMV, the ventilator provides a mandatory breath rate. If the patient breathes at a more rapid rate, the additional breaths

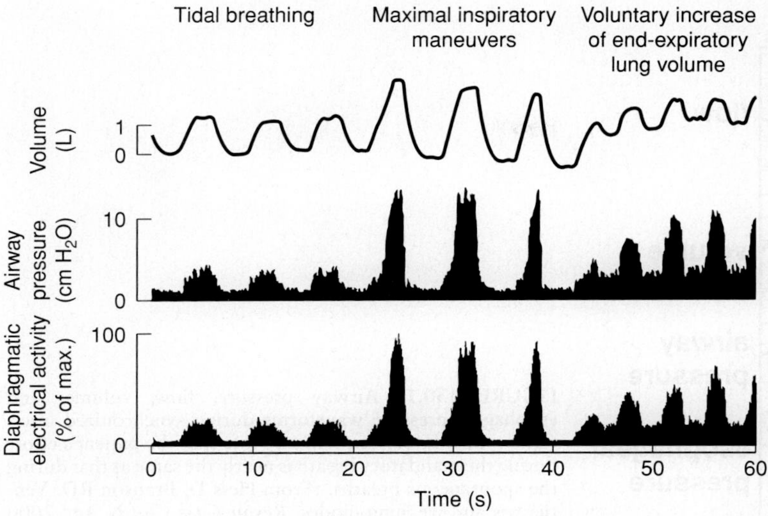

FIGURE 130.17. Neurally adjusted ventilatory assist (NAVA). There are continuous proportional adjustments of airway pressure (reflecting ventilatory assist) with changes in diaphragmatic electrical activity (reflecting neural drive) during changes in tidal and end-expiratory lung volumes. (From Sinderby C, Navalesi P, Beck J, et al. Neural control of mechanical ventilation in respiratory failure. *Nat Med.* 1999;5:1433, with permission.)

are unsupported. If the patient does not breathe at a rate more rapid than that set on the ventilator, SIMV and CMV are synonymous. The spontaneous breaths may or may not be pressure supported (Fig. 130.18). The mandatory breaths are synchronized to patient effort, and they can be volume controlled, pressure controlled, or dual controlled. It has been traditionally taught that the ventilator does the work for the mandatory breaths during SIMV, and that the patient does the work for the spontaneous breaths. However, this has not been supported by either physiologic studies or outcome studies. Inspiratory effort may be as great during mandatory breaths as spontaneous breaths (Fig. 130.19) (53,54). Moreover, dyssynchrony can occur because different breath types are delivered for the mandatory and spontaneous breaths. This dyssynchrony occurs because the patient's neural controller does not modulate its output based on an anticipated ventilator response.

Mandatory Minute Ventilation (MMV)

MMV is intended to guarantee the minute ventilation that the patient receives. If the patient's spontaneous ventilation does

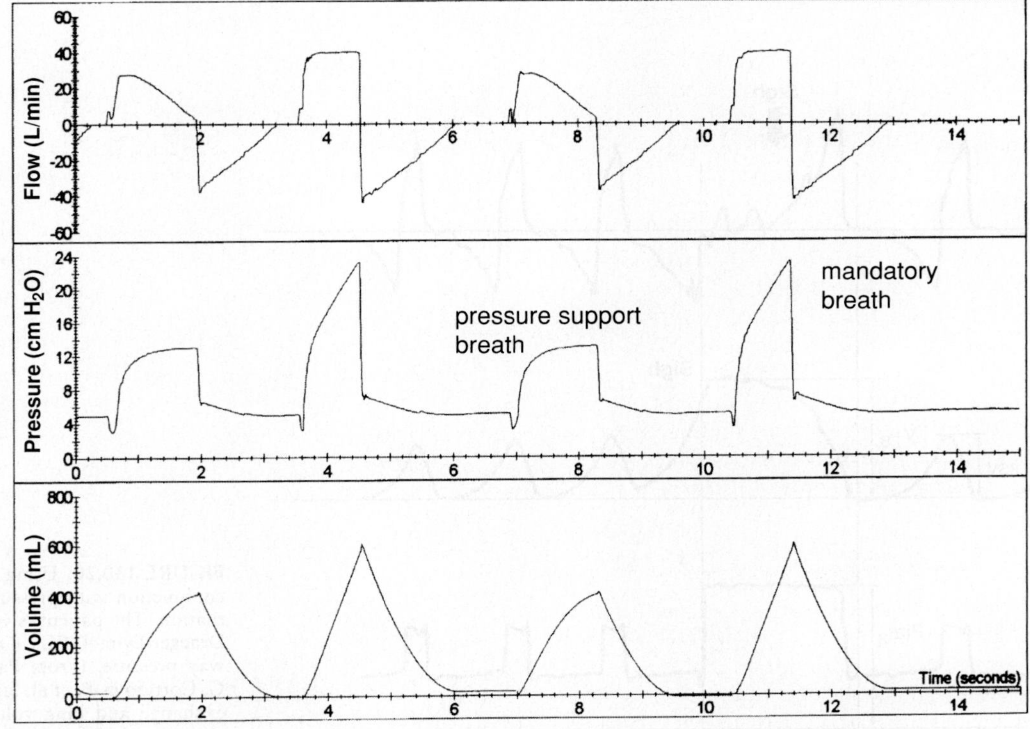

FIGURE 130.18. Airway pressure, flow, and volume waveforms for synchronized intermittent mandatory ventilation. Note that the mandatory breaths are constant flow, volume-controlled ventilation, and the spontaneous breaths are pressure supported.

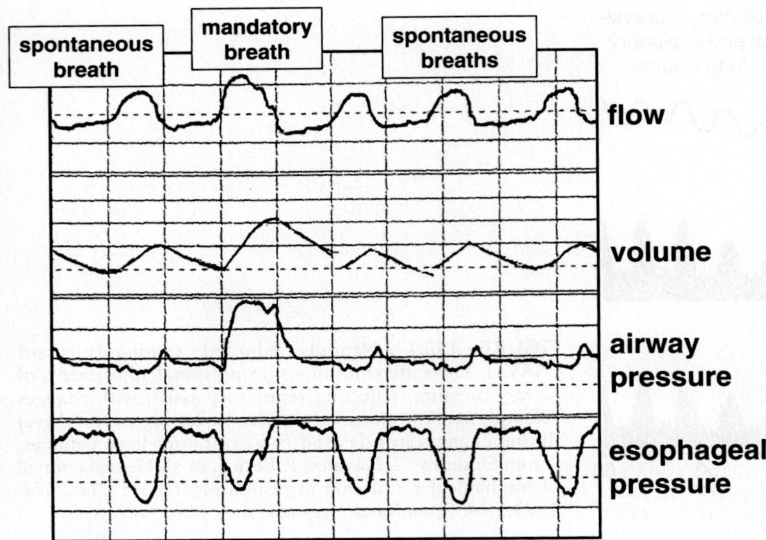

FIGURE 130.19. Airway pressure, flow, volume, and esophageal pressure waveforms during synchronized intermittent mandatory ventilation. Note that the patient's effort during the mandatory breath is nearly the same as that during the spontaneous breaths. (From Hess D, Branson RD. Ventilators and weaning modes. *Respir Care Clin N Am.* 2000 Sep;6[9]:407, with permission.)

not match the target minute ventilation set by the clinician, the ventilator supplies the difference between the patient's minute ventilation and the set minute ventilation. If the patient's spontaneous minute ventilation exceeds what is set, no ventilator support is provided. MMV can be provided by altering the rate or the tidal volume delivered from the ventilator. Some ventilators increase the mandatory breath rate if the minute ventilation falls below the target level, whereas others increase the level of pressure support when the minute ventilation falls below the set level.

Bilevel and PCV+

This mode is available on the Puritan-Bennett 840 (Bilevel) and the Draeger Evita 4 (PCV+). It is essentially a modification of SIMV that uses PCV for the mandatory breaths and PSV for the spontaneous breaths. This mode can be thought of as PSV with a sigh (55). The mandatory breath rate is set at 1 to 4 breaths/minute, with the pressure during the sigh set at 25 to 30 cm H_2O and a sigh duration of 2 to 4 seconds (Fig. 130.20). Because these ventilators have an active exhalation valve, the patient is able to breathe spontaneously when a

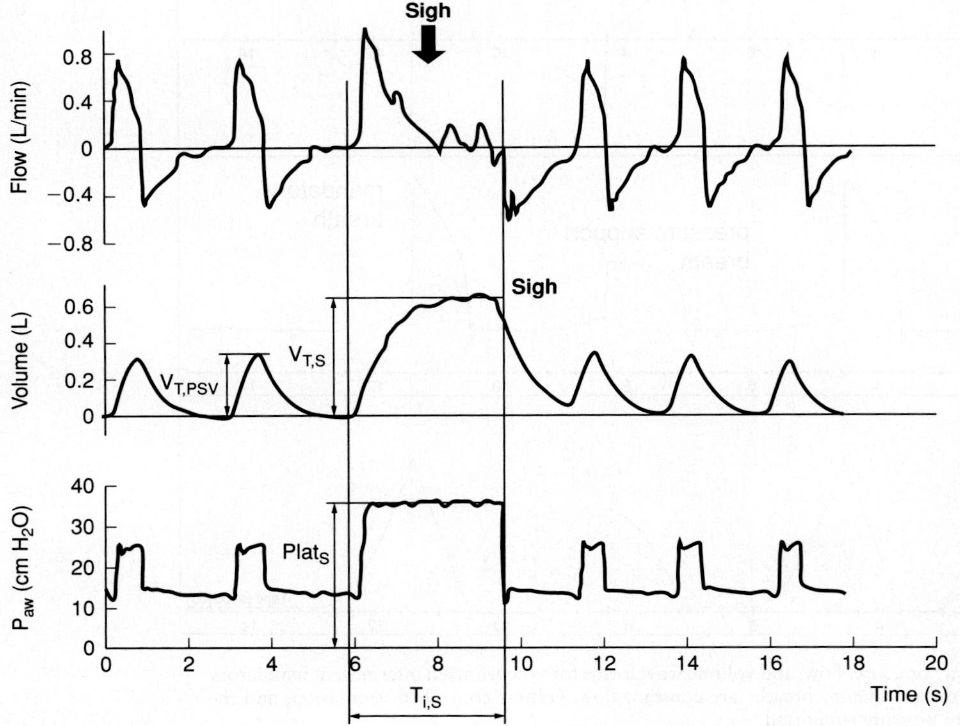

FIGURE 130.20. Using a sigh breath in conjunction with pressure support ventilation. The patient is ventilated with a Draeger Evita 4 (PCV+ mode). Paw, airway pressure. (From Patronati N, Foti G, Cortinovis B, et al. Sigh improves gas exchange and lung volume in patients with acute respiratory distress syndrome undergoing pressure support ventilation. *Anesthesiology.* 2002;96:788, with permission.)

pressure-controlled mandatory breath is delivered. This mode may be more comfortable than the sighs traditionally incorporated into ventilators because it is a pressure-controlled breath using an active exhalation valve.

SUMMARY

Various ventilator modes are available on modern ventilators. The plethora of settings available for the various modes on modern ventilators can be overwhelming. New modes are often based on technical and engineering capability rather than a clear clinical superiority over previously available modes. There is little evidence that any mode improves patient outcome. Patient outcomes are affected more by how the mode is used than by the mode *per se*.

TIPS AND PEARLS

1. Goals of invasive mechanical ventilation:
   a. Provide adequate oxygenation and ventilation.
   b. Maintain alveolar recruitment with adequate PEEP.
   c. Avoid overdistention by limiting the plateau pressure.
   d. Avoid auto-PEEP.
   e. Secure a possibly tenuous airway.
2. The result of any ventilator setting depends not only on what is set on the ventilator, but also on the physiologic characteristics of the patient—namely compliance and resistance, and any active inspiratory effort.
3. For any independent variable set on the ventilator (e.g., pressure), physiologic variables in the patient (compliance and resistance), and effort generated by the patient, there is only one possible result for the dependent variables (e.g., flow and tidal volume).
4. During fully controlled ventilation, bilevel is identical to pressure-controlled ventilation (PCV), and airway pressure release ventilation (APRV) is identical to pressure-controlled inverse ratio ventilation (PCIRV), which is a form of PCV.
5. During pressure ventilation (both pressure-controlled and pressure support), a fast time constant (i.e., low compliance and normal resistance), as is seen in acute lung injury/acute respiratory distress syndrome (ALI/ARDS), may result in a low mean airway pressure and low tidal volume; a slow time constant (i.e., normal or high compliance and high resistance) as is seen in asthma/COPD, may result in a high mean airway pressure, large tidal volumes, and auto-PEEP.

References

1. Chatburn RL. Classification of mechanical ventilators. *Respir Care.* 1992;37:1009.
2. Chatburn RL. A new system for understanding modes of mechanical ventilation. *Respir Care.* 2001;46:604.
3. Racca F, Squadrone V, Ranieri VM. Patient–ventilator interaction during the triggering phase. *Respir Care Clin N Am.* 2005;11:225.
4. Imanaka H, Nishimura M, Takeuchi M, et al. Autotriggering caused by cardiogenic oscillation during flow-triggered mechanical ventilation. *Crit Care Med.* 2000;28:402.
5. Richard JC, Carlucci A, Breton L, et al. Bench testing of pressure support ventilation with three different generations of ventilators. *Intensive Care Med.* 2002;28:1049.
6. Goulet R, Hess D, Kacmarek RM. Pressure vs. flow triggering during pressure support ventilation. *Chest.* 1997;111:1649.
7. Ranieri VM, Grasso S, Fiore T, et al. Auto-positive end-expiratory pressure and dynamic hyperinflation. *Clin Chest Med.* 1996;17:379.
8. Hudson LD, Hurlow RS, Craig KC, et al. Does intermittent mandatory ventilation correct respiratory alkalosis in patients receiving assisted mechanical ventilation? *Am Rev Respir Dis.* 1985;130:1071.
9. Nilsestuen JO, Hargett KD. Using ventilator graphics to identify patient–ventilator asynchrony. *Respir Care.* 2005;50:202.
10. Hess DR, Medoff BD, Fessler MB. Pulmonary mechanics and graphics during positive pressure ventilation. *Int Anesthesiol Clin.* 1999;37:15.
11. Marini JJ, Rodriguez RM, Lamb V. The inspiratory workload of patient-initiated mechanical ventilation. *Am Rev Respir Dis.* 1986;134:902.
12. The Acute Respiratory Distress Syndrome Network. Ventilation with lower tidal volumes as compared with traditional tidal volumes for acute lung injury and the acute respiratory distress syndrome. *N Engl J Med.* 2000;342:1301.
13. Hess DR, Thompson BT. Patient–ventilator dyssynchrony during lung protective ventilation: what's a clinician to do? *Crit Care Med.* 2006;34:231.
14. MacIntyre NR, McConnell R, Cheng KC, et al. Patient–ventilator flow dyssynchrony: flow-limited versus pressure-limited breaths. *Crit Care Med.* 1997;25:1671.
15. Uchiyama A, Imanaka H, Taenaka N. Relationship between work of breathing provided by a ventilator and patients' inspiratory drive during pressure support ventilation; effects of inspiratory rise time. *Anaesth Intensive Care.* 2001;29:349.
16. Esteban A, Alia I, Gordo F, et al. Prospective randomized trial comparing pressure-controlled ventilation and volume-controlled ventilation in ARDS. *Chest.* 2000;117:1690.
17. Davis K Jr, Branson RD, Campbell RS, et al. Comparison of volume control and pressure control ventilation: is flow waveform the difference? *J Trauma.* 1996;41:808.
18. Branson RD, Davis K Jr. Dual control modes: combining volume and pressure breaths. *Respir Care Clin N Am.* 2001;7:397.
19. Branson RD, Campbell RS, Davis K Jr. New modes of ventilatory support. *Int Anesthesiol Clin.* 1999;37:103.
20. Branson RD, Johannigman JA. What is the evidence base for the newer ventilation modes? *Respir Care.* 2004;49:742.
21. Branson RD, Johannigman JA. The role of ventilator graphics when setting dual-control modes. *Respir Care.* 2005;50:187.
22. Branson RD, Johannigman JA, Campbell RS, et al. Closed-loop mechanical ventilation. *Respir Care.* 2002;47:427.
23. Hess D, Branson RD. Ventilators and weaning modes. *Respir Care Clin N Am.* 2000;6:407.
24. D'Angio CT, Chess PR, Kovacs SJ, et al. Pressure-regulated volume control ventilation vs. synchronized intermittent mandatory ventilation for very low-birth-weight infants: a randomized controlled trial. *Arch Pediatr Adolesc Med.* 2005;159:868.
25. Jaber S, Delay JM, Matecki S, et al. Volume-guaranteed pressure-support ventilation facing acute changes in ventilatory demand. *Intensive Care Med.* 2005;31:1181.
26. Chan K, Abraham E. Effects of inverse ratio ventilation on cardiorespiratory parameters in severe respiratory failure. *Chest.* 1992;102:1556.
27. Mercat A, Titiriga M, Anguel N, et al. Inverse ratio ventilation (I/E = 2/1) in acute respiratory distress syndrome: a six-hour controlled study. *Am J Respir Crit Care Med.* 1997;155:1637.
28. Kacmarek RM, Hess D. Pressure-controlled inverse-ratio ventilation: panacea or auto-PEEP? *Respir Care.* 1990;35:945.
29. Habashi NM. Other approaches to open-lung ventilation: airway pressure release ventilation. *Crit Care Med.* 2005;33:S228.
30. McCunn M, Habashi NM. Airway pressure release ventilation in the acute respiratory distress syndrome following traumatic injury. *Int Anesthesiol Clin.* 2002;40(3):89.
31. Putensen C, Mutz NJ, Putensen-Himmer G, et al. Spontaneous breathing during ventilatory support improves ventilation-perfusion distributions in patients with acute respiratory distress syndrome. *Am J Respir Crit Care Med.* 1999;159:1241.
32. Putensen C, Zech S, Wrigge H, et al. Long-term effects of spontaneous breathing during ventilatory support in patients with acute lung injury. *Am J Respir Crit Care Med.* 2001;164:43.
33. Hess DR. Ventilator waveforms and the physiology of pressure support ventilation. *Respir Care.* 2005;50:166.
34. Chiumello D, Pelosi P, Croci M, et al. The effects of pressurization rate on breathing pattern, work of breathing, gas exchange and patient comfort in pressure support ventilation. *Eur Respir J.* 2001;18(1):107.
35. Chiumello D, Pelosi P, Taccone P, et al. Effect of different inspiratory rise time and cycling off criteria during pressure support ventilation in patients recovering from acute lung injury. *Crit Care Med.* 2003;31:2604.
36. Du HL, Yamada Y. Expiratory asynchrony. *Respir Care Clin N Am.* 2005;11:265.
37. Du HL, Amato MB, Yamada Y. Automation of expiratory trigger sensitivity in pressure support ventilation. *Respir Care Clin N Am.* 2001;7:503.
38. Yamada Y, Du HL. Analysis of the mechanisms of expiratory asynchrony in pressure support ventilation: a mathematical approach. *J Appl Physiol.* 2000;88:2143.
39. Tassaux D, Gainnier M, Battisti A, et al. Impact of expiratory trigger setting

on delayed cycling and inspiratory muscle workload. *Am J Respir Crit Care Med.* 2005;172:1283.
40. Tokioka H, Tanaka T, Ishizu T, et al. The effect of breath termination criterion on breathing patterns and the work of breathing during pressure support ventilation. *Anesth Analg.* 2001;92:161.
41. Brochard L, Pluskwa F, Lemaire F. Improved efficacy of spontaneous breathing with inspiratory pressure support. *Am Rev Respir Dis.* 1987;136:411.
42. Parthasarathy S, Tobin MJ. Effect of ventilator mode on sleep quality in critically ill patients. *Am J Respir Crit Care Med.* 2002;166:1423.
43. Dojat M, Brochard L. Knowledge-based systems for automatic ventilatory management. *Respir Care Clin N Am.* 2001;7:379.
44. Lellouche F, Mancebo J, Jolliet P, et al. A multicenter randomized trial of computer-driven protocolized weaning from mechanical ventilation. *Am J Respir Crit Care Med.* 2006;174:894.
45. Campbell RS, Branson RD, Johannigman JA. Adaptive support ventilation. *Respir Care Clin N Am.* 2001;7:425.
46. Guttmann J, Haberthur C, Mols G, et al. Automatic tube compensation (ATC). *Minerva Anestesiol.* 2002;68:369.
47. Guttmann J, Haberthur C, Mols G. Automatic tube compensation. *Respir Care Clin N Am.* 2001;7:475.
48. Haberthur C, Mols G, Elsasser S, et al. Extubation after breathing trials with automatic tube compensation, T-tube, or pressure support ventilation. *Acta Anaesthesiol Scand.* 2002;46:973.
49. Cohen JD, Shapiro M, Grozovski E, et al. Extubation outcome following a spontaneous breathing trial with automatic tube compensation versus continuous positive airway pressure. *Crit Care Med.* 2006;34:682.
50. Grasso S, Ranieri VM. Proportional assist ventilation. *Respir Care Clin N Am.* 2001;7:465.
51. Navalesi P, Costa R. New modes of mechanical ventilation: proportional assist ventilation, neurally adjusted ventilatory assist, and fractal ventilation. *Curr Opin Crit Care.* 2003;9:51.
52. Sinderby C, Navalesi P, Beck J, et al. Neural control of mechanical ventilation in respiratory failure. *Nat Med.* 1999;5:1433.
53. Marini JJ, Smith TC, Lamb VJ. External work output and force generation during synchronized intermittent mechanical ventilation. Effect of machine assistance on breathing effort. *Am Rev Respir Dis.* 1988;138:1169.
54. Imsand C, Feihl F, Perret C, et al. Regulation of inspiratory neuromuscular output during synchronized intermittent mandatory ventilation. *Anesthesiolog.* 1994;80:13.
55. Patroniti N, Foti G, Cortinovis B, et al. Sigh improves gas exchange and lung volume in patients with acute respiratory distress syndrome undergoing pressure support ventilation. *Anesthesiolog.* 2002;96:788.

CHAPTER 131 ■ BEDSIDE INTERPRETATION OF VENTILATORY WAVEFORMS

ETTORE CRIMI • DEAN R. HESS • LUCA M. BIGATELLO

Modern ventilators provide a continuous graphic display of the basic physiologic determinants of ventilation, i.e., pressure, flow, and volume. They also have the capability of performing diagnostic maneuvers to measure important physiologic variables such as plateau pressure and auto–positive end-expiratory pressure (PEEP) at the bedside. In addition, recognition of abnormal ventilator waveforms allows detection of conditions such as endobronchial intubation, missed triggering, and patient–ventilator dyssynchrony. This chapter focuses on the use of the waveforms displayed on ventilator screens to improve bedside assessment and management of patients with acute respiratory failure requiring mechanical ventilation.

BASICS OF VENTILATOR MONITORING

Ventilators can provide continuous measurement and display of pressure, flow, and volume. The ability of ventilators to display graphics and numeric data on their screen has become possible in recent years due to the availability of cost-effective sensor–transducer devices and the proliferation of microelectronic and digital technology. What used to be limited to expensive and delicate instruments used in the physiology laboratory is now compacted at relatively low cost in critical care ventilators.

How Ventilators Measure Pressure, Volume, and Flow

Airway pressure is measured in most ventilators by solid state transducers, such as piezoresistive or strain gauge transducers. Although airway pressure is best measured distal to the endotracheal tube (tracheal pressure) or at the airway, these locations tend to interfere with patient care and are not practical for continuous clinical monitoring. Hence, pressure transducers are generally located inside the ventilator at the inspiratory and expiratory valves, alternating measurements at the expiratory limb during inspiration and at the inspiratory limb during exhalation. These systems are reasonably accurate for clinical purposes but have potential flaws; for example, they will not accurately indicate proximal airway pressure if obstruction or kinking of the breathing circuit occur.

Gas flow to and from the patient during spontaneous and mechanical ventilation can be measured by various techniques (1,2). Screen and orifice pneumotachographs measure the pressure drop across a known resistance (a screen or an orifice) and derive the flow according to Ohm's law:

$$\text{Resistance} = \Delta\ \text{pressure/flow} \qquad [1]$$

and its modifications to account for laminar versus turbulent flow (2). Thermal cooling pneumotachographs estimate flow from the amount of heat loss produced by the flow across the device, applying the principle of thermal convection. They oppose minimal resistance to flow and show a rapid response to flow changes, but their accuracy is decreased by turbulence and moisture. Turbine spirometers work by vane displacement, where flow rate is derived from the rotations of the turbine blades. These devices are less accurate than pneumotachographs, particularly at low gas flow, but are sturdy and easy to clean; they have been of widespread use in anesthesia machines, but have been superseded by the newer pneumotachographs. As is the case for pressure measurements, most ventilators measure flow at the inspiratory and expiratory valves rather than at the airway. Flow sensors are calibrated for air/oxygen mixtures. Thus, inaccuracies can occur in the presence of other gases, such as heliox (3), unless the ventilator is designed to make appropriate corrections, as is the Viasys AVEA (Viasys Healthcare, Yorba Linda, CA).

Tidal volume is generally measured by time integration of the flow trace. When gas flow, as in most cases, is not measured at the proximal airway, there is a difference between volume output from the ventilator and the volume delivered to the patient due to the compressible volume of the ventilator circuit. The *compressible volume* is the volume of gas that is lost in the compliant structures of the system, mainly the corrugated tubing of the ventilator circuit. The size of this volume is determined by two main factors: the inspiratory pressure and the compliance of the tubing. Current ventilators compensate for this lost volume in different ways (4); commonly, they measure the compliance of the breathing circuit at the time of the initial automatic setup, and they calculate a factor in the range of 3 to 4 mL/cm H_2O, which is automatically added to the set tidal volume. Additional potential sources of error in volume measurements include gas conditioning by heating and humidification, which increases gas volume after the inspiratory flow sensor, as well as differences between the inspired and expired flow/volume due to oxygen consumption. Generally, these are small inaccuracies that fall within the margin of error of the flow sensors (±10%).

Additional Monitoring Functions

Common functions present in microprocessor-driven ventilators include the ability to perform diagnostic maneuvers that can be used to assess important physiologic variables at the bedside. The most common of these functions are the end-inspiratory and end-expiratory pauses (Fig. 131.1).

- An *end-inspiratory pause* is used to estimate alveolar pressure, respiratory compliance, and airways resistance. During volume-controlled ventilation with constant inspiratory flow, a manual or programmed end-inspiratory pause generates a characteristic pattern where the peak inspiratory pressure (PIP) is followed by a rapid descent to a plateau—the inspiratory plateau pressure (Pplat). When the inspiratory pause is of sufficient duration (0.5–2 seconds), it ensures cessation of gas flow and equilibration between the pressure at the proximal airway and alveolar pressure. Measurement of the Pplat requires full patient relaxation and the absence of spontaneous breathing efforts, because the consequent changes in intrathoracic pressure due to respiratory muscle

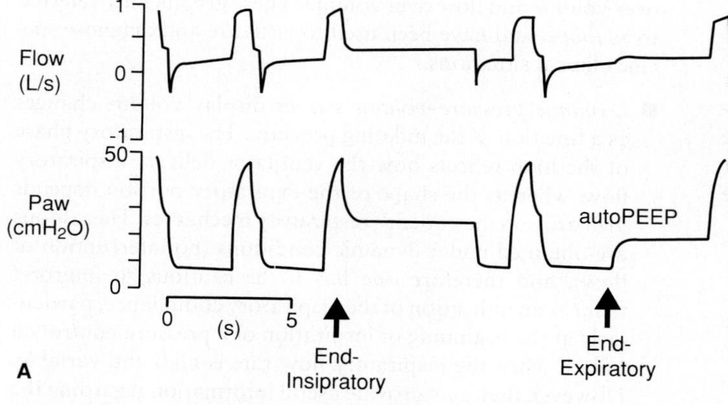

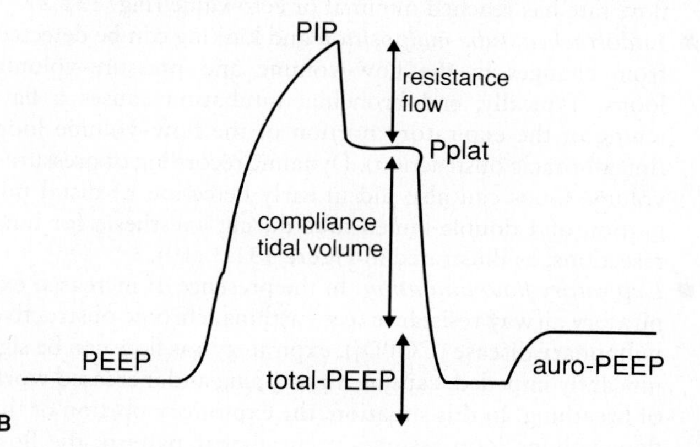

FIGURE 131.1. A: Flow and airway pressure (Paw) waveforms in a mechanically ventilated patient with chronic obstructive pulmonary disease, showing the performance of an end-inspiratory and an end-expiratory pause. (Modified from Putensen C, Mutz NJ, Putensen-Himmer G, et al. Spontaneous breathing during ventilatory support improves ventilation-perfusion distributions in patients with acute respiratory distress syndrome. *Am J Respir Crit Care Med.* 1999;159:1241. with permission.) **B:** Diagram of a typical airway pressure waveform during mechanical ventilation. The difference between peak inspiratory pressure (PIP) and plateau pressure (Pplat) is determined by airways resistance and end-inspiratory flow. The difference between plateau pressure and positive end-expiratory pressure (PEEP) is determined by compliance and tidal volume. (From Fisher D, Hess D. Respiratory monitoring. In: Bigatello LM, ed. *Critical Care Handbook of the Massachusetts General Hospital.* 4th ed. Philadelphia, PA: Lippincott Williams & Wilkins; 2006:33–52, with permission.)

activity would affect Pplat and invalidate compliance measurements. The presence of a leak in the system (within either the patient or the ventilator) will also not permit reaching a stable Pplat. The end-expiratory pause maneuver should be limited to a single breath at the time to avoid unnecessary prolongation of the inspiratory time and the development of auto-PEEP in patients at risk.

- An *end-expiratory pause* is used to estimate auto-PEEP when the lungs fail to empty to functional residual capacity (FRC) at end expiration. An end-expiratory pause of sufficient duration allows equilibration between alveolar and proximal airway pressure, and just as for the Pplat, this measurement is invalidated by the presence of spontaneous breathing efforts and by air leaks (5).

Additional monitoring functions, not universally available on ventilators, include the measurement of airway occlusion pressure ($P_{0.1}$) and the maximum inspiratory pressure (Pi_{max}).

- The $P_{0.1}$ is the value of negative airway pressure generated in the first 100 ms of an occluded inspiratory effort. Since the early part of inspiration is largely independent of the subject's voluntary effort, the $P_{0.1}$ is used as an index of ventilatory drive (6). Some ventilators can perform this measurement automatically, with seemingly equal accuracy as the manual measurement (7).
- The Pi_{max} is the most negative pressure generated during a maximal inspiratory effort against an occluded airway. It is an index of the strength of the inspiratory muscles and has been used as an index of readiness for ventilator weaning. The off-ventilator manual measurement technique uses a one-way valve, allowing exhalation but not inspiration and an occlusion for about 15 to 20 seconds, provided that no arrhythmias or desaturation occur (8). Some ventilators allow this measurement to be performed electronically by occluding both inspiratory and expiratory valves for a set time. Relevant differences between the manual and ventilator method include the starting lung volume, which is the residual volume (the subject is coached to exhale fully prior to the maneuver) in the manual method, and FRC in the automatic method.

SPECIFIC USES

Breath Delivery

Delivery of a ventilator breath is determined by the interaction between the machine's operation and the patient's physiology, which is described by the *equation of motion of the respiratory system*, discussed in more detail in Chapter 130:

$$P_{appl} = \text{Pvent} + \text{Pmus} = V_T/C + \dot{V} \times R \qquad [2]$$

Where P_{appl} is the pressure applied to generate the breath, Pvent is the pressure applied by the ventilator, Pmus is the pressure generated by the respiratory muscles, V_T is the tidal volume, C is the compliance, $\dot{V}$ is the gas flow, and R is the airway resistance. In essence, when a pressure (from the respiratory muscles, the ventilator, or both) is applied to the respiratory system, it generates a gas flow through the airways that is opposed by their resistance and causes a change in the volume of the respiratory system that is proportional to its compliance. Understanding the interaction between ventilator (P, V_T, and $\dot{V}$) and patient (C and R) variables greatly aids the understanding of the principles of ventilation. In the previous chapter (Chapter 130), we used this approach to describe how the ventilator delivers different types of breaths. Here, we will use the same basic approach to describe how these breaths can be affected by changes in ventilatory settings, changes in physiologic variables, and specific disease states. For example, if the ventilator measures pressure, volume, and flow at multiple times during the breath delivery, an iterative technique can be used to calculate resistance and compliance (least squares technique) (9). Note, however, that this technique assumes that the patient is making no active breathing effort (Pmus = 0).

Typical Pressure, Flow, and Volume Traces

Typically, a ventilator screen will display two graphic traces of pressure, flow, or volume over time. Most ventilators allow multiple graphic and numeric options that include displaying continuous measurements as well as—or as an alternative to—ventilator settings, alarm limits, and operational information. Graphic options may include adjusting scales, sweep speed, color coding of various ventilatory modes and breathing cycle phases, freezing of a desired screen, and performing precise measurements with a cursor. By convention, inspiratory events are displayed as positive and expiratory events as negative, and the baseline is the zero flow, volume, or pressure (or PEEP). Numerous typical traces obtained during different modes are shown in Chapter 130.

Loops

In addition to the time-based graphics of pressure, volume, and flow, ventilators can often display these variables as pressure over volume and flow over volume. These graphics are referred to as *loops*, and have been used to visualize and diagnose specific clinical situations.

- *Dynamic pressure–volume curves* display volume changes as a function of the inflating pressure. The inspiratory phase of the loop reflects how the ventilator delivers inspiratory flow, whereas the shape of the expiratory portion depends primarily on the patient's respiratory mechanics. These loops are obtained under dynamic conditions (no interruption of flow), and therefore one has to be cautious to interpret them as an indication of the respiratory compliance, particularly at the beginning of inspiration of a pressure-controlled breath when the inspiratory flow rate is high and variable. However, they may provide useful information regarding the state of lung inflation at end inspiration when the inspiratory flow rate has reached minimal or zero value (Fig. 131.2).
- *Endotracheal tube malposition* and kinking can be detected from changes in the flow–volume and pressure–volume loops. Typically, endobronchial intubation causes a flattening of the expiratory portion of the flow–volume loop (intrathoracic obstruction). Dynamic recording of pressure–volume loops can also aid in early detection of distal migration of a double-lumen tube during anesthesia for lung resections, as illustrated in Figure 131.3 (10).
- *Expiratory flow limitation*. In the presence of increased expiratory airway resistance (e.g., asthma, chronic obstructive pulmonary disease [COPD]), expiratory gas flow can be significantly impeded, causing air trapping and increased work of breathing. In this situation, the expiratory portion of the flow–volume loop assumes a curvilinear pattern: the flow

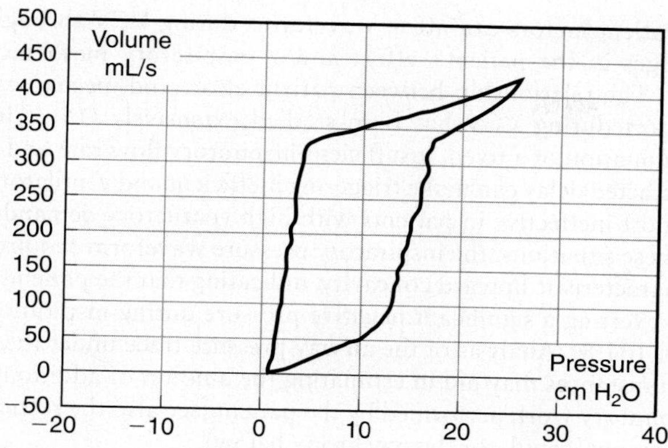

FIGURE 131.2. Pressure–volume loop showing hyperinflation as abrupt increase of pressure at the end of inspiration. (From Nilsestuen JO, Hargett KD. Using ventilator graphics to identify patient–ventilator asynchrony. *Respir Care.* 2005;50:202–234, with permission.)

decays rapidly after the beginning of exhalation and subsequently tapers off, ending with a prolonged low flow rate phase (Fig. 131.4). In addition, when expiratory flow persists through the end of exhalation, the flow–volume loop becomes truncated, indicating the presence of flow limitation and consequent auto-PEEP (11–13). Observation of the expiratory flow–volume loop can be used to assess response to a bronchodilator (Fig. 131.5).

- *Air leaks* cause a loss of volume with each breath, as well as a difference between the delivered and the exhaled tidal volume. Air leaks can occur within the ventilator system (e.g., at the ventilator circuit), between the ventilator and the patient (e.g., at connections between a thoracostomy tube and a drainage device), and within the patient, such as in the presence of a bronchopleural fistula. Regardless of their location, air leaks cause a characteristic failure of the flow–volume loop to close at the end of expiration, because a portion of the inspired tidal volume does not return to the site of volume measurement on the exhalation side (Fig. 131.6).

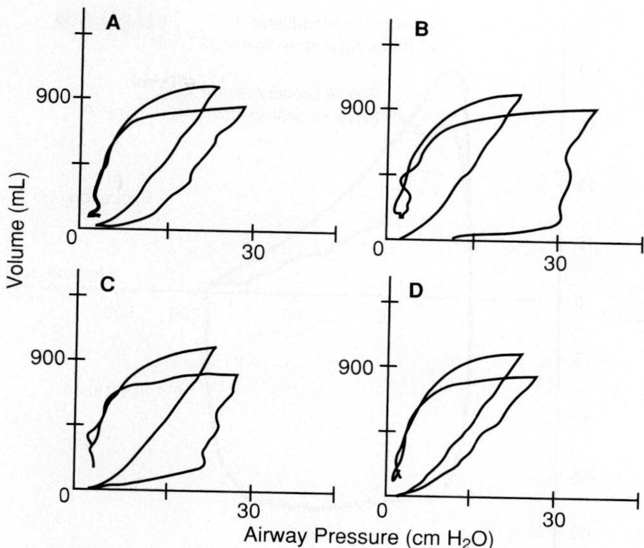

FIGURE 131.3. Pressure–volume curve during two-lung (*narrower loops*) and one-lung (*wider loops*) ventilation, using a double-lumen endotracheal tube. **A:** Baseline recording; on one-lung ventilation, the airway pressure is slightly higher than on two-lung ventilation for a similar volume, as expected. **B:** Acute change in inspiratory airway pressure. **C:** Partial reversal of the increase in airway pressure, as the endotracheal tube is withdrawn. **D:** Nearly full return to baseline after further withdrawal of the tube. (From Simon BA, Hurford WE, Alfille PH, et al. An aid in the diagnosis of malpositioned double-lumen tubes. *Anesthesiology.* 1992;76:862–863, with permission.)

Changes in Breath Delivery

Volume-controlled Ventilation (VCV)

During VCV, airway pressure waveforms can be affected by changes in the ventilator settings and changes in the patient's respiratory mechanics, as illustrated by equation [2]. Figure 131.7 shows how a change in peak inspiratory flow rate can affect the shape of the airway pressure trace during VCV at constant flow.

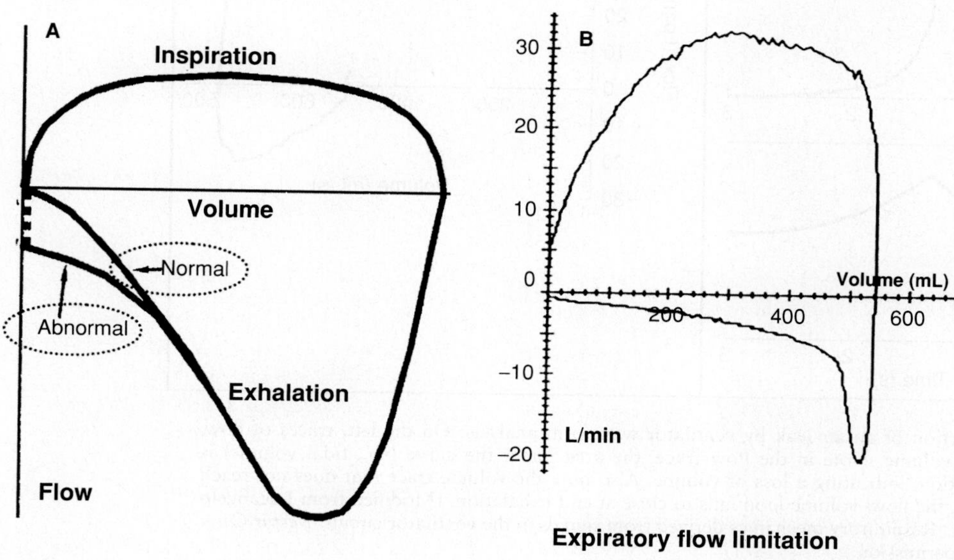

FIGURE 131.4. Flow–volume loops during mechanical ventilation. **A** shows a normal pattern (*shorter arrow*) and an expiratory obstruction pattern (*longer arrow*). Note how the expiratory flow is truncated at end expiration and does not reach the zero-flow line. (Modified from Dhand R. Ventilator graphics and respiratory mechanics in the patient with obstructive lung disease. *Respir Care.* 2005;50:246–261, with permission.) **B** also shows expiratory flow obstruction, where the flow decreases rapidly after the first few milliseconds and then continues for the rest of exhalation at a very slow rate, without ever reaching the zero-flow line.

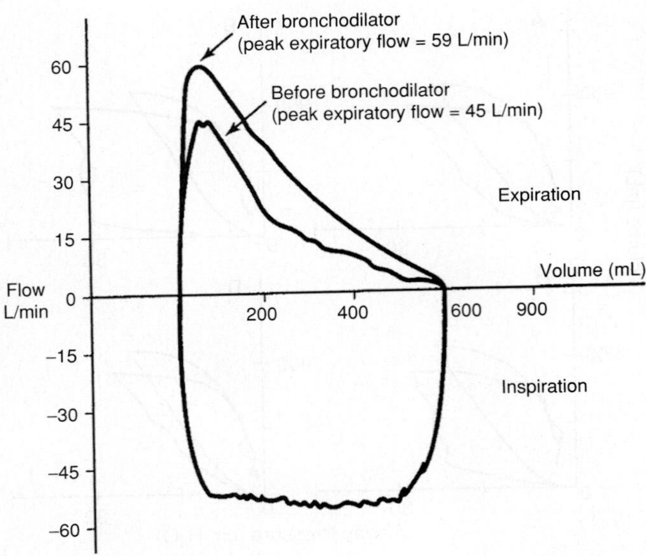

FIGURE 131.5. Flow–volume loops showing a response to pharmacologic bronchodilation. The expiratory limb is up in this figure (down in the previous figure) and it shows the concavity characteristic of flow limitation. The administration of a bronchodilator increased the peak expiratory flow rate and reduced the degree of concavity. (From Dhand R. Ventilator graphics and respiratory mechanics in the patient with obstructive lung disease. *Respir Care.* 2005;50:246–261, with permission.)

Patient factors can affect waveforms during VCV through changes in the patient's effort and/or respiratory mechanics (14). The relationship between patient effort and mechanical support during VCV has been studied extensively (15). The combination of a fixed, insufficient inspiratory flow rate and a protracted delay can make triggering inefficient and ventilatory support ineffective in patients with high ventilatory demands. In these situations, the inspiratory pressure waveform acquires a characteristic upward concavity, indicating that the patient is still exerting a significant negative pressure during inspiration (Fig. 131.8). Analysis of the airway pressure trace under these circumstances may aid in estimating the amount of additional respiratory work performed by the patient (see also the section on patient–ventilator dyssynchrony below).

During VCV, the breath can also be delivered with a descending ramp flow waveform. With such a flow pattern, the set peak inspiratory flow is reached early during the breath, after which the flow decreases in a linear fashion to a very low level—or zero—at end inspiration. For the same peak flow setting of a constant flow waveform, the descending ramp requires a substantially extended inspiratory time to provide the same area under the curve (the tidal volume). The descending ramp flow pattern also affects the shape of the pressure waveform, which increases more rapidly at the beginning of inspiration, resulting in a lower PIP, which approaches the Pplat (Fig. 131.9). The lower PIP is one reason why clinicians often favor the descending ramp over the constant flow waveform; in addition, the longer inspiratory time results in a higher mean airway pressure, which may be associated with enhanced lung recruitment (typically, in patients with ALI/ARDS [acute lung injury/acute

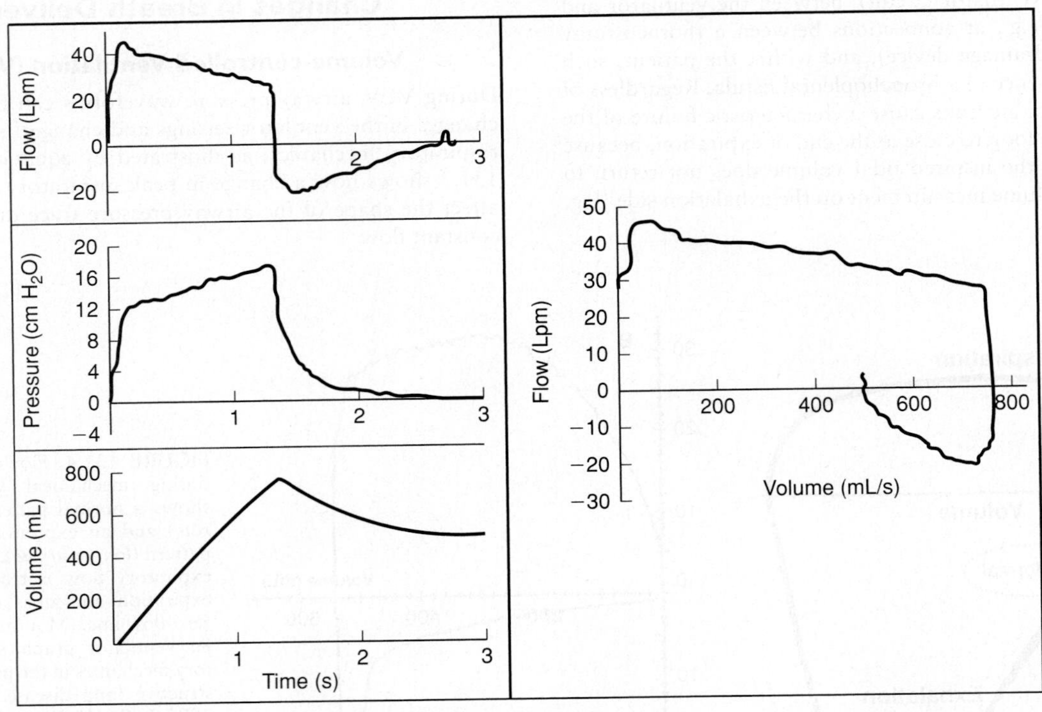

FIGURE 131.6. Detection of an air leak by ventilator waveform analysis. On the **left**, traces of flow, airway pressure, and volume. Note in the flow trace, the area under the curve (i.e., tidal volume) is smaller during exhalation, indicating a loss of volume. Also note the volume trace that does not reach baseline. On the **right**, the flow–volume loop fails to close at end exhalation. (Modified from Lucangelo U, Bernabe F, Blanch L. Respiratory mechanics derived from signals in the ventilator circuit. *Respir Care.* 2005;50:55–65, with permission.)

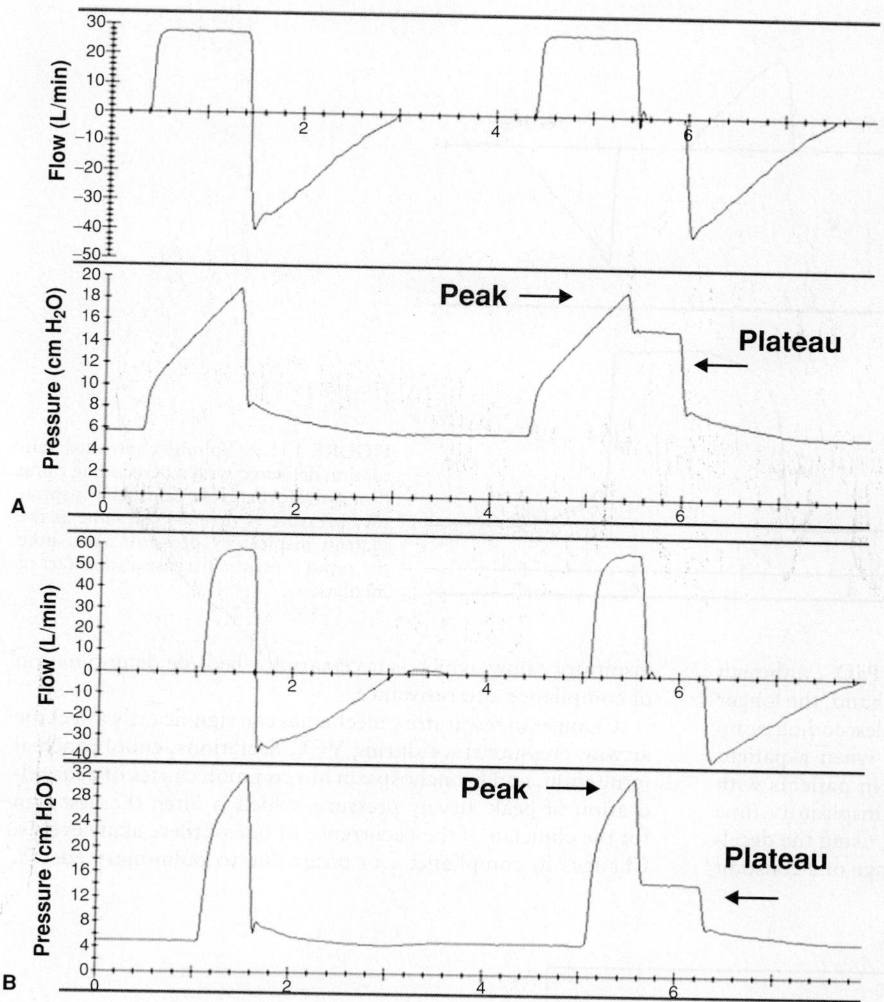

FIGURE 131.7. Changes in inspiratory airway pressure trace with different peak inspiratory flow rates during volume-controlled ventilation. A: Peak inspiratory flow rate = 30 L/min, tidal volume 500 mL. B: Peak inspiratory flow rate = 60 L/min, tidal volume 500 mL. The higher flow rate is associated with higher peak inspiratory airway pressure (but not plateau inspiratory pressure) and a shorter inspiratory time; the tidal volume is the same by default.

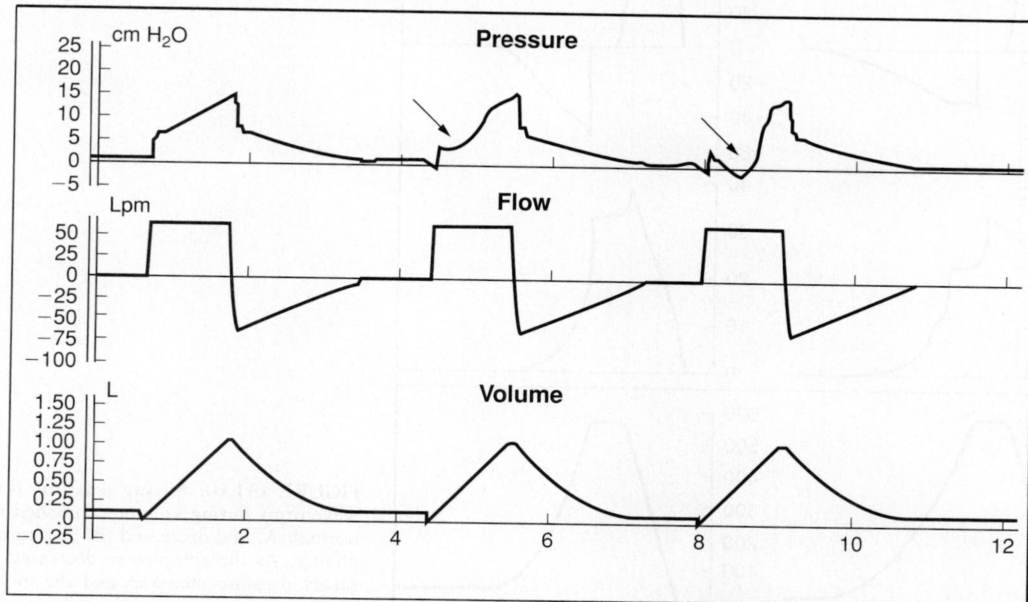

FIGURE 131.8. Examples of inadequate peak inspiratory flow rate during volume-controlled ventilation. The *arrows* point to the scooped appearance of the airway pressure waveform due to the patient's own inspiratory effort. (Modified from Nilsestuen JO, Hargett KD. Using ventilator graphics to identify patient-ventilator asynchrony. *Respir Care.* 2005;50:202–234, with permission.)

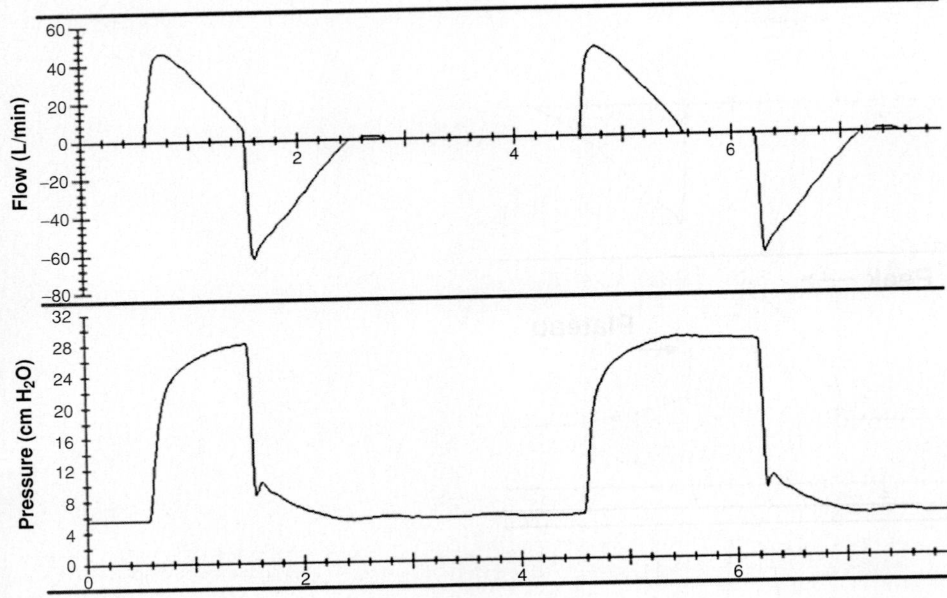

FIGURE 131.9. Volume-controlled ventilation delivered with a descending ramp flow waveform. Note that peak inspiratory pressure is virtually the same as the plateau inspiratory pressure. Also note the rapid pressure increase at the start of inhalation.

respiratory distress syndrome]) and a higher PaO_2, although the benefit is generally marginal. On the other hand, the longer inspiratory time may be a disadvantage of the descending ramp with respect to the constant flow waveform when a patient is at risk of developing auto-PEEP (typically, in patients with COPD and asthma) because it lengthens the inspiratory time and shortens the expiratory time. In addition, using the decelerating flow waveform takes away the advantage of a constant inspiratory flow, which is necessary for bedside determination of compliance and resistance.

Changes in respiratory mechanics can significantly affect the airway pressure trace during VCV. Secretions, endobronchial intubation, and bronchospasm are common causes of acute elevation of peak airway pressure, which is often the first sign for the clinician of the occurrence of one of these acute events. Changes in compliance can occur due to pulmonary edema,

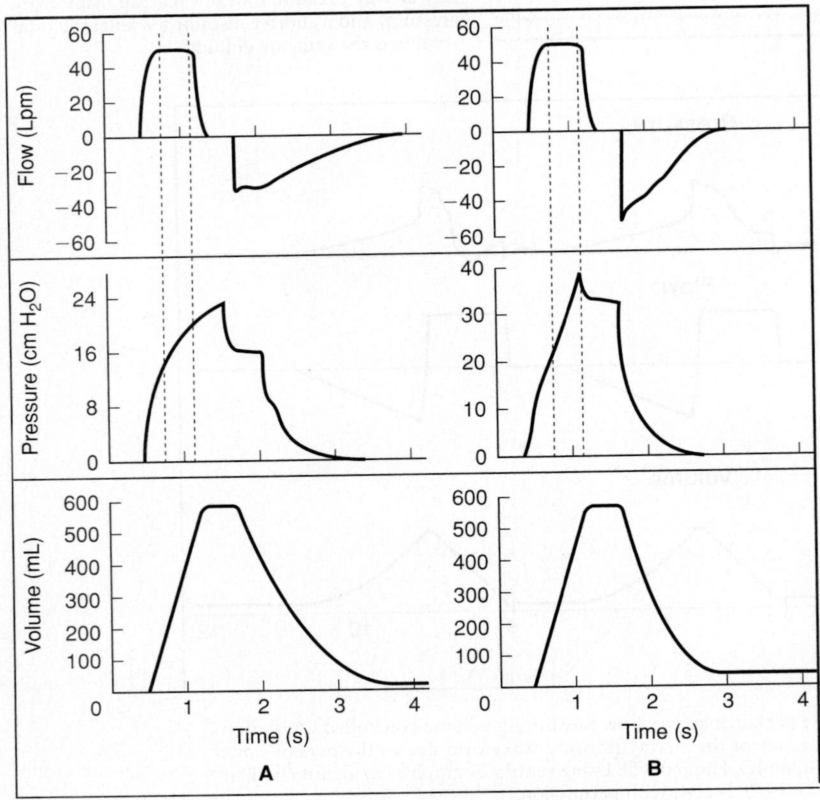

FIGURE 131.10. Airway pressure, flow, and volume waveforms during volume-controlled ventilation with normal (**A**) and decreased (**B**) respiratory system compliance. As the compliance decreases, the peak inspiratory pressure increases and the morphology of the airway pressure curve changes from concave to linear. (Modified from Lucangelo U, Bernabe F, Blanch L. Respiratory mechanics derived from signals in the ventilator circuit. *Respir Care.* 2005;50:55–65, with permission.)

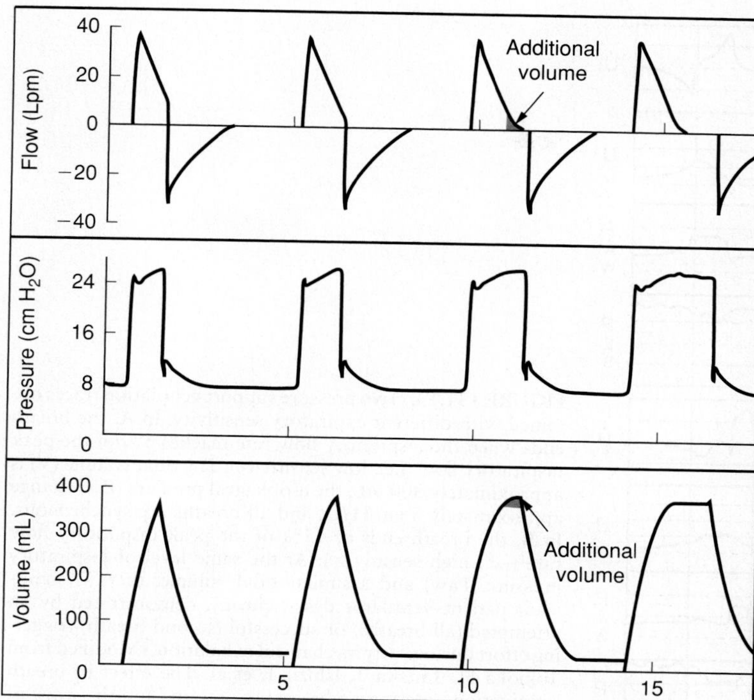

FIGURE 131.11. Effects of changes in the inspiratory time during pressure-controlled ventilation. As the duration of inspiration is progressively increased from the first breath on, the tidal volume increases (*arrows*). Once the inspiratory time is sufficiently long that the inspiratory flow reaches the zero line before the end of inspiration, no further volume is gained (last breath). (Modified from Lucangelo U, Bernabe F, Blanch L. Respiratory mechanics derived from signals in the ventilator circuit. *Respir Care.* 2005;50:55–65, with permission.)

increased abdominal pressure, and increased intrathoracic pressure (Fig. 131.10).

Pressure-controlled Ventilation (PCV)

During PCV, inspiratory airway pressure increases rapidly to the set value, resembling a square or rectangular wave. This airway pressure waveform is due to the unique way that inspiratory flow is delivered during pressure-controlled modes. The inspiratory flow rate is variable and is the result of a combination of several factors: the capability of the ventilator, the patient's effort, and the patient's respiratory mechanics (see also Chapter 130) (16). Once the set inspiratory pressure is reached, the flow rate decreases exponentially to maintain the set pressure for the desired time, and the decay of the flow rate (descending ramp) is largely determined by the time constant of the respiratory system, i.e., resistance times compliance. Therefore, the inspiratory flow waveform during PCV is variable (e.g., if the patient makes a greater effort, more flow will be delivered), and its analysis may be of use in understanding the individual patient's mechanics, as well as optimizing ventilatory settings. Figure 131.11 shows how the duration of the PCV breath may affect the size of tidal volume for a given set inspiratory pressure. When the breath ends before the inspiratory flow has reached the zero line, the tidal volume can be increased by prolonging the inspiratory time. Note also the change in the airway pressure trace, which did not reach a full plateau until the change was made and a new inspiratory pause (zero flow) created.

Changes of respiratory mechanics affect the flow waveform of PCV significantly (Fig. 131.12) and, with it, the efficiency of this mode of ventilation. Patients with a low compliance and normal resistance (fast time constant, such as in ALI/ARDS) show a steep descent of the inspiratory phase and will tend to have a low tidal volume. On the contrary, patients with a high compliance and high resistance (slow time constant, such as in asthma and COPD) show a flat slope and will tend to have problems of dyssynchrony in addition to tidal volume size. In addition, during PCV, inspiratory flow is increased by patient effort, which will increase the flow rate and the tidal volume delivered.

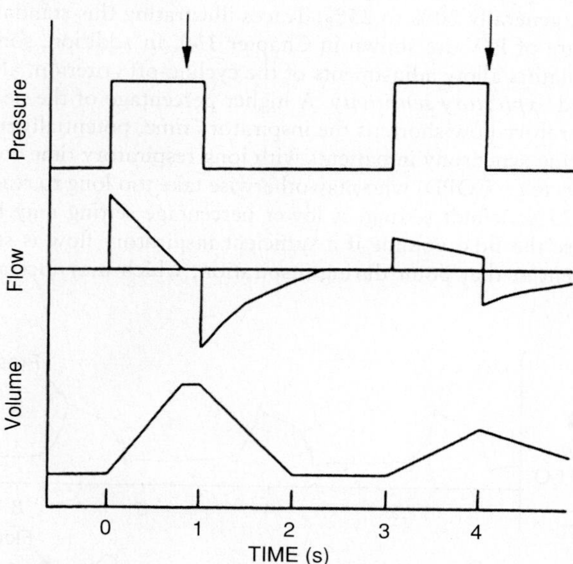

FIGURE 131.12. Changes of ventilator waveforms during pressure-controlled ventilation. An abrupt increase in airway resistance (second breath) causes a decrease in peak inspiratory flow rate and tidal volume. The arrows indicate the set end of inspiration: following the increase in resistance, the decay of the inspiratory flow rate is significantly slower and no longer reaches the zero-flow line before the end of inspiration, hence decreasing the tidal volume.

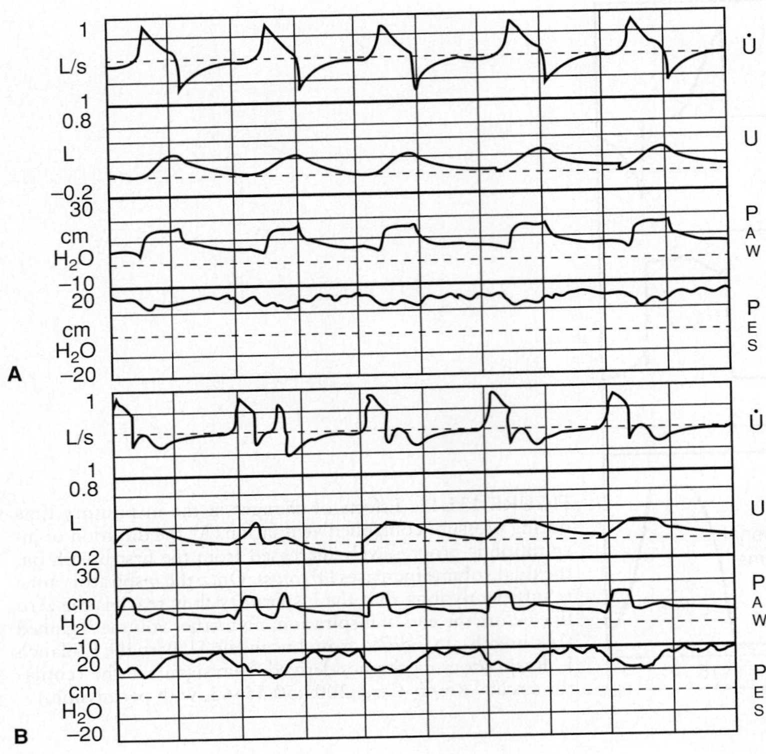

FIGURE 131.13. Two pressure support ventilation traces obtained with different expiratory sensitivity. In **A**, the breath ends when the inspiratory flow rate reaches 5% of the peak inspiratory flow (i.e., low sensitivity): The tidal volume (V) is approximately 300 mL, the esophageal pressure (Pes) change approximately 5 cm H_2O, and all breaths are synchronous. In **B**, the breath ends at 45% of the peak inspiratory flow rate (i.e., high sensitivity): At the same level of inspiratory pressure (Paw) and a similar tidal volume, there is significant patient–ventilator dyssynchrony, demonstrated by an attempted (all breaths) or successful (second breath) triggering effort during early mechanical exhalation. (Modified from Tokioka H, Tanaka T, Ishizu T, et al. The effect of breath termination criterion on breathing patterns and the work of breathing during pressure support ventilation. *Anesth Analg.* 2001;92:161–165, with permission.)

Pressure Support Ventilation (PSV)

With PSV, airway pressure during inspiration approximates a square wave in a way similar to PCV. However, the duration of a PSV breath is variable. Once the set inspiratory pressure is reached, the inspiratory flow decays similar to PCV (see above), except that the breath ends not at a set time, but when the inspiratory flow reaches a certain percentage of the peak inspiratory flow, generally 20% to 25%. Traces illustrating this standard feature of PSV are shown in Chapter 130. In addition, some ventilators allow adjustments of the cycling-off criterion, also called *expiratory sensitivity*. A higher percentage of the peak inspiratory flow shortens the inspiratory time, potentially improving synchrony in patients with long respiratory time constants (e.g., COPD) who may otherwise take too long to reach the 25% default setting. A lower percentage setting may increase the tidal volume if a sufficient inspiratory flow is still present at that point during inspiration, which may increase tidal volume and improve synchrony in patients with long respiratory time constants (Fig. 131.13) (17).

PSV allows two other criteria to end inspiration designed to minimize the chance of patient–ventilator dyssynchrony: a pressure-cycling and a time-cycling criterion. Figure 131.14 shows how inspiration can be terminated when the inspiratory pressure plateau rises above the set pressure by a certain level, generally 1 to 3 cm H_2O (18). A similar result can be reached with the second backup criterion, a time set duration of inspiration similar to PCV. This feature is particularly helpful in the presence of leaks; a leak of sufficient proportion may cause the inspiratory flow never to reach the predetermined cycling-off level, thus maintaining a constant flow as in continuous positive airway pressure (CPAP).

The *rise time* (or *pressurization rate*) is the time required for the ventilator to reach the pressure control level at the beginning of the inspiratory phase. A faster rise time delivers more

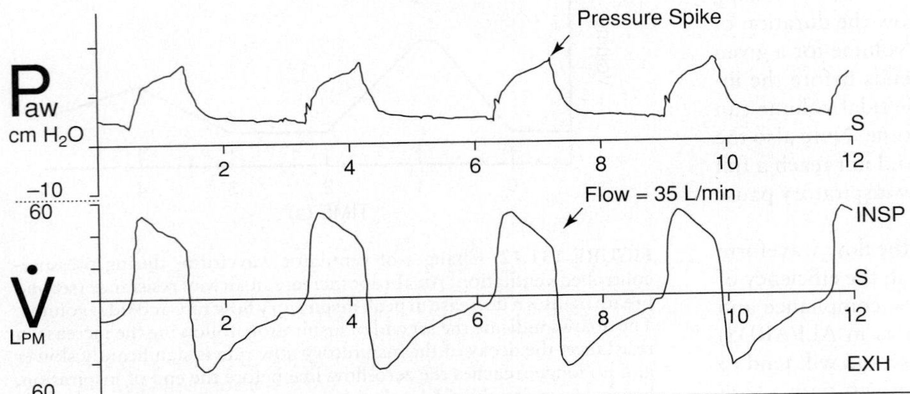

FIGURE 131.14. Termination of pressure support ventilation breaths by a pressure criterion. Once the set pressure is reached and maintained to begin a plateau, a further increase in pressure cycles the ventilator off. This setting is intended to decrease patient–ventilator dyssynchrony when a patients forces the end of inspiration (i.e., generates a positive airway pressure [Paw]) while the mechanical inspiration is not yet completed. This occurs typically in patients with long time constants, such as in COPD and asthma. (From Branson RD, Campbell RS. Pressure support ventilation, patient-ventilator synchrony, and ventilator algorithms. *Respir Care.* 1998;43:1045–1047, with permission.)

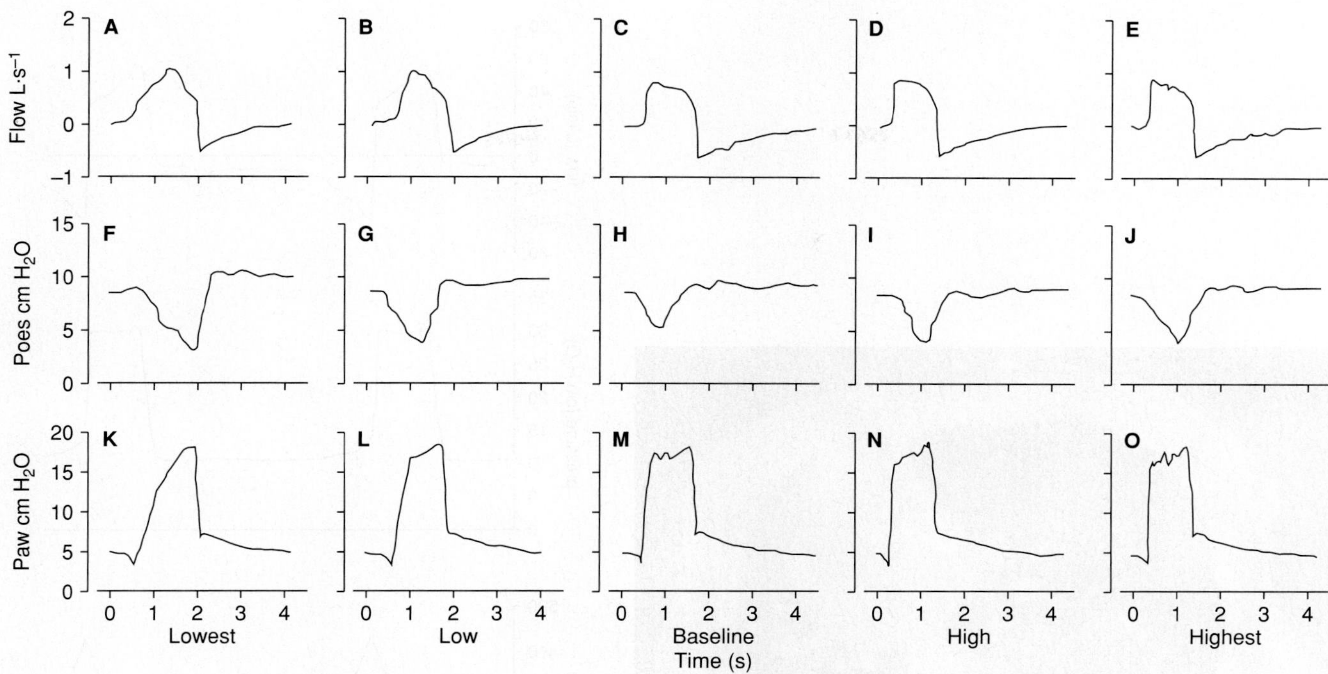

FIGURE 131.15. Effects of a progressive increase of the inspiratory pressurization rate during pressure support ventilation, from breath A to breath E. Note the different shapes of the flow and airway pressure (Paw) traces, and the variable esophageal pressure gradient (Poes), which suggests that the optimal (i.e., lowest inspiratory work) was obtained at the intermediate setting (breath C). (From Chiumello D, Pelosi P, Croci M, et al. The effects of pressurization rate on breathing pattern, work of breathing, gas exchange and patient comfort in pressure support ventilation. *Eur Respir J*. 2001;18:107–114, with permission.)

flow at the beginning of inspiration, which may relieve dyspnea in patients with high respiratory drive (Fig. 131.15). This feature can be expressed in absolute time: the higher the setting, the slower the rise time; or in percentage rate: the higher the setting, the faster the rise time (19).

Bedside Uses of Physiologic Measurements and Graphic Display

Assessment of Respiratory Mechanics

The electronic performance of end-inspiratory and end-expiratory pauses allows the measurement of respiratory compliance and resistance at the patient's bedside. The ventilator has to be set in the VCV mode, with a constant inspiratory flow pattern. Care must be paid to minimize the patient's own respiratory efforts, which would invalidate the measurements. This may be accomplished by overriding the patient's own drive by transiently hyperventilating, administering a short-acting sedative-hypnotic, or even by inducing pharmacologic neuromuscular blockade. A thorough risk–benefit evaluation has to be made before resorting to these interventions.

Compliance. Respiratory compliance (including both lungs and chest wall) is typically reduced in cases of atelectasis, pulmonary edema (cardiogenic and noncardiogenic), pneumonia, pulmonary fibrosis, pleural effusions, pneumothorax, and fibrothorax, and it is increased with asthma and emphysema. Respiratory compliance can be measured by applying an end-inspiratory pause. Following an end-inspiratory pause, the

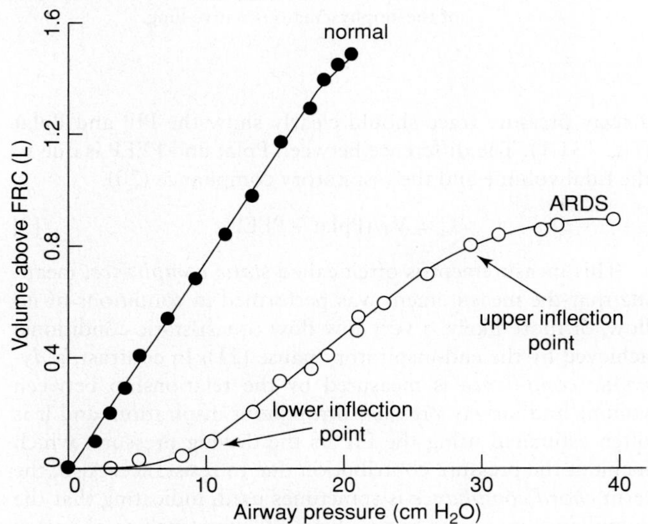

FIGURE 131.16. Idealized inflation pressure–volume (P-V) curves during passive mechanical ventilation. On the **left**, a normal trace, with a value of approximately 80 mL/cm H_2O. On the **right**, a P-V curve of a patient with acute respiratory distress syndrome, showing a lower and no longer linear compliance, with two distinct inflection points. ARDS, acute respiratory distress syndrome; FRC, functional residual capacity. (Modified from Fisher D, Hess D. Respiratory monitoring. In: Bigatello LM, ed. *Critical Care Handbook of the Massachusetts General Hospital*. 4th ed. Philadelphia, PA: Lippincott Williams & Wilkins; 2006:33–52, with permission.)

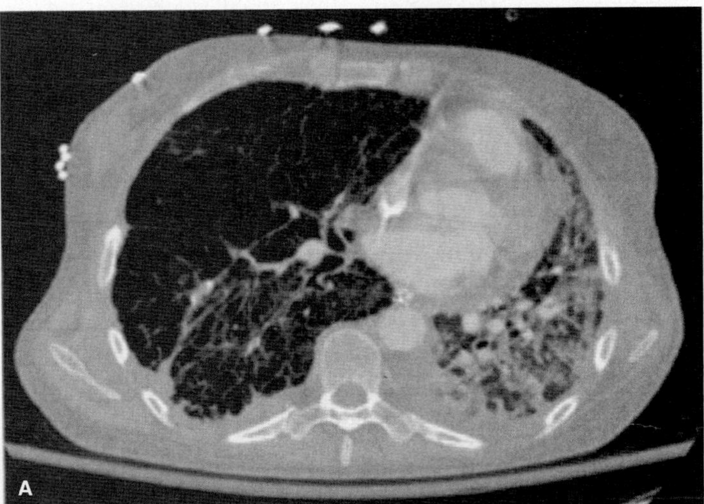

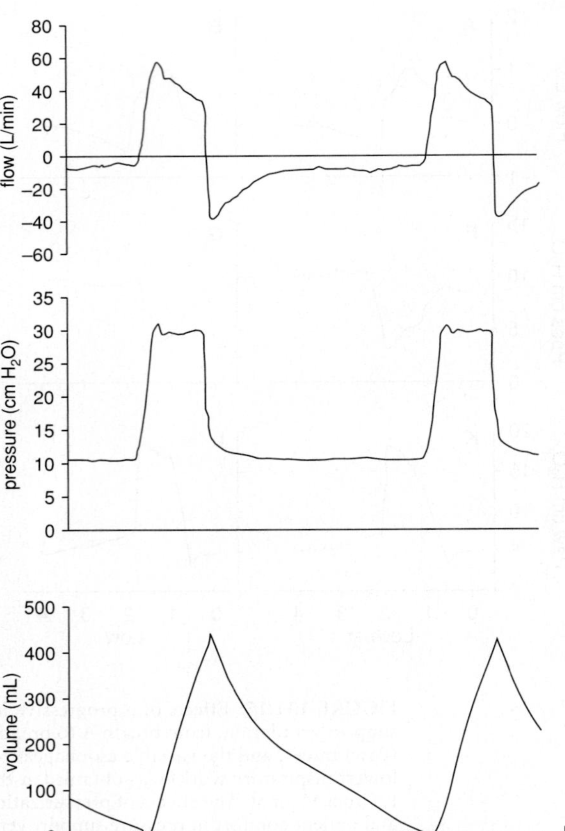

FIGURE 131.17. Acute lung injury in a transplanted lung. **A:** Computed tomogram showing severe emphysema of the right (native) lung and diffuse edema and consolidation of the left (transplanted) lung. **B:** Ventilator waveforms, compatible with a two-compartment model. The initial part of the breath, coming from the transplanted lung (seen best in the expiratory flow trace) has a fast time constant; the second part of the breath has a very slow time constant, because of the high resistance and high compliance of the emphysematous native lung.

airway pressure trace should clearly show the PIP and Pplat (Fig. 131.1). The difference between Pplat and PEEP is due to the tidal volume and the respiratory compliance (20).

$$C = V_T/(\text{Pplat} - \text{PEEP}) \quad [3]$$

This measurement is often called *static compliance*, meaning that the measurement was performed in conditions of no flow, or more likely, a very low flow (quasi-static conditions) achieved by the end-inspiratory pause (21). In contrast, a *dynamic compliance* is measured by the relationship between volume and airway pressure throughout inspiration, and it is often estimated using the PIP as the driving pressure, which includes the pressure contribution due to resistance. Also, the term *chord compliance* is sometimes used, indicating that the compliance measured at two lung volumes (such as above) is generally not linear (see below; *chord* is a line segment connecting two points on a curve). The *static compliance* measured with an end-inspiratory pause is relatively simple and valid for routine clinical use, but it also has several limitations:

- *It is measured at just one lung volume.* Although under normal circumstances, the pressure–volume (P-V) relationship of the respiratory system is linear within a physiologic range of lung volumes, pathologies such as ALI/ARDS may alter the P-V relationship so that compliance may vary significantly within a relatively narrow range of lung volumes (see below and Fig. 131.16) (22).
- *It assumes the respiratory system as a single compartment* which, in many cases, underestimates the complexity of regional compliances. In ALI/ARDS, pneumonia, or pneumothorax, the regional variation is significant (Fig. 131.17).
- *It does not distinguish between lung and chest wall*, the two mechanical components of the respiratory system. This distinction requires measuring intrathoracic (or pleural) pressure as described below. In the absence of a pleural pressure measurement, a significant contribution of the chest wall to a decreased compliance value can be suspected in the presence of abdominal distention, tight chest bandages, scars, and large pleural effusions (23).

Resistance. Common causes of increased resistance include bronchospasm, pulmonary edema, increased bronchial secretions, a low FRC, and a small inner diameter of an endotracheal tube. Following an end-inspiratory pause, inspiratory airway resistance can be estimated from the difference between PIP and Pplat (24,25):

$$R = (\text{PIP} - \text{Pplat})/\dot{V} \quad [4]$$

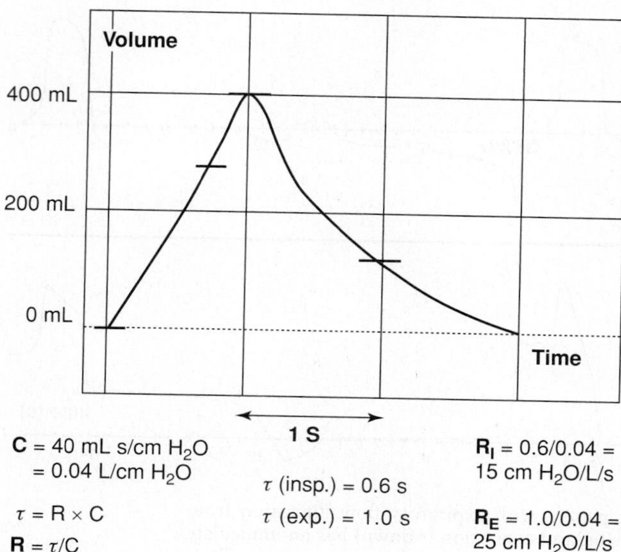

FIGURE 131.18. Measurement of inspiratory (R_I) and expiratory (R_E) resistance in a fully relaxed patient, based on the measurement of the time constant (τ), which equals compliance times resistance; one τ is the time necessary to inhale or exhale 63% of the final lung volume. The respiratory system compliance was 40 mL/cm H_2O; the inspiratory τ (time at 63% of inspiratory volume, *horizontal line*) was 0.6 s, and the expiratory τ (time at 63% of inspiratory volume, *horizontal line*) was 1 s. Values of R_I and R_E are shown. (From Nims RG, Conner EH, Comroe JH Jr. The compliance of the human thorax in anesthetized patients. *J Clin Invest*. 1955;34:744–750, with permission.)

For example, with a difference of 10 cm H_2O between PIP and Pplat and a dialed inspiratory flow rate of 60 L/min, R will be 10 cm H_2O/L/second. Measured as such, R reflects the resistance to ventilation imposed by the airways as well as the respiratory equipment, mainly the endotracheal tube.* However, the resistance of clean endotracheal tubes is known, and one can use this knowledge (26,27) and clinical judgment (presence of secretions within the tracheal or tracheostomy tube) in estimating the airway versus equipment contribution to resistance. Resistance changes with the flow rate, lung volume, and phase of respiration. Inspiratory resistance is typically lower than expiratory resistance due to the increased diameter of the airways during inspiration, particularly in patients with obstructive disease and dynamic airflow limitation (28). Airways resistance can also be estimated from the time constant ($\tau = R \times C$) of the respiratory system. This method permits one to calculate both inspiratory (R_I) and expiratory (R_E) resistance in fully relaxed patients (Fig. 131.18).

Auto-PEEP. Auto-PEEP is the result of incomplete emptying of the lung at end expiration, causing an increase in end-expiratory volume and alveolar pressure (28–31). This phenomenon is due to insufficient expiratory time and/or increased expiratory airflow resistance, in addition to decreased elastic recoil pressure, and it occurs chiefly in patients with asthma and COPD. Figure 131.19 shows a characteristic flow trace occurring in the presence of expiratory flow limitation and an end-expiratory pause to measure static auto-PEEP (Fig. 131.1). Following this maneuver, most ventilators will display a value that may correspond to the total PEEP, i.e., the absolute value measured, or to the auto-PEEP that will be calculated by subtracting the applied PEEP from the measured total PEEP. Because PEEP set on the ventilator can counterbalance auto-PEEP in patients with flow limitation, the measurement of auto-PEEP should ideally be made with the PEEP set on zero in patients with obstructive lung disease.

Intrathoracic or Pleural Pressure (Ppl). Pleural pressure is estimated by measuring the pressure in the midesophagus with an esophageal balloon catheter. Pleural pressure can be used to estimate lung and chest wall compliance to assess auto-PEEP and work of breathing during assisted modes of ventilation and to evaluate diaphragm dysfunction (21). The measurement of pleural pressure is of great value in the study of respiratory mechanics and can be used by experienced clinicians at the bedside (Fig. 131.20). However, its measurement is generally not performed and displayed by current ventilators, and it is obtained by using dedicated portable monitors or by means of home-built systems of recording that include sensor–transducers, analog-to-digital converters, a computer, and appropriate waveform analysis software (32).

Mean Airway Pressure ($\overline{Paw}$). Many of the desired and deleterious effects of mechanical ventilation are determined by the mean airway pressure ($\overline{Paw}$). Factors affecting the $\overline{Paw}$ are the PIP, PEEP, the inspiratory-to-expiratory (I:E) ratio, and the inspiratory pressure waveform. During pressure ventilation, the inspiratory pressure waveform is rectangular and $\overline{Paw}$ is estimated as follows: $\overline{Paw} = (PIP - PEEP)/(Ti/TT) + PEEP$, where Ti is inspiratory time and TT is total cycle time. For example, with a PIP of 40 cm H_2O, PEEP of 10 cm H_2O, Ti of 1 second, rate 15/minute (Ti/TT = 0.33), $\overline{Paw}$ is 20 cm H_2O. During constant flow volume ventilation, the inspiratory pressure waveform is triangular, and $\overline{Paw}$ can be estimated as $\overline{Paw} = 0.5 \times (PIP - PEEP)/(Ti/TT) + PEEP$. For example, with a PIP of 25 cm H_2O, PEEP 5 cm H_2O, Ti 1.5 seconds, rate 20/minute (Ti/TT = 0.5), $\overline{Paw}$ is 15 cm H_2O. Many current-generation microprocessor ventilators display $\overline{Paw}$ from integration of the airway pressure waveform. Typical $\overline{Paw}$ values for passively ventilated patients are 5 to 10 cm H_2O (normal), 10 to 20 cm H_2O (airflow obstruction), and 15 to 30 cm H_2O (ALI/ARDS).

Pressure–Time Waveforms. Measuring the overall pressure changes of the respiratory system throughout a breath (*dynamic compliance*, see above) may be a useful indicator of the mechanical behavior of the respiratory system during mechanical ventilation (33–36). For example, pressure changes measured over time under conditions of constant flow can provide information on alveolar recruitment and overdistention. A constant slope of the airway pressure suggests that there is no change in compliance during tidal ventilation; a progressive increase of the slope (upward concavity) indicates an increase in compliance (i.e., lung recruitment); and a progressive decrease in the slope (downward concavity) suggests a decrease in compliance (i.e., overdistention) (35,36) (Fig. 131.21).

*Modern ventilators do not include the resistance of the ventilator circuit in their resistance calculations. This is because they measure pressure during inhalation through the expiratory line and during exhalation through the inspiratory line (as described earlier in the chapter). So, this becomes *de facto* identical to putting the pressure transducer directly on the proximal airway.

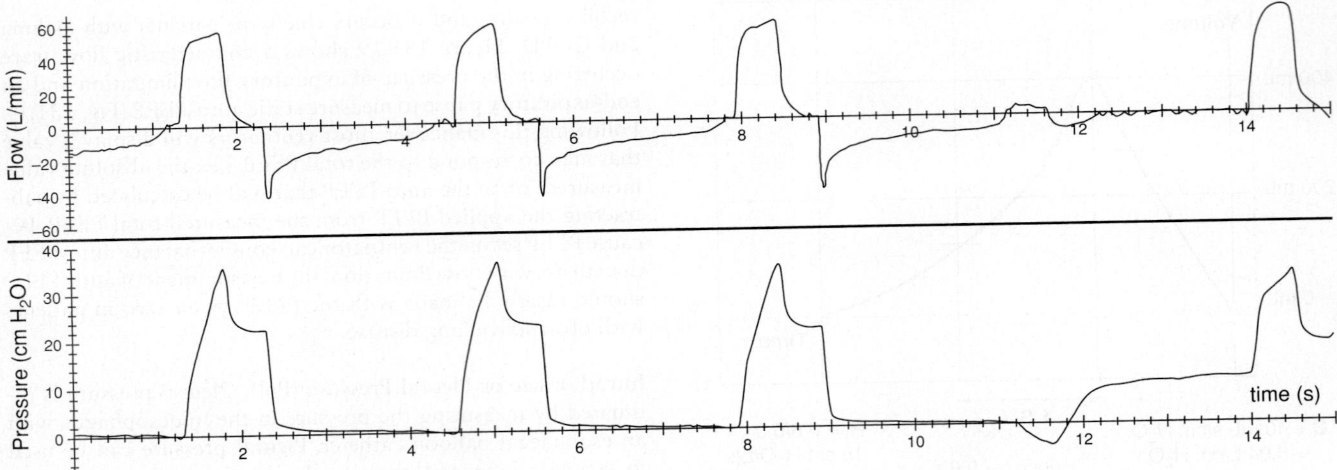

FIGURE 131.19. Airway pressure and flow traces in a patient with expiratory flow limitation from emphysema. The expiratory flow (**top** trace, inspiration is up and expiration is down) has an immediate sharp decrease in rate, then continues at a slow rate throughout expiration, and does not reach zero flow. During the last breath, an end-expiratory pause shows the presence of auto-PEEP.

Pressure–Volume (P-V) Curves in ALI/ARDS. ALI/ARDS is a syndrome of low lung compliance, but the measured value of compliance is the averaged approximation of different regional mechanics caused by inhomogeneous distribution of alveolar collapse and edema, as well as chest wall compliance and patient position (37,38). Compliance measurement at various lung volumes at the bedside has been advocated as a means to better evaluate the recruitment status of the lung and to assist in choosing the appropriate ventilator settings (39). The construction of a P-V curve over a range of lung volumes can be carried out in various ways. The manual method with a supersyringe is relatively simple but flawed, with low reproducibility and with the problem of having to disconnect the patient from the ventilator to perform the maneuver (22). Alternatively, a P-V curve can be performed automatically in selected ventilators without disconnecting the patient from the breathing circuit. The multiple occlusion method performs repeated end-inspiratory breath occlusions at different lung volumes, and the constant flow technique measures the change in airway opening pressure with a constant slow flow (≤10 L/min) (40,41). Several authors have used the analysis of the P-V curve to guide ventilator settings in patients with ALI/ARDS (42–47). Accordingly, setting the PEEP above the lower inflection point may optimize lung recruitment and reduce end-expiratory barotrauma. Setting the inspiratory airway pressure below an upper inflection point may avoid alveolar overdistention and inspiratory barotrauma (Fig. 131.16). Despite the theoretical appeal of this approach, its clinical use remains controversial. First, the two inflection points are often not as clear as one would like them to be, which will result in incorrect application of the physiologic principle behind this approach (48). Second, recent studies seem to indicate that the level of

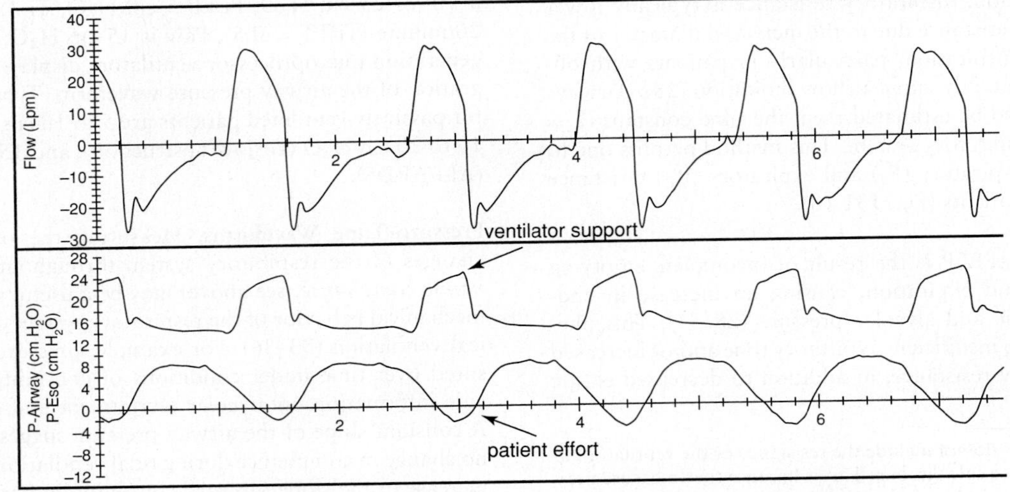

FIGURE 131.20. Flow, airway pressure, and esophageal pressure traces during pressure-controlled ventilation. At each breath, the esophageal pressure shows negative swings of approximately 10 cm H_2O, indicating active inspiratory efforts.

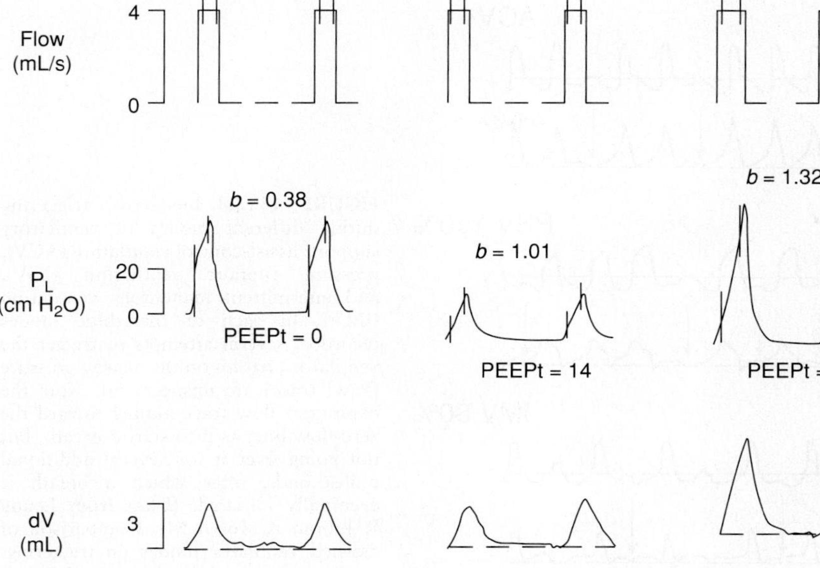

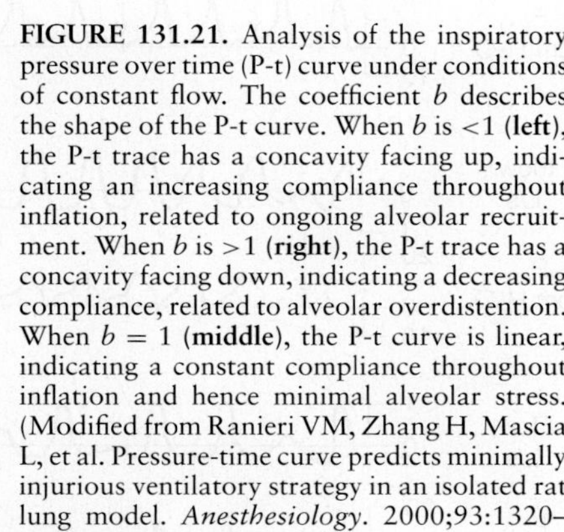

FIGURE 131.21. Analysis of the inspiratory pressure over time (P-t) curve under conditions of constant flow. The coefficient *b* describes the shape of the P-t curve. When *b* is <1 (**left**), the P-t trace has a concavity facing up, indicating an increasing compliance throughout inflation, related to ongoing alveolar recruitment. When *b* is >1 (**right**), the P-t trace has a concavity facing down, indicating a decreasing compliance, related to alveolar overdistention. When *b* = 1 (**middle**), the P-t curve is linear, indicating a constant compliance throughout inflation and hence minimal alveolar stress. (Modified from Ranieri VM, Zhang H, Mascia L, et al. Pressure-time curve predicts minimally injurious ventilatory strategy in an isolated rat lung model. *Anesthesiology*. 2000;93:1320–1328, with permission.)

PEEP does not make a significant difference in the outcome of patients with ALI/ARDS, and that a low inspiratory pressure (most of the time incompatible with a high PEEP) may be the most important ventilatory variable associated with a better outcome (49).

Patient–Ventilator Dyssynchrony

Dyssynchronous interactions between the patient's own effort and the machine's support may occur at any time in the course of mechanical ventilation for acute respiratory failure. Dyssynchrony may worsen gas exchange, cause hemodynamic instability, and generate additional mechanical load that may hinder ventilator weaning.

- *Insufficient gas flow support* can occur when the patient's ventilatory demand is higher than the inspiratory flow rate supplied by the ventilator. Increased inspiratory work during volume-assisted mechanical ventilation was demonstrated two decades ago (15), using the airway pressure trace to estimate the additional work of breathing imposed by ineffective machine support. By superimposing two airway pressure traces obtained during VCV at identical settings, with the patient fully relaxed and actively triggering the breath, the authors were able to extrapolate the amount of respiratory work performed by the patient (Fig. 131.22). Modern ventilators allow continuous assessment of these parameters, greatly enhancing our ability to identify optimal mechanical support. Patient–ventilator dyssynchrony can occur at multiple levels during the breathing cycle, and can be related both to patient's pathology and/or ventilator shortcomings. We will include here a few examples and we refer to other inclusive reviews (50–53).
- *Missed triggering* due to dynamic hyperinflation and auto-PEEP can occur with any mode of ventilatory support (54). Common to this phenomenon is the finding of the expiratory flow trace aiming toward the zero-flow line, as if to start a breath, but not going over it for several additional

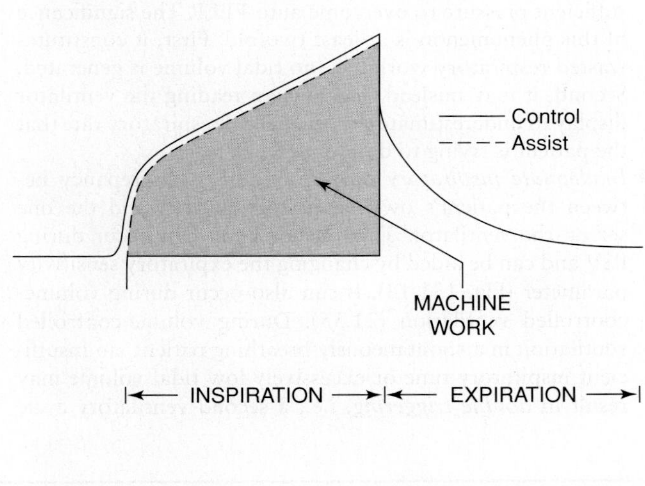

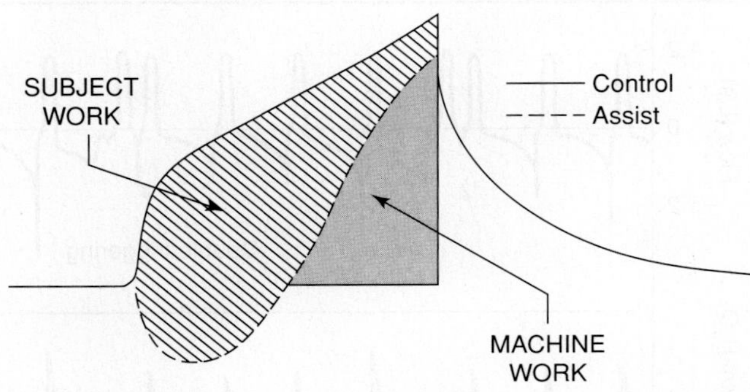

FIGURE 131.22. Airway pressure waveforms during controlled mechanical ventilation in the absence (**top**) and presence (**bottom**) of inspiratory muscle activity. In the **bottom** view, the *shaded* area represents the active work performed by the patient's inspiratory muscles. (From Marini JJ, Rodriguez RM, Lamb V. The inspiratory workload of patient-initiated mechanical ventilation. *Am Rev Respir Dis.* 1986;134:902–909, with permission.)

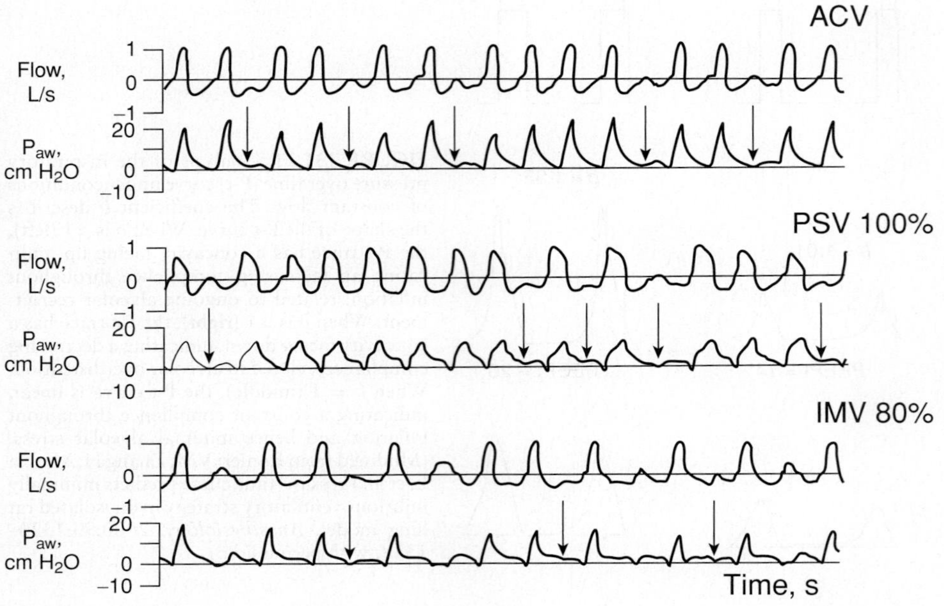

FIGURE 131.23. Ineffective triggering during different modes of ventilatory support: assist-control ventilation (ACV), pressure support ventilation (PSV), and intermittent mandatory ventilation (IMV). In each of the three modes recorded, several attempts to trigger the ventilator (*arrows* on the airway pressure [Paw] trace) are unsuccessful. Note the expiratory flow trace aiming toward the zero-flow line, as if to start a breath, but not going over it for several additional milliseconds, after which a breath is eventually initiated. (Data from Leung P, Jubran A, Tobin MJ. Comparison of assisted ventilator modes on triggering, patient effort, and dyspnea. *Am J Respir Crit Care Med.* 1997;155:1940–1948.)

milliseconds, after which a breath is eventually initiated. These "humps" on the expiratory flow trace (Fig. 131.23) indicate attempts to trigger a breath that do not generate sufficient pressure to overcome auto-PEEP. The significance of this phenomenon is at least twofold. First, it constitutes wasted respiratory work, i.e., no tidal volume is generated. Second, it may mislead the clinician reading the ventilator display to underestimate the true neural respiratory rate that the patient is trying to develop.

- *Inadequate inspiratory time* can cause a discrepancy between the patient's own ventilatory pattern and the one set on the ventilator. This phenomenon can occur during PSV and can be aided by changing the expiratory sensitivity parameter (Fig. 131.13). It can also occur during volume-controlled ventilation (21,55). During volume-controlled ventilation in a spontaneously breathing patient, an insufficient inspiratory time or excessively low tidal volume may result in *double triggering*, i.e., a second ventilatory cycle starts immediately after the previous one (Fig. 131.24). This phenomenon occurs because the patient's neural inspiration is longer than what is provided at that time by the ventilator; the patient's high demand is sufficient to close the expiratory valve early in exhalation and trigger a second inspiration before exhalation is completed.

SUMMARY

Modern ventilators measure and display physiologic information during mechanical ventilation. The observation of the pressure, volume, and flow traces may help clinicians to measure respiratory mechanics, adjust ventilator settings, and detect equipment abnormalities. In addition, it offers the opportunity to learn and teach applied respiratory physiology at the bedside.

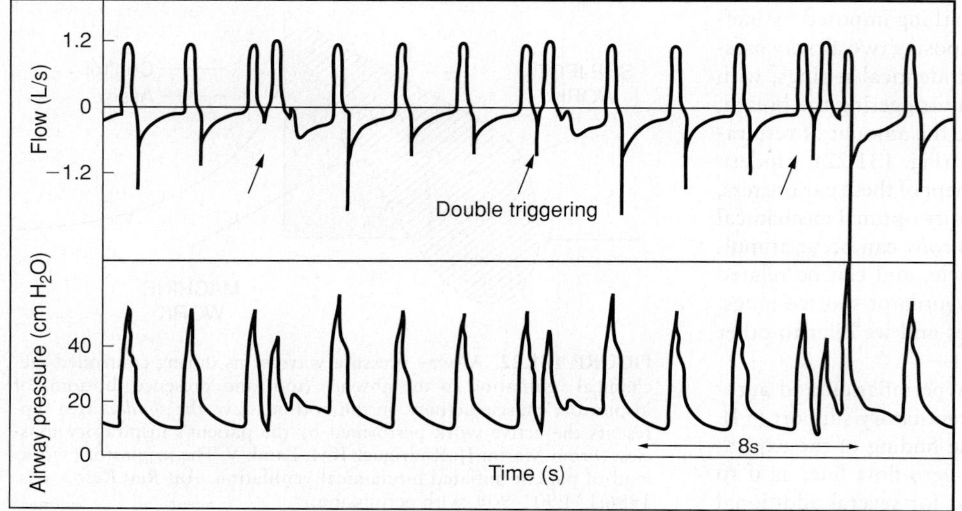

FIGURE 131.24. Double triggering during volume-controlled ventilation. Several breaths (*arrows*) start immediately after the previous breath, without allowing full exhalation. This phenomenon is characteristic of situations where the ventilator provides insufficient inspiratory flow, time, or volume to satisfy the patient's demand. (From Thille AW, Rodriguez P, Cabello B, et al. Patient-ventilator asynchrony during assisted mechanical ventilation. *Intensive Care Med.* 2006;32:1515–1522, with permission.)

TIPS AND PEARLS

1. The appropriate use of the end-inspiratory and end-expiratory pause functions on the ventilator can provide measurement and display of basic respiratory mechanics of use during mechanical ventilation for acute respiratory failure.
2. During volume-controlled ventilation, peak inspiratory airway pressure is determined by tidal volume, inspiratory flow rate, resistance, compliance, and PEEP.
3. With a large air leak from the lungs, the expiratory volume will be lower than the inspiratory volume.
4. Flow–volume loops can be used to assess endotracheal tube malposition, expiratory flow limitation, air leaks, and response to bronchodilators.
5. Attention to analysis of the pressure and flow waveforms during the most common modes of ventilation can reveal the presence of expiratory flow limitation, auto-PEEP, and missed breath triggering.
6. Insufficient inspiratory flow delivery during volume-controlled ventilation can be taxing to the patient and can be detected by the presence of an upward concavity in the early part of the pressure trace.
7. The value of the respiratory rate displayed on the ventilator screen may be deceiving. Missed triggering may occur due to expiratory flow limitation; the real respiratory rate is higher than the displayed respiratory rate. Double triggering may occur due to a set tidal volume that is too small, or a set inspiratory time that is too short for the patient's neural drive, and results in a higher respiratory rate.
8. Esophageal pressure changes reflect pleural pressure changes.

References

1. Sanborn WG. Monitoring respiratory mechanics during mechanical ventilation: where do the signals come from? *Respir Care.* 2005;50:28–52.
2. Sullivan WJ, Peters GM, Enright PL. Pneumotachographs: theory and clinical application. *Respir Care.* 1984;29:736–749.
3. Hess DR. Heliox and noninvasive positive-pressure ventilation: a role for heliox in exacerbations of chronic obstructive pulmonary disease? *Respir Care.* 2006;51:640–650.
4. Hess D, McCurdy S, Simmons M. Compression volume in adult ventilator circuits: a comparison of five disposable circuits and a non-disposable circuit. *Respir Care.* 1991;36:1113–1118.
5. Gottfried SB, Reissman H, Ranieri VM. A simple method for the measurement of intrinsic positive end-expiratory pressure during controlled and assisted modes of mechanical ventilation. *Crit Care Med.* 1992;20:621–629.
6. Brenner M, Mukai DS, Russell JE, et al. A new method for measurement of airway occlusion pressure. *Chest.* 1990;98:421–427.
7. Kuhlen R, Hausmann S, Pappert D, et al. A new method for P0.1 measurement using standard respiratory equipment. *Intensive Care Med.* 1995;21:554–560.
8. Marini JJ, Smith TC, Lamb V. Estimation of inspiratory muscle strength in mechanically ventilated patients: the measurements of maximal inspiratory pressure. *J Crit Care.* 1986;1:32–38.
9. Stahl CA, Moller K, Schumann S, et al. Dynamic versus static respiratory mechanics in acute lung injury and acute respiratory distress syndrome. *Crit Care Med.* 2006;34:2090–2098.
10. Simon BA, Hurford WE, Alfille PH, et al. An aid in the diagnosis of malpositioned double-lumen tubes. *Anesthesiology.* 1992;76:862–863.
11. Jubran A, Tobin MJ. Use of flow-volume curves in detecting secretions in ventilator-dependent patients. *Am J Respir Crit Care Med.* 1994;150:766–769.
12. Brown K, Sly PD, Milic-Emili J, et al. Evaluation of the flow-volume loop as an intra-operative monitor of respiratory mechanics in infants. *Pediatr Pulmonol.* 1989;6:8–13.
13. Dhand R. Ventilator graphics and respiratory mechanics in the patient with obstructive lung disease. *Respir Care.* 2005;50:246–261.
14. Kondili E, Prinianakis G, Georgopoulos D. Patient–ventilator interaction. *Br J Anaesth.* 2003;91:106–119.
15. Marini JJ, Rodriguez RM, Lamb V. The inspiratory workload of patient-initiated mechanical ventilation. *Am Rev Respir Dis.* 1986;134:902–909.
16. Bernasconi M, Ploysongsang Y, Gottfried SB, et al. Respiratory compliance and resistance in mechanically ventilated patients with acute respiratory failure. *Intensive Care Med.* 1988;14:547–553.
17. Tokioka H, Tanaka T, Ishizu T, et al. The effect of breath termination criterion on breathing patterns and the work of breathing during pressure support ventilation. *Anesth Analg.* 2001;92:161–165.
18. Branson RD, Campbell RS. Pressure support ventilation, patient–ventilator synchrony, and ventilator algorithms. *Respir Care* 1998;43:1045–1047.
19. Chiumello D, Pelosi P, Croci M, et al. The effects of pressurization rate on breathing pattern, work of breathing, gas exchange and patient comfort in pressure support ventilation. *Eur Respir J.* 2001;18:107–114.
20. D'Angelo E, Calderini E, Torri G, et al. Respiratory mechanics in anesthetized paralyzed humans: effects of flow, volume, and time. *J Appl Physiol.* 1989; 67:2556–2564.
21. Truwit JD, Marini JJ. Evaluation of the thoracic mechanics in the ventilated patients, I: primary measurements. *J Crit Care.* 1988;3:133–150.
22. Harris RS. Pressure-volume curves of the respiratory system. *Respir Care.* 2005;50:78–98.
23. Ranieri VM, Giuliani R, Mascia L, et al. Chest wall and lung contribution to the elastic properties of the respiratory system in patients with chronic obstructive pulmonary disease. *Eur Respir J.* 1996;9:1232–1239.
24. Lucangelo U, Bernabe F, Blanch L. Respiratory mechanics derived from signals in the ventilator circuit. *Respir Care.* 2005;50:55–65.
25. Hess D, Tabor T. Comparison of six methods to calculate airway resistance during mechanical ventilation in adults. *J Clin Monit.* 1993;9:275–282.
26. Rossi A, Gottfried SB, Higgs BD, et al. Respiratory mechanics in mechanically ventilated patients with respiratory failure. *J Appl Physiol.* 1985;58: 1849–1858.
27. Polese G, Lubli P, Poggi R, et al. Effects of inspiratory flow waveforms on arterial blood gases and respiratory mechanics after open heart surgery. *Eur Respir J.* 1997;10:2820–2824.
28. Smith TC, Marini JJ. Impact of PEEP on lung mechanics and work of breathing in severe airflow obstruction. *J Appl Physiol.* 1988;65:1488–1499.
29. Marini JJ, Culver BH, Kirk W. Flow resistance of exhalation valves and positive end-expiratory pressure devices used in mechanical ventilation. *Am Rev Respir Dis.* 1985;131:850–854.
30. Ranieri VM, Grasso S, Fiore T, et al. Auto-positive end-expiratory pressure and dynamic hyperinflation. *Clin Chest Med.* 1996;17:379–394.
31. Blanch L, Bernabe F, Lucangelo U. Measurement of air trapping, intrinsic positive end-expiratory pressure, and dynamic hyperinflation in mechanically ventilated patients. *Respir Care.* 2005;50:110–123.
32. Benditt JO. Esophageal and gastric pressure measurements. *Respir Care.* 2005;50:68–75.
33. Bates JH, Rossi A, Milic-Emili J. Analysis of the behavior of the respiratory system with constant inspiratory flow. *J Appl Physiol.* 1985;58:1840–1848.
34. Lichtwarck-Aschoff M, Kessler V, Sjostrand UH, et al. Static versus dynamic respiratory mechanics for setting the ventilator. *Br J Anaesth.* 2000;85:577–586.
35. Ranieri VM, Zhang H, Mascia L, et al. Pressure–time curve predicts minimally injurious ventilatory strategy in an isolated rat lung model. *Anesthesiology.* 2000;93:1320–1328.
36. Grasso S, Terragni P, Mascia L, et al. Airway pressure–time curve profile (stress index) detects tidal recruitment/hyperinflation in experimental acute lung injury. *Crit Care Med.* 2004;32:1018–1027.
37. Bigatello LM, Davignon KR, Stelfox HT. Respiratory mechanics and ventilator waveforms in the patient with acute lung injury. *Respir Care.* 2005;50: 235–245.
38. Pelosi P, Cereda M, Foti G, et al. Alterations of lung and chest wall mechanics in patients with acute lung injury: effects of positive end-expiratory pressure. *Am J Respir Crit Care Med.* 1995;152:531–537.
39. Amato MB, Barbas CS, Medeiros DM, et al. Effect of a protective-ventilation strategy on mortality in the acute respiratory distress syndrome. *N Engl J Med.* 1998;338:347–354.
40. Lu Q, Vieira SR, Richecoeur J, et al. A simple automated method for measuring pressure–volume curves during mechanical ventilation. *Am J Respir Crit Care Med.* 1999;159:275–282.
41. Servillo G, Svantesson C, Beydon L, et al. Pressure–volume curves in acute respiratory failure: automated low flow inflation versus occlusion. *Am J Respir Crit Care Med.* 1997;155:1629–1636.
42. Matamis D, Lemaire F, Harf A, et al. Total respiratory pressure–volume curves in the adult respiratory distress syndrome. *Chest.* 1984;86:58–66.
43. Hickling KG. The pressure–volume curve is greatly modified by recruitment. A mathematical model of ARDS lungs. *Am J Respir Crit Care Med.* 1998; 158:194–202.
44. Hickling KG. Best compliance during a decremental, but not incremental, positive end-expiratory pressure trial is related to open-lung positive end-expiratory pressure: a mathematical model of acute respiratory distress syndrome lungs. *Am J Respir Crit Care Med.* 2001;163:69–78.
45. Pelosi P, Goldner M, McKibben A, et al. Recruitment and derecruitment

during acute respiratory failure: an experimental study. *Am J Respir Crit Care Med.* 2001;164:122–130.

46. Crotti S, Mascheroni D, Caironi P, et al. Recruitment and derecruitment during acute respiratory failure: a clinical study. *Am J Respir Crit Care Med.* 2001;164:131–140.
47. Hickling KG. Reinterpreting the pressure–volume curve in patients with acute respiratory distress syndrome. *Curr Opin Crit Care.* 2002;8:32–38.
48. Harris RS, Hess DR, Venegas JG. An objective analysis of the pressure–volume curve in the acute respiratory distress syndrome. *Am J Respir Crit Care Med.* 2000;161:432–439.
49. Brower RG, Lanken PN, MacIntyre N, et al. Higher versus lower positive end-expiratory pressures in patients with the acute respiratory distress syndrome. *N Engl J Med.* 2004;351:327–336.
50. Nilsestuen JO, Hargett KD. Using ventilator graphics to identify patient–ventilator asynchrony. *Respir Care.* 2005;50:202–234.
51. Georgopoulos D, Prinianakis G, Kondili E. Bedside waveforms interpretation as a tool to identify patient–ventilator asynchronies. *Intensive Care Med.* 2006;32:34–47.
52. Younes M, Riddle W. Relation between respiratory neural output and tidal volume. *J Appl Physiol.* 1984;56:1110–1119.
53. Younes M. Patient–ventilator interaction with pressure-assisted modalities of ventilator support. *Semin Respir Med.* 1993;14:299–322.
54. Leung P, Jubran A, Tobin MJ. Comparison of assisted ventilator modes on triggering, patient effort, and dyspnea. *Am J Respir Crit Care Med.* 1997; 155:1940–1948.
55. Hess DR, Medoff BD, Fessler MB. Pulmonary mechanics and graphics during positive pressure ventilation. *Int Anesthesiol Clin.* 1999;37:15–34.
56. Thille AW, Rodriguez P, Cabello B, et al. Patient–ventilator asynchrony during assisted mechanical ventilation. *Intensive Care Med.* 2006;32:1515–1522.

CHAPTER 132 ■ WEANING FROM MECHANICAL VENTILATION

FRANCO LAGHI

Although often life-saving, mechanical ventilation can be associated with life-threatening complications (1). Accordingly, it is essential to safely discontinue mechanical ventilation at the earliest possible time. The process of discontinuing mechanical ventilation is known as *weaning*. Unfortunately, different investigators and clinicians mean different things with this word. For some, weaning is the gradual reduction in ventilator support when patients are recovering from respiratory failure but are clearly not ready yet for spontaneous respiration. For others, weaning is the act of disconnecting patients from the ventilator, and for yet others, weaning constitutes both discontinuation from mechanical ventilation and extubation.

A framework of seven stages of weaning has been recently proposed (Fig. 132.1) (2). *Stage 1* is preweaning, when patients are too ill to be considered ready for weaning—e.g., patients requiring high levels of oxygen (O_2) and positive end-expiratory pressure (PEEP). All ventilated patients begin at stage 1. In some large series, 13% to 26% of patients never go beyond stage 1 (3–5). During stage 1, measurement of weaning predictors is inappropriate and potentially dangerous.

Stage 2 is the period of diagnostic triggering. This is the time when a physician begins to consider that the patient *might* be ready to come off the ventilator. Failure to engage in this period of diagnostic triggering may be the greatest impediment to prompt weaning (2). In more than 75% of patients who are ventilated for a week—or longer—the ventilator can be successfully discontinued the same day weaning predictors are measured (6,7). This observation raises the possibility that, in many patients, discontinuation of mechanical ventilation could have occurred a day or so earlier if physicians had considered earlier that the patient might have been ready to come off the ventilator.

Stage 3 is the time to obtain physiologic measurements that serve as predictors (*weaning predictors*) and to interpret them in the context of each patient's unique clinical condition. During *stage 4* (*weaning trial*), ventilatory support is either gradually decreased over hours or days (e.g., gradual reduction in pressure support), or it is removed abruptly and completely (T-tube trial). In *stage 5*, patients who succeed the weaning trial are extubated. Patients who do not succeed the weaning trial are returned to ventilator support. Stages 6 and 7 apply to patients who do poorly after extubation. *Stage 6* is continuation of ventilator support with noninvasive ventilation. *Stage 7* is reintubation, usually accompanied by the reinstitution of mechanical ventilation (2).

This chapter will first review the pathophysiology of weaning failure, and then the clinical use of predictors of weaning outcome and techniques of weaning will be examined. Finally, extubation failure will be discussed. Areas of active research and controversial topics will be highlighted throughout the chapter.

PATHOPHYSIOLOGY OF WEANING FAILURE

Various disease states, alone or in combination, may cause weaning failure. From a pathophysiologic standpoint, it is useful to consider these disease states in terms of those characterized by a failure of the lungs as a gas exchange unit, and those characterized by a failure of the ventilatory pump. In a third group of patients, psychological factors may contribute to weaning failure.

Impaired Gas Exchange

Conditions characterized by failure of the lungs as a gas exchange unit include those associated with ventilation–perfusion mismatching and (less often) conditions associated with increased shunt (8). The typical consequence of impaired gas exchange is development of hypoxemia—or hypoxemia due to intrapulmonary pathologies (8). Impaired gas exchange is a common finding among patients considered for a trial of weaning. For example, the mean arterial-to-inspired oxygen ratio (PaO_2/FIO_2) in more than 600 patients enrolled in weaning studies of the Spanish Lung Failure Collaborative Group ranged from 200 to 335 mm Hg (7,9).

The ratio of dead space to tidal volume—an approximation of impaired gas exchange due to lung units with abnormally high ventilation–perfusion ratios—is normally about 0.30 at rest and less during exercise (10). In patients requiring prolonged mechanical ventilation, the ratio can increase to 0.74 or more (11). Patients can compensate for such an increase in dead space by increasing minute ventilation by as much as 2.5 times. Such an increase in minute ventilation poses a minor challenge when respiratory mechanics and respiratory muscles are normal; for example, hypercapnia is uncommon with pulmonary vascular disease (12). Likewise, in the presence of large shunts, increases in minute ventilation can be sufficient to prevent hypercapnia (13). Accordingly, an increase in dead space ventilation or shunt should not be considered the primary mechanisms responsible for weaning failure, unless there is a concurrent abnormality in the mechanical load of the respiratory muscles or in their contractile performance (8,12), or there are concurrent abnormalities in the control of breathing. For example, increases in dead space ventilation may develop

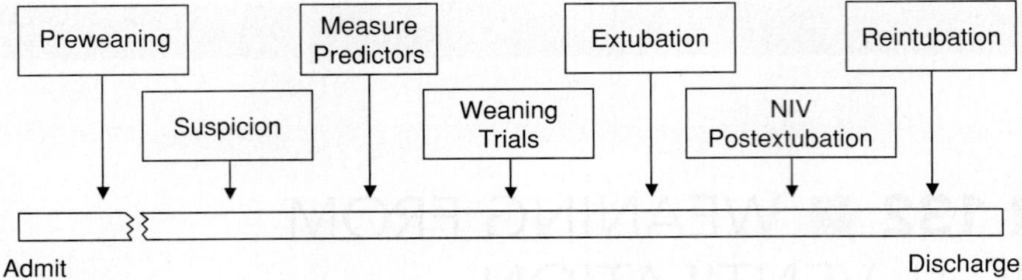

FIGURE 132.1. Seven stages of weaning. Stage 1 is preweaning, a stage that some patients never get beyond. Stage 2 is the period of diagnostic triggering, the time when a physician begins to think that the patient might be ready to come off the ventilator. Stage 3 is the time of measuring and interpreting weaning predictors. Stage 4 is the time of decreasing ventilator support (abruptly or gradually). Stage 5 is either extubation (of a weaning success patient) or reinstitution of mechanical ventilation (in a weaning failure patient). Stage 6 is use of noninvasive ventilation (NIV) after extubation. Stage 7 is reintubation. Failure to appreciate stage 2 probably leads to the greatest delays in weaning. (From Tobin MJ, Jubran A. Weaning from mechanical ventilation. In: Tobin MJ, ed. *Principles and Practice of Mechanical Ventilation*. New York, NY: McGraw-Hill; 2006:1185, with permission.)

during weaning trials as the result of rapid shallow breathing and dynamic hyperinflation (14,15). Finally, an increase in carbon dioxide production can probably only be a contributory factor and not a sole cause of weaning failure (16).

Impaired Ventilatory Pump

Impairment of the ventilatory pump can occur in conditions characterized by decreased respiratory drive, abnormal respiratory mechanics, diminished respiratory muscle performance, and impaired cardiovascular performance.

Decreased Respiratory Drive

Specific conditions such as central alveolar hypoventilation secondary to neurologic lesions (trauma, infections, infarction) can contribute to, or cause, weaning failure. In most weaning failure patients, however, estimations of respiratory drive indicate that drive is increased, and not decreased (17–20).

Purro et al. (21) measured airway occlusion pressure at 100 ms ($P_{0.1}$) during trials of spontaneous respiration in patients who had been mechanically ventilated for more than 3 weeks. All of the weaning failures—all of whom ended up being long-term ventilator dependent—had greater $P_{0.1}$ values than weaning successes. The high values of $P_{0.1}$ suggest an enhanced *neuromuscular** inspiratory drive (22–25). The high neuromuscular inspiratory drive, however, was poorly transformed into ventilatory output—the tidal volumes were lower in weaning failure patients than in weaning success patients—and it was associated with increased respiratory rate (21). It has been suggested that, by stimulating pulmonary or bronchial receptors (stretch or irritant), the increased mechanical load on the respiratory muscles could cause such a rapid and shallow breathing pattern (26). An elevated neuromuscular inspiratory drive in weaning failure patients does not necessarily translate into full respiratory muscle recruitment (Fig. 132.2).

In some patients, however, a decrease in drive relative to the ventilatory demands may still contribute to weaning failure. Jubran and Tobin (14) observed that 2 of 17 (12%) weaning

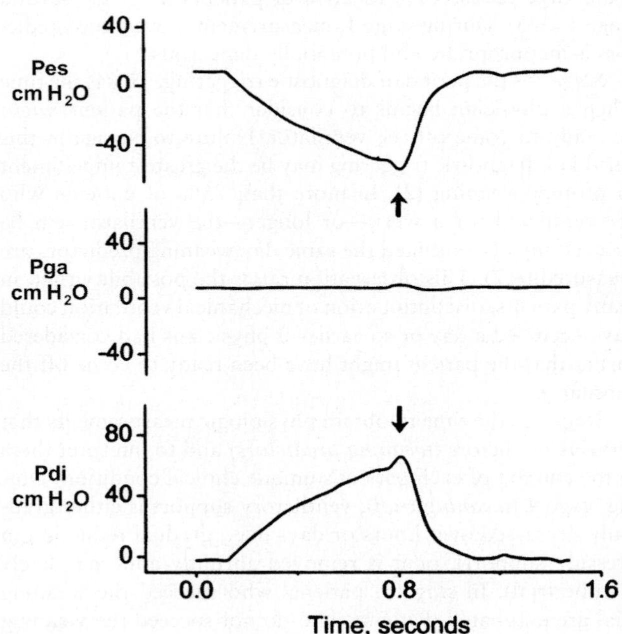

FIGURE 132.2. Continuous recordings of esophageal pressure (Pes), gastric pressure (Pga), and transdiaphragmatic pressure (Pdi) during airway occlusion in a patient after an unsuccessful trial of spontaneous breathing. Phrenic nerve stimulation (*arrow*) during the maximal inspiratory effort resulted in a detectable superimposed twitch. The presence of a superimposed twitch during a maximal effort indicates that voluntary activation of the diaphragm was incomplete. (From Laghi F, Cattapan SE, Jubran A, et al. Is weaning failure caused by low-frequency fatigue of the diaphragm? *Am J Respir Crit Care Med.* 2003;167:120, with permission.)

*$P_{0.1}$ is a function of both neural drive and capacity of the inspiratory muscles to generate pressure (22). The capacity to generate pressure depends on many factors including lung volume, respiratory muscle strength, and respiratory muscle fatigue (23). Because of the dual contribution (neural drive and capacity of the inspiratory muscles to generate pressure), $P_{0.1}$ cannot be considered a pure index of *neural inspiratory drive* but it is rather an index of *neuromuscular inspiratory drive* (pressure available to generate lung volume or ventilation) (22). In addition, $P_{0.1}$ will not result from pure inspiratory muscle contraction when patients relax their expiratory muscles after having recruited them during the preceding exhalation (24). During resting breathing, in healthy subjects, $P_{0.1}$ is about 0.5 to 1.5 cm H_2O (2).

failure patients developed acute hypercapnia during a trial of spontaneous respiration. Lung mechanics and the pressure output of the respiratory muscles of these weaning failure patients were within the range of the weaning success patients, suggesting that about 10% of patients who develop hypercapnia during a failed weaning trial may do so primarily because of (relative) respiratory center depression. Whether sleep deprivation decreases respiratory drive remains controversial (27,28).

Increased Mechanical Load

Patients who fail a weaning trial usually experience an increased mechanical load (14,15,21,29–32). The patients typically have a 30% to 50% greater inspiratory resistance (14,15, 32), 100% greater dynamic elastance (14,21), and 100% to 200% greater intrinsic PEEP (14,21,32) than do similar patients who are not in acute respiratory failure. Inspiratory effort is almost equally divided in offsetting intrinsic PEEP, elastic recoil, and inspiratory resistance (14,31). Abnormal mechanics arise from bronchoconstriction, bronchial edema, pulmonary edema (14), and lung inflammation (29,30). Rapid shallow breathing can aggravate the abnormalities in lung elastance, intrinsic PEEP, and carbon dioxide clearance (14,15). Expiratory muscle recruitment can also increase intrinsic PEEP (33) and breathing effort (32,34,35). Of interest, before the onset of a trial of spontaneous respiration (i.e., T-tube trial), Jubran and Tobin (36) reported that lung resistance, static elastance, and intrinsic PEEP (during passive ventilation) are equivalent in weaning failure and weaning success patients. The difference indicates that one or more factors associated with the act of spontaneous breathing is responsible for the marked difference between failure and success patients during a weaning trial (2).

Several lines of evidence support the likelihood that increased mechanical load contributes to weaning failure. First, during spontaneous respiration, mechanical load is greater in weaning failure patients than in weaning success patients (14,21,37). Second, among six patients who required mechanical ventilation for 6 to 70 days, progression to successful weaning was associated with improvement in work of breathing per liter of minute ventilation (38); values of work of breathing per liter of minute ventilation are a function of compliance, resistance, tidal volume, and minute ventilation (38). Third, in weaning failure patients, the mean inspiratory flow—or tidal volume to inspiratory time ratio—produced for a given level of neuromuscular inspiratory drive ($P_{0.1}$ to mean inspiratory flow ratio or *effective inspiratory impedance*) (22,39) is higher than in patients who are successfully weaned (Fig. 132.3) (21,37). The higher *effective inspiratory impedance* results entirely from a greater neuromuscular drive (21,37) and not from a reduced mean inspiratory flow (21). Given that, despite a greater neuromuscular drive (21,37) the mean inspiratory flow in weaning successes and weaning failures did not differ (21), indicates that for any given change in drive, the flow resistance and compliance characteristics of the respiratory system in weaning failure patients limits the capacity of neuromuscular drive to produce the otherwise expected changes in ventilation. Fourth, *effective inspiratory impedance* correlates with inspiratory pressure output (21). This correlation indicates a worse load-capacity balance in weaning failure patients than in weaning success patients (21).

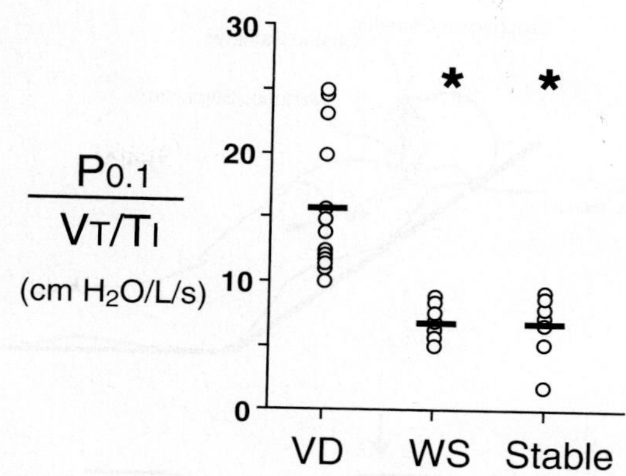

FIGURE 132.3. Effective inspiratory impedance ($P_{0.1}/V_T/T_I$) during periods of unassisted breathing in long-term ventilator-dependent (VD) patients with chronic obstructive pulmonary disease (COPD) ($n = 12$), in patients with COPD who were successfully weaned (WS) from mechanical ventilation after a period of prolonged ventilation ($n = 8$), and in stable patients with COPD ($n = 9$). Effective inspiratory impedance was less in weaning successes and in stable patients than in patients who were ventilator dependent. *Asterisks*, $p < 0.05$, VD versus WS and Stable; *horizontal bars*, average values. (Modified from Purro A, Appendini L, De Gaetano A, et al. Physiologic determinants of ventilator dependence in long-term mechanically ventilated patients. *Am J Respir Crit Care Med.* 2000;161:1115.)

Inadequate Performance of the Respiratory Muscles

Respiratory muscle weakness and respiratory muscle fatigue can decrease the capacity of these muscles to generate and sustain tension. Direct quantification of respiratory muscle tension is clinically impossible. Therefore, measurements of pressure produced by respiratory muscle contractions are used as an indirect means to determine whether inadequate performance of the respiratory muscles is responsible for weaning failure.

Respiratory Muscle Weakness

Detection of respiratory muscle weakness in critically ill patients. Measurements of airway pressure during maximal voluntary inspiratory efforts are used to evaluate global inspiratory muscle strength (40). In healthy subjects, maximum inspiratory airway pressure is usually more negative than -80 cm H_2O (40). In mechanically ventilated patients recovering from an episode or acute respiratory failure, maximum inspiratory airway pressure can range from less negative than -20 cm H_2O to about -100 cm H_2O (5,14,21). Values of maximal airway pressure during voluntary maneuvers depend greatly on a level of motivation and comprehension of the maneuver, often not obtainable in critically ill patients. Thus, it is not surprising that, in patients requiring short-term mechanical ventilation, measurements of maximum inspiratory airway pressure commonly do not differentiate between weaning successes and weaning failure patients (5,32,38,41–43).

In contrast to the voluntary nature of maximal voluntary inspiratory efforts, transdiaphragmatic pressures elicited by single stimulations of the phrenic nerves—or twitch pressure—are independent of patients' motivation and eliminate the influence of the central nervous system (40). Activation can be achieved with either an electrical stimulator (44) or a magnetic stimulator (44), though the latter is easier to use in a mechanically ventilated patient (Fig. 132.4) (32,45,46).

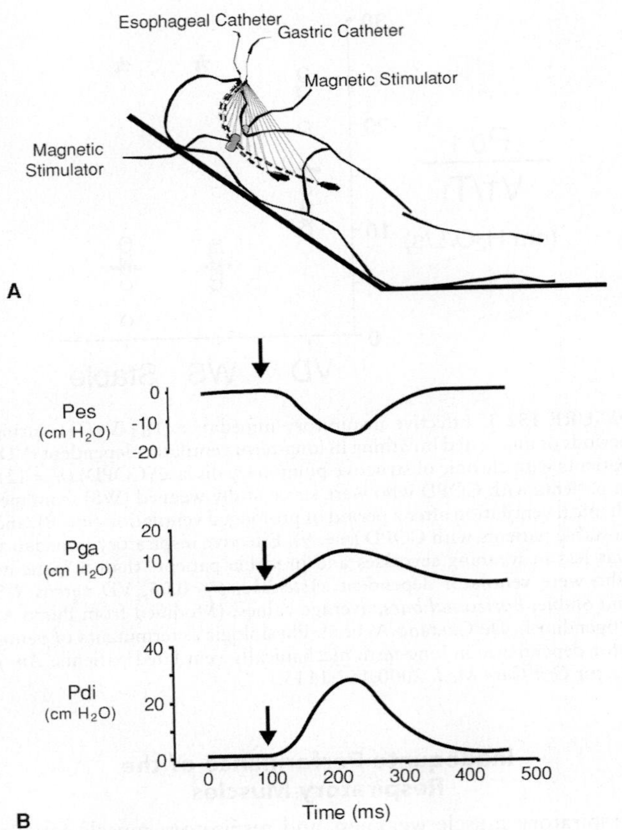

FIGURE 132.4. Twitch pressure recordings following magnetic stimulation of the phrenic nerves. **A:** An esophageal and a gastric balloon catheter are passed trough the nares. Magnetic stimulation of the phrenic nerves elicits diaphragmatic contraction. **B:** Continuous recordings of esophageal (Pes) and gastric pressures (Pga) and transdiaphragmatic pressure (Pdi), calculated by subtracting Pes from Pga. Phrenic nerve stimulation (*arrows*) results in contraction of the diaphragm with consequent fall in intrathoracic pressure (negative deflection of Pes) and rise in intra-abdominal pressure (positive deflection of Pga). These swings in pressure are responsible for transdiaphragmatic twitch pressure. The smaller the transdiaphragmatic twitch pressure, the smaller the force generating capacity of the diaphragm. (From Laghi F. Hypoventilation and respiratory muscle dysfunction. In: Parillo JE, Dellinger RP, eds. *Critical Care Medicine: Principles of Diagnosis and Management in the Adult*. St. Louis, MO: Mosby; 3rd ed.; 2008:829, with permission.)

In healthy volunteers, magnetic stimulation elicits twitch pressures that average 31 to 39 cm H_2O (40). In patients with severe chronic obstructive pulmonary disease (COPD), twitch pressures average 19 to 20 cm H_2O (47,48). The value of transdiaphragmatic twitch pressure in patients recovering from an episode of acute respiratory failure is about half of that recorded in ambulatory patients with severe COPD (Fig. 132.5) (32,45,46). This marked reduction in twitch pressure (45,46) indicates the presence of respiratory muscle weakness in most of these patients. Respiratory muscle weakness in critically ill patients can result from pre-existing conditions or from new onset conditions.

Weakness due to pre-existing conditions. Pre-existing conditions that can cause respiratory muscle weakness include disorders such as neuromuscular diseases, malnutrition, endocrine disorders, and hyperinflation. The existence of pre-existing conditions can be clinically recognized before instituting mechanical ventilation, when ventilator support is being delivered or when the patient fails a weaning trial.

NEUROMUSCULAR DISORDERS. According to the level of anatomic involvement, neuromuscular disorders can be grouped in those involving the central nervous system (e.g., multiple sclerosis, amyotrophic lateral sclerosis), motor neuron (e.g., spinal cord compression, postpolio syndrome, amyotrophic lateral sclerosis), peripheral nerves (e.g., Guillain-Barré syndrome), neuromuscular junction (e.g., botulism, myasthenia gravis), and peripheral muscles (e.g., inflammatory myopathies, myotonic dystrophy, Duchenne muscular dystrophy) (23).

Hypercapnic respiratory failure usually occurs when respiratory muscle strength falls to 39% of the predicted normal value (49). However, Gibson et al. (50) described several patients with neuromuscular disease who had a normal partial pressure of CO_2 despite decreases in respiratory muscle strength to less than 20% of predicted. Conversely, some patients with only moderate respiratory muscle weakness displayed hypercapnia (Fig. 132.6) (50). In other words, reductions in muscle strength do not consistently predict the degree of alveolar hypoventilation in this setting.

HYPERINFLATION. Hyperinflation is a common pre-existing problem in patients with obstructive lung diseases such as COPD (23), cystic fibrosis (51), bronchiolitis (52), and lymphangioleiomyomatosis (23). The severity of pre-existing hyperinflation commonly worsens in patients experiencing an exacerbation of COPD (15). Hyperinflation can also occur *de novo* in patients with pneumonia, acute respiratory distress syndrome, and chest trauma (15,53). Indirect evidence of hyperinflation has been reported in patients who fail a weaning trial (14,15,17,33,54,55).

Hyperinflation has several adverse effects on inspiratory muscle function: the inspiratory muscles operate at an unfavorable position of the length-tension relationship (Fig. 132.7) (56); flattening of the diaphragm decreases the size of the zone of apposition with the result that diaphragmatic contraction causes less effective rib cage expansion (23). Hyperinflation also has an adverse effect on the elastic recoil of the thoracic cage (23). This means that the inspiratory muscles must work not only against the elastic recoil of the lungs but also against that of the thoracic cage. The functional consequences of dynamic hyperinflation are probably the main causes of ventilatory failure in patients with COPD (57). Impairment of inspiratory muscle function as a consequence of hyperinflation, however, is less likely in patients with acute respiratory distress syndrome because these patients breathe at a low lung volume despite dynamic hyperinflation (53,58).

MALNUTRITION. Malnutrition is highly prevalent among critically ill patients requiring mechanical ventilation (59,60) and is associated with poor prognosis (60). Malnutrition decreases muscle mass and respiratory muscle strength both in humans (61,62) and laboratory animals (63–65).

In patients with COPD, inspiratory muscle strength is about 30% less in poorly nourished patients than in well-nourished patients with equivalent airway obstruction (66). Similarly, malnourished patients with anorexia nervosa can present with inspiratory muscle strength reduced to 35% to 50% of predicted (62), impaired respiratory muscle endurance (67), impaired hypercapnic ventilatory response (67), and, occasionally, with hypercapnia at rest (62). In malnourished patients,

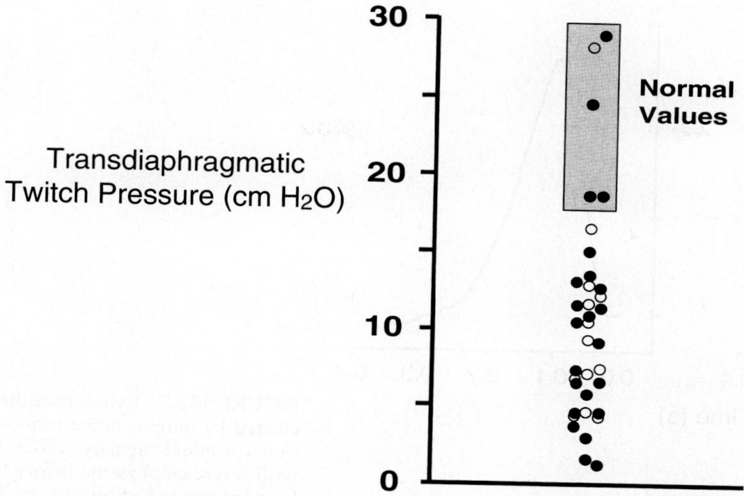

FIGURE 132.5. Transdiaphragmatic twitch pressure recorded in mechanically ventilated patients recovering from an episode of acute respiratory failure. Box represents range of transdiaphragmatic twitch pressures recorded in ambulatory patients with severe chronic obstructive pulmonary disease (COPD). Most mechanically ventilated patients had evidence of diaphragmatic weakness. (Data from Cattapan SE, Laghi F, Tobin MJ. Can diaphragmatic contractility be assessed by airway twitch pressure in mechanically ventilated patients? *Thorax*. 2003;58:58 [*open circles*]; and from Watson AC, Hughes PD, Louise HM, et al. Measurement of twitch transdiaphragmatic, esophageal, and endotracheal tube pressure with bilateral anterolateral magnetic phrenic nerve stimulation in patients in the intensive care unit. *Crit Care Med.* 2001;29:1325 [*closed circles*], with permission.) (Modified from Laghi F. Assessment of respiratory output in mechanically ventilated patients. *Respir Care Clin N Am.* 2005;11:173.)

inspiratory weakness (62,66,67), fatigability (66), and dyspnea (66) are partially reversible with nutritional support. The process is slow and, in laboratory animals, can take months of refeeding for muscle mass to return to normal values (68).

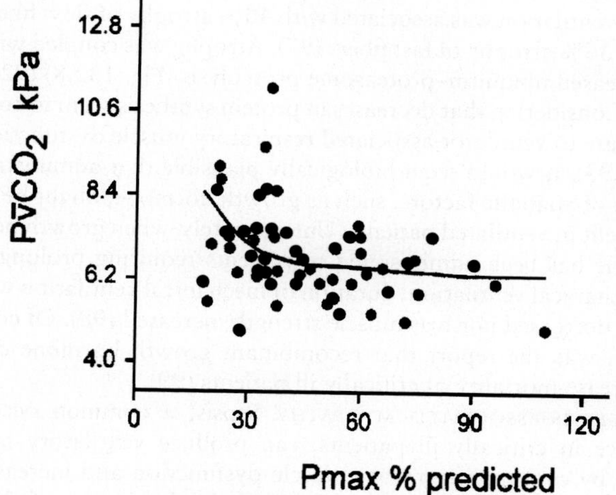

FIGURE 132.6. Relationship between muscle strength and mixed venous partial pressure of CO_2 ($PvCO_2$) in patients with respiratory muscle weakness due to myotonic dystrophy and a variety of nonmyotonic muscle diseases. Respiratory muscle strength is the arithmetic sum of maximum static inspiratory and expiratory mouth pressures (Pmax = PImax + PEmax). As respiratory muscle weakness became more severe $PvCO_2$ increased, although considerable variability was observed among patients. (Modified from Gibson GJ, Gilmartin JJ, Veale D, et al: Respiratory muscle function in neuromuscular disease. In Jones NL, Killian KJ, editors: *Breathlessness.* The Campbell Symposium. Hamilton, Ontario, 1992. Boehringer-Ingelheim)

To date, it remains unclear whether malnutrition by itself can cause sufficient respiratory muscle weakness to cause weaning failure. It is more likely for malnutrition to be a contributory factor and not a sole cause of weaning failure.

ENDOCRINE DISTURBANCES. Endocrine disturbances, such as hypothyroidism (69), hyperthyroidism (70–73), and acromegaly (74), can adversely affect respiratory muscle function. Proteolysis of myofibrillar proteins by the ubiquitin/proteasome proteolytic system (75) (Fig. 132.8) is probably responsible for respiratory muscle catabolism and weakness of hyperthyroidism (70). This mechanism is implicated in the muscle wasting associated with acidosis, renal failure, denervation, cancer, diabetes, AIDS, trauma, and burns (75). In contrast to other endocrine disturbances, respiratory muscle weakness is unusual in patients with Cushing syndrome (76).

Weakness due to new-onset conditions. New-onset respiratory muscle weakness in critically ill patients may result from conditions that are unique to these patients and that include ventilator-associated respiratory muscle dysfunction, sepsis-associated myopathy, and intensive care unit (ICU) acquired paresis. New-onset respiratory muscle weakness may also result from conditions that are not unique to critically ill patients and that include acid-base disorders, electrolyte disturbances, decreased oxygen delivery, or medications. Respiratory muscle weakness due to conditions that are unique to critically ill patients are often associated with alterations in respiratory muscle structure, whereas the others are not necessarily so associated. Recovery from respiratory muscle weakness, if it occurs at all, is slow when the weakness is caused by alterations in muscle structure. In contrast, recovery of respiratory muscle weakness in conditions that are not necessarily associated

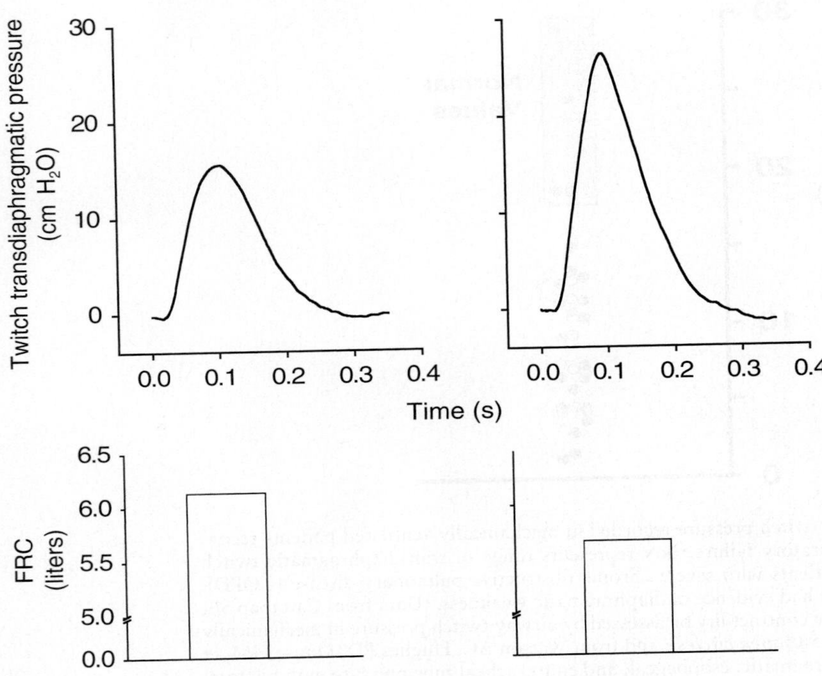

FIGURE 132.7. Twitch transdiaphragmatic pressure elicited by phrenic nerve stimulation (**top**) and functional residual capacity (FRC) (**bottom**) in a patient with severe emphysema before (**left**) and after (**right**) lung volume reduction surgery. The increase in transdiaphragmatic pressure after surgery was in part due to a decrease in the operating lung volume as demonstrated by the decrease in functional residual capacity. (Data from Laghi F, Jubran A, Topeli A, et al. Effect of lung volume reduction surgery on neuromechanical coupling of the diaphragm. *Am J Respir Crit Care Med.* 1998;157:475.)

with alterations in muscle structure is usually rapid once the underlying triggering factor has been corrected.

VENTILATOR-ASSOCIATED RESPIRATORY MUSCLE DYSFUNCTION. In laboratory animals, controlled mechanical ventilation delivered for 1 to 11 days can decrease diaphragmatic force generation by 20% to more than 50% (Fig. 132.9) (77–83) and it can cause similar decreases in diaphragmatic endurance (82). The reduction in force has been related to the extent of myofibril damage and mitochondrial swelling (rabbits) (79) and with a decrease in muscle fibers expressing type I myosin isoforms (rats) (Table 132.1) (78). Impaired membrane depolarization or impaired excitation/contraction coupling may contribute to ventilator-associated respiratory muscle dysfunction (81).

Several mechanisms, including structural injury (79,84,85), oxidative stress (86–89), muscle fiber remodeling (78,88,90), muscle atrophy (78,83,88,91,92)—with the attendant reduction in myofibril synthesis (93) and increased myofibril proteolysis (88,92)—appear to be responsible for ventilator-associated respiratory muscle dysfunction. Use of antioxidants may prevent the muscle damage that results from mechanical ventilation (86). For instance, in a study of more than 200 critically ill patients, 80% of whom required acute ventilator support, duration of mechanical ventilation was nearly 3 days shorter in those who completed a 10-day antioxidant supplementation protocol (vitamin E and vitamin C) than in those who completed a 10-day course of placebo (94). Similar results have been reported in critically ill surgical patients requiring mechanical ventilation (95). Whether the decrease in duration of mechanical ventilation in these studies was due, at least in part, to the (potential) positive effects of antioxidants on the respiratory muscles remains to be demonstrated.

It is unclear if ventilator-associated respiratory muscle dysfunction occurs in humans. In a retrospective study of 13 infants who received uninterrupted ventilator assistance for at least 12 days before death, most diaphragmatic fibers appeared atrophic (Fig. 132.10) (96). The development of atrophy was suggested by a smaller diaphragmatic muscle mass in these infants than in 26 infants who died after receiving mechanical ventilation for 7 days or less (96). These data are supported by a recent preliminary report of Levine et al. (97) who compared costal diaphragm biopsies of six brain-dead organ donors maintained on controlled mechanical ventilation for 18 to 72 hours with those of nine patients ventilated for less than 2 hours during surgery (to remove solitary pulmonary nodules). In this preliminary report, prolonged controlled mechanical ventilation was associated with 40% atrophy of slow fibers and 36% atrophy of fast fibers (97). Atrophy was coupled with increased ubiquitin–proteasome proteolysis (Fig. 132.8) (92).

Considering that decreases in protein synthesis seem to contribute to ventilator-associated respiratory muscle dysfunction (92,93), it would seem biologically plausible that administration of anabolic factors, such as growth hormone, might be of benefit in ventilated patients. Unfortunately, when growth hormone has been administered to patients requiring prolonged mechanical ventilation, duration of mechanical ventilation was not decreased nor was muscle strength increased (98). Of concern was the report that recombinant growth hormone can increase mortality of critically ill patients (99).

SEPSIS-ASSOCIATED MYOPATHY. Sepsis, a common occurrence in critically ill patients, can produce ventilatory failure by causing respiratory muscle dysfunction and increased metabolic demands (100). Septic animals develop failure of neuromuscular transmission (due to increased sarcolemmal electric potential) (101–103) and failure of excitation/contraction coupling (100,104). Mechanisms responsible for failure of excitation/contraction coupling include the cytotoxic effect of free radicals (105–108), ubiquitin/proteasome proteolysis (70,75,100,109–111), the cytotoxic effect of nitric oxide (Fig. 132.11) (102) and its metabolites (112,113), and a decrease in mitochondrial content with associated reduction in energy-rich phosphates (114).

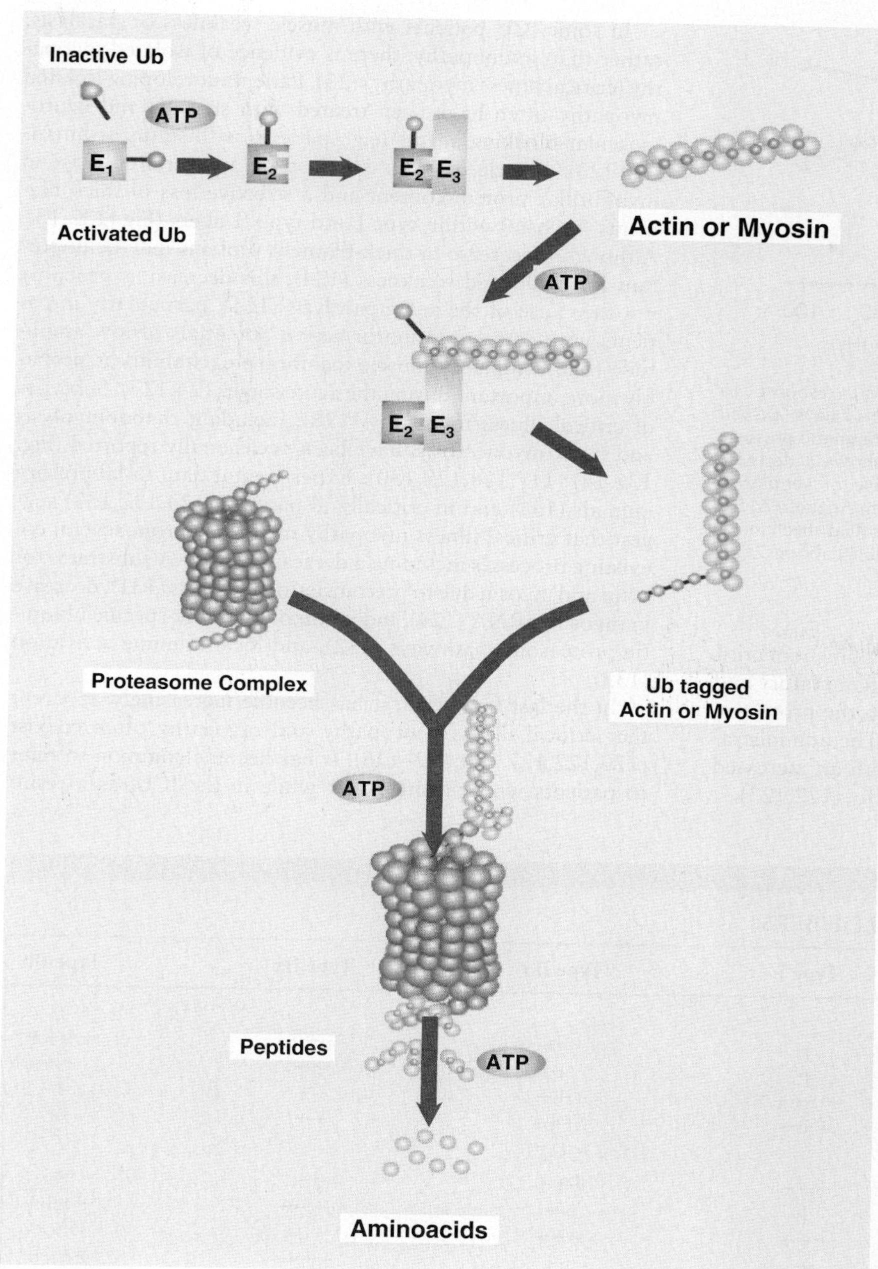

FIGURE 132.8. Ubiquitin/proteasome degradation of contractile proteins. The first step in degradation of actin and myosin is activation of ubiquitin (Ub) by a first enzyme, E1, a process requiring ATP (adenosine triphosphate). Activated ubiquitin interacts with a second enzyme, E2, a carrier protein. Ub and E2 join a third enzyme, E3. E3 transfers activated Ub to actin and myosin. The cycle is repeated until a chain of Ub is bound to the contractile proteins. The chain of Ub binds to one end of a proteasome complex in a process requiring ATP. The Ub chain is subsequently removed (allowing reuse of Ub), and actin and myosin are unfolded and pushed into the core of the proteasome. Multiple enzymes within the core degrade actin and myosin into small peptides. The peptides are extruded from the proteasome and degraded to amino acids by peptidases in the cytoplasm. The ubiquitin/proteasome system degrades myofibrillar proteins only after they have been cleaved and released by other proteolytic pathways—i.e., the ubiquitin/proteasome pathway cannot degrade intact myofibrillar proteins. (From Laghi F, Tobin MJ. Disorders of the respiratory muscles. *Am J Respir Crit Care Med.* 2003;168:10, with permission.)

To determine whether the inducible nitric oxide synthase pathway contributes to impaired skeletal muscle contractility in septic patients, Lanone et al. (115) obtained samples of the rectus abdominis in 16 septic patients and 21 control subjects. The muscles of the patients had lower contractile force and increases in inducible nitric oxide synthase expression (mRNA and protein) and activity. Immunohistochemical studies revealed the generation of peroxynitrite (a highly reactive oxidant formed by the reaction of nitric oxide with superoxide anion). Exposure of control muscles to the amount of peroxynitrite found in patients caused an irreversible decrease in force generation. These data suggest that one of the mechanisms by which sepsis decreases muscle force is through the production of nitric oxide and its toxic byproducts.

INTENSIVE CARE UNIT ACQUIRED PARESIS. While cared for in the ICU, critically ill patients can develop muscle weakness and, occasionally, paralysis. Some of these patients have evidence for axonal degeneration and denervation atrophy (Fig. 132.12) (23). This constellation of findings is known as *critical illness polyneuropathy* (Table 132.2) (116). Sensory involvement is usually more limited than motor involvement (117). Critical illness polyneuropathy has been considered one of the manifestations of multiple organ failure syndrome (118). Sepsis and multiple organ failure, though, are not essential prerequisites for the development of critical illness polyneuropathy (119,120). Tight control of hyperglycemia may reduce the risk of polyneuropathy and the duration of mechanical ventilation (121). It has been speculated that the known neurotoxic

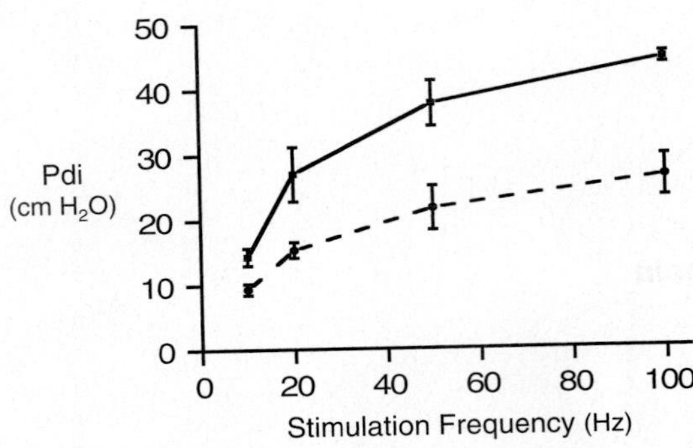

FIGURE 132.9. Transdiaphragmatic pressure (Pdi) response to phrenic nerve stimulation before (*solid line*) and after 11 days (*dashed line*) of mechanical ventilation. That the transdiaphragmatic pressure recorded after 11 days of mechanical ventilation shows a decrease response to all stimulation frequencies is suggestive of ventilator-associated diaphragmatic dysfunction. (Modified from Anzueto A, Peters JI, Tobin MJ, et al. Effects of prolonged controlled mechanical ventilation on diaphragmatic function in healthy adult baboons. *Crit Care Med,* 1997;25:1187.)

effects of hyperglycemia play a role in the development of critical illness polyneuropathy, and that the anti-inflammatory and neuroprotective effects of insulin contribute to the protective effects of tight hyperglycemic control (118). The administration of corticosteroids has not been linked with an increased risk of developing critical illness polyneuropathy (122,123).

In some ICU patients with muscle weakness or paralysis, rather than axonopathy, there is evidence of isolated myopathy (critical illness myopathy) (23). Patients developing isolated myopathy often have been treated with steroids and neuromuscular blocking agents (e.g., patients with status asthmaticus) (23). Muscle biopsies demonstrate a general decrease in myofibrillar protein content and a selective loss of thick filaments (myosin) within type I and type II fibers (Fig. 132.13). Although a decrease in thick-filament proteins may be important for prolonged weakness (124), this decrease is probably not the cause of the acute paralysis (125), particularly in patients with compound motor action potentials of low amplitude (126). Impaired muscle membrane excitability is probably more important during the acute stage (124,127). Subtypes of critical illness myopathy (128), including rhabdomyolysis and frank myonecrosis, have been occasionally reported (Fig. 132.14) (117,118,129,130). Experimental data in laboratory animals (131) and in critically ill patients (124,132,133) suggest that critical illness myopathy may result from several coexisting processes including a decrease in mRNA substrates for actin and myosin due to pretranslational defects (131), decrease in myosin mRNA (124), induction of myofiber-specific ubiquitin/proteasome pathways (132), and local immune activation (133).

In the last few years, it has become increasingly apparent that critical illness neuropathy and myopathy often coexist (120,122,127,130,132–136). It has become common to refer to patients who become weak while in the ICU, as a result

TABLE 132.1

CHARACTERISTICS OF TYPES OF MUSCLE FIBERS

	Type I	Type IIa	Type IIx	Type IIb
Contractile Properties				
Velocity of shortening	+	++	+++	++++
Tetanic force	+	+	++	++
Endurance	++++	+++	++	+
Work efficiency[a]	+++	++	++	+
Histochemistry				
Mitochondrial volume density	+++	+++	++	+
ATP consumption rate	+	++	+++	++++
Oxidative enzymes	+++	+++	++	+
Glycolytic enzymes	+	++	+++	++++
Glycogen	+	++	++	+++
Capillary Supply	+++	+++	++	+
Diameter	+	++	++	+++

ATP, adenosine triphosphate.
A single myosin heavy chain isoform is typically expressed within an adult skeletal muscle fiber. Fibers classified as type I, IIa, IIx, and IIb express myosin heavy chain isoform I (or slow), IIa, IIx, and IIb, respectively. Type IIx fibers have been reported in peripheral muscles of humans and animals and in the diaphragm of animals. Type IIx fibers have not been reported in the human diaphragm. More than one myosin heavy chain isoform is expressed in a few fibers (about 14% of adult rat diaphragm coexpresses myosin heavy chain isoforms IIb and IIx, and less than 1% coexpresses myosin heavy chain isoforms I and IIa) (337). Whereas the velocity of muscle contraction depends primarily on the myosin heavy chain isoform, the velocity of muscle relaxation is mainly determined by troponin C calcium binding and release and by calcium reuptake by the sarco-endoplasmic reticulum calcium–adenosine triphosphatase (SERCA). Several SERCA isoenzymes have been identified: SERCA 1 is expressed in type II fibers (fast calcium reuptake), and SERCA 2a is expressed in type I (slow calcium reuptake) (338). The density of pumping sites largely accounts for different rates of calcium uptake in fast- and slow-twitch muscle fibers (338). Despite this separation of tasks, velocity of contraction and velocity of relaxation tend to parallel each other; type II fibers contract and relax with a greater velocity than type I fibers. Slower velocity of relaxation allows fusion of repetitive twitches at lower frequencies of stimulation as compared with fast relaxations. Impairment of SERCA activity has been implicated in the development of fatigue and in disease states including heart failure and corticosteroid myopathy.
[a]Amount of work performed per unit of adenosine triphosphate consumed.
From Laghi F, Tobin MJ. Disorders of the respiratory muscles. *Am J Respir Crit Care Med.* 2003;168:10, with permission.

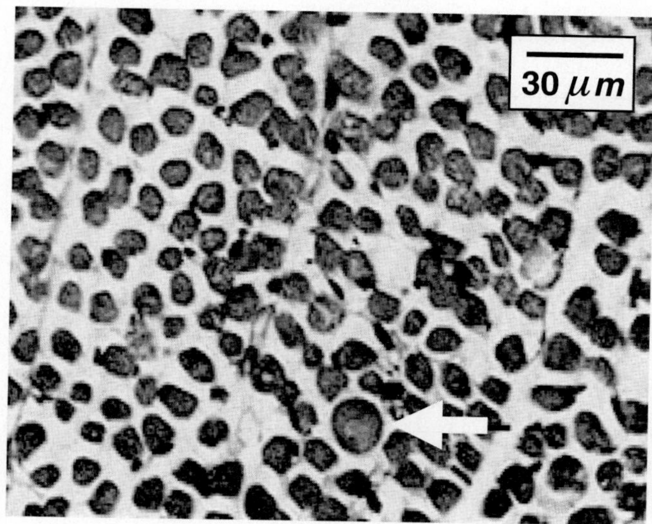

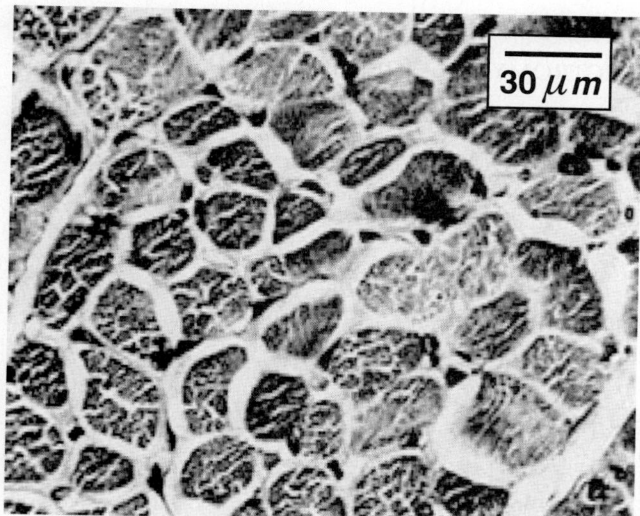

FIGURE 132.10. Photomicrographs of transverse sections of diaphragm from an infant ventilated from birth until death at day 47 (**left**) and from an infant ventilated from birth until accidental death at day 3 (**right**). Prolonged mechanical ventilation was associated with reduction in myofiber cross-sectional area. (The *arrow* in the left panel indicates a developing myofiber also known as Wohlfart myofiber.) (Modified from Knisely AS, Leal SM, Singer DB. Abnormalities of diaphragmatic muscle in neonates with ventilated lungs. *J Pediatr.* 1988;113:1074.)

of acquired neuropathy and/or myopathy (not associated with a known disorder), as simply having critical illness neuromyopathy or, more simply, ICU-acquired paresis (127,132,136). ICU-acquired paresis has been reported to be an independent risk factor of prolonged weaning (136,137) and to be associated with respiratory muscle weakness (138).

The functional outcome of ICU-acquired paresis is not uniform. Among long-term survivors of prolonged critical illness with an ICU stay of at least 4 weeks (117), neurophysiologic evidence of critical illness polyneuropathy has been recorded in 95% of patients up to 5 years following ICU discharge. Although all patients report extreme weakness after ICU and hospital discharge (117), 50% to 60% of them experience complete clinical recovery (ability to breathe spontaneously and to walk independently) over a period of 2 weeks to 6 months or longer (124,137,139). Yet, 10% to 30% experience severe

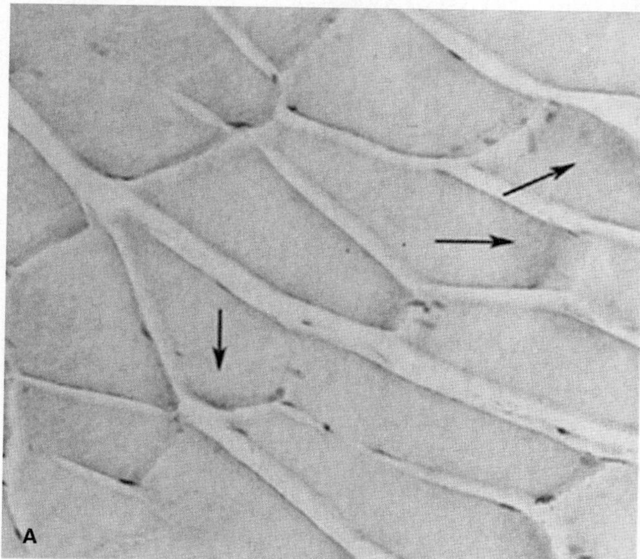

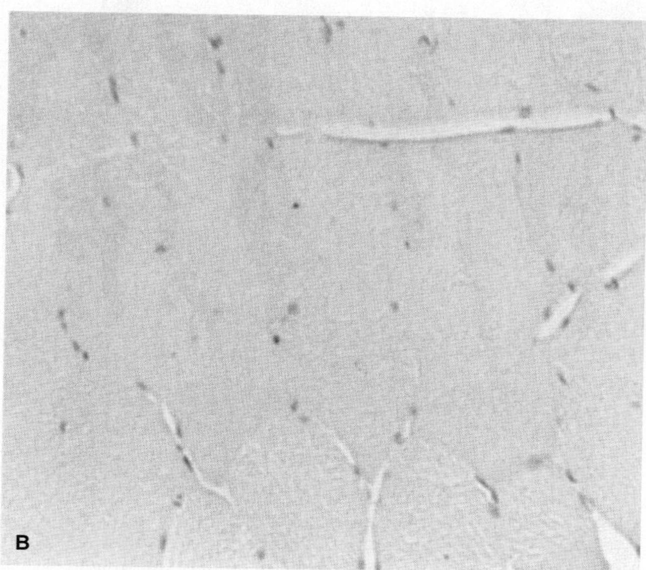

FIGURE 132.11. A: A sample of gastrocnemius muscle obtained from an adult Sprague-Dawley rat injected 12 hours earlier with *E. coli* endotoxin (20 mg/kg). The section was stained with an antibody to inducible nitric oxide synthase. Positive staining (*dark gray staining; arrows*) is evident inside the fibers. **B:** A sample of gastrocnemius muscle obtained from a rat injected 12 hours earlier with normal saline. No positive staining is evident. (Photomicrographs provided by Dr. Sabah N. Hussain, Royal Victoria Hospital, Montreal, Canada.) (From Laghi F, Tobin MJ. Disorders of the respiratory muscles. *Am J Respir Crit Care Med.* 2003;168:10, with permission.)

TABLE 132.2

ELECTROMYOGRAPHIC FINDINGS

	Axonal injury	Myelin injury	Neuromuscular conduction defect	Myopathy
Compound muscle action potential (amplitude)[a]	Reduced	Normal to slightly reduced	Normal[b]	Normal
Sensory nerve action potential (amplitude)[c]	Reduced	Normal to reduced	Normal	Normal
Conduction velocity	Normal to slightly reduced	Reduced	Normal	Normal
Spontaneous muscle depolarization[d]	Present	Absent	Absent	None to Present
Amplitude of compound muscle action potential with stimulation at 3 Hz[e]	Unchanged	Unchanged	Decreased	Unchanged
Motor unit activation	Decreased	Decreased	Normal	Increased

Examples of injuries and deficits: Axonal injury, critical illness myopathy; myelin injury, Guillain-Barré; neuromuscular conduction defect, myasthenia, prolonged neuromuscular blockade; myopathy, critical illness myopathy. Although features of myopathy can be recorded by electromyographic studies, electromyography cannot always distinguish critical illness myopathy from critical illness polyneuropathy, and muscle biopsies may be needed.

[a]Elicited by motor nerve stimulation.

[b]Decreased in the Lambert-Eaton syndrome.

[c]Elicited by sensory nerve stimulation.

[d]Spontaneous muscle depolarization (caused by denervation) is detected by presence of fibrillation potentials and positive sharp waves.

[e]Repetitive nerve stimulation is performed to exclude neuromuscular transmission defects such as prolonged neuromuscular paralysis.

From Laghi F, Tobin MJ. Disorders of the respiratory muscles. *Am J Respir Crit Care Med.* 2003;168:10, with permission.

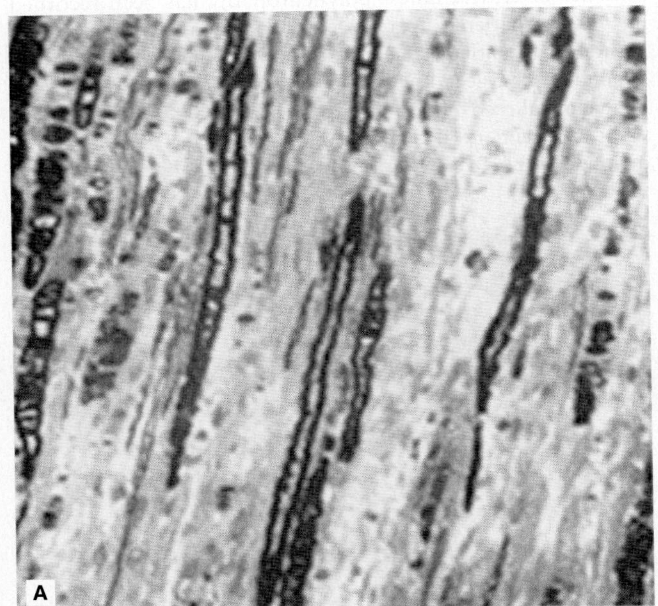

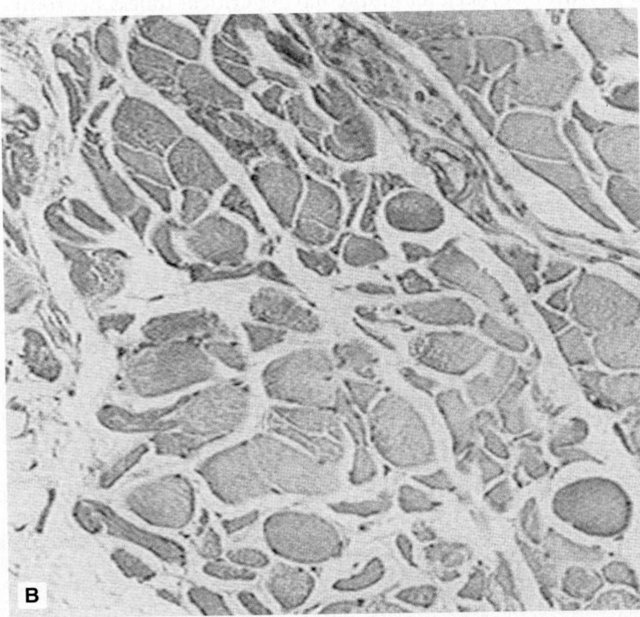

FIGURE 132.12. Transverse section of a peripheral motor nerve (deep peroneal nerve, **left**) and of a skeletal muscle (intercostal, **right**) in patients who developed profound weakness following a prolonged hospital course characterized by sepsis, multiple organ failure syndrome, and inability to wean from mechanical ventilation. **Left:** The long thin dark structures are myelin sheaths that contain axons. The axons are degenerating and dying. And, following death, they disintegrate. The myelin surrounding the disintegrating axons collapses around the axonal debris to form *ovoids of myelin*, seen better on the lateral portions of the micrograph. **Right:** Amid muscle fibers that are normal in size and shape there are atrophic ones that appear small and that have developed contours with acute angles. These findings are consistent with denervation atrophy secondary to axonal degeneration—so-called critical illness polyneuropathy. (Modified from Zochodne DW, Bolton CF, Wells GA, et al. Critical illness polyneuropathy. A complication of sepsis and multiple organ failure. *Brain.* 1987;110:819.)

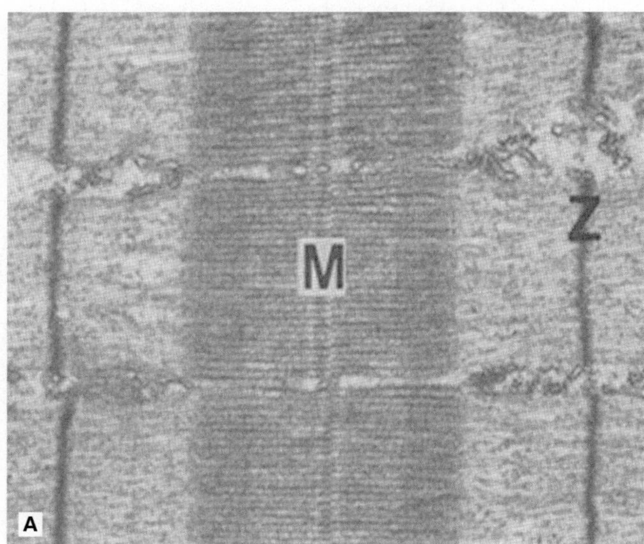

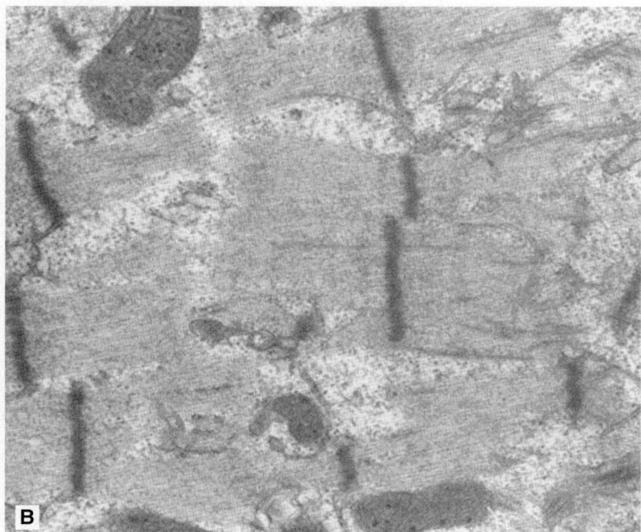

FIGURE 132.13. Electron micrographs of normal skeletal muscle (**left**) and skeletal muscle from a patient who received steroids and the neuromuscular blocking agent vecuronium during a hospitalization with status asthmaticus followed by flaccid quadriplegia (**right**). Compared with the normal structure, the patient developed extensive loss of thick (myosin) myofilaments and relative preservation of thin (actin) filaments. Muscle strength returned to normal 3 months after discontinuation of vecuronium. M, M-line formed by myosin filaments and M-line proteins; Z, Z-disk formed by a lattice of filaments that join the actin filaments of one sarcomere with the actin filaments of the adjacent sarcomere. (Modified from Eisenberg BR. In: Bradley WG, Gardner-Medwin D, Walton JN, eds. *Recent Advances in Myology*. Amsterdam, the Netherlands: Excerpta Med; 1975, with permission; and from Danon MJ, Carpenter S. Myopathy with thick filament (myosin) loss following prolonged paralysis with vecuronium during steroid treatment. *Muscle Nerv*. 1991;14:1131, with permission.)

persistent disability, and some patients continue to be paraparetic or paraplegic, or tetraparetic or tetraplegic (117,140). Other investigators report even worse outcome: only two of ten patients left the hospital in one study (130). Whether it is possible to prevent ICU-acquired paresis in patients recovering from severe acute illness and whether that would result in shorter duration of mechanical ventilation remains unknown.

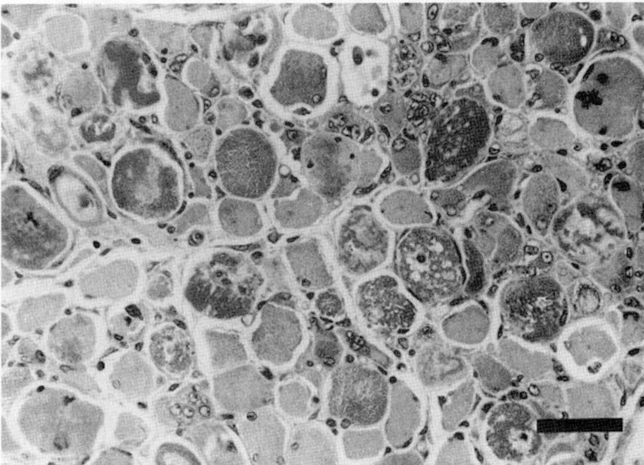

FIGURE 132.14. Transverse section of a peripheral skeletal muscle (rectus femoris) in a critically ill patient with necrotizing myopathy of the intensive care unit. Several muscle fibers demonstrate an obvious panfascicular destructive process. The destructive process is associated with myophagocytosis and small, regenerating muscle fibers that contain groups of vesicular nuclei and prominent nucleoli. Bar, 50 μm. (From Ramsay DA, Zochodne DW, Robertson DM, et al. A syndrome of acute severe muscle necrosis in intensive care unit patients. *J Neuropathol Exp Neurol*. 1993;52:387, with permission.)

ACID-BASE DISORDERS. Alkalosis, either metabolic or respiratory, does not affect skeletal muscle strength (141–143) and may improve endurance (141). Whether acidosis, either metabolic (144–152) or respiratory (142,143,145,153–156), impairs respiratory muscle function remains controversial.

ELECTROLYTE DISTURBANCES. Respiratory muscle function may be impaired by decreased levels of phosphate (157), calcium (158), magnesium (159), and potassium (160).

MEDICATIONS. Weakness can result from medications that have a direct myotoxic effect, such as blockade of myocyte glycoprotein synthesis and electron transport caused by statins (inhibitors of the hydroxy-methylglutaryl coenzyme A reductase) used in patients with hyperlipidemia or nucleoside analogues used in patients with human immunodeficiency virus (161–164). Weakness can also result with neuromuscular blocking agents and aminoglycosides, which interfere with neuromuscular transmission (165,166).

In acutely ventilated patients, paralysis (including the respiratory muscles) can persist after discontinuation of neuromuscular blocking agents (166–168). Prolonged blockade is estimated to occur in 12% to 44% of patients receiving pancuronium or vecuronium for 1 or more days (166–168). Accumulation of metabolites of the neuromuscular blocking agents is responsible for the prolonged blockade (166). Risk factors for prolonged blockade include renal and/or hepatic failure (depending on the agent used), hypermagnesemia, metabolic acidosis, female gender, and the concomitant use of various antibiotics, including aminoglycosides and clindamycin (118,166).

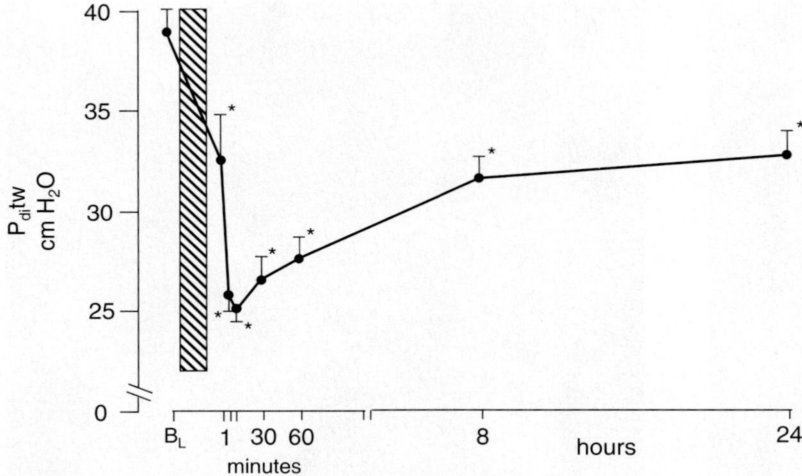

FIGURE 132.15. Induction of diaphragmatic fatigue (*vertical box*) produced a significant fall in transdiaphragmatic pressure (Pdi) elicited by twitch stimulation of phrenic nerves. Significant recovery of twitch pressure was noted in the first 8 hours after completion of the fatigue protocol; no further change was observed between 8 and 24 hours, and the 24-hour value was significantly lower than baseline. The delay in reaching the nadir of twitch transdiaphragmatic pressure probably results from twitch potentiation, induced by repeated contractions, which was present at the end of the protocol. Values are mean ± SE. *Significant difference compared with baseline value, $p < 0.01$. (From Laghi F, D'Alfonso N, Tobin MJ. Pattern of recovery from diaphragmatic fatigue over 24 hours. *J Appl Physiol.* 1995;79:539, with permission.)

Repetitive nerve stimulation demonstrates a decrement of the compound muscle action potential (Table 132.2). Recovery from prolonged neuromuscular blockade is usually reported to begin within 2 days of the last dose (166,167), which contrasts with the prolonged course of critical illness myopathy or neuropathy (124,139,140,169). It is thus unlikely, if not impossible, for prolonged neuromuscular blockade to cause long-term ventilator dependence (170,171). Dosing neuromuscular blocking agents with the assistance of a peripheral nerve stimulator (monitoring of train-of-four) (172) may be associated with faster recovery of neuromuscular function and spontaneous respiration (168). Treatment consists primarily of waiting for clearance of the neuromuscular blocking agents or their metabolites (118). Reversal of neuromuscular blockade with a cholinesterase has been used to establish a diagnosis. In the presence of high concentrations of neuromuscular blocking agents—or their metabolites—recovery is usually incomplete or transitory (118).

Limitations in the current classification of respiratory muscle weakness. When studying respiratory muscle weakness leading to weaning failure, it is necessary to bear in mind the current limited understanding of these conditions. First, the distinction between pre-existing conditions and new-onset conditions can be arbitrary. Second, conditions that are pre-existing—malnutrition and hyperinflation—can worsen during the course of an unrelated critical illness. Third, the nosology is often unsatisfactory: consider the nebulous distinction between ICU-acquired paresis and sepsis-associated myopathy, or between ICU-acquired paresis and ventilator-associated

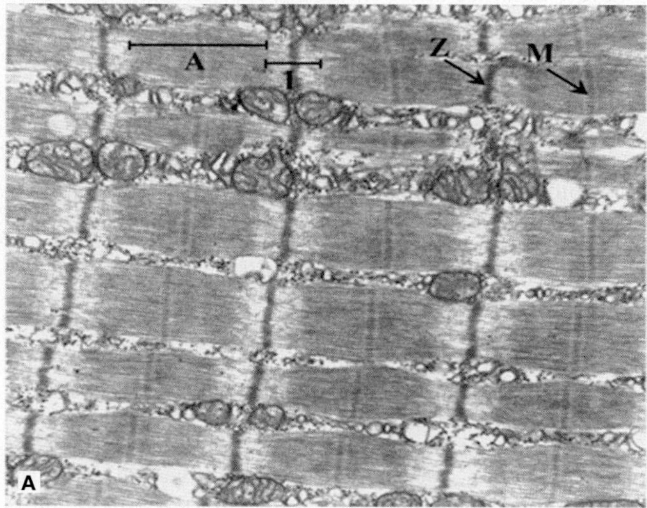

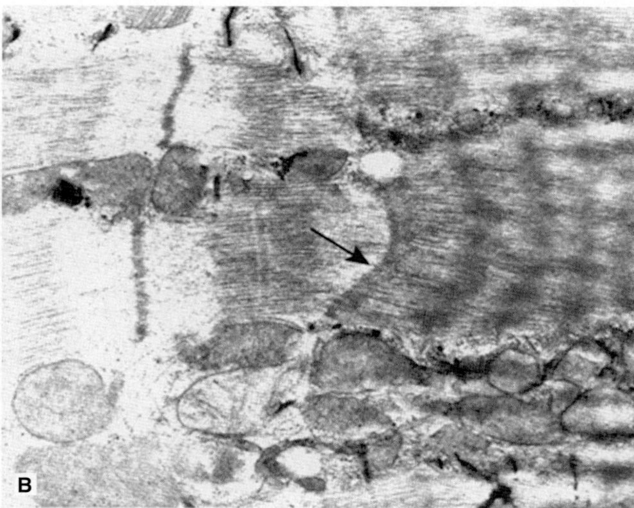

FIGURE 132.16. Electron micrographs of longitudinal sections from the costal diaphragm of a healthy control hamster (**left**) and a hamster exposed to 6 days of resistive loading (**right**). **Left:** Normal sarcomeres with distinct A-bands, I-bands, Z-bands, and M-lines that are aligned between adjacent myofibrils. **Right:** Load-induced damage recognizable by Z-band streaming (*arrow*) and disruption of sarcomeric structure (**right section**) with loss of distinct A-bands and I-bands. Z-band streaming is attributed to a loss of cytoskeletal protein elements such as desmin, alpha-actinin, and vimentin. Magnification for both micrographs: 16,500×. (Electron micrographs provided by Drs. David C. Walker and Darlene W. Reid, University of British Columbia, Vancouver, Canada.) (From Laghi F, Tobin MJ. Disorders of the respiratory muscles. *Am J Respir Crit Care Med.* 2003;168:10, with permission.)

respiratory muscle dysfunction. Fourth, conditions in which respiratory muscle weakness is associated with muscle damage can also display some degree of muscle atrophy: consider diaphragmatic atrophy in cases of ventilator-associated respiratory muscle dysfunction. Fifth, available diagnostic tools have limited specificity in differentiating the various conditions that may cause weakness in the ICU. Sixth, in any given patient, more than one mechanism may be responsible for respiratory muscle weakness. Last, respiratory muscle weakness can be combined with a depressed drive—for example, in the setting of hypercapnia-induced hypoventilation (23).

Respiratory Muscle Fatigue. Contractile fatigue occurs when a sufficiently large respiratory load is applied over a sufficiently long period (44,173–175). Contractile fatigue can be brief or prolonged (Fig. 132.15). Short-lasting fatigue results from accumulation of inorganic phosphate (176), failure of the membrane electrical potential to propagate beyond T tubes and, to a much lesser extent, intramuscular acidosis (177,178). Short-lasting fatigue appears to have a protective function because it can prevent injury to the sarcolemma caused by forceful muscle contractions (179). Long-lasting fatigue (174) is consistent with the development of, and recovery from, muscle injury (Fig. 132.16) (179,180). Several mechanisms may contribute to muscle injury. These include activation of calpain (a calcium-dependent nonlysosomal protease), increased muscle temperature, and excessive production of reactive oxygen species (23). Muscle injury can also be caused by eccentric contractions (contraction of a muscle while it is stretched by external forces) (23). Eccentric contractions can occur during ineffective inspiratory efforts, which have been associated with worse weaning outcome both in the acute (181) and chronic setting (182) and with ventilator dependence (21,182).

Whether critically ill patients develop short-lasting or long-lasting contractile fatigue of the respiratory muscles has not been clear. Patients who fail a trial of weaning from mechanical ventilation are at particular risk of developing fatigue because they experience marked increases in respiratory load (14,15,21). The addition of a new injury to the respiratory muscles (secondary to the development of contractile fatigue) might be the ultimate determinant of whether or not some patients are ever successfully weaned.

Laghi et al. (32) recently measured the contractile response of the diaphragm to phrenic nerve stimulation in nine patients who failed a weaning trial; seven patients who were successfully weaned served as control subjects. The weaning failure patients experienced a greater respiratory load. Moreover, the *tension-time index* of the diaphragm—an index of the ability of the diaphragm to sustain a given inspiratory load (183) calculated by multiplying two ratios: the respiratory duty cycle (inspiratory time divided by the time of a total respiratory cycle) and the mean inspiratory pressure per breath divided by maximum inspiratory pressure—was greater in the failure group than in the success group ($p = 0.01$). Nevertheless, not a single patient developed a decrease in transdiaphragmatic twitch pressure elicited by phrenic nerve stimulation (Fig. 132.17). The failure to develop fatigue is surprising because seven of the nine weaning failure patients had a tension-time index above 0.15 (the putative threshold for task failure and fatigue).

The increase in tension-time index over the course of the weaning trial (32) and predicted time to task failure (183) are shown in Figure 132.18. At the point that the physician reinstituted mechanical ventilation, patients were predicted to be an average of 13 minutes away from task failure. In other words, patients display clinical manifestations of severe respiratory distress for a substantial time before they develop fatigue. In an intensive care setting, these clinical signs will lead attendants to reinstitute mechanical ventilation before fatigue has time to develop.

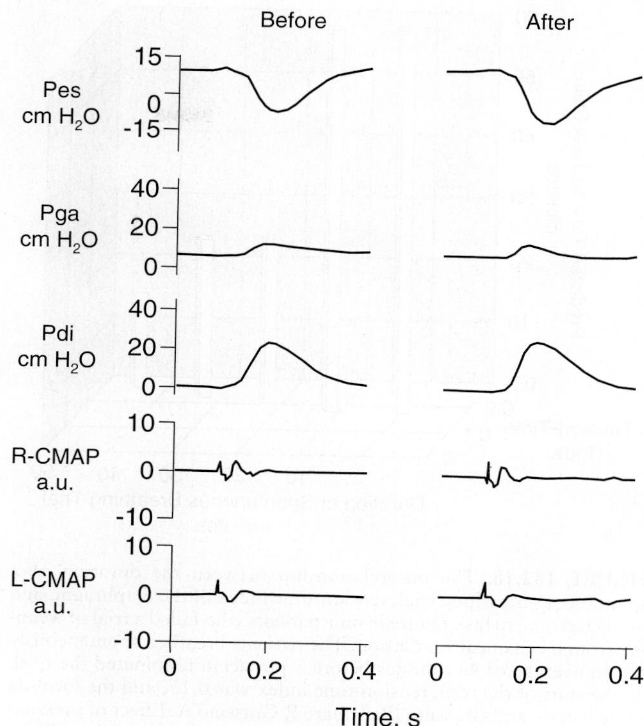

FIGURE 132.17. Esophageal pressure (Pes), gastric pressure (Pga), transdiaphragmatic pressure (Pdi), and compound motor action potentials (CMAP) of the right and left hemidiaphragms after phrenic nerve stimulation before (**left**) and after (**right**) a failed trial of weaning. The end-expiratory value of Pes and the amplitude of the right and left CMAPs were the same before and after the trial, indicating that the stimulations were delivered at the same lung volume and that the stimulations achieved the same extent of diaphragmatic recruitment. The amplitude of twitch Pdi elicited by phrenic nerve stimulation was the same before and after weaning. A.u., arbitrary units. (From Laghi F, Cattapan SE, Jubran A, et al. Is weaning failure caused by low-frequency fatigue of the diaphragm? *Am J Respir Crit Care Med.* 2003;167:120, with permission.)

Impaired Cardiovascular Performance

Spontaneous respiratory efforts decrease intrathoracic pressure, and thus increase the pressure gradient for systemic venous return (184). In addition, decreases in intrathoracic pressure increase left ventricular afterload, causing additional stress on the left ventricle (184). In patients with coronary artery disease, the increased stress can alter myocardial perfusion and cause transient left ventricular dilation (185). The occurrence of myocardial ischemia during periods of spontaneous respiration has been associated with a greater risk of weaning failure (186) and greater risk of ventilator dependence (187). Increases in transmural pulmonary artery occlusion pressure during spontaneous respiration (188) may be the central mechanism responsible for ventilator dependence in patients with

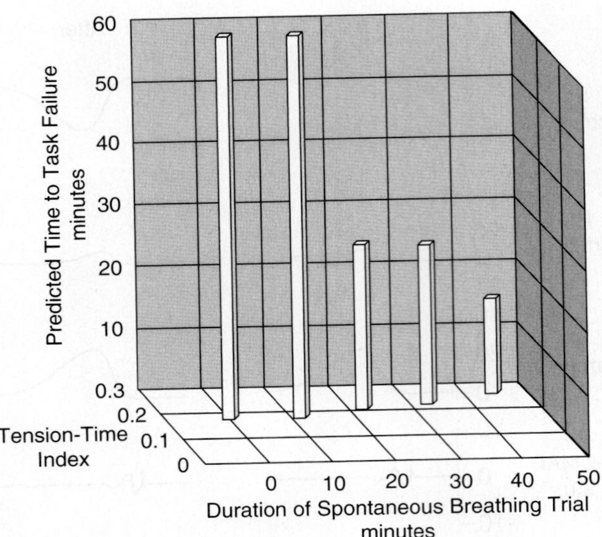

FIGURE 132.18. The interrelationship between the duration of a spontaneous breathing trial, tension-time index of the diaphragm, and predicted time to task failure in nine patients who failed a trial of weaning from mechanical ventilation. The patients breathed spontaneously for an average of 44 minutes before a physician terminated the trial. At the start of the trial, tension-time index was 0.17, and the formula of Bellemare and Grassino (Bellemare F, Grassino A. Effect of pressure and timing of contraction on human diaphragm fatigue. *J Appl Physiol.* 1982;53:1190) predicted that patients could sustain spontaneous breathing for another 59 minutes before developing task failure. As the trial progressed, tension-time index increased and predicted time to the development of task failure decreased. At the end of the trial, tension-time index reached 0.26; that patients were predicted to sustain spontaneous breathing for another 13 minutes before developing task failure clarifies why patients did not develop a decrease in diaphragmatic twitch pressure. In other words, physicians interrupted the trial based on clinical manifestations of respiratory distress before patients had sufficient time to develop contractile fatigue. (From Laghi F, Tobin MJ. Disorders of the respiratory muscles. *Am J Respir Crit Care Med.* 2003;168:10, with permission.)

myocardial ischemia (187) and in patients with impaired left ventricular function (189). Mechanisms by which increases in transmural pulmonary artery occlusion pressure could contribute to weaning failure include worsening pulmonary mechanics and decreased gas exchange.

In the acute setting, oxygen consumption at the completion of a weaning trial is equivalent in weaning-success and weaning-failure patients (190). The manner in which the cardiovascular system meets oxygen demands, however, differs between the two groups. In weaning successes, oxygen transport increases, mainly resulting from an increase in cardiac index; in weaning failures, the increase in demand is met by an increase in oxygen extraction, resulting in a decrease in mixed venous oxygen saturation (Fig. 132.19). A decrease in mixed venous oxygen saturation is consistent with a failing cardiovascular response to an increased metabolic demand (184).

High variability in hemodynamic response during failure to wean has been reported by Zakynthinos et al. (41). It is unclear whether the absent interaction between weaning failure and oxygen consumption in some of the patients studied by Zakynthinos et al. (41) was due to depression of the respiratory centers, limited capacity to extract oxygen, or limited cardiac reserve (191).

To date, detailed studies on the impact of cardiac factors in determining weaning outcome have not been performed. So far, few case reports have shown that successful diuresis and weight loss may be associated with weaning success (188,192). Whether intravenous inotropic agents such as dobutamine should be used in difficult-to-wean patients remains controversial (184,193).

Psychological Factors

Patients who require mechanical ventilation are commonly affected by psychological problems such as anxiety, agitation, delirium, depression, apathy, and posttraumatic stress disorder (PTSD) (194–198). Half of patients receiving prolonged ventilation experience delirium (199). In these patients, delirium has been associated with greater likelihood of discharge to a nursing home or long-term care facility and with increased mortality at 1 year (199). As with the high prevalence of delirium, PTSD has also been reported to be very common in acutely and chronically ventilated patients (200–202). Duration of mechanical ventilation, use of sedative agents, and presence and severity of PTSD appear causally linked and may influence duration of mechanical ventilation and psychological function after discharge (195). Last, in a preliminary report of 100 patients requiring prolonged ventilation, Dilling et al. (197) recorded an association between anxiety at the time of a spontaneous breathing trial and weaning failure.

Possible mechanisms for psychological dysfunction in mechanically ventilated patients include respiratory discomfort, severity of illness, sleep deprivation, sensory deprivation (Fig. 132.20), and medication side effects (196,201,203–205). The delivery of mechanical ventilation itself can cause psychological dysfunction (195,196). Mechanical ventilation limits mobility, fosters isolation, impairs communication, and interferes with or blocks patient control of the act of breathing (195,206). Anxiety and depression can decrease motivation, interfere with performing simple tasks, and decrease self-esteem (195).

Aggressive treatment of depression may increase the likelihood of weaning (207,208). Biofeedback (209,210), improving the patients' environment, communication, and mobility (195,211), and specialized weaning centers (212) have been used to decrease psychological problems in ventilated patients.

PREDICTION OF WEANING OUTCOME

Research on prediction of weaning outcome uses the tools of medical decision analysis (2). Therefore, before discussing weaning predictor tests, it is useful to review the principles of medical decision analysis.

Medical Decision Analysis

Diagnostic tests are designed to screen for a condition and to confirm the condition. The characteristics of screening tests and confirmatory tests differ, and only rarely will a single diagnostic test fulfill both functions (213).

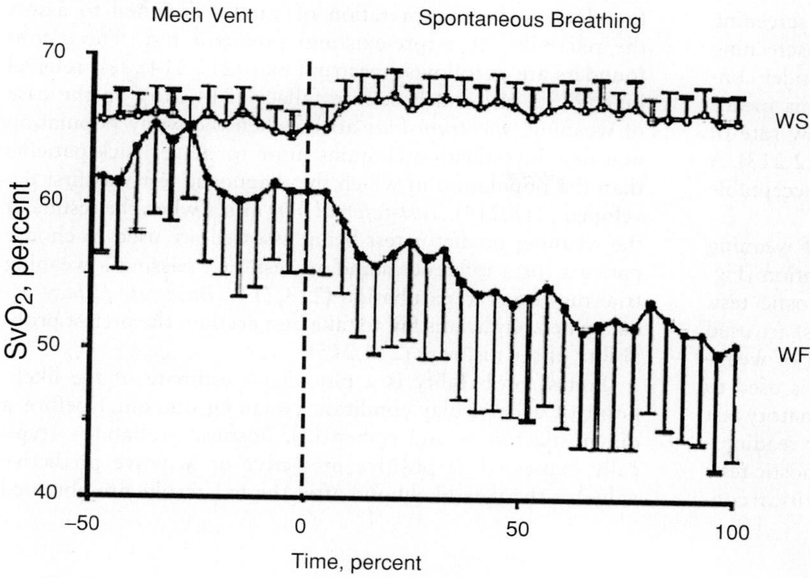

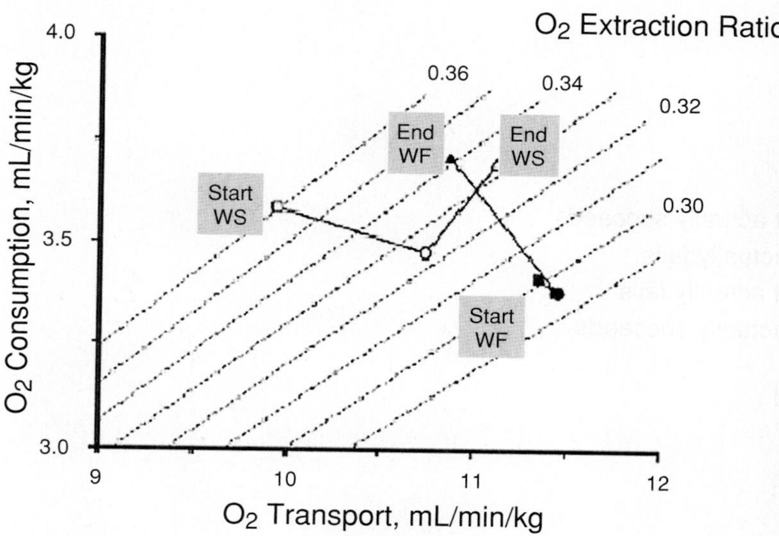

FIGURE 132.19. Top: Mixed venous oxygen saturation (SvO_2) during mechanical ventilation and a trial of spontaneous breathing in 11 weaning success (WS) patients (*open symbols*) and in 8 weaning failure (WF) patients (*closed symbols*). During mechanical ventilation, SvO_2 was similar in the two groups ($p = 0.28$). Between the onset (*dashed line*) and the end of the trial, SvO_2 decreased in the failure group ($p < 0.01$) whereas it remained unchanged in the success group ($p = 0.48$). Over the course of the trial, SvO_2 was lower in the failure group than in the success group ($p < 0.02$). Bars, SE, standard error. **Bottom:** Oxygen transport, oxygen consumption, and isopleths of oxygen extraction ratio in the success (WS, *open symbols*) and failure (WF, *closed symbols*) groups during mechanical ventilation (*squares*) and at the onset (*circles*) and end (*triangles*) of a spontaneous breathing trial. See text for details. (Modified from Jubran A, Mathru M, Dries D, et al. Continuous recordings of mixed venous oxygen saturation during weaning from mechanical ventilation and the ramifications thereof. *Am J Respir Crit Care Med.* 1998;158:1763.)

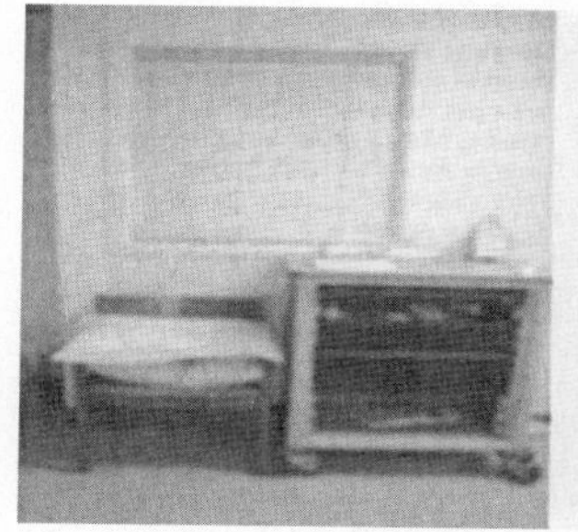

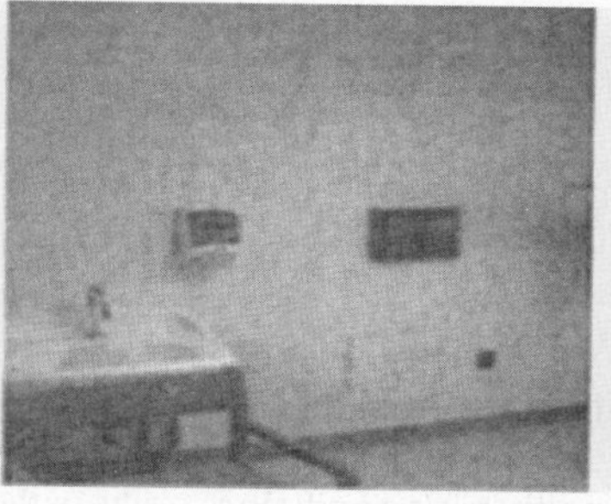

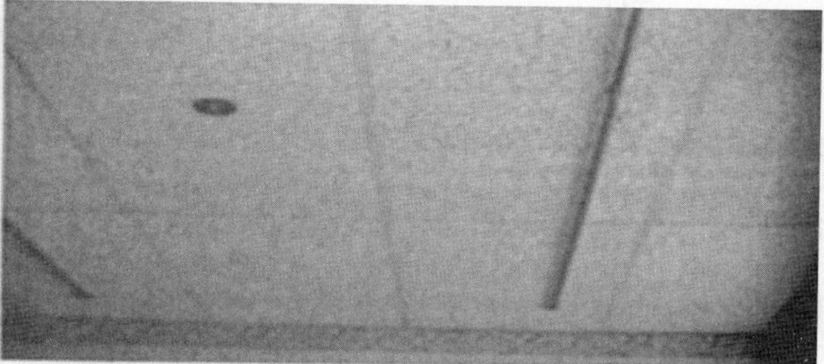

FIGURE 132.20. The environment where ventilated patients are being cared for can promote sensory deprivation through the lack of windows with a view (**left**), bare walls (**middle**), and tedious ceiling (**right**). (From Martin UJ, Criner GJ. Psychological problems in the ventilated patient. In: Tobin MJ, ed. *Principles and Practice of Mechanical Ventilation.* 2nd ed. New York, NY: McGraw-Hill; 2006:1142, with permission.)

The primary goal of weaning predictor tests is screening (2). A good weaning predictor test, like any good screening test, should miss no patient who has the condition under consideration, i.e., to be ready for a weaning trial. This means that a good weaning predictor test must have a low rate of false-negative results—high sensitivity (Fig. 132.21) (2,213). A high rate of false-positive results (low specificity) is acceptable (2,213).

The process of weaning entails measurement of weaning predictors, a trial of weaning, and a trial of extubation (Fig. 132.1) (2). Each step in this sequence is a diagnostic test. Measurements of weaning predictors (screening tests) are used to diagnose readiness for a weaning trial. The trial of weaning (confirmatory test of the screening tests) itself is used to screen for readiness to extubate. Extubation (confirmatory test of the weaning trial) is used to diagnose/screen for readiness to maintain spontaneous respiration. To apply diagnostic tests (screening or confirmatory) in sequence introduces critical confounders in the interpretation of studies designed to assess the reliability of a (pre-existing) predictor test. These confounders are as follows: spectrum bias (213,214), test-referral bias (213,214), and base-rate fallacy (214,215). In the case of weaning, *spectrum bias* arises when the study population in a new investigation contains more (or fewer) sick patients than the population in which the diagnostic test was first developed (213,214). *Test-referral bias* arises when the results of the weaning predictor test being assessed are used to choose patients for a reference-standard test, i.e., passing a weaning trial that leads to extubation (213,214). *Base-rate fallacy* occurs when physicians fail to take into account the pretest probability of the disorder (214,215).

Pretest probability is a physician's estimate of the likelihood of a particular condition (weaning outcome) before a diagnostic test is undertaken (2). Posttest probability (typically expressed as positive predictive or negative predictive value) is the new likelihood after the test results are obtained

		Gold Standard Success	Gold Standard Fail
Test (f/V_T)	Positive (≤100)	TP	FP
	Negative (>100)	FN	TN

TP = Test predicts weaning success and patient actually succeeds
TN = Test predicts weaning failure and patient actually fails
FP = Test predicts weaning success and patient actually fails
FN = Test predicts weaning failure and patient actually succeeds

$$\text{Sensitivity} = \frac{TP}{TP + FN} = TPR = [1 - FNR]$$

$$\text{Specificity} = \frac{TN}{TN + FP} = TNR = [1 - FPR]$$

$$PPV = \frac{TP}{TP + FP}$$

$$NPV = \frac{TN}{TN + FN}$$

FN Rate = 1 – Sensitivity

FP Rate = 1 – Specificity

Likelihood ratio for a positive test = TPR/FPR = sensitivity/(1 – specificity)

Likelihood ratio for a negative test = FNR/TNR = (1 – sensitivity)/specificity

Prevalence = TP + FN/(TP + TN + FP + FN)

Diagnostic accuracy = [TP + TN]/[TP + TN + FP + FN]

FIGURE 132.21. A 2 × 2 tabular display of the characteristics of diagnostic tests. The vertical columns represent the results of the gold standard test. The horizontal rows represent the results of the index test. Readings of f/Vt ≤100 are classified as positive test results and readings of >100 are classified as negative test results. The relationship of these binary results to the outcome of a T-tube weaning trial forms a decision matrix that has four possible combinations. (From Tobin MJ, Jubran A. Weaning from mechanical ventilation. In: Tobin MJ, ed. *Principles and Practice of Mechanical Ventilation.* New York, NY: McGraw-Hill; 2006:1185, with permission.)

(Fig. 132.21). A good diagnostic test achieves a marked increase (or decrease) in the posttest probability (over pretest probability). For every test in every medical subspecialty, the magnitude of change between pretest probability and postest probability is determined by Bayes' theorem (214). Three factors alone determine the magnitude of the pretest to posttest change: sensitivity, specificity, and pretest probability. It is commonly assumed that sensitivity and specificity remain constant for a test. In truth, test-referral bias, a common occurrence in studies of weaning tests, leads to major changes in sensitivity and specificity (213). Likewise, major changes in pretest probability arise as a consequence of spectrum bias (213). All of these factors need to be carefully considered when reading a study that evaluates the reliability of a weaning predictor test.

Weaning Predictor Tests

Several weaning predictor tests have been proposed and studied over the years. These tests include measurements of breathing pattern, pulmonary gas exchange, muscle strength, and neuromuscular drive. Their goal is to safely speed up the weaning process (2).

Respiratory Frequency to Tidal Volume Ratio (f/V_T)

The ratio of respiratory frequency to tidal volume (f/V_T)† is measured during 1 minute of spontaneous breathing (5) (Fig. 132.22). Measurements of f/V_T in the presence of pressure support or continuous positive airway pressure (CPAP) will result in inaccurate predictions of weaning outcome (2). The higher the f/V_T ratio, the more severe the rapid, shallow breathing and the greater the likelihood of unsuccessful weaning. An f/V_T ratio of 100 best discriminates between successful and unsuccessful attempts at weaning (5).

The initial evaluation of f/V_T was reported in 1991 (5). Since then, this test has been evaluated in more than 25 studies. Reported sensitivity ranges from 0.35 to 1.00 (214). Specificity ranges from 0.00 to 0.89 (214). At first glance, this wide scatter suggests that f/V_T is an unreliable predictor of weaning outcome. Many of the investigators, however, ignored the possibility of test-referral bias and spectrum bias (2). These problems were compounded by an Evidence-Based Medicine Task Force of the American College of Chest Physicians (ACCP), who recently undertook a meta-analysis of the studies (216).

The Task Force calculated pooled likelihood ratios for f/V_T and judged the summated values to signify that f/V_T was not a reliable predictor of weaning success (216,217). The studies included in the meta-analysis, however, exhibited significant heterogeneity in pretest probability of successful outcome (214). Such marked heterogeneity prohibits the undertaking of a reliable meta-analysis (218,219). When data from the studies (included in the meta-analysis) were entered into a Bayesian model with pretest probability as the operating point, the reported positive predictive values were significantly correlated with the values predicted by the original report (5) on f/V_T, $r = 0.86$ ($p < 0.0001$); likewise, reported negative predictive values were correlated with the values predicted, $r = 0.82$ ($p < 0.0001$) (Figs. 132.23 and 132.24) (214).

†For example, for a spontaneous respiratory rate of 25 breaths per minute, and a spontaneous tidal volume of 600 mL (0.6 L), the $f/V_T = 25/0.6 = 41.7 = 42$.

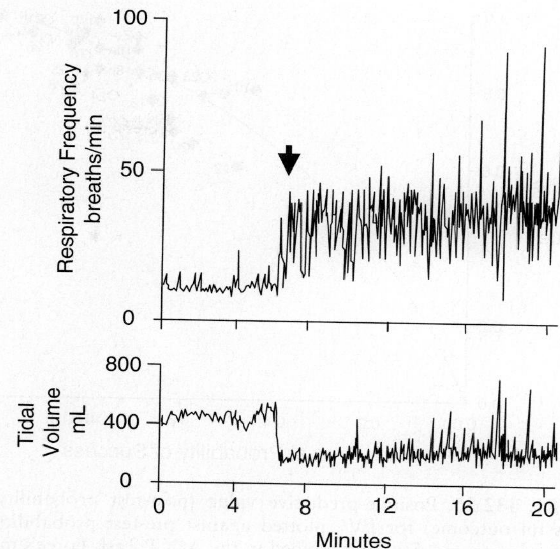

FIGURE 132.22. A time-series, breath-by-breath plot of respiratory frequency and tidal volume in a patient who failed a weaning trial. The *arrow* indicates the point of resuming spontaneous breathing. Rapid, shallow breathing developed almost immediately after discontinuation of the ventilator. (From Tobin MJ, Perez W, Guenther SM, et al. The pattern of breathing during successful and unsuccessful trials of weaning from mechanical ventilation. *Am Rev Respir Dis.* 1986;132:1111, with permission.)

The primary task of a weaning predictor test is screening, which requires a high sensitivity (2,213). The average sensitivity in all of the studies on f/V_T was 0.89, and 85% of the studies reveal sensitivities above 0.90 (214). This sensitivity compares well with commonly used diagnostic tests: creatine phosphokinase and troponin T for the diagnosis of acute myocardial infarction, sensitivity of 0.94 (2) and 0.98 (220), respectively; chest radiograph for lung cancer, 0.60 (2); stress electrocardiogram (ECG) for myocardial ischemia, 0.61 for women and 0.72 for men (221); and sensitivity to diagnose endocarditis of <0.60 to 0.70 with transthoracic echocardiography and between 0.75 and 0.95 with transesophageal echocardiography (222). The sensitivity of a spontaneous breathing trial is unknown.

Since screening is the primary purpose of a weaning predictor test, it is important that the test be performed early in a patient's ventilator course. Figures 132.23 and 132.24, however, reveal that pretest probability of weaning success was 75% or higher in more than half the studies of weaning predictor tests. In other words, most physicians are postponing (inappropriately) the undertaking of weaning predictor tests. A simple way for a physician to assess his or her own timeliness in initiating weaning is to estimate the number of times he or she obtained positive results on weaning predictor tests over the preceding 6 months. If a physician working in a typical medical ICU estimates that he or she obtained positive results 70% or more of the time, they should consider that they are being too slow in initiating weaning (2).

Pulmonary Gas Exchange

Mechanical ventilation is virtually never discontinued in a patient who has severe hypoxemia, such as arterial oxygen

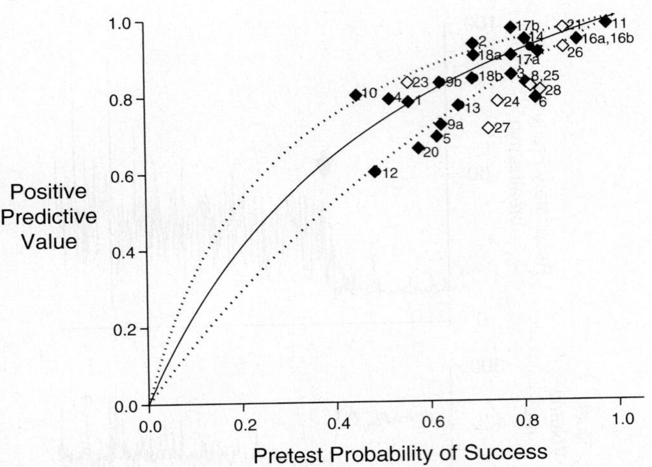

FIGURE 132.23. Positive-predictive value (post-test probability of successful outcome) for f/V_T plotted against pre-test probability of successful outcome. Studies included in the ACCP Task Force's meta-analysis (Meade M, Guyatt G, Cook D, et al. Predicting success in weaning from mechanical ventilation. *Chest,* 2001;120(6 Suppl):400S) are indicated by closed symbols; studies undertaken after publication of the Task Force's report are indicated by open symbols. The curve is based on the sensitivity, specificity originally reported by Yang and Tobin (Yang KL, Tobin MJ. A prospective study of indexes predicting the outcome of trials of weaning from mechanical ventilation. *N Engl J Med* 1991;324:1445) and Bayes' formula for 0.01-unit increments in pre-test probability between 0.00 and 1.00. The lines represent the upper and lower 95% confidence intervals for the predicted relationship of the positive predictive values against pre-test probability. The observed positive-predictive value in a study is plotted against the pre-test probability of weaning success (prevalence of successful outcome). Studies #5, #6, #11, #18a, #18b, and #24 include measurements of f/V_T obtained during pressure support. Studies #14 and #21 include measurements obtained in pediatric patients. Studies #7, #18a, #18b, and #28 used f/V_T threshold values <65. (**Modified from:** Tobin MJ, Jubran A. Variable performance of weaning-predictor tests: role of Bayes' theorem and spectrum and test-referral bias. *Intensive Care Med.* 2006;32:2002).

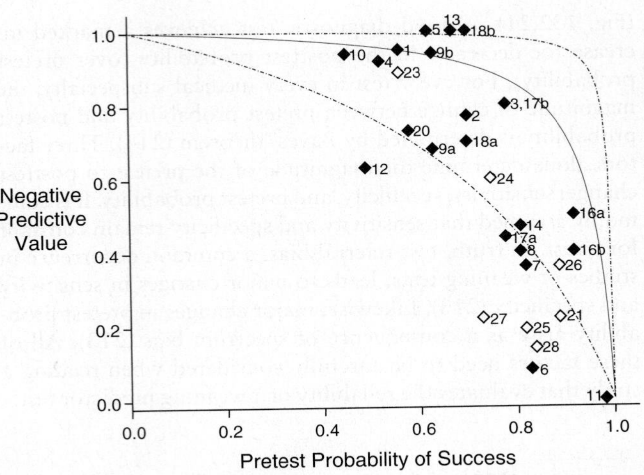

FIGURE 132.24. Negative-predictive value (post-test probability of unsuccessful outcome) for f/V_T. Studies included in the ACCP Task Force's meta-analysis (Meade M, Guyatt G, Cook D, et al. Predicting success in weaning from mechanical ventilation. *Chest,* 2001;120(6 Suppl):400S) are indicated by closed symbols; studies undertaken after publication of the Task Force's report are indicated by open symbols. The curve, its 95% confidence intervals, and placement of a study on the plot are described in the legend to Figure 132.23. The observed negative-predictive value in a study is plotted against the pre-test probability of weaning success (prevalence of successful outcome). Note study #11, which has a negative-predictive value of 0.00 and specificity of 0.00. These values suggest that f/VT is an unreliable test (and this will also be the natural conclusion reached by a meta-analysis of likelihood ratio). Instead, a negative-predictive value of 0.00 and specificity of 0.00 are the values predicted for the pre-test probability of weaning success of 98.2% reported in study #11. (**Modified from:** Tobin MJ, Jubran A. Variable performance of weaning-predictor tests: role of Bayes' theorem and spectrum and test-referral bias. *Intensive Care Med.* 2006;32:2002).

tension (PaO_2) less than 55 mm Hg with inspired oxygen fraction (FiO_2) greater than 0.40. Arterial-to-inspired oxygen ratio (PaO_2/FiO_2), alveolar-arterial oxygen tension gradient, and arterial/alveolar oxygen tension ratio (PaO_2/PAO_2) are indices derived from arterial blood gas measurements proposed as predictors of weaning outcome. Of these indices only PaO_2/PAO_2 has been prospectively evaluated, and it has performed poorly as a predictor of weaning outcome (5). The study (5) was marred by test-referral bias—i.e., patients with severe hypoxia were excluded from the study population. Therefore, it is not possible to conclude that the poor performance of PaO_2/PAO_2 means that indices derived from arterial blood gas measurements are of no value in predicting weaning outcome. While threshold values of the efficiency of indices derived from arterial blood gas measurements cannot be recommended for weaning prediction, weaning attempts are not recommended in patients with borderline hypoxemia.

Minute Ventilation

A minute ventilation of less than 10 L/minute was a classic index used to predict a successful weaning outcome (223). When prospectively assessed, however, minute ventilation has a high rate of false-negative and false-positive results and cannot be recommended as a predictor of weaning outcome (2).

Maximum Inspiratory Pressure

The use of maximum inspiratory pressure as a weaning predictor stems from a study by Sahn and Lakshminarayan (223). They found that all patients with a maximum inspiratory pressure value more negative than –30 cm H_2O were successfully weaned, whereas all patients with a maximum inspiratory pressure less negative than –20 cm H_2O failed a weaning trial. In most successive investigations, these threshold values have shown poor sensitivity and specificity (5,32,38,41–43).

Vital Capacity

The normal vital capacity is usually between 65 and 75 mL/kg, and a value of 10 mL/kg or more has been suggested to predict a successful weaning outcome (2). In a study of ten patients with Guillain-Barré syndrome, Chevrolet and Deleamont (224) reported that vital capacity was helpful in guiding the weaning process. Patients with a vital capacity of less than 7 mL/kg were unable to tolerate as few as 15 minutes of spontaneous breathing. As vital capacity increased to more than 15 mL/kg with recovery from the illness, patients were safely extubated. Apart from unique circumstances, such as patients with Guillain-Barré syndrome, vital capacity is rarely used as a weaning predictor, and it is often unreliable (2).

Airway Occlusion Pressure

Several investigators have evaluated the usefulness of $P_{0.1}$ as a predictor of weaning outcome (2). In these studies, $P_{0.1}$ values above 3.4 to 6.0 cm H_2O discriminated between weaning success and weaning failures (2). However, other investigators have found $P_{0.1}$ to be quite inaccurate (19). One mechanism that could contribute to the poor performance of $P_{0.1}$ is the limited reproducibility of the measurement. The within-individual coefficient of variation of $P_{0.1}$ is about 50% (225,226), and the interindividual coefficient of variation is as high as 60% (227).

Gastric Tonometry

The gastrointestinal mucosa becomes ischemic early with the development of either hemodynamic compromise or a redistribution of blood flow. One factor that leads to blood flow redistribution is an increase in respiratory muscle effort. Gastric tonometry is based on the principle that the carbon dioxide tension (PCO_2) of the fluid in the gastric lumen equilibrates with the PCO_2 of the mucosal layer, and that the recording of PCO_2 in gastric fluid provides a reliable estimate of the pH of the gut mucosa (228). The assumption that PCO_2 in the gastric lumen is similar to that in the tissues of the gastric wall, however, may not be true, especially in patients who experience an uneven distribution of gastric blood flow (2).

The accuracy of gastric tonometry as a predictor of weaning outcome has been investigated in five studies (229–233). These five studies differ in methodology, and they also reveal different patterns of abnormality for intramucosal pH and PCO_2 in patients undergoing weaning trials. Some investigators found that the measurements discriminated between the weaning-success and weaning-failure patients during mechanical ventilation (229,233), whereas others did not (230–232). If the ventilator was set at a level to achieve satisfactory muscle rest, it is difficult to see why gastric intramucosal pH should differ between the groups before the onset of spontaneous breathing. The studies reveal different levels of accuracy in predicting weaning outcome. The reported accuracy represents an overestimate because none of the investigators divided their data sets into training and validation subsets. Several investigators comment that the technique is simple. Yet it involves inserting a special intragastric tonometer, obtaining a radiograph to confirm location, the administration of histamine$_2$-receptor blockers, withholding enteral feeding, waiting a sufficient period of time for satisfactory equilibration, and withdrawing and analyzing a saline sample and an arterial blood gas (2).

WEANING TRIALS

When a screening test is positive—for example, a low f/V_T—the clinician proceeds to a confirmatory test (213), for example, pressure support of 6 to 8 cm H_2O or spontaneous respiration through a T tube. The goal of a positive result on a confirmatory test—no respiratory distress at the conclusion of the pressure support trial or T-tube trial—is to rule in a condition, in this case, a high likelihood that a patient will tolerate a trial of extubation (213). An ideal confirmatory test has a very low rate of false-positive results; that is, a high specificity (213). Unfortunately, the specificity of a spontaneous breathing trial is not known. Indeed, its specificity will never be known, because its determination would require an unethical experiment: extubating all patients who fail a weaning trial and counting how many require reintubation (2).

The major weaning techniques used include T-tube trial, pressure support ventilation, intermittent mandatory ventilation, or some combination of these three. Recently, noninvasive positive pressure ventilation has been used to facilitate extubation in selected patients.

Intermittent Mandatory Ventilation (IMV)

For many years, IMV was the most popular method of weaning from mechanical ventilation (234). With IMV weaning, the ventilator's mandatory rate is reduced in steps of one to three breaths per minute, and an arterial blood gas is obtained about 30 minutes after each rate change (235). Unfortunately, titrating the ventilator's mandatory rate according with the results of arterial blood gases can produce a false sense of security. As little as 2 to 3 IMV breaths per minute can achieve acceptable blood gases, but these values provide no information regarding the patient's work of breathing (2). At IMV rates of 14 breaths per minute or less, the patient's work of breathing may be excessive (236,237) both during the IMV breaths (ventilator-assisted breaths) and the intervening spontaneous breaths. The fact that, as the IMV rate is decreased, inspiratory work increases progressively not only for the spontaneous breaths, but also for the assisted breaths, is largely due to the inability of the respiratory center to adapt its output rapidly to intermittent support (237). By providing inadequate respiratory muscle rest, IMV is likely to delay, rather than facilitate, discontinuation of mechanical ventilation in difficult-to-wean patients (7). In easy-to-wean patients (patients who are successfully weaned at the first weaning attempt such as uncomplicated postoperative patients), weaning with IMV probably does not prolong the duration of mechanical ventilation (238).

Pressure Support

When pressure support is used for weaning, the level of pressure is reduced gradually and titrated on the basis of the patient's respiratory frequency (239). When the patient tolerates a minimal level of pressure support, he or she is extubated. What exactly constitutes a "minimal level of pressure support" has never been defined (240). For example, pressure support of 6 to 8 cm H_2O is widely used to compensate for the resistance imposed by the endotracheal tube and ventilator circuit (241). It is reasoned that a patient who can breathe comfortably at this level of pressure support will be able to tolerate extubation. However, if the upper airway is swollen because an endotracheal tube has been in place for several days, the work produced by breathing through the swollen airway is about the same as that caused by breathing through an endotracheal tube (241). Accordingly, any amount of pressure support may overcompensate for the resistance imposed by the endotracheal tube and ventilator circuit, and may give misleading information about the likelihood that a patient can tolerate extubation.

Recently, in a prospective, multicenter, randomized trial, Lellouche et al. (242) reported their experience with pressure support weaning using a computer-driven, closed-loop, knowledge-based algorithm. This algorithm included three basic functions. The first was an automatic gradual reduction in pressure support, with the goal of keeping the patient within a "comfort" zone (242). Comfort was defined as a respiratory rate ranging between 15 and 30 breaths/minute (up to 34 in patients with neurologic disease), a tidal volume above a minimum threshold (more than 250 mL if weight was less than 55 kg, and 300 mL otherwise), and end-tidal CO_2 level less than 55 mm Hg (less than 65 mm Hg in patients with COPD). The computerized system assesses the patient every 2 to 4 minutes, and, if considered necessary, it makes changes in the ventilator's output. The second function was an automatic performance of trials of minimal low-pressure support, which the investigators named "spontaneous breathing trials." The third was generation of an incentive message recommending separation from the ventilator when a spontaneous breathing trial was successfully passed. Of 1,014 eligible patients, 144 (14%) were included in the study—74 were randomized to the computer-driven weaning and 70 to physician-controlled weaning (T-tube trials, IMV trials, or trials of pressure support set at 7 to 12 cm H_2O). Computer-driven weaning reduced the median duration of weaning (3 vs. 5 days; $p = 0.01$), duration of mechanical ventilation (7.5 vs. 12 days, $p = 0.003$), and ICU stay (12 vs. 15.5 days, $p = 0.02$) (Fig. 132.25). Computer-driven weaning was not different from physician-driven weaning in terms of reintubation rate (16% vs. 23%, $p = 0.40$), hospital length of stay (30 vs. 35 days, $p = 0.22$), ICU mortality (22% vs. 23%, $p = 1.0$), and hospital mortality (38% vs. 29%, $p = 0.29$). As the investigators indicate, the study has some limitations including randomization of a small fraction of eligible patients, inability to blind the investigators to treatment assignment, and unclear knowledge of which patients may be poor candidates for computerized weaning. To this list should be included no record of tidal volume (243). The latter point is of relevance considering that in a preliminary study, Shannon et al. (244) reported that in one of ten patients, tidal volume during closed-loop pressure support ventilation was greater than 10 mL/kg. In the same preliminary study, Shannon et al. (244) reported that in two additional patients, closed-loop pressure support ventilation did not provide sufficient ventilatory assistance to unload the respiratory muscles and avoid sternocleidomastoid muscle contractions (244). Finally, in the study of Lellouche et al. (242), it was estimated that only half of the patients assigned to usual care underwent spontaneous breathing trials despite passing weaning criteria. This may have skewed the results in favor of computer-driven weaning. Despite its limitations, the promising investigation of Lellouche et al. (242) highlights the need for much earlier screening in weaning.

T-Tube Trials

The use of repeated T-tube trials several times a day is the oldest method for conducting a weaning trial (234). The patient receives an enriched supply of oxygen through a T-tube circuit. Initially 5 to 10 minutes in duration, T-tube trials are extended and repeated several times a day until the patient can sustain spontaneous ventilation for several hours. This approach has become unpopular because it requires considerable time on the part of the ICU staff.

Today, it is usual to limit a T-tube trial to once a day. Performing single daily T-tube trials is as effective as performing such trials several times a day (7) but much simpler. If the trial

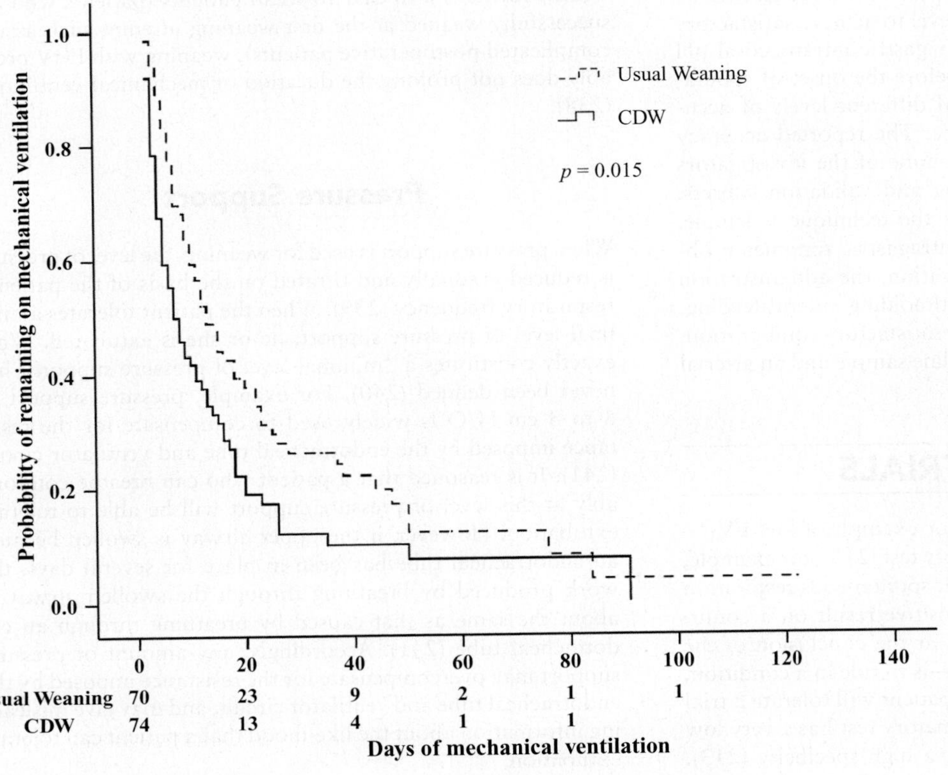

FIGURE 132.25. Kaplan-Meier analysis of weaning time until successful extubation or death in patients undergoing usual weaning ($n = 70$) and in patients undergoing computer-driven weaning (CDW)—i.e., computer-driven closed-loop knowledge-based algorithm ($n = 74$). The probability of remaining on mechanical ventilation was less with computer-driven weaning than with usual weaning (log-rank test, $p = 0.015$). (From Lellouche F, Mancebo J, Jolliet P, et al. A multicenter randomized trial of computer-driven protocolized weaning from mechanical ventilation. *Am J Respir Crit Care Med.* 2006;174:894, with permission.)

is successful, the patient is extubated. If the trial is unsuccessful, the patient is given at least 24 hours of respiratory muscle rest with full ventilator support before another trial is performed (2).

To assess whether the target duration of the single daily T-tube trials should be of 30 minutes or 120 minutes, Esteban et al. (9) conducted a prospective multicenter randomized trial of 526 patients who had received more than 48 hours of ventilation and who were considered ready for weaning. The rate of reintubation within 48 hours in patients randomized to trials lasting 30 minutes (14%) was equivalent to the rate of reintubation in patients randomized to trials lasting 120 minutes (13%). The two groups had similar ICU mortality rates and similar in-hospital mortality rates. The findings of this study suggest that, among patients with a high rate of weaning success (patients undergoing a first weaning attempt), a single daily T-tube trial with a target duration of 30 minutes is as effective in identifying patients who can be safely extubated as a single daily T-tube trial with target duration of 120 minutes. This study did not address the target duration of single daily T-tube trials in difficult-to-wean patients (patients who fail one or more weaning attempts).

Patients are judged to have failed a T-tube trial when they develop severe tachypnea, increased accessory muscle activity, diaphoresis, facial signs of respiratory distress, oxygen desaturation, tachycardia, arrhythmias, hypertension, or hypotension. The degree of change in these variables, however, varies from report to report. A standardized approach to patient monitoring during a T-tube trial does not exist. Indeed, there is no agreement as to whether the monitoring of any variable helps in deciding whether to continue a T-tube trial for an initially planned duration, prolong it, or curtail it (2).

Jubran et al. (245) investigated whether repeated measurements of esophageal pressure throughout a trial of spontaneous breathing might provide additional guidance over a single measurement obtained during the first minute of the trial. They quantified the change in esophageal pressure over the first 9 minutes of the trial using a multivariate adaptive regression spline procedure (Fig. 132.26). In a study of 60 patients (31 in the derivation data set and 29 in the prospective validation data set), an esophageal pressure trend index had a sensitivity of 0.91 and specificity of 0.89. Specifically, an esophageal pressure trend index reading of less than or equal to 0.44 was 8.2 times more likely to occur in weaning failure than in weaning success patients. These data suggest that, when available, the continuous monitoring of esophageal pressure swings during a T-tube trial may provide additional guidance in patient management over tests used for deciding when to initiate weaning.

Noninvasive Ventilation in Weaning

Noninvasive positive pressure ventilation (NIPPV) has been used to facilitate extubation in intubated patients with COPD and acute hypercapnic respiratory failure.

Nava et al. (246) studied 50 patients with COPD who had been intubated due to acute hypercapnic respiratory failure and who had failed a T-tube trial after 36 to 48 hours of mechanical ventilation. Patients were randomized to either immediate extubation with noninvasive pressure support ventilation via a face mask, or continued pressure support ventilation via the endotracheal tube. In both groups, the pressure support level was decreased by 2 to 4 cm H_2O per day as tolerated. In addition, all patients underwent trials of spontaneous breathing at least twice per day in an attempt to discontinue mechanical ventilation entirely. At the end of the trial, the investigators reported that noninvasive pressure support ventilation during weaning increased weaning rates at 60 days (88% vs. 68%), decreased the incidence of nosocomial pneumonia (0% vs. 28%), and significantly lowered 60-day mortality rates (8% vs. 28%). Noninvasive ventilation was generally well tolerated, although 14 of 25 patients developed nasal abrasions, and 2 developed gastric distention. By study design, patients were excluded if they had concomitant severe comorbidities—e.g., neurologic diseases, cancer, cardiogenic pulmonary edema, acute myocardial infarction, gastrointestinal bleeding, sepsis, trauma, diabetic ketoacidosis, coagulopathy, and other hematologic diseases. Postoperative patients were also excluded.

In a second trial, Girault et al. (247) studied 33 patients with either COPD, restrictive lung disease, or mixed obstructive-restrictive disease. Patients had been intubated due to acute-on-chronic respiratory failure and had failed a 2-hour T-piece

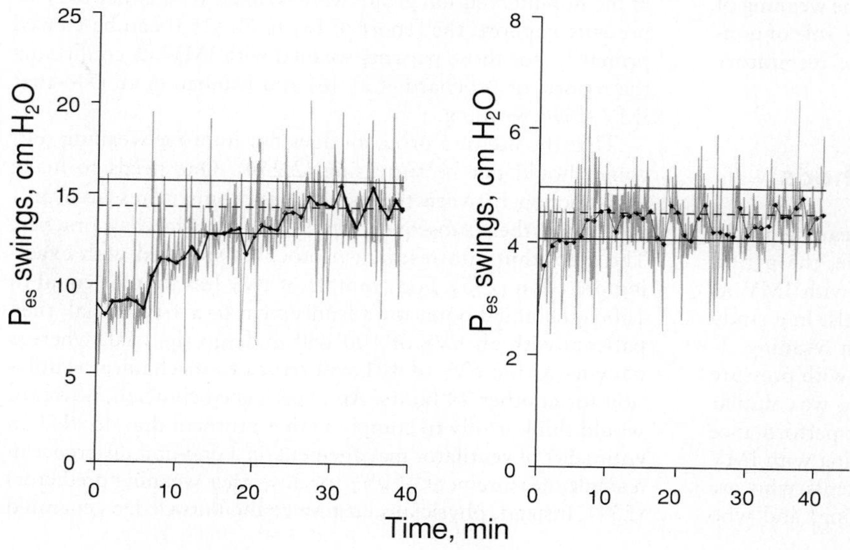

FIGURE 132.26. Time-series plot of swings in esophageal pressure (Pes) in a weaning failure (**left**) and a weaning success patient (**right**) during a trial of spontaneous breathing. *Black dots* represent 1-minute averages. The *solid line* indicates the average value of Pes swings of the final minute of the trial. The *dashed lines* indicate ±10% of the final minute values of Pes swings. The time taken to reach ±10% of the final value for Pes swings was 14 minutes for the failure patient and 6 minutes for the success patient. (From Jubran A, Grant BJ, Laghi F, et al. Weaning prediction: esophageal pressure monitoring complements readiness testing. *Am J Respir Crit Care Med.* 2005;171:1252, with permission.)

trial after an average of 4.5 days of mechanical ventilation. Patients were randomized to either immediate extubation and noninvasive ventilation—either assist-control ventilation or pressure support ventilation—via a face mask, or continued pressure support ventilation via the endotracheal tube. The noninvasive ventilation group had a shorter period of intubation (5 ± 2 vs. 8 ± 4 days, $p = 0.004$), but there were no differences in hospital and ICU lengths of stay or in mortality. By study design, patients were excluded if they had a history of difficult intubation at the start of invasive mechanical ventilation or had a history of recent gastrointestinal surgery or ileus. Patients with swallowing disorders, ineffective cough, or persistence of bronchial congestion at the time of weaning were also excluded.

A third randomized trial on the usefulness of noninvasive ventilation as a weaning aid was conducted by Ferrer et al. (248). They enrolled 43 patients who had failed once-daily T-tube trials for three consecutive days; 44% of patients had COPD. Twenty-one patients were assigned to extubation, followed by immediate noninvasive ventilation (inspiratory positive airway pressure [IPAP], 10 to 20 cm H_2O, and expiratory positive airway pressure [EPAP], 4 to 5 cm H_2O); 22 patients were reconnected to the ventilator and underwent conventional weaning with daily T-tube trials. An interim analysis after half the planned number of patients had been studied revealed a superior outcome in the noninvasive ventilation arm, and the study was stopped. Features of the better outcome in the noninvasive ventilation group—as compared to conventional weaning—included a higher ICU survival, 20% versus 14%; shorter duration of invasive ventilation, 10 versus 20 days; shorter ICU stay, 14 versus 25 days; shorter hospital stay, 28 versus 41 days; less frequent tracheotomy, 2% versus 14%; lower incidence of nosocomial pneumonia, 5% versus 14%; and lower incidence of septic shock, 2% versus 9%.

The three preceding studies suggest that noninvasive ventilation may be beneficial if instituted at the point when certain patients, in particular those with COPD, have just failed their first (246,247) or third T-tube trial (248). At this point, however, it is premature to recommend the routine use of noninvasive ventilation as weaning mode in patients with hypercapnic respiratory failure. Nonetheless, if the success of noninvasive ventilation is replicated in other trials, noninvasive ventilation may become an important adjunct in the weaning of such patients. Insufficient data are available on the role of noninvasive ventilation in weaning from hypoxemic respiratory failure.

Comparison of Weaning Methods

When assessed in difficult-to-wean patients, weaning methods are not equally effective (234). For example, the period of weaning is as much as three times as long with IMV as with T-tube trials (7) or pressure support (6) trials. In a study involving patients with respiratory difficulties on weaning, T-tube trials halved the weaning time as compared with pressure support (7); in another study, the weaning time was similar with the two methods (6). In contrast to the poor performance of IMV in difficult-to-wean patients (6,7), weaning with IMV in patients who are not difficult to wean (patients who are successfully extubated at the first trial of weaning) and who require short-term mechanical ventilation (less than 72 hours) is probably as effective as weaning with T-tube trials (238).

Weaning by Protocol versus Usual Care

The use of human-driven protocols for weaning versus usual care has been compared in six randomized controlled trials (3,249–253). The reports of Namen et al. (249), Randolph et al. (250), and Krishnan et al. (251) show no advantage for a protocol approach. The reports of Kollef et al. (3), Marelich et al. (252), and Ely et al. (253) are viewed as evidence for the superiority of a protocol approach to weaning.

In the trial of Kollef et al. (3), however, no advantage for weaning by protocol was observed in three of the four study ICUs. In the fourth unit, where a significant advantage for a protocol approach to weaning was observed, patients assigned to usual care were significantly sicker than the patients assigned to protocol management in that ICU; this confounding factor markedly weakens (if not destroys) any assertion that protocol weaning was superior (2).

Marelich et al. (252) studied weaning by protocol in two ICUs and found no significant advantage in one. The study of Ely et al. (253) does not consist of a straightforward comparison of protocol versus nonprotocol care. All of the patients in the intervention arm were weaned by T-tube or flow-by trials, whereas no patient in the nonintervention arm was weaned by T-tube or flow-by trials. Seventy-six percent of the patients in the nonintervention arm were managed by IMV alone or in combination with pressure support. Even if at the time of weaning all patients in the nonintervention arm happened to be managed with pressure support alone (and, unfortunately, this information is not provided in the manuscript) (253), the fact remains that the weaning techniques used in the intervention group (T tube) and in the nonintervention group were not the same. With this fundamental difference in techniques, it is impossible to use data from this study to form a judgment about the efficacy of a protocol *per se*. Instead, if all patients in the nonintervention group were weaned with pressure support, the report of Ely et al. (253) can be viewed primarily as confirming the report of Esteban et al. (7)—that T-tube weaning may be superior to pressure support weaning, and, if patients in the nonintervention group were weaned with either IMV or pressure support, the report of Ely et al. (253) can be viewed primarily (for those patients weaned with IMV) as confirming the reports of Brochard et al. (6) and Esteban et al. (7)—that IMV slows weaning.

That the use of a protocol does not improve weaning outcome should not be surprising (2,254). One needs to make a distinction between the use of algorithms in research protocols and their subsequent application in everyday practice. The algorithm in a research protocol is specified with exacting precision (255). For example, if f/V_T less than or equal to 100 is the nodal point for advancement to a T-tube trial, then patients with an f/V_T of 100 will undergo the trial, whereas patients with a f/V_T of 101 will return to mechanical ventilation for another 24 hours. An experienced clinician, however, would think it silly to comply with a protocol that decided an entire day of ventilator management on a one-unit difference in a single measurement of f/V_T (or any other weaning predictor) (254). Instead, physicians customize the knowledge generated by research to the particulars of each patient. The careful application of physiologic principles is likely to outperform an inflexible application of a protocol.

EXTUBATION

Decisions about weaning and extubation are commonly merged. Merging these two decisions, however, can cause patient mismanagement (256). When a patient tolerates a weaning trial without distress, a clinician feels reasonably confident that the patient will be able to sustain spontaneous ventilation after extubation. However, passing a weaning trial without distress is not the only consideration. The clinician also must consider whether the patient will be able to maintain a patent upper airway after extubation.

Removal of an endotracheal tube is typically performed under controlled conditions (256)—the patient has satisfactorily tolerated a weaning trial. Enteral feeding is temporally withheld for about 4 hours. When possible, the head of the bed should be at 30 to 90 degrees from the horizontal (257). The endotracheal tube, mouth, and upper airway are suctioned, paying attention to the collection of secretions above an inflated cuff, as inadequate clearing of secretions can result in postextubation laryngospasm (257). Some clinicians recommend keeping a suction catheter in place (aiming for the catheter to barely protrude from the distal end of the endotracheal tube) as the cuff is deflated; this step is taken in an attempt to capture any secretions sitting on top of an inflated cuff that may fall into the airway after deflating the cuff. Some clinicians inflate the lungs with an Ambu bag immediately before pulling out the endotracheal tube, hoping that the larger-than-usual ensuing exhalation will push secretions upward and outward (258). The cuff is then deflated, and the endotracheal tube is withdrawn. After removal of the endotracheal tube, the patient is given supplemental oxygen, titrated to oxygen saturation, being particularly cautious with a patient who is at risk of carbon dioxide retention. Patients may have impaired airway protection reflexes immediately after extubation (259,260), and aspiration can be silent—that is, aspiration can occur without coughing (261). If speech is impaired for more than 24 hours, indirect laryngoscopy should be undertaken to assess vocal cord function. Oral intake should be delayed in patients who have been intubated for a prolonged period (259,260).

In the hours following extubation, patients are carefully monitored for their ability to protect the upper airway and sustain ventilation. Most patients will display progressive improvement, allowing the discontinuation of supplemental oxygen and ultimate discharge from the ICU. Between 2% and 30% (232,242,262–266) of patients, however, experience respiratory distress in the postextubation period. Many, but not all, require reinsertion of the endotracheal tube and mechanical ventilation. These patients are commonly classified as *extubation failures*. In contrast to the relatively short time required to recognize that a patient is failing a weaning trial, the time course for the development of postextubation distress extends over a longer span. In the study of Epstein et al. (267), for example, 33% of reintubations occurred within the first 12 hours after extubation, and 42% occurred after 24 hours.

Causes of Postextubation Distress

The listed indications for reintubation vary considerably from study to study. Of these, postextubation upper airway obstruction has attracted the most attention.

Postextubation Upper Airway Obstruction

Upper airway obstruction is one of the most urgent and potentially lethal medical emergencies. Complete airway obstruction lasting for as little as 4 to 6 minutes can cause irreversible brain damage (13). The upper airway, which encompasses the passage between the nares and carina, can be obstructed by functional or anatomic causes. Among the first are vocal cord paralysis, paradoxical vocal cord motion, and laryngospasm (13,268,269). Among the second are trauma (including arytenoid dislocation) (270,271), burn, granulomas, infections, foreign bodies, tumors, tracheomalacia, compression by a hematoma in close proximity to the airway (272), and supraglottic, retroarytenoidal or subglottic edema (256,273,274). Edema can develop after only 6 hours of intubation (275). A thinner mucosa covering the cartilage of the vocal processes, less resistance to trauma, and smaller laryngeal diameter are probably responsible for the greater prevalence of laryngeal edema in female than male patients (276–279). Other risk factors associated with the development of laryngeal edema include traumatic intubation, excessive tube size, excessive tube mobility secondary to insufficient fixation, a patient fighting against the tube or trying to speak, excessive pressure in the cuff, too frequent or too aggressive tracheal suctioning, occurrence of infections or hypotension, and the presence of a nasogastric tube that predisposes to gastroesophageal reflux (273,278,280). It is also possible that a biochemical reaction between the tube material and the airway mucosa may cause laryngeal edema (273). Life-threatening obstruction, either functional or anatomic, can occur postoperatively in patients with redundant pharyngeal soft tissue—such as in sleep apnea—and loss of muscle tone related to the postanesthetic state (13).

Several investigators have reported that upper airway obstruction accounts for about 15% of patients requiring reintubation (9,267,281). When upper airway obstruction occurs, it typically becomes manifest within 3 to 12 hours after extubation (273,276,280). In the case of postextubation laryngeal edema, symptoms occur within 5 minutes postextubation in 47% of patients, within 6 to 30 minutes post extubation in 33% of patients, and after more than 30 minutes post extubation in 20% of patients (279). Symptoms rarely occur until 75% of the upper airway lumen has been obliterated (282,283). Occasionally, symptoms may not occur until the diameter of the airway is reduced to 5 mm (284).

Upper airway obstruction causes stridor only if the patient is capable of generating sufficient airflow; if airflow is insufficient, obstruction may cause hypercapnia, hypoxemia, or paradoxical breathing, but not stridor. Women are more susceptible to postextubation stridor than men (276–278). Among patients who develop stridor, 1% to 69% require reintubation (276,277,280,285). Many (276,278,280,285), but not all (277–279), investigators have noted that the rate of postextubation stridor increases in proportion to the duration of mechanical ventilation. Stridor usually occurs during inhalation in presence of extrathoracic airway obstruction and during exhalation in the presence of intrathoracic airway obstruction, and it can be biphasic with midtracheal stenosis (286, 287).

The first warning of airway obstruction in an unconscious patient may be failure of a jaw-thrust maneuver to open the airway or the inability to ventilate with a bag-valve. In a conscious patient, respiratory distress, stridor, altered voice—such as aphonia or dysphonia—snoring, dysphagia, odynophagia, prominence of neck veins, and neck and facial swelling all may indicate impending airway obstruction (13). Patients may bring their hands to their neck, a sign of choking. Other signs include suprasternal and intercostal retractions, and reduced or absent air movement on auscultation. Wheezing may be present or absent. Thoracoabdominal paradox may be prominent. Sympathetic discharge is high, and patients are diaphoretic, tachycardic, and hypertensive. As asphyxia progresses, bradycardia, hypotension, and death ensue (13). Arterial blood gases are not particularly helpful, because they are not specific to airway patency (288). They may show little change until a patient is *in extremis* (288).

Other Causes of Postextubation Distress

Conditions other than upper airway obstruction that cause postextubation distress include respiratory failure, congestive heart failure, aspiration or excessive secretions, encephalopathy, and other conditions (267). The frequency of a particular cause differs among studies. For example, cardiac failure accounted for 23% of the cases of Epstein et al. (267), 7% of the cases of Esteban et al. (9), but none of the cases of Smina et al. (281) or De Bast et al. (273).

Consequences of Postextubation Distress

Mortality among patients who require reintubation is more than six times as high as mortality among patients who can tolerate extubation (9); the reason for the higher mortality is unknown. It might be related to the development of new problems after extubation. In support of this possibility is the observation of Epstein et al. (267) that mortality increases in proportion to the time between extubation and reintubation: mortality of 24%, 39%, 50%, and 69% in patients reintubated between 0 and 2, 13 and 24, 25 and 48, and 49 and 72 hours after extubation, respectively. A second explanation is that the need for reintubation reflects greater severity of the underlying illness (256). In only a minority of patients, mortality is due to complications associated with reinsertion of a new tube (256).

In the subgroup of patients in whom postextubation distress results specifically from upper airway obstruction, complications include, but are not limited to, anoxic brain injury, cardiopulmonary arrest, and death (289,290). Upper airway obstruction can be complicated by pulmonary edema (13), with an incidence of 11% in one adult series (291), or pulmonary hemorrhage (292). Increased venous return, with more negative intrathoracic pressure and catecholamine-induced venoconstriction, contributes to pulmonary edema, but it cannot be the sole mechanism; as intrathoracic pressure becomes more negative, venous return to the right ventricle becomes flow limited (293). Other factors contributing to pulmonary edema include decreased left ventricular preload (leftward shift of interventricular septum), increased left ventricular afterload (increased negative intrathoracic pressure and catecholamine-induced elevation of systemic vascular resis-

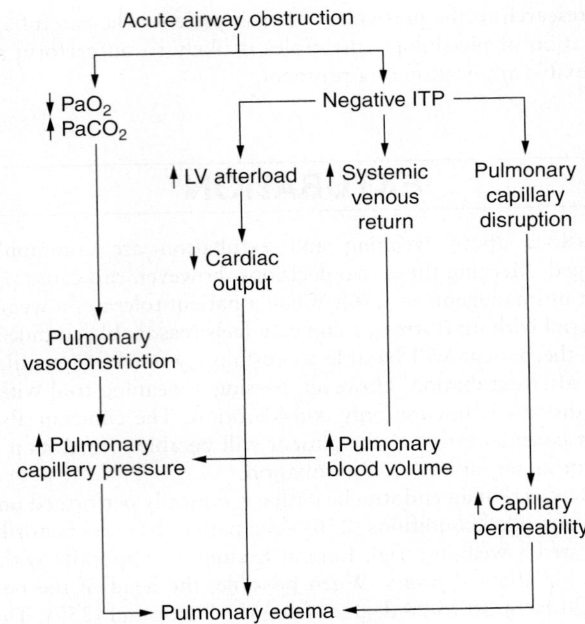

FIGURE 132.27. Mechanisms responsible for the development of pulmonary edema formation during acute airway obstruction. ITP, intrathoracic pressure; LV, left ventricle. (From Miro AM, Pinsky MR. Heart-lung interactions. In: Tobin MJ, ed. *Principles and Practice of Mechanical Ventilation*. 1st ed. New York, NY: McGraw-Hill; 1994:647, with permission.)

tance), pulmonary vasoconstriction (hypoxemia and acidosis), and, possibly, stress failure of the alveolar-capillary membrane (292) (Fig. 132.27).

Whether pulmonary edema develops during or after relief of upper airway obstruction may depend on whether the obstruction is fixed or variable (294). Fixed upper airway obstruction results in vigorous inspiratory efforts (Mueller maneuver), followed by vigorous expiratory efforts (Valsalva maneuver) (291,294). Exhalation against an obstructed airway raises intrathoracic and alveolar pressures. The positive expiratory pressure decreases pulmonary vascular filling and opposes the hydrostatic forces that favor transudation of fluid into the alveoli during inhalation (291). With a sudden relief of obstruction, positive expiratory pressure is lost; consequently, there is a massive transudation of fluid from the pulmonary interstitium into the alveoli, resulting in pulmonary edema over minutes to hours. In contrast to fixed obstruction, variable extrathoracic upper airway obstruction hinders inhalation, and exhalation is usually unaffected. In this situation, the hydrostatic forces that favor transudation of fluid into the alveoli during inhalation are unopposed, leading to edema before the obstruction is relieved (294).

Predictors of Postextubation Distress

Because reintubation causes serious complications in some patients, attempts are made to predict its likely occurrence. Several physiologic variables have been evaluated for their ability to predict this likelihood (Table 132.3). For some patients, the likelihood of reintubation is considered so high that a clinician

TABLE 132.3

POSSIBLE PREDICTORS OF POSTEXTUBATION DISTRESS

Ability to sustain spontaneous ventilation
Weaning predictor tests
Cuff-leak test
Laryngeal ultrasound
Secretions and cough
Neurologic assessment
Respiratory drive in the postextubation period

may proceed to tracheotomy without first attempting extubation (256).

Ability to Sustain Spontaneous Respiration

A true-positive result of a T-tube trial is defined as a patient who tolerates the trial without distress, is then extubated, and does not require reintubation (256). The usual rate of reintubation is 15% to 20%—sometimes lower—but higher reintubation rates have been reported by some investigators: 24% (295), 25% (231), 27% (232), 29% (264,265). These false-positive test results—that is, patients who tolerate the T-tube trial but require reintubation after extubation—mean that the positive predictive value and specificity of passing a T-tube trial in predicting that a patient will not require reintubation is less than 100%. To measure the false-negative rate (Fig. 132.21) would require extubation of patients who fail a T-tube trial and counting how many do *not* require reintubation. For obvious ethical reasons, this number is not known. Given the natural caution of physicians, it can be confidently assumed that it is higher than 0% (256).

Weaning Predictor Tests

Several investigators have examined the ability of weaning predictor tests to predict the development of distress after extubation. The question posed is along these lines: "Does f/VT, or some other predictor test, measured before a T-tube trial, predict the likelihood of reintubation?" To answer this question with scientific validity, it is imperative to avoid test-referral bias. This can be avoided if the investigators take steps to ensure that clinicians do *not* perform a T-tube trial or are *not* taking the results of the T-tube trial into account when deciding whether to extubate the study patients. In other words, a decision to extubate the patient must be taken before the T-tube trial, and must proceed even if the patient exhibits significant distress during the trial, a strategy that raises ethical concerns.

Zeggwagh et al. (296) are the only group of investigators who assessed the ability of weaning predictor tests to forecast development of distress after extubation without performing a weaning trial (after the weaning predictors had been recorded). The investigators prospectively studied 101 patients at the point that their ICU physicians contemplated weaning. They measured a series of physiologic measurements during 2 minutes of spontaneous breathing; the results of these measurements were not communicated to the primary team. The team then extubated the patients without first undertaking any form of weaning trial. The extubation decision was made by the ICU team based on the following criteria: improvement or resolution of the condition precipitating the need for mechanical ventilation; good level of consciousness with cessation of all sedative agents; temperature less than 38°C; respiratory frequency less than 35 breaths per minute; oxygen saturation greater than 90% on an FiO_2 less than or equal to 0.40; hemodynamic stability; and the absence of electrolyte disorders, acid-base disturbance, or anemia (defined as a hemoglobin less than 10 g/dL).

Reintubation was necessary in 37% of the patients. Several variables predicted the need for reintubation with a reasonable degree of accuracy. For example, f/VT had a sensitivity of 0.77 and a specificity of 0.79, with an area under a receiver operating curve (ROC) of 0.81 ± 0.06; maximum expiratory pressure had a sensitivity of 0.52 and a specificity of 0.92, with an area under a ROC of 0.73 ± 0.07. The investigators developed a model based on three variables: f/VT, maximum expiratory pressure, and vital capacity. The area under the ROC for the model was 0.91 ± 0.04 for a development data series and 0.86 ± 0.06 for a validation data series. The accuracy of weaning predictors to predict the development of distress after extubation in this study (296) contrasts sharply with their limited accuracy in studies where the investigators permitted a weaning trial (which altered clinician's extubation decisions) between measurement of the predictors and extubation (256). This difference in diagnostic accuracy is likely due to test-referral bias (2). An important aspect of this study (296) is that the results suggest that undertaking a weaning trial before extubation is useful; the rate of reintubation in the study of Zeggwagh et al. (296) was about double that reported in studies in which weaning trials preceded extubation (256).

Cuff-Leak Test

The presence of an endotracheal tube makes it extremely difficult to evaluate the structure and function of the airway before extubation. The amount of air leaking around the outside of an endotracheal tube on deflating the balloon cuff has been used by several investigators to predict upper airway obstruction after extubation (Fig. 132.28). The idea was first reported by Adderley and Mullins (297), who studied 31 planned extubations in 28 children with croup. After extubation, reintubation was required in 13% of children who had an audible leak

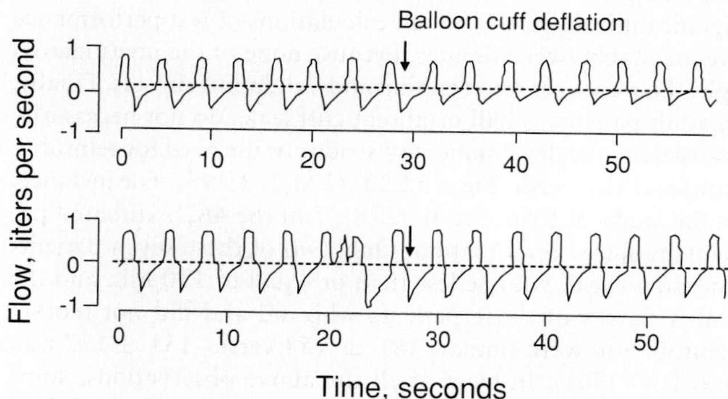

FIGURE 132.28. Tracings of inspiratory flow (*upgoing*) and expiratory flow (*downgoing*) in two patients before and after deflation of the cuff on the endotracheal tube (*arrow*). The patient in the upper panel had a large leak (positive test result): after deflation of the cuff, expiratory flow became substantially smaller than inspiratory flow. The patient in the lower tracing had a small leak (less than 12% of inspired tidal volume; negative test result): expiratory flow exhibited little if any decrease after cuff deflation. (**Modified from:** Jaber S, Chanques G, Matecki S, et al. Post-extubation stridor in intensive care unit patients. Risk factors evaluation and importance of the cuff-leak test. *Intensive Care Med.* 2003;29:69).

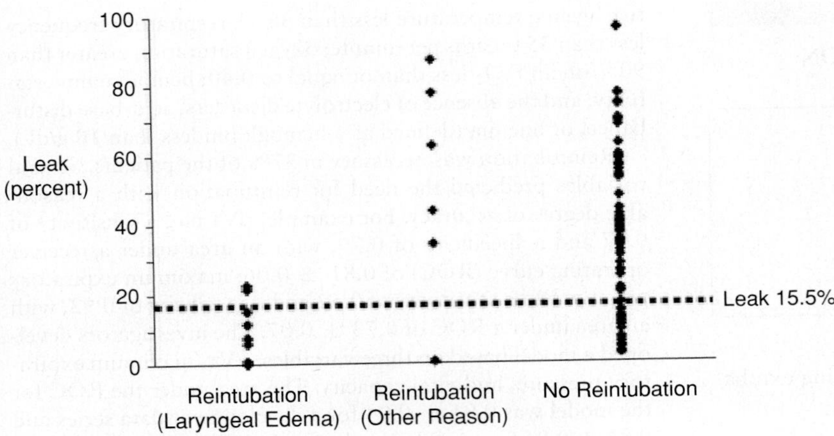

FIGURE 132.29. Cuff leak calculated as the percent difference between exhaled tidal volume when the cuff of the endotracheal tube was inflated and then deflated. Eight of 76 patients (11%) required reintubation for laryngeal edema. In this study, patients requiring reintubation for laryngeal edema had a smaller leak than the other patients. The best cut-off value for air leak was 15.5%. Small or absent cuff leaks, however, did not necessarily translate in reintubation. The positive predictive value of a leak less than 15.5% was only 25%—i.e., a patient with a small cuff leak still had 75% chance of being extubated without requiring reintubation for laryngeal edema. (**Modified from:** De Bast Y, De Backer D, Moraine JJ, et al. The cuff leak test to predict failure of tracheal extubation for laryngeal edema. *Intensive Care Med.* 2002;28:1267).

(on coughing or when plateau pressure was 40 cm H_2O), and reintubation was required in 38% of children without a leak. The cuff-leak test has since been evaluated by numerous investigators (273,278,280,285,298–300). For several reasons, however, it is difficult to provide general recommendations on how to perform and interpret a cuff-leak test (256).

First, the method for performing the test has not been standardized. In particular, none of the investigators addressed the setting of inspired tidal volume, which may influence the size of the leak; the method for quantifying the leak varies between absolute units (milliliters) and percentage of inspired tidal volume. Second, the outcome criterion is not always clearly stated: rate of reintubation for any reason, occurrence of stridor of any severity, or occurrence of stridor that requires reintubation. The rates of stridor vary considerably among studies, suggesting that investigators used different criteria; admittedly, it is not obvious that severity of stridor can be graded in any reproducible manner. Third, in some studies, it is not clear whether the investigators carefully excluded reasons for reintubation other than stridor. If a patient is reintubated because of left ventricular failure, it is not logical to expect the cuff-leak test to predict such an event. Fourth, the thresholds for defining a significant leak vary. Fifth, all calculations of test performance are inevitably overestimates, because none of the investigators split their data set into training and validation subsets. Finally, in adult patients, small or absent cuff leaks do not necessarily translate in the development of stridor or the need for reintubation, and vice versa (Fig. 132.29) (273,278,299). For instance, in the study of Kriner et al. (278), 7 of the 462 extubated patients required reintubation. Only two of these seven patients had an air leak volume less than or equal to 110 mL, and the leak volumes of those patients who did and did not require reintubation were similar: 181 ± 158 versus 131 ± 137 mL, $p = 0.47$ (301). In view of all the above observations, some investigators reason that in adult patients, failing a cuff-leak test should not be used as an indication for either delaying extubation or initiating other specific therapy (278,299,301) but, possibly, as an indicator of increasing vigilance at the time of extubation (301). Factors that may contribute to small or absent cuff leaks in patients who do not develop postextubation distress include the following: secretions located around the endotracheal tube, head and neck position, presence or absence of sedation, and large endotracheal tube relative to the size of the patient's larynx (278,302).

Laryngeal Ultrasound

In intubated patients, laryngeal ultrasonography can delineate the anatomic structures of the larynx, and it can record the shape and width of the column of air—both within and around the endotracheal tube—which passes through the vocal cords (302). Using laryngeal ultrasonography in 51 patients considered ready for extubation (4 developed postextubation stridor and 2 of them required reintubation), Ding et al. (302) measured the difference in width of the column of air passing through the vocal cords when the cuff of the endotracheal tube was inflated and the corresponding value when the cuff was deflated (Fig. 132.30). The smaller the difference in width, the greater the likelihood of postextubation stridor (302). As the investigators indicate, the study was not designed to assess how the column of air passing through the trachea, as detected by ultrasonography, could be affected by secretions located around the endotracheal tube, cross-sectional dimension of the endotracheal tube relative to the dimensions of the patient's airway, and wakefulness; all patients were studied while sedated to avoid the confounding effect of cough on ultrasound signals. Based on this single study, it is premature to recommend laryngeal ultrasonography as a screening tool before extubation.

Secretions and Cough

A proportion of patients fail either a weaning attempt or an extubation attempt because of excessive airway secretions. This proportion varies among reports, largely because there is no consistent definition of "excessive secretions" or even how best to quantify secretions (256). If one quantifies secretions according to the volume obtained by suctioning over a fixed time interval, a patient who coughs and expels secretions without difficulty may get classified as having a greater secretion problem than a patient who has thick viscid secretions that cannot be dislodged from the lower airways (256).

Investigators have recently evaluated measurements of secretions as predictors of postextubation distress (281,303–306). Khamiees et al. (303) attempted to quantify cough strength by placing a white card 1 to 2 cm from the end of the endotracheal tube and requesting the patient to cough as many as three or four times just before extubation. Any wetness on the card was classified as a positive test (assessment was made by a single observer). This test was seen as

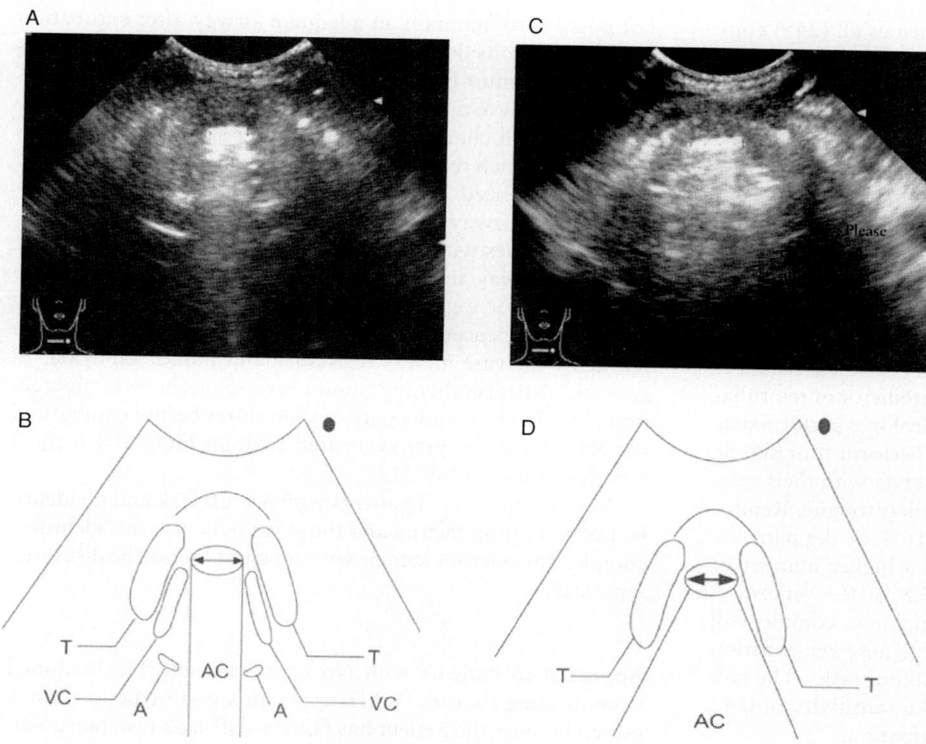

FIGURE 132.30. Laryngeal ultrasound in an intubated patient who did not develop postextubation stridor. When the cuff on the endotracheal tube is inflated—ultrasound (A) and schematic illustration (B)—the column of air (AC) passing trough the true vocal cords (VC) is square-shaped. The hypoechoic true vocal cords can be seen on both sides of the air column. The hyperechoic arytenoid cartilages are located behind the true vocal cords and next to the air column. When the cuff is deflated—ultrasound (C) and schematic illustration (D)—the column of air passing trough the true vocal cords becomes trapezoid and the air column width increases. In addition, the acoustic shadow of the laryngeal air column masks the arytenoid cartilages and part of the true vocal cords. *Arrow*, width of the air column; T, thyroid cartilage. (From Ding LW, Wang HC, Wu HD, et al. Laryngeal ultrasound: a useful method in predicting post-extubation stridor. A pilot study. *Eur Respir J.* 2006;27:384, with permission.)

a test of cough strength and not of the amount of secretions present. They studied 100 extubations in 91 patients; 18 patients were classified as extubation failures, and 11 were reintubated within 72 hours of extubation (the criteria for classifying the other seven patients as extubation failures are not clear). Extubation failure was three times more likely in patients with a negative white-card test (no secretions coughed onto the card). Three other measures also predicted extubation failure. Extubation failure was four times more likely among patients who had a weak or absent cough than in patients with a moderate or strong cough. Extubation failure was eight times more likely in patients classified as having moderate or abundant secretions by the nursing staff in the 4 to 6 hours preceding extubation than in patients with absent or mild secretions. Extubation failure was 16 times more likely among patients whose secretions required suctioning every 2 hours or less.

Salam et al. (304) of the same investigation group undertook a further study of predictors of reintubation in 88 patients who underwent 100 extubations; extubation failure was defined as reintubation. Reintubation within 72 hours was required in 16% of the patients. The cough peak flow was lower in reintubated patients than in patients successfully extubated (SE): 58 ± 5 (SE) versus 80 ± 4 L/minute. A threshold peak flow of less than or equal to 60 L/minute had a sensitivity 0.77, specificity 0.66, likelihood ratio of 2.3, and risk ratio of 4.8. The investigators also re-evaluated the white-card test described by Khamiees et al. (303) and found that it did not predict reintubation. Clearly, physicians in the study of Salam et al. (304) had reduced the number of extubations attempted in patients with larger volumes of secretions. The physicians had altered their pretest probability of extubation failure based on the need for frequent suctioning. The physicians refused to advance such patients to extubation (test-referral bias), and thus the results of the study give an erroneous impression that frequent suctioning is not a good predictor of reintubation. (A limitation of the white-card test is that it will be negative in patients with a strong cough who have few or no secretions.) The volume of secretions collected in the 2 to 3 hours before extubation was equivalent in reintubated and successfully extubated patients: 2.5 ± 0.9 versus 2.3 ± 0.4 mL/hour, respectively. A threshold of greater than 2.5 mL secretions per hour, however, did discriminate between the groups: sensitivity 0.71, specificity 0.62, likelihood ratio 1.9, and risk ratio 3.0.

Neurologic Assessment

Some ventilated patients demonstrate good respiratory function and tolerate a T-tube trial without distress, yet their physicians are reluctant to extubate them because they fear that the patients will not be able to protect their airway after extubation (256). Inability to protect the airway can be caused, among other factors, by unsatisfactory neural control over the upper airway, such that the tongue (in a recumbent patient) may fall back and occlude the airway lumen, as happens in patients with sleep apnea. It can also be caused by impaired laryngeal and other upper airway reflexes, placing patients at risk of aspiration of secretions or of ingested food.

Concern about protecting the airway most often arises in a patient with evidence of brain injury. Three groups of investigators—Coplin et al. (305), Namen et al. (249), and Salam et al. (304)—have studied the role of brain function in patients being considered for extubation. The most careful study is that by Coplin et al. (305), who studied 136 brain injury patients. Based on their data, these investigators (305) concluded that a depressed level of consciousness—quantified with the Glasgow coma scale score—and absence of a gag reflex should not be used as the sole indication for prolonged intubation.

In contrast to Coplin et al. (305), Namen et al. (249) concluded that a Glasgow coma scale score of greater than or equal to 8 helps in predicting successful extubation in brain injury patients. A fundamental problem with this second study (249) is that half of the extubations were part of the withdrawal of life-support therapy; hence, all of these patients died. Because these patients were not reintubated, it appears that the authors classified them as extubation successes. Irrespective of how these patients were classified, it is impossible to interpret data on extubation predictors where half of the extubations arose from a decision to withdraw life support.

The studies of Coplin et al. (305) and Namen et al. (249) were conducted in patients with brain injury, whereas Salam et al. (304) studied neurologic function as a predictor of reintubation in medical-cardiac ICU patients. Neurologic performance was quantified by requesting patients to perform four simple tasks (307): open their eyes, follow an observer with their eyes, grasp the observer's hand, and stick out their tongue. Reintubation within 72 hours was required in 16% of the patients. Patients tolerating extubation performed a higher number of tasks than did the reintubated patients: 3.8 ± 0.1 versus 2.9 ± 0.5, respectively. Patients who were unable to complete all four tasks were 4.3 times more likely to require reintubation than were patients who could complete all four tasks. The failure to perform any of the four tasks had a sensitivity of 0.42 and specificity of 0.91 in predicting reintubation.

Respiratory Neuromuscular Drive in the Postextubation Period

Increased neuromuscular drive ($P_{0.1}$ greater than 5 cm H_2O) 20 minutes into a T-tube weaning trial has been reported to predict the need for reintubation, with a sensitivity of 0.87 and a specificity 0.91 (308). In contrast to $P_{0.1}$ values recorded during a T-tube trial (308), measurements of $P_{0.1}$ during a pressure support weaning trial are less accurate in predicting the need of reintubation (309). In patients with COPD, a rise in $P_{0.1}$ 30 minutes after extubation (as compared to $P_{0.1}$ values before extubation) may predict the development of postextubation distress (310). Limitations of these studies include lack of prospective validation of $P_{0.1}$ thresholds and, for the latter study, the need to institute noninvasive ventilation for the sole purpose of measuring $P_{0.1}$ in all extubated patients.

Treatment of Postextubation Distress

When considering therapies for postextubation distress, it is useful to categorize patients into two groups: patients in whom upper airway obstruction is responsible for postextubation distress, and patients in whom postextubation distress is not due to upper airway obstruction.

Treatment of Postextubation Distress due to Upper Airway Obstruction

The clinical approach to patients with upper airway obstruction must be dictated by great caution, as difficulty or inability to reintubate a patient can cause excess morbidity, including anoxic brain injury and death (289,290). Each patient requires an individualized therapeutic approach; therefore, definite recommendations are problematic (290). Nevertheless, intensivists should have a preplanned strategy for extubation of the difficult airway, including plans to be implemented if it is not possible to maintain an adequate airway after extubation (290). Close consultation with an anesthesiologist and an otolaryngologist must be part of this strategy. Because recommendations on how to approach difficult extubations are essentially based on small clinical series or case reports, the appropriate weighting of each recommendation is a matter of judgment and may be influenced by specific expertise at particular institutions. Upper airway obstruction may worsen suddenly because resistance varies with the fourth power of the radius. A slight change in airway anatomy may dramatically increase resistive load (311). For example, manipulation of the upper airway by an inexperienced clinician may induce edema, which can markedly increase airway resistance and induce asphyxia. In general, pharmacotherapy cannot reverse mechanical obstruction (13). To ensure adequate oxygen stores before extubation, patients should be preoxygenated with an FiO_2 of 1.0 for 3 minutes or more (290,312).

Steps for the care of patients with no cuff leak and no identified complicating factors and those for patients with identified complicating factors with or without cuff leak will be discussed separately.

Approach to Patients with No Cuff Leak and No Identified Complicating Factors. When upper airway obstruction is suspected because the patient has failed a cuff-leak test, one possibility is to proceed with extubation while having an anesthesiologist at the bedside. Intubation equipment has to be readily accessible (313). If the patient develops postextubation distress, and reintubation is deemed necessary, the anesthesiologist is immediately available to proceed with reinsertion of the endotracheal tube.

Before extubation, the anesthesiologist may consider placement of an airway exchange catheter (AEC) through the endotracheal tube (Fig. 132.31) (314–317). Following extubation, the AEC is secured, and humidified oxygen can be insufflated through its central lumen. If the patient does not develop stridor or other signs of respiratory difficulty, the exchange catheter is removed after a variable period of time; exchange catheters have been left in place for up to 72 hours (314). If, however, the patient develops postextubation respiratory distress, and reintubation is deemed necessary, the AEC (with or without the help of laryngoscope) (257) can be used to facilitate reintubation (314–316). Should tracheal reintubation prove complicated, jet ventilation can be delivered through the AEC as a bridge to more definitive treatment (258,312,315). To avoid the risk of aspiration, patients should not be fed enterally while the AEC is in place (315).

Occasionally, extubation is performed over a bronchoscope. The bronchoscope provides the opportunity to visually assess the upper airway. When significant abnormalities are noted, the operator must decide whether to immediately reinsert the endotracheal tube or to withdraw the bronchoscope and treat the patient conservatively (see below, racemic epinephrine, heliox, and corticosteroids). Recently (272), the laryngeal mask airway device has been successfully used to rescue the airway in patients with upper airway obstruction when emergency tracheal intubation with direct laryngoscopy was impossible. When using laryngeal mask airway devices without grills, a flexible bronchoscope can be passed through the mask to assess the upper airway, and catheter-guided intubation can be performed through the device (272).

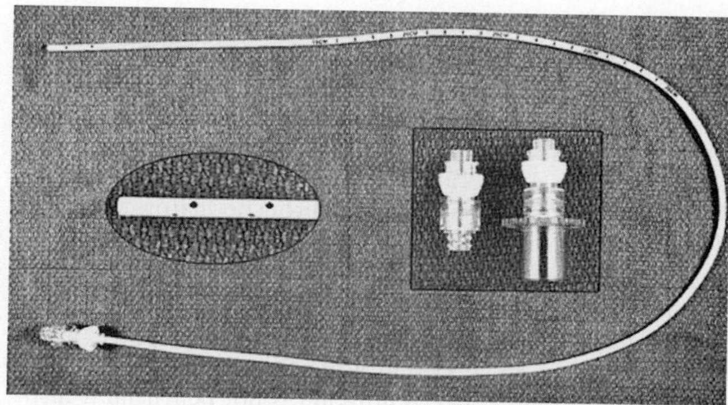

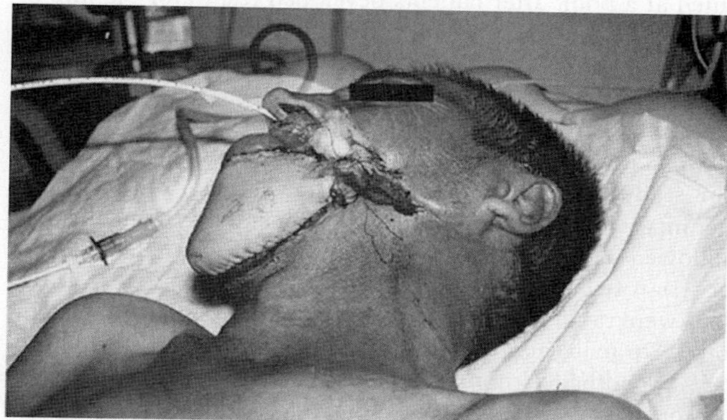

FIGURE 132.31. Top: The airway exchange catheter is a semirigid catheter designed to maintain airway access following tracheal extubation. **Left insert:** In the distal 3 cm several side holes are built into the catheter to allow delivery of gas if needed. **Right insert:** In the proximal end, a 15-mm connector for attachment to oxygen tubing (**right**) and a Luer lock connector (**left**) for attachment to jet ventilator circuit. (From Loudermilk EP, Hartmannsgruber M, Stoltzfus DP, et al. A prospective study of the safety of tracheal extubation using a pediatric airway exchange catheter for patients with a known difficult airway. *Chest.* 1997;111:1660, with permission.) **Bottom:** A representative patient following maxillofacial reconstructive surgery. The airway exchange catheter is emerging from the right nostril and is connected to an oxygen source. At the time of surgery, the endotracheal tube—through which the airway exchange catheter had been introduced at the time of extubation—was placed nasally. Airway exchange catheters have been used as stylets to facilitate reintubation of medical and surgical patients through the oral and nasal routes (see text for details). (From Dosemeci L, Yilmaz M, Yegin A, et al. The routine use of pediatric airway exchange catheter after extubation of adult patients who have undergone maxillofacial or major neck surgery: a clinical observational study. *Crit Care.* 2004;8:R385, with permission.)

When the patient develops postextubation distress with stridor, but immediate reintubation is not considered necessary, some intensivists administer aerosolized epinephrine or racemic epinephrine (as long as the compounds are not contraindicated) (258,315). In adults, aerosolized racemic epinephrine has been given at doses ranging from 0.25 to 0.75 mL of a 2.25% solution in 2.0 to 3.5 mL of normal saline (258,315,319). In patients with laryngeal edema, the response to aerosolized epinephrine or racemic epinephrine can be dramatic but short-lived (318). Therefore, if there is a positive response and patients do not develop side effects, nebulization of epinephrine or racemic epinephrine can be repeated every 1 to 4 hours (318,319); repeated doses of racemic epinephrine every 30 to 60 minutes have also been used (315). Racemic epinephrine consists of equal amounts of the dextro-isomers and levo-isomers. Most of epinephrine's pharmacologic action results from the levo-isomer, which is 30 times more potent than the dextro-isomer (256). Popularity of the more expensive racemic form is based on the supposition that it produces epinephrine's vasoconstrictor action without rebound vasodilation. In addition, less tachycardia, hypertension, and tremor are expected with aerosolized racemic epinephrine than with levo-epinephrine. The stated different actions, however, may have arisen from comparisons of inappropriate dosages (256). In children with postextubation stridor, levo-epinephrine is as effective as the more expensive racemic epinephrine (320).

High-dose corticosteroids—for example, dexamethasone 4 to 8 mg intravenously every 8 to 12 hours (321,322), tapered based on symptoms—may be administered alone or together with aerosolized racemic epinephrine. Whether corticosteroids should be administered before extubation in children (323,324) or in adults (276–279,300) remains controversial. In a recent investigation conducted in 761 adult patients who had been intubated for more than 36 hours, François et al. (279) reported that, compared to placebo, intravenous methylprednisolone started 12 hours before a planned extubation reduced the incidence of postextubation laryngeal edema from 22% to 3% (p <0.0001) and reduced the incidence of reintubation from 8% to 4% (p = 0.02). The investigators reason that the ineffectiveness of corticosteroids in preventing laryngeal edema reported in previous studies (276,277,325) probably resulted from incorrect timing of administration—all positive trials started corticosteroids 6 to 24 hours before planned extubation (279,300,324), whereas all negative trials started corticosteroids 30 minutes to 6 hours before extubation (276,277,323,325).

François et al. (279) assessed eligibility for extubation (by an unreported mechanism) and then left the patients intubated for a period lasting no less than 12 hours to allow for administration of corticosteroids (or placebo) before proceeding with planned extubation. This strategy was likely conducive to a conservative approach to extubation as supported by the low number of canceled extubations (five patients or 1.3% in the placebo group and three patients or 0.8% in the methylprednisolone group). If such delay indeed occurred in some patients, the extubation strategy of François et al. (279) would be a departure from what is the common practice of most intensivists—i.e., to extubate patients at the earliest feasible time to decrease the risk of iatrogenic complications including ventilator-associated pneumonia. Given the above considerations, it would seem premature to administer intravenous steroids 12 hours before planned extubation in every patient who has been intubated for more than 36 hours. However, for those patients in whom the intensivist has a high suspicion for laryngeal edema (and who do not have contraindications to steroids), the strategy of François et al. (279) seems justifiable.

For patients who do not require high FiO_2, helium-oxygen mixture (Heliox) may be tried (322,326–331). The goal of this low-density gas mixture is to reduce work of breathing by decreasing the pressure drop associated with turbulent flow across the obstruction.[‡] In most cases of airway obstruction, the response to heliox can be seen in minutes (327). If heliox

[‡]Mixtures of heliox and oxygen containing less than 70% helium are probably of little or no mechanical benefit (326).

is ineffective, it is likely that turbulent flow is not playing an important role in the patient's stridor. Even when effective, the use of helium-O_2 mixtures should not engender a false sense of security (311).

Finally, some authors have used noninvasive ventilation—CPAP (274) or bilevel positive airway pressure (BiPAP) (302,326,331)—alone or in combination with heliox (328). Neither heliox nor noninvasive ventilation have curative properties on their own. Yet, they may be able to "buy time" until the underlying cause of upper airway obstruction has resolved (e.g., laryngeal edema treated with high-dose corticosteroids). None of these pharmacologic and nonpharmacologic strategies has been studied systematically. If stridor does not respond to initial measures or recurs while patients are being treated with noninvasive ventilation, reintubation is usually necessary.

Racemic epinephrine, systemic corticosteroids, heliox, and noninvasive ventilation should be used only in carefully selected patients. Occasionally, the decision to defer intubation may give time to the obstruction of the upper airway to progress to a point at which intubation becomes more difficult, if not impossible (326). Similarly, pharmacologic strategies and noninvasive ventilation should not supplant endotracheal intubation when the upper airway obstruction is critical and expected to progress, e.g., upper airway infection, upper airway tumor awaiting surgery or radiation therapy (326).

Approach to Patients with Identified Complicating Factors with or without Cuff Leak. It may be prudent to have both an anesthesiologist and an otolaryngologist available at bedside–the latter with a tracheostomy tray open and ready to use–during extubation of patients with difficult airway. This category includes patients who fail a cuff-leak test and/or had stridor during the original intubation; have a history of self-extubation or in whom the original intubation was difficult or traumatic; patients who had undergone maxillofacial or major neck surgery; morbidly obese patients; or those with soft tissue swelling. Patients with cervical immobility or instability are also at risk of postextubation respiratory failure (315). If the patient develops postextubation distress, and he/she cannot be immediately be re-intubated, a surgical airway *via* cricothyrotomy or tracheostomy should be immediately considered. If time permits, and the patient is conscious and still ventilating and oxygenating adequately, some clinicians consider it best to transport the patient to the operating room (288), otherwise the procedure should be performed at the bedside. Although percutaneous tracheostomy is gaining in popularity, it is best performed in an already intubated patient and not as an emergency procedure (288). Jet ventilation through a 14-gauge angiocatheter passed through the cricothyroid membrane is occasionally used as a bridge for more definitive therapy (332,333). This technique is often marred with complications, and operator experience is usually limited (326). In selected patients, extubation should be performed in the operating room.

Unless upper airway tumor is considered as a possible cause of upper airway obstruction, endoscopic visualization of the upper airway before extubation has limited value (334), and it is usually not performed. In some high-risk patients, clinicians may decide to perform an elective tracheostomy (315). A patient with an obstructed airway should not be sedated until the airway has been secured, as minimal sedation may precipitate acute respiratory failure (13).

Treatment of Postextubation Distress Not due to Upper Airway Obstruction

As with patients developing postextubation distress due to upper airway obstruction, patients developing postextubation distress due to other causes require individualized therapy, e.g., chest tube for pneumothorax, bronchodilators for bronchoconstriction, and diuretics for volume overload or negative pressure pulmonary edema (13). In addition to specific therapies, noninvasive ventilation has also been used in patients developing postextubation distress not due to upper airway obstruction (266,335). Two groups of investigators, however, reported that noninvasive ventilation is not beneficial if instituted at a point after patients developed respiratory failure in the 48 hours after extubation (266,335). This contrasts with the accumulating data on the successful use of noninvasive ventilation in weaning (246–248).

Keenan et al. (335) studied patients who had received more than 48 hours of mechanical ventilation (overall, 4–5 days). In this study, one of the exclusion criteria was prior history of upper airway obstruction. All study patients were extubated and followed for 48 hours. Of 358 eligible patients, 23% developed criteria of respiratory distress. Of the patients with distress, half were randomly assigned to standard therapy (supplemental O_2 to maintain oxygen saturation greater than or equal to 95%), and half to noninvasive ventilation. The rate of reintubation was equivalent for the two groups: 72% for noninvasive ventilation and 69% for usual care, as was hospital mortality (31% for both groups). The duration of conventional mechanical ventilation tended to be shorter with noninvasive ventilation: 8 $\pm$ 7 versus 18 $\pm$ 28 days ($p = 0.11$). After the first year of the study, the investigators judged it unethical to withhold noninvasive ventilation in patients with COPD because of published data indicating the superior performance of patients with COPD with noninvasive ventilation. As a result, when the study was concluded, only 11% of the study population had COPD.

Like Keenan et al. (335) and Esteban et al. (266) also investigated the value of instituting noninvasive ventilation in patients after they have developed postextubation distress. All study patients were extubated and then followed for 48 hours. Of 980 eligible patients, 25% (244/980) developed criteria of respiratory distress. Urgent reintubation was necessary in 23 patients (2 patients were reintubated due to upper airway obstruction). Of the remaining patients, 114 were randomly assigned to noninvasive ventilation and 107 to usual care. Reintubation was required in 48% of patients in the noninvasive ventilation group and in 48% of patients in the usual care group. Reasons for reintubation included persistent respiratory distress, lack of improvement in pH or $PaCO_2$, hypoxemia, hypotension, copious secretions, and change in mental status; no patient was reintubated because of upper airway obstruction. Mortality in the ICU was higher with noninvasive ventilation, 25%, than with usual care, 14% ($p = 0.048$). The interval between extubation and reintubation was longer in the noninvasive ventilation group than in the usual care group: 12 versus 2.5 hours ($p = 0.02$).

An important aspect of this study (266) concerns the patients who were randomized to the usual care arm. When these patients developed distress and satisfied criteria for intubation, physicians had a choice to either reintubate them or manage them with noninvasive ventilation. Among the 28 patients who were crossed over to noninvasive ventilation, mortality was

11%. These 28 patients represent a sicker subgroup of the 107 patients in the usual care group, yet they had the lowest mortality of all groups requiring ventilator support. Of all patients receiving noninvasive ventilation in the study, these 28 patients were the only ones in whom it was instituted based on a physician's clinical judgment. Thus, it is possible that instituting noninvasive ventilation based on clinical judgment, as opposed to a random allocation, at the point of first observing respiratory distress has a major influence on the success of noninvasive ventilation.

COPD was not an exclusion criterion in the study of Esteban et al. (266). Yet, the fraction of patients with COPD in that study, 10%, was no higher than that in the study of Keenan et al. (335), 11%. The relatively low number of patients with COPD in both studies may have been a major factor in the failure to demonstrate a benefit with noninvasive ventilation. In the study of Esteban et al. (266), the average time between the institution of noninvasive ventilation (for postextubation distress) and reintubation was 12 hours. A substantial proportion of these patients had a decrease in oxygen saturation to less than 85%. It is perhaps not surprising that patients with significant respiratory failure of this magnitude over a prolonged period would experience a higher mortality after reintubation. Although the role of noninvasive ventilation in the management of postextubation distress in patients with COPD is not resolved by these studies, noninvasive ventilation does not appear to have a role in the treatment of other causes of postextubation distress.

A striking feature of the two negative studies is the limited inspiratory assistance that was provided. Patients received IPAP and EPAP settings of 9 and 4 cm H_2O, respectively, in the study of Keenan et al. (335), which is equivalent to pressure support of 5 cm H_2O. Delivered V_T was as little as 5 mL/kg in the study of Esteban et al. (266)—a tidal volume setting too low for most patients in acute respiratory failure, with the possible exception of patients with acute respiratory distress syndrome. The low assistance setting in these two negative studies contrasts with a pressure support setting of 19 ± 2 cm H_2O in the study of Nava et al. (246) and the IPAP and EPAP settings of 10 to 20 cm H_2O and 4 to 5 cm H_2O, respectively, in the study of Ferrer et al. (248). Application of a face mask connected to an inadequate level of positive pressure may pose an impediment for patients, and may have contributed to the negative outcomes in these two studies (266,335).

The only study that has addressed the role of noninvasive ventilation in the prevention of postextubation distress was conducted by Jiang et al. (336). They instituted noninvasive ventilation—initially at IPAP 12 cm H_2O and EPAP 5 cm H_2O—immediately after extubation. Reintubation was required in 13 of the 47 patients (28%) randomly assigned to noninvasive ventilation and in 7 of the 46 (15%) of patients assigned to usual care. The major problem with this study is that only 56 of the study patients were electively extubated after weaning; the other 37 (40%) patients were enrolled after unplanned extubation. Patients who experience unplanned extubation have a substantially higher rate of reintubation than electively extubated patients, yet the investigators did not state whether these patients were evenly distributed between the two arms of the study. They also do not state how many of their patients had COPD.

In summary, two studies (266,335) suggest that noninvasive ventilation is not beneficial in postextubated patients when instituted after they already have clinical manifestations of respiratory distress. It is possible, however, that noninvasive ventilation is beneficial in the subgroup with COPD. In the two negative studies, it is possible that an inadequate level of positive pressure was supplied to properly test its usefulness in postextubated patients. One can also argue that noninvasive ventilation was unlikely to be beneficial when instituted at such a late stage. An attempt has been made to address the question of whether noninvasive ventilation can prevent the development of postextubation distress (336), but it is not possible to form any conclusion because of the limitations of the study.

SUMMARY

In conclusion, to reduce the possibility of delayed weaning or premature extubation, clinicians should contemplate a two-step diagnostic strategy: first, measurement of weaning predictors and second, a weaning trial. Each step constitutes a diagnostic test, and therefore clinicians must be aware of the scientific principles of diagnostic testing when they interpret the information produced by each step (2). The key point is for physicians to consider the possibility that a patient *just may* be able to tolerate weaning. Such diagnostic triggering is facilitated through use of a screening test and is the rationale for measurement of weaning predictor tests (2). A positive result on a screening test (weaning predictor test) is followed by a confirmatory test (weaning trial) to increase the possibility that a patient will successfully tolerate extubation. It is important not to postpone the use of a screening test by waiting for a more complex diagnostic test, such as a T-tube trial. In contrast to our greater understanding of the pathophysiology of weaning failure, our understanding of the pathophysiology of severe respiratory distress in the postextubation period is rudimentary.

ACKNOWLEDGMENT

I am grateful to Dr. Martin Tobin for comments when discussing specific contents of this chapter with him.

Supported by a Merit Review Grant from the Veterans Administration Research Service

References

1. Epstein SK. Complications associated with mechanical ventilation. In: Tobin MJ, ed. *Principles and Practice of Mechanical Ventilation.* 2nd ed. New York, NY: McGraw-Hill: 2006:877–902.
2. Tobin MJ, Jubran A. Weaning from mechanical ventilation. In: Tobin MJ, ed. *Principles and Practice of Mechanical Ventilation.* 2nd ed. New York, NY: McGraw-Hill; 2006:1185–1220.
3. Kollef MH, Shapiro SD, Silver P, et al. A randomized, controlled trial of protocol-directed versus physician-directed weaning from mechanical ventilation. *Crit Care Med.* 1997;25(4):567–574.
4. Epstein SK. Etiology of extubation failure and the predictive value of the rapid shallow breathing index. *Am J Respir Crit Care Med.* 1995;152(2): 545–549.
5. Yang KL, Tobin MJ. A prospective study of indexes predicting the outcome of trials of weaning from mechanical ventilation. *N Engl J Med.* 1991;324(21):1445–1450.
6. Brochard L, Rauss A, Benito S, et al. Comparison of three methods of gradual withdrawal from ventilatory support during weaning from mechanical ventilation. *Am J Respir Crit Care Med.* 1994;150(4):896–903.

7. Esteban A, Frutos F, Tobin MJ, et al. A comparison of four methods of weaning patients from mechanical ventilation. Spanish Lung Failure Collaborative Group. *N Engl J Med.* 1995;332(6):345–350.
8. Rossi A, Poggi R, Roca J. Physiologic factors predisposing to chronic respiratory failure. *Respir Care Clin N Am.* 2002;8(3):379–404.
9. Esteban A, Alia I, Tobin MJ, et al. Effect of spontaneous breathing trial duration on outcome of attempts to discontinue mechanical ventilation. Spanish Lung Failure Collaborative Group. *Am J Respir Crit Care Med.* 1999;159(2):512–518.
10. West JB. *Pulmonary Pathophysiology: The Essentials.* 6th ed. Philadelphia, PA: Lippincott Williams & Wilkins; 2003:68.
11. Gluck EH. Predicting eventual success or failure to wean in patients receiving long-term mechanical ventilation. *Chest.* 1996;110(4):1018–1024.
12. Younes M. Mechanisms of ventilatory failure. *Curr Pulmonol.* 1993;14:243–292.
13. Laghi F, Tobin MJ. Indications for mechanical ventilation. In: Tobin MJ, ed. *Principles and Practice of Mechanical Ventilation.* 2nd ed. New York, NY: McGraw-Hill; 2006:129–162.
14. Jubran A, Tobin MJ. Pathophysiologic basis of acute respiratory distress in patients who fail a trial of weaning from mechanical ventilation. *Am J Respir Crit Care Med.* 1997;155(3):906–915.
15. Vassilakopoulos T, Zakynthinos S, Roussos C. The tension-time index and the frequency/tidal volume ratio are the major pathophysiologic determinants of weaning failure and success. *Am J Respir Crit Care Med.* 1998;158(2):378–385.
16. van den BB, Bogaard JM, Hop WC. High fat, low carbohydrate, enteral feeding in patients weaning from the ventilator. *Intensive Care Med.* 1994;20(7):470–475.
17. Tobin MJ, Perez W, Guenther SM, et al. The pattern of breathing during successful and unsuccessful trials of weaning from mechanical ventilation. *Am Rev Respir Dis.* 1986;132(6):1111–1118.
18. Sassoon CS, Te TT, Mahutte CK et al. Airway occlusion pressure. An important indicator for successful weaning in patients with chronic obstructive pulmonary disease. *Am Rev Respir Dis.* 1987;135(1):107–113.
19. Montgomery AB, Holle RH, Neagley SR, et al. Prediction of successful ventilator weaning using airway occlusion pressure and hypercapnic challenge. *Chest.* 1987;91(4):496–499.
20. Gandia F, Blanco J. Evaluation of indexes predicting the outcome of ventilator weaning and value of adding supplemental inspiratory load. *Intensive Care Med.* 1992;18(6):327–333.
21. Purro A, Appendini L, De Gaetano A, et al. Physiologic determinants of ventilator dependence in long-term mechanically ventilated patients. *Am J Respir Crit Care Med.* 2000;161(4 Pt 1):1115–1123.
22. Milic-Emili J, Aubier M. Some recent advances in the study of the control of breathing in patients with chronic obstructive lung disease. *Anesth Analg.* 1980;59(11):865–873.
23. Laghi F, Tobin MJ. Disorders of the respiratory muscles. *Am J Respir Crit Care Med.* 2003;168(1):10–48.
24. Tobin MJ, Gardner WN. Monitoring of the control of breathing. In: Tobin MJ, ed. *Principles and Practice of Intensive Care Monitoring.* New York, NY: McGraw-Hill; 1998:415–464.
25. Laghi F. Assessment of respiratory output in mechanically ventilated patients. *Respir Care Clin N Am.* 2005;11(2):173–199.
26. Murciano D, Boczkowski J, Lecocguic Y, et al. Tracheal occlusion pressure: a simple index to monitor respiratory muscle fatigue during acute respiratory failure in patients with chronic obstructive pulmonary disease. *Ann Intern Med.* 1988;108(6):800–805.
27. Cooper KR, Phillips BA. Effect of short-term sleep loss on breathing. *J Appl Physiol.* 1982;53(4):855–858.
28. Spengler CM, Shea SA. Sleep deprivation per se does not decrease the hypercapnic ventilatory response in humans. *Am J Respir Crit Care Med.* 2000;161(4 Pt 1):1124–1128.
29. Zakynthinos SG, Vassilakopoulos T, Roussos C. The load of inspiratory muscles in patients needing mechanical ventilation. *Am J Respir Crit Care Med.* 1995;152(4 Pt 1):1248–1255.
30. D'Angelo E, Calderini E, Robatto FM, et al. Lung and chest wall mechanics in patients with acquired immunodeficiency syndrome and severe *Pneumocystis carinii* pneumonia. *Eur Respir J.* 1997;10(10):2343–2350.
31. Appendini L, Purro A, Patessio A, et al. Partitioning of inspiratory muscle workload and pressure assistance in ventilator-dependent COPD patients. *Am J Respir Crit Care Med.* 1996;154(5):1301–1309.
32. Laghi F, Cattapan SE, Jubran A, et al. Is weaning failure caused by low-frequency fatigue of the diaphragm? *Am J Respir Crit Care Med.* 2003;167(2):120–127.
33. Parthasarathy S, Jubran A, Laghi F, et al. Sternomastoid, rib-cage and expiratory muscle activity during weaning failure. *J Appl Physiol.* 2007; 103(1):140–147. Epub 2007 Mar 29.
34. Zakynthinos SG, Vassilakopoulos T, Zakynthinos E, et al. Contribution of expiratory muscle pressure to dynamic intrinsic positive end-expiratory pressure: validation using the Campbell diagram. *Am J Respir Crit Care Med.* 2000;162(5):1633–1640.
35. Parthasarathy S, Jubran A, Tobin MJ. Cycling of inspiratory and expiratory muscle groups with the ventilator in airflow limitation. *Am J Respir Crit Care Med.* 1998;158(5 Pt 1):1471–1478.
36. Jubran A, Tobin MJ. Passive mechanics of lung and chest wall in patients who failed or succeeded in trials of weaning. *Am J Respir Crit Care Med.* 1997;155(3):916–921.
37. Capdevila X, Perrigault PF, Ramonatxo M, et al. Changes in breathing pattern and respiratory muscle performance parameters during difficult weaning. *Crit Care Med.* 1998;26(1):79–87.
38. Fiastro JF, Habib MP, Shon BY, et al. Comparison of standard weaning parameters and the mechanical work of breathing in mechanically ventilated patients. *Chest.* 1988;94(2):232–238.
39. Derenne JP, Couture J, Iscoe S, et al. Occlusion pressures in men rebreathing CO_2 under methoxyflurane anesthesia. *J Appl Physiol.* 1976;40(5):805–814.
40. Tobin MJ, Laghi F. Monitoring respiratory muscle function. In: Tobin MJ, ed. *Principles and Practice of Intensive Care Monitoring.* New York, NY: McGraw-Hill; 1998:497–544.
41. Zakynthinos S, Routsi C, Vassilakopoulos T, et al. Differential cardiovascular responses during weaning failure: effects on tissue oxygenation and lactate. *Intensive Care Med.* 2005;31(12):1634–1642.
42. Sassoon CS, Mahutte CK. Airway occlusion pressure and breathing pattern as predictors of weaning outcome. *Am Rev Respir Dis.* 1993;148(4 Pt 1):860–866.
43. Tahvanainen J, Salmenpera M, Nikki P. Extubation criteria after weaning from intermittent mandatory ventilation and continuous positive airway pressure. *Crit Care Med.* 1983;11(9):702–707.
44. Laghi F, Harrison MJ, Tobin MJ. Comparison of magnetic and electrical phrenic nerve stimulation in assessment of diaphragmatic contractility. *J Appl Physiol.* 1996;80(5):1731–1742.
45. Cattapan SE, Laghi F, Tobin MJ. Can diaphragmatic contractility be assessed by airway twitch pressure in mechanically ventilated patients? *Thorax.* 2003;58(1):58–62.
46. Watson AC, Hughes PD, Louise HM, et al. Measurement of twitch transdiaphragmatic, esophageal, and endotracheal tube pressure with bilateral anterolateral magnetic phrenic nerve stimulation in patients in the intensive care unit. *Crit Care Med.* 2001;29(7):1325–1331.
47. Polkey MI, Kyroussis D, Hamnegard CH, et al. Diaphragm strength in chronic obstructive pulmonary disease. *Am J Respir Crit Care Med.* 1996; 154(5):1310–1317.
48. Laghi F, Jubran A, Topeli A, et al. Effect of lung volume reduction surgery on diaphragmatic neuromechanical coupling at 2 years. *Chest.* 2004; 125(6):2188–2195.
49. Braun NM, Arora NS, Rochester DF. Respiratory muscle and pulmonary function in polymyositis and other proximal myopathies. *Thorax.* 1983;38(8):616–623.
50. Gibson GJ, Gilmartin JJ, Veale D, et al. Respiratory muscle function in neuromuscular disease. In: Jones NL, Killian KJ, eds. *Breathlessness. The Campbell Symposium.* Hamilton, Ontario: Boehringer-Ingelheim; 1992: 66–73.
51. Alison JA, Regnis JA, Donnelly PM, et al. End-expiratory lung volume during arm and leg exercise in normal subjects and patients with cystic fibrosis. *Am J Respir Crit Care Med.* 1998;158(5 Pt 1):1450–1458.
52. Bloch KE, Weder W, Boehler A, et al. Successful lung volume reduction surgery in a child with severe airflow obstruction and hyperinflation due to constrictive bronchiolitis. *Chest.* 2002;122(2):747–750.
53. Koutsoukou A, Armaganidis A, Stavrakaki-Kallergi C, et al. Expiratory flow limitation and intrinsic positive end-expiratory pressure at zero positive end-expiratory pressure in patients with adult respiratory distress syndrome. *Am J Respir Crit Care Med.* 2000;161(5):1590–1596.
54. Kimball WR, Leith DE, Robins AG. Dynamic hyperinflation and ventilator dependence in chronic obstructive pulmonary disease. *Am Rev Respir Dis.* 1982;126(6):991–995.
55. Tuxen DV, Lane S. The effects of ventilatory pattern on hyperinflation, airway pressures, and circulation in mechanical ventilation of patients with severe air-flow obstruction. *Am Rev Respir Dis.* 1987;136(4):872–879.
56. Laghi F, Jubran A, Topeli A, et al. Effect of lung volume reduction surgery on neuromechanical coupling of the diaphragm. *Am J Respir Crit Care Med.* 1998;157(2):475–483.
57. Coussa ML, Guerin C, Eissa NT, et al. Partitioning of work of breathing in mechanically ventilated COPD patients. *J Appl Physiol.* 1993;75(4):1711–1719.
58. Pelosi P, Cereda M, Foti G, et al. Alterations of lung and chest wall mechanics in patients with acute lung injury: effects of positive end-expiratory pressure. *Am J Respir Crit Care Med.* 1995;152(2):531–537.
59. Laaban JP, Kouchakji B, Dore MF, et al. Nutritional status of patients with chronic obstructive pulmonary disease and acute respiratory failure. *Chest.* 1993;103(5):1362–1368.
60. Faisy C, Rabbat A, Kouchakji B, et al. Bioelectrical impedance analysis in estimating nutritional status and outcome of patients with chronic obstructive pulmonary disease and acute respiratory failure. *Intensive Care Med.* 2000;26(5):518–525.
61. Kim J, Heshka S, Gallagher D, et al. Intermuscular adipose tissue-free skeletal muscle mass: estimation by dual-energy X-ray absorptiometry in adults. *J Appl Physiol.* 2004;97(2):655–660.
62. Murciano D, Rigaud D, Pingleton S, et al. Diaphragmatic function in

severely malnourished patients with anorexia nervosa. Effects of renutrition. *Am J Respir Crit Care Med.* 1994;150(6 Pt 1):1569–1574.
63. Ameredes BT, Watchko JF, Daood MJ, et al. Growth hormone restores aged diaphragm myosin composition and performance after chronic undernutrition. *J Appl Physiol.* 1999;87(4):1253–1259.
64. Lewis MI, Li H, Huang ZS, et al. Influence of varying degrees of malnutrition on IGF-I expression in the rat diaphragm. *J Appl Physiol.* 2003;95(2):555–562.
65. Lewis MI, Lorusso TJ, Zhan WZ, et al. Interactive effects of denervation and malnutrition on diaphragm structure and function. *J Appl Physiol.* 1996;81(5):2165–2172.
66. Schols AM, Soeters PB, Mostert R, et al. Physiologic effects of nutritional support and anabolic steroids in patients with chronic obstructive pulmonary disease. A placebo-controlled randomized trial. *Am J Respir Crit Care Med.* 1995;152(4 Pt 1):1268–1274.
67. Ryan CF, Whittaker JS, Road JD. Ventilatory dysfunction in severe anorexia nervosa. *Chest.* 1992;102(4):1286–1288.
68. Lanz JK Jr, Donahoe M, Rogers RM, et al. Effects of growth hormone on diaphragmatic recovery from malnutrition. *J Appl Physiol.* 1992;73(3):801–805.
69. Martinez FJ, Bermudez-Gomez M, Celli BR. Hypothyroidism. A reversible cause of diaphragmatic dysfunction. *Chest.* 1989;96(5):1059–1063.
70. Tawa NE, Jr., Odessey R, Goldberg AL. Inhibitors of the proteasome reduce the accelerated proteolysis in atrophying rat skeletal muscles. *J Clin Invest.* 1997;100(1):197–203.
71. Norrelund H, Hove KY, Brems-Dalgaard E, et al. Muscle mass and function in thyrotoxic patients before and during medical treatment. *Clin Endocrinol (Oxf).* 1999;51(6):693–699.
72. Goswami R, Guleria R, Gupta AK, et al. Prevalence of diaphragmatic muscle weakness and dyspnoea in Graves' disease and their reversibility with carbimazole therapy. *Eur J Endocrinol.* 2002;147(3):299–303.
73. Siafakas NM, Milona I, Salesiotou V, et al. Respiratory muscle strength in hyperthyroidism before and after treatment. *Am Rev Respir Dis.* 1992;146(4):1025–1029.
74. Iandelli I, Gorini M, Duranti R, et al. Respiratory muscle function and control of breathing in patients with acromegaly. *Eur Respir J.* 1997;10(5):977–982.
75. Mitch WE, Goldberg AL. Mechanisms of muscle wasting. The role of the ubiquitin-proteasome pathway. *N Engl J Med.* 1996;335(25):1897–1905.
76. Mills GH, Kyroussis D, Jenkins P, et al. Respiratory muscle strength in Cushing's syndrome. *Am J Respir Crit Care Med.* 1999;160(5 Pt 1):1762–1765.
77. Powers SK, Shanely RA, Coombes JS, et al. Mechanical ventilation results in progressive contractile dysfunction in the diaphragm. *J Appl Physiol.* 2002;92(5):1851–1858.
78. Yang L, Luo J, Bourdon J, et al. Controlled mechanical ventilation leads to remodeling of the rat diaphragm. *Am J Respir Crit Care Med.* 2002;166(8):1135–1140.
79. Sassoon CS, Ciaozzo VJ, Manka A, et al. Altered diaphragm contractile properties with controlled mechanical ventilation. *J Appl Physiol* 2002; 92(6):2585–2595.
80. Sassoon CS, Zhu E, Caiozzo VJ. Assist-control mechanical ventilation attenuates ventilator-induced diaphragmatic dysfunction. *Am J Respir Crit Care Med.* 2004;170(6):626–632.
81. Radell PJ, Remahl S, Nichols DG, et al. Effects of prolonged mechanical ventilation and inactivity on piglet diaphragm function. *Intensive Care Med.* 2002;28(3):358–364.
82. Anzueto A, Peters JI, Tobin MJ, et al. Effects of prolonged controlled mechanical ventilation on diaphragmatic function in healthy adult baboons. *Crit Care Med.* 1997;25(7):1187–1190.
83. Le Bourdelles G, Viires N, Boczkowski J, et al. Effects of mechanical ventilation on diaphragmatic contractile properties in rats. *Am J Respir Crit Care Med.* 1994;149(6):1539–1544.
84. Radell P, Edstrom L, Stibler H, et al. Changes in diaphragm structure following prolonged mechanical ventilation in piglets. *Acta Anaesthesiol Scand.* 2004;48(4):430–437.
85. Capdevila X, Lopez S, Bernard N, et al. Effects of controlled mechanical ventilation on respiratory muscle contractile properties in rabbits. *Intensive Care Med.* 2003;29(1):103–110.
86. Hussain SN, Vassilakopoulos T. Ventilator-induced cachexia. *Am J Respir Crit Care Med.* 2002;166(10):1307–1308.
87. Shanely RA, Coombes JS, Zergeroglu AM, et al. Short-duration mechanical ventilation enhances diaphragmatic fatigue resistance but impairs force production. *Chest.* 2003;123(1):195–201.
88. Shanely RA, Zergeroglu MA, Lennon SL, et al. Mechanical ventilation-induced diaphragmatic atrophy is associated with oxidative injury and increased proteolytic activity. *Am J Respir Crit Care Med.* 2002;166(10): 1369–1374.
89. Zergeroglu MA, McKenzie MJ, Shanely RA, et al. Mechanical ventilation-induced oxidative stress in the diaphragm. *J Appl Physiol.* 2003;95(3): 1116–1124.
90. Radell P, Edstrom L, Stibler H, et al. Changes in diaphragm structure following prolonged mechanical ventilation in piglets. *Acta Anaesthesiol Scand.* 2004;48(4):430–437.
91. Capdevila X, Lopez S, Bernard N, et al. Effects of controlled mechanical ventilation on respiratory muscle contractile properties in rabbits. *Intensive Care Med.* 2003;29(1):103–110.
92. Nguyen T, Friscia M, Kaiser LR, et al. Ventilator-induced proteolysis in human diaphragm myofibers. *Proc Am Thorac Soc.* 2006;3:A259.
93. Shanely RA, Van Gammeren D, DeRuisseau KC, et al. Mechanical ventilation depresses protein synthesis in the rat diaphragm. *Am J Respir Crit Care Med.* 2004;170(9):994–999.
94. Crimi E, Liguori A, Condorelli M, et al. The beneficial effects of antioxidant supplementation in enteral feeding in critically ill patients: a prospective, randomized, double-blind, placebo-controlled trial. *Anesth Analg.* 2004;99(3):857–863.
95. Nathens AB, Neff MJ, Jurkovich GJ, et al. Randomized, prospective trial of antioxidant supplementation in critically ill surgical patients. *Ann Surg.* 2002;236(6):814–822.
96. Knisely AS, Leal SM, Singer DB. Abnormalities of diaphragmatic muscle in neonates with ventilated lungs. *J Pediatr.* 1988;113(6):1074–1077.
97. Levine S, Nguyen T, Friscia M, et al. Ventilator-induced atrophy in human diaphragm myofibers. *Proc Am Thorac Soc.* 2006;3:A27.
98. Pichard C, Kyle U, Chevrolet JC, et al. Lack of effects of recombinant growth hormone on muscle function in patients requiring prolonged mechanical ventilation: a prospective, randomized, controlled study. *Crit Care Med.* 1996;24(3):403–413.
99. Takala J, Ruokonen E, Webster NR, et al. Increased mortality associated with growth hormone treatment in critically ill adults. *N Engl J Med.* 1999;341(11):785–792.
100. Hussain SN. Respiratory muscle dysfunction in sepsis. *Mol Cell Biochem.* 1998;179(1–2):125–134.
101. Leon A, Boczkowski J, Dureuil B, et al. Effects of endotoxic shock on diaphragmatic function in mechanically ventilated rats. *J Appl Physiol.* 1992;72(4):1466–1472.
102. Lin MC, Ebihara S, El Dwairi Q, et al. Diaphragm sarcolemmal injury is induced by sepsis and alleviated by nitric oxide synthase inhibition. *Am J Respir Crit Care Med.* 1998;158(5 Pt 1):1656–1663.
103. Aarli JA, Skeie GO, Mygland A, et al. Muscle striation antibodies in myasthenia gravis. Diagnostic and functional significance. *Ann N Y Acad Sci.* 1998;841:505–515.
104. Callahan LA, Nethery D, Stofan D, et al. Free radical-induced contractile protein dysfunction in endotoxin-induced sepsis. *Am J Respir Cell Mol Biol.* 2001;24(2):210–217.
105. Supinski G, Nethery D, DiMarco A. Effect of free radical scavengers on endotoxin-induced respiratory muscle dysfunction. *Am Rev Respir Dis.* 1993;148(5):1318–1324.
106. Taille C, Foresti R, Lanone S, et al. Protective role of heme oxygenases against endotoxin-induced diaphragmatic dysfunction in rats. *Am J Respir Crit Care Med.* 2001;163(3 Pt 1):753–761.
107. Javesghani D, Magder SA, Barreiro E, et al. Molecular characterization of a superoxide-generating NAD(P)H oxidase in the ventilatory muscles. *Am J Respir Crit Care Med.* 2002;165(3):412–418.
108. Fujimura N, Sumita S, Aimono M, et al. Effect of free radical scavengers on diaphragmatic contractility in septic peritonitis. *Am J Respir Crit Care Med.* 2000;162(6):2159–2165.
109. Tiao G, Fagan J, Roegner V, et al. Energy-ubiquitin-dependent muscle proteolysis during sepsis in rats is regulated by glucocorticoids. *J Clin Invest.* 1996;97(2):339–348.
110. Laghi F. Curing the septic diaphragm with the ventilator. *Am J Respir Crit Care Med.* 2002;165(2):145–146.
111. Klaude M, Fredriksson K, Tjader I, et al. Proteasome proteolytic activity in skeletal muscle is increased in patients with sepsis. *Clin Sci (Lond).* 2007;112(9):499–506.
112. Boczkowski J, Lisdero CL, Lanone S, et al. Endogenous peroxynitrite mediates mitochondrial dysfunction in rat diaphragm during endotoxemia. *FASEB J.* 1999;13(12):1637–1646.
113. El Dwairi Q, Comtois A, Guo Y, et al. Endotoxin-induced skeletal muscle contractile dysfunction: contribution of nitric oxide synthases. *Am J Physiol.* 1998;274(3 Pt 1):C770–C779.
114. Fredriksson K, Hammarqvist F, Strigard K, et al. Derangements in mitochondrial metabolism in intercostal and leg muscle of critically ill patients with sepsis-induced multiple organ failure. *Am J Physiol Endocrinol Metab.* 2006;291(5):E1044–E1050.
115. Lanone S, Mebazaa A, Heymes C, et al. Muscular contractile failure in septic patients: role of the inducible nitric oxide synthase pathway. *Am J Respir Crit Care Med.* 2000;162(6):2308–2315.
116. Bolton CF, Laverty DA, Brown JD, et al. Critically ill polyneuropathy: electrophysiological studies and differentiation from Guillain-Barré syndrome. *J Neurol Neurosurg Psychiatry.* 1986;49(5):563–573.
117. Fletcher SN, Kennedy DD, Ghosh IR, et al. Persistent neuromuscular and neurophysiologic abnormalities in long-term survivors of prolonged critical illness. *Crit Care Med.* 2003;31(4):1012–1016.
118. Deem S, Lee CM, Curtis JR. Acquired neuromuscular disorders in the intensive care unit. *Am J Respir Crit Care Med.* 2003;168(7):735–739.
119. Hund EF, Fogel W, Krieger D, et al. Critical illness polyneuropathy: clinical findings and outcomes of a frequent cause of neuromuscular weaning failure. *Crit Care Med.* 1996;24(8):1328–1333.

120. Latronico N, Fenzi F, Recupero D, et al. Critical illness myopathy and neuropathy. *Lancet.* 1996;347(9015):1579–1582.
121. Hermans G, Wilmer A, Meersseman W, et al. Impact of intensive insulin therapy on neuromuscular complications and ventilator dependency in the medical intensive care unit. *Am J Respir Crit Care Med.* 2007;175(5):480–489.
122. Khan J, Harrison TB, Rich MM, et al. Early development of critical illness myopathy and neuropathy in patients with severe sepsis. *Neurology.* 2006;67(8):1421–1425.
123. Bednarik J, Vondracek P, Dusek L, et al. Risk factors for critical illness polyneuromyopathy. *J Neurol.* 2005;252(3):343–351.
124. Larsson L, Li X, Edstrom L, et al. Acute quadriplegia and loss of muscle myosin in patients treated with nondepolarizing neuromuscular blocking agents and corticosteroids: mechanisms at the cellular and molecular levels. *Crit Care Med.* 2000;28(1):34–45.
125. Rich MM, Teener JW, Raps EC, et al. Muscle is electrically inexcitable in acute quadriplegic myopathy. *Neurology* 1996;46(3):731–736.
126. Rich MM, Bird SJ, Raps EC, et al. Direct muscle stimulation in acute quadriplegic myopathy. *Muscle Nerve.* 1997;20(6):665–673.
127. Lefaucheur JP, Nordine T, Rodriguez P, et al. Origin of ICU acquired paresis determined by direct muscle stimulation. *J Neurol Neurosurg Psychiatry.* 2006;77(4):500–506.
128. Bolton CF. Neuromuscular manifestations of critical illness. *Muscle Nerve.* 2005;32(2):140–163.
129. Ramsay DA, Zochodne DW, Robertson DM, et al. A syndrome of acute severe muscle necrosis in intensive care unit patients. *J Neuropathol Exp Neurol.* 1993;52(4):387–398.
130. Faragher MW, Day BJ, Dennett X. Critical care myopathy: an electrophysiological and histological study. *Muscle Nerve.* 1996;19(4):516–518.
131. Mozaffar T, Haddad F, Zeng M, et al. Molecular and cellular defects of skeletal muscle in an animal model of acute quadriplegic myopathy. *Muscle Nerve.* 2007;35(1):55–65.
132. Di Giovanni S, Molon A, Broccolini A, et al. Constitutive activation of MAPK cascade in acute quadriplegic myopathy. *Ann Neurol.* 2004;55(2):195–206.
133. de Letter MA, van Doorn PA, Savelkoul HF, et al. Critical illness polyneuropathy and myopathy (CIPNM): evidence for local immune activation by cytokine-expression in the muscle tissue. *J Neuroimmunol.* 2000;106(1–2):206–213.
134. De Jonghe B, Sharshar T, Lefaucheur JP, et al. Paresis acquired in the intensive care unit: a prospective multicenter study. *JAMA.* 2002;288(22):2859–2867.
135. Faragher MW, Day BJ. A practical approach to weakness in the intensive care unit. In: Cros D, ed. *Peripheral Neuropathy: A Practical Approach to Diagnosis and Management.* Philadelphia, PA: Lippincott Williams & Wilkins; 2001:370–386.
136. De Jonghe B, Bastuji-Garin S, Sharshar T, et al. Does ICU-acquired paresis lengthen weaning from mechanical ventilation? *Intensive Care Med.* 2004;30(6):1117–1121.
137. Latronico N, Shehu I, Seghelini E. Neuromuscular sequelae of critical illness. *Curr Opin Crit Care.* 2005;11(4):381–390.
138. De Jonghe B, Bastuji-Garin S, Durand MC, et al. Respiratory weakness is associated with limb weakness and delayed weaning in critical illness. *Crit Care Med.* 2007;35(9):2007–2015.
139. Leatherman JW, Fluegel WL, David WS, et al. Muscle weakness in mechanically ventilated patients with severe asthma. *Am J Respir Crit Care Med.* 1996;153(5):1686–1690.
140. de Seze M, Petit H, Wiart L, et al. Critical illness polyneuropathy. A 2-year follow-up study in 19 severe cases. *Eur Neurol.* 2000;43(2):61–69.
141. Roberts PA, Loxham SJ, Poucher SM, et al. Bicarbonate-induced alkalosis augments cellular acetyl group availability and isometric force during the rest-to-work transition in canine skeletal muscle. *Exp Physiol.* 2002;87(4):489–498.
142. Schnader JY, Juan G, Howell S, et al. Arterial CO_2 partial pressure affects diaphragmatic function. *J Appl Physiol.* 1985;58(3):823–829.
143. Juan G, Calverley P, Talamo C, et al. Effect of carbon dioxide on diaphragmatic function in human beings. *N Engl J Med* 1984;310(14):874–879.
144. Jackson DC, Arendt EA, Inman KC, et al. 31P-NMR study of normoxic and anoxic perfused turtle heart during graded CO_2 and lactic acidosis. *Am J Physiol.* 1991;260(6 Pt 2):R1130–R1136.
145. Yanos J, Wood LD, Davis K, et al. The effect of respiratory and lactic acidosis on diaphragm function. *Am Rev Respir Dis.* 1993;147(3):616–619.
146. Coast JR, Shanely RA, Lawler JM, et al. Lactic acidosis and diaphragmatic function in vitro. *Am J Respir Crit Care Med.* 1995;152(5 Pt 1):1648–1652.
147. Knuth ST, Dave H, Peters JR, et al. Low cell pH depresses peak power in rat skeletal muscle fibres at both 30 degrees C and 15 degrees C: implications for muscle fatigue. *J Physiol.* 2006;575(Pt 3):887–899.
148. Kristensen M, Albertsen J, Rentsch M, et al. Lactate and force production in skeletal muscle. *J Physiol.* 2005;562(Pt 2):521–526.
149. Posterino GS, Dutka TL, Lamb GD. L(+)-lactate does not affect twitch and tetanic responses in mechanically skinned mammalian muscle fibres. *Pflugers Arch.* 2001;442(2):197–203.
150. Degroot M, Massie BM, Boska M, et al. Dissociation of [H+] from fatigue in human muscle detected by high time resolution 31P-NMR. *Muscle Nerve.* 1993;16(1):91–98.
151. Westerblad H, Allen DG, Lannergren J. Muscle fatigue: lactic acid or inorganic phosphate the major cause? *News Physiol Sci.* 2002;17:17–21.
152. Nielsen OB, de Paoli F, Overgaard K. Protective effects of lactic acid on force production in rat skeletal muscle. *J Physiol.* 2001;536(Pt 1):161–166.
153. Rafferty GF, Lou HM, Polkey MI, et al. Effect of hypercapnia on maximal voluntary ventilation and diaphragm fatigue in normal humans. *Am J Respir Crit Care Med.* 1999;160(5 Pt 1):1567–1571.
154. Schnader J, Howell S, Fitzgerald RS, et al. Interaction of fatigue and hypercapnia in the canine diaphragm. *J Appl Physiol.* 1988;64(4):1636–1643.
155. Mador MJ, Wendel T, Kufel TJ. Effect of acute hypercapnia on diaphragmatic and limb muscle contractility. *Am J Respir Crit Care Med.* 1997;155(5):1590–1595.
156. Vianna LG, Koulouris N, Moxham J. Lack of effect of acute hypoxia and hypercapnia on muscle relaxation rate in man. *Rev Esp Fisiol.* 1993;49(1):7–15.
157. Aubier M, Murciano D, Lecocguic Y, et al. Effect of hypophosphatemia on diaphragmatic contractility in patients with acute respiratory failure. *N Engl J Med.* 1985;313(7):420–424.
158. Aubier M, Viires N, Piquet J, et al. Effects of hypocalcemia on diaphragmatic strength generation. *J Appl Physiol.* 1985;58(6):2054–2061.
159. Dhingra S, Solven F, Wilson A, et al. Hypomagnesemia and respiratory muscle power. *Am Rev Respir Dis.* 1984;129(3):497–498.
160. Stedwell RE, Allen KM, Binder LS. Hypokalemic paralyses: a review of the etiologies, pathophysiology, presentation, and therapy. *Am J Emerg Med.* 1992;10(2):143–148.
161. Rodriguez JA, Crespo-Leiro MG, Paniagua MJ, et al. Rhabdomyolysis in heart transplant patients on HMG-CoA reductase inhibitors and cyclosporine. *Transplant Proc.* 1999;31(6):2522–2523.
162. Masters BA, Palmoski MJ, Flint OP, et al. In vitro myotoxicity of the 3-hydroxy-3-methylglutaryl coenzyme A reductase inhibitors, pravastatin, lovastatin, and simvastatin, using neonatal rat skeletal myocytes. *Toxicol Appl Pharmacol.* 1995;131(1):163–174.
163. Sugiyama S. HMG CoA reductase inhibitor accelerates aging effect on diaphragm mitochondrial respiratory function in rats. *Biochem Mol Biol Int.* 1998;46(5):923–931.
164. Cote HC, Brumme ZL, Craib KJ, et al. Changes in mitochondrial DNA as a marker of nucleoside toxicity in HIV-infected patients. *N Engl J Med.* 2002;346(11):811–820.
165. Hasfurther DL, Bailey PL. Failure of neuromuscular blockade reversal after rocuronium in a patient who received oral neomycin. *Can J Anaesth.* 1996;43(6):617–620.
166. Segredo V, Caldwell JE, Matthay MA, et al. Persistent paralysis in critically ill patients after long-term administration of vecuronium. *N Engl J Med.* 1992;327(8):524–528.
167. de Lemos JM, Carr RR, Shalansky KF, et al. Paralysis in the critically ill: intermittent bolus pancuronium compared with continuous infusion. *Crit Care Med.* 1999;27(12):2648–2655.
168. Rudis MI, Sikora CA, Angus E, et al. A prospective, randomized, controlled evaluation of peripheral nerve stimulation versus standard clinical dosing of neuromuscular blocking agents in critically ill patients. *Crit Care Med.* 1997;25(4):575–583.
169. Hirano M, Ott BR, Raps EC, et al. Acute quadriplegic myopathy: a complication of treatment with steroids, nondepolarizing blocking agents, or both. *Neurology.* 1992;42(11):2082–2087.
170. Gooch JL, Suchyta MR, Balbierz JM, et al. Prolonged paralysis after treatment with neuromuscular junction blocking agents. *Crit Care Med.* 1991;19(9):1125–1131.
171. Whetstone Foster JG, Clark AP. Functional recovery after neuromuscular blockade in mechanically ventilated critically ill patients. *Heart Lung.* 2006;35(3):178–189.
172. Murray MJ, Cowen J, DeBlock H, et al. Clinical practice guidelines for sustained neuromuscular blockade in the adult critically ill patient. *Crit Care Med.* 2002;30(1):142–156.
173. Laghi F, Topeli A, Tobin MJ. Does resistive loading decrease diaphragmatic contractility before task failure? *J Appl Physiol.* 1998;85(3):1103–1112.
174. Laghi F, D'Alfonso N, Tobin MJ. Pattern of recovery from diaphragmatic fatigue over 24 hours. *J Appl Physiol.* 1995;79(2):539–546.
175. Travaline JM, Sudarshan S, Roy BG, et al. Effect of N-acetylcysteine on human diaphragm strength and fatigability. *Am J Respir Crit Care Med.* 1997;156(5):1567–1571.
176. Dahlstedt AJ, Katz A, Westerblad H. Role of myoplasmic phosphate in contractile function of skeletal muscle: studies on creatine kinase-deficient mice. *J Physiol.* 2001;533(Pt 2):379–388.
177. Radell PJ, Eleff SM, Nichols DG. Effects of loaded breathing and hypoxia on diaphragm metabolism as measured by ^{31}P-NMR spectroscopy. *J Appl Physiol.* 2000;88(3):933–938.
178. Westerblad H, Bruton JD, Lannergren J. The effect of intracellular pH on contractile function of intact, single fibres of mouse muscle declines with increasing temperature. *J Physi.* 1997;500:193–204.
179. Zhu E, Comtois AS, Fang L, et al. Influence of tension time on muscle fiber sarcolemmal injury in rat diaphragm. *J Appl Physiol.* 2000;88(1):135–141.

180. Jiang TX, Reid WD, Road JD. Delayed diaphragm injury and diaphragm force production. *Am J Respir Crit Care Med.* 1998;157(3 Pt 1):736–742.
181. Thille AW, Rodriguez P, Cabello B, et al. Patient-ventilator asynchrony during assisted mechanical ventilation. *Intensive Care Med.* 2006;32(10):1515–1522.
182. Chao DC, Scheinhorn DJ, Stearn-Hassenpflug M. Patient-ventilator trigger asynchrony in prolonged mechanical ventilation. *Chest.*1997;112(6):1592–1599.
183. Bellemare F, Grassino A. Effect of pressure and timing of contraction on human diaphragm fatigue. *J Appl Physiol.* 1982;53(5):1190–1195.
184. Pinsky MR. Effect of mechanical ventilation on heart-lung interactions. In: Tobin MJ, ed. *Principles and Practice of Mechanical Ventilation.* New York, NY: McGraw-Hill; 2006:729–757.
185. Hurford WE, Lynch KE, Strauss HW, et al. Myocardial perfusion as assessed by thallium-201 scintigraphy during the discontinuation of mechanical ventilation in ventilator-dependent patients. *Anesthesiology.* 1991;74(6):1007–1016.
186. Srivastava S, Chatila W, Amoateng-Adjepong Y, et al. Myocardial ischemia and weaning failure in patients with coronary artery disease: an update. *Crit Care Med.* 1999;27(10):2109–2112.
187. Hurford WE, Favorito F. Association of myocardial ischemia with failure to wean from mechanical ventilation. *Crit Care Med.* 1995;23(9):1475–1480.
188. Lemaire F, Teboul JL, Cinotti L, et al. Acute left ventricular dysfunction during unsuccessful weaning from mechanical ventilation. *Anesthesiology.* 1988;69(2):171–179.
189. Nozawa E, Azeka E, Ignez ZM, et al. Factors associated with failure of weaning from long-term mechanical ventilation after cardiac surgery. *Int Heart J.* 2005;46(5):819–831.
190. Jubran A, Mathru M, Dries D, et al. Continuous recordings of mixed venous oxygen saturation during weaning from mechanical ventilation and the ramifications thereof. *Am J Respir Crit Care Med.* 1998;158(6):1763–1769.
191. Richard C, Teboul JL. Weaning failure from cardiovascular origin. *Intensive Care Med.* 2005;31(12):1605–1607.
192. Scheinhorn D. Increase in serum albumin and decrease in body weight correlate with weaning from prolonged mechanical ventilation. *Am.Rev.Respir.Dis.* 1992;145:A522.
193. Beach T, Millen E, Grenvik A. Hemodynamic response to discontinuance of mechanical ventilation. *Crit Care Med.* 1973;1(2):85–90.
194. Indihar FJ. A 10-year report of patients in a prolonged respiratory care unit. *Minn Med.* 1991;74(4):23–27.
195. Martin UJ, Criner GJ. Psychological problems in the ventilated patient. In: Tobin MJ, ed. *Principles and Practice of Mechanical Ventilation.* 2nd ed. New York, NY: McGraw-Hill; 2006:1137–1151.
196. Banzett RB, Brown R. Addressing respiratory discomfort in the ventilated patient. In: Tobin MJ, ed. *Principles and Practice of Mechanical Ventilation.* 2nd ed. New York, NY: McGraw-Hill; 2006:1153–1162.
197. Dilling D, Duffner LA, Lawn G, et al. Anxiety levels in patients being weaned from mechanical ventilation. *Proc Am Thorac Soc.* 2005;2:A161.
198. Ramana RD, Lawn G, Kelly J, et al. Can anxiety be measured in patients weaning from prolonged mechanical ventilation? *Proc Am Thorac Soc.* 2006;3:A43.
199. Repetz N, Ciccolella DE, Criner GJ. Long-term outcome of patients with delirium on admission to a multidisciplinary ventilator rehabilitation unit (VRU). *Am.J Respir.Crit Care Med.* 2001;163:A889.
200. Yu BH, Dimsdale JE. Posttraumatic stress disorder in patients with burn injuries. *J Burn Care Rehabil.* 1999;20(5):426–433.
201. Kress JP, Gehlbach B, Lacy M, et al. The long-term psychological effects of daily sedative interruption on critically ill patients. *Am J Respir Crit Care Med.* 2003;168(12):1457–1461.
202. Cuthbertson BH, Hull A, Strachan M, et al. Post-traumatic stress disorder after critical illness requiring general intensive care. *Intensive Care Med.* 2004;30(3):450–455.
203. Hanly PJ. Sleep in the ventilated patient. In: Tobin MJ, ed. *Principles and Practice of Mechanical Ventilation.* 2nd ed. New York, NY: McGraw-Hill; 2006:1173–1183.
204. Dubois MJ, Bergeron N, Dumont M, et al. Delirium in an intensive care unit: a study of risk factors. *Intensive Care Med.* 2001;27(8):1297–1304.
205. Ely EW, Gautam S, Margolin R, et al. The impact of delirium in the intensive care unit on hospital length of stay. *Intensive Care Med.* 2001;27(12):1892–1900.
206. Bergbom-Engberg I, Haljamae H. Assessment of patients' experience of discomforts during respirator therapy. *Crit Care Med.* 1989;17(10):1068–1072.
207. Johnson CJ, Auger WR, Fedullo PF, et al. Methylphenidate in the 'hard to wean' patient. *J Psychosom Res.* 1995;39(1):63–68.
208. Rothenhausler HB, Ehrentraut S, von Degenfeld G, et al. Treatment of depression with methylphenidate in patients difficult to wean from mechanical ventilation in the intensive care unit. *J Clin Psychiatr.* 2000;61(10):750–755.
209. Holliday JE, Hyers TM. The reduction of weaning time from mechanical ventilation using tidal volume and relaxation biofeedback. *Am Rev Respir Dis.* 1990;141(5 Pt 1):1214–1220.
210. Acosta F. Biofeedback and progressive relaxation in weaning the anxious patient from the ventilator: a brief report. *Heart Lung.* 1988;17(3):299–301.
211. Martin UJ, Hincapie L, Nimchuk M, et al. Impact of whole-body rehabilitation in patients receiving chronic mechanical ventilation. *Crit Care Med.* 2005;33(10):2259–2265.
212. Elpern EH, Silver MR, Rosen RL, et al. The noninvasive respiratory care unit. Patterns of use and financial implications. *Chest.* 1991;99(1):205–208.
213. Feinstein AR. *Clinical Epidemiology: The Architecture of Clinical Research.* Philadelphia, PA: WB Saunders; 1985.
214. Tobin MJ, Jubran A. Variable performance of weaning-predictor tests: role of Bayes' theorem and spectrum and test-referral bias. *Intensive Care Med.* 2006;32(12):2002–2012.
215. Casscells W, Schoenberger A, Graboys TB. Interpretation by physicians of clinical laboratory results. *N Engl J Med.* 1978;299(18):999–1001.
216. Meade M, Guyatt G, Cook D, et al. Predicting success in weaning from mechanical ventilation. *Ches.* 2001;120(6 Suppl):400S–424S.
217. MacIntyre NR, Cook DJ, Ely EW Jr, et al. Evidence-based guidelines for weaning and discontinuing ventilatory support: a collective task force facilitated by the American College of Chest Physicians; the American Association for Respiratory Care; and the American College of Critical Care Medicine. *Chest.* 2001;120(6 Suppl):375S–395S.
218. Brand R, Kragt H. Importance of trends in the interpretation of an overall odds ratio in the meta-analysis of clinical trials. *Stat Med.* 1992;11(16):2077–2082.
219. Schmid CH, Lau J, McIntosh MW, et al. An empirical study of the effect of the control rate as a predictor of treatment efficacy in meta-analysis of clinical trials. *Stat Med.* 1998;17(17):1923–1942.
220. Engel G, Rockson SG. Rapid diagnosis of myocardial injury with troponin T and CK-MB relative index. *Mol Diagn Ther.* 2007;11(2):109–116.
221. Voigt GE. Biomechanics of blunt chest injuries especially of the thorax, aorta and heart. Contribution to the problem of the so-called internal safety of personal moor vehicles [in German]. *Hefte Unfallheilkd.* 1968;96:1–115.
222. Mylonakis E, Calderwood SB. Infective endocarditis in adults. *N Engl J Med.* 2001;345(18):1318–1330.
223. Sahn SA, Lakshminarayan S. Bedside criteria for discontinuation of mechanical ventilation. *Chest.* 1973;63(6):1002–1005.
224. Chevrolet JC, Deleamont P. Repeated vital capacity measurements as predictive parameters for mechanical ventilation need and weaning success in the Guillain-Barré syndrome. *Am Rev Respir Dis.* 1991;144(4):814–818.
225. Brenner M, Mukai DS, Russell JE, et al. A new method for measurement of airway occlusion pressure. *Chest.* 1990;98(2):421–427.
226. Burki NK. The effects of changes in functional residual capacity with posture on mouth occlusion pressure and ventilatory pattern. *Am Rev Respir Dis.* 1977;116(5):895–900.
227. Lederer DH, Altose MD, Kelsen SG, et al. Comparison of occlusion pressure and ventilatory responses. *Thorax.* 1977;32(2):212–220.
228. Brown SD, Gutierrez G. Gut mucosal pH monitoring. In: Tobin MJ, ed. *Principles and Practice of Intensive Care Monitoring.* 1st ed. New York, NY: McGraw-Hill; 1998:351–368.
229. Bouachour G, Guiraud MP, Gouello JP, et al. Gastric intramucosal pH: an indicator of weaning outcome from mechanical ventilation in COPD patients. *Eur Respir J.* 1996;9(9):1868–1873.
230. Bocquillon N, Mathieu D, Neviere R, et al. Gastric mucosal pH and blood flow during weaning from mechanical ventilation in patients with chronic obstructive pulmonary disease. *Am J Respir Crit Care Med.* 1999;160(5 Pt 1):1555–1561.
231. Uusaro A, Chittock DR, Russell JA, et al. Stress test and gastric-arterial PCO_2 measurement improve prediction of successful extubation. *Crit Care Med.* 2000;28(7):2313–2319.
232. Maldonado A, Bauer TT, Ferrer M, et al. Capnometric recirculation gas tonometry and weaning from mechanical ventilation. *Am J Respir Crit Care Med.* 2000;161(1):171–176.
233. Mohsenifar Z, Hay A, Hay J, et al. Gastric intramural pH as a predictor of success or failure in weaning patients from mechanical ventilation. *Ann Intern Med.* 1993;119(8):794–798.
234. Tobin MJ. Remembrance of weaning past: the seminal papers. *Intensive Care Med.* 2006;32(10):1485–1493.
235. Sassoon CS. Intermittent mechanical ventilation. In: Tobin MJ, ed. *Principles and Practice of Mechanical Ventilation.* 2nd ed. New York, NY: McGraw-Hil; 2006:201–220.
236. Marini JJ, Smith TC, Lamb VJ. External work output and force generation during synchronized intermittent mechanical ventilation. Effect of machine assistance on breathing effort. *Am Rev Respir Dis.* 1988;138(5):1169–1179.
237. Imsand C, Feihl F, Perret C, et al. Regulation of inspiratory neuromuscular output during synchronized intermittent mechanical ventilation. *Anesthesiology.* 1994;80(1):13–22.
238. Tomlinson JR, Miller KS, Lorch DG, et al. A prospective comparison of IMV and T-piece weaning from mechanical ventilation. *Chest.* 1989;96(2):348–352.
239. Brochard L. Pressure-support ventilation. In: Tobin MJ, ed. *Principles and Practice of Mechanical Ventilation.* 2nd ed. New York, NY: McGraw-Hill; 2006:221–250.

240. Jubran A, Van de Graaff WB, Tobin MJ. Variability of patient-ventilator interaction with pressure support ventilation in patients with chronic obstructive pulmonary disease. *Am J Respir Crit Care Med.* 1995;152(1):129–136.
241. Straus C, Louis B, Isabey D, et al. Contribution of the endotracheal tube and the upper airway to breathing workload. *Am J Respir Crit Care Med.* 1998;157(1):23–30.
242. Lellouche F, Mancebo J, Jolliet P, et al. A multicenter randomized trial of computer-driven protocolized weaning from mechanical ventilation. *Am J Respir Crit Care Med.* 2006;174(8):894–900.
243. Kager LM, Schultz MJ. Computer-driven protocolized weaning from mechanical ventilation. *Am J Respir Crit Care Med.* 2007;175(9):968–969.
244. Shannon J, Bonett S, Gabrielli A, et al. Evaluation of closed-loop ventilation for patient weaning. *Crit Care Med.* 2006;34:A91.
245. Jubran A, Grant BJ, Laghi F, et al. Weaning prediction: esophageal pressure monitoring complements readiness testing. *Am J Respir Crit Care Med.* 2005;171(11):1252–1259.
246. Nava S, Ambrosino N, Clini E, et al. Noninvasive mechanical ventilation in the weaning of patients with respiratory failure due to chronic obstructive pulmonary disease. A randomized, controlled trial. *Ann Intern Med.* 1998;128(9):721–728.
247. Girault C, Daudenthun I, Chevron V, et al. Noninvasive ventilation as a systematic extubation and weaning technique in acute-on-chronic respiratory failure: a prospective, randomized controlled study. *Am J Respir Crit Care Med.* 1999;160(1):86–92.
248. Ferrer M, Esquinas A, Arancibia F, et al. Noninvasive ventilation during persistent weaning failure: a randomized controlled trial. *Am J Respir Crit Care Med.* 2003;168(1):70–76.
249. Namen AM, Ely EW, Tatter SB, et al. Predictors of successful extubation in neurosurgical patients. *Am J Respir Crit Care Med.* 2001;163(3 Pt 1):658–664.
250. Randolph AG, Wypij D, Venkataraman ST, et al. Effect of mechanical ventilator weaning protocols on respiratory outcomes in infants and children: a randomized controlled trial. *JAMA.* 2002;288(20):2561–2568.
251. Krishnan JA, Moore D, Robeson C, et al. A prospective, controlled trial of a protocol-based strategy to discontinue mechanical ventilation. *Am J Respir Crit Care Med.* 2004;169(6):673–678.
252. Marelich GP, Murin S, Battistella F, et al. Protocol weaning of mechanical ventilation in medical and surgical patients by respiratory care practitioners and nurses: effect on weaning time and incidence of ventilator-associated pneumonia. *Chest.* 2000;118(2):459–467.
253. Ely EW, Baker AM, Evans GW, et al. The prognostic significance of passing a daily screen of weaning parameters. *Intensive Care Med.* 1999;25(6):581–587.
254. Tobin MJ. Of principles and protocols and weaning. *Am J Respir Crit Care Med.* 2004;169(6):661–662.
255. Morris AH. Algorithm-based decision making. In: Tobin MJ, ed. *Principles and Practice of Intensive Care Monitoring.* 1st ed. New York, NY: McGraw-Hill; 1998:1355–1381.
256. Tobin MJ, Laghi F. Extubation. In: Tobin MJ, ed. *Principles and Practice of Mechanical Ventilation.* 2nd ed. New York, NY: McGraw-Hill; 2006:1221–1237.
257. de la Linde Valverde CM. Extubation of the difficult airway [in Spanish]. *Rev Esp Anestesiol Reanim.* 2005;52(9):557–570.
258. Gal TG. Airway management. In: Miller RD, ed. *Miller's Anesthesia.* 6th ed. Philadelphia, PA: Elsevier, Churchill Livingstone; 2005:1617–1652.
259. Leder SB, Cohn SM, Moller BA. Fiberoptic endoscopic documentation of the high incidence of aspiration following extubation in critically ill trauma patients. *Dysphagia.* 1998;13(4):208–212.
260. El Solh A, Okada M, Bhat A, et al. Swallowing disorders post orotracheal intubation in the elderly. *Intensive Care Med.* 2003;29(9):1451–1455.
261. Barquist E, Brown M, Cohn S, et al. Postextubation fiberoptic endoscopic evaluation of swallowing after prolonged endotracheal intubation: a randomized, prospective trial. *Crit Care Med.* 2001;29(9):1710–1713.
262. Leitch EA, Moran JL, Grealy B. Weaning and extubation in the intensive care unit. Clinical or index-driven approach? *Intensive Care Med.* 1996;22(8):752–759.
263. Conti G, Montini L, Pennisi MA, et al. A prospective, blinded evaluation of indexes proposed to predict weaning from mechanical ventilation. *Intensive Care Med.* 2004;30(5):830–836.
264. Dojat M, Harf A, Touchard D, et al. Evaluation of a knowledge-based system providing ventilatory management and decision for extubation. *Am J Respir Crit Care Med.* 1996;153(3):997–1004.
265. Cohen JD, Shapiro M, Grozovski E, et al. Automatic tube compensation-assisted respiratory rate to tidal volume ratio improves the prediction of weaning outcome. *Chest.* 2002;122(3):980–984.
266. Esteban A, Frutos-Vivar F, Ferguson ND, et al. Noninvasive positive-pressure ventilation for respiratory failure after extubation. *N Engl J Med.* 2004;350(24):2452–2460.
267. Epstein SK, Ciubotaru RL. Independent effects of etiology of failure and time to reintubation on outcome for patients failing extubation. *Am J Respir Crit Care Med.* 1998;158(2):489–493.
268. Hammer G, Schwinn D, Wollman H. Postoperative complications due to paradoxical vocal cord motion. *Anesthesiology.* 1987;66(5):686–687.
269. Harbison J, Dodd J, McNicholas WT. Paradoxical vocal cord motion causing stridor after thyroidectomy. *Thorax.* 2000;55(6):533–534.
270. Rubin AD, Hawkshaw MJ, Moyer CA, et al. Arytenoid cartilage dislocation: a 20-year experience. *J Voice.* 2005;19(4):687–701.
271. Tolley NS, Cheesman TD, Morgan D, et al. Dislocated arytenoid: an intubation-induced injury. *Ann R Coll Surg Engl.* 1990;72(6):353–356.
272. Cook TM, Silsby J, Simpson TP. Airway rescue in acute upper airway obstruction using a ProSeal Laryngeal mask airway and an Aintree catheter: a review of the ProSeal Laryngeal mask airway in the management of the difficult airway. *Anaesthesia.* 2005;60(11):1129–1136.
273. De Bast Y, De Backer D, Moraine JJ, et al. The cuff leak test to predict failure of tracheal extubation for laryngeal edema. *Intensive Care Med.* 2002;28(9):1267–1272.
274. Sundaram RK, Nikolic G. Successful treatment of post-extubation stridor by continuous positive airway pressure. *Anaesth Intensive Care.* 1996;24(3):392–393.
275. Hartley M, Vaughan RS. Problems associated with tracheal extubation. *Br J Anaesth.* 1993;71(4):561–568.
276. Darmon JY, Rauss A, Dreyfuss D, et al. Evaluation of risk factors for laryngeal edema after tracheal extubation in adults and its prevention by dexamethasone. A placebo-controlled, double-blind, multicenter study. *Anesthesiology.* 1992;77(2):245–251.
277. Ho LI, Harn HJ, Lien TC, et al. Postextubation laryngeal edema in adults. Risk factor evaluation and prevention by hydrocortisone. *Intensive Care Med.* 1996;22(9):933–936.
278. Kriner EJ, Shafazand S, Colice GL. The endotracheal tube cuff-leak test as a predictor for postextubation stridor *Respir Car.* 2005;50(12):1632–1638.
279. François B, Bellissant E, Gissot V, et al. 12-h pretreatment with methylprednisolone versus placebo for prevention of postextubation laryngeal oedema: a randomised double-blind trial. *Lancet.* 2007;369(9567):1083–1089.
280. Jaber S, Chanques G, Matecki S, et al. Post-extubation stridor in intensive care unit patients. Risk factors evaluation and importance of the cuff-leak test. *Intensive Care Med.* 2003;29(1):69–74.
281. Smina M, Salam A, Khamiees M, et al. Cough peak flows and extubation outcomes. *Ches.* 2003;124(1):262–268.
282. Dane TE, King EG. A prospective study of complications after tracheostomy for assisted ventilation. *Ches.* 1975;67(4):398–404.
283. Pearson FG, Goldberg M, da Silva AJ. Tracheal stenosis complicating tracheostomy with cuffed tubes. Clinical experience and observations from a prospective study. *Arch Surg.* 1968;97(3):380–394.
284. Stauffer JL, Olson DE, Petty TL. Complications and consequences of endotracheal intubation and tracheotomy. A prospective study of 150 critically ill adult patients. *Am J Med.* 1981;70(1):65–76.
285. Sandhu RS, Pasquale MD, Miller K, et al. Measurement of endotracheal tube cuff leak to predict postextubation stridor and need for reintubation. *J Am Coll Surg.* 2000;190(6):682–687.
286. Ferrari LR, Gotta AW. Anesthesia for otolaringologic surgery. In: Barash PG, Cullen BF, Stoelting RK, eds. *Clinical Anesthesia.* 5th ed. Philadelphia, PA: Lippincott Williams & Wilkins; 2006:997–1012.
287. Patel A, Mitchell V. ENT and maxillofacial surgery. In: Calder I, Pearce A, editors. Core topics in Airway Management. Cambridge University Press, 2005:179.
288. Khosh MM, Lebovics RS. Upper airway obstruction. In: Parrillo JE, Dellinger PR, eds. *Critical Care Medicine. Principles of Diagnosis and Management in the Adult.* 2nd ed. St. Louis, MO: Mosby; 2001:808–825.
289. Cheney FW, Posner KL, Lee LA, et al. Trends in anesthesia-related death and brain damage: A closed claims analysis. *Anesthesiology.* 2006;105 (6):1081–1086.
290. Practice guidelines for management of the difficult airway: an updated report by the American Society of Anesthesiologists Task Force on Management of the Difficult Airway. *Anesthesiology.* 2003;98(5):1269–1277.
291. Tami TA, Chu F, Wildes TO, et al. Pulmonary edema and acute upper airway obstruction. *Laryngoscope.* 1986;96(5):506–509.
292. Schwartz DR, Maroo A, Malhotra A, et al. Negative pressure pulmonary hemorrhage. *Chest.* 1999;115(4):1194–1197.
293. Miro AM, Pinsky MR. Heart-lung interactions. In: Tobin MJ, ed. *Principles and Practice of Mechanical Ventilation.* 1st ed. New York, NY: McGraw-Hill; 1994:647–671.
294. Deepika K, Kenaan CA, Barrocas AM, et al. Negative pressure pulmonary edema after acute upper airway obstruction. *J Clin Anesth.* 1997;9(5):403–408.
295. Torres A, Gatell JM, Aznar E, et al. Re-intubation increases the risk of nosocomial pneumonia in patients needing mechanical ventilation. *Am J Respir Crit Care Med.* 1995;152(1):137–141.
296. Zeggwagh AA, Abouqal R, Madani N, et al. Weaning from mechanical ventilation: a model for extubation. *Intensive Care Med.* 1999;25(10):1077–1083.
297. Adderley RJ, Mullins GC. When to extubate the croup patient: the "leak" test. *Can J Anaesth.* 1987;34(3 (Pt 1)):304–306.
298. Miller RL, Cole RP. Association between reduced cuff leak volume and postextubation stridor. *Chest.* 1996;110(4):1035–1040.
299. Engoren M. Evaluation of the cuff-leak test in a cardiac surgery population. *Chest.* 1999;116(4):1029–1031.

300. Cheng KC, Hou CC, Huang HC, et al. Intravenous injection of methylprednisolone reduces the incidence of postextubation stridor in intensive care unit patients. *Crit Care Med.* 2006;34(5):1325–1350.
301. Deem S. Limited value of the cuff-leak test. *Respir Care.* 2005;50(12):1617–1618.
302. Ding LW, Wang HC, Wu HD, et al. Laryngeal ultrasound: a useful method in predicting post-extubation stridor. A pilot study. *Eur Respir J.* 2006;27(2):384–389.
303. Khamiees M, Raju P, DeGirolamo A, et al. Predictors of extubation outcome in patients who have successfully completed a spontaneous breathing trial. *Chest.* 2001;120(4):1262–1270.
304. Salam A, Tilluckdharry L, Amoateng-Adjepong Y, et al. Neurologic status, cough, secretions and extubation outcomes. *Intensive Care Med.* 2004;30(7):1334–1339.
305. Coplin WM, Pierson DJ, Cooley KD, et al. Implications of extubation delay in brain-injured patients meeting standard weaning criteria. *Am J Respir Crit Care Med.* 2000;161(5):1530–1536.
306. Vallverdu I, Calaf N, Subirana M, et al. Clinical characteristics, respiratory functional parameters, and outcome of a two-hour T-piece trial in patients weaning from mechanical ventilation. *Am J Respir Crit Care Med,* 1998;158(6):1855–1862.
307. Kress JP, O'Connor MF, Pohlman AS, et al. Sedation of critically ill patients during mechanical ventilation. A comparison of propofol and midazolam. *Am J Respir Crit Care Med.* 1996;153(3):1012–1018.
308. Capdevila XJ, Perrigault PF, Perey PJ, et al. Occlusion pressure and its ratio to maximum inspiratory pressure are useful predictors for successful extubation following T-piece weaning trial. *Chest.* 1995;108(2):482–489.
309. Fernandez R, Raurich JM, Mut T, et al. Extubation failure: diagnostic value of occlusion pressure (P0.1) and P0.1-derived parameters. *Intensive Care Med.* 2004;30(2):234–240.
310. Hilbert G, Gruson D, Portel L, et al. Airway occlusion pressure at 0.1 s (P0.1) after extubation: an early indicator of postextubation hypercapnic respiratory insufficiency. *Intensive Care Med.* 1998;24(12):1277–1282.
311. King EG, Sheehan GJ, McDonnell TJ. Upper airway obstruction. In: Hall JB, Schmidt GA, Wood LDH, eds. *Principles of Critical Care.* 1st ed. New York, NY: McGraw-Hill; 1992:1710–1718.
312. Cooper SD, Benumof JL. Airway algorithm: safety considerations. In: Murell RC, Eichhorn JH, eds. *Patient Safety in Anesthetic Practice.* New York, NY: Churchill Livingstone; 1997:221–262.
313. Practice guidelines for management of the difficult airway. A report by the American Society of Anesthesiologists Task Force on Management of the Difficult Airway. *Anesthesiology.* 1993;78(3):597–602.
314. Cooper RM. The use of an endotracheal ventilation catheter in the management of difficult extubations. *Can J Anaesth.* 1996;43(1):90–93.
315. Loudermilk EP, Hartmannsgruber M, Stoltzfus DP, et al. A prospective study of the safety of tracheal extubation using a pediatric airway exchange catheter for patients with a known difficult airway. *Chest.* 1997;111(6):1660–1665.
316. Dosemeci L, Yilmaz M, Yegin A, et al. The routine use of pediatric airway exchange catheter after extubation of adult patients who have undergone maxillofacial or major neck surgery: a clinical observational study. *Crit Care.* 2004;8(6):R385–R390.
317. Walz JM, Zayaruzny M, Heard SO. Airway management in critical illness. *Chest.* 2007;131(2):608–620.
318. Hartley M. Difficulties at tracheal extubation. In: Latto IP, Vaughan RS, eds. *Difficulties in Tracheal Intubation.* 2nd ed. London, UK: WB Saunders; 1997:347–359.
319. Grabovac MT, Kim K, Quinn TE, et al. Respiratory care. In: Miller RD, ed. *Miller's Anesthesia.* 6th ed. Philadelphia, PA: Elsevier, Churchill Livingstone; 2005:2811–2830.
320. Nutman J, Brooks LJ, Deakins KM, et al. Racemic versus l-epinephrine aerosol in the treatment of postextubation laryngeal edema: results from a prospective, randomized, double-blind study. *Crit Care Med.* 1994;22(10):1591–1594.
321. Schmidt GA, Hall JB. Management of the ventilated patient. In: Hall JB, Schmidt GA, Wood LDH, eds. *Principles of Critical Care Medicine.* 3rd ed. New York, NY: McGraw-Hill; 2005:481–468.
322. Donlon JV, Doyle DJ, Feldman MA. Anesthesia for eye, ear, nose and throat surgery. In: Miller RD, ed. *Miller's Anesthesia.* 6th ed. Philadelphi, PA: Elsevier, Churchill Livingstone; 2005:2527–2555.
323. Tellez DW, Galvis AG, Storgion SA, et al. Dexamethasone in the prevention of postextubation stridor in children. *J Pediatr.* 1991;118(2):289–294.
324. Anene O, Meert KL, Uy H, et al. Dexamethasone for the prevention of postextubation airway obstruction: a prospective, randomized, double-blind, placebo-controlled trial. *Crit Care Med.* 1996;24(10):1666–1669.
325. Ferrara TB, Georgieff MK, Ebert J, et al. Routine use of dexamethasone for the prevention of postextubation respiratory distress. *J Perinatol.* 1989;9(3):287–290.
326. Gehlbach B, Kress JP. Upper airway obstruction. In: Hall JB, Schmidt GA, Wood LDH, eds. *Principles of Critical Care Medicine.* 3rd ed. New York, NY: McGraw-Hil; 2005:455–464.
327. Orr JB. Helium-oxygen gas mixtures in the management of patients with airway obstruction. *Ear Nose Throat J.* 1988;67(12):866, 868–869.
328. Jaber S, Carlucci A, Boussarsar M, et al. Helium-oxygen in the postextubation period decreases inspiratory effort. *Am J Respir Crit Care Med.* 2001;164(4):633–637.
329. Skrinskas GJ, Hyland RH, Hutcheon MA. Using helium-oxygen mixtures in the management of acute upper airway obstruction. *Can Med Assoc J.* 1983;128(5):555–558.
330. Boorstein JM, Boorstein SM, Humphries GN, et al. Using helium-oxygen mixtures in the emergency management of acute upper airway obstruction. *Ann Emerg Med.* 1989;18(6):688–690.
331. Berkenbosch JW, Grueber RE, Graff GR, et al. Patterns of helium-oxygen (heliox) usage in the critical care environment. *J Intensive Care Med.* 2004;19(6):335–344.
332. Nakatsuka M, MacLeod AD. Hemodynamic and respiratory effects of transtracheal high-frequency jet ventilation during difficult intubation. *J Clin Anesth.* 1992;4(4):321–324.
333. Smith RB, Babinski M, Klain M, et al. Percutaneous transtracheal ventilation. *JACEP.* 1976;5(10):765–770.
334. Benjamin B. Prolonged intubation injuries of the larynx: endoscopic diagnosis, classification, and treatment. *Ann Otol Rhinol Laryngol Suppl.* 1993;160:1–15.
335. Keenan SP, Powers C, McCormack DG, et al. Noninvasive positive-pressure ventilation for postextubation respiratory distress: a randomized controlled trial. *JAMA.* 2002;287(24):3238–3244.
336. Jiang JS, Kao SJ, Wang SN. Effect of early application of biphasic positive airway pressure on the outcome of extubation in ventilator weaning. *Respirology.* 1999;4(2):161–165.
337. Sieck GC, Prakash YS. Cross-bridge kinetics in respiratory muscles. *Eur Respir J.* 1997;10(9):2147–2158.
338. Aubier M, Viires N. Calcium ATPase and respiratory muscle function. *Eur Respir J.* 1998;11(3):758–766.

CHAPTER 133 ■ HIGH-FREQUENCY VENTILATION: LESSONS LEARNED AND FUTURE DIRECTIONS

NIALL D. FERGUSON • ARTHUR S. SLUTSKY

Mechanical ventilation practices continue to evolve. In particular, the ventilatory care of patients with acute lung injury (ALI) and acute respiratory distress syndrome (ARDS) has been refocused on avoiding or minimizing further damage to the fragile, injured lung. Conventional ventilators have been used successfully to limit this ventilator-induced lung injury (VILI) (1–3), but questions remain regarding the optimal method for lung protection during mechanical ventilation. The recognition of the critical role that VILI can play in the outcome of adults with ALI/ARDS has, in part, spawned a renewed interest in alternative modes of ventilation that may be more lung protective.

High-frequency ventilation (HFV) is just such a modality. In this chapter, we briefly review the different subtypes of HFV and then concentrate on high-frequency oscillation as the mode with the most supporting data and promise. As will be seen, a great deal of experience with HFV has been accrued in the neonatal and pediatric settings. We will draw on this knowledge where relevant, but focus this chapter from the viewpoint of HFV as an emerging therapy in the adult intensive care unit (ICU).

DEFINITIONS, TERMINOLOGY, AND SUBTYPES OF HIGH-FREQUENCY VENTILATION

High-frequency ventilation is a collection of ventilatory modes, grouped together by their common property of employing high respiratory rates, all greater than 60 breaths per minute (4,5). In addition to high-frequency oscillation (HFO), other modes in this group include high-frequency jet ventilation (HFJV) and high-frequency percussive ventilation (HFPV).

High-frequency Jet Ventilation

HFJV is a mode of ventilation in which gas is delivered through a small-bore catheter into the lungs at rates of 100 to 150 breaths per minute (5,6). Delivered tidal volume is still small, but higher than just the volume exiting the jet, as the jets entrain an additional flow of gas by the *Venturi effect*. Exhalation is passive during HFJV, and gas trapping or dynamic hyperinflation can be an issue. In practice, a conventional ventilator is set up as a "slave" to the jet to provide positive end-expiratory pressure, along with basic monitoring and alarms.

HFJV is a very efficient mode for removing CO_2. Additionally, because of HFJV's very high flow rates and the differing pulmonary time constants in the clinical setting of bronchopleural fistulae, this mode of ventilation is purported to have beneficial effects in the presence of this disorder; however, these benefits have not been verified during objective testing (7,8). Concerns with HFJV relate to the delivery of high pressures (10–50 pounds per square inch), unpredictable tidal volumes, and the development of dynamic hyperinflation, all of which may worsen VILI rather than minimize it. In addition, problems with adequate humidification of inspired gas and the subsequent risks of tracheobronchitis have been noted and documented.

High-frequency Percussive Ventilation

HFPV is the newest and least well studied of the HFV modes. It combines a high-frequency rate of 200 to 900 breaths per minute superimposed on a conventional pressure mode of ventilation (9). HFPV is reported to enhance the clearance of respiratory secretions and has been successfully used in this regard in patients with burns and inhalational injury (9).

High-frequency Oscillation

HFO is a mode of mechanical ventilation that delivers very small tidal volumes around a set mean airway pressure at high respiratory rates of 3 to 15 Hz (equivalent to 180–900 breaths per minute, as 1 Hz = 60 breaths per minute) (10). HFO has been widely and effectively used in neonates and children for close to 20 years (11–15), but only recently has become available in the adult ICU; previous versions of this ventilator were only capable of generating sufficient flow so as to provide adequate CO_2 elimination in patients under 35 kg. In contrast to other HFV modes, humidification is less of an issue during HFO, as a continuous bias flow of humidified gas is passed in front of an oscillating membrane (Fig. 133.1). This oscillating membrane pushes the humidified gas into the patient and also provides active expiration, a factor that likely accounts for the lack of important gas trapping that is observed when HFO is employed at adequate airway pressures (16). The elegance of HFO is that it allows for "decoupling" of oxygenation and ventilation. Alveolar ventilation, and thus carbon dioxide elimination, are dependent on the frequency and tidal volume but are relatively independent of lung volume (17). In contrast, oxygenation is proportional to mean airway pressure and lung volume (18,19).

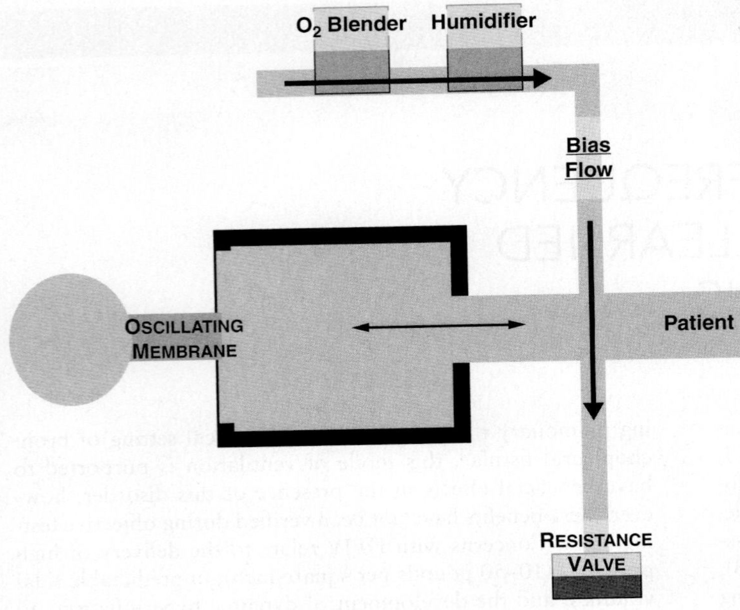

FIGURE 133.1. Schematic overview of the high-frequency oscillation (HFO) circuit. (Reused with permission from Ferguson ND, Stewart TE. New therapies for adults with acute lung injury: high-frequency oscillatory ventilation. *Crit Care Clin.* 2002;18:91–106.)

RATIONALE FOR THE USE OF HIGH-FREQUENCY VENTILATION IN ACUTE LUNG INJURY

Ventilator-induced Lung Injury

Mechanisms of Ventilator-induced Lung Injury

VILI is histologically indistinguishable from ARDS; three decades of experimental research has shown it to occur through a number of mechanisms, including (a) overdistention injury (*volutrauma*) (20–28), (b) collapse–reopening injury (*atelectrauma*) (1,2,20,29–34), and (c) oxygen toxicity (35–37). Each of these can lead, in turn, to further injury—termed *biotrauma*, the release of inflammatory mediators that may worsen pulmonary injury and propagate systemically to harm distant organs (1,2,31,32,38–45).

Numerous studies, performed using both small and large animals, consistently show that ventilatory high end-inspiratory stretch can cause a clinical and histologic picture similar to ARDS even in the absence of any other noxious stimulus (20–28). Patients with ARDS are at increased risk of regional lung overdistention because of the patchy nature of ARDS (46,47); the small areas of relatively normal lung (the so-called "baby lung") receive the bulk of the tidal volume and are at particular risk of volutrauma (48,49). Repeated opening and closing of alveolar units can also cause VILI. In the injured lung, alveolar damage and absolute, or qualitative, deficiencies in alveolar surfactant lead to alveolar instability and localized lung unit collapse. Through each respiratory cycle, these unstable alveoli undergo collapse and reopening, a process that generates injurious mechanical forces and causes further lung injury. There is a substantive body of animal evidence showing that efforts to limit lung unit closing on expiration by maintaining an adequate positive end-expiratory pressure (PEEP) are relatively protective against atelectrauma (1,2,20,30–34). Here, the paradigm is one of "opening the lung and keeping it open," thereby avoiding cyclic collapse and recruitment/derecruitment (2,50).

The major cause of death among ARDS patients is not refractory hypoxemia, as one might expect, but rather multiorgan dysfunction syndrome (MODS) (51). One hypothesis to explain the link between VILI and multiorgan failure is *biotrauma* (38,39)—the release of inflammatory mediators in response to injurious ventilation; these mediators may enter the systemic circulation, and hence lead to the development of MODS. Inflammatory mediators, such as interleukins, tumour necrosis factor-α, and platelet-activating factor, are released in response to VILI, oxygen-free radicals, and alveolar shearing. These mediators perpetuate the cascade of lung inflammation and worsen lung injury (31,32). Additionally, injurious ventilation has been shown to increase these inflammatory mediators in the peripheral blood of patients with ARDS (44,52). Through a variety of mechanisms, this inflammatory injury can lead to nonpulmonary organ dysfunction (41–43).

With an increased appreciation of the mechanisms of VILI, the next logical step is to employ ventilatory strategies that attempt to decrease overdistention, minimize shear injury, and limit oxygen toxicity (53–55). However, these aims may be competing; increasing PEEP may increase the risks of regional alveolar overdistention, while lowering tidal volumes can result in progressive alveolar collapse, a reduction in total lung volume, and higher oxygen requirements. The goals of mechanical ventilation in a patient at risk of VILI therefore should be to ventilate and oxygenate the patient while staying within a "safe window," avoiding both overdistention and derecruitment—collapse—as illustrated in the volume–pressure curve of the lung shown in Figure 133.2 (56).

Impact of Limiting Ventilator-induced Lung Injury with Conventional Ventilation

In the mid-1990s, given the expanding animal data on VILI outlined above and in light of initial promising, but uncontrolled,

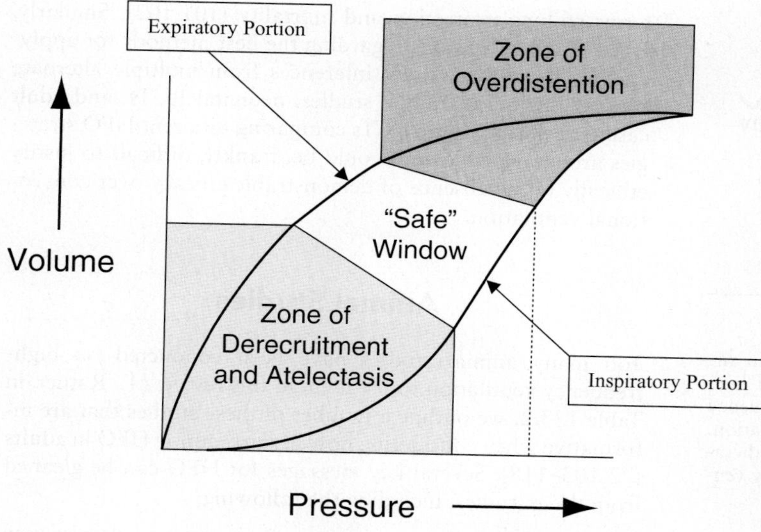

FIGURE 133.2. Volume–pressure curve of the injured lung. (Reused with permission from Froese AB. High-frequency oscillatory ventilation for adult respiratory distress syndrome: let's get it right this time. *Crit Care Med.* 1997;25[6]:906–908.)

human studies of lung-protective ventilation (57,58), a call was made for randomized trials (53). Initial trials focused on avoiding volutrauma, comparing strategies that limited tidal volumes and inspiratory pressures with traditional strategies, both using conventional ventilation. Three smaller studies did not find mortality differences between these approaches (59–61). However, a large, methodologically rigorous, and adequately powered trial conducted by the National Institutes of Health (NIH) ARDS Network did show important differences in mortality (3). In this study, 861 patients were randomly assigned to receive a low-stretch strategy with a targeted tidal volume of 6 mL/kg predicted body weight (PBW) and a plateau pressure limit of 30 cm H_2O, or to a higher-stretch strategy using a targeted tidal volume of 12 mL/kg PBW and a plateau pressure limit of up to 50 cm H_2O. The low-stretch strategy was associated with a mortality reduction from 40% in the control group to 31% in the experimental group (relative risk [RR] 0.78; 95% confidence interval [CI] 0.65–0.93). This trial clearly indicates that avoiding volutrauma saves lives in patients with acute lung injury. The trial has subsequently generated significant discussion regarding its mechanisms of benefit (62) and its choice of control strategy (63–66), but nevertheless, 6 mL/kg PBW has emerged as a standard for tidal volume limitation against which other strategies are compared (67,68).

Another early randomized controlled trial (RCT) published in the late 1990s demonstrated dramatic reductions in mortality using a lung-protective strategy whose goal was to limit both volutrauma and atelectrauma using low tidal volumes and higher PEEP compared with traditional ventilation (69). Amato et al. found a statistically significant reduction in 28-day mortality (11/29 [38%] vs. 17/24 [71%] deaths; RR 0.53; 95% CI 0.31–0.91) favoring patients exposed to the lung-protective strategy. In light of the subsequent positive ARDS Network trial noted above, interpretation of this trial is confounded by the use of both lower PEEP levels and higher tidal volumes and inspiratory pressures in the control group; the relative contribution of efforts to avoid cyclic collapse and reopening is unclear.

Drawing on the promise of the Amato trial, three RCTs have now been completed analyzing the effects of higher versus lower levels of PEEP, while limiting tidal volumes in all study patients. Two of these—the ExPress trial by Mercat et al. and the Lung Open Ventilation Study conducted by Meade et al.—are very recently completed and not yet published; both were presented at the 2006 European Society of Intensive Care Meeting. The one fully published trial, the ALVEOLI study, was conducted by the NIH ARDS Network investigators (70) and was stopped early, which likely contributed to the large baseline imbalance in age favoring the lower PEEP group. When we consider the relative risk after adjusting for baseline imbalances in prognostic factors (including age) from this trial, along with the preliminary findings from the two recent trials, a consistent trend favoring higher PEEP begins to emerge. Therefore, while no single trial has definitively shown an incremental mortality benefit with higher PEEP and attempts to limit atelectrauma while already avoiding overdistention injury, when viewed together, these trials suggest that this benefit may well exist. They also suggest that a higher level of PEEP with or without other maneuvers to open the lung, along with limited tidal volumes and inspiratory pressures, may be considered a very reasonable comparison strategy in future ventilation trials; this approach may be superior, and there is no suggestion of harm compared with lower PEEP levels. These studies clearly demonstrated that ventilatory strategy is important in patients with ARDS, and that lung-protective strategies can minimize VILI and decrease mortality in humans with ARDS. As such, and given the proposed mechanisms of lung protection (Fig. 133.2), a strategy that minimizes overdistention and allows the use of high PEEP should be the ideal mode in patients with ARDS. This is where HFO may have great clinical benefit.

Animal Studies Comparing Conventional Ventilation to High-frequency Oscillation in Acute Lung Injury

The very small delivered tidal volumes are the key to the lung-protective potential of HFO. Because cyclic alveolar stretch is minimal, clinicians are able to set the mean airway pressure (mP_{AW}) on HFO significantly higher than they are able to set PEEP on conventional ventilation, thereby avoiding cyclic collapse and atelectrauma—and yet they are still able to avoid very high peak inspiratory pressures and subsequent

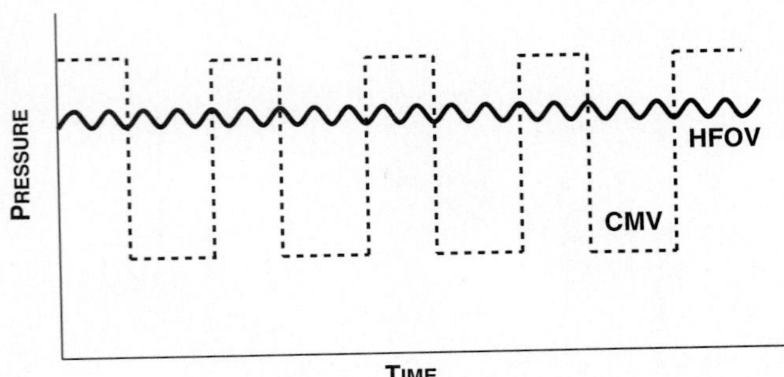

FIGURE 133.3. Pressure–time curve contrasts tidal variations in airway pressure associated with conventional ventilation (*dashed line*) and high-frequency oscillation (*solid line*). HFOV, high-frequency oscillation ventilation; CMV, conventional mechanical ventilation. (Reused with permission from Ferguson ND, Stewart TE. New therapies for adults with acute lung injury: high-frequency oscillatory ventilation. *Crit Care Clin.* 2002;18:91–106.)

volutrauma (Fig. 133.3). This should allow a larger margin of error and make it easier to stay within the "safe window" of lung protection (Fig. 133.2) (56). Since the first descriptions of HFO (71,72), numerous studies have examined the lung-protective potential of HFO using animal models (Table 133.1) (73–89). Perhaps not surprisingly, earlier studies that compared HFO with potentially injurious conventional ventilation uniformly found improvements in physiology, decreased inflammatory markers, and/or improved histology in animals treated with HFO (73–83). More relevant today, however, are recent studies that have compared HFO with lung-protective conventional ventilation, the majority of which continue to favor HFO in terms of physiology, inflammation, and pathology (Table 133.1) (86–89).

Mechanisms of Gas Transport during High-frequency Oscillation

Tidal volumes are extremely small with HFO, often smaller than the anatomic dead space, in the range of 1 to 2 mL/kg (90). In addition to relying on bulk flow, adequate CO_2 removal during HFO is achieved through a number of alternative mechanisms including convective streaming due to asymmetric velocity profiles, Pendelluft, cardiogenic mixing, and diffusion (Fig. 133.4). A full explanation of these physiologic principles is outside the scope of this chapter; the reader is referred to a number of papers reviewing this physiology in detail (5,91–99). The major message from these theoretical and experimental studies is that CO_2 elimination—which is inversely proportional to $PaCO_2$—is described by the relationship $f^aV_T{}^b$, where $a = \sim 1$ and $b = \sim 2$. This is important clinically in that it indicates that increases in frequency may lead to increased $PaCO_2$ if V_T falls (see below).

IMPLEMENTING AND OPTIMIZING HIGH-FREQUENCY OSCILLATION IN ADULTS

Because of the lack of an appropriate surrogate end point that correlates with mortality (3,100), a large multicenter trial will be needed to definitively determine the relative effects of HFO compared with conventional mechanical ventilation (CMV) in terms of lung protection and mortality (101,102). Similarly, when making decisions regarding the best methods for applying HFO, we must draw inferences from multiple alternate sources (including animal studies, neonatal RCTs, and adult case series), since large RCTs comparing different HFO strategies are unavailable and would be, frankly, difficult to justify ethically in the absence of demonstrable efficacy over conventional ventilation.

Animal Studies

Too many animal studies have been conducted on high-frequency ventilation to list them in this review (4). Rather, in Table 133.2, we outline a number of these studies that are informative when considering how best to employ HFO in adults (72,103–118). Several key messages for HFO can be gleaned from these studies, including the following:

1. At adequate mP_{AW}, gas trapping is not an issue despite very high respiratory rates.
2. Increasing mP_{AW} leads to improved oxygenation through lung recruitment.
3. Tidal pressure swings measured in the trachea can be increased with either underrecruitment or overdistention of the lung.
4. Recruitment maneuvers (sustained inflations) may be required to adequately recruit severely injured lungs.

Taken together, and in keeping with the current understanding of VILI mechanisms, these studies suggest that HFO in adults should be employed using an open-lung strategy, facilitated by higher mean airway pressures and lung recruitment maneuvers (56,119,120).

Neonatal Studies

The longest clinical experience and the most rigorous evaluation of HFO have both been in the neonatal population (121–130). The initial large RCT evaluating HFO in this setting raised safety concerns, but it later became evident that here, too, the safe and effective application of HFO requires lung volume recruitment (121,131,132). Subsequent RCTs of HFO with an open-lung approach have demonstrated HFO to be safe and effective in improving oxygenation and, as indicated by the current Cochrane systematic review, may reduce the risk of death or chronic lung disease (15). Interpreting the neonatal HFO literature is challenging due to differences in study populations (preterm vs. term), interventions (degree of lung recruitment targeted), the timing of HFO (immediately after birth vs. later), and by the introduction of exogenous surfactant as a standard therapy in the 1990s. In addition, it is important to realize that the baseline mortality rate in infant respiratory distress syndrome is an order of magnitude less than that seen in adults with severe ARDS. All of these factors mean that results from neonatal studies cannot be directly extrapolated to adult populations. Important lessons can be learned from the neonatal HFO literature, however, including the importance of thoroughly understanding the underlying physiologic mechanisms of the therapy, and the recognition that a learning curve may exist in the initiation of an HFO program (131,132).

TABLE 133.1

ANIMAL STUDIES COMPARING VILI WITH HFO VS. CMV

Author	Animal	Lung injury	HFO	CMV	LRM at onset	Duration	HFO effects on physiology	HFO effects on inflammation	HFO effects on pathology
HFO vs. potentially injurious (high volume/pressure) CMV									
Hamilton 1983	Rabbits	Saline lavage	$mP_{AW} = 15$, $f = 15$ Hz	PEEP 6, PIP 25	Both	5–20 h	↑ O_2	↓ Mortality in 20-h model	↓ Hyaline membranes
Tamura 1985	Rabbits	IV starch particle emboli	$f = 15$ Hz, V_T 1–2 mL/kg	PEEP 2, PIP 20	No	3 h	↑ O_2	↓ EVLW, ↓ protein leak	
McCulloch 1988	Rabbits	Saline lavage	High EELV	PEEP 8, PIP for CO_2	Both	7 h	↑ O_2, ↑ compliance		↓ Hyaline membranes
Bond 1993	Rabbits	Saline lavage	$mP_{AW} = 15$	PEEP 8, PIP for CO_2	Both	6 h	↑ O_2, ↑ compliance		
Imai 1994	Rabbits	Saline lavage	Intermittent LRM $mP_{AW} = 15$, $f = 15$ Hz	$mP_{AW} = 15$, PIP 25, PEEP 5	Both	4 h	↑ O_2, ↑ compliance	↓ PMN, PAF, TXB_2 in BAL	
Matsuoka 1994	Rabbits	Saline lavage	$mP_{AW} = 15$, $f = 15$ Hz	PEEP 5, PIP 25	Both	2–4 h	↑ O_2	↓ BAL PMN # and activation	↓ Intra-alveolar cellularity
Sugiura 1994	Rabbits	Saline lavage	$mP_{AW} = 15$ Hz	PEEP 5, PIP 23	Both	4 h	↑ O_2, ↑ compliance	↓ BAL PMN # and activation	↓ Lung injury
Takata 1997	Rabbits	Saline lavage	Intermittent LRM $mP_{AW} = 13$, $f = 15$ Hz	PEEP 5, PIP 28	Both	1–4 h	↑ O_2, ↑ compliance	↓ TNF-α mRNA, ↓ PMN in BAL	↓ Hyaline membranes
Gommers 1999	Rabbits	Saline lavage	$f = 10$ Hz mP_{AW} for PaO_2	PEEP 6, PIP 26	HFO only	5 h	↑ O_2		↓ Lung injury
Kerr 2001	Rabbits	NNMU lavage	$f = 15$ Hz $mP_{AW} = PIP-7$	PEEP 4, $V_T = 10$ mL/kg	No	1–2 h	↑ O_2, ↓ resp. acidosis	↓ LA surfactant conversion/loss	
Noda 2003	Rabbits	Saline lavage	$mP_{AW} = 15$, $f = 15$ Hz	PEEP 5, PIP 25	Both	4 h	↑ O_2	↓ TNF-α mRNA, ↓ BAL PMN #	
HFO vs. lung-protective CMV									
Vazquez de Anda 1999	Rats	Saline lavage	$f = 10$ Hz mP_{AW} for PaO_2	PEEP for PaO_2, V_T for CO_2	Both	3 h	Similar O_2	Similar BAL protein levels	
Rimensberger 2000	Rabbits	Saline lavage	$f = 15$ Hz $mP_{AW} = CCP + 4$	$V_T = 5$ mL/kg PEEP > CCP	Both	4 h	Similar O_2 and compliance	Similar MPO levels	Similar histology score
Rotta 2001	Rabbits	Saline lavage	$mP_{AW} = 16$, $f = 10$ Hz	PEEP > P_{flex}, $V_T = 6$ mL/kg	Both	4 h	↓ resp. acidosis, ↓ inotropes	Similar, elastase in BAL	↓ MDA in lung homogenate
Imai 2001	Rabbits	Saline lavage	$mP_{AW} = 15$, $f = 15$ Hz	PEEP 10, $V_T = 6$ mL/kg	Both	4 h	↑ O_2, ↓ CO_2, ↑ compliance	↓ TNF-α, ↓ PMN in BAL	↓ Alveolar path. score
Sedeek 2003	Sheep	Saline lavage	f = 8 Hz mP_{AW} = PMC	PIP <35; PEEP = PMC	Both; repeated	6 h	Similar O_2	Similar to ↓ cytokine mRNA	↓ Lung injury
Von der Hardt 2004	Piglets	Saline lavage	$mP_{AW} = 18$, $f = 15$ Hz	PEEP 4, PIP 20	No	8 h	↑ O_2	↓ mRNA of IL-8, IL-1β IL-6, etc.	↓ Macrophage IL-8 gene expr.

VILI, ventilator-induced lung injury; HFO, high-frequency oscillation; CMV, conventional mechanical ventilation; LRM, lung recruitment manoeuvre; mP_{AW}, mean airway pressure; *f*, frequency; PEEP, positive end-expiratory pressure; PIP, peak inspiratory pressure on CMV; EVLW, extravascular lung water; V_T, tidal volume; EELV, end-expiratory lung volume; PMN, polymorphonuclear cells; PAF, platelet-activating factor; TXB_2, thromboxane B_2; BAL, bronchoalveolar lavage; TNF, tumor necrosis factor; NNMU, *N*-nitroso-n-methylurethane; resp., respiratory; MDA, malondialdehyde (marker of lipid peroxidation); LA, large aggregate surfactant (i.e., functionally active surfactant); CCP, critical closing pressure (i.e., pressure on deflation limb of volume–pressure curve corresponding to 50% of total lung capacity); MPO, myeloperoxidase; PMC, point of maximal curvature (on the deflation limb of the volume–pressure curve); IL, interleukin; gene expr., gene expression; exog surf., exogenous surfactant.
Study selection criteria: Population: Animal models (excluding preterm animals) of acute lung injury; intervention: HFO vs. conventional ventilation, no additional cointerventions; outcome: any marker(s) of lung injury (not gas exchange alone); therefore, not crossover studies.

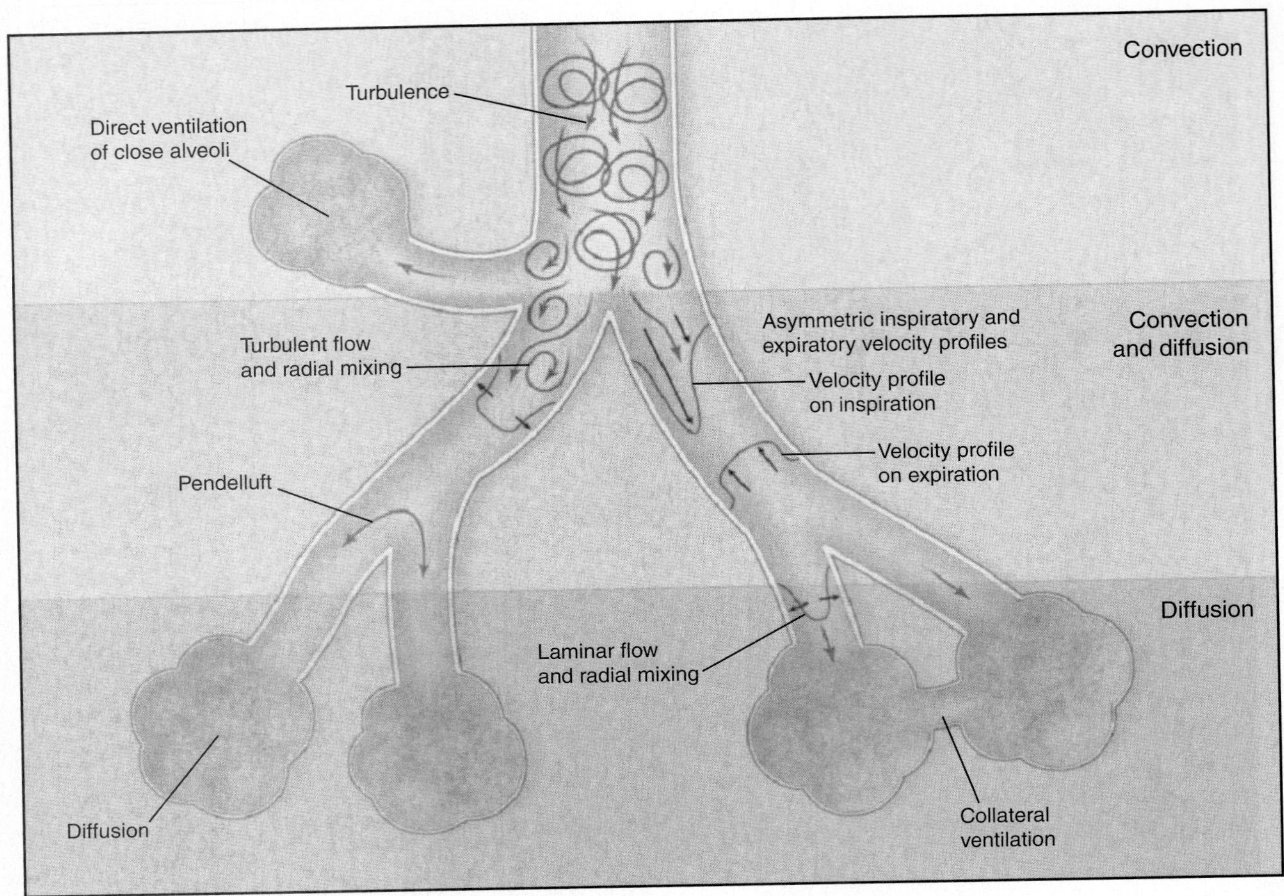

FIGURE 133.4. Alternative mechanisms of gas exchange with high-frequency oscillation (HFO). (Reused with permission from Slutsky AS, Drazen JM. Ventilation with small tidal volumes. *N Engl J Med.* 2002;347[9]:630–631.)

Uncontrolled Adult Studies

The studies reporting the clinical experience with HFO in adults, which are summarized in Table 133.3 (133–143), are also informative for optimizing an HFO protocol. Almost all of them studied HFO as rescue therapy for patients with extremely severe disease who were "failing" conventional ventilation. Despite being limited by their uncontrolled nature and by selection bias, consistent messages that arise from these rescue series include:

1. HFO is usually effective in improving oxygenation.
2. HFO appears safe, with no obvious increased rates of complications.
3. Both baseline oxygenation index and duration of CMV prior to HFO are associated with increased mortality.

One prospective, multicentered study from our group is unique in that it tested an explicit protocol for applying HFO early in the course of ARDS, incorporating lung recruitment maneuvers (RMs) and a descending titration of mean airway pressure to optimize lung volumes for gas exchange and lung protection (140). RMs—sustained inflation maneuvers with 30 to 40 cm H_2O pressures for 30 to 40 seconds—have been found to be safe in adults on CMV, but studies have shown mixed results in terms of efficacy and duration of their oxygenation effects (144–152). Because of the small tidal volumes generated with HFO, there is very little tidal recruitment of the lung, creating a more compelling rationale for RMs during HFO compared with CMV (19,50,102,153,154). The main finding from a physiologic standpoint in our study was that the combination of HFO and RMs was well tolerated and resulted in rapid and sustained lung recruitment (140). Furthermore, the explicit HFO protocol appeared feasible; adherence was excellent, and the method for weaning HFO and transitioning to CMV appeared practical and safe.

Tidal volume during HFO has always been assumed to be very low, but it is not routinely measured with currently available oscillators. Tidal volume is known to be inversely related to frequency due to a decreasing inspiratory time with increasing frequency (17), and in adults, typical frequencies have been significantly lower than those used in neonates (3–6 vs. 12–15 Hz) (132,139). Sedeek et al. explored this issue in a lung-injured sheep model, measuring tidal volumes of up to 4 mL/kg at high-pressure amplitudes and low frequencies (Table 133.2) (118). These tidal volume measurements may be overestimated because of technical reasons (155), but they do highlight the importance of efforts to minimize delivered tidal volumes with adult HFO, and they have spurred further investigation. Tidal volumes on HFO measured in adults using a very accurate device (156) were small—1.1 to 2.5 mL/kg—and strongly

(*text continues on page 2038*)

TABLE 133.2

ANIMAL STUDIES INFORMING OPTIMAL HFO IMPLEMENTATION

Author	Animal	Lung injury	Intervention	Design	Outcomes	Main findings	Comment
HFO proof of concept and basic settings							
Bohn 1980	Dogs	None	HFO at various frequencies	Single cohort	Gas exchange and airway pressures	First description of HFO showing safety and efficacy	HFO capable of supporting adequate gas exchange
Bryan 1986	Rabbits	Saline lavage	HFO at various mP_{AW}	Single cohort	Occlusion pressures	Gas trapping with HFO only seen at extremely low mP_{AW}	Gas trapping not an issue with HFO despite high frequencies
Bancalari 1987	Rabbits	Meconium aspiration	HFO (mP_{AW} = 11–22; f = 10–15 Hz) vs. HFJV	Crossover	Gas exchange, lung volumes (plethys.)	No significant gas trapping with HFO; yes with HFJV	Gas trapping not an issue with HFO despite high frequencies
Courtney 1992	Rabbits	Saline lavage	HFO at various I:E ratios (constant mP_{AW}, P and f)	Single cohort	Gas exchange and hemodynamics	Varying I:E ratios had no significant effect on PaO_2, $PaCO_2$, BP, or CO	At constant mP_{AW}, I:E ratio does not have a large effect on gas exchange
Pillow 1999	Rabbits	None	HFO at various I:E ratios	Single cohort	Airway–alveolar pressure difference	P_{ALV} was lower than mP_{AW} at I:E ratios below 1:1	With I:E of 1:2, alveolar pressures may be somewhat lower than set mP_{AW}
HFO volume-pressure and gas-exchange relationships							
Boynton 1991	Rabbits	Saline lavage	HFO at various mP_{AW}	Single cohort	Gas exchange, lung volumes (plethys.)	↑ mP_{AW} leads to ↑ O_2 through ↑lung volume; hysteresis present	Oxygenation response is a reasonable surrogate for recruitment
Goddon 2001	Sheep	Saline lavage	HFO at various mP_{AW}	Single cohort	Gas exchange and mechanics	Best O_2 was at mP_{AW} of P_{FLEX} + 6 also equal to PMC on deflation	Oxygenation response is a reasonable surrogate for recruitment
van Genderingen 2002 (ICM)	Pigs	Saline lavage	HFO with stepwise increases in mP_{AW}	Single cohort	Oxygenation index and shunt fraction	mP_{AW} with ↑ OI was close to ↑ shunt; large hysteresis	Oxygenation response is a reasonable surrogate for recruitment
Dembinski 2002	Pigs	Oleic acid infusion	HFO vs. CMV titrated to PaO_2	RCT	Airway pressures and shunt fraction	↑ mP_{AW} needed with HFO to match PaO_2 on CMV	High mP_{AW} needed for lung opening on HFO—may be reduced subsequently
Luecke 2003	Pigs	Saline lavage	HFO at various mP_{AW}	Single cohort	Gas exchange and mechanics	Increasing mP_{AW} mirrored volume on deflation limb of pressure–volume curve; no hysteresis on HFO	Lung opening may occur on HFO without RMs

(Continued)

TABLE 133.2

(CONTINUED)

Author	Animal	Lung injury	Intervention	Design	Outcomes	Main findings	Comment
Intrathoracic tidal pressure swings and lung recruitment during HFO							
Sakai 1999	Rabbits	Saline lavage	HFO at various mP_{AW} and V_T	Single cohort	Pressure swings in airway and pleura	At low mP_{AW} pressure swings are increased; decreased after an RM	Underrecruited lungs lead to higher pressure swings on HFO
van Genderingen 2002	Pigs	Saline lavage	HFO at various mP_{AW}	Single cohort	Oscillatory pressure ratio (OPR)[a]	OPR is increased when the lung is overdistended OR underrecruited	Underrecruited or overdistended lungs lead to higher pressure swings on HFO
Recruitment maneuver effects with HFO							
Byford 1988	Rabbits	Saline lavage + CMV	HFO + RMs with oscillator on and off	Crossover	Gas exchange, lung volumes (plethys.)	RMs with oscillator on yielded ↑ recruitment at ↓ pressures	RMs with oscillator not paused may be more effective
Sznajder 1988	Dogs	Oleic acid	HFO vs. high tidal volume CMV	Crossover	Gas exchange, lung volumes (plethys.)	Full lung recruitment on HFO only achieved after a RM to TLC	RMs on HFO needed for lung recruitment in severe lung injury model
Walsh 1988	Rabbits	Saline lavage	HFO + various RMs	Single cohort	Gas exchange and mechanics	RMs improve gas exchange and compliance on HFO	Lower pressures possible with HFO after RMs
Suzuki 1992	Rabbits	Saline lavage + CMV	HFO ± RMs	Single cohort	Lung volume and gas exchange	HFO without RMs was uniformly fatal; HFO + RMs improved gas exchange	RMs on HFO needed for lung recruitment in severe lung injury model
Delivered tidal volumes with "adult settings" on HFO							
Sedeek 2003	Sheep	Saline lavage	HFO at various ΔP and f	Single cohort	Delivered tidal volumes	At very low f and high ΔP, V_T may not be negligible on HFO	Need to target lowest V_T possible with HFO (use highest tolerated frequency)

[a] Oscillatory pressure ratio is the ratio of pressure swings at the proximal and distal end of the endotracheal tube during HFO.
HFO, high-frequency oscillation; mP_{AW}, mean airway pressure; f, frequency; HFJV, high-frequency jet ventilation; plethys., plethysmography; I:E, inspiratory:expiratory; BP, blood pressure; CO, cardiac output; P_{ALV}, alveolar pressure; P_{FLEX}, pressure at the lower inflexion point of the static volume–pressure curve; OI, oxygen index; RCT, randomized controlled trial; PMC, point of maximal curvature on the deflation limb of the static volume–pressure curve; CMV, conventional mechanical ventilation; V_T, tidal volume; RM, recruitment maneuver.

TABLE 133.3

UNCONTROLLED STUDIES HFO FOR ADULT ARDS

Author	*N*	Population	Baseline severity of illness	Design	Complications	Main findings	Comment
HFO as "rescue therapy"							
Fort 1997	17	ARDS	OI = 49 APACHE II = 23	Prospective	Barotrauma 6% ETT obstruction 6%	Improved oxygenation; mortality 53%	Baseline OI and duration of CMV associated with ↑ mortality
Claridge 1999	5	ARDS, trauma	P/F = 52 APACHE II = 28	Not reported	Not reported	Improved oxygenation; mortality 20%	HFO appears safe and improves O_2 in rescue setting
Mehta 1997	24	ARDS	OI = 33 APACHE II = 22	Prospective	Barotrauma 8% ETT obstruction 4%	Improved oxygenation; mortality 67%	HFO appears safe and improves O_2 in rescue setting
Andersen 2002	16	ARDS	OI = 28 APACHE II = 27	Retrospective	Barotrauma 6%	Improved oxygenation; mortality 31%	HFO appears safe and improves O_2 in rescue setting
David 2003	42	ARDS	OI = 23 APACHE II = 28	Prospective	Barotrauma 2%	Improved oxygenation; mortality 43%	HFO appears safe and improves O_2 in rescue setting
Cartotto 2004	25	ARDS, burns	OI = 27 APACHE II = 16	Retrospective	Barotrauma 0%	Improved oxygenation; mortality 28%	HFO appears safe and improves O_2 in rescue setting
Mehta 2004	156	ARDS	OI = 31 APACHE II = 24	Retrospective	Barotrauma 21%	Improved oxygenation; mortality 62%	Baseline OI and duration of CMV associated with ↑ mortality
Pachl 2006	30	ARDS	Not reported	Prospective	Not reported	Not reported	
Finkielman 2006	14	ARDS	OI = 35 APACHE II = 35	Retrospective	Barotrauma 0%	Improved oxygenation; mortality 57%	HFO appears safe and improves O_2 in rescue setting
Weiler 2006	5	ARDS	OI = 28 APACHE II = 25	Retrospective	Barotrauma 0%	Improved oxygenation; mortality not reported	HFO appears safe and improves O_2 in rescue setting
HFO for lung protection							
Ferguson 2005	25	Early ARDS	OI = 23 APACHE II = 24	Prospective, consecutive, protocolized	Barotrauma 8%–20%	Rapidly improved oxygenation; mortality 44%; excellent protocol adherence	Pilot study of an explicit protocol including conversion criteria to CMV

HFO, high-frequency oscillation; ARDS, acute respiratory distress syndrome; OI, oxygen index; ETT, endotracheal tube; CMV, conventional mechanical ventilation.

influenced by frequency (90). Cumulatively, these data are reassuring in that HFO in adults can be set to deliver very small tidal volumes, but at the same time they highlight the potential importance of targeting the lowest tidal volume possible (155). This could be achieved by increasing frequency as high as tolerated while avoiding severe respiratory acidosis, a strategy that has been proposed as physiologically sensible (157) and recently shown to be feasible in most patients (158).

Randomized Controlled Trials of High-frequency Oscillation in Adults

To date, only two RCTs have compared HFO with CMV in adults (101,159). Both of these trials were planned and started prior to the completion of the first ARDS Network study that showed benefit from strict control of tidal volumes (3). Neither RCT demonstrated safety concerns (the primary outcome); rates of barotrauma and other complications were similar between groups in both studies. The larger of the two RCTs shows an impressive trend toward a mortality benefit with HFO (RR 0.72; 95% CI 0.50–1.04) despite more than 10% of the control group crossing over to HFO (101). The second trial, which began accrual at the same time, was stopped because of slow enrollment. In fact, the enrollment rates per center per month were identical in both studies; the latter study simply highlights the need for extensive multicentered collaboration for a successful HFO RCT. Mortality results from the smaller study are less encouraging, but these are significantly confounded by large baseline differences favoring the control group, and by an almost 20% crossover rate. Nevertheless, pooled results from these trials still suggest a potentially important survival benefit with HFO (RR 0.899, 95% CI 0.51–1.58; random effects model). Inferences from these RCTs are limited, however, by their methodology, small sample sizes, and, importantly, by use of now dated, potentially injurious conventional ventilation strategies.

FUTURE DIRECTIONS

A research focus on the ventilatory care of ARDS patients has, to date, paid significantly greater dividends than the disappointing results of pharmacotherapy testing (160). Following the completion of the three conventional ventilation RCTs comparing a "lung open" approach with a lower PEEP approach, we believe that the study of HFO represents the next logical and important question to be addressed in ARDS research. We ground this belief in:

1. A strong physiologic rationale and database of animal studies
2. Experience from the neonatal and pediatric arenas
3. An expanding clinical experience with adult HFO
4. Promising results from small nondefinitive RCTs

Despite the very strong physiologic rationale and the encouraging clinical data to date, there are potential detrimental consequences of HFO. First, the physiologic benefit of HFO is likely derived from recruitment of the lung with higher mean airway pressures, while still not overdistending alveoli because of the very small tidal volumes. Hence, patients with mild disease and minimal collapsed or consolidated lung may not be good candidates for HFO (151). Second, the high mean airway pressures may negatively impact hemodynamics. Third, because the bias flow rate is insufficient to meet the inspiratory flow demands of adults in respiratory distress, all adults on HFO must have their respiratory efforts suppressed with intravenous sedation. This means that the majority of adults will be heavily sedated, and many may need transient neuromuscular blockade. Due to these concerns, and to target a population in need of recruitment, we believe that future studies should enroll patients with severe ARDS who are likely to have significant lung collapse and who frequently require significant amounts of sedation, with or without paralysis, on conventional ventilators.

In summary, we believe that HFO—and other forms of high-frequency ventilation—should currently be reserved for "rescue therapy" in patients who are failing conventional ventilation. We do not believe that HFO can be recommended for routine use in adults with ARDS at the current time because:

- There are potential detrimental physiologic and clinical consequences as described above
- This would represent premature dissemination of a complex technology without rigorous evaluation of its risks, benefits, and indications

A definitive RCT to establish the impact of HFO versus best current conventional ventilation on mortality is needed.

References

1. Pinhu L, Whitehead T, Evans T, et al. Ventilator-associated lung injury. *Lancet.* 2003;361:332–340.
2. Tremblay LN, Slutsky AS. Ventilator-induced lung injury: from the bench to the bedside. *Intensive Care Med.* 2006;32(1):24–33.
3. The Acute Respiratory Distress Syndrome Network. Ventilation with lower tidal volumes as compared with traditional tidal volumes for acute lung injury and the acute respiratory distress syndrome. *N Engl J Med.* 2000;342(18):1301–1308.
4. Froese AB, Bryan AC. High frequency ventilation. *Am Rev Resp Dis.* 1987;135(6):1363–1374.
5. Drazen JM, Kamm RD, Slutsky AS. High-frequency ventilation. *Physiol Rev.* 1984;64(2):505–543.
6. Klain M, Smith RB. High frequency percutaneous transtracheal jet ventilation. *Crit Care Med.* 1977;5(6):280–287.
7. Roth MD, Wright JW, Bellamy PE. Gas flow through a bronchopleural fistula. Measuring the effects of high-frequency jet ventilation and chest-tube suction. *Chest.* 1988;93(1):210–213.
8. Bishop MJ, Benson MS, Sato P, et al. Comparison of high-frequency jet ventilation with conventional mechanical ventilation for bronchopleural fistula. *Anesth Analg.* 1987;66(9):833–838.
9. Salim A, Martin M. High-frequency percussive ventilation. *Crit Care Med.* 2005;33(3 Suppl):S241–S245.
10. Chan KP, Stewart TE. Clinical use of high-frequency oscillatory ventilation in adult patients with acute respiratory distress syndrome. *Crit Care Med.* 2005;33(3 Suppl):S170–S174.
11. Froese AB, Butler PO, Fletcher WA, et al. High frequency oscillatory ventilation in premature infants with respiratory failure: a preliminary report. *Anesth Analg.* 1987;66:814–824.
12. Bryan AC. The Oscillations of HFO. *Am J Resp Crit Care Med.* 2001;163: 816–817.
13. Bollen CW, Uiterwaal CS, van Vught AJ. Cumulative metaanalysis of high-frequency versus conventional ventilation in premature neonates. *Am J Respir Crit Care Med.* 2003;168(10):1150–1155.
14. Arnold JH, Truog WE, Thompson JE, et al. High-frequency oscillatory ventilation in pediatric respiratory failure. *Crit Care Med.* 1993;21:272–278.
15. Henderson-Smart DJ. Elective high frequency oscillatory ventilation versus conventional ventilation for acute pulmonary dysfunction in preterm infants. *Cochrane Database Syst Rev.* 2006;2.
16. Bryan AC, Slutsky AS. Lung volume during high frequency oscillation. *Am Rev Resp Dis.* 1986;133(5):928–930.

17. Slutsky AS, Kamm RD, Rossing TH, et al. Effects of frequency, tidal volume, and lung volume on CO2 elimination in dogs by high frequency (2–30 Hz), low tidal volume ventilation. *J Clin Invest.* 1981;68(6):1475–1484.
18. Suzuki H, Papazoglou K, Bryan AC. Relationship between PaO_2 and lung volume during high frequency oscillatory ventilation. *Acta Paediatr Jpn.* 1992;34(5):494–500.
19. Kolton M, Cattran CB, Kent G, et al. Oxygenation during high-frequency ventilation compared with conventional mechanical ventilation in two models of lung injury. *Anesth Analg.* 1982;61(4):323–332.
20. Webb HH, Tierney DF. Experimental pulmonary edema due to intermittent positive pressure ventilation with high inflation pressures. Protection by positive end-expiratory pressure. *Am Rev Resp Dis.* 1974;110(5):556–565.
21. Dreyfuss D, Soler P, Basset G, et al. High inflation pressure pulmonary edema. Respective effects of high airway pressure, high tidal volume, and positive end-expiratory pressure. *Am Rev Resp Dis.* 1988;137(5):1159–1164.
22. Parker JC, Hernandez LA, Longenecker GL, et al. Lung edema caused by high peak inspiratory pressures in dogs. Role of increased microvascular filtration pressure and permeability. *Am Rev Resp Dis.* 1990;142(2):321–328.
23. Dreyfuss D, Basset G, Soler P, et al. Intermittent positive-pressure hyperventilation with high inflation pressures produces pulmonary microvascular injury in rats. *Am Rev Resp Dis.* 1985;132(4):880–884.
24. Kolobow T, Moretti MP, Fumagalli R, et al. Severe impairment in lung function induced by high peak airway pressure during mechanical ventilation. An experimental study. *Am Rev Resp Dis.* 1987;135(2):312–315.
25. Tsuno K, Miura K, Takeya M, et al. Histopathologic pulmonary changes from mechanical ventilation at high peak airway pressures. *Am Rev Resp Dis.* 1991;143(5 Pt 1):1115–1120.
26. Dreyfuss D, Saumon G. Ventilator-induced lung injury: lessons from experimental studies. *Am J Resp Crit Care Med.* 1998;157:294–323.
27. Hernandez LA, Peevy KJ, Moise AA, et al. Chest wall restriction limits high airway pressure-induced lung injury in young rabbits. *J Appl Physiol.* 1989;66(5):2364–2368.
28. Steinberg J, Schiller HJ, Halter JM, et al. Tidal volume increases do not affect alveolar mechanics in normal lung but cause alveolar overdistension and exacerbate alveolar instability after surfactant deactivation. *Crit Care Med.* 2002;30(12):2675–2683.
29. Slutsky AS. Lung injury caused by mechanical ventilation. *Chest.* 1999;116: 9S–15S.
30. Muscedere JG, Mullen JB, Gan K, et al. Tidal ventilation at low airway pressures can augment lung injury. *Am J Resp Crit Care Med.* 1994;149 (5):1327–1334.
31. Tremblay L, Valenza F, Ribeiro SP, et al. Injurious ventilatory strategies increase cytokines and c-fos m-RNA expression in an isolated rat lung model. *J Clin Invest.* 1997;99(5):944–952.
32. Tremblay L, Govindarajan A, Veldhuizen R, et al. TNFa levels are both time and ventilation strategy dependent in *ex vivo* rat lungs. *Am J Resp Crit Care Med.* 1998;157(3):A213.
33. Steinberg JM, Schiller HJ, Halter JM, et al. Alveolar instability causes early ventilator-induced lung injury independent of neutrophils. *Am J Resp Crit Care Med.* 2004;169(1):57–63.
34. Dos Santos CC, Slutsky AS. Cellular responses to mechanical stress: invited review: mechanisms of ventilator-induced lung injury: a perspective. *J Appl Physiol.* 2000;89(4):1645–1655.
35. Bryan CL, Jenkinson SG. Oxygen toxicity. *Clin Chest Med.* 1988;9(1):141–152.
36. Nash G, Blennerhassett JB, Pontoppidan H. Pulmonary lesions associated with oxygen therapy and artificial ventilation. *N Engl J Med.* 1967; 276(7):368–374.
37. Davis WB, Rennard SI, Bitterman PB, et al. Pulmonary oxygen toxicity. Early reversible changes in human alveolar structures induced by hyperoxia. *N Engl J Med.* 1983;309(15):878–883.
38. Tremblay LN, Slutsky AS. Ventilation-induced lung injury: from barotrauma to biotrauma. *Proc Assoc Am Phys.* 1998;110:482–488.
39. Slutsky AS, Tremblay LN. Multiple system organ failure. Is mechanical ventilation a contributing factor? *Am J Resp Crit Care Med.* 1998;157:1721–1725.
40. Chiumello D, Pristine G, Slutsky AS. Mechanical ventilation affects local and systemic cytokines in an animal model of acute respiratory distress syndrome. *Am J Respir Crit Care Med.* 1999;160(1):109–116.
41. Guery BP, Welsh DA, Viget NB, et al. Ventilation-induced lung injury is associated with an increase in gut permeability. *Shock.* 2003;19(6):559–563.
42. Choi WI, Quinn DA, Park KM, et al. Systemic microvascular leak in an in vivo rat model of ventilator-induced lung injury. *Am J Respir Crit Care Med.* 2003;167(12):1627–1632.
43. Imai Y, Parodo J, Kajikawa O, et al. Injurious mechanical ventilation and end-organ epithelial cell apoptosis and organ dysfunction in an experimental model of acute respiratory distress syndrome. *JAMA.* 2003;289:2104–2112.
44. Ranieri VM, Suter PM, Tortorella C, et al. Effect of mechanical ventilation on inflammatory mediators in patients with acute respiratory distress syndrome: a randomized controlled trial. *JAMA.* 1999;282(1):54–61.
45. Dos Santos CC, Slutsky AS. The contribution of biophysical lung injury to the development of biotrauma. *Annu Rev Physiol.* 2006;68:585–618.
46. Gattinoni L, Pelosi P, Vitale G, et al. Body position changes redistribute lung computed-tomographic density in patients with acute respiratory failure. *Anesthesiology.* 1991;74(1):15–23.
47. Gattinoni L, Caironi P, Pelosi P, et al. What has computed tomography taught us about the acute respiratory distress syndrome? *Am J Respir Crit Care Med.* 2001;164(9):1701–1711.
48. Roupie E, Dambrosio M, Servillo G, et al. Titration of tidal volume and induced hypercapnia in acute respiratory distress syndrome. *Am J Resp Crit Care Med.* 1995;152:121–128.
49. Gattinoni L, Pesenti A. The concept of "baby lung." *Intensive Care Med.* 2005;31(6):776–784.
50. Lachmann B. Open up the lung and keep it open. *Intensive Care Med.* 1992;18:319–321.
51. Montgomery AB, Stager MA, Carrico CJ, et al. Causes of mortality in patients with the adult respiratory distress syndrome. *Am Rev Resp Dis.* 1985;132(3):485–489.
52. Parsons PE, Eisner MD, Thompson BT, et al. Lower tidal volume ventilation and plasma cytokine markers of inflammation in patients with acute lung injury. *Crit Care Med.* 2005;33(1):1–6.
53. Slutsky AS. Mechanical ventilation. American College of Chest Physicians' Consensus Conference. *Chest.* 1993;104(6):1833–1859.
54. Stewart TE, Slutsky AS. Mechanical ventilation: a shifting philosophy. *Curr Sci.* 1995;1:49–56.
55. Stewart TE. Lung protection during mechanical ventilation. *Ontario Thorac Rev.* 1997;9:1–4.
56. Froese AB. High-frequency oscillatory ventilation for adult respiratory distress syndrome: let's get it right this time. *Crit Care Med.* 1997;25(6):906–908.
57. Hickling KG, Henderson SJ, Jackson R. Low mortality associated with low volume pressure limited ventilation with permissive hypercapnia in severe adult respiratory distress syndrome. *Intensive Care Med.* 1990;16(6):372–377.
58. Hickling KG, Walsh J, Henderson S, et al. Low mortality rate in adult respiratory distress syndrome using low-volume, pressure-limited ventilation with permissive hypercapnia: a prospective study. *Crit Care Med.* 1994;22(10):1568–1578.
59. Stewart TE, Meade MO, Cook DJ, et al. Evaluation of a ventilation strategy to prevent barotrauma in patients at high risk for acute respiratory distress syndrome. Pressure- and Volume-Limited Ventilation Strategy Group. *N Engl J Med.* 1998;338(6):355–361.
60. Brochard L, Roudot-Thoraval F, Roupie E, et al. Tidal volume reduction for prevention of ventilator-induced lung injury in acute respiratory distress syndrome. The Multicenter Trial Group on Tidal Volume reduction in ARDS. *Am J Resp Crit Care Med.* 1998;158(6):1831–1838.
61. Brower RG, Shanholtz CB, Fessler HE, et al. Prospective, randomized, controlled clinical trial comparing traditional versus reduced tidal volume ventilation in acute respiratory distress syndrome patients. *Crit Care Med.* 1999;27(8):1492–1498.
62. de Durante G, del Turco M, Rustichini L, et al. ARDSNet lower tidal volume ventilatory strategy may generate intrinsic positive end-expiratory pressure in patients with acute respiratory distress syndrome. *Am J Resp Crit Care Med.* 2002;165:1271–1274.
63. Eichacker PQ, Gerstenberger EP, Banks SM, et al. Meta-analysis of acute lung injury and acute respiratory distress syndrome trials testing low tidal volumes. *Am J Resp Crit Care Med.* 2002;166:1510–1514.
64. Brower RG, Matthay M, Schoenfeld D. Meta-analysis of acute lung injury and acute respiratory distress syndrome trials. *Am J Resp Crit Care Med.* 2002;166:1515–1517.
65. Steinbrook R. How best to ventilate? Trial design and patient safety in studies of the acute respiratory distress syndrome. *N Engl J Med.* 2003;348: 1393–1401.
66. Drazen JM. Controlling research trials. *N Engl J Med.* 2003;348:1377–1380.
67. Tobin MJ. Culmination of an era in research on the acute respiratory distress syndrome. *N Engl J Med.* 2000;342(18):1360–1361.
68. Stewart TE. Controversies around lung protective ventilation. *Am J Resp Crit Care Med.* 2002;166:1421–1422.
69. Amato MB, Barbas CS, Medeiros DM, et al. Effect of a protective-ventilation strategy on mortality in the acute respiratory distress syndrome. *N Engl J Med.* 1998;338(6):347–354.
70. Brower RG, Lanken PN, MacIntyre N, et al. Higher versus lower positive end-expiratory pressures in patients with the acute respiratory distress syndrome [see comment]. *N Engl J Med.* 2004;351(4):327–336.
71. Lunkenheimer PP, Rafflenbeul W, Keller H, et al. Application of transtracheal pressure oscillations as a modification of "diffusion respiration." *Br J Anaesth.* 1972;44:627.
72. Bohn DJ, Miyasaka K, Marchak BE, et al. Ventilation by high-frequency oscillation. *J Appl Physiol.* 1980;48(4):710–716.
73. Hamilton PP, Onayemi A, Smyth JA, et al. Comparison of conventional and high-frequency oscillatory ventilation: oxygenation and lung pathology. *J Appl Physiol.* 1983;55:131–138.
74. Tamura M, Kawano T, Fitz-James I, et al. High-frequency oscillatory

ventilation and pulmonary extravascular water. *Anesth Analg.* 1985;64 (11):1041–1046.
75. McCulloch PR, Forkert PG, Froese AB. Lung volume maintenance prevents lung injury during high frequency oscillatory ventilation in surfactant-deficient rabbits. *Am Rev Resp Dis.* 1988;137(5):1185–1192.
76. Bond DM, Froese AB. Volume recruitment maneuvers are less deleterious than persistent low lung volumes in the atelectasis-prone rabbit lung during high-frequency oscillation. *Crit Care Med.* 1993;21(3):402–412.
77. Imai Y, Kawano T, Miyasaka K, et al. Inflammatory chemical mediators during conventional ventilation and during high frequency oscillatory ventilation. *Am J Resp Crit Care Med.* 1994;150(6 Pt 1):1550–1554.
78. Matsuoka T, Kawano T, Miyasaka K. Role of high-frequency ventilation in surfactant-depleted lung injury as measured by granulocytes. *J Appl Physiol.* 1994;76(2):539–544.
79. Sugiura M, McCulloch PR, Wren S, et al. Ventilator pattern influences neutrophil influx and activation in atelectasis-prone rabbit lung. *J Appl Physiol.* 1994;77(3):1355–1365.
80. Takata M, Abe J, Tanaka H, et al. Intraalveolar expression of tumor necrosis factor-alpha gene during conventional and high-frequency ventilation. *Am J Resp Crit Care Med.* 1997;156(1):272–279.
81. Gommers D, Hartog A, Schnabel R, et al. High-frequency oscillatory ventilation is not superior to conventional mechanical ventilation in surfactant-treated rabbits with lung injury. *Eur Resp J.* 1999;14(4):738–744.
82. Kerr CL, Veldhuizen RA, Lewis JF. Effects of high-frequency oscillation on endogenous surfactant in an acute lung injury model. *Am J Resp Crit Care Med.* 2001;164(2):237–242.
83. Noda E, Hoshina H, Watanabe H, et al. Production of TNF-alpha by polymorphonuclear leukocytes during mechanical ventilation in the surfactant-depleted rabbit lung. *Pediatr Pulmonol.* 2003;36(6):475–481.
84. Vazquez de Anda GF, Hartog A, Verbrugge SJ, et al. The open lung concept: pressure-controlled ventilation is as effective as high-frequency oscillatory ventilation in improving gas exchange and lung mechanics in surfactant-deficient animals. *Intensive Care Med.* 1999;25(9):990–996.
85. Rimensberger PC, Pache JC, McKerlie C, et al. Lung recruitment and lung volume maintenance: a strategy for improving oxygenation and preventing lung injury during both conventional mechanical ventilation and high-frequency oscillation. *Intensive Care Med.* 2000;26(6):745–755.
86. Rotta AT, Gunnarsson B, Fuhrman BP, et al. Comparison of lung protective ventilation strategies in a rabbit model of acute lung injury. *Crit Care Med.* 2001;29(11):2176–2184.
87. Imai Y, Nakagawa S, Ito Y, et al. Comparison of lung protection strategies using conventional and high-frequency oscillatory ventilation. *J Appl Physiol.* 2001;91(4):1836–1844.
88. Sedeek KA, Takeuchi M, Suchodolski K, et al. Open-lung protective ventilation with pressure control ventilation, high-frequency oscillation, and intratracheal pulmonary ventilation results in similar gas exchange, hemodynamics, and lung mechanics. *Anesthesiology.* 2003;99(5):1102–1111.
89. von der Hardt K, Kandler MA, Fink L, et al. High frequency oscillatory ventilation suppresses inflammatory response in lung tissue and microdissected alveolar macrophages in surfactant depleted piglets. *Pediatr Res.* 2004;55(2):339–346.
90. Hager DN, Fessler HE, Fuld MK, et al. Effects of frequency and pressure amplitude on tidal volumes in adults with ARDS during high-frequency oscillatory ventilation. *Proc Am Thorac Soc.* 2006;3:A376.
91. Villar J, Slutsky AS. Alternative modalities for ventilatory support. In: Vincent JL, ed. *Update in Intensive Care and Emergency Medicine.* Brussels: Springer-Verlag; 1991:345–354.
92. Chang HK. Mechanisms of gas transport during ventilation by high-frequency oscillation. *J Appl Physiol.* 1984;56(3):553–563.
93. Ribeiro SP, Tremblay LN, Slutsky AS. High-frequency ventilation. In: Marini JJ, Slutsky AS, eds. *Physiological Basis of Ventilatory Support.* New York: Marcel Dekker; 1998:889–920.
94. Schmid ER, Knopp TJ, Rehder K. Intrapulmonary gas transport and perfusion during high-frequency oscillation. *J Appl Physiol Respir Environ Exerc Physiol.* 1981;51(6):1507–1514.
95. Slutsky AS. Gas mixing by cardiogenic oscillations: a theoretical quantitative analysis. *J Appl Physiol Respir Environ Exerc Physiol.* 1981;51(5):1287–1293.
96. Slutsky AS, Brown R. Cardiogenic oscillations: a potential mechanism enhancing oxygenation during apneic respiration. *Med Hypotheses.* 1982;8(4):393–400.
97. Cybulsky IJ, Abel JG, Menon AS, et al. Contribution of cardiogenic oscillations to gas exchange in constant-flow ventilation. *J Appl Physiol.* 1987;63(2):564–570.
98. Slutsky AS, Drazen JM. Ventilation with small tidal volumes. *N Engl J Med.* 2002;347(9):630–631.
99. Slutsky AS, Drazen FM, Ingram RH Jr, et al. Effective pulmonary ventilation with small-volume oscillations at high frequency. *Science.* 1980;209(4456):609–671.
100. Schoenfeld DA, Bernard GR, and the ARDS Network. Statistical evaluation of ventilator-free days as an efficacy measure in clinical trials of treatments for acute respiratory distress syndrome. *Crit Care Med.* 2002;30:1772–1777.
101. Derdak S, Mehta S, Stewart TE, et al. High frequency oscillatory ventilation for acute respiratory distress syndrome: a randomized controlled trial. *Am J Resp Crit Care Med.* 2002;166:801–808.
102. Froese AB. The incremental application of lung-protective high-frequency oscillatory ventilation. *Am J Resp Crit Care Med.* 2002;166:786–787.
103. Bryan AC, Slutsky AS. Long volume during high frequency oscillation. *Am Rev Resp Dis.* 1986;133(5):928–930.
104. Bancalari A, Gerhardt T, Bancalari E, et al. Gas trapping with high-frequency ventilation: jet versus oscillatory ventilation. *J Pediatr.* 1987;110(4):617–622.
105. Courtney SE, Weber KR, Spohn WA, et al. Cardiorespiratory effects of changing inspiratory to expiratory ratio during high-frequency oscillation in an animal model of respiratory failure. *Pediatr Pulmonol.* 1992;13(2):113–116.
106. Pillow JJ, Neil H, Wilkinson MH, et al. Effect of I/E ratio on mean alveolar pressure during high-frequency oscillatory ventilation. *J Appl Physiol.* 1999;87(1):407–414.
107. Boynton BR, Villanueva D, Hammond MD, et al. Effect of mean airway pressure on gas exchange during high-frequency oscillatory ventilation. *J Appl Physiol.* 1991;70(2):701–707.
108. Goddon S, Fujino Y, Hromi JM, et al. Optimal mean airway pressure during high-frequency oscillation: predicted by the pressure-volume curve. *Anesthesiology.* 2001;94(5):862–869.
109. van Genderingen HR, van Vught JA, Jansen JR, et al. Oxygenation index, an indicator of optimal distending pressure during high-frequency oscillatory ventilation? *Intensive Care Med.* 2002;28(8):1151–1156.
110. Dembinski R, Max M, Bensberg R, et al. High-frequency oscillatory ventilation in experimental lung injury: effects on gas exchange. *Intensive Care Med.* 2002;28(6):768–774.
111. Luecke T, Meinhardt JP, Herrmann P, et al. Setting mean airway pressure during high-frequency oscillatory ventilation according to the static pressure-volume curve in surfactant-deficient lung injury: a computed tomography study. *Anesthesiology.* 2003;99(6):1313–1322.
112. Sakai T, Kakizawa H, Aiba S, et al. Effects of mean and swing pressures on piston-type high-frequency oscillatory ventilation in rabbits with and without acute lung injury. *Pediatr Pulmonol.* 1999;27(5):328–335.
113. van Genderingen HR, van Vught AJ, Duval EL, et al. Attenuation of pressure swings along the endotracheal tube is indicative of optimal distending pressure during high-frequency oscillatory ventilation in a model of acute lung injury. *Pediatr Pulmonol.* 2002;33(6):429–436.
114. Byford LJ, Finkler JH, Froese AB. Lung volume recruitment during high-frequency oscillation in atelectasis-prone rabbits. *J Appl Physiol.* 1988;64(4):1607–1614.
115. Sznajder JI, Nahum A, Hansen DE, et al. Volume recruitment and oxygenation in pulmonary edema: a comparison between HFOV and CMV. *J Crit Care.* 1998;13(3):126–135.
116. Walsh MC, Carlo WA. Sustained inflation during HFOV improves pulmonary mechanics and oxygenation. *J Appl Physiol.* 1988;65(1):368–372.
117. Suzuki H, Papazoglou K, Bryan AC. Relationship between PaO_2 and lung volume during high frequency oscillatory ventilation. *Acta Paediatr Jpn.* 1992;34(5):494–500.
118. Sedeek KA, Takeuchi M, Suchodolski K, et al. Determinants of tidal volume during high-frequency oscillation. *Crit Care Med.* 2003;31(1):227–231.
119. Derdak S. High-frequency oscillatory ventilation for acute respiratory distress syndrome in adult patients. *Crit Care Med.* 2003;31:S317–S323.
120. Fessler HE, Brower RG. Protocols for lung protective ventilation. *Crit Care Med.* 2005;33(3 Suppl):S223–S227.
121. HIFI Study Group. High-frequency oscillatory ventilation compared with conventional mechanical ventilation in the treatment of respiratory failure in preterm infants. *N Engl J Med.* 1989;320(2):88–93.
122. Ogawa Y, Miyasaka K, Kawano T, et al. A multicenter randomized trial of high frequency oscillatory ventilation as compared with conventional mechanical ventilation in preterm infants with respiratory failure. *Early Hum Dev.* 1993;32(1):1–10.
123. HiFO Study Group. Randomized study of high-frequency oscillatory ventilation in infants with severe respiratory distress syndrome. *J Pediatr.* 1993;122(4):609–619.
124. Gerstmann DR, Minton SD, Stoddard RA, et al. The Provo multicenter early high-frequency oscillatory ventilation trial: improved pulmonary and clinical outcome in respiratory distress syndrome. *Pediatrics.* 1996;98 (6 Pt 1):1044–1057.
125. Moriette G, Paris-Llado J, Walti H, et al. Prospective randomized multicenter comparison of high-frequency oscillatory ventilation and conventional ventilation in preterm infants of less than 30 weeks with respiratory distress syndrome. *Pediatrics.* 2001;107:363–372.
126. Thome U, Kossel H, Lipowsky G, et al. Randomized comparison of high-frequency ventilation with high-rate intermittent positive pressure ventilation in preterm infants with respiratory failure. *J Pediatr.* 1999;135(1):39–46.
127. Rettwitz-Volk W, Veldman A, Roth B, et al. A prospective, randomized, multicenter trial of high-frequency oscillatory ventilation compared with conventional ventilation in preterm infants with respiratory distress syndrome receiving surfactant. *J Pediatr.* 1998;132(2):249–254.
128. Johnson AH, Peacock JL, Greenough A, et al. High-frequency oscillatory ventilation for the prevention of chronic lung disease of prematurity. *N Engl J Med.* 2002;347(9):633–642.

129. Courtney SE, Durand DJ, Asselin JM, et al. High-frequency oscillatory ventilation versus conventional mechanical ventilation for very-low-birth-weight infants. *N Engl J Med.* 2002;347(9):643–652.
130. Plavka R, Kopecky P, Sebron V, et al. A prospective randomized comparison of conventional mechanical ventilation and very early high frequency oscillatory ventilation in extremely premature newborns with respiratory distress syndrome. *Intensive Care Med.* 1999;25(1):68–75.
131. Bryan AC, Froese AB. Reflections on the HIFI trial. *Pediatrics.* 1991;87:565–567.
132. Froese AB, Kinsella JP. High-frequency oscillatory ventilation: lessons from the neonatal/pediatric experience. *Crit Care Med.* 2005;33(3 Suppl):S115–S121.
133. Fort P, Farmer C, Westerman J, et al. High-frequency oscillatory ventilation for adult respiratory distress syndrome-a pilot study. *Crit Care Med.* 1997;25(6):937–947.
134. Claridge JA, Hostetter RG, Lowson SM, et al. High-frequency oscillatory ventilation can be effective as rescue therapy for refractory acute lung dysfunction. *Am Surg.* 1999;65(11):1092–1096.
135. Mehta S, Lapinsky SE, Hallett DC, et al. A prospective trial of high frequency oscillatory ventilation in adults with acute respiratory distress syndrome. *Crit Care Med.* 2001;29:1360–1369.
136. Andersen FA, Guttormsen AB, Flaatten HK. High frequency oscillatory ventilation in adult patients with acute respiratory distress syndrome—a retrospective study. *Acta Anaesthesiol Scand.* 2002;46(9):1082–1088.
137. David M, Weiler N, Heinrichs W, et al. High-frequency oscillatory ventilation in adult acute respiratory distress syndrome. *Intensive Care Med.* 2003;29(10):1656–1665.
138. Cartotto R, Ellis S, Gomez M, et al. High frequency oscillatory ventilation in burn patients with the acute respiratory distress syndrome. *Burns.* 2004;30(5):453–463.
139. Mehta S, Granton J, MacDonald RJ, et al. High-frequency oscillatory ventilation in adults: the Toronto experience. *Chest.* 2004;126(2):518–527.
140. Ferguson ND, Chiche JD, Kacmarek RM, et al. Combining high-frequency oscillatory ventilation and recruitment maneuvers in adults with early acute respiratory distress syndrome: The Treatment with Oscillation and an Open Lung Strategy (TOOLS) Trial pilot study. *Crit Care Med.* 2005;33:479–486.
141. David M, Karmrodt J, Weiler N, et al. High-frequency oscillatory ventilation in adults with traumatic brain injury and acute respiratory distress syndrome. *Acta Anaesthesiol Scand.* 2005;49(2):209–214.
142. Pachl J, Roubik K, Waldauf P, et al. Normocapnic high-frequency oscillatory ventilation affects differently extrapulmonary and pulmonary forms of acute respiratory distress syndrome in adults. *Physiol Res.* 2006;55(1):15–24.
143. Finkielman JD, Gajic O, Farmer JC, et al. The initial Mayo Clinic experience using high-frequency oscillatory ventilation for adult patients: a retrospective study. *BMC Emerg Med.* 2006;6:2.
144. Villagra A, Ochagavia A, Vatua S, et al. Recruitment maneuvers during lung protective ventilation in acute respiratory distress syndrome. *Am J Resp Crit Care Med.* 2002;165(2):165–170.
145. Grasso S, Mascia L, Del Turco M, et al. Effects of recruiting maneuvers in patients with acute respiratory distress syndrome ventilated with protective ventilatory strategy. *Anesthesiology.* 2002;96:795–802.
146. Lapinsky SE, Aubin M, Mehta S, et al. Safety and efficacy of a sustained inflation for alveolar recruitment in adults with respiratory failure. *Intensive Care Med.* 1999;25(11):1297–1301.
147. Lim CM, Jung H, Koh Y, et al. Effect of alveolar recruitment maneuver in early acute respiratory distress syndrome according to antiderecruitment strategy, etiological category of diffuse lung injury, and body position of the patient. *Crit Care Med.* 2003;31(2):411–418.
148. The ARDS Clinical Trials Network. Effects of recruitment maneuvers in patients with acute lung injury and acute respiratory distress syndrome ventilated with high positive end-expiratory pressure. *Crit Care Med.* 2003; 31:2592–2597.
149. Tugrul S, Akinci O, Ozcan PE, et al. Effects of sustained inflation and postinflation positive end-expiratory pressure in acute respiratory distress syndrome: focusing on pulmonary and extrapulmonary forms. *Crit Care Med.* 2003;31(3):738–744.
150. Crotti S, Mascheroni D, Caironi P, et al. Recruitment and derecruitment during acute respiratory failure: a clinical study. *Am J Resp Crit Care Med.* 2001;164(1):131–140.
151. Gattinoni L, Caironi P, Cressoni M, et al. Lung recruitment in patients with the acute respiratory distress syndrome. *N Engl J Med.* 2006;354(17):1775–1786.
152. Borges JB, Okamoto VN, Matos GFJ, et al. Reversibility of lung collapse and hypoxemia in early acute respiratory distress syndrome. *Am J Respir Crit Care Med.* 2006;174(3):268–278.
153. Snyder JV, Froese AB. The open lung approach: concept and application. In: Snyder JV, Pinsky MR, eds. *Oxygen Transport in the Critically Ill.* Chicago: Yearbook Medical Publishers; 1987:358–373.
154. Froese AB. Role of lung volume in lung injury: HFO in the atelectasis-prone lung. *Acta Anaesthesiol Scand.* 1989;90(Suppl):126–130.
155. Gerstmann D. Major benefit of small tidal volumes during high-frequency ventilation. *Crit Care Med.* 2003;31(1):328–329.
156. Hager DN, Fuld M, Kaczka DW, et al. Four methods of measuring tidal volume during high-frequency oscillatory ventilation. *Crit Care Med.* 2006; 34(3):751–757.
157. Froese AB. The incremental application of lung-protective high-frequency oscillatory ventilation. *Am J Resp Crit Care Med.* 2002;166:786–787.
158. Fessler HE, Hager DN, Brower RG. Feasibility of very high frequencies during high-frequency oscillation in adults with acute respiratory distress syndrome. *Proc Am Thorac Soc.* 2006;3:A378.
159. Bollen CW, van Well GT, Sherry T, et al. High frequency oscillatory ventilation compared with conventional mechanical ventilation in adult respiratory distress syndrome: a randomized controlled trial. *Crit Care London.* 2005;9:R430–R439.
160. Ware LB, Matthay MA. The acute respiratory distress syndrome. *N Engl J Med.* 2000;342(18):1334–1349.

CHAPTER 134 ■ OXYGEN THERAPY AND BASIC RESPIRATORY CARE

ELAMIN M. ELAMIN • J. MICHAEL JAEGER • ANDREW C. MILLER

THE CHEMISTRY OF OXYGEN

Oxygen in air exists in a diatomic molecular form (O_2, molecular weight [MW] 16 g/mol) that, at standard temperature and pressure, is a colorless, odorless gas. The diatomic molecular state is the form that we administer to our patients as a respiratory gas, either pure oxygen or in mixtures with air or helium (heliox), and is that form most commonly referred to as *oxygen*. While the gaseous state of oxygen is most clinically relevant, it can be found in a liquid and solid state as well under appropriate conditions. However, molecular oxygen has additional chemical states that expand its impact on human physiology. The diatomic form ("oxygen") is essential for aerobic metabolism in animals but is toxic to obligate anaerobic organisms (a fact exploited in hyperbaric oxygen therapy). The triatomic form, ozone, is produced continuously by ultraviolet (UV) radiation in the upper layers of the atmosphere, and serves to shield the earth's surface from UV radiation. However, ozone is also produced by the immune system as an antimicrobial defense. Finally, *singlet oxygen* (several different forms exist) is a high-energy state of molecular oxygen in which all the electron spins are paired, resulting in extreme instability and exceptional reactivity toward common organic molecules. Such *oxygen-free radicals*, as they are collectively termed, have varied and increasingly important physiologic roles; therefore, their role in both normal and pathologic processes must be recognized and understood to allow the correct application of oxygen therapy.

In this chapter, we will discuss the various modalities for oxygen delivery in the critical care setting. In addition, we will address oxygen's diverse physiologic and possible pathologic effects, but in our discussion of oxygen-free radicals, we will confine it to their role in oxidative lung injury, while being cognizant of their potential impact on all tissues.

OXYGEN THERAPY DEVICES

Oxygen therapy is one of the basic modes of respiratory care. Yet, despite the fact that oxygen has been delivered to patients with lung disease for almost a century, it is commonly delivered in imprecise concentrations. Because oxygen is "invisible," it has often been downgraded to a position considerably less than the powerful drug that it is.

Delivery devices for oxygen therapy are typically classified into two groups: variable flow or fixed-flow equipment. The term *variable flow* relates to the fact that as the patient's respiratory pattern changes, delivered oxygen is diluted with room air. This results in a widely inconsistent and fluctuating fraction of inspired oxygen concentration (FiO_2). In fact, despite some commonly published figures for delivered FiO_2 at given flow rates, the actual FiO_2 delivered to the patient by various devices is neither precise nor predictable. Variable flow devices include nasal catheter, nasal cannulae, transtracheal oxygen catheter, and various oxygen masks.

Fixed-flow equipment, on the other hand, provides the entire patient's inspired gas with a precisely controlled FiO_2; when applied appropriately, the FiO_2 delivered to the patient is therefore constant, regardless of ventilatory pattern. Fixed-flow devices include air-entrainment masks, large-volume aerosol systems, and large-volume humidifier systems.

The following describes various oxygen delivery equipment and their proper placement, possible problems, and overall performance.

Variable Flow Equipment

Nasal Catheter

Description. The nasal catheter is the simplest oxygen delivery device. It is a soft, plastic, blind-end tube with numerous side holes at the distal tip. Nasal catheters typically come in French sizes, which is a reference to the outside diameter (OD) of the device. A French (Fr) size is three times the OD in millimeters, with typical adult sizes being 12 Fr to 14 Fr. Oxygen is delivered to the nasal catheter from a bubble humidifier through the oxygen tubing.

Placement. Before use, the catheter should be liberally lubricated with a water-soluble lubricant. The catheter is placed in the external naris and advanced along the floor of the nasal cavity into the oropharynx, stopping just behind the uvula. The appropriate size can be determined by inspection of the external naris and by measurement of the distance between the tip of the nose to the ipsilateral external ear.

To achieve proper placement, use a tongue blade and flashlight to observe the posterior pharynx, and then advance the catheter into the nasopharynx until it appears below the uvula. After identifying the catheter tip, withdraw the catheter until the tip of the catheter is no longer seen. Once proper placement is achieved, the catheter should be secured to the nose with tape.

Problems. Pain and discomfort during insertion have been described. In the presence of nasal pathologic conditions, including nasal polyps, deviated septum, and nasal congestion, placement may be particularly traumatic or impossible. Bleeding can occur resulting from mucosal irritation. For this reason, patients with coagulation disorders should not have a nasal catheter placed.

When in place, routine changing of the catheter is required to prevent blockage of the side holes with secretions in addition to subsequent reduction of oxygen flow.

Performance. Nasal catheters have been used for adults as well as infants (1). In adults, nasal catheters provide a relatively low FiO_2. The increase in FiO_2 through the nasal catheter is directly related to gas flow, and is enhanced at low flow rates by using the nasopharynx and oropharynx as a reservoir for oxygen. Accordingly, at flow rates of 6 to 10 L/minute, an FiO_2 of 0.69 to 0.82 can be delivered to the patient (2). However, like all variable performance equipment, delivered FiO_2 will vary with a change in respiratory rate or tidal volume.

The major advantage of using a nasal catheter is that it can be securely placed in obtunded patients. However, due to a long list of disadvantages, including discomfort, difficulty in insertion, and bleeding, nasal catheters are infrequently used today.

Nasal Cannula

Description. The nasal cannula is the most frequently utilized oxygen delivery device. It consists of a blind-end tube with two protruding "nasal prongs" that rest in the external naris. Cannulae come in a variety of designs for more comfortable or subtle application. Regardless of the design, the principle of oxygen delivery is the same. Cannulae are connected to an oxygen flowmeter through oxygen tubing without a humidification device for flow less than 4 L/minute and with a bubble humidifier for higher flow rates to prevent nasal drying (3).

Placement. Nasal cannulae are easily placed regardless of the type and brand.

Problems. The nasal cannula is relatively problem free. However, short-term use can result in drying of the nasal mucosa, while long-term use can cause pressure sores above the ears, under the chin, and above the upper lip. Gauze or foam padding can be placed between the cannula and irritation sites to limit this complication.

Performance. A nasal cannula is used with oxygen flow rates of 1 to 6 L/minute in adults and as low as 1/16 L/minute in infants. The exact FiO_2 delivered with a nasal cannula has been measured and estimated using a variety of methods and, as expected, yielded a variety of results.

An earlier method to predict FiO_2 through variable performance equipment and using a host of assumptions demonstrated a wide range of FiO_2 values delivered by nasal cannula at any given constant flow of oxygen (4). Another study in FiO_2 delivery through the nasal cannula utilized a model of the respiratory system (5). The model consisted of a lung placed inside a rigid container and attached to a rubber test lung through tubing that approximated tracheal volume. A ventilator producing a sine wave was connected to the container, and inspiratory flow varied from 12 to 40 L/minute at a constant rate and volume. The study illustrated that delivered FiO_2 varied 13% to 40% at a given oxygen flow when inspiratory flow varied from 12 to 40 L/minute.

The nasal cannula is commonly used as the first means to deliver oxygen to patients requiring long-term therapy. In theory, the nasal cannula increases FiO_2 by 0.04 for every liter of oxygen flow. Flow is typically set between 1 and 6 L/minute. Flow above 6 L/minute adds little to increased FiO_2, and may induce patient discomfort, including nasal mucosa dryness and bleeding.

Oxygen-conserving Devices

The wide use of nasal cannulae led to recognition of an important device limitation. Since there is lack of synchronization between the patient ventilation and continuous flow of oxygen through the cannula, there is wasted oxygen flow to the room during expiration. In an attempt to eliminate this waste and reduce the cost of oxygen delivery, several device modifications have been developed. However, the mechanism of oxygen conservation has centered on two main concepts.

Reservoir Cannula

Description. These devices use a mechanical reservoir or an increased anatomic reservoir that fills with 100% oxygen during exhalation and empties the oxygen into the lungs early in inspiration. This was achieved through the use of a collapsible chamber that empties on inspiration and fills during exhalation.

Moustache-style Cannula. This is among the most widely available reservoir devices. The cannula contains a soft, inflatable reservoir with a volume of approximately 20 mL. During patient exhalation, oxygen flow fills the expandable reservoir. Then, during early inspiration, the patient inspires first from the reservoir, causing the reservoir to begin to empty, and from the continuous flow once the reservoir is depleted.

Placement. The reservoir cannula rests directly beneath the nose.

Problems. The moustache-style cannula is larger, heavier, and more obvious than the traditional cannula. Hence, it is more obtrusive, and many patients in need of O_2 therapy at home may prefer not to wear it in public.

Performance. As expected, the reservoir cannula can achieve oxygenation equivalent to a conventional nasal cannula, but at a lower flow rate.

Pendant Reservoir Cannula

Description. The pendant reservoir cannula (Fig. 134.1) uses a pendant-like reservoir that is worn on the chest with a larger-diameter cannula and connecting tubing. The pendant contains an inflatable reservoir with a volume of approximately 40 mL that forces gas up the cannula tubing during expiration. Subsequently, during early inspiration, the gas stored in the tubing acts as a reservoir of oxygen, but as inspiration continues, the cannula begins to function like a conventional cannula.

Overall, most of the benefit appears to be derived from the oversized tubing between the patient and the pendant (6).

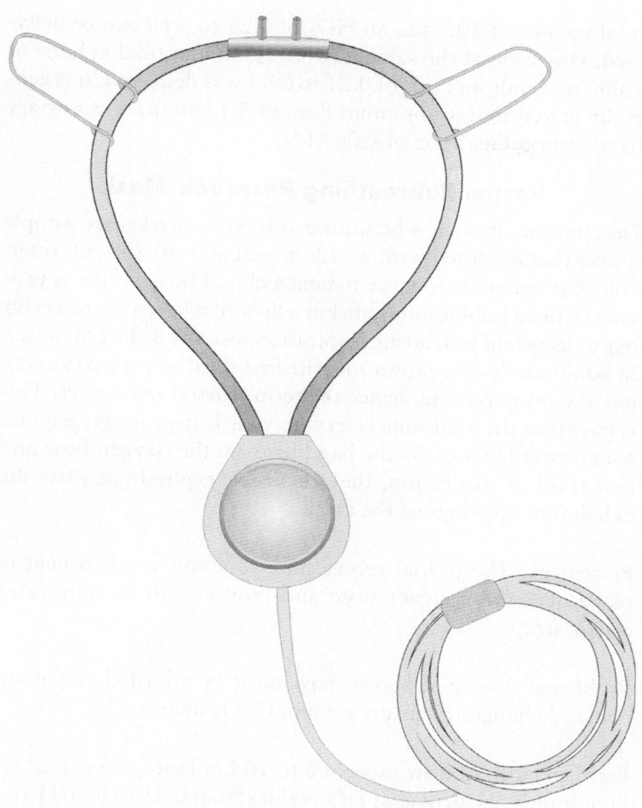

FIGURE 134.1. Pendant reservoir cannula.

Placement. The pendant reservoir is placed to the patient in a manner similar to a conventional cannula.

Problems. Tubing size makes the pendant cannula more prominent but less so than the moustache-style cannula.

Performance. Like the moustache-style cannula, the pendant reservoir cannula is capable of providing similar or higher oxygenation at the flow used with a conventional cannula (6). The cannula reservoir contains close to 80% oxygen at a flow rate of 0.5 L/minute, but increases to nearly 100% oxygen at a flow rate of 1 L/minute (7,8). In addition, at an inspiratory-to-expiratory ratio of 1:2 and a respiratory rate of 20 breaths/minute, the most efficacious FiO_2 delivery will occur during the first 0.5 seconds and the first 200 mL of inhalation (7,8).

Various studies compared the efficacy of reservoir cannulae with that of standard cannulae, and consistently indicated that the reservoir cannula at flow rates of 0.5, 1, and 2 L/minute will yield an FiO_2 equivalent to that delivered by flow rates of 2, 3, and 4 L/minute by the standard nasal cannulae, respectively (7,8).

Electronic Demand

Pulsed-dose Oxygen Delivery

Description. Electronic demand pulsed-dose oxygen therapy can be used in conjunction with a cannula, reservoir cannula, or transtracheal catheter. Pulsed-dose oxygen systems work by detecting patient effort and only provide gas during the early portion of inspiration (9,10).

During expiration, the demand device is referenced to the atmospheric pressure. Once the flow sensor detects patient effort, a solenoid valve opens and provides a "pulsed dose" of oxygen at the preselected flow setting. The pulsed dose is usually set to begin with every inspiratory effort or every second or third breath. The goal of these devices is to reduce oxygen usage while maintaining inspired oxygen concentration at a level that provides adequate oxygen saturation.

One of the major concerns about such devices is the effect of exercise and tachypnea on oxygen saturation. A device that produces adequate oxygen saturation while the patient is at rest may not produce adequate oxygen saturation when the patient is walking or becomes ill.

Placement. Pulsed-dose devices can be connected to any oxygen outlet, including cylinders and liquid oxygen systems. The device takes the place of a standard flowmeter or incorporates the flowmeter into the design.

Problems. Possible problems with such devices include displacement and improper sensing of patient effort. However, the device design incorporates an automatic alarm and default mechanism to allow continuous flow if patient effort is not sensed over a designated period. Also, the cost for the device can be a concern and must be weighed against the potential savings in oxygen usage.

Performance. Depending on the size and frequency of the oxygen pulse, the savings of such a device could be 4 to 1 or 7 to 1 compared with continuous flow oxygen. Equivalent oxygenation can also be accomplished at lower flow rates (10). On the other hand, it is important to remember that desaturation may occur in many patients during exercise. Hence, to ensure adequate oxygenation, they should be tested during various activities.

Transtracheal Oxygen Catheters

Description. Transtracheal oxygen catheters deliver oxygen directly into the trachea through small-bore catheters (Fig. 134.2). Direct delivery into the trachea prevents dilution of oxygen with room air, as seen with other appliances, and fills the upper respiratory tract with oxygen.

Placement. Under sterile technique and local anesthesia, a small incision is made in the skin. A tracheal stent is advanced through the incision into the trachea. This stent remains in place for 7 to 10 days to facilitate a permanent tract formation. Afterward, the stent is removed over a guidewire and a 9 Fr (3.0-mm OD) catheter is inserted over a guidewire and secured in place with external flange.

Problems. Problems may include subcutaneous emphysema, infection, hemoptysis, and malposition. However, the most common problem is mucous obstruction with a mucous ball at the tip of the catheter. Routine cleaning of the catheter with instillation of saline and a cleaning rod can help in avoiding such problem.

Performance. Transtracheal systems have been shown to increase oxygenation compared with conventional oxygen

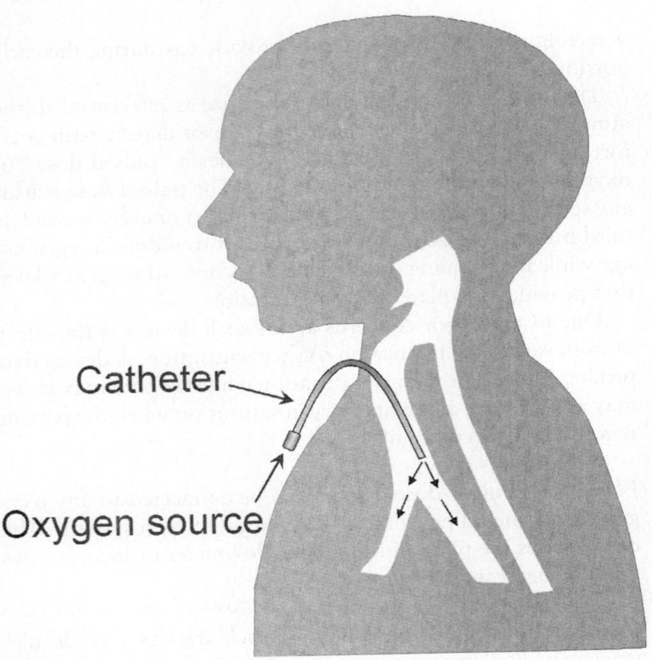

FIGURE 134.2. Transtracheal oxygen catheter.

therapy with a nasal cannula at equivalent flow rates, or can provide equivalent oxygenation at lower flow rates (11).

Patient acceptance is also reportedly improved because of the relatively hidden appearance of the equipment. Reduced oxygen usage, reduced costs, and increased life of portable gas sources have all been reported with transtracheal oxygen therapy. The use of transtracheal oxygen therapy can reduce required oxygen flow by close to 50% (12). The latter may even be enhanced with the additional use of demand pulsed-dose oxygen that can further increase the savings.

Masks

Simple Mask

Description. The simple mask is a disposable, lightweight plastic that increases FiO_2 by increasing the available reservoir by adding the volume of the mask. Oxygen is delivered to the mask through standard oxygen tubing at a flow rate of 5 to 12 L/minute. The mask allows room air to be drawn in around the mask edges and through side ports. A bubble humidifier may be used to provide comfort, especially with prolonged use.

Placement. Simple masks are held in place over the patient's nose and mouth with an adjustable elastic strap.

Problems. Patients wearing a mask may complain of claustrophobia or pain at the site of mask application. Also, it can interfere with eating and drinking.

Performance. Since it is a variable performance device, the actual FiO_2 delivered varies with mask fit, oxygen flow, and certainly patient respiratory effort. This was first suggested in a study by Bethune and Coffis (13), who investigated the relation of the flow and rebreathing of carbon dioxide (CO_2). They were able to demonstrate that, at flow rates of 1 to 8 L/minute and tidal volume of 500 mL, an FiO_2 of 0.21 to 0.60 can be delivered. However, at the same flow rates but at a tidal volume of 1,000 mL, only an FiO_2 of 0.21 to 0.43 was delivered. It is generally stated that a minimum flow of 5 L/minute is necessary to prevent rebreathing of CO_2 (14).

Partial Rebreathing Reservoir Mask

Description. Partial rebreathing reservoir masks are simple masks that are fitted with an additional 600- to 800-mL reservoir that extend below the patient's chin. Oxygen flow is provided from a bubble humidifier at a flow that keeps the reservoir bag at least half full during inspiration (usually 8–15 L/minute). In addition, during expiration, the first third of expired gas enters the reservoir bag, hence the term, *partial rebreather*. This is gas from the anatomic reservoir, so it is high in oxygen and contains little CO_2. As the bag fills from the oxygen flow and first third of expiration, the remaining expired gas exits the exhalation openings of the mask.

Placement. The partial rebreathing reservoir mask is held in place over the patient's nose and mouth with an adjustable elastic strap.

Problems. As stated above, flow must be adjusted as patient demand changes to ensure minimal FiO_2 delivery.

Performance. At flow rates of 6 to 10 L/minute, the partial rebreathing mask delivered FiO_2 values from 0.35 to 0.70 (15).

Nonrebreathing Reservoir Mask

Description. The Nonrebreathing Reservoir Mask incorporates one-way valves over one of the mask side ports and above the reservoir bag. The one-way valve over the reservoir bag prevents expired gas from entering into the bag. In addition, the one-way valve over the side port limits further entrainment of room air during inspiration, except if gas flow is inadvertently disconnected.

Placement. The nonrebreathing mask is held in place over the patient's nose and mouth with an adjustable elastic strap.

Problems. In addition to previously mentioned shortcomings of masks, the combined effects of time and moisture can cause one-way valves to stick in either the open or closed position.

Performance. The nonrebreathing mask requires minimum oxygen flow of 10 to 15 L/minute to prevent the reservoir bag from collapsing during inspiration. With that flow rate, it is estimated that an FiO_2 of 0.60 to 0.80 is delivered with a nonrebreathing mask (15). A FiO_2 of 0.57 to 0.70 is delivered when oxygen flow can be set greater than the patient minute ventilation. Contrary to common belief, FiO_2 values near 1.0 cannot be achieved using the commonly available disposable nonrebreathing masks.

Fixed-performance Devices

Air-entrainment Masks

Description. An air-entrainment mask consists of the mask, a jet nozzle, and entrainment ports. Oxygen under pressure is

TABLE 134.1

AIR-ENTRAINMENT MASK FiO_2 SETTINGS AND MINIMUM OPTIONAL OXYGEN FLOW RATES FOR VARIOUS SETTINGS

FiO_2 setting	Minimum oxygen flow (L/min)	Entrainment ratio O_2:Air	Total flow (L/min)
0.24	4	1:25	104
0.28	4	1:10	44
0.31	6	1:7	48
0.35	8	1:5	48
0.40	8	1:3	32
0.50	12	1:1.7	32
0.60	12	1:1	24
0.70	12	1:0.6	19

delivered through the jet nozzle just below the mask. As gas travels through the jet nozzle, its velocity increases dramatically. On exiting the nozzle, the gas at high velocity entrains or drags ambient air into the mask. This is due not to the Venturi principle, but rather to the viscous shearing forces between the gas traveling through the nozzle and the stagnant ambient air (16). Accordingly, the delivered FiO_2 is dependent on the size of the nozzle and entrainment ports, and the rate of oxygen flow. On average, an air-entrainment mask has six to eight FiO_2 settings as well as minimum optional oxygen flow rates for various settings (Table 134.1). To provide additional system humidity, an aerosol collar can be applied around the entrainment ports. The dry oxygen will then entrain air from an aerosol system, increasing the humidity delivered to the patient. However, the addition of aerosol particles to room air may increase gas density, which will reduce entrained volume, and may slightly increase the delivered FiO_2.

Placement. The mask is secured to the patient's face with an adjustable, elastic band.

Problems. The most important problem associated with the air-entrainment mask is obstruction of the entrainment port by various objects. This decreases total flow perceptibly and increases FiO_2.

Performance. The air-entrainment mask requires FiO_2 values <0.30 to maintain total flow 30% greater than peak inspiratory flow and continue to function as a fixed-performance system (17). At higher FiO_2, the total flow falls below 40 L/minute, and the air-entrainment mask becomes a variable performance device. The latter may occur if patient demand for flow increases and room air is drawn in around the mask (18).

To accommodate such a demand, masks with larger volumes (volume $\geq$ 300 mL) and extension tubes between the jet and the mask will act as reservoirs for blended gas, keeping delivered FiO_2 values more constant (19).

Overall, the air-entrainment mask is intended for patients with high or changing ventilatory demands, such as patients with chronic lung disease who may hypoventilate when exposed to high FiO_2 values.

The OxyMask

Description. The OxyMask is a recently introduced oxygen face mask for both hospital and home use. It uses a small diffuser to concentrate and direct oxygen toward the mouth or nose. This unique design enables the OxyMask to deliver oxygen more efficiently than a Venturi mask, especially in patients with chronic hypoxemia (20).

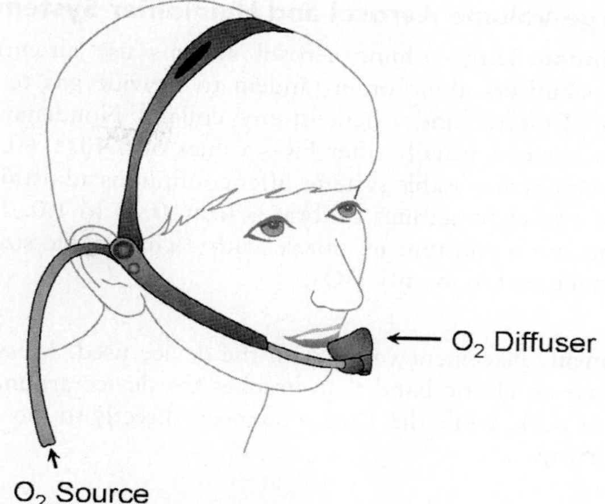

FIGURE 134.3. The OxyMask.

Placement. The OxyMask is an "open oxygen" system that does not require physical contact with the patient's face. The device resembles a hands-free telephone headset, with the speaker portion replaced with "an oxygen diffuser" for precise and comfortable oxygen delivery (Fig. 134.3). The oxygen diffuser can be directed toward the nose or mouth; however, it does not come in contact with either one. Consequently, the OxyMask will not interfere with various activities such as eating and talking (21).

Performance. A recent study compared the OxyMask versus the Venturi mask in 26 oxygen-dependent patients with chronic, stable respiratory disease in a randomized, single-blind, cross-over design (20). Oxygen delivery was titrated to maintain an oxygen saturation (SaO_2) 4% to 5% and 8% to 9% above baseline for two separate 30-minute periods of stable breathing. Oxygen flow rate, partial pressure of inspired and expired oxygen (PO_2) and carbon dioxide (PCO_2), minute ventilation, heart rate, nasal and oral breathing, SaO_2, and transcutaneous PCO_2 were recorded. The study reported lower oxygen flow rates, higher inspired PO_2, and lower expired PO_2 while using the OxyMask. In addition, minute ventilation and inspired and expired PCO_2 were significantly higher while using the OxyMask, whereas transcutaneous PCO_2, heart rate, and the ratio of nasal to oral breathing did not change significantly throughout the study. The study concluded that oxygen is delivered safely and more efficiently by the OxyMask than by the Venturi mask in stable oxygen-dependent patients.

Similar results were obtained in the early postoperative period, during which OxyMask delivered adequate levels of oxygen for most patients, with no patient experiencing an oxygen desaturation event less than 97.88% 4 minutes post extubation (21). In addition, patients and clinicians praised the OxyMask for its comfort and ease of use, allowing nurses to perform facial care without interrupting oxygen therapy.

Large-volume Aerosol and Humidifier Systems

Description. Large-volume aerosol systems use air-entrainment nebulizers alone or in tandem to provide gas to face masks, T-pieces, and tracheostomy collars. Nondisposable aerosol systems usually offer FiO_2 values of 0.40, 0.60, and 1.0, whereas disposable systems offer continuous adjustments, with six to eight settings calibrated from 0.28 to 1.0. These systems use a constant jet nozzle with a changeable size entrainment port to modify FiO_2.

Placement. Placement varies with the device used. Most systems use an elastic band that attaches the device around the head or neck, while the T-piece connects directly to the artificial airway.

Problems. The most common problem with the system is inadequate flow. Other common problems include the presence of water condensation in the delivery tubing that prevents room air entrainment and increases delivered FiO_2. In general, if mist from the aerosol escapes the oxygen delivery device during inspiration, flow is generally considered sufficient.

Performance. Under conditions of high patient ventilatory demand, these systems become variable performance devices (22). With decreased flow, room air becomes entrained in the mask, and therefore, despite the increase in set FiO_2 values, delivered FiO_2 decreases. Accordingly, when precise FiO_2 values are necessary at a high flow rate, a high-volume humidifier system is preferred. If delivery of oxygen is required in excess of 100 L/minute, a blender, air–oxygen flowmeter, or even a Venturi system can be used and directed through a heated humidifier. A reservoir is usually placed between the humidifier and the patient.

MIXING AIR AND OXYGEN

Oxygen Flowmeters and Blenders

Various commercially available oxygen flowmeters (Fig. 134.4) can be used to deliver precise oxygen concentrations. Gas is delivered from air and oxygen flowmeters and passes through a humidifier before being delivered to the nasal cannula or mask.

Air–oxygen blenders (Fig. 134.5) are more expensive compared with using two flowmeters, but with a 50-psig (pounds-force per square inch gauge) source, they can deliver more precise FiO_2 values. In general, blenders have three separate compartments where different functions are performed: the alarm, pressure-balancing, and proportioning compartments.

Air and oxygen enter the alarm compartment from two separate inlets. If the pressure differences between the two inlets are greater than 10 psig, the accuracy of FiO_2 will be compromised and a high-pitched alarm will sound (23). The pressure-balancing compartment will then use a diaphragm to balance the air and oxygen pressures. Finally, at the proportioning compartment, air and oxygen at similar pressures are adjusted in proportion to the desired FiO_2.

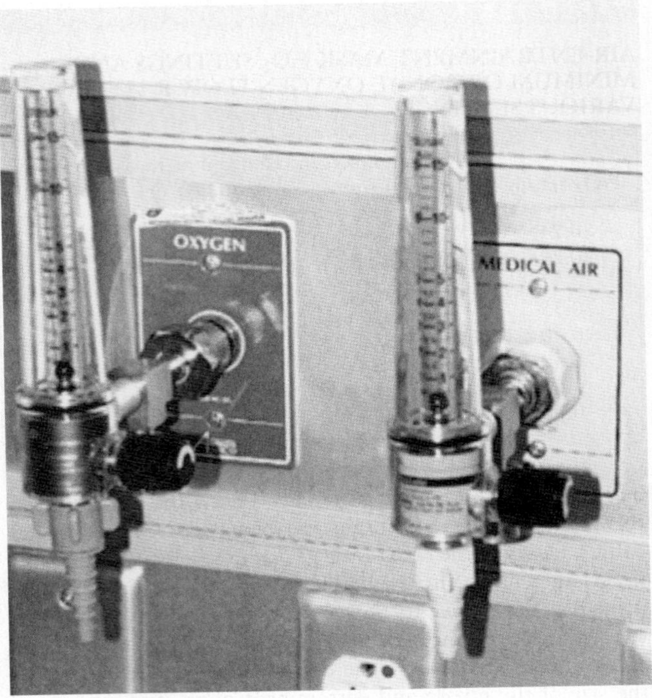

FIGURE 134.4. Oxygen and air flowmeters.

Postextubation Respiratory Therapy

Postextubation pulmonary complications are major causes of morbidity and mortality among intensive care unit (ICU) patients, especially after thoracic or upper abdominal surgeries. During normal respiration, healthy individuals inspire approximately ten times each hour and take large intermittent breaths—"sighing"—that are three times the normal tidal volume (24). However, postoperatively, such deep breaths are absent and replaced with a shallow, monotonous breathing pattern that decreases ventilation to the dependent lung regions, contributing—with the use of postoperative higher FiO_2—to the development of atelectasis. Factors such as residual

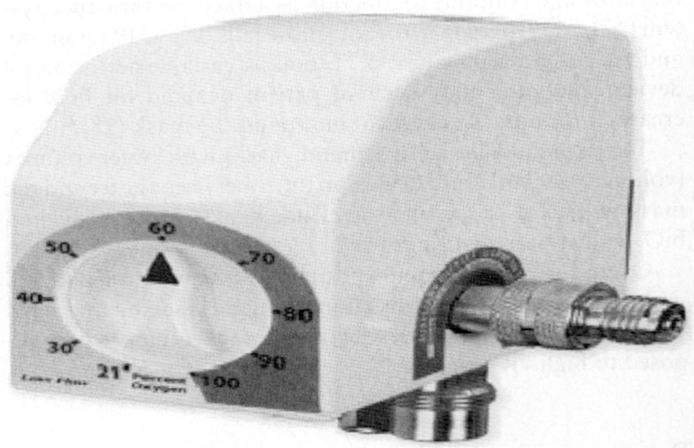

FIGURE 134.5. Oxygen blender.

anesthetic effects and incisional pain promote decreased resting lung volume. Furthermore, assuming a prolonged postoperative recumbent position, the diaphragmatic movement is limited and the functional residual capacity (FRC) decreased (25). The diminishing expiratory lung volume decreases lung compliance and eventually increases the elastic work of breathing. To minimize this work, patients take shallow, frequent breaths, which may further decrease lung volume (25). The primary goal of postoperative respiratory therapy is to increase FRC, reducing pulmonary atelectasis and their related complications.

A slight elevation of temperature and decrease in breath sounds over the lung bases may be useful in diagnosing atelectasis. However, these means are insensitive in detecting decreases in FRC. In addition, the large decline in the amount of air that can be maximally forced out of the lungs after a maximal inspiration (forced vital capacity [FVC]) and the forced expiratory volume in the first second (FEV_1) that occur after upper abdominal operations are patient effort dependent and cannot accurately predict a decrease in FRC. The same can be true regarding the interpretations of portable chest roentgenography in ICU patients, which is useful for identifying patients with atelectasis but does not predict FRC.

The use of postextubation positive pressure devices has been part of respiratory therapy management since intermittent positive pressure breathing (IPPB) was first introduced over 50 years ago (26). In addition to the incentive spirometer (IS), there are many positive pressure devices from which to choose; these include IPPB, continuous positive airway pressure (CPAP), positive expiratory pressure (PEP), and nasal intermittent positive pressure ventilation. In this section, we will review the physiologic effects and indications relating to the use of the IS and IPPB. However, the use of CPAP and noninvasive intermittent positive pressure ventilation will be discussed in detail elsewhere in the textbook.

Incentive Spirometer

Description. Compared to the many therapeutic maneuvers and devices that have been used to prevent postoperative pulmonary complications, the IS has gained the most popularity for its simplicity, and currently is a common mode of postoperative respiratory therapy worldwide.

The IS is designed to mimic natural sighing or yawning by encouraging the patient to maximally inflate the lungs and sustain that inflation. This is accomplished by using a device that provides patients with visual or other positive feedback when they inhale at a predetermined flow rate or volume and inspiratory time, the latter usually targeted at 3 seconds (27). The prolonged and forced lung inflations open collapsed alveoli, preventing or resolving atelectasis. Since the re-expanded alveoli remain inflated during expiration, the FRC increases.

Placement. The IS mouthpiece is placed in the mouth with the lips tightly sealed around it. The IS should be used five to ten breaths per session, or at a minimum every hour while awake (i.e., 100 times a day) (27).

Problems. The IS use may lead to discomfort secondary to inadequate incisional pain control and hypoxia secondary to interruption of prescribed oxygen therapy if a face mask or shield is being used. Furthermore, the IS is generally ineffective unless closely supervised or performed as ordered. In addition, although uncommon, it might result in barotrauma in patients with severely emphysematous lungs.

Performance. Four trials with 443 participants contributed to a recent Cochrane Database of Systematic Review about the benefits of the IS (28). In that review, there was no significant difference in pulmonary complications (atelectasis and pneumonia) between treatment with the IS and treatment with other positive pressure breathing techniques (CPAP, bilevel positive airway pressure [BiPAP], and IPPB), regardless of preoperative patient education. In addition, patients treated with the IS had worse pulmonary function and arterial oxygenation compared with positive pressure breathing (CPAP, BiPAP, IPPB). However, in view of the small number of patients in the included studies and the multiple methodologic and reporting shortcomings, these results should be interpreted cautiously.

Intermittent Positive Pressure Breathing

Description. IPPB is used in clinical practice, primarily to improve the lung volumes and to decrease the work of breathing. However, its role in clearing excessive secretions from the lungs is questionable and controversial. Commercially available devices are most commonly used for the delivery of IPPB. In general, all these devices are powered by compressed gas—either air or oxygen (29). Short-term humidification can be added to the driving gas. Since IPPB is a pressure-cycled device, the operator can select the pressure and flow rate of the gas and the sensitivity for the patient to trigger the system. Upon inspiration, a negative pressure is generated in the circuit, and inspiratory flow proceeds until the preset pressure is attained when flow ceases and the patient expires passively. The operator should adjust the machine settings until a desired maximal volume is delivered to the patient, in general "eyeballed" to 1 inch of chest excursion or approximately 6 to 8 mL/ideal body weight in kilograms (30,31).

Placement. The patient is connected to IPPB through a mouthpiece. The patient needs to be cooperative and spontaneously breathing to trigger the machine using the mouthpiece. Occasionally, a full face mask may be used for less conscious patients, as it is generally tolerated only for a brief period of time.

Problems. IPPB has been shown to increase tidal volume, and consequently minute ventilation, by passively ventilating the patient and hence improving arterial blood gases (29). However, this may lead to a decline in cardiac output as a result of increased intrathoracic pressure during delivery and decreased venous return.

Performance. A large body of literature has been published examining the efficacy of IPPB in different patient populations. The efficacy of IPPB in the management of chronic obstructive pulmonary disease (COPD) was found to be mainly unsupported (29). This can be partly explained by an inappropriate choice of patient populations, the frequency of IPPB used, and other confounding effects of concurrent chest physiotherapy techniques (32).

Another largely studied use of IPPB was in the prevention or management of postoperative respiratory complications (33). The comparative efficacy of IPPB with IS, deep breathing exercises, blow bottles, and physiotherapy has been studied.

Although this literature is overwhelmed by various methodologic problems, their outcomes demonstrated that the use of IPPB conferred no added benefit to patients following abdominal or cardiac surgery when compared to the other modalities (29). However, it is conceivable that in patients with excessive secretions, IPPB may need to be combined with gravity-assisted drainage and chest wall vibrations for more effective upward clearing of secretions (29).

The use of IPPB has declined over the past two decades, partly due to controversial research outcomes and partly as a result of the introduction of newer modes of positive pressure support. However, IPPB may still have a role—though reduced—in the management of patients with reduced lung volumes and respiratory insufficiency who cannot cooperate well with the use of IS.

OXYGEN: THE PHYSIOLOGIC IMPACT

The Fate of Oxygen in the Body

The predominant metabolic pathway for oxygen is as an electron acceptor in oxidative phosphorylation within the mitochondria (34). Oxidation of glucose and fatty acids shuttles electrons to special molecular carriers, which are either pyridine nucleotides or flavins within the mitochondria. The reduced forms of these carrier proteins, in turn, donate their high-potential electrons to molecular oxygen by means of an electron transport chain located in the inner membrane of the double-enveloped mitochondria. The transmembrane proton gradient generated as a by-product of this electron exchange and associated liberation of a large amount of free energy drives the synthesis of adenosine triphosphate (ATP) from adenosine diphosphate (ADP) and inorganic phosphate (P_i). Of the four protein complexes that form the electron transport chain, complex IV, also known as cytochrome *c* oxidase, is responsible for the transfer of four electrons, along with four hydrogen ions, to reduce molecular oxygen to two molecules of water. Cytochrome *c* oxidase has an extremely complex structure and contains 13 subunits, two heme groups (cytochrome *a* and cytochrome a_3), and multiple metal ion cofactors (three atoms of copper, one of magnesium, and one of zinc).

Although the transfer of four electrons and four protons reduces oxygen to water, the transfer of one or two electrons produces superoxide anion ($\bullet O_2^-$) and peroxide (O_2^{2-}), respectively. This occurs in about 1% to 2% of all cases (35). Superoxide anions need an additional electron to make them more stable, so they steal an electron from the nearest source such as mitochondrial DNA, the mitochondrial membrane (lipid peroxidation), protein, reductants such as vitamins C or E, or nonenzymatic antioxidants such as glutathione or thioredoxin. If too much mitochondrial damage occurs, the cell undergoes apoptosis, or programmed cell death (Fig. 134.6). The majority of superoxide anions produced is converted to hydrogen peroxide in the mitochondrial matrix or cytosol by one of three versions of superoxide dismutase. Hydrogen peroxide (H_2O_2) is a more stable compound; however, it also can cause cellular damage as a result of its further reduction to hydroxyl radicals ($\bullet OH$) by a series of iron-catalyzed reactions (36).

Oxygen-free radicals are produced in pulmonary smooth muscle cells, endothelial cells, alveolar cells, and leukocytes residing in the lungs. They are produced by both enzymatic and nonenzymatic (auto-oxidation) reactions. Enzymes capable of forming superoxide radicals include xanthine oxidase,

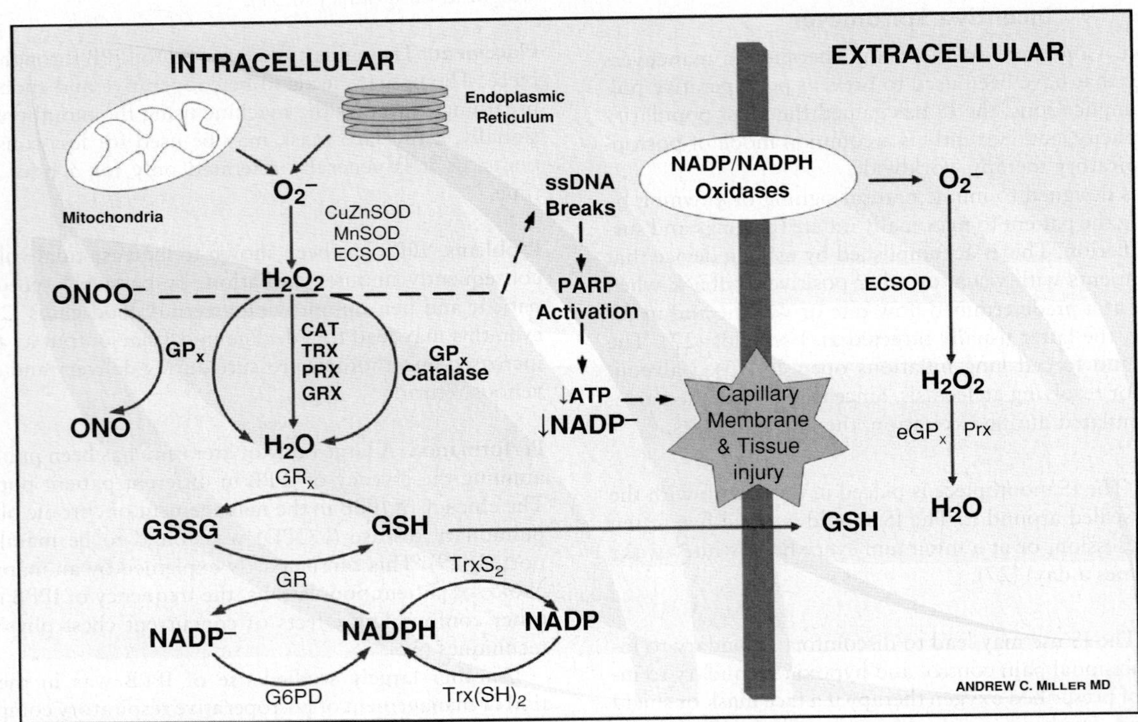

FIGURE 134.6. Oxidant and antioxidant systems.

arachidonic acid peroxidases, nitric oxide synthase, nicotinamide adenine dinucleotide phosphate (NADPH) oxidase, and nicotinamide adenine dinucleotide (NADH) oxidase (37,38). All of these enzymes are essential to the biochemical function of the cell. Phagocytic cells in the lung, such as neutrophils and alveolar macrophages, can form large quantities of superoxide anions during "respiratory bursts" (39,40). The most significant sources of free radicals in lung tissue are the mitochondria and endoplasmic reticulum, the sites of many of the aforementioned enzyme reactions.

The Antioxidants

To combat the excess accumulation of intracellular oxygen radicals, a system of enzymatic and nonenzymatic antioxidants exists in the lungs to prevent their formation and to facilitate the eradication of these reactive species (41,42). There are three primary enzymatic antioxidant systems, although other compounds serve as opportune scavengers. First is superoxide dismutase (SOD), which is found both intra- and extracellularly (42,43). It is present in the cytosol and the mitochondria on the plasma membrane surface, and in the extracellular plasma (44). The cytosolic form of SOD (CuZnSOD), which contains zinc and copper, is associated with pulmonary and endothelial vascular smooth muscle cells (45). The manganese-containing mitochondrial form (MnSOD) is abundant in pulmonary arterial smooth muscle and endothelium, and is felt to be the most active defense during times of pulmonary oxidative stress, catalyzing the dismutation of $\bullet O_2^-$ to H_2O_2.

Catalase and the glutathione antioxidant systems are the primary mechanisms for the reduction of hydrogen peroxide. Catalase is a hemoprotein found in peroxisomes that catalyzes the reduction of hydrogen peroxide to water. Its limited cellular distribution suggests that it has a specific role in managing hydrogen peroxide excess during inflammatory responses. The sulfur-containing antioxidant, glutathione, has a much broader distribution than catalase, and has been measured in the cytosol at millimolar concentrations (46). Exogenously administered glutathione has little effect on intracellular levels. However, N-acetylcysteine is a glutathione analogue capable of crossing the plasma membrane and enhancing glutathione activity, which may account for its purported beneficial effects in various forms of cellular injury. Glutathione peroxidase plays a role in eliminating lipid peroxidases formed from free radical–altered lipid membranes (46). Glutathione peroxidase enhances the reduction of H_2O_2 by first oxidizing glutathione (in its reduced form, GSH) and donating the pair of electrons to hydrogen peroxide to form water. The oxidized glutathione disulfide (GSSG) is subsequently reduced in a reaction that transfers the protons from NADPH + H^+ (Fig. 134.7) (47). Glutathione reductase activity is dependent on NADPH generated from the hexose monophosphate shunt (48). The activity of the glutathione peroxidase enzyme in humans is also dependent on the trace element selenium. The absence of selenium in the diet will markedly reduce the efficacy of the glutathione peroxidase system.

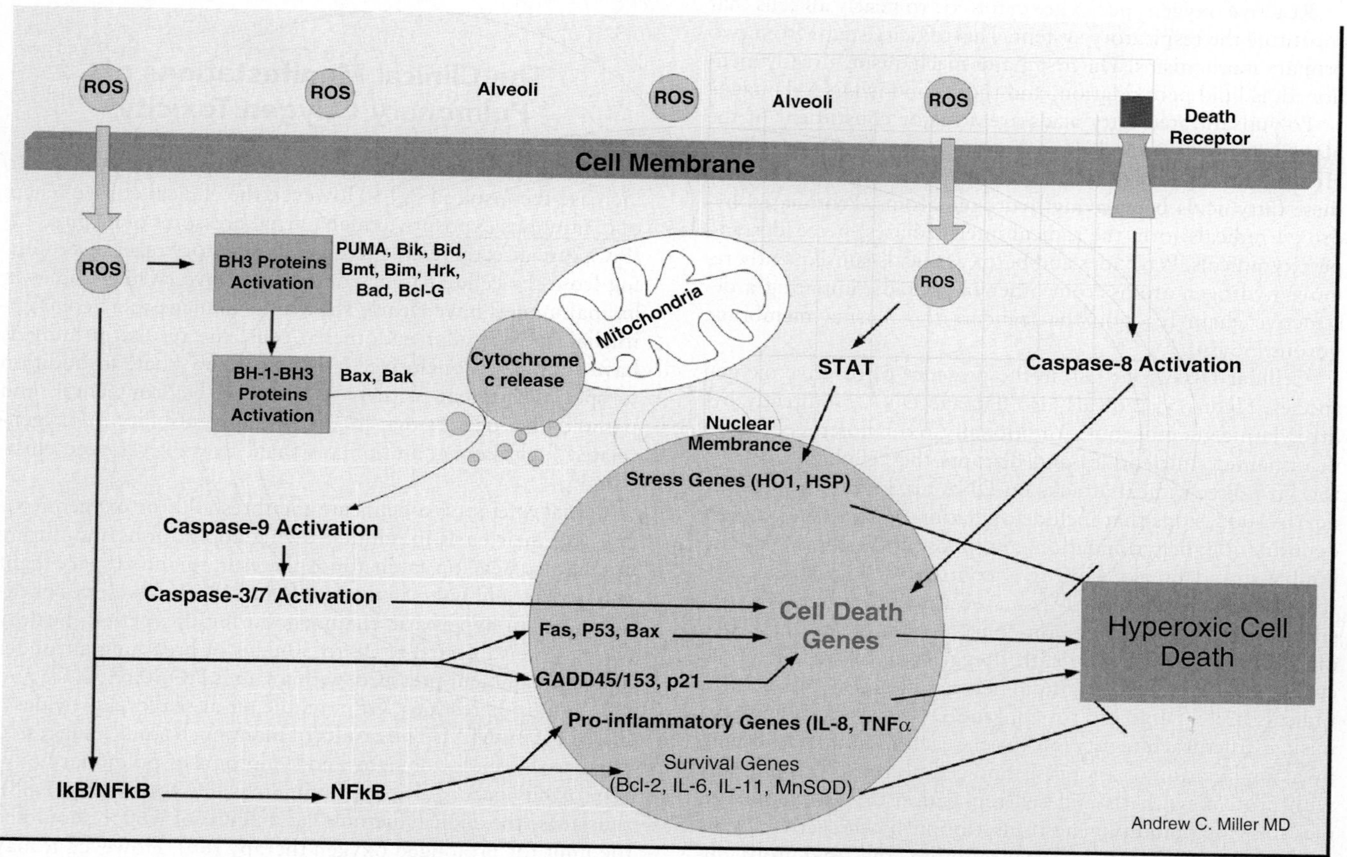

FIGURE 134.7. Hyperoxic cell death.

Other elements with antioxidant capacity include the lipid-soluble vitamin E and the water-soluble vitamin C. Vitamin E (α-tocopherol) is a plasma membrane constituent thought to play a role in inhibiting oxidative cell membrane injury, possibly by interfering with surfactant synthesis (49). Its deficiency in critically ill patients may lead to a susceptibility to pulmonary oxygen toxicity. Vitamin C, or ascorbic acid, is found primarily in the extracellular space and, given its water solubility, is best suited to protecting the respiratory airway mucosa from pollutant oxidants. Other purported nonenzymatic antioxidants include uric acid, β-carotene, taurine, albumin, and bilirubin. Newly discovered families of proteins, the thioredoxins, are located in the inner mitochondrial membrane of the airway epithelium. They may scavenge reactive oxygen species in response to oxidative stress and activate other intramitochondrial antioxidant systems such as MnSOD (50).

Pulmonary Oxygen Toxicity

It may appear paradoxical that oxygen could be a pulmonary toxin at nearly any concentration (51). The lung is well-prepared to cope with the insult when relatively low partial pressures of oxygen (e.g., 160 mm Hg at standard temperature and pressure (STP)) are breathed by virtue of the presence of abundant antioxidants. However, when these defense mechanisms are overwhelmed or depleted by prolonged exposure to an elevated PO_2, a progressive and potentially lethal inflammatory reaction takes place in the lungs (52).

Reactive oxygen species are cytotoxic to nearly all cells that constitute the respiratory system. This toxicity stems from two primary mechanisms. The first major mechanism, already mentioned, is lipid peroxidation, and the second is DNA damage.

Polyunsaturated fatty acids are a major constituent of the plasma membrane and mitochondrial membrane envelope. Hydroxyl-free radicals derived from molecular oxygen destroy these fatty acids by cleaving hydrogen atoms. Protonated hydroxyl radicals form the radical intermediates, peroxides and peroxyradicals. Peroxides and peroxyradicals subsequently remove hydrogen atoms from other fatty acids, initiating a destructive chain reaction that renders the plasma membrane porous (53,54).

Cellular DNA is at risk in the presence of reactive oxygen species. Hydroxyl radicals also damage DNA by directly hydroxylating guanine (55). Additionally, oxidant stress depletes nicotinamide nucleotides and disrupts the cellular cytoskeleton (56). Free radical attacks on DNA are known to produce nearly 100 lesions that include oxidation of bases and sugars, depurination, depyrimidation, and phosphodiester single- and double-strand breaks (57). It is controversial whether DNA strand breaks result directly from the attack of reactive oxygen species on DNA or are a consequence of nucleases activated during programmed cell death. Regardless, the reactive lipid compounds formed during lipid peroxidation by hydroxyl-free radicals are capable of cross-linking DNA proteins, compromising structural integrity (58). Such reactions induce cell death by a combination of apoptosis and cell necrosis, and interfere with protein synthesis and cell replication (59–61). Superoxides may also modify gene transcription by the activation of a potent regulator of gene transcription, the ubiquitous nuclear factor-κB (NF-κB) (62). It is unclear what impact this has on any specific protein synthesis, although one study provided some evidence of a negative feedback mechanism by inducing the expression of superoxide dismutase (63).

An additional primary target of oxygen-free radicals is pulmonary artery smooth muscle, resulting in vasoconstriction. Pulmonary artery smooth muscle contractility is affected through a variety of pathways, although most involve either the release of calcium from the sarcoplasmic reticulum or its sequestration via the enhanced activity of ATP-dependent Ca^{2+} uptake transporters. Superoxide anions also destroy nitric oxide produced by endothelial cells, in effect eliminating one of the most potent vasodilatory regulators in the lung (35).

A bimodal response to oxygen toxicity is seen in the lung. Initially, there is a proliferative phase where pulmonary artery endothelial cells replicate rapidly in response to the presence of superoxide anions. Superoxide anion production and release by these stimulated endothelial cells is far greater than that of quiescent endothelium. Thus begins a vicious cycle of superoxide radical generation and increased levels of exposure of surrounding lung parenchyma resulting in further DNA strand breakage, depletion of ATP, and enhanced membrane lipid peroxidation (64). This produces the inhibitory phase of endothelial proliferation. Other pulmonary cells such as bronchial and type I alveolar epithelial cells are also early victims in oxidant injury. Type I alveolar cells are replaced by hyperplasia of type II alveolar epithelial cells, resulting in the typical thickening of the alveolar epithelium seen in electron micrographs. Clara cells, which are nonciliated epithelial cells distributed throughout the airways and rich in cytochrome P450, are particularly sensitive to oxidant stress (65).

The Clinical Manifestations of Pulmonary Oxygen Toxicity

It is common to treat hypoxemia with supplemental oxygen to increase the inspired PO_2. However, the clinical consequences of continuous exposure to high partial pressures of inspired O_2 (PiO_2) are directly related to the inflammatory reactions resulting from the cellular injury described above. While studies in animal models have clearly shown the damage to alveolar epithelial and vascular endothelial cells, the results in humans have been less conclusive. It is very likely that, in addition to species differences, there are genetic, environmental, and pathologic processes that modify the susceptibility to oxygen-related lung damage in humans that have not yet been elucidated.

Initial attempts to delineate the threshold for oxygen toxicity had their basis in military diving applications and during attempts to develop cabin atmospheres for manned space flight and undersea habitats in the 1960s and 1970s. In a series of experiments in hyperbaric chambers during this period, healthy divers were subjected to 28 to 30 days of breathing air under increased ambient pressure, with a target PiO_2 0.51, 0.57, and 0.81 atmospheres (66). Of note, the air at sea level provides a PiO_2 of 0.21 ATM. The results of many such studies suggested that the threshold for signs and symptoms of pulmonary oxygen toxicity occurred at approximately a PiO_2 of 0.60 (67,68); thus arose the clinical dictum that an FiO_2 of $<60\%$ should be the limit for prolonged oxygen therapy (69). However, it may not be accurate to extrapolate such studies in healthy divers to sick patients with pre-existing parenchymal disease or the systemic inflammatory response syndrome (SIRS).

Normal individuals breathing 100% O_2 experience symptoms of tracheobronchitis within 12 to 24 hours (69). This initial phase of oxygen toxicity is marked by a decline in tracheobronchial clearance of particulates, substernal chest discomfort, tachypnea, and a nonproductive cough. Associated systemic symptoms include malaise, nausea, headache, and anorexia. While the decrease in particulate clearance may begin as early as 6 hours after such exposures, by 24 hours the vital capacity begins to decline significantly. Within 48 hours of exposure to 100% oxygen, decrements in static lung compliance and carbon monoxide–diffusing capacity are measurable. In a study of patients with irreversible brain damage and ventilated with 100% FiO_2, the alveolar-arterial gradient increased rapidly after 40 to 60 hours. Continued exposure of the lungs to high partial pressures of oxygen ultimately contributed to the development of the acute respiratory distress syndrome (ARDS) accompanied by severe dyspnea and subsequent pulmonary fibrotic changes. Chest radiographic findings are nonspecific and show increased interstitial markings or alveolar consolidation similar to a number of other causes of diffuse alveolar damage.

Hypercapnia

The wisdom of administering high partial pressures of oxygen to patients with chronic hypercarbia continues to be a source of debate among clinicians. The concern has been that the patient with CO_2 retention (e.g., COPD) relies predominantly on a hypoxic ventilatory drive and that increasing PaO_2 by the administration of oxygen will result in depression of this stimulus and a dangerous drop in minute ventilation with a rise in $PaCO_2$. $PaCO_2$ has been observed to rise in a subset of these patients suffering acute exacerbations of their COPD when treated with 100% O_2 (60). However, there have been several studies in both stable COPD and those with acute exacerbations that demonstrate only a transient decline in minute ventilation inadequate to explain the accompanying rise in CO_2 (70–72). Another explanation for a rise in $PaCO_2$ includes rightward displacement of the CO_2–hemoglobin dissociation curve in the presence of increased oxygen saturation, and a consequent reduction in carboxyhemoglobin formation and transport—the Haldane effect. More likely, there are relative increases in dead space ventilation via alterations in hypoxic pulmonary vasoconstriction. Hanson et al. modeled ventilation and perfusion in a computer simulation of the lung, and demonstrated that it was possible to account for the change in $PaCO_2$ by oxygen-induced relaxation of hypoxic pulmonary vasoconstriction (73). This pulmonary vascular response to hypoxia is capable of redirecting blood flow from alveoli that are poorly ventilated to those with a higher PaO_2. Blunting this response by artificially increasing the PaO_2 prevents appropriate matching between ventilation and pulmonary perfusion, and permits a rise in CO_2. A recent study examined a cohort of CO_2-retaining COPD patients recovering from an acute exacerbation after they had been weaned from mechanical ventilation to a baseline FiO_2 of 0.3 to 0.4 (72). Patients were re-exposed to an FiO_2 of 0.7 for 20 minutes, and no statistically significant changes in respiratory rate, tidal volume, dead space, or $PaCO_2$ were reported. Robinson et al. compared two groups of patients with acute COPD exacerbations, dividing them into CO_2-retaining and nonretaining groups (74). They found only modest declines in minute ventilation, with a rise in $PaCO_2$ averaging about 3 mm Hg in the CO_2 retainer group upon exposure to 100% O_2 face mask. The dispersion of alveolar ventilation/perfusion ratios increased nearly equally in both groups upon oxygen exposure, suggesting that hypoxic pulmonary vasoconstriction was affected equally in both groups. From these experiments, one must conclude that the mechanisms generating hypercapnia in individuals with COPD treated with supplemental oxygen are varied and complex. Close monitoring of respiratory parameters, including arterial oxygenation and carbon dioxide, is mandatory when oxygen therapy is employed to reverse severe hypoxemia.

Absorption Atelectasis

An individual spontaneously breathing a high inspired concentration of oxygen results in replacement of nitrogen with oxygen within the alveoli. This may cause absorption atelectasis secondary to oxygen diffusing into the alveolar capillary blood more rapidly than nitrogen can diffuse into the alveoli and inhaled oxygen can replace the lost volume (75). This may be more theoretical than practical, certainly in the short term where nitrogen will continue to diffuse into the blood from all tissues, and to some degree into the alveoli to re-establish an equilibrium. Nonetheless, it is potentially a problem in those regions of the lung experiencing low ventilation/perfusion ratios and subjected to large compressive forces (e.g., lower lobes from abdominal contents or weight of the heart in the supine individual). The rate of alveoli collapse may potentially be greater in those circumstances where there are increased metabolic demands and rates of oxygen uptake. Although the mechanism has not been fully elucidated, decrements in vital capacity of up to 20% have been recorded after exposure to 100% oxygen in patients, although oxygen-induced tracheobronchitis was presumed (76).

SUMMARY

The management of airway, breathing, and oxygen therapy in critically ill patients continues to be a challenging task. A comprehensive understanding of the various oxygen delivery modalities is of utmost importance in not only delivering the highest quality of care to the critically ill patients, but also avoiding major oxygen therapy–related consequences, including increased morbidity and even mortality.

References

1. Guilfojie T, Dabe K. Nasal catheter oxygen therapy for infants. *Respir Care.* 1981;26:35–39.
2. Kory RC, Bergman JC, Sweet RD, et al. Comparative evaluation of oxygen therapy techniques. *JAMA.* 1962;179:123–128.
3. AARC Clinical Practice Guideline: Oxygen Therapy for Adults in the Acute Care Facility—2002 Revision & Update. *Respir Care.* 2002;47(6):717–720.
4. Shapiro BA, Harrison RA, Kacmarek RM, et al. Oxygen therapy. In: Shapiro BA, Harrison RA, Kacmarek RM, et al., eds. *Clinical Application of Respiratory Care.* 3rd ed. Chicago, IL: Year Book Medical Publishers; 1985;176–191.
5. Ooi R, Joshi P, Soni N. An evaluation of oxygen delivery using nasal prongs. *Anesthesia.* 1992;47:591–593.

6. Domingo C, Roig J, Coll R, et al. Evaluation of the use of three different devices for nocturnal oxygen therapy in COPD patients. *Respiration.* 1996;63(4):230–235.
7. Tiep BL, Nicotra B, Carter R, et al. Evaluation of a low-flow oxygen-conserving nasal cannula. *Am Rev Respir Dis.* 1984;130:500–502.
8. Tiep BL, Lewis ML. Oxygen conservation and oxygen-conserving devices in chronic lung disease: a review. *Chest.* 1987;92:263–273.
9. Garrod R, Bestall JC, Paul E, et al. Evaluation of pulsed dose oxygen delivery during exercise in patients with severe chronic obstructive pulmonary disease. *Thorax.* 1999;54:242–244.
10. Fuhrman C, Chouaid C, Herigault R, et al. Comparison of four demand oxygen delivery systems at rest and during exercise for chronic obstructive pulmonary disease. *Respir Med.* 2004;98(10):938–944.
11. Blackmon GM, Johnson MC II, Plotkin E. Rapidly progressive extensive subcutaneous emphysema associated with an implantable intratracheal oxygen catheter. *Chest.* 1998;113(3):834–836.
12. Jackson M, King MA, Wells FC, et al. Clinical experience and physiologic results with an implantable intratracheal oxygen catheter. *Chest.* 1992;102:1413–1418.
13. Bethune DW, Coffis JM. Evaluation of oxygen therapy equipment. *Thorax.* 1967;22:221–225.
14. Jensen AG, Johnson A, Sandstedt S. Rebreathing during oxygen treatment with face mask. *Acta Anaesth Scand.* 1991;35:289–291.
15. Banjer NR, Govan JR. Long term transtracheal oxygen delivery through microcatheter in patients with hypoxaernia due to chronic obstructive airways disease. *BMJ.* 1986;293:111–114.
16. Redding JS, McAffee DD, Gross CW. Oxygen concentrations received from commonly used delivery systems. *South Med J.* 1978;71(2):169–172.
17. Woolner DF, Larkin J. An analysis of the performance of a variable Venturi-type oxygen mask. *Anaesth Intens Care.* 1980;8:44–51.
18. Campbell EJM, Minty KB. Controlled oxygen therapy at 60% concentration. *Lancet.* 1976;2:1199–1203.
19. Cox D, Gifibe C. Fixed performance oxygen masks. *Anaesthesia.* 1981;36:958–964.
20. Beecroft JM, Hanly PJ. Comparison of the OxyMask and Venturi mask in the delivery of supplemental oxygen: pilot study in oxygen-dependent patients. *Can Respir J.* 2006;13(5):247–252.
21. Futrell JW Jr, Moore JL. The OxyArm^{TM}: a supplemental oxygen delivery device *Anesth Analg.* 2006;102:491–494.
22. Foust GN, Potter WH, Wilson MD, et al. Shortcomings of using two jet nebulizer in tandem with an aerosol face mask for optimal oxygen therapy. *Chest.* 1991;99:1346–1351.
23. Barnes TA. Equipment for mixed gas and oxygen therapy. *Respir Care Clin N Am.* 2000;6(4):545–595.
24. Zikria BA, Spencer JL, Kinney JM, et al. Alterations in ventilatory function and breathing patterns following surgical trauma. *Ann Surg.* 1974;179:1–7.
25. Stock MC, Downs JB, Gauer PK, et al. Prevention of postoperative pulmonary and conservative therapy complications with CPAP, incentive spirometry, and conservative therapy. *Chest.* 1985;87:151–157.
26. Motley H, Cournand A, Richards D. Observations of the clinical use of intermittent positive pressure. *J Aviation Med.* 1947;18:417.
27. Marini JJ, Baker WL, Lamb VJ. Breath stacking increases the depth and duration of chest expansion by incentive spirometry. *Am Rev Respir Dis.* 1990;141:343–346.
28. Freitas ERFS, Soares BGO, Cardoso JR, et al. Incentive spirometry for preventing pulmonary complications after coronary artery bypass graft. Cochrane Database of Systematic Reviews 2007;3:CD004466. DOI: 10.1002/14651858. CD004466.pub2.
29. Denehy L, Berney S. The use of positive pressure devices by physiotherapists. *Eur Respir J.* 2001;7:821–829.
30. Webber BA, Pryor JA. Physiotherapy skills: techniques and adjuncts. In Webber BA, Pryor JA, ed. *Physiotherapy for Respiratory and Cardiac Problems.* London: Churchill Livingstone; 1993:113–172.
31. Bott J, Keilty S, Noone L. Intermittent positive pressure breathing—a dying art? *Physiotherapy.* 1992;78:656–660.
32. Ali J. Effect of post-operative intermittent positive pressure breathing on lung function. *Chest.* 1984;85:192–196.
33. Oikkonen M, Karjalainen K, Kahara V, et al. Comparison of incentive spirometry and intermittent positive pressure breathing after coronary artery bypass graft. *Chest.* 1991;99:60–65.
34. Stryer L. Oxidative phosphorylation. In *Biochemistry*. 4th ed. New York, W.H. Freeman and Co., 1995, 529–558.
35. Zhang DX, Gutterman DD. Mitochondrial reactive oxygen species-mediated signaling in endothelial cells. *Am J Physiol Heart Circ Physiol.* 2006;292:H2023.
36. Halliwell B, Gutteridge JM. Role of free radicals and catalytic metal ions in human disease: an overview. *Methods Enzymol.* 1990;186:1.
37. Marshall C, Mamary AJ, Verhoeven AJ, et al. Pulmonary artery NADPH-oxidase is activated in hypoxic pulmonary vasoconstriction. *Am J Resp Cell Mol Biol.* 1996;15:633.
38. Kukreja RC, Contos HA, Hess ML, et al. PGH synthase and lipoxygenase generate superoxide in the presence of NADH or NADPH. *Circ Res.* 1986;59:612.
39. Cross AR, Jones OT. Enzyme mechanisms of superoxide production. *Biochim Biophys Acta.* 1991;1057:281.
40. Forman HJ, Torres M. Reactive oxygen species and cell signaling: respiratory burst in macrophage signaling. *Am J Respir Crit Care Med.* 2002;166:S4.
41. Comhair SAA, Erzurum SC. Antioxidant responses to oxidant-mediated lung diseases. *Am J Physiol Lung Cell Mol Physiol.* 2002;283:L246.
42. Kinnula VL, Crapo JD. Superoxide dismutases in the lung and human lung diseases. *Am J Respir Crit Care Med.* 2003;167:1600.
43. Bowler RP, Crapo JD. Oxidative stress in airways: is there a role for extracellular superoxide dismutase? *Am J Respir Crit Care Med.* 2002;166:S38.
44. Sandstrom J, Karlsson K, Edlund T, et al. Heparin-affinity patterns and composition of extracellular superoxide dismutase in human plasma and tissues. *Biochem J.* 1993;294:853.
45. McCord JM, Fridovich I. Superoxide dismutase: an enzymic function for erythrocuprein (hemocuprein). *J Biol Chem.* 1969;244:6049.
46. Ross D, Norbeck K, Moldeus P. The generation and subsequent fate of glutathionyl radicals in biological systems. *J Biol Chem.* 1985;260:15028.
47. Deneke SM, Fanburg BL. Regulation of cellular glutathione. *Am J Physiol Lung Cell Mol Physiol.* 1989;257:L163.
48. Meister A, Anderson ME. Glutathione. *Am Rev Biochem.* 1983;52:711.
49. Kolleck I, Sinha P, Rustow B. Vitamin E as an antioxidant of the lung: mechanisms of vitamin E delivery to alveolar type II cells. *Am J Respir Crit Care Med.* 2002;166:S62.
50. Das KC, Guo XL, White CW. Induction of thioredoxin and thioredoxin reductase gene expression in lungs of newborn primates by oxygen. *Am J Physiol Lung Cell Mol Physiol.* 1991;276:L530.
51. Davies K. Oxidative stress: the paradox of aerobic life. *Biochem Soc Symp.* 1995;61:1.
52. Valko M, Leibfritz D, Moncol J, et al. Free radicals and antioxidants in normal physiological functions and human disease. *Int J Biochem Cell Biol.* 2007;39(1):44.
53. Doelman CJ, Bast A. Oxygen radicals in lung pathology. *Free Radic Biol Med.* 1990;9:381.
54. Van der Vliet A, Smith D, O'Neill CA, et al. Interactions of peroxynitrite with human plasma and its constituents: oxidative damage and antioxidant depletion. *Biochem J.* 1994;303:295.
55. Finkel T, Holbrook NJ. Oxidants, oxidative stress and the biology of ageing. *Nature.* 2000;408:239.
56. Rahman I, Biswas SK, Kode A. Oxidant and antioxidant balance in the airways and airway diseases. *Eur J Pharmacol.* 2006;533:222–239.
57. O'Reilly MA. DNA damage and cell cycle checkpoints in hyperoxic lung injury: braking to facilitate repair. *Am J Physiol Lung Cell Mol Physiol.* 2001;281(2):L291–305.
58. Wiseman H, Halliwell B. Damage to DNA by reactive oxygen and nitrogen species: role in inflammatory disease and progression to cancer. *Biochem J.* 1996;313:17.
59. Mantell LL, Lee PJ. Signal transduction pathways in hyperoxia-induced lung cell death. *Mol Genet Metab.* 2000;71(1–2):359–370.
60. Nanavaty UB, Pawliczak R, Doniger J, et al. Oxidant-induced cell death in respiratory epithelial cells is due to damage and loss of ATP. *Exp Lung Res.* 2002;28:591.
61. Volkert MR, Landini P. Transcriptional responses to DNA damage. *Curr Opin Microbiol.* 2001;4:178.
62. Shreck R, Baeuerle PA. Assessing oxygen radicals as mediators in activation of inducible eukaryotic transcription factor NF-kappa B. *Methods Enzymol.* 1994;234:151.
63. Demple D. Study of redox-regulated transcription factors in prokaryotes. *Methods.* 1997;11:267.
64. Li PF, Dietz R, von Harsdorf R. Differential effect of hydrogen peroxide and superoxide anion on apoptosis and proliferation of vascular smooth muscle cells. *Circulation.* 1997;96:3602.
65. Cho M, Chichester C, Plopper GC, et al. Biochemical factors important in Clara cell selective toxicity in the lung. *Drug Metab Rev.* 1995;27:369.
66. Dougherty JJH, Frayre RL, Miller DA, et al. Pulmonary function during shallow habitat air dives (SHAD I, II, III). In: Schilling CW, Beckett MW, eds. *Underwater Physiology VI: Proceedings of the Sixth Symposium on Underwater Physiology.* Bethesda, MD: FASEB; 1978:193.
67. Morgan TE Jr, Ulvedal F, Welch BE. Observations in the SAM two-man space cabin simulator. *II Biomedical aspects. Aerospace Med.* 1961;32:591.
68. Clark JM, Lambertsen CJ. *Pulmonary Oxygen Tolerance in Man and Derivation of Pulmonary Oxygen Tolerance Curves. Institute for Environmental Medicine Report.* Philadelphia: University of Pennsylvania; 1970:1.
69. Clark JM, Thom SR. Oxygen under pressure. In: Brubakk AO, Neuman TS, eds. *Bennett and Elliott's Physiology and Medicine of Diving.* 5th ed. Edinburgh: Saunders; 2003:358.
70. Aubier M, Murciano D, Milic-Emili J, et al. Effects of the administration of O_2 on ventilation and blood gases in patients with chronic obstructive pulmonary disease during acute respiratory failure. *Am Rev Respir Dis.* 1980;122:747.
71. Sassoon CSH, Hassell KT, Mahutte CK. Hyperoxic-induced hypercapnia in stable chronic obstructive pulmonary disease. *Am Rev Respir Dis.* 1987;135:907.
72. Crossley DJ, McGuire GP, Barrow PM, et al. Influence of inspired oxygen

concentration on deadspace, respiratory drive, and $PaCO_2$ in intubated patients with chronic obstructive pulmonary disease. *Crit Care Med.* 1997;25:1522.
73. Hanson CW, Marshall BE, Frasch HF, et al. Causes of hypercarbia with oxygen therapy in patients with chronic obstructive pulmonary disease. *Crit Care Med.* 1996;24:23.
74. Robinson TD, Freiberg DB, Regnis JA, et al. The role of hypoventilation and ventilation-perfusion redistribution in oxygen-induced hypercapnia during acute exacerbations of chronic obstructive pulmonary disease. *Am J Respir Crit Care Med.* 2000;161:1524.
75. Duggan M, Kavanagh BP. Pulmonary atelectasis: a pathogenic perioperative entity. *Anesthesiology.* 2005;102:838.
76. Carvalho CR, de Paula P, Schettino G, et al. Hyperoxia and lung disease. *Curr Opin Pulm Med.* 1998;4:300.

CHAPTER 135 ■ INDICATIONS FOR AND MANAGEMENT OF TRACHEOSTOMY

HAO CHIH HO • MIHAE YU

IMMEDIATE CONCERNS

Many critically ill patients require ventilator support for extended periods of time. Maintaining a safe and secure airway for these patients can be challenging, and the choice between continued translaryngeal intubation and tracheostomy is not always easy. Initially, most patients will have an endotracheal tube (ETT) in place. The main consideration for placement of a tracheostomy is the anticipated duration of ventilator support, need for airway access (suctioning), and patient comfort. Predicting the duration of ventilator support is difficult, and the optimal timing of tracheostomy in critically ill patients with acute respiratory failure is controversial. Tracheostomy should be an elective procedure and should not be performed on patients receiving high pressure ventilator support, except on rare occasions when there are mechanical problems with the ETT. With high-volume, low-pressure endotracheal tube cuffs, there is no time interval when conversion to a tracheostomy is mandatory because of potential damage to the trachea from pressure necrosis. The decision to perform a tracheostomy should not be based solely on the duration of endotracheal intubation, especially in patients requiring high pressure ventilator support where the risk of transport to the operating room or loss of airway pressure during percutaneous tracheostomy may cause significant morbidity.

OVERVIEW

Tracheostomy is one of the most commonly performed surgical procedures in critically ill patients (1). The modern surgical tracheostomy was first described in 1909 by Chevalier Jackson (2). Ciaglia et al. (3) first described the technique of percutaneous dilational tracheostomy (PDT) in 1985. Bedside PDT is now widely accepted in critical care units.

INDICATIONS AND TIMING

The primary indication for tracheostomy is the requirement for prolonged ventilator support and/or failure to wean from mechanical ventilation for 2 to 3 weeks (4). In 1989, the ACCP Consensus Conference on Artificial Airways in Patients Receiving Mechanical Ventilation recommended tracheostomy for patients whose anticipated need for artificial airway is greater than 21 days (5). Other indications are severe head injury with inability to protect the airway, high spinal cord injuries, laryngeal trauma, upper airway obstruction, and management of pulmonary secretions. The benefits of tracheostomy include sparing the larynx from further direct injury from the translaryngeal tube, improved comfort (6), ability to speak and eat, improved oral care, and possibly earlier transfer from the intensive care unit (ICU) (5). In patients with limited reserve, tracheostomy reduces the work of breathing (shorter length of tubing than the endotracheal tube) and may allow more flexibility in weaning (7,8).

There continues to be debate over the actual impact of tracheostomy on outcome. In two recent studies of patients requiring prolonged mechanical ventilation, Combes et al. (9) found that tracheostomy was associated with lower ICU and in-hospital mortality rates, whereas Clec'h et al. (10) found no reduction in mortality but increased post-ICU mortality if the tracheostomy was left in place.

Another controversial topic is the optimal timing of converting a translaryngeal intubation to a tracheostomy because there is no accurate way to predict the need for prolonged mechanical ventilation in the first few days. A high acuity of illness (Acute Physiology and Chronic Health Evaluation [APACHE] II scores greater than 25) and the presence of shock at the time of ICU admission are two of the best predictors (11–13). Pena et al. (14) reviewed 56 cases of subglottic stenosis and found that 86% had a history of tracheal intubation, with a mean duration of 17 days. The ACCP Consensus Conference recommends translaryngeal intubation for an anticipated need of the artificial airway up to ten days and tracheotomy for an anticipated need of the artificial airway for greater than 21 days. The ACCP Consensus Conference also recommends that the decision for tracheostomy be made as early as possible to minimize the duration of translaryngeal intubation (5).

Several studies have provided additional support for early tracheostomy. Rumbak et al. (15) randomized 128 medical patients to either early (within 48 hours) or late (14–16 days) percutaneous tracheostomy and found significantly shorter ICU stays, fewer days on the ventilator, and a lower mortality in the early tracheostomy group. A prospective review of trauma patients by Arabi et al. (16) also found that patients who received early tracheostomy (by day 7 of mechanical ventilation) had shorter ICU stays and fewer days on the ventilator. In a meta-analysis, Griffiths et al. (17) reviewed five clinical trails with a total of 406 patients that compared early (within 7 days) versus late tracheostomy in critically ill adult patients. Mortality and the risk of pneumonia were the same in the two groups, but early tracheostomy significantly reduced the duration of artificial ventilation and length of stay in the ICU.

PATIENT SELECTION

All patients requiring prolonged mechanical ventilation are candidates for tracheostomy. The main contraindications of tracheostomy are hemodynamic instability, uncorrected coagulopathy, active infection over the tracheostomy site, and emergency airway access. Other mitigating circumstances may include risk of infection to adjacent surgical wounds and central line sites (neck and upper chest incisions), and a high fraction of inspired oxygen (FiO_2) and/or positive end-expiratory pressure (PEEP) requirement.

OPEN VERSUS PERCUTANEOUS TRACHEOSTOMY

Surgical tracheostomy (ST) is usually performed in the operating room (OR). It can be performed in the ICU, but is not optimal in that setting because of inadequate lighting, suction, and cautery, as well as difficulty in maintaining a sterile field. PDT is usually performed in the ICU, eliminating the need to transport the patient to and from the operating room (OR), as well as the cost of the OR and possibly the cost of anesthesia. In a recent meta-analysis, Delaney et al. identified randomized clinical trials that compared PDT to ST. Seventeen studies involving 1,212 patients were reviewed, and the authors concluded that PDT reduced the incidence of wound infection and may further reduce clinically relevant bleeding and mortality when compared with ST performed in the OR (18). The choice between ST and PDT depends on the operator experience and individual patient issues.

Patient issues favoring surgical tracheostomy include:

1. Coagulation abnormalities—Larger blood vessels are more easily controlled under direct vision during ST, but the smaller wound opening and snug fit of the tracheostomy placed by PDT may help tamponade clinically relevant bleeding from small vessels at the wound edges.
2. High level of oxygenation support with a high FiO_2 and/or high PEEP—During PDT, the endotracheal tube is withdrawn until the tip is in the larynx. This often results in a substantial gas leak and possibly hypoxia in these patients. In ST, the endotracheal tube is only withdrawn when the tracheostomy tube is ready to be inserted, minimizing the gas leak and loss of PEEP.
3. Unstable cervical spine—Dilation and tracheostomy tube insertion during PDT requires a significant exertion of force that may result in excessive cervical spine motion which may be avoided with ST.
4. Unusual neck anatomy such as masses, previous surgery, or poor mobility—In these cases, it is safer to perform ST because of the direct visualization of the neck structures.

TECHNIQUES

Surgical Tracheostomy

ST can be performed in either the OR or the ICU. The patient usually has an endotracheal tube in place. A shoulder roll is placed to elevate the shoulders and extend the head, which elevates the larynx and exposes more of the upper trachea. The skin from the chin to below the clavicles is prepped. Sterile drapes are used to create an opening from the top of the larynx to the suprasternal notch. The thyroid notch and cricoid cartilage are identified by palpation (Fig. 135.1).

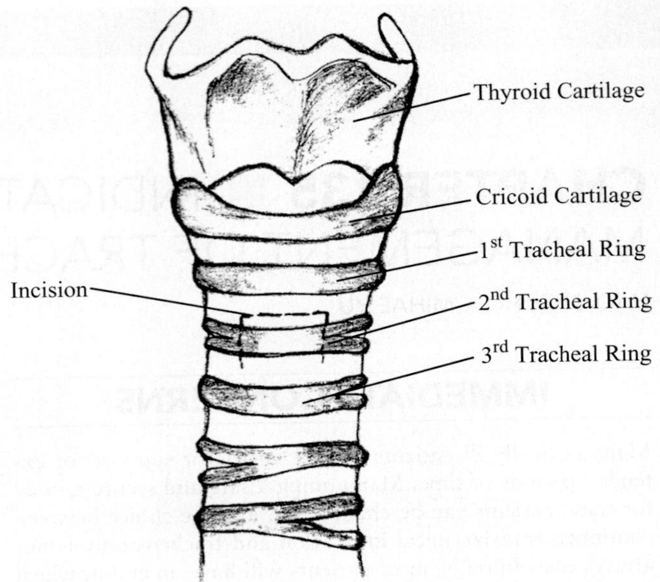

FIGURE 135.1. Tracheal anatomy and placement of incision.

Local anesthetic with a vasoconstrictor, such as epinephrine, is then injected into the skin and subcutaneous tissue overlying the second tracheal ring. A 2-cm midline vertical or horizontal incision is then made. The vertical incision extends from the inferior edge of the cricoid cartilage toward the suprasternal notch whereas the horizontal incision is made over the second tracheal ring. Dissection is carried sharply through the platysma muscle. Bleeding is controlled with cautery and/or hemostats and ties. Careful blunt dissection is then used to expose the thyroid isthmus, which is done by palpating the anatomy and using a curved hemostat to gently spread the submuscular tissues parallel to the long axis of the trachea. If the thyroid isthmus overlies the second and third tracheal rings, it may need to be partially or completely transected to expose the trachea.

Once the trachea is dissected free of the overlying tissues, the second ring is identified. An incision is made in the trachea between the first and second ring and extended laterally through the second ring (Fig. 135.1). This results in a tracheal flap (Fig. 135.2) that can be sutured to the inferior edge of the skin incision, creating a stoma. The endotracheal tube is withdrawn, and the tracheostomy tube is inserted into the trachea under direct vision. The creation of a stoma may facilitate reinsertion of the dislodged tube in the first few days when the fistula tract may not have stabilized. Another technique is to make a criss-cross incision on the trachea and simply insert the tracheostomy under direct vision after lifting the edges with a tracheal hook. Suturing the tracheostomy tube in place may help decrease the risk of accidental decannulation.

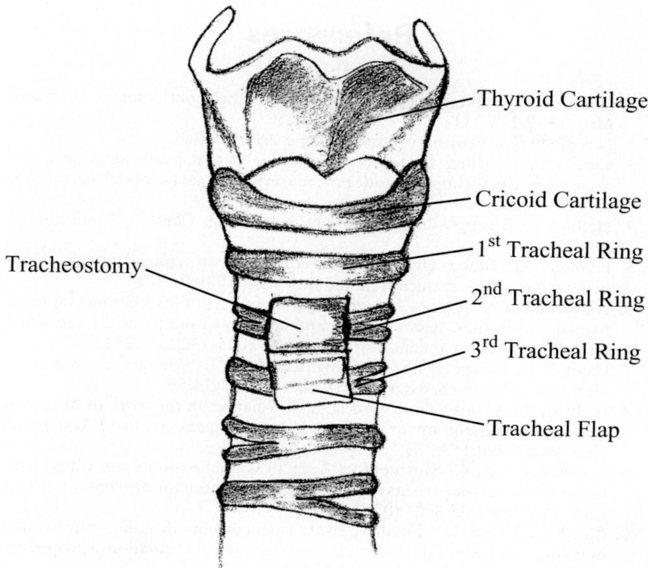

FIGURE 135.2. Tracheal flap created in open tracheostomy.

Percutaneous Dilational Tracheostomy

The most common technique for performing PDT is that of Ciaglia. Originally, the technique used sequential dilators (3), but it has since been simplified to using a single tapered dilator. This dilator has a hydrophilic coating that is activated by immersing it in sterile water or saline. This procedure can be performed blindly, although many clinicians use fiberoptic bronchoscopy to observe the placement, as well as to prevent inadvertent injury to the posterior wall of the trachea and/or misplacement of the tracheostomy (19,20).

The patient is positioned, and the neck is prepped and draped as described for the surgical technique. The neck is palpated to identify the thyroid notch and cricoid cartilage. Local anesthetic with a vasoconstrictor is then injected into the skin and subcutaneous tissue inferior to the cricoid cartilage, followed by a 1.5-cm incision made either horizontally or downward from the inferior edge of the cricoid cartilage. A curved hemostat is then used to dissect gently down to the anterior trachea. A fingertip is used to palpate the cricoid cartilage through the incision and to bluntly dissect any tissue overlying the trachea. The endotracheal tube is withdrawn until the upper tracheal rings are visualized with a bronchoscope. Additional local anesthetic is then injected into the tracheal wall. The trachea air column is located by directing the needle posterior and caudally in the midline. Entry into the trachea is visualized with the bronchoscope, and 1 mL of local anesthetic is injected into the lumen of the trachea. Thereafter, the partially filled local anesthetic syringe is attached to the sheathed introducer needle. Once again, the tracheal air column is found and verified with the bronchoscope. The goal is to place the needle between the first and second or the second and third tracheal rings (Fig. 135.1). Once free flow of air is obtained, the outer sheath is advanced slightly, and the inner needle is removed. The J-wire is then advanced through the sheath into the trachea, and the sheath is removed. The 14 French introducing dilator is advanced over the guidewire and is used to dilate the access site. Following the initial dilation, the large tapered dilator is used to dilate the track. Finally, the tracheostomy tube with a guide (the largest one that will fit inside the tracheostomy tube) is threaded over the sheath and guidewire, and then into the trachea. The dilation and tracheostomy tube insertion requires significant force, and visualization of the process with the bronchoscope is invaluable in minimizing the risk of an unidentified injury to the posterior wall of the trachea. After placement of the tracheostomy tube, the ETT is removed, and the bronchoscope is inserted into the fresh tracheostomy to confirm placement and remove blood and secretions. Fresh blood clots can cause acute airway obstruction; the bronchoscope allows direct visualization and removal of the clot.

COMPLICATIONS

The important complications of tracheostomy include infection, bleeding, inadvertent extubation, paratracheal placement, esophageal perforation, subcutaneous emphysema, pneumothorax, tracheal stenosis, tracheoinnominate fistula, tracheoesophageal fistula, tracheocutaneous fistula after decannulation, cardiopulmonary arrest, and death. In a meta-analysis of 1,212 patients, the most common clinically relevant complications noted were wound infections (6.6%) and bleeding (5.7%) (18). Inadvertent postoperative decannulation with inability to recannulate the trachea due to the absence of a formed tract may occur. Immediate endotracheal intubation is mandatory rather than attempting to push the tracheostomy tube back into a semioccluded orifice.

A specific complication of surgical tracheostomy is the risk of airway fire. This can occur when a spark from the electrocautery ignites the oxygen leaking from the opened trachea. This can be prevented by meticulous hemostasis during the pretracheal dissection, and avoiding the use of electrocautery to make the trachea incision and after the trachea is opened. Complications specific to PDT include extraluminal placement of the tracheostomy tube. Perforation of the esophagus or the pharynx has been described when a bronchoscope was not used. Cannulation of the mediastinum may result in catastrophe since the patient cannot be oxygenated or ventilated with acute asphyxiation. There is a learning curve using PDT, and it has been reported that complications are higher in the earlier cases of the operator (21). Using bronchoscopy to guide PDT should prevent extraluminal placement, and suturing the tracheostomy tube in place may decrease the risk of inadvertent decannulation of a freshly placed tube (21).

Obesity is associated with higher rates of complications in PDT, including posterior tracheal wall injury, malpositioning, and accidental decannulation (21,22); however, this technique may be safely used in experienced hands (23). The use of bronchoscopy and an extra-long tracheostomy may help minimize the incidence of these complications (21,24).

SUMMARY

Many tracheostomy procedures are performed in critically ill patients in the ICU. A high severity of injury and shock on admission are predictors of prolonged mechanical ventilation. If these patients do not show evidence of improvement in the first few days, the option of tracheostomy should be considered and discussed with the patient and/or medical decision makers. The choice between ST and PDT depends on local operator expertise and patient-specific issues. Bedside PDT is performed as safely as ST in the OR and may be associated with more efficient use of health care resources.

PEARLS

- There may be brisk bleeding from the skin edges or anterior jugular veins. Have sutures ready to ligate or oversew these sites.
- Make sure the bronchoscope and ET tube are withdrawn adequately to avoid impaling them with the needle. Place the end of the bronchoscope so that it remains in the ET tube, but leave the tip of the ET tube just visible. Withdraw the bronchoscope and ET tube as a unit until the upper tracheal rings are visualized. When they are withdrawn adequately, the light from the bronchoscope can be visualized through the neck incision, and pressure on the anterior trachea with a finger or hemostat at the anticipated tracheostomy site will result in an indentation that can be seen with the bronchoscope.
- Although seemingly easy, finding the airway with the needle is the most important and most difficult part of the procedure. Stabilize the trachea with the nondominant hand, and insert the needle perpendicular to the airway while carefully aspirating for air.
- Placing a finger on the tracheal opening between dilatation and tracheostomy tube insertion will minimize the gas leak and loss of PEEP.
- The track may require dilation with the curved hemostat to facilitate the insertion of the tracheostomy tube. A single-cannula tracheostomy tube has a smaller outer diameter and is easier to insert; the disadvantage is the lack of an inner cannula that can be removed and cleaned.
- For large necks, a longer tracheostomy tube—such as the Shiley XLT—may be necessary. Make sure the appropriate supplies are available before the procedure.
- Insert the bronchoscope into the newly placed tracheostomy tube to ensure placement and evacuate any blood from the procedure.
- Losing an airway can be life threatening. Any procedure of the airway should include personnel who are skilled at intubating and managing the airway emergently.
- Get a chest radiograph to make sure there is no pneumothorax and to document the tracheostomy tube placement.

References

1. Durbin GC Jr. Questions answered about tracheostomy timing? *Crit Care Med.* 1999;27:2024.
2. Jackson C. Tracheostomy. *Laryngoscope.* 1909;19:285.
3. Ciaglia P, Firsching R, Syniec C. Elective percutaneous dilational tracheostomy: a new simple bedside procedure; preliminary report. *Chest.* 1985;87:715.
4. Heffner JE. The role of tracheotomy in weaning. *Chest.* 2001;120(Suppl 6):477.
5. Plummer AL, Gracey DR. Consensus conference on artificial airways in patients requiring mechanical ventilation. *Chest.* 1989;96:178.
6. Nieszkowska A, Combes A, Luyt CE, et al. Impact of tracheotomy on sedative administration, sedation level, and comfort of mechanically ventilated intensive care unit patients. *Crit Care Med.* 2005;33:2527–2533.
7. Davis K Jr, Campbell RS, Johannigman JA, et al. Changes in respiratory mechanics after tracheostomy. *Arch Surg.* 1999;134:59.
8. Diehl JL, El Atrous S, Touchard D, et al. Changes in the work of breathing induced by tracheotomy in ventilator dependent patients. *Am J Respir Crit Care Med.* 1999;159:383.
9. Combes A, Luyt C, Nieszkowska A, et al. Is tracheostomy associated with better outcomes for patients requiring long-term mechanical ventilation? *Crit Care Med.* 2007;35:802–807.
10. Clec'h C, Alberti C, Vincent F, et al. Tracheostomy does not improve the outcome of patients requiring prolonged mechanical ventilation: a propensity analysis. *Crit Care Med.* 2007;35:132–138.
11. Heffner JE, Zamora CA. Clinical predictors of prolonged translaryngeal intubation in patients with the adult respiratory distress syndrome. *Chest.* 1990;97:447.
12. Estenssoro E, Gonzalez F, Laffaire E, et al. Shock on admission day is the best predictor of prolonged mechanical ventilation in the ICU. *Chest.* 2005;127:598.
13. Afessa B, Hogans L, Murphy R. Predicting 3-day and 7-day outcomes of weaning from mechanical ventilation. *Chest.* 1999;116:456.
14. Pena J, Cicero R, Marin J, et al. Laryngotracheal reconstruction in subglottic stenosis: an ancient problem still present. *Otolaryngol Head Neck Surg.* 2001;125:397.
15. Rumbak MJ, Newton M, Truncale T, et al. A prospective, randomized, study comparing early percutaneous dilational tracheotomy to prolonged translaryngeal intubation (delayed tracheotomy) in critically ill medical patients. *Crit Care Med.* 2004;32:1689.
16. Arabi Y, Haddad S, Shirawa N, et al. Early tracheostomy in intensive care trauma patients improves resource utilization: a cohort study and literature review. *Crit Care.* 2004;8:R347.
17. Griffiths J, Barber VS, Morgan L. Systematic review and meta-analysis of studies of the timing of tracheostomy in adult patients undergoing artificial ventilation. *BMJ.* 2005;330:1243.
18. Delaney A, Bagshaw SM, Nalos M. Percutaneous dilational tracheostomy versus surgical tracheostomy in critically ill patients: a systematic review and meta-analysis. *Crit Care.* 2006;10:R55.
19. Oberwalder M, Weis H, Nehoda H, et al. Videobronchoscopic guidance makes percutaneous dilational tracheostomy safer. *Surg Endosc.* 2004;18:839.
20. Fernandez L, Norwood S, Roettger R, et al. Bedside percutaneous tracheostomy with bronchoscopic guidance in critically ill patients. *Arch Surg.* 1996;131:129.
21. Kost K. Endoscopic percutaneous dilatational tracheotomy: a prospective evaluation of 500 consecutive cases. *Laryngoscope.* 2005;115(10 Pt 2):1–30.
22. Byhahn C, Lischke V, Meininger D, et al. Peri-operative complications during percutaneous tracheostomy in obese patients. *Anaesthesia.* 2005;60:12–15.
23. Heyrosa M, Melniczek D, Rovito P, et al. Percutaneous tracheostomy: a safe procedure in the morbidly obese. *J Am Coll Surg.* 2006;202:618–622.
24. Blankenship D, Kulbersh B, Gourin C, et al. High-risk tracheostomy: exploring the limits of the percutaneous tracheostomy. *Laryngoscope.* 2005;115:987–989.

CHAPTER 136 ■ ACUTE LUNG INJURY AND ACUTE RESPIRATORY DISTRESS SYNDROME

CARL W. PETERS • MIHAE YU • ROBERT N. SLADEN • ANDREA GABRIELLI • A. JOSEPH LAYON

IMMEDIATE CONCERNS

Major Problems

The acute respiratory distress syndrome (ARDS) is characterized by nonhydrostatic pulmonary edema and hypoxemia associated with a variety of etiologies that cause both direct and indirect insults to the lungs. The process develops acutely (usually within 72 hours of the precipitating event), requires immediate recognition, and often leads to death despite maximal medical support. The therapeutic goals in the setting of ARDS are to provide appropriate resuscitation measures and to quickly identify, address, and eliminate the precipitating event if possible. Adequate tissue perfusion and oxygenation must be maintained to support vital organs. Prevention of complications and the prompt recognition of their presence are critical to prevent late deaths (1).

Stress Points

1. ARDS is commonly seen with the systemic inflammatory response syndrome (SIRS) and the multiple organ dysfunction syndrome (MODS).
2. Risk factors for developing ARDS include SIRS, sepsis, pulmonary contusion, aspiration, inhalation of toxic substances, near-drowning, long bone fractures, pancreatitis, diffuse pneumonia, and multiple blood transfusions.
3. Most patients with ARDS demonstrate similar clinical and pathologic features, irrespective of the cause of the acute lung injury (ALI).
4. The lung's response to injury can be divided into an exudative phase, a proliferative phase, and a fibrotic phase.
5. A variety of inflammatory mediators have been implicated in the pathogenesis of ALI.
6. The neutrophil plays a central role in ALI.
7. The severe hypoxemia associated with this syndrome is caused by intrapulmonary shunting that occurs with interstitial edema, and alveolar flooding and collapse.
8. A reduction in functional residual capacity (FRC) and lung compliance are the hallmarks of ARDS.
9. Radiographic changes seen in patients with ARDS are characteristic but nonspecific, and rarely reveal the etiology of the syndrome.

Essential Diagnostic Tests and Procedures

1. History and physical examination
2. Chest radiograph
3. Arterial blood gas measurements
4. Further diagnostic tests based on the clinical circumstances

Initial Therapy

1. Most patients require early endotracheal intubation and positive pressure ventilation.
2. The goal of mechanical ventilation is to provide adequate oxygenation and carbon dioxide elimination while keeping complications, such as oxygen toxicity, ventilator-associated lung injury, and hemodynamic compromise, to a minimum.

OVERVIEW

ARDS is a devastating injury to the lungs, characterized by diffuse pulmonary inflammation, hypoxemia, and respiratory distress. ARDS was described by Ashbaugh et al. in 1967 (2), although the syndrome of acute pulmonary failure was recognized by military physicians during World War I (3). Initially described as acute respiratory failure, the constellation of the signs and symptoms were first termed "adult" respiratory distress syndrome (4). In 1994, the American-European Consensus Committee on ARDS changed the word "adult" back to "acute" because development of ARDS was not restricted to adults (5). The consensus meeting further defined diagnostic criteria to include (a) acute onset; (b) bilateral radiographic infiltrates; (c) pulmonary artery occlusion pressure (PAOP) $\leq$18 mm Hg, or no evidence of left atrial hypertension; and (d) PaO_2/FiO_2 ratio of $\leq$300 mm Hg for ALI and $\leq$200 mm Hg for ARDS.

This definition is far from perfect. Respiratory distress, characterized by tachypnea, dyspnea, and acute respiratory alkalosis not relieved by correcting hypoxemia, is common to many pulmonary processes. Bilateral radiographic infiltrates may be seen with cardiogenic edema, pneumonitis, and several other entities. The PaO_2/FiO_2 ratio may be influenced by therapy, especially positive end-expiratory pressure (PEEP) and the FiO_2 itself. It seems specious to separate "acute lung injury" from ARDS when the two terms reflect only somewhat different

TABLE 136.1

SYNONYMS OF ARDS

Adult hyaline membrane disease
Adult respiratory insufficiency syndrome
Congestive atelectasis
DaNang lung
Hemorrhagic atelectasis
Hemorrhagic lung syndrome
Hypoxic hyperventilation
Postperfusion lung
Posttraumatic atelectasis
Posttraumatic pulmonary insufficiency
Progressive pulmonary consolidation
Progressive respiratory distress
Pump lung
Shock lung
Traumatic wet lung
Transplant lung
White lung
Wet lung

ARDS, acute respiratory distress syndrome.
From Taylor RW, Duncan CA. The adult respiratory distress syndrome. *Res Med.* 1983;1:17.

severity of the same processes. Heart failure may be present at a PAOP <18 mm Hg and may coexist with ARDS, but heart failure may not be present with a PAOP of 18 mm Hg or higher. Nonetheless, although presently undergoing revision, this definition has stood the test of time and forms the basis for all investigation done on ARDS in the past decade.

A long list of synonyms of this syndrome exists in the literature, usually describing either the clinical situation or radiologic and pathologic changes (Table 136.1) (6). To better define the range of lung injury, Murray et al. in 1988 described the Lung Injury Score (LIS) based on chest radiographic findings, degree of hypoxemia (using PaO_2/FiO_2 values), compliance of the pulmonary system (if ventilated), and PEEP levels (7) (Table 136.2). A patient was considered to have ARDS if the score was >2.5. Whether this scoring system contributes additional descriptive value is debatable, since the mortality rate was impacted more by the comorbidities, such as sepsis or cirrhosis (8,9), than by the LIS value, and the LIS did not add accuracy to the definitions of the consensus statement (10).

Multiple risk factors for ALI/ARDS have been identified, with sepsis syndrome having the highest prevalence (30%–50%) (10–16). The pathogenesis for pulmonary and extrapulmonary causes for ALI may be different (17); the Consensus Committee categorized ARDS into direct versus indirect causes (Tables 136.3A and 136.3B) (5). Secondary predisposing factors described in the literature are alcohol abuse, chronic lung disease, and a low systemic pH (14).

While ARDS is usually considered a homogeneous entity, it should be considered the final common pathway of a very heterogeneous group of insults. Although the pulmonary injury is widespread, it does not uniformly affect lung tissue; this nonuniformity has important therapeutic consequences. There are also two broad etiologies of ARDS (17): In *pulmonary ARDS* (generally corresponding to "direct" disease), there is primary lung injury (e.g., pneumonia) that involves the alveolar epithelium, and may be confined to single organ failure.

TABLE 136.2

LUNG INJURY SCORE

Points	
Chest roentgenogram score	
0	No alveolar consolidation
1	Alveolar consolidation in one quadrant
2	Alveolar consolidation in two quadrants
3	Alveolar consolidation in three quadrants
4	Alveolar consolidation in four quadrants
Hypoxemia score	
0	$PaO_2/FiO_2 \geq 300$
1	PaO_2/FiO_2 225–299
2	PaO_2/FiO_2 175–224
3	PaO_2/FiO_2 100–174
4	$PaO_2/FiO_2 < 100$
Respiratory system compliance score (mL/cm H_2O)	
0	≥80
1	60–79
2	40–59
3	20–39
4	≤19
PEEP score (cm H_2O)	
0	≤5
1	6–8
2	9–11
3	12–14
4	≥15
Final value	
0	No lung injury
1–2.5	Acute lung injury (ALI)
>2.5	Severe lung injury (ARDS)

ARDS, acute respiratory distress syndrome.

TABLE 136.3A

MAJOR CATEGORIES OF ARDS RISK

DIRECT
- Pneumonia
- Aspiration
- Pulmonary contusion
- Fat emboli
- Near-drowning
- Inhalational injury
- Reperfusion after lung transplant or pulmonary embolectomy

INDIRECT
- Sepsis
- Severe trauma with shock
- Multiple transfusions
- Cardiopulmonary bypass
- Drug overdose
- Acute pancreatitis
- Multiple transfusions

ARDS, acute respiratory distress syndrome.
From Bernard GR, Artigas A, Brigham KL, et al. The American-European Consensus Conference on ARDS. *Am J Respir Crit Care Med.* 1994;149:818.

TABLE 136.3B

CONDITIONS ASSOCIATED WITH ARDS

SHOCK	
Hemorrhagic	Cardiogenic
Septic	Anaphylactic
TRAUMA	
Burns	Nonthoracic trauma
Fat emboli	(especially head trauma)
Lung contusion	Near-drowning
INFECTION	
Viral pneumonia	Gram-negative sepsis
Bacterial pneumonia	Tuberculosis
Fungal pneumonia	
INHALATION OF TOXIC GASES	
Oxygen	Cadmium
Smoke	Phosgene
NO_2, NH_3, Cl_2	
ASPIRATION OF GASTRIC CONTENTS (ESPECIALLY WITH A pH <2.5)	
DRUG INGESTION	
Cocaine	Fluorescein
Heroin	Propoxyphene
Methadone	Salicylates
Barbiturates	Chlordiazepoxide
Ethchlorvynol	Colchicine
Thiazides	Dextran 40
METABOLIC	
Uremia	Diabetic ketoacidosis
MISCELLANEOUS	
Pancreatitis	Leukoagglutinin reaction
Postcardiopulmonary bypass	Eclampsia
Postcardioversion	Air or amniotic fluid emboli
Multiple transfusions	Bowel infarction
DIC	Carcinomatosis

ARDS, acute respiratory distress syndrome; NO_2, nitrogen dioxide; NH_3, ammonia; Cl_2, chlorine; DIC, disseminated intravascular coagulation.
From Taylor RW, Duncan CA. The adult respiratory distress syndrome. *Res Med.* 1983;1:17.

In *extrapulmonary ARDS* (generally corresponding to "indirect" disease), the inflammatory effect of a remote insult—usually sepsis—reaches the capillary endothelium via a SIRS phenomenon, and lung failure becomes one more component of MODS. Although there are important differences in pathophysiology, the outcome between ARDS of pulmonary and extrapulmonary origin does not appear to differ greatly. While the vast majority of studies reviewed here consider ARDS to be a single entity, questions remain as to whether this is true.

The reported incidence of ARDS is variable. In 1972, the National Heart and Lung Institute Task Force on Respiratory Disease estimated the incidence to be 150,000 cases per year, or 71 patients per 100,000 people. Although the "true" incidence of ARDS as defined by the LIS may be lower—1.5 to 8 cases per 100,000 people—the incidence of ALI was found to be 89 cases per 100,000, which approximates the previous value (15,18). A more recent study reported the incidence of ALI to be 78.8 cases per 100,000 and for ARDS to be 58.7 cases per 100,000 (16).

OUTCOME

The cause of death in ARDS patients is more often associated with MODS than deficient oxygenation. The overall mortality rate has declined from 68% in the 1980s to 36% in 1993 (18), and presently ranges widely from 30% to 58% (4,13,16,18–24), depending on the specific patient group—based on age and etiology of lung injury—being studied. ARDS patients who leave the hospital seem to have no increased risk of subsequent death when matched for comorbidities (25).

Families and intensive care unit (ICU) patients frequently ask about the long-term outcomes and quality of life after ARDS. As with all heterogeneous diseases, outcome varies. Lung mechanics in ALI/ARDS survivors may return to normal in the year after hospital discharge, but pulmonary gas exchange abnormalities may persist (26). Spirometry is likely to be normal at 6 months, but the Short Form General Health Survey (SF-36) score was low in one study (27). Mild to moderate deterioration in health-related quality of life (QOL), as measured by the Sickness Impact Profile, has been reported (28). Thus, ARDS appears to add a functional burden of reduced QOL to survivors compared to non-ARDS patients who survived a major illness (29,30); nonetheless, as many as 78% of patients return to work (27). Determining whether the quality of life is "good" after a devastating illness is likely a personal decision.

Patients with ARDS who die within the first several days do so because of the underlying condition and respiratory failure. Many of those who survive the original insult succumb to sepsis or MODS. Of those who survive ARDS, most return to their premorbid state of respiratory function by about 6 months after extubation (28).

PATHOPHYSIOLOGY

The inciting process in ALI is the pathologic loss of integrity of the alveolar–capillary membrane complex associated with exuberant inflammation, with increased endothelial and epithelial permeability and leakage of proteinaceous edema and cellular components into the interstitial and alveolar spaces. This occurs in response to some provocative stimulus, which may arise from various disease processes or physical or chemical insults, including primary pulmonary or extrapulmonary events (Tables 136.3A and 136.3B). While the details of lung injury may differ between primary and secondary causes (31), the differences in overt clinical consequences are difficult to identify when comparing patients from either general category.

The initial acute event that induces disruption of the alveolar epithelial or capillary endothelial cells in the exudative phase of ARDS yields denuded alveolar basement membrane and dysfunctional or destroyed surfactant and type 1 and 2 pneumocytes (Table 136.4). Demarginated "activated" neutrophils within the pulmonary circulation release inflammatory mediators, degrading the integrity of capillary endothelial

TABLE 136.4

HISTOPATHOLOGIC CHANGES IN ARDS

	Exudative phase	Proliferative phase	Fibrotic phase
Macroscopic	■ Heavy, rigid, dark	■ Heavy, gray	■ Cobblestoned
Microscopic	■ Hyaline membranes ■ Edema ■ Neutrophils ■ Epithelial > endothelial damage	■ Barrier disruption ■ Edema ■ Alveolar type II cell proliferation ■ Myofibroblast infiltration ■ Neutrophils ■ Alveolar collapse ■ Alveoli filled with cells and organizing matrix ■ Epithelial apoptosis ■ Fibroproliferation	■ Fibrosis ■ Macrophages ■ Lymphocytes ■ Matrix organization ■ Deranged acinar architecture ■ Patchy emphysematous change
Vasculature	■ Local thrombus	■ Loss of capillaries ■ Pulmonary hypertension	■ Myointimal thickening ■ Tortuous vessels

cell junctions and allowing the influx of proteinaceous plasma fluid, erythrocytes, and inflammatory cells into the interstitium (32,33). Interstitial fluid volume eventually exceeds lymphatic clearance capabilities, flooding the alveoli with hemorrhagic plasma. Thickened interstitium is "stiffer" and worsens pulmonary compliance, yielding a scenario of restrictive physiology. Loss and dysfunction of surfactant (34) increases alveolar surface tension, thus producing alveolar collapse. Ongoing inflammation initiates the coagulation cascade within the microcapillaries, with platelet deposition (35) obliterating the capillary luminal cross-sectional area, disrupting blood flow, and raising pulmonary artery pressure. Further recruitment of activated neutrophils into the interstitium (32,33) augments the inflammatory cycle of capillary permeability, interstitial edema, and continuous alveolar macrophage activation (36) (Fig. 136.1).

Accumulation of proinflammatory mediators such as tumor necrosis factor-α (TNF-α), interleukin-1β (IL-1β), and IL-8 in the alveolar fluid of ARDS patients (37) portends the amplified production of cytokine and toxic reactive oxygen and nitrogen radical species (38,39) (Table 136.5). Activated complement components accumulate with fibrin and immunoglobulins to form alveolar hyaline membranes, further worsening compliance. Fibroproliferation and accelerated collagen deposition

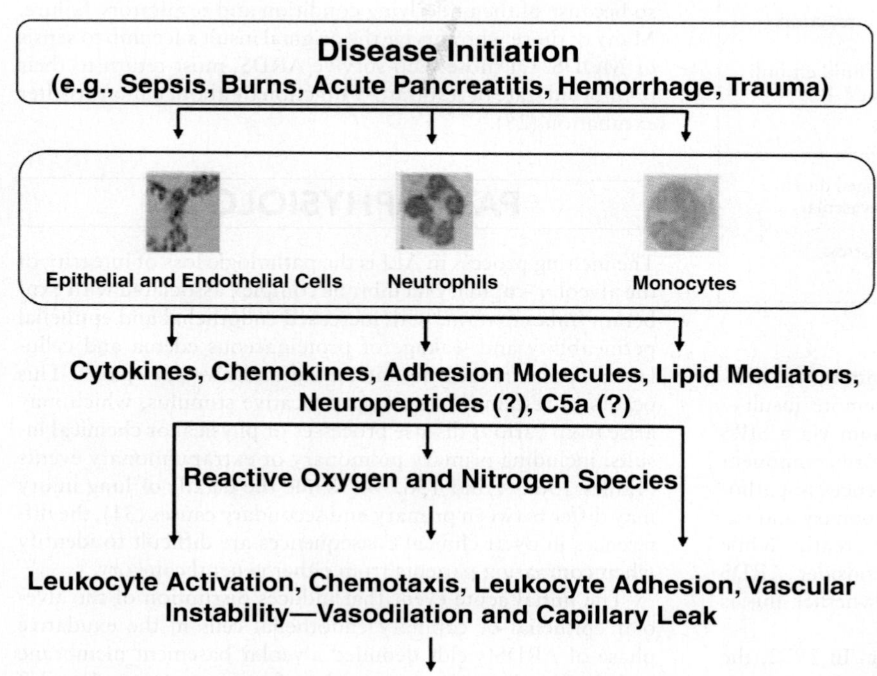

FIGURE 136.1. Pictorial detail of the pathogenesis of acute respiratory distress syndrome. (With permission from Bhatia M, Moochhala S. Role of inflammatory mediators in the pathophysiology of acute respiratory distress syndrome. *J Pathol.* 2004;202[2]:145–156.)

TABLE 136.5

INFLAMMATORY MEDIATORS IN ARDS

Inflammatory mediator	Function
TNF-α	Proinflammatory; neutrophil activation in ARDS
IL-1β	Proinflammatory; neutrophil activation in ARDS
IL-6	Leukocyte growth/activation; proliferation of myeloid progenitor cells; acute-phase response; pyrexia
IL-10	Anti-inflammatory; inhibits release of proinflammatory cytokines
TGF-β	Resolution of tissue injury; proinflammatory
GM-CSF	Host defense; hematologic growth factor
PAF	Platelet activation; neutrophil activation and chemotaxis
ICAM-I	Neutrophil adhesion
C5a	Leukocyte chemoattractant; dual pro- and anti-inflammatory role
Substance P	Proinflammatory
Chemokines	Leukocyte activation and chemotaxis
VEGF	Endothelial cytokine; plays a role in angiogenesis and vascular permeability
IGF-I	Alveolar macrophage-derived growth factor; profibrotic
KGF	Epithelial-specific growth factor; important for lung development repair
Reactive oxygen and nitrogen species	Regulation of vascular tone, antimicrobial action

may begin early in the inflammatory sequence and continue into the proliferative phase (7–21 days) (40,41), with thickening of the alveolar walls already denuded of type 1 pneumocytes (36,42).

While the original inciting event may resolve, judicious correction of persistent metabolic and infectious issues, and meticulous attention to appropriate ventilatory techniques, must continue in order to minimize iatrogenic contributions to self-sustaining inflammation (see Ventilator Associated Lung Injury below). Evolution into the *fibrotic phase* occurs, generally, after 3 to 4 weeks. Variable degrees of fibrosis and parenchymal tissue loss (40) yield "diffuse alveolar damage," the histologic correlate of advanced ARDS, characterized by widespread and severe damage to the alveolar–capillary unit (40). Micro- and macrocystic areas abut dilated ectatic bronchi, with fibrotic noncompliant septa and collapsed alveoli—no longer tethered open by healthy surrounding tissue—and interwoven with thrombosed capillaries that provide no capacity for gas exchange (i.e., dead space ventilation) (40). Hypoxemia from tenaciously collapsed, fibrotic, shunt-producing alveoli accompanies the hypercarbia and respiratory acidosis of large dead space fractions from non gas exchanging overdistended alveoli, dilated cystic areas, and thrombosed non–CO_2-excreting pulmonary capillaries.

CLINICAL PRESENTATION

Physical Examination

After the inciting event, several hours to a day may pass before clinically apparent respiratory failure ensues. Based on work by Gomez (43), the clinical findings in ARDS may be roughly grouped into four phases (Table 136.6). Tachypnea and tachycardia usually develop during the first 12 to 24 hours. The skin may appear moist and cyanotic. Intercostal and accessory respiratory muscles become actively involved in supporting ventilation. A dramatic increase in work of breathing can be appreciated at a glance from the bedside. High-pitched end-expiratory crackles are heard throughout all lung fields. Increasing agitation, lethargy, and obtundation may occur as the syndrome progresses. Because these clinical findings may

TABLE 136.6

PROGRESSION OF CLINICAL FINDINGS IN ARDS

PHASE 1: ACUTE INJURY
- Normal physical examination and chest radiograph
- Tachycardia, tachypnea, and respiratory alkalosis develop

PHASE 2: LATENT PERIOD
- Lasts approximately 6–48 h after injury
- Patient appears clinically stable
- Hyperventilation and hypocapnia persist
- Mild increase in work of breathing
- Widening of the alveolar-arterial oxygen gradient
- Minor abnormalities on physical examination and chest radiograph

PHASE 3: ACUTE RESPIRATORY FAILURE
- Marked tachypnea and dyspnea
- Decreased lung compliance
- Diffuse infiltrates on chest radiograph
- High-pitched crackles heard throughout all lung fields

PHASE 4: SEVERE ABNORMALITIES
- Severe hypoxemia unresponsive to therapy
- Increased intrapulmonary shunting
- Metabolic and respiratory acidosis

ARDS, acute respiratory distress syndrome.
From Taylor RW. The adult respiratory distress syndrome. In: Kirby RR, Taylor RW, eds. *Respiratory Failure*. Chicago: Year Book Medical Publishers; 1986:208.

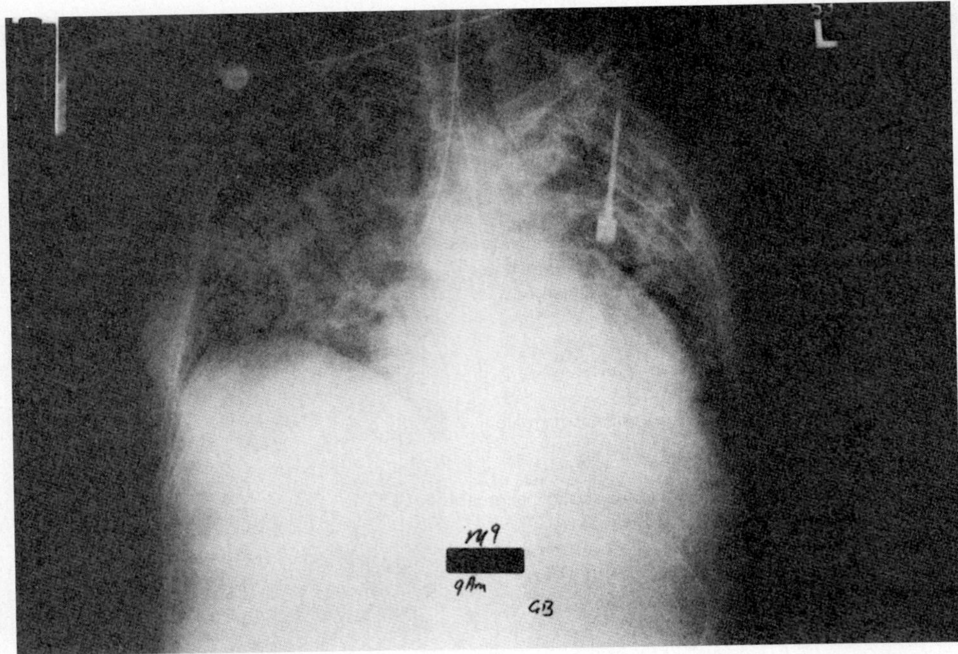

FIGURE 136.2. Diffuse interstitial and panacinar infiltrates are seen in a 36-year-old patient with acute respiratory distress syndrome. Also notice one of the complications of the respiratory support—a right mainstem intubation.

become apparent long after hypoxemia develops, careful attention to blood gas analysis is warranted in patients at risk for ARDS.

Lung Imaging

The changes seen on the chest radiograph in ARDS are characteristic but nonspecific, rarely revealing the etiology of the syndrome. Acutely, pulmonary edema is seen. Interstitial infiltrates progress to a diffuse, fluffy, panacinar pattern (Fig. 136.2). Although it may be difficult to differentiate from cardiogenic pulmonary edema, there is generally an absence of pulmonary vascular redistribution, pleural effusion, or cardiomegaly. The panacinar infiltrates may consolidate and, with time, take on a patchy or nodular pattern. If the patient improves, radiographic results may revert to normal. If the disorder progresses, a pattern of diffuse interstitial fibrosis may ensue (Fig. 136.3).

Therapeutic interventions may alter the radiographic findings. Pulmonary infiltrates may increase with injudicious fluid administration. Positive pressure ventilation and PEEP may lead to hyperinflation, and subcutaneous, mediastinal,

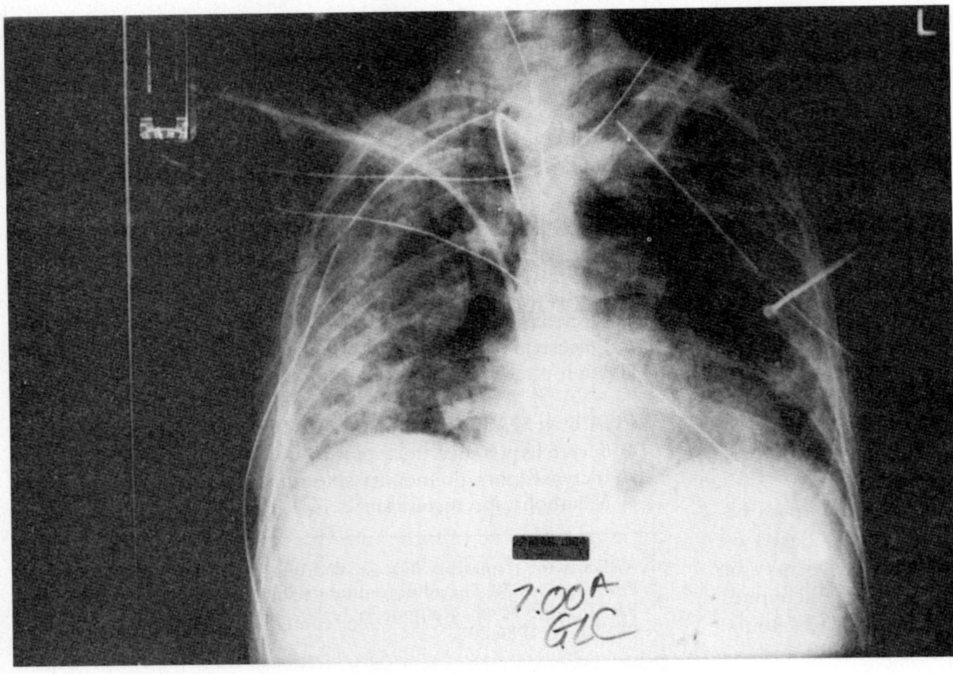

FIGURE 136.3. A pattern of diffuse interstitial fibrosis has developed in this 52-year-old patient with acute respiratory distress syndrome.

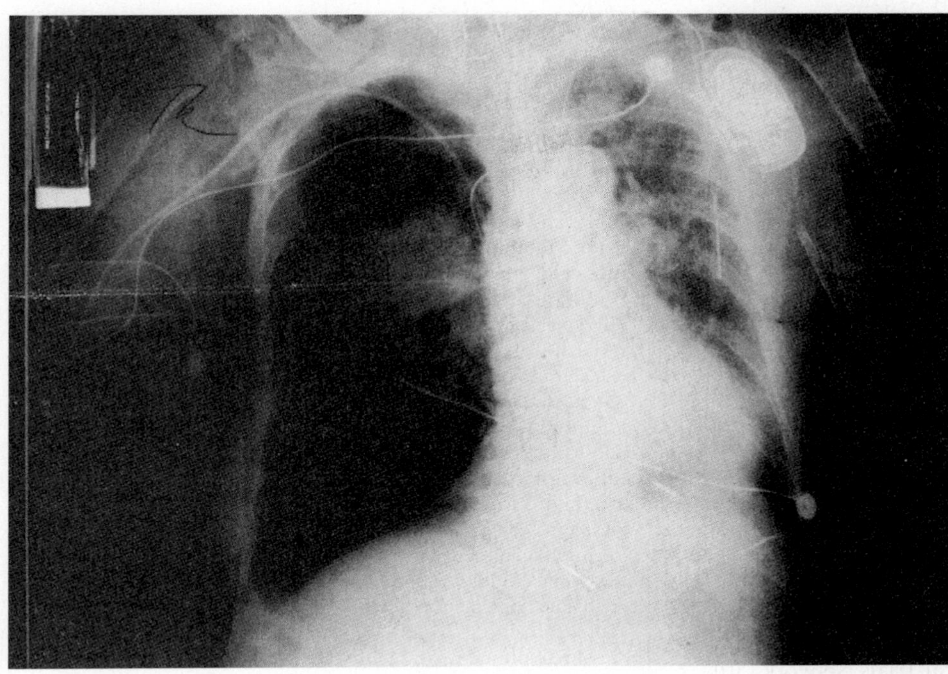

FIGURE 136.4. This 70-year-old patient with acute respiratory distress syndrome has a right tension pneumothorax and right mainstem intubation.

retroperitoneal, and intraperitoneal emphysema, or pneumothorax. Mainstem bronchus intubation may lead to ipsilateral pneumothorax or contralateral lung collapse (Fig. 136.4).

Whereas a two-dimensional chest radiograph may suggest diffuse homogeneous infiltrates, the chest computed tomography (CT) scan usually demonstrates remarkably inhomogeneous lung involvement. Dependent regions of the lung appear to be much more involved than nondependent regions. Although chest CT scanning is not always practical in the day-to-day management of patients with ARDS, in investigational trials, it has provided a vivid image of dramatically reduced lung volumes. The chest CT also may be useful in demonstrating the presence and magnitude of pneumothoraces and pleural effusions not well visualized on the standard chest radiograph. It is also useful for the positioning of thoracostomy tubes in patients with loculated pneumothoraces.

TREATMENT

General Therapeutic Measures

Nutritional Support

The gut serves a critical function beyond the absorption and transport of nutrients. Enteral nutrition seems to have an advantage over parenteral nutrition in preventing gastrointestinal atrophy, maintaining normal gut flora, and preserving immune function in surgical patients (44). Chapters 64 and 65 detail the importance of nutrition in the critically ill.

Fluid Management

Fluid management in ARDS has been controversial. As the permeability of the alveolar–capillary membrane increases, pulmonary edema develops at lower pulmonary capillary pressures. The Starling equation predicts mathematically what is seen clinically. When a strategy of fluid restriction and diuresis is undertaken, extravascular lung water (EVLW) is decreased, as is the duration of mechanical ventilation; mortality in ARDS seems to be associated with net fluid gain. Adequate intravascular volume must be maintained to avoid tissue hypoperfusion, although we recommend that the minimal amount of fluid be given, and that judicious attempts at diuresis be undertaken in the hemodynamically stable patient (45). A large study conducted by the National Heart, Lung, and Blood Institute (NHLBI) Acute Respiratory Distress Syndrome Clinical Trials Network (46) found no difference in 60-day mortality when comparing liberal and conservative fluid management strategies. Although the time allowed to enrollment was long (48 hours) and may not have captured the initial resuscitation, in light of the shorter ventilator and ICU days with conservative fluid management and associated improvement in pulmonary function when compared to liberal use of fluid, our routine practice is a conservative fluid strategy.

Bronchodilators

Multiple factors may lead to airflow obstruction in patients with ARDS, including mucosal and interstitial edema, airway secretions, and atelectasis. Airway hyperreactivity also contributes to increased airflow resistance in many patients with ARDS, in both the acute and chronic phases. Aerosolized β-agonists can decrease airway resistance, even in patients without underlying chronic obstructive pulmonary disease or asthma. By reducing airway resistance, the work of breathing can be decreased. We recommend a therapeutic trial of inhaled bronchodilators in patients with wheezing, in those with increased resistance as measured directly, or in patients with high peak airway pressures (47).

Steroids

The use of corticosteroids in the treatment of the various phases of ARDS is a basis of controversy and ongoing investigation.

The cytokine-mediated inflammatory response to an inciting event in ARDS intuitively suggests that suppression of that response would be therapeutic, but studies are equivocal in reporting benefit. Steroid use in different phases of ARDS has been meticulously investigated, but the dynamic nature of the inflammatory process has made the findings in individual studies difficult to extrapolate to varying illnesses at varying times. Furthermore, infectious risks of corticosteroid use aside, their prolonged use risks profoundly detrimental neuromuscular effects, even further compounded when employed with nondepolarizing neuromuscular blocking agents—often utilized in ARDS patients to facilitate efficient mechanical ventilation (48). Thus, routine use of corticosteroids is not advocated, especially in the acute phase of ARDS. During the late phase, fibroproliferation often occurs in response to tissue injury and is associated with persistent inflammation. In this setting, fever and SIRS are present in the absence of infection. A small uncontrolled trial suggested that improvement in "late" ARDS patients—those mechanically ventilated for ~15 days—with progressive fibroproliferation may be seen when corticosteroid treatment begins during that period (49). Proponents of this therapy recommend that a trial of corticosteroids be instituted in such patients *after* infection has been excluded. More recently, the NHLBI ARDS Clinical Trials Network (50) conducted a randomized multicenter controlled trial of steroid use in 180 patients with ARDS of at least 7 days' duration. While there was no difference overall in mortality at 60 and 180 days, steroids imparted a higher number of ventilator-free days and earlier departure from the ICU in the first 28 days. Those given methylprednisolone after day 13 of ARDS, however, had a higher mortality than controls. Meduri et al. (51) recently found reductions in length of mechanical ventilation and ICU stay and in mortality in early septic/ARDS patients receiving "low-dose" methylprednisolone infusions. While there have been several recent reviews and meta-analyses addressing corticosteroid use in ARDS (52–56), varying population groups and treatment regimens and differing end points and definitions of "success" in the studies make broadly inclusive recommendations difficult to formulate. Even the impact of steroids on mortality varies positively or negatively with different groups of patients. In general, corticosteroids are not effective in ameliorating cytokine-induced inflammation in ARDS in a clinically significant way, and routine use of corticosteroids is, therefore, not advocated, especially in the acute phase. There are, however, some subgroups of patients upon which corticosteroids may have a positive effect. One example may be the late phase, during which fibroproliferation often occurs in response to tissue injury. This response is damaging to the lung and is associated with persistent cytokine-mediated inflammation (57). Lung injury is characterized by endothelial and epithelial damage, as well as augmented fibroblast proliferation, which may be lessened by steroid treatment. Proponents of this therapy recommend that a trial of corticosteroids be instituted in patients with severe ARDS *after* infection has been excluded (49).

Monitoring

Monitoring the patient with ARDS is similar to that performed on other critically ill patients (Table 136.7). Chapters 16 through 22 detail descriptions of monitoring techniques that are essential to reduce or prevent the occurrence of significant complications. Careful titration of therapy is best guided by monitoring clinical, laboratory, and cardiorespiratory variables. Our standard practice is to always use a minimum of an arterial line, pulse oximetry, and capnography in patients with ALI/ARDS. More invasive devices—central venous pressure (CVP), pulmonary artery catheter—may be required based on the clinical situation.

TABLE 136.7

MONITORING THE PATIENT WITH ARDS[a]

LEVEL I
Temperature, heart rate, respiratory rate, arterial blood pressure, pulse oximetry, capnography
Weight
Intake and output
Caloric intake
Physical examination, with special emphasis on:
Skin (texture, turgor, perspiration, emphysema)
Respiratory (breathing pattern, lung examination)
Cardiovascular (heart examination, peripheral pulses)
Abdominal
Neurologic (mental status)
Continuous ECG monitoring
Chest radiography
Laboratory (CBC, electrolytes)
Arterial pressure monitoring/blood gases
Vital capacity
Negative inspiratory pressure
Dead space/tidal volume ratio (V_D/V_T)
Tracheal tube cuff pressures
Ventilator settings
Pressure–volume relationship
Lung and chest wall compliance and airways resistance
LEVEL II
Minimally invasive CO/CI with pulse waveform variability evaluation of preload
Pulmonary artery catheter
Pulmonary artery pressures, PAOP
waveforms, CI, mixed venous blood gases, stroke volume index, ventricular stroke work indices, systemic and pulmonary vascular resistance, arterial and mixed venous oxygen content, oxygen transport, arteriovenous content difference, oxygen consumption, oxygen extraction, venous admixture

ARDS, acute respiratory distress syndrome; ECG, electrocardiographic; CBC, complete blood cell count; CO/CI, cardiac output/cardiac index; PAOP, pulmonary artery occlusion pressure.
[a]Various monitoring techniques have been divided into three arbitrary levels. The levels are roughly ordered in terms of increasing invasiveness and sophistication. The exact monitoring modalities selected and the frequency with which measurements are made must be individualized.
From Taylor RW. The adult respiratory distress syndrome. In: Kirby RR, Taylor RW, eds. *Respiratory Failure.* Chicago: Year Book Medical Publishers; 1986:208.

Standard Management

Progress has been made in the management of ARDS, as suggested by the number of large studies and meta-analyses published in the last decade. Over this time, data have been gathered addressing modes of therapy and ancillary support techniques previously initiated and practiced empirically.

Despite considerable progress, however, many questions still await definitive resolution, as will become apparent in the discussion that follows. Due to the complex metabolic and pulmonary aberrations that characterize ARDS/ALI, treatment strategies can be divided into those directed toward respiratory support and all other therapeutic measures.

Respiratory Support

Mechanical ventilatory support, most often via an endotracheal tube, is fundamental to the management of ARDS, as perturbations of gas exchange and respiratory mechanics associated with this syndrome exceed the limits of compensation that most individuals are able to muster without mechanical assistance; it is as fundamental and integral to the management of the patient with ALI as is exogenous insulin to the diabetic or antibiotics to the treatment of infections. The indications for respiratory support are well defined (58), and include hemodynamic instability, protection and maintenance of the airway, inability to maintain PaO_2 above 55 mm Hg on an FiO_2 = 60%, need for positive airway pressure, and progressive ventilatory insufficiency with rising respiratory rate and hypercarbia. The presence of several or all of these features in most individuals with ALI mandates endotracheal intubation and mechanical ventilation to optimize gas exchange and minimize work of breathing. Noninvasive positive pressure ventilation (NIPPV) has been employed in some instances for those with less severe pulmonary impairment and preserved mental status (59), although studies are few with fairly high rates of eventual endotracheal intubation (60,61). Broad recommendations regarding the use of NIPPV in ARDS are difficult to make in the absence of large prospective studies due to the heterogeneity of patient populations, comorbidities, and diversity of the inciting pathophysiology (61).

Lung CT studies have demonstrated the distribution of areas of alveolar collapse and distention characteristic of ARDS to be regional rather than diffuse. Alveolar collapse predominates in dependent areas, producing venous admixture and hypoxemia, while nondependent areas manifest airway destruction with hyperinflation, often to the point of exclusion of pulmonary capillary blood flow (dead space) (62,63). These alveolar morphologies, however, are not strictly related to dependency within the chest cavity, as is clearly visible in Figure 136.5. Areas of atelectasis, producing shunt (*solid arrows*) and airway/alveolar destruction, and areas of overdistention, producing dead space (*dashed arrows*), may be randomly distributed and interspersed with areas of spared pulmonary tissue, thereby generating profound ventilation/perfusion mismatch.

The use of mechanical ventilation in ALI/ARDS has evolved dramatically over the last 30 years. Techniques of mechanical ventilation (MV) commonly employed through the decade of the 1980s led to use of what would now be described by most practitioners and investigators as "high" tidal volumes, with FiO_2 supplemented well above ambient. Subsequently, the observation was made (64,65) that ventilation of healthy laboratory animals with high tidal volumes induced profound clinical and histologic deterioration that was difficult to distinguish from those of ARDS. In 1990, Hickling et al. noted improved mortality in ARDS patients with lower than "traditional" tidal volumes (66). Subsequent investigations yielding conflicting results mandated the ARMA (Acute Respiratory Distress Syndrome Network Low Tidal Volume) trial of mechanical ventilation, with limited tidal volume and plateau

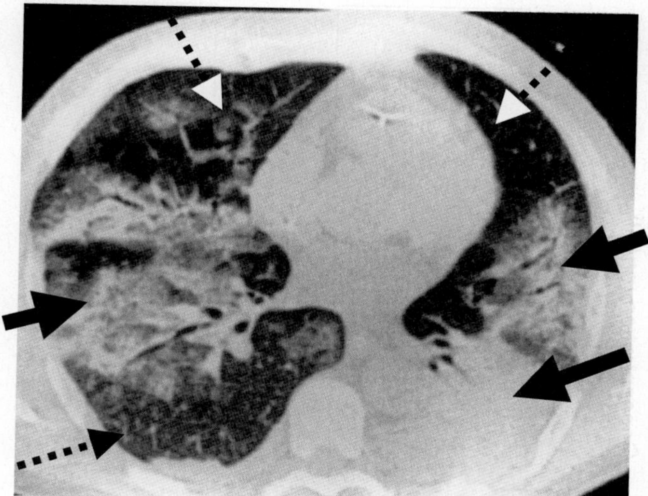

FIGURE 136.5. Computed tomography scan of the chest of a patient with acute respiratory distress syndrome. Solid arrows show dense parenchymal opacification resulting in shunt. The broken lines show relatively "normal"-appearing lung but that can suffer from overdistention, resulting in dead space. (With permission from Desai SR. Acute respiratory distress syndrome: imaging of the injured lung. *Clin Radiol.* 2002;57[1]:8–17.)

pressures compared to the higher values in common use at the time (67). The result was a reduction in mortality from 40% to 31% with the experimental protocol parameters. While the ARMA study has been criticized from a number of standpoints (68), none is sufficiently compelling to negate the persuasiveness of its results. In our practice, low tidal volume ventilation (V_t = 6–8 mL/kg ideal body weight) is considered standard, maintaining a plateau pressure <30 cm H_2O. Tidal volumes exceeding these parameters have been implicated in generating lung injury caused by mechanical ventilation itself. This phenomenon, termed *ventilator-associated lung injury* (VALI), is a by-product of the interaction of mechanical ventilation and the cytokine proliferation that is a fundamental pathophysiologic feature of ARDS (69,70). As described below, components of VALI include (a) *barotrauma*, the appearance of air outside the airways and alveoli, attributed to airway pressures that exceed certain thresholds (71,72); (b) *volutrauma,* increased alveolar and capillary permeability due to alveolar overdistention and leading to pulmonary edema (73); and (c) *atelectrauma*, the destructive repetitive opening and closing of stiff, collapsed, surfactant-depleted, fibrotic alveoli with thickened interstitium that are associated with cyclic positive pressure ventilation (74). Excessive alveolar stretch is associated with inflammatory cytokine proliferation, in particular during excursions into ranges of tidal volume that induce VALI (74,75) (Fig. 136.6). Of note, this cytokine proliferation can be limited by using a lung-protective ventilation strategy (using a pressure–volume curve to determine tidal volume and PEEP) (75).

The importance of limitation of tidal volume as a guide to appropriate MV in the acutely injured lung may be more easily understood when viewed within a conceptional framework of patchy, unevenly distributed alveolar injury. When such an injured lung receives a positive pressure breath, the gas distribution is impacted by the variability of compliance and resistance in the injured and healthy areas. Flow preferentially enters unaffected (i.e., low resistance, relatively high

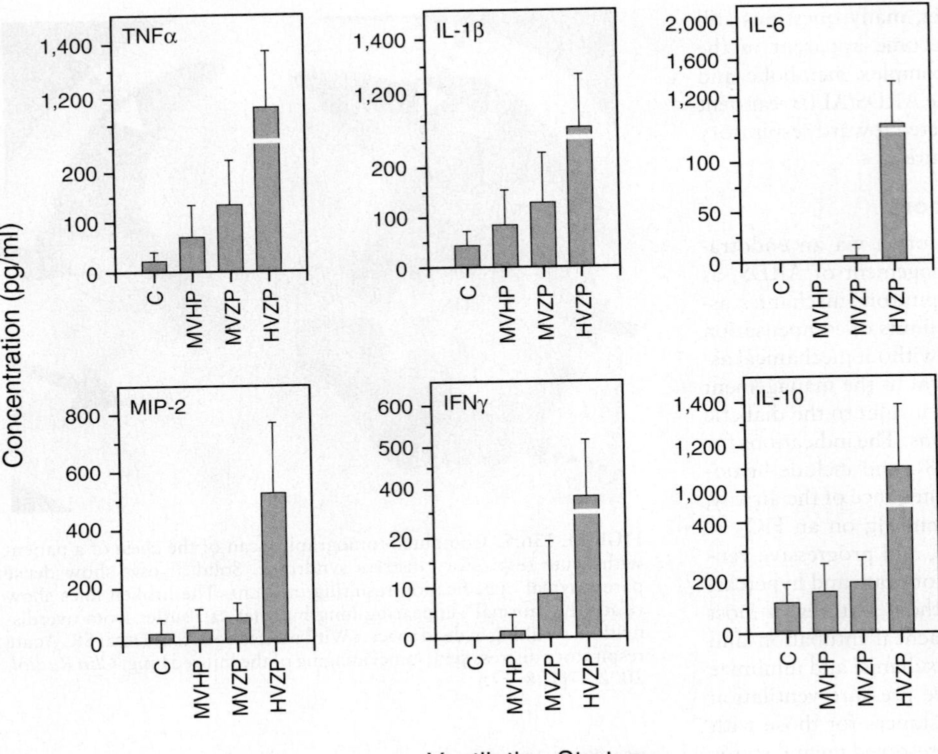

FIGURE 136.6. The effect of ventilation strategy on inflammatory mediator concentration. High tidal volume strategy resulted in higher levels. C, control: Vt = 7 mL/kg, PEEP = 3 cm H_2O; MVHP, moderate-volume, high PEEP: Vt = 15 mL/kg, PEEP = 10 cm H_2O; HVZP, high-volume, zero PEEP: Vt = 40 mL/kg; MVZP, moderate-volume, zero PEEP: Vt = 15 mL/kg. TNF-α, tumor necrosis factor-α; IL-1β, interleukin-1β; IL-6, = interleukin-6; MIP-2, macrophage inflammatory protein 2; IFNγ, interferon-γ. (With permission from Tremblay L, Valenza F, Ribeiro SP, et al. Injurious ventilatory strategies increase cytokines and c-fos m-RNA expression in an isolated rat lung model. *J Clin Invest.* 1997;99[5]:944–952.)

compliance) pulmonary tissue, risking unintentional overdistention and injury of these normal areas (76) despite inflation with an "appropriate" tidal volume based on body weight. This is often termed *the baby lung phenomenon* (77), since the volume of unaffected lung parenchyma within the ARDS patient's thorax more closely approximates that of a child than an adult. Delivered tidal volumes, therefore, must more closely approximate those appropriate for a smaller lung, usually on the order of 6 to 8 mL/kg; exceeding these volumes risks iatrogenic perpetuation of lung injury, since a positive pressure breath inflates a smaller volume of lung tissue than would be predicted by ideal body weight.

The importance of PEEP and recruitment maneuvers in providing efficient ventilator management of ARDS patients warrants further discussion. While the traditional approach of oxygen supplementation may improve the PaO_2 within the limits of a marginal FRC, such supplementation should be looked upon only as a temporizing measure. Prolonged high FiO_2 use risks toxicity and absorption atelectasis, while leaving the underlying cause of hypoxemia neither identified nor corrected. Recovery of FRC by reinflation of atelectatic areas using recruitment maneuvers and PEEP will restore gas flow to previously nonaerated areas of lung (78–82). These modalities of treatment are commonly utilized in the modern strategy of ARDS treatment (83,84). Areas of particularly tenacious atelectasis will often require an inspiratory time (T_i) equal to several inspiratory time-constants (one "time-constant" equals product of compliance and resistance, both easily measurable by current ventilators) to achieve inflation. Insufficient T_i may leave such areas persistently collapsed, worsening shunt fraction and compromising FRC and oxygenation. Despite the most heroic efforts, a substantial percentage of ARDS patients harbor lung tissue that is only variably "PEEP recruitable" (81). The benefit of recruitment maneuvers and PEEP can be understood within the context of the *Law of LaPlace* (actually the Young-LaPlace equation), which states that the pressure difference across a fluid interface is equal to the surface tension times the mean curvature of the surface. In pulmonary physiology and ARDS, this means that the pressure difference between alveolar gas and alveolar epithelium contracts the alveolus inward unless counteracted by surfactant. Furthermore, the relationship between surface tension and alveolar radius is inverse. Thus, the smaller the alveolar radius, the greater the force contracting it even further inward (i.e., toward collapse). Since surfactant decreases surface tension, the inward force within a collapsed alveolus is greater than that within its surfactant-replete, healthy, "noncollapsed" neighbor with lower surface tension, resulting in a temporary high-pressure requirement to open a collapsed alveolus. The alveolus may then be maintained open, with PEEP exceeding the alveolar closing pressure. Because low tidal volume (6 mL/kg) followed by PEEP in itself is generally ineffective in expanding collapsed alveoli, a "recruitment maneuver," the temporary application of airway pressure far above any possible alveolar retractive force, may be warranted to open and stabilize collapsed alveoli (85–87), preventing exposure to repetitive cyclic collapse and associated destructive shear forces by maintaining an "open lung" (Fig. 136.7).

The benefit of PEEP was recently addressed and revealed, surprisingly, that no difference was achieved in discharge or survival between ICU patients receiving high- or low-PEEP regimens (83). More recently, no significant improvement in all-cause mortality rates was noted in two studies of ARDS patients managed with an "open-lung" approach, involving the addition of modestly higher levels of PEEP and recruitment

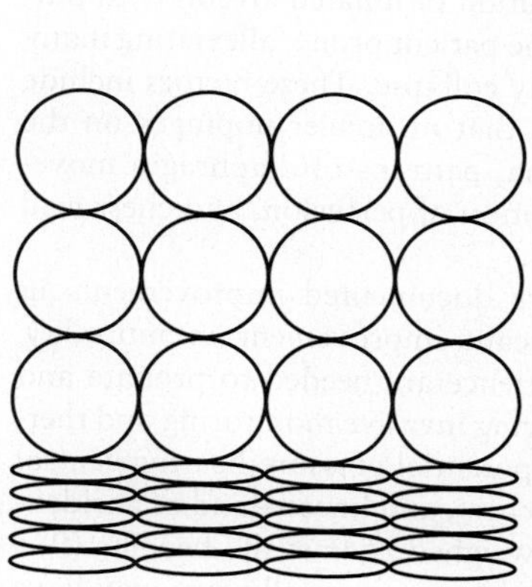

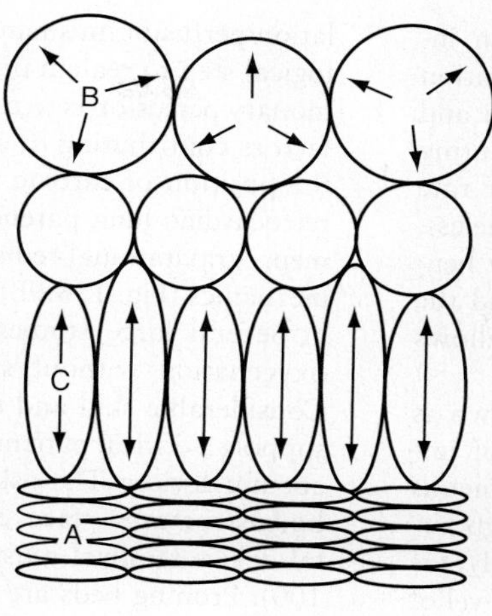

FIGURE 136.7. Atelectrauma and the interdependence of lung units. (With permission from Moloney ED, Griffiths MJ. Protective ventilation of patients with acute respiratory distress syndrome. *Br J Anaesth*. 2004;92[2]:261–270.)

maneuvers compared to a regimen utilizing a tidal volume of 6 mL/kg and approximately 10 cm H_2O PEEP (84). Nonetheless, most clinicians feel that utilizing a level of PEEP above the lower inflection point (LIP) on a pressure–volume curve (see below) improves FRC and oxygenation by inflating recruitable alveoli, and thus decreasing venous admixture.

The selection of tidal volume is intimately linked to the pressure–volume curve. Optimal gas exchange with minimal alveolar injury is achieved when the lung is positioned on the vertical portion of the pressure–volume curve (Fig. 136.8). This minimizes collapse in areas of high time-constants and overdistention in normal areas. Once alveolar re-expansion is optimized, which may take several hours of vigilance to titrate tidal volume and mean airway pressure, optimal inflation is maintained with PEEP as ventilation is then conducted along the expiratory limb of the curve, lowering mean pressures overall (Fig. 136.8). There is wide acceptance of the use of low tidal volume/limited plateau pressure ventilation techniques, directed toward gas exchange along the expiratory curve once inflation has been achieved, with the goal of preserving the

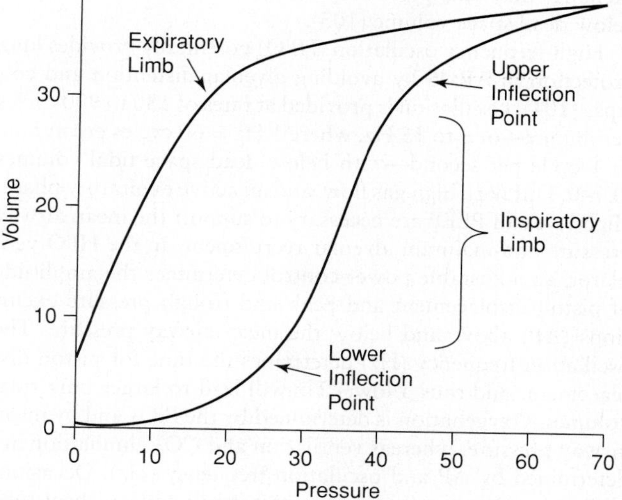

FIGURE 136.8. Pressure–volume curve of an idealized lung, showing both the inspiratory and expiratory limbs as well as the upper and lower inflection points.

integrity of pulmonary parenchyma not yet affected by inflammation and to allow healing of diseased areas. Since compliance varies between individual alveoli, a given inspiratory pressure may hold some in overdistention while others are minimally opened; the curve depicted in Figure 136.8 actually represents an averaged compliance. A not uncommon observation when monitoring gas exchange in ARDS is hypercarbia with mild acidemia, often more uncomfortable for the clinician to observe than the patient to experience. However, "permissive hypercapnia" is safe and acceptable (88) when not contraindicated by underlying medical condition (e.g., elevated intracranial pressure), though it often warrants protocol-delivered sedation. This may be understood by visualizing a variety of pressure–volume curves depicting compliance curves for variously distensible alveoli. The pressure to aerate sufficient numbers of tenaciously collapsed alveoli may overdistend more compliant areas such that the increased dead space precludes adequate ventilation.

The mode of mechanical ventilation used in ALI/ARDS is likely more dependent on the comfort level of the practitioner than on "best evidence." *Pressure control ventilation* (PCV) offers the theoretical advantages of limiting peak airway pressure, a component that may be associated with ventilator-induced lung injury (70). PCV may decrease work of breathing, possibly due to the variable flow rate (89). PCV is a ventilatory mode that is time initiated, pressure limited, and time cycled. PCV delivers a square pressure wave that provides tight control of the inflation pressure equal to the applied pressure plus PEEP. This mode also allows precise adjustment of inspiratory time at the expense of expiratory time—that is, increased inspiratory to expiratory (I:E) ratio, or "inverse ratio ventilation" (IRV). Mean airway pressure is substantially increased without an increase in peak airway pressure, promoting alveolar recruitment while—again, theoretically—attenuating barotrauma and volutrauma. With PC-IRV, mean airway pressures are typically increased from less than 10 to between 20 and 30 cm H_2O; inspiratory time—if the ventilator is set, for example, at 10 breaths per minute—between 3 and 5 seconds; and I:E ratio between 1:1 and 3:1. Indeed, IRV may be considered an alternative (or adjunct) to PEEP in providing airway pressure therapy during inspiration instead of expiration, and with limited peak airway pressure.

To date, the hypothesis that PC-IRV results in a better outcome than standard volume-limited ventilation has not been rigorously tested (90,91). Moreover, IRV may result in inadequate exhalation time, air trapping, and the generation of intrinsic PEEP ("auto-PEEP"), leading to barotrauma and CO_2 retention. Paradoxically, hypercarbia occurring during PC-IRV may be improved by decreasing the ventilator rate to allow additional time for CO_2 elimination. Nonetheless, high-time-constant, low-compliance lung segments may benefit from the ability to control the inspiratory time and the prolonged, but controlled, plateau pressures that PCV allows (92).

Airway pressure release ventilation (APRV), also known as invasive bilevel ventilation, combines the advantages of improved alveolar recruitment, lung protection, and spontaneous ventilation. In this mode, a sustained 3- to 4-second high airway pressure—the upper PEEP level—of 20 to 30 cm H_2O is intermittently released for about a second to the lower level of PEEP (5–10 cm H_2O), while allowing spontaneous breathing to occur throughout the cycle (93). This technique optimizes alveolar recruitment by increasing mean airway pressure while restricting the peak airway pressure to the upper PEEP level, and can maintain oxygenation and ventilation at lower airway pressures than conventional ventilation (93). This mode is useful in the transition from PC-IRV to ventilatory weaning with IMV or pressure support, but it has not been subjected to randomized outcome trials (94,95).

Advantageous aspects of both volume- and pressure-control ventilation can be combined in advanced circuitry ventilators in a mode termed *pressure-regulated volume control* (VC+). This mode allows the practitioner to select the mechanical rate, tidal volume, inspiratory time, pressure support level (if desired), FiO_2, PEEP level, and maximal values for peak inspiratory pressure and tidal volume. When VC+ is selected, the ventilator adjusts the pressure to deliver the desired tidal volume, changing the pressure by about 3 cm H_2O every third breath or so. As compliance worsens, tidal volume is maintained up to the maximal set peak inspiratory pressure, which will not be exceeded. When compliance improves, the ventilator automatically decreases the inspiratory pressure to keep the tidal volume within the set range. A single tidal volume delivered above the set maximal tidal volume generates a ventilator alarm. Thus, the potential problems one might see with standard volume ventilation (excessive peak pressure to deliver the target tidal volume) or PC ventilation (improving compliance, producing a dangerously high tidal volume) are obviated with this mode of ventilation.

Prone Positioning

The typical pattern of distribution of inflammatory edema and alveolar inflation in ARDS is noted in Figure 136.9A. A progressive decrease in transpulmonary pressure—the force distending the alveoli, defined as the difference between alveolar pressure (P_A) and pleural pressure (P_{pl})—with dependency manifests itself as airway collapse in the dependent portions of the inflamed lung. When proceeding from ventral to dorsal areas in the supine position, transpulmonary pressure—the outward traction force keeping the airways "tethered" open—no longer exceeds alveolar surface tension, and collapse occurs in dependent areas. In the absence of adequate PEEP, inflation of dependent alveoli, once achieved, cannot be maintained, and inspiratory volume is preferentially directed into nondependent areas of the lung (96). Preferential distribution of perfusion to dependent areas with collapsed alveoli contributes to ventilation/perfusion mismatch and intrapulmonary shunt (97). A logical step to realign distribution of inflated alveoli with pulmonary perfusion is to turn the patient prone, alleviating many factors contributing to airway collapse. These factors include the position of cardiac mass that no longer impinges on the retrocardiac lung parenchyma, patterns of diaphragm movement, gravitational redistribution of perfusion, and chest wall mechanics (Fig. 136.9B) (96).

Several large studies have documented improvements in oxygenation without significant improvement in mortality. Considerable skill and experience are needed to pronate and support a critical patient bearing invasive monitoring and therapeutic devices. The risks to potential pressure-bearing ventral body structures—face, eyes, chest, and knees—and of accidental device removal must be weighed against the benefits (98–100). Proning beds are available commercially, but may have certain restrictions such as cervical spine clearance and weight limits.

High-frequency Ventilation

High-frequency ventilation (HFV) is a technique that minimizes the risk of VALI and atelectrauma by avoiding both excessive inspiratory volumes and repetitive airway collapse produced by conventional cyclic ventilation in the noncompliant ARDS lung, while maintaining higher mean airway pressures (Fig. 136.10).

Subcategories of HFV include high-frequency positive pressure ventilation, high-frequency oscillatory ventilation, and high-frequency jet ventilation. Respiratory rates range from 50 to 2,400 breaths/minute, the latter rate produced in oscillatory ventilation. Gas transport and exchange occur through several mechanisms, some occurring simultaneously in a given patient. These include *bulk convection,* to a lesser degree than in conventional ventilation; *asymmetric velocity profiles*, causing a simultaneous, opposite directional flow of oxygen and carbon dioxide in different regions of the airways; *Pendelluft,* the asynchronous filling and emptying of alveoli with nonhomogeneous time constants; *Taylor dispersion,* wherein shear forces augment forward gas diffusion; and mixing due to *cardiogenic oscillations* and *molecular diffusion* (101,102). Effective gas exchange may take place despite the use of tidal volumes well below dead space volume (103).

High-frequency oscillation (HFO) potentially provides lung protection in ARDS by avoiding alveolar distention and collapse (104). Oscillation is provided at rates of 180 to 900 cycles per minute—or 3 to 15 Hz, where 1 Hz = 60 cycles per minute or 1 cycle per second—with below dead space tidal volumes (0.1–0.3 mL/kg), high gas flow, and an active expiratory phase. High levels of PEEP are necessary to support the mean airway pressure and maintain alveolar recruitment. In the HFO ventilator, an adjustable power control determines the amplitude of piston displacement and peak and trough pressure excursions (ΔP) above and below the mean airway pressure. The oscillation frequency (Hz) determines the time for piston displacement, and thus a lower Hz will lead to larger bulk tidal volumes. Oxygenation is determined by the FiO_2 and by mean airway pressure, whereas ventilation and CO_2 elimination are determined by ΔP and oscillation frequency (Hz). Occasionally, it may be necessary to create a small endotracheal tube cuff leak to facilitate CO_2 washout.

HFO provides a number of management challenges, including the necessity for a firm bed surface, with increased risk of

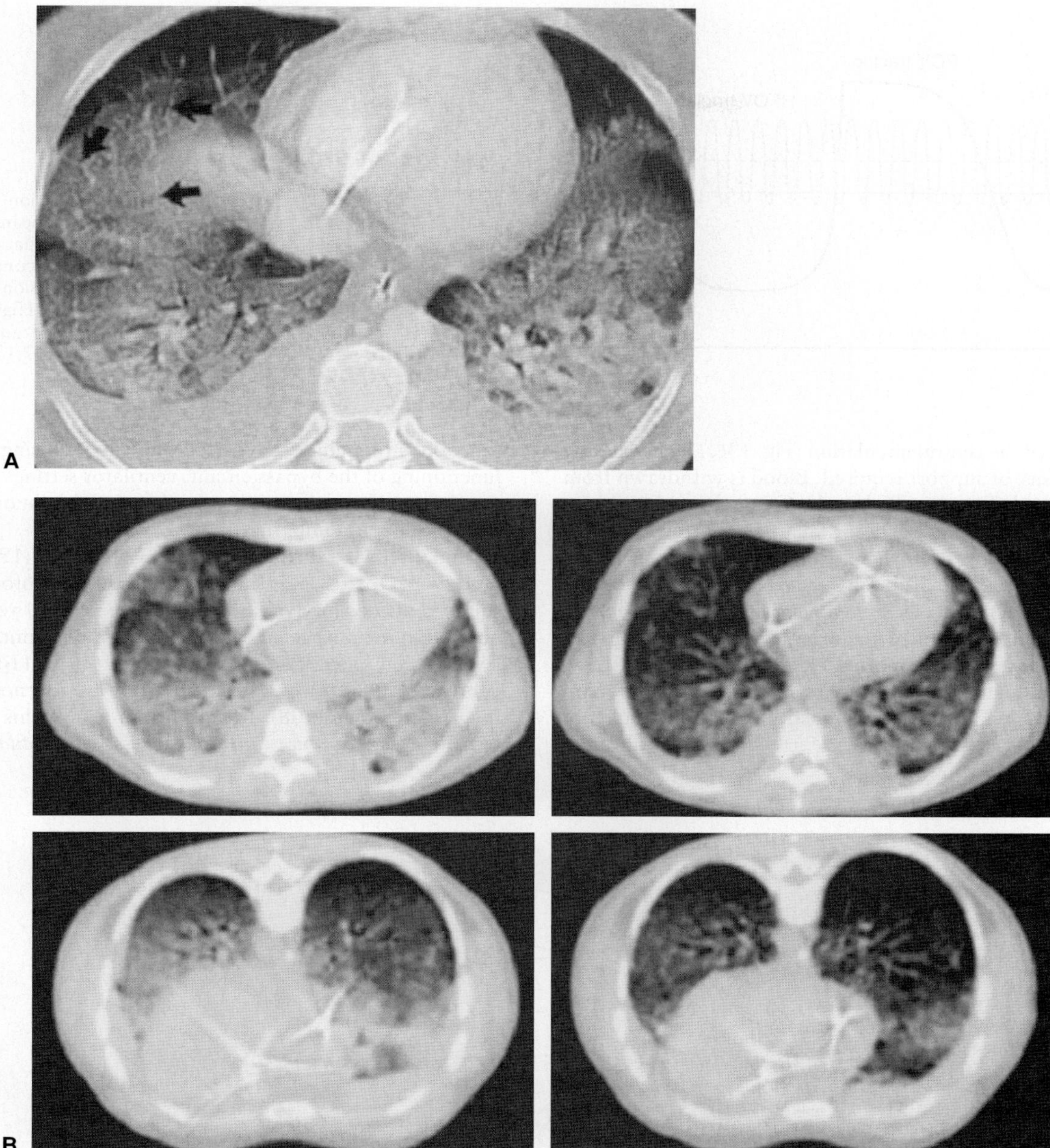

FIGURE 136.9. **A:** Consolidated lung in a patient with acute respiratory distress syndrome. Note the air bronchograms and dependent consolidation. (With permission from Ware LB, Matthay MA. The acute respiratory distress syndrome. *N Engl J Med.* 2000;342[18]:1334–1349.) **B:** Improvement in dependent consolidation once proning has occurred. (With permission from Pelosi P, Brazzi L, Gattinoni L. Prone position in acute respiratory distress syndrome. *Eur Respir J.* 2002;20[4]:1017–1028.)

pressure injury, and difficulty with humidification of inspired gas. Nonetheless, HFO has established itself as a ventilatory mode in pediatric ICUs and trauma units, where it facilitates ventilation in the presence of abdominal compartment syndrome and constrained lung volume (105). Thus far, only one large randomized trial has compared HFO with conventional ventilation in adults. After 2 to 4 days of conventional ventilation, 150 patients were randomized to HFO or PC-IRV (tidal volume 6–10 mL/kg) (106). Patients who received HFO had improved PaO_2/FiO_2 ratios at 24 hours, but there was no statistical difference in mortality—37% versus 52% ($p = 0.1$). Clearly, there is a need for a large randomized trial where HFO is instituted at an early stage of ARDS.

Extracorporeal Life Support

ARDS-related respiratory failure particularly refractory to the most aggressive support measures may warrant the temporary use of mechanical gas exchange devices for pulmonary support while native lung tissue recovers. The process, known as *extracorporeal life support* (ECLS) or ECMO (extracorporeal membrane oxygenation), employs a membrane oxygenator, blood warmer, and pump systems in parallel with

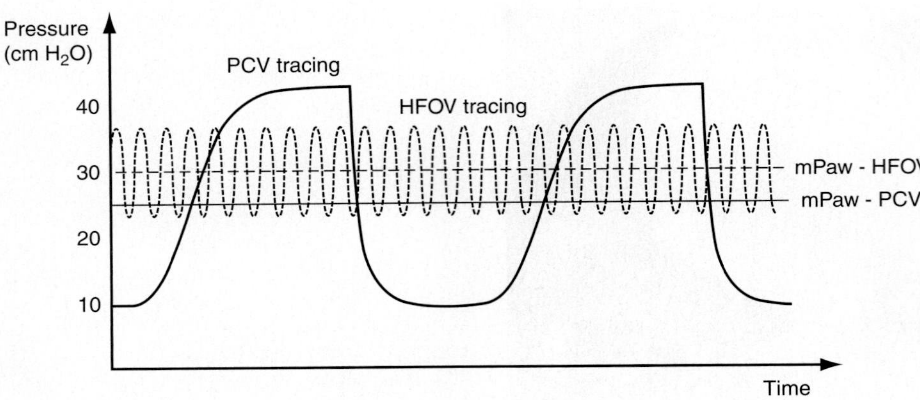

FIGURE 136.10. Depiction of airway pressures—peak and mean—in high-frequency oscillatory ventilation (HFOV) as compared to pressure control ventilation (PCV). (With permission from Chan KP, Stewart TE, Mehta S. High-frequency oscillatory ventilation for adult patients with ARDS. *Chest.* 2007;131[6]:1907–1916.)

components of the central circulation (Fig. 136.11), depending on the intensity of support required. Blood is withdrawn from the venous system—typically via the internal jugular vein—anticoagulated, oxygenated, decarbonated, adjusted to appropriate temperature, and then returned to the patient. Blood is returned via the femoral vein (venovenous ECLS) or the right carotid or femoral artery (venoarterial ECLS), depending on the physiologic system(s) requiring support (Fig. 136.11). Either function can be supported alone or together. ECLS is supportive only, bridging the patient's vital cardiopulmonary functions until definitive therapy is instituted. ECLS should not be used as a salvage procedure once irreversible loss of organ function is thought to have occurred (107). During the actual functioning of the bypass circuit, ventilator settings are turned to minimal, thereby avoiding the additional pulmonary insult that VALI would impart.

Initial studies, such as the U.S. ECMO trial (1974–1977), used ECMO with complete lung collapse; the unfortunate result was dismal survival (9%). Over the next 10 years, Gattinoni et al. demonstrated the effectiveness of maintaining low levels of lung ventilation (pressure limit 35 cmH_2O, rate 3–5 breaths/minute) by utilizing low flow venovenous ECMO for CO_2 removal (108). In Gattinoni's hands, this approach, termed *low-frequency positive pressure ventilation with*

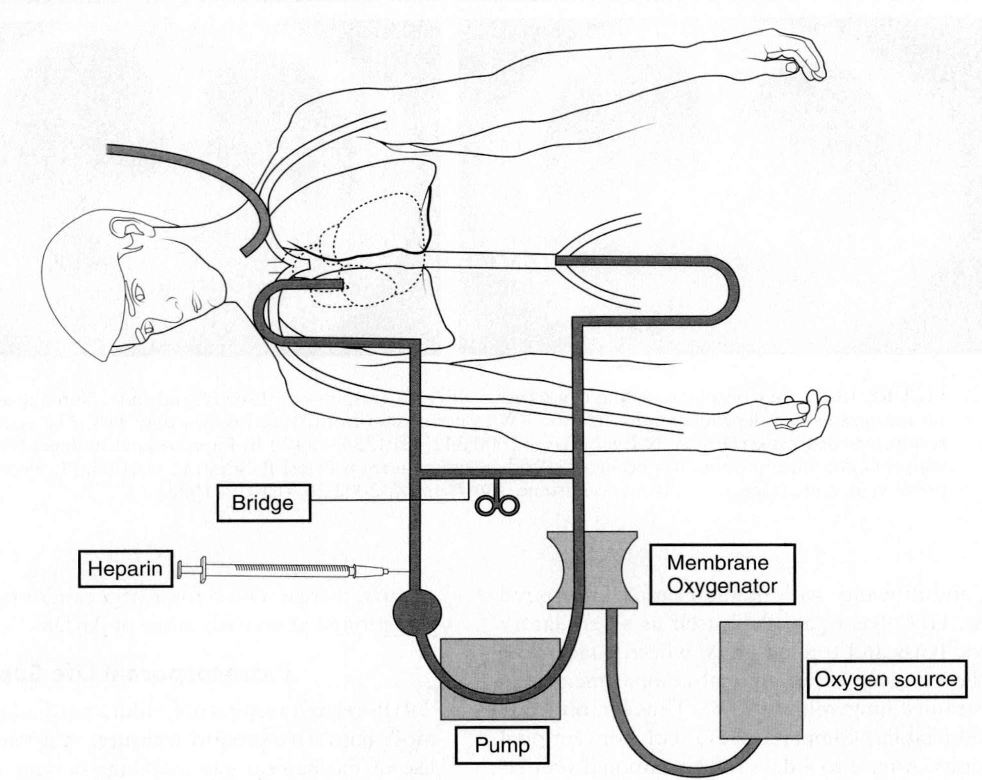

FIGURE 136.11. Depiction of extracorporeal membrane oxygenation. (With permission from Brown JK, Haft JW, Bartlett RH, et al. Acute lung injury and acute respiratory distress syndrome: extracorporeal life support and liquid ventilation for severe acute respiratory distress syndrome in adults. *Semin Respir Crit Care Med.* 2006;27[4]:416–425.)

extracorporeal CO_2 removal (LFPPV-$ECCO_2R$), was associated with a 49% survival in very severe ARDS patients (108). In survivors, lung function improved within 48 hours. In a subsequent randomized study carried out in the United States, Morris et al. compared LFPPV-$ECCO_2R$ with PC-IRV using computerized protocols in 40 patients (109). There was no statistical significance in 30-day survival—33% versus 42% ($p = 0.8$)—but the study size was small.

At present, ECLS is well established in neonatology and pediatrics (110,111), but use in the adult population is less widespread. In the most experienced center, the University of Michigan at Ann Arbor (http//www.med.umich.edu/ecmo/intro.htm), consideration is given to use of ECLS when all maximally supportive measures yield an arterial-alveolar DO_2 >600 with hypercarbia and persistently reduced compliance (107). Survival may exceed 50%, despite several potential complications, including coagulopathy with bleeding, stroke, pulmonary thromboembolism, ischemic bowel, sepsis, and MODS. Considerable experience and expertise in this complex, expensive, and resource-intensive procedure is required to maximize outcome. Venovenous ECMO may be a life-saving intervention in selected patients with primary ARDS, especially ischemic-perfusion injury after double lung transplantation. A salutary outcome is predicated on good cardiovascular function, the absence of MODS, and relatively rapid (<72-hour) improvement in lung function.

Inhaled Vasodilators

Fundamental to the pathophysiology of ALI/ARDS is the phenomenon of ventilation/perfusion mismatch–induced shunt-related hypoxemia. The phenomenon of hypoxic pulmonary vasoconstriction (HPV), which may be viewed evolutionarily as a mechanism to "isolate and exclude" the pathologic hypoxic collapsed alveoli, carries a price of right heart pressure elevation. The influence of HPV extends beyond the collapsed areas; well-aerated alveoli may abut remotely constricted vessels, increasing dead space ventilation and further straining the right ventricle. When airway inflation and stabilization via optimization of mechanical ventilation do not suffice to alleviate collapse, vasodilators may be employed. Intravenous agents, such as sodium nitroprusside, affect all vessels, frequently worsening hypoxemia by dilating and perfusing collapsed areas. Aerosolized vasoactive medications, such as nitric oxide or prostaglandin-I, diffuse from ventilated alveoli and result in relaxation of endothelial smooth muscle within remotely constricted vascular beds, thus improving ventilation/perfusion matching while vessels adjacent to collapsed alveoli remain unaffected. Selective vasodilation in ventilated areas decreases shunt fraction and contributes to alleviation of pulmonary hypertension (112,113) (Fig. 136.12).

Nitric oxide (NO) was discovered to be an endogenous compound with vasoactive properties in the late 1980s (114,115). The mechanism of action is through the generation of cyclic guanosine monophosphate (cGMP) (115). Its rapid absorption and inactivation by hemoglobin restrict its effects to the pulmonary circulation (116). While clinical trials have repeatedly documented improvement in pulmonary artery pressures and oxygenation with NO in ALI/ARDS, there is no evidence that overall mortality is reduced (117,118). Haphazard use of NO is inadvisable in that substantial potential toxicities exist, including free radical formation, production of nitrogen dioxide (NO_2) (119), and generation of methemoglobin. The rate of formation of NO_2 from oxygen and NO depends on the concentration of oxygen and the square of the NO concentrations. The Occupational Safety and Health Administration has set safety limits of 5 ppm for NO_2, as it can cause pathologic changes to the lungs at doses of 25 ppm. At extremely high doses, pulmonary edema, hemorrhage, and death have been seen in animal models. NO_2 levels should be monitored as closely as possible to the endotracheal tube (120). In clinical

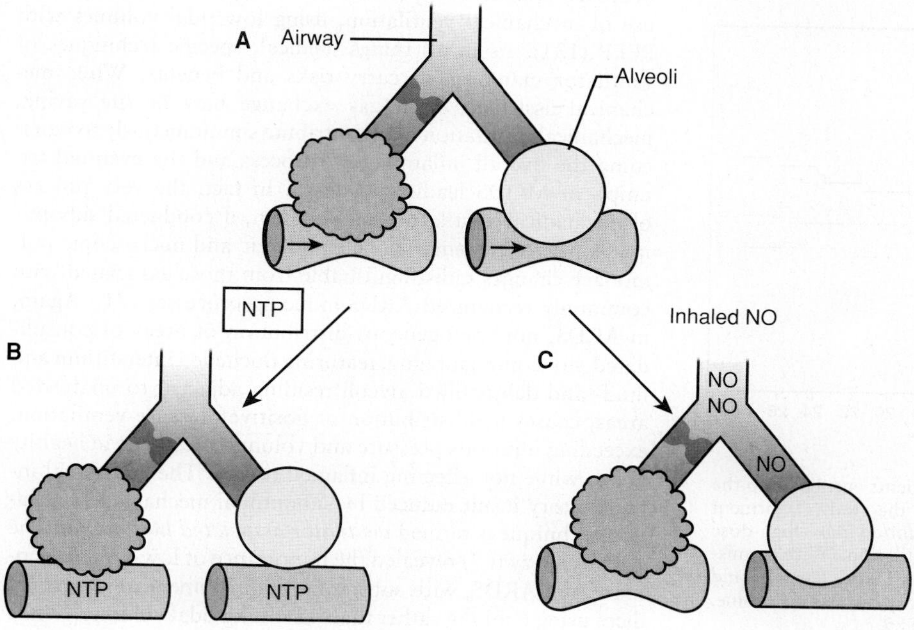

FIGURE 136.12. Intravenous versus inhaled vasodilator effects on pulmonary circulation. **A:** Shows two idealized alveoli, one occluded (left) and the other normal; both have hypoxic pulmonary vasoconstriction (HPV)-induced decreased pulmonary blood flow. **B:** Shows the result of using an intravenous vasodilator: HPV is removed to both the occluded and nonoccluded alveoli, resulting in significant shunt. **C:** Shows the result of utilization of inhaled nitric oxide (NO): HPV is reversed in the area of the ventilated alveolus, but not the obstructed one. NTP, nitroprusside. (With permission from Lunn RJ. Inhaled nitric oxide therapy. *Mayo Clin Proc.* 1995;70[3]:247–255.)

trials using NO at 5 to 40 ppm, NO_2 has not been a significant problem.

Methemoglobinemia is another potential but rare complication of NO administration. About 80% to 90% of inhaled NO is absorbed within the bloodstream, where it reacts with hemoglobin within the red blood cell to form nitrosylhemoglobin and methemoglobin. The primary factor determining the development of methemoglobinemia is the dose of NO, although the hemoglobin level, oxygen saturation, and methemoglobin reductase also play a role. In the United States, Native Americans more frequently have methemoglobin reductase deficiency—either partial or complete—and therefore are more susceptible to methemoglobinemia. Closer monitoring of such patients is warranted. In clinical trials using NO at 5 to 40 ppm, methemoglobinemia has not been a significant problem. Finally, the cost of inhaled NO is surprisingly steep (121), warranting the closest scrutiny of its use in "marginal" situations.

Liquid Ventilation

Pulmonary gas transport using complex low-surface tension, high vapor pressure fluorocarbon molecules in the liquid state has been investigated for use in patients with severe ALI. Respiratory gases are carried in solution, and either partial- or full-liquid ventilation is conducted with a conventional or "liquid ventilator," respectively. Perfluorocarbons possess anti-inflammatory properties and, by virtue of their liquid state, localize particularly in dependent areas where airway collapse is most prevalent and thus most in need of PEEP in the ARDS lung (122). These features of perfluorocarbons tend to stabilize collapsed dependent alveoli without the risks of high pressures associated with conventional ventilation. Animals have survived the imposition of liquid ventilation in experimental circumstances (123). Studies on adult humans, however, have not revealed a benefit to this form of treatment, with no overall improvement in outcome (124,125) (Fig. 136.13).

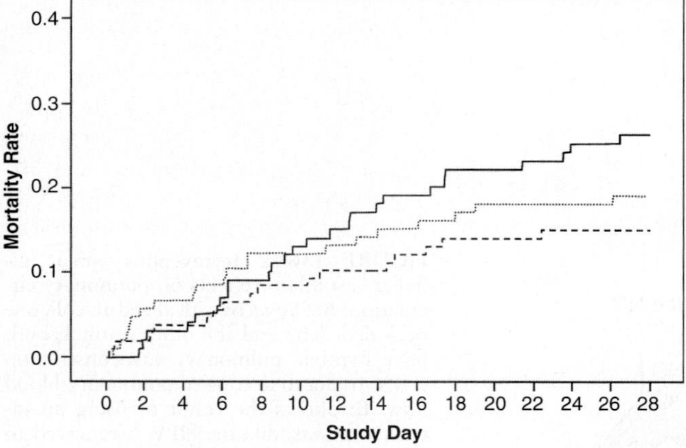

FIGURE 136.13. All-cause mortality for all patients enrolled into the three studied groups over the first 28 days of the study. Treatment groups: *solid line*—low-dose perfluorocarbon; *dotted line*—high-dose perfluorocarbon; *dashed line*—conventional ventilation. (With permission from Kacmarek RM, Wiedemann HP, Lavin PT, et al. Partial liquid ventilation in adult patients with acute respiratory distress syndrome. *Am J Respir Crit Care Med.* 2006;173[8]:882–889.)

Surfactant Replacement

Surfactant is a phospholipid, a protein material produced by type II epithelial pneumocytes, secreted along the alveolar surface and acting to decrease surface tension to prevent alveolar collapse. Hydrophilic surfactant proteins A and D contribute to the immune response (126), while hydrophobic types B and C facilitate monolayer formation within the alveolus (127). Pulmonary epithelial injury and surfactant dysfunction from direct or indirect injury destabilize alveoli, leading to the collapse, venous admixture, hypoxemia, and a decreased lung compliance characteristic of ARDS.

Surfactant replacement therapy in adults has been, thus far, unsuccessful. After an encouraging phase I/II trial of recombinant surfactant protein C–based surfactant supplement (128), a phase III trial of the same material improved oxygenation without lowering mortality or the number of ventilator days in adult patients with ARDS (129). Further investigation of this promising modality in adults is warranted based on its clear success in neonatology.

COMPLICATIONS

Significant morbidity or mortality may occur during supportive therapy for ALI/ARDS. Most aspects of supportive care transcend the specifics of ALI/ARDS, and the clinician should be aware of these potential complications, many of which are outlined by Pingleton (130) (Table 136.8). Attention to detail decreases complications and may improve outcome in ARDS. As suggested earlier, the ARDS patient is so exquisitely sensitive to the smallest subtleties of mechanical ventilation that discussion of the main potential sequela of suboptimal mechanical ventilation, namely VALI, is provided in detail below.

Ventilator-associated Lung Injury

To date, the only mode of management with which outcome in ARDS patients can predictably be improved is the optimal use of mechanical ventilation, using low tidal volumes with PEEP (131). As in all things medical, specific techniques of ventilator management carry risks and benefits. While mechanical assistance with gas exchange may be life saving, mechanical ventilation may contribute simultaneously to worsening the overall inflammatory process and the eventual triumph of MODS leading to death. In fact, the very process of mechanical ventilatory support can, if conducted suboptimally, provoke edematous morphologic and microscopic pulmonary changes indistinguishable from those associated with commonly recognized ARDS-inducing processes (71). Again, in ARDS, nonhomogeneous distribution of areas of consolidated, noncompliant lung, featuring thickened interstitium and fluid- and debris-filled alveoli residing adjacent to unaffected areas, causes maldistribution of positive pressure ventilation, exceeding injurious pressure and volume thresholds in healthy areas, while not affecting inflamed tissues. The additional inflammatory insult induced by suboptimal mechanical ventilation technique is termed *ventilator-associated lung injury.* The ARMA study (67) revealed the importance of low-volume ventilation in ARDS, with substantial improvement in several indices using 6 mL/kg rather than 12 mL/kg tidal volumes. While

TABLE 136.8

COMPLICATIONS ASSOCIATED WITH ARDS

PULMONARY Pulmonary emboli Pulmonary barotrauma Pulmonary fibrosis Oxygen toxicity **GASTROINTESTINAL** Gastrointestinal hemorrhage Ileus Gastric distention Pneumoperitoneum **RENAL** Renal failure Fluid retention **CARDIOVASCULAR** Invasive catheters Arrhythmia Hypotension Low cardiac output **INFECTION** Sepsis Nosocomial pneumonia **HEMATOLOGIC** Anemia Thrombocytopenia DIC **OTHER** Hepatic Endocrine Neurologic Psychiatric Malnutrition	**COMPLICATIONS ATTRIBUTABLE TO INTUBATION AND EXTUBATION** Prolonged attempt at intubation Intubation of a mainstem bronchus Premature extubation Self-extubation **COMPLICATIONS ASSOCIATED WITH ENDOTRACHEAL/TRACHEOSTOMY TUBES** Tube malfunction Nasal necrosis Paranasal sinus infection Tracheal stenosis Tracheomalacia Polyps Erosion Fistulae Airway obstruction Hoarseness **COMPLICATIONS ATTRIBUTABLE TO OPERATION OF THE VENTILATOR** Machine failure Alarm failure Alarms silenced Inadequate nebulization or humidification **COMPLICATIONS OCCURRING DURING POSITIVE AIRWAY PRESSURE THERAPY** Alveolar hypoventilation Alveolar hyperventilation Massive gastric distention Barotrauma Atelectasis Pneumonia Hypotension

ARDS, acute respiratory distress syndrome; DIC, disseminated intravascular coagulation.
From Taylor RW. The adult respiratory distress syndrome. In: Kirby RR, Taylor RW, eds. *Respiratory Failure.* Chicago: Year Book Medical Publishers; 1986:208.

criticized, the findings document the importance of avoiding several putative mechanisms of pathologic effect:

1. Excess alveolar hyperinflation with associated increased permeability and cytokine release
2. Escape of alveolar air outside the confines of alveoli
3. Destructive sheer-stress influence of repetitive inflation/collapse of unstable alveoli

Each of these phenomena contributes to pulmonary dysfunction and perpetuation of the inflammatory response in the ARDS patient, and thus each has been classified. *Barotrauma* refers to the presence of air outside the alveoli when receiving positive pressure ventilation. Air leaks track along the perivascular sheath to the mediastinum and pleural cavities, or along fascial planes to extrathoracic areas (132). It seems intuitive that such occurrences are related to pressures exceeding the limits of tissue structural integrity, but the issue is clearly more complicated, since musicians are repeatedly able to generate 150 cm H_2O airway pressure with no sequelae (133). It is speculated that barotrauma represents regional overinflation in areas of diseased lung, such areas thereby being particularly at risk for structural failure and air leak (133). *Volutrauma* occurs when excessive inspiratory volumes induce microvascular edema (134); the offending agent appears to be excessive *volume*, rather than the excessive *pressure* required to supply that volume (71). Resultant mechanical stretch triggers changes in the alveolar–capillary barrier (73) and in proliferation of inflammatory cytokines (75), resulting in interstitial and alveolar proteinaceous edema, decreased compliance, and hyaline membrane formation. Compromised surfactant production and function leads to increased surface tension, provoking alveolar collapse with increased venous admixture and subjecting alveolar epithelium to the tissue-destructive shear stresses of recruitment/derecruitment in the process known as *atelectrauma*. While the use of PEEP to maintain diseased distal alveoli splinted "open" has not definitively been demonstrated to improve outcome (75, and earlier discussion, above), improvements in oxygenation and pulmonary compliance with PEEP mandate its routine use in ARDS. Of note is the complex relationship between mechanical ventilation and patchy maldistribution throughout the lung in areas of varying ratios of ventilation and perfusion, with atelectatic areas abutting hyperinflated bullous and cystic areas. While collapsed noncompliant airways require high initial opening pressures consistent with the Law of Laplace (within the context of pulmonary physiology, the following formula is appropriate: $P = 2t/R$, where P = pressure, t = tension, and R = radius), such high pressure is transmitted throughout the lung, overdistending more compliant airways both through direct influence and by an unequally distributed traction force upon the adjacent airways, as depicted in Figure 136.7. Implicit in such heterogeneous patterns of gas distribution is the initiation of the destructive sequelae associated with inflation of each subregion of lung, as delineated above.

Furthermore, over the last few years, there has been recognition of the inflammatory cytokine release, as well as alveolar and interstitial neutrophil infiltration associated with ventilator-related pulmonary disruption, leading to MODS (69,135). While it is indisputable that "excessive" tidal volume ventilation augments systemic cytokine levels (75), the specific causal relationship with worse outcome has yet to be validated. The ALVEOLI study (83), which examined the variation of short-term indices—28-day mortality and number of ventilator-free days—with modulation of PEEP, was discontinued early based on lack of improvement in outcome with high PEEP levels. Thus, the optimal inspiratory pressure, or level of PEEP for a given ARDS patient's pressure–volume curve, can be exceedingly difficult to identify despite the potentially severe consequences of failure to do so. While dependent areas of tenaciously collapsed, high time-constant alveoli may require the equivalent of repeated and prolonged high-pressure recruitment maneuvers to achieve inflation and avoid atelectrauma, simultaneous transmission of such pressure to compliant alveoli incurs the risk of inducing volutrauma and inciting inflammation. Clearly, in those with advanced lung injury, the "optimal" inspiratory pressure, in reality, reflects a statistical bell curve of widely variable individual alveolar compliances. The clinician must vary inspiratory time, plateau pressure, PEEP, and tidal volume to inflate stiff alveoli while not persistently overdistending the normal ones. Such important actions are required because of the dynamic and changing compliance profiles of the inflamed lung.

References

1. Kollef MH, Schuster D. The acute respiratory distress syndrome. *N Engl J Med.* 1995;332:27.
2. Ashbaugh DG, Bigelow DB, Petty TL, et al. Acute respiratory distress in adults. *Lancet.* 1967;ii:319.
3. Simeone FA. Pulmonary complications of nonthoracic wounds: a historical perspective. *J Trauma.* 1968;8:625.
4. Petty TL, Ashbaugh DG. The adult respiratory distress syndrome: clinical features, factors influencing prognosis and principles of management. *Chest.* 1971;60:233.
5. Bernard GR, Artigas A, Brigham KL, et al. The American-European Consensus Conference on ARDS. *Am J Respir Crit Care Med.* 1994;149:818.
6. Balk R, Bone RC. The adult respiratory distress syndrome. *Med Clin North Am.* 1983;67:685.
7. Murray JF, Matthay MA, Luce JM, et al. An expanded definition of the adult respiratory distress syndrome. *Am Rev Respir Dis.* 1988;138:720.
8. Matthay MA. Conference summary—acute lung injury. *Chest.* 1999;116:119S–126S.
9. Zilberberg MD, Epstein SK. Acute lung injury in the medical ICU: comorbid conditions, age, etiology, and hospital outcome. *Am J Respir Crit Care Med.* 1998;157(Pt 1):1159–1164.
10. Moss M, Goodman PL, Heinig M, et al. Establishing the relative accuracy of three new definitions of the adult respiratory distress syndrome. *Crit Care Med.* 1995;23:1629.
11. Fowler AA, Hamman RF, Good JT, et al. Adult respiratory distress syndrome. Risk with common predisposition. *Ann Intern Med.* 1983;98:593.
12. Pepe PE, Potkin RT, Reus DH, et al. Clinical predictors of adult respiratory distress syndrome. *Am J Surg.* 1982;144:124.
13. Hudson LD, Milberg JA, Anardi D, et al. Clinical risks of the development of the acute respiratory distress syndrome. *Am J Respir Care.* 1995;151:293.
14. Hudson LD, Steinberg KP. Epidemiology of acute lung injury and ARDS. *Chest.* 1999;116:74S.
15. Ware LB, Matthay MA. The acute respiratory distress syndrome. *N Engl J Med.* 2000;342:1334.
16. Rubenfield GD, Caldwell E, Peabody E, et al. Incidence and outcomes of acute lung injury. *N Engl J Med.* 2005;353:1685.
17. Rocco PRM, Zin WA. Pulmonary and extrapulmonary acute respiratory distress syndrome: are they different? *Curr Opin Crit Care.* 2005;11:10.
18. Milberg JA, Davis DR, Steinberg KP, et al. Improved survival of patients with acute respiratory distress syndrome (ARDS): 1983–1993. *JAMA.* 1995;273(4):306–309.
19. Abel SJC, Finney SJ, Brett SJ, et al. Reduced mortality in association with acute respiratory distress syndrome (ARDS). *Thorax.* 1998;53:292.
20. Petty TL. Adult respiratory distress syndrome: definition and historical perspective. *Clin Chest Med.* 1982;3:3.
21. Taylor RW, Duncan CA. The adult respiratory distress syndrome. *Res Med.* 1983;1:17.
22. Brun-Buisson C, Minelli C, Bertolini G, et al. Epidemiology and outcome of acute lung injury in European intensive care units: results from the ALIVE study. *Intensive Care Med.* 2004;30:51–61.
23. Luhr OR, Antonsen K, Karlsson M, et al. Incidence and mortality after acute respiratory failure and acute respiratory distress syndrome in Sweden, Denmark, and Iceland: the ARF Study Group. *Am J Respir Crit Care Med.* 1999;159:1849–1861.
24. Bersten AD, Edibam C, Hunt T, et al. Incidence and mortality of acute lung injury and the acute respiratory distress syndrome in three Australian states. *Am J Respir Crit Care Med.* 2002;165:443–448.
25. Davidson TA, Rubenfeld GD, Caldwell ES, et al. The effect of acute respiratory distress syndrome on long-term survival. *Am J Respir Crit Care Med.* 1999;160:1838.
26. Luce JM. Acute lung injury and the acute respiratory distress syndrome. *Crit Care Med.* 1998;26(2):369–376.
27. Herridge MS, Cheung AM, Tansey CM, et al. One-year outcomes in survivors of the acute respiratory distress syndrome. *N Engl J Med.* 2003;348:683.
28. McHugh LG, Milberg JA, Whitecomb ME, et al. Recovery of function in survivors of the acute respiratory distress syndrome. *Am J Respir Crit Care Med.* 1994;150:90.
29. Davidson TA, Caldwell ES, Curtis JR, et al. Reduced quality of life in survivors of acute respiratory distress syndrome compared with critically ill control patients. *JAMA.* 1999;281:354.
30. Weinert CR, Gross CR, Kangas JR, et al. Health-related quality of life after acute lung injury. *Am J Respir Crit Care Med.* 1997;156:1120.
31. Pelosi P, D'Onofrio D, Chiumello D, et al. Pulmonary and extrapulmonary acute respiratory distress syndrome are different. *Eur Respir J (Suppl).* 2003;42:48s–56s.
32. Lee WL, Downey GP. Neutrophil activation and acute lung injury. *Curr Opin Crit Care.* 2001;7(1):1–7.
33. Abraham E. Neutrophils and acute lung injury. *Crit Care Med.* 2003;31(4 Suppl):S195–199.
34. Frerking I, Günther A, Seeger W, et al. Pulmonary surfactant: functions, abnormalities and therapeutic options. *Intensive Care Med.* 2001;27(11):1699–1717.
35. Idell S. Coagulation, fibrinolysis, and fibrin deposition in acute lung injury. *Crit Care Med.* 2003;31(4 Suppl):S213–220.
36. Pittet JF, Mackersie RC, Martin TR, et al. Biological markers of acute lung injury: prognostic and pathogenetic significance. *Am J Respir Crit Care Med.* 1997;155(4):1187–1205.
37. Park WY, Goodman RB, Steinberg KP, et al. Cytokine balance in the lungs of patients with acute respiratory distress syndrome. *Am J Respir Crit Care Med.* 2001;164(10 Pt 1):1896–1903.
38. Fink MP. Role of reactive oxygen and nitrogen species in acute respiratory distress syndrome. *Curr Opin Crit Care.* 2002;8(1):6–11.
39. Bhatia M, Moochhala S. Role of inflammatory mediators in the pathophysiology of acute respiratory distress syndrome. *J Pathol.* 2004;202(2):145–156.
40. Tomashefski JF Jr. Pulmonary pathology of acute respiratory distress syndrome. *Clin Chest Med.* 2000;21(3):435–466.
41. Bellingan GJ. The pulmonary physician in critical care: the pathogenesis of ALI/ARDS. *Thorax.* 2002;57(6):540–546.

42. Marshall RP, Bellingan G, Webb S, et al. Fibroproliferation occurs early in the acute respiratory distress syndrome and impacts on outcome. *Am J Respir Crit Care Med.* 2000;162(5):1783–1788.
43. Gomez AC: Pulmonary insufficiency in non-thoracic trauma [discussion]. *J Trauma.* 1968;8:666.
44. Moore FA, Feliciano DV, Andrassy RJ, et al. Early enteral feeding, compared with parenteral, reduces postoperative septic complications. *Ann Surg.* 1992;216:172.
45. Schuster D. Fluid management in ARDS: "keep them dry" or does it matter? *Intensive Care Med.* 1995;21:101.
46. National Heart, Lung, and Blood Institute Acute Respiratory Distress Syndrome (ARDS) Clinical Trials Network. Comparison of two fluid-management strategies in acute lung injury. *N Engl J Med.* 2006;354(24): 2564–2575.
47. Wright P, Carmichael L, Bernard G. Effect of bronchodilators on lung mechanics in the acute respiratory distress syndrome (ARDS). *Chest.* 1994;106:157.
48. Stoelting RK. *Pharmacology and Physiology in Anesthetic Practice.* 3rd ed. Philadelphia: Lippincott–Raven; 1999:196.
49. Meduri GU, Chinn AJ, Leeper KV, et al. Corticosteroid rescue treatment of progressive fibroproliferation in late ARDS. Patterns of response and predictors of outcome. *Chest.* 1994;105(5):1516–1527.
50. Steinberg KP, Hudson LD, Goodman RB, et al., and the National Heart, Lung, and Blood Institute Acute Respiratory Distress Syndrome (ARDS) Clinical Trials Network. Efficacy and safety of corticosteroids for persistent acute respiratory distress syndrome. *N Engl J Med.* 2006;354(16):1671–1684.
51. Meduri GU, Golden E, Freire AX, et al. Methylprednisolone infusion in early severe ARDS: results of a randomized controlled trial. *Chest.* 2007; 131(4):954–963.
52. Meduri GU, Marik PE, Chrousos GP, et al. Steroid treatment in ARDS: a critical appraisal of the ARDS network trial and the recent literature. *Intensive Care Med.* 2008;34(1):61–69.
53. Peter JV, John P, Graham PL, et al. Corticosteroids in the prevention and treatment of acute respiratory distress syndrome (ARDS) in adults: meta-analysis. *BMJ.* 2008;336(7651):1006–1009.
54. Calfee CS, Matthay MA. Nonventilatory treatments for acute lung injury and ARDS. *Chest.* 2007;131(3):913–920.
55. Hudson LD, Hough CL. Therapy for late-phase acute respiratory distress syndrome. *Clin Chest Med.* 2006;27(4):671–677.
56. Bream-Rouwenhorst HR, Beltz EA, Ross MB, et al. Recent developments in the management of acute respiratory distress syndrome in adults. *Am J Health Syst Pharm.* 2008;65(1):29–36.
57. Meduri GU, Headley S, Tolley E, et al. Plasma and BAL cytokine response to corticosteroid rescue treatment in late ARDS. *Chest.* 1995;103:1315.
58. Tobin MJ. *Principles and Practice of Mechanical Ventilation.* 2nd ed. New York: McGraw Hill; 2006:38, 129–154, 782–784.
59. Antonelli M, Conti G, Esquinas A, et al. A multiple-center survey on the use in clinical practice of noninvasive ventilation as a first-line intervention for acute respiratory distress syndrome. *Crit Care Med.* 2007;35(1):18–25.
60. Ferrer M, Esquinas A, Leon M, et al. Noninvasive ventilation in severe hypoxemic respiratory failure: a randomized clinical trial. *Am J Respir Crit Care Med.* 2003;168(12):1438–1444.
61. Keenan SP, Sinuff T, Cook DJ, et al. Does noninvasive positive pressure ventilation improve outcome in acute hypoxemic respiratory failure? A systematic review. *Crit Care Med.* 2004;32(12):2516–2523.
62. Rouby JJ, Puybasset L, Cluzel P, et al. Regional distribution of gas and tissue in acute respiratory distress syndrome. II. Physiological correlations and definition of an ARDS Severity Score. CT Scan ARDS Study Group. *Intensive Care Med.* 2000;26(8):1046–1056.
63. Puybasset L, Gusman P, Muller JC, et al. Regional distribution of gas and tissue in acute respiratory distress syndrome. III. Consequences for the effects of positive end-expiratory pressure. CT Scan ARDS Study Group. Adult Respiratory Distress Syndrome. *Intensive Care Med.* 2000;26(9): 1215–1227.
64. Kolobow T, Moretti MP, Fumagalli R, et al. Severe impairment in lung function induced by high peak airway pressure during mechanical ventilation. An experimental study. *Am Rev Respir Dis.* 1987;135(2):312–315.
65. Tsuno K, Prato P, Kolobow T. Acute lung injury from mechanical ventilation at moderately high airway pressures. *J Appl Physiol.* 1990;69(3):956–961.
66. Hickling KG, Henderson SJ, Jackson R. Low mortality associated with low volume pressure limited ventilation with permissive hypercapnia in severe adult respiratory distress syndrome. *Intensive Care Med.* 1990;16(6):372–377.
67. Acute Respiratory Distress Syndrome Network. Ventilation with lower tidal volumes as compared with traditional tidal volumes for acute lung injury and the acute respiratory distress syndrome. *N Engl J Med.* 2000; 342(18):1301–1308.
68. Tremblay LN, Slutsky AS. Ventilator-induced lung injury: from the bench to the bedside. *Intensive Care Med.* 2006;32(1):24–33.
69. Tremblay L, Valenza F, Ribeiro SP, et al. Injurious ventilatory strategies increase cytokines and c-fos m-RNA expression in an isolated rat lung model. *J Clin Invest.* 1997;99(5):944–952.
70. Slutsky AS. Lung injury caused by mechanical ventilation. *Chest.* 1999;116 (1 Suppl):9S–15S.
71. Webb HH, Tierney DF. Experimental pulmonary edema due to intermittent positive pressure ventilation with high inflation pressures. Protection by positive end-expiratory pressure. *Am Rev Respir Dis.* 1974;110(5):556–565.
72. Petersen GW, Baier H. Incidence of pulmonary barotrauma in a medical ICU. *Crit Care Med.* 1983;11(2):67–69.
73. Dreyfuss D, Saumon G. Ventilator-induced lung injury: lessons from experimental studies. *Am J Respir Crit Care Med.* 1998;157(1):294–323.
74. Belperio JA, Keane MP, Lynch JP 3rd, et al. The role of cytokines during the pathogenesis of ventilator-associated and ventilator-induced lung injury. *Semin Respir Crit Care Med.* 2006;27(4):350–364.
75. Ranieri VM, Suter PM, Tortorella C, et al. Effect of mechanical ventilation on inflammatory mediators in patients with acute respiratory distress syndrome: a randomized controlled trial. *JAMA.* 1999;282(1):54–61.
76. Terragni PP, Rosboch G, Tealdi A, et al. Tidal hyperinflation during low tidal volume ventilation in acute respiratory distress syndrome. *Am J Respir Crit Care Med.* 2007;175(2):160–166.
77. Gattinoni L, Pesenti A. The concept of "baby lung." *Intensive Care Med.* 2005;31(6):776–784.
78. Barbas CS, de Matos GF, Pincelli MP, et al. Mechanical ventilation in acute respiratory failure: recruitment and high positive end-expiratory pressure are necessary. *Curr Opin Crit Care.* 2005;11(1):18–28.
79. Amato MB, Barbas CS, Medeiros DM, et al. Effect of a protective-ventilation strategy on mortality in the acute respiratory distress syndrome. *N Engl J Med.* 1998;338(6):347–354.
80. Lachmann B. Open up the lung and keep the lung open. *Intensive Care Med.* 1992;18(6):319–321.
81. Gattinoni L, Caironi P, Cressoni M, et al. Lung recruitment in patients with the acute respiratory distress syndrome. *N Engl J Med.* 2006;354(17):1775–1786.
82. Dueck R. Alveolar recruitment versus hyperinflation: a balancing act. *Curr Opin Anaesthesiol.* 2006;19(6):650–654.
83. Brower RG, Lanken PN, MacIntyre N, et al., National Heart, Lung, and Blood Institute ARDS Clinical Trials Network. Higher versus lower positive end-expiratory pressures in patients with the acute respiratory distress syndrome. *N Engl J Med.* 2004;351(4):327–336.
84. Meade MO, Cook DJ, Guyatt GH, et al., Lung Open Ventilation Study Investigators. Ventilation strategy using low tidal volumes, recruitment maneuvers, and high positive end-expiratory pressure for acute lung injury and acute respiratory distress syndrome: a randomized controlled trial. *JAMA.* 2008;299(6):637–645.
85. Borges JB, Okamoto VN, Matos GF, et al. Reversibility of lung collapse and hypoxemia in early acute respiratory distress syndrome. *Am J Respir Crit Care Med.* 2006;174(3):268–278.
86. Lapinsky SE, Mehta S. Bench-to-bedside review: recruitment and recruiting maneuvers. *Crit Care.* 2005;9(1):60–65.
87. Medoff BD, Harris RS, Kesselman H, et al. Use of recruitment maneuvers and high-positive end-expiratory pressure in a patient with acute respiratory distress syndrome. *Crit Care Med.* 2000;28(4):1210–1216.
88. Laffey JG, O'Croinin D, McLoughlin P, et al. Permissive hypercapnia—role in protective lung ventilatory strategies. *Intensive Care Med.* 2004;30(3):347–356.
89. Kallet RH, Campbell AR, Alonso JA, et al. The effects of pressure control versus volume control assisted ventilation on patient work of breathing in acute lung injury and acute respiratory distress syndrome. *Respir Care.* 2000;45(9):1085–1096.
90. Shanholtz C, Brower R. Should inverse ratio ventilation be used in adult respiratory distress syndrome. *Am J Respir Crit Care Med.* 1994;149(5):1354–1358.
91. Mercat A, Graïni L, Teboul JL, et al. Cardiorespiratory effects of pressure-controlled ventilation with and without inverse ratio in the adult respiratory distress syndrome. *Chest.* 1993;104(3):871–875.
92. Esteban A, Alía I, Gordo F, et al. Prospective randomized trial comparing pressure-controlled ventilation and volume-controlled ventilation in ARDS. For the Spanish Lung Failure Collaborative Group. *Chest.* 2000;117(6):1690–1696.
93. Habashi NM. Other approaches to open-lung ventilation: airway pressure release ventilation. *Crit Care Med.* 2005;33(3 Suppl):S228–240.
94. Kaplan LJ, Bailey H, Formosa V. Airway pressure release ventilation increases cardiac performance in patients with acute lung injury/adult respiratory distress syndrome. *Crit Care.* 2001;5(4):221–226.
95. Putensen C, Zech S, Wrigge H, et al. Long-term effects of spontaneous breathing during ventilatory support in patients with acute lung injury. *Am J Respir Crit Care Med.* 2001;164(1):43–49.
96. Pelosi P, Brazzi L, Gattinoni L. Prone position in acute respiratory distress syndrome. *Eur Respir J.* 2002;20(4):1017–1028.
97. West JB, Dollery CT, Naimark A. Distribution of blood flow in isolated lung; relation to vascular and alveolar pressures. *J Appl Physiol.* 1964;19: 713–724.
98. Gattinoni L, Tognoni G, Pesenti A, et al., Prone-Supine Study Group. Effect of prone positioning on the survival of patients with acute respiratory failure. *N Engl J Med.* 2001;345(8):568–573.

99. Guerin C, Gaillard S, Lemasson S, et al. Effects of systematic prone positioning in hypoxemic acute respiratory failure: a randomized controlled trial. *JAMA.* 2004;292(19):2379–2387.
100. Mancebo J, Fernández R, Blanch L, et al. A multicenter trial of prolonged prone ventilation in severe acute respiratory distress syndrome. *Am J Respir Crit Care Med.* 2006;173(11):1233–1239.
101. Pillow JJ. High-frequency oscillatory ventilation: mechanisms of gas exchange and lung mechanics. *Crit Care Med.* 2005;33(3 Suppl):S135–141.
102. Chang HK. Mechanisms of gas transport during ventilation by high-frequency oscillation. *J Appl Physiol.* 1984;56(3):553–563.
103. Slutsky AS, Drazen FM, Ingram RH Jr, et al. Effective pulmonary ventilation with small-volume oscillations at high frequency. *Science.* 1980;209 (4456):609–671.
104. Derdak S. High-frequency oscillatory ventilation for acute respiratory distress syndrome in adult patients. *Crit Care Med.* 2003;31(4 Suppl):S317–323.
105. Wunsch H, Mapstone J, Takala J. High-frequency ventilation versus conventional ventilation for the treatment of acute lung injury and acute respiratory distress syndrome: a systematic review and Cochrane analysis. *Anesth Analg.* 2005;100(6):1765–1772.
106. Derdak S, Mehta S, Stewart TE, et al., Multicenter Oscillatory Ventilation For Acute Respiratory Distress Syndrome Trial (MOAT) Study Investigators. High-frequency oscillatory ventilation for acute respiratory distress syndrome in adults: a randomized, controlled trial. *Am J Respir Crit Care Med.* 2002;166(6):801–808.
107. Brown JK, Haft JW, Bartlett RH, et al. Acute lung injury and acute respiratory distress syndrome: extracorporeal life support and liquid ventilation for severe acute respiratory distress syndrome in adults. *Semin Respir Crit Care Med.* 2006;27(4):416–425.
108. Gattinoni L, Pesenti A, Mascheroni D, et al. Low-frequency positive-pressure ventilation with extracorporeal CO_2 removal in severe acute respiratory failure. *JAMA.* 1986;256:881–886.
109. Morris AH, Wallace CJ, Menlove RL, et al. Randomized clinical trial of pressure-controlled inverse ratio ventilation and extracorporeal CO_2 removal for adult respiratory distress syndrome. *Am J Respir Crit Care Med.* 1994;149:295–305.
110. Lequier L. Extracorporeal life support in pediatric and neonatal critical care: a review. *J Intensive Care Med.* 2004;19(5):243–258.
111. Skinner SC, Hirschl RB, Bartlett RH. Extracorporeal life support. *Semin Pediatr Surg.* 2006;15(4):242–250.
112. Pison U, López FA, Heidelmeyer CF, et al. Inhaled nitric oxide reverses hypoxic pulmonary vasoconstriction without impairing gas exchange. *J Appl Physiol.* 1993;74(3):1287–1292.
113. Rossaint R, Falke KJ, López F, et al. Inhaled nitric oxide for the adult respiratory distress syndrome. *N Engl J Med.* 1993;328(6):399–405.
114. Palmer RM, Ferrige AG, Moncada S. Nitric oxide release accounts for the biological activity of endothelium-derived relaxing factor. *Nature.* 1987;327(6122):524–526.
115. Moncada S, Palmer RM, Higgs EA. Nitric oxide: physiology, pathophysiology, and pharmacology. *Pharmacol Rev.* 1991;43(2):109–142.
116. Cooper CE. Nitric oxide and iron proteins. *Biochim Biophys Acta.* 1999;1411(2–3):290–309.
117. Taylor RW, Zimmerman JL, Dellinger RP, et al., Inhaled Nitric Oxide in ARDS Study Group. Low-dose inhaled nitric oxide in patients with acute lung injury: a randomized controlled trial. *JAMA.* 2004;291(13):1603–1609.
118. Adhikari NK, Burns KE, Friedrich JO, et al. Effect of nitric oxide on oxygenation and mortality in acute lung injury: systematic review and meta-analysis. *BMJ.* 2007;334(7597):779.
119. Lowson SM. Inhaled alternatives to nitric oxide. *Crit Care Med.* 2005;33(3 Suppl):S188–195.
120. Puybasset L, Rouby JJ, Mourgeon E, et al. Factors influencing cardiopulmonary effects of inhaled nitric oxide in acute respiratory failure. *Am J Respir Crit Care Med.* 1995;152(1):318–328.
121. Pierce CM, Peters MJ, Cohen G, et al. Cost of nitric oxide is exorbitant [Letter to the Editor]. *BMJ.* 2002;325(7359):336.
122. Wiedemann HP. Partial liquid ventilation for acute respiratory distress syndrome. *Clin Chest Med.* 2000;21(3):543–554.
123. Clark LC Jr, Gollan F. Survival of mammals breathing organic liquids equilibrated with oxygen at atmospheric pressure. *Science.* 1966;152(730):1755–1756.
124. Kacmarek RM, Wiedemann HP, Lavin PT, et al. Partial liquid ventilation in adult patients with acute respiratory distress syndrome. *Am J Respir Crit Care Med.* 2006;173(8):882–889.
125. Hirschl RB, Croce M, Gore D, et al. Prospective, randomized, controlled pilot study of partial liquid ventilation in adult acute respiratory distress syndrome. *Am J Respir Crit Care Med.* 2002;165(6):781–787.
126. Wright JR. Immunoregulatory functions of surfactant proteins. *Nat Rev Immunol.* 2005;5(1):58–68.
127. Stevens TP, Sinkin RA. Surfactant replacement therapy. *Chest.* 2007; 131(5):1577–1582.
128. Spragg RG, Lewis JF, Wurst W, et al. Treatment of acute respiratory distress syndrome with recombinant surfactant protein C surfactant. *Am J Respir Crit Care Med.* 2003;167(11):1562–1566.
129. Spragg RG, Lewis JF, Walmrath HD, et al. Effect of recombinant surfactant protein C-based surfactant on the acute respiratory distress syndrome. *N Engl J Med.* 2004;351(9):884–892.
130. Pingleton SK. Complications associated with the adult respiratory distress syndrome. *Clin Chest Med.* 1982;5:143.
131. Villar J, Kacmarek RM, Pérez-Méndez L, et al. A high positive end-expiratory pressure, low tidal volume ventilatory strategy improves outcome in persistent acute respiratory distress syndrome: a randomized, controlled trial. *Crit Care Med.* 2006;34(5):1311–1318.
132. Gammon RB, Shin MS, Buchalter SE. Pulmonary barotrauma in mechanical ventilation. Patterns and risk factors. *Chest.* 1992;102(2):568–572.
133. Bouhuys A. Physiology and musical instruments. *Nature.* 1969;221(5187): 1199–2004.
134. Dreyfuss D, Soler P, Saumon G. Mechanical ventilation-induced pulmonary edema. Interaction with previous lung alterations. *Am J Respir Crit Care Med.* 1995;151(5):1568–1575.
135. Kawano T, Mori S, Cybulsky M, et al. Effect of granulocyte depletion in a ventilated surfactant-depleted lung. *J Appl Physiol.* 1987;62(1):27–33.

CHAPTER 137 ■ EXTRACORPOREAL CIRCULATION FOR RESPIRATORY OR CARDIAC FAILURE

ROBERT H. BARTLETT • JONATHAN HAFT

You probably turned to this chapter because you are caring for a patient with acute heart or lung failure, and the patient is failing despite your best treatment. The risk of death for your patient is over 80% any way you measure it. The patient might be a woman with streptococcal pneumonia, a child who cannot come off cardiopulmonary bypass after a cardiac operation, a man with chest trauma, acute respiratory distress syndrome (ARDS), or massive pulmonary embolism, or an emergency room (ER) patient undergoing cardiopulmonary resuscitation (CPR). Your only option to improve survival is extracorporeal life support (ECLS) with mechanical artificial organs.

ECLS is the use of an artificial heart (pump) and lung (membrane oxygenator) to replace organ function for days or weeks, to allow time for diagnosis, treatment, and organ recovery or replacement. The indications for ECLS are acute, severe heart or lung failure, not improving on conventional management. In a patient with an 80% to 100% risk of dying, the healthy survival results with ECLS range from 40% in cardiac arrest with CPR to 95% in neonatal meconium aspiration. ECLS is routine treatment in every major neonatal ICU and pediatric cardiac surgery program. Why is ECLS not used routinely in every adult ICU and emergency room? The reasons are complexity, expense, the need for special equipment and experienced personnel, and education. Improvements in the technology for ECLS will solve some of these limitations. Intensivists in neonatology and pediatrics understand the principles of ECLS, so most of this discussion is devoted to adult patients.

BACKGROUND

The heart/lung machine was developed by John Gibbon, beginning in 1939 and culminating in the first successful heart operation using a heart–lung machine in 1954 (1). Dr. Gibbon's motivation was to develop a technique to treat massive pulmonary embolism, but what resulted instead was the entire field of intracardiac surgery. The artificial heart was simply a blood pump, and the artificial lung was direct exposure of the flowing blood to oxygen gas. For cardiac surgery all the venous return is diverted into the machine and pumped into the systemic circulation, leaving the heart empty long enough to repair intracardiac defects or operate on the coronary circulation. The opportunity to operate directly on the heart was miraculous, but the heart–lung machine itself caused damage to the fluid and solid elements of the blood, causing fatal complications if it was used for more than 4 hours. The major cause of blood damage was the direct exposure of blood to gas (2,3). Interposing a gas exchange membrane of plastic (4) or cellulose (5) between the flowing blood and the gas solved most of the blood-damage problems, but experimental devices required very large surface areas and were impractical for any clinical use (4–6). This changed when thin sheets of dimethyl polysiloxane polymer (commonly called silicone rubber) became available in the 1960s. Using silicone rubber membrane, artificial lungs with potential clinical application were designed and studied (7–10). By eliminating the gas interface it was possible to use a modified heart–lung machine for days at a time, and the physiology and pathophysiology of prolonged extracorporeal circulation was worked out in the laboratory (11–13).

The first successful use of prolonged life support with a heart–lung machine was conducted by J. Donald Hill et al. in 1971 (14). The patient was a young man suffering from ARDS, a newly recognized entity in those days and initially called "adult respiratory distress syndrome." The entire discipline we now call critical care was evolving at the same time. After Hill's case, several other successful cases were reported in children and adults with severe pulmonary and cardiac failure (15). At the same time there seemed to be an epidemic of ARDS, and it looked like extracorporeal support would be the answer. A multicenter clinical trial of prolonged extracorporeal circulation for adults with ARDS was commissioned by the National Institutes of Health in 1975. This was the first prospective randomized trial of a life-support technique in acute fatal illness in which the end point was death. There were many problems with the design and execution of that clinical trial, but from it we learned that the mortality for all patients with ARDS was 66%, and the mortality for severe ARDS was 90%, with or without ECLS. We learned that extracorporeal support attempted by inexperienced teams, in venoarterial mode for 1 week without protecting the lung from ventilator injury, did not improve the ultimate survival in severe ARDS. We learned (the hard way) the mistakes to avoid when conducting a prospective trial in acute fatal illness. And finally, we developed a name for the technology: extracorporeal membrane oxygenation (ECMO). The results of that study were published in 1979 (16). Laboratory and clinical research on ECLS in adults essentially stopped for a decade. However, the results in neonatal respiratory failure were very encouraging.

We reported the first successful case of ECLS for respiratory failure in a newborn infant in 1976 (17). Our laboratory had been studying membrane oxygenator development and prolonged extracorporeal circulation in animals for 10 years. We and others had used extracorporeal support for postoperative cardiopulmonary failure in children with the first successful pediatric cardiac case in 1972 (18). White et al. (19) and Dorson et al. (20) had initiated clinical trials in neonatal respiratory failure without success. We treated 40 newborn patients over the next 5 years with 50% survival (21). Neonatologists and surgeons from other institutions joined us to learn the technology. By 1986 eighteen neonatal centers had successful ECMO teams (22).

We conducted the first prospective randomized trial of ECMO in neonatal respiratory failure, using an adaptive design to correct some of the mistakes we had made in the earlier adult trial (23). Another prospective randomized trial was carried out by O'Rourke et al. at the Boston Children's Hospital (24). ECMO became standard treatment for severe neonatal respiratory failure by 1986, and standard treatment for severe cardiac failure in children by 1990.

Kolobow (25) showed that high ventilator inspiratory pressure (lung stretch) and high FiO_2 caused severe lung injury. Gattinoni et al. (26) and Kolobow (25) separated respiration from oxygenation by removing CO_2 by extracorporeal circulation (making ventilation unnecessary) and oxygenating by insufflation. Using extracorporeal CO_2 removal, they prevented stretch injury, and reported 56% survival in severe ARDS. These observations led to renewed interest in ECLS for adult respiratory failure. By the 1990s several groups reported similar results (27–29). The value of avoiding lung stretch injury has been verified in many studies (30–32), decreasing the incidence of iatrogenic lung injury (and decreasing the need for ECLS). Even with these and other improvements, the mortality for ARDS in otherwise healthy patients was still 30% (32).

The use of ECMO allows study of patients who would otherwise have died. This unveiled many aspects of respiratory pathophysiology and treatment, which in turn resulted in better understanding and the implementation of other simpler techniques. As the technology developed it was standardized, disseminated, studied, and improved in an organized fashion by the actual and potential users. This group of investigators and clinicians was formally organized as the Extracorporeal Life Support Organization (ELSO) in 1989. For the last 20 years that group has developed guidelines and practices, published the standard textbook in the field (33), and maintained a registry of ECLS cases.

ECLS TECHNIQUE AND PHYSIOLOGY

Extracorporeal life support is simply the use of a modified heart/lung machine to provide gas exchange (and systemic perfusion if necessary) to prolong the life of a patient when native heart and lung function is not adequate to sustain life. The technique, indications, methods, and results are described in detail in the book *ECMO: Extracorporeal Cardiopulmonary Support in Critical Care* published by the Extracorporeal Life Support Organization (www.elso.med.umich.edu) (33). The heart–lung machine used for cardiac surgery is modified, both in devices and technology, to be used for days or weeks in the intensive care unit, but the purpose is the same: to keep the body alive during heart or lung failure. The technique is invasive and complex. A large (23–30 French catheter) is inserted into the inferior vena cava or right atrium; venous blood is drained, passed through an artificial lung, and pumped back into the patient, either into the aorta (venoarterial [VA] bypass) or into the right atrium (venovenous [VV] bypass). VA bypass puts the artificial lung in parallel with the native lungs and substitutes for both heart and lung function. In VV bypass, the artificial lung is in series with the native lungs and the patient is reliant on his own hemodynamics for pulmonary and systemic perfusion. ECLS allows decreasing the ventilator to nondamaging "rest" settings (typically FiO_2 0.3, pressure 20/10, rate 4), decreasing vasoactive drugs, and optimizing other aspects of treatment.

Because the surfaces of the extracorporeal devices are plastic, it is necessary to anticoagulate the blood with a continuous infusion of heparin, titrated to a low but constant level of anticoagulation. This level of anticoagulation is measured by whole blood activated clotting time (ACT). The normal is 120 seconds, and during ECLS, ACT is maintained at approximately 180 seconds. Although this level of heparinization prevents thrombosis in the extracorporeal circuit, circulating platelets still adhere to the plastic surfaces, become activated which attracts more platelets, grow into platelet aggregates, and eventually break off and recirculate as effete platelets, which are removed by the reticuloendothelial system in the liver and spleen. Because heparinization and thrombocytopenia are necessary components of ECLS, the major risk of the procedure is bleeding. As currently practiced, significant bleeding is rarely a serious problem, but this requires the continuous bedside attendance of a specialist whose primary job is to measure the ACT and platelet count at very frequent intervals and titrate heparin dose and platelet infusions accordingly. Properly managed, ECLS can be used for weeks without hemolysis, device failure, clotting, or bleeding, but it is invasive and expensive. The technology not only must be learned and practiced by the intensive care unit team, but also must be endorsed by the entire hospital. Management of the patient during ECLS includes management of perfusion and gas exchange as above, but also attention to fluid balance, oxygen consumption and delivery, nutrition, position, and the monitoring and sustaining of function of other organs.

In *respiratory failure*, VV access is preferred. Gas exchange across the native lungs is usually minimal during the first several days of ECLS; therefore, the patient is totally dependent on the extracorporeal system. As native lung function returns, systemic blood oxygenation and CO_2 clearance improve, improved gas exchange can be measured at the airway, and the extracorporeal blood flow rate is gradually decreased, allowing the native lungs to assume a larger percentage of gas exchange. When the native lungs have improved, the patient is tried off ECLS at nondamaging ventilator settings. When this trial is successful, the cannulas are removed and recovery continues. Patients who are successfully weaned off ECLS have a 90% likelihood of complete recovery.

In *cardiac failure*, VA access is required (usually via the femoral vessels). Inotropes and pressors are weaned off, and systemic perfusion is maintained by extracorporeal flow. Lung function usually returns to normal in a day or two, and the patient can be awakened and extubated. When the patient is stable, and the function of other organs can be determined (especially the brain), a decision can be made regarding bridge to recovery or bridge to ventricular assist device (VAD) and transplantation. When ECLS is used for cardiac support, the pulmonary and left ventricular blood flow is decreased in proportion to the extracorporeal flow. This can lead to two problems. First, if the heart stops altogether, the left atrium and the left ventricle will gradually distend with bronchial venous blood, leading to high left atrial pressure and pulmonary edema. This condition is diagnosed by the lack of pulsatility in the systemic arterial system. If left ventricular (LV) function is inadequate to maintain emptying of the left heart, the left side of the heart must be drained into the venous line, either by direct catheterization of the left atrium or by creation of an atrial septal defect. The second problem with VA bypass in the totally failing heart is thrombosis in the left atrium or left ventricle. This will occur even in the presence of systemic heparinization. Thrombosis is diagnosed by echocardiography. If a patient has left atrial or left ventricle thrombus, it is important to avoid spontaneous left ventricular function. Usually such patients are candidates for VAD or cardiac replacement, and the clot is removed before embolism could occur.

CLINICAL RESULTS

The most recent data from the ELSO registry are shown in Table 137.1. Participation in the Extracorporeal Life Support Organization is voluntary, but almost all cases treated with ECLS in established centers are included in the registry. There are currently over 30,000 patients who have been managed with ECLS. Although there are extensive data on gas exchange, perfusion, coagulation, and so on, the only important statistic is hospital discharge survival because the technique is a life-support technique and it is applied only to patients who are not expected to survive otherwise with a high (80%–100%) risk of dying with continuing conventional treatment. The mortality risk is measured differently in different age groups.

Neonatal Respiratory Failure

The largest group of patients treated with ECLS is newborn infants with respiratory failure. There are only a few causes of severe respiratory failure in newborn infants. Survival after ECLS for meconium aspiration, infant respiratory distress syndrome (IRDS), primary pulmonary hypertension of the newborn (PPHN), and neonatal sepsis is 80% to 95%, and 60% for congenital diaphragmatic hernia. The reason for these excellent results is that the causes of respiratory failure in neonates do not destroy lung tissue. The primary pathophysiology is pulmonary hypertension with right-to-left shunting through the ductus arterious (persistent fetal circulation). During ECLS the pulmonary vasculature relaxes, the ductus closes, and lung recovery occurs promptly. The problem in congenital diaphragmatic hernia is that the hernia compresses the lungs and causes bilateral lung hypoplasia *in utero* in addition to pulmonary vasospasm. The hypoplastic lungs may be too small to support the infant.

The early neonatal ECMO patients are now adults with children of their own, and there is abundant information on long-term follow-up. About 10% of surviving patients have some neurologic disability; the most common is some degree of hearing loss. This is lower than the incidence of complications in critically ill infants not treated with ECLS, indicating that these are the complications of profound illness in the newborn. The use of ECLS in neonatal respiratory failure decreased after the initiation of nitric oxide inhalation to treat pulmonary hypertension. Approximately 1,000 per year are entered into the ELSO registry.

Pediatric Respiratory Failure

Severe respiratory failure in older children is relatively rare, compared to the incidence in newborn infants and adults. The most common cause is viral or bacterial pneumonia. Status asthmaticus is another life-threatening problem in children. ECLS is used when a patient is not responding to other methods of management. The survival rate is approximately 75%, varying to some extent with the primary condition. The effectiveness of ECLS in pediatric respiratory failure was

TABLE 137.1

OVERALL PATIENT OUTCOMES WITH ECLS FOR CARDIAC AND RESPIRATORY FAILURE

	Total	Surv ECLS		Surv to DC	
Neonatal					
Respiratory	20,993	17,889	85%	16,005	76%
Cardiac	2,898	1,684	58%	1,095	38%
ECPR	274	176	64%	109	40%
Pediatric					
Respiratory	3,390	2,173	64%	1,895	56%
Cardiac	3,658	2,199	60%	1,624	44%
ECPR	523	263	50%	200	38%
Adult					
Respiratory	1,255	740	59%	646	51%
Cardiac	671	300	45%	216	32%
ECPR	189	80	42%	59	31%
	33,851	25,504	75%	21,849	65%

ELSO registry data, December 2006. The data for 2006 are incomplete. ELSO, Extracorporeal Life Support Organization; Surv, survival; ECLS, extracorporeal life support; DC, discharge; ECPR, extracorporeal cardiopulmonary resuscitation.

demonstrated in a contemporary matched pairs study by Green et al. (34). Most children with respiratory failure can be managed successfully with venovenous access. In children who do not survive, the most common cause of death is progressive lung destruction from the primary infection, or brain damage from the period of hypoxia and ischemia that preceded ECLS. These children are all essentially normal in follow-up. Once the lung recovers, pulmonary function and exercise tolerance return to normal.

Adult Respiratory Failure

The cause of ARDS is a primary lung event in about half the cases (viral or bacterial pneumonia, aspiration, pulmonary vasculitis, etc.), and secondary to extrapulmonary causes in the others (shock, trauma, pancreatitis, sepsis). The overall mortality for ARDS is approximately 30% even with excellent management. ECLS is indicated for those patients who have a high mortality risk within the first week after intubation. These patients are relatively easy to identify. They have an alveolar-arterial (A-a) gradient for oxygen greater than 600 on day 2, 3, or 4 following initial intubation. The mortality risk for those patients is approximately 80%, and the recovery rate with ECLS in those patients is approximately 70% (35–38). Patients on the ventilator more than 5 days pre-ECLS have less chance of recovery; hence the overall survival rate for ECLS treatment of ARDS is approximately 55%. The University of Michigan has reported the largest experience with ECLS for ARDS. In that series, the overall survival rate was 52% and rose to 65% in 2002 (35). The series is large enough to characterize the patient population and identify the likelihood of recovery based on age and days on mechanical ventilation.

As technology for adult respiratory failure has evolved, ECLS is now practiced using primarily venovenous access, with high blood flow adequate to sustain oxygenation as well as CO_2 removal, lung rest, diuresis, and prone positioning. This approach leads to the 50% to 60% survival discussed above, but a new prospective randomized trial is clearly indicated, and is currently being conducted in the United Kingdom (UK), following the study design of the UK neonatal ECMO trial (39). This brilliant study design solves many of the logistic and ethical problems of prospective randomized trials of life support in which death is the end point. Patients who meet entry criteria in participating intensive care units throughout the country are randomized to continuing conventional care in that center or referral to an ECMO center. In the adult trial, there is one ECMO center in Leicester, England (40). With this approach, the best available care in the entire country will be compared to a specific algorithm in a specific center. The results of this study will be available in the fall of 2007, and preliminary results may be viewed at the Web site. (40) If ECLS is not used for adults in your intensive care unit, the answer to the question posed in the introduction is clear. Do the best you can with what you have, but do not try to set up an ECLS system on the spur of the moment.

Another important application for ECLS in children and adults is status asthmaticus. There are patients with acute asthmatic attacks unresponsive to bronchodilators, intubation, ventilation, sedation, heliox, general anesthesia, and the other extreme measures used to treat status asthmaticus. These patients have overexpansion, air trapping, normal oxygenation, and profound CO_2 retention. Pneumothorax often occurs and is usually a fatal complication. Approximately 4,000 people die of acute asthma in the United States every year. This condition is ideally treated with ECLS. Simple VV cannulation and relatively low blood flow is all that is required to achieve normal CO_2 clearance and return to normal blood gases. Once this occurs, bronchospasm invariably clears within a day or two (41). Because the risk of pneumothorax and death is significant, and because the risk of ECLS is low, ECLS should be considered in any patient who has a severe asthma attack with PCO_2 >80 despite mechanical ventilation and other optimal treatment. When ECLS is used for status asthmaticus, the gas flow to the membrane lung is slowly increased over hours to avoid potential complications of sudden changes in PCO_2 and pH.

Cardiac Failure in Children

Venoarterial ECLS is currently the only mechanical support system available for children in the United States. Most of the children treated with ECLS have cardiac failure following a cardiac operation, usually for congenital heart disease. These patients cannot be weaned from cardiopulmonary bypass in the operating room, or are weaned but remain in profound cardiac failure despite full inotropic support following operation. Patients who cannot be weaned from cardiopulmonary bypass are attached to the ECLS machine using the same cannulas used for cardiopulmonary bypass (CPB), typically in the right atrium and aorta. If the patient has been weaned off bypass and the chest is closed, vascular access is gained by cannulation of the right internal jugular vein and right common carotid artery, as in newborn respiratory failure. This same vascular access is used for children with myocarditis or myocardiopathy. Because ECLS is commonly used directly after cardiopulmonary bypass, bleeding is a more common occurrence in cardiac patients than in respiratory patients. This is best managed by maintaining the chest open with a sterile plastic sheet over the open wound and blood drainage tubes placed in the chest. In this way the amount of bleeding can be observed directly, and it is easy to reexplore the chest, which is often required every 8 to 12 hours for the first day on ECLS. Bleeding is managed by maintaining the heparinization at very low levels (1.25 times the upper limit of normal ACT), maintaining platelet count over 100,000, and adding aprotinin to enhance platelet function and Amicar to minimize fibrinolysis. A combination of Amicar, aprotinin, and low-level heparinization can lead to thrombus formation in the extracorporeal circuit. In these cases it is important to keep a primed extracorporeal circuit available so that the circuit can be changed if clotting occurs. Aprotinin has been removed from the market due to a higher incidence of renal failure, and further studies are being done.

Generalized fluid overload is a common problem associated with cardiac failure in children. Diuresis is begun immediately with ECLS. If satisfactory negative fluid balance cannot be achieved with continuous infusion of diuretics, continuous hemofiltration is instituted. Survival with ECLS in pediatric cardiac failure is 40% to 50% (42).

Cardiac Failure in Adults

The experience with ECLS for cardiac failure in adults is shown in Table 139.1. The most common indication for ECLS for cardiac support in adults is acute myocardial failure following myocardial infarction or heart failure following cardiac operation. Vascular access is usually achieved by cannulation of the right atrium via the right internal jugular or femoral vein with arterial return retrograde via the femoral artery. Intra-aortic balloon pumping is possible in adults and will support approximately 40% of the cardiac output. Most of the patients treated with ECLS have failed balloon pumping, as well as full inotropic support. If a balloon pump is in place through one of the femoral arteries, it is best left in place because of the risk of bleeding once the pump has been removed. The opposite femoral artery is used for arterial access.

Adult patients in acute cardiac failure are candidates for left ventricular assist device (LVAD) placement as a bridge to recovery or a bridge to transplantation. However, in the acute failure situation it is best to institute ECLS first, to stabilize the circulation and gas exchange, and to determine if other organs are functioning, specifically the brain. If severe brain injury has occurred during the period of acute cardiac failure, ECLS is discontinued, avoiding the futile thoracotomy and expense of LVAD placement. The survival for ECLS in adult cardiac failure is 40% to 50% (43–45).

EXTRACORPOREAL LIFE SUPPORT FOR CARDIOPULMONARY RESUSCITATION

ECLS can be used in association with resuscitation to support cardiac and pulmonary function in cardiac arrest or profound shock. In this application the ECLS circuit must be primed and available within minutes. Therefore, the extracorporeal life support for cardiopulmonary resuscitation (ECPR) cases are done primarily in established ECLS centers, which have both the equipment and the team to institute ECLS on a moment's notice. The limiting factor in establishing ECLS in these cases is vascular access. It is difficult to get rapid arterial and venous access in a patient in full cardiac arrest. Most successful ECPR cases have been in patients who arrested, then briefly resuscitated, with simple vascular access gained following initial resuscitation. Then ECLS cannulas can be placed over a wire through smaller catheters if and when the patient arrests again or proceeds to cardiogenic shock or intractable arrhythmias. In our institution we consider ECPR for patients who have been in cardiac arrest for less than 5 minutes. A few patients who have been arrested with full and well-documented resuscitation for over an hour have been treated successfully, but if the arrest has been prolonged and if profound metabolic acidosis exists, then establishing extracorporeal support is often futile. The overall results for successful, healthy survival after ECPR is approximately 40%, much better than the 5% successful results of external message only (46,47).

OTHER APPLICATIONS OF ECLS

The ability to totally control perfusion and gas exchange with an extracorporeal system offers unique opportunities in other aspects of acute medical care. Profound hypothermia can be treated by extracorporeal support. This is particularly important because patients who are hypothermic may develop ventricular fibrillation during external warming. Hypothermia associated with exsanguinating hemorrhage in the operating room can be treated successfully with ECLS. Perfusion is maintained during the period of bleeding, and hypothermia can be maintained to protect organ function. After bleeding is controlled, blood is returned to the patient associated with warming to avoid the coagulopathy caused by low temperature. Hyperthermic perfusion can be established, either for total body warming or for regional warming, as an adjunct to cancer chemotherapy.

Septic shock was once considered a contraindication to ECLS. However, sepsis often clears during ECLS, and this has become a standard indication in our institution. It is common for patients in septic shock to regain normal vascular tone and to come off all vasopressors within a day or two of instituting ECLS (48). This is partly related to establishing healthy perfusion and gas exchange, and partly related to adsorption of inflammatory mediators by the plastic in the circuit.

ECLS has also been used to support perfusion in potential organ donors, particularly in situations in which death prior to organ donation occurs because of cardiac arrest following elective withdrawal of ventilator support (49).

SUMMARY

Extracorporeal life support sustains cardiac and pulmonary function by mechanical means for patients with profound cardiac or respiratory failure. The technology includes extracorporeal vascular access, perfusion devices, and management of anticoagulation. ECLS does not treat cardiac or pulmonary failure, but offers hours or days of time to establish a diagnosis and allow time for organ recovery or replacement. Overall success is measured in survival because ECLS is used only in patients at a high risk of dying from acute heart or lung failure. Healthy survival ranges from 95% in some cases of newborn respiratory failure to 40% when ECLS is used as adjunct to cardiac resuscitation.

References

1. Gibbon JH. Application of a mechanical heart and lung apparatus to cardiac surgery. *Minn Med.* 1954;37:171.
2. Lee WH Jr, Krumhar D, Fonkalsrud EW, et al. Denaturation of plasma proteins as a cause of morbidity and death after intracardiac operations. *Surgery.* 1961;50:29–39.
3. Dobell ARC, Mitri M, Galva R, et al. Biological evaluation of blood after prolonged recirculation through film and membrane oxygenators. *Ann Surg.* 1965;161:617–622.
4. Clowes GHA Jr, Hopkins AL, Neville WE. An artificial lung dependent upon diffusion of oxygen and carbon dioxide through plastic membranes. *J Thorac Surg.* 1956;32:630–637.
5. Kolff WJ, Effler DB. Disposable membrane oxygenator (heart lung machine) and its use in experimental and clinical surgery while the heart is arrested with potassium citrate according to the Melrose technique. *Trans Am Soc Artif Intern Organs.* 1956;2:13–21.
6. Pierce EC II. Modification of the Clowes membrane lung. *J Thorac Cardiovasc Surg.* 1960;39:438.
7. Kolobow T, Bowman RL. Construction and evaluation of an alveolar membrane artificial heart-lung. *Trans Am Soc Artif Intern Organs.* 1963;9:238.
8. Bramson ML, Osborn JJ, Main FB, et al. A new disposable membrane oxygenator with integral heat exchanger. *J Thorac Cardiovasc Surg.* 1965;50:391.
9. Landé AJ, Dos SJ, Carlson RG, et al. A new membrane oxygenator-dialyzer. *Surg Clin North Am.* 1967;47:1461.
10. Bartlett RH, Isherwood J, Moss RA, et al. A toroidal flow membrane oxygenator: four day partial bypass in dogs. *Surg Forum.* 1969;20:152–153.

11. Kolobow T, Zapol W, Pierce J. High survival and minimal blood damage in lambs exposed to long term (1 week) veno-venous pumping with a polyurethane chamber roller pump with and without a membrane blood oxygenator. *Trans Am Soc Artif Intern Organs.* 1969;15:172–177.
12. Bartlett RH, Fong SW, Burns NE, et al. Prolonged partial venoarterial bypass: physiologic, biochemical and hematologic responses. *Ann Surg.* 1974;180: 850–856.
13. Fong SW, Burns NE, Williams G, et al. Changes in coagulation and platelet function during prolonged extracorporeal circulation (ECC) in sheep and man. *Trans Am Soc Artif Intern Organs.* 1974;20:239–246.
14. Hill JD, O'Brien TG, Murray JJ, et al. Extracorporeal oxygenation for acute post-traumatic respiratory failure (shock-lung syndrome): use of the Bramson membrane lung. *N Engl J Med.* 1972;286:629–634.
15. Bartlett RH. *Extracorporeal Life Support for Cardiopulmonary Failure. Current Problems in Surgery.* Vol. 27, No. 10. St. Louis, MO: Mosby-Year Book; 1990.
16. Zapol WM, Snider MT, Hill JD, et al. Extracorporeal membrane oxygenation in severe acute respiratory failure: A randomized prospective study. *JAMA.* 1979;242:2193–2196.
17. Bartlett RH, Gazzaniga AB, Jefferies R, et al. Extracorporeal membrane oxygenation (ECMO) cardiopulmonary support in infancy. *Trans Am Soc Artif Intern Organs.* 1976;22:80–88.
18. Bartlett RH, Gazzaniga AB, Fong SW, et al. Prolonged extracorporeal cardiopulmonary support in man. *J Thorac Cardiovasc Surg.* 1974;68:918–932.
19. White JJ, Andrews HG, Risemberg H, et al. Prolonged respiratory support in newborn infants with a membrane oxygenator. *Surgery.* 1971;70:288–296.
20. Dorson WJ, Baker E, Cohen ML, et al. A perfusion system for infants. *Trans Am Soc Artif Intern Organs.* 1969;15:155.
21. Bartlett RH, Andrews AF, Toomasian JM, et al. Extracorporeal membrane oxygenation (ECMO) for newborn respiratory failure: 45 cases. *Surgery.* 1982;92:425–433.
22. Toomasian JM, Snedecor SM, Cornell R, et al. National experience with extracorporeal membrane oxygenation (ECMO) for newborn respiratory failure: Data from 715 cases. *Trans Am Soc Artif Intern Organs.* 1988;34:140–147.
23. Bartlett RH, Roloff DW, Cornell RG, et al. Extracorporeal circulation in neonatal respiratory failure: a prospective randomized study. *Pediatrics.* 1985;4:479–487.
24. O'Rourke PP, Crone R, Vacanti J, et al. Extracorporeal membrane oxygenation and conventional medical therapy in neonates with persistent pulmonary hypertension of the newborn: a prospective randomized study. *Pediatrics.* 1989; 84:957–963.
25. Kolobow T. On how to injure healthy lungs (and prevent sick lungs from recovering). *Trans Am Soc Artif Intern Organs.* 1988;34:31–34.
26. Gattinoni L, Pesenti A, Mascheroni D, et al. Low frequency positive pressure ventilation with extracorporeal CO_2 removal in severe acute respiratory failure. *JAMA.* 1986;256:881–886.
27. Lewandowski K, Rossaint R, Pappert D, et al. High survival rate in 122 ARDS patients managed according to a clinical algorithm including extracorporeal membrane oxygenation. *Intensive Care Med.* 1997;23:819–835.
28. Ullrich R, Larber C, Roder G, et al. Controlled airway pressure therapy, nitric oxide inhalation, prime position, and ECMO as components of an integrated approach to ARDS. *Anesthesiology.* 1999;91:1577–1586.
29. Kolla S, Awad SA, Rich PB, et al. Extracorporeal life support for 100 adult patients with severe respiratory failure. *Ann Surg.* 1997;226:544–566.
30. Hickling K, Walsh J, Henderson S, et al. Low mortality in adult respiratory distress syndrome using low-volume, pressure-limited ventilation with permissive hypercapnia: a prospective study. *Crit Care Med.* 1994;22(10):1568.
31. Amato MB, Barbas CSV, Mederos DM, et al. Effect of a protective ventilator strategy on mortality in the acute respiratory distress syndrome. *N Eng J Med.* 1998;338(6):347–354.
32. The Acute Respiratory Distress Syndrome network. Ventilation with lower tidal volumes as compared with traditional volumes for ARDS. *N Engl J Med.* 2000;342:1301–1308.
33. Van Meurs K, Lally KP, Peek G, et al. *ECMO: Extracorporeal Support in Critical Care.* 3rd ed. Ann Arbor, MI: ELSO, 1996. www.elso.med.umich.edu.
34. Green TP, Timmons OD, Fackler JC, et al. The impact of extracorporeal membrane oxygenation on survival in pediatric patients with acute respiratory failure: Pediatric Critical Care Study. *Crit Care Med.* 1996;24:323–329.
35. Hemmila MR, Rowe SA, Boules TN, et al. Extracorporeal life support for severe acute respiratory syndrome in adults. *Ann Surg.* 2004;240(4).
36. Peek GJ, Moore HM, Sosnowski AW, et al. Extracorporeal membrane oxygenation for adult respiratory failure. *Chest.* 1997;112:759–764.
37. Ullrich R, Lorber C, Roder G, et al. Controlled airway pressure therapy, nitric oxide inhalation, prone position, and extracorporeal membrane oxygenation (ECMO) as components of an integrated approach to ARDS. *Anesthesiology.* 1999;91:1577–1586.
38. Linden V, Palmer K, Reinhard J, et al. High survival in adult patients with acute respiratory distress syndrome treated by extracorporeal membrane oxygenation, minimal sedation, and pressure supported ventilation. *Intensive Care Med.* 2000;26:1630–1637.
39. UK Neonatal ECMO Trial Group. UK collaborative randomized trial of neonatal extracorporeal membrane oxygenation. *Lancet.* 1996;348:75–82.
40. Conventional ventilation or ECMO for severe adult respiratory failure. http://www.cesar-trial.org/.
41. Shapiro MB, Kleaveland AC, Bartlett RH. Extracorporeal life support for status asthmaticus. *Chest.* 1993;103:1651–1654.
42. Thourani VH, Kirshbom PM, Kanter KR, et al. Venoarterial ECMO in pediatric cardiac support. *Ann Thorac Surg.* 2006;82:138–194.
43. Pagani FD, Aaronson KD, Dyke DB, et al. Assessment of an extracorporeal life support LVAD bridge to heart transplant strategy. *Ann Thorac Surg.* 2000;70(6):1977–1984; discussion 1984–1985.
44. Muehreke DD, McCarthy PM, Stewart RW, et al. Extracorporeal membrane oxygenation for postcardiotomy cardiogenic shock. *Ann Thorac Surg.* 1996;61:684–691.
45. Magovern GJ, Simpson KA. Extracorporeal membrane oxygenation for adult cardiac support: the Allegheny experience. *Ann Thorac Surg.* 1999;68: 655–661.
46. Younger JG, Schreiner RJ, Swaniker F, et al. Extracorporeal resuscitation of cardiac arrest. *Acad Emerg Med.* 1999;6(7):700–707.
47. Massetti M, Tasle M, Le Page O, et al. Back from irreversibility: extracorporeal life support for prolonged cardiac arrest. *Ann Thorac Surg.* 2005;79: 178–183.
48. MacLaren G, Butt W, Best D, et al. Extracorporeal membrane oxygenation for refractory septic shock in children: one institution's experience. *Pediatr Crit Care Med.* 2007;8(5):447–451.
49. Magliocca JF, Magee JC, Rowe SA, et al. Extracorporeal support for organ donation after cardiac death safely expands the donor pool. *J Trauma.* 2005;58(6):1095–1101.

CHAPTER 138 ■ DROWNING

ANDREA GABRIELLI • A. JOSEPH LAYON • AHAMED H. IDRIS • JEROME H. MODELL

DEFINITIONS AND DESCRIPTIONS

Several definitions and multiple terminology have appeared during the past half-century regarding the description of victims who suffer a fatal or near-fatal event from being submerged in water and other liquids. Some of the descriptors have had modifications placed on them and, furthermore, their meaning was somewhat lost when translated into some languages other than English. Because drowning is a global problem, at the World Congress on Drowning in Amsterdam, The Netherlands, on June 26 through 28, 2002, a group was convened from multiple countries to develop a definition of "drowning" that would be applicable in multiple languages worldwide (1). Although unanimity may not have been present on every term discussed, there clearly was a consensus to simplify the terminology for international application. What follows is the consensus of that group with comment and, in some cases, slight modification representing the bias of the authors of this chapter.

THE DROWNING PROCESS

Drowning is the process resulting from primary respiratory impairment from submersion or immersion in a liquid medium. Implicit in this definition is that a liquid-to-air interface must be present at the entrance to the victim's airway, thus precluding the possibility of the victim to breathe air. Although it is possible to suffer a drowning episode in multiple types of liquid, this chapter will be confined to the most common use of the terminology, namely, drowning in water.

The drowning process is a continuum that begins when the victim's airway is initially below the surface of the water. At this time, the victim first will voluntarily hold his or her breath. Some victims will swallow significant quantities of water during this time. This period of voluntary breath holding, which has been found in human volunteers to last an average of 87 seconds at rest and shorter with exercise (2), is followed by an involuntary period of laryngospasm secondary to water in the oropharynx or at the level of the larynx acting as a foreign body (3). During this period of breath-holding and laryngospasm, the patient cannot breathe; therefore, oxygen is depleted and carbon dioxide is not eliminated. This results in the patient becoming hypercarbic, hypoxic, and acidotic (4).

As the levels of carbon dioxide increase in the blood and levels of oxygen decrease, respiratory efforts become very active but no exchange of air occurs because of the obstruction at the larynx. Victims who subsequently recover and recall this period frequently describe it as being quite terrifying and painful as they struggle to create intense negative intrapleural pressure breathing against a closed glottis (5). As the patient's arterial oxygen tension drops further, laryngospasm abates, and the patient then actively breathes water. Further evidence of the magnitude of negative pressure created during laryngospasm is the fact that the lungs of drowning victims frequently demonstrate significant hyperinflation at autopsy (6).

The amount of liquid a drowning victim breathes varies considerably between victims (4). Studies comparing the biochemical changes occurring in humans after a drowning episode with those in experimental animals suggest that, while the volume of liquid actually inhaled varies considerably from one victim to another, only 15% of persons who die in the water aspirate in excess of 22 mL/kg of water (7), and the percentage is considerably less in those who survive (4). Changes occur in the lung, body fluids, and electrolyte concentrations, which are dependent on both the composition and volume of the liquid aspirated (8–10).

RESUSCITATION

A victim can be rescued at any time during the drowning process and given the appropriate resuscitation measures, in which case the process is interrupted. The victim may recover with the initial resuscitation efforts or after subsequent therapy aimed at eliminating hypoxia, hypercarbia, and acidosis and restoring normal organ function. If the patient is not removed from the water, then circulatory arrest will occur, and, in the absence of effective resuscitative efforts, multiple organ dysfunction and death will result, primarily from tissue hypoxia.

Although the tolerance to hypoxia of various tissues is different, it should be noted that the brain is the organ most at risk for permanent detrimental changes from relative brief periods of hypoxia. Frequently, the question is asked, How long can a person be submerged and still be rescued and resuscitated back to a normal life? While, obviously, there are no controlled human studies—nor should there be on this subject—the limiting time factor is likely the duration that cerebral hypoxia can be tolerated before irreversible changes occur. Irreversible damage to brain tissue is reported to begin approximately 3 minutes after the PaO_2 falls below 30 mm Hg under normothermic conditions in otherwise normal people (11). Such data suggest that if the victim is rescued and effective resuscitation efforts are applied within 3 minutes of the cessation of respiration (i.e., submersion in water), the vast majority of such victims should be able to be resuscitated and suffer no permanent brain damage. Further, because the period of voluntary breath holding and laryngospasm is thought to last for approximately 1½ to 2 minutes (2,12), persons who are retrieved within that time frame will likely not suffer lung damage secondary to the aspiration of liquid. Once the 3-minute time frame has been exceeded, although some normal survivors are reported, it becomes less likely that normal survival will result from resuscitation efforts. This time frame may be prolonged if hypothermia occurs rapidly because it decreases the cerebral requirement for oxygen.

Trained divers have been shown to be able to voluntarily hold their breath for much longer periods of time, approaching 4 to 5 minutes without complication (13). Persons who become hypothermic due to immersion or submersion in extremely cold water will rapidly develop hypothermia, which protects the brain by decreasing its oxygen requirement, and prolongs survival (14). In the latter case, seemingly miraculous recoveries of patients who have been submerged for over 20 minutes have been reported (15). It should be noted, however, that hypothermia is a two-edged sword; although it can protect the brain from oxygen deprivation, it also can cause death in the water secondary to its effect on the conduction system of the heart, resulting in circulatory arrest either by asystole or ventricular fibrillation (16).

The drowning process can be altered by the initiating event, such as if the victim suffers trauma, develops syncope or unconsciousness, has a circulatory arrest either by asystole or ventricular fibrillation as the precipitating event, hyperventilates prior to breath-holding under water, or has a convulsive disorder that leads him or her to become incapacitated, thereby becoming submerged, or if the victim's judgment and/or motor function is impaired by significant parenteral levels of depressant drugs, including alcohol. For example, in the victim who suffers a concussion from a blow to the head, subsequent recollection of the events is unlikely. If trauma results in a cervical fracture, disastrous damage to the spinal cord may occur acutely and, thus, motor function may be lost below that level. If the victim has a circulatory arrest either by asystole or ventricular fibrillation as a precipitating event, respiration will cease, and it is highly unlikely that significant amounts of water will be breathed into the lung given that active respiration is necessary for this to occur (17). If the victim hyperventilates prior to breath holding under water, it has been shown that the breath-holding breaking point can be extended until the level of hypoxia is so severe that consciousness is lost, and thus the victim actively breathes in water (2,12). The effect of drug usage is variable, depending on the level of depression and the patient's response. There is considerable variation in tolerance to depressant drugs and alcohol and their effects on performance and orientation. To better understand what to expect in each victim, the initiating event should be reported in every case if it is known.

When a person experiences a drowning episode, the result can be death or survival. Furthermore, the victim can survive without residual damage, or with residual damage to varying degrees (e.g., from minor neurologic difficulty to one that has no normal function other than continuation of an effective heart beat with or without spontaneous respiration).

CLASSIFICATIONS

The terms *drown* and *near-drown* have been used for decades in an attempt to separate these outcomes (18). At the World Congress on Drowning, however, it became apparent that their meaning was not felt to be clear when translated into some languages (1). Furthermore, a victim could have no signs of spontaneous physiologic function and, therefore, be "drowned"; however, once resuscitative efforts were applied, they would respond positively and survive to varying degrees and, thus, the term applied to them would have to be changed to "near-drown" (19). In addition, there is another group who do not die acutely, but die later of complications from their drowning episode. In this case, the question is, Were they "near-drowned" or were they "drowned"?

The definition of "drowned" we believe to be fairly clear—namely, death secondary to undergoing the drowning episode. "Near-drowned" presents a significantly greater problem of understanding. We believe that the term "drowned" should be retained for both those who die acutely in the water and those who die later of consequences directly resulting from the submersion episode. However, we agree with the consensus of the World Congress members that "near-drowned" may lead to unnecessary confusion and, therefore, should be replaced by terminology such as "the victim survived the drowning episode" and then describe the ultimate condition of the victim.

Other terms that have appeared in the literature over the past few decades that we believe are confusing and should be abandoned are as follows:

Dry versus wet drowning: Because all drowning occurs in liquid, by definition, they are all wet. This terminology has been used by some to categorize drowning victims into those who aspirate liquid into the lungs and those who do not. Frequently, it is not possible to determine at the scene of the accident whether the victim actually did aspirate water. This is particularly true when the quantity of water aspirated is small. Further, if evidence of fluid aspiration is not detected in the victim who dies or is discovered dead in the water, the diagnosis may be suspect (20). In these cases, one should look for other explanations such as acute mechanical standstill of the heart, from asystole or ventricular fibrillation, or, for that matter, whether the victim actually was alive when he or she first became submerged.

Active versus passive versus silent drowning: This terminology has been used by some to separate those victims who are observed to be struggling at the surface of the water from those who are first discovered when they are actually submerged and motionless. It has been shown with underwater cameras that even victims who were not seen to be in difficulty on the surface of the water by observers may have had unrecognized active motion while submerged. We believe, therefore, that these terms should be abandoned in favor of the terms "witnessed," when the episode is witnessed from the onset of submersion/immersion to the time of rescue, or "unwitnessed," when a body is found in the water without anybody seeing how it got there.

Secondary drowning: This terminology has been used by some to describe a situation when a precipitating event from another origin (e.g., syncope) causes a victim to be below the surface of the water, and then he or she drowns. On the other hand, some use this terminology to describe a victim who appears to be recovering from a drowning episode in the hospital and then develops adult respiratory distress syndrome. Not only is this terminology confusing but also, in the latter instance, a patient does not experience a second submersion or drowning episode, and therefore, this terminology should be abandoned.

PATHOPHYSIOLOGY

There have been extensive studies both in animals (7–9,14,18,21–34) and in humans (4,6,20,35–40) over the past century in an attempt to quantitate the changes that occur as a result of a drowning episode. What has consistently been shown over and over again is that, acutely, drowning produces asphyxia (i.e., hypoxia, hypercarbia, and acidosis). The hypercarbia is due to absent or ineffective ventilation, and is readily correctable when aggressive mechanical ventilation is instituted. The hypoxia that occurs initially is not as readily correctable and may be persistent for long periods of time (8–10). This hypoxia is first due to apnea, and then primarily to intrapulmonary shunting from alveoli that are perfused but not being ventilated, or not being ventilated adequately (32). The acidosis is mixed, and the respiratory component rapidly disappears with effective ventilation. The patient is, however, frequently left with significant metabolic acidosis due to anaerobic metabolism during the period of time that profound tissue hypoxia secondary to absent or ineffective respiration and cardiac output was present. The hallmark of this high anion gap metabolic acidosis is an increased level of serum lactic acid.

Pulmonary

While intrapulmonary shunting occurs after both fresh water and sea water aspiration, the etiology is different (33). In the case of fresh water, the aspirated water alters the surface tension properties of pulmonary surfactant. Thus, the alveoli become unstable and do not maintain their normal shape or patency, resulting in an increase in both absolute and relative intrapulmonary shunt (32,33). Sea water does not change the surface tension properties of pulmonary surfactant but, because it is hypertonic, it pulls fluid from the circulation into the alveoli, thus producing obstruction to gas exchange at the alveolar level. Bronchoconstriction also has been reported after aspiration of even small quantities of water (28).

Fresh water, being hypotonic, is absorbed very rapidly into the circulation and, because of the transient hypervolemia that occurs and the change in the surface tension properties of pulmonary surfactant, pulmonary edema results. The pulmonary edema is most commonly described as frothy or foamy and blood-tinged. This coloring is secondary to the presence of free plasma hemoglobin from the rupture of some red blood cells due to the absorption of hypotonic fluid into the circulation in the face of hypoxia (41). Pulmonary edema also occurs when sea water is aspirated, secondary to a semipermeable membrane effect because the sea water is hypertonic compared to plasma. Even though the etiology of the hypoxia is different between fresh water and sea water aspiration, the result of both is to increase intrapulmonary shunt, which requires aggressive therapy (32,42,43).

Extensive studies of serum electrolyte concentrations after drowning have shown that only 15% of victims who die in the water aspirate more than 22 mL/kg of water. In patients who survive, the percentage is much less and, thus, significant changes in serum electrolyte concentrations that require treatment are rarely observed (7), with the only exception being, perhaps, victims of drowning in the Dead Sea (44).

The treatment of the respiratory lesion requires providing mechanical ventilatory support in a fashion that will restore an adequate functional residual capacity and keep the alveoli open during all phases of the respiratory cycle, thus decreasing the intrapulmonary shunt. Obviously, if foreign material such as sand, silt, or plant life is aspirated into the lung, it may produce obstruction, and it should be removed via bronchoscopy.

Cardiovascular

The cardiovascular changes that occur during a drowning episode can best be ascribed to inadequate oxygenation. Although fatal arrhythmia such as ventricular fibrillation is rarely documented in human drowning victims, ventricular fibrillation can occur with profound hypoxia, especially if very significant changes in serum potassium and serum sodium result from the movement of fluid and rupture of red blood cells. Although a wide variety of cardiac arrhythmias have been reported (45), particularly in animal models, rarely do they require specific therapy other than improving oxygenation and correcting severe metabolic acidosis. More common problems are profound hypoxia and the leak of fluid into the lung as pulmonary edema, resulting in a relative hypovolemia in the patient. It has been shown by multiple investigators that to treat this hypovolemia, it may be necessary to infuse significant amounts of intravenous fluid to maintain an adequate effective circulating blood volume, even in the face of pulmonary edema (26,43). Without such therapy, even though the arterial oxygen tension might have improved with mechanical ventilatory support, the delivery of oxygen to the tissues remains compromised and incompatible with supplying adequate tissue oxygenation (43). Use of vasopressors and other pharmacologic agents may be indicated as a temporary crutch, so to speak, in these patients; however, they are not a substitute for providing adequate oxygenation and adequate intravascular fluid volume. If the latter are established, it is highly unlikely that pharmacologic support of the heart will be necessary.

Renal

Detrimental changes in renal function are rarely seen in persons recovering from near-drowning. However, when present, they likely are the result of inadequate perfusion and oxygenation rather than anything specifically related to the drowning episode *per se*. Some have emphasized the need for the kidneys to clear free plasma hemoglobin after fresh water drowning; however, significant levels of free plasma hemoglobin have rarely been reported in such patients. This is likely due to the fact that for red blood cells to rupture and release enough hemoglobin into the plasma during a drowning episode to require specific therapy for its clearance, it requires transfer of substantial volumes of free water into the circulation in the face of hypoxia (41). As stated above, this rarely occurs.

INITIAL RESCUE AND RESUSCITATION

To ensure survival after a drowning episode, it is imperative that one never lose sight of the fact that time is of the essence. The longer a person is without the ability to breathe air, the more profound are the hypoxia and permanent damage to vital tissues. Thus, those who are entrusted with guarding swimming facilities must never lose sight of the fact that continual vigilance is required to recognize a victim in distress, and that the victim must be removed from the water and resuscitative measures begun in a timely fashion. Frequently, bodies are discovered motionless in a pool, without anyone in attendance being able to pinpoint the length of time that the victim was submerged. In many cases, lifeguards report that they thought the victim was "fooling around" and, therefore, they did not effect a timely rescue. Also, lifeguards may be assigned other duties such as pool maintenance and tending to concession stands, thus precluding them from timely recognition of a victim in trouble and prompt rescue.

Frequently, bathers are permitted to deliberately hyperventilate on the side of the pool before becoming submerged to see "how long they can hold their breath" or "how far they can swim under water." These practices are to be condemned. If an individual is not noted to be making purposeful movements for more than 10 seconds, rescue attempts should be initiated (46). The individual responsible for safety at the pool should always be in proper attire and in position to effect such a rescue and complete it within 20 seconds of the recognition of the problem.

While removing the victim from the water, care should be taken to avoid complicating neck injuries when they are suspected. Routine stabilization of the neck is unnecessary unless the circumstances leading to the drowning episode suggest that trauma was likely (47). These circumstances include a history of diving, use of a water slide, signs of injury, or evidence of alcohol intoxication. If neck injury is suspected, gentle immobilization of the head should be accomplished, securing it in a neutral position. However, if the neck appears to be obviously deformed and the patient has pain with neck movement, the neck should be immobilized in the existing position.

If the victim is apneic, the airway should rapidly be cleared of foreign material, a patent airway secured, and mouth-to-mouth resuscitation started immediately. It is preferable to begin artificial ventilation in the water if it can be accomplished without jeopardizing the safety of the rescuer. It should be remembered that not all victims are in a state of cardiac arrest when the rescue attempt begins. They may be in a state of vasoconstriction or have a significant bradycardia, in which case, if effective ventilation is started, the myocardium will be reoxygenated, and increased cardiac activity will result in improved tissue perfusion.

Upon removing the victim from the water, he or she should rapidly be assessed for the presence of both spontaneous respiration and cardiac activity. In the absence of these, the airway should be inspected rapidly to ensure that there is no mechanical obstruction, and artificial respiration and cardiac compression should be instituted without delay. Chest compression alone—without artificial respiration—is an alternate resuscitation method that has been proposed for victims of dysrhythmic cardiac arrest. It must be emphasized that these recommendations do not apply to the drowning victim because the pathophysiologic lesion in the lungs requires active attempts at reinflation and stabilization of the alveoli. Therefore, cardiac arrest following drowning is more likely due to asphyxia, and thus, immediate provision of ventilation is recommended (47).

If equipment is available at the site for administering supplemental oxygen, it should be delivered in the highest concentration possible under the existing conditions. Electrical activity of the heart should quickly be evaluated and an automatic defibrillator applied if indicated. A pulse oximeter will frequently be of assistance in determining the effectiveness of oxygenation. However, many pulse oximeters do not work well if the victim is cold and vasoconstricted or if there is excessive movement.

Although the airway should rapidly be inspected for the presence of obstructing material, the abdominal thrust maneuver, which had been advocated by some in the past, has been thoroughly debated and found not to be of value in treating a drowning victim unless solid material is actually blocking the conducting airway (47,48). If the victim is apneic and a pulse is absent, chest compression should be initiated promptly (47). Chest compression alone can be effective in relieving airway obstruction.

PATIENT TRANSPORT AND EMERGENCY MEDICAL SERVICES

Neither equipment nor properly trained personnel are usually available at the site to provide advanced cardiac life support, including endotracheal intubation, intravenous access, drug therapy, and electrical defibrillation. However, these measures should be instituted when indicated and when the proper equipment and properly trained personnel are available. It is crucial that someone other than the individual rescuing and resuscitating the patient contact emergency medical services (EMS) as rapidly as possible so that they can respond in a timely fashion and perform advanced cardiac life support treatment on the victim.

Whenever a drowning victim has to be transported to a location or facility such as a hospital emergency room, it is important that a call be made promptly to inform the emergency room personnel of the exact circumstances, type of treatment instituted, and condition of the patient en route so that they will be prepared to accept the patient and render appropriate therapy immediately upon arrival.

When moving a critically ill drowning victim, it is imperative to remember the fragility of such patients because they can decompensate in a matter of a few seconds or minutes if appropriate therapy is withdrawn. Examples of such situations are movement (a) from the scene to the EMS vehicle, (b) from the EMS vehicle to the hospital emergency department, or (c) from the hospital emergency department to other hospital locations for testing, such as radiology, or for treatment, such as the intensive care unit (ICU). Thus, every attempt should be made to continue essential therapy at all times.

Treatment in the Emergency Department

In the emergency department, a thorough evaluation of the patient should be performed, keeping in mind that the most serious problems that require immediate therapy are pulmonary insufficiency and cardiovascular instability, which result in inadequate delivery of oxygen to vital tissues. If the victim is responding fully, does not require respiratory or cardiovascular support, and has a normal oxyhemoglobin saturation while breathing room air, it is unlikely that the victim has aspirated a significant amount of water, and observation may be all that is necessary. At the other extreme is the patient who is still unconscious and requires extensive pulmonary and cardiovascular support in an attempt to normalize vital signs and produce adequate cardiac output and tissue oxygenation. Thus, a cookbook-type treatment that would apply to *every* victim cannot be prescribed. However, the treating physician should keep in mind that increased intrapulmonary shunt and poorly matched ventilation-to-perfusion ratios are the rule rather than the exception for the victim who has aspirated a significant quantity of water.

Therapy must be aimed at improving ventilation-to-perfusion ratios and restoring adequate residual lung volume to optimally oxygenate the blood. A relative hypovolemia frequently is present due to fluid shifts between the lung and the circulation. These can be accentuated by the increase in mean intrathoracic pressure that occurs with mechanical ventilatory support. Thus, evaluation of effective circulating blood volume and replenishment of intravascular fluid volume to physiologic levels is important as a primary concern.

While currently some controversy exists regarding when to treat metabolic acidosis in persons who have suffered a cardiac arrest, we believe that the adverse effect of acidosis on the pulmonary vasculature and cardiac function is sufficient so that metabolic acidosis producing a pH of less than 7.20 should be treated with intravenous sodium bicarbonate. If the patient is a victim of sea water drowning and has aspirated sufficient water to produce hypernatremia, we might be better advised to use an agent such as tris (hydroxymethyl) aminomethane (Tris) buffer; 2-amino-2-hydroxyl-1.3-propandiol (THAM) to avoid compounding the hypernatremia. However, once again, it should be noted that the quantity of water aspirated is seldom sufficient to produce such significant changes in serum electrolyte concentrations, except perhaps when the drowning occurs in water of extreme hypersalinity such as the Dead Sea (44).

Changes in serum electrolyte concentrations and hemoglobin and hematocrit of sufficient magnitude to justify specific therapy are rare, as are alterations in renal function other than those that might be expected in the hypovolemic, hypoxic, or markedly acidotic patient.

The patient's level of consciousness on admission to the emergency room has been shown to markedly influence outcome (49,50). The most important consideration here is to provide adequate oxygenation and perfusion and to avoid producing increased intracranial pressure if possible. Treatments aimed specifically at preservation of cerebral function have not been shown to be particularly beneficial to date (50,51).

If the patient requires diagnostic testing in a distant location such as the radiology department, it is imperative that adequate personnel and equipment accompany the patient to ensure that optimum therapy is not interrupted at any time during transport or when performing the procedure. Likewise, transportation to the intensive care unit should be done with a "full team approach." Should optimum therapy be interrupted during any of these time periods, adverse consequences should be anticipated.

Drowning episodes in cold water may produce significant hypothermia. There are several methods of rewarming that have been recommended including, but not necessarily limited to, heating blankets, warmed intravenous fluids, warmed humidification of breathing circuits, gastric lavage, and cardiopulmonary bypass. The method used should be tailored to the resources available and the condition of the patient. It must be remembered, however, that rewarming peripheral tissues before the patient's circulation is capable of supplying adequate amounts of oxygenated blood can compound the situation and increase the degree of metabolic acidosis.

IN-HOSPITAL THERAPY: POSTRESUSCITATION CARE

Expert intensive care is vital to survival once optimal prehospital and emergency department management have been performed. Hemodynamic instability after cardiac arrest, respiratory insufficiency, and severe neurologic impairment are all criteria for admission to the intensive care unit. The administrative structure of the hospital's critical care service dictates the setting to which the patient is admitted. A recent attempt to classify survivors of drowning based on the severity of symptoms on a scale of 1 to 6 recommends ICU admission for all pediatric patients requiring high concentrations of oxygen, with or without the need for invasive ventilation (52).

Respiratory Support

Although the degree of intrapulmonary shunting after drowning is variable from one patient to the next, if the patient is breathing adequately to clear carbon dioxide, the single most important method of treatment in reversing hypoxemia is the application of continuous positive airway pressure (CPAP). The amount of CPAP applied must be individualized because the degree of atelectasis, the amount of pulmonary edema, and the magnitude of the intrapulmonary shunt varies between patients. In great measure, this will depend on the type and quantity of the water aspirated. Although the mechanism for producing the intrapulmonary shunt is different between fresh water and sea water (33), Lee found no statistically significant difference between the PaO_2/FiO_2 ratio in patients after the two types of aspiration (53).

The pathophysiologic mechanism involved in fresh water drowning is lowering of the sodium concentration in the alveolus, thus changing the surface tension characteristics of pulmonary surfactant (33,54). The alteration in the surface tension properties of pulmonary surfactant increases alveolar surface tension upon compression of the surfactant layer and results in alveolar volume loss. Also, pulmonary capillaries become more permeable, resulting in an increase in interstitial lung water that eventually compresses alveoli and promotes volume loss and causes pulmonary edema. Based on the severity of the acute respiratory derangement, this "abnormal surfactant state" has been termed *acute lung injury* (ALI) or acute respiratory distress syndrome (ARDS) (55).

ALI and ARDS represent a final common pathway that accompanies a number of physiologic insults that may occur after drowning, including respiratory obstruction, aspiration of water or gastric contents, and global hypoxemia from cardiovascular insufficiency or cardiac arrest. Unfortunately, ALI and ARDS often can be clinically and radiologically confused with acute pulmonary edema from left ventricular dysfunction or fluid overload of different etiologies.

Both CPAP and positive end-expiratory pressure (PEEP) have the capability to restore lung volume and improve oxygenation in many patients with decreased lung volume, especially functional residual capacity. However, there are some differences in their function. By definition, CPAP means that airway pressure remains positive during all phases of the respiratory cycle. With PEEP, during the inspiratory phase of a spontaneous breath, circuit pressures drop to zero or become negative as a result of a vigorous inspiratory effort by the patient. Because PEEP with spontaneous ventilation increases the work of breathing, it may increase pressure gradients between the pulmonary vasculature and the alveoli, thereby leading to more pulmonary edema. Also, it does not forcibly inflate alveoli with abnormal surfactant after fresh water drowning (32). Thus, CPAP is more beneficial than PEEP for spontaneously breathing drowning victims (42,56).

Both CPAP and PEEP increase expiratory pressure; thus, air is trapped within the lungs during the expiratory phase of respiration. This results in an increase in residual lung volume in many patients with ARDS. As alveolar units re-expand, intrapulmonary shunt decreases, and improvement is seen in oxygenation and compliance. The increase in compliance decreases the work of breathing (57). The degree of lung volume restoration roughly correlates with the improvement in oxygenation. As lung volume increases toward normal, gas exchange continues to improve. It has been shown, however, that while the above beneficial effect is found with CPAP in many victims of both fresh and sea water drowning (56,58), unless mechanical breaths are added, PEEP does not improve the ventilation-to-perfusion ratio after fresh water drowning (32,42,56). Also, in some fresh water drowning victims, CPAP alone does not produce an adequate response, and hence, mechanical breaths should be added (42).

When ARDS develops and oxygen desaturation occurs, an FiO_2 of 1.0 is recommended to attempt to restore adequate oxygenation. Increased work of breathing, severe hypoxemia, and hypercarbia are all indications for instituting mechanical ventilation. Ordinarily, CPAP is titrated to achieve an oxygen saturation greater than 95%, with the lowest possible inspired oxygen (FiO_2) levels down to an FiO_2 of 0.5 or less. We routinely increase CPAP at the bedside in increments of 3 to 5 cm H_2O in an attempt to achieve an oxygen saturation of 95%, and subsequently, the FiO_2 is gradually decreased to reach a PaO_2/FiO_2 of greater than 300 mm Hg. Increased dead-space ventilation and decreased preload are the two most important adverse effects that can limit the use of CPAP. Once adequate PaO_2/FiO_2 has been achieved, CPAP can slowly be weaned based on improvement of patient lung compliance and general clinical conditions.

Mechanical Ventilation

CPAP therapy alone is not sufficient in the case of the patient who is apneic, hypoventilating, or hypercarbic or shows little to no improvement in ventilation-to-perfusion matching while breathing spontaneously. In these patients, mechanical ventilatory breaths must also be provided. In general, mechanical ventilation in patients with ALI or ARDS can be applied either noninvasively or invasively (i.e., face mask vs. endotracheal tube, respectively). Noninvasive ventilation is reserved for milder cases of ARDS or pulmonary edema when the patient is awake, cooperative, triggering spontaneous ventilation, and has his or her swallowing and protective laryngeal reflexes intact. Although successful experience with noninvasive positive pressure ventilation (NPPV) for patients with respiratory failure other than from chronic obstructive pulmonary disease (COPD) is growing (59), potential complications include gastric distention, nasal congestion, regurgitation and aspiration of stomach contents, nasal bridge ulceration, and eye irritation (60). Several modes of mechanical ventilation and adjunct therapies are available; while not specifically used in drowning, their use has proven valuable in the ventilatory support of any patient with ALI or ARDS. A list of the most commonly used forms in drowning victims follows.

Controlled Mechanical Ventilation

Controlled mechanical ventilation (CMV) provides total ventilation, and it does not permit spontaneous breathing. It usually is indicated only in patients who are apneic, deeply comatose, deeply sedated, or paralyzed. All breaths delivered with CMV are positive pressure breaths; therefore, mean intrathoracic pressure is increased with potential deleterious hemodynamic effects. Most notable of these is the impedance of venous return, thus effectively causing a relative hypovolemia and decreased cardiac output (43).

Intermittent Mandatory Ventilation

Intermittent mandatory ventilation (IMV) combines mechanical ventilatory breaths with spontaneous breathing, and is better tolerated than CMV by most patients (61). Allowing some spontaneous breathing reduces mean intrathoracic pressure, which increases venous return and maintains better cardiac output. It also may reduce the incidence of barotrauma. The numbers of mechanical breaths used are those necessary to supplement the patient's own spontaneous ability to maintain adequate minute ventilation. As the patient is recovering, the ventilator rate is gradually reduced by one to two breaths per minute down to a minimum of two breaths per minute. IMV remains the mainstay of our ventilator support. It may be coupled with other modes such as pressure support ventilation (PSV).

Pressure Support Ventilation

The primary benefit of this ventilatory mode is to reduce the inspiratory work of breathing. The patient maintains control of the inspiratory-to-expiratory ratio, inspiratory time, and frequency during the spontaneous efforts. The mechanical breath delivered during PSV usually discontinues once flow decreases to 25% of peak inspiratory flow. Adjustable pressure support parameters include the time necessary to reach maximal flow or rate of rise of PSV. A shorter pressure rise time is generally used to reduce work of breathing in patients with the highest inspiratory flow demand.

PSV has the capability to reduce or eliminate both imposed (apparatus and airway resistance) and physiologic (lung and chest wall static compliance) work of breathing. Therefore, by choosing the appropriate level of PSV, the clinician may reduce or eliminate the extra imposed work of breathing and keep the physiologic work of breathing within tolerable limits.

In spite of a careful, stepwise approach to mechanical ventilation in ALI and ARDS, iatrogenic complications are frequent. Several potentially protective measures have been evaluated to reduce the incidence of barotrauma from increased peak airway pressure in patients with severely reduced total lung compliance; however, strong evidence in favor of their use is still lacking.

Nitric Oxide

Inhaled nitric oxide (NO) appears to act selectively on the pulmonary vascular bed and only in those areas associated with adequate ventilation, locally reversing hypoxic pulmonary vasoconstriction and increasing oxygenation. However, outcome in terms of mortality or number of days alive and off mechanical ventilation between patients treated with NO and those not treated has not changed when the effect of NO is studied in a prospective randomized fashion (62). Nevertheless, reducing the level of mechanical ventilatory support or FiO_2 needed to achieve adequate oxygenation is a potential benefit that could reduce barotrauma and the side effects of treatment.

Prone Positioning

Rotation of patients from supine to prone may cause rapid improvement in oxygenation that may last for up to 12 hours (63). With this maneuver, there is a relatively high risk of inadvertent extubation and removal of invasive monitors; nonetheless, oxygenation improves mainly because the nondependent dorsal portion of the lung has a higher air-to-tissue ratio (64). Obviously, the risks and benefits need to be considered before using this technique in any specific patient.

Bronchodilator Therapy

Small airway closure has been shown to occur even with aspiration of relatively small amounts of water (25). Thus, bronchodilator therapy should be considered in patients when bronchospasm is thought to be present.

Corticosteroids

The rationale for use of corticosteroids in ARDS seems to be limited to the fibroproliferative phase to reduce the incidence of pulmonary fibrosis (65). However, its efficacy for use in drowning victims has not been shown either in large retrospective clinical studies (4) or in prospective animal studies (66). Corticosteroids can interfere with normal pulmonary healing and increase the rate of sepsis. Corticosteroids have been associated with higher mortality in one study, probably due to the immunosuppressant effect in patients with sepsis (67). In another, their use has shown, after aspiration of gastric contents, to increase pulmonary granuloma formation (68,69).

Surfactant

ARDS from drowning involves both quantitative (sea water) and qualitative (fresh water) alterations in lung surfactant (33,70). Although the use of exogenous surfactant has been shown to lower mortality in neonates with respiratory distress syndrome (71), this effect in adults has been disappointing, and its prohibitive cost makes its use infrequent (72).

Prophylactic Antibiotics

The use of broad-spectrum antibiotics may enhance the emergence of resistant organisms. An exception represents survival from drowning in heavily contaminated water such as stagnant ponds or public spas, where *Pseudomonas* species are endemic. Our initial choice in this situation is usually a fourth-generation cephalosporin with broad Gram-negative coverage. In other patients, antibiotics are not recommended unless the patient develops evidence of infection, in which case cultures and sensitivities will guide the choice of antibiotics to be given.

Cardiovascular Support

By the time a drowning victim reaches the intensive care unit, cardiac arrhythmias are rarely a problem. If witnessed in the emergency department or the ICU, the most common cause of arrhythmias is severe hypoxia, and providing adequate ventilation and oxygenation will usually restore a normal rhythm. If not, drug therapy or, in the case of severe ventricular arrhythmias, electrical intervention is appropriate.

Hypotension may require initial pharmacologic support, but it should be remembered that the hypotension seen in drowning victims is predominantly due to fluid shifts resulting in hypovolemia (26,43). This hypovolemia may be accentuated when mechanical ventilatory techniques that increase mean intrathoracic pressure are used (43).

Experimental studies have shown that, whereas mechanical ventilation and CPAP will decrease intrapulmonary shunt and increase PaO_2, because of the detrimental effect on cardiac output, tissue perfusion is compromised. In one study, attempting to increase oxygen delivery by use of vasopressors and inotropes was not productive, but fluid administration to increase blood volume resulted in an increased cardiac output and oxygen delivery (43).

Precise fluid replacement is dependent on an accurate assessment of effective circulating blood volume. To this end, monitoring the patient with a pulmonary artery catheter or transesophageal echocardiography is extremely helpful.

Central Nervous System Support

The two most important factors influencing morbidity and mortality in victims surviving drowning are severe respiratory insufficiency and permanent neurologic impairment secondary to cerebral hypoxia. Despite improvement in emergency and intensive pulmonary and cardiovascular care, neurologic outcome in drowning patients is directly related to the initial duration of hypoxia from the onset of submersion until effective cardiopulmonary resuscitation (CPR) is provided. The Glasgow coma scale (GCS) score mirrors this relationship during the first few hours after submersion.

The most common cerebral lesion results from cytotoxic injury due to global central nervous system (CNS) hypoxemia. Cerebral edema, which usually is not clinically evident or is mild on presentation, reaches its peak by day 2 to 3 after the submersion event. It is understood that successful intensive care management of these patients reflects the ability to control the intracranial pressure (ICP) and limit secondary brain injury from inadequate cerebral perfusion and hypoxia through standard protocols. Therefore, monitoring of the intracranial pressure is often recommended in patients with a GCS score compatible with severe central nervous system injury (8 and below), in conjunction with what is described in detail in the neurosurgical guidelines for traumatic brain injury (73). Unfortunately, monitoring of ICP has not been shown to increase normal survival after drowning.

Seizure prophylaxis is immediately initiated in patients with CNS compromise, and ventilatory rate is titrated to achieve a $PaCO_2$ of 35 to 40 mm Hg. Although a chronic lower level of $PaCO_2$ has been often used in the past to decrease intracranial pressure, it is no longer recommended except for only a short period of time and only in patients with an acute increase of ICP refractory to pharmacotherapy or ventriculostomy drainage while a definitive imaging diagnosis is in process. In fact, chronic hyperventilation, while decreasing the ICP, can be accompanied by a reduction in cerebral blood flow (74), which can result in worsening cerebral ischemia (75). There are no data to support the use of barbiturates or steroids to lower refractory ICP (51). Despite adequate control of the intracranial pressure and maintenance of the cerebral perfusion pressure with aggressive brain resuscitation modalities, the majority of patients who were severely comatose upon arrival to the ICU died or left the ICU in a persistent vegetative state, because the damage from the initial event was so severe that it was irreversible (49,50).

Control of Blood Glucose Levels

Aggressive blood glucose control (less than 110 mg/dL) with insulin infusion has been associated with a reduced mortality, from 8% to 4.3%, when compared with intermittent doses of subcutaneous regular insulin in a heterogeneous large group of critically ill patients that were prospectively randomized (76). While this study included a variety of patients admitted to the intensive care unit with hypoxic or hypercapnic respiratory failure, the reduction in mortality from multiple organ failure suggests a possible benefit in patients surviving episodes of drowning who require prolonged ICU hospitalization. Interestingly, critical illness polyneuropathy was reduced 44% in the insulin infusion group. It is our practice to control the blood sugar level with an insulin infusion in any critically ill patient with a level above normal. A glucose-based crystalloid infusion is used when blood sugar is below 200 mg/dL to limit the risk of hypoglycemia. Blood glucose level is usually checked every 1 or 2 hours. Recent data (77), however, suggest that there may not be a positive difference if the glucose level is controlled at 110 mg/dL as compared to 150 mg/dL. Rather, the more intensive glucose control may lead to more episodes of hypoglycemia. While not advocating out-of-control glucose values, we are actively re-evaluating the appropriate level of control to values between 130 and 150 mg/dL.

Renal Support

Albuminuria, hemoglobinuria, oliguria, and anuria, while rare, have all been described in drowning victims secondary to acute tubular necrosis from hypoxemia, rhabdomyolysis, or both. Hypothermia leads to reduced blood flow to the skin and muscle, preserving core temperature and central organ perfusion. The acute pathophysiology of acute rhabdomyolysis is probably secondary to tissue hypoxia from acute vessel constriction due to the competitive need for heat conservation. Skeletal myolysis and increased circulating myoglobin will result. Acute renal failure may be aggravated by acute tubular necrosis secondary to hemodynamic instability.

Acute tubular necrosis and rhabdomyolysis require early and vigorous treatment directed at correcting hypovolemia, improving oxygenation, and enhancing heme protein elimination. Volume replacement therapy aims to restore normal blood flow and enhance renal oxygen supply. The medullary ascending limb of Henle loop is most vulnerable to hypoxic injury. Invasive monitoring may be necessary to provide adequate intravascular volume. A central venous pressure or pulmonary wedge pressure around 15 mm Hg is a reasonable hemodynamic goal if ventricular function is normal. Higher pressures may be necessary in patients with a significant increase in mean intrathoracic pressure. Right ventricular ejection fraction, a pulmonary artery catheter, or transthoracic or transesophageal echocardiography can be used if the interpretation of preload by invasive monitoring is difficult, as often is the case in patients requiring major ventilator support. The window of opportunity for restoration of intravascular volume and volume expansion is likely within 6 hours or less of the acute event.

If rhabdomyolysis is present, enhancing the elimination of heme protein helps to limit tubular damage. Systemic alkalinization of the urine with sodium bicarbonate increases the solubility and, therefore, the elimination of heme protein (78). A urine pH between 7 and 8 produces a myoglobin solubility of around 80% and is a reasonable goal. However, in a patient with low urine output, massive doses of sodium bicarbonate may be associated with volume overload secondary to an acute increase in intravascular osmolarity (79). In these cases, when the hemodynamic goal is mild hypervolemia, the weak diuretic acetazolamide may be a valid alternative. Acetazolamide increases the excretion of bicarbonate in urine as a result of the inhibition of the carbonic anhydrase enzyme; for regulatory reasons, the drug will no longer be available in the United States within the next year. However, diuretics, particularly in patients on significant ventilatory support, may adversely affect venous filling and cardiac output. Three other therapeutic agents have been used successfully to preserve renal function in patients with acute rhabdomyolysis: dopamine, loop diuretics, and mannitol. All three drugs enhance recovery of renal function by optimizing the relationship between renal oxygen supply and demand after a hypoxic insult (80).

Manipulating the renal output by means of significantly altering the effective circulating blood volume in drowning victims frequently has a detrimental effect on pulmonary and cardiovascular function. Therefore, a fine-tuned balancing act is frequently required to not adversely affect one organ system while treating another.

Other Concerns

Severe metabolic acidosis from low systemic oxygen delivery and resulting anaerobic metabolism should be corrected. We recommend correction of the base deficit with bicarbonate or acetate solutions to maintain a pH no lower than 7.20. Mechanical ventilation is adjusted frequently with the help of arterial blood gas determinations to maintain a $PaCO_2$ between 35 and 40 mm Hg. Lactic acid levels are checked frequently for a few hours after resuscitation. In fact, while base deficit and single absolute levels of lactic acidosis do not necessarily correlate with the development of multiple organ failure and survival, the rate of lactic acid clearance does (81). Because significant electrolyte abnormalities requiring specific therapy rarely are observed in the drowning victim, normal saline is given as replacement fluid in drowning victims. Isotonic solution also provides less chance of aggravating cerebral edema.

SUMMARY

An awareness of the hidden dangers of recreational activities in and around water, and close supervision of infants, children, and adolescents are the secrets to preventing a significant number of drowning incidents. Swimming pools should be enclosed by security fences to prevent small children from entering the water inadvertently or unsupervised. By identifying age-related drowning risks, communities can reduce drowning rates. Effective CPR and water safety skills should be encouraged in the community, particularly for parents with small children who own home pools. Furthermore, children who can swim should never do so alone or without adult supervision. Everyone participating in water sports should wear an approved personal flotation device. Adolescents need to be taught to swim and informed about the dangers of alcohol and other drug consumption during water sport activities. Between 13 and 19 years of age, risk-taking behavior increases significantly in boys; therefore, extra counseling is warranted. Alcohol should never be consumed, regardless of age, while swimming or engaging in water sports. Swimming with a partner is particularly important for individuals with medical conditions that may abruptly alter their level of consciousness, such as seizure disorders, cardiac disease, and several metabolic diseases. Emergency gear for rescuing and resuscitating drowning victims should be readily available at the poolside. The specific gear required may vary with the size, access, and ownership of the facility.

The community expects the government to enforce safety rules, promote health education through medical and nonmedical personnel, and punish individuals who transgress basic safety rules and regulations. Despite recent advances in cardiopulmonary resuscitation and more sophisticated intensive care medicine, drowning victims with poor Glasgow coma scale scores have a high likelihood of living in a vegetative state as a result of the initial injury. When this occurs, making life or death decisions regarding withdrawal of life support by relatives and health professionals represents a significant stressful event. At the time of this writing, prevention is still the most fundamental way to limit neurologic disasters from drowning.

References

1. Idris AH, Berg R, Bierens J, et al. Recommended guidelines for uniform reporting of data from drowing; the "Utstein style". *Circulation.* 2003 Nov 18; 108(20):2565–2574.
2. Craig AB Jr. Causes of loss of consciousness during underwater swimming. *J Appl Physiol.* 1961;16:583–586.
3. Swann HG. Resuscitation in semi-drowning. In: Whittenberg JF, ed. *Artificial Respiration: Theory and Application.* New York: Harper and Roe; 1962:202–224.
4. Modell JH, Graves SA, Ketover A. Clinical course of 91 consecutive near-drowning victims. *Chest.* 1976;70:231–238.
5. Lowson JA. Sensations in drowning. *Edinburgh Med J.* 1903;13:41–45.
6. Fuller RH. The 1962 Wellcome prize essay. Drowning and the post-immersion syndrome. A clinicopathologic study. *Milit Med.* 1963;129:22–36.
7. Modell JH, Davis JH. Electrolyte changes in human drowning victims. *Anesthesiology.* 1969;30:414–420.
8. Modell JH, Moya F, Newby EJ, et al. The effects of fluid volume and seawater drowning. *Ann Intern Med.* 1967;67:68–80.
9. Modell JH, Moya F. Effects of volume of aspirated fluid during chlorinated fresh water drowning. *Anesthesiology.* 1966;27:662–672.
10. Modell JH, Gaub M, Moya F, et al. Physiologic effects of near-drowning with chlorinated fresh water, distilled water and isotonic saline. *Anesthesiology.* 1966;27:33–41.
11. Leach RM, Treacher DS. ABC of oxygen: oxygen transport—2. Tissue hypoxia. *BMJ.* 1998;317:1370–1373.
12. Craig AB Jr. Underwater swimming and loss of consciousness. *JAMA.* 1961; 176:255–258.
13. Ferrett G, Costa M, Ferrigno M, et al. Alveolar gas composition exchange during deep breath-hold diving and dry breath holds in elite divers. *J Appl Physiol.* 1991;70:794–802.
14. Gray SW. Respiratory movement of rat during drowning and influence of water temperature upon survival after submersion. *Am J Physiol.* 1951;167:95–102.
15. Kvittingen TD, Naess A. Recovery from drowning in fresh water. *BMJ.* 1963;1:1315–1317.
16. Movritzen CV, Andersen MN. Myocardial temperature gradients and ventricular fibrillation during hypothermia. *J Thorac Cardiovasc Surg.* 1965; 49:937–944.
17. Cot C. *Les asphyxies accidentecelles (submersion, electrocution, intoxication, oxycarbonique) etude clinique, therapeutique et preventive.* Paris: Editions Medicales N. Maloine; 1931.
18. Modell JH. *The Pathophysiology and Treatment of Drowning and Near-drowning.* Springfield, IL: Charles C. Thomas; 1971:9.
19. Modell JH. Drown vs. near-drown: a discussion of definitions, editorial. *Crit Care Med.* 1981;9:341–352.
20. Modell JH, Bellefleur M, Davis JH. Drowning without aspiration: is this an appropriate diagnosis? *J Forensic Sci.* 1999;44(6):119–123.
21. Loughead DW, Janes JM, Hall GE. Physiological studies in experimental asphyxia and drowning. *Can Med Assoc J.* 1939;40:423–428.
22. Swann HG, Spafford NR. Body salt and water changes during fresh and sea water drowning. *Texas Rep Biol Med.* 1951;9:356–382.
23. Swann HG, Brucer M, Moore C, et al. Fresh water and sea water drowning. A study of the terminal cardiac and biochemical events. *Texas Rep Biol Med.* 1947;5:423–437.
24. Halmagyi DFJ, Colebatch HJH. Ventilation and circulation after fluid aspiration. *J Appl Physiol.* 1961;16:35–40.
25. Colebatch HJH, Halmagyi DFJ. Lung mechanics and resuscitation after fluid resuscitation. *J Appl Physiol.* 1961;16:684–696.
26. Redding JS, Voight GC, Safer P. Treatment of sea water aspiration. *J Appl Physiol.* 1960;15:1113–1116.
27. Colebatch HJH, Halmagyi DFJ. Reflex pulmonary hypertension of fresh water aspiration. *J Appl Physiol.* 1963;18:179–185.
28. Colebatch HJH, Halmagyi DFJ. Reflex airway reaction to fluid aspiration. *J Appl Physiol.* 1962;17:787–794.
29. Fainer DC, Martin CG, Ivy AC. Resuscitation of dogs from fresh water drowning. *J Appl Physiol.* 1951;3:417–426.
30. Redding JS, Cozine RA. Restoration of circulation after fresh water drowning. *J Appl Physiol.* 1961;16:1071–1074.
31. Redding JS, Voight GC, Safer P. Drowning treated with intermittent positive pressure breathing. *J Appl Physiol.* 1960;15:849–854.
32. Modell JH, Moya F, Williams HD, et al. Changes in blood gases and $AaDO_2$ during near-drowning. *Anesthesiology.* 1968;29:456–465.
33. Giammona ST, Modell JH. Drowning by total immersion. Effects on pulmonary surfactant of distilled water, isotonic saline and sea water. *Am J Dis Child.* 1967;114:612–616.
34. Spitz WV, Blanke RV. Mechanism of death in fresh-water drowning. I. An experimental approach to the problem. *Arch Path (Chicago).* 1961;71:661–668.
35. Modell JH, Davis JH, Giammona ST, et al. Blood gas and electrolyte changes in human near-drowning victims. *JAMA.* 1968;203:337–343.
36. Fainer DC. Near-drowning in sea water and fresh water. *Ann Intern Med.* 1963;59:537–541.
37. Hasan S, Avery WE, Fabian C, et al. Near-drowning in humans. A report of 36 cases. *Chest.* 1971;59:191–197.
38. Fuller RH. The clinical pathology of human near-drowning. *Proc Roy Soc Med.* 1963;56:33–38.
39. Moritz AR. Chemical methods for the determination of death by drowning. *Physiol Rev.* 1944;24:70–88.
40. Butt MP, Jalowayski A, Modell JH, et al. Pulmonary function after resuscitation from near-drowning. *Anesthesiology.* 1970;32:275–277.
41. Modell JH, Kuck EJ, Ruiz BC, et al. Effect of intravenous vs. aspirated distilled water on serum electrolytes and blood gas tensions. *J Appl Physiol.* 1972;32:579–584.
42. Bergquist RE, Vogelhut MM, Modell JH, et al. Comparison of ventilatory patterns in the treatment of fresh water near-drowning in dogs. *Anesthesiology.* 1980;52:142–148.
43. Tabeling BB, Modell JH. Fluid administration increases oxygen delivery during continuous positive pressure ventilation after freshwater near-drowning. *Crit Care Med.* 1983;11:693–696.
44. Yag IR, Stalnikowicz R, Michaeli J. Near-drowning in the Dead Sea—electrolyte imbalances and therapeutic implications. *Arch Intern Med.* 1985;145:50–53.
45. Modell JH. *The Pathophysiology and Treatment of Drowning and Near-drowning.* Springfield, IL: Charles C. Thomas; 1971:61–66.
46. Ellis J. *National Pool and Water Park Lifeguard Training Manual.* Boston: Jones & Bartlet; 2000.
47. 2005 American Heart Association guidelines for cardiopulmonary resuscitation and emergency cardiovascular care. *Circulation* 2005;112(24):IV-133–IV-135.
48. Rosen P, Stoto M, Harley J, et al., eds. *The Use of the Heimlich Maneuver in Near-Drowning.* Washington DC: Institute of Medicine Committee on the Treatment of Near-Drowning Victims.; 1994.
49. Conn A, Montes J, Barker G. Cerebral salvage in near-drowning following neurologic classification by triage. *Can J Anaesth.* 1980;27:201–210.
50. Modell JH, Graves SA, Kuck EJ. Near-drowning: correlation of level of consciousness and survival. *Can Anaesth Soc J.* 1980;27:211–215.

51. Bohn DJ, Biggart WD, Smith CR, et al. Influence of hypothermia, barbiturate therapy and intracranial pressure monitoring on morbidity and mortality after near-drowning. *Crit Care Med.* 1986;14:529–534.
52. Orlowski JP, Szpilman D. Pediatric critical care: drowning. Rescue, resuscitation and reanimation. A new millennium. *Pediatr Clin North Am.* 2001; 48:627–646.
53. Lee KH. A retrospective study of near drowned victims admitted to the intensive care unit. *Ann Acad Med Singapore.* 1998;27:344–346.
54. Goodwin SR. Aspiration syndromes. In: Civetta JM, Taylor RW, Kirby RR, eds. *Critical Care.* Philadelphia: Lippincott-Raven; 1997:1861–1875.
55. Bachofen M, Weibel ER. Alterations of the gas exchange apparatus in adult respiratory insufficiency associated with septicemia. *Am Rev Respir Dis.* 1977;116:589–615.
56. Ruiz BC, Calderwood HW, Modell JH. Effect of ventilatory patterns on arterial oxygenation after near-drowning with fresh water. A comparative study in dogs. *Anesth Analg.* 1973;52:570–576.
57. Suter PS, Fairley HB, Isenberg MD. Optimum end-expiratory airway pressure in patients with acute pulmonary failure. *N Engl J Med.* 1975;292:284–289.
58. Modell JH, Calderwood HW, Ruiz BC, et al. Effects of ventilatory patterns on arterial oxygenation after near-drowning in sea water. *Anesthesiology.* 1974;40:376–384.
59. Antonelli M, Conti G, Rocco M, et al. A comparison of noninvasive positive-pressure ventilation and conventional mechanical ventilation in patient with acute respiratory failure. *N Eng J Med.* 1998;339:429–435.
60. Rabatin JT, Gay PC. Noninvasive ventilation. *Mayo Clin Proc.* 1999;74: 817–820.
61. Downs JB, Klein EF Jr, Desautels D, et al. Intermittent mandatory ventilation: a new approach to weaning patients from mechanical ventilators. *Chest.* 1973;64:331–335.
62. Dellinger RP, Zimmerman JL, Taylor RW et al. Effects of inhaled nitric oxide in patients with acute respiratory distress syndrome: results of a randomized phase II trial. *Crit Care Med.* 1998;26:15–23.
63. Jolliet P, Bulpa P, Chevrolet J. Effects of the prone position on gas exchange and hemodynamics in severe acute respiratory distress syndrome. *Crit Care Med.* 1998;26:1977–1985.
64. Pelosi P, Tubiolo D, Mascheroni D, et al. Effects of the prone position on respiratory mechanics and gas exchange during acute lung injury. *Am J Respir Crit Care Med.* 1998;157:387–393.
65. Meduri GU, Headley AS, Golden E, et al. Effect of prolonged methylprednisolone therapy in unresolving acute respiratory distress syndrome: A randomized controlled trial. *JAMA.* 1998;280:159–165.
66. Calderwood HW, Modell JH, Ruiz BC. The ineffectiveness of steroid therapy for treatment of fresh-water near-drowning. *Anesthesiology.* 1975;43:642–650.
67. Bone RC, Fisher CJ Jr, Clemmer TP et al. Early methylprednisolone treatment for septic syndrome and the adult respiratory distress syndrome. *Chest.* 1987;92:1032–1036.
68. Wynne JW, Modell JH. Respiratory aspiration of stomach contents. *Ann Intern Med.* 1977;87:66–474.
69. Wynne JW, Reynolds JC, Hood CI, et al. Steroid therapy for pneumonitis induced in rabbits by aspiration of food stuff. *Anesthesiology.* 1979;51:11–19.
70. Petty TL, Reiss OK, Paul GW, et al. Characteristics of pulmonary surfactant in adult respiratory distress syndrome associated with trauma and shock. *Am Rev Respir Dis.* 1977;115:531–536.
71. Corbet A, Bucciarelli R, Goldman S, et al. Decreased mortality among small premature infants treated at birth with a single dose of synthetic surfactant: a multicenter controlled trial. *J Pediatr.* 1991;118:227–234.
72. Anzueto A, Baughman RP, Guntupalli KK, et al. Aerosolized surfactant in adults with sepsis-induced acute respiratory distress syndrome. *N Engl J Med.* 1996;334:1417–1421.
73. Bullock RM, Chestnut RM, Clifton GL, et al. Guidelines for the management of severe traumatic brain injury. *J Neurotrauma.* 2000;17:451–627.
74. Fortune JB, Feustel PJ, deLuna C, et al. Cerebral blood flow and blood volume in response to O2 and CO2 changes in normal humans. *J Trauma.* 1995;39:463–471.
75. Weckesser M, Posse S, Olthoff U, et al. Functional imaging of the visual cortex with bold contrast MRI: hyperventilation decreases signal response. *Magn Reson Med.* 1999;41:213–216.
76. Van den Berghe G, Wouters P, Weekers F, et al. Intensive insulin therapy in critically ill patients. *N Engl J Med.* 2001;345:1359–1367.
77. Brunkhorst FM, Engel C, Bloos F, et al. Intensive insulin therapy and pentastarch resuscitation in severe sepsis. *N Engl J Med.* 2008;358:125–139.
78. Better OS, Stein JH. Early management of shock and prophylaxis of acute renal failure in traumatic rhabdomyolysis. *N Engl J Med.* 1990;322:825–829.
79. Eneas JF, Schoenfeld PY, Humphreys MH. The Effect of infusion of mannitol-sodium bicarbonate on the clinical course of myoglobinuria. *Arch Intern Med.* 1979;139:801–805.
80. Gelman S. Preserving renal function during surgery. In: *International Anesthesia Research Society Review Course Lectures.* Baltimore: Williams and Wilkins; 1992:88–92.
81. Bakker J, Gris P, Coffernils M, et al. Serial blood lactate levels can predict the development of multiple organ failure following septic shock. *Am J Surg.* 1996;171:221–226.

CHAPTER 139 ■ ASPIRATION

HOLGER H. HASSELBRING • MICHAEL SYDOW

IMMEDIATE CONCERNS

Major Problems

Aspiration is a potentially critical event, occurring in patients often suffering from reduced consciousness with decreased protective airway reflexes. Signs and symptoms of aspiration depend on the quantity and the nature of the aspirate. Owing to a large number of aspiration events involving gastric contents, a high awareness is essential in those situations in which patients are at higher risk for this problem (i.e., ileus, trauma, pregnancy, etc.). The pulmonary pathophysiologic changes observed depend on the type of aspiration. In general, *particulate obstructive aspiration* results in significant hypoxemia, which rapidly progresses to cardiovascular collapse if the obstruction is unrelieved. As in any anoxic-ischemic event, the resultant sequelae depend on the degree and duration of the hypoxemia. *Particulate nonobstructive* and the various forms of *liquid aspiration* result in a broad spectrum of pathophysiologic changes. The initial major problem may only be bronchospasm. However, aspiration of particulate irritant, such as gastric acid, leads to an additional problem consisting of chemically induced pulmonary tissue injury with an associated inflammatory response. Thus, an initially mild hypoxemia and tachypnea may commonly progress to the acute respiratory distress syndrome (ARDS) and respiratory failure. On the other hand, microaspiration of oropharyngeal secretions in endotracheally intubated patients does not damage the lung directly, but is the major cause of ventilator-associated pneumonia (VAP).

This chapter deals only with pulmonary aspiration of substances other than water. Water aspiration (i.e., near-drowning) is discussed in Chapter 138. Furthermore, inhalational injury by noxious gases is discussed elsewhere.

Stress Points

1. Inhalation of any amount of fluid with a pH less than 2.5 is likely to damage lung tissue extensively by chemical inflammation.
2. Blood in the lungs may occur as a consequence of hematemesis, intrapulmonary hemorrhage, and surgical procedures involving the upper airway, pharynx, or maxillofacial areas. Immediately after aspiration of blood, patients will have an increased pulse and respiratory rate, and may become cyanotic if the amount of inhaled blood is sufficient to cause significant intrapulmonary shunting. Otherwise, blood is relatively harmless.
3. Ingestion of hydrocarbons such as kerosene, furniture polish, lighter fluid, gasoline, and other petroleum solvents account for 18% of accidental poisonings in children. Pulmonary toxicity occurs only if the hydrocarbon is aspirated either during ingestion or after it is regurgitated (1).

Essential Diagnostic Tests and Procedures

1. Success in diagnosing pulmonary aspiration depends on maintaining a high index of suspicion for its occurrence in at-risk patients. In 63% of cases, regurgitation is witnessed; 37% of patients have either silent or unwitnessed aspirations.
2. When clinical findings suggest pulmonary aspiration, further evaluation is essential. Arterial blood gas and pH analysis affords the most useful initial laboratory test.
3. Approximately 88% to 94% of people who aspirate gastric contents eventually demonstrate pulmonary infiltrates on chest radiograph (2). Thus, a normal finding on chest radiograph does not completely exclude the possibility of aspiration.
4. Because the initial physical findings and blood gas volumes may be identical in acid and nonacid aspiration, determination of the pH of any remaining gastric or pharyngeal fluid can be helpful. If the fluid is highly acidic, anticipate a worsening course.

Initial Therapy

1. Initial management depends on whether aspiration is imminent, occurring, or completed. When regurgitation occurs in an obtunded patient, the airway must be cleared, and the patient's head must be tilted down and to the side.
2. Suction equipment must be available and ready to use in areas where this problem is likely to occur (e.g., the operating, delivery, and emergency rooms; postanesthesia care unit; and intensive care unit [ICU]).
3. Oxygen should be administered immediately to all patients suspected of pulmonary aspiration.
4. The airway should be secured by intubating the trachea, and then one must attempt to clean the airway immediately by suctioning any particulate aspirate. Suctioning has no beneficial effect with acid aspiration because the injury is immediate.
5. No benefit is derived from alkaline tracheal lavage. In fact, the practice is detrimental.
6. Removal of large particulate matter usually requires rigid bronchoscopy. Fiberoptic techniques permit only the removal of small particles.

HISTORICAL BACKGROUND

Beginning with Aristotle's observation of the association between meconium staining of the amniotic fluid and a sleepy fetal state (3), aspiration pneumonia was recognized as a clinical problem as early as 400 BC when Hippocrates realized "Dangers of Aspiration" (4). More than 2,000 years later, in 1848, Simpson reported the first anesthetic death under chloroform caused by pulmonary aspiration and asphyxia (5). In 1946, Mendelson presented 66 cases of aspiration occurring among 44,016 obstetric patients undergoing general anesthesia for vaginal deliveries (6). His description was so complete that aspiration in this setting is commonly termed the "Mendelson syndrome." Subsequently, his laboratory investigations led him to the conclusion that two entirely separate clinical entities existed. One followed the aspiration of solid food and resulted in a clinical picture of laryngeal or bronchial obstruction, whereas the other resulted from direct acid injury to the lung and caused the "asthma-like" syndrome (7). Teabeaut, in 1952, showed that a liquid aspirate with a pH below 2.5 would produce pneumonitis in rabbits (8). The concept of a critical pH and a certain aspirate volume was introduced in 1974 by Roberts and Shirley from data obtained in rhesus monkeys (9). The results were calculated for humans in order to identify patients at risk of pulmonary aspiration. Subsequent animal studies demonstrated that larger volumes of acidic aspirates produced higher morbidity and mortality (10). The critical pH of 2.5 and critical volume of 0.4 mL/kg body weight (or approximately 25 mL in an adult) have since been challenged as inducing aspiration pneumonitis.

RISK FACTORS

In a healthy and conscious subject, effective protective laryngeal and cough reflexes prevent pulmonary aspiration. Since the reflex status depends on the level of consciousness, it is obvious that aspiration is predisposed by any reduction of consciousness, which, therefore, is *the* major risk factor for aspiration (11). Common causes of reduced consciousness include different kinds of neurologic pathology such as head injury, stroke, and cerebral hemorrhage, as well as infectious causes such as meningitis or sepsis, or metabolic sources such as diabetes or thyroid crisis, and so forth. Drug and alcohol overdose and the use of sedative medication increase the risk of pulmonary aspiration; interestingly, even during normal sleep, aspiration is not uncommon (12). Another group of patients with an increased risk of aspiration are those with laryngeal incompetence caused by neurologic disturbances such as multiple sclerosis or muscular dystrophy, or by surgery of the hypopharynx and larynx itself. The protecting closure reflex of the larynx against aspiration is also impaired with age (13).

General anesthesia not only reduces the level of consciousness, but also suppresses airway reflexes. Therefore, general anesthesia is a risk factor for aspiration, particularly in emergency cases. Certain patient conditions increase the risk of aspiration in the perioperative setting. Best known is pregnancy,

TABLE 139.1

RISK FACTORS FOR PULMONARY ASPIRATION

Increased gastric content	Tendency for regurgitation	Laryngeal incompetence	Other reasons
Small bowel obstruction Delayed gastric emptying Overdistended stomach Lack of fasting Obstetric patient/parturition	Depressed consciousness Drug overdose Metabolic coma CNS infections Seizures	Sedated patient Cerebral infarct/hemorrhage Head injury/trauma Neuromuscular disorders Traumatic or surgical pharynx, vocal cord, or hypopharynx disorders	Failed intubation Difficult airway Night-time surgery ASA III classification or higher Artificial airways: Tracheostomy or endotracheal tube
Emergencies Outpatients Nasogastric overfeeding Hiatal hernia Obesity (?)	Hypothermia Sepsis Anatomic esophageal disorders Gastroesophageal reflux	Advanced age	

CNS, central nervous system; ASA, American Society of Anesthesiologists.

with its associated increased abdominal pressure and delayed gastric emptying. Another condition is morbid obesity (14), with issues of increased gastric volume and increased abdominal pressure, at least in the supine position. However, more recent studies have questioned the assumption that obesity is a risk factor for pulmonary aspiration during anesthesia (15). An absolute high-risk situation is small bowel obstruction with high gastric pressure. In this condition, the stomach sometimes contains far more than 1 liter of bile and jejunal secretions, and the distended bowel causes abdominal hypertension. Other conditions predisposing to pulmonary aspiration include disorders resulting in (a) reduced lower esophageal sphincter tone, such as gastroesophageal reflux disease; (b) increased lower esophageal sphincter tone (achalasia); (c) increased pyloric tone, such as pyloric stenosis; and (d) diseases with delayed gastric emptying (e.g., diabetes). Each situation, leading to increased gastric pressures, may amplify the incidence of regurgitation and vomiting and, consequently, the risk of pulmonary aspiration.

In the perioperative period, aspiration occurs most often during the induction of anesthesia, when the patient is already unconscious and the endotracheal tube is not yet in place. Some measures can even increase the aspiration risk. For example, mask ventilation with high pressures can further insufflate the already full stomach with air and, thus, increase the intragastric pressure. The fast-acting muscle relaxant, succinylcholine, can cause abdominal muscle contractions and consequently increases the abdominal, and thus gastric, pressure if the patient has not been properly precurarized. A nasogastric tube in place at the time of induction of anesthesia reduces the patency of the esophageal sphincter and promotes gastroesophageal reflux. The body position of the patient influences the intra-abdominal pressure and, thus, affects the risk of regurgitation and aspiration as well. The flat, supine position is probably the worst position, whereas the semirecumbent position decreases abdominal pressure.

It seems obvious that the risk of aspiration is also increased at the end of anesthesia when the endotracheal tube has been removed but recovery of consciousness is not completed. Patients at special risk include those having undergone laryngeal or hypopharyngeal surgery, resulting in laryngeal incompetence. These patients need close observation postoperatively.

Critically ill patients with ventilatory insufficiency or failure are at particular risk of pulmonary aspiration. Muscle weakness, tachypnea, immobility, and impaired consciousness depress the normal airway-clearing mechanisms. Even in patients whose airway is protected by a cuffed endotracheal tube, aspiration is common. Although a properly inflated tube cuff can prevent macroaspiration, microaspiration of pooled subglottic secretions occurs because the cuff configuration does not provide complete sealing of the trachea; this may be obviated to a great extent by an endotracheal tube with a subglottic suction port incorporated into the tube. Other factors increasing the risk of aspiration in endotracheally intubated patients include reintubation, tracheostomy, frequent ventilator circuit changes, low intracuff pressure, and patient transport from the ICU (16). Further risk factors pertaining to the gastrointestinal tract include enteral nutrition, supine positioning, and stress ulcer prophylaxis with gastric pH-altering agents (17).

A nasogastric feeding tube not only promotes gastroesophageal reflux, but also eventually leads to oropharyngeal swallowing defects. An endotracheal tube causes vocal cord dysfunction and impairs the sensorimotor function of the pharynx and the larynx temporarily. After long-term intubation, swallowing defects are frequent, with a considerable risk of aspiration after extubation (18). A synopsis of the various risk factors is shown in Table 139.1.

INCIDENCE, MORBIDITY, AND MORTALITY

Aspiration in the Perioperative Period

Although general anesthesia is principally a risk factor for pulmonary aspiration, carefully developed strategies during the past decades have reduced the risk of aspiration during elective surgery. Several large studies were concerned primarily with the incidence of aspiration and its associated mortality during general anesthesia (19). In a retrospective study of 215,488 general anesthetics for elective and emergency surgery, Warner et al. (20) found an incidence of pulmonary aspiration of 1 in 3,216 (0.03%) and a mortality rate of 1 in 71,829 patients (0.0014%); the incidence of aspiration was found to be four times higher in patients undergoing emergency surgery. There was no serious morbidity from pulmonary aspiration in the immediate perioperative period in nearly 120,000 elective procedures and general anesthetics in American Society of Anesthesiologists (ASA) physical status I and II patients. The incidence of pulmonary aspiration and severity of pulmonary outcomes were highly associated with the presence of comorbidity (ASA physical status III and higher) and procedures performed emergently. Finally, Warner et al. concluded that patients with clinically apparent aspiration who do not develop symptoms within 2 hours of aspiration or completion of the procedure are unlikely to have respiratory sequelae.

Olsson et al. in 1986 (19) studied 185,385 patients undergoing general anesthesia and found an aspiration rate of 1 in 2,131 (0.05%). Forty-seven percent of the patients with reported aspiration developed aspiration pneumonitis, with a mortality rate of 1 in 45,454 (0.002%) (16). In 1996, Mellin-Olsen et al. studied 85,594 anesthetics prospectively. They reported 25 cases of aspiration, presenting an overall incidence of 1 in 3,424. All occurred in patients receiving general anesthesia, with an incidence of 1 in 2,106. Of the 25 aspiration cases, 13 occurred during elective procedures with an incidence of 1 in 3,303, and 12 in emergency procedures with an incidence of 1 in 809. There were no aspirative events in patients receiving regional anesthesia nor in those patients who were under IV sedation and analgesia but breathing spontaneously (21). In a report on the epidemiology and impact of aspiration pneumonia in patients undergoing surgery in Maryland between 1999 and 2000 (22), the prevalence of aspiration pneumonia was approximately 1% of hospitalized surgical patients, remarkably higher than in the other studies. However, in a letter to the editors (23), it was noted that the authors of the Maryland study did not distinguish between aspiration pneumonitis and aspiration pneumonia. The fact that all patients with postoperative nosocomial pneumonia were included in the aspiration group most likely explains the higher incidence of aspiration in this study.

Aspiration pneumonitis associated with pediatric anesthesia occurred in up to 1 in 1,162 (0.09%) children in Olsson's study (19). In a prospective study in 1999, Warner et al. reported an aspiration incidence of 3.8 per 10,000 (1:2,632; 0.04%) anesthetics in children (20). In a prospective survey carried out in France of 40,240 general anesthetics in children, only four aspirations were reported (0.01%). No morbidity or mortality was reported (24).

Aspiration in Obstetrics

Even though anesthesia-related maternal mortality rates have improved, anesthesia still remains prominent among the leading causes of maternal mortality; it is the seventh leading cause of maternal mortality in the United States (25). General anesthesia in the obstetric patient is more likely to be associated with maternal mortality than is regional anesthesia. Airway management tends to be more difficult in pregnant patients compared to the general population. Moreover, general anesthesia is indicated in emergency delivery surgery, with minimal time left for adequate preoperative evaluation and preparation for anesthesia. Several anatomic and physiologic alterations during pregnancy cause a difficult airway. Mucosal edema is common in expectant mothers due to hormonal effects and relative fluid overload, particularly in eclampsia (26).

The Closed Claims Analysis of the ASA revealed that respiratory events accounted for the single largest class of injury (27). According to the study by Chadwick et al., difficult tracheal intubation and esophageal intubation comprised 23% of harmful events associated with obstetric general anesthesia (28). Complications leading to anesthesia-related deaths due to airway management problems included aspiration of gastric contents, problems during intubation, esophageal intubation, and inadequate ventilation.

The pregnant woman is at special risk for aspiration of gastric contents for a variety of reasons, including mechanical, hormonal, and iatrogenic factors (26). The gravid uterus increases intra-abdominal and intragastric pressure, which may increase even more during delivery. The distortion of the esophagogastric junction and the stomach through the gravid uterus promotes esophageal reflux, and gastric emptying time is prolonged (29). Hormonal factors specific to pregnancy include higher levels of gastrin, which increases gastric acidity and volume, and progesterone, which can decrease gastroesophageal sphincter tone. Iatrogenic factors include the administration of sedatives and narcotics during labor, which further prolongs gastric emptying and also may depress protective airway reflexes. Moreover, the lithotomy position and manual abdominal compression for delivery additionally increase intragastric pressure. The incidence of aspiration in obstetric patients for cesarean section under general anesthesia was 1 in 1,431 (0.07%) in an Italian study (30). A Scandinavian report noted aspiration in 4 of 3,600 cesarean sections (0.11%) and in 4 of 36,800 parturients (0.01%), with no fatalities (31).

"Silent Aspiration" during Anesthesia

During the induction of anesthesia, when protective reflexes are diminished, the risk of aspiration is greatest. However, even after having successfully completed induction of anesthesia, pulmonary aspiration is not uncommon. Owing to the fact that this kind of aspiration is usually not detected by the anesthesiologist, it is called "silent" aspiration (32). Despite the tube being correctly placed in the trachea, with an appropriately inflated cuff to "seal" the airways, aspiration may still occur. Nevertheless, during short-term endotracheal intubation, the incidence of silent aspiration is relatively low. In older studies, an incidence of 8% to 25% during anesthesia was reported (33). In 1970, Blitt et al. detected "silent" aspiration in less than 1% of 900 studied anesthetized patients (34). These clinicians attributed the low incidence of aspiration to their use of cuffed endotracheal tubes and the exclusive use of fast-acting intravenous induction in contrast to the induction with inhalation anesthetics, which was still popular in those times. Moreover, they reported that only 1 out of the 900 patients (0.1%) may have developed pulmonary complications as a possible consequence of silent aspiration. However, even in this patient, the pulmonary complication may have been from other reasons (34). It is remarkable that there is no further, more recent study about silent aspiration during anesthesia. This fact and the very low incidence of serious consequences of aspiration underline that silent aspiration during short-term endotracheal intubation, as during anesthesia, is only of minor concern.

Aspiration in the Early Postoperative Period

There are no specific data about the incidence of aspiration in surgical patients in the early postoperative period or its sequel, aspiration pneumonia. Postoperative nausea and vomiting (PONV) is a frequent phenomenon after anesthesia and surgery (35) and has been well reviewed in large prospective multicenter studies. However, none of these studies revealed pulmonary aspiration associated with PONV as a significant problem. Nevertheless, as impaired consciousness is a major risk factor for pulmonary aspiration in all patients who are not fully recovered, the need for close observation is evident in the early postoperative period.

Pulmonary Aspiration in Critical Care

Pulmonary aspiration during induction of anesthesia or in an emergency case is generally witnessed, and the consequences of aspiration, such as bronchospasm and hypoxemia, develop early. In contrast, aspiration is usually silent in critical care patients and frequently chronic without early and clear signs of the event. Thus, estimating the incidence of aspiration in critical care patients is difficult. Markers like glucose, pepsin, radioisotope-labeled feeds, or dye in tracheobronchial secretions have been used to detect aspiration in these patients (36–38). With these methods, pulmonary aspiration was detected in up to 89% in mechanically ventilated, tube-fed patients (38). Other studies, reported in patients with tracheostomies, noted a positive aspiration rate between 33% (40) and 50% (39). The methods mentioned above identified minimal amounts of aspirated material, even if no clinical symptoms could be detected. In fact, 87% and 77% of the events, respectively, were classified as "silent aspiration" (39,40). Even in healthy subjects, tracheal aspiration during sleep is not uncommon (12). However, in healthy subjects, immune competence together with efficient airway-clearing mechanisms (coughing, mucociliary transport, etc.) and the low pathogenicity of the normal oropharyngeal flora prevent the development of airway infection. On the other hand, if the physiologic defense and clearing mechanisms are impaired—as in the critically ill and particularly in sedated, endotracheally intubated patients—pneumonia may follow, even if the amount of the aspirated substance is small and the number of bacteria low. Furthermore, recurrent aspiration of bacterially contaminated oropharyngeal secretions is frequent in these patients and increases the likelihood of respiratory tract infection. This explains the correlation between the duration of critical illness—and especially the time of intubation—with occurrence of respiratory tract infections. In a large European multicenter study, the incidence of pneumonia in endotracheally intubated patients was 15.8% at day 7 and 23.4% at day 14 (41). In critically ill patients, the immunocompromised state and previous antibiotic therapy lead to a shift of the oropharyngeal flora from physiologically less virulent bacteria to a pathogenic population consisting mostly of *Staphylococcus aureus,* Gram-negative enteric bacilli, *Pseudomonas aeruginosa,* and *Candida* species (42). Since aspiration pneumonia is one of the most common and relevant results of the aspiration of oropharyngeal secretions or gastric contents in critically ill patients, its occurrence can be used as a surrogate indicator of aspiration. However, the incidence of aspiration pneumonia is often submerged within the incidence of VAP. *VAP incidence*, as it is defined, refers only to endotracheally intubated, mechanically ventilated patients, and does not include the aspiration pneumonia of nonintubated patients, such as those having suffered a stroke or with swallowing defects of other origins. Thus, there is uncertainty as to the exact incidence of aspiration pneumonia. Even the incidence of VAP varies between 9% and 70%, depending upon the case mix of patients, the setting of the studies, and the criteria used for the diagnosis of pneumonia (43).

Pulmonary Aspiration in Medical Emergencies

Medical emergency situations are often accompanied by reduced consciousness and impaired protective reflexes. Thus, tracheobronchial aspiration is common in these cases. Although the exact incidence is uncertain, the overall risk of aspiration during emergency intubations is in the range of 20% (44). However, this number varies depending on the patient's condition—mainly the level of consciousness—and the situation during which airway management or airway protection measures are performed. Pulmonary aspiration during endotracheal intubation in emergency surgery, even though performed in the operating suite, takes place in 1 of 895 (0.1%) cases, which is about four times more frequent than in elective surgery (20). The risk of aspiration increases with the degree of unconsciousness, as measured by the Glasgow coma scale (45). In prehospital emergency care, aspiration prior to airway management occurs in about one third of severely head-injured patients—those with a Glasgow coma scale score between 3 and 8 (46,47). Although no specific data have been described in the patient with central nervous system (CNS) injury, some authors estimated the incidence of gastric aspiration to be up to 30-fold more likely in emergency—as compared to scheduled—cases (48). Another study revealed aspiration of gastric contents in 50% of the patients who needed to be intubated because of respiratory insufficiency in the prehospital setting, as opposed to 22% in those patients who required subsequent tracheal intubation in the emergency department (49). Even though different methods have been used to investigate the incidence of pulmonary aspiration in emergency care, it seems relatively clear that aspiration in emergencies occurs less frequently in a well-prepared setting such as the operating suite, with doctors highly skilled in airway management, as compared to the difficult situations seen in prehospital emergency care. Furthermore, it can be presumed that endotracheal intubation in an emergency situation *per se* might increase the risk of aspiration: if reflexes are not deeply suppressed, laryngoscopy stimulates the gag reflex caused by contact of the instrument with the pharyngeal wall and can induce vomiting.

Gastric contents will then be aspirated because of disturbed protective reflexes and discoordinated cough reflexes. In many trauma patients, the stomach is acutely dilated (50), which further promotes vomiting, regurgitation, and, finally, aspiration. Cardiopulmonary resuscitation also poses a high risk for aspiration. In an autopsy series of unsuccessfully resuscitated patients, nearly half of them had full stomachs, and the overall incidence of pulmonary aspiration was 29% (51). This underlines the high incidence of pulmonary aspiration in emergency patients.

PATHOPHYSIOLOGY OF PULMONARY ASPIRATION

Definition

Aspiration is defined as the misdirection of oropharyngeal or gastric contents into the larynx and lower respiratory tract (52). Aspiration of gastric contents results from either active vomiting or passive regurgitation, both associated with impairment or depression of protective laryngeal and cough reflexes. Aspiration can be composed of materials from the following groups, depending on the nature of the aspirated material (53):

1. Noxious fluids—acid, bile, jejunal secretions, and other chemical substances
2. Solid particles—food, teeth, and other foreign bodies
3. Miscellaneous fluids—blood, water, alcohol, meconium, milk, pus, etc.
4. Microbiologically contaminated secretions

Table 139.2 lists substances that are known to be aspirated.

TABLE 139.2

SUBSTANCES KNOWN TO BE ASPIRATED

GASTROINTESTINAL FLUIDS
Gastric acid
Bile
Jejunal secretions
Fluid enteral nutrition formula
SOLID PARTICLES
Food of any kind
Nuts (peanuts)
Teeth
Sand/small stones
MISCELLANEOUS FLUIDS
Blood
Alcohol
Hydrocarbons
Polyethylene glycol
Meconium
Milk
MICROBIOLOGICALLY CONTAMINATED SUBSTANCES
Oropharyngeal secretions
Pus

Aspiration Pneumonitis versus Aspiration Pneumonia

To better understand the problem of aspiration, it is important to distinguish between aspiration pneumonitis and aspiration pneumonia. Aspiration pneumonitis is caused by chemically injurious agents (e.g., acid). Such agents destroy the lung tissue directly, as by chemical burn. It most commonly occurs in patients with a decreased level of consciousness who aspirate gastric contents. By way of contrast, aspiration pneumonia occurs in a different group of patients, mainly elderly with dysphagia or gastric dysmotility, or in critically ill patients who are usually endotracheally intubated and mechanically ventilated. These patients often aspirate only small amounts of bacterially contaminated secretions. Furthermore, in this kind of aspiration, lung damage develops collaterally to aspiration, when bacterial invasion leads to pneumonia. Although the distinction is somewhat arbitrary, there clearly are different population groups at risk for the two potential aspiration-induced lung disorders. It is important to examine these two conditions separately to better define the prognosis and treatment of at-risk populations (54).

The outcome after pulmonary aspiration is dependent on the toxicity or virulence of the aspirate, the volume of the aspirate, and the effectiveness of the defense mechanisms of the organism. For example, small amounts of aspirated autologous blood will cause no harm to lung tissue. In contrast, a relatively small volume of gastric acid with low pH produces harmful damage to the alveolar tissue (i.e., pneumonitis). Although saliva is a neutral liquid and is aspirated only in small amounts, its bacterial contamination may cause serious pneumonia because of the impaired clearing mechanisms and decreased immune defense in critically ill patients.

Aspiration of Gastric Contents and Aspiration Pneumonitis

The major source of aspirated material is the stomach and upper gastrointestinal tract. The content is variable, consisting of gastric acid, food particles, or a mixture of both. In case of small bowel obstruction, the stomach may also contain jejunal secretions and bile. The aspect of solid food will be discussed in a later section.

Gastric acid is very deleterious to lung tissues. Most authors agree that a pH less than 2.5 and a volume of gastric aspirate greater than 0.4 mL/kg body weight—approximately 25 to 50 mL in adults—are required for the development of aspiration pneumonitis (6,8,10). Experimental studies have indicated that the instillation of low pH hydrochloric acid solutions results in a dose-related and pH-dependent acute lung injury (ALI). The severity of the injury is directly related to three variables: (a) the acidity of the instilled fluid, (b) the volume of the instilled fluid, and (c) the tonicity of the fluid (55). Hypotonic fluids cause a more severe lung injury than isotonic fluids; gastric contents have approximately one-third the osmolality of plasma. Most clinical and experimental studies demonstrate that there is an initial lung injury whose clinical presentation is airway constriction, arterial hypoxemia, and the development of pulmonary edema. In some experimental models, there is progression of the acid-induced lung injury, with the most serious injury seen at approximately 6 to 8 hours after the acid administration (56).

Small bowel obstruction often leads to massive (greater than 1 liter) reflux of bile and jejunal secretions into the stomach. This produces an increased gastric pressure with a high risk of regurgitation. Bile has an inflammatory potential comparable to acid (57). Owing to the direct chemical destruction of the lung tissue by aspiration of either gastric acid or bile, this kind of lung damage is termed *aspiration pneumonitis*.

Aspiration of Solid Particles

Aspirate containing large particles accounted for 7.5% of aspiration in Mendelson's series (6). While two of his five patients who aspirated solid material died of suffocation, most perioperative gastric aspirates do not contain large particles.

Solid particles obstruct the airways depending on their size. The bigger they are, the larger is the obstructed lung area behind the foreign body, and the higher the degree of the intrapulmonary right-to-left shunt, resulting in hypoxemia or even suffocation. In the zone around the foreign body, local inflammation will occur with infiltration of mononuclear cells and granulomatous reaction of the lung tissue. If the solid particle is not removed, permanent atelectasis and lung consolidation will develop downstream from the obstruction. Conversely, air trapping and emphysema may develop behind the obstruction (58). Depending on the bacterial content of the aspirate or of the airways behind the obstruction, local pneumonia or even a lung abscess may develop.

Teeth are sometimes accidentally aspirated in craniofacial trauma, and may be detected only by a routine chest radiograph postoperatively or during examination in the emergency room. Foreign body aspiration is a serious problem in children, with the ability to cause critical respiratory insufficiency (59). More than 17,000 children under the age of 14 were admitted to emergency departments in the United States in 2001, resulting in 160 deaths (60). More than 50% foreign body aspirations occur in children aged between 1 and 3 years, less than 10% in children younger than 1 year of age (61), and only occasionally in adults, usually secondary to impaired consciousness. A Medline search revealed that nearly anything that would fit into a pediatric trachea has been detected there. Aspiration of foreign bodies can occur very dramatically, with a full-blown picture of acute choking, or more subclinically with recurrent coughing or wheezing episodes mimicking respiratory infection or asthma (62). Nuts, especially peanuts, are occasionally aspirated by children and cause a special problem. These often break into small pieces when attempting to remove them bronchoscopically. Generally, removal of the aspirated foreign body by bronchoscopy is the therapy of choice.

Aspiration of Miscellaneous Fluids

Blood. During craniofacial trauma and, to a lesser extent, during ear–nose–throat surgery and maxillofacial surgery, the aspiration of blood is common. Blood is harmless in terms of its inflammatory property to tissue or mucosal structures. Depending on the volume aspirated, it will cause a certain degree of intrapulmonary right-to-left shunt and hypoxemia. About 400 mL of blood in the alveolar space may be sufficient to cause significant hypoxemia (63). Only a large amount of blood can obstruct the airways sufficiently to cause life-threatening hypoxemia and death through suffocation. Smaller volumes normally can easily be treated with the application of continuous positive airway pressure or positive end-expiratory pressure (PEEP) ventilation (64). Most often, the blood is reabsorbed without further harmful consequences, with the only hazard of aspirated blood being airway obstruction.

Alcohol. The pH of alcohol is similar to that of saliva—pH 6 to 7—and its destructive properties on lung tissue have been considered minimal. In an animal study, however, aspirated ethanol has been shown to produce marked pulmonary inflammation and bronchiolitis obliterans (65). How this might be adjudicated in the context of a human aspiration of alcohol is unclear, and only one study concerning ethanol aspiration in the literature underlines the fact that aspiration of ethanol is a rare event.

Hydrocarbons. Materials such as gasoline, kerosene, gasoil, furniture polish, and other light oil products are sometimes ingested—mainly accidentally—by children. If vomited or regurgitated, hydrocarbons can be aspirated, resulting in a rapid onset of hypoxemia caused by intrapulmonary shunt (66). The intrapulmonary shunt after aspiration of hydrocarbons results from pulmonary edema and mucosal bleeding (67).

Polyethylene Glycol. This material is generally used to clean the bowel prior to endoscopic examinations. Since it is given in relatively large quantities, pulmonary aspiration may occur in at-risk patients, such as children and the elderly (68). Polyethylene glycol induces mucosal inflammation, interstitial edema, and, consequently, hypoxemia.

Oropharyngeal Secretions. Oral secretions *per se* are innocuous to airway mucosa. If aspirated, oropharyngeal secretions are usually small in volume and will not cause significant obstruction of the airways. However, the oropharynx is heavily contaminated with a variety of microbes, which may cause a problem if aspirated. In healthy individuals, the normal oropharyngeal flora consists mostly of anaerobes and, to a small degree, aerobic bacteria (*Staphylococcus* and *Haemophilus* species, among others) (69), which only have a minor infectious potential in the immunocompetent subject. In the presence of an immunocompromised state, the normal flora may be overgrown by pathogens such as Gram-negative rods, *S. aureus,* and yeasts. Aspirated oropharyngeal secretions contaminated with these pathogenic microbes are usually the source of aspiration pneumonia. However, the development of pneumonia depends on the pathogen's virulence and the quantity aspirated, as well as the patient's defense mechanisms such as mucociliary clearance and cellular and humoral immunocompetence. Repeated aspiration of even small amounts of secretions from above the cuff of the endotracheal tube, as often takes place in mechanically ventilated patients, increases the likelihood of VAP.

Meconium. The aspiration of meconium (pH 5.5–7) in newborn infants can cause mechanical obstruction, depending on the amount and consistency of the material; it also induces a chemical pneumonitis (70). Meconium aspiration occurs in slightly less than 1% of the newborn infants (71). Of the infants who develop a meconium aspiration syndrome, more than 4% die, accounting for 2% of all perinatal deaths (72). In laboring women with thick meconium staining of the amniotic fluid, amnioinfusion did not reduce the risk of moderate to severe meconium aspiration syndrome, perinatal death, or other maternal or neonatal disorders (73). Routine oropharyngeal and nasopharyngeal suctioning during delivery of term newborns through meconium-stained amniotic fluid is a frequent therapy, but it has recently been suggested that this does not prevent the meconium aspiration syndrome (74).

Milk. Milk may be aspirated either directly after ingestion or subsequent to regurgitation or vomiting. The effects of pulmonary aspiration of milk have been studied in animals (75). Vomited milk is usually acidic due to gastric acid admixture. However, instillation of human breast milk into rabbit lung at a pH of 7 and 1.8 results in comparable tissue damage and pneumonitis, whereas instilled 5% dextrose solution at a pH of 1.8 did not cause significant lung injury. It appears, based on this study, that human breast milk may be harmful to the lung. Nevertheless, this interpretation from animal experimentation must been taken with caution, as no data exist on the effect of aspirated human breast milk on human lung tissue.

Pus. Aspiration of pus is a very rare event, occurring during surgery for lung abscess or rupture of a peritonsillar abscess. The consequence may be transmission of the infection to other regions of the respiratory tract.

DIAGNOSIS OF ASPIRATION AND ITS SEQUELAE

Patients who have aspirated gastric material may present with dramatic clinical signs and symptoms. The clinical features may include an abrupt onset of wheezing, coughing, dyspnea, and tachycardia. Patients may exhibit low-grade fever, bronchospasm, or cyanosis, with pink, frothy sputum. A severely decreased PaO_2 and hypoxemia also occur. If not witnessed, the diagnosis of acid pneumonitis is usually presumptive based upon the clinical picture. After an aspiration, the chest radiograph often shows localized or diffuse patchy alveolar infiltrates or, in severe cases, opacification of large lung fields; these changes are usually noted within 2 hours. Aspiration most often is localized in the right lower lobe, as this is the straightest path from the trachea, or in the most dependent lung area—frequently the right upper lobe in supine patients (76).

As a consequence of the aspiration-induced alveolar capillary membrane damage, capillary leak occurs with loss of intravascular fluid into the interstitial tissue of the lung, resulting in increased extravascular lung water, systemic hemoconcentration, hypotension, tachycardia, and, possibly, hypovolemic shock aggravating the hypoxemia. Pulmonary hypertension may occur secondary to bronchospasm, loss of alveolar function, and left ventricular dysfunction (77). In patients with neurologic injuries, pulmonary aspiration can contribute to secondary CNS injury through hypoxia, hypotension, and pulmonary hypertension, with decreased cerebral venous return causing an acute increase of intracranial pressure (48).

Interestingly, many patients do not have clinical progression to lung injury, only a cough or a wheeze. Some patients have silent aspiration, which may manifest only as arterial desaturation with subsequent radiologic evidence of aspiration or pneumonia (20). Subclinical aspiration can be detected only through additional measures. Several markers have been used to ascertain subclinical aspiration with various success. Such markers include glucose, radioisotope-labeled feeds, or dye (37,78,79). Recently, the presence of pepsin as a sensitive and specific marker of gastric contents has been suggested as a useful marker of occult aspiration (80,81).

If a patient is considered as having suffered clinically relevant aspiration, measuring the pH in the larynx may be used to confirm the diagnosis (82). We usually measure the pH with simple litmus paper, which is adequately sensitive, as gastric contents require a pH of less than 2.5 to produce chemical pneumonitis. Bronchoscopy supplies only limited additional information. If aspiration of solid particles is suspected or witnessed, bronchoscopy can confirm the type and size of the particle. However, for the removal of particles, rigid bronchoscopy may be necessary. In case of gastric acid aspiration, bronchoscopy is only able to show the amount of inflamed mucosa. It is useless to attempt to remove acid from the bronchi via bronchoscopic lavage and suctioning.

The diagnostic criteria of aspiration pneumonia (not to be confused with aspiration pneumonitis) are not different from the usual criteria of pneumonia, consisting of the typical clinical findings such as new pulmonary infiltrates, fever, deterioration of pulmonary function, and laboratory infectious findings such as leucocytosis and identification of the causative agent (83,84).

THERAPY FOR ASPIRATION

Witnessing the aspiration of gastric secretions into the pharynx should immediately prompt lateral head positioning, assuming integrity of the cervical spine, suctioning, and consideration of endotracheal intubation. The success of treatment may depend on immediate and vigorous measures to relieve airway obstruction. Tracheal suctioning may stimulate cough, bringing up some aspirated material, and thus help confirm a suspected diagnosis. Immediate bronchoscopy is performed only when solid particles, which may obstruct airways, are thought to have been aspirated. Removal of larger material requires rigid bronchoscopy. Bronchoscopic suctioning will not, however, protect the lungs from chemical injury, which essentially occurs immediately. Bronchial lavage may be deleterious, as it may result in surfactant washout and spread noxious aspirated material to uninvolved lung areas. Attempted neutralization of the acid aspirate is of no help, as the acid is rapidly neutralized physiologically.

The major therapeutic approach is to maintain pulmonary function, thus ensuring adequate gas exchange and minimizing further damage to the lungs. In an awake, alert, and cooperative patient, continuous positive airway pressure (CPAP) may be administered by mask, but more often, mechanical ventilation with PEEP in a lung-protective manner must be applied. Recent work also indicates that mechanical ventilation of acid-injured rat lungs with low tidal volumes of 6 mL/kg reduces the severity of lung injury compared to mechanical ventilation with higher tidal volumes of 12 mL/kg (85). These studies confirm the results of the ARDS Network trial in which low tidal volume ventilation decreased mortality in patients with ALI (86). Aerosolized β_2 agonists may reduce the severity of lung endothelial injury and augment active ion transport mechanisms, which are responsible for the removal of edema from distal alveoli and airways of the lung (87). Owing to the deleterious increase of pulmonary vascular resistance caused by acid injury, the use of selectively acting vasodilators, such as inhaled nitric oxide (iNO), sildenafil, and prostacyclin, may be helpful in improving lung function and cardiac performance.

Meconium aspiration syndrome (MAS) remains a relevant cause for respiratory distress syndrome in premature infants, and is characterized by severe impairment of pulmonary gas exchange, surfactant inactivation, and pronounced inflammatory changes. Surfactant replacement therapy has been established for years as one of the most important therapeutic interventions in the management of premature infants with ARDS (88,89). Owing to the fact that aspiration and ARDS include the loss of pulmonary surfactant function, there is considerable interest in surfactant replacement therapy in adult patients. An international, multicenter, industry-sponsored study showed no improvement in either oxygenation or mortality when replacement surfactant was used in these patients (90). The study had enrolled 498 patients when it was discontinued, after interim analysis revealed a 41% mortality rate in both groups. Clinical experience has shown exogenous surfactant inconsistent as a therapeutic modality for adult patients with ARDS. However, current data do suggest that patients with primary ARDS (e.g., pneumonia, aspiration) may benefit more from surfactant replacement therapy than patients with secondary ARDS (e.g., sepsis, trauma); there has been no large, randomized, clinical trial conclusively showing that exogenous surfactant improves outcome in ARDS (91). The value of surfactant replacement in near-drowning is discussed elsewhere.

Steroids in aspiration syndromes have been shown to be clinically ineffective and, indeed, impede recovery in animal models (92), and likely in humans as well (93–95).

Antibiotic Therapy

Aspiration Pneumonitis

Although common practice, the prophylactic use of antibiotics in patients with suspected or witnessed aspiration is not recommended (96). Prophylactic antibiotics may increase late mortality by promoting the growth of resistant bacteria (97). However, empiric antibiotic therapy is appropriate for patients who aspirate gastric contents consisting of small bowel secretions or in other conditions associated with high bacterial colonization of the aspirate. Specific antibiotic therapy should be initiated in the setting of a secondary bacterial infection and should also be considered for patients with aspiration pneumonitis that fails to recover within 48 hours after aspiration (23).

Aspiration Pneumonia

The antibiotic therapy of aspiration pneumonia depends on the expected causative agent. However, distinctions are made between early- and late-onset pneumonia, which have different epidemiology and pathogenesis, and thus each type requires different strategies for therapy and prevention.

Early-onset Pneumonia. Early-onset pneumonia occurs typically in trauma patients and acute illness a few days after admission (98). The mechanism is mostly aspiration of oropharyngeal secretions before or during endotracheal intubation. Thus, the causative microbial organisms of early-onset pneumonia are usually identical with those potentially pathogen microbes, which can frequently be found in the oropharyngeal flora of healthy subjects, such as methicillin-susceptible *S. aureus*, *Haemophilus influenzae*, or *Streptococcus pneumoniae*. Since these organisms are also responsible for community-acquired pneumonias, the antibiotic treatment of early-onset pneumonia is not different from that of community-acquired pneumonia.

Late-onset Pneumonia. As late-onset pneumonia occurs more than 4 to 7 days after admission (99), the spectrum of the causative organisms is usually nosocomial, often consisting of *Pseudomonas aeruginosa*, among others. The principles of antibiotic therapy of late-onset pneumonia are the same as those of nosocomial pneumonia. Both issues—therapy of community-acquired and nosocomial pneumonia—are discussed separately in Chapter 111.

PREVENTION OF ASPIRATION AND ITS SEQUELAE

Prevention of Aspiration in the Perioperative Period

The ritualistic preoperative fasting over the past decades has been questioned, given that fasting can cause dehydration, diminishes the energy reservoir, and increases patient anxiety. Moreover, the amount of gastric secretions may be increased through hunger and emotional stimuli (100–103).

Many studies have attempted to identify patients at risk before induction of general anesthesia with various fasting durations in various settings. It is generally agreed upon that clear fluid given up to 2 hours before elective surgery does not adversely affect gastric contents in healthy patients (100,104). This knowledge is one of the keystones of the "fast-track surgery" approach (105). One study found gastric volume and pH unchanged in children who had received 6 or 10 mL/kg apple juice 2.5 hours before anesthesia; in addition, they were less thirsty and less irritable than the control children who received no juice (107). However, the preoperative fast should not be lessened for anything other than clear liquids, as aspiration of particulate material (106) or human breast milk are grave, regardless of acidity (75), nor should fasting be abated in obstetric patients or patients awaiting emergency procedures. The current ASA guidelines for preoperative fasting (108) list fasting times for clear liquids, human breast milk, infant formula, nonhuman milk, and a light meal. Depending on the substance ingested, a preoperative fasting time between 2 and 6 hours is considered safe. However, the recommended fasting periods apply to healthy patients awaiting elective surgery; exceptions have been defined for other circumstances (Table 139.3).

Preoperative Administration of Antacids

The large retrospective review of 215,488 general anesthetics found no difference between patients who received or did not receive prophylaxis for acid aspiration. This leads to the author's question, "Should these medications have been used routinely?" (20). The potential value of the preoperative administration of antacids is based on the unproven presumption

TABLE 139.3

PRACTICE GUIDELINES FOR PREOPERATIVE FASTING[a]

Ingested material	Minimum fasting period[b] (h)
Clear liquids[c]	2
Breast milk	4
Infant formula	6
Nonhuman milk[d]	6
Light meal[e]	6

[a]These recommendations apply to healthy patients who are undergoing elective procedures. They are not intended for women in labor. Following the Guidelines does not guarantee complete gastric emptying.
[b]The fasting periods noted above apply to all ages.
[c]Examples of clear liquids include water, fruit juices without pulp, carbonated beverages, clear tea, and black coffee.
[d]Since nonhuman milk is similar to solids in gastric emptying time, the amount ingested must be considered when determining an appropriate fasting period.
[e]A light meal typically consists of toast and clear liquids. Meals that include fried or fatty foods or meat may prolong gastric emptying time. Both the amount and type of foods ingested must be considered when determining an appropriate fasting period.
From American Society of Anesthesiologists Task Force on Preoperative Fasting. Practice guidelines for preoperative fasting and the use of pharmacologic agents to reduce the risk of pulmonary aspiration: application to healthy patients undergoing elective procedures: a report by the American Society of Anesthesiologists Task Force on Preoperative Fasting. *Anesthesiology.* 1999;90:896–890.

that drug-induced increases in gastric pH will decrease the likelihood of severe acid pneumonitis (20). Despite the known ability of antacids to increase gastric fluid pH, it has not been documented that prophylactic administration to a high-risk patient population (e.g., parturients) decreases mortality (109,110). Furthermore, antacids and other drugs, such as H_2 antagonists or proton pump inhibitors, have no impact on the incidence of regurgitation and aspiration. The duration of antacid action highly depends on gastric emptying time, which can be shortened by prokinetic drugs like metoclopramide. However, this effect is blocked by atropine or opioids. Opioids slow gastric motility and thus prolong the pH-elevating effects of antacids. The administration of antacids (e.g., to the parturient who has also received opioids) may result in greatly increased gastric fluid volume at the time general anesthesia is induced. With this in mind, it seems more prudent to administer nonparticulate (clear) antacids, such as 15 to 30 mL sodium citrate as a single dose, approximately 30 minutes before the anticipated induction of general anesthesia (111–113).

The pH of a 0.3 molar sodium citrate solution is 8.4, which reliably increases gastric fluid pH in pregnant and nonpregnant patients. If time permits, aspiration prophylaxis should be considered in all patients with a so-called "full stomach." However, in emergency cases, neutralization of gastric secretion with sodium citrate shortly before intubation is often not possible if an adequate level of consciousness or a gag reflex is missing (48). Because of the slow onset of action, the use of H_2 antagonists or proton pump inhibitors does not provide adequate suppression of acid production, nor does metoclopramide enhance gastric emptying in these emergency cases.

Based on the arguments mentioned above, the ASA Task Force on Preoperative Fasting (108) does not recommend the routine administration of antacids, gastric acid secretion blockers, antiemetics, or anticholinergics in patients who have no apparent increased risk for aspiration. Only nonparticulate antacids should be used when indicated for selected patients to decrease gastric acidity during the perioperative period (e.g., prior to cesarean section).

Rapid Sequence Induction

Protection against acid aspiration in patients at risk relies mainly upon rapid sequence induction (RSI). Injection of intravenous agents and the simultaneous application of effective cricoid pressure are followed immediately by tracheal intubation. The Sellick maneuver should be used when regional anesthesia is not feasible in patients thought to be at high risk for aspiration. The cricoid pressure is used to produce a collapse of the esophageal lumen and should be maintained until the endotracheal tube is visualized passing through the vocal cords, the cuff has been inflated, appropriate breath sounds are confirmed, mist is noted to be present in the endotracheal tube, and end-tidal CO_2 presence is verified (29). Most anesthesiologists prefer an elevated head-up position during RSI. The rationale for this maneuver is that an intragastric pressure higher than 20 cm H_2O is required to overcome the lower esophageal sphincter. The head-up position exceeding this distance impedes passive regurgitation, as in the case of muscle paralysis. In contrast, the head-down, Trendelenburg position would enable the regurgitated gastric contents to drain out of the oropharynx passively or be suctioned actively with a suction system. However, since endotracheal intubation usually is easier with the patient in an elevated, semirecumbent position, we would recommend it rather than the head-down position.

Despite taking all precautions, aspiration may still occur regardless of the patient's position or the applied cricoid pressure. Moreover, the ability to maintain adequate cricoid pressure for the necessary length of time and the accuracy in the delivery of cricoid pressure are uncertain. The application of cricoid pressure is a nonevidence-based, but clinically widespread, method in aspiration prophylaxis. Although there is little scientific evidence to support the widely held belief that the application of cricoid pressure reduces the incidence of aspiration during RSI (114), we recommend its use because of the minimal detrimental effects of application.

Because of the drawbacks to general anesthesia, many anesthesiologists prefer regional anesthesia for cesarean section. The use of these techniques for cesarean delivery has greatly increased due to the far lower incidence of aspiration. Accordingly, the incidence of maternal pulmonary aspiration has decreased greatly in the past decades—from 43 per 100,000 live births to 1.7 per 100,000 live births (115). The absolute number of deaths due to regional anesthesia has been decreased by 80%, down to 1.9 per 1,000,000 regional anesthetics. However, when general anesthesia is thought necessary for any reason, RSI and insertion of a cuffed endotracheal tube are obligatory.

When general anesthesia is indicated in patients at risk for pulmonary aspiration, airway management is one of the most important issues. Failed intubation occurs in the general surgical population at a rate of 1 in 2,330 (0.04%) (116), and is approximately eightfold higher in the obstetric population (117). Most airway catastrophes occur when airway difficulty is not recognized before the induction of anesthesia, and the anesthesiologist is not prepared to manage the difficult airway. Thus, meticulous preanesthetic examination is necessary to identify the patient at risk for airway difficulty as well as for aspiration; additionally, every airway should be considered a difficult airway, and backup plans should be in place if needed. The difficult airway is discussed elsewhere (Chapter 38).

Prevention of Aspiration in Critical Care

Several studies have demonstrated that regurgitation and aspiration is increased in tube-fed, critically ill patients lying in the supine position, as compared to the semirecumbent position (118–120). A fourfold higher VAP incidence was found in the supine position (34%) as compared to the semirecumbent group (8%) (120); there was also a significant association with gastric feeding and the occurrence of VAP. However, the risks of enteral feeding have to be balanced against its benefits. Thus, it seems prudent to avoid large gastric volumes rather than abandon gastric feeding *per se* in critically ill patients (17).

Theoretically, a cuff sealing the endotracheal tube against the tracheal wall will prevent aspiration of even the smallest amounts of oropharyngeal secretions, so-called *microaspiration*. Low-volume, high-pressure cuffs increase the risk of tracheal mucosal damage and, thus, are not appropriate for long-term endotracheal intubation. Instead, endotracheal tubes with high-volume, low-pressure cuffs are preferred if long-term intubation is expected. However, an endotracheal tube with a high-volume, low-pressure cuff does not prevent microaspiration from the subglottic area (121). Leakage of subglottic secretions occurs down longitudinal channels caused by folds within the inflated cuff wall. The reason for these folds is that the cuff must be larger than the cross-section of the trachea so it can adjust to the tracheal wall. Over the past several years, attempts have been made to improve the fit of the cuff in the tracheal wall by changing the shape and material of the cuff (122). Although some laboratory studies have demonstrated decreased leakage using improved cuff configurations, the problem of VAP is still not clinically solved with this approach.

Since pooled, bacterially contaminated secretions above the cuff are the reservoir for microaspiration, drainage of these secretions should reduce the incidence of aspiration and, consequently, the risk for VAP. However, conventional oropharyngeal suctioning techniques are usually not able to access this subglottic area, which is below the vocal cords and above the cuff of the tube. The removal of secretions from the subglottic region requires a specially designed endotracheal tube with a separate dorsal suctioning lumen, which opens into the subglottic region just above the cuff (123). This extra dorsal lumen is connected to an evacuation system, and the subglottic region is either drained intermittently or continuously with a gentle negative pressure—about 30 mm Hg suction. In four randomized controlled trials, which included more than 800 patients, the use of subglottic suction tubes was compared to conventional endotracheal tubes in critically ill patients (124–127). Only two of the four trials revealed a significant reduction of VAP in the subglottic suction group. There was no decrease in either mortality, length of stay, or duration of mechanical ventilation by the method tested (128). Moreover, in a recent animal study, it was shown that continuous subglottic suctioning may even be deleterious to the tracheal mucosa, while only marginally lowering the bacterial colonization of the lung (129). A recently published study revealed that the use of continuous subglottic suctioning did not modify the level of oropharyngeal and tracheal colonization in long-term ventilated critically ill patients. Two of five patients who had received subglottic suctioning developed laryngeal edema immediately after extubation, and required reintubation (130). A recent meta-analysis (131) studied the effects of subglottic drainage by evaluating the four studies mentioned above (124–127) and a fifth study (132). Subglottic suctioning in patients expected to require more than 72 hours of mechanical ventilation resulted in a significant reduction of the incidence of early-onset pneumonia (that occurring 5–7 days after endotracheal intubation). Furthermore, the duration of mechanical ventilation was shortened by 2 days, and the length of stay in the ICU was shortened by 3 days in these patients. These results suggest that subglottic suctioning may play a role in patients expected to be ventilated for prolonged periods, and only by reducing the incidence of early-onset pneumonia. However, the method (i.e., the specially designed tube) is expensive and may damage the tracheal mucosa. This risk must be weighed against the expected reduction of the incidence of VAP.

Prevention of Aspiration Pneumonia

Pneumonia depends on lung contamination with pathogenic micro-organisms as well as their virulence (i.e., their ability to overcome the host defense and cause an infection). Thus, another approach to avoid aspiration pneumonia is to prevent the consequences of microaspiration in endotracheally intubated patients rather than the microaspiration itself. The aspiration of small amounts of oropharyngeal secretions would be harmless for the lung if the sputum was sterile or only contaminated with nonpathogenic microbes. However, several factors—mainly the immunosuppression caused by severe illness, as well as antibiotic therapy itself, etc.—disturb the physiologic microbial balance, causing a shift in the microbiology of the oropharynx. Within a few days, the low-pathogenic and physiologic oropharyngeal microflora changes into a high-pathogenic abnormal flora, consisting mainly of Gram-negative bacilli (133). Therefore, the oropharynx of critically ill patients, and particularly the pooled secretions in the subglottic region, is heavily contaminated with potentially pathogenic microorganisms. Aspiration of oropharyngeal secretions contaminated with these pathogenic microbes is usually the source of aspiration pneumonia (134–136). Therefore, any approach to reduce the bacterial burden of the aspirated oropharyngeal secretions, as well as the virulence of the abnormal microbial flora, might reduce the morbidity of microaspiration and decrease VAP. Topically administered antibiotics at the contamination site (i.e., the oropharynx and the airway) eradicate the micro-organisms, or at least reduce their number and, thus, impede the development of aspiration pneumonia. However, there is a considerable controversy about such prophylactic administration of antimicrobial agents given that it enhances the risk of developing resistant bacterial strains. During the last decades, two approaches have been used in mechanically ventilated, critical care patients. One method is the nebulization of antibiotics into the airways via the endotracheal tube to reduce the colonization of bacteria in the bronchial tract (137–139). The other approach is the decontamination of the sources of the pathogenic microbes (i.e., decontamination of the oropharynx as well as the gastrointestinal tract). Usually nonabsorbable antibiotics are used in both methods to allow the application of supra-high local antibiotic concentrations at the target site (i.e., the airways or the oropharynx and gastrointestinal tract) without unwanted systemic toxic side effects. The use of supra-high local antibiotic concentrations may prevent or, at least, impede the development of antibiotic resistance.

Most often, aminoglycosides have been used for nebulization. Besides their use in the critically ill, there is substantial experience in patients suffering from mucoviscidosis and cystic fibrosis with the application of nebulized aminoglycosides.

Although some data on the use of nebulized antibiotics in mechanically ventilated patients are promising, a final conclusion cannot be made because the studies vary in their methodology and are inadequately powered. Moreover, application of nebulized antibiotics is only effective in preventing pneumonia, and seems not to benefit patients with active pneumonia, particularly when compared to the use of potent systemic antibiotics (140). Mortality was not decreased by the use of nebulized antibiotics in mechanically ventilated patients. Three recently published reviews extensively discuss this topic (137–139).

Another approach to reduce the bacterial colonization of the respiratory tract is the decontamination of the patient's internal bacterial sources (i.e., the gut, the stomach, and the oropharynx). However, while total decontamination of the oropharyngeal cavity and the gastrointestinal tract is not possible, selective decontamination of the oropharynx and the digestive tract (SDD) has been shown to reduce aspiration pneumonia in critically ill patients (141). The concept of SDD is the elimination of the main pathogenic bacilli (especially Gram-negative bacteria and *S. aureus*) as well as yeasts by oral and enteral application of a combination of nonabsorbable antibiotics and antimycotics (142). These microbes are very often involved in major infections in critically ill patients, whereas they play virtually no role in the physiologic intestinal ecosystem. SDD, as a means of infection prophylaxis, should suppress/eliminate as many potentially pathogenic micro-organisms as possible, leaving the relatively harmless and even protective anaerobic microflora unchanged (143). SDD has been studied in various critically ill patient populations, and several meta-analyses have been published (141,144,145). To date, randomized controlled trials have only demonstrated a significant decrease of VAP and mortality in trauma and liver transplant patients (146–148). SSD requires meticulous microbial surveillance to monitor the effects of the applied agents (i.e., the successful selective decontamination), as well as the possible emergence of antibiotic resistance. Owing to the risk–benefit controversy, the use of SDD is not commonplace in the United States, and it is routinely used only in selected centers in Europe (149).

PEARLS

1. The major risk factor for aspiration is a reduced level of consciousness. General anesthesia is a risk factor, particularly in emergency cases. Furthermore, any situation that leads to increased gastric pressure or increased gastric content may amplify the incidence of regurgitation and vomiting and, consequently, the risk of pulmonary aspiration.
2. Critically ill patients with ventilatory insufficiency are at particular risk of pulmonary aspiration. Even in patients whose airway is protected by a cuffed endotracheal tube, microaspiration is common, because the cuff configuration does not provide a complete sealing of the trachea.
3. In general anesthetics, the overall incidence of pulmonary aspiration is approximately 1 in 3,000. The pregnant patient is at higher risk for aspiration of gastric contents (about 1 in 900 to 1 in 1,400) for a variety of reasons, including mechanical, hormonal, and iatrogenic factors.
4. Silent aspiration during *short-term endotracheal intubation,* such as during anesthesia, is only of minor concern.
5. Silent aspiration in *long-term intubated* and mechanically ventilated patients is common and has been detected in up to 90% of patients. Since aspiration is the main cause of pneumonia in critically ill patients, this issue is of major concern.
6. In emergency medicine, aspiration is a common event due to a reduced consciousness and the impaired protective reflexes of emergency patients. The less prepared, prehospital setting further increases the risk of aspiration.
7. It is important to distinguish between aspiration pneumonitis and aspiration pneumonia. Aspiration pneumonitis is caused by chemically injurious agents (e.g., acid). Such agents destroy the lung tissue directly (e.g., by chemical burn). In contrast, aspiration pneumonia occurs as a result of microaspiration of bacterially contaminated, subglottic secretions in critically ill patients who are usually endotracheally intubated and mechanically ventilated.
8. The pulmonary consequence of aspiration depends on the nature of the aspirated substance:
   a) Acid-related aspiration causes pneumonitis, a chemical injury to the lung parenchyma.
   b) Aspiration of solid particles leads to acute airway obstruction or reflex airway closure with arterial hypoxemia, depending on the size of the particles and the obstructed lung area downstream of the obstruction.
   c) Aspiration of blood is harmless in most circumstances.
   d) Microaspiration of subglottic secretions is the major cause of ventilator-associated pneumonia. The harm of microaspiration depends on the virulence and the amount of bacteria contaminating the oropharyngeal secretions.
9. Bronchoscopy, most effective rigid, should only be used to remove solid particles from the airway. Bronchoscopy does not improve the course and outcome of patients who aspirated only liquid acid gastric contents.
10. Bronchial lavage after aspiration of gastric acid is rather deleterious, because it may spread the aspirate to previously unaffected lung areas and can wash out surfactant.
11. Steroids in the treatment of aspiration pneumonitis have been shown to be clinically ineffective. The administration of corticosteroids is controversial and most likely does not yield benefit or improvement of long-term outcome after aspiration. Application of β_2 sympathomimetics improves bronchospastic symptoms and may improve the removal of airway edema.
12. The cornerstones of the treatment of the harmful consequences of pulmonary aspiration are symptomatic measures, such as oxygen application, mechanical ventilation with PEEP, and antibiotic therapy only in case of pneumonia.

13. Prevention of macroaspiration during general anesthesia include the following principles:
    a) Identification of the patient at risk
    b) Skilled and well-prepared personnel (staff anesthesiologist and specialized nurse)
    c) Relief of gastric pressure in case of increased contents (i.e., ileus)
    d) Maintaining lower esophageal sphincter competence (i.e., removal of the nasogastric tube before induction of anesthesia)
    e) In the obstetric patient, alkalization of gastric acid prior to induction
    f) Rapid sequence induction including application of cricoid pressure

References

1. Dice WH, Ward B, Kelly J, et al. Pulmonary toxicity following gastrointestinal absorption of kerosene. *Ann Emerg Med.* 1982;11:138.
2. Bynum K, Pierce AK. Pulmonary aspiration of gastric contents. *Am Rev Respir Dis.* 1976;114:1129.
3. Grand RJ, Watkins JB, Torti FM. Development of the human gastrointestinal tract. A review. *Gastroenterology.* 1976;70:790–810.
4. Chadwick J, Mann WN. *Medical Works of Hippocrates.* Oxford: C& J Adlard; 1950.
5. Simpson JY. Remarks on the alleged case of death from the action of chloroform. *Lancet.* 1848;1:175.
6. Mendelson CL. The aspiration of stomach contents into the lungs during obstetric anesthesia. *Am J Obstet Gynecol.* 1946;52:191.
7. Goodwin SR: Aspiration syndromes. In: Civetta JM, Taylor RW, Kirby RR, eds. *Critical Care.* 3rd ed. Philadelphia: Lippincott-Raven; 1997:1861–1873.
8. Teabeaut JR II. Aspiration of gastric contents: an experimental study. *Am J Pathol.* 1952;24:51.
9. Roberts RB, Shirley MA. Reducing the risk of acid aspiration during cesarean section [no abstract available]. *Anesth Analg.* 1974;53:859–868.
10. James CF, Modell JH, Gibbs CP, et al. Pulmonary aspiration—effects of volume and pH in the rat. *Anesth Analg.* 1984;63:665–668.
11. Bynum LJ, Pierce AK. Pulmonary aspiration of gastric contents. *Am Rev Respir Dis.* 1976;114:1129–1136.
12. Gleeson K, Eggli DF, Maxwell SL. Quantitative aspiration during sleep in normal subjects. *Chest.* 1997;111:1266.
13. Pontoppidan H, Beecher HK. Progressive loss of protective reflexes in the airway with the advance of age. *JAMA.* 1960;174:2209.
14. Vaughan RW, Bauer S, Wise L. Volume and pH of gastric juice in obese patients. *Anesthesiology.* 1975;43:686–689.
15. Illing L, Duncan PG, Yip R. Gastroesophageal reflux during anaesthesia. *Can J Anaesth.* 1992;39:466–470.
16. Cook D. Ventilator associated pneumonia: perspectives on the burden of illness [review]. *Intensive Care Med.* 2000;26(Suppl 1):S31–37.
17. McClave SA, DeMeo MT, DeLegge MH, et al. North American Summit on aspiration in the critically ill patient: consensus statement. *JPEN J Parenter Enteral Nutr.* 2002;26(6 Suppl):S80–85.
18. Barquist E, Brown M, Cohn S, et al. Postextubation fiberoptic endoscopic evaluation of swallowing after prolonged endotracheal intubation: a randomized, prospective trial. *Crit Care Med.* 2001;29:1710–1713.
19. Olsson GL, Hallen B, Hambraeus-Jonzon K. Aspiration during anaesthesia: a computer-aided study of 185,358 anaesthetics. *Acta Anaesthesiol Scand.* 1986;30:84–92.
20. Warner MA, Warner ME, Weber JG. Clinical significance of pulmonary aspiration during the perioperative period. *Anesthesiology.* 1993;78:56–62.
21. Mellin-Olsen J, Fasting S, Gisvold SE. Routine preoperative gastric emptying is seldom indicated. A study of 85,594 anaesthetics with special focus on aspiration pneumonia. *Acta Anaesthesiol Scand.* 1996;40:1184–1188.
22. Jeffrey H, Kozlow BA, Berenholtz SM, et al. Epidemiology and impact of aspiration pneumonia in patients undergoing surgery in Maryland, 1999–2000. *Crit Care Med.* 2003;31:1930.
23. Marik PE. Aspiration pneumonia: mixing apples with oranges and tangerines. *Crit Care Med.* 2004;32:1236.
24. Tiret L, Nivoche Y, Hatton F, et al. Complications related to anaesthesia in infants and children. A prospective survey of 40240 anaesthetics. *Br J Anaesth.* 1988;61:263–269.
25. Hawkins JL. Anesthesia-related maternal mortality [review; no abstract available]. *Clin Obstet Gynecol.* 2003;46:679–687.
26. Munnur U, de Boisblanc B, Suresh MS. Airway problems in pregnancy. *Crit Care Med.* 2005;33(10 Suppl):S259–S268.
27. Cheney FW. The American Society of Anesthesiologists Closed Claims Project: what have we learned, how has it affected practice, and how will it affect practice in the future? *Anesthesiology.* 1999;91:552.
28. Chadwick HS, Posner K, Caplan RA, et al. A comparison of obstetric and nonobstetric anesthesia malpractice claims. *Anesthesiology.* 1991;74:242–249.
29. James CF. Cesarean section. In: Lobato EB, Gravenstein N, Kirby RR, eds. *Complications in Anesthesiology.* Philadelphia: Lippincott Williams & Wilkins; 2008:673–690.
30. La Rosa M, Piva L, Ravanelli A, et al. Aspiration syndrome in cesarean section. Our experience from 1980 to 1990 [Italian]. *Minerva Anestesiol.* 1992;58:1213.
31. Soreide E, Bjornestad E, Steen PA. An audit of perioperative aspiration pneumonitis in gynaecological and obstetric patients. *Acta Anaesthesiol Scand.* 1996;40:14–19.
32. Berson W, Adriani J. Silent regurgitation and aspiration during anesthesia. *Anesthesiology.* 1954;15:644–649.
33. Stark DC. Aspiration in the surgical patient. *Int Anesthesiol Clin.* 1977;15:13–48.
34. Blitt CD, Gutmann HL, Cohen DD, et al. "Silent" regurgitation and aspiration during general anesthesia. *Anest Analg.* 1970;49:707–713.
35. Hirsch J. Impact of postoperative nausea and vomiting in the surgical setting. *Anaesthesia.* 1994;49(Suppl):30–33.
36. Kinsey GC, Murray MJ, Swensen SJ, et al. Glucose content of tracheal aspirates: implications for the detection of tube feeding aspiration. *Crit Care Med.* 1994;22:1557–1562.
37. Heyland DK, Drover JW, MacDonald S, et al. Effect of postpyloric feeding on gastroesophageal regurgitation and pulmonary microaspiration: results of a randomized controlled trial. *Crit Care Med.* 2001;29:1495–1501.
38. Metheny NA, Clouse RE, Chang YH, et al. Tracheobronchial aspiration of gastric contents in critically ill tube-fed patients: frequency, outcomes, and risk factors. *Crit Care Med.* 2006;34:1007–1015.
39. Elpern EH, Scott MG, Petro L, et al. Pulmonary aspiration in mechanically ventilated patients with tracheostomies. *Chest.* 1994;105:563–566.
40. Leder S-B. Incidence and type of aspiration in acute care patients requiring mechanical ventilation via a new tracheotomy. *Chest.* 2002;122:1721–1726.
41. Chevret S, Hemmer M, Carlet J, et al. Incidence and risk factors of pneumonia acquired in intensive care units. Results from a multicenter prospective study on 996 patients. European Cooperative Group on Nosocomial Pneumonia. *Intensive Care Med.* 1993;19:256–264.
42. Rello J, Diaz E. Pneumonia in the intensive care unit. *Crit Care Med.* 2003;31:2544–2551.
43. George DV. Epidemiology of nosocomial ventilator-associated pneumonia. *Infect Control Hosp Epidemiol.* 1993;14:163–169.
44. LoCicero J 3rd. Bronchopulmonary aspiration [review]. *Surg Clin North Am.* 1989;69:71–76.
45. Gentleman D, Dearden M, Midgley S, et al. Guidelines for resuscitation and transfer of patients with serious head injury [review; no abstract available]. *BMJ.* 1993;307(6903):547–552.
46. Vadeboncoeur TF, Davis DP, Ochs M, et al. The ability of paramedics to predict aspiration in patients undergoing prehospital rapid sequence intubation. *J Emerg Med.* 2006;30:131–136.
47. Lockey DJ, Coats T, Parr MJ. Aspiration in severe trauma: a prospective study. *Anaesthesia.* 1999;54:1097–1098.
48. Gabrielli A, Layon AJ. Airway management in the neurointensive care unit. In: Layon AJ, Gabrielli A, Friedman WA, eds. *Textbook of Neurointensive Care.* Philadelphia: Saunders; 2004:499–531.
49. Ufberg JW, Bushra JS, Karras DJ, et al. Aspiration of gastric contents: association with prehospital intubation. *Am J Emerg Med.* 2005;23:379–382.
50. Cogbill TH, Bintz M, Johnson JA, et al. Acute gastric dilatation after trauma. *J Trauma.* 1987;27:1113–1117.
51. Lawes EG, Baskett PJ. Pulmonary aspiration during unsuccessful cardiopulmonary resuscitation. *Intensive Care Med.* 1987;13:379–382.
52. Marik PE. Aspiration pneumonitis and aspiration pneumonia. *N Engl J Med.* 2001;344:665–671.
53. Engelhardt T, Webster NR. Pulmonary aspiration of gastric contents in anaesthesia. *Br J Anaesth.* 1999;83:453–460.
54. Isbister GK, Downes F, Sibbritt D, et al. Aspiration pneumonitis in an overdose population: frequency, predictors, and outcomes. *Crit Care Med.* 2004;32:88–93.
55. Mattay MA, Mednick G, Matthay ZA. Aspiration-induced lung injury: experimental and human studies. In: Vincent JL, ed. *Yearbook of Intensive Care and Emergency Medicine.* Berlin: Springer; 2006:349–365.
56. Folkesson HG, Matthay MA, Hebert CA, et al. Acid aspiration-induced lung injury in rabbits is mediated by interleukin-8-dependent mechanisms. *J Clin Invest.* 1995;96:107–116.
57. Porembka DT, Kier A, Sehlhorst S, et al. The pathophysiologic changes following bile aspiration in a porcine lung model. *Chest.* 1993;104:919–924.
58. Midulla F, Guidi R, Barbato A, et al. Foreign body aspiration in children. *Pediatr Int.* 2005;47:663–668.

59. Cotton E, Yasuda K. Foreign body aspiration. *Pediatr Clin North Am.* 1984;31:937–941.
60. Center for Disease Control (CDC). Nonfatal choking-related episodes among children—United States, 2001. *MMWR Morb Mortal Wkly Rep.* 2002;51:945–948.
61. Aytac A, Yurdakul Y, Ikizler C, et al. Inhalation of foreign bodies in children. Report of 500 cases. *J Thorac Cardiovasc Surg.* 1977;74:145–151.
62. Ayed AK, Jafar AM, Owayed A. Foreign body aspiration in children: diagnosis and treatment. *Pediatr Surg Int.* 2003;19:485–488.
63. Szidon JP, Fishman AP. Approach to the pulmonary patient with respiratory signs and symptoms. In: *Pulmonary Diseases and Disorders.* 2nd ed. New York: McGraw-Hill; 1988:346–351.
64. Perel A, Downs JB, Crawford CA, et al. Continuous positive airway pressure improves oxygenation in dogs after the aspiration of blood. *Crit Care Med.* 1983;11:868–871.
65. Moran TJ, Hellstrom HR. Experimental aspiration pneumonia. V. Acute pulmonary edema, pneumonia, and bronchiolitis obliterans produced by injection of ethyl alcohol. *Am J Clin Pathol.* 1957;27:300–308.
66. Dice WH, Ward G, Kelley J, et al. Pulmonary toxicity following gastrointestinal ingestion of kerosene. *Ann Emerg Med.* 1982;11:138–142.
67. Goodwin SR, Berman LS, Tabeling BB, et al. Kerosene aspiration: immediate and early pulmonary and cardiovascular effects. *Vet Hum Toxicol.* 1988;30:521–524.
68. de Graaf P, Slagt C, de Graaf JL, et al. Fatal aspiration of polyethylene glycol solution. *Neth J Med.* 2006;64:196–198.
69. Mackowiak PA. The normal microbial flora. *N Engl J Med.* 1982;307:83–93.
70. Vidyasagar D, Harris V, Pildes RS. Assisted ventilation in infants with meconium aspiration syndrome. *Pediatrics.* 1975;56(2):208–213.
71. Ross MG. Meconium aspiration syndrome-more than intrapartum meconium [no abstract available]. *N Engl J Med.* 2005;353:946–948.
72. Wiswell TE, Tuggle JM, Turner BS. Meconium aspiration syndrome: have we made a difference? *Pediatrics.* 1990;85:715–721.
73. Fraser WD, Hofmeyr J, Lede R, et al. Amnioinfusion Trial Group. Amnioinfusion for the prevention of the meconium aspiration syndrome. *N Engl J Med.* 2005;353:909–917.
74. Vain NE, Szyld EG, Prudent LM, et al. Oropharyngeal and nasopharyngeal suctioning of meconium-stained neonates before delivery of their shoulders: multicentre, randomised controlled trial. *Lancet.* 2004;364:597–602.
75. O'Hare B, Chin C, Lerman J, et al. Acute lung injury after instillation of human breast milk into rabbits' lungs: effects of pH and gastric juice. *Anesthesiology.* 1999;90:1112–1118.
76. Leighton BL. Intraoperative anesthetic complications. In: Noris MC, ed. *Obstetric Anesthesia.* 2nd ed. Philadelphia: Lippincott Williams & Wilkins; 1999:539–618.
77. Kinni ME, Stout MM. Aspiration pneumonitis: predisposing conditions and prevention. *J Oral Maxillofac Surg.* 1986;44:378–384.
78. Kinsey GC, Murray MJ, Swensen SJ, et al. Glucose content of tracheal aspirates: implications for the detection of tube feeding aspiration. *Crit Care Med.* 1994;22:1557–1562.
79. Metheny NA, Clouse RE, Chang YH, et al. Tracheobronchial aspiration of gastric contents in critically ill tube-fed patients: frequency, outcomes, and risk factors. *Crit Care Med.* 2006;34:1007–1015.
80. Badellino MM, Buckman RF Jr, Malaspina PJ, et al. Detection of pulmonary aspiration of gastric contents in an animal model by assay of peptic activity in bronchoalveolar fluid. *Crit Care Med.* 1996;24:1881–1885.
81. Ufberg JW, Bushra JS, Patel D, et al. A new pepsin assay to detect pulmonary aspiration of gastric contents among newly intubated patients. *Am J Emerg Med.* 2004;22:612–614.
82. Spurrier EJ, Clancy MJ, Deakin CD. Laryngopharyngeal pH measurement. *Emerg Med J.* 2004;21:493–494.
83. Artigas AT, Dronda SB, Vallés EC, et al. Risk factors for nosocomial pneumonia in critically ill trauma patients. *Crit Care Med.* 2001;29:304–309.
84. Torres A, Aznar R, Gatell JM, et al. Incidence, risk, and prognosis factors of nosocomial pneumonia in mechanically ventilated patients. *Am Rev Respir Dis.* 1990;142:523–528.
85. Frank JA, Gutierrez JA, Jones KD, et al. Low tidal volume reduces epithelial and endothelial injury in acid-injured rat lungs. *Am J Respir Crit Care Med.* 2002;165:242–249.
86. The Acute Respiratory Distress Syndrome Network. Efficacy of low tidal volume ventilation in patients with different clinical risk factors for acute lung injury and the acute respiratory distress syndrome. *Am J Respir Crit Care Med.* 2001;64:231.
87. McAuley DF, Frank JA, Fang X, et al. Clinically relevant concentrations of beta2-adrenergic agonists stimulate maximal cyclic adenosine monophosphate-dependent airspace fluid clearance and decrease pulmonary edema in experimental acid-induced lung injury. *Crit Care Med.* 2004;32:1470–1476.
88. Musante G, Schnitzler E. Different therapeutic perspectives for novel exogenous surfactant preparations. *Crit Care Med.* 2006;34:260–261.
89. Hilgendorff A, Doerner M, Rawer D, et al. Effects of a recombinant surfactant protein-C-based surfactant on lung function and the pulmonary surfactant system in a model of meconium aspiration syndrome. *Crit Care Med.* 2006;34:203–210.
90. Anzueto A, Baughman R, Guntupalli K, et al. An international randomized, placebo-controlled trial evaluating the efficacy of aerosolized surfactant in patients with sepsis-induced ARDS. *Am J Resp Crit Care.* 1994;149:A567.
91. Lauer S, Fischer L, Stubbe H, et al. (K)eine Surfactant-Therapie bei Patienten mit "acute respiratory distress syndrome"? *Der Anaesthesist.* 2006;55:433–442.
92. Wynne JW, DeMarco FJ, Hood CI. Physiological effects of corticosteroids in foodstuff aspiration. *Arch Surg.* 1981;116:46–49.
93. Lee M, Sukumaran M, Berger HW, et al. Influence of corticosteroid treatment on pulmonary function after recovery from aspiration of gastric contents [no abstract available]. *Mt Sinai J Med.* 1980;47:341–346.
94. Lowrey LD, Anderson M, Calhoun J, et al. Failure of corticosteroid therapy for experimental acid aspiration [no abstract available]. *J Surg Res.* 1982;32:168–172.
95. Bernard GR, Luce JM, Sprung CL, et al. High-dose corticosteroids in patients with the adult respiratory distress syndrome. *N Engl J Med.* 1987; 317:1565–1570.
96. Ott SR, Lode H. Diagnostik und Therapie der Aspirationspneumonie. *Dtsch Med Wochenschr.* 2006;131:624–628.
97. LeFrock JL, Clark TS, Davies B, et al. Aspiration pneumonia: a ten-year review. *Am Surg.* 1979;45:305–313.
98. Brun-Buisson C. Advances and controversies in the epidemiology, diagnosis, and prevention of nosocomial pneumonia in the ICU. *Curr Opin Crit Care.* 1995;1:341–348.
99. Ewig S, Torres A, El-Ebiary M, et al. Bacterial colonization patterns in mechanically ventilated patients with traumatic and medical head injury. Incidence, risk factors, and association with ventilator-associated pneumonia. *Am J Respir Crit Care Med.* 1999;159:188–198.
100. Kallar SK, Everett LL. Potential risks and preventive measures for pulmonary aspiration: new concepts in preoperative fasting guidelines. *Anesth Analg.* 1993;77:171–182.
101. Sutherland AD, Maltby JR, Sale JP, et al. The effect of preoperative oral fluid and ranitidine on gastric fluid volume and pH. *Can J Anaesth.* 1987; 34:117–121.
102. McGrady EM, Macdonald AG. Effect of the preoperative administration of water on gastric volume and pH. *Br J Anaesth.* 1988;60:803–805.
103. Hutchinson A, Maltby JR, Reid CR. Gastric fluid volume and pH in elective inpatients. Part I: coffee or orange juice versus overnight fast. *Can J Anaesth.* 1988;35:12–15.
104. Warner MA, Warner ME, Warner DO, et al. Perioperative pulmonary aspiration in infants and children. *Anesthesiology.* 1999;90:66–71.
105. Kehlet H, Wilmore DW. Multimodal strategies to improve surgical outcome. *Am J Surg.* 2002;183:630–641.
106. Schwartz DJ, Wynne JW, Gibbs CP, et al. The pulmonary consequences of aspiration of gastric contents at pH values greater than 2.5. *Am Rev Respir Dis.* 1980;121:119–126.
107. Splinter WM, Stewart JA, Muir JG. Large volumes of apple juice preoperatively do not affect gastric pH and volume in children. *Can J Anaesth.* 1990;37:36–39.
108. American Society of Anesthesiologist Task Force on Preoperative Fasting. Practice guidelines for preoperative fasting and the use of pharmacologic agents to reduce the risk of pulmonary aspiration: application to healthy patients undergoing elective procedures: a report by the American Society of Anesthesiologist Task Force on Preoperative Fasting. *Anesthesiology.* 1999; 90:896–905.
109. Taylor G. Acid pulmonary aspiration syndrome after antacids. A case report. *Br J Anaesth.* 1975;47:615–617.
110. Tompkinson J, Turnbull A, Robson R, et al. Report on confidential enquiries into maternal deaths in England and Wales 1976–1978. *London: Her Majesty's Stationery Office.* 1982;79.
111. Gibbs CP, Spohr L, Schmidt D. The effectiveness of sodium citrate as an antacid [no abstract available]. *Anesthesiology.* 1982;57:44–46.
112. Holdsworth JD, Johnson K, Mascall G, et al. Mixing of antacids with stomach contents. Another approach to the prevention of the acid aspiration (Mendelson's) syndrome. *Anaesthesia.* 1980;35:641–650.
113. Viegas OJ, Ravindran RS, Shumacker CA. Gastric fluid pH in patients receiving sodium citrate. *Anesth Analg.* 1981;60:521–523.
114. Butler J, Sen A. Best evidence topic report. Cricoid pressure in emergency rapid sequence induction [review]. *Emerg Med J.* 2005;22:815–816.
115. Hawkins JL, Koonin LM, Palmer SK, et al. Anesthesia-related deaths during obstetric delivery in the United States, 1979–1990. *Anesthesiology.* 1997; 86:277–284.
116. Samsoon GL, Young JR. Difficult tracheal intubation: a retrospective study. *Anaesthesia.* 1987;42:487–490.
117. Lyons G. Failed intubation. Six years' experience in a teaching maternity unit. *Anaesthesia.* 1985;40:759–762.
118. Torres A, Serra-Batlles J, Ros E, et al. Pulmonary aspiration of gastric contents in patients receiving mechanical ventilation: the effect of body position. *Ann Intern Med.* 1992;116:540–543.
119. Ibanez J, Penafiel A, Raurich JM, et al. Gastroesophageal reflux in intubated patients receiving enteral nutrition: effect of supine and semirecumbent positions. *JPEN J Parenter Enteral Nutr.* 1992;16:419–422.
120. Drakulovic MB, Torres A, Bauer TT, et al. Supine body position as a risk factor for nosocomial pneumonia in mechanically ventilated patients: a randomised trial. *Lancet.* 1999;354:1851–1858.

121. Seegobin RD, van Hasselt GL. Aspiration beyond endotracheal cuffs. *Can Anaesth Soc J.* 1986;33:273–279.
122. Young PJ, Blunt MC. Improving the shape and compliance characteristics of a high-volume, low-pressure cuff improves tracheal seal. *Br J Anaesth.* 1999;83:887–889.
123. Diaz E, Rodriguez AH, Rello J. Ventilator-associated pneumonia: issues related to the artificial airway. *Respir Care.* 2005;50:900–906; discussion 906–909.
124. Kollef MH, Skubas NJ, Sundt TM. A randomized clinical trial of continuous aspiration of subglottic secretions in cardiac surgery patients. *Chest.* 1999;116:1339–1346.
125. Mahul PH, Auboyer C, Jospe R, et al. Prevention of nosocomial pneumonia in intubated patients: respective role of mechanical subglottic secretions drainage and stress ulcer prophylaxis. *Intensive Care Med.* 1992;18:20–25.
126. Smulders K, van der Hoeven H, Weers-Pothoff I, et al. A randomized clinical trial of intermittent subglottic secretion drainage in patients receiving mechanical ventilation. *Chest.* 2002;121:858–862.
127. Valles J, Artigas A, Rello J, et al. Continuous aspiration of subglottic secretions in preventing ventilator-associated pneumonia. *Ann Intern Med.* 1995;122:179–186.
128. van Saene HK, Ashworth M, Petros AJ, et al. Do not suction above the cuff. *Crit Care Med.* 2004;32:2160–2162.
129. Berra L, De Marchi L, Panigada M, et al. Evaluation of continuous aspiration of subglottic secretion in an in vivo study. *Crit Care Med.* 2004;32: 2071–2078.
130. Girou E, Buu-Hoi A, Stephan F, et al. Airway colonisation in long-term mechanically ventilated patients. Effect of semi-recumbent position and continuous subglottic suctioning. *Intensive Care Med.* 2004;30:225–233.
131. Dezfulian C, Shojania K, Collard HR, et al. Subglottic secretion drainage for preventing ventilator-associated pneumonia: a meta-analysis. *Am J Med.* 2005;118:11–18.
132. Bo H, He L, Qu J. Influence of the subglottic secretion drainage on the morbidity of ventilator associated pneumonia in mechanically ventilated patients [in Chinese]. *Zhonghua Jie He He Hu Xi Za Zhi.* 2000;23:472–474.
133. Johanson WG, Pierce AK, Sanford JP. Changing pharyngeal bacterial flora of hospitalized patients. Emergence of gram-negative bacilli. *N Engl J Med.* 1969;281:1137–1140.
134. Johanson WG Jr, Pierce AK, Sanford JP, et al. Nosocomial respiratory infections with gram-negative bacilli. The significance of colonization of the respiratory tract. *Ann Intern Med.* 1972;77:701–706.
135. van Uffelen R, van Saene HK, Fidler V, et al. Oropharyngeal flora as a source of bacteria colonizing the lower airways in patients on artificial ventilation. *Intensive Care Med.* 1984;10:233–237.
136. Bonten MJ, Gaillard CA, de Leeuw PW, et al. Role of colonization of the upper intestinal tract in the pathogenesis of ventilator-associated pneumonia. *Clin Infect Dis.* 1997;24:309–319.
137. Cole PJ, et al. The role of nebulized antibiotics in treating serious respiratory infections. *J Chemother.* 2001;13:354–362.
138. Falagas ME, Siempos II, Bliziotis IA, et al. Administration of antibiotics via the respiratory tract for the prevention of ICU-acquired pneumonia: a meta-analysis of comparative trials. *Crit Care.* 2006;10(4):R123.
139. Wood GC, Boucher BA. Aerosolized antimicrobial therapy in acutely ill patients. *Pharmacotherapy.* 2000;20:166–181.
140. Schaad UB, Wedgwood-Krucko J, Suter S, et al. Efficacy of inhaled amikacin as adjunct to intravenous combination therapy (ceftazidime and amikacin) in cystic fibrosis. *Pediatrics.* 1987;111:599–605.
141. van Saene HK, Petros AJ, Ramsay G, et al. All great truths are iconoclastic: selective decontamination of the digestive tract moves from heresy to level 1 truth. *Intensive Care Med.* 2003;29:677–690.
142. van der Waaij D, Manson WL, Arends JP, et al. Clinical use of selective decontamination: the concept. *Intensive Care Med.* 1990;16(Suppl 3):S212–216.
143. van der Waaij D. History of recognition and measurement of colonization resistance of the digestive tract as an introduction to selective gastrointestinal decontamination. *Epidemiol Infect.* 1992;109:315–326.
144. Nathens AB, Marshall JC. Selective decontamination of the digestive tract in surgical patients: a systematic review of the evidence. *Arch Surg.* 1999; 134:170–176.
145. Safdar N, Said A, Lucey MR. The role of selective digestive decontamination for reducing infection in patients undergoing liver transplantation: a systematic review and meta-analysis. *Liver Transpl.* 2004;10:817–827.
146. Stoutenbeek CP, van Saene HK, Miranda DR, et al. The effect of selective decontamination of the digestive tract on colonisation and infection rate in multiple trauma patients. *Intensive Care Med.* 1984;10:185–192.
147. Ledingham IM, Alcock SR, Eastaway AT, et al. Triple regimen of selective decontamination of the digestive tract, systemic cefotaxime, and microbiological surveillance for prevention of acquired infection in intensive care. *Lancet.* 1988;1(8589):785–790.
148. de Jonge E, Schultz MJ, Spanjaard L, et al. Effects of selective decontamination of digestive tract on mortality and acquisition of resistant bacteria in intensive care: a randomised controlled trial. *Lancet.* 2003;362:1011–1016.
149. Misset B, Artigas A, Bihari D, et al. Short-term impact of the European Consensus Conference on the use of selective decontamination of the digestive tract with antibiotics in ICU patients. *Intensive Care Med.* 1996;22:981–984.

CHAPTER 140 ■ SEVERE ASTHMA EXACERBATION

PARASKEVI A. KATSAOUNOU • THEODOROS VASSILAKOPOULOS

DEFINITION AND CHARACTERISTICS OF SEVERE ASTHMA—DIFFERENT PHENOTYPES

It is imperative to use a recognized common definition of severe asthma and to distinguish other terms and definitions that are usually included in this definition or used as synonyms. This is because of the complexity of asthma as a disease, which is mostly a collection of different phenotypes, rather than a single, specific disease with a unifying pathogenic mechanism (1). Various clinical definitions have been proposed through national and international guidelines, working groups, and workshops, which incorporate symptoms, lung function, exacerbations, and, in many cases, specific use of high-dose corticosteroids (2–5). In the original European Network description, patients with severe asthma were defined as those who were difficult to control after evaluation and treatment by an asthma specialist for a year or more (4,6).

The NAEPP (National Asthma Educational and Prevention Program) (3) and GINA (Global Initiative for Asthma)

TABLE 140.1

TERMS AND DEFINITIONS IN SEVERE ASTHMA

Term	Definition
Severe persistent asthma (2)	Continual symptoms, frequent nocturnal symptoms, limited activity, frequent exacerbations, FEV_1 or PEV<60% predicted, PEF variability >30%.
Severe/refractory Asthma (5) Definition requires that at least one major criterion and two minor criteria are met, other disorders have been excluded, exacerbating factors have been treated, and patient is generally compliant.	MAJOR: 1. Treatment requires continuous or nearly continuous (≥50% of year) oral corticosteroids. 2. Treatment requires high-dose (>880 μg/d fluticasone or equivalent) inhaled corticosteroids. MINOR: 1. Asthma symptoms needing short-acting β-agonist use on a daily or near-daily basis. 2. Need for additional daily treatment with a controller medication (e.g., long-acting β-agonist, theophylline, or leukotriene antagonist). 3. Persistent airway obstruction (FEV_1<80% predicted, diurnal peak expiratory flow variability >20%). 4. One or more urgent care visits for asthma per year. 5. Three or more oral steroid bursts per year. 6. Prompt clinical deterioration with ≤25% reduction in oral or intravenous corticosteroid dose. 7. Near-fatal asthma event in the past.
Severe asthma (4)	Diagnosis requires at least three of the following: 1. Seen by a consultant in asthma >2 yr. 2. Has persistent symptoms and decreased quality of life. 3. Has received maximal asthma therapy (high-dose inhaled corticosteroids [ICS]) with documented adherence. 4. History of respiratory failure/intubation. 5. Has repeated low FEV_1 <70% predicted.
Status asthmaticus:	Severe airway obstruction and asthmatic symptoms persist despite the administration of standard acute asthma therapy.
Difficult-to-treat asthma:	Failure to achieve asthma control when maximally recommended doses of inhaled therapy are prescribed for at least 6–12 months.
Steroid-resistant Asthma[a]	Failure of FEV_1 or PEF to improve >15% after 14-d course of at least 40 mg/d of prednisone.
Steroid-dependent Asthma[a]	Asthma that can be controlled only with oral corticosteroids, but in contrast to corticosteroid-resistance there is a response to this agent, although only when high doses are given.
Irreversible asthma	Persistent airflow obstruction despite maximum controller therapy; presumably related to airway and parenchymal structural alterations.
Near-fatal asthma[b]	Attack associated with respiratory failure, intubation, and/or hemodynamic and metabolic compromise; usually requiring intensive care unit admission.
Fixed airway obstruction	Persistent airflow obstruction despite maximal controller therapy; presumably related to airway and parenchymal structural alterations.
Brittle asthma[a]	Unstable, unpredictable asthmatics with wide variability in PEF; type I—persistent PEF variability (>40%) despite controller therapy; type II—prone to sudden, dramatic falls in PEF.
Asthma related to specific triggers or circumstances	*Premenstrual asthma:* Worsening of asthma 7 days premenstrually. *Aspirin-induced asthma.*

FEV_1, forced expiratory volume in 1 second; PEV, peak expiratory velocity; PEF, peak expiratory flow; ICS, inhaled corticosteroids.
[a]Barnes PJ. Difficult asthma. *Eur Respir J.* 1998.
[b]Romagnoli M, Caramori G, Braccioni F, et al. Near-fatal asthma phenotype in the ENFUMOSA Cohort. Clin Exp Allergy. 2007;37:552–557.

(3) guidelines both assess disease severity on the basis of nocturnal symptoms, use of short-acting bronchodilators, frequency of exacerbations that affect daily activities, and baseline pulmonary function measurements before treatment (Table 140.1). Subjective elements (patient symptoms) and objective data (pulmonary function tests) are weighted equally in these classification schemes, yet respiratory symptoms have been shown to correlate poorly with objective measures of airway obstruction, such as forced expiratory volume in 1 second (FEV_1) (7–9). Multiple studies have shown that both patients and physicians inaccurately estimate disease severity, leading to *under*treatment of patients (9–11). A recent analysis

evaluating concordance between the NAEPP and GINA guideline classification found poor agreement among these methods of disease classification (11).

Perhaps the most comprehensive attempt at a definition was undertaken by an American Thoracic Society workshop, the proceedings of which were published in 2000 (5), on refractory asthma. In considering a term to describe this subgroup of asthmatic patients with troublesome disease, the workshop participants agreed on the term *refractory asthma*. They proposed to reserve the term, *severe asthma*, for those patients who have refractory asthma and remain difficult to control despite extensive re-evaluation of diagnosis, management, and observation by an asthma specialist for at least 6 months. Refractory asthma is not meant to describe only patients with "fatal" or "near-fatal" asthma, but it is meant to encompass the asthma subgroups previously described as "severe asthma," "steroid-dependent and/or resistant asthma," "difficult-to-control asthma," "poorly controlled asthma," "brittle asthma," or "irreversible asthma." Clinically, patients with refractory asthma may present with a variety of separate and/or overlapping conditions, including:

- Widely varying peak flows (brittle asthma)
- Severe but chronic airflow limitation
- Rapidly progressive loss of lung function
- Mucus production ranging from absent to copious
- Varying responses to corticosteroids

Whether these groups form distinct clinical, physiologic, and pathologic groups is unclear. The American Thoracic Society Workshop definition required one of two major criteria (Table 140.1), and two of seven additional minor criteria. The minor criteria included aspects of lung function, exacerbations, disease stability, and the use of one or more additional controller medications. However, this definition has not yet been subjected to prospective evaluation. The incorporation of health care use would strengthen the definition by identifying patients with the greatest morbidity (12). Interestingly, although severe or refractory asthma afflicts a small percentage—likely 10%—of the asthma population, it remains a frustrating disease for both patients and clinicians, proportionally reflecting >40% of total cost. Indeed, recent studies showed physician assessment of severity to be positively associated with emergency department visits and inpatient hospitalizations, and a previous hospital admission for asthma is reported to increase the risk of asthma mortality by tenfold (13). These studies suggest that measures of health care utilization are an important addition to the traditional measures of disease severity in asthma. The incorporation of these measures into the American Thoracic Society workshop definition should improve our ability to identify the subgroup of patients with severe asthma who are responsible for the morbidity and mortality associated with severe disease. The combination of two methods of severity assessment (NAEPP with physician assessment) in the Epidemiology and Natural History of Asthma: Outcomes and Treatment Regimens (TENOR), a study of nearly 5,000 "difficult-to-treat" patients with asthma cohort identified the patients with severe asthma who had the highest health care utilization (14).

A proportion of patients with severe asthma have a disease that is eminently treatable, but that remains misdiagnosed, underdiagnosed, or undertreated. Asthma severity can also result from poor adherence to treatment, most frequently because of fears related to side effects of inhaled corticosteroids or difficulties using inhaler devices (15). Patients should be evaluated for these factors prior to making the diagnosis of refractory disease. A trial of oral corticosteroids and careful supervision by a specialty clinic is usually sufficient to establish suboptimal treatment and correct this problem. Therefore, in conjunction with the previous criteria, patients must have had adherence and exacerbating factors fully addressed. This definition has recently been incorporated into a National Heart, Lung, and Blood Institute–sponsored network to study severe asthma. Although these definitions are a start, it is likely that objective investigations of populations with severe asthma, such as those undertaken by the National Heart, Lung, and Blood Institute, the European Network for Understanding Mechanisms of Severe Asthma (ENFUMOSA), and the follow-up to ENFUMOSA, BioAir, or pharmaceutical-sponsored studies such as TENOR, will markedly improve our ability to identify, study, and treat patients with severe asthma (6,7). Of note, severe asthma can be easily confused with poorly controlled asthma. Although distinctions are still being drawn, poorly controlled asthma may be a more transient state of the disease, in which the levels of symptoms can be improved when standard approaches to therapy are appropriately used. On the contrary, severe asthma represents disease that is not responsive to standard therapy, thus remaining poorly controlled despite vigorous attempts at management.

To clarify precisely which conditions are supposed to be aspects of severe/difficult-to-treat asthma, the terms and definitions are described (Table 140.1). Severe asthma is not a homogenous entity but a complex heterogeneous, multifaceted condition that can be subdivided into different subtypes (16–18). The value of phenotyping is to guide current therapy, increase understanding of the pathophysiology and natural history of the disease, and link specific phenotypes to genotypes in order to develop targeted treatments; the phenotyping can be done from very different perspectives. Numerous attempts at classifying potential phenotypes of severe asthma have been proposed, as shown in Table 140.2. Although these phenotypes may overlap, there is reasonable supporting evidence for the presence of at least six—and likely more—severe asthma phenotypes as defined by clinical parameters (natural history, clinical presentation, atopy, airflow obstruction), type of inflammation, and treatment-related parameters (13,17–23).

From a clinical point of view, three categories of severely asthmatic patients seem to be of particular importance:

- Those with frequent severe asthma exacerbations
- Those with fixed airway obstruction
- Those with oral steroid dependency

Together, these three categories encompass most of the patients referred with difficult-to-control asthma.

PATHOPHYSIOLOGY

Respiratory Mechanics

The main pathophysiologic mechanism of acute severe asthma is pulmonary hyperinflation (24) caused by a combination of factors (Fig. 140.1). The driving force for expiratory flow is reduced because of an abnormally low pulmonary elastic recoil, the etiology of which is uncertain (25,26). Persistent activation of the inspiratory muscles during expiration causes outward

TABLE 140.2

PHENOTYPES OF ASTHMA

Parameter	Description
Natural history	■ Early-onset (childhood-onset) ■ Late-onset (adult-onset)
Type of airway inflammation	■ Predominantly eosinophilic ■ Predominantly neutrophilic ■ Pauci-inflammatory phenotype
Response to treatment	■ Steroid-dependent ■ Steroid-resistant ■ Steroid-sensitive
Severity	■ Mild ■ Moderate ■ Severe ■ Near-fatal asthma ■ Fatal asthma
Pattern of bronchoconstriction	■ Brittle ■ Stable ■ Fixed obstruction
Presence or absence of atopy	■ Atopic ■ Nonatopic
Major trigger factor	■ Gastric asthma ■ Aspirin-sensitive asthma ■ Hormonal asthma

recoil of the chest wall, further reducing the driving force for expiration (27). At the same time, resistance to airflow is greatly augmented because of severely reduced airway caliber and, perhaps, also narrowing of the glottic aperture during expiration (28). Expiration is prolonged, so that the following inspiration starts before static equilibrium is reached. Consequently the end-expiratory alveolar pressure remains positive, a phenomenon known as *auto-PEEP* (positive end-expiratory pressure) or *intrinsic PEEP* (PEEPi) or static PEEPi (PEEPi, st) (29,30).

It should be noticed that the lung is extremely inhomogeneous during acute severe asthma. The distribution of bronchial obstruction is uneven because of both anatomic reasons—

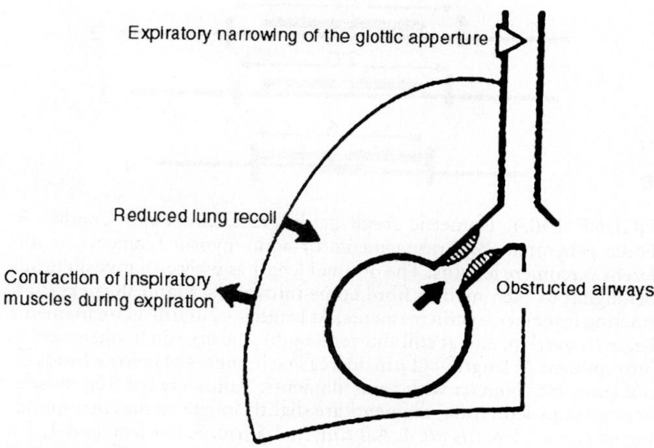

FIGURE 140.1. Mechanisms responsible for dynamic hyperinflation in asthma.

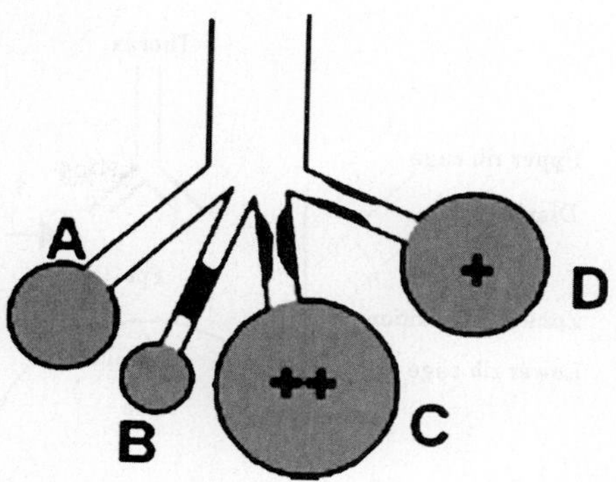

FIGURE 140.2. Effect of varying amounts of airway obstruction on end-expiratory alveolar volumes and pressures. (From Oddo M, Feihl F, Schaller MD, et al. Heliox improves pulsus paradoxus and peak expiratory flow in nonintubated patients with severe asthma. *Intensive Care Med.* 2006;32:501–510, with permission).

variable amounts of secretions, edema, bronchospasm—and variable external compression exerted on the distal airways by intrathoracic positive pressure during expiration (31). Thus, illustratively, four parallel compartments can be recognized (Fig. 140.2): compartment A represents the portion of the lung with neither bronchial obstruction nor hyperinflation; compartment B is the part of the lung where the airways are entirely obstructed during the whole respiratory cycle (mucous plugging); in compartment C, obstruction appears only during expiration, inducing alveolar hyperinflation and high PEEPi; and in compartment D, partial obstruction of the airways is present throughout the respiratory cycle, causing a lesser extent of alveolar hyperinflation and PEEPi than in compartment C.

Hyperinflation has several detrimental consequences (32, 33). First, the load the inspiratory muscles faces is increased for a variety of reasons. As already noted, expiration ends before the respiratory system reaches elastic equilibrium at functional residual capacity (FRC), and thus a positive elastic recoil pressure (PEEPi) remains. During the next inspiration, the inspiratory muscles have to develop an equal amount of pressure before the airway pressure becomes negative (subatmospheric), with subsequent initiation of airflow. Second, because of hyperinflation, tidal breathing occurs at a steeper portion of the pressure-volume curve of the lung, further increasing the load. Third, as FRC increases, tidal breathing may take place at that portion of the chest wall static pressure-volume curve where positive recoil pressure exists; that is, the chest wall tends to move inward. This is in contrast to the expanding tendency of the chest wall when tidal breathing begins from normal FRC.

Furthermore, with severe hyperinflation, the marked flattening of the diaphragm causes its costal and crural fibers to be arranged in series and perpendicularly to the chest wall. Contraction of these perpendicularly oriented fibers results in paradoxical inward movement of the lower rib cage. This distortion of the chest wall during inspiration elevates the elastic load. In summary, hyperinflation imposes a threshold load to initiate breathing and greatly augments the elastic load once breathing has started. Of course, acute severe asthma also increases the resistive load to breathe due to the obstruction of the airways caused by bronchoconstriction, copious secretions, and mucus plugging.

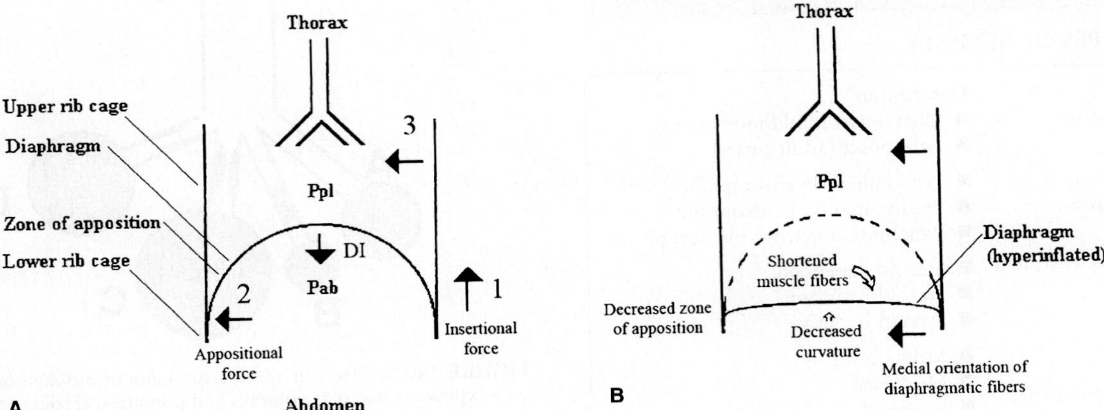

FIGURE 140.3. **A:** Actions of the diaphragm: When the diaphragm contracts, a caudally oriented force is being applied on the central tendon and the dome of the diaphragm descends (DI). Furthermore, the costal diaphragmatic fibers apply a cranially oriented force to the upper margins of the lower six ribs that has the effect of lifting and rotating them outward (insertional force, *arrow 1*). The zone of apposition makes the lower rib cage part of the abdomen and the changes in pressure in the pleural recess between the apposed diaphragm and the rib cage are almost equal to the changes in abdominal pressure. Pressure in this pleural recess rises rather than falls during inspiration because of diaphragmatic descent, and the rise in abdominal pressure is transmitted through the apposed diaphragm to expand the lower rib cage (*arrow* 2). All these effects result in expansion of the lower rib cage. On the upper rib cage, isolated contraction of the diaphragm causes a decrease in the anteroposterior diameter and this expiratory action is primarily due to the fall in pleural pressure (*arrow 3*). **B:** Deleterious effects of hyperinflation on the diaphragm.

At the same time that the load is severely increased, hyperinflation compromises the force-generating capacity of the diaphragm for a variety of reasons (Fig. 140.3) (32,33). First, the respiratory muscles, like other skeletal muscles, obey the length-tension relationship (Fig. 140.4). At any given level of activation, changes in muscle fiber length alter tension development. This is because the force-tension developed by a muscle depends on the interaction between actin and myosin fibrils, that is, the number of myosin heads attaching and thus pulling the actin fibrils closer within each sarcomere. The optimal fiber length (Lo) at which tension is maximal is the length at which all myosin heads attach and pull the actin fibrils. Below this length (as with hyperinflation, which shortens the diaphragm) actin-myosin interaction becomes suboptimal and tension development declines (Fig. 140.4). Second, as lung volume increases, the zone of apposition of the diaphragm decreases in size, and a larger fraction of the rib cage becomes exposed to pleural pressure (Fig. 140.3). Hence, the diaphragm's inspiratory action on the rib cage diminishes. When lung volume approaches total lung capacity, the zone of apposition all but disappears (Fig. 140.3), and the diaphragmatic muscle fibers become oriented horizontally internally. The insertional force of the diaphragm is then expiratory, rather than inspiratory, in direction. Third, the resulting flattening of the diaphragm increases its radius of curvature (Rdi) and thus diminishes its pressure-generating capacity (Pdi) for the same tension development (Tdi). This is because when a muscle contracts it generates tension, not pressure. Because of the geometry of the diaphragm, tension (Tdi) is transformed into pressure (Pdi), obeying the Laplace law, Pdi = 2 Tdi/Rdi, where Rdi is the radius of curvature of the diaphragm (Fig. 140.3B).

The imbalance between the load faced by the respiratory muscles and their capacity to develop force (32) results in dyspnea (32–35) and predisposes the respiratory muscle to the development of fatigue (32,33), which is a terminal event, likely

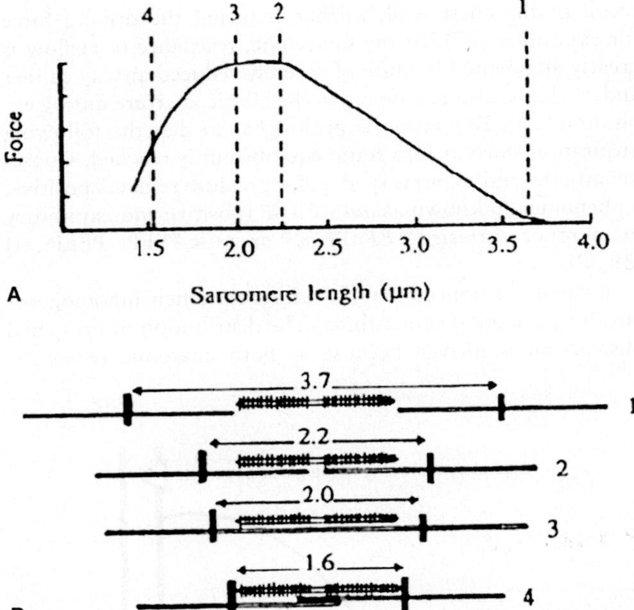

FIGURE 140.4. Isometric force at different sarcomere lengths. **A:** Force generated. **B:** Arrangements of actin-myosin filaments at different sarcomere lengths. The optimal length is where all myosin heads belonging to each myosin fibril come into contact (and thus exert attracting force) with actin filaments. At lengths <2.0 μm, actin filaments begin to overlap, and at still shorter lengths, the myosin filaments come into contact. At lengths >2 μm, increasing numbers of myosin heads do not come into contact with actin filaments. Values are for frog muscle. Mammalian actin (thin) filaments are slightly longer so the corresponding sarcomere lengths are 1, 4.0 μm; 2, 2.5 μm; 3, 2.4 μm; and 4, 1.6 μm. (Redrawn from Gordon AM, Huxley AF, Julian FJ. The variation in isometric tension with sarcomere length in vertebrate muscle fibres. *J Physiol.* 1966;184:170–192.)

to be present in an asthmatic crisis, necessitating intubation and mechanical ventilation.

Gas Exchange

Widespread occlusion of the airways leads to development of extensive areas of alveolar units in which ventilation (V) is severely reduced but perfusion (Q) is maintained; that is, areas with very low $\dot{V}/\dot{Q}$ ratios, frequently lower than 0.1. Intrapulmonary shunt appears to be rare in the majority of patients because of the collateral ventilation and the effectiveness of the hypoxic pulmonary vasoconstriction (36,37). Hypoxemia is therefore common in every asthmatic crisis of some severity; mild hypoxia is easily corrected with the administration of relatively low concentrations of supplemental oxygen. More severe hypoxemia and the need for higher concentrations of supplemental oxygen may relate to some contribution of shunt physiology.

Dead space increases substantially in most severe cases due to alveolar overdistention, that is, areas with very high $\dot{V}/\dot{Q}$ ratios (38). This is accompanied by increased CO_2 production from the increased work performed by the respiratory muscles. The respiratory muscles are unable to further increase minute ventilation, and thus hypercapnia ensues. However, even if minute ventilation were increased, it might not correct hypercapnia because it would lead to a vicious circle of worsening hyperinflation with more alveolar overdistention and thus increased dead space (38). It should be noted, nevertheless, that in milder attacks, reflex hyperventilation may lead to hypocapnia; however, as the severity of asthma attack increases, PCO_2 builds up first toward normal levels, and then, as respiratory failure impends, to supranormal values.

Cardiovascular System Effects

Acute severe asthma may also compromise hemodynamics. During expiration, because of the presence of dynamic hyperinflation, increased intrathoracic pressure impedes venous return. During the ensuing inspiration, forceful inspiratory muscle contraction renders intrathoracic pressure negative again, rapidly increasing venous return. Rapid filling of the right ventricle during inspiration shifts the interventricular septum toward the left ventricle, and leads to its incomplete filling during diastole, and thus to left ventricular diastolic dysfunction. The large negative intrathoracic pressure generated during inspiration increases left ventricular afterload and impairs systolic emptying (32).

Pulmonary artery pressure may also be increased by lung hyperinflation, thereby resulting in increased right ventricular afterload (32). These events in acute severe asthma may accentuate the normal inspiratory reduction in left ventricular stroke volume and systolic pressure, leading to the appearance of pulsus paradoxus, defined as a reduction of >10 mm Hg of the arterial systolic pressure during inspiration (39,40) (Fig. 140.5). A variation >12 mm Hg in systolic blood pressure between inspiration and expiration represents a sign of severity in asthmatic crisis. In advanced stages, when ventilatory muscle fatigue ensues, pulsus paradoxus (41) will decrease or disappear as force generation declines. Such status is a harbinger of impeding respiratory arrest.

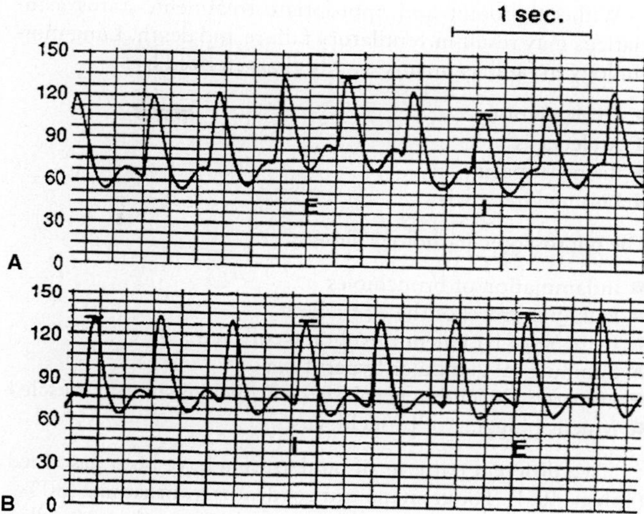

FIGURE 140.5. Arterial pressure of an asthmatic patient when breathing air (**A**) and heliox (**B**). Pulsus paradoxus was lower when the patient was breathing heliox. E, expiration; I, inspiration. (From Manthous CA, Hall JB, Caputo MA, et al. *Am J Respir Crit Care Med.* 1995;151:310–314, with permission.)

Clinicopathologic Patterns of Asthmatic Attacks

The time course of the asthmatic crisis, as well as the severity of airway obstruction, may vary broadly. Massive exposure to common allergens, sensitivity to nonsteroidal anti-inflammatory agents, and sensitivity to food allergens and sulphates are considered the main triggers in sudden asthma exacerbations. Patients at high risk of asthma-related death are described in Table 140.3.

TABLE 140.3

PATIENTS AT HIGH RISK OF ASTHMA-RELATED DEATH

- Patients with a history of near-fatal asthma requiring intubation and mechanical ventilation.
- Patients who have had a hospitalization or emergency care visit for asthma in the past year.
- Patients who are currently using or have recently stopped using oral glucocorticosteroids.
- Patients who are not currently using inhaled glucocorticosteroids.
- Patients who are overdependent on rapid-acting inhaled β_2-agonists, especially those who use more than one canister of salbutamol (or equivalent) monthly.
- Patients with a history of psychiatric disease or psychosocial problems, including the use of sedatives.
- Patients with a history of noncompliance with an asthma medication plan.

Global Initiative for Asthma. Global strategy for asthma management and prevention. Bethesda, MD: National Institutes of Health, National Heart, Lung, and Blood Institute; 2006.

Without prompt and appropriate treatment, status asthmaticus may result in ventilatory failure and death. Lung morphology in fatal asthma is mainly characterized by:

- Overinflation
- Atelectasis
- Bronchospasm
- Luminal narrowing

The microscopic pathology shows:

- Inflammation of bronchioles
- Patchy necrosis of the epithelium
- Increase of basement membrane collagen
- Submucosal glandular hyperplasia
- Hypertrophy and hyperplasia of bronchial smooth muscle
- Mucus plugging of bronchi, casts

Two different patterns of fatal asthma have been described (Table 140.4). The great majority of deaths from asthma (80%–85%) occur in patients with severe and poorly controlled disease who gradually deteriorate over days or weeks. Slow-onset asthma exacerbations are mainly related to faults in management—inadequate treatment, noncompliance to therapy, inappropriate control, coexisting psychological factors—that should be investigated and corrected in every patient in advance. An inappropriate response to dyspnea may be an important factor. This is the so-called slow onset–late arrival or *type I scenario of asthma death* (42,43). Repeated peak expiratory flow (PEF) measurements, when available, may document subacute worsening of expiratory flow over several days before the appearance of severe symptoms. This pattern of asthma death is generally considered preventable. A variation of this pattern is a history of unstable disease, which is partially responsive to treatment, on which a major attack is superimposed. In both situations, hypercapnic respiratory failure and mixed acidosis ensues and the patient succumbs to asphyxia or, if mechanical ventilation is applied, to complications such as barotrauma and ventilator-associated pneumonia.

Pathologic examination in such cases shows extensive plugging of the airways by dense and tenacious mucus mixed with inflammatory and epithelial cells ("endobronchial mucus suffocation"), epithelial denudation, mucosal edema, and an intense eosinophilic infiltration of the submucosa. In a small proportion of patients, lung function may deteriorate severely in <1 hour, leading to sudden and unexpected death from asthma, termed *sudden asphyxic asthma*, without obvious antecedent long-term deterioration of asthma control, the so-called sudden-onset asthma exacerbation, or type II, scenario of asthma death. Affected individuals rapidly develop severe hypercapnic respiratory failure with combined metabolic and respiratory acidosis, and succumb to asphyxia. If treated medically and/or with mechanical ventilation, however, they present a faster rate of improvement than patients with slow-onset asthmatic crisis. Pathologic examination in such cases shows "empty" airways (no mucus plugs) in some patients, and in almost all patients, there is a greater proportion of neutrophils than eosinophils infiltrating the submucosa. It is unclear whether the presence of neutrophils is an epiphenomenon or it directly contributes to the fatal attacks. A significant volume of research is currently dedicated to unraveling the characteristics of airway remodeling in patients with severe asthma (44), showing that smooth muscle alteration is the key structural alteration that distinguishes severe from moderate asthma. Phenotypic change in airway smooth muscle might contribute to the difficulty in obtaining adequate control in some patients with severe asthma. Sudden asphyxic asthma death is associated with inflammatory infiltrates both of proximal and distal lung tissues (45), with the outer wall of small membranous bronchioles being the main site of inflammatory changes (46).

TABLE 140.4

DIFFERENT PATTERNS OF FATAL ASTHMA

	Scenario of asthma death	
Variable	Type 1	Type 2
Time course	Subacute worsening (days). Slow onset–late arrival	Acute deterioration (hours). Sudden asphyxic asthma
Frequency	≈80%–85%	≈15%–20%
Airways	Extensive mucus plugging	More or less empty bronchi
Inflammation	Eosinophils	Neutrophils
Response to treatment	Slow	Faster
Prevention	Possible	(?)

Diagnosis

There are four parameters that should be investigated before the diagnosis of severe asthma is made for the first time, which are the following:

1. Incorrect diagnosis. The diagnosis of severe asthma is based on a solid confirmation of asthma. In case of doubt, alternative diagnoses (23,47) should be excluded (Tables 140.5 and 140.6).
2. Continuing exposure to sensitizing agents (Tables 140.5 and 140.6). Numerous factors such as ongoing (low-dose) allergen exposure at home or at work (48) can aggravate the inflammatory process in the airways and contribute to lack of control of the disease. Once the relationship with the sensitizing agent has been established, the patient must be encouraged to take avoidance measures. Smoking is another important factor that may contribute to the lack of adequate response, and therefore it is imperative that smoking cessation be encouraged.
3. Unrecognized aggravating comorbidities (Tables 140.5 and 140.6), such as chronic rhinosinusitis, recurrent respiratory tract infections (23,47,49–51), gastroesophageal reflux, obstructive sleep apnea, psychiatric problems, and obesity, should be treated.
4. Noncompliance with therapy.

If these four factors are excluded and the diagnosis remains consistent with severe asthma, an evaluation with a trial of systemic corticosteroid therapy, preferably intravenously or intramuscularly to circumvent the possibility of noncompliance, may be useful to assess the best attainable lung function, and to create the optimal condition for inhaled antiinflammatory treatment to penetrate deep into the airways.

TABLE 140.5

ALGORITHM OF POSSIBLE STRATEGIES AND RECOMMENDATIONS FOR MANAGING PATIENTS WITH DIFFICULT-TO-CONTROL ASTHMA DESPITE MAXIMUM COMBINATION TREATMENT

Patients with uncontrolled asthma symptoms with:

1. Persisting refractory symptoms and poor lung function (reduced FEV_1) despite high dose ICS + LABA
2. Frequent use of oral steroids
3. Regular use of health care resources (doctors' consultations, emergency services, hospital admissions)

POOR COMPLIANCE

YES →

1. **Review inhalation technique**
2. **Written self-management plan**
3. **Reassessment at next visit**

NO ↓

DIAGNOSTIC CONFIRMATION/VERIFICATION FOR

DISEASES THAT MIMIC ASTHMA	CONDITIONS ASSOCIATED WITH ASTHMA	UNUSUAL ASTHMA TRIGGER
• Bronchiectasis • Constrictive bronchiolitis • COPD • CHF • Dysfunctional breathlessness • Vocal cord dysfunction • Upper airway obstruction • ABPA • Chung-Strauss syndrome • Eosinophilic pneumonia • Thyrotoxicosis	• Chronic rhinosinusitis • Gastroesophageal reflux • Anxiety, panic-fear, depression • Dysfunctional breathlessness • Vocal cord dysfunction • Obesity • Obstructive sleep apnea	• Occupational exposure • Domestic irritants • Respiratory infections • Drugs (aspirin, NSAIDs, ACE inhibitors, beta-blockers) • Food (e.g., sulphite sensitivity) • Smoking • Inflamed upper airways • Acid reflux • Stress
1. Management of the condition 2. Reassess at next visit	1. Management of the condition 2. Reassess at next visit	1. Avoid triggers 2. Reassess at next visit

SHORT COURSE ORAL STEROIDS

NEGATIVE RESPONSE — **YES** → back to diagnostic confirmation/verification

NO ↓

1. Titrate down oral steroids (administer the lowest amount of oral steroid to control/stabilize symptoms).
2. Consider adding a steroid-sparing drug (e.g., azathioprine, methotrexate).
3. Add treatment for steroid-induced adverse effects (e.g., osteoporosis).
4. If uncontrolled, consider alternative therapeutic options (e.g., omalizumab, etanercept, high dose IVIG).
5. Frequent periodic re-evaluations.

FEV_1, forced expiratory volume in 1 second; ICS, inhaled corticosteroids; LABA, long-acting β-agonists; COPD, chronic obstructive pulmonary disease; CHF, congestive heart failure; ABPA, allergic bronchopulmonary aspergillosis; NSAIDs, nonsteroidal anti-inflammatory drugs; ACE, angiotensin-converting enzyme.

Adapted from Holgate ST, Polosa R. The mechanisms, diagnosis, and management of severe asthma in adults. *Lancet.* 2006;368(9537):780–793.

TABLE 140.6

HISTORY AND PHYSICAL EXAMINATION OF PATIENTS WITH DIFFICULT-TO-CONTROL ASTHMA

Medical history
History of asthma development
- Age of asthma onset
- Atopic syndrome and family history of asthma
- Management of disease and response to treatment
- Smoking history

Severity of disease
- Severe asthma exacerbations and hospitalization in past year
- Any admissions to asthma centers
- Any number of ICU admissions

Exogenous aggravating factors
- Exposure to allergens, occupational agents, chemicals
- Use of aspirin, NSAIDs, beta-blockers, ACE inhibitors, estrogens
- Influence of foods or food additives (nitrite, sulphate)

Endogenous aggravating factors
- Rhinosinusitis or previous surgery for nasal polyps
- Gastroesophageal reflux
- History of psychiatric disease
- Obstructive sleep apnea

Influence of menstruation
Miscellaneous
Adherence with medications
Adverse effects of treatment
Psychosocial circumstances

Physical examination (specific points of attention)
- Body mass index
- Evidence of comorbidities (e.g., nasal polyps)
- Evidence of alternative diagnoses (e.g., cardiac failure)
- Evidence of adverse effects of treatment

ICU, intensive care unit; NSAID, nonsteroidal anti-inflammatory drugs; ACE, angiotensin-converting enzyme.
Bel EH. Severe asthma. *Breathe*. December 2006;3(2):129–139.

CLINICAL PRESENTATION

Analysis of arterial blood gases is important in the management of patients with acute severe asthma and useful for decisions regarding hospital admission or tracheal intubation, but it is not predictive of outcome. In the early stages of acute severe asthma, analysis of arterial blood gases usually reveals mild hypoxemia, hypocapnia, and respiratory alkalosis. If the deterioration in the patient's clinical status lasts for a few days, there may be some compensatory renal bicarbonate loss (Table 140.7).

As the severity of airflow obstruction increases, $PaCO_2$ first normalizes (Table 140.8) and subsequently increases because of patient exhaustion, inadequate alveolar ventilation, and/or an increase in physiologic dead space. Hypercapnia is not usually observed for FEV_1 values higher than 25% of predicted normal; in general there is no correlation between airflow rates and gas exchange markers. Furthermore, paradoxical deterioration of gas exchange while flow rates improve after the administration of β-adrenergic agonists is not uncommon.

Respiratory acidosis is always present in hypercapnic patients who rapidly deteriorate, and in severe, advanced-stage disease, metabolic (lactic) acidosis may coexist. The pathogenesis of lactic acidosis in the acutely severe asthmatic patient remains to be fully elucidated. There are several mechanisms that are probably involved: the use of high-dose, parenteral β-adrenergic agonists; the increased work of breathing resulting in anaerobic metabolism of the ventilatory muscles and overproduction of lactic acid; the eventually coexisting tissue hypoxia; and the decreased lactate clearance by the liver because of hypoperfusion. A normal $PaCO_2$ in a distressed asthmatic patient should alert the physician to respiratory fatigue and the danger of respiratory arrest. This classification system is best applied after initial aggressive treatment of asthmatic patients and may be inappropriate if applied before initial therapy.

LABORATORY AND RADIOGRAPHIC DATA

Severe asthma may show right ventricular strain on electrocardiogram that resolves with clinical improvement. Table 140.9 presents further details.

THERAPEUTIC APPROACHES: MANAGEMENT OF ACUTE SEVERE ASTHMA

Most of the following management is recommended from GINA guidelines 2006 (2) and British Thoracic Society guidelines (52). The group of asthmatic patients that generally succumbs to fatal asthma are usually those with difficult-to-treat asthma, although, theoretically, all asthmatics may experience a severe exacerbation. Early diagnosis and treatment of asthma exacerbations should be the best strategy for management.

Early home management of asthma exacerbations is of paramount importance, as it avoids treatment delay and prevents clinical deterioration. The effectiveness of care depends on the abilities of the patients and/or their families, and on the availability of emergency care equipment—peak flow meter, appropriate medications, nebulizer, and, eventually, supplemental oxygen. Important elements for the prevention of exacerbations and for early asthma treatment include:

1. A written action plan for home self-management of asthma exacerbations, especially for those patients with severe asthma or a history of previous severe asthma attacks.
2. Patient should be instructed to recognize early signs of asthma worsening.
3. Clear instructions for appropriate intensification of therapy in case of deterioration.
4. Prompt communication between patient and clinician about any serious deterioration of asthma control.

Severe exacerbations are potentially life-threatening. Patients, their families, and their physicians, however, frequently underestimate the severity of asthma. Patients at high risk of asthma-related death require special attention, particularly intensive education, monitoring, and care, and should be encouraged to seek urgent care early in the course of their

TABLE 140.7

CLINICAL AND FUNCTIONAL ASSESSMENT OF SEVERE ASTHMA EXACERBATIONS[a]

Variable	Severe exacerbation	Imminent respiratory arrest
SYMPTOMS		
Dyspnea	At rest Hunched forward	
Speech	Single words, not sentences or phrases	
Alertness	Usually agitated	Drowsy or confused
SIGNS		
Respiratory rate	Often >30 breaths/min	
Heart rate	>120 beats/min	Bradycardia
Pulsus paradoxus	Often present >25 mm Hg	Absence suggests respiratory muscle fatigue
Use of accessory muscles and suprasternal reactions	Usually evident	Abdominal paradox (paradoxical thoracoabdominal movement)
Wheeze	Usually loud	Absence of wheeze "Silent chest"
FUNCTIONAL ASSESSMENT		
PEF (after initial bronchodilator, % predicted or % personal best)	<60% of predicted or personal best (<100 L/min adults) Or Response lasts <2 hours	
PaO_2	<60 mm Hg Possible cyanosis	
$PaCO_2$	>42 mm Hg Possible respiratory failure	
SpO_2	<90%	

PEF, peak expiratory flow.
[a]The presence of several parameters, but not necessarily all, indicates the general classification of the exacerbation.
Adapted from Global Initiative for Asthma. Global strategy for asthma management and prevention. Bethesda, MD: National Institutes of Health, National Heart, Lung, and Blood Institute; 2006.

exacerbation, meaning they should seek their physician promptly or—depending on the organization of local health services—proceed to the nearest clinic or hospital that provides emergency access for patients with acute asthma. These patients include those:

- With a history of near-fatal asthma requiring intubation and mechanical ventilation
- Who have had a hospitalization or emergency care visit for asthma in the last year
- Who are currently using or have recently stopped using oral glucocorticosteroids
- Who are not currently using inhaled glucocorticosteroids
- Who are overdependent on rapid-acting inhaled β_2-agonists, especially those who use more than one canister of salbutamol (or equivalent) monthly
- With a history of psychiatric disease or psychosocial problems, including the use of sedatives
- With a history of noncompliance with an asthma medication plan

The aims of treatment are to relieve airflow obstruction and hypoxemia as quickly as possible, and to plan the prevention of future relapses. Response to treatment may take time, and patients should be closely monitored using clinical as well as objective measurements. The increased treatment should

TABLE 140.8

STAGING SEVERE ASTHMA CRISIS BY ARTERIAL BLOOD GASES

	Stage 1	Stage 2	Stage 3	Stage 4	Stage 5
PaCO	Normal	↓ $PaCO_2$	↓ $PaCO_2$	Normal	↑ $PaCO_2$ (respiratory failure)
PaO_2	Normal	Normal PaO_2 (hyperventilation has led to normalization of PaO_2).	↓ PaO_2 (hyperventilation is now unable to compensate totally for a widened $P(A-a)O_2$.	↓↓↓ PaO_2 (inspiratory fatigue is now prominent).	↓↓↓PaO_2. These findings indicate an impending respiratory arrest.

TABLE 140.9

LABORATORY INVESTIGATIONS AND DIAGNOSTIC TESTS FOR PATIENTS WITH DIFFICULT-TO-CONTROL ASTHMA

Diagnostic tests
■ Peripheral blood
■ Erythrocyte sedimentation rate
■ Full blood count (eosinophils)
■ Total serum IgE
■ Specific IgE to common and less common allergens
■ Free-T4, thyroid-stimulating hormone
Lung function
■ Spirometry (pre- and postbronchodilator)
■ Lung volumes
■ Arterial blood gases
■ Histamine challenge test
Radiology
■ Chest radiography
■ Sinus CT scan
Additional tests for comorbidities and alternative diagnoses
■ Nasal endoscopy
■ 24-hour esophageal pH monitoring or trial with proton pump inhibitors
■ Polysomnography
■ Bronchoscopy
■ High-resolution CT scan of the thorax
■ D-dimer
■ ANCA
■ IgG against *Aspergillus fumigatus*

Ig, immunoglobulin; CT, computed tomography; ANCA, antineutrophilic cytoplasmic antibody.
Bel EH. Severe asthma. *Breathe*. December 2006;3(2):129–139.

continue until measurements of lung function (PEF or FEV_1) return to their previous best (ideally) or plateau, at which time a decision to admit or discharge can be made based on these values. Patients who can be safely discharged will have responded within the first 2 hours, at which time decisions regarding patient disposition can be made.

Schematically, a management plan of acute severe asthma in adults is shown in Table 140.10. In the emergency department, a brief history regarding time of onset, cause of exacerbation, severity of symptoms (especially in comparison to previous attacks), prior hospitalizations and/or emergency department visits for asthma, prior intubation or intensive care unit (ICU) admission, and complicating illness may be useful for treatment decisions. The primary therapies, the intensity of pharmacologic treatment and the patient's surveillance should correspond to the severity of the exacerbation. These, for acute severe asthma, include the therapies discussed in the following sections.

Oxygen

High-flow oxygen should be given to all patients with acute severe asthma as these individuals are hypoxemic. This may be corrected urgently using high concentrations of inspired oxygen by either nasal cannulae or mask. Unlike patients with chronic obstructive pulmonary disease, there is little danger of precipitating hypercapnia with high-flow oxygen. Hypercapnia indicates the development of near-fatal asthma and the need for emergency specialist/anesthetic intervention. An SpO_2 of at least 92% must be achieved and an SpO_2 >95% is desired in pregnant women, children, and in patients with coexistent cardiac disease. Oxygen therapy should be titrated against pulse oximetry to maintain satisfactory oxygen saturation.

β_2-Agonist Bronchodilators

Inhaled β_2-agonists are the cornerstone of asthma treatment. Continuous or repetitive nebulization of rapid-acting β_2-agonists is the safest and most effective means of reversing airflow obstruction, and should be administered as early as possible. In most cases of acute asthma, inhaled β_2-agonists given in high doses act quickly to relieve bronchospasm and have few side effects. There is no evidence for any difference in efficacy between salbutamol and terbutaline. In acute asthma without life-threatening features, β_2-agonists can be administered by repeated activations of a metered-dose inhaler via an appropriate large-volume spacer, or by wet nebulization. In view of the theoretical risk of oxygen desaturation while using air-driven compressors to nebulize β_2-agonist bronchodilators, oxygen-driven nebulizers are preferred.

Continuous nebulization of β_2-agonists is at least as efficacious as bolus nebulization in relieving acute asthma. Studies of intermittent versus continuous nebulized, short-acting β_2-agonists in acute asthma provide conflicting results. In a systematic review of six studies, there were no significant differences in bronchodilator effect or hospital admissions between the two treatments. In patients who require hospitalization, one study found that intermittent on-demand therapy led to a significantly shorter hospital stay, fewer nebulizations, and fewer palpitations when compared with intermittent therapy given every 4 hours. A reasonable approach to inhaled therapy in exacerbations, therefore, would be the initial use of continuous therapy, followed by intermittent on-demand therapy for hospitalized patients.

In severe asthma, with PEF <50% of personal best or FEV_1 <50% predicted, and asthma that is poorly responsive to an initial bolus dose of β_2-agonist, continuous nebulization should be considered. Continuous nebulization of β_2-agonists may also be more effective in children. Larger doses and more frequent dosing intervals for inhaled β_2-agonist therapy are needed in acute severe asthma because of decreased deposition at site of action, itself resultant from low tidal volumes and narrowed airways, alteration in dose-response curve, and altered duration of activity. Repeated doses of β_2-agonists should be given at 15- to 30-minute intervals, or continuous nebulization of salbutamol at 5 to 10 mg/hr used if there is an inadequate response to initial treatment. Higher bolus doses (e.g., 10 mg of salbutamol) are unlikely to be more effective.

Continuous or repetitive nebulization of salbutamol is preferred because of its potency, 4- to 6-hour duration of action, and β_2-selectivity. The usual dose is 2.5 mg of salbutamol (0.5 mL) in 2.5 mL of normal saline for each nebulization (Table 140.11). Nebulized β_2-agonists should be continued until a significant clinical response is achieved or serious side effects, such as severe tachycardia or dysrhythmias, appear. Prior ineffective use of β_2-agonists does not preclude their use and does not limit their efficacy.

TABLE 140.10

MANAGEMENT OF ACUTE SEVERE ASTHMA IN ADULTS IN THE EMERGENCY DEPARTMENT

INITIAL ASSESSMENT

Brief history (Exclude diagnoses other than asthma, time of onset, cause of exacerbation, severity of symptoms [especially in comparison to previous attacks], prior hospitalizations and/or emergency department visits for asthma, prior intubation or intensive care admission, complicating illness).

- **Focused physical examination** (auscultation, use of accessory muscles, heart rate, respiratory rate, color, alertness, vital signs).
- **Objective testing** (PEF or FEV_1, SpO_2, arterial blood gases if patient *in extremis*).

75%>PEF> 33% predicted or personal best

TIME

0 min

Features of severe asthma:

- PEF <50%
- Respiration ≥25/min
- Pulse ≥110/min
- Cannot complete sentence in one breath

IMPROVE AIRFLOW by 5 mg salbutamol by oxygen driven nebulizer

5 min

15-30 min

Clinically stable and PEF>75%	Clinically stable and PEF<75%	75%>PEF>50% Without any life-threatening features	Life-threatening features OR PEF<50%

Clinically stable and PEF>75% → possible discharge home (120 min).

Clinically stable and PEF<75% and **75%>PEF>50% without any life-threatening features** →

Repeat 5 mg salbutamol via oxygen-driven nebulizer PLUS 40–50 mg of prednisolone *per os*

- **Patient recovering and PEF>75%** → possible discharge home.
- **No signs of severe asthma and PEF<75%** → **OBSERVE:**
  - SpO_2
  - Respiratory rate
  - Heart rate
  - **Patient stable and PEF>50%** → possible discharge home.
  - **Signs of severe asthma OR PEF<50%** → hospitalize patient.
- **Signs of severe asthma OR PEF<50%**
  - Give/repeat 5 mg salbutamol plus 0.5 mg ipratropium via oxygen-driven nebulizer.
  - Decrease airway inflammation by 40–50 mg prednisolone *per os* or 100 mg hydrocortisone IV
  - Consider continuous salbutamol nebulizer 5–10 mg/h.
  - Consider improving airflow by 1,2–2gr $MgSO_4$ IV over 20 min.
  - Consider IV theophylline
  - Correct fluid/ electrolytes (especially K^+ disturbances)
  - Ancillary studies (CXR, laboratory test)

60 min

Life-threatening features OR PEF<50% → **IMMEDIATE MANAGEMENT**

- High concentration oxygen (VM>60% if possible)
- 5 mg salbutamol plus 0.5 mg ipratropium via oxygen driven nebulizer
- Decrease airway inflammation by 40–50 mg prednisolone *per os* or 100 mg hydrocortisone IV
- Consider continuous salbutamol nebulizer 5–10 mg/h.
- Consider improving airflow by 2g $MgSO_4$ IV over 20 min.
- Consider IV theophylline.
- Correct fluid/electrolytes (especially K^+ disturbances)
- Ancillary studies (CXR, laboratory tests)

120 min

Possible discharge home with:

- Consider adding a combination inhaler.
- If initial PEF<50% 40–50 mg prednisolone *per os* over 5 days.
- Check patient education (take medicine correctly, review action plan, close long-lasting medical follow-up).
- PEF>60% of predicted or personal best.

← IMPROVEMENT

HOSPITALIZE PATIENT

Patient should be accompanied by a nurse or doctor at all times

PEF <30% or any of life-threatening features (PaO_2 <92%, $PaCO_2$ normal or >40 mm Hg, PO_2 <60 mm Hg, low pH, severe drowsiness, confusion, coma, exhaustion, bradycardia, dysrhythmia, silent chest, cyanosis, poor respiratory effort, risk factors for near-fatal asthma)

ADMISSION TO INTENSIVE CARE

Possible intubation and mechanical ventilation

PEF, peak expiratory flow; FEV_1, forced expiratory volume in 1 second IV, intravenously; CXR, chest x-ray; VM, ventimask.

TABLE 140.11

PHARMACOLOGIC TREATMENT IN THE EMERGENCY DEPARTMENT

Agent	Dose
Salbutamol	2.5 mg (0.5 mL) in 2.5 mL normal saline by nebulization continuously, or every 15–20 min until a significant clinical response is achieved or serious side effects appear.
Epinephrine	0.3–0.4 mL of a 1:1,000 solution SC every 20 min for three doses.
Terbutaline	Preferable to epinephrine in pregnancy.
β-Agonists IV	IV administration should be considered in patients who have not responded to inhaled or SC, in whom respiratory arrest is imminent.
Corticosteroids	Methylprednisolone 60–125 mg IV or prednisone 40 mg *per os*.
Anticholinergics	Ipratropium bromide 0.5 mg by nebulization every 1–4 hours, combined with salbutamol.
Methylxanthines	Theophylline 5 mg/kg IV over 30 min—loading dose in patients not already taking theophylline, followed by 0.4 mg/kg/h IV maintenance dose. Serum levels should be checked within 6 h.
Magnesium sulfate	Usually given as a single 2-g infusion IV over 20 min, only following consultation with senior medical staff. Nebulized salbutamol administered in isotonic magnesium sulfate provides greater benefit than if it is delivered in normal saline.

SC, subcutaneously; IV, intravenously.

Inhaled therapy with β_2-agonists appears to be equal to, or even better than, intravenous (IV) infusion in treating airway obstruction in adults with severe asthma (meta-analysis has excluded subcutaneous trials). Intravenous β_2-agonists should be reserved for those patients in whom inhaled therapy cannot be used reliably.

Although most rapid-acting β_2-agonists have a short duration of effect, the long-acting bronchodilator, formoterol, which has both a rapid onset of action and a long duration of effect, has been shown to be equally effective without increasing side effects, although it is considerably more expensive. The importance of this feature of formoterol is that it provides support and reassurance regarding the use of a combination of formoterol and budesonide early in asthma exacerbations.

Two types of nebulizer systems are available for inhalation therapy: the face mask and the hand-held nebulizer with a mouthpiece. The mouthpiece is preferred because it delivers more drug, but it requires more patient cooperation because a good seal must be maintained around the mouthpiece. In the severely ill asthmatic patient, the face mask system may be necessary.

When β_2-selective agents are delivered parenterally or orally, they lose much of their β_2-selectivity, so terbutaline loses its β-selectivity and offers no advantages over epinephrine. When subcutaneous terbutaline is compared with subcutaneous epinephrine, equal cardiac side effects are seen. Terbutaline administered subcutaneously should be used only in pregnancy because it appears safer. Oral β_2-selective agents should not be used as primary treatment for patients with acute asthma because the therapeutic-to-toxicity ratio is less than that with inhaled agents. Subcutaneous β-agonist therapy—epinephrine or terbutaline—also has a disadvantageous therapeutic-to-toxicity ratio when compared with inhaled β_2-selective agonists.

Subcutaneous epinephrine or terbutaline might, however, be useful in several situations and should be considered:

- In children in whom inhaled agents are often difficult to administer. In addition, the pediatric population has a reduced susceptibility to β_1 toxicity, making subcutaneous administration a useful route of drug delivery.
- In seriously ill asthmatic patients with impending respiratory arrest in whom rapid delivery of β-agonists to the airway is desirable. The combination of inhaled and subcutaneously administered β-agonists in this circumstance could enhance bronchodilation by delivering the drug both by the airway and by the circulation. However, no clear data support this concept. There is also a concern, although again not documented, that subcutaneous adrenergic therapy is indicated in patients with severe bronchospasm because inhaled agents may not be adequately delivered to the peripheral sites of action. The fact that many patients with severe asthma present in extreme distress with a PEF rate <60 L/min and respond very briskly to continuous nebulized β-agonist therapy seems to refute this contention. If patients do not respond to initial inhaled therapy, particularly if the attack has lasted several days and mucus plugging is a possibility, subcutaneous therapy could be attempted.
- In patients unable to cooperate secondary to depression of mental status, apnea, coma.

Subcutaneously, 0.3 to 0.4 mL of a solution of 1:1,000 (1 mg/mL) epinephrine can be administered every 20 minutes for three doses (Table 140.11). Terbutaline can be administered subcutaneously (0.25 mg) or as IV infusion starting at 0.05 to 0.10 mg/kg/min (Table 140.11). Subcutaneous administration of epinephrine or terbutaline should not be avoided or delayed as it is well tolerated even in patients older than 40 to 50 years of age with no history of cardiovascular disease, such as angina or recent myocardial infarction. Intravenous administration of the β-agonists, epinephrine or salbutamol, is also an option in extreme situations and should be considered in the treatment of patients who have not responded to inhaled or subcutaneous treatment and in whom respiratory arrest is imminent. Finally, it is critical to remember that drug dosing should be individualized according to severity and patient response.

Steroids

Systemic corticosteroids in adequate doses should be administered in all cases of acute asthma, especially if:

- The initial rapid-acting inhaled β_2-agonist therapy fails to achieve lasting improvement
- The exacerbation develops even though the patient was already taking oral glucocorticosteroids
- Previous exacerbations required oral glucocorticosteroids

Systemic corticosteroids are used to accelerate the resolution of the exacerbation. They reduce the risk of relapses, rehospitalization, requirement for β_2-agonist therapy, all-cause mortality in elderly asthmatics, and more generally reduce mortality from asthma. The earlier they are given in the acute attack, the better the outcome.

Minimal or no side effects occur with a single large dose of IV steroid. Some enhancement of β-agonist effect may be seen as early as 1 hour; however, 4 to 6 hours are required for anti-inflammatory activity. The benefit derived by the asthmatic is probably from a combination of enhancement of β_2-receptor responsiveness, interruption of arachidonic acid inflammatory pathways, decrease in capillary basement membrane permeability, decreased leukocyte attachment, modulation of calcium migration intracellularly, reduction in airway mucus production, and suppression of immunoglobulin E receptor binding. Oral glucocorticosteroids are usually as effective—provided tablets can be swallowed and retained—as those administered intravenously and are preferred because this route of delivery is less invasive and less expensive. The optimal dose and dosing frequency of systemic corticosteroids in severe hospitalized asthmatics are not clearly established. One common approach is the IV administration of 60 to 125 mg of methylprednisolone every 6 hours during the initial 24 to 48 hours of treatment (Table 140.11), followed by 60 to 80 mg daily in improving patients, with gradual tapering during the next 2 weeks.

In addition to well-known side effects of corticosteroid administration—hyperglycemia, hypertension, hypokalemia, psychosis, susceptibility to infections—myopathy should be considered in the intubated and mechanically ventilated patient (see later discussion). The intensification of a patient's corticosteroid therapy should begin as early as possible, at the first sign of loss of asthma control. Because benefits from corticosteroid treatment are not usually seen before 6 to 12 hours, early administration is necessary. Daily doses of systemic glucocorticosteroids equivalent to 60 to 80 mg of methylprednisolone as a single dose, or 40 to 50 mg of prednisolone daily, or parenteral hydrocortisone 400 mg daily, often delivered in a dosage of 100 mg IV 4 times daily, are as effective as higher doses. In fact, 40 mg of methylprednisolone or 200 mg of hydrocortisone is probably adequate in most cases. For convenience, steroid tablets may be given as 2 × 25 mg tablets daily rather than 8 to 12 × 5 mg tablets. Prednisolone 40 to 50 mg daily should be continued for at least 5 days or until recovery. A 7-day course in adults has been found to be as effective as a 14-day course. There is no benefit in tapering the dose of oral glucocorticosteroids, either in the short term or over several weeks. So, apart from patients on maintenance steroid treatment or rare instances in which steroids are required for 3 or more weeks, steroid tablets can be stopped abruptly following recovery from the acute exacerbation provided the patient receives inhaled steroids.

There is no firm evidence to suggest that inhaled steroids can substitute for steroid tablets in treating patients with acute severe or life-threatening asthma despite some promising results. Inhaled steroids should be started as soon as possible, or continued, at the beginning of the chronic asthma management plan, as they can be as effective as oral steroids at preventing relapses. Patients discharged from the emergency department with prednisone and inhaled budesonide have a lower rate of relapse than those receiving prednisone alone. A high dose of inhaled glucocorticosteroid, for example, 2.4 mg of budesonide daily in four divided doses, achieves a relapse rate similar to 40 mg of oral prednisone daily.

Anticholinergics

Although ipratropium produces less bronchodilatation at peak effect than a β-agonist and is associated with a less predictable clinical response, literature in general supports the use of ipratropium as adjunctive therapy in patients with acute severe asthma. Ipratropium bromide appears to reliably augment the bronchodilating effect of β-agonists in acute asthma and is particularly useful in the presence of β-blockade. Combining nebulized ipratropium bromide with a nebulized β_2-agonist has been shown to produce significantly greater bronchodilation than a β_2-agonist alone, leading to a faster recovery, a shorter duration of admission, lower hospitalization rates, greater improvement in PEF and FEV_1, and should be administered before methylxanthines are considered. Recommended dose is 0.25 to 0.5 mg by nebulizer. This can be combined with an albuterol dose. Contrary to what occurs in patients with chronic stable disease, ipratropium may produce a clinically significant response within minutes of administration. A paradoxical bronchoconstrictive response to ipratropium, although much rarer than initially reported, may occur and is due to the preservative in the solution. Anticholinergic treatment is not necessary and may not be beneficial in milder exacerbations of asthma or after stabilization. Without any doubt, nebulized ipratropium bromide in a dose of 0.5 mg every 4 to 6 hours should be added to β_2-agonist treatment for patients with acute severe or life-threatening asthma or those with a poor initial response to β_2-agonist therapy.

The hand-held mouthpiece nebulizer system should be used if anticholinergic medication is being administered. Contamination of the ocular area with precipitation of narrow-angle glaucoma may occur in susceptible individuals if a face mask is used for delivery of an anticholinergic agent.

Magnesium

Intravenous magnesium sulfate, usually given as a single 1.2- to 2-g infusion over 20 minutes, can help reduce hospital admission rates in certain patients. A single dose of IV magnesium sulphate should be considered for patients with:

- Acute severe asthma, with FEV_1 25% to 30% predicted at presentation
- Adults and children who fail to respond to initial treatment
- Life-threatening or near-fatal asthma

Magnesium's potential to reverse bronchoconstriction is multifactorial and is based on characteristics of inhibition of the calcium channel and decreased acetylcholine release.

Considerable controversy exists as to the potential benefit of magnesium sulfate as adjunctive therapy in acute asthma. A single dose of IV magnesium sulphate is safe and sometimes effective in acute severe asthma, although the responsive patients cannot be predicted. The safety and efficacy of repeated doses have not been assessed in patients with asthma. Repeated doses could give rise to hypermagnesemia with muscle weakness and respiratory failure. More studies are needed to determine the optimal frequency and dose of IV magnesium sulphate therapy.

Methylxanthines

In the emergency department, methylxanthines are of debated efficacy and not generally recommended (Tables 140.10 and 140.11). Theophylline, when compared with a placebo, is clearly an effective bronchodilator in the patient with acute bronchospasm, but in view of the effectiveness and relative safety of rapid-acting β_2-agonists, has a minimal role in the management of acute asthma. The question, however, is whether theophylline plus adequate dosing of an inhaled β-agonist produces greater bronchodilation than adequate dosing of β-agonist alone in the patient with acute asthma. The majority of studies have demonstrated no significant additional improvement in physiologic or outcome variables when theophylline is added to full doses of inhaled β-agonist therapy. In addition, theophylline toxicity is a concern. Its use is associated with severe and potentially fatal side effects, particularly in those on long-term therapy with sustained-release theophylline. However, in one study of children with near-fatal asthma, IV theophylline provided additional benefit to patients also receiving an aggressive regimen of inhaled and IV β_2-agonists, inhaled ipratropium bromide, and IV systemic glucocorticosteroids. Additionally, extrapolating data from short-term studies showing no additional benefit of theophylline may be problematic because other studies have noted evidence for the use of theophylline as adjunctive therapy, demonstrating improvement in ventilatory function at 1 and 24 hours, improvement in FEV_1 during the first 3 hours and at 48 hours, and improvement in FEV_1 at 4 hours. Therefore, there are no data to definitively support or reject the use of theophylline in this setting.

Theophylline has been demonstrated *in vitro* and *in vivo* to have nonbronchodilator effects of potential clinical benefit. It increases diaphragmatic endurance and is a respiratory muscle inotrope and a nonspecific respiratory stimulant. It is doubtful, however, that any of these effects exert a significant clinical impact. The anti-inflammatory effects of theophylline are noted in concentrations of $<10\ \mu g/mL$.

All patients evaluated for acute bronchospasm who have been receiving a theophylline preparation should have a theophylline level determined, the results of which are useful in later dosing decisions. The theophylline levels correlate, however, only roughly with toxicity. Patient symptoms are unreliable in predicting theophylline level. The longer acting the oral theophylline compound, the more likely it is to be associated with a higher initial level. If aminophylline is to be used, a decreased loading dose (2 mg/kg) is recommended in the severely bronchospastic asthmatic patient who admits to poor or partial compliance in taking medications. A therapeutic range of serum theophylline at 8 to 12 $\mu g/mL$ minimizes risk for toxicity.

Conclusively, some individual patients with near-fatal or life-threatening asthma, as well as patients admitted to the ICU with a poor response to initial therapy, may gain additional benefit from IV aminophylline, with a 5 mg/kg loading dose administered over 20 minutes unless on maintenance oral therapy, followed by an infusion of 0.5 to 0.7 mg/kg/h, added to full-dose inhaled β-agonist; higher doses may be used in children. A 1 mg/kg IV aminophylline dose increases the serum level roughly by 2 $\mu g/mL$, with considerable scatter. A 5-mg/kg dose is, therefore, estimated to give a level of approximately 10 $\mu g/mL$. This relationship of loading dose to incremental increase in blood level can also be used for additional dosing considerations after the theophylline level is known. The rate of metabolism is highly variable and may be affected by many factors. Factors that decrease aminophylline clearance and necessitate lowering of infusion rates include use of cimetidine, erythromycin, upper respiratory tract infections, pneumonia, and so forth. If IV aminophylline is given to patients receiving oral aminophylline or theophylline, blood levels should be checked on admission. Levels should be checked daily for all patients receiving aminophylline infusions.

Leukotriene Modifiers

There are little data to suggest a role for leukotriene modifiers in acute asthma and, therefore, these agents are not recommended in the management of acute asthma.

Antibiotics

Routine administration of antibiotics is not indicated and should be reserved for those with evidence of infection such as pneumonia or sinusitis. When an infection precipitates an exacerbation of asthma, it is likely to be viral in nature.

Helium–Oxygen Therapy

A blended mixture of helium and oxygen (heliox) is available in mixtures of 60:40, 70:30, and 80:20. Heliox is less dense than air and can be delivered through a tight-fitting nonrebreathing mask or, in the intubated patient, through the ventilatory circuit. This less dense gas mixture results in decreased airway resistance. Studies have shown the ability of heliox to decrease pulsus paradoxus and improve both inspiratory and expiratory flows. Heliox may have potential benefit in delaying need for intubation while bronchodilators exert their effect, as well as decreasing peak airway pressures in the mechanically ventilated patient. In the latter case, its potential to decrease auto-PEEP may be particularly useful. A mixture of 60:40 of heliox can be used as initial therapy with careful monitoring of oxygenation. Recalibration of gas blenders and flowmeters is required to obtain accurate measures of oxygen concentration and tidal volumes when this mixture is used in the mechanically ventilated patient.

It must be remembered that, despite reported anecdotal success, no controlled trials have demonstrated an alteration of outcome variables and, therefore, the use of heliox in adults with acute asthma cannot be recommended as standard therapy on the basis of present evidence. The mixture might be considered for patients who do not respond to standard therapy.

Intravenous Fluids

There are no controlled trials, or even observational or cohort studies, of differing fluid regimens in acute asthma. Some patients with acute asthma require rehydration and correction of electrolyte imbalance. Hypokalemia can be caused or exacerbated by β_2-agonist and/or steroid treatment and must be corrected. Aggressive hydration is not recommended for adults or older children but may be indicated for infants and young children. Chest physical therapy and mucolytics are not recommended.

Sedatives

Sedation should be strictly avoided during exacerbations of asthma because of the respiratory depressant effect of anxiolytic and hypnotic drugs. An association between the use of these drugs and avoidable asthma deaths has been demonstrated.

REFERRAL TO THE INTENSIVE CARE UNIT

All patients transferred to the ICU should be accompanied by a physician suitably equipped and skilled to perform endotracheal intubation, if necessary. Indications for admission to intensive care facilities or a high-dependency unit include patients requiring ventilatory support and those with severe acute or life-threatening asthma who are failing to respond to therapy, as evidenced by:

- Deteriorating PEF
- Persisting or worsening hypoxia
- Hypercapnia
- Worsening acidosis
- Exhaustion, feeble respiration
- Drowsiness, confusion
- Coma or respiratory arrest

Admission Decisions

Criteria for Discharge from the Emergency Department versus Hospitalization

Criteria for determining whether a patient should be discharged from the emergency department or admitted to the hospital have been succinctly reviewed and stratified based on consensus. Patients with a pretreatment FEV_1 or PEF <25% of predicted/personal best, or those with a posttreatment FEV_1 or PEF <40% of predicted/personal best, require hospitalization.

Patients with posttreatment FEV_1 or PEF of 40% to 60% of predicted/personal best may be discharged, provided that adequate follow-up is available in the community and that compliance is assured. Patients with posttreatment FEV_1 or PEF >60% of predicted/personal best can be discharged with significantly less immediate concern. For patients discharged from the emergency department:

- At a minimum, a 7-day course of oral glucocorticosteroids for adults and a shorter course (3–5 days) for children should be prescribed, along with continuation of bronchodilator therapy.
- The bronchodilator can be used on an as-needed basis, based on both symptomatic and objective improvement, until the patient returns to his or her pre-exacerbation use of rapid-acting inhaled β_2-agonists.
- Ipratropium bromide is unlikely to provide additional benefit beyond the acute phase and may be quickly discontinued.
- The patient's inhaler technique and use of peak flow meter to monitor therapy at home should be reviewed. Patients discharged from the emergency department with a peak flow meter and action plan have a better response than patients discharged without these resources.
- The factors that precipitated the exacerbation should be identified and strategies for their future avoidance implemented.
- The patient's response to the exacerbation should be evaluated. The action plan should be reviewed and written guidance provided.

Indications for Intubation

Careful and repeat assessment of patients with severe exacerbations is mandatory. Not all patients admitted to the ICU need invasive mechanical ventilation. The exact time to intubate is based mainly on clinical judgment (53–55):

- Patients presenting with apnea or coma should be intubated immediately.
- Progressive exhaustion, patient fatigue, and worsening hypercapnia despite maximal therapy, together with altered level of consciousness, are indications for intubation.
- Maintaining adequate oxygenation (and oxygen transport) with supplemental oxygen is seldom a problem even in very severe asthma and is a relatively uncommon reason for intubation.
- If the patient is cooperative, hypercapnia and fatigue do not necessarily mandate intubation because noninvasive ventilation may be an option (see later discussion).

Intubation

Intubation may be performed by either the nasal or the oral route, the latter allowing for the insertion of a larger tube that facilitates suctioning, which is important for removing tenacious mucus plugs mobilized during recovery, and offers less resistance to flow. A larger endotracheal tube reduces flow-resistive pressure during inspiration, but this is not important during controlled mechanical ventilation. Given the

TABLE 140.12

DRUGS USED FOR INTUBATION IN ACUTE SEVERE ASTHMA

Agents	Dose	Advantages	Side effects	Contraindications
Midazolam	1 mg (intravenous) slowly, every 2–3 min until the patient allows positioning and airways inspection	Amnesia Muscle relaxation	Hypotension Respiratory depression	—
Ketamine	1–2 mg/kg (intravenous) at a rate of 0.5 mg/kg/min	No respiratory depression No hypotension Short-term bronchodilation	Increased laryngeal reflexes Increased laryngeal secretions Sympathomimetic effects (hypertension, tachycardia) Increased intracranial pressure Delirium Hallucinations (prevented by midazolam coadministration)	Atherosclerosis Hypertension Increased intracranial pressure
Propofol	60–80 mg/min initial intravenous infusion up to 2.0 mg/kg	Rapid onset and resolution of sedation Bronchodilation	Hypotension Respiratory depression	Hemodynamic instability

extraordinary high resistance of the patient's airways, the effect of the larger-bore tube on expiratory flow is also trivial (38). Intubation should be performed by the most skilled operator available to avoid repeated airway manipulation, which may induce laryngospasm and bronchoconstriction. Satisfactory local anesthesia of the oropharynx, nasopharynx, and larynx is essential. Table 140.12 summarizes drugs used to facilitate intubation of patients with severe asthma (38,56). It should be stressed that many of these drugs reduce vascular tone and may cause profound hypotension if combined with decreased venous return because of hyperinflation. This may require rapid infusion of IV fluids and manual ventilation via a bag/valve/mask device at a slow rate or even temporary apnea to decrease hyperinflation. Lack of response suggests the presence of tension pneumothorax (38).

Mechanical Ventilation

Noninvasive Positive Pressure Ventilation

Noninvasive positive pressure ventilation (NIPPV) can be considered in asthmatic patients at risk for endotracheal intubation from progressive exhaustion (57). However, there is only one prospective randomized controlled trial in normocapnic asthmatic patients showing that a short trial of NIPPV in the emergency department decreases hospitalization rate, respiratory frequency, and improves spirometric indices of pulmonary function (58). Other observational studies, without a rigorous prospective randomized control design, suggest that even in hypercapnic (59) asthmatic patients, a trial of NIPPV may be beneficial. However, the NIPPV trial should not unnecessarily delay endotracheal intubation (60). Absolute contraindications for the use of NIPPV in asthma are emergency intubation for cardiorespiratory resuscitation, hemodynamic and electrocardiographic instability, life-threatening hypoxemia, and an altered state of consciousness. The presence of severe hypercapnia on hospital admission should alert the clinician to the high risk of endotracheal intubation despite not being, per se, a contraindication to NIPPV. Interestingly, among severe asthmatics admitted to the ICU, patients successfully treated with NIPPV had less hypercapnia (mean $PaCO_2$ 53 ± 13 mm Hg; mean pH 7.28 ± 0.008) than those who eventually underwent endotracheal intubation (mean $PaCO_2$ 89 ± 29 mm Hg; mean pH 7.05 ± 0.21) (54).

When used, NIPPV should be started with low levels of inspiratory pressure support (5–10 cm H_2O) and PEEP (3–5 cm H_2O). Pressure support should be progressively increased by 2 cm H_2O every 15 minutes, the goal being to reduce respiratory rate below 25 breaths per minute, while keeping peak inspiratory pressure below 25 cm H_2O. Future prospective randomized controlled trials are required to definitely establish the role of NIPPV in acute severe asthma (55).

Invasive Mechanical Ventilation

The goal of mechanical ventilation is to buy time until pharmacotherapy can reverse the underlying pathophysiologic features of airway inflammation, mucus plugging, and bronchoconstriction. The main strategy of ventilatory support is to minimize hyperinflation and avoid excessive airway pressure development (overdistention) (38,61). Thus, controlled hypoventilation or permissive hypercapnia is often required (62, 63).

Controlled ventilation is often used because of the need for deep sedation—with or without muscle paralysis—to avoid patient–ventilator asynchrony and to achieve controlled hypoventilation (38,61). Volume-controlled ventilation is usually preferable to pressure control, as the latter carries the risk of delivering variable tidal volume with sometimes unacceptably low alveolar ventilation in conditions of fluctuating high airway resistance and hyperinflation (38,61).

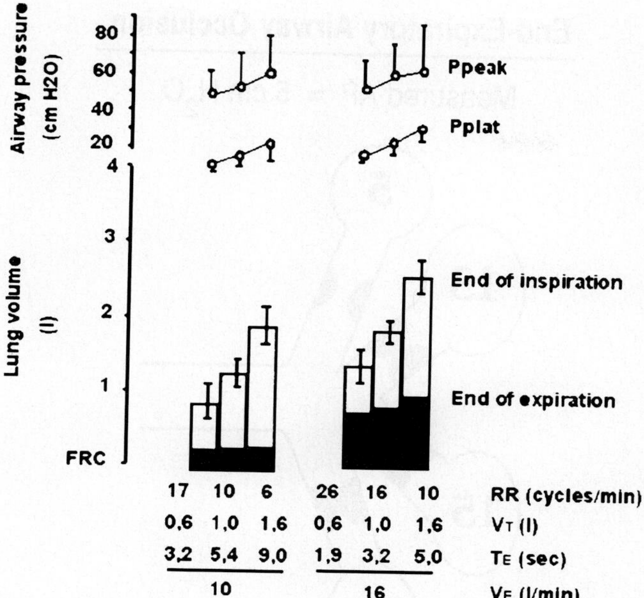

FIGURE 140.6. Effect of respiratory rate and tidal volume variations on airway pressures and lung volumes during mechanical ventilation of acute severe asthma. FRC, functional residual capacity; Ppeak, peak inspiratory pressure; Pplat, end-inspiratory plateau pressure; RR, respiratory rate; V_T, tidal volume; T_E, expiratory time; V_E, minute ventilation. All conditions are for a square inspiratory flow of 100 L/min. (From Tuxen D, Lane S. The effects of ventilatory pattern on hyperinflation, airway pressures, and circulation in mechanical ventilation of patients with severe air-flow obstruction. *Am Rev Respir Dis.* 1987;136:872–879, with permission.)

The most important parameter to achieve the goal of reducing end-expiratory lung volume (i.e., hyperinflation) is a reduction in the administered minute ventilation (i.e., <10 L/min) (Figs. 140.6 and 140.7) (64). For a given level of minute ventilation, the end-expiratory lung volume will be similar regardless of the combination of tidal volume and respiratory rate. However, for any level of minute ventilation and with constant (square wave) inspiratory flow rate, end-inspiratory lung distention is minimized by a combination of low tidal volume (V_T) and high respiratory rate (Fig. 140.6). This is because in the inhomogeneous asthmatic lung, most of the tidal volume delivered by positive pressure ventilation goes to the parts of lung parenchyma with almost normal mechanical characteristics (compartment A, Fig. 140.2). Because such "mechanically normal" areas represent only a small fraction of the total asthmatic lung, they become overdistended. Thus, the lower tidal volume would cause less end-inspiratory lung overdistention.

When keeping minute ventilation, tidal volume, and respiratory rate constant, increasing inspiratory flow allows inspiratory time (T_I) to be reduced and thus expiratory time (T_E) to be increased. When minute ventilation is high (>10 L/min), increasing inspiratory flow and thus reducing T_I allows a decrease in lung hyperinflation (Fig. 140.7). It should be stressed, however, that prolonging T_E is not very effective in decreasing dynamic hyperinflation when minute ventilation is <10 L/min (65). This is because flow progressively decreases during expiration, so prolonging expiration will allow additional time for expiration at a point at which expiratory flows are low, and thus the additional volume that could be exhaled (the integral of flow over time) is modest; this decrease in dynamic hyperinflation is even less when respiratory rate is low. Thus, at any given minute ventilation, inspiratory flow should be 60 to 80 L/min (Table 140.13), as further prolonging T_E by greater inspiratory flow will not significantly reduce hyperinflation.

The optimal inspiratory flow waveform with volume-controlled ventilation is not entirely clear. For a given tidal volume, T_I will be shorter and thus T_E longer when constant flow (square wave) rather than decelerating flow is used. However, the effect of this on reducing hyperinflation is clinically insignificant (see previous discussion). At identical levels of V_T, T_I, and P_{plat}, a square wave results in a higher peak inspiratory pressure (Ppeak) than does a decelerating wave. This consideration has limited clinical relevance because Ppeak is highly dependent on inspiratory flow-resistive properties; therefore, Ppeak does not reflect alveolar distention pressure in most of the lung (59) (i.e., increased airway resistance combined with

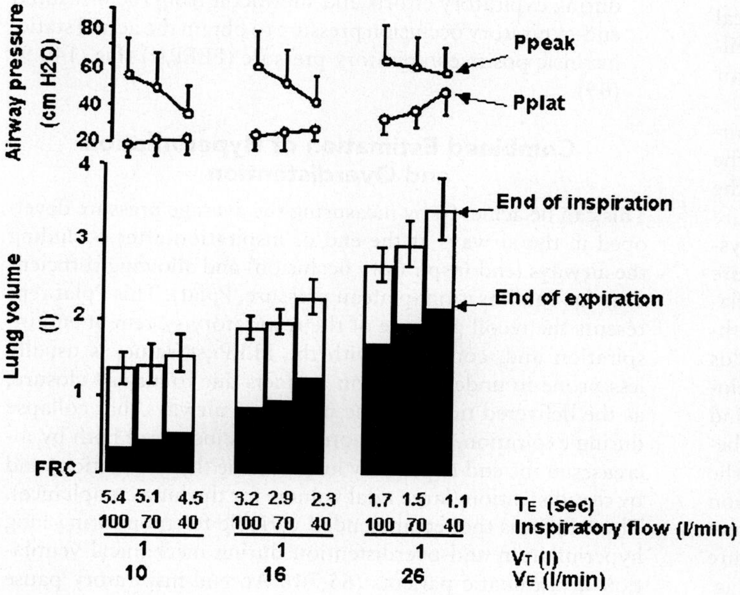

FIGURE 140.7. Effect of inspiratory flow variations on airway pressures and lung volumes during mechanical ventilation in acute severe asthma. FRC, functional residual capacity; Ppeak, peak inspiratory pressure; Pplat, end-inspiratory plateau pressure; RR, respiratory rate; V_T, tidal volume; T_E, expiratory time; V_E, minute ventilation. (From Tuxen D, Lane S. The effects of ventilatory pattern on hyperinflation, airway pressures, and circulation in mechanical ventilation of patients with severe air-flow obstruction. *Am Rev Respir Dis.* 1987;136:872–879, with permission.)

TABLE 140.13

INITIAL VENTILATORY SETTINGS IN STATUS ASTHMATICUS

Setting	Recommendation
Mode	Volume control ventilation
Minute ventilation	<10 L/min
Respiratory rate	10–15 breaths/min
PEEP	Titration trial (increments of 2 cm H_2O)
Expiratory time	>4 sec
Inspiratory flow	60–80 L/min
FIO_2	Maintain SpO_2 >90%
Pplat	<30 cm H_2O

PEEP, positive end-expiratory pressure; FIO_2, fraction of inspired oxygen; Pplat, end-inspiratory plateau pressure; SaO_2, oxygen saturation.

high inspiratory flow rate may result in Ppeak above 50 cm H_2O but without increased risk of barotraumas). Nevertheless, a lower Ppeak may mean less overdistention of alveoli distal to the least obstructed airways, as these are the most exposed to high pressure in the central airways. Another reason to minimize Ppeak, and thus to prefer the decelerating over the square waveform, is that delivery of the full V_T is less easily interrupted by opening of the pop-off safety valve of the ventilator, securing a steadier minute ventilation (58).

Monitoring of Hyperinflation and Overdistention

Dynamic hyperinflation can be monitored in two different ways:

1. By measuring the volume passively exhaled from end-inspiration to the static functional residual capacity in the course of a prolonged (38) apnea and subtracting the delivered tidal volume (V_{EI}) (64). Although this is the most accurate way of measuring dynamic hyperinflation and estimating the attendant risks of hypotension and barotrauma (57,66), the need for complete muscle relaxation, with its potential complications (see later discussion), and practical aspects of the measurement reduce its clinical applicability (61). Furthermore, it cannot measure the volume of air trapped behind closed airways (compartment and C).
2. By measuring the average pressure developed in the airways at the end of expiration (PEEPi) after occluding the airways and allowing sufficient time for equilibration (the end-expiratory occlusion technique) (29,67). This pressure represents the average recoil pressure of the respiratory system at the end of expiration, and is an indirect measure of the end expiratory lung volume and thus of hyperinflation. However, it should be kept in mind that, in acute asthmatic crisis, the measurement of PEEPi sometimes yields unexpectedly low values, presumably reflecting airway closure (67). This is because the pressure developed behind noncommunicating airways (which might be quite high because of regional hyperinflation) does not contribute to the static PEEPi measurement by the end-expiratory occlusion technique (Fig. 140.8). Thus, the average airway pressure at the end of expiration might underestimate the pressure that corresponds to the end-expiratory lung volume (Fig. 140.8). Absence of respiratory muscle activity is required for a valid measurement because expiratory efforts can artifactually increase the measured end-expiratory occlusion pressure (68). In such cases, insertion of a gastric balloon is required to measure the increase in the gastric pressure during expiratory efforts and subtract it from the measured end-expiratory occlusion pressure to obtain the actual static, intrinsic positive expiratory pressure (PEEP,st) (Fig. 140.9) (69).

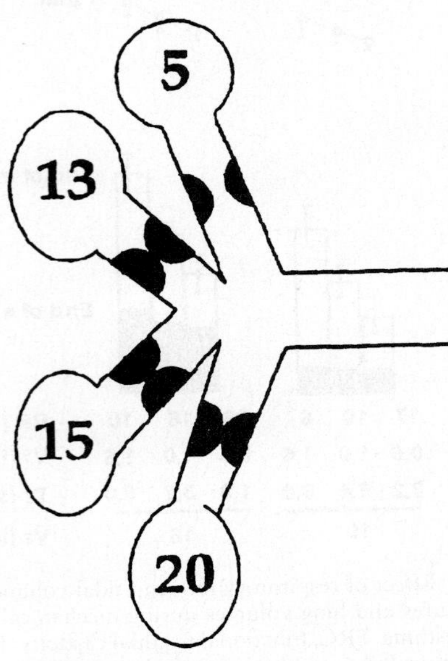

FIGURE 140.8. Hypothetical model suggesting a mechanism whereby measured auto-PEEP (positive end-expiratory pressure) by the end-expiratory occlusion technique may underestimate the severity of hyperinflation because of widespread airway closure at end-expiration. Measured auto-PEEP reflects only the end-expiratory alveolar pressure in lung units that are in communication with the proximal airway at end expiration. (From Leatherman JW, Ravenscraft SA. Low measured auto-positive end-expiratory pressure during mechanical ventilation of patients with severe asthma: hidden auto-positive end-expiratory pressure. *Critical Care Med.* 1996;24:541–546, with permission.)

Combined Estimation of Hyperinflation and Overdistention

This can be achieved by measuring the average pressure developed in the airways at the end of inspiration after occluding the airways (end-inspiratory occlusion) and allowing sufficient time for equilibration (plateau pressure, Pplat). This Pplat represents the recoil pressure of the respiratory system at end inspiration and, compared with the PEEPi,st value, is usually less prone to underestimation artifacts due to airway closure, as the delivered tidal volume may open airways that collapse during expiration. Furthermore, Pplat is increased both by increases in the end-expiratory lung volume (hyperinflation) and by overdistention (large tidal volume for the lung compliance). Thus, Pplat is the recommended variable for monitoring lung hyperinflation and overdistention during mechanical ventilation in asthmatic patients (65,70). An end-inspiratory pause

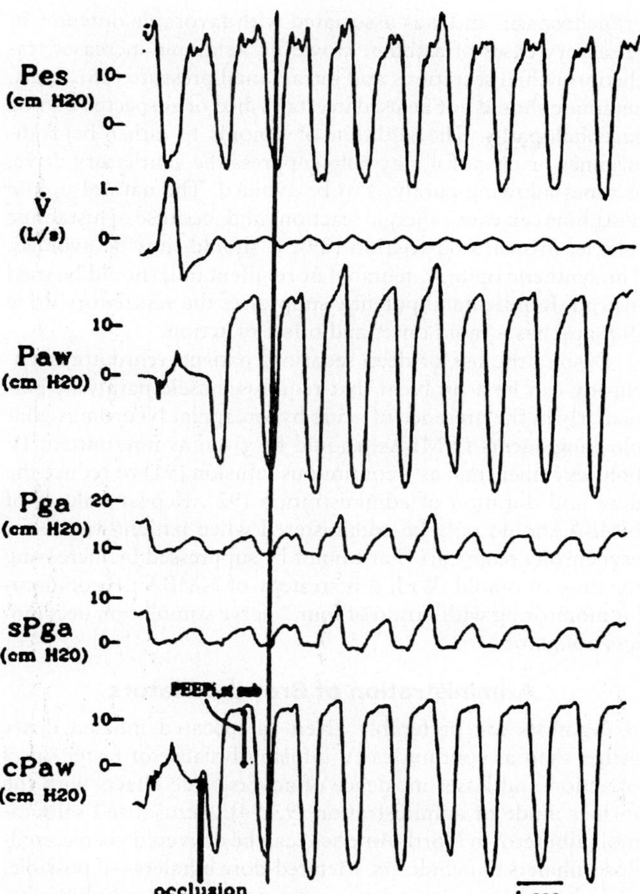

FIGURE 140.9. Correction of PEEPi,st measurement for expiratory muscle contraction with the use of a gastric balloon. Recordings of esophageal (Pes), airway (Paw), gastric (Pga), "suppressed" gastric pressure (sPga), and online "corrected" airway pressure (cPaw) in a representative actively expiring patient during airway occlusion. sPga is the Pga tracing suppressed to zero at its lowest value at the end-inspiratory level (*vertical line*) where expiratory muscle activity is nil, that is, at this level it was given the value of zero irrespective of its true value relative to atmospheric pressure. cPaw is obtained by subtracting sPga from Paw. Note a consistent end-expiratory plateau in cPaw despite marked variability in Pga swings. From this plateau PEEPi,st sub was measured. (From Zakynthinos SG, Vassilakopoulos T, Zakynthinos E, et al. Correcting static intrinsic positive end-expiratory pressure for expiratory muscle contraction. Validation of a new method. *Am J Respir Crit Care Med.* 1999;160:785–790, with permission.)

of several seconds is required for an accurate measurement of Pplat because of the prolonged equilibration time of the extremely heterogeneous asthmatic lung (56,61). Pplat should not exceed 30 cm H_2O (67). Ppeak, in contrast to Pplat, is not useful for assessing lung hyperinflation in asthmatic patients because it depends strongly on airway resistance and inspiratory flow (Fig. 140.4).

The Role of Extrinsic PEEP

Controlled Mechanical Ventilation. The addition of PEEP during controlled mechanical ventilation in asthma patients results in a variable and unpredictable response (68–70). In some patients, extrinsic PEEP (PEEPe) causes overinflation (71,72); in others, FRC and PEEPi (72,73) are decreased; and in still others no response to PEEP is observed until PEEPe exceeds baseline PEEPi (72). This might be due to the great heterogeneity of the asthmatic lung with various combinations of the previously described compartments in each patient.

- If the predominant site of increased resistance to airflow is located in the central, noncollapsible airways, and the transmural pressure of peripheral, collapsible bronchi and bronchioles remains positive throughout expiration, passive exhalation is not flow-limited (74), and the applied PEEPe extends all the way up to the alveoli, increasing end-expiratory lung volume (61,75).
- If the prevailing pathophysiology is flow limitation of peripheral, collapsible bronchi and bronchioles, the addition of PEEP will not affect end-expiratory lung volume until PEEPe exceeds baseline PEEPi. This is explained by the classic waterfall theory of flow limitation, which suggests that expiratory flow is determined by pressure gradients up to the choke point (point of flow limitation) and that conditions downstream from the choke point have no influence on expiratory flow (76–78). By analogy, the level of the lake downstream from a waterfall is said to have no influence on the water flow falling into it (provided that the lake level does not exceed the waterfall's edge). The water flow would be determined basically by the difference in level between the headspring and the edge of the waterfall. Because PEEPe represents the level of the downstream lake in such an analogy, it follows that PEEPe application either should have no influence on expiratory flow or should only impair it when PEEPi is approached (69).
- If the prevailing pathophysiology is sticky airway closure during exhalation, leaving trapped behind some highly pressurized air, application of PEEPe—associated with transiently high end-inspiratory pressures—might reopen such a disconnected lung unit and then, because of airway hysteresis, this PEEPe might be enough to prevent expiratory airway re-collapse in the next breaths, promoting appropriate progressive deflation of overinflated lung (a recruiting effect analogous to that described in acute respiratory distress syndrome) (72,79).

Thus, a PEEPe trial—a stepwise application of PEEP in increments of 2 cm H_2O every 5 minutes—with measurement of the plateau pressure at each step might be a useful bedside approach. If Pplat decreases, application of PEEPe is deflating the lung and is beneficial (72); if Pplat increases, PEEPe should be withdrawn.

Assisted Mechanical Ventilation. At the resolution phase, when inspiratory muscle activity resumes and the patient triggers the ventilator, low levels of PEEPe may be useful because PEEPe may decrease muscle effort required to trigger the ventilator by providing part of the threshold pressure that PEEPi represents, which the inspiratory muscles have to overcome before airway pressure becomes negative and the ventilator is triggered (80). Keeping in mind that the existence of the waterfall effect is not guaranteed, and also that flow-limited and flow-unlimited pathways may coexist in these conditions, a prudent trial of PEEPe to a level lower than PEEPi is worth pursuing, with titration for patient comfort under close monitoring of airway and blood pressures (75). Frequent reassessment is essential because the adequate level of PEEPe is subject to change as lung mechanics and ventilatory requirements evolve.

Permissive Hypercapnia

The ventilatory strategy described is accompanied by variable levels of hypercapnia with values averaging between 60 and 70 mm Hg, but sometimes exceeding 100 mm Hg (38). At times hypercapnia is unavoidable rather than permissive (see "Pathophysiology: Gas Exchange").

The physiologic and untoward effects of hypercapnia are related to acute reduction of intracellular pH (due to high CO_2 diffusibility; the interested reader should consult excellent detailed reviews (63). However, effective compensatory mechanisms return intracellular pH to nearly normal within 1 to 3 hours, which explains why even extreme degrees of normoxic hypercapnia are well tolerated. Except in patients with raised intracranial pressure or severe myocardial depression, the respiratory acidosis induced by permissive hypercapnia does not need to be treated (38,62). In ventilated asthmatic patients, CO_2 production should be reduced by the use of sedation, analgesia, and antipyretics to reduce hypercapnia (61). If these measures are insufficient, muscle relaxants may be considered (61). In acute asthma, hypercapnia usually improves within the first 12 hours of mechanical ventilation (probably as a result of the time-dependent effect of corticosteroids).

Hypercapnia depresses myocardial contractility, relaxes systemic arterioles, and increases the tone in venous capacitance vessels. In the absence of β-blockade, reflex sympathetic stimulation offsets the depressed contractility (63). The integrated hemodynamic response to acute hypercapnia in patients with normal cardiac function is an increase in cardiac output accompanied by decreased systemic vascular resistance (63). In patients with underlying left ventricular dysfunction, adverse hemodynamic effects may ensue, including severe hypotension and dysrhythmias, so cautious use of permissive hypercapnia is suggested in this situation (38).

Hypercapnia reversibly increases cerebral blood flow and intracranial pressure (63), which may prove disastrous in patients with intracranial pathology (59,62). A clinical challenge is presented by patients who have experienced profound cerebral anoxia secondary to respiratory arrest before intubation, in which clinicians face the therapeutic dilemma of brain protection versus controlled hypoventilation for addressing the asthmatic crisis. Although not supported by strong clinical data, blood alkalinization may be considered in this context. A slow infusion of sodium bicarbonate should be used, as rapid bicarbonate administration in the context of suppressed ventilatory drive may transiently raise the $PaCO_2$, thus worsening intracellular and cerebrospinal acidosis. Other buffers such as *tris*-hydroxymethyl aminomethane (tromethamine, Tham) or Carbicarb (a mixture of sodium carbonate and bicarbonate) do not have these disadvantages, but clinical experience with these agents is quite limited (81).

Sedation

Hypercapnia stimulates the respiratory center, increasing the drive to the respiratory muscles (63). Thus, controlled hypoventilation requires deep sedation to suppress respiratory muscle activity. Benzodiazepines can be safely used (66,82), as can propofol with its rapid onset of action and—with short-term use—lack of accumulation and bronchodilating action (83,84); there is a risk of hypotension with propofol, particularly in hypovolemic patients (85). Ketamine has anesthetic, sedative, analgesic, and bronchodilating effects (86). In anesthetic (87) or subanesthetic (88) doses, ketamine reduced bronchospasm and was associated with favorable outcome in refractory cases of asthma. However, ketamine increases tracheobronchial secretions and intracranial pressure (86). Thus, ketamine should not be used in established or suspected anoxic encephalopathy. The addition of opioids to either benzodiazepines or propofol may help suppress the ventilatory drive, at times allowing paralysis to be avoided. The natural opioid morphine can cause allergic reactions and, because of histamine release, bronchoconstriction (89); it should thus be avoided. The synthetic opioids, fentanyl or remifentanil, should be used instead. Remifentanil potently suppresses the ventilatory drive (90) and has a rapid onset and offset of action.

Despite the use of deep sedation, patient–ventilator asynchrony can be a problem that requires muscle paralysis, particularly in the presence of acute hypercapnia. Neuromuscular blocking agents (NMBAs) should be given as intermittent IV boluses rather than as a continuous infusion (91) to reduce the dose and duration of administration (92). Repeat boluses of NMBA should only be administered when patient–ventilator asynchrony reappears that cannot be suppressed by increasing the dose of opioid. With this strategy of NMBA neuromuscular monitoring with "train of four," nerve stimulation becomes less obligatory.

Administration of Bronchodilators

β_2-Agonists are preferably given as repeated inhaled doses rather than as continuous IV infusion because of faster onset of action and lesser incidence of adverse side effects with the former mode of administration (93,94). Aerosolized salbutamol (albuterol in North America) can be delivered via metered-dose inhalers or nebulizers. Metered-dose inhalers—if possible, with the use of a spacer device—are preferred to nebulizers because of less cost and inconvenience of use, lower risk of bacterial contamination, better reproducibility of dosing, and faster maximal bronchodilatation (95,96).

Humidification

Heated wire humidifiers are preferable to heat and moisture exchangers. The latter add to expiratory airway resistance and increase dead space—being inserted between the endotracheal tube and the Y-piece of ventilator tubing—and therefore contribute to hypercapnia (61).

Weaning

Once dynamic hyperinflation has abated sufficiently, as assessed by a substantial resolution of wheezing on chest auscultation and decrease of Pplat and PEEPi, weaning should be initiated using standard procedures (97). Suppression of respiratory muscle activity with controlled hypoventilation should be maintained as short as possible to prevent ventilator-induced diaphragmatic dysfunction (98). Weaning is normally rapidly achieved in patients with acute severe asthma (99). Weaning difficulty in the absence of persistent severe airway obstruction must raise the suspicion of myopathy induced by previous administration of NMBAs and corticosteroids (see later discussion).

COMPLICATIONS AND MORTALITY

Controlled hypoventilation for acute severe asthma has significantly reduced complications and mortality compared with conventional mechanical ventilation aimed at normalizing blood gases (66,82,83,99,100). The mortality of patients mechanically ventilated for acute severe asthma has been <10% in all studies after 1990 except two (100,101). A frequently reported cause of death is cerebral anoxia secondary to prehospital cardiac arrest (38,61).

Hypotension

The most frequent complication of mechanical ventilation in asthmatic patients is hemodynamic instability manifested as hypotension (38,61,66,101), usually occurring at the initiation of ventilation (see previous discussion), which can occasionally be life-threatening (101). This mechanism is easily verified by temporarily disconnecting the patient from the ventilator (1 minute, under close monitoring of SpO_2) and documenting an immediate increase in blood pressure. Ventilation should be resumed with lower tidal volume and respiratory rate, and adequate volume expansion should rapidly follow. When hypotension is unresponsive to ventilator disconnection, tension pneumothorax must be suspected (38,61).

Pneumothorax

Barotrauma is the second most frequently reported complication. Controlled hypoventilation does not confer complete protection against pneumothorax, but decreases its incidence from 30% to <10% (66). Although usually not reported as a direct cause of mortality when rapidly diagnosed and adequately treated, barotrauma can still be life-threatening (100).

Myopathy

Diffuse paresis of voluntary muscles (frequently termed *acute quadriplegic myopathy*) has been observed on cessation of NMBA administration in asthmatic patients, lasting from a few hours to months, sometimes involving the respiratory muscles and thus delaying ventilator weaning (102–106). A deleterious interaction of combined treatment with NMBAs and corticosteroids has been implicated in the pathogenesis of this complication (107). The duration of muscle relaxation (100) and the cumulative dose of NMBAs increase the risk (108). Electromyography typically shows acute myopathy confirmed by usually mildly elevated levels of creatine-phosphokinase and thick filament necrosis on muscle biopsy, which is often seen on light microscopy but found more definitely on electron microscopy (106–108). There is no specific treatment. The best approach is to avoid NMBAs and steroids, or to use these medications as sparingly as possible.

CLINICAL PEARLS

1. Lessons learned from asthmatic deaths include:
   - Most deaths can be avoided, because severe asthma crisis requiring hospitalization usually progresses over >6 hours.
   - Factors that lead to death are nonreferral to a specialist and inadequate steroid dosage and monitoring of disease.
   - Patients with severe asthma and psychiatric disease or psychosocial problems may experience near-fatal asthma.
   - Patients with a history of near-fatal asthma or unstable asthma should be treated only by specialists who should closely follow these patients for at least 1 year after admission.
2. Early identification and treatment of asthma is essential.
3. Severe asthma is usually resistant to treatment.
4. After establishing the diagnosis of severe asthma, all exacerbating factors should be identified and treated.
5. Aggressive use of inhaled bronchodilator therapy plus systemic anti-inflammatory therapy (although not immediately effective) are fundamental elements of therapy.
6. The primary cause of respiratory demise in the patient with severe asthma is acute respiratory acidosis and ventilatory insufficiency. Acute respiratory acidosis may lead to depressed level of consciousness and loss of airway protection.
7. Patients with status asthmaticus may be unresponsive to initial therapeutic intervention and may require prolonged and aggressive therapy.
8. Patients failing drug therapy should be considered early for intubation and mechanical ventilation.
9. Avoidance of hyperinflation and overdistention at the expense of minute ventilation—permissive hypercapnia—are the cornerstones of ventilatory management.
10. After patients recover and return to the general medical ward, the treating team should address the prevention and treatment of subsequent asthma attacks.

References

1. Wenzel S. Severe asthma in adults. *Am J Respir Crit Care Med.* 2005; 172:149–160.
2. Global Initiative for Asthma. Global strategy for asthma management and prevention. Bethesda, MD: National Institutes of Health, National Heart, Lung, and Blood Institute; 2006.
3. National Asthma Education and Prevention Program expert panel report 2: guidelines for the diagnosis and management of asthma. Washington, DC: U.S. Department of Health and Human Services; NAEPP Publication 1997;97:4051.
4. Chung KF, Godard P, Adelroth E, et al. Difficult/therapy-resistant asthma: the need for an integrated approach to define clinical phenotypes, evaluate risk factors, understand pathophysiology and find novel therapies. ERS Task Force on Difficult/Therapy-Resistant Asthma. *Eur Respir J* 1999; 13:1198–1208.
5. Proceedings of the ATS Workshop on Refractory Asthma: current understanding, recommendations and unanswered questions. *Am J Respir Crit Care Med.* 2000;162:2341–2351.
6. European Network for Understanding Mechanisms of Severe Asthma. The ENFUMOSA cross-sectional European multicentre study of the clinical phenotype of chronic severe asthma. *Eur Respir J.* 2003;22:470–477.
7. Colice GL. Categorizing asthma severity: an overview of national guidelines. *Clin Med Res.* 2004;2:155–163.
8. Bacharier LB, Strunk RC, Mauger D, et al. Classifying asthma severity in children: mismatch between symptoms, medication use and lung function. *Am J Respir Crit Care Med.* 2004;170:426–432.
9. Teeter JG, Bleecker ER. Relationship between airway obstruction and respiratory symptoms in adult asthmatics. *Chest.* 1998;113:272–277.
10. Boulet LP, Phillips R, O'Byrne P, et al. Evaluation of asthma control by physicians and patients: comparison with current guidelines. *Can Respir J.* 2002;9:417–423.
11. Wolfenden LL, Diette GB, Krishnan JA, et al. Lower physician estimate of underlying asthma severity leads to undertreatment. *Arch Intern Med.* 2003;163:231–236.

12. Moore WC, Peters SP. Severe asthma: an overview. *J Allergy Clin Immunol.* 2006;117:487–494.
13. Tough SC, Hessel PA, Ruff M, et al. Features that distinguish those who die from asthma from community controls with asthma. *J Asthma.* 1998;35:657–665.
14. Miller MK, Johnson C, Miller DP, et al, for the TENOR Study Group. Severity assessment in asthma: an evolving concept. *J Allergy Clin Immunol.* 2005;116:990–995.
15. Harrison BDW. Difficult asthma in adults: recognition and approaches to management. *Int Med J.* 2005;35:543–547.
16. Bel EH. Clinical phenotypes of asthma. *Curr Opin Pulm Med.* 2004;10:44–50.
17. Fabbri LM, Romagnoli M, Corbetta L, et al. Differences in airway inflammation in patients with fixed airflow obstruction due to asthma or chronic obstructive pulmonary disease. *Am J Respir Crit Care Med.* 2003;167:418–424.
18. Wenzel SE. Asthma: defining of the persistent adult phenotypes. *Lancet.* 2006;368:804–813.
19. Wenzel S. Mechanisms of severe asthma. *Clin Exp Allergy.* 2003;33:1622–1628.
20. Busse WW, Banks-Schlegel S, Wenzel SE. Pathophysiology of severe asthma. *J Allergy Clin Immunol.* 2000;106:1033–1042.
21. Wenzel S. Pathology of difficult asthma. *Paediatr Respir Rev.* 2003;4:306–311.
22. Gaga M, Papageorgiou N, Yiourgioti G, et al; on behalf of the ENFUMOSA study group. Risk factors and characteristics associated with severe and difficult to treat asthma phenotype: an analysis of the ENFUMOSA group of patients based on the ECRHS questionnaire. *Clin Exp Allergy.* 2005;35:954–959.
23. Bel EH. Severe asthma. *Breathe.* December 2006;3(2):129–139.
24. McFadden ER Jr, Kiser R, DeGroot WJ. Acute bronchial asthma. Relations between clinical and physiologic manifestations. *N Engl J Med.* 1973;288:221–225.
25. McCarthy DS, Sigurdson M. Lung elastic recoil and reduced airflow in clinically stable asthma. *Thorax.* 1980;35:298–302.
26. Colebatch HJ, Finucane KE, Smith MM. Pulmonary conductance and elastic recoil relationships in asthma and emphysema. *J Appl Physiol.* 1973;34:143–153.
27. Martin J, Powell E, Shore S, et al. The role of respiratory muscles in the hyperinflation of bronchial asthma. *Am Rev Respir Dis.* 1980;121:441–447.
28. Collett PW, Brancatisano T, Engel LA. Changes in the glottic aperture during bronchial asthma. *Am Rev Respir Dis.* 1983;128:719–723.
29. Pepe PE, Marini JJ. Occult positive end-expiratory pressure in mechanically ventilated patients with airflow obstruction: the auto-PEEP effect. *Am Rev Respir Dis.* 1982;126:166–170.
30. Briscoe WA, McLG Jr. Ventilatory function in bronchial asthma. *Thorax.* 1952;7:66–77.
31. Oddo M, Feihl F, Schaller MD, et al. Management of mechanical ventilation in acute severe asthma: practical aspects. *Intensive Care Med.* 2006;32:501–510.
32. Vassilakopoulos T, Zakynthinos S, Roussos Ch. Respiratory muscles and weaning failure. *Eur Respir J.* 1996;9:2383–2400.
33. Vassilakopoulos T, Zakynthinos S, Roussos Ch. Muscle function: basic concepts. In: Marini JJ, Slutsky A, eds. *Physiologic Basis of Ventilator Support.* New York: Marcel Dekker; 1998:103–152.
34. Lougheed DM, Webb KA, O'Donnell DE. Breathlessness during induced lung hyperinflation in asthma: the role of the inspiratory threshold load. *Am J Respir Crit Care Med.* 1995;152:911–920.
35. Lougheed MD, Lam M, Forkert L, et al. Breathlessness during acute bronchoconstriction in asthma. Pathophysiologic mechanisms. *Am Rev Respir Dis.* 1993;148:1452–1459.
36. Rodriguez-Roisin R. Acute severe asthma: pathophysiology and pathobiology of gas exchange abnormalities. *Eur Respir J.* 1997;10:1359–1371.
37. Rodriguez-Roisin R, Ballester E, Roca J, et al. Mechanisms of hypoxemia in patients with status asthmaticus requiring mechanical ventilation. *Am Rev Respir Dis.* 1989;139:732–739.
38. Leatherman JW. Mechanical ventilation for severe asthma. In: Tobin MJ, ed. *Principles and Practice of Mechanical Ventilation.* 2nd ed. New York: McGraw Hill; 2006:649–662.
39. Shim C, Williams MH Jr. Pulsus paradoxus in asthma. *Lancet.* 1978;1:530–531.
40. Martin J, Jardim J, Sampson M et al. Factors influencing pulsus paradoxus in asthma. *Chest.* 1981;80:543–549.
41. Manthous CA, Hall JB, Caputo MA, et al. Heliox improves pulsus paradoxus and peak expiratory flow in nonintubated patients with severe asthma. *Am J Respir Crit Care Med.* 1995;151:310–314.
42. Papiris S, Kotanidou A, Malagari K et al. Clinical review: severe asthma. *Crit Care.* 2002;6:30–44.
43. McFadden ER Jr. Fatal and near-fatal asthma. *N Engl J Med.* 1991; 324:409–411.
44. Pepe C, Foley S, Shannon J, et al. Differences in airway remodeling between subjects with severe and moderate asthma. *J Allergy Clin Immunol.* 2005;116:544–549.
45. Faul JL, Tormey VJ, Leonard C, et al. Lung immunopathology in cases of sudden asthma death. *Eur Respir J.* 1997;10:301–307.
46. Simoes S, dos Santos M, Oliveiraw M, et al. Inflammatory cell mapping of the respiratory tract in fatal asthma. *Clin Exp Allergy.* 2005;35:602–611.
47. Holgate ST, Polosa R. The mechanisms, diagnosis, and management of severe asthma in adults. *Lancet.* 2006;368:780–793.
48. Eisner MD, Yelin EH, Katz PP, et al. Risk factors for work disability in severe adult asthma. *Am J Med.* 2006;119:884–891.
49. Pasternack R, Huhtala H, Karjalainen J. *Chlamydophila (Chlamydia) pneumoniae* serology and asthma in adults: a longitudinal analysis. *J Allergy Clin Immunol.* 2005;116:1123–1128.
50. ten Brinke A, Sterk PJ, Masclee AA, et al. Risk factors of frequent exacerbations in difficult-to-treat asthma. *Eur Respir J.* 2005;26:812–818.
51. ten Brinke A, van Dissel JT, Sterk PJ, et al. Persistent airflow limitation in adult-onset -REF>nonatopic asthma is associated with serologic evidence of *Chlamydia pneumoniae* infection. *J Allergy Clin Immunol.* 2001;107:449–454.
52. British guideline on the management of asthma. *Thorax.* 2003;58(Suppl I): 32–47.
53. Tuxen DV, Williams TJ, Scheinkestel CD, et al. Use of a measurement of pulmonary hyperinflation to control the level of mechanical ventilation in patients with acute severe asthma. *Am Rev Respir Dis.* 1992;146:1136–1142.
54. Fernandez MM, Villagra A, Blanch L, et al. Non-invasive mechanical ventilation in status asthmaticus. *Intensive Care Med.* 2001;27:486–492.
55. Ram FS, Wellington S, Rowe B, et al. Non-invasive positive pressure ventilation for treatment of respiratory failure due to severe acute exacerbations of asthma. *Cochrane Database Syst Rev.* 2005 Jul 20;(3):CD004360.
56. Corbridge TC, Hall JB. The assessment and management of adults with status asthmaticus. *Am J Respir Crit Care Med.* 1995;151:1296–1316.
57. McFadden ER Jr. Acute severe asthma. *Am J Respir Crit Care Med.* 2003;168:740–759.
58. Soroksky A, Stav D, Shpirer I. A pilot prospective, randomized, placebo-controlled trial of bilevel positive airway pressure in acute asthmatic attack. *Chest.* 2003;123:1018–1025.
59. Meduri GU, Cook TR, Turner RE, et al. Noninvasive positive pressure ventilation in status asthmaticus. *Chest.* 1996;110:767–774.
60. International Consensus Conferences in Intensive Care Medicine: noninvasive positive pressure ventilation in acute Respiratory failure. *Am J Respir Crit Care Med.* 2001;163:283–291.
61. Oddo M, Feihl F, Schaller MD, et al. Management of mechanical ventilation in acute severe asthma: practical aspects. *Intensive Care Med.* 2006;32:501–510.
62. Darioli R, Perret C. Mechanical controlled hypoventilation in status asthmaticus. *Am Rev Respir Dis.* 1984;129:385–387.
63. Feihl F, Perret C. Permissive hypercapnia. How permissive should we be? *Am J Respir Crit Care Med.* 1994;150:1722–1737.
64. Tuxen DV, Lane S. The effects of ventilatory pattern on hyperinflation, airway pressures, and circulation in mechanical ventilation of patients with severe air-flow obstruction. *Am Rev Respir Dis.* 1987;136:872–879.
65. Leatherman JW, McArthur C, Shapiro RS. Effect of prolongation of expiratory time on dynamic hyperinflation in mechanically ventilated patients with severe asthma. *Crit Care Med.* 2004;32:1542–1545.
66. Williams TJ, Tuxen DV, Scheinkestel CD, et al. Risk factors for morbidity in mechanically ventilated patients with acute severe asthma. *Am Rev Respir Dis.* 1992;146:607–615.
67. Leatherman JW, Ravenscraft SA. Low measured auto-positive end-expiratory pressure during mechanical ventilation of patients with severe asthma: hidden auto-positive end-expiratory pressure. *Crit Care Med.* 1996;24:541–546.
68. Ninane V, Yernault JC, de Troyer A. Intrinsic PEEP in patients with chronic obstructive pulmonary disease. Role of expiratory muscles. *Am Rev Respir Dis.* 1993;148:1037–1042.
69. Zakynthinos S, Vassilakopoulos T, Roussos C, et al. Correcting static intrinsic PEEP for expiratory muscle contraction: Validation of a new method. *Am J Respir Crit Care Med.* 1999;160:785–790.
70. Slutsky AS. Consensus conference on mechanical ventilation, January 28–30, 1993 at Northbrook, Illinois, USA. Part 2. *Intensive Care Med.* 1994;20:150–162.
71. Tuxen DV. Detrimental effects of positive end-expiratory pressure during controlled mechanical ventilation of patients with severe airflow obstruction. *Am Rev Respir Dis.* 1989;140:5–9.
72. Caramez MP, Borges JB, Tucci MR, et al. Paradoxical responses to positive end-expiratory pressure in patients with airway obstruction during controlled ventilation. *Crit Care Med.* 2005;33:1519–1528.
73. Qvist J, Andersen JB, Pemberton M, et al. High-level PEEP in severe asthma. *N Engl J Med.* 1982;307:1347–1348.
74. McFadden ER Jr, Ingram RH Jr, Haynes RL, et al. Predominant site of flow limitation and mechanisms of postexertional asthma. *J Appl Physiol.* 1977;42:746–752.
75. Marini JJ. Should PEEP be used in airflow obstruction?. *Am Rev Respir Dis.* 1989;140:1–3.
76. Pride NB, Permutt S, Riley RL, et al. Determinants of maximal expiratory flow from lungs. *J Appl Physiol.* 1967;23:643–662.

77. Tobin MJ, Lodato RF. PEEP, auto-PEEP, and waterfalls. *Chest*. 1989;96: 449–451.
78. Dawson SV, Elliott EA. Wave-speed limitation on expiratory flow: a unifying concept. *J Appl Physiol*. 1977;43:498–515.
79. Marini JJ. Positive end-expiratory pressure in severe airflow obstruction: more than a "one-trick pony"?. *Crit Care Med*. 2005;33:1652–1653.
80. Smith TC, Marini JJ. Impact of PEEP on lung mechanics and work of breathing in severe airflow obstruction. *J Appl Physiol*. 1988;65:1488–1499.
81. Levraut J, Grimaud D. Treatment of metabolic acidosis. *Curr Opin Crit Care*. 2003;9:260–265.
82. Bellomo R, McLaughlin P, Tai E, et al. Asthma requiring mechanical ventilation. A low morbidity approach. *Chest*. 1994;105:891–896.
83. Kearney SE, Graham DR, Atherton ST. Acute severe asthma treated by mechanical ventilation: a comparison of the changing characteristics over a 17 yr period. *Respir Med*. 1998;92:716–721.
84. Conti G, Ferretti A, Tellan G, et al. Propofol induces bronchodilation in a patient mechanically ventilated for status asthmaticus. *Intensive Care Med*. 1993;19:305.
85. Mirenda J, Broyles G. Propofol as used for sedation in the ICU. *Chest*. 1995;108:539–548.
86. Reves J, Glass P, Lubarsky D. Nonbarbiturate intravenous anesthetics. In: Miller R, ed. *Anesthesia*. New York: Churchill Livingstone; 1994: 259–264.
87. Hemming A, MacKenzie I, Finfer S. Response to ketamine in status asthmaticus resistant to maximal medical treatment. *Thorax*. 1994;49: 90–91.
88. Sarma VJ. Use of ketamine in acute severe asthma. *Acta Anaesthesiol Scand*. 1992;36:106–107.
89. Golembiewski JA. Allergic reactions to drugs: implications for perioperative care. *J Perianesth Nurs*. 2002;17:393–398.
90. Bouillon T, Bruhn J, Radu-Radulescu L, et al. A model of the ventilatory depressant potency of remifentanil in the non-steady state. *Anesthesiology*. 2003;99:779–787.
91. Shapiro BA, Warren J, Egol AB, et al. Practice parameters for sustained neuromuscular blockade in the adult critically ill patient: an executive summary. Society of Critical Care Medicine. *Crit Care Med*. 1995;23:1601–1605.
92. Lemos JM de, Carr RR, Shalansky KF, et al. Paralysis in the critically ill: intermittent bolus pancuronium compared with continuous infusion. *Crit Care Med*. 1999;27:2648–2655.
93. Travers AH, Rowe BH, Barker S, et al. The effectiveness of IV beta-agonists in treating patients with acute asthma in the emergency department: a meta-analysis. *Chest*. 2002;122:1200–1207.
94. Rodrigo GJ. Inhaled therapy for acute adult asthma. *Curr Opin Allergy Clin Immunol*. 2003;3:169–175.
95. Duarte AG. Inhaled bronchodilator administration during mechanical ventilation. *Respir Care*. 2004;49:623–634.
96. Duarte AG, Momii K, Bidani A. Bronchodilator therapy with metered-dose inhaler and spacer versus nebulizer in mechanically ventilated patients: comparison of magnitude and duration of response. *Respir Care*. 2000;45:817–823.
97. Vassilakopoulos T, Roussos C, Zakynthinos S. Weaning from mechanical ventilation. *J Crit Care*. 1999;14:39–62.
98. Vassilakopoulos T. Ventilator-induced diaphragm dysfunction: the clinical relevance of animal models. *Intensive Care Med*. 2008;34:7–16.
99. Mansel JK, Stogner SW, Petrini MF, et al. Mechanical ventilation in patients with acute severe asthma. *Am J Med*. 1990;89:42–48.
100. Afessa B, Morales I, Cury JD. Clinical course and outcome of patients admitted to an ICU for status asthmaticus. *Chest*. 2001;120:1616–1621.
101. Rosengarten PL, Tuxen DV, Dziukas L, et al Circulatory arrest induced by intermittent positive pressure ventilation in a patient with severe asthma. *Anaesth Intensive Care*. 1991;19:118–121.
102. David WS, Roehr CL, Leatherman JW. EMG findings in acute myopathy with status asthmaticus, steroids and paralytics. Clinical and electrophysiologic correlation. *Electromyogr Clin Neurophysiol*. 1998;38:371–376.
103. Griffin D, Fairman N, Coursin D, et al. Acute myopathy during treatment of status asthmaticus with corticosteroids and steroidal muscle relaxants. *Chest*. 1992;102:510–514.
104. Danon MJ, Carpenter S. Myopathy with thick filament (myosin) loss following prolonged paralysis with vecuronium during steroid treatment. *Muscle Nerve*. 1991;14:1131–1139.
105. Adnet F, Dhissi G, Borron SW, et al. Complication profiles of adult asthmatics requiring paralysis during mechanical ventilation. *Intensive Care Med*. 2001;27:1729–1736.
106. Leatherman JW, Fluegel WL, David WS, et al. Muscle weakness in mechanically ventilated patients with severe asthma. *Am J Respir Crit Care Med*. 1996;153:1686–1690.
107. Behbehani NA, Al-Mane F, D'Yachkova Y, et al. Myopathy following mechanical ventilation for acute severe asthma: the role of muscle relaxants and corticosteroids. *Chest*. 1999;115:1627–16231.
108. Douglass JA, Tuxen DV, Horne M, et al. Myopathy in severe asthma. *Am Rev Respir Dis*. 1992;146:517–519.

CHAPTER 141 ■ ACUTE RESPIRATORY FAILURE IN CHRONIC OBSTRUCTIVE PULMONARY DISEASE

MARCELO AMATO

Chronic obstructive pulmonary diseases (COPDs) are a group of disorders characterized by airflow limitation that is not fully reversible (1). There are several diseases under this designation (Table 141.1), the most common of which are chronic bronchitis and emphysema. These two disorders represent the extremes of the COPD spectrum and usually coexist in COPD patients. Bronchitis is predominantly a disease of the airways and presents as a chronic productive cough for at least 3 months during 2 consecutive years, while emphysema is a disease of the parenchyma and consists of permanent airspace enlargement associated with rupture of the alveolar septa.

The common final pathway leading to COPD is an increased inflammatory response to inhaled particles or gases, of which the most common is cigarette smoke. This inflammatory process involves the airways and the lung parenchyma, leading to mucosal gland hypertrophy and disruption of alveolar septa with loss of elastic recoil. These alterations ultimately lead to the obstructive ventilatory defect that defines COPD (2,3). Some patients develop pulmonary hyperinflation caused by the loss of elastic recoil and increased airway resistance. During exacerbations, there might be a secondary dynamic pulmonary hyperinflation (2,4) caused by the increased ventilatory requirement and shortened expiratory time (5). The capacity of the respiratory muscles to generate inspiratory pressure is limited by their shortened operating length and impaired geometric arrangement (6). Long-term steroid use and/or malnutrition

TABLE 141.1

DISEASES ASSOCIATED WITH CHRONIC OBSTRUCTIVE PULMONARY DISEASE

Chronic bronchitis	Tuberculosis
Emphysema	α_1-Trypsin deficiency
Bronchiolitis	
Bronchiectasis	

also contribute to strength impairment in many patients with severe chronic disease (7).

Only about 15% of all smokers will develop the full-blown syndrome with overt clinical symptoms, although a much higher proportion will develop some degree of airway obstruction. Rarely, the disease results from an inborn imbalance between the proteases and antiproteases present in the lung, as occurs in the autosomal recessive α_1-antitrypsin deficiency (8).

CLINICAL FINDINGS

The clinical manifestations of COPD appear late in the course of the disease. There is initially a slow decline in lung function that goes unnoticed over the years (9). Cough is the first finding, usually after the patient has been a smoker for many years. After about 20 years of smoking, some patients begin to notice shortness of breath on exertion, reflecting the progressive airflow limitation that is characteristic of the disease. The dyspnea worsens slowly over time, although sometimes patients deny the deterioration of lung function because they slowly adapt their level of activity to their exercise capacity. The decrease in lung function might become steeper during exacerbations, with a slow recovery to baseline levels after resolution of the decompensation.

Spirometry

Spirometry is the most important functional test for the diagnosis and the classification of severity of the disease. It consists of a forced exhalation after a deep inspiration while the patient is connected to a pneumotachograph. The ratio of the forced expiratory volume in the first second of the exhalation (FEV_1) to the forced vital capacity is diagnostic of an obstructive ventilatory defect if <0.7 (1). The FEV_1 is a useful marker of the disease severity (Table 141.2) and is well suited as a longitudinal monitor of lung function (9).

Lung Volume

Lung volumes can be measured using whole-body plethysmography or gas dilution (helium or nitrogen washout) techniques. In emphysema, both total lung capacity and residual volume may be increased because of loss of lung elastic recoil. The carbon monoxide diffusing capacity may be diminished with the progression of the disease, reflecting the loss of the functional parenchyma.

TABLE 141.2

CLASSIFICATION OF SEVERITY ACCORDING TO GOLD

Stage	Characteristics
0: At risk	Normal spirometry Chronic symptoms (cough, sputum production)
I: Mild COPD	$FEV_1/FVC < 70\%$ $FEV_1 = 80\%$ predicted With or without chronic symptoms (cough, sputum production)
II: Moderate COPD	$FEV_1/FVC < 70\%$ $50\% = FEV_1 < 80\%$ predicted With or without chronic symptoms (cough, sputum production)
III: Severe COPD	$FEV_1/FVC < 70\%$ $30\% = FEV_1 < 50\%$ predicted With or without chronic symptoms (cough, sputum production)
IV: Very severe COPD	$FEV_1/FVC < 70\%$ $FEV_1 < 30\%$ predicted or $FEV_1 < 50\%$ predicted plus chronic respiratory failure

GOLD, Global Initiative for Chronic Obstructive Lung Disease; COPD, chronic obstructive pulmonary disease; FEV_1, forced expiratory volume in the first second of the exhalation; FVC, forced vital capacity. From Rabe KF, Hurd S, Anzueto A, et al. Global Strategy for the Diagnosis, Management, and Prevention of Chronic Obstructive Pulmonary Disease: Gold Executive Summary. *Am J Respir Crit Care Med.* 2007;176:532–555.

Chest Radiographic Findings

Chest radiographic alterations usually occur late in the course of the disease, and there is no alteration pathognomonic of COPD. The radiograph is usually normal in mild disease; changes reflecting airway disease and hyperinflation may appear with progression of COPD. Sometimes it is possible to see enlarged bronchial walls reflected as an increase in bronchovascular markings. Emphysema is manifested by an increased lucency of the lungs. In smokers, these changes are more prominent in the upper lobes, while in α_1-antitrypsin deficiency, they are more likely in basal zones. With hyperinflation, the chest becomes vertically elongated with low, flattened diaphragms. The heart shadow is also vertical and narrow. The retrosternal airspace is increased on the lateral view, and the sternal-diaphragmatic angle exceeds 90 degrees. Radiographic computerized tomography is more sensitive and specific for the presence of emphysema, but it is rarely required. It is most useful in the preoperative evaluation for lung volume reduction surgery.

EXACERBATION

COPD exacerbation can be defined as an increase in dyspnea, cough, or sputum production that requires therapy (10). The two most commonly identified precipitating factors are infection—viral, such as *Rhinovirus* spp. or influenza, and bacterial, such as *Haemophilus influenzae, Streptococcus pneumoniae, Moraxella catarrhalis, Enterobacteriaceae* spp., or *Pseudomonas* spp.—as well as environmental exposure to air pollutants. However, in about one third of cases, no underlying cause is identified. Infectious agents can also be recovered from some patients with stable COPD, indicating that in some instances, their presence in decompensated COPD represents an epiphenomenon. On the other hand, Sethi et al. (11) have recently recognized that the acquisition of a new strain of a bacterial species colonized with a pathogenic bacteria might lead to an exacerbation in stable COPD patients. All exacerbations should be evaluated carefully for their potential to lead to or worsen respiratory failure that requires hospitalization. In the following section, we discuss the hospital treatment of COPD exacerbations.

Treatment of Exacerbations

The goals of the treatment of COPD exacerbations are to eliminate or control the cause of the exacerbation, provide optimum bronchodilator therapy, assure adequate oxygenation, and correct respiratory acidemia, all the while avoiding tracheal intubation when possible. Most patients with mild exacerbations can be treated at home, but those with a more severe presentation require hospitalization.

Admission criteria according to the American Thoracic Society/European Respiratory Society guidelines (12) include:

- High-risk comorbidities including pneumonia, cardiac arrhythmia, congestive heart failure, diabetes mellitus, renal failure, or liver failure
- Inadequate response of symptoms to outpatient management
- Marked increase in dyspnea
- Inability to eat or sleep because of symptoms
- Worsening hypoxemia
- Worsening hypercapnia
- Changes in mental status
- Inability to care for oneself (i.e., lack of home support)
- Uncertain diagnosis

Pharmacologic

The mainstay of pharmacologic treatment is the use of bronchodilators, corticosteroids, and antibiotics which are discussed below.

Bronchodilators.

1. β_2-Agonists: The bronchodilators most commonly used are the inhaled short-acting β_2-agonists because of their rapid onset of action. They can be administered via a nebulizer or through metered dose inhalers (MDIs). Typically, two puffs of albuterol or salbutamol are given every 4 hours, or an equivalent dose via nebulizer. During mechanical ventilation, the use of a spacer interposed in the circuit between the tube and the Y-piece is recommended. An unresolved issue relates to dosage when MDIs are used with intubated patients. Fernandez et al. (13) used two puffs, Gay et al. (14) used three puffs, and Fuller et al. (15) used four puffs in their studies. Because the MDI dose deposited in the lungs of intubated patients is, at best, half of the dose deposited in the lungs of ambulatory patients, it seems reasonable to at least double the number of MDI puffs in intubated patients (i.e., at least four puffs). In some patients, this dose will be inadequate, and a greater number of puffs (e.g., 10 to 20) can be safely and effectively used. Long-acting β_2-agonists can also be considered. Subcutaneous or intravenous administration should not be used unless there is contraindication for the inhaled route because of their increased systemic effects.
2. Anticholinergics: Ipratropium bromide can be used in association with the β_2-agonists as needed. It is available both via nebulization (500 μg) or MDI (two puffs every 2 to 4 hours). There are no clinical studies that have evaluated the use of the long-acting anticholinergic tiotropium bromide during COPD exacerbations.
3. Methylxanthines: Methylxanthines are currently not indicated in the treatment of exacerbations of COPD.

Corticosteroids. Steroids are usually recommended for exacerbations of COPD. If feasible, prednisone can be given orally at a dose of 30 to 40 mg/day for 10 to 14 days. If the oral route is not an option, hydrocortisone or methylprednisolone can be substituted in equivalent doses. Some investigators advocate the use of much higher doses (methylprednisolone, 125 mg intravenously 4 times daily) (16), but as no studies have been designed to find the optimal dose, we favor the lower dose. More recent studies (17,18) have proposed the use of inhaled steroids for the treatment of acute exacerbations. The combination of salmeterol, 50 μg, and fluticasone, 500 μg, given twice daily, has been compared with placebo and resulted in a reduction in mortality of 3 years ($p = 0.052$), fewer exacerbations, and improved health status and lung function. Nebulized budesonide, 1,500 μg 4 times daily, was compared with prednisolone 40 mg and demonstrated equal efficacy and potentially fewer side effects, especially less hyperglycemia.

Antibiotics. Antibiotics decrease mortality during exacerbations. These agents are indicated when there is increased production or change in the color of the sputum. For mild exacerbations, amoxicillin, sulfamethoxazole-trimethoprim, or doxycycline for 7 to 10 days is usually adequate. Patients requiring hospitalizations should receive penicillin/penicillinase (e.g., amoxicillin/clavulanate), a respiratory quinolone (levofloxacin, gatifloxacin, moxifloxacin), or a third-generation cephalosporin together with a macrolide (e.g., ceftriaxone plus clarithromycin). In addition to their antimicrobial activity, macrolides possess anti-inflammatory and mucoregulatory properties that may confer beneficial effects to patients with COPD (19).

Respiratory Support

The goal of respiratory support in patients with exacerbations of COPD is to correct hypoxemia/acidemia and reduce the respiratory work, thus avoiding respiratory muscle fatigue (20,21). In the acute setting, oxygen therapy alone is able to revert hypoxemia, but not acidemia and respiratory distress. For this reason, invasive or noninvasive mechanical ventilation are frequently needed (2,20).

Oxygen Therapy. To improve the hypoxemia commonly present in exacerbations of COPD, controlled oxygen therapy is the cornerstone of hospital treatment (2). Long-term oxygen therapy is established as the standard of care for selected patients with advanced chronic stable hypoxemia due to COPD (22,23). However, in the acute setting, some patients have an impaired response to hypercapnia when treated with supplementary oxygen, leading to worsening of CO_2 retention (24,25). The precise mechanism of this impairment is not well understood, but ventilation/perfusion (26–29) and respiratory drive (30,31) disturbances have been implicated. Some evidence suggests that the relief of hypoxic vasoconstriction due to the higher oxygen content in poorly ventilated areas may be the culprit of the acute CO_2 retention. The increased perfusion of such poorly ventilated, previously hypoxic areas might suddenly increase the shunt effect, transferring a great part of the venous CO_2 content directly to the arterial compartment.

There is no individual risk factor that identifies patients with COPD who will evolve to hypercapnia after oxygen exposure (2,24,25); therefore, the National Heart, Lung, Blood Institute/World Health Organization Global Initiative for Chronic Obstructive Lung Disease (GOLD) Workshop summary has recommended controlled oxygen therapy for the exacerbations, where adequate levels of oxygenation—$Pao_2 \geq 60$ mm Hg or $Sao_2 \geq 90\%$—are easy to achieve in uncomplicated exacerbations. Notwithstanding, CO_2 retention can occur insidiously with little change in symptoms; hence, measuring arterial blood gases 30 minutes after oxygen therapy, as recommended, is started. Venturi masks are more accurate sources of oxygen than are nasal prongs, but are more likely to be removed by the patient (2). Controlled oxygen therapy must be started at a low inspiratory oxygen fraction—0.24 to 0.28—and titrated upward to reach a $Pao_2 \geq 60$ mm Hg or $Sao_2 \geq 90\%$ without significant retention of CO_2. A clinically significant increase in $Paco_2$ has been arbitrarily defined as a raise in CO_2 of 6.5 mm Hg, especially if clinical mental deterioration occurs (24).

One must always remember that most of these patients have some degree of chronic vascular disease associated with their smoking history, and cardiovascular complications may be frequent during prolonged hypoxic episodes; for example, acute coronary syndromes, atrial fibrillation, cerebral ischemia, and pulmonary congestion. Therefore, the quick reversal of severe hypoxemia is frequently a priority.

Noninvasive Mechanical Ventilation. Patients with COPD are prone to acute hypercapnic respiratory failure, often resulting in emergency admission to the hospital. Between 20% and 30% of patients admitted with hypercapnic respiratory failure secondary to acute exacerbation of COPD will die in the hospital (32–35). Traditionally, patients who do not respond to conventional treatment are given invasive mechanical ventilation despite its well-known risks. Tracheal intubation and assisted ventilation have been associated with high morbidity and mortality rates, in addition to the difficulties during the weaning process from the ventilator (36,37). Many clinical complications seem to arise from the intubation procedure itself, or during the course of mechanical ventilation. The most common complications have been nosocomial infections, aspiration, pulmonary embolism, muscle atrophy, polyneuropathies, electrolyte imbalance, and gastrointestinal bleeding, as well as prolonging the stay in the intensive care unit (38,39).

In view of such difficulties, noninvasive positive pressure ventilation is an alternative treatment for patients admitted to the hospital with hypercapnic respiratory failure secondary to acute exacerbation of COPD. With this ventilatory modality, the patient receives air, or a mixture of air and oxygen, from a flow generator or a special ventilator through a facial/nasal mask, thus avoiding the need for tracheal intubation (32–34,40–42). Many studies have shown that noninvasive positive pressure ventilation increases pH, reduces $Paco_2$, reduces the severity of breathlessness in the first 4 hours of treatment, and decreases the length of hospital stay (32–34). More importantly, mortality and the intubation rate are consistently reduced by this intervention (32–34). Some studies suggest that the use of proper noninvasive ventilation can reduce the chances of an eventual endotracheal intubation to less than half (0.42, 95% confidence interval of 0.31 to 0.59) when compared with the conventional treatment with oxygen mask. This alternative has been also associated to a reduced mortality rate (0.41, 95% confidence interval [CI] of 0.26 to 0.64). In clinical-physiological terms, the expected elevation of pH after one hour of treatment should be around 0.03 (95% CI 0.02 to 0.04) and the expected reduction in $Paco_2$ in the same interval around –3.0 mm Hg (95% CI –5.1 to –0.2) (43).

Unfortunately, noninvasive ventilation is not appropriate for all patients (2). Failure rates between 9% and 50% have been reported (44,45). One important signal that this procedure is not working for a patient is the progression—even slight—of hypercapnia or acidosis 30 to 60 minutes after the procedure, and deterioration of the mental status.

The classic indications for noninvasive mechanical ventilation in exacerbated COPD patients are (1) respiratory distress with respiratory rate above 30 to 35 breaths per minute; (2) respiratory acidosis with a pH <7.35, and with normal or high standard base excess; and (3) a Pao_2 below 45 mm Hg. These measurements are made after the patient has been breathing room air for at least 10 minutes (32,33,46). Noninvasive mechanical ventilation is contraindicated for patients with profound bradypnea, defined as a respiratory rate below 12 breaths per minute, severe hypercapnic encephalopathy with Glasgow Coma Scale score below 10, cardiac and/or respiratory arrest, and hemodynamic instability (32,33,46). Some authors, however, have successfully applied noninvasive mechanical ventilation in comatose COPD patients with a Glasgow Coma Scale score below 8, with other causes of coma being ruled out (47). This latter use of noninvasive mechanical ventilation is not widely accepted (46).

Adjustments of noninvasive ventilation. Among the studies on noninvasive mechanical ventilation and COPD exacerbation, some used an exclusive inspiratory pressure support (33) or inspiratory volume support (32); most used an associated positive end-expiratory pressure (PEEP) in consonance with the rationale that the use of PEEP/continuous positive airway pressure (CPAP) further reduces the inspiratory work in patients with COPD exacerbation, especially the extra load generated by high levels of intrinsic PEEP (48–50).

There are many approaches to set the noninvasive ventilation. An easy way is to set the expiratory pressure at 5 cm H_2O, the inspiratory pressure at 10 cm H_2O—resulting in a "delta P" of 5 cm H_2O—and to increase the delta P in increments of 5 cm H_2O, up to 20 to 25 cm H_2O or the maximum tolerated, over 1 hour (42). An alternative approach is to adjust the inspiratory pressure in order to obtain a tidal volume of 6 to 8 mL/kg and a respiratory rate of 25 to 30 breaths per minute, setting the end-expiratory pressure to 5 cm H_2O to offset the inspiratory threshold induced by intrinsic PEEP.

If inspiratory comfort is not achieved, especially when wasted inspiratory efforts are visible without a prompt response from the ventilator, meaning that the patient effort is not enough to easily trigger the assisted breath, trials of 2 cm H_2O elevations in the PEEP/CPAP levels must be performed in order to further reduce the extra load imposed by the intrinsic PEEP. During these trials of augmentation of external PEEP, the minimum inspiratory pressure should be provided that maintains a stable tidal volume (51). Oxygen should be offered to keep oxygen saturation above 85% to 90% (2,42,51).

Theoretically, pure CPAP support in these patients might be of some help, offsetting part of the inspiratory threshold load imposed on COPD patients. The appeal of such a strategy is the possibility of using low-cost CPAP systems. This approach, however, has not been tested systematically and should be reserved for very special conditions under close supervision. Whenever possible, some level of inspiratory support should always be added to a CPAP strategy.

Taking all the studies into account, there is evidence to support the use of noninvasive mechanical ventilation in these patients, with documented success rates of 80% to 85% (52). Nevertheless, it is important that those patients who will fail the noninvasive ventilation trial be recognized early. Confalonieri et al. (53) evaluated the risk of failure of noninvasive ventilation in 1,033 consecutive patients with exacerbation of COPD admitted to experienced hospital units. The identified risk factors were Glasgow Coma Scale score <11, Acute Physiology and Chronic Health Evaluation (APACHE) II score ≥ 29, respiratory rate ≥ 30 breaths per minute, and arterial pH on admission of <7.25. The presence of all these risk factors resulted in a predicted risk of failure $>70\%$. An arterial pH <7.25 after 2 hours of ventilation greatly increased the risk of failure to $>90\%$. All these numbers and thresholds should be taken as relative reference points, because the success of noninvasive mechanical ventilation depends on a learning curve of the whole staff. The less experienced the staff, the more conservative we should be with these limits, not waiting for further deterioration of the patient before deciding on invasive ventilation.

After hospital admission, the correct timing for starting noninvasive ventilatory support is either immediately or at any time the patient shows worsening of the respiratory distress, a fall in Pa_{O_2}, or an increase in Pa_{CO_2} (42,51). Noninvasive ventilatory support can be applied in any area of the hospital where close monitoring of the patient by trained personnel is available, such as intensive care units, emergency departments, high-dependency units, and respiratory wards. The duration of the noninvasive ventilation and the number of possible interruptions for oral and facial cleaning varies according to the patient need. Ventilatory periods lasting at least 40 minutes are warranted (33), and some patients will require uninterrupted use (42,51).

The choice for an appropriate mask is an important aspect of noninvasive mechanical ventilation. In general, patients benefit from a facial mask that covers the mouth and the nose; this is more efficient than the nasal type to deliver effective inspiratory pressures. Leaks directed at the eyes, sores in the nasal area, and a dry mouth are frequent causes of extreme discomfort to patients. The total face mask may be better tolerated by some patients, but not all, and greatly reduces the skin sores. However, one has to be aware that the anatomic dead space may increase a bit with this mask, which also imposes some challenges to the mechanical ventilator in terms of synchrony and PEEP maintenance.

The helmet interface is not yet appropriate to use in COPD patients; it warrants further technical improvements. Although efficient in maintaining the end-expiratory pressure, this device usually results in poor inspiratory support because of the high compliance of the whole system.

Invasive Mechanical Ventilation. Invasive mechanical ventilation can be either the initial choice in patients with COPD exacerbation or the strategy to be applied after failure of a trial of noninvasive ventilation (2). Mechanical ventilation can reduce or eliminate the work of breathing and improve gas exchange, while allowing the respiratory function to return to baseline through the treatment of the precipitating causes of the acute decompensation (4).

Assuming that all appropriate measures to improve airflow obstruction have already been taken (see previous discussion), minimization of dynamic hyperinflation is a key objective of the ventilatory support of these COPD patients. At the bedside, dynamic hyperinflation is typically detected by the presence of nonzero end-expiratory flow at the flow-time curve, or by effectively measuring the end-expiratory pressure (auto-PEEP) after an expiratory pause. Precise quantification of the auto-PEEP, however, is problematic in patients with spontaneous breathing efforts (54).

In some patients, especially in those with predominant emphysema, the airway obstruction in the expiratory phase is disproportionally higher than in the inspiration. In these patients, the measured auto-PEEP is higher than expected when considering the calculated inspiratory airway resistance. This situation can be anticipated by looking at the flow-volume curve available on most ventilators. The slope of this curve is proportional to the time constant of the respiratory system, and the differences between inspiratory and expiratory airway resistances can thus be determined (Fig. 141.1) (55).

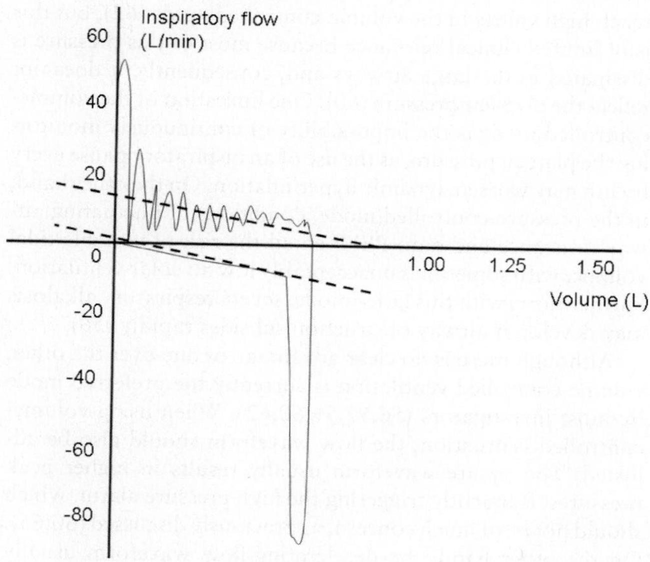

FIGURE 141.1. Example of a flow-volume curve of a patient mechanically ventilated with severe and equivalent inspiratory and expiratory flow limitation. The *dashed lines* represent the slope of the curves and are proportional to the inspiratory and expiratory time constants.

To reduce the hyperinflation, several concepts that have emerged from the recently published literature should be employed (4,56). The most effective strategy is controlled hypoventilation (57), which decreases dynamic hyperinflation through the reduction of the minute volume. Hypoventilation, with a fixed inspiratory time, decreases the expiratory flow requirement and consequently reduces air trapping and plateau pressures (57–59). An appropriate clinical goal at present is to keep the plateau pressures $\leq$30 cm H_2O, a strategy associated with lower rates (4%) of barotrauma (60,61). Adequate sedation and analgesia help by lowering the production of CO_2 and allowing further reduction of the minute volume (4). At the bedside, the general rules to minimize hyperinflation are (1) keep the minute volume $\leq$8 L/min, and (2) keep the expiratory time $\geq$4 seconds; low respiratory rates should be used, for example, 8 to 12 breaths per minute, with 5 to 8 mL/kg of tidal volume. Once these goals have been achieved, there is probably little gain from further adjusting the ventilator. For example, Leatherman et al. (62) showed that halving minute ventilation from 7.4 to 3.7 L/min, and more than doubling expiratory time from 4.5 to 9.5 seconds had no significant effect on auto-PEEP and plateau pressure (56). Although controlled hypoventilation is the most effective measure to decrease hyperinflation, this ventilatory strategy frequently worsens CO_2 retention. The hypercapnia and acidosis are generally well tolerated and considered acceptable by most clinicians (4,56,57), provided that such levels of hypoventilation are essential to keep plateau pressures below 30 cm H_2O.

Metabolic acidosis may also accompany the respiratory acidosis seen in COPD exacerbations, resulting in amplification of the acidemia (63). The underlying mechanism of such acidosis is not clear (63), but its buffering may accentuate coexistent pulmonary injury in hypoxemic patients (64). The treatment of metabolic acidosis in these hypercapnic patients should be directed to the etiology of the process, and not to the metabolic acidosis per se.

There is no optimal ventilation modality to support exacerbated COPD patients (56). The peak airway pressure may reach high values in the volume-controlled mode (62), but this is of limited clinical relevance because most of this pressure is dissipated in the large airways and, consequently, it does not reflect the alveolar pressure (60). One limitation of the volume-controlled mode is the impossibility of continuously monitoring the plateau pressure, as the use of an inspiratory pause every breath may worsen dynamic hyperinflation. On the other hand, in the pressure-controlled mode, conditions of fluctuating airway resistance and auto-PEEP entail the risk of variable tidal volume, with sometimes unacceptably low alveolar ventilation. Furthermore, with this latter mode, severe respiratory alkalosis may develop if airway obstruction subsides rapidly (56).

Although there is no clear advantage of one over the other, volume-controlled ventilation is currently the preferred mode by most investigators (56,57,59,60,62). When using volume-controlled ventilation, the flow waveform should also be adjusted. The square waveform usually results in higher peak pressures, frequently triggering the high pressure alarm, which should not be of much concern, as previously discussed (60,65). On the other hand, the decelerating-flow waveform usually minimizes peak pressure, allowing full delivery of the tidal volume, with less interruption by opening of the pop-off safety valve (56). By forcing a slower flow at the end of inspiration, this flow waveform could result in two theoretical benefits: (1) less overdistention of alveoli distal to the least obstructed airways, and (2) slightly better CO_2 exchange. Whenever possible, and provided that peak pressures are effectively reduced (this must be tested), this flow pattern thus should be preferred. During controlled mechanical ventilation with volume-controlled ventilation, the inspiratory pause should be used with extreme caution, and mainly for monitoring purposes to check whether hyperinflation is improving.

When initiating mechanical ventilation in the pressure-controlled mode, one must keep in mind that the inspiratory time should be set in proportion to the inspiratory time constant in order to deliver the desired tidal volume with the lowest possible plateau pressure (66). Thus, patients with increased airways resistance will need a longer inspiratory time. For a fixed respiratory rate, the increase in inspiratory time always occurs at the expense of a shortening of the expiratory time, which might aggravate pulmonary hyperinflation. Therefore, the ideal inspiratory time would optimize delivery of tidal volume without increasing air trapping. That will occur if, when looking at the flow-volume curve, both end-inspiratory and end-expiratory flows are equal or close to zero (4,56,60).

After choosing the best respiratory rate and inspiratory and expiratory times, the physician has to decide on how much PEEP to apply. During controlled mechanical ventilation, PEEP can be detrimental to paralyzed patients with severe airflow obstruction, raising the functional pulmonary capacity (67). Based on this information, some authors have advocated the use of zero PEEP or no more than 5 cm H_2O (56,67). However, some patients show a paradoxical response to an increase in PEEP with relief of the air trapping (Fig. 141.2) (68). There are two ways to identify these patients:

1. Using volume-control mode, with an inspiratory pause of 1 to 2 seconds, tidal volume of 5 to 8 mL/kg, and a respiratory rate of 10 breaths per minute (with the lowest inspiratory:expiratory ratio possible, e.g. <1:4), increase the external PEEP in steps of 2 cm H_2O every 10 to 20 respiratory cycles, starting from ZEEP (baseline). The best PEEP is the highest level associated with a plateau pressure equal to or less than the baseline.
2. In pressure-control mode, start with ZEEP, driving pressure, and inspiratory time to achieve a tidal volume of 5 to 8 mL/g. Raise the external PEEP in steps of 2 cm H_2O every 10 to 20 respiratory cycles, keeping the plateau pressure constant. If there is an increase in tidal volume during the upward PEEP titration, it means there was recruitment of the airway. PEEP should be kept at the highest level before the tidal volume begins to fall (4).

As soon as possible, the ventilation mode should be switched from controlled to assisted ventilation in order to decrease muscle atrophy. There are no objective indicators of the best moment to start assisted ventilation; therefore, at least daily trials of assisted ventilation should be made, with close monitoring of patient comfort and plateau pressure (4,56). Adding external PEEP during assisted ventilation can reduce the inspiratory work by means of eliminating the offset of inspiratory pressure threshold induced by auto-PEEP (4). Appendini et al. (69) demonstrated that 41% of the inspiratory muscle effort was expended to overcome auto-PEEP in patients with COPD during spontaneous breathing. Adding external PEEP at an average of 80% of the measured auto-PEEP is well tolerated, with no increase of total PEEP or plateau pressure (70), improving

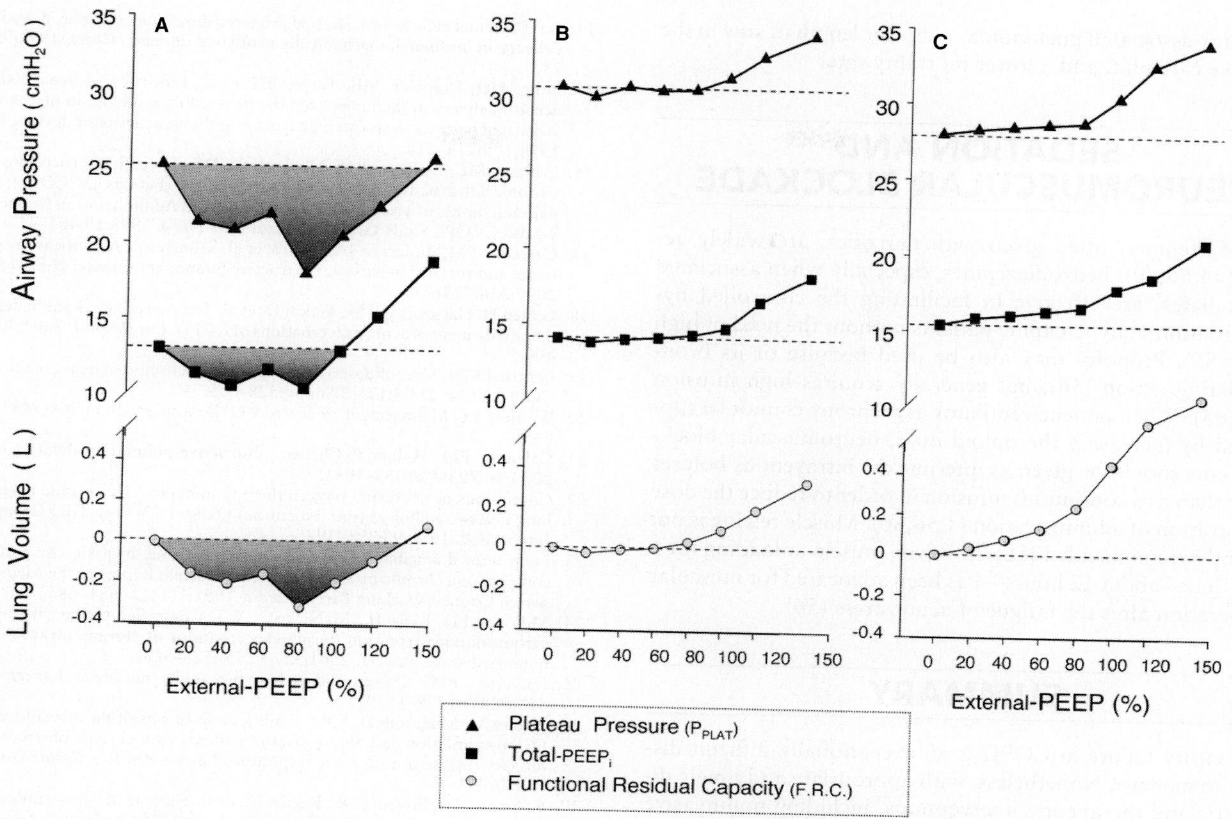

FIGURE 141.2. Three of the possible responses observed in plateau pressure (PPLAT), total intrinsic positive end-expiratory pressure ($PEEP_i$), and functional residual capacity (F.R.C.) with the application of external-PEEP (represented as percentage of $PEEP_i$ measured at zero external-PEEP). The FRC measured at zero external-PEEP was considered as the reference. **A,** Paradoxical response (patient 4), observed with a tidal volume (V_T) of 6 mL/kg and respiratory rate (RR) of 9 breaths/min; **B,** biphasic response (patient 7), observed with V_T of 9 mL/kg and RR of 6 breaths/min; **C,** classic overinflation response (patient 5), observed with a V_T of 9 mL/kg and RR of 9 breaths/min. (From Caramez MP, Borges JB, Tucci MR, et al. Paradoxical responses to positive end-expiratory pressure in patients with airway obstruction during controlled ventilation. *Crit Care Med.* 2005;33:1519–1528, with permission.)

synchrony between patient and ventilator (48–50). Frequent reassessments are essential because the adequate level of external PEEP is subject to change as lung mechanics and ventilatory requirements change.

Humidification should be achieved with a heated humidifier, not with heat and moisture exchangers. The latter devices are undesirable for three reasons: (1) they increase expiratory airway resistance, which would hardly be of any help to reduce hyperinflation (71); (2) when inserted between the tracheal tube and the Y-piece of ventilator tubing, they increase dead space and therefore contribute unnecessarily to hypercapnia (72,73); and (3) the efficacy of any inhalational medication will be blunted by the heat and moisture exchanger (56).

Weaning from the ventilator should be initiated as soon as possible in order to avoid mechanical ventilator-associated complications (74). According to recent published experiences of two specialized weaning units, 19% of patients with COPD exacerbation remained partially dependent on the ventilator (75,76). The classic rapid shallow breathing criterion—<80 breaths per minute per liter—was met by 56% of COPD patients who failed the weaning trial (77). General patient condition and subjective dyspnea seemed to be more effective predictors of success of extubation than quantifiable indexes (78).

Using spontaneous breathing trials or progressive reduction in pressure support is equally effective to wean the patient from the ventilator (79). Automatic algorithms for pressure support reduction are available today, which resulted in a faster weaning process when compared with the physician-driven approach (80,81).

If the spontaneous breathing trial is chosen, it can be applied for at least 30 minutes, up to 2 hours once a day (36). After tracheal decannulation, the use of intermittent or continuous support with noninvasive mechanical ventilation for at least 24 hours is strongly recommended, using settings similar to those used during conventional ventilation weaning. The last technique is associated with higher rates of extubation success, lower length of stay in the intensive care unit and/or hospital, and a lower mortality at 60 days (82,83). Nava et al. (84) have described a strategy in which patients are ventilated and sedated for 6 to 8 hours after intubation; an assisted mode is subsequently started using pressure support. After 48 hours of conventional mechanical ventilation, if the patient is not hypersecretory or hemodynamically unstable, he or she is extubated and supported with noninvasive mechanical ventilation using the same ventilatory settings as before tracheal decannulation. This approach is associated with less ventilator-associated pneumonia, a shorter length of stay in the intensive care unit, and a lower mortality rate.

SEDATION AND NEUROMUSCULAR BLOCKADE

Benzodiazepines, often given with narcotics, are widely accepted (4,56,60). Benzodiazepines, especially when associated with opiates, are effective in facilitating the controlled hypoventilation in hypercapnic patients without the need of high doses (85). Propofol may also be used because of its bronchodilating action (56), but generally requires high infusion rates (85). When patient-ventilator asynchrony cannot be suppressed by increasing the opioid dose, neuromuscular blocking agents should be given as intermittent intravenous boluses rather than as a continuous infusion in order to reduce the dose and duration of administration (4,56,60). Muscle resting is not currently recommended (86); however, muscle unloading for a short time—about 12 hours—has been advocated for muscular recuperation after the fatigue of acute stress (56).

SUMMARY

Respiratory failure in COPD is an exceptionally difficult disorder to manage. Nonetheless, with appropriate and timely diagnostic and therapeutic interventions, including noninvasive ventilation in the proper clinical setting, our hope is that the mortality rate can be decreased from its approximate 20% to 30%.

References

1. Rabe KF, Hurd S, Anzueto A, et al. Global Strategy for the Diagnosis, Management, and Prevention of Chronic Obstructive Pulmonary Disease: GOLD Executive Summary. *Am J Respir Crit Care Med.* 2007;176:532–555.
2. Pauwels RA, Buist AS, Calverley PM, et al. Global strategy for the diagnosis, management, and prevention of chronic obstructive pulmonary disease. NHLBI/WHO Global Initiative for Chronic Obstructive Lung Disease (GOLD) Workshop summary. *Am J Respir Crit Care Med.* 2001;163:1256–1276.
3. Barnes PJ. Chronic obstructive pulmonary disease. *N Engl J Med.* 2000; 343:269–280.
4. Peigang Y, Marini JJ. Ventilation of patients with asthma and chronic obstructive pulmonary disease. *Curr Opin Crit Care.* 2002;8:70–76.
5. Rossi A, Ganassini A, Polese G, et al. Pulmonary hyperinflation and ventilator-dependent patients. *Eur Respir J.* 1997;10:1663–1674.
6. Marchand E, Decramer M. Respiratory muscle function and drive in chronic obstructive pulmonary disease. *Clin Chest Med.* 2000;21:679–692.
7. Perez T, Becquart LA, Stach B, et al. Inspiratory muscle strength and endurance in steroid-dependent asthma. *Am J Respir Crit Care Med.* 1996;153: 610–615.
8. Eriksson S. Pulmonary emphysema and alpha1-antitrypsin deficiency. *Acta Med Scand.* 1964;175:197–205.
9. Burchfiel CM, Marcus EB, Curb JD, et al. Effects of smoking and smoking cessation on longitudinal decline in pulmonary function. *Am J Respir Crit Care Med.* 1995;151:1778–1785.
10. Rodriguez-Roisin R. Toward a consensus definition for COPD exacerbations. *Chest.* 2000;117(5 Suppl 2):398S–401S.
11. Sethi S, Evans N, Grant BJ, et al. New strains of bacteria and exacerbations of chronic obstructive pulmonary disease. *N Engl J Med.* 2002;347:465–471.
12. Celli BR, Macnee W. Standards for the diagnosis and treatment of patients with COPD: a summary of the ATS/ERS position paper. *Eur Respir J.* 2004; 23:932–946.
13. Fernandez A, Lazaro A, Garcia A, et al. Bronchodilators in patients with chronic obstructive pulmonary disease on mechanical ventilation. Utilization of metered-dose inhalers. *Am Rev Respir Dis.* 1990;141:164–168.
14. Gay PC, Patel HG, Nelson SB, et al. Metered dose inhalers for bronchodilator delivery in intubated, mechanically ventilated patients. *Chest.* 1991;99:66–71.
15. Fuller HD, Dolovich MB, Turpie FH, et al. Efficiency of bronchodilator aerosol delivery to the lungs from the metered dose inhaler in mechanically ventilated patients. A study comparing four different actuator devices. *Chest.* 1994;105:214–218.
16. Erbland ML, Deupree RH, Niewoehner DE. Systemic Corticosteroids in Chronic Obstructive Pulmonary Disease Exacerbations (SCCOPE): rationale and design of an equivalence trial. Veterans Administration Cooperative Trials SCCOPE Study Group. *Control Clin Trials.* 1998;19:404–417.
17. Calverley PM, Anderson JA, Celli B, et al. Salmeterol and fluticasone propionate and survival in chronic obstructive pulmonary disease. *N Engl J Med.* 2007;356:775–789.
18. Gunen H, Hacievliyagil SS, Yetkin O, et al. The role of nebulised budesonide in the treatment of acute exacerbations of COPD. *Eur Respir J.* 2007;30:399–400.
19. Gotfried MH. Macrolides for the treatment of chronic sinusitis, asthma, and COPD. *Chest.* 2004;125(2 Suppl):52S–60S.
20. Wouters EF. Management of severe COPD. *Lancet.* 2004;364(9437):883–895.
21. Calverley PM, Walker P. Chronic obstructive pulmonary disease. *Lancet.* 2003;362(9389):1053–1061.
22. Continuous or nocturnal oxygen therapy in hypoxemic chronic obstructive lung disease: a clinical trial. Nocturnal Oxygen Therapy Trial Group. *Ann Intern Med.* 1980;93:391–398.
23. Long term domiciliary oxygen therapy in chronic hypoxic cor pulmonale complicating chronic bronchitis and emphysema. Report of the Medical Research Council Working Party. *Lancet.* 1981;1(8222):681–686.
24. Moloney ED, Kiely JL, McNicholas WT. Controlled oxygen therapy and carbon dioxide retention during exacerbations of chronic obstructive pulmonary disease. *Lancet.* 2001;357(9255):526–528.
25. Calverley PM. Oxygen-induced hypercapnia revisited. *Lancet.* 2000; 356(9241):1538–1539.
26. Aubier M, Murciano D, Milic-Emili J, et al. Effects of the administration of O_2 on ventilation and blood gases in patients with chronic obstructive pulmonary disease during acute respiratory failure. *Am Rev Respir Dis.* 1980; 122:747–754.
27. Robinson TD, Freiberg DB, Regnis JA, et al. The role of hypoventilation and ventilation-perfusion redistribution in oxygen-induced hypercapnia during acute exacerbations of chronic obstructive pulmonary disease. *Am J Respir Crit Care Med.* 2000;161:1524–1529.
28. Hanson CW, III, Marshall BE, Frasch HF, et al. Causes of hypercarbia with oxygen therapy in patients with chronic obstructive pulmonary disease. *Crit Care Med.* 1996;24:23–28.
29. Sassoon CS, Hassell KT, Mahutte CK. Hyperoxic-induced hypercapnia in stable chronic obstructive pulmonary disease. *Am Rev Respir Dis.* 1987;135: 907–911.
30. Dunn WF, Nelson SB, Hubmayr RD. Oxygen-induced hypercarbia in obstructive pulmonary disease. *Am Rev Respir Dis.* 1991;144(3 Pt 1):526–530.
31. Dick CR, Liu Z, Sassoon CS, et al. O_2-induced change in ventilation and ventilatory drive in COPD. *Am J Respir Crit Care Med.* 1997;155:609–614.
32. Bott J, Carroll MP, Conway JH, et al. Randomised controlled trial of nasal ventilation in acute ventilatory failure due to chronic obstructive airways disease. *Lancet.* 1993;341(8860):1555–1557.
33. Brochard L, Mancebo J, Wysocki M, et al. Noninvasive ventilation for acute exacerbations of chronic obstructive pulmonary disease. *N Engl J Med.* 1995; 333:817–822.
34. Foglio C, Vitacca M, Quadri A, et al. Acute exacerbations in severe COLD patients. Treatment using positive pressure ventilation by nasal mask. *Chest.* 1992;101:1533–1538.
35. Ambrosino N, Foglio K, Rubini F, et al. Non-invasive mechanical ventilation in acute respiratory failure due to chronic obstructive pulmonary disease: correlates for success. *Thorax.* 1995;50:755–757.
36. Esteban A, Frutos F, Tobin MJ et al. A comparison of four methods of weaning patients from mechanical ventilation. Spanish Lung Failure Collaborative Group. *N Engl J Med.* 1995;332:345–350.
37. Brochard L, Rauss A, Benito S, et al. Comparison of three methods of gradual withdrawal from ventilatory support during weaning from mechanical ventilation. *Am J Respir Crit Care Med.* 1994;150:896–903.
38. Guerin C, Girard R, Chemorin C, et al. Facial mask noninvasive mechanical ventilation reduces the incidence of nosocomial pneumonia. A prospective epidemiological survey from a single ICU. *Intensive Care Med.* 1997;23: 1024–1032.
39. Nourdine K, Combes P, Carton MJ, et al. Does noninvasive ventilation reduce the ICU nosocomial infection risk? A prospective clinical survey. *Intensive Care Med.* 1999;25:567–573.
40. Meduri GU, Abou-Shala N, Fox RC, et al. Noninvasive face mask mechanical ventilation in patients with acute hypercapnic respiratory failure. *Chest.* 1991;100:445–454.
41. Celikel T, Sungur M, Ceyhan B, et al. Comparison of noninvasive positive pressure ventilation with standard medical therapy in hypercapnic acute respiratory failure. *Chest.* 1998;114:1636–1642.
42. Plant PK, Owen JL, Elliott MW. Early use of non-invasive ventilation for acute exacerbations of chronic obstructive pulmonary disease on general

respiratory wards: a multicentre randomised controlled trial. *Lancet.* 2000; 355(9219):1931–1935.
43. Lightowler JV, Wedzicha JA, Elliott MW, et al. Non-invasive positive pressure ventilation to treat respiratory failure resulting from exacerbations of chronic obstructive pulmonary disease: Cochrane systematic review and meta-analysis. *BMJ.* 2003;326(7382):185.
44. Kramer N, Meyer TJ, Meharg J, et al. Randomized, prospective trial of noninvasive positive pressure ventilation in acute respiratory failure. *Am J Respir Crit Care Med.* 1995;151:1799–1806.
45. Soo Hoo GW, Santiago S, Williams AJ. Nasal mechanical ventilation for hypercapnic respiratory failure in chronic obstructive pulmonary disease: determinants of success and failure. *Crit Care Med.* 1994;22:1253–1261.
46. Evans TW. International Consensus Conferences in Intensive Care Medicine: non-invasive positive pressure ventilation in acute respiratory failure. Organised jointly by the American Thoracic Society, the European Respiratory Society, the European Society of Intensive Care Medicine, and the Societe de Reanimation de Langue Francaise, and approved by the ATS Board of Directors, December 2000. *Intensive Care Med.* 2001;27:166–178.
47. Diaz GG, Alcaraz AC, Talavera JC, et al. Noninvasive positive-pressure ventilation to treat hypercapnic coma secondary to respiratory failure. *Chest.* 2005;127:952–960.
48. Goldberg P, Reissmann H, Maltais F, et al. Efficacy of noninvasive CPAP in COPD with acute respiratory failure. *Eur Respir J.* 1995;8:1894–1900.
49. Appendini L, Patessio A, Zanaboni S, et al. Physiologic effects of positive end-expiratory pressure and mask pressure support during exacerbations of chronic obstructive pulmonary disease. *Am J Respir Crit Care Med.* 1994; 149:1069–1076.
50. Smith TC, Marini JJ. Impact of PEEP on lung mechanics and work of breathing in severe airflow obstruction. *J Appl Physiol.* 1988;65:1488–1499.
51. Conti G, Antonelli M, Navalesi P, et al. Noninvasive vs. conventional mechanical ventilation in patients with chronic obstructive pulmonary disease after failure of medical treatment in the ward: a randomized trial. *Intensive Care Med.* 2002;28:1701–1707.
52. International Consensus Conferences in Intensive Care Medicine: noninvasive positive pressure ventilation in acute respiratory failure. *Am J Respir Crit Care Med.* 2001;163:283–291.
53. Confalonieri M, Garuti G, Cattaruzza MS, et al. A chart of failure risk for noninvasive ventilation in patients with COPD exacerbation. *Eur Respir J.* 2005;25:348–355.
54. Gladwin MT, Pierson DJ. Mechanical ventilation of the patient with severe chronic obstructive pulmonary disease. *Intensive Care Med.* 1998;24:898–910.
55. Dhand R. Ventilator graphics and respiratory mechanics in the patient with obstructive lung disease. *Respir Care.* 2005;50:246–261.
56. Oddo M, Feihl F, Schaller MD, et al. Management of mechanical ventilation in acute severe asthma: practical aspects. *Intensive Care Med.* 2006;32:501–510.
57. Darioli R, Perret C. Mechanical controlled hypoventilation in status asthmaticus. *Am Rev Respir Dis.* 1984;129:385–387.
58. Darioli R, Domenighetti G, Perret C. Mechanical ventilation in the treatment of acute respiratory insufficiency in asthma [in German]. *Schweiz Med Wochenschr.* 1981;111:194–196.
59. Tuxen DV. Permissive hypercapnic ventilation. *Am J Respir Crit Care Med.* 1994;150:870–874.
60. Leatherman JW. Mechanical ventilation in obstructive lung disease. *Clin Chest Med.* 1996;17:577–590.
61. Leatherman J. Life-threatening asthma. *Clin Chest Med.* 1994;15:453–479.
62. Leatherman JW, McArthur C, Shapiro RS. Effect of prolongation of expiratory time on dynamic hyperinflation in mechanically ventilated patients with severe asthma. *Crit Care Med.* 2004;32:1542–1545.
63. Mountain RD, Heffner JE, Brackett NC Jr, et al. Acid-base disturbances in acute asthma. *Chest.* 1990;98:651–655.
64. Laffey JG, Engelberts D, Kavanagh BP. Buffering hypercapnic acidosis worsens acute lung injury. *Am J Respir Crit Care Med.* 2000;161:141–146.
65. Guerin C, Lemasson S, La Cara MF, et al. Physiological effects of constant versus decelerating inflation flow in patients with chronic obstructive pulmonary disease under controlled mechanical ventilation. *Intensive Care Med.* 2002;28:164–169.
66. Marini JJ, Crooke PS III, Truwit JD. Determinants and limits of pressure-preset ventilation: a mathematical model of pressure control. *J Appl Physiol.* 1989;67:1081–1092.
67. Tuxen DV. Detrimental effects of positive end-expiratory pressure during controlled mechanical ventilation of patients with severe airflow obstruction. *Am Rev Respir Dis.* 1989;140:5–9.
68. Caramez MP, Borges JB, Tucci MR, et al. Paradoxical responses to positive end-expiratory pressure in patients with airway obstruction during controlled ventilation. *Crit Care Med.* 2005;33:1519–1528.
69. Appendini L, Purro A, Patessio A, et al. Partitioning of inspiratory muscle workload and pressure assistance in ventilator-dependent COPD patients. *Am J Respir Crit Care Med.* 1996;154:1301–1309.
70. Guerin C, Milic-Emili J, Fournier G. Effect of PEEP on work of breathing in mechanically ventilated COPD patients. *Intensive Care Med.* 2000;26:1207–1214.
71. Verkerke GJ, Geertsema AA, Schutte HK. Airflow resistance of heat and moisture exchange filters with and without a tracheostoma valve. *Ann Otol Rhinol Laryngol.* 2002;111:333–337.
72. Hinkson CR, Benson MS, Stephens LM, et al. The effects of apparatus dead space on $P(aCO_2)$ in patients receiving lung-protective ventilation. *Respir Care.* 2006;51:1140–1144.
73. Moran I, Bellapart J, Vari A, et al. Heat and moisture exchangers and heated humidifiers in acute lung injury/acute respiratory distress syndrome patients. Effects on respiratory mechanics and gas exchange. *Intensive Care Med.* 2006;32:524–531.
74. Pingleton SK. Complications of acute respiratory failure. *Am Rev Respir Dis.* 1988;137:1463–1493.
75. Dasgupta A, Rice R, Mascha E, et al. Four-year experience with a unit for long-term ventilation (respiratory special care unit) at the Cleveland Clinic Foundation. *Chest.* 1999;116:447–455.
76. Bagley PH, Cooney E. A community-based regional ventilator weaning unit: development and outcomes. *Chest.* 1997;111:1024–1029.
77. Purro A, Appendini L, De Gaetano A, et al. Physiologic determinants of ventilator dependence in long-term mechanically ventilated patients. *Am J Respir Crit Care Med.* 2000;161(4 Pt 1):1115–1123.
78. Afessa B, Hogans L, Murphy R. Predicting 3-day and 7-day outcomes of weaning from mechanical ventilation. *Chest.* 1999;116:456–461.
79. Vitacca M, Vianello A, Colombo D, et al. Comparison of two methods for weaning patients with chronic obstructive pulmonary disease requiring mechanical ventilation for more than 15 days. *Am J Respir Crit Care Med.* 2001;164:225–230.
80. Bouadma L, Lellouche F, Cabello B, et al. Computer-driven management of prolonged mechanical ventilation and weaning: a pilot study. *Intensive Care Med.* 2005;31:1446–1450.
81. Lellouche F, Mancebo J, Jolliet P, et al. A multicenter randomized trial of computer-driven protocolized weaning from mechanical ventilation. *Am J Respir Crit Care Med.* 2006;174:894–900.
82. Ferrer M, Valencia M, Nicolas JM, et al. Early noninvasive ventilation averts extubation failure in patients at risk: a randomized trial. *Am J Respir Crit Care Med.* 2006;173:164–170.
83. Nava S, Gregoretti C, Fanfulla F, et al. Noninvasive ventilation to prevent respiratory failure after extubation in high-risk patients. *Crit Care Med.* 2005; 33:2465–2470.
84. Nava S, Ambrosino N, Clini E, et al. Noninvasive mechanical ventilation in the weaning of patients with respiratory failure due to chronic obstructive pulmonary disease. A randomized, controlled trial. *Ann Intern Med.* 1998; 128:721–728.
85. Vinayak AG, Gehlbach B, Pohlman AS, et al. The relationship between sedative infusion requirements and permissive hypercapnia in critically ill, mechanically ventilated patients. *Crit Care Med.* 2006;34:1668–1673.
86. Vassilakopoulos T, Zakynthinos S, Roussos C. Bench-to-bedside review: weaning failure—should we rest the respiratory muscles with controlled mechanical ventilation? *Crit Care.* 2006;10:204.

CHAPTER 142 ■ PULMONARY EMBOLISM

KENNETH E. WOOD • AARON JOFFE

Despite significant advances in prophylaxis, diagnostic approaches, and therapeutic modalities for pulmonary embolism (PE), this disease process still remains an underrecognized and lethal entity. Contemporary estimates suggest that PE affects more than 600,000 patients per year in the United States and reportedly causes or contributes to 50,000 to 200,000 deaths. The incidence of PE causing, contributing to, or accompanying death in hospitalized patients has remained relatively constant at 15% for the past 40 years. Disconcertingly, the antemortem diagnosis of fatal PE has remained fixed at approximately 30% over the same time period. Large contemporary observational studies of PE have reported unexpectedly high mortality rates. In the Management Strategies and Determinants of Outcome in Acute Major PE (MAPPET) series, the overall 3-month mortality in patients with PE was 17% with an in-hospital mortality of 31% when PE was associated with hemodynamic instability. PE-attributable mortality was 45% and 91% in the respective groups (1). In the International Cooperative Pulmonary Embolism Registry (ICOPER), the 90-day mortality was 14.5% in hemodynamically stable PE patients and 51.9% in those with hemodynamic instability. PE-attributable mortality was 34% and 62.5% in the respective groups (2).

In fatal cases of PE, it has long been appreciated that two thirds of PE deaths will occur within 1 hour of presentation and that anatomically massive PE will account for only one half of the deaths as the remainder can be attributed to smaller submassive or recurrent emboli. There are several important implications of these observations. First, an evidenced-based approach is nearly impossible to define for hemodynamically unstable PE. Second, it is reasonable to propose that outcome from PE is related to the size of the embolism and the underlying cardiopulmonary function. There is a dynamic interaction between the patient's underlying cardiopulmonary status and the embolism size; similar hemodynamic and clinical outcomes will manifest from an anatomically massive PE in a patient with normal cardiopulmonary function and an anatomically submassive embolism in a patient with impaired cardiopulmonary function. Third, an implicit understanding of the physiology of PE will allow for the application of physiologic risk stratification that can be used for diagnostic evaluation and therapeutics. Figure 142.1 represents a proposed risk stratification model defined by the relationship between mortality and severity characterized by the integration of cardiopulmonary status and embolism size. The combination of embolism size and underlying cardiopulmonary status that produces cardiac arrest is associated with a predicted mortality of 70%; this implies that 30% of arrested PE patients will survive and warrants continued use of chest compressions to mechanically fracture the embolism and consideration toward thrombolysis or embolectomy even without a definitive diagnosis when PE is highly suspected. At the opposite extreme, the combination of embolism size and cardiopulmonary status that fails to produce right ventricular (RV) dilatation is associated with a 0% to 1% mortality provided therapeutic anticoagulation is achieved. The combination of embolism size and cardiopulmonary status that produces hemodynamic instability or shock is associated with a 30% mortality rate. Consequently, the presence of shock has traditionally defined the threshold for thrombolysis. As depicted in Figure 142.1, there is likely a broad spectrum of PE patients that are hemodynamically stable with RV dysfunction ranging from those with a minimal embolic burden and a low predicted mortality to patients with incipient shock and a predicted mortality just under 30%. The use of thrombolytics in this heterogeneous group is controversial as the constitutive characteristics of the mortality inflection point remain elusive. Syncope represents an intermediary position between shock and cardiac arrest as failure to recover consciousness results in cardiac arrest, and patients who regain consciousness have a high incidence of hemodynamic instability. The outcomes and mortality associated with emboli in transit and PE patients with a patent foramen ovale (PFO) have not been well reported and likely have severity as depicted in Figure 142.1.

The spectrum of PE most likely to confront the intensivist is predominantly confined to two situations; first, the patient presenting with undifferentiated shock or respiratory failure, and second, an established hospital or ICU patient who develops PE after admission. In either situation, the diagnostics and therapeutics are challenging. Differentiating PE from other life-threatening cardiopulmonary disorders can be exceedingly difficult; logistic constraints can jeopardize definitive diagnostic testing, and hemorrhagic risks in the critically ill can significantly alter the therapeutic approach and compromise the ability to anticoagulate or institute thrombolytic therapy. This chapter will review a structured physiologic approach to diagnostic, resuscitative, and management strategies as well as discuss prophylaxis and ICU-specific PE issues.

PREVENTION OF VENOUS THROMBOEMBOLISM

Principles of Prophylaxis

Prophylaxis is defined as any measure "designed to preserve health and prevent the spread of disease." Insofar as venous thromboembolic disease (VTE) (3) is prevalent among acutely ill hospitalized patients and unprevented VTE may lead to adverse consequences, the use of pharmacologic, mechanical, or vena caval interruption as a means for reducing the occurrence of VTE certainly qualifies as a measure intended to preserve health. In fact, based on strength of evidence, the Agency for

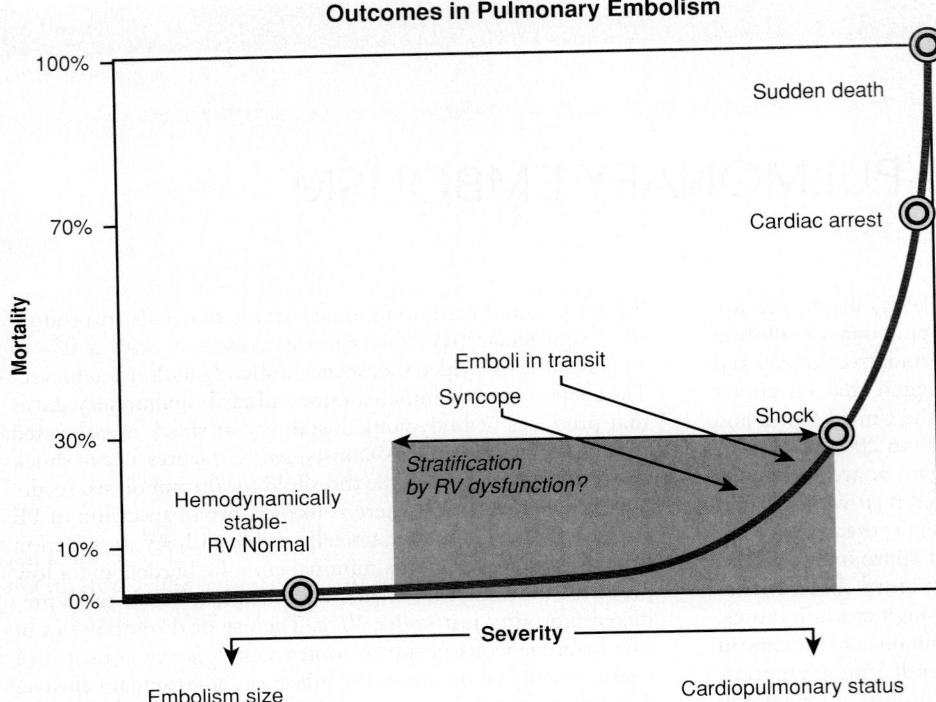

FIGURE 142.1. Outcomes in pulmonary embolism. RV, right ventricle.

Healthcare Research and Quality (AHRQ) has identified "appropriate use of prophylaxis to prevent venous thromboembolism in patients at risk" as the number one opportunity for improvement of patient safety, supporting more widespread implementation (1). The choice of primary prophylaxis is based on the patient's risk of bleeding and thrombosis and is presented in Table 142.1.

Risk Factors

The Virchow triad of stasis, vessel trauma, and hypercoagulability remain fundamental risk factors for VTE. Furthermore, risk factors can be considered clinical (i.e., multiple trauma or major abdominal surgery, acute myocardial infarction or stroke, need for mechanical ventilation) or patient-related (prior history of VTE, malignancy, inherited coagulopathy).

TABLE 142.1

VENOUS THROMBOEMBOLISM PROPHYLAXIS OF CRITICAL CARE PATIENT

Bleeding risk	Thrombosis risk	Prophylaxis recommendation
Low	Moderate	LDH 5000 units sq bid
Low	High	LMWH ■ Dalteparin ■ Enoxaparin
High	Moderate	GCS or IPC → LMWH when bleeding risk subsides
High	High	GCS or IPC → LMWH when bleeding risk subsides

LDH, low dose heparin; LMWH, low molecular-weight heparin; GCS, graded compression stockings; IPC, intermittent pneumatic compression devices.
Adapted from Geerts CHEST 2003;124(6)S:357S–363S.

With respect to lower extremity deep venous thrombosis (DVT), observational studies of medical-surgical ICU patients have identified mechanical ventilation, treatment with neuromuscular blockers, and presence of a central venous catheter (CVC) as risk factors for DVT (4). Central venous catheterization, in particular, has been reported to confer an increased relative risk (RR) of 1.04 for each day the catheter was in place (5). Among 261 medical-surgical ICU patients, multivariate regression analysis defined exposure to platelet transfusions and the use of vasopressors to be independent risk factors for ICU-acquired DVT (6).

The two most powerful patient-related risk factors are a prior history of VTE and malignancy. Malignancy is perhaps the most common acquired hypercoagulable state encountered in the ICU and likely will become more prevalent as the general population continues to age. Additionally, end-stage renal disease has been identified as an independent risk factor for ICU-acquired DVT (6). Activated protein C resistance from factor V Leyden (FVL) is the most common hereditary defect predisposition for DVT. In order of descending prevalence among the general population, prothrombin gene mutation 20210A, antithrombin, protein C and S deficiency, elevations in homocysteine, and coagulation factors VIII, IX, and XI may predispose the patient to developing DVT (4). Although uncommon, heparin-induced thrombocytopenia (HIT), an acquired platelet disorder, results in increased risk of both venous and arterial thrombosis (7).

Cancer and the presence of a CVC are the two most powerful risk factors for upper extremity DVT (UEDVT). In the report of Mustafa et al., a CVC at the site of the upper extremity DVT was present in 60% of patients and 46% were diagnosed with cancer. Underscoring the possible additive nature of these two risk factors, 76% of the patients with cancer also had an indwelling CVC (8). In a review of cancer patients who had an indwelling CVC, the reported prevalence of upper extremity DVT, either symptomatic or asymptomatic, ranged from 6.7 to 48% (9). In a prospective registry of 592 patients with upper extremity DVT, the presence of an indwelling CVC was the strongest independent predictor of occurrence (odds ratio, 7.3) (10). It is important to note that nearly 30% of patients will develop an UEDVT with no apparent cause. In these patients, inherited thrombophilia, particularly FVL, prothrombin G20210A mutation, and anticoagulant protein deficiencies may be causative. Evaluated prospectively for a median follow-up of 5.1 years, recurrence of primary UEDVT was reported to be 4.4% in those with inherited thrombophilia compared to 1.6% in those without (11).

Prevalence/Incidence

DVT in the setting of critical illness is underappreciated. Systematic screening has shown 10% of medical-surgical ICU patients to have an existing proximal lower extremity DVT on admission to the ICU. When no form of prophylaxis is used, the incidence of DVT during the ICU stay is variable but high.

Patients undergoing major general surgery have an event rate of 25% without DVT prophylaxis; 9% of patients will have clinically detectable DVT, and 7% will have proximal DVT. In a study of trauma patients who did not receive prophylaxis, 58% of patients developed a DVT, one third of which were proximal. Similarly, in patients undergoing elective hip surgery and not receiving prophylaxis, the incidence of DVT is 50%, with 23% being clinically detectable and 20% proximal (12). The pooled incidence of detectable DVT in neurosurgical patients is 22%, and the incidence in acute spinal cord injury patients is as high as 90% when prophylaxis is not used (4). The incidence of DVT in critically ill medical patients is reported to be 1% to 15% depending on which screening technique was used. No studies specific to the critically ill have been performed regarding upper extremity DVT, and no prospective studies using systematic screening techniques are available to assess the prevalence or incidence. Nonetheless, there has been an increase over the last several decades attributed to the greater use of transvenous pacemakers and central venous catheters. Symptomatic PE is reported to occur in 7–9% of these patients (13,14), and studies using systematic ventilation/perfusion scanning in those previously diagnosed with upper extremity DVT have reported high-probability scans in 13% (15).

Pharmacologic Prophylaxis

A paucity of data is available regarding anticoagulant prophylaxis in the critical care setting. To date, two published randomized trials of thromboprophylaxis versus placebo in medical-surgical ICU patients are available. In a prospective, double-blind, randomized control trial (RCT) of unfractionated heparin (UFH), 5,000 U administered subcutaneously (SQ) twice daily versus placebo, the rate of objectively confirmed DVT was reduced from 29% to 13% (16). In patients requiring mechanical ventilation ≥48 hours for exacerbations of chronic obstructive pulmonary disease (COPD), treatment with the low-molecular-weight heparin (LMWH) nadroparin once daily versus placebo decreased DVT rates from 29% to 16% (17). Another prospective trial, published in abstract form only, also demonstrated the efficacy of UFH versus placebo as thromboprophylaxis, reducing the DVT rates from 31% to 11% (18).

Despite limited generalizability to the critical care setting, thromboprophylaxis trials of acutely ill hospitalized medical patients and high-risk surgical patients are relevant. A comparison of enoxaparin, 40 mg or 20 mg, with placebo administered once daily for 6 to 14 days (MEDENOX) resulted in fewer DVTs in those receiving the 40-mg dose (19). In a randomized, placebo-controlled trial of dalteparin for the prevention of VTE (PREVENT), dalteparin, 5,000 IU once daily, halved the rate of VTE with a low risk of bleeding (20). Questions have been raised, however, as to whether or not SQ administration of LMWH has sufficient bioavailability to achieve therapeutic plasma levels (≥0.3 IU/mL) in the critically ill. In a prospective, controlled, open-labeled study of enoxaparin, 40 mg once daily, critically ill patients with normal renal function demonstrated significantly lower anti-Xa levels when compared with medical patients in the normal ward (21). This difference does not appear to be associated with vasopressor administration. On the contrary, body weight does seem to have a negative correlation with anti-Xa levels. More recently, a pilot study did not find clinically relevant differences in anti-Xa activity after subcutaneous administration of 2,500 IU dalteparin for venous thromboembolism prophylaxis between ICU patients with and without subcutaneous edema but again demonstrated critically ill patients to have lower anti-Xa activity levels than healthy volunteers (22). These findings call into question whether once-daily dosing is appropriate for the critically ill.

Last, fondaparinux, a synthetic factor Xa inibitor in doses of 2.5 mg SQ daily, has been reported to decrease VTE rates by half versus placebo in older acutely ill medical patients (ARTEMIS) (23); to be more effective than enoxaparin, 30 mg twice daily, for VTE prophylaxis after elective major knee surgery (24); and equivalent to dalteparin, 5,000 IU daily, for the prevention of VTE in high-risk abdominal surgery (PEGASUS) (25). Of note, patients requiring mechanical ventilation and those with severe sepsis and septic shock were excluded from these trials and most were not in the ICU. Nevertheless, the notion that these drugs are superior to placebo in the prevention of VTE is indeed supported.

Mechanical Prophylaxis

Graded compression stockings (GCS), intermittent pneumatic compression devices (IPC), and venous foot pumps (VFP) are attractive insofar as they are without bleeding risk. To date, no RCTs are available to guide their use in medical-surgical ICU patients. In an unblended study of 422 trauma patients, more DVT occurred in patients in whom IPC devices were used than with LMWH (2.7% vs. 0.5%) (26). Only a trend toward significance was found among 2,551 consecutive patients undergoing cardiac surgery treated with either UFH, 5,000 U SQ twice daily, or a combined prophylactic regimen of IPC and UFH; the incidence of objectively confirmed PE decreased from 4% to 1.5% (27). Use of IPC did not appear to have any additional benefit when used with either UFH or LMWH in a randomized pilot trial for VTE prophylaxis in patients undergoing craniotomy (28). IPC was less effective in preventing PE when used in addition to UFH versus LMWH alone in a prospective, randomized, multicenter trial involving acute spinal cord injury patients (29). Additionally, poor fitting GCS may lead to undue constriction and stasis of the limb on which it is applied, increasing risk of subsequent clot. As a preventative measure, most garments are manufactured with a more highly elasticized portion at the upper end as an aid to keeping the hosiery in position. It is important to realize that mechanical prophylaxis in isolation has not been shown to reduce the risk of death or PE. Mechanical VTE prophylaxis alone is not likely to be effective in the ICU and unless bleeding is of great concern, these devices should be deferred in favor of pharmacologic prophylaxis.

IVC Filters

The idea of interrupting the inferior vena cava (IVC) to prevent transit of lower extremity thromboses to the pulmonary circulation is attributed to Trousseau in 1868 (30). Today, IVC interruption is most often carried out by percutaneous insertion of a filter or "umbrella" via the femoral or jugular vein. As a result of technical refinements and ever-increasing expertise in performing the procedure, this one-time surgical technique is performed nearly 50,000 times a year (31). Categorical indications for IVC filter (IVCF) placement include contraindications to anticoagulation (absolute or relative), complications of previously instituted anticoagulation (failure, bleeding, thrombocytopenia, drug reactions), as a prophylactic adjunct to anticoagulation in patients thought to be unable to withstand another embolic event, failure of a previous IVCF, or in association with another procedure (thrombectomy, embolectomy, or thrombolysis). Unfortunately, methodologically sound literature in support of specific indications for filter placement is lacking. This paucity of evidence is highlighted by a systematic MEDLINE search for vena cava filters from 1975–2000, which produced 568 references (32). Only one RCT was identified, and only 15 prospective studies included $\geq$100 patients. The remainder were retrospective or case reports (65%) or reported on miscellaneous topics (8.1%). This is supported by a more recent Cochrane review (33). Consequently, recommendations for filter placement are largely a matter of opinion.

Decousus et al. (34) reported the first and only RCT of IVCFs for the prevention of PE in patients with documented proximal LEDVT. Patients were followed for 2 years in the initial report, and results of a longer-term follow-up in the same patients were reported after 8 years (35). In the initial report, 400 patients were randomized to receive a filter or no filter in addition to anticoagulation with UFH or LMWH. At 12 days, fewer patients suffered symptomatic or asymptomatic PE in the filter group while bleeding and mortality were unaffected. At 2 years, the number of patients suffering symptomatic PE was no longer significantly different (as a result of more symptomatic PE between years 1 and 2 in the filter group), and the recurrence of DVT was significantly higher in the filter group. Placement of an IVCF had no effect on survival. At 8-year follow-up, patients with filters still had higher DVT rates, but symptomatic PE was lower than in patients without a filter. Mortality was still unaffected. These reports suggest that DVT patients with or without PE may derive limited benefit from an IVCF in addition to anticoagulation alone. Placement of a filter in PE patients who have failed anticoagulation are at higher risk for a decrease in IVC patency or frank occlusion over time when compared to those with other indications for filter placement (36). However, no differences in edema formation, occurrence of varicose veins, trophic disorders, ulcer formation, or postthrombotic syndrome have been shown between those with and without a filter (35). Percutaneous filter placement in the superior vena cava may also be considered for prevention of symptomatic PE due to acute upper extremity DVT in patients in whom therapeutic anticoagulation has failed or is contraindicated. Limited observational data support its safety and efficacy in this setting (37,38).

IVCF use has not been systematically studied in critical care outside the setting of major trauma, where the deployment of retrievable IVCFs (R-IVCF) has been favored. Allen et al. (39) reported that retrievable filters are safe and effective in the prevention of PE in high-risk trauma patients with contraindications to anticoagulation. Interpretation of their findings is hampered by several factors: lack of anticoagulated patients as a comparator, small numbers (53 devices placed in 2,426 patients), and a low overall incidence of thromboembolic events (2.1% with DVT, 0.2% with nonfatal PE, no fatal PE). Others have cautioned that liberal application of these filters in the trauma population does not alter rates of VTE and may lead to a greater incidence of filter and retrieval-related complications (40). Furthermore, two recent studies reported that only about one in five of these devices is, in fact, retrieved, suggesting that they have simply become permanent filters (40,41). A small study of morbidly obese patients undergoing R-IVCF placement prior to gastric bypass surgery reported a 95% success rate when filter retrieval was attempted. Still, 21% developed VTE postoperatively (42).

In sum, no RCT of IVCF for the prevention of PE, generalizable to the critically ill, has yet been published. Currently, their use can only be recommended for those in whom anticoagulation is contraindicated or failed altogether. Consideration may be given to using a R-IVCF in the highest-risk surgical patients with contraindications to anticoagulation, with the emphasis on retrieval and commencement of anticoagulation as soon as is feasible.

Diagnosis of DVT

Validated prediction rules have been published and are useful in patients able to communicate their symptoms. However, many ICU patients will be incapable of effectively communicating any symptoms due to altered mental status, requirement for mechanical ventilation and/or infusions of sedatives, analgesics, or neuromuscular blocking drugs. Physical exam is equally unhelpful. The gold standard for DVT is lower limb venography (43). Adequately performed, it is able to detect all clinically important forms of DVT, including calf thrombosis, thrombosis of the pelvis, and the inferior vena cava. Due to the technical nature of the test, risk of radiocontrast-induced nephrotoxicity, and need to transport the patient from the ICU, it is rarely performed outside research settings. Consequently, compression ultrasound (CUS) is the most commonly reported method of detecting DVT in the ICU setting (44). For symptomatic patients, the reported pooled sensitivity for CUS in excluding a proximal DVT is 97%, but only 62% in asymptomatic patients. Furthermore, CUS lacks sensitivity in the detection of distal DVT, yielding pooled sensitivities of 73% and 53% for symptomatic and asymptomatic patients, respectively (45). Negative serial CUS over a 7- to 10-day period may effectively rule out clinically important DVT, but thus far has only been validated in symptomatic outpatients (43). An alternative to both venography and CUS is computed tomography venography (CTV) of the lower extremities and the pelvic veins as a continuation of CT angiography of the pulmonary arteries. In the setting of diagnostic workup for PE, CTV has a reported sensitivity and specificity of 70% and 96%, respectively, for all DVT, comparable to CUS in one study (46) and was superior to CUS for detection of iliofemoral DVT in a second report, yielding 100% sensitivity and specificity (47). Most recently, the PIOPED investigators reported that CTV and CUS are diagnostically equivalent, reporting a 95.5% concordance between CTV and CUS for diagnosis or exclusion of LEDVT (48). Thus the choice of imaging technique can be made on the basis of safety, expense, and time constraints. Limitations of the test are the same as for those previously mentioned for CT angiography of the pulmonary arteries.

In the case of upper extremity DVT, the first-line diagnostic test is color duplex ultrasound with a three-step protocol involving compression, color, and color Doppler with reported sensitivity and specificity ranging from 78% to 100% and 82% to 100%, respectively (9). In the event of vessel incompressibility but the presence of isolated flow abnormalities in combination with persistent clinical likelihood, contrast venography should be considered. Magnetic resonance venography (MRV) has been studied but with disappointing results. Reported sensitivities are 50% and 71% for MRV with and without gadolinium enhancement, respectively (47).

Treatment of DVT

The mainstay of therapy for all forms of VTE is anticoagulation. The reader is referred to the section for treatment of PE for further details. For larger clot burden involving the iliofemoral system, some suggest administration to thrombolytics. Indeed, a Cochrane review concluded that thrombolysis reduces post-thrombotic syndrome and maintains venous patency after DVT when compared to traditional anticoagulation (49). However, the optimum drug, dose, and route of administration have yet to be determined. Endovascular catheter-directed thrombolysis is another promising treatment for acute iliofemoral thrombosis. A more definitive report of any benefits over other therapies will await completion of a recently initiated multicenter RCT for DVT (50).

PULMONARY EMBOLISM

Contemporary risk stratification for the diagnosis, resuscitation, and treatment of PE is predicated on an implicit understanding of the pathophysiology of PE. The vicious pathophysiologic sequence of events related to the impaction of the embolic material on the pulmonary outflow is depicted in Figure 142.2. The combination of mechanical obstruction and neurohumoral factors combined with the patients underlying cardiopulmonary status results in an increase in pulmonary vascular impedance and the induction of pressure load on the right ventricle. Although the impact of the mechanical obstruction is well appreciated, the effect of neurohumoral influence is significantly underappreciated. The release of factors from platelets in the imbedded clot, which include serotonin, adenosine diphosphate (ADP), and thrombin, all precipitate vasoconstriction in the pulmonary artery system (51). The development of a pressure load will precipitate right ventricular decompensation, which decreases right ventricular output. Because the heart is two hydraulic pumps linked in series,

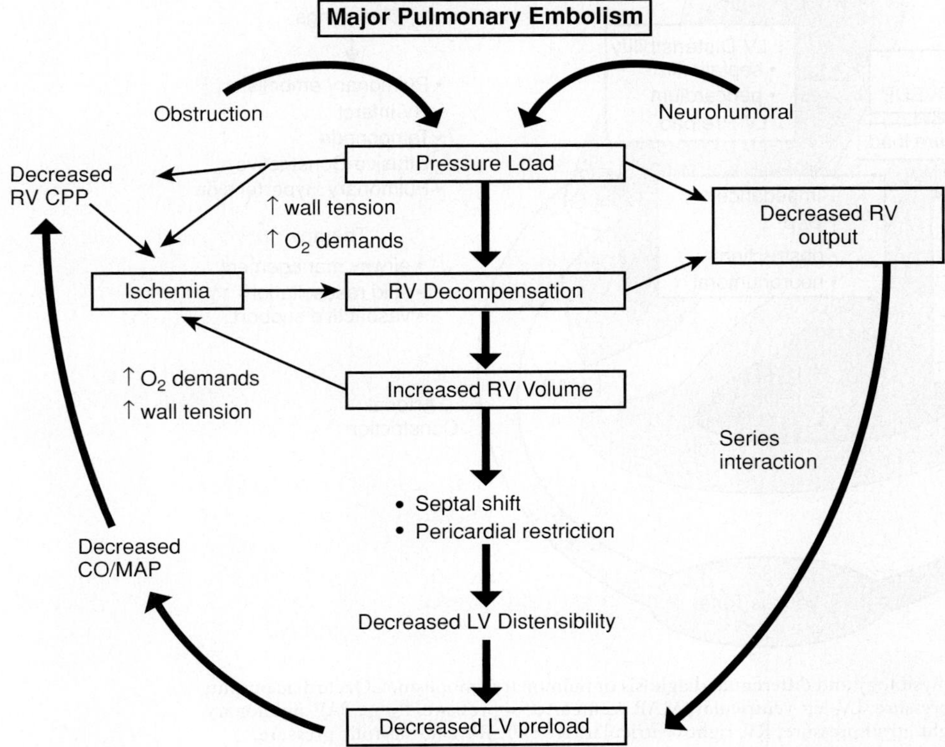

FIGURE 142.2. Pathophysiology of pulmonary embolism. CO/MAP, cardiac output/mean arterial pressure; CPP, cardiopulmonary pressure; LV, left ventricular; RV, right ventricular.

diminished output of the right ventricle will result in diminished left ventricular preload. The consequence of diminished left ventricular preload is a decrease in cardiac output and a resultant loss of mean arterial pressure. The perfusion pressure gradient for the right ventricular subendocardium is the difference between the mean arterial pressure and the right ventricular end-diastolic pressure. PE precipitates an increase in right ventricular end-diastolic pressure through the induction of a right ventricular pressure load and the development of right ventricular decompensation. This increases right ventricular myocardial oxygen demands because of the diminished gradient between the mean arterial pressure and the right ventricular subendocardium. This induces further right ventricular decompensation and resultant right ventricular ischemia. The right ventricle compensates through the use of the Starling mechanism and increases right ventricular volume. This results in a left septal shift of the intraventricular septum and further jeopardizing of left ventricular filling. Pericardial restraint, further limits of left ventricular filling, and further impairments of left ventricular distensibility additionally decrease left ventricular preload. This pathophysiologic sequence results in a vicious cycle of ventricular decompensation that manifests as hemodynamic instability and shock. It is important to recognize that PE is a spectrum of presentations and that the most extreme form of PE will result in gross hemodynamic instability and cardiac arrest. Figure 142.3 illustrates a diagrammatic overview of the sequence of events that occur in PE.

The care of the critically ill patient often proceeds along two parallel pathways; physiologic resuscitation and generation of a differential diagnosis that eventually leads to a definitive diagnosis and treatment. Consequently, the use of a universally applicable model of the circulatory system is of substantial utility in characterizing the physiologic elements for resuscitation and assisting in the differential diagnosis generation. Figure 142.4 represents a three-compartmental model of the circulatory system that is characterized by two hydraulic pumps linked in series. Each hydraulic pump has its own capacitance (volume reservoir) and impedance (resistive element) system. Insofar as the pumps are aligned in series, the output of one pump can never exceed the output of the other. Consequently, hydraulic pumps may be conceptualized as a single hydraulic unit. Using this model, the circulatory system can be viewed as a venous capacitance reservoir that provides volume to a hydraulic pump that generates flow into an impedance bed. Any hemodynamic abnormality, such as hypovolemia, ventricular failure, sepsis, or major PE, may be characterized by defining one or more of the variables in this hydraulic pump. The surrogates for venous capacitance pressure, hydraulic pump function, and impedance are right arterial pressure (RAP), cardiac output (CO), and systemic venous resistance (SVR), respectively. Oftentimes invasive monitoring or echocardiographic assessment is not immediately available on patient presentation in the intensive care unit. Consequently, it is frequently necessary to assess the model elements from physical exam; the venous capacitance reservoir may be estimated from examination

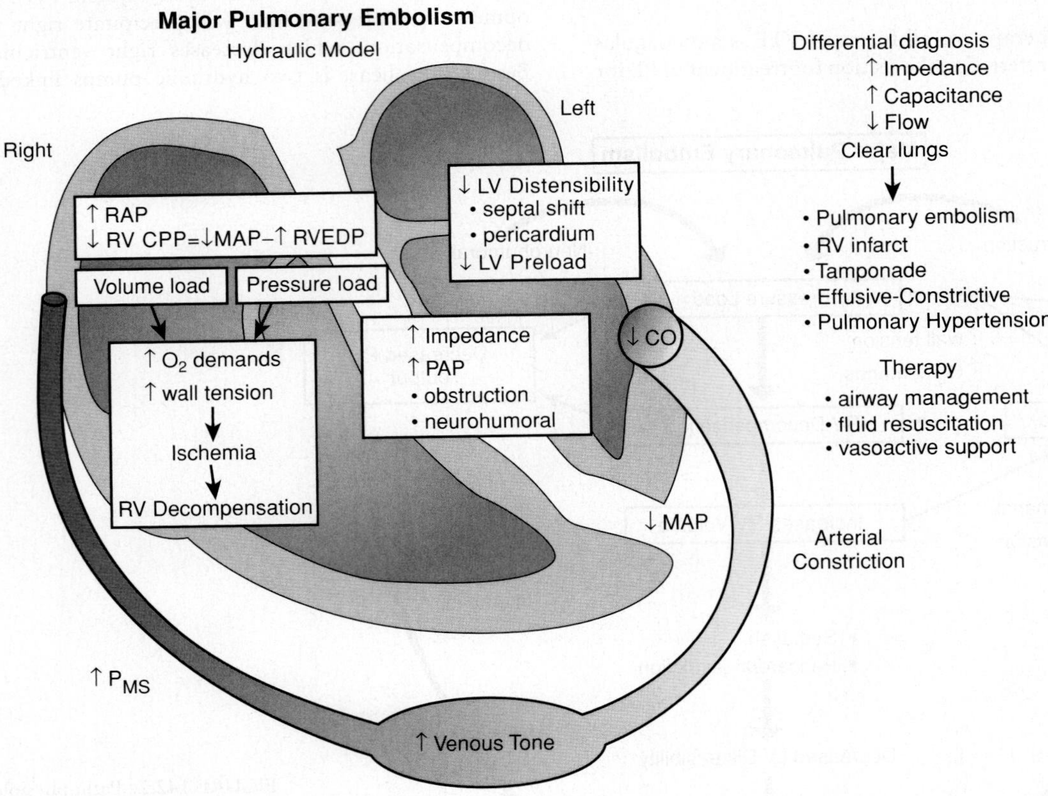

FIGURE 142.3. Pathophysiology and differential diagnosis of pulmonary embolism. CO, cardiac output; CPP, cardiopulmonary pressure; LV, left ventricular; MAP, mean arterial pressure; P_{MS}, , PAP, pulmonary artery pressure; RAP, right atrial pressure; RV, right ventricular; RVEDP, RV end-diastolic pressure.

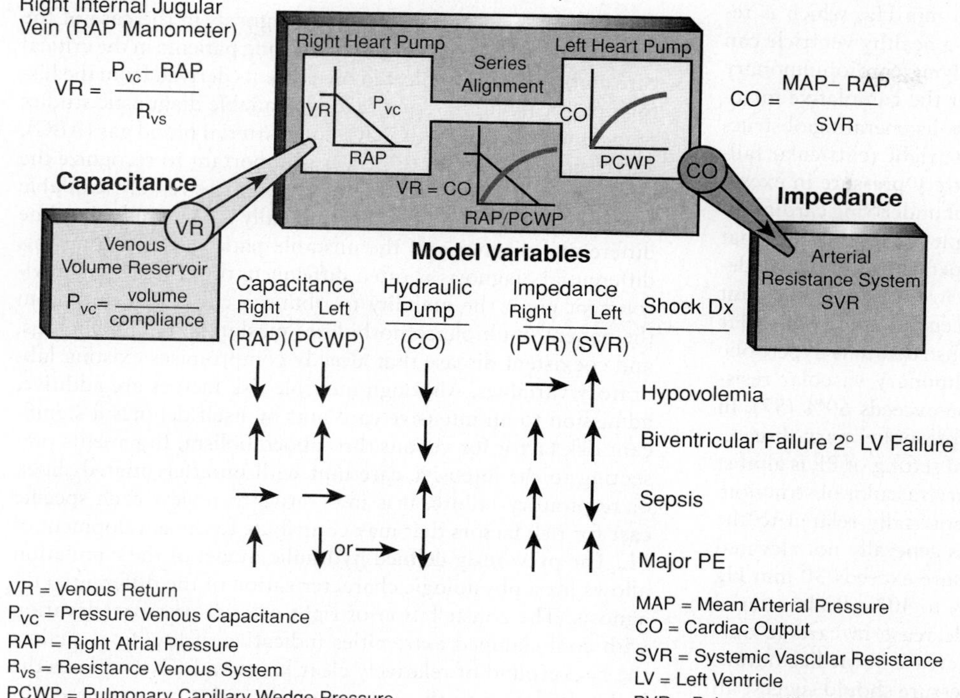

FIGURE 142.4. Three-compartment circulatory shock model.

the right internal jugular vein, and the pulse character and temperature of extremities maybe relied on to approximate the arterial impedance. Characteristically, a reciprocal relationship between flow and impedance is present in most disease states. Warm flushed extremities with a very wide pulse pressure indicate low vascular impedance and a correspondingly high flow state, whereas cool constricted extremities with a thready narrow pulse pressure suggest a state of high vascular impedance resulting from the compensatory increase in catecholamines to maintain perfusion pressure gradients. Recognizing that flow and impedance are almost uniformly reciprocal, one can exploit this relationship to assist with the differential diagnosis of shock patients. Therefore, the initial assessment of impedance (resistance) allows for the inferential derivation of flow. Cool clamped hypoperfused extremities reflect a catecholamines surge and low flow state. Given the hydraulic pump alignment in series, the presence of an elevated jugular venous pressure against the background of clinical and radiographically clear lungs isolates the hemodynamic lesion to the right ventricle. The differential diagnosis of increased impedance, increased capacitance pressure, and decreased flow against the background of clear lungs is illustrated in Figure 142.3 and includes PE, right ventricular infarct, and pericardial tamponade. Impaired gas exchange in conjunction with the preceding is strongly suggestive of PE. Given the potential likelihood of anticoagulation and thrombolytic therapy in this patient population, invasive monitoring should be selectively used when the circulatory model variables cannot be well characterized from physical exam. A characterization of model variables for various shock states are depicted in Figure 142.4.

The gas exchange abnormalities in PE are exceedingly complex and a function of the size and character of the embolic material, the magnitude of the occlusion against the background of the patients underlying cardiopulmonary status, and the interval time since the embolic event (52). The multiple causes of hypoxia have been attributed to an increase in alveolar dead space, ventilation perfusion abnormalities, right-to-left shunting, and in the case of cardiogenic shock, a low mixed venous O_2. Although seemingly counterintuitive, the multiple inert gas technique suggests that a low V/Q relationship develops and precipitates hypoxia in PE consequent to the redistribution of blood flow away from the embolized area, resulting in excessive perfusion in the unembolized lung regions and subsequent reperfusion through the atelectatic area of the previous clot.

It is especially instructive to exam the clinical manifestation of PE patients without underlying cardiac pulmonary disease because it permits the assessment of the effects of the embolic event and specific compensatory responses. In this particular population, the clinical and physiologic implications of PE are directly correlated to the size of embolism (53–55). In these studies, there is significant correlation observed between the magnitude of the angiographic obstruction and the mean pulmonary artery pressure (mPAP) RAP, PaO_2, and pulse. It has been suggested that a pulmonary vascular resistance (PVR) of greater than 500 dyne.s.cm^{-5} is correlative with a degree of obstruction exceeding 50% (56). It is interesting to note that depression in oxygen saturation is common and may occur with as little as 13% angiographic obstruction and commonly is the only clinical manifestation when the obstruction is less than 25% (55). When the extent of pulmonary vascular obstruction is 25% to 30%, pulmonary hypertension begins to develop (normal mPAP, 20 mmHg). It is important to recognize that this represents an increase in excess to similarly described nonembolic experimental obstruction, which further illustrates the relative contribution of the neurohumoral mechanism to pulmonary vascular impedance. Patients without underlying cardiopulmonary disease are unable to generate a mean pulmonary artery pressure in excess of 40 mm Hg, which is reported to be the maximal pressure that a healthy ventricle can generate. In patients without an underlying cardiopulmonary disease, either a large single embolus or the cumulative incremental effects of multiple recurrent emboli generating obstructions over 50% are needed to precipitate right ventricular failure. Consequently, mean pulmonary artery pressure in excess of 40 mm Hg represents either significant underlying cardiopulmonary disease or the effects of multiple embolic events that have occurred over a prolonged time period enabling the development of the right ventricular hypertrophy. It is important to recognize that the relationship between pulmonary vascular resistance and the extent of anatomic obstruction is hyperbolic and not linear. Direct increases in pulmonary vascular resistance occur when anatomic obstruction exceeds 60% (57). In the population with no underlying cardiopulmonary disease, an increase in right arterial pressure and setting of PE is almost uniformly indicative of severe pulmonary vascular obstruction. The right arterial pressure is characteristically related to the mean pulmonary artery pressure but is generally not elevated until the mean pulmonary artery pressure exceeds 30 mm Hg and anatomic obstruction exceeds 35% to 40%. Right arterial pressure can be elevated without a decrease in cardiac output in patients with PE. However, a decrease in cardiac output without an increase in right arterial pressure should suggest an alternative non–PE-related diagnosis.

In contrast to patients without an underlying cardiopulmonary disease, patients with previous cardiopulmonary disease characteristically will manifest a significantly greater degree of cardiovascular impairment with less anatomic vascular obstruction (58). This is perhaps best exemplified in the European Pulmonary Embolism Trial where 90% of the patients who presented in shock had prior cardiopulmonary disease and 56% of those with prior cardiopulmonary disease presented in shock compared to only 2% of patients without cardiopulmonary disease (59). In this population of patients with prior cardiac disease, the level of mean pulmonary artery pressure is disproportionately elevated compared to that of anatomic obstruction, which strongly suggests that underlying cardiopulmonary hemodynamics dominates the presentation process. With a mean angiographic obstruction of only 23%, significant elevations in mean pulmonary artery pressure were reported in a population with previous cardiopulmonary disease, and the increment in the mean pulmonary artery pressure was directly related to the pulmonary capillary wedge pressure (PCWP) (58). This level of anatomic obstruction would be below the threshold to elicit an increase in mean pulmonary artery pressure in patients without cardiopulmonary disease. In patients with prior cardiopulmonary disease, the right arterial pressure was reported to be an unreliable indicator of the magnitude of the embolic event and limited its usefulness in the assessment of extensive vascular obstruction and life-threatening disease. Therefore, it appears that there is no consistent relationship between the extent of embolic obstruction and right ventricular impairment in patients with previous cardiopulmonary disease. Hemodynamic and right ventricular function can be misleading as measurements of the effect of the embolic event, which clearly underscores that the assessment of the severity is predicated on the pre-embolic status of the patient as illustrated in Figure 142.1.

Readily Available Diagnostic Studies

The development of a differential diagnosis in the case of the undifferentiated shock patient or existing patients in the critical care unit is usually predicated on elements derived from the history, physical findings, and readily available diagnostic studies to include a chest x-ray (CXR) study, arterial blood gas (ABG), and electrocardiogram (ECG). It is important to recognize the physiologic footprint that PE makes on these readily available studies to ensure that PE is hierarchically incorporated into the differential diagnosis of the unstable patient. Generating this differential diagnosis is often difficult in the critical care environment given the inability to obtain a current history from the patient, multiple comorbidities masking physical findings, and coexistent disease that already compromises existing laboratory variables. Although multiple risk factors are additive, admission to an intensive care unit by itself denotes a significant risk factor for venous thromboembolism. In patients presenting to the intensive care unit with undifferentiated shock or respiratory failure, it is imperative to review each specific case for risk factors that may contribute to the development of PE. The previously defined hydraulic model of the circulation allows for a physiologic characterization of the differential diagnosis. The constellation of right arterial pressure elevation with cool clamped extremities indicative of low flow against the background of relatively clear lungs and CXR isolates the hydraulic lesion to the right ventricle with a very limited differential diagnosis as illustrated in Figure 142.3. Occasionally, invasive hemodynamic measurements will be available, which should reflect an increase in the right arterial pressure, a low cardiac output state in the shock population, associated with a low pulmonary capillary wedge pressure and a high SVR.

Electrocardiogram

Since the sentinel description in 1935 by McGinn and White (60) of the $S_1Q_3T_3$ pattern in a limited number of patients with PE-induced cor pulmonale, a plethora of ECG manifestation have been reported. However, several important points from large series regarding the ECG findings for PE may be helpful: First, a normal ECG is distinctly unusual and it is reported in only in a minority of patients in the UPET Trial without cardiopulmonary disease (14%) (61) and was similarly appreciated in only 30% of patients in the PIOPED Trial (62). Rhythm disturbances are uncommon, and the incidence of atrial fibrillation and flutter as a presenting component of PE is exceedingly small as are first-, second-, or third-degree heart blocks. The most common ECG findings are related to abnormalities in the ST-T wave segment. In UPET (61) and PIOPED (62), these changes occurred in 42% and 49% of patients, respectively. Recently, it has been shown that the anterior T-wave inversion pattern is the most common abnormality in PE, occurring in 68% of patients. It was the ECG sign that was most correlative with the severity of the underlying embolic event as 90% of the patients with anterior T-wave inversion had a Miller Score exceeding 50% (mean 60%), and 81% of those had a mean pulmonary artery pressure elevation exceeding 30 mm Hg (54). The early appearance of the T-wave inversion was reported to be an even stronger marker of the severity of the event and similarly correlative with the efficacy of thrombolytic therapy given the T-wave normalization that occurred in patients who had successful thrombolytic therapy (63).

Chest Radiograph

Although the chest radiograph cannot be effectively used to include and exclude PE, it is helpful in contributing to the diagnostic assessment by excluding other diseases that may mimic PE and defining abnormalities that necessitate further evaluation, and it may provide a crude assessment of severity (64). Similar to the ECG, a normal chest radiograph in patients with angiographic-proven PE is unusual and occurred in only 16% and 34% of patients in the PIOPED (62) and UPET (61), respectively, who did not have cardiopulmonary disease. In PIOPED, there appeared to be an association between severity of the thromboembolic event and the radiographic findings defined by the relationships between pulmonary artery pressure (PAP), oxygen saturation, and CXR findings when normal chest x-ray views were compared to those with parenchymal and vascular abnormalities (64). Vascular abnormalities including relative oligemia in the area of embolic event were correlative with the severity of PE. Other findings on CXR suggestive of PE include abrupt cutoff of the pulmonary artery, relative or focal oligemia, and distention of the proximal portion of the pulmonary artery.

Arterial Blood Gas

It is important to recognize that hypoxia in PE is not uniform as PaO_2 readings greater than 80 mm Hg were seen in approximately 12% of UPET patients and 19% of PIOPED patients (65,66). It is similarly important to recognize that a normal PaO_2 does not exclude PE and occurred in approximately 14% of patients in the PIOPED Trial (62,67). In patients without underlying cardiopulmonary disease, it is likely that these small changes in oxygen saturation reflect low levels of severity in PE. In contrast to the almost linear relationship between PE severity and arterial oxygen saturation levels in patients without cardiopulmonary disease, there appears to be no correlation between the arterial oxygen saturation or PaO_2 and magnitude of the embolic event in patients with cardiopulmonary disease. Given that many patients in intensive care units have significant gas impairment and are maintained on mechanical ventilation, it is the change in the oxygen saturation or the requirement of escalating levels of inspired oxygen that should prompt the consideration toward evaluation for PE. In intensive care units that are capable of measuring dead space (Vd/Vt) or end-tidal CO_2, these should similarly be used given the physiologic imprint of increased dead space with PE.

DIAGNOSTIC THERAPEUTIC APPROACH

Risk Stratification

The contemporary approach to physiologic risk stratification is depicted in Figure 142.1. The combination underlying cardiopulmonary status and embolic size that precipitates cardiac arrest is surprisingly associated with a mortality of only 70% in reported series. This underscores the necessity of aggressively pursuing patients with suspected underlying PE presenting with cardiac arrest because approximately 30% of those patients with PE and cardiac arrest will survive. At the other extreme, it is equally underappreciated that the predicted mortality of patients with hemodynamically stable PE and normal right ventricle is very low when treated with appropriate anticoagulation. The combination of embolic size and cardiopulmonary status that precipitates decompensation resulting in shock is associated with a 30% mortality. Although not well reported, syncope and emboli in transit have predicted mortalities just below that of a shock patient. Echocardiography is frequently used to risk-stratify patients with PE who are hemodynamically stable. However, it is important to recognize that the vast overwhelming majority of patients with right ventricular dysfunction and hemodynamic stability will do well with anticoagulation alone. As is evident in Figure 142.1, there is a spectrum of presentations related to hemodynamically stable patients with PE that may include patients with incipient shock and those with insignificant dilatation of the right heart. It is important to recognize that an anatomic obstruction of approximately 30% is necessary to provoke elevations in pulmonary artery pressure. Similarly literature related to echocardiography reveals that an obstruction of 30% is needed to precipitate right ventricular dilatation.

The presence of hemodynamic deterioration or shock in a patient with PE represents the failure of both compensatory mechanisms to maintain forward flow and is associated with significant increases in mortality. Consequently, the presence of shock has traditionally been used as a discriminator to define the likelihood of survivorship from PE. The presence of shock in patients with PE is associated with a threefold to sevenfold increase in mortality (68,69). It is underappreciated that the vast majority of patients with anatomically massive PE do not present in shock. Case series have reported a majority of patients without underlying cardiopulmonary disease and associated anatomically massive PE present with a normal cardiac output (70). Similarly, it is important to recognize that hemodynamically stable patients who are not in shock, who have experienced submassive or massive PE, have similar mortality rates (68,69). An anatomically massive PE, unless accompanied by physiologic decompensation resulting in shock and hemodynamic instability, does not appear to be associated with increased mortality.

Figure 142.5 represents a diagnostic/therapeutic algorithm based on the presence or absent of shock. In all patients presenting with PE, therapeutic anticoagulation should be undertaken on presentation provided there are no contradictions to anticoagulation. The therapeutic effect of heparin is related to the ability to prevent further clot propagation and the prevention of recurrent of PE. Insofar as the risk of recurrent thromboembolic event is highest in the period immediately after PE, and because recurrent thromboembolic events are the most common cause of death in hemodynamic stable patients, it is pivotal to adequately and appropriately achieve a therapeutic level of anticoagulation as soon as feasible. Given the risks of bleeding associated with critical illness, unfractionated intravenous heparin is recommended because of the short half-life and the ability to reverse the therapeutic effect of heparin with protamine. Low-molecular-weight heparin, although appealing in

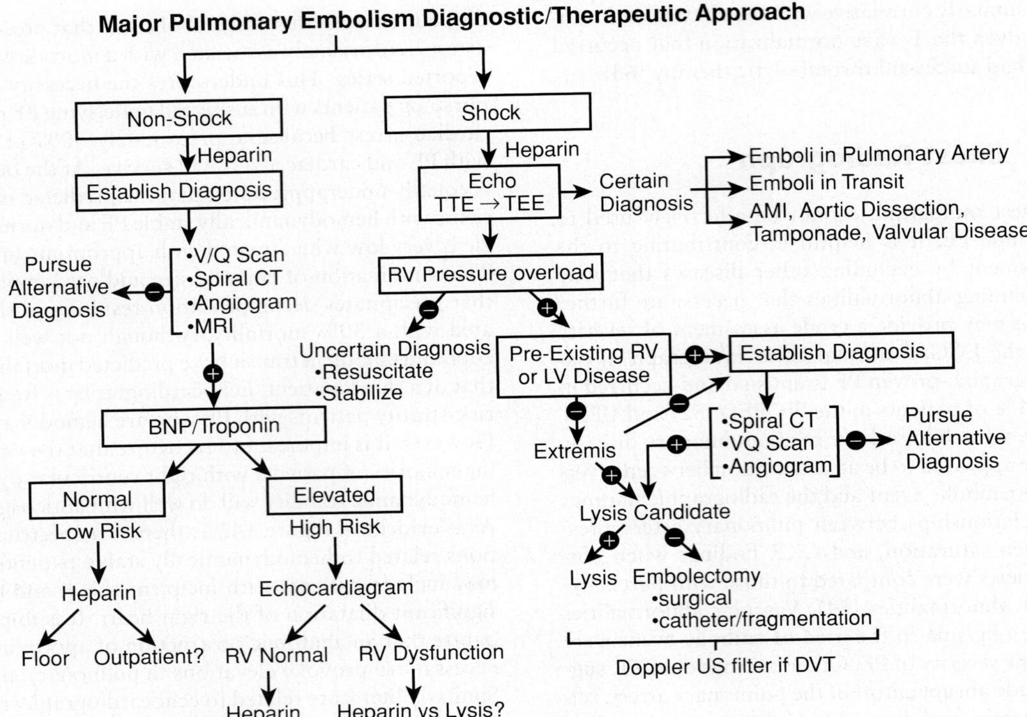

FIGURE 142.5. Diagnostic therapeutic approach to pulmonary embolism. AMI, acute mesenteric ischemia; CT, computed tomography; DVT, deep vein thrombus; LV, left ventricle; RV, right ventricle; TEE, transesophageal echocardiography; TTE, transthoracic echocardiography; US, ultrasound; V/Q, ventilation/perfusion.

the outpatient treatment of DVT and stable PE patients cannot be readily reversed.

In patients without evidence of hemodynamic stability, spiral CT scanning has supplanted ventilation perfusion scanning as a diagnostic modality of choice in PE. In patients with elevated creatinine or inability to tolerate a CT scan, Ventilation/perfusion (V/Q) scanning represents a reasonable alternative given the overwhelming experience using this technique. Pretest probability characterizations are pivotal in the diagnosis of PE whether CT scanning or ventilation/perfusion scanning is used. Pretest probability can be characterized by the use of scoring systems or based on clinical judgment. The combination of a high pretest probability with a high-probability V/Q scan confirms the diagnosis of PE. Similarly, a low-probability V/Q scan in conjunction with a low clinical pretest probability effectively excludes PE. Any other combination of pretest probability and scan probability requires further testing to include and exclude PE. Similarly, it is imperative to characterize a pretest probability for PE using CT scanning as a diagnostic modality. In patients with a high pretest probability and a negative spiral CT scan, further diagnostic studies should be undertaken. Although spiral CT scanning has been used to either exclude or confirm PE, there is an evolving literature that suggests spiral CT scanning can be used to define the severity of PE. Recent reports have been able to characterize the extent of pulmonary artery obstruction (71,72). Similar to the Miller and Walsh scores, which defined the extent of anatomic obstruction, there has been variability in reports of outcome related to the extent of obstruction. Measurements that are available from the CT scan include the calculation of the RV/LV axis ratio, the diameter of the right ventricular chamber, assessment of pulmonary artery diameter, and reflux of contrast material into the inferior vena cava (73). Although there are no prospective studies that have been conducted to assess the utility of spiral CT scanning as a predictor for severity stratification, it has been reported that the probability of death is significantly correlative with the RV/LV ratio. It appears that spiral CT scanning is evolving as the modality of choice for the diagnosis of PE and will be used to define severity stratification (73).

Further risk stratification of hemodynamically stable patients with PE may be undertaken using brain natriuretic peptide (BNP) and troponin levels. In patients with hemodynamic stability and confirmed PE that presents with a normal BNP and troponin levels, the predicted outcomes are excellent, and many of these patients may be treated as outpatient in the future. The presence of elevation in BNP and troponin define a high-risk population of patients with hemodynamic stability and warrant admission and close observation. The approach to this population will be discussed subsequently in this chapter.

In contrast to the patient presenting without hemodynamic instability, patients with suspected PE and hemodynamic instability are at high risk for rapid deterioration and sudden death. This demands an expeditions approach to the diagnosis, resuscitation, and therapy of this population. Echocardiography is an ideal first assessment of the hemodynamically unstable patient because it is becoming readily available, an integral part of critical care medicine, repeatable, and useful in recognition and differentiation of PE along with assessing the severity of the embolic event and the patient's response to therapy

(74–76). Characteristic findings suggestive of PE include right-sided thrombi, right ventricular dilatation, hypokinesis, tricuspid regurgitation, and paradoxical shifting of the ventricular septum. Similarly, the echocardiographic findings of acute myocardial infarction, tamponade, aortic dissection, or valvular disease may be equally useful in confirming the diagnosis and excluding PE. In patients without underlying cardiopulmonary disease, the magnitude of the abnormalities seen on echocardiogram correlate with the degree of pulmonary artery outflow obstruction (77). Similar to the original data related to angiographic measurement of pressure generation with PE, it appears that an obstruction of 30% is necessary to produce right ventricular dilatation. Degrees of obstruction less than 30% will not characteristically present with right ventricular dilatation. Consequently, right ventricular dilatation has been used for severity stratification as the outcome of patients who do not have right ventricular dysfunction is excellent with therapeutic anticoagulation. It is crucial to recognize that the presence of right ventricular function is not specific for PE. Patients with previous cardiopulmonary disease may have evidence of right ventricular dysfunction at baseline. In this setting, right ventricular function might be a representative of a spectrum of diseases that range from RV infarct with cardiomyopathy to cor pulmonale and antecedent pulmonary hypertension. Several echocardiographic findings have been reported to be useful in differentiating PE from non-PE events. Patients with baseline cor pulmonale or recurrent PE characteristically have evidence of hypertrophy in the right ventricle with a thickness measuring greater than 5 mm (76,78) and a minimal septal shift, whereas acute right ventricular failure secondary to PE should not be associated with right ventricular hypertrophy nor accompanied by a septal shift (77,79). In patients with pre-existing cardiopulmonary disease, it is imperative to establish the diagnosis of PE, which may be undertaken with diagnostic studies previously discussed in a nonshock patient. Spiral CT scanning has supplanted V/Q scans in the critically ill population. In patients with evidence of PE that is confirmed on the diagnostic studies, candidacy for either medical thrombectomy with thrombolytic therapy or surgical embolectomy should be undertaken. It is crucial to recognize that the absence of right ventricular pressure overload in the unstable patient in whom PE is being considered effectively excludes PE as a culprit cause of the hemodynamic instability. Occasionally, and in the appropriate clinical context, patients without underlying cardiopulmonary disease in extremis and with anticipated arrest with evidence of right ventricular dilatation and high pretest probability for PE may be considered as candidates for medical embolectomy with thrombolytic therapy or surgical embolectomy, given the time necessary to perform confirmatory studies, which may jeopardize effective treatment.

Resuscitation and Stabilization

Throughout the diagnostic evaluation, patients with suspected PE often require aggressive resuscitation and attempts at stabilization. In these patients, marginal hemodynamic stability is often maintained by intense catecholamine release. Frequently, escalating oxygen requirements necessitate intubation and mechanical ventilation. Intubation may precipitate cardiovascular collapse in patients with major PE for several reasons: sedative hypnotics that are used for intubation can mitigate the catecholamine surge on which the patient is dependent and similarly produce vasodilatation, which impairs the perfusion pressure gradient to the right ventricular subendocardium, provoking further ischemia and cardiac decompensation. Excessive lung ventilation on initial intubation may create air trapping and diminish venous return. Initiation of mechanical ventilation can increase the pulmonary vascular resistance and further jeopardize right ventricular function. Consequently, intubation should be carefully undertaken, weighing the risk and benefits of a conscience awake technique with topical or local anesthesia in conjunction with a rapid-sequence approach using neuromuscular blockade and/or fiberoptic intubation. Etomidate is an ideal sedative hypnotic insofar as it preserves hemodynamic status.

Conventionally, volume expansion with 1 to 2 L of crystalloid solution is initial treatment for hypotension in patients with undifferentiated shock. However, in patients with PE-related shock, increases in right ventricular pressure and volume generate significant increases in systolic wall stress, provoking myocardial ischemia. Excessive fluid resuscitation further dilates the right ventricle and produces increased wall stress, resulting in further right ventricular decompensation. In patients with anatomically massive PE and low cardiac output who were normotensive and required vasopressors on presentation, Mercat et al. (80) reported increases in cardiac output with a 500-mL fluid challenge. The authors reported that the increase in cardiac output was consistently proportional to the baseline right ventricular and diastolic volume index. Therefore, fluid may be used judicially in normotensive patients without evidence of significant right ventricular dysfunction. In patients with echocardiographic evidence of severe right ventricular dysfunction, fluid resuscitation may provoke increased wall stress, ischemia, and right ventricular dysfunction. When measured right ventricular pressure are high or there is evidence of severe right ventricular dysfunction, early consideration should be given to vasopressor therapy.

Although there are no controlled human trials related to vasoactive support in PE, extrapolation from animal models suggests that norepinephrine improves right ventricular dysfunction through vasoconstriction that augments mean arterial pressure and enhances perfusion pressure gradients to the right ventricular subendocardium. In addition, norepinephrine possesses modest inotropic properties that have been shown to provide complementary enhancement of right ventricular function (81,82). Given the previously described vasoconstrictive effects of the neurohumoral response to PE, it may be reasonable to consider the use of inhaled nitric oxide to decrease pulmonary vascular afterload in patients with evidence of severe right ventricular dysfunction who are pressor dependent. Small reports have suggested that inhaled prostacyclin and nitric oxide will increase cardiac output, decrease pulmonary artery pressures, and improve gas exchange in cases of shock-related PE (83,84).

The presence of shock or hemodynamic decompensation in patients with proven PE is an indication for either medical embolectomy with thrombolytic therapy or surgical embolectomy. Although the use of thrombolytic therapy is controversial in patients who are hemodynamically stable, it is acknowledged as the therapeutic choice in hemodynamically unstable patients in whom there is no contraindication to thrombolytic therapy. The PIOPED investigators considered thrombolytic therapy the standard of care for patients with "shock or major disability"

TABLE 142.2

RATE AND EXTENT OF PERFUSION SCAN RESOLUTION IN UROKINASE PULMONARY EMBOLISM TRIAL (UPET)

	Heparin (82) 25.4%		Urokinase (78) 26.2%	
	Absolute resolution	% Resolution	Absolute resolution	% Resolution
24 hours	2.7%	8.1%	6.2%	22.1%
Day 2	4.9%	17%	8.0%	25.8%
Day 5	9.3%	35.5%	11.3%	40.6%
Day 14	14.7%	58.2%	14.9%	52.0%
1 year		77.2%		78.8%
No CPD → 90% resolution		91% of patients		88% of patients
CPD → 90% resolution		72% of patients		77% of patients

CPD, cardiopulmonary disease.
From Urokinase pulmonary embolism trial. Phase 1 results: a cooperative study. *JAMA.* 1970;214:2163–2172; and Urokinase pulmonary embolism trial. *Circulation.* 1973;47(Suppl):1–108.

and considered it unethical to treat patients with hemodynamic stability with heparin alone in the research trial (85). Several points regarding the use of thrombolytic therapy in PE patients should be emphasized. First, in virtually all studies, there is greater rapidity in the rate of resolution when comparing heparin to thrombolytic therapy in terms of the percent resolution detected by perfusion scanning and angiography. Second, no reported clinical trial has defined any difference in the degree of embolic resolution after day 7. This is perhaps best illustrated in the original UPET Trial conducted in 1970 (68). In this landmark publication related to the use of thrombolytic therapy and PE, the baseline angiographic defect in the heparin group was 25% and 26% in the urokinase group. Within the first 24 hours, the percent of angiographic resolution in the heparin group was 8.1% and 22.1% in the urokinase-treated group. However, by day 5, the extent of the degree of angiographic resolution in the heparin and urokinase groups was equivalent at 36% and 40%, respectively. By 1 year, the extent of angiographic resolution was 77% in the heparin group and 78% in the urokinase group (Table 142.2). A comparison of clinical trials conducted comparing lytic therapy to heparin reveals similar findings as there is no reported difference in any physiologic or imaging modality after day 5 when comparing the two therapeutic options (Table 142.3). However appealing the rapidity of resolution may be, only one small trial (86) has demonstrated a mortality benefit. This small trial consisted of only eight patients with benefit confined only to those who received thrombolytic therapy. It is important to note that the patients randomized to heparin had previously been treated with heparin and experienced recurrent PE and were subsequently

TABLE 142.3

RANDOMIZED TRIALS—LYSIS VERSUS HEPARIN

	Early				
Study	Angio	Scan	Hemodyn	Echo	Late
UPET 1970	↑ 24 h	↑ 24 h	↑ 24 h	—	Scan, day 5; pulmonary HTN
Tibbutt 1974	↑ 72 h	—	↑ 72 h	—	Limited
Arnesen 1978	↑ 72 h	—	—	—	—
Ly 1978	↑ 72 h	—	—	—	—
Marini 1988	→ 7 day	→ 24 h	→ 7 day	—	No difference, 1 yr
PIOPED 1990	→ 2 h	→ 24, 48 h	↑ PVR 1.5 day	—	No difference
Giuntini 1984	—	↑ 24 h	—	—	Scan, day 3
Levine 1990	—	↑ 24 h	—	—	Scan, day 7
PAIMS 1992	↑ 2 h	→ 7 day	↑ 2 h PAP/CI	—	Scan/angio, day 7
Goldhaber 1993	—	↑ 24 h	—	↑ 3, 24 h	—

HTN, hypertension; PVR, pulmonary vascular resistance; PAP/CI, pulmonary artery pressure/cardiac index.

randomized to the heparin treatment. Third, there does not appear to be any difference related to the effectiveness of thrombolytic agents provided that they are given in equivalent doses over a similar time frame (70,87). This is best exemplified in trials that compared rT-PA given over 2 hours and urokinase given in the same time interval (70). Fourth, bleeding complications from thrombolytic therapy remain a substantial concern with major hemorrhage report occurring in approximately 12% of patients and fatal hemorrhage occurring in 1% to 2% of patients (88). Intracranial hemorrhage rates have been reported from 1.2% to 2.1% (89) and is fatal in at least half of the cases (90). Last, there does not appear to be a difference between intrapulmonary thrombolytic therapy and peripheral IV thrombolytic therapy (91).

Assessing the efficacy of thrombolytic therapy can be difficult in the first several hours. Echocardiographic studies undertaken prior to the use of thrombolytic therapy have suggested that there are two types of morphologic characteristics of PE that may assist in defining the efficacy of therapy. Thrombi that are long, mobile, and hypoechoic/heterogeneous seem to be more susceptible to thrombolytic therapy. In contrast, echocardiographically defined emboli that are immobile and hyperechoic/homogeneous seem less susceptible to thrombolytic therapy. In a small case report series of patients who received thrombolytic therapy and had the previous characterizations made by echocardiography, long mobile hypoechoic emboli had higher cardiac outputs, lower central venous pressures, and diminished peripheral vascular resistance compared to the group with echocardiographically defined immobile embolism after the use of thrombolytic therapy. It is important to note that the mortality in the group that underwent successful embolectomy was 0% compared to a 30% mortality in the group that failed to respond to thrombolytic therapy (92). Monitoring the efficacy of thrombolytic therapy can similarly be challenging as continuous echocardiography and imaging studies are not available. Monitoring of end-tidal CO_2 has been proposed to monitor the efficacy of thrombolytic therapy. End-tidal CO_2 was found to significantly increase in patients who survived with thrombolytic therapy compared to those with no appreciable change in end-tidal CO_2 measurements in patients who did not survive. This would suggest that continuous monitoring of end-tidal CO_2 enables assessment of the efficacy of thrombolytic therapy and may be used as a barometer to define the need of subsequent thrombolytic or embolectomy in cases of failed thrombolytic therapy (93). Unsuccessful thrombolysis is reported to occur in approximately 8% of patients undergoing therapy. This may be defined as persistent clinical instability or significant residual echocardiographic dysfunction. In the limited literature that compares repeat thrombolysis to surgical thromboembolectomy, there appears to be significant survival benefit in undertaking surgical embolectomy. The mortality in patients undergoing surgical embolectomy after failed thrombolytic therapy was reported to be 7% compared to 38% of patients who underwent repeat thrombolysis. Recurrent PE was significantly higher in patients who underwent repeat thrombolysis and was the cause of death in a significant number of patients. It should be noted that patients who underwent surgical thromboembolectomy also had the placement of vena cava filters (94).

Thrombolytic therapy in hemodynamically stable patients remains a continuing and controversial topic. Multiple reviews and meta-analyses are available to assist with the use of thrombolytic therapy (95–97) (Cochrane Collaboration 2006, issue 3). The long-term outcome of patients with thrombolytic therapy is not well described but it appears that most patients undergo an uneventful course, the mortality is approximately 8%, and major bleeding is reported to occur in 9.6% with recurrent PE reported in 7.6%. The mean vascular obstruction diminished from 64% to 29% within 48 hours, and right ventricular function was reversible within 48 hours in 80% of the patients, while lung scan improved 45% within 6 to 8 days of therapy. This contemporary review of thrombolytic therapy similarly reported that predictive indicators of a poor hospital course in patients receiving thrombolytic therapy were an initial pulmonary vascular obstruction greater than 70% and hemodynamic instability at presentation associated with persistence of paradoxical septal motion on echocardiography. Long-term mortality was related to older age, persistence of vascular obstruction more than 30% after thrombolytic therapy, and cancer (98).

Surgical embolectomy is indicated for patients presenting in shock or cardiopulmonary instability and an inability to tolerate thrombolytic therapy. Ideally, these emboli are large and located centrally and consideration of embolectomy is undertaken prior to cardiac arrest. This requires preoperative localization via CT documentation and ideally echocardiographic of right heart function (99). In the era of modern surgical embolectomy, outstanding results have been reported by multiple investigators. In a study that undertook surgical embolectomy with most patients having a contraindication to thrombolytic therapy and significant right ventricular dysfunction, there was a 6% operative mortality and only 12% late deaths from disease other than PE (100). The overall improvement in operative mortality related to surgical thromboembolectomy most likely relates to preop selection of patients who had not experienced cardiac arrest and the use of cardiopulmonary bypass (99).

The approach to hemodynamically stable patients with PE and right ventricular dysfunction remains a controversial and contentious topic. Recently, the use of BNP, which is indicative of right ventricular stress, and troponin levels, which are indicative of myocardial ischemia, have been used in the stratification of this population. These biomarkers have been reported to allow for severity characterization of patients with PE. In instances where there is an absence of an elevation in BNP or troponin levels, the predicted outcome is excellent and these patients do not warrant intensive care evaluation. In contrast, elevations in BNP and troponin levels are associated with a higher mortality and are evolving as discriminators for the use of thrombolytic therapy in patients with PE.

In summary, PE remains a common and lethal problem that usually confronts the intensivist in the form of undifferentiated respiratory failure and shock. Diagnosis is difficult and challenging in the intensive care unit because of the patient complexity and coexistent illnesses. The use of spiral CT scans and echocardiography is evolving to define severity stratification in the ICU population and facilitate the timely diagnosis of PE. It is imperative to incorporate PE into the differential diagnosis of patients with undifferentiated shock, and the use of a structure model for shock diagnosis and therapy is helpful to ensure that PE is expeditiously diagnosed and optimal treatment is undertaken. Thrombolytic therapy is recognized as the treatment of choice for hemodynamically unstable patients, and the optimal approach to the hemodynamically stable patient with right ventricular dysfunction remains to be defined.

References

1. Kasper W, Konstantinides S, Geibel A, et al. Management strategies and determinants of outcome in acute major pulmonary embolism: results of a multicenter registry. *J Am Coll Cardiol.* 1997;30:1165–1171.
2. Goldhaber SZ, Visani L, De Rosa M. Acute pulmonary embolism: clinical outcomes in the international cooperative pulmonary embolism registry (icoper). *Lancet.* 1999;353:1386–1389.
3. Quality AfHRa. Making health care safer: a critical analysis of patient safety practices. April 28, 2008.
4. Cook DJ, Crowther MA, Meade MO, et al. Prevalence, incidence, and risk factors for venous thromboembolism in medical-surgical intensive care unit patients. *J Crit Care.* 2005;20:309–313.
5. Ibrahim EH, Iregui M, Prentice D, et al. Deep vein thrombosis during prolonged mechanical ventilation despite prophylaxis. *Crit Care Med.* 2002;30:771–774.
6. Cook D, Crowther M, Meade M, et al. Deep venous thrombosis in medical-surgical critically ill patients: prevalence, incidence, and risk factors. *Crit Care Med.* 2005;33:1565–1571.
7. Warkentin TE, Greinacher A. Heparin-induced thrombocytopenia and cardiac surgery. *Ann Thor Surg.* 2003;76:638–648.
8. Mustafa S, Stein PD, Patel KC, et al. Upper extremity deep venous thrombosis. *Chest.* 2003;123:1953–1956.
9. Gaitini D, Beck-Razi N, Haim N, et al. Prevalence of upper extremity deep venous thrombosis diagnosed by color Doppler duplex sonography in cancer patients with central venous catheters. *J Ultrasound Med.* 2006; 25:1297–1303.
10. Joffe HV, Kucher N, Tapson VF, et al. Upper-extremity deep vein thrombosis: a prospective registry of 592 patients. *Circulation.* 2004;110:1605–1611.
11. Martinelli I, Battaglioli T, Bucciarelli P, et al. Risk factors and recurrence rate of primary deep vein thrombosis of the upper extremities. *Circulation.* 2004;110:566–570.
12. Murray MT, Coursin DB, Pearl RG, et al., eds. *Critical Care Medicine: Perioperative Management.* 2nd ed. Philadelphia, PA: Lippincott Williams & Wilkins; 2002.
13. Becker DM, Philbrick JT, Walker FB 4th. Axillary and subclavian venous thrombosis. Prognosis and treatment. *Arch Intern Med.* 1991;151:1934–1943.
14. Hingorani A, Ascher E, Lorenson E, et al. Upper extremity deep venous thrombosis and its impact on morbidity and mortality rates in a hospital-based population. *J Vasc Surg.* 1997;26:853–860.
15. Monreal M, Lafoz E, Ruiz J, et al. Upper-extremity deep venous thrombosis and pulmonary embolism. A prospective study. *Chest.* 1991;99:280–283.
16. Fraisse F, Holzapfel L, Couland JM, et al. Nadroparin in the prevention of deep vein thrombosis in acute decompensated COPD. The association of non-university affiliated intensive care specialist physicians of France. *Am J Resp Crit Care Med.* 2000;161:1109–1114.
17. Cade JF. High risk of the critically ill for venous thromboembolism. *Crit Care Med.* 1982;10:448–450.
18. Kappor M KY, Tessler S. Subcutaneous heparin prophylaxis significantly reduces the incidence of venous thromboembolic events in the critically ill. *Crit Care Med.* 1999;27:A69.
19. Samama MM, Cohen AT, Darmon JY, et al. A comparison of enoxaparin with placebo for the prevention of venous thromboembolism in acutely ill medical patients. Prophylaxis in medical patients with enoxaparin study group. *N Engl J Med.* 1999;341:793–800.
20. Leizorovicz A, Cohen AT, Turpie AG, et al. Randomized, placebo-controlled trial of dalteparin for the prevention of venous thromboembolism in acutely ill medical patients. *Circulation.* 2004;110:874–879.
21. Priglinger U, Delle Karth G, Geppert A, et al. Prophylactic anticoagulation with enoxaparin: is the subcutaneous route appropriate in the critically ill? *Crit Care Med.* 2003;31:1405–1409.
22. Rommers MK, Van der Lely N, Egberts TC, et al. Anti-xa activity after subcutaneous administration of dalteparin in ICU patients with and without subcutaneous oedema: a pilot study. *Crit Care (London, England.)* 2006;10:R93.
23. Cohen AT, Davidson BL, Gallus AS, et al. Efficacy and safety of fondaparinux for the prevention of venous thromboembolism in older acute medical patients: Randomised placebo controlled trial. *BMJ.* 2006;332:325–329.
24. Bauer KA, Eriksson BI, Lassen MR, et al. Fondaparinux compared with enoxaparin for the prevention of venous thromboembolism after elective major knee surgery. *N Engl J Med.* 2001;345:1305–1310.
25. Agnelli G, Bergqvist D, Cohen AT, et al. Randomized clinical trial of postoperative fondaparinux versus perioperative dalteparin for prevention of venous thromboembolism in high-risk abdominal surgery. *Br J Surg.* 2005;92:1212–1220.
26. Ginzburg E, Cohn SM, Lopez J, et al. Randomized clinical trial of intermittent pneumatic compression and low molecular weight heparin in trauma. *Br J Surg.* 2003;90:1338–1344.
27. Ramos R, Salem BI, De Pawlikowski MP, et al. The efficacy of pneumatic compression stockings in the prevention of pulmonary embolism after cardiac surgery. *Chest.* 1996;109:82–85.
28. Macdonald RL, Amidei C, Baron J, et al. Randomized, pilot study of intermittent pneumatic compression devices plus dalteparin versus intermittent pneumatic compression devices plus heparin for prevention of venous thromboembolism in patients undergoing craniotomy. *Surg Neurol.* 2003;59:363–372; discussion 372–364.
29. Prevention of venous thromboembolism in the acute treatment phase after spinal cord injury: a randomized, multicenter trial comparing low-dose heparin plus intermittent pneumatic compression with enoxaparin. *J Trauma.* 2003;54:1116–1124; discussion 1125–1116.
30. Trousseau A. Phlegmatia alba dolens: Clinique medicale de l'hotel-dieu de paris. *JB Baillere et Fils.* 1868:652–695.
31. Ansell J. Vena cava filters: do we know all that we need to know? *Circulation.* 2005;112:298–299.
32. Girard P, Stern JB, Parent F. Medical literature and vena cava filters: so far so weak. *Chest.* 2002;122:963–967.
33. Young T, Tang H, Aukes J, et al. Vena caval filters for the prevention of pulmonary embolism. *Cochrane Database Syst Rev.* 2007 Oct 17;(4): CD006212.
34. Decousus H, Leizorovicz A, Parent F, et al. A clinical trial of vena caval filters in the prevention of pulmonary embolism in patients with proximal deep-vein thrombosis. Prévention du Risque d'Embolie Pulmonaire par Interruption Cave Study Group. *N Engl J Med.* 1998;338:409–415.
35. PREPIC Study Group. Eight-year follow-up of patients with permanent vena cava filters in the prevention of pulmonary embolism: the PREPIC (Prévention du Risque d'Embolie Pulmonaire par Interruption Cave) Randomized Study. *Circulation.* 2005;112:416–422.
36. Crochet DP, Stora O, Ferry D, et al. Vena Tech-LGM filter: long-term results of a prospective study. *Radiology.* 1993;188:857–860.
37. Ascher E, Hingorani A, Tsemekhin B, et al. Lessons learned from a 6-year clinical experience with superior vena cava Greenfield filters. *J Vasc Surg.* 2000;32:881–887.
38. Spence LD, Gironta MG, Malde HM, et al. Acute upper extremity deep venous thrombosis: safety and effectiveness of superior vena caval filters. *Radiology.* 1999;210:53–58.
39. Allen TL, Carter JL, Morris BJ, et al. Retrievable vena cava filters in trauma patients for high-risk prophylaxis and prevention of pulmonary embolism. *Am J Surg.* 2005;189:656–661.
40. Antevil JL, Sise MJ, Sack DI, et al. Retrievable vena cava filters for preventing pulmonary embolism in trauma patients: a cautionary tale. *J Trauma.* 2006;60:35–40.
41. Karmy-Jones R, Jurkovich GJ, Velmahos GC, et al. Practice patterns and outcomes of retrievable vena cava filters in trauma patients: an AAST multicenter study. *J Trauma.* 2007;62:17–24; discussion 24–15.
42. Schuster R, Hagedorn JC, Curet MJ, et al. Retrievable inferior vena cava filters may be safely applied in gastric bypass surgery. *Surg Endosc.* 2007;21:2277–2279.
43. Cook D, Douketis J, Crowther MA, et al. The diagnosis of deep venous thrombosis and pulmonary embolism in medical-surgical intensive care unit patients. *J Crit Care.* 2005;20:314–319.
44. Cook D, McMullin J, Hodder R, et al. Prevention and diagnosis of venous thromboembolism in critically ill patients: a Canadian survey. *Crit Care (London, England).* 2001;5:336–342.
45. Kearon C, Gent M, Hirsh J, et al. A comparison of three months of anticoagulation with extended anticoagulation for a first episode of idiopathic venous thromboembolism. *N Engl J Med.* 1999;340:901–907.
46. Taffoni MJ, Ravenel JG, Ackerman SJ. Prospective comparison of indirect CT venography versus venous sonography in ICU patients. *AJR Am J Roentgenol.* 2005;185:457–462.
47. Lim KE, Hsu WC, Hsu YY, et al. Deep venous thrombosis: comparison of indirect multidetector CT venography and sonography of lower extremities in 26 patients. *Clin Imag.* 2004;28:439–444.
48. Goodman LR, Stein PD, Beemath A, et al. CT venography for deep venous thrombosis: continuous images versus reformatted discontinuous images using PIOPED II data. *AJR Am J Roentgenol.* 2007;189:409–412.
49. Watson LI, Armon MP. Thrombolysis for acute deep vein thrombosis. *Cochrane Database Syst Rev.* 2004 Oct 18;(4):CD002783.
50. Enden T, Sandvik L, Klow NE, et al. Catheter-directed Venous Thrombolysis in acute iliofemoral vein thrombosis–the CaVenT study: rationale and design of a multicenter, randomized, controlled, clinical trial (nct00251771). *Am Heart J.* 2007;154:808–814.
51. Stratmann G, Gregory GA. Neurogenic and humoral vasoconstriction in acute pulmonary thromboembolism. *Anesth Analg.* 2003;97:341–354.
52. D'Alonzo GE, Dantzker DR. Gas exchange alterations following pulmonary thromboembolism. *Clin Chest Med.* 1984;5:411–419.
53. Dalen JE, Banas JS Jr., Brooks HL, et al. Resolution rate of acute pulmonary embolism in man. *N Engl J Med.* 1969;280:1194–1199.
54. McDonald IG, Hirsh J, Hale GS, et al. Major pulmonary embolism, a correlation of clinical findings, haemodynamics, pulmonary angiography, and pathological physiology. *Br Heart J.* 1972;34:356–364.
55. McIntyre KM, Sasahara AA. The hemodynamic response to pulmonary

embolism in patients without prior cardiopulmonary disease. *Am J Cardiol.* 1971;28:288–294.

56. Dalen JE, Grossman W. *Profiles in pulmonary embolism: cardiac catheterization and angiography.* Philadelphia, PA: Lea & Febiger; 1980.
57. Petitpretz P, Simmoneau G, Cerrina J, et al. Effects of a single bolus of urokinase in patients with life-threatening pulmonary emboli: a descriptive trial. *Circulation.* 1984;70:861–866.
58. McIntyre KM, Sasahara AA. Determinants of right ventricular function and hemodynamics after pulmonary embolism. *Chest.* 1974;65:534–543.
59. The UKEP study: multicentre clinical trial on two local regimens of urokinase in massive pulmonary embolism. The UKEP Study Research Group. *Eur Heart J.* 1987;8:2–10.
60. McGinn S, White P. Acute cor pulmonale resulting from pulmonary embolism. *JAMA.* 1935;104:1473–1480.
61. Stein PD, Dalen JE, McIntyre KM, et al. The electrocardiogram in acute pulmonary embolism. *Progr Cardiovasc Dis.* 1975;17:247–257.
62. Stein PD, Terrin ML, Hales CA, et al. Clinical, laboratory, roentgenographic, and electrocardiographic findings in patients with acute pulmonary embolism and no pre-existing cardiac or pulmonary disease. *Chest.* 1991;100:598–603.
63. Ferrari E IA, Darcourt J. No scintigraphic evidence of myocardial abnormality in severe pulmonary embolism with electrocardiographic signs of anterior ischemia *Eur Heart J.* 1995;16(Suppl):269 abstract.
64. Stein PD, Athanasoulis C, Greenspan RH, et al. Relation of plain chest radiographic findings to pulmonary arterial pressure and arterial blood oxygen levels in patients with acute pulmonary embolism. *Am J Cardiol.* 1992;69:394–396.
65. Urokinase pulmonary embolism trial. *Circulation.* 1973;47(Suppl):1–108.
66. Stein PD, Goldhaber SZ, Henry JW, et al. Arterial blood gas analysis in the assessment of suspected acute pulmonary embolism. *Chest.* 1996;109:78–81.
67. Stein PD, Goldhaber SZ, Henry JW. Alveolar-arterial oxygen gradient in the assessment of acute pulmonary embolism. *Chest.* 1995;107:139–143.
68. Urokinase pulmonary embolism trial. Phase 1 results: a cooperative study. *JAMA.* 1970;214:2163–2172.
69. Alpert JS, Smith R, Carlson J, et al. Mortality in patients treated for pulmonary embolism. *JAMA.* 1976;236:1477–1480.
70. Meneveau N, Schiele F, Metz D, et al. Comparative efficacy of a two-hour regimen of streptokinase versus alteplase in acute massive pulmonary embolism: immediate clinical and hemodynamic outcome and one-year follow-up. *J Am Coll Cardiol.* 1998;31:1057–1063.
71. Mastora I, Remy-Jardin M, Masson P, et al. Severity of acute pulmonary embolism: evaluation of a new spiral CT angiographic score in correlation with echocardiographic data. *Eur Radiol* 2003;13:29–35.
72. Qanadli SD, El Hajjam M, Vieillard-Baron A, et al. New CT index to quantify arterial obstruction in pulmonary embolism: comparison with angiographic index and echocardiography. *AJR Am J Roentgenol.* 2001; 176:1415–1420.
73. Ghaye B, Ghuysen A, Willems V, et al. Severe pulmonary embolism: pulmonary artery clot load scores and cardiovascular parameters as predictors of mortality. *Radiology.* 2006;239:884–891.
74. Come PC. Echocardiographic evaluation of pulmonary embolism and its response to therapeutic interventions. *Chest.* 1992;101 (Suppl):151S–162S.
75. Konstantinides S GA, Kasper W. Role of cardiac ultrasound in the detection of pulmonary embolism. *Semin Respir Crit Care Med.* 1996;17:39–49.
76. Torbicki A, Tramarin R, Morpurgo M. Role of echo/Doppler in the diagnosis of pulmonary embolism. *Clin Cardiol.* 1992;15:805–810.
77. Jardin F, Dubourg O, Bourdarias JP. Echocardiographic pattern of acute cor pulmonale. *Chest.* 1997;111:209–217.
78. Kasper W, Geibel A, Tiede N, et al. Distinguishing between acute and subacute massive pulmonary embolism by conventional and Doppler echocardiography. *Br Heart J.* 1993;70:352–356.
79. Kasper W, Geibel A, Tiede N, et al. Echocardiography in the diagnosis of lung embolism [in German]. *Herz.* 1989;14:82–101.
80. Mercat A, Diehl JL, Meyer G, et al. Hemodynamic effects of fluid loading in acute massive pulmonary embolism. *Crit Care Med.* 1999;27:540–544.
81. Angle MR, Molloy DW, Penner B, et al. The cardiopulmonary and renal hemodynamic effects of norepinephrine in canine pulmonary embolism. *Chest.* 1989;95:1333–1337.
82. Hirsch LJ, Rooney MW, Wat SS, et al. Norepinephrine and phenylephrine effects on right ventricular function in experimental canine pulmonary embolism. *Chest.* 1991;100:796–801.
83. Capellier G, Jacques T, Balvay P, et al. Inhaled nitric oxide in patients with pulmonary embolism. *Intens Care Med.* 1997;23:1089–1092.
84. Webb SA, Stott S, van Heerden PV. The use of inhaled aerosolized prostacyclin (IAP) in the treatment of pulmonary hypertension secondary to pulmonary embolism. *Intens Care Med.* 1996;22:353–355.
85. Tissue plasminogen activator for the treatment of acute pulmonary embolism. A collaborative study by the PIOPED investigators. *Chest.* 1990; 97:528–533.
86. Jerjes-Sanchez C, Ramirez-Rivera A, de Lourdes Garcia M, et al. Streptokinase and heparin versus heparin alone in massive pulmonary embolism: a randomized controlled trial. *J Thromb Thrombol.* 1995;2:227–229.
87. Goldhaber SZ, Kessler CM, Heit JA, et al. Recombinant tissue-type plasminogen activator versus a novel dosing regimen of urokinase in acute pulmonary embolism: a randomized controlled multicenter trial. *J Am Coll Cardiol.* 1992;20:24–30.
88. Levine MN. Thrombolytic therapy for venous thromboembolism. Complications and contraindications. *Clin Chest Med.* 1995;16:321–328.
89. Dalen JE, Alpert JS, Hirsh J. Thrombolytic therapy for pulmonary embolism: is it effective? Is it safe? When is it indicated? *Arch Int Med.* 1997;157:2550–2556.
90. Arcasoy SM, Kreit JW. Thrombolytic therapy of pulmonary embolism: a comprehensive review of current evidence. *Chest.* 1999;115:1695–1707.
91. Verstraete M, Miller GA, Bounameaux H, et al. Intravenous and intrapulmonary recombinant tissue-type plasminogen activator in the treatment of acute massive pulmonary embolism. *Circulation.* 1988;77:353–360.
92. Podbregar M, Krivec B, Voga G. Impact of morphologic characteristics of central pulmonary thromboemboli in massive pulmonary embolism. *Chest.* 2002;122(3):973–979.
93. Wiegand UK, Kurowski V, Giannitsis E, et al. Effectiveness of end-tidal carbon dioxide tension for monitoring thrombolytic therapy in acute pulmonary embolism. *Crit Care Med.* 2000;28:3588–3592.
94. Meneveau N, Seronde MF, Blonde MC, et al. Management of unsuccessful thrombolysis in acute massive pulmonary embolism. *Chest.* 2006;129:1043–1050.
95. Agnelli G, Becattini C, Kirschstein T. Thrombolysis vs heparin in the treatment of pulmonary embolism: a clinical outcome-based meta-analysis. *Arch Int Med.* 2002;162:2537–2541.
96. Thabut G, Thabut D, Myers RP, et al. Thrombolytic therapy of pulmonary embolism: a meta-analysis. *J Am Coll Cardiol.* 2002;40:1660–1667.
97. Wan S, Quinlan DJ, Agnelli G, et al. Thrombolysis compared with heparin for the initial treatment of pulmonary embolism: a meta-analysis of the randomized controlled trials. *Circulation.* 2004;110:744–749.
98. Meneveau N, Ming LP, Seronde MF, et al. In-hospital and long-term outcome after sub-massive and massive pulmonary embolism submitted to thrombolytic therapy. *Eur Heart J.* 2003;24:1447–1454.
99. Aklog L. Emergency surgical pulmonary embolectomy. *Semin Vasc Med.* 2001;1:235–246.
100. Leacche M, Unic D, Goldhaber SZ, et al. Modern surgical treatment of massive pulmonary embolism: results in 47 consecutive patients after rapid diagnosis and aggressive surgical approach. *J Thor Cardiovasc Surg.* 2005;129:1018–1023.

CHAPTER 143 ■ OTHER EMBOLIC SYNDROMES (AIR, FAT, AMNIOTIC FLUID)

MURAT SUNGUR • KÜRSAT UZUN

Pulmonary embolism usually results from the mobilization of blood clots from lower extremity or pelvis thromboses. However, embolization of other materials, including air, fat, and amniotic fluid, can also obstruct the pulmonary vessels. While these emboli are uncommon, they are generally associated with clear risk factors or precipitating events. In this chapter, the pathophysiology, clinical course, and treatment of these "other" embolic phenomena are discussed.

GAS EMBOLISM

Gas embolism is defined as the entrance of gas into the vascular compartment. Air and other gases—such as carbon dioxide and nitrogen—may result in gas emboli. The gas may reach any organ, but the most significant damage is to the organs with high oxygen consumption rates, such as brain and heart. Gas embolism can be venous or arterial and, most frequently, it is an iatrogenic problem that may be fatal (1). Hence, prevention of gas embolism is an important patient safety issue that necessitates physician awareness.

Given that, most often, gas embolism is an iatrogenic problem (Table 143.1), the highest-risk surgical procedures for venous air embolism (VAE) are sitting neurosurgical operations, posterior fossa and neck surgery, laparoscopic procedures, total hip arthroplasty, cesarean section, and central venous line procedures—both placement and removal. In addition to these factors, there are numerous case studies reporting emboli during different procedures.

During a neurosurgical procedure in the sitting position, air usually enters through the noncollapsing veins, including the dural venous sinuses and emissary veins (2). While the true incidence of VAE is unknown—because most cases are asymptomatic and the sensitivity of detection methods differs significantly—the incidence is reported to be between 7% and 50% using Doppler detection methodology (3,4). However, one study that used the transesophageal detection method reported an incidence of 76% (5).

Pathophysiology

The severity of gas embolism is related to the volume of gas entering the circulation as well as the rate of gas accumulation. In a neurologic surgery case performed in the sitting position, the volume and rate of air entry are determined by the position of the patient, venous pressure, and height of the vein above the heart. The fatal gas volume in humans is unknown, but in a canine model, it is 7.5 mL/kg (6); the *estimated* fatal volume for humans is between 200 and 300 mL (7). A patient's underlying cardiac disease may impact the volume of air necessary for lethality. For example, with underlying impaired cardiac contractility, the volume of air needed to cause cardiac arrest is less than in adults with normal cardiac function (7).

Entry of air into the pulmonary venous system acutely increases pulmonary artery pressure, degrades gas exchange, and provokes cardiac dysrhythmias (8,9). Mean arterial pressure (MAP) decreases rapidly, perhaps secondary to an immediate decrease in cardiac output or due to a reflex mechanism resulting in the release of vasoactive substances (8,9). A "paradoxical" gas embolism can occur in the presence of a right-to-left shunt, such as in a patient with a patent foramen ovale. The term *paradoxical* is used, as the right-sided pressures need be higher than those on the left side for passage of the gas from the right to the left heart. Right-sided heart pressures may be increased with the application of positive end-expiratory pressure (PEEP), the Valsalva maneuver, and/or a VAE, creating a right-to-left shunt (10).

The lung acts like a filter to prevent gas bubbles from moving through the circulation, but this system can be overwhelmed by a significant load of gas bubbles (11). In animals, it has been noted that at loads of less than 0.15 mL/kg, the lung can totally handle oxygen and nitrogen bubbles, but above this level, gas emboli can transverse the pulmonary bed (11). During mechanical ventilation, depending on the degree of embolization, pulmonary gas embolism impairs pulmonary gas exchange. How far a steady-state phase in gas exchange can be reached during continuous venous gas infusion depends on whether the circulation can adapt; circulation—as well as gas exchange—can become deficient with significant embolization (12). The hypoxemia and hypercapnia that may be seen with gas embolism are primarily related to significant ventilation-to-perfusion inequality (12).

Arterial gas embolism (AGE) is caused by entry of gas into the arterial system. AGE can be caused by venous gas embolism entering the arterial circulation *via* a right-to-left shunt or directly *via* the pulmonary capillary bed by overloading of the pulmonary filtering capacity. In compressed air diving, the cause of AGE is pulmonary overpressurization by failing to exhale or due to regional gas trapping during ascent, leading to alveolar rupture and entry of gas into pulmonary capillaries. Iatrogenic causes include accidental air injection during cardiopulmonary bypass or angiography. AGE can also be caused by pulmonary barotrauma during mechanical ventilation (13,14) and, although rare, may be a complication of thoracic trauma and lung surgery (15,16). Gas distribution to the organs is dependent upon their blood flow; gas entering the coronary circulation may result in a typical infarct, while gas

TABLE 143.1

ETIOLOGY OF GAS EMBOLISM

Decompression injury	
Vascular entrance of gas	Central line placement and removal Arterial catheterization Invasive radiologic procedures Intra-aortic balloon rupture IV fluid administration Rapid IV infusion systems
Gastrointestinal procedures	Gastrointestinal endoscopy Laparoscopic surgery Endoscopic retrograde cholangiopancreatography
Neurosurgical procedures	Sitting-position craniotomies Posterior fossa surgery Cervical laminectomy Spinal fusion Deep brain stimulator placement Lumbar puncture Epidural catheter placement
Neck procedures	Radical neck dissection Thyroidectomy Nd:YAG laser surgery
Ophthalmologic procedures	Eye surgery
Cardiac procedures	Extracorporeal bypass Coronary angiography
Obstetric and gynecologic procedures	Cesarean section Intravaginal, intrauterine gas insufflation during pregnancy
Orthopedic procedures	Hip surgery Spinal surgery Gas insufflation during arthroscopic surgery
Urologic procedures	Transurethral prostatectomy Radical prostatectomy
Thoracic procedures	Lung biopsy Lung trauma Thoracoscopy Chest tube placement

passing into the cerebral circulation may cause an ischemic stroke.

Diagnosis

The most important diagnostic tool is the patient history. If the patient has undergone a high-risk procedure, a high index of suspicion for gas embolism is required. Symptoms have a wide range, depending on the severity of gas embolism and presence of cerebral embolus. The most common symptoms and signs are acute dyspnea and hemodynamic instability. There are numerous nonspecific symptoms and signs including nausea, vomiting, respiratory distress, tachypnea, wheezing, chest tightness, pallor, sweating, tachycardia, bradycardia, hypotension, and sudden cardiac arrest (17–23). Neurologic symptoms may include acute dizziness, unconsciousness, paresthesias, paraparesis, paraplegia, and/or seizures (17–22). The so-called "mill-wheel murmur" can be auscultated in the precordial area, and is secondary to the presence of air in the cardiac chambers (23). Hemodynamic changes may be the initial signs of gas embolism. Hypotension and an acute increase in pulmonary artery pressure can be observed at early periods of gas embolism (8,9). Central venous pressure may increase, along with a right ventricular pressure increase due to elevated pulmonary artery pressure or air in the right ventricle. The differential diagnosis is very important, as the signs and symptoms of gas embolism are fairly nonspecific (Table 143.2).

Monitoring of end-tidal CO_2 ($PetCO_2$) is routinely used in the operating room and is increasingly available for intubated patients in the intensive care unit (ICU). There are case reports of—and animal studies have shown—a sudden and severe drop in $PetCO_2$ values in cases of gas embolism (19,24). A rapid progressive fall in $PetCO_2$ can be a sign of gas embolism in spite of a normal blood pressure. Thus, capnography should be used in both the operating room and ICU whenever air embolism is a risk (25); in our ICUs, the use of capnography is standard. However, a sudden or progressive drop in $PetCO_2$ is not necessarily a specific sign of gas embolism, even if it indicates the potential presence of an important complication, such as pulmonary thromboembolism, pneumothorax, or airway

TABLE 143.2

DIFFERENTIAL DIAGNOSIS OF GAS EMBOLISM

Pulmonary embolism	Thromboembolism Fat embolism
Respiratory failure	Pulmonary edema Acute bronchospasm Pneumothorax
Stroke	
Cardiac events	Myocardial infarction Pericardial tamponade Arrhythmias with hemodynamic compromise
Shock	Cardiogenic Septic Hypovolemic
Hypoglycemia	

obstruction. In the nonintubated patient, $PetCO_2$ monitoring is neither easy nor routine.

Pulse oximetry is a standard of care for procedures performed in the operating room as well as for ICU patients. A sudden drop in arterial oxygen saturation is a very common finding of gas embolism and typically indicates a severe disturbance of pulmonary function (21,26). Simple chest radiography can also show air in the vascular compartments and heart (1). Electrocardiographic (ECG) changes may be observed related to myocardial ischemia. Often, the first change noted is peaking of the P wave; S-T segment depression can follow peaking of P wave, depending on the severity of gas embolism (27). Hemoconcentration, possibly related to a shift of intravascular fluid to extravascular space, may be observed in patients with gas embolism (28,29).

A precordial Doppler is a sensitive indicator that can be used to detect gas embolism (27). It is placed on the left parasternal border (second or third intercostal space) during a high-risk procedure and appears to be very accurate in diagnosing gas embolism. Transesophageal echocardiography (TEE) is perhaps the most sensitive method for detecting gas embolism (30,31) and is considered the gold standard, but it is costly and more invasive than precordial Doppler monitoring. TEE is increasingly used for routine intraoperative monitoring for detection of VAE during high-risk surgeries such as sitting craniotomies (31). A patent foramen ovale (PFO) can be detected with TEE, which may allow the identification of patients at high risk for paradoxical gas embolism (32). Moreover, TEE can be used as a clinical guide to patient positioning. Esophageal Doppler has been shown to be a sensitive indicator of air embolism; the optimal position for VAE detection has been determined to be at the level of the superior vena cava above its junction with the right atrium (33).

Prevention and Treatment

Gas embolism in the ICU is mostly iatrogenic and is preventable in most cases. The effect of patient positioning after suspected VAE is a controversial issue. It was claimed that dogs subjected to air emboli were more tolerant of air infusion, as indicated by measurement of the hemodynamic variables, while lying on their left sides (34). Investigators speculated that the left lateral recumbent (LLR) position placed the right ventricular outflow tract in a position inferior to the right ventricular cavity, allowing the air bolus to migrate superiorly and removing the obstruction to blood flow (34). The Trendelenburg position is also claimed to prevent the gas embolism from occluding the outflow tract by placing the right ventricular cavity in a more superior position (35). However, recent studies that compared different positions in canine models of VAE showed no benefit of LLR and LLR head-down over supine positions (36,37). Moreover, it was claimed that placing patients with suspected VAE in the supine position might afford physicians a better opportunity to administer supportive therapy, including ventilatory support and oxygen, to establish access for catecholamine delivery and perform cardiopulmonary resuscitation (23). Furthermore, the Trendelenburg position may not decrease the incidence of cerebral microembolism compared to the supine position (38).

Positioning of the patients during central venous line placement and removal is also a matter of debate for the same reasons discussed above. While we recommend following local hospital policy, our practice is to place patients who will have a subclavian or internal jugular venous line inserted in the head-down position. The only situation in which this may not be appropriate is if the patient has elevated intracranial pressure or severely compromised pulmonary function. This policy is also utilized for the removal of central lines. Of course, the placement or removal of femoral venous lines would indicate that the patient be placed in reverse Trendelenburg. Placement or removal of central venous lines (CVLs) should essentially never be done while the patient is in a sitting position.

Patients should be observed when in Trendelenburg position for signs of respiratory distress and anxiety. Spontaneously breathing patients may have a higher risk of VAE compared to mechanically ventilated patients because of negative intrathoracic pressures during inspiration. If cooperative, the patient may be asked to perform a Valsalva maneuver (i.e., breath holding during expiration and humming), which can increase venous pressure (39). Air embolism after catheter removal through the residual tract has also been reported many times in the literature (40,41); thus, proper maintenance of the entrance site should be performed. VAE via a disconnected line or fractured catheter hub may also occur, and maximum attention should be paid to prevent this possibility.

Carbon dioxide (CO_2) embolism can occur during laparoscopic surgery. Most commonly, CO_2 embolism occurs when a pneumoperitoneum is created through a tear in a vessel in the abdominal wall or peritoneum (42). If CO_2 embolism is suspected, insufflation of the gas should be discontinued.

The application of PEEP is not helpful in preventing air embolism during sitting-position craniotomies; furthermore, it may be harmful (2). Low central venous pressure may increase the negative pressure gradient between the atrium and wound site and, thus, the risk for VAE. Increasing central venous pressure to upper normal limits can decrease the risk for VAE (2).

Aggressive resuscitation and cardiopulmonary resuscitation (CPR) should be started immediately following the collapse of the patient. Aggressive volume resuscitation is recommended to increase right atrial pressure, which can prevent further air entry into the venous circulation (23). High-concentration oxygen (100%) maximizes oxygenation of the patient and can also decrease the volume of the embolus via elimination of the nitrogen component of the embolus. Aspiration of air from the right atrium with an existing central venous catheter may remove up to 60% of air (43,44); however, our experience with this technique has not been uniformly positive. Catheter type and position are very important for the successful removal of air; multiorifice catheters are superior to single-lumen catheters (45).

Treatment for Arterial Gas Embolism

Mechanical ventilation in intubated patients can decrease the time it takes to eliminate air from cerebral arteries if performed at a FiO_2 of 1.0 (46); hyperventilation is currently not recommended in mechanically ventilated patients (47). Seizures after cerebral embolism may not respond to benzodiazepines (48), although barbiturates can suppress seizure activity in these patients (49). Hypotension should be avoided, as this can increase bubble entrapment and decrease cerebral blood flow (50). A short period of hypertension can facilitate bubble redistribution through the arterioles to the capillaries and veins (48).

Hyperbaric Oxygen Therapy

Hyperbaric oxygen (HBO) therapy is recommended for cerebral air embolism, and is the gold standard for AGE (51). Patients breathe 100% oxygen above atmospheric pressures with HBO therapy, and the pressure in the chamber decreases the volume of air bubbles and creates significant hyperoxia. With HBO, alveolar PO_2 can reach 2,000 mm Hg. The hyperoxia creates a diffusion gradient for oxygen and nitrogen in the air bubble (52), and the majority of oxygen is dissolved in plasma. These high levels of oxygen that are carried to the tissues can help to reduce cerebral ischemia. HBO can prevent further brain edema development by reducing vascular permeability (53).

The optimal time to start HBO therapy is unclear. Immediate HBO treatment has the best response (52), although delayed therapy—more than 6 hours after injury—may still have benefits (54). The decision for HBO therapy for delayed cases should be based on the clinical status of the patient and the risk of transportation.

FAT EMBOLISM

Fat embolism in a patient with severe crush injury was first described by Zenker in 1862 (55) and, despite the passage of time, there is still no single definition for fat embolism syndrome (FES). Fat embolus is a pathophysiologic condition, and FES is a clinical condition that occurs with fat embolus. The classic presentation of FES is petechial rash, respiratory distress, and confusion, with an onset of 24 to 48 hours following pelvic or long bone fracture. However, the clinically most crucial part of fat embolism syndrome is respiratory insufficiency. Respiratory insufficiency alone can easily be confused with other concomitant problems such as lung contusion, aspiration, and pulmonary edema. Mental status changes may be secondary to cerebral contusion, drugs, and systemic inflammatory response syndrome (SIRS), in addition to FES. If petechial rash is delayed or absent, diagnosis may be very difficult. FES resulted in a 10% to 20% mortality rate in the 1960s and, although it has declined since then, mortality still remains high (56).

TABLE 143.3

CLINICAL FEATURES OF FAT EMBOLISM

Major	Petechial rash
	Respiratory symptoms and bilateral infiltrates on chest radiograph
	Altered mental status
Minor	Tachycardia
	Fever
	Retinal fat or petechia
	Anuria, oliguria, fat globules in urine
	Sudden drop in hemoglobin level
	Sudden thrombocytopenia
	High erythrocyte sedimentation rate
	Fat globules in sputum

While FES has been reported to occur most commonly with long bone fractures, it is also associated with bone marrow transplantation, sickle cell disease, pancreatitis, liposuction, soft tissue injuries, extracorporeal circulation, burns, decompression sickness, high altitude, osteomyelitis, fatty liver, and epilepsy (57). Diagnostic criteria for FES proposed by Gurd are widely used, although not universally accepted (58). The clinical features of FES are divided into major and minor features (Table 143.3). The diagnosis of fat embolism syndrome requires the presence of one major and four minor criteria according to Gurd's study (58). A fat embolism index score has been defined by Schonfeld et al. for predetermined and designated clinical signs and symptoms (59) (Table 143.4). A score of 5 or more is diagnostic of FES, and negative if less than 5.

Epidemiology

It is difficult to estimate the true incidence of fat embolism, as there is no universal definition, and many cases with fat embolus may not develop FES. The true incidence of FES is probably higher than the reported rates—19% in patients with major trauma (60). The occurrence of fat embolism in autopsy reports in trauma patients ranges between 52% and 96% (61–63), whereas only 1% to 5% of patients develop FES (64). The incidence of FES related to femoral shaft fractures has been

TABLE 143.4

FAT EMBOLISM INDEX SCORE

Symptom or Sign	Points
Petechiae	5
Diffuse alveolar infiltrates	4
Hypoxemia (PaO_2 <70 mm Hg)	3
Confusion	1
Fever ≥38.5°C	1
Tachycardia ≥120 beats/min	1
Tachypnea ≥30 breaths/min	1

A positive fat embolism syndrome score is ≥5 points.

reported as 0.9% to 13.2%, depending on the type of fracture and time of stabilization (65–68), although the most recent data suggest an even lower incidence of FES—0.9% to 11% among trauma patients with long bone fractures (66,70). FES seldom occurs with fractures of the upper limb (69).

Patients undergoing nailing of a lower extremity were found to have embolic showers in 41% of cases, but only 16% were defined as severe (66). Fat emboli were noted by TEE in 94% of pathologic femur fractures (59% severe, defined as fat embolism syndrome with respiratory distress), 62% of femur fractures (6% severe), and 94% of tibial fractures (none severe) (71). Paradoxical embolus may occur in patients with a PFO and increases the mortality risk (72); hypoxemia can be seen in 35% to 74% of these patients (73,74). An alveolar-arterial gradient above 20 mm Hg is observed in nearly all patients with uncomplicated long bone and pelvic fractures (75).

The incidence of full-blown FES decreased from 22% to 1.4% after implementation of internal fixation in patients with long bone fractures (75). Timing of fracture fixation has an important impact on the incidence of FES, with early surgery resulting in lesser risk—by as much as fivefold—of FES. While current recommendations suggest that some fractures require earlier skeletal stabilization (75–78), the effect of the fixation method on the incidence of FES has not been extensively studied, and initial reports have shown no difference between plating versus nailing (79). The incidence of FES increases with the number of fractures (78) and, in military situations, in those with femoral shaft fractures from high-velocity missile wounds of the thigh; it is absent in those with low-velocity missile wounds without fracture (80).

Pathophysiology

The two explanations of the pathophysiologic mechanisms of FES are the mechanical and the biochemical theories; in fact, these are likely intimately related.

When bones fracture, or their medullary channel is manipulated or pressurized, fat cells are disrupted and enter the venous circulation. Large fat globules and spongiosa bone fragments can obstruct the pulmonary capillaries. Smaller fat globules bypass the pulmonary circulation and enter the systemic circulation. Major systemic emboli can occur with migration of fat globules through the pulmonary capillary circuit (81,82). As previously mentioned, in the presence of an intracardiac defect—such as a PFO, seen in 20% to 30% of the population (83,84)—there can be direct access of fat particles to the systemic circulation.

Bone marrow fragments have been seen in autopsy specimens of lung tissue from trauma patients (85) and in lung biopsies from similar trauma populations (86). The highest number of obstructed capillaries is seen after 24 hours of the initial injury, and vascular congestion and pulmonary edema follow the obstruction of capillaries (87,88). The amount of fat is an important indicator for the emergence of a full-blown FES because, as the number of fractures increases, the risk for FES does so as well. Mechanical obstruction of the pulmonary artery with fat may be an important reason for immediate death after trauma (82), and obstruction of the cerebral capillaries may be the cause of the altered mental status observed in FES. Petechial hemorrhages may be secondary to the presence of fat emboli in the subcutaneous capillaries.

Manipulation of the bone medulla during surgery increases intramedullary pressure, which normally ranges between 30 and 50 mm Hg. In animal models, if intramedullary pressure increases to 300 to 400 mm Hg, even when the bone is intact, vena cava blood shows large fat emboli (89); this effect is also observed in patients undergoing long bone surgery (90). According to the biochemical theory, increased levels of free fatty acids (FFAs) after bone fracture or manipulation have a direct toxic effect on pneumocytes. These FFAs can either be freely moving in the circulation or accumulate in pulmonary capillaries. Capillary leakage, clot formation, and platelet adhesion resulting from the toxic effects of FFAs lead to organ damage. It is thought that lipase released from pneumocytes breaks down bone marrow fat to glycerol and free fatty acids, the latter in toxic concentrations. FFA damage to the pulmonary endothelium results in capillary damage and nonhydrostatic pulmonary edema (64,91,92).

The role of polymorphonuclear neutrophils (PMNLs) in FES is not clear. Intravenous injection of fat may result in accumulation of PMNLs in the pulmonary capillaries (87). Lung tissue damage, as well as neutrophil and platelet activation, leads to the release of vasoactive substances such as histamine, serotonin, and bradykinin. The result is inflammation and edema, with resultant respiratory distress and multiorgan system failure (93). Orthopedic surgery has a greater influence on the coagulation system than does general surgery. Manipulation of bone, with resultant fat embolism, is the reason for the hypercoagulable state seen after orthopedic surgery. This includes increased platelet aggregation (94) and tissue factor release, both of which stimulate the coagulation system (94) and result in capillary clot formation in the pulmonary circulation; activation of monocytes induces pericellular fibrin deposition, which further increases the hypercoagulable state (95,96).

NO, phospholipase (PL)-A_2, O_2-free radicals, and proinflammatory cytokines such as tumor necrosis factor (TNF)-α, interleukin (IL)-1β, and IL-10 play a role in the pathogenesis of FES-induced acute respiratory distress syndrome (ARDS). Alveolar macrophages are probably the major source of inducible NO synthase, producing NO in the lung (97).

Neurologic signs of FES likely occur via several mechanisms, including cerebral blood vessel occlusion by fat emboli, disruption of the blood–brain barrier due to toxic FFAs, and obstruction due to alteration in the solubility of fat in blood (98,99).

Clinical Presentation and Diagnosis

Unfortunately, there is no universal definition for FES. The diagnosis of FES requires a high index of suspicion in the proper setting, and is a diagnosis of exclusion. The severity of symptoms and signs depends on the size of the fat embolus. The classical triad for fat embolism includes respiratory insufficiency, altered mental status, and upper extremity and thoracic petechiae; unfortunately, all three are seldom seen together. The most commonly used criteria for FES were defined by Gurd (58). According to these criteria, there are major and minor signs and symptoms. At least one major and four minor criteria are required for the diagnosis of FES (Table 143.3) (58). Clinical signs do not usually appear within 12 hours after the injury, and the major signs appear within 24 hours in 65% and within 48 hours in 85% of patients (56).

The most common signs and symptoms of FES are hypoxia, fever, tachycardia, anemia, and altered mental status (66). Early fever, >38.5°C, is a common sign and may be seen at presentation to the emergency department (56). In trauma patients with fractures, early fever should provoke a suspicion of fat embolism. Petechiae are very important findings, but only present in one third of patients (66); microscopic examination of petechiae reveal fat droplets obstructing capillaries (56).

Respiratory involvement is the most common feature, with tachypnea, dyspnea, and bilateral diffuse infiltrates evident on chest radiograph (61). Cyanosis can be observed if hypoxia is significant, but anemia along with FES can prevent the occurrence of cyanosis even with significant hypoxia. The $PaCO_2$ initially decreases secondary to hyperventilation; however, if pulmonary deterioration continues, it may rise. Chest radiography shows diffuse bilateral pulmonary infiltrates; 70% of the patients demonstrate chest radiographic changes no later than 48 hours—and usually within 24 hours—after injury (100).

The early clinical signs of FES are actually the signs of SIRS. The clinical presentation of FES is also very similar to ARDS with multiple organ failure. Thus, in the presence of multiple injuries, the clinicopathologic features of FES and acute lung injury (ALI)/ARDS overlap to such an extent that absolute distinction is usually not possible (101).

With FES, cardiac output can decrease, and ventilation–perfusion mismatch will occur (102). Hemodynamic compromise secondary to fat embolism can be severe enough to cause cardiac arrest (103). Pulmonary artery pressure increases after femoral and tibial pressurization, and fat globules can be seen in the lungs, kidneys, and brain parenchyma (89). Blood drawn from the right atrium or pulmonary artery may show fat globules; however, fat droplets in plasma can be observed in more than half of trauma patients without FES (104,105). A retinal exam may reveal exudates, hemorrhages, and, rarely, fat globules (58).

High-resolution chest computed tomography (CT) scan findings of FES include ground glass opacities, which may be associated with thickened interlobular septa. A patchy distribution resulting in a "geographic" appearance, which represents the existence of normal and abnormal lung areas with sharp borders and nodular patterns, can also be observed. Resolution of the abnormalities occurs within 2 weeks (105).

Cerebral manifestations can occur with a wide range of symptoms ranging from confusion, drowsiness, and lethargy to convulsions and coma (106–109). Pulmonary contusion along with long bone fractures may increase the risk for cerebral fat embolism (110).

Typically in FES, a cerebral CT scan reveals no abnormalities, even in patients with neurologic symptoms (111). Cerebral magnetic resonance imaging (MRI) may demonstrate hypointense lesions, disruption of the blood–brain barrier, and multiple diffuse foci of hyperintensity in the white matter of the subcortical, periventricular, and centrum semiovale regions, as well as changes related to vasogenic edema, petechial hemorrhages, or hemorrhagic infarcts involving gray and white matter ranging in size from a few millimeters to several centimeters (112,113). Transcranial Doppler study in trauma patients with long bone fractures can detect cerebral fat embolism (114).

Identification of fat droplets within cells recovered with bronchoalveolar lavage is another diagnostic tool that may be used. However, such findings are also frequently observed in trauma patients without FES (115,116).

Treatment

As there is no specific treatment for FES, therapy is mostly supportive. The general goals for hypoxic respiratory failure should be instituted for presumed FES. Methylprednisolone given prophylactically may reduce the incidence of FES and can reduce the degree of hypoxemia associated with long bone fractures of the lower extremity (117,118). High-dose prophylactic steroids with aspirin can result in significant normalization of blood gases, coagulation proteins, and platelet numbers; however, prophylactic steroids did not improve mortality in any of the studies. Fluid loading, which dilutes the amount of free fatty acids, or increased glucose intake, which decreases free fatty acid mobilization, has not been found to be helpful (117,119). FES may lead to cerebral edema and increased intracranial pressure (ICP) and, if there are signs of cerebral edema, intracranial pressure monitoring is recommended (120). Sedation and analgesia should be appropriately titrated to allow for frequent neurologic examinations of the patient. Ethanol with its antilipolytic effect has also been studied, but did not show any benefit in the prevention of fat embolism (121).

Early fixation of long bone fractures can be helpful to prevent the occurrence of FES. However, it should be kept in mind that, in addition to fat embolization from the initial trauma, long bone fixation may result in additional embolizations and FES (122). Delayed stabilization of the fracture in the patient with multiple injuries increases the incidence of pulmonary complications (ARDS, fat embolism, and pneumonia), as well as the hospital and ICU stay. The cost of hospital care also significantly increases for patients who had delayed treatment of the fractures compared with those who were stabilized early (123, 124). Early femur fracture fixation in patients with chest and head trauma is associated with an improved outcome (125).

Increased intramedullary pressure increases the risk of fat embolism. Reaming before nailing the femur was considered as a possible way to prevent this effect, although the reaming procedure itself increases intramedullary pressure. Reaming before femoral nail insertion did not decrease fat embolism compared to the unreamed technique (126).

AMNIOTIC FLUID EMBOLISM

Ricardo Meyer first described the entry of amniotic fluid into the maternal circulation in 1926 (127). However, amniotic fluid embolism (AFE) was not recognized as a syndrome until Steiner and Luschbaugh's study in 1941. They reported a sudden death of a woman during labor with fetal mucin, amorphous eosinophilic material, and squamous cells in pulmonary vessels (128).

Amniotic fluid embolism is an uncommon and catastrophic syndrome that occurs during pregnancy or shortly after delivery. Although the pathophysiology was thought to involve the embolization of amniotic fluid, investigations showed that the syndrome results from biochemical mediators released after the embolization occurs (129). It has been suggested that the syndrome be renamed as the "anaphylactoid syndrome of pregnancy" because of similarities among the characteristics of AFE, septic shock, and anaphylactic shock (130).

Amniotic fluid embolism is an important cause of maternal death in developed countries, with a high morbidity and mortality rate. The associated mortality and morbidity has dramatically decreased to approximately 16% in recent years (131). The decline in mortality may be due to improved recognition of the disorder, so that even mild cases are included in the analysis, as well as to improvements in resuscitation.

Epidemiology

While the true incidence is not known because of inaccuracies in reporting maternal deaths, lack of data from mild cases, and the fact that AFE is difficult to identify and remains a diagnosis of exclusion, AFE is thought to account for up to 10% of all maternal deaths in the United States (130,132). The UK AFE registry investigated maternal and fetal morbidity and mortality rates between 1997 and 2004. In this registry, the data of 44 women with AFE were studied. The maternal death rate was 29.5% (13 patients) (133). The incidence of pulmonary emboli (PE) cases associated with pregnancy and/or delivery was 0.8% of the total PE cases in Japan. Among them, AFE was found in 73.3% (33 of 45) of the PE cases with vaginal delivery and in 21.2% (7 of 33) of PE cases with cesarean delivery (134). AFE was identified in 19 patients between 1971 and 1988 in Swedish studies (135,136). AFE occurred during labor in 70% of the women, after vaginal delivery in 11%, and during cesarean section in 19%. Kramer et al. (137) conducted an epidemiologic study evaluating the relationship between AFE and the medical induction of labor for the Maternal Health Study Group of the Canadian Perinatal Surveillance System between 1991 and 2002. In this study, the total rate of AFE was 14.8 per 100,000 multiple deliveries and 6.0 per 100,000 singleton deliveries. The mortality rate was 0.8 per 100,000 singleton deliveries, but none was fatal in multiple deliveries (137). Gilbert and Danielsen (138) investigated 1,094,248 deliveries during a 2-year period. Fifty-three singleton pregnancies had the diagnosis of AFE, for a population frequency of 1 per 20,646 pregnancies. Burrows and Khoo (139) published a series of ten cases of AFE with a maternal mortality rate of 22%; neonatal survival rate was 95% and routine discharge was reported as 72% in this study (139).

Pathophysiology

The pathophysiology of AFE remains unclear. Uterine contractions during normal labor force amniotic fluid into the maternal venous circulation through small tears in the lower uterine segment or high endocervical canal (139). In order for AFE to occur, there must be a pressure gradient favoring the entry of amniotic fluid from the uterus into the maternal circulation, as well as ruptured membranes. Small tears in the lower uterine segment and endocervix are common during labor and delivery, and are now thought to be the most likely entry site (140). Two separate life-threatening processes seem to occur either simultaneously or in sequence: cardiorespiratory collapse and coagulopathy.

Cardiorespiratory Collapse

The conventional explanation states that particulate matter such as fetal squamous cells, lanugo, and meconium contained in the amniotic fluid produce pulmonary vascular obstruction, leading to pulmonary hypertension, right- and left-sided heart failure, hypotension, and death. However, current evidence suggests that a mechanical origin is less likely than an immunologic reaction. In this model, pulmonary vasospasm causes physiologic pulmonary artery obstruction as a reaction to abnormal substances such as leukotrienes and metabolites of arachidonic acid in the amniotic fluid (141). Arachidonic acid metabolites have been implicated in the inflammatory response, and may in part be responsible for AFE. The presence of these metabolites in AFE suggests a possible humoral mechanism.

Humoral pathways invoking a proinflammatory response with release of cytokines and arachidonic acid metabolites in AFE, anaphylaxis, and shock may be responsible for the similar clinical presentation. This complex inflammatory cascade with mediator release will lead to a systemic inflammatory response and the development of multiple organ system failure (142).

Mild to moderate elevations in pulmonary artery pressures are only transiently noted in AFE (143). In an attempt to reconcile clinical and experimental findings, a biphasic model is proposed to explain the hemodynamic abnormalities that occur with amniotic fluid emboli (144). Acute pulmonary hypertension and vasospasm may be the initial hemodynamic response. The resulting right heart failure and accompanying hypoxia could account for the cases of sudden death or severe neurologic impairment. The limited hemodynamic data obtained by invasive pulmonary artery monitoring or echocardiography during the hyperacute phase of AFE demonstrated left ventricular failure as the dominant finding (144). Myocardial dysfunction may be the result of a sudden increase in maternal plasma endothelin levels that occurs with the introduction of amniotic fluid, which contains a high concentration of endothelin (145).

Disseminated Intravascular Coagulation

Disseminated intravascular coagulation (DIC), commonly observed as a late sequela, may be attributed to antithrombin- or thromboplastin-type effects of amniotic fluid or even complement activators. Amniotic fluid has highly potent, total thromboplastinlike activity; this procoagulant activity increases with the duration of gestation. Additionally, amniotic fluid has relatively strong antifibrinolytic activity, which causes nonspecific inhibition of the fibrinolytic system; this activity of amniotic fluid also increases during gestation. The fibrinolytic inhibition activity may predispose a patient to DIC and diffuse thrombosis by inhibiting or dampening the usual secondary fibrinolytic response seen in DIC patients. The secondary fibrinolytic response that usually occurs in DIC is responsible for hemorrhage due to plasmin digestion of numerous clotting factors; however, this secondary fibrinolytic response also serves to help keep the circulation free of thrombi (146).

Clinical Presentation

The symptoms of AFE commonly occur during labor (80%) and delivery, or in the immediate postpartum period. AFE can also develop 4 to 48 hours postpartum or after cesarean delivery, amniocentesis, or removal of the placenta, or with first- and second-trimester abortions (147–150). The risk factors associated for AFE are older age, multiparity, marked exaggeration of uterine contraction following rupture of the uterine membranes, or markedly exaggerated uterine contraction due to the use of oxytocin or other uterine stimulatory agents, prolonged

TABLE 143.5

RISK FACTORS OF AMNIOTIC FLUID EMBOLISM

Older age
Multiparity
Physiologic intense uterine contractions
Medical induction of labor
Instrumental vaginal delivery
Prolonged gestation
Cesarean section
Uterine rupture
Polyhydramnios
High cervical tear
Premature placental separation
Intrauterine fetal death
Large fetal size
Meconium staining of the amniotic fluid
Placental abruption
Eclampsia
Fetal distress
Trauma to abdomen
Surgical intervention
Saline amnioinfusion

gestation, instrumented vaginal delivery, eclampsia, polyhydramnios, fetal distress, large fetal size, meconium staining of the amniotic fluid, cesarean section, uterine rupture, high cervical laceration, premature separation of the placenta, and intrauterine fetal death (137,140,146). Blunt abdominal trauma, surgical intervention, cervical suture removal, and saline amnioinfusion are other rare causes of AFE (151–155) (Table 143.5).

The classic clinical presentation of AFE is the sudden onset of dyspnea, respiratory failure, and hypotension, followed by cardiovascular collapse and DIC (128). Cardiorespiratory collapse is almost invariably present. However, the presenting symptom in 51% of patients was respiratory distress, hypotension in 27%, coagulopathy in 12%, and seizures in 10%; fetal bradycardia (17%) and hypotension (13%) are also common presenting features (145).

Typically, the patient is in active labor with intact amnion and develops sudden respiratory failure and circulatory collapse, followed by a systemic thrombohemorrhagic disorder (146). However, in some women, postpartum consumptive coagulopathy appears to be the sole presenting sign. Abrupt fetal bradycardia followed by coagulopathy can occur (156). The exact progression of maternal signs and symptoms in the initial phase of AFE is difficult to identify because of the rarity of the condition and lack of monitoring during the event (138). Acute hypoxia immediately followed by an initial increase in blood pressure, with subsequent hypotension, which is suggestive of left atrial and ventricular failure, can be observed in AFE (157).

Cardiogenic pulmonary edema due to left ventricular failure can occur (158). Seizures occur in 10% to 20% of patients. Profound hypoxia and right-sided heart failure follow pulmonary arterial spasm and may account for the 50% mortality rate within the first hour (159). DIC is a common finding—seen in up to 83%—in most of the women with AFE, and half of these patients develop coagulopathy within 4 hours of initial presentation (130). Typically, the presenting manifestation of DIC is profound hemorrhage, prompting an extensive search for anatomic causes of bleeding. The onset of DIC is variable, and may be seen in either the early phase or later phases of the syndrome (160). There are three identified phases of AFE in humans:

- Phase 1: Pulmonary—Respiratory distress and cyanosis
- Phase 2: Hemodynamic—Pulmonary edema and hemorrhagic shock
- Phase 3: Neurologic—Confusion and coma

These manifestations can occur in combination, separately, and in different magnitudes. If patients survive the initial cardiorespiratory insult, 40% to 50% progress into phase 2, which is characterized by coagulopathy, hemorrhage, and shock. In phase 2, left-sided heart failure is evident and is the most reported sign in humans. Increased pulmonary capillary wedge pressure and central venous pressure are characteristics of pulmonary edema. In phase 3, acute symptoms disappear, and injury to the brain, lung, and renal systems is noted. Phase 3 may last weeks, and patients may die as a result of severe brain and lung injury; infection and multiple organ system failure may also cause death (159).

Diagnosis

AFE is largely a diagnosis of exclusion. The differential diagnosis includes air or thrombotic pulmonary emboli, septic shock, acute myocardial infarction, cardiomyopathy, anaphylaxis, aspiration, placental abruption, eclampsia, uterine rupture, transfusion reaction, and local anesthetic toxicity (161). The diagnosis of amniotic fluid embolism should be considered when a pregnant woman with one or more risk factors suddenly develops respiratory distress, bleeding, or shock. Several methods have been suggested for diagnosing amniotic fluid embolism, but none of these diagnostic tests is reliable (162).

The initial presenting signs are often seen on the ECG and the pulse oximeter. The former may show tachycardia with a right-heart strain pattern and ST-T–wave changes; pulse oximetry may reveal a sudden drop in oxygen saturation (163). The clinical diagnosis is made most frequently in 65% to 70% of cases during labor and much less frequently in 11% of cases in the postpartum period (160).

Initial laboratory data should include an arterial blood gas analysis to determine the adequacy of ventilation and degree of hypoxemia (160). Diagnostic markers for amniotic fluid embolism based on peripheral blood samples have also been introduced. These include sialyl Tn (STN), a mucin-associated disaccharide antigen carried by apomucins, zinc coproporphyrin, and complement factor consumption (164,165). Significantly higher serum STN levels were found in patients with clinically apparent AFE (166). It has been demonstrated that the monoclonal antibody THK-2, an antibody directed to STN, may be a specific pathologic marker for amniotic fluid embolism (166,167). Fetal megakaryocytes and syncytiotrophoblastic cells can be found in maternal pulmonary circulation by monoclonal antibodies (CD-61—GPIIIa, β-hCG, and factor VIII-vW hPL antibodies) and may be diagnostic (168). Laboratory tests to evaluate the development of DIC are the anti–thrombin III level, fibrinopeptide A level, D-dimer level, prothrombin fragment 1.2 (PF 1.2), thrombin precursor protein, and platelet count. More global tests, including the prothrombin time (PT), partial thromboplastin time (PTT), and fibrinogen level, are helpful (146).

When correlated with clinical signs and symptoms, other diagnostic tools may be employed to support the presumptive diagnosis of AFE. Echocardiography may show severe pulmonary hypertension and right ventricular dilatation, with a displaced intraventricular septum pressing on the left ventricle (169). TEE may show right ventricular failure with leftward deviation of the interventricular septum and severe tricuspid regurgitation (170). Chest radiography is a helpful diagnostic tool, but it is limited by a lack of specificity. In mothers with AFE, 24% to 93% of chest radiographs show a pulmonary edema pattern (171); however, multiple patchy, nodular infiltrates and small pleural effusion may also be seen (169).

Histologic examination demonstrates foreign material in the pulmonary capillaries, arterioles, and arteries (172). Special stains such as TKH-2, a monoclonal antibody to fetal glycoprotein sialyl Tn antigen, have been applied to pathologic specimens (172).

Treatment

Treatment is supportive. Despite the decline in mortality, no new therapies have emerged. Aggressive resuscitation may be indicated depending on the clinical presentation. Management strategies include improving oxygenation, support of circulation, and correcting coagulopathy. Arterial and pulmonary artery catheters should be placed to help guide the therapy when hemodynamic deterioration is severe (173). If the fetus is sufficiently mature and is undelivered at the time of maternal cardiac arrest, cesarean section should be instituted as soon as possible (145). Maternal oxygenation up to an arterial oxygen tension of more than 60 mm Hg should be achieved by administering oxygen via a face mask to all nonintubated patients. Tracheal intubation and mechanical ventilation should be instituted in patients with refractory hypoxemia or seizures, or in the comatose individual (174). Vasoactive drug therapy must be tailored to the clinical situation. Dopamine is suggested to enhance cardiac output and support blood pressure, although in severe shock, epinephrine or norepinephrine may be required (175).

In less than 4 hours, half of the patients who survive develop DIC, with massive hemorrhage (128). Therefore, blood products should be prepared ahead of time, and replacement with typed-and-crossed packed red blood cells, or with O-negative blood, is essential (176). Treatment of DIC requires the transfusion of packed red blood cells and blood products. Large-bore IV access is essential because massive transfusion may be required (177). Platelets, cryoprecipitate, and fresh frozen plasma should be administered as guided by laboratory assessment of the thromboelastogram (TEG) or international normalized ratio (INR)/PT/PTT, fibrinogen, and fibrin and fibrin degradation products. Plasma exchange, cardiopulmonary bypass, aprotinin, and recombinant activated factor VII (rVIIa) in the management of the associated coagulopathy are used to treat AFE (178–180). The successful use of uterine arterial embolization to control massive bleeding in two cases of AFE has been described (181). During cardiopulmonary resuscitation and chest compressions, and before delivery, the uterus should be displaced to the left to avoid compressing of the aorta and inferior cava which would compromise maternal venous return to the heart. The uterus can be displaced manually or by placing a wedge under the patient's right hip (160).

Prognosis

AFE remains one of the most feared and lethal complications of pregnancy. The prognosis and mortality of AFE have improved significantly with early diagnosis and prompt and early resuscitative measures. A parturient with a known history of atopy or anaphylaxis is also at a high risk of AFE (182). In the National Amniotic Fluid Embolism Registry, a known history of drug allergy and atopy was found in 41% of the 46 patients with AFE (130). The mainstay of a successful outcome remains the identification of high-risk patients. In some cases, death is inevitable despite early and appropriate management. Neonatal survival is reported as 70%. Although there are many new developments with respect to our knowledge of the diseases, AFE continues to be a catastrophic illness.

SUMMARY

The entry of gas into the arterial or venous system has severe clinical consequences, including death. Gas embolism is mostly an iatrogenic problem, which can be prevented most of the time. Inadvertent entry of air is the major cause of gas embolism, although medical gases such as carbon dioxide, nitrogen, and helium can be responsible. Optimal patient positioning during procedures is the mainstay of the prevention strategies for gas embolism. Hospital-wide protocols for central line placement and removal are of the utmost importance. Aggressive volume resuscitation, administration of 100% oxygen, suctioning of gas from the right side of the heart, and avoiding further entry of gas into the circulation are essential for treating and preventing venous gas embolism. Further measures include transfer of the patient to the critical care unit, vasopressor treatment, and mechanical ventilatory support. Hyperbaric oxygen administration after initial stabilization of the patient with cerebral arterial gas embolism should be performed, if available.

Fat embolism syndrome frequently occurs in trauma patients. Making the diagnosis is rather difficult, and criteria have remained unchanged for the last three decades. Fat embolism becomes clinically apparent with classic signs of respiratory failure, petechial rash, and fever. Treatment is mainly supportive. Early fracture fixation and modern critical care should help minimize the impact of fat embolism. The cornerstone of treatment is preventing hypovolemia and hypoxia, followed by operative stabilization of fractures. Further studies are required to improve our ability to diagnose and treat FES.

AFE is a catastrophic complication, which can lead to death. The etiology and pathophysiology of AFE remain unclear despite many new research developments. A high index of suspicion is required for diagnosis, which remains one of exclusion. Right heart failure that progresses to left heart dysfunction, rapidly developing pulmonary edema, neurologic symptoms, and hematologic abnormalities are the main clinical features of AFE; aggressive supportive treatment should be performed. DIC is a very frequent complication of AFE. Blood and blood products should be prepared in advance for potential major hemorrhages. Tracheal intubation and mechanical ventilation should be instituted in patients with refractory hypoxemia or seizures.

References

1. Novitsky YW, Mostafa G, Sing RF, et al. Fatal cardiac air embolism. *Injury.* 2006;37:78–80.
2. Porter JM, Pidgeon C, Cunningham AJ. The sitting position in neurosurgery: a critical appraisal. *Br J Anaest.* 1999;82:117–128.
3. Voorhies RM, Fraser RA, Van Poznak A. Prevention of air embolism with positive end expiratory pressure. *Neurosurgery.* 1983;12:503–506.
4. Standefer M, Bay JW, Trusso R. The sitting position in neurosurgery: a retrospective analysis of 488 cases. *Neurosurgery.* 1984;14:649–658.
5. Papadopoulos G, Kuhly P, Brock M, et al. Venous and paradoxical air embolism in the sitting position. A prospective study with transoesophageal echocardiography. *Acta Neurochir.* 1994;126:140–143.
6. Oppenheimer MJ, Durant TM, Lynch P. Body position related to venous air embolism and associated cardiovascular-respiratory changes. 1953;225:362–373.
7. Toung TJ, Rossberg MI, Hutchins GM. Volume of air in a lethal venous air embolism. *Anesthesiology.* 2001;94:360–361.
8. Verstappen FT, Bernards JA, Kreuzer F. Effects of pulmonary gas embolism on circulation and respiration in the dog. I. Effects on circulation. *Pflugers Arch.* 1977;368:89–96.
9. Vik A, Brubakk AO, Hennessy TR, et al. Venous air embolism in swine: transport of gas bubbles through the pulmonary circulation. *J Appl Physiol.* 1990;69:237–244.
10. Lynch JJ, Schuchard GH, Gross CM, et al. Prevalence of right-to-left atrial shunting in a healthy population: detection by Valsalva maneuver contrast echocardiography. *Am J Cardiol.* 1984;53(10):1478–1480.
11. Spencer MP, Oyama Y. Pulmonary capacity for dissipation of venous gas emboli. *Aerosp Med.* 1971;42:822–827.
12. Verstappen FT, Bernards JA, Kreuzer F. Effects of pulmonary gas embolism on circulation and respiration in the dog. II. Effects on respiration. *Pflugers Arch.* 1977;368:97–104.
13. Neuman TS. Arterial gas embolism and decompression sickness. *News Physiol Sci.* 2002;17:77–81.
14. Moon RE. Bubbles in the brain: what to do for arterial gas embolism? *Crit Care Med.* 2005;33:909–910.
15. Lion F, Cochard G, Arvieux J, et al. Arterial gas embolism originating from the lung in anaesthesia and intensive care. *Ann Fr Anesth Reanim.* 2007;26:77–80.
16. Hilbert P, Liedke H, Heyne G, et al. Arterial air embolism following multiple injuries after a fall from the tenth floor. *Unfallchirurg.* 2007;110:711–715.
17. Hill BF, Jones JS. Venous air embolism following orogenital sex during pregnancy. *Am J Emerg Med.* 1993;11:155–157.
18. Voorhies RM, Fraser RA. Cerebral air embolism occurring at angiography and diagnosed by computerized tomography. Case report. *J Neurosurg.* 1984;60:177–178.
19. Mattei P, Tyler DC. Carbon dioxide embolism during laparoscopic cholecystectomy due to a patent paraumbilical vein. *J Pediatr Surg.* 2007;42:570–572.
20. Truhlar A, Cerny V, Dostal P, et al. Out-of-hospital cardiac arrest from air embolism during sexual intercourse: case report and review of the literature. *Resuscitation.* 2007;73:475–484.
21. Grifols JR, Ferra C, Sancho JM, et al. A case of non-lethal pulmonary air embolism after leukapheresis catheter removal. *J Clin Apher.* 2005;20:93–94.
22. Turgeman Y, Antonelli D, Atar S, et al. Massive transient pulmonary air embolism during pacemaker implantation under mild sedation: an unrecognized hazard of snoring. *Pacing Clin Electrophysiol.* 2004;27:684–685.
23. Muth CM, Shank E. Gas Embolism. *N Engl J Med.* 2000;342:476–482.
24. Drummond JC, Prutow RJ, Scheller MS. A comparison of the sensitivity of pulmonary artery pressure, end-tidal carbon dioxide, and end-tidal nitrogen in the detection of venous air embolism in the dog. *Anesth Analg.* 1985;64:688–692.
25. Simo Moyo J, Adnet P, Wambo M. Detection of gas embolism in neurosurgery by capnography. Apropos of 32 patients surgically treated in seated position. *Cah Anesthesiol.* 1995;43:77–79.
26. Green BT, Tendler DA. Cerebral air embolism during upper endoscopy: case report and review. *Gastrointest Endosc.* 2005;61:620–623.
27. Gildenberg PL, O'Brien RP, Britt WJ, et al. The efficacy of Doppler monitoring for the detection of venous air embolism. *J Neurosurg.* 1981;54:75–78.
28. Smith RM, Van Hoesen KB, Neuman TS. Arterial gas embolism and hemoconcentration. *J Emerg Med.* 1994;12:147–153.
29. Levin LL, Stewart GJ, Lynch PR, et al. Blood and blood vessel wall changes induced by decompression sickness in dogs. *J Appl Physiol.* 1981;50:944–949.
30. Furuya H, Suzuki T, Okumura F, et al. Detection of air embolism by transesophageal echocardiography. *Anesthesiology.* 1983;58:124–129.
31. Himmelseher S, Pfenninger E, Werner C. Intraoperative monitoring in neuroanesthesia: a national comparison between two surveys in Germany in 1991 and 1997. *Anesth Analg.* 2001;92:166–171.
32. Kwapisz MM, Deinsberger W, Müller M, et al. Transesophageal echocardiography as a guide for patient positioning before neurosurgical procedures in semi-sitting position. *J Neurosurg Anesthesiol.* 2004;16:277–281.
33. Martin RW, Colley PS. Evaluation of transesophageal Doppler detection of air embolism in dogs. *Anesthesiology.* 1983;58:117–123.
34. Durant TM, Long JH, Oppenheimer MJ. Pulmonary (venous) air embolism. *Am Heart J.* 1947;33:269–281.
35. Lambert MJ 3rd. Air embolism in central venous catheterization: diagnosis, treatment, and prevention. *South Med J.* 1982;75:1189–1191.
36. Mehlhorn U, Burke EJ, Butler BD, et al. Body position does not affect the hemodynamic response to venous air embolism in dogs. *Anesth Analg.* 1994;79:734–739.
37. Geissler HJ, Allen SJ, Mehlhorn U, et al. Effect of body repositioning after venous air embolism: an echocardiographic study. *Anesthesiology.* 1997;86:710–717.
38. Rodriguez RA, Cornel G, Weerasena NA, et al. Effect of Trendelenburg head position during cardiac deairing on cerebral microemboli in children: a randomized controlled trial. *J Thorac Cardiovasc Surg.* 2001;121:3–9.
39. Wysoki MG, Covey A, Pollak J, et al. Evaluation of various maneuvers for prevention of air embolism during central venous catheter placement. *J Vasc Interv Radiol.* 2001;12:764–766.
40. Deceuninck O, Roy LD, Moruzi S, et al. Massive air embolism after central venous catheter removal. *Circulation.* 2007;116:e516–518.
41. Mennim P, Coyle CF, Taylor JD. Venous air embolism associated with removal of central venous catheter. *BMJ.* 1992;305:171–172.
42. Joshi GP. Complications of laparoscopy. *Anesthesiol Clin North Am.* 2001;19:89–105.
43. Colley PS, Artru AA. Bunegin-Albin catheter improves air retrieval and resuscitation from lethal venous air embolism in upright dogs. *Anesth Analg.* 1989;68:298–301.
44. Bedford RF, Marshall WK, Butler A, et al. Cardiac catheters for diagnosis and treatment of venous air embolism: a prospective study in man. *J Neurosurg.* 1981;55:610–614.
45. Hanna PG, Gravenstein N, Pashayan AG. *In vitro* comparison of central venous catheters for aspiration of venous air embolism: Effect of catheter type, catheter tip position, and cardiac inclination. *J Clin Anesth.* 1991;3:290–294.
46. Annane D, Troche G, Delisle F, et al. Effects of mechanical ventilation with normobaric oxygen therapy on the rate of air removal from cerebral arteries. *Crit Care Med.* 1994;22:851–857.
47. Van Hulst RA, Haitsma JJ, Lameris TW, et al. Hyperventilation impairs brain function in acute cerebral air embolism in pigs. *Intensive Care Med.* 2004;30:944–950.
48. Tovar EA, Del Campo C, Borsari A, et al. Postoperative management of cerebral air embolism: gas physiology for surgeons. *Ann Thorac Surg.* 1995;60:1138–1142.
49. Bleck TP. Management approaches to prolonged seizures and status epilepticus. *Epilepsia.* 1999;40(Suppl 1):S59–63.
50. Helps SC, Parsons DW, Reilly PL, et al. The effect of gas emboli on rabbit cerebral blood flow. *Stroke.* 1990;21:94–99.
51. Ziser A, Adir Y, Lavon H, et al. Hyperbaric oxygen therapy for massive arterial air embolism during cardiac operations. *J Thorac Cardiovasc Surg.* 1999;117:818–821.
52. Moon RE, de Lisle Dear G, Stolp BW. Treatment of decompression illness and iatrogenic gas embolism. *Respir Care Clin North Am.* 1999;5:93–135.
53. Mink RB, Dutka AJ. Hyperbaric oxygen after global cerebral ischemia in rabbits reduces brain vascular permeability and blood flow. *Stroke.* 1995;26:2307–2312.
54. Mader JT, Hulet WH. Delayed hyperbaric treatment of cerebral air embolism. *Arch Neurol.* 1979;36:504–505.
55. Zenker FA. *Beitrage zur normalen und pathologischen Anatomie der Lunge.* Dresden: Schönfeld; 1862.
56. ten Duis HJ. The fat embolism syndrome. *Injury.* 1997;28:77–85.
57. Peltier LF, Collins JA, Evarts CM, et al. A panel by correspondence. Fat embolism. *Arch Surg.* 1974;109:12–16.
58. Gurd AR. Fat embolism: an aid to diagnosis. *J Bone Joint Surg.* 1970;52:732–737.
59. Schonfeld SA, Ploysongsang Y, Dilisio R, et al. Fat embolism prophylaxis with corticosteroids. A prospective study in high-risk patients. *Ann Intern Med.* 1983;99:438–443.
60. Gurd AR, Wilson RI. The fat embolism syndrome. *J Bone Joint Surg.* 1974;56:408–416.
61. Behn C, Hopker WW, Puschel K. [Fat embolism a too infrequently determined pathoanatomic diagnosis]. *Versicherungsmedizin.* 1997;49:89–93.
62. Emson HE. Fat embolism studied in 100 patients dying after injury. *J Clin Pathol.* 1958;11:28–35.
63. Palmovic V, McCarroll JR. Fat embolism in trauma. *Arch Pathol.* 1965;80:630–635.
64. Peltier LF, Sevitt S. Trauma workshop report: fat embolism. *J Trauma.* 1970;10:1074–1077.
65. Allardyce DB, Meek RN, Woodruff B, et al. Increasing our knowledge of the pathogenesis of fat embolism: a prospective study of 43 patients with fractured femoral shafts. *J Trauma.* 1974;14:955–962.
66. Bulger EM, Smith DG, Maier RV, et al. Fat embolism syndrome. A 10-year review. *Arch Surg.* 1997;132:435–439.

67. Pinney SJ, Keating JF, Meek RN. Fat embolism syndrome in isolated femoral fractures: does timing of nailing influence incidence? *Injury.* 1998;29:131–133.
68. ten Duis HJ, Nijsten MW, Klasen HJ, et al. Fat embolism in patients with an isolated fracture of the femoral shaft. *J Trauma.* 1988;28:383–390.
69. Wildsmith JA, Masson AH. Severe fat embolism: a review of 24 cases. *Scott Med J.* 1978;23:141–148.
70. Fabian TC, Hoots AV, Stanford DS, et al. Fat embolism syndrome: prospective evaluation in 92 fracture patients. *Crit Care Med.* 1990;18:42–46.
71. Pell AC, Christie J, Keating JF, et al. The detection of fat embolism by transoesophageal echocardiography during reamed intramedullary nailing. A study of 24 patients with femoral and tibial fractures. *J Bone Joint Surg Br.* 1993;75:921–925.
72. Christie J, Robinson CM, Pell AC, et al. Transcardiac echocardiography during invasive intramedullary procedures. *J Bone Joint Surg Br.* 1995;77:450–455.
73. Moed BR, Boyd DW, Andring RE. Clinically inapparent hypoxemia after skeletal injury. The use of the pulse oximeter as a screening method. *Clin Orthop Relat Res.* 1993;293:269–273.
74. McCarthy B, Mammen E, Leblanc LP, et al. Subclinical fat embolism: a prospective study of 50 patients with extremity fractures. *J Trauma.* 1973;13:9–16.
75. Riska EB, Myllynen P. Fat embolism in patients with multiple injuries. *J Trauma.* 1982;22:891–894.
76. Talucci RC, Manning J, Lampard S, et al. Early intramedullary nailing of femoral shaft fractures: a cause of fat embolism syndrome. *Am J Surg.* 1983;146:107–111.
77. Meek RN, Vivoda EE, Pirani S. Comparison of mortality of patients with multiple injuries according to type of fracture treatment—a retrospective age- and injury-matched series. *Injury.* 1986;17:2–4.
78. Goris RJ, Gimbrere JS, van Niekerk JL, et al. Early osteosynthesis and prophylactic mechanical ventilation in the multitrauma patient. *J Trauma.* 1982;22:895–903.
79. Bosse MJ, MacKenzie EJ, Riemer BL, et al. Adult respiratory distress syndrome, pneumonia, and mortality following thoracic injury and a femoral fracture treated either with intramedullary nailing with reaming or with a plate. A comparative study. *J Bone Joint Surg Am.* 1997;79:799–809.
80. Collins JA, Gordon WC Jr, Hudson TL, et al. Inapparent hypoxemia in causalities with wounded limbs: pulmonary fat embolism? *Ann Surg.* 1968;167:511–520.
81. Moylan JA, Bimbaum M, Katz A, et al. Fat embolism syndrome. *J Trauma.* 1976;16:341–347.
82. Bierre AR, Koelmeyer TD. Pulmonary fat and bone marrow embolism in aircraft accident victims. *Pathology.* 1983;15:131–135.
83. Pell AC, Hughes D, Keating J, et al. Brief report: fulminating fat embolism syndrome caused by paradoxical embolism through a patent foramen ovale. *N Engl J Med.* 1993;329:926–929.
84. Etchells EE, Wong DT, Davidson G, et al. Fatal cerebral fat embolism associated with a patent foramen ovale. *Chest.* 1993;104:962–963.
85. Kramer M, Penners BM. Postmortem tissue embolisms. Report of 3 cases. *Arch Kriminol.* 1989;183:29–36.
86. Kerstell J. Pathogenesis of post-traumatic fat embolism. *Am J Surg.* 1971; 121:712–715.
87. Jacobovitz-Derks D, Derks CM. Pulmonary neutral fat embolism in dogs. *Am J Pathol.* 1979;95:29–42.
88. Joachim H, Riede UN, Mittermayer C. The weight of human lungs as a diagnostic criterium (distinction of normal lungs from shock lungs by histologic, morphometric and biochemical investigations). *Pathol Res Pract.* 1978;162:24–40.
89. Schemitsch EH, Turchin DC, Anderson GI, et al. Pulmonary and systemic fat embolization after medullary canal pressurization: a hemodynamic and histologic investigation in the dog. *J Trauma.* 1998;45:738–742.
90. Kropfl A, Berger U, Neureiter H, et al. Intramedullary pressure and bone marrow fat intravasation in unreamed femoral nailing. *J Trauma.* 1997;42:946–954.
91. Peltier LF. Fat embolism. A perspective. *Clin Orthop Relat Res.* 1988;232:263–270.
92. Baker PL, Pazell JA, Peltier LF. Free fatty acids, catecholamines, and arterial hypoxia in patients with fat embolism. *J Trauma.* 1971;11:1026–1030.
93. Goodman RB, Pugin J, Lee JS, et al. Cytokine-mediated inflammation in acute lung injury. *Cytokine Growth Factor Rev.* 2003;14:523–535.
94. Gierckskу KE. The procoagulant activity of adipose tissue. *Scand J Haematol.* 1977;19:385–395.
95. Dahl OE, Pedersen T, Kierulf P, et al. Sequential intrapulmonary and systemic activation of coagulation and fibrinolysis during and after total hip replacement surgery. *Thromb Res.* 1993;70:451–458.
96. Hogevold HE, Lyberg T, Kierulf P, et al. Generation of procoagulant (thromboplastin) and plasminogen activator activities in peripheral blood monocytes after total hip replacement surgery. Effects of high doses of corticosteroids. *Thromb Res.* 1991;62:449–457.
97. Kao SJ, Yeh DY, Chen HI. Clinical and pathological features of fat embolism with acute respiratory distress syndrome. *Clin Sci.* 2007;113:279–285.
98. Drew PA, Smith E, Thomas PD. Fat distribution and changes in the blood brain barrier in a rat model of cerebral arterial fat embolism. *J Neurol Sci.* 1998;156:138–143.
99. Kim HJ, Lee CH, Lee SH, et al. Early development of vasogenic edema in experimental cerebral fat embolism in cats: correlation with MRI and electron microscopic findings. *Invest Radiol.* 2001;36:460–469.
100. Muangman N, Stern EJ, Bulger EM, et al. Chest radiographic evolution in fat embolism syndrome. *J Med Assoc Thai.* 2005;88:1854–1860.
101. Robinson CM. Current concepts of respiratory insufficiency syndromes after fracture. *J Bone Joint Surg.* 2001;83:781–791.
102. Ereth MH, Weber JG, Abel MD, et al. Cemented versus noncemented total hip arthroplasty—embolism, hemodynamics, and intrapulmonary shunting. *Mayo Clin Proc.* 1992;67:1066–1074.
103. Fallon KM, Fuller JG, Morley-Forster P. Fat embolization and fatal cardiac arrest during hip arthroplasty with methylmethacrylate. *Can J Anesth.* 2001;48:626–629.
104. Adolph MD, Fabian HF, el-Khairi SM, et al. The pulmonary artery catheter: a diagnostic adjunct for fat embolism syndrome. *J Orthop Trauma.* 1994;8:173–176.
105. Malagari K, Economopoulos N, Stoupis C, et al. High-resolution CT findings in mild pulmonary fat embolism. *Chest.* 2003;123:1196–1201.
106. Evarts CM. The fat embolism syndrome: a review. *Surg Clin North Am.* 1970;50:493–507.
107. Bortone E, Bettoni G, Giorgi C, et al. Adult postanoxic "erratic" status epilepticus. *Epilepsia.* 1992;33:1047–1050.
108. King MB, Harmon KR. Unusual forms of pulmonary embolism. *Clin Chest Med.* 1994;15:561–580.
109. Bolesta MJ. Fat embolism syndrome without adult respiratory distress syndrome. *N C Med J.* 1986;47:257.
110. Aydin MD, Akçay F, Aydin N, et al. Cerebral fat embolism: pulmonary contusion is a more important etiology than long bone fractures. *Clin Neuropathol.* 2005;24:86–90.
111. Sakamoto T, Sawada Y, Yukioka T, et al. Computed tomography for diagnosis and assessment of cerebral fat embolism. *Neuroradiology.* 1983;24:283–285.
112. Simon AD, Ulmer JL, Strottmann JM. Contrast-enhanced MR imaging of cerebral fat embolism: case report and review of the literature. *AJNR Am J Neuroradiol.* 2003;24(1):97–101.
113. Chen JJ, Ha JC, Mirvis SE. MR imaging of the brain in fat embolism syndrome. *Emerg Radiol.* 2007.
114. Forteza AM, Koch S, Romano JG, et al. Transcranial Doppler detection of fat emboli. *Stroke.* 1999;30:2687–2691.
115. Chastre J, Fagon JY, Soler P, et al. Bronchoalveolar lavage for rapid diagnosis of the fat embolism syndrome in trauma patients. *Ann Intern Med.* 1990;113:583–588.
116. Roger N, Xaubet A, Agustí C, et al. Role of bronchoalveolar lavage in the diagnosis of fat embolism syndrome. *Eur Respir J.* 1995;8:1275–1280.
117. Stoltenberg JJ, Gustilo RB. The use of methylprednisolone and hypertonic glucose in the prophylaxis of fat embolism syndrome. *Clin Orthop Relat Res.* 1979;143:211–221.
118. Babalis GA, Yiannakopoulos CK, Karliaftis K, et al. Prevention of posttraumatic hypoxaemia in isolated lower limb long bone fractures with a minimal prophylactic dose of corticosteroids. *Injury.* 2004;35:309–317.
119. Shier MR, Wilson RF, James RE, et al. Fat embolism prophylaxis: a study of four treatment modalities. *J Trauma.* 1977;17:621–629.
120. Sie MY, Toh KW, Rajeev K. Cerebral fat embolism: an indication for ICP monitor? *J Trauma.* 2003;55:1185–1186.
121. White T, Petrisor BA, Bhandari M. Prevention of fat embolism syndrome. *Injury.* 2006;37(Suppl 4):S59–67.
122. Habashi NM, Andrews PL, Scalea TM. Therapeutic aspects of fat embolism syndrome. *Injury.* 2006;37(Suppl 4):S68–73.
123. Bone LB, Johnson KD, Weigelt J, et al. Early versus delayed stabilization of femoral fractures. A prospective randomized study. *J Bone Joint Surg Am.* 1989;71:336–340.
124. Behrman SW, Fabian TC, Kudsk KA, et al. Improved outcome with femur fractures: early vs. delayed fixation. *J Trauma.* 1990;30:792–797.
125. Brundage SI, McGhan R, Jurkovich GJ, et al. Timing of femur fracture fixation: effect on outcome in patients with thoracic and head injuries. *J Trauma.* 2002;52:299–307.
126. Coles RE, Clements FM, Lardenoye JW, et al. Transesophageal echocardiography in quantification of emboli during femoral nailing: reamed versus unreamed techniques. *J South Orthop Assoc.* 2000;9:98–104.
127. Meyer JR. Embolia pulmonary amino caseosa. *Bras Med.* 1926;2:301–303.
128. Steiner PE, Lauschbaugh C. Landmark article, Oct. 1941: Maternal pulmonary embolism by amniotic fluid as a cause of obstetric shock and unexpected deaths in obstetrics. *JAMA.* 1986;255:2187–2203.
129. Cromley MG, Taylor PJ, Cumming DC. Probable amniotic fluid embolism after first trimester termination. A case report. *J Reprod Med.* 1983;28:209–211.
130. Clark SL, Hankins GD, Dudley DA, et al. Amniotic fluid embolism: analysis of the national registry. *Am J Obstet Gynecol.* 1995;172:1158–1167.
131. Tuffnell DJ. Amniotic fluid embolism. *Curr Opin Obstet Gynecol.* 2003;15: 119–122.

132. Schandl CA, Collins KA. Maternal autopsy. In: Collins KA, Hutchins GM, eds. *Autopsy Performance & Reporting*. 2nd ed. Northfield, IL: College of American Pathologists; 2003:135–147.
133. Tuffnell DJ. United Kingdom Amniotic fluid embolism register. *BJOG*. 2005;112:1625–1629.
134. Sakuma M, Sugimura K, Nakamura M, et al. Unusual pulmonary embolism-septic pulmonary embolism and amniotic fluid embolism. *Circ J*. 2007;71:772–775.
135. Hogberg U. Maternal deaths in Sweden, 1971–1980. *Acta Obstet Gynecol Scand*. 1986;65:161–167.
136. Hogberg U, Innala E, Sandstrom A. Maternal mortality in Sweden, 1980–1988. *Obstet Gynecol*. 1994;84:240–244.
137. Kramer MS, Rouleau J, Baskett TF, et al. Amniotic-fluid embolism and medical induction of labour: a retrospective, population-based cohort study. *Lancet*. 2006;368:1444–1448.
138. Gilbert WM, Danielsen B. Amniotic fluid embolism: decreased mortality in a population-based study. *Obstet Gynecol*. 1999;93:973–977.
139. Burrows A, Khoo SK. The amniotic fluid embolism syndrome: 10 years' experience at a major teaching hospital. *Aust N Z J Obstet Gynaecol*. 1995;35:245–250.
140. Christiansen LR, Collins KA. Pregnancy-associated deaths: a 15-year retrospective study and overall review of maternal pathophysiology. *Am J Forensic Med Pathol*. 2006;27:11–19.
141. Rossi SE, Goodman PC, Franquet T. Nonthrombotic pulmonary emboli. *AJR Am J Roentgenol*. 2000;174:1499–1508.
142. Aurangzeb I, George L, Roof S. Amniotic fluid embolism. *Crit Care Clin*. 2004;20:643–650.
143. Hankins GDV, Snyder RR, Clark SL, et al. Acute hemodynamic and respiratory effects of amniotic fluid embolism in the pregnant goat model. *Am J Obstet Gynecol*. 1993;168:1113–1129.
144. Clark SL, Cotton DB, Gonik B, et al. Central haemodynamic alterations in amniotic fluid embolism. *Am J Obstet Gynecol*. 1988;158:1124–1126.
145. Davies S. Amniotic fluid embolus: a review of literature. *Can J Anesth*. 2001;48:88–98.
146. Bick RL. Disseminated intravascular coagulation: a review of etiology, pathophysiology, diagnosis, and management: guidelines for care. *Clin Appl Thromb Hemost*. 2002;8:1–31.
147. Hassart Th, Essed GG. Amniotic fluid embolism after transabdominal amniocentesis. *Eur J Obstet Gynecol Reprod Biol*. 1983;16:25–30.
148. Malhotra P, Agarwal R, Awasthi A, et al. Delayed presentation of amniotic fluid embolism: lessons from a case diagnosed at autopsy. *Respirology*. 2007;12:148–150.
149. Tramoni G, Valentin S, Robert MO, et al. Amniotic fluid embolism during caesarean section. *Int J Obstet Anesth*. 2004;13:271–274.
150. Ray BK, Vallejo MC, Creinin MD, et al. Amniotic fluid embolism with second trimester pregnancy termination: a case report. *Can J Anesth*. 2004;51(2):139–144.
151. Rainio J, Penttila A. Amniotic fluid embolism as cause of death in a car accident—a case report. *Forensic Sci Int*. 2003;137:231–234.
152. Ellingsen CL, Eggebo TM, Lexow K. Amniotic fluid embolism after blunt abdominal trauma. *Resuscitation*. 2007;75:180–183.
153. Pluymakers C, De Weerdt A, Jacquemyn Y, et al. Amniotic fluid embolism after surgical trauma: two cases reports and review of the literature. *Resuscitation*. 2007;72:324–332.
154. Haines J, Wilkes RG. Non-fatal amniotic fluid embolism after cervical suture removal. *Br J Anesth*. 2003;90:244–247.
155. Dorairajan G, Soundararaghavan S. Maternal death after intrapartum saline amnioinfusion—report of two cases. *BJOG*. 2005;112:1331–1333.
156. Levy R, Furman B, Hagay ZJ. Fetal bradycardia and disseminated coagulopathy: atypical presentation of amniotic fluid emboli. *Acta Anaesthesiol Scand*. 2004;48:1214–1215.
157. Fava S, Galizia AC. Amniotic fluid embolism. *Br J Obstet Gynaecol*. 1993; 100:1049–1050.
158. Huybrechts W, Jorens PG, Jacquemyn Y, et al. Amniotic fluid embolism: a rare cause of acute left-sided heart failure. *Acta Cardiol*. 2006;61:643–649.
159. Gilmore DA, Wakim J, Secrets J, et al. Anaphylactoid syndrome of pregnancy: a review of the literature with latest management and outcome data. *AANA J*. 2003;71:120–126.
160. Moore J, Baldisseri MR. Amniotic fluid embolism. *Crit Care Med*. 2005;33(Suppl l):S279–285.
161. Masson RG. Amniotic fluid embolism. *Clin Chest Med*. 1992;13:657–665.
162. Moore J. Amniotic fluid embolism: on the trail of an elusive diagnosis. *Lancet*. 2006;368:1399–1401.
163. O'Shea A, Eappen S. Amniotic fluid embolism. *Int Anesthesiol Clin*. 2007;45:17–28.
164. Kanayama N, Yamazaki T, Naruse H, et al. Determining zinc coproporphyrin in maternal plasma—a new method for diagnosing amniotic fluid embolism. *Clin Chem*. 1992;38:526–529.
165. Harboe T, Benson MD, Oi H, et al. Cardiopulmonary distress during obstetrical anaesthesia: attempts to diagnose amniotic fluid embolism in a case series of suspected allergic anaphylaxis. *Acta Anaesthesiol Scand*. 2006;50:324–330.
166. Oi H, Kobayashi H, Hirashima Y, et al. Serological and immunohistochemical diagnosis of amniotic fluid embolism. *Semin Thromb Hemost*. 1998;24:479–484.
167. Kobayashi H, Ooi H, Hayakawa H, et al. Histological diagnosis of amniotic fluid embolism by monoclonal antibody TKH-2 that recognizes NeuAc alpha 2-6GalNAc epitope. *Hum Pathol*. 1997;28:428–433.
168. Lunetta P, Penttila A. Immunohistochemical identification of syncytiotrophoblastic cells and megacaryocytes in pulmonary vessels in a fatal case of amniotic fluid embolism. *Int J Legal Med*. 1996;108:210–214.
169. Hussain SA, Sondhi DS, Munir A, et al. Amniotic fluid embolism with late respiratory failure. *Hosp Physician*. 2001;37:40–43.
170. Porat S, Leibowitz D, Mildwidsky A, et al. Transient intracardiac thrombi in amniotic fluid embolism. *BJOG*. 2004;111:506–510.
171. Demianczuk CE, Corbett TF. Successful pregnancy after amniotic fluid embolism: a case report. *J Obstet Gynaecol Can*. 2005;27:699–701.
172. Shapiro JM. Critical care of the obstetric patient. *J Intensive Care Med*. 2006;21:278.
173. Capan LM, Miller SM. Monitoring for suspected pulmonary embolism. *Anesthesiol Clin North Am*. 2001;19:673–703.
174. Rodgers L, Dangel-Palmer MC, Berner N. Acute circulatory and respiratory collapse in obstetrical patients: a case report and review of the literature. *Am Assoc Nurse Anesthetists J*. 2000;68:444–450.
175. Sprung J, Cheng EY, Patel S, et al. Understanding and management of amniotic fluid embolism. *J Clin Anesth*. 1992;4:235–240.
176. Waters JH, Biscotti C, Potter PS, et al. Amniotic fluid removal during cell salvage in the Cesarean section patient. *Anesthesiology*. 2000;92:1531–1536.
177. Davies S. Amniotic fluid embolism and isolated disseminated intravascular coagulation. *Can J Anaesth*. 1999;46:456–459.
178. Stanten RD, Iverson LI, Daugharty TM, et al. Amniotic fluid embolism causing catastrophic pulmonary vasoconstriction: diagnosis by transesophageal echocardiogram and treatment by cardiopulmonary bypass. *Obstet Gynecol*. 2003;102:496–498.
179. Stroup J, Haraway D, Beal JM. Aprotinin in the management of coagulopathy associated with amniotic fluid embolus. *Pharmacotherapy*. 2006;26:689–693.
180. Prosper SC, Goudge CS, Lupo VR. Recombinant factor VIIa to successfully manage disseminated intravascular coagulation from amniotic fluid embolism. *Obstet Gynecol*. 2007;109:524–525.
181. Goldazmidt E, Davies S. Two cases of hemorrhage secondary to amniotic fluid embolus managed with uterine artery embolisation. *Can J Anaesth*. 2003;50:917–921.
182. Stiller RJ, Siddiqui D, Laifer SA, et al. Successful pregnancy after suspected anaphylactoid syndrome of pregnancy (amniotic fluid embolus)—a case report. *J Reprod Med*. 2000;45:1007–1009.

CHAPTER 144 ■ PLEURAL DISEASE IN THE INTENSIVE CARE UNIT

MICHAEL A. JANTZ • VEENA B. ANTONY

Pleural disease itself is an unusual cause for admission to the intensive care unit (ICU). Conditions potentially requiring ICU admission include a large pleural effusion causing acute respiratory failure, hemothorax producing respiratory or hemodynamic compromise, secondary spontaneous pneumothorax with respiratory failure, empyema with sepsis, and re-expansion pulmonary edema. Pleural complications of disease processes and procedures performed in the ICU are common, however, and the changes in respiratory physiology are additive to that of the underlying lung disease. The development of a pneumothorax in a critically ill patient, particularly in mechanically ventilated patients, may be a life-threatening event. Pleural effusions may be overshadowed by the illness requiring ICU admission in the critically ill patient. Pleural effusions and pneumothoraces may not be detected on chest radiographs because the radiologic appearance may differ in the supine patient.

PLEURAL EFFUSIONS IN THE INTENSIVE CARE UNIT

Radiologic Evaluation

In the normal pleural space, air and fluid tend to distribute following gravitational influences, with air initially accumulating between the superior portion of the lung and the apex of the thorax, while fluid accumulates between the inferior margin of the lung and the diaphragm. Pleural air and fluid collections shift location when radiographs are obtained in positions other than the erect position. Because radiographs in critically ill patients are taken in the supine or semierect position, the radiographic appearance of air and fluid in the pleural space may thus change.

In normal humans in the supine position, the radiolucency of the lung base is equal to or greater than that of the lung apex due to the anteroposterior diameter of the lung being greatest at the lung base. In addition, in the supine patient, breast and pectoral tissues will tend to move laterally away from the lung base. A pleural effusion should be suspected when increased homogeneous density is present over the lower lung fields as compared with the upper lung fields. Patient rotation, an off-center x-ray beam, prior lobectomy, or a pleural or chest wall mass may produce a unilateral homogenous density that simulates the appearance of a pleural effusion (1). Cardiomegaly, a prominent epicardial fat pad, and lobar collapse or consolidation may obscure the detection of a pleural effusion on a supine radiograph.

Approximately 175 to 525 mL of pleural fluid will produce blunting of the costophrenic angle on an erect chest radiograph (2). This quantity of pleural fluid can usually be detected on a supine radiograph as an increased density over the lower lung zone. Blunting of the costophrenic angle (meniscus sign), silhouetting of the hemidiaphragm, and apical capping may be seen with larger effusions (3). An apparent elevation of the hemidiaphragm may be secondary to a subpulmonic collection of pleural fluid. A diffuse increase in the radiodensity of the hemithorax, or "veiling," may be seen with very large effusions in the supine radiograph. Thus, the major radiographic finding of a pleural effusion in the supine patient is an increased homogeneous density over the lower lung field that does not obliterate normal bronchovascular markings, does not demonstrate air bronchograms, and does not produce hilar or mediastinal displacement until the effusion is massive. If a pleural effusion is suspected in the supine patient, obtaining an erect or lateral decubitus radiograph may be helpful.

Because the critically ill patient often has underlying parenchymal lung disease, the diagnosis of pleural effusion can be problematic. Ultrasonography (US) or computed tomography (CT) scanning may be required to confirm or exclude the presence of a pleural effusion. US provides good characterization of pleural disease and has an advantage of being able to be performed at the bedside in critically ill patients who are not stable for transport to the radiology department for CT. Disadvantages include impedance of the ultrasound wave by air in the lung or pleural space, a restricted field of view, inferior evaluation of the lung parenchyma compared to CT, and operator dependence (1). In one study of 74 ICU patients evaluated by both chest radiograph and US, the latter detected a pleural effusion that was not appreciated on chest radiograph in 10 additional patients (29% of patients determined to have a pleural effusion) (4). In another study, US was helpful in making a diagnosis in 27 of 41 (66%) patients and influenced treatment planning in 17 of 41 critically ill patients (41%) (5). US-guided thoracentesis at the bedside was successful in 24 of 25 patients in that same study. Other studies have noted the usefulness of US to safely guide bedside thoracentesis in mechanically ventilated patients (6–8). The presence of complex septated, complex nonseptated, and homogeneously echogenic patterns within pleural fluid collections are typically indicative of an exudative pleural effusion (9). Homogeneously echogenic effusions suggest hemorrhagic effusions or empyemas whereas US evidence of fibrin septae suggests a parapneumonic effusion, empyema, hemothorax, or malignant effusion (9).

CT may also be helpful in assessing pleural processes in the critically ill patient, and has the advantages of better lung parenchymal imaging, evaluation of the mediastinum, and ability to distinguish pleural from parenchymal abnormalities (1). On CT, free-flowing pleural fluid produces a sickle-shaped opacity in the most dependent part of the thorax (10). Loculated pleural fluid collections are seen as lenticular or rounded opacities in a fixed position with a relatively homogeneous water density (10). CT may be particularly helpful in the diagnosis and management of loculated pleural effusions (11). The most reliable sign of empyema, the split pleura sign, is usually identified during the organizing phase. Following administration of intravenous contrast, the parietal and visceral pleura will be thickened and enhanced and will be noted to be separated, and the extrapleural fat between the empyema and the chest wall may be increased in size (12,13). In one study, this sign was present in only 68% of patients, however (12). CT may be helpful in assessing inadequately drained fluid collections in patients with persistent fevers or sepsis due to malpositioned chest tubes (14).

Diagnostic Thoracentesis

Pleural effusions are common in the ICU. In one prospective study of 100 consecutive patients admitted to a medical ICU, pleural effusions were found on chest radiographs and/or by US in 62% of patients (4). Patients with a pleural effusion provide the opportunity to diagnose, at least presumptively, the underlying process responsible for the accumulation of pleural fluid. Although disease of any organ system can cause a pleural effusion in critically ill patients, the diagnoses listed in Table 144.1 represent most causes in the ICU.

When a pleural effusion is suspected on physical exam and confirmed radiologically, a diagnostic thoracentesis should be considered to establish the cause of the effusion. Observation alone may be reasonable in situations in which the clinical diagnosis is reasonably secure and a small amount of pleural fluid is present, such as in atelectasis or uncomplicated heart failure (15). Thoracentesis should be performed, however, if the patient's clinical condition changes. When the distance from the pleural fluid line to the inside of the chest wall is less than 1 cm on lateral decubitus radiograph, the risk of thoracentesis probably outweighs the value of pleural fluid analysis. If the underlying disease causing the pleural effusion becomes clinically problematic, the effusion will often increase in size and allow for safe thoracentesis. When sampling of a small-volume pleural effusion is indicated, thoracentesis should be performed with US guidance.

The indications for diagnostic thoracentesis are not different in the ICU patient, and receiving mechanical ventilation is not a contraindication. Establishing the diagnosis quickly in critically ill patients may be more important than in the noncritically ill. The reported incidence of pneumothorax in nonventilated patients ranges from 4% to 30% (16–20). Various risk factors for developing a pneumothorax after thoracentesis have been reported, although operator inexperience, baseline lung disease, and use of positive pressure mechanical ventilation appear to be the most established risk factors. Several earlier studies have demonstrated that the incidence of pneumothorax after blind thoracentesis in mechanically ventilated patients, 5% to 10%, is similar to that of nonventilated patients, and it is thus safe to perform blind thoracentesis in mechanically ventilated patients (21–23). If the patient on mechanical ventilation does develop a pneumothorax, however, a significant risk of progression to a life-threatening tension pneumothorax exists. As such, some authors have advocated the routine use of ultrasound guidance for all thoracentesis procedures in mechanically ventilated patients given the observed pneumothorax rates of 0% to 3% with ultrasound guidance in nonventilated patients (20,24), as well as in patients receiving mechanical ventilation (6–8). Strong consideration should be given to using US guidance in patients with small or moderate effusions, although large effusions may be sampled relatively safely unless the operator is inexperienced. US or CT guidance should be used to sample loculated pleural fluid collections. There are no absolute contraindications to diagnostic thoracentesis. The major relative contraindications are a bleeding diathesis or anticoagulation. In one study of 207 patients with mild to moderate coagulopathy, defined as a prothrombin time (PT) or partial thromboplastin time (PTT) up to twice normal or a platelet count from 50,000 to 100,000 cells/μL, no increase in bleeding complications was noted (25). Thoracentesis should not be performed through an area of active skin infection.

TABLE 144.1

CAUSES OF PLEURAL EFFUSIONS IN ICU PATIENTS

Abdominal surgery
Acute respiratory distress syndrome (ARDS)
Atelectasis
Chylothorax
Congestive heart failure
Coronary artery bypass surgery
Empyema
Esophageal rupture
Esophageal sclerotherapy
Hemothorax
Hepatic hydrothorax
Hypoalbuminemia
Iatrogenic
Central venous catheter placement
Nasogastric tube placement
Vascular erosion by central venous catheter
Intra-abdominal abscess
Malignancy
Pancreatitis/Pancreatic pseudocyst
Pneumonia
Postcardiac injury syndrome
Pulmonary embolism
Uremia

Therapeutic Thoracentesis and Physiologic Effects

The primary indication for therapeutic thoracentesis or chest tube drainage of a pleural effusion is relief of dyspnea, although pulmonary mechanics and oxygenation may be improved in some patients (26). Contraindications to therapeutic thoracentesis are similar to those of diagnostic thoracentesis. Complications from therapeutic thoracentesis are similar to that of diagnostic thoracentesis, with the additional complications of hypoxemia, re-expansion pulmonary edema, and hypovolemia. An increased risk of pneumothorax compared to diagnostic thoracentesis has been noted with therapeutic thoracentesis in some studies (18,20,27) although not others (19,28).

We would recommend the use of a catheter-over-needle system in performing therapeutic thoracentesis to reduce the risk of developing a pneumothorax. In patients with pleural effusion and ipsilateral shift suggesting endobronchial obstruction or a trapped lung, the risk of re-expansion pulmonary edema may be increased, and the patient may be less likely to experience a beneficial effect. In addition, patients with initial negative pleural pressures and those with more precipitous falls in pleural pressures with fluid removal also likely have trapped lung or endobronchial obstruction and are less likely to benefit from therapeutic thoracentesis (29).

Pleural effusions compress the lung, causing atelectasis, ventilation/perfusion mismatch, and shunt physiology with resultant hypoxemia (30). Pleural fluid tends to enlarge the volume of the hemithorax more than it compresses lung volume. Studies in humans have shown that total lung capacity following thoracentesis increases by only approximately one third of the thoracentesis fluid volume, and forced vital capacity increases by approximately one half of the increase in total lung capacity (31). Studies evaluating gas exchange in nonventilated patients have been mixed. One study found a decrease in PaO_2 (32), one study found no change in PaO_2 (33), and one study showed a mild increase in PaO_2 (34). More recent studies have also shown variable results, with one study reporting a small increase in PaO_2 and decrease in alveolar-arterial O_2 gradient (35), although another noted no change in PaO_2, alveolar-arterial O_2 gradient or shunt, while the amount of blood flow to low ventilation/perfusion units increased slightly (30).

Despite these mixed results, some patients requiring mechanical ventilation may benefit from pleural fluid drainage. Talmor et al. (26) reported that 19 patients with acute respiratory failure and pleural effusions who had a poor response to positive end-expiratory pressure (PEEP)—defined as the inability to wean FiO_2 to 0.5 with PEEP up to 20 cm H_2O—benefited from chest tube drainage of the pleural effusions. The PaO_2 increased from 125 to 199 mm Hg, and the PaO_2/FiO_2 ratio increased from 151 to 254. Fourteen patients had a unilateral effusion, and five patients had bilateral effusions necessitating bilateral chest tube placement. More recently, Doelken et al. (36) studied the effects of thoracentesis on respiratory mechanics and gas exchange in eight mechanically ventilated patients. Following removal of 800 to 1,950 mL (mean 1,495 mL), no significant change in PaO_2 or dead space ventilation was observed. No significant changes were noted for peak and plateau pressures, dynamic and effective static compliance, respiratory system resistance, and intrinsic PEEP. Mean work performed by the ventilator did significantly decrease, however. Further studies are required to confirm these results, although in patients who are difficult to wean from mechanical ventilation, we would consider a trial of therapeutic thoracentesis.

Abdominal Surgery

Approximately one half of patients undergoing abdominal surgery will develop small unilateral or bilateral pleural effusions 24 to 48 hours following surgery (37,38). The incidence of pleural effusions is higher in procedures involving the upper abdomen, in patients having ascitic fluid at time of surgery, and in patients who have postoperative atelectasis (29). Larger left-sided effusions are common following splenectomy. The effusion after abdominal surgery is usually exudative* with a normal glucose level, pH >7.40, and less than 10,000 nucleated cells/μL (37). Small effusions generally do not require diagnostic thoracentesis and resolve spontaneously without becoming clinical significant. Thoracentesis is indicated to exclude empyema if the effusion is relatively large or loculated or if the possibility of a subdiaphragmatic abscess related to the surgery exists.

Acute Respiratory Distress Syndrome

The presence of pleural effusions in acute respiratory distress syndrome (ARDS) has not been well appreciated or studied. In a retrospective study of 25 patients with ARDS, 36% were found to have pleural effusions (39). All patients had extensive alveolar infiltrates in addition to pleural effusions. Pleural effusions have been observed in animal models of ARDS using α-naphthylthiourea, oleic acid, and ethchlorvynol (40,41). In the oleic acid model, 35% of the excess lung water collected in the pleural spaces (40). Effusions are likely underdiagnosed in ARDS because the patient has bilateral alveolar infiltrates and the radiograph is taken in the supine position. In experimental models of ARDS, the effusions are serous to serosanguineous with a predominance of polymorphonuclear leukocytes (PMNs) (41). These effusions resolve as the ARDS resolves and require no specific therapy.

Atelectasis

Atelectasis is a common cause of small pleural effusions in the ICU due to patients being immobile (4). Atelectasis and small effusions are commonly observed following cardiothoracic or abdominal surgery. Other potential causes include endobronchial obstruction from tumor, foreign body, or mucus plugging as well as extrinsic airway compression from malignancy. With lung collapse, local areas of increased negative pressure are created by the separation of the lung and chest wall. The decrease in pleural pressure favors the movement of fluid into the pleural space, presumably from the surface of the parietal pleura (15).

Pleural effusions from atelectasis are serous transudates with a few mononuclear cells, a glucose concentration equal to serum, and a pH of 7.45 to 7.55. The pleural effusions dissipate over several days when the atelectasis resolves.

Chylothorax

A chylothorax is defined as the accumulation of chyle in the pleural space. The predominant mechanisms of chylothorax formation include disruption of the thoracic duct, extravasation from pleural lymphatics, and transdiaphragmatic efflux from chylous ascites (42). The most common cause of chylothorax is lymphoma, accounting for 37% of chylothoraces in

*Effusions are termed exudative—or not—by lactate dehydrogenase (LDH) and protein criteria. Only LDH and protein values are used in the Light criteria although cholesterol level is used by some. pH, glucose, and cell counts are not part of the classification of transudate versus exudate.

a series of 191 patients (43). The second most frequent cause is surgical trauma, which represented 25% of cases in the same series of 191 patients (43). The incidence of chylothorax following thoracic surgery has been reported to be 0.36% to 0.42% (44,45) and 1.9% following lower neck surgery (46). A higher proportion of chylothoraces are noted following esophagectomy (44,45). Virtually all intrathoracic surgical procedures, including lobectomy, pneumonectomy, and coronary artery bypass grafting, have been reported to cause chylothorax (43). Nonsurgical trauma, including blunt and penetrating injuries to the neck, thorax, and upper abdomen as well as obstruction of the superior vena cava or thrombosis of the left subclavian vein from indwelling central venous catheters, may produce chylothoraces in ICU patients (47).

The patient may be asymptomatic if the effusion is small and unilateral, or may be dyspneic with a large unilateral effusion or bilateral effusions. The pleural fluid is usually milky but can be serous, serosanguineous, or bloody. The fluid may not have a milky appearance if the patient is malnourished or not eating (48). The pleural fluid typically has less than 7,000 nucleated cells/μL which are greater than 80% lymphocytes. The pH is alkaline (7.40–7.80), and the triglyceride levels exceed plasma levels (15). A pleural fluid triglyceride concentration greater than 110 mg/dL makes the diagnosis of chylothorax highly likely, whereas a concentration less than 50 mg/dL makes the diagnosis highly unlikely. With triglyceride concentrations of 50 to 110 mg/dL, lipoprotein electrophoresis is indicated to demonstrate the presence of chylomicrons, which confirms the diagnosis of chylothorax (48).

Up to 2 to 3 L of chyle may drain daily, causing loss of fluid, electrolytes, protein, fat, fat-soluble vitamins, and lymphocytes. Severe nutritional depletion and immunodeficiency may result if these losses are not addressed. In addition to chest tube drainage, initial conservative management consists of intravenous hydration and a nonfat, high-protein, high-calorie diet with medium-chain triglycerides, which are absorbed directly into the portal system, or discontinuing all oral feeding and initiating total parenteral nutrition. If the chylothorax fails to resolve with conservative measures after 7 to 14 days, then surgery with thoracic duct ligation may be considered (44,45), although pleuroperitoneal shunting has also been used.

Congestive Heart Failure

Congestive heart failure (CHF) is the most common cause of all transudative pleural effusions and in one study was the most common cause of pleural effusions in a medical ICU (4). Pleural effusions due to CHF are associated with increases in pulmonary venous pressure. In a study of 37 patients admitted for CHF, the mean pulmonary capillary wedge pressure (PCWP) was higher in patients with pleural effusions than in those without—24.1 versus 17.2 mm Hg, respectively (49). Isolated increases in right heart pressures were not associated with pleural effusions. Patients with chronic obstructive pulmonary disease (COPD) and cor pulmonale, in the absence of left ventricular dysfunction, thus rarely have pleural effusions, and other causes for pleural effusions should be sought in these patients.

Most patients with pleural effusion secondary to CHF have the usual signs and symptoms. The chest radiograph classically demonstrates cardiomegaly and bilateral small to moderate pleural effusions of similar size, with right-sided effusions often being slightly greater than the left. Radiographic evidence of pulmonary edema is usually present, with the severity of pulmonary edema correlating with the presence of effusions. In patients who have been hospitalized, records will usually show intake greater than output for several days, weight gain, an increasing alveolar-arterial O_2 gradient, and decreasing compliance in those patients requiring mechanical ventilation. Some patients without a history of CHF may not be suspected of having CHF until intravenous hydration produces pleural effusions and subsequent echocardiograms demonstrate left ventricular dysfunction (4).

Pleural effusions from CHF are transudates and have less than 1,000 nucleated cells/μL, which are mainly mesothelial cells and lymphocytes. Acute diuresis may increase the protein concentration of the pleural fluid and thus change the classification of the fluid from transudative to exudative in 8% to 38% of patients (50). In the afebrile patient with clinical CHF and cardiomegaly with bilateral effusions of relatively equal size on chest radiograph, the diagnosis is reasonably secure and observation is appropriate. In patients who are febrile, have pleuritic chest pain, or are noted on chest radiograph to have effusions of disparate size, unilateral effusions, a larger effusion on the left than the right, or absence of cardiomegaly, thoracentesis should be considered to evaluate for other causes of the effusion(s).

Treatment consists of decreasing preload and improving cardiac output with diuretics, inotropes, and afterload-reducing agents. With appropriate management, the pleural effusions will resolve over days to weeks.

Coronary Artery Bypass Surgery

A small left pleural effusion is virtually always present following coronary artery bypass surgery. The effusion is associated with left lower lobe atelectasis and elevation of the left hemidiaphragm on chest radiograph. A few patients may have moderate to large pleural effusions, which may be bloody (51). These effusions tend to be associated with internal mammary artery grafting, which causes exudation from the bed where the internal mammary artery is harvested.

The pleural fluid is an exudate, may or may not be hemorrhagic, and has a low nucleated cell count, with glucose level similar to serum and a pH greater than 7.40. Rarely, a loculated hemothorax may develop with a trapped lung, resulting in clinically significant restriction (52). If a large effusion that qualifies as a hemothorax is present, the fluid should be drained by chest tube thoracostomy. It is unclear if a large hemorrhagic effusion with a pleural fluid/blood hematocrit less than 50% needs to be drained to avoid later necessity for decortication. Treatment with anti-inflammatory agents and possibly chemical pleurodesis may be required for patients with recurrent nonbloody effusions (51).

Esophageal Rupture

Spontaneous esophageal rupture—Boerhaave syndrome—is a potentially life-threatening event and requires immediate diagnosis and therapy. Esophageal rupture or perforation may rarely occur with blunt thoracic trauma or as a complication of endoscopy and nasogastric/orogastric tube placement. The history in spontaneous esophageal rupture is usually severe retching or vomiting; however, activities that generate a Valsalva maneuver can cause esophageal rupture, and in some patients the perforation may be silent (53). The findings on chest radiograph may vary depending on the time between perforation and obtaining of the chest radiograph, the site of perforation, and integrity of the mediastinal pleura. Mediastinal emphysema is present in less than half of patients and may take 1 to 2 hours to be observed, whereas mediastinal widening may take several hours. Pneumothorax, indicating rupture of the mediastinal pleura, is present in 75% of patients; 70% of pneumothoraces are on the left, 20% are on the right, and 10% are bilateral (54). Pleural effusion, with or without associated pneumothorax, occurs in 75% of patients. A presumptive diagnosis should be confirmed radiographically with an esophagram as soon as possible. Because rapid passage of the contrast in the upright patient may not demonstrate a small perforation, the study should be done with the patient in the appropriate lateral decubitus position.

Pleural fluid findings depend on the degree of perforation and the timing of thoracentesis. Early thoracentesis without mediastinal perforation shows a sterile serous exudate with a predominance of PMNs and a pH greater than 7.30. Amylase of salivary origin appears in the fluid in high concentration following disruption of the mediastinal pleura. With the seeding of the pleural space by anaerobic bacteria, the pH falls rapidly and progressively to approach 6.00. The presence of food particles and squamous epithelial cells in the pleural fluid also suggests esophageal rupture (55). Management is usually operative intervention in conjunction with pleural space drainage and antibiotics. Nonoperative therapy with antibiotics and chest tube drainage alone may be considered in a nontoxic patient with small perforations due to instrumentation.

Esophageal Sclerotherapy

Pleural effusions are found in approximately 50% of patients 48 to 72 hours following esophageal sclerotherapy (56). Effusions may be unilateral or bilateral, with no predilection for side. The effusions tend to be small serous exudates with variable nucleated (38,000–90,000 cells/μL) and red cell counts (126,000 to 160,000 cells/μL) and glucose concentrations similar to serum. The mechanism for development of these effusions is likely extravasation of the sclerosant beyond the esophageal mucosa, resulting in mediastinal and mediastinal pleural inflammation. An effusion that is not associated with fever, chest pain, or signs of perforation is not important clinically, and will usually resolve over several days to weeks without specific therapy. A diagnostic thoracentesis should be performed and an esophagram considered in patients with symptomatic effusions for 24 to 48 hours to exclude empyema and esophageal perforation.

Hemothorax

Hemothorax needs to be differentiated from a hemorrhagic pleural effusion, as the latter can be the result of only a few drops of blood in serous pleural fluid. The arbitrary definition of a hemothorax is a pleural fluid to blood hematocrit ratio greater than 50%. Most hemothoraces result from blunt or penetrating thoracic trauma (57). Hemothorax can also result from invasive procedures, pulmonary infarction, malignancy, and ruptured aortic aneurysms. Anticoagulation therapy or coagulopathy may rarely cause a spontaneous hemothorax. Hemothorax should be suspected in any patient with blunt or penetrating chest trauma with a pleural effusion on chest radiograph. Chest tube thoracostomy with a 28 to 32 French chest tube should be performed in these patients and pleural fluid hematocrit measured. In the patient with suspected iatrogenic or spontaneous hemothorax, thoracentesis should be performed, and if positive, a chest tube should be inserted. Chest tube drainage allows the monitoring of the rate of bleeding, may potentially tamponade the bleeding, and will evacuate the pleural space, thus decreasing the risk of developing empyema or a subsequent fibrothorax (57,58). Indications for surgical exploration vary between clinicians, but general guidelines are hemodynamic instability despite adequate resuscitation, initial drainage greater than 1,500 mL, continued bleeding of greater than 200 mL/hour for 3 consecutive hours, continued bleeding of greater than 1,500 mL/day, and radiographic evidence of significant retained clot (greater than one third of the pleural space).

Hepatic Hydrothorax

Pleural effusions are present in approximately 6% of patients with cirrhosis and clinically apparent ascites (59,60). The effusions result from movement of ascitic fluid through congenital or acquired diaphragmatic defects. Rarely, a hepatic hydrothorax may be found in a patient without clinical ascites but with ascites demonstrated only by US, implying the presence of a large diaphragmatic defect. With a small pleural effusion, the patient may be asymptomatic, whereas with large to massive effusions, the patient may have varying degrees of dyspnea. The chest radiograph usually demonstrates a normal cardiac silhouette and a right-sided pleural effusion in 70% of patients, which can vary from small to massive. Effusions are less commonly isolated to the left pleural space (15%) or are bilateral (15%). The pleural fluid is a serous transudate with a low nucleated cell count and a predominance of mononuclear cells, pH greater than 7.40, a glucose level similar to serum, and an amylase less than serum amylase (15). The diagnosis is substantiated by demonstrating that the pleural fluid and ascitic fluid have similar chemistries. If the diagnosis is still in question, injection of a radionuclide into the ascitic fluid with subsequent detection on chest imaging supports the diagnosis (61).

Treatment of hepatic hydrothorax is directed at resolution of the ascites with sodium restriction, diuretics, and paracentesis. It is not uncommon for the effusion to persist until all of the ascitic fluid is mobilized. If the patient is acutely dyspneic or hypoxemic, therapeutic thoracentesis may be done as a temporizing measure. Chest tube drainage should be avoided, as it can cause infection of the fluid, and the prolonged drainage can lead to volume depletion, protein and lymphocyte depletion, and may precipitate renal failure. Chemical pleurodesis is usually unsuccessful due to rapid movement of ascitic fluid into the pleural space. Transjugular intrahepatic portal systemic shunt (TIPS) has been used to treat symptomatic hepatic hydrothorax refractory to medical management (59,60), as has video-assisted thoracoscopic surgery to patch the diaphragmatic defect followed by pleural abrasion or talc poudrage (62).

Hepatic hydrothorax may occasionally be complicated by spontaneous bacterial empyema (SBE) (63). The formation of SBE is a result of either bacterial translocation from infected ascitic fluid or bacteremia and seeding of a hepatic hydrothorax. The criteria for diagnosing SBE are similar to that for diagnosing spontaneous bacterial peritonitis and include a positive Gram stain, positive pleural fluid culture, or total neutrophil count greater than 500 cells/μL. Treatment of SBE is conservative with antibiotic therapy alone, unless frank pus is present, in which case chest tube thoracostomy should be considered.

Hypoalbuminemia

Many patients admitted to the medical ICU have chronic illnesses and associated hypoalbuminemia. Pleural effusions may be observed when the serum albumin is less than 1.8 g/dL. In one study evaluating the association of pleural effusions with hypoalbuminemia, 3 of 21 (14%) patients with serum albumin less than 2.0 g/dL had pleural effusions (64). Since the normal pleural space has an effective lymphatic drainage system, pleural fluid tends to be the last site of collection of extravascular fluid in patients with low oncotic pressure. It is, therefore, unusual to find a pleural effusion solely due to hypoalbuminemia in the absence of anasarca. The chest radiograph usually shows small to moderate bilateral effusions with a normal heart size. The pleural fluid is a serous transudate with less than 1,000 nucleated cells/μL, predominantly mesothelial cells and lymphocytes. The pH ranges from 7.45 to 7.55, and the glucose level is similar to serum. Diagnosis is presumptive if other causes of transudative effusions are sufficiently excluded. The effusions resolve when the hypoalbuminemia is corrected.

Iatrogenic

Insertion of a central venous catheter or extravascular migration of a central venous catheter can cause a pneumothorax, hemothorax, chylothorax, or transudative pleural effusion (65,66). Extravascular migration of a catheter, occurring in approximately 0.4% to 1.0% of insertions, is more common with insertion into the left subclavian and internal jugular veins due to the horizontal orientation of the left brachiocephalic vein in relation to the superior vena cava (58). The postprocedure chest radiograph should always be assessed for proper catheter placement, with catheter positioning parallel to the long axis of the superior vena cava and tip positioning at the right tracheobronchial angle indicating proper placement (67).

In the conscious patient, acute infusion of intravenous fluid into the mediastinum usually results in chest pain and dyspnea. Depending on the volume and rate of infusion of fluid into the mediastinum, tachypnea, respiratory distress, and cardiac tamponade may occur. The chest radiograph demonstrates the catheter tip in an abnormal position, a widened mediastinum, and unilateral or bilateral effusions. The effusion can have characteristics similar to the infusate (milky if lipid is being given), and may be hemorrhagic and neutrophil predominant due to trauma and inflammation. If a glucose-containing solution is being infused, the pleural fluid to serum glucose ratio is greater than 1.0 (66). The central venous catheter should be removed immediately. Observation is sufficient if the effusion is small. If the effusion is large or causes respiratory distress, thoracentesis or tube thoracostomy should be performed. If a hemothorax is discovered, a chest tube should be placed.

Pancreatitis

Pleural effusions are commonly associated with pancreatitis due to the close proximity of the pancreas to the diaphragm. Pleural effusions have been noted in 3% to 20% of patients with pancreatitis (68). The chest radiograph usually demonstrates a small to moderate left-sided effusion (60%), although effusions may be isolated to the right side (30%) or occur bilaterally (10%) (69). The patient usually presents with abdominal symptoms of pancreatitis. The diagnosis is confirmed by an elevated pleural fluid amylase concentration that is greater than serum, although a normal pleural fluid amylase may be found early in the course of acute pancreatitis. The pleural fluid is an exudate with 10,000 to 50,000 nucleated cells/μL, predominantly PMNs. The pleural fluid pH is usually 7.30 to 7.35, and the glucose level is similar to serum (15).

No specific treatment is necessary for pleural effusions associated with acute pancreatitis. The effusion resolves as the pancreatic inflammation subsides. If the pleural effusion does not resolve in 2 to 3 weeks, pancreatic abscess or pseudocyst should be suspected. Recent studies suggest that the presence of pleural effusions in acute pancreatitis is correlated with increased morbidity and mortality (68,70).

Parapneumonic Effusions and Empyema

Patients with severe community-acquired pneumonia admitted to the ICU and patients who develop nosocomial pneumonia often develop parapneumonic effusions, with progression to empyema being less common. An *empyema* is defined as the presence of pus in the pleural space, although many clinicians extend the definition to include pleural fluid that has a positive Gram stain for bacteria or a positive bacterial culture. *Complicated parapneumonic effusions* are defined as pleural effusions that will not respond to antibiotic therapy alone and require drainage for resolution, whereas *uncomplicated parapneumonic effusions* do not require drainage and respond to antibiotic therapy alone for the underlying pneumonia (71–74).

The usual presentation is similar to the non-ICU patient with fever, dyspnea, chest pain, purulent sputum, leukocytosis, and a new alveolar infiltrate on chest radiograph. In the elderly, debilitated, or immunosuppressed patient, however, many of these findings may be absent. Although pleural space infections most commonly occur in association with pneumonia, it should also be recognized that pleural space infections may result from thoracic surgery, chest tube placement, penetrating chest trauma, esophageal perforation, mediastinitis, subdiaphragmatic abscesses, spontaneous bacterial peritonitis, and bacteremic seeding of a pre-existing effusion (71).

The pleural fluid protein concentration, nucleated cell count, or percentage of PMNs is not helpful in differentiating a complicated from an uncomplicated effusion. When the effusion is free-flowing, as demonstrated by lateral decubitus views or US, and thoracentesis shows a nonpurulent PMN-predominant exudate with a glucose level greater than 60 mg/dL, lactate dehydrogenase (LDH) less than 1,000 IU/L, and pH greater than 7.20, the patient has a high likelihood of pleural fluid resolution with antibiotics alone over 7 to 14 days (uncomplicated effusion). If pus is aspirated on thoracentesis, the diagnosis of empyema is established and immediate drainage is needed. Most clinicians would also advocate drainage of the effusion if the Gram stain or bacterial culture is positive, regardless of the fluid chemistries. If the pH is less than 7.20 in the absence of a positive Gram stain or culture, or if glucose is less than 40 mg/dL and LDH is greater than 1,000 IU/L, particularly with a loculated effusion, most clinicians would advocate drainage (complicated effusion) (72–75).

In nonloculated complicated parapneumonic effusions and empyemas, drainage can be accomplished by standard chest tube thoracostomy or image-guided percutaneous catheters. Controversy exists concerning the optimal treatment of multiloculated parapneumonic pleural effusions, and it is beyond the scope of this chapter to discuss each approach in detail. Single chest tubes or multiple blindly placed chest tubes are unlikely to be successful. Potential strategies include image-guided catheters with intrapleural fibrinolytic agents or video-assisted thoracic surgery (VATS) as initial therapy (72–80). If these measures fail, then empyemectomy and decortication will be required. In the absence of Gram stain or cultures to direct antibiotic therapy, broad-spectrum antibiotics should be used initially. Empyemas are often mixed infections, including anaerobes, and a regimen that includes coverage for anaerobes should be chosen. Aminoglycosides may have poor clinical activity in empyemas and probably should not be used (81).

Postcardiac Injury Syndrome

Postcardiac injury syndrome (PCIS) is characterized by the onset of fever, pleuropericarditis, and parenchymal infiltrates typically 3 weeks (2 to 86 days) following injury to the myocardium or pericardium (82,83). PCIS has been reported following myocardial infarction, cardiac surgery, blunt chest trauma, and pacemaker implantation. The incidence following myocardial infarction has been estimated at up to 4% and up to 30% following cardiac surgery. Based on available data, it appears that PCIS results from an autoimmune reaction following myocardial or pericardial injury (84).

Pleuritic chest pain is reported by virtually all patients, whereas one half of patients will be noted to have dyspnea, fever, pericardial rub, and rales. Half of the patients have a leukocytosis, and almost all have an elevated erythrocyte sedimentation rate. The chest radiograph is abnormal in most patients, with the most common abnormality being left-sided and bilateral pleural effusions (83). Pulmonary infiltrates are present in 75% of patients and are most commonly seen in the left lower lobe (82). The pleural fluid is a serosanguineous or bloody exudate with pH greater than 7.30 and glucose level greater than 60 mg/dL. Nucleated cells range from 500 to 39,000 cells/μL, with a predominance of PMNs early in the course (15). The finding of pericardial fluid on echocardiogram suggests PCIS. The diagnosis is made clinically after pulmonary embolism and parapneumonic effusion have been excluded. An antimyocardial antibody titer in pleural fluid greater than in serum further supports the diagnosis (85).

PCIS is usually self-limited and may not require treatment if symptoms are minor. PCIS usually responds to aspirin or nonsteroidal anti-inflammatory agents, although some patients may require corticosteroids for resolution. Following treatment, the pleural effusion resolves within 1 to 3 weeks. It is important to not misdiagnose PCIS as a pulmonary embolism, as anticoagulation therapy may lead to pericardial hemorrhage and tamponade.

Pulmonary Embolism

Pleural effusions occur in up to 50% of patients with pulmonary embolism (86). The pathogenesis of pleural effusions in pulmonary embolism includes ischemia and inflammatory mediator-induced increased pleural capillary permeability, imbalance in microvascular and pleural space hydrostatic pressures, pleuropulmonary hemorrhage, and atelectasis. With pulmonary infarction, necrosis and hemorrhage into the lung and pleural space may result. More than 80% of patients with pulmonary infarction will have bloody pleural effusions, while up to 40% of patients without radiographic evidence of infarction will also have hemorrhagic fluid (86). Ipsilateral pleuritic chest pain occurs in most patients with pleural effusions complicating pulmonary embolism. A coexistent pulmonary infiltrate is noted on chest radiograph in approximately half of patients with pulmonary embolism and pleural effusion.

Pleural fluid analysis is variable and may demonstrate either an exudate or a transudate (15,87). A bloody pleural effusion in the absence of chest trauma, recent cardiac injury, asbestos exposure, or malignancy should increase the suspicion of pulmonary embolism (88). The pleural fluid is hemorrhagic in two thirds of patients, although the number of red blood cells exceeds 100,000 cells/μL in less than 20% (15). The nucleated cell count ranges from less than 100 (presumably atelectatic transudates) to 50,000 cells/μL (pulmonary infarction). When thoracentesis is performed near the time of acute symptoms, PMNs are predominant; with later thoracentesis, lymphocytes represent the majority of cells, and eosinophils may be present as well. The effusion from pulmonary embolism is usually apparent (92%) on the initial chest radiograph and reaches a maximum volume during the first 72 hours. In patients who demonstrate progression of effusions after 72 hours of therapy, recurrent embolism, hemothorax secondary to anticoagulation, an infected infarction, or an alternative diagnosis should be considered. The effusions usually resolve in 1 week in the absence of an infiltrate on chest radiograph. When an infiltrate is present, presumably representing a pulmonary infarction, the resolution time is longer, typically 2 to 3 weeks (86).

The association of a pleural effusion with pulmonary embolism does not alter therapy. The presence of a bloody effusion is not a contraindication to full-dose anticoagulation, since hemothorax is a rare complication of heparin therapy for pulmonary embolism (89,90). An enlarging pleural effusion on therapy necessitates thoracentesis to exclude hemothorax, empyema, or another cause. The development of a hemothorax during therapy requires discontinuation of anticoagulation, chest tube thoracostomy, and placement of a vena cava filter.

Uremia

Uremic pleural effusions have been reported in 3% to 5% of patients undergoing chronic dialysis (91). In one study evaluating the cause of pleural effusions in 100 patients requiring long-term hemodialysis, uremic pleurisy accounted for 16% of cases (92). Patients may manifest fever, cough, chest pain, and pleural friction rubs. The chest radiograph usually shows a moderate unilateral effusion, although massive and bilateral pleural effusions have been reported (93–95). The pleural effusion is a serosanguineous or bloody exudate, with less than 1,500 nucleated cells/μL, predominantly lymphocytes. The creatinine concentration is high, although the pleural fluid to serum creatinine ratio is less than 1.0, unlike in urinothorax (15). The effusions generally resolve with continued dialysis over several weeks but may recur. Uremic pleuritis may cause pleural fibrosis and restriction, requiring decortication in some patients (96,97).

PNEUMOTHORAX IN THE INTENSIVE CARE UNIT

Pneumothorax, defined as accumulation of air in the pleural space, represents one form of extra-alveolar air. Other forms of extra-alveolar air include pulmonary interstitial emphysema, pneumomediastinum, pneumopericardium, pneumoperitoneum, pneumoretroperitoneum, and systemic air embolism. Three pathologic processes may give rise to extra-alveolar air: (1) generation by gas-forming micro-organisms during an infectious process, (2) direct introduction following trauma to cutaneous or mucosal barriers, and (3) alveolar rupture due to pressure gradients between alveoli and the surrounding interstitial space (barotrauma) (98).

The mechanisms of spontaneous generation of extra-alveolar air were first delineated by Macklin and Macklin (99). In situations in which intra-alveolar pressure is increased, a gradient is produced between the alveolus and the adjacent vascular sheath, causing the alveoli to rupture at their bases. Following rupture, air is introduced in the perivascular adventitia, resulting in interstitial emphysema. The air then dissects proximally to the lung hilum and mediastinum due to a lower mean pressure in the mediastinum compared to that of the lung parenchyma. Once in the mediastinum, the accumulated air may decompress along paths of least resistance into the subcutaneous tissues or, less commonly, into the pericardium, peritoneum, and retroperitoneum. If mediastinal pressure increases abruptly or if decompression via these routes is not sufficient, the mediastinal parietal may rupture, resulting in pneumothorax. Alternatively, air from ruptured alveoli may dissect to the periphery of the lung and rupture via subpleural blebs through the visceral pleura into the pleural space (100).

Pneumothoraces are classified as spontaneous, which occur without preceding trauma or other obvious causes, and traumatic, which occur as a result of direct or indirect trauma to the chest. Spontaneous pneumothoraces can be subdivided into primary spontaneous, which occur in otherwise healthy patients without clinical lung disease, and secondary spontaneous, which occur in patients with underlying lung disease. Traumatic pneumothoraces can be subdivided into the categories of iatrogenic and related to blunt or penetrating chest trauma. In addition, pneumothoraces can be classified as simple or complicated, with complicated pneumothoraces consisting of tension pneumothorax, hemopneumothorax, pyopneumothorax, and open pneumothorax in which the integrity of the chest wall is disrupted. The potential causes of pneumothoraces in critically ill patients are listed in Table 144.2. We will focus mainly on iatrogenic pneumothoraces and pneumothoraces resulting from barotrauma, as these are the most common causes of pneumothoraces in ICU patients.

TABLE 144.2

CAUSES OF PNEUMOTHORACES IN ICU PATIENTS

SECONDARY SPONTANEOUS
Airway diseases
Chronic obstructive pulmonary disease (COPD)
Status asthmaticus
Cystic fibrosis
Parenchymal lung diseases
Idiopathic pulmonary fibrosis
Sarcoidosis (stage IV)
Langerhans cell histiocytosis (histiocytosis-X)
Malignancy
Pulmonary infections
Pneumocystis jiroveci
Necrotizing bacterial pneumonia
Tuberculosis
Fungal pneumonia
BAROTRAUMA/VOLUTRAUMA
Mechanical ventilation
Acute respiratory disease syndrome (ARDS)
Status asthmaticus
COPD
Inhalational drug usage
Decompression injury
TRAUMA
Blunt chest trauma
Penetrating chest trauma
Tracheobronchial injuries
Rib fractures
Esophageal rupture
IATROGENIC
Endotracheal intubation
Tracheostomy
Central venous catheter placement
Thoracentesis
Nasogastric tube placement
Bronchoscopy with bronchoalveolar lavage (BAL) or biopsies
Postoperative
Bag/valve/mask ventilation
Cardiopulmonary resuscitation

Radiologic Evaluation

The radiographic signs of pneumothorax in the supine patient frequently differ from the classic visceral pleural line seen on erect views. In a review of 88 critically ill patients with 112 pneumothoraces, only 22% of pneumothoraces were in the classic apicolateral location (101). In this same study, 30% of pneumothoraces were not detected initially, and of these, half progressed to a tension pneumothorax. The anteromedial position is the most common location for pneumothoraces in the supine patient since this area is the least dependent pleural recess (102). With anteromedial collections of air above the level of the pulmonary hilum, the lucency sharply outlines adjacent vascular structures such as the ascending aorta, superior vena cava, and azygous vein. Below the hilum, the lateral cardiac borders are sharply outlined and paralleled by zones of radiolucency. Increased lucency in the region of the anterior cardiophrenic sulcus may also result from air below the hilar level (102).

In addition to the anteromedial and apicolateral locations, pneumothoraces in supine patients can also occur in the subpulmonic and posteromedial locations (101). A subpulmonic pneumothorax may be recognized as a basilar hyperlucency, most commonly in the left hemithorax (103,104). A pleural line defining the base of the lung may be apparent in some cases, allowing for diagnosis of pneumothorax. Other features that may help in the recognition of a subpulmonic pneumothorax include lucency extending deep into the costophrenic sulcus (deep sulcus sign), depression of the hemidiaphragm, and visualization of an unusually distinct cardiac apex (105,106).

An erect or decubitus radiograph should be obtained if possible to confirm or refute the presence of a pneumothorax. In problematic cases, CT or US can be diagnostic. Several studies have demonstrated the presence of pneumothoraces on CT that were not apparent or not appreciated on conventional radiographs (14,107). Occasionally, a pneumothorax may be confused with a large bulla in patients with COPD and other pulmonary diseases that generate cystic changes. In these instances, a CT may be helpful in making the correct diagnosis (100). If the patient is too unstable to obtain a CT, bedside US can be used to evaluate for the presence of a pneumothorax by determining the presence or absence of "lung sliding." In patients without pneumothorax, the lung–chest wall interface, which represents a to-and-fro movement synchronized with respiration, can be identified. In one study, the disappearance of lung sliding was 95% sensitive for detecting pneumothorax, although false positives did occur (108).

Primary and Secondary Spontaneous Pneumothorax

Patients with pneumothorax have a decrease in vital capacity and an increase in the alveolar-arterial oxygen gradient, with hypoxemia being present in some patients. The hypoxemia is thought to be secondary to development of both anatomic shunts and areas of low ventilation/perfusion in the atelectatic lung. Patients with primary spontaneous pneumothorax rarely require admission to the ICU, as the contralateral lung can maintain the necessary alveolar ventilation and hypoxemia can be managed with supplemental oxygen. Patients with secondary spontaneous pneumothoraces may need ICU admission because the gas exchange abnormality caused by the pneumothorax is superimposed on pre-existing gas exchange abnormalities and, thus, severe hypoxemia can occur. Patients with secondary spontaneous pneumothoraces are more likely to develop hypercapnic respiratory failure than are patients with primary spontaneous pneumothorax (109,110).

Iatrogenic Pneumothorax

Insertion of central venous catheters (CVC) is the most common cause of iatrogenic pneumothoraces in the ICU. In two studies of mechanical complications of central venous catheters, 1.1% of 534 patients and 1.0% of 713 patients suffered a pneumothorax (111,112). Cannulation of the subclavian vein is associated with a higher risk of pneumothorax than cannulation of the internal jugular vein (113,114). Most pneumothoraces occur at the time of the procedure from direct lung puncture, but delayed pneumothoraces have been noted. Bilateral pneumothoraces have been reported to occur from unilateral cannulation attempts (115). A postprocedure chest radiograph should be obtained following placement of a central venous catheter, regardless of the site cannulated, to assess for pneumothorax and proper catheter tip position.

Cardiopulmonary resuscitation has been reported as a cause of iatrogenic pneumothorax. Pneumothorax in this setting may arise either from barotrauma as a consequence of bag-ventilation or from rib fractures sustained during the resuscitation. Hillman and Albin (116) described three patients who developed subcutaneous emphysema and pneumothoraces, one of whom had bilateral pneumothoraces following cardiopulmonary resuscitation with bag-ventilation. Shulman et al. (117) reported two patients in whom barotrauma was observed following resuscitation. One of the patients was ventilated with an Ambu-bag whereas the other was ventilated with a positive pressure demand valve. Other cases of pneumothorax related to cardiopulmonary resuscitation or malfunctioning valves in self-inflating bags have been reported (118,119).

Based on these observations, a chest radiograph should be obtained on all patients after a successful resuscitation to evaluate for pneumothorax. During cardiopulmonary resuscitation, if the patient is difficult to ventilate, subcutaneous emphysema is noted, or pulseless electrical activity (electromechanical dissociation) is present, the diagnosis of pneumothorax, particularly tension pneumothorax, should be suspected. In a study analyzing postmortem chest radiographs, only 40 of 77 patients had been clinically diagnosed as having a pneumothorax. In this study, procedures most frequently associated with pneumothorax were mechanical ventilation and cardiopulmonary resuscitation. Rib fractures were noted in 23 of the 77 cases (120).

Pneumothoraces may rarely occur following endotracheal intubation, usually due to rupture of the posterior membranous portion of the trachea (121). In a prospective study of translaryngeal intubation in 297 critically ill patients in a teaching hospital, pneumothorax occurred in 1% of patients (122). Pneumothoraces may also result from tracheostomy, either from open procedures or bedside percutaneous dilatational tracheostomy (123). The incidence of pneumothorax after tracheostomy in adults has been reported to be between 0% and 4% (124).

Bronchoscopy in critically ill patients may also cause pneumothoraces. The risk is higher when transbronchial biopsies are obtained, although the degree of increased risk compared to nonventilated patients and the influence of high airway pressures and positive end-expiratory pressure (PEEP) is unknown. It should be recognized that performing bronchoalveolar lavage (BAL) alone may produce a pneumothorax (125–127).

Pneumothorax Associated with Mechanical Ventilation

Pneumothorax is a frequent, potentially lethal complication of mechanical ventilation. The pathogenesis of pneumothorax associated with mechanical ventilation—barotrauma—is related to the decompression of extra-alveolar air contained in the mediastinum through the mediastinal pleura or rupture of subpleural blebs through the visceral pleura, as previously described. Conditions associated with an increased risk of pneumothorax while patients undergo mechanical ventilation include ARDS, COPD, asthma, fibrotic lung diseases, aspiration pneumonia, necrotizing pneumonia, and right mainstem bronchus intubation (100).

More recently conducted studies in mechanically ventilated patients with acute lung injury or ARDS have reported pneumothorax occurrence rates between 7% and 42% (128–133). The relationship of barotrauma and pneumothoraces to ventilatory pressures in patients with ARDS continues to be debated given earlier studies that suggested a causal relationship. Gammon et al. (128) observed that of 139 patients requiring mechanical ventilation for various diagnoses, the group with pneumothoraces had higher peak inspiratory pressure (PIP) (55 vs. 44 cm H_2O) and levels of PEEP (7.7 vs. 3.3 cm H_2O). When patients with ARDS and those with other diagnoses were analyzed separately, however, no differences in airway pressures were found between patients with and without pneumothoraces. In a subsequent study by Gammon et al. (129) of 168 patients, trends toward higher airway pressures were observed; however, multivariate analysis revealed that only the presence of ARDS was independently correlated with the development of a pneumothorax. Weg et al. (131), in their study of 725 patients with ARDS, observed no differences in PIP, mean airway pressure, levels of PEEP, or delivered tidal volumes between patients who had a pneumothorax and/or air leak and those who did not. In the study by Amato et al. (132), however, the pneumothorax rate in conventionally ventilated patients with a tidal volume of 12 mL/kg and average plateau pressure of 38 cm H_2O was 42% compared to patients ventilated with a lung protective strategy with a tidal volume of 6 mL/kg and average plateau pressure of 24 cm H_2O.

The patient requiring mechanical ventilation usually becomes symptomatic after developing a pneumothorax because of the underlying lung parenchymal disease, and this complication should be suspected whenever a sudden clinical deterioration occurs. If conscious, the patient becomes dyspneic and tachypneic and may become dyssynchronous with the ventilator; worsening oxygenation is often seen. Peak inspiratory pressures may increase with a coexisting decrease in lung compliance. A significant percentage of patients will develop a tension pneumothorax. A heightened suspicion for development of a pneumothorax should be maintained in patients who exhibit other forms of barotrauma, such as subcutaneous emphysema, pneumomediastinum, and subpleural air cysts.

Tension Pneumothorax

A tension pneumothorax occurs when intrapleural pressure exceeds atmospheric pressure throughout expiration, and often inspiration as well. This develops when a break in the visceral or parietal pleura produces a one-way valve that is open during inspiration, allowing air to enter the pleural space, but is closed during expiration, preventing the egress of air collecting in the pleural space (92). Tension pneumothoraces most commonly develop as a complication of mechanical ventilation—barotrauma or volutrauma—or as a result of blunt and penetrating thoracic trauma, although tension pneumothoraces can occur in 1% to 4% of patients with spontaneous pneumothoraces (134,135). Attempts at CVC placement in patients receiving positive pressure ventilation may also cause tension pneumothoraces, with delayed presentations having been reported (136). It is important to consider the presence of a tension pneumothorax in the differential diagnosis of a patient with pulseless electrical activity (electromechanical dissociation) undergoing cardiopulmonary resuscitation (CPR).

Tension pneumothorax usually presents as an acute cardiopulmonary emergency beginning with respiratory distress and, if unrecognized and untreated, progresses to cardiovascular collapse and death. Conscious patients with tension pneumothorax appear acutely ill with dyspnea, tachypnea, tachycardia, diaphoresis, and cyanosis. Patients with tension pneumothorax often exhibit decreased ipsilateral breath sounds, hyperresonance to percussion, distended neck veins, tracheal deviation to the contralateral side, and hypotension. Caveats to the aforementioned findings are that severe parenchymal disease or airway obstruction, coupled with the noise generated by ventilator cycling, may cause difficulty in appreciating differences between the hemithoraces, and distension of the neck veins may not be present in patients who are volume depleted. The absence of physical exam findings does not completely exclude the diagnosis of a tension pneumothorax. In the unconscious or critically ill patient, worsening oxygenation may be one of the earliest signs. Increases in airway peak and plateau pressures and decreases in compliance are often observed in mechanically ventilated patients. During hand bagging of the patient, increased pressure requirements to deliver breaths and difficulty in delivering adequate tidal volume may be noted. Increases in pulmonary artery diastolic pressures may be seen in patients who have a Swan-Ganz catheter in place (137).

On the chest radiograph in a patient with tension pneumothorax, in addition to the pneumothorax, there is often shift of the trachea and mediastinum to the contralateral side, ipsilateral diaphragmatic depression, and increased distance between contiguous ribs compared to the unaffected side. It should be emphasized, however, that tension pneumothorax is a clinical diagnosis, and these radiographic findings may be observed in patients without physiologic evidence of a tension pneumothorax. It should also be noted that patients may have cardiopulmonary compromise due to a tension pneumothorax without observing tracheal or mediastinal shift on chest radiograph (138,139).

In one study of 16 ARDS patients with tension pneumothorax, only 5 patients had subtle mediastinal shift (138). Of these 16 patients, 11 had flattening of the diaphragm and 8 had depression of the diaphragm. Diaphragmatic abnormalities may therefore be a more sensitive indicator of tension pneumothorax in patients with ARDS. In 15 of the 16 patients, the location of a loculated tension pneumothorax was subpulmonic or paracardiac. Potential explanations for these observations include the presence of adhesions between the parietal and visceral pleura, as documented in patients with ARDS, which prevent lung collapse and spread of air throughout the pleural space. In addition, the noncompliance of lungs in patients with ARDS may prevent collapse of the ipsilateral lung and compression of the contralateral lung, allowing a small volume of air to significantly increase intrapleural pressure (138,139).

It is important to note that patients with ARDS can develop tension pneumothoraces despite the presence of a chest tube on the ipsilateral side being placed for a previous pneumothorax (138–141). In the 16 patients reported by Gobien et al. (138) and the 3 patients reported by Ross et al. (139), all patients had a functional ipsilateral chest tube and had localized pneumothoraces. In a study by Heffner et al. (140), 14 patients had recurrent pneumothoraces despite ipsilateral chest tubes, with 9 of the 14 having tension pneumothoraces. In the latter study, 12 of the 14 chest tubes had horizontal as opposed to vertical placement on chest radiograph. The chest tubes in all 9 patients with tension pneumothoraces had horizontal placement. Seven of the 14 patients had subsequent CT scans, with the finding that all 7 chest tubes were placed within interlobar fissures. Thus, chest tubes placed into interlobar or posterior locations may not drain anterior gas loculations, the most common location of pneumothoraces in ARDS patients (101,142), allowing for development of localized tension pneumothoraces. In the patient reported by McConaghy and Kennedy (141), the chest tube was intraparenchymal.

Management of Pneumothoraces and Tension Pneumothoraces

Most critically ill patients in the ICU will have poor cardiopulmonary reserves and may be unable to tolerate a pneumothorax, even in the absence of tension physiology. In nonventilated patients who are hemodynamically stable and have adequate oxygenation and ventilation, simple pneumothoraces that occur as a result of a procedure and are small may reasonably be managed with close observation and monitoring with serial radiographs. Patients with secondary pneumothoraces who require ICU care will usually require chest tube placement because of their poor pulmonary reserve. Patients who are not receiving positive pressure ventilation, but are hemodynamically unstable, should be treated with chest tube thoracostomy, since the additive effects of development of hypoxia or early tension physiology could quickly precipitate cardiopulmonary arrest.

In general, chest tube thoracostomy should be performed in mechanically ventilated patients with a pneumothorax of any size given the significant risk of progression to a tension pneumothorax. Attempts to decrease plateau airway pressures, tidal volumes, and PEEP should be considered if possible after development of a pneumothorax in patients receiving mechanical ventilation. Controlled hypoventilation with the use of neuromuscular blockers or deep sedation may be required in some patients to achieve these goals. For patients with ARDS and recurrent pneumothoraces, the chest tube attempts should be made to place anteriorly where the loculation is most likely to occur. In those patients with recurrent pneumothoraces who are stable for transport to the radiology department, we advocate the use of CT-guided percutaneous drainage, as blind placement of chest tubes into loculi may be difficult (143,144). When extra-alveolar gas is observed in the absence of a pneumothorax, similar attempts to decrease plateau pressure, tidal volume, and PEEP should be considered. No evidence exists that placement of "prophylactic" chest tubes will prevent these patients from suffering a subsequent pneumothorax. These patients should be closely monitored for development of a tension pneumothorax, and equipment to perform an emergent bedside tube thoracostomy should be available.

The development of a tension pneumothorax represents a medical emergency, and the deteriorating patient should be treated based on clinical presentation without waiting for radiographic confirmation. In one series of 74 patients with tension pneumothorax, a diagnosis was made clinically in 45 patients (61%), and these patients had an attributable mortality of 7%. In the remaining 29 patients, diagnosis was delayed between 30 minutes and 8 hours; 31% of these patients died of pneumothorax (145). If a chest tube is not immediately available, a large-bore needle or intravenous catheter should be inserted into the pleural space through the second intercostal space at the midclavicular line. Escape of air from the needle confirms the diagnosis. After decompression, the needle or catheter should be left in place and in communication with the atmosphere until definitive chest tube thoracostomy is performed. As previously mentioned, a high index of suspicion for tension pneumothorax should be maintained for patients who are in cardiac arrest and exhibit pulseless electrical activity.

BRONCHOPLEURAL FISTULA IN THE INTENSIVE CARE UNIT

A bronchopleural fistula (BPF) represents a communication between the bronchial tree and the pleural space. Bronchopleural fistulae (BPFs) most commonly result from surgical procedures including pneumonectomy, segmentectomy, and wedge resections of the lung, with an incidence of 1.6% to 6.8% (146). The mortality in patients with BPFs following surgical resection is reported to be between 23% and 71%, usually due to infectious complications (146–148). BPFs may also result from blunt or penetrating chest trauma, pulmonary infarction, and as a complication of pulmonary and pleural infections such as tuberculosis, necrotizing pneumonia, lung abscess, or empyema (149,150). Last, BPFs may result as a complication of mechanical ventilation for acute respiratory failure, particularly in patients with ARDS, and, as such, represent a form of barotrauma/volutrauma (149,151). For this discussion, we will focus primarily on BPFs in the setting of patients requiring mechanical ventilation.

BPF in the ventilated patient is defined as an air leak that persists for more than 24 hours following placement of a chest tube. BPFs in patients receiving mechanical ventilation may present acutely with the development of a pneumothorax, with or without tension, or with sudden expectoration of potentially infected material from the pleural space, with flooding of the ipsilateral and contralateral airways leading to respiratory compromise.

Several potential adverse effects of a BPF in the mechanically ventilated patient have been noted. Depending on the size of the fistula, flow resistance through the fistula versus the airways and lung parenchyma, and pressure gradient between the airways and pleural space, air may be redirected from normal intrapulmonary routes to the BPF (152). This can cause loss of effective tidal volume, which may lead to difficulty in oxygenating and ventilating the patient and subsequent development of life-threatening hypoxemia and respiratory acidosis (151). If incomplete lung expansion due to the BPF is present, ventilation/perfusion mismatching and shunt may occur. There may be difficulty in maintaining PEEP with further decrements in oxygenation (153,154). If a high level of chest tube suction is used, the negative pressure may be transmitted to the proximal airways, causing inappropriate ventilator cycling (153,155). Last, BPFs may cause pleural space infection or contamination of the airways.

The amount of air flow through a BPF is typically estimated by subtracting the expired tidal volume from the inspired tidal volume as measured by the ventilator. This method, however, becomes increasingly inaccurate as the size of the leak decreases, particularly when the size of the leak is less than 200 mL/breath (156). More accurate, albeit cumbersome, methods have been developed to quantify the amount of flow through a BPF (157–160). Air flows through BPFs have been reported up to 22 L/min (157). It has been recognized that the air escaping from a BPF does not flow passively from the airways into the pleural space, but instead participates to some degree in physiologic gas exchange. In two studies evaluating CO_2 excretion by BPF in 15 patients, the percent of minute ventilation lost through the BPF ranged from 4% to 53%, with 3% to 44% of CO_2 excretion occurring *via* the BPF (161,162).

The development of a BPF has been regarded as a serious and life-threatening complication of mechanical ventilation. In one of the largest series reported—1,700 consecutive patients receiving mechanical ventilation—Pierson et al. (163) observed that 39 (2.3%) patients developed a BPF. In that study, overall mortality in patients with BPF was 67%. Mortality was higher in patients who developed a BPF late in their illness (94%) than when it occurred within 24 hours of admission (45%). Patients with air leaks greater than 500 mL/breath had a mortality of 100% compared with a mortality of 57% in patients with air leaks less than 500 mL/breath. Mortality was also higher in patients with ARDS than in patients without—81% versus 50%—and in patients with pleural space infections compared to those without said infection—87% versus 54%. A more recent ARDS study by Weg et al. (131), however, suggested that mortality was not different between patients with or without air leaks, 46% versus 39%, respectively. In that study, however, the duration of mechanical ventilation was 4.3 ± 1.3 days, which may not be typical for many patients with BPF, and the subset of patients with BPF was not analyzed separately. It may be that the presence of a BPF is a marker for severity of lung injury and by itself does not directly contribute to mortality.

Management of Bronchopleural Fistulae

Numerous interventions, listed in Table 144.3, have been proposed in the management of BPFs. Many of these are based on the concept of decreasing the pressure gradient between the airways and the pleural space, with decreased air flow through the fistula allowing for earlier closure. Although the various manipulations theoretically make sense, they have not been evaluated in controlled trials. The suggested changes in ventilator settings may actually worsen oxygenation and ventilation in some patients with ARDS. We will discuss those interventions for which some data are available in the following sections. In the absence of difficulty oxygenating or ventilating the patient, it is unknown if active measures to close the BPF affects outcome. Definitive therapy for BPFs includes surgical procedures such as bronchial stump closure with thoracoplasty, myoplasty, or omentoplasty, or completion pneumonectomy (146,148). Unfortunately, most critically ill patients will not be sufficiently stable to undergo these procedures and must be managed medically. Adequate pleural space drainage, antibiotic therapy for pleural space infections, and support of nutritional status is vital in these patients.

TABLE 144.3

POTENTIAL OPTIONS FOR MANAGEMENT OF BRONCHOPLEURAL FISTULA IN MECHANICALLY VENTILATED PATIENTS

CHEST TUBE DRAINAGE
Adequate size chest tube
Drainage system with adequate ability to handle air leak
Additional chest tube placement if lung not fully expanded
REDUCE AIRWAY PRESSURES
Reduce delivered tidal volume
Use synchronized intermittent mandatory ventilation (SIMV) instead of assist-control mode
Decrease level of positive end-expiratory pressure (PEEP)
Decrease inspiratory time (I:E ratio)
Avoid inspiratory pause
Minimize auto-PEEP
ALTERNATIVE MODES OF MECHANICAL VENTILATION
High-frequency jet ventilation
High-frequency oscillatory ventilation
Independent lung ventilation
CHEST TUBE MANIPULATION
Decrease chest tube suction
Apply PEEP to chest tube
Inspiratory chest tube occlusion
DIRECT CLOSURE/OCCLUSION OF BRONCHOPLEURAL FISTULA (BPF)
Surgical closure or resection
Endobronchial occlusion of BPF
Cyanoacrylate-based tissue adhesives
Fibrin sealants
One-way endobronchial valves
Stent placement
Pleurodesis
Blood patch
Talc
Doxycycline

Adequate chest tube drainage and full expansion of the lung should be assessed in patients with BPF. An appropriately sized chest tube should be placed, recognizing that air flow through a chest tube is inversely proportional to the length and radius to the fifth power of the tube. It has been suggested that a tube with an internal diameter of 6 mm (18 Fr) is the smallest acceptable size because it will allow a maximum possible flow rate of 15 L/minute at –10 cm H_2O (164). Our preference is to use at least a 28 Fr chest tube in these patients. Placement of additional chest tubes or CT-guided percutaneous catheters—if the pleural space is complicated—should be considered if the lung is not fully expanded. As with the chest tube, resistance to flow of air through a chest tube drainage system may need to be considered. In an animal model of BPF, when the size of air leak reached 4 to 5 L/minute, the Thora-Klex and Sentinel Seal systems become clinically impractical. The Pleur-Evac system can handle flow rates up to 34 L/minute, although its use with rates greater than 28 L/min is impractical due to intense bubbling in the control chamber. The Emerson pump, which can be set to deliver chest tube suction greater than –20 cm H_2O, is capable of handling air flows up to 35 L/min and is the system of choice for BPFs with extremely high flow rates (164).

Manipulation of the level of chest tube suction may affect BPF air flow, and some authors have suggested using the least amount of suction that maintains lung inflation (151,152). An animal model demonstrated that increasingly negative intrapleural pressures increased air flow in large BPFs but had no effect on small BPFs (165). Roth et al. (160) reported that increasing chest tube suction from 0 to 22.5 cm H_2O increased BPF flow in a patient from 24.6 to 26.7 L/minute. In a study of six patients by Powner et al. (158), increasing chest tube suction from 0 to 25 cm H_2O increased BPF flow in two patients, had no effect in two patients, and decreased flow in two patients. To decrease air loss through the BPF and applied PEEP, some investigators have applied PEEP to the chest tube (154,166,167), while others have devised systems to synchronously occlude the chest tube during inspiration (168,169). A lack of success using these methods has been noted by other investigators, however (163). These techniques may pose a risk of increasing the size of the pneumothorax or causing a tension pneumothorax; thus, the patient should be closely monitored.

The goals of mechanical ventilation in patients with a BPF are to maintain adequate oxygenation and ventilation while reducing fistula flow. In general, strategies for conventional mechanical ventilation that limit airway pressure and tidal volumes may reduce the amount of air flow escaping through the BPF and allow the fistulous site to heal. As such, it has been recommended to use the lowest possible tidal volume, fewest mechanical breaths per minute, lowest level of PEEP, and shortest inspiratory time.

Alternative methods of mechanical ventilation have been used in a few patients. High-frequency jet ventilation (HFJV) and high-frequency oscillatory ventilation (HFOV) have been used based on the principle that lower airway pressures may be generated in these modes of ventilation and should, therefore, decrease BPF air flow. In one animal model of BPF, an increase in fistula flow was seen with increasing mean airway pressures, and effects on flow were similar whether mean airway pressure was changed by manipulating peak inspiratory pressure, PEEP, or inspiratory:expiratory (I:E) ratios (165). In another animal model, a nonsignificant trend toward increasing BPF flow with increasing peak inspiratory pressures, and a significant increase in BPF flow with increasing PEEP was observed (170).

Several studies comparing HFJV and HFOV with conventional ventilation using animal models have shown less BPF air flow during HFJV and HFOV (171–174), although one study using HFJV demonstrated no difference (175). In studies reporting blood gases, improved oxygenation was seen during HFJV and HFOV compared with conventional ventilation (172–174). Increasing levels of PEEP were also noted to increase BPF flow in two studies (171,175). It is problematic to extrapolate these studies to patients in the ICU because the animal models were cannulated in more proximal bronchi and the lung parenchyma was relatively normal.

HFJV has been used successfully in BPF patients failing conventional therapy (176–180). The two case series comparing the use of HFJV with conventional ventilation have reported disappointing results. In one study, HFJV was of clinical value in only two of the seven patients (159). In that study, no change in the air leak was observed in three patients; one had an unacceptable decline in oxygenation, and one patient disliked the sensation of HFJV and refused further therapy. In the other series of seven patients, no significant decrease in BPF flow was seen, while three patients had an increase in the air leak despite a decrease in peak airway pressures (181). Oxygenation deteriorated in six of the seven patients when switched to HFJV.

Other modes of mechanical ventilation have also been used in patients with BPF. Case reports have reported independent lung ventilation to be of benefit (182–184). Case reports of combining independent lung ventilation with high-frequency, low tidal volume ventilation of the affected lung (185) and HFJV of the affected lung have been published (186,187). Differential lung ventilation using a single ventilator and a variable resistance valve attached to one lumen of a bifurcated endotracheal tube has also been described (188,189). Discussion of the techniques of independent lung ventilation and its attendant difficulties is beyond the scope of this chapter, and the reader is referred to other reviews (190,191).

Because many critically ill patients are unable to tolerate a major thoracic procedure, bronchoscopic techniques may provide viable alternatives for closure of BPFs. Endobronchial occlusion of BPFs has been reported with cyanoacrylate-based tissue adhesives (Histoacryl, Bucrylate), fibrin sealants (Tisseal, Hemaseal, thrombin plus fibrinogen or cryoprecipitate), absorbable gelatin sponge (Gelfoam), vascular occlusion coils, doxycycline and blood, Nd:YAG laser, silver nitrate, and lead shot (192–194). The agent initially seals the leak by acting as a plug and subsequently induces an inflammatory process with fibrosis and mucosal proliferation, permanently sealing the area. Of these techniques, the uses of cyanoacrylate tissue adhesives and fibrin sealants have been most widely reported. Airway stents may be used to cover and seal the fistula in selected patients depending on the location of the fistula. BPFs due to breakdown of a stump after lobectomy or pneumonectomy, or bronchial dehiscence after lung transplantation or bronchoplastic procedures are the most amenable to successful closure with airway stenting. More recently, the successful closure of BPFs using bronchoscopic placement of endobronchial valves designed for emphysema has been described (195–197).

Pleurodesis with various agents has also been tried to effect closure of BPFs. Autologous "blood patch" pleurodesis has been described to be effective in some patients (198–200). Pleurodesis with fibrin glue has also been reported (201,202). However, none of these patients was undergoing mechanical ventilation at the time of pleurodesis.

COMPLICATIONS OF THORACENTESIS AND CHEST TUBE THORACOSTOMY

Thoracentesis

The most common complication of diagnostic or therapeutic thoracentesis is pneumothorax. The rate of pneumothorax with blind thoracentesis in nonventilated patients has been reported to be between 4% and 30% in prospective studies

(16–20). As previously noted, the 5% to 10% rate of pneumothorax in mechanically ventilated patients undergoing blind thoracentesis is similar to that of nonventilated patients (21–23). Pneumothorax may be more common following therapeutic thoracentesis than diagnostic thoracentesis, although this was not confirmed in other studies. The incidence of pneumothorax following thoracentesis appears to be less with ultrasound guidance in both nonventilated and mechanically ventilated patients (6–8,20,24). Hemothorax has been reported in 0.8% and 1.2% of patients (17,203). Other infrequent complications with an incidence less than 1% include laceration of intercostal vessels, liver and splenic puncture, intra-abdominal hemorrhage, catheter shearing with retained catheter in the pleural space, and systemic air embolism (17,18,203).

Chest Tube Thoracostomy

The complication rate for chest tube placement, excluding recurrent pneumothorax, is low, ranging from 1% to 3% when placed for acute trauma (204–206). Reported complications in these studies were empyema (1%–3%), lung parenchyma perforation (0.2%–0.6%), diaphragmatic perforation (0.4%), and subcutaneous placement (0.6%). In an analysis of 126 chest tube placements by pulmonologists at a teaching hospital, the complication rate was 11%, although 10 of the 14 reported complications were related to clotting, kinking, or dislodgment of the chest tube (207). Pulmonary laceration was reported in one patient (0.8%), and subcutaneous placement was noted in one patient (0.8%).

In addition to empyema, chest tube malposition is the most common complication of chest tube thoracostomy. In a study of 77 chest tubes placed emergently in 51 trauma patients, subsequent assessment by CT scanning revealed malpositioning in 20 of the 77 (26%) chest tubes (208). Two chest tubes were subcutaneous, five were intraparenchymal, and nine were intrafissural. Insufficient information was available to determine intraparenchymal versus intrafissural tube placement in four patients. Sixteen of the 20 (80%) chest tube malpositions were associated with persistent pneumothoraces and hemothoraces, including 2 under tension. Of the five intraparenchymal chest tubes documented at CT, only one could be diagnosed by chest radiograph, and only four of the nine intrafissural chest tubes were noted on chest radiograph. Delayed pulmonary perforation by a chest tube has been reported (209), and autopsies have noted perforations that were not clinically suspected (210).

In addition to perforation of the lung, perforation of diaphragm and intra-abdominal organs (spleen, liver, stomach, and colon) has been reported (205,211). These complications are more likely with the use of a trocar. We and others (211) believe that the trocar should never be used. Exploration of the pleural space with a finger should be done prior to tube insertion to confirm placement into the pleural space and to assess for the presence of pleural adhesions and adhesion of the lung to the chest wall, which increases the risk of pulmonary perforation. Other complications include perforation of the right ventricle and right atrium (212,213), cardiogenic shock due to chest tube compression of the right ventricle (214), mediastinal perforation and contralateral hemothorax and pneumothorax (215,216), bleeding from intercostal artery injury (217), and infection at the chest tube site.

Re-expansion Pulmonary Edema

Re-expansion pulmonary edema (RPE) represents one of the most potentially life-threatening complications of therapeutic thoracentesis and chest tube thoracostomy for pleural effusion and pneumothorax. RPE has also been reported following re-expansion of atelectasis from endobronchial obstruction and right mainstem bronchus intubation (218–220). Patients developing significant hypoxemia from RPE will often require admission to the ICU. The precise incidence of RPE is unknown. In two series of 400 and 375 cases of spontaneous pneumothorax, no cases of RPE were noted (221,222). Matsuura et al. (223), however, reported that 14% of 146 patients treated for spontaneous pneumothorax developed RPE. In a series of 320 patients with spontaneous pneumothorax, Rozenman et al. (224) observed a 0.9% incidence of RPE, which is likely to best represent the clinical occurrence of RPE. To our knowledge, no studies have been done evaluating the incidence or clinical course of RPE in ICU patients undergoing thoracentesis or chest tube placement. In the study by Matsuura et al. (223), 8 of the 21 patients with RPE were reported as having tension pneumothoraces.

Clinical signs and symptoms include cough, chest tightness or chest pain, dyspnea, tachypnea, tachycardia, and ipsilateral crackles. Patients may produce pink frothy sputum or have frank hemoptysis. The onset of symptoms is immediate or within 1 hour of thoracentesis or chest tube placement in two thirds of patients but may be delayed up to 24 hours (225). Infiltrates are almost always ipsilateral to the side of the pneumothorax or effusion, although contralateral infiltrates alone and bilateral infiltrates have been reported (226). Focal infiltrates corresponding to areas of atelectasis produced by the effusion or pneumothorax have also been reported. RPE has been reported to occur primarily in chronically collapsed lungs. In a review of reported cases by Mahfood et al. (225), however, 8 of 47 (17%) patients and 9 of the 21 (43%) patients in the series of Matsuura et al. (223) had pneumothoraces for less than 24 hours.

Although hypoxemic respiratory failure is a well-recognized complication of RPE, it may not be appreciated that RPE may cause hypotension and cardiovascular collapse. Several case reports have noted severe hypotension with RPE despite adequate oxygenation in some patients (227–230). In patients in whom a Swan-Ganz catheter was placed, a low cardiac output, a low or normal PCWP, and normal systemic vascular resistance were uniformly observed (227–230). Hemoconcentration was noted in some patients, suggesting that third-spacing of fluids into the lung accounted for part of the hypotension (230). Many of these patients remained hypotensive despite administration of large amounts of intravenous fluids and vasopressor agents, however, and mortality was 40% (four of ten patients).

Treatment of RPE is mainly supportive, with mechanical ventilation and PEEP being the mainstay of therapy. Diuretics and corticosteroids have been used by some clinicians, although evidence that they are of benefit is lacking. In patients with hypotension, administration of intravenous fluids and vasopressor agents may be necessary. The development of RPE carries a substantial mortality. In a review of 53 reported cases of RPE, Mahfood et al. (225) noted an observed mortality of 20%.

References

1. Wiener MD, Garay SM, Leitman BS, et al. Imaging of the intensive care unit patient. *Clin Chest Med.* 1991;12:169.
2. Collins JD, Burwell D, Furmanksi S, et al. Minimal detectable pleural effusions: a roentgen pathology model. *Radiology.* 1972;105:51.
3. Woodring JH. Recognition of pleural effusion of supine radiographs: how much fluid is required? *AJR Am J Roentgenol.* 1984;142:59.
4. Mattison LE, Coppage L, Alderman DF, et al. Pleural effusions in the Medical ICU: prevalence, causes, and clinical implications. *Chest.* 1997;111:1018.
5. Yu CJ, Yang PC, Chang DB, et al. Diagnostic and therapeutic use of chest sonography: value in critically ill patients. *AJR Am J Roentgenol.* 1992;159:695.
6. Mayo PH, Goltz HR, Tafreshi M, et al. Safety of ultrasound-guided thoracentesis in patients receiving mechanical ventilation. *Chest.* 2004;125:1059.
7. Lichtenstein D, Hulot JS, Rabiller A, et al. Feasibility and safety of ultrasound-aided thoracentesis in mechanically ventilated patients. *Intensive Care Med.* 1999;25:955.
8. Petersen S, Freitag M, Albert W, et al. Ultrasound-guided thoracentesis in surgical intensive care patients. *Intensive Care Med.* 1999;25:1029.
9. Yang PC, Luh KT, Chang DB, et al. Value of sonography in determining the nature of pleural effusion: analysis of 320 cases. *AJR Am J Roentgenol.* 1992;159:29.
10. McLoud TC, Flower CDR. Imaging the pleura: sonography, CT, and MR imaging. *AJR Am J Roentgenol.* 1991;156:1145.
11. McLoud TC. CT and MR in pleural disease. *Clin Chest Med.* 1998;19:261.
12. Stark DD, Federle MP, Goodman PC, et al. Differentiating lung abscess and empyema: radiography and computed tomography. *AJR Am J Roentgenol.* 1983;141:163.
13. Waite RJ, Carbonneau RJ, Balikian JP, et al. Parietal pleural changes in empyema: appearances at CT. *Radiology.* 1990;175:145.
14. Mirvis SE, Tobin KD, Kostrubiak I, et al. Thoracic CT in detecting occult disease in critically ill patients. *AJR Am J Roentgenol.* 1987;148:685.
15. Sahn SA. The pleura: state of the art. *Am Rev Respir Dis.* 1988;138:184.
16. Barter T, Mayo PD, Pratter MR, et al. Lower risk and higher yield for thoracentesis when performed by experienced operators. *Chest.* 1993;103:1873.
17. Seneff MG, Corwin W, Gold LH, et al. Complications associated with thoracentesis. *Chest.* 1986;90:97.
18. Collins TR, Sahn SA. Thoracocentesis: clinical value, complications, technical problems, and patient experience. *Chest.* 1987;91:817.
19. Colt HG, Brewer N, Barbur E. Evaluation of patient-related and procedure-related factors contributing to pneumothorax following thoracentesis. *Chest.* 1999;116:134.
20. Grogan DR, Irwin RS, Channick R, et al. Complications associated with thoracentesis: a prospective, randomized study comparing three different methods. *Arch Intern Med.* 1990;150:873.
21. LeMense GP, Sahn SA. Safety and value of thoracentesis in medical ICU patients. *J Intensive Care Med.* 1998;13:144.
22. Godwin JE, Sahn SA. Thoracentesis: a safe procedure in mechanically ventilated patients. *Ann Intern Med.* 1990;113:800.
23. McCartney JP, Adams JW II, Hazard PB. Safety of thoracentesis in mechanically ventilated patients. *Chest.* 1993;103:1920.
24. Jones PW, Moyers JP, Rogers JT, et al. Ultrasound-guided thoracentesis: is it a safer method? *Chest.* 2003;123:418.
25. McVay PA, Toy PTCY. Lack of increased bleeding after paracentesis and thoracentesis in patients with mild coagulation abnormalities. *Transfusion.* 1991;31:164.
26. Talmor M, Hydo L, Gershenwald JG, et al. Beneficial effects of chest tube drainage of pleural effusion in acute respiratory failure refractory to positive end-expiratory pressure ventilation. *Surgery.* 1998;123:137.
27. Raptopoulos V, Davis LM, Lee G, et al. Factors affecting the development of pneumothorax associated with thoracentesis. *AJR Am J Roentgenol.* 1991;156:917.
28. Petersen WG, Zimmerman R. Limited utility of chest radiograph after thoracentesis. *Chest.* 2000;117:1038.
29. Light RW, Jenkinson SG, Minh V, et al. Observations on pleural pressures as fluid is withdrawn during thoracentesis. *Am Rev Respir Dis.* 1980;121:799.
30. Agusti AG, Cardus J, Roca J, et al. Ventilation-perfusion mismatch in patients with pleural effusion: effects of thoracentesis. *Am J Respir Crit Care Med.* 1997;156:1205.
31. Judson MA, Sahn SA. Pulmonary physiologic abnormalities caused by pleural disease. *Semin Respir Crit Care Med.* 1995;16:346.
32. Brandsletter RD, Cohen RP. Hypoxemia after thoracentesis: a predictable and treatable condition. *JAMA.* 1979;242:1060.
33. Karetzky MS, Kothari GA, Fourre JA, et al. Effect of thoracentesis on arterial oxygen tension. *Respiration.* 1978;36:96.
34. Brown NE, Zamel N, Aberman A. Changes in pulmonary mechanics and gas exchange following thoracocentesis. *Chest.* 1978;540.
35. Wang J-S, Tseng CH. Changes in pulmonary mechanics and gas exchange after thoracentesis on patients with inversion of a hemidiaphragm secondary to large pleural effusion. *Chest.* 1995;107:1610.
36. Doelken P, Abreu R, Sahn SA, et al. Effect of thoracentesis on respiratory mechanics and gas exchange in the patient receiving mechanical ventilation. *Chest.* 2006;130:1354.
37. Light RW, George RB. Incidence and significance of pleural effusion after surgery. *Chest.* 1976;69:621.
38. Nielsen PH, Jepsan SB, Olsen AD. Postoperative pleural effusion following upper abdominal surgery. *Chest.* 1989;96:1133.
39. Aberle DR, Wiener-Kronish JP, Webb WR, et al. Hydrostatic vs. increased permeability pulmonary edema: diagnosis based on radiographic criteria in critically ill patients. *Radiology.* 1988;168:73.
40. Wiener-Kronish JP, Broaddus VC, Albertine KH, et al. Relationship of pleural effusions to increased permeability pulmonary edema in anesthetized sheep. *J Clin Invest.* 1988;82:1422.
41. Miller KS, Harley RA, Sahn SA. Pleural effusions associated with ethchlorvynol lung injury result from visceral pleural leak. *Am Rev Respir Dis.* 1989;140:764.
42. Doerr CH, Miller DL, Ryu JH. Chylothorax. *Semin Respir Crit Care Med.* 2001;22:617.
43. Valentine VG, Raffin TA. The management of chylothorax. *Chest.* 1992;102:586.
44. Ferguson MK, Little AG, Skinner DB. Current concepts in the management of postoperative chylothorax. *Ann Thorac Surg.* 1985;40:542.
45. Cerfolio RJ, Allen MS, Deschamps C, et al. Postoperative chylothorax. *J Thorac Cardiovasc Surg.* 1996;112:1361.
46. Spiro JD, Spiro RH, Strong EW. The management of chyle fistula. *Laryngoscope.* 1990;100:771.
47. Teba L, Dedhia HV, Bowen R, et al. Chylothorax review. *Crit Care Med.* 1985;13:49.
48. Staats BA, Ellefson RD, Budhan LL, et al. The lipoprotein profile of chylous and non-chylous pleural effusions. *Mayo Clin Proc.* 1980;55:700.
49. Wiener-Kronish JP, Matthay MA, Callen PW, et al. Relationship of pulmonary hemodynamics to pleural effusions in patients with heart failure. *Am Rev Respir Dis.* 1985;132:1253.
50. Shinto RA, Light RW. Effects of diuresis on the characteristics of pleural fluid in patients with congestive heart failure. *Am J Med.* 1990;88:230.
51. Light RW, Rogers JT, Cheng D-S, et al. Large pleural effusions occurring after coronary artery bypass grafting. *Ann Intern Med.* 1999;130:891.
52. Kollef MH. Trapped-lung syndrome after cardiac surgery: a potentially preventable complication of pleural injury. *Heart Lung.* 1990;19:671.
53. Henderson JAM, Peloquin AJM. Boerhaave revisited: spontaneous esophageal perforation as a diagnostic masquerader. *Am J Med.* 1989;86:559.
54. O'Connell ND. Spontaneous rupture of the esophagus. *Am J Roentgen.* 1967;99:186.
55. Drury M, Anderson W, Heffner JE. Diagnostic value of pleural fluid cytology in occult Boerhaave's syndrome. *Chest.* 1992;102:976.
56. Bacon BR, Bailey-Newton RS, Connors AF. Pleural effusions after endoscopic variceal sclerotherapy. *Gastroenterology.* 1985;88:1910.
57. Symbas PN. Cardiothoracic trauma. *Curr Probl Surg.* 1991;28:741.
58. Feliciano DV. The diagnostic and therapeutic approach to chest trauma. *Semin Thorac Cardiovasc Surg.* 1992;4:156.
59. Gur C, Ilan Y, Shibolet O. Hepatic hydrothorax—pathophysiology, diagnosis and treatment—review of the literature. *Liver Int.* 2004;24:281.
60. Cardenas A, Arroyo V. Management of ascites and hepatic hydrothorax. *Best Pract Res Clin Gastroenterol.* 2007;21:55.
61. Verreault J, Lepage S, Bisson G, et al. Ascites and right pleural effusion: demonstration of a peritoneo-pleural communication. *J Nucl Med.* 1986;27:1706.
62. Mouroux J, Perrin C, Venissac N, et al. Management of pleural effusion of cirrhotic origin. *Chest.* 1996;109:1093.
63. Xiol X, Castellvi JM, Guardiolo J, et al. Spontaneous bacterial empyema in cirrhotic patients: a prospective study. *Hepatology.* 1996;23:719.
64. Eid AA, Keddissi JI, Kinasewitz GT. Hypoalbuminemia as a cause of pleural effusions. *Chest.* 1999;115:1066.
65. Scott WL. Complications associated with central venous catheters: a survey. *Chest.* 1988;94:1221.
66. Duntley P, Siever J, Korwes ML, et al. Vascular erosion by central venous catheters: clinical features and outcome. *Chest.* 1992;101:1633.
67. Aslamy Z, Dewald CL, Heffner JE. MRI of central venous anatomy: implications for central venous catheter insertion. *Chest.* 1998;114:820.
68. Maringhini A, Ciambra M, Patti R, et al. Ascites, pleural, and pericardial effusions in acute pancreatitis: a prospective study of incidence, natural history, and prognostic role. *Dig Dis Sci.* 1996;41:848.
69. Kaye MD. Pleuropulmonary complications of pancreatitis. *Thorax.* 1968;23:297.
70. Lankisch PG, Droge M, Becher R. Pleural effusions: a new negative prognostic parameter for acute pancreatitis. *Am J Gastroenterol.* 1994;89:1849.
71. Strange C, Sahn SA. The definitions and epidemiology of pleural space infection. *Semin Respir Infect.* 1999;14:3.
72. Rahman NM, Chapman SJ, Davies RJ. The approach to the patient with a parapneumonic effusion. *Clin Chest Med.* 2006;27:253.

73. Schiza S, Siafakas NM. Clinical presentation and management of empyema, lung abscess and pleural effusion. *Curr Opin Pulm Med.* 2006;12:205.
74. Light RW. Parapneumonic effusions and empyema. *Proc Am Thorac Soc.* 2006;3:75.
75. Heffner JE. Indications for draining a parapneumonic effusion: an evidence-based approach. *Semin Respir Infect.* 1999;14:48.
76. Sahn SA. Use of fibrinolytic agents in the management of complicated parapneumonic effusions and empyemas. *Thorax.* 1998;53(Suppl 2):S65.
77. Moulton JS. Image-guided drainage techniques. *Semin Respir Infect.* 1999;14:59.
78. Landreneau RJ, Keenan RJ, Hazelrigg SR, et al. Thoracoscopy for empyema and hemothorax. *Chest.* 1995;109:18.
79. Ferguson MK. Surgical management of intrapleural infections. *Semin Respir Infect.* 1999;14:73.
80. Cremonesini D, Thomson AH. How should we manage empyema: antibiotics alone, fibrinolytics, or primary video-assisted thoracoscopic surgery (VATS)? *Semin Respir Crit Care Med.* 2007;28:322.
81. Everts RJ, Reller LB. Pleural space infections: microbiology and antimicrobial therapy. *Semin Respir Infect.* 1999;14:18.
82. Dressler W. The post-myocardial-infarction syndrome: a report on forty-four cases. *Arch Intern Med.* 1959;103:28.
83. Stelzner TJ, King TE, Antony VB, et al. The pleuropulmonary manifestations of the postcardiac injury syndrome. *Chest.* 1983;84:383.
84. Khan AH. The postcardiac injury syndromes. *Clin Cardiol.* 1992;15:67.
85. Kim S, Sahn SA. Postcardiac injury syndrome: an immunologic pleural fluid analysis. *Chest.* 1996;109:570.
86. Bynum LJ, Wilson JE III. Radiographic features of pleural effusions in pulmonary embolism. *Am Rev Respir Dis.* 1978;117:829.
87. Bynum LJ, Wilson JE III. Characteristics of pleural effusions associated with pulmonary embolism. *Arch Intern Med.* 1976;136:159.
88. Sahn SA. Pleural fluid analysis: narrowing the differential diagnosis. *Semin Respir Med.* 1987;9:22.
89. Simon HB, Daggett WN, DeSanctis RW. Hemothorax as a complication of anticoagulant therapy in the presence of pulmonary infarction. *JAMA.* 1969;208:1830.
90. Brathwaite CE, Mure AJ, O'Malley KF, et al. Complications of anticoagulation for pulmonary embolism in low risk trauma patients. *Chest.* 1993;104:718.
91. Berger HW, Rammohan G, Neff MS, et al. Uremic pleural effusion: a study in 14 patients on chronic dialysis. *Ann Intern Med.* 1975;82:362.
92. Jarratt MJ, Sahn SA. Pleural effusions in hospitalized patients receiving long-term hemodialysis. *Chest.* 1995;108:470.
93. Galen MA, Steinberg SM, Lowrie EG, et al. Hemorrhagic pleural effusion in patients undergoing chronic hemodialysis. *Ann Intern Med.* 1975;82:359.
94. Bakirci T, Sasak G, Ozturk S, et al. Pleural effusion in long-term hemodialysis patients. *Transplant Proc.* 2007;39:889.
95. Yoshii C, Morita S, Tokunaga M, et al. Bilateral massive pleural effusions caused by uremic pleuritis. *Intern Med.* 2001;40:646.
96. Rodelas R, Rakowski TA, Argy WP, et al. Fibrosing uremic pleuritis during hemodialysis. *JAMA.* 1980;243:2424.
97. Maher JF. Uremic pleuritis. *Am J Kidney Dis.* 1987;10:19.
98. Maunder RJ, Pierson DJ, Hudson LD. Subcutaneous and mediastinal emphysema: pathophysiology, diagnosis, and management. *Arch Intern Med.* 1984;144:1447.
99. Macklin MT, Macklin CC. Malignant interstitial emphysema of the lungs and mediastinum as an important occult complication in may respiratory diseases and other conditions: an interpretation of the clinical literature in the light of laboratory experiment. *Medicine.* 1944;23:281.
100. Jantz MA, Pierson DJ. Pneumothorax and barotrauma. *Clin Chest Med.* 1994;15:75.
101. Tocino IM, Miller MH, Fairfax WR. Distribution of pneumothorax in the supine and semirecumbent critically ill adult. *AJR Am J Roentgenol.* 1985;144:901.
102. Buckner CB, Harmon BH, Plallin JS. The radiology of abnormal intrathoracic air. *Curr Probl Diagn Radiol.* 1988;17:37.
103. Tocino IM. Pneumothorax in the supine patient: radiographic anatomy. *Radiographics.* 1985;5:557.
104. Ziter FM, Westcott JL. Supine subpulmonary pneumothorax. *AJR Am J Roentgenol.* 1981;137:699.
105. Gordon R. The deep sulcus sign. *Radiology.* 1980;136:25.
106. Rhea JT, van Sonnenberg E, McLoud TC. Basilar pneumothorax in the supine adult. *Radiology.* 1979;133:593.
107. McGonigal MD, Schwab CW, Kauder DR, et al. Supplemental emergent chest computed tomography in the management of blunt torso trauma. *J Trauma.* 1990;30:1431.
108. Lichtenstein DA, Menu Y. A bedside ultrasound sign ruling out pneumothorax in the critically ill. *Chest.* 1995;108:1345.
109. Dines DE, Clagett OT, Payne WS. Spontaneous pneumothorax and emphysema. *Mayo Clin Proc.* 1970;45:481.
110. George RB, Herbert SJ, Shames JM, et al. Pneumothorax complicating pulmonary emphysema. *JAMA.* 1975;234:389.
111. Hagley MT, Martin B, Gast P, et al. Infectious and mechanical complications of central venous catheters placed by percutaneous venipuncture and over guidewires. *Crit Care Med.* 1992;20:1426.
112. Giuffrida DJ, Bryan-Brown CW, Lumb PD, et al. Central vs peripheral venous catheters in critically ill patients. *Chest.* 1986;90:806.
113. Eerola R, Kaukinen L, Kaukinen S. Analysis of 13,800 subclavian catheterizations. *Acta Anesthesiol Scand.* 1985;29:193.
114. Tyden H. Cannulation of the internal jugular vein—500 cases. *Acta Anesthesiol Scand.* 1982;26:485.
115. Weiner P, Sznajder I, Plavnick L, et al. Unusual complications of subclavian vein catheterization. *Crit Care Med.* 1984;12:538.
116. Hillman K, Albin M. Pulmonary barotrauma during cardiopulmonary resuscitation. *Crit Care Med.* 1986;14:606.
117. Shulman D, Beilin B, Olshwang D. Pulmonary barotrauma during cardiopulmonary resuscitation. *Resuscitation.* 1987;15:201.
118. Myers DP, de Leon-Casasola OA, Bacon DR, et al. Bilateral pneumothoraces from a malfunctioning resuscitation valve. *J Clin Anesth.* 1993;5:433.
119. Silbergleit R, Lee DC, Blank-Reid C, et al. Sudden severe barotrauma from self-inflating bag-valve devices. *J Trauma.* 1996;40:320.
120. Ludwig J, Kienzle GD. Pneumothorax in a large autopsy population: a study of 77 cases. *Am J Clin Pathol.* 1978;70:24.
121. McCulloch TM, Bishop MJ. Complications of translaryngeal intubation. *Clin Chest Med.* 1991;12:507.
122. Schwartz DE, Matthay MA, Cohen NH. Death and other complications of emergency airway management in critically ill adults: a prospective investigation of 297 tracheal intubations. *Anesthesiology.* 1995;82:367.
123. Berroushot J, Oeken J, Steiniger L, et al. Perioperative complications of percutaneous dilatational tracheostomy. *Laryngoscope.* 1997;107:1538.
124. Myers EN, Carrau RL. Early complications of tracheotomy: incidence and management. *Clin Chest Med.* 1991;12:589.
125. Steinberg KP, Mitchell DR, Maunder RJ, et al. Safety of bronchoalveolar lavage in patients with adult respiratory distress syndrome. *Am Rev Respir Dis.* 1993;148:556.
126. Ruiz F, Casado T, Monso E. Pneumothorax during bronchoalveolar lavage. *Chest.* 1989;96:1441.
127. Cazzadori A, Di Perri G, Bonora S, et al. Fatal pneumothorax complicating BAL in a bone marrow transplant recipient with bronchiolitis obliterans. *Chest.* 1997;111:1468.
128. Gammon RB, Shin MS, Buchalter SE. Pulmonary barotrauma in mechanical ventilation: patterns and risk factors. *Chest.* 1992;102:568.
129. Gammon RB, Shin MS, Groves RH Jr, et al. Clinical risk factors for pulmonary barotrauma: a multivariate analysis. *Am J Respir Crit Care Med.* 1995;152:1235.
130. Schnapp LM, Chin DP, Szaflarski N, et al. Frequency and importance of barotrauma in 100 patients with acute lung injury. *Crit Care Med.* 1995;23:272.
131. Weg JG, Anzuetto A, Balk RA, et al. The relationship of pneumothorax and other air leaks to mortality in the acute respiratory distress syndrome. *N Engl J Med.* 1998;338:341.
132. Amato MBP, Barbas CSV, Medeiros DM, et al. Effect of a protective-ventilation strategy on mortality in the acute respiratory distress syndrome. *N Engl J Med.* 1998;338:347.
133. Stewart TE, Meade MO, Cook DJ, et al. Evaluation of a ventilation strategy to prevent barotrauma in patients at high risk for acute respiratory distress syndrome. *N Engl J Med.* 1998;338:355.
134. Moxon RK. Spontaneous pneumothorax: observations on twenty-six cases. *U S Armed Forces Med J.* 1950;1:1157.
135. Myers JA. Simple spontaneous pneumothorax. *Dis Chest.* 1954;26:120.
136. Plewa MC, Ledrick D, Sferra JJ. Delayed tension pneumothorax complicating central venous catheterization and positive pressure ventilation. *Am J Emerg Med.* 1995;13:532.
137. Yu PYH, Lee LW. Pulmonary artery pressures with tension pneumothorax. *Can J Anaesth.* 1990;37:584.
138. Gobien RP, Reines HD, Schabel SI. Localized tension pneumothorax: unrecognized form of barotrauma in adult respiratory distress syndrome. *Radiology.* 1982;142:15.
139. Ross IB, Fleiszer DM, Brown RA. Localized tension pneumothorax in patients with adult respiratory distress syndrome. *Can J Surg.* 1994;37:415.
140. Heffner JE, McDonald J, Barbieri C. Recurrent pneumothoraces in ventilated patients despite ipsilateral chest tubes. *Chest.* 1995;108:1053.
141. McConaghy PM, Kennedy N. Tension pneumothorax due to intrapulmonary placement of intercostal chest drain. *Anaesth Intensive Care.* 1995;23:496.
142. Tagliabue M, Casella T, Zincone G, et al. CT and chest radiography in the evaluation of adult respiratory distress syndrome. *Acta Radiol.* 1994;35:230.
143. Kaplan LJ, Trooskin SZ, Santora TA, et al. Percutaneous drainage of recurrent pneumothoraces and pneumatoceles. *J Trauma.* 1996;41:1069.
144. Klein JS, Schultz S, Heffner JE. Interventional radiology of the chest: image-guided percutaneous drainage of pleural effusions, lung abscess, and pneumothorax. *AJR Am J Roentgenol.* 1995;164:581.
145. Steier M, Ching N, Roberts EB, et al. Pneumothorax complicating continuous ventilatory support. *J Thorac Cardiovasc Surg.* 1974;67:17.
146. Gall SA Jr, Wolfe WG. Management of microfistula following pulmonary resection. *Chest Surg Clin North Am.* 1996;6:543.

147. Hollaus PH, Lax F, El-Nashef BB, et al. Natural history of bronchopleural fistula after pneumonectomy: a review of 96 cases. *Ann Thorac Surg.* 1997;63:1391.
148. Puskas JD, Mathisen DJ, Grillo HC, et al. Treatment strategies for bronchopleural fistula. *J Thorac Cardiovasc Surg.* 1995;109:989.
149. Baumann MH, Sahn SA. Medical management and therapy of bronchopleural fistulas in the mechanically ventilated patient. *Chest.* 1990;97:721.
150. Calhoon JH, Grover FL, Trinkle JK. Chest trauma: approach and management. *Clin Chest Med.* 1992;13:55.
151. Pierson DJ. Persistent bronchopleural air leak during mechanical ventilation: a review. *Respir Care.* 1982;27:408.
152. Powner DJ, Grenvik A. Ventilatory management of life-threatening bronchopleural fistulae. *Crit Care Med.* 1981;9:54.
153. Zimmerman JE, Colgan DL, Mills M. Management of bronchopleural fistula complicating therapy with positive end expiratory pressure (PEEP). *Chest.* 1973;64:526.
154. Downs JB, Chapman RL. Treatment of bronchopleural fistula during continuous positive pressure ventilation. *Chest.* 1976;69:363.
155. Tilles RB, Don HF. Complications of high pleural suction in bronchopleural fistulas. *Anesthesiology.* 1975;43:486.
156. Larson RP, Capps JS, Pierson DJ. A comparison of three devices used for quantitating bronchopleural air leak. *Respir Care.* 1986;31:1065.
157. Ritz R, Benson M, Bishop MJ. Measuring gas leakage from bronchopleural fistulas during high-frequency jet ventilation. *Crit Care Med.* 1984;12: 836.
158. Powner DJ, Cline D, Rodman GH Jr. Effect of chest-tube suction on gas flow through a bronchopleural fistula. *Crit Care Med.* 1985;13:99.
159. Albelda SM, Hansen-Flaschen JH, Taylor E, et al. Evaluation of high-frequency jet ventilation in patients with bronchopleural fistulas by quantitation of the airleak. *Anesthesiology.* 1985;63:551.
160. Roth MD, Wright JW, Bellamy PE. Gas flow through a bronchopleural fistula: measuring the effects of high-frequency jet ventilation and chest-tube suction. *Chest.* 1988;93:210.
161. Bishop MJ, Benson MS, Pierson DJ. Carbon dioxide excretion via bronchopleural fistulas in adult respiratory distress syndrome. *Chest.* 1987;91: 400.
162. Benson MS, Bishop MJ, Pierson DJ. Determination of dead-space ventilation and CO_2 production in the presence of gas leak from bronchopleural fistula complicating ARDS. *Respir Care.* 1986;31:398.
163. Pierson DJ, Horton CA, Bates PW. Persistent bronchopleural air leak during mechanical ventilation: a review of 39 cases. *Chest.* 1986;90:321.
164. Rusch VW, Capps JS, Tyler ML, et al. The performance of four pleural drainage systems in an animal model of bronchopleural fistula. *Chest.* 1988;93:859.
165. Walsh MC, Carlo WA. Determinants of gas flow through a bronchopleural fistula. *J Appl Physiol.* 1989;67:1591.
166. Philips YY, Lonigan RM, Joyner LB. A simple technique for managing a bronchopleural fistula while maintaining positive pressure ventilation. *Crit Care Med.* 1979;7:351.
167. Crawford CA, Downs JB. Chest tube pressurization for bronchopleural fistula: a case report. *Respir Care.* 1979;24:932.
168. Blanch PB, Koens JC Jr, Layon AJ. A new device that allows synchronous intermittent inspiratory chest tube occlusion with any mechanical ventilator. *Chest.* 1990;97:1426.
169. Gallagher TJ, Smith RA, Kirby RR, et al. Intermittent inspiratory chest tube occlusion to limit bronchopleural cutaneous airleaks. *Crit Care Med.* 1976;4:328.
170. Dennis JW, Eigen H, Ballantine TVN, et al, The relationship between peak inspiratory pressure and positive end expiratory pressure on the volume of air lost through a bronchopleural fistula. *J Pediatr Surg.* 1980;15:971.
171. Barringer M, Meredith J, Prough D, et al. Effectiveness of high-frequency jet ventilation in management of an experimental bronchopleural fistula. *Am Surg.* 1982;48:610.
172. Sjostrand UH, Smith RB, Hoff BH, et al. Conventional and high-frequency ventilation in dogs with bronchopleural fistula. *Crit Care Med.* 1985;13:191.
173. Orlando R III, Gluck EH, Cohen M, et al. Ultra-high frequency jet ventilation in a bronchopleural fistula model. *Arch Surg.* 1988;123:591.
174. Mayers I, Long R, Breen PH, et al. Artificial ventilation of a canine model of bronchopleural fistula. *Anesthesiology.* 1986;64:739.
175. Spinale FG, Linker RW, Crawford FA, et al. Conventional versus high frequency jet ventilation with a bronchopleural fistula. *J Surg Res.* 1989;46:147.
176. Carlon GC, Ray C Jr, Klain M, et al. High-frequency positive-pressure ventilation in management of a patient with bronchopleural fistula. *Anesthesiology.* 1980;52:160.
177. Carlon GC, Khan RC, Howland WS, et al. Clinical experience with high-frequency jet ventilation. *Crit Care Med.* 1981;9:1.
178. Derderian SS, Rajogopal KR, Abbrecht PH, et al. High frequency positive pressure jet ventilation in bilateral bronchopleural fistulae. *Crit Care Med.* 1982;10:119.
179. Schmale TJ, Brown M, Brown EM. High-frequency jet ventilation in a patient with sarcoidosis and bilateral bronchopleural fistulae. *J Natl Med Assoc.* 1984;76:193.
180. Rubio JJ, Algora-Weber A, Dominguez-de Villota E, et al. Prolonged high-frequency jet ventilation in a patient with bronchopleural fistula: an alternative mode of ventilation. *Intensive Care Med.* 1986;12:161.
181. Bishop MJ, Benson MS, Sato P, et al. Comparison of high-frequency jet ventilation with conventional mechanical ventilation for bronchopleural fistula. *Anesth Analg.* 1987;66:833.
182. Dodds CP, Hillman KM. Management of massive air leak with asynchronous independent lung ventilation. *Intensive Care Med.* 1982;8:287.
183. Wendt M, Hachenberg T, Winde G, et al. Differential ventilation with low-flow CPAP and CPPV in the treatment of unilateral chest trauma. *Intensive Care Med.* 1989;15:209.
184. Lohse AW, Klein O, Hermann E, et al. Pneumatoceles and pneumothoraces complicating staphylococcal pneumonia: treatment by synchronous independent lung ventilation. *Thorax.* 1993;48:578.
185. Feeley TW, Keating D, Nishimura T. Independent lung ventilation using high-frequency ventilation in the management of a bronchopleural fistula. *Anesthesiology.* 1988;69:420.
186. Crimi G, Candiani A, Conti G, et al. Clinical applications of independent lung ventilation with unilateral high-frequency jet ventilation (ILV-UHFJV). *Intensive Care Med.* 1986;12:90.
187. Mortimer AJ, Laurie PS, Garrett H, et al. Unilateral high frequency jet ventilation: reduction of leak in bronchopleural fistula. *Intensive Care Med.* 1984;10:39.
188. Charan NB, Carvalho CG, Hawk P, et al. Independent lung ventilation with a single ventilator using a variable resistance valve. *Chest.* 1995;107:256.
189. Carvalho P, Thompson WH, Riggs R, et al. Management of bronchopleural fistula with a variable-resistance valve and a single ventilator. *Chest.* 1997;111:1452.
190. Thomas AR, Bryce TL. Ventilation in the patient with unilateral lung disease. *Crit Care Clin.* 1998;14:743.
191. Ost D, Corbridge T. Independent lung ventilation. *Clin Chest Med.* 1996;17:591.
192. Sippel JM, Chesnutt MS. Bronchoscopic therapy for bronchopleural fistulas. *J Bronchol.* 1998;5:61.
193. McManigle JE, Fletcher GL, Tenholder MF. Bronchoscopy in the management of bronchopleural fistula. *Chest.* 1990;97:1235.
194. Lois M, Noppen M. Bronchopleural fistulas: an overview of the problem with special focus on endoscopic management. *Chest.* 2005;128:395.
195. Toma TP, Kon OM, Oldfield W, et al. Reduction of persistent air leak with endoscopic valve implants. *Thorax.* 2007;62:830.
196. Feller-Kopman D, Bechara R, Garland R, et al. Use of a removable endobronchial valve for the treatment of bronchopleural fistula. *Chest.* 2006;130:273.
197. Ferguson JS, Sprenger K, Van Natta T. Closure of a bronchopleural fistula using bronchoscopic placement of an endobronchial valve designed for the treatment of emphysema. *Chest.* 2006;129:479.
198. Andreetti C, Venuta F, Anile M, et al. Pleurodesis with an autologous blood patch to prevent persistent air leaks after lobectomy. *J Thorac Cardiovasc Surg.* 2007;133:759.
199. Droghetti A, Schiavini A, Muriana P, et al. Autologous blood patch in persistent air leaks after pulmonary resection. *J Thorac Cardiovasc Surg.* 2006;132:556.
200. Lang-Lazdunski L, Coonar AS. A prospective study of autologous 'blood patch' pleurodesis for persistent air leak after pulmonary resection. *Eur J Cardiothorac Surg.* 2004;26:897.
201. Matar AF, Hill JG, Duncan W, et al. Use of biologic glue to control pulmonary air leaks. *Thorax.* 1990;45:670.
202. Nicholas JM, Dulchavsky SA. Successful use of autologous fibrin gel in traumatic bronchopleural fistula: case report. *J Trauma.* 1992;32:87.
203. Doyle JJ, Hnatiuk OW, Torrington KG, et al. Necessity of routine chest roentgenography after thoracentesis. *Ann Intern Med.* 1996;124:816.
204. Daly RC, Mucha P, Pairolero PC, et al. The risk of percutaneous chest tube thoracostomy for blunt thoracic trauma. *Ann Emerg Med.* 1985;14:865.
205. Millikan JS, Moore EE, Steiner E, et al. Complications of tube thoracostomy for acute trauma. *Am J Surg.* 1980;140:738.
206. Helling TS, Gyles NR III, Eisenstein CL, et al. Complications following blunt and penetrating injuries in 216 victims of chest trauma requiring tube thoracostomy. *J Trauma.* 1989;29:1367.
207. Collop NA, Kim S, Sahn SA. Analysis of tube thoracostomy performed by pulmonologists at a teaching hospital. *Chest.* 1997;112:709.
208. Baldt MM, Bankier AA, Germann PS, et al. Complications after emergency tube thoracostomy: assessment with CT. *Radiology.* 1995;195:539.
209. Resnick DK. Delayed pulmonary perforation: a rare complication of tube thoracostomy. *Chest.* 1993;103:311.
210. Fraser RS. Lung perforation complicating tube thoracostomy: pathologic description of three cases. *Hum Pathol.* 1988;19:518.
211. Symbas PN. Chest drainage tubes. *Surg Clinics North Am.* 1989;69:41.
212. Kopec SE, Conlan AA, Irwin RS. Perforation of the right ventricle: a complication of blind placement of a chest tube into the postpneumonectomy space. *Chest.* 1998;114:1213.
213. Meisel S, Ram Z, Priel I, et al. Another complication of thoracostomy-perforation of the right atrium. *Chest.* 1990;98:772.
214. Kollef MH, Dothager DW. Reversible cardiogenic shock due to chest tube compression of the right ventricle. *Chest.* 1991;99:976.

215. Rashid MA, Wikstrom T, Ortenwall P. Mediastinal perforation and contralateral hemothorax by a chest tube. *Thorac Cardiovasc Surg.* 1998;46:375.
216. Gerard PS, Kaldawi E, Litani V, et al. Right-sided pneumothorax as a result of a left-sided chest tube. *Chest.* 1993;103:1602.
217. Muthuswamy P, Samuel J, Mizock B, et al. Recurrent massive bleeding from an intercostal artery aneurysm through an empyema chest tube. *Chest.* 1993;104:637.
218. Smolle-Juettner FM, Prauser G, Ratzenhofer B, et al. The importance of early detection and therapy of reexpansion pulmonary edema. *Thorac Cardiovasc Surg.* 1991;39:162.
219. Kramer MR, Melzer E, Sprung C. Unilateral pulmonary edema after intubation of the right mainstem bronchus. *Crit Care Med.* 1989;17:472.
220. Ravin CE, Dahmash NS. Re-expansion pulmonary edema. *Chest.* 1980;77:709–710.
221. Mills M, Balsch BF. Spontaneous pneumothorax: a series of 400 cases. *Ann Thorac Surg.* 1965;1:286.
222. Brooks JW. Open thoracotomy in the management of spontaneous pneumothorax. *Ann Surg.* 1973;177:798.
223. Matsuura Y, Nomimura T, Murakami H, et al. Clinical analysis of reexpansion pulmonary edema. *Chest.* 1991;100:1562.
224. Rozenman J, Yellin A, Simansky DA, et al. Re-expansion pulmonary oedema following spontaneous pneumothorax. *Respir Med.* 1996;90:235.
225. Mahfood S, Hix WR, Aaron BL, et al. Reexpansion pulmonary edema. *Ann Thorac Surg.* 1988;45:340.
226. Ragozzino MW, Greene R. Bilateral reexpansion pulmonary edema following unilateral pleurocentesis. *Chest.* 1991;99:506.
227. Kernodle DS, DiRaimondo CR, Fulkerson WJ. Reexpansion pulmonary edema after pneumothorax. *South Med J.* 1984;77:318.
228. Sprung CL, Loewenherz JW, Baier H, et al. Evidence for increased permeability in reexpansion pulmonary edema. *Am J Med.* 1981;71:497.
229. Gascoigne A, Appleton A, Taylor R, et al. Catastrophic circulatory collapse following re-expansion pulmonary oedema. *Resuscitation.* 1996;31:265.
230. Pavlin DJ, Raghu G, Rogers TR, et al. Reexpansion hypotension: a complication of rapid evacuation of prolonged pneumothorax. *Chest.* 1986;89:70.

CHAPTER 145 ■ MASSIVE HEMOPTYSIS

MICHAEL A. JANTZ • VEENA B. ANTONY

Hemoptysis is defined as the expectoration of blood that originates from the lower respiratory tract. Pseudohemoptysis is the expectoration of blood from a source other than the lower respiratory tract such as the nares, oropharynx, larynx, or the gastrointestinal tract. Massive hemoptysis is defined as expectoration of blood exceeding 200 to 1,000 mL over a 24-hour period, with expectoration of greater than 600 mL in 24 hours being the most commonly used definition (1).

In practice, the rapidity of bleeding and ability to maintain a patent airway are critical factors; life-threatening hemoptysis can alternatively be defined as the amount of bleeding that compromises ventilation (2). Only 3% to 5% of patients with hemoptysis have a massive bleed, with the mortality rate ranging from 20% to as high as 80% in some case series (3–6). Most patients who die from massive hemoptysis do so from asphyxiation secondary to airway occlusion by clot and blood—not from exsanguination. Prognostic factors associated with an increased risk of death from massive hemoptysis include bleeding in excess of 1,000 mL/24 hours, hemoptysis due to neoplasms, radiographic evidence of aspiration, and hemodynamic instability (3,7,8).

ETIOLOGY OF MASSIVE HEMOPTYSIS

The causes of massive hemoptysis are listed in Table 145.1. Virtually all causes of hemoptysis may result in massive hemoptysis. Infections associated with bronchiectasis, tuberculosis, lung abscess, and necrotizing pneumonia are commonly responsible for the massive bleeding. Other common causes include bronchogenic carcinoma, mycetoma, invasive fungal diseases, chest trauma, cystic fibrosis, pulmonary infarction, and coagulopathy. Although massive hemoptysis is usually due to bleeding from the bronchial circulation, alveolar hemorrhage due to conditions such as Wegener granulomatosis and Goodpasture syndrome may occasionally cause massive hemoptysis (Table 145.2).

ANATOMIC SOURCES OF HEMPOTYSIS

The sources of lower respiratory tract bleeding include the pulmonary and bronchial circulations. The pulmonary circulation is a low-pressure circuit when normal pulmonary artery pressures are present. The pulmonary arteries supply blood to the pulmonary parenchyma. The bronchial circulation consists of the bronchial arteries, which originate from the aorta and have systemic arterial pressures, and the bronchial veins, which drain into the systemic veins to the right side of the heart. The bronchial and pulmonary circulations are normally interconnected by a bronchopulmonary anastomosis near the junction of the terminal and respiratory bronchioles. The bronchial arteries are the main source of blood to the airways, large branches of the pulmonary vessels, and supporting structures of the lung. The bronchial arteries feeding the proximal airways, such as the trachea and mainstem bronchi, drain into bronchial veins, which empty into the right side of the heart. Bronchial arteries serving the intrapulmonary airways and lung parenchyma drain through the bronchopulmonary anastomosis into the pulmonary veins, which empty into the left side of the heart. Angiographic studies of patients with active hemoptysis have demonstrated that the bronchial artery circulation

TABLE 145.1

POTENTIAL CAUSES OF MASSIVE HEMOPTYSIS

NEOPLASM
Bronchogenic cancer
Metastasis (parenchymal or endobronchial)
Carcinoid
Leukemia
INFECTIOUS
Lung abscess
Bronchiectasis
Tuberculosis
Necrotizing pneumonia
Fungal pneumonia
Septic pulmonary emboli
Mycetoma (aspergilloma)
PULMONARY
Bronchiectasis
Cystic fibrosis
Sarcoidosis (fibrocavitary)
Diffuse alveolar hemorrhage
Airway foreign body
CARDIAC/VASCULAR
Mitral stenosis
Pulmonary embolism/infarction
Arteriovenous malformation
Bronchoarterial fistula
Ruptured aortic aneurysm
CONGESTIVE HEART FAILURE
Pulmonary arteriovenous fistula
IATROGENIC/TRAUMATIC
Blunt or penetrating chest trauma
Tracheal/bronchial tear or rupture
Tracheoinnominate artery fistula
Bronchoscopy
Pulmonary artery rupture from pulmonary artery catheter
Endotracheal tube suctioning trauma
HEMATOLOGIC
Coagulopathy
Disseminated intravascular coagulation
Thrombocytopenia
DRUGS/TOXINS
Anticoagulants
Antiplatelet agents
Thrombolytic agents
Crack cocaine

is responsible for bleeding in approximately 90% of cases (9). Bronchial arteries arise directly or indirectly from the thoracic aorta at the level of the third through the eighth thoracic vertebrae, originating most commonly at the level of the fifth and sixth vertebrae.

The bronchopulmonary anastomosis may increase in size due to chronic inflammatory conditions such as bronchiectasis, cystic fibrosis, and tuberculosis (10). New collateral vessels from bronchial arteries or other intrathoracic systemic arteries may also develop in chronic inflammatory conditions.

TABLE 145.2

CAUSES OF ALVEOLAR HEMORRHAGE

Goodpasture syndrome
Vasculitis/collagen vascular disease
Wegener granulomatosis
Microscopic polyangiitis
System lupus erythematosus
Mixed connective tissue disorder
Systemic sclerosis (scleroderma)
Rheumatoid arthritis
Henoch-Schonlein purpura
Mixed cryoglobulinemia
Behçet syndrome
Diffuse alveolar damage
Antiphospholipid syndrome
Idiopathic pulmonary hemosiderosis
Hematopoietic stem cell/bone marrow transplantation
Coagulopathy
Mitral stenosis
Lymphangioleiomyomastosis
Drugs/toxins
Isocyanates
Trimellitic anhydride
D-penicillamine
Nitrofurantoin
All-trans retinoic acid
Crack cocaine

INITIAL EVALUATION

A detailed history and physical examination should be performed. Patients with a history of tuberculosis may have bleeding from rupture of a pulmonary artery aneurysm in the cavity lumen, known as a Rasmussen aneurysm, or by breakdown of bronchopulmonary anastomoses within the wall of old cavities (11). Bronchogenic carcinoma should be suspected in smokers older than 40 years of age. Repeated episodes of hemoptysis over months to years suggest bronchiectasis or a carcinoid tumor. Chronic sputum production predating the hemoptysis implies a diagnosis of chronic bronchitis, bronchiectasis, or cystic fibrosis. Pulmonary embolism should be suspected in patients with a history of deep venous thrombosis or risk factors for pulmonary thromboembolism. A febrile illness with sputum production, night sweats, and weight loss suggests a lung abscess or tuberculosis. Excessive anticoagulation, thrombolytic therapy, and coagulopathy may also cause hemoptysis (12,13). In children with hemoptysis, the most likely diagnoses are carcinoid tumors, vascular anomalies, and aspiration of foreign bodies (14,15). Alveolar hemorrhage should be suspected in patients with dyspnea, hypoxemia, and diffuse pulmonary infiltrates. The triad of upper airway disease, lower airway disease, and renal disease suggests Wegener granulomatosis (16). Goodpasture syndrome should be suspected in young men with alveolar hemorrhage and microscopic or macroscopic hematuria (17). Patients with a history of systemic lupus erythematosus may develop alveolar hemorrhage at any time during the course of their disease, and alveolar hemorrhage may be the initial manifestation (18). Alveolar hemorrhage should be considered in patients with diffuse pulmonary infiltrates who have recently undergone hematopoietic stem cell or bone marrow transplantation (19). Although an uncommon cause of hemoptysis, a tracheoinnominate artery fistula is an important consideration in patients with tracheostomy (20,21). The peak incidence is between the first and second week, although hemorrhage can occur as early as 48 hours and as late as 18 months after the procedure. A sentinel self-limited bleed is observed in 35% to 50% of patients. Trauma from suctioning, particularly in the setting of abnormal coagulation, may also cause hemoptysis in patients with a tracheostomy tube or in those who are intubated with an endotracheal tube. The possibility of traumatic rupture of a pulmonary artery should be considered in patients with a pulmonary artery catheter in place (22,23).

Physical Examination

The physical examination may provide clues to the diagnosis of massive hemoptysis. A saddle nose deformity and/or septal perforation suggest Wegener granulomatosis. Stridor or unilateral wheezing indicates a possible laryngeal tumor, tracheobronchial tumor, or airway foreign body. Pulmonary embolism should be considered in patients with tachypnea, a pleural friction rub, and lower extremity phlebitis. Diffuse rales on examination raise the possibility of diffuse alveolar hemorrhage, diffuse parenchymal lung disease, or cardiac disease as the cause of the hemoptysis. The presence of telangiectasias of the skin or mucous membranes suggests hereditary hemorrhagic telangiectasia or a connective tissue disease as the cause. Ecchymoses or petechiae suggest a hematologic abnormality or coagulopathy. Clubbing of the fingers may be a sign of a lung carcinoma, bronchiectasis, and cystic fibrosis. The finding of pulsation of the tracheostomy tube is of concern for the development of a tracheoinnominate fistula.

Laboratory Studies

Laboratory studies, including a complete blood count (CBC), coagulation studies, urinalysis, and chest radiograph, should be obtained in all patients. The CBC may suggest an infectious process or hematologic disorder as the cause of hemoptysis and indicates the need for blood transfusion. Coagulation studies may provide evidence for a hematologic disorder as the cause for the hemoptysis, or may identify a coagulopathy that is causing or contributing to the bleeding from another disease. Hematuria may be noted on urinalysis, which suggests the diagnosis of Goodpasture syndrome, Wegener granulomatosis, or another systemic vasculitis.

Chest Radiograph

The chest radiograph is an important study to identify the cause and side of bleeding. The chest radiograph may demonstrate abnormalities such as lung masses, cavitary lesions, atelectasis, focal infiltrates, and diffuse infiltrate. Single or multiple pulmonary cavities suggest neoplasm, tuberculosis, fungal disease, lung abscess, septic pulmonary emboli, parasitic infection, or Wegener granulomatosis as the cause for hemoptysis. The presence of a mass within a cavitary lesion indicates a possible mycetoma (aspergilloma). The appearance of a new air–fluid level in a cavity or infiltrate around a cavity is suggestive of the site of bleeding. A solitary pulmonary nodule that has vessels going toward the nodule may be an arteriovenous malformation. Diffuse pulmonary infiltrates suggest diffuse alveolar hemorrhage (Table 145.2), bleeding from coagulopathy, lung contusions from blunt chest trauma, hemorrhage with multiple areas of aspiration, or pulmonary edema with a cardiac cause for hemoptysis. Chest radiographs may be normal or nonlocalizing in 20% to 45% of patients (24,25).

Computed Tomography

The role of computed tomography (CT) in the management of massive hemoptysis is somewhat controversial. CT may demonstrate abnormalities that are not visible on the chest radiograph. It is helpful in the diagnosis of bronchiectasis (26), although abnormalities from bronchiectasis can usually be appreciated on the chest radiograph. CT with contrast may detect pulmonary emboli, thoracic aneurysms, or arteriovenous malformations. CT scans may also demonstrate cavitation with a surrounding infiltrate, the halo sign, which suggests a necrotizing infection such as aspergillosis or mucormycosis (27,28). Some studies have noted that CT scanning before bronchoscopy may increase the yield of bronchoscopy (29). In one retrospective study of 80 patients with large or massive hemoptysis, chest CT was superior to chest radiograph or bronchoscopy in determining the cause of bleeding and was similar to bronchoscopy in successfully localizing the site of bleeding (30). Some authors have argued that transport of the potentially unstable patient with massive hemoptysis may not be judicious, however. The patient should be adequately stabilized prior to obtaining a chest CT.

Angiography

Angiography can determine the site of bleeding in 90% to 95% of cases. However, in one case series, the routine use of diagnostic angiography provided a diagnosis not identified on bronchoscopy in only 4% of patients (31). Angiography can be helpful in detecting a pseudoaneurysm that has formed after healing of a pulmonary artery tear from pulmonary artery catheterization (32). As previously noted, the bronchial arteries and other collateral systemic arteries account for the source of bleeding in most cases of massive hemoptysis. Pulmonary angiography is usually performed only when there is suspicion for pulmonary aneurysms, arteriovenous malformations, and pulmonary embolism. Technetium-labeled red blood cell or colloid studies rarely provided any information that is not obtained by bronchoscopy and chest CT. The use and timing of bronchoscopy will be discussed in a subsequent section.

Other Studies

Depending on the suspected causes of massive hemoptysis, additional studies may be indicated. For potential infections, sputum and bronchoscopic specimens should be sent for bacterial cultures, fungal stains and cultures, viral cultures, acid-fast bacilli stains, and mycobacterial cultures. Bronchoalveolar lavage (BAL) specimens may also be sent for cytology, with special stains to evaluate for fungi, *Pneumocystis*, viruses, protozoa, and parasites. Bronchoscopic specimens should be obtained if a neoplasm if suspected. Echocardiography may be performed if a cardiac cause is possible. If diffuse alveolar hemorrhage syndromes are suspected, laboratory testing, including antiglomerular basement membrane antibody, antineutrophilic cytoplasmic antibody, antinuclear antibody, rheumatoid factor, complement levels, cryoglobulins, rheumatoid factor, and antiphospholipid antibodies, should be performed depending on the causes that are being considered. Transbronchial lung biopsy, open lung biopsy, or kidney biopsy may be indicated in some cases of alveolar hemorrhage to establish a diagnosis.

MANAGEMENT OF MASSIVE HEMOPTYSIS

Airway Protection and Stabilization

Once the diagnosis of massive hemoptysis is established, the initial priorities are to protect the airway and stabilize the patient. In general, the patient with massive hemoptysis should be monitored in the ICU setting, even if intubation and mechanical ventilation are not required. Large-bore IV access should be established and supplemental oxygen provided. Blood should be drawn for a CBC, arterial blood gas analysis, coagulation studies, electrolytes, renal function tests, and liver function tests. The patient should be type and cross-matched for blood, and 4 to 6 units of packed red blood cells should always be available. Correction of thrombocytopenia and coagulopathy, if present, with appropriate blood products should be considered. Attempts to lateralize the site of bleeding should be made in anticipation of steps to prevent aspiration into the nonbleeding lung. The patient may be positioned in a lateral decubitus position with the bleeding lung down.

Airway patency must be ensured in patients with massive hemoptysis, as deaths from this process are predominantly due to asphyxiation. Most patients with ongoing massive hemoptysis will require intubation and mechanical ventilation, although select patients who are not hypoxemic and are able to keep the airway clear on their own may not require intubation. Although intubation generally preserves oxygenation and facilitates blood removal from the lower respiratory tract, the endotracheal tube (ET) can become obstructed by blood clots, leading to the inability to oxygenate and ventilate the patient. The largest possible ET should be inserted to allow the use of bronchoscopes with a 2.8 to 3.0 mm working channel for more effective suctioning and to allow for better ventilation with the bronchoscope in the airway for prolonged periods of time. In severe cases, the mainstem bronchus of the nonbleeding lung can be selectively intubated under bronchoscopic guidance to preserve oxygenation and ventilation from the normal lung.

Some authors have recommended the use of a double-lumen ET to isolate the normal lung and permit selective intubation. Although double-lumen endotracheal tubes have been used successfully in the airway management of massive hemoptysis, there are several potential pitfalls. First, placement of a double-lumen ET is difficult for less-experienced operators, particularly with a large amount of blood in the larynx and oropharynx. Second, the individual lumens of the ET are significantly smaller than a standard ET and are at significant risk of being occluded by blood and blood clots. Last, positioning of the double-lumen ET and subsequent bronchoscopic suctioning of the distal airways requires a small pediatric bronchoscope with working channels of 1.2 to 1.4 mm. Adequate suctioning of large amounts of blood and blood clots through such bronchoscopes is extremely problematic. In one series of 62 patients with massive hemoptysis, death occurred in 4 of 7 patients managed with a double-lumen ET due to loss of tube positioning and aspiration (33). In general, we do not recommend the use of double-lumen ETs for airway management in massive hemoptysis. As an alternative to selective mainstem bronchial intubation or intubation with a double-lumen ET, an ET that incorporates a bronchial blocker, such as the Univent tube, may be used.

Localization of Source and Cause of Hemoptysis

Once the patient is stabilized and airway patency is achieved, the source of bleeding should be localized as precisely as possible, and the cause of bleeding should be determined. Identification of the cause and location of the bleeding potentially allows for more specific therapy. Methods of localization include patient history, physical examination, chest radiograph, chest CT, bronchoscopy, and angiography. In one study of 105 patients with hemoptysis, patients themselves were able to localize the side of bleeding in 10% of cases but with an accuracy of 70% when able to do so (34). Localization by a physical examination performed by a physician was possible in 43% of patients. Chest radiographs were able to localize bleeding in 60% of cases. Bronchoscopy was accurate in localizing the source of bleeding in 86% of patients. In another study, 9 of 24 patients were able to accurately localize the side of their bleeding (35). Chest radiographs should be routinely obtained to help localize the source of bleeding and determine the cause. As discussed earlier, chest CT may provide additional information beyond the chest radiograph, and may be more accurate in localizing the bleeding and determining the cause, although concerns about transporting a potentially unstable patient out of the ICU exist (36,37). Bronchoscopy and angiography remain the modalities for localizing the source of hemoptysis and offer potential therapeutic intervention.

Early—rather than delayed—bronchoscopy should be performed to increase the likelihood of localizing the source of bleeding. Bronchoscopy performed within 48 hours of bleeding onset successfully localized bleeding in 34% to 91% of patients, depending on the case series, as compared to successful localization in 11% to 52% of patients if delayed bronchoscopy was performed (38). Bronchoscopy performed within 12 to 24 hours may provide an even higher yield. Bedside flexible bronchoscopy should not be performed to establish a diagnosis of a tracheoarterial fistula such as a tracheoinnominate fistula (39,40). Bronchoscopy may be performed in the patient with a tracheostomy tube and hemoptysis to exclude bleeding from suction trauma, tracheitis, granulation tissue, and lower respiratory tract disorders. If no other causes for hemoptysis can be found, or if the observation that anterior and downward pressure on the cannula at the level of the stomal site or overinflation of the tracheostomy tube slows down the bleeding, a surgical consultation should be obtained. The tracheostomy balloon should not be deflated, and the tracheostomy tube should not be removed without protecting the airway below the tracheostomy tube. The patient should be brought to the operating room for further examination with preparations for surgical repair in place.

Bronchoscopic Therapies to Control Hemoptysis

Endobronchial tamponade via flexible bronchoscopy can prevent aspiration of blood into the contralateral lung and preserve gas exchange in patients with massive hemoptysis. Endobronchial tamponade can be achieved with a 4 French Fogarty balloon-tipped catheter. The catheter may be passed directly through the working channel of the bronchoscope, or the catheter can be grasped with biopsy forceps placed though the working channel of the bronchoscope prior to introduction into the airway of the bronchoscope and catheter. The catheter is held in place adjacent to the bronchoscope by the biopsy forceps, and both are then inserted as a unit into the airway. Care must be taken not to perforate the catheter or balloon by the forceps. The catheter tip is inserted into the bleeding segmental orifice, and the balloon is inflated. If passed through the suction channel, the proximal end of the catheter is clamped with a hemostat, the hub cut off, and a straight pin inserted into the catheter channel proximal to the hemostat to maintain inflation of the balloon catheter. The clamp is removed, and the bronchoscope is carefully withdrawn from the bronchus with the Fogarty catheter remaining in position, thus providing endobronchial hemostasis (41–43). The catheter can safely remain in position until hemostasis is ensured by surgical resection of the bleeding segment or bronchial artery embolization. Right heart balloon catheters have been used in a similar fashion (44). A modified technique for placement of a balloon catheter has been described using a guidewire for insertion. A 0.035-inch soft-tipped guidewire is inserted through the working channel of the bronchoscope into the bleeding segment. The bronchoscope is withdrawn, leaving the guidewire in place. A balloon catheter is then inserted over the guidewire and placed under direct visualization after reintroduction of the bronchoscope (45). The use of endobronchial blockers developed for unilateral lung ventilation during surgery may hold promise for management of massive hemoptysis in tamponading bleeding and preventing contralateral aspiration of blood (46). The Arndt endobronchial blocker is placed through a standard ET and directly positioned with a pediatric bronchoscope. Suctioning and injection of medications can be performed through the lumen of the catheter after placement. The Cohen tip-deflecting endobronchial blocker is also placed through a standard ET and directed into place with a self-contained steering mechanism under bronchoscopic visualization. At this time, there is limited published experience with these blockers in the setting of massive hemoptysis, although the author has successfully used them for this application. The prolonged use of endobronchial blockers may cause mucosal ischemic injury and postobstructive pneumonia.

Additional bronchoscopic techniques may be useful as temporizing measures in patients with massive hemoptysis. Bronchoscopically administered topical therapies, such as iced sterile saline lavage or topical 1:10,000 or 1:20,000 epinephrine solution, may be helpful (47). Direct application of a solution of thrombin or a fibrinogen-thrombin combination solution has been used (48). The use of bronchoscopy-guided topical hemostatic tamponade therapy using oxidized regenerated cellulose mesh has recently been described (49). Although anecdotal, the author has had success with topical application of a sodium bicarbonate solution.

For patients who have hemoptysis due to endobronchial lesions, particularly endobronchial tumors, hemostasis may be achieved with the use of neodymium-yttrium-aluminum-garnet (Nd:YAG) laser phototherapy, electrocautery, or cryotherapy via the bronchoscope.

Angiography and Embolization

Angiography can identify the bleeding site in more than 90% of cases. As noted, the bronchial arteries are the most frequent source of bleeding in massive hemoptysis. In some cases, systemic vessels other than the bronchial arteries can be the source of bleeding (50). The pulmonary arteries may be the source for massive hemoptysis in 8% to 10% of cases (9). Visualization of extravasated dye from a vessel is relatively uncommon. Signs that suggest a particular vessel is the source of bleeding include vessel tortuosity, increased vessel diameter, and aneurysmal dilatation.

Bronchial artery embolization is considered the most effective nonsurgical modality for treatment of massive hemoptysis. The immediate success rates from bronchial artery embolization range from 51% to 100% (3,51–65). Embolization has been performed with Gelfoam, polyurethane particles, polyvinyl alcohol particles, and vascular coils. Sclerosing agents may cause subsequent lung necrosis and should be avoided. Recurrence of bleeding, although usually nonmassive, has been noted in 16% to 46% of patients (51,52). Repeat embolization may be required in some patients (57,60,62,66). Complications include chest pain, fever, vessel perforation and intimal tears, and embolization of material to mesenteric and extremity arteries. The most serious complication is embolization of the anterior spinal artery, which may arise from the bronchial artery, with subsequent spinal artery infarction and paraparesis. The risk of this occurrence is less than 1%.

Rupture of the Pulmonary Artery

The pulmonary artery may potentially be ruptured from right heart catheterization. This complication should be suspected in patients who develop hemoptysis with a pulmonary artery catheter in place. Balloon tamponade and contralateral selective intubation should be performed (67). The catheter should be withdrawn 5 cm with the balloon deflated, and the balloon is then inflated with 2 mL of airway and allowed to float back into the ruptured vessel to occlude it. Patients who stop bleeding should undergo angiographic evaluation to localize the tear and identify the formation of a pseudoaneurysm (32,68). If a pseudoaneurysm is identified, embolization of the affected vessel should be considered to prevent subsequent hemorrhage.

perfusion can be assessed with xenon computed tomography (CT) or perfusion CT imaging. Invasive techniques can be used to continuously monitor brain oxygenation. Combined monitoring of arterial oxygen saturation and the oxygen saturation in the internal jugular vein allows the calculation of the arteriojugular oxygen content difference ($AJDO_2$), which is dependent on the amount of oxygen consumed by the brain ($CMRO_2$) and on CBF by the formula $CMRO_2$/CBF. An increased $AJDO_2$ indicates a deficiency of flow relative to the metabolic needs of the brain. Brain oxygenation can also be monitored continuously in a local region of the brain by inserting an invasive probe to measure the brain tissue oxygen tension (PbO_2). Continuous global monitoring provides an overall assessment of brain oxygenation but can miss local changes (5). Continuous local monitoring with an invasive probe provides information on a specific portion of the brain but is dependent on probe location and may not reflect overall brain perfusion (6).

Clinical Pearl. Maintenance of oxygenation of brain tissue is of paramount importance in the injured brain. Cerebral blood flow (CBF) must be maintained at levels high enough to deliver sufficient oxygen. Below a CBF of 20 mL/100 g of brain per minute, the brain does not function normally. Below a CBF of 8 mL/100 g of brain per minute, the neurons die.

COMMONLY MONITORED PARAMETERS IN PATIENTS WITH ELEVATED ICP

Intracranial Pressure

Elevated ICP can be both measured and treated. Normal ICP in the adult is less than 10 mm Hg. An ICP value of 20 to 30 mm Hg is mild intracranial hypertension, and values above 40 mm Hg are severe, life-threatening intracranial hypertension. The goal of treatment should be to maintain ICP below 20 to 25 mm Hg. Studies of traumatic brain injury patients have demonstrated that patients with elevated ICP have a worse outcome than those with ICP below 20 (7–10).

The gold standard for monitoring ICP is a ventriculostomy catheter inserted through a burr hole into one of the lateral ventricles. The ventriculostomy catheter is connected to a drainage system and can be used to monitor the ICP through a fluid-coupled external pressure transducer. This system provides the most accurate measurement of ICP and is stable over time (11). A ventriculostomy catheter will also allow drainage of CSF for control of ICP. Problems associated with ventriculostomy catheters include blockage of the catheter, displacement of the catheter from the ventricle, and infection. Antibiotic-impregnated ventriculostomy catheters reduce the risk of infection from 9.4% to 1.3% (12).

Other invasive monitors for ICP include intraparenchymal, subdural, and epidural monitors. These probes use either a strain gauge or a fiberoptic probe. These probes require zeroing prior to insertion and are subject to drift over time. Of these probes, intraparenchymal probes are the most accurate with the least amount of drift. The advantage of these probes is that they do not have to be inserted into the ventricle, which may be difficult to locate if it is collapsed or if there is significant midline shift.

Clinical Pearl. A ventriculostomy catheter placed into one of the lateral ventricles is the gold standard for ICP monitoring. ICP should be maintained at less than 20 to 25 mm Hg.

Cerebral Perfusion Pressure

Cerebral perfusion pressure (CPP) is defined as the mean arterial pressure (MAP) minus the ICP. It can be measured using a combination of an ICP monitor and either an arterial line or a noninvasive blood pressure monitor. CPP is a second major parameter that can be both monitored and treated in the patient with elevated intracranial pressure. CPP can be supported by maintaining MAP with intravenous fluids and vasopressors and by lowering ICP. CPP should be maintained at a level that will allow adequate perfusion of the brain. For most patients, a CPP of at least 60 mm Hg is adequate (13).

Brain Oxygenation

Brain tissue oxygenation can be measured either using PET imaging techniques to obtain a single time point sample of oxygenation across the entire brain or by using probes to continuously monitor brain tissue pO_2 (PbO_2) and/or jugular venous oxygen saturation (SjO_2). PET imaging is not widely available for ICU patients, but has provided important insights into the pathophysiology of brain injury. PbO_2 and SjO_2 monitoring can be used in any ICU setting.

Brain Tissue Oxygen Tension

Insertion of a PbO_2 probe allows continuous monitoring of oxygenation in a local region of the brain. The location of the probe is critical and determines the nature of the pO_2 information that will be obtained (Fig. 146.2). If the probe is inserted near a focal lesion, oxygenation can be monitored in the tissue at greatest risk should the injury expand. Insertion of the probe in uninjured brain allows monitoring of a local area that should be representative of the overall less-injured oxygenation status of the brain. This pO_2 value provides information that is similar to SjO_2 monitoring (6). Both monitoring strategies have been successfully used.

Normal values and critical threshold values for PbO_2 are somewhat less accepted. In anesthetized subjects, PbO_2 in normal brain ranges from 20 to 40 mm Hg. Recent studies comparing PbO_2 values to PET measurements of oxygen extraction fraction (OEF) found that the PbO_2 value associated with an OEF of 40% (the mean value for OEF in normal subjects) was 14 mm Hg (14). Values of PbO_2 that indicate tissue hypoxia/ischemia are probably considerably less than 14 mm Hg. Serial measurements of both SjO_2 and PbO_2 suggest that a PbO_2 of 8.5 mm Hg indicates a similar level of oxygenation as a SjO_2 of 50% (15).

Prospective studies have demonstrated that PbO_2 less than 15 mm Hg is associated with poor outcome (16). Some studies have suggested that a treatment protocol aimed at keeping brain pO_2 higher than 25 mm Hg may reduce mortality when compared to patients treated similarly with no brain pO_2 probe (17).

Jugular Venous Oxygen Saturation

Oxygen saturation in the jugular bulb can be measured by inserting a catheter into the internal jugular vein and advancing

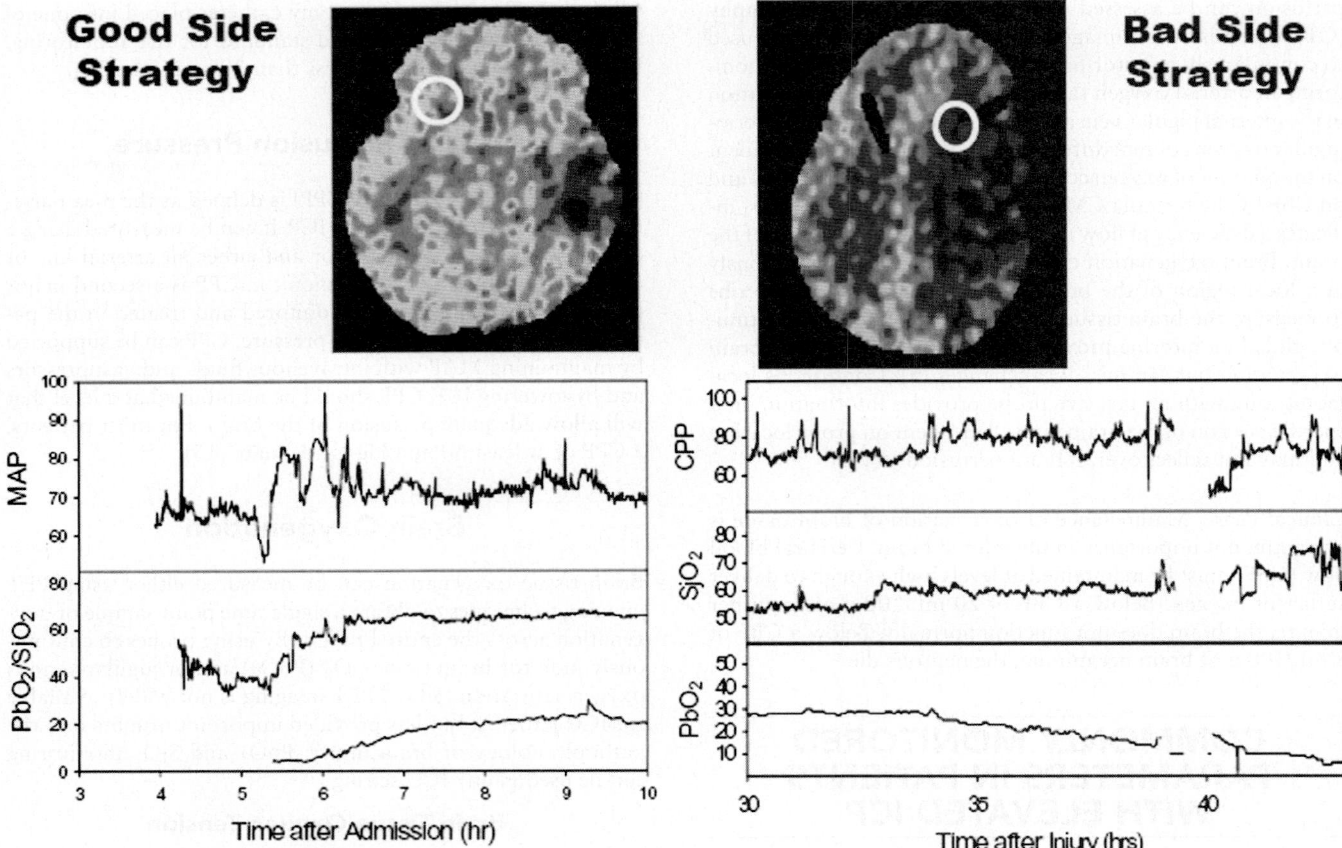

FIGURE 146.2. Location of the brain tissue oxygen tension (PbO_2) catheter relative to the injured brain determines the nature of the pO_2 information that will be obtained. On the left is a patient where the PbO_2 catheter was placed in relatively normal brain opposite a temporal contusion. The PbO_2 reflected the global oxygenation of the brain measured with jugular venous oxygen saturation (SjO_2). On the right is a patient where the PbO_2 catheter was placed near a contusion. As this contusion evolved, the PbO_2 decreased even though the global measures (SjO_2 and cerebral perfusion pressure [CPP]) remained unchanged. MAP, mean arterial pressure.

it to the skull base. This allows measurement of the oxygen saturation of the blood exiting the brain, which provides information on the adequacy of cerebral blood flow and oxygen delivery to the brain (5). Episodes of jugular venous oxygen desaturation are associated with worse neurologic outcome (18). Increased SjO_2 may indicate decreased oxygen uptake in the brain (19). The major limitation of SjO_2 monitoring is that it cannot detect local ischemia within the brain.

Normal values for SjO_2 are better established than for PbO_2. Gibbs et al. (20) studied 50 normal young males and observed that their SjO_2 ranged from 55% to 71% (mean of 61.8%). Some studies suggest that normal SjO_2 values may be as low as 45% (21). Normal SjO_2 is lower than normal mixed venous oxygen saturation, indicating that the brain normally extracts oxygen more completely from arterial blood than do many other organs.

Clinical Pearl. Brain oxygenation can be measured globally at a single time point using PET imaging. Global brain oxygenation can be monitored continuously using a catheter inserted into the internal jugular vein to measure the oxygen saturation of venous blood from the brain. Local brain oxygen tension can be measured continuously by inserting a pO_2 probe directly into the brain parenchyma.

WHAT IS THE MOST IMPORTANT PHYSIOLOGIC END POINT (ICP, CPP, OR BRAIN OXYGENATION)?

As it has become possible to measure additional brain-specific physiologic parameters in the ICU, different management strategies have evolved that place special emphasis on parameters other than ICP. For example, some have advocated that ICP is not important as long as CPP is maintained. This philosophy led to the use of CPP-directed therapy where induced hypertension was used to drive CPP to high levels even though ICP was also increased by the therapy (22). However, all of these physiologic parameters are related to outcome, and there is no clear evidence that one parameter is more important than the others. Table 146.1 presents normal values and treatment thresholds for these parameters.

The best circumstance occurs when ICP, CPP, and brain oxygenation are all maintained in normal ranges, and this should

TABLE 146.1

NORMAL VALUES AND TREATMENT THRESHOLDS FOR PHYSIOLOGIC PARAMETERS

	Normal	Treatment threshold
ICP	0–10 mm Hg	20–25 mm Hg
CPP	50 mm Hg	60 mm Hg
SjO_2	55%–71%	50%
PbO_2	20–40 mm Hg	8–10 mm Hg

ICP, intracranial pressure; CPP, cerebral perfusion pressure; SjO_2, jugular venous oxygen saturation; PbO_2, brain tissue oxygen tension.

probably be the goal of management. When this is not possible, it is important to understand the limitations of each of the monitors when making therapeutic decisions. Additionally, clinical studies are needed to demonstrate what management strategies may best improve neurologic outcome.

IMMEDIATE CONCERNS FOR TREATMENT

Identification of Patients with Increased ICP

A patient with mildly increased ICP can present with complaints of headache and blurred vision. Further increases in ICP are associated with decreased level of consciousness and symptoms of herniation. Herniation of the temporal lobe over the edge of the tentorium can compress cranial nerve III causing ipsilateral pupillary dilation and decreased reaction to light. Direct compression of the brainstem can cause contralateral posturing or hemiparesis, although if the brainstem is displaced and compressed against the opposite side of the tentorium, there may be ipsilateral symptoms, called Kernohan notch phenomenon. Further symptoms of herniation are hypertension, bradycardia, and widening pulse pressure, which make up the Cushing triad. Respiratory abnormalities may be present, including Cheyne-Stokes respiration, hypoventilation, and central neurogenic hyperventilation. Any patient in whom elevated ICP is suspected should undergo noncontrast CT scan of the brain to evaluate for mass lesions, hydrocephalus, subarachnoid hemorrhage, or other treatable causes.

Clinical Pearl. Symptoms concerning for elevated ICP include decreased level of consciousness, a fixed and dilated pupil, decorticate or decerebrate posturing, or hemiparesis.

Initial Stabilization and Management of Patients with Elevated ICP

The initial steps in managing any patient with elevated ICP (Fig. 146.3) are defined by the ABCs of trauma resuscitation. Episodes of hypoxemia (arterial pO_2 <60 mm Hg) or hypotension (systolic blood pressure <90 mm Hg) have been associated with significantly worse outcome in patients with traumatic brain injury (10,23–26).

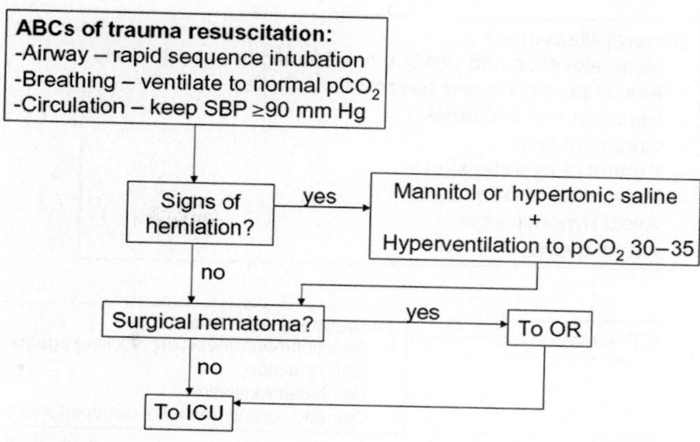

FIGURE 146.3. Algorithm for initial management of patient with elevated intracranial pressure. ICU, intensive care unit; OR, operating room; SBP, systolic blood pressure.

Airway protection is essential (27). All patients with a Glasgow coma score (GCS) of 8 or less should be intubated to protect the airway. Patients with GCS above 8 may also need intubation if they cannot adequately protect their airway (28). Supplemental oxygen and mechanical ventilation may be necessary to avoid hypoxemia.

Ideally, airway protection should start in the field. However, some studies have suggested that intubation of brain-injured patients in the field results in higher mortality rates (29). Paramedics must be adequately trained in the technique of rapid-sequence intubation, excessive hyperventilation should be avoided following intubation, and this procedure should not significantly delay transport of the patient (30).

Blood pressure should be supported with fluid resuscitation and vasopressors as necessary. Hypotension should not be attributed to the brain injury unless all other possible causes have been excluded. Patients with elevated ICP should be cared for in a dedicated neurologic intensive care unit with a neurosurgeon included in the care team (31,32).

Immediate aggressive management of elevated ICP should be initiated in patients who demonstrate signs and symptoms of herniation. Mild hyperventilation, to a $paCO_2$ of 30 to 35 mm Hg, can reduce intracranial pressure by constricting cerebral blood vessels. Once fluid resuscitation has been completed, osmotic therapy with either mannitol or hypertonic saline should be initiated. The standard dose for mannitol is an intravenous bolus of 1 g/kg. In patients with a subdural hematoma and signs of herniation, early preoperative administration of high-dose mannitol (1.4 g/kg) significantly improved outcome in one study (33). Mannitol should only be given once fluid resuscitation has been completed as it does result in an osmotic diuresis and can cause hypotension in the incompletely resuscitated patient. An alternative osmotic agent is hypertonic saline, which may have an advantage in the hypotensive patient since it does not induce diuresis. Resuscitation with hypertonic saline has been demonstrated to result in less hypotension when compared with mannitol but has not clearly been shown to result in an improved outcome.

If a surgical lesion is identified, the patient should be immediately taken to the operating room for evacuation of the lesion. Invasive monitoring devices can be inserted either at the bedside or in the operating room if surgery is required. At a minimum, an ICP monitor, preferably a ventriculostomy

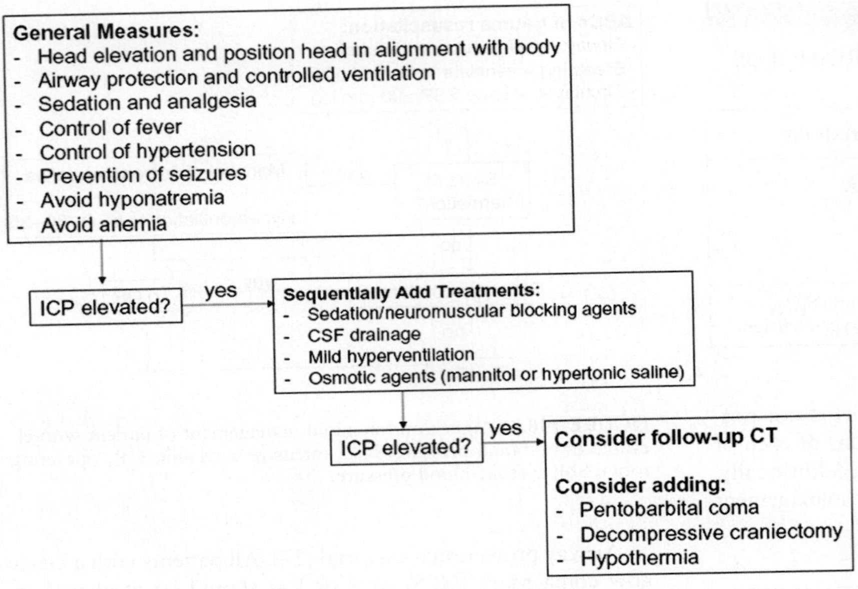
General Measures:
- Head elevation and position head in alignment with body
- Airway protection and controlled ventilation
- Sedation and analgesia
- Control of fever
- Control of hypertension
- Prevention of seizures
- Avoid hyponatremia
- Avoid anemia
ICP elevated?
yes
Sequentially Add Treatments:
- Sedation/neuromuscular blocking agents
- CSF drainage
- Mild hyperventilation
- Osmotic agents (mannitol or hypertonic saline)
ICP elevated?
yes
Consider follow-up CT
Consider adding:
- Pentobarbital coma
- Decompressive craniectomy
- Hypothermia

FIGURE 146.4. Algorithm for treatment of elevated intracranial pressure (ICP). CT, computed tomography; CSF, cerebrospinal fluid.

drain, should be inserted. Other monitoring devices that can be used if available include a brain PbO_2 monitor and a SjO_2 catheter. An arterial line and a Foley catheter should also be placed. A central venous catheter may be needed, especially if hypotension is present or large doses of mannitol are needed.

Clinical Pearl. Initial management of the patient with elevated ICP should focus on the ABCs of the Advanced Trauma Life Support (ATLS) system. When signs of herniation are present, mannitol or hypertonic saline should be given. Early administration of high-dose mannitol (1.4 g/kg) may improve outcome for patients with subdural hematoma and signs of herniation. Surgical mass lesions should be identified and promptly evacuated.

TREATMENT OF ELEVATED INTRACRANIAL PRESSURE—PRINCIPLES OF CNS RESUSCITATION

Principles of management of intracranial hypertension (Fig. 146.4) include general measures that are used in all patients to minimize factors that exacerbate ICP, first-line therapies that are applied to patients who subsequently have elevated ICP, and additional treatments that can be used if elevated ICP is refractory to these first-line measures.

General Measures

Prevention or treatment of factors that may aggravate or precipitate intracranial hypertension is the cornerstone of central nervous system (CNS) resuscitation. Specific factors that may aggravate intracranial hypertension include obstruction of venous return (head position, agitation), respiratory problems (airway obstruction, hypoxia, hypercapnia), fever, severe hypertension, hyponatremia, anemia, and seizures. Routine critical care management of the patient at risk for intracranial hypertension should include measures to prevent these factors. Also important are general strategies for maintaining normal brain oxygenation and cerebral perfusion pressure.

Minimize Obstruction to Venous Return

Elevation of the head of the bed and keeping the head in a neutral position to minimize compression of venous return from the brain has been standard neurosurgery practice for management of ICP. Elevation of the head to 30 degrees results in a reduction in ICP without a reduction in either CPP or CBF in most patients (34,35). If head elevation is used, it is important to remember that both the ICP and blood pressure transducers should be zeroed at the same level, i.e., at the level of the foramen of Monro (36).

In multiple-trauma patients, where abdominal injury may also be present, an increased intra-abdominal pressure may also impede venous return from the brain, decrease blood pressure (BP), and increase ICP. Abdominal decompression can improve control of ICP when abdominal compartment syndrome is present (37).

Prevent Fever

Fever is common during the recovery from a head injury. In experimental studies, postinjury fever worsens the outcome from fluid percussion injury (38). Fever is a potent cerebral vasodilator and can raise ICP. In addition, fever can raise cerebral metabolic requirements. Efficient external cooling systems as well as intravascular cooling devices are available and can maintain normal body temperature. When fever occurs, infectious causes should be investigated with appropriate cultures and treated with antibiotics.

Prevent Seizures

Seizures occur in approximately 15% of patients with head injury (39). The risk of seizures is related to the severity of injury.

In a study of 4,541 patients with head injury, the standardized incidence ratio for developing seizures was 1.5 after mild injuries but with no increase over the expected number after 5 years, 2.9 after moderate injuries, and 17.0 after severe injuries (40).

Since patients are often sedated and pharmacologically paralyzed to treat intracranial hypertension, clinical monitoring is often not helpful. Continuous electroencephalogram (EEG) monitoring may be useful for this high-risk group of patients (41).

The use of anticonvulsants to prevent seizures is controversial. Although seizures can dramatically increase cerebral metabolic rate, there is not a clear relationship between the occurrence of early seizures and a worse neurologic outcome (42). Young et al. (43) found no difference in the incidence of seizures with prophylactically administered phenytoin. Temkin et al. (44) recently reported results from a double-blind study in which 404 severely head-injured patients randomly received phenytoin or placebo for 1 year. Phenytoin reduced the incidence of seizures during the first week but not thereafter.

Maintain Brain Oxygenation

Oxygen delivery to the brain is dependent on oxygen content of the blood and cerebral blood flow. Oxygen content of the blood can be increased by ensuring an adequate hemoglobin concentration and by increasing arterial pO_2. The optimal hemoglobin concentration for tissue oxygenation is approximately 10 g/dL (45). A lower hemoglobin concentration reduces the oxygen-carrying capacity of the blood more than it improves viscosity. A higher hemoglobin concentration increases viscosity and reduces CBF even though it increases oxygen-carrying capacity.

Increasing arterial pO_2 after hemoglobin is nearly 100% saturated increases arterial oxygen content only by a small amount, i.e., by the amount of oxygen dissolved in the blood. However, if tissues are ischemic, even small increases in oxygen content can be important. In addition, studies using PET imaging have suggested that there may be impaired diffusion of oxygen in injured brain tissue (46). Other studies demonstrate mitochondrial dysfunction in injured brain (47). Hyperoxia may improve tissue oxygenation under these conditions. Menzel et al. (48) have observed an increase in PbO_2 and a decrease in extracellular lactate concentration in the brain, measured by microdialysis, when patients with very low baseline PbO_2 were placed on 100% oxygen. The reduction in lactate accumulation with this therapy suggests that the increase in PbO_2 altered ischemic cerebral metabolism favorably.

Maintain Cerebral Perfusion Pressure

Initial volume resuscitation should be aimed at achieving euvolemia. Once an ICP monitor is in place, further blood pressure management should be aimed at maintaining a CPP of at least 60 mm Hg (13). Boluses of intravenous fluid can be used as initial treatment of low CPP. All intravenous fluids given should be isotonic to avoid worsening cerebral edema. If fluid resuscitation is not sufficient to maintain CPP, treatment with pressors should be initiated. Some studies have suggested that treatment with norepinephrine results in a more predictable blood pressure response than treatment with dopamine (49). Treating to a CPP higher than 60 mm Hg has not been shown to improve outcome but does increase the risk of ARDS (50).

First-line Therapies of Intracranial Hypertension

When ICP becomes elevated despite measures to remove exacerbating factors, the first-line therapies include sedation and neuromuscular blockade, osmotic therapy, CSF drainage, and mild hyperventilation.

Sedation and Paralysis

Sedative/analgesic drugs blunt the effect that the routine nursing care of patients has on intracranial pressure. Routine paralysis of all patients with severe head injury increases the risk of pulmonary complications and prolongs the ICU stay (51). However, ICP raised by agitation, posturing, or coughing should be prevented by narcotics and nondepolarizing muscle relaxants that do not alter cerebrovascular resistance. A reasonable regimen is morphine and lorazepam for analgesia/sedation and cisatracurium or vecuronium as a muscle relaxant, with the dose titrated by twitch response to stimulation (52). Although the neurologic examination cannot be closely monitored while the patient is paralyzed, muscle relaxants can be withheld once a day, usually before morning rounds, to obtain a brief neurologic examination.

Osmotic Therapy to Reduce Intracranial Pressure

One of the mainstays of treatment of elevated ICP is osmotic therapy with either mannitol or hypertonic saline. This treatment can be initiated prior to insertion of an ICP monitor if signs and symptoms of herniation are present. The initial dose of mannitol is 1g/kg. Once an ICP monitor has been inserted, further bolus doses can be given to maintain ICP <20 to 25 mm Hg. Bolus dosing of 0.25 mg to 0.5 mg per kg every 2 to 6 hours can be given if the serum osmolality is less than 320. Dosing to a serum osmolality of greater than 320 has not been demonstrated to improve outcome and increases the risk of acute renal failure.

Mannitol is thought to reduce ICP through two mechanisms (53). The first mechanism of action is an immediate expansion of the intravascular volume, resulting in reduced hematocrit and reduced blood viscosity that causes decreased ICP and increased cerebral blood flow and oxygen delivery. The second mechanism of action involves the establishment of osmotic gradients between the plasma and the cells, resulting in decreased cellular volume. Long-term treatment with mannitol can result in build-up of mannitol within the cells. This effect is more marked with continuous infusion of mannitol.

Although mannitol has been more widely studied, some studies have suggested that hypertonic saline is more effective at lowering intracranial pressure. These studies have been small and have not demonstrated a statistically significant difference in outcome. The usual dose form is boluses of 7.5% hypertonic saline (54). Other agents that are under investigation include hypertonic saline hetastarch, with studies comparing bolus doses of 7.2% hypertonic saline hetastarch 200/0.5 with 15% mannitol showing some improved reduction in ICP with the hypertonic saline hetastarch but no significant difference in outcome (55). Another study comparing 7.5% hypertonic saline/6% dextran solution to bolus dosing of 20% mannitol showed improved reduction of ICP but no difference in outcome (56). Further large randomized controlled studies are necessary to define the role of hypertonic saline in the treatment of increased ICP.

Clinical Pearl. Osmotic therapy is one of the mainstays of treatment for elevated ICP. Mannitol can be dosed with an initial bolus of 1 g/kg. Further bolus doses of 0.25 to 0.5 g/kg can be given as necessary. Hypertonic saline is another agent that can be used.

Drainage of Cerebrospinal Fluid

Placement of a ventriculostomy catheter allows drainage of CSF during episodes of increased ICP. Drainage of 3 to 5 mL of CSF can reduce ICP. CSF drainage is a mainstay of therapy for hydrocephalus but may be useful in more diffuse processes where the ventricles are effaced by brain swelling. If CSF is to be drained continuously, the drainage system should not be set lower than 10 cm above the level of foramen of Monro, which is approximated by the external auditory canal.

Hyperventilation

Hyperventilation, to a $paCO_2$ of 30 to 35 mm Hg, can reduce intracranial pressure by constricting cerebral blood vessels and reducing cerebral blood volume. The effect of changes in $paCO_2$ on cerebral vessels is mediated by the change in pH induced in the extracellular fluid (57). The effects of hyperventilation on ICP are immediate, but the duration of the effect is brief because the pH of the brain, at least in normal individuals, soon equilibrates to the lower pCO_2 level.

Long-term hyperventilation (to $paCO_2$ of 25–30 mm Hg) has been demonstrated to result in worse outcomes after traumatic brain injury, possibly secondary to reduction in CBF (58). The authors of this study recommended using hyperventilation only in patients with intracranial hypertension rather than as a routine in all head-injured patients.

In patients who have been chronically hyperventilated, abruptly returning the pCO_2 to normal can result in a dramatic increase in ICP. In experimental studies, this phenomenon occurs after 24 hours of hyperventilation and is associated with vasodilation of cerebral vessels as the CSF pH equilibrates at the new lower pCO_2 level (59). Hyperventilation should be withdrawn over several days to avoid this increase in ICP.

Additional Treatments for Refractory Intracranial Hypertension

All of the treatments outlined below have been shown in clinical studies to significantly reduce ICP, even when the ICP is refractory to initial treatments. However, none of these treatments have been demonstrated to improve neurologic outcome. There are also no data to suggest which of these treatments is most effective or has the least morbidity. For these reasons, such additional therapies are usually applied selectively to patients who are judged to have some potential for neurologic recovery if their ICP can be controlled.

When refractory intracranial hypertension occurs, it is also important to consider whether a delayed intracranial hematoma may have developed. A follow-up CT scan may be indicated before advancing to these additional treatments of elevated ICP. Any surgical intracranial hematoma should be evacuated.

Pentobarbital Coma

If CSF drainage and mannitol fail to control elevated ICP, other techniques need to be considered. One intervention that can lower ICP is administration of pentobarbital to achieve burst suppression on EEG. However, routine use of barbiturates in unselected patients has not been consistently effective in reducing morbidity or mortality after severe head injury (60,61). A randomized multicenter trial demonstrated that instituting barbiturate coma in patients with refractory intracranial hypertension resulted in a twofold greater chance of controlling the ICP (62).

A simple dosing scheme from the randomized clinical trial is a loading dose of 10 mg/kg intravenously (IV) over 30 minutes followed by 5 mg/kg per hour for three doses followed by a maintenance dose of 1 mg/kg per hour (62). The maintenance dose rate should be titrated to achieve a level of 3.5 to 5.0 mg% (35–50 *ug*/mL). If available, continuous EEG may be used to monitor for burst suppression to ensure maximal therapeutic effect. Significant hypotension may develop during administration of the loading dose (61). Consideration should be given to placement of a Swan-Ganz catheter for continuous cardiac monitoring during loading. The initial loading dose should be given by slow intravenous push with close monitoring of the blood pressure. Hypotension during induction of barbiturate coma usually responds to fluid bolus. Higher doses of pentobarbital can cause myocardial depression and require inotropic or even vasopressor support. Laboratory studies suggest that for the treatment of hypotension associated with barbiturate coma, volume resuscitation may be better than dopamine (63). In these studies, dopamine infusion increased cerebral metabolic requirements and partially offset the beneficial effects of barbiturates on metabolism.

The goal of treatment is to reduce ICP to $<$20 to 25 mm Hg. After ICP has been controlled for 24 to 48 hours, pentobarbital can be weaned and stopped. If ICP increases during reduction of pentobarbital, stop titration and increase the dose until ICP is controlled. Pentobarbital is thought to work through multiple mechanisms, including alterations in vascular tone, decreased cerebral metabolism, and decreased free radical production (64,65).

Pentobarbital coma is associated with significant morbidity. Hypotension is a common complication (61) and may require concomitant administration of vasopressors, which should be available when loading. Pentobarbital coma increases the risk of pneumonia, pressure ulcers, and paralytic ileus.

Several studies have tried to predict which patient would be most likely to respond to pentobarbital coma. Characteristics that may indicate a favorable ICP response to barbiturates include younger age, diffuse rather than focal brain injury, a relatively high level of brain electrical activity, and a high cerebral metabolic rate prior to treatment (66,67). Preservation of CO_2 reactivity predicted a good ICP response to barbiturates in one study (68).

Clinical Pearl. Routine use of barbiturate coma does not improve neurologic outcome. If CSF drainage and osmotic therapy are not sufficient to control elevated ICP, barbiturate coma has been shown to double the chances of controlling ICP. Hypotension is the most common complication of barbiturate coma.

Decompressive Craniectomy

Initially described by Kocher in 1901, craniectomy for control of elevated intracranial pressure has a long history. Studies in the 1970s initially showed improved outcome (69) resulting in increased usage of the procedure, but follow-up studies did not demonstrate the same improved outcome (70) and craniectomy became less popular. More recent studies have demonstrated benefit (71) and craniectomy is being used more often for control of elevated ICP. Craniectomy can be considered in patients with elevated intracranial pressure uncontrolled by CSF drainage and osmotic therapy. If the injury primarily involves a single hemisphere of the brain, a hemicraniectomy can provide adequate decompression. A large bone flap should be removed with particular focus on decompressing the anterior temporal lobe and visualization of the floor of the middle fossa. Diffuse injury involving both hemispheres may necessitate bifrontal craniectomy, with removal of a large bone flap and decompression of both temporal lobes and both frontal lobes.

Craniectomy has been demonstrated to result in a significant decrease in ICP and in retrospective review has been suggested to improve outcome (72), although further prospective trials are needed. Two randomized clinical trials of decompressive craniectomy, Rescue ICP (73) and DECRAN, for traumatic brain injury are currently underway. Craniectomy can also be useful in treatment of elevated ICP secondary to malignant middle cerebral artery stroke, with significant reduction in mortality and improved outcome if performed prior to the development of symptoms of herniation (74–76).

Hypothermia

Hypothermia has several potentially neuroprotective effects, including reducing cerebral metabolism and decreasing ICP. Although a randomized, controlled trial in humans did not show a significant improvement in neurologic outcome, ICP was better controlled during hypothermia (77). Routine induction of hypothermia is not indicated at present, but hypothermia may be an effective adjunctive treatment for increased ICP refractory to other medical management.

Steroids

Multiple randomized, controlled studies have demonstrated no benefit in treating patients with traumatic brain injury with steroids (78). The recently completed Corticosteroid Randomization After Significant Head injury (CRASH) trial observed an increased risk of death in patients receiving methylprednisolone for 48 hours after injury (79). As a result, steroids are not recommended for treatment of head injury. Steroids are also not recommended for treatment of the cellular edema accompanying stroke.

Steroids, however, can be useful in treating vasogenic edema associated with brain tumors or selected infections such as neurocysticercosis (80). Dosing schemes are relatively arbitrary with a typical dosing scheme for a patient with significant symptomatic vasogenic edema from a tumor being dexamethasone, 4 mg IV every 6 hours.

Completion of Treatment

Treatment should be titrated off once ICP has been controlled below 20 mm Hg for 24 to 48 hours. ICP monitors can be removed if ICP is stable below 20 mm Hg for 48 hours off any intervention. It is important to remember that patients may develop delayed increase in ICP secondary to blossoming of contusions, evolution of a stroke, or development of new mass lesions.

OUTCOME WITH INTRACRANIAL HYPERTENSION

Patients with traumatic brain injury can be classified based on initial GCS. Patients with mild head injury, with a GCS of 13 to 15, have a minimal chance (3%) of deteriorating into a coma and developing elevated ICP. Patients with moderate head injury, with a GCS from 9 to 12, have a moderate chance (10%–20%) of deteriorating into a coma and developing elevated ICP. Patients with a GCS of 8 or less, defined as a severe head injury, have the highest chance of developing elevated ICP and also have the worst outcome. Patients classified as having a severe head injury are more likely to develop increased ICP if they have an abnormal head CT or if they meet two of the three criteria of age older than 40 years, unilateral or bilateral motor posturing, or SBP <90 mm Hg (81).

No study clearly demonstrates that monitoring and treating ICP improves neurologic outcome, but there are strong associations between intracranial hypertension and a poor outcome, and the development of refractory intracranial hypertension has a very high mortality rate (7–10,60). In the randomized trial of pentobarbital coma for refractory intracranial hypertension, control of the elevated ICP determined the outcome, with 92% of patients where ICP was controlled surviving, and 83% of patients where ICP was not controlled dying (62).

Historically, institution of treatment protocols aimed at controlling elevated intracranial pressure has significantly improved outcome in traumatic brain injury. Jennett et al. (82) in 1977 reported a mortality rate of 50% in comatose patients (GCS <8) in a cohort treated without ICP monitoring. Becker et al. (83) reported significantly lower mortality of 30% in a similar patient cohort using ICP monitoring. Mortality rates at 30 days for patients with severe brain injury have been slowly declining with mortality of patients in the Traumatic Coma Data Bank reduced from 39% in 1984 to 27% in 1996 (84).

The availability of multiple monitoring modalities has provided more information on which patients have poor outcomes and has provided treatment goals. Treatment strategies are now aimed at maintaining ICP less than 20–25 mm Hg, maintaining CPP greater than 60 mm Hg, and maintaining brain tissue oxygenation at greater than 10 mm Hg. Even with these advances in treatment, traumatic brain injury is still associated with significant morbidity and mortality in both the short and long term.

SUMMARY

Elevated intracranial pressure can be caused by multiple injuries, including stroke, subarachnoid hemorrhage, mass lesion, hydrocephalus, and traumatic brain injury. Initial management is focused on maintaining oxygenation and perfusion using the ABCs of resuscitation. If signs of herniation are present, an initial bolus of mannitol should be given. Surgical mass lesions should be identified and evacuated. A ventriculostomy catheter should be inserted to allow monitoring of ICP. Treatment should be initiated with the goal of maintaining ICP below 20 to 25 mm Hg. Cerebral perfusion pressure should be maintained at 60 mm Hg. Initial treatments of elevated ICP include sedation and paralysis, drainage of CSF, mild hyperventilation, and bolus administration of osmotic agents such as mannitol. If ICP is not controlled with these measures, additional treatments including pentobarbital coma, hypothermia, or decompressive craniectomy can be considered. Other parameters that can be monitored and treated include jugular venous oxygen saturation and brain tissue oxygenation. Therapy should be continued until ICP is controlled at less than 20 mm Hg for 24 to 48 hours. Mortality rates for severe head injury have shown a steady decrease but are still 27%.

References

1. Marmarou A, Signoretti S, Fatouros PP, et al. Predominance of cellular edema in traumatic brain swelling in patients with severe head injuries. *J Neurosurg.* 2006;104:720.
2. Hlatky R, Furuya Y, Valadka AB, et al. Dynamic autoregulatory response after severe head injury. *J Neurosurg.* 2002;97:1054.
3. Bouma GJ, Muizelaar JP, Choi SC, et al. Cerebral blood flow and metabolism after severe traumatic brain injury: the elusive role of ischemia. *J Neurosurg.* 1991;75:685.
4. Hlatky R, Contant CF, Diaz Marchan P, et al. Significance of a reduced CBF during the first 12 hours following traumatic brain injury. *Neurocrit Care.* 2004;1:69.
5. Robertson CS, Gopinatb SP, Goodman JC, et al. $SjvO_2$ monitoring in head-injured patients. *J Neurotrauma.* 1995;12:891.
6. Gopinath SP, Valadka A, Uzura M, et al. Comparison of brain tissue pO_2 and jugular venous oxygen saturation as monitors of cerebral oxygenation. *Crit Care Med.* 1999;27:2337.
7. Marshall LF, Smith RW, Shapiro HM. The outcome with aggressive treatment in severe head injuries, I: significance of intracranial pressure monitoring. *J Neurosurg.* 1979;50:20.
8. Miller JD, Butterworth J, Gudeman SK, et al. Further experience in the management of severe head injury. *J Neurosurg.* 1981;54:289.
9. Saul TG, Ducker TB. Effect of intracranial pressure monitoring and aggressive treatment on mortality in severe head injury. *J Neurosurg.* 1982;56: 498.
10. Marmarou A, Anderson RL, Ward JD, et al. Impact of ICP instability and hypotension on outcome in patients with severe head injury. *J Neurosurg.* 1991;75:S59.
11. Bullock RM, Chesnut R, Clifton GL, et al. Management and prognosis of severe traumatic brain injury, 1: guidelines for the management of severe traumatic brain injury: recommendations for intracranial pressure monitoring technology. *J Neurotrauma.* 2000;17:497.
12. Zabramski JM, Whiting D, Darouiche RO, et al. Efficacy of antimicrobial-impregnated external ventricular drain catheters: a prospective, randomized, controlled trial. *J Neurosurg.* 2003;98:725.
13. Robertson CS, Valadka AB, Hannay HJ, et al. Prevention of secondary insults after severe head injury. *Crit Care Med.* 1999;27:2086.
14. Johnston AJ, Steiner LA, Coles JP, et al. Effect of cerebral perfusion pressure augmentation on regional oxygenation and metabolism after head injury. *Crit Care Med.* 2005;33:189.
15. Kiening KL, Unterberg AW, Bardt TF, et al. Monitoring of cerebral oxygenation in patients with severe head injuries: brain tissue PO_2 versus jugular vein oxygen saturation. *J Neurosurg.* 1996;85:751.
16. Valadka A, Gopinath SP, Contant CF, et al. Critical values for brain tissue PO_2 to outcome after severe head injury. *Crit Care Med.* 1998;26:1576.
17. Stiefel MF, Spiotta A, Gracias VH, et al. Reduced mortality rate in patients with severe traumatic brain injury treated with brain tissue oxygen monitoring. *J Neurosurg.* 2005;103:805.
18. Gopinath SP, Robertson CS, Contant CF, et al. Jugular venous desaturation and outcome after head injury. *J Neurol Neurosurg Psych.* 1994;57:717.
19. Cormio M, Valadka AB, Robertson CS. Elevated jugular bulb oxygen saturation after severe head injury. *J Neurosurg.* 1999;90:9.
20. Gibbs EL, Lennox WG, Nims LF, et al. Arterial and cerebral venous blood. Arterial-venous differences in man. *J Biol Chem.* 1942;144:325.
21. Chieregato A, Calzolari F, Trasforini G, et al. Normal jugular bulb oxygen saturation. *J Neurol Neurosurg Psychiatry* 2003;74:784.
22. Rosner MJ, Daughton S. Cerebral perfusion pressure management in head injury. *J Trauma.* 1993;30:933.
23. Fearnside MR, Cook RJ, McDougall P, et al. The Westmead Head Injury Project outcome in severe head injury. A comparative analysis of pre-hospital, clinical and CT variables. *Br J Neurosurg.* 1993;7:267.
24. Chesnut RM, Marshall LF, Klauber MR, et al. The role of secondary brain injury in determining outcome from severe head injury. *J Trauma.* 1993; 34:216.
25. Miller JD. Head injury and brain ischaemia—implications for therapy. *Br J Anaesth.* 1985;57:120.
26. Pigula FA, Wald SL, Shackford SR, et al. The effect of hypotension and hypoxia on children with severe head injuries. *J Pediatr Surg.* 1993;28:310.
27. Winchell RJ, Hoyt DB. Endotracheal intubation in the field improves survival in patients with severe head injury. *Trauma Research and Education Foundation of San Diego. Arch Surg.* 1997;132:592.
28. Hsiao AK, Michelson SP, Hedges JR. Emergent intubation and CT scan pathology of blunt trauma patients with Glasgow Coma Scale scores of 3-13. *Prehosp Disaster Med.* 1993;8:229.
29. Davis DP, Hoyt DB, Ochs M, et al. The effect of paramedic rapid sequence intubation on outcome in patients with severe traumatic brain injury. *J Trauma.* 2003;54:444.
30. Davis DP, Fakhry SM, Wang HE, et al. Paramedic rapid sequence intubation for severe traumatic brain injury: perspectives from an expert panel. *Prehosp Emerg Care.* 2007;11:1.
31. American College of Surgeons Committee on Trauma. Resources for the Optimal Care of the Injured Patient. Chicago: American College of Surgeons. 2006.
32. Bullock RM, Chesnut R, Clifton GL, et al. Management and prognosis of severe traumatic brain injury, 1: guidelines for the management of severe traumatic brain injury: trauma systems. *J Neurotrauma.* 2000;17:457.
33. Cruz J, Minoja G, Okuchi K. Improving clinical outcomes from acute subdural hematomas with the emergency preoperative administration of high doses of mannitol: a randomized trial. *Neurosurgery.* 2001;49:864.
34. Feldman Z, Kanter MJ, Robertson CS, et al. Effect of head elevation on intracranial pressure, cerebral perfusion pressure, and cerebral blood flow in head-injured patients. *J Neurosurg.* 1992;76:207.
35. Meixensberger J, Baunach S, Amschler J, et al. Influence of body position on tissue-pO_2, cerebral perfusion pressure and intracranial pressure in patients with acute brain injury. *Neurol Res.* 1997;19:249.
36. Rosner MJ, Coley IB. Cerebral perfusion pressure, intracranial pressure, and head elevation. *J Neurosurg.* 1986;65:636.
37. Bloomfield GL, Dalton JM, Sugerman HJ, et al. Treatment of increasing intracranial pressure secondary to the acute abdominal compartment syndrome in a patient with combined abdominal and head trauma. *J Trauma.* 1995;39:1168.
38. Dietrich WD, Alonso O, Halley M, et al. Delayed posttraumatic brain hyperthermia worsens outcome after fluid percussion brain injury: a light and electron microscopic study in rats. *Neurosurgery.* 1996;38:533.
39. Jennett B. *Epilepsy after Nonmissile Head Injuries.* 2nd ed. London, England: Heineman; 1976.
40. Annegers JF, Hauser WA, Coan SP, et al. A population-based study of seizures after traumatic brain injuries. *N Engl J Med.* 1998;338:20.
41. Vespa PM, Nenov V, Nuwer MR. Continuous EEG monitoring in the intensive care unit: early findings and clinical efficacy. *J Clin Neurophysiol.* 1999;16:1.
42. Lee ST, Lui TN, Wong CW, et al. Early seizures after severe closed head injury. *Can J Neurol Sci.* 1997;24:40.
43. Young B, Rapp RP, Norton NA, et al. Failure of prophylactically administered phenytoin to prevent early posttraumatic seizures. *J Neurosurg.* 1983; 58:231.
44. Temkin NR, Dikmen SS, Wilensky AJ, et al. A randomized, double-blind study of phenytoin for the prevention of post-traumatic seizures. *N Engl J Med.* 1990;323:497.
45. Kee DB, Wood JH. Rheology of the cerebral circulation. *Neurosurgery.* 1984;15:125.
46. Menon DK, Coles JP, Gupta AK, et al. Diffusion limited oxygen delivery following head injury. *Crit Care Med.* 2004;32:1384.
47. Daugherty WP, Levasseur JE, Sun D, et al. Effects of hyperbaric oxygen therapy on cerebral oxygenation and mitochondrial function following moderate lateral fluid-percussion injury in rats. *J Neurosurg.* 2004;101:499.
48. Menzel M, Doppenberg EMR, Zauner A, et al. Increased inspired oxygen concentration as a factor in improved brain tissue oxygenation and tissue lactate levels after severe human head injury. *J Neurosurg.* 1999;91:1.
49. Steiner LA, Johnston AJ, Czosnyka M, et al. Direct comparison of cerebrovascular effects of norepinephrine and dopamine in head-injured patients. *Crit Care Med.* 2004;32:1049.
50. Contant CF, Valadka AB, Hannay HJ, et al. ARDS as a complication of induced hypertension after severe head injury. *J Neurosurg.* 2003;95:560.
51. Hsiang J, Chesnut RM, Crisp CB, et al. Early, routine paralysis for ICP control in severe head injury: Is it necessary? *Crit Care Med.* 1994;22:1471.
52. Schramm WM, Jesenko R, Bartunek A, et al. Effects of cisatracurium on cerebral and cardiovascular hemodynamics in patients with severe brain injury. *Acta Anaesthesiol Scand.* 1997;41:1319.

53. Muizelaar JP, Lutz HA, Becker DP. Effect of mannitol on ICP and CBF and correlation with pressure autoregulation in severely head-injured patients. *J Neurosurg.* 1984;61:700.
54. Vialet R, Albanese J, Thomachot L, et al. Isovolume hypertonic solutes (sodium chloride or mannitol) in the treatment of refractory posttraumatic intracranial hypertension: 2 mL/kg 7.5% saline is more effective than 2 mL/kg 20% mannitol. *Crit Care Med.* 2003;31:1683.
55. Harutjunyan L, Holz C, Rieger A, et al. Efficiency of 7.2% hypertonic saline hydroxyethyl starch 200/0.5 versus mannitol 15% in the treatment of increased intracranial pressure in neurosurgical patients—a randomized clinical trial [ISRCTN62699180]. *Crit Care.* 2005;9:R530.
56. Battison C, Andrews PJ, Graham C, et al. Randomized, controlled trial on the effect of a 20% mannitol solution and a 7.5% saline/6% dextran solution on increased intracranial pressure after brain injury. *Crit Care Med.* 2005;33:196.
57. Kontos HA, Wei EP, Raper AJ, et al. Local mechanism of CO_2 action on cat pial arterioles. *Stroke.* 1977;8:226.
58. Muizelaar JP, Marmarou A, Ward JD, et al. Adverse effects of prolonged hyperventilation in patients with severe head injury: a randomized clinical trial. *J Neurosurg.* 1991;75:731.
59. Muizelaar JP, van der Poel HG, Li ZC, et al. Pial artery diameter and CO_2 reactivity during prolonged hyperventilation in the rabbit. *J Neurosurg.* 1988;69:923.
60. Schwartz ML, Tator CH, Rowed DW, et al. The University of Toronto Head Injury Treatment Study: A prospective, randomized comparison of pentobarbital and mannitol. *Can J Neurol Sci.* 1984;11:434.
61. Ward JD, Becker DP, Miller JD, et al. Failure of prophylactic barbiturate coma in the treatment of severe head injury. *J Neurosurg.* 1985;62:383.
62. Eisenberg HM, Frankowski RF, Contant CF, et al. High-dose barbiturate control of elevated intracranial pressure in patients with severe head injury. *J Neurosurg.* 1988;69:15.
63. Sato M, Niiyama K, Kuroda R, et al. Influence of dopamine on cerebral blood flow, and metabolism for oxygen and glucose under barbiturate administration in cats. *Acta Neurochir (Wien).* 1991;110:174.
64. Goodman JC, Valadka AB, Gopinath SP, et al. Lactate and excitatory amino acids measured by microdialysis are decreased by pentobarbital coma in head-injured patients. *J Neurotrauma.* 1996;13:549.
65. Kassell NF, Hitchon PW, Gerk MK, et al. Alterations in cerebral blood flow, oxygen metabolism, and electrical activity produced by high dose sodium thiopental. *Neurosurgery.* 1980;7:598.
66. Miller JD, Piper IR, Dearden NM. Management of intracranial hypertension in head injury: matching treatment with cause. *Acta Neurochir Suppl (Wien).* 1993;57:152.
67. Cormio M, Gopinath SP, Valadka AB, et al. Cerebral hemodynamic effects of pentobarbital coma in head injured patients. *J Neurotrauma.* 1999;16:927.
68. Messeter K, Nordstrom CH, Sundbarg G, et al. Cerebral hemodynamics in patients with acute severe head trauma. *J Neurosurg* .1986;64:231.
69. Ransohoff J, Benjamin V. Hemicraniectomy in the treatment of acute subdural haematoma. *J Neurol Neurosurg Psychiatry.* 1971;34:106.
70. Cooper PR, Rovit RL, Ransohoff J. Hemicraniectomy in the treatment of acute subdural hematoma: a re-appraisal. *Surg Neurol.* 1976;5:25.
71. Aarabi B, Hesdorffer DC, Ahn ES, et al. Outcome following decompressive craniectomy for malignant swelling due to severe head injury. *J Neurosurg.* 2006;104:469.
72. Sahuquillo J, Arikan F. Decompressive craniectomy for the treatment of refractory high intracranial pressure in traumatic brain injury. *Cochrane Database Syst Rev.* 2006 Jan 25;(1):CD003983.
73. Hutchinson PJ, Corteen E, Czosnyka M, et al. Decompressive craniectomy in traumatic brain injury: the randomized multicenter RESCUEicp study (www.RESCUEicp.com). *Acta Neurochir Suppl.* 2006;96:17.
74. Mori K, Nakao Y, Yamamoto T, et al. Early external decompressive craniectomy with duroplasty improves functional recovery in patients with massive hemispheric embolic infarction: timing and indication of decompressive surgery for malignant cerebral infarction. *Surg Neurol.* 2004;62:420.
75. Cho DY, Chen TC, Lee HC. Ultra-early decompressive craniectomy for malignant middle cerebral artery infarction. *Surg Neurol.* 2003;60:227.
76. Schwab S, Steiner T, Aschoff A, et al. Early hemicraniectomy in patients with complete middle cerebral artery infarction. *Stroke.* 1998;29:1888.
77. Clifton GL, Miller ER, Choi SC, et al. Lack of effect of induction of hypothermia after acute brain injury. *N Engl J Med.* 2001;344:556.
78. Bullock RM, Chesnut R, Clifton GL, et al. Management and prognosis of severe traumatic brain injury, 1: guidelines for the management of severe traumatic brain injury: role of steroids. *J Neurotrauma.* 2000;17:531.
79. Edwards P, Arango M, Balica L, et al. Final results of MRC CRASH, a randomised placebo-controlled trial of intravenous corticosteroid in adults with head injury-outcomes at 6 months. *Lancet.* 2005;365:1957.
80. French LA, Galicich JH. The use of steroids for control of cerebral edema. *Clin Neurosurg.* 1964;10:212.
81. Narayan RK, Kishore PRS, Becker DP, et al. Intracranial pressure: to monitor or not to monitor? A review of our experience with severe head injury. *J Neurosurg.* 1982;56:650.
82. Jennett B, Teasdale G, Galbraith S, et al. Severe head injuries in three countries. *J Neurol Neurosurg Psychiatry.* 1977;40:291.
83. Becker DP, Miller JD, Ward JD, et al. The outcome from severe head injury with early diagnosis and intensive management. *J Neurosurg.* 1977;47:491.
84. Lu J, Marmarou A, Choi S, et al. Mortality from traumatic brain injury. *Acta Neurochir Suppl.* 2005;95:281.

CHAPTER 147 ■ ALTERED CONSCIOUSNESS AND COMA IN THE INTENSIVE CARE UNIT

EELCO F. M. WIJDICKS

Impaired consciousness is a very common neurologic problem in the Intensive Care Unit (ICU). Neurologists are commonly consulted for "altered mental status," often after sedation has been discontinued, after cardiopulmonary resuscitation and failure to awaken, and in patients with multisystem trauma to address the extent of traumatic brain injury and assist in management. With the emergence of transplantation intensive care units, neurologic complications have surfaced with many involving altered awareness.

The assessment of impaired consciousness or coma is a complex undertaking. Obviously, there are multiple factors in play, but simply denoting the cause of impaired consciousness as multifactorial would be counterproductive and, most likely, inaccurate. Some patterns, however, are apparent. First, prolonged accumulation of sedative agents in patients with impaired renal or hepatic function is common, and allowance of time for these agents to metabolize would lead to improvement. Second, hypoxic/ischemic injury to the brain is probably more likely than commonly appreciated. The circumstances for episodic hypoxemia and shock are commonly present, and therefore, the brain is at risk. Third, the clinical spectrum of the neurologic aspect of critical illness has become better defined. In many circumstances, with a plethora of potential causes of coma, it is possible to localize the lesion and diagnose the cause of coma. The more frequent use of MRI technology has increased, providing not only important diagnostic findings, but also prognostic pointers. This chapter provides the essentials of neurologic examination and places it into the context of the different ICUs.

ANATOMY OF COMA

In general, structural lesions interrupt the ascending reticular activating system. This system consists of the reticular formation, a network of neurons that signals the thalamus and cortex. The thalamus, with its complex circuitry connecting the cortex and basal forebrain, participates in arousal. Without this neuronal network, the person cannot be aroused. The thalamus, through the interlaminar nuclei, maintains arousal and relays sensory, motor, and critical cortical circuits. As a general principle, altered consciousness is caused by lesions that are dorsally located in the pons and thalamus, or are bihemispheric (1,2). Bilateral lesions of the thalamus, bilateral white matter lesions, or bilateral cortical lesions are necessary to impair consciousness. Alternatively, a mass in one hemisphere could produce bilateral injury when brain shift occurs or when the ventricular system become obstructed, resulting in an acute hydrocephalus.

The mechanism of acute physiologic derangement of the brain in acute metabolic abnormalities is not as well understood, and not uncommonly, a structural lesion is at play. Examples are patients with rapid sodium correction that causes osmotic demyelination, central pontine myelinolysis, or extensive white matter disease. Cerebral edema may also occur in patients with acute ketoacidosis or in those with fulminant hepatic failure. In these circumstances, it would appear that the laboratory derangement is the cause of coma, but, in fact, a structural abnormality is present.

DEFINITIONS

The major categories of altered level of consciousness can be arbitrarily defined to facilitate interphysician communication. Many patients in the ICU are in an *acute confusional state.* This is a condition in which there is impairment of attention, inability to retain memory, and incoherent conversation. The patient is not following any commands, including simply tracking a finger. When hallucinations occur and are accompanied by signs of autonomic hyperactivity that may include tachycardia, hypertension, and sweating, the term *delirium* is used. Some patients may be combative, noisy, and have a markedly abnormal sleep pattern (3–6). Hallucinations can be vivid and often visual, particularly in cyclosporin toxicity. A delirium tremens should be recognized and is probably more common than appreciated. The warning signs are increased pulse to more than 120 beats per minute, systolic blood pressure more than 160 mm Hg, respiratory rate of more than 30 breaths per minute, fever, new-onset seizures, and a need for incremental doses of lorazepam or other benzodiazepines to control confusion.

Patients who are *comatose* are unresponsive, have their eyes closed, and do not respond to painful stimuli. In this condition, painful stimuli should not produce a localizing response to the pain stimulus, nor eye opening, grimacing, nor—in the absence of an endotracheal tube—speech. Additionally, the patient is unable to fixate on an object. Patients who remain in a comatose state for a prolonged period will eventually open their eyes, start to fixate on persons around the bedside, and then, in a gradual fashion, show improvement by following commands and uttering a few words.

Patients with pathologic motor responses, such as extensor (decerebrate posturing) or flexor (decorticate posturing) motor responses, who remain comatose may open their eyes, but then typically start to develop sleep-and-wake cycles. There will be periods during which the patient has the eyes open without fixation and periods in which the eyes are closed and the patient is in a deep sleep. These patients do not recognize any external stimuli, and there is no meaningful expression and no visual tracking, but brainstem function, including respiration, is preserved. These patients are termed as being in a persistent *vegetative state.* If a vegetative state persists for a sufficient amount of time—a year after traumatic brain injury and 3 months after anoxic ischemic injury, the adjective *permanent* has been used, indicating the virtual impossibility of recovery and awakening (7). Anoxic-ischemic encephalopathy after cardiopulmonary resuscitation or asphyxia spares the brainstem but damages the cortex, and is a common cause of the vegetative state. After a traumatic brain injury, there is often some improvement in the level of consciousness; for these patients, the term *minimally conscious state* has been used. Some communication is possible, but the disability is profound.

When all brain function is lost, the patient fulfills the clinical criteria for *brain death* (8). Irreversible loss of all brain and brainstem function occurs in patients with catastrophic neurologic injury, often with a sudden increase in intracranial pressure due to a traumatic injury or cerebral hemorrhage. Using certain criteria, the clinical diagnosis of brain death can be made, allowing for the legal declaration of the patient's death.

Physicians should recognize these different comatose states but should also be aware of the states that mimic coma, the most common of which is known as *locked-in syndrome* (9). In this state, patients have normal consciousness but complete body paralysis, except for vertical eye movements. These patients cannot move their limbs, grimace, or swallow but are able to look up and down and blink. The lesion is typically in the base of the pons—often an embolus to the basilar artery—but due to sparing of the ascending reticular formation, consciousness is not impaired, and patients are fully alert.

CLINICAL EXAMINATION

The neurologic examination consists of two parts. The first is to evaluate the patient in a broad manner using coma scales. The Glasgow coma scale has been in use for many years and continues to be a useful means of conducting such an examination; however, in the ICU, with a high proportion of patients who are ventilated, the scale becomes largely useless. This has been recognized, and a new scale—the FOUR score—has been devised and validated both in emergency departments, medical and surgical ICUs (10–12).

FOUR Score

The FOUR (Full Outline of UnResponsiveness) score, not surprisingly, has four components, each of which has 4 as the maximal grade. The FOUR score is shown in Figure 147.1.

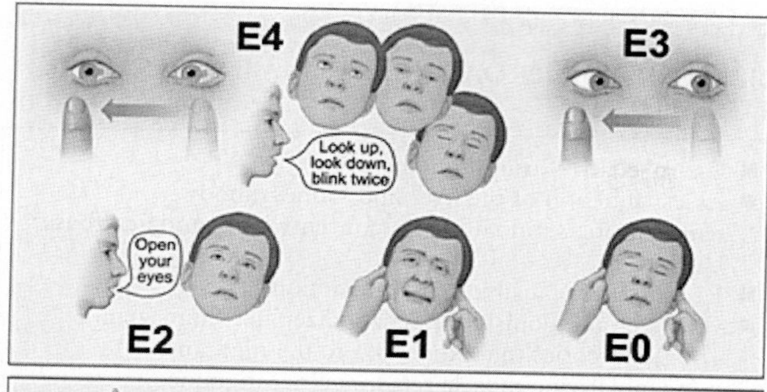

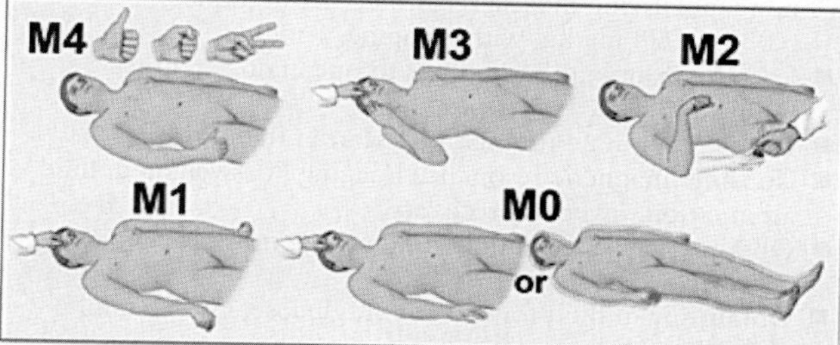

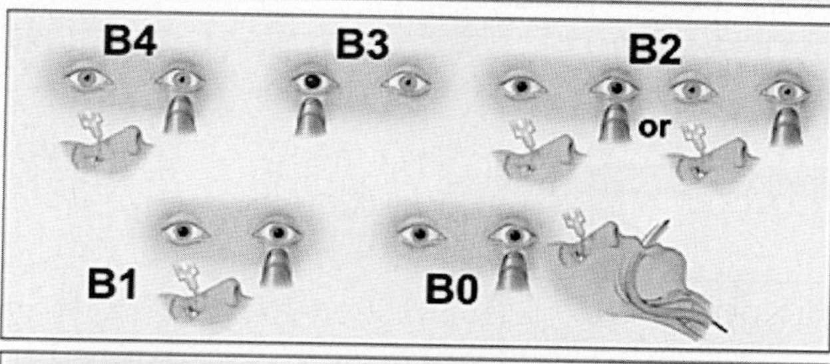

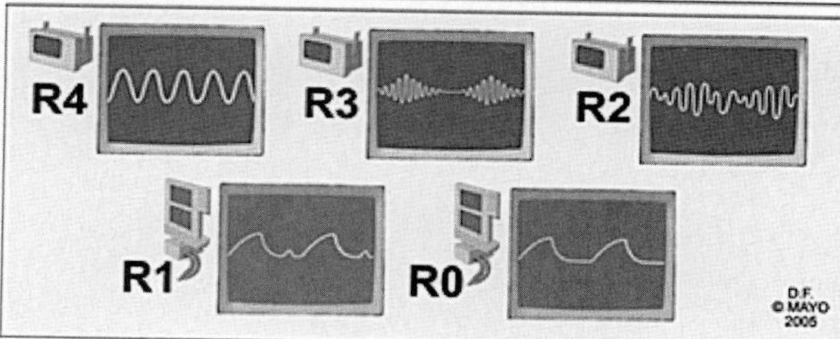

FIGURE 147.1. The FOUR score components are eye response, motor response, brainstem reflexes, and respiration. The eye responses are E0 for eyelids that remain closed with pain; E1 for eyelids closed but open to pain; E2 for eyelids closed but open to loud voice; E3 for eyelids open but not tracking; E4 for eyelids open or open to tracking or blinking to commands. The motor responses are M0 for no response to pain or a generalized myoclonic status epilepticus; M1 for extension response to pain; M2 for flexion response to pain; M3 for localizing to pain; M4 for thumbs up, fist, or peace sign. The brainstem reflexes are B0 for absent pupil, corneal, or cough reflex; B1 for pupil and corneal reflexes absent; B2 for pupil or corneal reflexes absent; B3 for one pupil wide and fixed; B4 for pupil and corneal reflexes present. And finally, respiration responses are R0 for breathes at a ventilator rate or apnea; R1 for breathes above ventilator rate; R2 for not intubated and irregular breathing; R3 for not intubated and Cheyne-Stokes breathing pattern; and R4 for not intubated, regular breathing pattern.

This score is simple to use and has significant advantages. It is able to recognize signs that suggest increased intracranial pressure and uncal herniation. It also recognizes respiratory patterns that not only indicate a need for ventilatory support but are also indicative of a declining level of consciousness and abnormal respiratory pattern. A recent validation study also found that the score is predictive of in-hospital death (10).

This score can be used to communicate between nurses, staff and residents, and indicates the depth of coma.

Neurological Examination

The next step in the neurologic examination is the examination of the brainstem reflexes (11,12). The pupillary responses are typically present; very few patients in the ICU have an abnormality in pupil diameter. Bilateral myosis is often seen because most patients are treated with opioids. A unilateral myosis represents a Horner syndrome when ptosis is present. In the ICU, it commonly reflects damage to the sympathetic pathway after placement of an internal jugular vein catheter. Extensive thoracic surgery or brachial plexopathies are also causes for unilateral myosis; (it is surprisingly common that the consult is for a "dilated eye" on the opposite side). Bilateral mydriasis with good light responses is due to delirium or anxiety. A fixed, dilated pupil indicates a third cranial nerve involvement. This could be due to direct compression from herniated brain tissue, but more likely is due to shift of the brainstem in which the third nerve is tethered. This is an important clinical sign that indicates brainstem distortion and immediately indicates the presence of a new structural mass. However, a major pitfall in the ICU is that unilateral pupillary dilatation can be seen with aerosolized anticholinergics and may cause alarm. The mist condenses on eyelids and then touches the cornea, causing a dilated pupil.

Gaze deviation is an important clinical sign, although it has very little localizing value, and can be seen in acute hepatic or renal failure without a structural brain lesion. *Downward gaze* indicates a lesion in the thalamus or dorsal midbrain and is frequently seen after hypoxic/ischemic injury. Traditionally, *gaze preference* indicates a lesion in one hemisphere, which, most of the time, is a lesion of the frontal lobe. The eyes turn *toward* the abnormality because one eye field is unopposed. *Skew deviation*, in which the eyes at rest are not lined up correctly, is a classic sign of a midbrain or pons lesion.

Spontaneous eye movement abnormalities have been noted. Common eye movements are the following:

- ***Ping pong:*** Horizontal conjunctive deviation of the eyes alternating every few seconds
- ***Convergence nystagmus:*** Ocular divergence in slow motion followed by rapid convergent jerk
- ***Ocular bobbing:*** Rapid downward conjugate movement with slow return to baseline
- ***Ocular dipping:*** Slow downward conjunctive movements with rapid return

These spontaneous eye movement abnormalities are indicative of a bihemispheric lesion and are rarely observed in toxic encephalopathie.

The motor tone is then investigated, and the patient is observed for the presence of rigidity or flaccidity. Marked flaccidity often indicates the presence of poisoning or drug intoxication. In patients who have been in the ICU for many months, a critical illness polyneuropathy should be considered. Twitching of the face and mouth may indicate seizures but, more often, will represent myoclonus status epilepticus. Myoclonus status epilepticus, with repetitive twitching in face, arm, and legs, is an important clinical sign. It has been seen in drug intoxications but also after cardiopulmonary resuscitation, and is a poor prognostic indication.

LOCALIZATION PRINCIPLES

It is important to make several decisions after certain neurologic findings have presented themselves. First, is the lesion structural or metabolic? Second, is the lesion in the cerebral hemispheres or brainstem? To achieve this objective, it is important to have a systematic diagnostic approach to coma in critical illness. The major categories of coma are as follows: hemispheric lesions with brain shift; diffuse bihemispheric structural lesion; diencephalon lesion involving both thalami; cerebellar lesion with brainstem compression or ischemia; primary brainstem lesion in the mesencephalon or pons; or a diffuse physiologic brain dysfunction from acute metabolic derangement, drugs, or intoxication; and, much less likely, a psychogenic unresponsiveness. Table 147.1 shows the common causes of these major categories of coma; a systematic diagnostic approach is shown in Table 147.2.

TABLE 147.2

DIAGNOSTIC APPROACH TO COMA IN CRITICAL ILLNESS

- Chart sedative drugs and doses
- Assess function of the liver and kidneys, body temperature, serum albumin concentration, and acid-base balance
- Reconstruct plausible drug interactions
- Consider antagonists for benzodiazepines (flumazenil, 1 mg), narcotics (naloxone, 0.1 to 0.4 mg), and nondepolarizing muscle relaxants (neostigmine, 0.035–0.070 mg/kg, with atropine, 1 mg)
- Localize examination findings to one main category (Table 147.1)
- Obtain computed tomography scan of the brain
- Consider magnetic resonance imaging (T2-weighted, fluid attenuation, inversion recovery)
- Obtain electroencephalogram and somatosensory potentials (optional)
- Obtain spinal fluid for cell count, glucose, Gram stain, and cultures (optional)

TABLE 147.1

CLASSIFICATION AND MAJOR CAUSES OF COMA

STRUCTURAL BRAIN INJURY
Hemisphere
Unilateral (with displacement)
- Intraparenchymal hematoma
- Middle cerebral artery occlusion
- Hemorrhagic contusion
- Cerebral abscess
- Brain tumor

Bilateral
- Penetrating traumatic brain injury
- Multiple traumatic brain contusions
- Anoxic-ischemic encephalopathy
- Multiple cerebral infarcts
- Bilateral thalamic infarcts
- Lymphoma
- Meningitis/encephalitis
- Gliomatosis
- Acute disseminated encephalomyelitis
- Cerebral edema
- Multiple brain metastases
- Acute hydrocephalus
- Acute leukoencephalopathy

Brainstem
- Pontine hemorrhage
- Basilar artery occlusion
- Central pontine myelinolysis
- Brainstem hemorrhagic contusion

Cerebellum (with displacement of brainstem)
- Cerebellar infarct
- Cerebellar hematoma
- Cerebellar abscess
- Cerebellar glioma

ACUTE METABOLIC-ENDOCRINE DERANGEMENT
- Hypoglycemia
- Hyperglycemia (nonketotic hyperosmolar)
- Hyponatremia
- Hypernatremia
- Addison disease
- Hypercalcemia
- Acute hypothyroidism
- Acute panhypopituitarism
- Acute uremia
- Hyperbilirubinemia
- Hypercapnia

DIFFUSE PHYSIOLOGIC BRAIN DYSFUNCTION
- Generalized tonic-clonic seizures
- Poisoning, illicit drug use
- Hypothermia
- Gas inhalation
- Basilar migraine
- Idiopathic recurrent stupor

PSYCHOGENIC UNRESPONSIVENESS
- Acute (lethal) catatonia, malignant neuroleptic syndrome
- Hysterical coma
- Malingering

From Wijdicks EFM. *Catastrophic Neurologic Disorders in the Emergency Department*. 2nd ed. Oxford University Press; 2004, with permission.

TABLE 147.3

FREQUENT ABNORMALITIES ON NEUROIMAGING STUDIES IN COMA

FINDINGS	SUGGESTED DISORDERS
Computed Tomography	
Mass lesion (brain shift, herniation)	Hematoma, hemorrhagic contusion, MCA territory infarct
Hemorrhage in basal cisterns	Aneurysmal SAH
Intraventricular hemorrhage	Arteriovenous malformation
Multiple hemorrhagic infarcts	Cerebral venous thrombosis
Multiple cerebral infarcts	Endocarditis, coagulopathy, CNS vasculitis
Diffuse cerebral edema	Cardiac arrest, fulminant meningitis, acute hepatic necrosis, encephalitis
Acute hydrocephalus	Aqueduct obstruction, colloid cyst, pineal region tumor
Pontine or cerebellum hemorrhage	Hypertension, arteriovenous malformation
Shear lesions in the white matter	Head injury
Magnetic Resonance Imaging	
Bilateral caudate and putaminal lesions	Carbon monoxide poisoning, methanol
Hyperdense signal along sagittal, straight, and transverse sinuses	Cerebral venous thrombosis
Lesions in corpus callosum, white matter	Severe head injury
Diffuse confluent hyperintense lesions in white matter, basal ganglia	Acute disseminated encephalomyelitis immunosuppressive agent, or chemotherapeutic agent toxicity, metabolic leukodystrophies
Pontine trident-shaped lesion	Central pontine myelinolysis
Thalamus, occipital, pontine lesions	Acute basilar artery occlusion
Temporal, frontal lobe hyperintensities	Herpes simplex encephalitis

MCA, middle cerebral artery; SAH, subarachnoid hemorrhage; CNS, central nervous system.
From Wijdicks EFM. *Neurologic Complications in Critical Illness.* Contemporary Neurology Series 2nd ed. Oxford University Press; 2002.

After the cause of the coma state has been localized on examination, computed tomography (CT), magnetic resonance imaging (MRI) scan, cerebrospinal fluid testing, or electrodiagnostic tests may be helpful. An MRI scan is able to document certain abnormalities and can be very helpful in determining not only the cause but also the immediate action to undertake. The MRI scan has become extremely important in the diagnosis of coma, but it requires anesthesia support in many patients and, therefore, is cumbersome in certain circumstances. A summary of the abnormalities seen on neuroimaging studies of comatose patients is shown in Table 147.3. This can be used as a reference of the most common causes of coma seen in the ICU. The electroencephalograph (EEG) has lost much of its value, largely because MRI scans are able to clearly show the lesion. EEGs can be performed to detect nonconvulsive status epilepticus (NCSE), a rare condition in which the patient has subtle eye blinking or eye movements or gaze preference that is associated with epileptic discharges. The EEG can detect these abnormalities, and the patient can sometimes be successfully treated. Most often, the EEG is the reflection of significant brain injury, and aggressive treatment has not led to a marked improvement in outcome (13). The major EEG abnormalities include delta or theta activity, in which there is marked slowing of the activity that is typically seen in sedation, meningitis, encephalitis, or other diffuse injuries. Triphasic waves are typically associated with hepatic or renal failure. Burst suppression patterns are seen most likely after anoxic ischemic injury. EEG-defined patterns, such as alpha, theta, or spindle coma, have little prognostic value.

Laboratory tests are typically available on a daily basis in a critically ill patient, and therefore, these parameters should be known. Nevertheless, several essential laboratory studies are needed to exclude acute metabolic derangements in coma and certainly should be obtained if acute new changes have occurred in neurologic examination (Table 147.4).

FAILURE TO AWAKEN AFTER SURGERY

A common problem is patients who fail to awaken after a general surgical or vascular surgical procedure. In the vast majority of patients, anoxic/ischemic injury or multiple infarcts are detected. Failure to awaken after surgery may also be due to multiple emboli to the brain. The risk of embolization is most significant in patients with severe atherosclerotic disease of the ascending aorta and thus is applicable to patients with major cardiovascular surgeries (14). However, not uncommonly, patients do not awaken because of the accumulation of narcotic and sedative agents. Many of these patients have underlying liver dysfunction that further increases accumulation of these

TABLE 147.4

LABORATORY TESTS IN THE EVALUATION OF COMA

Hematocrit, white blood cell count
Electrolytes (Na, KCl, CO_2, Ca, PO_4)
Glucose
Urea, creatinine
Aspartate transaminase (AST) and γ-glutamyltransferase (GGT)
Osmolality
Arterial blood gases (pH, PCO_2, PO_2, HCO_3, HbCO) (optional)
Platelets, smear, fibrinogen degeneration products, activated partial thromboplastin time, prothrombin time (optional)
Plasma thyrotropin (optional)
Blood and cerebrospinal fluid cultures (optional)
Toxic screen in blood and urine (optional)
Cerebrospinal fluid (protein, cells, glucose, India ink stain, and cryptococcal antigen, viral titers) (optional)

PO_2/PCO_2, partial pressure of O_2/CO_2; HbCO, carbon monoxide hemoglobin.
From: Wijdicks EFM. *Neurologic Complications in Critical Illness.* Contemporary Neurology Series 64. 2nd ed. Oxford University Press; 2002.

drugs. Finally, acute postoperative hyponatremia, due to administration of a large volume of hypertonic fluid to patients, may be a cause of failure to awaken.

FAILURE TO AWAKEN AFTER TRANSPLANTATION

Changes in consciousness have been recognized in patients having undergone major organ transplantation (15). This is most commonly seen with cardiac or liver transplantation. Although in the vast majority of patients, a delirium that may evolve to coma develops due to the toxicity of immunosuppressive agents, other reasons for loss of consciousness are hypoxic ischemic encephalopathy, central pontine myelinolysis, air embolization, acute uremia, acute graft failure, or multiple intracranial abscesses from aspergillosis. Immunosuppressive agents such as cyclosporin and tacrolimus can produce a marked neurotoxicity in which patients evolve from rambling speech and visual hallucinations into a stuporous stage that is associated with marked MRI abnormalities. The MRI scan often shows diffuse lesions in the white matter that are fully reversible with discontinuation of the medication. Both tacrolimus and cyclosporin are known offenders in this context; a new drug, sirolimus, has been found to be much less frequently associated with neurotoxicity (15).

Central nervous system infections are often serious and may be caused by opportunistic infections. Cytomegalovirus is the most common viral infection after organ transplantation but rarely results in cytomegalovirus encephalitis. In most of these patients, there is slow onset of abnormalities. Serious complications result from infection with *Cryptococcus neoformans* or *Aspergillus fumigatus* that leave not only multiple brain abscesses but also multiple intracranial hemorrhages. The outcome from these infections is very poor.

Sudden loss of consciousness may indicate a new onset of seizures in transplant recipients; the incidence in liver transplantation is recognized to be about 20%. An acute metabolic derangement—such as hypernatremia or hyperglycemia—may be implicated, but in a large proportion of patients, an intracranial hemorrhage or bacterial abscess is the causative factor. Seizures in cardiac transplantation occur in 10% to 15% of transplanted patients and most of the time are associated with an ischemic stroke.

FAILURE TO AWAKEN IN MULTISYSTEM TRAUMA

Trauma units commonly admit patients with not only multiple fractures but also with traumatic brain injury (TBI). The initial attention paid to the patient with TBI may be less in patients with severe shock due to blood loss and, since many of these patients require urgent exploration, they are taken to the operating room with an inadequate evaluation of their brain function. Multitrauma patients are at high risk of TBI, so close observation is important. In fact, these patients may need intracranial pressure monitoring, particularly if they do not localize to pain or open their eyes to pain, or have brainstem reflex abnormalities. Many traumatic parenchymal lesions are localized in the frontal and temporal lobes, and there is a significant risk of secondary deterioration from swelling. In the most severe circumstances, diffuse axonal injury is present, in which the injury itself causes swelling with multiple so-called *shear lesions* in the brain. These are typically in the frontal cortex, white matter, basal ganglia, thalamus, and internal capsule. Rarely, failure to awaken after trauma is due to the fat embolization syndrome; these patients often have axillary or subconjunctival petechiae, are markedly hypoxemic, and frequently have pulmonary edema. These patients have large bone fractures and often present 12 to 75 hours after the initial traumatic injury.

MANAGEMENT OF COMA

Initial management is determined by the presence or absence of increased intracranial pressure (ICP). Patients with a supratentorial mass lesion or diffuse edema are best treated with placement of an ICP monitor, followed by the brief (hours) use of hyperventilation, with a target of a $PaCO_2$ of 30 mm Hg (Table 147.5). Mannitol is a more effective method. Mannitol is typically administered at a dose of 1 gm/kg using a 20% solution, with the goal of increasing plasma osmolality to 310 mOsmols/L. Mannitol decreases brain volume by extracting water from brain tissue, which is generated through an osmotic gradient. It is an important initial intervention and can bridge the patient to neurosurgical evacuation. Hypertonic saline (7.5 or 23.4%) may be more effective (30 cc bolus) but requires infusion through a central line. Surgical evacuation of the mass is indicated before further brainstem compression occurs and all brainstem function is lost. The use of corticosteroids is highly questionable and may have a role only in patients who have edema surrounding a metastatic lesion or primary brain tumor. It has no role in closed-head injury, cerebral infarction, or cerebral abscess. Patients presenting in coma from an infectious disease such as acute bacterial meningitis need immediate IV infusion with antibiotics. The empiric treatment is discussed

TABLE 147.5

MANAGEMENT OF ACUTE SUPRATENTORIAL MASS WITH BRAIN SHIFT

STABILIZING MEASURES
Protect airway: Intubate
Correct hypoxemia with O_2 nasal cannulae, 3–4 L/min, or face mask
Elevate head to 30 degrees
Treat extreme agitation with lorazepam, 2 mg intravenously, or propofol, 0.3 mg/kg/h
Correct coagulopathy with fresh frozen plasma, vitamin K (if applicable), consider factor VIIa

SPECIFIC MEDICAL MEASURES
Hyperventilation: Increase respiratory rate to 20 breaths/min, aim for a $PaCO_2$ of 25–30 mm Hg
Mannitol 20%, 1 g/kg; if no effect, 2 g/kg; aim for a plasma osmolality of 310 mOsm/L
Dexamethasone, 100 mg intravenously (in tumors only)

SPECIFIC SURGICAL MEASURES
Evacuation of hematoma
Placement of drain in abscess
Decompressive craniotomy in brain swelling of one hemisphere

$PaCO_2$, arterial partial pressure of CO_2.

TABLE 147.6

MANAGEMENT OF ACUTE SUBTENTORIAL MASS OR BRAIN STEM LESION

STABILIZING MEASURES
Intubation and mechanical ventilation
Correct hypoxemia with 3 L of O_2/min
Flat body position (in acute basilar artery occlusion)

SPECIFIC MEDICAL MEASURES
Intra-arterial tpa (in basilar artery occlusion)
Mannitol 20%, 1 g/kg (in acute cerebellar mass)
Hyperventilation to $PaCO_2$ of 25–50 mm Hg (in acute cerebellar mass)

SPECIFIC SURGICAL MEASURES
Ventriculostomy
Suboccipital craniotomy

$PaCO_2$, arterial partial pressure of CO_2.

elsewhere but includes cefotaxime (2 g intravenously (IV) every 6 hours), vancomycin (2 g IV every 12 hours), and corticosteroids. If herpes simplex encephalitis is considered, acyclovir (10 mg/kg IV every 8 hours) is administered. In practice, in most patients with an infectious cause but no clear etiologic factors, both antibacterial and antiviral treatments are initiated until the spinal fluid examination reveals the true cause of infection.

The neurosurgeon's role in the treatment of comatose patients includes removal of the mass and placement of a ventriculostomy, particularly in patients with a subtentorial mass or brainstem lesion. A craniotomy to remove a bone flap can be performed to allow for swelling. This is an option in patients with massive middle cerebral artery infarction or those with a swollen traumatic contusion. In patients with a brain abscess in the setting of organ transplantation, a drain can be placed in the abscess. The management of patients in coma from a subtentorial lesion is noted in Table 147.6.

PROGNOSIS

Prognosis may be determined before hospital admission. Time without circulation and poor airway control may all play an important role in outcome; in TBI, outcome is related to prehospital hypoxemia. Many guidelines have been proposed to determine the futility of care (16–20). Certain neurologic conditions may be associated with no hope for good recovery. These include patients with myoclonus status epilepticus and brain swelling after cardiac arrest; patients with multiple territorial infarcts and brain swelling after cardiac surgery; occlusion of the basilar artery and coma; multiple intracranial hemorrhages associated with tissue plasminogen activator (tPA); pontine hemorrhages with hypertension and extension to the midbrain and thalamus; multiple hemorrhagic contusion and associated extradural hematomas; patients with gunshot wounds; and intraventricular extension. In any of these circumstances, outcome is poor and the level of care should be discussed with family members. Major reasons for consultation in the ICU are prognostication in a comatose patient after cardiopulmonary resuscitation. Recent guidelines have been proposed by the American Academy of Neurology (17). An evidence-based evaluation has determined that myoclonus status epilepticus, the absence of corneal and pupillary reflexes, and absent N20 potentials on somatosensory evoked potentials (SSEP) are important indicators of poor outcome (Fig. 147.2). MRI and CT scan are useful diagnostic tests but have not been investigated thoroughly to be used as prognosticating tools. Outcome in TBI is very difficult to assess with certainty in young individuals, who can make a substantial improvement despite neuroimaging indicators of severe brain damage.

BRAIN DEATH

Loss of all brain function is not frequently noted but may occur after traumatic brain injury, severe anoxic/ischemic injury, and cardiac resuscitation. Patients with catastrophic intracranial hemorrhages and massive hemispheric infarcts, cerebral edema, and fulminant hepatic failure are other major examples (8). Brain death is equivalent to death, where the time of its determination is the time of death. Definition of brain death implies documentation of loss of consciousness, no motor response to painful stimuli, no brainstem reflexes, and apnea. A structural lesion on CT scan is commonly found.

The diagnosis of brain death is made in the following steps:

1. First, the cause has to be identified, and coma has to be irreversible.
2. Major confounding factors have to be excluded, and there should be no reversible medical illness.
3. The core temperature should be at least 32°C, and no confounding pharmaceutical agents should have been administered or lingering on.

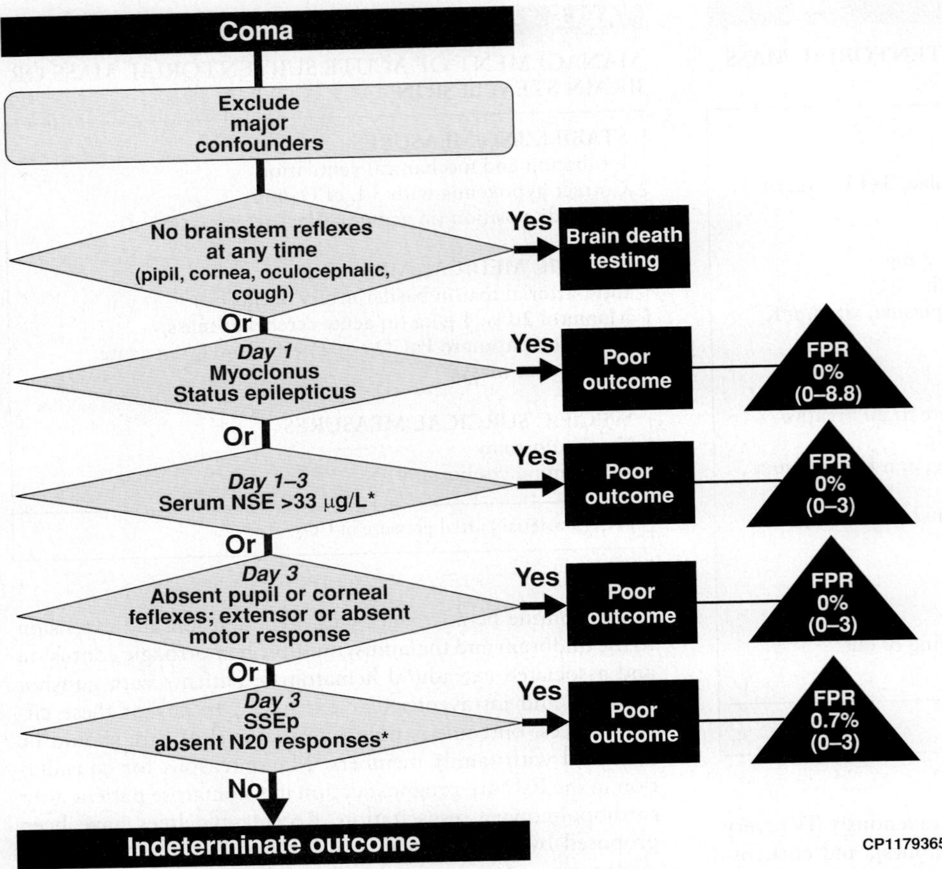

FIGURE 147.2. Algorithm for determination of prognosis of coma after cardiopulmonary resuscitation. FPR, false positive ratio; NSE, neuron-specific enolase; SSEP, somatosensory evoked potentials. *These laboratory tests may not be available on a timely basis.

4. On examination, there is no motor response to pain applied to the face and limbs. Any movement that is seen must be attributable only to a spinal cord response.
5. There should be absent pupil response, absent cold caloric oculovestibular response, absent corneal reflex, absent cough to bronchial suctioning, and
6. Apnea with a $PaCO_2$ of 60 mm Hg—or a 20 mm Hg increase from pretest baseline. The apnea test is done under controlled circumstances using the oxygen diffusion method.

If a patient fulfills all these criteria, brain death can be diagnosed. It is useful to have two examinations 6 hours apart, although the American Academy of Neurology considers this optional. In younger children, electrophysiologic tests are required.

WITHDRAWAL OF CARE

In the discussion of withdrawal of care, it is important to have a neurologist involved to explain to the family members the findings and how they play a role in their assessment. Palliative care includes use of lorazepam and phosphenytoin to prevent seizures but also involves the use of propofol to reduce myoclonus status epilepticus, which can be a dreadful sight to family members. Neurologic complications in critically ill patients are often major setbacks, certainly when the patient has lapsed into coma. Failure to awaken after 1 week in a structural coma is often associated with a high mortality rate due to withdrawal of support, either instigated by directives of the patient or by family members.

References

1. Young GB, Pigott SE. Neurobiological basis of consciousness. *Arch Neuro.* 1999;56:153–157.
2. Wÿdicks EFM. The Comatose Patient. Oxford, England: Oxford University Press; 2008.
3. van der Mast RC, Roest FH. Delirium after cardiac surgery: a critical review. *J Psychosom Res.* 1996;41:13–30.
4. Dyer CB, Ashton CM, Teasdale TA. Postoperative delirium. A review of 80 primary data-collection studies. *Arch Intern Med.* 1995;155:461–465.
5. Brown TM. Drug-induced delirium. *Semin Clin Neuropsychiatry.* 2000;5: 113–124.
6. O'Keeffe ST, Ni Chonchubhair A. Postoperative delirium in the elderly. *Br J Anaesth.* 2004;73:673–687.
7. Wÿdicks EFM, Crawford RE. Clinical diagnosis of prolonged states of impaired consciousness in adults. *Mayo Clinic Proceedings.* 2005;80:1037–1045.
8. Wijdicks EFM. The diagnosis of brain death. *N Engl J Med.* 2001;344:1215.
9. Smith E, Delargy M. Locked-in syndrome. *BMJ.* 2005;330:406–409.
10. Wijdicks EF, Bamlet WR, Maramattom BV, et al. Validation of a new coma scale: The FOUR score. *Ann Neurol.* 2005;58(4):585–93.
11. Wijdicks EFM. *Neurologic Complications of Critical Illness.* Contemporary Neurology Series 64. 2nd ed. Oxford, England: Oxford University Press; 2002.
12. Wijdicks EF. Neurologic complications in critically ill patients. *Anesth Analg.* 1996;83(2):411–419.
13. Kaplan PW. The EEG in metabolic encephalopathy and coma. *J Clin Neurophysiol.* 2004;21:307–318.
14. Gootjes EC, Wijdicks EF, McClelland RL. Postoperative stupor and coma. *Mayo Clin Proc.* 2005;80(3):350–354.
15. Wijdicks EF. Neurotoxicity of immunosuppressive drugs. *Liver Transpl.* 2001;7(11):937–942.
16. Wijdicks EF, Rabinstein AA. Absolutely no hope? Some ambiguity of

futility of care in devastating acute stroke. *Crit Care Med.* 2004;32(11): 2332–2342.
17. Wijdicks EF, Hijdra A, Young GB, et al; Quality Standards Subcommittee of the American Academy of Neurology. Practice parameter: prediction of outcome in comatose survivors after cardiopulmonary resuscitation (an evidence-based review): report of the Quality Standards Subcommittee of the American Academy of Neurology. *Neurology.* 2006;67(2):203–210.
18. Bates D. The prognosis of medical coma. *J Neurol Neurosurg Psychiatry.* 2001;71(Suppl 1):i20–i23.
19. Bateman DE. Neurological assessment of coma. *J Neurol Neurosurg Psychiatry.* 2001;71(Suppl 1):i13–i17.
20. Chi JH, Knudson MM, Vassar MJ, et al. Prehospital hypoxia affects outcome in patients with traumatic brain injury: a prospective multicenter trial. *J Trauma.* 2006;61(5):1134–1141.

CHAPTER 148 ■ SEIZURES AND STATUS EPILEPTICUS

GEORGES A. GHACIBEH

Status epilepticus (SE) is defined as continuous or rapidly repeating seizures, and should be viewed as a life-threatening medical and neurologic emergency requiring prompt therapeutic intervention. The frequency of SE in the United States is estimated at 152,000 cases per year, with roughly 55,000 related deaths annually. SE can be the presenting sign of epilepsy in up to 30% of patients. Therefore, it is essential for all health care providers to be able to identify and treat patients with SE adequately.

DEFINITIONS AND CLASSIFICATIONS

Epileptic Seizure

According to the International League Against Epilepsy (ILAE), an *epileptic seizure* is defined as a transient occurrence of signs and/or symptoms due to abnormally excessive or synchronous neuronal activity in the brain (1). There are two components in this definition: The first component is the occurrence of clinical signs and symptoms, which are usually neurologic, and the second component is the presence of abnormal neuronal activity. Therefore, classification schemes of seizures can follow either of these two components. Seizures can be classified based on either their semiology or the pattern of neuronal activity. Neuronal activity is measured as neurophysiologic electrical signals seen as tracings on an electroencephalogram (EEG).

Seizures are divided into two types, depending on whether the abnormal neuronal activity starts in a specific region of the brain or diffusely in the entire brain. A seizure is called *focal* (previously called partial) when the electrical activity starts in a specific region of the brain. This can be a well-defined focus, a large brain region, or even an entire hemisphere. A seizure is called *generalized* when the electrical activity starts diffusely, involving the entire brain at onset. It is important to note that a seizure that starts focally can spread to involve the entire brain. In this case, the seizure is called *secondarily generalized.*

Classification based on semiology is more complicated due to the wide variety of clinical features. Although the division of seizures into focal and generalized does not take into account the clinical semiology, specific clinical features occur in each seizure type.

There are six distinct types of generalized seizures: Tonic-clonic (grand mal), tonic, clonic, atonic, myoclonic, and absence (petit mal). The clinical features of focal epilepsy are more varied, depending on the primary function of the brain region where the abnormal electrical activity occurs. For example, if the seizure focus is in the motor cortex, repeated contractions are expected to occur. The older classification divided focal seizures into three types, depending on the degree of impairment in consciousness. Seizures are considered *simple partial* if consciousness is not impaired; *complex partial* if consciousness is impaired; and secondarily generalized when a secondary generalized tonic-clonic seizure occurs after a focal onset. The distinction between simple partial and complex partial is sometimes difficult, especially when language remains intact. For this reason, the new classification proposed by the ILAE removed simple partial and complex partial from the focal seizure subtype. However, this classification remains widely used and can be clinically useful.

Epilepsy

According to the ILAE, epilepsy is a disorder of the brain characterized by an enduring predisposition to generate epileptic seizures and by the neurobiologic, cognitive, psychological, and social consequences of this condition. The definition of epilepsy requires the occurrence of at least one epileptic seizure (1). Several epileptic syndromes have been proposed by the ILAE based on genetic, etiologic, and clinical features. However, for practical reasons, epileptic disorders can be best classified and understood depending on the type of seizures that occur. Focal epilepsy (previously called partial epilepsy) is a disorder characterized by the occurrence of focal seizures, and generalized epilepsy is a disorder characterized by the occurrence of generalized seizures. The terms primary and secondary are frequently used to distinguish between idiopathic syndromes (primary) and syndromes with a known cause (secondary). Primary generalized epilepsy (PGE) refers to a set of epilepsy syndromes with different combinations of generalized seizures that have, in general, a good prognosis. Symptomatic (or secondary) generalized epilepsy refers to a set of heterogeneous disorders characterized by severe intractable epilepsy and several seizure types, and are associated with significant mental retardation and poor prognosis. Lennox-Gastaut syndrome is a common type of secondary, generalized epilepsy.

Status Epilepticus

Status epilepticus is defined as recurrent epileptic seizure activity lacking full recovery of neurologic function between seizures, or continuous clinical and/or electrical seizure activity that lasts 30 minutes or longer, whether or not consciousness is impaired (2). This original definition has been changed several times over the years, and the duration of continuous seizure activity that is accepted as SE has gradually decreased due to several factors. Research with animals shows that repetitive seizures become self-sustaining and resistant to medical treatment within 15 to 30 minutes (3,4). In addition, irreversible neuronal injury and death are likely to occur with prolonged seizure activity (5). Furthermore, it is extremely important to emphasize early aggressive treatment. Therefore, an operational definition was introduced by several experts, suggesting that 5 minutes of continuous seizure activity should be enough to define SE (6,7). This new definition has become widely accepted; however, the choice of 5 minutes is empirical and is dictated by the need to treat early and not wait until seizure activity becomes refractory to treatment and/or neuronal injury has occurred. The problem is that not all patients who have continuous seizures for 5 minutes are in established SE. In one study (8), more than 40% of the seizures lasting from 10 to 29 minutes stopped spontaneously without treatment, and overall mortality was 2.6% versus 19% for status epilepticus lasting over 30 minutes. For this reason, the term, *impending status epilepticus* (9), was recently introduced to describe those patients who have continuous seizure activity for at least 5 minutes but less than 30 minutes. The 5-minute cut-off is in agreement with the operational definition of status, and is based in part on the fact that the great majority of secondarily generalized tonic-clonic seizures terminate spontaneously after approximately 1 minute (10). However, this definition also takes into account the fact that there is a significant difference in terms of natural progression, response to treatment, and mortality between seizures lasting more than 30 minutes and those lasting less than 30 minutes (8,11,12). The term, *established status epilepticus*, was therefore used to describe seizures lasting more than 30 minutes (9). While this definition can be useful both in clinical practice and in clinical trials, it is important to remember that the transition from impending to established SE is a continuum.

Classification of status epilepticus follows the same scheme as the classification of seizures and, theoretically, any seizure can become SE if it does not terminate spontaneously. According to the ILAE, SE is divided into generalized and focal, depending on the mode of onset of the abnormal neuronal activity. However, it is important to note that a focal seizure can evolve either into focal or into generalized SE, depending on whether there is progression into secondary generalization.

The most commonly used classification scheme divides SE into convulsive, nonconvulsive, and subtle, depending on the presence or absence of motor manifestations. Nonconvulsive status epilepticus (NCSE) manifests most commonly with impairment of consciousness of varying degrees, ranging from mild confusion to deep coma. The concept of subtle status epilepticus was introduced (13) to emphasize the point that prolonged convulsive SE changes in character with time, and the motor manifestations become less evident. Patients usually remain unconscious and have subtle motor manifestations, such as nystagmus, eyelid twitching, and finger twitching. However, the prognostic and therapeutic implications remain very similar to the convulsive state. Although this classification is somewhat simplistic and does not take into account the complexities of clinical and electrographic manifestations of various types of SE, it is very practical and useful in the clinical setting. In general, uncontrolled convulsive status is considered a life-threatening condition with a high morbidity rate, requiring prompt and aggressive treatment.

EPIDEMIOLOGY

The incidence of status epilepticus ranges from 10 to 41 per 100,000 individuals per year in various studies (14–17). All studies showed a significantly higher incidence in the elderly, especially after 60 years of age, raising a concern that the overall incidence may rise as the population ages. In addition, only 40% to 50% of patients presenting with first-time SE have a previous diagnosis of epilepsy (15,16). NCSE represents about 30% to 40% of all cases of SE, with an estimated incidence of 5 to 9 per 100,000 individuals per year. However, the true incidence of NCSE may be underestimated. In fact, various studies reported an incidence of NCSE in patients in the intensive care unit (ICU) with altered mental status ranging from 8% to 37% (18–22). Even when all patients with clinical evidence or history of seizures were excluded, the incidence of NCSE was 8% (18); in patients with intracerebral hemorrhage, the incidence rises to 28% (21). Diagnosis requires clinical suspicion and long-term EEG monitoring, which is not routinely performed on critically ill patients in many institutions.

Mortality from SE, estimated in most studies at 10% to 20%, rises significantly with age (23), reaching 38% in elderly people (14). One of the primary predictors of poor outcome is prolonged seizure. When seizure activity lasts more than 1 hour, mortality reaches 32% compared to 2.7% with shorter seizures (23,24). Mortality from NCSE seems to be higher, averaging 50% (25).

ETIOLOGY

In about 30% of cases, status epilepticus occurs in patients with chronic epilepsy and is due to withdrawal, or low blood concentrations, of antiepileptic drugs (9,23,26). Hence, in the majority of cases, SE occurs in patients with no history of epilepsy and may be due to a variety of causes, most commonly intracranial pathology, such as ischemic stroke, intracerebral and subarachnoid hemorrhage, central nervous system (CNS) infections, head trauma, and brain tumors. Other etiologies include cardiac arrest and hypoxic/anoxic brain injury, alcohol withdrawal, metabolic disturbances, and toxic causes. In some patients, no cause can be identified (9,26).

Both acute and chronic intracranial pathology can cause seizures. Seizures and SE may actually be the presenting signs of several neurologic conditions. This is true for intracranial hemorrhage, including subarachnoid and intracerebral hemorrhage, acute embolic stroke, and brain tumors. Approximately 50% of patients with brain tumors experience seizures (27,28), and a seizure is the presenting sign of a tumor in 23% of cases (29). Seizures can also be the presenting sign of an acute stroke (30) and frequently occur in the first 2 weeks after a stroke. It is estimated that seizures occur in up to 6% of patients with ischemic stroke, up to 18% of patients with intracerebral hemorrhage, and up to 26% of patients with subarachnoid hemorrhage (30,31). Up to 2.8% of patients with stroke go into SE either at presentation or within 2 weeks of their stroke (32). The risk of chronic epilepsy is 17 times higher after an ischemic stroke than the general population (33), and the risk of having a seizure or developing chronic epilepsy after any type of stroke is 11.5% (34). In subarachnoid hemorrhage, generalized tonic-clonic seizures have been reported in up to 26% of patients at the time of onset or shortly after onset (31,35), and nonconvulsive status epilepticus occurred in 8% of patients who survived the first 48 hours and had an unexplained decline in their level of consciousness (36).

Metabolic disturbances that may cause seizures include hyponatremia, hypoglycemia, hypocalcemia, hypomagnesemia, uremia, hepatic encephalopathy, and hyperosmolar states (26). However, it is important to note that metabolic encephalopathies can frequently cause EEG abnormalities that can be difficult to distinguish from subtle seizure activity, such as high-amplitude slowing and triphasic waves. Therefore, extra care should be taken to avoid both over- and underdiagnosing patients as having SE when they have a clear metabolic dysfunction. Response to treatment may be critical in these situations.

Several drugs can cause seizures at toxic levels, including some analgesics such as meperidine, propoxyphene, and tramadol; some psychiatric medications such as bupropion, tricyclic antidepressants, lithium, olanzapine, selective serotonin reuptake inhibitors (SSRIs), venlafaxine, and clozapine; in addition to other drugs such as theophylline, isoniazid, lidocaine, phenothiazines, and some antibiotics such as imipenem/cilastatin, penicillins, and ciprofloxacin. Furthermore, several commonly abused drugs can cause seizures, most notably cocaine, amphetamines, phencyclidine, and γ-hydroxybutyric acid (37,38).

PATHOPHYSIOLOGY AND MECHANISMS

The great majority of seizures stop spontaneously in less than 2 minutes (39). This is most likely due to inhibitory mechanisms that attempt to deter any excessive, abnormal neuronal activity. This inhibition is evident on the EEG as postictal slowing and attenuation. It is believed that status epilepticus occurs when inhibitory mechanisms fail, resulting in a self-sustaining and prolonged seizure activity; the exact cause of this failure is not well understood. A large number of elegant experiments done on animal models of SE tried to shed some light on the underlying mechanisms causing SE. Review of these studies is beyond the scope of this chapter; however, two points are worth discussing, since they have important implications on treatment strategy.

Self-sustaining status can be easily triggered in animal models using electrical stimulation (40). However, this can be blocked by many drugs that increase inhibition or reduce excitation only if administered early, prior to the development of a self-sustained seizure (41). In contrast, once a self-sustaining state is established, it becomes more difficult to stop the seizure (42), and much higher dosages of inhibitory drugs are required, leading to significant toxicity, including cardiovascular depression (43). Another important feature of self-sustaining status is the progressive development of resistance to antiepileptic drugs. The anticonvulsant potency of benzodiazepines can decrease by 20 times within 30 minutes of self-sustaining status epilepticus (44). The same phenomenon was observed with other anticonvulsants, such as phenytoin; however, the decline in potency was slower (12).

Pathophysiologically, SE produces a number of changes, which can be divided into neurologic and systemic. Primary neurologic complications occur in both convulsive and nonconvulsive status, and are time dependent and probably preventable with early termination of the seizure. In animal models of SE, neuronal injury occurs even in the absence of convulsive activity (45,46), and cell death is thought to result from excessive neuronal firing through excitotoxic mechanisms (47). It is impossible to replicate these experiments in human beings; however, there is widespread belief—supported by some anecdotal evidence—that neuronal injury and death occur after prolonged seizures. For example, brain damage and decreased hippocampal neuronal density are often seen in patients who die from status epilepticus (48,49). Furthermore, cerebral edema and chronic brain atrophy seen on neuroimaging studies have been reported after status epilepticus (50–53).

Systemic complications of prolonged seizures are seen primarily in convulsive SE, and are due to autonomic hyperactivity and excessive muscle activity. Therefore, systemic complications can potentially be prevented, or minimized, with early termination of seizure activity or induction of muscle paralysis and artificial ventilation (46). Pathophysiologic manifestations include increased systemic blood pressure, tachycardia, and cardiac arrhythmias; increased pulmonary blood pressure; increase in cerebral blood flow; elevation of body temperature; increased peripheral white cell count; transient pleocytosis in the spinal fluid; and a marked metabolic acidosis (4,45,54). Epinephrine levels are elevated and reach the arrhythmogenic range; these may play a role in sudden death (54). With prolonged status—defined as lasting 30 minutes or more, systemic blood pressure and cerebral blood flow can drop significantly (45). Additionally, blood glucose is initially elevated in response to excessive adrenergic stimulation. However, after 30 minutes of SE, hypoglycemia may occur (45). Both hypoglycemia and decreased cerebral blood flow contribute to further neuronal injury (55). Excessive muscle contraction often causes severe metabolic acidosis, breakdown of muscle tissue, and hyperkalemia (4,45,46). Arterial pH has been reported to fall below 7.0 (56) and contribute, along with hyperkalemia, to cardiac arrhythmias. Rhabdomyolysis and myoglobinuria can also occur and may lead to acute renal failure (57).

EVALUATION

Clinical Presentation

Obtaining a focused history and examination may be very helpful for diagnosis and management (Table 148.1). Convulsive and nonconvulsive SE have very different clinical presentations. Convulsive SE frequently occurs outside the hospital, and management may start in the ambulance before patients arrive to the emergency room. The diagnosis is usually evident, unless there is a strong clinical suspicion of psychogenic nonepileptic seizure (PNES). Convulsive SE usually starts as a focal seizure with secondary generalization. Rarely, primary generalized seizures evolve into SE. The generalized convulsion either becomes continuous, or stops and recurs before the patient regains full consciousness. In either case, the tonic-clonic activity changes in character with time and often patients go into a continuous clonic phase where clonic activity persists and gradually slows down and becomes more subtle. With time, the only persistent motor activity may consist of small-amplitude twitching of the face, hands, or feet or nystagmoid jerking of the eyes (13,58). Sometimes the motor activity subsides completely, and patients remain stuporous or comatose. In this case, patients evolve from convulsive to nonconvulsive SE (20).

By the time patients arrive to the emergency room, they may already be in established SE. If there is strong clinical suspicion of PNES, an EEG is essential to confirm the diagnosis. The average duration of a PNES is approximately 5 minutes (59), and therefore, it is unlikely that a PNES could mimic convulsive status. However, patients with PNES may have repeated seizures and remain unresponsive between them, creating a diagnostic challenge. Although rare, one should always keep in mind the possibility of PNES in a patient presenting with SE. However, treatment should not be delayed, unless the diagnosis of PNES is certain.

Nonconvulsive SE has a different clinical presentation. It may occur either outside the hospital or, frequently, in the hospital, in patients already admitted for other reasons such as stroke, intracranial hemorrhage, brain tumors, or metabolic disturbances. As mentioned earlier, NCSE may also occur in partially treated convulsive SE, when the convulsive activity is controlled (20). In either case, the common clinical presentation is that of decline in mental status that cannot be completely explained by other causes. Frequently, the underlying etiology may account in part for the impairment in consciousness; however, patients frequently have an unexplained decline of mental status after a period of clinical improvement. Therefore, clinical suspicion should be strong, and evaluation for NCSE should be undertaken in any patient with unexplained impairment in mental status.

Electroencephalogram

The EEG is the only diagnostic tool that can confirm or refute the diagnosis of SE. In convulsive status, an EEG may not be necessary initially, unless PNES needs to be excluded. However, if convulsive activity stops and patients do not recover their baseline level of consciousness, evaluation with an EEG is important to exclude the continuous presence of seizure activity. In NCSE, the EEG is essential. However, a single routine EEG of 20 minutes' duration may not be adequate and may only capture seizure activity in 20% of cases. A longer EEG recording of at least 1 hour increases the sensitivity to 50%. More prolonged EEG monitoring is recommended if shorter-duration EEGs are nondiagnostic. Long-term EEG monitoring of 24 to 48 hours can increase the diagnostic accuracy to over 90% (22). Several EEG patterns have been described during status epilepticus, reflecting probably different stages of brain activity (13). In addition, several patterns have been described in NCSE. Discussion of these different EEG patterns is beyond the scope of this chapter; however, an important issue needs to be emphasized. Some EEG patterns can be difficult to distinguish from epileptiform activity, such as diffuse triphasic waves in metabolic encephalopathies (Fig. 148.1) and breach rhythms after a craniotomy (Fig. 148.2). These patterns can be very deceiving and can often be misinterpreted as epileptiform. Therefore, it is very important for the EEG to be interpreted by an experienced electroencephalographer. Response to intravenous benzodiazepines has been suggested as a means to distinguish these rhythms from true epileptiform activity. Relying on changes in EEG activity alone in these cases can be dangerous, since intravenous benzodiazepines usually cause diffuse slowing of the EEG signal and may attenuate patterns of activity that are not necessarily epileptiform. On the other hand, if a clear clinical response is observed after the administration of intravenous benzodiazepines (i.e., improved level of consciousness), the diagnosis of seizure is therefore more evident, since patients with metabolic dysfunction are likely to become more drowsy if given sedatives. Newer techniques of quantitative EEG analysis, such as compressed spectral arrays, are now offered by many manufacturers and can be helpful in online monitoring. Experienced ICU nursing staff can be trained to recognize certain patterns that may indicate the occurrence of a nonconvulsive seizure. Review of the raw EEG data by

TABLE 148.1

HISTORY AND PHYSICAL EXAMINATION

	Comment
History of epilepsy	Current antiepileptic drugs, missed doses, compliance
List of current medications	Toxic ingestion of medications or other agents
History of psychiatric illness	Suicidal ideations or attempts
Trauma	Evidence of scalp laceration and bruises
Focal neurologic signs	May be difficult to assess; look for obvious signs
Signs of medical illness	Hepatic or renal disease, infection
Signs of substance abuse	Alcohol withdrawal, cocaine intoxication

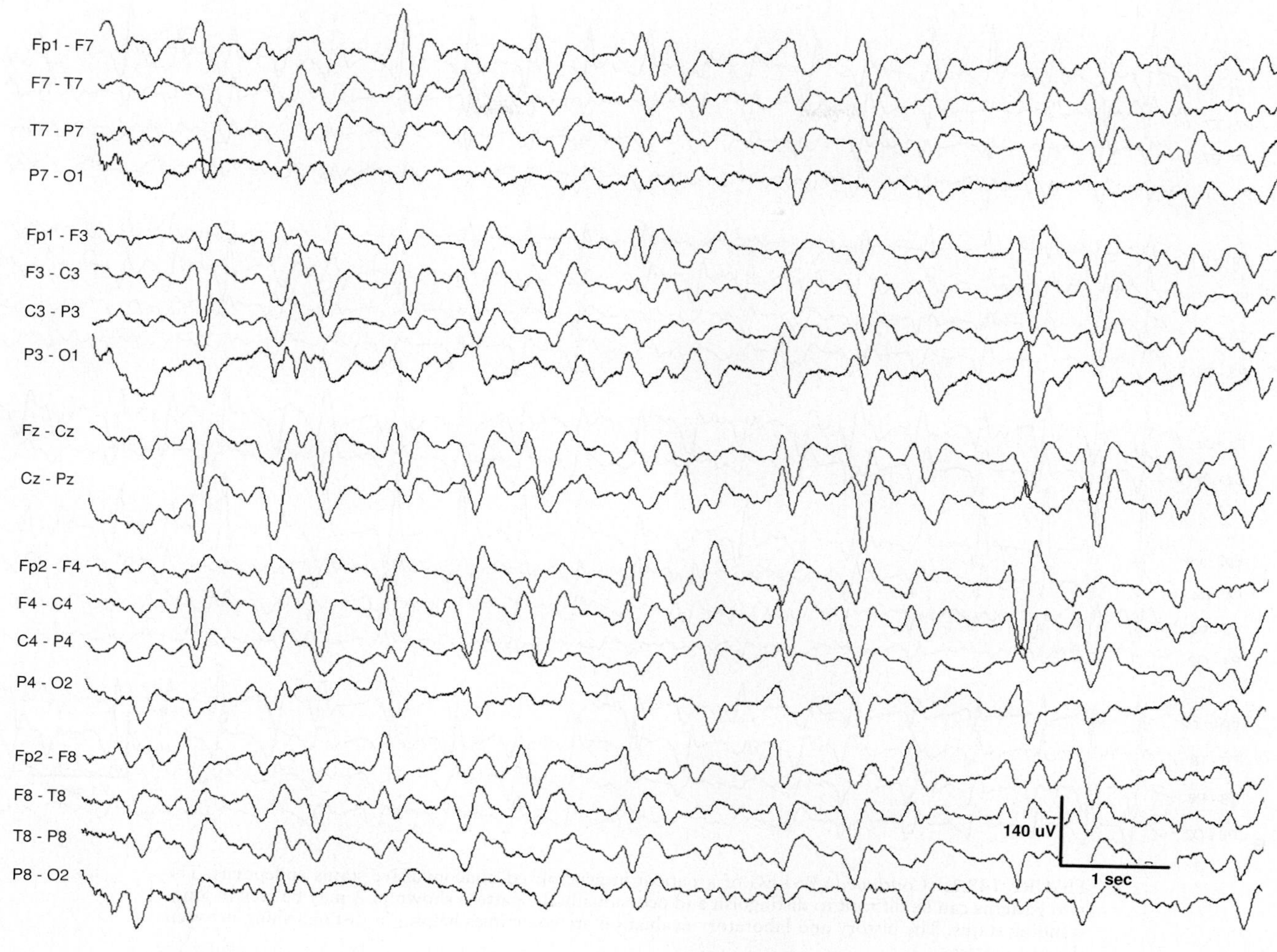

FIGURE 148.1. Generalized status versus generalized slowing with triphasic waves. **A:** Electroencephalogram (EEG) of a patient in hepatic encephalopathy showing diffuse background slowing and prominent triphasic waves. (*Continued*)

the electroencephalographer can then confirm the presence of seizure activity.

Neuroimaging

Neuroimaging studies are always recommended to assess for the presence of intracranial pathology. Even in patients with known pathologies, such as tumors or stroke, repeat imaging is recommended to exclude progression or complications of the underlying disease. For example, a stable tumor can become necrotic or hemorrhagic, or a stable acute or subacute infarct can turn hemorrhagic. Unenhanced computed tomography (CT) of the brain is adequate in the acute setting; however, magnetic resonance imaging (MRI) is much more sensitive and may detect lesions not seen on CT.

Laboratory Evaluation

Full laboratory evaluation is always recommended (Table 148.2), including blood cell count, renal function, liver function, electrolytes, calcium, magnesium, and antiepileptic drug levels. Toxicology should be performed when there is a clinical suspicion of intoxication or substance abuse. This is especially important in patients with a psychiatric illness at risk of suicide and in children who may have access to adult medications. Lumbar puncture is indicated if there is any consideration of an infectious etiology. Also, a lumbar puncture should be considered when subarachnoid hemorrhage, not seen on CT scan, is suspected. However, in the presence of any sign of intracranial hypertension, lumbar puncture should be avoided, since it may increase the risk of transtentorial herniation. It is important to note that patients with convulsive SE often exhibit clinical features suggestive of meningitis, such as elevated temperatures, increased peripheral white blood cell counts, and pleocytosis in the cerebrospinal fluid (54). These abnormalities have been reported in up to 18% of patients with convulsive status, without any evidence of infection (54), and are thought to result from breakdown of the blood–brain barrier. Usually, the total white blood cell count in the cerebrospinal fluid (CSF) remains under 100 and glucose level remains normal. Treatment with antimicrobials should be initiated if there is clinical suspicion for a CNS infection.

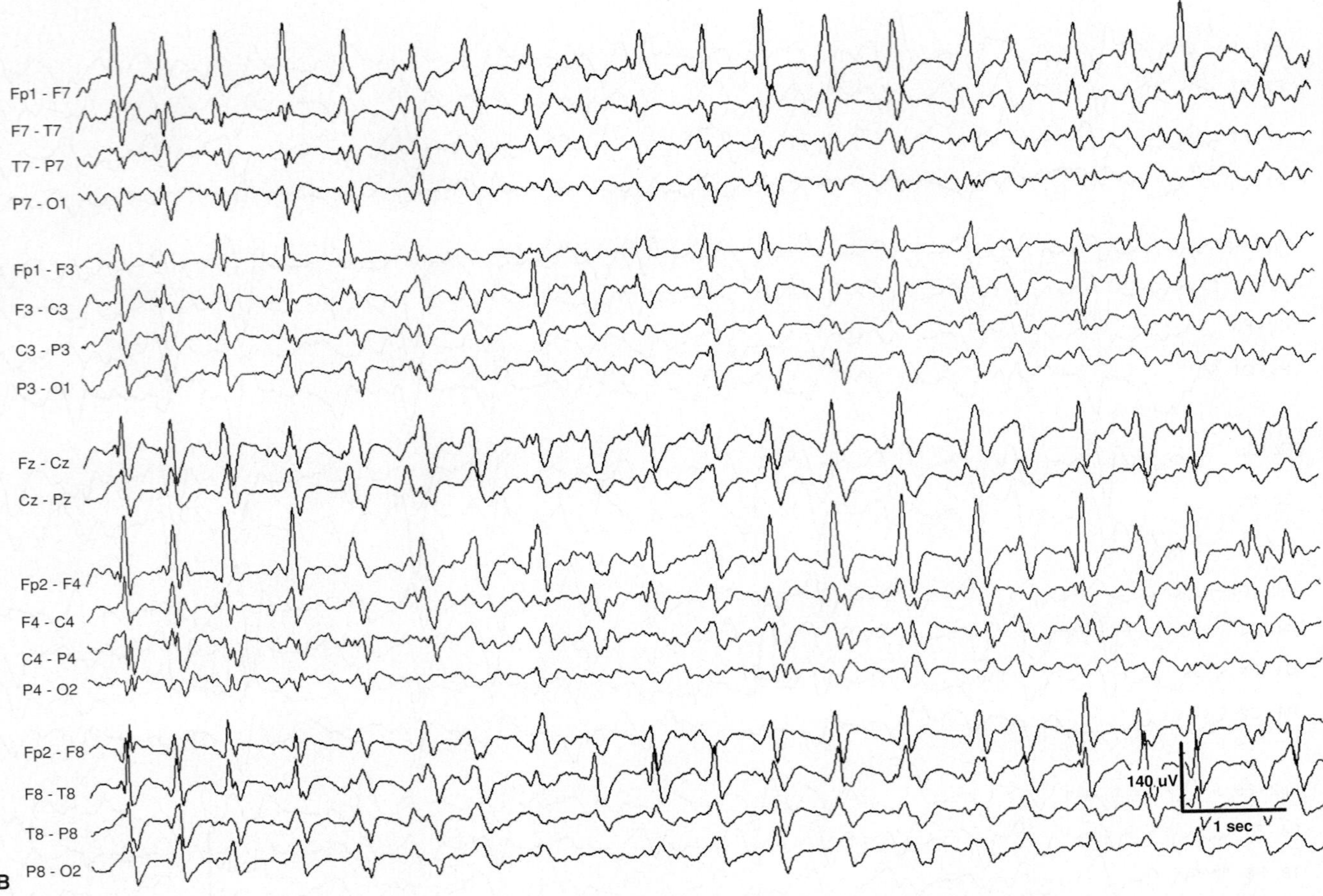

FIGURE 148.1. (*Continued*) B: EEG of a patient in generalized nonconvulsive status epilepticus. The two patterns can be difficult to distinguish and occasionally the pattern shown in A may be seen in long-standing status. The history and laboratory evaluation are sometimes helpful in distinguishing between the two patterns.

TREATMENT

Seizures and Epilepsy

Treatment with antiepileptic drugs (AEDs) is not recommended after a single unprovoked seizure (60); however, after a second unprovoked seizure, the likelihood of recurrent seizures is high, and treatment is recommended (60). Treatment with AEDs is successful and prevents the occurrence of seizures in about 70% of patients (61). Patients who continue to have breakthrough seizures despite adequate treatment with AEDs are believed to have medically refractory epilepsy. Other treatment options are then considered, including vagus nerve stimulation and epilepsy surgery (62). In addition, newer experimental approaches are currently under investigation. There are several antiepileptic drugs available. The choice of AED depends on several factors, including the type of epilepsy, side effect profile, comorbid conditions, drug interactions, previous treatment, cost, approved Food and Drug Administration (FDA) indications, and guidelines published by national and international societies (63–66). In the acute setting, treatment with intravenous benzodiazepine is indicated only if the seizure lasts more than 5 minutes, fulfilling the definition of impending status epilepticus.

Convulsive Status Epilepticus

Treatment Principles

Status epilepticus is a medical emergency and should be dealt with as such. Therapies are aimed at early termination of seizure activity, identification and correction of the cause, prevention of seizure recurrence, and treatment of pathophysiologic complications. There is ample evidence that delayed treatment leads to poor outcome (23,67). In addition, there is a time-dependent loss of efficacy of anticonvulsant medications (12,44). Therefore, early initiation of aggressive treatment is essential in the management of SE. It is highly recommended that every emergency department and intensive care unit have a well-defined and clear treatment protocol. This helps avoid many of the pitfalls leading to delayed and insufficient treatment of status (68).

Prehospital Management

In many cases, patients with convulsive SE are brought into the emergency room by ambulance, making prehospital treatment possible. Initiation of treatment in the ambulance is highly recommended, when possible, given the importance of early intervention. Both rectal diazepam (69,70) and intravenous diazepam and lorazepam (71) can be safely and effectively

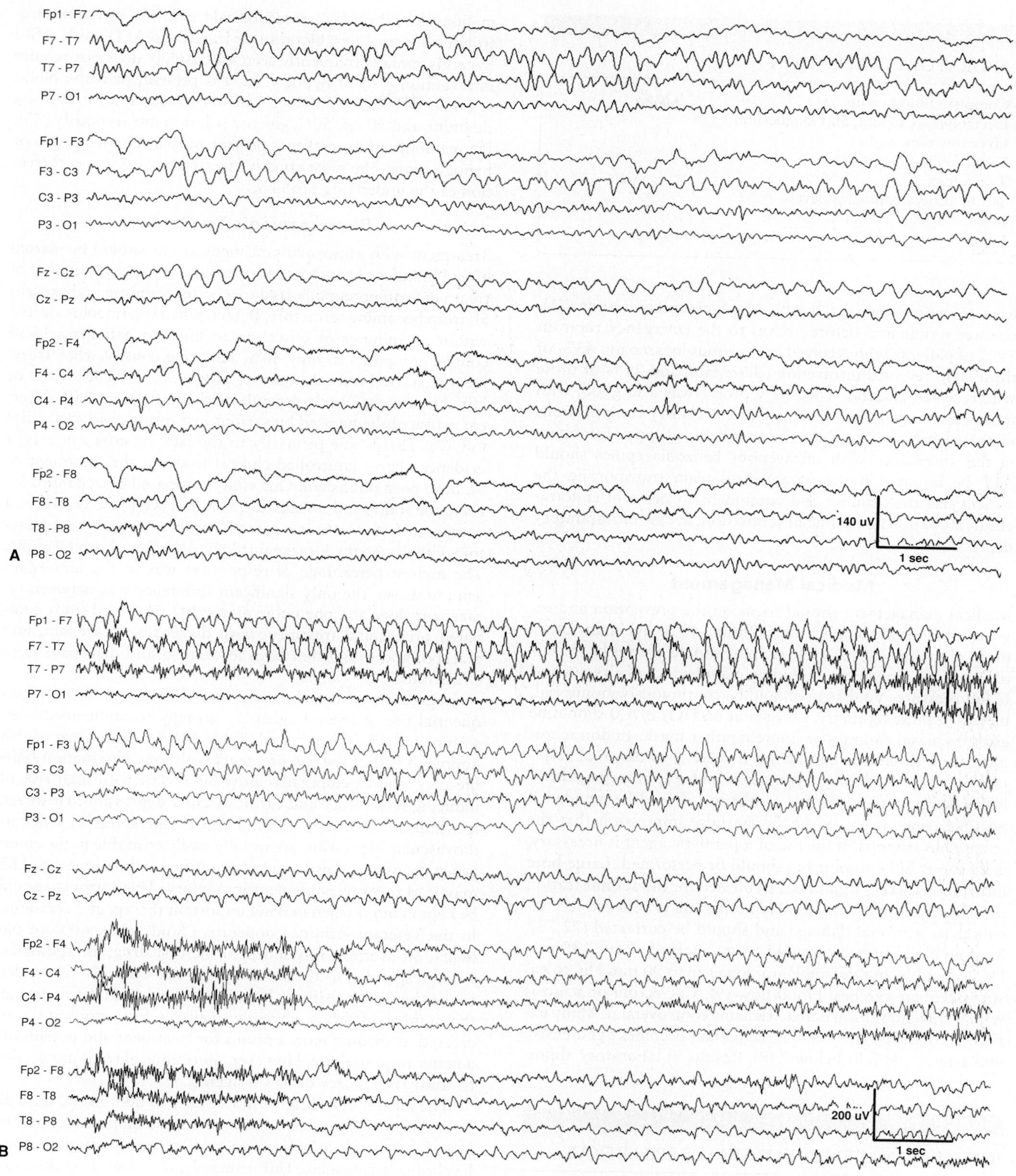

FIGURE 148.2. Focal status versus focal slowing and breach rhythm. A: Electroencephalogram (EEG) of a patient with a history of left temporal benign tumor, surgically resected several years ago. The high-amplitude slowing seen focally from the left temporal and frontal regions represents a breach rhythm, believed to result from the loss of resistance to electrical flow after a craniotomy. B: EEG of a patient having a left temporal lobe seizure. Note the presence of well-organized rhythmic activity compared to A, where the rhythmic slowing is more random and intermittent.

TABLE 148.2

LABORATORY EVALUATION

Complete blood count
Electrolytes, calcium, and magnesium
Liver function studies
Renal function studies
Toxicology
Serum antiepileptic drug levels
Brain imaging as soon as possible
Lumbar puncture if strong suspicion of meningitis

used. In one randomized, double-blind, prospective study (71), seizures terminated before arrival to the emergency room in 59% of patients who received intravenous lorazepam, 43% of those who received intravenous diazepam, and 21% of those who received placebo. The safety profile was also good, with more patients having respiratory or circulatory complications in the placebo group than the treatment groups. Treatment in the ambulance with intravenous benzodiazepines should only be initiated if the paramedical team transporting the patient has the training and equipment to perform endotracheal intubation and artificial ventilation, in case of respiratory depression.

Medical Management

Medical management should focus on the prevention and reversal of medical complications (Table 148.3). As in any other medical emergency, basic life support should always be the initial step in management, including maintenance of airways and blood pressure. Vital signs should be continuously monitored, including pulse oximetry. Oxygen at an FiO_2 of 1.0 should be given by nasal cannula or nonrebreather mask. Endotracheal intubation should be considered if there is evidence of respiratory failure, including hypoxemia and respiratory acidosis. Pharmacologic paralysis for intubation should be avoided if possible, since it can result in the false impression that the seizure has stopped. If the use of a paralytic agent is necessary, continuous EEG monitoring should be performed. Large-bore intravenous access should be established for the administration of intravenous medications. Hyperthermia is believed to contribute to neuronal damage and should be corrected (72,73). Systolic blood pressure should be maintained above 120 mm Hg if possible, but definitely not lower than 90 mm Hg, to ensure adequate cerebral blood flow (9). Correction of acidosis with intravenous bicarbonate remains controversial. Many experts recommend treatment if the patient becomes hypotensive and arterial pH falls below 7 (9). Results of laboratory abnormalities should guide further medical treatment, including electrolyte abnormalities, blood sugar levels, and AED levels. Mild hyperglycemia is frequently seen and usually does not require intervention (74). If hypoglycemia is present, or if the blood sugar level is not available, patients should receive 100 mg thiamine and 50 mL 50% glucose solution intravenously (75). If a metabolic abnormality is present, such as hyponatremia or hypoglycemia, the most effective treatment of status is correction of the underlying problem.

TABLE 148.3

INITIAL MANAGEMENT OF STATUS EPILEPTICUS

1. ABC	Airways, vital signs, pulse oximetry, and cardiac rhythm
2. Blood glucose	Intravenous infusion of thiamine 100 mg and 50 mL of glucose 50%
3. Antiepileptic drugs	See Table 148.4
4. Evaluation	History and examination (Table 148.1) and laboratory (Table 148.2)

Pharmacologic Treatment

Treatment with anticonvulsant medications should be started after 5 minutes of continuous seizure activity. Early initiation of treatment can potentially lead to a better response and prevent SE from becoming refractory. In fact, when treatment is started within 30 minutes of onset, up to 80% of patients achieve control compared to only 40% achieving control when treatment is started after 2 hours of onset (26,76). The choice of initial treatment largely depends on the institution, with different protocols being used by various institutions and specialists (68,77). This is due primarily to the lack of sufficient class I evidence. Three controlled clinical trials on the treatment of SE have been published. One study compared diazepam to lorazepam and found no significant difference (78). The second compared four treatment protocols: phenytoin alone, phenytoin with diazepam, lorazepam alone, and phenobarbital alone. The highest percentage of responders was in the lorazepam arm; however, the only significant difference was between lorazepam alone and phenytoin alone (11). The third study compared prehospital treatment with diazepam, lorazepam, and placebo, and found that both lorazepam and diazepam were efficacious (71).

Regardless of the choice of initial therapy, the rapid sequential use of several agents is strongly recommended until seizure activity is terminated (Table 148.4). The caveat of this approach is that the use of agents with long elimination half-life may lead to cumulative adverse effects, with high risk of inducing respiratory and cardiovascular depression. However, it is important to keep in mind that both respiratory and cardiovascular depression are usually easily treatable in the emergency room or intensive care unit settings, while prolonged SE may lead to irreversible neuronal injury. This formula should be kept in mind when making important therapeutic decisions. In the Veterans Affairs Cooperative Study (11), 60% of patients, on average, responded to the first drug; an additional 7.3% responded to the second drug; and only 2% responded to the third drug. Although these numbers seem discouraging, the number of drugs currently available has significantly increased, providing more options for treatment and potentially a better response rate. However, more clinical trials are needed to study the efficacy of newer agents.

The ideal initial drug would be easy to administer, have an immediate and long-lasting seizure-suppressing action, and be free of serious adverse effects on cardiorespiratory function and level of consciousness. Unfortunately, the ideal drug does not exist. Benzodiazepines and barbiturates depress consciousness and respiratory drive and may lower blood pressure; phenytoin can cause hypotension and cardiac arrhythmias, which limits the rate of intravenous infusion.

Benzodiazepines are the most commonly used first-line agents due to their potency and fast-acting effect. Pharmacologically, they enhance inhibitory γ-aminobutyric acid (GABA)

TABLE 148.4

SUGGESTED PROTOCOL FOR ANTIEPILEPTIC DRUG TREATMENT

Step	Medication	Dosage	Route	Maximum rate	Comment
1	Lorazepam	0.1 mg/kg	IV bolus	2 mg/min	May repeat once if seizure activity continues after 5 min If seizure activity stops, additional medications may not be required
2	Phenytoin Fosphenytoin	20 mg/kg 20 mg/kg PE	IV bolus IV bolus	50 mg/min 150 mg/min	May give additional 5–10 mg/kg if seizure continues Consider valproate in patients with epilepsy on valproate, especially with subtherapeutic level
3	Phenobarbital Valproate	20 mg/kg 25 mg/kg	IV bolus IV bolus	50 mg/min 200 mg/min	Skip this stage and go straight to general anesthesia if status started more than 60 min ago May give additional 5–10 mg/kg if seizure continues
4	Pentobarbital				
	Initial bolus	5–10 mg/kg	IV bolus	50 mg/min	Repeat 5 mg/kg every 5–10 min until seizures stop
	Maintenance	1 mg/kg/h	IV infusion		Titrate up to 10 mg/kg/h, until desired EEG pattern attained[a]
	Midazolam				
	Initial bolus	0.2 mg/kg	IV bolus	—	Repeat 0.2–0.4 mg/kg every 5 min until seizures stop, maximum 2 mg/kg
	Maintenance	0.1 mg/kg/h	IV infusion		Titrate up to 2 mg/kg/h until desired EEG pattern attained[a]
	Propofol				
	Initial bolus	1 mg/kg	IV bolus	—	Repeat 1–2 mg/kg every 5 min until seizures stop, maximum 10 mg/kg
	Maintenance	1 mg/kg/h	IV infusion		Titrate up to 1 mg/kg/h = 16 microgram/kg/min, until desired EEG pattern attained[a]
5	Ketamine Inhalation anesthetic				

[a]Usually burst-suppression pattern.
PE, phenytoin equivalent; EEG, electroencephalogram.

transmission. The three most commonly used agents are lorazepam, diazepam, and midazolam. Direct comparison between lorazepam and diazepam revealed no significant difference (78). Diazepam is more lipid soluble, and may cross the blood–brain barrier and reach higher concentrations in the cerebrospinal fluid more rapidly than lorazepam. However, this increased lipid solubility may be disadvantageous, and leads to a higher rate of redistribution in peripheral adipose tissue. Therefore, despite having a longer elimination half-life of 48 hours, the effective duration of action of diazepam is actually shorter—15 to 30 minutes—than that of lorazepam, which has a duration of action of 12 to 24 hours. This may lead to increased incidence of seizure recurrence after initial termination of SE when diazepam is used alone. The rapid onset of action and prolonged duration of seizure-suppressing effect has made lorazepam the preferred first-line agent by many neurologists. Midazolam has never been used in a double-blind study. Like diazepam and lorazepam, midazolam has a rapid onset of action, but its extremely short elimination half-life makes it more appropriately used as a continuous intravenous infusion in refractory SE.

The routine concomitant or sequential use of a second agent is advocated by many experts. It is recommended to use an agent with a different mechanism of action, such as phenytoin or fosphenytoin. However, as shown by the Veterans Affairs Cooperative Study (11), lorazepam alone may be sufficient in many cases, especially when SE is caused by a known and reversible process, such as low serum concentration of antiepileptic drugs or acute metabolic disturbances. Some experts argue that the early use of phenytoin or fosphenytoin is important to prevent seizure recurrence. This is based on the experimental evidence that benzodiazepines are subject to rapid time-dependent loss of potency as opposed to phenytoin, which loses its potency at a much slower rate (12,44). This claim, however, remains to be proven in controlled clinical trials.

The recommended dose of intravenous phenytoin is 20 mg/kg. The common practice of administering a standard loading dose of 1,000 mg of phenytoin is inadequate for most patients, and some patients require as much as 30 mg/kg to stop seizure activity (79). Phenytoin should be administered at a maximum infusion rate of 50 mg/minute. A faster administration rate may result in cardiovascular complications, including hypotension, bradycardia, and ectopic beats. These effects are more common in elderly patients and patients with pre-existing cardiac disease. Cardiovascular complications are not due to phenytoin itself, but to the propylene glycol diluent (80). For this reason, fosphenytoin, a water-soluble prodrug of phenytoin, was introduced and has gained broad popularity. Fosphenytoin is rapidly converted to phenytoin, and is dosed in phenytoin equivalents. Because of its water solubility, fosphenytoin can be administered at a much faster infusion rate than phenytoin—up to 150 mg/minute. Theoretically, the risk of cardiovascular adverse effects should be lower with fosphenytoin; however, this was never proven in clinical trials. In fact, in one study, the rate of complications was similar for intravenous phenytoin and fosphenytoin (81) as long as the recommended maximum rate of administration is followed, although infusion site reactions (phlebitis and soft tissue damage) were less common with fosphenytoin. The main advantage of fosphenytoin in the treatment of SE seems to be related to the rapidity of infusion. The question of whether fosphenytoin reaches its peak concentration in the brain faster than phenytoin is not known. Fosphenytoin has to be converted to phenytoin by liver enzymes, a process that may delay its true bioavailability. One study found that when phenytoin or fosphenytoin are administered at the maximum recommended infusion rate, the therapeutic serum concentration of phenytoin for either drug is attained within 10 minutes (82). Thus, fosphenytoin and phenytoin may very well have an equivalent onset of action; however, this will need to be studied in controlled clinical trials.

Phenobarbital is another effective treatment for SE; however, because of its powerful depressant effect on respiratory drive, level of consciousness, and blood pressure, it should be used only after benzodiazepines and phenytoin fail. The usual recommended loading dose is 20 mg/kg at an infusion rate of 50 mg/minute.

Intravenous valproic acid is another viable option for the acute treatment of SE, and may offer a significant advantage over phenobarbital, with a much safer side effect profile (83). Although the recommended infusion rate is 20 mg/minute, much faster infusion rates up to 555 mg/minute have been safely used (84). Several anecdotal reports and uncontrolled trials were initially published, suggesting a potential usefulness for valproate in the treatment of SE (85–87). A single double-blind controlled trial was published comparing phenytoin to valproic acid in acute convulsive SE (88), and found a higher rate of seizure termination with valproic acid as a first-line agent (66% vs. 43% for phenytoin). After failure of the first agent, valproic acid was also superior to phenytoin when used as a second agent. The current evidence and clinical experience are insufficient to recommend valproate as first-line treatment for SE; however, it may be safely and effectively used as a third- or fourth-line treatment when other agents are unsuccessful and before resorting to general anesthesia (89). The question of whether intravenous valproic acid should replace phenytoin as a second-line agent remains unanswered.

Topiramate has been reported to be useful in some patients with refractory SE (90,91), including children (92). It is administered as suspension via a nasogastric tube, with a good rate of seizure termination and an excellent safety profile. Although intravenous formulations are most likely more effective, topiramate may be a safe alternative to more aggressive treatments. Controlled clinical trials are needed to establish its efficacy and safety in this setting.

Intravenous levetiracetam was recently introduced and seems to have a good safety profile (93). There are no published studies about its use in SE, and therefore, no recommendations can be made. Levetiracetam has, overall, very good pharmacokinetic properties and a good safety profile, and may offer another option for the treatment of SE in the future.

Refractory Status Epilepticus

Status epilepticus is considered refractory if it does not respond to two or three first-line treatments (94). In practice, if seizure activity continues after the administration of a benzodiazepine, phenytoin, or phenobarbital, status is considered refractory and more aggressive treatment should be pursued. In the Veterans Affairs Cooperative Study (11), failure of the first two agents was seen in 38% of patients presenting with convulsive SE and 82% of patients presenting with subtle SE. Patients with refractory SE are at higher risk of developing complications (95), including respiratory failure, fever, pneumonia, hypotension, sepsis, and requiring blood transfusion. In addition, the clinical outcome is worse than nonrefractory SE, with a mortality of 23% compared to 14% in nonrefractory cases (95).

In a survey conducted among neurologists (77), there was strong agreement for the use of benzodiazepines and phenytoin or fosphenytoin as first- and second-line therapies for SE. However, there was less consistency for the choice of third- and fourth-line therapy. Treatment options include intravenous phenobarbital or valproate, or continuous infusion of pentobarbital, propofol, or midazolam. It is important to note that once the choice of continuous infusion of antiseizure medications—often termed "general anesthesia," although this is a bit of a misnomer—is made, patients are committed to undergo endotracheal intubation and artificial ventilation for a period of time. While it is extremely important to terminate seizure activity as rapidly as possible, intubation and ventilation are not, of course, complication free, which should be kept in mind when making such a decision. Although there is no consensus agreement on the treatment approach, I and others recommend trying at least one third-line agent before resorting to general anesthesia, especially given the safety profiles of intravenous valproate and levetiracetam.

Continuous intravenous infusion of pentobarbital, propofol, and midazolam at anesthetic doses is the treatment of choice for refractory SE. A published meta-analysis provides useful information on the relative advantages and disadvantages of each drug (94). Overall, pentobarbital appears to be more effective in stopping seizures and preventing seizure recurrence. However, pentobarbital is associated with more severe hemodynamic instability and hypotension, often requiring the use of vasopressors and, even in young individuals, mandating the placement of invasive monitoring devices to manage the significant negative inotropic state-induced inadequate oxygen delivery. Of importance, there is no difference in mortality among the three treatments. Propofol and midazolam have become the preferred agents for refractory SE mainly because of their rapid onset of action and short half-life, with rapid clearance. However, a review of a number of articles reporting data about the use of propofol in refractory SE raised several concerns about the safety of propofol in this setting (96). In contrast, more recent emerging evidence suggests propofol to be superior and safer than pentobarbital (97), even in children (98).

Once continuous infusion of an anesthetic agent is initiated, a multidisciplinary approach, including an experienced neurologist and a critical care team, is crucial to ensure adequate treatment. Continuous EEG monitoring is strongly recommended, and can provide online information about the presence of seizure activity and the success of treatment. This is especially true if convulsive activity stops, since often patients continue to have NCSE after the cessation of motor activity. Once seizure activity is completely suppressed and the desired level of anesthesia is attained—most often a 90% burst-suppression pattern on EEG—the infusion is maintained for 12 to 24 hours and is then gradually withdrawn. It is extremely important to make sure that patients are on adequate standing dosages and have adequate serum levels of other AEDs prior to withdrawal of the coma-inducing agent(s). If seizure activity recurs, therapy should be resumed for progressively longer periods, and the depth of anesthesia may be increased. In this situation, some experts advocate—and in this I agree—attaining electrocerebral silence in severely refractory cases. If infusion of one agent is not successful in stopping seizure activity despite high dosages, and significant side effects, then a second agent should be tried, either alone or in combination. Prolonged treatment with midazolam may lead to tachyphylaxis, leading to the need of very high dosages.

Other treatment options for refractory status epilepticus include inhalation anesthetic agents and ketamine. Both isoflurane and desflurane have been reported to rapidly suppress all electrographic seizure activity in patients who failed treatment with propofol, midazolam, and pentobarbital (99). However, the risk of complications is high and these agents should only be used as a last resort. Ketamine is another agent that has been advocated as a potential treatment option for patients with refractory SE (100). Ketamine offers the advantage of being neuroprotective and can increase blood pressure due to its sympathomimetic properties (67). The clinical experience with ketamine is very limited, and the potential for serious complications is unknown (101). Therefore, its use should be limited to severely refractory cases.

Nonconvulsive Status Epilepticus

There are two types of NCSE: absence and complex partial. The two subtypes can only be distinguished based upon the EEG pattern. Absence status is relatively rare and does not result in permanent neuronal injury. It usually occurs in patients with known primary generalized epilepsy due to low serum levels of AEDs. Most cases of absence status respond to intravenous benzodiazepines, with rapid return to baseline of the mental status. More recently, the use of intravenous valproate has been proposed, since valproate is in general an effective treatment for absence epilepsy.

Complex partial status is both more common and more difficult to diagnose and treat. It often occurs in patients without a history of epilepsy. NCSE either occurs *de novo* or can be a late manifestation of untreated or partially treated convulsive SE. NCSE occurs frequently in patients who are critically ill due to metabolic disturbances or neurologic disease, most frequently acute brain injury due to stroke, trauma, tumor, infection, or intracranial hemorrhage.

Initial therapy of NCSE should be identical to that of convulsive SE: intravenous benzodiazepines, followed by phenytoin or fosphenytoin, intravenous valproate or levetiracetam, or even oral topiramate. There is little question that seizures should be stopped as quickly as possible. The controversial issue remains whether more aggressive treatment is necessary or not (102). It is unclear if NCSE leads to brain damage. Some studies reported that in the absence of acute brain injury, the majority of patients with NCSE return to their baseline after cessation of seizure activity (103); other studies reported the presence of permanent neurologic impairment after prolonged NCSE (104); and still other studies were inconclusive (21).

In the absence of class I evidence and consensus guidelines, it is difficult to make definite recommendations. If NCSE is a late manifestation of convulsive SE, then it should be treated as refractory SE, and aggressive management is recommended. NCSE that results from metabolic dysfunction will most likely subside once the metabolic disturbance is corrected, and therefore aggressive treatment may not be necessary. The difficult question involves patients with acute brain injury, such as intracranial hemorrhage, trauma, brain surgery, or stroke, who have impaired consciousness and continuous or intermittent seizure activity on EEG, without any evidence of motor activity. These patients have a poor prognosis regardless of the treatment, with a high mortality rate and high risk of permanent neurologic impairment. The exact contribution of seizure activity to permanent neuronal injury is not known. The controversy arises from the fact that the aggressive coma-inducing treatment of SE is associated with high morbidity and mortality (94). A large number of these patients die from ICU complications, especially infections (43,105). It is not yet known whether aggressive treatment will shorten or lengthen the stay in the ICU and the duration of intubation. Even more importantly, it is not yet known whether aggressive treatment will have any impact on prognosis. Our approach is to treat with multiple nonsedating AEDs, such as phenytoin, levetiracetam, and valproate at high dosages, and only resort to coma-inducing agents if seizure activity persists or progresses despite more conservative management. A team approach in these cases is necessary, and decisions should be made on a case-by-case basis, taking into consideration several factors, such as the underlying etiology, age, and comorbidities.

PROGNOSIS

Status epilepticus is associated with significant morbidity and mortality. Several factors influence outcome, including etiology, age, and the duration of seizure activity (23,56). The overall mortality rate among adults is approximately 20% but rises significantly with age (23), reaching 38% in those older than 60 (14). Longer duration of SE usually leads to worse outcome, especially in the presence of severe physiologic disturbances. Mortality for seizures lasting more than 1 hour is 32%, compared to 2.7% when seizures are less than 1 hour long (23,24). Among survivors, the risk of developing chronic epilepsy and subsequent episodes of status is very high (76).

Patients with refractory SE tend to have a worse outcome (67). This is likely due to a combination of factors, including a more serious etiology and longer duration of seizure activity, which usually leads to increased duration of stay in the ICU, and subsequently, an increased rate of complications (95,106). Furthermore, patients with refractory SE are at significantly higher risk of developing chronic epilepsy than those with nonrefractory SE (106).

Patients with acute neurologic disease, such as infection, stroke, intracranial hemorrhage, or trauma, and patients with concomitant systemic illnesses tend to have worse outcomes (107); patients with anoxic brain injury have a very poor outcome (108). However, in these patients, the etiology and comorbid conditions are most likely the major determinants of outcome, with SE playing an additional complicating role. In contrast, patients with a history of chronic epilepsy who develop SE because of AED withdrawal, or patients with no history of epilepsy who develop SE because of alcohol withdrawal, tend to have a good outcome, often with return to their baseline level of functioning (106).

Mortality from NCSE seems to be higher overall, averaging 50% (25). Several factors can influence prognosis, including etiology and the level of consciousness at presentation. Patients presenting with minimal obtundation have a better outcome than those presenting with deep stupor or coma (107). Again, it is impossible to sort out which is the major determinant of prognosis—the severity of the status itself or the severity of the underlying condition.

PEARLS

- Status epilepticus is defined as continuous or rapidly repeating seizures.
- Any seizure type can turn into status epilepticus.
- Every institution should have a well-defined treatment protocol to avoid delays and inadequate treatment.
- In the majority of cases, status epilepticus develops in patients without any history of seizures or epilepsy.
- In patients with a history of epilepsy, the most common cause is low serum concentration of antiepileptic drugs.
- Intracranial pathology and metabolic disturbances can cause status epilepticus.
- When possible, correction of the underlying etiology is the most effective treatment.
- Status epilepticus is a medical emergency requiring aggressive and immediate therapeutic intervention.
- Mortality and morbidity increase significantly if seizure activity persists longer than 60 minutes.
- Delayed treatment may cause the status to become refractory to therapy.
- Rapid sequential use of several anticonvulsive medications is strongly recommended.
- In refractory cases, general anesthesia is the recommended therapy.
- Nonconvulsive status epilepticus is frequently underdiagnosed in comatose patients, especially those with acute neurologic injury.
- Continuous EEG monitoring is strongly recommended in most cases.

References

1. Fisher RS, Boas WvE, Blume W, et al. Epileptic seizures and epilepsy: definitions proposed by the International League Against Epilepsy (ILAE) and the International Bureau for Epilepsy (IBE). *Epilepsia.* 2005;46:470.
2. Treatment of convulsive status epilepticus. Recommendations of the Epilepsy Foundation of America's Working Group on Status Epilepticus. *JAMA.* 1993;270:854.
3. Mazarati AM, Wasterlain CG, Sankar R, et al. Self-sustaining status epilepticus after brief electrical stimulation of the perforant path. *Brain Res.* 1998;801:251.
4. Wasterlain CG. Mortality and morbidity from serial seizures. An experimental study. *Epilepsia.* 1974;15:155.
5. Fujikawa DG. The temporal evolution of neuronal damage from pilocarpine-induced status epilepticus. *Brain Res.* 1996;725:11.
6. Lowenstein DH, Bleck T, Macdonald RL. It's time to revise the definition of status epilepticus. *Epilepsia.* 1999;40:120.
7. Meldrum BS. The revised operational definition of generalised tonic-clonic (TC) status epilepticus in adults. *Epilepsia.* 1999;40:123.
8. DeLorenzo RJ, Garnett LK, Towne AR, et al. Comparison of status epilepticus with prolonged seizure episodes lasting from 10 to 29 minutes. *Epilepsia.* 1999;40:164.
9. Chen JW, Wasterlain CG. Status epilepticus: pathophysiology and management in adults. *Lancet Neurol.* 2006;5:246.
10. Theodore WH, Porter RJ, Albert P, et al. The secondarily generalized tonic-clonic seizure: a videotape analysis. *Neurology.* 1994;44:1403.
11. Treiman DM, Meyers PD, Walton NY, et al. A comparison of four treatments for generalized convulsive status epilepticus. Veterans Affairs Status Epilepticus Cooperative Study Group. *N Engl J Med.* 1998;339:792.
12. Mazarati AM, Baldwin RA, Sankar R, et al. Time-dependent decrease in the effectiveness of antiepileptic drugs during the course of self-sustaining status epilepticus. *Brain Res.* 1998;814:179.
13. Treiman DM, Walton NY, Kendrick C. A progressive sequence of electroencephalographic changes during generalized convulsive status epilepticus. *Epilepsy Res.* 1990;5:49.
14. DeLorenzo RJ, Hauser WA, Towne AR, et al. A prospective, population-based epidemiologic study of status epilepticus in Richmond, Virginia. *Neurology.* 1996;46:1029.
15. Knake S, Rosenow F, Vescovi M, et al. Incidence of status epilepticus in adults in Germany: a prospective, population-based study. *Epilepsia.* 2001;42:714.
16. Coeytaux A, Jallon P, Galobardes B, et al. Incidence of status epilepticus in French-speaking Switzerland: (EPISTAR). *Neurology.* 2000;55:693.
17. Hesdorffer DC, Logroscino G, Cascino G, et al. Incidence of status epilepticus in Rochester, Minnesota, 1965–1984. *Neurology.* 1998;50:735.
18. Towne AR, Waterhouse EJ, Boggs JG, et al. Prevalence of nonconvulsive status epilepticus in comatose patients. *Neurology.* 2000;54:340.
19. Privitera M, Hoffman M, Moore JL, et al. EEG detection of nontonic-clonic status epilepticus in patients with altered consciousness. *Epilepsy Res.* 1994;18:155.
20. DeLorenzo RJ, Waterhouse EJ, Towne AR, et al. Persistent nonconvulsive status epilepticus after the control of convulsive status epilepticus. *Epilepsia.* 1998;39:833.
21. Vespa PM, O'Phelan K, Shah M, et al. Acute seizures after intracerebral hemorrhage: a factor in progressive midline shift and outcome. *Neurology.* 2003;60:1441.
22. Claassen J, Mayer SA, Kowalski RG, et al. Detection of electrographic seizures with continuous EEG monitoring in critically ill patients. *Neurology.* 2004;62:1743.
23. Towne AR, Pellock JM, Ko D, et al. Determinants of mortality in status epilepticus. *Epilepsia.* 1994;35:27.
24. Lawn ND, Wijdicks EF. Progress in clinical neurosciences: status epilepticus: a critical review of management options. *Can J Neurol Sci.* 2002;29:206.
25. Ruegg SJ, Dichter MA. Diagnosis and treatment of nonconvulsive status epilepticus in an intensive care unit setting. *Curr Treat Options Neurol.* 2003;5:93.
26. Lowenstein DH, Alldredge BK. Status epilepticus at an urban public hospital in the 1980s. *Neurology.* 1993;43:483.
27. Schaller B, Ruegg SJ. Brain tumor and seizures: pathophysiology and its implications for treatment revisited. *Epilepsia.* 2003;44:1223.
28. Sperling MR, Ko J. Seizures and brain tumors. *Semin Oncol.* 2006;33:333.
29. Liigant A, Haldre S, Oun A, et al. Seizure disorders in patients with brain tumors. *Eur Neurol.* 2001;45:46.
30. Labovitz DL, Hauser WA, Sacco RL. Prevalence and predictors of early seizure and status epilepticus after first stroke. *Neurology.* 2001;57:200.
31. Hart RG, Byer JA, Slaughter JR, et al. Occurrence and implications of seizures in subarachnoid hemorrhage due to ruptured intracranial aneurysms. *Neurosurgery.* 1981;8:417.
32. Afsar N, Kaya D, Aktan S, et al. Stroke and status epilepticus: stroke type, type of status epilepticus, and prognosis. *Seizure.* 2003;12:23.
33. So EL, Annegers JF, Hauser WA, et al. Population-based study of seizure disorders after cerebral infarction. *Neurology.* 1996;46:350.
34. Burn J, Dennis M, Bamford J, et al. Epileptic seizures after a first stroke: the Oxfordshire Community Stroke Project. *BMJ.* 1997;315:1582.
35. Hasan D, Schonck RS, Avezaat CJ, et al. Epileptic seizures after subarachnoid hemorrhage. *Ann Neurol.* 1993;33:286.
36. Dennis LJ, Claassen J, Hirsch LJ, et al. Nonconvulsive status epilepticus after subarachnoid hemorrhage. *Neurosurgery.* 2002;51:1136.
37. Kunisaki TA, Augenstein WL. Drug- and toxin-induced seizures. *Emerg Med Clin North Am.* 1994;12:1027.
38. Wills B, Erickson T. Drug- and toxin-associated seizures. *Med Clin North Am.* 2005;89:1297.
39. Jenssen S, Gracely EJ, Sperling MR. How long do most seizures last? A systematic comparison of seizures recorded in the epilepsy monitoring unit. *Epilepsia.* 2006;47:1499.
40. Vicedomini JP, Nadler JV. A model of status epilepticus based on electrical stimulation of hippocampal afferent pathways. *Exp Neurol.* 1987;96:681.
41. Wasterlain CG, Mazarati AM, Naylor D, et al. Short-term plasticity of hippocampal neuropeptides and neuronal circuitry in experimental status epilepticus. *Epilepsia.* 2002;43(Suppl 5):20.
42. Mazarati AM, Wasterlain CG. N-methyl-D-aspartate receptor antagonists

abolish the maintenance phase of self-sustaining status epilepticus in rat. *Neurosci Lett.* 1999;265:187.
43. Krishnamurthy KB, Drislane FW. Relapse and survival after barbiturate anesthetic treatment of refractory status epilepticus. *Epilepsia.* 1996; 37:863.
44. Kapur J, Macdonald RL. Rapid seizure-induced reduction of benzodiazepine and Zn2+ sensitivity of hippocampal dentate granule cell GABAA receptors. *J Neurosci.* 1997;17:7532.
45. Meldrum BS, Horton RW. Physiology of status epilepticus in primates. *Arch Neurol.* 1973;28:1.
46. Meldrum BS, Vigouroux RA, Brierley JB. Systemic factors and epileptic brain damage. Prolonged seizures in paralyzed, artificially ventilated baboons. *Arch Neurol.* 1973;29:82.
47. Sloviter RS. Decreased hippocampal inhibition and a selective loss of interneurons in experimental epilepsy. *Science.* 1987;235:73.
48. Corsellis JA, Bruton CJ. Neuropathology of status epilepticus in humans. *Adv Neurol.* 1983;34:129.
49. DeGiorgio CM, Correale JD, Gott PS, et al. Serum neuron-specific enolase in human status epilepticus. *Neurology.* 1995;45:1134.
50. Chu K, Kang DW, Kim JY, et al. Diffusion-weighted magnetic resonance imaging in nonconvulsive status epilepticus. *Arch Neurol.* 2001;58: 993.
51. Walker MT, Lee SY. Profound neocortical atrophy after prolonged, continuous status epilepticus. *AJR Am J Roentgenol.* 1999;173:1712.
52. Lansberg MG, O'Brien MW, Norbash AM, et al. MRI abnormalities associated with partial status epilepticus. *Neurology.* 1999;52:1021.
53. Lazeyras F, Blanke O, Zimine I, et al. MRI, (1)H-MRS, and functional MRI during and after prolonged nonconvulsive seizure activity. *Neurology.* 2000;55:1677.
54. Simon RP. Physiologic consequences of status epilepticus. *Epilepsia.* 1985; 26(Suppl 1):S58.
55. Meldrum BS, Brierley JB. Prolonged epileptic seizures in primates. Ischemic cell change and its relation to ictal physiological events. *Arch Neurol.* 1973; 28:10.
56. Aminoff MJ, Simon RP. Status epilepticus. Causes, clinical features and consequences in 98 patients. *Am J Med.* 1980;69:657.
57. Winocour PH, Waise A, Young G, et al. Severe, self-limiting lactic acidosis and rhabdomyolysis accompanying convulsions. *Postgrad Med J.* 1989;65:321.
58. Lowenstein DH, Aminoff MJ. Clinical and EEG features of status epilepticus in comatose patients. *Neurology.* 1992;42:100.
59. Jedrzejczak J, Owczarek K, Majkowski J. Psychogenic pseudoepileptic seizures: clinical and electroencephalogram (EEG) video-tape recordings. *Eur J Neurol.* 1999;6:473.
60. Musicco M, Beghi E, Solari A, et al. Treatment of first tonic-clonic seizure does not improve the prognosis of epilepsy. First Seizure Trial Group (FIRST Group). *Neurology.* 1997;49:991.
61. Kwan P, Brodie MJ. Early identification of refractory epilepsy. *N Engl J Med.* 2000;342:314.
62. Devinsky O. Patients with refractory seizures. *N Engl J Med.* 1999;340: 1565.
63. Glauser T, Ben-Menachem E, Bourgeois B, et al. ILAE treatment guidelines: evidence-based analysis of antiepileptic drug efficacy and effectiveness as initial monotherapy for epileptic seizures and syndromes. *Epilepsia.* 2006;47:1094.
64. Wilby J, Kainth A, Hawkins N, et al. Clinical effectiveness, tolerability and cost-effectiveness of newer drugs for epilepsy in adults: a systematic review and economic evaluation. *Health Technol Assess.* 2005;9:1.
65. French JA, Kanner AM, Bautista J, et al. Efficacy and tolerability of the new antiepileptic drugs II: treatment of refractory epilepsy: report of the Therapeutics and Technology Assessment Subcommittee and Quality Standards Subcommittee of the American Academy of Neurology and the American Epilepsy Society. *Neurology.* 2004;62:1261.
66. French JA, Kanner AM, Bautista J, et al. Efficacy and tolerability of the new antiepileptic drugs I: treatment of new onset epilepsy: report of the Therapeutics and Technology Assessment Subcommittee and Quality Standards Subcommittee of the American Academy of Neurology and the American Epilepsy Society. *Neurology.* 2004;62:1252.
67. Lowenstein DH. The management of refractory status epilepticus: an update. *Epilepsia.* 2006;47(Suppl 1):35.
68. Walker MC, Smith SJ, Shorvon SD. The intensive care treatment of convulsive status epilepticus in the UK. Results of a national survey and recommendations. *Anaesthesia.* 1995;50:130.
69. Cloyd JC, Lalonde RL, Beniak TE, et al. A single-blind, crossover comparison of the pharmacokinetics and cognitive effects of a new diazepam rectal gel with intravenous diazepam. *Epilepsia.* 1998;39:520.
70. Collins M, Marin H, Rutecki P, et al. A protocol for status epilepticus in a long-term care facility using rectal diazepam (Diastat). *J Am Med Dir Assoc.* 2001;2:66.
71. Alldredge BK, Gelb AM, Isaacs SM, et al. A comparison of lorazepam, diazepam, and placebo for the treatment of out-of-hospital status epilepticus. *N Engl J Med.* 2001;345:631.
72. Lundgren J, Smith ML, Blennow G, et al. Hyperthermia aggravates and hypothermia ameliorates epileptic brain damage. *Exp Brain Res.* 1994;99: 43.
73. Liu Z, Gatt A, Mikati M, et al. Effect of temperature on kainic acid-induced seizures. *Brain Res.* 1993;631:51.
74. Swan JH, Meldrum BS, Simon RP. Hyperglycemia does not augment neuronal damage in experimental status epilepticus. *Neurology.* 1986;36: 1351.
75. Pang T, Hirsch LJ. Treatment of convulsive and nonconvulsive status epilepticus. *Curr Treat Options Neurol.* 2005;7:247.
76. Lowenstein DH, Alldredge BK. Status epilepticus. *N Engl J Med.* 1998; 338:970.
77. Claassen J, Hirsch LJ, Mayer SA. Treatment of status epilepticus: a survey of neurologists. *J Neurol Sci.* 2003;211:37.
78. Leppik IE, Derivan AT, Homan RW, et al. Double-blind study of lorazepam and diazepam in status epilepticus. *JAMA.* 1983;249:1452.
79. Osorio I, Reed RC. Treatment of refractory generalized tonic-clonic status epilepticus with pentobarbital anesthesia after high-dose phenytoin. *Epilepsia.* 1989;30:464.
80. Cranford RE, Leppik IE, Patrick B, et al. Intravenous phenytoin: clinical and pharmacokinetic aspects. *Neurology.* 1978;28:874.
81. Coplin WM, Rhoney DH, Rebuck JA, et al. Randomized evaluation of adverse events and length-of-stay with routine emergency department use of phenytoin or fosphenytoin. *Neurol Res.* 2002;24:842.
82. Kugler A, Knapp L, Eldon M. Attainment of therapeutic phenytoin concentration following administration of loading doses of fosphenytoin: a metaanalysis [abstract]. *Neurology.* 1996;46(Suppl):A176.
83. Ramsay RE, Cantrell D, Collins SD, et al. Safety and tolerance of rapidly infused Depacon. A randomized trial in subjects with epilepsy. *Epilepsy Res.* 2003;52:189.
84. Limdi NA, Faught E. The safety of rapid valproic acid infusion. *Epilepsia.* 2000;41:1342.
85. Limdi NA, Shimpi AV, Faught E, et al. Efficacy of rapid IV administration of valproic acid for status epilepticus. *Neurology.* 2005;64:353.
86. Sinha S, Naritoku DK. Intravenous valproate is well tolerated in unstable patients with status epilepticus. *Neurology.* 2000;55:722.
87. Yu KT, Mills S, Thompson N, et al. Safety and efficacy of intravenous valproate in pediatric status epilepticus and acute repetitive seizures. *Epilepsia.* 2003;44:724.
88. Misra UK, Kalita J, Patel R. Sodium valproate vs. phenytoin in status epilepticus: a pilot study. *Neurology.* 2006;67:340.
89. Hodges BM, Mazur JE. Intravenous valproate in status epilepticus. *Ann Pharmacother.* 2001;35:1465.
90. Towne AR, Garnett LK, Waterhouse EJ, et al. The use of topiramate in refractory status epilepticus. *Neurology.* 2003;60:332.
91. Bensalem MK, Fakhoury TA. Topiramate and status epilepticus: report of three cases. *Epilepsy Behav.* 2003;4:757.
92. Perry MS, Holt PJ, Sladky JT. Topiramate loading for refractory status epilepticus in children. *Epilepsia.* 2006;47:1070.
93. Ramael S, Daoust A, Otoul C, et al. Levetiracetam intravenous infusion: a randomized, placebo-controlled safety and pharmacokinetic study. *Epilepsia.* 2006;47:1128.
94. Claassen J, Hirsch LJ, Emerson RG, et al. Treatment of refractory status epilepticus with pentobarbital, propofol, or midazolam: a systematic review. *Epilepsia.* 2002;43:146.
95. Mayer SA, Claassen J, Lokin J, et al. Refractory status epilepticus: frequency, risk factors, and impact on outcome. *Arch Neurol.* 2002;59:205.
96. Niermeijer JM, Uiterwaal CS, Van Donselaar CA. Propofol in status epilepticus: little evidence, many dangers? *J Neurol.* 2003;250:1237.
97. Rossetti AO, Reichhart MD, Schaller MD, et al. Propofol treatment of refractory status epilepticus: a study of 31 episodes. *Epilepsia.* 2004;45:757.
98. van Gestel JP, Blusse van Oud-Alblas HJ, Malingre M, et al. Propofol and thiopental for refractory status epilepticus in children. *Neurology.* 2005; 65:591.
99. Mirsattari SM, Sharpe MD, Young GB. Treatment of refractory status epilepticus with inhalational anesthetic agents isoflurane and desflurane. *Arch Neurol.* 2004;61:1254.
100. Sheth RD, Gidal BE. Refractory status epilepticus: response to ketamine. *Neurology.* 1998;51:1765.
101. Ubogu EE, Sagar SM, Lerner AJ, et al. Ketamine for refractory status epilepticus: a case of possible ketamine-induced neurotoxicity. *Epilepsy Behav.* 2003;4:70.
102. Jordan KG, Hirsch LJ. In Nonconvulsive status epilepticus (NCSE), treat to burst-suppression: pro and con. *Epilepsia.* 2006;47(Suppl 1):41.
103. Drislane FW. Evidence against permanent neurologic damage from nonconvulsive status epilepticus. *J Clin Neurophysiol.* 1999;16:323.
104. Krumholz A, Sung GY, Fisher RS, et al. Complex partial status epilepticus accompanied by serious morbidity and mortality. *Neurology.* 1995; 45:1499.
105. Yaffe K, Lowenstein DH. Prognostic factors of pentobarbital therapy for refractory generalized status epilepticus. *Neurology.* 1993;43:895.
106. Holtkamp M, Othman J, Buchheim K, et al. Predictors and prognosis of refractory status epilepticus treated in a neurological intensive care unit. *J Neurol Neurosurg Psychiatry.* 2005;76:534.
107. Shneker BF, Fountain NB. Assessment of acute morbidity and mortality in nonconvulsive status epilepticus. *Neurology.* 2003;61:1066.
108. Drislane FW, Schomer DL. Clinical implications of generalized electrographic status epilepticus. *Epilepsy Res.* 1994;19:111.

CHAPTER 149 ■ NEUROMUSCULAR DISORDERS

EDWARD VALENSTEIN • MATTHEW MUSULIN

Neuromuscular disorders are commonly encountered in the critical care setting. Patients with known neuromuscular disorders, such as Guillain-Barré syndrome or myasthenia gravis, are admitted when weakness compromises the patient's ability to protect his or her airway or threatens ventilatory failure. Patients admitted with ventilatory failure of unknown cause may be diagnosed with a neuromuscular disorder such as amyotrophic lateral sclerosis or myasthenia gravis. Rarely, treatment may unmask a pre-existing neuromuscular disorder, as when drugs with neuromuscular blocking properties are given to patients with myasthenia gravis. Finally, patients with nonneuromuscular critical illnesses frequently develop neuromuscular weakness as a result of their illness or its treatment (1).

Intensive care physicians need to be familiar with the principles underlying diagnosis and management of patients with neuromuscular disease. Because electrophysiologic testing is often necessary to diagnose neuromuscular disorders in the intensive care setting, they should also have a basic appreciation of the techniques and indications for these studies. They should be familiar with the common neuromuscular disorders that require intensive care; Guillain-Barré syndrome and myasthenia gravis are considered in some detail because they are prevalent and treatable, and because, with proper treatment, they often carry a favorable prognosis. Finally, the intensive care physician will be responsible for recognizing and managing neuromuscular disorders that result from critical illness, which are now the neuromuscular disorders most commonly encountered in the intensive care setting (2).

GENERAL CONSIDERATIONS IN THE DIAGNOSIS OF NEUROMUSCULAR DISORDERS

As with central nervous system (CNS) disorders, the first step in the diagnosis of neuromuscular disorders is localization. Neuromuscular disorders comprise disorders of the anterior horn cell, the peripheral nervous system (PNS), the neuromuscular junction, and muscle (Fig. 149.1). Disorders of the PNS are further subdivided into disorders of roots, plexus, and peripheral nerve; and disorders of peripheral nerve are further subdivided into focal neuropathies, multifocal neuropathies, and polyneuropathies. Polyneuropathies, in turn, can be either length dependent or non–length dependent. Each of these nine major localizations has a characteristic pattern of symptoms and physical findings (Table 149.1). Localization is not just an academic exercise; each localization allows the physician to narrow the range considerably of likely diagnoses (Fig. 149.1). For example, if deficits are restricted to the distribution of a single nerve, the diagnosis is probably nerve entrapment, compression, or trauma. Multiple individual peripheral nerve involvement, in the absence of multiple trauma, should suggest an autoimmune neuropathy, often a vasculitis. Length-dependent polyneuropathy affects the longest nerves first, and consequently presents with deficits in the feet and legs before affecting the hands. Proximal strength is preserved until late. The differential diagnosis is wide, but comprises principally metabolic, toxic, or inherited neuropathies. Non–length-dependent localization is suggested when proximal weakness is greater than would be expected with a length-dependent polyneuropathy. Non–length-dependent polyneuropathies are overwhelmingly caused by autoimmune processes, including Guillain-Barré syndrome, but critical illness polyneuropathy may also be considered non–length dependent.

Recognition that a patient's problem is related to a disorder of nerve, neuromuscular junction, or muscle is relatively straightforward in patients who can give a history of their illness, and who can be adequately examined. If the problem is exclusively neuromuscular, features suggestive of central nervous system localization should be absent. These include mental status changes, hemibody weakness, or numbness suggestive of hemispheric or lateralized brainstem lesions; truncal motor or sensory level suggestive of spinal cord localization; increased muscle tone; hyperactive tendon reflexes; and pathologic reflexes such as the Babinski response. Features consistent with localization to the peripheral nervous system include weakness, atrophy, decreased or absent tendon reflexes, and sensory loss. Most acquired myopathies present with symmetric proximal weakness, and sensory loss is not a feature of either myopathy or disorders of neuromuscular transmission. Fatigable ptosis, weakness of extraocular movement, dysphagia, dysarthria, and neck, respiratory, and proximal limb weakness should suggest myasthenia gravis, the most common nonpharmacologic disorder of neuromuscular transmission.

Rarely, the presentation of a neuromuscular disorder may be so restricted as to first suggest a nonneurologic problem. Acute pandysautonomia presents with autonomic failure that can mimic cardiovascular, gastrointestinal, or urinary disorders (3). Diabetic truncal neuropathy can present with abdominal pain that often leads to extensive evaluation for nonneurological abdominal disorders, including exploratory surgery (4). Respiratory failure can be the presenting feature of a number of neuromuscular diseases, including amyotrophic lateral sclerosis (ALS) (5,6), myasthenia gravis (7), and myopathies such as adult-onset acid maltase deficiency (8). These patients may be admitted for respiratory support before the cause is

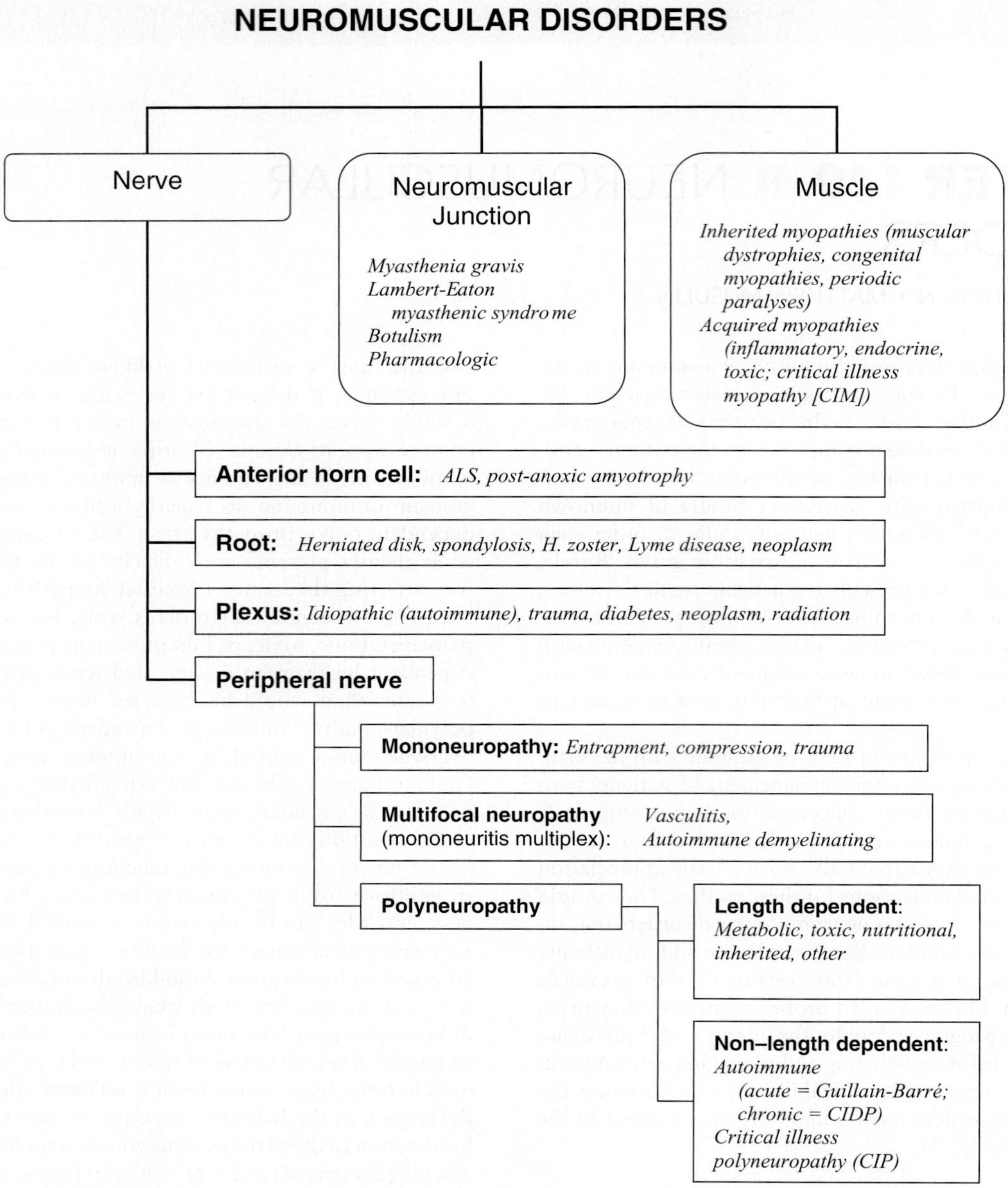

FIGURE 149.1. Localization of neuromuscular disorders, with the most important exemplars for each of the nine localizations. ALS, amyotrophic lateral sclerosis; CIDP, chronic inflammatory demyelinating polyneuropathy.

understood; it is left to the intensive care physician to suspect the correct diagnosis.

Diagnosing neuromuscular disorders that develop in critically ill patients can be challenging, since the patients are often unable to provide a history or to cooperate with the examination. Neuromuscular problems are usually first suspected when patients recovering from critical illness cannot be weaned from the respirator or are not moving their limbs; both central and neuromuscular causes of weakness need to be considered. Central causes of weakness may be suggested by the history and physical examination. Hemiparesis should always suggest a central localization; however, bilateral weakness can also result from central causes. A history of severe hypotension suggests the possibility of bilateral watershed infarction (9); rapid correction of hyponatremia predisposes to central pontine myelinolysis (CPM), an osmotic demyelination syndrome that presents with bulbar weakness and quadriparesis (10); patients after cardiac surgery may have multiple cerebral emboli; and patients with aortic dissection may suffer spinal cord infarction. Brain imaging may help establish a diagnosis in stroke or CPM; in other conditions, such as hypoxia or even acute spinal cord ischemia, imaging may be normal or nondiagnostic. If the cause of apparent weakness remains in question, electrodiagnostic testing is of value in suggesting or helping to exclude a neuromuscular localization.

TABLE 149.1

SALIENT FEATURES OF NEUROMUSCULAR DISORDERS

Localization	Pain	Sensory loss	Tendon reflexes	Distribution of weakness
Muscle	Variable (myalgia)	No	Normal or ↓	Symmetric, proximal
Neuromuscular junction				
Myasthenia gravis	No	No	Normal	EOM, bulbar, respiratory, proximal
Lambert-Eaton	No	No	↓	Bulbar, proximal
Nerve				
Anterior horn cell	No	No	**↓, (↑ in ALS)**	**Diffuse (begins focally); spares EOMs, bladder**
Root	Yes	Variable	Focally ↓	Root
Plexus	Yes	Variable	Focally ↓	Plexus
Mononeuropathy	Variable	Usual	Often normal	**Single nerve**
Multiple mononeuropathy	Variable	Usual	Often normal	**2 or more single nerves**
Length-dependent polyneuropathy	Variable	Usual	Ankle jerks ↓	**Distal (feet → legs → hands)**
Non–length-dependent polyneuropathy	Variable	Variable	Often areflexic	**Proximal as well as distal**

ALS, amyotrophic lateral sclerosis; EOM, extraocular muscle. The most important salient features are indicated in **bold typeface.**

Electrodiagnostic Studies

Although it requires the expertise of a physician trained in both the clinical and electrophysiologic diagnosis of neuromuscular disorders to decide what studies are appropriate and to interpret the results, it is important for the treating physician to appreciate how these studies can assist in diagnosis and management. Electrodiagnostic studies can help to answer the following questions:

1. Is there a neuromuscular disorder causing weakness?
2. Is this a disorder of nerve, neuromuscular junction, or muscle?
3. If there is a disorder of nerve, is the pathology primarily demyelinating or axonal?
4. What is the distribution of the deficits?

Nerve conduction studies, late wave analysis, needle electromyography (EMG), and repetitive stimulation are the standard procedures available to assist in the diagnosis of neuromuscular disorders, and can be performed using portable equipment in the intensive care setting. Table 149.2 summarizes the typical electrodiagnostic findings in disorders of nerve, neuromuscular junction, and muscle.

Motor Nerve Conduction Studies

Figure 149.2A illustrates the typical motor nerve conduction procedure and normal response from stimulation of the tibial nerve. The nerve is stimulated at two or more sites, and the response is recorded with surface electrodes over a muscle innervated by that nerve. The muscle response is called a *compound muscle action potential* (CMAP), because it is the sum of all muscle fiber action potentials activated by nerve stimulation. The stimulus at each site is gradually increased until no further increase in CMAP amplitude is seen. This indicates that all of the motor neurons capable of generating an action potential have been activated. The latency to the onset of the CMAP reflects the speed of conduction in the fastest nerve fibers. Motor nerve conduction velocity is calculated by measuring the distance between the sites of stimulation, and dividing that distance by the proximal minus the distal latency, which is the time it takes for the stimulus to traverse that nerve segment. By itself, motor nerve conduction can be diagnostic of focal or generalized demyelinating neuropathy (Fig. 149.2C,D). Interpreting a low-amplitude response (Fig. 149.2B) requires additional studies, since low CMAP amplitude can reflect not only loss of nerve axons or conduction block, but also defective neuromuscular transmission or loss of muscle fibers.

Sensory Nerve Conduction Studies

In orthodromic sensory nerve conduction studies, the skin is stimulated and a response is recorded over the nerve. Antidromic studies are more commonly performed by stimulating the nerve and recording over the skin. The result in either case is a sensory nerve action potential (SNAP), with a latency that reflects conduction in the fastest nerve fibers, and an amplitude that is proportional to the number of functioning nerve fibers. The normal SNAP amplitude is small and measured in microvolts. Abnormal SNAPs are indicative of pathology distal to dorsal root ganglion—either plexopathy or neuropathy. SNAPs are normal in radiculopathy if the pathology spares the dorsal root ganglia in CNS disorders as well as in disorders of neuromuscular transmission and muscle. In a patient with weakness and abnormal motor nerve conduction studies, small or absent SNAPs suggest sensorimotor neuropathy or plexopathy.

F-wave Studies

Action potentials in motor neurons are normally generated at the axon hillock and travel distally to nerve terminals in muscle; but when the nerve is stimulated in the course of nerve conduction studies, action potentials travel both orthodromically (distally) and antidromically (proximally) from the point

TABLE 149.2

ELECTRODIAGNOSTIC FEATURES IN NONFOCAL NEUROMUSCULAR DISORDERS

	Anterior horn cell	Axonal neuropathy	Demyelinating neuropathy	Neuromuscular junction disorder	Myopathy
MOTOR NERVE CONDUCTION STUDIES					
CMAP amplitude to distal stimulation	Small	**Small**	**Larger than to proximal stimulation**	Normal (MG) or small (MG, LEMS)	Normal or small
CMAP amplitude to proximal stimulation	Same as to distal stimulation	Same as to distal stimulation	**Smaller than to distal stimulation**	Same as to distal stimulation	Same as to distal stimulation
Conduction velocity	Over 70% LLN	**Over 70% LLN**	**Can be <70% LLN**	Normal	Normal
F-WAVE STUDIES					
F-wave latency	Normal or increased latency	Normal or increased latency	Absent or increased latency	Normal	Normal
SENSORY NERVE CONDUCTION STUDIES					
Sensory nerve action potentials	**Normal**	**Can be reduced or absent (normal in pure motor forms)**	Often reduced or absent (normal in pure motor forms)	**Normal**	**Normal**
NEEDLE EMG					
Spontaneous activity	**Increased**	Increased	Normal	Normal	Normal or increased
MUP morphology	**Normal or large**	Normal or large	Normal or large	Variable MUP morphology	**Small amplitude, polyphasic**
Recruitment	**Decreased**	Decreased	Decreased	Normal or "increased"	**Full recruitment produces little force**
REPETITIVE STIMULATION					
2–3 Hz stimulation	Usually normal	Usually normal	Usually normal	**>10% decrement in MG, LEMS**	Usually normal
20–50 Hz stimulation	Normal	Normal	Normal	**>50% increment in LEMS**	Normal

CMAP, compound muscle action potential (the potential recorded in motor nerve conduction studies); EMG, electromyography; MG, myasthenia gravis; LLN, lower limits of normal; LEMS, Lambert-Eaton myasthenic syndrome; MUP, motor unit potential.
The most salient features for each localization are indicated in **bold typeface.**

of stimulation. The antidromic action potential depolarizes the axon hillock and, in a minority of neurons, this depolarization generates another action potential that travels orthodromically down the nerve. This produces a small, late, muscle action potential, called the *F wave*, which can be recorded from most muscles. Increased F-wave latency, when combined with normal distal motor nerve conduction, indicates disease in the proximal portions of the nerve. Abnormal or absent F waves are the earliest electrophysiologic manifestation of Guillain-Barré syndrome (11,12).

Needle Electromyography

Needle EMG entails inserting a recording needle electrode into a muscle and observing (a) insertional activity consisting of action potentials generated by mechanical deformation of muscle fibers as the needle is inserted; (b) resting activity, which in normal muscles is only seen when the needle is near an end plate; and (c) voluntary activity, which consists of motor unit action potentials (MUPs). The motor unit consists of a motor neuron and all the muscle fibers innervated by it. The MUP is the sum of action potentials of all the muscle fibers in the vicinity of the recording needle electrode that are activated by a single motor neuron. Insertional and resting activity do not require patient cooperation, and can be observed in comatose or uncooperative patients. One to three weeks after denervation associated with axon damage, denervated muscle membranes become hypersensitive and discharge both spontaneously and in response to needle insertion, causing increased insertional activity and the appearance of positive sharp waves and fibrillations, which are spontaneous or needle movement–induced discharges of single muscle fibers. Similar abnormal spontaneous activity can be seen in disorders of muscle,

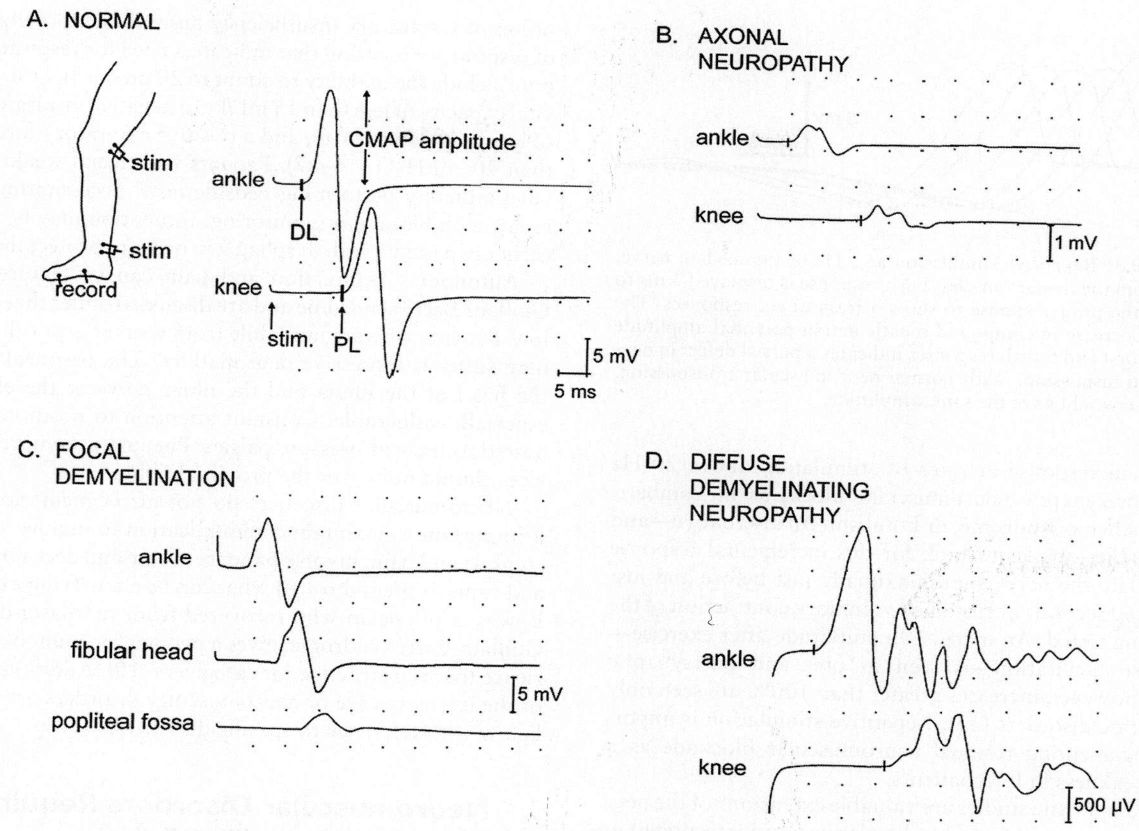

FIGURE 149.2. Typical motor nerve conduction findings. The sweep speed is 5 ms/div in all traces, but the gain is 5 mV/div in A and C, 1 mV/div in B, and 500 μV/div in D. **A:** Tibial motor nerve conduction in a normal subject. The drawing shows the two sites of stimulation over the posterior tibial nerve at the ankle and knee, and the sites of surface electrodes recording the response of the medial plantar muscle group. The two waveforms are the responses to stimulation at the ankle and knee. Conduction velocity is calculated as the distance between proximal and distal sites of stimulation divided by the time it takes for the stimulus to travel between the sites of stimulation (PL minus DL). **B:** Tibial motor nerve conduction in a patient with axonal sensorimotor neuropathy. CMAP amplitudes are less than 2 mV, with normal being greater than 4 mV. The amplitudes are similar with proximal (knee) and distal (ankle) stimulation. The conduction velocity is slightly slow, but is greater than 80% of the lower limits of normal. **C:** Peroneal motor nerve conduction study in focal nerve compression. CMAP amplitude drops sharply with nerve stimulation above the site of compression, at the fibular head. This conduction block is caused by focal nerve demyelination. Because there is no damage to axons, the nerve responds normally to stimulation distal to the area of demyelination. Conduction velocity is slow across the fibular head. **D:** Acquired diffuse demyelinating polyradiculoneuropathy. Multifocal demyelination affects some neurons more than others, resulting in prolonged and irregular CMAPs. Conduction velocities less than 70% of the lower limits of normal are also diagnostic of demyelination. DL, distal latency; PL, proximal latency; CMAP, compound muscle action potential.

particularly in the inflammatory myopathies, perhaps as a result of functional denervation caused by muscle fiber damage. If the patient is cooperative or happens to activate the muscle during the needle EMG study, additional information can be obtained by observing MUP activity. MUP morphology is of diagnostic value: high-amplitude, long-duration motor unit potentials indicate denervation with reinnervation, and low-amplitude, polyphasic motor unit potentials suggest primary disease of muscle or neuromuscular junction. Observation of motor unit recruitment with increasing effort can be diagnostic of denervation in the absence of any other abnormality. With denervation, MUP firing frequency increases with increasing effort, but insufficient numbers of different MUPs are recruited. Conversely, rapid recruitment of small polyphasic MUPs suggests myopathy or a disorder of neuromuscular transmission. Increased variability of the shape of a single MUP suggests a disorder of neuromuscular transmission.

Repetitive Stimulation

Disorders of neuromuscular transmission may be postsynaptic, as is the case in myasthenia gravis or most pharmacologic neuromuscular blocking agents, or presynaptic, as in Lambert-Eaton myasthenic syndrome and with exposure to botulinum toxin. Repetitive supramaximal stimulation of a motor nerve at a constant rate for five to ten stimuli is a simple way to assess for deficits of neuromuscular transmission. The resultant CMAP amplitudes should be constant. Progressive decrements in amplitude across the first four to five responses with 3-Hz stimulation is seen in both postsynaptic and presynaptic disorders of neuromuscular transmission (Fig. 149.3). Progressive

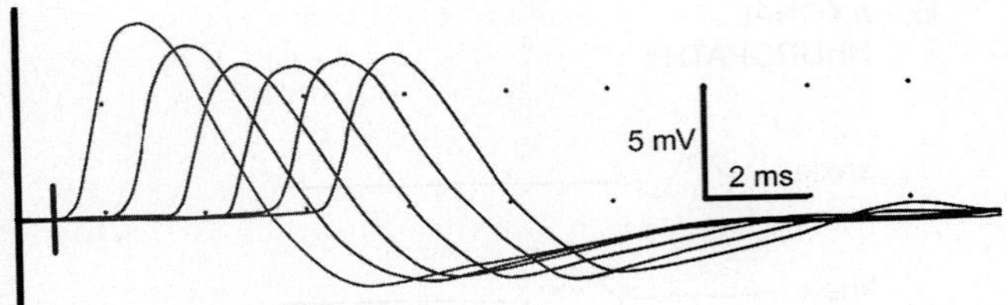

FIGURE 149.3. Repetitive stimulation at 3 Hz of the median nerve, recording from the thenar muscles. Each response is displayed 1 ms to the right of the prior response to show a train of six responses. The progressive decrease in compound muscle action potential amplitude between the first and fourth responses indicates a partial defect in neuromuscular transmission. With normal neuromuscular transmission, each response would have the same amplitude.

increments in response at rates of stimulation above 20 Hz suggest a presynaptic neuromuscular block, as in Lambert-Eaton myasthenic syndrome, or botulism. An alternative—and more tolerable—means to look for this incremental response is to stimulate the nerve supramaximally just before and just after 10 to 60 seconds of sustained voluntary contraction of the muscle being tested. An increase in amplitude after exercise—postexercise facilitation—is seen in pre- and postsynaptic disorders; however, increases greater than 100% are seen only in presynaptic disorders (13). Repetitive stimulation is important in documenting residual neuromuscular blockade as a cause of weakness in ICU patients.

Electrodiagnostic studies are valuable extensions of the neurologic assessment, and need to be planned and interpreted in the context of the history and neurologic examination. For example, in some contexts, absent sensory nerve responses provide evidence that weakness is related to an acute disorder of nerve, but in other circumstances may reflect prior sensory neuropathy, focal entrapment, or technical difficulties when recording very small potentials in an electrically noisy environment. Well-trained technicians can perform routine nerve conduction and repetitive stimulation studies; however, needle EMG must be performed by a knowledgeable physician, and study planning and interpretation must be the responsibility of physicians expert in both clinical neurophysiology and the clinical assessment of neuromuscular disorders.

GENERAL PRINCIPLES FOR THE INTENSIVE CARE OF PATIENTS WITH NEUROMUSCULAR DISORDERS

Indications for intensive care of patients with neuromuscular disorders include airway protection, ventilatory failure, and autonomic instability. Principles of evaluation and care are covered elsewhere in this book; however, it is worth pointing out here that many of the signs typically associated with respiratory failure in patients with obstructive pulmonary disorders, such as increased airway noises and increased respiratory excursion, may not be seen in patients with neuromuscular causes of respiratory failure. Instead, air hunger, tachypnea, shallow breaths, and staccato speech are characteristic. An inability to lay supine and paradoxical respirations are manifestations of diaphragmatic weakness. Confusion and somnolence with rising $PaCO_2$ may lessen respiratory distress and make recognition of respiratory insufficiency more difficult. Bedside tests of respiratory function that indicate a need for respiratory support include the inability to count to 20 on one breath, a forced vital capacity of less than 15 mL/kg, a negative inspiratory force of less than 25 cm H_2O, and a positive expiratory force of less than 40 cm H_2O (14–17). Patients with facial weakness may have difficulty performing bedside tests, necessitating greater reliance on blood gas monitoring. Intubation may be required earlier in patients with dysphagia in order to protect the airway.

Autonomic dysfunction and pain can be features of the Guillain-Barré syndrome and are discussed under that topic below. Patients who are immobile from weakness or other causes may suffer compressive neuropathies. The peroneal nerve at the head of the fibula and the ulnar nerve at the elbow are especially vulnerable. Constant attention to positioning is required to prevent pressure palsies. Pneumatic compression devices should not cover the proximal fibula.

Neuromuscular disorders do not affect mentation, and it is important to maintain communication to inquire about discomfort and pain, involve patients in care and decision making, and support them through what can be a terrifying experience. Bowes, a physician who recovered from ventilator-dependent Guillain-Barré syndrome, gives a personal account of her experience that is instructive for caregivers (18). Additional aspects of the intensive care of neuromuscular disorders are discussed below with reference to specific disorders.

Neuromuscular Disorders Requiring Intensive Care

Table 149.3 lists some of the neuromuscular conditions that can cause respiratory failure. In many of these conditions, weakness develops gradually, and management does not require intensive care, except when intercurrent illness, such as aspiration pneumonia, causes decompensation. ALS inevitably leads to respiratory failure, but alternative arrangements for care usually preclude intensive care admission. In a minority of patients with ALS, however, respiratory insufficiency is the presenting symptom, and leads to intensive care admission before the diagnosis is made. The diagnosis is suggested by finding fasciculations, atrophy, weakness, and hyperactive reflexes in the absence of sensory loss, extraocular muscle weakness, or autonomic dysfunction, and by excluding alternative causes, such as spinal cord compression or neuropathy. Electrophysiologic studies can be helpful. Nerve conduction studies document normal sensory nerve action potentials, and needle EMG reveals denervation in muscle of three or more extremities, or two extremities and bulbar muscles. Needle EMG can also document diaphragm denervation. Early in the course, clinical and electrophysiologic findings may not suffice for definitive diagnosis.

Respiratory weakness is seen in some muscle disorders, and is a terminal event in Duchenne muscular dystrophy. Respiratory weakness can be the presenting feature of adult-onset acid maltase deficiency, a glycogen storage disease (19), and it is a feature of some of the congenital myopathies and muscular dystrophies. Respiratory weakness can occur in inflammatory myopathies in the context of severe proximal limb weakness, and polymyositis associated with Jo-1 antibodies can be associated with interstitial pulmonary disease (20).

The two neuromuscular disorders that most commonly lead to admission for intensive care are Guillain-Barré syndrome

TABLE 149.3

NEUROMUSCULAR CAUSES OF RESPIRATORY FAILURE

DISORDERS OF NERVE
Amyotrophic lateral sclerosis (ALS)
Guillain-Barré syndrome
Toxic neuropathies
Critical illness polyneuropathy
Phrenic neuropathy (brachial plexus neuropathy, radiation trauma, postthoracotomy)
DISORDERS OF NEUROMUSCULAR JUNCTION
Myasthenia gravis
Acetylcholine receptor antibody associated
Muscle-specific kinase (MuSK) antibody associated
Lambert-Eaton myasthenic syndrome
Botulism
Pharmacologic neuromuscular blockade
DISORDERS OF MUSCLE
Polymyositis/dermatomyositis
Muscular dystrophies (dystrophinopathies, limb girdle types 2A and 2I, myotonic muscular dystrophy, myofibrillar myopathies)
Congenital myopathies (nemaline rod, centronuclear)
Glycogen storage disorders (acid maltase deficiency, debrancher enzyme deficiency)
Other inherited myopathies (mitochondrial myopathies, distal muscular dystrophy with respiratory weakness)
Metabolic myopathies

and myasthenia gravis. They are both autoimmune disorders and can cause rapidly progressive weakness; they are both treatable and, with appropriate management, most affected patients recover.

Guillain-Barré Syndrome

History. In 1859, Landry (21) described ascending paralysis progressing to respiratory paralysis and death. Guillain, Barré, and Strohl described the classic features of progressive weakness, sensory symptoms without signs, and loss of tendon reflexes, but their patients recovered. They also described increased cerebrospinal fluid protein without cells (albuminocytologic dissociation), a finding that helped to distinguish this disorder from poliomyelitis (22). An association with prior infection was established (23,24), and the concept that the disease was of autoimmune pathogenesis was supported by the development of an animal model—experimental allergic neuritis, in which inflammation and demyelination of peripheral nerves followed exposure to components of peripheral nerves (25).

Definition and Subtypes. Guillain-Barré syndrome is an autoimmune disorder of peripheral nerves with progression over less than 4 weeks, which is manifested by weakness, reduced or absent tendon reflexes, and variable sensory and autonomic dysfunction (26). Subtypes have been distinguished based on the presence or absence of motor, sensory, and/or autonomic involvement, and on whether the predominant damage is to myelin sheaths or axons. Acute inflammatory demyelinating polyradiculoneuropathy (AIDP) is by far the most common subtype, accounting for more than 85% of cases in the United States (27). Patients have weakness and reflex loss, with varying degrees of sensory and autonomic involvement, and there is electrophysiologic and pathologic evidence of peripheral nerve demyelination. Patients who have no sensory loss and electrodiagnostic studies suggesting axonal rather than demyelinating pathology have acute motor axonal neuropathy (AMAN). This variety of Guillain-Barré syndrome was first described in Asia, where it occurs epidemically following gastroenteritis caused by *Campylobacter jejuni* (28). Acute motor sensory axonal neuropathy (AMSAN) is diagnosed when there is both motor and sensory involvement and nerve conduction studies are consistent with early axonal dysfunction (29). The axonal forms of Guillain-Barré comprise less than 5% of cases in Europe and North America, but up to 47% of cases in China, Japan, and Central and South America (30). Acute pandysautonomia (31,32) and some forms of acute sensory neuropathy (33) are sometimes considered to be subtypes of Guillain-Barré syndrome even though weakness is not a feature, since they run a similar time course, and are presumed to be autoimmune. The Miller-Fisher variant of Guillain-Barré syndrome features ophthalmoplegia, ataxia, and areflexia (34). The Miller-Fisher variant may overlap with other forms of Guillain-Barré syndrome (30,35).

Epidemiology and Pathogenesis of Guillain-Barré Syndrome. The incidence of Guillain-Barré is less than 1 in 100,000 in children, averages 1 to 2 per 100,000 in adults, and increases to 4 in 100,000 in adults over 75 years of age (36,37). In about two thirds of patients, the disease follows an infection, most often a flulike syndrome or gastroenteritis, by 1 to 8 weeks (38). When serologic studies are performed, evidence of infection with *C. jejuni*, cytomegalovirus, Epstein-Barr virus, *Haemophilus influenzae,* and *Mycoplasma pneumoniae* are found to account for the majority of cases (39,40); 5% follow surgery (24). Although 3% of cases are attributed to vaccination (38), only rabies vaccine is associated with a definite increase in the incidence of Guillain-Barré (41); influenza vaccination causes little, if any, increase (41,42).

The pathology of AIDP consists of a multifocal inflammation of peripheral nerves, in which macrophages destroy the myelin sheath (43–46). This response is mediated by activated T cells (47). Direct binding of antibodies to Schwann cell membranes with subsequent complement-mediated destruction and secondary macrophage invasion may also play a role (48). Similar pathologic findings characterize experimental allergic neuritis (EAN), which is considered to be a good experimental model for Guillain-Barré syndrome (49). EAN can be initiated by injections of several myelin components, including myelin proteins P0 and P2, myelin basic protein, peripheral myelin protein-22 (PMP-22), and myelin-associated glycoprotein (MAG) (47). No specific myelin antibodies have been identified in the pathogenesis of AIDP.

The pathology of AMAN differs from that of AIDP in that macrophages target the axonal membrane in ventral (motor) roots and nerves at nodes of Ranvier, resulting in axonal rather than myelin damage (50,51). The pathology in AMSAN is similar to that of AMAN, except that the disorder affects both motor and sensory roots and nerves (29). Recent evidence suggests that AMAN may result from molecular mimicry. The capsule of the strains of *C. jejuni* implicated in patients with Guillain-Barré syndrome contains a lipopolysaccharide with a structure similar to the GM_1 ganglioside present in peripheral nerves. Antibodies to these strains of *C. jejuni* cross-react with peripheral nerve GM_1 ganglioside, resulting in axonal dysfunction in experimental animals (52). Similarly, many patients with the Miller-Fisher variant have GQ1b and GT1a antibodies (53) that cross-react with *Campylobacter* lipopolysaccharides (54,55). Anti-GD1b antibodies have been associated with acute and chronic sensory neuropathies (30). Although there is evidence that molecular mimicry is a plausible explanation for some patients with Guillain-Barré polyneuropathy, the relationships are complex. Patients may have antibodies to several gangliosides, antibodies to a particular ganglioside can be associated with several different types of neuropathy, and infections with a specific organism may be followed by more than one kind of neuropathy (30).

Clinical Presentation and Diagnosis. AIDP, the most common form of Guillain-Barré, presents with weakness and decreased or absent tendon reflexes. It is a non–length-dependent polyneuropathy, with proximal as well as distal weakness that usually begins in the legs and ascends, but can affect other regions first. Bilateral facial weakness occurs in half of the patients. Since symptoms can progress to oropharyngeal and respiratory weakness in 33% of patients, all patients require careful monitoring, as discussed below. Eye movements are usually spared, the exception being the Miller-Fisher variant. Sensory symptoms occur in 80% of patients. Sensory signs are less frequent and often mild, but, when prominent, can contribute significantly to disability (56). Pain and temperature sensation mediated by small unmyelinated neurons may be affected less than position and vibratory sensation, mediated by large myelinated fibers. Fifty percent have pain, either back and muscle pain that can be aggravated by movement, or neuropathic pain, such as burning paresthesias, sometimes with allodynia (pathologic sensitivity to touch). Tendon reflexes are lost early in the course of the disease; indeed, the diagnosis should be questioned if reflexes are retained. Autonomic dysfunction is present in 66% of patients, and can manifest with tachyarrhythmias or bradyarrhythmias, spontaneous or orthostatic hypotension, paroxysmal hypertension, abnormalities of sweating, urinary retention, or ileus (57). Guillain-Barré syndrome is a subacute process: 50% of patients stop progressing in less than 2 weeks, 80% by 3 weeks, and more than 90% by 4 weeks (58).

The much less common axonal variants of Guillain-Barré are distinguished from AIDP by electrophysiologic studies. Nerve conduction studies should show low-amplitude motor CMAPs without marked conduction slowing, conduction block, or dispersion in both AMAN and AMSAN. AMAN is distinguished from AMSAN by preservation of sensory nerve action potential amplitudes (59).

The differential diagnosis of patients presenting with subacute weakness includes disorders of the CNS, PNS, neuromuscular junction, and muscle. Although Babinski responses, brisk reflexes, and sensory level will usually distinguish spinal cord from peripheral nerve diseases, there is overlap because reflexes may be depressed acutely in CNS disorders; bladder dysfunction, while suggestive of CNS lesions, can be seen in Guillain-Barré; and CNS demyelination may occasionally accompany Guillain-Barré syndrome (60). Conversely, Guillain-Barré syndrome should be in the differential of patients with the locked-in syndrome when tendon reflexes are depressed. Toxic, drug-induced, and metabolic neuropathies may occasionally present over a similar time course as Guillain-Barré syndrome. In patients without sensory disturbances, disorders of neuromuscular junction and muscle should be considered. Muscle disorders that can present with severe subacute or acute weakness include the periodic paralyses, hypokalemic myopathy, drug-induced myopathies, and inflammatory myopathies.

Evaluation should include appropriate imaging to exclude CNS disorders, routine laboratory studies, and lumbar puncture. The cerebrospinal fluid (CSF) is normal during the first days of illness, after which there is a transient elevation of protein with minimal or no pleocytosis. A significant pleocytosis should raise the question of infection such as Lyme disease or West Nile virus (61); when the clinical picture is otherwise classic for Guillain-Barré, CSF pleocytosis should suggest human immunodeficiency virus (HIV) infection in which immune dysregulation increases the incidence of autoimmune disorders (62). Blood should be sent for basic metabolic profile, B_{12}, porphyrins, tests for Lyme disease and HIV, and heavy metal levels. Electrodiagnostic studies must be interpreted in the context of the clinical findings. Early in Guillain-Barré, nerve conduction and F-wave studies may be normal if recorded from a limb without severe weakness. Delayed or absent F waves, sometimes replaced by axon reflex waves, are the earliest abnormalities (63). When recorded from a paralyzed muscle, normal motor nerve conduction studies with normal F waves indicate that the weakness does not result from a peripheral cause, and should direct attention toward an alternative diagnosis with localization to the central nervous system.

Management of Guillain-Barré Syndrome. Patients with Guillain-Barré syndrome should be admitted and carefully monitored for respiratory function, swallowing ability, and autonomic function. Specific treatment can hasten recovery and reduce hospital costs, and is recommended for all patients whose weakness threatens loss of ambulation (64). Plasma exchange was the first treatment demonstrated to be effective in Guillain-Barré syndrome. Treated patients demonstrated greater improvement at 4 weeks than untreated controls, and treatment reduced the proportion of patients requiring mechanical ventilation at 4 weeks from 27% to 14% (28,65–67). Every-other-day treatment to a total of five plasma volumes is usually employed. Complications include pneumothorax and sepsis related to central venous access, hypocalcemia, coagulopathy, and hypotension. Intravenous immunoglobulin treatment (IVIG) was shown to be equally effective as plasma exchange in controlled trials (68), and has become the preferred treatment because of greater ease of administration and lesser risk of serious complications. The usual dose is 0.4 g/kg/day infused slowly for 5 days to a total dose of 2 g/kg. Complications include hypersensitivity in patients with immunoglobulin A (IgA) deficiency, acute renal failure, congestive failure, hypercoagulable state, and aseptic meningitis. Treatment is indicated in all but the mildest cases, and is best instituted early in the course of the disease. Treatment after 4 weeks is unlikely to be of benefit. High-dose corticosteroids are of no proven benefit, and in several trials treated patients had more disability than controls (69).

Patients with rapidly progressive weakness should be transferred to the ICU. Respiratory failure is often preceded by progression of weakness to involve the upper extremities, shoulders, neck, and face, but may occur before this weakness is evident. Tachypnea, paradoxical respirations, hypophonia, staccato speech, and a marked increase in respiratory dysfunction when supine are clinical indications of respiratory failure (14). Confusion from carbon dioxide retention is a late manifestation. Respiratory function should be monitored with bedside spirometry, and heart rate and blood pressure should be closely monitored. Indications for intubation are reviewed under General Principles, above.

Autonomic instability is common and usually not life threatening, unless it is manifested by asystole or ventricular fibrillation. Hypertension should be treated cautiously, as patients may be unusually sensitive to antihypertensive medications. Paroxysmal hypertension may sometimes be a manifestation of pain, in which case adequately treating the pain can be curative. Neuropathic pain can be treated with antiepileptic medications such as gabapentin (70), antidepressants such as amitriptyline, or analgesics.

The prognosis for recovery is good in all types of Guillain-Barré syndrome, but is poorest for patients with severe AMSAN. Poor recovery is correlated with age, severity of deficits at the nadir of the disease, more rapid progression of deficits (30), and, in some studies, evidence of axonal damage on electrophysiologic studies (71); however, even the most severely afflicted patients may recover fully. About half of patients with otherwise good recovery are left with mild sensory disturbances (72–74).

Myasthenia Gravis

History. The first description of myasthenia gravis is variously credited to Wilks in 1867 or to Erb in 1879, although Sir Thomas Willis provided a description of the symptoms more than 200 years earlier (75). Freidreich Jolly, who first described the decremental response to repetitive stimulation, called this disorder myasthenia gravis pseudoparalytica (76). Mary Walker, a physician working at St. Alfege's Hospital in Greenwich, was the first to use acetylcholinesterase inhibitors to treat myasthenic patients (77). The dramatic, albeit temporary, reversal of weakness by physostigmine was called the "Miracle of St. Alfege's Hospital." The transient weakness manifested by infants born to myasthenic mothers, and the association of myasthenia with thymic tumors and with thyroiditis, led to the theory that myasthenia was an autoimmune disease (78). This was confirmed in the early 1970s with the demonstration that animals injected with concentrated acetylcholine receptor produced antibodies that caused weakness (79), as well as with the discovery of antibodies to acetylcholine receptors in the sera of myasthenic patients (80). Immunotherapy and improved critical care have lessened overall mortality from 20% to 30% in the 1950s (81) to nearly zero (82).

Epidemiology. Myasthenia gravis has a current prevalence of about 20 per 100,000 population. There are about 60,000 patients with myasthenia in the United States (83). Myasthenia gravis occurs throughout life with bimodal peaks in the second and third decade in women and in the fifth and six decades in men (84). As the population ages, the average age of onset has increased and men are now more often affected than women (83). Myasthenic crisis occurs in about 20% of patients with myasthenia; almost 33% of these patients can experience a second crisis (85,86).

Pathophysiology. The neuromuscular junction is composed of a presynaptic motor neuron membrane, the synaptic cleft, and the postsynaptic muscle membrane. In the normal neuromuscular junction, the arrival of an action potential at the nerve terminal leads to the influx of calcium through voltage-gated calcium channels, which triggers release of acetylcholine into the synaptic cleft (87). Acetylcholine diffuses across the synaptic cleft to bind with acetylcholine receptors on the postsynaptic muscle membrane. This binding generates end-plate potentials that depolarize the muscle membrane. When the depolarization exceeds threshold, a muscle action potential is generated, which leads to a cascade of events that results in muscle contraction (88). Neuromuscular transmission fails if the end-plate potential fails to reach the threshold for muscle action potential generation. In Lambert-Eaton myasthenic syndrome, the end-plate potential is small because antibodies to voltage-gated calcium channels on the presynaptic membrane interfere with acetylcholine release. In myasthenia gravis, the end-plate potential is small because antibodies to the acetylcholine receptor or related sites on the postsynaptic membrane decrease the depolarization caused by normal amounts of acetylcholine.

The acetylcholine receptor is composed of four subunits (89). Antibodies to the acetylcholine receptor can be found in 80% to 90% of patients with generalized myasthenia (90). These antibodies can cause neuromuscular transmission failure by binding to the acetylcholine receptor and altering function, by increasing the rate of degradation of the receptors, and by complement-mediated destruction of the postsynaptic membrane (91). About 30% of patients with generalized myasthenia who are seronegative for acetylcholine receptor antibodies have antibodies to muscle-specific kinase (MuSK) (92). Patients with MuSK antibodies demonstrate more severe disease than patients with antibodies against the acetylcholine receptor (93).

The thymus gland has been implicated in the pathogenesis of myasthenia gravis. Thymic abnormalities are seen in 75% of patients with myasthenia gravis. Of these, 75% have lymphoid follicular hyperplasia and 15% have thymomas (94). Acetylcholine receptors are found on myoid cells of the thymus (95). The majority of myasthenic thymuses contain B cells that can produce antibodies to the acetylcholine receptor (96). Anti-striated muscle antibodies in patients with myasthenia gravis correlate highly with thymoma (97).

Patients with myasthenia gravis often have other autoimmune disorders, including thyroiditis, scleroderma, Sjögren syndrome, rheumatoid arthritis, pernicious anemia, polymyositis, and lupus erythematosus (98).

Clinical Presentation. Patients with myasthenia gravis present with fluctuating weakness that improves with rest. The most common complaints are ocular—namely, ptosis and diplopia related to weakness of the levator palpebrae and the extraocular muscles, respectively. Ptosis is the presenting symptom in 50% to 90% of patients, and 90% to 95% of patients complain of diplopia during the disease. Weakness can remain purely ocular in up to 15% of cases, but the majority of patients with myasthenia gravis develop generalized symptoms (76). Dysarthria and dysphagia are common complaints. Neck extensors and flexors are often more involved than other muscles in generalized disease (76). Patients may have to support their chin with their hand to prevent head drop because of neck extensor weakness or to keep their jaw shut because of weakness of the temporalis and masseter muscles. Proximal limb weakness is usually present when the disease is not purely ocular. It is sometimes asymmetric, is occasionally very focal, and

TABLE 149.4

MYASTHENIC WEAKNESS

DRUGS THAT COMMONLY WORSEN MYASTHENIC WEAKNESS
Neuromuscular blocking agents
Aminoglycoside antibiotics (gentamicin, neomycin, tobramycin, kanamycin, and others)
Telithromycin (Ketek) (100)
Procainamide, quinidine, quinine
Penicillamine[a]
α-Interferon[a]
Magnesium salts
DRUGS THAT MAY WORSEN MYASTHENIC WEAKNESS (SELECTIVE LIST)
Macrolide antibiotics (erythromycin, azithromycin, and others)
Other antibiotics: Nitrofurantoin, fluoroquinolones
β-Blockers
Calcium channel blockers
Anticonvulsants (Dilantin, gabapentin, carbamazepine, and others)
Narcotic analgesics
Estrogen therapy
Timolol, betaxolol hydrochloride (ophthalmic solutions)
Phenothiazines
Chloroquine
Iodinated contrast agents

[a]May cause autoimmune myasthenia gravis.
From Pascuzzi RM. Medications and myasthenia gravis (A reference for health care professionals). Myasthenia Gravis Foundation of America. 2007. http://www.myasthenia.org/hp_edmaterials.cfm. Accessed June 12, 2007.

can affect distal muscles. In less than 10% of cases, myasthenia presents with proximal weakness without bulbar or ocular weakness.

Myasthenic crisis is diagnosed when weakness progresses to cause dysphagia with loss of airway protection or hypoventilation. Myasthenic crisis can be precipitated by infection, surgical procedures, pregnancy, treatment with corticosteroids, sepsis, cholinergic crisis, and the rapid withdrawal of immune-suppressing medications (86). Pulmonary system infection, including aspiration pneumonia, is the most common identifiable precipitating factor (86). Many medications can also worsen myasthenic symptoms (Table 149.4) (99), often because they impair neuromuscular transmission. Aminoglycoside antibiotics, quinidine, and procainamide are particularly likely to cause weakness, and should be avoided in patients with myasthenia. Limited experience with telithromycin suggests that it should also be avoided (100). Penicillamine and α-interferon may cause autoimmune myasthenia. Evidence that other medications exacerbate myasthenia gravis is less convincing, but in patients with increasing weakness, all medications must be scrutinized against the long list of potentially offending agents (99).

Myasthenic crisis can involve muscles of inspiration, including the diaphragm and the external intercostals, along with accessory muscles of inspiration, including the scalene and sternocleidomastoid muscles. Respiratory strength can be measured by vital capacity and negative inspiratory force (101). As respiratory weakness leads to ventilatory failure, tidal volumes decline. Patients in myasthenic crisis have an intact respiratory drive, and therefore respond to the decrease in tidal volume with an increase in respiratory rate (102). Oropharyngeal muscle weakness may result in obstruction with upper airway collapse. Secretions can be difficult to control and can also obstruct the airway and lead to aspiration. In the 1950s and 1960s, mortality from myasthenic crisis was as high as 70% to 80% (103,104). In more recent reports, mortality is closer to 4% (85,86), related to improvements in intensive care as well as effective immunomodulatory treatment.

Diagnosis. The history and examination often strongly suggest the diagnosis. A history of fluctuating ptosis, diplopia, fatigable dysarthria, dysphagia, and neck weakness are highly suggestive. Sometimes the presentation may be misleading, as when ocular myasthenia presents with isolated eye muscle weakness or with a pattern of eye movements that mimics internuclear ophthalmoplegia from brainstem lesions, or when patients have proximal limb weakness without eye or bulbar weakness, suggesting a primary disorder of muscle. Conversely, patients with purely ocular findings should be worked up for other causes of ophthalmoplegia, including thyroid eye disease and retrobulbar or cavernous sinus lesions. ALS may present with bulbar symptoms, but patients with ALS do not have ptosis or eye movement weakness, and often have pseudobulbar dysarthria, characterized by slow labored speech and poorly modulated emotional expression, with laughing or crying that is disproportionate to the situation.

Many tests are available to confirm the diagnosis of myasthenia. Definitive diagnosis is important, as most patients will require years of immunomodulatory therapy. Pharmacologic testing with edrophonium (Tensilon), a rapid-acting, short-duration acetylcholinesterase, can result in transient increase in strength. Caution should be used in using edrophonium because anticholinergic side effects, such as bradycardia and bronchospasm, can develop. A test dose of 2 mg of edrophonium, given intravenously, should be administered, followed by increments of 2 mg, for a total dose of 10 mg. Atropine should be available to counteract muscarinic side effects (105). Definite improvement in strength, as demonstrated by improvement in ptosis, dysarthria, or resistance against the examiner's testing, is supportive of the diagnosis. The test is, therefore, most helpful in patients with clear weakness that can be evaluated in an objective manner (105). In patients with cardiac disease, especially those on β-blockers or drugs that cause atrioventricular block, edrophonium should be avoided, as it can cause asystole (106). Fortunately, there are many alternative tests to confirm the diagnosis of myasthenia.

Serum acetylcholine receptor antibodies are found in 80% to 90% of patients with generalized myasthenia gravis, and have very high diagnostic specificity. Increased titers are also found in patients with thymoma without myasthenia, and rarely in other diseases, including systemic lupus, ALS, liver disease, and inflammatory neuropathies, and in patients with Lambert-Eaton myasthenic syndrome (107). Antibodies to striated muscle are present in about 30% of patients with myasthenic gravis, and are highly associated with thymoma (108). About 30% of patients with myasthenia gravis who lack antibodies to acetylcholine receptor have antibodies to MuSK. Other antibodies directed against muscle antigens can be found in patients with myasthenia gravis (109).

Repetitive nerve stimulation can be performed to rule out a decrement in the amplitude or area of the fourth or fifth potential compared to the first potential (Fig. 149.3). A train of five to ten stimuli is delivered at a rate of 2 to 3 Hz. If the decrement is more than 10%, it is considered abnormal. The yield can be increased by testing clinically weak muscles and with repeat testing after exercise of the specific muscle. Because typically myasthenia affects proximal more than distal muscles, the test is more likely to be abnormal when testing proximal or facial muscles than when testing hand muscles (110). Single-fiber EMG is abnormal in nearly all patients with generalized myasthenia (111), but it is not widely available because it is time consuming, is technically demanding, and requires expensive needle electrodes.

Patients diagnosed with myasthenia should have additional testing for associated conditions. Computed tomography (CT) or magnetic resonance imaging (MRI) of the chest is required to evaluate for thymoma (82). Tests of thyroid function are important, because about 10% of myasthenics have associated autoimmune thyroid disease, and because proximal weakness and restriction of extraocular movements can be caused by thyroid disease. Antinuclear antibody (ANA) and rheumatoid factor may detect much less commonly associated autoimmune disorders. Tuberculin test and fasting glucose should be obtained prior to treatment with steroids.

Management. The majority of myasthenic patients respond well to treatment and never require intensive care. Although anticholinesterase medications can produce dramatic improvement in strength, they do not address the underlying autoimmune pathogenesis of the disease, and tend to become ineffective as the disease progresses. They may be sufficient, however, for patients with mild, nonprogressive disease, and they can be helpful as adjunctive treatment in patients on immunomodulatory treatment. Pyridostigmine, which does not cross the blood–brain barrier, is the most commonly used oral agent. Sustained-release pyridostigmine is appropriate for use at bedtime to mitigate weakness during the night and in the morning; however, multiple daytime doses of sustained-release preparations should be avoided, as accumulation may lead to cholinergic weakness.

Oral prednisone is the most commonly used agent to induce remission in myasthenic patients, and is effective in 80% to 90% of patients. High-dose prednisone—60 to 100 mg/day—may cause transient worsening of myasthenia, and should not be initiated unless patients can be closely observed. Lower doses appear safer, but are not entirely free from this complication. Most patients experience gradual improvement in strength beginning 2 or 3 weeks after initiation of therapy. Once a good response has been achieved, the dose can be tapered over several months to low-dose alternate-day treatment. Doses less than 40 mg every other day are generally well tolerated. Doses of 40 mg or above every other day are associated with many long-term side effects, including diabetes, hypertension, cataracts, avascular necrosis, and increased susceptibility to infection. Azathioprine may reduce steroid dependence. Treatment with IVIG can produce rapid improvement in strength, and may be useful to provide short-term improvement while waiting for steroids to become effective.

Myasthenic weakness can progress very rapidly; therefore, patients with worsening myasthenic symptoms should be hospitalized for definitive management. Patients with progressive bulbar weakness who have difficulty controlling secretions, an ineffective cough, or vital capacities less than 20 to 25 mL/kg should be admitted to the ICU (112,113). When the vital capacity reaches 15 mL/kg, endotracheal intubation should be strongly considered. Elective intubation can help patients avoid abrupt respiratory failure and mucous plugging (114). Intermittent mandatory ventilation with pressure support is used to reduce alveolar collapse or atelectasis. Positive end-expiratory pressure can reduce complications related to atelectasis (115). If mechanical ventilation is required for more than 2 weeks, tracheostomy should be considered. The most common complications of myasthenic crisis are fever, pneumonia, and atelectasis (86). Aggressive respiratory treatment with suctioning, bronchodilator treatments, sighs, chest physiotherapy, and intermittent positive pressure can reduce the complications of mechanical ventilation and shorten the period that patients are in the intensive care unit (116). Weaning trials should be attempted with patients who show clear improvement of respiratory muscle strength, with the goal to eliminate mandatory ventilation and then reduce the amount of pressure support. Cholinesterase inhibitors are generally discontinued after intubation because of increased secretions and the potential for depolarization blockade. After a definite response to treatment, cholinesterase inhibitors can be restarted at a low dose.

Plasma exchange has been shown to be effective for the treatment of myasthenic crisis and to prepare patients for surgery (117). Many different protocols are used, but a series of five to six exchanges of 2 to 4 liters every other day is most commonly employed. Improvement can usually be seen in 3 to 4 days and can last for several weeks, but is not sustained without the addition of an immune suppressant agent. Side effects of plasma exchange, which can be life threatening, include hypotension, bradycardia, congestive heart failure, venous thrombosis, infection, and dramatic shifts in electrolytes, including calcium. Controlled randomized trials have demonstrated that IVIG is as effective as plasma exchange in patients with myasthenic crises (118). This trial used 1.2 and 2.0 g/kg of IVIG over 2 to 5 days. Patients who fail to respond to IVIG may subsequently respond to plasma exchange (119). Intravenous steroids have been used in high doses in myasthenic crisis in patients who do not respond to IVIG or plasma exchange (120), but this may be complicated by transient worsening of myasthenic weakness that may precipitate the need for, or prolong, mechanical ventilation. Other immune-suppressant medications can be useful as steroid-sparing drugs and as sole therapy for myasthenia, but they take weeks or months to produce improvement, and therefore are not appropriate choices to treat myasthenic crisis.

Thymectomy is indicated in patients with thymoma, and is also accepted therapy for myasthenia gravis without thymoma, particularly in younger patients without thymic involution. However, the absence of class I evidence and the shortcomings of existing case-control or cohort trials have led to a call for prospective randomized controlled clinical trials (121).

Perioperative Care. Myasthenic crisis is common in patients undergoing surgical procedures. The main risk factors for postoperative complications include severe bulbar weakness, chronic myasthenia, respiratory illness, and decreased vital capacity preoperatively (122). Whenever possible, preoperative treatment to improve strength should be undertaken. Plasma exchange or IVIG can be performed preoperatively in patients with bulbar weakness or generalized myasthenia. A response is often seen within 3 to 6 days, although preoperative IVIG has shown a variable time to maximal response (123). Preoperative pulmonary function testing can be performed to assess respiratory function. Drugs that are known to exacerbate myasthenia (Table 149.4) should be avoided whenever possible.

Critical Illness Polyneuropathy and Myopathy

History. Although earlier references are cited (see Lindsay et al. [124,125]), recognition that critically ill patients frequently develop new neuromuscular dysfunction was not widespread until the last decade of the 20th century. In 1984, Bolton et al. (126) described five patients who failed to wean from the ventilator after treatment of sepsis, and were found to have neuromuscular weakness related to an axonal sensorimotor polyneuropathy. They called this *critical illness polyneuropathy* (CIP). In 1992, Sagredo et al. (127) attributed prolonged paralysis, seen in patients in whom vecuronium had been weaned, to persistent plasma levels of vecuronium metabolites in those patients with impaired renal function. Hirano et al. (128) described severe weakness in two critically ill asthmatic patients treated with steroids and nondepolarizing blocking agents. Muscle biopsy demonstrated depletion of thick myosin filaments. They called this *acute quadriplegic myopathy*. Other terms for the same or similar illness have included hydrocortisone myopathy, necrotizing myopathy, thick filament myopathy, postparalysis syndrome, and acute myopathy of intensive care; we will refer to it by the most common designation: critical illness myopathy (CIM). The term *critical illness neuromyopathy* (CINM) is used to refer to patients in whom both neuropathy and myopathy coexist, or when it is uncertain which condition is causing the patient's weakness. The term CINM could also be applied to patients with persistent neuromuscular blockade; however, electrophysiologic studies should exclude this as a contributing factor in most patients.

Epidemiology. The incidence of critical illness neuromyopathy is estimated to be as high as 70% of mechanically ventilated ICU patients with sepsis and multiorgan failure. Witt et al. (129) found, in a prospective study, that 70% of 43 ICU patients with sepsis and failure of more than two organs developed electrophysiologic evidence of peripheral neuropathy, and half of these patients had clinically evident neuropathy with difficulty being weaned from the ventilator. De Jonghe et al. (130) found that 25.3% of ICU patients intubated for 7 or more days developed neuromuscular weakness. All had sensorimotor axonopathy, and all who were biopsied also had myopathy. Bednarik et al. (131) prospectively studied 61 ICU patients with evidence of multiorgan failure; 27% had clinical and 54% electrophysiologic evidence for critical illness neuromyopathy. Bercker et al. (132) found that 60% of 50 consecutive patients with acute respiratory distress syndrome studied retrospectively developed critical illness neuromyopathy.

Pathophysiology

Critical Illness Polyneuropathy. Sepsis and multiorgan failure are the major risk factors for CIP (131,133,134); other risk factors include duration of mechanical ventilation, hyperglycemia, hyperosmolality, and decreased serum albumin (129). The peripheral nervous system is one of the organ systems damaged in systemic inflammatory response syndrome (SIRS). Decreased capillary flow and increased capillary permeability related to sepsis-related cytokine release, and other factors such as a generally high catabolic rate, result in a reduced supply of nutrients, decreased clearance of toxic factors (including medications), and tissue edema. Pathologically, there is axonal degeneration without inflammation, and there is an increase in adhesion molecule expression in nerve (133).

Critical Illness Myopathy. Risk factors for CIM overlap with those for CIP; however, there is more emphasis on primary pulmonary disease (asthma and acute respiratory distress syndrome [ARDS]) and on the use of neuromuscular blocking agents and corticosteroids (130,135). Apoptotic activity may be increased. High corticosteroid levels may increase expression of ubiquitin, leading to increased proteolytic activity (136). Denervation from coexisting CIP may also make the muscle more susceptible. Muscle biopsy shows loss of thick (myosin) filaments; there may also be fiber-type atrophy and/or necrosis (128,137). Whether the different pathologies represent a spectrum of severity or different entities remains unsettled.

Most patients on ventilators are given neuromuscular blocking agents. Normally, the effects of these agents wear off within hours of discontinuation; however, it is not unusual for residual blockade to last 1 to 2 days (127). Early reports of more prolonged weakness after neuromuscular blockade did not consider the effects of CIP and CIM. In a recent review, Murray et al. (135) concluded that nondepolarizing neuromuscular blocking agents may potentiate muscle weakness by a number of mechanisms, including up-regulation of acetylcholine receptors with fetal-type receptors that are less responsive to acetylcholine, presynaptic inhibition of exocytosis of acetylcholine, and potentiation of muscle damage by corticosteroids and by sepsis-induced ischemia.

Clinical Presentation. CIP is preceded by sepsis and failure of more than one organ. Sepsis leads to SIRS, which is manifested by two or more of the following (138):

- Elevated (greater than 38°C) or reduced (less than 36°C) temperature
- Tachycardia (greater than 90 beats/minute)
- Tachypnea (greater than 20 breaths/minute)
- $PaCO_2$ less than 32 mm Hg
- High (greater than 12,000) or low (less than 4,000 cells/μL) white blood cell count

Most patients have a septic encephalopathy manifested by confusion and reduced responsiveness, and most require ventilatory assistance. With antibiotic treatment, sepsis and septic encephalopathy improve, and patients awaken, tracking the examiner with the eyes and demonstrating comprehension with eye movements or weak limb movements; in patients who cannot cooperate for the examination, weakness is manifested by decreased or absent spontaneous limb movement and difficulty weaning from the ventilator. The diagnosis of CIP is further supported if reflexes are absent and if a sensory loss can be demonstrated; however, not all patients with CIP have absent reflexes or sensory loss on examination, and, in many patients, an accurate sensory examination cannot be done. Electrodiagnostic studies are, therefore, key to diagnosis.

CIM may have similar antecedents, but is more likely in the setting of ventilatory failure from asthma (128,137) or ARDS (132). The use of neuromuscular blocking agents (139) and corticosteroids (130) appears to predispose to CIM, although CIM has been reported without either one (140). Clinically, the presentation is similar to that of CIP. Sensation is normal if neuropathy does not coexist, but often confusion and poor communication make it difficult to assess sensation. Here again, electrophysiologic testing is key to diagnosis.

Diagnosis. Critical illness neuromyopathy should be suspected in any critically ill patient whose medical condition is improving but who appears to have trouble moving or cannot be weaned from the ventilator. A diagnostic algorithm is presented in Figure 149.4. The diagnosis is likely in patients with risk factors, particularly sepsis, SIRS, multiorgan failure, prolonged artificial ventilation, hyperglycemia, and exposure to neuromuscular blocking agents or corticosteroids (141). Alternative causes for weakness in the ICU must be considered and, if possible, excluded. These include medications that cause myopathy, neuromuscular blockade, or neuropathy; electrolyte disorders such as hypokalemia or hypophosphatemia; undiagnosed neuromuscular disorders such as myasthenia gravis, Guillain-Barré syndrome, or ALS; and a variety of central nervous system disorders, including ischemic myelopathy, anterior horn cell loss from hypoxia (142), central pontine myelinolysis that most often follows rapid correction of hyponatremia (143), and hemispheric stroke from hypotension, emboli, or hemorrhage (144). West Nile encephalitis (WNE) should be considered in patients who present with fever and encephalopathy, and in those who develop neuromuscular weakness, since WNE can affect anterior horn cells and, less often, peripheral nerves (145). Depending on clinical suspicions, imaging of the brain and spinal cord may be appropriate. If clinical findings suggest neuromuscular weakness rather than a CNS disorder, it may be more efficient to confirm with electrodiagnostic studies than to pursue studies for CNS disorders.

Laboratory studies should include a basic metabolic profile to assess blood sugar and electrolytes. Elevation of creatine kinase (CK) may suggest myopathy, and very high CK suggests rhabdomyolysis. Normal CK does not exclude critical illness myopathy, and mild elevations in CK can be seen with acute denervation. Tests for myasthenia (see above) are indicated when there is a clinical suspicion. Spinal fluid findings are not often reported in CIP. Lumbar puncture is indicated principally if there is clinical suspicion of infection.

Electrodiagnostic testing is helpful to confirm a neuromuscular disorder and to distinguish among disorders of nerve, neuromuscular junction, and muscle (for a more detailed synopsis, see Dhand [146]). Repetitive nerve stimulation at 2 to 3 Hz will show a decremental response (Fig. 149.3) in patients with disorders of neuromuscular transmission. If the patient has been given neuromuscular blocking agents, repeat testing in 1 to 2 days should demonstrate resolution of neuromuscular blockade. Other causes of neuromuscular blockade should be considered if decremental responses persist. Motor nerve conduction studies will show a decreased amplitude CMAP in patients with CIP within several days of the onset of weakness (to allow for Wallerian degeneration). In patients with CIM, the CMAP is also of low amplitude, but may also be prolonged (147). Sensory nerve action potentials are often reduced or absent in CIP, and should be normal in CIM, unless there is coexistent CIP. It should be kept in mind that preexisting neuropathy may account for some of the deficits found on electrophysiologic testing, as, for example, in patients with diabetic neuropathy. Guillain-Barré polyneuropathy can follow surgery or trauma, and could therefore occur in settings similar to the critical illness neuromyopathies. Electrophysiologic findings diagnostic of demyelinating neuropathy—not found in CIP or CIM—would suggest this possibility, leading to a trial of IVIG or plasma exchange. In theory, an axonal form of Guillain-Barré would be electrophysiologically indistinguishable from CIP. This highly unlikely occurrence should be considered in patients who lack the usual risk factors for CIP. Needle EMG studies may show abnormal spontaneous activity in patients with neuropathy, but only after 2 to 3 weeks of denervation. Voluntary activity may be difficult to study in poorly cooperative patients; however, when the patient can make a full effort, there will be reduced recruitment in neuropathy and small polyphasic motor unit potentials in myopathy, helping to differentiate CIP from CIM.

Additional electrodiagnostic studies that may be useful in diagnosis include phrenic nerve stimulation, diaphragmatic EMG, and direct muscle stimulation. While these studies do not require specialized equipment, many electromyographers do not have sufficient experience with them to be confident in their performance or interpretation. Phrenic nerve stimulation in the neck with surface recording over the diaphragm shows a normal response in patients with pulmonary causes of respiratory failure, but a low amplitude or absent response in patients with neuromuscular respiratory weakness. Needle EMG of the diaphragm can be done in patients without severe chronic obstructive pulmonary disease (COPD), ileus, or coagulopathy, and may diagnose denervation or myopathy affecting the diaphragm (148). CIP and CIM may be distinguished by comparing the muscle response to direct muscle stimulation with the response to nerve stimulation. If the response to muscle stimulation is larger than to nerve stimulation, CIP is likely; when both are small, CIM is likely (149,150).

In patients suspected of having CINM, nerve and muscle biopsy may document axonal neuropathy or myopathy with loss of myosin filaments; however, they will only change management if they demonstrate an alternative diagnosis that may be amenable to treatment, such as a demyelinating or vasculitic neuropathy, or an inflammatory myopathy. In patients whose neuromuscular deficits are clearly related to the usual risk factors for CINM, treatable conditions are not sufficiently likely to warrant biopsy (151).

Management. Of the factors that may contribute to the development of CINM, many—like the response to sepsis and the incidence of multiorgan failure—are related to the severity of the presenting critical illness, and are not easily modifiable. It remains to be demonstrated whether the reduced use of corticosteroids or neuromuscular blocking agents will result in a decreased incidence of CIM. It makes sense, however, to eliminate continued exposure to either type of agent whenever possible. It also makes sense to avoid medications that can be neurotoxic, or those that can interfere with neuromuscular transmission. Intensive insulin therapy in critically ill patients has been demonstrated to reduce the risk of CIP by 49% over standard therapy (152). The safety and efficacy of intensive insulin therapy remains controversial, however (153,154), and is currently the subject of several prospective controlled multicenter studies.

Patients with neuropathy will be more prone to pressure palsies, and thus, great care must be taken in positioning and support to avoid this complication. Physical therapy should be directed toward avoiding contractures until the patient is able to participate in strengthening exercises.

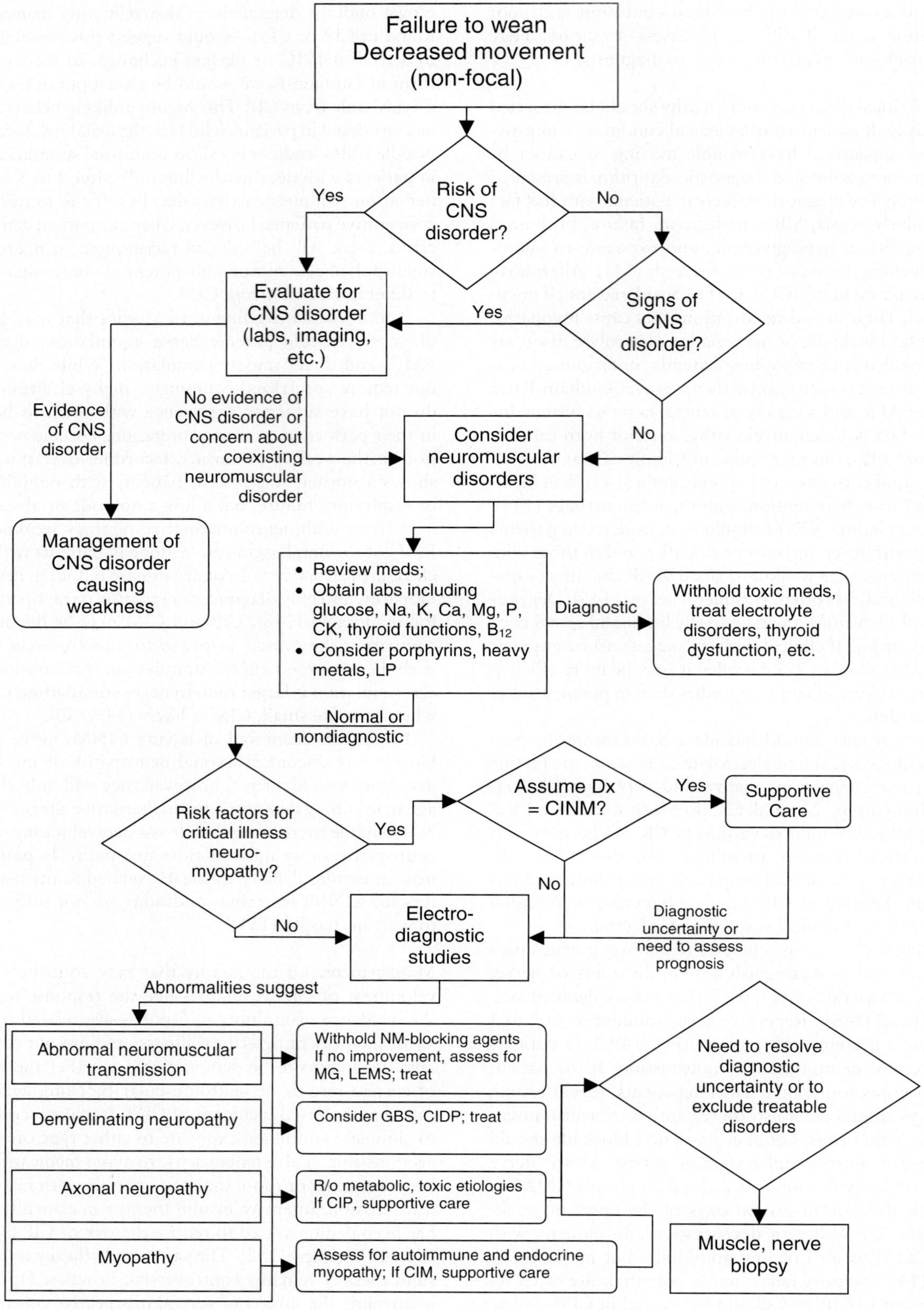

FIGURE 149.4. Algorithm for diagnostic evaluation and management of weakness developing in the intensive care setting. CIDP, chronic inflammatory demyelinating polyneuropathy; CIM, critical illness myopathy; CINM, critical illness neuromyopathy; CIP, critical illness polyneuropathy; CK, creatine kinase; CNS, central nervous system; GBS, Guillain-Barré syndrome; LEMS, Lambert-Eaton myasthenic syndrome; LP, lipid peroxidation; MG, myasthenia gravis; NM, neuromuscular.

Prognosis. There is no comprehensive study on prognosis in CINM. Mortality is high early in the course, and is related to the underlying critical illness (155). Patients with CINM who survive the acute illness and who begin to recover strength are likely to continue to recover over the weeks to months that follow; it is sufficient to monitor improvement with clinical assessment of strength. Patients with CINM who fail to show clinical improvement in strength can be evaluated with repeat electrophysiologic testing. Patients with electrophysiologic evidence of severe axonal loss, with small or absent responses to nerve stimulation and abundant positive waves and fibrillations on needle EMG, will recover slowly if at all, and are likely to have residual deficits—sometimes severe (129,155–157). Although the task of regenerating severely damaged axons may be more daunting than regenerating muscle, it is not clear whether the prognosis for recovery from CIM is better than from CIP (158,159).

SUMMARY

Neuromuscular diseases may necessitate admission for intensive care to provide airway protection and respiratory support. Disorders such as Guillain-Barré syndrome and myasthenia gravis can lead to precipitous weakness, and require careful monitoring so that assistance can be given before hypoxemia occurs. Management must also address autonomic dysfunction, sensory loss, pain, and psychological distress. Neuromuscular disorders of autoimmune pathogenesis often respond to specific treatment, and a favorable outcome can be expected for the majority of such patients. The critical illness neuromyopathies have become the most common cause of weakness that develop in the intensive care setting, requiring critical care physicians to be familiar with their presentation, diagnosis, and management. Although no specific treatment is available for CINM, most patients improve with supportive care. A minority, however, are left with irreversible weakness. Attempts to address the factors that predispose to CINM may eventually reduce the burden of this recently discovered group of neuromuscular disorders.

References

1. Bolton CF, Gilbert JJ, Hahn AF, et al. Polyneuropathy in critically ill patients. *J Neurol Neurosurg Psychiatry.* 1984;47:1223.
2. Lacomis D, Petrella JT, Giuliani MJ. Causes of neuromuscular weakness in the intensive care unit: a study of ninety-two patients. *Muscle Nerve.* 1998;21:610.
3. Young RR, Asbury AK, Corbett JF, et al. Pure pandysautonomia with recovery: description and discussion of diagnostic criteria. *Brain.* 1975;98:613.
4. Waxman SG, Sabin TD. Diabetic truncal polyneuropathy. *Arch Neurol.* 1981;38:46.
5. Fromm GB, Wisdom PJ, Block AJ. Amyotrophic lateral sclerosis presenting with respiratory failure: diaphragmatic paralysis and dependence on mechanical ventilation in two patients. *Chest.* 1977;71:612.
6. Chen R, Grand'Maison F, Strong MJ, et al. Motor neuron disease presenting as acute respiratory failure. A clinical and pathological study. *J Neurol Neurosurg Psychiatry.* 1996;60:455.
7. Dushay KM, Zibrak JD, Jensen WA. Myasthenia gravis presenting as isolated respiratory failure. *Chest.* 1990;97:232.
8. Rosenow EC 3rd, Engel AG. Acid maltase deficiency in adults presenting as respiratory failure. *Am J Med.* 1978;64:485.
9. Mohr JP. Distal field infarction. *Neurology.* 1969;12:279.
10. Riggs JE. Neurologic manifestations of electrolyte disturbances. *Neurol Clin.* 2002;20:227.
11. Kimura J, Butzer JF. F-wave conduction velocity in Guillain-Barré syndrome. Assessment of nerve segment between axilla and spinal cord. *Arch Neurol.* 1975;32:524.
12. Kuwabara S, Ogawara K, Mizobuchi K, et al. Isolated absence of F waves and proximal axonal dysfunction in Guillain-Barré syndrome with antiganglioside antibodies *J Neurol Neurosurg Psychiatry.* 2000;68:191.
13. Maddison P, Newsom-Davis J, Mills KR. Distribution of electrophysiological abnormality in Lambert-Eaton myasthenic syndrome. *J Neurol Neurosurg Psychiatry.* 1998;65:213.
14. Chalela JA. Pearls and pitfalls in the intensive care management of Guillain-Barré syndrome. *Semin Neurol.* 2004;21:399.
15. Borel CO, Guy J. Ventilatory management in critical neurologic illness. In: Jordan KG ed. *Neurologic Clinics.* Philadelphia: WB Saunders; 1995:627.
16. Ropper AJ, Wijdicks EFM, Truax BT. General care. In: Ropper AH, Wijdicks EFM, Truax BT, eds. *Guillain-Barré Syndrome.* Philadelphia: FA Davis; 1991:237.
17. Fulgham JR, Wijdicks EFM. Guillain-Barré syndrome. In: Diringer M, ed. *Critical Care Clinics: Update on Neurologic Critical Care.* Philadelphia: WB Saunders; 1997:1.
18. Bowes D. The doctor as a patient: an encounter with Guillain-Barré syndrome. *Can Med Assoc J.* 1984;131:1343.
19. Winkel LP, Hagemans ML, van Doom PA, et al. The natural course of non-classic Pompe's disease; a review of 225 published cases. *J Neurol.* 2005;252:875.
20. Dalakas MC, Hohlfeld R. Polylmyositis and dermatomyositis. *Lancet.* 2003;362:1762.
21. Landry O. Note sur la paralysie ascendante aiguë. *Gaz Hebd Med Paris.* 1859;6:472.
22. Guillain G, Barré JA, Strohl A. Sur un syndrome de radiculonévrite avec hyperalbuminose du liquide céphalo-rachidien sans réaction cellulaire. Remarques sur les caractéres cliniques et graphiques des réflexes tendineux. *Bull Mem Soc Med Hop Paris.* 1916;40:1462.
23. Melnick SC, Flewett TH. Role of infection in the Guillain-Barre syndrome. *J Neurol Neurosurg Psychiatry.* 1964;27:385.
24. Hurwitz ES, Holman RC, Nelson DB, et al. National surveillance for Guillain-Barre syndrome: January 1978–March 1979. *Neurology.* 1983; 33:150.
25. Waksman BH, Adams RD. A comparative study of experimental allergic neuritis in the rabbit, guinea pig, and mouse. *J Neuropathol Exp Neurol.* 1956;15:293.
26. National Institute of Neurological and Communicative Disorders and Stroke ad hoc Committee (NINCDS). Criteria for diagnosis of Guillain-Barré syndrome. *Ann Neurol.* 1978;3:565.
27. Griffin JW, Sheikh K. The Guillain-Barré syndromes. In: Dyck PJ, Thomas PK, eds. *Peripheral Neuropathy.* 4th ed. Philadelphia: Elsevier Saunders; 2005:2197.
28. McKhann GM, Cornblath DR, Griffin JW, et al. Acute motor axonal neuropathy: a frequent cause of acute flaccid paralysis in China. *Ann Neurol.* 1993;33:333.
29. Griffin JW, Li CY, Ho TW, et al. Pathology of the motor-sensory axonal Guillain-Barré syndrome. *Ann Neurol.* 1996;39:17.
30. Hughes RAC, Cornblath DR. Guillain-Barré syndrome. *Lancet.* 2005; 366:1653.
31. Young RR, Asbury AK, Adams RD, et al. Pure pandysautonomia with recovery. *Trans Am Neurol Assoc.* 1969;94:355.
32. Young RR, Asbury AK, Corbett JL, et al. Pure pandysautonomia with recovery: description and discussion of diagnostic criteria. *Brain.* 1975; 98:613.
33. Pan CL, Yuki N, Koga M, et al. Acute sensory ataxic neuropathy associated with monospecific anti-GD1b IgG antibody. *Neurology.* 2001;57:1316.
34. Fisher CM. An unusual variant of acute idiopathic polyneuritis: syndrome of ophthalmoplegia, ataxia and areflexia. *N Engl J Med.* 1956;255:57.
35. Shimamura H, Miura H, Iwaki Y, et al. Clinical, electrophysiological, and serological overlap between Miller Fisher syndrome and acute sensory ataxic neuropathy. *Acta Neurol Scand.* 2002;105:411.
36. Chio A, Cocito D, Leone M, et al. Guillain-Barré syndrome: a prospective, population-based incidence and outcome survey. *Neurology.* 2003; 60:1146.
37. Alter M. The epidemiology of Guillain-Barré syndrome. *Ann Neurol.* 1990; 27(Suppl):S7.
38. Hadden RDM, Karch H, Hartung H-P, et al. Preceding infections, immune factors, and outcome in Guillain-Barre syndrome. *Neurology.* 2001;56:758.
39. Van Koningsveld R, Schmitz PIM, Ang CW, et al. Infections and course of disease in mild forms of Guillain-Barre syndrome. *Neurology.* 2002;58:610.
40. Hemachudha T, Griffin DE, Chen WW, et al. Immunologic studies of rabies vaccination-induced GBS. *Neurology.* 1988;38:375.
41. Kaplan JE, Katona P, Hurwitz ES, et al. Guillain-Barré syndrome in the United States, 1989–1980 and 1980–1981. Lack of an association with influenza vaccination. *JAMA.* 1982;248:698.
42. Lasky T, Terracciano GJ, Magder L, et al. The Guillain-Barré syndrome and the 1992–1993 and 1993–1994 influenza vaccines. *N Engl J Med.* 1998;339:1797.
43. Asbury AK, Arnason BG, Adams RD. The inflammatory lesion in idiopathic polyneuritis. Its role in pathogenesis. *Medicine.* 1969;48:173.
44. Prineas JW. Acute idiopathic polyneuritis. An electronmicroscope study. *Lab Invest.* 1972;26:133.
45. Prineas JW. Pathology of the Guillain-Barré syndrome. *Ann Neurol.* 1981; 9(suppl):6.

46. Lampert PW. Electron microscopic studies on ordinary and hyperacute experimental allergic encephalomyelitis. *Acta Neuropathol.* 1967;9:99.
47. Kieseier BC, Kiefer R, Gold R, et al. Advances in understanding and treatment of immune-mediated disorders of the peripheral nervous system. *Muscle Nerve.* 2004;30:131.
48. Waksman NH, Adams RD. Allergic neuritis: an experimental disease in rabbits induced by the injection of peripheral nervous tissue and adjuvant. *J Exp Med.* 1955;102:213.
49. Hafer-Macko CE, Sheikh KA, Li CY, et al. Immune attack on the Schwann cell surface in acute inflammatory demyelinating polyneuropathy. *Ann Neurol.* 1996;39:627.
50. Griffin JW, Li CY, Macko C, et al. Early nodal changes in the acute motor axonal neuropathy pattern of the Guillain-Barré syndrome. *J Neurocytol.* 1996;25:33.
51. Hafer-Macko C, Hsieh ST, Li CY, et al. Acute motor axonal neuropathy: an antibody-mediated attack on axolemma. *Ann Neurol.* 1996;40:635.
52. Yuki N, Susuki K, Koga M, et al. Carbohydrate mimicry between human ganglioside GM1 and *Campylobacter jejuni* lipooligosaccharide causes Guillain-Barré syndrome. *Proc Natl Acad Sci U S A.* 2004;101:11404.
53. Chiba A, Kusunoki S, Shimizu T, et al. *Ann Neurol* 1992;31:6779.
54. Willison HJ. The immunobiology of Guillain-Barre syndromes. *J Peripher Nerv Syst.* 2005;10:94.
55. Koga M, Gilbert M, Li J, et al. Antecedent infections in Fisher syndrome: a common pathogenesis of molecular mimicry. *Neurology.* 2005;64:1605.
56. Bernsen RAJAM, de Jager AEJ, Schmitz PIM, et al. Long-term sensory deficit after Guillain-Barré syndrome. *J Neurol.* 2001;248:483.
57. Ropper AH, Wijdicks EFM, Truax, BT. *Guillain-Barré Syndrome.* Philadelphia: FA Davis; 1991.
58. Masucci EF, Kurtzke JG. Diagnostic criteria for the Guillain-Barré syndrome. An analysis of 50 cases. *J Neurol Sci.* 1971;13:483.
59. Kuwabara S, Ogawara K, Misawa S, et al. Sensory nerve conduction in demyelinating and axonal Guillain-Barre syndromes. *Eur Neurol.* 2004; 51:196.
60. Maier H, Schmidbauer M, Pfausler B, et al. Central nervous system pathology in patients with the Guillain-Barré syndrome. *Brain.* 1997;120:451.
61. Jeha LE, Sila CA, Lederman RJ, et al. West Nile virus infection: a new acute paralytic illness. *Neurology.* 2003;61:55.
62. Brannagan TH, Zhou Y. HIV-associated Guillain-Barré syndrome. *J Neurol Sci.* 2003;208:39.
63. Olney RK, Aminof MJ. Electrodiagnostic features of the Guillain-Barré syndrome: the relative sensitivity of different techniques. *Neurology.* 1990; 40:471.
64. Hughes RAC, Wijdicks E, Barohn RJ, et al. Practice parameter: immunotherapy for Guillain-Barré syndrome: report of the Quality Standards Subcommittee of the American Academy of Neurology. *Neurology.* 2003;61:736.
65. Osterman PO, Fagius J, Lundemo G, et al. Beneficial effects of plasma exchange in acute inflammatory polyradiculoneuropathy. *Lancet.* 1984; 2:1296.
66. The Guillain-Barré Syndrome Study Group. Plasmapheresis and acute Guillain-Barré syndrome. *Neurology.* 1985;35:1096.
67. Raphaël JC, Chevret S, Hughes RA, et al. Plasma exchange for Guillain-Barré syndrome. *Cochrane Database Syst Rev.* 2002;2:CD001798.
68. van der Meché FGA, Schmitz PIM, Dutch Guillain-Barré Study Group. A randomized trial comparing intravenous immune globulin and plasma exchange in Guillain-Barré syndrome. *N Engl J Med.* 1992;326:1123.
69. Hughes RAC, van der Meché FG. Corticosteroids for treating Guillain-Barré syndrome. *Cochrane Database Syst Rev.* 2000;2:CD001446.
70. Pandey CK, Bose N, Garg G, et al. Gabapentin for the treatment of pain in Guillain-Barré syndrome: a double-blinded, placebo-controlled, crossover study. *Anesth Analg.* 2002;95:1719.
71. Cornblath DR, Mellits ED, Griffin JW, et al. Motor conduction studies in Guillain-Barré syndrome: description and prognostic value. *Ann Neurol.* 1988;23:354.
72. De la Cour CD, Jakobsen J. Residual neuropathy in long-term population-based follow-up of Guillain-Barré syndrome. *Neurology.* 2005;64:246.
73. Bernsen RAJAM, de Jager AEJ, Schmitz PIM, et al. Long-term sensory deficits after Guillain-Barré syndrome. *J Neurol.* 2001;248:483.
74. Forsberg A, Pressc R, Einarssonb U, et al. Impairment in Guillain-Barré syndrome during the first 2 years after onset: a prospective study. *J Neurol Sci.* 2004;227:131.
75. Pearce JMS. Mary Broadfoot Walker (1888–1974): a historic discovery in myasthenia gravis. *Eur Neurol.* 2005;53:51.
76. Drachman DB. Myasthenia gravis: an illustrated history (book review). *N Engl J Med.* 2003;348:181.
77. Walker MB. Treatment of myasthenia gravis with physostigmine. *Lancet.* 1934;i:1200.
78. Simpson JA. Immunological disturbances in myasthenia gravis with a report of Hashimoto's disease developing after thymectomy. *J Neurol Neurosurg Psychiatry.* 1964;27:485.
79. Patrick J, Lindstrom J. Autoimmune response to acetylcholine receptor. *Science.* 1973;180:871.
80. Almon RR, Andrew CG, Appel SH. Serum globulin in myasthenia gravis: inhibition of a-bungarotoxin binding to acetylcholine receptors. *Science.* 1974;186:55.
81. Oosterhuis HJ. The natural course of myasthenia gravis: a long-term follow-up study. *J Neurol Neurosurg Psychiatry.* 1989;52:1121.
82. Drachman DB. Myasthenia gravis. *N Engl J Med.* 1994;330:1797.
83. Phillips LH II. The epidemiology of myasthenia gravis. *Ann N Y Acad Sci.* 2003;998:407.
84. Richman DP, Agius MA. Myasthenia gravis: pathogenesis and treatment. *Semin Neurol.* 1994;14:106.
85. Gracy DR, Divertie MB, Howard FM. Mechanical ventilation for respiratory failure in myasthenia gravis: two-year experience with 22 patients. *Mayo Clin Proc.* 1983;58:597.
86. Thomas CE, Mayer SA, Gungor Y, et al. Myasthenic crisis: clinical features, mortality, complications, and risk factors for prolonged intubation. *Neurology.* 1997;48:1253.
87. Engel AG. Anatomy and molecular architecture of the neuromuscular junction. In: Engel Ag, ed. *Myasthenia Gravis and Myasthenic Disorders.* Oxford: Oxford University Press; 1999:2.
88. Ruff RL. Neurophysiology of the neuromuscular junction: overview. *Ann N Y Acad Sci.* 2003;998:1.
89. Lindrstrom J. Acetylcholine receptor structure. In: Kaminiski HL, ed. *Myasthenia Gravis and Related Disorders.* Totowa, NJ: Humana Press; 2003:15.
90. Lindstrom JM, Seybold MD, Lennon VA, et al. Antibody to acetylcholine receptor in myasthenia gravis: prevalence, clinical correlates, and diagnostic value. *Neurology.* 1976;26:1054.
91. Drachman D, Angus CW, Adams RN, et al. Effect of myasthenic patients' immunoglobulin on acetylcholine receptor turnover: selectivity of degradation process. *Proc Natl Acad Sci U S A.* 1978;75:3422.
92. Hoch W, McConville J, Helms S, et al. Auto-antibodies to the receptor tyrosine kinase MuSK in patients with myasthenia gravis without acetylcholine receptor antibodies. *Nat Med.* 2001;7:365.
93. Evoli A, Tonali PA, Padua L, et al. Clinical correlates with anti-MuSk antibodies in generalized myasthenia gravis. *Brain.* 2003;126:2304.
94. Hohlfeld R, Wekerle H. The thymus in myasthenia gravis. *Neurol Clin.* 1994;12:331.
95. Kao I, Drachman DB. Thymic muscle cells bear acetylcholine receptors: possible relation to myasthenia gravis. *Science.* 1977;195:74.
96. Kaminski HJ, Fenstermaker RA, Abdul-Karim FW, et al. Acetylcholine receptor subunit gene expression in thymic tissue. *Muscle Nerve.* 1993; 16:1332.
97. Iwasa K. Striational autoantibodies in myasthenia gravis mainly react with ryanodine receptor. *Muscle Nerve.* 1997;20:753.
98. Behan PO. Immune disease and HLA associations with myasthenia gravis. *J Neurol Neurosurg Psychiatry.* 1980;43:611.
99. Pascuzzi RM. Medications and myasthenia gravis (A reference for health care professionals). Myasthenia Gravis Foundation of America. 2007. http://www.myasthenia.org/hp_edmaterials.cfm. Accessed June 12, 2007.
100. Perrot X, Bernard N, Vial C, et al. Myasthenia gravis exacerbation or unmasking associated with telithromycin treatment. *Neurology.* 2006;67: 2256.
101. Garrity ER. Respiratory failure due to disorders of the chest wall and respiratory muscles. In: MacDonnell KF, Fahey PJ, Segal MS, eds. *Respiratory Intensive Care.* Boston: Little Brown; 1987:312.
102. Borel CO, Teitelbaum JS, Hanley DF. Ventilatory failure and carbon monoxide response in ventilatory failure due to myasthenia gravis and Guillain-Barre syndrome. *Crit Care Med.* 1993;21:1717.
103. Tether JE. Management of myasthenic and cholinergic crisis. *Am J Med.* 1955;19:740.
104. Ashworth B, Hunter AR. Respiratory failure in myasthenia gravis. *Proc R Soc Med.* 1971;64:489.
105. Daroff RB. The office Tensilon test for ocular myasthenia gravis. *Arch Neurol.* 1986;43:843.
106. Okun MS, Charriez CM, Bhatti MR, et al. Asystole induced by edrophonium following beta blockade. *Neurology.* 2001;57:739.
107. Lennon VA. Serological diagnosis of myasthenic gravis and Lambert-Eaton myasthenic syndrome. In: Lisak RP, ed. *Handbook of Myasthenic Gravis and Myasthenic Syndromes.* New York: Marcel Dekker; 1994:149.
108. Cikes N, Momi MY, Williams CL, et al. Striational autoantibodies: quantitative detection by enzyme immunoassay in myasthenia gravis, thymoma, and recipients of D-penicillamine or allogenic bone marrow. *Mayo Clinic Proc.* 1998;63:474.
109. Skeie Go, Romi F, Aarli JA, et al. Pathogenesis of myositis and myasthenia associated with titin ryanodine receptor antibodies. *Ann N Y Acad Sci.* 2003;998:343.
110. Howard JF, Sanders DB, Massey JM. The electrodiagnosis of myasthenia gravis and the Lambert-Eaton myasthenic syndrome. *Neurol Clin.* 1994; 12:305.
111. Oh SJ, Kim DE, Kuruoglu R, et al. Diagnostic sensitivity of the laboratory tests in myasthenia gravis. *Muscle Nerve.* 1992;15:720.
112. Bedlack RS, Sanders DB. On the concept of myasthenic crisis. *J Clin Neuromusc Dis.* 2002;4:40.
113. Rabinstein AA, Wijdicks EFM. Warning signs of imminent respiratory failure in neurological patients. *Semin Neurol.* 2003;23:97.
114. Bennet DA, Bleck TP. Recognizing impending respiratory failure from neuromuscular causes. *J Crit Illness.* 1998;3:46.
115. Juel VC. Myasthenia gravis: management of myasthenic crisis and perioperative care. *Semin Neurol.* 2004;24:75.

116. Varelas PN, Chua HC, Natterman J, et al. Ventilatory care in myasthenia gravis crisis: assessing the baseline adverse event rate. *Crit Care Med.* 2002;30:2663.
117. Antozzi C, Gemma M, Regi B, et al. A short plasma exchange protocol is effective in severe myasthenia gravis. *J Neurol.* 1991;238:103.
118. Gajdos P, Chevert S, Clair B, et al. Myasthenia Gravis Clinical Study Group. Clinical trial of plasma exchange and high-dose intravenous immunoglobulin in myasthenia gravis. *Ann Neurol.* 1997;41:789.
119. Stricker RB, Kwiatkowska BJ, Habis JA, et al. Myasthenic crisis: response to plasmapheresis following failure of intravenous gamma-globulin. *Arch Neurol.* 1993;50:837.
120. Arsura El, Brunner NG, Namba T, et al. High-dose intravenous methylprednisolone in myasthenia gravis. *Arch Neurol.* 1985;42:1149.
121. Gronseth GS, Barohn RJ. Practice parameter: thymectomy for autoimmune myasthenia gravis (an evidence-based review): report of the Quality Standards Subcommittee of the American Academy of Neurology. *Neurology.* 2000;55:7.
122. Leventhal SR, Orkin FK, Hirsh RA. Prediction for postoperative mechanical ventilation in myasthenia gravis. *Anesthesiology.* 1980;53:26.
123. Huang C-s, Hsu H-s, Kao K-P, et al. Intravenous immunoglobulin in the preparation of thymectomy for myasthenia gravis. *Acta Neurol Scand.* 2003;108:136.
124. Lindsay AE, Dimachkie M, Pulley MT, et al. Critical illness myopathy and polyneuropathy. *Medlink Neurol.* 2006.
125. Gorson KC. Approach to neuromuscular disorders in the intensive care unit. *Neurocrit Care.* 2006;3:195.
126. Bolton CF, Gilbert JJ, Hahn AF, et al. Polyneuropathy in critically ill patients. *J Neurol Neurosurg Psychiatry.* 1984;47:1223.
127. Sagredo V, Caldwell JE, Matthay MA, et al. Persistent paralysis in critically ill patients after long-term administration of vecuronium. *N Engl J Med.* 1992;327:524.
128. Hirano M, Ott BR, Raps EC. Acute quadriplegic myopathy: complication of treatment with steroids, nondepolarizing blocking agents, or both. *Neurology.* 1992;42:2082.
129. Witt NJ, Zochodne DW, Bolton CF, et al. Peripheral nerve function in sepsis and multiple organ failure. *Chest.* 1991;99:176.
130. De Jonghe B, Sharshar T, Lefaucheur J-P, et al. Paresis acquired in the intensive care unit. A prospective multicenter study. *JAMA.* 2002;288:2859.
131. Bednarik J, Vondracek P, Dusek L, et al. Risk factors for critical illness polyneuropathy. *J Neurol.* 2005;252:343.
132. Bercker S, Weber-Carstens S, Deja M, et al. Critical illness polyneuropathy and myopathy in patients with acute respiratory distress syndrome. *Crit Care Med.* 2005;33:711.
133. Zochodne DW, Bolton CF, Wells GA, et al. Critical illness polyneuropathy: a complication of sepsis and multiple organ failure. *Brain.* 1987;110: 819.
134. de Letter MA, Schmitz PI, Visser LH, et al. Risk factors for the development of polyneuropathy and myopathy in critically ill patients. *Crit Care Med.* 2001;29:2281–2286.
135. Murray MJ, Brull SJ, Bolton CF. Brief review: nondepolarizing neuromuscular blocking drugs and critical illness myopathy. *Can J Anesth.* 2006;53:1148.
136. Minetti C, Hirano M, Morreale G, et al. Ubiquitin expression in acute steroid myopathy with loss of thick myosin filaments. *Muscle Nerve.* 1996; 19:94.
137. Danon MJ, Carpenter S. Myopathy and thick filament (myosin) loss following prolonged paralysis with vecuronium during steroid treatment. *Muscle Nerve.* 1991;14:1131.
138. Bone RC, Sprung CL, Sibbald WJ. Definitions for sepsis and organ failure. *Crit Care Med.* 1992;20:724.
139. Adnet F, Dhissi G, Borron SW, et al. Complication profiles of adult asthmatics requiring paralysis during mechanical ventilation. *Intensive Care Med.* 2001;27(11):1729.
140. Hoke A, Rewcastle NB, Zochodne DW. Acute quadriplegic myopathy unrelated to steroids or paralyzing agents: quantitative EMG studies. *Can J Neurol Sci.* 1999;26:325.
141. Deem S. Intensive-care-unit-acquired muscle weakness. *Respir Care.* 2006; 51:1042.
142. Azzarelli B, Roessmann U. Diffuse "anoxic" myelopathy. *Neurology.* 1977; 27:1049.
143. Riggs JE. Neurological manifestations of electrolyte disturbances. *Neurol Clin.* 2002;30:227.
144. Maramattom BV, Wijdicks EFM. Acute neuromuscular weakness in the intensive care unit. *Crit Care Med.* 2006;34:2835.
145. Glass JD, Samuels O, Rich MM. Poliomyelitis due to West Nile virus. *N Engl J Med.* 2002;347:1280.
146. Dhand UK. Clinical approach to the weak patient in the intensive care unit. *Respir Care.* 2006;51:1024.
147. Parak EJ, Nishida T, Sufit RL, et al. Prolonged compound muscle action potential duration in critical illness myopathy. Report of nine cases. *J Clin Neuromusc Dis.* 2004;5:176.
148. Bolton CF. AAEM minimonograph #40: clinical neurophysiology of the respiratory system. *Muscle Nerve.* 1993;16:809.
149. Rich MM, Teener JW, Raps EC, et al. Muscle is electrically inexcitable in acute quadriplegic myopathy. *Neurology.* 1996;46:731.
150. Lefaucheur JP, Nordine T, Rodriguez P, et al. Origin of ICU acquired paresis determined by direct muscle stimulation. *J Neurol Neurosurg Psychiatry.* 2006;77:500.
151. Lacomis D, Zochodne D, Bird SJ. Critical illness myopathy. *Muscle Nerve.* 2000;23:1785.
152. Van den Berghe G, Schoonheydt K, Becx P, et al. Insulin therapy protects the central and peripheral nervous system of intensive care patients. *Neurology.* 2005;64:1348.
153. Malhotra A. Intensive insulin in intensive care. *N Engl J Med.* 2006; 354:516.
154. Brunkhorst FM, Kuhnt E, Engel C, et al. Intensive insulin therapy in patient with severe sepsis and septic shock is associated with an increased rate of hypoglycemia: results from a randomized multicenter study (VISEP). *Infection.* 2005;33(Suppl):19.
155. Lacomis D, Petrella JT, Giuliani MJ. Causes of neuromuscular weakness in the intensive care unit: a study of ninety-two patients. *Muscle Nerve.* 1998;21:610.
156. Zifko UA. Long-term outcome of critical illness polyneuropathy. *Muscle Nerve.* 2000;9(Suppl):S49.
157. Latronico N, Shehu I, Seghelini E. Neuromuscular sequelae of critical illness. *Curr Opin Crit Care.* 2005;11:381.
158. Latronico N, Fenzi F, Boniotti C, et al. Acute reversible paralysis in critically ill patients. *Acta Anaesthesiol Ital.* 1993;44:157.
159. Latronico N, Fenzi F, Recupero D, et al. critical illness myopathy and neuropathy. *Lancet.* 1996;347:1579.

CHAPTER 150 ■ BEHAVIORAL DISTURBANCES IN THE INTENSIVE CARE UNIT

RAMONA O. HOPKINS • JAMES C. JACKSON

Advances in critical care have led to improved survival rates among those admitted to intensive care units (ICUs). In the United States approximately 55,000 patients are treated in ICUs each day (1). At least 40% of adult ICU patients require mechanical ventilation (2). Patients who require long-term mechanical ventilation (>3 days) represent 4% to 10% of critical care admissions and consume 30% to 50% of critical care resources (3). Critical illness often results in multiple system organ dysfunction, including neurologic dysfunction, and is associated with poor neurologic outcomes (4). Investigations of the effects of critical illness on neurologic dysfunction have been relatively neglected compared to other organ systems. The incidence of neurologic dysfunction or injury has been underestimated, underreported, and only recently studied in critically ill patients. The only study that assessed neurologic organ dysfunction in critically ill patients found that a higher severity of the initial neurologic dysfunction (e.g., lower Glasgow coma score) was associated with higher 30-day mortality. No change or worsening of the severity of the Glasgow coma score from the first to third ICU day was also associated with higher 30-day mortality (5). Neurologic injury following critical illness involves both the central and peripheral nervous systems and contributes to mortality and morbidity (6). Neurologic morbidities include polyneuropathy, encephalopathy, delirium, and cognitive impairments.

Medical and surgical management of critical illnesses can, and frequently does, result in *de novo* behavioral disturbances, including delirium and cognitive impairments. This chapter will focus on behavioral disturbances associated with critical illness, with an emphasis on delirium and chronic cognitive impairments.

DELIRIUM: AN ACUTE BEHAVIORAL DISTURBANCE

Delirium is a neurobehavioral syndrome characterized by acute confusion, inattention, disorganized thinking, and a fluctuating course of mental status changes (7,8). Although delirium is often thought of as a unitary construct, such a concept is simplistic and potentially misleading. The motoric subtypes of delirium are hypoactive, hyperactive, and mixed (8). *Hypoactive* or "quiet" delirium is characterized by reduced mental and physical activity and inattention (8). In contrast, *hyperactively* delirious patients are agitated, combative, and at risk for self-extubation, reintubation, pulling out central lines, and falls. Delirium is a dynamic condition and often fluctuates between the hypoactive or hyperactive delirium (9). In ICU populations, a mixed clinical picture is common (10). Given the multiple possible presentations, it is not uncommon for clinicians to miss the diagnosis of delirium (11). A large survey found delirium to be underdiagnosed by 80% of physicians (12). Standardized ICU examinations using the reliable, sensitive, and specific CAM (Confusion Assessment Method)-ICU (13) allows for accurate detection and analysis of delirium.

As others have observed (14), delirium may be the most common psychiatric condition experienced by hospitalized elderly, affecting between 15% and 20% of hospitalized medical patients (15,16), 25% to 65% of surgical patients (17), and as many as 80% of patients in ICU settings (13,18). Although once considered benign (19), recent evidence has linked delirium with various adverse outcomes, including prolonged hospitalization (20–22), poor surgical recovery (23), and increased morbidity and mortality (24). Delirium is also associated with adverse cognitive outcomes in critically ill patients (25) (see section on the association between delirium and cognitive outcomes below). Although delirium may be a sign of emerging cognitive impairment, it is clearly *not* the case that the cognitive decline experienced by many patients with delirium is solely or primarily related to pre-existing cognitive impairment. For example, Jackson et al. (25) excluded patients with probable early dementia and found nearly one third of the ICU patients (all with delirium) with cognitive impairments at 6 months. Thus, delirium is not simply a marker of pre-existing subclinical or early dementia.

CHRONIC COGNITIVE IMPAIRMENTS

Critical illness and its medical and surgical management can and frequently do result in *de novo* cognitive impairments. Cognitive processes or functions are defined as ways of experiencing and thinking about the world and include intelligence, attention, learning, memory, language, visual spatial abilities, and executive function (e.g., reasoning, decision making, planning, problem solving, working memory, sequencing, and executive control). Research is limited regarding cognitive outcomes in survivors of critical illness; however, these patients are at risk to develop long-term or chronic cognitive impairments (25–29). In ICU survivors, approximately one third or more will develop chronic cognitive impairment (25). Although it is difficult to make comparisons across studies due to different definitions of cognitive sequelae, neuropsychological tests administered, time to follow-up, patient population, study design (prospective vs. retrospective), or inclusion of a control group, current data suggest that cognitive impairments are common in survivors of critical illness.

NATURE OF COGNITIVE IMPAIRMENTS

Currently, there are 10 cohorts totaling approximately 455 patients that have assessed long-term cognitive impairments following critical illness (30–40). The populations of the patient cohorts include five studies in acute respiratory distress syndrome (ARDS) patients (30,34,35,38,41,42)—one study of acute lung injury (40), one study in patients with respiratory failure (42), one study in medical ICU patients (39), and two studies in general ICU patients (32,36). The time to cognitive assessment is variable, with most of the cognitive follow-up occurring during the first year post hospital discharge (43). The evidence suggests that 25% to 78% of ICU survivors experience cognitive impairments (30,31,33–40,42). Among specific populations, such as patients with ARDS, the prevalence of cognitive impairments is as high as 78% at hospital discharge, 46% at 1 year (30), and 25% at 6 years (40). A prospective study found cognitive impairments in 70% of ARDS patients at hospital discharge, 45% at 1 year, and 47% at 2 years (42), with almost half of the patient scores falling below the sixth percentile of the normal distribution of cognitive function. The cognitive impairments occur in various cognitive domains (Table 150.1). The cognitive impairments in critically ill patients are similar to those reported in other populations such as carbon monoxide poisoning (44) and following elective coronary artery bypass graft surgery (45).

In the general population of critically ill patients, Jackson et al. (25) found that 33% had chronic cognitive impairments

TABLE 150.1

COGNITIVE IMPAIRMENTS OBSERVED FOLLOWING CRITICAL ILLNESS

COGNITIVE DOMAINS	SPECIFIC COGNITIVE IMPAIRMENTS
Attention	Divided attention Focused attention Sustained attention
Memory	Explicit or declarative Recall (verbal and nonverbal) Recognition (verbal and nonverbal) Short-term memory
Intelligence	Verbal intelligence Performance intelligence Full-scale (general) intelligence
Language	Verbal fluency
Visual spatial	Apraxia Visuoconstruction
Executive function	Decision making Executive control Impulsivity Perseveration Planning Problem solving Shifting sets Working memory
Mental processing speed	Slow mental processing speed
Motor	Grip strength

(defined using a very conservative definition of impairment of 2 test scores 2 standard deviations below the mean or 3 test scores 1.5 standard deviations below the mean). The cognitive deficits were mild to moderate in severity. Although 34 patients completed a 6-month cognitive follow-up, 128 patients, all without pre-existing cognitive impairment assessed using the Informant Questionnaire of Cognitive Decline in the Elderly (IQCODE), were administered an initial Mini Mental State Exam (MMSE) at ICU discharge. Of the critically ill survivors who did not complete cognitive follow-up, mean MMSE scores were below the impairment cutoff of 24 and were significantly lower than those of the patients who completed follow-up. This finding suggests that cognitive impairments may be more common than reported in current outcome studies, as the patients with the lowest MMSE scores were lost to follow-up (25). Similar findings of cognitive impairments come from a prospective cohort of 32 critically ill medical patients who underwent long-term mechanical ventilation (5 or more days). Of the patients with long-term mechanical ventilation, 91% at hospital discharge and 41% at 6 months had cognitive impairments (33).

Cognitive impairments in ICU survivors occur in various cognitive domains, although information regarding the nature and severity of the impairments is incomplete. Studies conducted to date have inconsistently assessed cognitive domains, with some investigations focusing on a wide range of cognitive functioning and others focusing on a narrower range of capacities. The neuropsychological test batteries used to assess cognitive function in critically ill survivors have generally been fairly brief (they were designed to accommodate the fatigue that is common in ICU survivors) rather than comprehensive neuropsychological test batteries designed to investigate a complete range of cognitive abilities. The cognitive domains impaired in survivors of critical illness may depend on the nature of the insults experienced and their treatment, the presence of pre-existing neurologic abnormalities, and individual vulnerabilities such as older age or comorbid disorders that might render specific domains more vulnerable to critical illness–induced brain injury. For example, hypoxia is associated with impaired memory and hippocampal damage (46).

In general, memory is the most frequently observed deficit, followed by impaired executive function and attention (43). For example, a memory questionnaire administered to a prospective cohort of 87 ARDS survivors found 20% of patients rated their memory as poor 18 months after ICU discharge (38). One study predominately assessed executive function in general ICU survivors at 3 and 9 months and found that 35% of the patients had impaired executive function (36). Similar findings were found in mechanically ventilated, nondelirious patients who had impaired memory and problem-solving abilities (i.e., executive dysfunction) during ICU treatment, during hospital treatment, and at 2-month follow-up (32). While in the ICU, 100% of the patients had impaired executive function and 67% had impaired memory. At 2-month follow-up, 50% had impaired executive function and 31% had impaired memory (32).

In addition to impairments in specific cognitive domains, Hopkins et al. (42) compared ARDS patients' premorbid estimated intelligence quotient (IQ) to their measured IQ. The ARDS patients had a significantly lower measured IQ compared to their premorbid estimated IQ at hospital discharge. However, the measured IQ returned to the premorbid level at 1 year follow-up, with no additional improvement in IQ at 2 years. The finding that general intellectual function recovered over time, however, does not necessarily suggest a comparable recovery in all cognitive domains, as data from the traumatic and anoxic brain injury literature suggest that some cognitive abilities are more likely to improve than others.

DURATION OF THE COGNITIVE IMPAIRMENTS

Many critically ill patients have significant chronic cognitive impairments that persist for long periods of time. Cognitive impairments have been reported at 2 months (32), 6 months (33,39), 9 months (36), 1 year (30,34,38), 2 years (42), and up to 6 years (35,40). Cognitive post hospital discharge impairments appear to improve during the first 6 to 12 months post hospital discharge. For example, 70% of ARDS survivors had cognitive impairments at hospital discharge, whereas only 45% had cognitive impairments at 1 year, with no additional improvement at 2 years (42). A retrospective cohort study ($N =$ 46) found 25% of ARDS survivors had cognitive impairments 6 years following ICU treatment; only 21 patients returned to full-time employment, and all patients with cognitive impairments were disabled (40). A second study in ARDS survivors found impaired memory, attention, concentration, executive dysfunction, and motor impairments from 6 months to more than 6 years post hospital discharge (35). The above studies suggest that the cognitive impairments in survivors of critical illness are long lasting and likely permanent. The persistent effects of critical illness on cognitive function may be particularly striking in geriatric patients with pre-existing mild cognitive impairment or dementia, as critical illness–related neurologic insults may serve to heighten their cognitive decline and lead to what could be characterized as "ICU-accelerated dementia or cognitive decline." Such a pattern (e.g., medical illness accelerating the trajectory of dementia or cognitive decline) has been observed in other populations but has not been investigated in critically ill cohorts (47,48).

INDICATORS OF COGNITIVE IMPAIRMENTS

A consistent finding across investigations is the lack of association between some indicators of illness severity and the development of cognitive impairments. Cognitive impairments in survivors of critical illness have not been associated with ICU length of stay, Acute Physiology and Chronic Health Evaluation II (APACHE II) scores, tidal volume, or number of days receiving sedative, narcotic, or paralytic medications (39,42). The above finding suggests that the cognitive impairments experienced by ICU survivors cannot be explained simply in terms of the degree of acute illness severity, as one might intuitively conclude. Alternatively, Jones et al. (32) found that impaired executive function measured *during* ICU treatment was associated with ICU and hospital length of stay, and impaired memory measured during ICU and hospital treatment was associated with admission APACHE II scores; however, these relationships were not present by 2-month follow-up. One limitation of the current data are the small sample sizes, which can result in insufficient power to detect real differences when they may actually exist. Thus, new studies with larger samples may find relationships between cognitive impairments or indicators of illness severity.

Similar to indicators of illness severity, age has not been associated with cognitive impairments (30,39,40), although most of the patients in the 10 cohorts studied to date were young or middle-aged adults (mean age, 54 years). Several studies used demographically corrected scores that account for the possible effects of age, gender, and education (30,34,42,49), and other studies used multivariable analysis to adjust for age (39). Elderly patients (age >65 years) were included in all studies (30,31,33–40,42); however, only one study included a predominately older population (36). Data from the existing studies indicate that age is not associated with cognitive outcomes, likely due to a restricted range. Additional studies in larger and older ICU cohorts are needed to confirm this finding. Although critical illness may affect cognitive functioning regardless of age, patients of an advanced age may be more vulnerable to the development of cognitive impairment due to pre-existing age-related vulnerabilities.

DELIRIUM AND ITS RELATION TO ADVERSE COGNITIVE OUTCOMES

Studies of the association between delirium and adverse cognitive outcomes have generally been carried out in non-ICU populations, although data from these investigations likely apply to intensive care unit cohorts. One important difference between delirium and cognitive impairments is that delirium fluctuates, whereas cognitive impairments do not. Table 150.2 shows a comparison of characteristics of delirium, dementia, and cognitive impairments. A total of nine studies have explored the relationship between new-onset delirium and subsequent development of cognitive decline. Four of these investigations found a greater cognitive decline at follow-up among hospitalized patients who experienced delirium compared to matched controls. Geriatric patients with hip fractures who developed delirium (excluding those with a diagnosis of dementia) were almost twice as likely to have cognitive impairment 2 years post surgery (21). In hospitalized, community-dwelling geriatric patients, patients with delirium had slightly lower Mini Mental Status Examination (MMSE) scores at 6-month follow-up and experienced further cognitive decline over the next 18 months (50). In hospitalized geriatric medical patients following treatment in the emergency department (excluding patients with pre-existing dementia), MMSE scores were nearly 5 points lower in patients with delirium compared to patients without delirium at 1 year after adjusting for premorbid function, comorbid diseases, and illness severity (51). Finally, geriatric nursing home and assisted-living residents who developed delirium during medical hospitalization had a significant decline in cognitive function, including lower MMSE scores (52).

Four studies found a higher incidence of dementia in hospitalized elderly patients with a history of delirium at follow-up evaluations. Of nondemented community-dwelling patients older than 65 years who were hospitalized due to acute delirium, 14 were diagnosed with dementia immediately following delirium, and 14 additional patients developed dementia at 2-year follow-up (53). Rahkonen et al. (54) studied patients 85 years or older, excluding those with dementia, and found that patients with an episode of delirium during hospitalization were significantly more likely to be diagnosed with dementia

TABLE 150.2

COMPARISONS BETWEEN COMPONENTS OF DELIRIUM, DEMENTIA, AND COGNITIVE IMPAIRMENTS

	Delirium	Dementia	Cognitive Impairments
Mental status	Marked fluctuation	Chronically impaired—appears stable but deteriorates over time	Normal
Cognitive function	Sudden onset Acute cognitive impairment characterized by disorientation and confusion	Insidious onset Chronic cognitive impairment Often memory is the first observed cognitive impairment Progressive loss of cognitive functions (impaired judgment, executive function, etc.) Progressive decline over time Interferes with daily functioning and work May include changes in personality, mood, and behavior	Sudden onset Chronic cognitive impairment May affect one or multiple cognitive domains, with memory, executive function, and information processing most commonly affected Initially there may be some recovery or improvement of cognitive function Stable over time May interfere with daily functioning and work
Duration	Temporary	Permanent	Permanent

at 3-year follow-up compared to patients without delirium. Over a 3-year period, 60% of geriatric medical patients with delirium at hospital admission (after evaluating for dementia at baseline) developed dementia compared to only 18.5% of the patients without delirium. The incidence of dementia was 18.1% per year for patients with delirium compared to 5.6% per year for patients without delirium (55). Koponen et al. (56) in 1989 reported MMSE scores at 1-year follow-up in 70 patients diagnosed with delirium during psychiatric hospitalization which revealed that one third evidenced cognitive deterioration (56).

Only one study assessed delirium and cognitive outcomes in critically ill patients. This study found that one in three patients with delirium had cognitive impairments at 6-month follow-up (25). The patients were not primarily geriatric (mean age of 53 years) as were the patients in the other studies cited above (25). The above findings suggest that the presence of delirium may be critical in predicting adverse long-term cognitive outcome.

BRAIN IMAGING FINDINGS IN ASSOCIATION WITH DELIRIUM AND COGNITIVE IMPAIRMENTS

Neuroimaging data are lacking in critically ill patients with delirium or those who develop long-term cognitive impairments. However, various central nervous system insults, such as stroke and traumatic brain injury, can cause delirium and cognitive impairments, suggesting that widely distributed central nervous system abnormalities can occur (57). A study using brain computed tomography (CT) scans found significant ventricular enlargement and generalized atrophy in elderly delirious patients admitted to a psychiatric ward compared to controls (58). Greater brain atrophy correlated with lower MMSE scores in these patients. Focal lesions (infarcts and hemorrhage) have also been observed in the right frontal and parietal regions in the delirious patients (58). Delirium induced by electroconvulsive therapy is associated with basal ganglia lesions and subcortical white matter hyperintensities (59). A study in critically ill patients who underwent CT brain imaging for a diminished level of consciousness, confusion, altered mental status, or prolonged delirium showed that 61% had abnormalities on brain imaging, including generalized brain atrophy, ventricular enlargement, white matter lesions/hyperintensities, and cortical and subcortical lesions (60). Similarly, significant brain atrophy was found in critically ill ARDS patients. The ARDS patients underwent brain CT imaging during ICU treatment and had significant brain atrophy, ventricular enlargement, and a large ventricle-to-brain ratio compared to age- and sex-matched normal control subjects (61). In addition to generalized brain atrophy, radiologic reports identified structural lesions in the central pons and left parietal lobe, subcortical white matter hyperintensities in the right frontal lobe, and hippocampal atrophy (61). These findings parallel those reported by Koponen et al. in patients with delirium. Although the data are limited, future studies using brain imaging may help advance our understanding of the neurologic effects of delirium and cognitive impairments following critical illness and its treatment.

IMPACT OF COGNITIVE IMPAIRMENTS

The relationship between cognitive impairments and quality of life following critical illness has only recently been studied. Two studies found that cognitive impairments were not related to a decreased quality of life in ARDS patients (34) and in medical critically ill patients (36). In contrast, other studies indicate that ARDS patients with cognitive impairments had a worse quality of life compared to patients without cognitive impairments (31,40). Cognitive impairments have been linked to a worse quality of life following stroke (62,63), multiple trauma resulting in ICU treatment (64), traumatic brain injury (65), and carbon monoxide poisoning (66,67). Cognitive impairments can lead to the inability to return to work, poor work productivity, and decreased life satisfaction following ALI (acute lung injury)/ARDS (40).

The impact of critical illness on patients and their families is substantial and frequently includes significant financial burdens. The Study to Understand Prognoses and Preferences for Outcomes and Risks of Treatment examined 2,661 patients hospitalized with a serious illness regarding the impact of returning home. Twenty percent of patients reported that a family member had to quit work, 29% lost the major source of family income, and 31% lost most of the family savings (68). The financial implications of a growing population of survivors of critical illness with cognitive and emotional sequelae are enormous. For example, cognitive decline in a previously high-functioning older person predicts institutionalization (69,70) and carries an eightfold risk of hospitalization (71). The annual per-patient societal cost burden is estimated to be approximately $15,000 for mild cognitive impairment and $35,000 for more severe impairments (72). Over half of critically ill survivors require caregiver support 1 year after treatment, resulting in an additional $18 billion (U.S. dollars) annual financial burden (73).

LACK OF RECOGNITION OF COGNITIVE IMPAIRMENTS

Studies suggest that in non-ICU clinical settings, many physicians fail to recognize (or assess) cognitive impairment in 35% to 90% of patients (74). Cognitive impairments are rarely evaluated in critically ill patients (25) and may be overlooked in one of every two cases (75). For example, in 42% of ARDS survivors who underwent rehabilitation therapy, most were not evaluated for cognitive impairments, and only 12% of the patients were identified as having cognitive impairments by the clinical rehabilitation team (42). Thus, cognitive impairments appear to be underrecognized by both ICU and rehabilitation providers. This may be partly because the manifestations of cognitive impairments are often subtle, and patients may experience impairment in select cognitive domains even if they are alert, oriented, and appear generally cognitively intact. Education of clinical care providers regarding clinical manifestations of cognitive impairments in patients prior to ICU discharge may help increase the identification rates (76). Increased identification of cognitive impairment may benefit patients by raising physician awareness, potentially leading to increased referrals to rehabilitation specialists, neuropsychologists, speech and language therapists, and other health care providers who can provide interventions such as cognitive remediation. There is a paucity of data regarding interventions for cognitive impairments or the potential benefit of such interventions in critically ill patients.

The consequences of cognitive impairments are far-reaching and may contribute to decreased ability to perform activities of daily living and the inability to return to work. Two years after hospital discharge, 34% of ARDS survivors had returned to full-time work or were full-time students, 34% were receiving disability payments started after hospital discharge for ARDS, and 32% (20 of 62) were not working or were retired (42). An investigation that focused on 1-year outcomes found 51% of ARDS survivors had not returned to work; most of these individuals reported physically as opposed to cognitively related reasons for failure to return to work (27).

POTENTIAL MECHANISMS OF DELIRIUM AND LONG-TERM COGNITIVE IMPAIRMENTS

Many physiologic and pharmacologic perturbations affect the central nervous system in critically ill patients. Although the precise mechanisms that contribute to delirium and cognitive impairment or both are unknown, various theories have been proposed. The theories include the following:

- The potentially adverse effects of medical illness on cognition (77,78)
- Pathologic processes underlying delirium and cognitive impairments (79,80)
- The impact of psychoactive medications, including sedatives and analgesics (81,82)

Delirium and cognitive impairments rarely have one causal mechanism, and they are thought to be multifactorial (83); as such, the pathogeneses are likely due to interactions between patient vulnerability and precipitating factors or insults (84), including critical illness and its treatment. Studies have not focused on putative mechanisms, and a number of studies address and, in some cases, offer opinions regarding potential mechanisms. The investigation of the mechanisms of delirium and long-term cognitive impairments remains a promising area of neuroscientific study.

Psychoactive Medications

The role of certain medications such as sedatives, narcotics, and paralytics in the development of delirium are well known (85). Many medications used for sedation or pain control—including those used in the ICU setting—are known to cause or worsen delirium, although findings from some studies are negative or equivocal (86). An association exists between the high delirium prevalence rates in surgical and critically ill populations and the use of sedatives and narcotics (87–89). Although data on the impact of anesthetics and sedatives on long-term cognitive functioning are conflicting, reports suggest they may have neurotoxic effects, particularly for high-risk groups such as the very old (>75 years) and/or those with a recent history of cognitive impairment (90,91).

In some individuals, the effects of medications on cognition may be mediated by genetic factors. For example, the apolipoprotein E4 (APOE4) allele is one probable genetic factor that may affect individual sensitivity to drug effects. The APOE4 allele is a significant risk factor for the development of certain forms of Alzheimer disease (92), hippocampal atrophy (93), worse recovery of neurologic function following traumatic brain injury (94), cognitive decline following cardiopulmonary bypass surgery (95), and delirium (96). Although more research is needed, it appears that certain anticholinergic agents may have particularly adverse effects on cognition when administered to patients possessing the APOE4 allele. In particular, lorazepam—commonly used in ICU settings—increases susceptibility to impaired verbal learning and related cognitive deficits in patients with the APOE4 allele compared to patients without this polymorphism (97).

DELIRIUM AS A MECHANISM OF COGNITIVE IMPAIRMENTS

The findings of cognitive decline among hospitalized patients, particularly the older patients, are consistent with the literature showing that medical illnesses in general and cumulative illnesses in particular may signal the beginning of cognitive deterioration (77,98). For the so-called frail elderly (99) who are in an unstable state of vulnerability due to factors such as diminished physical status and compromised nutrition and immune system functioning, even minor insults can have a profound impact and lead to cognitive impairment and functional disability (100). Delirium may be such an insult.

Some researchers have speculated that delirium is a marker of subclinical dementia or cognitive impairment, which might not otherwise develop for years or decades. Data suggest that common pathogenic mechanisms might underlie both Alzheimer disease and delirium (79) although, from a clinical standpoint, there are similarities and differences. For example, inflammatory processes contribute to the development of delirium and are present in the brains of patients with Alzheimer disease (101). Other studies have suggested that elevated cytokines (interleukin-1) may play a central role in the pathogenesis of delirium (102) and cognitive impairments (103,104). Another possible connection between delirium and Alzheimer disease is diminishing neuroplasticity acting as an effect modifier, leading to greater neurodegeneration and cognitive deficits (105,106). Evidence suggests that the greater the neuronal loss or dysfunction, the higher the risk of cognitive impairments (49,61,106,107). Delirium may directly result in structural neural damage to vital brain regions, particularly subcortical regions (e.g., brainstem and thalamus) (108), limbic structures (e.g., hippocampus), and prefrontal and right parietal cortex (83). These brain regions are involved in attention, memory, and executive function, cognitive domains in which survivors of critical illness frequently experience impairments (25,42).

COGNITIVE REHABILITATION

Cognitive rehabilitation has been used widely with patients following traumatic brain injury, stroke, and other neurologic insults (109). Evidence suggests that cognitive rehabilitation can be highly effective, which may be mediated by factors such as the cause of the brain injury and the cognitive domain (i.e., memory, executive functioning, etc.) of focus (110). For example, patients with hypoxic brain injuries may be less responsive to cognitive rehabilitation than those with traumatic brain injury or stroke (111). Questions exist regarding the applicability of the cognitive rehabilitation literature to critically ill populations, as ICU-related cognitive impairment is rarely due to a brain injury, as classically defined. However, there is no inherent reason to imagine that the potential benefits of cognitive rehabilitation would not apply to those experiencing neuropsychological dysfunction following critical illness and ICU treatment. Although previous and ongoing studies have focused on the identification of modifiable risk factors as a way of reducing cognitive impairment after critical illness, future trials should focus not only on modifiable risk factors, but also on development and implementation of cognitive rehabilitation interventions. Along with this venue, physicians should consider referring patients for specialized cognitive rehabilitation when possible, particularly cases in which patients are referred to physical rehabilitation facilities where such treatments are widely available.

EMOTIONAL DISORDERS

Psychiatric morbidity following critical illness is common and includes depression, anxiety, and posttraumatic stress disorder (PTSD). The prevalence and severity of depression, anxiety, and PTSD in survivors of critical illness are heterogenous (26,40,112,113). It is unclear whether emotional disorders are a psychological reaction to extraordinary emotional and physiologic stress, sequelae of brain injury sustained due to critical illness and its treatment, or all of the above. The combination of medications, physiological changes, pain, altered sensory inputs, and an unfamiliar environment may contribute to emotional changes (113–115). Recent evidence suggests that mood disorders secondary to medical illness constitute discrete entities in which the symptoms are similar to primary mood disorders, but there is a male predominance and earlier onset (116).

Posttraumatic Stress Disorder (PTSD)

Estimates of PTSD prevalence in critically ill cohorts are as high as 63% (117) and generally exceed those of other high-risk populations. Although alarming, caution should be used when interpreting these findings due to some methodologic shortcomings of investigations of PTSD in critically ill populations, such as overreliance on screening tools (as opposed to diagnostic tools), questionable interpretation of available data, the lack of evaluation of non-ICU-related causes of PTSD, low follow-up rates, and other limitations. With these caveats, PTSD clearly occurs and persists in a subset of ICU survivors.

Among critically ill subjects, general medical ICU cohorts have been shown to have both the lowest and highest rates of PTSD compared to more specialized populations. In studies of general medical ICU patients, reported prevalence rates of PTSD range from 9.7% (118) to 63% (117), with rates of PTSD in specialized populations ranging from 18.5% (119) to 43% (120). Risk factors for the development of PTSD and related symptoms have not been systematically studied; however, several probable risk factors have been identified. One risk factor of interest is delusional memories, with two investigations reporting associations between delusional memories and development of PTSD in survivors of critical illness (112,121). Other risk factors include younger age, the existence of a prior mental health history (122), anxiety (123), and female gender (124).

Although the clinical impact of PTSD on the quality of life and overall functioning of ICU survivors has not been explored, the real-world impact of PTSD has been extensively studied in wide-ranging clinical samples. Although a survey of this literature is beyond the scope of this chapter, the effects of PTSD can be far-reaching and profound. Individuals with PTSD have lower rates of employment (125), decreased quality of life (126), increased rates of depression (127), and increased use of health care services (128). For these and other reasons, the identification and early treatment of ICU survivors with PTSD should be a priority.

Depression and Anxiety

Depression is common among medically ill cohorts due both to the specific physical effects of certain illnesses and/or the effects of illness on quality of life, independence, employment, and other factors (129–131). Depression occurs in 25% (42) to over 50% of ARDS survivors (26). For example, 43% of ALI patients and 50% of ARDS survivors had symptoms of depression following ICU treatment (26). The Toronto ARDS outcomes group found that 58% of ARDS survivors had depressive symptoms 2 years after ICU discharge (38). In the most comprehensive study conducted to date, Weinert (131) administered 105 interviews using a comprehensive diagnostic tool (Structured Clinical Interview for DSM-IV Disorders) 2 months after hospital discharge in survivors of acute respiratory failure. Weinert reported prevalence and incident rates of major depressive disorder (MDD) of 15% and 11%, respectively. He further noted that another 16% of patients met criteria for a diagnosis of adjustment disorder with depressed mood. The investigators found antidepressant use was widespread (37%), while observing that the safety and efficacy of antidepressants is unknown in critically ill patients (131).

Although the evidence up to the present suggests that depression is indeed a concern in ICU survivors, much remains unknown. In particular, the rates of pre-existing depressive symptoms or clinical depression in critically ill populations are unknown but may be high due to the many medical comorbidities experienced by a high percentage of these patients. Key questions remain about the nature of depressive symptoms following critical illness. Although the study by Weinert et al. used a diagnostic interview, most studies have merely used brief self-report instruments. Such instruments often fail to distinguish between cognitive and somatic symptoms. Thus, it may be the case that some of the depressive complaints expressed by ICU survivors (i.e., fatigue, sleeping difficulties) may actually be manifestations of physical illness.

Although data are accumulating regarding depression following critical illness, less is known regarding anxiety, with the exception of PTSD. Anxiety occurs in 4% to 41% of ARDS survivors (120,132). Anxiety has been reported in 24% of ARDS survivors at 1 and 2 years (34,42). Possible factors that may be associated with development of depression and anxiety following critical illness include a current smoking status or prior alcohol abuse. In ARDS survivors, smokers had higher depression scores at 1 year but not at 2 years compared to nonsmokers. There was no difference in anxiety for smokers at 1 year, but at 2 years, smokers reported significantly more anxiety than nonsmokers. The ARDS patients with a history of alcohol abuse had higher depression and anxiety scores at 1 and 2 years compared to nonabusers. Thus, smoking and alcohol abuse may be related to symptoms of depression and anxiety in ARDS survivors (133).

SIGNIFICANCE OF COGNITIVE AND BEHAVIORAL SEQUELAE

The significance of cognitive and behavioral sequelae in the intensive care unit is becoming increasingly clear. Cognitive and behavioral sequelae have a negative impact on the patients' quality of life, return to work, emotional state, and financial impact. Although the treatment and management of serious medical conditions is of obvious importance, it is not the only goal. Intensive care unit clinicians should be aware of the impact of critical illness on emotional and neuropsychological functioning and be prepared to respond in a sensitive and informed fashion to the problems that patients present. In particular, they may consider building formal relationships with specialists from other disciplines, such as psychology and psychiatry, and possibly including them as members of ICU treatment teams. Intensive care unit clinicians may wish to develop unit-wide programs and protocols that involve the routine assessment and monitoring of common conditions such as delirium as well as mental status and mood. Furthermore, they should inquire about cognitive and emotional functioning at follow-up (76).

Intensive care unit researchers should follow the lead of their counterparts in other medical disciplines such as cardiac surgery, oncology, and infectious disease, and make the investigation of cognitive and emotional outcomes in critical care survivors a priority. Fruitful areas of emphasis may include determining the causes and modifiable risk factors for conditions such as ICU-related depression and cognitive impairment. Other explorations might focus on whether critical illness accelerates and/or alters the trajectory of pre-existing cognitive impairment and whether cognitive rehabilitation might enhance long-term cognitive outcomes. The nature of the impact of cognitive and emotional difficulties on daily functioning in survivors of critical illness is an extremely important topic, yet it has rarely been explored (134).

Although technologic and medical advances have saved the lives of thousands of critically ill patients who would have died a decade or two ago, the cognitive and emotional problems encountered by ICU survivors are real and long lasting. Through careful attention to such problems and through the development of clinical interventions and research programs, it may be possible to alleviate a measure of the suffering associated with critical illness. During patient follow-up, on a more personal level, clinicians should be careful to express the same degree of concern about patients' cognitive and emotional complaints as their medical complaints.

SUMMARY

Physicians and other health care providers need to be mindful of adverse behavioral outcomes in critically ill patients. Current data suggest that the delirium, cognitive impairments, and emotional morbidity are common following critical illness. Cognitive and emotional morbidity may persist years after ICU discharge. Cognitive impairments are ubiquitous at hospital discharge and appear to improve during the first 12 months, but a significant percent of patients still have chronic cognitive impairments years after ICU treatment. The adverse behavioral impairments can have a significant impact on the quality of life and the ability to return to work, in addition to substantial economic consequences. Research is needed to determine strategies for the early identification of patients with cognitive impairments and emotional sequelae, mechanisms of neural injury, and treatments to prevent or decrease the frequency and severity of cognitive and emotional sequelae. Such research will likely yield valuable insights into identification, natural history, prognosis, potential mechanisms, and treatment of behavioral impairments in survivors of critical illness.

References

1. Schmitz R, Lantin M, White A. *Future Workforce Needs in Pulmonary and Critical Care Medicine*. Cambridge, MA: Abt Associates; 1998.
2. Esteban A, Anzueto A, Alia I, et al. How is mechanical ventilation employed in the intensive care unit? An international utilization review. *Am J Respir Crit Care Med*. 2000;161:1450–1458.
3. Cohen IL, Booth FV. Cost containment and mechanical ventilation in the United States. *New Horiz*. 1994;2:283–290.
4. Vincent JL, Moreno R, Takala J, et al. The SOFA (Sepsis-related Organ Failure Assessment) score to describe organ dysfunction/failure. On behalf of the Working Group on Sepsis-Related Problems of the European Society of Intensive Care Medicine. *Intensive Care Med*. 1996;22:707–710.
5. Russell JA, Singer J, Bernard GR, et al. Changing pattern of organ dysfunction in early human sepsis is related to mortality. *Crit Care Med*. 2000;28:3405–3411.
6. Young B. Neurologic complications of systemic critical illness. *Neurol Clin*. 1995;13:645–658.
7. Justic M. Does "ICU psychosis" really exist? *Crit Care Nurse*. 2000;20:28–37; quiz 38–29.
8. Meagher DJ, O'Hanlon D, O'Mahony E, et al. Relationship between symptoms and motoric subtype of delirium. *J Neuropsychiatry Clin Neurosci*. 2000;12:51–56.
9. Ely EW, Inouye SK, Bernard GR, et al. Delirium in mechanically ventilated patients: validity and reliability of the confusion assessment method for the intensive care unit (CAM-ICU). *JAMA*. 2001;286:2703–2710.
10. Peterson JF, Pun BT, Dittus RS, et al. Delirium and its motoric subtypes: a study of 614 critically ill patients. *J Am Geriatr Soc*. 2006;54:479–484.
11. Inouye SK, Foreman MD, Mion LC, et al. Nurses' recognition of delirium and its symptoms: comparison of nurse and researcher ratings. *Arch Intern Med*. 2001;161:2467–2473.
12. Ely EW, Stephens RK, Jackson JC, et al. Current opinions regarding the importance, diagnosis, and management of delirium in the intensive care unit: a survey of 912 healthcare professionals. *Crit Care Med*. 2004;32:106–112.
13. Ely EW, Gautam S, Margolin R, et al. Evaluation of delirium in critically ill patients: validation of the confusion assessment method for the intensive care unit (CAM-ICU). *Crit Care Med*. 2001;29:1370–1379.
14. Meagher DJ. Delirium: optimising management. *Br Med J*. 2001;322:144–149.
15. Levkoff SE, Evans DA, Liptzin B, et al. Delirium: the occurrence and persistence of symptoms among elderly hospitalized patients. *Arch Intern Med*. 1992;152:334–340.
16. Lipowski ZJ. Delirium in the elderly patient. *N Engl J Med*. 1989;320:578–582.
17. Galanakis P, Bickel H, Gradinger R, et al. Acute confusional state in the elderly following hip surgery: incidence, risk factors and complications. *Int J Geriatr Psychiatry*. 2001;16:349–355.
18. Ely EW, Siegel MD, Inouye SK. Delirium in the intensive care unit: an under-recognized syndrome of organ dysfunction. *Semin Respir Crit Care Med*. 2001;22:115–126.
19. McGuire BE, Basten CJ, Ryan CJ, et al. Intensive care unit syndrome: a dangerous misnomer. *Arch Intern Med*. 2000;160:906–909.
20. Ely EW, Shintani A, Bernard G, et al. Delirium in the ICU is associated with prolonged length of stay in the hospital and higher mortality. *Am J Respir Crit Care Med*. 2002;165:A23.
21. Dolan MM, Hawkes WG, Zimmerman SI, et al. Delirium on hospital admission in aged hip fracture patients: Prediction of mortality and 2-year functional outcomes. *J Gerontol A Biol Sci Med Sci*. 2001;55A:M527–M534.
22. Uldall KK, Ryan R, Berghuis JP, et al. Association between delirium and death in AIDS patients. *Aids Patient Care STDS*. 2000;14:95–100.
23. Marcantonio ER, Flacker JM, Michaels M, et al. Delirium is independently associated with poor functional recovery after hip fracture. *J Am Geriatr Soc*. 2000;48:618–624.
24. McCusker J, Cole M, Abrahamowicz M, et al. Delirium predicts 12-month mortality. *Arch Intern Med*. 2002;162:457–463.
25. Jackson JC, Hart RP, Gordon SM, et al. Six-month neuropsychological outcome of medical intensive care unit patients. *Crit Care Med*. 2003;31:1226–1234.
26. Angus DC, Musthafa AA, Clermont G, et al. Quality-adjusted survival in the first year after the acute respiratory distress syndrome. *Am J Respir Crit Care Med*. 2001;163:1389–1394.
27. Herridge MS, Cheung AM, Tansey CM, et al. One-year outcomes in survivors of the acute respiratory distress syndrome. *N Engl J Med*. 2003; 348:683–693.
28. Orme JF Jr, Romney JS, Hopkins RO, et al. Pulmonary function and health-related quality of life in survivors of acute respiratory distress syndrome. *Am J Respir Crit Care Med*. 2003;167:690–694.
29. Weinert CR, Gross CR, Kangas JR, et al. Health-related quality of life after acute lung injury. *Am J Respir Crit Care Med*. 1997;156:1120–1128.
30. Hopkins RO, Weaver LK, Pope D, et al. Neuropsychological sequelae and impaired health status in survivors of severe acute respiratory distress syndrome. *Am J Respir Crit Care Med*. 1999;160:50–56.
31. Christie J, DeMissie E, Gaughan C, et al. Validity of a brief telephone-administered battery to assess cognitive function in survivors of the adult respiratory distress syndrome (ARDS). *Am J Respir Crit Care Med*. 2004; 169:A781.
32. Jones C, Griffiths RD, Slater T, et al. Significant cognitive dysfunction in non-delirious patients identified during and persisting following critical illness. *Intensive Care Med*. 2006;32:923–926.
33. Hopkins RO, Jackson JC, Wallace CJ. Neurocognitive impairments in ICU patients with prolonged mechanical ventilation. In: *International Neuropsychological Society 33rd Annual Meeting Program and Abstracts*. St. Louis, MO. 2005:61.
34. Hopkins RO, Weaver LK, Chan KJ, et al. Quality of life, emotional, and cognitive function following acute respiratory distress syndrome. *J Int Neuropsychol Soc*. 2004;10:1005–1017.
35. Suchyta MR, Hopkins RO, White J, et al. The incidence of cognitive dysfunction after ARDS. *Am J Respir Crit Care Med*. 2004;169:A18.
36. Sukantarat KT, Burgess PW, Williamson RC, et al. Prolonged cognitive dysfunction in survivors of critical illness. *Anaesthesia*. 2005;60:847–853.
37. Marquis K, Curtis J, Caldwell E, et al. Neuropsychological sequelae in survivors of ARDS compared with critically ill control patients. *Am J Respir Crit Care Med*. 2000;161:A383.
38. Al-Saidi F, McAndrews MP, Cheunt AM, et al. Neuropsychological sequelae in ARDS survivors. *Am J Respir Crit Care Med*. 2003;167:A737.
39. Jackson JC, Gordon SM, Burger C, et al. Acute respiratory distress syndrome and long-term cognitive impairment: a case study. *Arch Clin Neuropsychol*. 2003;18:688.
40. Rothenhausler HB, Ehrentraut S, Stoll C, et al. The relationship between cognitive performance and employment and health status in long-term survivors of the acute respiratory distress syndrome: results of an exploratory study. *Gen Hosp Psychiatry*. 2001;23:90–96.
41. Christie JD, Biester RC, Taichman DB, et al. Formation and validation of a telephone battery to assess cognitive function in acute respiratory distress syndrome survivors. *J Crit Care*. 2006;21:125–132.
42. Hopkins RO, Weaver LK, Collingridge D, et al. Two-year cognitive, emotional, and quality-of-life outcomes in acute respiratory distress syndrome. *Am J Respir Crit Care Med*. 2005;171:340–347.
43. Hopkins RO, Jackson JC. Long-term neurocognitive function after critical illness. *Chest*. 2006;130:869–878.
44. Weaver LK, Hopkins RO, Chan KJ, et al. Hyperbaric oxygen for acute carbon monoxide poisoning. *N Engl J Med*. 2002;347:1057–1067.
45. Newman M, Kirchner J, Phillips-Bute B, et al. Longitudinal assessment of neurocognitive function after coronary-artery bypass surgery. *N Engl J Med*. 2001;344:395–402.
46. Hopkins RO, Myers CE, Shohamy D, et al. Impaired probabilistic category learning in hypoxic subjects with hippocampal damage. *Neuropsychologia*. 2004;42:524–535.
47. Lee TA, Wolozin B, Weiss KB, et al. Assessment of the emergence of Alzheimer's disease following coronary artery bypass graft surgery or percutaneous transluminal coronary angioplasty. *J Alzheimers Dis*. 2005;7:319–324.
48. Lyketsos CG, Toone L, Tschanz J, et al. Population-based study of medical comorbidity in early dementia and "cognitive impairment, no dementia (CIND)": association with functional and cognitive impairment: the Cache County Study. *Am J Geriatr Psychiatry*. 2005;13:656–664.
49. Hopkins RO, Tate DF, Bigler ED. Anoxic versus traumatic brain injury: amount of tissue loss, not etiology, alters cognitive and emotional function. *Neuropsychology*. 2005;19:233–242.
50. Francis J, Kapoor WN. Prognosis after hospital discharge of older medical patients with delirium. *J Am Geriatr Soc*. 1992;40:601–606.
51. McCusker J, Cole M, Dendukuri N, et al. Delirium in older medical inpatients and subsequent cognitive and functional status: a prospective study. *Can Med Assoc J*. 2001;165:575–583.
52. Katz IR, Curyto KJ, TenHave T, et al. Validating the diagnosis of delirium and evaluating its association with deterioration over a one-year period. *Am J Geriatr Psychiatry*. 2001;9:148–159.
53. Rahkonen T, Luukkainen-Markkula R, Paanilla S, et al. Delirium episode as a sign of undetected dementia among community dwelling subjects: a 2 year follow up study. *J Neurol Neurosurg Psychiatr*. 2000;69:519–521.
54. Rahkonen T, Eloniemi-Sulkava U, Halonen P, et al. Delirium in the non-demented oldest old in the general population: risk factors and prognosis. *Int J Geriatr Psychiatry*. 2001;16:415–421.
55. Rockwood K, Cosway S, Carver D, et al. The risk of dementia and death after delirium. *Age Ageing*. 1999;28:551–556.
56. Koponen H, Stenback U, Mattila E, et al. Delirium among elderly persons admitted to a psychiatric hospital: clinical course during the acute stage and one-year follow-up. *Acta Psychiatr Scand*. 1989;79:579–585.

57. Lerner DM, Rosenstein DL. Neuroimaging in delirium and related conditions. *Semin Clin Neuropsychiatry*. 2000;5:98–112.
58. Koponen H, Hurri L, Stenback U, et al. Computed tomography findings in delirium. *J Nerv Ment Dis*. 1989;177:226–231.
59. Figiel GS, Coffey CE, Djang WT, et al. Brain magnetic resonance imaging findings in ECT-induced delirium. *J Neuropsychiatry Clin Neurosci*. 1990; 2:53–58.
60. Suchyta MR, Jephson A, Hopkins RO. Brain MR and CT findings associated with critical illness [abstract]. *Proc Am Thorac Soc*. 2005;2: A426.
61. Hopkins RO, Gale SD, Weaver LK. Brain atrophy and cognitive impairment in survivors of acute respiratory distress syndrome. *Brain Inj*. 2006;20:263–271.
62. Kwa VI, Limburg M, de Haan RJ. The role of cognitive impairment in the quality of life after ischaemic stroke. *J Neurol*. 1996;243:599–604.
63. Kwa VI, Limburg M, Voogel AJ, et al. Feasibility of cognitive screening of patients with ischaemic stroke using the CAMCOG. A hospital-based study. *J Neurol*. 1996;243:405–409.
64. Thiagarajan J, Miranda DR. Quality of life after multiple trauma requiring intensive care. *Anaesthesia*. 1995;49:211–218.
65. Warren L, Wrigley JM, Yoels WC, et al. Factors associated with life satisfaction among a sample of persons with neurotrauma. *J Rehabil Res Dev*. 1996;33:404–408.
66. Churchill S, Hopkins RO, Weaver LK, et al. Health related quality of life (HRQL) following carbon monoxide poisoning. *Undersea Hyperb Med*. 2002;29:139–140.
67. McSweeny AJ, Labuhn KT. The relationship of neuropsychological functioning to life quality in systemic medical disease: the example of chronic obstructive pulmonary disease. In: Grant I, Adams KM, eds. *Neuropsychological Assessment in Neuropsychiatry*. New York, NY: Oxford University Press; 1996:577–602.
68. Covinsky KE, Goldman L, Cook EF, et al. The impact of serious illness on patients' families. SUPPORT Investigators. Study to Understand Prognoses and Preferences for Outcomes and Risks of Treatment. *JAMA*. 1994;272:1839–1844.
69. Strain LA, Blandford AA, Mitchell LA, et al. Cognitively impaired older adults: risk profiles for institutionalization. *Int Psychogeriatr*. 2003;15: 351–366.
70. Aguero-Torres H, von Strauss E, Viitanen M, et al. Institutionalization in the elderly: the role of chronic diseases and dementia. Cross-sectional and longitudinal data from a population-based study. *J Clin Epidemiol*. 2001;54:795–801.
71. Chodosh J, Seeman TE, Keeler E, et al. Cognitive decline in high-functioning older persons is associated with an increased risk of hospitalization. *J Am Geriatr Soc*. 2004;52:1456–1462.
72. Rockwood K, Brown M, Merry H, et al. Societal costs of vascular cognitive impairment in older adults. *Stroke*. 2002;33:1605–1609.
73. Langa KM, Chernew ME, Kabeto MU, et al. National estimates of the quantity and cost of informal caregiving for the elderly with dementia. *J Gen Intern Med*. 2001;16:770–778.
74. Callahan CM, Hendrie HC, Tierney WM. Documentation and evaluation of cognitive impairment in elderly primary care patients. *Ann Intern Med*. 1995;122:422–429.
75. Wilkes MM, Navickis RJ. Patient survival after human albumin administration. A meta-analysis of randomized, controlled trials. *Ann Intern Med*. 2001;135:149–164.
76. Gordon SM, Jackson JC, Ely EW, et al. Clinical identification of cognitive impairment in ICU survivors: insights for intensivists. *Intensive Care Med*. 2004;30:1997–2008.
77. Patrick L, Gaskovski P, Rexroth D. Cumulative illness and neuropsychological decline in hospitalized geriatric patients. *Clin Neuropsychol*. 2002;16:145–156.
78. Sands LP, Yaffe K, Lui LY, et al. The effects of acute illness on ADL decline over 1 year in frail older adults with and without cognitive impairment. *J Gerontol*. 2002;57:M449–454.
79. Eikelenboom P, Hoogendijk WJ. Do delirium and Alzheimer's dementia share specific pathogenetic mechanisms? *Dement Geriatr Cogn Disord*. 1999;10:319–324.
80. Gibson GE, Blass JP, Huang HM, et al. The cellular basis of delirium and its relevance to age-related disorders including Alzheimer's disease. *Int Psychogeriatr*. 1991;3:373–395.
81. Moore AR, O'Keeffe ST. Drug-induced cognitive impairment in the elderly. *Drugs Aging*. 1999;15:15–28.
82. Fong HK, Sands LP, Leung JM. The role of postoperative analgesia in delirium and cognitive decline in elderly patients: a systematic review. *Anesth Analg*. 2006;102:1255–1266.
83. Trzepacz PT. Update on the neuropathogenesis of delirium. *Dement Geriatr Cogn Disord*. 1999;10:330–334.
84. Inouye SK, Rushing JT, Foreman MD, et al. Does delirium contribute to poor hospital outcomes? A three-site epidemiologic study. *J Gen Intern Med*. 1998;13:234–242.
85. Morrison RS, Magaziner J, Gilbert M, et al. Relationship between pain and opioid analgesics on the development of delirium following hip fracture. *J Gerontol*. 2003;58:76–81.
86. Gaudreau JD, Gagnon P, Roy MA, et al. Association between psychoactive medications and delirium in hospitalized patients. A critical review. *Psychosomatics*. 2005;46:302–316.
87. Granberg Axell AI, Malmros CW, Bergbom IL, et al. Intensive care unit syndrome/delirium is associated with anemia, drug therapy and duration of ventilation treatment. *Acta Anaesthesiol Scand*. 2002;46:726–731.
88. Somprakit P, Lertakyamanee J, Satraratanamai C, et al. Mental state change after general and regional anesthesia in adults and elderly patients, a randomized clinical trial. *J Med Assoc Thai*. 2002;85:S875–883.
89. Winawer N. Postoperative delirium. *Med Clin North Am*. 2001;85:1229–1239.
90. Ancelin ML, de Roquefeuil G, Ledesert B, et al. Exposure to anaesthetic agents, cognitive functioning and depressive symptomatology in the elderly. *Br J Psychiatry*. 2001;178:360–366.
91. Dodds C, Allison J. Postoperative cognitive deficit in the elderly surgical patient. *Br J Anaesth*. 1998;81:449–462.
92. Saunders AM, Strittmatter WJ, Schmechel D, et al. Association of apolipoprotein E allele epsilon 4 with late-onset familial and sporadic Alzheimer's disease. *Neurology*. 1993;43:1467–1472.
93. den Heijer T, Oudkerk M, Launer LJ, et al. Hippocampal, amygdalar, and global brain atrophy in different apolipoprotein E genotypes. *Neurology*. 2002;59:746–748.
94. Friedman G, Froom P, Sazbon L, et al. Apolipoprotein E-epsilon4 genotype predicts a poor outcome in survivors of traumatic brain injury. *Neurology*. 1999;52:244–248.
95. Tardiff BE, Newman MF, Saunders AM, et al. Preliminary report of a genetic basis for cognitive decline after cardiac operations. The Neurologic Outcome Research Group of the Duke Heart Center. *Ann Thorac Surg*. 1997;64:715–720.
96. Ely EW, Girard TD, Shintani AK, et al. Apolipoprotein E4 polymorphism as a genetic predisposition to delirium in critically ill patients. *Crit Care Med*. 2007;35(1):112–117.
97. Pomara N, Facelle TM, Roth AE, et al. Dose-dependent retrograde facilitation of verbal memory in healthy elderly after acute oral lorazepam administration. *Psychopharmacology (Berl)*. 2006;185:487–494.
98. Doraiswamy PM, Leon J, Cummings JL, et al. Prevalence and impact of medical comorbidity in Alzheimer's disease. *J Gerontol*. 2002;57A:M173–177.
99. Hamerman D. Toward an understanding of frailty. *Ann Intern Med*. 1999;130:945–950.
100. Nourhashemi F, Andrieu S, Gillette-Guyonnet S, et al. Instrumental activities of daily living as a potential marker of frailty: a study of 7364 community-dwelling elderly women (the EPIDOS study). *J Gerontol A Biol Sci Med Sci*. 2001;56:M448–453.
101. McGeer PL, Schulzer M, McGeer EG. Arthritis and anti-inflammatory agents as possible protective factors for Alzheimer's disease: a review of 17 epidemiologic studies. *Neurology*. 1996;47:425–432.
102. Stefano GB, Bilfinger TV, Fricchione GL. The immune-neuro-link and the macrophage: postcardiotomy delirium, HIV-associated dementia and psychiatry. *Prog Neurobiol*. 1994;42:475–488.
103. Wilson CJ, Finch CE, Cohen HJ. Cytokines and cognition—the case for a head-to-toe inflammatory paradigm. *J Am Geriatr Soc*. 2002;50:2041–2056.
104. Meyers CA, Albitar M, Estey E. Cognitive impairment, fatigue, and cytokine levels in patients with acute myelogenous leukemia or myelodysplastic syndrome. *Cancer*. 2005;104:788–793.
105. Blennow K, Gottfries CG. Neurochemistry of aging. In: Nelson JG, ed. *Geriatric Psychopharmacology*. New York, NY: Marcel Dekker Inc; 1998.
106. Gunther ML, Morandi A, Ely EW. Pathophysiology of delirium in the intensive care unit. *Critical Care Clinics*. 2008;24:45–65.
107. Jackson JC, Gordon SM, Hart RP, et al. The association between delirium and cognitive decline: a review of the empirical literature. *Neuropsychol Rev*. 2004;14:87–98.
108. Trzepacz PT. The neuropathogenesis of delirium. A need to focus our research. *Psychosomatics*. 1994;35:374–391.
109. Cicerone KD, Dahlberg C, Malec JF, et al. Evidence-based cognitive rehabilitation: updated review of the literature from 1998 through 2002. *Arch Phys Med Rehabil*. 2005;86:1681–1692.
110. Salmond CH, Sahakian BJ. Cognitive outcome in traumatic brain injury survivors. *Curr Opin Crit Care*. 2005;11:111–116.
111. Groswasser Z, Cohen M, Costeff H. Rehabilitation outcome after anoxic brain damage. *Arch Phys Med Rehabil*. 1989;70:186–188.
112. Kress JP, Gehlbach B, Lacy M, et al. The long-term psychological effects of daily sedative interruption on critically ill patients. *Am J Respir Crit Care Med*. 2003;168:1457–1461.
113. Szokol JW, Vender JS. Anxiety, delirium, and pain in the intensive care unit. *Crit Care Clin*. 2001;17:821–842.
114. McCartney JR, Boland RJ. Anxiety and delirium in the intensive care unit. *Crit Care Clin*. 1994;10:673–680.
115. Skodol AE. Anxiety in the medically ill: nosology and principles of differential diagnosis. *Semin Clin Neuropsychiatry*. 1999;4:64–71.
116. Clayton PJ, Lewis CE. The significance of secondary depression. *J Affect Disord*. 1981;3:25–35.
117. Schelling G, Briegel J, Roozendaal B, et al. The effect of stress doses of hydrocortisone during septic shock on posttraumatic stress disorder in survivors. *Biol Psychiatry*. 2001;50:978–985.

118. Nickel M, Leiberich P, Nickel C, et al. The occurrence of posttraumatic stress disorder in patients following intensive care treatment: a cross-sectional study in a random sample. *J Intensive Care Med.* 2004;19:285–290.
119. Schelling G, Stoll C, Kapfhammer HP, et al. The effect of stress doses of hydrocortisone during septic shock on posttraumatic stress disorder and health-related quality of life in survivors. *Crit Care Med.* 1999;27:2678–2683.
120. Kapfhammer HP, Rothenhausler HB, Krauseneck T, et al. Posttraumatic stress disorder and health-related quality of life in long-term survivors of acute respiratory distress syndrome. *Am J Psychiatry.* 2004;161:45–52.
121. Jones C, Skirrow P, Griffiths RD, et al. Rehabilitation after critical illness: a randomized, controlled trial. *Crit Care Med.* 2003;31:2456–2461.
122. Cuthbertson BH, Hull A, Strachan M, et al. Post-traumatic stress disorder after critical illness requiring general intensive care. *Intensive Care Med.* 2004;30:450–455.
123. Jones C, Griffiths RD, Humphris G, et al. Memory, delusions, and the development of acute posttraumatic stress disorder-related symptoms after intensive care. *Crit Care Med.* 2001;29:573–580.
124. Eddleston JM, White P, Guthrie E. Survival, morbidity, and quality of life after discharge from intensive care. *Crit Care Med.* 2000;28:2293–2299.
125. Smith MW, Schnurr PP, Rosenheck RA. Employment outcomes and PTSD symptom severity. *Ment Health Serv Res.* 2005;7:89–101.
126. Kiely JM, Brasel KJ, Weidner KL, et al. Predicting quality of life six months after traumatic injury. *J Trauma.* 2006;61:791–798.
127. Shalev AY, Freedman S, Peri T, et al. Prospective study of posttraumatic stress disorder and depression following trauma. *Am J Psychiatry.* 1998;155:630–637.
128. Leserman J, Whetten K, Lowe K, et al. How trauma, recent stressful events, and PTSD affect functional health status and health utilization in HIV-infected patients in the south. *Psychosom Med.* 2005;67:500–507.
129. Sobel RM, Lotkowski S, Mandel S. Update on depression in neurologic illness: stroke, epilepsy, and multiple sclerosis. *Curr Psychiatry Rep.* 2005;7:396–403.
130. Lustman PJ, Clouse RE. Depression in diabetic patients: the relationship between mood and glycemic control. *J Diabetes Complications.* 2005;19:113–122.
131. Weinert C. Epidemiology and treatment of psychiatric conditions that develop after critical illness. *Curr Opin Crit Care.* 2005;11:376–380.
132. Granja C, Teixeira-Pinto A, Costa-Pereira A. Quality of life after intensive care–evaluation with EQ-5D questionnaire. *Intensive Care Med.* 2002;28:898–907.
133. Hopkins RO, Weaver LK, Orme JF Jr, et al. Two-year cognitive, emotional, and quality-of-life outcomes in acute respiratory distress syndrome: response to correspondence. *Am J Respir Crit Care Med.* 2005;172:786–787.
134. Jackson JC, Gordon SM, Ely EW, et al. Research issues in the evaluation of cognitive impairment in intensive care unit survivors. *Intensive Care Med.* 2004;30:2009–2016.

CHAPTER 151 ■ ICU DISCHARGE CRITERIA AND REHABILITATION POTENTIAL FOR SEVERE BRAIN INJURY PATIENTS

RITA FORMISANO • MARIA MATTEIS • UMBERTO BIVONA • MARIA PAOLO CIURLI • R. ZAFONTE

DEFINITION OF ALTERED MENTAL STATUS AFTER SEVERE TRAUMATIC BRAIN INJURY

Severe brain injury is defined as a condition with coma, scored by the Glasgow coma scale (GCS) (1) as equal to or less than 8 for at least 6 hours (2). Severe brain injury has also been defined as a coma condition with a GCS equal to or less than 8, either initially or after deterioration, within 48 hours of injury (3). In the acute phase, the severity of coma is universally scored by means of the GCS, which differentiates mild, moderate, and severe brain injury, respectively, with scores of 13 to 15, 9 to 12 and ≤8 for severe brain injury. Although this scale is the most commonly used in the intensive care unit (ICU), other severity indexes such as the Innsbruck coma scale (ICS) have demonstrated a higher predictive power for mortality because of the inclusion of brainstem reflexes as a predictive value (4). For a detailed description of the most commonly used coma scales, see Frowein and Firsching (5) and Dolce and Sazbon (6).

Coma

The definition of coma includes the clinical triad of "closed eyes, not obeying simple commands, no comprehensible verbal utterances" (7). Coma has also been defined as a complete failure of the arousal system, with no spontaneous eye opening in patients who are unable to be awakened by application of vigorous sensory stimulation (8).

Although the assessment of impaired consciousness has been greatly facilitated by the development of the GCS, the presence of an artificial airway and ocular swelling often prevents assessment of the verbal score and complicates evaluation of eye opening; for these reasons, the grading of severely injured patients is largely, if not entirely, dependent on the motor score (9).

Coma can be associated with respiratory insufficiency, dysautonomic syndrome, and immunologic depression, especially during severe and prolonged disturbances of consciousness (6,10,11). Furthermore, specific clinical features can be observed during the rehabilitation phase, such as muscular hypertonia, dysautonomic symptoms, psychomotor agitation, and tracheopharyngeal dysfunction (12,13).

Recurrent respiratory failure is not uncommon. Although appropriate ICU discharge guidelines should include liberation from mechanical ventilation for at least 48 hours (14), 25% of the patients will require re-establishment of some form of assisted ventilation (15,16).

Severe brain injury patients often need a central venous access, an enteral feeding tube, or a percutaneous endoscopic gastrostomy (PEG). Comatose patients in the rehabilitation phase generally do not have a neurologic bladder, although only data of the acute phase are available (17,18). Therefore, the Foley catheter, a common cause of infection, should be removed as soon as possible and substituted with a condom catheter as needed.

Prolonged immobilization in the ICU may cause pressure skin decubitus, muscle contractures, ankylosis, and para-articular ossification (19–22), together with muscular atrophy and critical illness polyneuropathy (CIP) (23,24); the latter complication is commonly associated with sepsis. Immediate motor rehabilitation should be applied by means of adequate positioning, which should contrast pathologic postures and promote passive range of motion and basal stimulation.

Sensorial deprivation related to a long stay in ICU may also reduce a patient's interaction with the environment in the early phases of coma recovery, especially in the presence of behavioral disturbances, such as psychomotor agitation or inertia, aggravated by the limited contact of the patient with the family. A friendly environment can significantly improve a patient's interactions. For example, a music-based therapeutic approach (25) has been associated with improved neurophysiologic parameters (26).

The term *prolonged coma* (PC) may be an indicator of very severe brain injury for those patients with unconsciousness duration of at least 15 days (27,28). Arousal and vigilance (eyes opening) is generally noted after 3 to 4 weeks from coma onset, either with recovery of awareness (awakening) or without recovery of consciousness (vegetative state) (29,30).

Vegetative State

The vegetative state (VS) is a condition that follows coma, when the patient recovers the vigilance or alertness (eyes opening) but not the awareness, i.e., the ability to obey simple commands. The patient, in fact, is unable to interact with the surroundings, in spite of the eyes opening and the recovery of the sleep/wake cycle. The terms "persistent" or "permanent" are no longer used to avoid inaccurate prognostic adjectives (31). In fact, consciousness recovery after 1 year has been reported in up to 10% of the cases in traumatic VS and 5% of the cases in nontraumatic VS (32). Similarly, misdiagnosis of VS has been frequently described (33), as secondary to sedative drugs or subclinical seizures, with 6.3% of them displaying a nonconvulsive status epilepticus (34).

The locked-in syndrome (LIS) is defined as a condition apparently similar to VS, because of the presence of quadriplegia, mutism, and paralysis of the mouth, lips, and tongue, but it is distinguished from VS since the patients are fully aware of self and their surroundings and are able to communicate by means of vertical gaze and upper eyelid movements (8). This condition is generally caused by a complete deafferentation at the level of the ventral pons with normal electroencephalographic (EEG) activity.

VS patients may occasionally evolve to a locked-in syndrome during recovery of consciousness, especially in the presence of brainstem lesions or diffuse axonal injury with a functional disconnection syndrome.

As synonymous of VS, the term *apallic syndrome* (AS) has been recently reproposed (35) in the European guidelines for quality management of severe brain injury patients (36). In these guidelines, the clinical picture of the patient with VS/apallic syndrome is described as more complex and comprehensive of mutism, severe dysautonomic syndrome inclusive of hyperdynamic state (37), extrapyramidal symptoms such as akinesia, rigidity, parkinsonian posture, hypomimia, not extinguishable glabellar reflex, hypersalivation (sialorrhea), and facial seborrhea (38). Parkinsonian symptoms during recovery from prolonged posttraumatic coma or VS after severe traumatic brain injury (TBI) are very common, although they are rarely reported in the literature (39–41). These parkinsonian features generally improved after levodopa treatment together with different degrees of consciousness recovery, especially if used early in the first remission phases (42). We recently found a significant correlation between the motor slowness of some severe TBI patients and specific motor-evoked potentials (Bereits-Schaft potentials) (43). These parkinsonian motor deficits frequently show neuroradiologic features of diffuse axonal injury (43–46). Similarly, cerebellar signs can be very common in survivors of prolonged posttraumatic coma or VS because of the anatomic or functional involvement of the brainstem and the afferent/efferent pathways to and from the cerebellum (47).

Minimally Conscious State

The term *minimally conscious state* (MCS) (48), previously called "minimally responsive state" (49), has been recently introduced to identify those patients who are occasionally able to obey simple commands (50,51). This clinical state may follow either coma or VS as a transitional or permanent condition between VS and severe disability (52–54).

MCS patients demonstrate discernible behavioral evidence of consciousness but remain unable to reproduce this behavior consistently (50,51,55,56). Nevertheless, the distinction between VS and MCS is not always so clear, because of possible oscillations of the disturbance of consciousness due to different coexisting neurologic (34) and neurosurgical (57) conditions (34) or drug side effects (58,59).

Psychomotor agitation, aggressiveness, and sexual disinhibition (Klüver-Bucy syndrome) are frequent behaviors in severe brain injury patients who are not able to reliably follow simple commands, and their early occurrence is a positive predictor of consciousness recovery (59,60). Few published cases suggest that clinical examination may not be sufficient to frame the patient's unconsciousness state.

As for the differential diagnosis between VS, MCS, and LIS, Owen et al. (61) recently described the case of a young woman who sustained a severe head injury in a traffic accident with clinical evolution to VS. Though the VS persisted (48), an investigation by means of magnetic resonance imaging (MRI) scans 5 months after the accident showed a retained ability to process language and maintain complex visual imagery as in healthy subjects (61,62). Since it has also been reported that occasional LIS patients are not able to communicate by eyelid movements because of an extended palsy to ocular motility (63), in such cases a clinical differentiation between VS and LIS becomes and should be supported at least by an EEG, an examination not reported in this last case (62).

In the postacute phase of the patient with VS and MCS, the disability rating scale (DRS) (64), the Rancho Los Amigos scale, also defined as levels of cognitive functioning (LCF) (65) (Appendix), the Coma Recovery Scale (CRS) (49), and the Wessex

Head Injury Matrix (66) are among the scales able to monitor minimal behavioral changes during consciousness recovery.

For a more extensive description of the coma and disability scales for the evaluation of severe brain injury patients, see Gill-Thwaites and Munday (67), Formisano et al. (68), Dolce and Sazbon (6), and Koren et al. (69).

EPIDEMIOLOGY

Intensive care units (ICUs) often admit patients suffering from coma not only of traumatic cause, but also of different causes such as hypoxemic or dysrhythmic cardiac arrest, ischemic or hemorrhagic stroke, central nervous system (CNS) infections and intoxications, and organic brain diseases. Epidemiologic data on coma incidence and prevalence are very poor because of the various causes of coma and the different evolution toward recovery.

Severe traumatic brain injury (TBI), mainly secondary to road accidents, represents the first cause of disability in the young population between 15 and 35 years of age, which is the more productive age range, with longer life expectancy (70–72). Data collected in Europe (Italy) report that TBI affects 300 new cases every 100,000 subjects per year, with a total of 1,500,000 new cases every year (73–75). One percent to 2% of the patients persist in coma for longer than 1 month. Data extrapolated from the United Kingdom (76) estimate a prevalence of disability secondary to traumatic coma of 35,000 individuals every year. In the United States, the number of individuals who sustain severe TBI with prolonged loss of consciousness each year is estimated to be between 56 and 170 per one million population (PMP) (55,76,77). In the United States, of the nearly 400,000 individuals with a head injury who are admitted to a hospital each year, at least 98,000 will be significantly disabled (78,79).

The incidence of VS continuing for at least 6 months after the accident rises at a rate between 5 and 25 PMP, whereas the prevalence of VS in adults is reported to be between 40 and 168 PMP; the incidence and the prevalence of MCS have yet to be established (52).

Official national statistics are not available for these conditions, since neither VS nor MCS is a formal diagnosis under *DSM*-IV-TR (80) or ICD-10 (81). Conversely, VS has been included and coded in the International Classification of Functioning (ICF) (82). More recent data from an Italian study group (83) calculated an incidence for VS at 6 months after brain injury, ranging from 0.5 to 4/100,000 inhabitants, with a mean survival rate from 6 months to 15 years.

Neurologic Aspects of Postcomatose TBI Patients

Early Clinical Predictive Features

The prognostic role of age in the recovery process has been widely reported in the literature (84–89). In fact, a coma duration of 15 days or longer never leads to a complete functional recovery in subjects older than 50 years (59,90).

As for the premorbid personality, alcohol and drug abuse, together with previous psychiatric disorders, have been reported as a possible risk factor for TBI (85). In our experience, survivors of severe TBI sometimes improve in their previous depressive syndrome or get over drug addiction/substance abuse and dependence, likely because of the affective mood flattening due to an electroshocklike effect of the TBI, which frequently involves the frontal lobes.

Among the most important admission prognostic factors, hypoxia—either hypotensive or ischemic—significantly worsens the final outcome (46,91–93). Several authors have, in fact, reported a 20% increase in mortality or evolution to VS in those patients who were hypoxic in the acute phase (94,95) and of 30% in those with shock at the time of admission (96). We have observed that most of the patients who developed VS lasting longer than 1 year had sustained a further secondary hypoxic damage. In fact, it has been reported that 90% of adults who sustained severe brain injury can show evidence of brain hypoxic ischemia at autopsy (97). GCS and duration of coma are universally considered clinical predictive indicators of the final outcome (2,53).

As soon as the patient becomes responsive, in the early phases after coma recovery, agitation and restlessness are frequent and typical of delirium complaints, which generally are a specific characteristic of posttraumatic amnesia (PTA) and coincides with level 4 of the LCF scale (confused-agitated). PTA is defined as the period of time after coma recovery when the patient is not able to memorize everyday events of the last 24 hours (98). This period may last from twice to four times the coma duration (72) and is universally considered one of the most significant predictive factors for the final outcome of severe brain injury patients (9,99). Added behavioral features of PTA may include aggression, akathisia, disinhibition, and emotional lability (100).

The presence of brainstem reflexes in the acute phase have also been reported as important clinical prognostic factors (2,9,101). The 1-year mortality after severe TBI is reported to be 86% with absent pupillary response and 90% when both pupillary reaction and oculocephalic response are absent. When both responses are absent for more than 24 hours, the death rate is 100% (102). Eye movements are a useful diagnostic discriminant (103–105), and the absence of the normal oculocephalic reflex is widely considered a sign of very poor prognosis (105,106).

In the acute and postacute phase, possible endocrinologic disorders should be investigated since hypopituitarism may need specific hormone replacement therapy (107,108). Vigilance disorders, hydroelectrolytic alterations, immunologic deficits, dysautonomic vegetative symptoms, and cognitive and behavioral disturbances may be secondary to selective or total dysfunction of the hypothalamic-pituitary axis (109–119).

Other predictors of poor long-term functional prognosis include decortication and decerebration postures (6,35) and vegetative dysautonomia (6,11,37). The result is difficulty in the passive range of motion, with muscle contractures and ankylosis at the level of the major joints frequently complicated by periarticular ossification (PAO) and tendon retractions or shortenings (19–22,120).

In VS patients, the appearance of primitive oral automatisms, such as chewing, sucking, and yawning, may be negative predictive features for consciousness recovery (6). Conversely, psychomotor agitation and bulimia during recovery from coma and VS may be considered good prognostic indicators for the final outcome (59), as is the presence of the Klüver-Bucy syndrome, a transitory behavioral disinhibition, increased primitive oral automatisms, and hypersexuality (60,121,122). Motor recovery, when present, generally starts from the distal to proximal limb, likely because of the relative sparing of the cerebral cortex, where the hand and foot are largely controlled.

Asymmetric motor recovery can also represent undiagnosed spinal cord injury, or CIP, or it may be linked to hydrocephalus (57), especially if associated to epileptic seizures, and cognitive and behavioral disturbances poorly responsive to pharmacologic and rehabilitative treatment. Finally myoclonic jerks may be secondary to cortical or brainstem lesions or cerebral hypoxic damage with unfavorable prognosis for long-lasting disability (6).

Instrumental Prognostic Investigations

Electrophysiologic techniques (EEG and evoked potentials [EP]) carry out an important role in the management of severe brain injury patients and should be integrated with neuroimaging techniques (computed tomography [CT] and MRI).

Electroencephalogram

Electroencephalogram (EEG) reactivity seems to be a very significant parameter, being minimally influenced by mild sedation (123,124). The presence of alpha-coma, theta-coma, triphasic waves, and spontaneous not reagent burst suppression are considered signs of an unfavorable outcome both in terms of survival and in quality of life (125). A possible predictive index for posttraumatic coma and VS prognosis that has raised interest in the past few years is the pattern of sleep organization. EEG patterns similar to those of sleep have been considered good prognostic markers (126–130).

Somatosensory Evoked Potentials

The International Federation of Clinical Neurophysiology (IFCN) (131) published guidelines on the interpretation of somatosensory evoked potentials (SEP) believed to be highly reliable from the prognostic standpoint (132).

Acoustic Evoked Potentials

Absent or abnormal brainstem acoustic evoked potentials (BAEPs) are universally poor predictors; in fact, 98% of these patients die or will remain in VS (132). Conversely, a delayed P300 component, which is a cognitive response, was observed in all patients with LIS, all MCS patients, and in three of five patients in a VS (133), whereas the presence of N400 event-related evoked potentials were able to differentiate VS, near VS, and patients not in VS (134).

In general, BAEPs have a better predictive value in terms of predicting survival, whereas SEPs are able to better predict quality of outcome. Outcome can become extremely accurate (98%) when EP and EEG are combined (124).

Computed Tomography

The Marshall classification (135) is widely used in the acute phase of a comatose patient as a discriminant of cerebral edema, focal or diffuse damage, and severity of diffuse axonal injury (DAI). Whereas hemorrhagic axonal injury can be seen on computed tomography (CT) as multiple foci of high attenuation, nonhemorrhagic injury can be missed. In fact, CT is abnormal in less than half of all patients with DAI (136).

Magnetic Resonance Imaging

Magnetic resonance imaging (MRI) can predict recovery from posttraumatic VS when brainstem damage is present (137,138). Proton MRI spectroscopy can detect the amount of creatine, choline, myoinositol, and N-acetylaspartate (NAA) in a selected tissue volume (139). NAA can be assumed to be a marker of neuronal loss. Several investigators have found that a lower NAA-to-creatine ratio correlates with poorer outcome after TBI (140–148). More recent studies correlated spectroscopic MRI with histologic changes, severity of TBI, and VS prediction (149–155). Functional MRI (fMRI) is currently being explored as a method to predict the recovery of consciousness in those VS patients who will evolve toward MCS (61,62).

Single Photon Emission Computed Tomography

Since MRI detects lesions missed by single photon emission computed tomography (SPECT) and vice versa, a combination of MRI and SPECT may enhance or correct a prognostic prediction (156,157). Experience in this field is accumulating as the technology becomes more widely available.

Positron Emission Tomography

The reduction of cerebral metabolism by positron emission tomography (PET) can be useful to diagnose the extent of DAI (158). Recent PET studies in VS patients indicated altered activity in a critical frontoparietal cortical network, the restoration of which can be linked to a recovery of consciousness (159).

REHABILITATION PROTOCOL IN THE ACUTE PHASE

The ICU hospital course of severe brain injury patients may last from a few days to several weeks, but rehabilitation should start as soon as possible. Besides the evolution of the primary injury, infections are the most common impediment to early rehabilitation. The comatose patient frequently shows a high proneness to infections, secondary to central immunodepression (10) or peripheral facilitating factors such as the presence of a central venous catheter, tracheostomy tube, bladder catheter, pressure decubitus, and resistant nosocomial infections (160).

The utility of a passive range of motion in the acute phase is confirmed by experimental studies in animals, where it was demonstrated that a satisfying articular and muscle tendinous range of motion may be maintained in subjects after prolonged immobility, only if every joint is mobilized daily and for 2 hours (161). Similarly, prevention of muscle contractures or ankylosis can be prevented by dynamic positioning splinting (120,162,163).

State-of-the-art prevention of bed rest contractures include the following:

a. Early mobilization of the limbs to avoid joint contractures and para-articular ossification, osteoporosis, and nonuse muscular atrophy
b. Venous thrombosis prophylaxis at the lower limbs by means of elastic compression and specific pharmacotherapy (subcutaneous low-dose heparin)
c. Early recovery of the sitting position to counteract extensor muscle spasms and limit the tonic labyrinthic reflex (163)

The stabilization of the medical conditions and vital functions represents a fundamental requisite for the patient's transfer potential from the ICU to the intensive rehabilitation unit.

Besides the obvious requirement for hemodynamic stability, a diagnostic/therapeutic protocol for severe brain injury patients scheduled for transfer to a rehabilitation unit should include the following:

- Cerebral CT or MRI to rule out late neurosurgical complications such as chronic hematoma, hygroma, and hydrocephalus (57,164)
- Tracheobronchoscopy to rule out tracheal stenosis or esophagotracheal fistula, even in the absence of obvious respiratory stridor (165–168)
- Properly functioning enteral tube feeding, or a percutaneous endoscopic gastrostomy (PEG), when tube feeding has to be continued for >1 month
- Complete fever workup in case of recurrent and persistent hyperpyrexia
- Endocrinologic investigation of possible hypopituitarism (107,108)
- Echo Doppler of the lower limbs to rule out silent venous thrombosis secondary to the prolonged bed rest (169–171)
- Electromyography and electroneurography of the upper and lower limbs in case of early muscular atrophy to rule out critical illness polyneuropathy (CIP) (24,172) or compressive neuropathies, secondary to articular ankylosis, pathologic postures, and inadequate positioning

Postacute Rehabilitation

The first rehabilitation goal after discharge from the ICU is the gradual recovery of the sitting position, with monitoring of the cardiovascular parameters, prevention of arterial orthostatic hypotension, and facilitation of exercises to improve head and trunk control in assisted sitting and passive standing positions.

An early phoniatric evaluation investigates respiratory air space by means of fibro-laryngoscopy, whereas a speech therapist examines daily oromotor abilities and dysphagia (173), including an evaluation of deglutition initiative, cough reflex elicitation, and risk of pulmonary aspiration. The first oral meal of adequate consistency has to be assisted by a phoniatric therapist, who has a specific expertise in swallowing training, compensatory posturing of the head during deglutition, and suctioning techniques. Winstein (174) reported that approximately 25% of the head-injured adults admitted to a rehabilitation facility demonstrated swallowing or oral motor problems on admission. Ninety-four percent of this group ultimately became successful oral feeders within 3 months, associated with a concomitant improvement of cognitive functions, primitive oral motor reflexes, and neurogenic dysphagia.

Respiratory training includes thorax clapping, bronchial secretions suctioning, cough elicitation, and forced expiratory exercises. Gradual downsizing of the tracheostomy tube size to closure should be monitored by pulse oximetry. Complications and setbacks are frequent in this phase, often requiring transferring of the patient to a higher acuity ward for events such as:

- Recurrent acute respiratory failure
- Recurrent infections or severe hyperthermia
- Progressive tracheal stenosis or tracheoesophageal fistula
- Plastic surgery of sacral and pressure calcaneal ulcers
- Stabilization of limb fractures or early excision of periarticular ossification
- Hydrocephalus or malfunctioning ventriculoperitoneal/atrial shunting (57)
- Worsening of chronic posttraumatic hematomas or hygromas requiring emergency craniotomy or early cranioplasty, since the latter may determine some clinical improvement (175–178)

Neuropsychological Approach to Severe Brain Injury Patients and their Family

Caregiver

At the beginning of the rehabilitation process, the patient's family (caregiver) often complains of the lack of information while their relative is in the acute phase. A professional intervention by a psychologist is often necessary to reconcile the family with the intensive care experience, which includes close and honest communication and reassurance (179–182). Emotional support and practical advice and educational brochures are highly valued by family members during the first year after injury (179,183–185).

Patient Assessment

The levels of cognitive functioning scale (LCF) (65) (Appendix 1) assesses behavioral and cognitive patient functioning—from onset of coma to recovery of consciousness and cognition.

In addition to qualitative measurement methods, quantitative measures are also available and have been widely used. A short list is indicated below:

- Coma Recovery Scale (CRS) (49) and CRS-Revised (CRS-R) (186);
- Coma/Near Coma Scale (CNC) (187);
- Sensory Stimulation Assessment Measure (SSAM) (188);
- Western Neuro Sensory Stimulation Profile (WNSSP) (189);
- Wessex Head Injury Matrix (WHIM) (66).

Other custom-made scales, such as the one proposed by Whyte (190), are founded on an individualized protocol that is able to assess *specific* behaviors for *each* patient. In the early stage of coma recovery, these tools define *intentionality, frequency,* and *consistency* of the behavioral reactions of the patient. In the first phase of coma recovery, the patient's performance is erratic and may depend on the general clinical condition, the arousal state, and the external conditions. Creating a quiet environment that avoids distractions and performing very short and frequent yet comprehensive evaluations are fundamental.

Neuropsychological Support

Specific neuropsychological interventions may promote recovery, particularly in patients in MCS. For example, in our experience, music therapy may improve collaboration, reducing behavioral disorders and improving initiative and calm (191). However, the standards of care have not been established to guide rehabilitative treatment in patients with disorders of consciousness (DOC), and the effect of rehabilitative treatment in restoring consciousness, cognition, or functional capacity is still highly debated (51,192,193).

In conclusion, clinical experience in postacute rehabilitation suggests the importance of a global approach to the TBI patient and the need to involve the family in the rehabilitation treatment. Adequate exchange with the family by means of psychosocial interviews may, in fact, allow a better understanding of the patient's premorbid personality and social network.

PHARMACOTHERAPY

An adequate pharmacologic treatment during coma and its remission phases may accelerate the recovery process and improve symptoms and emerging syndromes (68). Although agitated severe brain injury patients often need sedation in the ICU, traditional neuroleptics should be avoided in the acute phase because of severe side effects such as vigilance reduction, extrapyramidal effects, epileptogenesis, and impairment of neural plasticity (194). Agitation may be controlled with fewer side effects by antiepileptic drugs such as carbamazepine and valproic acid (195,196). Similarly, the beta-blocker propranolol at low dosage is the only drug that demonstrated a significant efficacy in agitated patients according to the Cochrane Review (197). Propranolol should also be used for the control of vegetative dysautonomic symptoms, especially tachycardia and tachypnea, arterial hypertension, and severe sweating, all signs of sympathetic nervous system hyperactivity and hyperfunction of basal metabolism up to 180% (198, 199).

Tricyclic antidepressant agents such as amitriptyline, even if epileptogenic, have been used for agitation (194,200); they may also be useful in the presence of spastic laughing and crying, chronic pain, depressive mood, or food refusal in the awakening phase, as well as activating agents (201). Benzodiazepines such as diazepam may be used when severe spasticity compromises spontaneous motility. Unfortunately, benzodiazepines and other commonly used drugs in these patients—such as clonidine, phenobarbital, cortisone, and haloperidol—have all shown adverse effects when used in the ICU (194). Recently, the minor tranquilizer zolpidem has been reported as facilitating consciousness recovery in chronic VS and MVS patients (202). Zolpidem is a GABA-A–enhancing agent acting on omega receptors and is generally used for insomnia. Some antiepileptic drugs, such as oxcarbazepine, gabapentin, clonazepam, and more recently, pregabalin, may be used for the treatment of epilepsy, myoclonic jerks, tremor, hyperpathia or dysesthesia, agitation, and dystonia (oral trismus). Restlessness and agitation may also be treated by atypical neuroleptics, such as clozapine, risperidone, olanzapine, quetiapine, and in some cases buspirone (68,203). One agent, quetiapine, has the advantage of causing less iatrogenic parkinsonism and to be less epileptogenic than the other neuroleptics (204,205) in patients already at risk for secondary epilepsy and posttraumatic parkinsonism (39,40,41,43,206,207). Unfortunately, all antiepileptics and atypical neuroleptics may worsen vigilance and delay consciousness recovery.

Antidepressant drugs such as tricyclics and serotoninergic (SSRI), mixed serotoninergic, and noradrenergic agents have been occasionally used and found effective for motor, neuropsychological, and psychological recovery of TBI patients (208–210). Drugs such as baclofen, tizanidine, and diazepam are often used as muscle relaxant agents or antispasticity drugs. Among them, disodium dantrolene has the advantage of having a less sedative effect. Another more recent alternative is the botulinum toxin, used as a local infiltration for patients with segmental spasticity (211,212), whereas the continuous intrathecal infusion of baclofen (ITB) (baclofen pump) is used for diffuse spasticity, contractures, pain, and dysautonomic syndrome (213,214)—sometimes with responsivity improvement after ITB (215). The most common side effects of ITB, even if rarely reported, include hypotonia, asthenia, nystagmus, dizziness, drowsiness, disorientation, nausea, vomiting, urine retention, constipation, and more rarely, cardiorespiratory depression, seizures, and paralytic ileus (216–218). The latter complication should be suspected especially in cases of brainstem injury, because baclofen acts directly over vegetative nuclei but can be easily minimized by reducing the total daily dose of the drug (210,212).

Despite the widespread use of antiepileptic drugs for prevention of posttraumatic epilepsy (PTE) (219–221), controlled studies and international guidelines demonstrated the lack of efficacy and recommend against their prophylactic use (222–225). Interestingly, the use of prophylactic antiepileptic therapy seems to increase the risk of late PTE during the discontinuation of treatment (226). Myoclonic jerks may be successfully treated by piracetam, clonazepam, and more recently, by levetiracetam (227–229).

A survey of 127 neurosurgical clinics showed that penetrating injuries, intracranial hemorrhages, rise in ICP, and electroencephalographic (EEG) abnormalities were the most frequent reasons why antiepileptic prophylaxis was initiated in the neurologic ICU (230–232). Since traditional antiepileptic drugs may further compromise the vigilance state, carbamazepine or valproic acid should be used only when restlessness or agitation are present during the ICU hospital course or in the case of late PTE.

As for the treatment of early PTE, phenytoin is one of the drugs of choice in the ICU. The first-choice drugs among the traditional antiepileptics for late PTE are carbamazepine and valproic acid, whereas among the new antiepileptic drugs lamotrigine, topiramate, oxcarbazepine, and especially levetiracetam seem to have less detrimental effects on cognitive function (233,234).

Restlessness is frequently associated with chronic pain in severe brain injury patients, and it may be secondary to the central hyperpathia (thalamic syndrome) or peripheral dysesthesias (critical illness polyneuropathy [CIP]). The new antiepileptic drugs such as lamotrigine, topiramate, gabapentin, and pregabalin may also be useful for the treatment of chronic pain and for increasing tolerance to passive range of motion.

The use of inotropic agents may be useful for counteracting somnolence and the iatrogenic soporous state induced by antiepileptic agents. In particular, piracetam, a cyclic derivative of gamma-aminobutyric acid (GABA), has been used for its inhibitory action on the excitatory amino acids (235,236).

Among the drugs with activating action, L-dopa showed electroencephalographic and behavioral effects of awakening, counteracting the hypnogenic effect of 5-hydroxytryptophan (42,237–240). Newman et al. (241), as well, reported an improvement in cognitive functions including logical association after L-dopa and carbidopa. Amantadine and dopaminergic drugs may improve both parkinsonian features and consciousness recovery (242–245). Similarly, Weinberg et al. (246) obtained good results in the recovery of cognitive functions in patients with sequelae of TBI after dopaminergic drugs were given. Other authors reported an interesting positive effect of L-dopa and bromocriptine in the motor and cognitive recovery of postcomatose patients (247–249).

Amantadine, which exerts a dopaminergic effect and an inhibitory action on excitatory amino acids, demonstrated a significant efficacy in the improvement of attention, psychomotor speed, mobility, vocalization, motivation, and agitation in severe TBI patients (245,250–254). Finally, methylphenidate has demonstrated some effects on attention deficits after TBI, with associated improvement on restlessness and agitation (255).

In summary, the sequential pharmacotherapeutic protocol of severe brain injury patients should include the treatment of vegetative dysautonomia by means of beta-blockers (199). The reduction of muscle tone and the improvement of the passive range of motion ultimately prevent joint ankylosis and tendon shortening (120,256). Preventive therapy for PAO includes etidronate and nonsteroid antiphlogistic agents, especially indomethacin given at the dosage of 75 mg daily together with gastric protection (257–261).

Psychomotor agitation significantly impairs the potential for neurorehabilitation, especially when associated with pain and antagonistic behavior. The drugs of choice for controlling agitation are propranolol (197), carbamazepine, and valproic acid, as well as new antiepileptic drugs such as oxcarbazepine and lamotrigine. When antiepileptics are not effective against agitation and restlessness, amantadine (251) and amitriptyline (200) may be useful. Quetiapine can be introduced during propofol discontinuation in the ICU or when aggressiveness and delirium persist for longer periods of time (205). L-Dopa and dopaminergic drugs may enhance consciousness and verbal communication recovery, improving cognitive functions and parkinsonian symptoms (39,42,262).

APPENDIX

Appendix 1

Levels of Cognitive Functioning

(Personal communication: Chris Hagen, Ph.D.; Denise Malkmus, MA; Patricia A. Durham, MS; Rancho Los Amigos Hospital). (www.calpoly.edu/~lklooste/levels.htm).

1. No response
   Patient appears to be in a deep sleep and completely unresponsive to any stimuli.
2. Generalized response
   Patient reacts inconsistently and nonpurposefully to stimuli. Responses are limited in nature and are often the same regardless of the stimulus presented. Responses may be physiologic, gross body movements, and vocalization. Responses are likely to be delayed. The earliest response is to deep pain.
3. Localized response
   Patient reacts specifically but inconsistently to stimuli. Responses are directly related to the type of stimulus presented, as in turning the head toward a sound or focusing on an object presented. The patient may withdraw an extremity and vocalize when exposed to a painful stimulus. He or she may follow simple commands in an inconsistent, delayed manner, such as closing the eyes, squeezing, or extending an extremity. Once external stimuli are removed, the patient may lie quietly. He or she may also show a vague awareness of self and body by responding to discomfort by pulling at nasogastric tube or catheter, or resisting restraints. The patient may show a bias toward responding to some persons, especially family and friends, but not to others.
4. Confused-agitated
   Patient is in a heightened state of activity with severe impairment to process information. Behavior is frequently bizarre and nonpurposeful relative to the immediate environment. He or she does not discriminate among persons or objects and is unable to cooperate directly with treatment efforts. Verbalization is frequently incoherent or inappropriate to the environment. Confabulation and hostility may be present. Being unaware of present events, the patient lacks short-term recall and may be reacting to past events. He or she is unable to perform self-care activities without maximum assistance. If not motor-disabled, the patient may perform automatic motor activities such as sitting, reaching, and ambulating as part of the agitated state but not necessarily as a purposeful act or on request.
5. Confused-inappropriate
   Patient appears alert and is able to respond to simple commands fairly consistently. However, with increased complexity of commands or lack of any external structure, responses are nonpurposeful, random, or at best, fragmented toward any desired goal. With structure, the patient may be able to converse on a social-automatic level for short periods of time. Verbalization is often inappropriate; confabulation may be triggered by present events. The patient can usually perform self-care activities with assistance and may accomplish feeding with supervision. If the patient is physically mobile, he or she may wander off, either randomly or with vague intention of "going home."
6. Confused-appropriate
   Patient shows goal-directed behavior, but is dependent on external input for direction. He or she follows simple directions consistently and shows carryover for learned tasks, e.g., self-care. Responses may be incorrect due to memory problems but are appropriate to the situation. Selective attention to tasks may be impaired, especially with difficult tasks and in unstructured settings, but patient is now functional for common daily activities.
7. Automatic-appropriate
   Patient appears oriented and acts appropriately within hospital and home settings, and goes through a daily routine automatically but robotlike, with minimal to absent confusion, and has shallow recall for what he or she has been doing. Patient is independent in self-care activities and supervised in home and community skills for safety. With structure, the patient is able to initiate tasks or social and recreation activities in which he or she now has interest. The patient's judgment remains impaired.
8. Purposeful-appropriate
   Patient is alert and oriented, able to recall and integrate past and recent events, and is aware of and responsive to his or her culture. Within the patient's physical capabilities, he or she is independent in home and community skills. The patient's social, emotional, and intellectual capacities may continue to be at a decreased level from baseline but functional within society.

SUMMARY

In the intensive care unit (ICU), the hospital course of severe brain injury patients may last from a few days to several weeks. The reasons for a more prolonged length of stay include the persistent need of vital functions support and the recurrence of infections or hyperpyrexia of central or peripheral cause (10). Timing of when best to transfer the patient from the ICU to rehabilitation facilities often represents the most delicate phase of the history of the comatose patient.

Many complications may be avoided by adequate nursing care and early rehabilitation approach in the ICU (161–163). Adequate nursing care including correct hygiene and early passive range of motion of severe brain injury patients may reduce the occurrence and severity of the early and late complications and facilitate the transfer from the ICU to rehabilitation.

Finally, a focused pharmacologic approach should focus on the possible adverse effects in selected cases and only by experienced clinicians. Since severe brain injury carries a great deal of social disability and cost for the society, randomized multicenter controlled studies on clinical and pharmacologic intervention efficacy should be encouraged.

References

1. Teasdale G, Jennett B. Assessment of coma and impaired consciousness. A practical scale. *Lancet.* 1974;2(7872):81.
2. Jennett B, Teasdale G, Braakman R, et al. Prognosis of patients with severe head injury. *Neurosurgery.* 1979;4:283.
3. Marshall LF, Becker DP, Bowers SA, et al. The National Traumatic Coma Data Bank, I: design, purpose, goals and results. *J Neurosurg.* 1983;59:276.
4. Benzer A, Mitterschiffthaler G, Marosi M, et al. Prediction of non-survival after trauma: Innsbruck Coma Scale. *Lancet.* 1991;338:125.
5. Frowein RA, Firsching R. Classification of head injury. In: Vinken PJ, Bruyn GW, Klawans HL. *Handbook of Clinical Neurology.* Vol. 57. Amsterdam, the Netherlands: Elsevier Science; 1990:101.
6. Dolce G, Sazbon L. *The Post-traumatic Vegetative State.* Stuttgart, Germany: Thieme Medical Publishers; 2002.
7. Jennett B. Clinical assesment of consciousness. Introduction. *Acta Neurochir.* 1986;(Suppl 36):90.
8. Plum F, Posner J. *The Diagnosis of Stupor and Coma.* 3rd ed., Philadelphia, PA: FA Davis Co; 1982.
9. Levin HS, Hamilton WJ, Grossman RG. Outcome after head injury. In: Vinken PJ, Bruyn GW, Klawans HL. *Handbook of Clinical Neurolgy.* Vol. 57. Amsterdam, the Netherlands: Elsevier Science; 1990:367.
10. Formisano R, Grelli S, Matteucci C, et al. Immunological and endocrinological disturbances in patients after prolonged coma following head injury. *Eur J Neurol.* 1998;5(2):151.
11. Intiso D, Formisano R, Grasso MG, et al. Neurovegetative disorders after severe head injury. *J Auton Nerv Syst.* 1993;43(Suppl):86.
12. Kazandjian MS, Dikeman KJ, Bach JR. Assessment and management of communication impairment in neuromuscular disease. *Semin Neurol.* 1995;15(1):52.
13. Eubenks DH, Bone R. *Comprehensive Respiratory Care: A learning System.* St. Louis, MO: Mosby; 1990.
14. Taricco M, De Tanti A, Boldrini P, et al. National Consensus Conference, Guidelines. *Eura Medicophys.* 2006;42:73. www.minervamedica.it/pdf/R33Y2006/R33Y2006N01A0073.pdf.
15. Capdevila X, Perrigault PF, Ramontxo M, et al. Changes in breathing pattern and respiratory muscle performance parameters during difficult weaning. *Crit Care Med.* 1998;26:79.
16. Amini S, Gabrielli A, Layon J. Respiratory function and mechanical ventilation in the patient with neurological impairment. In: Layon AJ, Gabrielli A, Friedman NA, eds. *Textbook of Neurointensive Care.* Philadelphia, PA: Saunders Elsevier; 2004:579–605.
17. Wyndaele JJ. Micturition in comatose patients. *J Urol.* 1986;135:1209.
18. Wyndaele JJ. Urodynamics in comatose patients. *Neurol Urodyn.* 1990; 9:43.
19. Sazbon L, Najenson T, Tartakovsky M, et al. Widespread periarticular newbone formation in long-term comatose patients. *J Bone Joint Surg Br.* 1981 Feb;63-B(1):120.
20. Ippolito E, Formisano R, Caterini R, et al. Resection of elbow ossification and continuous passive motion in post-comatose patients. *J Hand Surg.* 1999;24-A(3):546.
21. Ippolito E, Formisano R, Farsetti P, et al. Excision for the treatment of periarticular ossification of the in patients who have a traumatic brain injury. *J Bone Joint Surg.* 1999;81-A(6):783.
22. Ippolito E, Formisano R, Caterini R, et al. Operative treatment of heterotopic hip ossification in patients with coma after brain injury. *Clin Orthop Relat Res.* 1999;(365):130.
23. Latronico N, Fenzi F, Recupero D, et al. Critical illness myopathy and neuropathy. *Lancet.* 1996;347:1579.
24. Latronico N, Peli E, Botteri M. Critical illness myopathy and neuropathy. *Curr Opin Crit Care.* 2005;11(2):126.
25. Nordoff P, Robbins C. *Creative Music Therapy.* New York, NY: Day J ed.; 1977.
26. Gustorff D. Lieder ohne Worte. *Musiktherapeutische Umschau.* 1990;11: 120.
27. Formisano R, Voogt RD, Buzzi MG, et al. Time interval of oral feeding recovery as a prognostic factor in severe traumatic brain injury. *Brain Inj.* 2004;18(1):103.
28. Formisano R, Carlesimo GA, Sabbadini M, et al. Clinical predictors and neuropsychological outcome in severe traumatic brain injury patients. *Acta Neurochir (Wien).* 2004;146:457.
29. Danze F. Coma and the vegetative states [in French]. *Soins.* 1993;(569):4.
30. Jennett B, Plum F. Persistent vegetative state after brain damage. A syndrome in search of a name. *Lancet,* 1972;1:734–737.
31. International Working Party. *Report on the Vegetative State.* London, England: Royal College of Physicians; 1996.
32. Borthwick C. The permanent vegetative state: ethical crux, medical fiction. *Issues Law Med.* 1996;12(2):167.
33. Childs NL, Mercer WN, Childs HW. Accuracy of diagnosis of persistent vegetative state. *Neurology.* 1993;43(8):1457.
34. Vespa PM, Nuwer MR, Nenov V, et al. Increased incidence and impact of nonconvulsive and convulsive seizures after traumatic brain injury as detected by continuous electroencephalographic monitoring. *J Neurosurg.* 1999;91(5):750.
35. Gerstenbrand F. *Das Traumatische Apallische Syndrom.* Vienna-New York: Springer; 1967.
36. von Wild K, Gerstenbrand F, Dolce G, et al. Guidelines on quality management of patients in apallic syndrome (vegetative state). *Eur J Trauma.* 2007;33(3):268–292.
37. Baguley IJ, Nicholls JL, Felmingham KL, et al. Dysautonomia after traumatic brain injury: a forgotten syndrome? *J Neurol Neurosurg Psychiatry.* 1999;67(1):39.
38. Binder H, Gerstenbrand F, Grunberger J, et al. Experience with a L-dopa retard preparation in the peroral long-term therapy of the parkinsonian syndrome. *Nervenarzt.* 1976;47(11):656.
39. Jellinger KA. Parkinsonism and persistent vegetative state after head injury. *J Neurol Neurosurg Psychiatry.* 2004;75:1082.
40. Matsuda W, Matsumura A, Komatsu Y, et al. Awakenings from persistent vegetative state: report of three cases with parkinsonism and brain stem lesions on MRI. *J Neurol Neurosurg Psychiatry.* 2003;74:1571.
41. Matsuda W, Komatsu Y, Matsumura A, et al. Authors' reply. 2004. http://jnnp.bmj.com/cgi/content/full/75/7/1082-a.
42. Haig AJ, Ruess JM. Recovery from vegetative state of six months duration associated with Sinemet (levodopa/carbidopa). *Arch Phys Med Rehab.* 1990;71(13):1081.
43. Di Russo F, Incoccia C, Formisano R, et al. Abnormal motor preparation in severe traumatic brain injury with good recovery. *J Neurotrauma.* 2005;22:297.
44. Tomaiuolo F, Carlesimo GA, Di Paola M, et al. Gross morphology and morphometric sequelae in the hippocampus, fornix and corpus callosum of patients with severe non missile traumatic brain injury without macroscopic detectable lesions: a T1 weighted MRI study. *J Neurol Neurosurg Psychiatry.* 2004;75 (9):1314.
45. Adams RD, Victor M. *Principles of Neurology.* 3rd ed. New York, NY: McGraw-Hill; 1976.
46. Graham DI, Mclellan D, Adams JH, et al. The neuropathology of the vegetative state after severe disability after non-missile head injury. *Acta Neurochir.* 1983;32:65–67.
47. Formisano R, Saltuari L, Sailer U, et al. Post-traumatic cerebellar syndrome. *New Trends Clin Neuropharmacol.* 1987;(1–2):115.
48. Medical aspects of the persistent vegetative state (1). The Multi-Society Task Force on PVS. *N Engl J Med.* 1994;330(21):1499.
49. Giacino JT, Kezmarsky MA, De Luca J, et al. Monitoring rate of recovery to predict outcome in minimally responsive patients. *Arch Phys Med Rehab.* 1991;72:897.
50. Giacino JT. The vegetative and minimally conscious state: consensus-based criteria for establishing diagnosis and prognosis. *NeuroRehabilitation.* 2004;19(4):293.
51. Giacino JT, Trott CT. Rehabilitative management of patients with disorders of consciousness. *J Head Trauma Rehabil.* 2004;19(3):254.
52. Beaumont JG, Kenealy PM. Incidence and prevalence of the vegetative and minimally conscious states. *Neuropsychol Rehabil.* 2005;15(3–4):184.
53. Jennett B, Bond M. Assessment of outcome after severe brain damage. *Lancet.* 1975;1(7905):480.

54. Jennett B, McMillan R. Epidemiology of head injury. *BMJ.* 1981;282:101.
55. Giacino JT, Ashwal S, Childs N, et al. The minimally conscious state: definition and diagnostic criteria. *Neurology.* 2002;58:349.
56. Giacino JT. Disorders of consciousness: differential diagnosis and neuropathologic features. *Semin Neurol.* 1997;17(2):105.
57. Missori P, Miscusi M, Formisano R, et al. Magnetic resonance imaging flow void changes after cerebrospinal fluid shunt in post-traumatic hydrocephalus: clinical correlations and outcome. *Neurosurg Rev.* 2006;29:224.
58. Strens LH, Mazibrada G, Duncan JS, et al. Misdiagnosing the vegetative state after severe brain injury: the influence of medication. *Brain Inj.* 2004; 18(2):213.
59. Formisano R, Bivona U, Penta F, et al. Early clinical predictive factors during coma recovery. *Acta Neurochir Suppl.* 2005; 93:201.
60. Formisano R, Saltuari L, Gerstenbrand F. Presence of Klüver-Bucy syndrome as a positive prognostic feature for the remission of traumatic prolonged disturbances of consciousness. *Acta Neurol Scand.* 1995;91:54.
61. Owen AM, Coleman MR, Boly M, et al. Detecting awareness in the vegetative state. *Science.* 2006;313:1402.
62. Owen AM, Coleman MR, Boly M, et al. Supporting online material (SOM). 2006. www.sciencemag.org/cgi/content/full/313/5792/1402/DCI.
63. Smith E, Delargy M. Locked-in syndrome. *BMJ.* 2005;330:406.
64. Rappaport M, Hall KM, Hopkins K, et al. Disability rating scale for severe head trauma: coma to community. *Arch Phys Med Rehab.* 1982;63:132.
65. Hagen C, Malkmus D, Durham P. Levels of cognitive functioning. In: *Rehabilitation of the Head Injured Adult. Comprehensive Physical Management.* Downey, CA: Professional Staff Association of Rancho Los Amigos Hospital, Inc; 1979.
66. Shiel A, Horn SA, Wilson BA, et al. The Wessex Head Injury Matrix (WHIM) main scale: a preliminary report on a scale to assess and monitor patient recovery after severe head injury. *Clin Rehab.* 2000;14:408.
67. Gill-Thwaites H, Munday R. The Sensory Modality Assessment and Rehabilitation Technique (SMART): a comprehensive and integrated assessment and treatment protocol for the vegetative state and minimally responsive patient. *Neuropsychol Rehab.* 1999;9(3–4):305.
68. Formisano R, Penta F, Bivona U, et al. Protocollo diagnostico-terapeutico del grave traumatizzato cranico con coma prolungato post-traumatico. Rome, Italy: Istituto Superiore di Sanitá, Rapporti Istisan. Published January 26, 2001. http://www.iss.it/iss3/publ/rapp/index.php?lang=1&tipo=5&anno=2001.
69. Koren C, Gil M, Sazbon L. Assessment of the vegetative state. In: Dolce G, Sazbon L, eds. *The Post-traumatic Vegetative State.* Stuttgart, Germany: Thieme Medical Publishers; 2002:46–59.
70. Klauber RK, Barret-Connor E, Marshall LF et al. The epidemiology of head injury: a prospective study of an entire community, San Diego County, California, 1978. *Am J Epidemiol.* 1981;113:50.
71. Annegers JF, Grabow JD, Kurland TL. The incidence, causes and secular trends of head trauma in Olmsted Country, Minnesota, 1935–74. *Neurology.* 1980;30:919.
72. Jennett B, Frankowski RF. The epidemiology of head injury. In: Vinken PJ, Bruyn GW, Klawans HL. *Handbook of Clinical Neurology.* Vol. 57. Amsterdam, the Netherlands: Elsevier Science; 1990:1.
73. National Institute of Statistics - ISTAT 1986. www.istat.it.
74. Servadei F, Verlicchi A, Soldano F, et al. Descriptive epidemiology of head injury in Romagna and Trentino. Comparison between two geographically different Italian regions. *Neuroepidemiology.* 2002;21(6):297.
75. Bryden J. How many head injured? The epidemiology of post head injury disability. In: Wood RL, Eames P. *Models of Brain Injury Rehabilitation: 17.* London, England: Chapman & Hall; 1990.
76. Giacino JT, Zasler ND. Outcome after severe traumatic brain injury: coma, the vegetative state and the minimally responsive state. *J Head Trauma Rehab.* 1995;10:40.
77. Tresch DD, Sims FH, Duthie EH, et al. Clinical characteristics of patients in the persistent vegetative state. *Arch Intern Med.* 1991;151(5):930.
78. Johnson R, Gleave J. Counting the people disabled by head injury. *Injury.* 1987;18:7.
79. Kraus JF. Epidemiology of head injury. In: Cooper PR, ed. *Head Injury.* 2nd ed. Baltimore, MD: Williams & Wilkins; 1987:1.
80. American Psychiatric Association. *Diagnostic and Statistical Manual of Mental Disorders.* 4th ed. Washington, DC: American Psychiatric Association; 2000.
81. World Health Organisation. *The ICD-10 Classification of Mental and Behavioural Disorders: Clinical Descriptions and Diagnostic Guidelines.* Geneva, Switzerland: World Health Organisation; 1992.
82. International classification of functioning—ICF, WHO 2001. http://www3.who.int/icf/icftemplate.cfm.
83. Ministero della Salute. Stato vegetativo e stato di minima coscienza. *Ital J Rehab Med-MR.* 2007;21:5–25.
84. Jennett B, McMillan R. Epidemiology of head injury. *BMJ.* 1981;282:101.
85. Rimel RW, Jane JA, Bond MR. Characteristics of the head injured patient. In: Rosenthal M, Griffith E, Kreutzer J, et al., eds. *Rehabilitation of the Adult with Traumatic Brain Injury.* 2nd ed. Philadelphia, PA: FA Davis Co; 1991:8.
86. Harrison-Felix C, Newton C, Hall KM, et al. Descriptive findings from the traumatic brain injury model systems national data base. *J Head Trauma Rehabil.* 1996;11:1.
87. Carlsson C, Von Essen C, Lofgreen J. Factors affecting the clinical course of patients with severe head injury. *J Neurosurg.* 1968;29:242–251.
88. Pazzaglia P, Frank G, Frank F, et al. Clinical course and prognosis of acute post-traumatic coma. *J Neurol Neurosurg Psychiatry.* 1975;38:149.
89. Luerssen F, Klauber M, Marshall L. Outcome from head injury related to patient's age. *J Neurosurg.* 1988;68:409–416.
90. Frowein RA, Therhaag P, Firsching R. Long lasting coma after head injury: late results. *Adv Neurosurg.* 1989b;17:36.
91. Miller JD, Becker DP. Secondary insults to the injured brain. *J R Coll Surg Edinb.* 1982;27(5):292.
92. Overgaard J, Mosdal C, Tweed WA. Cerebral circulation after head injury, III: does reduced regional cerebral blood flow determine recovery of brain function after blunt head injury? *Neurosurgery.* 1981;55:63–74.
93. Obrist WD, Gennarelli TA, Segava H, et al. Relation of cerebral blood flow to neurological status and outcome in head injured patients. *J Neurosurg.* 1979;51:292–300.
94. Price DJ, Murray A. The influence of hypoxia and hypotension on recovery from head injury. *Injury.* 1972;3:218–225.
95. Miller JD. Head injury and brain ischemia, implication for therapy. *Br J Anaesthesiol.* 1985;57:120–129.
96. Newfield P, Pitts L, Kaktis J. The influence of shock on mortality after head trauma. *Crit Care Med.* 1980;8:254.
97. Graham DI, Ford I, Hume-Adams J, et al. Ischemic brain damage is still common in fatal non-missile head injury. *J. Neurol Neurosurg. Psychiatry.* 1989;52:346.
98. Russel WR, Smith A. Post traumatic amnesia in closed head injury. *Arch Neurol.* 1961;5:4.
99. Jennett B, Teasdale G, Braakman R, et al. Prediction of outcome in individual patients after severe head injury. *Neurosurgery.* 1976;4:283.
100. Sandel ME, Mysiw WJ. The agitated brain injured patient, 1: definitions, differential diagnosis, and assessment. *Arch Phys Med Rehab.* 1996;77:617.
101. Braakman R, Gelpke GJ, Habbema JDF, et al. Systematic selection of prognostic features in patients with severe head injury. *Neurosurgery.* 1980; 6:362.
102. Levati A, Farina ML, Vecchi G, et al. Prognosis of severe head injuries. *J Neurosurgery.* 1982;57:779.
103. Avezaat CJJ, van den Berge HJ, Braakman R. Eye movements as a prognostic factor. *Acta Neurochir Suppl (Wien).* 1979; 28:26.
104. Plum F, Posner JB. Ocular movements. In: Plum F, ed. Diagnosis of stupor and coma. 3rd ed. Philadelphia, PA: FA Davis Co; 1980:47–53.
105. Choi S, Ward JD, Becker DP. Chart for outcome prediction in severe head injury. *J Neurosurg.* 1983;59:294.
106. Mendelow AD. Clinical examination in traumatic brain damage. In: Vinken PJ, Bruyn GW, Klawans HL. *Handbook of Clinical Neurology.* Vol. 57. Amsterdam, the Netherlands: Elsevier Science; 1990:123.
107. Kelly DF, Gonzalo IT, Cohan P, et al. Hypopituitarism following traumatic brain injury and aneurysmal subarachnoid hemorrhage: a preliminary report. *J Neurosurg.* 2000;93(5):743.
108. Benvenga S, Campenni A, Ruggeri RM, et al. Clinical review 113: hypopituitarism secondary to head trauma. *J Clin Endocrinol Metab.* 2000; 85(4):1353.
109. Masel BE. Rehabilitation and hypopituitarism after traumatic brain injury. *Growth Horm IGF Res.* 2004;14(Suppl A):S108.
110. Agha A, Rogers B, Sherlock M, et al. Anterior pituitary dysfunction in survivors of traumatic brain injury. *J Clin Endocrinol Metab.* 2004;89(10): 4929.
111. Agha A, Phillips J, O'Kelly P, et al. The natural history of post-traumatic hypopituitarism: implications for assessment and treatment. *Am J Med.* 2005;118:1416.
112. Agha A, Thompson C. Anterior pituitary dysfunction following traumatic brain injury (TBI). *Clin Endrocrinol.* 2006;64:481.
113. Aimaretti G, Ghigo E. Traumatic brain injury and hypopituitarism. *Scientific World Journal.* 2005;5:777.
114. Aimaretti G, Ambrosio MR, Di Somma C, et al. Hypopituitarism induced by traumatic brain injury in the transition phase. *J Endocrinol Invest.* 2005; 28:984.
115. Bondanelli M, Ambrosio MR, Zatelli MC, et al. Hypopituitarism after traumatic brain injury. *Eur J Endocrinol.* 2005;152:679.
116. Leal-Cerro A, Flores JM, Rincon M, et al. Prevalence of hypopituitarism and growth hormone deficiency in adults long-term after severe traumatic brain injury. *Clin Endrocrinol.* 2005;62:525.
117. Popovic V. GH deficiency as the most common pituitary defect after TBI: clinical implications. *Pituitary.* 2005;8:239.
118. Popovic V, Aimaretti G, Casanueva FF, et al. Hypopituitarism following traumatic brain injury (TBI): call for attention. *J. Endocrinol. Invest.* 2005;28:61.
119. Schneider HJ, Schneider M, Saller B, et al. Prevalence of anterior pituitary insufficiency 3 and 12 months after traumatic brain injury. *Eur J Endocrinol.* 2006;154:259.
120. Singer BJ, Singer KP, Allison GT. Evaluation of extensibility, passive torque and stretch reflex responses in triceps surae muscles following serial casting to correct spastic equinovarus deformity. *Brain Inj.* 2003;17(4):309–324.
121. Gerstenbrand F, Poewe W, Aichner F, et al. Klüver-Bucy syndrome in man: experiences with posttraumatic cases. *Neurosci Biobehav Rev.* 1983;7:413–417.

122. Goscinski I, Kwiatkowski S, Polak J, et al. The Klüver-Bucy syndrome. *J Neurosurg Sci.* 1997;41(3):269.
123. Synek VM. EEG abnormality grades and subdivision of prognostic importance in traumatic and anoxic coma in adults. *Clin Electroencephalogr.* 1998;19(3):160.
124. Gutling E, Gonser A, Imof HG, et al. EEG reactivity in the prognosis of severe head injury. *Neurology.* 1995;45:915.
125. Klein HJ, Rath SA, Goppel F. The use of EEG spectral analysis after thiopental bolus in the prognostic evaluation of comatose patients with brain injures. *Acta Neurochir Suppl (Wien).* 1988;42:31.
126. Bergamasco B, Bergamini L, Doriguzzi T. Clinical value of the sleep electroencephalographic patterns in post-traumatic coma. *Acta Nerol Scand.* 1968;44:495.
127. Rumpl E, Prugger M, Bauer G, et al. Incidence and prognostic value of spindles in posttraumatic coma. *Electroencephalogr Clin Neurophisiol.* 1983; 56:420.
128. Giubilei F, Formisano R, Fiorini M, et al. Sleep abnormalities in traumatic apallic syndrome. *J Neurol Neurosurg Psychiatry.* 1995;58:484.
129. Ron S, Algom D, Hary D, et al. Time-related changes in the distribution of sleep stages in brain injured patients. *Electroencephalogr Clin Neurophysiol.* 1980;48:432.
130. Valente M, Placidi F, Oliveira AJ, et al. Sleep organization pattern as a prognostic marker at the subacute stage of post-traumatic coma. *Clin Neurophisiol.* 2002;113:1798.
131. Chatrian GE, Bergamasco B, Bricolo A, et al. IFCN recommended standards for electrophysiologic monitoring in comatose and other unresponsive states. Report of an IFCN committee. *Electroencephalogr Clin Neurophysiol.* 1996;99:103.
132. Greenberg RP, Becher DP, Miller DJ, et al. Evaluation of brain function in severe human head trauma with multimodality evoked potentials, II: localization of brain dysfunction and correlation with posttraumatic neurological conditions. *J Neurosurgery.* 1977;47:163.
133. Perrin F, Schnakers C, Schabus M, et al. Brain response to one's own name in vegetative state, minimally conscious state, and locked-in syndrome. *Arch Neurol.* 2006 Apr;63(4):562.
134. Schoenle PW, Witzke W. How vegetative is the vegetative state? Preserved semantic processing in VS patient-evidence from N400 event-related potentials. *Neuro Rehabilitation.* 2004;19(4):329.
135. Marshall LF, Marshall SB, Klauber MR, et al. The diagnosis of head injury requires a classification based on computed axial tomography. *J Neurotrauma.* 1992;9(Suppl 1):S287.
136. Mittl RL, Grossman RI, Hiehle JF, et al. Prevalence of MR evidence of diffuse axonal injury in patients with mild head injury and normal head CT findings. *AJNR Am J Neuroradiol.* 1994;15:1583.
137. Kampfl A, Schmutzhard E, Pfausler B, et al. Prediction of recovery from post-traumatic vegetative state with cerebral magnetic resonance imaging. *Lancet.* 1998;351:1763.
138. Firsching R, Woiscneck D, Dietrich M, et al. Early magnetic resonance imaging of brainstem lesions after severe head injury. *J Neurosurg.* 1998; 89(5):707.
139. Lin A, Ross BT, Harris K, et al. Efficacy of proton magnetic resonance spectroscopy in neurological diagnosis and neurotherapeutic decision making. *NeuroRx.* 2005;2:197.
140. Barzo P, Marmarou A, Fatouros P, et al. MRI diffusion-weighted spectroscopy of reversible and irreversible ischemic injury following closed head injury. *Acta Neurochir Suppl.* 1997;70:115.
141. Ross BD, Ernst T, Kreis R, et al. 1H MRS in acute traumatic brain injury. *J Magn Reson Imaging.* 1998;8(4):829.
142. Cecil KM, Hills EC, Sandel ME, et al. Proton magnetic resonance spectroscopy for detection of axonal injury in the splenium of the corpus callosum of brain-injured patients. *J Neurosurg.* 1998;88(5):795.
143. Sinson G, Bagley LJ, Cecil KM, et al. Magnetization transfer imaging and proton MR spectroscopy in the evaluation of axonal injury: correlations with clinical outcome after traumatic brain injury. *AJNR Am J Neuroradiol.* 2001;22:143.
144. Macmillan CS, Wild JM, Wardlaw JM, et al. Traumatic brain injury and subarachnoid hemorrhage: *in vivo* occult pathology demonstrated by magnetic resonance spectroscopy may not be "sischaemic." A primary study and review of the literature. *Acta Neurochir (Wien).* 2002;144(9):853.
145. Ashwal S, Holshouser B, Tong K, et al. Proton MR spectroscopy detected glutamate/glutamine is increased in children with traumatic brain injury. *J Neurotrauma.* 2004;21(11):1539.
146. Holshouser BA, Tong KA, Ashwal S. Proton MR spectroscopic imaging depicts diffuse axonal injury in children with traumatic brain injury. *AJNR Am J Neuroradiol.* 2005;26(5):1276.
147. Tavazzi B, Signoretti S, Lazzarino G, et al. Cerebral oxidative stress and depression of energy metabolism correlate with severity of diffuse brain injury in rats. *Neurosurgery.* 2005;56(3):582.
148. Soustiel JF, Glenn TC, Shik V, et al. Monitoring of cerebral blood flow and metabolism in traumatic brain injury. *J Neurotrauma.* 2005;22(9):955.
149. Friedman SD, Brooks WM, Jung RE, et al. Quantitative proton MRS predicts outcome after traumatic brain injury. *Neurology.* 1999;52(7):1384.
150. Brooks WM, Stidley CA, Petropoulos H, et al. Metabolic and cognitive response to human traumatic brain injury: a quantitative proton magnetic resonance study. *J Neurotrauma.* 2000;17(8):629.
151. Garnett MR, Blamire AM, Corkill RG, et al. Early proton magnetic resonance spectroscopy in normal-appearing brain correlates with outcome in patients following traumatic brain injury. *Brain.* 2000;123(Pt 10):2046.
152. Schuhmann MU, Stiller D, Skardelly M, et al. Metabolic changes in the vicinity of brain contusions: a proton magnetic resonance spectroscopy and histology study. *J Neurotrauma.* 2003;20(8):725.
153. Ashwal S, Holshouser B, Tong K, et al. Proton spectroscopy detected myoinositol in children with traumatic brain injury. *Pediatr Res.* 2004; 56(4):630.
154. Holshouser BA, Tong KA, Ashwal S, et al. Prospective longitudinal proton magnetic resonance spectroscopic imaging in adult traumatic brain injury. *J Magn Reson Imaging.* 2006;24(1):33.
155. Carpentier A, Galanaud D, Puybasset L, et al. Early morphologic and spectroscopic magnetic resonance in severe traumatic brain injuries can detect "invisible brain stem damage" and predict "vegetative states." *J Neurotrauma.* 2006;23(5):674.
156. Mitchener A, Wyper DJ, Patterson J, et al. SPECT, CT, and MRI in head injury: acute abnormalities followed up at six months. *J Neurol Neurosurg Psychiatry.* 1997;62:633.
157. Boly M, Faymonville ME, Peigneux P, et al. Auditory processing in severely brain injured patients : differences between the minimally conscious state and the persistent vegetative state. *Arch Neurol.* 2004;61(2):233.
158. Beuthien-Baumann B, Handrick W, Schmidt T, et al. Persistent vegetative state: evaluation of brain metabolism and brain perfusion with PET and SPECT. *Nucl Med Commun.* 2003;24(6):643.
159. Laureys S. Functional neuroimaging in the vegetative state. *NeuroRehabilitation.* 2004;19(4):335.
160. Feingold DS. Hospital acquired infections. *New Engl J Med.* 1970;283: 1384.
161. Medical Disability Society. *The Management of Traumatic Brain Injury. Development Trust for the Young Disabled.* London, England: ; 1988.
162. Feldman PA. Upper extremity casting and splinting. In: Glenn MB, Whyte J, ed. *The Practical Management of Spasticity in Children and Adults.* Philadelphia, PA: Lea & Febiger; 1990.
163. Hallenborg SC. Positioning. In: Glenn MB, Whyte J, ed. *The Practical Management of Spasticity in Children and Adults.* Philadelphia, PA: Lea & Febiger; 1990.
164. Marmarou A, Foda MA, Bandoh K, et al. Posttraumatic ventriculomegaly: hydrocephalus or atrophy? A new approach for diagnosis using CSF dynamics. *J Neurosurg.* 1996;85(6):1026.
165. Citta-Pietrolungo TJ, Alexander MA, Cook SP, et al. Complications of tracheostomy and decannulation in pediatric and young patients with traumatic brain injury. *Arch Phys Med Rehabil.* 1993;74(9):905.
166. Law JH, Barnhart K, Rowlett W, et al. Increased frequency of obstructive airway abnormalities with long-term tracheostomy. *Chest.* 1993; 104(1):136.
167. Grillo HC. The history of tracheal surgery. *Chest Surg Clin N Am.* 2003; 13(2):175.
168. Ciccone AM, De Giacomo T, Venuta F. Operative and non-operative treatment of benign subglottic laryngotracheal stenosis. *Eur J Cardiothorac Surg.* 2004;26(4):818.
169. Kaufman HH, Satterwhite T, McConnell BJ, et al. Deep vein thrombosis and pulmonary embolism in head injured patients. *Angiology.* 1983; 34:627.
170. Geerts W, Code K, Jay R, et al. Prospective study of venous thromboembolism after major trauma. *N Engl J Med.* 1994;331:1601.
171. Meythaler JM, Fisher WS, Rue LW, et al. Screening for venous thromboembolism in traumatic brain injury: limitations of D-dimer assay. *Arch Phys Med Rehabil.* 2003;84(2):285.
172. Tenilla A, Salmi T, Petilla V, et al. Early signs of critical illness polyneuropathy in ICU patients with systemic inflammatory response syndrome or sepsis. *Intensive Care Med.* 2000;26:1360.
173. Cot F, Deshairnais G. La dysphagie chez l'adult. Evaluation et traitment. Parigi: Ed. Maloine; 1985. Courjon J. A longitudinal electro-clinical study of 80 cases of post-traumatic epilepsy observed from the time of the original trauma. *Epilepsia.* 1970;11(1):29.
174. Winstein CJ. Neurogenic dysphagia. Frequency, progression, and outcome in adults following head injury. *Phys Ther.* 1983;63(12):1992.
175. Suzuki N, Suzuki S, Iwabuchi T. Neurological improvement after cranioplasty. Analysis by dinamic CT scan. *Acta Neurochir (Wien).* 1993;122(1–2):49.
176. Dujovny M, Aviles A, Agner C, et al. Cranioplasty: cosmetic or therapeutic? *Surg Neurol.* 1997;47(3):238.
177. Agner C, Dujovny M, Gaviria M. Neurocognitive assessment before and after cranioplasty. *Acta Neurochir (Wien).* 2002;144(10):1033.
178. Masur H, Papke K. *Scales and Scores in Neurology: Quantification of Neurological Deficits in Research and Practice.* New York, NY: Thieme Medical Publishers; 2003.
179. Serio CD, Kreutzer JS, Witol AD. Family needs after traumatic brain injury: a factor analytic study of the Family Needs Questionnaire. *Brain Inj.* 1997;11(1):1.
180. Mauss-Clum N, Ryan M. Brain injury and the family. *J Neurosurg Nurs.* 1981;13:165.
181. Mathis M. Personal needs of families of critically ill patients with and without brain injury. *J Neurosurg Nurs.* 1984;16:36.

182. Campbell C. Needs of relatives and helpfulness of support groups in severe head injury. *Rehab Nurs.* 1988;13:320.
183. Wood RL, Yurdakul LK. Change in relationship status following traumatic brain injury. *Brain Inj.* 1997;11:491.
184. Sinnakaruppan I, Williams DM. Family careers and the adult head-injured: a critical review of carers' needs. *Brain Inj.* 2001;15(8):653.
185. Morris KC. Psychological distress in carers of head injured individuals: the provision of written information. *Brain Inj.* 2001;(3):239.
186. Giacino JT, Kalmar K, Whyte J. The JFK Coma Recovery Scale-Revised: measurement characteristics and diagnostic utility. *Arch Phys Med Rehabil.* 2004;85(12):2020.
187. Rappaport M, Dougherty AM, Kelting DL. Evaluation of coma and vegetative states. *Arch Phys Med Rehab.* 1992;73(7):628.
188. Rader MA, Alston JB, Ellis DW. Sensory stimulation of severely brain injured patients. *Brain Inj.* 1989;3(2):141.
189. Ansell BJ, Keeman JE. The Western Neurosensory Stimulation Profile: a tool for assessing slow to recover head injured patients. *Arch Phys Med Rehab.* 1989;70:104.
190. Whyte J. Clinical trials in rehabilitation: what are the obstacles? *Am J Phys Med Rehabil.* 2003;82(10 Suppl):S16.
191. Formisano R, Vinicola V, Penta F, et al. Active music therapy in the rehabilitation of severe brain injured patients during coma recovery. *Ann Ist Super Sanitá.* 2001;37(4):627.
192. Lombardi F, Taricco M, De Tanti A, et al. The effectiveness of sensory stimulation programs in patients with severe brain injury. *Cochrane Database Syst Rev.* 2002;(2):CD001427.
193. Elliot L, Walker L. Rehabilitation interventions for vegetative and minimally conscious patients. *Neuropsychol Rehab.* 2005;15 (3/4):480.
194. Feeney DM, Sutton RL. Pharmacotherapy for recovery of function after brain injury. *Crit Rev Neurobiol.* 1987;3(2):135.
195. Fugate LP, Spacek LA, Kresty LA, et al. Mesurement and treatment of agitation following traumatic brain injury, II: a survey of the Brain Injury Special Interest Group of the American Academy of Physical Medicine and Rehabilitation. *Arch Phys Med Rehab.* 1997;78:924.
196. Mysiw WJ, Sandel ME. The agitated brain injured patient, 2: pathophysiology and treatment. *Arch Phys Med Rehab.* 1997;78:213.
197. Fleminger S, Greenwood RJ, Oliver DL. Pharmacological management for agitation and aggression in people with acquired brain injury. *Cochrane Database Syst Rev.* 2006 Oct 18;(4):CD003299. www.theCochraneLibrary.com.
198. Haider W, Benzer H, Krystof G, et al. Urinary catecholamine excretion and thyroid hormone blood level in the course of severe acute brain damage. *Eur J Intensive Care Med.* 1975;1(3):115.
199. Hörtnagl H, Hammerle AF, Hackl JM. Hypermetabolism in head injury and tetanus: patho-physiological and new therapeutic conceptions [in German]. *Infusionsther Klin Ernahr.* 1980;7(6):312.
200. Mysiw WJ, Jackson RD, Corrigan JD. Amitriptyline for post traumatic agitation. *Am J Phys Med Rehab.* 1988;67(1):29.
201. Lipton MA, DiMascio A, Killam KF, eds. *Psychopharmacology: a generation of progress.* New York, NY: Raven Press; 1978.
202. Clauss R, Nel W. Drug induced arousal from the permanent vegetative state. *Neuro Rehabilitation.* 2006;21(1):23.
203. Brooke M, Patterson D, Questad K, et al. The treatment of agitation during initial hospitalization after traumatic brain injury. *Arch Phys Med Rehabil.* 1992;73:917.
204. DelBello MP, Kowatch RA, Adler CM, et al. A double-blind randomized pilot study comparing quetiapine and divalproex for adolescent mania. *J Am Acad Child Adolesc Psychiatry.* 2006;45(3):305.
205. Kim E, Bijlani M. A pilot study of quetiapine treatment of aggression due to traumatic brain injury. *J Neuropsychiatry Clin Neurosci.* 2006;18(4):547.
206. Pohlmann-Eden B, Bruckmeir J. Predictors and dynamics of posttraumatic epilepsy. *Acta Neurol Scand.* 1997;95(5):257.
207. Peppe A, Stanzione P, Pierantozzi M, et al. Does pattern electroretinogram spatial tuning alteration in Parkinson's disease depend on motor disturbances or retinal dopaminergic loss? *Electroencephalogr Clin Neurophysiol.* 1998;106(4):374.
208. Fann JR, Uomoto JM, Katon WJ. Sertraline in the treatment of major depression following mild traumatic brain injury. *J Neuropsychiatry Clin Neurosci.* 2000;12:226.
209. Zafonte RD, Cullen N, Lexell J. Serotonin agents in the treatment of acquired brain injury. *J Head Trauma Rehab.* 2002;17(4):322.
210. Horsfield SA, Rosse RB, Tomasino V, et al. Fluoxetine's effects on cognitive performance in patients with traumatic brain injury. *Int J Psych Med.* 2002;32(4):337.
211. Francisco GE, Boake C, Vaughn A. Botulinum toxine in upper limb spasticity after acquired brain injury: a randomized trial comparing dilution tecniques. *Am J Phys Med Rehabil.* 2002;81:355.
212. Thompson AJ, Jarrett L, Lockley L, et al. Clinical management of spasticity. *J Neurol Neurosurg Psychiatry.* 2005;76(4):459.
213. Stokic DS, Yablon SA, Hayes A. Comparison of clinical and neurophysiologic responses to intrathecal baclofen bolus administration in moderate to severe spasticity after acquired brain injury. *Arch Phys Med Rehabil.* 2005;86(9):1801.
214. Nuttin B, Ivanhoe C, Albright L, et al. Intratecal baclofen therapy for spasticity of cerebral origin: cerebral palsy and brain injury. *Neuromodulation.* 1999;2:120.
215. Sara M, Sacco S, Cipolola F, et al. An unexpected recovery from permanent vegetative state. *Brain Inj.* 2007;21(1):101–103.
216. Morant A, Noè E, Boyer J, et al. Paralytic ileus: a complication after intrathecal baclofen therapy. *Brain Inj.* 2006;20(13–14):1451.
217. Albright AL, Gillmartin RG, Swift D, et al. Long-term intrathecal baclofen therapy for severe spasticity of cerebral origin. *J Neurosurg.* 2003;98:291.
218. Kofler M, Matzak H, Saltuari L. The impact of intrathecal baclofen on gastrointestinal function. *Brain Inj.* 2002;16:825.
219. Rapport RL 2nd, Penry JK. A survey of attitudes toward the pharmacological prophylaxis of posttraumatic epilepsy. *J Neurosurg.* 1973;38(2):159.
220. Caveness WF, Meirowsky AM, Rish BL, et al. The nature of posttraumatic epilepsy. *J Neurosurg.* 1979;50(5):545.
221. Caveness WF. Incidence of craniocerebral trauma in the United States in 1976 with trend from 1970 to 1975. *Adv Neurol.* 1979;22:1.
222. Penry JK, Newmark ME. The use of antiepileptic drugs. *Ann Intern Med.* 1979;90(2):207.
223. Young B, Rapp RP, Norton JA, et al. Failure of prophylactically administered phenytoin to prevent late posttraumatic seizures. *J Neurosurg.* 1983;58 (2):236.
224. Temkin NR, Dikmen S, Machamer J, et al. General versus disease-specific measures. Further work on the Sickness Impact Profile for head injury. *Med Care.* 1989;27(Suppl 3):S44.
225. Temkin NR. Antiepileptogenesis and seizure prevention trials with antiepileptic drugs: meta-analysis of controlled trials. *Epilepsia.* 2001; 42(4):515–524.
226. Formisano R, Barba C, Buzzi MG, et al. The impact of prophylactic treatment on post-traumatic epilepsy after severe traumatic brain injury. *Brain Inj.* 2007;21(5):499–504.
227. Van Vleymen B, Van Zandijcke M. Piracetam in the treatment of myoclonus: an overview. *Acta Neurol Belg.* 1996;96(4):270.
228. Ben-Menachem E, Falter U, for the European Levetiracetam Study Group. Efficacy and tolerability of levetiracetam 3000 mg/day in patients with refractory partial seizures: a multicenter, double-blind, responder-selected study evaluating monotherapy. *Epilepsia.* 2000;41:1276–1283.
229. Cereghino JJ, Biton V, Abou-Khalil B, et al. The United States Levetiracetam Study Group. Levetiracetam for partial seizures: results of a double-blind, randomized clinical trial. *Neurology.* 2000;55:236–242.
230. Marienne J. Post-traumatic acute rise in ICP related to subclinical epileptic seizures. *Acta Neurochir.* 1979;28:89.
231. Roberts I. Barbiturates for acute traumatic brain injury. *Cochrane Database Syst Rev.* 2000;(2):CD000033.
232. Dauch WA, Schutze M, Guttinger M, et al. Post-traumatic seizure prevention-results of a survey of 127 neurosurgery clinics. *Zentralbl Neurochir.* 1996;57(4):190.
233. Shorvon SD, Lowenthal A, Janz D, et al., for the European Levetiracetam Study Group. Multicenter, double-blind, randomized, placebo controlled trial of levetiracetam as add-on therapy in patients with refractory partial seizures. *Epilepsia.* 2000;41:1179–1186.
234. Genton P, Sadzot B, Fejerman N, et al. Levetiracetam in a broad population of patients with refractory epilepsy: interim results of the international SKATE trial. *Acta Neurol Scand.* 2006 Jun;113(6):387.
235. Giurgea C, Moyersoons F. The pharmacology of callosal transmission: a general survey. In: Russel I, Van Hof M, Berlucchi G, eds. *Structure and Function of Cerebral Commissures.* London, England: Macmillan; 1979: 283.
236. Rago LK, Allikmets LH, Zarkovsky AM. Effect of piracetam on the central dopaminergic transmission. *Naunyn Schmiedebergs Arch Pharmacol.* 1981;318:36.
237. Key B, Marley E. The effect of sympathomimetic amines on behaviour and electrocortical activity of the chicken. *Electroencephalogr Clin Neurophysiol.* 1962;14:90.
238. Mc Greer P, Mc Greer E, Wada J. Central aromatic amine level and behaviour. Serotonin and catecholamine levels in various cat brain areas following administration of psychoactive drugs or amine precursors. *Arch Neurol.* 1963;9:81.
239. Eames P. The use of Sinemet and bromocriptine. *Brain Inj.* 1989;3(3):319.
240. Kneale TA, Eames P. Pharmacology and flexibility in the rehabilitation of two brain-injured adults. *Brain Inj.* 1991;5(3):327.
241. Newman R, Weingartner H, Smallberg SA, et al. Effortful and automatic memory: effects of dopamine. *Neurology.* 1984;34:805.
242. Kraus MF, Maki PM. Effect of amantadine hydrochloride on symptoms of frontal lobe disfunction in brain injury: case studies and review. *Neuropsychiatry Clin Neurosci.* 1997;9(2):222.
243. Orient-Lopez F, Terre-Boliart R, Bernabeu-Guitart M, et al. The usefulness of dopaminergic drugs in traumatic brain injury. *Rev Neurol.* 2002; 35(4):362.
244. Krimchansky BZ, Keren O, Sazbon L, et al. Differential time and related appearance of signs, indicating improvement in the state of consciousness in vegetative state traumatic brain injury (VS-TBI) patients after initiation of dopamine treatment. *Brain Inj.* 2004;18(11):1099.
245. Hughes S, Colantonio A, Santaguida PL, et al. Amantadine to enhance readiness for rehabilitation following severe traumatic brain injury. *Brain Inj.* 2005;19(14):1197.

246. Weinberg RM, Auerbach SH, Moore S. Pharmacologic treatment of cognitive deficits: a case study. *Brain Inj.* 1987;1(1):57.
247. Powell JH, Al-Adawi S, Morgan J, et al. Motivational deficits after brain injury: effects of bromocriptine in 11 patients. *J Neurol Neurosurg Psychiatry.* 1996;60(4):416.
248. Karli DC, Burke DT, Kim HJ, et al. Effects of dopaminergic combination therapy for frontal lobe dysfunction in traumatic brain injury rehabilitation. *Brain Inj.* 1999;13:63.
249. Smaïl DB, Samuel C, Rouy-Thenaisy K, et al. Bromocriptine in traumatic brain injury. *Brain Inj.* 2006;20(1):111.
250. Gualtieri T, Chandler M, Coons TB, et al. Amantadine: a new clinical profile for traumatic brain injury. *Clin Neuropharmacol.* 1989;12 (4):258.
251. Chandler MC, Barnhill JL, Gualtieri CT. Amantadine for the agitated head injured patient. *Brain Inj.* 1988;2:309.
252. Nickels JL, Schneider WN, Dombovy ML, et al. Clinical use of amantadine in brain injury rehabilitation. *Brain Inj.* 1994;8:709.
253. Van Reekum L, Bayley M, Garner S, et al. N of 1 study: amantadine for the amotivational syndrome in a patient with traumatic brain injury. *Brain Inj.* 1995;9(1):49.
254. Leone H, Polsonetti BW. Amantadine for traumatic brain injury: does it improve cognition and reduce agitation? *J Clin Pharm Ther.* 2005;30:101.
255. Whyte J, Hart T, Vaccaro M, et al. The effects of methyphenidate on attention deficits after traumatic brain injury: a multi-dimensional randomized controlled trial. *Am J Phys Med Rehabil.* 2004;83(6):401.
256. Zafonte R, Elovic EP, Lombard L. Acute care management of post-TBI spasticity. *J Head Trauma Rehabil.* 2004;19(2):89–100.
257. Singer BJ, Jegasothy GM, Singer KP, et al. Incidence of ankle contracture after moderate to severe acquired brain injury. *Arch Phys Med Rehabil.* 2004 Sep;85(9):1465–1469.
258. Stover SL, Hahn HR, Miller JM 3rd. Disodium etidronate in the prevention of heterotopic ossification following spinal cord injury (preliminary report). *Paraplegia.* 1976;14(2):146.
259. Spielman G, Gennarelli TA, Rogers CR. Disodium etidronate: its role in preventing heterotopic ossification in severe head injury. *Arch Phys Med Rehabil.* 1983;64(11):539.
260. Mital MA, Garber JE, Stinson JT. Ectopic bone formation in children and adolescents with head injuries: its management. *J Pediatr Orthop.* 1987;7(1):83.
261. Hurvitz EA, Mandac BR, Davidoff G, et al. Risk factors for heterotopic ossification in children and adolescents with severe traumatic brain injury. *Arch Phys Med Rehabil.* 1992;73(5):459.
262. Matsuda W, Komatsu Y, Yanaka K, et al. Levodopa treatment for patients in persistent vegetative or minimally conscious states. *Neuropsychol Rehabil.* 2005;15(3–4):414–427.

CHAPTER 152 ■ UPPER GASTROINTESTINAL BLEEDING

GÖKHAN M. MUTLU • ECE A. MUTLU

Acute gastrointestinal (GI) bleeding is a common indication for admission to the intensive care unit (ICU) in the United States, with over 300,000 admissions per year (1). Most (75%) of these arise from the upper GI tract. Despite advances in critical care medicine, the mortality associated with upper GI bleeding has not changed and remains about 10%, likely due to aging of the population and increasing comorbidities (2,3). In this chapter, we will summarize the causes of upper GI bleeding, review the principles of a diagnostic approach, and outline the therapeutic modalities available for management of these patients. Last, we will provide an overview of stress-related mucosal damage.

EPIDEMIOLOGY

The annual incidence of hospital admission for upper GI bleeding in the United States is approximately 100 per 100,000 (1,4). The incidence is twice more common in males than females and increases with age. Patients rarely die from blood loss; rather, death is due to decompensation of other underlying conditions. Mortality for patients younger than 60 years in the absence of malignancy or organ failure is less than 1%.

Peptic ulcer disease is the most common cause of upper GI bleeding, accounting for half of cases (5) (Table 152.1). There are four major risk factors for peptic ulcers, including nonsteroidal anti-inflammatory drugs (NSAIDs), *Heliobacter pylori* infection, stress, and gastric acid (6,7). Among ulcers, those in the duodenum are more common than those found in the stomach (gastric ulcers) (Fig. 152.1). Recent data showed a decline in the proportion of cases caused by peptic ulcer disease—down to 21%—with nonspecific mucosal abnormalities being the most common cause (42%) (8).

Mallory-Weiss tears account for 5% to 15% of cases, while the proportion of patients bleeding from varices varies widely, depending on the population, from about 5% to 30%. Hemorrhagic or erosive gastropathy (usually from NSAIDs or alcohol) and erosive esophagitis often cause mild upper GI bleeding, but major hemorrhage should not occur from erosions (Fig. 152.2). As the prevalence of *H. pylori* has decreased in developed countries and the use of NSAIDs has increased, the *incidence* of bleeding ulcers has decreased, and the *proportion* of bleeding ulcers due to NSAID—rather than *H. pylori*—has increased.

Esophagogastric varices are also a common cause of upper GI bleeding and usually develop as a consequence of systemic or segmental portal hypertension (Fig. 152.3). The development of massive bleeding from gastroesophageal varices is indicative of advanced liver disease, and liver transplantation is the only treatment that improves the long-term prognosis in these patients. Isolated gastric varices can occur due to segmental portal hypertension secondary to obstruction of the splenic vein or as a consequence of obliteration of esophageal varices with endoscopic intervention. Active variceal bleeding occurs in about 50% of patients with decompensated cirrhosis, accounting for about one third of all cirrhosis-related deaths. The outcome of an episode of active variceal hemorrhage depends on the control of active bleeding and the avoidance of complications associated with bleeding and its treatment. Establishing the correct diagnosis is also important.

CLINICAL PRESENTATION

Upper GI bleeding commonly presents with hematemesis and/or melena. The clinical presentation provides clues pointing to the presence of upper GI bleeding. Hematemesis or coffee-ground emesis indicates an upper GI source of bleeding, which is above the ligament of Treitz, at the junction of the duodenum and jejunum. Melena suggests a minimum blood loss of 200 mL. The presence of melena is indicative of blood being present in the digestive tract for at least 12 to 14 hours. Although the more proximal the bleeding site in the upper GI tract, the more likely the patient will have melena, a significant percentage of patients with ascending colon sources of bleeding may also present with melena. Hematochezia is usually a presentation of lower GI bleeding, but an upper GI source that bleeds rapidly may also present with hematochezia (9). Patients with upper GI bleeding who have hematochezia usually have hemodynamic instability and rapidly dropping hemoglobin. Vomiting, retching, or coughing preceding hematemesis—especially in an alcoholic patient—should increase suspicion for a Mallory-Weiss tear. In addition to symptoms, a detailed history should include use of aspirin or other NSAID intake, alcohol consumption, presence of liver disease or variceal bleeding, history of peptic ulcer disease, weight loss, dysphagia, reflux, aortic aneurysm, or abdominal aortic vascular graft.

DIAGNOSTIC EVALUATION

Gastric Lavage

Nasogastric lavage is important for confirmation of the diagnosis and may be predictive of a high-risk lesion if bright red

TABLE 152.1

ETIOLOGY OF UPPER GASTROINTESTINAL BLEEDING

MUCOSAL (EROSIVE OR ULCERATIVE)
1. Peptic ulcer disease
   a. Idiopathic
   b. Aspirin- or NSAID-induced
   c. Infectious (*Heliobacter pylori,* Cytomegalovirus, *Herpes simplex virus*)
2. Stress-related mucosal disease
3. Zollinger-Ellison
4. Esophagitis
   a. Peptic
   b. Infectious (*Candida albicans, H. simplex virus,* Cytomegalovirus)
   c. Medication-related (aspirin, NSAIDs, alendronate)

VASCULAR
1. Dieulafoy lesion
2. Idiopathic angiomas
3. Osler-Weber-Rendu syndrome
4. Watermelon stomach
5. Radiation-induced telangiectasia
6. Blue rubber bleb nevus syndrome

PORTAL HYPERTENSION
1. Esophageal varices
2. Gastric varices
3. Portal hypertensive gastropathy

TUMORS
1. Benign (leiomyoma, polyp, lipoma)
2. Malignant

TRAUMATIC
1. Mallory-Weiss tear
2. Nasogastric tube (usually while in the intensive care unit)
3. Foreign body ingestion

OTHER
1. Hemobilia
2. Hemosuccus pancreaticus

blood is present in the lavage (10). A nasogastric tube may also decrease the risk of aspiration in patients with active hematemesis. A nonbloody nasogastric aspirate may be seen in up to 16% of patients with upper GI bleeding, usually if bleeding has ceased or if from a duodenal source, particularly if the pylorus is closed (11). Even the presence of bile in the aspirate is often (50%) misleading and does not necessarily rule out a postpyloric source of bleeding (11). Testing stool or emesis for blood during an acute episode of bleeding is not usually helpful (12). Testing of gastric contents can frequently be misleading because of nasogastric tube-related trauma. In addition, the low pH of gastric contents may interfere with the guaiac test's design for occult blood testing in stool, giving false results.

Laboratory evaluation may provide clues to the location of GI bleeding (upper versus lower). An elevated blood urea nitrogen (BUN)-to-creatinine ratio usually indicates an upper GI source as well as major blood loss (13). Patients without renal disease who have a BUN greater than 25 mg/dL have lost a minimum of 1 L of blood. Persistent azotemia (for more than 24 hours) is an indication of hypovolemia because volume loss contributes quantitatively more than the digestion of blood in raising BUN, and is the sole determinant of azotemia 24 hours after cessation of bleeding (14).

Amount of Blood Loss

Determination of estimated blood loss is the single, most important aspect of care in patients with upper GI bleeding. This estimation helps with the aggressiveness of volume resuscitation and triage to an appropriate level of care (i.e., transfer to ICU). Most complications associated with blood loss result from the adverse effects of hypovolemia and hemorrhagic shock on organs, and are compounded by the presence of pre-existing atherosclerosis or previous organ damage. Estimation of blood loss is often incorrect and requires an accurate assessment of vital signs, central venous pressure, hemoglobin and hematocrit, and a degree of clinical experience. Most of the indicators of clinically significant blood loss are derived from clinical data, which are summarized in Table 152.2.

Severe hemorrhage is usually defined as greater than 1,000 mL of blood loss. Initial hematocrit may be misleading due to loss of whole blood, which results in equal loss of plasma and erythrocytes. Redistribution of plasma from the extracellular to intravascular space, within 24 to 48 hours of the initial hemorrhage, results in dilution of red cell mass and a fall in hematocrit. The hematocrit fall may occur even more rapidly with volume replacement with crystalloid or nonheme colloid.

Physiologic changes in the cardiovascular system in response to blood loss are helpful in determining the severity of GI bleeding. *Acute* responses to blood loss represent a spectrum of changes, including resting tachycardia, orthostasis, peripheral vasoconstriction (cold, clammy skin), and acute end-organ dysfunction (mental status changes, oliguria). *Chronic* blood loss is usually associated with stable hemodynamic responses, retention of hypotonic fluid, and an absence of impaired organ function due to compensatory changes in the cardiovascular system. Many factors may impair or unmask normal responses to blood loss, including drugs, pre-existing dehydration, oxygen desaturation from pulmonary disease, the state of the cardiovascular system (particularly atherosclerotic cerebrovascular disease), abnormal concentration of plasma proteins, and miscellaneous conditions such as spinal cord disease, neuropathy, renal dysfunction, shock, and congestive heart failure.

Diagnostic Workup

Upper GI endoscopy is the diagnostic modality of choice for further evaluation of upper GI bleeding (5,15). Endoscopy helps in localization and identification of the bleeding lesion in the upper GI tract, and can be therapeutic in establishing hemostasis and preventing recurrent bleeding. Upper GI studies with radiocontrast material such as barium are contraindicated in the setting of acute upper GI bleeding due to interference with subsequent endoscopic intervention, angiography, and surgery (5).

Other diagnostic tests for workup of upper GI bleeding include angiography and tagged red blood cell scan (16). Angiographic diagnosis of the source of upper GI bleeding

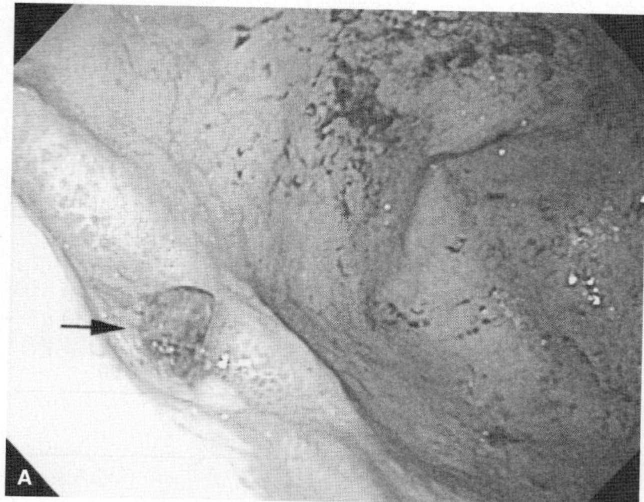

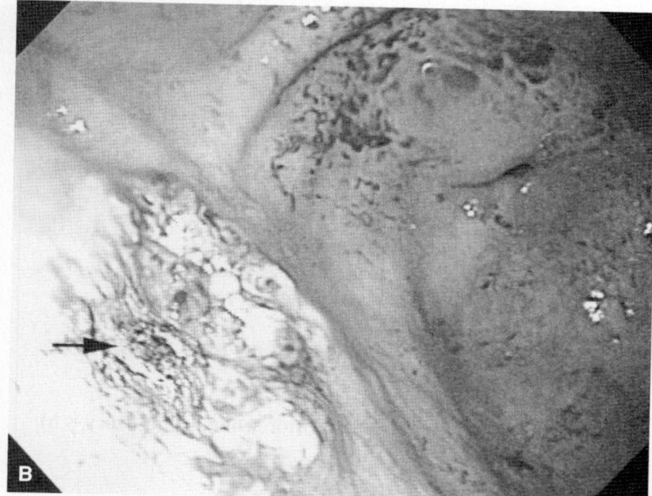

FIGURE 152.1. Peptic ulcer disease. Endoscopic view of a gastric ulcer with a visible vessel (*arrow*) before (A) and after (B) endoscopic intervention with gold probe cautery.

is made by extravasation of contrast material. The bleeding must be brisk, with a rate of about 0.5 to 1 mL/minute. Angiography can be helpful in establishing the diagnosis in 75% of patients; about 85% of bleeding originates from a branch of the left gastric artery (17). Nuclear medicine studies using ^{99m}Tc-pertechnetate-labeled red blood cell scan may also aid in localization of the bleeding site and has the ability to detect bleeding at lower rates (less than 0.5 mL/minute) than contrast angiography.

Endoscopy is the diagnostic method of choice for esophagogastric varices. In cases where endoscopy is nondiagnostic and gastric variceal bleeding is suspected, studies such as endoscopic ultrasound, portal venography, or computed tomography (CT) angiography can be used. Cirrhotic patients with upper GI bleeding should be administered a prophylactic antibiotic—usually a fluoroquinolone—preferably prior to endoscopy (18,19).

PREDICTORS OF OUTCOME AND RISK STRATIFICATION

Three clinical parameters that are independent predictors of death and rebleeding are (i) hemodynamic instability, (ii) older age, and (iii) presence of comorbidities (Table 152.3). In addition to clinical features, endoscopic assessment provides further prognostic information and may guide subsequent management decisions.

Upper endoscopy should be performed as soon as possible in patients who present with hemodynamic instability because endoscopic intervention in patients with major bleeding may reveal high-risk findings, such as varices, ulcers with active bleeding, or visible vessel. On the contrary, early endoscopy increases costs without a change in outcomes in patients with low-risk clinical and endoscopic features. Thus, patients with

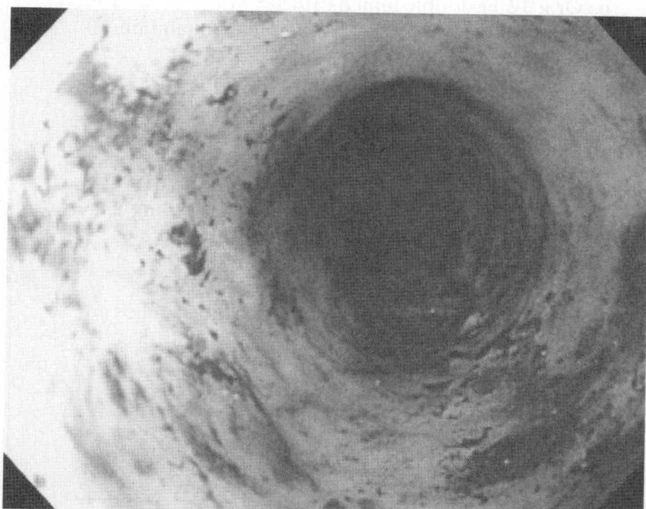

FIGURE 152.2. Severe esophagitis. Endoscopic view of severe esophagitis.

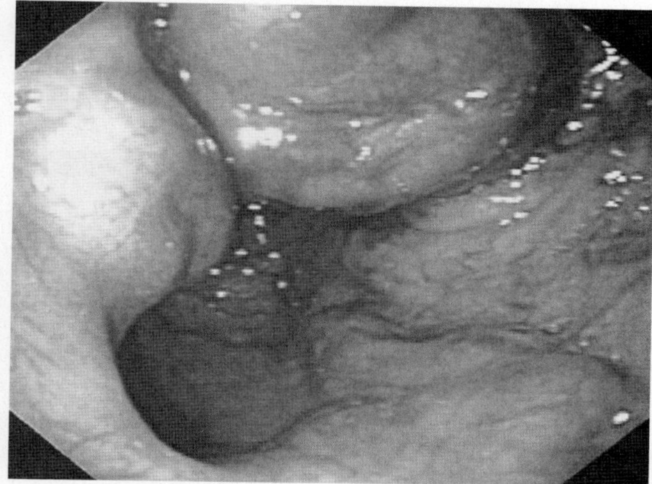

FIGURE 152.3. Esophageal varices. Endoscopic view of a large esophageal varix at the gastroesophageal junction. (Courtesy of Dr. Martin Cohen)

TABLE 152.2

CLINICAL AND LABORATORY DETERMINANTS OF SIGNIFICANT BLOOD LOSS

CLINICAL
1. Resting tachycardia (>100 beats/min or 20 beat increase from baseline if baseline heart rate >100 beats/min)
2. Orthostasis:
   a. Pulse increase greater than 20 beat/min
   b. Systolic BP decrease more than 20 mm Hg
   c. Diastolic BP decrease more than 10 mm Hg
3. Hematochezia
4. Failure to clear bright red blood from gastric lavage

LABORATORY
1. High transfusion requirement (more than 1 unit every 8 h)
2. Lactic acidosis
3. Azotemia

BP, blood pressure.

clean-base ulcers, nonbleeding Mallory-Weiss tears, and erosive or hemorrhagic gastropathy who have no hemodynamic or hemoglobin instability and no other medical problems can be considered for discharge to home.

Risk stratification may be useful in that it may allow the identification of low-risk patients who can be managed safely without the need for hospitalization. Risk stratification of patients with upper GI bleeding can be done using clinical and laboratory data, and endoscopic findings (20). Endoscopic risk stratification depends on findings that predict the risk of rebleeding (20) (Table 152.4). Although several scoring systems based on these findings have been proposed, they have not been validated in large studies and, thus, are not routinely used in most centers (21–26).

MANAGEMENT

The initial evaluation of a patient with upper GI bleeding includes the assessment of hemodynamic stability and need for aggressive resuscitation, if necessary (27). Management of upper GI bleeding can be complex, requiring that additional complications associated with blood loss be considered, particularly if the latter is severe and associated with hemodynamic instability. Table 152.5 summarizes the general principles of management.

TABLE 152.3

CLINICAL INDICATORS OF SIGNIFICANT UPPER GI BLEEDING

PATIENT CHARACTERISTICS
Older age (greater than 60 y)
Severe comorbidities (i.e., cardiopulmonary disease)
Onset of hemorrhage after hospitalization

RELATED TO AMOUNT OF BLEEDING
Hematemesis of bright red blood
Hematochezia
Gastric lavage with bright red blood
Hemorrhagic shock
High transfusion requirement

TABLE 152.4

ENDOSCOPIC FINDINGS THAT PREDICT RECURRENT UPPER GI BLEEDING

ENDOSCOPIC STIGMATA OF BLEEDING	PREVALENCE (%)	RISK OF BLEEDING (%)
Clean ulcer base	35	3–5
Flat spot	10	7–10
Oozing without visible vessel	10	10–20
Adherent clot	10	25–30
Nonbleeding visible vessel	25	50
Active arterial bleeding	10	90

(Adapted from Reference 20)

Hemodynamic Resuscitation

The initial management of upper GI bleeding should be directed at restoring blood/volume loss to maintain hemodynamic stability. Hemodynamic stabilization with adequate volume and blood resuscitation prior to endoscopic evaluation also helps to minimize treatment-associated complications (28). Intravenous access with two large-bore (14- to 16-gauge) catheters should be maintained at all times. In cases where peripheral

TABLE 152.5

PRINCIPLES OF TREATMENT FOR UPPER GASTROINTESTINAL BLEEDING

GENERAL
1. Close monitoring in the ICU if bleeding is significant
2. Place a large nasogastric tube
3. Large bore IV access
   a. At least two 14- or 16-gauge peripheral IVs
   b. Or a 12 Fr double lumen catheter or a 9 Fr introducer
4. Volume resuscitation with crystalloids to maintain hemodynamic stability
5. Transfuse PRBCs to maintain hemoglobin
   a. Greater than 7 g/dL in healthy, young individuals
   b. Greater than 10 g/dL in elderly with comorbidities such as ischemic heart disease
6. Correct coagulopathy
7. Consult gastroenterology and surgery if bleeding severe

SPECIFIC (BASED ON THE CAUSE/LESION)
1. Acid suppression
2. Splanchnic vasoconstrictors for variceal bleeding
   a. Octreotide
   b. Vasopressin analogues
3. Antibiotics (fluoroquinolones) for variceal bleeding
4. Upper GI endoscopy
5. Angiography (as indicated)
6. Surgery

ICU, intensive care unit; IV, intravenous; Fr, French; PRBCs, packed red blood cells; GI, gastrointestinal.

intravenous (IV) catheters cannot be placed, a large-bore central line (9 to 12 French) should be inserted; triple-lumen catheters have one 16- and two 18-gauge ports and are long and should therefore be avoided due to unacceptably high resistance to flow. Hypovolemia and hypotension from GI blood loss should be treated promptly with fluid resuscitation using crystalloid and packed red blood cells (PRBCs).

All patients with hemodynamic instability or a hematocrit drop of more than 6%, a transfusion requirement greater than two units of PRBCs, or significant active bleeding as evidenced by continued hematemesis with bright red blood from gastric lavage or hematochezia should be admitted to ICU for close observation and resuscitation. High-risk patients, including the elderly or those with severe comorbidities such as ischemic heart disease or congestive heart failure, should be transfused to maintain their hemoglobin greater than 10 g/dL. On the contrary, unnecessary transfusion should be avoided in young, healthy individuals in whom maintenance of hemoglobin above 7 g/dL may be sufficient.

In hemorrhagic shock, close monitoring of end-organ perfusion (coronary, central nervous system, and renal) and preventing ischemic organ injury improves survival. In addition to a baseline electrocardiogram (ECG) and telemetry monitoring, urine output should be monitored continuously. In patients with massive hemorrhage or variceal bleeding, monitoring of preload via a central venous or pulmonary artery catheter may be useful; less invasive monitoring, including those devices using pulse-wave form variability (LidCO, PICCO, Flow Track) to evaluate preload, may also be useful in these situations.

Coagulopathy should be corrected as needed to maintain platelet count greater than 50,000 cells/μL and prothrombin time within 2 seconds of the upper level of normal. After replacement of factors and platelets, recombinant activated factor VII can rapidly correct severe coagulopathy in hepatic failure (29). Elective intubation should be considered in patients with ongoing hematemesis or altered mental status to facilitate endoscopy and decrease the risk of aspiration. Gastroenterology and, in cases of severe bleeding, surgery consultations should be requested (30).

Pharmacologic Treatment

Gastric Acid Suppression

Acid-suppressive therapy with proton pump inhibitors (PPI) is an essential adjunct to therapeutic endoscopy for management of patients with peptic ulcer disease–related upper GI bleeding (31). Acid suppression is beneficial, especially after endoscopic intervention (31,32). Other acid-suppressing agents, including H_2-receptor antagonists (H_2RA), have not been shown to reduce the rate of rebleeding or transfusion requirement in peptic ulcer disease (31,33–35). High-dose proton pump inhibitor infusion following a bolus injection significantly reduces the rate of rebleeding compared to standard therapy in patients with bleeding from peptic ulcer disease (31,36). It is unknown whether oral PPI will provide benefits similar to intravenous PPI. The superiority of PPI over H_2RAs has been attributed to better maintenance of gastric pH above 6.0, which may lead to clot stabilization by prevention of fibrinolysis, and thus rebleeding (37). Current recommended doses of IV PPI therapy are lansoprazole, 90- to 120-mg bolus followed by 6 to 9 mg/hour infusion, and pantoprazole, 80 mg bolus followed by 8 mg/hour infusion. The infusion is usually continued for 48 to 72 hours and, if there is no further bleeding, switched to a twice daily dose.

Other Therapies

Splanchnic vasoconstrictors are important adjunct therapies to variceal hemorrhage. The current agent of choice in the United States is the somatostatin analogue, octreotide. Somatostatin and its analogues inhibit the release of vasodilator hormones such as glucagon, thereby indirectly causing splanchnic vasoconstriction and decreased portal inflow. For octreotide, the recommended dose is a 50-μg IV bolus followed by an infusion of 50 μg/hour for 5 days. Additionally, a longer-acting analogue of vasopressin, terlipressin, may also be used. Its efficacy is similar to octreotide and endoscopic sclerotherapy (38). Octreotide may also be considered as an adjunct therapy in the management of nonvariceal bleeding (39).

Cirrhotic patients with upper GI bleeding should be administered a prophylactic antibiotic—usually a fluoroquinolone—preferably prior to endoscopy (18,19). If a vasopressor is needed temporarily for the maintenance of blood pressure, medications that have β_2-adrenergic activity, such as dopamine or albuterol, should be avoided due to potential risk of splanchnic vasodilation.

Endoscopic Treatment

Identification and hemostasis of the source of upper GI bleeding is critical in the patient's outcome. In cases for which hemodynamic stability can be established quickly with volume resuscitation, endoscopy can be performed within 24 hours. Emergent endoscopy with therapeutic intervention is needed in patients who remain hemodynamically unstable and continue to bleed (27,40,41).

Several endoscopic therapeutic techniques have been developed to achieve hemostasis in nonvariceal upper GI bleeding, including thermal contact devices, bipolar electrocoagulation, heater probe, and injection therapy (epinephrine, alcohol, sclerosing agents such as polidocanol) (Fig. 152.4). The two most commonly used techniques in the United States are injection therapy with epinephrine (1:10,000) and contact thermal devices, which stop bleeding by producing vasoconstriction of bleeding vessels and coagulation, with subsequent destruction of bleeding vessels, respectively (42). Combination therapy with injection and thermal coagulation are superior to monotherapy in patients with major endoscopic stigmata such as active bleeding or adherent clot (43,44). Visible vessels should be treated with thermal coagulation, whereas endoscopic intervention is not required for low-risk lesions such as a clean-base ulcer or a flat spot.

Upper GI endoscopy is associated with potential complications, including aspiration, adverse reactions to conscious sedation, viscus perforation, and increased hemorrhage during therapeutic intervention. In patients with recent ischemic cardiac events, the risks of endoscopy may outweigh its benefits, and it should therefore be used judiciously (45). Contraindications to endoscopy include suspected GI perforation, unstable angina, severe coagulopathy, and severe agitation. Complications of endoscopic therapy include mucosal ulceration, motility abnormalities, stricture formation, esophageal perforation, and mediastinitis, as well as portal hypertensive gastropathy due to shunting of blood to the gastric mucosa.

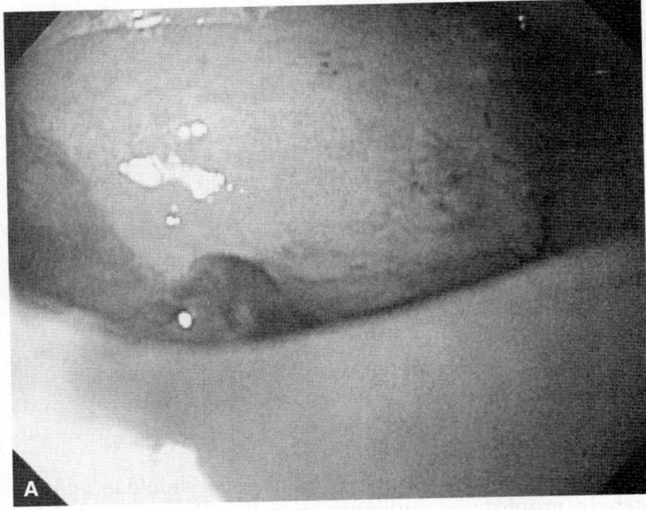

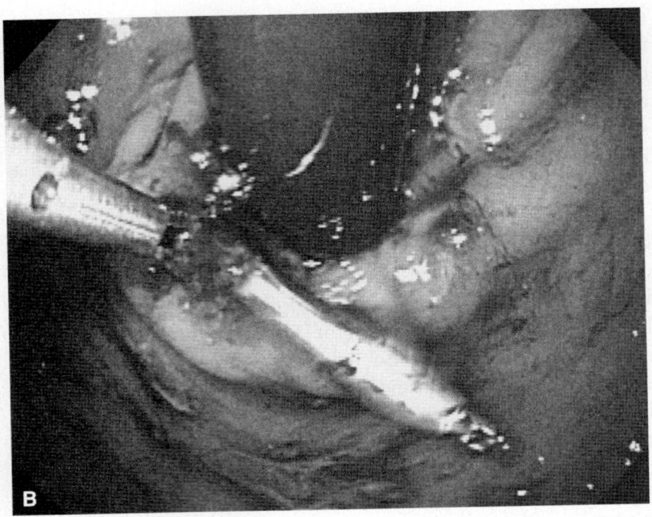

FIGURE 152.4. Endoscopic management of upper gastrointestinal bleeding. Bleeding Dieulafoy lesion before (A) and after (B) endoscopic intervention (clipping). (Courtesy of Dr. Sri Komanduri)

Nonvariceal Bleeding

Early therapeutic endoscopic intervention has an important role in achieving hemostasis, reducing rebleeding rates, and improving morbidity and mortality in peptic ulcer–related upper GI bleeding (27,40,46). One third of patients with active bleeding or a nonbleeding visible vessel require urgent surgery; further bleeding is possible if treated conservatively. These patients clearly benefit from endoscopic intervention with reduction in further bleeding, hospital stay, mortality, and costs; newer information suggests that higher-risk patients also benefit from PPI therapy (31). Patients with recurrent bleeding after endoscopic therapy were shown, in a randomized controlled trial, to have benefited from repeat endoscopic therapy. Most patients avoided surgery, and the rate of complication was significantly lower than in the group who underwent surgery (31).

Treatment of adherent clots is controversial. Two small endoscopic trials, which were terminated prematurely, showed better results with endoscopic therapy than conservative therapy (44,47). The control groups had a rebleeding rate of about 35%, whereas patients who were treated endoscopically had rebleeding rates of 0% (44) to 4.8% (47). Double-blind trials of PPI therapy without endoscopic therapy showed extremely low rates of recurrent bleeding (48,49). A recent meta-analysis showed marked heterogeneity among the trials, indicating that aggregating the trials for a summary statistic may not be appropriate. Nonetheless, the summary statistics did not show any significant benefit of endoscopic therapy. Vigorous irrigation to remove the clot may be recommended. If the clot is adherent, perhaps endoscopic therapy is not needed, but the use of a bolus plus a high-dose constant infusion of PPI may be used. Patients with underlying comorbidities may benefit from endoscopic intervention even if the clot is adherent.

A Mallory-Weiss tear is a self-limited disease and therefore does not usually require therapeutic intervention. Bleeding from these tears, which are usually on the gastric side of the gastroesophageal junction, stops spontaneously in 80% to 90% of patients, and recurs only in up to 5% of patients. Endoscopic intervention is effective in actively bleeding Mallory-Weiss tears but is not necessary if active bleeding is not present. Angiographic therapy with intra-arterial infusion of vasopressin or embolization may be useful. Rarely, surgery may be required to repair the tear. Massive bleeding can be seen if the Mallory-Weiss tear occurs in a patient with portal hypertension (50).

Variceal Bleeding

Compared to nonvariceal causes of upper GI bleeding, which stop spontaneously in 90% of cases, variceal bleeding subsides spontaneously in only 50% of patients. The mortality is very high, ranging between 70% and 80% in patients with continued variceal bleeding or rebleeding; each episode of bleeding is associated with a 30% risk of mortality (51). Variceal hemorrhage can predispose patients to hepatic encephalopathy, hepatorenal syndrome, and systemic infection, all of which increase the mortality in these patients. The risk of rebleeding remains high, ranging between 60% and 70%, unless endoscopic intervention is instituted to obliterate the varices. The greatest risk of rebleeding is within the first 48 to 72 hours, although it can occur as late as 6 weeks. Table 152.6 summarizes the risk factors for rebleeding from esophageal varices.

TABLE 152.6

RISK FACTORS FOR EARLY (LESS THAN 6 WEEKS) RECURRENT VARICEAL BLEEDING

CLINICAL
Age greater than 60 years
Severity of initial bleed
Severity of chronic liver disease
Presence of ascites
Renal failure
ENDOSCOPIC
Active bleeding during endoscopy
Clot on varices
Red color signs (i.e., cherry red spot)
Increasing size of varices

Esophageal variceal bleeding is usually amenable to endoscopic therapy, which is done to cease blood flow through the venous collateral system in the distal esophageal mucosa and cardia. Cessation of blood flow and obliteration of varices is achieved by either sclerotherapy (induction of thrombosis) or band ligation (direct occlusion). Endoscopic band ligation is the procedure of choice based on the results from a meta-analysis that showed superiority of band ligation over sclerotherapy in initial hemostasis, rate of recurrent bleeding, complications, and mortality (52). Sclerotherapy may be indicated in cases where visualization is poor, but is usually followed by band ligation.

Unlike esophageal varices, endoscopic management of gastric varices is less effective due to deeper localization of varices in the submucosa. Injection of cyanoacrylate tissue glue and thrombin are promising therapies in the endoscopic management of gastric varices (53,54). These patients may usually require nonendoscopic therapies such as balloon tamponade (Sengstaken-Blakemore tube), transjugular portosystemic shunt (TIPS), and surgery. The TIPS procedure is done as salvage therapy to artificially create a portosystemic shunt to decompress the portal venous system and, consequently, variceal vasculature. It is recommended in patients with variceal bleeding refractory to pharmacologic and endoscopic therapy, regardless of the severity of cirrhosis.

Angiographic Treatment

In a few patients with nonvariceal upper GI bleeding, angiographic localization may be necessary, with the option of hemostasis using a vasoconstrictor (i.e., intra-arterial vasopressin) or embolization (i.e., gelatin sponge). Embolization carries the risk of bowel ischemia, infarction, and necrosis, which is seen less in the duodenum than in the stomach due to the dual circulation from celiac and superior mesenteric arteries.

Surgery

Surgical indications for the management of nonvariceal hemorrhage are life-threatening hemorrhage refractory to pharmacologic and endoscopic intervention, failure of medical therapy to resolve or prevent the recurrence of peptic ulcer disease, and related complications such as bleeding. The surgical procedure depends on the location of the ulcer and the clinical status of the patient. Mortality from surgical intervention for peptic ulcer disease can be as high as 30%.

The TIPS procedure has decreased the need for surgical shunt, which is indicated for patients with variceal hemorrhage and preserved hepatic synthetic function (55). Distal esophageal transaction, with or without devascularization, is another surgical option in patients with massive, refractory variceal hemorrhage, but is associated with high mortality.

STRESS-RELATED MUCOSAL DAMAGE

Upper GI bleeding, in addition to being a cause for admission to the ICU, can also develop as a complication of critical illness while the patient is being treated in the ICU. Stress-related mucosa damage (SRMD), also known as stress ulcers, occurs as a consequence of critical illness and is the most common cause of GI bleeding in the ICU (56). The critical care environment is characterized by invasive monitoring and vasoactive and other drugs that affect mesenteric perfusion and oxygen delivery. Additionally, positive pressure ventilation, particularly positive end-expiratory pressure, and conditions such as left heart failure and sepsis can have profound effects on GI epithelial function (56). Impaired splanchnic perfusion plays a pivotal role in the pathogenesis of SRMD (Fig. 152.5). The splanchnic vasculature lacks vasomotor autoregulation, leading to persistent vasoconstriction that continues even after resolution of hemodynamic instability. Gastric acid and pepsin also play a role in the pathogenesis.

Acute respiratory failure requiring mechanical ventilation for longer than 48 hours and coagulopathy are the two strongest independent risk factors for clinically significant GI bleeding due to SRMD (57,58). Mechanically ventilated patients almost invariably develop SRMD and subepithelial hemorrhage within 24 hours of admission to the ICU (59,60). SRMD occurs within a few hours of critical illness and can present as lesions ranging from subepithelial petechiae to superficial erosions that can progress into true ulcers (56). These lesions are usually multiple and occur predominantly in the fundus of the stomach, typically sparing the antrum (60).

Most SRMD lesions are asymptomatic and clinically insignificant, although some patients may develop clinically evident bleeding, presenting with hematemesis, coffee-ground emesis, melena, and hematochezia. Clinically evident bleeding due to SRMD occurs in up to 25% of critically ill patients who do not receive prophylactic therapy, with approximately 20%—corresponding to about 5% of all patients—having clinically significant bleeding, that is, associated with hemodynamic changes or necessitating transfusion (57,60,61). Clinically significant, SRMD-related bleeding is associated with an increased length of ICU stay and morbidity and mortality (62).

Treatment

The treatment of stress ulcer bleeding is supportive. Efforts should be focused on reversing the precipitating factors. Acid suppression with H_2RA or PPIs is routinely used as adjunct therapy, given that luminal acidity is an essential factor in the pathogenesis of SRMD (63). Bleeding from SRMD is usually not amenable to endoscopic intervention because the lesions are diffuse. In cases of severe bleeding, endoscopy may be indicated and successful if hemorrhage is from one or several lesions. Since the gastric mucosa has a rich collateral blood supply, angiographic treatment—including embolization or intra-arterial vasopressin—may be considered for bleeding refractory to endoscopic therapy.

Prophylaxis

The incidence of stress ulcer bleeding has been decreasing as a result of more aggressive fluid resuscitation and prophylactic therapy (64). Most deaths in patients with stress ulcer bleeding are not due to GI hemorrhage. Therefore, the contribution of stress ulcer bleeding to overall ICU mortality does not appear to

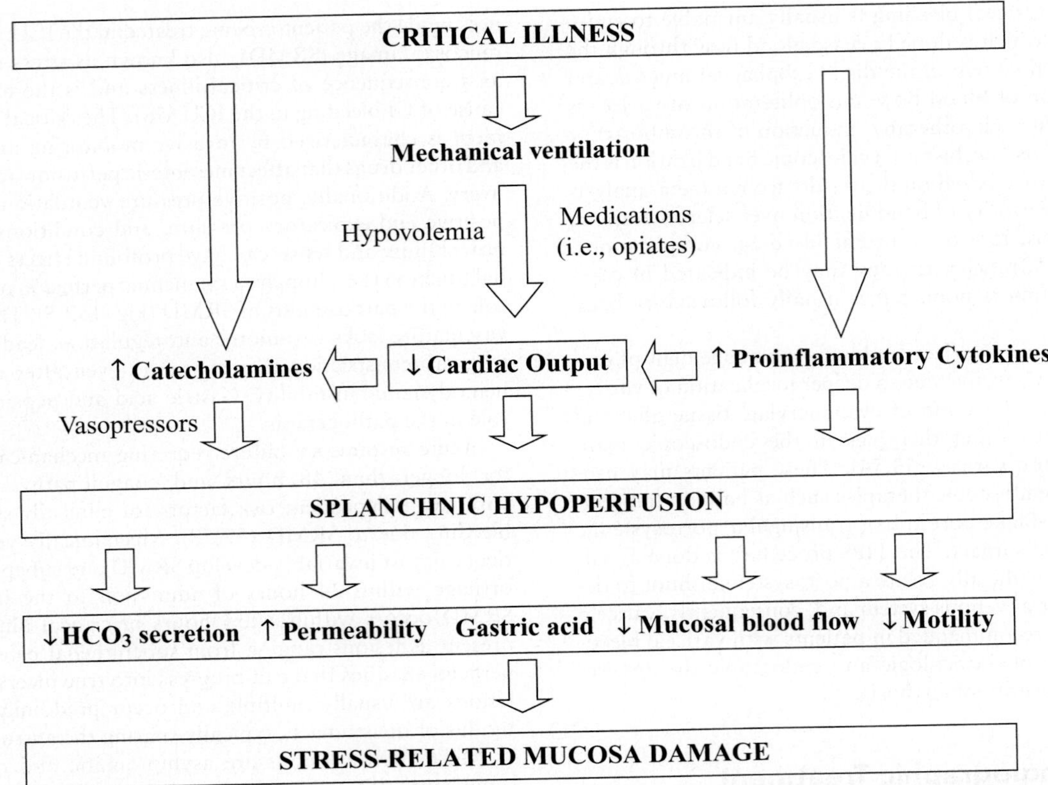

FIGURE 152.5. Mechanisms important in the pathogenesis of stress-related mucosa damage. Splanchnic hypoperfusion leading to diminished mucosal blood flow and other changes in gastrointestinal epithelial function plays a pivotal role in development of stress ulceration. (Adapted from Mutlu GM, Mutlu EA, Factor P. GI complications in patients receiving mechanical ventilation. *Chest.* 2001;119[4]:1222–1241, with permission.)

be significant in unselected ICU populations, and, as such, routine prophylaxis in all patients is not warranted. Identification of patients at risk for stress ulcer bleeding is more important than the particular medication used and can reduce unnecessary medication use and cost. Table 152.7 summarizes the risk factors for bleeding from stress ulcers.

Although gastric acid production is not increased in the most critically ill patients, except those with increased intracranial pressure or severe burns, it is essential in the pathogenesis of SRMD, and thus, therapies targeting gastric acid have been the mainstay of prophylaxis. Medications that suppress gastric acid, such as H_2RAs and PPIs, prevent SRMD by raising the gastric fluid pH, ideally above 4.0. Continuous infusion of H_2RAs may provide more effective acid suppression compared to intermittent dosing, but the relevance of this practice remains unclear (65). Gastric pH-altering agents, as well as sucralfate, decrease the incidence of clinically significant bleeding by approximately 50%—the absolute rate decreases from about 4% to about 1.7% to 2%—and are effective in preventing clinically evident and significant stress ulcer bleeding (66,67). However, a more recent study showed the superiority of H_2RAs over sucralfate in the prevention of SRMD-related bleeding (58).

Theoretically, PPIs may provide better prophylaxis due to more consistent pH control; however, their superiority over H_2RAs in stress ulcer prophylaxis has not been proven (68,69). In critically ill patients, IV PPI has been shown to achieve and maintain gastric pH greater than or equal to 4 within a few hours of initiation, with a progressive increase within the first 48 hours (70). The continuous administration of IV H_2RA was not able to maintain pH control by day 2 despite achieving a gastric pH greater than or equal to 4 initially. However, there have been no large trials specifically investigating the role of IV PPI in SRMD prophylaxis or whether more consistent increases in pH translate into better outcomes. Both H_2RAs and PPIs, despite a lack of strong clinical data, are the first-line drugs for

TABLE 152.7

RISK FACTORS FOR STRESS ULCER BLEEDING

1. Respiratory failure requiring mechanical ventilation for more than 48 h
2. Coagulopathy
   a. Thrombocytopenia (less than 50,000 cells/μL)
   b. INR (greater than 1.5)
   c. PTT (greater than 2 times the upper limit of normal)
3. *OTHER RISK FACTORS*
   Severe sepsis syndrome
   Shock
   Liver failure
   Renal failure
   Major trauma
   Extensive burns
   Intracranial hypertension

stress ulcer prophylaxis, with the route of administration—oral versus IV—determined based on the availability of the GI tract.

The major concern about using pH-altering medications is their association with gastric colonization with the Enterobacteriaceae due to an increased gastric pH and subsequent retrograde gastro-oropharyngeal contamination resulting in an increased risk of ventilator-associated pneumonia (71–73). Based on available data, the risk of pneumonia attributable to pH-altering drugs can be minimized via the implementation of preventive measures such as maintenance of the semirecumbent position, avoidance of high gastric residuals, and the administration of tube feeds into the small bowel whenever possible (74,75).

Enteral feeding also decreases the risk of clinically evident GI bleeding (62,76,77). The beneficial effects of enteral feeding are probably multifactorial, including dilutional alkalinization of gastric fluid and mucosal cytoprotection through the restoration of gastric epithelial energy stores (62,78). However, due to limited data, the use of enteral nutrition as the sole "therapy" for stress ulcer prophylaxis should be discouraged. Initiation and discontinuation of pharmacologic prophylaxis should be independent of enteral nutrition.

PEARLS

- Peptic ulcer disease is the most common cause of upper GI bleeding.
- Most (greater than 90%) nonvariceal upper GI bleeding subsides spontaneously.
- Hemodynamic resuscitation is critical for management of upper GI bleeding.
- Three clinical characteristics that are independent predictors of death and rebleeding of upper GI bleeding are hemodynamic instability, older age, and the presence of comorbidities.
- Endoscopy is the diagnostic modality of choice for further evaluation of upper GI bleeding.
- Early therapeutic endoscopic intervention plays an important role in achieving hemostasis, reducing the rebleeding rate, and improving morbidity and mortality in peptic ulcer–related upper GI bleeding.
- A high-dose infusion of proton pump inhibitor following a bolus injection significantly reduces the rate of rebleeding compared to standard therapy in patients with bleeding from peptic ulcer disease.
- Variceal bleeding subsides spontaneously in only 50% of patients.
- Mortality is very high—between 70% and 80%—in patients with continued variceal bleeding or rebleeding.
- The greatest risk of rebleeding is within the first 48 to 72 hours, although it can occur as late as 6 weeks.
- Splanchnic hypoperfusion plays a pivotal role in the pathogenesis of stress-related mucosal damage.
- Stress-related mucosal damage may occur in most critically ill patients within 24 hours of admission to the intensive care unit.
- Mechanical ventilation and coagulopathy are the most important risk factors for stress ulcer bleeding.
- Use of prophylaxis against stress-related mucosal damage should be restricted to critically ill patients with risk factors.
- The treatment of stress ulcer bleeding is supportive.

References

1. Zimmerman HM, Curfman K. Acute gastrointestinal bleeding. *AACN Clin Issues.* 1997;8(3):449–458.
2. Pitcher JL. Therapeutic endoscopy and bleeding ulcers: historical overview. *Gastrointest Endosc.* 1990;36(5 Suppl):S2–S7.
3. Farrell JJ, Friedman LS. Gastrointestinal bleeding in older people. *Gastroenterol Clin North Am.* 2000;29(1):1–36, v.
4. Longstreth GF. Epidemiology of hospitalization for acute upper gastrointestinal hemorrhage: a population-based study. *Am J Gastroenterol.* 1995;90(2):206–210.
5. Jutabha R, Jensen DM. Management of upper gastrointestinal bleeding in the patient with chronic liver disease. *Med Clin North Am.* 1996;80(5):1035–1068.
6. Hunt RH, Malfertheiner P, Yeomans ND, et al. Critical issues in the pathophysiology and management of peptic ulcer disease. *Eur J Gastroenterol Hepatol.* 1995;7(7):685–699.
7. Hallas J, Lauritsen J, Villadsen HD, Gram LF. Nonsteroidal anti-inflammatory drugs and upper gastrointestinal bleeding, identifying high-risk groups by excess risk estimates. *Scand J Gastroenterol.* 1995;30(5):438–444.
8. Boonpongmanee S, Fleischer DE, Pezzullo JC, et al. The frequency of peptic ulcer as a cause of upper-GI bleeding is exaggerated. *Gastrointest Endosc.* 2004;59(7):788–794.
9. Jensen DM, Machicado GA. Diagnosis and treatment of severe hematochezia. The role of urgent colonoscopy after purge. *Gastroenterology.* 1988;95(6):1569–1574.
10. Aljebreen AM, Fallone CA, Barkun AN. Nasogastric aspirate predicts high-risk endoscopic lesions in patients with acute upper-GI bleeding. *Gastrointest Endosc.* 2004;59(2):172–178.
11. Cuellar RE, Gavaler JS, Alexander JA, et al. Gastrointestinal tract hemorrhage. The value of a nasogastric aspirate. *Arch Intern Med.* 1990;150(7):1381–1384.
12. Schaffner J. Acute gastrointestinal bleeding. *Med Clin North Am.* 1986;70(5):1055–1066.
13. Felber S, Rosenthal P, Henton D. The BUN/creatinine ratio in localizing gastrointestinal bleeding in pediatric patients. *J Pediatr Gastroenterol Nutr.* 1988;7(5):685–687.
14. Stellato T, Rhodes RS, McDougal WS. Azotemia in upper gastrointestinal hemorrhage. A review. *Am J Gastroenterol.* 1980;73(6):486–489.
15. Adang RP, Vismans JF, Talmon JL, et al. Appropriateness of indications for diagnostic upper gastrointestinal endoscopy: association with relevant endoscopic disease. *Gastrointest Endosc.* 1995;42(5):390–397.
16. Barth KH. Radiological intervention in upper and lower gastrointestinal bleeding. *Baillieres Clin Gastroenterol.* 1995;9(1):53–69.
17. Irving JD, Northfield TC. Emergency arteriography in acute gastrointestinal bleeding. *Br Med J.* 1976;1(6015):929–931.
18. Soriano G, Guarner C, Tomas A, et al. Norfloxacin prevents bacterial infection in cirrhotics with gastrointestinal hemorrhage. *Gastroenterology.* 1992;103(4):1267–1272.
19. Hou MC, Lin HC, Liu TT, et al. Antibiotic prophylaxis after endoscopic therapy prevents rebleeding in acute variceal hemorrhage: a randomized trial. *Hepatology.* 2004;39(3):746–753.
20. Katschinski B, Logan R, Davies J, et al. Prognostic factors in upper gastrointestinal bleeding. *Dig Dis Sci.* 1994;39(4):706–712.
21. Rockall TA, Logan RF, Devlin HB, et al. Risk assessment after acute upper gastrointestinal haemorrhage. *Gut.* 1996;38(3):316–321.
22. Rockall TA, Logan RF, Devlin HB, et al. Selection of patients for early discharge or outpatient care after acute upper gastrointestinal haemorrhage. National Audit of Acute Upper Gastrointestinal Haemorrhage. *Lancet.* 1996;347(9009):1138–1140.
23. Kollef MH, O'Brien JD, Zuckerman GR, et al. BLEED: a classification tool to predict outcomes in patients with acute upper and lower gastrointestinal hemorrhage. *Crit Care Med.* 1997;25(7):1125–1132.
24. Corley DA, Stefan AM, Wolf M, et al. Early indicators of prognosis in upper gastrointestinal hemorrhage. *Am J Gastroenterol.* 1998;93(3):336–340.
25. Church NI, Dallal HJ, Masson J, et al. Validity of the Rockall scoring system after endoscopic therapy for bleeding peptic ulcer: a prospective cohort study. *Gastrointest Endosc.* 2006;63(4):606–612.
26. Bjorkman DJ, Zaman A, Fennerty MB, et al. Urgent vs. elective endoscopy for acute non-variceal upper-GI bleeding: an effectiveness study. *Gastrointest Endosc.* 2004;60(1):1–8.
27. Barkun A, Bardou M, Marshall JK. Consensus recommendations for managing patients with nonvariceal upper gastrointestinal bleeding. *Ann Intern Med.* 2003;139(10):843–857.
28. Baradarian R, Ramdhaney S, Chapalamadugu R, et al. Early intensive resuscitation of patients with upper gastrointestinal bleeding decreases mortality. *Am J Gastroenterol.* 2004;99(4):619–622.
29. Ejlersen E, Melsen T, Ingerslev J, et al. Recombinant activated factor VII (rFVIIa) acutely normalizes prothrombin time in patients with cirrhosis during bleeding from oesophageal varices. *Scand J Gastroenterol.* 2001;36(10):1081–1085.
30. Kolkman JJ, Meuwissen SG. A review on treatment of bleeding peptic ulcer: a

collaborative task of gastroenterologist and surgeon. *Scand J Gastroenterol.* 1996;218(Suppl):16–25.
31. Lau JY, Sung JJ, Lee KK, et al. Effect of intravenous omeprazole on recurrent bleeding after endoscopic treatment of bleeding peptic ulcers. *N Engl J Med.* 2000;343(5):310–316.
32. Jensen DM, Cheng S, Kovacs TO, et al. A controlled study of ranitidine for the prevention of recurrent hemorrhage from duodenal ulcer. *N Engl J Med.* 1994;330(6):382–386.
33. Gisbert JP, Gonzalez L, Calvet X, et al. Proton pump inhibitors versus H_2-antagonists: a meta-analysis of their efficacy in treating bleeding peptic ulcer. *Aliment Pharmacol Ther.* 2001;15(7):917–926.
34. Kaviani MJ, Hashemi MR, Kazemifar AR, et al. Effect of oral omeprazole in reducing re-bleeding in bleeding peptic ulcers: a prospective, double-blind, randomized, clinical trial. *Aliment Pharmacol Ther.* 2003;17(2):211–216.
35. Collins R, Langman M. Treatment with histamine H_2 antagonists in acute upper gastrointestinal hemorrhage. Implications of randomized trials. *N Engl J Med.* 1985;313(11):660–666.
36. Lin HJ, Lo WC, Lee FY, et al. A prospective randomized comparative trial showing that omeprazole prevents rebleeding in patients with bleeding peptic ulcer after successful endoscopic therapy. *Arch Intern Med.* 1998;158(1):54–58.
37. Green FW, Kaplan MM, Curtis LE, et al. Effect of acid and pepsin on blood coagulation and platelet aggregation. A possible contributor prolonged gastroduodenal mucosal hemorrhage. *Gastroenterology.* 1978;74(1):38–43.
38. Escorsell A, Ruiz del Arbol L, Planas R, et al. Multicenter randomized controlled trial of terlipressin versus sclerotherapy in the treatment of acute variceal bleeding: the TEST study. *Hepatology.* 2000;32(3):471–476.
39. Imperiale TF, Birgisson S. Somatostatin or octreotide compared with H_2 antagonists and placebo in the management of acute nonvariceal upper gastrointestinal hemorrhage: a meta-analysis. *Ann Intern Med.* 1997;127(12):1062–1071.
40. Rollhauser C, Fleischer DE. Ulcers and nonvariceal bleeding. *Endoscopy.* 1999;31(1):17–25.
41. ASGE Standards of Practice Committee. An annotated algorithmic approach to upper gastrointestinal bleeding. *Gastrointest Endosc.* 2001;53:853– 858.
42. ASGE Technology Status Evaluation Report: Endoscopic hemostatic devices. *Gastrointest Endosc.* 2001;54:833–840.
43. Chung SS, Lau JY, Sung JJ, et al. Randomised comparison between adrenaline injection alone and adrenaline injection plus heat probe treatment for actively bleeding ulcers. *BMJ.* 1997;314(7090):1307–1311.
44. Jensen DM, Kovacs TO, Jutabha R, et al. Randomized trial of medical or endoscopic therapy to prevent recurrent ulcer hemorrhage in patients with adherent clots. *Gastroenterology.* 2002;123(2):407–413.
45. Cappell MS, Iacovone FM Jr. Safety and efficacy of esophagogastroduodenoscopy after myocardial infarction. *Am J Med.* 1999;106(1):29–35.
46. Laine L, Peterson WL. Bleeding peptic ulcer. *N Engl J Med.* 1994;331(11):717–727.
47. Bleau BL, Gostout CJ, Sherman KE, et al. Recurrent bleeding from peptic ulcer associated with adherent clot: a randomized study comparing endoscopic treatment with medical therapy. *Gastrointest Endosc.* 2002;56(1):1–6.
48. Sung JJ, Chan FK, Lau JY, et al. The effect of endoscopic therapy in patients receiving omeprazole for bleeding ulcers with nonbleeding visible vessels or adherent clots: a randomized comparison. *Ann Intern Med.* 2003;139(4):237–243.
49. Khuroo MS, Yattoo GN, Javid G, et al. A comparison of omeprazole and placebo for bleeding peptic ulcer. *N Engl J Med.* 1997;336(15):1054–1058.
50. Schuman BM, Threadgill ST. The influence of liver disease and portal hypertension on bleeding in Mallory-Weiss syndrome. *J Clin Gastroenterol.* 1994;18(1):10–12.
51. Smith JL, Graham DY. Variceal hemorrhage: a critical evaluation of survival analysis. *Gastroenterology.* 1982;82(5 Pt 1):968–973.
52. Laine L, Cook D. Endoscopic ligation compared with sclerotherapy for treatment of esophageal variceal bleeding. A meta-analysis. *Ann Intern Med.* 1995;123(4):280–287.
53. Lo GH, Lai KH, Cheng JS, et al. A prospective, randomized trial of butyl cyanoacrylate injection versus band ligation in the management of bleeding gastric varices. *Hepatology.* 2001;33(5):1060–1064.
54. Yang WL, Tripathi D, Therapondos G, et al. Endoscopic use of human thrombin in bleeding gastric varices. *Am J Gastroenterol.* 2002;97(6):1381–1385.
55. Henderson JM, Nagle A, Curtas S, et al. Surgical shunts and TIPS for variceal decompression in the 1990s. *Surgery.* 200;128(4):540–547.
56. Mutlu GM, Mutlu EA, Factor P. GI complications in patients receiving mechanical ventilation. *Chest.* 2001;119(4):1222–1241.
57. Schuster DP, Rowley H, Feinstein S, et al. Prospective evaluation of the risk of upper gastrointestinal bleeding after admission to a medical intensive care unit. *Am J Med.* 1984;76(4):623–630.
58. Cook D, Guyatt G, Marshall J, et al. A comparison of sucralfate and ranitidine for the prevention of upper gastrointestinal bleeding in patients requiring mechanical ventilation. Canadian Critical Care Trials Group. *N Engl J Med.* 1998;338(12):791–797.
59. Lucas CE, Sugawa C, Riddle J, et al. Natural history and surgical dilemma of "stress" gastric bleeding. *Arch Surg.* 1971;102(4):266–273.
60. Peura DA, Johnson LF. Cimetidine for prevention and treatment of gastroduodenal mucosal lesions in patients in an intensive care unit. *Ann Intern Med.* 1985;103(2):173–177.
61. Gurman G, Samri M, Sarov B, et al. The rate of gastrointestinal bleeding in a general ICU population: a retrospective study. *Intensive Care Med.* 1990;16(1):4449.
62. Cook D, Heyland D, Griffith L, et al. Risk factors for clinically important upper gastrointestinal bleeding in patients requiring mechanical ventilation. Canadian Critical Care Trials Group. *Crit Care Med.* 1999;27(12):2812–2817.
63. Skillman JJ, Gould SA, Chung RS, et al. The gastric mucosal barrier: clinical and experimental studies in critically ill and normal man, and in the rabbit. *Ann Surg.* 1970;172(4):564–584.
64. Haglund U. Stress ulcers. *Scand J Gastroenterol Suppl.* 1990;175:27–33.
65. Baghaie AA, Mojtahedzadeh M, Levine RL, et al. Comparison of the effect of intermittent administration and continuous infusion of famotidine on gastric pH in critically ill patients: results of a prospective, randomized, crossover study. *Crit Care Med.* 1995;23(4):687–691.
66. Cook DJ, Witt LG, Cook RJ, et al. Stress ulcer prophylaxis in the critically ill: a meta-analysis. *Am J Med.* 1991;91(5):519–527.
67. Cook DJ, Reeve BK, Guyatt GH, et al. Stress ulcer prophylaxis in critically ill patients. Resolving discordant meta-analyses. *JAMA.* 1996;275(4):308–314.
68. Levy MJ, Seelig CB, Robinson NJ, et al. Comparison of omeprazole and ranitidine for stress ulcer prophylaxis. *Dig Dis Sci.* 1997;42(6):1255–1259.
69. Kantorova I, Svoboda P, Scheer P, et al. Stress ulcer prophylaxis in critically ill patients: a randomized controlled trial. *Hepatogastroenterology.* 2004;51(57):757–761.
70. Morris JA, Karlstadt R, Blatcher D, et al. Intermittent intravenous pantoprazole rapidly achieves and maintains gastric pH ≥ 4 compared with continuous infusion H_2-receptor antagonist in intensive care unit. *Crit Care Med* 31st Annual congress of the Society of Critical Care Medicine (SSCM) 26-30 January, 2002, San Diego, CA. 30:Abstract 143.
71. Heyland D, Mandell LA. Gastric colonization by Gram-negative bacilli and nosocomial pneumonia in the intensive care unit patient. Evidence for causation. *Chest.* 1992;101(1):187–193.
72. du Moulin GC, Paterson DG, Hedley-Whyte J, et al. 1982. Aspiration of gastric bacteria in antacid-treated patients: a frequent cause of postoperative colonisation of the airway. *Lancet.* 1982;1(8266):242–245.
73. Craven DE, Steger KA, Barat LM, et al. Nosocomial pneumonia: epidemiology and infection control. *Intensive Care Med.* 1992;18(Suppl 1):S3–S9.
74. Kollef MH. Ventilator-associated pneumonia. A multivariate analysis. *JAMA.* 1993;270(16):1965–1970.
75. Drakulovic MB, Torres A, Bauer TT, et al. 1999. Supine body position as a risk factor for nosocomial pneumonia in mechanically ventilated patients: a randomised trial. *Lancet.* 1999;354(9193):1851–1858.
76. Pingleton SK, Hadzima SK. Enteral alimentation and gastrointestinal bleeding in mechanically ventilated patients. *Crit Care Med.* 1983;11(1):13–16.
77. Raff T, Germann G, Hartmann B. The value of early enteral nutrition in the prophylaxis of stress ulceration in the severely burned patient. *Burns.* 1997;23(4):313–318.
78. Ruiz-Santana S, Ortiz E, Gonzalez B, et al. Stress-induced gastroduodenal lesions and total parenteral nutrition in critically ill patients: frequency, complications, and the value of prophylactic treatment. A prospective, randomized study. *Crit Care Med.* 1991;19(7):887–891.

CHAPTER 153 ■ APPROACH TO LOWER GASTROINTESTINAL BLEEDING

HSIU-PO WANG

IMMEDIATE CONCERNS

Lower gastrointestinal (LGI) bleeding (LGIB) may be the primary cause of admission to the intensive care unit (ICU) or occurs during the course of ICU care for disorders other than LGIB. The initial approach to patients with LGIB, whether occult or acutely overt, is resuscitation to maintain organ perfusion. ICU physicians must maintain adequacy of airway and circulation, including ensuring an open airway and adequate intravenous access. Thereafter, the severity of bleeding should be graded to determine whether urgent diagnostic and interventional procedures need be initiated immediately. The consequences of LGIB should be prevented or treated, just as would an acute myocardial infarction (AMI) induced by anemia or unstable hemodynamic status. A summary approach to ICU patients is noted in Table 153.1 and Figure 153.1.

Evaluation

1. Is there true gastrointestinal (GI) bleeding (for suspicious cases with anemia in the ICU)?
2. Is the bleeding from the lower or upper GI tract?
3. Are there any adverse consequences caused by the LGIB?
4. What are the effective diagnostic and interventional tools to use for the workup of patients with LGIB?

Essential Diagnostic Tests and Procedures

1. History taking, including previous operative interventions and medications
2. Physical examination, including digital examination
3. Stool guaiac for anemic patients with suspicious GI blood loss
4. Complete blood count
5. Endoscopic procedures: sigmoidoscopy, colonoscopy, enteroscopy, and capsule endoscopy
6. Barium study
7. Bedside ultrasound (US)
8. Radiologic procedures: angiography
9. Nuclear scintigraphy: technetium-labeled red blood cell scan
10. Other examinations for affected organs due to unstable hemodynamics, such as electrocardiogram (ECG) for AMI

Treatment

1. Ensure stable hemodynamic status, using fluids and transfusion of blood components.
2. Endoscopic therapies include local injection, electrocoagulation, hemoclipping, argon plasma coagulation, and elastic banding according to the nature of the bleeding.
3. Radiologic interventions include angiography with intra-arterial vasopressin infusion, embolization, and glue.
4. The adverse events caused by treatment modalities, such as perforation caused by endoscopic thermocoagulation or bowel infarction due to angiographic embolization, should be monitored and managed.
5. Surgical consultation is warranted for severe LGIB in which the patient cannot be resuscitated, or if all available therapeutic modalities fail.

OVERVIEW

Gastrointestinal diseases are often encountered in the ICU setting, either as the major cause of admission to the ICU or as a comorbid complication of another primary disease process. The consequences of LGIB in the ICU—anemia and hypovolemia—may delay the weaning or extubation of patients, which can prolong the ICU course. LGIB is defined as a bleeding source distal to the ligament of Treitz, thus involving the small bowel and colon, and accounts for an estimated 20% to 24% of all major GI bleeding (1,2). It has been estimated that the annual incidence of LGIB is approximately 0.03% in the adult population (3). Longstreth estimated the annual incidence of hospitalization for LGIB to be 20 to 30 cases per 100,000 persons (4). LGIB is more common in men than women, and the incidence increases with age, with a greater than 200-fold increase from the third to ninth decades of life (2). The true incidence of LGIB during ICU hospitalization is not precisely clear; the incidence for ICU patients with acquired hemorrhage (not primarily due to LGIB) was reported as 0.94% (5).

LGIB is clinically distinct from upper gastrointestinal (UGI) bleeding (UGIB) in epidemiology, management, and outcome. LGIB is approximately 20% to 33% as common as UGIB (2,6,7). LGIB generally has a lower mortality rate than does UGIB (8), but mortality is markedly higher in patients who begin bleeding after admission: 2.4% versus 23% (4). Most deaths are not the direct result of uncontrolled bleeding, but rather exacerbation of an underlying disorder or development of a nosocomial complication. Lin et al. (5) noted a 53%

TABLE 153.1

SUMMARY OF AN APPROACH TO ICU PATIENTS WITH LOWER GASTROINTESTINAL BLEEDING

1. Immediately assess and stabilize the patient's hemodynamic status The ABCs of resuscitation 2. Determine presence of lower gastrointestinal bleeding By history, physical examination, and sometimes nasogastric aspiration 3. Arrange appropriate diagnostic and therapeutic interventions to stop any active bleeding 4. Treat any underlying lesions, and monitor and manage the comorbid illness
ICU, intensive care unit.

mortality in 55 patients, but this outcome was attributable to LGIB in only two patients. In another study, Lin et al. noted that patients with LGIB and comorbid illness had a higher mortality rate than those without: 29.5% versus 4.3% (9). No matter whether reported in the general population or in an ICU-based study, LGIB remains a difficult diagnostic and treatment problem for several reasons:

1. Bleeding can originate from any part of the lower GI tract.
2. Blood loss is often intermittent in nature, and it is difficult to identify the source in the absence of active bleeding, especially angiographically.
3. The colon preparation before urgent colonoscopy is, obviously, needed but often incomplete (10).
4. Recurrent bleeding due to angiodysplasia (7) or diverticula (8,11) may be seen with LGIB.
5. Unlike UGIB, there are no evidence-based and effective pharmacologic therapies for LGIB.

Among the many causes of LGIB (Table 153.2), diverticular bleeding, angiodysplasia, colitis, and neoplasm have been reported to be the most frequent (4,12). While the data from most reports are mixed with both non-ICU and ICU patients, the spectrum of LGIB from ICU patients should be different from others. Data from a study limited to medical ICU patients have shown ischemic colitis and acute hemorrhagic rectal ulcers to be the most frequent causes of LGIB, followed by colitis and diverticular bleeding (5). Our unpublished data—from surgical, trauma, and medical ICUs—showed acute hemorrhagic rectal ulcers followed by ischemic colitis to be the most frequently encountered causes (Table 153.3).

Patient age is a very important factor in the differential diagnosis of GI bleeding. Patients younger than 40 years are more likely to suffer from small bowel tumors, such as lymphomas, carcinoid tumors, and adenocarcinomas; anatomic anomalies such as Meckel diverticulum and Dieulafoy lesions; genetic problems such as polyps from a hereditary polyposis syndrome; or Crohn disease and ulcerative colitis, which are common in Western countries and, recently, increasing in Asia. Patients older than 40 years are more prone to bleeding from vascular lesions and neoplasm (12). Lewis et al., while evaluating small bowel bleeding, noted that in patients between 30 and 50 years, tumors were the most common abnormalities; in patients younger than 25 years, Meckel diverticulum was the most common source of small bowel bleeding, whereas vascular ectasias predominated in the elderly (13).

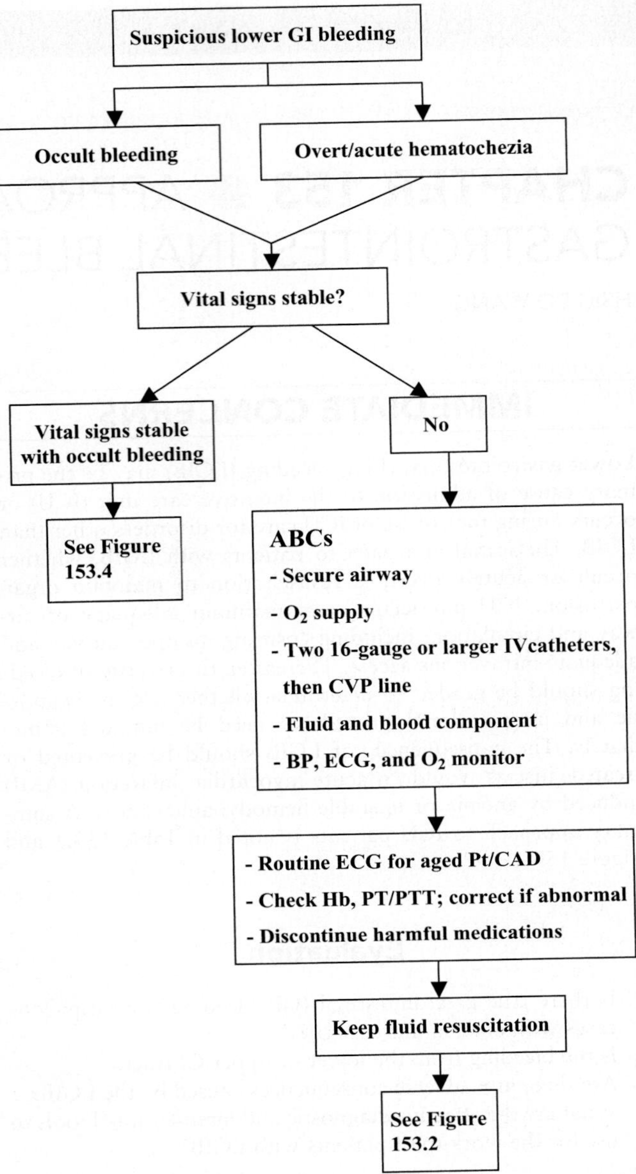

FIGURE 153.1. General approach to lower gastrointestinal bleeding. GI, gastrointestinal; CVP, central venous pressure; BP, blood pressure; ECG, electrocardiogram; Pt, patient; CAD, coronary artery disease; Hb, hemoglobin; PT, prothrombin time; PTT, partial thromboplastin time.

Presentation

Specific groups may have specific causes of LGIB. In the immunosuppressed patient, such as those with human immunodeficiency virus (HIV) infection and renal or pancreatic transplant patients, LGIB is often caused by cytomegalovirus (CMV) ulcers. Renal failure is a well-known risk factor for angiodysplasia (14); this is also prone to occur in patients with aortic valvular stenosis (15). Radiation colitis should be considered

TABLE 153.2

CAUSES OF LOWER GASTROINTESTINAL BLEEDING

COLONIC SOURCES
- Vascular ectasia
- Diverticulosis
- Ischemic colitis
- Acute hemorrhagic rectal ulcer syndrome
- Neoplasia
- Postpolypectomy
- Inflammatory bowel disease
- Infectious colitis and ulcer
- NSAID-induced colopathy
- Radiation colitis
- Hemorrhoids
- Dieulafoy lesions
- Colon varices
- Aortoenteric fistula

SMALL BOWEL SOURCES
- Vascular ectasia
- Focal active bleeding small bowel tumor:
  - Lymphoma
  - Adenocarcinoma
  - GIST
  - Other tumors
- NSAID-induced enteropathy
- Crohn disease
- Meckel diverticulum
- Vasculitis: SLE, Behçet disease, Schönlein-Henoch purpura
- Infection related ulcer: CMV, and so forth
- Small bowel varices
- Aortoenteric fistula

NSAID, nonsteroidal anti-inflammatory drugs; GIST, gastrointestinal stromal tumor; SLE, systemic lupus erythematosus; CMV, cytomegalovirus.

TABLE 153.3

CAUSES OF LOWER GASTROINTESTINAL BLEEDING IN SURGICAL, TRAUMA, AND MEDICAL ICUS

Causes	%
Acute hemorrhagic rectal ulcer syndrome (AHRUS)	26.7
Ischemic colitis	17.1
Colitis other than ischemia	8.6
Vascular ectasia (angiodysplasia)	6.7
Diverticular bleeding	5.7
Malignancy	5.7
Colonic polyp	3.8
Solitary ulcer	3.8
Hemorrhoid	2.9
Dieulafoy lesions	1.9
Radiation colitis	1
Small bowel bleeding	6.7
Undetermined	9.4

ICU, intensive care unit.
From Wang HP. Unpublished data.

in patients with LGIB and a history of radiation therapy for cervical or prostate malignancy. Although some lesions (i.e., diverticula) are common in the left colon, most bleeding sites are noted in the right colon. In approximately 76% of patients, a definitive site of bleeding will be diagnosed (16). Bleeding in most patients with LGIB will stop spontaneously, although continued or recurrent bleeding during an acute episode occurs in 10% to 40% of patients (17–19). Finally, 2% to 15% of patients with presumed LGIB will have UGIB (20); the cause of overt GI bleeding remains undetermined in 4% to 15% of cases, even after upper GI endoscopy and colonoscopy (21).

LGIB may present in multiple ways, including occult fecal blood; iron deficiency anemia; melena; intermittent scant hematochezia; or acute, massive, and overt bleeding (22). Patients with chronic LGIB may only present with anemia, whereas those with acute LGIB may complain of passing bright red blood per rectum, dark blood with clots, or, less commonly, melena. Patients with brown or infrequent stools are unlikely to have brisk bleeding, and those with frequent passage of red or maroon stool may have aggressive ongoing bleeding (23). Pallor, fatigue, chest pain, palpitations, dyspnea, tachypnea, tachycardia, posture-related dizziness, and syncope are suggestive of hemodynamic compromise and demand aggressive care. The severity of LGIB may be underestimated due to compensatory mechanisms that delay the onset of hypotension. Careful history taking and physical examination are essential to the care of LGIB patients.

Modern management of LGIB encompasses emergency medicine, intensive care medicine, gastroenterology, interventional radiology, and surgery. The approach to LGIB patients is initially aimed at immediate assessment and stabilization of the hemodynamic status, followed by identifying the source of bleeding, stopping any active bleeding, treating any underlying lesions, monitoring and managing comorbid illness, and preventing recurrent bleeding.

The first phase of management adheres to the ABCs of resuscitation, governed by the same priorities that apply to all acutely ill patients. Of course, resuscitation and diagnosis must proceed simultaneously. To identify the source of bleeding, endoscopy, mesenteric arteriography, and radionuclide scintigraphy are the major tools, in addition to history taking and physical examination. Endoscopy, the gold-standard procedure for LGIB, includes:

- Sigmoidoscopy
- Colonoscopy
- Capsule endoscopy
- Push enteroscopy
- Double-balloon enteroscopy

Endoscopic local hemostasis can be performed at the same time the diagnosis is made. Mesenteric arteriography and radionuclide scintigraphy may be used in difficult LGIB cases, with the former providing the ability for embolization or delivering pharmacotherapy. Advances in endoscopic and radiologic hemostasis techniques appear to decrease the rates of rebleeding and surgical intervention (24,25). Transabdominal ultrasound (US) has become popular as a first-line diagnostic tool in a GI emergency. Details of these procedures are noted below. The limited pharmacologic treatments available for LGIB—estrogen and octreotide for angiodysplasia, and topical formalin for intractable bleeding from radiation colitis—are strongly supported (26,27). Even with the advances in localization studies, approximately 10% of patients still require surgical intervention without having their bleeding source identified (28).

ANATOMIC CONSIDERATIONS OF LOWER GASTROINTESTINAL BLEEDING

LGIB is anatomically defined as bleeding located from the ligament of Treitz to the anus, and may include the jejunum, ileum, ileocecal valve, colon (ascending, transverse, descending, sigmoid, rectum), and anus. Given the length of lower GI tract (the small bowel averages 6.7 meters), as well as the special anatomic problem for the small bowel, such as its free intraperitoneal location, multiple overlying loops, and active contractility, there are several management issues for LGIB; these include choice of tests for fecal occult blood, the necessity of nasogastric (NG) tube placement, and the application of endoscopy, radiologic procedures, and US.

Fecal Occult Blood

This is the most common form of GI bleeding. In the ICU, patients suspected of having GI blood loss, secondary to findings of persistent anemia, will have a fecal occult blood study as the first investigative step. While there are numerous types of fecal occult blood tests, the test used determines the location in the GI tract where blood is likely to be detected (29).

Guaiac-based Tests

Guaiac-based tests, the classic fecal occult blood study, utilizes hemoglobin's pseudoperoxidase activity. Guaiac turns blue after oxidation by oxidants or peroxidases in the presence of an oxygen donor such as hydrogen peroxide. Because hemoglobin is degraded in the GI tract, guaiac-based tests are more sensitive for detecting bleeding in the lower than upper GI tract (21). However, the characteristics of specific guaiac-based tests from different companies vary. Whether a guaiac-based test will be positive or not is related to the quantity of blood present in the stool, which is related to the size and location of the bleeding lesion (30,31). Because bleeding colonic lesions are more likely to lead to undegraded blood and heme in the stool, guaiac-based tests are best at detecting these distal lesions (29). Various factors influence guaiac test results; for example, fecal rehydration affects the reactivity of guaiac-based tests, and may raise sensitivity but reduce specificity (32). Additionally, foods that contain peroxidases or animal hemoglobin can cause false-positive guaiac test results. False-negative guaiac-based tests may be seen with hemoglobin degradation, sample storage, and vitamin C ingestion (21). Orally administered iron, even in large amounts, does not cause a positive guaiac reaction (33). Bismuth-containing antacids and antidiarrheals cause dark stool, which should not be confused with a positive guaiac reaction. Guaiac-based tests are rapid bedside studies.

Immunochemical Fecal Occult Blood Tests

Immunochemical fecal occult blood tests detect human globin epitopes, and are highly sensitive for the detection of stool blood (34). These tests do not detect UGI blood because globin molecules are degraded by UGI tract enzymes. Theoretically, these tests have a higher specificity for the detection of colonic lesions than guaiac-based tests. However, they are limited by technical problems and the need for more intensive laboratory processing. A false negative may occur from hemoglobin degradation and sample storage.

Heme-porphyrin Test

The heme-porphyrin test provides a highly accurate determination of total stool hemoglobin based on a spectrofluorometric method that measures porphyrin derived from heme. The heme-porphyrin test is the most sensitive method of detecting occult blood loss of either the upper or lower GI tract. The results of the heme-porphyrin test are neither affected by intraluminal degradation of hemoglobin nor by the interference of peroxidase-producing substances. False positives result from animal hemoglobin and red meats, which contain myoglobin, a heme-containing protein; false negatives are a consequence of sample storage. In summary, guaiac-based tests and immunochemical fecal occult blood tests focus on LGIB, especially from the colon. The heme-porphyrin tests cannot discriminate between bleeding from the upper and lower GI tract.

In the cardiac ICU, warfarin or low-dose aspirin is used frequently. Neither of these alone appears to cause positive guaiac-based, fecal occult blood tests (35). A positive fecal occult blood test in this setting should raise the possibility of a GI tract abnormality, and requires appropriate evaluation. Jaffin et al., prospectively evaluating the GI tract in anticoagulated patients with positive guaiac-based fecal occult blood tests, showed that 20% of these results were associated with malignancy (36).

Nasogastric Tube Placement

The necessity of NG tube placement and gastric lavage for acute LGIB to exclude a UGI source has not been studied prospectively. Theoretically, blood originating from the LGI tract will not retropulse across the ligament of Treitz to the duodenum or stomach, and there should be no blood content in the nasogastric aspirate. Nonetheless, approximately 2% to 15% of patients presenting with acute severe hematochezia have an upper GI source of bleeding identified on upper GI endoscopy (20). Therefore, some favor the routine use of the NG tube to exclude the possibility of a UGI bleed, although this is controversial and, overall, nasogastric aspiration localizes bleeding accurately only in 66% of attempts (37). In the American Society for Gastrointestinal Endoscopy (ASGE) guideline, NG tube placement to rule out a UGI source of bleeding may be considered if a source is not identified on colonoscopy, particularly if there is a history of UGI symptoms or anemia (38). Patients with hemodynamic compromise and hematochezia should have an NG tube placed (39). The absence of blood in NG aspirate is not sufficient to exclude UGI bleeding—16% of patients with bleeding secondary to a duodenal ulcer have a negative NG tube lavage. The presence of bile without blood is considered as the most reassuring result of a negative NG aspirate, and indicates the absence of active UGIB (40).

In spite of the length of the LGI tract, there are anatomically fixed portions, such as the ascending and descending colon and rectum, which makes a US survey of part of the LGI tract possible. The proximal jejunum and terminal ileum can be traced from the fixed duodenum and cecum, respectively (41). US may be considered as a screening tool for LGIB, or applied when the bleeding source cannot be identified by other modalities.

The small bowel is a problematic area to evaluate because of the limitations of standard upper GI endoscopy and colonoscopy. The length of the small intestine and its loosely supported and looped structure on the mesentery make conventional endoscopic techniques difficult and, frequently, inadequate. Push enteroscopy can reach only the proximal jejunum. Even with the maximal depth of insertion, approximately 160 cm beyond the ligament of Treitz, most of the small intestine still remains unexamined. The distal ileum, the small intestine closest to the colon, can be surveyed occasionally with traditional colonoscopy retrograde examination via the ileocecal valve. Initially introduced by Yamamoto in 2001, double-balloon enteroscopy (DBE) has been implemented as a method of deeper intubation of the small bowel (42). By combining oral intubation and anal intubation, a complete study of the small bowel can be achieved.

Blood supply to the LGI tract is separated into the superior mesentery artery (SMA) and inferior mesentery artery (IMA) territories. The SMA territory includes the jejunum, ileum, ascending colon, and transverse colon, while the IMA territory covers the descending colon, sigmoid colon, and rectum. The territory of the mesentery vessels is very important for interventional angiography or second-look endoscopy if the first endoscopic survey fails.

APPROACH TO LOWER GASTROINTESTINAL BLEEDING

Resuscitation

Approximately 85% of GI bleeding episodes stop spontaneously, whereas the remainder require aggressive resuscitation, diagnostic modalities, and often intense medical and/or surgical management. The first management step for a patient presenting with overt LGIB is the ABCs of resuscitation. Resuscitation is imperative to restore euvolemia and prevent complications of blood loss in the cardiac, pulmonary, renal, or neurologic systems. This takes place in parallel with the initial evaluation of the patient; resuscitation must not be withheld or delayed for diagnostic procedures. The patient's respiratory and heart rates, and blood pressure, including orthostatic measurements, should be assessed. Attention to the airway is important when the LGIB is caused by an obstructive lesion, which may lead to vomiting with the consequent high risk of aspiration. Postural hemodynamic changes, chest pain, palpitations, syncope, pallor, dyspnea, and tachycardia suggest hemodynamic compromise (43); the severity of bleeding is easy to underestimate due to compensatory mechanisms. An orthostatic decrease in systolic blood pressure greater than 10 mm Hg or an increase in heart rate greater than 10 beats/minute indicates an acute loss of at least 15% of blood volume (44). With hemodynamic compromise, two 16-gauge or larger intravenous (IV) catheters should be secured immediately; central venous access can be established in unstable patients. Packed red blood cells should be utilized in hemodynamically unstable patients, with the goal of maintaining a hematocrit of approximately 30% in the elderly and in those with heart disease or who are otherwise compromised physiologically, and 20% to 25% in younger patients (45). The initial hematocrit may not be the true value, requiring up to 72 hours for equilibration with the intravascular space (46). The presence of coagulopathy (international normalized ratio [INR] greater than 1.5) or thrombocytopenia (less than 50,000 cells/μL) should be corrected with fresh frozen plasma or platelet transfusions, respectively. Oxygen should be administered to keep the SpO_2 between 93% and 95% at a minimum, and vital signs and urine output should be closely monitored. In the elderly or those with a history of cardiac disease, an ECG and cardiac enzyme analysis should be considered. Approaches for LGIB with hemodynamic instability and hemodynamically stable LGIB are noted, respectively, in Figures 153.2 and 153.3.

Determination of Bleeding Site: Noninstrumental

History

Careful history taking is helpful for determining the level of bleeding from the GI tract and to work out a differential diagnosis of the LGIB. Included should be the duration, frequency, and color of the stool; related symptoms of the GI tract such as constipation, fever, or location of pain; medical or surgical history; and history of medications. Except for asymptomatic patients with only anemia due to GI bleeding, the *color of the stool* is always queried. The patient presenting with acute LGIB may complain of passing bright red blood per rectum, dark blood with clots, or, less commonly, melena. The stool appearance, largely dependent on blood transit time, may be suggestive of the location of bleeding. Blood that has been in the GI tract for <5 hours is usually red, whereas blood present for >20 hours is usually melenic. Upper GI, small bowel bleeding, or slow oozing from the right colon usually produces melena, whereas patients with hematochezia typically have left colonic or rectal lesions (47). If the blood coats the surface of stool, the left colon—especially the rectum and anus—is more likely to be the bleeding source. Blood dripping into the toilet may occur with hemorrhoidal bleeding. If the stool is mixed with blood, the source may be in the right colon. Of course, massive UGIB can occasionally masquerade as lower GI bleeding in 10% to 15% of patients presenting with severe hematochezia (20). This may happen when massive bleeding originates from esophageal or gastric varices; insertion of an NG tube may be helpful in this situation if the patient does not have hematemesis.

The duration and frequency of bleeding may help in determining the severity of the problem. Related GI tract symptoms may lead to the diagnosis of LGIB. Severe constipation should prompt an investigation for colon cancer or a stercoral ulcer; diarrhea may indicate enterocolitis; and fever or local pain may indicate an inflammation-related bleeding source, such as infectious colitis or inflammatory bowel disease. The medical or surgical history may provide clues to the causes of LGIB. A previous history of colonic polyps, diverticulosis, or colonic tumor should be considered as a possible source of LGIB during the initial evaluation. Renal failure is a well-known risk factor for angiodysplasia or arteriovenous malformation (AVM) (48), as is aortic stenosis (15). Note should be made of patients with renal impairment or who are being dialyzed, as these patients may have platelet abnormalities, resulting in a tendency to bleed if a lesion is present. Ischemic bowel may be present

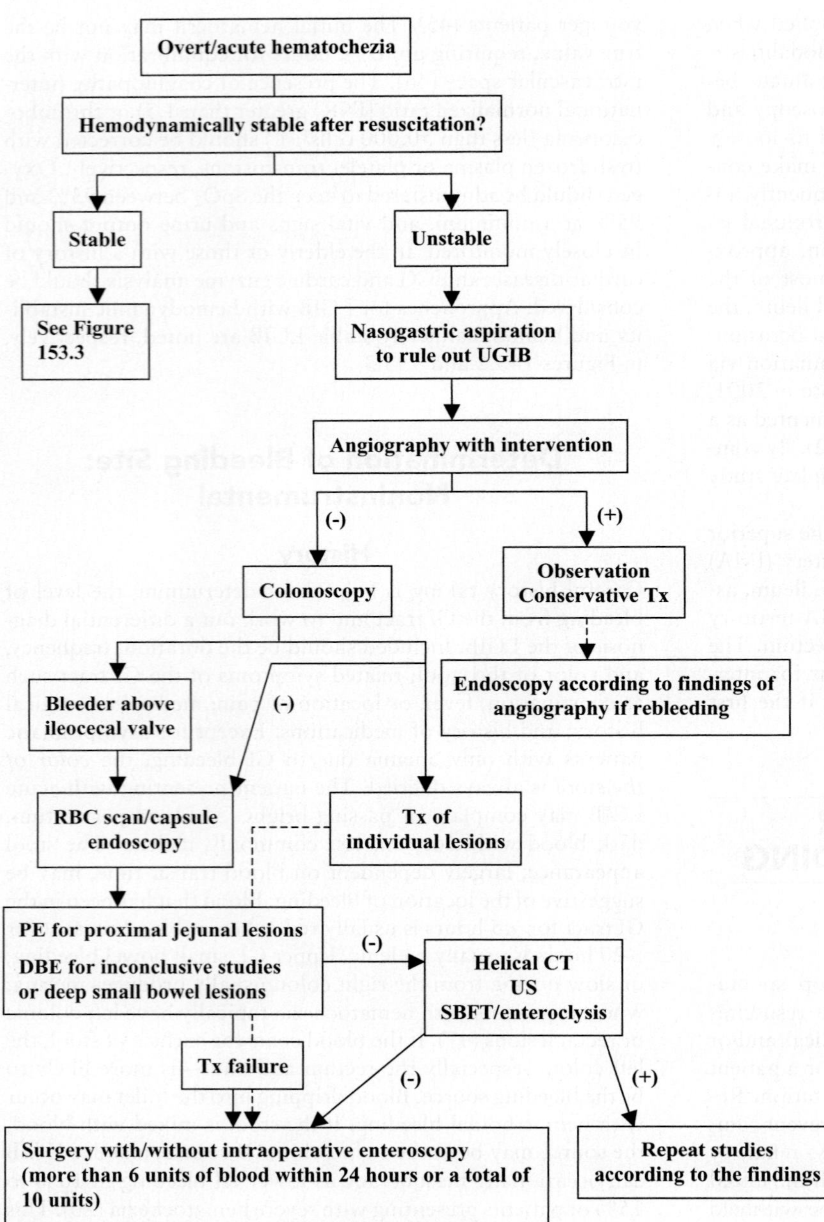

FIGURE 153.2. Approach for lower gastrointestinal bleeding with hemodynamic instability. UGIB, upper gastrointestinal bleeding; Tx, treatment; RBC, red blood cell; PE, push-type enteroscopy; DBE, double-balloon enteroscopy; CT, computed tomography; US, ultrasound; SBFT, small bowel follow-through.

when severe abdominal pain and bloody stool occur in patients with severe atherosclerotic vascular disease, atrial fibrillation, or hypotension. Radiation therapy for prostate or pelvic cancer induces inflammatory changes of the rectum, and can produce radiation proctitis, presenting months or even years after the radiation exposure. A history of recent colonoscopy with polypectomy indicates postpolypectomy bleeding as the likely source. In patients who have undergone aortoiliac reconstructive surgery, the frequency of significant postoperative colonic ischemia ranges between 1% and 7% (49–51).

Medication history is also important. Medications that can damage the GI mucosa or exacerbate bleeding include nonsteroidal anti-inflammatory drugs (NSAIDs), alendronate, potassium chloride, and anticoagulants. Patients admitted with GI bleeding were more likely to be taking selective serotonin reuptake inhibitors (SSRIs) than controls; this association exists for LGIB as well as UGIB (52). Concurrent anticoagulation or use of NSAIDs may be important cofactors in potentiating bleeding (53). The use of aspirin or NSAIDs is strongly associated with both LGIB—chiefly from diverticula—and UGIB (54,55). NSAID enteropathy has been increasingly reported, and can be a potential cause of LGIB (56,57). A family history of colon cancer increases the likelihood of a colorectal neoplasm, and generally calls for a complete colonic examination in patients with hematochezia (58,59).

Physical Examination

A thorough physical examination is essential to assess loss of blood volume, a possible bleeding source, and comorbid conditions (especially for ICU patients). The comorbid conditions may affect the suitability for interventions, such as urgent colonoscopy. The physical examination should also include complete vital signs and heart, lung, and abdominal assessment, as well as an examination of the conjunctiva and

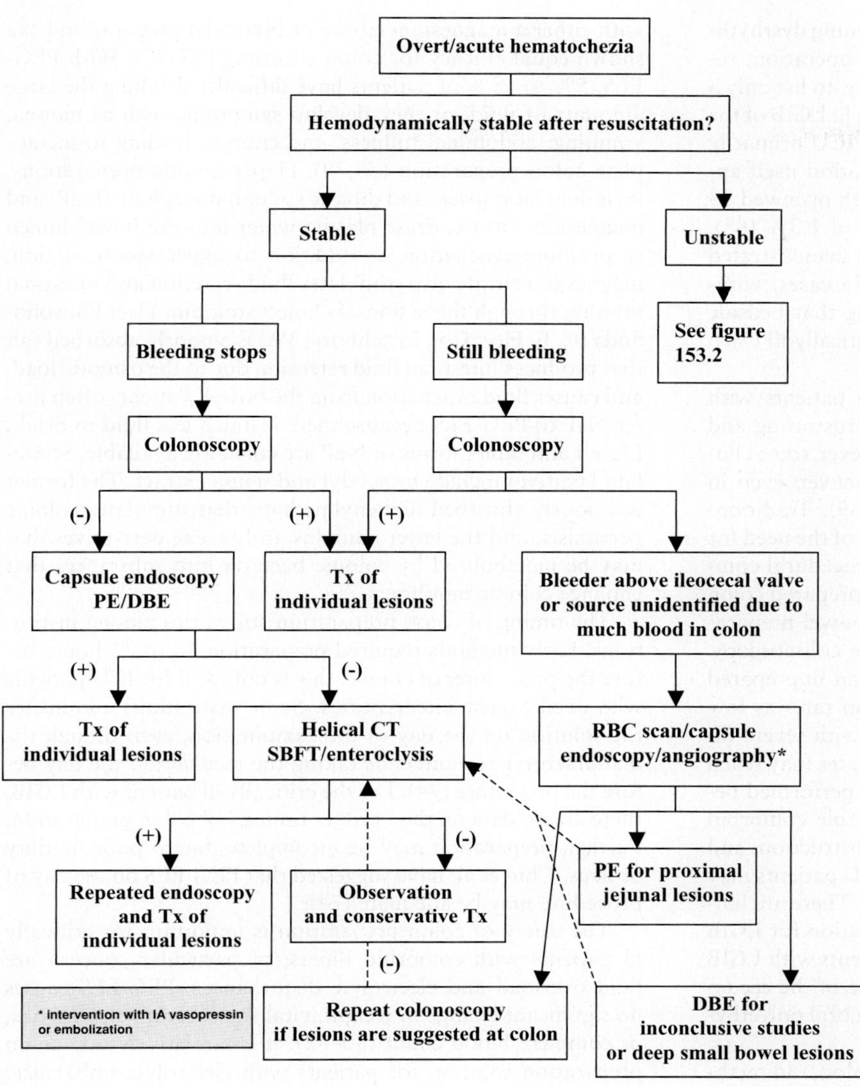

FIGURE 153.3. Approach for hemodynamically stable lower gastrointestinal bleeding. PE, push-type enteroscopy; DBE, double-balloon enteroscopy; Tx, treatment; SBFT, small bowel follow-through.

skin. Pale conjunctiva indicate anemia. Cutaneous manifestations may suggest disorders causing GI bleeding; those caused by celiac sprue may indicate dermatitis herpetiformis. The polyposis syndromes (Peutz-Jeghers syndrome, Gardner syndrome, and Cronkite-Canada syndrome) often have cutaneous abnormalities, such as lip pigmentation in Peutz-Jeghers syndrome. Orthostatic vital signs are an important complement to standard monitoring in a patient with severe bleeding but without overt hemodynamic instability. Abdominal tenderness on examination may indicate an inflammatory process, such as ischemic colitis or inflammatory bowel disease (60). The rectal examination serves to identify anorectal lesions and confirm the stool color described by the patient. In addition, approximately 40% of rectal carcinomas are palpable during a digital rectal examination (61). Regardless of the presenting features and findings on physical examination, most patients with LGIB still warrant a full examination of the colon.

Laboratory Examination

Initial laboratory studies should include a complete blood count, serum urea nitrogen, creatinine, coagulation profile (prothrombin time, INR, and partial thromboplastin time), liver tests, blood type and cross-match, and electrolytes. As discussed above, positive fecal occult tests (guaiac-based tests and immunochemical fecal occult blood tests) may favor LGIB. The blood urea nitrogen–to–creatinine ratio has been used as a noninvasive test to help distinguish UGIB from colonic sources of bleeding (62–64). In the study of Chalasani et al., a ratio of 33 or higher had a sensitivity of 96% for UGIB, although overlap was observed with LGIB, especially in patients with UGIB without hematemesis (62).

Determination of the Bleeding Site: Diagnostic Approach

Endoscopic Approach: General

Safety of Endoscopic Procedures for Critically Ill Patients. Colonoscopy remains the procedure of choice for evaluating patients with acute LGIB, and enteroscopy is considered for proximal small bowel bleeding. However, for ICU patients with acquired bleeding and hemodynamic instability, questions remain due to the possibility of severe comorbid illness, including respiratory distress, aortic aneurysm, life-threatening dysrhythmias, AMI, history of GI tract perforation or operation, severe lower GI obstruction, and bleeding tendency, to list only a few conditions. Colonoscopy complication rates in LGIB of the general population or patients admitted to the ICU primarily for hemorrhage are low, and the bowel preparation itself appears to be safe (65–67). Zuckerman and Prakash reviewed 13 studies and found an overall complication rate of 1.3% (68). A study of 55 ICU patients with acquired LGIB demonstrated an acceptable diagnostic rate of 67% (37 of 55 cases) without procedure-related complications, suggesting that bedside colonoscopy after preparation is safe for the critically ill (5).

Preparation before Endoscopic Procedures. In patients with massive active bleeding, colonoscopy is often frustrating and nonproductive, and sometimes dangerous. However, some clinicians still consider it the first diagnostic maneuver, even in the patient with severe ongoing bleeding (20,69). Traditionally, colonoscopy for LGIB was delayed because of the need for bowel preparation and the fear of increased procedural complications. Indeed, urgent colonoscopy in an unprepared colon can be challenging, or even dangerous. Good bowel preparation is important for an adequate and sensitive colonoscopy. Studies of urgent colonoscopies performed in an unprepared colon to evaluate for LGIB revealed completion rates as low as 35% (70,71). Jensen et al. studied patients with severe diverticular hemorrhage, noting that completion rates may reach up to 100% if aggressive bowel preparation is performed before urgent colonoscopy (24). Because of variable comorbid conditions, such as decreased bowel motility, obstruction, and electrolyte disturbance, colon preparation in ICU patients may not be as thorough as in the general population. There are limited studies of the effectiveness of colon preparation for LGIB in ICU patients. Lin et al. (5) noted that for patients with LGIB occurring after admission to ICU, the reach rate of the cecum with a colonoscope was 58% after enemas or an oral polyethylene glycol solution were administered.

In spite of providing a relatively feces-free colon, old methods for colon preparation with clear liquids, laxatives, and enemas or peroral gut lavage 48 to 72 hours before colonoscopy are time consuming, uncomfortable, and inconvenient for patients. For those in the ICU or with active LGIB, these methods are clearly not useful. Peroral gut lavage with saline or balanced electrolyte solutions have been proposed and were found to provide rapid, effective cleansing of the colon; however, the method is not tolerated in 11% of patients due to the high fluid volume—7 to 12 L—and might cause fluid and electrolyte disturbances (72). Recently, development of osmotically balanced solutions may provide minimal water absorption or secretion into the bowel lumen. Generally speaking, there are isoosmotic preparations, hyperosmotic preparations, and stimulant laxatives for colon cleansing. Polyethylene glycol electrolyte lavage solution (PEG-ELS) is an isotonic, nonabsorbable electrolyte solution that clears the bowel by washing out ingested fluid without significant fluid and electrolyte shifts. Rapid purge is best accomplished with polyethylene glycol-based solutions. They can be administered by a nasogastric tube or by drinking 1 L every 30 to 45 minutes, to a median dose of 5.5 L (range 4–14 L); 3 to 4 hours are required to cleanse the colon (73). Two liters of PEG-ELS plus bisacodyl or magnesium citrate have also been suggested for colon preparation (74). The studies comparing a standard 4-L PEG-ELS with 2 PEG-ELS with either a magnesium citrate or bisacodyl preparation have shown equal efficacy for colon cleansing (75–77). With PEG-ELS, 5% to 15% of patients have difficulty drinking the large amounts of fluid, or they develop symptoms such as nausea, vomiting, abdominal fullness, and cramps, leading to incomplete colon preparation (78,79). Hyperosmotic preparations, including monobasic and dibasic sodium phosphate (NaP) and magnesium citrate, draw plasma water into the bowel lumen to promote evacuation. In addition to hyperosmotic action, magnesium citrate also stimulates fluid secretion and intestinal motility through the action of cholecystokinin. Fleet Phospho-Soda (C. B. Fleet Co., Lynchburg, VA) is a poorly absorbed salt that produces intestinal fluid retention due to the osmotic load, and causes fluid evacuation from the bowel. Patients often prefer NaP to PEG-ELS because there is much less fluid to drink. Liquid and tablet forms of NaP are currently available. Stimulant laxatives include bisacodyl and senna extract. The former is a poorly absorbed diphenylmethane that stimulates colonic peristalsis, and the latter contains anthracene derivatives that may be metabolized by colonic bacteria into substances that enhance colonic motility.

The timing of colon preparation still varies among institutions. Early methods required preparation 48 to 72 hours before the procedure; of course, this is not ideal for ICU patients who need urgent interventions. Some institutions administer the solution on the day of the examination, even though the manufacturer recommends taking the medication the day before the procedure (74). For the critically ill patient with LGIB, there are no data on the "proper timing" of colon preparation. Further, preparation may be incomplete due to poor motility or ileus. Chiu et al. have suggested that PEG-ELS on the day of procedure may be adequate (74).

The safety of colon preparation is important for critically ill patients with comorbid illness; of particular concern are fluid overload and electrolyte disturbances. PEG-ELS causes no significant change in weight, vital signs, serum electrolytes, or complete blood count (80–82). It is a relatively safe colon preparation solution for patients with electrolyte imbalance, advanced liver disease, poorly compensated congestive heart failure, or renal failure, although in the study of Granberry et al., exacerbation of congestive heart failure after PEG-ELS administration was noted (83). NaP, a hyperosmotic preparation, may cause alterations in serum electrolytes and extracellular fluid status (84,85). Asymptomatic hyperphosphatemia is seen in up to 40% of patients, but clinically significant hyperphosphatemia is rare and usually limited to patients with renal failure (86–88). Twenty percent of patients had abnormally low serum potassium levels after bowel preparation with NaP (84). It is suggested that NaP is contraindicated in patients with renal failure, acute myocardial infarction or unstable angina, congestive heart failure, ileus, intestinal malabsorption, and significant ascites. Gremse et al. reported that the degree of asymptomatic hyperphosphatemia in children was greater than in adults, and recommended avoiding NaP in children with renal failure, congestive heart failure, ileus, and ascites (88).

Colonoscopy for Critically Ill Patients

Three primary diagnostic tools for LGIB are colonoscopy, radionuclide scintigraphy, and mesenteric arteriography.

Advances in endoscopic technology have brought colonoscopy to the forefront of the management of LGIB. Colonoscopy as the first choice for occult or stable LGIB is not in dispute. However, for brisk LGIB or LGIB with hemodynamic compromise, whether the attending physicians consider colonoscopy as the first diagnostic maneuver for brisk LGIB or LGIB with hemodynamic compromise is controversial. Colonoscopy in patients with severe hematochezia is impractical because of inadequate visualization caused by brisk blood loss (2,68). Some are reluctant to perform colonoscopy in hemodynamically unstable patients with ongoing bleeding, suggesting that these patients are best served by urgent angiography, perhaps in conjunction with surgical consultation (73,89). However, there is a reason to favor colonoscopy for acute LGIB. In addition to affording a rapid diagnosis, colonoscopy may indicate specific therapy (when [and if] the bleeders are found [24,90–92], although the rate for intervention in an ICU study was low [5]). Rapid endoscopic identification of a bleeding source, regardless of whether therapy is administered, may contribute to the clinical management of recurrent bleeding, if it occurs. Finally, compared with angiography, urgent colonoscopy has a higher diagnostic yield and a lower complication rate. In a retrospective study of 107 patients with severe LGIB, colonoscopy was diagnostic in 90% of patients and angiography in 48%; the former was therapeutic in 12% versus 22% for the latter (19). In another study, the diagnostic yield of colonoscopy was 82% versus 12% for angiography (20). Interestingly, most patients undergoing radiographic evaluation for LGIB—regardless of findings and interventions—will subsequently require a colonoscopy to establish the cause of bleeding. In addition to diagnosis, occasional therapy, and management planning, earlier colonoscopy does contribute to a shorter length of hospital stay (93). Hemodynamic instability, higher comorbidity, performance of a tagged red blood cell nuclear scan, and surgery for hemostasis were significantly associated with a decreased likelihood of discharge (93).

While most episodes of LGIB will stop spontaneously, 10% to 15% of patients undergoing urgent colonoscopy received endoscopic therapy. The lesions most amenable to colonoscopic treatment of LGIB, in most studies, are usually angiodysplasia or diverticulosis. Once it is identified as the source of bleeding, angiodysplasia is usually coagulated by methods including the following (5,24,94,95):

- Injection therapy (epinephrine, saline, or ethanol)
- Heater probe
- Monopolar and multipolar electrocoagulation
- Argon plasma coagulation
- Hemoclips
- Band ligation

In a study of ICU patients with nonprimary LGIB, spontaneous cessation occurred in 53% of patients; 29% achieved hemostasis with endoscopy, but had a higher rate (19%) of recurrent bleeding (5). Other studies, not limited to ICU patients, have reported rebleeding rates of 13% to 53%, and many patients may require more than one treatment (94,95).

Timing of Colonoscopy

The use of colonoscopy is controversial for critically ill patients with LGIB. Some believe that colonoscopy is best utilized in patients whose bleeding has stopped or slowed down (73,89), and others agree with early colonoscopy for LGIB. Evidence suggests that earlier intervention leads to more diagnostic and therapeutic opportunities (24,96). It has further been noted that early colonoscopy reduces the length of hospital stay, and therefore should decrease treatment costs (97,98). Urgent colonoscopy after bowel preparation with endoscopic treatment of patients with active diverticular bleeding or stigmata of bleeding has been shown to be highly effective in decreasing the need for surgical intervention (24,73).

In conclusion, prompt intervention may decrease the need for surgical exploration, as well as the rate of recurrent bleeding and length of hospital stay. Who needs urgent colonoscopy? Early identification of high-risk patients would allow the more selective delivery of urgent therapeutic interventions to those who will benefit. Clinical high-risk predictors in the first hour of evaluation in patients with severe LGIB have been proposed, and included an initial hematocrit of no more than 35%, the presence of abnormal vital signs 1 hour after initial medical evaluation, and gross blood on initial rectal examination (99). How early should the urgent colonoscopy be performed? The definition of *urgent colonoscopy* varies widely in the literature—from within 8 hours to 24 hours of presentation (5,20,24,100–104). Most definitions consider the procedure within 12 to 24 hours; more recently, the literature defines urgent colonoscopy as within 12 hours (20,24).

Sigmoidoscopy or Colonoscopy?

In studies of the general population with LGIB, diverticular and angiodysplastic bleeding are the most frequent events. Although anatomically prone to be located in the left colon, bleeding most often occurs in the right colon; thus, most endoscopists prefer a total colonoscopy. Flexible sigmoidoscopy can be performed in the initial evaluation of patients with LGIB, but the diagnostic yield of flexible sigmoidoscopy in LGIB is low, ranging from 9% to 58% (10). Regardless of presentation, flexible sigmoidoscopy may miss serious proximal pathology (105). However, in the study of ICU patients with acquired bleeding, 78% of responsible lesions were in the left colon (5). If the critical situation precludes use of total colonoscopy, sigmoidoscopy as the first maneuver may be acceptable for this patient group. Nonetheless, unless a definite and compatible bleeding source is identified with flexible sigmoidoscopy, the study of LGIB should proceed to a full colonoscopy in most patients.

In 2005, the ASGE offered the following guidelines regarding LGIB (38):

1. Colonoscopy is effective in the diagnosis and treatment of LGIB (prospective controls).
2. Colonoscopy is recommended in the early evaluation of severe acute LGIB (prospective controls).
3. Thermal contact modalities, including heat probe, and bipolar/multipolar coagulation and/or epinephrine injection can be used in the treatment of bleeding diverticula, vascular ectasia, or postpolypectomy bleeding (prospective controls).

Enteroscopy and Capsule Endoscopy for Critically Ill Patients

The small bowel has traditionally been a problematic area to evaluate because of the long length, looping, free intraperitoneal location, active contractility, and limits of standard endoscopy. It is estimated that 10% to 25% of LGIB originates in the small bowel and can pose a diagnostic dilemma for clinicians (106–108). Small bowel sources account for 0.9% to 7% of cases presenting with blood per rectum (19,20,109), and comprises approximately 5% of obscure GI bleeding (110). Upper endoscopy and colonoscopy appear to have limited roles in the investigation of small bowel bleeding, and are only useful when the bleeding source is the duodenum or the most distal segment of the small intestine (terminal ileum), respectively (53). Some clinicians have utilized peroral intubation with a standard colonoscope, reaching a point 20 to 60 cm distal to the ligament of Treitz; this may increase the diagnostic yield of GI bleeding of obscure origin by 17% to 46%—not an insignificant proportion (13,111–113). Small bowel enteroscopy is currently the best endoscopic investigative modality. Indeed, it has become the cornerstone of management in patients with obscure GI bleeding. Current tools for ruling out small bowel diseases include push-type enteroscopy (PE), double-balloon enteroscopy (DBE), intraoperative enteroscopy, and capsule endoscopy.

Small bowel evaluation may be performed with PE, which allows endoscopic evaluation of the proximal 60 cm of the jejunum or 150 cm distal to the pylorus. PE is probably the most commonly performed small bowel procedure today, and is often pursued when upper GI endoscopy and colonoscopy have failed to find the source for blood loss. PE may be performed using an enteroscope or pediatric colonoscope. The obvious limitation of push enteroscopy is the inability to reach lesions distal to the middle jejunum. PE can only examine a relatively short portion of the small bowel, even under fluoroscopy, and the true depth of insertion is unreliable. Some experts consider it complementary to capsule endoscopy, and believe that it should be performed only if capsule endoscopy or other modalities are positive for a proximal small bowel lesion. The use of an overtube to prevent looping of the instrument in the stomach increases the insertion depth by 10 to 25 cm (114). Prototype, variable stiffness enteroscopes are emerging in an attempt to achieve maximal insertion depth without the use of an overtube (115,116). Although PE cannot investigate the entire small bowel, an important benefit of PE is the ability to provide diagnostic and therapeutic capabilities with one procedure *if* the bleeder can be found.

The diagnostic yield of PE is between 38% and 65% of patients in whom upper and lower endoscopy are negative (117). Multivariate analysis in a retrospective, two-center study by Lepère et al. showed that melena and chronic renal failure increase the diagnostic yield of PE in patients with unexplained GI bleeding (123). The positive findings noted with PE for patients with renal failure were most often in the distal duodenum or jejunum, including ulcers (17%) and AVMs (41%). Others have shown similar results in that most small bowel lesions diagnosed by PE are vascular in nature (angiodysplasia/AVM) (119–121), followed by ulcerations and malignancies (122). A delay between the bleeding and PE (less than or more than 4 days) and a history of recurrent intestinal bleedings before PE were not associated with positive findings; thus, rapid performance of PE may not be necessary, except in patients with continuous active bleeding (123). Another benefit of PE is that it provides a "second look" for lesions that may have been missed on original endoscopy. Interestingly, 25% to 40% of lesions found on PE are within reach of a standard upper endoscopy (124,125). Complications of PE are infrequent, occurring in less than 1% of cases. Most complications, including bleeding and perforation, are related to the use of an overtube (126,127). The data of effectiveness and safety of PE for ICU patients are limited.

Even when PE reaches a maximal depth of insertion of 160 cm below the ligament of Treitz, there is still over 250 cm of small intestine remaining unexamined. It is possible to close this gap with a newly developed DBE system (128). The newest modality for imaging the small bowel was introduced in 2001, when Yamamoto et al. reported their results using a double-balloon method in four patients (129). The DBE represents the first successful provision of both diagnostic and therapeutic intervention to the entire small bowel. The goal is to reach the ileocecal valve, but this often is not possible. The total inspection of the small bowel is usually attainable with the peroral approach and retrograde approach per rectum. On average, approximately 250 cm is achieved via the oral route and 130 cm via the anal route, with a mean examination time of 75 min (130). If total enteroscopy is necessary, it can be achieved in 60% to 86% of cases, depending on the experience of the endoscopist (131,132). Yamamoto et al. performed 50% of the studies in an antegrade fashion, with the remainder being retrograde. The bleeding source was found in 76%, and hemostasis using electrocautery was performed successfully in 18% (131). Multicenter experience with DBE in the United States showed that the mean procedure time was 115 minutes, and the yield of DBE for a GI bleed ranged between 52% and 75% (130,133). Oral DBE requires no specific preparation other than a 6- to 8-hour fast before the procedure. If a retrograde (anal) approach is undertaken, standard colonic preparation is necessary. Conscious sedation or general anesthesia may be utilized. Endoscopic hemostasis using injection therapy, argon plasma coagulation, electrocautery, and hemoclipping may be used as is done in routine upper GI endoscopy and colonoscopy. Complications of DBE are noted in 1.1% to 8.5% (131,133), and include aspiration pneumonia, abdominal pain, perforation, and acute pancreatitis (130,131,133–135). The effectiveness and safety of DBE for critically ill patients are unknown.

Before the advent of capsule endoscopy and DBE, intraoperative endoscopy was the only way to detect and treat lesions beyond the reach of push enteroscopy. Now the role of diagnostic intraoperative enteroscopy is likely to decrease with introduction of the less invasive capsule endoscopy and DBE; however, it still plays a role in specific clinical situations. Intraoperative endoscopy is performed in conjunction with a surgeon in the operating room, and with the patient under general anesthesia. Intubation may be achieved transorally, transanally, or through an operative enterotomy, depending on the clinical circumstance and physicians' preference.

During laparotomy combined with intraoperative enteroscopy, the endoscopist carefully inspects the intestinal lumen with a push enteroscope, while the surgeon slowly guides the bowel over the endoscope using the air-trapping technique and examines the external wall with palpation and transillumination (136). Lesions can be treated endoscopically or marked with a tattoo for surgical resection. The terminal ileum is reached in more than 90% of patients (137). The yield in detecting bleeding lesions reaches 70% to 100% (53,138), making intraoperative endoscopy the most sensitive method of diagnosing small bowel disorders. However, the high sensitivity comes at the cost of extreme invasiveness, making it a procedure of last resort. The complication rate is estimated at about

3%, including mucosal tears and bleeding of the mesentery due to traction (133).

Capsule endoscopy is a safe and promising diagnostic tool for GI bleeding of unknown origin, focusing especially on the small bowel; it may obviate the need for angiography in some difficult patients. The idea of wireless imaging of the small intestine was conceived simultaneously by Paul Swain, a British gastroenterologist, and Gavriel Iddan, an Israeli scientist. They merged research efforts in 1998 and soon developed a pill-sized camera with sufficient battery life to image the entire small intestine (139). Capsule endoscopy was introduced into clinical practice in 2001 and made it possible for the first time to visualize intraluminal conditions throughout the entire small bowel. The first commercially available video capsule (Given) is composed of three main subsystems: an ingestible capsule endoscope, a data recorder, and a workstation. The PillCam SB capsule measures 11 × 26 mm in size, and weighs less than 4 g, with a miniaturized image-capturing system, battery, light source, and transmitter. After an overnight fast, the patient swallows the capsule, which travels through the GI tract by means of the actions of normal peristalsis. The capsule device captures two images per second and has a battery life of approximately 6 to 8 hours. Captured images are transmitted by a digital radio-frequency communication channel to an external data recorder unit.

Studies comparing capsule endoscopy with other diagnostic procedures, including enteroclysis, PE, computed tomography (CT) scan, and intraoperative enteroscopy, showed that capsule endoscopy was clearly superior in the diagnosis of occult/obscure/overt small bowel bleeding (127,140–149). Capsule endoscopy has proven superior to enteroclysis (144–147) and PE (140,142,143). In a series of 60 patients comparing the wireless capsule to PE, Saurin et al. showed that the use of the capsule raised the diagnostic yield from 38% to 69% (143). However, one study did not show the superiority of capsule endoscopy over PE. Van Gossum et al. noted that, with obscure GI bleeding, no significant difference in diagnostic yield was found between push and wireless-capsule endoscopy (150). Capsule endoscopy, compared to CT scanning, is reported to be superior in detecting small bowel lesions (144,146,147). In a study of 42 patients with obscure GI bleeding, capsule endoscopy sensitivity and intraoperative enteroscopy was not significantly different. Furthermore, no additional diagnoses were made with intraoperative enteroscopy (149).

The overall diagnostic yield rate of capsule endoscopy in patients with GI bleeding ranges from 45% to 66% (141,144,151,152,153). The timing of capsule endoscopy has been addressed in two studies and appears related to diagnostic yield. When administered to patients with ongoing overt bleeding, the diagnostic yield is higher—87% to 92%—than in those with previous overt bleeding or iron deficiency anemia—46% to 56% (151,154). Hartmann et al. noted that capsule endoscopy identified lesions in 100% of patients with ongoing overt bleeding, 67% of patients with previous overt bleeding, and 67% of patients with obscure/occult bleeding (148). To increase the diagnostic yield of capsule endoscopy, prokinetic agents (155), oral bowel preparation (oral sodium phosphate and polyethylene glycol), simethicone, and erythromycin have been recommended. Prokinetic agents prompt the passage of the capsule and prevent the exhaustion of batteries before study completion. Bowel preparation with oral sodium phosphate has been suggested to offer better visualization than overnight fasting alone, and is associated with fewer disturbances by intraluminal turbid fluid (156). However, there are concerns that increasing bowel motility may result in missing a lesion. Fireman et al. showed that erythromycin markedly reduced gastric emptying time and had a negative effect on the small bowel images. Preparation of elderly subjects with PEG or sodium phosphate also had a negative effect on small bowel transit time (157). PEG increased the visibility in the proximal small bowel in one study, but had no effect in a second investigation (158,159). Presently, bowel preparation is preferred by most practitioners. Erythromycin leads to faster gastric emptying at the expense of small bowel transit time and poorer visualization (160). Bowel preparation with simethicone, which can decrease intraluminal gas bubbles, resulted in significantly better visibility (161). Simethicone may be added to the routine preparation for capsule endoscopy to improve visualization of the small bowel mucosa. A delay in bowel transit time may result in an incomplete study due to capsule battery drainage.

Despite the higher diagnostic yield, capsule endoscopy limitations are evident: biopsy specimens cannot be obtained, therapeutic intervention cannot be performed, and localization of some lesions is imprecise (162). Capsule endoscopy, however, is regarded as a low-risk procedure that is well tolerated (163). The primary risk with capsule endoscopy is capsule entrapment within the GI tract; this occurs in 0.75% to 5% of cases. Most entrapment occurs in the small intestine, although case studies report impaction at the cricopharyngeus, tracheal aspiration, and retention in diverticula (10). Risk factors for entrapment include NSAID-induced strictures, prior abdominal radiation, Crohn enteritis, prior major abdominal surgery, and known diverticula. A trapped capsule may be retrieved endoscopically or surgically. In cases where the colon is not visualized on capsule endoscopy and the patient does not see the capsule pass, an abdominal radiograph should be obtained to document passage. Absolute contraindications to its use include GI obstruction and pseudo-obstruction—meaning ileus. Relative contraindications include a history of GI motility disorders, such as gastroparesis; history of intestinal strictures or fistulae; pregnancy; history of multiple small bowel diverticula; history of Zenker diverticulum; history of abdominal surgeries or radiation; and an active swallowing disorder or dysphagia. Although there is concern about the use of capsule endoscopy in patients with pacemakers, new evidence suggests that capsule endoscopy may be safely utilized in these patients (164).

Capsule endoscopy has been reported to change patient management in up to 75% of cases (142), although the studies focused solely on small bowel lesions. Colonic bleeding is difficult to evaluate via capsule endoscopy because of retained stool, limited battery life, and poor visual field due to the colon's large diameter. A recently developed PillCam Colon capsule endoscopy appears promising for colonic evaluation (165), although in comparison to conventional colonoscopy, false-positive findings were recorded in 33% cases (166).

The use of capsule endoscopy in critically ill patients has been limited. These patients often cannot ingest the capsule by themselves, especially if endotracheally intubated; an endoscopic technique of capsule placement has been described for such patients (167). In addition to swallowing problems, bowel transit time may be delayed due to sepsis, electrolyte imbalance, medication use, and anatomic changes due to surgeries. Abnormal bowel transit time affects the diagnostic yield of capsule endoscopy. The utilization of capsule endoscopy for small bowel or obscure bleeding must be made on a case-by-case basis.

Nonendoscopic Approach

Nuclear Medicine

As mentioned previously, for LGIB, endoscopy, nuclear medicine, and mesentery angiography are three main diagnostic modalities. The two techniques of radionuclide scanning commonly use either ^{99m}Tc-labeled red blood cells or ^{99m}technetium sulfur colloid. A ^{99m}Tc-labeled red blood cell scan is the preferred technique, with images that can be detected for up to 12 to 24 hours after injection. If the rate of bleeding is insufficient to give an immediate positive test, or if the bleeding is intermittent, the labeled red blood cells can sometimes accumulate to detect the site of bleeding—when rescanned—up to 24 hours after injection. This technique can detect bleeding at a rate as low as 0.1 to 0.5 mL/minute, and is thought to be a sensitive diagnostic tool for LGIB (168). ^{99m}Technetium sulfur colloid is rapidly cleared by the reticuloendothelial system after injection, with a half-life of only 2 to 3 minutes. Therefore, if there is no active bleeding when administered, the ^{99m}technetium sulfur colloid is quickly cleared, with a resultant nondiagnostic test.

Timing the Use of Radionuclide Scanning. Radionuclide scanning, often performed repeatedly during a hospital course, may be used as the screening test, followed by angiography, small bowel enteroscopy, or surgery to definitively localize and treat the bleeding lesion. Because of its high sensitivity—it has the ability to detect bleeding as low as 0.1 to 0.5 mL/minute—radionuclide scanning has been utilized as a guide for surgical resection, and as a screening test prior to angiography when colonoscopy fails to find the LGI bleeder. As a guide for surgical resection, localization of the bleeding site is essential. The literature suggests that the localization accuracy of radionuclide scanning is quite variable, ranging from 24% to 94% (169–171). Contrarily, a review by Hunter and Pezim suggested that a localization rate with the red blood cell scan was estimated to be 25% to 75% (172). In the same study, nearly half of patients studied (42%) underwent an incorrect surgical procedure based on red blood cell scan results (172); other studies have noted that radionuclide scanning did not alter surgical management in any manner (173–175). Thus, most clinicians use radionuclide scanning as a guide for further diagnostic studies, such as enteroscopy/colonoscopy, rather than for surgical intervention (176).

Reportedly requiring 10-fold less hemorrhage to achieve a positive study than angiography, the sensitivity of a radionuclide scan for active bleeding has been noted to be greater than 90%, and is superior to that of angiography (177–179). Pennoyer et al. showed that radionuclide scans increased the yield of angiography from 22% to 53% (180). Other studies have had contrary results (180–182), and radionuclide scanning may potentially delay therapeutic interventions (183). Therefore, although there is no strong evidence supporting radionuclide scanning prior to mesentery angiography, it may demonstrate low-flow bleeders, leading to better management.

Another role for radionuclide scanning is in the evaluation for Meckel diverticulum, especially in young patients presenting with LGIB (184). The Meckel scan uses a technetium pertechnetate tracer, which has affinity to accumulate in the gastric mucosa. It is quite useful in the pediatric population, with sensitivity as high as 81% to 90% (185,186). Due to insufficient gastric mucosa in the diverticulum, the sensitivity of the Meckel scan is much lower in the adult population, estimated to be approximately 62% (187,188). Several techniques that are reported to increase the diagnostic yield of the Meckel scan, administered before the study, include pentagastrin, histamine blockers, and saline lavage of the stomach and bladder (189–192).

Angiography

Angiography, first employed in the diagnosis of GI bleeding more than 40 years ago, provides imaging of the entire mesenteric system, localizes the sites of hemorrhage, and affords the opportunity for transcatheter interventions. It now holds an established place in dealing with difficult GI bleeding, both for diagnosis and treatment. Mesenteric angiography is more invasive than technetium-labeled red blood cell scanning, and requires a bleeding rate of at least 0.5 to 1.0 mL/minute to detect bleeding (193). Unfortunately, bleeding is frequently intermittent and may occur at a much lower rate, resulting in the inability to detect the causative lesion (194). Angiography is usually undertaken when patients have clinical indicators of severe bleeding (e.g., tachycardia and/or syncope). Although colonoscopy is the diagnostic modality of first choice for LGIB, many endoscopists are reluctant to perform colonoscopy in hemodynamically unstable patients with ongoing bleeding; these patients usually undergo radiographic studies. In addition, the bleeding of colonic lesions, such as vascular abnormalities, can be too massive for colonoscopic visualization, thus precluding the procedure. In some centers, a radionuclide scan is requested before mesenteric angiography, because a negative radionuclide scan is unlikely to have a positive angiogram. Angiography has been reported to be especially useful in patients presenting with postoperative GI hemorrhage (195).

Angiography will localize the site of bleeding in 40% to 86% of patients with LGIB (118,183,196,197). Even if a bleeding site is identified on angiography, localizing the site intraoperatively can be difficult; angiography has a specificity of 100% but a sensitivity of only 30% to 47% (198). Diverticula and angiodysplasia are the most common findings when angiography is positive, with 50% to 80% of the bowel bleeding sites being supplied by the superior mesenteric artery (199). Diverticular hemorrhage is most likely to produce extravasation on angiography (200). Following the injection of contrast media, bleeding and nonbleeding angiodysplastic lesions are characteristically seen as ectatic slowly emptying veins, vascular tufts, or small veins, with early filling in the arterial phase (201). Angiography is more sensitive than colonoscopy for detecting angiodysplasia (202), and when angiography identifies a bleeding site, treatment with embolization therapy or directed infusion of vasopressin may be performed. The overall rate of complication for mesenteric angiography is similar to most selective angiography, and is acceptable at less than 5% (203). Complications include hematoma or bleeding at the catheter site; access site thrombosis; contrast reactions; injury to the target vessels, including dissection and distal embolization; and renal failure (204). The injured vessels usually involve the SMA, IMA, and celiac artery.

In addition to its diagnostic role, angiography offers therapeutic possibilities via pharmacologic vasoconstriction or selective embolization (transcatheter arterial embolization [TAE]), and therefore may reduce the need for surgical resection. Once the bleeder is confirmed with contrast injection, embolization of the vessel is performed, usually with one of three embolic agents: microcoils, polyvinyl alcohol sponge particles, or gelatin sponge particles, alone or in combination (205). Pharmacologic vasoconstriction is achieved with intra-arterial vasopressin infusion.

TAE may be a more definitive means of controlling bleeding, but is associated with a risk of intestinal infarction. Selective embolization initially controls bleeding in up to 100% of patients, but rebleeding rates have been reported to be 15% to 40% (206,207). The major complication rate was 10% to 20% and included dysrhythmias, pulmonary edema, hypertension, and ischemia (206,207). The bowel infarction or colonic necrosis rate from embolization ranged from 10% to 20% (208–210). Superselective TAE may decrease the incidence of ischemia and rebleeding (209,211,212). A literature review of 144 cases by Kuo et al. showed a minor complication rate of 9% and 0% for major complications (205).

In the past, embolization has been reserved for treatment of UGIB, whereas LGIB has been controlled with vasopressin infusion. The reason is based on reports in the older literature in which infarction frequently occurred after LGI embolization. With advances in superselective embolization techniques, clinically significant bowel ischemia has become an uncommon complication (213,214). Although the efficacies of vasopressin and embolization are reasonably comparable, embolization allows more rapid completion of therapy and a decreased likelihood of systemic complications. Embolization should be considered a primary option for LGIB, although vasopressin is still preferable for diffuse lesions and cases in which superselective catheterization is not technically possible.

Pharmacologic vasoconstriction for LGIB involves an intra-arterial infusion of vasopressin, started at a rate of 0.2 units/minute. If the bleeding continues, the rate of infusion can be increased up to maximal dose of 0.4 units/minute. A repeat angiogram can be performed after 20 to 30 minutes to assess whether the bleeding is continuing or slowing down. If the bleeding seems to stop, infusion continues at the same rate for 12 hours, and subsequently, the dose of vasopressin is decreased by 50% provided that no bleeding recurs. After 12 hours of only saline infusion, the catheters are removed (169). Success rates for hemostasis are variable, with some reports as low as 36% and others as high as 100% (183,196,215,216). Bleeding recurrence is high, and may occur in up to 50% of patients after cessation of the infusion (183). Vasopressin should not be used in patients with significant coronary artery disease or peripheral vascular disease; mesenteric thrombosis, intestinal infarction, and death have been reported with its use (196). During the vasopressin infusion, patients need to be in an ICU setting where they can be monitored for myocardial, bowel, and peripheral ischemia; hypertension; dysrhythmias; and hyponatremia. Nitroglycerin reverses the vasopressin-induced coronary vasoconstriction without affecting the therapeutic vasoconstriction of the mesenteric artery (217). If standard angiography is negative, provocative angiography has been suggested with anticoagulants, vasodilators, and thrombolytics; of course, their use may cause bleeding (122) and is not routine. The use of provocative angiography should be reserved for selected patients at competent centers with well-trained radiologists.

For critically ill patients, ensuring the adequacy of intravascular volume is very important before mesentery angiography. Dehydration may exacerbate the nephrotoxicity of the contrast medium.

Computed Tomography Scan and Magnetic Resonance Imaging

CT scans are not usually considered diagnostic tools for LGIB, except in the context of bleeding bowel tumors. Several recent reports suggest that helical CT scans may be useful (218–220) in that this mode of scanning has the potential to detect hemorrhage rates of 0.5 mL/minute or less (221,222)—between 72% and 79% (218,219). In the evaluation of colonic vascular lesions, helical CT has a sensitivity of 70% and specificity of 100% compared to colonoscopy and conventional angiography (223).

Helical CT angiogram is a modified form of angiography. A rapid-acquisition CT scan is performed 30 seconds after contrast is injected into the abdominal aorta. The images are taken in 10-mm slices, 5 mm apart. A positive result is seen as extravasation of contrast medium into the intestinal lumen. Helical CT angiography reports a 70% sensitivity in the diagnosis of colonic angiodysplasia through the demonstration of vessel accumulation in the colon wall, early filling vein, and enlarged supplying artery (223). Currently, there is no role for the use of magnetic resonance imaging (MRI) in the evaluation of LGIB.

Ultrasound

Ultrasonography is a convenient, noninvasive, nonradiation-emitting, and easily available diagnostic tool in the emergency department and ICU. Data regarding the use of US for LGIB have been limited. Yamaguchi et al. noted that the colonic bleeding site was localized by US in 59 of the 90 (66%) patients compared with 81% by colonoscopy. When the bleeding site was in the rectum, the US detection rate was only 30% (10 of 33 patients), but the US detection rate was 82% to 100% when the bleeding site was elsewhere. These clinicians concluded that rectal and diverticular bleeding were difficult to diagnose by US, but for the other diseases, diagnosis by US was possible in 91% to 100% of cases (224). In our experience, angiodysplasia cannot be detected by US, while diverticulitis—but not diverticular bleeding—can. Other causes of bleeding, especially due to tumors, enteropathy, and colitis, can also be detected by US. In contrast to Yamaguchi's study (224), we think rectal lesions may be visualized via US through a urinary bladder window. We have proposed the "ultrasonographic bisection approximation method" to localize and detect GI obstructive lesions. The accuracy of US in predicting obstructive levels in the gastric outlet and duodenum, the jejunum and ileum, and the colon were 100%, 74%, and 98%, respectively (225).

Other Modalities

Small bowel follow-through (SBFT) and enteroclysis are used to detect small lesions, while barium enema is the image study for the colon. All of these are less sensitive for superficial lesions such as angiodysplasia, a common bleeder of LGIB. SBFT is of little use in evaluating obscure GI bleeding, with a diagnostic yield that may be as low as 0% (226). For patients with a high index of suspicion for the presence of small bowel diseases, such as small bowel tumor or Crohn disease, the diagnostic yield will be higher; SBFT detected 83% of small bowel tumors. In patients with suspected Crohn disease, SBFT may have a sensitivity of over 90% (227,228).

Enteroclysis is a modified form of SBFT in which a 10 French catheter is inserted into the distal duodenum or proximal jejunum under fluoroscopy, followed by the infusion under high pressure of a double-contrast solution with barium and air, water, or methylcellulose. This rapid rate of infusion allows better distention and visualization of the small bowel. Studies revealed that enteroclysis seems superior to SBFT for evaluation of the small bowel (229–231). Small bowel tumors seem to be the most common diagnosis made by enteroclysis, followed by Meckel diverticulum and Crohn disease of the terminal ileum (232,233). Angiodysplasia is not detected by enteroclysis. With the advent of capsule endoscopy, the use of SBFT or enteroclysis for GI bleeding has declined.

Barium enema cannot detect superficial lesions or confirm a definitive bleeding source of the colon. Furthermore, it may complicate subsequent colonoscopy or angiography, and is less useful for critically ill patients with LGIB.

TREATMENT OF LOWER GASTROINTESTINAL BLEEDING

Pharmacologic Therapy

Unlike pharmacologic therapies for UGIB, there are no medications with a strong evidence base for LGIB. The medications for the different causes of LGIB include estrogen/progesterone compounds, octreotide, aminocaproic acid (an antifibrinolytic), and tranexamic acid (an antifibrinolytic, marketed as Cyklokapron in the United States and as Transamin in Asia). Hormonal therapy with estrogen/progesterone compounds, previously used to treat bleeding associated with hereditary hemorrhagic telangiectasia, has been tried in patients with GI bleeding from angiodysplasia. For diffuse ectasias or angiodysplasia refractory to conservative and endoscopic therapy, estrogen/progesterone compound use is controversial, and has been noted to be ineffective in recent studies (234–237). Although the true mechanism is unknown, estrogen/progesterone compounds are thought to improve coagulation, alter microvascular circulation, and improve endothelial integrity. Adverse effects include breast tenderness and vaginal bleeding in women, gynecomastia and loss of libido in men, fluid retention, and stroke (238).

Octreotide has been used in patients with bleeding from diffuse vascular ectasia (238–240). At a dose of 0.05 to 1 mg/day subcutaneously, it was reported to be effective and without adverse effects (238,239). Nardone et al. noted that octreotide may lead to decreased transfusion requirements (239), but unfortunately, carefully controlled trials are not available. Other agents, including aminocaproic acid and tranexamic acid, may be helpful, but studies with controlled data are not forthcoming.

Steroids, 5-aminosalicylic acid compounds, and sucralfate (per mouth or per rectum) have been used to treat radiation proctitis, but there are little data supporting their effectiveness (241–244).

Ulcerative colitis (UC) and Crohn disease can cause severe LGIB (245). A recent review of acute major GI hemorrhage in inflammatory bowel disease suggests that bleeding is much more common in Crohn disease than UC (245). Bleeding from inflammatory diseases is usually self-limited and responds to medical therapy. An endoscopically treatable lesion is uncommon. Steroid and 5-aminosalicylic acid compounds are frequently used for active lesions. Infliximab, known as a "chimeric monoclonal antibody," reduces the amount of active tumor necrosis factor-*a* (TNF-*a*) in the body. It has been used successfully to avoid emergency surgery in Crohn patients with severe bleeding (246,247).

Endoscopic Procedures

Endoscopic therapy has been the major modality for LGIB, including the small bowel and colon, as long as the endoscopes reach the lesions. Endoscopic therapy for LGIB includes injection therapy (epinephrine, saline, or ethanol), heater probe, monopolar and multipolar electrocoagulation, argon plasma coagulation (APC), hemoclips, and band ligation (Table 153.4). An alternative treatment for hemorrhagic radiation-induced proctitis, by topical application of formalin, was first described by Rubinstein et al. in 1986 (248). Topical application of formalin for hemorrhagic radiation-induced proctitis can be performed with or without endoscopy in the operating room. It is simple, effective, inexpensive, and without major systemic

TABLE 153.4

ENDOSCOPIC PROCEDURES FOR BLEEDING

LGIB lesions	Endoscopic procedures
Ulcer	Injection therapy Heater probe Electrocoagulation Hemoclips Band ligation[a] APC[b]
Angiodysplasia	APC Heater probe Electrocoagulation
Diverticulum	Hemoclips APC Injection therapy Heater probe Electrocoagulation
Radiation proctitis	APC Topical formalin
Postpolypectomy bleeding	Hemoclips Band ligation APC Injection therapy Heater probe

LGIB, lower gastrointestinal bleeding.
[a]Especially for Dieulafoy lesions.
[b]APC, argon plasma coagulation. Not recommended for ulcers with big exposed vessels.

TABLE 153.5

COMPARISON BETWEEN TAE AND INTRA-ARTERIAL VASOPRESSIN INFUSION FOR LGIB

	TAE	Vasopressin infusion
Completion of Tx	Quick	Slow
Definite Tx	Yes	No
Diffuse lesions	Discouraged	Favored
Complications	Bowel infarct	Myocardial ischemia, bowel ischemia, peripheral ischemia, hypertension, arrhythmias, hyponatremia

TAE, transcatheter arterial embolization; LGIB, lower gastrointestinal bleeding; Tx, therapy. −, depend; +, Yes; ×, No.

side effects. Monitoring and management of the adverse events caused by endoscopic treatment are essential, such as perforation caused by endoscopic thermocoagulation and abdominal distention caused by argon gas after APC.

Radiologic Interventions (See Also Angiography)

In addition to its diagnostic role, angiography offers therapeutic possibilities via pharmacologic vasoconstriction with vasopressin or selective embolization (TAE) with microcoils, polyvinyl alcohols sponge particles, or gelatin sponge particles, alone or in combination. Comparison between embolization and intra-arterial vasopressin infusion is listed in Table 153.5. Recently, superselective intra-arterial embolization with tissue glue, *N*-butyl-2-cyanoacrylate, has been applied in UGIB (249); further study is needed in LGIB.

Surgery

Despite the advances of interventional modalities, an emergency surgical procedure for LGIB is ultimately required in 10% to 25% of patients (250), and is indicated for uncontrolled, massive, or recurrent bleeding. An emergency procedure is suggested for patients who require more than 6 units of blood within 24 hours, or a total of 10 units (73). Among the causes of LGIB, the most challenging are vascular ectasias and angiodysplasia. These lesions are usually multiple, and localize in different segments of bowel, making management difficult.

Surgery should be considered in patients in whom a bleeding source has clearly been identified. Blind segmental resection is contraindicated, as it is associated with a rebleeding rate of 42% and excessive rates of morbidity and mortality as high as 83% and 57%, respectively (251). If the bleeder cannot be clearly identified, intraoperative enteroscopy may be a management option. Recurrent bleeding from colon diverticula occurs in 20% to 40% of patients and is generally considered an indication for surgery (11). The operative mortality of diverticula bleeding is 10%, even with accurate localization, and up to 57% with blind subtotal colectomy (108,251,252). Most cases of colonic ischemia resolve with conservative treatment. However, 15% to 20% of patients who develop infarction will require surgical intervention, with a substantial risk of death (253). Until recently, surgery was the only effective management for Dieulafoy lesions in up to 5% of patients (254). Surgery is usually not recommended on the basis of nuclear red blood cell scans alone because of variable accuracy of nuclear red blood cell scans.

ASSESSMENT OF SEVERITY IN LOWER GASTROINTESTINAL BLEEDING

Acute LGIB ceases spontaneously in 80% to 85% of patients (68), but the overall mortality rate may be as high as 12% (255). A reliable predictive or scoring system can accurately and quickly forecast the severity of an episode of acute LGIB, risk of recurrent bleeding, need for therapeutic intervention, and related mortality. Moreover, a scoring system is potentially of great benefit to the clinician at the point that initial triage is performed to ensure appropriate levels of care. Unfortunately, in contrast to acute UGIB, there are few scoring systems developed and validated to predict the outcome of patients with acute LGIB.

The BLEED classification system was proposed for evaluation of acute UGIB and LGIB by Kollef et al. (256) utilizing five items, including ongoing bleeding, systolic blood pressure <100 mm Hg, prothrombin time greater than 1.2 times control, altered mental status, and unstable comorbid disease. The BLEED classification system triages patients with acute LGIB into those at high and low risk of adverse in-hospital outcome—defined as recurrent hemorrhage, need for surgery for control of hemorrhage, and death. A second study by the same group found that it could predict outcome in patients hospitalized with acute LGIB when the BLEED classification system was applied at the point of initial evaluation in the emergency department (257). In a retrospective chart review of 252 consecutive, hospitalized patients, Strate et al. analyzed 24 clinical, nonendoscopic variables that were available within 4 hours of medical evaluation (60). They identified seven independent clinical risk factors for severe, acute LGIB: tachycardia, low systolic blood pressure, syncope, nontender abdominal examination, bleeding per rectum within the first 4 hours of medical assessment, use of aspirin, and more than two active comorbid conditions. The investigators speculated that such clinical data may be used to risk-stratify patients with acute LGIB who may benefit from urgent intervention. Based on these factors, patients were stratified into three risk groups: (a) those with more than three risk factors—an 84% risk of severe bleeding; (b) those with one to three risk factors—a 43% risk; and (c) those with no risk factors—a 9% risk. Das et al. developed and validated artificial neural networks (ANNs), computer-based decision support systems, for the prediction of recurrent bleeding, need for intervention, and death with LGIB (258). ANNs performed well in predicting death (97%), recurrent bleeding (93%), and the need for intervention (94%). Velayos et al. prospectively studied patients admitted with LGIB, and identified three predictors of severity and adverse outcome in the first hour of evaluation: initial hematocrit less than 35%, presence of abnormal vital signs 1 hour after initial medical evaluation,

TABLE 153.6

RISK FACTORS USED IN DIFFERENT SCORING SYSTEMS FOR SEVERITY OF LGIB

Scoring system	Risk factors
The BLEED classification system (performed at point of initial evaluation in the emergency department)	■ Ongoing bleeding ■ Systolic blood pressure less than 100 mm Hg ■ Prothrombin time greater than 1.2 times control ■ Altered mental status ■ Unstable comorbid disease
Scoring system of Strate et al. (performed within 4 h of initial evaluation)	■ Tachycardia ■ Low systolic blood pressure ■ Syncope ■ Nontender abdominal examination ■ Bleeding per rectum within the first 4 h of medical assessment ■ Use of aspirin ■ More than two active comorbid conditions
Scoring system of Velayos et al. (performed within the first hour of initial evaluation)	■ Initial hematocrit less than 35% ■ Presence of abnormal vital signs 1 h after initial medical evaluation ■ Gross blood on initial rectal examination

LGIB, lower gastrointestinal bleeding.

and gross blood on initial rectal examination. These predictive tools may help guide the initial triage and approach to the patient with LGIB (259). The scoring system elements are summarized in Table 153.6; however, an ideal risk scoring system does not yet exist.

Which factors are most predictive of adverse patient outcome? The presence of comorbidity, evidence of acute hemodynamic instability, and presence of high-risk endoscopic stigmata of recent hemorrhage are considered most predictive of an adverse outcome. The initial hemoglobin level may be an inaccurate marker of the severity of GI bleeding. Which risk stratification system is better—endoscopic or nonendoscopic? It has been suggested that endoscopic triage in acute LGIB may *not* be as efficacious as with acute UGIB (255).

OBSCURE LOWER GASTROINTESTINAL BLEEDING

Upper GI endoscopy and colonoscopy are the usual initial evaluation tools for GI bleeding; they will be negative in the patient with a source in the small intestine. If, despite the initial evaluation, no source is found and bleeding continues, the patient meets the definition of *obscure GI bleeding*, defined as ongoing or recurrent intestinal bleeding without a cause found at original endoscopic studies. Approximately 5% of patients have recurrent bleeding of unclear etiology, and need extensive and repetitive testing (260,261). Furthermore, even after extensive localization studies, approximately 10% of patients require surgical intervention without having identified the bleeding source (262). A missed diagnosis may occur secondary to bleeding that has stopped during endoscopic examination; very slow or intermittent bleeding leading to negative endoscopic and nuclear scans; significant anemia and volume contraction causing lesions to appear less obvious; and lesions in the small bowel that are not detected by routine examinations (263). When repeated endoscopy of the upper or lower GI tract is negative, investigation should rapidly focus on the small intestine. However, before surveying the small bowel, one needs to ensure that a repeat upper GI endoscopy has been performed, as 25% to 64% of patients with a negative upper GI endoscopy and colonoscopy are found to have UGI tract lesions at the time of repeat UGI endoscopy (264–267). Interestingly, the source of obscure GI bleeding may be identified in up to 58% of cases within a month from the last bleeding episode, even if previous investigations did not allow identification (268).

Clinically, the age of the patient is very important in the differential diagnosis of GI bleeding. Patients younger than 40 are more likely to suffer from small bowel tumors, anatomic anomalies, genetic problems, or Crohn disease/ulcerative colitis. Patients older than 40 are more prone to bleeding from vascular lesions and neoplasm (12). A special group of patients may have the specific causes of LGIB. In populations with immunosuppression, such as patients with HIV infection, renal transplant, or pancreatic transplant, LGIB often is caused by CMV ulcers. Renal failure and aortic valvular stenosis are well-known risk factors for angiodysplasia (14,15). Radiation colitis should be considered in patients with a history of radiation therapy for cervical or prostate cancer. Aortoenteric fistulae may be considered in patients with obscure GI bleeding and prior aortic aneurysm repair. The approach to the evaluation of the obscure bleeder is listed in Table 153.7 and Figure 153.4.

Bleeding from the small intestine that occurs between the ligament of Treitz and the ileocecal valve represents a challenging problem because of the relative inaccessibility of traditional endoscopy to the long, looping small intestine. Small

TABLE 153.7

APPROACH TO THE EVALUATION OF OBSCURE BLEEDING

Elderly patients Renal disease Aortic valvular stenosis Connective tissue disease von Willebrand disease	Higher risk for vascular lesions
Surgical patients	Higher risk for anastomotic bleeding or aortoenteric fistulae
NSAID drug use	Increased risk of small bowel ulcerations.
Immune-compromised patients	Cytomegalovirus ulcers
History of radiation to pelvis	Radiation colitis

NSAID, nonsteroidal anti-inflammatory drug.

bowel bleeding comprises approximately 5% of obscure GI bleeding (110). The utilization of resources was reported to be significantly higher in this group of LGI bleeders, with a higher number of diagnostic procedures and blood transfusions, longer hospitalization, and a higher cost of hospitalization when compared with patients with upper or distal lower GI bleeding (269). Small bowel examination can be divided into radiographic, endoscopic, and surgical modalities (Table 153.8). Radiographic techniques include barium studies, such as SBFT and enteroclysis; radionuclide scanning, such as tagged red blood cell scans and Meckel scan; cross-sectional imaging, such as CT and MRI; and mesenteric angiography. Endoscopic examinations include push enteroscopy, double-balloon enteroscopy, and capsule endoscopy. Surgical procedures include exploratory laparotomy, with and without assistance of intraoperative enteroscopy. The details of each diagnostic tool have been given above. Among these modalities, available data suggest that SBFT has little use in the evaluation of obscure GI bleeding unless a tumor or Crohn disease is suspected (270).

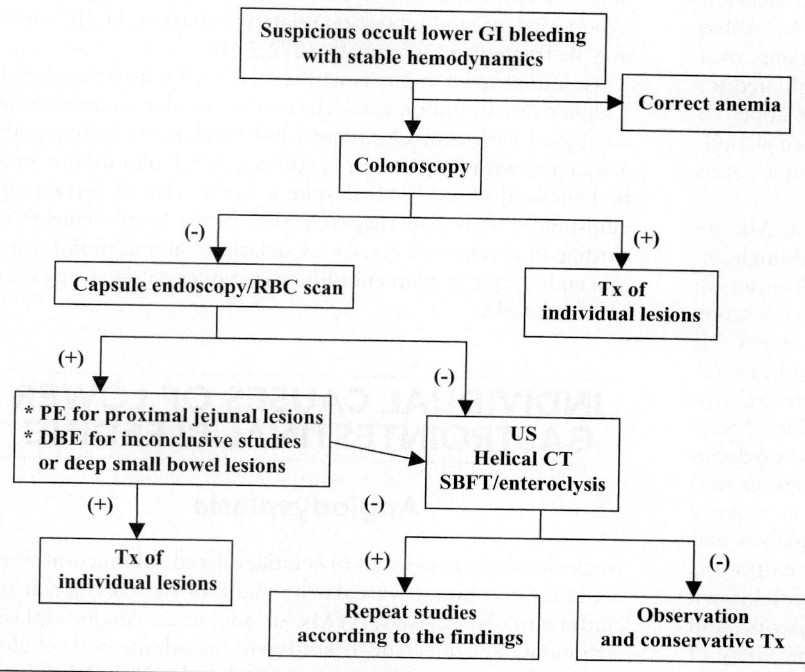

FIGURE 153.4. Approach for occult lower gastrointestinal bleeding. GI, gastrointestinal; RBC, red blood cell; Tx, treatment; PE, push-type enteroscopy; DBE, double-balloon enteroscopy; CT, computed tomography; SBFT, small bowel follow-through; US, ultrasound.

LOWER GASTROINTESTINAL BLEEDING AND ACUTE MYOCARDIAL INFARCTION

GI bleeding may occur after myocardial infarction (MI) due to both medications and interventions, or it can induce an MI secondary to hemodynamic instability and anemia. For the critical care practitioner, management of coexisting GI bleeding and coronary arterial events includes how to predict and detect an MI that occurs after GI bleeding, how to prevent and manage GI bleeding associated with interventions related to the acute MI, and the necessity/safety/timing of endoscopic procedures.

The prevalence of acute MI in patients with GI bleeding ranges from 1% to 14% (271–274). Conversely, acute MI seen with significant upper or lower GI bleeding occurs in 30% to 49% of patients admitted to the ICU, with an overall mortality rate of 5% to 10% (271,272). Significant GI bleeding deleteriously affects myocardial function, as massive blood loss may cause hypovolemia, hypoperfusion, and decreased oxygenation delivery to the myocardium, eventually leading to an acute MI. Elderly and patients with a history of coronary artery disease (CAD) are candidates for acute MI after a significant GI bleed. On occasion, the overt symptoms of GI bleeding may mask the typical symptoms of an evolving MI. Therefore, cardiac enzymes, including troponin-I, and an electrocardiogram are routinely suggested in high-risk patients with GI bleeding, even when the patient has no chest pain, to avoid a delay in diagnosis

TABLE 153.8

IMAGING STUDIES FOR SMALL BOWEL BLEEDING

	Studies		Tx
Radiographic techniques	Barium studies	Small bowel follow-through Enteroclysis	N
	Nuclear studies	Tagged red blood cell scans Meckel scan	N
	Cross-sectional imaging	CT MRI	N
	Angiography		Y
Endoscopic techniques	Push enteroscopy Double-balloon enteroscopy		Y
	Capsule endoscopy		N
Surgical procedures	Exploratory laparotomy with and without endoscopic assistance		Y

Tx, treatment; Y, yes; N, no; CT, computed tomography; MRI, magnetic resonance imaging.

of myocardial ischemia or acute MI (273). Although GI bleeding occurring after an acute MI carries significant mortality (275), an acute MI after a GI bleed does not seem to alter the risk of in-hospital mortality (271,272).

GI bleeding occurs after an acute MI, owing to the use of antiplatelet agents, anticoagulants, and thrombolytic agents. In a recent meta-analysis of 6,300 patients receiving low-dose aspirin (less than 325 mg/day) for secondary prevention of coronary artery disease, it was found that the aspirin group was 2.5 times more likely to have GI bleeding than the placebo group (276). Another antiplatelet agent, clopidogrel, was noted to have a significant association with GI bleeding when used in patients with a history of GI bleeding (277); however, clopidogrel incited fewer cases of GI bleeding compared with aspirin in the Clopidogrel versus Aspirin in Patients at Risk of Ischemic Events trial (278). In the study of 3,130 patients by Abbas et al., GI bleeding was more likely to occur in patients over 70 years old (276). In spite of many studies that evaluated for GI bleeding after acute MI, most lesions were in the upper GI tract; data on LGIB after acute MI are limited. When sigmoidoscopy is performed within 30 days of an MI, ischemic colitis is the most frequent diagnosis of LGIB (279).

Whether LGIB occurs before or after the acute MI, selecting an endoscopic procedure is a dilemma. Although endoscopy has been applied widely in managing GI disorders in the general population, the risks versus benefits of endoscopy must be carefully considered in patients with a recent MI because of the potential for cardiopulmonary complications, including myocardial ischemia, hypotension, cardiac arrhythmias, and hypoxia. Underlying heart disease, lower blood pressure on arrival in the emergency department, lower hemoglobin level on arrival, and persistent shock before endoscopic examination are all associated with higher risk of MI after emergency endoscopy (280). Establishment of stable hemodynamics and oxygen delivery before emergency endoscopy may reduce the risk of procedure-related MI, especially in patients with known heart disease. Sigmoidoscopy, colonoscopy, enteroscopy, and capsule endoscopy may be arranged for LGIB. The safety of enteroscopy and capsule endoscopy for small bowel bleeding complicated by an MI is unknown, although, theoretically, capsule endoscopy should be safer than the enteroscopy, because it is less invasive. Cappell has suggested that sigmoidoscopy is relatively safe and often beneficial after MI, even in moderately ill patients, but should be undertaken with pulse oximetry and continuous electrocardiography (279). In the same study, the complication rate of sigmoidoscopy was lower than that of UGI endoscopy (7.5%) after an MI, probably because sigmoidoscopy is less invasive, is less painful, and does not affect the airway. Cappell also suggested that sigmoidoscopy should be deferred in unstable patients, such as those in shock, for several weeks after myocardial infarction unless an emergent indication for the procedure exists. Urgent sigmoidoscopy may be indicated in the patient with LGIB related to anticoagulant or thrombolytic therapy (281,282), or LGIB related to colonic ischemia from systemic hypotension due to MI, myocardial hypoperfusion, and infarction related to massive LGIB, which may be treated endoscopically (272,273).

Colonoscopy in patients with a recent MI is associated with a higher rate of minor, transient cardiovascular complications compared with control patients, but is relatively infrequently associated with major complications (283). Colonoscopy may be beneficial after an MI despite a higher risk in certain circumstances. It is also suggested that recent improvements in cardiac interventions, conscious sedation, patient monitoring, and endoscopic instrumentation may render colonoscopy even safer after MI.

INDIVIDUAL CAUSES OF LOWER GASTROINTESTINAL BLEEDING

Angiodysplasia

Angiodysplasia composed of ectatic, dilated submucosal veins is the most common vascular anomaly of the GI tract. It includes vascular ectasias, AVMs, or angiomas. Angiodysplasia is thought to be due to degeneration of the submucosal venules, and thus is seen predominately in the elderly (284). It has been reported as a common cause of acute major LGIB and slow intermittent blood loss (285,286). The percentage of acute LGIB that has been attributed to angiodysplasia varies from 3% to 40%, depending on the study (287,288). Angiodysplasia is also the most common cause of small bowel bleeding, accounting for 70% to 80% of episodes (289). Angiodysplasia may be a clinically challenging problem, as it frequently has multiple lesions that may be difficult to identify, and bleeding associated with angiodysplasia is more likely to be intermittent than diverticular bleeding. Furthermore, angiodysplasia is the most common cause of recurrent LGIB of the elderly, with recurrent bleeding rates reported between 10% and 30% (285,286,290). The lesions of angiodysplasia are predominantly located in the right colon (cecum and ascending colon, 54%), followed by the sigmoid colon (18%) and rectum (14%) (291), whereas angiodysplasia can be found throughout the small intestine. Overt bleeding from angiodysplasia is typically brisk, painless, and intermittent. Modalities for diagnosing angiodysplasia as a cause of LGIB include colonoscopy, mesentery angiography, enteroscopy, capsule endoscopy, and, sometimes, helical CT angiography. The sensitivity of colonoscopy for detecting angiodysplasia exceeds 80% (202). At colonoscopy, angiodysplastic lesions have a characteristic appearance: red, flat, ectatic blood vessels radiating from a central feeding vessel. A pale halo may typically be seen around the lesion. Use of narcotic medications for sedation and analgesia have been reported to decrease the sensitivity of colonoscopy for detecting angiodysplasia because of a transient decrease in mucosal blood flow. Additionally, colonoscopy can provide a therapeutic function; this mode of therapy is safe and effective for angiodysplasia. Argon plasma coagulation is increasingly popular for the treatment of bleeding colonic angiodysplastic lesions and angiodysplasia located in the small bowel (292,293). Other methods include heater probe, bipolar coagulation, and injection therapy. If no other cause of bleeding is identified in a patient with recurrent or persistent GI bleeding requiring transfusions, the presence of angiodysplasia is an indication for treatment. Angiography is the other diagnostic modality for angiodysplasia. After injection of contrast, angiodysplasia is seen as ectatic slowly emptying veins, vascular tufts, or small veins with early filling. When angiography identifies a bleeding angiodysplasia, treatment with embolization therapy or infusion of vasopressin may be performed. Helical CT angiography had 70% sensitivity in the diagnosis of colonic angiodysplasia by the demonstration of vessel accumulation in the colon wall, early filling vein, and enlarged supplying artery (259). Pharmacologic therapy for diffuse angiodysplasia includes hormonal therapy with estrogen/progesterone and octreotide analogues. Octreotide has been tried in patients with bleeding caused by diffuse angiodysplasia, at a dose of 0.05 to 1 mg/day subcutaneously, and was reported to be effective and without adverse effects (239). However, so far, no randomized, double-blinded studies have demonstrated the effectiveness of these agents. Adverse effects seen with hormonal therapy include vaginal bleeding, fluid retention, and stroke (294). Surgery should be considered in patients with a bleeding source clearly identified and in whom conservative therapies have failed.

Colonic Diverticular Bleeding

Colonic diverticular bleeding results from rupture of the intramural branches (vasa recta) of the marginal artery at the dome of a diverticulum or at the antimesenteric margin (295,296). Diverticula are the second most common source, if not the most common, of acute LGIB in some studies, and have been reported to comprise 20% to 55% of all cases of LGIB. Although greater than 75% of diverticula are found in the left colon, the right colon is the source of diverticular bleeding in 50% to 90% of patients. Most of the diverticula are not symptomatic, whereas approximately 20% develop diverticulitis and 3% to 5% develop acute severe bloody stool (11). Clinical presentation in LGIB generally is acute, painless hematochezia (295–297). Diverticulosis is rare in patients under 40 years of age. Age and NSAIDs have been shown to be associated with diverticular bleeding (298,299). At least 75% of diverticular bleeding will stop spontaneously, but up to 25% will require emergent intervention (300). Recurrent bleeding from diverticula occurs in 14% to 38% of patients (4,11,169,297). Colonoscopy and angiography are used to diagnose diverticular bleeding. Endoscopic therapy utilized includes epinephrine injection, bipolar coagulation, band ligation, and placement of hemoclips; the latter has been more popular in recent years. Diverticular hemorrhage is most likely to produce extravasation on angiography (200). Vasopressin infusion and embolization have also been used to stop bleeding. The traditional management of diverticular bleeding has largely been supportive. Nonsurgical therapy may be performed with angiography or colonoscopy. Surgical intervention is required when hemodynamic instability persists despite aggressive resuscitation. Surgical intervention may be necessary in 18% to 25% of cases. In the elderly patient with comorbid conditions, diverticular bleeding results in morbidity and mortality rates of 10% to 20% (301,302).

Ischemic Colitis

Ischemic colitis, resulting from a sudden, often temporary, reduction in mesenteric blood flow, is increasingly recognized as a cause of acute LGIB. Ischemic colitis accounts for approximately 1% to 19% of LGIB (303), and may be transient and reversible. Data from a study limited to medical ICU patients has shown that ischemic colitis, not angiodysplasia or diverticula, is one of the most frequent causes of LGIB (5). Ischemic colitis is usually caused by "low-flow states" and occlusion of small, rather than large, vessels. Mesenteric hemodynamics may be compromised by changes in the systemic circulation or by anatomic or functional changes in the mesenteric vasculature. In patients who have undergone aortoiliac reconstructive surgery, the frequency of postoperative colonic ischemia is 1% to 7% (304–306). The typical segments affected by nonocclusive colonic ischemia are the "'watershed" areas of the colon: the splenic flexure and the rectosigmoid junction. Clinically, ischemic colitis most frequently involves the splenic flexure, the descending colon, and the sigmoid colon. Ischemic colitis with segmental distribution has an abrupt transition between damaged and normal mucosa at colonoscopy. Clinically, ischemic colitis presents with the sudden onset of mild, left lower quadrant, crampy abdominal pain with infrequent hemodynamic alterations. The pain may be accompanied or followed by bright red blood per rectum or bloody diarrhea. Conditions that compromise colonic blood flow can lead to ischemia, and include cardiovascular insults; aortic bypass surgery; aneurysmal rupture; vasculitis; inherited or acquired hypercoagulable states, such as pregnancy and oral contraceptives; intense exercise (304); and medications or drugs that reduce colonic motility or blood flow, such as catecholamines. Among them, intense exercise results in blood being shunted from the viscera to the working muscles, resulting in decreased splanchnic blood flow by as much as 80% (305). Colonoscopy or flexible sigmoidoscopy have replaced barium enema as the choice for colonic ischemia. Edema, hemorrhage, and ulceration with a sharp demarcation between normal and abnormal mucosa can be shown at endoscopy. Histologically, submucosal hemorrhages, intravascular thrombus, and hyalinization of the lamina propria are seen, in addition to inflammatory cell infiltrates. In contrast to acute mesenteric ischemia, angiography is not necessary for ischemic colitis. Most cases of colonic ischemia resolve with conservative treatment. The 15% to 20% of patients who develop gangrene will require surgical intervention (306). A minority of patients will develop chronic ischemic colitis or stricture. Treatment is supportive with bowel rest, intravenous fluids, optimization of hemodynamic status, and correction of the precipitating conditions (307). When surgery is necessary, it is often because of transmural infarction with necrosis rather than bleeding.

Nonsteroidal Anti-inflammatory Drug–induced Enteropathy and Colonopathy

NSAID enteropathy and colonopathy are lesions related to the use of NSAIDs. NSAIDs have been demonstrated to exacerbate inflammatory bowel disease, cause colitis that resembles inflammatory bowel disease, and complicate diverticular diseases by increasing the risk of perforation and severe hematochezia (308,309). The terminal ileum and cecum are particularly susceptible to NSAID-induced injury. This is because the pills may be static for a longer period of time in the terminal ileum and cecum than in other segments of the bowel. History of use of NSAIDs and endoscopy (colonoscopy and enteroscopy) are essential for diagnosing NSAID enteropathy and colonopathy. The diaphragm-like stricture is pathognomonic of NSAID injury as a result of a scarring reaction secondary to ulceration. They are most frequently found in the midsection of the small intestine, but have also been reported to occur in the terminal ileum and colon (310–313). Treatment of NSAID-induced mucosal injury is discontinuation of the NSAIDs. Performance of a repeat colonoscopy has been suggested 6 to 8 weeks after cessation of the NSAID in order to check for resolution of the ulcers or colitis. Surgical intervention is rarely required for NSAID-induced bleeding or perforation (310).

Radiation Colitis

Radiation therapy to the colon may induce inflammatory changes and can produce radiation colitis. A history of prior radiation therapy for prostate or pelvic cancer may indicate radiation proctitis, no matter how distant from radiation exposure. Argon plasma coagulation is the most effective treatment (314–316). Complications of argon plasma coagulation were reported, such as severe bleeding, extensive necrosis of the rectum, or perforation, which occurred in 10% of patients. Treatment of hemorrhagic, radiation-induced proctitis by topical application of formalin can be simple, effective, and inexpensive. No major systemic side effects have been described. Other treatments of radiation colitis include steroids, hyperbaric oxygen, 5-aminosalicylic acid compounds, and sucralfate, but little data support their effectiveness.

Dieulafoy Lesions

Dieulafoy lesions are unpredictable and life threatening, because bleeding is often massive and recurrent (317,318). Dieulafoy lesions should always be included in the differential diagnosis of GI bleeding, especially when a definitive source is not found on routine investigation (i.e., in the presence of obscure GI bleeding). In the colon, solid bowel content can contribute to mucosal stercoral ulceration over an abnormally dilated submucosal arteriole and subsequent rupture and bleeding. Endoscopic diagnosis and treatment of enteric Dieulafoy lesions beyond the duodenal bulb are difficult. In colonic Dieulafoy lesions, massive bleeding makes endoscopic diagnosis and treatment more problematic; angiography can be quite useful in localizing the source of bleeding in these situations. Once the Dieulafoy lesions are found by endoscopy, they can be treated with heater probe, electrocoagulation, sclerotherapy, band ligation, or hemoclips; failure of endoscopic treatment is not uncommon. Angiography can also be therapeutic, providing access for such treatments as embolization or tissue glue. Surgery is now reserved for lesions that cannot be controlled by endoscopic or angiographic techniques, estimated at up to 5% of patients.

Postpolypectomy Bleeding

Postpolypectomy bleeding is the cause of 2% to 5% of acute LGIB. A history of recent colonoscopy with polypectomy leads to the diagnosis of postpolypectomy bleeding as the most likely source. Most of this bleeding stops spontaneously. Persistent bleeding can be treated with various endoscopic techniques, including injection of epinephrine followed by thermal therapy, band ligation of the remaining polyp stalk, and hemoclips (39). Endoscopic therapy was successful in treating over 95% of patients in a retrospective case review study (319).

Ulcerative Colitis and Crohn Disease

Bleeding due to ulcerative colitis and Crohn disease is usually self-limited and responds to medical therapy, but can sometimes cause severe LGIB (245). An endoscopically treatable lesion is uncommon, and surgical intervention may be necessary, especially in patients with recurrent bleeding. Bleeding is much more common in Crohn disease than in ulcerative colitis (245). Infliximab has been used successfully to avoid emergency surgery in Crohn patients with severe bleeding (246,247).

Less Common Causes of Lower Gastrointestinal Bleeding

There are less common causes of LGIB. Neoplastic lesions are the cause of acute LGIB in 2% to 26% of cases (2); if limited to ICU patients, the incidence may be even lower. Severe constipation should prompt an investigation for a stercoral ulcer. Hemorrhoids are common and account for 2% to 9% of cases of acute severe hematochezia (3,4). Conservative management with sitz baths, avoidance of straining, and dietary modification are usually effective. However, surgical hemorrhoidectomy and rubber band ligation are options for refractory cases. Colitis, including pseudomembranous colitis, can be caused by different diseases, each a potential cause of LGIB. Numerous infectious agents can penetrate and injure the colonic mucosa and cause acute LGIB. The major role of endoscopy is to visualize the mucosa and obtain biopsies to guide the use of antimicrobial agents. There are no reports of endoscopic therapy for bleeding due to colitis, although sometimes an actively bleeding ulcer or a visible vessel may warrant an attempt endoscopic therapy.

Acute Hemorrhagic Rectal Ulcer or Acute Hemorrhagic Rectal Ulcer Syndrome

Acute hemorrhagic rectal ulcer (AHRU) or acute hemorrhagic rectal ulcer syndrome (AHRUS) has attracted the attention of ICU practitioners. AHRUS has been reported as one of the most frequent causes of LGIB in the ICU (5). AHRUS was first introduced in 1981, and was recognized as a syndrome later; so far, there are reports only from Japan and Taiwan (320–323). AHRUS accounts for 2.8% of the patients with massive LGIB (321). AHRUS characteristically occurs suddenly, with painless, massive, fresh rectal bleeding in elderly, bedridden patients with severe comorbid illness (321,322). It is prone to occur in patients with diabetes mellitus who are using anticoagulant or antiplatelet agents (323). Lesions of AHRUS locate at the lower rectum. Endoscopically, they were characteristically solitary or multiple rectal ulcers with round, circumferential, geographic, or Dieulafoy-like lesions located within a mean distance of 4.7 ± 1.5 cm from the dentate line. Histopathologically, the lesions appear as necrosis, with denudation of the covering epithelium, hemorrhage, and multiple thrombi in the vessels of the mucosa and underlying stroma (320). Lesions of AHRUS are considered to be similar to stress-related mucosal injury. Therapies for AHRUS include injection therapy, heater probe, hemoclips, and per anal suturing (322,323). As a hemostatic strategy, hemoclipping alone showed a favorable result, with a hemostatic success rate as high as 76.9% (323). There is no established pharmacologic treatment. Risk factors associated with recurrent bleeding were severity of comorbid disease and abnormal coagulation status. The prognosis of AHRUS depends on the state of the underlying diseases and achievement of hemostasis (322).

PEARLS

- The consequences of LGIB in the ICU, anemia and hypovolemia, may prevent weaning and extubation, thus prolonging ICU length of stay.
- Data indicating the true incidence of LGIB during ICU hospitalization are lacking.
- Patients who develop LGIB while hospitalized for another disease process have a higher risk of death than those admitted with LGIB.
- LGIB patients with comorbid illness have higher mortality than those without.
- Two to 15% of patients with presumed LGIB will have UGIB.
- Studies limited to ICU patients show that ischemic colitis and acute hemorrhagic rectal ulcers are the most frequent causes of LGIB, followed by colitis and diverticula.
- Pallor, fatigue, chest pain, palpitations, dyspnea, tachypnea, tachycardia, posture-related dizziness, and syncope are suggestive of hemodynamic compromise, and demand aggressive care.
- For detecting occult blood loss from the lower GI tract, guaiac-based tests and immunochemical fecal occult blood tests are optimal choices. Heme-porphyrin tests cannot discriminate between UGIB and LGIB.
- NG tube placement to rule out a UGI source of bleeding should be considered in patients with hemodynamic compromise and hematochezia, or if a source is not identified on colonoscopy.
- The absence of blood in NG aspirate is not sufficient to refute UGI bleeding, but the presence of bile without blood indicates the absence of an active UGIB.
- The past medical history may help to elucidate a specific bleeding source. Key points include antecedent constipation or diarrhea, the presence of diverticulosis, radiation therapy, recent polypectomy, and vascular disease/systemic hypotension/atrial fibrillation/aortoiliac reconstructive surgery.
- A rectal exam is essential in LGIB, serving to identify anorectal lesions and confirm the stool color described by the patient.
- Evaluation of the small bowel is indicated for those patients in whom UGI endoscopy and colonoscopy are negative.
- Current endoscopic tools for small bowel diseases include PE, DBE, intraoperative enteroscopy, and capsule endoscopy.
- The diagnostic yield of PE is between 38% to 65% in patients with negative upper and lower endoscopy.
- The diagnostic yield of DBE is between 52% and 76%.
- Intraoperative endoscopy provides the highest diagnostic and therapeutic yield (70%–100%) in patients with chronic or acute recurrent LGIB.
- The use of capsule endoscopy for small bowel or obscure bleeding must be made on a case-by-case basis.
- The timing of capsule endoscopy appears related to the diagnostic yield. A high yield may be possible in ongoing overt bleeding.
- Evidence suggests that capsule endoscopy may be safely used in patients with pacemakers.
- Radionuclide scanning or angiography may be appropriate in patients with massive bleeding that precludes colonoscopy or in whom a bleeding source is not identified on colonoscopy.
- Radionuclide scanning detects active bleeding at rates of 0.1 to 0.5 mL/minute, and is more sensitive than angiography, but less specific than a positive endoscopic or angiographic study.
- Radionuclide scanning is normally not used as a definitive study before surgical therapy, but rather as a tool to guide further diagnostic studies or therapeutic interventions.
- Angiography may be a useful diagnostic and therapeutic tool in patients with active bleeding.

- Angiography may be used in patients with massive LGIB and unstable hemodynamic status, or after a failed endoscopy or a positive radionuclide scan.
- Angiography offers therapeutic options via pharmacologic vasoconstriction with vasopressin or selective embolization (TAE) with microcoils, polyvinyl alcohol sponge particles, or gelatin sponge particles, alone or in combination.
- Intra-arterial vasopressin infusion is preferred in diffuse or multiple lesions.
- During the vasopressin infusion, patients need to be in an ICU setting.
- For critically ill patients, maintenance of adequate intravascular volume is very important to prevent contrast nephrotoxicity.
- In general, the presence of comorbidity, acute hemodynamic instability, and high-risk endoscopic stigmata of recent bleeding are considered most predictive of an adverse outcome.

References

1. Gostout CJ. Acute lower GI bleeding. In: Brandt LJ, ed. *Current Medicine. Clinical Practice of Gastroenterology.* Philadelphia: Churchill Livingstone; 1998:651–662.
2. Peura DA, Lanza FL, Gostout CJ, et al. The American College of Gastroenterology Bleeding Registry: preliminary findings. *Am J Gastroenterol.* 1997;92:924–928.
3. Bramley PN, Masson JW, McKnight G, et al. The role of an open-access bleeding unit in the management of colonic haemorrhage: a 2-year prospective study. *Scand J Gastroenterol.* 1996;31:764–769.
4. Longstreth GF. Epidemiology and outcome of patients hospitalized with acute lower gastrointestinal hemorrhage: a population-based study. *Am J Gastroenterol.* 1997;92:419–424.
5. Lin CC, Lee YC, Lee H, et al. Bedside colonoscopy for critically ill patients with acute lower gastrointestinal bleeding. *Intensive Care Med.* 2005;31:743–746.
6. Velayos FS, Williamson A, Sousa KH, et al. Early predictors of severe lower gastrointestinal bleeding and adverse outcomes: a prospective study. *Clin Gastroenterol Hepatol.* 2004;2:485–490.
7. Santos JCM, Apilli F, Guimaraes AS, et al. Angiodysplasia of the colon: endoscopic diagnosis and treatment. *Br J Surg.* 1988;75:256–258.
8. Farrell JJ, Friedman LS. Gastrointestinal bleeding in the elderly. *Gastroenterol Clin North Am.* 2001;30:377–407.
9. Lin CC, Wang HP, Wu MS, et al. The etiology and clinical characteristics of acute lower gastrointestinal bleeding in patients hospitalized for comorbid illnesses. *Hepato-Gastroenterology.* 2006;52:391–394.
10. Strate LL. Lower GI bleeding: epidemiology and diagnosis. *Gastroenterol Clin North Am.* 2005;34:643–664.
11. McGuire HH. Bleeding colonic diverticula. A reappraisal of natural history and management. *Ann Surg.* 1994;220:653–656.
12. Mujica VR, Barkin JS. Occult gastrointestinal bleeding: general overview and approach. *Gastrointest Endosc Clin N Am* 1996;6:833–845.
13. Lewis BS, Kornbluth A, Waye JD. Small bowel tumours: yield of enteroscopy. *Gut.* 1991;32:763–765.
14. Marcuard S, Weinstock J. Gastrointestinal angiodysplasia in renal failure. *J Clin Gastroenterol.* 1988;10:482–484.
15. Imperiale T, Ransohoff D. Aortic stenosis, idiopathic gastrointestinal bleeding and angiodysplasia: is there an association? A methodologic critique of the literature. *Gastroenterology.* 1988;95:1670–1676.
16. Rossini FP, Ferrari A, Spandre M, et al. Emergency colonoscopy. *World J Surg.* 1989;13:190–192.
17. Angtuaco TL, Reddy SK, Drapkin S, et al. The utility of urgent colonoscopy in the evaluation of acute lower gastrointestinal tract bleeding: a 2-year experience from a single center. *Am J Gastroenterol.* 2001;96:1782–1785.
18. McGuire HH. Bleeding colonic diverticula. A reappraisal of natural history and management. *Ann Surg.* 1994;220:653–656.
19. Richter JM, Christensen MR, Kaplan LM, et al. Effectiveness of current technology in the diagnosis and management of lower gastrointestinal hemorrhage. *Gastrointest Endosc.* 1995;41:93–98.
20. Jensen DM, Machicado GA. Diagnosis and treatment of severe hematochezia. The role of urgent colonoscopy after purge. *Gastroenterology.* 1988;95:1569–1574.
21. Rockey DC. Occult gastrointestinal bleeding. *N Engl J Med.* 1999;341:38–46.
22. Proctor DD. Critical issues in digestive diseases. *Clin Chest Med.* 2003;24:623–632.
23. Green BT, Rockey DC. Acute gastrointestinal bleeding. *Semin Gastrointest Dis.* 2003;14:44–65.
24. Jensen DM, Machicado GA, Jutabha R, et al. Urgent colonoscopy for the diagnosis and treatment of severe diverticular hemorrhage. *N Engl J Med.* 2000;342:78–82.
25. Patel TH, Cordts PR, Abcarian P, et al. Will transcatheter embolotherapy replace surgery in the treatment of gastrointestinal bleeding? *Curr Surg.* 2001;58:323–327.
26. Seow-Choen F, Goh H, Eu K, et al. A simple and effective treatment for hemorrhagic radiation proctitis using formalin. *Dis Colon Rectum.* 1993;36:135–138.
27. Mathai V, Seow-Choen F. Endoluminal formalin therapy for haemorrhagic radiation proctitis. *Br J Surg.* 1995;82:190.
28. Klas JV, Madoff RD. Surgical options in lower gastrointestinal bleeding. *Semin Colon Rectal Surg.* 1997;8:172–177.
29. Rockey DC. Occult gastrointestinal bleeding. *Gastroenterol Clin North Am.* 2005;34:699–718.
30. Dybdahl JH, Daae LN, Larsen S, et al. Occult faecal blood loss determined by a 51Cr method and chemical tests in patients referred for colonoscopy. *Scand J Gastroenterol.* 1984;19:245–254.
31. Herzog P, Holtermuller KH, Preiss J, et al. Fecal blood loss in patients with colonic polyps: a comparison of measurements with 51chromium-labeled erythrocytes and with the haemoccult test. *Gastroenterology.* 1982;83:957–962.
32. Mandel JS, Bond JH, Church TR, et al. Reducing mortality from colorectal cancer by screening for fecal occult blood. Minnesota Colon Cancer Control Study. *N Engl J Med.* 1993;328:1365–1371.
33. Laine LA, Bentley E, Chandrasoma P. Effect of oral iron therapy on the upper gastrointestinal tract. A prospective evaluation. *Dig Dis Sci.* 1988;33:172–177.
34. Saito H. Screening for colorectal cancer by immunochemical fecal occult blood testing. *Jpn J Cancer Res.* 1996;87:1011–1024.
35. Greenberg PD, Cello JP, Rockey DC. Asymptomatic chronic gastrointestinal blood loss in patients taking aspirin or warfarin for cardiovascular disease. *Am J Med.* 1996;100:598–604.
36. Jaffin BW, Bliss CM, LaMont JT. Significance of occult gastrointestinal bleeding during anticoagulation therapy. *Am J Med.* 1987;83:269–272.
37. Witting MD, Magder L, Heins AE, et al. Usefulness and validity of diagnostic nasogastric aspiration in patients without hematemesis. *Ann Emerg Med.* 2004;43:525–532.
38. ASGE Guideline: the role of endoscopy in the patient with lower-GI bleeding *Gastrointest Endosc.* 2005;62(5):656–660.
39. Green BT, Rockey DC. Lower gastrointestinal bleeding—management. *Gastroenterol Clin North Am.* 2005;34:665–678.
40. Cuellar RE, Gavaler JS, Alexander JA, et al. Gastrointestinal tract hemorrhage: the value of a nasogastric aspirate. *Arch Intern Med.* 1990;150:1381–1384.
41. Lin CK, Chiu HM, Lien WC, et al. Ultrasonographic bisection approximation method for gastrointestinal obstruction in ER. *Hepato-Gastroenterology.* 2006;53:547–551.
42. Yamamoto H, Sekine Y, Sato Y, et al. Total enteroscopy with a nonsurgical steerable double-balloon method. *Gastrointest Endosc.* 2001;53:216–220.
43. Rockey DC. Gastrointestinal bleeding. In: Feldman M, Friedman LS, Sleisenger MH, eds. *Sleisenger and Fordra's Gastrointestinal and Liver Disease.* 7th ed. Philadelphia: Saunders; 2002:211–248.
44. Committee on Trauma. American College of Surgeons. *Advanced Trauma Life Support.* 5th ed. Chicago: American College of Surgeons; 1993:84.
45. Proctor DD. Critical issues in digestive diseases *Clin Chest Med.* 2003;24:623–632.
46. Ebert RA, Stead EA, Gibson JG. Response of normal subjects to acute blood loss. *Arch Intern Med.* 1940;68:578–580.
47. Hilsman JH. The color of blood-containing feces following the instillation of citrated blood at various levels of the small intestine. *Gastroenterology.* 1950;15:131–134.
48. Marcuard S, Weinstock J. Gastrointestinal angiodysplasia in renal failure. *J Clin Gastroenterol.* 1988;10:482–484.
49. Ernst CB, Hagihara PF, Daughtery ME, et al. Ischemic colitis incidence following abdominal aortic reconstruction: a prospective study. *Surgery.* 1976;80:417–421.
50. Hagihara PF, Ernst CB, Griffen WO Jr. Incidence of ischemic colitis following abdominal aortic reconstruction. *Surg Gynecol Obstet.* 1979;149:571–573.
51. Brewster DC, Franklin DP, Cambria RP, et al. Intestinal ischemia complicating abdominal aortic surgery. *Surgery.* 1991;109:447–454.
52. Wessinger S, Kaplan M, Choi L, et al. Increased use of selective serotonin reuptake inhibitors in patients admitted with gastrointestinal haemorrhage: a multicentre retrospective analysis. *Aliment Pharmacol Ther.* 2006;23:937–944.
53. Zuckerman GR, Prakash C, Askin MP, et al. Technical review: the evaluation and management of occult and obscure GI bleeding. *Gastroenterology.* 2000;118:201–221.
54. Aldoori WH, Giovannucci EL, Rimm EB, et al. Use of acetaminophen and nonsteroidal anti-inflammatory drugs: a prospective study and the risk

of symptomatic diverticular disease in men. *Arch Fam Med.* 1998;7:255–260.

55. Laine L, Connors LG, Reicin A, et al. Serious lower gastrointestinal clinical events with nonselective NSAID or coxib use. *Gastroenterology.* 2003;124:288–292.
56. Kwo PY, Tremaine WJ. Nonsteroidal anti-inflammatory drug-induced enteropathy: case discussion and review of the literature. *Mayo Clin Proc.* 1995;70:55–61.
57. Lang J, Price AB, Levi AJ, et al. Diaphragm disease: pathology of disease of the small intestine induced by non-steroidal anti-inflammatory drugs. *J Clin Pathol.* 1988;41:516–526.
58. Bjarnason I, Hayllar J, MacPherson AJ, et al. Side effects of nonsteroidal antiinflammatory drugs on the small and large intestine in humans. *Gastroenterology.* 1993;104:1832–1847.
59. Foutch PG. Diverticular bleeding: are nonsteroidal anti-inflammatory drugs risk factors for hemorrhage and can colonoscopy predict outcome for patients? *Am J Gastroenterol.* 1995;90:1779–1784.
60. Strate LL, Orav EJ, Syngal S. Early predictors of severity in acute lower intestinal tract bleeding. *Arch Intern Med.* 2003;163:838–843.
61. Steer ML, Silen W. Diagnostic procedures in gastrointestinal hemorrhage. *N Engl J Med.* 1983;309:646–650.
62. Chalasani N, Clark WS, Wilcox CM. Blood urea nitrogen to creatinine concentration in gastrointestinal bleeding: a reappraisal. *Am J Gastroenterol.* 1997;92:1796–1799.
63. Richards RJ, Donica MB, Grayer D. Can the blood urea nitrogen/creatinine ratio distinguish upper from lower gastrointestinal bleeding? *J Clin Gastroenterol.* 1990;12:500–504.
64. Snook JA, Holdstock GE, Bamforth J. Value of a simple biochemical ratio in distinguishing upper and lower sites of gastrointestinal haemorrhage. *Lancet.* 1986;1:1064–1065.
65. Cook DJ, Guyatt GH, Salena BJ, et al. Endoscopic therapy for acute nonvariceal upper gastrointestinal hemorrhage: a meta-analysis. *Gastroenterology.* 2000;102:139–148.
66. Van Dam J, Brugge WR. Endoscopy of upper gastrointestinal tract. *N Engl J Med.* 1999;341:1738–1748.
67. Lewis JD, Shin EJ, Metz DC. Characterization of gastrointestinal bleeding in severely ill hospitalized patients. *Crit Care Med.* 2000;28:46–50.
68. Zuckerman GR, Prakash C. Acute lower intestinal bleeding: part I: clinical presentation and diagnosis. *Gastrointest Endosc.* 1998;48:606–617.
69. Wright HK. Massive colonic hemorrhage. *Surg Clin North Am.* 1980;60: 1297–1304.
70. Tada M, Shimizu S, Kawai K. Emergency colonoscopy for the diagnosis of lower intestinal bleeding. *Gastroenterol Jpn.* 1991;26(Suppl 3):121–124.
71. Vellacott KD. Early endoscopy for acute lower gastrointestinal haemorrhage. *Ann R Coll Surg Engl.* 1986;68:243–244.
72. Tooson JD, Gates LK. Bowel preparation before colonoscopy choosing the best lavage regimen. *Postgrad Med.* 1996;100:203–214.
73. Elta GH. Urgent colonoscopy for acute lower-GI bleeding. *Gastrointest Endosc.* 2004;59:402–408.
74. Chiu HM, Lin JT, Wang HP, et al. The impact of colon preparation timing on colonoscopic detection of colorectal neoplasms—a prospective endoscopist-blinded randomized trial. *Am J Gastroenterol.* 2006;101: 2719–2725.
75. Sharma VK, Chockalingham SK, Ugheoke EA, et al. Prospective, randomized, controlled comparison of the use of polyethylene glycol electrolyte lavage solution in four-liter versus two-liter volumes and pretreatment with either magnesium citrate or bisacodyl for colonoscopy preparation. *Gastrointest Endosc.* 1998;47:167–171.
76. Sharma VK, Steinberg EN, Vasudeva R, et al. Randomized, controlled study of pretreatment with magnesium citrate on the quality of colonoscopy preparation with polyethylene glycol electrolyte lavage solution. *Gastrointest Endosc.* 1997;46:541–543.
77. Adams WJ, Meagher AP, Lubowski DZ, et al. Bisacodyl reduces the volume of polyethylene glycol solution required for bowel preparation. *Dis Colon Rectum.* 1994;37:229–234.
78. Marshall JB, Pineda JJ, Barthel JS, et al. Prospective, randomized trial comparing sodium phosphate solution with polyethylene glycol-electrolyte lavage for colonoscopy preparation. *Gastrointest Endosc.* 1993;39:631–634.
79. Golub RW, Kerner BA, Wise WE, et al. Colonic bowel preparations—which one? A blinded, prospective, randomized trial. *Dis Colon Rectum.* 1995;58:594–597.
80. Ernstoff JJ, Howard DA, Marshall JB, et al. A randomized blinded clinical trial of a rapid colonic lavage solution (Golytely) compared with standard preparation for colonoscopy and barium enema. *Gastroenterology.* 1983;84:1512–1516.
81. DiPalma JA, Brady CE, Pierson WP. Colon cleansing: acceptance by older patients. *Am J Gastroenterol.* 1986;81:652–655.
82. Fordtran JS, Santa Ana CA, Cleveland MvB. A low-sodium solution for gastrointestinal lavage. *Gastroenterology.* 1990;98:11–16.
83. Granberry MC, White LM, Gardner SF. Exacerbation of congestive heart failure after administration of polyethylene glycol-electrolyte lavage solution. *Ann Pharmacother.* 1995;29:1232–1234.
84. Clarkston WK, Tsen TN, Dies DF, et al. Oral sodium phosphate versus sulfate-free polyethylene glycol electrolyte lavage solution in outpatient preparation for colonoscopy: a prospective comparison. *Gastrointest Endosc.* 1996;43:42–48.
85. Kolts BE, Lyles WE, Achem SR, et al. A comparison of the effectiveness and patient tolerance of oral sodium phosphate, castor oil, and standard electrolyte lavage for colonoscopy or sigmoidoscopy preparation. *Am J Gastroenterol.* 1993;88:1218–1223.
86. Afridi SA, Barthel JS, King PD, et al. Prospective, randomized trial comparing a sodium phosphate-biscodyl regimen with conventional PEG-ES lavage for outpatient colonoscopy preparation. *Gastrointest Endosc.* 1995; 41:485–489.
87. Lieberman DA, Ghormley J, Flora K. Effect of oral sodium phosphate colon preparation on serum electrolytes in patients with normal serum creatinine. *Gastrointest Endosc.* 1996;43:467–469.
88. Gremse DA, Sacks AI, Raines S. Comparison of oral sodium phosphate to polyethylene glycol-based solution for bowel preparation for colonoscopy in children. *J Pediatr Gastroenterol Nutr.* 1996;23:586–590.
89. Strate LL, Syngal S. Predictors of utilization of early colonoscopy vs. radiography for severe lower intestinal bleeding *Gastrointest Endosc.* 2005;61:46–52.
90. Ohyama T, Sakurai Y, Ito M, et al. Analysis of urgent colonoscopy for lower gastrointestinal tract bleeding. *Digestion.* 2000;61:189–192.
91. Strate LL, Syngal S. Timing of colonoscopy: impact on length of hospital stay in patients with acute lower intestinal bleeding. *Am J Gastroenterol.* 2003;98:317–322.
92. Garcia Sanchez M, Gonzalez Galilea A, Lopez Vallejos P, et al. Role of early endoscopy in severe acute lower gastrointestinal bleeding. *Gastroenterol Hepatol.* 2001;24:327–332.
93. Schmulewitz N, Fisher DA, Rockey DC. Early colonoscopy for acute lower GI bleeding predicts shorter hospital stay: a retrospective study of experience in a single center. *Gastrointest Endosc.* 2003;58:841–846.
94. Kovacs TO, Jensen DM. Recent advances in the endoscopic diagnosis and therapy of upper gastrointestinal, small intestinal, and colonic bleeding. *Med Clin North Am.* 2002;86:1319–1356.
95. Vernava AM, Moore BA, Longo WE, et al. Lower gastrointestinal bleeding. *Dis Colon Rectum.* 1997;40:846–858.
96. Colacchio TA, Forde KA, Patsos TJ, et al. Impact of modern diagnostic methods on the management of active rectal bleeding. Ten-year experience. *Am J Surg.* 1982;143:607–610.
97. Jiranek GC, Kozarek RA. A cost-effective approach to the patient with peptic ulcer bleeding. *Surg Clin North Am.* 1996;76:83–103.
98. Lee JG, Turnipseed S, Romano PS, et al. Endoscopy-based triage significantly reduces hospitalization rates and costs of treating upper GI bleeding: a randomized controlled trial. *Gastrointest Endosc.* 1999;50:755–761.
99. Velayos FS, Williamson A, Sousa KH, et al. Early predictors of severe lower gastrointestinal bleeding and adverse outcomes: a prospective study. *Clin Gastroenterol Hepatol.* 2004;2(6):485–490.
100. Farrell JJ, Friedman LS. Review article: the management of lower gastrointestinal bleeding. *Aliment Pharmacol Ther.* 2005;21:1281–1298.
101. Chaudhry V, Hyser MJ, Gracias VH, et al. Colonoscopy: the initial test for acute lower gastrointestinal bleeding. *Am Surg.* 1998;64:723–728.
102. Kok KY, Kum CK, Goh PM. Colonoscopic evaluation of severe hematochezia in an Oriental population. *Endoscopy.* 1998;30:675–680.
103. Angtuaco TL, Reddy SK, Drapkin S, et al. The utility of urgent colonoscopy in the evaluation of acute lower gastrointestinal tract bleeding: a 2-year experience from a single center. *Am J Gastroenterol.* 2001;96(6):1782–1785.
104. Green BT, Rockey DC, Portwood G, et al. Urgent colonoscopy for evaluation and management of acute lower gastrointestinal hemorrhage: a randomized controlled trial. *Am J Gastroenterol.* 2005;100:2395–2402.
105. Fine KD, Nelson AC, Ellington RT, et al. Comparison of the color of fecal blood with the anatomical location of gastrointestinal bleeding lesions: potential misdiagnosis using only flexible sigmoidoscopy for bright red blood per rectum. *Am J Gastroenterol.* 1999;94:3202–3210.
106. Farrands PA, Taylor I. Management of acute lower gastrointestinal hemorrhage in a surgical unit over a four year period. *J R Soc Med.* 1987;80:79–82.
107. Leitman IM, Paul DE, Shires GT. Evaluation and management of massive lower gastrointestinal hemorrhage. *Ann Surg.* 1989;209:175–180.
108. Wagner HE, Stain SC, Gilg M, et al. Systematic assessment of massive bleeding of the lower part of the gastrointestinal tract. *Surg Gynecol Obstet.* 1992;175:445–449.
109. Zuckerman GR, Prakash C. Acute lower intestinal bleeding. Part I: clinical presentation and diagnosis. *Gastrointest Endosc.* 1998;48:606–616.
110. Lewis BS. Small intestinal bleeding. *Gastrointest Endosc Clin N Am.* 1994; 23:67–69.
111. Foutch PG, Sanowski RA, Kelly S. Enteroscopy: a method for detection of small bowel tumors. *Am J Gastroenterol.* 1985;80:887–890.
112. Goff JS. Peroral colonoscopy: technique, depth, and yield of lesions. *Gastrointest Endosc Clin N Am.* 1996;6:753–758.
113. Pennazio M, Arrigoni A, Risio M, et al. Clinical evaluation of push enteroscopy. *Endoscopy.* 1995;27:164–170.
114. TaylorAC, Chen RY, Desmond PV. Use of an overtube for enteroscopy: does it increase depth of insertion? A prospective study of enteroscopy with and without an overtube. *Endoscopy.* 2001;33:227–230.

115. Harewood GC, Gostout CJ, Farrell MA, et al. Prospective controlled assessment of variable stiffness enteroscopy. *Gastrointest Endosc.* 2003;58:267–271.
116. Keizman D, Brill S, Umansky M, et al. Diagnostic yield of routine push enteroscopy with a graded-stiffness enteroscope without overtube. *Gastrointest Endosc.* 2003;57:877–881.
117. Wilmer A, Rutgeerts P. Push enteroscopy: technique, depth, and yield of insertion. *Gastrointest Endosc Clin N Am.* 1996;6:759–776.
118. Koval G, Benner KG, Rosch J, et al. Aggressive angiographic diagnosis in acute lower gastrointestinal hemorrhage. *Dig Dis Sci.* 1987;32:248–253.
119. Chak A, Koehler MK, Sundaram SN, et al. Diagnostic and therapeutic impact of push enteroscopy: analysis of factors associated with positive findings. *Gastrointest Endosc.* 1998;47:18–22.
120. Schmit A, Gay F, Adler M, et al. Diagnostic efficacy of push-enteroscopy and long-term follow-up of patients with small bowel angiodysplasias. *Dig Dis Sci.* 1996;41:2348–2352.
121. Hayat M, Axon AT, O'Mahony S. Diagnostic yield and effect on clinical outcomes of push enteroscopy in suspected small-bowel bleeding. *Endoscopy.* 2000;32:369–372.
122. Lin S, Rockey DC. Obscure gastrointestinal bleeding. *Gastroenterol Clin North Am.* 2005;34:679–698.
123. Lepère C, Cuillerier E, Van Gossum A, et al. Predictive factors of positive findings in patients explored by push enteroscopy for unexplained GI bleeding. *Gastrointest Endosc.* 2005;61:709–714.
124. Berner JS, Mauer K, Lewis BS. Push and sonde enteroscopy for the diagnosis of obscure gastrointestinal bleeding. *Am J Gastroenterol.* 1994;89(12): 2139–2142.
125. Perry SD, Welfare MR, Cobden I, et al. Push enteroscopy in a UK district general hospital: experience of 51 cases over 2 years. *Eur J Gastroenterol Hepatol.* 2002;14:305–309.
126. Landi B, Tkoub M, Gaudric M, et al. Diagnostic yield of push-type enteroscopy in relation to indication. *Gut.* 1998;42:421–425.
127. Ell C, Remke S, May A, et al. The first prospective controlled trial comparing wireless capsule endoscopy with push enteroscopy in chronic gastrointestinal bleeding. *Endoscopy.* 2002;34(9):685–689.
128. May A, Nachbar L, Wardak A, et al. Double-balloon enteroscopy: preliminary experience in patients with obscure gastrointestinal bleeding or chronic abdominal pain. *Endoscopy.* 2003;35:985–991.
129. Yamamoto H, Sekine Y, Sato Y, et al. Total enteroscopy with a nonsurgical steerable double balloon method. *Gastrointest Endosc.* 2001;53(2):216–220.
130. May A, Ell C. Push-and-pull enteroscopy using the double-balloon technique/double-balloon enteroscopy. *Dig Liver Dis.* 2006;38:932–938.
131. Yamamoto H, Kita H, Sunada K, et al. Clinical outcomes of double-balloon endoscopy for the diagnosis and treatment of small-intestinal diseases. *Clin Gastroenterol Hepatol.* 2004;2:1010–1016.
132. May A, Nachbar L, Schneider M, et al. Double-balloon enteroscopy (push-and-pull enteroscopy) of the small bowel: feasibility, diagnostic and therapeutic yield in patients with suspected small bowel disease. *Gastrointest Endosc.* 2005;62:62–70.
133. Carey EJ, Fleischer DE. Investigation of the small bowel in gastrointestinal bleeding—enteroscopy and capsule endoscopy. *Gastroenterol Clin North Am.* 2005;34:719–734.
134. Heine GDN, Hadithi M, Groenen MJM, et al. Double-balloon enteroscopy: indications, diagnostic yield, and complications in a series of 275 patients with suspected small bowel disease. *Endoscopy.* 2006;38:42–48.
135. Groenen MJM, Moreels TGG, Orlent H, et al. Acute pancreatitis after double-balloon enteroscopy: an old pathogenetic theory revisited as a result of using a new endoscopic tool. *Endoscopy.* 2006;38:82–85.
136. Delmotte JS, Gay GJ, Houcke PH, et al. Intraoperative endoscopy. *Gastrointest Endosc Clin N Am.* 1999;9:61–69.
137. Zaman A, Sheppard B, Katon RM. Total peroral intraoperative enteroscopy for obscure GI bleeding using a dedicated push enteroscope: diagnostic yield and patient outcome. *Gastrointest Endosc.* 1999;50:506–510.
138. Swain P, Fritscher-Ravens A. Role of video endoscopy in managing small bowel disease. *Gut.* 2004;53:1866–1875.
139. Iddan GJ, Swain CP. History and development of capsule endoscopy. *Gastrointest Endosc Clin N Am.* 2004;14:1–9.
140. Hartmann D, Schilling D, Bolz G, et al. Capsule endoscopy versus push enteroscopy in patients with occult gastrointestinal bleeding. *Z Gastroenterol.* 2003;41:377–382.
141. Lewis BS, Swain P. Capsule endoscopy in the evaluation of patients with suspected small bowel intestinal bleeding: results of a pilot study. *Gastrointest Endosc.* 2002;56:349–353.
142. Mylonaki M, Fritscher-Ravens A, Swain P. Wireless capsule endoscopy: a comparison with push enteroscopy in patients with gastroscopy and colonoscopy negative gastrointestinal bleeding. *Gut.* 2003;52:1122–1126.
143. Saurin JC, Delvaux M, Gaudin JL, et al. Diagnostic value of endoscopic capsule in patients with obscure digestive bleeding: blinded comparison with video push-enteroscopy. *Endoscopy.* 2003;35:576–584.
144. Costamagna G, Shah SK, Riccioni ME, et al. A prospective trial comparing small bowel radiographs and video capsule endoscopy for suspected small bowel disease. *Gastroenterology.* 2002;123:999–1005.
145. Liangpunsakul S, Chadalawada V, Rex DK, et al. Wireless capsule endoscopy detects small bowel ulcers in patients with normal results from state of the art enteroclysis. *Am J Gastroenterol.* 2003;98:1295–1298.
146. Eliakim R, Fischer D, Suissa A, et al. Wireless capsule video endoscopy is a superior diagnostic tool in comparison to barium followthrough and computerized tomography in patients with suspected Crohn's disease. *Eur J Gastroenterol Hepatol.* 2003;15:363–367.
147. Hara AK, Leighton JA, Sharma VK, et al. Small bowel: preliminary comparison of capsule endoscopy with barium study and CT. *Radiology.* 2004;230:260–265.
148. Hartmann D, Schilling D, Bolz G, et al. A prospective two-center study comparing wireless capsule endoscopy with intraoperative enteroscopy in patients with obscure GI bleeding. *Gastrointest Endosc.* 2005;61:826–832.
149. Bolz G, Schmitt H, Hartmann D, et al. Prospective controlled trial comparing wireless capsule endoscopy with intraoperative enteroscopy in patients with chronic gastrointestinal bleeding: ongoing multicenter study. Presented at the 3rd International Conference on Capsule Endoscopy, Miami, FL, March 1, 2004.
150. Van Gossum A, Hittelet A, Schmit A, et al. A prospective comparative study of push and wireless-capsule enteroscopy in patients with obscure digestive bleeding. *Acta Gastroenterol Belg.* 2003;66:199–205.
151. Pennazio M, Santucci R, Rondonotti E, et al. Outcome of patients with obscure gastrointestinal bleeding after capsule endoscopy: report of 100 consecutive patients. *Gastroenterology.* 2004;126:643–653.
152. Triester SL, Leighton JA, Fleischer DE, et al. Yield of capsule endoscopy compared to other modalities in patients with obscure GI bleeding: a meta-analysis. *Am J Gastroenterol.* 2004;99:A941.
153. Enns R, Go K, Chang H, et al. Capsule endoscopy: a single centre experience with the first 226 capsules. *Can J Gastroenterol.* 2004;18(9):555–558.
154. Carey EJ, Leighton JA, Heigh RI, et al. Single center outcomes of 260 consecutive patients undergoing capsule endoscopy for obscure GI bleeding. *Gastroenterology.* 2004;126(4):A96.
155. Rosch T. DDW Report 2004 New Orleans: capsule endoscopy. *Endoscopy.* 2004;36(9):763–769.
156. Niv Y, Niv G, Wiser K, Demarco DC. Capsule endoscopy—comparison of two strategies of bowel preparation. *Aliment Pharmacol Ther.* 2005; 22(10):957–962.
157. Fireman Z, Paz D, Kopelman Y. Capsule endoscopy: improving transit time and image view. *World J Gastroenterol.* 2005;11(37):5863–5866.
158. Chong A, Miller A, Taylor A, et al. Randomised controlled trial of polyethylene glycol administration prior to capsule endoscopy [Abstract]. *Gastrointest Endosc.* 2004;59(5):AB179.
159. Soussan EB, Antonietti M, Lecleire S, et al. Influence of bowel preparation for capsule endoscopy: quality of examination and transit time [Abstract]. *Gastrointest Endosc.* 2004;59(5):AB178.
160. Coumaros D, Claudel L, Levy P, et al. Diagnostic value of capsule endoscopy (CE) in obscure digestive bleeding (ODB) and effect of erythromycin injection [Abstract]. *Gastrointest Endosc.* 2004;59(5):AB177.
161. Albert J, Gobel CM, Lesske J, et al. Simethicone for small bowel preparation for capsule endoscopy: a systematic, single-blinded, controlled study. *Gastrointest Endosc.* 2004a;59:487–491.
162. Adler DG, Knipschield M, Gostout C. A prospective comparison of capsule endoscopy and push enteroscopy in patients with GI bleeding of obscure origin *Gastrointest Endosc.* 2004;59:492–498.
163. Scapa E, Jacob H, Lewkowicz S, et al. Initial experience of wireless-capsule endoscopy for evaluating occult gastrointestinal bleeding and suspected small bowel pathology. *Am J Gastroenterol.* 2002;97:2776–2779.
164. Leighton JA, Sharma VK, Srivathsan K, et al. Safety of capsule endoscopy in patients with pacemakers. *Gastrointest Endosc.* 2004;59:567–569.
165. Schoof N, Deviere J, Van Gossum A. PillCam colon capsule endoscopy compared with colonoscopy for colorectal tumor diagnosis: a prospective pilot study. *Endoscopy.* 2006;38(10):971–977.
166. Eliakim R, Fireman Z, Gralnek IM, et al. Evaluation of the PillCam Colon capsule in the detection of colonic pathology: results of the first multicenter, prospective, comparative study. *Endoscopy.* 2006;38(10):963–970.
167. Carey EJ, Heigh RI, Fleischer DE. Endoscopic capsule endoscope delivery for patients with dysphagia, anatomical abnormalities, or gastroparesis. *Gastrointest Endosc.* 2004;59(3):423–426.
168. McKusick KA, Froelich J, Callahan RJ, et al. 99mTc red blood cells for detection of gastrointestinal bleeding: experience with 80 patients. *AJR Am J Roentgenol.* 1981;137:1113–1118.
169. Bounds BC, Friedman LS. Lower gastrointestinal bleeding. *Gastroenterol Clin North Am.* 2003;32:1107–1125.
170. Nicholson ML, Neoptolemos JP, Sharp JF, et al. Localization of lower gastrointestinal bleeding using in vivo technetium-99m-labeled red blood cell scintigraphy. *Br J Surg.* 1989;76:358–361.
171. Suzman MS, Talmor M, Jennis R, et al. Accurate localization and surgical management of active lower gastrointestinal hemorrhage with technetium-labeled erythrocyte scintigraphy. *Ann Surg.* 1996;224:29–36.
172. Hunter JM, Pezim MR. Limited value of technetium 99m-labeled red cell scintigraphy in localization of lower gastrointestinal bleeding. *Am J Surg.* 1990;59:504–506.
173. Levy R, Barto W, Gani J. Retrospective study of the utility of nuclear scintigraphic-labelled red cell scanning for lower gastrointestinal bleeding. *ANZ J Surg.* 2003;73:205–209.

174. Rantis PC Jr, Harford FJ, Wagner RH, et al. Technetium-labelled red blood cell scintigraphy: is it useful in acute lower gastrointestinal bleeding? *Int J Colorectal Dis.* 1995;10:210–215.
175. Garofalo TE, Abdu RA. Accuracy and efficacy of nuclear scintigraphy for the detection of gastrointestinal bleeding. *Arch Surg.* 1997;132:196–199.
176. Nusbaum M, Baum S. Radiographic demonstration of unknown sites of gastrointestinal bleeding. *Surg Forum.* 1963;14:374–375.
177. Szasz IJ, Morrison RT, Lyster DM. Technetium-99m-labelled red blood cell scanning to diagnose occult gastrointestinal bleeding. *Can J Surg.* 1985;28:512–514.
178. Voeller GR, Bunch G, Britt LG. Use of technetium-labeled red blood cell scintigraphy in the detection and management of gastrointestinal hemorrhage. *Surgery.* 1991;110:799–804.
179. Smith R, Copely DJ, Bolen FH. 99mTc RBC Scintigraphy: correlation of gastrointestinal bleeding rates with scintigraphic findings. *AJR Am J Roentgenol.* 1987;148:869–874.
180. Pennoyer WP, Vignati PV, Cohen JL. Mesenteric angiography for lower gastrointestinal hemorrhage: are there predictors for a positive study? *Dis Colon Rectum.* 1997;40:1014–1018.
181. Hyman N, Waye JD. Endoscopic four quadrant tattoo for the identification of colonic lesions at surgery. *Gastrointest Endosc.* 1991;37:56–58.
182. Bentley DE, Richardson JD. The role of tagged red blood cell imaging in the localization of gastrointestinal bleeding. *Arch Surg.* 1991;126:821–824.
183. Browder W, Cerise EJ, Litwin MS. Impact of emergency angiography in massive lower gastrointestinal bleeding. *Ann Surg.* 1986;204:530–536.
184. Zuccaro G Jr. Management of the adult patient with acute lower gastrointestinal bleeding. American College of Gastroenterology. Practice Parameters Committee. *Am J Gastroenterol.* 1998;93:1202–1208.
185. Kong MS, Chen CY, Tzen KY, et al. Technetium-99m pertechnetate scan for ectopic gastric mucosa in children with gastrointestinal bleeding. *J Formos Med Assoc.* 1993;92:717–720.
186. Sfakianakis GN, Conway JJ. Detection of ectopic gastric mucosa in Meckel's diverticulum and in other aberrations by scintigraphy: II. Indications and methods—a 10-year experience. *J Nucl Med.* 1981;22:732–738.
187. Schwartz MJ, Lewis JH. Meckel's diverticulum: pitfalls in scintigraphic detection in the adult. *Am J Gastroenterol.* 1984;79:611–618.
188. Lin S, Suhocki PV, Ludwig KA, et al. Gastrointestinal bleeding in adult patients with Meckel's diverticulum: the role of technetium 99m pertechnetate scan. *South Med J.* 2002;95:1338–1341.
189. Heyman S. Meckel's diverticulum: possible detection by combining pentagastrin with histamine H2 receptor blocker. *J Nucl Med.* 1994;35:1656–1658.
190. Treves S, Grand RJ, Eraklis AJ. Pentagastrin stimulation of technetium-99m uptake by ectopic gastric mucosa in a Meckel's diverticulum. *Radiology.* 1978;128:711–712.
191. Diamond RH, Rothstein RD, Alavi A. The role of cimetidine-enhanced technetium-99m-pertechnetate imaging for visualizing Meckel's diverticulum. *J Nucl Med.* 1991;32:1422–1424.
192. Singh PR, Russell CD, Dubovsky EV, et al. Technique of scanning for Meckel's diverticulum. *Clin Nucl Med.* 1978;3:188–192.
193. Nusbaum M, Baum S, Blakemore WS. Clinical experience with the diagnosis and management of gastrointestinal haemorrhage by selective mesenteric catheterization. *Ann Surg.* 1969;170:506–514.
194. Zuckerman DA, Bocchini TP, Birnbaum EH. Massive hemorrhage in the lower gastrointestinal tract in adults: diagnostic imaging and intervention. *AJR Am J Roentgenol.* 1993;161:703–711.
195. Ng BL, Thompson JN, Adam A, et al. Selective visceral angiography in obscure postoperative gastrointestinal bleeding. *Ann R Coll Surg Engl.* 1987;69:237–240.
196. Leitman IM, Paull DE, Shires GT III. Evaluation and management of massive lower gastrointestinal hemorrhage. *Ann Surg.* 1989;209:175–180.
197. Britt LG, Warren L, Moore OF III. Selective management of lower gastrointestinal bleeding. *Am Surg.* 1983;49:121–125.
198. Fiorito JJ, Brandt LJ, Kozicky O, et al. The diagnostic yield of superior mesenteric angiography: correlation with the pattern of gastrointestinal bleeding. *Am J Gastroenterol.* 1989;84:878–881.
199. Reinus JF, Brandt LJ. Vascular ectasias and diverticulosis: common causes of lower intestinal bleeding. *Gastroenterol Clin North Am.* 1994;23:1–20.
200. Casarella WJ, Galloway SJ, Taxin RN, et al. Lower gastrointestinal tract hemorrhage: new concepts based on arteriography. *AJR Am J Roentgenol.* 1974;121:357–368.
201. Baum S, Athanasoulis CA, Waltman AC, et al. Angiodysplasia of the right colon: a cause of gastrointestinal bleeding. *AJR Am J Roentgenol.* 1977;129:789–794.
202. Richter JM, Hedberg SE, Athanasoulis CA, et al. Angiodysplasia. Clinical presentation and colonoscopic diagnosis. *Dig Dis Sci.* 1984;29:481–485.
203. Miller M Jr, Smith TP. Angiographic diagnosis and endovascular management of nonvariceal gastrointestinal hemorrhage. *Gastroenterol Clin North Am.* 2005;34:735–752.
204. Cohn SM, Moller BA, Zieg PM, et al. Angiography for preoperative evaluation in patients with lower gastrointestinal bleeding: are the benefits worth the risks? *Arch Surg.* 1998;133:50–5.
205. Kuo WT, Lee DE, Saad WE, et al. Superselective microcoil embolization for the treatment of lower gastrointestinal hemorrhage. *J Vasc Interv Radiol.* 2003;14:1503–1509.
206. Ledermann HP, Schoch E, Jost R, et al. Super selective coil embolization in acute gastrointestinal hemorrhage: personal experience in 10 patients and review of the literature. *J Vasc Interv Radiol.* 1998;9:753–760.
207. Peck DJ, McLoughlin RF, Hughson MN, et al. Percutaneous embolotherapy of lower gastrointestinal hemorrhage. *J Vasc Interv Radiol.* 1998;9:747–751.
208. Rosenkrantz H, Bookestein JJ, Bosen RJ, et al. Postembolic colonic infarction. *Radiology.* 1982;142:47–51.
209. Guy GE, Shetty PC, Sharma RP, et al. Acute lower gastrointestinal hemorrhage: treatment by superselective embolization with polyvinyl alcohol particles. *AJR Am J Roentgenol.* 1992;159:521–526.
210. Funaki B. Endovascular intervention for the treatment of acute arterial gastrointestinal bleeding. *Gastroenterol Clin North Am.* 2002;31:701–713.
211. Gordon R, Ahl K, Kerlan R, et al. Selective arterial embolization for the control of lower gastrointestinal bleeding. *Am J Surg.* 1997;174:24–28.
212. Luchtefeld MA, Senagore AJ, Szomstein M, et al. Evaluation of transarterial embolization for lower gastrointestinal bleeding. *Dis Colon Rectum.* 2000;43:532–534.
213. Patel TH, Cordts PR, Abcarian P, et al. Will transcatheter embolotherapy replace surgery in the treatment of gastrointestinal bleeding? *Curr Surg.* 2001;58:323–327.
214. Darcy M. Treatment of lower gastrointestinal bleeding: vasopressin infusion versus embolization *J Vasc Interv Radiol.* 2003;14:535–543.
215. Baum S, Rosch J, Dotter CT, et al. Selective mesenteric arterial infusions in the management of massive diverticular hemorrhage. *N Engl J Med.* 1973;288:1269–1272.
216. Clark RA, Colley DP, Eggers FM. Acute arterial gastrointestinal hemorrhage: efficacy of transcatheter control. *AJR Am J Roentgenol.* 1981;136:1185–1189.
217. Bush HL Jr, Nabseth DC. Intravenous nitroglycerin to improve coronary blood flow and left ventricular performance during vasopressin therapy. *Surg Forum.* 1979;30:226–228.
218. Ettorre GC, Francioso G, Garribba AP, et al. Helical CT angiography in gastrointestinal bleeding of obscure origin. *AJR Am J Roentgenol.* 1997;168:727–731.
219. Ernst O, Bulois P, Saint-Drenant S, et al. Helical CT in acute lower gastrointestinal bleeding. *Eur Radiol.* 2003;13:114–117.
220. Yamaguchi T, Yoshikawa K. Enhanced CT for initial localization of active lower gastrointestinal bleeding. *Abdom Imaging.* 2003;28:634–636.
221. Kuhle WG, Sheiman RG. Detection of active colonic hemorrhage with use of helical CT: findings in a swine model. *Radiology.* 2003;228:743–752.
222. Summers RM. Science to practice: detection of active colonic hemorrhage with use of helical CT: findings in a swine model. *Radiology.* 2003;228:599–600.
223. Junquera F, Quiroga S, Saperas E, et al. Accuracy of helical computed tomographic angiography for the diagnosis of colonic angiodysplasia. *Gastroenterology.* 2000;119:293–299.
224. Yamaguchi T, Manabe N, Hata J, et al. The usefulness of transabdominal ultrasound for the diagnosis of lower gastrointestinal bleeding. *Aliment Pharmacol Ther.* 2006;23:1267–1272.
225. Lin CK, Chiu HM, Lien WC, et al. Ultrasonographic bisection approximation method for gastrointestinal obstruction in ER. *Hepato-Gastroenterology.* 2006;53:547–551.
226. Fried AM, Poulos A, Hatfield DR. The effectiveness of the incidental small-bowel series. *Radiology.* 1981;140:4–6.
227. Kusumoto H, Takahashi I, Yoshida M, et al. Primary malignant tumors of the small intestine: analysis of 40 Japanese patients. *J Surg Oncol.* 1992;50:139–143.
228. Ott DJ, Chen YM, Gerlfand DW, et al. Detailed per-oral small bowel examination vs. enteroclysis. Part I: expenditures and radiation exposure. *Radiology.* 1985;155:29–31.
229. Maglinte DD, Chernish SM, Kelvin FM, et al. Crohn disease of the small intestine: accuracy and relevance of enteroclysis. *Radiology.* 1992;184:541–545.
230. Chernish SM, Maglinte DD, O'Connor K. Evaluation of the small intestine by enteroclysis for Crohn's disease. *Am J Gastroenterol.* 1992;87:696–701.
231. Vallance R. An evaluation of the small bowel enema based on an analysis of 350 consecutive examinations. *Clin Radiol.* 1980;31:227–232.
232. Moch A, Herlinger H, Kochman ML, et al. Enteroclysis in the evaluation of obscure gastrointestinal bleeding. *AJR Am J Roentgenol.* 1994;163:1381–1384.
233. Rex DK, Lappas JC, Maglinte DDT, et al. Enteroclysis in the evaluation of suspected small intestinal bleeding. *Gastroenterology.* 1989;97:58–60.
234. Barkin JS, Ross BS. Medical therapy for chronic gastrointestinal bleeding of obscure origin. *Am J Gastroenterol.* 1998;93:1250–1254.
235. van Cutsem E, Rutgeerts P, Vantrappen G. Treatment of bleeding gastrointestinal vascular malformations with oestrogen-progesterone. *Lancet.* 1990;335:953–955.
236. Lewis BS, Salomon P, Rivera-MacMurray S, et al. Does hormonal therapy have any benefit for bleeding angiodysplasia? *J Clin Gastroenterol.* 1992;15:99–103.
237. Barkin JS, Ross BS. Medical therapy for chronic gastrointestinal bleeding of obscure origin. *Am J Gastroenterol.* 1998;93:1250–1254.
238. Szilagyi A, Ghali MP. Pharmacological therapy of vascular malformations of the gastrointestinal tract. *Can J Gastroenterol.* 2006;20(3):171–178.

239. Nardone G, Rocco A, Balzano T, et al. The efficacy of octreotide therapy in chronic bleeding due to vascular abnormalities of the gastrointestinal tract. *Aliment Pharmacol Ther.* 1999;13:1429–1436.
240. Szilagyi A, Ghali MP. Pharmacological therapy of vascular malformations of the gastrointestinal tract. *Can J Gastroenterol.* 2006;20(3):171–178.
241. Kochhar R, Sharma SC, Gupta BB, et al. Rectal sucralfate in radiation proctitis. *Lancet.* 1988;2:400.
242. Sasai T, Hiraishi H, Suzuki Y, et al. Treatment of chronic post-radiation proctitis with oral administration of sucralfate. *Am J Gastroenterol.* 1998; 93:1593–1595.
243. Stockdale AD, Biswas A. Long-term control of radiation proctitis following treatment with sucralfate enemas. *Br J Surg.* 1997;84:379.
244. Denton AS, Andreyev HJ, Forbes A, et al. Systematic review for nonsurgical interventions for the management of late radiation proctitis. *Br J Cancer.* 2002;87:134–143.
245. Pardi DS, Loftus EV, Tremaine WJ, et al. Acute major gastrointestinal hemorrhage in inflammatory bowel disease. *Gastrointest Endosc.* 1999;49:153–157.
246. Tsujikawa T, Nezu R, Andoh A, et al. Infliximab as a possible treatment for the hemorrhagic type of Crohn's disease. *J Gastroenterol.* 2004;39(3):284–287.
247. Papi C, Gili L, Tarquini M, et al. Infliximab for severe recurrent Crohn's disease presenting with massive gastrointestinal hemorrhage. *J Clin Gastroenterol.* 2003;36(3):238–241.
248. Rubinstein E, Ibsen T, Rasmussen RB, et al. Formalin treatment of radiation-induced hemorrhagic proctitis. *Am J Gastroenterol.* 1986;81:44–45.
249. Lee CW, Liu, MD KL, Wang HP, et al. Transcatheter arterial embolization with N-butyl-2-cyanoacrylate in acute upper gastrointestinal bleeding. *J Vasc Interv Radiol.* 2007;18:209–216.
250. Jensen DM, Machicado GA. Colonoscopy for diagnosis and treatment of severe lower gastrointestinal bleeding. Routine outcomes and cost analysis. *Gastrointest Endosc Clin N Am.* 1997;7:477–498.
251. Parkes BM, Obeid FN, Sorensen VJ, et al. The management of massive lower gastrointestinal bleeding. *Am Surg.* 1993;59:676–678.
252. Bokhari M, Vernava AM, Ure T, et al. Diverticular hemorrhage in the elderly—is it well tolerated? *Dis Colon Rectum.* 1996;39:191–195.
253. Scharff JR, Longo WE, Vartanian SM, et al. Ischemic colitis: spectrum of disease and outcome. *Surgery.* 2003;134:624–629.
254. Reilly HF, Al-Kawas FH. Dieulafoy's lesion. Diagnosis and management. *Dig Dis Sci.* 1991;36:1702–1707.
255. Das A, Wong RC. Prediction of outcome of acute GI hemorrhage: a review of risk scores and predictive models. *Gastrointest Endosc.* 2004;60:85–93.
256. Kollef MH, Canfield DA, Zuckerman GR. Triage considerations for patients with acute gastrointestinal hemorrhage admitted to a medical intensive care unit. *Crit Care Med.* 1995;23:1048–1054.
257. Kollef MH, O'Brien JD, Zuckerman GR, et al. BLEED: a classification tool to predict outcomes in patients with acute upper and lower gastrointestinal hemorrhage. *Crit Care Med.* 1997;25:1125–1132.
258. Das A, Ben-Menachem T, Cooper GS, et al. Prediction of outcome in acute lower-gastrointestinal haemorrhage based on an artificial neural network: internal and external validation of a predictive model. *Lancet.* 2003;362:1261–1266.
259. Velayos FS, Williamson A, Sousa KH, et al. Early predictors of severe lower gastrointestinal bleeding and adverse outcomes: a prospective study. *Clin Gastroenterol Hepatol.* 2004;2:485–490.
260. Spiller RC, Parkins RA. Recurrent gastrointestinal bleeding of obscure origin: report of 17 cases and a guide to logical management. *Br J Surg.* 1983;70:489–493.
261. Thompson JN, Salem RR, Hemingway AP, et al. Specialist investigation of obscure gastrointestinal bleeding. *Gut.* 1987;28:47–51.
262. Klas JV, Madoff RD. Surgical options in lower gastrointestinal bleeding. *Semin Colon Rectal Surg.* 1997;8:172–177.
263. Leighton JA, Goldstein J, Hirota W, et al. Obscure gastrointestinal bleeding. *Gastrointest Endosc.* 2003;58:650–655.
264. Chak A, Cooper GS, Canto MI, et al. Enteroscopy for the initial evaluation of iron deficiency. *Gastrointest Endosc.* 1998;47:144–148.
265. Landi B, Tkoub M, Gaudric M, et al. Diagnostic yield of push-type enteroscopy in relation to indication. *Gut.* 1998;42:421–425.
266. Zaman A, Katon RM. Puch enteroscopy for obscure gastrointestinal bleeding yields a high incidence of proximal lesions within reach of a standard endoscope. *Gastrointest Endosc.* 1998;47:372–376.
267. Descamps C, Schmit A, Van Gossum A. "Missed" upper gastrointestinal tract lesions may explain "occult" bleeding. *Endoscopy.* 1999;31:452–455.
268. Sturniolo GC, Leo VD, Vettorato MG, et al. Small bowel exploration by wireless capsule endoscopy: results from 314 procedures. *Am J Med.* 2006; 119:341–347.
269. Prakash C, Zuckerman GR. Acute small bowel bleeding: a distinct entity with significantly different economic implications compared with GI bleeding from other locations. *Gastrointest Endosc.* 2003;58:330–335.
270. Fried AM, Poulos A, Hatfield DR. The effectiveness of the incidental small-bowel series. *Radiology.* 1981;140:45–46.
271. Emenike E, Srivastava S, Amoateng-Adjepong Y, et al. Myocardial infarction complicating gastrointestinal hemorrhage. *Mayo Clin Proc.* 1999; 74:235–241.
272. Bhatti N, Amoateng-Adjepong Y, Qamar A, et al. Myocardial infarction in critically ill patients presenting with gastrointestinal hemorrhage: retrospective analysis of risks and outcomes. *Chest.* 1998;114:1137–1142.
273. Bellotto F, Fagiuoli S, Pavei A, et al. Anemia and ischemia: myocardial injury in patients with gastrointestinal bleeding. *Am J Med.* 2005;118:548–551.
274. Cappell MS. A study of the syndrome of simultaneous acute upper gastrointestinal bleeding and myocardial infarction in 36 patients. *Am J Gastroenterol.* 1995;90:1444–1449.
275. Cappell MS. Gastrointestinal bleeding associated with myocardial infarction. *Gastroenterol Clin North Am.* 2000;29:423–444.
276. Abbas AE, Brodie B, Dixon S, et al. Incidence and prognostic impact of gastrointestinal bleeding after percutaneous coronary intervention for acute myocardial infarction *Am J Cardiol.* 2005;96:173–176.
277. Ng FH, Wong SY, Chang CM, et al. High incidence of clopidogrel-associated gastrointestinal bleeding in patients with previous peptic ulcer disease. *Aliment Pharmacol Ther.* 2003;18:443–449.
278. The Clopidogrel in Unstable Angina to Prevent Recurrent Events Trial Investigators. Effects of clopidogrel in addition to aspirin in patients with acute coronary syndromes without ST-segment elevation. *N Engl J Med.* 2001;345:494–502.
279. Cappell MS. Risks versus benefits of flexible sigmoidoscopy after myocardial infarction: an analysis of 78 patients at three medical centers. *Am J Med.* 2004;116:707–710.
280. Lee CT, Huang SP, Cheng TY, et al. Factors associated with myocardial infarction after emergency endoscopy for upper gastrointestinal bleeding in high risk patients: a prospective observational study. *Am J Emerg Med.* 2007;25(1):49–52.
281. van Es RF, Jonker JJ, Verheught FW, et al. Aspirin and coumadin after acute coronary syndromes (the ASPECT-2 Study): a randomized controlled trial. *Lancet.* 2002;360:109–113.
282. Choudari CP, Rajgopal C, Palmer KR. Acute gastrointestinal haemorrhage in anticoagulated patients: diagnoses and response to endoscopic treatment. *Gut.* 1994;35:464–466.
283. Cappell MS. Safety and efficacy of colonoscopy after myocardial infarction: an analysis of 100 study patients and 100 control patients at two tertiary cardiac referral hospitals. *Gastrointest Endosc.* 2004;60:901–909.
284. Boley SJ, Sammartano R, Adams A, et al. On the nature and etiology of vascular ectasias of the colon. Degenerative lesions of aging. *Gastroenterology.* 1977;72:650–660.
285. Boley SJ, DiBase A, Brandt LJ. Lower intestinal bleeding in the elderly. *Am J Surg.* 1979;137:57–64.
286. Welch CE, Athanasoulis CA, Galdibini JJ. Hemorrhage from the large bowel with special reference to angiodysplasia and diverticular disease. *World J Surg.* 1978;2:73–83.
287. Boley SJ, Sammartano R, Brandt LJ, et al. Vascular ectasias of the colon. *Surg Gynecol Obstet.* 1979;149:353–359.
288. Rogers RH. Endoscopic diagnosis and therapy of mucosal vascular abnormalities of the gastrointestinal tract occurring in elderly patients and associated with cardiac, vascular and pulmonary disease. *Gastrointest Endosc.* 1980;26:134–138.
289. Lewis B, Waye JD. Bleeding from the small intestine. In: Suguwa C, Schuman BM, Lucas CE, eds. *Gastrointestinal Bleeding.* New York: Lgaku-Shoin; 1992:178–188.
290. Santos JCM, Apilli F, Guimaraes AS, et al. Angiodysplasia of the colon: endoscopic diagnosis and treatment. *Br J Surg.* 1988;75:256–258.
291. Hochter W, Weingart J, Kuhner W, et al. Angiodysplasia in the colon and rectum: endoscopic morphology, localisation and frequency. *Endoscopy.* 1985;17:182–185.
292. Wahab PJ, Mulder CJ, den Hartog G, et al. Argon plasma coagulation in flexible gastrointestinal endoscopy: pilot experiences. *Endoscopy.* 1997; 29:176–181.
293. Johanns W, Luis W, Janssen J, et al. Argon plasma coagulation (APC) in gastroenterology: experimental and clinical experiences. *Eur J Gastroenterol Hepatol.* 1997;9:581–587.
294. Szilagyi A, Ghali MP. Pharmacological therapy of vascular malformations of the gastrointestinal tract. *Can J Gastroenterol.* 2006;20(3):171–178.
295. Meyers MA, Alonso DR, Gray GF, et al. Pathogenesis of bleeding colonic diverticulosis. *Gastroenterology.* 1976;71:577–583.
296. Meyers MA, Alonso DR, Baer JW. Pathogenesis of massively bleeding colonic diverticulosis: new observations. *AJR Am J Roentgenol.* 1976;127: 901–908.
297. Gostout CJ, Wang KK, Ahlquist DA, et al. Acute gastrointestinal bleeding: experience ofa specialized management team. *J Clin Gastroenterol.* 1992;14:260–267.
298. Aldoori WH, Giovannucci EL, Rimm EB, et al. Use of acetaminophen and nonsteroidal anti-inflammatory drugs: a prospective study and the risk of symptomatic diverticular disease in men. *Arch Fam Med.* 1998;7: 255–260.
299. Laine L, Connors LG, Reicin A, et al. Serious lower gastrointestinal clinical events with nonselective NSAID or coxib use. *Gastroenterology.* 2003;124:288–292.
300. McGuire HH, Haynes BW. Massive hemorrhage for diverticulosis of the colon: guidelines for therapy based on bleeding patterns observed in fifty cases. *Ann Surg.* 1972;175:847–855.

301. Browder W, Cerise EJ, Litwin MS. Impact of emergency angiography in massive lower gastrointestinal bleeding. *Ann Surg.* 1986;204:530–536.
302. Uden P, Jiborn H, Jonsson K. Influence of selective mesenteric arteriography on the outcome of emergency surgery for massive, lower gastrointestinal hemorrhage: a 15-year experience. *Dis Colon Rectum.* 1986;29:561–566.
303. Newman JR, Cooper MA. Lower gastrointestinal bleeding and ischemic colitis. *Can J Gastroenterol.* 2002;16:597–600.
304. Heer M, Repond F, Hany A, et al. Acute ischaemic colitis in a female long-distance runner. *Gut.* 1987;28:986–989.
305. Qumar M, Read A. Effects of mesenteric blood flow in man. *Gut.* 1987;28:583–587.
306. Scharff JR, Longo WE, Vartanian SM, et al. Ischemic colitis: spectrum of disease and outcome. *Surgery.* 2003;134:624–629.
307. Green BT, Tendler DA. Ischemic colitis: a clinical review. *South Med J.* 2005;98:217–222.
308. Bjarnason I, Hayllar J, MacPherson AJ, et al. Side effects of nonsteroidal anti-inflammatory drugs on the small and large intestine in humans. *Gastroenterology.* 1993;104:1832–1847.
309. Foutch PG. Diverticular bleeding: are nonsteroidal anti-inflammatory drugs risk factors for hemorrhage and can colonoscopy predict outcome for patients? *Am J Gastroenterol.* 1995;90:1779–1784.
310. Kaufman HL, Fischer AH, Carroll M, et al. Colonic ulceration associated with nonsteroidal anti-inflammatory drugs: report of three cases. *Dis Colon Rectum.* 1996;39:705–710.
311. Lang J, Price AB, Levi AJ, et al. Diaphragm disease: pathology of disease of the small intestine induced by non-steroidal anti-inflammatory drugs. *J Clin Pathol.* 1988;41:516–526.
312. Huber T, Ruchti C, Halter F. Nonsteroidal antiinflammatory drug-induced colonic strictures: a case report. *Gastroenterology.* 1991;100:1119–1122.
313. Matsuhashi N, Yamada A, Hiraishi M, et al. Multiple strictures of the small intestine after long-term nonsteroidal anti-inflammatory drug therapy. *Am J Gastroenterol.* 1992;87:1183–1186.
314. Lee J. Radiation proctitis—a niche for the argon plasma coagulator. *Gastrointest Endosc.* 2002;56:779–781.
315. Denton AS, Andreyev HJ, Forbes A, et al. Systematic review for nonsurgical interventions for the management of late radiation proctitis. *Br J Cancer.* 2002;87:134–143.
316. Taieb S, Rolachon A, Cenni JC, et al. Effective use of argon plasma coagulation in the treatment of severe radiation proctitis. *Dis Colon Rectum.* 2001;44:1766–1771.
317. Franko E, Chardavoyne R, Wise L. Massive rectal bleeding from a Dieulafoy's type ulcer of the rectum: a review of this unusual disease. *Am J Gastroenterol.* 1991;86:1545–1547.
318. Abdulian JD, Santoro MJ, Chen YK, et al. Dieulafoy-like lesion of the rectum presenting with exsanguinating hemorrhage: successful endoscopic sclerotherapy. *Am J Gastroenterol.* 1993;88:1939–1941.
319. Parra-Blanco A, Kaminaga N, Kojima T, et al. Hemoclipping for post-polypectomy andpostbiopsy colonic bleeding. *Gastrointest Endosc.* 2000;51:37–41.
320. Tseng CA, Chen LT, Tsai KB, et al. Acute hemorrhagic rectal ulcer syndrome: a new clinical entity? Report of 19 cases and review of the literature. *Dis Colon Rectum.* 2004;47(6):895–903.
321. Takeuchi K, Tsuzuki Y, Ando T, et al. Clinical characteristics of acute hemorrhagic rectal ulcer. *J Clin Gastroenterol.* 2001;33(3):226–228.
322. Hung HY, Changchien CR, You JF, et al. Massive hematochezia from acute hemorrhagic rectal ulcer in patients with severe comorbid illness: rapid control of bleeding by per anal suturing of bleeder using anoretractor. *Dis Colon Rectum.* 2006;49(2):238–243.
323. Oku T, Maeda M, Ihara H, et al. Clinical and endoscopic features of acute hemorrhagic rectal ulcer. *J Gastroenterol.* 2006;41(10):962–970.

CHAPTER 154 ■ LIVER FAILURE: ACUTE AND CHRONIC

R. TODD STRAVITZ • ANDREAS H. KRAMER

ACUTE LIVER FAILURE

Definitions and Immediate Concerns

Acute liver failure (ALF) may be defined as the development of hepatic encephalopathy (HE) and coagulopathy in a patient with no history of previous liver disease, with the onset HE within 26 weeks of jaundice (1). It should be stressed that ALF is not a disease, but rather a clinical syndrome triggered by numerous etiologic agents; consequently, ALF is extremely heterogeneous, and its management has not been well defined.

Overview

There are three possible outcomes after ALF: spontaneous survival without orthotopic liver transplantation (OLT), OLT, or death. In the U.S. Acute Liver Failure Study cohort consisting of more than 1,000 enrollees with ALF between 1998 and 2006, one third of patients died, one quarter underwent OLT, and the remainder (42%) recovered spontaneously (W. M. Lee, personal communication) (2). The dismal overall survival of patients with ALF, 25% in the 1970s, has improved to approximately 65% with the advent of OLT as a rescue treatment and improvements in intensive care management (3).

Etiology, Prevalence, and Initial Testing

In the U.S. ALF Study Group (SG) Cohort, acetaminophen (APAP) accounts for approximately 45% of cases (3), half of those due to ingestion of a single large dose with suicidal intent, and the other half as "therapeutic misadventures" (4,5). Patients in the latter group frequently ingest large doses of APAP in combination with narcotic preparations, and ingestions tend to be multiple over time (5). The second most common cause of ALF remains indeterminate even after extensive serologic and historical evaluation (15% of cases), followed by idiosyncratic drug reactions (13%) and acute hepatitis B (7%), with autoimmune hepatitis, acute hepatitis A, hepatic vein thrombosis (Budd-Chiari syndrome), hypotension ("shock liver"), fulminant Wilson disease, malignant infiltration of the liver, and pregnancy-associated ALF (acute fatty liver and HELLP [hemolysis, elevated liver enzymes, and low platelets] syndrome) constituting fewer than 5% of cases each.

TABLE 154.1

CAUSE, PREVALENCE, AND EVALUATION OF ACUTE LIVER FAILURE

Cause	Prevalence[a] (%)	Evaluation
APAP	45	History; APAP level
HBV	7	anti-HBc (IgM and total), HBsAg, anti-HBs, HBV DNA, anti-HDV
AIH	5	ANA, ASMA, anti-LKM, immunoglobulins
HAV	4	anti-HAV (IgM and total)
Shock liver	4	Echocardiogram, brain natriuretic peptide
Wilson disease	3	Serum ceruloplasmin and copper; urine copper; slitlamp eye exam
BCS	2	Doppler ultrasound of liver
Malignancy	1	Contrast-enhanced CT; MRI (preferred)
AFLP/HELLP	1	Pregnancy test
HSV	0.5	Anti-HSV 1/2, HSV DNA
Other	4	Anti-HCV/HCV RNA, anti-CMV/CMV DNA, anti-EBV/EBV DNA, toxicology screen
Indeterminate	14	All of above negative
Idiosyncratic drug	13	History; all of above negative

APAP, acetaminophen; HBV, hepatitis B virus; HDV, hepatitis D virus; AIH, autoimmune hepatitis; ANA, anti-nuclear antibody; ASMA, anti-smooth muscle antibody; anti-LKM, anti-liver kidney microsomal antibody; HAV, hepatitis A virus; BCS, Budd-Chiari syndrome; CT, computed tomography; MRI, magnetic resonance imaging; AFLP/HELLP, acute fatty liver of pregnancy/hemolysis-elevated liver enzymes–low platelet syndrome; HSV, herpes simplex virus; HCV, hepatitis C virus; CMV, cytomegalovirus; EBV, Epstein-Barr virus.
N = approximately 1,000 at the time of publication. (W.M. Lee, personal communication.)
Suggested evaluation of patients with idiosyncratic drug hepatotoxicity and indeterminate ALF should include all of the tests listed, since these are diagnoses of exclusion.
[a]Prevalence of causes are estimates based on the U.S. Acute Liver Failure Study Group Cohort. (personal communication).

It remains doubtful that acute hepatitis C virus infection causes ALF, but chronic hepatitis C may increase a patient's susceptibility to ALF after a different acute insult (6). The initial laboratory and procedural evaluation of patients with ALF to determine cause is indicated in Table 154.1 (7).

Assessment of Prognosis

Outcomes of ALF

Two general rules improve the prediction of outcome in patients with ALF. First, the cause of ALF is the single, most important prognostic factor. In patients with APAP overdose, spontaneous recovery is the rule (63% in the ALFSG cohort). Patients with acute hepatitis A, shock liver, and pregnancy-related ALF—assuming prompt delivery of the fetus—also have relatively high rates of spontaneous survival (more than 50%). Patients with ALF from all other causes have very poor rates of recovery without OLT, approximately 25% for those with indeterminate cause, acute hepatitis B, and idiosyncratic drug reactions (2). Second, the shorter the interval between jaundice and the development of HE, the higher the likelihood of spontaneous survival; conversely, the longer this interval, the more likely is death without OLT (8). Patients with APAP overdose and acute hepatitis A usually have hyperacute progression (jaundice-HE interval within 7 days) and have a relatively good prognosis, whereas most idiosyncratic drug reactions have a more subacute presentation (jaundice-HE interval of more than 28 days) and dismal prognosis without OLT.

Prognostication Schemes

To anticipate the need for OLT, prognostic schemes have been developed to predict death without OLT in patients with ALF. The most time-honored scheme, the King's College Criteria (9), retrospectively analyzed outcomes in patients with ALF according to cause and subsequently validated the model in a test population. For patients with APAP-induced ALF, predictors of death included acidosis on admission (arterial pH less than 7.30), or azotemia, severe coagulopathy, and high-grade HE (grade 3 or 4). In patients with ALF due to other causes, severe coagulopathy or any three of the criteria listed in Table 154.2 also predicted death. Although the original series using these criteria reported a predictive accuracy for death without OLT of more than 85%, subsequent analyses have suggested that they are less accurate (10). Consequently, other prognostic parameters continue to be applied to individual patients with ALF during the weighty decision of whether to proceed with OLT.

Complications and Treatment

General Management

ALF commonly causes multiorgan dysfunction, such that management requires close collaboration between intensivists, hepatologists, transplant surgeons, and other specialists (11). Improvements in critical care practice have resulted in improved mortality over past decades, even in patients who do not

TABLE 154.2

SCHEMES FOR PREDICTING POOR PROGNOSIS AND THE NEED FOR ORTHOTOPIC LIVER TRANSPLANTATION IN PATIENTS WITH ACUTE LIVER FAILURE (ALF)

Scheme	Cause of ALF	Criteria for liver transplantation	Reference
King's College criteria	APAP	Arterial pH <7.30 *or* all of the following: 1. PT >100 s 2. Creatinine >3.4 mg/dL 3. Grade 3/4 encephalopathy	O'Grady et al., 1989 (9)
	Non-APAP	PT >100 s (INR >6.5) *or* any 3 of the following: 1. NANB/drug/halothane etiology, 2. Jaundice to encephalopathy >7 d 3. Age <10 or >40 y 4. PT >50 s 5. Bilirubin >17.4 mg/dL	
Factor V	Viral	Age <30 y: factor V <20% *or* Any age: Factor V <30% and grade 3/4 encephalopathy	Bernuau et al., 1986; 1991 (202,203)
Factor VIII/V ratio	APAP	Factor VIII/V ratio >30	Pereira et al., 1992 (204)
Liver biopsy	Mixed	Hepatocyte necrosis >70%	Donaldson et al., 1993 (205)
Arterial phosphate	APAP	>1.2 mmol/L	Schmidt and Dalhoff, 2002 (206)
Arterial lactate	APAP	>3.5 mmol/L	Bernal et al., 2002 (207)
Arterial ammonia	Mixed	>150–200 μmol/L	Clemmesen et al., 1999 (24)
APACHE II/III score	APAP	>15	Bernal et al., 1998; Mitchell et al., 1998 (208,209)
MELD score	Non-APAP	>30	Rossaro et al., 2005 (210)

Abbreviations per legend of Table 154.1, as well as: PT, prothrombin time; INR, international normalized ratio; NANB, non-A, non-B viral hepatitis; APACHE, Acute Physiology and Chronic Health Evaluation; MELD, model for end-stage liver disease.
Modified from Sanyal AJ, Stravitz RT. Acute liver failure. In: Boyer TD, Wright T, Manns MP, eds. *Hepatology—A Textbook of Liver Disease*. 5th ed. Philadelphia, PA: Elsevier; 2006:383–415; and Stravitz RT, Kramer AH, Davern T, et al., and the Adult Acute Liver Failure Study Group. Management of acute liver failure: recommendations of the Acute Liver Failure Study Group. *Crit Care Med*. 2007;35:2498–2508.

undergo OLT (12,13). Since the progression of complications can be rapid, patients should be transferred to a liver transplant center; in general, higher-volume centers have superior outcome. Sedation should initially be minimized to avoid confusing the effects of drugs with deteriorating mental status. Worsening hepatic encephalopathy (HE) is a clear indication for admission to the ICU; the likelihood of spontaneous survival decreases with a worsening coma grade at admission (9,14).

Cause-Specific Management

Acetaminophen. The administration of *N*-acetylcysteine (NAC) has become widely applied to patients with ALF due to APAP on the basis of both laboratory and clinical data (15,16); however, randomized, placebo-controlled studies documenting the efficacy of NAC in APAP overdose have never been performed. Several rules of administration require emphasis. First, although nomograms describing the probability of hepatotoxicity after a single APAP ingestion have been used widely to determine whether NAC should be administered, the time of ingestion frequently cannot be determined accurately, and ingestions are multiple. Therefore, NAC should be administered "whenever there is doubt concerning the timing, dose ingested, or plasma concentration, since the use of the antidote is much less hazardous than the consequences of withholding it" (17). Second, intravenous NAC should be administered when a patient has higher than grade 1 HE, or in patients who do not tolerate oral dosing (16). Finally, since the administration of NAC, even late after ingestion, appears to confer survival benefit, dosing should continue until evidence of severe liver injury resolves (international normalized ratio [INR] less than 1.5 and resolution of HE), rather than by completion of a set number of doses of the drug (18).

Other Cause-Specific Treatments. Specific medications that should be considered in patients with ALF due to other causes are outlined in Table 154.3. It should be emphasized that randomized, controlled studies to support these therapies do not exist, and most of these recommendations are made only on the basis of case reports, expert opinion, and a high therapeutic threshold.

Management of Specific Complications of ALF

Neurologic Complications

Pathophysiology. By definition, patients with ALF develop varying degrees of HE (Table 154.4). Worsening mental status

TABLE 154.3

CAUSE-SPECIFIC THERAPY OF PATIENTS WITH ACUTE LIVER FAILURE

Cause	Therapy	References
APAP	NAC Oral: 140 mg/kg load, then 70 mg/kg every 4 hrs	Smilkstein et al., 1988 (15)
	NAC IV: 150 mg/kg load, then 12.5 mg/kg/h × 4 hrs, then 6.25 mg/kg/hr	Buckley et al., 1999 (212), Smilkstein et al., 1991 (16)
Amanita	Penicillin G: 1 g/kg/d IV & NAC (as in APAP overdose)	Broussard et al., 2001 (213)
HSV	Acyclovir: 30 mg/kg/d IV	Peters et al., 2000 (214)
AIH	Methylprednisolone 60 mg/d IV	Kessler et al., 2004 (215)
HBV	Lamivudine 100 to 150 mg/d PO	Tillmann et al., 2006 (216)
Wilson disease	? Plasmapheresis, D-penicillamine	Rodriguez et al., 2003 (217)
AFLP/HELLP	Delivery of fetus	Castro et al., 1999 (218)

APAP, acetaminophen; NAC, *N*-acetylcysteine; *Amanita* refers to mushroom intoxication; HSV, herpes simplex virus; AIH, autoimmune hepatitis; HBV, hepatitis B virus; AFLP/HELLP, acute fatty liver of pregnancy/hemolysis-elevated liver enzymes–low platelet syndrome.

may be a consequence of progression to cerebral edema, which is present in 38% to 81% of cases of grade 3 or 4 encephalopathy and becomes increasingly likely as the level of consciousness declines (19,20). The pathophysiology of cerebral edema in ALF has been studied extensively and is unique compared with other causes of raised intracranial pressure (ICP) (Fig. 154.1). Although both cytotoxic (intracellular) and vasogenic (extracellular) edema coexist; the former predominates, coinciding with the observation that most swelling localizes to gray matter astrocytes. Although there may be increased permeability to water and various other molecules, there is no widespread breakdown of the blood–brain barrier (21–23).

Elevated serum ammonia, produced primarily by gut microorganisms and inadequately cleared by the liver, has long been recognized to contribute to the development of cerebral edema in ALF. Patients who develop cerebral herniation have substantially higher serum ammonia levels—usually more than 200 μmol/L—and greater cerebral ammonia uptake. Conversely, herniation rarely occurs when serum ammonia levels remain below 150 μmol/L (24). Ammonia readily crosses the blood–brain barrier and is taken up by astrocytes, where it combines with glutamate to form glutamine, which in turn contributes to an osmotic gradient that draws water into the intracellular space (25). Although the brain usually compensates for such an

TABLE 154.4

HEPATIC ENCEPHALOPATHY GRADES AND RELATIONSHIP TO CEREBRAL EDEMA AND PROGNOSIS IN ACUTE LIVER FAILURE

Stage	Mental status	Cerebral edema	Spontaneous recovery without liver transplantation
I	Euphoria, mild confusion, dysarthria, abnormal sleep rhythm	Rare	52% overall 87% APAP 35% drug reaction 18% indeterminate cause 38% other cause
II	Accentuation of stage I, lethargy, moderate confusion, incontinence		
III	Stupor, severe confusion, incoherent speech	40%–80%	33% overall 50% APAP 12% drug reaction 16% indeterminate cause 27% other cause
IV	Coma or near coma		

APAP, acetaminophen.
Data modified from Trey C, Davidson C. The management of fulminant hepatic failure. *Prog Liver Dis.* 1970;3:282–298; Gazzard BG, Portmann B, Murray-Lyon IM, et al. Causes of death in fulminant hepatic failure and relationship to quantitative histological assessment of parenchymal damage. *Q J Med.* 1975;44(176):615–626; and Ostapowicz G, Fontana RJ, Schiodt FV, et al. Results of a prospective study of acute liver failure at 17 tertiary care centers in the United States. *Ann Intern Med.* 2002;137(12):947–954.

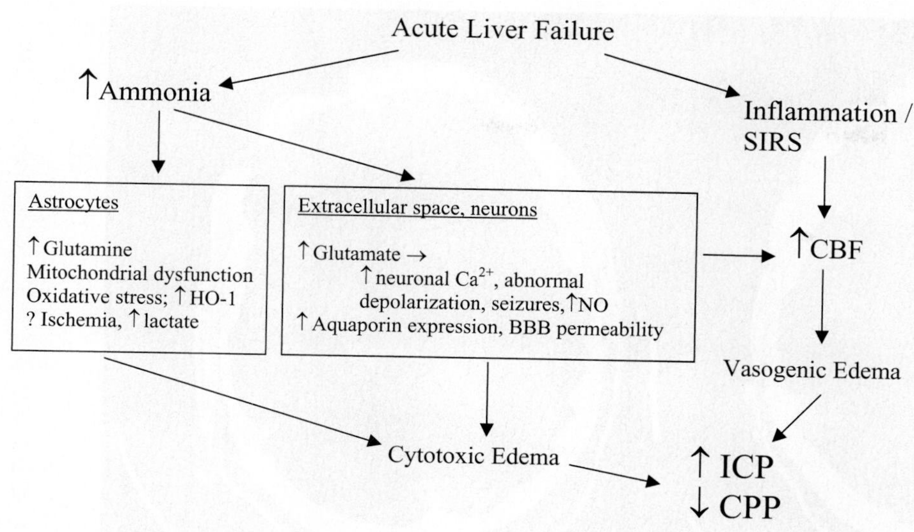

FIGURE 154.1. Pathogenesis of cerebral edema and intracranial hypertension in acute liver failure. BBB, blood–brain barrier; Ca^{2+}, calcium; CBF, cerebral blood flow; CPP, cerebral perfusion pressure; HO-1, heme-oxidase-1; ICP, intracranial pressure; NO, nitric oxide; SIRS, systemic inflammatory response syndrome.

osmotic challenge by extruding organic osmolytes—for example, myoinositol—the rapidity of its development in ALF often does not allow time for compensation to occur, as it would with chronic liver failure (26). Ammonia also interferes with cerebral energy metabolism, leading to the accumulation of lactate (27). Inhibition of glutamate uptake by astrocytes and the resulting high extracellular levels leads to excessive activation of N-methyl-D-aspartate (NMDA) receptors (28), which in turn stimulates neuronal calcium influx, abnormal membrane depolarization, promotion of seizures, and increased nitric oxide (NO) production (29).

Despite the relative lack of vasogenic edema, and the observation that the blood–brain barrier remains grossly intact, increased cerebral blood flow (CBF) remains an important factor in the formation of cerebral edema. Although the cerebral metabolic rate is low in patients with ALF, CBF rises with the accumulation of ammonia and is frequently excessive relative to energy expenditure (30–32). Early in the course of disease, CBF may be appropriately low to match the reduced cerebral metabolic rate, but with progression of hepatic failure, hyperemia ensues (33). Systemic inflammation often coincides with increases in CBF and ICP, suggesting that it may have a pathogenic role (34,35). Abnormal CBF in patients with ALF also results from impairment in cerebrovascular autoregulation. Rather than remaining constant in the face of varying levels of cerebral perfusion pressure (CPP = mean arterial pressure [MAP] − ICP), CBF tends to vary directly with blood pressure (36,37). Thus, although excessive CBF contributes to worsening cerebral edema (38), patients are also especially vulnerable to ischemia if hypotension occurs. Furthermore, despite global increases in CBF, there may be important regional variations, such that blood flow is excessive in some areas and insufficient in others (39). Thus, it is important that CPP be carefully controlled, and extremes avoided.

Management of HE, Cerebral Edema, and Seizures. Considering the central importance of ammonia in the pathogenesis of hepatic encephalopathy and cerebral edema, clinicians often use therapies aimed at lowering serum ammonia levels in patients with ALF. The most commonly used agents in chronic liver disease, nonabsorbable disaccharides (e.g., lactulose) and oral antibiotics (neomycin, rifaximin, or metronidazole), have not been adequately studied in patients with ALF but appear to have little effect on outcome (40). Nevertheless, if lactulose is administered, the dose should be adjusted to achieve no more than three to four bowel movements per day, and care must be taken to avoid excessive abdominal distention, volume depletion, and hypernatremia. Even though oral neomycin is minimally absorbed from the gastrointestinal tract, it has been reported to cause acute renal failure and is therefore not recommended (41).

A computed tomography (CT) scan of the head should be considered early in the course of ALF to exclude other causes of altered mental status, especially intracerebral hemorrhage. Although a head CT may also detect cerebral edema, a normal scan does not rule out clinically important intracranial hypertension (Fig. 154.2) (42,43). Since ICP cannot accurately be determined noninvasively and carries important prognostic implications for spontaneous survival and neurologic recovery after OLT, many experts advocate ICP monitor placement in OLT candidates with stage III or IV HE (7,44). Although there is a perception that ICP monitoring significantly improves the outcome of patients with ALF, no prospective, randomized studies exist to support the practice, and retrospective studies in fact refute this perception (45). The invariable presence of coagulopathy in patients with ALF increases the bleeding risk of ICP monitor placement, and earlier studies reported bleeding complications in up to 20% (45). However, the clinical significance of many of these bleeding complications was probably negligible (44,45), and more recent series have found lower bleeding rates with the use of recombinant factor VIIa (rFVIIa) shortly before insertion of the device (46). The burr hole for an ICP monitor is usually placed over the frontal lobe of the nondominant cerebral hemisphere, and ventriculostomies are generally not recommended because of a higher risk of bleeding and infection. Although placement of ICP monitors into the epidural space may minimize the risk of hemorrhage (45,47), the accuracy of this practice, compared with other methods of ICP monitoring, has not been well studied.

The specific management of cerebral edema in patients with ALF resembles that of other causes of intracranial hypertension, with the important caveat that hyperemia plays an

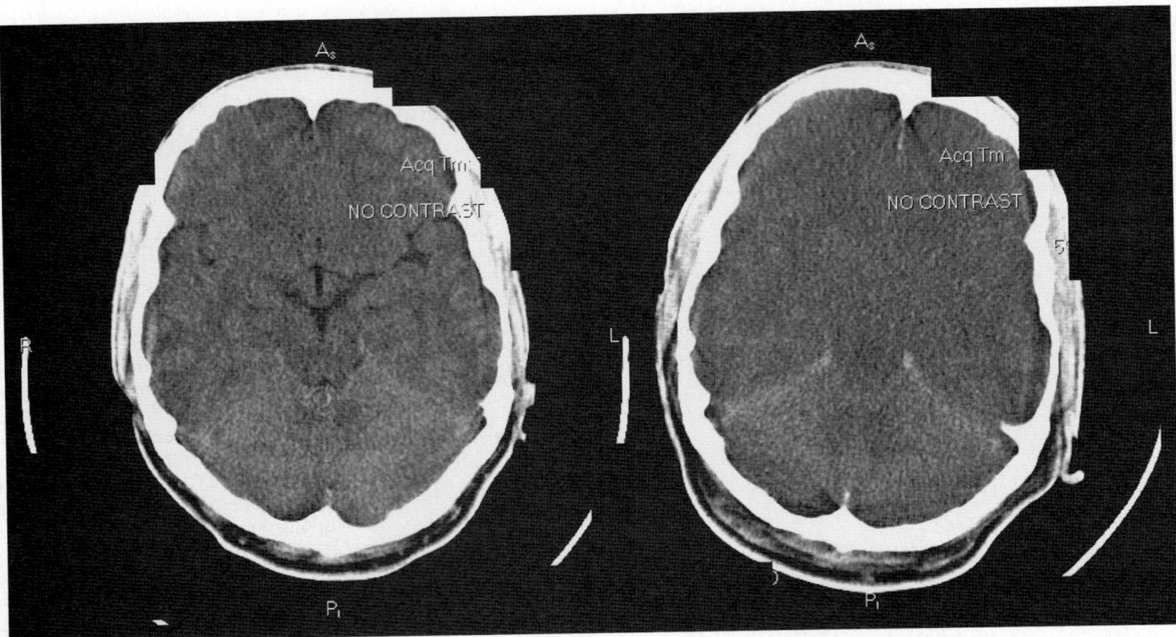

FIGURE 154.2. Head computed tomography (CT) scans of a 32-year-old man with acute liver failure who died of progressive cerebral edema. At admission **(left)**, the CT scan was normal; 48 hours later **(right)**, there was diffuse loss of gray-white differentiation, effacement of sulci, and obliteration of the basal cisterns, consistent with severe diffuse edema and transtentorial herniation with brainstem compression.

important additional pathogenic role in the former (Fig. 154.3). Patients should be cared for in a calm, quiet environment, with limited stimulation. Chest physiotherapy and suctioning should be temporarily minimized. The head of the bed should be elevated to at least 30°, as this reduces ICP and decreases the risk of hospital-acquired pneumonia (48–50). The duration of time that a patient is placed supine or in Trendelenburg position for procedures should be minimized, especially if ICP is not monitored. Endotracheal intubation and mechanical ventilation must be implemented in a timely fashion to avoid the potentially injurious effects of hypoxemia and hypercapnia, while also reducing aspiration risk and facilitating management of intracranial hypertension. Laryngoscopy and intubation may cause transient elevations in ICP and fluctuations in blood pressure. Appropriate measures should be taken to minimize these physiologic derangements, including the appropriate use of sedation and neuromuscular blockade. Although controversial, intravenous lidocaine may further attenuate the rise in ICP from laryngoscopy (51,52).

Adequate analgesia and sedation must be administered to manage intracranial hypertension in ALF. In general, shorter-acting agents are preferred, such that patients can be more quickly awakened and re-examined. Increased levels of endogenous benzodiazepinelike molecules and GABA-ergic neurotransmission have been implicated in the pathogenesis of HE (53). Therefore, sedatives with GABA-ergic properties may exacerbate HE; propofol is preferred over benzodiazepines by some authors (54). However, if used over several days, the dose of propofol should be limited to less than 5 mg/kg per hour to decrease the risk of the potentially fatal propofol infusion syndrome, and appropriate adjustments to the patient's caloric intake should be made (55).

Hyperventilation causes cerebral vasoconstriction and a reduction in cerebral blood volume, effects that can be used therapeutically to reduce ICP. Patients with hepatic encephalopathy often spontaneously hyperventilate, with resultant respiratory alkalosis (56). If the $PaCO_2$ suddenly normalizes because of sedation or respiratory exhaustion, rebound vasodilatation may occur, with consequent elevated ICP (57). Thus, initial ventilator settings should probably be set to match the previous, spontaneous minute ventilation of the patient, and either arterial blood gases or end-tidal CO_2 should be closely monitored. The major concern with using hyperventilation as a means to lower ICP is that vasoconstriction may be severe enough to cause cerebral ischemia. In fact, this effect has been demonstrated even with moderate hyperventilation in patients with traumatic brain injury, a condition where CBF is usually reduced (58,59). In the setting of cerebral hyperemia, one might expect that hyperventilation would be particularly effective in controlling ICP; indeed, one study found that hyperventilation improved CBF autoregulation in ALF (60).

Jugular venous oximetry may be useful to guide therapy, with a high jugular venous oxygen saturation (or low arteriojugulovenous oxygen difference [$AVjDO_2$]) used as evidence that hyperventilation is safe (61). While this method provides a more objective approach to gauging the effects of hyperventilation, jugular venous oximetry has proven relatively insensitive to the detection of even relatively large areas of cerebral ischemia (60,62). Since heterogeneity of CBF may sensitize some regions of the brain to ischemia in ALF (39) and another controlled trial found no clinical benefit (63), the routine use of hyperventilation in the management of ALF patients with HE cannot be advocated. However, spontaneous hyperventilation of patients with ALF should not be discouraged.

Osmotic agents, including mannitol and hypertonic saline (HTS), lower ICP most effectively in the setting of global (rather than unilateral) cerebral edema with an intact blood–brain barrier (64,65), which characterizes ALF. In small human and

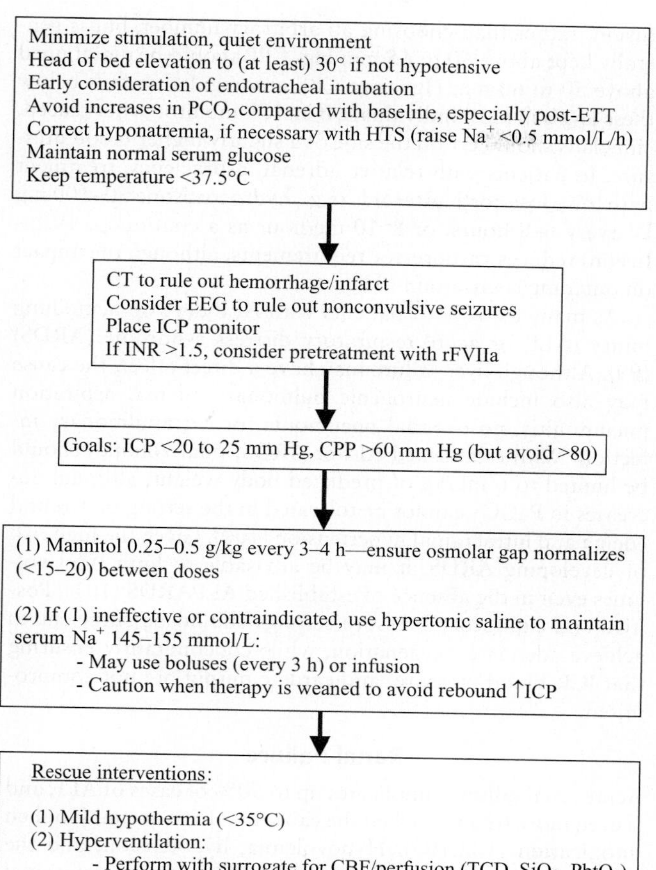

Minimize stimulation, quiet environment
Head of bed elevation to (at least) 30° if not hypotensive
Early consideration of endotracheal intubation
Avoid increases in PCO_2 compared with baseline, especially post-ETT
Correct hyponatremia, if necessary with HTS (raise Na^+ <0.5 mmol/L/h)
Maintain normal serum glucose
Keep temperature <37.5°C
CT to rule out hemorrhage/infarct
Consider EEG to rule out nonconvulsive seizures
Place ICP monitor
If INR >1.5, consider pretreatment with rFVIIa
Goals: ICP <20 to 25 mm Hg, CPP >60 mm Hg (but avoid >80)
(1) Mannitol 0.25–0.5 g/kg every 3–4 h—ensure osmolar gap normalizes (<15–20) between doses
(2) If (1) ineffective or contraindicated, use hypertonic saline to maintain serum Na^+ 145–155 mmol/L:
- May use boluses (every 3 h) or infusion
- Caution when therapy is weaned to avoid rebound ↑ICP
Rescue interventions:
(1) Mild hypothermia (<35°C)
(2) Hyperventilation:
- Perform with surrogate for CBF/perfusion (TCD, SjO_2, $PbtO_2$)
- If SjO_2 used, keep >60%; if $PbtO_2$, keep >15–20 mm Hg
(3) Deeper sedation with goal of burst suppression
- EEG to guide dosing
(4) Indomethacin?

FIGURE 154.3. Algorithm for management of cerebral edema and raised intracranial pressure in acute liver failure (ALF) (see text for details). CBF, cerebral blood flow; CPP, cerebral perfusion pressure; CT, computed tomography; EEG, electroencephalogram; ETT, endotracheal tube; rFVIIa, recombinant factor 7 activated; HTS, hypertonic saline; ICP, intracranial pressure; INR, international normalized ratio; $PbtO_2$, brain tissue oxygen tension; SjO_2, jugular venous saturation; TCD, transcranial Doppler.

animal studies, mannitol effectively lowered ICP and appeared to improve survival (66,67). A general indication for the administration of mannitol includes persistently (>10 minutes) elevated ICP (more than 20 mm Hg) after ensuring proper calibration of the ICP monitor. The optimal dose of mannitol remains untested, but smaller boluses (e.g., 0.25–0.5 g/kg every 4 to 6 hours) appear to be as effective as larger ones (68). Apart from potentially causing hypovolemia, the accumulation of mannitol may be nephrotoxic, an important consideration given that many patients with ALF have abnormal renal function. It is often stated that the serum osmolality should be kept below 320 mOsm/L, but this threshold is arbitrary, is frequently exceeded without adverse effect in other neurocritical care patients, and does not predict an increased risk of renal failure. Since most hospital laboratories do not assay mannitol concentrations, a useful surrogate is the osmolar gap, which more reliably predicts the risk of renal failure and should be allowed to normalize (e.g, less than 15–20) between doses (69).

HTS is increasingly being used in various settings as an alternative to mannitol to treat cerebral edema (64,70). Theoretical advantages over mannitol include the following: (a) the blood–brain barrier is less permeable to HTS (making it a more effective osmotic agent); (b) it is a volume expander rather than a diuretic; and (c) there is no proven nephrotoxicity. HTS can be administered as boluses of 3% to 30% saline every 3 to 4 hours, or as a continuous infusion. In one randomized, controlled trial of patients with ALF and high-grade encephalopathy, a HTS infusion (30% saline, 5–20 mL/hour) to maintain serum sodium levels of 145 to 155 mmol/L effectively acted as prophylaxis against intracranial hypertension (71). However, great caution must be taken when HTS is weaned or discontinued to ensure that the serum sodium falls very slowly to avoid precipitating rebound cerebral edema. Apart from the potentially beneficial effects of inducing mild hypernatremia, it is perhaps more important to avoid hyponatremia. Approximately two thirds of patients with ALF present with serum sodium levels less than 135 mmol/L and one third have levels less than 130 mmol/L. The presence of hyponatremia may contribute to the development of cerebral edema early in the course of ALF (72) and is an independent predictor of worse outcome (73,74). Hyponatremia should therefore be corrected, but serum sodium levels should not be raised more quickly than 0.3 to 0.5 mmol/L/hour to minimize the risk of osmotic demyelination. HTS can cause local tissue damage and phlebitis, and therefore—whenever possible—should be administered through a central venous catheter.

High-dose barbiturates (pentobarbital [3–5 mg/kg IV loading bolus followed by 1–3 mg/kg per hour IV infusion], or thiopental [5–10 mg/kg loading bolus followed by 3–5 mg/kg per hour]) can be used as rescue therapy when other interventions have been maximized but the ICP remains more than 20 mm Hg (75). Electroencephalography (EEG) should be performed to guide dosing, with the goal being to achieve a burst-suppression pattern. Although effective at reducing ICP, barbiturates have numerous deleterious effects, including hypotension, electrolyte disturbances, and immunosuppression. It is also unclear that there is any additional benefit to using barbiturates when an EEG already demonstrates burst suppression with the use of other sedatives (e.g., propofol). Indomethacin (25 mg IV bolus) constricts intracerebral blood vessels and has also been reported to be effective at lowering ICP. Considering the potential of untoward gastric mucosal and renal side effects, however, the use of indomethacin requires further study (76). Corticosteroids are of no value in treating intracranial hypertension in ALF and should not be used for this purpose (66).

Fever increases ICP (77) and is an independent predictor of worse outcome in brain-injured patients (78), such that euthermia should be maintained. Conversely, the induction of mild hypothermia is a promising intervention in ALF, since it interferes with several steps in the pathogenesis of cerebral edema. Specifically, hypothermia attenuates the osmotic gradient created by increased astrocytic glutamine (79), normalizes extracellular glutamate and lactate (80), decreases CBF (81), restores autoregulation (82), and reduces ICP (83). Temperatures of 32°C to 33°C have been used to control intracranial hypertension in patients with ALF refractory to standard care (84). Several novel methods of maintaining hypothermia, both surface-based and intravascular, are available to achieve consistent temperature control (85,86). Important potential adverse effects of hypothermia in the setting of ALF include interference with coagulation and an increased risk of infection.

Current models of hepatic encephalopathy suggest that early in the course, cerebral edema is largely due to ammonia-induced cytotoxic edema, whereas subsequent increases in ICP are associated with increased CBF and hyperemia (33). In the former case, osmotic therapy may be most appropriate and effective, whereas in the latter situation, various measures to reduce CBF, including hyperventilation, deeper sedation, greater head-of-bed elevation, or hypothermia may be preferred. Thus, knowledge of CBF potentially helps predict deterioration and guide therapy. Determining CBF has long been largely a research tool, but an increasing number of bedside monitors have been developed, although it is important for clinicians to be familiar with their limitations. Transcranial Doppler (TCD) flow velocities are easiest to measure over the middle cerebral artery (MCA) and are dependent on CBF, vessel caliber, and the angle of insonation (operator technique) (87). Jugular venous oximetry is relatively simple to perform, with normal saturation levels (SjO_2) having a relatively broad range from as low as 55% to as high as 75% ($AVjDO_2 = 5$–6 mL/100 mL). Assuming that cerebral oxygen consumption remains constant, one would expect SjO_2 to vary with CBF, with levels more than 75% suggestive of hyperemia, and less than 55%, ischemia (88). However, as discussed earlier, there is a wide range of "normal" values, and this is a global measure that cannot exclude regional ischemia. If parenchymal ICP monitors are used, there is little additional risk in placing a brain PO_2 ($PbtO_2$) monitor or microdialysis catheter, although experience with these modalities specifically in the setting of ALF is limited (76).

Nonconvulsive seizures are a potential cause of worsening cerebral edema and secondary brain injury. A small study using 2-channel—rather than the usual 16 to 20 channels—EEG suggested that nonconvulsive seizures are relatively common with ALF, although the criteria used for electrographic seizures were not described (89). Given the frequency of nonconvulsive seizures and status epilepticus among comatose patients in general, routinely obtaining an EEG in patients with hepatic encephalopathy, particularly when there is a clinical change in neurologic status, may be useful (90). However, there is currently insufficient evidence to justify the routine use of prophylactic phenytoin (89,91). Furthermore, sedation with propofol or benzodiazepines is likely to provide more effective antiseizure prophylaxis than phenytoin.

Cardiopulmonary Complications

Patients with ALF frequently develop systemic inflammatory response syndrome (SIRS), regardless of whether or not their course is complicated by infection (35). Hypotension is typical of patients with ALF and can be ascribed to low systemic vascular resistance, the use of sedatives, mechanical ventilation, and relative adrenal insufficiency (92,93). Even though overall energy expenditure is increased (94), peripheral oxygen extraction may be impaired (95). Lactic acidosis is an important prognostic marker in ALF, but the mechanism is not primarily dysoxia, but rather impaired hepatic clearance and increased splanchnic production (96).

Dopamine and norepinephrine are currently the preferred vasopressors for vasodilatory shock (97). Most patients with severe ALF will require an arterial catheter, and various tools are available to optimize volume status and cardiac output (98). The goal MAP should be individualized to optimize organ perfusion, rather than choosing an arbitrary number, but is generally kept above 60 to 65 mm Hg. CPP should be maintained above 50 to 60 mm Hg, since CBF autoregulation fails below these levels in most individuals; if an ICP monitor is not placed, clinicians should err on the side of a slightly higher blood pressure. In patients with relative adrenal insufficiency, treatment with low-dose corticosteroids (e.g., hydrocortisone 50–100 mg IV every 6–8 hours, or 8–10 mg/hour as a continuous IV infusion) reduces vasopressor requirements, although the impact on outcome is uncertain (93).

As many as 37% of patients with ALF develop acute lung injury (ALI) or acute respiratory distress syndrome (ARDS) (99). Although liver failure may have a direct effect, the cause may also include neurogenic pulmonary edema, aspiration pneumonitis, nosocomial pneumonia, or extrapulmonary infection. With established ALI or ARDS, tidal volumes should be limited to 6 mL/kg of predicted body weight, although increases in $PaCO_2$ cannot be tolerated in the setting of cerebral edema and intracranial hypertension (100). Given the high risk of developing ARDS, it may be advisable to limit tidal volumes even in the absence of established ALI/ARDS (101). Positive end-expiratory pressure settings should be sufficient to achieve adequate oxygenation, while concomitantly ensuring that ICP, blood pressure, and cardiac output are not compromised.

Renal Failure

Acute renal failure complicates up to 50% of cases of ALF, and is even more frequent when the cause of ALF is acetaminophen intoxication (102,103). Hypovolemia, hypotension, and the use of nephrotoxins—including aminoglycosides, nonsteroidal anti-inflammatory drugs, and intravenous contrast—should be minimized. Patients with ALF can develop hepatorenal syndrome (HRS) as a consequence of intense renal vasoconstriction (104) (see Chronic Liver Failure, below). The decision to initiate renal replacement therapy (RRT) must consider the magnitude of renal dysfunction, metabolic derangements, and volume overload. Continuous renal replacement therapy (CRRT) is preferred over intermittent hemodialysis (IHD) by many clinicians, largely because of more stable volume management and greater time-averaged dialysis dose (105). Even transient hypotension is poorly tolerated in patients with cerebral edema; not only does the CPP decrease, but cerebral vasodilatation may increase, with further increases in CBF and ICP (106). Excessively rapid correction of metabolic acidosis with bicarbonate-based dialysate may transiently increase cerebrospinal fluid CO_2, reduce central nervous system (CNS) pH, and promote more cerebral vasodilatation (107). Good results have been achieved with CRRT in patients with ALF (108). However, when performed using carefully designed protocols, hemodynamic stability can also be achieved with IHD (109). Regardless of the mode of RRT, an adequate hemofiltration or dialysis dose should be used (110), while blood pressure—and preferably ICP—are carefully monitored and maintained. With CRRT, regional, rather than systemic, anticoagulation is most often used to improve filter longevity, most often with citrate. Since citrate accumulates with poor hepatic function, ionized calcium levels must be regularly monitored (111).

Infections

ALF is associated with reticuloendothelial dysfunction and impaired immunity, with reduced complement levels, abnormal opsonization, and ineffective phagocytosis (112,113). ALF patients are, therefore, at high risk of nosocomial infections with both bacterial and fungal pathogens, which occur in almost 40% of these patients (114). Early diagnosis can be difficult since patients often have subtle manifestations of infection but is vital because of the high associated morbidity and mortality (34,115). Daily surveillance cultures (urine, blood, sputum) and chest radiography should be considered, as they may improve early diagnosis of infection and guide selection of antimicrobial agents (115). Although prophylactic antibiotics (enteral and parenteral) decrease the risk of infection in ALF, they have not been shown to improve survival and may promote infection with resistant pathogens (116). Nevertheless, many clinicians prefer to use them, especially in patients listed for transplantation. Empiric broad-spectrum antibiotics (including vancomycin and an antifungal agent, as indicated) should be administered to any patient with ALF who develops significant isolates on surveillance cultures (114), unexplained progression of HE (34), or signs of SIRS (35), as these frequently predict sepsis in patients with ALF.

Coagulopathy

Despite a deficiency of clotting factors, low fibrinogen, thrombocytopenia, and platelet dysfunction, clinically important spontaneous bleeding is relatively infrequent in patients with ALF, being seen in less than 10% of patients. Therefore, the routine use of blood products to correct these abnormalities is not justified since they are unnecessary, ineffective, and interfere with the prognostic utility of the INR. Correction of coagulopathy should be performed in the setting of significant hemorrhage, or in anticipation of invasive procedures (117). Vitamin K deficiency has been reported to contribute to the coagulopathy of ALF (118) and should be repleted parenterally (10 mg subcutaneously [SC] or slow [over 30 minutes] IV). rFVIIa (40 μg/kg) may be considered in patients with life-threatening bleeding and prior to placement of an ICP monitor or performance of a liver biopsy (46,119). If fibrinogen levels are low (less than 100 mg/dL), cryoprecipitate should be given prior to rFVIIa. The risk of thrombosis with rFVIIa is increasingly being documented (120), even among patients with ALF (121). Coagulopathy and mechanical ventilation are well-established indications for gastrointestinal (GI) stress ulcer prophylaxis, which has been shown to decrease the risk of GI bleeding in ALF patients (122,123). Mechanical methods of deep venous thrombosis prophylaxis are recommended in place of low-dose unfractionated heparin or low-molecular-weight heparin.

Metabolic Derangements

ALF is a catabolic state, with increased energy requirements and negative nitrogen balance, which may in turn contribute to immunosuppression (94). Higher-than-usual caloric intake is therefore recommended, with 35 to 40 kcal/kg per day and 0.8 to 1 g/kg per day of protein, preferably provided via the enteral route. Reduced hepatic glycogen stores and impaired gluconeogenesis are responsible for the frequent development of hypoglycemia, which often requires treatment with intravenous dextrose (94). Conversely, hyperglycemia may contribute to increases in ICP and other complications (124,125). Thus, blood glucose values must be closely monitored and maintained within the normal range with intravenous short-acting insulin.

Liver Transplantation for ALF

OLT remains the treatment of last resort for ALF. The decision to list a patient with ALF for OLT requires careful clinical and psychosocial assessment and should be started immediately on recognition of poor prognosis as discussed above. In addition to usual clinical evaluation, patients with ALF due to APAP overdose often present with histories of suicidal ideation or substance abuse (5), which may preclude their consideration as viable OLT candidates. Since OLT candidates with ALF are generally younger and healthier than their counterparts with chronic liver disease, the pretransplant evaluation can usually be abbreviated to include echocardiography, duplex ultrasonography of the liver, and routine pretransplant laboratories (e.g., total anti-CMV, HIV antibody).

Criteria for listing a patient with ALF for OLT change and current criteria may be found at UNOS.ORG in Policy 3.6. Presently, patients with ALF are given priority to receive a cadaveric organ over all patients with chronic liver disease (status 1). Candidates must have a life expectancy without OLT of less than 7 days, have onset of hepatic encephalopathy within 8 weeks of the first symptoms of liver disease, and no history of pre-existing liver disease. In addition, patients must be in the ICU and must fulfill one of the following three criteria: (i) be ventilator dependent; (ii) require dialysis or CRRT; or (iii) have an INR more than 2.0. Patients with acute decompensated Wilson disease may also be listed as status 1 in consideration with their extremely poor prognosis for spontaneous survival. Before transporting a patient with ALF to the operating room for OLT, a detailed rereview of the patient's neurologic status must be made so that OLT is not performed when likelihood of neurologic recovery is poor. Specifically, it has been observed that severe, sustained intracranial hypertension predicts brainstem herniation during OLT or poor neurologic recovery after OLT, and patients with ICP greater than 40 mm Hg or CPP less than 40 mm Hg for more than 2 hours appear to be particularly vulnerable to these disastrous outcomes (126).

Early (3-month) mortality after OLT for ALF is higher than for patients transplanted for all causes of chronic liver disease—about 20% versus 10%, respectively (127), reflecting the acuity and severity of disease at the time of transplant. Thereafter, however, 5- and 10-year survival after OLT for ALF approximates 70% and 65%, respectively (127).

CHRONIC LIVER FAILURE

Definitions and Immediate Concerns

Almost all patients with chronic liver failure have underlying cirrhosis, the fibroinflammatory alteration of hepatic architecture that results from numerous chronic insults to the liver. Immediate concerns regarding every patient with chronic liver failure on presentation to the ICU include assessment for possible infection and upper gastrointestinal bleeding, which precipitate most admissions (128).

Overview

Patients with chronic liver disease develop liver failure (decompensation) as a result of portal hypertension and hepatocellular insufficiency. Complications of portal hypertension include hemodynamic alterations, functional renal failure, ascites, and gastrointestinal bleeding, most commonly from variceal hemorrhage. Complications of hepatocellular insufficiency include coagulopathy and hepatic encephalopathy, although it should be appreciated that the latter occurs also as a result of portosystemic shunting. An important trend in recent management of patients admitted to the hospital for decompensated cirrhosis has been an increasing use of ICUs (from 18%–28% of hospitalizations in one major center over 10 years) (128).

Etiology

According to the Scientific Registry of Transplant Recipients, the most common cause of end-stage liver disease in the United States is chronic hepatitis C, with or without a contribution from alcohol abuse (about 40% of cases) (129). Patients with alcoholic cirrhosis and indeterminate (cryptogenic) causes, many of whom have nonalcoholic steatohepatitis (NASH), occupy second and third most frequent causes, respectively. Other less common causes include chronic hepatitis B, immune-mediated liver diseases (autoimmune hepatitis, primary biliary cirrhosis, primary sclerosing cholangitis), and hereditary liver diseases (hemochromatosis, alpha-1-antitrypsin deficiency).

Assessment of Prognosis in Cirrhotic Patients Admitted to the ICU

The assessment of prognosis in cirrhotic patients admitted to the ICU is essential to identify patients in whom aggressive treatment is likely futile. Several prognostic schemes have been assessed (Table 154.5), and those using general organ system assessments, such as the Sequential Organ Failure Assessment (SOFA) score, appear to be more accurate than liver-specific schemes (130–132). Indeed, the number of organ systems (cardiovascular, respiratory, hepatic, renal, coagulation, and neurologic) failing 24 hours after ICU admission strongly predicts in-hospital mortality, from 33% in patients with failure of one organ to 97% in those with failure of three or more organs (131,132). It should be emphasized that, in the absence of OLT as a therapeutic option, cirrhotic patients admitted to the ICU have a very poor long-term prognosis, with 69% 1-year mortality and median survival of only 1 month (133). In such patients, a high APACHE III score, vasopressor use, mechanical ventilation, and jaundice predict in-hospital mortality (133,134).

Management of Complications of Chronic Liver Failure in the ICU

Evaluation of Abdominal Pain

The development of abdominal pain in a patient with end-stage liver disease often denotes a life-threatening complication of cirrhosis or portal hypertension. Certain causes of abdominal pain have increased prevalence in patients with cirrhosis and deserve particular emphasis because of high morbidity and mortality, as well as often subtle presentation (Table 154.6). A diagnostic paracentesis should be performed immediately in any patient with ascites and abdominal pain to diagnose spontaneous bacterial peritonitis (SBP), and look for evidence of gastrointestinal tract perforation into ascites. The latter may be distinguished from SBP by its higher total protein and LDH concentration, the isolation of more than one organism (including anaerobes and *Candida*), lower glucose, and trend toward higher white blood cell (WBC) and polymorphonuclear (PMN) leucocyte counts (135). Hemoperitoneum from spontaneous rupture of a mesenteric varix (136) or hepatocellular carcinoma (137) may also be rapidly detected by diagnostic paracentesis, in which case the patient should be referred for emergent interventional angiography.

The diagnosis and treatment of intra-abdominal catastrophes in patients with cirrhosis remains challenging. Specifically, complicated gallstone and peptic ulcer disease may present

TABLE 154.5

CALCULATION OF THE SEQUENTIAL ORGAN FAILURE ASSESSMENT (SOFA) SCORE TO PREDICT IN-HOSPITAL MORTALITY IN PATIENTS WITH CIRRHOSIS ADMITTED TO THE ICU

Organ system (criterion)	0 Points	1 Point	2 Points	3 Points	4 Points
Respiratory (PaO_2/FiO_2)	>400	301–400	201–300	101–200 (ventilated)	≤100 (ventilated)
Hemostatic (platelets [$\times 10^3/mm^3$])	>150	101–150	51–100	21–50	≤20
Hepatic (bilirubin [mg/dL])	<1.2	1.2–1.9	2.0–5.9	6.0–11.9	>12.0
Cardiovascular[a] (hypotension)	MAP ≥0 mm Hg	MAP <70 mm Hg	Dopamine ≤5 or dobutamine[a]	Dopamine >5 or epi/norepi ≤0.1	Dopamine >15 or epi/norepi >0.1
Neurologic (Glasgow coma score)	15	13–14	10–12	6–9	<6
Renal (creatinine [mg/dL])	<1.2	1.2–1.9	2.0–3.4	3.5–4.9	>5.0

PaO_2/FiO_2, arterial oxygen tension/fractional inspired oxygen; MAP, mean arterial pressure; epi, epinephrine; norepi, norepinephrine.
A SOFA score with a cutoff of 8 points had a sensitivity of 95%, specificity of 88%, overall correctness of 91%, PPV of 87%, and NPV of 96% for predicting in-hospital mortality.
[a] Adrenergic agents in μg/kg/min.
Modified from Wehler M, Kokoska J, Reulbach U, et al. Short-term prognosis in critically ill patients with cirrhosis assessed by prognostic scoring systems. *Hepatology*. 2004;34(2):255–261.

TABLE 154.6

DIFFERENTIAL DIAGNOSIS OF ABDOMINAL PAIN IN PATIENTS WITH CIRRHOSIS

Cause of abdominal pain	Etiologic associations	Clinical presentation	References
Spontaneous bacterial peritonitis	Low protein ascites	Fever, rebound tenderness, HE, azotemia	Runyon, 2004 (150)
Incarcerated hernia (umbilical, inguinal)	Ascites, recanalization of the umbilical vein	Localized pain, bowel obstruction	Carbonell et al., 2005 (219)
Cholelithiasis and complications	Pigmented gallstones	Localized pain, jaundice, fever, pancreatitis	Silva and Wong, 2005 (138); Perkins et al., 2004 (220)
Peptic ulcer and complications	Decompensated cirrhosis, *Helicobacter* infection	UGI bleeding, perforated viscous	Calvet et al., 1998 (221); Lehnert and Herfarth, 1993 (139); Mosnier et al., 1992 (222)
Hepatocellular carcinoma	Spontaneous rupture	Hemoperitoneum (rare)	Castells et al., 2001 (137)
Portal/mesenteric venous thrombosis	Hepatocellular carcinoma	Bowel ischemia, GI bleeding, ileus	Amitrano et al., 2004 (140)
Rupture of mesenteric varix	Recent large-volume paracentesis	Hemoperitoneum	Akriviadis, 1997 (223); Arnold et al., 1997 (136)

HE, hepatic encephalopathy; UGI, upper gastrointestinal; GI, gastrointestinal.
In addition to the usual causes of abdominal pain and acute abdomen in the general ICU population, all of the above have been described with higher prevalence in patients with cirrhosis. Appropriate screening tests for the above include diagnostic paracentesis, duplex ultrasonography, contrast-enhanced abdominal computerized tomography (CT), and/or upper endoscopy.

less acutely in patients with cirrhosis, delaying diagnosis; in those requiring surgical intervention, morbidity and mortality remain very high (138,139). Acute portal vein thrombosis, which may complicate cirrhosis and often denotes development of hepatocellular carcinoma (HCC), should be suspected in patients with abdominal pain, GI bleeding, and ileus (140), and should prompt screening with Doppler ultrasound. However, if the thrombus propagates acutely into the superior mesenteric vein, bowel ischemia and infarction, and death, usually ensue.

Cardiovascular Complications

The resting hemodynamic state in decompensated cirrhosis consists of systemic hypotension due to systemic and splanchnic arterial dilation (141,142). Consequently, patients with decompensated cirrhosis have marked arterial underfilling of systemic vascular beds in the renal arterial and hypothalamic circulations, resulting in the elaboration of compensatory neurohumoral hormones such as renin, vasopressin, and norepinephrine. The primary pathogenic mechanism underlying this hyperdynamic state includes release of vasodilatory mediators such as endothelins and nitric oxide by the portal endothelium.

In addition, patients with decompensated cirrhosis have impaired cardiac contractility in response to stress, in particular, infection or GI bleeding (143). Such myocardial failure was formerly ascribed to the myocardial toxicity of ethanol or iron in patients with cirrhosis due to alcohol abuse or hemochromatosis, respectively. Recently, cirrhotic cardiomyopathy, depressed myocardial contractility as a complication of cirrhosis *per se*, has been proposed to explain the hemodynamic collapse in cirrhotics who experience a complication of their disease (143). Diagnostic criteria include blunted inotropic and chronotropic responses to stress, diastolic dysfunction, and prolonged QT interval on electrocardiogram (ECG). A pathogenic role of cirrhotic cardiomyopathy has also been documented in patients with the hepatorenal syndrome (144), particularly in the setting of infection (145), and in the circulatory dysfunction after large volume paracentesis without adequate plasma expansion (143,146). The treatment of heart failure in the setting of decompensated cirrhosis remains poorly defined; due to the underlying hemodynamic abnormalities, afterload reduction with angiotensin-converting enzyme inhibitors may precipitate profound hypotension and renal failure, and cardiac glycosides and β-adrenergic agonists have been shown to be relatively ineffective (143).

Ascites and Renal Complications

Acute renal failure (ARF) in patients with decompensated cirrhosis is an independent predictor of death in the ICU (147) and frequently denotes the onset of infection (148). The differential diagnosis of acute renal failure in a decompensated cirrhotic includes prerenal azotemia, hepatorenal syndrome (HRS), and acute tubular necrosis (ATN). Analysis of urine sediment and sodium differentiate the above possibilities: the former two diagnoses present with normal urine sediment and low (less than 10 mEq/L) urine sodium, and the latter with renal tubular cell debris and high urine sodium. The distinction of these causes of renal failure remains paramount, since in its late stages, HRS portends a very poor prognosis and is generally irreversible without OLT, in contrast to prerenal azotemia and ATN. In practical terms, the diagnosis of HRS is often made after the exclusion of septic shock, intrinsic renal disease, obstructive uropathy, and most important, prerenal azotemia, the latter after a 1.5-L IV fluid (normal saline with or without colloid) challenge (Table 154.7) (104).

HRS and cirrhotic ascites have the same basic pathogenesis (Fig. 154.4). As outlined above, renal arterial constriction occurs in normal compensation for systemic hypotension. Poor renal perfusion results in sodium retention, plasma volume expansion, and, in the presence of hepatic sinusoidal

TABLE 154.7

DIAGNOSTIC CRITERIA OF HEPATORENAL SYNDROME (HRS)

Major criteria
Low GFR (creatinine >2.5 mg/dL; CrCl <20 mL/min)
Absence of shock, infection, nephrotoxins
Absence of improvement after 1.5 L fluid challenge
Absence of intrinsic renal disease
Proteinuria <500 mg/d
Normal renal ultrasound
Minor criteria
Oliguria (<500 mL/d)
Urine sodium <10 mEq/L
Serum sodium <130 mEq/L

GFR, glomerular filtration rate; CrCl, creatinine clearance
Adapted from Arroyo V, Gines P, Gerbes AL, et al. Definition and diagnostic criteria of refractory ascites and hepatorenal syndrome in cirrhosis. International Ascites Club. *Hepatology*. 1996;23(1): 164–176.

hypertension, the transudation of lymph across the Glisson capsule as low-protein ascites (149). HRS can be considered an exaggeration of this renal vasoconstriction, often in the setting of cardiac hypocontractility (144).

The treatment of ascites in the ICU should include judicious administration of diuretics in subjects without marked azotemia (creatinine >2 g/dL), electrolyte abnormalities, or hypotension. A combination of furosemide and spironolactone has been shown to better effect a diuresis than either agent alone; a ratio of 40 mg of the former to 100 mg of the latter administered by mouth has been shown empirically to preserve potassium balance in most patients with cirrhosis (150), and the administration of IV albumin (12.5 g/day) may improve the efficacy of diuretics (151). Large-volume paracentesis should be performed if ascites interferes with ventilation of the patient or if diuretics result in azotemia or electrolyte abnormalities. IV colloid administration (albumin 6–8 g for each liter of ascites removed) should accompany paracentesis of greater than or equal to 5 L to prevent postparacentesis circulatory dysfunction (152). The insertion of a transjugular intrahepatic portosystemic shunt (TIPS) may be considered in patients who have failed medical therapy (104). In an ICU setting, however, patients are often too ill to consider TIPS for this indication (153), and it is important for intensivists to recognize when TIPS placement is inappropriate (Table 154.8).

TABLE 154.8

RELATIVE CONTRAINDICATIONS AND ADVERSE OUTCOMES ASSOCIATED WITH PLACEMENT OF TIPS FOR SALVAGE THERAPY OF ACUTE VARICEAL HEMORRHAGE, REFRACTORY ASCITES, OR REFRACTORY HEPATIC HYDROTHORAX

Relative Contraindications
Severe liver failure (MELD ≥20; PT >20 s; creatinine >2.0 mg/dL; bilirubin >3.0 mg/dL)
Active systemic infection (risk of TIPS infection ["endo-TIPSitis"])
Recurrent/severe hepatic encephalopathy
Current hemodynamic instability
Congestive heart failure
Chronic renal failure
Pulmonary hypertension
Adverse Outcomes
Does not improve long-term patient survival for any indication
TIPS-induced hemolytic anemia
Worsening or precipitation of hepatic encephalopathy
TIPS stenosis (>50% at 1 y; lower with covered stents)
Failure of TIPS to prevent recurrence of indication for placement (for rescue in variceal bleeding about 5%, refractory ascites 15%–60%, hepatic hydrothorax 30%–40%)

TIPS, transjugular intrahepatic portosystemic shunt; MELD, model for end-stage liver disease; PT, prothrombin time.
The above relative contraindications and adverse outcomes need to be taken in the context of the risk of immediate death as they assume less importance in the setting of rescue therapy for acute variceal bleeding.
Data adapted from Laberge JM. Transjugular intrahepatic portosystemic shunt-role in treating intractable variceal bleeding, ascites, and hepatic hydrothorax. *Clin Liver Dis*. 2006;10(3): 583–598; Sanyal AJ. The use and misuse of transjugular intrahepatic portasystemic shunts. *Curr Gastroenterol Rep*. 2000;2(1): 61–71; and Sanyal AJ. Pros and cons of TIPS for refractory ascites. *J Hepatol*. 2005;43(6):924–925.

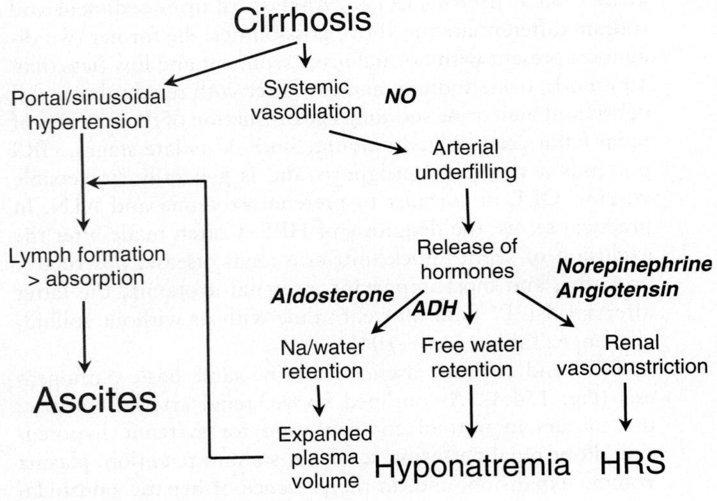

FIGURE 154.4. Pathogenesis of ascites, hepatorenal syndrome, and hyponatremia in patients with decomposed cirrhosis. Vasoactive substances are shown in *italics*. ADH, antidiuretic hormone/vasopressin; HRS, hepatorenal syndrome; NO, nitric oxide. (Adapted from Sandhu BS, Sanyal AJ. Management of ascites in cirrhosis. *Clin Liver Dis*. 2005;9[4]:715–732, viii.)

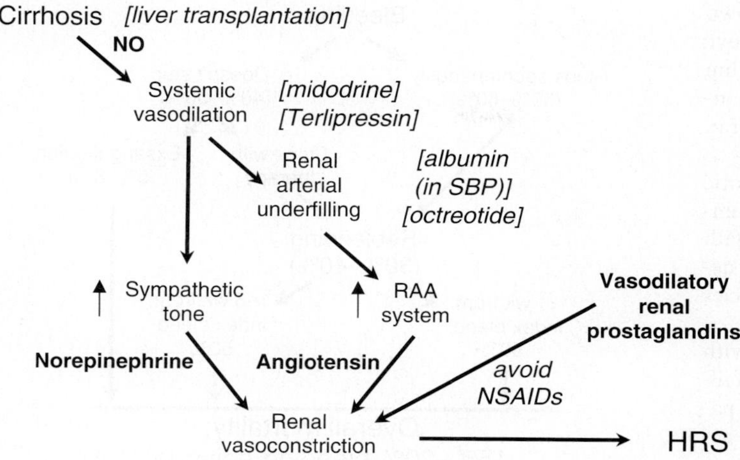

FIGURE 154.5. Pathogenesis and treatment of hepatorenal syndrome (HRS). Interventions are indicated in *bracketed italics*. HRS, hepatorenal syndrome; NO, nitric oxide; NSAIDs, nonsteroidal anti-inflammatory drugs; RAA, renin–angiotensin–aldosterone axis; SBP, spontaneous bacterial peritonitis.

The optimal treatment of HRS remains undefined (154). Figure 154.5 outlines potential treatments, not mutually exclusive, related to the pathogenetic mechanism of HRS. The ultimate treatment of the hemodynamic abnormalities of cirrhosis is OLT, which can completely reverse HRS if performed relatively soon after its onset (155). Vasoconstrictor therapy holds promise for reversing HRS by reversing the state of systemic vasodilation. The oral α-adrenergic agonist midodrine (5–10 mg orally thrice daily) was found to be effective in one widely cited but preliminary study, when used in combination with octreotide (100 μg subcutaneously twice daily), which increases systemic blood volume and thus renal blood flow by counteracting splanchnic vasodilation (156). Terlipressin, an intravenously administered vasopressin analogue with fewer ischemic complications, also reverses systemic vasodilation and has been found to effectively reverse HRS in Europe, but is not yet available in the United States (154). The administration of intravenous colloid, specifically albumin, serves to improve renal vascular perfusion (154–156). Finally, patients with decompensated cirrhosis should not receive even small therapeutic doses of NSAIDs (e.g., for fever), since these agents exacerbate renal vasoconstriction by inhibiting production of endogenous vasodilatory renal prostaglandins.

Electrolyte abnormalities frequently accompany ARF in cirrhosis and complicate the treatment of ascites. Hyponatremia and hypomagnesemia result from furosemide administration, and hyponatremia and hyperkalemia from spironolactone administration. Hyponatremia also results from hemodilution in the setting of high vasopressin release from the neurohypophysis and portends a poor prognosis (157).

Infectious Complications

Bacterial infections represent the most common cause of admission of cirrhotic patients to the ICU and remain one of the two primary causes of death (158). Risk factors for bacterial infections in hospitalized patients with cirrhosis include ICU admission and GI bleeding (159). Patients with cirrhosis are relatively immunocompromised as a result of portal hypertension and immune dysfunction. Portal hypertension results in the formation of a low-protein ascites, which is susceptible to infection because of its low complement concentration and, thus, low opsonic activity (160). In addition, gut congestion from portal hypertension increases the likelihood of bacterial translocation into blood, which seeds the ascites secondarily, so-called spontaneous bacterial peritonitis (SBP) (150).

Most studies of bacterial infections in patients with cirrhosis were performed in the 1980s, during which community-acquired, Gram-negative infections (urinary tract infections and SBP) predominated. More recent studies, however, have documented an evolution of the epidemiology of infection in patients with cirrhosis. SBP remains the most common bacterial infection in patients admitted to the ICU, but a shift toward Gram-positive infections has occurred. In one major hepatic diseases ICU, 77% of isolates were Gram-positive, which was ascribed to the widespread use of prophylactic fluoroquinolones in cirrhotic patients with low-protein ascites (161), and to the frequent use of invasive procedures, including IV catheter insertion and variceal band ligation (128). Therefore, any patient admitted to an ICU with clinical suspicion of sepsis should be empirically given IV antibacterial agents to cover Gram-positive as well as Gram-negative organisms until cultures and sensitivities allow narrowing of the regimen; empiric vancomycin should be considered in patients who have been instrumented. The choice of coverage for Gram-negative bacilli should be a third-generation cephalosporin (e.g., cefotaxime [2 g IV every 8 hours] or ceftriaxone [1 g IV every 24 hours]) (162); aminoglycosides should be avoided except in serious infections with a multiply-resistant organism because of the susceptibility of cirrhotic patients to aminoglycoside nephrotoxicity (163).

Diagnostic paracentesis should be performed on all cirrhotic patients admitted to the ICU with ascites and renal failure, HE, or any evidence of infection. Localizing symptoms and signs of peritonitis—abdominal pain, fever, rebound tenderness—may be absent in up to 30% of patients with this process. Blood and ascites should be immediately inoculated into culture bottles at the bedside, which has been shown to increase culture yields (164). However, even with bedside inoculation of a large volume of ascetic fluid (20 mL), culture yields may be as low as 40% (128). Therefore, the diagnosis of SBP should rely solely on a PMN leukocyte count of greater than or equal to 250 cells/μL, and culture-negative neutrocytic ascites—that is, with more than 250 PMNs/μL—should be considered the equivalent of SBP (165). Patients with ascetic fluid PMN count of equal to or more than 250 cells/μL should receive a third-generation cephalosporin (as above) and IV albumin (1.5 g/kg at diagnosis and 1.0 g/kg 48 hours after diagnosis), which has been shown both to decrease the incidence of HRS after SBP and to improve mortality (166). A similar diagnostic and therapeutic algorithm should be followed for spontaneous bacterial empyema, the infectious equivalent of SBP in patients with hepatic hydrothorax (see below) (167).

The incidence of fungal infections also increases in cirrhotic patients admitted to the ICU. Although not classically as immunosuppressed as after cancer chemotherapy, patients with Child's C cirrhosis have been reported to spontaneously develop invasive aspergillosis in the ICU (168). *Candida* species also rarely infect cirrhotic ascites, with disastrous outcome.

The mortality of cirrhotic patients admitted to the ICU with infection remains high, with death usually from hepatic failure, HRS, or refractory septic shock (128,169). As with patients with ALF, relative adrenal insufficiency commonly accompanies decompensated cirrhosis and sepsis, and refractory shock in such patients may respond to stress doses of corticosteroids (see Cardiovascular Complications, in ALF section above) (170).

Gastrointestinal Bleeding

Acute upper gastrointestinal (UGI) bleeding, presenting as hematemesis and/or melena, remains one of the three most common indications for admission of patients with cirrhosis to the ICU (171). Esophageal varices account for most UGI bleeds in patients with cirrhosis, with gastric varices accounting for approximately 5% to 10%, and nonvariceal UGI pathology (gastric or duodenal mucosal lesions) noted in up to 30% (172). Other uncommon causes of UGI bleeding associated with cirrhosis include portal hypertensive gastropathy and gastric antral vascular ectasia, which more often present with occult GI bleeding and anemia (173). Therefore, upper endoscopy must be performed in all patients admitted to the ICU with acute UGI bleeding to identify its source as well as administer therapy.

Patients with cirrhosis who present with acute UGI bleeding should be considered for ICU admission to deliver intensive nursing care and to manage the bleed as well as its complications. Despite the trend toward improved survival after variceal hemorrhage in the last two decades (174), each episode still carries a mortality risk of 10% to 20%, and the risk of rebleeding remains highest during the first few days after the index event (Fig. 154.6). General resuscitative measures on admission to the ICU should include correction of hypotension, repletion of blood (not to exceed a hemoglobin of approximately 8–9 g/dL), and consideration of endotracheal intubation before endoscopy (Table 154.9). A recent retrospective study has shown that endotracheal intubation prior to endoscopy may decrease the risk of fatal massive aspiration of blood, but does not decrease the risk of aspiration pneumonia (175). Factors that should contribute to the decision of whether to intubate a cirrhotic patient with an UGI bleed should include the rate of bleeding, hemodynamic instability, and degree of hepatic encephalopathy. Suppression of gastric acid secretion with proton pump inhibitors has been shown to decrease the number, size,

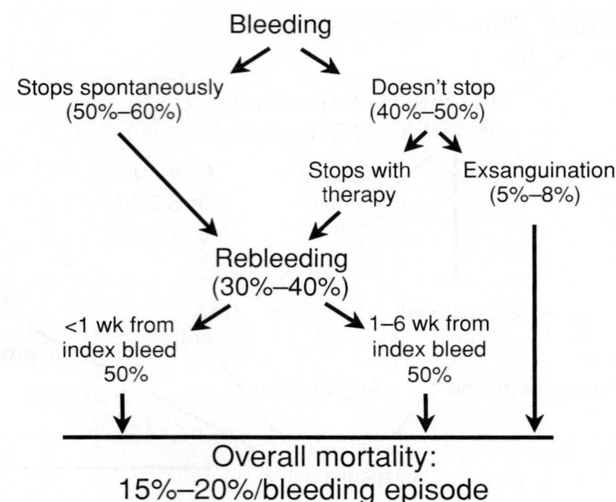

FIGURE 154.6. Natural history of acute esophageal variceal hemorrhage in patients with cirrhosis. (Adapted from de Franchis R, Primignani M. Natural history of portal hypertension in patients with cirrhosis. *Clin Liver Dis.* 2001;5[3]:645–663.)

TABLE 154.9

SPECIFIC MANAGEMENT OF ACUTE VARICEAL HEMORRHAGE AND ITS COMPLICATIONS

Therapeutic maneuver	Dose/route/indication	References
Transfusion of RBC	To hemoglobin of 8–9 g/dL	Bosch et al., 2003 (226)
Octreotide	100 μg IV bolus, then 50 μg/h for 5 d	Corley et al., 2001 (178)
Endoscopy	EVL preferred over EVS	De Franchis and Primignani, 1999 (180)
Proton pump inhibitors	Pantoprazole 40 mg IV or PO/d for 9 d	Shaheen et al., 2005 (176)
Antibiotic prophylaxis	Norfloxacin 400 mg/d for 7 d, or ceftriaxone 1 g/d for 7 d	Bernard et al., 1999 (184); Fernandez et al., 2006 (185)
TIPS	After two failed therapeutic endoscopies	Mihas and Sanyal, 2004 (181)

RBC, red blood cells; EVL, esophageal variceal ligation; EVS, endoscopic variceal sclerotherapy; TIPS, transjugular intrahepatic porto-sytemic shunt.

and complications from post–band ligation esophageal ulcers (176).

In the last 20 years, three major improvements in the management of acute variceal hemorrhage have increased survival of patients with cirrhosis: the early administration of vasoactive agents to decrease portal pressure, the widespread use of variceal band ligation, and antibiotic prophylaxis at the time of acute bleed (Table 154.9). Vasopressin, formerly used for lowering portal pressure for this indication, has fallen from favor due to vasospastic adverse effects; although the vasopressin analogue terlipressin has a better safety profile and appears to improve control of acute variceal bleeding (177), it has not yet been approved for use in the United States. The somatostatin analogue octreotide (100 μg IV bolus followed by 50 μg/hour as an IV infusion; Table 154.9) also has a favorable safety profile, and meta-analysis has demonstrated improved rates of sustained bleeding control after acute hemorrhage from esophageal varices (178). Octreotide should be administered as early as possible in a cirrhotic patient with acute UGI bleeding, preferably during transport to the hospital.

Endoscopic therapy after stabilization of the patient remains the definitive treatment for bleeding esophageal varices and controls active bleeding in more than 75% of cases when combined with vasoactive therapy (179). Endoscopic band ligation and sclerotherapy yield similar rates of control of active bleeding, but band ligation results in fewer local complications (esophageal ulcers, recurrent bleeding) and is therefore preferred (180). Recurrent bleeding should prompt a second attempt at endoscopic treatment in most cases (181). In patients with recurrence after a second endoscopic treatment, or in any recurrence with hemodynamic instability, emergent insertion of a TIPS should be considered (181). In such dire situations, the relative contraindications for TIPS placement, outlined in Table 154.7, become less important. Patients with acute hemorrhage from fundic gastric varices present a particular therapeutic challenge because the bleeding is more profuse and interventions have been less successful in controlling the acute bleed (172). Vasoactive therapy should be administered as for bleeding from esophageal varices, and sclerotherapy may be attempted. Cyanoacrylate glue injection has been shown to control acute bleeding from varices in the gastric fundus or cardia but is not widely available in the United States (182); in the absence of endoscopic and vasoactive control of gastric variceal bleeding, insertion of a large tamponade balloon (Linton tube) can temporize control before insertion of a TIPS (172).

In previous periods, bacterial infection complicated acute variceal bleeding in 40% of patients (174) and contributed to renal failure and recurrent early bleeding (183). Antibiotic prophylaxis after variceal hemorrhage has been shown to decrease the incidence of infection as well as variceal rebleeding, resulting in improved survival (183,184). Although oral or IV fluoroquinolones (norfloxacin 400 mg orally/day or ofloxacin 200 mg IV twice daily) have been more thoroughly studied for this purpose, a recent randomized trial has suggested superior efficacy of cephalosporins (for example, ceftriaxone, 1 g IV daily) because of the widespread development of resistance to the former (185); however, local resistance patterns should be considered.

Pulmonary Complications

Respiratory failure accounts for up to 40% of admissions of cirrhotic patients to the ICU (132). The differential diagnosis of respiratory distress in patients with cirrhosis may be categorized into complications of cirrhosis, pulmonary vascular diseases resulting from portal hypertension, and primary liver diseases with cardiopulmonary manifestations (Table 154.10) (186). Complications of cirrhosis include massive ascites, and hepatic hydrothorax (HH), the accumulation of extracellular fluid with similar protein characteristics as ascites (low-protein, high-albumin gradient as compared to serum) within the pleural space (167). HH usually occurs in the right pleural space (85%) and may occur in the absence of obvious ascites as a result of negative intrathoracic pressure during inspiration. The treatment of HH includes diuretic administration as for ascites, and therapeutic thoracentesis. Placement of a TIPS in patients with refractory HH may be considered but is not universally effective, and relapsefree 1-year survival is only 35% (187,188). Chest tube placement and pleurodesis are relatively contraindicated in refractory HH as they often contaminate the pleural space, precluding OLT. An infectious complication of HH, spontaneous bacterial empyema, should be diagnosed and managed similarly to SBP, but has a high mortality (167).

Two relatively uncommon, insidiously presenting pulmonary vascular complications may cause respiratory failure in patients with cirrhosis. The hepatopulmonary syndrome (HPS) may be defined as a widened alveolar-arterial oxygen due to intrapulmonary vasodilation in a patient with liver disease. The pathogenesis of HPS remains obscure but likely results from the release of vasoactive mediators from the liver, which increase intrapulmonary nitric oxide production (Fig. 154.7) (186). In a patient with cirrhosis and resting hypoxemia (PaO_2 less than 70 mm Hg while breathing an FiO_2 of 0.21), the diagnosis is confirmed by a contrast echocardiogram, in which agitated saline administered intravenously delivers microbubbles into the left ventricle at least three heartbeats after their appearance in the right ventricle (186). Supplemental oxygen usually bridges patients with HPS to OLT, which improves or reverses the process in 85% of patients (189). Patients with HPS have increased transplant waiting list mortality when compared to patients with normal gas exchange; consequently, patients with

TABLE 154.10

DIFFERENTIAL DIAGNOSIS OF RESPIRATORY DISTRESS AND HYPOXEMIA IN PATIENTS WITH CIRRHOSIS

Complications of cirrhosis
Massive ascites
Hepatic hydrothorax
Muscle wasting
Aspiration pneumonia
Pulmonary vascular disorders due to portal hypertension
Hepatopulmonary syndrome
Portopulmonary hypertension
Liver diseases with cardiopulmonary manifestations
Alpha-1-antitrypsin deficiency (basilar emphysema)
Sarcoidosis (restrictive lung disease, cardiomyopathy)
Hemochromatosis (cardiomyopathy)
Ethanol (cardiomyopathy)

Adapted from Arguedas MR, Fallon MB. Hepatopulmonary syndrome. *Clin Liver Dis.* 2005;9(4):733–746.

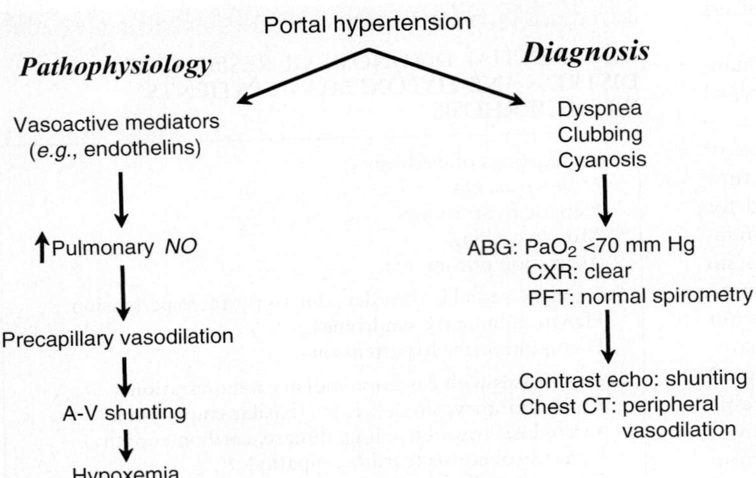

FIGURE 154.7. Pathophysiology and diagnostic algorithm of hepatopulmonary syndrome. ABG, arterial blood gas; A-V, arteriovenous; CT, computed tomography; CXR, chest x-ray film; echo, echocardiogram; NO, nitric oxide; PFT, pulmonary function testing.

HPS and PaO_2 less than 60 mm Hg on room air are allowed increased priority for OLT under the current organ allocation system in the United States (190). Perioperative mortality after OLT in patients with HPS varies according to the degree of shunting and hypoxemia (190,191).

In contrast to HPS, portopulmonary hypertension (PPH) is the development of increased pulmonary vascular resistance due to vasoconstriction and subsequent vascular remodeling in a patient with portal hypertension (Fig. 154.8) (192). Screening with transthoracic echocardiography reveals evidence of pulmonary hypertension (right ventricular systolic pressure greater than 50 mm Hg), but the diagnosis must be confirmed with right heart catheterization showing elevated mean pulmonary artery pressure (PAP more than 25 mm Hg), as well as high pulmonary vascular resistance (greater than 240 dynes/second per cm^{-5}) and normal pulmonary capillary wedge pressure (192,193). The treatment of PPH—indicated when mean PAP is more than 35 mm Hg—has not been well defined (192); prostacyclin analogues (epoprostenol titrated via pulmonary artery [PA] catheter; inhaled iloprost [5 μg six times daily]), phosphodiesterase inhibitors (sildenafil, 20 mg PO thrice daily), or combination therapy appear to be effective in small case series (192). Unfortunately, the prognosis of patients with PPH is sufficiently poor after OLT that many patients with a mean PAP more than 35 mm Hg are not offered transplant.

Neurologic Complications

Changes in mental status frequently accompany admission of patients with cirrhosis to the ICU and should not automatically suggest the presence of hepatic encephalopathy (HE) (Table 154.11). Usually, HE presents as a global decline in cognition and intellect, but focal neurologic deficits and signs of cerebral edema—decerebrate posturing and seizures—have also been described rarely (194). After screening for toxic and metabolic derangements, a severely obtunded patient should undergo non–contrast-enhanced head CT to rule out intracranial bleeding. HE may then be diagnosed on clinical grounds after ruling out the above; high serum ammonia levels may help confirm, but are not necessary to make, the diagnosis. Most important, the presentation of a patient with advanced-grade HE to the ICU should prompt a search for precipitating factors, particularly infection and UGI bleeding (Table 154.12). The

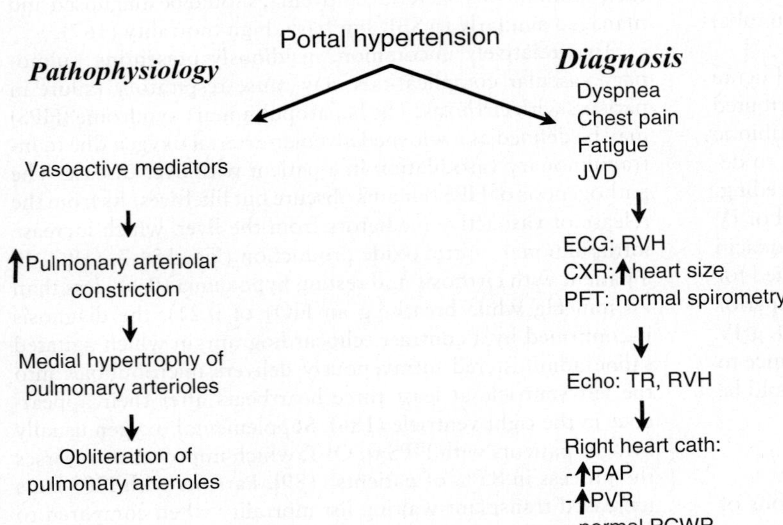

FIGURE 154.8. Pathophysiology and diagnostic algorithm of portopulmonary hypertension. ECG, electrocardiogram; JVD, jugular venous distention; PAP, pulmonary artery pressure; PCWP, pulmonary capillary wedge pressure; PFT, pulmonary function testing; PVR, pulmonary vascular resistance; RVH, right ventricular hypertrophy; TR, tricuspid valve regurgitation.

TABLE 154.11

DIFFERENTIAL DIAGNOSIS OF ALTERED MENTAL STATUS IN PATIENTS WITH CIRRHOSIS

Hepatic encephalopathy
Electrolyte abnormalities
hyponatremia
hypokalemia
hypomagnesemia
Hypoglycemia
Uremia
Intracranial bleeding
subdural hematoma
subarachnoid hemorrhage
Alcohol and/or drugs
intoxication
withdrawal

administration of broad-spectrum antibiotics (e.g., ceftriaxone) should be considered until cultures have returned negative, and fluid and electrolyte abnormalities should be corrected. If sedation is required for procedures, benzodiazepines should be used with caution, since they exacerbate even subclinical HE (195).

The specific treatment of HE poses special challenges in the ICU. The standard therapy, oral lactulose, must be administered via nasogastric tube in an intubated patient, cannot be given if there is an ileus, and its overzealous administration risks aspiration pneumonia, gaseous distention of the bowel, toxic megacolon, and electrolyte imbalance. Rectal lactulose offers an alternative route of administration, but its efficacy over tap water or saline enemas is unknown. The "nonabsorbable" antibiotic neomycin should be avoided, as the absorption of even small quantities from the gut risks renal injury. Rifaximin, a rifampin derivative that also decreases gut flora production of neurotoxins, appears to be as effective as lactulose, and has a good safety profile (196). The benzodiazepine receptor antagonist flumazenil (1 mg IV) improves HE, but the benefit wanes within 2 hours (197). Extracorporeal albumin dialysis also improves HE in refractory cases and may be considered as a bridge to OLT (198).

TABLE 154.12

PRECIPITATING EVENTS AND MECHANISMS OF HEPATIC ENCEPHALOPATHY IN PATIENTS WITH CIRRHOSIS

Event	Mechanism
Excessive protein ingestion Constipation GI bleed	↑ Gut ammonia production
Portosystemic shunting Fever, infection	↓ Neurotoxin clearance (ammonia, endogenous BZD)
Dehydration, azotemia Hypokalemia	↓ Renal excretion of ammonium
Sedatives (BZD)	↑ Inhibitory neurotransmission (GABA)

GI, gastrointestinal; BZD, benzodiazepines; GABA, gamma aminobutyric acid.

Liver Transplantation for Patients with Chronic Liver Failure in the ICU

ICUs have been increasingly used to care for patients with decompensated cirrhosis partly due to expansion of the indications for OLT. Therefore, intensivists must have a working understanding of the indications and contraindications for listing cirrhotic patients for OLT (Table 154.13). To decrease waiting list mortality, the United States has adopted a "sickest-first" policy for OLT prioritization since 1997, initially using the Child-Turcotte-Pugh (CTP) score, which is based on serum bilirubin, prothrombin time, albumin, HE, and ascites. In 2002, a new allocation system, the model of end-stage liver disease (MELD) score, was adopted by all OLT centers in the United States, based on studies that predicted a 3-month mortality in patients being considered for TIPS (199). The MELD may be calculated from serum bilirubin, creatinine, and INR, most easily on-line at UNOS.ORG. Subsequent studies have demonstrated the superiority of the MELD over the CTP system in predicting waiting list mortality (200). A minimal MELD score of 15 points for activating patients on the liver transplant waiting list has been adopted by most programs based on the observation that a MELD of 15 points predicts a 90-day mortality of about 10% without transplant, the same short-term mortality associated with transplant (201). Many patients in the ICU reach very high MELD scores (e.g., 35–40) with the onset of renal failure and are often removed from the OLT waiting list after developing infection and/or multiorgan system failure.

TABLE 154.13

INDICATIONS AND CONTRAINDICATIONS FOR LISTING PATIENTS WITH DECOMPENSATED CIRRHOSIS FOR ORTHOTOPIC LIVER TRANSPLANTATION (OLT)

Indications	Contraindications
MELD $\geq$15	Active infection outside the liver
CTP score >7	Advanced cardiopulmonary disease
Hepatopulmonary syndrome (PO_2 <60 mm Hg)	Recent or metastatic malignancy
HCC (tumor stage 2)	Uncontrolled HIV infection/AIDS
Hyponatremia (<130 mEq/L)	Cholangiocarcinoma
Ascites refractory to medical therapy[a]	Active substance abuse
Hepatic hydrothorax Hepatorenal syndrome	Psychosocial issues that would jeopardize posttransplant compliance

MELD, model for end-stage liver disease; CTP, Child-Turcotte-Pugh; HCC, hepatocellular carcinoma; HIV, human immunodeficiency virus; AIDS, acquired immunodeficiency syndrome.
[a]Refractory ascites may be functionally defined as an inadequate response to, or adverse effects (hyponatremia, hyperkalemia, azotemia) from, maximal medical therapy (104).

SUMMARY

In the United States, patients with chronic liver failure constitute an increasing proportion of ICU admissions, principally due to the maturation of the hepatitis C epidemic, which is not expected to peak until 2018. The trend may accelerate as a new wave of patients with cirrhosis due to nonalcoholic steatohepatitis decompensates, since obesity and the metabolic syndrome affect approximately one third of the U.S. population. Therefore, intensivists can expect to manage more patients with chronic liver failure to bridge them to OLT, which remains the only effective long-term therapy. In contrast to chronic liver failure, ALF patients constitute a small and numerically stable minority of patients admitted to the ICU. For intensivists, the importance of a thorough understanding of the management of ALF lies in its very high morbidity and mortality, which can be improved by vigilant intensive care as a bridge to OLT.

Stress Points: Acute Liver Failure

1. ALF is a clinical syndrome with a high mortality that affects almost every organ system.
2. The three most common causes of death in patients with ALF are cerebral edema/intracranial hypertension/brainstem herniation, infection, and multiorgan system failure.
3. OLT is a highly effective treatment for ALF but must be judiciously applied, as many patients recover spontaneously, organs are scarce, and long-term complications of OLT remain considerable (4). Therefore, prediction of death without OLT is of paramount importance.

Stress Points: Chronic Liver Disease

1. Patients with chronic liver disease are admitted to the ICU most commonly as the result of infection and/or upper GI bleeding, which results in hepatic decompensation.
2. Iatrogenic injury to a patient with decompensated chronic liver disease admitted to the ICU represents a major source of preventable morbidity and mortality. Sources of significant iatrogenic injury include nephrotoxic medications (e.g., aminoglycosides, NSAIDs) and unnecessary invasive procedures, particularly insertion of central venous and indwelling urinary catheters.
3. The prognosis of patients with cirrhosis admitted to the ICU is poor, with in-hospital mortality paralleling the degree of multiorgan system failure. Long-term prognosis of cirrhotic patients admitted to the ICU is also poor without OLT.

References

1. Trey C, Davidson C. The management of fulminant hepatic failure. *Prog Liver Dis.* 1970;3:282–298.
2. Lee WM. Acute liver failure in the United States. *Semin Liver Dis.* 2003; 23(3):217–226.
3. Williams R, Wendon J. Indications for orthotopic liver transplantation in fulminant liver failure. *Hepatology.* 1994;20:S5–10S.
4. Sethi A, Stravitz RT. Review article: medical management of the liver transplant recipient - a primer for non-transplant doctors. *Aliment Pharmacol Ther.* 2007;25:229–245.
5. Larson AM, Polson J, Fontana RJ, et al. Acetaminophen-induced acute liver failure: results of a United States multicenter, prospective study. *Hepatology.* 2005;42(6):1364–1372.
6. Vento S, Garofano T, Renzini C, et al. Fulminant hepatitis associated with hepatitis A virus superinfection in patients with chronic hepatitis C. *N Engl J Med.* 1998;338(5):286–290.
7. Polson J, Lee WM. AASLD position paper: the management of acute liver failure. *Hepatology.* 2005;41(5):1179–1197.
8. O'Grady JG, Schalm SW, Williams R. Acute liver failure: redefining the syndromes. *Lancet.* 1993;342:273–275.
9. O'Grady JG, Alexander GJ, Hayllar KM, et al. Early indicators of prognosis in fulminant hepatic failure. *Gastroenterology.* 1989;97(2):439–445.
10. Anand AC, Nightingale P, Neuberger JM. Early indicators of prognosis in fulminant hepatic failure: an assessment of the King's criteria. *J Hepatol.* 1997;26(1):62–68.
11. Stravitz RT, Kramer AH, Davern T, et al., and the Adult Acute Liver Failure Study Group. Management of acute liver failure: recommendations of the Acute Liver Failure Study Group. *Crit Care Med.* 2007;35:2498–2508.
12. Schiodt FV, Lee WM. Fulminant liver disease. *Clin Liver Dis.* 2003;7(2): 331–349.
13. Ostapowicz G, Fontana RJ, Schiodt FV, et al. Results of a prospective study of acute liver failure at 17 tertiary care centers in the United States. *Ann Intern Med.* 2002;137(12):947–954.
14. Gazzard BG, Portmann B, Murray-Lyon IM, et al. Causes of death in fulminant hepatic failure and relationship to quantitative histological assessment of parenchymal damage. *Q J Med.* 1975;44(176):615–626.
15. Smilkstein MJ, Knapp GL, Kulig KW, et al. Efficacy of oral N-acetylcysteine in the treatment of acetaminophen overdose. Analysis of the national multicenter study (1976 to 1985). *N Engl J Med.* 1988;319(24):1557–1562.
16. Smilkstein MJ, Bronstein AC, Linden C, et al. Acetaminophen overdose: a 48-hour intravenous N-acetylcysteine treatment protocol. *Ann Emerg Med.* 1991;20(10):1058–1063.
17. Makin A, Williams R. Acetaminophen-induced acute liver failure. In: Lee WM, Williams R, eds. *Acute Liver Failure.* 1st ed. Cambridge, England: Cambridge University Press; 1997:32–42.
18. Harrison PM, Keays R, Bray GP, et al. Improved outcome of paracetamol-induced fulminant hepatic failure by late administration of acetylcysteine. *Lancet.* 1990;335:1572–1573.
19. Ware AJ, D'Agostino AN, Combes B. Cerebral edema: a major complication of massive hepatic necrosis. *Gastroenterology.* 1971;61(6):877–884.
20. Jalan R. Intracranial hypertension in acute liver failure: pathophysiological basis of rational management. *Semin Liver Dis.* 2003;23(3):271–282.
21. Blei AT. The pathophysiology of brain edema in acute liver failure. *Neurochem Int.* 2005;47(1–2):71–77.
22. Kato M, Hughes RD, Keays RT, et al. Electron microscopic study of brain capillaries in cerebral edema from fulminant hepatic failure. *Hepatology.* 1992;15(6):1060–1066.
23. Ranjan P, Mishra AM, Kale R, et al. Cytotoxic edema is responsible for raised intracranial pressure in fulminant hepatic failure: in vivo demonstration using diffusion-weighted MRI in human subjects. *Metab Brain Dis.* 2005;20(3):181–192.
24. Clemmesen JO, Larsen FS, Kondrup J, et al. Cerebral herniation in patients with acute liver failure is correlated with arterial ammonia concentration. *Hepatology.* 1999;29(3):648–653.
25. Swain M, Butterworth RF, Blei AT. Ammonia and related amino acids in the pathogenesis of brain edema in acute ischemic liver failure in rats. *Hepatology.* 1992;15(3):449–453.
26. Cordoba J, Gottstein J, Blei AT. Glutamine, myo-inositol, and organic brain osmolytes after portocaval anastomosis in the rat: implications for ammonia-induced brain edema. *Hepatology.* 1996;24(4):919–923.
27. Lai JC, Cooper AJ. Neurotoxicity of ammonia and fatty acids: differential inhibition of mitochondrial dehydrogenases by ammonia and fatty acyl coenzyme A derivatives. *Neurochem Res.* 1991;16(7):795–803.
28. Butterworth RF. Glutamate transporters in hyperammonemia. *Neurochem Int.* 2002;41:81–85.
29. Hermenegildo C, Monfort P, Felipo V. Activation of N-methyl-D-aspartate receptors in rat brain in vivo following acute ammonia intoxication: characterization by in vivo brain microdialysis. *Hepatology.* 2000;31(3):709–715.
30. Wendon JA, Harrison PM, Keays R, et al. Cerebral blood flow and metabolism in fulminant liver failure. *Hepatology.* 1994;19(6):1407–1413.
31. Master S, Gottstein J, Blei AT. Cerebral blood flow and the development of ammonia-induced brain edema in rats after portacaval anastomosis. *Hepatology.* 1999;30(4):876–880.
32. Aggarwal S, Kramer D, Yonas H, et al. Cerebral hemodynamic and metabolic changes in fulminant hepatic failure: a retrospective study. *Hepatology.* 1994;19(1):80–87.
33. Aggarwal S, Obrist W, Yonas H, et al. Cerebral hemodynamic and metabolic profiles in fulminant hepatic failure: relationship to outcome. *Liver Transpl.* 2005;11(11):1353–1360.
34. Vaquero J, Polson J, Chung C, et al. Infection and the progression of hepatic encephalopathy in acute liver failure. *Gastroenterology.* 2003;125(3):755–764.
35. Rolando N, Wade J, Davalos M, et al. The systemic inflammatory response syndrome in acute liver failure. *Hepatology.* 2000;32:734–739.
36. Strauss G, Hansen BA, Kirkegaard P, et al. Liver function, cerebral blood

flow autoregulation, and hepatic encephalopathy in fulminant hepatic failure. *Hepatology.* 1997;25(4):837–839.
37. Larsen FS, Ejlersen E, Hansen BA, et al. Functional loss of cerebral blood flow autoregulation in patients with fulminant hepatic failure. *J Hepatol.* 1995;23(2):212–217.
38. Dethloff T, Knudsen GM, Hansen BA, et al. Effects of porta-systemic shunting and ammonia infusion on cerebral blood flow autoregulation in the rat. *Neurocrit Care.* 2005;3(1):86–90.
39. Strauss GI, Hogh P, Moller K, et al. Regional cerebral blood flow during mechanical hyperventilation in patients with fulminant hepatic failure. *Hepatology.* 1999;30(6):1368–1373.
40. Alba L, Hay JE, Angullo P, et al. Lactulose therapy in acute liver failure [abstract]. *Hepatology.* 2002;36:33A.
41. Greenberg LH, Momary H. Audiotoxicity and nephrotoxicity due to orally administered neomycin. *JAMA.* 1965;194(7):827–828.
42. Munoz SJ, Robinson M, Northrup B, et al. Elevated intracranial pressure and computed tomography of the brain in fulminant hepatocellular failure. *Hepatology.* 1991;13(2):209–212.
43. Wijdicks EF, Plevak DJ, Rakela J, et al. Clinical and radiologic features of cerebral edema in fulminant hepatic failure. *Mayo Clin Proc.* 1995;70(2): 119–124.
44. Vaquero J, Fontana RJ, Larson AM, et al. Complications and use of intracranial pressure monitoring in patients with acute liver failure and severe encephalopathy. *Liver Transpl.* 2005;11(12):1581–1589.
45. Blei AT, Olafsson S, Webster S, et al. Complications of intracranial pressure monitoring in fulminant hepatic failure. *Lancet.* 1993;341:157–158.
46. Shami VM, Caldwell SH, Hespenheide EE, et al. Recombinant activated factor VII for coagulopathy in fulminant hepatic failure compared with conventional therapy. *Liver Transpl.* 2003;9(2):138–143.
47. Keays RT, Alexander GJ, Williams R. The safety and value of extradural intracranial pressure monitors in fulminant hepatic failure. *J Hepatol.* 1993;18(2):205–209.
48. Herrine S, Northup B, Bell R, et al. The effect of head elevation on cerebral perfusion pressure in fulminant hepatic failure [abstract]. *Hepatology.* 1995;22:289A.
49. Ng I, Lim J, Wong HB. Effects of head posture on cerebral hemodynamics: its influences on intracranial pressure, cerebral perfusion pressure, and cerebral oxygenation. *Neurosurgery.* 2004;54(3):593–597.
50. Dodek P, Keenan S, Cook D, et al. Evidence-based clinical practice guideline for the prevention of ventilator-associated pneumonia. *Ann Intern Med.* 2004;141(4):305–313.
51. Yano M, Nishiyama H, Yokota H, et al. Effect of lidocaine on ICP response to endotracheal suctioning. *Anesthesiology.* 1986;64(5):651–653.
52. Robinson N, Clancy M. In patients with head injury undergoing rapid sequence intubation, does pretreatment with intravenous lignocaine/lidocaine lead to an improved neurological outcome? A review of the literature. *Emerg Med J.* 2001;18(6):453–457.
53. Basile AS, Hughes RD, Harrison PM, et al. Elevated brain concentrations of 1,4-benzodiazepines in fulminant hepatic failure. *N Engl J Med.* 1991; 325(7):473–478.
54. Wijdicks EF, Nyberg SL. Propofol to control intracranial pressure in fulminant hepatic failure. *Transplant Proc.* 2002;34(4):1220–1222.
55. Cremer OL, Moons KG, Bouman EA, et al. Long-term propofol infusion and cardiac failure in adult head-injured patients. *Lancet.* 2001;357:117–118.
56. Mazzara JT, Ayres SM, Grace WJ. Extreme hypocapnia in the critically ill patient. *Am J Med.* 1974;56(4):450–456.
57. Stocchetti N, Maas AI, Chieregato A, et al. Hyperventilation in head injury: a review. *Chest.* 2005;127(5):1812–1827.
58. Marion DW, Puccio A, Wisniewski SR, et al. Effect of hyperventilation on extracellular concentrations of glutamate, lactate, pyruvate, and local cerebral blood flow in patients with severe traumatic brain injury. *Crit Care Med.* 2002;30(12):2619–2625.
59. Coles JP, Minhas PS, Fryer TD, et al. Effect of hyperventilation on cerebral blood flow in traumatic head injury: clinical relevance and monitoring correlates. *Crit Care Med.* 2002;30(9):1950–1959.
60. Strauss G, Hansen BA, Knudsen GM, et al. Hyperventilation restores cerebral blood flow autoregulation in patients with acute liver failure. *J Hepatol.* 1998;28(2):199–203.
61. Raghavan M, Marik PE. Therapy of intracranial hypertension in patients with fulminant hepatic failure. *Neurocrit Care.* 2006;4(2):179–189.
62. Coles JP, Fryer TD, Coleman MR, et al. Hyperventilation following head injury: effect on ischemic burden and cerebral oxidative metabolism. *Crit Care Med.* 2007;35:568–578.
63. Ede RJ, Gimson AE, Bihari D, et al. Controlled hyperventilation in the prevention of cerebral oedema in fulminant hepatic failure. *J Hepatol.* 1986; 2(1):43–51.
64. Ogden AT, Mayer SA, Connolly ES Jr. Hyperosmolar agents in neurosurgical practice: the evolving role of hypertonic saline. *Neurosurgery.* 2005;57(2):207–215.
65. Diringer MN, Zazulia AR. Osmotic therapy: fact and fiction. *Neurocrit Care.* 2004;1(2):219–233.
66. Canalese J, Gimson AE, Davis C, et al. Controlled trial of dexamethasone and mannitol for the cerebral oedema of fulminant hepatic failure. *Gut.* 1982;23(7):625–629.
67. Hanid MA, Davies M, Mellon PJ, et al. Clinical monitoring of intracranial pressure in fulminant hepatic failure. *Gut.* 1980;21(10):866–869.
68. Marshall LF, Smith RW, Rauscher LA, et al. Mannitol dose requirements in brain-injured patients. *J Neurosurg.* 1978;48(2):169–172.
69. Gondim FA, Aiyagari V, Shackleford A, et al. Osmolality not predictive of mannitol-induced acute renal insufficiency. *J Neurosurg.* 2005;103(3):444–447.
70. White H, Cook D, Venkatesh B. The use of hypertonic saline for treating intracranial hypertension after traumatic brain injury. *Anesth Analg.* 2006;102(6):1836–1846.
71. Murphy N, Auzinger G, Bernel W, et al. The effect of hypertonic sodium chloride on intracranial pressure in patients with acute liver failure. *Hepatology.* 2004;39(2):464–470.
72. Cordoba J, Gottstein J, Blei AT. Chronic hyponatremia exacerbates ammonia-induced brain edema in rats after portacaval anastomosis. *J Hepatol.* 1998;29(4):589–594.
73. Tandon BN, Joshi YK, Tandon M. Acute liver failure. Experience with 145 patients. *J Clin Gastroenterol.* 1986;8(6):664–668.
74. Srivastava KL, Mittal A, Kumar A, et al. Predictors of outcome in fulminant hepatic failure in children. *Indian J Gastroenterol.* 1998;17(2):43–45.
75. Forbes A, Alexander GJ, O'Grady JG, et al. Thiopental infusion in the treatment of intracranial hypertension complicating fulminant hepatic failure. *Hepatology.* 1989;10(3):306–310.
76. Tofteng F, Larsen FS. The effect of indomethacin on intracranial pressure, cerebral perfusion and extracellular lactate and glutamate concentrations in patients with fulminant hepatic failure. *J Cereb Blood Flow Metab.* 2004; 24(7):798–804.
77. Diringer MN, Reaven NL, Funk SE, et al. Elevated body temperature independently contributes to increased length of stay in neurologic intensive care unit patients. *Crit Care Med.* 2004;32(7):1489–1495.
78. Munoz SJ, Moritz MJ, Bell R, et al. Factors associated with severe intracranial hypertension in candidates for emergency liver transplantation. *Transplantation.* 1993;55(5):1071–1074.
79. Zwingmann C, Chatauret N, Rose C, et al. Selective alterations of brain osmolytes in acute liver failure: protective effect of mild hypothermia. *Brain Res.* 2004;999(1):118–123.
80. Chatauret N, Zwingmann C, Rose C, et al. Effects of hypothermia on brain glucose metabolism in acute liver failure: a H/C-nuclear magnetic resonance study. *Gastroenterology.* 2003;125(3):815–824.
81. Jalan R, Olde Damink SW, Deutz NE, et al. Moderate hypothermia prevents cerebral hyperemia and increase in intracranial pressure in patients undergoing liver transplantation for acute liver failure. *Transplantation.* 2003;75(12):2034–2039.
82. Jalan R, Olde Damink SW, Deutz NE, et al. Restoration of cerebral blood flow autoregulation and reactivity to carbon dioxide in acute liver failure by moderate hypothermia. *Hepatology.* 2001;34(1):50–54.
83. Jalan R, Damink SW, Deutz NE, et al. Moderate hypothermia for uncontrolled intracranial hypertension in acute liver failure. *Lancet.* 1999;354: 1164–1168.
84. Jalan R, Olde Damink SW, Deutz NE, et al. Moderate hypothermia in patients with acute liver failure and uncontrolled intracranial hypertension. *Gastroenterology.* 2004;127(5):1338–1346.
85. Mayer SA, Kowalski RG, Presciutti M, et al. Clinical trial of a novel surface cooling system for fever control in neurocritical care patients. *Crit Care Med.* 2004;32(12):2508–2515.
86. Diringer MN. Treatment of fever in the neurologic intensive care unit with a catheter-based heat exchange system. *Crit Care Med.* 2004;32(2):559–564.
87. White H, Venkatesh B. Applications of transcranial Doppler in the ICU: a review. *Intensive Care Med.* 2006;32(7):981–994.
88. Dunn IF, Ellegala DB, Kim DH, Litvack ZN. Neuromonitoring in neurological critical care. *Neurocrit Care.* 2006;4(1):83–92.
89. Ellis AJ, Wendon JA, Williams R. Subclinical seizure activity and prophylactic phenytoin infusion in acute liver failure: a controlled clinical trial. *Hepatology.* 2000;32(3):536–541.
90. Claassen J, Mayer SA, Kowalski RG, et al. Detection of electrographic seizures with continuous EEG monitoring in critically ill patients. *Neurology.* 2004;62(10):1743–1748.
91. Bhatia V, Batra Y, Acharya SK. Prophylactic phenytoin does not improve cerebral edema or survival in acute liver failure—a controlled clinical trial. *J Hepatol.* 2004;41(1):89–96.
92. Harry R, Auzinger G, Wendon J. The clinical importance of adrenal insufficiency in acute hepatic dysfunction. *Hepatology.* 2002;36(2):395–402.
93. Marik PE, Gayowski T, Starzl TE. The hepatoadrenal syndrome: a common yet unrecognized clinical condition. *Crit Care Med.* 2005;33(6):1254–1259.
94. Schneeweiss B, Pammer J, Ratheiser K, et al. Energy metabolism in acute hepatic failure. *Gastroenterology.* 1993;105(5):1515–1521.
95. Bihari D, Gimson AE, Waterson M, et al. Tissue hypoxia during fulminant hepatic failure. *Crit Care Med.* 1985;13(12):1034–1039.
96. Clemmesen O, Ott P, Larsen FS. Splanchnic metabolism in acute liver failure and sepsis. *Curr Opin Crit Care.* 2004;10(2):152–155.
97. Beale RJ, Hollenberg SM, Vincent JL, Parrillo JE. Vasopressor and inotropic support in septic shock: an evidence-based review. *Crit Care Med.* 2004;32(11 Suppl):S455–S465.

98. Pinsky MR. Hemodynamic monitoring over the past 10 years. *Crit Care.* 2006;10(1):117.
99. Trewby PN, Warren R, Contini S, et al. Incidence and pathophysiology of pulmonary edema in fulminant hepatic failure. *Gastroenterology.* 1978; 74(5 Pt 1):859–865.
100. [No authors listed.] Ventilation with lower tidal volumes as compared with traditional tidal volumes for acute lung injury and the acute respiratory distress syndrome. The Acute Respiratory Distress Syndrome Network. *N Engl J Med.* 2000;342(18):1301–1308.
101. Gajic O, Dara SI, Mendez JL, et al. Ventilator-associated lung injury in patients without acute lung injury at the onset of mechanical ventilation. *Crit Care Med.* 2004;32(9):1817–1824.
102. Ring-Larsen H, Palazzo U. Renal failure in fulminant hepatic failure and terminal cirrhosis: a comparison between incidence, types, and prognosis. *Gut.* 1981;22(7):585–591.
103. Moore K. Renal failure in acute liver failure. *Eur J Gastroenterol Hepatol.* 1999;11(9):967–975.
104. Arroyo V, Gines P, Gerbes AL, et al. Definition and diagnostic criteria of refractory ascites and hepatorenal syndrome in cirrhosis. International Ascites Club. *Hepatology.* 1996;23(1):164–176.
105. Kellum J, Palevsky PM. Renal support in acute kidney injury. *Lancet.* 2006; 368:344–345.
106. Davenport A, Will EJ, Davidson AM. Improved cardiovascular stability during continuous modes of renal replacement therapy in critically ill patients with acute hepatic and renal failure. *Crit Care Med.* 1993;21(3):328–338.
107. Davenport A. Renal replacement therapy for patients with acute liver failure awaiting orthotopic hepatic transplantation. *Nephron.* 1991;59(2):315–316.
108. Naka T, Wan L, Bellomo R, et al. Kidney failure associated with liver transplantation or liver failure: the impact of continuous veno-venous hemofiltration. *Int J Artif Organs.* 2004;27(11):949–955.
109. Schortgen F, Soubrier N, Delclaux C, et al. Hemodynamic tolerance of intermittent hemodialysis in critically ill patients: usefulness of practice guidelines. *Am J Respir Crit Care Med.* 2000;162(1):197–202.
110. Ronco C, Bellomo R, Homel P, et al. Effects of different doses in continuous veno-venous haemofiltration on outcomes of acute renal failure: a prospective randomised trial. *Lancet.* 2000;356(9223):26–30.
111. Meier-Kriesche HU, Finkel KW, Gitomer JJ, et al. Unexpected severe hypocalcemia during continuous venovenous hemodialysis with regional citrate anticoagulation. *Am J Kidney Dis.* 1999;33(4):e8.
112. Wyke RJ, Rajkovic IA, Eddleston AL, et al. Defective opsonisation and complement deficiency in serum from patients with fulminant hepatic failure. *Gut.* 1980;21(8):643–649.
113. Canalese J, Gove CD, Gimson AE, et al. Reticuloendothelial system and hepatocytic function in fulminant hepatic failure. *Gut.* 1982;23(4):265–269.
114. Rolando N, Philpott-Howard J, Williams R. Bacterial and fungal infection in acute liver failure. *Semin Liver Dis.* 1996;16(4):389–402.
115. Rolando N, Harvey F, Brahm J, et al. Prospective study of bacterial infection in acute liver failure: an analysis of fifty patients. *Hepatology.* 1990; 11(1):49–53.
116. Rolando N, Gimson A, Wade J, et al. Prospective controlled trial of selective parenteral and enteral antimicrobial regimen in fulminant liver failure. *Hepatology.* 1993;17(2):196–201.
117. Gazzard BG, Henderson JM, Williams R. Early changes in coagulation following a paracetamol overdose and a controlled trial of fresh frozen plasma therapy. *Gut.* 1975;16(8):617–620.
118. Pereira SP, Rowbotham D, Fitt S, et al. Pharmacokinetics and efficacy of oral versus intravenous mixed-micellar phylloquinone (vitamin K1) in severe acute liver disease. *J Hepatol.* 2005;42(3):365–370.
119. Jeffers L, Chalasani N, Balart L, et al. Safety and efficacy of recombinant factor VIIa in patients with liver disease undergoing laparoscopic liver biopsy. *Gastroenterology.* 2002;123(1):118–126.
120. O'Connell KA, Wood JJ, Wise RP, et al. Thromboembolic adverse events after use of recombinant human coagulation factor VIIa. *JAMA.* 2006; 295(3):293–298.
121. Pavese P, Bonadona A, Beaubien J, et al. FVIIa corrects the coagulopathy of fulminant hepatic failure but may be associated with thrombosis: a report of four cases. *Can J Anaesth.* 2005;52(1):26–29.
122. MacDougall BR, Williams R. H2-receptor antagonist in the prevention of acute upper gastrointestinal hemorrhage in fulminant hepatic failure: a controlled trial. *Gastroenterology.* 1978;74(2 Pt 2):464–465.
123. Cook DJ, Fuller HD, Guyatt GH, et al. Risk factors for gastrointestinal bleeding in critically ill patients. Canadian Critical Care Trials Group. *N Engl J Med.* 1994;330(6):377–381.
124. Kodakat S, Gopal P, Wendon J. Hyperglycaemia is associated with intracranial hypertension in patients with acute liver failure [abstract]. *Liver Transpl.* 2001;7(6):C-21.
125. Van den BG, Schoonheydt K, Becx P, et al. Insulin therapy protects the central and peripheral nervous system of intensive care patients. *Neurology.* 2005;64(8):1348–1353.
126. Lidofsky SD, Bass NM, Prager MC, et al. Intracranial pressure monitoring and liver transplantation for fulminant hepatic failure. *Hepatology.* 1992; 16(1):1–7.
127. Roberts MS, Angus DC, Bryce CL, et al. Survival after liver transplantation in the United States: a disease-specific analysis of the UNOS database. *Liver Transpl.* 2004;10(7):886–897.
128. Fernandez J, Navasa M, Gomez J, et al. Bacterial infections in cirrhosis: epidemiological changes with invasive procedures and norfloxacin prophylaxis. *Hepatology.* 2002;35(1):140–148.
129. Shiffman ML, Saab S, Feng S, et al. Liver and intestine transplantation in the United States, 1995–2004. *Am J Transplant.* 2006;6:1170–1187.
130. Ho YP, Chen YC, Yang C, et al. Outcome prediction for critically ill cirrhotic patients: a comparison of APACHE II and Child-Pugh scoring systems. *J Intensive Care Med.* 2004;19(2):105–110.
131. Wehler M, Kokoska J, Reulbach U, et al. Short-term prognosis in critically ill patients with cirrhosis assessed by prognostic scoring systems. *Hepatology.* 2004;34(2):255–261.
132. Cholongitas E, Senzolo M, Patch D, et al. Risk factors, sequential organ failure assessment and model for end-stage liver disease scores for predicting short term mortality in cirrhotic patients admitted to intensive care unit. *Aliment Pharmacol Ther.* 2006;23(7):883–893.
133. Gildea TR, Cook WC, Nelson DR, et al. Predictors of long-term mortality in patients with cirrhosis of the liver admitted to a medical ICU. *Chest.* 2004;126(5):1598–1603.
134. Aggarwal A, Ong JP, Younossi ZM, et al. Predictors of mortality and resource utilization in cirrhotic patients admitted to the medical ICU. *Chest.* 2001;119(5):1489–1497.
135. Runyon BA, Hoefs JC. Ascitic fluid analysis in the differentiation of spontaneous bacterial peritonitis from gastrointestinal tract perforation into ascitic fluid. *Hepatology.* 1984;4(3):447–450.
136. Arnold C, Haag K, Blum HE, et al. Acute hemoperitoneum after large-volume paracentesis. *Gastroenterology.* 1997;113(3):978–982.
137. Castells L, Moreiras M, Quiroga S, et al. Hemoperitoneum as a first manifestation of hepatocellular carcinoma in western patients with liver cirrhosis: effectiveness of emergency treatment with transcatheter arterial embolization. *Dig Dis Sci.* 2001;46(3):555–562.
138. Silva MA, Wong T. Gallstones in chronic liver disease. *J Gastrointest Surg.* 2005;9:739–746.
139. Lehnert T, Herfarth C. Peptic ulcer surgery in patients with liver cirrhosis. *Ann Surg.* 1993;217:338–346.
140. Amitrano L, Guardascione MA, Brancaccio V, et al. Risk factors and clinical presentation of portal vein thrombosis in patients with liver cirrhosis. *J Hepatol.* 2004;40(5):736–741.
141. Schrier RW, Arroyo V, Bernardi M, et al. Peripheral arterial vasodilation hypothesis: a proposal for the initiation of renal sodium and water retention in cirrhosis. *Hepatology.* 1988;8(5):1151–1157.
142. Liu H, Gaskari SA, Lee SS. Cardiac and vascular changes in cirrhosis: pathogenic mechanisms. *World J Gastroenterol.* 2006;12(6):837–842.
143. Gaskari SA, Honar H, Lee SS. Therapy insight: cirrhotic cardiomyopathy. *Nat Clin Pract Gastroenterol Hepatol.* 2006;3(6):329–337.
144. Ruiz-del-Arbol L, Monescillo A, Arocena C, et al. Circulatory function and hepatorenal syndrome in cirrhosis. *Hepatology.* 2005;42(2):439–447.
145. Ruiz-del-Arbol L, Urman J, Fernàndez J, et al. Systemic, renal, and hepatic hemodynamic derangement in cirrhotic patients with spontaneous bacterial peritonitis. *Hepatology.* 2003;38:1210–1218.
146. Ruiz-del-Arbol L, Monescillo A, Jimenez W, et al. Paracentesis-induced circulatory dysfunction: mechanism and effect on hepatic hemodynamics in cirrhosis. *Gastroenterology.* 1997;113(2):579–586.
147. du Cheyron D, Bouchet B, Parienti JJ, et al. The attributable mortality of acute renal failure in critically ill patients with liver cirrhosis. *Intensive Care Med.* 2005;31(12):1693–1699.
148. Terra C, Guevara M, Torre A, et al. Renal failure in patients with cirrhosis and sepsis unrelated to spontaneous bacterial peritonitis: value of MELD score. *Gastroenterology.* 2005;129(6):1944–1953.
149. Runyon BA, Montano AA, Akriviadis EA, et al. The serum-ascites albumin gradient is superior to the exudate-transudate concept in the differential diagnosis of ascites. *Ann Intern Med.* 1992;117(3):215–220.
150. Runyon BA. Management of adult patients with ascites due to cirrhosis. *Hepatology.* 2004;39(3):841–856.
151. Gentilini P, Casini-Raggi V, Di FG, et al. Albumin improves the response to diuretics in patients with cirrhosis and ascites: results of a randomized, controlled trial. *J Hepatol.* 1999;30(4):639–645.
152. Gines P, Tito L, Arroyo V, et al. Randomized comparative study of therapeutic paracentesis with and without intravenous albumin in cirrhosis. *Gastroenterology.* 1988;94(6):1493–1502.
153. Sanyal AJ. Pros and cons of TIPS for refractory ascites. *J Hepatol.* 2005; 43(6):924–925.
154. Arroyo V, Terra C, Gines P. New treatments of hepatorenal syndrome. *Semin Liver Dis.* 2006;26(3):254–264.
155. Cardenas A, Gines P. Therapy insight: management of hepatorenal syndrome. *Nat Clin Pract Gastroenterol Hepatol.* 2006;3(6):338–348.
156. Angeli P, Volpin R, Gerunda G, et al. Reversal of type 1 hepatorenal syndrome with the administration of midodrine and octreotide. *Hepatology.* 1999;29(6):1690–1697.
157. Heuman DM, bou-Assi SG, Habib A, et al. Persistent ascites and low serum sodium identify patients with cirrhosis and low MELD scores who are at high risk for early death. *Hepatology.* 2004;40(4):802–810.

158. Caly WR, Strauss E. A prospective study of bacterial infections in patients with cirrhosis. *J Hepatol.* 1993;18(3):353–358.
159. Deschenes M, Villeneuve JP. Risk factors for the development of bacterial infections in hospitalized patients with cirrhosis. *Am J Gastroenterol.* 1999;94(8):2193–2197.
160. Runyon BA, Morrissey RL, Hoefs JC, et al. Opsonic activity of human ascitic fluid: a potentially important protective mechanism against spontaneous bacterial peritonitis. *Hepatology.* 1985;5(4):634–637.
161. Gines P, Rimola A, Planas R, et al. Norfloxacin prevents spontaneous bacterial peritonitis recurrence in cirrhosis: results of a double-blind, placebo-controlled trial. *Hepatology.* 1990;12:716–724.
162. Runyon BA, McHutchison JG, Antillon MR, et al. Short-course versus long-course antibiotic treatment of spontaneous bacterial peritonitis. A randomized controlled study of 100 patients. *Gastroenterology.* 1991; 100(6):1737–1742.
163. Hampel H, Bynum GD, Zamora E, et al. Risk factors for the development of renal dysfunction in hospitalized patients with cirrhosis. *Am J Gastroenterol.* 2001;96(7):2206–2210.
164. Runyon BA, Antillon MR, Akriviadis EA, et al. Bedside inoculation of blood culture bottles with ascitic fluid is superior to delayed inoculation in the detection of spontaneous bacterial peritonitis. *J Clin Microbiol.* 1990;28(12): 2811–2812.
165. Runyon BA, Hoefs JC. Culture-negative neutrocytic ascites: a variant of spontaneous bacterial peritonitis. *Hepatology.* 1984;4(6):1209–1211.
166. Sort P, Navasa M, Arroyo V, et al. Effect of intravenous albumin on renal impairment and mortality in patients with cirrhosis and spontaneous bacterial peritonitis. *N Engl J Med.* 1999;341(6):403–409.
167. Garcia N Jr, Mihas AA. Hepatic hydrothorax: pathophysiology, diagnosis, and management. *J Clin Gastroenterol.* 2004;38(1):52–58.
168. Meersseman W, Vandecasteele SJ, Wilmer A, et al. Invasive aspergillosis in critically ill patients without malignancy. *Am J Respir Crit Care Med.* 2004; 170(6):621–625.
169. Follo A, Llovet JM, Navasa M, et al. Renal impairment after spontaneous bacterial peritonitis in cirrhosis: incidence, clinical course, predictive factors and prognosis. *Hepatology.* 1994;20(6):1495–1501.
170. Fernandez J, Escorsell A, Zabalza M, et al. Adrenal insufficiency in patients with cirrhosis and septic shock: effect of treatment with hydrocortisone on survival. *Hepatology.* 2006;44(5):1288–1295.
171. de Franchis R, Primignani M. Natural history of portal hypertension in patients with cirrhosis. *Clin Liver Dis.* 2001;5(3):645–663.
172. Ryan BM, Stockbrugger RW, Ryan JM. A pathophysiologic, gastroenterologic, and radiologic approach to the management of gastric varices. *Gastroenterology.* 2004;126(4):1175–1189.
173. Payen JL, Cales P, Voigt JJ, et al. Severe portal hypertensive gastropathy and antral vascular ectasia are distinct entities in patients with cirrhosis. *Gastroenterology.* 1995;108(1):138–144.
174. Carbonell N, Pauwels A, Serfaty L, et al. Improved survival after variceal bleeding in patients with cirrhosis over the past two decades. *Hepatology.* 2004;40(3):652–659.
175. Rudolph SJ, Landsverk BK, Freeman ML. Endotracheal intubation for airway protection during endoscopy for severe upper GI hemorrhage. *Gastrointest Endosc.* 2003;57(1):58–61.
176. Shaheen NJ, Stuart E, Schmitz SM, et al. Pantoprazole reduces the size of postbanding ulcers after variceal band ligation: a randomized, controlled trial. *Hepatology.* 2005;41(3):588–594.
177. Ioannou GN, Doust J, Rockey DC. Systematic review: terlipressin in acute oesophageal variceal haemorrhage. *Aliment Pharmacol Ther.* 2003; 17(1):53–64.
178. Corley DA, Cello JP, Adkisson W, et al. Octreotide for acute esophageal variceal bleeding: a meta-analysis. *Gastroenterology.* 2001;120(4):946–954.
179. Cardenas A, Gines P. Management of complications of cirrhosis in patients awaiting liver transplantation. *J Hepatol.* 2005;42(Suppl 1):S124–S133.
180. de Franchis R, Primignani M. Endoscopic treatments for portal hypertension. *Semin Liver Dis.* 1999;19(4):439–455.
181. Mihas AA, Sanyal AJ. Recurrent variceal bleeding despite endoscopic and medical therapy. *Gastroenterology.* 2004;127(2):621–629.
182. Sarin SK, Jain AK, Jain M, et al. A randomized controlled trial of cyanoacrylate versus alcohol injection in patients with isolated fundic varices. *Am J Gastroenterol.* 2002;97(4):1010–1015.
183. Hou MC, Lin HC, Liu TT, et al. Antibiotic prophylaxis after endoscopic therapy prevents rebleeding in acute variceal hemorrhage: a randomized trial. *Hepatology.* 2004;39(3):746–753.
184. Bernard B, Grange JD, Khac EN, et al. Antibiotic prophylaxis for the prevention of bacterial infections in cirrhotic patients with gastrointestinal bleeding: a meta-analysis. *Hepatology.* 1999;29(6):1655–1661.
185. Fernandez J, Ruiz del AL, Gomez C, et al. Norfloxacin vs ceftriaxone in the prophylaxis of infections in patients with advanced cirrhosis and hemorrhage. *Gastroenterology.* 2006;131(4):1049–1056.
186. Arguedas MR, Fallon MB. Hepatopulmonary syndrome. *Clin Liver Dis.* 2005;9(4):733–46.
187. Siegerstetter V, Deibert P, Ochs A, et al. Treatment of refractory hepatic hydrothorax with transjugular intrahepatic portosystemic shunt: long-term results in 40 patients. *Eur J Gastroenterol Hepatol.* 2001;13(5):529–534.
188. Therapondos G, Wong F. Miscellaneous indications for transjugular intrahepatic portosystemic stent-shunt. *Eur J Gastroenterol Hepatol.* 2006; 18(11):1161–1166.
189. Lange PA, Stoller JK. The hepatopulmonary syndrome. Effect of liver transplantation. *Clin Chest Med.* 1996;17(1):115–123.
190. Mandell MS. The diagnosis and treatment of hepatopulmonary syndrome. *Clin Liver Dis.* 2006;10(2):387–405.
191. Collisson EA, Nourmand H, Fraiman MH, et al. Retrospective analysis of the results of liver transplantation for adults with severe hepatopulmonary syndrome. *Liver Transpl.* 2002;8(10):925–931.
192. Krowka MJ. Evolving dilemmas and management of portopulmonary hypertension. *Semin Liver Dis.* 2006;26(3):265–272.
193. Krowka MJ, Swanson KL, Frantz RP, et al. Portopulmonary hypertension: results from a 10-year screening algorithm. *Hepatology.* 2006;44(6):1502–1510.
194. Cadranel JF, Lebiez E, Di Martino V, et al. Focal neurological signs in hepatic encephalopathy in cirrhotic patients: an underestimated entity? *Am J Gastroenterol.* 2001;96(2):515–518.
195. Vasudevan AE, Goh KL, Bulgiba AM. Impairment of psychomotor responses after conscious sedation in cirrhotic patients undergoing therapeutic upper GI endoscopy. *Am J Gastroenterol.* 2002;97(7):1717–1721.
196. Mas A, Rodes J, Sunyer L, et al. Comparison of rifaximin and lactitol in the treatment of acute hepatic encephalopathy: results of a randomized, double-blind, double-dummy, controlled clinical trial. *J Hepatol.* 2003;38(1):51–58.
197. Barbaro G, Di LG, Soldini M, et al. Flumazenil for hepatic encephalopathy grade III and IVa in patients with cirrhosis: an Italian multicenter double-blind, placebo-controlled, cross-over study. *Hepatology.* 1998;28(2):374–378.
198. Heemann U, Treichel U, Loock J, et al. Albumin dialysis in cirrhosis with superimposed acute liver injury: a prospective, controlled study. *Hepatology.* 2002;36:949–958.
199. Kamath PS, Wiesner RH, Malinchoc M, et al. A model to predict survival in patients with end-stage liver disease. *Hepatology.* 2001;33(2):464–470.
200. Wiesner R, Edwards E, Freeman R, et al. Model for end-stage liver disease (MELD) and allocation of donor livers. *Gastroenterology.* 2003;124(1):91–96.
201. Merion RM, Schaubel DE, Dykstra DM, et al. The survival benefit of liver transplantation. *Am J Transplant.* 2005;5(2):307–313.
202. Bernuau J, Rueff B, Benhamou JP. Fulminant and subfulminant liver failure: definitions and causes. *Semin Liver Dis.* 1986;6(2):97–106.
203. Bernuau J, Samuel D, Durand F. Criteria for emergency liver transplantation in patients with acute viral hepatitis and factor V below 50% of normal: a prospective study [abstract]. *Hepatology.* 1991;14:49A.
204. Pereira LM, Langley PG, Hayllar KM, et al. Coagulation factor V and VIII/V ratio as predictors of outcome in paracetamol induced fulminant hepatic failure: relation to other prognostic indicators. *Gut.* 1992;33(1):98–102.
205. Donaldson BW, Gopinath R, Wanless IR, et al. The role of transjugular liver biopsy in fulminant liver failure: relation to other prognostic indicators. *Hepatology.* 1993;18(6):1370–1376.
206. Schmidt LE, Dalhoff K. Serum phosphate is an early predictor of outcome in severe acetaminophen-induced hepatotoxicity. *Hepatology.* 2002;36(3): 659–665.
207. Bernal W, Donaldson N, Wyncoll D, et al. Blood lactate as an early predictor of outcome in paracetamol-induced acute liver failure: a cohort study. *Lancet.* 2002;359:558–563.
208. Bernal W, Wendon J, Rela M, et al. Use and outcome of liver transplantation in acetaminophen-induced acute liver failure. *Hepatology.* 1998;27(4): 1050–1055.
209. Mitchell I, Bihari D, Chang R, et al. Earlier identification of patients at risk from acetaminophen-induced acute liver failure. *Crit Care Med.* 1998; 26(2):279–284.
210. Rossaro L, Chambers C, Polson J, et al. Performance of MELD in predicting outcome in acute liver failure [abstract]. *Am J Transpl.* 2005;5:A248.
211. Sanyal AJ, Stravitz RT. Acute liver failure. In: Boyer TD, Wright T, Manns MP, eds. *Hepatology—Textbook of Liver Disease.* 5th ed. Philadelphia, PA: Elsevier Science; 2006:383–415.
212. Buckley NA, Whyte IM, O'Connell DL, et al. Oral or intravenous N-acetylcysteine: which is the treatment of choice for acetaminophen (paracetamol) poisoning? *J Toxicol Clin Toxicol.* 1999;37(6):759–767.
213. Broussard CN, Aggarwal A, Lacey SR, et al. Mushroom poisoning—from diarrhea to liver transplantation. *Am J Gastroenterol.* 2001;96(11):3195–3198.
214. Peters DJ, Greene WH, Ruggiero F, et al. Herpes simplex-induced fulminant hepatitis in adults: a call for empiric therapy. *Dig Dis Sci.* 2000;45(12): 2399–2404.
215. Kessler WR, Cummings OW, Eckert G, et al. Fulminant hepatic failure as the initial presentation of acute autoimmune hepatitis. *Clin Gastroenterol Hepatol.* 2004;2(7):625–631.
216. Tillmann HL, Hadem J, Leifeld L, et al. Safety and efficacy of lamivudine in patients with severe acute or fulminant hepatitis B, a multicenter experience. *J Viral Hepat.* 2006;13(4):256–263.
217. Rodriguez FE, Tremosa LG, Xiol Q, et al. D-penicillamine and plasmapheresis in acute liver failure secondary to Wilson's disease. *Rev Esp Enferm Dig.* 2003;95(1):60–65.

218. Castro MA, Fassett MJ, Reynolds TB, et al. Reversible peripartum liver failure: a new perspective on the diagnosis, treatment, and cause of acute fatty liver of pregnancy, based on 28 consecutive cases. *Am J Obstet Gynecol.* 1999;181(2):389–395.
219. Carbonell AM, Wolfe LG, DeMaria EJ. Poor outcomes in cirrhosis-associated hernia repair: a nationwide cohort study of 32,033 patients. *Hernia.* 2005;9(4):353–357.
220. Perkins L, Jeffries M, Patel T. Utility of preoperative scores for predicting morbidity after cholecystectomy in patients with cirrhosis. *Clin Gastroenterol Hepatol.* 2004;2(12):1123–1128.
221. Calvet X, Navarro M, Gil M, et al. Epidemiology of peptic ulcer disease in cirrhotic patients: role of Helicobacter pylori infection. *Am J Gastroenterol.* 1998;93(12):2501–2507.
222. Mosnier H, Farges O, Vons C, et al. Gastroduodenal perforation in the patient with cirrhosis. *Surg Gynecol Obstet.* 1992;174:297–301.
223. Akriviadis EA. Hemoperitoneum in patients with ascites. *Am J Gastroenterol.* 1997;92(4):567–575.
224. Laberge JM. Transjugular intrahepatic portosystemic shunt-role in treating intractable variceal bleeding, ascites, and hepatic hydrothorax. *Clin Liver Dis.* 2006;10(3):583–598.
225. Sanyal AJ. The use and misuse of transjugular intrahepatic portasystemic shunts. *Curr Gastroenterol Rep.* 2000;2(1):61–71.
226. Bosch J, Abraldes JG, Groszmann R. Current management of portal hypertension. *J Hepatol.* 2003;38(Suppl 1):S54–S68.
227. Sandhu BS, Sanyal AJ. Management of ascites in cirrhosis. *Clin Liver Dis.* 2005;9(4):715–732, viii.

CHAPTER 155 ■ PANCREATIC DISEASE

FELICIA A. IVASCU • GEORGE D. GARCIA • DANNY SLEEMAN

OVERVIEW

Acute pancreatitis has an annual incidence of 5 to 40 per 100,000 (1,2) with an overall mortality of 1.5 per 100,000 (1). The clinical course of acute pancreatitis is often self-limited and results in little, if any, structural alteration of the gland and requires no intervention. Approximately one third of patients, however, develop pancreatic necrosis, which has an associated mortality rate that can be as high as 30% (1,3). All complications of this disease are potentially lethal and may require aggressive intervention to control or abort the process, and support the patient until the condition is resolved. Because of this, acute pancreatitis can be among the most difficult of clinical entities to treat. Very few, if any, other conditions present with such a myriad of origins, diagnostic difficulties, clinical manifestations, risk of multisystem involvement, and indeterminate prognosis for such a prolonged period. Severe acute pancreatitis often demands an extended stay in the intensive care unit and hours on hours of multidisciplinary care. Numerous causative factors of acute pancreatitis have been recognized. The most important risk factors for pancreatitis in adults are gallstones and excessive alcohol use, although clinically detectable pancreatitis never develops in most persons with these risk factors. The incidence of gallstone pancreatitis is increased among white women older than the age of 60 years (4,5) and is highest in patients with gallstones <5 mm in diameter (5,6). Other causes include metabolic derangements such as hypertriglyceridemia, duct obstruction (for example, related to tumor or pancreas divisum), medications (i.e., azathioprine, thiazides, and estrogens), and trauma. About 20% of cases remain idiopathic, although this classification is expected to become less common as factors of genetic predisposition and environmental susceptibility are elucidated (7).

Trypsin is the key enzyme in the activation of pancreatic zymogens. Underlying the pathophysiology of acute pancreatitis is the inappropriate conversion of trypsinogen to trypsin and a lack of prompt elimination of active trypsin inside the pancreas (7). Activation of other pancreatic enzymes causes injury to the gland and results in an inflammatory process that seems to be out of proportion to the response of other organs to a similar insult, possibly due to disturbances in the microcirculation of the pancreas and the exquisite sensitivity of the pancreas to ischemia (8). In addition to further significant tissue damage as a direct result, the inflammatory process may extend beyond the pancreas and result in the systemic inflammatory response syndrome, multiorgan failure, and ultimately, death.

DIAGNOSIS OF THE DISEASE PROCESS

At times, diagnosing acute pancreatitis may be as difficult as predicting the course or defining the treatment. Even with history, physical examination, laboratory values, radiographic studies, and special procedures, a conclusive diagnosis of acute pancreatitis and its complications is often elusive. The best approach may be to elucidate the history of a similar attack or hospitalization and identify associated etiologic factors, most commonly alcohol abuse or biliary tract disease.

The recurrence rate of acute pancreatitis has been reported to be as high as 33% (9) and can be even higher in the alcoholic population (10). Disease isolated to the head or tail of the pancreas may result in pain localized to the right or left upper quadrant with diaphragmatic irritation and referred pain to the subcapsular areas. The classic presentation of epigastric pain that radiates through to the back may be present in only 50% of patients presenting with acute pancreatitis. After the patient develops peritoneal signs, pancreatitis can mimic all other acute abdominal crises, especially those necessitating emergent surgery.

Laboratory Testing

Of the biochemical diagnostic criteria, the most commonly used is the serum amylase level (11). Serum amylase levels that are more than three times the upper limit of normal are almost always caused by acute pancreatitis given the appropriate clinical presentation (12). Although the serum amylase concentration begins to rise shortly after onset of the disease, it may return to normal levels in 2 to 4 days. However, a normal serum amylase level does not exclude the disease. In one series, up to 19% of patients with an attack of acute pancreatitis had a normal serum amylase level and an abnormal computerized tomography scan (13). Acute pancreatitis with normal serum amylase levels is often characterized by a high prevalence of patients with an alcoholic etiology and a longer duration of symptoms before admission (14). Other factors that may contribute to the absence of elevated serum amylase levels include return to normal levels prior to presentation or the inability of an inflamed or chronically diseased pancreas to produce a significant quantity of amylase. Pancreatitis secondary to biliary tract disease will often present with some of the highest serum amylase levels. In addition, an elevated alanine aminotransferase level in a patient without alcoholism who has pancreatitis is the single best predictor of biliary pancreatitis with a level more than three times the upper limit of normal having a positive predictive value of 95% for gallstone pancreatitis (15). The clinician must remain aware that an elevated serum amylase is not necessarily diagnostic of acute pancreatitis. The differential diagnosis of hyperamylasemia includes perforated or penetrating gastric ulcer, ruptured ectopic pregnancy, and intestinal obstruction or infarction. Measuring urinary amylase, amylase-to-creatinine ratios (16), and amylase isoenzymes (17) have shown little clinical advantage, with the exception of ruling out macroamylasemias.

An elevated concentration of serum lipase, however, is quite sensitive for diagnosis of acute pancreatitis secondary to alcohol abuse (18). Lipase levels tend to remain elevated longer than amylase concentrations. Therefore, an elevated lipase level can be useful information for patients who present later in the course of disease and who may have a normal amylase concentration. Serum lipase levels, although thought to be more specific for pancreatic destruction, have little, if any, role in predicting severity of disease.

Although elevated serum amylase and lipase levels are most widely used for the diagnosis of acute pancreatitis, as stated, they have little, if any, value in predicting the severity of disease. In an attempt at early prediction of severity of pancreatitis, the four most reliable serum markers are polymorphonuclear (PMN) elastase, albumin, C-reactive protein, and pancreatic amylase (14). An acute phase reactant, C-reactive protein, is most widely used. While elevated levels of C-reactive protein have been associated with pancreatic necrosis (19,20), a 24- to 48-hour latency for C-reactive protein to reach optimal predictability is well recognized (21–24), perhaps limiting its use as an early predictor of disease severity. Measuring levels of trypsinogen activation peptide (25) and trypsinogen-2 (26) are more specific for acute pancreatitis but are not widely available. Of the many cytokines that have been evaluated in an attempt to predict severity, interleukin (IL)-6 appears to hold the most promise, although further studies are needed (27) regarding its potential use as a clinically relevant predictor of disease severity.

Except for differentiation of other bacterial sources of peritonitis or diagnosis of complications of pancreatitis that would necessitate surgery, diagnostic peritoneal lavage has had little or no role in our institution in making the definitive diagnosis or assessing the prognosis of a given episode of pancreatitis.

Radiologic and Diagnostic Studies

Numerous radiologic findings are suggestive of, but not specific for, pancreatitis. These include dilatation of the first portion of the duodenum (duodenal ileus), dilatation of the first loop of the jejunum (jejunal ileus or sentinel loop), dilatation of the transverse colon or colon cutoff sign (secondary to a transverse colonic ileus), and elevated hemidiaphragm and pleural effusion, especially on the left side (secondary to diaphragmatic irritation and sympathetic pleural effusions).

Transabdominal pancreatic ultrasonography is not sensitive in the diagnosis of acute pancreatitis, often because of gas in the bowel. Ultrasonography frequently provides an incomplete view of the pancreas and the peripancreatic area, especially in patients who are obese with severe disease and excessive bowel gas secondary to ileus. In addition, if imaging of the tail of the pancreas in necessary, an incomplete view may occur because of poor sonic window. It can, however, be helpful in detection of early complications of pancreatitis and identification of associated biliary tract disease (28). Transabdominal ultrasound is more sensitive than either computerized tomography or magnetic resonance imaging for identifying cholelithiasis and sludge and for detecting dilatation of the biliary ducts, but is insensitive for the detection of distal biliary duct stones (4,5). Endoscopic ultrasonography may be the most accurate test for diagnosing or ruling out biliary causes of acute pancreatitis and may guide the use of endoscopic retrograde cholangiopancreatography (ERCP) (29).

Persistent biliary obstruction worsens the outcome and increases the severity of acute pancreatitis and predisposes the patient to progression to bacterial cholangitis. ERCP is used with endoscopic sphincterotomy to extract impacted gallstones and to drain infected bile in severe acute pancreatitis (30–33). Although ERCP has recognized risk, including bleeding and either causing or exacerbating pancreatitis, complications are uncommon when performed by experienced endoscopists. Three randomized trials involving a total of 511 patients with gallstone pancreatitis compared conservative management with ERCP and endoscopic sphincterotomy within 24 to 72 hours after admission. The studies showed a significantly lower risk of pancreatitis-associated complications in the ERCP group (31). Based on this evidence, it is recommended that patients with severe acute gallstone pancreatitis undergo early ERCP and, if indicated, endoscopic sphincterotomy (30). ERCP can also demonstrate ductal disruptions in traumatic pancreatitis and may also allow identification of pancreas divisum, thought to be a rare cause of acute pancreatitis.

In patients with abdominal pain of unclear cause, computerized tomography can confirm the diagnosis of acute pancreatitis and either rule out or confirm other causes of abdominal pain. When the use of intravenous radiocontrast material is contraindicated, the diagnosis of acute pancreatitis can be inferred from homogenous glandular enlargement and the presence of peripancreatic fluid collections (34). In the absence of contraindication, computerized tomography with radiocontrast is preferred, as contrast-enhanced computed tomography (CT) remains the gold standard in the diagnosis of pancreatic necrosis (35). Determination of the extent of pancreatic necrosis correlates with prognosis as mortality increases markedly in patients with necrosis involving more than 30% of the gland (36–39). Radiocontrast allows the identification of pancreatic necrosis, which appears as focal or diffuse zones of nonenhanced parenchyma. Areas of necrosis may not be present, however, for 48 to 72 hours after presentation. In the clinically stable patient with a contraindication to intravenous contrast, magnetic resonance imaging (MRI) is an alternative method to diagnose and evaluate the extent of pancreatic necrosis. MRI may also identify early duct disruption that is not visible on CT scan (40). Although contrast-enhanced CT allows the identification of pancreatic necrosis, there are no imaging techniques that allow precise and reliable identification of infected pancreatic necrosis. The appearance of air in the pancreatic parenchyma, caused by gas-producing bacteria, is not common in patients with infected pancreatic necrosis; however, when present it usually indicates infection. Fine-needle aspiration, under CT or ultrasound guidance, with Gram staining and culture of the aspirate is the gold standard for the diagnosis of infected pancreatic necrosis (41–44). Most series report sensitivity for the prediction of infected necrosis that ranges from 90% to 100% and specificity between 96% and 100% (41,45,46).

Although angiography does not have a role among the usual diagnostic techniques for pancreatitis, it has become useful for localizing hemorrhagic complications of the disease and extremely useful for nonoperative or preoperative control of bleeding vessels.

CLASSIFICATION

The Marseilles classification recognized four types of pancreatitis: (i) acute pancreatitis, (ii) recurrent acute pancreatitis, (iii) relapsing chronic pancreatitis, and (iv) chronic pancreatitis (47). This classification system has been useful to characterize the pathology of the gland and clinical episodes. The result of a 1992 International Symposium, the classification by Bradley (48) identified seven clinical entities: (i) acute pancreatitis, (ii) severe acute pancreatitis, (iii) mild acute pancreatitis, (iv) acute fluid collection, (v) pancreatic necrosis, (vi) pseudocysts, and (vii) pancreatic abscess.

The most relevant classification to the intensivist determines the degree of severity and progress of an individual episode of pancreatitis. Ranson et al. (49,50) established 11 clinical criteria, 5 of which were assessed on admission and 6 within 48 hours. They are well correlated with morbidity, number of days' stay in the ICU, and eventual mortality. The admission criteria are as follows: age older than 55 years, blood glucose level greater than 200 mg/dL, leukocyte count greater than 16,000/mm^3, serum lactate dehydrogenase (LDH) level greater than 350 IU/L, and serum glutamic-oxaloacetic transaminase (SGOT) greater than 250 Sigma Frankel units. The criteria to be determined within 48 hours are as follows: serum calcium level less than 8 mg/dL, PaO_2 less than 60 mm Hg, base deficit greater than 4 mEq/L, increase in blood urea nitrogen (BUN) of more than 5 mg/dL, decrease in hematocrit of more than 10 percentage points and more than 6 L fluid sequestration. The presence of fewer than 3 of these 11 criteria within 48 hours of admission usually correlates with a more benign form and course of disease, with an eventual mortality rate of 3%. The presence of three or more of these parameters on admission or within 48 hours usually implies a more severe form of pancreatitis and is associated with high risk of death and major complication.

The list of 11 numeric parameters proposed by Ranson et al. has suffered little discussion. With a single exception, the patients' age, these time-honored criteria are the result of the statistical analysis of 43 parameters. These parameters were gathered retrospectively from three overlapping series totaling 450 patients with acute pancreatitis (49,51,52). Of these 450 patients, however, only 94 (21%) had acute pancreatitis definitively confirmed by surgery or postmortem exam. Furthermore, the 13 parameters retained in the essentially statistical study of 1977 (51) were available in only 113 (38%) of the 300 patients studied, possibly representing a selection bias. Nevertheless, the Ranson scale has been used since the 1980s in virtually all studies relating to acute pancreatitis.

TREATMENT OF ACUTE PANCREATITIS

An overall approach to the therapy for acute pancreatitis should include placing the pancreas "at rest," supporting the patient's nutritional and metabolic needs, correcting the acute causes of morality (i.e., cardiovascular collapse, respiratory insufficiency, and renal failure), detecting those complications of disease that require surgical intervention, and preventing and treating delayed causes of mortality (i.e., septic complications).

Gland Suppression

Suppression of the secretory function of the pancreas has been attempted by elimination of oral fluids (53,54), suppression of acid secretion with various H_2 blockers (55,56) and antacids, and use of anticholinergics (47,57) and proteolytic enzyme inhibitors (58). Calcitonin (59) and somatostatin (60), which are potent inhibitors of pancreatic enzyme secretion, have also been subjected to clinical trials. Although there may be a good physiologic rationale, controlled randomized studies have not shown significant improvement.

Historically, it was felt that early feeding may increase the severity of the disease and re-exacerbate the inflammatory process. It was felt that most patients admitted to the ICU had pancreatitis of sufficient severity and associated ileus to prohibit enteral intake. Gut rest, with or without parenteral nutrition, had become regarded as the standard of care. However, it is now known that acute pancreatitis results in a hypermetabolic, hyperdynamic systemic inflammatory response syndrome that results in a catabolic state (61). Recent evidence suggests that enteral nutrition is not only feasible but may be desirable in such patients. The most severe complication of acute pancreatitis is pancreatic infection. The finding that the micro-organisms causing pancreatic infection are common enteric pathogens implies that bacterial translocation from the intestinal tract to the pancreas may have a role in the pathogenesis of infected pancreatic necrosis (62–68). Lack of enteral feeding results in atrophy of the gastrointestinal mucosa, bacterial overgrowth, increased gut permeability, and translocation of bacteria or bacterial products into the circulation. Total parenteral nutrition may, therefore, promote bacterial translocation in patients with pancreatitis.

Animal studies have shown that the site in the gastrointestinal tract to which feedings are delivered determines to what extent the pancreas is stimulated. Jejunal feedings have been shown to result in negligible increases in enzyme, bicarbonate, and volume output from the pancreas (69,70). This observation has been confirmed in humans (71). It has been suggested that enteral feeding stimulates lysosomal movement to the cell surface, minimizing the intracellular release of pancreatic enzymes and may, in fact, be therapeutic in acute pancreatitis (61). In addition, enteral nutrition reduces production of proinflammatory mediators that may also have therapeutic potential in such patients.

Several studies have now shown jejunal feeding to be not only less expensive than total parenteral nutrition but associated with fewer septic complications, possible modulation of the acute phase response (72–78), and shorter length of stay (61). Few studies, however, have addressed the potential problems associated with placement of nasojejunal tubes and the resulting delay in initiation of feeding. From studies of enteral feeding in burn patients, it seems that initiating enteral feeding within 48 hours of admission helps to maintain gut function, allowing improved tolerance and fewer problems with ileus and gastric stasis compared with feeding delayed by 4 or 5 days (79,80). In a small case series without controls, Eatock et al. (81) found that nasogastric feeding was well tolerated and did not appear to exacerbate pancreatitis. To confirm this, in the largest study to date of enteral feeding in patients with objectively graded acute pancreatitis, Eatock et al. compared the nasogastric route with the use of the nasojejunal route (82). He found that there was no evidence of exacerbation of disease with the nasogastric route, supporting the use of enteral feeding and challenging the commonly held belief that enteral feedings must be delivered distal to the ligament of Treitz.

Hypocalcemia in acute pancreatitis has many possible causes, including hypoalbuminemia (83) with decreased protein binding, formation of calcium soaps in the presence of fat necrosis (84), stimulation of calcitonin secretion (85) by increased serum glucagons (86), and decreased parathormone secretion by various mechanisms (87), but rarely is there a clinically significant decrease in ionized calcium. If deficits are found, however, calcium and magnesium are easily replaced.

Cardiovascular Collapse, Renal Failure, and Respiratory Insufficiency

One of the most important determinants of poor outcome in severe acute pancreatitis is the early development and persistence of organ dysfunction. Although various scoring systems, biomarkers, and radiologic findings can help identify patients at risk of organ dysfunction, these do not substitute for frequent clinical assessment and monitoring. Several clinical findings including thirst, poor urine output, progressive tachycardia, tachypnea, hypoxemia, agitation, confusion, a rising hematocrit level, and a lack of improvement within the first 48 hours are warning signs of impending severe disease (12). The cornerstone of management in early pancreatitis is fluid resuscitation and close monitoring for early manifestations of organ dysfunction. In addition to the frequent assessment of vital signs, the intravascular volume status should be monitored by means of physical exam and urinary output. Early identification of hypoxemia via either pulse oximetry or arterial blood gas measurement is also paramount.

Hypovolemia is easy to explain as a result of the chemical peritonitis that develops in these patients; the associated increased capillary permeability, relative lymphatic obstruction, and partial splanchnic venous obstruction can account for sequestration of up to 40% of the patient's circulatory plasma volume in just a few hours. Renal insufficiency may be a result of this massive fluid loss. If it is present, the association of renal failure in acute pancreatitis markedly increases the mortality in these patients (88).

Whether or not there is a myocardial depressant factor associated with severe pancreatitis (89), inotropic agents may be required to improve cardiac function if cardiac output remains low despite adequate filling pressures.

The respiratory insufficiency associated with severe pancreatitis is much more complex and is probably a combination of a decrease in functional residual capacity and shunting, which may be related to elevated paralyzed hemidiaphragms, basilar atelectasis, pleural effusion, empyema, pneumonia, micropulmonary emboli, or alveolar collapse secondary to the decrease in pulmonary surfactant, which is degraded by circulating pancreatic enzymes. Respiratory assistance with positive end-expiratory pressure (PEEP) is required until the process resolves and the patient can maintain adequate minute ventilation and oxygenation.

Patients with severe acute pancreatitis who meet conventional criteria should be admitted to the intensive care unit, as well as those patients who are at high risk of rapid deterioration such as the elderly (90), patients requiring ongoing volume resuscitation, those with renal failure, respiratory compromise, and evidence of substantial pancreatic necrosis (greater than 30%) (30). In addition, it has been recognized that morbidly obese patients are at increased risk for developing the severe form of acute pancreatitis. When compared to normal-weight patients, patients with a body mass index (BMI) of greater than or equal to 25 kg/m^2 and less than 30 kg/m^2 (overweight) or greater than 30 kg/m^2 (obese), the number and type of complications increased as the body mass index increased (91) in a study of 250 patients with biliary pancreatitis.

It is not known if the outcome of severe acute pancreatitis is affected by the model of critical care delivery, as there are currently no studies examining this relationship. However, a review of 26 observational studies showed that a heterogenous group of critically ill patients, when cared for by an intensivist or using an intensivist consultant in a closed ICU, had a shorter length of stay and a lower mortality rate than similar patients cared for in units without such staffing patterns (92). It is not clear whether admission of all patients with severe acute pancreatitis to the ICU will result in better outcomes, as this has not been studied. The remaining challenge is the development of a more accurate predictor of organ failure so that patients who truly need intensive care can be admitted to the ICU without delay.

Therapeutic Peritoneal Lavage

Short-term (48–96 hour) therapeutic peritoneal lavage has clearly been demonstrated by Ranson and Spencer (52) to improve the early clinical condition of patients with acute pancreatitis. In their randomized, prospective studies, the mortality rate during the first 10 days decreased from 45% in control subjects to 0% in patients treated with peritoneal lavage. Cardiovascular instability and respiratory insufficiency improved and did not result in early mortality. The overall survival rate, however, was not significantly improved; the cause of death only shifted from cardiovascular and respiratory insufficiency to late infection of devitalized pancreatic and peripancreatic tissue. When compared to short-term lavage, long-term (7-day) peritoneal lavage in severe acute pancreatitis showed a reduction in both the incidence of pancreatic sepsis and its associated mortality rate (93). This therapy, however, is a major undertaking as it involves hourly lavage for at least 7 days with an antibiotic-containing isotonic balanced electrolyte solution.

More recently a meta-analysis of peritoneal lavage for acute pancreatitis was undertaken (94). This study identified eight randomized, prospective clinical trials evaluating the use of continuous lavage in patients with pancreatitis. The duration of lavage ranged from 1 to 12 days. In contrast to the studies referred to above and several uncontrolled prospective and retrospective reviews that almost universally supported its use based on comparisons with historical controls (95–103), the results of this study indicate that continuous peritoneal lavage with crystalloid solutions in patients with acute pancreatitis has not been associated with any significant improvement in morbidity or mortality. Despite the inherent limitations, the meta-analysis supported the findings of the individual studies, as none of these found a significant difference in either morbidity or mortality between treatment or control groups.

There are several reasons to explain why continuous lavage may not be of benefit in patients with acute pancreatitis. The presence of large volumes of fluid within the peritoneal cavity may degrade the peritoneal defense mechanisms due to the inability to localize the source of contamination through local fibrinous adhesions between omentum, loops of bowel, and the abdominal wall. The lavage may, in addition, enhance the absorption of inflammatory mediators into the systemic circulation via diaphragmatic stomata (104). The lavage may also potentially remove important local inflammatory mediators and thereby impair peritoneal defense mechanisms (105,106). Last, the peritoneal mesothelial cells are usually lost in association with peritonitis, and their regeneration may be important in the resolution of the inflammation (94). Lavage, with either crystalloid or peritoneal dialysis solutions, has been found to inhibit the rate of mesothelial healing (107).

To improve the efficacy of lavage in pancreatitis, studies have focused on the benefit of adding protease inhibitors to the lavage solution, and in experimental work on animal models of pancreatitis this has been found to improve prognosis (108). Based on the apparent success of this technique, there have been two randomized clinical trials of patients with acute fulminant pancreatitis (109,110). Patients were randomized to receive either lavage containing aprotinin (a protease inhibitor) or standard lavage solution. There was no significant difference in morbidity or mortality in either trial. Aprotinin is currently not available until further safety studies are done.

Despite several early, initially enthusiastic reports, the use of continuous lavage in patients with acute pancreatitis is not supported by the currently available evidence.

Antibiotics

Bacterial infection plays an important role in the course and the management of acute pancreatitis. In the mild, self-limited form of the disease, mortality rates are less than 1% and septic complications are rare. The past decade has seen a considerable increase in our understanding and management of necrotizing pancreatitis. The natural course of severe acute pancreatitis progresses in two phases (111). The first 14 days are characterized by the systemic inflammatory response syndrome as a result of the release of multiple inflammatory mediators. The second phase, beginning roughly 2 weeks after the onset of disease, is dominated by sepsis-related complications resulting from infection of pancreatic necrosis (112,113). In the natural course of the disease, infection of pancreatic necrosis occurs in up to 70% of patients and has become the most important risk factor for death from necrotizing pancreatitis (114–116). Several factors have been associated with the infection rate of pancreatic necrosis. It has been demonstrated that the frequency of infected necrosis correlates with the duration of disease. In patients with necrotizing pancreatitis, the proportion of patients with proven infected necrosis at the time of surgery increased from 22% to 24% after the first week to 36% to 55% after the second week and up to 72% after the third week (112,114). The extent of pancreatic necrosis may also be a risk factor for infection. Beger et al. (112) reported the highest infection rates in patients with more than 50% necrosis of the pancreas. This finding is supported by the data of other investigators (117). It appears, therefore, that the presence of a significant amount of necrosis (over 50% on CT scan) may be predictive of severe disease and help identify those patients at risk of developing septic complications.

Among patients with sterile necrotizing pancreatitis, mortality rates of 10% to 15% are reported (118), whereas infected pancreatic necrosis carries with it a mortality rate of up to 50% (62,112,119). Supporting the concept that infection is the major determinant of outcome, it has been demonstrated that in patients with sterile necrosis, the extent of necrosis correlated with the frequency of organ failure, whereas infected necrosis was associated with organ failure regardless of the extent of necrosis (120).

Interest has focused on the prophylactic use of antibiotics to prevent infectious complications and reduce the associated morbidity and mortality. Initial uncontrolled studies using prophylactic antibiotics in acute pancreatitis failed to demonstrate any effect on morbidity or mortality (121–123). However, ampicillin, the most commonly used drug in those trials, failed to reach its effective minimum inhibitory concentration (MIC) in normal or necrotic pancreatic tissue (124,125). Further animal and human studies have shown that third-generation cephalosporins, piperacillin, mezlocillin, 4-quinolone, metronidazole, and imipenem can achieve their MIC in pancreatic tissue, whereas, the aminopenicillins, first-generation cephalosporins, and aminoglycosides cannot (126). The choice of antibiotic agent is critical as the agent must have a spectrum of activity against the most commonly encountered organisms found in infected necrosis and must penetrate the pancreas adequately. Buchler et al. (127,128) and Bassi et al. (129) have identified imipenem as the antibiotic agent of first choice because it reached higher pancreatic tissue levels and provided higher bactericidal activity against most of the bacteria present in pancreatic infection compared with other types of antibiotics. In a comparison between meropenem and imipenem, there were no significant differences in septic complications, indication for surgery, or mortality (130), indicating that meropenem is equally effective. The combination of quinolones and metronidazole is not an effective antibiotic prophylaxis (131). Maravi-Poma et al., in a prospective, randomized, multicenter trial (132), compared two imipenem regimens for the prevention of septic complications in patients with severe acute necrotizing pancreatitis. Patients were randomized to receive antibiotic prophylaxis either for 14 days or at least 14 days and as long as major systemic complications of the disease persisted. They found that compared to a 14-day course, longer antibiotic administration in patients with acute necrotizing pancreatitis is not associated with a reduction in the incidence of septic complications of the disease. However, prolonged imipenem administration in patients with persisting systemic complications tends to reduce mortality in acute necrotizing pancreatitis compared to a 14-day regimen.

The issue of prophylactic antibiotics was revisited in a multicenter trial (133) of 74 patients with acute necrotizing pancreatitis diagnosed by computerized tomography. Patients were randomized to intravenous imipenem or no antibiotic prophylaxis. Pancreatic infection was diagnosed either by CT-guided aspiration or culture obtained at laparotomy. Among those receiving prophylactic antibiotics, there was a numeric reduction in local pancreatic infection and in mortality. In addition, there were significantly fewer episodes of sepsis among the prophylactic antibiotic group. In a study randomizing 60 patients with acute necrotizing pancreatitis to either prophylactic cefuroxime or no antibiotic prophylaxis, there was no reduction in local pancreatic infection or sepsis (134). However, there was a significant reduction in mortality in the prophylactic group.

More recently, a prospective single-center trial by Buchler et al. (111) evaluated the role of nonsurgical management, which included the use of early antibiotics, of necrotizing pancreatitis. This study confirmed that the conservative treatment of sterile necrosis using early antibiotics (imipenem–cilastatin) is safe and effective. Of 56 patients with sterile necrosis managed without surgery, only 1 died of acute respiratory distress syndrome not responsive to treatment. This trial also demonstrated an infection rate of 34% in necrotizing pancreatitis treated with early antibiotics, which is lower than prevalence data of up to 70% observed in patients who were not treated with prophylactic antibiotics (112,135,136). Nordback et al. (137) conducted a randomized study to compare the use of early versus delayed imipenem–cilastatin in the treatment of necrotizing pancreatitis. Ninety patients with acute necrotizing pancreatitis were randomized within 48 hours to either early imipenem–cilastatin or control. The primary end point was indication for necrosectomy due to infection. In the control group, imipenem–cilastatin was started when the operative indication was fulfilled. Early imipenem–cilastatin therapy significantly reduced the need for surgery and the overall number of major organ complications in acute necrotizing pancreatitis. Furthermore, the mortality rate was reduced by half. Likewise, a meta-analysis of prophylactic antibiotic administration in acute necrotizing pancreatitis (138) revealed a significant improvement in sepsis and mortality in patients with acute necrotizing pancreatitis receiving antibiotic prophylaxis and a trend toward a reduction in local pancreatic infection.

The bacterial spectrum of infection in acute necrotizing pancreatitis has been described as primarily Gram negative and, in part, anaerobic with the predominant pathogens including *Escherichia coli*, *Pseudomonas* species, *Enterobacter*, *Bacteroides*, and *Proteus* (139). Bacterial translocation from the gut has been demonstrated to be the main cause of infection in necrotizing pancreatitis (140–143). In addition to the safety and efficacy of early antibiotic treatment in necrotizing pancreatitis, a second major finding of Buchler et al. (111) was that early antibiotic treatment of necrotizing pancreatitis changes the spectrum of bacteria in those patients who develop infection. After the administration of antibiotics with primary efficacy against Gram-negative and anaerobic bacteria, more than half of patients who developed pancreatic infection were found to have Gram-positive infection.

Similarly, Howard and Temple (144) compared operative cultures from 61 consecutive patients with pancreatic necrosis treated during routine prophylactic antibiotic use to 34 consecutive patients with necrosis prior to the use of prophylactic antibiotics. They demonstrated a dramatic shift in bacteriology between the two time periods with 56% of isolates being Gram-negative organisms in the control group to only 26% in the antibiotic treatment group. *Enterobacter*, *Pseudomonas*, and *Proteus* made up 38% of the isolates in the control group, but *Klebsiella* was the predominant Gram-negative isolate in the control group. *Enterococcus* was found in similar percentages in both groups. But in the antibiotic group, other Gram-positive cocci, including *S. epidermidis*, *S. aureus*, and *Corynebacterium* species, made up 31% of all bacterial isolates. It is likely that these infections do not originate in the gut, but rather, are nosocomial infections acquired via venous catheters, urinary catheters, or endotracheal tubes. The argument that these infections are hospital acquired is supported by the fact that these infections tend to occur much later (typically after 20 days) whereas infections with Gram-negative organisms are seen much sooner, usually within 2 weeks of admission (111).

In addition to a shift from predominantly Gram-negative to Gram-positive organisms, the question arises as to whether antibiotic prophylaxis predisposes patients to fungal infection. De Waele et al. (145) reviewed data from an 8-year period for 46 patients with severe acute pancreatitis and infected pancreatic necrosis to determine the incidence of fungal infection and to identify risk factors for the development of fungal infection. They found an overall incidence for *Candida* infection of 37% and, excluding patients who received early antifungal prophylaxis, the incidence of *Candida* infection was as high as 50%, the highest figure ever described (145). Despite the fact that the total duration of antibiotic prophylaxis was very long and multiple types of antibiotics were administered to individual patients, both described as risk factors for the development of *Candida* infection (146), they failed to identify any risk factor for fungal infection among their patients.

Buchler et al. (111) found an incidence of fungal infection of 29% among patients receiving early antibiotic treatment for necrotizing pancreatitis. However, up to 25% of patients with necrotizing pancreatitis who do not receive antibiotics also develop fungal infection (147,148). Four of the randomized trials on antibiotic prophylaxis included the incidence of fungal superinfection (133,134,149,150). The incidence of fungal infection was below seven percent in three trials (133,134,150), whereas it exceeded 20% in one small study (149). These trials were recently meta-analyzed (131). The fungal infection rate was not different between patients receiving prophylactic antibiotics (4.9%) and those in the control group (6.7%). The conclusion of this meta-analysis was that antibiotic prophylaxis does not result in increased incidence of fungal infections.

SURGICAL MANAGEMENT

Most episodes of acute pancreatitis are mild and self-limiting, resolving spontaneously within 3 to 5 days. The mortality rate in these patients is less than 1%, and these patients do not routinely require intensive care or surgical management. However, there are several absolute indications for operative intervention in patients with severe acute pancreatitis, including prevention of recurrence and treatment of complications. As the conservative management of infected pancreatic necrosis associated with multiple organ failure has a mortality rate of up to 100% (151), proven infected pancreatic necrosis, as well as septic complications directly resulting from pancreatic infection, are indications for surgical intervention (132).

Treatment of Biliary Pancreatitis

Biliary pancreatitis is most often associated with the passage of a small common bile duct stone. Typically, the highest serum amylase levels may be present initially, but they return to normal, as do the patient's clinical signs and symptoms. Occasionally, a stone may become impacted at the ampulla of Vater. In this case, rapid progressive deterioration of the patient's clinical course may soon follow. For patients with severe acute gallstone pancreatitis, urgent biliary drainage and clearance of the common bile duct must be considered. There is general agreement that open cholecystectomy with supraduodenal bile duct exploration and insertion of a T tube is an unacceptable emergency procedure in patients with severe gallstone pancreatitis, as both higher morbidity and mortality rates have been shown following early surgery (132). There is general consensus that patients with signs and symptoms consistent with cholangitis and patients with severe acute gallstone pancreatitis and obstructive jaundice should undergo urgent endoscopic retrograde cholangiopancreatography (ERCP), and, if choledocholithiasis is confirmed, endoscopic sphincterotomy should be performed (30).

In patients with severe acute pancreatitis due to suspected or proven cholelithiasis but without obstructive jaundice, the role of ERCP and endoscopic sphincterotomy is less well defined. Three trials have examined the role of emergency ERCP and endoscopic sphincterotomy (defined as within 24 hours of admission or 72 hours of onset of symptoms) as compared to conservative management (152) or planned interval ERCP (152,153) in patients with biliary pancreatitis. In all three trials, endoscopic sphincterotomy and stone extraction were performed only if common bile duct stones were identified on ERCP.

Neoptolemos et al. (153) demonstrated significantly lower morbidity rates following emergency ERCP. There was an equal distribution of patients with cholangitis in both treatment groups, and the complication rate was significantly lower after emergency ERCP, even after exclusion of these patients. Patients with biliary obstruction were excluded in the Fölsch et al. (152) trial, and median bilirubin levels were equal in both groups in the Fan et al. (154) trial. These two trials failed to demonstrate significant effects on morbidity and mortality rates.

Both Neoptolemos et al. (153) and Fan et al. (154) evaluated the outcome for severe disease separately. Neither found a significant difference in complication and mortality rates in patients with mild biliary pancreatitis. In contrast, both trials demonstrated a significantly lower complication rate in patients with severe acute pancreatitis, but the difference in mortality rates did not reach statistical significance. Fan et al. (154) also found a decrease in the incidence of biliary sepsis in patients with severe biliary pancreatitis. A recent meta-analysis (30) of the trials of Fan et al. (154), Neoptolemos et al. (153) and Fölsch et al. (152) found that emergency ERCP and endoscopic sphincterotomy significantly reduced the overall complication rate without a significant effect on the mortality rate. Subgroup analyses of patients with mild biliary pancreatitis revealed no differences in overall complications or mortality. In contrast, ERCP significantly reduced both the overall complication and mortality rates in patients with severe biliary pancreatitis. In a meta-analysis of four randomized trials (48,152–154) by Sharma and Howden (155), they found a significantly lower morbidity and mortality rate following early ERCP when compared with interval ERCP. However, in this meta-analysis, patients with severe pancreatitis were not examined separately.

ERCP and endoscopic sphincterotomy have no influence on the outcome of mild biliary pancreatitis. Based on lower morbidity and reduced mortality rates, emergency ERCP and endoscopic sphincterotomy should be strongly considered in patients with severe biliary pancreatitis as well as in patients with standard indications for ERCP and endoscopic sphincterotomy such as obstructive jaundice and cholangitis.

Recurrence of acute pancreatitis in patients with cholelithiasis has been reported in 29% to 63% of cases if the patient is discharged from the hospital without additional treatment. The rationale for cholecystectomy and clearance of the common bile duct in these patients is to prevent recurrent biliary pancreatitis. The timing of cholecystectomy, however, depends on the clinical circumstances. In mild gallstone pancreatitis, cholecystectomy should be performed as soon as the patient has recovered from the attack and, preferably, during the same hospital stay. In severe gallstone pancreatitis, cholecystectomy should be performed once the inflammatory process has subsided and with sufficient clinical recovery to make the procedure technically easier and safer for the patient. Although the optimal timing for cholecystectomy is still under debate, if endoscopic sphincterotomy was performed, cholecystectomy should be performed within 6 weeks (156). Cholecystectomy can be performed safely after an episode of gallstone pancreatitis via the laparoscopic approach with a reported conversion to open rate of 0 to 16% (157–159).

Vascular Complications

Vascular complications of pancreatitis may be divided into systemic and local. The systemic vascular effects of acute pancreatitis are probably related to the release of pancreatic proteases, such as trypsin, which locally and distally may activate complement C5a and precipitate the coagulation cascade (160). This causes microscopic and physiologic changes in granulocytes that induce a cell-to-cell interaction and clumping. The clumps may then embolize and set the stage for further fibrin deposition and thrombosis. This phenomenon explains the leukoembolic damage of the posterior fundus of the eye in the syndrome of sudden blindness associated with sever trauma and pancreatitis (Purtscher retinopathy) (161). Other systemic effects of C5a may be granulocyte aggregation and leukoembolization of other vital tissues, such as the lung, kidney, and splanchnic and systemic vascular beds, which may explain some of the respiratory distress syndromes, renal insufficiency, splanchnic venous thrombosis, and incidence of pulmonary emboli in these patients (160).

There are both arterial and venous local vascular effects and complications of pancreatitis. Bleeding from pancreatic pseudocysts and ruptured pseudoaneurysms is the most often fatal complication of pancreatitis, carrying a mortality rate of 25% to 40% (162–164). Bleeding may present as melena from erosion into the proximal gastrointestinal tract or as hypovolemia and abdominal pain if there is rupture into the peritoneal cavity. Diagnosis is usually made late in the patient's clinical course or only at postmortem examination. Most patients with gastrointestinal tract bleeding secondary to acute or chronic pancreatitis are alcoholics, and the cause of the bleeding is usually missed because of more common causes of serious bleeding in this patient population (i.e., peptic ulcer disease, gastritis, varices, Mallory-Weiss tears). The development of aneurysms is probably related to the severe inflammation and enzymatic autodigestion of the pancreatic and peripancreatic arteries with eventual formation of a pseudoaneurysm. With growth and expansion, the pseudoaneurysms may rupture into pseudocysts, adjacent viscera, the peritoneal cavity, or the pancreatic duct.

The most common vessel involved in splanchnic pseudoaneurysms related to pancreatitis is the splenic artery, followed by the gastroduodenal and the inferior pancreaticoduodenal, but such involvement may occur with any of the adjacent splanchnic vessels (165). Patients with chronic pancreatitis may have as high as a 10% incidence of pseudoaneurysms demonstrated on angiographic studies, but bleeding from these rarely occurs unless they are associated with pseudocysts (166). The treatment of ruptured pseudoaneurysms requires that the diagnosis be recognized; therefore, the clinician must know of it, must have a high index of suspicion, and must have a well-defined diagnostic and therapeutic plan, including emergency upper endoscopy, selective visceral angiography, ultrasonography, and CT scanning. Control can be rendered by either selective arterial infusion of vasopressin (166) or angioembolization with Gelfoam (167), detachable intravascular balloons (168), Gianturco coils (169), or polymerizing adhesives (169). Surgical control is indicated only for immediate life-threatening bleeding or failure of interventional control of bleeding.

Hemoductal pancreatitis or hemosuccus pancreatitis is the complication of pseudoaneurysm rupture into the pancreatic duct and usually encompasses the triad of gastrointestinal bleeding, pancreatitis with epigastric pain, and partial common bile duct obstruction (170). The diagnosis can be confirmed by selective visceral angiography or ERCP. The treatment of this rare complication requires ligation of the pseudoaneurysm and possible pancreatic resection.

Venous complications of acute pancreatitis, although not as dramatic, may be just as lethal as their arterial counterparts. Venous thrombosis of the portal vein is a potential complication of acute or chronic pancreatitis. The patient's course is complicated by acute decompensation, hypotension with sequestration in the vascular bed, acidosis, hepatic enzyme elevation, alteration in clotting studies, and venous infarction of the bowel. Patients who survive this insult all develop portal hypertension, and some present months to years later with bleeding esophageal varices. Selective splenic venous thrombosis occurs more frequently, and patients usually present with an increased spleen size, unexplained blood loss, pain in the left upper quadrant and subscapular area, and possibly, hypotension and cardiovascular collapse because the subscapular hematoma ruptured into the free peritoneal cavity. The treatment is splenectomy with preoperative vascular control by angiographic techniques and balloons.

During drainage procedures for pancreatic pseudocysts in the presence of associated splenic venous thrombosis, the transgastric approach should be avoided to decrease postoperative bleeding from the rich submucosal plexus of high-pressure veins. In the absence of bleeding gastric varices, one may elect to leave the spleen *in situ* even with splenic vein thrombosis, because not all patients develop bleeding from gastric varices.

Pancreatic Pseudocyst

Peripancreatic fluid collections can occur as a result of acute pancreatitis, chronic pancreatitis, surgery (either pancreatic or other abdominal surgery), trauma, or neoplasia. With the exception of a cystic neoplasm, peripancreatic fluid collections form either as a result of a disruption in the pancreatic ductal system with subsequent fluid leakage or the maturation of peripancreatic necrosis. The terminology for acute pancreatitis and its complications has historically been confusing and often conflicting. The result is a difficulty interpreting literature dealing with treatment of pancreatic pseudocyst as often the term "pseudocyst" was applied when perhaps "acute fluid collection" would have been more appropriate, or vice versa. In response to this confusion, and in an attempt to dispel it, an International Symposium on Acute Pancreatitis was convened in 1992. The result is a standardized classification system (49) of acute pancreatitis and its complications.

According to these published definitions, an acute fluid collection is located in or near the pancreas, occurs early in the course of acute pancreatitis, and *always* lacks a wall of granulation or fibrous tissue (49). Acute fluid collections are common in patients with severe acute pancreatitis, occurring in up to 50% of cases (171,172). However, more than half of these lesions regress spontaneously (171,172). Rarely on the demonstrable on physical exam and are usually found with imaging techniques. The precise composition of these collections is not known. *The critical clinical distinction between an acute fluid collection and a pseudocyst (or pancreatic abscess) is the lack of a defined wall.*

Pseudocyst formation is a frequent complication of pancreatitis with a reported incidence of 10% to 20% in acute pancreatitis and 20% to 40% in chronic pancreatitis (173). Formation of an acute pseudocyst requires four or more weeks from the onset of acute pancreatitis. In contrast, chronic pseudocysts have a well-defined wall but arise in patients with chronic pancreatitis without a preceding episode of acute pancreatitis. It is defined as a collection of pancreatic juice that arises as a consequence of acute or chronic pancreatitis or pancreatic trauma that is enclosed by a nonepithelialized wall composed of either fibrous or granulation tissue. Pseudocysts in patients with acute pancreatitis are usually diagnosed with imaging studies, either CT scan or ultrasound, although they are occasionally palpable. The contents are usually rich in pancreatic enzymes and are most often sterile. Bacteria may be present in pseudocysts but often are of no clinical significance since they represent contamination and not clinical infection. When pus is present, the lesion is more correctly termed a *pancreatic abscess*. The distinction between pancreatic abscess and infected necrosis is critical for two reasons: the mortality risk for infected necrosis is double that for pancreatic abscess (174), and specific therapy for each condition may be markedly different.

The traditional management of pancreatic pseudocyst has been based for decades on a sentinel report by Bradley et al. (175), who studied 93 patients using ultrasound. They found spontaneous resolution of the pseudocyst in 24 of 54 patients studied, but all resolution took place before 6 weeks and was almost exclusively seen in collections less than 6 cm in size. They also found the incidence of complications increased after 6 weeks of follow-up. Thus, standard therapy became treatment if the pseudocyst persisted beyond 6 weeks and/or was larger than 6 cm. With improved imaging techniques, the criteria for intervention eventually were modified to include imaging confirming cyst wall "maturity." Operative intervention was the mainstay, and the procedure performed was internal drainage via a cyst-enteric anastomosis, primarily cystgastrostomy or cystojejunostomy, depending on the location of the pseudocyst. The morbidity rate ranges from 7% to 37%, and mortality rates vary from 0 to 6% (176,177). The recurrence rate with the operative technique is approximately 10% (178). However, the traditional method of surgical drainage has been challenged by the introduction of less invasive techniques.

Percutaneous drainage was first introduced in the 1970s. Unfortunately, simple aspiration of the cyst has been associated with a recurrence rate of more than 70% and can, therefore, not be regarded as a definitive treatment (179,180). Continuous catheter drainage has shown better short-term results, with an 84% success rate and an average 7% recurrence rate (179,181,182). However, the prolonged presence of an indwelling catheter for several weeks and frequent fistula formation remain disadvantages of this technique.

Endoscopic drainage has been increasingly used during the last 10 years, either via a transpapillary route or through the gastrointestinal wall. The short-term results appear to be encouraging. Analyses of collective data indicate that resolution of cysts can be achieved in nearly 90% of patients, with morbidity rates of 9% to 25% and mortality rates of 0 to 1% (176,183). Data regarding long-term results to this point, however, remain scarce.

The question, then, arises as to which method to use. Nealon and Walser (184) have shown that the anatomy of the main pancreatic duct can be used to guide the choice of modality for treating pancreatic pseudocyst. In patients scheduled for either elective operation or percutaneous drainage of the pseudocyst, they performed endoscopic retrograde cholangiopancreatography 1 day prior to the procedure. They categorized the main pancreatic duct as either normal, normal with stricture, or normal with complete cutoff at some portion of the duct (184). A "normal" duct was meant to represent a duct without evidence of chronic pancreatitis. Patients were segregated for analysis into either normal, stricture with communication to the pseudocyst, stricture without communication, or complete cutoff. They found that pancreatic ductal anatomy correlated well with outcomes in patients treated with percutaneous drainage. Among failures of percutaneous drainage, all patients either had complete cutoff of the pancreatic duct or stricture with communication to the cyst. In either case, percutaneous catheter drainage would have a poor likelihood of success as no amount of long-term drainage could be expected to re-establish normal ductal drainage.

Likewise, determination of ductal anatomy has been used to determine the best route of endoscopic drainage. In a review (173) of 92 consecutive patients who underwent endoscopic drainage of pancreatic pseudocyst, the method was based on visualization of the pancreatic duct. If a connection between the pseudocyst and the pancreatic duct was confirmed, the transpapillary route was preferred and a single stent with multiple side holes was placed in the pancreatic duct, with the distal end of the stent positioned just proximal to the cyst. In all other cases, the transgastric or transduodenal route was chosen, depending on the position of the cyst and its relationship to the gut lumen. The technical success rate of the drainage procedure was 97%, and the mortality rate was 1% (173). Overall, endoscopic drainage was successful in treating the pseudocyst in 71% of patients (173).

It appears, then, that either percutaneous or endoscopic drainage techniques are comparable to the outcome of surgical drainage techniques in the appropriately selected patients. At our institution, patients are routinely treated with either percutaneous or endoscopic drainage, depending on the ductal anatomy, and surgical drainage is reserved for failure or complication of these methods.

Biliary Obstruction Due to Pancreatic Inflammation

Biliary obstruction may be found in as many as 25% of cases presenting with acute pancreatitis (185), and this obstruction, caused by pancreatic swelling, can be confused with a stone lodged at the ampulla. The intrapancreatic portion of the common bile duct becomes involved in the inflammatory process, but this usually resolves over the course of the disease (186). If the biliary obstruction does not resolve, a workup including ultrasonography, ERCP, or transhepatic cholangiography may be necessary to define the problem and the anatomy so that an appropriate decompressive procedure can be performed. If the patient develops cholangitis and becomes septic from infected bile in the obstructed duct, transhepatic cholangiography and drainage may be life-saving to provide decompression without subjecting the patient in septic shock to an emergency operation.

Pancreatic Necrosis, Infected Pancreatic Necrosis, and Abscess

Little is known of what triggers the release of activated pancreatic enzymes that autodigest the gland and surrounding retroperitoneal tissue and convert acute interstitial or edematous pancreatitis to pancreatic necrosis. If venous thrombosis and erosion to the small peripancreatic vessels occur, the combination is hemorrhagic necrotizing pancreatitis. Enteric bacterial contamination results in combined abscess and infected necrosis, which carries the highest mortality rate. The timing of this sequence of presentations in important. It is rare to see septic complications within the first week of presentation but not unusual after the second week, and they are almost universally present if the patient's course requires therapy for more than 3 weeks. Clinical signs of abdominal pain, fever, leukocytosis, associated severe systemic manifestations of hypotension, cardiovascular collapse, pulmonary insufficiency, renal failure, and mental status changes all strongly suggest the onset of this complication. The problem is rarely that of making the diagnosis of sepsis, but rather, of differentiating pancreatic necrosis and abscess formation from other sources of systemic sepsis such as pneumonia, urinary tract infection, and intravascular catheter-related infection.

Sequential contrast-enhanced computerized tomography is the best tool available for diagnosing and following this disease process. The study is diagnostic of abscess formation if air is seen in the phlegmon. Percutaneous fine-needle aspiration of the intrapancreatic or peripancreatic fluid collections can be used to confirm bacterial contamination in the absence of air. If necrosis is demonstrated on CT scan, aspirates are sterile, and the patient is not toxic, a conservative approach may be attempted. At present there is general agreement that surgery for severe pancreatitis should be deferred as long as the patient continues to respond favorably to conservative management. Early operation directed toward debridement of devitalized tissue to prevent septic complications has only led to increased morbidity and incidence of sepsis. Optimal surgical timing should occur, at the minimum, 2 to 3 weeks after the onset of pancreatitis to allow a sequestrum to form. The rationale for delaying surgical therapy is to permit proper demarcation of pancreatic and peripancreatic necrosis to occur, limiting the extent of surgery that is needed to facilitate debridement. This approach decreases the risk of bleeding and minimizes the surgery-related loss of vital tissue that predisposes to endocrine and exocrine pancreatic insufficiency.

In most studies published over the last decade, indication for surgery was defined by necrosis formation on CT scan and positive fine-needle aspiration. In the unstable patient, CT-guided percutaneous aspiration and drainage of pancreatic abscesses used as a temporizing measure before surgery may improve the patient's overall condition. Surgical techniques are still necessary for debridement and drainage if percutaneous drainage does not improve the septic course. The goal of surgery in patients with necrotizing pancreatitis is to remove all areas of necrotic tissue including necrotic pancreatic tissue and any infected necrotic tissue. In so doing, the risk of further complications may be minimized by reducing the progress of spreading necrosis and/or infection and the release of proinflammatory mediators. Resective procedures, such as partial or total pancreatectomy that also remove vital pancreatic tissue and healthy organs, are associated with high mortality rates.

The surgical techniques for the treatment of pancreatic necrosis are varied, and the ideal method is still debated. Generally agreed-on principles of surgical management include an organ-preserving approach that involves debridement or necrosectomy, minimization of intraoperative hemorrhage, and maximization of postoperative removal of retroperitoneal debris and exudate (132). Traditionally, three techniques have been used with comparable results; these include the following: (1) open necrosectomy with closed continuous lavage of the retroperitoneum, (ii) open necrosectomy that may or may not be staged with planned relaparotomies followed by delayed primary closure and drainage or with multiple drainage and relaparotomy as required, and (iii) open necrosectomy, often with marsupialization, with open packing and planned relaparotomies. It is reported that these approaches are associated with a postoperative mortality of less than 15%, but there has never been a trial that has prospectively compared these techniques (132). However, with the improvement in intensive care and success of conservative management, open surgery for infected pancreatic necrosis is becoming less frequent, and many young surgeons have likely never performed these procedures.

Minimal-access surgical approaches have been described in an attempt at reducing the mortality and substantial morbidity of open surgery for infected necrotizing pancreatitis (187). These approaches have used either an endoscopic or a videoscopic retroperitoneal approach for draining infected fluid. Because in most cases, the sequestrum is limited to the lesser sac, minimal-access retroperitoneal techniques have significant limitations for primary debridement. The use of a transperitoneal approach similar to that used for open debridement of necrotic pancreatic and peripancreatic necrosis has been largely anecdotal.

Recently, however, Parekh (187) reported the largest series of laparoscopic debridement for pancreatic necrosis. A hand-assisted laparoscopic (HAL) technique was used for the debridement of necrotizing pancreatitis. Hand-assisted laparoscopic surgery is useful for complex abdominal procedures since the benefits of traditional laparoscopic surgery are retained. In this series, 19 patients underwent laparoscopic evacuation of pancreatic necrosis, and in 18 patients, the procedure was completed. Four patients required reoperations, two using HALs and two open. There were no postoperative complications related to the HAL procedure itself, such as major wound infections, intestinal fistulae, or postoperative hemorrhage. Postoperative computed tomography confirmed adequacy of debridement. Although currently largely limited to a few specialized centers, HALs may provide a new option for the surgical treatment of selected patients with severe necrotizing pancreatitis.

We have become increasingly aggressive in our use of percutaneous debridement of infected pancreatic tissue. Early reports on the use of percutaneous drainage of infected pancreatic tissue were not encouraging. Lee et al. (188) reported a 33% mortality and a failure rate of over 50% with drainage alone. Kam et al. (189) reported three cases where catheter drainage was found to be inadequate and inappropriate. Szentkereszty et al. (190) reported a success rate of only 25% in 12 patients. The poor success rate likely reflects the inability to drain infected tissue and debris with relatively small drains. Van Sonnenberg et al. (191) reported a success rate of 86% when dealing with an abscess and not infected tissue.

In contrast to drainage alone where no debridement is undertaken, we use active debridement and removal of infected tissue at multiple settings. Shonnard et al. (192) reported the use of Nitrol snares for active debridement and removal of pancreatic tissue. Gouzi et al. (193), using lavage techniques, reported a 15% mortality rate and a success rate of 70%. Freeny et al. (194) reported a series of 34 patients. Their success rate was 47% with debridement alone and a mortality rate of 12%. Our group (195) reported an initial experience with 20 patients. We had a 0% mortality and a success rate of 100%. We have recently reviewed our experience, which includes 34 patients divided into two groups: critically ill patients who are intubated in the intensive care unit and stable patients who are on the surgical floor.

The overall mortality was 2.9%, and the success rate was 63%. The success rate was markedly different between the two groups. The critically ill group had a 100% failure rate, and the stable group had a success rate of 83%. Our conclusion was that debridement and lavage is an ineffective form of therapy in the critically ill patient. These results were comparable to those of Freeny et al. (194), who also found that the critically ill patients responded poorly. The technique of debridement varies; however, they generally include the placement of one to five catheters into the pancreatic and peripancreatic areas and the paracolic gutters. These catheters are gradually increased in size up to 16 French. An aggressive irrigation is then performed, and active removal of infected pancreatic tissue is undertaken two to three times per week. The catheters are removed once the drainage becomes minimal and the cavity becomes small. This approach is a slow process and requires an intensive time-consuming approach. This may be one of the reasons of its failure in the critically ill patient. However, when successful, this approach may avoid a major operative debridement.

References

1. Toouli J, Brooke-Smith M, Bassi C, et al. Guidelines for the management of acute pancreatitis. *J Gastroenterol Hepatol.* 2002;17(Suppl):S15.
2. Beckingham I, Bornman P. ABC of diseases of liver, pancreas, and biliary system. Acute pancreatitis. *BMJ.* 2001;322:595.
3. Mitchell R, Byren M, Baillie J. Pancreatitis. *Lancet.* 2003;361:1447.
4. Chwistek M, Roberts I, Amoateng-Adjepong Y. Gallstone pancreatitis: a community teaching hospital experience. *J Clin Gastroenterol.* 2001;33:41.
5. Levy P, Boruchowicz A, Hatier P, et al. Diagnostic criteria in predicting a biliary origin of acute pancreatitis in the era of endoscopic ultrasound: multicentre prospective evaluation of 213 patients. *Pancreatology.* 2005;5:450.
6. Venneman N, Buskens E, Besselink M, et al. Small gallstones are associated with increased risk of acute pancreatitis: potential benefits of prophylactic cholecystectomy? *Am J Gastroenterol.* 2005;100:2540.
7. Whitcomb D. Value of genetic testing in management of pancreatitis. *Gut.* 2004;53:1710.
8. Cuthbertson C, Christophi C. Disturbances of the microcirculation in acute pancreatitis. *Br J Surg.* 2006;93:518.
9. Satiani B, Stone H. Predictability of present outcome and future recurrence in acute pancreatitis. *Arch Surg.* 1979;114:711.
10. Trapnell J, Duncan E. Patterns of incidence in acute pancreatitis. *Br Med J.* 1975;1:179.
11. Salt W, Schenker S. Amylase—its clinical significance: a review of the literature. *Medicine.* 1976;55:269.
12. Whitcomb D. Acute pancreatitis. *N Engl J Med.* 2006;354:2142.
13. Clavien P, Robert J, Meyer P, et al. Acute pancreatitis and normoamylasemia: not an uncommon combination. *Ann Surg.* 1989;210:614.
14. Robert J, Frossard J, Mermillod B, et al. Early predictors of acute pancreatitis: prospective study comparing computed tomography scans, Ranson, Glasgow, Acute Physiology and Chronic Health Evaluation II scores, and various serum markers. *World J Surg.* 2002;26:612.
15. Tenner S, Dubner H, Steinberg W. Predicting gallstone pancreatitis with laboratory parameters: a meta-analysis. *Am J Gastroenterol.* 1994;89:1863.
16. Warshaw A, Fuller F. Specificity of increased renal clearance of amylase in diagnosis of acute pancreatitis. *N Engl J Med.* 1975;292:325.
17. Levitt M. Clinical use of amylase clearance and isoamylase measurements. *Mayo Clin Proc.* 1979;54:428.
18. Gumaste V. Diagnostic tests for acute pancreatitis. *Gastroenterologist.* 1994;2:119.
19. Wilson C, Heads A, Shenkin A, et al. C-reactive protein, antiproteases and complement factors as objective markers of severity in acute pancreatitis. *Br J Surg.* 1989;76:177.
20. Puolakkainen P, Valtonen V, Paanenen A, et al. C-reactive protein (CRP) and serum phospholipase A2 in the assessment of the severity of acute pancreatitis. *Gut.* 1987;28:764.
21. Gudgeon A, Heath D, Hurely P, et al. Trypsinogen activation peptides assay in the early prediction of severity of acute pancreatitis. *Lancet.* 1990;1:4.
22. Puolakkainen P. Early assessment of acute pancreatitis: a comparative study of computed tomography and laboratory tests. *Acta Chir Scand.* 1989;155:25.
23. Viedma J, Perez-Mateo M, Dominguez J, et al. Inflammatory response in the early prediction of severity in human AP. *Gut.* 1994;35:822.
24. Buchler M, Malfertheiner P, Schoetensack C, et al. Sensitivity of antiproteases, complement factors and C-reactive protein in detecting pancreatic necrosis: results of a prospective clinical study. *Int J Pancreatol.* 1986;1:227.
25. Neoptolemos J, Kemppainen E, Mayer J, et al. Early prediction of severity in acute pancreatitis by urinary trypsinogen activation peptide: a multicentre study. *Lancet.* 2000;355:1955.
26. Kemppainen E, Hedstrom J, Puolakkainen P, et al. Increased serum trypsinogen 2 and trypsin 2-alpha 1 antitrypsin complex values identify endoscopic retrograde cholangiopancreatography induced pancreatitis with a high accuracy. *Gut* 1997;41:690.
27. Frossard J, Hadengue A, Pastor C. New serum markers for the detection of severe acute pancreatitis in humans. *Am J Respir Crit Care Med.* 2001; 164:162.
28. Lawson T. Acute pancreatitis and its complications: computed tomography and sonography. *Radiol Clin North Am.* 1983;21:495.
29. Romagnuolo J, Currie G. Noninvasive vs. selective invasive biliary imaging for acute biliary pancreatitis: an economic evaluation by using decision tree analysis. *Gastrointest Endosc.* 2005;61:86.
30. Nathens A, Curtis J, Beale R, et al. Management of the critically ill patient with severe acute pancreatitis. *Crit Care Med.* 2004;32:2524.
31. Ayub K, Imada R, Slavin J. Endoscopic retrograde cholangiopancreatography in gallstone-associated acute pancreatitis. *Cochrane Database Syst Rev.* 2004;4:CD003630.
32. Working Party of the British Society of Gastroenterology, Association of Surgeons of Great Britain and Ireland, Pancreatic Society of Great Britain and Ireland, Association of Upper GI Surgeons of Great Britain and Ireland. UK guidelines for the management of acute pancreatitis. *Gut.* 2005;54(Suppl 3):iii1.
33. NIH state-of-the-science statement on endoscopic retrograde cholangiopancreatography (ERCP) for diagnosis and therapy. *NIH Consens State Sci Statements.* 2002;19:1.
34. Balthazar E. Acute pancreatitis: assessment of severity with clinical and CT evaluation. *Radiology.* 2002;223:603.
35. Beger H, Isenmann R. Acute pancreatitis: who needs an operation? *J Hepatobiliary Pancreat Surg.* 2002;9:436.
36. Balthazar E, Robinson D. Megibow A. Acute pancreatitis: value of CT in establishing prognosis. *Radiology.* 1990;174:331.
37. Paulson E, Vitellas K, Keogan M, et al. Acute pancreatitis complicated by gland necrosis: spectrum of findings on contrast-enhanced CT. *Am J Roentgenol.* 1999;172:609.
38. Johnson C, Stephens D, Sarr M. CT of acute pancreatitis: correlation between lack of contrast enhancement and pancreatic necrosis. *Am J Roentgenol.* 1991;156:93.
39. Vitellas K, Paulson E, Enns R, et al. Pancreatitis complicated by gland necrosis: evolution of findings on contrast-enhanced CT. *Comput Assist Tomogr.* 1999;23:898.
40. Arvanitakis M, Delhaye M, De Maertelaere V, et al. Computed tomography and magnetic resonance imaging in the assessment of acute pancreatitis. *Gastroenterology.* 2004;126:715.
41. Buchler M, Uhl W, Malfertheiner P. Therapie der akuten pankreatitis. *Dtsch Med Wochenschr.* 1994;119:1739.
42. Bradley E, Murphy F, Ferguson C. Prediction of pancreatic necrosis by dynamic pancreatography. *Ann Surg.* 1989;210:495.
43. Foitzik T, Bassi D, Schmidt J, et al. Intravenous contrast medium accentuates the severity of acute necrotizing pancreatitis in rat. *Gastroenterology.* 1994;106:207.
44. London N, Leese T, Lavelle J, et al. Rapid-bolus contrast-enhanced dynamic computed tomography in acute pancreatitis: a prospective study. *Br J Surg.* 1991;78:1452.
45. Rau B, Pralle U, Mayer J, et al. Role of ultrasonographically guided fine-needle aspiration cytology in the diagnosis of infected pancreatic necrosis. *Br J Surg.* 1998;85:179.
46. Paye F, Rotman N, Radier C, et al. Percutaneous aspiration for bacteriological studies in patients with necrotizing pancreatitis. *Br J Surg.* 1998;85: 755.
47. Sarles H. Pancreatitis: symposium of Marseilles, 1963. Basel, Switzerland: Skarger; 1965.
48. Bradley E. A clinically based classification system for acute pancreatitis. *Arch Surg.* 1993;128:586.
49. Ranson J, Rifkind K, Turner J. Prognostic signs and nonoperative peritoneal lavage in acute pancreatitis. *Surg Gynecol Obstet.* 1976;143:209.
50. Ranson J, Spencer F. The role of peritoneal lavage in severe acute pancreatitis. *Ann Surg.* 1978;187:565.
51. Ranson J, Pasternack B. Statistical methods for quantifying the severity of clinical pancreatitis. *J Surg Res.* 1977;22:79.
52. Ranson J, Spencer F. The role of peritoneal lavage in severe acute pancreatitis. *Ann Surg.* 1978;187:565.
53. Levant J, Secrist D, Resin H, et al. Nasogastric suction in the treatment of alcoholic pancreatitis: a controlled study. *JAMA.* 1974;229:51.
54. Sarr M, Sanfey H, Cameron J. Prospective randomized trial of nasogastric suction in patients with acute pancreatitis. *Surgery.* 1986;100:500.
55. Meshkinpour H, Molinari M, Gardner L, et al. Cimetidine in the treatment of acute alcoholic pancreatitis. *Gastroenterology.* 1979;77:687.
56. Bore P, Zinner M, Cameron J. A clinical trial of cimetidine in acute pancreatitis. *Surg Gynec Obstet.* 1982;154:13.
57. Switz D, Vlahcevic J, Ferrar J. The effect of anticholinergic and/or nasogastric suction on the outcome of acute alcoholic pancreatitis: a controlled trial. *Gastroenterology.* 1975;68:994.
58. Trapnell J, Rigby C, Talbot C, et al. A controlled trial of Trasylol in the treatment of acute pancreatitis. *Br J Surg.* 1974;61:177.
59. Goebell H, Ammann R, Herfarth C, et al. A double-blind trial of synthetic salmon calcitonin in the treatment of acute pancreatitis. *Scand J Gastroenterol.* 1979;14:881.
60. Usadel K, Leuschner U, Uberla K. Treatment of acute pancreatitis with somatostatin: a multicenter double-blind trial. *N Engl J Med.* 1980;303:999.

61. Marik P, Zaloga G. Meta-analysis of parenteral nutrition versus enteral nutrition in patients with acute pancreatitis. *BMJ.* 2004;328:1407.
62. Renner I, Savage W, Pantoja J, et al. Death due to acute pancreatitis. A retrospective analysis of 405 autopsy cases. *Dig Dis Sci.* 1985;30:1005.
63. Lumsden A, Bradley E. Secondary pancreatic infections. *Surg Gynecol Obstet.* 1990;170:459.
64. Beger H, Bittner R, Block S, et al. Bacterial contamination of pancreatic necrosis. A prospective clinical study. *Gastroenterology.* 1986;91:433.
65. Medich D, Lee T, Melhem M, et al. Pathogenesis of pancreatic sepsis. *Am J Surg.* 1993;165:46.
66. Runkel N, Moody F, Smith G, et al. The role of the gut in the development of sepsis in acute pancreatitis. *J Surg Res.* 1991;51:18.
67. Cicalese L, Sahai A, Sileri P, et al. Acute pancreatitis and bacterial translocation. *Dig Dis Sci.* 2001;46:1127.
68. Nettelbladt C, Katouli M, Bark T, et al. Evidence of bacterial translocation in fatal hemorrhagic pancreatitis. *J Trauma.* 2000;48:314.
69. Ragins H, Levenson S, Signer R, et al. Intrajejunal administration of an elemental diet at neutral pH avoids pancreatic stimulation. Studies in dog and man. *Am J Surg.* 1973;126:606.
70. Cassim M, Allardyce D. Pancreatic secretion in response to jejunal feeding of elemental diet. *Ann Surg.* 1974;180:228.
71. Vu M, van der Veek P, Frolich M, et al. Does jejunal feeding activate exocrine pancreatic secretion? *Eur J Clin Invest.* 1999;29:1053.
72. Abou-Assi S, Craig K, O'Keefe S. Hypocaloric jejunal feeding is better than total parenteral nutrition in acute pancreatitis: results of a randomized comparative study. *Am J Gastroenterol.* 2002;97:2255.
73. McClave S, Greene L, Snider H, et al. Comparison of the safety of early enteral vs parenteral nutrition in mild acute pancreatitis. *J Parenter Enteral Nutr.* 1997;21:14.
74. Nakad A, Piessevaux H, Marot J, et al. Is early enteral nutrition in acute pancreatitis dangerous? About 20 patients fed by an endoscopically placed nasogastrojejunal tube. *Pancreas.* 1998;17:187.
75. Olah A, Pardavi G, Belagyi T, et al. Early nasojejunal feeding in acute pancreatitis is associated with a lower complication rate. *Nutrition.* 2002;18:259.
76. Windsor A, Kanwar S, Li A, et al. Compared with parenteral nutrition, enteral feeding attenuates the acute phase response and improves disease severity in acute pancreatitis. *Gut.* 1998;42:431.
77. Kalfarentzos F, Kehagias J, Mead N, et al. Enteral nutrition is superior to parenteral nutrition in severe acute pancreatitis: results of a randomized prospective trial. *Br J Surg.* 1997;84:1665.
78. Powell J, Murchison J, Fearon K, et al. Randomized controlled trial of the effect of early enteral nutrition on markers of the inflammatory response in predicted severe acute pancreatitis. *Br J Surg.* 2000;87:1375.
79. Hansbrough W, Hansbrough J. Success of immediate intragastric feeding of patients with burns. *J Burn Care Rehabil.* 1993;14:512.
80. McArdle A, Palmason C, Brown R, et al. Early enteral feeding of patients with major burns: prevention of catabolism. *Ann Plast Surg.* 1984;13:396.
81. Eatock F, Brombacher G, Steven A, et al. Nasogastric feeding in severe acute pancreatitis may be practical and safe. *Int J Pancreatol.* 2000;28:23.
82. Eatock F, Chong P, Menezes N, et al. A randomized study of early nasogastric versus nasojejunal feeding in severe acute pancreatitis. *Am J Gastroenterol.* 2005;100:432.
83. Imrie C, Allam B, Ferguson J. Hypocalcemia of acute pancreatitis: the effect of hypoalbuminemia. *Curr Med Res Opin.* 1976;4:101.
84. Storck G, Bjorntorp P. Chemical composition of fat necrosis in experimental pancreatitis in the rat. *Scand J Gastroenterol.* 1971;6:225.
85. Canale D, Donabedian R. Hypercalcitoninemia in acute pancreatitis. *J Clin Endocrinol Metab.* 1975;40:738.
86. Donowitz M. Glucagon secretion in acute and chronic pancreatitis. *Ann Intern Med.* 1975;83:778.
87. Robertson G. Inadequate parathyroid response in acute pancreatitis. *N Engl J Med.* 1976;294:512.
88. Balslov J, Jorgensen H, Nielsen R. Acute renal failure complicating severe pancreatitis. *Acta Chir Scand.* 1962;124:348.
89. Ito K, Ramirez-Schon G, Shah P, et al. The myocardial depressant factor in acute hemorrhagic pancreatitis. *Trans Am Soc Artif Intern Organ.* 1980;26:149.
90. McKay C, Evans S, Sinclair M, et al. High early mortality rate from acute pancreatitis in Scotland, 1984–1995. *Br J Surg.* 1999;86:1302.
91. De Waele B, Vanmierlo B, Van Nieuwenhove Y, et al. Impact of body overweight and class I, II and III obesity on the outcome of acute biliary pancreatitis. *Pancreas.* 2006;32:343.
92. Pronovost P, Angus D, Dorman T, et al. Physician staffing patterns and clinical outcomes in critically ill patients: a systematic review. *JAMA.* 2002;288:2151.
93. Ranson J, Berman R. Long peritoneal lavage decreases pancreatic sepsis in acute pancreatitis. *Ann Surg.* 1990;211:708.
94. Platell C, Cooper D, Hall J. Acute pancreatitis: effects of somatostatin analogs and peritoneal lavage. A meta-analysis of peritoneal lavage for acute pancreatitis. *J Gastroenterol Hepatol.* 2001;16:689.
95. Hwang T, Chiu C, Chen H, et al. Surgical results for severe acute pancreatitis—comparison of the different surgical procedures. *Hepatogastroenterology.* 1995;42:1026.
96. Cogliandolo A, Manganaro T, Saitta F, et al. The role of necrosectomy and continuous peritoneal lavage in the treatment of acute necrotic-hemorrhagic pancreatitis. *Chir Ital.* 1995;47:58.
97. Borie D, Frileux P, Levy E, et al. Surgery of acute necrotizing pancreatitis. Active prolonged drainage in 157 consecutive patients. *Presse Med.* 1994;23:1064.
98. Pederzoli P, Bassi C, Vesentini S, et al. Necrosectomy by lavage in the surgical treatment of severe necrotizing pancreatitis. Results in 263 patients. *Acta Chir Scand.* 1990;156:775.
99. Pederzoli P, Bassi C, Vesentini S, et al. Retroperitoneal and peritoneal drainage and lavage in the treatment of severe necrotizing pancreatitis. *Surg Gynecol Obstet.* 1990;170:197.
100. Larvin M, Chalmers A, Robinson P, et al. Debridement and closed cavity irrigation for the treatment of pancreatic necrosis. *Br J Surg.* 1989;76:465.
101. Lasson A, Balldin G, Genell S, et al. Peritoneal lavage in severe acute pancreatitis. *Acta Chir Scand.* 1982;150:479.
102. Fagniez P, Bonnet F, Rotman N. Treatment of acute necrotizing pancreatitis with peritoneal lavage. 12 cases. *Nouv Presse Med.* 1982;11:3555.
103. Currie D. Continuous peritoneal lavage. *Surg Gynecol Obstet.* 1972;135:951.
104. Dunn D, Barke R, Ahrenholz D, et al. The adjuvant effect of peritoneal fluid in experimental peritonitis. Mechanism and clinical implications. *Ann Surg.* 1984;199:37.
105. Maddaus M, Ahrenholz D, Simmons R. The biology of peritonitis and implications for treatment. *Surg Clin North Am.* 1988;68:431.
106. Lamperi S, Carozzi S. Immunologic patters in CAPD patients with peritonitis. *Clin Nephrol.* 1988;30(Suppl):S41.
107. Breborowicz A, Rodela H, Oreopoulos D. Toxicity of osmotic solutes on human mesothelial cells in vitro. *Kidney Int.* 1992;41:1280.
108. Niederau C, Crass R, Silver G, et al. Therapeutic regimens in acute experimental hemorrhagic pancreatitis. Effects of hydration, oxygenation, peritoneal lavage, and a potent protease inhibitor. *Gastroenterology.* 1988;95:1648.
109. Balldin G, Borgstrom A, Genell S, et al. The effect of peritoneal lavage and aprotinin in the treatment of severe acute pancreatitis. *Res Exp Med.* 1983;183:203.
110. Berling R, Borgstrom A, Ohlsson K. Peritoneal lavage with aprotinin in patient with severe acute pancreatitis. Effects on plasma and peritoneal levels of trypsin and leukocyte proteases and their major inhibitors. *Int J Pancreatol.* 1998;24:9.
111. Buchler M, Bloor B, Muller C, et al. Acute necrotizing pancreatitis: treatment strategy according to the status of infection. *Ann Surg.* 2000;232:619.
112. Beger H, Bittner R, Block S, et al. Bacterial contamination of pancreatic necrosis. A prospective clinical study. *Gastroenterology.* 1986;91:433.
113. Uhl W, Schrag H, Wheatley A, et al. The role of infection in acute pancreatitis. *Dig Surg.* 1994;11:214.
114. Gerzof S, Banks P, Robbins A, et al. Early diagnosis of pancreatic infection by computed tomography-guided aspiration. *Gastroenterology.* 1987;93:1315.
115. Beger H, Rau B, Mayer J, et al. Natural course of acute pancreatitis. *World J Surg.* 1997;21:130.
116. Bassi C, Falconi M, Girelli F, et al. Microbiological findings in severe pancreatitis. *Surg Res Comm.* 1989;5:1.
117. Gotzinger P, Wamser P, Barlan M, et al. Candida infection of local necrosis in severe acute pancreatitis is associated with increased mortality. *Shock.* 2000;14:320.
118. Uomo G, Visconti M, Manes G, et al. Nonsurgical treatment of acute necrotizing pancreatitis. *Pancreas.* 1996;2:142.
119. Banks P. Infected necrosis: morbidity and therapeutic consequences. *Hepatogastroenterology.* 1991;38:116.
120. Isenmann R, Rau B, Beger H. Bacterial infection and extent of necrosis are determinants of organ failure in patients with acute necrotizing pancreatitis. *Br J Surg.* 1999;86:1020.
121. Craig R, Dordal E, Myles L. The use of ampicillin in acute pancreatitis [letter]. *Ann Intern Med.* 1975;83:831.
122. Howes R, Zuidema G, Cameron J. Evaluation of prophylactic antibiotics in acute pancreatitis. *J Surg Res.* 1975;18:197.
123. Finch W, Sawyers J, Schenker S. A prospective study to determine the efficacy of antibiotics in acute pancreatitis. *Ann Surg.* 1976;183:667.
124. Roberts E, Williams R. Ampicillin concentrations in pancreatic fluid bile obtained at endoscopic retrograde cholangiopancreatography (ERCP). *Scand J Gastroenterol.* 1979;14:669.
125. Trudel J, Wittnich C, Brown R. Antibiotics bioavailability in acute experimental pancreatitis. *J Am Coll Surg.* 1994;178:475.
126. Powell J, Miles R, Siriwardena A. Antibiotic prophylaxis in the initial management of severe acute pancreatitis. *Br J Surg.* 1998;85:582.
127. Buchler M, Malfertheiner P, Friess H, et al. The penetration of antibiotics into human pancreas. *Infection.* 1989;17:20.
128. Buchler M, Malfertheiner P, Friess H, et al. Human pancreatic tissue concentration of bactericidal antibiotics. *Gastroenterology.* 1992;103:1902.
129. Bassi C, Pederzoli P, Vesentini S, et al. Behavior of antibiotics during human necrotizing pancreatitis. *Antimicrob Agents Chemother.* 1994;38:830.
130. Manes G, Rabitti P, Menchise A, et al. Prophylaxis with meropenem of septic complications in acute pancreatitis: a randomized, controlled trial versus imipenem. *Pancreas.* 2003;27:e79.

131. Heinrich S, Schafer M, Rousson V, et al. Evidence-based treatment of acute pancreatitis. A look at established paradigms. *Ann Surg.* 2006;243:154.
132. Uhl W, Warshaw A, Imrie C, et al. IAP guidelines for the surgical management of acute pancreatitis. *Pancreatology.* 2002;2:565.
133. Pederzoli P, Bassi C, Vesentini S, et al. A randomized multicenter clinical trial of antibiotic prophylaxis of septic complications in acute necrotizing pancreatitis with imipenem. *Surg Gynecol Obstet.* 1993;176:480.
134. Sainio V, Kemppainen E, Puolakkainen P, et al. Early antibiotic treatment in acute necrotizing pancreatitis. *Lancet.* 1995;346:663.
135. Rattner D, Warshaw A. Surgical intervention in acute pancreatitis. *Crit Care Med.* 1988;16:89.
136. Frey C, Bradley E, Beger H. Progress in acute pancreatitis. *Surg Gynecol Obstet.* 1988;167:282.
137. Nordback I, Sand J, Saaristo R, et al. Early treatment with antibiotics reduces the need for surgery in acute necrotizing pancreatitis—a single-center randomized study. *J Gastrointest Surg.* 2001;5:113.
138. Sharma V, Howden C. Prophylactic antibiotic administration reduces sepsis and mortality in acute necrotizing pancreatitis: a meta-analysis. *Pancreas.* 2001;22:28.
139. Hartwig W, Werner J, Uhl W, et al. Management of infection in acute pancreatitis. *J Hepatobiliary Pancreat Surg.* 2002;9:423.
140. Moody F, Haley-Russell D, Muney D. Intestinal transit and bacterial translocation in obstructive pancreatitis. *Dig Dis Sci.* 1995;40:1798.
141. Runkel N, Moody F, Smith G, et al. The role of the gut in the development of sepsis in acute pancreatitis. *J Surg Res.* 1991;51:18.
142. Widdison A, Karanjia N, Reber H. Routes of spread of pathogens into the pancreas in a feline model of acute pancreatitis. *Gut.* 1994;35:1306.
143. Widdison A, Alvarez C, Chang Y, et al. Sources of pancreatic pathogens in acute pancreatitis in cats. *Pancreas.* 1994;9:536.
144. Howard T, Temple M. Prophylactic antibiotics alter the bacteriology of infected necrosis in severe acute pancreatitis. *J Am Coll Surg.* 2002;195:759.
145. De Waele J, Vogelaers D, Blot S, et al. Fungal infections in patients with severe acute pancreatitis and the use of prophylactic therapy. *Clin Infect Dis.* 2003;37:208.
146. Wey S, Mori M, Pfaller M, et al. Risk factors for hospital-acquired candidemia: a matched case-control study. *Arch Intern Med.* 1989;149:2349.
147. Hoerauf A, Hammer S, Muller-Myhsok B, et al. Intra-abdominal *Candida* infection during acute necrotizing pancreatitis has a high prevalence and is associated with increased mortality. *Crit Care Med.* 1998;26:2010.
148. Gotzinger P, Wamser P, Barlan M, et al. Candida infection of local necrosis in severe acute pancreatitis is associated with increased mortality. *Shock.* 2000;14:320.
149. Schwarz M, Isenmann R, Meyer H, et al. Antibiotic use in necrotizing pancreatitis: results of a controlled study. *Dtsch Med Wochenschr.* 1997;122:356.
150. Isenmann R, Schwarz M, Rau B, et al. Characteristics of infection with *Candida* species in patients with necrotizing pancreatitis. *World J Surg.* 2002;26:372.
151. Widdison A, Karanjia N. Pancreatic infection complicating acute pancreatitis. *Br J Surg.* 1993;80:148.
152. Mangiante G, Canepari P, Colucci G, et al. A probiotic as an antagonist of bacterial translocation in experimental pancreatitis [in Italian]. *Chir Ital.* 1999;51:221.
153. Olah A, Belagyi T, Issekutz A, et al. Randomized clinical trial of specific lactobacillus and fibre supplement to early enteral nutrition in patients with acute pancreatitis. *Br J Surg.* 2002;89:1103.
154. Hallay J, Kovacs G, Szatmari K, et al. Early jejunal nutrition and change in the immunological parameters of patients with acute pancreatitis. *Hepatogastroenterology.* 2001;48:1488.
155. Ockenga J, Borchert K, Rifai K, et al. Effect of glutamine-enriched total parenteral nutrition in patients with acute pancreatitis. *Clin Nutr.* 2002;21:409.
156. Boerma D, Rauws E, Keulemans Y, et al. Wait-and-see policy or laparoscopic cholecystectomy after endoscopic sphincterotomy for bile-duct stones: a randomized trial. *Lancet.* 2002;360:761.
157. Uhl W, Muller C, Krahenbuhl L, et al. Acute gallstone pancreatitis: timing of laparoscopic cholecystectomy in mild and severe disease. *Surg Endosc.* 1999;13:1070.
158. Tang E, Stain S, Tang G, et al. Timing of laparoscopic surgery in gallstone pancreatitis. *Arch Surg.* 1995;130:496.
159. Soper N, Brunt L, Callery M, et al. Role of laparoscopic cholecystectomy in the management of acute gallstone pancreatitis. *Am J Surg.* 1994;167:42.
160. Jacob H, Craddock P, Hammerschmidt D, et al. Complement-induced granulocyte aggregation: an unsuspected mechanism of disease. *N Engl J Med.* 1980;302:789.
161. Jones W. Purtscher's retinopathy associated with acute pancreatitis. *Am J Optom Physiol Opt.* 1981;58:855.
162. Frey C. Pancreatic pseudocyst: operative strategy. *Ann Surg.* 1978;188:652.
163. Gadacz T, Trunkey D, Kieffer R. Visceral vessel erosion associate with pancreatitis. *Arch Surg.* 1978;113:1438.
164. Stanley J, Frey C, Miller T, et al. Major arterial hemorrhage: a complication of pancreatic pseudocysts and chronic pancreatitis. *Arch Surg.* 1976;111:435.
165. Stabile B, Wilson S, Debas H. Reduced mortality from bleeding pseudocysts and pseudoaneurysms caused by pancreatitis. *Arch Surg.* 1983;118:45.
166. White A, Baum S, Buranasiri S. Aneurysms secondary to pancreatitis. *AJR Am J Roentgenol.* 1976;127:393.
167. Vujic I, Anderson M, Meredith H, et al. Successful embolization of the dorsal pancreatic artery to control massive upper gastrointestinal hemorrhage. *Ann Surg.* 1980;46:184.
168. Kaufman S, Strandberg J, Barth K, et al. Therapeutic embolization with detachable silastic balloons: long term effects in swine. *Invest Radiol.* 1979;14:156.
169. Wallace S, Gianturco C, Anderson H, et al. Therapeutic vascular occlusion utilizing steel coil technique: clinical application. *Am J Roentgenol.* 1976;127:381.
170. Harper P, Gamelli R, Kaye M. Recurrent hemorrhage into the pancreatic duct from a splenic artery aneurysm. *Gastroenterology.* 1984;87:417.
171. Bradley E, Gonzalez A, Clements J. Acute pancreatic pseudocysts: incidence and implications. *Ann Surg.* 1976;184:734.
172. Siegelman S, Copeland B, Saba G, et al. CT of fluid collections associate with pancreatitis. *AJR Am J Roentgenol.* 1980;134:1121.
173. Cahen D, Rauws E, Fockens P, et al. Endoscopic drainage of pancreatic pseudocysts: long-term outcome and procedural factors associated with safe and successful treatment. *Endoscopy.* 2005;37:977.
174. Bittner R, Block S, Buchler M, et al. Pancreatic abscess and infected pancreatic necrosis: different local septic complications in acute pancreatitis. *Dig Dis Sci.* 1987;32:1082.
175. Bradley E, Clements J, Gonzales A. The natural history of pancreatic pseudocysts: a unified concept of management. *Am J Surg.* 1979;137:135.
176. Lehman G. Pseudocysts. *Gastrointest Endosc.* 1999;49:S81.
177. Boerma D, van Gulik T, Obertop H, et al. Internal drainage of infected pancreatic pseudocysts: safe or sorry? *Dig Surg.* 1999;16:501.
178. Lohr-Happe A, Peiper M, Lankisch P. Natural course of operated pseudocysts in chronic pancreatitis. *Gut.* 1994;35:1479.
179. Gumaste U, Dave P. Pancreatic pseudocyst drainage: the needle or the scalpel? *J Clin Gastroenterol.* 1991;13:500.
180. Hancke S, Pedersen J. Percutaneous pancreatic cyst puncture guided by ultrasound. *Ugeskr Laeger.* 1977;139:700.
181. Spivak H, Galloway J, Amerson J, et al. Management of pancreatic pseudocysts. *J Am Coll Surg.* 1998;186:507.
182. Boggi U, di Candio G, Campatelli A, et al. Nonoperative management of pancreatic pseudocysts: problems in differential diagnosis. *Int J Pancreatol.* 1999;25:123.
183. Vitale G, Lawhon J, Larson G, et al. Endoscopic drainage of the pancreatic pseudocyst. *Surgery.* 1999;126:616.
184. Nealon W, Walser E. Main pancreatic ductal anatomy can direct choice of modality for treating pancreatic pseudocysts (surgery versus percutaneous drainage). *Ann Surg.* 2002;235:751.
185. Frieden J. The significance of jaundice in acute pancreatitis. *Arch Surg.* 1965;90:422.
186. Bradley E, Salam A. Hyperbilirubinemia in inflammatory pancreatic disease: natural history and management. *Ann Surg.* 1978;188:626.
187. Parekh D. Laparoscopic-assisted pancreatic necrosectomy. *Arch Surg.* 2006;141:895.
188. Lee M, Rattner D, Legemate D, et al. Acute complicated pancreatitis: redefining the role of interventional radiology. *Radiology.* 1992;183:171.
189. Kam A, Young N, Markson G, et al. Case report: inappropriate use of percutaneous drainage in the management of pancreatic necrosis. *J Gastroenterol Hepatol.* 1999;14:699.
190. Szentkereszty Z, Halay J, Czako D, et al. CT guided percutaneous peripancreatic drainage: a possible therapy in acute necrotizing patients. *Hepatogastroenterology.* 2002;49:1696.
191. Van Sonnenberg E, Wittich G, Chon K, et al. Percutaneous radiologic drainage of pancreatic abscesses. *Am J Roentgenol.* 1997;168:979.
192. Shonnard K, McCarter D, Lyon R. Percutaneous debridement of infected pancreatic necrosis with nitinol snares. *J Vasc Interv Radiol.* 1997;124:31.
193. Gouzi J, Bloom E, Julio C, et al. Percutaneous drainage of infected pancreatic necrosis: an alternative to surgery. *Chirurgie.* 1999;124:31.
194. Freeny P, Althaus S, Traverso L, et al. CT-guided catheter drainage of infected acute necrotizing pancreatitis: techniques and results. *AJR Am J Roentgenol.* 1998;170:969.
195. Echenique A, Sleeman D, Yrizarri J, et al. Percutaneous catheter-directed debridement of infected pancreatic necrosis: results in 20 patients. *J Vasc Interv Radiol.* 1998;9:565.

CHAPTER 156 ■ INFLAMMATORY BOWEL DISEASE AND TOXIC MEGACOLON

NIMISHA K. PAREKH • STEPHEN B. HANAUER

FULMINANT COLITIS

Ulcerative colitis is characterized by a diffuse, continuous inflammatory process usually limited to the superficial mucosa of the colon. *Crohn disease* entails a more focal, transmural inflammation that can affect the colon either alone or accompanied by small bowel involvement. Both have the potential for severe, fulminating or toxic colitis (1). Since the original classification was published by Truelove and Witts in 1955, severe, acute, ulcerative colitis has been defined by the presence of six or more bloody bowel movements per day associated with temperature greater than 37.8°C, heart rate greater than 90 beats/minute, hemoglobin less than 10.5 g/dL, and/or an erythrocyte sedimentation rate (ESR) greater than 30 mm/hour (2). It has long been recognized that these criteria are indications for hospitalization and intravenous corticosteroid therapy (3,4).

However, it is apparent that the spectrum of ulcerative colitis extends beyond the severity to necessitate hospitalization to *fulminant colitis* and *toxic megacolon,* implying progression of mucosal inflammation into deeper layers of the colon wall (5), which is a medical emergency requiring more intense and combined medical and surgical management (6). In addition to the symptomatic criteria set forth by Truelove and Witts, patients with fulminant colitis or toxic megacolon have evidence of transmural inflammation, including more profound tachycardia (heart rate greater than 120 beats/minute), fever (greater than 38°C), hypoactive bowel sounds, hypoalbuminemia, and metabolic alkalosis, accompanied by radiologic and endoscopic evidence of transmural disease and circular muscle paralysis, which precipitates dilatation (7) (Table 156.1). Approximately 15% of patients with ulcerative colitis will have a severe flare-up that will require hospitalization (3,8). Between 6.3% and 9% will have severe colitis as their initial presentation (8). Mortality from severe colitis is less than 2%, with a colectomy rate of about 30% (2,3). The risks of surgery or colectomy with fulminant colitis or toxic megacolon have not been independently assessed, but their prognosis is, most certainly, worse than patients presenting with criteria for severe colitis alone (7).

Clinical Features

In contrast to patients with severe colitis, those with fulminant colitis are characterized by having more than ten bowel movements per day, rectal urgency, continuous bleeding, abdominal pain and distention, fevers, weight loss, and dehydration (5). On physical examination, patients present with fever, tachycardia, abdominal tenderness and mild distention, tympany, and decreased bowel sounds (9). Laboratory abnormalities include leukocytosis, anemia (hemoconcentration must be taken into account), hypoalbuminemia, hypokalemia, hyponatremia, and elevated sedimentation rate and C-reactive protein (CRP). The degree of metabolic alkalosis correlates with the severity of colitis (7).

A plain abdominal radiograph can determine the extent of ulcerative colitis by the absence of fecal material distal to the margin of disease and the presence of air outlining normal haustrations proximal to the disease margin (10,11). Radiologic features of fulminant colitis include wall thickening, with islands of edematous mucosa surrounded by deep ulcerations (9,12,13). The presence of colonic dilatation greater than 5.5 cm is predictive of the presence of—or evolution to—toxic megacolon (9).

A limited proctoscopic examination or flexible sigmoidoscopy with minimal air insufflation may be performed safely to evaluate the mucosa for pseudomembranes or ischemia (11). Examination generally shows extensive ulceration with friable, bleeding mucosa. In rare instances, however, such as with rectal enema therapy or in the setting of Crohn disease, the rectum may be normal. In patients whose initial presentation of inflammatory bowel disease is severe colitis, biopsies should be performed to evaluate for Crohn disease and to rule out acute self-limited colitis. In those with an exacerbation of known diagnosis, biopsies can help to exclude *Clostridium difficile* or cytomegalovirus (14). More extensive endoscopic examinations (15) are generally contraindicated due to the risk of perforation or inducing toxic megacolon. However, they have been performed safely in some experienced centers (7). If performed, the presence of severe colitis (deep penetrating ulcers) in conjunction with clinical features of severe disease is a poor prognostic sign (9,13,15,16). Similarly, the presence of extensive and deep ulcerations is a poor prognostic marker in Crohn disease (12). Stool analysis for ova and parasites, *C. difficile, Escherichia coli* O157:H7, *Campylobacter, Salmonella,* and *Shigella* should be performed as part of the diagnostic workup (7,17).

Management

Few medical emergencies require as close cooperation between medical and surgical personnel as does fulminant colitis. A team approach with early management and continuous assessment by both groups is vital not only to determine whether surgery is indicated, but also to support critically ill patients preoperatively and postoperatively. Early recognition and

TABLE 156.1

DETERMINATION OF SEVERITY OF BOWEL DISEASE: CLINICAL/LABORATORY FINDINGS

	DISEASE SEVERITY	
	Severe disease	Fulminant disease
Stools (number/d)	More than 6	More than 10
Blood in stool	Frequent	Continuous
Temperature (Celsius)	Greater than 37.5°	Greater than 37.5°
Pulse	Greater than 90 bpm	Greater than 90 bpm
Hemoglobin	Less than 75% of normal	Transfusion required
Erythrocyte sedimentation rate	More than 30	More than 30
Radiographic features	Colon wall edema Thumbprinting	Dilated colon
Clinical examination	Abdominal tenderness	Abdominal distention and tenderness

institution of therapy by an experienced team can alter the outcome of this life-threatening illness (3,4,7,17).

Medical Treatment

Resuscitative measures, including vigorous fluid, electrolyte, and blood replacement to maintain the serum hematocrit at approximately 30%, are paramount. The goal of fluid replacement should be to restore previous losses and continue replenishing those that are ongoing from diarrhea, fever, and third spacing of fluids (7). Despite the fact that bowel rest is an ineffective primary therapy for severe colitis, oral intake of fluids should be discontinued in fulminant colitis or once colonic dilatation is recognized (18). Parenteral nutritional support in attempts to correct malnutrition and electrolyte and acid-base balance—including repletion of phosphate, calcium, and magnesium—should be initiated. Although severe hypokalemia may not be present, total body potassium depletion is common and may be exacerbated by glucocorticoids such that resuscitative measures should include adequate potassium replacement (7).

Aminosalicylates, a mainstay of maintenance therapy and the treatment of mild to moderate disease, have no role in the treatment of fulminant colitis (3,4,7,17). Their limited activity on superficial inflammation is insufficient to abort or control the transmural disease, and potential adverse effects (e.g., nausea, vomiting, or worsening colitis) may confuse the clinical picture. These drugs should be withheld until the patient has recovered and resumed a normal diet.

Corticosteroids have long been used in the management of ulcerative colitis as well as in Crohn colitis (3,7,17). There is no general agreement regarding which corticosteroid preparation or dose should be given. Usual doses employed for severe fulminant colitis range from 40 to 80 mg of methylprednisolone (in Europe, often 1 mg/kg) or 400 mg of hydrocortisone provided in divided doses or continuous infusion (3,4,7,17,19). Prednisone, 25 mg intravenously every 6 hours, and prednisolone sodium phosphate have been used successfully. In the United States, hydrocortisone, 100 mg every 6 hours, and methylprednisolone, 6 to 15 mg every 6 hours, are both available for intravenous administration. There is no advantage to doses greater than 60 mg of methylprednisolone daily (19,20). A continuous infusion of corticosteroids may be beneficial to maintain steady plasma levels; however, a recent trial did not identify a difference between twice-daily intravenous dosing versus continuous infusions (21). The use of adrenocorticotropic hormone (ACTH) has not been shown to be superior to corticosteroids and, although it may be preferred in patients not previously exposed to corticosteroids, at a dose of 100 to 150 U per day (22), its use has become an anachronism.

The response to corticosteroids in the setting of severe fulminant colitis has remained constant for the past several decades (19), with approximately 75% of patients responding (11,19,23) and less than half failing to achieve remission (17). Mechanisms of steroid resistance have not been fully elucidated (24). The most critical assessment in the setting of fulminant colitis is the response to therapy within the first 5 days (11). The presence of hypoalbuminemia, high CRP, short duration of illness, and prior corticosteroid use are predictors of medical failure (25, 26). In addition, ex-smokers have a worse prognosis (27). Short-term prognosis to corticosteroids in severe disease can be predicted as early as 24 hours. Persistence of more than nine stools per day, an albumin less than 3 g/dL, or a pulse rate greater than 90 beats/minute was predictive of greater than 60% risk of colectomy (9). Patients with greater than eight stools per day and a CRP greater than 4.5 mg/dL by day 3 had an 85% likelihood of requiring colectomy (11) or cyclosporine therapy. Continuation of intravenous corticosteroids beyond 7 to 10 days does not provide any additional benefits (19,28) and may increase morbidity and surgical risks (29).

Patients who improve, as evidenced by restitution of formed bowel movements with the absence of bleeding and ability to pass flatus without using the toilet, are then transitioned to oral prednisone at the same daily dose used to achieve the clinical remission. They may be discharged from the hospital when tolerating a low-residue diet with formed stools without blood or rectal urgency; premature discharge is doomed to failure and readmission. Aminosalicylates are added as a maintenance therapy once patients are tolerating oral steroids and a full diet. The long-term prognosis after hospitalizations for severe colitis requiring corticosteroid therapy is not as promising as once considered (30–32). The impact of the addition of immunomodulators or biologics has not been assessed in this population.

Cyclosporin A, administered as a continuous IV infusion, either alone (33) or in combination with corticosteroids, has been effective in treating severe ulcerative colitis (28). Although initial studies employed a 4 mg/kg dose as a continuous infusion (28), subsequent trials have confirmed similar results and less toxicity with doses of 2 mg/kg (34). Immediate response rates up to 85% to 92% have been reported (35) and, similar to the experience with the "intensive intravenous corticosteroid" regime, failure to improve—as defined by having eight or more stools per day or persistence of CRP elevation after 3 days of cyclosporine—is predictive of the need for colectomy (11). Careful daily monitoring for serious side effects of nephrotoxicity, infection, and seizures must be carried out when using cyclosporine (36).

Once patients have responded to intravenous cyclosporine with achievement of a clinical remission—again, defined as formed bowel movements without bleeding or rectal urgency—they are transitioned to oral cyclosporine by doubling the intravenous dose for twice-daily oral administration (e.g., if the intravenous dose is 100 mg/24 hours, the oral dose would be 100 mg twice daily) (36). Patients receiving a combination of corticosteroids and cyclosporine should receive *Pneumocystis* prophylaxis with sulfamethoxazole-trimethoprim three times weekly (37). Forty to fifty percent of patients treated with intravenous cyclosporine experience long-term remission (37–40). Improved outcomes are reported for patients who have been transitioned to oral cyclosporine with the addition of 6-MP or azathioprine (37,41).

Most recently, infliximab, a chimeric anti tumor necrosis factor (TNF) monoclonal antibody, has been shown to be effective as outpatient therapy for patients with moderate to severe ulcerative colitis (42). The role of infliximab in fulminant ulcerative colitis has been debated; the controversy is likely related to the severity of the disease (43–45). The largest clinical trial enrolled outpatients with moderate to severe disease. Subsequent, smaller trials in hospitalized patients have demonstrated conflicting results (46–49). It appears that infliximab will be more effective for patients in the moderate to severe spectrum (47–49), whereas the results with fulminant disease are less convincing (43,47,48). In choosing between infliximab and cyclosporine therapy, the former has been more effective and easily administered (less therapeutic monitoring), whereas the results with cyclosporine have been more consistent in the sicker group of patients (7,17,44).

Surgical Management

Persistence of medical therapy in the setting of fulminant colitis must be balanced against the potential for a surgical "cure" of the disease. Indications for surgery in fulminant colitis include clinical deterioration or failure to respond to medical therapy (3,4,7,17). Although the medical management of fulminant colitis is similar to that for toxic megacolon, the absence of acute colonic dilatation may permit delay of surgical intervention. However, the timing of surgical intervention in these less urgent cases requires experienced clinical judgment. Early intervention to reduce mortality must be balanced against the potential for intensive medical management to control the inflammatory process and complications, thereby potentially preventing the psychosocial and medical stigmata of colectomy. Generally, in the absence of colonic dilatation, medical management may be continued for 5 to 7 days in a further attempt to reverse transmural inflammation, as long as the patient is stable and improving. Patients with fulminant colitis who do not begin to respond to the intensive intravenous steroid regimen, as described above, should be referred to a center experienced in cyclosporin therapy or undergo colectomy.

The type of operation performed for treatment of fulminant colitis depends on the clinical status of the patient and experience of the surgeon (7,17,50–52). A one-stage procedure that cures ulcerative colitis without the need for a second operation is appropriate for older patients or those not desiring restorative ileal pouch–anal anastomosis. Most surgeons prefer a limited abdominal colectomy with ileostomy, leaving the rectosigmoid as a mucous fistula or the rectum alone, using a Hartmann procedure (53). This approach has the advantages of limiting the lengthy pelvic dissection in acutely ill patients while allowing for the option of a subsequent restorative, sphincter-saving procedure (ileoanal anastomosis) (54). In patients with indeterminate colitis or Crohn disease, preservation of the rectum may provide the opportunity for an eventual ileorectal or ileoanal anastomosis to preserve anal continence after temporary diversion and pathologic review of the colectomy specimen (1,55).

TOXIC MEGACOLON

Toxic megacolon refers to acute nonobstructive dilatation of the colon, generally as a complication of ulcerative colitis, but it may occur with any severe inflammatory colitis (56). This condition has been described with idiopathic and infectious colitis, including ulcerative colitis, Crohn disease (57), amebic colitis (58), pseudomembranous colitis (59), and other infections (*Shigella*, *Salmonella*, Chagas disease, and cytomegalovirus [CMV]) (14,60). Toxic megacolon has been reported to complicate 1% to 13% of all ulcerative colitis cases (61,62) and 2% to 3% of Crohn colitis cases (62). Although mortality in early series was as high as 25%, reaching 50% if colonic perforation occurred, early recognition and management of toxic megacolon has substantially lowered mortality to below 15% (62) generally and, in experienced centers, usually below 2% (63). Factors associated with increased mortality include age older than 40 years, the presence of colonic perforation, and delay of surgery (62). Colonic perforation, whether free or localized, is the greatest risk factor leading to increased morbidity or death.

Predisposing Factors

The severity of disease activity is the most important predictor of toxic megacolon, which is more common in extensive colitis than in proctitis or proctosigmoiditis (64). However, limited right- or left-sided segmental colitis (61,62) has been associated with toxic megacolon (64,65).

Toxic megacolon typically occurs early in the course of ulcerative colitis, usually within the first 5 years of disease; 25% to 40% of cases present with the initial attack (62,64–66). The onset of toxic megacolon has been temporally linked to diagnostic examinations such as barium enemas or colonoscopy, suggesting that manipulation of the inflamed bowel or vigorous laxative preparation may exacerbate the process, possibly through electrolyte imbalance (62,64).

Certain drug therapies have been implicated in the development of toxic megacolon. Diphenoxylate atropine sulfate (Lomotil), loperamide, and other inhibitors of colonic motility such as opiates and narcotics may contribute to the development of toxic megacolon by inhibiting colon muscle function in severe transmural disease. Electrolyte and pH disturbances are risk factors for toxic megacolon (7). Severe potassium depletion, secondary to significant diarrhea or corticosteroid therapy, or both, is known to inhibit colonic motility. Despite early speculations regarding the role of corticosteroids in inducing toxic megacolon (67,68), most no longer accept the implication that corticosteroids or adrenocorticotropic hormone are precipitating factors (7,17,66,69,70). Concern remains, however, that corticosteroids may suppress signs of perforation, thereby delaying surgical therapy.

CMV infection may contribute to fulminant colitis or toxic megacolon (71–74). There are no controlled trials regarding the utility of treating CMV and, often, in the absence of systemic manifestations of CMV (e.g., fever, hepatitis), no treatment is necessary (7,17), although there are reports of successful intervention targeting CMV if identified in colon biopsies.

Clinical Features

Toxic megacolon usually occurs in the background of chronic inflammatory bowel disease (66,68,75). Jalan et al. described the most accepted clinical criteria based on signs, symptoms, and diagnostic abnormalities for toxic megacolon (56,62) (Table 156.2). The presentation typically evolves with progressive diarrhea, bloody stools, cramping abdominal pain, and abdominal distention. Impaired consciousness and lethargy may be present and are ominous signs (62). Occasionally, in chronically treated patients, a paradoxical decrease in stool frequency with passage of only bloody discharge or bloody membranes may be an ominous sign. Thereafter, clinical signs of toxemia, including pyrexia (temperature greater than 38.5°C) and tachycardia, develop as abdominal pain and distention become progressive and bowel sounds diminish or cease. On physical examination, peritoneal irritation, including rebound tenderness and abdominal guarding, represent transmural inflammation with serosal involvement, even in the absence of free perforation. Conversely, peritoneal signs may be minimal or absent in elderly patients or those receiving high-dose or prolonged corticosteroid therapy. In such patients, loss of hepatic dullness may be the first clinical indication of colonic perforation. Mental status changes, including confusion, agitation, and apathy, are occasionally noted (66). Leukocytosis, defined as total white blood cell count greater than 10,500 cells/μL, with a left shift, anemia, hypokalemia, and hypoalbuminemia are common laboratory findings (56).

TABLE 156.2

JALAN'S CRITERIA FOR DIAGNOSIS OF TOXIC MEGACOLON

1. Radiographic evidence of colonic dilatation
2. At least three of the following:
   a. Temperature greater than 38.5°C
   b. Heart rate greater than 120 bpm
   c. White blood cell count greater than 10.5 ($\times 10^3/\mu$L)
   d. Anemia
3. At least one of the following:
   a. Dehydration
   b. Mental status changes
   c. Electrolyte disturbances
   d. Hypotension

Jalan KN, et al. An experience of ulcerative colitis. I. Toxic dilation in 55 cases. *Gastroenterology.* 1969;57(1):68–82.

Diagnosis

Plain films of the abdomen are usually sufficient radiographic studies, revealing loss of haustration with segmental or total colonic dilatation (76) (Table 156.2). Clinical studies have demonstrated a strong correlation between colonic dilatation and deep ulceration involving the muscle layers (13). The magnitude of dilatation may not be severe, averaging 8 to 9 cm (normal is less than 5–6 cm), although colonic diameter may reach 15 cm before rupture. Maximal dilatation can occur in any part of the colon. Accompanying mucosal thumbprinting or pneumatosis cystoides coli reflects severe transmural disease. Free peritoneal air should serve as an immediate indication for surgery (62,66). Infrequently, retroperitoneal tracking of air from a colonic perforation may produce subcutaneous emphysema and pneumomediastinum without pneumoperitoneum (77). In patients with severe colitis, small bowel ileus may herald toxic megacolon (78,79) and is a bad prognostic sign for medical success (63). Discrepancies may exist between physical and radiographic findings. Abdominal distention by physical examination can be minimal despite massive colonic dilatation. Conversely, physical findings may dominate the presentation, and peritoneal signs in the absence of free air or dilatation should not be ignored.

Management

Just as in fulminant colitis, a coordinated team approach between medical and surgical services to management and monitoring is necessary in patients with toxic megacolon.

Medical Treatment

The initial treatment is supportive and similar to treatment outlined for fulminant colitis. Aggressive resuscitation with fluids, electrolytes, and blood is necessary. Patients with nausea and vomiting or significant abdominal pain should be on complete bowel rest. Anticholinergic and narcotic agents should be discontinued immediately. In the presence of small bowel ileus, a nasogastric tube is usually placed, and despite a lack of clear evidence for the placement of long intestinal tubes, they are advocated by some (80). Patient repositioning from front to back or prone knee–elbow position may redistribute colonic air and assist in decompression (81,82). Rarely, patients with dilatation in the absence of toxic signs or symptoms may benefit from rectal tube decompression.

Broad-spectrum antibiotics, with adequate Gram-negative and anaerobic coverage, are considered standard therapy and should be administered without delay once transmural inflammation or toxic megacolon is suspected (56). Antibiotics should be continued until the patient stabilizes over several days to a week or through the initial postoperative period. Whether antibiotics help avert progression of toxic megacolon is not known.

Generally, most patients with inflammatory bowel disease (IBD) will have been receiving corticosteroids before toxic megacolon developed, in which case they should be continued. There is no evidence that corticosteroids precipitate or worsen outcome in toxic megacolon. Similar to therapy for fulminant colitis, augmented doses of corticosteroids should be administered in view of the additional stress of the toxic state. There is concern that corticosteroids could mask signs of perforation or peritonitis, so close monitoring is necessary. In cases of toxic megacolon caused by infectious etiologies, corticosteroids should not be used. Just as in fulminant colitis, there is no consensus regarding the corticosteroid preparation for treatment in toxic megacolon.

Surgical Management

After 12 to 24 hours of intensive medical management, if no improvement or deterioration occurs, surgical intervention is required for toxic megacolon. Some physicians actually view early surgical management of toxic megacolon as the conservative approach, noting that delay of operative therapy may promote higher mortality.

Evidence of colonic perforation is an unequivocal indication for emergent surgery. If physical signs of perforation are absent, 12- to 24-hour radiographic surveillance is necessary. Perforation is associated with severe complications, including peritonitis, extreme fluid and electrolyte imbalance, and hemodynamic instability. Early recognition of perforation should lessen morbidity or mortality. Other indications for emergent surgery precluding protracted medical management include signs of septic shock, multiorgan dysfunction (7), and imminent transverse colon rupture (diameter greater than 12 cm) (56). Hypoalbuminemia, persistently elevated C-reactive protein or erythrocyte sedimentation rate, small bowel ileus, and deep colonic ulcers are poor prognostic factors for successful medical therapy (11,63,83,84).

The surgical management of toxic megacolon must be individualized for each patient. The type of operation is dependent on the clinical condition of the patient and the experience of the surgeon (51,52,85). The types of surgery are outlined in the fulminant colitis section. Rarely, "blow-hole" colotomies may be useful in highly selected individuals with poor operative prognoses (86).

COMPLICATING SCENARIOS IN INFLAMMATORY BOWEL DISEASE

Thrombosis

Inflammatory bowel disease is associated with an increased risk of arterial and venous thromboembolism (87). The prevalence of thromboembolism in IBD patients is as low as 1% to 8% (88) and as high as 39% in a postmortem study (87). The mechanism is unclear, but systemic inflammation is considered a potent prothrombotic stimulus. In addition, coagulation factor abnormalities—factor V Leiden, decreased antithrombin III, protein C and S, increased levels of factors V and VIII, fibrinogen, and plasminogen activator inhibitor—contribute to the hypercoagulable state (89–91). Another risk factor is recent abdominal surgery. In a case series of 83 patients who underwent total colectomy for inflammatory bowel disease, 4.8% developed mesenteric vein thrombosis (92). Deep vein thrombosis and pulmonary embolism are the most common presentation of thrombosis in IBD (87). Portal vein thrombosis in IBD has 50% mortality and occurs in 9% of patients with deep vein thrombus (93). Approximately 10% of thromboembolisms in IBD manifest as cerebral vascular accidents (94).

The treatment of deep vein thrombosis in IBD patients is similar to non-IBD patients. Options include unfractionated heparin, low-molecular-weight heparins, and warfarin for venous thrombosis (95). Those with contraindications to anticoagulation will require an inferior vena cava filter to prevent pulmonary embolus. Thrombolytics can be used for large pulmonary emboli. Arterial thrombosis treatment in IBD includes surgical thrombectomy or fibrinolysis (96,97).

Managing Pregnant Women with Inflammatory Bowel Disease

The treatment of fulminant colitis and toxic megacolon in the pregnant woman is similar to the nonpregnant patient. Continued severe illness poses a greater risk to the fetus than the medical or surgical intervention (98). Diagnostic modalities of ultrasound and magnetic resonance imaging (MRI) are safe and can be used for detection of abscess or colonic wall thickening and dilation. Low-dose radiographs (less than 5 rads) have minimal risk to fetus (99).

Flexible sigmoidoscopy is a valuable tool to assess the severity of disease and anatomic extent of disease. It is considered a safe procedure to perform when indicated (100). Full colonoscopy is rarely indicated. Polyethylene glycol solution has not been studied in pregnancy; thus, fetal outcomes are unknown. Generally, oral bowel preparations are not recommended and, if a full colonoscopy is necessary, tap water enemas are recommended (101). The indications for surgery—medically refractory severe colitis, obstruction, perforation, and intractable bleeding—are the same as in the nonpregnant IBD patient. Surgery for an acute indication in the setting of pregnancy carries a high risk of fetal loss (102), but case reports of deliveries of healthy infants following colectomy for fulminant colitis are reported (103,104). There is no evidence that therapeutic abortion improves the outcome of fulminant colitis, so it is not indicated. A team approach with early management and continuous assessment by the obstetrician, surgeon, and gastroenterologist is vital for the patient.

Gastrointestinal Bleeding

Massive gastrointestinal bleeding is an unusual complication in inflammatory bowel disease, occurring in 0.9% to 6% of patients (105,106). The general management is the same as in non-IBD patients. Resuscitation is the first step, followed by diagnostic evaluation—usually with endoscopy—to localize the site of bleeding. In one case series, colonoscopy identified the source of bleeding in 60% of IBD patients, and angiography was used in cases where colonoscopy was not diagnostic (107). Conservative therapy has been advocated, but surgery is indicated when bleeding is not stabilized by transfusions or if recurrent massive bleeding is present. Principles of management of gastrointestinal bleeding are discussed elsewhere in this text.

PEARLS

Management of Fulminant Colitis and Toxic Megacolon

- Team approach including medical and surgical personnel
- Intravenous fluid resuscitation
- Supplemental parenteral nutrition
- Bowel rest in the presence of vomiting, abdominal pain, or colonic dilatation
- Evaluate for enteric pathogens, *C. difficile*, and CMV
- Abdominal girth measurement
- Decompression
  - Nasogastric tube (ileus)
  - Repositioning maneuvers (colonic dilatation)
- Medical treatments
- Specific treatments for infections
- Intravenous corticosteroids for inflammatory bowel disease
- Cyclosporin or infliximab in selected patients not responding to intravenous corticosteroids after 3 to 7 days
- Broad-spectrum antibiotics if toxic
- Blood transfusions to maintain hematocrit at about 30%
- Radiology
  - Daily to frequent abdominal radiographs
  - Computed tomographic scan as needed for management
- Surgical indications
  - Failed medical therapy
  - Progressive dilatation or toxicity
  - Shock or multiorgan dysfunction
  - Persistent hemorrhage
  - Evidence of perforation

References

1. Swan NC, et al. Fulminant colitis in inflammatory bowel disease: detailed pathologic and clinical analysis. *Dis Colon Rectum.* 1998;41(12):1511–1515.
2. Truelove S, Witts L. Cortisone in ulcerative colitis. Final report on a therapeutic trial. *BMJ.* 1955;2:1041.
3. Carter MJ, Lobo AJ, Travis SP, Guidelines for the management of inflammatory bowel disease in adults. *Gut.* 2004;53(Suppl 5):V1–16.
4. Kornbluth A, Sachar DB. Ulcerative colitis practice guidelines in adults (update): American College of Gastroenterology, Practice Parameters Committee. *Am J Gastroenterol.* 2004;99(7):1371–1385.
5. Hanauer SB. Inflammatory bowel disease. *N Engl J Med.* 1996;334(13):841–848.
6. Stein R, Hanauer SB. Life-threatening complications of IBD: how to handle fulminant colitis and toxic megacolon. *J Crit Illness.* 1998;13(8):518–525.
7. Caprilli R, Viscido A, Latella G. Current management of severe ulcerative colitis. *Nature Clin Pract.* 2007;4(2):92–101.
8. Durai D, Hawthorne A. Review article: how and when to use ciclosporin in ulcerative colitis. *Aliment Pharmacol Ther.* 2005;22:907.
9. Lennard-Jones JE, et al. Assessment of severity in colitis: a preliminary study. *Gut.* 1975;16(8):579–584.
10. Prantera C, et al. The plain abdominal film accurately estimates extent of active ulcerative colitis. *J Clin Gastroenterol.* 1991;13(2):231–234.
11. Travis SP, et al. Predicting outcome in severe ulcerative colitis. *Gut.* 1996;38(6):905–910.
12. Allez M, et al. Long term outcome of patients with active Crohn's disease exhibiting extensive and deep ulcerations at colonoscopy. *Am J Gastroenterol.* 2002;97(4):947–953.
13. Buckell NA, et al. Depth of ulceration in acute colitis: correlation with outcome and clinical and radiologic features. *Gastroenterology.* 1980;79(1):19–25.
14. Cottone M, et al. Prevalence of cytomegalovirus infection in severe refractory ulcerative and Crohn's colitis. *Am J Gastroenterol.* 2001;96(3):773–775.
15. Carbonnel F, et al. Colonoscopy of acute colitis. A safe and reliable tool for assessment of severity. *Digest Dis Sci.* 1994;39(7):1550–1557.
16. Carbonnel F, et al. Predictive factors of outcome of intensive intravenous treatment for attacks of ulcerative colitis. *Aliment Pharmacol Ther.* 2000;14(3):273–279.
17. Jakobovits SL, Travis SP. Management of acute severe colitis. *Br Med Bull.* 2005;75–76:131–144.
18. McIntyre PB, et al. Controlled trial of bowel rest in the treatment of severe acute colitis. *Gut.* 1986;27(5):481–485.
19. Turner D, et al. Response to corticosteroids in severe ulcerative colitis: a systematic review of the literature and a meta-regression. *Clin Gastroenterol Hepatol.* 2007;5(1):103–110.
20. Rosenberg W, Ireland A, Jewell DP. High-dose methylprednisolone in the treatment of active ulcerative colitis. *J Clin Gastroenterol.* 1990;12(1):40–41.
21. Bossa F, et al. Continuous infusion versus bolus administration of steroids in severe attacks of ulcerative colitis: a randomized, double-blind trial. *Am J Gastroenterol.* 2007;102(3):601–608.
22. Meyers S, et al. Corticotropin versus hydrocortisone in the intravenous treatment of ulcerative colitis. A prospective, randomized, double-blind clinical trial. *Gastroenterology.* 1983;85(2):351–357.
23. Truelove SC, et al. Further experience in the treatment of severe attacks of ulcerative colitis. *Lancet.* 1978;2:1086–1088.
24. Creed TJ, Probert CS. Review article: steroid resistance in inflammatory bowel disease—mechanisms and therapeutic strategies. *Aliment Pharmacol Ther.* 2007;25(2):111–122.
25. Lindgren SC, et al. Early predictors of glucocorticosteroid treatment failure in severe and moderately severe attacks of ulcerative colitis. *Eur J Gastroenterol Hepatol.* 1998;10(10):831–835.
26. Kumar S, et al. Severe ulcerative colitis: prospective study of parameters determining outcome. *J Gastroenterol Hepatol.* 2004;19(11):1247–1252.
27. Odes HS, et al. Effects of current cigarette smoking on clinical course of Crohn's disease and ulcerative colitis. *Dig Dis Sci.* 2001;46(8):1717–1721.
28. Lichtiger S, et al. Cyclosporine in severe ulcerative colitis refractory to steroid therapy (see comment). *N Engl J Med.* 1994;330(26):1841–1845.
29. Poritz LS, et al. Intravenous cyclosporine for the treatment of severe steroid refractory ulcerative colitis: what is the cost? *Dis Colon Rectum.* 2005;48(9):1685–1690.
30. Faubion WA Jr, et al. The natural history of corticosteroid therapy for inflammatory bowel disease: a population-based study. *Gastroenterology.* 2001;121(2):255–260.
31. Ho GT, et al. The efficacy of corticosteroid therapy in inflammatory bowel disease: analysis of a 5-year UK inception cohort. *Aliment Pharmacol Ther.* 2006;24(2):319–330.
32. Tung J, et al. A population-based study of the frequency of corticosteroid resistance and dependence in pediatric patients with Crohn's disease and ulcerative colitis. *Inflamm Bowel Dis.* 2006;12(12):1093–1100.
33. D'Haens G, et al. Intravenous cyclosporine versus intravenous corticosteroids as single therapy for severe attacks of ulcerative colitis. *Gastroenterology.* 2001;120(6):1323–1329.
34. Van Assche G, et al. Randomized, double-blind comparison of 4 mg/kg versus 2 mg/kg intravenous cyclosporine in severe ulcerative colitis. *Gastroenterology.* 2003;125(4):1025–1031.
35. Pham CQ, Efros CB, Berardi RR. Cyclosporine for severe ulcerative colitis. *Ann Pharmacother.* 2006;40(1):96–101.
36. Kornbluth A, et al. Cyclosporin for severe ulcerative colitis: a user's guide. *Am J Gastroenterol.* 1997;92(9):1424–1428.
37. Cohen RD, Stein R, Hanauer SB. Intravenous cyclosporin in ulcerative colitis: a five-year experience (see comment). *Am J Gastroenterol.* 1999;94(6):1587–1592.
38. Arts J, et al. Long-term outcome of treatment with intravenous cyclosporin in patients with severe ulcerative colitis. *Inflamm Bowel Dis.* 2004;10(2):73–78.
39. Rayner CK, et al. Long-term results of low-dose intravenous ciclosporin for acute severe ulcerative colitis. *Aliment Pharmacol Ther.* 2003;18(3):303–308.
40. Campbell S, Travis S, Jewell D. Ciclosporin use in acute ulcerative colitis: a long-term experience. *Eur J Gastroenterol Hepatol.* 2005;17(1):79–84.
41. Moskovitz DN, et al. Incidence of colectomy during long-term follow-up after cyclosporine-induced remission of severe ulcerative colitis. *Clin Gastroenterol Hepatol.* 2006;4(6):760–765.
42. Rutgeerts P, et al. Infliximab for induction and maintenance therapy for ulcerative colitis. *N Engl J Med.* 2005;353(23):2462–2476.
43. Regueiro M, Curtis J, Plevy S. Infliximab for hospitalized patients with severe ulcerative colitis. *J Clin Gastroenterol.* 2006;40(6):476–481.
44. Hanauer SB. Infliximab or cyclosporine for severe ulcerative colitis. *Gastroenterology.* 2005;129(4):1358–1359; author reply 1359.
45. Jarnerot G. Infliximab or cyclosporine for severe ulcerative colitis. *Gastroenterology.* 2006;130(1):286; author reply 287.
46. Sands BE, et al. Infliximab in the treatment of severe, steroid-refractory ulcerative colitis: a pilot study (see comment). *Inflamm Bowel Dis.* 2001;7(2):83–88.
47. Actis GC, et al. Infliximab for treatment of steroid-refractory ulcerative colitis (see comment). *Digest Liver Dis.* 2002;34(9):631–634.
48. Jarnerot G, et al. Infliximab as rescue therapy in severe to moderately severe ulcerative colitis: a randomized, placebo-controlled study. *Gastroenterology.* 2005;128(7):1805–1811.

49. Probert CS, et al. Infliximab in moderately severe glucocorticoid resistant ulcerative colitis: a randomised controlled trial. *Gut.* 2003;52(7):998–1002.
50. Berg DF, et al. Acute surgical emergencies in inflammatory bowel disease. *Am J Surg.* 2002;184(1):45–51.
51. Cohen JL, et al. Practice parameters for the surgical treatment of ulcerative colitis. *Dis Colon Rectum.* 2005;48(11):1997–2009.
52. Larson DW, Pemberton JH. Current concepts and controversies in surgery for IBD. *Gastroenterology.* 2004;126(6):1611–1619.
53. Ritchie JK, et al. Management of severe acute colitis in district hospitals. *J Royal Soc Med.* 1984;77(6):465–471.
54. Mowschenson P. New surgical approaches. *Semin Colon Rectal Surg.* 1993;4:25.
55. Stewenius J, et al. Operations in unselected patients with ulcerative colitis and indeterminate colitis: a long-term follow-up study. *Eur J Surg.* 1996;162:131.
56. Gan SI, Beck PL. A new look at toxic megacolon: an update and review of incidence, etiology, pathogenesis, and management. *Am J Gastroenterol.* 2003;98(11):2363–2371.
57. Greenstein AJ, Kark AE, Dreiling DA. Crohn's disease of the colon. III. Toxic dilatation of the colon in Crohn's colitis. *Am J Gastroenterol.* 1975; 63(2):117–128.
58. Stein D, Bank S, Louw JH. Fulminating amoebic colitis. *Surgery.* 1979;85 (3):349–352.
59. Brown CH, Ferrante WA, Davis WD Jr. Toxic dilatation of the colon complicating pseudomembranous enterocolitis. *Am J Digest Dis.* 1968;13(9):813–821.
60. Schofield PF, Mandal BK, Ironside AG. Toxic dilatation of the colon in salmonella colitis and inflammatory bowel disease. *Br J Surg.* 1979;66(1): 5–8.
61. Greenstein AJ, et al. Outcome of toxic dilatation in ulcerative and Crohn's colitis. *J Clin Gastroenterol.* 1985;7(2):137–143.
62. Jalan KN, et al. An experience of ulcerative colitis. I. Toxic dilation in 55 cases. *Gastroenterology.* 1969;57(1):68–82.
63. Hyde GM, Jewell DP. Review article: the management of severe ulcerative colitis. *Aliment Pharmacol Ther.* 1997;11(3):419–424.
64. Farmer RG, Easley KA, Rankin GB. Clinical patterns, natural history, and progression of ulcerative colitis. A long-term follow-up of 1116 patients. *Digest Dis Sci.* 1993;38(6):1137–1146.
65. Kisloff B, Adkins JC. Toxic megacolon developing in a patient with long-standing distal ulcerative colitis. *Am J Gastroenterol.* 1981;75(6):451–453.
66. Norland CC, Kirsner JB. Toxic dilatation of colon (toxic megacolon): etiology, treatment and prognosis in 42 patients. *Medicine.* 1969;48(3):229–250.
67. Marshak R, Lester L, Frideman A. Megacolon, a complication of ulcerative colitis. *Gastroenterology.* 1950;16:768.
68. Binder HJ. Steroids and toxic megacolon. *Gastroenterology.* 1979;76(4): 888–889.
69. Truelove SC, Marks CG. Toxic megacolon. Part I: pathogenesis, diagnosis and treatment. *Clin Gastroenterol.* 1981;10(1):107–117.
70. Meyers S, Janowitz HD. The place of steroids in the therapy of toxic megacolon. *Gastroenterology.* 1978;75(4):729–731.
71. Kotanagi H, et al. A case of toxic megacolon in ulcerative colitis associated with cytomegalovirus infection. *J Gastroenterol.* 1994;29(4):501–505.
72. Kambham N, et al. Cytomegalovirus infection in steroid-refractory ulcerative colitis: a case-control study. *Am J Surg Pathol.* 2004;28(3):365–373.
73. Hommes DW, et al. The pathogenicity of cytomegalovirus in inflammatory bowel disease: a systematic review and evidence-based recommendations for future research. *Inflamm Bowel Dis.* 2004;10(3):245–250.
74. Maconi G, et al. Prevalence, detection rate and outcome of cytomegalovirus infection in ulcerative colitis patients requiring colonic resection. *Dig Liver Dis.* 2005;37(6):418–423.
75. Binder SC, Miller HH, Deterling RA Jr. Emergency and urgent operations for ulcerative colitis. The procedure of choice. *Arch Surg.* 1975;110(3):284–289.
76. Almer S, et al. Plain X-ray films and air enema films reflect severe mucosal inflammation in acute ulcerative colitis. *Digestion.* 1995;56(6):528–533.
77. Mogan GR, et al. Toxic megacolon in ulcerative colitis complicated by pneumomediastinum: report of two cases. *Gastroenterology.* 1980;79(3):559–562.
78. Caprilli R, et al. Early recognition of toxic megacolon. *J Clin Gastroenterol.* 1987;9(2):160–164.
79. Chew CN, Nolan DJ, Jewell DP. Small bowel gas in severe ulcerative colitis. *Gut.* 1991;32(12):1535–1537.
80. Present DH. Toxic megacolon. *Med Clin North Am.* 1993;77(5):1129–1148.
81. Present DH. The knee-elbow position relieves distension (comment). *Gut.* 1994;35(8):1150; author reply 1151.
82. Panos MZ, Wood MJ, Asquith P. Toxic megacolon: the knee-elbow position relieves bowel distension (see comments). *Gut.* 1993;34(12):1726–1727.
83. Chakravarty BJ. Predictors and the rate of medical treatment failure in ulcerative colitis. *Am J Gastroenterol.* 1993;88(6):852–855.
84. Lindgren SC, et al. Early predictors of glucocorticosteroid treatment failure in severe and moderately severe attacks of ulcerative colitis. *Eur J Gastroenterol Hepatol.* 1998;10(10):831–835.
85. D'Amico C, et al. Early surgery for the treatment of toxic megacolon. *Digestion.* 2005;72(2–3):146–149.
86. Remzi FH, et al. Current indications for blow-hole colostomy:ileostomy procedure. A single center experience. *Int J Colorectal Dis.* 2003;18(4): 361–364.
87. Talbot RW, et al. Vascular complications of inflammatory bowel disease. *Mayo Clin Proc.* 1986;61(2):140–145.
88. Koutroubakis IE. Role of thrombotic vascular risk factors in inflammatory bowel disease. *Digest Dis.* 2000;18(3):161–167.
89. Lake AM, Stauffer JQ, Stuart MJ. Hemostatic alterations in inflammatory bowel disease: response to therapy. *Am J Digest Dis.* 1978;23(10):897–902.
90. Lam A, et al. Coagulation studies in ulcerative colitis and Crohn's disease. *Gastroenterology.* 1975;68(2):245–251.
91. Liebman HA, et al. The factor V Leiden mutation increases the risk of venous thrombosis in patients with inflammatory bowel disease (see comment). *Gastroenterology.* 1998;115(4):830–834.
92. Fichera A, et al. Superior mesenteric vein thrombosis after colectomy for inflammatory bowel disease: a not uncommon cause of postoperative acute abdominal pain (see comment). *Dis Colon Rectum.* 2003;46(5):643–648.
93. Capron J, et al. Gastrointestinal bleeding due to chronic portal vein thrombosis in ulcerative colitis. *Digest Dis Sci.* 1979;24:232.
94. Schneiderman JH, Sharpe JA, Sutton DM. Cerebral and retinal vascular complications of inflammatory bowel disease. *Ann Neurol.* 1979;5(4):331–337.
95. Koutroubakis IE. Therapy insight: vascular complications in patients with inflammatory bowel disease. *Nat Clin Pract Gastroenterol Hepatol.* 2005;2(6):266–272.
96. Szychta P, et al. Aortic thrombosis and ulcerative colitis. *Ann Vasc Surg.* 2001;15(3):402–404.
97. Lengle SJ, Nadler P, Jordan GW. Arterial thrombosis in ulcerative colitis. Transcatheter thrombolytic therapy. *West J Med.* 1995;162(6):543–547.
98. Kane S. Inflammatory bowel disease in pregnancy. *Gastroenterol Clin North Am.* 2003;32(1):323–340.
99. American College of Obstetricians and Gynecologists. Guidelines for diagnostic imaging during pregnancy. *Int J Gynecol Obstet.* 1995;48:331.
100. Cappell MS, Colon VJ, Sidhom OA. A study at 10 medical centers of the safety and efficacy of 48 flexible sigmoidoscopies and 8 colonoscopies during pregnancy with follow-up of fetal outcome and with comparison to control groups. *Digest Dis Sci.* 1996;41(12):2353–2361.
101. Mahadevan U, Kane S. American gastroenterological association institute technical review on the use of gastrointestinal medications in pregnancy. *Gastroenterology.* 2006;131(1):283–2311.
102. Hill J, Clark A, Scott N. Surgical treatment of acute manifestations of Crohn's disease during pregnancy. *J Royal Soc Med.* 1998;90:64.
103. Boulton R, et al. Fulminant ulcerative colitis in pregnancy (see comment). *Am J Gastroenterol.* 1994;89(6):931–933.
104. Watson WJ, Gaines TE. Third-trimester colectomy for severe ulcerative colitis. A case report. *J Reprod Med.* 1987;32(11):869–872.
105. Robert JR, Sachar DB, Greenstein AJ. Severe gastrointestinal hemorrhage in Crohn's disease. *Ann Surg.* 1991;213(3):207–211.
106. Driver CP, Anderson DN, Keenan RA. Massive intestinal bleeding in association with Crohn's disease. *J Royal Coll Surg Edin.* 1996;41(3):152–154.
107. Belaiche J, et al. Acute lower gastrointestinal bleeding in Crohn's disease: characteristics of a unique series of 34 patients. Belgian IBD Research Group. *Am J Gastroenterol.* 1999;94(8):2177–2181.

CHAPTER 157 ■ ESOPHAGEAL DISORDERS

JACK A. DI PALMA • CODY B. BARNETT

IMMEDIATE CONCERNS

Various esophageal disorders may require intensive care or may develop in the critically ill. This chapter briefly reviews some of these disorders with attention to those that require emergency evaluation and treatment. As a rule, esophageal disorders become emergent when the airway is compromised either by the initial insult or by a high risk of aspiration. Protection of the airway is of major importance. Disorders of the esophagus that require emergency evaluation and treatment include obstruction, foreign bodies, corrosive injury, perforation, trauma, esophagitis in the immunocompromised host, medication injury, and bleeding. Esophageal bleeding is reviewed in another chapter; however, the other disorders may have subtle presentations, and the patient, at first glance, may not appear very ill.

Stress Points

1. Protection of the airway from aspiration
2. Consideration of aspiration and secondary pulmonary insult occurring *before* presentation
3. Elimination of ongoing damage (as in the case of corrosives)
4. Avoidance of long-term complications by careful initial management

ESOPHAGEAL OBSTRUCTION

Pearls

- It is not unusual for patients to present with sudden onset of the inability to swallow food, liquids, or saliva.
- Most are not critically ill, but life-threatening complications may develop.
- Occasionally, they may be orthostatic or dehydrated or may have aspirated gastrointestinal (GI) contents.
- The goal of management is to relieve the obstruction and to prevent potential complications such as aspiration, bleeding, or esophageal perforation.
- Most authors recommend immediate esophagoscopy to confirm the suspicion of obstruction and the use of endoscopic techniques to remove the impacted bolus or foreign body.
- Several nonendoscopic removal techniques and pharmacologic interventions are used as alternative approaches, particularly when endoscopy is not available or is considered risky.
- After obstruction is relieved, subsequent management is directed at evaluation of underlying esophageal pathology.

Presentation

Most patients with food impaction and esophageal obstruction present with acute onset of dysphagia and complete inability to swallow food or liquids, even their own saliva. It is not unusual for these persons to delay presentation for 24 to 96 hours and have resultant dehydration or orthostasis. Pulmonary aspiration of esophageal contents may occur before they seek treatment. Some may have experienced minor, transient episodes in the past and expected this prolonged event to resolve similarly. Typically, symptoms are temporarily related to swallowing a poorly chewed food bolus, usually meat. The descriptive names "steakhouse syndrome" or "backyard barbecue syndrome," therefore, have been applied (1). Many patients admit concurrent alcohol use or inebriation. Steakhouse syndrome is more common in older persons who may be edentulous or have poorly fitting dentures. Chest pain, odynophagia, hypersalivation, retching, and vomiting are associated complaints.

Physical examination should determine the consequences of fluid or electrolyte depletion or pulmonary aspiration.

Diagnostic Approach

Immediate esophagoscopy is the current approach recommended for diagnostic evaluation and treatment. It may be necessary to lavage the obstructed esophagus before the procedure, particularly if long delays occurred before the patient appeared for care. Esophagoscopy with flexible fiberoptic instruments is safe and rapid in the hands of experienced endoscopists. Most patients tolerate endoscopy well. It is probably the most acceptable approach to food impaction, allowing rapid confirmation of the esophageal obstruction, treatment, and, in most cases, evaluation for underlying esophageal pathology. Barium contrast radiographs can also be used to confirm obstruction and define the nature or location of the impaction. Figure 157.1 shows an esophagram with esophageal obstruction and impacted food bolus in the distal esophagus seen as a large filling defect. Contrast studies are neither necessary nor desirable because the presence of barium in the esophagus complicates removal of the bolus by compromising endoscopic visualization (2). Meglumine diatrizoate (Gastrografin) is avoided because it is hypertonic and results in severe pneumonitis if aspirated. If contrast radiographs are performed, an attempt should be made to carefully aspirate residual loose food, fluids, and

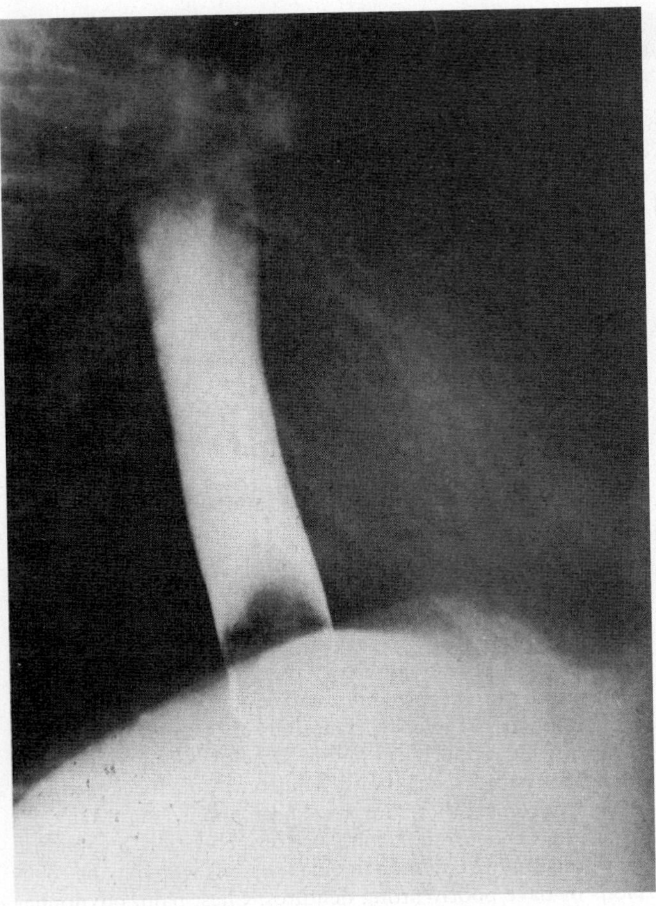

FIGURE 157.1. Barium esophagram shows food bolus impaction obstructing the distal esophagus.

barium before endoscopy. In cases where perforation is a concern, water-soluble contrast media may be used.

Management

Therapeutic options are endoscopic bolus retrieval, pharmacologic interventions to relieve obstruction, and nonendoscopic retrieval techniques. We prefer endoscopic management.

Endoscopy allows relief of bolus impaction to be attempted under direct visual guidance. The bolus can be retrieved and extracted using endoscopy forceps, graspers, or polyp retrieval devices. The bolus can also be desiccated by visually guided catheter lavage or broken up with enzyme-containing lavage solutions. The bezoar should not, however, be forced into the stomach until the nature of any underlying esophageal lesion is known.

Several alternatives to the endoscopic approach can be tried when a competent endoscopist is not available or when the planned endoscopic procedure and necessary sedation pose an unacceptable risk to the patient. The traditional approach has been to confirm impaction and obstruction with a barium sulfate contrast radiograph. Occasionally, the weight of the barium column above the impaction may relieve the obstruction. If the impaction is persistent, hormonal relaxation using 1 mg glucagon or 0.4 mg atropine intravenously given slowly may be tried (3). Sublingual nitroglycerin and oral hydralazine have been used as smooth muscle relaxants. The calcium channel blocker nifedipine has been suggested for esophageal spasm and obstruction. Nifedipine in doses of 20 mg given orally or buccally dramatically decreases distal esophageal and lower sphincter pressures in normal volunteers. In patients with achalasia, sphincter pressures after 20 mg nifedipine may be reduced more than 60%. These reductions are similar to those seen in patients who undergo surgical cardiomyotomy. We have had varying success using nifedipine for the food-obstructed esophagus. Doses of 20 mg of nifedipine are necessary because in the distal esophagus the pharmacologic effect of the commonly used 10-mg dose is minimal. Caution is advised when nifedipine doses of 20 mg or more are used, because blood pressure may be reduced and should be monitored carefully. Experience with other calcium blockers is limited.

Enzymatic therapy using papain or meat tenderizers has long been used in attempts to dissolve the food bolus (4). Such approaches are time consuming and specifically not advised in patients who have had obstruction for more than 24 hours. Patients with prolonged obstruction have some element of esophageal ischemia, and dissolution enzymes pose a risk in this situation.

Nonendoscopic procedures for food bolus removal have involved tubes for suction or retrieval with radiographically guided graspers or balloons to pull out the bolus. We have removed a food bolus using a 34F large-bore tube modified by cutting off the distal 8 to 9 cm with the side holes and making sure that the cut end is smooth (5). The patient's hypopharynx is anesthetized with lidocaine spray or gargle. We then put the patient in a left lateral decubitus position and pass the tube through the mouth to the level of the bolus. The procedure is guided by fluoroscopy, if available. Suction is applied using the 120-mL lavage syringe supplied in the tube kit. The food bolus is partially aspirated into the end of the large-bore tube and carefully extracted. Special caution is advised because the bolus could potentially be dropped while passing through the hypopharynx, posing a risk of tracheal aspiration and obstruction. This suction technique should be attempted only by personnel experienced in gastrointestinal tube placement and airway management.

Special Considerations for Subsequent Management and "Steakhouse Spasm"

Most authors have approached steakhouse syndrome and esophageal obstruction as disorders in which a food bolus impacts in or above a pre-existing esophageal lesion. Reported lesions include neoplastic, peptic, or caustic strictures, webs, distal rings, and vascular anomalies. Food impaction is also a common presentation of eosinophilic esophagitis (6). However, we reported data on several patients with food impaction and complete obstruction for 72 to 96 hours who had no underlying anatomic lesions (7). Subsequent endoscopy and barium radiographs were normal, but esophageal motility disorders were defined by esophageal manometry. A careful review of previous literature revealed that most reported cases of steakhouse syndrome had no anatomic explanation for obstruction, and we call this variant "steakhouse spasm" to emphasize the spastic nature of the obstruction. Before endoscopic bolus retrieval is attempted in these patients, we recommend correcting the fluid and electrolyte imbalance and using 20 mg buccal or sublingual nifedipine.

FOREIGN BODIES

Capsule

Foreign bodies other than meat bolus are a common cause of esophageal injury. Endoscopic removal is the preferred management. Special attention should be made to protect the airway.

Presentation

It has been reported that over 1,500 people die yearly because of foreign body ingestions (2,8). In this condition, the flexible fiberoptic endoscope has had a significant impact on management. Commonly ingested items include coins, batteries, sharp and pointed objects, and cocaine packets. As previously discussed, food impaction is probably the most common upper GI foreign body that requires medical management. Over 75% of foreign body obstructions occurs in pediatric patients (8). Children more often ingest coins and toys, whereas adults have problems with meat and bones. Prisoners and psychiatric patients have been known to ingest multiple and unusual objects (2).

Management

Most objects pass spontaneously, but approximately 10% to 20% need to be removed endoscopically, and about 1% may require surgery (8).

The preferred management for most foreign body obstructions of the upper GI tract is removal with a flexible endoscope. As a rule, pushing agents into the stomach is not recommended. An overtube or some other protective device is recommended to protect the upper GI mucosa from damage or perforation from sharp or pointed foreign bodies, particularly razor blades (9). Although less than 1% of foreign bodies may perforate the gut, all sharp and pointed objects should be removed before they pass the stomach in an attempt to avoid distal intestinal perforation. Batteries, particularly the small button battery type, may cause caustic mucosal injury. In the esophagus, esophagoaortic fistula has been reported. Batteries that reach the stomach do not pose as serious a risk of mucosal damage because of the acid milieu. Batteries in the stomach may be followed radiographically with endoscopic removal if symptoms develop or if the battery remains in the stomach for more than 36 to 48 hours. After the object is beyond the reach of the upper endoscope, it usually passes without difficulty. If it fails to progress or if the patient becomes symptomatic, surgical intervention may be necessary. In recent years, drugs (most commonly cocaine) have been swallowed in packet form for transport or other reasons for concealment. Endoscopy is not recommended in these conditions because of the risk of packet rupture. Surgery is the safest way to remove these agents.

Foreign bodies lodged in the hypopharynx or proximal esophagus may require rigid esophagoscopy. Most other objects are amenable to removal with a flexible endoscope. It must be emphasized that the airway should be protected because of the risk of dropping and aspirating the object as it passes the hypopharynx. When there is any doubt or risk, tracheal intubation or rigid esophagoscopy with general anesthesia can be used.

CORROSIVE INJURY

Pearls

- When presented with a patient who has ingested a caustic substance, immediate attention is focused on the overall condition, presence of systemic complications, status of oropharynx and airway, nature of the offending agent, and extent of injury (10,11).
- If the victim is seen within 1 hour of ingestion, neutralization of alkali with water or dilute vinegar, and neutralization of acids with milk or antacids can be tried.
- Emetics are contraindicated. If 1 hour has lapsed from ingestion of the substance, the patient should be kept NPO (nothing by mouth) and vigorously hydrated intravenously.
- The oropharynx should be examined carefully and radiographs of the chest and abdomen obtained.
- The extent and severity of damage should be assessed early using fiberoptic endoscopy.
- The value of antibiotics or steroid therapy is controversial, but antibiotics should be used for suspected aspiration or perforation and steroids for laryngeal edema.
- After initial stabilization, the goals of management are to observe the patient for complications such as infection or perforation and to prevent late sequelae of stricture formation.

Presentation

The clinical presentation of a patient with corrosive injury is dependent on the type (alkali or acid) and nature (solid or liquid) of the caustic substance (12). Liquid alkali is swallowed rapidly, causing less oropharyngeal injury but extensive damage to the esophagus and stomach. Solid alkali causes severe burns to the oropharynx and induces severe pain and expectoration such that little corrosive is actually swallowed. Acid ingestion injury is more localized to the gastric antrum, but systemic acidosis and toxicity have been reported. Thus, mouth pain, hoarseness, dysphagia, odynophagia, or abdominal pain can occur as determined by the agent ingested and location of the injury. Stridor, aphonia, dyspnea, and hoarseness suggest laryngeal edema. Substernal, abdominal, or back pain raises concern for mediastinitis or peritonitis.

Physical examination of the lips, mouth, and pharynx can reveal a spectrum of injuries from mild erythema to erosions, ulcers, and obvious severe burns. Some authors have graded the injury by the presence and severity of oropharyngeal findings at the time of admission. It is often possible to estimate the degree of esophageal injury from the state of the oropharynx and type of agent ingested, but esophageal damage has been seen in patients without oropharyngeal burns.

Diagnostic Approach

After the history and physical examination have been obtained, with particular attention devoted to the oropharyngeal and airway status, laboratory evaluation is directed at determining complications of the ingestion such as renal or hepatic insufficiency or anemia. Chest and abdominal radiographs should be performed to look for evidence of aspiration, visceral perforation, or mediastinal air. After the patient has been stabilized, the extent and severity of disease can be evaluated by fiberoptic endoscopy. Caustic injuries are graded similarly to skin burns (grades 1, 2, and 3 [worst]). When endoscopy was initially introduced as a diagnostic procedure for evaluating caustic ingestions, concern was raised about the risk of perforation. Authors opposed using early endoscopy or recommended not passing the endoscope beyond the first burned area. Recent work suggests that endoscopy can be safely performed early in the course and provides information about severity and extent of damage that may influence management (11,13) When possible, a complete endoscopic examination evaluating the esophagus, stomach, and duodenum should be accomplished. Recent data suggest that endoscopic ultrasound may help predict risk of subsequent stricture formation (14).

Radiographic examination can be helpful, particularly when endoscopy is not available or is dangerous because of suspected perforation. In these situations, water-soluble contrast agents should be used.

Complications

Chemical injury to the gastrointestinal tract and resultant complications depend on the nature of the agent, the quantity and concentration of the agent, and the contact time duration. Liquid alkali such as Liquid Plumber was a 20% sodium hydroxide solution when introduced in the late 1960s and was subsequently reduced to a 5% solution after being implicated in 20% of reported caustic ingestions. Liquid alkalis have a high specific gravity and pass rapidly through the esophagus to the stomach. In dogs, violent regurgitation of gastric contents and pyloric and cricopharyngeal spasm cause a seesaw action that prolongs contact time. Solid alkali is usually in crystal form and causes severe pain that limits further ingestion. Crystals adhere to mucous membranes of mouth, pharynx, and upper esophagus, causing predominantly proximal burns. Alkali produces injury by liquefaction necrosis. This type of injury enhances alkali penetration and prevents surface neutralization that results in full-thickness burns.

Concentrated acids produce a coagulative necrosis that forms eschar, which, with the coagulum, limits penetration to deeper muscular coats. Surface sloughing and perforation are therefore common problems. Late complications relate to location and extent of injury. Gastric injury may result in pyloric obstruction, antral stenosis, or hourglass deformity. Esophageal stricture may be proximal or distal, and despite careful management, develops in 10% to 20% of patients with caustic ingestion. In these patients, esophageal cancer has an estimated incidence of 2% to 4%, with a 1,000-fold increase over normal persons more than 20 years after the caustic burn. Acid ingestion, particularly glacial acetic acid, has been associated with higher frequency of complications and mortality rate than alkali ingestion (14).

In attempts to avoid cicatricial esophageal stenosis, several interventions have been tried with controversial results. Traditional approaches have used antibiotics, steroids, and early "prophylactic" dilations, but these cannot be supported by any well-controlled studies. Corticosteroids, in particular, have been shown not to be of benefit in treating children who have ingested caustic substances (15). Total parenteral nutrition, agents that impair collagen synthesis, penicillamine, and intraluminal splinting with large-bore Silastic tubes or nasogastric tubes have also been used, but the role of these techniques in stricture prevention remains unclear. Prophylactic stenting for severe caustic injury is not recommended, but self-expanding plastic stents may have some benefit in selected cases (16).

Management

Initial efforts are directed toward stabilizing the patient and replacing fluids and blood as appropriate (17). The need for careful assessment of the airway cannot be overemphasized. Translaryngeal intubation or tracheostomy may be necessary. Evidence of esophageal perforation requires early surgical intervention. The corrosive should be neutralized only when the patient is seen within 1 hour of ingestion. Milk or antacids are used for acid ingestions and water or vinegar for alkali ingestions. Nasogastric intubation should be avoided unless the tube is placed under direct vision.

Early endoscopy is used when feasible. Complete examination of the esophagus, stomach, and duodenum should be attempted. If no significant injury is found, the patient can be discharged. In patients with significant injury, hospitalization and careful management are necessary. The use of steroids or antibiotics is not routinely advocated. Broad-spectrum antibiotic coverage is used for signs of aspiration, infection, or suspected perforation, or it may be used when deep ulcers are present and perforation seems imminent. Laryngeal edema is treated with short courses of high-dose steroids. Early bougienage using mercury-weighted rubber (Maloney) or polyvinyl dilators can be used in an attempt to prevent strictures and is usually started 2 to 3 weeks after the ingestion. Patients are kept NPO until they can swallow their saliva. Then clear liquids are allowed, advancing the diet thereafter as tolerated. Parenteral nutrition should be started early after stabilization.

It must be remembered that corrosive injuries are often severe, causing full-thickness mucosal destruction and perforation. The patients must be carefully observed for the need of surgical intervention as it is often the best option in severe cases (18,19).

ESOPHAGEAL PERFORATION

Pearls

- Esophageal perforation is a catastrophic event that is uniformly fatal if left untreated.
- Despite improved understanding, potent antibiotics, and advances in surgical technique, the mortality remains at 15% to 20%.
- Identified poor prognostic factors are delayed treatment, severe underlying esophageal disease, the need for major extirpative procedures, and thoracic location of perforation.

- Early recognition and prompt diagnosis are essential because treatment delays greater than 12 hours are associated with increased mortality.
- Plain radiographs are valuable and suggestive of perforation in 90% of cases.
- Contrast radiographs using barium sulfate or water-soluble contrast agents provide pertinent information about the site and extent of perforation.
- Management includes broad-spectrum antibiotics, NPO status, intravenous hydration, nasogastric suction, and parenteral nutrition.
- Definitive treatment is usually surgical, but there is a place for conservative, nonoperative management of small, contained, instrumental injuries or pharyngeal perforations.

Presentation

Esophageal perforations may be iatrogenic or noniatrogenic. Iatrogenic causes occur as complications of instrumentation such as esophagoscopy, attempts at endotracheal intubation or obturator airway placement, or esophageal tubes or stents. Dilatation procedures and surgical misadventures or leaks also lead to perforation of the esophagus. Noniatrogenic causes are usually barogenic ruptures. The most well-known "spontaneous" rupture occurred in the gluttonous Dutch admiral Baron Van Wassanaer. The admiral gorged himself and induced forceful vomiting for relief. His autopsy by Hermann Boerhaave was published in 1724 and described the pathologic findings of barogenic esophageal rupture. Resultant signs and symptoms are similar for Boerhaave syndrome and iatrogenic perforations. Pain is a near-universal experience, and 30% of patients develop acute pain. Fever and leukocytosis are also common.

Other presentations are influenced by the site of perforation. Patients with abdominal esophageal segment tears have had retroperitoneal air and vague epigastric pain. Patients with thoracic perforations often complain of abdominal and back pain. Cervical perforations are associated with subcutaneous emphysema and chest pain. Symptoms that occur during or shortly after an esophageal procedure should raise concern for iatrogenic perforations. Other clinical findings in patients with esophageal tears include pleural effusion, pneumothorax, dysphagia, cervical crepitus, hematemesis, and shock. However, asymptomatic perforations have been demonstrated radiographically, which emphasizes the importance of an accurate history and a high index of suspicion.

Diagnostic Approach

The diagnosis of esophageal perforation may be fairly obvious, particularly in the iatrogenic group. Plain chest radiographs may suggest perforation in over 90% of patients (Fig. 157.2) (20). Findings include mediastinal air, pneumothorax, pleural effusion, infiltrate, or subcutaneous emphysema. Hyperextended neck films can reveal widened spaces, air, or esophageal displacement. Fears of barium mediastinitis have traditionally led to the use of water-soluble contrast media (21). Recent reports indicate that iodinated water-soluble contrast radiographs may be normal in 20% to 25% of thoracic and 50% of cervical perforations (20). Therefore, negative or equivocal findings on water-soluble studies should be immediately re-examined with barium sulfate contrast radiographs. Other authors believe that barium does not potentiate mediastinal inflammation. Because it is more palatable than water-soluble agents and less dangerous if aspirated into the bronchial tree, many use dilute barium in the initial examination to take advantage of its better coating and definition. Regardless of the agent used, it is important to examine the entire esophagus in multiple positions.

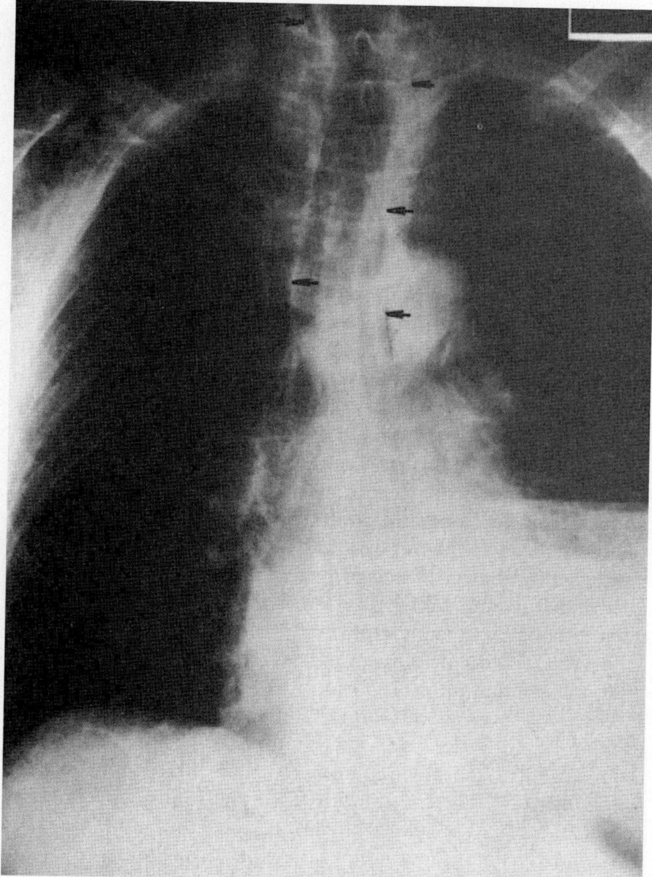

FIGURE 157.2. Chest radiograph in Boerhaave syndrome. Note left pleural effusion, esophageal deviation, and presence of mediastinal and subcutaneous air (*arrows*).

Management

Early diagnosis of esophageal perforation is essential for successful management. Intravenous access should be obtained and intravenous hydration initiated. The patient is placed NPO, and high-dose, broad-spectrum antibiotic therapy is started. Nasogastric suction and parenteral nutrition are used. Some authors recommend treating small instrumental tears or pharyngeal perforations nonoperatively, but most large instrument tears, trauma, or spontaneous perforations require surgery (22). Prompt neck exploration is advised for large cervical perforations. Absolute indications for operative intervention are sepsis, shock, respiratory failure, pneumothorax, pneumoperitoneum, and mediastinal emphysema. Most thoracic surgeons advise exploration with primary repair and drainage as the procedure of choice (23). Spontaneous esophageal perforation requires early surgical exploration with drainage and irrigation of mediastinum and pleural cavity. Most cervical perforations can be treated nonoperatively with therapy. Perforations often require surgical intervention (24).

Special Considerations

The development of small-bore fiberoptic endoscopy techniques has dramatically decreased the incidence of iatrogenic instrumental perforation from esophagoscopy (22). Previously used rigid esophagoscopy had a perforation rate of 0.2% to 1.9%. Perforation during esophagoscopy performed with modern flexible fiberscopes is approximately 0.01%. However, current palliative therapy for esophageal and gastric cardia neoplasms may have perforation rates above 10%. Aggressive therapeutic endoscopy techniques use laser photocoagulation and bipolar electrocoagulation, dilatation, or intubation with prosthetic stents. One report of 34 perforations occurring after palliative intubation notes favorable experience with nonsurgical management, particularly for pharyngeal tears, and advocates conservative management (25).

Before World War II, traumatic external injury to the esophagus was uncommonly reported (26). In an approach similar to that for spontaneous or instrumental perforations to the esophagus, early detection and prompt surgical exploration is emphasized. It must be remembered that with esophageal injury, both esophagoscopy and the radiographic esophagram can give false-negative results (26). Both studies have been recommended as a preoperative evaluation for ideal management in a patient in stable condition.

MEDICATION INJURY

Pearls

- In the critical care unit, we cannot ignore esophageal injury from prescribed medications.

Presentation

Accidental or suicidal injury with caustic agents has been previously discussed, but typical therapeutic doses of commonly used medications can cause significant esophageal injury. Patients predisposed to injury are those who are supine and who do not receive concurrent ingestion of adequate amounts of fluids. Such patients are frequent residents of the critical care unit. The American College of Gastroenterology (ACG) Committee on Food and Drug Administration (FDA)-related matters published a review of 127 cases of drug-induced esophagitis in 1987 (27). Eighty-nine percent of the cases were related to quinidine, potassium chloride, emepronium bromide, and tetracycline and its derivatives. The remaining 11% were caused by 14 other medications. Serious sequelae, including death, were linked to esophageal injury from medications, particularly those that may be potassium induced.

In the ACG report, the most common presenting symptoms of medication injury were retrosternal pain, odynophagia, and dysphagia. Retrosternal pain was seen in 61%, odynophagia in 50%, and dysphagia in 40%. Hematemesis and low-grade fever occurred, and complete aphagia with the inability to swallow oral secretions was not uncommon. Medication injury should be suspected in critically ill patients with unexplained esophageal symptoms. The diagnosis can be offered and made by clinical history alone, but radiographic or endoscopic diagnostic studies can add additional information concerning the nature of the injury.

TABLE 157.1

DRUGS IMPLICATED IN DRUG-INDUCED ESOPHAGEAL MUCOSAL INJURY

Commonly reported	Miscellaneous drugs
Emepronium bromide	Aspirin
Doxycycline	Nonsteroidal anti-inflammatory drugs
Tetracycline	Cromolyn
Minocycline	Theophylline
Potassium chloride	Phenobarbital
Quinidine	Ascorbic acid
	Alprenolol
	Naftidrofuryl
	Ferrous sulfate
	Clindamycin
	Bisphosphonates
	Lincomycin

Drugs implicated in medication esophageal injury are outlined in Table 157.1. Emepronium bromide is a quaternary ammonium anticholinergic agent with a peripheral effect similar to that of atropine. It is used predominantly in Great Britain for women with urinary frequency and urgency in an attempt to reduce muscular tone of the urinary bladder. Tetracycline, doxycycline, and minocycline are also frequent offenders. Sustained-release potassium chloride preparations were involved in 18 of the 127 cases of drug-induced esophagitis reported by the ACG. Potassium chloride solution and nonenteric preparations of potassium chloride are also reported to cause esophageal injury. A common area for esophageal stricture from these agents is at the level of the compression of the esophagus by the aortic arch or left antrum. In the group of patients reported, six deaths were related to potassium esophageal injury. Two patients developed fistulas from the esophagus to the aorta or left antrum. One patient had perforation to the mediastinum and died from sepsis. Another patient died from a bleeding esophageal ulcer. Quinidine is also a commonly reported agent of esophageal mucosal injury. In some of the reported cases, the patients were also taking medications that may have contributed to the injury, and some patients had underlying esophageal obstruction disease.

Management

Most cases of medication esophageal injury resolve without sequelae when the medication is discontinued (28). Liquid preparations may be substituted when it is not possible to discontinue the offending medication. Antacids, H_2 receptor antagonists, proton pump inhibitors, and cytoprotective agents can be given, although it is not clear if specific therapy is required or even effective. Severe odynophagia may be treated with a topical anesthetic agent. Esophageal stricture may be treated with bougienage.

In the critical care unit, prevention of esophageal injury is the best approach to the problem. If possible, patients should have the head of the bed elevated during oral medication administration with sufficient quantities of water given afterward. Certain medicines should be used with caution in patients with cardiomegaly or in those who are elderly or have known or suspected underlying esophageal obstruction. Oral potassium should be avoided in critically ill patients.

References

1. Palmer ED. Backyard barbecue syndrome: steak impaction in the esophagus. *JAMA.* 1976;125:277.
2. Brady PG. Management of esophageal and gastric foreign bodies. *A/S/G/E Clinical Update.* 1994;2:1.
3. Ferrucci JT, Long JA. Radiologic treatment of foreign food impaction using intravenous glucagon. *Radiology.* 1977;135:25.
4. Goldner F, Danley D. Enzymatic digestion of esophageal meat impaction—a study of Adolph's Meat Tenderizer. *Dig Dis Sci.* 1985;30:456.
5. Kozarek RA, Sanowski RA. Esophageal food impaction: description of a new method for bolus removal. *Dig Dis Sci.* 1980;25:100.
6. Desai TK, Stecevic V, Chang CH, et al. Association of eosinophilic inflammation with esophageal food impactions in adults. *Gastrintest Endosc.* 2005;61(7):795–801.
7. DiPalma JA, Brady CE III. Steakhouse spasm. *J Clin Gastroenterol.* 1987;9:274.
8. Webb WA. Management of foreign bodies in the upper gastrointestinal tract. *Gastroenterology.* 1988;94:204.
9. Marcon NE. Overtubes and foreign bodies. *Can J Gastroenterol.* 1990;4:599.
10. Goldman LP, Weigert JM. Corrosive substance ingestion: a review. *Am J Gastroenterol.* 1984;79:85.
11. Zargar SA, Kochhar R, Nagi B, et al. Ingestion of strong corrosive alkalis: spectrum of injury to upper gastrointestinal tract and natural history. *Am J Gastroenterol.* 1992;87:337.
12. Oakes DD, Sherck JP, Mark JBD. Lye ingestion—clinical patterns and therapeutic implications. *J Thorac Cardiovasc Surg.* 1982;83:194.
13. Poley JW, Steyerberg EW, Kuipers EJ, et al. Ingestion of acid and alkaline agents: outcome and prognostic value of early upper endoscopy. *Gastrointest Endosc.* 2004;60(3):372-377.
14. Kamijo Y, Kondo I, Kokuto M, et al. Miniprobe ultrasonography for determining prognosis in corrosive esophagitis. *Am J Gastroenterol.* 2004;99(5):851-854.
15. Anderson KD, Rouse TM, Randolph JG. A controlled trial of corticosteroids in children with corrosive injury of the esophagus. *N Engl J Med.* 1990;323:637.
16. Evrard S, Le Moine O, Lazaraki G, et al. Self-expanding metal stents for benign esophageal lesions. *Gastrointest Endosc.* 2004;60(6):894–900.
17. Tucker JA, Yarington CT. The treatment of caustic ingestion. *Otolaryngol Clin North Am.* 1979;12:343.
18. DiCostanzo J, Noirclerc M, Jouglard J, et al. New therapeutic approach to corrosive burns of the upper gastrointestinal tract. *Gut.* 1980;21:370.
19. Han Y, Cheng QS, Li XF, et al. Surgical management of esophageal strictures after caustic burns: a 30 year experience. *World J Gastroenterol.* 2004;10(19):2846–2849.
20. Phillips LG, Cunningham J. Esophageal perforation. *Radiol Clin North Am.* 1984;22:607.
21. Foley MJ, Ghahremani GG, Rogers LF. Reappraisal of contrast media used to detect upper gastrointestinal perforations—comparison of ionic water-soluble media with barium sulfate. *Radiology.* 1982;144:231.
22. Beck DE, DiPalma JA. Complications of gastrointestinal procedures. In: DiPalma JA, ed. *Problems in Critical Care: Gastrointestinal Complications.* Philadelphia, PA: JB Lippincott Co; 1989:361.
23. Richardson JD, Martin LF, Borzotta AP, et al. Unifying concepts in treatment of esophageal leaks. *Am J Surg.* 1985;149:157.
24. Amir A, van Dullemen H, Plukker JT, et al. Selective approach in the treatment of esophageal perforations. *Scand J Gastroenterol.* 2004;39(5):418–422.
25. Hine KR, Atkinson M. The diagnosis and management of perforations of esophagus and pharynx sustained during intubation of neoplastic esophageal strictures. *Dig Dis Sci.* 1986;31:571.
26. Cheadle W, Richardson JD. Options in management of trauma of the esophagus. *Surg Gynecol Obstet* 1982;155:380.
27. Bott S, Prakasah C, McCallum RW, et al. Medication-esophageal injury: survey of the literature. *Am J Gastroenterol.* 1987;82:758.
28. Abid S, Mumtaz K, Jafri W, et al. Pill-induced esophageal injury: evaluation, features, and clinical outcomes. *Endosurgery.* 2005;37(8):740–744.

CHAPTER 158 ■ GASTROINTESTINAL MOTILITY DISORDERS

NICHOLAS VERNE • JOHN G. LIEB, II

Motility is fundamental to the function of the gastrointestinal (GI) system such that alterations may lead to many gastrointestinal disorders, such as gastroesophageal reflux disease (GERD), irritable bowel syndrome, chronic constipation/diarrhea, and adynamic ileus. Although only the rare patient will be admitted to the intensive care unit (ICU) solely on the basis of a GI motility disorder, motility is a significant contributor to several ICU admission diagnoses such as aspiration pneumonia, Ogilvie syndrome, sigmoid volvulus, and so forth. In addition, disorders of gastrointestinal motility may complicate a patient's ICU course as in oropharyngeal dysfunction, gastroparesis, and enteral nutrition failures, a topic that is covered elsewhere. In this chapter, the major motility disorders that affect ICU management will be discussed starting at the esophagus and ending in the hindgut.

ESOPHAGUS

For several reasons, the esophagus is the ideal introductory topic to a chapter on GI motility. First, the esophagus is vulnerable to various insults in the ICU. Second, many of the principles of esophageal motility and dysmotility are fundamental to an understanding of other GI organs. Third, these principles are the best studied of any GI organ because of easy access to the esophagus.

The principal role of the esophagus is propulsion of sustenance towards the stomach, i.e., motility. The body of the esophagus, essentially a propulsive tube, accomplishes this role. A second role of the esophagus is to prevent unwanted material from entering the airway. In this role, two other suborgans of the esophagus, the upper esophageal sphincter (UES) and the lower esophageal sphincter (LES), are integral. Although the process of propulsion from oropharynx to stomach, i.e., *primary peristalsis*, appears simple, it requires a remarkably coordinated series of actions; for example, striated and smooth muscle must coordinate. Also, nitric oxide and acetylcholine—seemingly antagonistic neurotransmitters—must act synergistically. That the esophagus can accomplish these roles without the aid of, and even against, gravity, is all the more remarkable.

A brief review of normal esophageal physiology will assist in later discussions of esophageal motility disorders in the ICU. As in the rest of the GI tract, esophageal motility depends on intact function of the muscular layers of the esophageal wall and an intact local and central nervous system. The thickest and strongest contractile element of the esophagus is the muscular wall. In the proximal esophagus, including the UES, this muscle wall is striated, whereas in the distal two thirds of the esophagus, the muscle wall consists of two smooth muscle layers: longitudinal and circular. These smooth muscle layers are mostly under the control of the vagus nerve and the enteric nervous system, a "second brain," whose neural tissue weighs almost as much as the brain. This second brain consists of a neural plexus throughout the gut wall that regulates wall movement through the activation of local reflexes. These reflexes and the vagus coordinate the formation of a peristaltic wave, which consists of a contractile wave and a relaxation "bubble." For example, the power of the contractile wave depends on acetylcholine-mediated, lumen-occluding contraction of the circular smooth muscle proximal to the bolus of food. This contractile wave propels food down the esophagus, achieving pressures as high as 53 mm Hg in the upper, 35 mm Hg in the middle, and 69 mm Hg in the lower third of the esophagus. Equally as important, nitric oxide (NO) and vasoactive intestinal peptide (VIP) relax smooth muscle caudad to the bolus, creating a zone of lower pressure, that is a "bubble" of relaxation. This relaxation bubble also travels the length of the esophagus just ahead of the contractile wave and helps propagate the contractile wave toward the stomach. Together, the contractile wave and relaxation bubble form the *peristaltic wave*. To further propagate the peristaltic wave, the longitudinal smooth muscle layer contracts to shorten the length of the esophagus (1–5). The peristaltic wave of contraction and relaxation propels the food bolus and eventually reaches a point just above the LES (6). This is termed *primary peristalsis*, whereas *secondary peristalsis* occurs when a pressure stimulus is applied to the esophagus, such as from residual food left from an unsuccessful primary peristalsis or from refluxed gastric contents (7).

The LES is defined by esophageal manometry as a 2- to 4-cm zone of high resting pressure at the gastroesophageal junction (GEJ). This high resting pressure is formed by an extrinsic component of the surrounding crural diaphragm and an intrinsic smooth muscle component. Motilin and intra-abdominal pressure also cause LES contraction, which is abolished by atropine (8).

Relaxation of the LES is crucial to the pathophysiology of many motility disorders in the ICU and occurs under several circumstances. The first is a result of primary peristalsis from esophageal distention just proximal to the LES. With primary peristalsis and relaxation of the LES, a bolus is propelled into the stomach within 8 to 10 seconds (9). A second type of relaxation is transient LES relaxation, the primary motility disorder in GERD. This occurs in eructation and vomiting, and is activated through partly local and brainstem mechanisms. It may be elicited by pharyngeal stimulation, proximal gastric distention, and introduction of fat into the duodenum. Several common pharmacologic agents affect the function of the LES (Table 158.1).

With this background, we can now initiate a discussion of some of the most common esophageal motility disorders encountered in the ICU.

Oropharyngeal Motility Disorders

Any disorder of the upper esophagus inevitably involves the entire oropharyngeal system, including the oropharynx, thyroid cartilage, upper esophageal sphincter (UES), and more remnants of the "gill arches" such as the larynx, hyoid bone, and several cranial nerves (V, VII, IX, X, XII). The muscle of the oropharynx is exclusively striated and therefore requires nicotinic-acetylcholine and myelinated innervation as opposed to the muscarinic cholinergic smooth muscle of the distal two thirds of the esophagus. The advantage of striated muscle is its speed. However, measuring disorders of this speed necessitates testing inaccessible to most ICU patients: solid-state manometry in the UES and upper esophagus, or a cinemetric esophagram with higher-speed fluoroscopic imaging—for example, a "rehab swallow"—than that used for a routine barium swallow. Another disadvantage of striated muscle is that the upper esophagus is subject to the same damage as other striated muscle in the body. For example, rhabdomyolysis, polymyositis, hyperthyroidism, and myopathic drugs such as amiodarone, alcohol, vincristine, steroids, and statins can all disrupt the normal functioning of the oropharyngeal system.

The extensive neurologic innervation and coordination is a second Achilles heel of this system and explains why so many disorders of this system are neurologic in origin. For example, one third of stroke, Parkinson, and Alzheimer patients have oropharyngeal dysphagia (10–13). Oropharyngeal dysfunction affects the outcome of acute stroke, probably through increasing the risk of aspiration pneumonia (14). The risk of aspiration is best assessed by video barium swallow; clinical assessments are less sensitive (15,16).

Typical symptoms and signs include choking and gagging during meals; repeated (often unsuccessful) attempts at swallowing, nasal regurgitation of food and drink, and immediate regurgitation of the swallowed bolus—or in the case of a Zenker diverticulum, regurgitation of old undigested food. Other bulbar signs and symptoms such as vertigo, hiccup, tinnitus, ataxia, diplopia, horizontal ophthalmoplegia, and drop attacks may indicate brainstem and cranial nerve dysfunction such as from vertebrobasilar insufficiency, stroke, the Miller-Fisher variant of Guillain-Barré syndrome, or paraneoplastic cerebellar degeneration. Muscle fatigability and nasal voice would point to myasthenia gravis. Generalized weakness would point to a rhabdomyolysis, myositis, a steroid or drug-induced myopathy, or a motor neuron degenerative process such as amyotrophic lateral sclerosis (ALS). Symptoms of dry mouth should point to anticholinergic side effects of ICU

TABLE 158.1

AGENTS THAT AFFECT THE LOWER ESOPHAGEAL SPHINCTER (LES)

	Elevated LES pressure	Decreased LES pressure
Drugs	α-agonists β-antagonists (especially β2) Cholinergics (bethanecol) Suxamethonium (142) Metoclopramide Domperidone Cisapride Vecuronium (142) (not pancuronium)	α-antagonists β-agonists Anticholinergics Calcium channel blockers Theophylline Diazepam Meperidine Morphine Barbiturates Nitrates Dopamine ETOH Caffeine
Endogenous modifiers	Gastrin Motilin Substance P Prostaglandin F2-α	Cholecystokinin Secretin Glucagon Progesterone VIP
Food	Protein	Fat Chocolate Peppermint

ETOH, ethanol; VIP, vasoactive intestinal peptide.
Modified from van der Hoeven CW, Attia A, Deen L, et al. The influence of anaesthetic drugs on the lower oesophageal sphincter in propofol/nitrous oxide anaesthetized dogs. Pressure profilometry in an animal model. *Acta Anaesthesiol Scand.* 1995;39(6):822–826, with permission.

drugs or the sicca syndrome of rheumatoid arthritis or Sjögren syndrome (17).

Some other disorders that may impair oropharyngeal function, and hence render the patient vulnerable to aspiration, include radiation-induced neuronal and myopathic damage, postcricoid webs, and cervical osteophytes. Some of the most common devices in the ICU, e.g., nasogastric or nasoduodenal tubes, can further disturb oropharyngeal and upper esophageal motility, and lead to aspiration (18).

The treatment of oropharyngeal disorders is guided by three principles: (a) a multidisciplinary approach is vital, (b) treatment must be tailored to the cause of the disorder, and (c) treatment is chronic and progress can be slow. In particular, involvement of the speech and swallow therapists is essential. They teach swallowing exercises, dietary modifications, and techniques tailored to the disorder to help the patient improve swallowing function. Also, rheumatologists can assist in the treatment of connective tissue disease with anti-inflammatory therapies. Additionally, neurologists can assist in the diagnosis and medical management of myasthenia gravis with acetylcholinesterase inhibitors and Parkinson disease with prodopaminergic drugs. They can also rule out immediate concerns such as vertebrobasilar stroke and drug effects. Finally, radiologists and gastroenterologists can assist with ruling out other diagnoses and offer means of long-term feeding access.

Diffuse Esophageal Spasm

In contrast to disorders of the oropharynx, which are often multisystem in origin and treatment, the first disorder of the intrinsic esophagus is mostly a primary esophageal disorder. In the ICU, diffuse esophageal spasm may manifest as chest pain with workup negative for acute myocardial infarction, pulmonary embolus, or aortic dissection. The hallmark of diffuse esophageal spasm (DES) is uncoordinated esophageal contraction, often unprovoked by swallowing. In DES, peristalsis is haphazard, with multiple—sometimes spontaneous—and nearly simultaneous high-amplitude contractions.

Nitric oxide sequestration and donation have been shown to induce and inhibit, respectively, the contractions seen in DES (19,20), pointing to disorganized, nitric oxide–dependent esophageal body relaxation in this disorder. This disordered contraction is either primary or may be secondary to GERD, as evidenced by the disproportionate prevalence of GERD in patients with DES. In addition, some patients are hyperresponsive to the contractile effects of cholinergic stimuli during edrophonium testing (21).

Clinical Presentation

Chest pain is the cardinal feature of DES. This can be difficult to distinguish from angina pectoris, especially since the majority of patients are older than age 50 years. Pain may be provoked by swallowing, emotional distress, cholinergic stimuli, or rarely, exercise, and lasts seconds to minutes, and sometimes hours. Some patients may also present with dysphagia.

Diagnosis

Spasm may be present on barium radiographs showing multiple, unprovoked nonlumen-occluding contractions that may propel the barium both caudad and cephalad. However, manometry is considered the gold standard for diagnosis.

Although much debate surrounds the definition of DES, most authorities believe a few of the following manometric criteria—especially numbers 1, 2, and 3—would rule in the diagnosis:

1. Nonpropulsive contractions on at least 10% of test swallows
2. High-amplitude contractions greater than 30 mm Hg
3. Triple-peaked contractions
4. Hypertensive LES

Treatment

Because many patients have DES secondary to GERD, most physicians advocate that the first treatment should be an empiric course of antireflux therapy. Trials using twice-daily proton pump inhibitors (PPIs) for patients with chest pain may demonstrate close to 90% efficacy with comparable diagnostic accuracy to ambulatory pH monitoring. Antispasmodics such as sublingual nitroglycerine (22), nifedipine, and anticholinergics may be used but are inconsistent at relieving pain (23,24), probably because they also relax the LES and perpetuate reflux. Therefore, anticholinergics should be used only for PPI failure. Some patients respond to attempts at decreasing visceral pain sensation with antidepressants such as trazodone, 100 to 150 mg, or low-dose tricyclic antidepressants (25).

Nutcracker Esophagus

A variant of esophageal spasm that presents with chest pain, almost always during swallowing, and high-amplitude but coordinated contractions is called *nutcracker esophagus*. Manometrically, nutcracker esophagus is defined as greater than 80% of contractions effective and peristaltic, with an amplitude greater than 180 mm Hg. In theory, this pressure may be enough to decrease blood supply to the esophagus, and may be the cause of pain in this disorder. However mucosal integrity is almost universally intact due to the redundant blood supply to the esophagus (26). Treatment focuses on GERD and is similar to that of diffuse spasm.

Achalasia

Classic or idiopathic achalasia, as its Greek root for "lack of relaxation" implies, is defined by two key abnormalities: poor relaxation of the LES, and aperistalsis of the esophageal body (27,28). It is a rare disorder, occurring in 1 in 10,000 (29)—common enough for most gastroenterologists to have seen a few cases, but uncommon enough to make its diagnosis and treatment challenging. For example, years may pass between the development of symptoms and the diagnosis of achalasia. Therefore, it is not uncommon of for achalasia to be diagnosed in the ICU in a patient with an unexplained wide mediastinum (Fig. 158.1) or aspiration.

The cause of idiopathic achalasia is unknown, but several hypotheses have been suggested, including viral (30), neurodegenerative (31), genetic (32), autoimmune (33), or, more likely, a combination of the above. Regardless, the end pathophysiologic event is destruction of nitric oxide and VIP neurons in the myenteric plexus, preventing effective LES relaxation and causing esophageal body aperistalsis.

The symptoms of achalasia include dysphagia to solids *and* liquids (like most motility disorders as opposed to structural disorders), weight loss, and regurgitation of phlegm (especially

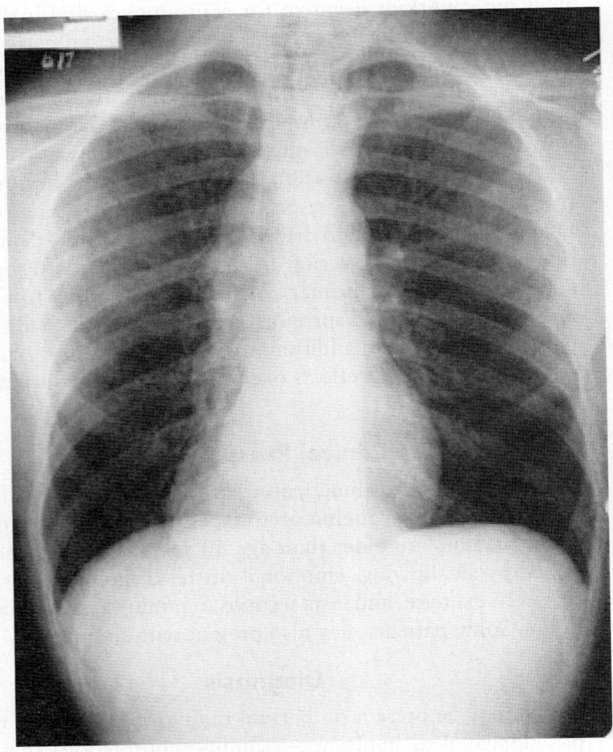

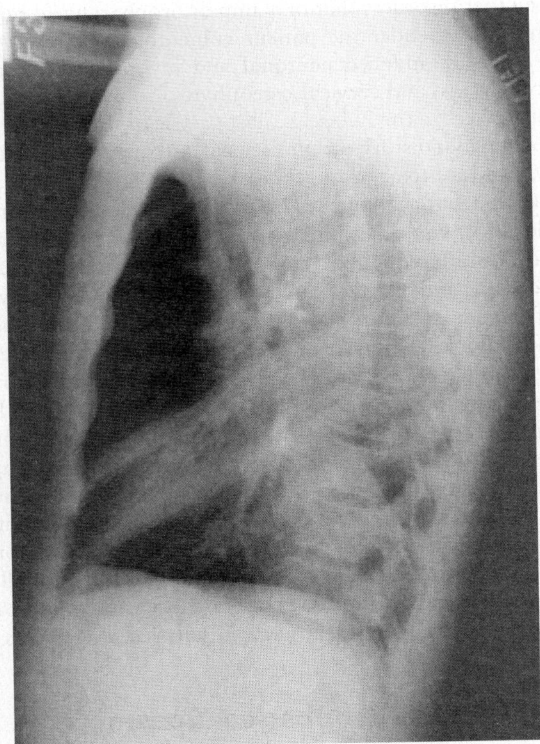

FIGURE 158.1. A wide mediastinum can result from achalasia. (Courtesy of Department of Radiology, Detroit Receiving Hospital, Detroit, Michigan.)

in the morning) and undigested food, often several days old. Some patients may present with pneumonia or food impaction (described later). A few case reports in the literature have described acute postprandial airway obstruction in patients with classic achalasia (34) combined with "upper achalasia," i.e., inability of the upper esophageal sphincter to relax. In those cases, swallowed air cannot be released and the resultant dilatation of the esophagus compresses the airway. Emergent nasogastric tube (NGT) decompression of the esophagus is the immediate treatment of choice (35). For chronic therapy of upper achalasia, a cricopharyngeal myotomy or Botox to the UES by otolaryngology may be effective.

Some diagnostic features of classical achalasia include the bird's beak—a long and narrow LES on barium swallow—and characteristic manometric findings. Other possible presenting features include a retrocardiac mass or mediastinal air fluid level on plain chest radiographs and an epiphrenic esophageal diverticulum, which can be perforated by Dobbhoff or NGT placement.

Secondary causes of achalasia should be ruled out, including gastroesophageal, lung, or breast cancer; lymphoma; amyloidosis; sarcoidosis; paraneoplastic syndromes; and Chagas disease caused by a trypanosome protozoan prevalent in South America and resulting in megaesophagus and megacolon (see below) due to inflammation in the myenteric plexus.

Treatment aims to relax the LES, including endoscopic Botox injection or balloon dilation (36), and Heller myotomy. Botox works by poisoning acetylcholine (ACh)-containing neurons, thus restoring a balance in the LES between ACh and nitric oxide—between contraction and relaxation. Various medications have been tried, such as oral nitrates (37) and sildenafil (38), as well as calcium channel blockers, especially the dihydropyridine calcium channel blockers; the nondihydropyridines, such as diltiazem and verapamil, may be somewhat less effective (39). Unfortunately, tachyphylaxis limits the clinical utility of these oral antispasmodics in the treatment of achalasia.

Hypotonic Lower Esophageal Sphincter

A hypotonic LES, defined by a manometric pressure less than 10 mm Hg, may also be suggested radiographically by a patulous (i.e., wide open, or gaping) gastroesophageal junction (GEJ). Many studies over decades have typically associated these findings with GERD, often with a sliding hiatal hernia.

For the ICU, the hypotonic LES may assume great importance during cardiopulmonary arrest. In animal models, the LES pressure drops from a baseline of 20 cm H_2O to 5 cm H_2O (3.8 mm Hg) (40).* In simulations of cardiac arrest during ventilation with bag-valve-mask device, this low pressure leads to stomach ventilation (41), diaphragm elevation, reduced respiratory system compliance (42), aspiration, and poor outcomes (43). Several investigators have shown acute drops in LES pressure during cardiopulmonary arrest (44).

Several techniques may limit the impact of hypotonic LES during arrest. We propose that first responders minimize peak airway pressure to less than 5 cm H_2O, lower tidal volumes to 300 to 500 mL with a higher FiO_2 (45), and decrease peak inspiratory flow (46). Pressure can be applied over the cricoid to seal off the esophagus (47). Arguably, several of these techniques could be extrapolated to patients on noninvasive ventilation.

*1 mm Hg = 1.33 cm H_2O.

Impaired Esophageal Motility

Weak esophageal body motility has more recently been termed *ineffective esophageal motility* (IEM). Manometrically, IEM has more than two swallows out of ten associated with esophageal body contraction amplitudes less than 30 mm Hg, which is the minimum required to propel a barium bolus. Some patients with IEM may complain of dysphagia secondary to slow transit through the esophagus. Much controversy surrounds whether GERD and acid exposure are the cause, or the result, of IEM. Patients may develop secondary overgrowth with *Candida*, or may develop one of the most common causes of GI bleeding in the ICU: esophagitis. Dobbhoff and NG tubes, which lower LES pressure, can be especially dangerous in these patients, facilitating acid-induced esophageal damage. If ICU clinicians require gastroduodenal access, ruling out *epiphrenic diverticula* is advised before nasogastric or nasoduodenal tube placement in IEM, as in the case of achalasia.

Conditions that predispose to IEM, other than GERD, include many of the connective tissue diseases such as scleroderma, CREST, hypothyroidism, mixed connective tissue disease, rheumatoid arthritis, Raynaud's phenomenon, systemic lupus erythematosus, chronic intestinal pseudoobstruction, amyloidosis, diabetes mellitus, and multiple sclerosis. Scleroderma, CREST (calcinosis, Raynaud phenomenon, esophageal motility disorders, sclerodactyly, and telangiectasia), and mixed connective tissue disease often have additional factors that predispose to GERD and esophageal damage including decreased LES pressure, gastroparesis, and colonic inertia. Mechanisms are controversial but likely include spasm and vasculitis of the vasa nervorum (capillaries around nerve bodies), periaxonal collagen deposition, and even antimyenteric plexus antibodies. All of these mechanisms may eventually progress to atrophy and fibrosis of smooth muscle in the esophagus. Fundoplication may improve esophageal motility in some patients with IEM but can be risky in connective tissue disease patients due to the high incidence of postoperative dysphagia (48). Therefore, the principal management is twice-daily proton pump inhibitors and antireflux measures, such as avoiding drugs that relax the LES, and elevation of the head of the bed.

Some investigators have tried promotility drugs effective elsewhere in the GI tract such as metoclopramide and, more recently, tegaserod in the management of IEM. Unfortunately, no one has shown a clear-cut clinical benefit from these agents as of yet (49). However, anecdotal experience at our institution suggests that erythromycin, tegaserod, and an older procholinergic prokinetic, formerly used in surgical patients with postoperative gastroparesis and bladder stasis, bethanecol, may be useful. In diabetic or connective disease patients, treatment other than twice-a-day proton pump inhibitor and avoidance of Dobbhoff and NG tubes is aimed at the systemic disease.

Food Impaction in the Esophagus

Abnormal motility may contribute to an important esophageal emergency: food impaction. The three typical areas of impaction, in order of increasing frequency, include the upper esophageal sphincter, the level of the aortic arch, and the distal esophagus. Predisposition varies depending on the location. In the upper esophagus, neurologic disease or Zenker diverticula can be factors, whereas in the middle esophagus, extrinsic compression by aortic aneurysm and malignant lymph nodes predominate. In the most common location, the distal esophagus, many disorders may predispose to impaction, such as Schatzki ring, achalasia, spasm, and cancer. In some series, approximately 50% of patients with food impaction have underlying motility disturbance such as eosinophilic esophagitis (50). Patients may present with choking or foreign body sensation, neck pain, and sudden onset of the inability to swallow food or saliva. Inability to speak, or hoarseness, may imply supralaryngeal impaction or compression of the larynx by a distended esophagus, and may necessitate an otolaryngologic consult to rule out impaction that could endanger the airway before an endoscopy is performed. Most patients with food impaction are not critically ill, but occasionally they may be dehydrated or may have aspirated. Immediate management aims to relieve the obstruction and prevent potential complications such as aspiration, bleeding, or esophageal perforation. Most authors recommend immediate endoscopic removal of the impacted bolus or foreign body to prevent edema and fibrosis, and to restore patency of the lumen.

STOMACH AND SMALL INTESTINE

Motility disorders of the stomach and small bowel are common in the ICU. To understand these disorders, we must review normal physiology.

The physiology of the stomach and small bowel is intimately linked. Specifically, the stomach functions as three suborgans: (a) a body/fundus for storage, (b) an antrum for grinding, and (c) a pacemaker for the entire GI tract, usually along the greater curve. This pacemaker governs the *migrating motor complex* (MMC), an essential GI motility pattern that links stomach and small bowel. Disorders in any of the suborgans can have profound symptomatology, such as distention and intolerance to tube feeds, increased aspiration risk, decreased absorption of drugs, increased risk for stress ulceration, and so forth.

The suborgans of the stomach monitor food content and regulate the speed of gastric emptying. For example, the second suborgan, the antrum, is the area primarily responsible for grinding of solid food particles in the fed state. This grinding better prepares the food for absorption in the small intestine (51). However, the drawback of this grinding is a delay of gastric emptying of solids, which is significantly slower than that of liquids. Furthermore, under normal circumstances, only particles less than 1 mm pass the pylorus, so that particles larger than that may have delayed emptying. For example, on average, the stomach clears 1-cm pieces of calf liver after 5 hours, whereas most 2- to 3-mm pieces are emptied within 2 hours, and homogenized liver empties within 30 minutes (52). However, erythromycin, a propulsive agent, can stimulate the passage of particles larger than 1 mm through the pylorus.

The third suborgan of the stomach, the pacemaker for the MMC, plays a crucial role in the emptying of solids. This pacemaker is located in 80% of patients on the greater curve of the stomach and the remainder in the duodenum (53). Several times daily in the normal fasting state, massive motor waves, dubbed the *activity front* of the MMC (Fig. 158.2), stimulate emptying of large particles through the pylorus and into the small intestine. Disruption of the pacemaker of the MMC may in part explain the high rate of GI symptoms after partial gastrectomy/bariatric surgery. For example, without a pacemaker and MMC to clear particles greater than 1 mm, bezoars may form; in theory, bezoars may predispose to aspiration.

In addition, these activity fronts of phase III of the MMC are essential in the function and coordination of the stomach and entire small bowel. The activity front of phase III is the "gastrointestinal housekeeper" and propagates all the way to the ileum. In addition to assisting gastric emptying of large

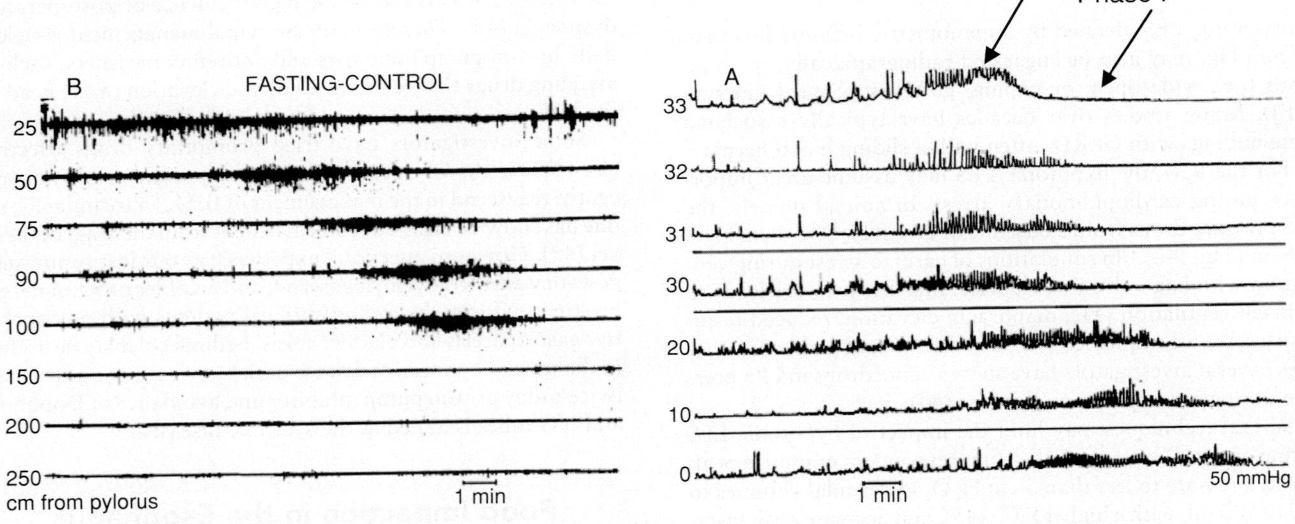

FIGURE 158.2. Activity front of the MMC seen by antroduodenal manometry. The *y* axis is the distance from the pylorus at multiple leads, and the *x* axis is time. Phase III is the Activity Front (AF) of the MMC. MMC, migrating motor complex. (From *Braz J Med Biol Res.*1998;31(7):889–900, with permission.)

particles, these waves clear bacteria from the proximal small bowel to prevent the syndrome of *bacterial overgrowth*. These waves also clear the entire GI tract of shed epithelial cells. Interestingly, caloric intake of as little as 200 kcal inhibits these important waves. This is the principle why an astute public speaker will eat a candy bar to prevent stomach "growling" on the lecture circuit. Theoretically in the ICU, patients receiving continuous enteral feedings may have less frequent or diminished activity fronts of the MMC. This lack of a GI housekeeper could predispose to tube-feed diarrhea, bloating, abdominal pain, bacterial overgrowth and translocation, poor stomach emptying, and aspiration.

The best studied method of measuring the activity fronts of the MMC is by antroduodenal (small bowel) manometry. Manometry requires insertion of a pressure-sensitive catheter in a cooperative patient, under fluoroscopy, into the proximal small bowel. Three leads are antral and three are duodenal. In only extraordinary cases, manometry can be accomplished in the ICU. However, in outpatients, the antroduodenal manometry catheter monitors fed and fasting states and responses to various prokinetic agents. Generally, low-dose octreotide—50 μg at bedtime—is the best stimulant of MMC activity fronts in ambulatory patients. However, in gastroparetics, our anecdotal experience with small bowel manometry favors azithromycin liquid, 400 mg each morning (which has *virtually* no risk of prolonging QT), or erythromycin liquid, 200 mg every 6 hours, 30 min before meals if the Q-Tc is less than 440 msec. The risk of sudden death with erythromycin is highly controversial (see below, Gastroparesis).

The first-mentioned suborgan of the stomach, the fundus, accounts for differences between liquid and solid emptying. Relaxation and enlargement of the fundus are crucial to the digestion of large liquid meals or solid meals that contain liquid. The vagus nerve mediates this relaxation of the fundus (54). Diabetics may have a vagal neuropathy and, together with surgical vagotomy patients, often lack this ability of the stomach to accommodate, leading to rapid liquid emptying, postprandial pain, and diarrhea. The effect of metoclopramide in the symptom relief of gastroparesis may be due to procholinergic stimulation of fundic relaxation and compliance.

The nutritional content of gastric contents also regulates how the stomach processes food. For example, isotonic materials empty quickest, whereas hypertonic ones empty slowest, with hypotonic materials emptying at intermediate speed. Proteins and carbohydrates empty equally well and much better than fats, which stimulate cholecystokinin, thought to perturb gastric emptying in such disorders as chronic pancreatitis (55). Delays in the gastric clearance of fat may have profound importance: common diabetic drinks and enteral formulations are usually low in carbohydrates, but their high fat content in theory may decrease gastric emptying. High-glucose concentrations, at a threshold of 8%, may also empty slower than 1% glucose solutions, which empty quickly, at about the same rate as 0.9% NaCl (56).

The stomach and small bowel are also in close communication via the gastroileal reflex. When high-nutrient contents reach the ileum, normal patients have a feedback reflex that delays release of stomach contents into the duodenum and decreases gastric emptying. In animals, this can be induced by instillation of fat into the ileum. The gastroileal reflex, in theory, may partly explain the paradox of the typical ICU patient: intolerant of tube feeds, with simultaneous diarrhea—due to poor absorption and high nutrient contents reaching the bacteria of the large bowel—and bloating/distention due to gastroparesis.

In the following text, we will investigate disorders of gastric and small intestinal motility.

Gastroparesis

Definitions of gastroparesis vary but, in general, the hallmark of gastroparesis is a delay in the emptying of solids. Patients complain of nausea (93%), abdominal pain (90%), early satiety (86%), and vomiting (68%) (57). Another common complaint is bloating, either perceived or frankly visible; patients may describe changing belt or pant size after meals.

Gastroparesis may contribute to aspiration pneumonia by two mechanisms. The first is by increasing gastroesophageal reflux. For example, up to 15% of ambulatory patients with refractory GERD have gastroparesis (58), leading one to speculate that gastroparesis may predispose to aspiration pneumonia in the ICU (59). In addition to promoting more frequent reflux in the ICU, gastroparesis stimulates colonization of the stomach with Gram-negative enteric and nosocomial flora, putting patients in the ICU with gastroparesis at increased risk for Gram-negative pneumonia (60).

The diagnosis of gastroparesis can be problematic. Barium studies lack caloric content and are liquid based. Therefore, they are a poor reflection of gastric or, for that matter, small bowel motility. Evidence suggests noncaloric liquids empty based only on the pressure they apply to the luminal wall (61). However, gastric scintigraphy with a technitium-99 labeled egg sandwich more accurately measures gastric emptying, especially of solids. Unfortunately, nearly every large medical center in this country seems to have its own protocol, controls, and standards for this test. In addition, a single patient's gastric emptying can vary from day to day due to nicotine intake or to recent narcotic or prokinetic ingestion. Male and female populations have different standards for gastric emptying, but generally a half-time of emptying of greater than 90 minutes implies gastroparesis. More specificity can be gained by extending the amount of time the patient remains in the scanner. For example, the gastric residual at 2 hours is the most common measurement in community hospitals, and although sensitivity may be 100%, specificity is only 20%. The 4-hour measurement is more accurate with 100% sensitivity and 70% specificity (62). However, even the 2-hour measurement is impractical for the ICU setting, and gold standards to compare against scintigraphy are lacking. In addition, clinicians often encounter the quandary of a patient with borderline emptying at 100 minutes. One way to handle such a case is to recollect that, in our hands, most patients with symptomatic gastroparesis have emptying half-times greater than 120 minutes. However, many patients with normal half-times clinically benefit from prokinetics. Therefore, in borderline cases, we move to antroduodenal manometry or treat empirically.

Causes for gastroparesis are similar to almost all motility disorders and are quite diverse, including metabolic disorders: diabetes, hypothyroidism, uremia; drug-induced emptying disorders: narcotics; infiltrative processes: amyloid, scleroderma; and backflow-related disorders such as portal hypertension, right-sided congestive heart failure (CHF), or hypoalbuminemia; nonetheless, many remain idiopathic. Diabetics presenting with gastroparesis often have evidence of neuropathy. Indeed, a vagal neuropathy is believed to be the fundamental problem in diabetic gastroparesis. Due to the rising incidence of type 2 diabetes, the number of gastroparesis patients with type 2 diabetes now equals that with type 1 diabetes. Idiopathic patients are more often female of childbearing age. The hormone progesterone may be responsible for hyperemesis gravidarum and idiopathic gastroparesis.

A hallmark of gastroparesis treatment is medical management. *Erythromycin*, a motilin agonist, is one of the strongest pharmacologic stimulants of gastric emptying (63,64). Unfortunately, it is short acting, limited by tachyphylaxis, and must be given in intravenous (IV) form immediately before eating, or in PO (oral) form about 30 minutes before each meal. Given the fast-paced environment in today's intensive care units, it may be impractical to dose this medicine at the exact time it is needed. Because gastric emptying to solids is slower than that of liquids, we prefer the suspension over the tablet form, 100 to 200 mg three times daily and before meals. However, IV administration may be more effective, and we have some experience with outpatients who require a PICC (peripherally inserted central catheter) line with chronic four-times-daily IV erythromycin. Another use of erythromycin in the ICU was found in one study to increase the tolerance of enteral nutrition in critically ill patients (66).

Much controversy surrounds the dangers of QTc prolongation in patients taking erythromycin. One methodologically problematic study found several deaths due to dysrhythmias in patients taking chronic erythromycin (67). Although these risks may be overstated, to be cautious, we recommend avoiding P450 inhibitors and other medications that also prolong the QTc while on erythromycin, such as several of the antidepressants and antidysrhythmics, including common ICU drugs such as fluconazole, quinidine, amiodarone, procainamide, and haloperidol. Fortunately, another option is *azithromycin* which does not prolong the QT interval (65). During antroduodenal manometry, we see pronounced antral contractions from azithromycin at a dose of 400 mg liquid orally 30 min before breakfast (unpublished data). However, like all macrolides, azithromycin can cause significant diarrhea. This side effect can be useful in the patient with adynamic ileus, chronic colonic inertia, or constipation-predominant irritable bowel syndrome, but can be problematic in ICU patients with antibiotic or tube-feed–associated diarrhea. Another drawback of the macrolides is some patients will develop abdominal pain and nausea. Part of this phenomenon can be explained by experiments showing that overdrive pacing the stomach faster than its baseline contraction rate of three waves per minute can sometimes delay gastric emptying (68). Therefore, it is not unreasonable to start low, at 100 mg liquid orally three times daily 30 minutes before meals.

Another agent in the treatment of gastroparesis is *metoclopramide*, a mixed dopamine antagonist and procholinergic. This drug has fallen out of favor in recent years for several reasons. First, 20% of patients develop Parkinsonism early or sometimes very late into treatment. Usually, this is reversible. However, 3% of patients taking metoclopramide will develop irreversible tardive dyskinesia (69). In addition, many patients experience restlessness and agitation. Metoclopramide is not as potent a stimulant of gastric emptying as the macrolides, and stimulates colon and esophageal motility very poorly. The typical dose is 5 to 10 mg three times daily, 30 min before meals IV or PO.

Because of the difficulties with macrolides and metoclopramide, gastroenterologists have sought other agents. One of those was *cisapride*, which is a very strong stimulant of all enteric motility. Unfortunately, several deaths due to torsades de pointes occurred, and it is no longer available for use (70). However, on a compassionate basis, it is still available from the manufacturer.

Zelnorm (*tegaserod*) is often used off-label to supplement other therapies for gastroparesis, but in rare patients can be used as monotherapy (71). It is a partial 5HT4 agonist. We typically crush 6 mg mixed with 2 to 3 ounces of liquid or applesauce three times daily 30 minutes before eating. Side effects are relatively rare but include diarrhea and headaches. As the side effects indicate, it is useful for chronic constipation and FDA approved for women with constipation-predominant irritable bowel syndrome and men and women with chronic constipation. However, it has not been well tested in patients with creatinine (Cr) clearance less than 40 mL/minute. Unfortunately, in February 2007, the FDA took tegaserod off the market due to a very low absolute risk of cardiac events.

Bethanecol is an older drug, formerly used in postsurgical ileus and bladder stasis, but may be useful in the gastroparetic patient who is intolerant of macrolides (72). As bethanecol is a procholinergic agent, one must monitor for potentially life-threatening reactions such as reactive airways disease, bradycardia, prostate obstruction, and diarrhea. The typical dose for gastroparesis is 25 mg orally four times daily.

Serum glucose is a strong inhibitor of gastric emptying (73,74); therefore, tight control of glucose is fundamental to treating gastroparesis. We aim for a glucose less than 200 mg/dL, even postprandially, especially in patients admitted for nausea and vomiting of gastroparesis. In addition, hyperglycemia attenuates the effects of prokinetics (75). Hyperglycemia also reduces the frequency of MMCs and affects small bowel motility (76). Therefore, tight glucose control may benefit other motility disturbances, especially postoperative ileus.

In ambulatory gastroparesis patients, the choice of narcotic may help patients considerably for not only gastroparesis, but all the slow motility disorders. For example, we prefer Ultram and propoxyphene, which have fewer effects on motility than traditional mu-agonists such as morphine, fentanyl, and Dilaudid (77). A promising treatment in gastroparesis—and in all motility, for that matter—is a mu-opiate antagonist that does not cross the blood–brain barrier. A recent study showed benefit in postoperative ileus patients receiving an investigational opiate antagonist agent (78). However, although other investigators have successfully used agents similar to this in dog models of gastroparesis, results in humans have been disappointing (79–81).

In addition to changing opiates, discontinuing other antimotility agents such as calcium channel blockers, anticholinergics, and alpha-2 antagonists such as clonidine is important in the management of gastroparesis (82).

Dumping Syndrome

Dumping syndrome is a constellation of postprandial symptoms in patients who have undergone surgical vagotomy and gastric drainage procedures such as pyloroplasty, antrectomy, or gastric resections (83,84). Inadvertent damage to the vagal nerve as in esophageal surgery or from neuropathy can also cause dumping syndrome. Therefore, ICU clinicians may encounter this disorder. In the dumping syndrome, abnormally rapid emptying of gastric contents leads to early delivery of osmotically rich food into the small intestine, resulting in volume shifts and the excessive release of vasoactive peptides and insulin. Symptoms include adrenergic discharge with symptoms such as tachycardia, diaphoresis, agitation or confusion, diarrhea, abdominal cramps, and even hypotension. Measurable hypoglycemia was once thought to be common in dumping syndrome, but further studies have not concurred; perhaps the autonomic nervous system provides sufficient counterregulation to insulin surge in most patients to prevent frank hypoglycemia. A key historical point in the diagnosis of dumping syndrome is that patients are free of these symptoms under fasting conditions. The symptoms are classified as early dumping, within the first 30 to 60 minutes after meal ingestion, and less commonly, late dumping, within 90 to 240 minutes after meals. Liquids and foods rich in carbohydrates are generally not well tolerated, and patients may lose weight due to fear of eating meals (84).

Dietary adjustments are fundamental to the management of the dumping syndrome (85). Patients should divide their caloric intake over at least six meals per day and minimize intake of fluids with solids. Meals rich in carbohydrates, such as Boost or Ensure, commonly induce dumping symptoms. Therefore, dumping patients should eat meals high in protein and fat and low in carbohydrates. Because lactose is absorbed in the jejunum, many patients experience milk intolerance after gastrojejunostomy and respond to restriction of lactose-containing products. The addition of agents like pectin or guar gum that increase the meal viscosity may help patients with dumping symptoms, although these supplements are not universally well tolerated. Dietary fiber may be effective in dumping syndrome (86,87). Acarbose, which delays carbohydrate absorption, may prevent late dumping (88,89). However, diarrhea due to fermentation of unabsorbed carbohydrates limits long-term use.

Mechanical Ventilation/Pressors and Stomach and Small Intestine Motility

Two very common ICU treatments, mechanical ventilation and pressors, cause profound motility disturbances of the stomach and small bowel. Two observational studies measured antroduodenal manometry in mechanically ventilated ICU patients, most on opiate sedation and dopamine. These studies found marked disruptions in the normal fed state and increased phase III activity fronts—which should be off to facilitate mixing and absorption in the fed state—leading to poor tolerance of enteral feeding (90,91). Low-dose dopamine causes a similar effect in healthy volunteers (92) and, in a recent randomized controlled trial, in hemodynamically stable ICU patients (93). Perhaps this effect causes the diarrhea and malabsorption so often seen in critically ill patients on initiation of enteral nutrition. In the latter trial, despite the exclusion of opiate use, the dopamine group also had significantly fewer fasting antral contractions. Thus, dopamine may delay gastric emptying independent of opiate use in the ICU. However, the astute reader may recognize a possible confounder in this study: Most of the patients received IV propofol, which has a high fat content and can delay gastric emptying. However, a second study of critically ill patients also found delayed absorption of acetaminophen, a marker of gastric emptying (94). In the acetaminophen study, significantly higher volumes of gastric contents were aspirated while on dopamine. Dopamine may also prevent the normal fundic relaxation that is essential to prevent aspiration during ingestion of large volumes (95). Perhaps metoclopramide, a dopamine antagonist, which primarily stimulates fundic relaxation and accommodation, could reverse this effect of dopamine (see gastroparesis section for pitfalls of metoclopramide use). Vasopressin may also delay gastric emptying (96). Overall, mechanical ventilation and pressor use may decrease antral motility and reduce fundic relaxation, perhaps accounting for the bloating and high gastric tube outputs sometimes seen in enterally fed ICU patients.

Intestinal Ileus (Acute Intestinal Pseudo-obstruction)

Although many ICU patients have the aberrant, fed-state stimulation of MMCs demonstrated above, a more common scenario is inhibition of small intestinal motility in the ICU, leading to the condition of the small intestinal ileus, or paralytic ileus, an acute delay in caudad passage of intestinal contents in the absence of obstruction.

Patients with ileus present with distention, poorly localized abdominal pain, nausea, vomiting, obstipation, and decreased bowel sounds. Differentiating ileus from mechanical obstruction can be challenging, and an obstruction series abdominal film can be suggestive. However, passage of computed tomography (CT) contrast into the colon within 4 hours virtually excludes mechanical obstruction (97).

Recent surgery or bowel manipulation can decrease bowel motility, leading to ileus. Normally, small intestinal motility returns within 24 hours after surgery, whereas gastric motility returns after 48 hours and that of the colon after 3 to 5 days. Various surgical factors are thought to account for differences in length of postoperative ileus, such as vagotomy, degree of intestinal manipulation, and presence of enterotomy, but these have not been proven (98,99). Several investigators have shown that activity of the left colon is key to recovery from postoperative ileus (100,101).

Causes of ileus are often multifactorial. Laparotomy decreases the amplitude of MMCs; activation of the sympathetic nervous system is likely a major factor. Similarly, inflammation plays an important role and may account for decreases in postoperative ileus in laparoscopic, as compared to open, surgeries (102). Epidural anesthesia may decrease the incidence of ileus compared to conventional narcotic analgesia (103). Sepsis, mesenteric ischemia, myocardial infarction, lower lobe pneumonia, lower rib fractures, chronic mesenteric ischemia, phenothiazines, calcium channel blockers (especially the nondihydropyridines), hypokalemia, hypomagnesemia and hypermagnesemia, hyponatremia, hypercalcemia—please note that because many ICU patients are hypoalbuminemic, an ionized calcium value is crucial here—and thyroid disorders have all been associated with intestinal ileus (104). Hypoalbuminemia may lead to bowel edema, which may account for part of the decreased motility seen in portal hypertension (105).

Most patients can be managed conservatively by identifying and treating/removing contributors to ileus. In patients with marked distention, pain, or respiratory compromise, NG suctioning should be initiated. In our practice, we recommend physical therapy and turning or sitting patients upright every shift. Some have advocated serial rectal exams, a brief trial of a rectal tube, or gentle tap water or 1 to 2 Fleet enemas (although, because these contain sodium phosphate, they should not be used in hypernatremic, hyperphosphatemic patients) to stimulate motility. Oral and stimulant laxatives should be avoided, especially lactulose, which releases hydrogen gas that can add to the problem, especially if mechanical obstruction has not definitively been ruled out. Unfortunately, prokinetic agents have so far been disappointing in the treatment of intestinal ileus. Metoclopramide is more potent in the foregut than hindgut. Erythromycin, a more potent foregut agent, is also active in the hindgut, but has not been shown to be effective in postoperative patients (106). The latter agent and tegaserod may have roles in the medical patient with ileus. Many agents are being tested in this exciting area of motility research.

Chronic Intestinal Pseudo-obstruction

Although it would be quite rare to diagnose chronic intestinal pseudo-obstruction in the ICU, for completeness, we will review the presentation, pathophysiology, causes, and treatments of this family of disorders. These rare motility disorders are characterized by symptoms and signs of chronic nonmechanical intestinal obstruction. Many of these disorders can affect the GI tract in several areas, causing megacolon, megaesophagus, megaduodenum, and so forth. The presence of small bowel diverticula should prompt a search for one of these disorders. Patients can present with steatorrhea from small bowel overgrowth, alternating constipation and diarrhea depending on recent antibiotic use, feculent vomiting and halitosis, gastroparesis, pseudoachalasia, or even GI hemorrhage.

Generally these disorders are characterized as either myopathic or neuropathic, and can be congenital or acquired.

The visceral myopathies involve degeneration and fibrosis of the muscularis propria, which can involve the smooth muscle of the bowel (enlarged esophagus, megaduodenum, redundant colon); iris (mydriasis); face (ptosis, ophthalmoplegia); bladder (megacystitis); and uterus (uterine inertia). They can present at any age, genetically or sporadically (107). Histology may show absence of actin, degenerating myofibrils, and mitochondrial abnormalities (108). Systemic disorders can cause visceral myopathy such as scleroderma and amyloidosis. Barium enema may show lack of haustrations, unlike the neuropathic disorders reviewed below. Antroduodenal manometery may show low-amplitude or absent MMCs (109).

In contrast, the visceral neuropathies are degenerative disorders of the myenteric plexus but can also be familial or sporadic. Histologically, these disorders display degeneration and/or inflammation of axons, dendrites, and absence of silver staining, occasionally with viral inclusions of cytomegalovirus (CMV) (110) or Epstein-Barr virus (EBV) (111). Other systemic contributors to visceral neuropathy include myxedema, Parkinson, narcotic bowel syndrome, late-stage Chagas disease, tumor or stroke of the medulla, acute encephalitis, and paraneoplastic neuronal degeneration, often from occult small cell carcinoma. This association is important to recognize because the time from diagnosis of extraintestinal primary small cell tumor to death is less than 1 year (112). In contrast to the myopathic disorders, the neuropathic disorders show uncoordinated bursts of activity, and abnormal propagation and configuration of MMCs (113). As in the myopathic disorders, suction biopsy can sometimes be diagnostic, but often a full thickness biopsy is required (113).

Treatment of visceral myopathy and neuropathy can be medical with erythromycin (115) or low-dose octreotide, 50 μg at bedtime, especially in scleroderma (114,115), nutritional with addition of B_{12} and fat-soluble vitamins with or without TPN, or surgical with resection of involved segments (116).

LARGE INTESTINE

Diarrhea

Diarrhea is a common ICU problem. Although a comprehensive approach to acute and chronic diarrhea is too expansive for this chapter, several important ICU diagnoses need to be ruled out, including *Clostridium difficile* toxemia, medication-induced diarrhea, acute mesenteric ischemia, pseudodiarrhea, and malabsorption.

The diagnosis of *C. difficile* infection is covered in depth elsewhere in this text, but is important to mention because of several common pitfalls. First, *C. difficile* can rarely be toxin negative, even when the standard three samples are sent for analysis, with colonoscopy serving as the gold standard (117). Therefore, if clinical suspicion for *C. difficile* colitis or enteritis is high, antibiotic therapy and isolation should be initiated before toxin results come back, and should be continued until at least three samples are toxin negative—potentially longer if GI consultation recommends. Second, care must be taken in interpreting a single positive toxin, especially in the patient at risk for antibiotic-associated non–*C. difficile* diarrhea. For example, 20% of patients have a false-positive *C. difficile* toxin. These patients actually have medication-related, antibiotic-associated diarrhea or simple colonization, without signs of serious illness such as fever, abdominal pain, leukocytosis, and acute hypoalbuminemia (118). Removing the offending agent, often a macrolide, is the definitive management of antibiotic-associated diarrhea and is also important in *C. difficile* diarrhea. Recall that the diarrhea of *C. difficile* is often hemoccult positive. For patients who must remain on antibiotics, much controversy surrounds the use of probiotic agents such as lactobacillus and *Saccharomyces boulardii* in the prevention and treatment of antibiotic-associated diarrhea. These agents are generally safe but are not FDA-regulated, and there have been several case reports of *S. cerevisiae* fungemia and lactobacillus bacteremia in immunocompromised patients due to handling of central catheters after placing the medication in feeding tubes (119).

Other bacterial infectious enteritides are quite rare in the patient who develops diarrhea. However, in the ICU patient with diarrhea admitted from the emergency department (ED) for other reasons, it is reasonable to test for the most common causes of acute infectious bacterial enteritis, such as *Campylobacter*, salmonella, shigella, and *Escherichia coli* 0157:H7. Recall that these patients can appear toxic, and any of these enteroinvasive bacteria can present with hemolytic-uremic syndrome or toxic megacolon. *Campylobacter jejuni,* as its name implies, can present with jejunal thickening on CT resembling mesenteric ischemia. Recall that a classic finding of salmonellosis is fever without tachycardia, one of the rare infections other than mycoplasma that give that presentation.

The diarrhea of acute mesenteric ischemia is important to recognize. It is often heme positive and can appear maroon or melenic. Sloughing of mucosa may be seen and, in addition to sudden distention, may portend infarction. In the patient with pain out of proportion to physical exam early in the course, many signs are absent, and a high clinical suspicion must be maintained. A rancid odor may be appreciated but can be stifled by a rectal tube with balloon, only to be noticed when the bag is changed. Patients may not appear toxic until late in the course when bowel infarction, peritonitis, and lactic acidosis occur. In our experience, patients at highest risk are vascular surgery patients, those undergoing cardiopulmonary bypass, patients with embolic risk whose anticoagulants are held for bleeding, and severely hypotensive patients. Digoxin can decrease mesenteric flow in patients on multiple pressors (120).

Another common cause of diarrhea in ICU patients is iatrogenic diarrhea, which is important to recognize. Oral magnesium, selective serotonin reuptake inhibitors (SSRIs), proton pump inhibitors (PPIs), H_2 blockers, caffeine/theophylline, antibiotics, nonsteroidal anti-inflammatory agents (NSAIDS), colchicine, gastroparesis therapies, ursodeoxycholic acid (URSO), senna/colace orders from the patient's time on the general ward, and Kayexalate are common offenders. Some common surgical procedures that cause diarrhea are cholecystectomy, partial pancreatectomy, long bowel resections, partial ileal resections, and ileoanal anastomoses. Diarrhea post cholecystectomy and after ileal resections less than 100 cm in length can be treated with cholestyramine, a bile salt binder three times daily (121). This drug can bind and interfere with the absorption of most other medications, so it must be given at least 1 to 2 hours after other drugs. The rare patient with a less than 100-cm ileal resection can develop bile salt depletion and malabsorption if given cholestyramine, although this is common in ileal resections greater than 100 cm. Pancreatic exocrine insufficiency is common after a Whipple procedure because many patients have some degree of chronic pancreatitis prior to the operation. Enteric-coated pancreatic enzyme supplementation, such as with Creon or Ultrase-20, two tabs with meals, is curative.

Another cause of iatrogenic diarrhea is small bowel bacterial overgrowth. In this case, anaerobic bacteria from the colon reflux into the small bowel and prevent absorption of bile salts and nutrients. This is the mechanism behind the diarrhea after ileocecal valve resection. Occasionally, PPIs can cause overgrowth by suppressing the protective effect of stomach acid. Because these bacteria produce folate, blood levels of this B vitamin are often elevated. The D-xylose breath test is the most convenient and sensitive substitute for endoscopic aspiration and culture of duodenal contents (122). However, both tests are inconvenient in ICU patients, and empirical therapy with tetracycline, amoxicillin/clavulanate, trimethoprim/sulfamethoxazole with metronidazole, or quinolones for 1 week is often effective.

Initiation of *tube feeds*—total enteral nutrition or TEN—can cause diarrhea in the ICU. Patients with low oncotic pressures, with hypotension and/or pressor requirements, and elevated lactic acid are most susceptible. If a patient is at less than average risk for pulmonary aspiration, these feeds can be diluted 50% to improve gastric emptying. In addition, high-glucose containing products such as Ensure or Boost can be exchanged for higher fat content such as Glucerna and vice versa. In the hypoalbuminemic patient, TEN may have to be withheld while total parental nutrition (TPN) temporarily restores oncotic pressure. In the patient with new diarrhea after percutaneous endoscopic gastric tube (PEG) placement, one must be vigilant to rule out inadvertent placement through the colon. If this tube is inserted through the transverse colon, in critically ill patients on broad-spectrum antibiotics, the presence of unaltered tube feeds in the stool may be the only sign. The diagnosis of a colonic perforation during PEG requires a CT scan with PEG-instilled contrast, as a kidney, ureters, and bladder (KUB) will show some free air even in normal post-PEG patients. In the patient with new tube feeds and diarrhea, the ICU clinician may need to rule out jejunal ischemia, as there have been several case reports (123). If, in fact, tube feed diarrhea is idiopathic, a possible treatment is adding soluble partly hydrolyzed guar as a source of fiber. In one randomized controlled trial in mechanically ventilated and septic patients, guar significantly reduced—from 32% to 9%—the percentage of tube feed–induced diarrhea (124). The only enteral formula with fiber is Jevity, but even this may not be sufficient. Elemental or semielemental formulas such as Peptimen may be easier to absorb, especially in ICU patients, but are expensive.

Pseudodiarrhea is important to rule out. Spinal cord patients, diabetic patients, patients with neuropathies/strokes/anticonvulsant therapy, patients with prior episiotomy or prostate surgery, and sedated patients may have baseline low anal sphincter pressure. They may be unable to sense the urge to defecate. If the stool is looser because of tube feeds or antibiotic therapy, the critical care team may start an exhaustive and expensive search for all the causes of diarrhea when a simple rectal exam may be suggestive (125). Treatment is outpatient biofeedback and pelvic floor muscle strengthening.

Hirschsprung Disease

A prototypic, but rare, disorder of constipation is congenital aganglionosis of the colon, also known as congenital megacolon. Although it would be rare to diagnose a patient in the ICU, save for the pediatric ICU (PICU), the physiology of Hirschsprung disease is worthy of a brief discussion and illustrates several broadly applicable motility principles.

Hirschsprung disease results from failure of the neural crest cells to migrate into and from the myenteric plexus in a contiguous region of the left colon. Patients present with severe constipation without palpable stool in the rectal vault, without fecal soiling, but with a narrowed, *diseased* colon segment and a more proximally dilated, but *normal*, colonic segment.

Patients suspected of having Hirschsprung disease should undergo anorectal manometry in the gastrointestinal laboratory, an impossibility in most ICU patients. Lack of compensatory rectal relaxation to distention of the rectal balloon is suggestive. These patients should undergo colonic suction biopsy, which can sometimes reach the muscularis propria and rule out visceral neuropathy, myopathy, and amyloidosis. However, lack of myenteric plexus neurons on endoscopic suction biopsy does not entirely prove Hirschsprung disease, and often a laparoscopic full thickness biopsy is required (126).

The lack of nitric oxide–containing neurons, which prevent rectal relaxation, may be the principal mechanism of disease. Chagas disease can even result in a Hirschsprunglike presentation in adults even in the United States (127). Some have found that 70% of adults with acute megacolon may have some histologic features of congenital neurologic disease (128).

Colonic Inertia

Probably the most common cause of refractory constipation in adults is colonic inertia due to generalized decreased colonic motility. A subset of patients may present with obstipation, evidence of colonic dilation, and even respiratory compromise from diaphragmatic impingement. In patients without a prior radiograph, it may be difficult to rule out acute processes such as megacolon. Patients may have a long history of chronic stimulant laxative use. However, much controversy exists over whether this is in fact the cause or the result of colonic inertia.

Less controversial causes include opiates, dehydration/diuretics, calcium channel blockers, clonidine, hypothyroidism, electrolyte imbalance (see ileus section), and immobility. For diagnosis, ambulatory patients can swallow a capsule filled with radio-opaque beads (also known as Sitz markers) and be followed with daily radiographs of the abdomen (KUBs) (129). Markers that are evenly distributed throughout the colon—more than 5 out of 20 at 4 days—are diagnostic of colonic inertia, whereas those that "pile up" can indicate obstruction or pelvic floor dyssynergia.

Ruling out *C. difficile* in the patient presenting with constipation, bloating, and colonic distention, sometimes with hemoglobin-positive rectal exams as well, is essential. In immunocompromised patients, CMV can present similarly. Although colonic amebiasis would be a rare cause of this presentation (130), the southeastern United States has a higher prevalence than the rest of the nation, especially among individuals at high risk such as travelers to endemic areas and homosexual men. Other causes of infectious colitis can rarely cause toxic megacolon but are in the differential diagnosis.

Treatment is aimed at removing offending agents and gently stimulating bowel movements with tap water or Fleets enemas (see section on ileus). Most acute presentations can be treated with manual disimpaction. Rarely would a patient benefit from emergency colonoscopy, unless manual disimpaction and enemas have failed, and colonic dilation proximal to the impaction exceeds 10 cm in the cecum. Prokinetics and oral or stimulant laxatives should not be used until the impaction has been removed. After relief, patients should be maintained on a chronic, safe bowel regimen to prevent impaction, such as once-daily Miralax, or, in patients with normal renal function, with milk of magnesia or magnesium citrate, 1 to 2 teaspoons daily.

Ogilvie Syndrome

One of the most important motility associated diseases is acute colonic pseudo-obstruction. When this condition coincides with recent orthopedic, trauma, gynecologic, or other surgery, it is classically known as Ogilvie syndrome. This is important to distinguish from simple small bowel ileus or from acute colonic obstruction from stool impaction, and so forth, which require different management.

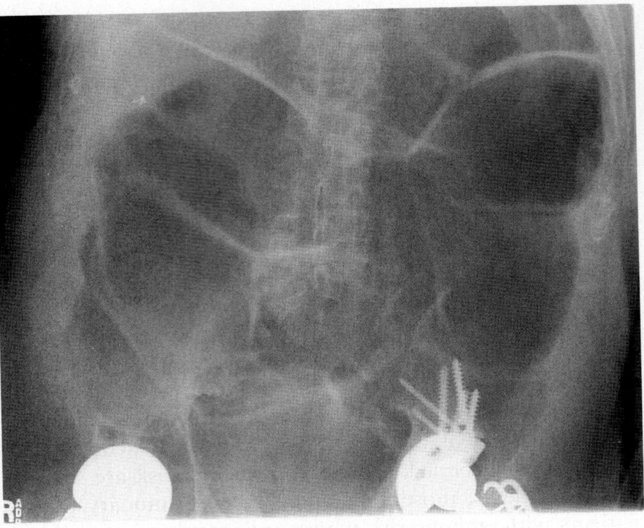

FIGURE 158.3. Ogilvie syndrome. This 95-year-old veteran presented with distention, obstipation, and self-elicited tympany. Note extremely dilated loops of colon. Note hip hardware, a common comorbidity. (Courtesy of Veterans Administration Hospital, Gainesville, Florida.)

Typical Ogilvie patients present on initiation of diet several days after surgery with acute or subacute colonic dilation, distention, often with lack of gas passage, sometimes with nausea, vomiting, or respiratory compromise due to diaphragmatic compression. Generally, not much stool and no transition point is seen (Fig. 158.3). Massive dilation can occur and may lead to perforation, especially when cecal diameter approaches 11 to 12 cm. The cecum is most susceptible to baro-induced ischemia and perforation, as it is the thinnest walled area of the colon. Laplace's law states that transmural pressure is highest across the thinnest portion of a wall. Once pressure inside the cecum exceeds that of the superior mesenteric vein, ischemia can occur (131). Predisposing factors to Ogilvie syndrome include colonic inertia, age, immobility, electrolyte imbalance, or neurologic conditions, such as strokes or parkinsonism with dysautonomia.

If the colon is dangerously dilated, the patient should undergo nasogastric tube suctioning, conversion to nothing-by-mouth status, perhaps with total parenteral nutrition, and gentle stimulation with serial rectal exams and enemas. In some patients, a carefully placed rectal tube can release some of the gas buildup if the dilation extends to the rectum. As in the case of fecal impaction, lactulose, which produces more gas, and other oral laxatives should be avoided. The gold standard in management for many years was an emergency water-soluble contrast enema in the radiology suite. The hyperosmolarity of the enema often induces evacuation and at the same time rules out obstruction. The waning of expertise in this technique, as well as the widespread and emergency availability of colonoscopy, has resulted in a shift in this paradigm. Careful colonoscopy without oral bowel lavage and with minimal insufflation can decompress a severely dilated colon, but is associated with a 1% or higher risk of perforation in this setting. Placement of a decompression tube has a debatable effect on recurrence (132). Therefore, since 1999, some proponents have advocated pharmacologic management with erythromycin (133), cisapride (134)—a mixed procholinergic and 5HT4 agonist no longer available in the United States, and neostigmine, a potent acetylcholinesterase blocker that has many of the side effects, albeit much more temporary, of acute nerve gas poisoning. Therefore, patients receiving neostigmine in our institution must be at the intermediate care unit (IMC) or higher level of care, with atropine instantly available. We do not use neostigmine in actively wheezing patients, those on oxygen for chronic obstructive pulmonary disease (COPD), patients with coronary artery disease, or those at higher-than-average risk of bradycardia and asystole, such as those on several atrioventricular (AV) nodal-blocking agents such as amiodarone or a calcium channel blocker with a beta-blocker. We typically notify cardiology or the critical care team of impending neostigmine use and ask patients to sign a consent form. The standard dose is 2.5 mg IV slow infusion over 1 to 3 minutes. An effect is generally seen within 2 to 20 minutes. The response can be dramatic, with massive evacuation of stool and gas and instant relief. The dose may be repeated 2 to 3 times very carefully. A prospective trial showed a 91% response rate compared to 0% with placebo (135). Nevertheless, many patients may have improved on more aggressive nonneostigmine medical therapy (136).

In the presence of peritonitis, leukocytosis, fever, or a cecal diameter of greater than 12 cm, surgery may be necessary, which, if ischemia is present, usually includes right hemicolectomy, ileostomy, and mucous fistula formation.

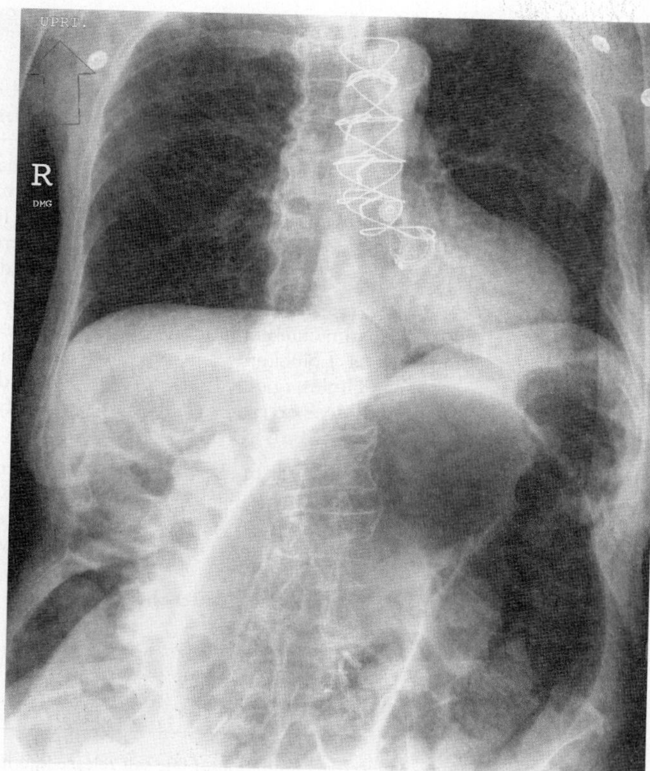

FIGURE 158.4. Sigmoid volvulus. KUB showing a dilated loop of sigmoid displaced to the periumbilical region with the appearance of a C or bent inner tube. Note fecal material in descending colon. KUB, kidney, ureters, and bladder. (Courtesy of Veterans Administration Hospital, Gainesville, Florida.)

Sigmoid Volvulus

Similar principals can be applied to the management of sigmoid volvulus, the "medical" volvulus; many patients are elderly with a history of chronic constipation and other comorbid diseases (137). In one series, up to 13% were in chronic institutions. Most present with distension and obstipation, but about 30% report pain. Significant tenderness on exam may portend ischemia and peritonitis. Radiographically, a sigmoid volvulus may appear as a markedly dilated, ahaustral, sigmoid colon, with paucity of gas in the rectum. The dilated sigmoid loop may extend into the right upper quadrant, assuming a C or bent inner tube shape (Fig. 158.4). In nontoxic patients without signs of peritonitis, emergent sigmoidoscopy is the procedure of choice, using minimal air insufflation, and is successful 60% of the time (139). Once the transition point is passed, a visible untwisting can be seen, associated with massive passage of stool and gas. Our practice is to do a colonoscopy, or at least reach the transverse colon whenever possible, to look for an underlying stricturing lesion. However, because of poor preparation, emergency sigmoidoscopy cannot rule out small areas of ischemic mucosa and may delay definitive surgery in some patients. Careful placement of a rectal tube may decrease recurrence, which is quite high, on the order of 50%. Therefore, after emergent sigmoidoscopy, our practice is to continue to cleanse the bowel with enemas and, if tolerated, with gentle oral lavage to permit more accurate exam of the colon at the time of recurrence. Overall mortality of sigmoid volvulus is 8% (140), mostly due to the 20% of patients with ischemia who have a mortality rate of 80% in an older study (138), but a more recently reported rate is 25% (137).

SUMMARY

The ICU is home to many motility disorders. Some universal principles of diagnosis include ruling out emergencies such as impending colonic perforation, intestinal ischemia, food impaction, and so forth. In managing these disorders, some basic principles apply: (a) in the "slow disorders" such as gastroparesis, ileus, constipation, Ogilvie's etc., correct electrolytes, rule out occult thyroid disease, keep glucose less than 150 mg/dL, minimize tubes and drains—especially in the upper GI tract, and remove offending agents (Table 158.2) such as calcium channel blockers, central alpha 2 antagonists, and pure mu-opiates; (b) in the "fast disorders," such as diarrhea, avoid magnesium-containing medications, SSRIs, PPIs, and unnecessary antibiotics. In patients that fail TEN, consider motility as a cause. Consider guar for diarrhea and changing fat and sugar content for distention. Rule out hypoalbuminemia and lactic acidosis. In colonic distention, distinguish among fecal impaction (perhaps from chronic inertia) versus Ogilvie versus sigmoid volvulus. Basic management is the same: (i) use clinical assessment to rule out impending infarction; (ii) rule out cecal diameter greater than 10 cm; (iii) apply gentle enemas and rectal tube if the patient is nontoxic; (iv) consider promotility agents only in Ogilvie (the only case in which neostigmine is used) or *decompressed* volvulus or disimpacted colonic inertia.

TABLE 158.2

FACTORS AFFECTING MOTILITY

	Decelerate	Accelerate
Luminal Contents	Fat High level of simple sugars Hyperosmolar Hypo-osmolar Solids	Normal saline Fat (in colon) High level of simple sugar (in colon) Hyperosmolar (in colon) Liquids
Drugs	Opiates Calcium channel blockers Alpha-2 blockers Anticholinergics High-dose octreotide (50–200 μg SQ tid[a])	Opiate antagonists Procholinergics Motility drugs (see text) Low-dose octreotide (small bowel only, 50 μg SQ at hour of sleep)
Metabolic Factors	Hypothyroidism Hypercalcemia Hypokalemia Hypomagnesemia Hyponatremia Hyperglycemia (greater than 150 mg/dL) Acidosis Uremia Hypoalbuminemia	Hyperthyroidism Hypoalbuminemia (if receiving enteral feeds) (colon and small bowel)

[a]Unless malabsorption is induced via inhibition of bile salt release into lumen.

PEARLS

Motility Disorders of the Esophagus

- Oropharyngeal disorders predispose to aspiration and may be due to stroke, medications, and neurodegenerative or striated muscle disorders. Obtain rehab barium swallow and speech pathology consults early.
- Do not insert a Dobbhoff or NGT into a patient with a distal esophageal hypomotility disorder until epiphrenic diverticula have been ruled out by barium swallow.
- A wide mediastinum may be GI in origin.
- The mucosa of the esophagus is almost never affected by ischemia.
- Be aware of the disorders and drugs that affect LES pressure, as these may contribute to aspiration.
- NGT and Dobbhoff tubes lower LES and predispose to aspiration and esophagitis.
- During cardiac arrest, remember the importance of the LES and maneuvers to decrease gastric ventilation.
- Patients with connective tissue disease, especially those with esophageal dysmotility, are more vulnerable than the average patient to esophageal damage and aspiration.
- A food impaction must be removed immediately by endoscopy. Many are due to motility disturbances.

Motility Disorders of the Stomach

- Remember the stomach is the origin of the MMC in 80% of patients.
- Gastroparesis can predispose to aspiration of nosocomial Gram-negative bacteria and TEN intolerance.
- Secondary causes of gastroparesis, as in most motility disorders, include hyperglycemia, hypothyroidism, hypokalemia, hypercalcemia, uremia, high progesterone states, portal hypertension, connective tissue disease, right-sided CHF, and hypoalbuminemia.
- Treat by keeping blood glucose level less than 150 mg/dL, correcting electrolytes, avoiding precipitants such as opiates, calcium channel blockers, and clonidine.
- If possible, use propoxyphene and/or tramadol for pain control in gastroparetics and other patients with slow motility disorders.
- Erythromycin is the mainstay: start low at 100 mg liquid 30 minutes before meals or IV 10 minutes before meals, titrating to 200 four times daily if QTc is acceptable. Watch for P450 inhibitors and long QTc interactions.
- Some patients may benefit from azithromycin, which does not prolong the QTc, instead of erythromycin.
- Any drug that stimulates gastric emptying can cause diarrhea.
- Gastroparesis is worsened by high salt, sugar, fat, and fiber content. Thus, in outpatients, where aspiration is not a risk, tube feeds can be diluted 50% with water.
- In contrast, patients with dumping benefit from low-carbohydrate, high-fat, high-fiber diets.

Motility Disorders of the Small Bowel

- Recognize why some patients on pressors fail enteral nutrition.

- In the management of ileus:
  - ☐ Correct electrolytes.
  - ☐ Increase patient mobility.
  - ☐ Use gentle enemas but not oral-stimulant laxatives or lactulose.
  - ☐ Avoid calcium channel blockers, clonidine, anticholinergics, and opiates.
  - ☐ Consider oral opiate antagonists, prokinetics, and epidural anesthesia in patients at high risk for postop ileus.
- Rule out small cell carcinoma in susceptible patients with new and unexplained constipation, gastroparesis, small or large bowel dysmotility.

Motility Disorders of the Large Intestine

- Common causes of diarrhea include magnesium salts, SSRIs, PPIs, antibiotics, TEN.
- In TEN diarrhea, consider changing or diluting formula if aspiration is not likely. Also rule out jejunal ischemia and misplaced PEG, and consider adding guar-based fiber.
- Be able to distinguish false-positive *C. difficile* toxin in antibiotic-associated diarrhea from patients with *C. difficile* disease and false-negative toxin.
- Distinguish Ogilvie syndrome from sigmoid volvulus and from fecal impaction with megacolon.
- The initial approach to nontoxic Ogilvie and sigmoid volvulus patients is rectal tube placement, gentle enemas, correction of electrolytes, serial KUBs, and removal of antimotility agents such as narcotics, anticholinergics, and calcium channel blockers.
- Ogilvie patients can also be started on erythromycin if QTc interval is acceptable.
- If the patient fails to improve or if cecal diameter rises to about 10 cm or enough to cause respiratory insufficiency, urgent sigmoid or colonoscopy is required.
- Toxic patients should go the operating room (OR) or undergo cecostomy in the case of Ogilvie. Gastrografin enema in the radiology suite and IV neostigmine are other options, the cecostomy, only if the patient is not wheezing, bradycardic, and does not have coronary artery disease, or is in an IMC or higher level of care with atropine and resuscitation equipment for asystole easily available.

References

1. Weisbrodt NW, Christianson J. Gradients of contractions in the opossum esophagus. *Gastroenterology.* 1972;62:1159–1166.
2. Yamato S, Saha JK, Goyal RK. Role of nitric oxide in lower esophageal sphincter relaxation to swallowing. *Life Sci.* 1992;50:1263–1272.
3. Diamant NE, El Sharkawy TY. Neural control of esophageal peristalsis. A conceptual analysis. *Gastroenterology.* 1977;72:546–556.
4. Dodds WJ, Christianson J, Dent J, et al. Pharmacologic investigation of primary peristalsis in smooth muscle portion of opossum esophagus. *Am J Physiol.* 1979;237:E561–E566.
5. Gidda JS, Boyinski JP. Swallow evoked peristalsis in opossum esophagus: role of cholinergic mechanisms. *Am J Physiol.* 1986;251:G779–G781.
6. Richter JE, Wu WC, Johns DN, et al. Esophageal manometry in 95 healthy volunteers. Variability of pressures with age and frequency of abnormal contractions. *Dig Dis Sci.* 1987;32:583–592.
7. Paterson WG, Rattan S, Goyal RK. Esophageal responses to transient and sustained esophageal distension. *Am J Physiol.* 1988;255:G587–G595.
8. Katz PO, Richter JE, Cowan R, et al. Apparent complete lower esophageal sphincter relaxation in achalasia. *Gastroenterology.* 1986;90:978–983.
9. Kahrilas PJ, Dodds WJ, Dent J, et al. Upper esophageal sphincter function during deglutition. *Gastroenterology.* 1988;95:52–62.
10. Horner J, Massey EW, Riski JE, et al. Aspiration following stroke: clinical correlates and outcome. *Neurology.* 1988;38:1359–1362.
11. Logeman JA, Blonsky ER, Boshes B. Dysphagia in parkinsonism. *JAMA.* 1975;231(1):69–70.
12. Siebens H, Trupe E, Siebens A, et al. Correlates and consequences of eating dependency in the institutionalized elderly. *J Am Geriatr Soc.* 1986;34:192–198.
13. Goher ME. The prevalence of swallowing disorders in two teaching hospitals. *Dysphagia.* 1986;1:3–6.
14. Smithard DG, O'Neill PA, Park C, et al. Complications and outcome after acute stroke: does dysphagia matter? *Stroke.* 1996;27:1200–1204.
15. Splaingard ML, Hutchins B, Sulton LD, et al. Aspiration in rehabilitation patients: videofluoroscopy vs bedside clinical assessment. *Ach Phys Med Rehabil.* 1988;69:637–640.
16. Logemann JA. The role of the modified barium swallow in management of patients with dysphagia. *Otolaryngol Head Neck Surg.* 1997;116(3):335–338.
17. Cook IJ. Chapter 10. Disorders causing oropharyngeal dysphagia In: Castell DO, Richter J, eds. *The Esophagus.* 4rd ed. Philadelphia, PA: Lippincott Williams & Wilkins; 2003:197–198.
18. Norton B, Homer WM, Donnelly MT, et al. A randomized, prospective comparison of percutaneous endoscopic gastrostomy and nasogastric tube feeding after acute dysphagic stroke. *BMJ.* 1996;312(7022):13–16.
19. Murray JA, Ledlow A, Launspach J, et al. The effects of recombinant human hemoglobin on esophageal motor function in humans. *Gastroenterology.* 1995;109:1241–1248.
20. Konturek JW, Gillessen A, Domschke W. Diffuse esophageal spasm: a malfunction that involves nitric oxide? *Scand J Gastroenterol.* 1995;30:1041–1045.
21. Richter JE, Hackshaw BT, Wu WC, et al. Edrophonium: a useful provocative test for esophageal chest pain. *Ann Int Med.* 1985;103:14–21.
22. Orlando RC, Bozymski EM. Clinical and manometric effects of nitroglycerin in diffuse esophageal spasm. *N Engl J Med.* 1973;289:23–25.
23. Hongo M, Traube M, McCallum RW. Comparison of effects of nifedipine, propantheline bromide, and the combination on esophageal motor function in normal volunteers. *Dig Dis Sci.* 1984;29:300–304.
24. Davies HA, Lewis MJ, Rhoads J, et al. Trial of nifedipine for prevention of esophageal spasm. *Digestion.* 1987;36:81–83.
25. Cannon RO 3rd, Quyyumi AA, Mincemoyer R, et al. Imipramine in patients with chest pain despite normal coronary angiograms. *N Engl J Med.* 1994;330:1411–1417.
26. Richter JE, Dalton C, Bradley L, et al. Oral nifedipine in the treatment of noncardiac chest pain in patients with the nutcracker esophagus. *Gastroenterology.* 1987;93:21.
27. Ali GN, Hunt DR, Jorgensen JE, et al. Esophageal achalasia and coexistent upper esophageal sphincter relaxation disorder presenting with airway obstruction. *Gastroenterology.* 1995;109:1328–1332.
28. Cohen S, Lipschutz W. Lower esophageal sphincter dysfunction in patients with achalasia. *Gastroenterology.* 1971;61:814–820.
29. Mayberry JF. Epidemiology and demographics of achalasia. *Gastrointest Endosc Clin N Am.* 2001;11:235–247.
30. Niwamoto H, Okamoto E, Fujimoto J, et al. Are human herpes viruses or measles virus associated with esophageal achalasia? *Dig Dis Sci.* 1995;859–864.
31. Cassella RR, Ellis FH Jr, Brown AL Jr. Fine structure changes in achalasia of the esophagus, I: vagus nerves. *Am J Pathol.* 1965;279:46–54.
32. Goldblum JR, Rice TW, Richter JE. Histopathologic features in esophagomyotomy specimens from patients with achalasia. *Gastroenterology.* 1996; 111:648–654.
33. Verne GN, Hahn AB, Pineau BC, et al. Association of LSA-DR and -DQ alleles with idiopathic achalasia. *Gastroenterology.* 1999;117:26–31.
34. Wagh MS, Matloff DS, Carr-Locke DL. Life-threatening acute airway obstruction in achalasia. *Med Gen Med.* 2004;6(3):12.
35. Arcos E, Medina C, Mearin F, et al. Achalasia presenting as acute airway obstruction. *Dig Dis Sci.* 2000;45(10):2079–2083.
36. Vaezi MJ, Richter JE, Wilcox CM. Botulinum toxin versus balloon dilation in the treatment of achalasia: a randomized trial. *Gut.* 1999;44;231–239.
37. Gelfand M, Rozen P, Gilat T. Isosorbide dinitrate and nifedipine treatment of achalasia. *Ann Intern Med.* 1982;83:963–969.
38. Eherer AJ, Schwetz I, Hammer HF, et al. Effect of sildenafil on esophageal motor function in healthy subjects and in patients with esophageal motility disorders. *Gut.* 2002;50:758–764.
39. Becker BS, Burakoff R. The effect of verapamil on the lower esophageal sphincter in normal subjects and in achalasia. *Am J Gastroenterol.* 1983;78: 773–776.
40. Bowman FP, Mengazzi JJ, Check BD, et al. The lower esophageal sphincter pressure during prolonged cardiac arrest and resuscitation. *Ann Emerg Med.* 1995;26:216–219.
41. Wenzel V, Idris AH, Banner MJ, et al. Influence of volume on the distribution of gas between the lungs and stomach in the unintubated patient receiving positive pressure ventilation. *Crit Care Med.* 1998;26:264–268.
42. Wenzel V, Idris AH, Banner MJ, et al. Respiratory system compliance decreases after cardiopulmonary resuscitation and stomach inflation: impact of large and small tidal volumes on calculated peak airway pressure. *Resuscitation.* 1998;38:113–118.

43. Lawes EG, Baskett PJF. Pulmonary aspiration during unsuccessful cardiopulmonary resuscitation. *Intensive Care Med* 1987;13:379–382.
44. Gabrielli A, Wenzel V, Layon J, et al. Lower esophageal sphincter pressure measurement during cardiac arrest in humans: potential implications for ventilation of the unprotected airway. *Anesthesiology.* 205;103:897–899.
45. Dorges V, Ocker H, Hagelberg S, et al. Smaller tidal volumes with room air are not sufficient to ensure adequate oxygenation during basic life support. *Resuscitation.* 2000;44:37–41.
46. Wagner-Berger HG, Wenzel V, Stallinger A, et al. Decreasing peak flow rate with a new bag-valve mask device: effects of respiratory mechanics and gas distribution in a bench model of the unprotected airway. *Resuscitation.* 2003;57:193–197.
47. Baskett PJ, Baskett TF. Resuscitation great. Brian Sellick, cricoid pressure and the Sellick maneuver. *Resuscitation.* 2004;61:5–7.
48. Cohen S, Lauffer I, Snape WJ et al. The gastrointestinal manifestations of scleroderma: pathogenesis and management. *Gastroenterology.* 1980;79:155.
49. Lieb JG II, Katzka D. Motility disorders of the esophagus. In: Parkman HP, Fisher RS, eds. Lichtenstein G, series ed. *A Clinician's Guide to Acid Peptic and Motility Disorders.* Thorofare, NJ: Slack Publishers; 2006.
50. Desai TK, Stecevic V, Chang CH, et al. Association of eosinophilic inflammation with esophageal food impaction in adults. *Gastrointest Endosc.* 2005;61(7):795–801.
51. Camilleri M, Malagelada JR, Brown ML, et al. Relation between antral motility and gastric emptying of solids and liquids in humans. *Am J Physiol.* 1985;249(5 Pt 1):G580–585.
52. Meyer JH, Thomson JB, Cohen MB, et al. Sieving of solid food by the canine stomach and sieving after gastric surgery. *Gastroenterology.* 1979; 76(4):804–813.
53. Tanaka M, Sarr MG, Van Lier Ribbink JA Gastrointestinal motor patterns: motilin as a coordinating factor. *J Surg Res.* 1989;47(4):325–331.
54. Fich A, Neri M, Camilleri M, et al. Stasis syndromes following gastric surgery: clinical and motility features of 60 symptomatic patients. *J Clin Gastroenterol.* 1990;12(5):505–512.
55. Chowdhury RS, Forsmark CE, Davis RH, et al. Prevalence of gastroparesis in patients with small duct chronic pancreatitis. *Pancreas.* 2003;26:235–238.
56. McHugh PR, Moran TH: Calories and gastric emptying: a regulatory capacity with implications for feeding. *Am J Physiol.* 1979;236:R254–R260.
57. Hoogerwerf WA, Pasricha PJ, Kalloo AN, et al. Pain: the overlooked symptom in gastroparesis. *Am J Gastroenterol.* 1999;94(4):1029–1033.
58. Maddern J, Jamieson G, Myers J. Effect of cisapride on delayed gastric emptying in gastroesophageal reflux disease. *Gut.* 1991;32:470–474.
59. Drakulovic MB, Torres A, Bauer TT, et al. Supine body position as a risk factor for nosocomial pneumonia in mechanically ventilated patients: a randomised trial. *Lancet.* 1999;354:1851–1858.
60. Heyland D, Mandell L. Gastric colonization by Gram negative bacilli and nosocomial pneumonia in the intensive care unit patient: evidence of causation. *Chest.* 1992;101(1):187–193.
61. Kelly KA. Gastric emptying of liquids and solids: roles of proximal and distal stomach. *Am J Physiol.* 1980;239:G71–G76.
62. Thomforde GM, Camilleri M, Phillips SF, et al. Evaluation of an inexpensive screening scintigraphic test of gastric emptying. *J Nucl Med.* 1995; 36(1):93–96.
63. Urbain JLC, Vantrappen G, Janssens J, et al. Intravenous erythromycin dramatically accelerates gastric emptying in gastroparesis diabeticorum and normals and abolishes the emptying discrimination between solids and liquids. *J Nucl Med.* 1990;31:1490–1493.
64. Fraser R, Shearer T, Fuller J, et al. Intravenous erythromycin overcomes small intestinal feedback on antral, pyloric, and duodenal motility. *Gastroentrerology.* 1992;103:114–119.
65. Iannini PB. Cardiotoxicity of macrolides, ketolides, and fluoroquinolones that prolong the QTc. *Expert Opin Drug Saf.* 2002;1(2):121–128.
66. Booth CM, Heyland DK, Paterson WG. Gastrointestinal promotility drugs in the critical care setting: a systematic review of the evidence. *Crit Care Med.* 2002;30:1429–1435.
67. Ray WA, Murray KT, Meredith S, et al. Oral erythromycin and the risk of sudden death from cardiac causes. *N Engl J Med.* 2004;351(11):1089–1096.
68. Ouyang H, Xing J, Chen JD. Tachygastria induced by gastric electrical stimulation is mediated via alpha- and beta-adrenergic pathway and inhibits antral motility in dogs. *Neurogastroenterol Motil.* 2005;17(6):846–853.
69. Ganzini L, Casey DE, Hoffman WF, et al. The prevalence of metoclopramide-induced tardive dyskinesia and acute extrapyramidal movement disorders. *Arch Intern Med.* 1993;153:1469–475.
70. Wysowski DK, Corken A, Gallo-Torres H, et al. Postmarketing reports of QT prolongation and ventricular arrhythmia in association with cisapride and Food and Drug Administration regulatory actions. *Am J Gastroenterol.* 2001;96:1698–1703.
71. Beglinger C. Tegaserod: a novel, selective 5-HT_4 receptor partial agonist for irritable bowel syndrome. *Int J Clin Pract.* 2002;56:47–51.
72. Regional gastric contractility alterations in a diabetic gastroparesis mouse model: effects of cholinergic and serotonergic stimulation. *Am J Physiol Gastrointest Liver Physiol.* 2004;287(3):G612–619.
73. Fraser RJ, Horowitz M, Maddox AF, et al. Hyperglycaemia slows gastric emptying in type 1 (insulin-dependent) diabetes mellitus. *Diabetologia.* 1990;33(11):675–680.
74. Schvarcz E, Palmer M, Aman J, et al. Physiological hyperglycemia slows gastric emptying in normal subjects and patients with insulin-dependent diabetes mellitus. *Gastroenterology.* 1997;113(1):60–66.
75. Petrakis IE, Kogerakis N, Vrachassotakis N, et al. Hyperglycemia attenuates erythromycin-induced acceleration of solid-phase gastric emptying in healthy subjects. *Abdom Imaging.* 2002;27(3):309–314.
76. Bjomsson ES, Urbanavicius V, Eliasson B, et al. Effects of hyperglycemia on interdigestive gastrointestinal motility in humans. *Scand J Gastroenterol.* 1994;29:1096–1104.
77. A comparison of the abuse liability of tramadol, NSAIDs, and hydrocodone in patients with chronic pain. *J Pain Symptom Manage.* 2006;31(5):465–476.
78. Taguchi A, Sharma N, Saleem R, et al. Selective postoperative inhibition of gastrointestinal opioid receptors. *N Engl J Med.* 2001;345:13.
79. Yuan CS, Foss JE. Oral methylnaltrexone for opioid-induced constipation. *JAMA.* 2000;284:1383–1384.
80. Foss JF, Yuan CS, Roizen MF, et al. Prevention of apomorphine- or cisplatin-induced emesis in the dog by a combination of methylnaltrexone and morphine. *Cancer Chemother Pharmacol.* 1998;42:287–291.
81. Moerman I, Franck P, Camu F. Evaluation of methylnaltrexone for the reduction of postoperative vomiting and nausea incidences. *Acta Anaesthesiol Belg.* 1995;46:127–132.
82. Jones KL, Russo A, Stevens JE, et al. Predictors of delayed gastric emptying in diabetes. *Diabetes Care.* 2001;24:1264–1269.
83. Carvajal SH, Mulvihill SJ. Postgastrectomy syndromes/dumping and diarrhea. *Gastroenterol Clin North Am.* 1994;23:61–79.
84. Vecht J, Masclee AA, Lamers CB. The dumping syndrome. Current insights into pathophysiology, diagnosis and treatment. *Scand J Gastroenterol Suppl.* 1997;223:21–27.
85. Cuschieri A. Surgical management of severe intractable post-vagotomy diarrhoea. *Br J Surg.* 1986;73:981–984.
86. Bouras EP, Scolapio JS. Gastric motility disorders. Management that optimizes nutritional status. *J Clin Gastroenterol.* 2004;38:549–557.
87. Kneepkens CM, Fernandes J, Vonk RJ. Dumping syndrome in children. Diagnosis and effect of glucomannan on glucose tolerance and absorption. *Acta Paediatr Scand.* 1988;7:279–286.
88. Speth PAJ, Jansen JB, Lamers CB. Effect of acarbose, pectin, a combination of acarbose with pectin, and placebo on postprandial reactive hypoglycemia after gastric surgery. *Gut.* 1983;24:798–802.
89. Lyons TJ, McLoughlin JC, Shaw C, et al. Effect of acarbose on biochemical responses and clinical symptoms in dumping syndrome. *Digestion.* 1985; 31:89–96.
90. Dive A, Moulart M, Mahieu P. Gastroduodenal motility in mechanically ventilated critically ill patients. A manometric study. *Crit Care Med.* 1994; 22:441–447.
91. Dive A, Miesse C, Jamart J. Duodenal motor response to continuous enteral feeding is impaired in mechanically ventilated patients. *Clin Nutr.* 1994; 13:302–306.
92. Marzio L, Neri M, Cuccurullo F, et al. Dopamine interrupts gastrointestinal fed motility pattern in humans. Effect on motilin and somatostatin blood levels . *Dig Dis Sci.* 1990;35:327–332.
93. Dive A, Foret F, Jamart J, et al. Effect of dopamine on gastrointestinal motility during critical illness. *Intens Car Med.* 2000;26:901–907.
94. Tarling M, Toner C, Withington P, et al. A model of gastric emptying using paracetamol absorption in intensive care patients. *Intensive Care Med.* 1997;23:256–260.
95. Hartley M, Sarginson R, Green C. Gastric pressure response to low dose dopamine infusion in normal man. *Clin Nutr.* 1992;11:23–29.
96. Xing J, Qian L, Chen J. Experimental gastric dysrhythmias and its correlation with *in vivo* gastric muscle contractions. *World J Gastroenterol.* 2006;12(25):3994–3998.
97. Peck J, Milleson T, Phelan J. The role of CT with contrast and SBFT in the management of small bowel obstruction. *Am J Surg.* 1999;177:375.
98. Graber J, Schulte W, Condon R, et al. Relationship of the duration of postoperative ileus to extent and site of operative dissection. *Surgery.* 1982;92: 87.
99. Condon R, Cowles V, Schulte W, et al. Resolution of postoperative ileus in humans. *Gut.* 1986;203:574.
100. Waldhausen J, Shaffrey M, Skenderis B, et al. Gastrointestinal, myoelectric, and clinical patterns of recovery after laparotomy. *Ann Surg.* 1990;211: 777.
101. Cordon R, Cowels V, Ferraz A, et al. Human colonic smooth muscle electrical activity during and after recovery from postoperative ileus. *Am J Physiol.* 1995;269:G408.
102. Kehlet H. Postoperative ileus. *Gut.* 2000;47:iv85.
103. Holte K, Kehlet H. Postoperative ileus, a preventable event. *Br J Surg.* 2000; 87:1480.
104. Turnage R, Bergen C. Intestinal obstruction and ileus. In: *Sleisinger and Fordtran's Gastrointestinal and Liver Disease.* 7th ed. Philadelphia, PA: WB Saunders; 2003.
105. Reilly JA Jr, Forst CF, Quigley EM, Rikkers LF. Gastric emptying of liquids and solids in the portal hypertensive rat. *Dig Dis Sci.* 1990;35(6):781–786.

106. Brungard T, Kale-Pradhan P. Prokinetic agents for the treatment of postoperative ileus in adults: a review of the literature. *Pharmacotherapy.* 1999; 19:419.
107. Schuffler M, Lowe M, Bill A. Studies of idiopathic chronic intestinal pseudoobstruction, I: hereditary hollow visceral myopathy: clinical and pathological studies. *Gastroenterology.* 1979;77:664.
108. Smith V, Lake B, Kamm M, et al. Intestinal pseudoobstruction with deficient smooth muscle *a*-actin. *Histopathology.* 1992;21:535.
109. Verne GN, Sninski C. Chronic intestinal pseudoobstruction. *Dig Dis Sci.* 1995;13:163.
110. Krisnamurthy S, Schuffler M. pathology of the neuromuscular disorders of the small intestine and colon. *Gastroenterology.* 1987;93:610.
111. Besnard M, Faure C, Fromont-Hankard G, et al. Intestinal pseudoobstruction and acute pandysautonomia associated with Epstein-Barr infection. *Am J Gastroenterol.* 2000;95:280.
112. Chinn J, Schuffler M. Paraneoplastic visceral myopathy as a cause of severe gastrointestinal motor dysfunction. *Gastroenterology.* 1988;95:1279.
113. Barenet J, McDonnell W, Appleman H, et al. Familial visceral neuropathy with neuronal intranuclear inclusions: diagnosis by rectal biopsy. *Gastroenterology.* 1992;102:684.
114. Soudah H, Hasler W, Owyang C. Effect of octreotide on intestinal motility and bacterial overgrowth in scleroderma. *N Engl J Med.* 1991;325:1461.
115. Verne GN, Eaker E, Hardy E, et al. Effect of octreotide and erythromycin on idiopathic and scleroderma-associated intestinal pseudo-obstruction. *Dig Dis. Sci.* 1995;40:1892.
116. Schuffler M, Leon S, Krishnamurthy S. Intestinal pseudoobstruction caused by a new form of visceral neuropathy. Palliation by radical small bowel resection. *Gastroenterology.* 1985;89:1152.
117. Borriello S, Larson H, Welch A. Enterotoxigenic *Clostridium perfringens*: a possible cause of antibiotic associated diarrhea. *Lancet.* 1984;(1):305.
118. Bartlett J. *Clostridium difficile*. Clinical considerations. *Rev Infect Dis.* 1990;12:S244.
119. Burkhardt O, Köhnlein T, Pletz M, et al. *Saccharomyces boulardii* induced sepsis: successful therapy with voriconazole after treatment failure with fluconazole. *Scand J Infect Dis.* 2005;37(1):69–72.
120. Kurland B, Brandt L, Delany H. Diagnostic tests for intestinal ischemia. *Surg Clin N Am.* 1992;72:85.
121. Arrambride K, Santa Ana C, Schiller L, et al. Loss of absorptive capacity for sodium chloride as a cause of diarrhea following partial ilial and right colon resection. *Dig Dis Sci.* 1989;34:193.
122. King C, Toskes P, Guilarte T, et al. Detection of small bowel bacterial overgrowth by means of a C14 -D-xylose breath test. *Gastroenterology.* 1979;77:75.
123. Schunn CD, Daly JM. Small bowel necrosis associated with postoperative jejunal tube feeding. *J Am Coll Surg.* 1995;180:410–416.
124. Spapen H, Diltoer M, Van Malderen C, et al. Soluble fiber reduces the incidence of diarrhea in septic patients receiving total enteral nutrition: a prospective, double-blind, randomized, and controlled trial. *Clin Nutr.* 2001;20:301–305.
125. Tatar EL.Trivedi C. Pseudodiarrhea caused by vaginal pessary in an elderly patient. *J Am Geriatr Soc.* 2005;53:1083.
126. Preston D, Lennard-Jones J, Thomas B. Towards a radiographic definition of idiopathic megacolon. *Gastrointest Radiol.* 1985;10:167.
127. Holbert R, Magiris E, Hirsch C. Chagas' disease: a case in south Mississippi. *J Miss State Med Assoc.* 1995;36:1.
128. Basilova T, Vorob'ev G, Nasyrina T. Changes in the intramural nervous system in idiopathic megacolon in adults [in Russian]. *Arkh Patol.* 1995;57: 28.
129. Metcalf A, Phillips S, Zinsmeister A, et al. A simplified assessment of segmental colonic transit. *Gastroenterology.* 1987;92:40.
130. Suarez Artacho G, Olano Acosta MC, Vazquez Monchul J, et al. Acute fulminant colitis caused by intestinal amebiasis. *Rev Esp Enferm Dig.* 2006;98(7):559–560.
131. Sleisenger, page 2126.
132. Stephenson K, Rodrigues-Bigas M. Decompression of the large intestine in Oglivie's syndrome by a colonoscopically placed long intestinal tube. *Surg Endosc.* 1994;8:116.
133. Armstrong D, Ballantyne G, Modlin I. Erythromycin for reflex ileus in Ogilvie's syndrome. *Lancet.* 1991;337:378.
134. MacColl C, MacConnell K, Baylis B, et al. Treatment of acute colonic pseudoobstruction (Ogilvie's syndrome) with cisapride. *Gastroenterology.* 1990;98:773.
135. Pronec R, Saunders M, Kimmey M. Neostigmine for the treatment of acute colonic pseudoobstruction. *N Engl J Med.* 1999;341:137.
136. Sloyer A, Panella V, Demas B, et al. Ogilvie's syndrome. Successful management without colonoscopy. *Dig Dis Sci.* 1988;33:1391.
137. Grossman E, Longo W, Stratton M, et al. Sigmoid volvulus in the department of veterans affairs medical centers. *Dis Colon Rectum.* 2000;43:414.
138. Arnold G, Nance F: Volvulus of the sigmoid colon. *Ann Surg.* 1973;177:527.
139. Brothers T, Strodel W, Eckhauser F. Endoscopy in colonic volvulus. *Ann Surg.* 1987;206:1.
140. Ballantyne G. Review of sigmoid volvulus. History and results of treatment. *Dis Colon Rectum.* 1982;25;494.
141. McNally P. GERD. In: *GI/Liver Secrets.* 2nd ed. Philadelphia, PA: Hanley & Belfus; 2001:9.
142. van der Hoeven CW, Attia A, Deen L, et al. The influence of anaesthetic drugs on the lower oesophageal sphincter in propofol/nitrous oxide anaesthetized dogs. Pressure profilometry in an animal model. *Acta Anaesthesiol Scand.* 1995;39(6):822–826.

CHAPTER 159 ■ MESENTERIC ISCHEMIA

THOMAS S. HUBER

Mesenteric ischemia is a generic term that implies inadequate blood flow to the intestines. It is relevant from a clinical standpoint as two separate disease processes: acute mesenteric ischemia (AMI) and chronic mesenteric ischemia (CMI). Although the underlying process is similar (i.e., inadequate intestinal blood flow), the clinical presentation, diagnostic concerns, and treatment algorithms are different. CMI is almost exclusively related to visceral artery occlusive disease from atherosclerosis and is relevant to intensive care physicians primarily because of the multiple organ dysfunction that occurs after revascularization. AMI results from a broad spectrum of underlying conditions including arterial emboli, *in situ* thrombosis in the setting of visceral arterial occlusive disease, mesenteric venous thrombosis, nonocclusive mesenteric ischemia (NOMI), and acute aortic dissections. AMI is relevant to intensivists not only because of the early postoperative concerns, but also because it can occur in critically ill patients with other active problems (e.g., post coronary artery bypass, acute pancreatitis). A thorough understanding of both clinical entities is essential for all intensive care physicians. The underlying pathophysiology and treatment of CMI will be discussed first to provide a foundation for addressing AMI. Although not traditionally considered AMI, isolated colon ischemia will also be discussed for completeness.

CHRONIC MESENTERIC ISCHEMIA

Pathophysiology

The underlying pathophysiology of CMI is the inability to achieve postprandial hyperemic intestinal blood flow. Intestinal

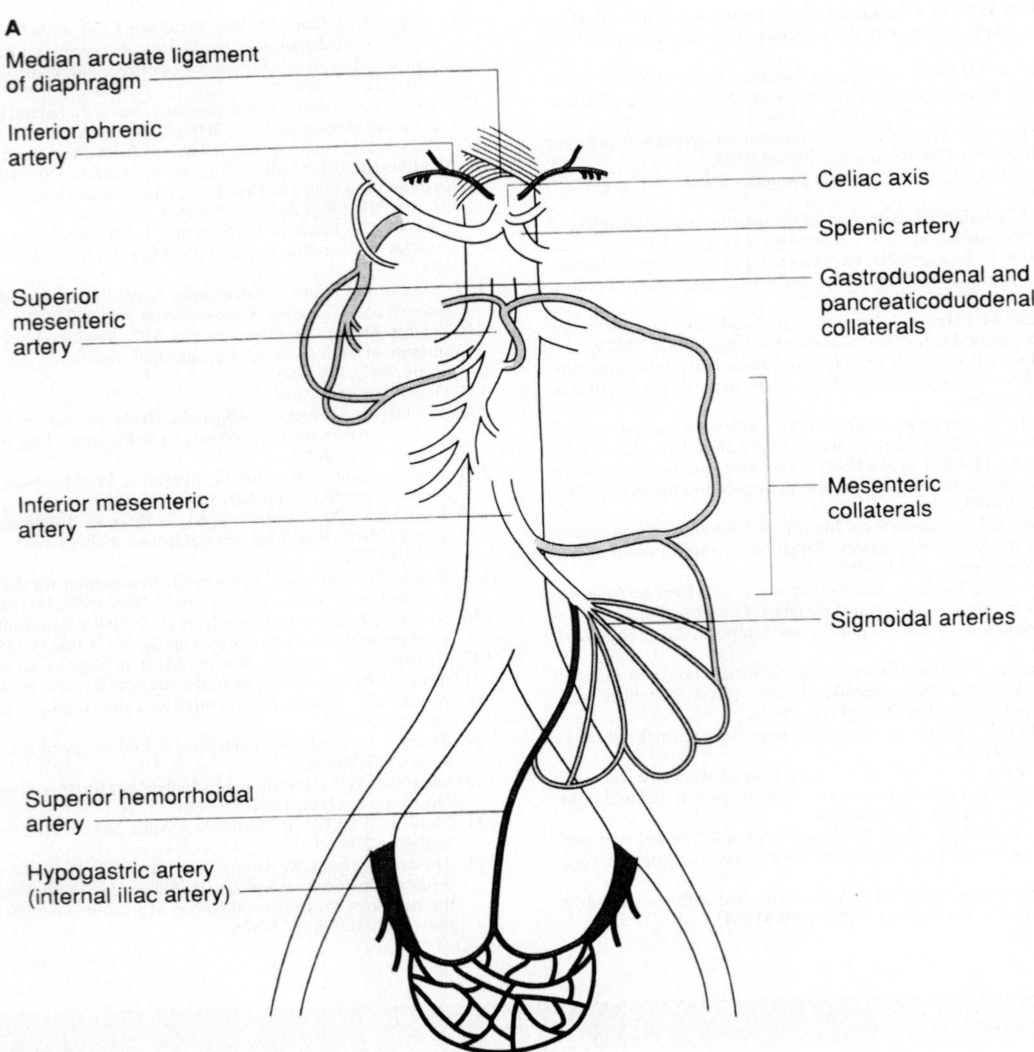

FIGURE 159.1. A diagram of the collateral pathways for the mesenteric vessels is shown. The celiac axis and superior mesenteric arteries communicate through the superior and inferior pancreaticoduodenal arteries, respectively. The superior and inferior mesenteric arteries communicate through the meandering artery and the marginal artery of Drummond with the meandering artery serving as the dominant collateral. The inferior mesenteric artery communicates with the internal iliac artery through the hemorrhoidal vessels. (From Zelenock GB. Visceral occlusive disease. In Greenfield LJ, ed. *Surgery: Scientific Principles and Practice*. Philadelphia, PA: Lippincott Williams & Wilkins; 2001:1691, with permission.)

blood flow in the normal fasting state is fairly modest but increases markedly postprandially with the magnitude contingent on the size and composition of the meal. Most of the hyperemic changes occur in the pancreas and small bowel and peak within 30 to 60 minutes after eating (1,2). In the presence of significant arterial occlusive disease, this postprandial hyperemia is not possible and patients develop ischemic pain similar to angina pectoris appropriately termed *mesenteric angina*.

The normal visceral circulation is fairly redundant and has a rich collateral network (Fig. 159.1). The celiac axis communicates with the superior mesenteric artery through the superior and inferior pancreaticoduodenal arteries. The superior mesenteric artery communicates with the inferior mesenteric artery via the meandering mesenteric artery that runs within the proximal mesentery. This collateral has multiple eponyms, but should be differentiated from the less significant collateral known, the marginal artery of Drummond, located in the distal mesentery. Last, the inferior mesenteric artery communicates with the internal iliac artery via the superior and middle hemorrhoidal arteries. The symptoms of mesenteric ischemia usually do not occur unless two of the three visceral vessels (i.e., celiac axis, superior mesenteric artery, inferior mesenteric artery) are significantly diseased because of this rich collateral network. However, symptoms may occur with isolated disease in the superior mesenteric artery in the absence of adequate collaterals (3).

The overwhelming majority of visceral artery stenoses are due to atherosclerosis. Various other causes have been reported including neurofibromatosis, fibromuscular disease, rheumatoid disorders, aortic dissection, radiation, Buerger disease, and certain drugs, although these are collectively less common. Symptomatic visceral artery occlusive disease (i.e., CMI) is relatively rare despite the prevalence of visceral artery stenoses. Indeed, a hemodynamically significant visceral artery stenosis (>50% diameter reduction) has been reported in up to 27% of patients with peripheral arterial occlusive disease undergoing arteriography (4) and in up to 5 to 10% of unselected patients at autopsy (5). The atherosclerotic process usually involves just the origin of the visceral vessels. Patients with occlusive disease in the celiac axis and superior mesenteric artery frequently have renal artery lesions (and vice versa). The risk factors for visceral artery atherosclerosis are the same as those for the other vascular beds.

Clinical Presentation and Diagnosis

The appearance and presentation of patients with CMI is fairly characteristic. Most patients are cachectic, elderly women with strong smoking histories. Indeed, CMI is one of the few cardiovascular problems more common in women with a reported ratio of approximately 3:1 (6). The mean age (± SD) of patients undergoing repair in a recent national series was 66 ± 11 although the disease process is not exclusive to the elderly and is frequently found in patients in their fourth and fifth decades of life (6).

Abdominal pain is usually the presenting symptom. It initially occurs postprandially but may progress to a persistent nature in the latter stages of the disease process. Unfortunately, the pain has no specific characteristics. As a result of the pain, patients develop a fear of food and avoid eating. The net result is a predictable weight loss with a mean of 20 to 30 lb in several recent clinical series (7–9). It should be noted that the cause of the weight loss is poor nutrition rather than an abnormality of intestinal absorption. Patients may develop nausea/vomiting, constipation, or diarrhea. Indeed, AMI is a fairly strong cathartic, and motility symptoms rather than pain may be the predominate symptom. Patients with CMI frequently have evidence of systemic vascular disease although there are no characteristic physical findings.

The diagnosis of CMI requires the appropriate clinical history and the presence of significant visceral artery occlusive disease. The diagnostic approach is a stepwise one with consideration of the more common problems first. Although the appearance and clinical presentation of patients with CMI is fairly characteristic, the differential diagnosis of patients with abdominal pain and weight loss is extensive and includes gastrointestinal malignancy first and foremost. Indeed, CMI is usually not even considered by most primary care providers, and this is reflected by the fact that the mean duration from presentation to diagnosis exceeds a calendar year and 2.8 diagnostic tests (10). The initial diagnostic workup for patients with abdominal pain and weight loss should include esophagogastroduodenoscopy, colonoscopy, abdominal ultrasound, and an abdominal/pelvic computed tomography (CT) scan. Notably, gastric ulcers are relatively common in patients with CMI and likely result from ischemia (11). A surprising number of patients are subjected to cholecystectomy as part of their workup before the definitive diagnosis of CMI is made.

Mesenteric duplex scan is an excellent *screening* tool for visceral artery stenosis with reported sensitivity and specificity rates of approximately 80% (12). However, it is technically challenging, operator dependent, and not available in all centers. Various criteria have been proposed to grade the severity of stenoses based on the systolic/diastolic velocities or frequency shifts (12,13). The various criteria are probably equivalent as far as their accuracy in grading the degree of stenosis. However, it is imperative that they be validated at each institution by comparison with the institutional gold standard (i.e., CT arteriogram, contrast arteriogram). Various provocative tests have been proposed to unmask clinically significant visceral artery stenoses, although their utility is unclear and they have not achieved widespread use (14,15).

CT arteriography has largely replaced catheter-based contrast arteriography as the *diagnostic* study of choice for patients with CMI (Fig. 159.2) and is usually sufficient to plan open surgical revascularization (16–18). CT arteriography is safe, noninvasive, and almost universally available. It is very good for identifying occlusive disease in the superior mesenteric artery and celiac axis. Furthermore, it is useful for identifying the presence of collateral vessels between the visceral vessels (i.e., celiac axis, superior mesenteric, inferior mesenteric) and/or the internal iliac arteries that suggest hemodynamically significant stenoses. Additionally, it is very good for evaluating other intra-abdominal processes.

Catheter-based contrast arteriography is very useful for evaluating the visceral circulation and has traditionally been used as the definitive *diagnostic* test for CMI (Fig. 159.3A). The major advantage of contrast arteriography over CT arteriography is that therapeutic interventions can be performed at the time of the diagnostic procedure. However, it is an invasive procedure with a small but finite complication rate. A lateral arteriogram is mandatory as part of the examination to accurately assess the origins of the celiac axis and superior mesenteric artery due to their anterior/posterior orientation. The significant findings on arteriogram include ostial stenoses of the celiac axis and superior mesenteric artery, the presence of visceral collaterals, and the presence of central aortic atherosclerotic disease. A small percentage of patients with CMI may have visceral artery aneurysms, presumably from increased flow through the collateral vessels.

Magnetic resonance (MR) arteriography has been used as a diagnostic study for patients with CMI and offers many of the advantages of CT arteriography (19,20). However, it is not as universally available as CT arteriography. Furthermore, it is not practical and may be contraindicated for many patients including those in the intensive care unit. Last, MR arteriography tends to overestimate the degree of stenosis in the visceral vessels.

Treatment Strategies

All patients with CMI require treatment. The natural history of the untreated disease process is death either from inanition or bowel infarction. The theoretical treatment options include medical management with total parenteral nutrition or revascularization by either endovascular or open surgical techniques. The role of long-term parenteral nutrition is very limited given its complexity, expense, and complications, particularly those associated with the infusion catheters. Additionally, patients with CMI may not be able to metabolize the parenteral nutrition. Endovascular treatment (angioplasty with or without stenting) has emerged as the initial revascularization option for most patients with CMI but should be viewed as an alternative to the open surgical approach (21–27). Endovascular treatment

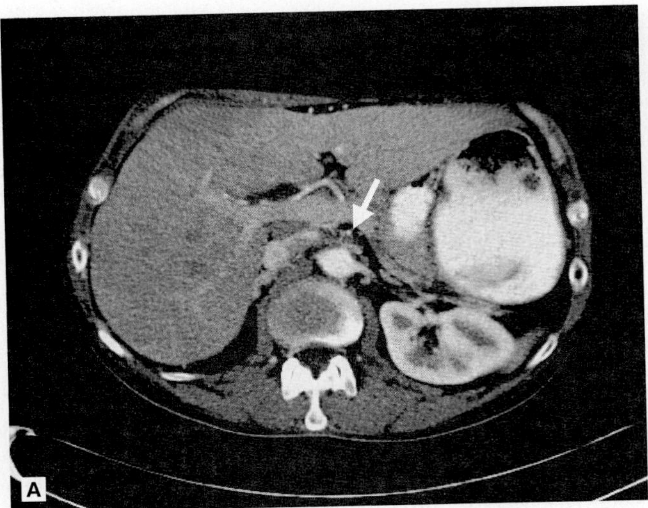

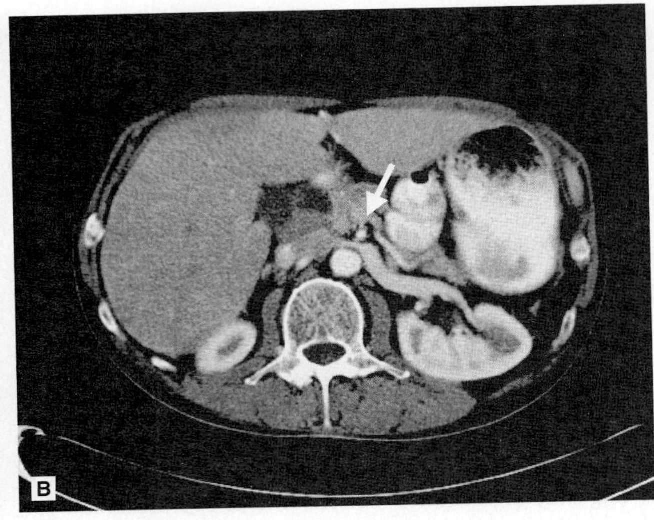

FIGURE 159.2. Two CT arteriograms are shown in a patient with chronic mesenteric ischemia (CMI) and an occluded celiac axis and superior mesenteric artery. **A:** The origin of the superior mesenteric artery is shown with the *arrow*. There is no contrast within the lumen of the vessel at this cross section. **B:** The superior mesenteric artery is shown with the *arrow* in this cross section that is 10 mm caudal to the first image. The artery is patent at this level as reflected by the contrast within the lumen.

has consistently been shown to have a lower mortality rate, a lower complication rate, and shorter hospital length of stay when compared to open surgical revascularization. However, the patency rates for the endovascular approach are lower. Notably, this has not been associated with a decrease in survival, and vessel thrombosis and/or recurrent stenosis has not necessarily resulted in AMI. The endovascular approach can serve as an excellent bridge to open surgical revascularization for debilitated patients who are poor initial candidates for a major surgical procedure. The recent development of lower-profile (i.e., smaller-diameter) angioplasty balloon/stent systems has further extended the applications of the endovascular approach (25), and reasonable short-term results have been reported for patients with even occluded (versus stenotic) vessels (23).

Endovascular Revascularization

The preoperative evaluation prior to endovascular treatment is essentially the same for all catheter-based contrast arteriography. Patients with a contrast allergy should be treated with an appropriate steroid preparation. Patients with elevated serum creatinine levels (serum creatinine 1.5–2.0 mg/dL) should

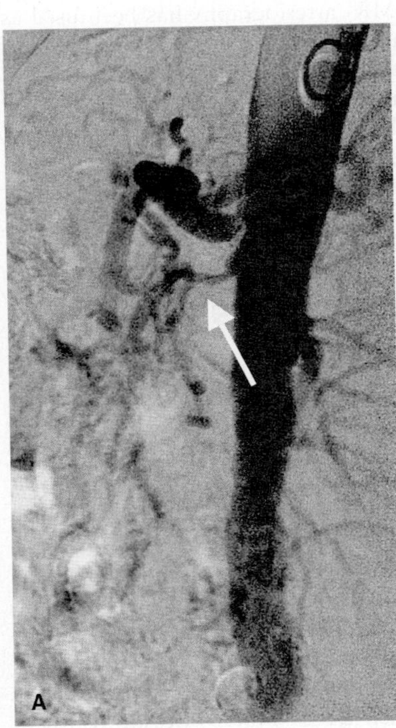

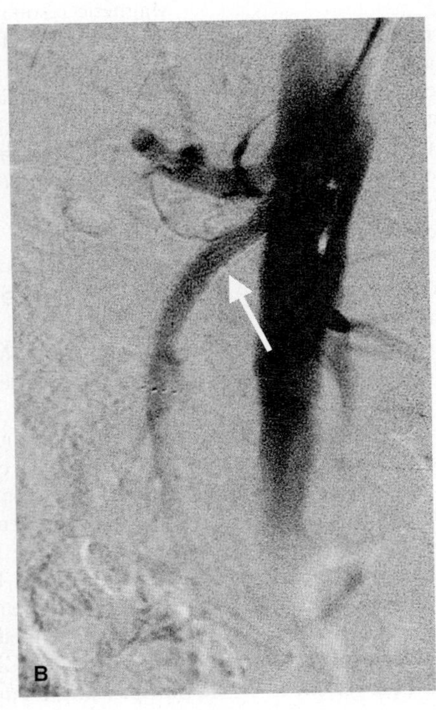

FIGURE 159.3. A lateral aortogram of a patient with chronic mesenteric ischemia (CMI) is shown. **A:** There is a moderate stenosis in the proximal superior mesenteric artery as shown with the *arrow*. **B:** No residual stenosis is seen in the superior mesenteric artery after placement of an intraluminal stent.

receive gentle hydration and acetylcysteine, although admittedly their benefits are somewhat unsubstantiated.

Percutaneous access can be obtained through either the femoral or brachial arteries although the latter is favored for therapeutic procedures given the vector forces associated with the catheters/sheaths. A flush aortogram is performed in both the anteroposterior and lateral projections. Since most lesions in the superior mesenteric artery and celiac axis are orificial and located in the proximal 2 cm, selective catheterization is not usually necessary unless a distal lesion is suspected or the extent of the lesion cannot be determined. A >50% diameter reduction of the superior mesenteric artery is usually considered clinically significant regardless of whether or not the celiac axis is involved. In contrast, the diagnosis of CMI should be questioned in the presence of an isolated celiac axis stenosis. Symptomatic stenoses can be treated at the time of the diagnostic arteriogram (Fig. 159.3B). The orificial stenoses in the mesenteric vessels are refractory to angioplasty alone, and primary stenting is recommended. Balloon angioplasty with selective stenting is reserved for midsegment lesions. Balloon-expandable stents (vs. self-expanding stents) are preferred for the orificial stenoses due to their superior radial forces and controlled deployment mechanism.

The postoperative care after mesenteric angioplasty/stenting is comparable to that for other peripheral endovascular procedures. Patients are admitted to the general care hospital ward for overnight observation and started on clopidogrel. Most patients notice a marked improvement of their postprandial symptoms shortly after the procedure. A fasting mesenteric duplex ultrasound scan is obtained on the morning after the procedure to serve as a baseline. Elevated velocities are occasionally noted in the duplex scan despite a technically satisfactory arteriographic result and complete resolution of the preoperative symptoms. The explanation for these abnormal duplex findings is unclear although we have elected to follow the patient's clinical course in this setting and only repeat the arteriogram and/or intervention if there is a significant change. A repeat duplex examination is performed at 1 month and aspirin (325 mg/day) is substituted for the clopidogrel at that time. The subsequent follow-up with serial duplex examination is comparable to that outlined for open revascularization.

Open Surgical Revascularization

The preoperative workup for patients undergoing open mesenteric revascularization is comparable to that for other major vascular surgical procedures and includes optimization of all organ systems. Multiple algorithms have been developed to reduce the cardiac risk for vascular surgical patients undergoing noncardiac procedures (28) although their utility is unclear given the results of several recent publications (29,30). Regardless of the specific preoperative cardiac evaluation, all patients should likely be on aspirin, a beta-blocker (if not contraindicated), and a cholesterol-lowering agent (preferably a statin/HMG Co-A reductase inhibitor) (31). A CT or contrast arteriogram is mandatory to both confirm the diagnosis and plan the operative procedure. There is no clear-cut role for extended preoperative parenteral alimentation to replete the nutritional stores, and, indeed, it may actually be detrimental.

Various open surgical procedures have been reported although the antegrade aortoceliac/superior mesenteric artery bypass (159.4) and the retrograde aortosuperior mesenteric artery bypass (Fig. 159.5) are the most common. Unfortunately, the relative infrequency of the problem has prevented the requisite randomized controlled trials. The advantages of the antegrade aortoceliac/superior mesenteric bypass are that both visceral vessels are revascularized and that the supraceliac aorta (the origin of the bypass) is usually free of atherosclerotic occlusive disease. The major disadvantage is the complexity of the procedure. In contrast, retrograde aortosuperior mesenteric artery bypass is relatively straightforward, although only a single vessel is revascularized and the graft is prone to kinking given its obligatory retrograde course that traverses both caudal to cephalad and posterior to anterior. The optimal choice for a specific patient is contingent on his or her comorbidities with the retrograde bypass generally reserved for patients who will not tolerate the more complex antegrade procedure.

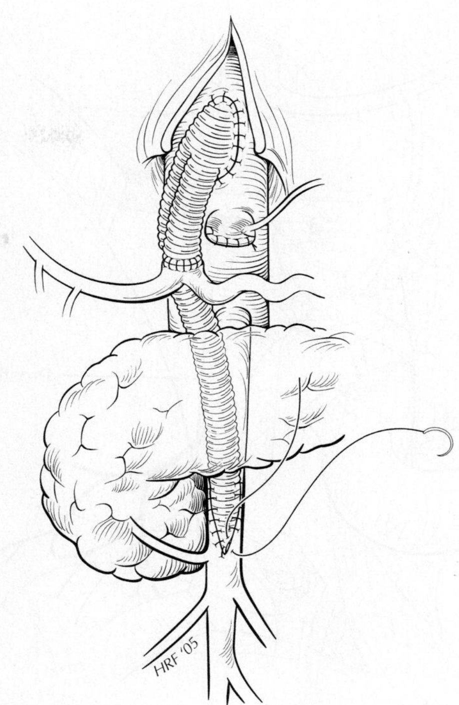

FIGURE 159.4. The completed antegrade bypass from the supraceliac aorta to both the celiac axis and the superior mesenteric artery is shown. (From Huber TS, Lee WA. Revascularization for chronic mesenteric ischemia. In: Zelenock GB, Huber TS, Messina LM, et al., eds. *Mastery of Vascular and Endovascular Surgery*. Philadelphia, PA: Lippincott Williams & Wilkins; 2006:301, with permission.)

The immediate postoperative care for patients undergoing revascularization for CMI is frequently complicated by the development of multiple organ dysfunction and is distinctly different from that associated with most other abdominal vascular surgical procedures such as aortobifemoral bypass for aortoiliac occlusive disease. This propensity to develop multiple organ dysfunction likely accounts for the prolonged intensive care and total hospital length of stays and is one of the leading causes of death in the postoperative period (32). The responsible mechanism for this multiple organ dysfunction is likely the visceral ischemia and reperfusion phenomenon inherent to the revascularization. This process has been reported to induce a complex response involving several interrelated inflammatory mediators that have the potential to

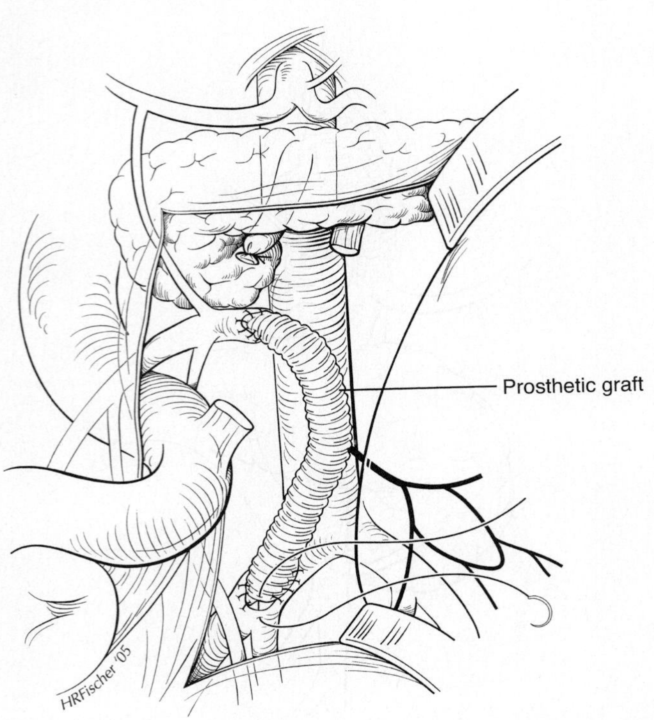

FIGURE 159.5. The completed retrograde bypass from the terminal aorta/proximal right common iliac artery to the superior mesenteric artery bypass is shown. (From Huber TS, Lee WA. Revascularization for chronic mesenteric ischemia. In Zelenock GB, Huber TS, Messina LM, et al., eds. *Mastery of Vascular and Endovascular Surgery*. Philadelphia, PA: Lippincott Williams & Wilkins; 2006:301, with permission.)

cause both local and distant organ injury (33). In a detailed study, Harward et al. (32) characterized the individual organ system dysfunction after revascularization for both AMI and CMI. They reported that the serum hepatic transaminases (i.e., serum glutamic-oxaloacetic transaminase [SGOT], serum glutamic-pyruvic transaminase [SGPT]) increased 90- to 100-fold immediately postoperatively and did not normalize for 7 to 10 days, the platelet counts fell below 40,000 per microliter within 12 to 24 hours and remained abnormal for the first 3 to 6 days, and the prothrombin (PT) and partial thromboplastin (PTT) times became elevated and stayed elevated also for 3 to 6 days. Perhaps most notably, they reported that the overwhelming majority of patients developed a significant pulmonary injury characterized by an elevated mean shunt fraction and a radiographic picture of the acute respiratory distress syndrome that manifested between 1 to 3 days and persisted for 5 to 8 days. Jimenez et al. (7) documented a 64% incidence of multiple organ dysfunction and a 53% incidence of prolonged mechanical ventilation after antegrade revascularization for CMI and further corroborated the findings by Harward et al. (32).

The optimal management strategy for patients in the early postoperative period after mesenteric revascularization is to simply support the individual organ systems until the dysfunction resolves. Admittedly, not all patients develop organ dysfunction, but the incidence is quite high and somewhat unpredictable. The optimal ventilator management remains unresolved. We have usually extubated patients in the early postoperative period when they satisfy the various weaning criteria and have been reluctant to maintain them on mechanical ventilation in anticipation that they may develop a lung injury. However, it is not infrequent that they need to be reintubated and started back on mechanical ventilation. The thrombocytopenia and coagulopathy are usually managed expectantly with platelet and/or plasma transfusions reserved for severely depressed platelet counts and/or any clinical evidence of bleeding. Notably, the report by Harward et al. (32) suggested that the inherent coagulopathy after mesenteric revascularization was not responsive to vitamin K. Patients should be maintained on total parenteral nutrition throughout the postoperative period until their bowel function returns. This is particularly important given the fact that most patients are severely compromised from a nutritional standpoint. Unfortunately, patients may have a prolonged ileus after revascularization and parenteral nutrition is required for some time. The bypass should be interrogated prior to discharge to confirm the technical adequacy of the reconstruction. Essentially the same imaging studies used to make the diagnosis are options. Our preference is mesenteric duplex although examination in the early postoperative period is frequently compromised by the persistent ileus and the presence of bowel gas. Patients with acute changes in their clinical status should also undergo visceral imaging to confirm that their bypass is patent. It can be difficult to differentiate multiple organ dysfunction that is a sequelae of the ischemia and reperfusion injury from AMI secondary to graft thrombosis. Serum lactate levels may be helpful in this setting.

All patients who undergo revascularization for CMI require long-term follow-up. Patients are usually seen frequently in the early postoperative period until all their active issues resolve and then every 6 months thereafter with a mesenteric duplex to confirm graft patency and to identify any graft or anastomotic related problems. Objective assessment of graft patency is critical and significantly better than the return of symptoms that has been used as a surrogate marker (34). All abnormalities on duplex imaging merit further investigation with additional imaging and/or intervention.

Diarrhea is a common complaint after revascularization for CMI and can persist for several months. It is more common in patients with preoperative diarrhea and can be so severe that it necessitates total parenteral nutrition. Notably, Jimenez et al. (7) reported that 33% of the patients in their series experienced significant postoperative diarrhea and that it persisted greater than 6 months in 24%. Furthermore, Kihara et al. (35) reported that patients had almost two stools/day (1.9 ± 0.4) after revascularization for CMI. The cause of the diarrhea is unclear but may be related to intestinal atrophy, bacterial overgrowth, or disruption of the mesenteric neuroplexus.

Outcome

The outcome after mesenteric revascularization for CMI is quite good. The perioperative mortality rate after open surgical revascularization is <15% (6–8,10,34–39) whereas that for the endovascular treatment is <5% (9,21–24,26,27,40–49). The corresponding complication rates are approximately 30% and 15% for the open and endovascular treatments, respectively. The initial technical success rate for the endovascular treatment is approximately 90%. The objectively documented 5-year patency rates after open revascularization are approximately 75%; patency rates after endovascular treatment are not as well described, but likely fall short of those reported for the open treatment. The 5-year survival after either treatment is approximately 75%, and most patients return to their presymptoms weight.

PEARLS

- The underlying pathophysiology of CMI is the inability to achieve postprandial hyperemic intestinal blood flow.
- The symptoms of mesenteric ischemia usually do not occur unless two of the three visceral vessels are significantly diseased because of the rich collateral network.
- Patients presenting with abdominal pain and weight loss should initially undergo an evaluation to rule out a gastrointestinal malignancy.
- CT arteriography has largely replaced catheter-based contrast arteriography as the *diagnostic* study of choice for patients with CMI.
- Endovascular treatment has emerged as the initial revascularization option for most patients with CMI, but should be viewed as an alternative to open surgical revascularization.
- The immediate postoperative care for patients undergoing revascularization for CMI is frequently complicated by the development of multiple organ dysfunction.
- The optimal management strategy for patients in the early postoperative period after mesenteric revascularization is to support the individual organ systems until the dysfunction resolves.

ACUTE MESENTERIC ISCHEMIA

Acute mesenteric ischemia (AMI) is the end point for several distinct disease processes. Mesenteric emboli and *in situ* thrombosis are the most common among these and account for approximately 50% and 25% of the cases, respectively (50,51). Nonocclusive mesenteric ischemia (NOMI, 20%), mesenteric venous thrombosis (5%), and aortic dissections account for the balance (50,51). The underlying pathophysiology of AMI is that the impaired intestinal perfusion leads to mucosal compromise. This results in the release of the intracellular contents and the influx of substances (including bacteria) from the lumen of the bowel. This can lead to the activation of the systemic inflammatory response, resulting in both local and distant organ dysfunction (e.g., lung injury). If the impaired perfusion persists, bowel infarction with perforation and peritonitis ensues. The immediate clinical concerns for patients with AMI are to reverse the underlying clinical condition and prevent bowel infarction. The clinical presentation, diagnostic approach, and treatment for the various causes of AMI are similar, but there are distinct differences that mandate individual consideration. AMI from an embolus will be discussed in depth given the fact that it is the most common cause, and the respective differences will be highlighted for the other causes. Fortunately, the underlying cause can usually be determined from the history and clinical setting. Not surprisingly, the morbidity and mortality associated with AMI are significant. The optimal therapy requires prompt diagnosis and definitive treatment although this is often difficult given the susceptible patient population and common clinical scenarios. Indeed, AMI may be either the cause or the effect of the patient's critical illness.

Embolus

Pathophysiology

The emboli responsible for AMI usually lodge in the superior mesenteric artery and originate from the heart. The intracardiac thrombus is related to either atrial fibrillation, an acute myocardial infarction, or a ventricular aneurysm. Patients frequently have prior embolic events from the same source although they are not necessarily limited to the superior mesenteric artery (e.g., common femoral artery bifurcation presenting with acute lower extremity ischemia). Notably, the material that constitutes these macroemboli is actually quite large as might be predicted from the size of the arteries involved. This is in contradistinction to the micron-sized atheroembolic particles that commonly cause blue toes after invasive arteriographic procedures (i.e., artery–artery emboli). The extent of bowel ischemia and/or infarction after an embolus to the superior mesenteric artery is contingent on the extent of the collateral circulation, the pattern of the arterial occlusion, and the duration of the ischemia. In this setting, the bowel progresses from ischemia to infarction in a time-dependent fashion although it may remain viable for 6–12 hours. Acute embolic occlusion of the superior mesenteric usually results in ischemia/infarction of the bowel from the proximal jejunum to the transverse colon. The duodenum and descending colon are usually spared because they are supplied by branches of the celiac axis and inferior mesenteric artery, respectively.

Clinical Presentation and Diagnosis

The diagnosis of AMI from an embolus (or other causes of AMI) may be difficult. The differential list of diagnoses includes all the more common causes of acute abdominal pain. The diagnosis is confounded by the fact that the patients are often critically ill, and thus, their history/physical examination may not be reliable. Diagnosis requires a high index of suspicion and an aggressive approach since delays in diagnosis adversely affect outcome. This requires an appreciation of the types of patients and clinical scenarios in which AMI occurs including post myocardial infarction, end-stage renal disease (52), and post coronary artery bypass grafting (53–55).

Patients with AMI from an embolus usually present with diffuse abdominal pain. The classic description of the pain secondary to AMI is pain out of proportion to the physical findings although this scenario is not always present. Unfortunately, the pain is neither specific nor localized to a particular abdominal quadrant. Peritoneal signs can be present, but they usually occur late in the process and suggest bowel perforation. Patients often experience nausea/vomiting and/or diarrhea, but again these are fairly nonspecific complaints. Notably, AMI is a potent cathartic. Similar to the physical examination, the routine chemistry and hematologic laboratory studies are usually nonspecific and insensitive. Patients frequently have mild abnormalities of their laboratory values including an elevated white blood count, a decreased platelet count, an elevated hematocrit, and a mildly elevated amylase level. The hemodynamic status of the patients at the time of presentation ranges from normovolemia to profound hypovolemic shock with acidosis and is contingent on the status of the bowel and the duration of symptoms.

Various diagnostic studies are available to help make the diagnosis of AMI secondary to an embolus. Plain abdominal radiographs have been used traditionally for patients with acute abdominal pain and can be helpful to demonstrate free air from an intestinal perforation or identify other causes of abdominal pain. However, patients with AMI frequently have either normal plain radiographs or demonstrate nonspecific findings (e.g., ileus). CT arteriography with 1- to 2-mm cuts has emerged as the diagnostic study of choice for patients with AMI secondary to an embolus (56–58). Notably, the study is performed using only intravenous contrast since both oral and rectal contrast potentially interfere with the arteriogram itself. Both stenoses and occlusions in the visceral vessels are well demonstrated on CT arteriography. In patients with AMI secondary to an embolus, a meniscus sign can often be seen in the mid/distal superior mesenteric artery. The images obtained using the CT arteriogram protocol are also excellent for the nonvascular structures. The significant nonvascular findings of AMI include bowel wall thickening, bowel wall gas, bowel/solid organ infarction, and hepatic/portal venous gas. Indeed, Paran et al. (57) reported that most patients with portal/mesenteric venous gas had mesenteric ischemia and that the associated mortality rate was 86%. Mesenteric duplex, although an excellent screening test for CMI, is not usually helpful in patients with AMI because abdominal distention/gas precludes the accurate interrogation of the visceral vessels.

Standard contrast arteriography can be used as an alternative to CT arteriography, and indeed, has been the traditional imaging study for the visceral vessels in the setting of AMI from an embolus or *in situ* thrombosis. Similar to studies in patients with CMI, it can potentially serve as both a diagnostic test and therapeutic modality since an intervention can be performed at the same time. The major disadvantages are the obligatory time required to obtain the procedure and the small, but finite, complications associated with the contrast agent and vessel cannulation. Given the new treatment algorithms with vascular surgeons assuming the traditional roles of the interventional radiologists, it is conceivable that the diagnostic contrast arteriogram could be performed in an operating room with a fixed imaging unit. The definitive operative procedure could be performed at the same setting if the arteriogram confirmed the diagnosis.

Laparoscopy offers an additional diagnostic modality for patients with AMI (59,60). It can be used to assess the viability of the bowel and confirm the diagnosis. Furthermore, it can be performed in the intensive care unit with sedation and, therefore, is feasible for unstable patients with a suspected intra-abdominal process. Notably, the authors of the evidence-based guidelines from the European Association for Endoscopic Surgery concluded that laparoscopy had an unclear or limited role in the setting of AMI (61). However, they did state that it may be indicated if the routine diagnostic studies are inconclusive. Laparotomy remains the definitive diagnostic test for patients with AMI. However, the diagnostic studies outlined above are usually sufficient.

Treatment Strategies

Patients should be taken emergently to the operating room for definitive treatment once the diagnosis of AMI from an embolus is made. An extensive preoperative evaluation is unnecessary and potentially harmful in light of the narrow window for salvaging the bowel. There is essentially no role for medical management alone in this setting. Patients should be systemically anticoagulated with heparin to prevent further clot development and started on broad-spectrum antibiotics against enteric organisms. Importantly, patients with AMI are frequently hypovolemic and should be volume resuscitated prior to the induction of anesthesia. This can be performed fairly expeditiously and should not delay transfer to the operating room.

Both midline and transverse abdominal incisions provide adequate exposure to the visceral vessels, and the choice is contingent on surgeon preference. The diagnosis of AMI from an embolus is usually confirmed by the distribution of the ischemic/infarcted bowel that extends from the proximal jejunum to the transverse colon. However, the diagnosis should be further substantiated by interrogating the visceral vessels with continuous wave Doppler. The embolus may be extracted from the superior mesenteric artery using a Fogarty thromboembolectomy catheter. Although there are several approaches to the superior mesenteric artery, the easiest approach is to incise the base of the transverse mesocolon after retracting the transverse colon itself cephalad. The arteriotomy in the superior mesenteric artery may be performed either longitudinally or horizontally. Although the longitudinal arteriotomy needs to be closed with a vein patch to prevent narrowing its lumen, it is the preferred approach because it affords greater flexibility in case a bypass procedure is necessary.

The management of the bowel for patients with AMI merits further comment. All of the bowel that is obviously dead should be resected, and intestinal anastomoses should be avoided in favor of proximal and distal stomas. This mandates a second procedure to restore bowel continuity, but it allows the bowel (i.e., mucosa of the stoma) to be examined at the bedside during the postoperative period. Furthermore, it avoids using ischemic or borderline ischemic tissues for the anastomosis. Bowel that is ischemic though not frankly necrotic should be revascularized and then re-examined before any final decision about resection. A conservative approach is justified in this setting because many of the borderline areas will remain viable after revascularization. Admittedly, the differentiation between viable and nonviable bowel is difficult. Various complicated modalities have been described to help differentiate viable from nonviable bowel in this setting although they have not been universally adopted. Simple adjuncts include visual inspection for peristalsis, use of continuous wave Doppler to detect arterial signals within the mesentery, and intravenous fluorescein in combination with a Wood lamp. Notably, approximately 100 to 150 cm of small bowel is necessary for nutritional absorption.

A decision to perform a second-look operation to reassess the viability of the bowel should be made at the time of the initial procedure. This is routinely performed 24 to 48 hours after the first procedure, a time usually sufficient for the marginal bowel to declare itself. A recent retrospective review has questioned the role of the second-look operation and reported that survival was actually greater in those patients in whom it was not performed (62). Admittedly, there was a tremendous selection bias in this review and the authors conceded that the experience of the surgeon is likely the key factor regarding the decision to perform a second look. A "damage control" operation may be justified in a small subset of unstable patients with AMI as suggested by Freeman and Graham (63). This includes emergent laparotomy, resection of obviously dead bowel, and creation of proximal/distal stomas, leaving the abdomen open and deferring the definitive vascular/gastrointestinal procedure until later.

Despite its definitive role for patients with CMI, there is likely little role for endovascular therapies in patients with AMI secondary to an embolus. The obligatory time for endovascular treatment, including chemical lysis, is too long given the threatened bowel and the potential to progress from ischemic bowel to infarcted bowel. Furthermore, it does not allow direct assessment of the bowel, and the chemical lysis may cause intestinal bleeding from mucosal sloughing. A recent systematic review of the literature examining the role of thrombolysis for acute superior mesenteric artery occlusion found insufficient evidence to support the practice despite a few case reports (64–70).

The postoperative course after embolectomy for AMI is similar to that after revascularization for CMI although the incidence of postoperative complications and multiple organ dysfunction are greater. As noted above, revascularization may cause an ischemia/reperfusion injury that affects both local and distant organ systems. Accordingly, patients are at risk for developing an abdominal compartment syndrome. Bladder pressures can be measured, and the abdomen closure can be dissembled as necessary. Patients should be continued on broad-spectrum antibiotics throughout the early postoperative period. Furthermore, they need to be anticoagulated long term due to the potential for recurrent emboli.

Outcome

The mortality rate for patients with AMI is approximately 70%, and this rate has changed very little over the past several decades (51,68,71,72). Unfortunately, most of the case series tend to encompass all of the causes rather than a specific one (e.g., embolus). A recent systematic review by Schoots et al. (68) reported that the mortality rates for AMI from mesenteric venous thrombosis were better than those for arterial problems and that the mortality rates for mesenteric emboli were better than those for *in situ* thromboses. The aggregate mortality rates in their study by cause are listed: mesenteric venous thrombosis, 32%; embolus, 54%; NOMI, 74%; *in situ* thrombosis, 77%. Several predictable factors have been associated with mortality in the various case series including patient age, time to definitive surgery, shock, acidosis, leukocytosis, cardiac status, and coagulopathy (71,73,74). Most deaths in a recent report were due to multiple organ failure (75).

In Situ Thrombosis

Patients with visceral artery occlusive disease may also present with AMI secondary to *in situ* thrombosis. The presentation is superimposed on the symptoms of CMI in more than 50% of the patients (76) and can usually be differentiated from the other causes of AMI by the history and clinical setting. However, it is important to emphasize that patients may present with AMI as the initial symptom of their visceral occlusive disease. The clinical presentation, diagnostic approach, and immediate postoperative care of patients with AMI secondary to *in situ* thrombosis is similar to that outlined above for emboli although the operative approach is somewhat different.

Patients with AMI secondary to *in situ* thrombosis require a mesenteric bypass. Although antegrade aortoceliac/superior mesenteric artery bypass is probably the optimal bypass for CMI, retrograde bypass from the infrarenal aorta or common iliac artery is likely the optimal procedure for AMI (Fig. 159.5). The objectives and treatment are somewhat different in the acute setting (i.e., AMI vs. CMI). The main objective is to restore blood flow to the ischemic vascular bed as safely and expeditiously as possible. This usually requires only bypass to the superior mesenteric artery. Patients with isolated celiac axis stenosis rarely develop AMI because the collateral blood flow to the foregut is so good and the liver may be sustained on portal blood flow alone. Prosthetic conduits are relatively contraindicated in the setting of bowel infarction and/or perforation due to the potential for postoperative graft infection. Autogenous conduits with either saphenous or superficial femoral vein are suitable although the latter may be more durable.

The role of endovascular treatment for patients with AMI secondary to *in situ* thrombosis is likely limited for the reasons noted above for AMI secondary to an embolus. Wyers et al. (77) have reported a small case series using novel hybrid open/endovascular approach in which a stent is placed retrograde through the superior mesenteric artery at the time of laparotomy. This approach allows assessment of the bowel and is potentially less morbid than the more traditional open revascularization.

Occasionally patients will undergo bowel resection for infarction by a nonvascular surgeon, and the diagnosis of mesenteric ischemia will be missed both preoperatively and intraoperatively. It is important to emphasize that infarction of the bowel is not a spontaneous event, but rather an end-stage complication of another disease process; it is imperative that the cause of all bowel infarctions be established in an attempt to prevent recurrences. An appropriate imaging study (i.e., CT arteriogram, contrast arteriogram) should be obtained in the early postoperative period, and the necessary treatment including anticoagulation and revascularization implemented in a timely fashion.

Nonocclusive Mesenteric Ischemia

Pathophysiology

Nonocclusive mesenteric ischemia (NOMI) represents an abnormal or paradoxical mesenteric vasoconstriction characterized by the loss of autoregulation. Shock or circulatory stress normally causes mesenteric vasoconstriction in an attempt to maintain cerebral and/or cardiac perfusion. The mesenteric vasoconstriction ordinarily resolves when the underlying circulatory disorders are corrected; persistent vasoconstriction results in NOMI. There are multiple potential causes for NOMI including cardiogenic shock, sepsis, burn injury, trauma, pancreatitis, digitals, vasopressors, and renal failure (78–83). Indeed, almost any underlying condition that can precipitate shock or circulatory stress may precipitate NOMI.

Clinical Presentation and Diagnosis

Similar to the other causes of AMI, the diagnosis of NOMI requires a high index of suspicion and the proper clinical setting. Patients may develop abdominal pain, although the physical examination is frequently unreliable due to the other active medical issues and altered sensorium. Laboratory abnormalities are common including acidosis, leukocytosis, elevated lactate levels, and hyperamylasemia, but these are all relatively nonspecific markers of the underlying shock state. Contrast arteriography has traditionally been the diagnostic study of choice and is also potentially therapeutic. The significant findings on arteriogram for patients with NOMI include segmental stenosis/narrowing of the superior mesenteric artery in a string-of-beads appearance. Furthermore, there is narrowing of the branches of the superior mesenteric artery at their origins, spasm of the mesenteric arcades, and impaired filling of the intramural branches. The contrast arteriogram can also be helpful to rule out the other potential causes of AMI. The published experience with CT arteriography in the setting of NOMI is limited, although it likely affords the same advantages as contrast arteriography with fewer risks.

Treatment Strategies

The initial treatment of patients with NOMI is nonoperative and directed at correcting the underlying condition that precipitated the circulatory stress. Specifically, patients should be resuscitated in an attempt to improve their cardiac output and systemic perfusion. All vasoactive drugs should be stopped (if possible), and patients should be started on broad-spectrum antibiotics directed against enteric organisms. Furthermore, patients should be systemically anticoagulated unless contraindicated. Despite these efforts, the characteristic mesenteric vasoconstriction may persist. Continuous intra-arterial papaverine, administered through an infusion catheter placed into the superior mesenteric artery, may reverse the vasoconstriction (84,85). A 45-mg test dose of papaverine (i.e., short-acting calcium channel blocker) should be given over 15 minutes, and a continuous infusion of 30 to 60 mg/hour should be started if no adverse reactions are encountered. Serial mesenteric arteriograms should be performed to monitor the response to the papaverine with the first performed 1 hour after initiating therapy. The intra-arterial infusion may be continued up to 24 hours. It should be noted that the infusion will reverse the mesenteric vasoconstriction only if the underlying hemodynamic instability is corrected. Operative treatment of NOMI should be reserved only for the clinical scenario when bowel infarction is suspected.

Mesenteric Venous Thrombosis

Pathophysiology

Mesenteric venous thrombosis may also result in AMI and is considered in this section for completeness. However, the associated degree of bowel ischemia is usually less than with arterial occlusion from either an embolus or *in situ* thrombosis. The pathophysiology is similar to venous thrombosis in other vascular beds and may be explained in terms of the Virchow classic triad of stasis, intimal injury, and hypercoagulable states. Mesenteric venous thrombosis results in edema in the bowel and mesentery with significant third-space fluid losses. This may result in bloody ascites and, indeed, a bloody tap at the time of paracentesis may be diagnostic. Progression to bowel infarction is contingent on the magnitude of the clot load and its distribution. Clot localized to the portal or superior mesenteric vein does not usually lead to bowel infarction because of the collateral channels whereas clot in the peripheral mesenteric veins is more likely to do so. The natural history of untreated mesenteric venous thrombosis is poor and almost universally progresses from bowel infarction to perforation and death.

Mesenteric venous thrombosis may result from abnormalities in any of the components of the Virchow triad (i.e., stasis, intimal injury, hypercoagulable state). Stasis may result from congestive heart failure or portal hypertension whereas intimal injury may result from general anesthesia or any number of intra-abdominal infectious processes. A hypercoagulable state is perhaps the strongest of the contributory factors and has been identified in up to 90% of patients with mesenteric venous thrombosis (86).

Clinical Presentation and Diagnosis

Patients with mesenteric venous thrombosis usually present with vague, mild abdominal pain. The pain is usually insidious in onset and frequently present for some time before the patients seek medical attention. Furthermore, the pain is not usually localized to any specific quadrant. Physical examination is notable only for mild, diffuse abdominal pain. Peritoneal signs suggest bowel infarction, but are found only later in the disease process. An abdominal CT scan is the diagnostic study of choice (87,88). The significant findings include bowel edema and thrombus within the mesenteric veins with inflammation of the vessel wall (Fig. 159.6). Plain abdominal radiographs may suggest abdominal wall edema and are helpful to rule out other causes of the abdominal pain. Standard catheter-based contrast arteriography may be helpful but is inferior to CT. The arteriographic findings that suggest mesenteric venous thrombosis include arterial spasm with a prolonged arterial phase, opacification of the bowel wall, extravasations of the contrast into the bowel lumen, and visualization of the venous thrombus.

Treatment Strategies

The primary treatment of patients with mesenteric venous thrombosis is anticoagulation. Patients should be aggressively anticoagulated with heparin when the diagnosis is made and

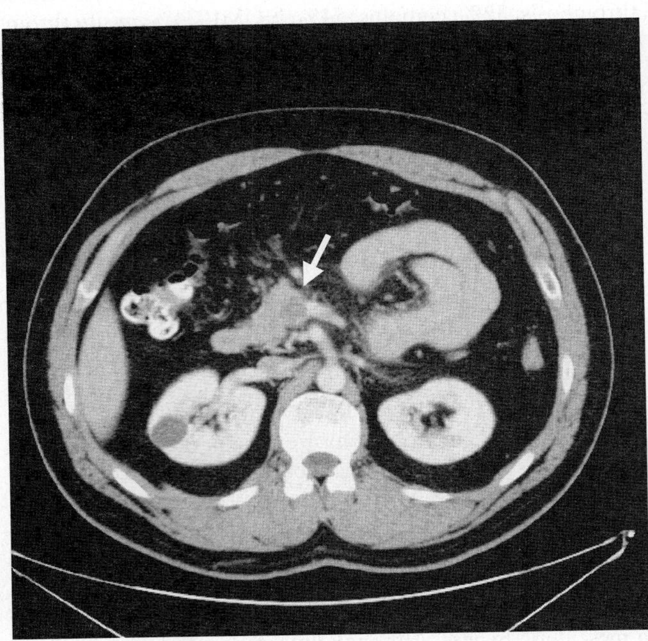

FIGURE 159.6. A CT scan of a patient with mesenteric venous thrombosis is shown. Note the thrombus in the superior mesenteric vein at its confluence with the splenic vein as shown with the *arrow*.

should be maintained on long-term oral anticoagulation. Similar to patients with massive iliofemoral deep venous thrombosis, it may be difficult to achieve effective anticoagulation initially using the standard dosing schedules for heparin (i.e., 80 units/kg bolus, 18 units/kg per hour drip), presumably secondary to the clot burden. Larger doses of heparin may be required, and the adequacy of heparinization (e.g., partial thromboplastin time) may need to be monitored more frequently. Although the required dosage of heparin may be unsettling, the potential clot propagation and its associated complications likely exceed any increased risk from bleeding. A hypercoagulable workup for the standard hematologic abnormalities should be performed prior to initiation of anticoagulation. However, long-term anticoagulation should be continued even in the absence of an *identifiable* hypercoagulable state since it is likely that many of these patients have some type of hypercoagulable disorder even though it may not be characterized on initial screening. Additionally, patients frequently require fluid resuscitation at the time of diagnosis due to the significant third-space losses from the bowel edema.

Exploratory laparotomy should be reserved for cases in which bowel infarction is suspected. The intraoperative findings include edematous/rubbery bowel, bloody ascites, and thrombus within the mesentery. A wide resection of the bowel should be performed in the presence of infarction. Primary enteric anastomosis is probably safe if the margins of resection are free of thrombus within the mesentery. Proximal and distal stomas are advisable if the viability of the bowel at the margins of resection is questionable. Patients are at risk for additional or ongoing thrombosis with the most common site being the margins of the resection and/or the anastomosis. Mechanical thrombectomy is not advocated at the time of laparotomy because of the extensive clot burden.

Endovascular treatment including chemical lysis likely has a limited role for patients with mesenteric venous thrombosis despite several case reports (89–91). Similar to the concerns with mechanical thrombectomy, the clot burden is very significant and usually extends from the small peripheral collaterals in the mesentery to the portal and mesenteric veins.

Outcome

As noted above, the mortality rate (approximately 30%) for mesenteric venous thrombosis is significantly less than for the arterial causes of AMI (68). Death has been associated with portal vein thrombosis, systemic venous thromboembolism, and obesity. The increased mortality rate associated with venous thromboembolism underscores the importance of early, adequate anticoagulation.

Aortic Dissection

Patients with acute aortic dissection can present with visceral malperfusion and AMI. The management of acute aortic dissections is beyond the scope of this chapter, but the topic is included to emphasize the importance of evaluating the status of the visceral vessels in all patients presenting with acute dissections. The presence of visceral malperfusion significantly increases the mortality rate (92,93). Various endovascular approaches have been used to treat the visceral malperfusion in this setting (94,95). Endovascular revascularization is probably superior to the open approach provided the patients are candidates from an anatomic and technical standpoint.

Protocols and Algorithms

See Fig. 159.7.

PEARLS

- The impaired intestinal perfusion associated with AMI leads to mucosal compromise that can lead to the activation of the systemic inflammatory and bowel infarction with perforation.
- The immediate clinical concerns for patients with AMI are to reverse the underlying clinical condition and prevent bowel infarction.
- The cause of AMI (i.e., embolus, *in situ* thrombosis, NOMI, mesenteric venous thrombosis, dissection) can usually be determined from the history and clinical setting.
- The emboli responsible for AMI usually lodge in the superior mesenteric artery and originate from the heart as a result of atrial fibrillation, an acute myocardial infarction, or a ventricular aneurysm.
- In patients with *in situ* thrombosis, the presentation of AMI is superimposed on the symptoms of CMI in more than 50% of the patients.
- NOMI represents an abnormal or paradoxical mesenteric vasoconstriction characterized by the loss of autoregulation.
- Mesenteric venous thrombosis is associated with a high incidence of hypercoagulable states and merits long-term anticoagulation even in the absence of an identifiable condition.
- CT arteriography with 1- to 2-mm cuts has emerged as the diagnostic study of choice for patients with AMI.
- Patients with AMI from an embolus or *in situ* thrombosis require emergent operative treatment.
- Operative treatment for patients with NOMI and mesenteric venous thrombosis is reserved for cases in which bowel infarction is suspected.

COLON ISCHEMIA

Isolated colon ischemia can occur after both open and endovascular aneurysm repair. Furthermore, it can develop as a complication of hemodynamic shock, similar to NOMI. Ischemic colitis has been reported to occur in approximately 2% to 13% of open aneurysm repairs (96). The reported incidence depends on the diagnostic algorithm and modality (routine sigmoidoscopy vs. selective sigmoidoscopy) and is dramatically increased after ruptured aneurysm repair. Indeed, the incidence of colonic ischemia after ruptured aneurysm repair in patients undergoing routine colonoscopy is approximately 25 to 40% (96,97). The sigmoid colon is affected most frequently, although all the sections of the colon may be involved. The ischemia may result from inadequate resuscitation, disruption of collaterals, and/or failure to revascularize a hemodynamically significant inferior mesenteric artery. Interestingly, routine reimplantation of the inferior mesenteric artery at the time of aortic reconstruction does not prevent colon ischemia (98). The ischemic colitis associated with endovascular aneurysm repair is more commonly

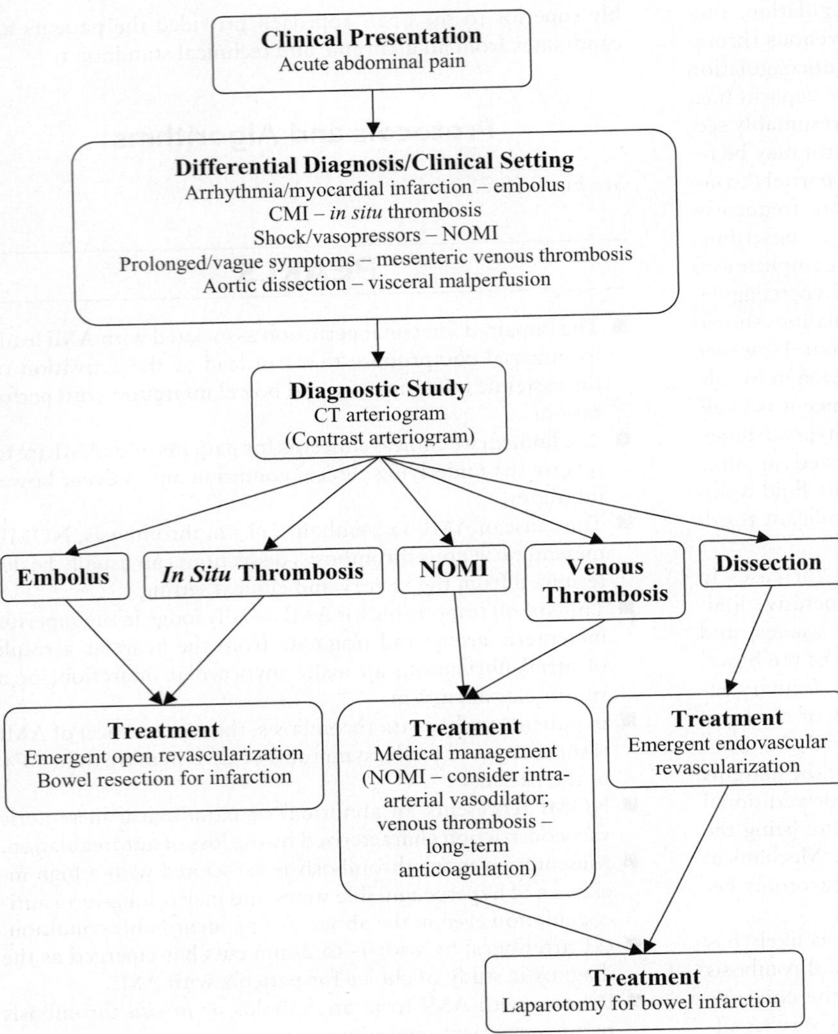

FIGURE 159.7. A flow diagram for the evaluation of patients with acute mesenteric ischemia (AMI) is shown. Although patients frequently present with abdominal pain, their sensorium may be altered. The diagnosis should be considered in the critical care setting when patients decompensate acutely. The differential diagnosis should be framed within the appropriate clinical setting. A computed tomography (CT) arteriogram is the diagnostic test of choice although a contrast arteriogram can be used. The CT findings are fairly characteristic for each of the diagnoses. Emergent, open revascularization is required in the setting of an embolus and *in situ* thrombosis; the bowel should be resected as necessary for ischemia/infarction. Preoperative evaluation should include broad-spectrum antibiotics, anticoagulation, and resuscitation. Medical management alone is usually adequate for patients with nonocclusive mesenteric ischemia (NOMI) and mesenteric venous thrombosis. Intra-arterial vasodilation may be required for persistent vasoconstriction in patients with NOMI. Lifetime anticoagulation is required for mesenteric venous thrombosis. Emergent endovascular revascularization is required for patients with acute aortic dissections and visceral malperfusion. Exploratory laparotomy and bowel resection should be reserved in patients with NOMI, mesenteric venous thrombosis, and aortic dissections for presumed bowel infarction. CMI, chronic mesenteric ischemia.

related to atheroembolism than acute internal iliac artery occlusion as might be suspected. The prognosis for ischemic colitis after endovascular aneurysm repair is worse than that for open repair (99).

Patients with ischemic colitis usually present with bloody diarrhea in contrast to patients with AMI who usually present with abdominal pain. In the most common scenario, patients develop bloody diarrhea on the first or second postoperative day after aortic reconstruction. However, the diagnosis should be considered after aortic reconstruction in the absence of bloody diarrhea in patients with thrombocytopenia, multiple-organ dysfunction, increasing abdominal pain/peritonitis, and generalized failure to thrive. The diagnosis may be confirmed by endoscopy. Although sigmoidoscopy is used most frequently, a complete colonoscopy is likely optimal due to the potential involvement of the other colon segments.

Treatment depends on the endoscopic findings and clinical setting. The endoscopic findings range from mucosal ischemia to transmural necrosis. Unfortunately, it is often difficult to differentiate diffuse mucosal ischemia from transmural necrosis. Patients with mucosal ischemia alone should be treated with bowel rest, broad-spectrum antibiotics, total parenteral nutrition, and serial endoscopic examinations. Many of these lesions resolve spontaneously without long-term sequelae although colonic strictures may develop in a small subset of patients. Patients with transmural colonic necrosis should undergo laparotomy with resection of the involved segment, a proximal diverting colostomy, and a distal Hartmann pouch.

The reported mortality rate in patients with transmural colon necrosis after aortic reconstruction is approximately 85% (96). Maintaining antegrade flow through the internal iliac vessels, routinely implanting the inferior mesenteric artery, and preserving the colonic collateral circulation may reduce or prevent this adverse outcome.

References

1. Fara JW. Postprandial mesenteric hyperemia. In: Shepard AP, Granger DN, eds. *Physiology of the Intestinal Circulation*. New York, NY: Raven Press; 1984:99.
2. Moneta GL, Taylor DC, Helton WS, et al. Duplex ultrasound measurement of postprandial intestinal blood flow: effect of meal composition. *Gastroenterology.* 1988;95(5):1294–1301.
3. Carrick RP, Borge MA, Labropolous N, et al. Chronic mesenteric ischemia resulting from isolated lesions of the superior mesenteric artery—a case report. *Angiology.* 2005;56(6):785–788.
4. Valentine RJ, Martin JD, Myers SI, et al. Asymptomatic celiac and superior

mesenteric artery stenoses are more prevalent among patients with unsuspected renal artery stenoses. *J Vasc Surg.* 1991;14(2):195–199.
5. Croft RJ, Menon GP, Marston A. Does 'intestinal angina' exist? A critical study of obstructed visceral arteries. *Br J Surg.* 1981;68(5):316–318.
6. Derrow AE, Seeger JM, Dame DA, et al. The outcome in the United States after thoracoabdominal aortic aneurysm repair, renal artery bypass, and mesenteric revascularization. *J Vasc Surg.* 2001;34(1):54–61.
7. Jimenez JG, Huber TS, Ozaki CK, et al. Durability of antegrade synthetic aortomesenteric bypass for chronic mesenteric ischemia. *J Vasc Surg.* 2002;35(6):1078–1084.
8. Johnston KW, Lindsay TF, Walker PM, et al. Mesenteric arterial bypass grafts: early and late results and suggested surgical approach for chronic and acute mesenteric ischemia. *Surgery.* 1995;118(1):1–7.
9. Matsumoto AH, Angle JF, Spinosa DJ, et al. Percutaneous transluminal angioplasty and stenting in the treatment of chronic mesenteric ischemia: results and longterm followup. *J Am Coll Surg.* 2002;194(1 Suppl):S22–S31.
10. Mateo RB, O'Hara PJ, Hertzer NR, et al. Elective surgical treatment of symptomatic chronic mesenteric occlusive disease: early results and late outcomes. *J Vasc Surg.* 1999;29(5):821–31.
11. Van Damme H, Jacquet N, Belaiche J, et al. Chronic ischaemic gastritis: an unusual form of splanchnic vascular insufficiency. *J Cardiovasc Surg (Torino).* 1992;33(4):451–453.
12. Moneta GL, Lee RW, Yeager RA, et al. Mesenteric duplex scanning: a blinded prospective study. *J Vasc Surg.* 1993;17(1):79–84.
13. Zwolak RM, Fillinger MF, Walsh DB, et al. Mesenteric and celiac duplex scanning: a validation study. *J Vasc Surg.* 1998;27(6):1078–1087.
14. Boley SJ, Brandt LJ, Veith FJ, et al. A new provocative test for chronic mesenteric ischemia. *Am J Gastroenterol.* 1991;86(7):888–891.
15. Gentile AT, Moneta GL, Lee RW, et al. Usefulness of fasting and postprandial duplex ultrasound examinations for predicting high-grade superior mesenteric artery stenosis. *Am J Surg.* 1995;169(5):476–479.
16. Cademartiri F, Raaijmakers RH, Kuiper JW, et al. Multi-detector row CT angiography in patients with abdominal angina. *Radiographics.* 2004; 24(4):969–984.
17. Wildermuth S, Leschka S, Alkadhi H, et al. Multislice CT in the pre- and postinterventional evaluation of mesenteric perfusion. *Eur Radiol.* 2005; 15(6):1203–1210.
18. Zandrino F, Musante F, Gallesio I, et al. Assessment of patients with acute mesenteric ischemia: multislice computed tomography signs and clinical performance in a group of patients with surgical correlation. *Minerva Gastroenterol Dietol.* 2006;52(3):317–325.
19. Hagspiel KD, Leung DA, Angle JF, et al. MR angiography of the mesenteric vasculature. *Radiol Clin North Am.* 2002;40(4):867–886.
20. Laissy JP, Trillaud H, Douek P. MR angiography: noninvasive vascular imaging of the abdomen. *Abdom Imaging.* 2002;27(5):488–506.
21. Brown DJ, Schermerhorn ML, Powell RJ, et al. Mesenteric stenting for chronic mesenteric ischemia. *J Vasc Surg.* 2005;42(2):268–274.
22. Landis MS, Rajan DK, Simons ME, et al. Percutaneous management of chronic mesenteric ischemia: outcomes after intervention. *J Vasc Interv Radiol.* 2005;16(10):1319–1325.
23. Resch T, Lindh M, Dias N, et al. Endovascular recanalisation in occlusive mesenteric ischemia—feasibility and early results. *Eur J Vasc Endovasc Surg.* 2005;29(2):199–203.
24. Schaefer PJ, Schaefer FK, Mueller-Huelsbeck S, et al. Chronic mesenteric ischemia: stenting of mesenteric arteries. *Abdom Imaging.* 2007;32(3):304–309. Epub 2006 Sep 6.
25. Schaefer PJ, Schaefer FK, Hinrichsen H, et al. Stent placement with the monorail technique for treatment of mesenteric artery stenosis. *J Vasc Interv Radiol.* 2006;17(4):637–643.
26. Silva JA, White CJ, Collins TJ, et al. Endovascular therapy for chronic mesenteric ischemia. *J Am Coll Cardiol.* 2006;47(5):944–950.
27. Sivamurthy N, Rhodes JM, Lee D, et al. Endovascular versus open mesenteric revascularization: immediate benefits do not equate with short-term functional outcomes. *J Am Coll Surg.* 2006;202(6):859–867.
28. Eagle KA, Berger PB, Calkins H, et al. ACC/AHA guideline update for perioperative cardiovascular evaluation for noncardiac surgery—executive summary a report of the American College of Cardiology/American Heart Association Task Force on Practice Guidelines (Committee to Update the 1996 Guidelines on Perioperative Cardiovascular Evaluation for Noncardiac Surgery). *Circulation.* 2002;105(10):1257–1267.
29. McFalls EO, Ward HB, Moritz TE, et al. Coronary-artery revascularization before elective major vascular surgery. *N Engl J Med.* 2004;351(27):2795–2804.
30. Poldermans D, Bax JJ, Schouten O, et al. Should major vascular surgery be delayed because of preoperative cardiac testing in intermediate-risk patients receiving beta-blocker therapy with tight heart rate control? *J Am Coll Cardiol.* 2006;48(5):964–969.
31. Smith SC Jr, Blair SN, Bonow RO, et al. AHA/ACC Guidelines for Preventing Heart Attack and Death in Patients with Atherosclerotic Cardiovascular Disease: 2001 update. A statement for healthcare professionals from the American Heart Association and the American College of Cardiology. *J Am Coll Cardiol.* 2001 Nov 1;38(5):1581–1583.
32. Harward TR, Brooks DL, Flynn TC, et al. Multiple organ dysfunction after mesenteric artery revascularization. *J Vasc Surg.* 1993;18(3):459–467.
33. Kagan SA, Myers SI. Acute embolic and thrombotic mesenteric ischemia. In: Ernst CB, Stanley JC, eds. *Current Therapy in Vascular Surgery.* 4th ed. St. Louis, MO: Mosby; 2001:675.
34. McMillan WD, McCarthy WJ, Bresticker MR, et al. Mesenteric artery bypass: objective patency determination. *J Vasc Surg.* 1995;21(5):729–740.
35. Kihara TK, Blebea J, Anderson KM, et al. Risk factors and outcomes following revascularization for chronic mesenteric ischemia. *Ann Vasc Surg.* 1999;13(1):37–44.
36. Cho JS, Carr JA, Jacobsen G, et al. Long-term outcome after mesenteric artery reconstruction: a 37-year experience. *J Vasc Surg.* 2002;35(3):453–460.
37. Foley MI, Moneta GL, Abou-Zamzam AM Jr, et al. Revascularization of the superior mesenteric artery alone for treatment of intestinal ischemia. *J Vasc Surg.* 2000;32(1):37–47.
38. Moawad J, McKinsey JF, Wyble CW, et al. Current results of surgical therapy for chronic mesenteric ischemia. *Arch Surg.* 1997;132(6):613–618.
39. Park WM, Cherry KJ Jr, Chua HK, et al. Current results of open revascularization for chronic mesenteric ischemia: a standard for comparison. *J Vasc Surg.* 2002;35(5):853–859.
40. Allen RC, Martin GH, Rees CR, et al. Mesenteric angioplasty in the treatment of chronic intestinal ischemia. *J Vasc Surg.* 1996;24(3):415–421.
41. Cognet F, Ben Salem D, Dranssart M, et al. Chronic mesenteric ischemia: imaging and percutaneous treatment. *Radiographics.* 2002;22(4):863–879.
42. Hallisey MJ, Deschaine J, Illescas FF, et al. Angioplasty for the treatment of visceral ischemia. *J Vasc Interv Radiol.* 1995;6(5):785–791.
43. Kasirajan K, O'Hara PJ, Gray BH, et al. Chronic mesenteric ischemia: open surgery versus percutaneous angioplasty and stenting. *J Vasc Surg.* 2001; 33(1):63–71.
44. Maspes F, Mazzetti dP, Gandini R, et al. Percutaneous transluminal angioplasty in the treatment of chronic mesenteric ischemia: results and 3 years of follow-up in 23 patients. *Abdom Imaging.* 1998;23(4):358–363.
45. Nyman U, Ivancev K, Lindh M, et al. Endovascular treatment of chronic mesenteric ischemia: report of five cases. *Cardiovasc Intervent Radiol.* 1998;21(4):305–313.
46. Pietura R, Szymanska A, El Furah M, et al. Chronic mesenteric ischemia: diagnosis and treatment with balloon angioplasty and stenting. *Med Sci Monit.* 2002;8(1):R8–R12.
47. Sharafuddin MJ, Olson CH, Sun S, et al. Endovascular treatment of celiac and mesenteric arteries stenoses: applications and results. *J Vasc Surg.* 2003; 38(4):692–698.
48. Sheeran SR, Murphy TP, Khwaja A, et al. Stent placement for treatment of mesenteric artery stenoses or occlusions. *J Vasc Interv Radiol.* 1999; 10(7):861–867.
49. Steinmetz E, Tatou E, Favier-Blavoux C, et al. Endovascular treatment as first choice in chronic intestinal ischemia. *Ann Vasc Surg.* 2002;16(6):693–699.
50. Lock G. Acute mesenteric ischemia: classification, evaluation and therapy. *Acta Gastroenterol Belg.* 2002;65(4):220–225.
51. Safioleas MC, Moulakakis KG, Papavassiliou VG, et al. Acute mesenteric ischaemia, a highly lethal disease with a devastating outcome. *Vasa.* 2006;35(2):106–111.
52. Bassilios N, Menoyo V, Berger A, et al. Mesenteric ischaemia in haemodialysis patients: a case/control study. *Nephrol Dial Transplant.* 2003;18(5):911–917.
53. Bolcal C, Iyem H, Sargin M, et al. Gastrointestinal complications after cardiopulmonary bypass: sixteen years of experience. *Can J Gastroenterol.* 2005;19(10):613–617.
54. Edwards MS, Cherr GS, Craven TE, et al. Acute occlusive mesenteric ischemia: surgical management and outcomes. *Ann Vasc Surg.* 2003;17(1):72–79.
55. Ghosh S, Roberts N, Firmin RK, et al. Risk factors for intestinal ischaemia in cardiac surgical patients. *Eur J Cardiothorac Surg.* 2002;21(3):411–416.
56. Lee R, Tung HK, Tung PH, et al. CT in acute mesenteric ischaemia. *Clin Radiol.* 2003;58(4):279–287.
57. Paran H, Epstein T, Gutman M, et al. Mesenteric and portal vein gas: computerized tomography findings and clinical significance. *Dig Surg.* 2003;20(2):127–132.
58. Schindera ST, Triller J, Vock P, et al. Detection of hepatic portal venous gas: its clinical impact and outcome. *Emerg Radiol.* 2006;12(4):164–170.
59. Gagne DJ, Malay MB, Hogle NJ, et al. Bedside diagnostic minilaparoscopy in the intensive care patient. *Surgery.* 2002;131(5):491–496.
60. Jaramillo EJ, Trevino JM, Berghoff KR, et al. Bedside diagnostic laparoscopy in the intensive care unit: a 13-year experience. *JSLS.* 2006;10(2):155–149.
61. Sauerland S, Agresta F, Bergamaschi R, et al. Laparoscopy for abdominal emergencies: evidence-based guidelines of the European Association for Endoscopic Surgery. *Surg Endosc.* 2006;20(1):14–29.
62. Kaminsky O, Yampolski I, Aranovich D, et al. Does a second-look operation improve survival in patients with peritonitis due to acute mesenteric ischemia? A five-year retrospective experience. *World J Surg.* 2005;29(5):645–648.
63. Freeman AJ, Graham JC. Damage control surgery and angiography in cases of acute mesenteric ischaemia. *ANZ J Surg.* 2005;75(5):308–314.
64. Calin GA, Calin S, Ionescu R, et al. Successful local fibrinolytic treatment and balloon angioplasty in superior mesenteric arterial embolism: a case report and literature review. *Hepatogastroenterology.* 2003;50(51):732–734.

65. Lim RP, Dowling RJ, Mitchell PJ, et al. Endovascular treatment of arterial mesenteric ischaemia: a retrospective review. *Australas Radiol.* 2005; 49(6):467–475.
66. Milner R, Woo EY, Carpenter JP. Superior mesenteric artery angioplasty and stenting via a retrograde approach in a patient with bowel ischemia—a case report. *Vasc Endovascular Surg.* 2004;38(1):89–91.
67. Russo MJ, Chaer RA, Lin SC, et al. Percutaneous endovascular treatment of acute sequential systemic emboli. *J Vasc Surg.* 2006;43(2):388–392.
68. Schoots IG, Koffeman GI, Legemate DA, et al. Systematic review of survival after acute mesenteric ischaemia according to disease aetiology. *Br J Surg.* 2004;91(1):17–27.
69. Schoots IG, Levi MM, Reekers JA, et al. Thrombolytic therapy for acute superior mesenteric artery occlusion. *J Vasc Interv Radiol.* 2005;16(3):317–329.
70. Wakabayashi H, Shiode T, Kurose M, et al. Emergent treatment of acute embolic superior mesenteric ischemia with combination of thrombolysis and angioplasty: report of two cases. *Cardiovasc Intervent Radiol.* 2004;27(4):389–393.
71. Ritz JP, Germer CT, Buhr HJ. Prognostic factors for mesenteric infarction: multivariate analysis of 187 patients with regard to patient age. *Ann Vasc Surg.* 2005;19(3):328–334.
72. Moore EM, Endean EC. Treatment of acute intestinal ischemia caused by arterial occlusions. In: Rutherford RB, ed. *Vascular Surgery.* 6th ed. Philadelphia, PA: Elsevier Saunders; 2005:1718–1727.
73. Yasuhara H, Niwa H, Takenoue T, et al. Factors influencing mortality of acute intestinal infarction associated with SIRS. *Hepatogastroenterology.* 2005;52(65):1474–1478.
74. Costa-Merida MA, Marchena-Gomez J, Hemmersbach-Miller M, et al. Identification of risk factors for perioperative mortality in acute mesenteric ischemia. *World J Surg.* 2006;30(8):1579–1585.
75. Park WM, Gloviczki P, Cherry KJ Jr, et al. Contemporary management of acute mesenteric ischemia: factors associated with survival. *J Vasc Surg.* 2002;35(3):445–452.
76. Kaleya RN, Sammartano RJ, Boley SJ. Aggressive approach to acute mesenteric ischemia. *Surg Clin North Am.* 1992;72(1):157–182.
77. Wyers MC, Powell RJ, Nolan BW, et al. Retrograde mesenteric stenting during laparotomy for acute occlusive mesenteric ischemia. *J Vasc Surg.* 2007;45(2):269–275.
78. Ceppa EP, Fuh KC, Bulkley GB. Mesenteric hemodynamic response to circulatory shock. *Curr Opin Crit Care.* 2003;9(2):127–132.
79. Hirota M, Inoue K, Kimura Y, et al. Non-occlusive mesenteric ischemia and its associated intestinal gangrene in acute pancreatitis. *Pancreatology.* 2003;3(4):316–322.
80. Imanaka K, Kyo S, Ban S. Possible close relationship between non-occlusive mesenteric ischemia and cholesterol crystal embolism after cardiovascular surgery. *Eur J Cardiothorac Surg.* 2002;22(6):1032–1034.
81. Katz MG, Schachner A, Ezri T, et al. Nonocclusive mesenteric ischemia after off-pump coronary artery bypass surgery: a word of caution. *Am Surg.* 2006;72(3):228–231.
82. Ori Y, Chagnac A, Schwartz A, et al. Non-occlusive mesenteric ischemia in chronically dialyzed patients: a disease with multiple risk factors. *Nephron Clin Pract.* 2005;101(2):c87–c93.
83. Weil J, Sen GR, Herfarth H. Nonocclusive mesenteric ischemia induced by digitalis. *Int J Colorectal Dis.* 2004;19(3):277–280.
84. Klotz S, Vestring T, Rotker J, et al. Diagnosis and treatment of nonocclusive mesenteric ischemia after open heart surgery. *Ann Thorac Surg.* 2001;72(5):1583–1586.
85. Luckner G, Jochberger S, Mayr VD, et al. Vasopressin as adjunct vasopressor for vasodilatory shock due to non-occlusive mesenteric ischemia. *Anaesthesist.* 2006;55(3):283–286.
86. Harward TR, Green D, Bergan JJ, et al. Mesenteric venous thrombosis. *J Vasc Surg.* 1989;9(2):328–333.
87. Bradbury MS, Kavanagh PV, Chen MY, et al. Noninvasive assessment of portomesenteric venous thrombosis: current concepts and imaging strategies. *J Comput Assist Tomogr.* 2002;26(3):392–404.
88. Bradbury MS, Kavanagh PV, Bechtold RE, et al. Mesenteric venous thrombosis: diagnosis and noninvasive imaging. *Radiographics.* 2002;22(3):527–541.
89. Zhou W, Choi L, Lin PH, et al. Percutaneous transhepatic thrombectomy and pharmacologic thrombolysis of mesenteric venous thrombosis. *Vascular.* 2007;15(1):41–45.
90. Lopera JE, Correa G, Brazzini A, et al. Percutaneous transhepatic treatment of symptomatic mesenteric venous thrombosis. *J Vasc Surg.* 2002;36(5):1058–1061.
91. Stein M, Link DP. Symptomatic spleno-mesenteric-portal venous thrombosis: recanalization and reconstruction with endovascular stents. *J Vasc Interv Radiol.* 1999;10(3):363–371.
92. Sandridge L, Kern JA. Acute descending aortic dissections: management of visceral, spinal cord, and extremity malperfusion. *Semin Thorac Cardiovasc Surg.* 2005;17(3):256–261.
93. Yagdi T, Atay Y, Engin C, et al. Impact of organ malperfusion on mortality and morbidity in acute type a aortic dissections. *J Card Surg.* 2006;21(4):363–369.
94. Vedantham S, Picus D, Sanchez LA, et al. Percutaneous management of ischemic complications in patients with type-B aortic dissection. *J Vasc Interv Radiol.* 2003;14(2 Pt 1):181–194.
95. Leprince P, Cluzel P, Bonnet N, et al. An endovascular stent relieves celiac and mesenteric ischemia in acute aortic dissection. *Ann Thorac Surg.* 2004;78(1):e3–e5.
96. Tollefson DF, Ernst CB. Colon Ischemia following Aortic Reconstruction. Basic Data Underlying Clinical Decision Making. *Vascular Surgery.* St. Louis, MO: Quality Medical; 1994:111–115.
97. Champagne BJ, Darling RC III, Daneshmand M, et al. Outcome of aggressive surveillance colonoscopy in ruptured abdominal aortic aneurysm. *J Vasc Surg.* 2004;39(4):792–796.
98. Mitchell KM, Valentine RJ. Inferior mesenteric artery reimplantation does not guarantee colon viability in aortic surgery. *J Am Coll Surg.* 2002;194(2):151–155.
99. Geraghty PJ, Sanchez LA, Rubin BG, et al. Overt ischemic colitis after endovascular repair of aortoiliac aneurysms. *J Vasc Surg.* 2004;40(3):413–418.

CHAPTER 160 ■ ACUTE RENAL FAILURE

SEAN M. BAGSHAW • RINALDO BELLOMO

Acute renal failure (ARF) remains a major diagnostic and therapeutic challenge for the critical care physician. The term, *acute renal failure,* describes a syndrome characterized by a rapid—that is, hours to days—decrease in the kidney's ability to eliminate waste products. Such loss of function is clinically manifested by the accumulation of end products of nitrogen metabolism such as urea and creatinine. Other typical clinical manifestations include decreased urine output (although this is not always present), accumulation of nonvolatile acids, and an increased concentration of potassium and phosphate.

DEFINITION AND CLASSIFICATION OF ACUTE RENAL FAILURE

Depending on the criteria used to define its presence, ARF has been reported in 5% to 25% of critically ill patients (1–5). Recently, a consensus definition and classification for ARF has been developed and validated in hospitalized and critically ill patients (6–8). This definition, which goes by the acronym of *RIFLE*, divides renal dysfunction into the categories of risk, injury, and failure (Fig. 160.1) and is likely to be the dominant approach to defining ARF in the intensive care unit (ICU) for the next 5 to 10 years. Using this classification, the incidence of at least some degree of renal dysfunction has been reported as high as 67% in a recent study of more than 5,000 critically ill patients (8). The development of renal dysfunction with a maximum RIFLE category failure has been reported in up to 28% of critically ill patients and is associated with an increased risk of in-hospital death by severalfold (7,8).

ASSESSMENT OF RENAL FUNCTION

Renal function is complex, involving acid-base balance, water balance, tonicity control, regulation of calcium and phosphate, erythropoiesis, disposal of some cytokines, lactate removal, and so forth. In the clinical context, however, monitoring of renal function is reduced to the indirect assessment of glomerular filtration rate (GFR) by the measurement of serum creatinine and urea. These waste products are insensitive markers of GFR and are heavily modified by numerous factors such as age, gender, muscle mass, nutritional status, the use of steroids, the presence of gastrointestinal blood, or muscle injury. Furthermore, they generally start becoming abnormal only when GFR is reduced by more than 50%, they fail to reflect dynamic changes in GFR, and can be grossly modified by aggressive fluid resuscitation. The use of creatinine clearance via a 2- or 4-hour urine collection or of calculated clearance by means of formulae might increase the accuracy of GFR estimation but rarely changes clinical management. The use of more sophisticated radionuclide-based tests is cumbersome in the ICU and useful only for research purposes.

Urine output is another commonly measured parameter of renal function and is often more sensitive to changes in renal hemodynamics than biochemical markers of solute clearance. However, urine output alone is of limited value; patients are capable of developing severe ARF—as detected by a markedly elevated serum creatinine—while maintaining normal urine output—so-called *nonoliguric ARF.* Since nonoliguric ARF has a lower mortality rate than oliguric ARF, urine output is frequently used to differentiate ARF (9). Classically, oliguria has been defined approximately as urine output less than 5 mL/kg/day or 0.5 mL/kg/hour. The recent RIFLE classification has incorporated oliguria as an important measure for categories of severity of ARF (Fig. 160.1).

EPIDEMIOLOGY

A degree of acute renal injury—manifested by either albuminuria or loss of small tubular proteins; inability to excrete a water, sodium, or amino acid load; or any combination of the above—can be demonstrated in most ICU patients. The syndrome of ARF, however, occurs in 5% to 8% of all hospitalized patients (9,10). The incidence is even greater in ICU patients, occurring in 5% to 25%, depending on the operative definition and specific population being studied (1–5). Recent trends have suggested that the incidence and mortality of ARF may be increasing, in particular in critically ill patients despite advances in our understanding of the pathophysiology and treatment. This may be attributable to a major shift from single-organ ARF to the multiorgan dysfunction syndrome now typically seen in ICU patients (3).

Several risk factors for ARF in ICU patients have been identified (1,4) including

- Older age
- Male gender
- Pre-existing comorbid illness
- Diagnosis of sepsis
- Major surgery
- Specifically cardiac surgery
- Cardiogenic shock
- Hypovolemia
- Exposure to nephrotoxic drugs.

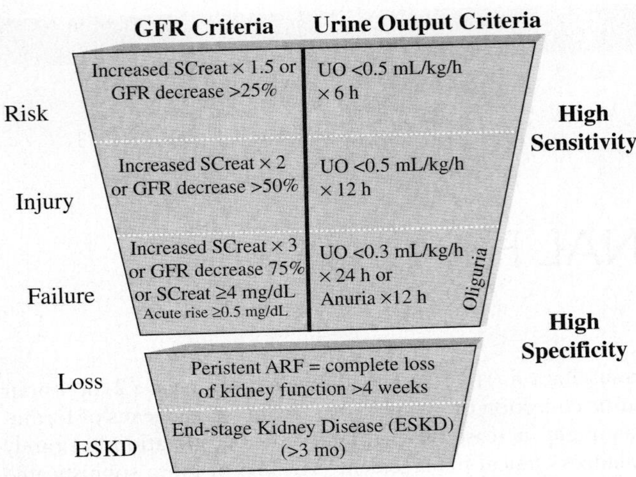

FIGURE 160.1. RIFLE (Risk, Injury, Failure, Loss, End-stage) classification scheme for acute renal failure. The classification system includes separate criteria for creatinine and urine output. The criteria that lead to the worst possible classification should be used. Note that RIFLE-F (F = failure) is present even if the increase in serum creatinine concentration (SCreat) is less than threefold so long as the new SCreat is greater than 4.0 mg/dL (350 μmol/L) in the setting of an acute increase of at least 0.5 mg/dL (44 μmol/L). The designation RIFLE-FC should be used in this case to denote acute-on-chronic disease. Similarly when RIFLE-F classification is reached by urine output criteria only, a designation of RIFLE-FO should be used to denote oliguria. The shape of the figure denotes the fact that more patients (high sensitivity) will be included in the mild category, including some without actually having renal failure (less specificity). In contrast, at the bottom, the criteria are strict and therefore specific, but some patients with renal dysfunction might be missed. GFR, glomerular filtration rate; ARF, acute renal failure; UO, urine output.

In addition, multiorgan dysfunction—specifically concomitant acute circulatory, pulmonary, and hepatic organ dysfunction—is commonly associated with ARF (2,11,12).

APPROACH TO CLINICAL CLASSIFICATION

The most practical and useful approach to the etiologic diagnosis of ARF is to divide its causes according to the probable source of renal injury: prerenal, renal (parenchymal), and postrenal.

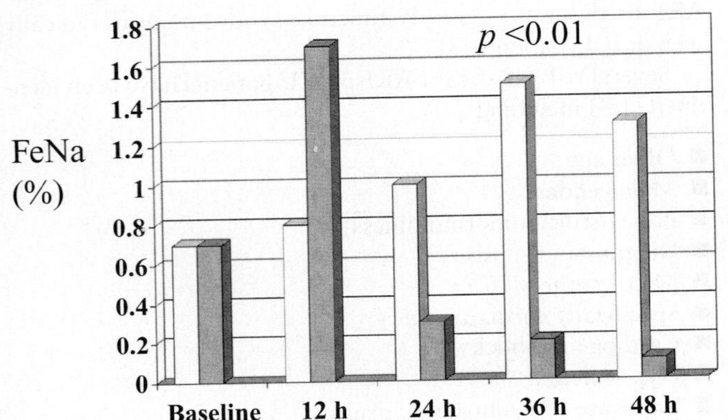

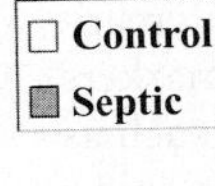

FIGURE 160.2. Histogram showing the effect of experimental sepsis in sheep on the fractional excretion of sodium (FeNa). FeNa decreased in sepsis as would be expected during decreased perfusion. In fact, all experimental animals had a twofold to threefold increase in renal blood flow, providing proof of the concept that FeNa cannot be used to infer renal hypoperfusion.

Prerenal Renal Failure

This form of ARF is by far the most common in the ICU. The term indicates that the kidney malfunctions predominantly because of systemic factors that decrease GFR. For example, GFR may be decreased if renal blood flow (RBF) is diminished by decreased cardiac output, hypotension, or raised intra-abdominal pressure. Such elevated intra-abdominal pressure is suspected on clinical grounds and confirmed by measuring bladder pressure with a urinary catheter. A pressure of greater than 25 to 30 mm Hg above the pubis should prompt consideration of decompression. If the systemic cause of renal failure is rapidly removed or corrected, renal function improves and relatively rapidly returns to near normal levels. However, if intervention is delayed or unsuccessful, renal injury becomes established, and several days or weeks are then necessary for recovery. Several tests—measurement of urinary sodium, fractional excretion of sodium, and other derived indices—have been promoted to help clinicians identify the development of such established ARF. Unfortunately, their accuracy and significance are questionable (13,14) (Fig. 160.2). The clinical value of these tests in ICU patients who receive vasopressors, massive fluid resuscitation, and loop diuretics is low. Furthermore, it is important to bear in mind that prerenal ARF and established ARF are part of a continuum and that their separation has limited clinical implications. The principles of management are essentially the same: treatment of the cause while promptly resuscitating the patient by using invasive hemodynamic monitoring to guide therapy.

Parenchymal Renal Failure

Parenchymal renal failure is a term used to define a syndrome where the principal source of damage is within the kidney and where typical structural changes can be seen on microscopy. Numerous disorders that affect the glomerulus or the tubule may be responsible (Table 160.1). Among these, nephrotoxins are particularly important, especially in hospitalized patients (10). The most common nephrotoxic drugs affecting ICU patients are listed in Table 160.2. Many cases of drug-induced ARF rapidly improve on removal of the offending agent. Accordingly, a careful history of drug administration is mandatory in all patients with ARF.

More than a third of patients who develop ARF in ICU have chronic renal dysfunction due to factors such as age-related

TABLE 160.1

CAUSES OF PARENCHYMAL ARF

Glomerulonephritis
Vasculitis
Renovascular
Interstitial nephritis
Nephrotoxins
Tubular deposition/obstruction
Renal allograft rejection
Trauma

changes, long-standing hypertension, diabetes mellitus, or atheromatous disease of the renal vessels. Such chronic renal disease may be manifest by an elevated serum creatinine. However, this is not always the case. Often, what may seem to the clinician to be a relatively trivial insult that does not fully explain the onset of ARF in a normal patient is sufficient to unmask a lack of renal functional reserve in a patient with chronic renal disease.

Post-renal Failure

Obstruction to urine outflow is the most common cause of functional renal impairment in the community (15) but is uncommon in the ICU. The pathogenesis of obstructive ARF involves several humoral responses as well as mechanical factors. Typical causes of obstructive ARF include bladder neck obstruction from an enlarged prostate, ureteric obstruction from pelvic tumors or retroperitoneal fibrosis, papillary necrosis, or large calculi. The clinical presentation of obstruction may be acute or acute on chronic in patients with long-standing renal calculi. It may not always be associated with oliguria. If obstruction is suspected, ultrasonography can be easily performed at the bedside. However, not all cases of acute obstruction have an abnormal ultrasound, and in many cases, obstruction occurs in conjunction with other renal insults such as staghorn calculi and severe sepsis of renal origin. Assessment of the role of each factor and overall management should be conducted in conjunction with a urologist. Finally, the sudden and unexpected development of anuria in an ICU patient should always suggest obstruction of the urinary catheter as the cause. Appropriate flushing or changing of the catheter should be implemented in this setting.

TABLE 160.2

DRUGS THAT MAY CAUSE ACUTE RENAL FAILURE IN THE INTENSIVE CARE UNIT

Radiocontrast media
Aminoglycosides
Amphotericin
Nonsteroidal anti-inflammatory drugs
β-Lactam antibiotics (interstitial nephropathy)
Sulphonamides
Acyclovir
Methotrexate
Cisplatin
Cyclosporin A
FK-506 (tacrolimus)
Sirolimus

PATHOGENESIS OF SPECIFIC SYNDROMES

Hepatorenal Syndrome

Hepatorenal syndrome is a form of ARF that typically occurs in the setting of advanced cirrhosis; however, it can occur with severe liver dysfunction due to alcoholic hepatitis or other forms of acute hepatic failure (16).

The pathogenesis of hepatorenal syndrome (HRS) is incompletely understood; however, several potential mechanisms may contribute to HRS, including: (a) activation of the renin-angiotensin system in response to systemic hypotension; (b) activation of the sympathetic nervous system in response to systemic hypotension and increased intrahepatic sinusoidal pressure; (c) increased release of arginine vasopressin due to systemic hypotension; and (d) reduced hepatic clearance of various vascular mediators such as endothelin, prostaglandins, and endotoxin (16,17).

Although HRS can occur spontaneously in patients with advanced cirrhosis, it is important to recognize that other precipitants are much more common. These include sepsis—specifically, spontaneous bacterial peritonitis (SBP)—raised intra-abdominal pressure due to tense ascites, gastrointestinal bleeding, and hypovolemia due to paracentesis, diuretics and/or lactulose administration, or any combination of these factors. Likewise, other contributing factors for ARF should be routinely ruled out, including cardiomyopathy due to alcoholism, nutritional deficiencies, viral infection, and exposure to nephrotoxins.

Typically, HRS develops in patients with advanced cirrhosis and evidence of portal hypertension with ascites in the absence of other apparent causes of ARF. It generally presents as oligo-anuria, with progressive increases in serum creatinine and/or urea, along with a bland urinary sediment. These patients develop profound sodium and water retention, with evidence of hyponatremia, a urine osmolality higher than that of plasma, and a very low urinary sodium concentration (less than 10 mmol/L).

Management of the patient with HRS can be challenging. However, it should include the systematic identification and prompt treatment of potential reversible precipitants. The attenuation of hypovolemia by albumin administration in patients with SBP has been shown to decrease the incidence of ARF in a randomized controlled trial (18). These causes must be investigated and promptly treated. Recent studies suggest that vasopressin derivatives (terlipressin) may improve GFR in this condition (19,20).

Placement of a transjugular intrahepatic, portosystemic stent-shunt (TIPS) has been associated with modest improvements in kidney function in those with HRS, as well as improvement in outcome, and represent a palliative measure for those who are not candidates for—or are awaiting—transplant (21,22). In general, the ideal solution for reversal of ARF in these patients is to improve hepatic function with therapy for the underlying primary liver disease and/or referral for successful liver transplantation.

ARF with Rhabdomyolysis

The incidence of rhabdomyolysis-induced ARF is estimated at 1% in hospitalized patients, but, in critically ill patients, may account for close to 5% to 7% of cases of ARF, depending on the setting (10,23). Its pathogenesis involves the interplay of prerenal, renal, and postrenal factors, including concurrent hypovolemia, ischemia, direct tubular toxicity mediated by the heme pigment in myoglobin, and intratubular obstruction (24). The causes of muscle injury that can result in rhabdomyolysis include major trauma; drug overdose such as occurs with narcotics, cocaine, or other stimulants; vascular embolism; prolonged seizures; malignant hyperthermia; neuroleptic malignant syndrome; various infections such as pyomyositis, necrotizing fasciitis, influenza, HIV; severe exertion; alcoholism; and a result of various agents that can interact to induce major muscle injury, such as the combination of macrolide antibiotics or cyclosporin and statins.

The clinical manifestations of rhabdomyolysis include an elevated serum creatine kinase, evidence of pigmented granular casts, and red-to-brown coloring of the urine. Patients can also have various electrolyte disorders as a result of muscle breakdown including hyperphosphatemia, hyperkalemia, hypocalcemia, and hyperuricemia.

The principles of prevention of ARF include (a) identification and elimination of potential causative agents and/or correction of underlying compartment syndromes; (b) prompt and aggressive fluid resuscitation and maintenance of polyuria—that is, greater than or equal to 1.5 to 2 mL/kg ideal or adjusted body weight/hour, usually more than about 300 mL/hour to restore vascular volume and potentially flush obstructing cellular casts; and (3) urine alkalinization to a goal of pH more than 6.5 to reduce renal toxicity by myoglobin-induced lipid peroxidation and improve the solubility of myoglobin (24). Experimental studies have suggested that mannitol may act as a scavenger of free radicals and reduce cellular toxicity; however, the role of forced diuresis with mannitol remains controversial.

ARF Due to Nephrotoxins

Several mechanisms have been reported to play a role in the development of renal injury after exposure to nephrotoxins. Particular drugs can often invoke various pathophysiologic effects on the kidney that, collectively, contribute to ARF. Alterations in intrarenal hemodynamics are an important initial consequence of many nephrotoxins. These changes to regional renal blood flow may occur through the increased activity of local vasoconstrictors such as angiotensin II, endothelin, adenosine; at the same time, there is diminished activity of important vasodilators such as nitric oxide and prostaglandins. This imbalance can lead to renal vasoconstriction and ischemia, particularly to susceptible regions such as the outer medulla, for example, in response to radiocontrast media, or can induce humorally mediated vasoconstriction of afferent arterioles, for example, as a result of exposure to NSAIDs and cyclosporine (25). The end result of a reduction in regional blood flow is a critical reduction in oxygen delivery, thus predisposing to tubular hypoxia (25). In addition, nephrotoxins can directly contribute to impaired tubular metabolism and oxygen usage. They lead to generation of oxygen-free radical species including superoxide anions, hydrogen peroxide, hydroxyl radicals, reduction in intrinsic antioxidant enzyme activity, accumulation of intracellular calcium, mitogen-activated protein kinases, and phospholipase A_2, for example, after exposure to aminoglycosides (26–28).

These responses to nephrotoxins can induce tubular cell vacuolization, interstitial inflammation, altered cell membrane properties, and disruption of normal tubular adhesion to basement membranes. Failure of these mechanisms contributes to tubular cell apoptosis and necrosis, as well as tubular sloughing into the luminal space, cast formation, and obstruction (26). Raised intraluminal pressures due to obstruction, altered cellular permeability, and interstitial inflammation can contribute to backup diffusion of fluid and secondary edema formation.

Radiocontrast media and aminoglycosides are leading agents contributing to nephrotoxin-induced ARF (29,30). Radiocontrast media–induced toxicity is believed to occur from the interplay of alterations in renal hemodynamics due to vasoconstriction, increased intravascular viscosity and erythrocyte aggregation, direct tubular epithelial cell toxicity, and concomitant atheroembolic microshowers in the renovasculature. Aminoglycosides are taken up *via* organic anion transport systems in the proximal tubules where they accumulate and generate oxygen-free radical species and increased intracellular calcium, which lead to tubular apoptosis, necrosis, and nonoliguric ARF.

Radiocontrast Nephropathy

Radiocontrast nephropathy is the leading cause of iatrogenic ARF in hospitalized patients, and results in prolonged hospitalization, higher mortality rates, excessive health care costs, and potentially long-term kidney impairment (10). Radiocontrast nephropathy presents with an acute rise in serum creatinine within 24 to 48 hours following injection of radiocontrast media. The serum creatinine level generally peaks within 3 to 5 days and returns towards baseline within 7 to 10 days; however, in some patients, kidney function may not return to baseline, and a persistent reduction in function may occur. Radiocontrast nephropathy is often associated with pre-existing risk factors, in particular, pre-existing chronic kidney disease—that is, a GFR less than 60 mL/minute/1.73 m^2—a diagnosis of diabetes mellitus, and use of large quantities of radiocontrast media.

There are few evidence-based prophylactic or therapeutic interventions shown to reduce the occurrence of radiocontrast nephropathy, and no therapy has proven effective once it is established (31). Strategies for prevention include early identification of patients at risk and consideration either to delay the investigation or to use an alternative modality until kidney function can be optimized. Likewise, every effort should be made to correct volume depletion and discontinue potential nephrotoxins. There is no evidence to support the routine use of diuretics, mannitol, or dopamine. Recent studies have shown that periprocedure hydration and use of nonionic iso-osmolar (for example, iodixanol) radiocontrast media can reduce the risk (32–35). Several randomized trials and meta-analyses have suggested a potential benefit with use of N-acetylcysteine (36,37). As these preventive measures

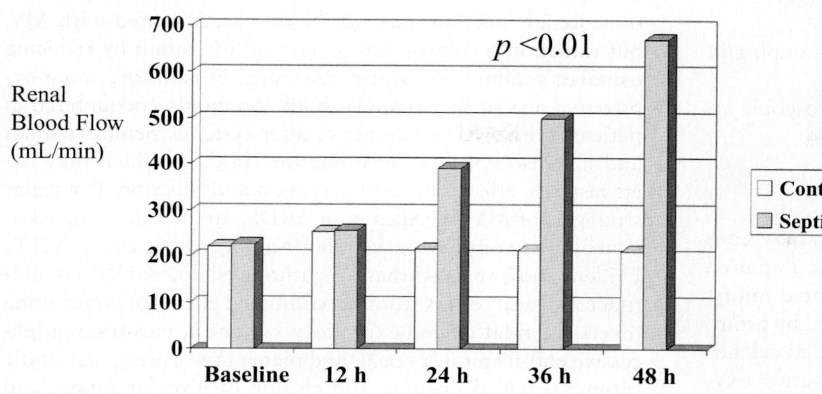

FIGURE 160.3. Histogram showing the effect on renal blood flow of experimental sepsis in sheep. Renal blood flow increased threefold while creatinine increased from 80–400 μmol/L, providing evidence that acute renal failure in sepsis can occur during renal hyperemia.

have minimal risk, their use should be considered whenever a patient is scheduled for the administration of intravenous radiocontrast media. Their effectiveness in already fluid-resuscitated ICU patients, however, remains unknown.

Septic ARF

Sepsis is a leading predisposing factor to ARF in critically ill patients (4). Epidemiologic studies estimate between 45% to 70% of all ARF encountered in the ICU is associated with sepsis (1,4,23). The distinction between septic and nonseptic ARF may have particular clinical relevance, considering recent evidence to suggest that septic ARF may be characterized by a unique pathophysiology (38–40).

The classic teaching is that sepsis brings about hypotension, leading to a reduction in critical organ blood flow, including to the kidney, causing ischemic injury and ARF. Furthermore, sepsis would lead to activation of the sympathetic nervous system, stimulating release of potent vasoconstrictors that induce renal vasoconstriction and aggravate kidney ischemia, thus worsening ARF. However, recent data raise serious questions about this ischemic-induced paradigm of septic ARF (38,39). A recent experimental study in a large mammalian model of hyperdynamic sepsis found that RBF was markedly increased above baseline despite significant reductions in kidney excretory function (40) (Fig. 160.3). These findings are supported by small clinical studies of resuscitated patients with septic ARF who also show increases in RBF (41–43). The implications are that in hyperdynamic sepsis, ARF is hyperemic rather than ischemic, with global RBF considerably increased. Moreover, experimental studies have shown that regional cortical and medullary RBF is preserved in sepsis and can be further augmented by infusion of norepinephrine (44) (Fig. 160.4). This concept of hyperemic ARF in sepsis is consistent with the relative paucity of renal histopathologic evidence of tubular necrosis in patients with septic ARF (45).

Thus, evolving evidence suggests that the pathogenesis of septic ARF predominantly involves toxic and immune-mediated mechanisms. Sepsis is known to release a vast array of proinflammatory and anti-inflammatory mediators such as cytokines, arachidonic acid metabolites, and thrombogenic agents, all of which may participate in the development of ARF (46). Similarly, experimental studies have found evidence of renal tubular cell apoptosis in response to inflammatory mediators in endotoxemia (47,48). Renal tubular apoptosis may prove to be an important mechanism of septic ARF in critically ill patients (45,49,50). No studies exist to tell us which of the above mechanisms are most important and when they might be active in the course of an episode of septic ARF. However, interventions with antiapoptotic properties such as intensive insulin therapy, human recombinant activated protein C, or selective caspase inhibitors may aid in attenuating renal injury and promote recovery of function (46). To date, however, no human randomized controlled trials have assessed the impact of these interventions on kidney function, and their value is unknown.

ARF in Association with Major Surgery

Acute renal failure is a common complication following major surgery (4). The incidence is variable and dependent on the prevalence of pre-existing comorbid illnesses, preoperative kidney function, and the type and urgency of surgery being performed. Numerous intraoperative events can act to negatively affect kidney function, including the following:

- Hemodynamic instability (e.g., intravenous or inhaled anaesthetic agents)

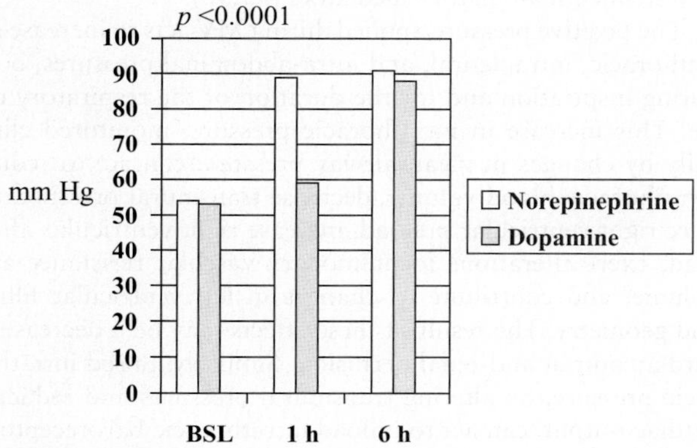

FIGURE 160.4. Histogram showing the effect of norepinephrine on mean arterial blood pressure (MAP) compared to high-dose dopamine in a randomized controlled trial in humans. MAP is more reliably restored using norepinephrine when given alone as an alternative to high-dose dopamine or after high-dose dopamine has failed. BSL, baseline.

- Hypovolemia due to blood loss or third spacing
- Details of the operative field (e.g., aortic cross-clamping in major vascular surgery)
- Increases in intra-abdominal pressure (e.g., laparoscopic insufflation of CO_2)
- Concomitant sepsis
- Use of nephrotoxin drugs

Any of these factors, alone or in combination, may contribute to a critical reduction in RBF and ischemia, impaired oxygen delivery, and toxin- or inflammatory-mediated injury. Postoperative ARF is believed to be, in part, mediated by proinflammatory mechanisms such as increased endothelial cell adhesion, tubular cell infiltration, generation of reactive oxygen species, proinflammatory cytokines, and reperfusion injury (51,52). Cardiac surgery with cardiopulmonary bypass (CPB) commonly induces early postoperative renal injury. The mechanisms whereby CPB causes injury are incompletely understood, although there is a suggestion that CPB is proinflammatory, activating components of the nonspecific immune system. In turn, this leads to oxidative stress with the generation of oxygen-free radical species and serum lipid peroxidation products (53). In addition, CPB has been shown to deplete serum antioxidative capacity for a prolonged duration after surgery. Such oxidant stress has been shown to directly induce renal injury in experimental studies (54).

ARF in Association with Mechanical Ventilation

Most critically ill patients require mechanical ventilation (MV), either for disease-specific indications such as acute respiratory distress syndrome (ARDS) or simply for routine postoperative care. The application of positive pressure MV, particularly with positive end-expiratory pressure (PEEP), can have important physiologic effects on kidney function. Experimental and clinical studies have clearly established an association between MV and PEEP and alterations in kidney function. This can occur through several mechanisms including (a) alterations in cardiovascular function, (b) alterations in neurohormonal activation, (c) abnormalities in gas exchange, and (d) alterations in systemic inflammatory mediators (55,56).

The positive pressure applied during MV acts to increase intrathoracic, intrapleural, and intra-abdominal pressures, both during inspiration and for the duration of the respiratory cycle. This increase in intrathoracic pressure, monitored clinically by changes in mean airway pressure, can act to reduce intrathoracic blood volume, decrease transmural pressure, reduce right ventricular preload, increase right ventricular afterload, exert alterations to pulmonary vascular resistance and volume, and contribute to changes in left ventricular filling and geometry. The result of these effects may be a decrease in cardiac output and renal perfusion. Similarly, raised intrathoracic pressure, by altering transmural pressures and reducing cardiac output, can act to unload intrathoracic baroreceptors. This initiates a cascade of compensatory neurohormonal events characterized by increased systemic and renal sympathetic nervous activity, increased activation of the renin–angiotensin–aldosterone system, increased secretion of vasopressin, and a reduction in release of atrial natriuretic peptide. These culminate in altered renal perfusion and kidney excretory function. Renal function may not be, *per se*, impaired with MV, but rather, may appropriately respond to stimuli by reducing osmolar, sodium, and water clearance. In addition, acute hypoxemia and/or hypercapnia, both commonly encountered in patients with ARDS, can act to alter systemic hemodynamics and increase systemic inflammation, both of which may exert negative effects on renal perfusion and function. Particular strategies of MV, specifically in ARDS, are now recognized to contribute to or provoke ventilator-induced lung injury (VILI). Evidence now suggests that the pathophysiology of VILI is multifactorial and results from the combined effects of volutrauma (excessive tidal or end-expiratory volumes), barotrauma (excessive end-inspiratory peak and plateau pressures), atelectatic trauma (cyclical opening and closing of alveolar units), and biotrauma (local release of inflammatory mediators from injured lung) (57). Such injurious MV can initiate a cascade of events that increase systemic inflammation and adversely affect kidney function (58).

THE CLINICAL PICTURE

The most common clinical picture seen in the ICU is that of a patient who has sustained or is experiencing a major systemic insult such as trauma, sepsis, myocardial infarction, severe hemorrhage, cardiogenic shock, or major surgery. When the patient arrives in the ICU, resuscitation is typically well underway, or surgery may have just been completed. Despite such efforts, the patient is already anuric or profoundly oliguric, and the serum creatinine is rising, and a metabolic acidosis is developing; serum potassium and phosphate levels may be rapidly rising as well. In these critically ill patients with ARF, multiple organ dysfunction—with the need for mechanical ventilation and vasoactive drugs—is common. Fluid resuscitation is typically undertaken in the ICU with the guidance of invasive hemodynamic monitoring. Vasoactive drugs are often used to restore mean arterial pressure (MAP) to acceptable levels, typically greater than 65 to 70 mm Hg (Fig. 160.4). The patient may improve over time, and urine output may return with or without the assistance of diuretic agents (Fig. 160.5). If urine output does not return, however, renal replacement therapy (RRT) needs to be considered. If the cause of ARF has been removed, and the patient has become physiologically stable, slow recovery occurs within 4 to 5 days to as long as 3 or 4 weeks. In some cases, urine output can be above normal for several days. If the cause of ARF has not been adequately remedied, the patient remains gravely ill, the kidneys do not recover, and death from multiorgan failure may occur.

PREVENTING ARF

The fundamental principle of ARF prevention is to treat its cause. If prerenal factors contribute, these must be identified and hemodynamic resuscitation quickly instituted.

Fluid Resuscitation

Intravascular volume must be maintained or rapidly restored; this is often best done using invasive hemodynamic monitoring, such as with an arterial cannula and central venous

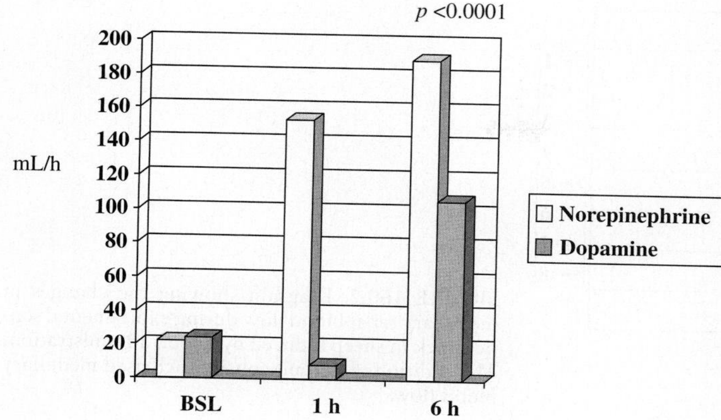

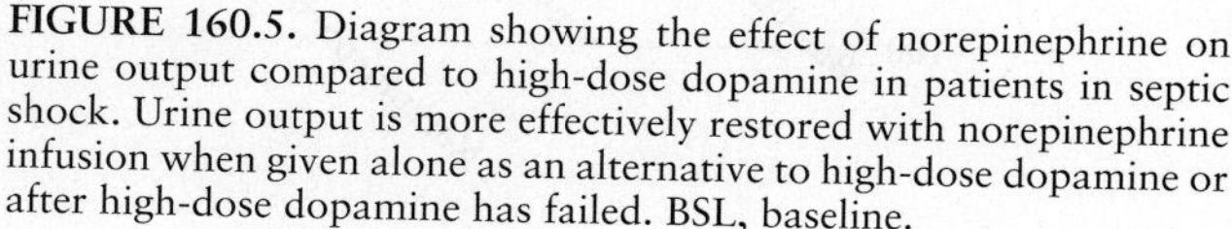
FIGURE 160.5. Diagram showing the effect of norepinephrine on urine output compared to high-dose dopamine in patients in septic shock. Urine output is more effectively restored with norepinephrine infusion when given alone as an alternative to high-dose dopamine or after high-dose dopamine has failed. BSL, baseline.

catheter, pulmonary artery catheter, or pulse contour cardiac output catheter. Oxygenation must be maintained. An adequate hemoglobin concentration, usually at least more than about 7.0 g/dL, must be maintained or immediately restored. Once intravascular volume has been restored, some patients remain with a MAP less than 70 mm Hg. In these patients, autoregulation of RBF may be lost, and restoration of MAP to near normal levels may increase GFR (59–61). Such elevations in MAP, however, require the addition of vasopressor drugs (59–61). In patients with pre-existing hypertension or renovascular disease, a MAP of 75 to 80 mm Hg may still be inadequate. Experimental evidence suggests that vasopressor support in hypotensive sepsis increases renal blood flow (Fig. 160.6) and renal medullary blood flow (Fig. 160.7). The renal protective role of additional fluid therapy in a patient with a normal or increased cardiac output and blood pressure is questionable. Despite these resuscitation measures, renal failure may still develop if cardiac output is inadequate. This may require various interventions, from the use of inotropic drugs to the application of ventricular assist devices.

Fluid Therapy

Fluid therapy is the cornerstone in resuscitation of the critically ill patient, and is the primary strategy for preservation of kidney function in the setting of increases in serum creatinine and/or urea, and oliguria. However, evolving evidence has suggested there may be negative consequences to overly aggressive fluid therapy for both renal and nonrenal organ function.

A large multicenter study found no significant difference in the incidence of ARF when comparing fluid resuscitation with crystalloid to albumin in critically ill patients (62). However, some synthetic colloid therapies, such as with the use of hydroxyethyl starches, have been associated with higher rates of ARF in critically ill patients after resuscitation for severe sepsis (63). Although the exact mechanism(s) remain uncertain, the hydroxyethyl starches may influence intrarenal hemodynamics or glomerular filtration through alterations in vascular oncotic pressure.

In critically ill patients, once apparent optimization of hemodynamics and intravascular volume status has been achieved, there is little evidence to support continued aggressive fluid resuscitation to improve kidney function (64). Rather, there is evidence from recent studies to suggest that such continued fluid administration and a positive cumulative balance can contribute to notable deteriorations in nonrenal organ function, in particular that of the lung (65,66). The ARDS Clinical Trials Network has completed the largest randomized trial assessing fluid therapy in patients with lung injury (67). This trial compared restrictive and liberal strategies for fluid management in 1,000 critically ill patients, mostly in those with pneumonia or sepsis with evidence of acute lung injury. At 72 hours, those receiving a restrictive fluid strategy had a near neutral fluid balance, whereas those in the liberal strategy were positive with more than 5 L. Although the study failed to show a difference in mortality between the strategies, a restrictive strategy improved lung function, increased ventilator-free days, and reduced ICU length of stay. Moreover, those in the restrictive group had a trend toward a reduced need for RRT.

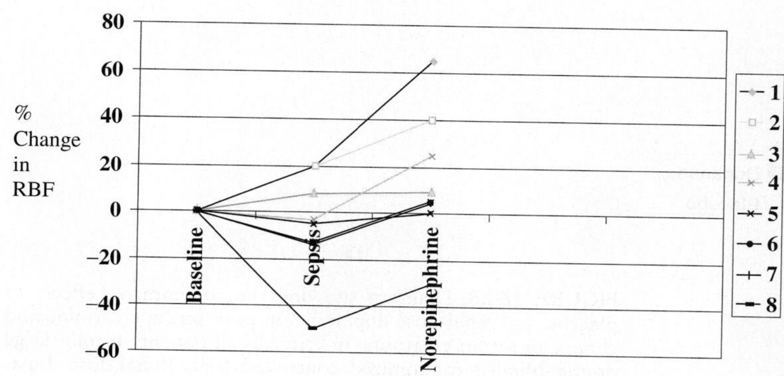

FIGURE 160.6. Diagram showing the changes in renal blood flow (RBF) during experimental *E. coli*–induced septic shock in sheep. The addition of norepinephrine increased renal blood flow.

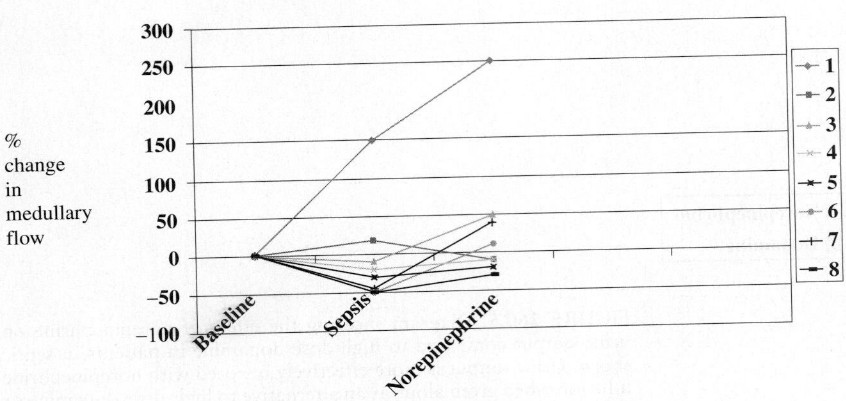

FIGURE 160.7. Diagram showing the changes in medullary renal blood flow during experimental septic shock in sheep induced by *E. coli* administration. The addition of norepinephrine increased medullary blood flow.

Renal Protective Drugs

Following hemodynamic resuscitation and removal of nephrotoxins, it is unclear whether the use of additional pharmacologic measures is of further benefit to the kidneys.

Renal Dose or Low-Dose Dopamine

Evidence of the efficacy or safety of the administration of dopamine in critically ill patients is lacking. However, this agent is a tubular diuretic and occasionally increases urine output. This may be incorrectly interpreted as an increase in GFR. Furthermore, a recent large phase III trial in critically ill patients showed low-dose dopamine to be as effective as placebo in the prevention of renal dysfunction (68) (Fig. 160.8).

Mannitol

A biologic rationale exists for the use of mannitol, as is the case for dopamine. However, no controlled human data exist to support its clinical use. The effect of mannitol as a renal protective agent remains questionable.

Loop Diuretics

These agents may protect the loop of Henle from ischemia by decreasing its transport-related workload. Animal data are encouraging, as are *ex vivo* experiments. There are no double-blind randomized controlled studies of suitable size to prove that these agents reduce the incidence of renal failure. However, some studies support the view that loop diuretics may decrease the need for RRT in patients developing ARF (69). They appear to achieve this by inducing polyuria, which allows for easier control of volume overload, acidosis, and hyperkalemia, the three major triggers for RRT in the ICU. Because avoiding dialysis simplifies treatment and reduces the cost of care, loop diuretics are occasionally used in patients with renal dysfunction, especially in the form of continuous infusion.

Other Agents

Other agents such as theophylline, urodilatin, and anaritide, a synthetic atrial natriuretic factor, have also been proposed. Studies so far, however, have been either experimental or underpowered, or have shown no beneficial effect. In a randomized double-blind, placebo-controlled trial, fenoldopam was shown to attenuate the deterioration in serum creatinine typically seen in septic patients (70). Studies of fenoldopam in other situations, however, have failed to show similar benefit (71). Thus, its role in ARF remains uncertain. Similarly, in a single-center study, recombinant human atrial natriuretic factor (rhANF) has been shown to attenuate renal injury in higher-risk patients undergoing cardiac surgery (72), but a large multicenter study of ARF failed to show a benefit (73). Many more investigations are urgently needed in this field.

DIAGNOSTIC INVESTIGATIONS

An etiologic diagnosis of ARF must always be established (Fig. 160.9). Although such diagnosis may be obvious on clinical grounds, in many patients it is best to consider all possibilities and exclude common treatable causes by simple investigations. One such investigation includes microscopic examination of the urinary sediment. Urinalysis is a simple and noninvasive test that yields important diagnostic information and patterns suggestive of specific syndromes. The finding of dysmorphic red

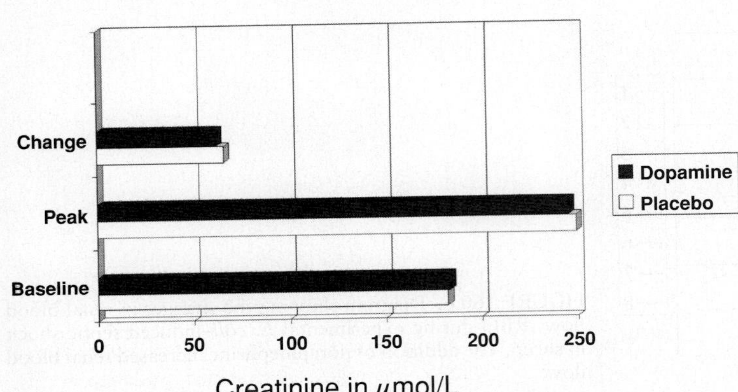

FIGURE 160.8. Diagram showing the comparative effects of placebo and renal-dose dopamine on peak serum creatinine and change in serum creatinine in critically ill patients from a large double-blinded randomized controlled trial. Renal-dose dopamine had no effect on serum creatinine.

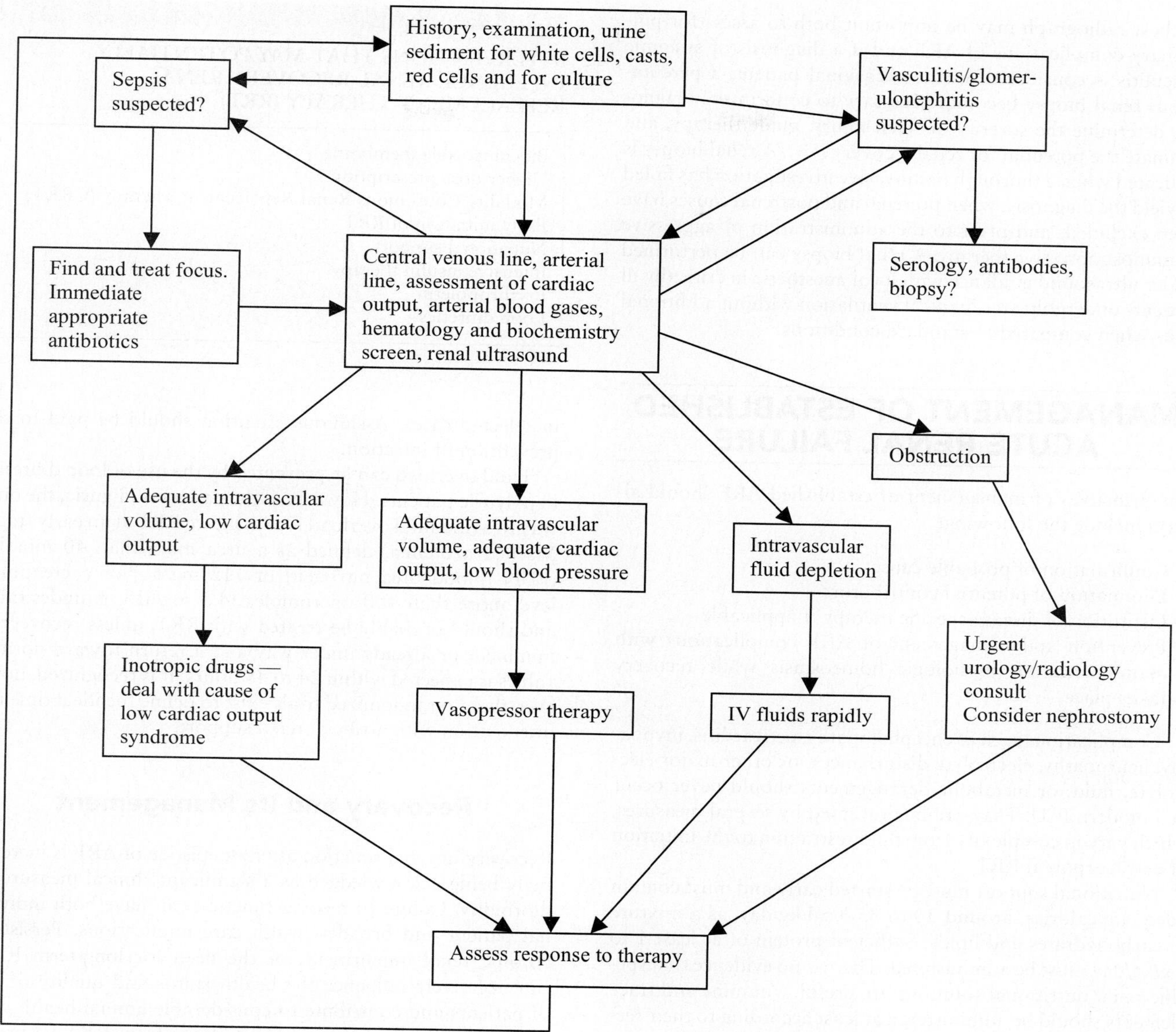

FIGURE 160.9. Diagnostic and treatment approach to an intensive care unit patient presenting with acute renal failure.

blood cells (RBC) or RBC casts is virtually diagnostic of active glomerulonephritis or vasculitis. Heavy proteinuria suggests some form of glomerular disease. White blood cell casts can suggest either interstitial nephropathy or infection. Similarly, a normal urinalysis can provide important information and can suggest that ARF is due to a prerenal or obstructive cause. Finally, examination of urine will provide evidence of whether a urinary tract infection is present.

Several additional investigations may be necessary to establish the diagnosis. Evidence of marked anemia in the absence of blood loss may suggest acute hemolysis, thrombotic microangiopathy, or paraproteinemia related to malignancy. In microangiopathic hemolytic anemia, a peripheral blood smear will typically show evidence of hemolysis with the presence of schistocytes; the additional measurement of lactic dehydrogenase, haptoglobin, unconjugated bilirubin, and free hemoglobin are needed. If paraproteinemia due to multiple myeloma or lymphoma is suspected, serum and urine protein electrophoresis and serum calcium should be measured. A history of recent cancer diagnosis or chemotherapy should prompt the measurement of uric acid for tumor lysis syndrome.

In patients with a possible mechanism for muscle injury, creatine kinase and free myoglobin for possible rhabdomyolysis should be determined. If an elevated anion gap metabolic acidosis is present with suggestion of a toxic ingestion, ethylene glycol, methanol, and salicylates should be measured.

Systemic eosinophilia may be a clue suggesting systemic vasculitis, allergic interstitial nephritis, or atheroembolic disease. The measurement of specific antibodies—antiglomerular basement membrane (GBM), antineutrophil cytoplasmic antibodies (ANCA), antinuclear antibodies (ANA), anti-DNA, antismooth muscle, and so forth—or cryoglobulins are extremely useful screening tests to support the diagnosis of vasculitis or certain types of collagen vascular diseases or glomerulonephritis.

Imaging by renal ultrasonography is a rapid noninvasive investigation principally designed to rule out evidence of obstruction, stones, cysts, masses, or overt renovascular disease.

A chest radiograph may be important both to assess for pulmonary complications of ARF and if a diagnosis of systemic vasculitis is considered. In the occasional patient, a percutaneous renal biopsy becomes necessary to confirm the diagnosis, determine the severity of renal injury, guide therapy, and estimate the potential for renal recovery (74). A renal biopsy is indicated when a thorough noninvasive investigation has failed to yield the diagnosis, when prerenal and postrenal causes have been excluded, and prior to the administration of aggressive immunosuppressive therapy. A renal biopsy can be performed under ultrasound guidance with local anesthetic in critically ill patients undergoing mechanical ventilation without additional risks when compared to standard conditions.

MANAGEMENT OF ESTABLISHED ACUTE RENAL FAILURE

The principles of management of established ARF should always include the following:

- Confirmation of probable cause
- Elimination of potential contributors
- Institution of disease-specific therapy if applicable
- Prevention and management of ARF complications with maintenance of physiologic homeostasis while recovery takes place

Complications such as encephalopathy, pericarditis, myopathy, neuropathy, electrolyte disturbances, or other major electrolyte, fluid, or metabolic derangements should never occur in a modern ICU. They can be prevented by several measures, which vary in complexity from fluid restriction to the initiation of extracorporeal RRT.

Nutritional support must be started early and must contain adequate calories, around 30 to 35 Kcal/kg/day, as a mixture of carbohydrates and lipids. Sufficient protein of at least 1 to 2 g/kg/day must be administered. There is no evidence that specific renal nutritional solutions are useful. Vitamins and trace elements should be administered at least according to their recommended daily allowance. The role of newer immunonutritional solution remains controversial. The enteral route is preferred to the use of parenteral nutrition.

Hyperkalemia—a serum potassium level of greater than 6 mmol/L—must be promptly treated either with insulin and dextrose administration, the infusion of bicarbonate if acidosis is present, the administration of nebulized salbutamol, or all of the above combined. If the "true" serum potassium is more than 7 mmol/L, or if electrocardiographic signs of hyperkalemia appear, calcium gluconate—10 mL of 10% solution administered IV—should also be used. The above measures are temporizing actions while RRT is being arranged. The presence of hyperkalemia is a major indication for the immediate institution of RRT.

Metabolic acidosis, almost always present, rarely requires treatment *per se*. Anemia requires correction to maintain a hemoglobin greater than about 7.0 g/dL; more aggressive transfusion may be needed based on individual patient assessment (75). Drug therapy must be adjusted to take into account the effect of the decreased clearances associated with loss of renal function. Stress ulcer prophylaxis is advisable and should be based on H_2-receptor antagonists or proton pump inhibitors in selected cases. Assiduous attention should be paid to the prevention of infection.

TABLE 160.3

INTERVENTIONS THAT MAY POTENTIALLY INFLUENCE RENAL RECOVERY RENAL REPLACEMENT THERAPY (RRT)

Biocompatible membrane
Higher-dose prescription
Modality Continuous Renal Replacement Therapy (CRRT)
Early initiation of RRT
Nutritional support
Intensive insulin therapy
Erythropoietin
Loop diuretics

Fluid overload can be prevented by the use of loop diuretics in polyuric patients. However, if the patient is oliguric, the only way to avoid fluid overload is to institute RRT at an early stage. Marked azotemia, defined as a urea more than 40 mmol/L (BUN [blood urea nitrogen] of 112 mg/dL) or a creatinine level more than 400 micromoles (4.5 mg/dL), is undesirable and should probably be treated with RRT, unless recovery is imminent or already under way and a return toward normal values is expected within 24 to 48 hours. It is recognized, however, that no randomized trials exist to define the ideal time for intervention with artificial renal support.

Recovery and Its Management

Recovery of renal function after an episode of ARF is increasingly being acknowledged as a significant clinical measure of morbidity. Failure to recover function can have both individual patient and broader health care implications. Persistent chronic renal impairment, or the need for long-term RRT, can negatively influence the health status and quality of life of patients and contribute to considerable annual health care expenditures. Recovery to independence from RRT occurs in an estimated 68% to 85% of critically ill patients by hospital discharge and generally peaks by 90 days (1,4). Studies have shown that older patients and those with pre-existing comorbid illnesses, such as chronic kidney disease or advanced cardiovascular disease, are less likely to recover function, whereas those with septic ARF may be more likely to recover function. Several other potentially modifiable factors have been linked with improved rates of recovery, including early and aggressive initiation of RRT when indicated, use of continuous rather than intermittent RRT, early and adequate nutritional support, and intensive insulin therapy (Table 160.3). Whether adjuvant erythropoietin and routine use of loop diuretics can influence renal prognosis and promote early recovery remain controversial.

PROGNOSIS

Acute renal failure can independently influence both short- and long-term prognosis. In hospitalized patients, mortality is estimated at 20% among all those developing ARF;

however, this rate is greatly influenced by the severity of renal injury. The prognosis is worse for critically ill patients and those in whom RRT becomes necessary. The in-hospital mortality for critically ill patients with ARF is estimated at 50% to 60%, yet, depending on the case mix, can range between 40% to 80% (1,3,4,76,77). It is frequently stated that patients die *with* renal failure rather than *of* renal failure. However, growing evidence suggests that better uremic control and more intensive artificial renal support may improve survival (78,79). Such evidence supports a careful and proactive approach to the treatment of critically ill patients with ARF, which is based on the prevention of uncontrolled uremia and the maintenance of low urea levels throughout the patient's illness.

In those who survive an episode of ARF associated with critical illness, the long-term health status, including health-related quality of life (HRQoL), functional status, and hospital discharge location, are also now considered important indicators of morbidity. These patients frequently describe limitations in daily activities, defficulties with mobility, and high levels of sleep disturbance, fatigue, anxiety, and depression. However, HRQoL is generally good and perceived as acceptable, despite evidence that their quality of life is considerably lower than that of the general population (80).

FUTURE DEVELOPMENTS

The discipline of nephrology concerned with ARF and RRT in critically ill patients has undergone remarkable progress in recent years; however, mortality rates for ARF remain unacceptably high. A consensus definition has now been developed and published that will guide research and, it is hoped, translate into improved patient outcome (6). Such research is needed to explore the relationship between survival and subsequent morbidity—specifically, recovery of kidney function, health-related quality of life, and the economic consequences of decisions made during care of critically ill patients with ARF.

Some recent advances have been made, particularly in the prevention of ARF associated with radiocontrast nephropathy with use of N-acetylcysteine. Although studies with fenoldopam are provocative, in general, no specific drugs have been found to help. Apoptosis has recently been shown as an important mechanism of renal tubular injury in ARF (47–49,86). There is therapeutic potential for molecular targets, such as selective inhibitors of pro-apoptotic proteins (e.g., capsase inhibitors), involved in ARF that may attenuate injury or promote recovery; however, at present, no evidence in humans has emerged.

PEARLS

- Restoring mean arterial pressure (MAP) within the autoregulatory range for blood flow to the kidney—65 to 110 mm Hg—is important in maintaining the glomerular filtration rate. Once the patient has been adequately fluid resuscitated, with a CVP at least greater than 8 mm Hg, and the cardiac output is known to be adequate or high, MAP should be corrected within autoregulation with the use of norepinephrine.
- Low-dose dopamine has been extensively studied, meta-analyzed, and assessed for the treatment of acute renal failure. Although it probably increases urine output through its tubular diuretic effect, it does not maintain or improve the glomerular filtration rate.
- Once a patient has been fluid resuscitated as described above, if the cardiac output is adequate or high, and the mean arterial pressure is adequate or normal, there is no renal benefit to be gained by giving more intravenous fluids. Such fluids often precipitate pulmonary congestion and have no sustained beneficial effect on glomerular filtration. They should not be given.

References

1. Bagshaw SM, Laupland KB, Doig CJ, et al. Prognosis for long-term survival and renal recovery in critically ill patients with severe acute renal failure: a population-based study. *Crit Care.* 2005;9(6):R700–R709.
2. de Mendonca A, Vincent JL, Suter PM, et al. Acute renal failure in the ICU: risk factors and outcome evaluated by the SOFA score. *Intensive Care Med.* 2000;26(7):915–921.
3. Liano F, Junco E, Pascual J, et al. The spectrum of acute renal failure in the intensive care unit compared with that seen in other settings. The Madrid Acute Renal Failure Study Group. *Kidney Int Suppl.* 1998;66:S16–24.
4. Uchino S, Kellum JA, Bellomo R, et al. Acute renal failure in critically ill patients: a multinational, multicenter study. *JAMA.* 2005;294(7):813–818.
5. Metnitz PG, Krenn CG, Steltzer H, et al. Effect of acute renal failure requiring renal replacement therapy on outcome in critically ill patients. *Crit Care Med.* 2002;30(9):2051–2058.
6. Bellomo R, Ronco C, Kellum JA, et al. Acute renal failure—definition, outcome measures, animal models, fluid therapy and information technology needs: the Second International Consensus Conference of the Acute Dialysis Quality Initiative (ADQI) Group. *Crit Care.* 2004;8(4):R204–212.
7. Uchino S, Bellomo R, Goldsmith D, et al. An assessment of the RIFLE criteria for acute renal failure in hospitalized patients. *Crit Care Med.* 2006;34:1913–1917.
8. Hoste EA, Clermont G, Kersten A, et al. RIFLE criteria for acute kidney injury are associated with hospital mortality in critically ill patients: a cohort analysis. *Crit Care.* 2006;10(3):R73.
9. Hou SH, Bushinsky DA, Wish JB, et al. Hospital-acquired renal insufficiency: a prospective study. *Am J Med.* 1983;74(2):243–248.
10. Nash K, Hafeez A, Hou S. Hospital-acquired renal insufficiency. *Am J Kidney Dis.* 2002;39(5):930–936.
11. McCarthy JT. Prognosis of patients with acute renal failure in the intensive-care unit: a tale of two eras. *Mayo Clin Proc.* 1996;71(2):117–126.
12. Tran DD, Cuesta MA, Oe PL. Acute renal failure in patients with severe civilian trauma. *Nephrol Dial Transplant.* 1994;9(Suppl 4):121–125.
13. Bagshaw SM, Langenberg C, Bellomo R. Urinary biochemistry and microscopy in septic acute renal failure—a systematic review. *Am J Kidney Dis.* 2006;48(5):695–705.
14. Langenberg C, Wan L, Bagshaw SM, et al. Urinary biochemistry in experimental septic acute renal failure. *Nephrol Dial Transplant.* 2006;21(12):3389–3397.
15. Feest T, Round A, Hamad S. Incidence of severe acute renal failure in adults: results of a community based study. *BMJ.* 1993;306:481–483.
16. Gines P, Guevara M, Arroyo V, et al. Hepatorenal syndrome. *Lancet.* 2003;362(9398):1819–1827.
17. Arroyo V, Guevara M, Gines P. Hepatorenal syndrome in cirrhosis: pathogenesis and treatment. *Gastroenterology.* 2002;122(6):1658–1676.
18. Sort P, Navasa M, Arroyo V, et al. Effect of intravenous albumin on renal impairment and mortality in patients with cirrhosis and spontaneous bacterial peritonitis. *N Engl J Med.* 1999;341(6):403–409.
19. Guevara M, Gines P, Fernandez-Esparrach G, et al. Reversibility of hepatorenal syndrome by prolonged administration of ornipressin and plasma volume expansion. *Hepatology.* 1998;27(1):35–41.
20. Fabrizi F, Dixit V, Martin P. Meta-analysis: terlipressin therapy for the hepatorenal syndrome. *Aliment Pharmacol Ther.* 2006;24(6):935–944.
21. Guevara M, Gines P, Bandi JC, et al. Transjugular intrahepatic portosystemic shunt in hepatorenal syndrome: effects on renal function and vasoactive systems. *Hepatology.* 1998;28(2):416–422.
22. Brensing KA, Textor J, Perz J, et al. Long term outcome after transjugular intrahepatic portosystemic stent-shunt in non-transplant cirrhotics with hepatorenal syndrome: a phase II study. *Gut.* 2000;47(2):288–295.
23. Silvester W, Bellomo R, Cole L. Epidemiology, management, and outcome of severe acute renal failure of critical illness in Australia. *Crit Care Med.* 2001;29(10):1910–1915.
24. Holt SG, Moore KP. Pathogenesis and treatment of renal dysfunction in rhabdomyolysis. *Intensive Care Med.* 2001;27(5):803–811.

25. Heyman SN, Brezis M, Reubinoff CA, et al. Acute renal failure with selective medullary injury in the rat. *J Clin Invest.* 1988;82(2):401–412.
26. Bonventre JV. Mechanisms of ischemic acute renal failure. *Kidney Int.* 1993;43(5):1160–1178.
27. di Mari JF, Davis R, Safirstein RL. MAPK activation determines renal epithelial cell survival during oxidative injury. *Am J Physiol.* 1999;277(2 Pt 2):F195–203.
28. Portilla D, Mandel LJ, Bar-Sagi D, Millington DS. Anoxia induces phospholipase A2 activation in rabbit renal proximal tubules. *Am J Physiol.* 1992;262(3 Pt 2):F354–360.
29. Bennett WM, Luft F, Porter GA. Pathogenesis of renal failure due to aminoglycosides and contrast media used in roentgenography. *Am J Med.* 1980;69(5):767–774.
30. Cunha MA, Schor N. Effects of gentamicin, lipopolysaccharide, and contrast media on immortalized proximal tubular cells. *Ren Fail.* 2002;24(6):687–690.
31. Bagshaw SM, Culleton BF. Contrast-induced nephropathy: epidemiology and prevention. *Minerva Cardioangiol.* 2006;54(1):109–129.
32. Aspelin P, Aubry P, Fransson SG, et al. Nephrotoxic effects in high-risk patients undergoing angiography. *N Engl J Med.* 2003;348(6):491–499.
33. Merten GJ, Burgess WP, Gray LV, et al. Prevention of contrast-induced nephropathy with sodium bicarbonate: a randomized controlled trial. *JAMA.* 2004;291(19):2328–2334.
34. Mueller C, Seidensticker P, Buettner HJ, et al. Incidence of contrast nephropathy in patients receiving comprehensive intravenous and oral hydration. *Swiss Med Wkly.* 2005;135(19–20):286–290.
35. Stevens MA, McCullough PA, Tobin KJ, et al. A prospective randomized trial of prevention measures in patients at high risk for contrast nephropathy: results of the P.R.I.N.C.E. Study. Prevention of Radiocontrast Induced Nephropathy Clinical Evaluation. *J Am Coll Cardiol.* 1999;33(2):403–411.
36. Bagshaw SM, Ghali WA. Acetylcysteine for prevention of contrast-induced nephropathy after intravascular angiography: a systematic review and meta-analysis. *BMC Med.* 2004;2:38.
37. Tepel M, van der Giet M, Schwarzfeld C, et al. Prevention of radiographic-contrast-agent-induced reductions in renal function by acetylcysteine. *N Engl J Med.* 2000;343(3):180–184.
38. Langenberg C, Bellomo R, May C, et al. Renal blood flow in sepsis. *Crit Care.* 2005;9(4):R363–3674.
39. Langenberg C, Bellomo R, May CN, et al. Renal vascular resistance in sepsis. *Nephron Physiol.* 2006;104(1):1–11.
40. Langenberg C, Wan L, Egi M, et al. Renal blood flow in experimental septic acute renal failure. *Kidney Int.* 2006;69(11):1996–2002.
41. Lucas CE, Rector FE, Werner M, et al. Altered renal homeostasis with acute sepsis. Clinical significance. *Arch Surg.* 1973;106(4):444–449.
42. Rector F, Goyal S, Rosenberg IK, et al. Renal hyperemia in associated with clinical sepsis. *Surg Forum.* 1972;23:51–53.
43. Brenner M, Schaer GL, Mallory DL, et al. Detection of renal blood flow abnormalities in septic and critically ill patients using a newly designed indwelling thermodilution renal vein catheter. *Chest.* 1990;98(1):170–179.
44. Di Giantomasso D, Morimatsu H, May CN, et al. Intrarenal blood flow distribution in hyperdynamic septic shock: effect of norepinephrine. *Crit Care Med.* 2003;31(10):2509–2513.
45. Hotchkiss RS, Swanson PE, Freeman BD, et al. Apoptotic cell death in patients with sepsis, shock, and multiple organ dysfunction. *Crit Care Med.* 1999;27(7):1230–1251.
46. Wan L, Bellomo R, Di Giantomasso D, et al. The pathogenesis of septic acute renal failure. *Curr Opin Crit Care.* 2003;9(6):496–502.
47. Jo SK, Cha DR, Cho WY, et al. Inflammatory cytokines and lipopolysaccharide induce Fas-mediated apoptosis in renal tubular cells. *Nephron.* 2002;91(3):406–415.
48. Messmer UK, Briner VA, Pfeilschifter J. Tumor necrosis factor-alpha and lipopolysaccharide induce apoptotic cell death in bovine glomerular endothelial cells. *Kidney Int.* 1999;55(6):2322–2337.
49. Bonegio R, Lieberthal W. Role of apoptosis in the pathogenesis of acute renal failure. *Curr Opin Nephrol Hypertens.* 2002;11(3):301–308.
50. Imai Y, Parodo J, Kajikawa O, et al. Injurious mechanical ventilation and end-organ epithelial cell apoptosis and organ dysfunction in an experimental model of acute respiratory distress syndrome. *JAMA.* 2003;289(16):2104–2112.
51. Gueler F, Rong S, Park JK, et al. Postischemic acute renal failure is reduced by short-term statin treatment in a rat model. *J Am Soc Nephrol.* 2002;13(9):2288–2298.
52. Noiri E, Nakao A, Uchida K, et al. Oxidative and nitrosative stress in acute renal ischemia. *Am J Physiol Renal Physiol.* 2001;281(5):F948–957.
53. Starkopf J, Zilmer K, Vihalemm T, et al. Time course of oxidative stress during open-heart surgery. *Scand J Thorac Cardiovasc Surg.* 1995;29(4):181–186.
54. Ishizuka S, Nagashima Y, Numata M, et al. Regulation and immunohistochemical analysis of stress protein heme oxygenase-1 in rat kidney with myoglobinuric acute renal failure. *Biochem Biophys Res Commun.* 1997;240(1):93–98.
55. Kuiper JW, Groeneveld AB, Slutsky AS, et al. Mechanical ventilation and acute renal failure. *Crit Care Med.* 2005;33(6):1408–1415.
56. Pannu N, Mehta RL. Mechanical ventilation and renal function: an area for concern? *Am J Kidney Dis.* 2002;39(3):616–624.
57. Ricard JD, Dreyfuss D, Saumon G. Ventilator-induced lung injury. *Curr Opin Crit Care.* 2002;8(1):12–20.
58. Ranieri VM, Suter PM, Tortorella C, et al. Effect of mechanical ventilation on inflammatory mediators in patients with acute respiratory distress syndrome: a randomized controlled trial. *JAMA.* 1999;282(1):54–61.
59. Albanese J, Leone M, Garnier F, et al. Renal effects of norepinephrine in septic and nonseptic patients. *Chest.* 2004;126(2):534–539.
60. Bellomo R, Kellum JA, Wisniewski SR, et al. Effects of norepinephrine on the renal vasculature in normal and endotoxemic dogs. *Am J Respir Crit Care Med.* 1999;159(4 Pt 1):1186–1192.
61. Bourgoin A, Leone M, Delmas A, et al. Increasing mean arterial pressure in patients with septic shock: effects on oxygen variables and renal function. *Crit Care Med.* 2005;33(4):780–786.
62. Finfer S, Bellomo R, Boyce N, et al. A comparison of albumin and saline for fluid resuscitation in the intensive care unit. *N Engl J Med.* 2004;350(22):2247–2256.
63. Schortgen F, Lacherade JC, Bruneel F, et al. Effects of hydroxyethylstarch and gelatin on renal function in severe sepsis: a multicentre randomised study. *Lancet.* 2001;357(9260):911–916.
64. Van Biesen W, Yegenaga I, Vanholder R, et al. Relationship between fluid status and its management on acute renal failure (ARF) in intensive care unit (ICU) patients with sepsis: a prospective analysis. *J Nephrol.* 2005;18(1):54–60.
65. Sakr Y, Vincent JL, Reinhart K, et al. High tidal volume and positive fluid balance are associated with worse outcome in acute lung injury. *Chest.* 2005;128(5):3098–3108.
66. Simmons RS, Berdine GG, Seidenfeld JJ, et al. Fluid balance and the adult respiratory distress syndrome. *Am Rev Respir Dis.* 1987;135(4):924–929.
67. Wiedemann HP, Wheeler AP, Bernard GR, et al. Comparison of two fluid-management strategies in acute lung injury. *N Engl J Med.* 2006;354(24):2564–2575.
68. Bellomo R, Chapman M, Finfer S, et al. Low-dose dopamine in patients with early renal dysfunction: a placebo-controlled randomised trial. Australian and New Zealand Intensive Care Society (ANZICS) Clinical Trials Group. *Lancet.* 2000;356(9248):2139–2143.
69. Shilliday IR, Quinn KJ, Allison ME. Loop diuretics in the management of acute renal failure: a prospective, double-blind, placebo-controlled, randomized study. *Nephrol Dial Transpl.* 1997;12(12):2592–2596.
70. Morelli A, Ricci Z, Bellomo R, et al. Prophylactic fenoldopam for renal protection in sepsis: a randomized, double-blind, placebo-controlled pilot trial. *Crit Care Med.* 2005;33(11):2451–2456.
71. Bove T, Landoni G, Calabro MG, et al. Renoprotective action of fenoldopam in high-risk patients undergoing cardiac surgery: a prospective, double-blind, randomized clinical trial. *Circulation.* 2005;111(24):3230–3235.
72. Sward K, Valsson F, Odencrants P, et al. Recombinant human atrial natriuretic peptide in ischemic acute renal failure: a randomized placebo-controlled trial. *Crit Care Med.* 2004;32(6):1310–1315.
73. Chertow GM, Lazarus JM, Paganini EP, et al. Predictors of mortality and the provision of dialysis in patients with acute tubular necrosis. The Auriculin Anaritide Acute Renal Failure Study Group. *J Am Soc Nephrol.* 1998;9(4):692–698.
74. Korbet SM. Percutaneous renal biopsy. *Semin Nephrol.* 2002;22(3):254–267.
75. Hebert PC, Wells G, Blajchman MA, et al. A multicenter, randomized, controlled clinical trial of transfusion requirements in critical care. Transfusion Requirements in Critical Care Investigators, Canadian Critical Care Trials Group. *N Engl J Med.* 1999;340(6):409–417.
76. Mehta RL, Pascual MT, Soroko S, et al. Spectrum of acute renal failure in the intensive care unit: the PICARD experience. *Kidney Int.* 2004;66(4):1613–1621.
77. Ympa YP, Sakr Y, Reinhart K, et al. Has mortality from acute renal failure decreased? A systematic review of the literature. *Am J Med.* 2005;118(8):827–832.
78. Schiffl H, Lang SM, Fischer R. Daily hemodialysis and the outcome of acute renal failure. *N Engl J Med* 2002;346:305–310.
79. Phu NH, Hien TT, Hoang NT, et al. Hemofiltration and peritoneal dialysis in infection-associated acute renal failure in Vietnam. *N Engl J Med* 2002;347:895–902.
80. Ronco C, Bellomo R, Homel P, et al. Effects of different doses in continuous veno-venous haemofiltration on outcomes of acute renal failure: a prospective randomised trail. *Lancet* 2000;355:26–30.

CHAPTER 161 ■ RENAL REPLACEMENT THERAPIES IN THE CRITICALLY ILL PATIENT

CLAUDIO RONCO • ZACCARIA RICCI

Despite recent advances in acute renal failure (ARF) definition, diagnosis, and treatment many aspects remain subject to controversy and lack of consensus. Renal replacement therapies (RRT) are an important part of this ongoing debate, and although modern technology has made a vast pool of different strategies of extracorporeal renal support easily available, it is still not clear which one is superior to the other in terms of efficacy and outcome. Moreover, evidence-based medicine has not yet defined the best time to prescribe RRT and when and how patients should be weaned from this therapy. This chapter will review most of these aspects and will provide some theoretical and practical bases for RRT prescription with the goal of helping intensive care unit (ICU) clinicians understand critical care nephrology.

ACUTE RENAL FAILURE AND THE CRITICALLY ILL PATIENT

A recent multinational, multicenter prospective epidemiologic survey of ARF was conducted in ICU patients who either were treated with RRT or fulfilled at least one of the predefined criteria for ARF (1). Predefined ARF criteria were oliguria, defined as urine output less than 200 mL in 12 hours, and/or marked azotemia, defined as a blood urea nitrogen level higher than 30 mmol/L. The data were collected at 54 hospitals in 23 countries. Of 29,269 critically ill patients admitted during the 16 month study period, 1,738 (5.9%) had ARF during their ICU stay, including 1,260 (4.3%) who were treated with RRT. Overall hospital mortality was 60.3%. The most common contributing factor to ARF was septic shock (47.5%). Approximately 30% of patients had preadmission renal dysfunction; 86.2% survivors were independent from dialysis at hospital discharge. Independent risk factors for hospital mortality included the use of vasopressors, mechanical ventilation, septic shock, cardiogenic shock, and hepatorenal syndrome.

Crude mortality assessment shows that the overall hospital outcome of ARF has remained high today, and it has not changed in the last 30 years; nevertheless, such analysis is profoundly misleading. Patients with ARF 30 years ago were mostly treated outside the ICU, did not require or receive mechanical ventilation or vasopressor drugs, were 20 to 30 years younger in age, and their outcome was typically assessed retrospectively and in academic centers. Despite such profound differences that indicate a much greater illness severity for patients treated in 2005, the mortality of ARF has not increased, and perhaps has slightly decreased. The duration of treatment has clearly decreased in terms of need for dialysis, as well as the patient's stay in the ICU and hospital, and the techniques of artificial renal support have also changed markedly (2). It is a matter of fact, however, that 50% to 60% crude mortality associated with ARF will remain unchanged in the next decade. In fact, as therapeutic capability improves and the system continues to accept a mortality of 50% as reasonable for these very sick patients, the health care system will progressively admit and treat sicker and sicker patients with ARF.

In modern health care systems, hence, ARF and the requirement for acute RRT have become an established reality. It has been estimated that the incidence of ARF requiring extracorporeal support is 11.0 per 100,000 population/year. The annual mortality rate is 7.3 per 100,000 residents, with the highest rates in males older than 65 years. Renal recovery occurs in 78% (68/87) of survivors at 1 year, meaning that, although a great number of patients with severe ARF will proceed to die, most survivors will become independent from RRT within a year (3). The number of acute dialytic treatments has grown up to the development of a new specialized branch of nephrology in the last 10 years: however, it is important to emphasize that a critically ill patient with ARF is not a patient with isolated renal dysfunction. ARF requires a multidisciplinary approach with intensivists and nephrologists sharing their respective knowledge. Fluid balance, vasopressor dosage, mechanical ventilation support, and arterial blood gas exchange—including PaO_2/F_IO_2 (partial pressure of oxygen/inspired fraction of oxygen) ratio—need to be associated to RRT prescription, dialysis dose, ultrafiltration requirement, and anticoagulation strategy. Younger ICU clinicians need an in-depth understanding in their routine practice of all theoretical and technical aspects of critical care nephrology.

HISTORICAL NOTES

From the initial description of continuous arteriovenous hemofiltration (CAVH) in 1977 by Peter Kramer et al. (4), RRT has progressively evolved in the ICU from a last-chance therapy for ARF to a standardized, widely used, fully independent form of artificial kidney support. Hardware and software technology supporting the application of RRT has greatly improved. The trend of this evolution and the potential of RRT have grown to a point in which multiple organ support therapy (MOST) is envisaged as a possible therapeutic approach in the critical care setting.

CAVH was the first example of artificial renal support applied to critically ill patients (Fig. 161.1A); this mode was capable of overcoming the traditional hemodialysis side effects, making possible the treatment of critically ill patients who previously could not be treated because of severe instability.

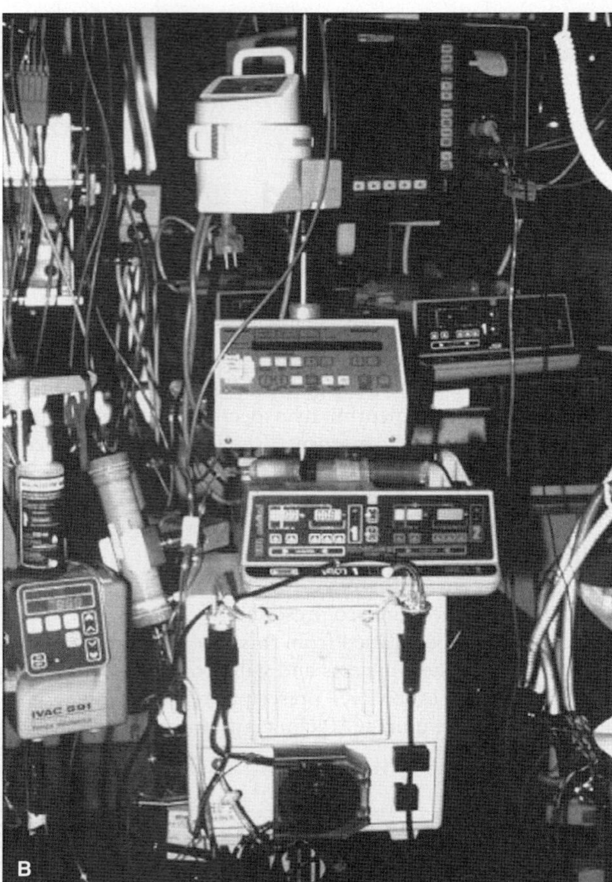

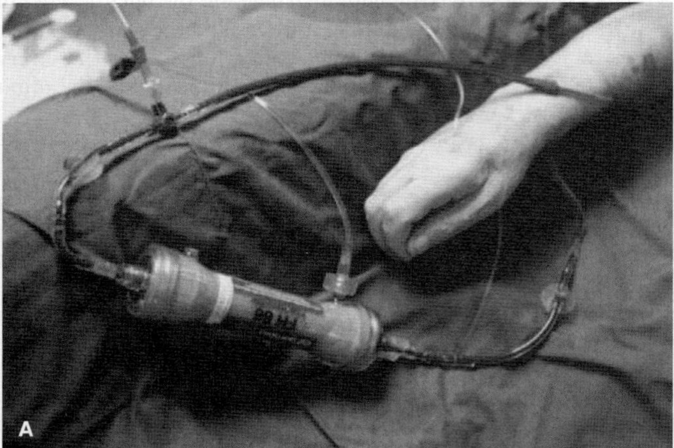

FIGURE 161.1. A: Continuous arteriovenous hemofiltration: artery and vein are cannulated; blood flow depends on pressure gradient; ultrafiltration is spontaneous and is mostly a function of ultrafiltrate column from the patient level to the effluent bag. **B:** Early example of pump systems applied to renal replacement therapy: the "Christmas tree–like effect".

Hypotension due to rapid fluid removal, arrhythmias caused by rapid electrolytes and intravascular volume shifts, and cerebral edema in head-injured patients were just some of the typical complications occurring during traditional dialysis therapies. The clinical picture was further worsened by the fast reduction of plasma osmolality induced by hemodialysis. CAVH provided slow, continuous fluid removal while maintaining steady solute concentrations and preventing peaks of toxic substances. At the same time, the advent of CAVH coincided with the establishment of fully staffed, independent intensive care units. In some of these units, renal replacement therapy could even be performed in the absence of a nephrology or a dialysis team. CAVH, however, had serious limitations. It required arterial access routinely associated with technical problems and high morbidity. Solute clearance was limited by the low rates of ultrafiltration and the pure convective nature of the treatment. Ultrafiltration limitation was imposed by the relatively low blood flow in the circuit, driven by a spontaneous arteriovenous pressure gradient and low transmembrane pressure (TMP) gradient. The first was dependent on the mean arterial pressure of the patient and the intrinsic resistance of the circuit; the second was determined by the hydrostatic pressure drop inside the filter and the negative suction provided by the ultrafiltrate column from the patient level to the ground. This meant that the most hemodynamically unstable patients achieved the lowest clearances and presented early clotting of the circuit. Technical improvements of CAVH (suction in the ultrafiltrate side, predilution, supplementation of countercurrent dialysate flow) allowed it to exceed 20 mL/minute of clearance, hardly sufficient to meet the needs of severely catabolic patients. To overcome such technical limitations, new filters were designed with an increased cross-sectional area and inner hollow fiber diameter, reduced unit length, and lower resistance to blood flow; by these measures, the phenomenon of filtration pressure equilibrium and easy clotting due to poorly optimized ultrafiltration profile was diminished, if not avoided. Another option explored in those days was the use of highly biocompatible membranes mounted on parallel plate devices. These filters presented lower intrinsic resistance (ensuring higher extracorporeal blood flows at a given arteriovenous pressure gradient), and they were equipped with a second port in the filtrate compartment so that countercurrent dialysate flow could be programmed in the newly conceived continuous arteriovenous hemodiafiltration (CAVHD) mode.

The evolution of technology and the progress experienced in the ICU made it possible to activate renal replacement therapy programs in several institutions, even in the absence of a chronic dialysis facility or a trained nephrologic team. Initial limitations and drawbacks of CAVH stimulated nurses and physicians to explore new avenues for better outcome of the therapy. The logical evolution was to apply a peristaltic pump to the extracorporeal circuit. It must be reminded that the use of a blood pump in the ICU was considered in those days as a proprietary technology of the dialysis team (nurses and nephrology consultants) and a technology that required a specific expertise. Eventually, the knowledge of pumped systems began to be disseminated in the critical care world, making venovenous hemofiltration a reality. The need of hardware evolution in CAVH was not limited to blood pumps, but it was also extended to fluid delivery systems and ultrafiltration control mechanisms such that it allowed delivery of dialysate or replacement solutions with an acceptable degree of accuracy.

The first step toward continuous venovenous renal replacement therapies was the advent of double lumen catheters that made possible the puncture of a single vein, thus decreasing the high rate of complications due to the need of arterial cannulation. The driving force was no longer produced by the patient's mean arterial pressure, but resulted from the mechanical action of the roller pumps. Blood flows could finally be programmed and delivered with adequate precision. Nevertheless, the new configuration of the extracorporeal circuit brought with it the requirement for new accessories and new safety features that were mostly borrowed from the chronic hemodialysis technology. The continuous venovenous therapy setup required negative pressure measurement and alarm in the arterial line before the pump, as well as positive pressure measurement and alarm in the venous return line. In this line, a bubble trap had to be inserted to prevent air embolism (this was not necessary in CAVH where the circuit operated at positive pressure along the entire length of the system). The higher blood flows induced higher filtration rates and the possibility to exploit higher clearances because of increased dialysate flow rates. For this reason, roller pumps were also applied to the dialysate or fluid replacement delivery section of the circuit, and external scales had to be frequently used to provide sufficiently accurate fluid balance during treatment.

The benefits induced by the new adaptive technology were soon counterbalanced by the gross inaccuracy of the systems and the limited integration between the extracorporeal circuit and the fluid balance devices. Furthermore, the fact that these combined devices were mostly derived from the chronic dialysis world conflicted with the possibility of their adequate usage in continuous and prolonged treatment. Finally, the need of obtaining additional information or performing additional functions led physicians and nurses to include in the system several other devices often poorly integrated, with the final result of a cumbersome Christmas tree–like effect (Fig. 161.1B). Safety and performance were definitely not optimized. Blood pumps were often inaccurate, circuit tubing was damaged over time, uncontrolled filtration fractions resulted because of pressure and flow fluctuations, intrafilter hematocrit and platelet count consequently increased beyond safe values, and filter clotting typically occurred. Accurate ultrafiltration control is mandatory in modern RRT. Early machines did not have scales or pumps, and when volumetric pumps started to be used to drive dialysate and ultrafiltrate in and out from the filters, inaccuracies close to 10% were observed, an unacceptable error during 24-hour-long therapies. Furthermore, when the membrane was clogged and approaching failure, the ultrafiltrate volumetric pump was increasing its inaccuracy because of the wide fluctuation in the membrane ultrafiltration coefficient. It soon became evident that an ideal extracorporeal circuit should have incorporated continuous pressure measurements of the inlet and outlet lumen of the catheter, inlet and outlet of the filter, and ultrafiltrate and dialysate ports. When this information was integrated with adequate alarms, it resulted of crucial importance, and allowed the ICU staff to maintain filter efficiency and circuit patency, detect potential sources of clotting, and ensure patient safety.

INDICATIONS FOR INITIATION AND CESSATION OF RENAL REPLACEMENT THERAPY

General Indications

Uremic complications of ARF such as pulmonary edema, severe fluid overload, hyperkalemia-induced arrhythmias, and uncontrolled metabolic acidosis have long been described. Nonetheless, there are no predefined established indications on when to start RRT. Medical management attempts to prevent renal dysfunction include the use of diuretics, bicarbonate, fluid restriction, and nutritional restriction to control hyperkalemia. When these attempts fail, treatment is escalated to RRT. In recent times, a more aggressive blood purification approach has been advocated, with the maintenance of homeostasis and prevention of complications being a priority for the critically ill patient (5). Now that multiple RRT options are easily available in the ICU and little morbidity is described in association with the administration of extracorporeal renal support, early blood purification is desirable, and a prevention-based algorithm for initiation of RRT can be used (Table 161.1). Unfortunately, once RRT has started, there is no scientifically established biochemical or clinical marker that should be targeted by the therapy. A routine clinical practice is to maintain urea concentration below 30 mg/dL, creatinine below 2.5 mg/dL, and electrolytes within normal values.

Techniques and timing of weaning patients from RRT are poorly described in the literature. Again, following practical clinical concepts, it is recommended that when the patient has

TABLE 161.1

INDICATIONS FOR STARTING RRT

The presence of one indication ***suggests***, two indications ***strongly suggest***, three indications ***mandate*** initiation of RRT.

- Anuria/oliguria (diuresis ≤200 mL in 12 h)
- Severe metabolic acidosis (pH <7.10)
- Hyperazotemia (BUN ≥80 mg/100 mL) or creatinine >4 mg/dL
- Hyperkalemia (K^+ ≥6.5 mEq/L)
- Clinical signs of uremic toxicity
- Severe dysnatremia (Na^+ ≤115 or ≥160 mEq/L)
- Hyperthermia (temperature >40°C without response to medical therapy)
- Anasarca or severe fluid overload
- Multiple organ failure with renal dysfunction and/or systemic inflammatory reaction syndrome, sepsis or septic shock with renal dysfunction

reached hemodynamic stability, and/or the need for vasopressors has been reduced and/or the severity of illness has decreased, intensity of the blood purification can be decreased. If the patient was on a continuous schedule, he or she can be switched to an intermittent or semicontinuous modality. This process can be accelerated when urine output and fluid balance become adequate. Current research focuses on the possibility of classifying ARF according to multilevel classification (see below) and applying it to administer renal supportive therapies, depending on the level of the disease.

Controversies

A clear ARF consensus definition is needed that would allow clinicians to better classify epidemiology, randomizing patients in controlled trials, testing therapies in similar groups of patients, developing animal models, and validating diagnostic tests. To make consensus-based recommendations and delineate key questions for future studies, the Acute Dialysis Quality Initiative (ADQI) work group in 2004 identified the need for a definition/classification system for ARF as a topic related to the field of ARF and ranked this need first for importance and clinical impact (6). The work group considered that the definition of ARF necessarily required the following features:

- Ease of use and clinical applicability across different centers
- High sensitivity and specificity for different populations and research questions

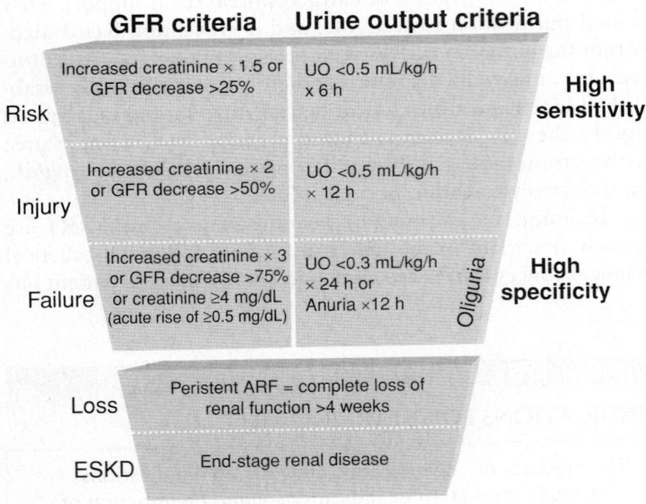

FIGURE 161.2. The RIFLE classification separates criteria for serum creatinine and urine output (UO). The criteria that lead to the worst possible classification should be used. RIFLE-F is present even if the increase in serum creatinine is below threefold, as long as the new serum creatinine is 4.0 mg/dL (350 mmol/L) or above in the setting of an acute increase of at least 0.5 mg/dL (44 mmol/L). The shape of the figure denotes the fact that more patients (high sensitivity) will be included in the mild category, including some not actually having renal failure (less specificity). In contrast, at the bottom, the criteria are strict and therefore specific, but some patients will be missed. ARF, acute renal failure; GFR, glomerular filtration rate. (From Bellomo R, Ronco C, Kellum JA, et al., and the ADQI workgroup. Acute renal failure—definition, outcome measures, animal models, fluid therapy and information technology needs: the Second International Consensus Conference of the Acute Dialysis Quality Initiative [ADQI] Group. *Crit Care.* 2004;8:R204–R212, with permission.)

- Consideration of creatinine changes from baseline
- A classification for acute or chronic renal disease

Such a classification would include and separate mild and severe as well as early or late cases, and would allow the detection of patients in whom renal function is mildly affected (high sensitivity for the detection of kidney malfunction but limited specificity for its presence) and patients in whom renal function is markedly affected (high specificity for true renal dysfunction but limited sensitivity in picking up early and more subtle loss of function). Accordingly, a multilevel classification system was proposed for a wide range of conditions such as Renal dysfunction, Injury to the kidney, Failure or Loss of kidney function, and End-stage kidney disease; these criteria are identified by the acronym RIFLE (Fig. 161.2).

When such classification achieves sufficient clinical validation (7), it will be reasonable to couple each level of ARF severity to a specific management plan (medical or artificial) and/or to identify a RRT modality/prescription for that level of renal dysfunction. In our experience, a RIFLE-F level (Fig. 161.2) of ARF severity could be a reasonable trigger to start RRT apart from any previously attempted medical therapy.

CONTINUOUS, INTERMITTENT, DIFFUSIVE, CONVECTIVE: AN ONGOING MATTER

RRT Modalities: Description and Nomenclature

Renal replacement consists of the purification of blood by semipermeable membranes. A wide range of molecules, from water to urea to low-, middle-, and high-molecular-weight solutes, is transported across such membranes by the mechanism of ultrafiltration (water), convection, and diffusion (solutes) (Fig. 161.3).

During *diffusion,* the movement of solutes depends on their tendency to reach the same concentration on each side of the membrane; the practical result is the passage of solutes from the compartment with the highest concentration to the compartment with the lowest concentration. Other components of the semipermeable membrane deeply affect diffusion: thickness and surface, temperature, and diffusion coefficient. *Dialysis* is a modality of RRT and is predominantly based on the principle of diffusion: a dialytic solution flows through the filter countercurrent to blood flow to maintain the highest solute gradient from inlet to outlet port.

During *convection,* the movement of solute across a semipermeable membrane takes place in conjunction with significant amounts of *ultrafiltration* (water transfer across the membrane). In other words, as the solvent (plasma water) is pushed across the membrane in response to the transmembrane pressure (TMP) by ultrafiltration (UF), solutes are carried with it, as long as the porosity of the membrane allows the molecules to be sieved from blood. The process of UF is governed by the UF rate (Qf), the membrane UF coefficient (Km), and the TMP gradient generated by the pressures on both sides of the membrane, according to the following formula:

$$Qf = Km \times TMP$$

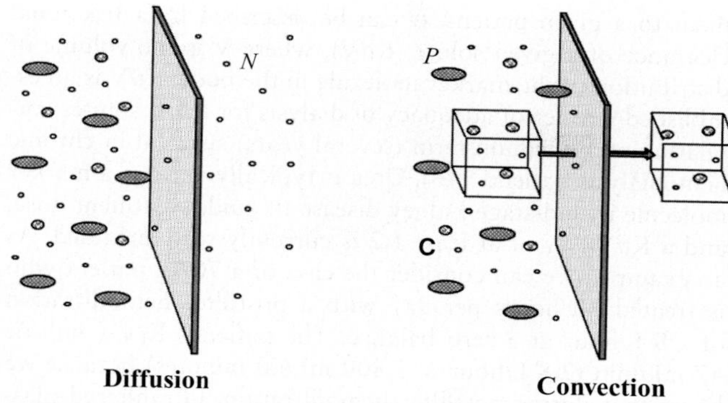

FIGURE 161.3. Diffusion and convection are schematically represented. During diffusion, solutes flux (Jx) is a function of solutes concentration gradient (dc) between the two sides of the semipermeable membrane, temperature (T), diffusivity coefficient (D), membrane thickness (dx), and surface area (A) according to the following equation:

$$Jx = DTA(dc/dx) \quad (1)$$

Convective flux of solutes (Jf) requires instead a pressure gradient between the two sides of the membrane (transmembrane pressure, TMP) that moves a fluid (plasma water) with its crystalloid content (a process called ultrafiltration, whose entity is also dependent on the membrane permeability coefficient (Kf). Colloids and cells will not cross the semipermeable membrane, depending on the pores' size.

$$Jf = Kf \times TMP \quad (2)$$

$TMP = Pb - Pd - \pi$, where Pb is blood hydrostatic pressure, Pd is hydrostatic pressure on the ultrafiltrate side of the membrane, and π is blood oncotic pressure).

The hydrostatic pressure in the blood compartment is dependent on blood flow (Qb). The greater the Qb, the greater the TMP. In modern RRT machines, UF control throughout the filter is obtained by applying a pump that generates suction to the UF side of the membrane. Modern systems are optimally designed to maintain a constant Qf; it is worth noting that, when the filter is fresh, the initial effect of UF pumps is to retard UF production, generating a positive pressure on the UF side. Thus, TMP is initially dependent only on Qb. As the membrane fibers foul, a negative pressure is necessary to achieve a constant Qf. In this case, a progressive increase of TMP can be observed up to a maximal level in which clotting is likely, membrane rupture may occur, and, above all, solute clearance may be significantly compromised. In fact, if it is true that the size of molecules cleared during convection exceeds that during diffusion, because they are physically dragged to the UF side, it is also true that this feature is seriously limited by the protein layer that progressively closes filter pores during convective treatments (8). A peculiar membrane capacity, defined as *adsorption*, has been shown to have a major role in higher-molecular-weight toxins (9); however, it should be considered that membrane adsorptive capacity is generally saturated in the first hours from the beginning of the treatment. This observation reflects the minimal impact of the adsorption component on solute clearance, and suggests relying only on the relatively minor effects of mass separation processes such as diffusion and convection (10).

As UF proceeds and plasma water and solutes are filtered from blood, hydrostatic pressure within the filter is lost and oncotic pressure is gained because blood concentrates and hematocrit increases. The fraction of plasma water that is removed from blood during UF is called *filtration fraction*; it should be kept in the range of 20% to 25% to prevent excessive hemoconcentration within the filtering membrane and to avoid the critical point at which oncotic pressure is equal to TMP and a condition of filtration/pressure equilibrium is reached. Finally, replacing plasma water with a substitution solution completes the *hemofiltration* (HF) process and returns purified blood to the patient. The replacement fluid can be administered after the filter, with a process called *postdilution HF*. Otherwise, the solution can be infused before the filter to obtain predilution HF, whereas predilution plus postdilution replacement is obtained on mixed infusion of substitution fluids both before and after filtering the membrane. Although postdilution allows a urea clearance equivalent to therapy delivery (i.e., 2,000 mL/hour—see below), predilution, in spite of theoretical reduced solute clearances, prolongs the circuit life span, reducing the hemoconcentration and protein caking effects occurring within filter fibers. Conventional hemofiltration is performed with a highly permeable membrane with a surface area of about 1 m^2, steam sterilized, with a cutoff point of 30 kd (Fig. 161.4).

The Concept of RRT Dose

The conventional view of RRT dose is that it is a measure of the quantity of blood purification achieved by means of

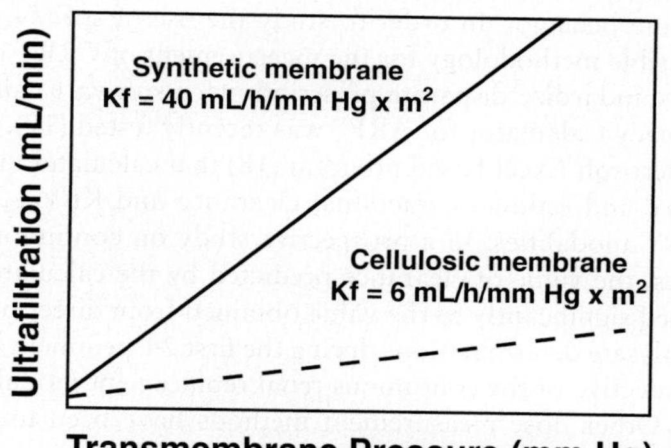

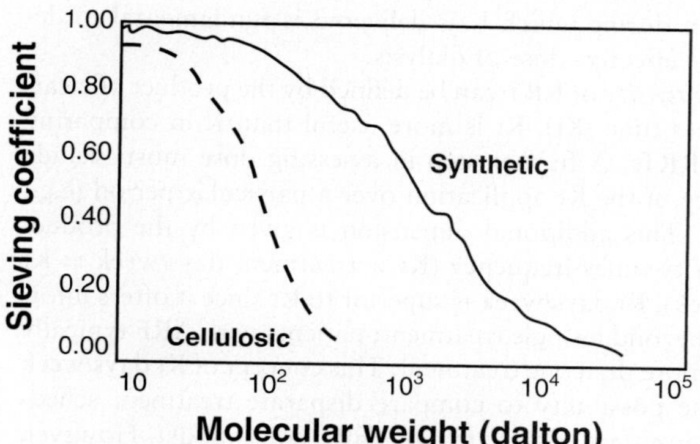

FIGURE 161.4. Membranes are classified based on their permeability or filtration coefficient (Kf – mL/h/mm Hg) and their sieving coefficient. A high flux (synthetic membrane) will have a higher permeability to water, with optimal use during hemofiltration or hemodiafiltration (prevalently convective treatments) and bigger pore size to let higher–molecular-weight molecules cross the membrane.

extracorporeal techniques. As this broad concept is too difficult to measure and quantify, the *operative* view of RRT dose is that it is a measure of the quantity of a representative marker solute that is removed from a patient. This marker solute is considered to be reasonably representative of similar solutes, which require removal for blood purification to be considered adequate. This premise has several major flaws; the marker solute cannot and does not represent all the solutes that accumulate in renal failure. Its kinetics and volume of distribution are also different from those of such solutes. Finally, its removal during RRT is not representative of the removal of other solutes. This is true both for end-stage renal failure and acute renal failure. However, a significant body of data in the end-stage renal failure literature (11–16) suggests that, despite all of the above major limitations, a single solute marker assessment of dialysis dose appears to have a clinically meaningful relationship with patient outcome, and therefore clinical utility. Nevertheless, the HEMO (hemodialysis) Study Group, examining the effect of intermittent hemodialysis (IHD) doses, enforced the concept that "less dialysis is worse," but failed to confirm the intuition that "more dialysis is better" (16). Thus, if this premise seems useful in end-stage renal failure, it is accepted to be potentially useful in ARF for operative purposes. Hence, the amount (measure) of delivered dose of RRT can be described by various terms: efficiency, intensity, frequency, and clinical efficacy. Each will be discussed below.

The *efficiency* of RRT is represented by the concept of clearance (K), i.e., the volume of blood cleared of a given solute over a given time. K does not reflect the overall solute removal rate (mass transfer) but, rather, its value normalized by the serum concentration. Even when K remains stable over time, the removal rate will vary if the blood levels of the reference molecule change. K depends on solute molecular size and transport modality (diffusion or convection), as well as circuit operational characteristics (blood flow rate [Qb], dialysate flow rate [Qd], ultrafiltration rate [Qf], and hemodialyzer type and size). K can be normally used to compare the treatment dose during each dialysis session, but it cannot be used as an absolute dose measure to compare treatments with different time schedules. For example, K is typically higher in intermittent hemodialysis (IHD) than continuous renal replacement therapy (CRRT) and sustained low-efficiency daily dialysis (SLEDD). This is not surprising, since K represents only the instantaneous efficiency of the system. However, mass removal may be greater during SLEDD or CRRT. For this reason, the information about the time span during which K is delivered is fundamental to describe the effective dose of dialysis.

The *intensity* of RRT can be defined by the product of clearance times time (Kt). Kt is more useful than K in comparing various RRTs. A further step in assessing dose must include frequency of the Kt application over a particular period (e.g., a week). This additional dimension is given by the product of intensity times frequency (Kt $\times$ treatment days/week $=$ Kt days/week). Kt days/week is superior to Kt since it offers information beyond a single treatment; patients with ARF typically require more than one treatment. This concept of Kt days/week offers the possibility to compare disparate treatment schedules (intermittent, alternate day, daily, continuous). However, it does not take into account the size of the pool of solute that needs to be cleared. This requires the dimension of efficacy.

The *efficacy* of RRT represents the effective solute removal outcome resulting from the administration of a given treatment to a given patient. It can be described by a fractional clearance of a given solute (Kt/V), where V is the volume of distribution of the marker molecule in the body. Kt/V is an established marker of adequacy of dialysis for small solutes correlating with medium-term (several years) survival in chronic hemodialysis patients (16). Urea is typically used as a marker molecule in end-stage kidney disease to guide treatment dose, and a Kt/V_{UREA} of at least 1.2 is currently recommended. As an example, we can consider the case of a 70-kg patient who is treated 20 hours per day with a postfilter hemofiltration of 2.8 L/hour at a zero balance. The patient's K_{UREA} will be 47 mL/min (2.8 L/hour $=$ 2,800 mL/60 minutes) because we know that during postfilter hemofiltration, ultrafiltered plasmatic water will drag all urea across the membrane, making its clearance identical to UF flow. The treatment time (t) will be 1,200 minutes (60 minutes for 20 hours). The urea volume of distribution will be approximately 42,000 mL (60% of 70 kg, 42 L $=$ 42,000 mL)—that is, roughly equal to total body water. Simplifying our patient's Kt/V_{UREA}, we will have $47 \times 1{,}200/42{,}000 = 1.34$.

However, Kt/V_{UREA} application to patients with ARF has not been rigorously validated. In fact, although the application of Kt/V to the assessment of dose in ARF is theoretically intriguing, many concerns have been raised because problems intrinsic to ARF can hinder the accuracy and meaning of such dose measurement. These include the lack of a metabolic steady state, uncertainty about the volume of distribution of urea (V_{UREA}), a high protein catabolic rate (PCR), labile fluid volumes, and possible residual renal function, which changes dynamically during the course of treatment. Furthermore, delivery of the prescribed dose in ARF can be limited by technical problems such as access recirculation, poor blood flows with temporary venous catheters, membrane clotting, and machine malfunction. In addition, clinical issues such as hypotension and vasopressor requirements can be responsible for solute disequilibrium within tissues and organs.

These aspects are particularly evident during IHD, less so during SLEDD, and even less during CRRT. This difference is due to the fact that, after some days of CRRT, the patient's urea levels approach a real steady state. Access recirculation is also an issue of lesser impact during low efficiency continuous techniques. Finally, because the therapy is applied continuously, the effect of compartmentalization of solutes is minimized and, from a theoretical point of view, single pool kinetics can be applied (spKt/V) with a reasonable chance of approximating true solute behavior. In order to study the use of $spKt/V_{UREA}$ as a feasible methodology for the measurement of CRRT dose and to standardize disparate prescriptions, a software called "Adequacy Calculator for ARF" was recently tested (17). This is a Microsoft Excel-based program (18) that calculates urea clearance and estimates fractional clearance and Kt/V_{UREA} for all RRT modalities. In a prospective study on continuous therapies, the value of clearance predicted by the calculator correlated significantly to the value obtained from direct blood and dialysate determinations during the first 24 treatment hours, irrespective of the continuous renal replacement modality used.

Other dose measurement methods have been used in patients with end-stage renal failure but have not been sufficiently investigated in the setting of ARF. The time-averaged blood urea concentration (TAC_{UREA}) is the area under the sawtooth curve produced by intermittent dialysis sessions. TAC_{UREA} is a function of dialysis dose and urea generation rate (G) from protein intake. As such, it is not a good indicator of RRT dose, *per se*. Emerging evidence from patients with end-stage renal failure suggests the importance of using equivalent renal clearance (EKRc). If G and TAC_{UREA} are known, EKRc can be calculated by the ratio of total urea removal (equal to G at steady state) and TAC_{UREA}. A modification of this equation was described by Gotch as standardized Kt/V (stdKt/V), and it is calculated as the ratio of G and mean weekly urea pretreatment concentrations (MPC) normalized for V_{UREA} (19–21). These formulas allow comparisons among the dose measurements of disparate therapies and different frequencies of RRT. However, G, MPC, and TAC_{UREA} calculations are less immediate than K, t and V_{UREA}, which seem easier to achieve without formal modeling. Furthermore, G is likely to be extremely variable from day to day in ARF patients. Finally, in patients who might receive only three or four sessions of IHD, the concept of MPC, which requires a parametric distribution of values, is simply statistically incorrect. V_{UREA} is also dynamic and not as easily estimated using anthropometric calculations.

To evaluate V_{UREA} in patients with ARF, Himmelfarb et al. (22) undertook a systematic study in a cohort of 28 patients with ARF. They found that determination of V_{UREA} by different approaches to anthropometric measurements (Watson, 42.5 $\pm$ 7.0 L; Hume-Weyer, 43.6 $\pm$ 7.1 L; Chertow, 46.8 $\pm$ 8.1 L) yielded significantly lower values compared to V_{UREA} determined by physiologic formulae and by bioimpedance (51.1 $\pm$ 11.6 L and 51.1 $\pm$ 13.3 L, respectively). Finally and more importantly, all measures of V_{UREA} by blood-based kinetics exceeded measurements by any method (7% to 50% difference). These investigators inevitably concluded that estimates of V_{UREA} cannot be reliably used in patients with ARF.

These observations highlight the gross inadequacies of applying end-stage renal failure paradigms to patients with ARF. They also indicate that, unlike in the field of chronic hemodialysis, only major changes in the application of dose (e.g., changing from twice-a-day to daily dialysis) can be reasonably believed to truly deliver a different dose in the setting of ARF. More subtle adjustments, such as prescribing a calculated Kt/V of 1 versus 1.2, can easily be criticized as being within the calculation error for each prescription and not necessarily representing a reliable change in dose delivery. The major shortcoming of the traditional solute marker–based approach to dialysis dose in ARF lies well beyond any methodologic critique of single-solute kinetics-based prescriptions. In patients with ARF, most of whom are in intensive care, a restrictive (solute-based only) concept of dialysis dose seems grossly inappropriate. In these patients, the therapeutic needs that can be, or need to be, affected by the dose of renal replacement therapy are more than the simple control of small solutes as represented by urea. They include control of acid-base value, tonicity, potassium, magnesium, calcium, phosphate, intravascular volume, extravascular volume, temperature, and the avoidance of unwanted side effects associated with the delivery of solute control. In the critically ill patient, it is much more important (e.g., in the setting of coagulopathic bleeding after cardiac surgery) for 10 units of fresh frozen plasma, 10 units of cryoprecipitate, and 10 units of platelets to be administered rapidly without inducing fluid overload (because 1 to 1.5 L of ultrafiltrate are removed in 1 hour) than for Kt/V to be of any particular value. A dose of RRT is aimed toward prophylactic volume control. In a patient with right ventricular failure, ARF, and ARDS who is receiving lung-protective ventilation with permissive hypercapnia and with acidemia, inducing a further life-threatening deterioration in pulmonary vascular resistance, the dose component of RRT that matters immediately is acid-base control and normalization of pH 24 hours/day. The Kt/V (or any other solute-centric concept of dose) is almost just a by-product of such dose delivery. In a young man with trauma, rhabdomyolysis, and a rapidly rising serum potassium already at 7 mmol/L, the dialysis dose is selected to control hyperkalemia. In a patient with fulminant liver failure, ARF, sepsis, and cerebral edema awaiting urgent liver transplantation, and whose cerebral edema is worsening because of fever, the RRT dose is centered on lowering the temperature without any tonicity shifts that might increase intracranial pressure. Finally, in a patient with pulmonary edema after an ischemic ventricular septal defect requiring emergency surgery, along with ARF, ischemic hepatitis, and the need for inotropic and intra-aortic balloon counterpulsation support, the RRT dose mostly concerns removing fluid gently and safely so that the extravascular volume falls while the intravascular volume remains optimal. Solute removal is simply a by-product of fluid control. These aspects of dose must explicitly be considered when discussing the dose of RRT in ARF, for it is likely that patients die more often from incorrect dose delivery of this type than incorrect dose delivery of the Kt/V type. Although each aspect of this broader understanding of dose is difficult to measure, clinically relevant assessment of dose in critically ill patients with ARF should include all dimensions of such a dose, and not one dimension picked because of a similarity with end-stage renal failure. There is no evidence in the acute field that such solute control data are more relevant to clinical outcomes than volume control, acid-base control, or tonicity control.

RRT Prescription

Theoretical Aspects

Despite all the uncertainty surrounding its meaning and the gross shortcomings related to its accuracy in patients with ARF, the idea that there might be an optimal dose of solute removal continues to have a powerful hold in the literature. This is likely due to evidence from ESRD, where a minimum Kt/V of 1.2 three times weekly is indicated as standard (16). However, the benefits of greater Kt/V accrue over years of therapy. In ARF, any difference in dose would apply for days to weeks. The view that it would still be sufficient to alter clinical outcomes remains somewhat optimistic.

Nonetheless, the hypothesis that higher doses of dialysis may be beneficial in critically ill patients with ARF must be considered by analogy and investigated. Several reports in the literature deal with this issue. Furthermore, the concept of a predefined dose is a powerful tool to guide clinicians to a correct prescription and to at least avoid undertreatment.

Brause et al. (23), using continuous venovenous hemofiltration (CVVH), found that higher Kt/V values (0.8 vs. 0.53) correlated with improved uremic control and acid-base balance; this would be expected. No clinically important outcome was affected. Investigators from the Cleveland clinic (24) retrospectively evaluated 844 patients with ARF requiring CRRT or IHD over a 7-year period. They found that, when patients were stratified for disease severity, the dialysis dose did not affect outcome in patients with very high or very low scores but did correlate with survival in patients with intermediate degrees of illness. A mean Kt/V greater than 1.0 or TAC_{UREA} less than 45 mg/dL was associated with increased survival. This study was retrospective with a clear *post hoc* selection bias. Therefore, the validity of these observations remains highly questionable.

Daily IHD compared to alternate-day dialysis also seemed to be associated with improved outcome in a recent trial (25). Daily hemodialysis resulted in significantly improved survival (72% vs. 54%, $p = 0.01$), better control of uremia, fewer hypotensive episodes, and more rapid resolution of ARF. However, several limitations affected this study: sicker, hemodynamically unstable patients were excluded and underwent CRRT instead. Furthermore, according to reported mean TAC_{UREA}, it appears that patients receiving conventional IHD were underdialyzed. In addition, this study was a single-center study with all the inherent limitations in regard to external validity. Furthermore, twice-daily dialysis was associated with significant differences in fluid removal and dialysis-associated hypotension, suggesting that other aspects of dose beyond solute control (inadequate and episodic volume control) may have explained the findings. These observations suggest that further studies should be undertaken to assess the most effective dose of IHD on outcome.

In a randomized controlled trial of CRRT dose, continuous venovenous postdilution hemofiltration (CVVH) at 35 mL/kg/hour or 45 mL/kg/hour was associated with improved survival when compared to 20 mL/kg/hour in 425 critically ill patients with ARF (26). Applying Kt/V dose assessment methodology to CVVH, at a dose of 35 mL/kg/hour in a 70-kg patient treated for 24 hours, a treatment day would be equivalent to a Kt/V of 1.4 applied daily. Despite the uncertainty regarding the calculation of V_{UREA}, CVVH at 35 mL/kg/hour would still provide an effective *daily* delivery of 1.2, even in the presence of an underestimation of V_{UREA} by 20%. Many technical and/or clinical problems, however, can make it difficult in routine practice to apply such strict protocol by pure postdilution hemofiltration. These problems include filter clotting; high filtration fraction in the presence of access dysfunction and fluctuations in blood flow; and circuit downtime during surgery, radiologic procedures, and filter changes. Equally important are the observations that this study was conducted over 6 years in a single center, uremic control was not reported, the incidence of sepsis was low compared to that of the typical populations reported to develop ARF in the world, and that its final outcome was not the accepted 28-day or 90-day mortality typically used in ICU trials. Thus, the external validity of this study remains untested.

Another prospective randomized trial conducted by Bouman et al. (27) assigned patients to three groups: (i) early high-volume hemofiltration (72 to 96 L per 24 hours); (ii) early low-volume hemofiltration (24 to 36 L per 24 hours); and (iii) late low-volume hemofiltration (24 to 36 L per 24 hours). These investigators found no difference in terms of renal recovery or 28-day mortality. Unfortunately, prescribed doses were not standardized by weight, making the potential variability in RRT dose large. Furthermore, the number of patients was small, making the study insufficiently powered, and, again, the incidence of sepsis was low compared to that of the typical populations reported to develop ARF in the world.

All of these studies, however, must be seen in the light of an absolute lack of any previous attempt to adjust ARF treatment dose to specific target levels. During the third International Course on Critical Care Nephrology held in Vicenza, Italy, a survey on various aspects of ARF was conducted, including treatment prescription, among about 550 participants (equally distributed between nephrologists and intensivists) from about 500 centers (28). More than one third of responders declared not prescribing any specific RRT dose for ARF patients, and 75% of responders did not monitor the RRT-delivered dose. In fact, although a clear understanding of the adequate dose of RRT has not yet been achieved, it is also true that, as is true for antibiotic blood levels during severe infections, adequate prescription should be followed by adequate administration. The differences between delivered and prescribed dose in patients with ARF undergoing IHD were analyzed by Evanson et al. (29). The authors found that high patient weight, male gender, and low blood flow were limiting factors affecting RRT administration, and that about 70% of dialysis delivered a Kt/V of less than 1.2. A retrospective study by Venkataraman et al. (30) also showed that, similarly, patients received only 67% of prescribed CRRT therapy. Furthermore, the use of the Adequacy Calculator allowed us (17) to strictly monitor treatments during the study period, and an average 10.7% ($p < 0.05$) reduction of therapy delivery was found when compared to the prescribed dose. This delivery reduction was sometimes due to Calculator overestimation and, more often, to an operative treatment time that was shorter than prescribed (during bag substitution, alarms troubleshooting, and filter change, CRRT is not administered). Of note in the CVVH dose trial (26), only patients who achieved more than 85% of the prescribed dose were included. To obtain this goal, compensation for interruptions in treatment due to ICU procedures was made by increasing effluent flow rates in the subsequent hours. These observations underline that RRT prescriptions for ARF patients in the ICU should be monitored closely if one wishes to ensure adequate delivery of the prescribed dose.

Practical Aspects

During RRT, clearance depends on circuit blood flow (Qb), hemofiltration (Qf), or dialysis (Qd) flow, solute molecular weights, and hemodialyzer type and size. Qb, as a variable in delivering RRT dose, is mainly dependent on vascular access and the operational characteristics of machines used in the clinical setting. Qf is strictly linked to Qb during convective techniques by filtration fraction. Filtration fraction does not limit Qd, but when the Qd/Qb ratio exceeds 0.3, it can be estimated that dialysate will not be completely saturated by blood-diffusing solutes. The search for specific toxins to be cleared, furthermore, has not been successful despite years of research, and urea and creatinine are generally used as reference solutes to measure renal replacement clearance for renal failure. Although available evidence does not allow the direct correlation of the degree of uremia with outcome in chronic renal disease, in the absence of a specific solute, clearances of urea and creatinine blood levels are used to guide treatment dose. During UF, the driving pressure jams solutes, such as urea and creatinine, against the membrane and into the pores, depending on the membrane-sieving coefficient (SC) for that molecule. SC expresses a dimensionless value, and is estimated by the ratio of the concentration of the solutes in the filtrate divided by that in the plasma water or blood. A SC of 1.0, as is the case for urea and creatinine, demonstrates complete permeability, and a value of 0 reflects complete rejection. Molecular size over approximately 12 kd and filter porosity are the major

TABLE 161.2

GUIDELINES FOR RRT PRESCRIPTION

Clinical variables	Operational variables	Setting
Fluid balance	Net ultrafiltration	A continuous management of negative balance (100–300 mL/h) is preferred in hemodynamically unstable patients. A complete monitoring (CVC, S-G, arterial line, ECG, pulse oximeter) is recommended.
Adequacy and dose	Clearance/modality	2,000–3,000 mL/h K (or 35 mL/kg/h) for CRRT; consider first CVVHDF. If IHD is selected, a prescription of every day for 4 h is recommended. Prescribe a Kt/V >1.2.
Acid-base balance	Solution buffer	Bicarbonate buffered solutions are preferable to lactate buffered solutions in case of lactic acidosis and/or hepatic failure.
Electrolyte	Dialysate/replacement	Consider solutions without K^+ in case of severe hyperkalemia. Accurately manage $MgPO_4$.
Timing	Schedule	Early and intense RRT is suggested.
Protocol	Staff/machine	Well-trained staff should routinely use RRT monitors according to predefined institutional protocols.

CVC, central venous catheter; S-G, Swan-Ganz catheter; ECG, electrocardiogram; CRRT, continuous renal replacement therapy; CVVHDF, continuous venovenous hemodiafiltration; IHD, intermittent hemodialysis.

determinants of SC. The K during convection is measured by the product of Qf times SC. Thus, different from diffusion, there is a linear relationship between K and Qf, SC being the changing variable for different solutes. During diffusion, the linear relationship is lost when Qd exceeds about one third of Qb. As a rough estimate, we can consider that during continuous low-efficiency treatments, the RRT dose is a direct expression of ultrafitrative (Qf) and dialysis (Qd), independent of which solute must be removed from blood. During continuous treatment, it has now been suggested to deliver at least a urea clearance of 2 L/hour, with the clinical evidence that 35 mL/kg/hour may be the best prescription (i.e., about 2.8 L/hour in a 70-kg patient). Other authors suggest a prescription based on patient requirements, in turn based on the urea generation rate and catabolic state of the single patient. It has been shown, however, that during continuous therapy, a clearance less than 2 L/hour will almost definitely be insufficient in an adult critically ill patient. For more exact estimations, simple computations have been shown to adequately estimate clearance (17,31). Tables 161.2 and 161.3 provide details that could be followed each time a RRT prescription is indicated.

TABLE 161.3

EXAMPLE OF A POSSIBLE PRESCRIPTION FOR CONTINUOUS TREATMENT IN A 70-kg PATIENT (V_{UREA}: 42 L) DURING AN IDEAL SESSION OF 24 HOURS (t: 1,440 MINUTES) (NET ULTRAFILTRATION [PATIENT FLUID LOSS] IS CONSIDERED ZERO IN K_{CALC} FOR SIMPLICITY)

	Estimated urea clearance (K_{CALC})	Notes	Value of Q to obtain 35 mL/kg/h	Value of Q to obtain a Kt/V of 1
CVVH postdilution	K_{CALC} = Qrep	Always keep filtration fraction <20% (Qb must be 5 times Qrep)	Qrep: 41 mL/min or 2,450 mL/h	Qrep: 29 mL/min or 1,750 mL/h
CVVH predilution	K_{CALC} = Quf/ [1 + (Qrep/Qb)]	Filtration fraction computation changes (keep <20%)	For a Qb of 200 mL/min, Qrep: 53 mL/min or 3,200 mL/h	For a Qb of 200 mL/min, Qrep: 35 mL/min or 2,100 mL/h
CVVHD	K_{CALC} = Qdo	Keep Qb at least thrice Qdo	Qdo: 41 mL/min or 2,450 mL/h	Qdo: 29 mL/min or 1,750 mL/h
CVVHDF postdilution (50% convective and diffusive K)	K_{CALC} = Qrep + Qdo	Consider notes of both CVVH and CVVHD	Qrep: 20 mL/min + Qdo: 21 mL/min	Qrep: 14 mL/min replacement solution + Qdo: 15 mL/min

CVVH, continuous venovenous hemofiltration; Qrep, replacement solution flow rate; Qb, blood flow rate; Quf, ultrafiltration flow rate (Quf = Qrep + Qnet); CVVHD, continuous venovenous hemodialysis; Qdo, dialysate solution flow rate; CVVHDF, continuous venovenous hemodiafiltration; Qnet, patient's net fluid loss.
Urea volume of distribution V (L): patient's body weight (Kg) × 0.6.
Estimated fractional clearance (Kt/V_{CALC}): K_{CALC} (mL/min) × prescribed treatment time (min)/V (mL).
A quantity of 35 mL/kg/h roughly corresponds to a Kt/V of 1.4. A Kt/V of 1 corresponds to approximately 25 mL/kg/h.
Filtration fraction calculation (postdilution): Qrep/Qb × 100. Filtration fraction calculation (predilution): Qrep/Qb + Qrep × 100.

From Continuous to Intermittent: One Treatment Fits All?

Clearance-based dose quantification methods may not be adequate to compare effectiveness. For example, peritoneal dialysis (PD), traditionally providing less urea clearance per week than IHD, has comparable patient outcomes. Furthermore, when EKRc is used to compare intermittent and continuous therapies, it does not appear to be equivalent in terms of outcome: typically, PD patients have better outcomes with less EKRc than IHD patients (32). When the critical parameter is metabolic control, an acceptable mean blood urea nitrogen level of 60 mg/dL—easily obtainable in a 100-kg patient with a 2 L/hour CVVH in a computer-based simulation—has been shown to be very difficult to reach, even by intensive IHD regimens (31). In addition to the benefits specifically pertaining to the kinetics of solute removal, increased RRT frequency results in decreased ultrafiltration requirements per treatment. The avoidance of volume swings related to rapid ultrafiltration rates may also represent another dimension of dose where comparability is difficult.

Despite the development of new membranes, sophisticated dialysis machinery, tailored dialysate composition, and continuous dialysis therapies, a relationship with the frequency of RRT (continuous versus intermittent) delivery has not been fully established. Most recently, the Surviving Sepsis Campaign guidelines for management of severe sepsis and septic shock (33) concluded that, based on present scientific evidence, continuous RRT should be considered equivalent to IHD for the treatment of ARF. In a large comparative trial randomizing 166 critically ill patients with ARF to either CRRT or IHD, Mehta et al. (34) found that the CRRT population, despite randomization, had significantly greater severity of illness scores. This could, in part, explain why, despite better control of azotemia and a greater likelihood of achieving the desired fluid balance, CRRT had increased mortality. Another more recent smaller trial at the Cleveland Clinic (35) failed to find a difference in outcome between one therapy and another. In recent years, a meta-analysis on this issue has been unable to solve the debate of continuous versus intermittent treatment. A meta-analysis of 13 studies conducted by Kellum et al. (36) concluded that, after the stratification of 1,400 patients according to disease severity, when similar patients were compared, CRRT was associated with a significant decrease in the risk of death. However, when the same data were analyzed the same year by Tonelli et al. (37), no difference in outcome could be detected. Thus, it remains uncertain whether the choice of RRT modality (intermittent or continuous) actually matters to patient outcome. A recent randomized controlled trial comparing IHD and continuous venovenous hemodiafiltration concluded that, provided strict guidelines to improve tolerance and metabolic control are used, almost all patients with ARF as part of their multiorgan dysfunction syndrome can be treated with intermittent hemodialysis (38).

Given the lack of clear outcome data, the community of nephrologist intensivists might then consider compromise solutions. One such solution could be represented by hybrid techniques, which have been given various names such as sustained low-efficiency daily dialysis (SLEDD), prolonged daily intermittent RRT (PDIRRT), extended daily dialysis (EDD), or simply extended dialysis (39–43), depending on variations in schedule and type of solute removal (convective or diffusive). Theoretically speaking, the purpose of such therapy would be the optimization of the advantages offered by either CRRT or IHD, including efficient solute removal with minimum solute disequilibrium, reduced ultrafiltration rate with hemodynamic stability, optimized delivery to a prescribed ratio, low anticoagulant need, diminished cost of therapy delivery, efficiency of resource use, and improved patient mobility. Initial case series have shown the feasibility and high clearances potentially associated with such approaches. A single short-term, single-center trial comparing hybrid therapies to CRRT has shown satisfying results in terms of dose delivery and hemodynamic stability. New technology that can be used in the ICU by nurses to deliver SLEDD with convective components offers further options from a therapeutic, logistic, and cost-effectiveness point of view.

TECHNICAL NOTES

RRT Modalities: Description and Nomenclature

Apart from what evidence-based medicine dictates, continuous therapies are used in 80% of ICUs worldwide, whereas intermittent hemodialysis (17%) and peritoneal dialysis (3%) have less common use (1). In the 1980s, a passionate debate between simple CAVH and complex early CVVH lasted for about 10 years, stimulating the industries to produce increasingly effective machines and monitoring systems. Accurate ultrafiltration control is now obtained by integrated roller volumetric pumps (blood, replacement dialysate, and effluent) and scales. These monitors display pressure measurements of all crucial segments of the circuit (catheter inlet and outlet, filter inlet and outlet, UF and dialysate ports). This information, integrated with adequate alarm systems, has allowed the ICU staff to increase filter efficiency and lengthen circuit patency, with the ability to detect potential sources of clotting, thereby improving patient safety. A complete monitoring of fluid balance is also provided by continuous recording of the history of the last 24 hours of treatment. When an alarm occurs, a "smart" message on the screen suggests the most appropriate intervention required. A complete range of ICU RRT therapeutic modalities includes slow continuous ultrafiltration (SCUF), continuous venovenous hemofiltration (CVVH), continuous venovenous hemodialysis (CVVHD), continuous venovenous hemodiafiltration (CVVHDF), and therapeutic plasma exchange (TPE) described below in detail (Fig. 161.5).

Intermittent Hemodialysis

Intermittent hemodialysis (IHD) is a prevalently diffusive treatment in which blood and dialysate are circulated in countercurrent mode, and generally, a low permeability, cellulose-based membrane is used. Dialysate must be pyrogen-free but not necessarily sterile, since dialysate-blood contact does not occur. The ultrafiltration rate is equal to the scheduled weight loss. This treatment can typically be performed 4 hours three times a week or daily. Our group prefers to start with Qb of 150 to 300 mL/minute; Qd, 300 to 500 mL/minute.

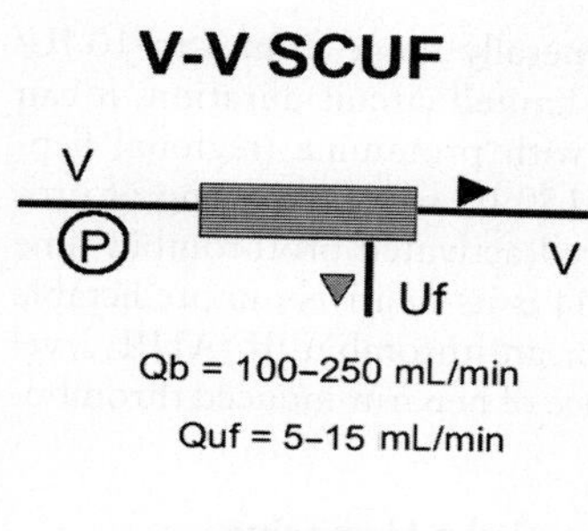

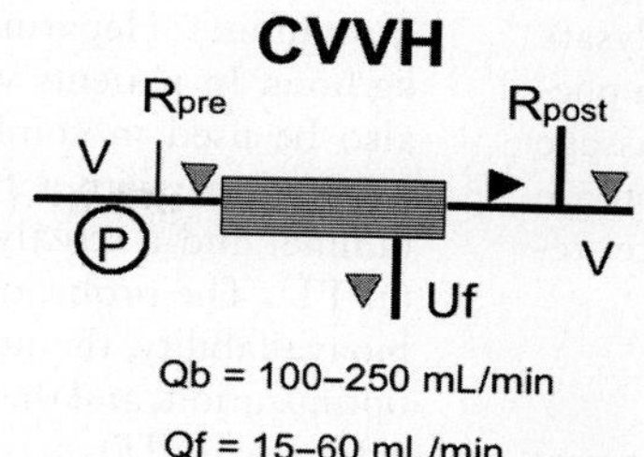

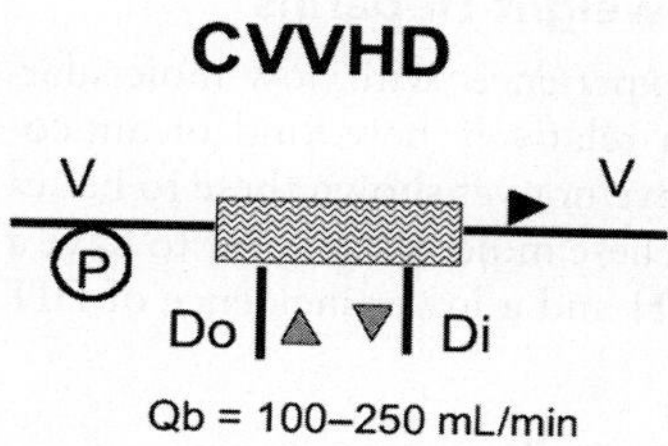

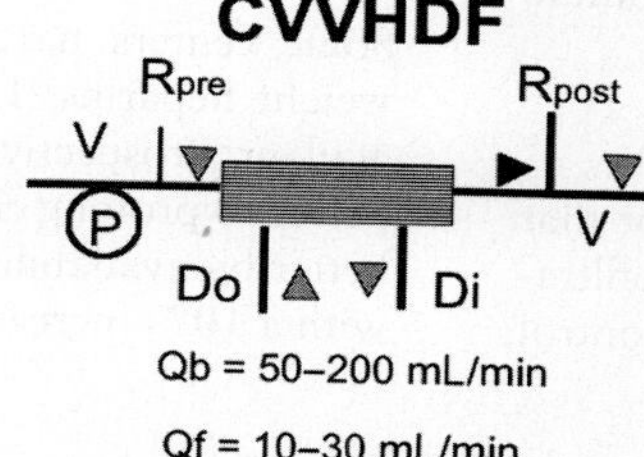

FIGURE 161.5. Schematic representation of the most common continuous renal replacement therapy (RRT) setups. A *black triangle* represents blood flow direction; a *gray triangle* indicates dialysate/replacement solutions flows. CVVH, continuous venovenous hemofiltration; CVVHD, continuous venovenous hemodialysis; CVVHDF, continuous venovenous hemodiafiltration; Di, dialysate in; Do, dialysate out; Qb, blood flow; Qd, dialysate solution flow; Qf, replacement solution flow; Quf, ultrafiltration flow; Rpost, replacement solution postfilter; Rpre, replacement solution prefilter; Uf, ultrafiltration; V-V SCUF, venovenous slow continuous ultrafiltration.

Peritoneal Dialysis

Peritoneal dialysis (PD) is a predominantly diffusive treatment in which blood circulating along the capillaries of the peritoneal membrane is exposed to dialysate. Access is obtained by the insertion of a peritoneal catheter, which allows the abdominal instillation of dialysate. Solute and water movement is achieved by means of variable concentration and tonicity gradients generated by the dialysate. This treatment can be performed continuously or intermittently.

Slow Continuous Ultrafiltration

Slow continuous ultrafiltration (SCUF) is a technique by which blood is driven through a highly permeable filter via an extracorporeal circuit in venovenous mode. The ultrafiltrate produced during membrane transit is not replaced and corresponds to weight loss. It is used only for fluid control in overloaded patients (i.e., congestive heart failure patients who do not respond to diuretic therapy). Our group prefers to start with Qb of 100 to 250 mL/minute; Quf, 5 to 15 mL/minute.

Continuous Venovenous Hemofiltration

Continuous venovenous hemofiltration (CVVH) is a technique by which blood is driven through a highly permeable filter via an extracorporeal circuit in venovenous mode. The ultrafiltrate produced during membrane transit is replaced, in part or completely, to achieve blood purification and volume control. If replacement fluid is delivered after the filter, the technique is defined as *postdilution hemofiltration*. If it is delivered before the filter, the technique is defined as *predilution hemofiltration*. The replacement fluid can also be delivered both prefilter and postfilter. Clearance for all solutes is convective and equals the ultrafiltration rate. Our group prefers to start with Qb of 100 to 250 mL/minute; Quf, 15 to 60 mL/minute.

Continuous Venovenous Hemodialysis

Continuous venovenous hemodialysis (CVVHD) is a technique by which blood is driven through a low-permeability dialyzer via an extracorporeal circuit in venovenous mode, and a countercurrent flow of dialysate is delivered in the dialysate compartment. The ultrafiltrate produced during membrane transit corresponds to the patient's weight loss. Solute clearance is mainly diffusive, and efficiency is limited to small solutes only. Our group prefers to start with Qb of 100 to 250 mL/minute; Qd, 15 to 60 mL/minute.

Continuous Venovenous Hemodiafiltration

Continuous venovenous hemodiafiltration (CVVHDF) is a technique by which blood is driven through a highly permeable dialyzer via an extracorporeal circuit in venovenous mode, and a countercurrent flow of dialysate is delivered in the dialysate compartment. The ultrafiltrate produced during membrane transit is in excess of the patient's desired weight loss. A replacement solution is needed to maintain fluid balance. Solute clearance is both convective and diffusive. Our group prefers to start with Qb of 100 to 250 mL/minute; Qd, 15 to 60 mL/minute; Qf, 15 to 60 mL/minute.

Hemoperfusion

By hemoperfusion (HP), blood is circulated on a bed of coated charcoal powder to remove solutes by adsorption. The technique is specifically indicated in cases of poisoning or intoxication with agents that can be effectively removed by charcoal. This treatment may cause platelet and protein depletion.

Plasmapheresis

Plasmapheresis (PP) is a treatment that uses specific plasmafilters. Molecular-weight cutoff of the membrane is much higher than that of hemofilters (100,000 to 1,000,000 kd); plasma as a whole is filtered and blood is reconstituted by the infusion of plasma products such as frozen plasma or albumin. This technique is performed to remove proteins or protein-bound solutes.

High-flux Dialysis

High-flux dialysis (HFD) is a treatment that uses highly permeable membranes in conjunction with an ultrafiltration control system. Due to the characteristics of the membrane, ultrafiltration occurs in the proximal part of the filter that is counterbalanced by positive pressure applied to the dialysate compartment. This causes, in the distal part of the filter, a phenomenon called *backfiltration*, which is the convective passage of the dialysate into the blood. Diffusion and convection are combined, but due to the use of a pyrogenfree dialysate, replacement is avoided.

High-volume Hemofiltration

High-volume hemofiltration (HVHF) is a treatment that uses highly permeable membranes and hemofiltration with a high volume setting. Our suggested settings are Qb >200 mL/minute and Qf >45 mL/kg/hour (44).

High-permeability Hemofiltration

High-permeability hemofiltration (HPHF) is a treatment that uses high-cutoff (60 kd) permeable membranes and hemofiltration. High treatment flows are not necessary, but strict control of bigger molecules, like albumin, is recommended (45).

Anticoagulation

The need for anticoagulation of the CRRT circuit arises from the fact that the contact between blood and the tubing of the circuit and the membrane of the filter induces activation of the coagulation cascade. This extracorporeal activation inevitably results in filter or circuit clotting. It is evident that the anticoagulation strategy will change depending on the prescribed RRT schedule, being a priority feature of continuous treatments where blood–artificial surface interaction is maximized. The aims of anticoagulation are as follows: maintenance of extracorporeal circuit and dialyzer patency; reduction of off-treatment time (downtime) that could have a clinical impact on the overall RRT clearance; reduction of treatment cost by the use of as little material as possible; and achievement of the above aims with minimal risk for the patient. This last concept should perhaps be the first to rule anticoagulation management: under no circumstances should the patient be put at risk of bleeding to prolong circuit life.

Circuit Setup Optimization and No Anticoagulation

Several technical features of the RRT circuit are likely to affect the success of any anticoagulant approach. Vascular access must be of adequate size; tubing kinking should be avoided; blood flow rate should exceed 100 mL/minute; pump flow fluctuations must be prevented (in modern machines this event is mainly due to increased circuit resistances rather than flow rate inaccuracies); and venous bubble trap, where air/blood contact occurs, must be accurately monitored. Another component of circuit setup has to be addressed: the plasma filtration fraction should be kept as far as possible below 20%, and when possible or considered correct, predilutional hemofiltration should be selected. There is evidence that, when setup is perfectly optimized, anticoagulants are only a relatively minor component of circuit patency; in fact, whenever the patient's clinical features present risk factors for bleeding (prolonged clotting times, thrombocytopenia), RRT can be safely performed without the use of any anticoagulant (46).

Unfractionated Heparin

Unfractionated heparin (UFH) is a commonly available anticoagulant. It is easy to use, and an antidote is available (protamine). Heparin doses generally range from 5 to 10 IU/kg/hour. In patients with very limited circuit duration, it can also be used in combination with protamine (regional heparinization), with a 1:1 ratio (150 IU of UFH per mg of protamine) and a strictly monitored activated prothrombin time (aPTT). The problem with UFH is its relatively unpredictable bioavailability, the necessity for antithrombin III (ATIII) level optimization, and the occurrence of heparin-induced thrombocytopenia (HIT).

Low-molecular-weight Heparins

Some centers have gained experience with low-molecular-weight heparins (LMWH)s, a relatively new kind of anticoagulant. Prospective studies have not yet shown these to be superior to prolong circuit life. These molecules appear to have a better bioavailability than UFH and a lower incidence of HIT with a 10% increased cost.

Prostacyclin

Prostacyclin (PGI_2) is a potentially useful drug for RRT anticoagulation, being the most potent inhibitor of platelet aggregation with the shortest half-life. PGI_2 is infused at a dose of 4 to 8 ng/kg/hour, with or without the adjunct of a low dose of UFH. Hypotension may be induced by higher doses of PGI_2. Some studies have demonstrated PGI_2 efficacy, but its high cost and harmful side effects might limit the use of this agent to patients with short circuit duration (47).

Citrate

Citrate provides a form of regional anticoagulation that depends on the ability of citrate to chelate calcium. The chelation of calcium prevents clot formation. Briefly, a calcium-free sodium citrate containing replacement solution and/or dialysate solution is prepared and administered at the appropriate rate to achieve the desired activated PTT (aPTT) (60 to 90 seconds). Calcium chloride is then administered to replace chelated/dialyzed calcium and maintain normocalcemia. This approach is effective in maintaining excellent filter patency and compares favorably with heparin. It also avoids the risk for HIT and does not lead to systemic anticoagulation. The relative drawbacks of this anticoagulation management strategy include the risk for hypocalcemia and metabolic alkalosis, and the use of cumbersome replacement/dialysate fluid preparation (48,49).

Other Strategies

Alternatives to the techniques presented above are listed in Table 161.4 for completeness.

Vascular Access

The fundamental role played by vascular access must be emphasized. In fact, circuit failure is more often due to inadequate vascular access than insufficient anticoagulation. Thus, the optimal dialysis catheter can save the patient from inappropriate increases of the anticoagulation dose. Venovenous RRT relies on the use of a temporary double-lumen catheter. Such catheters are inserted in a central vein and available in different brands, shapes, and sizes (Fig. 161.6). The site of insertion of double-lumen catheters implies several considerations (clinician expertise, body habitus of the patient, the presence of

TABLE 161.4

ANTICOAGULATION STRATEGIES

Drug	PRO	CON
No anticoagulation	High risk of bleeding in patients	Relatively shorter circuit life span
Unfractionated heparin	Routine	HIT
Low-molecular-weight heparin	Routine (alternative to UH)	HIT
Prostacyclin	Very short circuit life span	Hypotension
Citrate	Routine/very short circuit life span	Hypocalcemia
Danaparoid	HIT	Insufficient data available
Argatroban	HIT	Insufficient data available
Irudine	HIT	Insufficient data available
Nafamostat mesilate	HIT	Insufficient data available
Heparin-coated circuits	Routine	Insufficient data available

HIT, heparin-induced thrombocytopenia; UH, unfractionated heparin.

other intravenous catheters). The femoral vein is generally the first choice of vascular access; internal jugular or subclavian accesses are often associated with inadequate performance, and the inguinal puncture is safer and easier to perform in coagulopathic critically ill patients. A valid alternative may be achieved by cannulation of the right jugular internal vein with the tip of the catheter reaching the right atrium; circuit blood flow rates with this approach can reach 300 mL/minute. Catheter sizes for adult patients range from 12 to 14 French and length from 16 to 25 cm; the bigger and shorter the catheter, the higher the performance. Nonetheless, when the femoral vein is selected, a 20-cm-long catheter has its tip positioned close to the inferior vena cava, allowing optimal flows within the circuit. When an inadequate blood flow or a catheter malfunction is suspected, venous

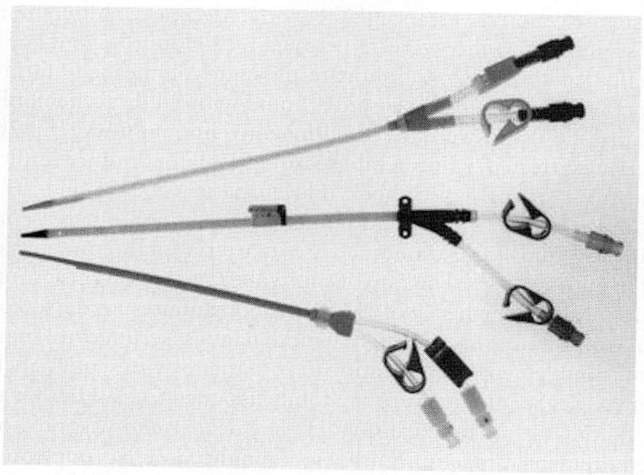

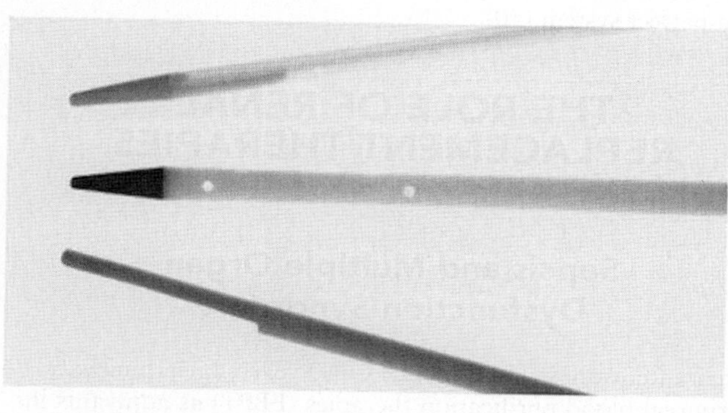

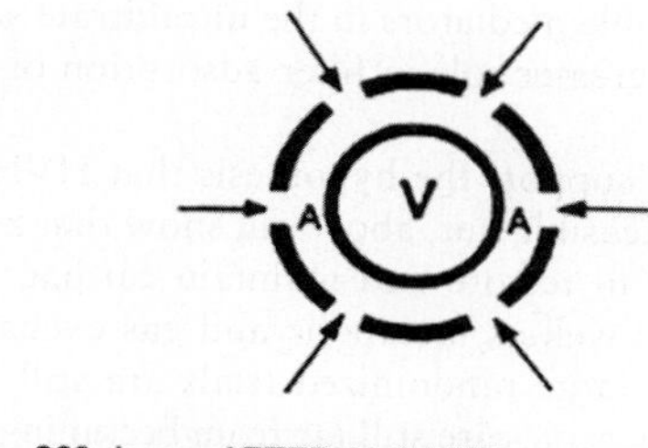

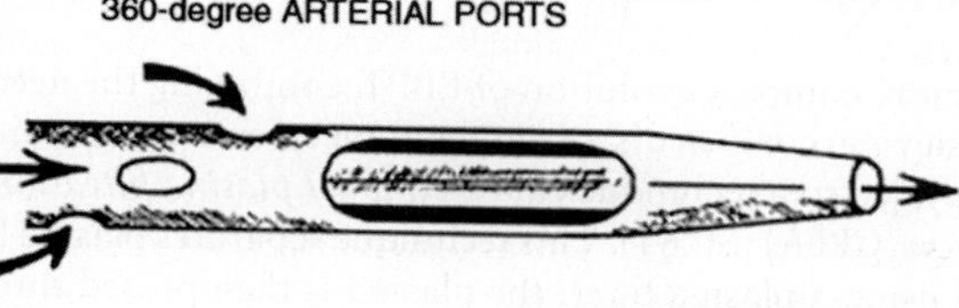

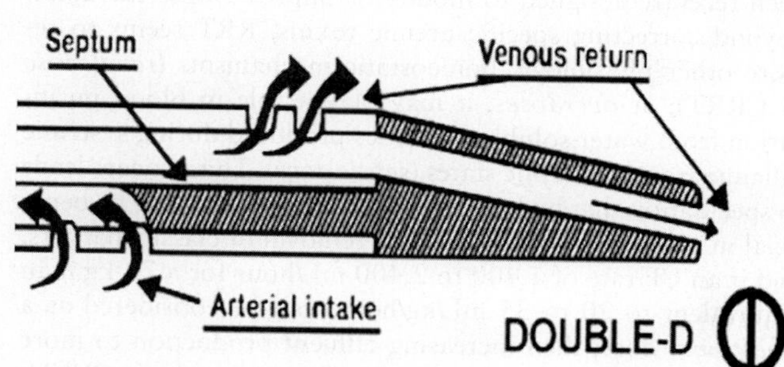

FIGURE 161.6. Representation of some double-lumen catheter shapes and details of blood intake and outflow on their tips

and arterial lumens should be flushed with saline, with the goal of testing resistance to injection and aspiration. Limb clotting of the line versus kinking due to the patient's position must be distinguished. In the first case, a switching of arterial and venous limb can be attempted. This maneuver increases circuit recirculation, but clinical consequences are negligible. In the second case, a heparin or urokinase lock can be tried for a few hours. Another approach is a catheter (guidewire) exchange.

Perspective for the Future

The ideal RRT machine for the future should self-set the right RRT technique, modality, and prescription after the clinician has provided all the information for the specific patient. Monitors and materials of the future will further increase ease of use, safety measures, and the accuracy of each component of the integrated system, reducing the labor involved. The minimal safety standards should allow operators to manually control circuit pressure, de-aerate the chamber and/or bubble sensor and integrated ultrafiltration, with the possibility of consulting/saving the history of treatment settings, events, and pressure trends. However, when described features and alarms are manipulated by human operators, the opportunity for errors will always be present. Physicians and nurses involved in the prescription and delivery of RRT should have precise protocols and defined procedure checkpoints to prevent major clinical problems. Unfortunately, there is no solution to the unwise use of a perfect system (50).

THE ROLE OF RENAL REPLACEMENT THERAPIES IN DIFFERENT SETTINGS

Sepsis and Multiple Organ Dysfunction Syndrome

Great interest has arisen in the last 10 years concerning extracorporeal blood purification therapies (EBPT) as adjuvants in the complex therapy of sepsis and multiple organ dysfunction syndrome (MODS). RRT was the first and still is the most used and effective type of EBPT. Evidence is growing about its ability to maintain homeostatic balance in critically ill patients—specifically, septic patients with MODS. Clinical trials have been recently designed to modify or improve these therapies. Beyond correcting specific uremic toxins, RRT seems to restore other physiologic homeostatic mechanisms (*renal dose* of CRRT); at *overdoses*, it may play a role in blood purification from water-soluble cytokines produced during systemic inflammatory and septic states (*sepsis dose*). This concept leads to speculation that higher-volume hemofiltration may be beneficial in septic patients beyond the removal of classic markers, and if an UF rate of 1,400 to 2,400 mL/hour for a 70-kg man (equivalent to 20 to 35 mL/kg/hour) can be considered as a *traditional dose*, then increasing effluent production to more than 45 mL/kg/hour can be considered as high-volume CVVH. Based on this speculation, a further increase in UF has been suggested, and high-volume hemofiltration (HVHF) protocols have been developed by several authors. Unlike with purely continuous therapies, one of the main challenges of HVHF is the technical limit of currently available machines (UF ranges from 4 L/hour to 9 or 10 L/hour), so that sessions are often intermittent or interrupted by traditional CVVH after 2 to 8 hours. Animal models of severe sepsis (51–53) clearly demonstrated a beneficial effect of HVHF on hemodynamics, proportional to the intensity of ultrafiltration. These experiments have triggered great interest in HVHF as a potential "ideal model of therapy to be started when endotoxemia is present or suspected, or even before it occurs" (53). In the experimental setting, the UF rate is increased up to a level equivalent to 12 L/hour in a 70-kg human being. Journois et al. (54) conducted a randomized controlled study of zero-balanced HVHF in 20 children (UF rate equivalent to 7 to 9 L/hour in a 70-kg adult) undergoing cardiac surgery and demonstrated a significant reduction in postoperative blood loss, time to extubation, and improvements in alveolar-arterial oxygen gradient. The first reports of application of HVHF to the treatment of septic shock in humans with MODS have appeared recently. Lonnemann (55) demonstrated a beneficial effect on macrophage function with restoration of the ability to produce tumor necrosis factor-α (TNF-α) in response to endotoxin exposure, showing the potential of EBPT for immunomodulation at a cellular and humoral level in sepsis. Oudemans-van Straaten et al. (56) conducted a prospective cohort analysis in 306 patients who received HVHF at a mean UF rate of 4 L/hour. They found an improvement in cardiac index (CI), blood pressure (BP), and stroke volume (SV) in hypodynamic patients, and increase in systemic venous resistance (SVR) with a decrease in dopamine dose in those who were hyperdynamic. Honore et al. (57) evaluated the effects of short-term, high-volume hemofiltration (STHVH). Sessions lasted 4 hours with 9 L/hour hemofiltration flow and were followed by conventional CVVH in 20 patients affected by intractable cardiocirculatory failure resulting from severe septic shock. Eleven patients ("responders") attained all therapeutic end points (increase in CI; increase in mixed venous saturation; increase in arterial pH; reduction in epinephrine dose). The rate of survival to 28 days in this group was markedly higher (9 of 11) than among nonresponders (0 of 9). Cole et al. (58) measured hemodynamics, serum cytokines, and complement concentration in 11 patients with septic shock and MODS. Patients were randomly assigned to HVHF (8 h at 6 L/hour) or to standard CVVH. The decrease in vasopressor requirement was significantly higher in the HVHF group. Cole et al. also noted that in the HVHF group, the concentration of the measured soluble mediators in the ultrafiltrate was negligible, indicating a greater role in filter adsorption of studied mediators.

All of these data support the hypothesis that HVHF techniques are safe and feasible but, above all, show that adequate blood purification can restore and maintain cardiac and circulatory function as well as metabolic and gas exchange parameters. However, large randomized trials are still lacking, and these types of therapies are still far from becoming routine (59).

A more complex evolution of EBPT, combining the need for high sieving coefficients of larger molecules and continuous therapy, led to a technique called *coupled plasma filtration adsorption* (CPFA) (60,61). This technique separates plasma from blood using a plasma filter; the plasma is then passed through a synthetic resin cartridge and returned to the blood. A second blood filter is used to remove excess fluid and low-molecular-weight toxins. The resin was chosen based on its adsorption capacity for important inflammatory mediators, low levels of extractable toxins, and good pressure flow performance. In a randomized clinical trial, the adsorbent removed almost 100% of TNF-α and interleukin-β (IL-β), allowing a significant reduction of vasopressor dosage when compared to CVVH alone.

Congestive Heart Failure

Fluid overload may occur in patients with congestive heart failure. Under normal conditions, this is treated with inotropic support and diuretics. However, when diuretics fail, fluid removal becomes uncontrolled, and other therapeutic options must be undertaken. Extracorporeal ultrafiltration is a possible solution to restore the status of fluid balance close to normal. Several new technologies have made ultrafiltration available today in all centers and are easy to institute. Acute isolated schedules of ultrafiltration may, however, be too aggressive and could result in severe hemodynamic instability. For this reason, continuous extracorporeal techniques have been applied in such patients, and the therapy is generally carried out with success. Excellent hemodynamic stability, a good cardiovascular response, and, often, diuresis restoration are the most common effects encountered using continuous forms of extracorporeal fluid removal.

One specific comment must be made concerning the difference between CVVH and all other techniques, including dialysis and the use of diuretics. In all pharmacologic and dialytic techniques, the removal of sodium and water cannot be dissociated, and the mechanisms are strictly correlated. In particular, the diuretic effect is based on a remarkable natriuresis, while ultrafiltration during dialysis may result in hypotonia or hypertonia, depending on the interference with diffusion and removal of other molecules such as urea and other electrolytes. In such circumstances, water removal is linked to other solutes in proportions that are dependent on the technique used. In SCUF, the mechanism of ultrafiltration produces a fluid that is substantially similar to plasma water except for a minimal interference due to Donnan effects. In such a technique, ultrafiltration is basically iso-osmotic and isonatremic, and water and sodium removal cannot be dissociated, with sodium elimination linked to the sodium plasma water concentration. In CVVH and hemofiltration in general, the ultrafiltrate composition is definitely similar to plasma water, but the sodium balance can be significantly affected by the sodium concentration in the replacement solution. Sodium removal can be dissociated from water removal in CVVH, thus obtaining a real manipulation of the sodium pool in the body. This effect cannot be achieved with any other technique. The advantage is that not only plasma concentrations can be normalized but also the electrolyte content in the extracellular—and possibly intracellular—volume (62).

Contrast-induced Nephropathy

Radiocontrast-induced nephropathy (RCIN) causes acute kidney injury and increases mortality. Several studies have examined the capacity of various forms of extracorporeal blood purification therapies for the prevention of RCIN, with conflicting results. A recent systematic review of published trials to determine whether periprocedural extracorporeal blood purification prevents RCIN revealed that the incidence of RCIN, defined as an increase in serum creatinine concentration (>0.5 mg/dL [>44 mmol/L]), was 35.2% in the standard medical therapy group and 27.8% in the extracorporeal blood purification group. Extracorporeal blood purification did not decrease the incidence of RCIN significantly as compared with standard medical therapy (risk ratio, 0.97; 95% confidence interval, 0.44–2.14); however, the patients' heterogeneity was high. Limiting analysis to only randomized trials did not eliminate heterogeneity, but limiting analysis to only hemodialysis trials did. Periprocedural hemodialysis did not decrease the incidence of RCIN (63).

RRT for Children

There are some important differences in the RRT indications, methods, and prescription between children and adult patients; nevertheless, the technique is essentially the same. The main indication is the correction of water overload; different from the adult setting, where solute control may play a key role, it has been shown that restoring adequate water content in small children is the main independent variable for outcome prediction (64,65). This concept is much more important in critically ill, smaller children, in whom a relatively larger amount of fluid must be administered to deliver an adequate amount of drug infusion, parenteral/enteral nutrition, blood derivates, and so on. Corrections of acid-base imbalance and electrolyte disorders are also strong indications for RRT prescription in children. Catheter size ranges from 6.5 French (10 cm long) for patients weighing less than 10 kg to 8 French (15 cm long) for patients weighing 11 to 15 kg. Blood priming may be indicated if more than 8 mL/kg of patient's blood volume are necessary to fill a RRT circuit. Full anticoagulation must always be maintained to avoid excessive blood loss in case of circuit clotting. Predilution hemofiltration is generally the preferred modality and is delivered in a continuous fashion. Fluid balance requires strict monitoring and highest accuracy due to the risk of excessive patient dehydration. Prescription of RRT clearance should be titrated based on the patient body surface area, an approach that will usually lead to relatively higher doses for small children with respect to adult patients when considered per kilogram (66). Critically ill children weighing below 10 kg and neonates with ARF are often treated with peritoneal dialysis (PD); this discussion goes beyond the scope of this chapter. An important exception to this general approach is the case of children with ARF during an extracorporeal membrane oxygenation treatment (ECMO). In this case, the RRT circuit is placed in parallel to the ECMO circuit, and it is possible to let a significant blood flow run into the filter even in the smallest patients.

SUMMARY

The mechanisms involved in RRT are founded on the principle of water and solute transport according to two fundamental mechanisms: diffusion and convection. These mechanisms can be applied to clinical practice as different techniques (intermittent, extended, or continuous RRT) and modalities (hemofiltration, hemodialysis, hemodiafiltration, plasmafiltration, hemoperfusion, coupled plasmafiltration and adsorption). A precise understanding of technical and clinical implications of such therapies seems important in deriving a correct RRT prescription since, so far, no consensus exists about which modality should be administered to critically ill patients with ARF. Different RRT prescriptions, modalities, and schedules can be administered to critically ill patients with acute kidney injury. Clinical effects on critically ill patients depend on the selected RRT strategy and on the severity/complexity of the patient's clinical picture. Modern versatile machines and flexible operative prescriptions allow the operators to range from highly intermittent high-efficiency therapies to slow continuous hemofiltration, depending on the patient's hemodynamic stability, fluid balance needs, acid-base balance, and electrolyte derangements. A specific dose of RRT has not been adopted in clinical practice; a standard dose prescription and strict control of the delivered dose should be monitored if one wishes to ensure the adequate delivery of a prescribed dose. The best evidence to date supports a renal replacement therapy dose of at least 35 mL/kg/hour—spKt/V of 1.4—for CVVH, CVVHDF, or daily IHD.

ACKNOWLEDGMENTS

Dr. Zaccaria Ricci wishes to thank Dr. Stefano De Paulis from the Cardiac Surgery Department of Cardiovascular Medicine, Division of Cardiac Anesthesia and Intensive Care, Policlinico Gemelli, Università Cattolica del Sacro Cuore, Rome, Italy, for his highly valued critical revision of the manuscript.

References

1. Uchino S, Kellum JA, Bellomo R, et al., for the Beginning and Ending Supportive Therapy for the Kidney (BEST Kidney) Investigators. Acute renal failure in critically ill patients: a multinational, multicenter study. *JAMA.* 2005; 294:813–818.
2. Bellomo R. The epidemiology of acute renal failure: 1975 versus 2005. *Curr Op Crit Care.* 2006;12:557–560.
3. Bagshaw SM, Laupland KB, Doig CJ, et al. Prognosis for long-term survival and renal recovery in critically ill patients with severe acute renal failure: a population-based study. *Crit Care.* 2005,9:R700–R709.
4. Kramer P, Wigger W, Rieger J, et al. Arteriovenous haemofiltration: a new simple method for treatment of overhydrated patients resistant to diuretics [in German]. *Klin Wochenschr.* 1977;55:1121–1122.
5. Burchardi H. Renal replacement therapy in the ICU: criteria for initiating RRT. *Contrib Nephrol.* 2001;132:171–180.
6. Bellomo R, Ronco C, Kellum JA, et al., and the ADQI workgroup. Acute renal failure—definition, outcome measures, animal models, fluid therapy and information technology needs: the Second International Consensus Conference of the Acute Dialysis Quality Initiative (ADQI) Group. *Crit Care.* 2004; 8:R204–R212.
7. Hoste EAJ, Kellum JA. Acute kidney injury: epidemiology and diagnostic criteria. *Curr Op Crit Care.* 2006;12:531–537.
8. Ronco C, Bellomo R. Principles of solute clearance during continuous renal replacement therapy. In: *Critical Care Nephrology.* Philadelphia, PA: Kluwer Academic Publishers; 1213–1223.
9. Cole L, Bellomo R, Davenport P, et al. Cytokine removal during continuous renal replacement therapy: an ex vivo comparison of convection and diffusion. *Int J Artif Organs.* 2004;27(5):388–397.
10. Ricci Z, Ronco C, Bachetoni A, et al. Solute removal during continuous renal replacement therapy in critically ill patients: convection versus diffusion. *Crit Care.* 2006;10:R67.
11. Owen W, Lew N, Liu Y, et al. The urea reduction ratio and serum albumin concentrations as predictors of mortality in patients undergoing hemodialysis. *N Engl J Med.* 1993;329:1001–1006.
12. Collins AJ, Ma JZ, Umen A, et al. Urea index and other predictors of long term outcome in hemodialysis patient survival. *Am J Kidney Dis.* 1994;23: 272–282.
13. Hakim R, Breyer J, Ismail N, et al. Effects of dose of dialysis on morbidity and mortality. *Am J Kidney Dis.* 1994;23:661–669.
14. Parker T, Hushni L, Huang W, et al. Survival of hemodialysis patients in the United States is improved with a greater quantity of dialysis. *Am J Kidney Dis.* 1994;23:670–680.
15. Eknoyan G, Levin N. NKF-K/DOQI clinical practice guidelines: update 2000. *Am J Kidney Dis.* 2001;38:917.
16. Arabed G, Knoyan E, Erald G, et al. Effect of dialysis dose and membrane flux in maintenance hemodialysis. *N Engl J Med.* 2002;347:2010–2019.
17. Ricci Z, Salvatori G, Bonello M, et al. In vivo validation of the adequacy calculator for continuous renal replacement therapies. *Crit Care.* 2005;9:R266–R273.
18. Pisitkun T, Tiranathanagul K, Poulin S, et al. A practical tool for determining the adequacy of renal replacement therapy in acute renal failure patients. *Contrib Nephrol.* 2004,144:329–349.
19. Gotch FA. Daily dialysis is a complex therapy with unproven benefits. *Blood Purif.* 2001;19:211–216.
20. Casino FG, Lopez T. The equivalent renal clearance: a new parameter to assess dialysis dose. *Nephol Dial Transplant.* 1996;11:1574–1581.
21. Gotch FA. The current place of urea kinetic modelling with respect to different dialysis modalities. *Nephrol Dial Transplant.* 1998;13(Suppl 6):10–14.
22. Himmelfarb J, Evanson J, Hakim RM, et al. Urea volume of distribution exceeds total body water in patients with acute renal failure. *Kidney Int.* 2002; 61:317–323.
23. Brause M, Neumann A, Schumacher T, et al. Effect of filtration volume of continuous venovenous hemofiltration in the treatment of patients with acute renal failure in intensive care units. *Crit Care Med.* 2003;31:841–846.
24. Paganini EP, Tapolyai M, Goormastic M, et al. Establishing a dialysis therapy/patient outcome link in intensive care unit/acute dialysis for patients with acute renal failure. *Am J Kidney Dis.* 1996;28(Suppl 3):S81–S89.
25. Schiffl H, Lang SM, Fischer R. Daily hemodialysis and the outcome of acute renal failure. *N Engl J Med.* 2002;346:305–310.
26. Ronco C, Bellomo R, Homel P, et al. Effects of different doses in continuous veno-venous haemofiltration on outcomes of acute renal failure: a prospective randomised trial. *Lancet.* 2000;356:26–30.
27. Bouman C, Oudemans-van Straaten H, Tijssen J, et al. Effects of early high-volume continuous veno-venous hemofiltration on survival and recovery of renal function in intensive care patients with acute renal failure: a prospective randomized trial. *Crit Care Med.* 2002;30:2205–2211.
28. Ricci Z, Ronco C, D'amico G, et al. Practice patterns in the management of acute renal failure in the critically ill patient: an international survey. *Nephrol Dial Transplant.* 2006;21(3):690–696.
29. Evanson JA, Himmelfarb J, Wingard R, et al. Prescribed versus delivered dialysis in acute renal failure patients. *Am J Kidney Dis.* 1998;32:731–738.
30. Venkataraman R, Kellum JA, Palevsky P. Dosing patterns for CRRT at a large academic medical center in the United States. *J Crit Care.* 2002;17:246–250.
31. Clark WR, Mueller BA, Kraus MA, et al. Renal replacement quantification in acute renal failure. *Nephrol Dial Transplant.* 1998;13(Suppl 6):86–90.
32. Depner TA. Benefits of more frequent dialysis: lower TAC at the same Kt/V. *Nephrol Dial Transplant.* 1998;13(Suppl 6):20–24.
33. Dellinger RP, Carlet JM, Masur H, et al. Surviving Sepsis Campaign guidelines for management of severe sepsis and septic shock. *Crit Care Med* 2004; 32:858–873.
34. Mehta RL, McDonald B, Gabbai FB, et al. A randomized clinical trial of continuous versus intermittent dialysis for acute renal failure. *Kidney Int.* 2001;60:1154–1163.
35. Augustine JJ, Sandy D, Seifert TH, et al. A randomized controlled trial comparing intermittent with continuous dialysis in patients with ARF. *Am J Kidney Dis.* 2004;44:1000–1007.
36. Kellum J, Angus DC, Johnson JP, et al. Continuous versus intermittent renal replacement therapy: a meta-analysis. *Intensive Care Med.* 2002;28:29–37.
37. Tonelli M, Manns B, Feller-Kopman D. Acute renal failure in the intensive care unit: a systematic review of the impact of dialytic modality on mortality and renal recovery. *Am J Kidney Dis.* 2002;40:875–885.
38. Vinsonneau C, Camus C, Combes A, et al., for the Hemodiafe Study Group. Continuous venovenous haemodiafiltration versus intermittent haemodialysis for acute renal failure in patients with multiple-organ dysfunction syndrome: a multicentre randomised trial. *Lancet.* 2006;368:379–385.
39. Butler R, Keenan SP, Inman KJ, et al. Is there a preferred technique for weaning the difficult-to-wean patient? A systematic review of the literature. *Crit Care Med.* 1999;27:2331–2336.
40. Marshall MR, Golper TA, Shaver MJ, et al. Urea kinetics during sustained low efficiency dialysis in critically ill patients requiring renal replacement therapy. *Am J Kidney Dis.* 2002;39:556–570.
41. Naka T, Baldwin I, Bellomo R, et al. Prolonged daily intermittent renal replacement therapy in ICU patients by ICU nurses and ICU physicians. *Int J Artif Organs.* 2004;27:380–387.
42. Kumar VA, Craig M, Depner T, et al. Extended daily dialysis: a new approach to renal replacement for acute renal failure in the intensive care tnit. *Am J Kidney Dis.* 2000;36:294–300.
43. Kielstein JT, Kretschmer U, Ernst T, et al. Efficacy and cardiovascular tolerability of extended dialysis in critically ill patients: a randomized controlled study. *Am J Kidney Dis.* 2004;43:342–349.
44. Bellomo R, Baldwin I, Ronco C. High volume vemofiltration. *Contrib Nephrol.* 2001;132:375–382.

45. Morgera S, Haase M, Kuss T, et al. Pilot study on the effects of high cutoff hemofiltration on the need for norepinephrine in septic patients with acute renal failure. *Crit Care Med.* 2006;34(8):2099–2104.
46. Tan HK, Baldwin I, Bellomo R. Continuous veno-venous hemofiltration without anticoagulation in high-risk patients. *Intensive Care Med.* 2000;26:1652–1657.
47. Fiaccadori E, Maggiore U, Rotelli C, et al. Continuous haemofiltration in acute renal failure with prostacyclin as the sole anti-haemostatic agent. *Intensive Care Med.* 2002;28:586–593.
48. Kutsogiannis DJ, Gibney N, Stollery D, et al. Regional citrate versus systemic heparin anticoagulation for continuous renal replacement in critically ill patients. *Kidney Int.* 2005;67:2361–2367.
49. Monchi M, Berghmans D, Ledoux D, et al. Citrate vs. heparin for anticoagulation in continuous venovenous hemofiltration: a prospective randomized study. *Intensive Care Med.* 2004;30:260–265.
50. Ronco C, Ricci Z, Bellomo R, et al. Management of fluid balance in CRRT: a technical approach. *Int J Artif Organs.* 2005;28(8):765–776.
51. Groodendorst AF. High volume hemofiltration improves haemodynamics of endotoxin-induced shock in the pig. *J Crit Care.* 1992;7:67–75.
52. Rogiers P. Continuous veno-venous hemofiltration improves cardiac performance by mechanism other than tumor necrosis factor alpha attenuation during endotoxic shock. *Crit Care Med.* 1999;27:1848–1855.
53. Bellomo R. The effect of intensive plasma water exchange by hemofiltration on haemodynamics and soluble mediators in canine endotoxemia. *Am J Respir Crit Care. Med.* 2000;161:1429–1436.
54. Journois D, Israel-Biet D, Pouard P, et al. High volume, zero-balanced hemofiltration to reduce delayed inflammatory response to cardiopulmonary bypass in children. *Anesthesiology.* 1996;85:965–976.
55. Lonneman G: Tumor necrosis factor alpha during continuous high-flux hemodialysis in sepsis with acute renal failure. *Kidney Int.* 1999;56:S84–S87.
56. Oudemans-van Straaten HM, Bosman RJ, van der Spoel JI, et al. Outcome of critically ill patients treated with high volume hemofiltration: a prospective cohort analysis. *Intensive Care Med.* 1999;25:814–821.
57. Honore PM, Jamez J, Wauthier M, et al. Prospective evaluation of short-term, high volume isovolemic hemofiltration on the hemodynamic course and outcome in patients with intractable circulatory failure resulting from septic shock. *Crit Care Med.* 2000;28(11):3581–3587.
58. Cole L, Bellomo R, Journois D, et al. High-volume hemofiltration in human septic shock. *Intensive Care Med.* 2001;27:978–986.
59. Cole L, Bellomo R, Hart G, et al. A phase II randomized, controlled trial of continuous hemofiltration in sepsis. *Crit Care Med.* 2002;30:100–106.
60. Ronco C, Brendolan A, Lonnemann G, et al. A pilot study of coupled plasma filtration with adsorption in septic shock. *Crit Care Med.* 2002;30(6):1250–1255.
61. Formica M, Olivieri C, Livigni S, et al. Hemodynamic response to coupled plasmafiltration-adsorption in human septic shock. *Intensive Care Med.* 2003;29:703–708.
62. Ronco C, Ricci Z, Bellomo R, et al. Extracorporeal ultrafiltration for the treatment of overhydration and congestive heart failure. *Cardiology.* 2001;96:155–168.
63. Cruz D, Perazella MA, Bellomo R, et al. Extracorporeal blood purification therapies for prevention of radiocontrast-induced nephropathy: a systematic review. *Am J Kidney Dis.* 2006;48:361–371.
64. Goldstein SL, Currier H, Graf C, et al. Outcome in children receiving continuous veno-venous hemofiltration. *Pediatrics.* 2001;107:1309–1312.
65. Foland JA, Fortenberry JD, Warshaw BL, et al. Fluid overload before continuous hemofiltration and survival in critically ill children: a retrospective analysis. *Crit Care Med.* 2004;32:1771–1776.
66. Brophy PD, Bunchman TE. References and overview for hemofiltration in pediatrics and adolescents. www.pcrrt.com. Accessed August 25, 2006.

CHAPTER 162 ■ ENDOCRINOPATHY IN THE ICU

ADRIEN BOUGLE • DJILLALI ANNANE

During critical illness, the stressors are multiple and include emotional and physical stress such as trauma or infection, and various therapeutic or diagnostic interventions such as surgery, arterial or venous catheterization, laryngeal intubation and mechanical ventilation, and drugs. It is also paramount to recognize that stress is sustained at a certain level of intensity for several days with additive and unpredictable surges. Thus, the host has to adapt to counteract prolonged stress while maintaining ability to adjust to unpredictable surges of stress. The integrity and flexibility of host response to these stressors is essential to survive critical illness.

The development of molecular biology has provided scientists with tools to demonstrate the close interaction between the neuroendocrine and immune system. It is now recognized that the "stress system" has two main components: the corticotropin-releasing hormone/vasopressin neurons of the hypothalamus and the locus ceruleus noradrenaline/autonomic neurons of the brainstem (1). In this chapter, we will summarize recent knowledge on how immune molecules such as interleukin or nitric oxide signal the brain to generate both neurologic and hormonal responses aimed at downgrading the immune system when the inflammatory response is no longer needed. Abbreviations used in this chapter are presented in Table 162.1.

PHYSIOLOGY OF THE ENDOCRINE RESPONSE

Two pathways are used by the organism for interorgan communication. First the central nervous system and its peripheral arms allow rapid communication between different tissues. The endocrine system is made of several organs or tissues distributed throughout the body. All endocrine tissues are directly linked to the pituitary and the hypothalamus. The anatomic organization of the endocrine system highlights its pivotal role in the interorgan communication. After Claude Bernard discovered that glucose is delivered from the liver to the blood, Bayliss and Starling in 1904 identified for the first time that chemical substances can be secreted by one organ (e.g., secretin from the intestinal mucosa) and carried by the bloodstream to act on specific distant tissues. They introduced the term *hormone* to characterize such chemical substances. In the vertebrates, the endocrine organs include anterior and posterior pituitary, ovary and testis, adrenal cortex and medulla, thyroids and parathyroids, islets of Langerhans in the pancreas, and various parts of the intestinal mucosa (Fig. 162.1). The pineal and thymus can also be considered endocrine organs. In addition, many other organs have some endocrine properties. For example, the kidney secretes rennin and angiotensin, and the heart secretes natriuretic factors. The main known hormones are listed in Table 162.2 including the organ from which they are secreted, their carrier in the bloodstream (if any), their target tissues, and main actions. Hormones are divided into steroids (cholesterol-derived proteins), peptides, and amines.

General Organization of the Endocrine System

The pituitary gland (hypophysis) can be considered a pivotal endocrine organ. It is connected to the central nervous system by the pituitary stalk and is divided into two parts: the anterior pituitary (adenohypophysis) as it originates from the Rathke pouch, and the posterior pituitary (neurohypophysis), which is developed from the brain (Fig. 162.2). The anterior pituitary is made up of the *pars distalis* which is richly vascular and has three cell types (chromophobe and two types of chromophil cells), the *pars intermedia* which is the least vascular part and contains only a few cells, and the *pars tuberalis*. The anterior pituitary produces seven hormones: gonadotropic hormones (follicle-stimulating hormones (FSH), luteinizing hormone (LH) and luteotropic hormone (LTH)), thyrotropic (thyroid-stimulating) hormone (TSH), adrenocorticotropic hormone (ACTH), growth hormone (GH), and prolactin (PRL). The posterior pituitary has three parts: the median eminence, infundibular stem, and infundibular process or neural lobe. Its tissues consist of unmyelinated fibers, fusiform cells, neurons, and mast cells. The posterior pituitary produces mainly vasopressin, also called the antidiuretic hormone (ADH). It is obvious from this brief description that the anterior pituitary exerts control of most endocrine organs, and insufficiency of the anterior pituitary results in atrophy of ovary or testis, adrenal cortex, and thyroid.

The thyroid and adrenal cortex have no specific target organ, and the hormones they secrete act broadly to contribute to homeostasis. The gonads also produce hormones that act on tissues in general and on specific target organs (urogenital apparatus). The adrenal medulla secretes adrenalin and noradrenalin, which are released during stressed states enhancing the sympathetic system in a "fight or flight" response. It is possible that the release of these hormones depends on direct sympathetic activation rather than on ACTH stimulation.

TABLE 162.1

ABBREVIATIONS

ACTH	adrenocorticotropic hormone
ADH	antidiuretic hormone
AVP	arginine vasopressin
CO	carbon monoxide
CRH	corticotropin-releasing hormone
FSH	follicle-stimulating hormone
FSHRF	FSH-releasing factor
GABA	gamma-aminobutyric acid
GH	growth hormone
GHRF	GH-releasing factor
GHRH	GH-releasing hormone
GHRP	GH-releasing peptide
GLUT	glucose transporter isoform 4
GNRH	gonadotropin-releasing hormone
HMGB	high mobility group box
IGF	insulinlike growth factor
IL	interleukin
iNOS	inducible nitric oxide synthase
IRR	insulin receptor-related receptor
LH	luteinizing hormone
LHRH	LH-releasing hormone
LTH	luteotrophic hormone
MIF	macrophage migration inhibitory factor
NO	nitric oxide
NTIS	non-thyroidal illness syndrome
PRL	prolactin
T3	tri-iodothyronine
T4	serum thyroxine
Th1	helper T cell 1
Th2	helper T cell 2
TNF	tumor necrosis factor
TRH	thyrotropin-releasing hormone
TSH	thyroid-stimulating hormone

Physiologic Control of the Endocrine System

There is probably no uniform mechanism for the regulation of hormone activity. For example, there is no evidence that parathormone is released from the parathyroid glands on innervating nerve stimulation or action of a specific trophic hormone. This is in contrast to the thyroid, adrenals, and gonads. We will focus on the main hormones involved in response to stress, i.e., steroids, catecholamines, and vasopressin (Fig. 162.3). One has to consider two main mechanisms of regulation of the endocrine activity: feedback loops, and interaction with the central nervous system. Experiments in which peripheral glands are disconnected from the pituitary showed full cessation of gonad function whereas the thyroid and adrenal cortex continue to secrete hormones at a lower level depicting their intrinsic activity. Similarly, the anterior pituitary has an intrinsic activity specific to thyroid and adrenal cortex function.

The feedback mechanisms allow circulating hormones from the target organs as well as from the anterior pituitary to down- or up-regulate the release of hypothalamic molecules. The feedback loop also involves the central nervous structures such as the hippocampus, which contains the highest concentration of glucocorticoid receptors in the central nervous system. This self-balancing system stabilizes the endocrine activity under resting conditions but is insufficient in case of enhanced endocrine activity. In the latter case, the neurologic control is the key regulator of the endocrine activity, and the hypothalamus plays a key role in the regulation of these hormones. First, it is directly connected to the posterior pituitary and the adrenal medulla. Second, it influences the anterior pituitary by releasing in synchronous pulses (approximately hourly) stimulatory or inhibitory hormones in the hypophyseal portal vessels of the pituitary stalk. This hypothalamic influence is demonstrated by dramatic falls in hormone activity when the pituitary gland is disconnected from the hypothalamus.

The hypothalamus is organized into three regions including the lateral, medial, and periventricular hypothalamus with each having distinct morphologic and functional features. The paraventricular nuclei is organized into three cellular divisions: a medial group that produces corticotropin-releasing hormone (CRH) that is released into the hypophyseal portal system; an intermediate group that secretes vasopressin in association with the supraoptic nuclei that is stored in the posterior pituitary gland; and a lateral group that produces CRH and innervates noradrenergic neurons in the brainstem. Hypothalamic-derived peptides that stimulate the pituitary gland include corticotropin-releasing hormone (CRH), LH-releasing hormone (LHRH), FSH-releasing factor (FSHRF), GH-releasing factor (GHRF), prolactin (PRL)-stimulating factor, and thyrotropin-releasing hormone (TRH). Other peptides are inhibiting factors such as GH-inhibiting hormone (somatostatin) and PRL-inhibiting hormone (2). Vasopressin, natriuretic peptides, and catecholamines also influence the pituitary function by direct action on the gland. The effect of CRH on ACTH release by the pituitary is permissive, and vasopressin acts in synergy with CRH. There are tight interconnections between projections of CRH-synthesizing neurons from the parvocellular nuclei to the brainstem, and reciprocally noradrenergic projections originating from the locus coeruleus and ending in the parvocellular reticular nuclei. Thereby, noradrenaline, CRH, and vasopressin can stimulate each other. Through collateral fibers, ultrashort negative feedback loops allow permanent adaptation of the synergy between the two systems. Finally, CRH, vasopressin, and noradrenaline are on the stimulatory control of the serotoninergic, cholinergic, and histaminergic systems, and are inhibited by the gamma-aminobutyric acid, benzodiazepine, and opioids.

POTENTIAL MECHANISMS OF REGULATION OF THE ENDOCRINE ACTIVITY DURING CRITICAL ILLNESS

The Stressors

Critical illness is a condition involving multiple stressors of both emotional and physical types. Critically ill patients are unexpectedly faced with a life-threatening situation and a hostile environment (the intensive care unit). Physical stressors can be classified into disease related (e.g., infection, burns, trauma) and interventions related (e.g., surgery, invasive diagnostic or therapeutic procedures, drugs). The unpredictable nature,

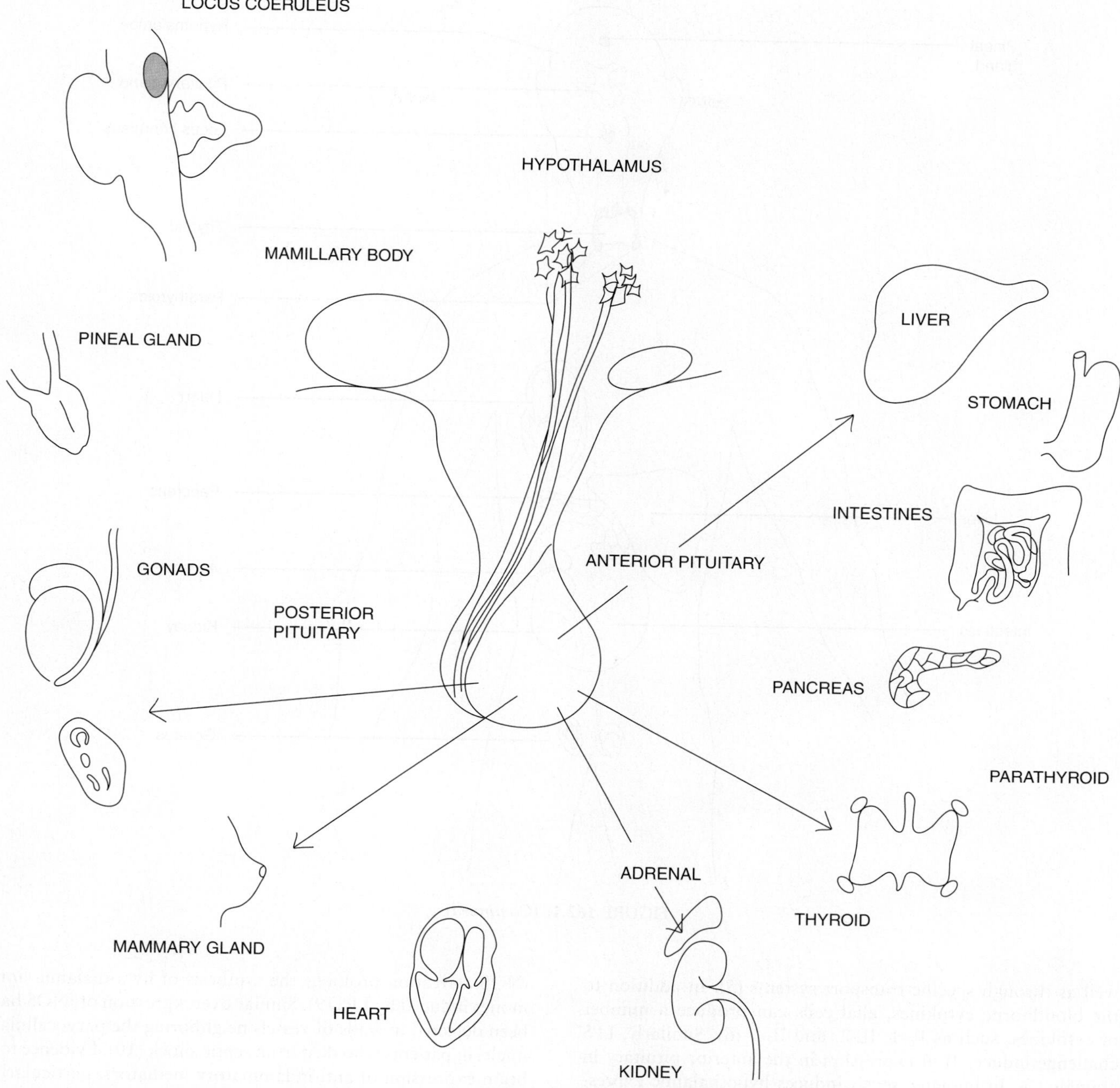

FIGURE 162.1. The endocrine organs are distributed throughout the body. There is an electrochemical connection from the hypothalamus to all organs, controlling body metabolism, growth and development, and reproduction. (*Continued*)

duration, and intensity of the stressors renders the host response more problematic.

Mechanisms of Neuroendocrine Activation in Acute Inflammation

Signals Sent to the Hypothalamic-Pituitary Axis

Acute inflammatory response to insults such as lipopolysaccharide (LPS) include the release of a number of mediators such as tumor necrosis factor alpha (TNF-α), interleukin (IL)-1, IL-6, IL-8, nitric oxide (NO), and the late mediators, macrophage migration-inhibiting factors (MIF), and high mobility group box (HMGB)-1 (3) (Fig. 162.4). These mediators reach the hypophyseal portal capillaries in the median eminence via the anterior hypophyseal arteries. Cytokines can diffuse into the pituitary as these areas are free of blood–brain barrier (4) and be carried to the hypothalamus and the brain areas lacking a blood–brain barrier (organum vasculosum lamina terminalis, subfornical organ, subcommissural organ, area postrema, pineal gland, and probably the plexus choroids), as

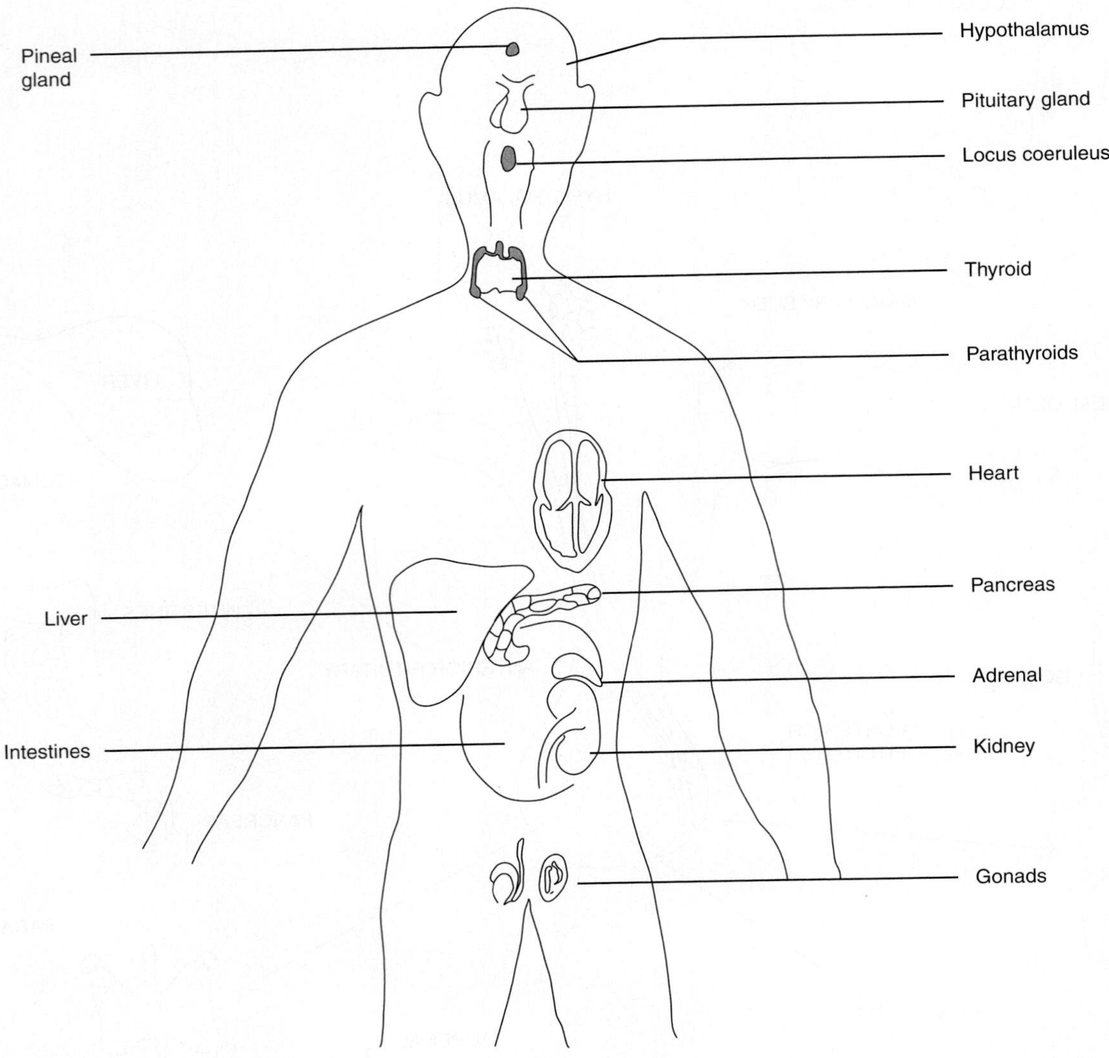

FIGURE 162.1. *(Continued)*

well as through specific transport systems (5). In addition to the bloodborne cytokines, glial cells can produce a number of cytokines, such as IL-1, IL-2, and IL-6 (6). Similarly, LPS challenge induces IL-6 expression in the anterior pituitary in animals (7). In humans, sepsis induces hypothalamic expression of TNF and IL-1β within the parvocellular and supraoptic nuclei (8). Intraperitoneal injection of LPS induces IL-1β followed by inducible NO synthase (iNOS) mRNA within 2 hours, peaking in 4 to 6 hours and then returning to basal values by 24 hours (9). The induction of IL-1β and iNOS occur in the meninges, areas lacking a blood–brain barrier, and also in the parvocellular nuclei and the arcuate nucleus, which contain the hypothalamic-releasing and -inhibiting hormones. Because the latter nuclei are inside the blood–brain barrier, active transport of cytokines is required (5). Alternately, the neurons from the parvocellular and arcuate nuclei may have projections to the median eminence and may express LPS receptors on their surface (9). LPS can also be carried by the cerebrospinal fluid to the third ventricle where it crosses the ependyma or acts on projections from parvocellular neurons. Thus, it is likely that delayed overexpression of NO through iNOS activation prolongs the synthesis of hypothalamic hormones induced by LPS (9). Similar overexpression of iNOS has been detected in walls of vessels neighboring the parvocellular nuclei in patients who died from septic shock (10). Evidence for brain expression of anti-inflammatory mediators, particularly IL-10, IL-13, and IL-1 receptor antagonists in the pituitary and pineal gland, suggest that they antagonize the stimulatory effects of the proinflammatory mediators on the neurohormones (11). In addition, cytokines, via activation of GABAergic neurons, block NO-induced LHRH but not FSH release, inhibit GHRH release, and stimulate somatostatin and prolactin release (9). The regulatory action of NO is mediated by the combined activation of guanylate cyclase, cyclo-oxygenase, and lipoxygenase (12). Cytokines can also directly act on the anterior pituitary, particularly to stimulate ACTH synthesis and release (13).

A second pathway of activation of the hypothalamic-pituitary axis is the neural route. Various afferent neurons of the peripheral system sense the threat at the inflammatory sites and stimulate the noradrenergic system and the hypothalamus (1). Stimulation of vagal afferent fibers by LPS results in

(text continues on page 2418)

TABLE 162.2

LIST OF HORMONES

Hormones	Organ	Carrier in bloodstream	Target tissues	Main actions
Insulin	Pancreas: β cells of the islets of Langerhans	Free	Liver, muscle, fat	Decreases blood glucose level Decreases gluconeogenesis, proteinolysis, lipolysis Increases fatty acid and glycogen synthesis
Glucagon	Pancreas: α cells of the islets of Langerhans	Free	Liver	Increases blood glucose level by increasing glycogenolysis and gluconeogenesis
Somatostatin	Hypothalamus cells and cells of pancreas, intestine, stomach	Free	Pancreas	Suppresses gastrointestinal hormone secretion Inhibits insulin and glucagon secretion Inhibits GH and TSH release
Thrombopoietin	Liver, kidney, striated muscle, stromal cells of the bone marrow	Free	Bone marrow	Regulates the differentiation of megakaryocytes and platelets
Angiotensinogen	Liver	Free	Plasma	Releases aldosterone Causes vasoconstriction
Insulin growth factor	Liver	IGF-binding proteins	Muscle, cartilage, bone, liver, kidney, nerves, skin, and lungs	Regulates cell proliferation and apoptosis
Tri-iodothyronine (T3) Thyroxine (T4) Calcitonin	Thyroid	Thyroxine-binding globulin (TBG 70%) Thyroxine-binding prealbumin (TBPA 10%–15%) Albumin (15%–20%) Free	Whole body Intestines, bone, kidney, central nervous system	Increases metabolic rate Promotes growth Metabolic effects: stimulates carbohydrate metabolism, fat metabolism; decreases cholesterol, phospholipid, and triglyceride plasma levels Prohormone for the active T3 Reduces blood calcium levels Regulates vitamin D and bone mineral metabolism Controls satiety
Adrenocorticotropin hormone (ACTH)	Anterior pituitary	Free	Adrenal cortex	Produces glucocorticoids and mineral corticoids
Luteinizing hormone (LH)		Free	In females, granulosa cells and theca cells In males, Leydig cells of the testis	Reproduction: - In females, triggers ovulation and maintains luteal function during the first 2 weeks of menstruation. - In males, increases testosterone production
Follicle-stimulating hormone (FSH)		Free	In females, graafian cells In males, Sertoli cells of the testes	Reproduction: - In females, initiates follicular growth - In males, enhances androgen-binding protein and acts in the spermatogenesis
Thyroid-stimulating hormone (TSH)		Free	Thyroid gland	Secretes thyroxine (T4) and tri-iodothyronine (T3)

(continued)

TABLE 162.2

(CONTINUED)

Hormones	Organ	Carrier in bloodstream	Target tissues	Main actions
Growth hormone (GH)		Free	Liver, chondrocytes, and whole body	Anabolic hormone: promotes lipolysis, increases protein synthesis, reduces liver uptake of glucose Enables height growth in childhood Increases calcium retention and increases bone mineralization Stimulates the immune system
Prolactin		Free	Mammary glands	Stimulates lactation
Oxytocin	Posterior pituitary	Free	Brain, mammary gland, myometrium, endometrium, kidney, heart	Peripheral actions: - Letdown reflex in lactating - Uterine contraction - Reduces diurese and stimulates sodium excretion - Embryonal development of heart Brain actions: - Sexual arousal - Social behavior - Maternal behavior - Increases trust and reduces fear
Antidiuretic hormone (ADH)		Free	Vessels, liver, pituitary gland, kidney, brain	Peripheral actions: - V1a: vasoconstriction, gluconeogenesis, platelet aggregation and release of factor VIII and von Willebrand factor - V1b: ACTH secretion - V2: water reabsorption in the collecting ducts Brain actions: - memory formation - response to stress
Cortisol	Adrenal cortex	Corticosteroid-binding globulin (CBG 90%) Albumin Free (about 4%)	Liver, vessels, immune system, hippocampus	Metabolic properties: - Enhances hepatic gluconeogenesis and glycogenolysis - Induces peripheral insulin resistance - Induces free-fatty acid and amino-acid release Cardiovascular properties: - Maintains vascular tone - Maintains endothelial and vascular permeability Anti-inflammatory and immunosuppressive actions
Aldosterone		Free	Collecting ducts of the kidney	Reabsorption of sodium and excretion of potassium H^+ secretion

Estrogen	Ovary, placenta	Free	Uterus, coagulation system, liver, gastrointestinal tract	Promotes development of female secondary sex characteristics Regulates the menstrual cycle Causes thickening of the endometrium Promotes lipid metabolism, protein synthesis, fluid balance
Progesterone		Free	Endometrium, vaginal epithelium, brain, smooth muscle, immune system, thyroid, skeleton	Reproduction Neurosteroid: involved in myelinization, synaptic function
Testosterone	Testes of males and ovaries of females	Sex hormone binding globulin (SHBG)	In males,	Anabolic effects: - Growth of muscle mass - Increases bone density and maturation Virilizing effects: - Maturation of sex organs - Development of male secondary sex characteristics
Parathormone	Parathyroid	Free	Skeleton, gastrointestinal tract, kidney	Increases blood calcium concentration in three ways: - Enhances calcium release from the bone - Enhances calcium reabsorption from renal tubules - Enhances calcium absorption in the intestine
Human chorionic gonadotropin (HCG)	Placenta	Free	Uterus	Maintains the corpus luteum and progesterone production during pregnancy
Atrial natriuretic peptide (ANP) Brain natriuretic peptide (BNP)	Atrial myocytes of the heart Cardiac ventricles	Free	Kidney, vessels, adrenal, adipose tissue	Reduces blood volume, central venous pressure, cardiac output, arterial blood pressure Increases renal sodium secretion and excretion Increases lipolysis
Melatonin	Pineal gland, retina, gastrointestinal tract	Free	Brain	Circadian rhythms Antioxidant Immune system: increases T-cell response
Renin	Kidney	Free	Plasma	Activates the renin–angiotensin–aldosterone system by cleaving angiotensinogen to angiotensin 1
Calcitriol	Kidney	Free	Intestinal epithelium	Increases calcium absorption from the gastrointestinal tract

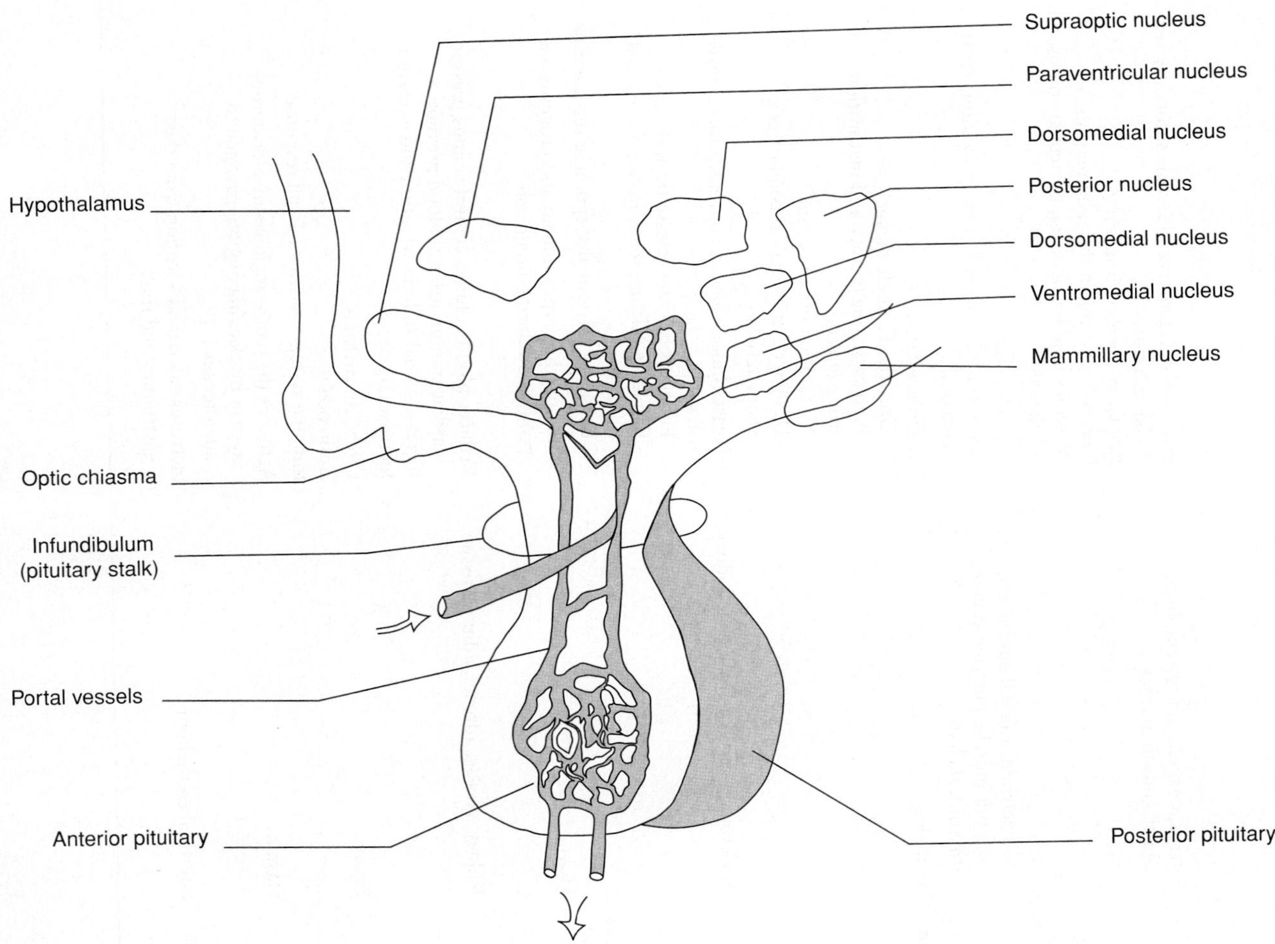

FIGURE 162.2. The hypothalamus lies directly above the pituitary gland. The hypothalamic neurohypophysial tract defines the neuronal system terminating in the posterior pituitary and is best known for its secretion of vasopressin and oxytocin into the peripheral circulation. The pars distalis of the anterior pituitary is supplied by venous blood delivered through the long portal veins that descend along the ventral surface of the pituitary stalk and interconnect capillary beds in the pars distalis with specialized capillary beds of the portal capillary system in the base of the hypothalamus called the *median eminence*. Venous drainage from the anterior pituitary to the systemic circulation is through adenohypophyseal veins.

activation of the locus coeruleus where neurons have projections that synapse on cholinergic interneurons in the parvocellular nucleus (14). It has been shown that CRH is released on acetylcholine stimulation of muscarinic receptors (15), and that this effect is prevented by nonspecific NO antagonists (14). Nitric oxide diffuses in the parvocellular cells and induces the generation of both cyclo-oxygenase and lipoxygenase, which in turn stimulate CRH synthesis (12).

More recently, the role of endogenous gas in the modulation of the hypothalamic pituitary response to stress has been suggested. The effects of carbon monoxide (CO) are inconsistent with data showing that incubation of hypothalamic cells with a CO-enriched milieu resulted in huge release of CRH (16), but another study reported inhibitory effects (17). Carbon monoxide generation was shown to prevent the release of vasopressin from hypothalamic explants (18). Hydrogen sulfide is another endogenous gaseous neuromodulator that was shown both *in vitro* and *in vivo* to inhibit CRH and vasopressin release (19).

Factors Influencing Cytokine-Induced Activation of the Hypothalamic-Pituitary Axis

All cytokines do not exert the same effect on CRH release. IL-1 was the first cytokine that was shown to activate the hypothalamus to release CRH (20). IL-1 injection is associated with a strong and sustained activation of the hypothalamic-pituitary axis, whereas IL-6 and TNF induce weak and transient hypothalamic responses, and IL-2 and interferon alpha have no effect (21). The route of cytokine administration also influences their stimulatory effects on the hypothalamus. IL-1 given intravenously increased ACTH and corticosterone in plasma within 15 minutes and the effect lasted 1 hour (22), whereas when given intraperitoneally, ACTH and corticosterone increased within 30 minutes and peaked after 2 hours (20). Cyclo-oxygenase inhibitors prevented hypothalamic response to intravenous IL-1 challenge but prevented only the early response to intraperitoneal IL-1 challenge, suggesting a biphasic response to IL-1 (20,23). Cyclo-oxygenase inhibitors

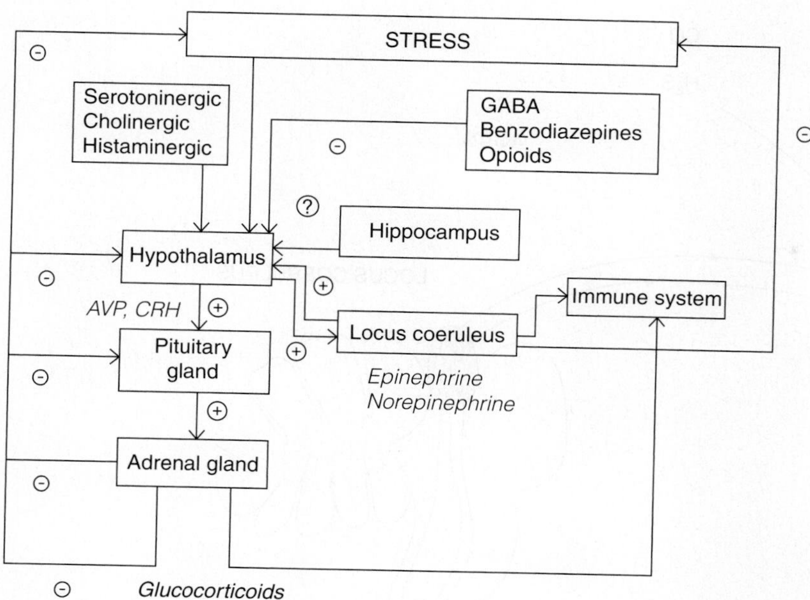

FIGURE 162.3. Integrative approach of the endocrine system. AVP, arginine vasopressin; CRH, corticotropin-releasing hormone; GABA, gamma-aminobutyric acid.

also attenuated hypothalamic response to TNF but not to IL-6 (21). The noradrenergic system, mainly substance P, neuropeptides Y, or galanin, modulate the hypothalamic response to IL-1 whereas the serotoninergic system has no effect (24).

PATTERNS OF ENDOCRINE ACTIVITY DURING CRITICAL ILLNESS

Infection, LPS challenge, major surgery, trauma, or burns elicit very similar patterns of pituitary hormone secretion. Plasma ACTH and prolactin increase within a few minutes following the insult and are associated with a rapid inhibition of LH and TSH but not FSH. Growth hormone secretion is also stimulated in humans but inhibited in rats (13).

Hypothalamic-Pituitary-Adrenal Axis

Acute stress is associated with an immediate increase in the amplitude of hypothalamic hormones, mainly CRH and vasopressin, resulting in increases in amplitude and frequency of ACTH and cortisol pulses and the loss of the circadian rhythm (1). To achieve this enhanced and accelerated release of hormones, the host recruits additional secretagogues of CRH, vasopressin, and ACTH, mainly magnocellular vasopressin and angiotensin II. In addition, catecholamines, neuropeptides Y, and to a lesser extent CRH released from the adrenal medulla, as well as direct autonomic neural input to the adrenal cortex, stimulate glucocorticoid secretion. The common feature is characterized by high circulating levels of ACTH and cortisol, which remain in plateau as long as the stressful condition is maintained. However, in critical illness, circulating levels of cortisol reflect not only cortisol release, but also cortisol clearance from plasma (25). In critically ill patients, cortisol levels may vary from less than 5 μg/dL to more than 100 μg/dL and do not reflect the hypothalamic-pituitary-adrenal (HPA) axis function (26).

Vasopressin (ADH)

Circulating vasopressin levels are regulated through various stimuli including changes in blood volume or blood pressure, plasma osmolality (27), cytokines, and other neuromediators (as discussed above). Acute illness may be associated with inappropriately high circulating levels of vasopressin resulting in water retention and hyponatremia (28). In sepsis, vasopressin levels in plasma seem to follow a biphasic response with initially high concentrations, probably related to the release from posterior pituitary stores on strong baroreflex activation, followed by a decline in 72 hours with relative vasopressin insufficiency occurring in about one third of cases (29). The delayed decrease in vasopressin levels in plasma is not related to altered hormone clearance from plasma (29) and may result from NO overexpression in the parvocellular nuclei (10).

The Hypothalamic-Pituitary Thyroid Axis

Low T3-T4 syndrome has been described for more than 20 years in fasting conditions and in a wide variety of diseases (e.g., sepsis, surgery, myocardial infarction, transplantation, heart, renal and hepatic failure, cancers, malnutrition, inflammatory diseases) and is also called euthyroid sick syndrome or nonthyroidal illness syndrome (NTIS) (30). In the early phase following an acute stress, there is a decrease in serum triiodothyronine (T3) level, an increase in rT3 level. Then serum thyroxine (T4) levels decrease within 24 to 48 hours, and TSH levels remain within normal range without a circadian rhythm (31). Underlying mechanisms include the following: (i) a decrease in conversion of T4 and T3 in extrathyroid tissues due to inhibition of the hepatic 5′-monodeiodination; (ii) the lack of substrates due to the presence of transport protein inhibitors preventing T4 fixation on the protein; (iii) a dysfunction of the thyrotrophic negative feedback on the hypothalamic-pituitary axis; (iv) cytokines (IL-1, IL-6, TNF-α, IFN-γ) inhibiting the thyrotrophic centers and/or affecting the expression of thyroid

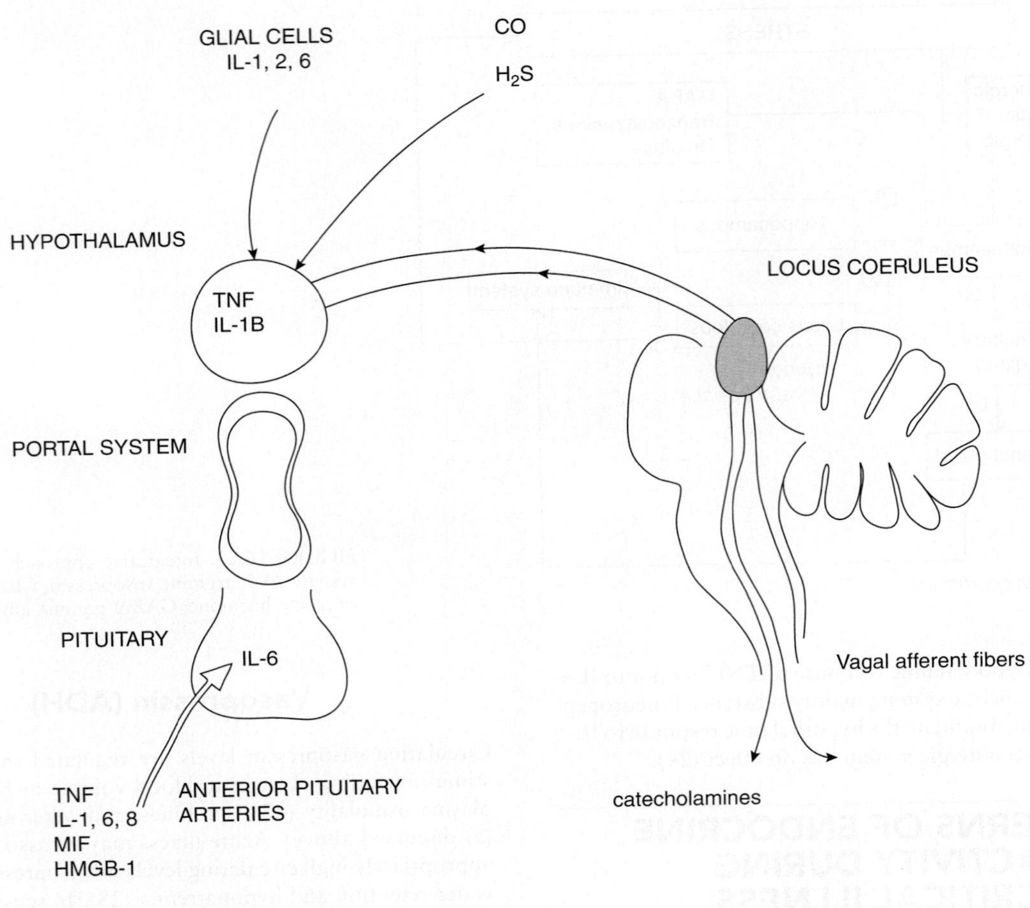

FIGURE 162.4. Signals to the hypothalamus–pituitary axis. There are two different pathways of activation of the hypothalamus–pituitary axis. The humoral pathway acts by (a) cytokines produced in the blood and carried to the hypothalamus and the areas of the brain lacking a blood-brain barrier, (b) cytokines produced by glial cells, and (c) cytokines produced in the pituitary gland and the hypothalamus. The second pathway is the neural route. It acts by activation of various afferent neurons of the peripheral system such as vagal fibers. Finally, endogenous gas such as hydrogen sulfide (H_2S) or carbon monoxide (CO) may play a role. Refer to Table 162.1 for definitions of abbreviations.

hormone nuclear receptors (32); (v) the presence of other inhibitory substances such as dopamine. Prolonged critical illness is associated with centrally induced hypothyroidism as suggested by restoration of T3 and T4 pulses by exogenous TRH infusion (33). In addition, as compared with patients who died from acute illness, postmortem examination of patients who died from chronic critical illness showed diminished thyroid gland weight and follicular size (34), low expression of TRH mRNA in the hypothalamic paraventricular nuclei, and low concentrations of tissue T3 (35,36).

Growth Hormone

The acute phase of critical illness is characterized by high growth hormone levels with attenuated oscillatory activity associated with low levels of insulinlike growth factor (IGF)-1 (37). Serum concentrations of GH effectors IGF-1 are low during this phase (38). This pattern is interpreted as a state of resistance to GH that is mainly related to decreased expression of GH receptors (39). This GH resistance seems to be beneficial: the direct lipolysis and anti-insulin effects may be enhanced, liberating metabolic substrates such as free fatty acids and glucose to vital organs, while costly metabolism mediated by IGF-1 is postponed. When critical illness–related stress is sustained, the pattern of GH secretion shows less pulsatile fraction and elevated nonpulsatile fraction (40). It correlates with the low circulating levels of peripheral effectors such as IGF-1. However, contrary to the acute phase of critical illness, this reduced secretion of IGF-1 does not reflect resistance to GH, but rather, suggests a hypothalamic origin as confirmed by the restoration of the pulsatile GH secretion pattern by infusion of GH secretagogues (41).

Adrenal Medulla Hormones

It is well known that under resting conditions very small amounts of adrenaline and noradrenaline are released from

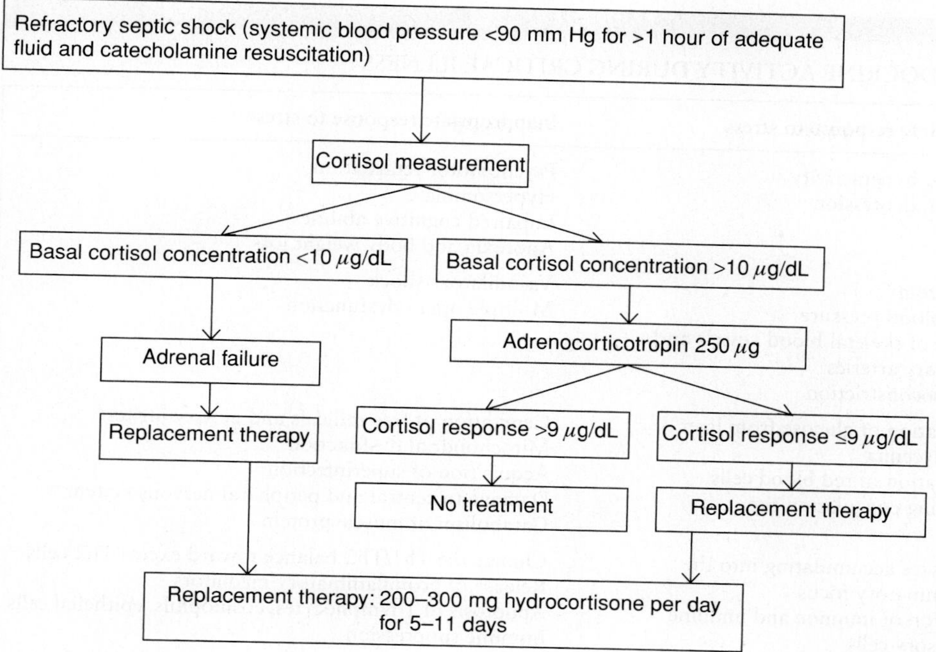

FIGURE 162.5. Decision tree for the diagnosis and treatment of adrenal insufficiency.

the adrenal medulla (i.e., less than 50 ng/kg per minute in the dog). Therefore, removing the adrenal medulla allows an animal to survive indefinitely (42). However, exposure to stressors like fright, pain, anesthesia, exercise, cold, or endotoxin cause within seconds an increase in circulating adrenaline and noradrenaline concentrations by 2 to 3 logs, an effect that was prevented by removal of the adrenal medulla. The release of the catecholamines in the circulation account for the tachycardia, pupillary dilation, pilar erection, and spitting observed in the stressed animals (43). Following his experiments in the early twentieth century, Cannon introduced the concept of "fight or flight" and established its relationship with catecholamines release. Catecholamine synthesis results from an enzymatic cascade starting from the hydroxylation of the amino acid tyrosine leading to the production of dihydroxyphenylalanine (dopa). Dopa is decarboxylated to form dopamine. Dopamine is then hydroxylated in the side chain to form noradrenaline. Finally, noradrenaline is *N*-methylated by phenylethanolamine-*N*-methyltransferase to form adrenaline. Adrenaline is stored in the adrenal medulla in vesicles. Noradrenaline is present in the subcellular granules of the sympathetic nervous endings. Catecholamines have a very short half-life (10–20 seconds for adrenaline) and are metabolized through captation, enzymatic inactivation (methylation in liver or kidney; oxidative deamination by monoamine oxydase), or renal excretion. The regulation of catecholamine secretion involves hormonal and nervous factors, and negative feedback through calcium channels. The hormonal regulation depends on cortisol, which is necessary for the enzymatic degradation of catecholamine synthesis. This interaction relies on nerve transmission, paracrine effect, and the local vascular system. The neurogenic regulation involves the cholinergic preganglionic parasympathetic nervous system through the splanchnic nerves. Like cortisol, catecholamine levels in plasma can remain elevated as long as the stress is maintained, even up to a few months after recovery. Nonetheless, obtaining circulating plasma levels of adrenaline and noradrenaline is useless to assess the appropriateness of the catecholamine response to critical illness.

Insulin

Insulin is involved in glucose metabolism through (i)) mobilization of the store of glucose transport molecules in target cells such as muscle and fat tissue, (ii) activation of hepatic glucokinase gene transcription, and (iii) activation of glycogen synthetase and inhibition of glycogen phosphorylase. Other actions of insulin include growth stimulation, cellular differentiation, intracellular traffic, increased lipogenesis, glycogenesis, and protein synthesis. These effects result from insulin fixation to a ubiquitous membrane receptor belonging to the tyrosine kinase family, the insulinlike growth factor receptor (IGF-1) and insulin receptor–related receptor (IRR). Insulin levels in plasma are rapidly increased following an acute stress as a result of both increased secretion and tissue resistance. Insulin suppresses and antagonizes the effects of TNF (44), macrophage migration inhibitory factor (MIF), and superoxide anions (45), and decreases the synthesis of the acute phase reactants (46). Moreover, insulin modulates leptin and other adipokine release from fat cells (47).

CLINICAL CONSEQUENCES OF ENDOCRINE ACTIVITY DURING CRITICAL ILLNESS

The main objective of the neuroendocrine response to critical illness is fight or flight. The immediate activation for the endocrine system, mainly the sympathoadrenal hormones, results in alertness, insomnia, hyperactivity, pupillary dilation, pilar erection, sweating, salivary secretion, tachycardia, rise in blood pressure with vasodilation of skeletal muscle and

TABLE 162.3

CLINICAL CONSEQUENCES OF ENDOCRINE ACTIVITY DURING CRITICAL ILLNESS

	Appropriate response to stress	Inappropriate response to stress
Behavioral changes	Alertness, hyperactivity Insomnia, depression	Psychomotor retardation Hypersomnia Impaired cognitive abilities Anorexia and body weight loss
Cardiovascular changes	Tachycardia Rise in blood pressure Dilation of skeletal blood vessels and coronary arteries Skin vasoconstriction	Vasodilatory shock Multiple organ dysfunction
Metabolic changes	Mobilization of glucose from liver Hyperglycemia Mobilization of red blood cells Shortening coagulation time	Generation of free radicals and peroxynitrites Mitochondrial dysfunction Acquisition of superinfection Damage to central and peripheral nervous system Catabolism of muscle protein
Immune changes	Leukocytes accumulating into the inflammatory focus Activation of immune and immune accessory cells Generation of cytokines, neuropeptides, and lipid mediators of inflammation	Change the Th1/Th2 balance toward excess Th2 cells Release of proinflammatory mediators Apoptosis of T lymphocytes, eosinophils, epithelial cells Immune suppression

coronary arteries, bronchiolar dilation, skin vasoconstriction, mobilization of glucose from liver with hyperglycemia, increased oxygen capacity of the blood via spleen constriction and mobilization of red blood cells, and shortening of coagulation time. However, in the intensive care unit where flight is not possible, fighting is the only option, and the appropriateness of the neuroendocrine activity to the intensity and duration of the stress determines host survival and recovery (Table 162.3). The clinical consequences of the stress system activation include behavioral changes and cardiovascular, metabolic, and immune adaptations.

Behavioral Changes

In animals, infections are associated with anorexia and body weight loss, hypersomnia, psychomotor retardation, fatigue, and impaired cognitive abilities (48). Similar behavioral changes are consistently reported in humans after cytokine or LPS challenge (49). The so-called depression due to a general medical condition is likely mediated through release of peripheral and brain cytokines. When glucocorticoids and catecholamine responses are insufficient, critically ill patients will develop brain dysfunction that can result to coma.

Cardiovascular Changes

The cardiovascular adaptation is mainly driven by the sympathoadrenal hormones even though thyroid hormones and vasopressin contribute to cardiac adaptation, blood volume, and vasomotor tone regulation. Corticosteroids exert important actions of the various elements of the cardiovascular system including the capillaries, the arterioles, and the myocardium. Numerous studies in various animal models, in healthy volunteers challenged with LPS, and in patients consistently showed that corticosteroids enhanced vessel responsiveness to various vasoactive agents, particularly catecholamines (50). The underlying mechanisms are not fully understood and may involve direct mobilization of intracellular calcium, enzymatic metabolism of adrenaline, increased binding affinity of adrenaline for its receptor, or facilitation of the intracellular signalization that follows the coupling of adrenaline to its receptor. Corticosteroids also have catecholamine-independent effects on the heart and the vessels, and by retaining salt and water contribute to maintain an appropriate blood volume. This results in the fight or flight response: tachycardia, high blood pressure, oliguria, skin vasoconstriction, and cardiac output being redistributed toward the brain, the heart, the liver, and skeletal muscles.

However, whenever the hypothalamic-pituitary adrenal axis or the noradrenergic responses are inappropriate, critically ill patients will develop cardiovascular dysfunction. It has been shown that septic shock patients with adrenal insufficiency, as defined by an increase in cortisol of 9 μg/dL or less to ACTH challenge, have more pronounced hypotension than those with presumed normal function and are more likely to develop refractory shock (51). Adrenal failure also resulted in a more prolonged cardiovascular dysfunction and death in the septic patients (52). Although more common in septic shock, adrenal insufficiency can develop in other critical illnesses (26), particularly in chronically ventilated patients where an association with weaning failure has been observed (53). Adrenal insufficiency is at best diagnosed in critically ill patients by either low baseline cortisol levels (of 10 μg/dL or less) or cortisol increment after 250 μg of corticotropin (ACTH) of 9 μg/dL or less (26). Failure of the noradrenergic system will also result in cardiovascular dysfunction during critical illness. Both animal and human studies have shown that LPS challenge or sepsis is associated with decrease in the noradrenergic activity that precedes cardiovascular dysfunction (54–56). The decrease of the pulsatile activity of the HPA axis and the noradrenergic system result in regularity within the circulatory and respiratory function enabling the subject to adjust to stressful conditions, losing the interorgan communications resulting in multiple organ dysfunction and death (57). Finally, inappropriately low vasopressin levels contribute to the vasodilatory shock associated with many critical illnesses (58).

Metabolic Changes

The net result from the activation of the endocrine system is hyperglycemia. The rise in blood glucose follows the activation of the so-called counterregulatory hormones (glucocorticoids, adrenaline, and glucagon) and results in mobilization of glucose mainly from the liver. Subsequently, tissues that are insulin dependent cannot uptake glucose which is then available for insulin-independent tissues like the brain or inflammatory cells (47). The main reason for critical illness–associated insulin resistance is impairment in glucose transporter isoform (GLUT)-4 metabolism (59). Proinflammatory cytokines such as TNF result in the generation of intracellular ceramides that block the transcription of the gene coding for GLUT-4, preventing the translocation of GLUT-4 to the cell's membrane and entry of glucose into the cells (60). Hyperglycemia has been shown to increase mortality in critical illness (61,62). The mechanisms underlying glucose toxicity for the cells is still unknown and may include an overloading of the insulin-independent cells such as neurons. Subsequent to low ATP levels in the cells, the excess of intracellular glucose cannot enter the Krebs cycle and result in the generation of free radicals and peroxynitrites, which in turn block complex IV of the mitochondria. By destroying the mitochondria of insulin-independent cells, hyperglycemia may facilitate acquisition of superinfection, damage the central and peripheral nervous system and the liver, and eventually cause multiple organ dysfunction (62). Excess in the catabolic hormones (cortisol, adrenaline, and glucagon) will also elicit an imbalance between muscle protein breakdown rate and the rate of muscle protein synthesis, resulting in a net catabolism of muscle protein (63), which may contribute to critical illness–induced muscle weakness and affect long-term prognosis (64).

Immune Changes

The changes in the immune function are mainly related to the sympathoadrenal hormones even though insulin and vasopressin can also influence immunity. Glucocorticoids suppress most, if not all, T-cell–derived cytokines and change the T-helper (Th)1/Th2 balance toward excess Th2 cells (50). Glucocorticoids up-regulate lymphocyte-derived IL-10 but do not effect IL-10 synthesis. They also inhibit the synthesis of many other inflammatory mediators such as cyclo-oxygenase and inducible NOS and down-regulate cell surfaces markers such as endotoxin receptor and adhesion molecules. Finally, they enhance the occurrence of apoptosis of thymocytes, mature T lymphocytes, eosinophils, epithelial cells, and precursors of dermal/interstitial dendritic cells, but delay apoptosis of neutrophils (50). Catecholamines also drive a Th2 shift in both antigen-presenting cells and Th1 cells. In LPS-stimulated human blood cultures, noradrenaline and adrenaline inhibit IL-12 synthesis and enhance IL-10 release, an effect that is mediated via beta-adrenergic receptors (65). These effects of beta-adrenergic stimulation on the Th1/Th2 balance are also observed *in vivo*. However, through alpha-adrenergic stimulation, catecholamines increase TNF and IL-1 synthesis from LPS-stimulated peritoneal macrophages or lung mononuclear cells (1). Thus, while the stress hormones glucocorticoids and catecholamines induce systemically a shift of the Th1/Th2 balance in favor of Th2 cells, catecholamines also promote locally at the level of inflamed tissues the synthesis of proinflammatory mediators. In addition, at the inflammatory sites, tight cross talk between cytokines and the cortisone/cortisol shuttle, with TNF and IL-1 converting cortisone to cortisol and IL-4 and IL-13 inactivating cortisol into cortisone, helps balance the proinflammatory and anti-inflammatory responses (66).

When critical illness is associated with an impaired HPA axis, the Th1/Th2 shift favors the release of proinflammatory mediators in the circulation and in body tissues, allowing cytokine-induced cell deaths either through ischemic or apoptotic mechanisms. In acute lung injury, sepsis, or trauma, or in patients with an adrenal insufficiency, there are large amounts of circulating proinflammatory cytokines that contribute to the development of multiple organ dysfunction and death (67,68). By contrast, too high circulating cortisol levels, such as after a bolus of a high dose of methylprednisolone, may eventually induce systemic immune suppression and favor superinfection and death (69).

MANIPULATION OF ENDOCRINE ACTIVITY DURING CRITICAL ILLNESS

The use of exogenous hormones in critical illness has become a standard of care (Table 162.4). It was shown a long time ago that hypotension can be corrected by administration of catecholamines. Even though there are no randomized controlled trials of adrenaline, noradrenaline, or dopamine versus a placebo or no treatment, these drugs are routinely administered in critically ill patients with cardiovascular dysfunction (70). A recent multicenter randomized trial has shown that adrenaline and noradrenaline are equally effective in restoring cardiovascular homeostasis during septic shock (71). Several trials have also demonstrated that administration of vasopressin can improve cardiovascular function in vasodilatory shock (58,72,73). Vasopressin administration increases systemic vascular resistance and mean arterial pressure and improves cardiac performance and renal function. Although it is clear that exogenous administration of catecholamines or vasopressin can restore hemodynamic stability in critical illness, whether manipulating these hormones helps survival remains uncertain.

The effects of corticosteroid administration have been studied, particularly in patients with severe infections. There is enough evidence in the literature supporting the benefit of corticosteroids on hemodynamic and systemic inflammation (74). In a meta-analysis of all randomized controlled trials of

TABLE 162.4

MANIPULATION OF ENDOCRINE ACTIVITY DURING CRITICAL ILLNESS

Endocrine intervention	Main effects
Vasopressin	Increases systemic vascular resistance and mean arterial pressure Improves cardiac performance Improves renal function
Corticosteroids	Improves systemic hemodynamics and hastens shock recovery Improves organ dysfunction and mortality
Insulin	Improves morbidity and mortality in both surgical and medical patients
Thyroid hormones	Improves hemodynamics No evidence of survival benefit
Growth hormone	High doses associated with increased morbidity and mortality
Coadministration of GHRP-2, TRH, and GNRH	Beneficial metabolic effects?

Refer to Table 162.1 for abbreviations.

hydrocortisone for septic shock, it was demonstrated that hydrocortisone at a dose of 200 to 300 mg per day for 5 to 11 days improved systemic hemodynamic instability and hastened shock recovery. The benefit of treatment on systemic inflammation during sepsis was characterized by prompt and important reduction in circulating proinflammatory mediators, in expression of adhesion molecules, in endothelial activation, and in cell capacity to produce late inflammatory mediators such as MIF (75,76). It is well recognized that a short course of high-dose glucocorticoids should be avoided (74). In contrast, combined administration of low doses of glucocorticoid and mineralocorticoid improved survival in septic shock patients with demonstrable failure of the HPA axis (77) although there are conflicting results.

In another prospective randomized trial (Corticus trial), there was no difference in the 28-day mortality between steroid recipients and the placebo group (78). The use of corticosteroids in patients with septic shock has been controversial for several decades and continues to be controversial despite these two large well-performed studies (77,78). The two studies evaluated different patient populations and came to opposite conclusions. Similarities between the two studies included steroids' beneficial effects on time to shock reversal, and no evidence for increased risk of neuromuscular weakness and hyperglycemia. Differences between the two studies include the following for Annane et al. (77) and Sprung et al. (78), respectively: entry window (8 vs. 72 hours; systolic blood pressure [SBP] <90 mm Hg [>1 hour vs. <1 hour]); additional treatment (fludrocortisone vs. no fludrocortisone); treatment duration (7 vs. 11 days); weaning (none vs. present); SAPS II scores (Simplified Acute Physiology Score) (59 vs. 49); nonresponders to corticotropin (77% vs. 47%); differences in steroid effects according to the response to corticotropin (yes vs. no); increased risk of superinfection (no vs. yes), and the study occurred after practice guidelines recommended steroids (no vs. yes). The updated Surviving Sepsis campaign has given the following recommendation: "We suggest intravenous hydrocortisone be given only to adult septic shock patients after blood pressure is identified to be poorly responsive to fluid resuscitation and vasopressor therapy" (79). Additional recommendations are as follows: fludrocortisone is optional when hydrocortisone is used, and steroid therapy should not be guided by the corticotropin test results (79). In fact, another international task force came up with similar recommendations: "Hydrocortisone should be considered in the management strategy of patients with septic shock, particularly those patients who have responded poorly to fluid resuscitation and vasopressor agents" (80). The benefit of hydrocortisone in refractory shock can also be seen in neonates (81). Finally, in critically ill patients who failed to wean from the ventilator because of adrenal insufficiency, hydrocortisone replacement significantly improved outcome (53).

Recently, intensive treatment with insulin targeting a blood glucose of 4.4 to 6 mmol/L was shown to significantly improve morbidity and mortality in both surgical (82) and medical (83) patients. The benefit is mainly observed in the chronic phase of critical illness (after 72 hours) and may be related to protection of cells from glucose toxicity rather than from direct anti-inflammatory effects of insulin. However, this manipulation of glucose metabolism is extremely difficult and limited by the risk of hypoglycemia. A recent multicenter study did not find any benefit for a tight glucose control with intensive insulin therapy in patients with severe sepsis (84), but the problem may have been in the method of glucose measurement since capillary samples may not read similar levels as whole blood samples, particularly in critically ill patients. One may also suggest that the very early increase in blood glucose mainly relates to stress hormones and should not be counteracted whereas later hyperglycemia relates more to cytokine-induced insulin resistance and should be treated. In other words, the lack of benefit observed in the VISEP study may result from a too-early intervention (84).

Other attempts to manipulate the endocrine system during critical illness have been less successful. Many studies have tried to replace thyroid hormones in various critical illnesses including in patients with cardiac disease, sepsis, acute respiratory distress syndrome, or with burn and trauma patients. Although hormone replacement was associated with some hemodynamic improvement, there was evidence for side effects–related increased risk of death (85). Similarly, the attempt to treat critically ill patients with growth hormone was associated with increased mortality (86), although there is speculation that elevation of blood sugars may have contributed to increased mortality. Nonetheless, it was suggested that combined activation of the GH and thyroid axis with treatment with GH-releasing peptide, TRH, and GNRH elicited beneficial metabolic effect in chronic critically ill patients (87).

SUMMARY

The neuroendocrine response to critical illness is the determinant of host survival and recovery. The sympathoadrenal hormones are the key actors in maintaining homeostasis, and they are very tightly controlled by the brain. When the neuroendocrine response to an acute event such as trauma, infection, burns, and surgery is appropriate both in time and in intensity, then critical illness does not develop and recovery is easy. Otherwise, if the neuroendocrine response is insufficient for the intensity or duration of the stressful episode-related inflammation, then multiple organ failure syndrome develops. By contrast, if the host response is too excessive when compared to the intensity or duration of the inflammatory process, then persistent changes in behavior and mood, in metabolic state, and in immune function cause increased susceptibility to superinfection, risk for chronic muscle fatigue, and posttraumatic stress disorders. Whether the neuroendocrine system can be manipulated to be adjusted to the inflammatory process remains a controversial issue.

PEARLS

Physiology of the endocrine system:
Interorgan communication depends on:

- The noradrenergic and vagal systems
- Hormones

The pituitary is made of:

- Anterior pituitary, which produces:
  1. Gonadotrophic hormones (follicle-stimulating hormones, luteinizing hormone, and luteotrophic hormone)
  2. Thyrotrophic hormone
  3. Adrenocorticotropic hormone
  4. Growth hormone
  5. Prolactin
- Posterior pituitary, which produces mainly vasopressin

Physiologic control of the endocrine activity:

- Feedback loops modulate hormone synthesis and release under resting conditions
- Hypothalamus regulates the endocrine activity in stress conditions

Signalization to the hypothalamic-pituitary axis involves five mechanisms:

- Bloodborne cytokines diffuse into the hypothalamic pituitary axis through areas lacking blood–brain barriers, mainly circumventricular organs
- Bloodborne cytokines are actively transported across the blood–brain barrier via specific carriers
- Cells inside the blood–brain barrier can produce cytokines
- Activated afferent vagal fibers activate the locus ceruleus with subsequent cholinergic-mediated release of CRH
- Gaseous neuromediators such as carbon monoxide and hydroxide sulphide modulate vasopressin and CRH release

Patterns of endocrine activity during critical illness:

- Loss of pulsatile release of hypothalamic hormones
- Increased and sustained ACTH and cortisol levels in plasma
- Increased and sustained circulating catecholamine levels
- Biphasic response in vasopressin with initial high circulating levels and subsequent progressive decline
- Inhibition of TRH release, normal TSH levels with low T3 and T4 concentrations in plasma
- High GH levels and low IGF-1 levels in plasma
- High insulin levels and high blood glucose levels

Endocrine system failure contributes to cardiovascular dysfunction and exaggerated immune response in critical illness:

- Abnormal cortisol response is associated with loss in pressure sensitivity to catecholamines
- Loss in noradrenergic-mediated cardiovascular variability precedes shock in sepsis and contributes to multiple organ dysfunction
- Low vasopressin levels aggravate the impaired noradrenergic system–related vasodilatory shock
- Impaired cortisol and autonomic nervous system induce a shift of the Th1/Th2 balance in favor of Th1 response

Excessive endocrine response to critical illness results in organ dysfunction and immune suppression:

- Excess in counterregulatory hormones induces glucose overload in insulin-independent cells
- Subsequently, via generation of peroxynitrites, mitochondrial function is stopped, predisposing to cell death and organ dysfunction, mainly long-term sequels such as neurologic impairment
- Excess activation of cortisol and autonomic nervous system induces a systemic shift of the Th1/Th2 balance toward excessive Th2 response resulting in immune suppression and predisposing to superinfection

References

1. Chrousos GP. The stress response and immune function: clinical implications. The 1999 Novera H. Spector Lecture. *Ann N Y Acad Sci.* 2000;917:38.
2. McCann SM, Ojeda SR. The anterior pituitary and hypothalamus. In: Griffin JE, Ojeda SR, eds. *Textbook of Endocrine Physiology.* 3rd ed. Oxford, England: Oxford University Press; 1996:101–133.
3. Annane D, Bellissant E, Cavaillon JM. Septic shock. *Lancet.* 2005;365:63.
4. Porter JC, Sisom JF, Arita J, et al. The hypothalamic-hypophysial vasculature and its relationship to secretory cells of the hypothalamus and pituitary gland. *Vitam Horm.* 1983;40:145.
5. Banks WA, Kastin AJ, Huang W, et al. Leptin enters the brain by a saturable system independent of insulin. *Peptides.* 1996;17:305.
6. Koenig JI. Presence of cytokines in the hypothalamic-pituitary axis. *Prog Neuroendocrinoimmunol.* 1991;4:143.
7. Spangelo BL, MacLeod RM, Isakson PC. Production of interleukin-6 by anterior pituitary cells *in vitro*. *Endocrinology.* 1990;126:582.
8. Sharshar T, Annane D, Lorin de la Grandmaison G, et al. The neuropathology of septic shock. *Brain Pathol.* 2004;14:21.
9. McCann SM, Kimura M, Karanth S, et al. The mechanism of action of cytokines to control the release of hypothalamic and pituitary hormones in infection. *Ann N Y Acad Sci.* 2000;917:4.
10. Sharshar T, Gray F, Lorin de la Grandmaison G, et al. Apoptosis of neurons in cardiovascular autonomic centres triggered by inducible nitric oxide synthase after death from septic shock. *Lancet.* 2003;362:1799.
11. Wong ML, Bongiorno PB, Rettori, et al. Interleukin (IL) 1b, IL-1 receptor antagonist, IL-10, IL-13 gene expression in the central nervous system and anterior pituitary during systemic inflammation: pathophysiological implications. *Proc Natl Acad Sci U S A.* 1997;93:227.
12. Lyson K, McCann SM. Involvement of arachidonic acid cascade pathways in interleukin-6 stimulated corticotropin-releasing factor release *in vitro*. *Neuroendocrinology.* 1992;55:708.
13. Rettori V, Dees WL, Hiney JK, et al. An interleukin-1a-like neuronal system in the preoptic-hypothalamic region and its induction by bacterial lipopolysaccharide in concentrations which alter pituitary hormone release. *Neuroimmunomodulation.* 1994;1:251.
14. Karanth S, Lyson K, McCann SM. Role of nitric oxide in interleukin 2 induced corticotropin-releasing factor release from incubated hypothalami. *Proc Natl Acad Sci U S A.* 1993;90:3383.
15. Karanth S, Lyson K, McCann SM. Effects of cholinergic agonists and antagonists on interleukin-2-induced corticotropin-releasing hormone release from the mediobasal hypothalamus. *Neuroimmunomodulation.* 1999;6:168.
16. Parkes D, Kasckow J, Vale W. Carbon monoxide modulates secretion of corticotropin-releasing factor (CRF) from rat hypothalamic cell cultures. *Brain Res.* 1993;646:315.
17. Pozzoli G, Mancuso C, Mirtella A, et al. Carbon monoxide as a novel neuroendocrine modulator: inhibition of stimulated corticotropin-releasing

hormone release from acute rat hypothalamic explants. *Endocrinology.* 1994;135:2314.
18. Kostoglou-Athanassiou I, Forsling ML, Navarra P, et al. Oxytocin release is inhibited by the generation of carbon monoxide from the rat hypothalamus—further evidence for carbon monoxide as a neuromodulator. *Mol Braisn Res.* 1996;42:301.
19. Dello Russo C, Tringali G, Ragazzoni N, et al. Evidence that hydrogen sulfide can modulate hypothalamo-pituitary-adrenal axis function: *in vitro* and *in vivo* studies in the rat. *J Neuroendocrinol.* 2000;12:225.
20. Besedovsky HO, Del Rey A, Sorkin E, et al. Immunoregulatory feedback between interleukin-1 and glucocorticoid hormones. *Science.* 1986;233:652.
21. Dunn AJ. Cytokine activation of the HPA axis. *Ann N Y Acad Sci.* 2000;917:608.
22. Dunn AJ, Chuluyan H. The role of cyclo-oxygenase and lipoxygenase in the interleukin-1 induced activation of the HPA axis: dependence on the route of the injection. *Life Sci.* 1992;51:219.
23. Rivier C, Vale W. Stimulatory effect of interleukin-1 on adrenocorticotropin secretion in the rat: is it modulated by prostaglandins? *Endocrinology.* 1991;129:384.
24. Dunn AJ. Endotoxin-induced activation of cerebral catecholamine and serotonin metabolism: comparison with interleukin-1. *J Pharmacol Exp Ther.* 1992;261:964.
25. Melby JC, Spink WW. Comparative studies on adrenal cortical function and cortisol metabolism in healthy adults and in patients with shock due to infection. *J Clin Invest.* 1958;37:1791.
26. Annane D, Maxime V, Ibrahim F, et al. Diagnosis of adrenal insufficiency in severe sepsis and septic shock. *Am J Respir Crit Care Med.* 2006; 174(12):1319–1326. Epub 2006 Sep 14.
27. Holmes CL, Patel BM, Russell JA, et al. Physiology of vasopressin relevant to management of septic shock. *Chest.* 2001;120:989.
28. Dreyfuss D, Leviel F, Paillard M, et al. Acute infectious pneumonia is accompanied by a latent vasopressin-dependent impairment of renal water excretion. *Am Rev Respir Dis.* 1988;138:583.
29. Sharshar T, Blanchard A, Paillard M, et al. Circulating vasopressin levels in septic shock. *Crit Care Med.* 2003;31:1752.
30. De Groot LJ. Dangerous dogmas in medicine: the nonthyroidal illness syndrome. *J Clin Endocrinol Metab.* 1999;84:151.
31. Romijn JA, Wiersinga WM. Decreased nocturnal surge of thyrotropin in nonthyroidal illness. *J Clin Endocrinol Metab.* 1990;70:35.
32. Michalaki M, Vagenakis AG, Makri M, et al. Dissociation of the early decline in serum T(3) concentration and serum IL-6 rise and TNFalpha in nonthyroidal illness syndrome induced by abdominal surgery. *J Clin Endocrinol Metab.* 2001;86:4198.
33. De Jongh FE, Jobsis AC, Elte JW. Thyroid morphology in lethal nonthyroidal illness: a post-mortem study. *Eur J Endocrinol.* 2001;144:221.
34. Van den Berghe G, de Zegher F, Baxter RC, et al. Neuroendocrinology of prolonged critical illness: effects of exogenous thyrotropin-releasing hormone and its combination with growth hormone secretagogues. *J Clin Endocrinol Metab.* 1998;83:309.
35. Fliers E, Guldenaar SE, Wiersinga WM, et al. Decreased hypothalamic thyrotropin-releasing hormone gene expression in patients with nonthyroidal illness. *J Clin Endocrinol Metab.* 1997;82:4032.
36. Arem R, Wiener GJ, Kaplan SG, et al. Reduced tissue thyroid hormone levels in fatal illness. *Metabolism.* 1993;42:1102.
37. Ross R, Miell J, Freeman E, et al. Critically ill patients have high basal growth hormone levels with attenuated oscillatory activity associated with low levels of insulin-like growth factor-I. *Clin Endocrinol (Oxf).* 1991;35:47.
38. Baxter RC, Hawker FH, To C, et al. Thirty-day monitoring of insulin-like growth factors and their binding proteins in intensive care unit patients. *Growth Horm IGF Res.* 1998;8:455.
39. Hermansson M, Wickelgren RB, Hammarqvist F, et al. Measurement of human growth hormone receptor messenger ribonucleic acid by a quantitative polymerase chain reaction-based assay: demonstration of reduced expression after elective surgery. *J Clin Endocrinol Metab.* 1997;82:421.
40. Van den Berghe G, de Zegher F, Lauwers P, et al. Growth hormone secretion in critical illness: effect of dopamine. *J Clin Endocrinol Metab.* 1994;79:1141.
41. Van den Berghe G, de Zegher F, Veldhuis JD, et al. The somatotropic axis in critical illness: effect of continuous growth hormone (GH)-releasing hormone and GH-releasing peptide-2 infusion. *J Clin Endocrinol Metab.* 1997;82: 590.
42. Witek-Janusek L, Yelich MR. Role of the adrenal cortex and medulla in the young rats' glucoregulatory response to endotoxin. *Shock.* 1995;3:434.
43. Cannon WB. *Am J Physiol.* 1914;33:356.
44. Satomi N, Sakurai A, Haranaka K. Relationship of hypoglycemia to tumor necrosis factor production and antitumor activity: role of glucose, insulin, and macrophages. *J Natl Cancer Inst.* 1985;74:1255.
45. Das UN. Is insulin an antiinflammatory molecule? *Nutrition.* 2001;17:409.
46. Seshadri V, Fox PL, Mukhopadhyayi CK. Dual role of insulin in transcriptional regulation of the acute phase reactant ceruloplasmin. *J Biol Chem.* 2002;277:27903.
47. Saltiel AR, Kahn CR. Insulin signaling and the regulation of glucose and lipid metabolism. *Nature.* 2001;414:799.
48. Maier SF, Watkins LR. Cytokines for psychologists: implications of bidirectional immune-to-brain communication for understanding behaviour, mood, and cognition. *Psychol Rev.* 1998;105:83.
49. Meyers CA. Mood and cognitive disorders in cancer patients receiving cytokine therapy. In: Dantzer R, Wollman EE, Yirmiya R, eds, *Cytokines, Stress and Depression.* New York, NY: Kluwer Academic/Plenum Publishers; 1999;75–82.
50. Annane D, Cavaillon JM. Corticosteroids in sepsis: from bench to bedside? *Shock.* 2003;20:197.
51. Annane D, Bellissant E, Lesieur O, et al. Impaired pressor sensitivity to norepinephrine in septic shock patients with and without impaired adrenal function reserve. *Br J Clin Pharmacol.* 1998;46:589.
52. Annane D, Sébille V, Troché G, et al. A three-level prognostic classification in septic shock based on cortisol levels and cortisol response to corticotropin. *JAMA.* 2000;283:1038.
53. Huang CJ, Lin HC. Association between adrenal insufficiency and ventilator weaning. *Am J Respir Crit Care Med.* 2006;173:276.
54. Goldstein B, Kempski MH, Stair D, et al. Autonomic modulation of heart rate variability during endotoxin shock in rabbits. *Crit Care Med.* 1995;23:1694.
55. Godin PJ, Fleisher LA, Eidsath A, et al. Experimental human endotoxemia increases cardiac regularity: results from a prospective, randomized, crossover trial. *Crit Care Med.* 1996;24:1117.
56. Annane D, Trabold F, Sharshar T, et al. Inappropriate sympathetic activation at onset of septic shock : a spectral analysis approach. *Am J Respir Crit Care Med.* 1999;160:458.
57. Godin PJ, Buchman TG. Uncoupling of biological oscillators: a complementary hypothesis concerning the pathogenesis of multiple organ dysfunction syndrome. *Crit Care Med.* 1996;24:1107.
58. Landry DW, Levin HR, Gallant EM, et al. Vasopressin deficiency contributes to the vasodilation of septic shock. *Circulation.* 1997;95:1122.
59. Minokoshi Y, Kahn CR, Kahn BB. Tissue-specific ablation of the GLUT4 glucose transporter or the insulin receptor challenges assumptions about insulin action and glucose homeostasis. *J Bio Chem.* 2003;278:33609.
60. QI C, Pekala PH. Tumor necrosis factor-alpha-induced insulin resistance in adipocytes. *Proc Soc Exp Biol Med.* 2000;223:128.
61. Umpierrez JE, Isaacs SD, Bazargan N, et al. Hyperglycemia: an independent marker of in-hospital mortality in patients with undiagnosed diabetes. *J Clin Endocrinol Metab.* 2002;87:978.
62. Van den Berghe G. How does blood glucose control with insulin save lives in intensive care? *J Clin Invest.* 2004;114:1187.
63. Gore DC, Jahoor F, Wolfe RR, et al. Acute response of human muscle protein to catabolic hormones. *Ann Surg.* 1993;218:679.
64. Herridge MS, Cheung AM, Tansey CM, et al. One-year outcomes in survivors of the acute respiratory distress syndrome. *N Engl J Med.* 2003;348:683.
65. Elenkov IJ, Papanicolaou RL, Wilder GP, et al. Modulatory effects of glucocorticoids and catecholamines on human interleukin-12 and interleukin-10 production: clinical implications. *Proc Assoc Am Physiol.* 1996;108:374.
66. Rook G, Baker R, Walker B, et al. Local regulation of glucocorticoid activity in sites of inflammation: insights from the study of tuberculosis. *Ann N Y Acad Sci.* 2000;917:913.
67. Hoen S, Asehnoune K, Brailly-Tabard S, et al. Cortisol response to corticotropin stimulation in trauma patients: influence of hemorrhagic shock. *Anesthesiology.* 2002;97:807.
68. Annane D, Sebille V, Bellissant E, et al. Effect of low doses of corticosteroids in septic shock patients with or without early acute respiratory distress syndrome. *Crit Care Med.* 2006;34:22.
69. Bone RC, Fischer CJ Jr, Clemmer TP, et al. A controlled clinical trial of high-dose methylprednisolone in the treatment of severe sepsis and septic shock. *N Engl J Med.* 1987;317:653.
70. Hollenberg SM, Ahrens TS, Annane D, et al. Practice parameters for hemodynamic support of sepsis in adult patients: 2004 update. *Crit Care Med.* 2004;32:1928.
71. Annane D, Vignon P, Bollaert PE, et al. Norepinephrine plus dobutamine versus epinephrine alone for the management of septic shock [abstract]. *Intensive Care Med.* 2005;31:S18.
72. Argenziano M, Choudhry AF, Oz MC, et al. A prospective randomized trial of arginine vasopressin in the treatment of vasodilatory shock after left ventricular assist device placement. *Circulation.* 1997;96(Suppl 9):286.
73. Dunser MW, Mayr AJ, Ulmer H, et al. Arginine vasopressin in advanced vasodilatory shock: a prospective, randomized, controlled study. *Circulation.* 2003;107:2313.
74. Annane D, Bellissant E, Bollaert PE, et al. Corticosteroids for severe sepsis and septic shock: a systematic review and meta-analysis. *BMJ.* 2004;329:480.
75. Keh D, Boehnke T, Weber-Cartens S, et al. Immunologic and hemodynamic effects of "low-dose" hydrocortisone in septic shock: a double-blind, randomized, placebo-controlled, crossover study. *Am J Respir Crit Care Med.* 2003;167:512.
76. Maxime V, Fitting C, Annane D, et al. Corticoids normalize leukocyte production of macrophage migration inhibitory factor in septic shock. *J Infect Dis.* 2005;191:138.
77. Annane D, Sebille V, Charpentier C, et al. Effect of treatment with low doses of hydrocortisone and fludrocortisone on mortality in patients with septic shock. *JAMA.* 2002;288:862.

78. Sprung CL, Annane D, Keh D, et al. Hydrocortisone therapy for patients with septic shock. *N Engl J Med.* 2008;358:111.
79. Dellinger EP, Levy MM, Carlet JM, et al. Surviving Sepsis Campaign: International guidelines for management of severe sepsis and septic shock: 2008. *Crit Care Med.* 2008;36:296.
80. Marik PE, Pastores SM, Annane D, et al. Clinical practice guidelines for the diagnosis and management of corticosteroid insufficiency in critical illness: recommendations of an international task force. Submitted for publication.
81. Ng PC, Lee CH, Bnur FL, et al. A double-blind, randomized, controlled study of a "stress dose" of hydrocortisone for rescue treatment of refractory hypotension in preterm infants. *Pediatrics.* 2006;117:367.
82. Van den Berghe G, Wouters P, Weekers F, et al. Intensive insulin therapy in the critically ill patients. *N Engl J Med.* 2001;345:1359.
83. Van den Berghe G, Wilmer A, Hermans G, et al. Intensive insulin therapy in the medical ICU. *N Engl J Med.* 2006;354:449.
84. Brunkhorst FM, Engel C, Bloos F, et al. Intensive insulin therapy and pentastarch resuscitation in severe sepsis. *N Engl J Med.* 2008;358:125.
85. Stathatos N, Levetan C, Burman KD, et al. The controversy of the treatment of critically ill patients with thyroid hormone. *Best Pract Res Clin Endocrinol Metab.* 2001;15:465.
86. Takala J, Ruokonen E, Webster NR, et al. Increased mortality associated with growth hormone treatment in critically ill adults. *N Engl J Med.* 1999;341:785.
87. Van den Berghe G, Baxter RC, Weekers F, et al. The combined administration of GH-releasing peptide-2 (GHRP-2), TRH and GnRH to men with prolonged critical illness evokes superior endocrine and metabolic effects compared to treatment with GHRP-2 alone. *Clin Endocrinol (Oxf).* 2002;56:655.

CHAPTER 163 ■ DISORDERED GLUCOSE METABOLISM

JACK D. SHANNON • KEVIN W. HATTON • ELAMIN M. ELAMIN

PEARLS

- Diabetic ketoacidosis (DKA) and hyperosmolar hyperglycemic nonketotic syndrome (HHS) result from dysregulation of normal glucose homeostasis caused by one of many precipitating conditions in patients with diabetes mellitus.
- DKA (minimal intrinsic insulin secretion) is associated with hyperglycemia and ketone body formation, whereas HHS (intact intrinsic insulin secretion) is associated with hyperglycemia without ketone body formation.
- Both DKA and HHS may present with various and vague complaints and progress to severe shock with cardiovascular collapse, severe metabolic acidosis, and death.
- The treatment of DKA and HHS involves intravascular fluid resuscitation and insulin replacement with additional electrolyte supplementation.
- Patients, during treatment of DKA and HHS, should be closely monitored for evidence of hypoglycemia, hyperglycemia, electrolyte disturbances, worsening lactic acidosis, intravascular volume overload, cerebral edema, acute respiratory distress syndrome (ARDS), severe coagulopathy, rhabdomyolysis, and thromboembolism.
- Recent evidence has suggested that intensified glycemic control of intensive care unit (ICU) patients by using intravenous insulin infusions results in improved outcomes, including decreased mortality rate. While these observations led to dramatic changes in the management of diabetic patients in the ICU, the optimal range of glycemic control for patients without systemic disorders of glucose metabolism and the clinical implication of the increased risk of iatrogenic hypoglycemia are currently under investigation.

Disordered glucose metabolism is a significant medical problem in patients in the outpatient, emergency room, ward, and intensive care settings. Diabetes mellitus (DM), the most important group of medical conditions resulting from disordered glucose metabolism, results in significant short-term and chronic morbidity, and is increasing in prevalence around the globe. In the United States alone, nearly 6% of the population (18.2 million people) is estimated to have this disease (1). Additionally, a significant number of these patients may not be diagnosed, which can further negatively impact their health. Despite increasing public awareness over the last few years, the prevalence of diabetes continues to increase (2).

Due to a combination of the sheer volume of patients with DM and the associated chronic health conditions, the disease is important for physicians, nurses, health care administrators, insurers, and public health advocates. More than 3.8 million hospitalizations per year are associated with diabetes, which is an increase of more than 70% over the last 20 years (3). Of note, the average length of stay is 6.5 days for these hospitalizations (3). Undeniably, these facts alone place an enormous economic and workforce burden on the entire health care system.

In addition to the many associated chronic health conditions developed by patients with DM, there are several acute and life-threatening conditions that also develop in these patients. Hyperglycemic emergencies, such as DKA and HHS, are important causes of morbidity and mortality in patients with DM who are admitted to the intensive care unit. Additionally, new research indicates that the prevention of hyperglycemia—with or without the diagnosis of diabetes—may be a key component of appropriate intensive care support of patients with numerous medical and surgical conditions.

DIABETIC KETOACIDOSIS

Since the discovery of insulin by Frederick Banting in 1921, outcomes for patients with diabetic ketoacidosis have steadily improved. Nevertheless, DKA remains a serious and potentially fatal complication of DM. Overall mortality from DKA is less than 5%; however, mortality increases substantially with extremes of age, the presence of coma, or the development of hypotension (4).

Hospital and ICU admissions for DKA and related conditions are increasing, and cause a significant burden on current health care delivery systems (5). With an annual incidence of 4.6 to 8 episodes per 1,000 patients with diabetes, DKA is the initial presentation of DM in up to 30% of patients overall, with approximately 40% of children and 17% of adults presenting in DKA without prior diagnosis of DM (4,5). While most patients presenting with DKA have type 1 DM, those with type 2 DM can also develop DKA during times of significant physiologic stress.

Pathophysiology

DKA results from a serious dysregulation of normal glucose homeostasis, leading to hyperglycemia and ketone body formation. Excess glucose and ketones launch a host of subsequent systemic sequelae. A deficiency, either relative or absolute, in insulin production, combined with an excess production of certain insulin counterregulatory hormones—glucagon, catecholamines, cortisol, and growth hormone, is responsible for these changes in serum glucose control. Most patients with type 1 DM who develop DKA have an absolute or near-absolute insulin deficiency, whereas most patients with type 2 DM have either normal or elevated insulin levels (6,7). Because of the aberrant hormonal milieu, protein, lipid, and carbohydrate metabolism are all disrupted, and culminate in the production of proinflammatory cytokines, such as interleukin-6, interleukin-1β, interleukin-8, and tumor necrosis factor-α; free fatty acids; and plasminogen activator inhibitor-1, resulting in significant morbidity and mortality (8).

Normal glucose metabolism is typically tightly regulated to maintain a serum glucose concentration between 70 and 115 mg/dL (about 3.9–6.4 mm/L) by carefully balancing glucose production in the liver and glucose utilization in peripheral tissues (9). Insulin, a 51-amino-acid peptide, is mainly responsible for this tight glucose control by stimulating hepatic glucose uptake and storage (glycogen synthesis), and suppressing hepatic gluconeogenesis and glycogenolysis. Insulin also affects peripheral muscle tissue by promoting peripheral glucose uptake, promoting glycogen synthesis, and inhibiting peripheral glycogenolysis.

In DKA, either relative or absolute insulin deficiency combined with increased counterregulatory hormones (CRHs) promotes metabolic pathways opposite to insulin in both hepatic and peripheral tissues (10–13). These changes are typically the result of a precipitating event in patients with severely imbalanced DM (Table 163.1). Infection accounts for 30% to 50% of precipitating causes of DKA, with urinary tract and pulmonary infections making up the vast majority (14). Myocardial infarction, cerebrovascular accident, pulmonary embolism, pancreatitis, trauma, alcohol abuse, and drugs that affect carbohydrate metabolism can also precipitate DKA (15).

The end result of these changes is a substantial increase in serum glucose—through increased hepatic gluconeogenesis, glycogenolysis, and lipolysis—with inappropriately decreased peripheral insulin uptake (Fig. 163.1). DKA is also associated with ketosis, an additional product of worsening glucose homeostatic decompensation, which occurs as a result of increased lipolysis from increased action of hormone-sensitive lipase, an enzyme that causes increased triglyceride breakdown and free fatty acid release into the systemic circulation. Hormone-sensitive lipase is highly up-regulated during periods of insulin deficiency and elevations in CRH. Hepatic oxidation of free fatty acids induced by hormone-sensitive lipase produces ketone bodies, mainly β-hydroxybutyrate (β-OHB) and acetoacetic acid, strong acids that present a large hydrogen ion load to the body. The normal buffering systems are rapidly overwhelmed by the ongoing hydrogen load, and an anion gap acidosis develops.

Hyperglycemia and ketonemia produce a hypertonic intravascular environment, resulting in an intracellular water shift into the intravascular and interstitial compartments. The ensuing cellular dehydration is accompanied by electrolyte shifts as well. When the renal glucose reabsorption rate is exceeded, an osmotic diuresis of water and electrolytes occurs. Sodium, potassium, magnesium, calcium, chloride, and phosphate are all lost during this osmotic diuresis. Commonly, water and electrolyte deficits are compounded by poor oral intake and protracted vomiting. The effects of hypovolemia are responsible for the clinical picture as the depletion of the intravascular space produces the life-threatening signs and symptoms. The body's response is a further increase in CRH, and the cycle is perpetuated.

TABLE 163.1

PRECIPITATING FACTORS IN DIABETIC KETOACIDOSIS AND HYPEROSMOLAR HYPERGLYCEMIC NONKETOTIC SYNDROME

INFECTION
- Urinary tract infection
- Pneumonia
- Dental infection
- Cellulitis

COEXISTING CONDITIONS
- Acute myocardial infarction
- Cerebral vascular accident
- Pancreatitis
- Pulmonary embolism
- Hyperthermia
- Hypothermia
- Renal failure/dialysis
- Severe thermal injury
- Thyrotoxicosis
- Cushing syndrome
- Mesenteric thrombosis

MEDICATIONS
- Calcium-channel blockers
- β-Blockers
- Chlorpromazine
- Cimetidine
- Diazoxide
- Diuretics
- Ethacrynic acid
- Phenytoin
- Steroids
- Total parenteral nutrition

SUBSTANCE ABUSE
- Alcohol
- Cocaine

UNDIAGNOSED DIABETES MELLITUS

Presentation and Diagnosis

The presentation and diagnosis of DKA is typically straightforward and relies on a thorough patient history, focused physical examination, and appropriate laboratory analysis. Patients typically report a history of poor glucose control and symptoms associated with hyperglycemia, such as polyuria, polydipsia, weight loss, and lethargy that may progress over the course of days to weeks. Nausea, vomiting, and abdominal pain are also common presenting complaints and frequently signify the progression from symptomatic hyperglycemia to overt DKA. Physical examination may reveal evidence of dehydration—for example, tachycardia, hypotension, prolonged capillary refill time, poor skin turgor, dry mucous membranes, and weight loss. Additionally, Kussmaul respirations (very deep, gasping breaths taken in response to severe metabolic acidosis), an acetone or fruity breath odor, depressed mental status, and even focal neurologic deficits or coma may also be seen.

Laboratory analysis is usually confirmatory of DKA in these patients (Table 163.2). A complete blood count, blood

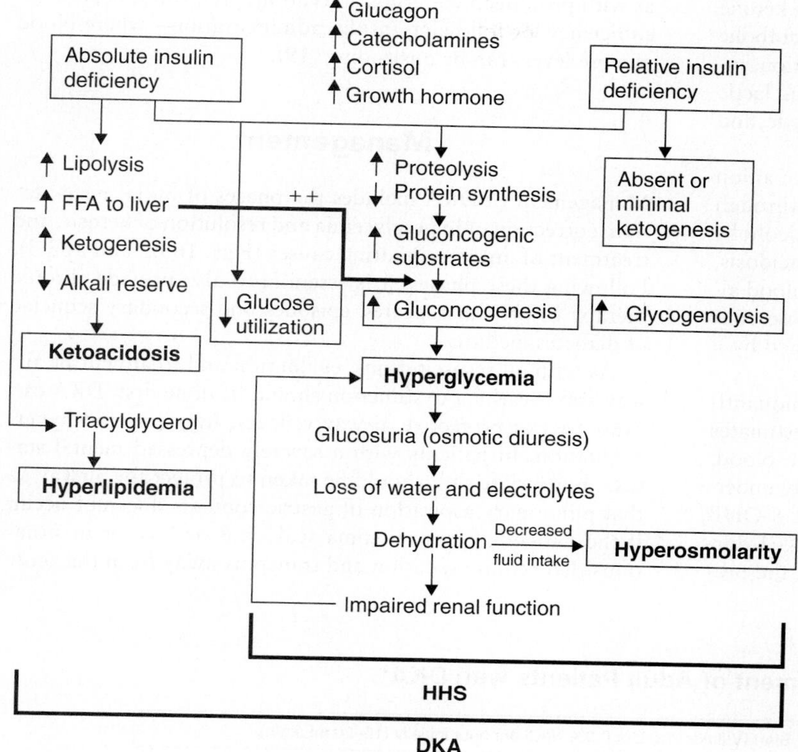

FIGURE 163.1. Pathogenesis of diabetic ketoacidosis (DKA) and hyperosmolar hyperglycemic nonketotic syndrome (HHS). FFA, free fatty acid. (Copyright © 2001, American Diabetes Association, from *Diabetes Care* 2001;24:131–153. Reprinted with permission from the American Diabetes Association.)

glucose, serum electrolytes, serum osmolality, blood urea nitrogen, serum creatinine, arterial or venous blood gas, serum ketones, and urinalysis should be ordered in patients with suspected DKA. Caution should be exercised when using the serum sodium levels in patients with DKA, as the reported laboratory value can be artificially low, normal, or elevated, depending on the spurious effects of glucose and triglycerides in these patients and the relative loss of water compared to sodium. In the presence of hyperglycemia, serum sodium measurement can be corrected by adding 1.6 mg/dL to the measured serum sodium for each 100 mg/dL increase of glucose above normal (16). Appropriate cultures should be requested if infectious triggers of DKA are suspected. Other tests, such as serum lactate, β-human chorionic gonadotropin (β-HCG), electrocardiography, chest radiography, and computed tomography may be indicated, depending on the clinical scenario.

A plasma anion gap–associated metabolic acidosis is typically seen in laboratory analysis of patients with DKA, as ketosis and ketone body accumulation are responsible for an increase in the anion gap. However, in up to 11% of patients, a

TABLE 163.2

DIAGNOSTIC CRITERIA FOR DIABETIC KETOACIDOSIS (DKA) AND HYPEROSMOLAR HYPERGLYCEMIC NONKETOTIC SYNDROME (HHS)

Parameter	Normal range	DKA	HHS
Plasma glucose (mmol/L)	<6.7	>13.9	>33
Arterial pH	7.35–7.45	<7.30	>7.30
Serum bicarbonate (mmol/L)	22–28	<15	>15
Anion gap	>10	>12	<12
Serum osmolality (mOsm/kg)	Variable	Variable	>320
Serum ketones	Negative	Moderate to high	None
Urine ketones	Negative	Moderate to high	None

Adapted from Kitabchi AE, Umpierrez GE, Murphy MB, et al. Management of hyperglycemic crises in patients with diabetes. *Diabetes Care.* 2001;24:131–153; and Chiasson JL, Aris-Jilwan N, Belanger R, et al. Diagnosis and treatment of diabetic ketoacidosis and the hyperglycemic hyperosmolar state. *CMAJ.* 2003;168:859–866.

nongap hyperchloremic metabolic acidosis may occur instead (17). Typically, the normal anion gap is between 7 and 9 mEq/L and reflects unmeasured ions in the serum. In patients with DKA, an elevated anion gap occurs because of the high ketone concentration. Other causes of anion gap–associated metabolic acidosis, which must be excluded during DKA evaluation, include alcoholic ketoacidosis, starvation ketoacidosis, and lactic acidosis, as well as methanol, ethylene glycol, paraldehyde, and salicylate ingestion.

In patients with possible DKA, these other causes of anion gap–associated metabolic acidosis should be excluded through further history and laboratory analysis. For example, alcoholic ketoacidosis may present with profound metabolic acidosis, but typically has a characteristic history, an elevated blood alcohol content, and only mildly elevated serum glucose concentrations. Likewise, starvation ketosis is accompanied by a significant history and only mild acidosis.

Ketonemia and ketonuria can both be assessed semiquantitatively with the nitroprusside reaction test. This test estimates the relative levels of acetoacetate and acetone in the blood, but does not detect the presence of β-OHB, potentially underestimating the degree of ketosis. Because the ratio of β-OHB to acetoacetate may increase from 1:1 to as much as 5:1 during the development of DKA, β-OHB may represent the predominant ketone during illness (18). Of note, β-OHB monitoring may significantly improve the diagnostic specificity in DKA patients with euglycemia or only mild hyperglycemia—as with prolonged vomiting, starvation, pregnancy, hepatic insufficiency, or following insulin administration—where blood glucose levels can be misleading (19).

Management

Management of DKA includes the phases of initial resuscitation, correction of hyperglycemia and resolution of ketosis, and treatment of any precipitating causes (Figs. 163.2 and 163.3). Following these phases, it is essential to also provide chronic therapy to prevent repeated episodes and secondary sequelae of diabetes mellitus.

As with all resuscitations, evaluation and treatment of airway and breathing dysfunction should be done first. DKA can cause loss of protective airway reflexes, hypoxia, and hyperventilation. In patients with a severely depressed mental status, appropriate care should be taken to protect the airway so that pulmonary aspiration of gastric contents does not occur. If the patient's Glasgow coma scale is 8 or less, or in situations that require sedation and transport away from the acute

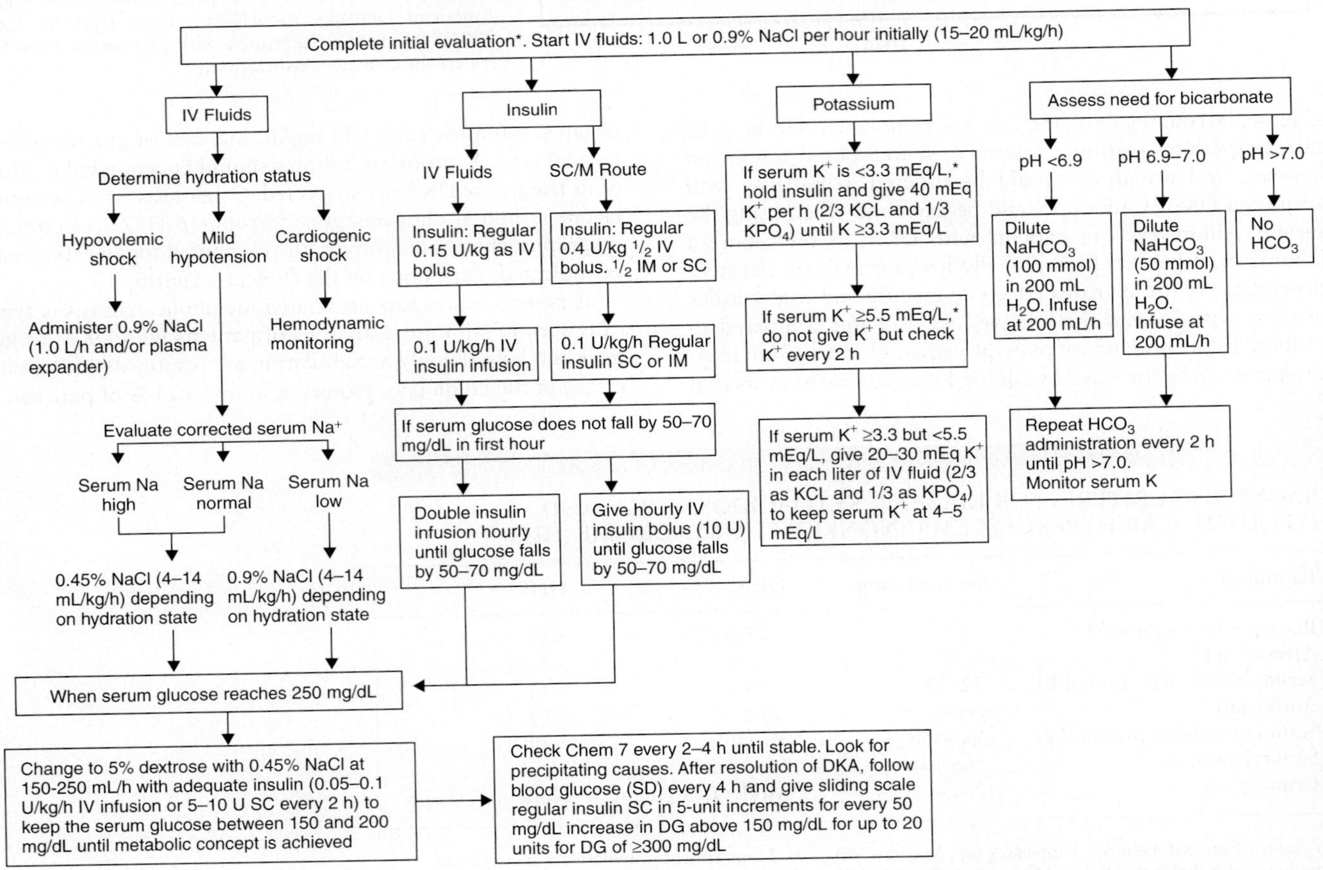

FIGURE 163.2. Management of adult patients with diabetic ketoacidosis (DKA). DG,; SD, . (Copyright © 2001, American Diabetes Association, from *Diabetes Care* 2001;24:131–153. Reprinted with permission from the American Diabetes Association.)

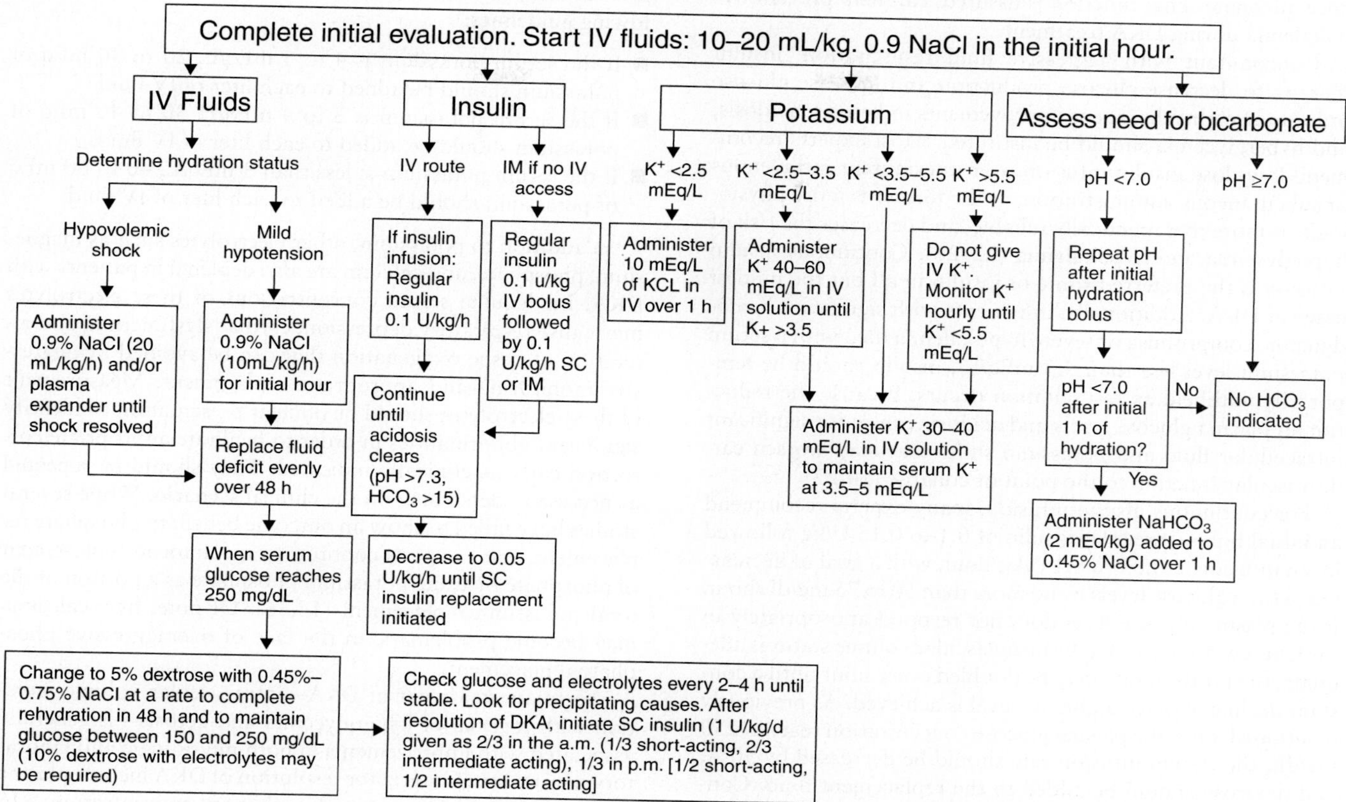

FIGURE 163.3. Management of pediatric patients with diabetic ketoacidosis (DKA) or hyperosmolar hyperglycemic nonketotic syndrome (HHS). (Copyright © 2001, American Diabetes Association, from *Diabetes Care* 2001;24:131–153. Reprinted with permission from the American Diabetes Association.)

care environment for further evaluation, tracheal intubation may be necessary to ensure adequate airway protection and ventilation. Because these patients have a high incidence of gastroparesis, the placement of a decompressive gastric tube may also be warranted in the presence of an altered level of consciousness, and elevation of the head of bed to between 30 and 40 degrees may serve to prevent passive regurgitation. Mechanical ventilation, if utilized, should be set to maintain respiratory compensation of the accompanying severe metabolic acidosis initially and adjusted appropriately as the acidosis corrects.

Following airway and respiratory care, initial therapy should be directed at restoring adequate blood volume and organ perfusion with intravascular volume resuscitation. In addition to correcting the hemodynamic insults associated with severe hypovolemia, appropriate volume administration can also decrease CRH levels and plasma glucose concentration (20,21). The goal during this phase is to replace the fluid deficit over the first 24 hours, half of which should be replaced in the first 6 to 8 hours. Estimation of fluid deficit can be based on body weight or general guidelines and response characteristics. Typically 1 to 2 liters of isotonic saline in the first 1 to 2 hours is sufficient for initial resuscitation; however, in more severe cases the resuscitation may require larger volumes, and some prefer to add colloids. The following clinical estimations of volume deficit using orthostatic blood pressure and heart rate may also be used to guide initial fluid replacement, although these criteria may be less reliable in patients with neuropathy and/or impaired cardiovascular reflexes (14):

- An increase in pulse without change in blood pressure with orthostatic position change indicates approximately a 10% decrease in extracellular volume (i.e., 2 liters).
- A decrease in blood pressure (>15/10 mm Hg) with position change indicates approximately a 15% to 20% decrease in extracellular volume (i.e., 3–4 liters).
- Supine hypotension indicates a decrease of >20% in extracellular fluid volume (i.e., >4 liters).

After the initial resuscitation phase, both the rate of infusion and type of intravenous fluid must be adjusted. Current recommendations are to decrease the infusion rate to 250 mL/hour or to 4 to 14 mL/kg/hour, depending on the patient's hydration status and goal replacement volume. Depending on the patient's corrected serum sodium, isotonic saline is continued or changed to hypotonic saline. If the patient's corrected serum sodium is low, 0.9% saline solution should be continued as the replacement fluid; however, if the patient's corrected serum sodium is normal or elevated, the fluid should be changed to 0.45% saline solution in order to continue free water deficit replacement. Additionally, once plasma glucose levels reach 250 mg/dL, either 5% or 10% dextrose solution should be added to the replacement fluids to maintain serum glucose levels between 150 and 200 mg/dL, allow the insulin infusion to continue until ketosis is reversed, and prevent the too rapid correction of serum glucose levels. The addition of potassium to the fluids, once adequate renal function is assured, can help prevent hypokalemia during DKA treatment.

Concomitant with aggressive fluid resuscitation, insulin therapy to decrease glucose production and increase glucose utilization with subsequent improvements in ketosis, acidosis, and hyperglycemia should be instituted. Most experts recommend low-dose insulin infusion over intermittent intravenous or subcutaneous administration, as the former is more physiologic, is more therapeutically reliable, and decreases the risk of hypoglycemia and hypokalemia (22–26). Continuous insulin infusion is the preferred route of insulin in all but the mildest cases of DKA. Additionally, in patients with significant hemodynamic compromise or severe hypokalemia (i.e., with a serum potassium level less than 3.3 mEq/L), insulin should be temporarily withheld as resuscitation occurs, because the reduction in plasma glucose levels and acidosis can cause significant intracellular fluid and potassium shifts that may worsen cardiovascular function to the point of collapse (14,27).

For continuous insulin infusion, many experts recommend an initial bolus of regular insulin of 0.1 to 0.15 U/kg followed by an infusion at 0.05 to 0.1 U/kg/hour, with a goal of decreasing plasma glucose levels by no more than 50 to 75 mg/dL/hour. If the plasma glucose level does not respond appropriately in the first few hours, and if the intravascular volume status is adequate, the infusion rate may be doubled every hour until a constant decline in plasma glucose level is achieved. As previously mentioned, once the plasma glucose concentration reaches 250 mg/dL, the insulin infusion rate should be decreased by 50%, and dextrose should be added to the replacement fluid. Continuous adjustment of the insulin infusion rate and dextrose concentration is required to maintain appropriate plasma glucose concentration.

In addition to serum glucose and bicarbonate levels, the American Diabetic Association recommends evaluation of β-OHB levels as the preferred method of monitoring DKA, which may become the preferred method for rapid diagnosis. Typically, β-OHB concentrations are less than 1 mmol/L; however, in patients with DKA, plasma β-OHB concentration can be elevated to concentrations in excess of 4 to 12 mmol/L (mean 7 mmol/L). Adequate DKA treatment should prompt a decrease in β-OHB concentration by approximately 1 mmol/L/hour, and should return to baseline (<1 mmol/L) (18,29–33). As has been documented, serum bicarbonate levels are slower to correct, and β-OHB is a more appropriate measure of therapy. It is also noted that as appropriate treatment progresses, β-OHB is oxidized to acetoacetate, which may worsen the results of the nitroprusside reaction test and lead to incorrect conclusions. For these reasons, it is now recommended to directly measure β-OHB for diagnosis and treatment monitoring in DKA (14,28).

Despite massive potassium losses (3–5 mEq/kg) in patients presenting with DKA, the serum potassium concentration may be normal due to intravascular volume contraction and intracellular electrolyte shifts, and should not be used as an indicator of potassium homeostasis in the early phases of treatment. As insulin is provided and acidosis is corrected, potassium may quickly shift back into the intracellular compartment. Additionally, initial resuscitation with normal saline may lower the serum potassium concentration. Severe hypokalemia may potentially cause life-threatening cardiac dysrhythmias and respiratory muscle weakness (13,34,35). Potassium replacement should begin once the serum potassium concentration falls below 5.5 mEq/L, assuming adequate urine output, using the following guidelines:

- If the serum potassium is 4 to 5 mEq/L, 20 to 30 mEq of potassium should be added to each liter of IV fluid.
- If the serum potassium is 3 to 4 mEq/L, 30 to 40 mEq of potassium should be added to each liter of IV fluid.
- If the serum potassium is less than 3 mEq/L, 40 to 60 mEq of potassium should be added to each liter of IV fluid.

In addition to potassium, other electrolytes such as magnesium, phosphate, and calcium are also depleted in patients with DKA. Inadequate serum concentrations of these electrolytes may cause respiratory depression, cardiac dysfunction, and alteration of tissue oxygenation that can be avoided by aggressive monitoring and appropriate replacement. Measurement of these electrolytes should be done at presentation to identify significant abnormalities in order to facilitate appropriate correction early as clinically indicated. They should be repeated as necessary, depending on the clinical scenario. While several studies have failed to show an outcome benefit to phosphate replacement, some experts continue to recommend replacement of phosphate by using potassium phosphate as a portion of the total potassium replacement (14,36). Of note, hypocalcemia may become problematic in the face of overaggressive phosphate replacement.

Adequate treatment of DKA—intravascular volume repletion with reversal of hyperglycemia and ketosis—is generally associated with improvements in both physiologic and laboratory parameters. Criteria for resolution of DKA include plasma glucose <200 mg/dL, serum bicarbonate concentration $\geq$18 mEq/L, venous pH >7.3, anion gap <12 mEq/L, and, recently, β-OHB <1 mmol/L (19). After resolution of the DKA episode, when the patient is able to tolerate enteral nutrition, a multidose subcutaneous insulin regimen that includes a combination of short- and intermediate- or long-acting insulin should be instituted. To allow for sufficient insulin plasma levels, intravenous insulin should be continued for 1 to 2 hours following the first dose of subcutaneous insulin. Patients with previously diagnosed diabetes may restart their previous insulin schedule with additional adjustment and coverage as needed.

These treatments should ideally be provided in an environment that has adequate nursing care and monitoring capabilities, as well as rapid turnaround of laboratory tests. Invasive monitoring should be provided as necessary; patients with mild to moderate DKA may require only noninvasive blood pressure monitoring, continuous electrocardiography, pulse oximetry, and a urinary catheter, whereas patients with the most severe disease states and comorbidities may, in addition, require arterial and central venous catheterization. Additionally, patients with oliguria or hypotension refractory to initial rehydration, mental obtundation, sepsis, respiratory insufficiency, pregnancy, or significant comorbidities or precipitating events, such as myocardial infarction or decompensated congestive heart failure, should be managed in a critical care environment (14,34).

Complications

Common complications encountered during DKA treatment include hypoglycemia and hyperglycemia, various electrolyte

TABLE 163.3

COMPLICATIONS OF DIABETIC KETOACIDOSIS AND HYPEROSMOLAR HYPERGLYCEMIC NONKETOTIC SYNDROME TREATMENT

- Hyperglycemia
- Hypoglycemia
- Electrolyte disturbances (hypokalemia, hyperkalemia)
- Hyperchloremic metabolic acidosis
- Cerebral edema
- Intravascular volume overload
- Hypoxemia
- Noncardiogenic pulmonary edema
- Acute respiratory distress syndrome
- Rhabdomyolysis
- Thromboembolism
- Pancreatitis

disturbances, lactic acidosis, intravascular volume overload, cerebral edema, acute respiratory distress syndrome, coagulopathy, rhabdomyolysis, and thromboembolism (Table 163.3).

Hypoglycemia and hyperglycemia are common complications of DKA treatment. Because intensive intravenous insulin therapy intentionally decreases blood glucose levels, reverses ketone body formation, and improves insulin sensitivity, it also places the patient at significant risk for hypoglycemia and its associated serious complications, including significant cognitive dysfunction, coma, and death. The incidence of serious hypoglycemic episodes associated with DKA treatment can be substantially decreased with the institution of low-dose insulin protocols, the addition of dextrose-containing solutions to intravenous fluid management when the blood glucose concentration reaches 250 to 300 mg/dL, and the institution of frequent blood glucose monitoring with frequent insulin infusion rate titration (4,34). Additionally, hyperglycemia—with the potential for DKA to recur—can be seen following the resolution of DKA, due in large part to abrupt termination of the intravenous insulin infusion without adequate overlap of nonintravenous therapies, including subcutaneous insulin.

Hypokalemia may be regularly encountered in the treatment phase of DKA due to intracellular translocation of potassium during insulin treatment with inadequate replacement. This electrolyte abnormality may be responsible for associated dysrhythmias, skeletal muscle weakness, and ileus. Treatment of the acidemic state with bicarbonate and inadequate potassium replacement predisposes patients to hypokalemia.

Cerebral edema is a rare, but devastating, complication of DKA therapy. It occurs more commonly in pediatric populations, and may be seen in up to 1% of the patients treated for DKA (4). The exact reason for the development of cerebral edema during DKA treatment remains unproven; however, it is felt to be related to an overly rapid correction of the hyperosmolar state. For this reason, current recommendations state that the change in serum osmolality resultant from therapy should not exceed 3 mOsm/kg/hour, and, in patients with concomitant cardiac and renal compromise, serum osmolality should be monitored frequently (22,37–40); we check serum osmolality every 4 to 6 hours, depending on the severity of the episode of DKA and underlying disease.

With worsening cerebral edema, intracranial pressure may significantly increase—occasionally to the point of brainstem herniation with associated respiratory arrest and cardiovascular derangements. For this reason, careful monitoring should be done during DKA treatment for signs of cerebral edema and brainstem herniation such as the acute onset of headache, changes in the level of consciousness, the development of papilledema, or the onset of seizures. Additionally, sodium and water deficits are slowly corrected, and rapid decreases in blood glucose levels are avoided. Treatment of this condition is largely supportive, and may be improved with the use of mannitol as an osmotic diuretic to decrease the amount of cerebral edema.

Acute respiratory distress syndrome is also a rare but potentially fatal complication that may occur at any time during the process of DKA. The disorder may be linked to the underlying cause of DKA as a source of infection, or the treatment phase with associated fluid resuscitation, fluid shifts, and changing osmotic gradients. Pulmonary aspiration of gastric secretions may also be responsible for the respiratory involvement. Patients with hypoxemia, widened alveolar-to-arterial oxygen gradients, or other pre-existing cardiorespiratory conditions warrant close monitoring and possibly more judicious fluid resuscitation (14,41).

HYPEROSMOLAR HYPERGLYCEMIC NONKETOTIC SYNDROME

HHS is a medical emergency that develops in response to one of many precipitating conditions (Table 163.1) in patients with type 2 DM. Among adults in the United States, the incidence of HHS is approximately 17.5 cases per 100,000 persons per year, and results in significant morbidity and mortality (42). The mortality rate from HHS is related directly to patient age, considering that mortality is, for example, less than 10% in patients younger than 75 years of age compared to 35% in patients older than 84 years of age (43,44).

In approximately 20% of patients presenting with HHS, this diagnosis is their initial presentation with type 2 diabetes (42). Additionally, the diagnosis is usually made after significant delay, and is made more complex because HHS can coexist with DKA in approximately 30% of patients (44).

Pathophysiology

The basic pathophysiologic abnormality in HHS is a relative insulin deficiency caused by both an increase in peripheral insulin resistance and an increase in blood levels of counterregulatory hormones (Fig. 163.1) (44–46). These hormones—glucagon, cortisol, and growth hormone—and various catecholamines increase hepatic and renal glucose production, and further worsen peripheral tissue glucose utilization (44,45). Together, these defects cause an insidious but dramatic rise in serum glucose concentration, typically over days to weeks (45).

With increasing serum glucose concentration, an osmotic gradient develops between the intravascular and extravascular compartment (47). Because water moves from the extravascular compartment down this osmotic gradient, both intracellular dehydration and a transiently increased intravascular volume with relative serum hyponatremia can occur. As the serum glucose concentration continues to rise, osmotic diuresis causes profound decreases in intravascular volume, coupled with losses of vital electrolytes such as sodium, potassium, phosphate, and magnesium (43). This large intravascular volume loss can result in life-threatening end-organ hypoperfusion and nonketotic metabolic acidosis.

Compared to DKA, ketones are minimally produced in patients with HHS likely due to the ability of the pancreas to secrete insulin. The amount of insulin, while not sufficient to prevent hyperglycemia in these patients, does prevent fatty acid lipolysis and the formation of ketone bodies and development of ketoacidosis.

Presentation and Diagnosis

Because patients with HHS typically fail to develop ketoacidosis, the time from onset to diagnosis and treatment can be significantly longer than in patients with DKA (45). The clinical diagnosis of these patients, therefore, requires a high clinical suspicion to promptly recognize the signs and symptoms of HHS and institute appropriate diagnostic and treatment modalities.

Patients with suspected HHS may initially exhibit nausea/vomiting, visual disturbances, muscle weakness, and leg cramps (48). Left untreated, these patients eventually develop confusion, lethargy, hemiparesis, seizures, and coma (49). Physical examination may reveal both signs of profound dehydration—such as decreased skin turgor and dry mucous membranes—as well as abdominal distension from gastroparesis (50).

Initial laboratory evaluation in patients with suspected HHS should include serum glucose, ketones, electrolytes, and creatinine concentration; serum measured and calculated osmolality; urinalysis; and appropriate empiric bacterial and fungal cultures (Table 163.2) (45). Because these patients can have significantly elevated serum glucose concentrations—as high as or higher than 1,000 mg/dL, the serum osmolality can be quite high and seems to correlate with neurologic symptoms (51).

Management

The treatment goals for HHS include aggressive intravascular fluid replacement, insulin administration to correct hyperglycemia, appropriate electrolyte replacement, and, if indicated, respiratory system support (Fig. 163.4). Ultimately, effective patient education and long-term patient support are also important.

HHS treatment is typically undertaken in two phases. The first is the acute—emergency—phase and consists of rapid restoration of circulatory volume and electrolyte deficits with

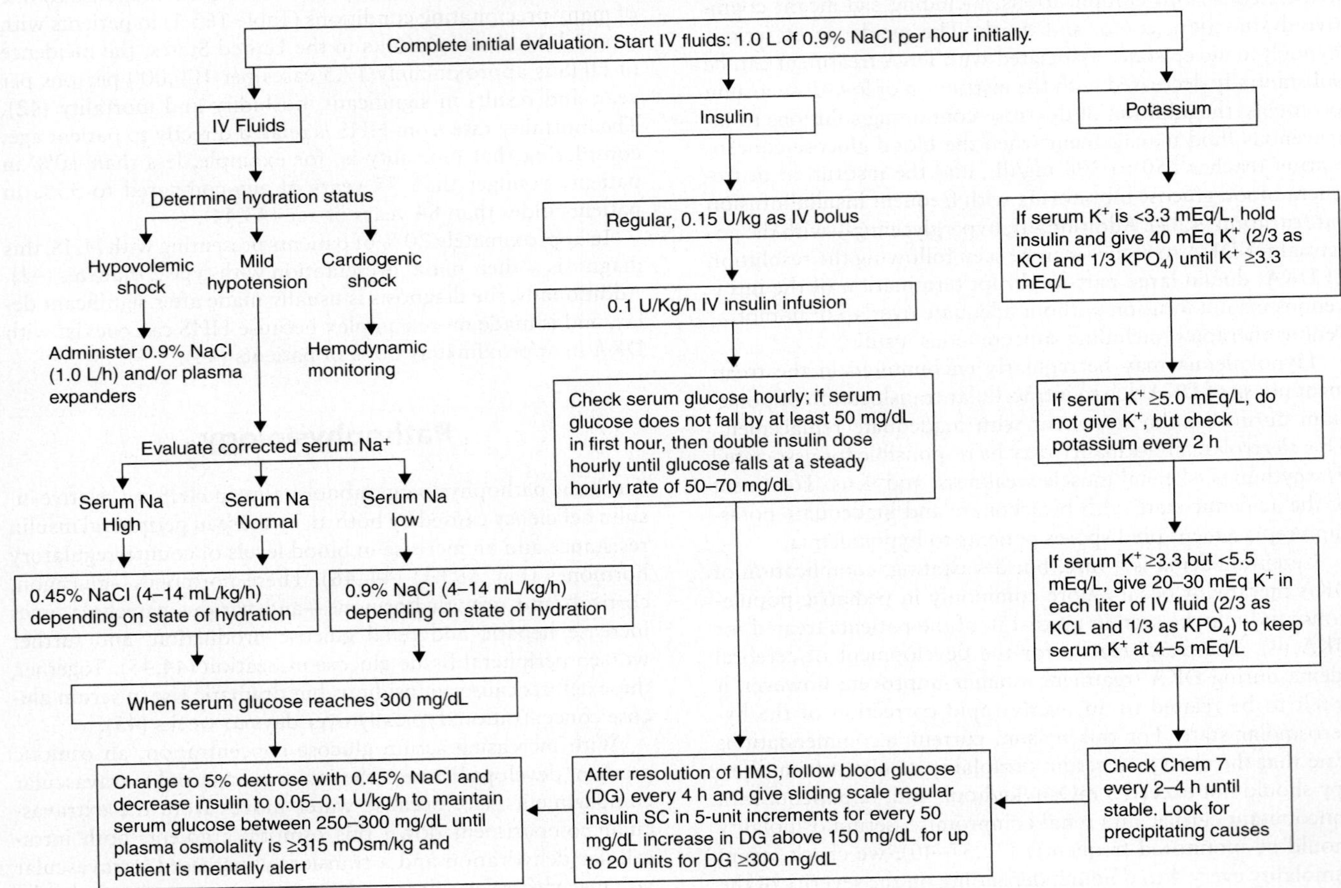

FIGURE 163.4. Management of adult patients with hyperosmolar hyperglycemic nonketotic syndrome (HHS). DG,; HMS,. (Copyright © 2001, American Diabetes Association, from *Diabetes Care* 2001;24:131–153. Reprinted with permission from the American Diabetes Association.)

concomitant insulin administration to correct serum hyperglycemia and hyperosmolality. Additionally, treatment of the triggering disorder should be started. This phase ends with near-correction of hyperglycemia and metabolic acidosis. The second phase is a transitional phase centered on changing insulin replacement to appropriate chronic diabetes therapy (i.e., subcutaneous or oral hypoglycemic regimen), as well as patient education and support.

In patients with HHS, the total body water deficit can be as high as 100 to 200 mL/kg in adults; thus, fluid replacement is the mainstay therapy for intravascular collapse and poor organ perfusion, and can lower glucose concentration independent of insulin administration. Initially, 0.9% saline solution should be infused at 15 to 20 mL/kg total body weight per hour to restore extracellular fluid volume deficit. Normal saline infusion should continue until blood pressure and end-organ perfusion have been normalized. The intravenous solution should then be changed to 0.45% saline solution at a reduced rate to restore the intracellular fluid deficit. The overall fluid resuscitation goal should be replacement of one half of the estimated fluid deficit over the first 8 hours, and the other half of the estimated fluid deficit over the next 16 hours. Care should be taken to ensure that the serum osmolality does not decrease more than 3 mOsm/kg/hour to reduce the risk of acute cerebral edema.

The cornerstone of therapy for HHS is intravenous insulin given to restore normal peripheral glucose uptake, suppress lipolysis, and decrease hepatic gluconeogenesis. Complications of insulin therapy include hypoglycemia, hypokalemia (insulin infusion should not begin with serum potassium less than 3.5 mEq/dL), and hypophosphatemia. Insulin should be initially given as an intravenous bolus of 0.15 units/kg, followed by a continuous infusion of 0.1 unit/kg/hour with a goal glucose decrease of 50 to 75 mg/dL/hour. While the patient is receiving intravenous insulin, the glucose should be monitored every 1 to 2 hours via either capillary or serum samples. Once the serum glucose decreases to 250 mg/dL, dextrose should be added to the intravenous fluid administration, and the insulin infusion should be decreased to 0.05 to 0.1 unit/kg/hour.

Electrolyte replacement is also an important component to the management of HHS. Hypokalemia can develop during HHS treatment because insulin administration causes an intracellular shift of potassium ions from the extracellular compartment. Additionally, the ongoing osmotic diuresis can cause a dramatic depletion of total body potassium stores; this loss can exceed 400 mEq in severe HHS. For this reason, electrocardiographic monitoring should be utilized during this phase of therapy, and aggressive potassium replacement—with up to 40 mEq/hour—may be necessary. Hypophosphatemia may also develop secondary to the ongoing osmotic diuresis. Replacement of phosphate during HHS treatment seems prudent; however, several prospective randomized studies have failed to show a definitive benefit to phosphate replacement in the absence of decreased cardiac or respiratory function and anemia (36,52). If phosphate replacement is necessary, potassium phosphate may be an ideal replacement infusion to correct both hypokalemia and hypophosphatemia.

Complications

In addition to the electrolyte abnormalities discussed above, complications from HHS include pancreatitis, rhabdomyolysis, thromboembolism, hyperchloremic metabolic acidosis, cerebral edema, acute gastric dilatation, and ARDS (Table 163.3). Patients with HHS are at increased risk for thromboembolism, and thus, subcutaneous heparin administration may be warranted to prevent thromboembolic complications (43,53). Complications of HHS treatment include intravascular volume overload and acute cerebral edema from overaggressive intravenous fluid administration. Intravascular volume overload is seen as hypoxemic respiratory failure—often with pulmonary edema—and lower extremity pitting edema. Acute cerebral edema is manifested by headache, lethargy, and depressed levels of consciousness that can rapidly progress to brainstem herniation. Treatment of this potentially devastating complication consists of administering an osmotic diuretic such as mannitol and supportive care.

SUMMARY

Future directions in DKA and HHS therapy involve further refinements in protocols and therapies aimed to improve the hyperglycemia, acidosis, and electrolyte imbalances while minimizing risks such as volume overload, ARDS, and cerebral edema. Additionally, ongoing efforts to provide patients and caregivers with the tools for early identification and the need for aggressive treatment of these hyperglycemic emergencies may ultimately have the largest impact on long-term morbidity and mortality.

GLYCEMIC CONTROL AND INSULIN THERAPY IN THE INTENSIVE CARE UNIT

Over the last decade, multiple published studies (Table 163.4) (54–58) suggested that intensified glycemic control of ICU patients by using intravenous insulin infusion results in improved outcomes, including decreased mortality rate. While these observations led to dramatic changes in the management of ICU blood glucose control in both Europe and North America, concerns have been raised about the optimal range of glycemic control for ICU patients and the clinical implication of the increased risk of iatrogenic hypoglycemia (59,60).

The recommendation that glucose levels be maintained no higher than 4.4 to 6.1 mmol/L (1 mmol/L of glucose = 18 mg/dL) has its origins in a key study conducted in Leuven, Belgium, by Van den Berghe et al. and published in 2001 (54). In this large randomized, single-center trial of predominantly cardiac surgery ICU patients, there was a reduction in ICU mortality with intensive intravenous insulin protocol targeting blood glucose to 4.4 to 6.1 mmol/L (for all patients, a 43% relative and 3.4% absolute mortality reduction; for those with >5 days in the ICU, a 48% relative and 9.6% absolute mortality reduction). In addition, the study demonstrated a reduction in organ dysfunction and ICU length of stay (LOS) in the subset with ICU LOS >5 days from a median of 15 to 12 days.

Although there were significant differences in design, blood sugar target, and patient population among all studies listed in Table 163.4, the results were, for the most part, fairly similar. Intensive therapy with intravenous insulin produced a consistent decrease in mortality rate in a variety of patient

TABLE 163.4

RELATION BETWEEN INTENSIVE INSULIN THERAPY AND OUTCOME IN CRITICALLY ILL PATIENTS

Study	DIGAMI	Leuven I	Portland	Stamford	Leuven II
Patient population	Acute MI (N = 620)	Surgical (N = 1,548)	CABG (N = 3,554)	Medical ICU (N = 1,600)	Medical ICU (N = 767)
Diabetes	100%	13%	100%	17%	15%
Decrease in mortality rate	30%	34%	53%	29%	18%
Reason for reduced mortality rate	N/K	Sepsis	HF, VT, VF	N/K	Multiple
Hypoglycemia (%) (glucose level, mmol/L)[a]	17 (<3.0)	5.2 (<2.2)	0.8 (<3.3)	1.3 (<3.3)	25 (<2.2)
Mean glucose (mmol/L):					
Intensive treatment	9.2	5.7	9.8	7.3	5.8
Conventional treatment	12.0	8.5	11.8	8.4	8.6

CABG, coronary artery bypass graft; HF, heart failure; ICU, intensive care unit; MI, myocardial infarction; VF, ventricular fibrillation; VT, ventricular tachycardia; N/K, unknown.
[a]1 glucose mmol/L = 18 mg/dL.

populations. However, several important differences should be noted. In some cases, all the participants had diabetes, whereas in others, most participants were nondiabetic. In addition, there were remarkable differences in the range of blood glucose levels achieved. For instance, the glucose levels of the control group of the Leuven studies were similar to—and in some cases, lower than—the levels in the intensive treatment groups of the other studies. However, the differences in blood glucose levels between the control and intensive treatment groups were similar in all five studies. Furthermore, there was a comparable improvement in mortality rate in the critically ill patients targeted to reach a serum glucose goal of 6.1 mmol/L and 7.3 to 9.8 mmol/L.

Another important observation is that the two studies that achieved by far the lowest glucose levels in the intensively treated patients were also the only two studies in which parenteral nutrition (PN) was often associated with hyperglycemia and hypertriglyceridemia (62). Furthermore, there is considerable evidence that PN can be responsible for other adverse outcomes in critically ill patients. In a meta-analysis of 27 studies comparing PN with enteral nutrition and involving >1,800 patients, Braunschweig et al. found a >50% higher incidence of infection in participants receiving PN, but no difference in mortality rate (62). The implications of these findings in interpreting the Leuven I study are obvious. Patients in the Leuven I study received PN, a treatment known to increase infection rates, and when glucose level was lowered with insulin infusion to an average of 5.7 mmol/L, an improvement in mortality rate, based mostly on a reduction in infection rate, was observed. Hence, the administration of intravenous insulin in this study merely reduced infectious complications to a level that would have been observed if PN had not been otherwise given.

Furthermore, one of the mechanisms that may explain an increased rate of infection in diabetic individuals and hospitalized patients with hyperglycemia is impaired immune function secondary to a defect in the adherence properties of polymorphonuclear leukocytes (63,64). An analysis of data from the 363 patients who remained in intensive care for >7 days in the Leuven I study revealed a strong relationship between serum triglyceride (TG) and ICU mortality rate by univariate analysis (an approximate 400% increase in mortality rate in patients with TAG >3.4 mmol/L compared with individuals with TAG <1.1 mmol/L). Accordingly, an alternative explanation for the benefits of insulin infusion is that they were not a direct consequence of lowering glucose, but rather due to effects of insulin on lipid control, especially in patients who received PN (65).

Most recently, two additional multicenter randomized control trials (RCTs) of intensive insulin therapy—one focused on patients with severe sepsis (VISEP) and the second on medical and surgical ICU patients—failed to demonstrate improvement in mortality, though they are not yet fully published (66,67). Nevertheless, both were stopped earlier than planned because of high rates of hypoglycemia and adverse events in the intensive insulin groups. This finding is particularly important for ICU patients who are commonly sedated and mechanically ventilated since aggressive lowering of serum glucose levels may

TABLE 163.5

THE SURVIVING SEPSIS CAMPAIGN 2008 CONSENSUS RECOMMENDATION ON GLUCOSE CONTROL DURING SEVERE SEPSIS

1. Following initial stabilization, intensive care unit patients with severe sepsis and hyperglycemia to receive intravenous insulin therapy to reduce blood glucose levels (grade 1B)
2. Validated protocol to be used for insulin dose adjustments and targeting glucose levels to the <150 mg/dL range (grade 2C)
3. All patients receiving intravenous insulin to receive a glucose calorie source in addition to monitoring blood glucose values every 1–2 h until glucose values and insulin infusion rates are stable, then every 4 h thereafter (grade 1C)
4. Caution taken if using point-of-care testing for capillary blood glucose as it may overestimate arterial blood or plasma glucose values (grade 1B)

Adapted from Dellinger P, Levy MM, Jean M, et al. Surviving Sepsis Campaign: international guidelines for management of severe sepsis and septic shock: 2008. *Crit Care Med.* 2008;36(1):296–327.

carry the risk of hypoglycemia, which is potentially more difficult to detect (59).

To address the above concerns, a large RCT in 20 ICUs in Australia and New Zealand is currently under way to compare target serum glucose levels of 4.5 to 6.0 mmol/L (80–110 mg/dL) versus 8 to 10 mmol/L (140–180 mg/dL) (68). This trial will provide information about the effect of normoglycemia in a heterogeneous group of critically ill patients. In addition, it will recruit >6,000 patients and most likely will produce ≥500,000 glucose measurements that subsequently can be used to reveal some of the many unknown dimensions of glycemic control and its consequences in ICU patients.

In the meantime, several recommendations for glycemic control in the ICU have been suggested in the most current Surviving Sepsis Campaign (Table 163.5) (69). These recommendations are intended to provide some direction for the clinician caring for ICU patients with severe sepsis while awaiting results from the ongoing studies on potential differences in outcomes with different glucose targets and various insulin protocols.

Until the full results of the ongoing studies become available, intensive insulin therapy to *all ICU patients* remains unsupported, and should be viewed with a healthy degree of scientific skepticism.

SUMMARY

The weight of available data indicates that intensified insulin treatment of the critically ill is associated with impressive reductions in mortality rate. Therefore, the value of intensive insulin treatment should not be in doubt. However, the question remains if the available data justify a glycemic target of 6.1 mmol/L. As pointed out above, the reduction in mortality reported in Leuven I can be secondary to lipid, rather than glucose, control. Since these are mere associations, additional research will be required in which lipid levels are maneuvered more directly in order to assess whether nonglucose effects of insulin are, in fact, responsible for the apparent benefits of insulin. In addition, since the use of PN in the Leuven I study may impose additional constraints on its subjects, intensive insulin treatment in this study may merely have counteracted the adverse effects of PN. Finally, considering that the Leuven I study was not designed to compare different glycemic targets with intensive insulin treatment, judgments concerning whether a goal of 6.1 mmol/L will produce better outcomes than a higher goal must await the results of ongoing studies.

Furthermore, since hypoglycemia is likely to be more frequent and more severe with lower glucose targets, it seems prudent to adjust the dose of intravenous insulin to target glucose levels ≥5.0 and <8.3 mmol/L.

References

1. American Diabetes Association. Report of the expert committee on the diagnosis and classification of diabetes mellitus. *Diabetes Care.* 2003;26:S5.
2. Burke JP, Williams K, Gaskill SP, et al. Rapid rise in the incidence of type 2 diabetes from 1987 to 1996: results from the San Antonio heart study. *Arch Intern Med.* 1999;159:1450–1456.
3. Currie CJ, Morgan CL, Peters JR. The epidemiology and cost of inpatient care for peripheral vascular disease, infection, neuropathy, and ulceration in diabetes. *Diabetes Care.* 1998;21:42–48.
4. Kitabchi AE, Umpierrez GE, Murphy MB, et al. Hyperglycemic crises in diabetes. *Diabetes Care.* 2004;27:S94–102.
5. Fishbein H, Palumbo PJ. *Acute Metabolic Complications in Diabetes.* Bethesda, MD: National Institutes of Health; 1995 #NIH 95–1468. 9. Centers for Disease Control, Division of Diabetes Translations. Diabetes Surveillance, 1991. Washington, DC: US Government Printing Office; 1992:635–1150.
6. White NH. Diabetic ketoacidosis in children. *Endocrinol Metab Clin North Am.* 2000;29:657–682.
7. Kitabchi AE, Wall BM. Diabetic ketoacidosis. *Med Clin North Am.* 1995; 79:9–37.
8. Stentz FB, Umpierrez GE, Cuervo R, et al. Proinflammatory cytokines, markers of cardiovascular risks, oxidative stress, and lipid peroxidation in patients with hyperglycemic crises. *Diabetes.* 2004;53:2079–2086.
9. Merimee TJ, Tyson JE. Stabilization of plasma glucose during fasting: normal variations in two separate studies. *N Engl J Med.* 1974;291:1275–1278.
10. Gerich JE, Lorenzi M, Bier DM, et al. Effects of physiologic levels of glucagon and growth hormone on human carbohydrate and lipid metabolism: studies involving administration of exogenous hormone during suppression of endogenous hormone secretion with somatostatin. *J Clin Invest.* 1976;57:875–884.
11. Felig P, Sherwin RS, Soman V, et al. Hormonal interactions in the regulation of blood glucose. *Recent Prog Horm Res.* 1979;35:501–532.
12. McGarry JD, Woeltje KF, Kuwajima M, et al. Regulation of ketogenesis and the renaissance of carnitine palmitoyltransferase. *Diabetes Metab Rev.* 1989;5:271–284.
13. DeFronzo RA, Matzuda M, Barret E. Diabetic ketoacidosis: a combined metabolic nephrologic approach to therapy. *Diabetes Rev.* 1994;2:209–238.
14. Kitabchi AE, Umpierrez GE, Murphy MB, et al. Management of hyperglycemic crises in patients with diabetes. *Diabetes Care.* 2001;24:131–153.
15. Faich GA, Fishbein HA, Ellis SE. The epidemiology of diabetic acidosis: a population-based study. *Am J Epidemiol.* 1983;117:551–558.
16. Katz MA. Hyperglycemia-induced hyponatremia: calculation of expected sodium depression. *N Engl J Med.* 1973;289:843–844.
17. Adrogue HJ, Wilson H, Boyd AE, et al. Plasma acid-base patterns in diabetic ketoacidosis. *N Engl J Med.* 1982;307:1603–1610.
18. Stephens JM, Sulway MJ, Watkins PJ. Relationship of blood acetoacetate and 3-hydroxybutyrate in diabetes. *Diabetes.* 1971;20:485–489.
19. Wallace TM, Matthews DR. Recent advances in the monitoring and management of diabetic ketoacidosis. *Q J Med.* 2004;97:773–780.
20. Waldhausl W, Kleinberger G, Korn A, et al. Severe hyperglycemia: effects of rehydration on endocrine derangements and blood glucose concentration. *Diabetes.* 1979;28:577–584.
21. Owen OE, Licht JH, Sapir DG. Renal function and effects of partial rehydration during diabetic ketoacidosis. *Diabetes.* 1981;30:510–518.
22. Kitabchi AE, Fisher JN, Murphy MB, et al. Diabetic ketoacidosis and hyperglycemic, hyperosmolar nonketotic state. In: Kahn CR, Weir GC, eds. *Joslin's Diabetes Mellitus Textbook.* Philadelphia: Lea & Febiger; 1993: 753–760.
23. Foster DW, McGarry JD. The metabolic derangements and treatment of diabetic ketoacidosis. *N Engl J Med.* 1983;309:159–169.
24. Fleckman AM. Diabetic ketoacidosis. *Endocrinol Metab Clin North Am.* 1993;22:181–207.
25. Kitabchi AE. Low-dose insulin therapy in diabetic ketoacidosis: fact or fiction? *Diabetes Metab Rev.*1989;5:337–363.
26. Burghen GA, Etteldorf JN, Fisher JN, et al. Comparison of high dose and low-dose insulin by continuous intravenous infusion in the treatment of diabetic ketoacidosis in children. *Diabetes Care.* 1980;3:15–20.
27. Magee MF, Bankim AB. Management of decompensated diabetes. Diabetic ketoacidosis and hyperosmolar hyperglycemic syndrome. *Crit Care Clin.* 2001;17:75–106.
28. Naunheim R, Jang TJ, Banet G, et al. Point-of-care test identifies diabetic ketoacidosis at triage. *Acad Emerg Med.* 2006;13:683–685.
29. Wallace TM, Meston NM, Gardner SG, et al. The hospital and home use of a 30-second hand-held blood ketone meter: guidelines for clinical practice. *Diabetes Med.* 2001;18:640–645.
30. Foster KJ, Alberti KG, Hinks L, et al. Blood intermediary metabolite and insulin concentrations after an overnight fast: reference ranges for adults, and interrelations. *Clin Chem.* 1978;24:1568–1572.
31. Umpierrez GE, Watts NB, Phillips LS. Clinical utility of b-hydroxybutyrate determined by reflectance meter in the management of diabetic ketoacidosis (Letter). *Diabetes Care.* 1995;18:137–138.
32. Luzi L, Barrett EJ, Groop LC, et al. Metabolic effects of low-dose insulin therapy on glucose metabolism in diabetic ketoacidosis. *Diabetes.* 1988; 37:1470–1477.
33. Sulway MJ, Malins JM. Acetone in diabetic ketoacidosis. *Lancet.* 1970; 2:736–740.
34. Umpierrez GE, Kitabchi AE. Diabetic ketoacidosis: risk factors and management strategies. *Treat Endocrinol.* 2003;2:95–108.
35. Abramson E, Arky R. Diabetic acidosis with initial hypokalemia: therapeutic implications. *JAMA.* 1966;196:401–403.
36. Fisher JN, Kitabchi AE. A randomized study of phosphate therapy in the treatment of diabetic ketoacidosis. *J Clin Endocrinol Metab.* 1983;57:177–180.
37. Ennis ED, Stahl E, Kreisberg RA. The hyperosmolar hyperglycemic syndrome. *Diabetes Rev.* 1994;2:115–126.

38. Hillman K. Fluid resuscitation in diabetic emergencies—a reappraisal. *Intensive Care Med.* 1987;13:4–8.
39. Marshall SM, Walker M, Alberti KGM. Diabetic ketoacidosis and hyperglycemic non-ketotic coma. In: Alberti KGM, Zimmet P, DeFronzo RA, eds. *International Textbook of Diabetes Mellitus.* New York: John Wiley; 1997:1215–1229.
40. Ennis ED, Stahl EJ, Kreisberg RA. Diabetic ketoacidosis. In: Porte D Jr, Sherwin RS, eds. *Diabetes Mellitus: Theory and Practice.* Amsterdam: Elsevier; 1997:827–844.
41. Carroll P, Matz R. Adult respiratory distress syndrome complicating severely uncontrolled diabetes mellitus: report of nine cases and a review of the literature. *Diabetes Care.* 1982;5(6):574–580.
42. Yared Z, Chiasson JL. Ketoacidosis and the hyperosmolar hyperglycemic state in adult diabetic patients. *Minerva Med.* 2003;94:909–913.
43. Venkatraman R, Singhi SC. Hyperglycemic hyperosmolar nonketotic syndrome. *Ind J Pediatr.* 2006;73(1):55–60.
44. Gaglia JL, Wyckoff J, Abrahamson MJ. Acute hyperglycemic crisis in the elderly. *Med Clin N Am.* 2004;88(4):1063–1084.
45. American Diabetes Association. Hyperglycemic crises in patients with diabetes mellitus. *Diabetes Care.* 2001;24:1988–1996.
46. Chiasson JL, Aris-Jilwan N, Belanger R, et al. Diagnosis and treatment of diabetic ketoacidosis and the hyperglycemic hyperosmolar state. *CMAJ.* 2003;168:859–866.
47. Brenner ZR. Management of hyperglycemic emergencies. *AACN Clin Issues.* 2006;17:56–65.
48. Stoner GD. Hyperosmolar hyperglycemic state. *Am Fam Physician.* 2005; 71:1723–1730.
49. Ting JY. Hyperosmolar diabetic non-ketotic coma, hyperkalaemia and an unusual near death experience. *Eur J Emerg Med.* 2001;8:57–63.
50. Delaney MF, Zisman A, Kettyle WM. Diabetic ketoacidosis and hyperglycemic hyperosmolar nonketotic syndrome. *Endocrinol Metab Clin North Am.* 2000;29:683–705.
51. Siperstein MD. Diabetic ketoacidosis and hyperosmolar coma. *Endocrinol Metab Clin North Am.* 1992;21:415–432.
52. Wilson HK, Keuer SP, Lea AS, et al. Phospate therapy in diabetic ketoacidosis. *Arch Intern Med.* 1982;142:517–520.
53. Mather HM. Management of hyperosmolar coma. *J Royal Soc Med.* 1980; 73:134–138.
54. Van den Berghe G, Wouters P, Weekers F, et al. Intensive insulin therapy in critically ill patients. *N Engl J Med.* 2001;345:1359–1367.
55. Malmberg K. Prospective randomised study of intensive insulin treatment on long term survival after acute myocardial infarction in patients with diabetes mellitus. DIGAMI (Diabetes Mellitus, Insulin Glucose Infusion in Acute Myocardial Infarction) Study Group. *BMJ.* 1997;314:1512–1515.
56. Furnary AP, Gao G, Grunkemeier GL, et al. Continuous insulin infusion reduces mortality in patients with diabetes undergoing coronary artery bypass grafting. *J Thorac Cardiovasc Surg.* 2003;125:1007–1021.
57. Krinsley JS. Effect of an intensive glucose management protocol on the mortality of critically ill adult patients. *Mayo Clin Proc.* 2004;79:992–1000.
58. Van den Berghe G, Wilmer A, Hermans G, et al. Intensive insulin therapy in the medical ICU. *N Engl J Med.* 2006;354:449–461.
59. Cryer PE. Hypoglycaemia: the limiting factor in the glycaemic management of the critically ill?. *Diabetologia.* 2006;49:1722–1725.
60. Bhatia A, Cadman B, Mackenzie I. Hypoglycemia and cardiac arrest in a critically ill patient on strict glycemic control. *Anesth Analg.* 2006;102:549–551.
61. Klein CJ, Stanek GS, Wiles CE 3rd. Overfeeding macronutrients to critically ill adults: metabolic complications. *J Am Diet Assoc.* 1998;98:795–806.
62. Braunschweig CL, Levy P, Sheean PM, et al. Enteral compared with parenteral nutrition: a meta-analysis. *Am J Clin Nutr.* 2001;74:534–542.
63. Bagdade JD, Root RK, Bulger RJ. Impaired leukocyte function in patients with poorly controlled diabetes. *Diabetes.* 1974;23:9–15.
64. McMahon MM, Bistrian BR. Host defenses and susceptibility to infection in patients with diabetes mellitus. *Infect Dis Clin North Am.* 1995;9:1–9.
65. Mesotten D, Swinnen JV, Vanderhoydonc F, et al. Contribution of circulating lipids to the improved outcome of critical illness by glycemic control with intensive insulin therapy. *J Clin Endocrinol Metab.* 2004;89:219–226.
66. Brunkhorst FM, Kuhnt E, Engel C, et al. Intensive insulin therapy in patient with severe sepsis and septic shock is associated with an increased rate of hypoglycemia—results from a randomized multicenter study (VISEP). *Abstr Infect.* 2005;33:19–20.
67. Preiser JC. Intensive glycemic control in medsurg patients (European Glucontrol trial). Program and abstracts of the Society of Critical Care Medicine 36th Critical Care Congress, February 17–21, 2007, Orlando, FL.
68. Normoglycemia in Intensive Care Evaluation and Survival Using Glucose Algorithm Regulation (NICE-SUGAR). Current controlled trials: a multicentre, open label, randomised controlled trial of two target ranges for glycaemic control in intensive care unit (ICU) patients. http://controlled-trials.com/isrctn/trial/ISRCTN04968275/0/04968275. Accessed June 10, 2008.
69. Dellinger P, Levy MM, Jean M, et al. Surviving Sepsis Campaign: international guidelines for management of severe sepsis and septic shock: 2008. *Crit Care Med.* 2008;36(1):296–327.

CHAPTER 164 ■ THE ADRENAL GLAND IN CRITICAL ILLNESS

MARK S. COOPER

IMMEDIATE CONCERNS

Major Problems

The most important adrenal problem affecting the intensivist is impaired production of adrenal steroids. Individuals with impaired capacity to produce adrenal steroids can become critically ill with illnesses that are otherwise trivial and are unlikely to improve in the absence of steroid replacement. Critically ill patients may also develop adrenal insufficiency in the course of an intensive care unit (ICU) admission secondary to the effects of the underlying disease, or its treatment, on either the pituitary or adrenal gland. Furthermore, it has been suggested that conditions such as septic shock and acute respiratory distress syndrome (ARDS) might frequently be associated with a relative deficiency of adrenal steroids and, thus, patients with these conditions might benefit from steroid treatment, even in the absence of pre-existing adrenal disease. Other adrenal problems present rarely in the critical care setting; however, unrecognized pheochromocytoma can present as either severe hypertension or circulatory collapse on removal of the tumor.

Stress Points

1. The most important hormones synthesized by the adrenal gland are cortisol (the main glucocorticoid) and aldosterone (the main mineralocorticoid). Cortisol production is regulated by adrenocorticotropin hormone (ACTH) secretion whereas aldosterone secretion is primarily regulated by the renin–angiotensin system.
2. Corticosteroid insufficiency (hypoadrenalism) is the most important clinical problem involving the adrenal gland in the ICU setting. It can occur as a result of diseases that directly affect the adrenal gland (primary adrenal insufficiency) or those that impair ACTH production from the pituitary (secondary adrenal insufficiency). Corticosteroid insufficiency can be difficult to recognize since its clinical features are similar to those of other severe illnesses, and some features are masked by ICU interventions. Unrecognized, corticosteroid insufficiency is associated with a high mortality. The clinical findings associated with adrenal insufficiency are shown in Table 164.1.
3. The diagnosis of adrenal insufficiency is difficult in critically ill patients due to the insensitivity of clinical features and the dramatic and variable changes that occur normally in the hypothalamic-pituitary-adrenal (HPA) axis during severe illness. The interpretation of biochemical tests is difficult and will depend on the clinical context. Where there is uncertainty, empiric glucocorticoid replacement is indicated.
4. When the possibility of adrenal insufficiency during critical illness has been raised, definitive testing to determine whether it is present, persistent, and its nature—e.g., pituitary versus adrenal—will be needed, but only when the patient's condition has improved so as to safely allow the studies.

Essential Diagnostic Tests and Procedures

1. The symptoms, physical signs, and laboratory findings traditionally associated with hypoadrenalism are not sufficiently sensitive to be reliable in making the diagnosis of adrenal insufficiency. Rather, these may suggest the need for biochemical testing.
2. The diagnosis will usually be made on either a random serum cortisol level, the level of cortisol achieved after a short ACTH test, or (in the specific situation of septic shock) a poor increment in cortisol across a short ACTH test (Figs. 164.1 and 164.2).

Initial Therapy

For critically ill individuals with known or suspected structural defects in the HPA axis, treatment should be with 100 mg hydrocortisone every 6 hours. With improvement, this dose can be progressively reduced to replacement doses (typically 20 mg hydrocortisone a.m. and 10 mg p.m.). Patients with adrenal disease will also require fludrocortisone when the daily hydrocortisone dose drops below 50 mg per day. In septic shock, the recommended replacement dose for patients with suspected relative adrenal insufficiency is 50 mg hydrocortisone every 8 hours.

PHYSIOLOGY OF THE ADRENAL GLAND

The adrenal gland is composed of a cortex and a medulla. The adrenal cortex is the site of synthesis of adrenal corticosteroids, whereas the medulla synthesizes catecholamines (primarily adrenaline). The cortex is structurally and functionally divided into layers (zones) that secrete mineralocorticoids, glucocorticoids, and adrenal androgens. Adrenal hormones are synthesized rapidly from cholesterol with very little hormone being stored within the gland.

TABLE 164.1

CLINICAL FINDINGS IN ADRENAL INSUFFICIENCY

Symptoms
Weakness/fatigue
Anorexia
Nausea, vomiting, abdominal pain
Salt craving[a]
Postural dizziness
Myalgias/arthralgias
Signs
Weight loss
Hyperpigmentation[a]
Hypotension
Vitiligo[a]
Clinical findings
Hyponatremia
Hyperkalemia[a]
Hypoglycemia
Uremia
Anemia
Eosinophilia
Vasopressor insensitivity
Systemic inflammatory response in absence of infection

[a]Features usually present in primary adrenal insufficiency but not secondary adrenal insufficiency.

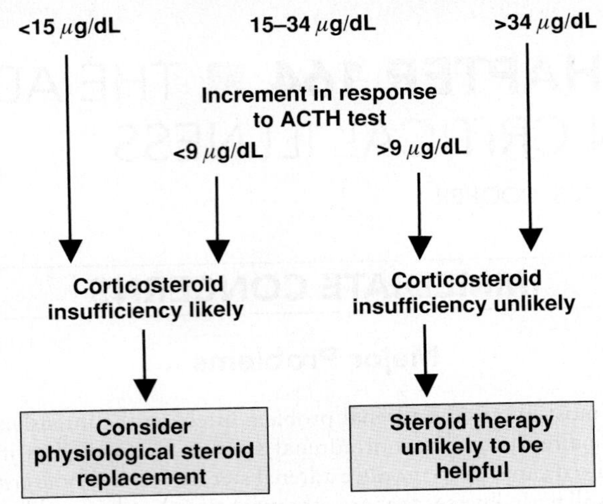

FIGURE 164.2. An adequate basal response is required to rule out central causes of corticosteroid insufficiency whereas an adequate increment has been reported to be needed to exclude relative adrenal insufficiency. The use of an incremental response outside of the setting of septic shock is not recommended. (Adapted from Cooper MS, Stewart, PM. Corticosteroid insufficiency in acutely ill patients. *N Engl J Med*. 2003;348:727–734.)

Adrenal Hormones

The main hormones synthesized by the adrenal cortex are aldosterone (the main mineralocorticoid), cortisol (the main glucocorticoid), and dehydroepiandrosterone (the main adrenal androgen). In conjunction with cortisol, aldosterone regulates salt and water balance. The main action of aldosterone is to increase sodium resorption within the distal nephron; it also regulates sodium excretion from the skin (in sweat), the pancreas, and the colon. Cortisol action affects almost all tissues in the body. These actions are important in maintaining homeostasis under resting conditions and also during stress. Many of these actions are evident only in states of glucocorticoid deficiency or excess. Cortisol levels in the circulation have a pronounced diurnal rhythm, being high in the morning and very low in the late evening. Cortisol in the circulation is heavily bound to serum proteins—corticosteroid-binding globulin (CBG) and albumin—such that only a small fraction is available in a tissue in free form (1). Adrenal androgens are the most abundantly produced adrenal steroids, but their clinical significance is minor compared to the other adrenal steroids, and they are not routinely substituted in patients with adrenal insufficiency.

Adrenaline is the main catecholamine secreted from the adrenal medulla. Although this hormone may modify some aspects of the stress response, the relative normality of individuals who have had both adrenal medullas removed suggests that this action is of limited importance in most situations. The focus of this chapter will therefore be on the adrenal cortex.

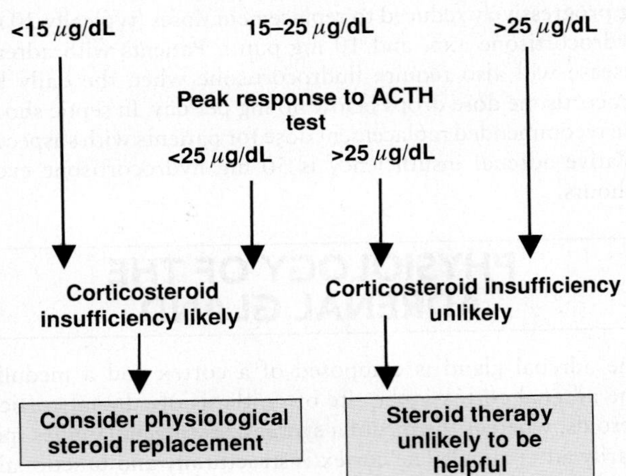

FIGURE 164.1. The combination of basal values and peak responses to ACTH tests is intended to avoid missing corticosteroid insufficiency of either central or adrenal origin.

Regulation of Adrenal Hormone Synthesis

Glucocorticoids and mineralocorticoids are regulated differently. Cortisol is synthesized in response to ACTH, which is released from the anterior pituitary. ACTH release is controlled by hypothalamic corticotrophin-releasing hormone (CRH) secretion. Central activation of the HPA axis occurs with all physiologic stressors and also entrains the diurnal rhythm of cortisol secretion. ACTH has an important trophic action on the adrenal cortex, and continued ACTH secretion is essential to maintain the structural integrity of the cortex and the capacity to generate cortisol. Impairment of ACTH secretion leads to a prolonged reduction in the capacity of the adrenal to respond to exogenous ACTH. This is most evident in pituitary disease but is also seen commonly in patients who take supraphysiologic doses of therapeutic glucocorticoids on a prolonged basis since these drugs inhibit ACTH secretion through negative feedback.

During severe illness, factors such as hypotension, pain, anxiety, and endotoxin substantially increase ACTH and cortisol secretion. The level of CBG also decreases rapidly due to a combination of reduced synthesis and increased breakdown (1). These combined effects lead to increased cortisol levels and a higher proportion of bioactive cortisol to protein-bound cortisol. These factors increase cortisol levels within target tissues.

Although the synthesis of the early precursors for aldosterone synthesis are under control of ACTH, the rate-limiting step is regulated by angiotensin II. The activity of the renin–angiotensin system is thus the most important factor in regulating aldosterone synthesis. This explains why aldosterone secretion is still maintained in patients with pituitary disease and consequent ACTH deficiency (2). Although aldosterone secretion does increase during the early phase of critical illness, its importance is probably minor because cortisol, when present at high levels, has a substantial mineralocorticoid effect.

Glucocorticoid Action

The range of actions of glucocorticoids is vast. These actions are sometimes apparent only when glucocorticoid levels are very low or high. Most of the side effects of therapeutic glucocorticoids result from an exaggeration of the physiologic effects that are normally protective during short-term stress.

Metabolic Effects

Glucocorticoids strongly influence most of the metabolic pathways involved in energy homeostasis. Glucocorticoids induce enzymes responsible for hepatic gluconeogenesis and antagonize the anabolic actions of insulin on glycogen deposition. Glucocorticoids also increase the production of fuels for gluconeogenesis by stimulating muscle amino acid generation and adipose tissue fatty acid synthesis. These combined effects ensure that glucose is readily available as a fuel, an effect likely to be of importance for immune cells and in damaged tissues. When prolonged, however, these effects result in adverse outcomes. Increased gluconeogenesis increases the risk of glucose intolerance and frank diabetes mellitus. Continued breakdown of protein leads to myopathy, skin thinning, easy bruising, and poor wound healing. Increased peripheral lipolysis leads to loss of fat on limbs but accumulation of central fat.

Cardiovascular Effects

Glucocorticoids have important effects on salt and water balance, which are likely to be an important part of the stress response protecting against hemorrhage or sepsis. Glucocorticoids contribute to renal sodium reabsorption, even though the dominant regulatory pathway is *via* aldosterone, and also have a major impact on the capacity to excrete water through the kidney. A deficiency of glucocorticoids can induce a state of excessive water retention and hyponatremia that is clinically indistinguishable from the syndrome of inappropriate antidiuretic hormone secretion (SIADH). The reason for the high prevalence of hypotension and circulatory collapse during adrenal insufficiency is the permissive effect glucocorticoids have on the vascular action of catecholamines. In the absence of glucocorticoids, the vasculature can become insensitive to the pressor effects of catecholamines; this feature is an important clue to the presence of corticosteroid insufficiency.

Immunologic Effects

Glucocorticoids have a broad spectrum of effects on inflammation and the immune system, including an impact on the development, migration, and survival of leukocytes, and a reduction of the synthesis of proinflammatory cytokines by immune cells and blockade of tissue production of eicosanoids such as prostaglandins and leukotrienes. While excessive glucocorticoid action can lead to immunosuppression, glucocorticoid deficiency states are also associated with impaired resistance to microbial infection.

Other Effects

In addition to those effects noted above, glucocorticoids also have a wide range of other clinical actions. For example, a common problem seen with the administration of glucocorticoids is a disturbance of bone metabolism leading to osteoporosis and fractures. The hormone may also induce a range of neuropsychiatric symptoms ranging from sleep disturbance to frank psychosis.

CORTICOSTEROID INSUFFICIENCY

Corticosteroid insufficiency can occur with diseases or interventions that involve the adrenal gland directly (primary adrenal insufficiency), or secondary to reduced stimulation by ACTH of an otherwise normal adrenal gland due to hypothalamic or pituitary disease (secondary adrenal insufficiency). Glucocorticoid replacement is similar in the two conditions, but important clinical features may differ; biochemical testing will provide different results depending on setting, and the pattern of deficiency of other hormones will be different. In septic shock, it has been suggested that a relative deficiency of corticosteroids either at the tissue level or within the circulation might occur, and that low-dose corticosteroid treatment may improve outcome; this remains, however, an area of great debate (1,3,4).

Causes of Corticosteroid Insufficiency

In outpatient endocrine practice, the differential diagnosis of hypoadrenalism is wide, with the most common causes of primary hypoadrenalism in the United States being autoimmune adrenalitis and that of secondary hypoadrenalism being partial or complete hypopituitarism. On the other hand, worldwide, the most common cause of permanent hypoadrenalism is tuberculous adrenalitis. By contrast, in the general population, adrenal insufficiency is most frequently encountered in patients who have developed hypoadrenalism secondary to recent oral glucocorticoid usage.

During critical illness, reversible adrenal insufficiency may develop secondary to many factors, including the use of anesthetic agents and antibiotics, central nervous system (CNS) disease, and adrenal insults that may comprise hemorrhage, infection, and hypoperfusion (Table 164.1) (3,5,6). Increased proinflammatory cytokine production during sepsis can also induce systemic glucocorticoid resistance such that normal adrenal responses may be insufficient to control systemic inflammation. The term, *relative adrenal insufficiency*, has been used to describe this situation (4,6). Adrenal insufficiency can profoundly influence the chances of survival from critical illness, as demonstrated by the increased mortality associated with prolonged etomidate administration when this agent was used as an ICU sedative. The effect was due to the drug's potent action to inhibit the enzyme systems needed to synthesize cortisol, especially 11-β-hydroxylase (7,8).

An underappreciated problem is secondary hypoadrenalism due to recent exogenous glucocorticoid therapy. Such therapy suppresses the HPA axis, with consequent adrenal atrophy that may last for months after cessation of glucocorticoid treatment. Adrenal atrophy and subsequent deficiency depends on both the dose and duration of treatment but should be anticipated in any subject taking (or having recently stopped) more than 30 mg hydrocortisone per day (7.5 mg prednisolone, 0.75 mg dexamethasone) for greater than 3 weeks. In such subjects, hypoadrenalism may be precipitated by failure to give adequate glucocorticoid replacement for intercurrent stress.

Clinical Presentation

Adrenal insufficiency may present with either the classical symptoms of this syndrome, symptoms related to other hormone deficiencies, or symptoms relating to the underlying cause of adrenal insufficiency. It may also present with few specific features. The clinical presentation of adrenal insufficiency also differs greatly between the endocrine outpatient setting and the intensive care unit, as might be expected. In an outpatient setting, clinical features depend on rate of onset and severity of adrenal deficiency. The onset may be insidious, with presenting symptoms such as weakness, weight loss, nausea, abdominal pain, arthralgia, and postural syncope, and the diagnosis being made only with the development of an acute crisis during an intercurrent illness. Acute adrenal insufficiency (addisonian crisis) is a medical emergency manifesting as hypotension and circulatory failure. Anorexia, nausea, vomiting, diarrhea, and abdominal pain may occur, and fever and hypoglycemia may be present. Skin pigmentation usually differentiates primary from secondary hypoadrenalism, reflecting the persistently high circulating ACTH concentrations in the former condition. In autoimmune Addison disease, there may be associated vitiligo. In secondary adrenal insufficiency due to hypopituitarism, the presentation may relate to symptom complexes due to deficiency of hormones other than ACTH, notably leuteinizing hormone (LH)/follicle-stimulating hormone (FSH)—presenting with infertility, oligomenorrhea/amenorrhea, and/or poor libido—and thyroid-stimulating hormone (TSH)—presenting with weight gain and cold intolerance. Rarely, presentation may be more acute in patients with pituitary apoplexy.

In critically ill patients, these features may be masked, and the only signs may be hemodynamic instability despite adequate fluid resuscitation, usually with a hyperdynamic circulation and decreased systemic vascular resistance, or ongoing evidence of inflammation without an obvious source or response to empiric treatment.

Biochemical Diagnosis

The biochemical diagnosis of hypoadrenalism can be straightforward in an outpatient setting but is often much more difficult in the critical care unit. In established primary hypoadrenalism, hyponatremia is present in 90% of cases and hyperkalemia in 65%. Hyperkalemia occurs due to aldosterone deficiency, and is therefore usually absent in secondary hypoadrenalism. Hyponatremia may be depletional in addisonian crisis, but elevated vasopressin levels can cause dilutional hyponatremia in secondary adrenal insufficiency. Usually, free thyroxine concentrations are low or normal, but TSH values are frequently elevated. This is a direct effect of glucocorticoid deficiency and reverses with glucocorticoid replacement. Thyroxine levels may also be low in secondary hypoadrenalism. Thyroid hormone administration without glucocorticoids in these situations can precipitate adrenal insufficiency and should be avoided. Eosinophilia may be seen and can occasionally alert the astute clinician to the diagnosis (9).

Clinical suspicion of hypoadrenalism should be confirmed biochemically and, in the outpatient setting, there is a general consensus on the appropriate way to diagnose adrenal insufficiency; in the critical care unit setting, this is a bit more of a problem. Although a low 0900 hour—or even random—cortisol level may be highly suggestive of hypoadrenalism, the marked diurnal variation in serum cortisol levels and response of the serum cortisol level to stress generally require that stimulation tests be used. The gold standard stimulation test is the insulin tolerance test (ITT), which assesses the integrity of the whole HPA axis (10,11). However, it cannot be performed in patients with ischemic heart disease, epilepsy, or severe cortisol deficiency (an 0900 hour cortisol less than 7 μg/dL). In normal subjects, peak plasma cortisol exceeds 18 μg/dL. However, the cortisol response to hypoglycemia can be reliably predicted by the ACTH stimulation test—a safer, quicker, and less expensive study. The ACTH stimulation test involves intramuscular or intravenous administration of 250 μg tetracosactin (Synacthen, Cosyntropin; 1-24 ACTH) (12). In critically ill patients, the intravenous (IV) route is preferred due to the reduced reliability of intramuscular (IM) absorption. In outpatient endocrine practice, plasma cortisol levels are measured at 0 and 30 minutes post-ACTH infusion, and a normal response is defined by peak plasma cortisol greater than 20 μg/dL. In critically ill patients, an additional sample 60 minutes after baseline is often used, with the peak value defined as the higher of the 30- and 60-minute values. The use of the 60-minute sample is not standard practice when basing decisions on peak levels but is reasonable when an increment is being used, e.g., septic shock (as described below). The peak value is unaffected by the time of day, but the basal value varies with the diurnal rhythm, so the incremental response in this setting should not be used as a measure of adrenal function. The test can still be performed in patients who have recently commenced corticosteroid replacement therapy with dexamethasone, as it does not cross-react in the cortisol assay. In primary adrenal insufficiency, ACTH levels are disproportionately elevated relative to plasma cortisol. Since the cortisol response is dependent on endogenous ACTH trophic drive to the adrenal cortex, impaired pituitary ACTH secretion will result in an impaired cortisol response. The ACTH test should, therefore, not be used after a recent pituitary insult (surgery, apoplexy), as it may take 2 to 3 weeks for the adrenal cortex to readjust to the reduced level of ACTH secretion (13). A low-dose (1 μg) ACTH stimulation test has been proposed, with the suggestion that it may be more sensitive than the 250-μg test; at this time, it is not widely used (14).

In patients found to have abnormal responses to the 250-μg study, further tests will usually be required to determine the cause, for example, studies for adrenal autoantibodies, abdominal imaging for primary adrenal failure, and/or pituitary MRI and other anterior pituitary function tests for secondary adrenal failure.

In a critically ill patient, the testing regimen is more complex and more difficult, thus making it—at this juncture—perhaps technically impossible to robustly diagnose adrenal insufficiency. This is largely due to the dramatic and variable changes at all levels of the HPA axis, the difficulty of performing dynamic tests in critically ill patients, and the complex pathogenesis and heterogeneity of clinical causes (6). Consequently, no test has proven reliable in the diagnosis of adrenal insufficiency (1,6). Since cortisol levels are normally elevated during critical illness, random cortisol levels below 20 μg/dL might be considered suggestive of adrenal insufficiency. Cortisol responses during stress, however, are usually much higher than those seen during the short ACTH test, and thus higher cutoff levels have been proposed (15). The use of the short ACTH is controversial in critical illness but remains the test that is most useful to intensivists. In patients with suspected primary adrenal insufficiency, the peak value obtained during an ACTH test should be at least 20 μg/dL, but in patients with hypotension or sepsis, it would be reasonable to expect values to exceed 25 μg/dL. This test, however, has clear limitations when hypoadrenalism occurs secondary to recent hypothalamic or pituitary insults, and thus should not be relied on in patients with possible recent-onset secondary adrenal insufficiency.

A general scheme for investigating adrenal insufficiency in critical illness, combining basal and stimulated tests, is given in Figure 164.1. Specifically, in vasopressor-dependent septic shock, the incremental response post-ACTH administration—in contrast to that in noncritically ill patients—may have prognostic implications, with a limited increment (less than 9 μg/dL) being associated with increased mortality (16). Furthermore, there is some evidence that glucocorticoid supplementation improves mortality in this setting (17). A scheme for investigating adrenal insufficiency in septic shock is given in Figure 164.2. It is currently unclear which critically ill patients should be investigated for adrenal insufficiency, but there should always be a clear indication to undergo testing. It seems reasonable to assess HPA-axis function using the acute ACTH test in critically ill patients with severe inflammation, those previously treated with glucocorticoids, and those with clinical or biochemical features suggestive of adrenal insufficiency. In these complex cases, testing may be required on more than one occasion in any individual. Clinical improvement with hydrocortisone replacement is good evidence for adrenal insufficiency when the diagnosis is uncertain.

Management

In addition to measurement of plasma electrolytes and blood glucose, samples for ACTH and cortisol should be taken before initiating corticosteroid therapy. If the patient is not critically ill, an ACTH stimulation test can be performed. In critically ill patients, intravenous hydrocortisone should be given in a dose of 100 mg every 6 hours either as a bolus dose or a continuous infusion. This additional corticosteroid is given to try to mimic the normal production of adrenal steroid during severe illness. Hydrocortisone is the pharmaceutical name for cortisol (the difference in name when measured by assay or when given as a drug is purely historical). Hydrocortisone is used in preference to other glucocorticoids, e.g., prednisone, prednisolone, methylprednisolone, or dexamethasone, because it is a physiologic replacement and because in previous trials of septic shock, use of the other glucocorticoids did not improve survival. In the patient suffering from shock, intravenous 0.9% saline solution should be given initially; adding 5% dextrose to this solution may be required if hypoglycemia is present. Subsequent saline and dextrose therapy will depend on clinical

TABLE 164.2

RELATIVE POTENCY OF GLUCOCORTICOIDS AND APPROXIMATE DOSE EQUIVALENTS WHEN USED FOR GLUCOCORTICOID REPLACEMENT

	Relative glucocorticoid potency[a]	Replacement dose (mg)
Hydrocortisone[b]	1	30[d]
Cortisone[b,c]	0.8	37.5
Prednisolone	4.5	5–7.5
Prednisone[c]	4.5	5–7.5
Methylprednisolone	5	4
Dexamethasone	35	0.75

[a]Relative glucocorticoid potency varies with the parameter studied so is only approximate and refers predominantly to glucocorticoid replacement in Addison.
[b]Physiologic glucocorticoids that are preferred for replacement purposes.
[c]These steroids are inactive prodrugs so are used only *via* the oral route.
[d]This is the standard initial replacement dose in patients with possible adrenal insufficiency but can often be reduced to 15–20 mg when needed long term.

and biochemical monitoring. Clinical improvement, especially in blood pressure, should be evident within 6 hours if the diagnosis is correct. It is important to recognize and treat any precipitating condition, such as infection.

After 24 hours, the hydrocortisone dose can be reduced, usually to 50 mg every 6 hours and subsequently, if possible, to oral hydrocortisone, 40 mg in the morning and 20 mg at 1800 hours. This can then be rapidly reduced to standard replacement doses of 20 mg on wakening and 10 mg at 1800 hours. Although synthetic glucocorticoids have been used in adrenal replacement—their relative potencies and dose equivalents are given in Table 164.2—they have no advantage over hydrocortisone and are more frequently associated with adverse effects with long-term use. Mineralocorticoid replacement is not required during high-dose hydrocortisone therapy, but patients with adrenal disease will also require fludrocortisone when daily hydrocortisone dose drops below 50 mg per day.

In septic shock, the recommended replacement is 50 mg of hydrocortisone every 8 hours. This lower dose reflects the following facts: (a) most people treated with replacement glucocorticoids have only relative adrenal insufficiency; (b) the clearance of hydrocortisone appears to be reduced in septic shock compared to other conditions; and (c) this is the dose that has been most widely studied in clinical trials (17–19). This dose does lead to supraphysiologic levels of hydrocortisone in the circulation, but it is unclear whether this is important either in terms of leading to adverse effects or in accounting for any benefit through overcoming tissue resistance to corticosteroids. In the largest trial that examined glucocorticoid replacement in septic shock, fludrocortisone was given orally for 1 week in addition to glucocorticoids (17). On the basis of the mineralocorticoid activity of hydrocortisone and experience in patients with Addison disease, it is unlikely that fludrocortisone accounts for any of the benefits of low-dose corticosteroid supplementation, and thus would not normally be needed in the acute setting. When relative adrenal insufficiency has been diagnosed during a critical illness, this relative deficiency is most often transient. Nonetheless, low doses of corticosteroids should continue until definite testing has been carried out after resolution of illness.

ADRENAL HORMONE EXCESS (CUSHING SYNDROME)

States of endogenous corticosteroid excess are rare. Cushing disease is due to an ACTH-secreting pituitary adenoma and has an incidence of approximately 1 per million of population. Endogenous Cushing *syndrome* is otherwise from a cortisol-secreting adrenal adenoma or ectopic ACTH secretion, often from a benign or malignant pulmonary tumor. The diagnosis of Cushing disease/syndrome and the determination of the site of the lesion are difficult to make, involving dynamic suppression tests, imaging, and venous sampling (20). It is unlikely that states of endogenous cortisol excess will present initially to critical care physicians, so their management is outside the scope of this chapter.

Much more common is iatrogenic Cushing syndrome caused by therapeutic glucocorticoids. Patients with this disorder are likely to have the classic features of Cushing syndrome—namely, central obesity, myopathy, skin fragility, glucose intolerance, osteoporosis, and hypertension—but the main clinical issue in this situation is to ensure that a physiologic replacement dose of steroid is maintained during intercurrent stress. In any patient on long-term oral steroid doses above 5 to 7.5 mg prednisolone or its equivalent, intravenous steroid replacement should be administered if the patient is unable to continue the oral dose, since it is likely that he or she will have a variable degree of adrenal atrophy secondary to prolonged ACTH suppression.

OTHER ADRENAL DISEASES

Hyperaldosteronism

Other adrenal diseases are uncommon or do not present significant problems in the critical care setting. Primary hyperaldosteronism was previously thought to be uncommon, but is increasingly recognized as a major cause of hypertension. This form of mineralocorticoid-mediated hypertension is associated with hypokalemia and a raised aldosterone-to-renin ratio (21). The use of this ratio has increased the number of diagnoses of primary hyperaldosteronism, mainly due to an increased incidence of bilateral adrenal hyperplasia. Treatment is with surgery or with long-term spironolactone.

Pheochromocytoma

Pheochromocytoma is an adrenal medullary tumor that secretes excessive amounts of catecholamines (22). This tumor is rare and sporadic, but is a common feature of some inherited endocrine syndromes such as multiple endocrine neoplasia type 2, von Hippel-Lindau, and neurofibromatosis. The symptoms of pheochromocytoma are vague and include palpitations, sweating, headaches, and overwhelming anxiety in association with sustained or paroxysmal hypertension. Although hypertensive crisis is a risk, especially during handling of the tumor or with administration of beta-blockers, sustained catecholamine release leads to vasoconstriction and contraction of the intravascular volume. Removal of the tumor can lead to a dramatic *reduction* in blood pressure due to vasodilatation. These effects may be prevented by preoperative treatment, initially with increasing doses of an alpha-blocker such as phenoxybenzamine and followed, if needed, by a beta-blocker. If postural hypotension develops, volume replacement with IV normal saline is indicated.

ADRENAL FUNCTION TESTS

The following section describes important common biochemical tests for evaluating patients with adrenal disease.

Serum Cortisol

Procedure. Serum is collected for a standard radioimmunoassay or ELISA (enzyme-linked immunosorbent assay). It is important to note the time of collection, because cortisol levels vary throughout the day.

Normal Values

Unstressed patient:	0800 value usually 5 to 25 μg/dL.
During critical illness:	Random value less than 7 μg/dL strongly suggests adrenal insufficiency (AI). Value less than 15 μg/dL in possible secondary AI suggests deficiency. Value greater than 34 μg/dL associated with a poor prognosis but AI unlikely.

Comments. Serum cortisol levels normally vary in a circadian pattern, with peak levels in the early morning and nadirs late at night. During critical illness, this diurnal rhythm is lost and cortisol levels increase broadly with the degree of stress. Basal cortisol levels alone are not very useful in the evaluation of adrenal disease, but are the only useful test in recent-onset secondary AI. Refinements on serum cortisol measurement include estimation of serum-free cortisol, taking into account CBG and albumin levels (23), but these assays are not widely available or tested thoroughly in critical care settings.

Short ACTH Stimulation Test

Procedure. Serum samples are obtained just before and 30 (and/or 60) minutes after an IV injection of 250 μg of tetracosactin (Synacthen, Cosyntropin, 1-24 ACTH).

Interpretation

Unstressed patient:	Peak cortisol value less than 20 μg/dL suggests AI
During critical illness:	Peak cortisol less than 20 μg/dL suggests AI (patients without sepsis or hypotension) Peak cortisol less than 25 μg/dL suggests AI (patients with sepsis or hypotension) Cortisol increment less than 9 μg/dL indicates relative AI (of use *only* in vasopressor-dependent septic shock)

Comments. The diagnosis of AI in the ICU usually depends on the short ACTH stimulation test, but its interpretation is difficult and depends on clinical context. Peak cortisol values of either 20 or 25 μg/dL have been proposed and should be used depending on the severity of the illness. In septic shock, the use of the increment has been proposed for diagnosing relative adrenal insufficiency and may identify patients likely to benefit from glucocorticoid replacement; however, it should *not* be used outside this setting without evidence. The test does not differentiate between primary and secondary hypoadrenalism, and is unreliable in recent-onset secondary AI.

Insulin Tolerance Test

Procedure. An intravenous cannula is inserted, and 0.1 to 0.15 U/kg regular insulin given IV, with measurement of plasma cortisol at 0, 30, 45, 60, 90, and 120 minutes. Adequate hypoglycemia—blood glucose less than 40 mg/dL (2.2 mmol/L) with signs of neuroglycopenia, e.g., sweating and tachycardia—is essential.

Interpretation

Peak cortisol greater than 18 μg/dL rules out deficiency. ACTH levels can indicate whether deficiency is due to primary or secondary AI.

Comments. Contraindicated in patients with epilepsy, ischemic heart disease, and in patients with serum cortisol levels less than 7 μg/dL. Unsuitable for use in the critical care setting.

References

1. Arafah BM. Hypothalamic pituitary adrenal function during critical illness: limitations of current assessment methods. *J Clin Endocrinol Metab.* 2006;91:3725–3745.
2. Cooper MS, Stewart PM. Diagnosis and treatment of ACTH deficiency. *Rev Endocr Metab Disord.* 2005;6:47–54.
3. Annane D. Glucocorticoids in the treatment of severe sepsis and septic shock. *Curr Opin Crit Care.* 2005;11:449–453.
4. Beishuizen A, Thijs LG. Relative adrenal failure in intensive care: an identifiable problem requiring treatment? *Best Pract Res Clin Endocrinol Metab.* 2001;15:513–531.
5. Burchard K. A review of the adrenal cortex and severe inflammation: quest of the "eucorticoid" state. *J Trauma.* 2001;51:800–814.
6. Cooper MS, Stewart PM. Corticosteroid insufficiency in acutely ill patients. *N Engl J Med.* 2003;348:727–734.
7. Watt I, Ledingham IM. Mortality amongst multiple trauma patients admitted to an intensive therapy unit. *Anaesthesia.* 1984;39:973–981.
8. Jackson WL Jr. Should we use etomidate as an induction agent for endotracheal intubation in patients with septic shock?: a critical appraisal. *Chest.* 2005;127:1031–1038.
9. Beishuizen A, Vermes I, Hylkema BS, et al. Relative eosinophilia and functional adrenal insufficiency in critically ill patients. *Lancet.* 1999;353:1675–1676.
10. Stewart PM, Corrie J, Seckl JR, et al. A rational approach for assessing the hypothalamo-pituitary-adrenal axis. *Lancet.* 1988;1:1208–1210.
11. Galloway PJ, McNeill E, Paterson WF, et al. Safety of the insulin tolerance test. *Arch Dis Child.* 2002;87:354–356.
12. Dickstein G, Shechner C, Nicholson WE, et al. Adrenocorticotropin stimulation test: effects of basal cortisol level, time of day, and suggested new sensitive low dose test. *J Clin Endocrinol Metab.* 1991;72:773–778.
13. Clark PM, Neylon I, Raggatt PR, et al. Defining the normal cortisol response to the short Synacthen test: implications for the investigation of hypothalamic-pituitary disorders. *Clin Endocrinol (Oxf).* 1998;49:287–292.
14. Abdu TA, Elhadd TA, Neary R, et al. Comparison of the low dose short Synacthen test (1 microg), the conventional dose short Synacthen test (250 microg), and the insulin tolerance test for assessment of the hypothalamo-pituitary-adrenal axis in patients with pituitary disease. *J Clin Endocrinol Metab.* 1999;84:838–843.
15. Marik PE, Zaloga GP. Adrenal insufficiency during septic shock. *Crit Care Med.* 2003;31:141–145.
16. Annane D, Sebille V, Troche G, et al. A 3-level prognostic classification in septic shock based on cortisol levels and cortisol response to corticotropin. *JAMA.* 2000;283:1038–1045.
17. Annane D, Sebille V, Charpentier C, et al. Effect of treatment with low doses of hydrocortisone and fludrocortisone on mortality in patients with septic shock. *JAMA.* 2002;288:862–871.
18. Briegel J, Forst H, Haller M, et al. Stress doses of hydrocortisone reverse hyperdynamic septic shock: a prospective, randomized, double-blind, single-center study. *Crit Care Med.* 1999;27:723–732.
19. Bollaert PE, Charpentier C, Levy B, et al. Reversal of late septic shock with supraphysiologic doses of hydrocortisone. *Crit Care Med.* 1998;26:645–650.
20. Newell-Price J, Bertagna X, Grossman AB, et al. Cushing's syndrome. *Lancet.* 2006;367:1605–1617.
21. Mulatero P, Dluhy RG, Giacchetti G, et al. Diagnosis of primary aldosteronism: from screening to subtype differentiation. *Trends Endocrinol Metab.* 2005;16:114–119.
22. Lenders JW, Eisenhofer G, Mannelli M, et al. Phaeochromocytoma. *Lancet.* 2005;366:665–675.
23. Hamrahian AH, Oseni TS, Arafah BM. Measurements of serum free cortisol in critically ill patients. *N Engl J Med.*2004;350:1629–1638.

CHAPTER 165 ■ PHEOCHROMOCYTOMA

DANIEL T. RUAN • QUAN-YANG DUH

IMMEDIATE CONCERNS

Major Problems

Pheochromocytoma is a rare catecholamine-secreting tumor with a wide spectrum of presentations ranging from minimal symptoms (1) to sudden death (2). Although early diagnosis can lead to a curative treatment course (3), outcomes are often fatal when the condition is unrecognized (4). Pheochromocytoma should be included in the differential diagnosis for patients with poorly controlled hypertension, heart failure, and cerebrovascular events. Furthermore, critical care physicians should be familiar with pheochromocytoma crisis, as it is a medical emergency requiring the highest level of specialty care.

Stress Points

1. The diagnosis of pheochromocytoma should be considered in any patient who presents with severe hypertension or the classic symptoms of episodic headache, palpitations, and diaphoresis.
2. Fractionated plasma metanephrines or 24-hour urine metanephrines are the initial laboratory studies to rule out pheochromocytoma.
3. α-Blockade with phenoxybenzamine should be started as soon as the biochemical diagnosis of pheochromocytoma is established.
4. After adequate α-blockade is established, β-blockers can be used as an adjuvant means of controlling tachycardia.
5. Pheochromocytoma crisis is a medical emergency requiring immediate α-blockade and invasive hemodynamic monitoring; additional pharmacologic agents, such as β-blockers, calcium channel blockers, and intravenous nitrates, are often needed to control heart rate and blood pressure.
6. The only curative therapy for pheochromocytoma is surgical resection; however, this should be attempted only on an elective basis after several weeks of adrenergic blockade.

PATHOPHYSIOLOGY

Although approximately 90% of pheochromocytomas are histologically benign, the morbidity of pheochromocytoma is primarily related to the cardiovascular impact of unregulated systemic catecholamine excess. Pheochromocytomas originate from chromaffin cells, and by definition, are located in the adrenal medulla. Although extra-adrenal pheochromocytomas are often termed paragangliomas, these terms will be considered synonymous for the purposes of this chapter.

Intermittent and unregulated catecholamine release is the hallmark pathophysiologic feature of pheochromocytoma. There are three sequential products synthesized in the adrenal medulla from the precursor L-tyrosine—dopamine, norepinephrine, and epinephrine. The rate-limiting step in catecholamine synthesis is the production of the precursor peptide L-DOPA, a process catalyzed by the enzyme tyrosine hydroxylase. By decarboxylation, L-DOPA is converted to dopamine, which is then converted to norepinephrine by β-hydroxylase. Ultimately, norepinephrine is converted to epinephrine by phenylethanolamine-N-methyltransferase.

Although norepinephrine is the predominant catecholamine secreted by most pheochromocytomas, there are reports of rare tumors that secrete dopamine (5), adrenocorticotropic hormone (6), vasoactive intestinal peptide (7), and calcitonin gene-related peptide (8). The highly varied presentation of pheochromocytoma may, in part, be explained by the variety of secretory products that have been reported. Vasoactive intestinal peptide can cause abdominal discomfort and a secretory diarrhea. Calcitonin, a gene-related peptidelike vasoactive intestinal peptide, is a potent vasodilator that can cause hypotension.

Because phenylethanolamine-N-methyltransferase is found only in the adrenal medulla and the organ of Zuckerkandl, epinephrine-secreting tumors are typically located in these two locations. Although some evidence suggests that patients in pheochromocytoma crisis have tumors that secrete primarily epinephrine, this has not been substantiated (9).

The diagnostic laboratory tests rely primarily on the detection of the metabolic products of the catecholamines. Monoamine oxidase catalyzes the conversion of catecholamines into vanillylmandelic acid and homovanillic acid. Furthermore, carboxyl-O-methyl transferase converts norepinephrine to normetanephrine and epinephrine into metanephrine.

EPIDEMIOLOGY OF PHEOCHROMOCYTOMA

Pheochromocytoma is a rare tumor with an incidence ranging from 0.1% (10) to 0.25% (11) in large autopsy studies. The prevalence in hypertensive patients is in the range of 0.1% to 1%. Pheochromocytoma can occur sporadically or in association with several familial syndromes. Although approximately 84% of cases are estimated to be sporadic (12), up to 24% of nonsyndromic pheochromocytoma patients have specific germ line mutations, including RET (MEN-2), VHL (von Hippel-Lindau), and succinate dehydrogenase subunit D (SDHD) and B (SDHB) (13).

Approximately 40% of MEN 2 patients develop pheochromocytoma. While bilateral and multicentric tumors are more common in these patients, extra-adrenal and malignant lesions are uncommon. Because of the relatively high incidence of pheochromocytoma, patients known to have the RET protooncogene mutation should be routinely screened for elevation in serum or urine metanephrines.

VHL disease is inherited in an autosomal dominant fashion and is characterized by retinal hemangiomatosis, pancreatic tumors, cerebellar hemangioblastoma, kidney lesions, and epididymal cystadenoma. Pheochromocytoma can be found in up to 20% of people with VHL disease. As in MEN 2, bilateral disease is more common than in sporadic cases.

SDHB and SDHD are susceptibility genes for pheochromocytoma associated with extra-adrenal lesions (14). Whereas SDHD mutation carriers are more likely to have multifocal extra-adrenal pheochromocytomas, SDHB mutation carriers are more likely to develop malignancy and may be associated with kidney and thyroid cancer.

Other rare familial disorders that are associated with pheochromocytoma include von Recklinghausen disease (15) and Carney syndrome (16).

CLINICAL PRESENTATION

Signs and Symptoms

The symptoms of pheochromocytoma are highly variable (17), which has earned this tumor the nickname "the great mimic" (18). The classic symptoms include episodic headache, palpitations, diaphoresis, and visual blurring. Other complaints may include tremors, anxiety, dizziness, nausea, diarrhea, abdominal discomfort, Raynaud phenomenon, and weight loss (19). In addition, observers often note intermittent pallor and weight loss in those affected.

Although some pheochromocytomas are discovered incidentally on radiographic scans performed for other reasons (20), on specific questioning, many of these patients report symptoms referable to the hyperadrenergic state. Up to 23% of all "incidentalomas" are discovered during abdominal imaging in trauma patients, further underscoring the significance of this tumor in the critical care setting (21). Moreover, among patients with a known history of another malignancy, up to a fourth of radiologically discovered adrenal tumors are pheochromocytomas and not metastatic disease (22).

Hypertension is the most common feature of pheochromocytoma and occurs in up to 90% of patients. Patients may be normotensive between episodes of catecholamine excess, and postural tachycardia and hypotension is another commonly seen feature of pheochromocytoma. Anecdotal reports indicate that peripheral vasoconstriction can be severe to a point that blood pressure cannot be measured with a traditional cuff and sphygmomanometer. Conversely, some patients can be normotensive for many years (23) and only suffer a hypertensive crisis after being stressed (24). Less commonly, some present with diastolic hypertension and postural hypotension, in the absence of antihypertensive therapy. Notably, some ophthalmologists have diagnosed pheochromocytoma by identifying severe retinopathy on routine eye examination.

ESSENTIAL DIAGNOSTIC TESTS

Biochemical Identification

The biochemical diagnosis of pheochromocytoma is dependent on the detection of elevated levels of catecholamines or their metabolites. Because functional pheochromocytomas release catecholamines heterogeneously and intermittently (25), spot checks of norepinephrine, epinephrine, or dopamine are often within a normal range and cannot reliably exclude the diagnosis of pheochromocytoma.

Conversely, free metanephrines are continuously elevated in patients with functional pheochromocytomas. Total metanephrine measurement is less sensitive than determining the fractionated amount of normetanephrine, metanephrine, and methoxytyramine, which are the metabolites of norepinephrine, epinephrine, and dopamine, respectively.

Fractionated plasma metanephrine measurement is also more sensitive than 24-hour urinary total metanephrines and catecholamines, but is less specific (26). In the critically ill patient with clinical characteristics that are highly suspicious for pheochromocytoma, measurement of fractionated plasma metanephrines is the most appropriate test. Conversely, when low-risk patients are screened, 24-hour urinary studies will yield the lowest proportion of false-positive results.

Furthermore, certain medications and radiographic contrast agents can interfere with the laboratory results and should be withheld before the draw. Clinicians should be aware of these medications, as they can affect the secretion or metabolism of catecholamines. The list of medications that can affect the biochemical testing for pheochromocytoma is long and includes the following: acetaminophen, beta-blockers, vasodilators, alpha-blockers, stimulants, antipsychotics, antidepressants, and calcium channel blockers.

In the elective setting when the diagnosis is equivocal, these medications should be withheld prior to biochemical testing. Provocative tests with agents such as histamine, glucagon, and naloxone are no longer recommended, as they can be dangerous and are ineffective in patients with normal urinary studies (27).

Tumor Localization

Although biochemical diagnosis is essential to diagnose and start treatment for the critically ill patient with pheochromocytoma, tumor localization will not change the therapeutic plan for patients in the intensive care unit. The identification of extra-adrenal pheochromocytoma may not be predictive of malignancy or prognosis (28). However, localization studies are important for surgical planning (29) and can confirm the diagnosis.

Ultrasound is particularly useful in critically ill patients, as it can be done at the bedside without exposing them to nephrotoxic contrast agents or ionizing radiation. Although ultrasound can be performed quickly and can accurately rule out a large adrenal lesion, it can also be highly user dependent.

Magnetic resonance imaging is another effective way to identify pheochromocytoma lesions and can delineate the anatomy important for surgical planning. Pheochromocytomas have a characteristic high-intensity signal on T2-weighted MR images. The drawbacks of MR imaging are the high cost and the lack of available scanners at some institutions.

CT scanning is available at more centers than MRI or nuclear medicine studies. Although most pheochromocytomas occur in the adrenal glands, patients should be scanned from the chest to the pelvis to evaluate for extra-adrenal lesions. Drawbacks to consider include (a) the possibility of exacerbating a pheochromocytoma crisis from contrast injection; (b) the exposure to ionizing radiation, which may be important in some obstetric or pediatric patients; and (c) the obscuring artifacts that can occur from implanted devices and surgical clips.

Meta-[^{131}]iodobenzylguanidine (MIBG) is concentrated within adrenergic vesicles, which allow sensitive scintigraphic imaging of the whole body. It is particularly useful in patients at risk for multiple or extra-adrenal tumors, such as in young children, and in patients with a family history or familial syndrome associated with pheochromocytoma. Although MIBG scanning can localize extra-adrenal lesions, multicentric lesions, and malignant tumors with good specificity, it is less sensitive than CT or MRI.

Workup of Incidental Lesions

Subclinical or mild cases of pheochromocytoma are sometimes discovered when incidental lesions are found on CT scans or MR images obtained for other reasons. Although many clinicians continue to perform fine-needle aspiration biopsy and selective venous sampling for patients with adrenal tumors, these interventional studies may precipitate a pheochromocytoma crisis and are relatively contraindicated. The finding of an adrenal "incidentaloma" should prompt the biochemical workup described above, as well as the measurement of plasma aldosterone, renin activity, and 24-hour urine cortisol. These studies will rule out aldosteronoma and Cushing syndrome. All functioning adrenal lesions, including pheochromocytoma, should be resected electively.

MANAGEMENT

Treatment of Nonemergent Pheochromocytoma

Although pheochromocytoma is uncommon, it is a potential cause of cardiovascular emergencies such as heart failure (30), myocardial infarction (31), and stroke (32). When pheochromocytoma is the cause of these events, appropriate therapy to control the hyperadrenergic state can often reverse or minimize disability. Most patients with pheochromocytoma who succumb to myocardial infarction or cerebrovascular catastrophe have undiagnosed tumors (33).

Although surgical intervention remains the only curative therapy for pheochromocytoma, the tumor should be resected only after appropriate preoperative steps are undertaken. Preoperative preparation for elective resection includes α-blockade to control hypertension, prevent cardiac arrhythmias, and allow adequate volume resuscitation before resection. Effective preoperative preparation and α-blockade reduces operative mortality (34). Even in the normotensive patient, complete α-blockade will prevent hemodynamic instability caused by operative stress and tumor manipulation during elective resection.

Phenoxybenzamine is an ideal α-blocker for preoperative patients because it has a relatively long half-life. The starting dose is 10 mg every 12 hours and should be titrated upward, as tolerated. The highest tolerable level of blockade is preferable, and dose escalation can be halted when the patient has postural hypotension. Most patients complain of nasal congestion during adequate α-blockade, but this need not prompt adjustment in dosage.

β-Blockers are sometimes needed to control heart rate before the resection. They should be given only after adequate α-blockade, to avoid severe hypertension from unopposed α-stimulation. Metyrosine, an inhibitor of tyrosine hydroxylase, reduces catecholamine production and can be added to the preoperative regimen (35). Narcotics should generally be avoided, as they may stimulate histamine release, which may in turn trigger a crisis.

Although surgical resection is the only curative intervention for patients with pheochromocytoma, appropriate preoperative measures help to avoid unfavorable events, such as intraoperative hemodynamic instability. α-Blockade must be attained before elective resection of pheochromocytoma. β-Blockade is used selectively in patients with persistent tachycardia, but only after adequate α-blockade.

Managing the Postoperative Patient

Perioperative complications are either related to inadequate adrenergic blockade, lack of appropriate intravascular volume expansion, or to a technical problem. Surgical complications include bleeding, infection, and damage to nearby structures, such as the spleen or renal vessels.

Most pheochromocytomas smaller than 6 cm can be resected using the laparoscopic technique. Larger tumors may require laparotomy or thoracoabdominal access for safe resection.

Despite preoperative α-blockade, many patients have either arrhythmias or some form of hemodynamic instability during adrenalectomy. Some compensatory hypotension often results after tumor extirpation. Typically, this drop in blood pressure is minimized when blood volume is restored appropriately and when α-blockade is adequate preoperatively. Sometimes, intravenous boluses of crystalloid and colloid, or catecholamines, are required to maintain blood pressure after resection.

Although many patients with pheochromocytoma are hyperglycemic before resection, because of chronic catecholamine excess, they may be profoundly hypoglycemic in the early postoperative period. Intravenous glucose and frequent blood sugar checks are required in many of these patients.

Essential hypertension may persist after resection. Disease may recur from the contralateral adrenal gland or metastases years after surgery. Reoperative resection is the treatment of choice when complete extirpation is feasible. Furthermore, palliative debulking is often desirable in patients with disease that cannot be completely resected, as it can improve symptoms and the effectiveness of medical therapy. An uncommon surgical complication of adrenalectomy is renovascular hypertension, a result of injury to, or thrombosis of, the renal artery or vein.

Treatment of Pheochromocytoma Crisis

Pheochromocytoma crisis is an uncommon event that requires prompt diagnosis and emergent medical intervention. The clinical presentation of pheochromocytoma crisis includes (i) multisystem organ failure; (ii) fever, often exceeding 40°C; (iii) encephalopathy; and (iv) hemodynamic instability (36). A common error is the misdiagnosis of sepsis in patients whose condition continues to decline despite empiric antibiotic therapy.

Episodes of pheochromocytoma crisis are typically precipitated by traumatic stress, which is often iatrogenic. Furthermore, crises usually develop in undiagnosed or untreated patients without α-blockade. Patients in pheochromocytoma crisis should be transferred urgently to an intensive care unit, or to the highest level of care available.

Phentolamine, an intravenous α-blocker, should be given in 2-mg boluses. Larger doses can result in hypotension. Phenoxybenzamine and prazosin can also be used but can be more difficult to titrate.

β-Blockade, without α-blockade, can precipitate hemodynamic instability, as unopposed α-stimulation can cause peripheral vasoconstriction (37). However, after initial α-blockade is started, β-blockade can effectively control heart rate and blood pressure. Labetalol, which has both α- and β-blocker effects, can be given intravenously during crisis situations.

Other useful medications include nitrates, such as sodium nitroprusside and nitroglycerine. These agents result in prompt venodilation, which can decrease cardiac preload and cause an immediate decline in blood pressure. Side effects from sodium nitroprusside include cyanide accumulation after long-term use. Ultimately, these agents should be used as adjuvant therapies after α-adrenergic blockade is achieved.

Ideally, real-time arterial pressure should be monitored with the placement of a radial artery arterial line. Measurement of urinary output with a bladder catheter is simple, quick, and useful. Central venous monitoring is not an essential component in the initial care of patients in pheochromocytoma crisis, and central venous catheter placement should not delay pharmacologic treatment. However, many pharmacologic agents require central venous delivery, and central venous catheters are useful for monitoring volume status.

Emergent adrenalectomy should be avoided in patients with pheochromocytoma crisis. After the patient is stabilized and α-blockade instituted, planning should begin for elective adrenalectomy with curative intent. This can be performed during the same admission after preoperative planning, including the completion of localization studies and at least 2 weeks of α-blockade.

Pregnancy and Pheochromocytoma

The stress of pregnancy and labor can prompt pheochromocytoma crisis and elicit symptoms in patients with unrecognized pheochromocytoma (38). On rare occasions, symptoms are minimal during gestation and manifest only after delivery (39). Obstetric outcomes are exceptionally poor when maternal pheochromocytoma is unrecognized; fetal and maternal mortality rates exceed 50% in such cases (40). However, others have reported favorable results when the diagnosis is established and the mother is adequately treated antenatally (41). Although the presenting symptoms and the biochemical workup are no different in obstetric patients, maternal hypertension is often erroneously attributed to pre-eclampsia or eclampsia. Because of the grave consequences related to this missed diagnosis, pheochromocytoma should be considered in any hypertensive gravid woman.

The localization of pheochromocytoma lesions in pregnant women should avoid fetal exposure to ionizing radiation. Ultrasound and MRI are safe, but CT and MIBG scanning result in some fetal exposure to radiation.

Both α- and β-blockade can be given safely in the obstetric patient. The timing of surgical resection should be carefully planned. Emergent adrenalectomy is not required and should be delayed until delivery, which should be accomplished by cesarean section, or thereafter. If the diagnosis is made early in the gestational period and medical therapy is poorly tolerated, the second trimester is the ideal time period for elective laparoscopic resection. Surgery in the first trimester is associated with fetal loss, and resection in the third trimester can be technically challenging because of the larger uterus, and can cause premature labor.

SUMMARY

The diagnosis of pheochromocytoma should be considered in any patient with the classic symptoms of headache and diaphoresis with severe hypertension. Furthermore, pheochromocytoma should be included in the differential diagnosis in any patient with an unexplained cardiovascular event, including congestive heart failure, myocardial infarction, or stroke. The cornerstone of diagnosis is biochemical evaluation by either plasma-fractionated metanephrines or 24-hour collection of urine metanephrines. Pheochromocytoma crisis is a medical emergency that is often misdiagnosed as severe sepsis. Clinical outcomes are uniformly fatal when pheochromocytoma crisis is undiagnosed. The initial therapy includes α-blockade titrated to orthostatic hypotension. Both β-blockade and intravenous nitrates are useful adjuvant therapies to control tachycardia and hypertension, respectively. Ultimately, curative outcomes depend on complete surgical resection, which is most safely performed after a 2-week period of α-blockade and subsequent resuscitation.

References

1. Cohen DL, Fraker D, Townsend RR. Lack of symptoms in patients with histologic evidence of pheochromocytoma: a diagnostic challenge. *Ann NY Acad Sci.* 2006;1073:47–51.
2. Preuss J, Woenckhaus C, Schwesinger G, et al. Non-diagnosed pheochromocytoma as a cause of sudden death in a 49-year-old man: a case report with medico-legal implications. *Forensic Sci Int.* 2006;156:223–228.
3. Khorram-Manesh A, Ahlman H, Nilsson O, et al. Long-term outcome of a large series of patients surgically treated for pheochromocytoma. *J Intern Med.* 2005;258:55–66.
4. Sutton MG, Sheps SG, Lie JT. Prevalence of clinically unsuspected pheochromocytoma. Review of a 50-year autopsy series. *Mayo Clin Proc.* 1981;56:354–360.
5. Dubois LA, Gray DK. Dopamine-secreting pheochromocytomas: in search of a syndrome. *World J Surg.* 2005;29:909–913.
6. Otsuka F, Miyoshi T, Murakami K, et al. An extra-adrenal abdominal pheochromocytoma causing ectopic ACTH syndrome. *Am J Hypertens.* 2005;18:1364–1368.
7. Herrera MF, Stone E, Deitel M, et al. Pheochromocytoma producing multiple vasoactive peptides. *Arch Surg.* 1992;127:105–108.

8. Takami H, Shikata J, Kakudo K, et al. Calcitonin gene-regulated peptide in patients with endocrine tumors. *J Surg Oncol.* 1990;43:28–32.
9. Newell KA, Prinz RA, Pickleman J, et al. Pheochromocytoma multisystem crisis: a surgical emergency. *Arch Surg.* 1988;123:956–959.
10. Minno AM, Bennett WA, Kvale WF. Pheochromocytoma: a study of 15 cases diagnosed at autopsy. *N Engl J Med.* 1954;251:959–965.
11. Berkheiser SW, Rappoport AE. Unsuspected pheochromocytoma of the adrenal. *Am J Clin Path.* 1951;21:657–665.
12. Goldstein RE, O'Neill JA Jr, Holcomb GW 3rd, et al. Clinical experience over 48 years with pheochromocytoma. *Ann Surg.* 1999;229:755–764.
13. Neumann HPH, Bausch B, McWhinney SR, et al. Germ-line mutations in nonsyndromic pheochromocytoma. *N Engl J Med.* 2002;346:1459–1466.
14. Neumann HPH, Pawlu C, Peczkowska M, et al. Distinct clinical features of paraganglioma syndromes associated with SDHB and SDHD gene mutations. *JAMA.* 2004;292:943–951.
15. Mezitis SGE, Geller M, Bocchieri E, et al. Association of pheochromocytoma and ganglioneuroma: usual finding in neurofibromatosis type 1. *Endocr Pract.* 2007;13:647–651.
16. Margulies KB, Sheps SG. Carney's triad: guidelines for management. *Mayo Clin Proc.* 1988;63:496–502.
17. Baguet JP, Hammer L, Mazzuco TL, et al. Circumstances of discovery of phaeochromocytoma: a retrospective study of 41 consecutive patients. *Eur J Endocrinol.* 2004;150:681–686.
18. Mitchell L, Bellis F. Phaeochromocytoma—"the great mimic": an unusual presentation. *Emerg Med J.* 2007;24:672–673.
19. Kebebew E, Duh Q-Y. Benign and malignant pheochromocytoma: diagnosis, treatment, and follow-up. *Surg Oncol Clin N Am.* 1998;7:765–789.
20. Kudva Y, Young WF, Thompson GB, et al. Adrenal incidentaloma: an important component of the clinical presentation spectrum of benign sporadic adrenal pheochromocytoma. *Endocrinologist.* 1999;9:77.
21. Kirshtein B, Pagliarello G, Yelle JD, et al. Incidence of pheochromocytoma in trauma patients during the management of unrelated illness: a retrospective review. *Int J Surg.* 2007;5:332–5.
22. Adler JT, Mack E, Chen HC, Isolated adrenal mass in patients with a history of cancer: remember pheochromocytoma. *Ann Surg Oncol.* 2007;14:2358–2362.
23. Agarwal A, Gupta S, Mishra AK, et al. Normotensive pheochromocytoma: institutional experience. *World J Surg.* 2005;29:1185–1188.
24. Kizer JR, Koniaris LS, Edelman JD, et al. Pheochromocytoma crisis, cardiomyopathy, and hemodynamic collapse. *Chest.* 2000;118:1221–1223.
25. Graham PE, Smythe GA, Edwards GA, et al. Laboratory diagnosis of pheochromocytoma: which analytes should we measure? *Ann Clin Biochem.* 1993;30:129–134.
26. Sawka A, Jaeschke R, Singh R, et al: A comparison of biochemical tests for pheochromocytoma: measurement of fractionated plasma metanephrines compared with the combination of 24-hour urinary metanephrines and catecholamines. *J Clin Endocrinol Metab.* 2003;88:553–558.
27. Young W. Phaeochromocytoma: how to catch a moonbeam in your hand. *Eur J Endocrinol.* 1997;136:28.
28. Goldstein RE, O'Neill JA Jr, Holcomb GW III, et al. Clinical experience over 48 years with pheochromocytoma. *Ann Surg.* 1999;229:755–766.
29. Plouin PF, Duclos JM, Soppelsa F, et al. Factors associated with perioperative morbidity and mortality in patients with pheochromocytoma: analysis of 165 operations at a single center. *J Clin Endocrinol Metab.* 2001;86:1480–1486.
30. Brukamp K, Goral S, Townsend RR, et al. Rapidly reversible cardiogenic shock as a pheochromocytoma presentation. *Am J Med.* 2007;120:e1–e2.
31. Boulkina LS, Newton CA, Drake AJ, et al. Acute myocardial infarction attributable to adrenergic crises in a patient with pheochromocytoma and neurofibromatosis 1. *Endocr Pract.* 2007;13:269–273.
32. Lin PC, Hsu JT, Chung, CM, et al. Pheochromocytoma underlying hypertension, stroke, and dilated cardiomyopathy. *Tex Heart Inst J.* 2007;34:244–246.
33. Sutton MG, Sheps SG, Lie JT. Prevalence of clinically unsuspected pheochromocytoma. Review of a 50-year autopsy series. *Mayo Clin Proc.* 1981;56: 354–360.
34. Freier DT, Eckhouser FE, Harrison TS. Pheochromocytoma: a persistently problematic and still potentially lethal disease. *Arch Surg.* 1980;115:388–391.
35. Steinsapir J, Carr AA, Prisant LM, et al. Metyrosine and pheochromocytoma. *Arch Intern Med.* 1997;157:901–906.
36. Newell KA, Prinz RA, Pickleman J, et al. Pheochromocytoma multisystem crisis. A surgical emergency. *Arch Surg.* 1988;123:956–959.
37. Sibal L, Jovanovic A, Agarwal SC, et al. Phaeochromocytomas presenting as acute crises after beta blockade therapy. *Clin Endocrinol (Oxf).* 2006;65: 186–190.
38. Kamari Y, Sharabi Y, Leiba A, et al. Peripartum hypertension from pheochromocytoma: a rare and challenging entity. *Am J Hypertens.* 2005;18:1306–1312.
39. Kisters K, Franitza P, Hausberg M. A case of pheochromocytoma symptomatic after delivery. *J Hypertens.* 2007;25:1977.
40. Ellison GT, Mansberger JA, Mansberger AR Jr. Malignant recurrent pheochromocytoma during pregnancy. *Surgery.* 1988;103:484–489.
41. Harper AM, Munaghan GA, Kennedy L, et al. Pheochromocytoma in pregnancy: five cases and a review of the literature. *Br J Obstet Gynecol.* 1989;96: 594–606.

CHAPTER 166 ■ THYROID DISEASE IN THE INTENSIVE CARE UNIT

JENNIFER A. SIPOS • WILLIAM G. CANCE

The purpose of this chapter is to discuss thyroid disease as it may present in an intensive care unit (ICU). Interpretation of thyroid function tests in a critically ill patient requires knowledge of the perturbations of hormone synthesis that may occur with illness and certain medications. This text will also discuss the diagnosis and treatment of thyroid emergencies: myxedema coma, thyroid storm, postthyroidectomy hypocalcemia, and airway obstruction by goiter.

THYROID FUNCTION TESTS

There are a myriad of tests that may be ordered to evaluate thyroid function, so finding the right test or set of tests can confound many physicians. Further compounding the complexity is interpreting these values once they are obtained. The purpose of this section is to provide an overview of the most commonly ordered labs. A later section will delineate how to interpret these values in the critically ill patient.

Serum Thyroid-stimulating Hormone/Free Thyroxine

Measurement of serum thyroid-stimulating hormone (TSH) and free thyroxine (FT_4) is sufficient to diagnose most thyroid disorders. It is recommended to use the now widely available ultrasensitive TSH (1). The normal reference range for this test

TABLE 166.1

INTERPRETATION OF THYROID FUNCTION TESTS

	TSH	Free T_4	Total T_3	T_3U	rT_3
Hypothyroidism					
Primary	High	Low	Normal	Low	Low/normal
Secondary	Low/normal	Low	Normal	Low	Low/normal
Hyperthyroidism	Low	High/normal	High	High	Low/normal
Sick euthyroid	Low/normal	Low/normal	Low	High	High

TSH, thyroid-stimulating hormone; T_4, thyroxine; T_3, triiodothyronine; T_3U, T_3 resin uptake; rT_3, reverse T_3.

is an extensively debated issue among endocrinologists. Currently, the most widely accepted range of 0.45 to 4.12 mIU/L is based on values from the NHANES III (National Health and Nutrition Examination Survey) database (2). Fueling the controversy, however, was a study revealing that exclusion of patients with thyroid dysfunction and those taking medications known to affect thyroid tests yields an upper limit of normal at 2.5 mIU/L (3). The issue will require further investigation with larger studies. In this chapter, the normal range will be based on the NHANES data: 0.45 to 4.12 mIU/L.

Total T_4 Measurement

Total T_4 (TT_4) measurement includes both bound and free thyroxine. Therefore, conditions or medications that affect serum levels of thyroid-binding globulin will also affect the total T_4 value; use of FT_4 can eliminate this shortcoming. However, if FT_4 is not available, this level can be estimated by looking at the FT_4 index, FTI. This number is calculated by multiplying the total T_4 by the T_3 resin uptake, (T^3RU) (see below for explanation). Many laboratories use this value when reporting a FT_4.

Serum Tri-iodothyronine (T_3)

Similar to thyroxine, serum tri-iodothyronine (T_3) may be measured in the free and bound fractions, although it is generally recommended that the total T_3 be used, as only a minute fraction of T_3 is free (4). T_3 levels should be measured in patients suspected of having hyperthyroidism, as some patients may have excess secretion of only T_3 early in the course of thyrotoxicosis. As a result, patients may have a suppressed TSH, normal free T_4, and an elevated total T_3 (T_3 toxicosis). Measurement of this hormone is not helpful, however, in hypothyroidism, as the elevated TSH stimulates preferential formation of T_3, typically maintaining these levels in the normal range (5,6).

T_3 Resin Uptake

T_3 resin uptake is an indirect, inverse test to estimate the number of unoccupied serum protein-binding sites. Radiolabeled T_3 is added to the patient's serum and distributed between unoccupied T_4-binding sites on thyroid-binding globulin (TBG) in the serum and an adsorbent that has been added to the solution. ^{125}I-T_3 binding to the adsorbent is increased if the number of unoccupied binding sites is decreased. This may be due to either low TBG levels such as in nephrotic syndrome or chronic liver disease, or increased thyroid hormone levels as in hyperthyroidism (7). In contrast, the T_3RU is low if the number of unoccupied binding sites is increased. Low thyroid hormone concentrations (hypothyroidism or high TBG concentrations) estrogen therapy, or pregnancy may lead to a low T_3RU (8).

Reverse T_3

Reverse T_3 differs from T_3 in that the iodine is missing from the inner ring instead of the outer ring of T_4. It is largely bound to proteins in the serum. Its half-life in the serum is quite short (9), and furthermore, the biologic function of rT_3 is not completely understood in humans. The clinical utility of measuring these levels is chiefly in the setting of sick euthyroidism and will be discussed in greater detail in the section dealing with interpretation of thyroid function in critically ill patients. Table 166.1 details the interpretation of thyroid function tests.

DRUGS AND THYROID FUNCTION

There are a number of drugs commonly used in the ICU that will interfere with thyroid homeostasis. Although many of these actions are viewed as detrimental, some effects may also be used for a therapeutic benefit, particularly in thyrotoxicosis. The vast majority of the effects of pharmacologic agents on thyroid hormone homeostasis may be divided into four different categories. First, they may alter the synthesis or secretion of thyroid hormones. Second, they may alter hormone concentration by changing serum levels of binding proteins or by competing for their binding sites. Third, the pharmacologic agents may modify the cellular uptake and metabolism of thyroid hormones. Fourth, drugs may interfere with thyroid hormone action at the tissue level. Typically these effects on thyroid hormone metabolism are transient, but they may complicate the interpretation of the thyroid function tests (10). The more commonly used compounds interfering with thyroid function and their mechanisms of action are listed in Table 166.2.

TABLE 166.2

COMMONLY USED DRUGS THAT AFFECT THYROID FUNCTION

Drug	Mode of action	Thyroid function abnormality
Amiodarone	Inhibits cellular hormone uptake Alters hormone secretion Alters intracellular metabolism	Hyperthyroidism Hypothyroidism (10)
Lithium	Reduced hormone secretion (acute) Autoantibody immune response (chronic)	Hypothyroidism (acute) Hyperthyroidism (chronic) (10)
Dopamine	Reduced hormone secretion	Reduced TSH, T_4 (11)
Cholestyramine *Ferrous sulfate* *Charcoal* *Sucralfate*	Reduced absorption from gut	Elevated TSH, reduced T_4 (12)
Propranolol	Altered hormone synthesis	Reduced T_4-to-T_3 conversion (13)
Phenobarbital	Alters intracellular metabolism	Reduced total T_4 (13)
Sodium ipodate *Iopanoic acid*	Reduced hormone secretion Altered hormone synthesis	Reduced T_4-to-T_3 conversion (14)
Glucocorticoids	Reduced TSH secretion Altered hormone synthesis	Reduced total T_4 Reduced T_4-to-T_3 conversion (15)
Heparin	Inhibits T_4 binding to TBG	Transient increase in fT_4 (13)
Lasix	Inhibits T_4 binding to TBG	Reduced total T_3, total T_4 (16)
Salicylates	Inhibits T_4 binding to TBG	Reduced total T_3, total T_4 (13) Increased free T_3, free T_4
Carbamazepine	Alters intracellular metabolism	Reduced total T_4 (17)
Radiographic contrast agents	Alters hormone secretion	Increased free T_4 Decreased free T_3 (10)
Cytokines	Autoantibody immune response	Transient hypothyroidism or hyperthyroidism (18)

Thyrotoxicosis

Clinical Presentation

In the ICU, patients with thyrotoxicosis may have an atypical presentation, with tachyarrhythmias or central nervous system disturbance as the primary sign. It is important for the intensivist to consider thyroid dysfunction in the differential diagnosis of such patients, since treatment with beta-blockers and antithyroid medications can rapidly improve the clinical course (19). The diagnosis may need to be a clinical one, as results of laboratory testing can take days. Table 166.3 lists the symptoms and signs that may be seen in a patient with thyrotoxicosis.

Cardiovascular Manifestations

Sinus tachycardia and atrial fibrillation are the most commonly seen cardiovascular disorders in hyperthyroidism. Since atrial fibrillation may be the only indication of thyrotoxicosis, it is important to screen such patients with a TSH and FT_4. Congestive heart failure typically occurs only in patients with underlying heart disease, but may also manifest as a result of chronic tachycardia-induced cardiomyopathy (20). Physical examination findings in a thyrotoxic patient include widened pulse pressure, hyperdynamic precordium, tachycardia, and systolic ejection murmur. The pathogenesis of cardiovascular diseases from exposure to excessive thyroid hormone is not entirely understood. Thyroid hormone has both indirect and direct effects on vascular smooth muscle tone and increases cardiac output. Thyroxine also regulates expression of myocardial genes involved in the handling of calcium (21).

The typical electrocardiographic changes seen in thyrotoxicosis are sinus tachycardia and atrial fibrillation (20). Patients may also present with complete heart block, and cases have been reported that showed reversal with treatment of the underlying thyroid disorder (22–25).

TABLE 166.3

SIGNS AND SYMPTOMS OF THYROTOXICOSIS

Symptoms	Signs
Anxiety	Goiter
Hyperdefecation	Lid lag/lid retraction
Sweating/heat intolerance	Proximal muscle weakness
Palpitations	Tremor
Weight loss	Tachycardia/arrhythmias
Weakness	Hyperreflexia
Increased appetite	Thyroid bruit
Scant/absent menses	Dermopathy

Pulmonary Manifestations

Dyspnea on exertion is a common presenting symptom of patients with hyperthyroidism. Respiratory muscle strength is significantly reduced in thyrotoxicosis and improves with reduction of thyroid hormone levels (26). Several studies have also shown that thyrotoxicosis is a risk factor for the development of pulmonary hypertension (27–29). Pulmonary emboli may be seen in patients with atrial fibrillation who are not on anticoagulation therapy (30). Furthermore, pulmonary edema has been described in uncontrolled thyrotoxic patients (31–34).

Laboratory Findings

The laboratory findings in hyperthyroidism are the combination of a low TSH and a high FT_4 (35) (Table 166.1). If the FT_4 is normal and TSH suppressed in a patient suspected of having thyrotoxicosis, it is important to check a T_3 level, as this may be elevated in early Graves disease or in T_3-secreting toxic adenomas. In the event that the patient presents with an elevated T_4 or T_3 and a detectable or "normal" TSH, the clinician should consider the effects of nonthyroidal illness (see below) or drugs (Table 166.2) on thyroid function testing. Rarely, the patient may have a TSH-secreting pituitary tumor or thyroid hormone resistance (35). Consultation with an endocrinologist may be warranted if the patient has unusual thyroid function tests that cannot be readily corroborated with the entire clinical picture.

Etiology

The two most common causes of thyrotoxicosis in the outpatient setting are Graves disease and toxic multinodular goiter. Elderly patients tend to have a solitary or multiple nodules that become autonomously functioning and lead to hypersecretion of thyroid hormone. The goiter may not always be palpable if the offending nodule is small or if the patient has a substernal goiter. Tracheal deviation on chest radiograph may be the only finding to alert the physician of the underlying disease process. By way of contrast, young women are more likely to present with the classic stigmata of Graves disease: thyroid bruit, ophthalmopathy, and diffuse goiter. In the ICU, however, it is important to consider other causes of hyperthyroidism. Factitious thyrotoxicosis is rare but should be considered in a patient with a history of taking herbal supplements or over-the-counter weight loss medications (36). Surreptitious use of thyroid hormone may be diagnosed by measurement of serum thyroglobulin levels. If low, this would indicate that the patient is self-medicating (37). Typically, the thyroglobulin levels are high in patients with true thyroid disorders. Iodinated contrast media as used with computed tomography or cardiac catheterization may also cause hyperthyroidism because these agents contain free iodine (38). Generally, patients with normal thyroid function are not at risk of this complication. However, patients with a history of Graves disease, multinodular goiter, or even subclinical hyperthyroidism may develop frank thyrotoxicosis several days after the administration of contrast media (see below for further discussion of contrast media and thyroid function) (38,39).

Treatment

The treatment of thyrotoxicosis is based on the underlying pathophysiology. Patients with Graves disease, toxic multinodular goiter, or toxic adenoma should be started on a thionamide, such as methimazole (MMI) or propylthiouracil (PTU). The dosage of antithyroid medication should be tailored to the degree of thyrotoxicosis; hence, consultation with an endocrinologist is advisable. Patients with peripheral manifestations of hyperthyroidism may also benefit from the addition of a β-adrenergic antagonist drug. This agent will assist with the symptoms of agitation, tremor, palpitations, and diarrhea. Propranolol is the drug most commonly used in the United States. Patients who have overdosed on thyroid hormone or are taking a supplement with thyroid hormone extract should be counseled regarding the complications of taking thyroid hormone supplements in excess, and the offending agent should be discontinued. If the patient requires treatment, β-adrenergic antagonists and bile acid sequestrants—for example, cholestyramine—may be used.

Thyroid Storm

Thyroid storm is a rare but life-threatening syndrome of exaggerated clinical manifestations of thyrotoxicosis. There are no universally accepted criteria for its diagnosis, and consequently, the incidence is unknown. Laboratory testing is unreliable in distinguishing patients with thyrotoxicosis and thyroid storm; thus the diagnosis of thyroid storm is primarily a clinical one. It is a medical emergency typically caused by exacerbation of hyperthyroidism following a precipitating event or illness; Table 166.4 lists the precipitants of thyroid storm. The clinical picture is one of decompensation of one or more organ systems (40). There are four main features noted in thyroid storm: tachycardia, fever, central nervous system disturbances, and gastrointestinal symptoms. The CNS symptoms vary from marked hyperirritability and anxiety, to confusion and coma. Mortality rates range from 20% to 100%, so prompt, multifaceted therapy is essential (41).

Management

The treatment of thyroid storm takes a four-pronged approach (Table 166.5). First, an antithyroid drug must be given to

TABLE 166.4

PRECIPITANTS OF THYROID STORM

Infection
Parturition
Nonthyroid surgery
Radioactive iodine therapy
Postthyroidectomy
Vigorous palpation of the thyroid
Iodine therapy/radiographic contrast agents
Diabetic ketoacidosis
Hypoglycemia
Withdrawal of antithyroid drug therapy
Myocardial infarction
Cerebrovascular accident
Pulmonary embolus
Trauma
Medications
Thyroxine
Haldol (42)
Pseudoephedrine (43)

TABLE 166.5

SUMMARY OF TREATMENT FOR THYROID STORM

Medication	Dose and route of administration	Action
Propranolol	0.5–1 mg IV over 10 min, then 1–3 mg IV as needed 80–120 mg PO q6h	β-Adrenergic blockade and inhibition of T_4-to-T_3 conversion
Thionamides		
PTU	200–400 mg PO/NG/PR q4h	Inhibit hormone synthesis and block conversion of T_4 to T_3
Methimazole	20 mg PO/NG q4h	Inhibits hormone synthesis
Iodine[a]		Blocks release of thyroid hormone
SSKI	5 drops POo/NG q6h	
Lugol solution	10 drops PO/NG q8h	
Iodinated contrast agents[a]		Blocks release of thyroid hormone and conversion of T_4 to T_3
Sodium ipodate or iopanoic acid	0.5 g PO/NG q12h	
Glucocorticoids		
Hydrocortisone	200 mg IV load, then 100 mg IV q8h	Stress-dose steroids and blocks conversion of T_4 to T_3
Dexamethasone	2 mg PO/NG/IV q6h	
Lithium	300 mg PO/NG q6h titrate to lithium level of 1 mEq/L	Inhibits hormone synthesis
Cholestyramine	4 g PO/NG q6h	Lowers serum T_3 and T_4

IV, intravenously; PO, orally; PTU, propylthiouracil; NG, nasogastrically; SSKI, saturated solution of potassium iodide.
[a]Either iodine or iodinated contrast agents should be used, but not both. Administration of iodine should be preceded by PTU by 2–3 hours to avoid enhancement of thyroid hormone synthesis.

reduce thyroid hormone production and peripheral conversion of T_4 to T_3. Second, supportive care must be administered against the systemic disturbances of fever, hypovolemia, and cardiovascular compromise. Third, the peripheral actions of thyroid hormone should be blocked. Finally, any precipitating factors should be addressed.

A thionamide is given to block synthesis of T_3 and T_4. PTU is the favored agent because it also inhibits peripheral conversion of T_4 to T_3. By reducing T_3 concentrations in the serum, it is postulated that the manifestations of thyrotoxicosis are more rapidly improved with PTU than with MMI (41). Neither of these drugs is available parenterally, so administration is typically by mouth or nasogastric (NG) tube. In patients with altered mental status, or in whom an NG cannot be placed, rectal administration of PTU has been reported to be used successfully in a few patients (44,45). It is conventional to use high doses of antithyroid drugs, such as 200 to 400 mg PTU every 4 hours or 20 mg MMI every 4 hours.

Thionamides do not inhibit the release of preformed T_3 and T_4 from the thyroid. Inorganic iodide, however, can accomplish this goal. It may be administered orally as Lugol solution (ten drops every 8 hours) or as saturated solution of potassium iodide (SSKI, five drops every 6 hours). Oral radiographic contrast agents, sodium ipodate or iopanoic acid, may be substituted for iodine. These drugs block the release of preformed thyroid hormone from the gland and inhibit the extrathyroidal conversion of T_4 to T_3 (14). It is critical to administer thionamide therapy about an hour before the iodide or contrast agent is given, because the sudden influx of iodide into the thyroid can lead to increased thyroid hormone production and thereby prolong the thyrotoxicosis (46). However, when the iodide or contrast agent is given after the antithyroid drug, serum T_3 and T_4 levels are substantially reduced in 2 to 3 days and may reach the normal range in 5 to 7 days (41,47).

If the patient has an allergy to iodide or cannot tolerate thionamides, lithium may be substituted to inhibit T_3 and T_4 synthesis (48). It may be given initially at a dose of 300 mg every 6 hours and titrated to maintain serum lithium concentrations around 1 mEq/L.

Supportive care should also be provided. Fever is preferentially treated with acetaminophen. Salicylates should not be used as they competitively inhibit T_3 and T_4 binding to serum proteins and thus increase serum free T_3 and T_4 levels (49). The patient's fluid losses should be appropriately replaced, bearing in mind the insensible losses from high fever and, if present, diarrhea. Hypercalcemia, if present, will usually be reversed by adequate hydration. High-dose glucocorticoids have been given historically for empiric treatment of relative adrenal insufficiency. Such treatment also has the added benefit of inhibition of peripheral conversion of T_4 to T_3. In patients with Graves disease, glucocorticoids also directly inhibit secretion of thyroid hormone. A loading dose of hydrocortisone 200 mg may be given initially followed by 100 mg every 8 hours; this therapy can be tapered rapidly after 2 to 3 days. Dexamethasone or methylprednisolone at equivalent doses may be substituted for hydrocortisone if preferred.

Therapy directed against the peripheral actions of thyroid hormone should be administered as well. β-Adrenergic antagonist drugs can provide rapid amelioration of many of the symptoms of thyroid storm and should be dispensed immediately. Propranolol is the most commonly used agent, and may be given intravenously or orally depending on the clinical setting. If the oral route is used, the patient may be given between 80 and 120 mg every 6 hours. It is important to consider that in the thyrotoxic state, drug clearance is increased and higher-than-usual doses are necessary to achieve the desired effect. If rapid beta-blockade is necessary to reduce heart rate, or if the patient's mental status precludes oral drugs, intravenous

(IV) administration is preferred. The initial dose should be 0.5 to 1 mg given over 10 minutes while continuously monitoring the patient's cardiac rhythm, and subsequently, 1 to 3 mg may be given over 10 minutes every several hours as needed. Propranolol attenuates the effects of catecholamines and weakly inhibits the peripheral conversion of T_4 to T_3. This inhibition occurs over a period of a week, however, and thus does not solely account for the beneficial effects of propranolol in the thyrotoxic patient.

In extreme cases, it may be beneficial to use a method to remove T_3 and T_4 from the patient's serum. The simplest approach is to administer oral cholestyramine. This drug binds the hormones in the GI tract, interrupting the enterohepatic circulation (50). Plasmapheresis has also been used successfully to lower T_3 and T_4 levels (51,52), although other studies were unable to confirm the beneficial effects (53).

Finally, it is important to search for and treat underlying illnesses that may have precipitated the thyroid storm. This process can be difficult in obtunded patients, but a systematic approach is usually successful in uncovering the cause.

Patients treated with the above regimen usually recover in 12 to 24 hours if the syndrome is recognized and treated in a timely fashion. As the patient's condition stabilizes, it is important to wean the glucocorticoids, switch to oral rehydration, and taper the beta-blocking drugs. Long-term treatment of hyperthyroidism is required if the patient has Graves disease or toxic multinodular goiter. In patients with Graves disease, it may be preferable to treat with thionamides, as there is a chance of remission of the autoimmune condition. However, if a patient's disease is severe enough to lead to thyroid storm, others advocate total thyroidectomy. Radioiodine ablation is not an option for several months because the inorganic iodide used in treatment of the thyroid storm saturates the gland and precludes further uptake of iodide.

Drug-induced Alterations in Thyroid Function

Amiodarone

Amiodarone is a lipophilic drug that contains 75 mg iodine per 200-mg tablet. The drug has a half-life of several months, and, during that time, it releases approximately 9 mg of inorganic iodine per day. In euthyroid patients, chronic administration of the drug results in increased serum TT_4, FT_4, and rT_3 levels; lower T_3 concentrations; and normal TSH (54). The reason for these changes is the drug's strong inhibition of 5′-deiodinase, the enzyme responsible for conversion of T_4 to T_3 and rT_3 to T_2. Most patients remain euthyroid while on amiodarone despite the hormonal derangements that may be seen; on the other hand, about 14% to 18% of patients develop either hypothyroidism or hyperthyroidism while on amiodarone (55). Hypothyroidism is more commonly encountered in iodine-replete areas, such as the United States (56). Treatment is aimed at normalization of the TSH with levothyroxine replacement while the amiodarone therapy is continued. On discontinuation of the amiodarone, most patients return to euthyroidism, although it may take several months because of the prolonged half-life of the drug.

In iodine-deficient regions, it is more common to see hyperthyroidism as a result of amiodarone therapy (56). There are two mechanisms (Table 166.6) of amiodarone-induced thyrotoxicosis (AIT). Distinction of these two disorders is relevant because their treatment differs. Type I AIT occurs in glands with an underlying abnormality. Areas of autonomy, such as a toxic nodule or autoimmune disease in the thyroid, produce increased levels of hormone in response to the excess iodine released from the amiodarone (55). Type II AIT develops as a result of a direct cytotoxic effect of amiodarone on the thyrocyte (57). Treatment of type I AIT is difficult because most patients do not respond to thionamides, as these drugs have decreased efficacy in states of iodine excess (58). Use of potassium perchlorate ($KClO_4$) blocks further iodine entry into the thyrocyte and may enhance the efficacy of thionamides (54). It is important to note that both thionamides and $KClO_4$ may cause agranulocytosis, so serial monitoring of blood counts is advisable. If possible, it is also important to discontinue the amiodarone. The treatment of type II AIT is primarily with glucocorticoids and by discontinuation of the amiodarone, although in some cases, it is reasonable to continue the antiarrhythmic medication (59). In patients in whom chronic therapy with amiodarone is essential, thyroidectomy is a potential option for treatment of AIT (54). Radioiodine ablation is not an option given the low iodine uptake as a result of the iodine excess from the amiodarone.

TABLE 166.6

FEATURES OF AMIODARONE-INDUCED THYROTOXICOSIS

	Iodine-induced thyrotoxicosis (Type I)	Destructive thyrotoxicosis (Type II)
Underlying thyroid abnormality	Yes	No
Goiter	Diffuse or multinodular usually present	Occasionally small, firm goiter
RAIU	Low/normal/high	Low
Serum IL-6 concentrations	Slightly elevated	Markedly elevated
Pathogenic mechanism	Excessive thyroid hormone synthesis	Excessive hormone release (destructive thyroiditis)
Treatment	Thionamides and $KClO_4$	Glucocorticoids
Subsequent hypothyroidism	Unlikely	Possible
Color flow Doppler sonography	Normal or increased blood flow	Decreased blood flow

RAIU, radioactive iodine uptake; IL-6, interleukin-6; $KClO_4$, potassium perchlorate.

CONTRAST MEDIA AND THYROID FUNCTION

Another potential source of excess iodine is radiographic contrast media. As noted in the section about the management of thyroid storm, the oral cholecystographic agents, iopanoic acid and sodium ipodate, may be used short-term in thyrotoxic patients for their side effect of decreasing peripheral conversion of T_4 to T_3 and blocking hormone secretion from the thyroid. Used over a longer period of time, however, such agents will only exacerbate the underlying hyperthyroidism (14). Many other agents are available that have variable effects on the thyroid gland. Typically, patients with no underlying thyroid disease will not be affected by the use of these agents (60), but patients with Graves disease, multinodular goiter, or the elderly are at risk to develop thyrotoxicosis after their use (38). The lipid-soluble agents used for myelography, bronchography, and uterosalpingography are cleared slowly and release inorganic iodine for months to years. Newer water-soluble preparations used in arteriography and computed tomography are cleared from the plasma more quickly, but the iodine they release during these procedures can still affect thyroid function. The degree of thyroid dysfunction can range from mild transient subclinical hyperthyroidism to thyroid storm (61–65). Most patients experience only transient thyrotoxicosis, and the syndrome resolves when the excess iodine is cleared. If treatment is required, thionamides and β-adrenergic blockade may be used until the thyrotoxicosis resolves (65).

THYROTOXIC PERIODIC PARALYSIS

Thyrotoxic periodic paralysis (TPP) is a complication of hyperthyroidism characterized by localized or generalized attacks of weakness or flaccid paralysis and hypokalemia (66). Although it has been reported in Western countries and in women, it is more common in Asian men, where the incidence is 1.9% in thyrotoxic patients (67). The clinical presentation is identical to familial hypokalemic periodic paralysis, but the pathophysiology is distinct. Although the mechanism of the syndrome is not clearly defined, hypokalemia alone is not enough to elicit the paralysis. Hypokalemia sufficient to create the paralysis in a hyperthyroid patient has no effect on the same patient when euthyroid (68). This finding points to the importance of thyroid hormone excess in the pathophysiology of this process. It is most commonly associated with Graves disease but may be seen with any form of thyrotoxicosis (69).

Clinical Presentation

The clinical presentation is one of flaccid weakness that is symmetrical; lower extremities are generally affected more than the upper extremities. Breathing may be impaired if the patient has a more generalized weakness. The onset of the attacks is usually sudden and may be preceded by cramping. Ingestion of alcohol or carbohydrates and strenuous physical exercise commonly precipitate the episodes of weakness. Patients have decreased or absent deep-tendon reflexes. The symptoms may last from a few hours to several days (68).

Treatment

Treatment is aimed at correction of the hyperthyroidism. If hypokalemia is present, replacement should be given. Some patients are given a potassium-sparing diuretic in addition to the potassium supplementation until euthyroidism is achieved. β-Adrenergic antagonists also decrease the frequency of attacks in these patients (67).

Preoperative Management

Adequate preparation for surgery in thyrotoxic patients is critical to the successful outcome of the procedure. Surgery in a hyperthyroid patient can precipitate thyroid storm, with high morbidity and mortality if preoperative care is inadequate. The type of treatment will depend on the amount of time before the surgery. Elective procedures should be postponed until the T_3 and T_4 levels are normalized with thionamides and β-adrenergic blockade. This can usually be achieved within approximately 2 weeks. It is important to note that a suppressed TSH may not normalize for months, and this value should not be used as the criteria to assess the thyroid status. Urgent or emergent procedures may be safely done after initiation of PTU and a β-adrenergic antagonist. Iodide, as either SSKI, Lugol solution, or an oral radiographic contrast agent—sodium ipodate or iopanoic acid—should also be administered to block release of thyroid hormone and decrease peripheral conversion of T_4 to T_3 (70). Finally, a glucocorticoid, such as hydrocortisone or dexamethasone, should also be used if the patient is suspected of having concomitant adrenal insufficiency, or additional inhibition of extrathyroidal conversion of T_4 to T_3 is needed (71). Considerable lowering of T_3 and T_4 levels can be achieved within 1 to 3 days and normalization within 3 to 5 days, if the above regimen is used (71,72).

HYPOTHYROIDISM

Hypothyroidism is a common clinical problem, affecting approximately 4.6% of the population in the United States (73). It is important to recognize the clinical features and potential complications of a patient with hypothyroidism. Nonthyroidal illness, surgery, or diagnostic testing can lead to metabolic decompensation in patients with undiagnosed or untreated hypothyroidism. Additionally, it is important to note that untreated hypothyroidism may slow the metabolism of certain drugs, thereby increasing the risk of problematic side effects. Hypothyroidism is most often caused by autoimmune thyroiditis, also known as *Hashimoto thyroiditis*. Other common causes of hypothyroidism are noted in Table 166.7.

The clinical manifestations of hypothyroidism are manifold. Most of the symptoms are nonspecific, which can lead to a delay in the diagnosis. In elderly patients, the diagnosis may be missed because the patient may be asymptomatic or the signs attributed to aging (74). Patients in the ICU may present with severe central nervous system (CNS) disturbances, cardiovascular derangements, hyponatremia, or respiratory failure. Table 166.8 notes the signs and symptoms of hypothyroidism.

TABLE 166.7

CAUSES OF HYPOTHYROIDISM

Autoimmune, Hashimoto thyroiditis
Postthyroidectomy
Postradiation
^{131}I treatment
External beam radiation
Iodine deficiency
Drugs
Lithium
Iodine-containing drugs (amiodarone, radiocontrast agents)
Secondary hypothyroidism
Pituitary tumor, irradiation, empty sella syndrome, infiltrative disorders
Hypothalamic disease
Transient disorders
Silent, subacute thyroiditis

Cardiovascular Manifestations

The symptoms of cardiovascular dysfunction are much less pronounced in patients with hypothyroidism compared to their thyrotoxic counterparts. These cardiovascular changes may manifest themselves in the hypothyroid patient who is undergoing the stress of anesthesia and surgery. Cardiovascular hemodynamics are affected by hypothyroidism in several ways. In particular, patients have decreased cardiac output, mediated by reduced contractility and heart rate (75). This reduction in cardiac output contributes to the dyspnea on exertion seen in many hypothyroid patients. These patients also have increased systemic vascular resistance, predisposing them to hypertension (76). Diastolic filling and compliance are reduced, leading to diastolic dysfunction (77). Patients may have an elevation of diastolic pressure out of proportion to systolic pressure, leading to a reduction in pulse pressure (78).

The presence of decreased cardiac output, diastolic hypertension, and increased systemic vascular resistance suggests that hypothyroidism can cause congestive heart failure. It is rare, however, for hypothyroidism to be the sole causative agent in the development of heart failure (79). Typically, patients have underlying cardiac disease that is exacerbated by hypothyroidism. Pericardial effusion associated with hypothyroidism may also compromise cardiac function (80). Angina may also worsen in patients with hypothyroidism. Patients without preexisting cardiac dysfunction typically do not manifest symptoms and signs of congestive heart failure or coronary artery syndrome unless the hypothyroidism is profound (81).

TABLE 166.8

CLINICAL MANIFESTATIONS OF HYPOTHYROIDISM

Symptoms	Signs
Fatigue and weakness	Delayed relaxation of tendon reflexes
Cold intolerance	Bradycardia
Weight gain	Hypoventilation
Constipation	Diastolic hypertension
Dyspnea on exertion	Reduced pulse pressure
Depression	Pericardial and pleural effusions
Menorrhagia	Generalized and periorbital edema
Myalgia	Macroglossia
Dry skin and hair	Loss of eyebrows

Pulmonary Manifestations

Dyspnea on exertion is a common presenting complaint in patients with hypothyroidism, in part due to the impaired cardiac function and reduced pulmonary function. Respiratory muscle weakness also appears to play a role in this dyspnea (82–84). There is a reduction in central pulmonary drive in response to hypoxia and hypercapnia, leading to hypoventilation (34,85). Upper airway obstruction may occur as a result of goiter (see below: Acute Airway Obstruction) (86). Sleep apnea may occur as a result of macroglossia (87). Patients may thus require continuous positive airway pressure in addition to replacement of the thyroid hormone. Finally, a restrictive pattern of disease may be seen in the presence of a pulmonary effusion (34).

Gastrointestinal Manifestations

Peristalsis is slowed in patients with hypothyroidism. Most patients have normal bowel motility, but a small proportion with hypothyroidism requires laxative use. Patients may report vague abdominal pain and distention. Rarely, severe cases may present with ileus (88–90). Severely hypothyroid patients may also have malabsorption. The mechanism of this abnormal absorption is not clearly defined; theories include myxedematous infiltration of the mucosa, associated autoimmunity (91), and decreased intestinal motility (92).

Metabolic Manifestations

Hypothyroidism may lead to decreased free water clearance and subsequent hyponatremia. The magnitude of sodium derangement is directly related to the severity of hypothyroidism; most patients with hyponatremia have myxedema coma (93). The mechanism of the development of hyponatremia in these patients is unclear (94–96). Hyperlipidemia is a more commonly seen metabolic derangement than hyponatremia. Lipid clearance is decreased in patients with hypothyroidism, resulting in elevated levels of free fatty acids, low-density lipoprotein (LDL), and total cholesterol (97). Treatment of the hypothyroidism results in improvement of the lipid panel (98,99).

Treatment

Thyroid hormone is preferentially replaced with T_4. Levothyroxine is then converted to T_3 intracellularly, and thus, it is unnecessary to administer T_3 in most situations. In adults, the starting dose of T_4 is typically 1.7 μg/kg/day (based on ideal body weight). Elderly patients or those with coronary disease should be started at lower doses and titrated based on TSH levels every 6 weeks.

Complications

Myxedema Coma

Myxedema coma is a rare but life-threatening complication of hypothyroidism. It may occur after severe long-standing hypothyroidism or after an acute precipitating event such as surgery or infection. It is more likely to occur in elderly women during the winter months (100). Any of the usual causes of hypothyroidism (Table 166.6) may induce myxedema coma. Prompt recognition and treatment are essential, even before laboratory results are available. Mortality rates are improving due to early diagnosis and treatment, but mortality remains at 30% to 40%. Patients with cardiac complications and the elderly are at greatest risk (101,102).

Clinical Presentation. Most patients with myxedema coma have had symptoms of hypothyroidism for many months. There is a gradual onset of lethargy, progressing to stupor, which is precipitated by cold exposure, infection, or medications. Other precipitating events are stroke, congestive heart failure, trauma, or gastrointestinal bleeding. The patient is typically an obese elderly woman with yellow discoloration of the skin. The principal features of myxedema are hypothermia, bradycardia, and decreased mental status or coma (40). Patients also characteristically have a decreased respiratory rate as a result of reduced hypoxic ventilatory drive (103). The resultant carbon dioxide retention can exacerbate the altered mental status. Similar to the patient with profound hypothyroidism, the respiratory muscle weakness and pleural effusions, if present, can make ventilating these patients difficult (83,103).

Hypothermia is present in nearly all patients with myxedema coma (100). Temperature may be quite low (less than 80°F, [20°C]); values below 90°F [32°C] predict a poorer prognosis (102). The hypothermia may go unrecognized if the proper thermometer is not used; many thermometers may not be able to measure below 93°F [34°C]. The diagnosis of myxedema coma should be considered in any unconscious patient with infection who does not have a fever. Warming should be gradual, using ordinary hospital blankets. Electric heating blankets should not be used, as they may cause peripheral vasodilation and subsequent hypotension.

The cardiovascular abnormalities seen in myxedema coma are similar to those associated with severe hypothyroidism. Patients can present with bradycardia, reduced cardiac output, and decreased cardiac contractility, which may lead to hypotension. Signs of congestive heart failure may be found. In patients with diminished heart sounds, low-voltage ECG, or cardiomegaly on chest radiograph, an investigation for pericardial effusion should be performed (104).

This profound level of hypothyroidism may lead to impaired free water excretion. As a result, over half of patients can have hyponatremia (100,105). Severely reduced sodium levels can also exacerbate the altered mental status. The impaired free water clearance may be manifested by generalized nonpitting edema and periorbital swelling. Patients should be managed by free water restriction; the condition will improve with thyroid hormone replacement.

Additional clinical features of myxedema include ileus or megacolon as a result of decreased intestinal motility (90). Bladder atony may occur so patients should be monitored for residual volumes postvoiding. Hypoglycemia is a common feature that is the result of the hypothyroidism or concomitant adrenal insufficiency.

Diagnosis. The diagnosis of myxedema coma is initially made based on historical and clinical clues. It is important to investigate other causes of altered mental status, such as cerebrovascular accident and infection. Serum should be obtained for measurement of TSH, free T_4, and cortisol. If the clinical picture is consistent with myxedema coma, treatment should be initiated before laboratory confirmation of the diagnosis.

Treatment. Because of the high mortality rate of this endocrine emergency, patients with myxedema coma should be treated aggressively (106). Patients should be presumed to have adrenal insufficiency and treated with stress-dose steroids (hydrocortisone, 100 mg IV every 8 hours) until laboratory data exclude the diagnosis. The administration of levothyroxine prior to glucocorticoids in such patients can provoke an adrenal crisis.

The optimal replacement strategy for levothyroxine is unknown because of the rarity of the condition. Clinical judgment must be used to weigh the risk of rapid administration of thyroid hormone—with the possibility of precipitation of myocardial infarction—against the risk of not replacing the thyroid hormone fast enough in light of the high mortality of undertreated myxedema coma. Whether to administer T_3 or T_4 alone or in combination and the dose of these agents is a subject of much debate among endocrinologists. It is preferable to administer thyroid hormone intravenously in patients with myxedema because of the possibility of impaired gastrointestinal absorption. One regimen is to begin 200 to 300 μg of T_4 intravenously (4 μg/kg ideal body weight), followed by 100 μg 24 hours later. The patient can then be maintained on 50 μg IV or orally (PO) daily. T_3 is also given at an initial dose of 10 μg and can be given every 8 to 12 hours until the patient can take oral medications (100).

Supportive care should be directed to the coexisting medical conditions. Hyponatremia can usually be managed with free water restriction, but 3% saline may be given in extreme circumstances. Hypotension will usually improve with initiation of levothyroxine. Refractory hypotension should be treated with vasopressor agents until the thyroid hormone has had time to act. Patients may require mechanical ventilation because of respiratory muscle weakness, depressed mental status, or decreased hypoxic ventilatory drive. Warming should be accomplished as noted above. Finally, it is important to address the underlying medical illness that precipitated the myxedema coma.

Preoperative Management of Hypothyroidism

Patients with mild to moderate hypothyroidism may proceed to surgery, as no convincing evidence exists to show that there is an adverse effect on outcomes (107–110); if the procedure is elective, it is optimal to begin replacement with thyroid hormone and delay the surgery until the patient is euthyroid. The exception to this rule is a patient with coronary artery disease awaiting bypass or stenting. Such patients should have their coronary vasculature addressed first, and then have their thyroid hormone replaced postoperatively. Evidence suggests that replacement of thyroid hormone before restoring coronary blood flow could tax an already ischemic myocardium (111). A patient with severe hypothyroidism—for example, very low levels of thyroid hormone, or myxedema coma, or clinical symptoms of chronic thyroid hormone deficiency such as altered mentation, pericardial effusion, or heart failure—who requires urgent surgery should be given a loading dose of intravenous T_4 and possibly T_3. In addition, stress-dose glucocorticoids should be given if adrenal or pituitary function is uncertain, as replacement of thyroxine in a patient with adrenal insufficiency can precipitate adrenal crisis. The patient may be given an initial dose of T_4 at 200 to 300 μg IV, followed by 50 μg daily. Depending on the patient's age and cardiac risk factors, T_3 may be given simultaneously at 10 μg every 8 to 12 hours (112).

THYROID FUNCTION IN NONTHYROIDAL ILLNESS

Aberrations in thyroid function during illness occur along a continuum, with wider deviations from the mean as the patient becomes more severely ill. Several names have been ascribed to the condition, including euthyroid sick syndrome, low T_3 syndrome, low T_4 syndrome, and nonthyroidal illness. Considerable debate exists as to whether this syndrome represents a pathologic process marked by hypothyroidism or an adaptive response to systemic illness that allows the body to lower its tissue energy requirements. In light of this controversy, it is understandable that no consensus exists on whether or how to treat this entity.

Interpretation of thyroid function tests in critically ill patients is complex. For this reason, thyroid function should not be measured in this setting unless a thyroid disorder is strongly suspected. When it is deemed appropriate to evaluate the hypothalamic-pituitary-thyroid axis, the clinician should check a TSH, total T_4, free T_4, and total T_3.

The most commonly seen change in thyroid hormone function tests in hospitalized patients is a low serum T_3 concentration (113). Most T_3 in the serum is produced by deiodination of T_4 to T_3 in the peripheral tissues. The levels of the enzyme responsible for this conversion, 5′-monodeiodinase, are decreased with even mild illness (114). As described in the above section about drugs and thyroid function, many commonly used medications in the ICU may also decrease the peripheral conversion of T_4 to T_3, further lowering the circulating T_3 levels. Glucocorticoids and β-adrenergic antagonists are the most common offending agents. In addition, free fatty acids inhibit the deiodinase activity (115). Cytokines have also been shown to have a role in the development of the sick euthyroid syndrome by their role in decreasing the conversion of T_4 to T_3 (116).

Concomitant with the decline in T_3 levels is a rise in rT_3 (reverse T_3) in nonthyroidal illness. Fasting may produce this clinical picture within 24 to 36 hours and is reversed as quickly with refeeding (117). This pattern of low T_3/high rT_3 is found in many patients with various acute and chronic illnesses, whether due to infection, surgery, cancer, cardiovascular diseases, pulmonary processes, burns, or trauma. The metabolic rate of formation of rT_3 is unchanged in the setting of illness. The increase in this value is, instead, a reflection of the attenuated rates of clearance of rT_3 (118). The complicating factor with routinely measuring the rT_3 levels in patients suspected of having nonthyroidal illness is that it may take up to a week to process the test in the laboratory.

Thyroxine (T_4) levels may also be reduced in up to 20% of hospitalized patients and 50% of critically ill patients (119). These low T_4 levels are correlated with a higher mortality rate (120). The reduction in T_4 can, in part, be attributed to decreased concentrations of one of the three thyroid hormone-binding proteins: thyroxine-binding globulin (TBG), transthyretin, and albumin. Agents that inhibit the T_4-binding protein interaction have also been identified as responsible for the lowering of T_4 levels in the serum of critically ill patients. Some data point to high levels of free fatty acids as a causative agent in this process (121).

Serum TSH levels are typically normal in most patients with nonthyroidal illness, although during the recovery phase of the illness, thyrotropin concentrations may rise (122). In more critically ill patients, the TSH may simultaneously fall with the decline in T_4 levels. Such findings have led some to suggest that some patients may have an acquired transient central hypothyroidism during the nonthyroidal illness. Thyroid hormone replacement, however, has not been shown to improve outcomes in critically ill patients (123). Medications may also alter TSH levels (Table 166.2). Dopamine infusions are frequently associated with a reduction in serum thyrotropin concentration.

When measuring TSH levels in the ICU, it is important to use a high-sensitivity assay with a lower detection limit of at least 0.01 mU/L. The vast majority of hospitalized patients with low, but detectable, TSH by this assay have sick euthyroid syndrome. In contrast, patients with undetectable thyrotropin are more likely to be hyperthyroid. Finally, those patients with high TSH (up to 20 mU/L) are likely recovering from a nonthyroidal illness and should be reassessed 6 weeks after the hospitalization.

Acute Airway Obstruction and Goiter

Acute airway obstruction is a life-threatening complication of an enlarged thyroid gland. Typically, development of a goiter is a gradual process, but rapid growth of the gland may occur in certain circumstances. Fortunately quite rare, but important to consider, is anaplastic thyroid cancer. Patients with this disease may present with considerable growth of the thyroid within a few weeks (124). Thyroid lymphoma can also show a rapid growth pattern but will quickly respond to appropriate chemotherapy and/or radiation therapy. Riedel thyroiditis, also rare, with a prevalence of 0.06% to 0.3%, may present with a rapidly enlarging, hard neck mass that must be differentiated from thyroid cancer or lymphoma. The fibrous tissue may invade soft tissue and muscle and lead to tracheal compression (125). The more common scenario is a patient who presents with a nodule that rapidly increases in size over several minutes to hours. In these cases, the patient has underlying nodular disease that has encroached on a nearby blood vessel and bled into a cystic compartment of the nodule. Typically, patients have regression of such a nodule over the ensuing weeks.

The clinical presentation of a compressive goiter is varied. Patients may present with complaints of a pressure sensation in the neck, particularly with movement of the head. Difficulty swallowing and vocal cord paralysis also may be encountered. The Pemberton sign, facial flushing and jugular venous distention on raising the arms over the head, is an indication of obstruction of venous outflow from the head (126). Many patients with a goiter have a mild degree of airway obstruction when screened with pulmonary function tests. Additionally, although chest radiographs accurately indicate retrosternal extension of goiters, they cannot predict airway obstruction as reliably as flow-volume loops (86). It is critical to recognize that a patient presenting with new-onset wheezing or stridor may have a substernal goiter (127).

The management of acute airway compromise is primarily surgical (128). If airway collapse is imminent, it is critical to protect the airway with intubation (129). The type of surgery necessary depends on the size of the goiter and whether there is an associated malignancy. Radioiodine treatment can take months to years to shrink the goiter (130).

Postthyroidectomy Hypocalcemia

Hypoparathyroidism

The most common cause of hypoparathyroidism is surgery on the neck, with resultant removal of, or injury to, the parathyroid glands. This is typically seen after cancer surgery, total thyroidectomy, or parathyroidectomy. It is most often a transient condition with symptoms occurring 1 to 2 days postoperatively. Symptoms may vary from subtle perioral numbness and tingling to profound fatigue to tetany. Table 166.9 lists the symptoms and signs that may be seen in patients with hypocalcemia. Risk of hypocalcemia is dependent on the extent of surgery, localization and preservation of the parathyroids, and skill of the surgeon. Incidence rates of postoperative, transient hypocalcemia range from 1.6% up to greater than 50%, but most of these patients will regain parathyroid function over the ensuing months. The risk of permanent hypoparathyroidism is variable, between zero and 10% (131). During nonparathyroid neck surgery, it is critical for the surgeon to recognize a compromised parathyroid gland and autotransplant the gland into the adjacent neck muscle to ensure the gland will regain function.

TABLE 166.9

SYMPTOMS AND SIGNS OF ACUTE HYPOCALCEMIA

Symptoms	Signs
Perioral numbness and tingling	Chvostek sign
Tingling paresthesias in distal extremities	Trousseau sign
Muscle cramps	Hypotension
Hyperreflexia	Bradycardia
Carpopedal spasm	Prolonged QT interval
Seizures	Arrhythmias

Treatment. Treatment is aimed at normalization of the serum calcium. Many surgeons begin thrice-daily prophylactic oral calcium supplementation the night of the surgery (132). If the patient develops progressive symptoms, tetany, or seizures, the use of IV calcium gluconate is warranted. In life-threatening situations, 10 mL of calcium gluconate may be administered intravenously over a 5- to 10-minute period and repeated as necessary. In less acute situations, a continuous calcium infusion may be used by mixing ten ampules of calcium gluconate in 500 mL of 5% dextrose in water. The infusion rate may vary between 0.3 mg/kg/hour to 2 mg/kg/hour, depending on the clinical setting. The goal of therapy is to reverse hypocalcemic symptoms and restore calcium levels to the low-normal range. Chronic management of permanent hypoparathyroidism is beyond the scope of this chapter.

Hungry Bone Syndrome

Hungry bone syndrome, HBS, is a well recognized complication of surgical correction of severe hyperparathyroidism. Patients with very high levels of parathyroid hormone (PTH) may develop significant hypocalcemia after surgical removal of the offending parathyroid adenoma(s). The mechanism of this metabolic derangement is rapid skeletal mineralization. Less commonly seen is HBS after thyroidectomy for thyrotoxicosis. Patients with hyperthyroidism may develop secondary osteoporosis and resultant hypercalcemia from the increased bone resorption. After surgical removal of the thyroid gland, patients have a reversal of the thyrotoxic osteodystrophy and, instead, have a net flux of calcium and phosphorous deposition into bone. In extreme thyrotoxicosis, the patient may develop hypocalcemia. This condition typically resolves within a few days to weeks with treatment of the hypocalcemia (133).

References

1. los Santos ET, Mazzaferri EL. Sensitive thyroid-stimulating hormone assays: clinical applications and limitations. *Compr Ther.* 1988;14(9):26–33.
2. Hollowell JG, Staehling NW, Flanders WD, et al. Serum TSH, T(4), and thyroid antibodies in the United States population (1988 to 1994): National Health and Nutrition Examination Survey (NHANES III). *J Clin Endocrinol Metab.* 2002;87(2):489–499.
3. Wartofsky L, Dickey RA. The evidence for a narrower thyrotropin reference range is compelling. *J Clin Endocrinol Metab.* 2005;90(9):5483–5488.
4. Stockigt JR. Free thyroid hormone measurement. A critical appraisal. *Endocrinol Metab Clin North Am.* 2001;30(2):265–289.
5. Stepanas AV, Mashiter G, Maisey MN. Serum triiodothyronine: clinical experience with a new radioimmunoassay kit. *Clin Endocrinol (Oxf).* 1977;6(3):171–183.
6. Adami HO, Rimsten A, Thoren L, et al. Thyroid disease and function in breast cancer patients and non-hospitalized controls evaluated by determination of TSH, T3, rT3 and T4 levels in serum. *Acta Chir Scand.* 1978; 144(2):89–97.
7. Afrasiabi MA, Vaziri ND, Gwinup G, et al. Thyroid function studies in the nephrotic syndrome. *Ann Intern Med.* 1979;90(3):335–338.
8. Swanson MA, Custer TR, Suey CM. Free thyroxine and free thyroxine index in women taking oral contraceptives. *Clin Nucl Med.* 1981;6(4):168–171.
9. Schimmel M, Utiger RD. Thyroidal and peripheral production of thyroid hormones. Review of recent findings and their clinical implications. *Ann Intern Med.* 1977;87(6):760–768.
10. Gittoes NJ, Franklyn JA. Drug-induced thyroid disorders. *Drug Saf.* 1995; 13(1):46–55.
11. Kaptein EM, Spencer CA, Kamiel MB, et al. Prolonged dopamine administration and thyroid hormone economy in normal and critically ill subjects. *J Clin Endocrinol Metab.* 1980;51(2):387–393.
12. Rosenberg R. Malabsorption of thyroid hormone with cholestyramine administration. *Conn Med.* 1994;58(2):109.

13. Davies PH, Franklyn JA. The effects of drugs on tests of thyroid function. *Eur J Clin Pharmacol.* 1991;40(5):439–451.
14. Braga M, Cooper DS. Clinical review 129: oral cholecystographic agents and the thyroid. *J Clin Endocrinol Metab.* 2001;86(5):1853–1860.
15. Nicoloff JT, Fisher DA, Appleman MD Jr. The role of glucocorticoids in the regulation of thyroid function in man. *J Clin Invest.* 1970;49(10):1922–1929.
16. Lim CF, Bai Y, Topliss DJ, et al. Drug and fatty acid effects on serum thyroid hormone binding. *J Clin Endocrinol Metab.* 1988;67(4):682–688.
17. Surks MI, DeFesi CR. Normal serum free thyroid hormone concentrations in patients treated with phenytoin or carbamazepine—a paradox resolved. *JAMA.* 1996;275:1495–1498.
18. Bohbot NL, Young J, Orgiazzi J, et al. Interferon-alpha-induced hyperthyroidism: a three-stage evolution from silent thyroiditis towards Graves' disease. *Eur J Endocrinol.* 2006;154(3):367–372.
19. Ringel MD. Management of hypothyroidism and hyperthyroidism in the intensive care unit. *Crit Care Clin.* 2001;17(1):59–74.
20. Roffi M, Cattaneo F, Brandle M. Thyrotoxicosis and the cardiovascular system. *Minerva Endocrinol.* 2005;30(2):47–58.
21. Moolman JA. Thyroid hormone and the heart. *Cardiovasc J S Afr.* 2002;13(4):159–163.
22. Jalal S, Khan KA, Rauoof MA, et al. Thyrotoxicosis presenting with complete heart block. *Saudi Med J.* 2004;25(12):2057–2058.
23. Osman F, Ayuk J, Dale J, et al. Thyrotoxicosis with heart block. *J R Soc Med.* 2001;94(7):346–348.
24. Zargar AH, Bashir MI, Wani AI, et al. Reversible complete heart block in Grave's disease. *J Assoc Physicians India.* 1999;47(11):1120–1121.
25. Kernoff LM, Rossouw JE, Kennelly BM. Complete heart block complicating thyrotoxicosis. *S Afr Med J.* 1974;47(12):513–515.
26. McElvaney GN, Wilcox PG, Fairbarn MS, et al. Respiratory muscle weakness and dyspnea in thyrotoxic patients. *Am Rev Respir Dis.* 1990;141(5 Pt 1):1221–1227.
27. Armigliato M, Paolini R, Aggio S, et al. Hyperthyroidism as a cause of pulmonary arterial hypertension: a prospective study. *Angiology.* 2006;57(5):600–606.
28. Ma RC, Chow CC. Thyrotoxicosis as a risk factor for pulmonary arterial hypertension. *Ann Intern Med.* 2006;144(3):222–223.
29. Ma RC, Cheng AY, So WY, et al. Thyrotoxicosis and pulmonary hypertension. *Am J Med.* 2005;118(8):927–928.
30. Werner D, Misfeld M, Regenfus M, et al. Emergency coronary angiography with gadolinium in a patient with thyrotoxicosis, pulmonary embolism and persistent right atrial thrombi. *Clin Res Cardiol.* 2006;95(8):418–421.
31. Glikson M, Freimark D, Leor R, et al. Unstable anginal syndrome and pulmonary oedema due to thyrotoxicosis. *Postgrad Med J.* 1991;67(783):81–83.
32. Blasco PF, Perez MR, Roman GF, et al. High output heart failure and pulmonary acute edema as presentation of thyrotoxicosis secondary to toxic multinodular goiter [in Spanish]. *Rev Clin Esp.* 2004;204(11):608–609.
33. Wald DA, Silver A. Cardiovascular manifestations of thyroid storm: a case report. *J Emerg Med.* 2003;25(1):23–28.
34. Brussel T, Matthay MA, Chernow B. Pulmonary manifestations of endocrine and metabolic disorders. *Clin Chest Med.* 1989;10(4):645–653.
35. Surks MI, Chopra IJ, Mariash CN, et al. American Thyroid Association guidelines for use of laboratory tests in thyroid disorders. *JAMA.* 1990;263(11):1529–1532.
36. Ohye H, Fukata S, Kanoh M, et al. Thyrotoxicosis caused by weight-reducing herbal medicines. *Arch Intern Med.* 2005;165(8):831–834.
37. Cohen JH, III, Ingbar SH, Braverman LE. Thyrotoxicosis due to ingestion of excess thyroid hormone. *Endocr Rev.* 1989;10(2):113–124.
38. van der Molen AJ, Thomsen HS, Morcos SK. Effect of iodinated contrast media on thyroid function in adults. *Eur Radiol.* 2004;14(5):902–907.
39. Chen CC, Huang WS, Huang SC, et al. Thyrotoxicosis aggravated by iodinated contrast medium: a case report. *Zhonghua Yi Xue Za Zhi (Taipei).* 1994;53(6):379–382.
40. Burger AG, Philippe J. Thyroid emergencies. *Baillieres Clin Endocrinol Metab.* 1992;6(1):77–93.
41. Burch HB, Wartofsky L. Life-threatening thyrotoxicosis. Thyroid storm. *Endocrinol Metab Clin North Am.* 1993;22(2):263–277.
42. Hoffman WH, Chodoroff G, Piggott LR. Haloperidol and thyroid storm. *Am J Psychiatry.* 1978;135(4):484–486.
43. Wilson BE, Hobbs WN. Case report: pseudoephedrine-associated thyroid storm: thyroid hormone-catecholamine interactions. *Am J Med Sci.* 1993;306(5):317–319.
44. Zweig SB, Schlosser JR, Thomas SA, et al. Rectal administration of propylthiouracil in suppository form in patients with thyrotoxicosis and critical illness: case report and review of literature. *Endocr Pract.* 2006;12(1):43–47.
45. Cansler CL, Latham JA, Brown PM Jr, et al. Duodenal obstruction in thyroid storm. *South Med J.* 1997;90(11):1143–1146.
46. Livadas DP, Koutras DA, Souvatzoglou A, et al. The toxic effect of small iodine supplements in patients with autonomous thyroid nodules. *Clin Endocrinol (Oxf).* 1977;7(2):121–127.
47. Bal C, Nair N. The therapeutic efficacy of oral cholecystographic agent (iopanoic acid) in the management of hyperthyroidism. *J Nucl Med.* 1990;31(7):1180–1182.
48. Ng YW, Tiu SC, Choi KL et al. Use of lithium in the treatment of thyrotoxicosis. *Hong Kong Med J.* 2006;12(4):254–259.
49. Faber J, Waetjen I, Siersbaek-Nielsen K. Free thyroxine measured in undiluted serum by dialysis and ultrafiltration: effects of non-thyroidal illness, and an acute load of salicylate or heparin. *Clin Chim Acta.* 1993;223(1-2):159–167.
50. Solomon BL, Wartofsky L, Burman KD. Adjunctive cholestyramine therapy for thyrotoxicosis. *Clin Endocrinol (Oxf).* 1993;38(1):39–43.
51. Tshirch LS, Drews J, Liedtke R, Schemmel K. Treatment of thyroid storm with plasmapheresis (author's transl) [in German]. *Med Klin.* 1975;70(18):807–811.
52. Ashkar FS, Katims RB, Smoak WM III, et al. Thyroid storm treatment with blood exchange and plasmapheresis. *JAMA.* 1970;214(7):1275–1279.
53. Ligtenberg J, Tulleken J, Zijlstra J. Plasmapheresis in thyrotoxicosis. *Ann Intern Med.* 1999;131(1):71–72.
54. Newman CM, Price A, Davies DW, et al. Amiodarone and the thyroid: a practical guide to the management of thyroid dysfunction induced by amiodarone therapy. *Heart.* 1998;79(2):121–127.
55. Martino E, Bartalena L, Bogazzi F, et al. The effects of amiodarone on the thyroid. *Endocr Rev.* 2001;22(2):240–254.
56. Martino E, Safran M, Aghini-Lombardi F, et al. Environmental iodine intake and thyroid dysfunction during chronic amiodarone therapy. *Ann Intern Med.* 1984;101(1):28–34.
57. Bartalena L, Grasso L, Brogioni S, et al. Serum interleukin-6 in amiodarone-induced thyrotoxicosis. *J Clin Endocrinol Metab.* 1994;78(2):423–427.
58. Bogazzi F, Bartalena L, Gasperi M, et al. The various effects of amiodarone on thyroid function. *Thyroid.* 2001;11(5):511–519.
59. Loh KC. Amiodarone-induced thyroid disorders: a clinical review. *Postgrad Med J.* 2000;76(893):133–140.
60. Woeber KA. Iodine and thyroid disease. *Med Clin North Am.* 1991;75(1):169–178.
61. Weber C, Scholz GH, Lamesch P, et al. Thyroidectomy in iodine induced thyrotoxic storm. *Exp Clin Endocrinol Diabetes.* 1999;107(7):468–472.
62. Lorberboym M, Mechanick JI. Accelerated thyrotoxicosis induced by iodinated contrast media in metastatic differentiated thyroid carcinoma. *J Nucl Med.* 1996;37(9):1532–1535.
63. Shimura H, Takazawa K, Endo T, et al. T4-thyroid storm after CT-scan with iodinated contrast medium. *J Endocrinol Invest.* 1990;13(1):73–76.
64. Blum M, Kranjac T, Park CM, et al. Thyroid storm after cardiac angiography with iodinated contrast medium. Occurrence in a patient with a previously euthyroid autonomous nodule of the thyroid. *JAMA.* 1976;235(21):2324–2325.
65. Martin FI, Tress BW, Colman PG, et al. Iodine-induced hyperthyroidism due to nonionic contrast radiography in the elderly. *Am J Med.* 1993;95(1):78–82.
66. Kung AW. Clinical review: thyrotoxic periodic paralysis: a diagnostic challenge. *J Clin Endocrinol Metab.* 2006;91(7):2490–2495.
67. Hsieh CH, Kuo SW, Pei D, et al. Thyrotoxic periodic paralysis: an overview. *Ann Saudi Med.* 2004;24(6):418–422.
68. Ober KP. Thyrotoxic periodic paralysis in the United States. Report of 7 cases and review of the literature. *Medicine (Baltimore).* 1992;71(3):109–120.
69. Lin SH. Thyrotoxic periodic paralysis. *Mayo Clin Proc.* 2005;80(1):99–105.
70. Langley RW, Burch HB. Perioperative management of the thyrotoxic patient. *Endocrinol Metab Clin North Am.* 2003;32(2):519–534.
71. Baeza A, Aguayo J, Barria M, et al. Rapid preoperative preparation in hyperthyroidism. *Clin Endocrinol (Oxf).* 1991;35(5):439–442.
72. Pandey CK, Raza M, Dhiraaj S, et al. Rapid preparation of severe uncontrolled thyrotoxicosis due to Graves' disease with iopanoic acid–a case report. *Can J Anaesth.* 2004;51(1):38–40.
73. Hollowell JG, Staehling NW, Flanders WD et al. Serum TSH, T(4), and thyroid antibodies in the United States population (1988 to 1994): National Health and Nutrition Examination Survey (NHANES III). *J Clin Endocrinol Metab.* 2002;87(2):489–499.
74. Wallace K, Hofmann MT. Thyroid dysfunction: how to manage overt and subclinical disease in older patients. *Geriatrics.* 1998;53(4):32–38, 41.
75. Forfar JC, Muir AL, Toft AD. Left ventricular function in hypothyroidism. Responses to exercise and beta adrenoceptor blockade. *Br Heart J.* 1982;48(3):278–284.
76. Klein I. Thyroid hormone and the cardiovascular system. *Am J Med.* 1990;88(6):631–637.
77. Wieshammer S, Keck FS, Waitzinger J, et al. Acute hypothyroidism slows the rate of left ventricular diastolic relaxation. *Can J Physiol Pharmacol.* 1989;67(9):1007–1010.
78. Danzi S, Klein I. Thyroid hormone and blood pressure regulation. *Curr Hypertens Rep.* 2003;5(6):513–520.
79. Ladenson PW. Recognition and management of cardiovascular disease related to thyroid dysfunction. *Am J Med.* 1990;88(6):638–641.
80. Karu AK, Khalife WI, Houser R, et al. Impending cardiac tamponade as a primary presentation of hypothyroidism: case report and review of literature. *Endocr Pract.* 2005;11(4):265–271.

81. Ladenson PW, Sherman SI, Baughman KL, et al. Reversible alterations in myocardial gene expression in a young man with dilated cardiomyopathy and hypothyroidism. *Proc Natl Acad Sci U S A*. 1992;89(12):5251–5255.
82. Weiner M, Chausow A, Szidon P. Reversible respiratory muscle weakness in hypothyroidism. *Br J Dis Chest*. 1986;80(4):391–395.
83. Siafakas NM, Salesiotou V, Filaditaki V, et al. Respiratory muscle strength in hypothyroidism. *Chest*. 1992;102(1):189–194.
84. Laroche CM, Cairns T, Moxham J, et al. Hypothyroidism presenting with respiratory muscle weakness. *Am Rev Respir Dis*. 1988;138(2):472–474.
85. Duranti R, Gheri RG, Gorini M, et al. Control of breathing in patients with severe hypothyroidism. *Am J Med*. 1993;95(1):29–37.
86. Miller MR, Pincock AC, Oates GD, et al. Upper airway obstruction due to goitre: detection, prevalence and results of surgical management. *Q J Med*. 1990;74(274):177–188.
87. Skatrud J, Iber C, Ewart R, et al. Disordered breathing during sleep in hypothyroidism. *Am Rev Respir Dis*. 1981;124(3):325–329.
88. Bassotti G, Pagliacci MC, Nicoletti I, et al. Intestinal pseudoobstruction secondary to hypothyroidism. Importance of small bowel manometry. *J Clin Gastroenterol*. 1992;14(1):56–58.
89. Thompson M, Fischer PM. Ileus with hypothyroidism. *J Fam Pract*. 1986; 23(3):269–270.
90. Abbasi AA, Douglass RC, Bissell GW, et al. Myxedema ileus. A form of intestinal pseudo-obstruction. *JAMA*. 1975;234(2):181–183.
91. Siurala M, Varis K, Lamberg BA. Intestinal absorption and autoimmunity in endocrine disorders. *Acta Med Scand*. 1968;184(1-2):53–64.
92. Misra GC, Bose SL, Samal AK. Malabsorption in thyroid dysfunctions. *J Indian Med Assoc*. 1991;89(7):195–197.
93. Croal BL, Blake AM, Johnston J, et al. Absence of relation between hyponatraemia and hypothyroidism. *Lancet*. 1997;350(9088):1402.
94. Macaron C, Famuyiwa O. Hyponatremia of hypothyroidism. Appropriate suppression of antidiuretic hormone levels. *Arch Intern Med*. 1978;138(5): 820–822.
95. Schmitz PH, de Meijer PH, Meinders AE. Hyponatremia due to hypothyroidism: a pure renal mechanism. *Neth J Med*. 2001;58(3):143–149.
96. Nakano M, Higa M, Ishikawa R, et al. Hyponatremia with increased plasma antidiuretic hormone in a case of hypothyroidism. *Intern Med*. 2000;39(12):1075–1078.
97. Diekman T, Lansberg PJ, Kastelein JJP, et al. Prevalence and correction of hypothyroidism in a large cohort of patients referred for dyslipidemia. *Arch Intern Med*. 1995;155:1490–1495.
98. Pucci E, Chiovato L, Pinchera A. Thyroid and lipid metabolism. *Int J Obes Relat Metab Disord*. 2000;24(Suppl 2):S109–S112.
99. O'Brien T, Dinneen SF, O'Brien PC, et al. Hyperlipidemia in patients with primary and secondary hypothyroidism. *Mayo Clin Proc*. 1993;68(9):860–866.
100. Wartofsky L. Myxedema coma. *Endocrinol Metab Clin North Am*. 2006; 35(4):687–98, vii–viii.
101. Yamamoto T, Fukuyama J, Fujiyoshi A. Factors associated with mortality of myxedema coma: report of eight cases and literature survey. *Thyroid*. 1999;9(12):1167–1174.
102. Hylander B, Rosenqvist U. Treatment of myxoedema coma–factors associated with fatal outcome. *Acta Endocrinol (Copenh)*. 1985;108(1):65–71.
103. Behnia M, Clay AS, Farber MO. Management of myxedematous respiratory failure: review of ventilation and weaning principles. *Am J Med Sci*. 2000;320(6):368–373.
104. Benvenga S, Squadrito S, Saporito F, et al. Myxedema coma of both primary and secondary origin, with non-classic presentation and extremely elevated creatine kinase. *Horm Metab Res*. 2000;32(9):364–366.
105. Wall CR. Myxedema coma: diagnosis and treatment. *Am Fam Physician*. 2000;62(11):2485–2490.
106. Yamamoto T, Fukuyama J, Fujiyoshi A. Factors associated with mortality of myxedema coma: report of eight cases and literature survey. *Thyroid*. 1999;9(12):1167–1174.
107. Jones TH, Hunter SM, Price A, et al. Should thyroid function be assessed before cardiopulmonary bypass operations? *Ann Thorac Surg*. 1994;58(2): 434–436.
108. Connery LE, Coursin DB. Assessment and therapy of selected endocrine disorders. *Anesthesiol Clin North Am*. 2004;22(1):93–123.
109. Weinberg AD, Brennan MD, Gorman CA, et al. Outcome of anesthesia and surgery in hypothyroid patients. *Arch Intern Med*. 1983;143(5):893–897.
110. Ladenson PW, Levin AA, Ridgway EC, et al. Complications of surgery in hypothyroid patients. *Am J Med*. 1984;77(2):261–266.
111. Stathatos N, Wartofsky L. Perioperative management of patients with hypothyroidism. *Endocrinol Metab Clin North Am*. 2003;32(2):503–518.
112. Schiff RL, Welsh GA. Perioperative evaluation and management of the patient with endocrine dysfunction. *Med Clin North Am*. 2003;87(1):175–192.
113. McIver B, Gorman CA. Euthyroid sick syndrome: an overview. *Thyroid*. 1997;7(1):125–132.
114. Davidson MB, Chopra IJ. Effect of carbohydrate and noncarbohydrate sources of calories on plasma 3,5,3'-triiodothyronine concentrations in man. *J Clin Endocrinol Metab*. 1979;48(4):577–581.
115. Chopra IJ, Huang TS, Beredo A, et al. Evidence for an inhibitor of extrathyroidal conversion of thyroxine to 3,5,3'-triiodothyronine in sera of patients with nonthyroidal illnesses. *J Clin Endocrinol Metab*. 1985;60(4): 666–672.
116. van der PT, Romijn JA, Wiersinga WM, et al. Tumor necrosis factor: a putative mediator of the sick euthyroid syndrome in man. *J Clin Endocrinol Metab*. 1990;71(6):1567–1572.
117. Wartofsky L, Burman KD. Alterations in thyroid function in patients with systemic illness: the "euthyroid sick syndrome." *Endocr Rev*. 1982;3(2): 164–217.
118. Papanicolaou DA. Euthyroid sick syndrome and the role of cytokines. *Rev Endocr Metab Disord*. 2000;1(1–2):43–48.
119. Arem R, Deppe S. Fatal nonthyroidal illness may impair nocturnal thyrotropin levels. *Am J Med*. 1990;88(3):258–262.
120. Slag MF, Morley JE, Elson MK, et al. Hypothyroxinemia in critically ill patients as a predictor of high mortality. *JAMA*. 1981;245(1):43–45.
121. Lim CF, Curtis AJ, Barlow JW, et al. Interactions between oleic acid and drug competitors influence specific binding of thyroxine in serum. *J Clin Endocrinol Metab*. 1991;73(5):1106–1110.
122. Hamblin PS, Dyer SA, Mohr VS, et al. Relationship between thyrotropin and thyroxine changes during recovery from severe hypothyroxinemia of critical illness. *J Clin Endocrinol Metab*. 1986;62(4):717–722.
123. Brent GA, Hershman JM. Thyroxine therapy in patients with severe nonthyroidal illnesses and low serum thyroxine concentration. *J Clin Endocrinol Metab*. 1986;63(1):1–8.
124. Nel CJ, van Heerden JA, Goellner JR, et al. Anaplastic carcinoma of the thyroid: a clinicopathologic study of 82 cases. *Mayo Clin Proc*. 1985;60:51–58.
125. Few J, Thompson NW, Angelos P, et al. Riedel's thyroiditis: treatment with tamoxifen. *Surgery*. 1996;120:993–998.
126. Anders H, Keller C. Pemberton's maneuver—a clinical test for latent superior vena cava syndrome caused by a substernal mass. *Eur J Med Res*. 1997;2(11):488–490.
127. Katlic MR, Grillo HC, Wang CA. Substernal goiter. Analysis of 80 patients from Massachusetts General Hospital. *Am J Surg*. 1985;149(2):283–287.
128. Ben Nun A, Soudack M, Best LA. Retrosternal thyroid goiter: 15 years experience. *Isr Med Assoc J*. 2006;8(2):106–109.
129. Nielsen VM, Lovgreen NA, Elbrond O. Intrathoracic goitre. Surgical treatment in an ENT department. *J Laryngol Otol*. 1983;97(11):1039–1045.
130. Huysmans D, Hermus A, Edelbroek M, et al. Radioiodine for nontoxic multinodular goiter. *Thyroid*. 1997;7(2):235–239.
131. Pattou F, Combemale F, Fabre S, et al. Hypocalcemia following thyroid surgery: incidence and prediction of outcome. *World J Surg*. 1998;22(7): 718–724.
132. Carty SE. Prevention and management of complications in parathyroid surgery. *Otolaryngol Clin North Am*. 2004;37(4):897–907, xi.
133. Dembinski TC, Yatscoff RW, Blandford DE. Thyrotoxicosis and hungry bone syndrome—a cause of posttreatment hypocalcemia. *Clin Biochem*. 1994;27(1):69–74.

SECTION XVIII ■ SKIN AND MUSCLE DISEASE AND DYSFUNCTION

CHAPTER 167 ■ CRITICAL CARE OF AUTOIMMUNE AND CONNECTIVE TISSUE DISORDERS: RHEUMATOLOGIC DISEASES IN THE INTENSIVE CARE UNIT

HARAKH V. DEDHIA • RONALD A. MUDRY

Emergencies resulting from autoimmune processes or connective tissue diseases (CTDs) are relatively uncommon in critical care medicine; nonetheless, they can be life threatening. The term *autoimmune* describes a number of disorders whose basic underlying pathophysiology is a derangement of the immune system's ability to recognize "self." Virtually any organ system may be subject to an inflammatory assault by one's own immune system (1–8). Such disease processes may range from relatively mild and indolent to fulminant and life threatening. The following are scenarios that may be encountered by the critical care provider:

1. A patient may be admitted to the intensive care unit (ICU) because of CTD complications or the complications of drug therapy. Sometimes a patient may present with an acute crisis without a past history of CTDs.
2. Clinical manifestations can affect every major organ.
3. Clinical presentations vary and may include stridor, acute or progressive respiratory failure, life-threatening hemoptysis, acute renal failure, paralysis, cerebritis, mesenteric ischemia, or unstable spine. Septic shock due to an infected joint may occur.
4. Placing an arterial line or obtaining a reliable pulse oximetric signal in a patient with systemic sclerosis or severe vasculitis may be a problem.
5. Some of the drugs used to treat these diseases may cause acute or chronic respiratory failure as well as mimic infection.

Even though the exact causes and pathophysiology of many CTDs remain unclear, our understanding of the immunologic alteration and its manipulation by drugs has improved significantly in the last decade. New immune modulators have arguably altered the clinical manifestations of rheumatologic disease, but have caused new complications as well (9–18).

RHEUMATOID ARTHRITIS

Rheumatoid arthritis (RA), a systemic debilitating autoimmune disease affecting up to 1% of the population, is characterized by chronic synovial and periarticular inflammation that leads to the erosion of joints and bones. In addition, there are significant extra-articular systemic manifestations (1–9). It is likely that the interaction of genetic and environmental factors with endogenous antigenic stimuli is the key to the development of the disease. Cytokines important in the perpetuation of the inflammation and tissue damage include tumor necrosis factor-α (TNF-α) and interleukins-1, -2, -13, -15, -17, and -18. The disease may involve many other mediators and cytokines in complex interactions (9–21). Proteolytic enzymes have the ability to degrade components of the extracellular matrix and damage joints. The clinical features of RA are divided into articular and nonarticular manifestations. The American Rheumatology Association has established criteria for diagnosis of RA that include morning stiffness, arthritis of hand joints, symmetric arthritis, rheumatoid nodules, positive serum rheumatoid factor (RF), and radiologic changes. Generalized fatigue, weakness, and involvement of other organs are common in patients with positive RF. Extra-articular manifestations of RA are common, but variable; they appear to be immune mediated and can shorten survival. The systemic manifestations of RA and their management present a unique challenge to the intensivist.

Pulmonary Manifestations of Rheumatoid Arthritis

The noncardiac thoracic manifestations of RA are protean and complex, and can lead to significant morbidity and mortality (9,22–35). The exact incidence of lung disease is unknown because the pathology may be due to RA, may be a complication of drug therapy, or may be associated with comorbidities. Even though RA is more common in women, rheumatoid lung disease occurs more frequently in those men with long-standing RA, positive rheumatoid factor, and subcutaneous nodules. A classification of RA affecting the respiratory system and its relative frequency is shown in Tables 167.1 and 167.2.

Airway Disease in Rheumatoid Arthritis

Upper Airway Problems and Obstruction. The clinical presentation of upper airway obstruction is variable. Symptoms of odynophagia, hoarseness of voice, throat soreness, and cough occur early. Mild obstruction may progress to exertional dyspnea and stridor. Erythema, vocal cord edema, or stridor may

TABLE 167.1

PULMONARY MANIFESTATIONS OF RHEUMATOID ARTHRITIS

1. Airway disease
2. Interstitial lung disease
3. Rheumatoid nodules
4. Pleural disease
5. Vasculitis
6. Drug-induced lung disease
7. Infections
8. Chest wall; limitations of thoracic cage
9. Respiratory failure from spinal cord injury
10. Sleep apnea

occur secondary to local infection or previous intubation. It is essential to suspect and diagnose these conditions early to avoid an emergent situation. Diagnosis of subtle upper airway obstruction can be made by direct laryngoscopy or flow volume loops during forced inspiration, which will show variable extrathoracic obstruction. Ankylosis of the cricoarytenoid (CA) joint can lead to upper airway obstruction (25–30). Evaluation of the upper airway should include cervical spine examination, as instability may also be present. The laryngeal problems may be from CA joint inflammation, arthritis, or ankylosis, or from vasculitis affecting the vagus or recurrent laryngeal nerve, all of which may cause upper airway obstruction (8,21,25–30). In patients with RA, Brazeau-Lamontagne et al. showed various laryngeal problems and abnormalities in 75% of patients by direct fiberoptic laryngoscopy and in 72% with high-resolution computed tomography (HR-CT) of the neck and chest (25). Tracheal deviation due to severe cervical spine disease or laryngeal abnormality can make direct laryngoscopic endotracheal intubation difficult or impossible in some patients. It is advisable to use a small-caliber tube when intubating patients with laryngeal disease. The inhalation of a helium–oxygen mixture (e.g., 75% He and 25% O_2) may help in dyspneic patients. In others, emergent tracheostomy may be necessary to establish an airway.

Small Airway Obstruction. Abnormalities in the lower airways in RA can occur due to obstructive disease or bronchial hyperresponsiveness. Treatment of hyperresponsiveness with β agonists, inhaled steroids, and anticholinergics is similar to the management of asthma or chronic obstructive pulmonary disease (COPD).

Bronchiolitis Obliterans with Organizing Pneumonia, Obliterative Bronchiolitis, and Bronchiectasis

An association between bronchiectasis and rheumatoid arthritis has been noted, but the incidence is relatively low, varying from 0% to 10%, and remains clinically insignificant in the majority of the cases. Some patients with acute infection or decompensation may require treatment. It is similar to that used for other forms of bronchiectasis, including antibiotics and bronchodilators. It presents no unusual challenges to an intensivist. Patients with obliterative bronchiolitis (OB) or bronchiolitis obliterans with organizing pneumonia (BOOP) may present with progressive dyspnea, cough, and fever or weight loss. These airway abnormalities in patients with RA or systemic lupus erythematosus (SLE) are similar to those seen in conventional BO or BOOP. Spirometry may show an obstructive, restrictive, or mixed pattern. In patients with BO, the chest radiograph is often normal, but HR-CT will show a mosaic pattern. BO is confirmed by lung biopsy. Both BO and BOOP can

TABLE 167.2

FREQUENCY OF PULMONARY COMPLICATIONS IN RHEUMATOLOGIC DISEASE

Clinical manifestation	RA	SLE	SSc	PM-DM	AS	SjS	MCTD
ILD	3+	2+	4+	3+	1+	3+	2+
DAH	1+	2+	1+	1+	0	0	1+
BOOP	2+	1+	1+	3+	0	1+	1+
OB	2+	0	0	0	0	1+	0
Lung nodules	2+	0	0	0	0	1+	0
Plural effusion	3+	2+	1+	0	0	1+	2+
Aspiration Pn.	0	0	3+	3+	0	2+	2+
Vasculitis	2+	2+	0	1+	0	0	1+
Pulm. HTN	1+	2+	4+	1+	0	0	2+
Respiratory muscle involvement	1+	2+	0	2+	0	0	1+

Explanations for the keys: 1+ some, 4+ maximal.
RA, rheumatoid arthritis; SLE, systemic lupus erythematosus; SSc, systemic sclerosis; PM-DM, polymyositis–dermatomyositis; AS, ankylosing spondylitis; SjS, Sjögren syndrome; MCTD, mixed connective tissue disease; ILD, interstitial lung disease; DAH, diffuse alveolar hemorrhage; BOOP, bronchiolitis obliterans with organizing pneumonia; OB, obliterative bronchiolitis; Aspiration Pn., aspiration pneumonia; Pulm. HTN, pulmonary hypertension.
Modified from Tanoue L. Pulmonary manifestations of collagen vascular disease. In: Fishman AP, Elias JA, Fishman JA, et al., eds. *Fishman's Manual of Pulmonary Disease and Disorders*. 3rd ed. New York: McGraw Hill; 2002.

TABLE 167.3

CLINICAL FEATURES OF OB AND BOOP

	OB	BOOP
Onset	Slow; progressive dyspnea and cough	Relatively rapid; cough and progressive dyspnea
Chest exam	Generalized ↓ air entry and breath sounds, ± inspiratory squeak	Bibasilar crackles, clubbing, cor pulmonale in advanced cases
Chest radiographs	Normal or hyperinflation	Alveolar infiltrates, patchy and peripheral, sometimes diffuse
Chest HR-CT	Adjacent area of ↓ and ↑ attenuation	
PFT	Air flow obstruction and normal or ↓ lung diffusion Occasionally restrictive defect	Restrictive impairment and ↓ lung diffusion
Treatment and prognosis	Corticosteroids but response poor; progressive respiratory failure	Good response to steroids and immunosuppressive drugs

OB, obliterans bronchiolitis; BOOP, bronchiolitis obliterans organizing pneumonia; HR-CT, high-resolution computed tomograph; PFT, pulmonary function test.

be treated with high-dose steroids or other immunosuppressive drugs (Table 167.3).

Interstitial Lung Disease

Some degree of interstitial lung disease (ILD) occurs in the majority of patients with RA, but the limitations imposed by the musculoskeletal and joint disease often limit activities and the exercise capacity of these patients, and may not allow the pulmonary symptoms to manifest until the ILD has significantly advanced. At this point, symptoms of dyspnea may occur with minimal activities or at rest. The clinical presentation and histologic and radiologic manifestations are similar to other idiopathic interstitial lung diseases or idiopathic pulmonary fibrosis (IPF). Histopathologic specimens may show a pattern of usual interstitial pneumonia (UIP), desquamative interstitial pneumonia (DIP), nonspecific interstitial pneumonia (NSIP), organizing pneumonia (OP), or lymphocytic interstitial pneumonia (LIP). The clinical course of ILD in RA is slower than that of IPF; however, cor pulmonale and respiratory failure may occur (8,19–21). Chest radiography shows bilateral basilar parenchymal infiltrates and ground glass appearance. Honeycombing is seen in advanced disease (Fig. 167.1). Pulmonary function tests show restrictive impairment with low lung diffusion. Treatment with corticosteroids and other immunosuppressive therapy is similar to that of IPF. Once the ILD is established, it is associated with a poor prognosis and 5-year survival around 50%.

Rheumatoid Lung Nodules

Rheumatoid nodules occur in many patients, most frequently in the subcutaneous tissues, but can develop in other tissues including the lung. Pulmonary rheumatoid nodules (PRNs) are seen occasionally and are associated with rheumatoid nodules elsewhere in the body. Rheumatoid pulmonary nodules are generally located in subpleural areas or along interlobular septa. The histology of a PRN is similar to that of nodules seen in nonpulmonary sites. Generally, the nodules cause no major symptoms, and are simply followed by periodic chest radiographs. Sometimes, nodules cavitate or rupture, and can cause hemoptysis, pneumothorax, pleural effusion, infection, or pyopneumothorax. In a patient with a high risk for cancer, biopsy may be necessary. Caplan syndrome is a form of rheumatoid pulmonary nodules occurring with pneumoconiosis related to mining dust (Fig. 167.2). The pathology is comparable to other rheumatic nodules in addition to pigmented cells seen due to pneumoconiosis. The nodules may rapidly break down or necrose, and can cause airflow obstruction. Nodules may complicate progressive massive fibrosis. Otherwise, the prognosis is good, and treatment is primarily symptomatic.

Pleural Disease

Pleural effusions occur frequently in patients with RA and may precede joint disease. They are more common in men, especially those with long-standing RA. Patients may present

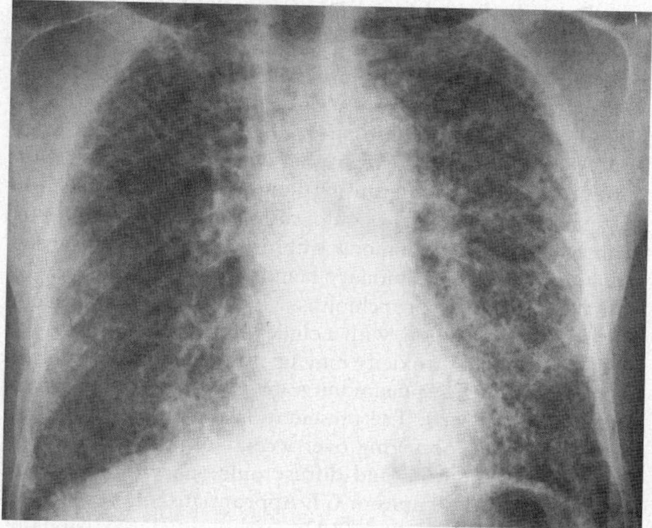

FIGURE 167.1. Chest radiograph showing severe interstitial lung disease and honeycomb appearance in a patient with rheumatoid arthritis.

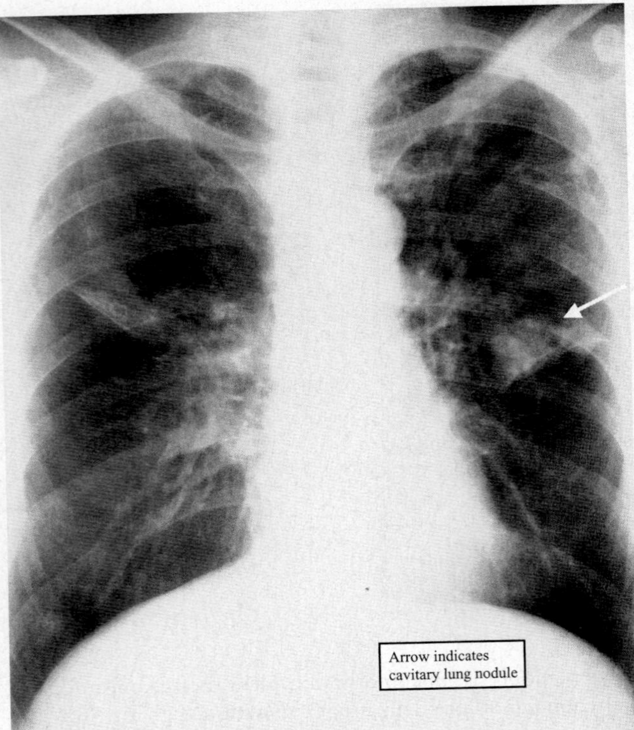
Arrow indicates
cavitary lung nodule

FIGURE 167.2. Chest radiograph of a patient with Caplan syndrome.

TABLE 167.4

PULMONARY COMPLICATIONS OF DRUGS USED TO TREAT RHEUMATOLOGIC DISEASES

1. **Noncardiogenic pulmonary edema (ARDS)**
    - Aspirin
    - NSAIDs
    - Opiates, sedatives, and hypnotic agents
    - Colchicine
2. **Bronchospasm**
    - Aspirin
    - NSAIDs
    - Sulfasalazine
    - β-Adrenoreceptor antagonist (some)
3. **Alveolar hemorrhage**
    - d-Penicillamine
4. **Interstitial lung disease**
    - Gold
    - Methotrexate
    - Penicillamine
    - Azathioprine
    - Cyclophosphamide
5. **Hypersensitivity lung disease**
    - Gold
    - Methotrexate
    - NSAIDs
    - Penicillamine
    - β-Lactam and sulfa antibiotics
6. **Bronchiolitis obliterans**
    - Gold
    - Penicillamine
    - Sulfasalazine

ARDS, acute respiratory distress syndrome; NSAIDs, nonsteroidal anti-inflammatory drugs.

with cough, dyspnea, fever, or pleuritic chest pain. The pleural fluid is exudative, with a low pH, low glucose, and white cell count less than 5,000 cells/μL, with a lymphocytic predominance. The level of rheumatoid factor in pleural fluid parallels that in the serum. Symptoms may mimic pulmonary embolism. Empyema can occur, particularly in patients on corticosteroids. Noninfectious pleurisy can be treated with nonsteroidal anti-inflammatory drugs (NSAIDs), and occasionally with fluid drainage. In recurrent and symptomatic effusions, pleural sclerosis may be required.

Drug-induced Lung Disease and Infections

The lungs are commonly affected by drugs used for treatment of RA. The immunosuppressive therapy can predispose patients to systemic complications including infection (Table 167.4). Treatment with disease-modifying antirheumatic drugs (DMARDs) is associated with a high incidence of sepsis. If the current drug therapy is causing lung toxicity, withdrawal of the agent is necessary. The complications include pneumonitis, bronchospasm, ILD–pulmonary fibrosis, infection, noncardiac pulmonary edema, pulmonary hemorrhage, drug-induced lupus, and obliterative bronchiolitis. Methotrexate-induced lung disease is very common, with a clinical presentation that is not specific. Pulmonary toxicity may be associated with a mortality rate up to 20%; pneumonitis may be, potentially, a fatal complication as well. The presentation often consists of dyspnea and cough, occurring over weeks to months. Rales are heard on auscultation, and diffuse pulmonary infiltrates are seen on chest radiographs or CT. Appropriate cultures, including bronchoalveolar lavage (BAL), are essential. Occasionally, lung biopsy may be necessary. The diagnosis must be made after exclusion of other causes of pulmonary diseases. Another possible complication of antirheumatic drug therapy is noncardiogenic pulmonary edema (NCPE). This may be seen in patients taking high-dose aspirin, NSAIDs, methotrexate, and cyclophosphamide, or in the setting of colchicine overdose. NCPE must be included in the differential diagnosis of any patient presenting with respiratory failure and a history of taking these drugs.

Acute Respiratory Failure in Rheumatoid Arthritis

Acute respiratory failure can occur in RA patients from a variety of causes. Common causes include pneumonia, pulmonary edema, pulmonary embolism, sepsis, progression of the RA lung disease, or cervical spine disease. Unusual cases of cardiopulmonary arrest have been reported. Proposed causes have included acute laryngeal stridor, CA arthritis with or without ankylosis, vocal cord immobility, spinal cord compression, cervicomedullary compression causing respiratory muscle weakness and paralysis, and instability of the atlantoaxial joint (26–36). Sleep apnea due to RA has been reported as well (36).

Neurologic Complications and Cervical Spine Involvement in Rheumatoid Arthritis

The involvement of cervical spine joints in RA, and clinical presentation thereof, is highly variable but clinically important to the intensivist (37–39). Instability of the cervical spine is the most critical problem. Risk factors include older age at onset of RA, active synovitis, and progressive erosive peripheral joint disease. Clinical symptoms include neck pain, stiffness, radicular pain, and hyperreflexia. Among the findings that require immediate evaluation and intervention are:

- Loss of sphincter control
- Respiratory impairment
- "Drop attacks"
- Dysphagia
- Dysarthria
- Vertigo
- Convulsions
- Hemiplegia
- Nystagmus
- Alteration in the levels of consciousness
- Sensation of the head falling forward upon flexion of the cervical spine

Clinical examination may reveal abnormal findings. Pain, discomfort, or resistance to passive cervical spine movement; loss of occipitocervical lordosis; or abnormal protrusion of the axial arch felt in the posterior pharyngeal wall each might suggest atlantoaxial subluxation. Abnormal gait, muscle weakness or atrophy, increased deep tendon reflexes, and abnormal plantar response may be seen. These may be severe enough for urgent surgery to stabilize the cervical spine and reduce the threat of cervical spinal cord compression.

Routine preoperative cervical spine radiography for all RA patients undergoing surgery has been suggested since subluxation may be asymptomatic. Neck positioning required for intubation can be fatal in patients with unrecognized C1-C2 disease (37–40). Involvement of the bursa around the odontoid process can cause erosion and weakness of the ligaments, which can lead to subluxation of the atlantoaxial joint. It is important to remember that subluxation occurs with the flexion of the cervical spine and, hence, should be minimized or avoided altogether. Cases of sudden death have been reported due to the compression of the upper cervical cord and medulla (41–45). Preliminary radiologic evaluation consists of plain radiograph—anteroposterior (AP) and lateral—with a neck flexion view of the cervical spine. A separation between the odontoid peg and the C1 arch or between C1 and C2 (anterior subluxation) may be seen. Neck CT can show spinal cord compression. Magnetic resonance imaging (MRI) allows better visualization of the cord and bone and, thus, is more helpful in assessing cord compression in the cervical spine (40). Therapy for cervical spine instability may be as simple as cervical collars to maintain the spine stable, while in others, halo traction may be necessary. Patients with subluxation and signs of spinal cord compression have a poor prognosis without surgery (41–43). Spinal manipulation should be avoided.

Airway Management and Anesthesia Implications in Rheumatoid Arthritis

Airway management in a patient with upper airway, cervical spine, or laryngeal disease is both a concern and a challenge for the anesthesiologist and intensivist (21,44–47). Airway problems may result from various causes, as discussed earlier. Laryngeal involvement is more common than previously thought (22,26,29,35). Drugs used to treat RA also affect anesthesia and postoperative care. Neck positioning required for intubation may potentially be fatal due to unrecognized disease at cervical spine levels 1 and 2 (C1-C2). Tracheal intubation using a direct laryngoscopic technique may be very difficult or potentially dangerous in some of these patients. During translaryngeal intubation of the trachea, it is important to stabilize the cervical spine and avoid flexion or hyperextension of the neck. In difficult cases, it is better to use topical anesthesia in the upper airway and intubate the patient with a flexible fiberoptic bronchoscope (FOB) or laryngoscope (23,35,44–46); such patients may be gently sedated, but are allowed to breathe spontaneously. Adequate clinical neurologic observation for possible spinal cord compression, weakness, or paralysis of the extremities must be done during the procedure. This usually consists of asking the patient for development of new or sudden tingling or numbness in the hands or feet while manipulating the airway or neck. Perceived or observed muscle weakness or paralysis of a limb is equally important, as this may imply spinal cord compression. This intubation technique has a favorable influence on the safety of the airway management of patients with RA. Blind nasotracheal intubation technique can be done as well, but may cause laryngeal edema and contribute to postextubation airway problems. It is advisable to avoid this technique, if possible, in a patient with the laryngeal disease.

Cardiovascular Manifestations of Rheumatoid Arthritis

The prevalence of cardiovascular involvement in RA may be as high as 35% (3,48–55) and contributes to a high mortality. Clinically significant manifestations are not common, but autopsy series and echocardiographic studies have shown a high prevalence of pericardial disease with or without effusion. The occurrence of pericardial disease is more common during a flare-up of RA. Occasionally, symptomatic pericarditis may lead to chronic disease, requiring surgical intervention. Inflammatory nodules can occur in the myocardium and on the valves, causing valvular dysfunction, embolic phenomena, and conduction changes. The mitral valve is affected most often, followed by the aortic, tricuspid, and pulmonary valves.

Additionally, the risk for coronary artery disease is high. Ischemic heart disease may be unmasked by the use of NSAIDs or cyclo-oxygenase (COX)-2 inhibitors. Some newer biologic DMARDs can increase mortality if used in patients with significant congestive heart failure. The initial treatment for pericarditis includes the use of NSAIDs; prednisone (1 mg/kg) may be necessary in some patients. High-dose corticosteroids may be of benefit in myocarditis.

Vascular Disease and Vasculitis

Rheumatoid inflammation may induce a vasculitis, which commonly involves the skin, and is generally without the features of a coexistent systemic vasculitis. Inflammation may damage the exocrine glands, resulting in secondary Sjögren syndrome (xerostomia and keratoconjunctivitis sicca). These manifestations suggest a systemic defect in immune homeostasis. Patients with active extra-articular disease and high rheumatoid factor titer can develop vasculitis, which can manifest as muscle pain or weakness, infarcts of the nail beds, and gangrene of the fingertips due to distal arteritis, cutaneous ulcerations, sensory neuropathy, or mononeuritis multiplex. Arteritis of visceral vessels may manifest as abdominal pain; the lung, heart, and spleen may also be involved.

Muscle Involvement

Muscle weakness in a patient with RA is common and multifactorial, and may be due to synovitis and joint disease, deformed joints, myositis, or polymyositis, and occasionally it may be due to drug-induced myopathy. Corticosteroids, HMG-CoA inhibitors, and antimalarial drugs can cause muscle weakness or myopathy.

Osteoporosis, Osteopenia, and Skin Involvement

Osteoporosis and osteopenia of the hip or lumbar spine are common in patients with RA, usually resulting in stress fractures of long bones and vertebral compression deformities. Skin changes include atrophy and ecchymosis due to steroid use, and ulceration due to chronic stasis, arterial insufficiency, or neutrophilic dermatoses.

Renal Involvement

Glomerulonephritis or vasculitis may occasionally occur in patients with RA. However, many of the drugs used to treat RA, especially NSAIDs, gold, cyclosporine, and penicillamine, may also damage the kidneys; secondary amyloidosis may also occur.

Hematologic Involvement

Many patients with active disease have anemia of chronic disease, a normocytic hypochromic pattern with hemoglobin hovering around 10 g/dL. The degree of anemia correlates with disease activity and the erythrocyte sedimentation rate (ESR).

Felty syndrome is a clinical condition characterized by an enlarged spleen, anemia, and thrombocytopenia. These patients may come to the ICU post splenectomy. Pseudo-Felty syndrome, or "large granular lymphocyte (LGL) syndrome," is characterized by splenomegaly, circulating LGLs, and neutropenia; these patients are prone to repeated infections. Lymphoproliferative disease can occur in patients with RA and, in some, may be due to therapeutic interventions—especially methotrexate and the newer biologic DMARDs.

Central Nervous System Involvement

The central nervous system (CNS) is usually not affected in RA, although vasculitis of peripheral nerves can cause mononeuritis multiplex.

TABLE 167.5

CURRENT THERAPY OF RHEUMATOID ARTHRITIS: TRADITIONAL DISEASE-MODIFYING ANTIRHEUMATIC DRUGS

Methotrexate
Hydroxychloroquine
Leflunomide
Cyclosporin
Azathioprine
Oral/parenteral gold
d-Penicillamine
Minocycline

Treatment of Rheumatoid Arthritis

The therapy of RA has evolved significantly in the past few years. The proper management of RA requires the identification of the stage, activity, and severity of disease (6–18). Early aggressive therapy (Table 167.5) is given to minimize the severe disability commonly seen in patients with advanced RA, but a goal of complete remission is elusive. A clear, optimal drug treatment algorithm is lacking. In general, the drugs can be divided into three classes: (a) NSAIDs, (b) glucocorticoids, and (c) DMARDs, both traditional and biologic. In general, physicians use the above-mentioned drug classes sequentially. Traditional treatment is started with NSAIDs for symptomatic relief of stiffness and pain. The traditional DMARDs are started if there is no clinical response to this first-line therapy. Corticosteroids are used for flare-ups, although, like the DMARDs, their side effect profile is significant (Table 167.6).

Aggressive biologic therapy targets specific components of the immune response such as inhibition of TNF by monoclonal antibodies, inhibition of interleukin-1, inhibition of T-cell activation, and B-cell depletion (Table 167.7). Specific guidelines have been developed for TNF inhibitors. TNF inhibitors are given when a satisfactory response is not seen by conventional DMARDs in a patient with active RA; it is followed by other biologic DMARDs, anticytokine treatment, and sometimes combination therapy (8–18). The newer biologic DMARDs are very expensive and associated with serious risks of infection, cancer, and death (16–18). The long-term efficacy of the biologic DMARDs is unknown. TNF inhibitors should be avoided in a patient with significant heart failure, as it may increase mortality. Besides local infusion side effects, development of serious infections occur in 3% to 6% of cases; these agents should be stopped in the presence of an active infection. Reactivation of tuberculosis is a major concern; hence, patients should be screened for tuberculosis before initiating therapy. Other drugs have shown benefits in patients who have not responded to conventional DMARDs and TNF inhibitors. For example, rituximab was recently approved for use in RA. It is an anti-CD20 monoclonal antibody that depletes B lymphocytes (17). The risk of serious infection, including tuberculosis, remains high with the use of this drug. Interestingly, patients with chronic obstructive lung disease have more adverse pulmonary effects. Serious side effects, including fever, chills, urticaria, bronchospasm, bronchopneumonia, hypotension, *Staphylococcus aureus* sepsis, angioedema, and even death, have been reported with use of this drug.

TABLE 167.6

COMPLICATIONS OF RHEUMATIC DRUGS COMMONLY SEEN IN THE INTENSIVE CARE UNIT

Drug	GI tract	Hematology, dermatology, others
NSAIDs	Upper GI bleeding Peptic ulcer disease	Anemia
Azathioprine	Enterocolitis, cholestasis, jaundice, hepatic vein thrombosis, transaminase elevations	Low WBC count
Methotrexate	Enterocolitis, elevation of ALT and AST	Low platelet and WBC count
Cyclophosphamide	Hemorrhagic cystitis	
Corticosteroids	Peptic ulcer disease, osteoporosis, acute psychosis	Fatty liver, DM, pancreatitis
Allopurinol	Hepatitis	Steven-Johnson syndrome
Colchicine	Diarrhea/dehydration, gastritis hepatic injury	Hypersensitivity vasculitis, interstitial nephritis
Sulfasalazine	Hepatitis, pancreatitis	Aplastic anemia, Stevens-Johnson syndrome, agranulocytosis, hemolysis, methemoglobinemia
Gold	Enterocolitis, intrahepatic cholestasis	Exfoliative dermatitis
Penicillamine	Hemolysis	Arrhythmia, cardiomyopathy, pemphigus, seizures

GI, gastrointestinal; NSAIDs, nonsteroidal anti-inflammatory drugs; WBC, white blood cell; ALT, alanine aminotransferase; AST, aspartate aminotransferase; DM, diabetes mellitus.

Diagnosis, Treatment, and Monitoring of Lung Disease in Rheumatoid Arthritis

The treatment of lung disease in RA is empiric, based upon the underlying problem. Usually, the pulmonary manifestations of RA respond well to corticosteroids; other immunosuppressive drugs are often added when pulmonary disease progresses and/or steroid side effects appear. It is important to differentiate between the pulmonary effects of the underlying connective tissue disease and complications due to treatment, such as opportunistic infections, and toxic and idiosyncratic drug reactions. Unrelated primary pulmonary disease such as COPD may also be present.

If histologic investigation is needed to establish or exclude a diagnosis of lung involvement, open lung biopsy is the gold

TABLE 167.7

CURRENT THERAPY OF RHEUMATOID ARTHRITIS: BIOLOGIC DISEASE-MODIFYING ANTIRHEUMATIC DRUGS

Drug	Dose/route	Class	Other considerations
Methotrexate	7.5–25 mg/wk	Dihydrofolate reductase	Generic, drug of choice oral/SC/IM
Leflunomide (Arava)	10–20 mg qd oral	Pyrimidine synthesis inhibitor	Very long half-life, enterohepatic recirculation
Etarercept (Enbrel)	50 mg/wk SC	TNF receptor blockade	No live vaccine, careful in CHF
Adalimumab (Humira)	40 mg q2wk SC	Anti-TNF monoclonal antibody	No live vaccines, careful in CHF
Infliximab (Remicade)	3 mg/kg q4–8wk IV	TNF monoclonal antibody	No live vaccines, careful in CHF
Anakinra (Kineret)	100 mg qd SC	IL-1 receptor antagonist	No live vaccines
Rituximab (Rituxan)	1,000 mg IV q2–4wk; single, short course	Anti-CD20 monoclonal antibody, B-cell depletion	Given with methotrexate Avoid in pregnancy, death reported
Abatacept (Orencia)	500–1,000 mg/wt based dose, variable interval	T-lymphocyte modulator	No live vaccines Test for TB, limited to refractory disease

SC, subcutaneous; IM, intramuscular; TNF, tumor necrosis factor; CHF, congestive heart failure; IL, interleukin.

standard (8,20). As the natural history is variable, clear guidelines for monitoring lung disease do not exist. Obtaining baseline pulmonary function tests (PFTs), including spirometry, lung diffusion, and lung volumes, is important, and follow-up tests can be tailored based on the patient's symptoms. Once abnormalities are detected, or a patient is on treatment, appropriate follow-up with PFTs and chest CT can be done. High-resolution chest CT appears more sensitive than PFTs for detecting small airway disease (22).

Preoperative Evaluation of Rheumatoid Arthritis Patients

Surgery should be undertaken after an overall assessment of general health, status of the arthritis, and preparedness for rehabilitation. Attention must be given to organs that may be affected by RA. Sites requiring specific review include the cervical spine, lungs, airway, bone, and bone marrow. The patient with RA may require supplementary corticosteroids and an adjustment of the dose of their antirheumatic medications.

Intensive Care Unit and Postoperative Care and Outcomes

Patients with RA may be admitted to the ICU due to non–RA-related medical or surgical diseases requiring ICU care (53–57). Medical complications from the drug treatment of RA can occur, including severe sepsis and shock, gastrointestinal (GI) bleeding, airway compromise due to sedative and narcotic use, respiratory failure from lung disease, or spinal cord compression and neurologic impairment. Careful administration of the drugs and close monitoring are essential. Respiratory failure due to restrictive or obstructive lung disease also makes these patients susceptible to pulmonary complications. Close neurologic monitoring of these patients is important.

The studies evaluating ICU admission and outcome of patients with RA are limited and retrospective in nature (53–57). All appear to show a high mortality. Such analyses are good for predicting outcome in a research setting, but are difficult to use in predicting outcome of an individual patient. Short-term mortality correlates with a higher simplified acute physiologic score (SAPS), poor health status, prior corticosteroid therapy, and infection. Acute infection, the main reason for ICU admission, is a negative predictor for survival.

Invasive Monitoring Catheter Placement

Placing a radial arterial catheter may be difficult in advanced cases of RA due to flexion joint deformities at the wrist. In addition, arteries may be small and calcified. Patients may have severe peripheral arterial disease, vasculitis, or carpal tunnel syndrome, and may be at risk of increased complications of the radial artery arterial line placed (12,13). It is better to avoid inserting a peripheral arterial catheter in a patient with Raynaud phenomenon. If a patient needs continuous blood pressure (BP) monitoring, one should preferably insert a femoral arterial line. Central line placement in the neck may be a problem due to fusion or flexion deformities of the cervical spine.

Use of Immunosuppressive Drugs in the Perioperative Period

The use of immunosuppressive drug therapy in the perioperative period remains controversial (52). A survey of 200 physicians was conducted regarding the use of methotrexate in the preoperative period in RA patients undergoing surgery. Many physicians were concerned about the increased risk of postoperative complications from its use; newer biologic DMARDs should be avoided in the perioperative period.

Mixed Connective Tissue Diseases

Mixed rheumatologic conditions have features of polymyositis, dermatomyositis, SLE, and scleroderma. A high incidence of pulmonary complications is seen with these variants, including pulmonary hypertension, pleural effusions, aspiration, respiratory muscle dysfunction, and varying degrees of ILD.

ANKYLOSING SPONDYLITIS

Ankylosing spondylitis (AS) primarily affects young adults, with an average onset of age between 20 and 30 years. It is associated with chronic backache, fatigue, malaise, impaired sleep due to back or joint pain, and, occasionally, fever. AS is considered primarily a spinal disease, but the hip joints, eyes, lungs, and heart may also be involved (49,58–67). The diagnosis of AS is a clinical one; however, finding sacroiliitis on imaging can be supportive. Neurologic symptoms, such as paresis and variable impairment, can occur with spinal cord or spinal nerve compression. Some may develop vertebral fractures with trivial trauma. The most common site of compression of the spinal cord is at the C5-C6 level. Sometimes, clinically significant spontaneous subluxation of the atlantoaxial joint can occur. Ramos-Remus et al., in a study of 103 patients, observed anterior or posterior atlantoaxial subluxation in 21% and 2%, respectively, of individuals with AS (60). After 2 years, progression of anterior subluxation was observed in about 50%. This problem is managed similar to that seen in RA. A higher incidence of compression fractures of the thoracic lumbar spine is also noted due to premature osteoporosis. The "cauda equina syndrome" can occur due to advanced lumbosacral ankylosis.

Pulmonary involvement consists of restrictive disease. Cough with dyspnea due to chest wall fixation and stiffness can occur, but diaphragmatic function is usually preserved (58); lung diffusion is impaired (63). The incidence of ILD is very low in AS but may appear as a late complication of chronic AS. ILD has a predilection for upper lobes and causes fibrocystic changes which may mimic pulmonary tuberculosis; there is no specific therapy. The potential for infection and life-threatening hemoptysis due to *Aspergillus* species remains high.

Asymptomatic cardiovascular disease secondary to AS is common (49). An echocardiographic study showed cardiac abnormalities in 29%, including aortic regurgitation, pericardial effusion, mitral valve prolapse, and electrocardiogram (ECG) changes. Transesophageal echocardiography has shown valvular abnormalities in up to 80%, mostly of no clinical significance. Aortic regurgitation can occur, and is managed like any other incidence of aortic regurgitation.

Renal disease associated with AS includes problems due to analgesic use or abuse, IgA nephropathy, and secondary amyloidosis. End-stage renal disease may result, and the prognosis is poor.

Asymptomatic ileal and colonic mucosal ulcerations have been detected by endoscopic examination. In one study, endoscopic lesions were found in 44% of patients with spondyloarthropathy versus only 6% of patients with other inflammatory arthritides (65). Treatment is with DMARDs (66,67). Uveitis, cataracts, glaucoma, intraocular pressure, and macular edema may also occur.

SYSTEMIC SCLEROSIS: SCLERODERMA

Systemic sclerosis (SSc) is a systemic inflammatory disease that leads to extensive fibrotic changes affecting the musculoskeletal, kidney, lung, and circulatory systems, as well as the GI tract (68–76). SSc is divided into diffuse (DcSSc) and limited cutaneous systemic sclerosis (LcSSc). Patients with DcSSc are characterized by skin sclerosis of the chest, abdomen, or upper arms and shoulders, and are more likely to have, or develop, internal organ damage due to ischemic injury or fibrosis than are those with LcSSc. LcSSc is generally associated with the CREST syndrome, and consists of calcinosis cutis, Raynaud phenomenon, esophageal dysmotility, sclerodactyly, and telangiectasia.

Raynaud phenomenon (RP) is due to an episodic, reversible arterial vasospasm in the digits, characterized by sequential color changes of pallor ("white"), acrocyanosis ("blue"), and reperfusion hyperemia ("red"). It is precipitated by changes in temperature or stress. Some patients with SSc can develop progressive structural changes in the small blood vessels, with permanently impaired flow, digital ulceration, or infarction. RP is also seen in other connective tissue diseases. Vascular injury and subsequent chronic damage underlies other serious complications of systemic sclerosis, including pulmonary arterial hypertension, scleroderma renal crisis, and gastric antral vascular ectasia, and contributes to the pathogenesis of cardiac and gastrointestinal complications.

The lungs are involved in the majority of the patients, with a variety of abnormalities being present (Table 167.2). The majority of the patients will develop progressive dyspnea, cough, and respiratory failure. Even in an asymptomatic patient with a normal chest radiograph, a chest CT may demonstrate ILD. The ILD in SSc is common and progressive, and eventually leads to end-stage fibrosis and honeycombing. The course of the disease is slower than idiopathic UIP; otherwise, the clinical presentation and treatment are similar to that of other causes of ILD. The results of therapy are variable. The risk of lung cancer is increased as well.

Pulmonary vascular disease occurs in approximately 10% of patients with SSc. It resembles idiopathic pulmonary hypertension, and is often complicated by cor pulmonale, dyspnea with exertion, and low exercise tolerance; it is progressive and often fatal within 5 years. However, with recent new drugs, the course of the disease may be altered favorably for some patients.

The majority of patients with SSc will have some degree of gastrointestinal involvement—esophageal hypomotility, gastroesophageal reflux, chronic esophagitis, stricture formation—all of which may result in aspiration pneumonia. Pseudo-obstruction, malabsorption, and fecal incontinence can occur. Vascular ectasia in the stomach is not uncommon and may cause chronic GI bleeding and anemia.

Kidney disease is very common in SSc and may be asymptomatic (71–73). Autopsy data suggest that 60% to 80% of patients with DcSSc have pathologic evidence of kidney damage. Acute onset of renal failure with moderate or malignant hypertension may be noted. Microangiopathic hemolytic anemia, pulmonary edema, headache, blurred vision, hypertensive encephalopathy, or seizures may occur. Treatment with calcium channel blockers, such as nifedipine, diltiazem, or amlodipine, may show benefit in RP, and angiotensin-converting enzyme inhibitors may be helpful in improving local blood flow. Sildenafil and other phosphodiesterase V inhibitors and bosentan, an inhibitor of the potent vasoconstrictor endothelin-1, are being used for improvement of the peripheral and pulmonary circulation.

SJÖGREN SYNDROME

Sjögren syndrome (SjS)—a disease with a predilection for women—consists of a triad of polyarthritis, keratoconjunctivitis, and xerostomia. The secondary form can be associated with any of the connective tissue diseases, most commonly with RA (77–79). Patients with SjS developed inspissated airway secretions, cough, hoarseness of voice, recurrent aspiration pneumonia, and, eventually, bronchiectasis (77). The risk of ILD remains high in the secondary form of SjS. Lymphoproliferation can occur, resulting in lymphocytic ILD or lymphomatous transformation. Pseudolymphoma may be difficult to differentiate from malignant lymphoma, and may appear as one or multiple masses on chest images. The lymphocytes infiltrate into the alveoli and interstitium, causing restrictive impairment on PFTs. The disease responds well to immunosuppressive treatment. The development of enlarged thoracic lymph nodes or pleural effusion suggests lymphoma (77,79).

POLYMYOSITIS–DERMATOMYOSITIS

In this process, difficulties with swallowing and with airway protection are significant problems, and aspiration is a common occurrence. Patients usually have significant skin and muscle involvement prior to developing aspiration (80–82). Maximal airway pressures during inspiration and exhalation are usually decreased; respiratory failure due to muscle weakness can occur. The serial analysis of airway pressure measurement can be used to assess response to medical therapy. Occasionally, patients may need mechanical ventilatory support during an acute crisis or in the presence of respiratory failure precipitated by recurrent aspiration.

SYSTEMIC LUPUS ERYTHEMATOSUS

General Considerations and Epidemiology

SLE is characterized in the laboratory by the presence of antibodies directed against nuclear antigens. Clinically, it is a multisystem disorder that may be organ or life threatening, and patients may have a variety of presentations. Over 90% of patients with SLE have positive antinuclear antibodies (with a titer greater than 1:80). While this test is sensitive for the diagnosis, it is nonspecific; antibodies to double-stranded DNA and nucleosomes are more specific for SLE. The American Rheumatologic Association (ARA) has published diagnostic criteria (83). The diagnosis of SLE is made when four or more of the criteria are present, either simultaneously or serially, as shown in Table 167.8. The etiology of SLE is likely multifactorial—genetic, hormonal, environmental, and immunologic factors all have a role. SLE affects adult women approximately ten times more frequently than men, with a predilection for females in their 20s or 30s. The course of SLE may be indolent or explosive. Important clinical manifestations are discussed below.

Lupus Nephritis

Lupus nephritis occurs due to formation of immune deposits in the glomerulus. It remains the most feared complication and carries the highest risk of death or morbidity. Significant renal disease affects approximately 30% of patients with SLE. Proteinuria (greater than 0.5 g/24 hours) and/or red blood cell casts

TABLE 167.8

AMERICAN RHEUMATOLOGIC ASSOCIATION CRITERIA FOR THE DIAGNOSIS OF SYSTEMIC LUPUS ERYTHEMATOSUS

Criterion	Definition
Malar rash	Fixed erythema over the malar eminences, tending to spare the nasolabial folds
Discoid rash	Erythematous raised scaly patches with follicular plugging; atrophic scarring may occur in older lesions
Photosensitivity	Skin rash as a result of unusual reaction to sunlight
Oral ulcers	Oral or nasopharyngeal ulceration, usually painless
Arthritis	Nonerosive arthritis involving two or more joints, characterized by tenderness, swelling, or effusion
Serositis	a) Pleuritis with history of pain, rub heard by physician, or effusion OR b) Pericarditis as evident on electrocardiogram, or the presence of a rub or pericardial effusion
Renal disorder	a) Persistent proteinuria greater than 0.5 g/d or greater than 3+ qualitatively OR b) Cellular casts (red cell, hemoglobin, granular, tubular, or mixed)
Neurologic disorder	Seizures or psychosis—in the absence of offending drugs or metabolic derangements
Hematologic disorders	a) Hemolytic anemia with reticulocytosis OR b) Leukopenia—less than 4,000 cells/μL on two or more occasions OR c) Lymphopenia—less than 1,500 cells/μL on two or more occasions OR d) Thrombocytopenia—less than 150,000 cells/μL in the absence of offending drugs
Immunologic disorders	a) Positive antiphospholipid antibody OR b) Anti-DNA antibody in abnormal titer OR c) Anti-Sm antibody OR d) False-positive serologic test for syphilis known to be positive for at least 6 mo and confirmed by a negative *Treponema pallidum* immobilization or fluorescent treponemal antibody absorption test
Antinuclear antibody (ANA)	An abnormal titer of ANA by immunofluorescence or an equivalent assay at any point in time and in the absence of drugs known to be associated with "drug-induced lupus" syndrome

Adapted from Tan EM, Cohen AS, Fries JF, et al. The 1982 revised criteria for the classification of systemic lupus erythematosus (SLE). *Arthritis Rheum.* 1982;25:1271–1277.

TABLE 167.9

CLASSIFICATION OF GLOMERULONEPHRITIS IN SYSTEMIC LUPUS ERYTHEMATOSUS

Class I	**Minimal mesangial lupus nephritis:** Normal on light microscopy; mesangial immune deposits on immunofluorescence
Class II	**Mesangial proliferative lupus nephritis:** Mesangial hypercellularity or matrix expansion, with mesangial immune deposits on immunofluorescence
Class III	**Focal lupus nephritis:** Glomerulonephritis involving less than 50% of glomeruli, typically with subendothelial immune deposits
Class IV	**Diffuse lupus nephritis:** Glomerulonephritis involving greater than 50% of glomeruli, typically with subendothelial immune deposits; can be segmental or global
Class V	**Membranous lupus nephritis:** Global or segmental subendothelial immune deposits
Class VI	**Advanced sclerotic lupus nephritis:** greater than 90% of glomeruli globally sclerosed without residual activity

Modified from Weening JJ, D'Agati VD, Schwartz MM, et al. The classification of glomerulonephritis in systemic lupus erythematosus revisited. *J Am Soc Nephrol.* 2004;15(2):241–250.

suggest renal involvement. Table 167.9 displays the revised classification of lupus glomerulonephritis. Even though most patients with SLE are asymptomatic, renal involvement on biopsy exceeds 90% with most having class II to IV glomerulonephritis. Aggressive immunosuppressive therapy is always indicated for class IV, class V, and severe class III glomerulonephritis to avoid progression to renal failure.

Most induction regimens involve the use of high-dose pulse steroids (methylprednisolone 0.5–1 g daily for 3 days) in combination with cyclophosphamide. The latter may take 10 to 14 days to work. Monthly IV cyclophosphamide boluses may be less toxic than, and as effective as, daily oral drug (84–86). In addition to the well-known side effects of corticosteroids, cyclophosphamide use may result in significant morbidity, including hemorrhagic cystitis, life-threatening infections, increased risk of malignancy, and gonadal toxicity, in premenopausal women. More recently, induction regimens using mycophenolate mofetil have shown encouraging results (87–91).

Pulmonary Manifestations of Systemic Lupus Erythematosus

The lung parenchyma, pleura, vasculature, and/or diaphragm may be affected in SLE. Infection, including opportunistic organisms and tuberculosis, should be considered (92).

Pleuritis and Effusion

Pleural effusions in SLE are generally small to moderate, recurrent, often bilateral, and characterized by an elevated pleural fluid lactate dehydrogenase (LDH), a slightly low pleural fluid glucose, and low protein. An elevated pleural fluid antinuclear antibody (ANA) suggests the diagnosis; however, this test adds little to the finding of an elevated serum ANA, and is not necessary (93). The presence of a pleural rub or radiographic evidence of a pleural effusion helps to make the diagnosis of lupus pleurisy. Treatment includes drainage if the patient is dyspneic. Effusions often respond to therapy with NSAIDs. In nonresponders, moderate- to high-dose corticosteroids are usually effective; immunosuppressive agents are rarely needed. Fibrothorax, or trapped lung, is a rare complication that may require decortication (94).

Acute and Chronic Pneumonitis

Acute lupus pneumonitis, an uncommon manifestation of SLE, presents as fever, cough, dyspnea, hypoxemia, pleurisy, basilar rales, and occasionally hemoptysis and pleural effusion (95,96). Chest radiographs show diffuse acinar infiltrates, especially in the lower lung zones. Lung biopsy reveals acute alveolar wall injury, edema, hemorrhage, hyaline membrane formation, and immunoglobulin and complement deposition (97). The HR-CT scan shows ground-glass opacification and/or fibrosis. BAL may show either a lymphocytosis or granulocytosis. An open or video-assisted thoracoscopic lung biopsy may be necessary to establish the diagnosis. Distinguishing between lupus pneumonitis and alveolar hemorrhage may be difficult, but the treatment is the same.

In patients with long-standing SLE, chronic pneumonitis with fibrosis can occur, often preceded by an episode of acute pneumonitis. Patients may have an insidious onset of dyspnea, chronic dry cough, and recurrent pleuritic chest pain. PFTs show a restrictive impairment with a reduced diffusing capacity of the lung for carbon monoxide (DLCO) and high alveolar-arterial (A-a) gradient. The clinical and pathologic features resemble that of IPF. The differential diagnosis includes bilateral pneumonia, congestive heart failure, acute respiratory distress syndrome (ARDS), occupational lung disease, malignancy, eosinophilic pneumonia, and other interstitial lung diseases. Diagnostic tools that may be helpful include BAL, HR-CT, and occasionally, open lung biopsy. The treatment regimen generally tried—prednisone 1 mg/kg/day and cyclophosphamide—is similar to that used in treating fibrosing alveolitis (96–98).

Vanishing Lung Syndrome

This peculiar syndrome is seen in some patients with SLE; it is characterized by a progressive decrease in lung volume without evidence of interstitial fibrosis or significant pleural disease.

Symptoms include progressive dyspnea and episodes of pleuritic chest pain (99–101). It should be suspected in patients with dyspnea, a clear chest radiograph, and elevated diaphragms. The pathogenesis of this disorder has been debated. One possible mechanism is poor function and elevation of the diaphragm secondary to myositis or myopathy (102,103). However, other reports have documented restrictive lung volumes with normal diaphragmatic strength (100,104). Theophylline, corticosteroids, and/or immunosuppressive therapy may improve symptoms and lung function (99,105,106). Nocturnal and/or intermittent noninvasive bilevel ventilation may prove to be useful.

Diffuse Alveolar Hemorrhage in Systemic Lupus Erythematosus

Diffuse alveolar hemorrhage (DAH), with or without hemoptysis, is a rare but serious manifestation of SLE. The etiology is unknown (107,108). Patients typically present acutely ill with dyspnea, cough, and sometimes hemoptysis. Bleeding may be severe enough to produce anemia. Chest radiograph and CT frequently show bilateral alveolar infiltrates that may mimic pulmonary edema or infection (Figs. 167.3 and 167.4). BAL fluid may be increasingly bloody on consecutive BAL specimens; hemosiderin-laden macrophages may also be present. T2-weighted MRI images may also be useful in establishing the diagnosis (109). An elevated DLCO is strongly suggestive of pulmonary hemorrhage but is nonspecific. Definitive diagnosis can be established only by open lung biopsy (108–111). Diffuse alveolar hemorrhage in SLE is associated with a very high mortality, even with treatment. However, improved outcomes may be seen with the use of high-dose corticosteroids (e.g., methylprednisolone 500–2,000 mg/day), cyclophosphamide, mechanical ventilation, and antibiotics (111). Plasmapheresis has been used with success (112).

Pulmonary Hypertension in Systemic Lupus Erythematosus

Mild to moderate pulmonary hypertension is frequently seen in SLE. Patients may present with dyspnea, chest pain, syncope, fatigue, edema, palpitations, or increased abdominal girth. Physical findings include jugular venous distention (JVD), a right ventricular heave, fixed splitting of S_2, a right ventricular S_3, hepatomegaly, ascites, peripheral edema, and murmurs of tricuspid regurgitation or pulmonic insufficiency. Mild hypoxemia, enlarged pulmonary arteries with clear lung fields on chest radiograph, reduced DLCO, and ECG evidence of right ventricular hypertrophy may be seen. The histopathology shows plexiform angiomatous lesions, thickening of the media layer of the pulmonary arteries, and immunoglobulin and complement deposition in the walls, and, rarely, vasculitis (113–115). The diagnosis is made by echocardiography and right heart catheterization, during which vasodilator testing may be performed. Ventilation/perfusion scanning to rule out chronic thromboemboli should be done since patients with SLE may have antiphospholipid antibodies, putting them at risk for thrombosis. Treatment of pulmonary hypertension in patients with SLE is similar to that of patients with idiopathic pulmonary hypertension. Patients may benefit from the use of oxygen, anticoagulants, vasodilators (prostacyclin, calcium channel blockers), bosentan, sildenafil, and intermittent IV cyclophosphamide (116,117). The treatment of pulmonary hypertension is discussed in detail elsewhere. Further investigation is needed to clarify the role of cytotoxic agents in SLE-related pulmonary hypertension. In general, pulmonary hypertension associated with SLE is resistant to treatment and has a poor prognosis (117).

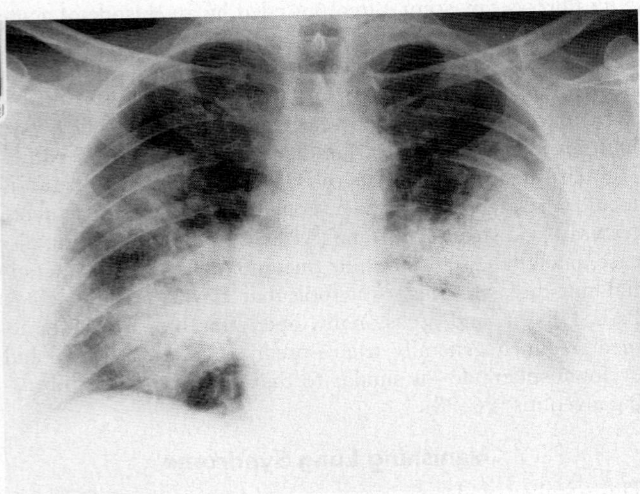

FIGURE 167.3. Chest radiograph showing pulmonary edema–like picture in a case of systemic lupus erythematosus with pulmonary alveolar hemorrhage.

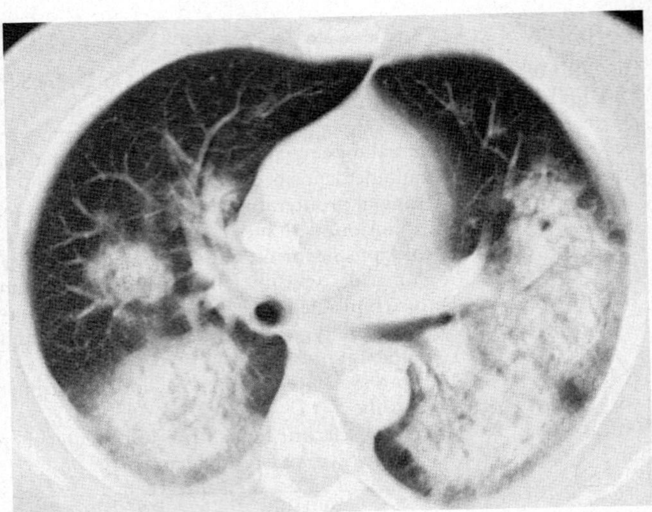

FIGURE 167.4. Chest computed tomography showing pulmonary edema–like picture in a case of systemic lupus erythematosus with pulmonary alveolar hemorrhage.

Acute Reversible Hypoxemia

Acute unexplained hypoxemia is a recognized phenomenon in SLE (118). Chest radiographs are negative, and pulmonary emboli are not identified. Plasma C3a levels have been noted to be markedly elevated, suggesting the role of pulmonary leukoaggregation and complement activation in this disorder. Further supporting this theory of leuko-occlusive vasculopathy is the noted up-regulation of adhesion molecules, E-selectin, VCAM-1, and ICAM-1. Treatment includes corticosteroids alone or in combination with aspirin. Gas exchange has been shown to improve within 3 days (118–120).

Pulmonary Embolism in Systemic Lupus Erythematosus

Patients with SLE and antiphospholipid antibodies can suffer from a variety of thromboembolic events, including deep venous thrombosis, acute pulmonary embolism and/or infarction, and chronic thromboemboli causing pulmonary hypertension. Most patients are treated with anticoagulation. Immunosuppressive regimens are generally ineffective.

Bronchiolitis Obliterans with Organizing Pneumonia

BOOP is seen in SLE and RA, among other disorders, and is discussed above (Table 167.3). Therapy with prednisone is usually effective; however, the addition of cyclophosphamide may be necessary in some cases (121).

Catastrophic Antiphospholipid Antibody Syndrome

Antiphospholipid antibody syndrome (APS) is characterized by recurrent arterial and/or venous thrombosis or pregnancy loss, in association with antibodies directed against plasma proteins that are bound to anionic phospholipids. Antibodies that may be detected include anticardiolipin antibodies, lupus anticoagulants, and anti-B_2 glycoprotein-I antibodies. APS is often associated with SLE or other autoimmune disease, but may also occur alone. A patient with APS may present with widespread thrombotic disease and end-organ damage, referred to as "catastrophic" APS. Diagnostic criteria include involvement of three or more organ systems, abrupt onset, and confirmation by histopathology of small vessel occlusion in at least one organ or tissue, and the presence of antiphospholipid antibodies. Without treatment, the prognosis is poor. The recommended management includes the treatment of any precipitating factor (i.e., infection), anticoagulation with heparin followed by long-term

TABLE 167.10

CLASSIFICATION OF VASCULITIS

Vasculitis	Sites of involvement/description
Large vessel vasculitis	
Takayasu arteritis	Aorta and its primary branches
Giant cell or temporal arteritis	May be generalized but primarily involves the cranial branches of vessels originating from the aortic arch
Medium-sized vessel vasculitis	
Polyarteritis nodosa	Systemic necrotizing vasculitis typically affecting small and medium-sized muscular arteries
Kawasaki disease	Large, medium, and small arteries, particularly the coronaries
Isolated central nervous system vasculitis	Medium and small arteries of the central nervous system
Small vessel vasculitis	
Churg-Strauss arteritis	Most often lungs and skin, but may be generalized
Wegener granulomatosis	Systemic vasculitis of the medium and small arteries, as well as arterioles and venules Most often involves upper and lower respiratory tract and kidneys Associated with positive ANCA, hemoptysis, and cavitary lung lesions
Microscopic polyarteritis	Capillaries, venules, or arterioles
Henoch-Schönlein purpura	Systemic vasculitis characterized by deposition of IgA-containing immune complexes
Essential cryoglobulinemic vasculitis	Immune complex deposition in the walls of capillaries, venules, and arterioles most often secondary to hepatitis C infection
Hypersensitivity vasculitis	A leukocytoclastic vasculitis most prominent in postcapillary venules; usually secondary to drugs
Vasculitis secondary to connective tissue disorder	Involves small muscular arteries, arterioles, and venules May occur in RA, SLE, relapsing polychondritis, and Behçet disease among others.
Vasculitis secondary to viral infection	Vasculitis of medium and/or small vessel Associated with hepatitis B and C, HIV, CMV, EBV, and Parvo B19 virus.

ANCA, antineutrophil cytoplasmic antibodies; RA, rheumatoid arthritis; SLE, systemic lupus erythematosus; HIV, human immunodeficiency virus; CMV, cytomegalovirus; EBV, Epstein-Barr virus.

warfarin, and high-dose corticosteroids (methylprednisolone 1 g daily for 3 days) followed by prednisone 1 to 2 mg/kg/day and cyclophosphamide. Plasma exchange and/or intravenous immunoglobulin (IVIG) (400 mg/kg/day for 5 days) are used if there are features of microangiopathy (122–126).

Cardiac Manifestations in Systemic Lupus Erythematosus

Pericardial Disease

Cardiac disease is common in patients with SLE. Pericardial, myocardial, valvular, coronary, and conduction system involvement may occur (127–134). Pericardial involvement, the most common cardiac manifestation, may be asymptomatic or present with positional substernal chest pain and an audible rub on auscultation. On histopathologic specimens, the pericardium may reveal foci of inflammatory lesions with immune complexes. Large effusions, tamponade, and constrictive pericarditis are rare (129). Pericardiocentesis may be indicated in patients in whom there is a suspicion of infection. This is especially true for those who are febrile, are immunocompromised, or have persistent symptoms or effusion despite treatment. Pericardiocentesis may be necessary to rule out purulent, tuberculous, or malignant pericarditis, or if tamponade is present. Symptomatic patients generally respond to an NSAID such as indomethacin.

Valvular Disease

Structural valvular disease is common in SLE; the mitral valve is involved most frequently (129). In addition, Libman-Sacks (verrucous) endocarditis is fairly common in patients with SLE. Verrucae consist of accumulations of immune complexes, mononuclear cells, hematoxylin bodies, and fibrin and platelet thrombi. If the lesions are extensive, the healing process may lead to valve deformity and regurgitation.

Myocarditis

Myocarditis is often asymptomatic, but global hypokinesis may result (131). Conduction defects can occur from active or past myocarditis. Myocardial biopsy may be necessary to distinguish myocarditis from other causes of cardiomyopathy. Improvement in systolic function has been noted with the use of high-dose corticosteroids, azathioprine, cyclophosphamide, or IVIG (130–132).

Coronary Artery Disease

It is becoming increasingly apparent that SLE may predispose to premature coronary artery disease (CAD). Chronic use of glucocorticoids, which can cause or exacerbate hyperlipidemia, diabetes, and obesity, may be one contributing factor in the development of CAD. Furthermore, the autoimmune vascular injury present in SLE may also predispose to atherosclerotic plaque formation by a number of mechanisms (134).

Neurologic Manifestations of Systemic Lupus Erythematosus

Neurologic and/or psychiatric symptoms occur in 10% to 80% of SLE patients either before or after their diagnosis (135–137). Neuropsychiatric manifestations seen in SLE (from most to least prevalent) include cognitive dysfunction, headache, mood disorder, cerebrovascular disease, seizures, polyneuropathy, anxiety, and psychosis.

THE VASCULITIDES

Vasculitis is defined by the presence of leukocytes in the vessel wall with reactive damage to mural structures. The various vasculitides, in general, vary by the size and location of affected vessels (Table 167.10). Illness may be severe and life threatening, warranting the need for prompt recognition and treatment. Unfortunately, the diagnosis of vasculitis is often delayed because the clinical manifestations can be mimicked by a number of other disorders. Radiologic manifestations are variable as well, from normal to lung nodule, pulmonary hemorrhage, or mediastinal lymphadenopathy. Figure 167.5 shows a lung nodule with cavitation in a case of Wegner granulomatosis. Therapy depends on the nature and severity of the vasculitis. A mild cutaneous hypersensitivity vasculitis due to a drug reaction may resolve spontaneously by discontinuing the offending drug. However, the systemic vasculitic involvement usually requires glucocorticoid treatment. Corticosteroids alone are usually sufficient to induce remission in giant cell arteritis. However, rapidly progressive diseases, such as Wegener granulomatosis and polyarteritis nodosa, are likely to require steroids plus cytotoxic therapy, usually cyclophosphamide.

PEARLS

- An adequate history and physical examination is essential in the accurate diagnosis of suspected rheumatic disease. Appropriate serologic testing can be requested. Early consultation of a rheumatologist can be very helpful rather than ordering a wide variety of serologic tests.

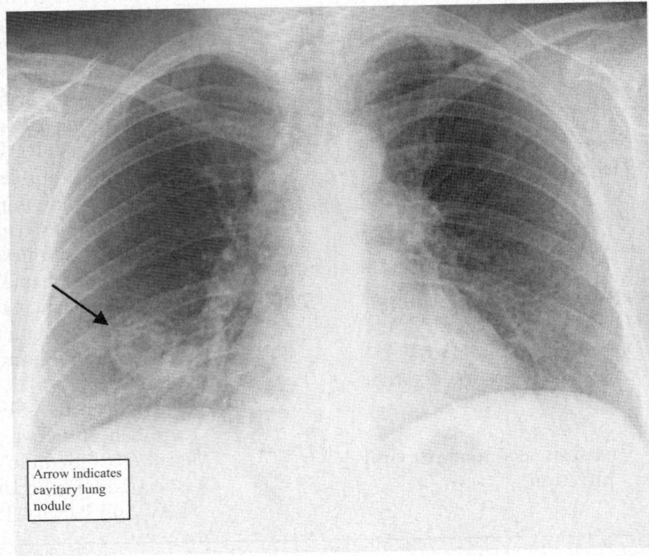
Arrow indicates
cavitary lung
nodule

FIGURE 167.5. Lung nodule with cavitation in Wegner granulomatosis.

- The morbidity and mortality of a person with a rheumatologic emergency remains high. Prompt recognition and treatment are essential for a better outcome.
- Extra care and proper stabilization must be done in patients with cervical spine problems. Use fiberoptic instrument for endotracheal intubation in a patient with a compromised airway.
- The presence of mononeuritis multiplex, pulmonary-renal involvement, and palpable purpura is strongly suggestive of an underlying vasculitic process.
- The prompt evaluation and therapy of vasculitis is critical for better outcome.
- Aspiration and respiratory failure is frequent in Sjögren syndrome and polymyositis.
- Placement of an arterial catheter should be avoided in patients with Raynaud phenomenon.
- SLE, the disease itself, as well as available treatments, predispose to infection.
- Many clinical manifestations of SLE may mimic infectious etiologies. To avoid potentially disastrous outcomes, infection must be excluded before starting immunosuppressive therapy for a presumed "lupus flare."

References

1. Lawrence RC, Felson DT, Helmick CG, et al. Estimates of the prevalence of arthritis and other rheumatic conditions in the United States. Part II. *Arthritis Rheum.* 2008;58(1):26–35.
2. Aletaha D, Ward MM, Machold KP, et al. Remission and active disease in rheumatoid arthritis. Defining criteria for disease activity states. *Arthritis Rheum.* 2005;52:2625.
3. Goronzy JJ, Weyand CM. Rheumatoid arthritis. Epidemiology, pathology, and pathogenesis. In: Klippel JH, Weyand CM, Wortmann RL, eds. *Primer on the Rheumatic Diseases.* 11th ed. Atlanta, GA: Arthritis Foundation; 1997:155.
4. Haringman JJ, Ludikhuize J, Tak PP. Chemokines in joint disease: the key to inflammation? *Ann Rheum Dis.* 2004;63:1186.
5. Kirkham BW, Lassere MN, Edmonds JP, et al. Synovial membrane cytokine expression is predictive of joint damage progression in rheumatoid arthritis: a two-year prospective study (the DAMAGE study cohort). *Arthritis Rheum.* 2006;54:1122.
6. Firestein GS. Evolving concept of rheumatoid arthritis. *Nature.* 2003;423 356.
7. Mitchell DM, Spitz PW, Young DY, et al. Survival, prognosis, and causes of death in rheumatoid arthritis. *Arthritis Rheum.* 1986;29(6):706.
8. Du Bois RM, Wells AU. The lung and connective tissue diseases In: Murray JF, Nadel JA, Mason RJ, et al., eds. *Textbook of Respiratory Medicine.* 3rd ed. Philadelphia: W. B. Saunders Company; 2000:691.
9. Guidelines for the management of rheumatoid arthritis: 2002 update. American College of Rheumatology Ad Hoc Committee on Clinical Guidelines. *Arthritis Rheum.* 2002;46:328.
10. McInnes IB, Liew FY. Cytokine networks—towards new therapies for rheumatoid arthritis. *Nat Clin Pract.* 2005;1.
11. Edwards CJ. Immunological therapies for rheumatoid arthritis. *Br Med Bull.* 2005;73–74:71.
12. Dendooven A, De Rycke L, Verhelst X, et al. Leflunomide and methotrexate combination therapy in daily clinical practice. *Ann Rheum Dis.* 2006; 65:833–834.
13. Baghai M, Osmon DR, Wolk DM, et al. Fatal sepsis in a patient with rheumatoid arthritis treated with etanercept. *Mayo Clin Proc.* 2001;76(6)653.
14. Scott DL, Kingsley GH. Tumor necrosis factor inhibitors for rheumatoid arthritis. *N Engl J Med.* 2006;355:704.
15. Edwards JCW, Szczepanski L, Szechinski J, et al. Efficacy of B-cell-targeted therapy with rituximab in patients with rheumatoid arthritis. *N Engl J Med.* 2004;350:2572–2581.
16. Tsokos GC. B cell be gone—B cells depletion in the treatment of rheumatoid arthritis. *N Engl J Med.* 2004;350:25, 2546–2548.
17. The Medical Letter on Drugs and Therapeutics. Rituximab (Rituxan) for rheumatoid arthritis. *Med Lett.* 2006;48(1233):34–35.
18. The Medical Letter on Drugs and Therapeutics. Abatacept (Orencia) for rheumatoid arthritis. *Med Lett.* 2006;48(1229):17–18.
19. Doyle JJ, Eliasson AH, Argyros GJ, et al. Prevalence of pulmonary disorders in patients with newly diagnosed rheumatoid arthritis. *Clin Rheumatol.* 2000;19(3):217–221.
20. Grubben MJ, Kerstens PJ, Wiersma JM, et al. Pleuro-pulmonary involvement in patients with connective tissue disease. The role of open lung biopsy. *Neth J Med.* 1993;43(5–6):269.
21. Dedhia HV, DiBartolomeo A. Rheumatoid arthritis. In: Guntupalli K, Bandi V, eds. *Critical Care Clinics: Rheumatological Emergencies.* Philadelphia: WB Saunders; 2002:841–854.
22. Perez T, Remy-Jardin M, Cortet B. Airways involvement in rheumatoid arthritis: clinical, functional, and HRCT findings. *Am J Respir Crit Care Med.* 1998;157:1658.
23. Hakala M. Poor prognosis in patients with rheumatoid arthritis hospitalized for interstitial lung fibrosis. *Chest.* 1988;93(1):114–118.
24. Harris ED Jr. *Rheumatoid Arthritis.* Philadelphia: WB Saunders Co; 1997.
25. Brazeau-Lamontagne L, Charlin B, Levesque RY, et al. Cricoarytenoiditis: CT assessment in rheumatoid arthritis. *Radiology.* 1986;158(2):463–466.
26. Geterud A, Bake B, Berthelsen B, et al. Laryngeal involvement in rheumatoid arthritis. *Acta Otolaryngol.* 1991;111(5):990–998.
27. Guerra LG, Lau KY, Marwah R. Upper airway obstruction as the sole manifestation of rheumatoid arthritis. *J Rheumatol.* 1992;19(6):974–976.
28. Redlund-Johnell I. Upper airway obstruction in patients with rheumatoid arthritis and temporomandibular joint destruction. *Scand J Rheumatol.* 1988;17(4):273–279.
29. Vergnenegre A, Pugnere N, Antonini MT, et al. Airway obstruction and rheumatoid arthritis. *Eur Respir J.* 1997;10(5):1072–1078.
30. Andora TF, Gilmore IM, Sorber JA, et al. Cricoarytenoid arthritis presenting as cardiopulmonary arrest. *Ann Emerg Med.* 1985;14(7):700–702.
31. Shannon TM, Gale ME. Noncardiac manifestations of rheumatoid arthritis in the thorax. *J Thorac Imaging.* 1992;7(2):19–29.
32. Link D, McCaffrey TV, Krauss WE, et al. Cervicomedullary compression: an unrecognized cause of vocal cord paralysis in rheumatoid arthritis. *Ann Otol Rhinol Laryngol.* 1998;107(6):462–471.
33. Nanke Y, Kotake S, Yonemoto K, et al. Cricoarytenoid arthritis with rheumatoid arthritis and systemic lupus erythematosus. *J Rheumatol.* 2001; 28(3):624–626.
34. Thompson LD, McCaffrey TV, Krauss WE, et al. Cervicomedullary compression: an unrecognized cause of vocal cord paralysis in rheumatoid arthritis. *Ann Otol Rhinol Laryngol.* 1998;107(6):462.
35. Wattenmaker I, Concepcion M, Hibberd P, et al. Upper-airway obstruction and perioperative management of the airway in patients managed with posterior operations on the cervical spine for rheumatoid arthritis. *J Bone Joint Surg Am.* 1994;76(3):360–365.
36. Pepin JL, Della Negra E, Grosclaude S, et al. Sleep apnea syndrome secondary to rheumatoid arthritis. *Thorax.* 1995;50(6):697.
37. Campbell RS, Wou P, Watt I. A continuing role for pre-operative cervical spine radiography in rheumatoid arthritis? *Clin Radiol.* 1995;50(3):157–159.
38. Zikou AK, Alamanos Y, Argyropoulou MI, et al. Radiological cervical spine involvement in patients with rheumatoid arthritis: a cross sectional study. *J Rheumatol.* 2005;32:801.
39. Neva MH, Hakkinen A, Makinen H, et al. High prevalence of asymptomatic cervical spine subluxation in patients with rheumatoid arthritis waiting for orthopedic surgery. *Ann Rheum Dis.* 2006;65:884.
40. Stiskal MA, Neuhold A, Szolar DH, et al. Rheumatoid arthritis of the craniocervical region by MR imaging: detection and characterization. *AJR Am J Roentgenol.* 1995;165:585.
41. Hamilton JD, Gordon M, McInnes IB, et al. Improved medical and surgical management of cervical spine disease in patients with rheumatoid arthritis over 10 years. *Ann Rheum Dis.* 2000;59:434.
42. Zygmunt SC, Christensson D, Saveland H, et al. Occipito-cervical fixation in rheumatoid arthritis—an analysis of surgical risk factors in 163 patients. *Acta Neurochir (Wien).* 1995;135:25.
43. Christensson D, Saveland H, Rydholm U. A cervical spine surgery in rheumatoid arthritis. *Scand J Rheumatol.* 2000;29(5):314–319.
44. Matti MV, Sharrock NE. Anesthesia on the rheumatoid patient. *Rheum Dis Clin North Am.* 1998;24:19.
45. Crosby ET, Lui A. The adult cervical spine: implications for airway management. *Can J Anaesth.* 1990;37(1):77.
46. Hakala P, Randell T. Intubation difficulties in patients with rheumatoid arthritis. A retrospective analysis. *Acta Anaesthesiol Scand.* 1998;42(2) 195–198.
47. Khanam T. Anaesthetic risks in rheumatoid arthritis. *Hosp Med.* 1994; 52(7):320.
48. John JT Jr, Hough A, et al. Pericardial disease in rheumatoid arthritis. *Am J Med.* 1979;66:385–390.
49. Roldan CA. Valvular disease associated with systemic illness. *Cardiol Clin.* 1998;16:531–550.
50. Goodson N. Coronary artery disease and rheumatoid arthritis. *Curr Opin Rheumatol.* 2002;14:115.
51. Steuer A, Keat AC. Perioperative use of methotrexate—a survey of clinical practice in the UK. *Br J Rheumatol.* 1997;36(9):1009–1011.
52. Goodson N. Coronary artery disease and rheumatoid arthritis. *Curr Opin Rheumatol.* 2002;14:115–120. PMID: 11845015.
53. Wolfe F, Michaud K, Gefeller O, et al. Predicting mortality in patients with rheumatoid arthritis. *Arthritis Rheum.* 2003;48:1530–1542. PMID: 12794820.

54. Van Doornum S, McColl G, Wicks IP. Accelerated atherosclerosis: an extraarticular feature of rheumatoid arthritis? *Arthritis Rehum.* 2002;46862–873. PMID: 11953961.
55. Godeau B, Boudjadja A, Dhainaut JF, Schlemmeret B, et al. Outcome of patients with systemic rheumatic disease admitted to medical intensive care units. *Ann Rheum Dis.* May 1992;51:627–631.
56. Godeau B, Mortie E, Roy P-M, et al. Short Bertand G, Emmanuel M, Pierre-Marie R et al in Short and Long term Outcomes for Patients with Systemic Rheumatic Diseases Admitted to Intensive Care Units: A Prognostic Study of 181 Patients. *The Journal of Rheumatology.* 1997;23(7):1317–1323.
57. Kollef MH, Enzenauer RJ. Predicting outcome from intensive care for patients with rheumatologic diseases. *J Rheumatol.* 1992;19(9):1260.
58. Fisher LR, Lawley MI. Relation between chest expansion, pulmonary function and exercise tolerance in patients with ankylosing spondylitis. *J Rheuma Dis.* 1990;49:9215.
59. Vosse D, Feldtkeller E, Erlendsson J, et al. Clinical vertebral fractures in patients with ankylosing spondylitis. *J Rheumatol.* 2004;31:1981.
60. Ramos-Remus C, Gomez-Vargas A, Guzman-Guzman JL, et al. Frequency of atlantoaxial subluxation and neurologic involvement in patients with ankylosing spondylitis. *J Rheumatol.* 1995;22:2120.
61. Boushea DK, Sundstrom WR. The pleuropulmonary manifestations of ankylosing spondylitis. *Semin Arthritis Rheum.* 1989;18:277.
62. Leirisalo-Repo M, Turunen U, Stenman S, et al. High frequency of silent inflammatory bowel disease in spondyloarthropathy. *Arthritis Rheum.* 1994;37:23.
63. Godfrin B, Zabraniecki L, Lamboley V, et al. Spondyloarthropathy with entheseal pain. A prospective study in 33 patients. *Joint Bone Spine.* 2004;71:557.
64. Lee CC, Lee SH, Chang IJ, et al. Spontaneous pneumothorax associated with ankylosing spondylitis. *Rheumatology (Oxford).* 2005;44:1538.
65. Bulkley BH, Roberts WC. Ankylosing spondylitis and aortic regurgitation. Description of the characteristic cardiovascular lesion from study of eight necropsy patients. *Circulation.* 1973;48:1014.
66. Khan MA. Update on spondylo arthropathics. *Ann Intern Med.* 2002; 136:896–907. PMID: 12069564.
67. Gorman JD, Sack KE, Davis JC Jr. Treatment of ankylosing spondiyities by inhibition of tumor necrosis factor alpha. *N Engl J Med.* 2002;346:1349–1356.
68. Legerton CW, Smith EA, Silver RM. Systemic sclerosis: clinical management of its major complications. *Rheum Dis Clin North Am.* 1995;21:203.
69. Van den Hoogen FHJ, van de Putte LBA. Treatment of systemic sclerosis. *Curr Opin Rheumatol.* 1994;6:637.
70. Troshinsky MB, Kane GC, Varga J, et al. Pulmonary function and gastroesophageal reflex in systemic sclerosis. *Ann Int Med.* 1994;121:6–10.
71. Steen VD, Medsger TA. Scleroderma renal crisis. In: Mandell BF, ed. *Acute Rheumatic and Immunological Disease.* New York: Markel Dekker; 1994:353.
72. Medsger TA Jr, Masi AT. Survival with scleroderma. II. A life-table analysis of clinical and demographic factors in 358 male U.S. veteran patients. *J Chronic Dis.* 1973;26:647.
73. Traub YM, Shapiro AP, Rodnan GP, et al. Hypertension and renal failure (scleroderma renal crisis) in progressive systemic sclerosis. Review of a 25-year experience with 68 cases. *Medicine (Baltimore).* 1983;62:335.
74. Akesson A, Wollheim FA. Organ manifestations in 100 patients with progressive systemic sclerosis: a comparison between the CREST syndrome and diffuse scleroderma. *Br J Rheumatol.* 1989;28:281.
75. Frust DE. Rational therapy in the treatment of systemic sclerosis. *Curr Opin Rheumatol.* 2000;12:540–544.
76. Rubin LJ, Badesch DB, Barst RJ, et al. Bosentan therapy for pulmonary arterial hypertension. *N Engl J Med.* 2002;346:896.
77. Block KG, Buchanan WW, Wohl MJ, et al. Sjogren's syndrome. *Medicine.* 1965;44:187–231.
78. Newball HH, Brahim SA. Chronic obstructive airway disease in patients with Sjogren's syndrome. *Am Rev Respir Dis.* 1977;115:295–304.
79. Kadota J, Kusano S, Kawakami K, et al. Usual interstitial pneumonia associated with primary Sjogren syndrome. *Chest.* 1995;108:1756–1758.
80. Dunne JA, Sabanthan S. Use of metallic stents in relapsing polychondritis. *Chest.* 1994;105:864–867. PMID: 8131553.
81. Tso AS, Chung HS, Wu Cy, et al. Anesthetic management of a patient with relapsing polychondritis—a case report. *Acta Anesthesiol Sin.* 2001;39:189–194.
82. Mastaglia FL, Phillips BA, Zilko PJ. Immunoglobulin therapy in inflammatory myopathies. *J Neuro Neurosurg Psychiatry.* 1998;65:107.
83. Hochberg MC. Updating the American College of Rheumatology revised criteria for the classification of systemic lupus erythematosus. *Arthritis Rheum.* 1997;40:1725.
84. Kimberly RP, Lockshin MD, Sherman RL, et al. High-dose intravenous methylprednisolone pulse therapy in SLE. *Am J Med.* 1981;70:817.
85. Steinberg AD. The treatment of lupus nephritis. *Kidney Int.* 1986;30:769.
86. Felson DT, Anderson J. Evidence for the superiority of immunosuppressive drugs and prednisone over prednisone alone in lupus nephritis. Results of a pooled analysis. *N Engl J Med.* 1984;311:1528.
87. Ginzler EM, Dooley MA, Aranow C, et al. Mycophenolate mofetil or intravenous cyclophosphamide for lupus nephritis. *N Engl J Med.* 2005;353:2219.
88. McCune WJ. Mycophenolate mofetil for lupus nephritis. *N Engl J Med.* 2005;353:2282.
89. Chan TM, Li FK, Tang CS, et al. Efficacy of mycophenolate mofetil in patients with diffuse proliferative lupus nephritis. Hong Kong-Guangzhou Nephrology Study Group. *N Engl J Med.* 2000;343:1156.
90. Chan TM, Tse KC, Tang CS, et al. Long-term study of mycophenolate mofetil as continuous induction and maintenance treatment for diffuse proliferative lupus nephritis. *J Am Soc Nephrol.* 2005;16:1076.
91. Ong LM, Hooi LS, Lim TO, et al. Randomized controlled trial of pulse intravenous cyclophosphamide versus mycophenolate mofetil in the induction therapy of proliferative lupus nephritis. *Nephrology (Carlton).* 2005;10:504.
92. Kim HY, Im JG, Goo JM, et al. Pulmonary tuberculosis in patients with systemic lupus erythematosus. *AJR Am J Roentgenol.* 1999;173:1639.
93. Small P, Frank H, Kreisman H, et al. An immunological evaluation of pleural effusions in systemic lupus erythematosus. *Ann Allergy.* 1982;49:101.
94. Sharma S, Smith R, Al-Hameed F. Fibrothorax and severe lung restriction secondary to lupus pleuritis and its successful treatment by pleurectomy. *Can Respir J.* 2002;9:335.
95. Matthay RA, Schwarz MI, Petty TL, et al. Pulmonary manifestations of systemic lupus erythematosus: review of twelve cases of acute lupus pneumonitis. *Medicine.* 1975;54:397.
96. Wiedemann HP, Matthay RA. Pulmonary manifestations of systemic lupus erythematosus. *J Thorac Imag.* 1992;7:1.
97. Lawrence EC. Systemic lupus erythematosus and the lung. In: Lahita RG, ed. *Systemic Lupus Erythematosus.* New York: John Wiley and Sons; 1987.
98. Weinrib L, Sharma OP, Quismorio FP Jr. A long-term study of interstitial lung disease in systemic lupus erythematosus. *Semin Arthritis Rheum.* 1990;20:48.
99. Karim MY, Miranda LC, Tench CM, et al. Presentation and prognosis of the shrinking lung syndrome in systemic lupus erythematosus. *Semin Arthritis Rheum.* 2002;31:289.
100. Laroche CM, Mulvey DA, Hawkins PN, et al. Diaphragm strength in the shrinking lung syndrome of SLE. *Q J Med.* 1989;71:429.
101. Warrington KJ, Moder KG, Brutinel WM. The shrinking lungs syndrome in systemic lupus erythematosus. *Mayo Clin Proc.* 2000;75:467.
102. Rubin LA, Urowitz MB. Shrinking lung syndrome in SLE—a clinical pathologic study. *J Rheumatol.* 1983;10:973.
103. Hawkins P, Davison AG, Dasgupta B, et al. Diaphragm strength in acute systemic lupus erythematosus in a patient with paradoxical abdominal motion and reduced lung volumes. *Thorax.* 2001;56:329.
104. Walz-Leblanc BA, Urowitz MB, Gladman DN, et al. The "shrinking lungs syndrome" in systemic lupus erythematosus—improvement with corticosteroid therapy. *J Rheumatol.* 1992;19:1970.
105. Soubrier M, Dubost JJ, Piette JC, et al. Shrinking lung syndrome in SLE. A report of three cases. *Rev Rhum Engl Ed.* 1995;62:395.
106. Badsha H, Teh CL, Kong KO, et al. Pulmonary hemorrhage in systemic lupus erythematosus. *Semin Arthritis Rheum.* 2004;33:414.
107. Zamora MR, Warner ML, Tuder R, et al. Diffuse alveolar hemorrhage and systemic lupus erythematosus. *Medicine.* 1997;76:192.
108. Hsu BY, Edwards DK III, Trambert MA. Pulmonary hemorrhage complicating SLE: role of MR imaging in diagnosis. *AJR Am J Roentgenol.* 1992;158:519.
109. Myers JL, Katzenstein AA. Microangiitis in lupus-induced pulmonary hemorrhage. *Am J Clin Pathol.* 1986;85:852.
110. Schwab EP, Schumacher HR Jr, Freundlich B, et al. Pulmonary alveolar hemorrhage in SLE. *Semin Arthritis Rheum.* 1993;23:8.
111. Erickson RW, Franklin WA, Emlen W. Treatment of hemorrhagic lupus pneumonitis with plasmapheresis. *Semin Arthritis Rheum.* 1994;24;114.
112. Winslow TM, Ossipov MA, Fazio GP, et al. Five-year follow-up study of the prevalence and progression of pulmonary hypertension in systemic lupus erythematosus. *Am Heart J.* 1995;129:510.
113. Rubin LA, Geran A, Rose TH, et al. A fatal pulmonary complication of lupus in pregnancy. *Arthritis Rheum.* 1995;38:710.
114. Roncoroni AJ, Alvarez C, Molinas F. Plexogenic arteriopathy associated with pulmonary vasculitis in systemic lupus erythematosus. *Respiration.* 1992;59:52.
115. Rubin LJ, Barst RJ, Kaiser LR, et al. Primary pulmonary hypertension. ACCP Consensus Report. *Chest.* 1993;104:236.
116. Gonzalez-Lopez L, Cardona-Munoz EG, Celis A, et al. Therapy with intermittent pulse cyclophosphamide for pulmonary hypertension associated with systemic lupus erythematosus. *Lupus.* 2004;13:105.
117. Abramson SB, Dobro J, Eberle MA, et al. Acute reversible hypoxemia in systemic lupus erythematosus. *Ann Intern Med.* 1991;114:941.
118. Belmont HM, Buyon J, Giorno R, et al. Up-regulation of endothelial cell adhesion molecules characterizes disease activity in systemic lupus erythematosus. *Arthritis Rheum.* 1994;37:376.
119. Martinez-Taboada VM, Blanco R, Armona J, et al. Acute reversible hypoxemia in SLE: a new syndrome or an index of disease activity. *Lupus.* 1995;4:259.
120. Godeau B, Cormier C, Menkes CJ. Bronchiolitis obliterans in systemic lupus erythematosus: beneficial effect of intravenous cyclophosphamide. *Ann Rheum Dis.* 1991;50:956.

121. Asherson RA, Cervera R, de Groot PG, et al. Catastrophic antiphospholipid syndrome: international consensus statement on classification criteria and treatment guidelines. *Lupus.* 2003;12:530.
122. Erkan D, Cervera R, Asherson RA. Catastrophic antiphospholipid syndrome: where do we stand? *Arthritis Rheum.* 2003;48:3320.
123. Asherson RA, Cervera R, Piette JC, et al. Catastrophic antiphospholipid syndrome. Clinical and laboratory features of 50 patients. *Medicine (Baltimore).* 1998;77:195.
124. Bucciarelli, Espinosa G, Cervera R, et al. Mortality in the catastrophic antiphospholipid syndrome: causes of death and prognostic factors in a series of 250 patients. *Arthritis Rheum.* 2006;54:2568.
125. Lockshin MD, Erkan D. Treatment of the antiphospholipid antibody syndrome. *N Engl J Med.* 2003;349:1177.
126. Kahl LE. The spectrum of pericardial tamponade in systemic lupus erythematosus. *Arthritis Rheum.* 1992;35:1343.
127. Mandell BF. Cardiovascular involvement in systemic lupus erythematosus. *Semin Arthbitis Rheum.* 1987;17:126.
128. Galve E, Candell-Riera J, Pigrau C, et al. Prevalence, morphologic types, and evolution of cardiac valvular disease in systemic lupus erythematosus. *N Engl J Med.* 1988;319:817.
129. Wijetunga M, Rockson S. Myocarditis in systemic lupus erythematosus. *Am J Med.* 2002;113:419.
130. Borenstein DG, Fye WB, Arnett FC, et al. The myocarditis of systemic lupus erythematosus. *Ann Intern Med.* 1978;89:619.
131. Sherer Y, Levy Y, Shoenfeld Y. Marked improvement of severe cardiac dysfunction after one course of intravenous immunoglobulin in a patient with systemic lupus erythematosus. *Clin Rheumatol.* 1999;18:238.
132. Law WG, Thong BY, Lian TY, et al. Acute lupus myocarditis: clinical features and outcome of an oriental case series. *Lupus.* 2005;14:827.
133. Bruce IN. 'Not only... but also': factors that contribute to accelerated atherosclerosis and premature coronary heart disease in systemic lupus erythematosus. *Rheumatology (Oxford).* 2005;44:1492.
134. Sibley JT, Olszynski WP, Decoteau WE, et al. The incidence and prognosis of central nervous system disease in systemic lupus erythematosus. *J Rheumatol.* 1992;19:47.
135. Wong KL, Woo EK, Yu YL, et al. Neurologic manifestations of systemic lupus erythematosus: a prospective study. *Q J Med.* 1991;81:857.
136. Bruyn GA. Controversies in lupus: nervous system involvement. *Ann Rheum Dis.* 1995;54:159.
137. Tan EM, Cohen AS, Fries JF, et al. The 1982 revised criteria for the classification of systemic lupus erythematosus (SLE). *Arthritis Rheum.* 1982;25:1271–1277.
138. Weening JJ, D'Agati VD, Schwartz MM, et al. The classification of glomerulonephritis in systemic lupus erythematosus revisited. *J Am Soc Nephrol.* 2004;15(2):241–250.

CHAPTER 168 ■ DERMATOLOGIC CONDITIONS

MARIONA BADIA • JOSE JAVIER TRUJILLANO

IMMEDIATE CONCERNS

This chapter will consider the skin-related problems that may be found in intensive care units (ICUs). Within the area of intensive care medicine, dermatologic problems are often forgotten in the course of daily clinical practice (1). The characteristics of patients in the ICU—for example, the sedated patient—can cause dermatologic problems to go unnoticed, as the patient may be reliant on ICU staff to make note of the integumentary issue for them. Nevertheless, the emergence of skin problems affecting ICU patients can reach up to 10% of those admitted (2).

The definition of dermatologic disorders (DD) refers to problems found in the skin, which, due to their magnitude, need for treatment, or the fact that they may be indicators of potentially serious diseases, need a medical diagnosis. With the collaboration of ICU staff, a simple visual inspection of the patient's skin, in some cases, may help to make an effective early diagnosis. A definitive diagnosis may then be made by an intensivist and, in many cases, finalized by a dermatology consultant (Table 168.1). Due to the potential severity of its consequences, it is essential that this pathology be handled by a critical care specialist (3).

The most expansive organ in the human body, the skin, comprises various strata:

1. *Epidermis, squamous epithelium*: Stratified in continual regeneration; acts as a protective wall to the exterior
2. *Dermis*: Can be found below the forma stratum, supplying it with circulation, sensation, and communication with other systems
3. *Hypodermis*: Subcutaneous fatty tissue, which acts as a padding with the underlying layer (4)

Dermatologic disorders that produce alterations in the normal structure of the skin can become severe due to the loss or deterioration in the cutaneous functions. The definition of DDs that will be used in this chapter is not that used in conventional studies of dermatology but follows a perspective based in intensive care medicine (Table 168.2).

LIFE-THREATENING DERMATOLOGIC DISORDERS

Some dermatologic diseases produce a loss of cutaneous functions due to an alteration in the stratum corneum, which protects us from physical, chemical, and microbiologic assault and also helps to maintain corporal temperature and homeostasis (5). The destruction of the stratum corneum, which provides the skin's barrier function, produces a significant loss in fluids, causes disorders in thermoregulation, and favors infection. The term, *acute skin failure*, was born out of the need to define those dermatologic diseases that, owing to their severity and involvement of cutaneous tissue, can lead to multiple systemic complications which may be life threatening (6). Some of these dermatologic diseases, by nature of their own severity, may also be life-threatening for the patient and require treatment in the intensive care unit.

Skin failure has various causes—apart from the most common pathologies such as thermal injury, which are discussed

TABLE 168.1

THE USUAL LEXICON USED TO "READ" SKIN CONDITIONS

Term	Definition
GENERAL SKIN AFFLICTIONS	
Exanthem	Skin eruption
Rash	A widespread eruption of lesions
Erythema	Blanchable redness of the skin by dilation of superficial blood vessels and capillaries
Purpura	Nonblanching violaceous or purple discoloration of the skin due to extravasation of blood into the tissue. May be palpable or nonpalpable
Nikolsky sign	A detachment of the skin when tangential pressure is applied with a finger or other object
BASIC SKIN LESIONS	
Macule	A circumscribed change in skin color without elevation or depression
Papule	A well-circumscribed, elevated, solid lesion less than 1 cm in diameter
Plaque	A well-circumscribed, elevated, superficial, solid lesion greater than 1 cm in size
Wheal	An edematous papule or plaque caused by swelling in the dermis
Nodule	A palpable solid lesion greater than 0.5 cm and less than 2 cm present in the epidermis, dermis, or subcutaneous tissue
Vesicle	A circumscribed elevated lesion that contains free fluid, less than 0.5 cm in size
Pustule	A circumscribed elevated lesion that contains purulent material, less than 0.5 cm in size
Bulla	A circumscribed elevated lesion that contains free fluid, greater than 0.5 cm in size
Petechia	Small nonblanching purpuric macules, less than 0.5 cm in size due to extravasated blood in the skin
Ecchymosis	Nonblanching purpuric macules greater than 0.5 cm in size due to extravasated blood in the skin
SYMPTOMATOLOGY	
Pruritus and Pain	Common symptoms of skin disorder, but in the critically ill patient, it may not be possible to evaluate the symptoms due to use of sedation or the comatose state

elsewhere—and include cutaneous disorders (i.e., immunobullous disorders, pustular psoriasis, erythroderma, etc.), drug reactions, and infectious disorders, which can produce systemic complications (7) (Table 168.3).

Specific Skin Diseases

Pemphigus

Pemphigus is a disease that produces severe blistering of the skin and mucous membranes. Pemphigus vulgaris is the most common form of this group of disorders. It is characterized by the loss of intracellular adhesion (acantholysis) of the keratinocytes induced by the IgG immunoglobulins that act against the desmoglein 1 and 3 (Dsg1 and 3) markers that are responsible for the intercellular adhesion of the desmosomes (8).

Pemphigus is related to various factors that can condition an immunologic reaction against epidermal desmosomes. The disorder has been associated with drugs such as penicillamine and captopril, viruses—especially herpes virus (9), pregnancy, and malignancies such as lymphoma and other lymphoproliferative disorders (10). Pemphigus may also be related to other autoimmune diseases, such as rheumatoid arthritis, myasthenia gravis, and pernicious anemia (11).

Clinical Presentation. In most patients, the lesions start in the oral mucous membranes, which represent the first indication of the disease. The blisters found in the oral mucous membranes

TABLE 168.2

CLASSIFICATION OF DERMATOLOGIC DISORDERS IN INTENSIVE CARE MEDICINE

Classification
Life-threatening dermatologic disorders
Dermatologic disorders that are manifestations of a systemic disease
Dermatologic disorders developed during ICU stay
Dermatologic disorders in specific situations
Prior dermatologic disorders

TABLE 168.3

LIFE-THREATENING DERMATOLOGIC DISORDERS

SPECIFIC SKIN DISEASES
Pemphigus vulgaris
Bullous pemphigoid
Acute generalized pustular psoriasis
Erythroderma
SEVERE DRUG ERUPTIONS
Toxic epidermal necrolysis (TEN)
Stevens-Johnson Syndrome (SJS)
INFECTIOUS DERMATOLOGIC DISORDERS
Staphylococcal scalded skin syndrome (SSSS)

are very fragile, easily bursting and leaving very painful denuded areas. Later, flaccid bullae develop over large areas of the patient, especially the trunk, scalp, and flexor surfaces (Fig. 168.1). The epidermal fragility shows itself with the Nikolsky sign, consisting of detachment of the skin when tangential pressure is applied with a finger or the eraser of a pencil. Despite the intensity of the clinical picture, pruritus is not a part of the presentation.

Diagnosis. The diagnosis of pemphigus is based on three criteria: clinical signs, histologic examination, and immunologic studies. When treating a patient with erosions and mucocutaneous blisters, one should consider pemphigus. The routine histopathologic examination reveals a suprabasilar blister, acantholysis, and a mild superficial dermal inflammatory infiltration (Fig. 168.2). Direct immunofluorescence, using the perilesional skin as a substrate, reveals IgG and C3 deposition in the intercellular spaces of the keratinocytes. Indirect immunofluorescence confirms the existence of antibodies circulating in more than 90% of the patients with active illness, and the enzyme-linked immunosorbent assay (ELISA) detects antibodies against the Dsg 1 and 3 (12).

Management. Several therapies are available; however, they have rarely been evaluated in randomized studies. Pemphigus is a fairly uncommon disease, and its severity and response to treatment vary from patient to patient. However, without treatment, it is a progressive disease with an almost 100% mortality, although, currently, the prognosis has been greatly improved by steroid therapy (13).

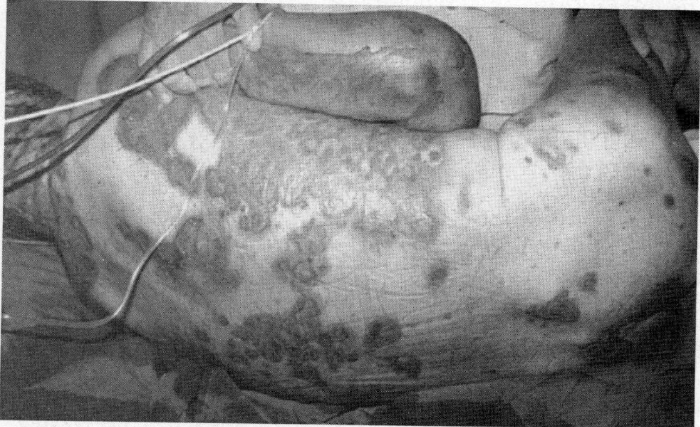

FIGURE 168.1. Severe life-threatening pemphigus vulgaris. Extensive erosions caused acute skin failure.

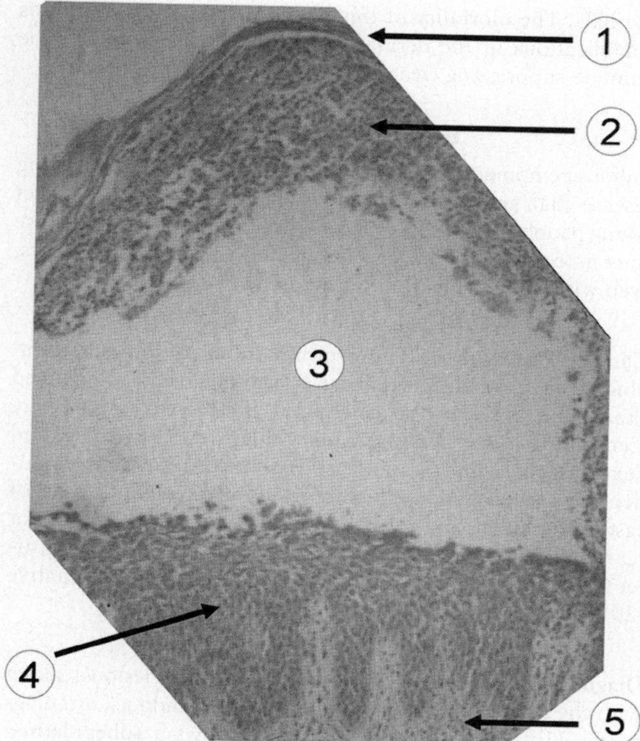

FIGURE 168.2. Histopathology of pemphigus vulgaris. Intraepidermic blister containing acantholytic cells. 1. Stratum corneum. 2. Granular and spinous layers. 3. Suprabasilar blister. 4. Basal layer. 5. Dermis. Hematoxylin-eosin stain.

The treatment of pemphigus is adjusted according to progression of the lesions. Oral lesions will respond partially to topical or intralesional treatment with corticosteroids or other immunosuppressants (14). The standard treatment for pemphigus vulgaris includes the administration of oral prednisone at a dose of 70 to 90 mg daily; the dose is increased until control is achieved. The use of steroids with other immunosuppressants—for example, azathioprine—allows the steroid dosage to be reduced (15). For those patients with more than 50% of the total body surface area involved, it is appropriate to use pulse steroids, for example, 1 g of methylprednisolone daily for 5 days. Another therapeutic option is the use of plasmapheresis, which acts by removing the pathogenic antibodies. However, due to the risk of infection, the administration of intravenous immunoglobin, at a dose of 2 g/kg for 3 to 5 days, which decreases the concentrations of circulating pathogenic antibodies, is the treatment of choice (16). Alternative adjuvant treatments used with steroids, apart from azathioprine, are cyclophosphamide, mycophenolate mofetil, methotrexate, gold, and dapsone. Rituximab, an anti-CD20 antibody, is in the experimental phase but has shown promising results (17,18).

Patients with pemphigus may require admission to the ICU based on the extensiveness of their lesions; the disorder itself will have usually been diagnosed by a dermatologist. Organ failure is another reason that these patients are placed in the ICU. The mortality of this disease is related to infectious complications of the dermatologic disorder itself and of the immune-suppressing treatment (10).

Bullous Pemphigoid

Bullous pemphigoid is an autoimmune, subepidermal blistering disease that generally affects the elderly but can also affect young people and children. The natural evolution of the disease runs its course with exacerbations and relapses, but it halts, even without treatment, in most patients after 5 years (19).

Clinical Presentation. The typical lesions of bullous pemphigoid are tense blisters that can appear on normal or inflamed skin. The lesions may be generalized, but most commonly are seen on the lower abdomen, inner thighs, groin, axillae, and flexor aspects of arms and legs. The mucous membrane, particularly the oral mucous membrane, is affected in one third of cases. The bullae are normally full of clear liquid and do not scar. Unlike pemphigus vulgaris, the lesions are pruritic and, after their rupture, are not painful. The Nikolsky sign is negative (20).

Diagnosis. The clinical characteristics of the lesions, along with the histopathologic and immunologic findings, are diagnostic. Histologic study of the lesion shows a subepidermal blister with fibrinoid material and inflammatory cell infiltration in its interior, with a predominance of eosinophils. Direct immunofluorescence (IF) will show deposits of IgG and C3 in the dermoepidermal junction, and indirect IF shows autoantibodies circulating against proteins of the basal membrane.

Management. Corticosteroids are the mainstay of therapy for bullous pemphigoid, although the prognosis is good even without treatment. Localized bullous pemphigoid usually responds to topical corticoid treatment. Other treatments that are used with steroids are azathioprine, dapsone, tetracycline, or plasmapheresis, although these adjunctive therapies are of doubtful value (21). As noted with pemphigus, these patients are admitted to the ICU after they have been diagnosed; ICU admission is mandated based on the extent of the lesions and the presence of organ failure.

Acute Generalized Pustular Psoriasis

Acute generalized pustular psoriasis (Von Zumbusch type) is an acute variant of the psoriasis that is characterized by widespread erythema and pustules. Precipitating factors have been detailed and include infection, pregnancy, hypocalcemia, lithium, and the withdrawal of steroids (22).

Clinical Presentation. The disorder is characterized by a high fever, followed by the sudden appearance of sterile pustules 2 to 3 mm in diameter. These are initially noted in pre-existing psoriatic plaques but rapidly generalize to the trunk and extremities, including palms and soles, and are associated with generalized erythema.

At a systemic level, the disorder manifests itself with hypovolemia and renal and/or hepatic failure. It presents a high risk of infection and sepsis, with *Staphylococcus* species a common causative agent (23).

Diagnosis. The diagnosis is clinical, based on previous history of psoriasis with the appearance of marked erythema and pinpoint pustules.

Management. Oral retinoids seem to be the most effective treatment for clearing the lesions in the shortest time. To avoid recurrences, the treatment should be continued over a period of 3 or 4 months. Methotrexate and cyclosporine have also been shown to be effective in the treatment of this disorder. Topical triamcinolone ointment plus wet dressings reduces scaling, tenderness, pruritus, and discomfort, and helps to re-establish the barrier function of the skin (24).

Erythroderma

Erythroderma is defined as a cutaneous inflammation affecting more than 90% of the body surface area, with a loss of normal integumentary function. It is the clinical manifestation of diverse dermatologic or systemic diseases (Table 168.4). The most frequent causes are psoriasis, spongiotic dermatitis, drug reaction, and cutaneous T-cell lymphoma, although, on occasion, it is not possible to identify the underlying disease, and the disorder is classified as idiopathic erythroderma (25).

TABLE 168.4

PRINCIPAL CAUSES OF ERYTHRODERMA

DERMATOSES
- Psoriasis
- Atopic dermatitis
- Spongiotic dermatitis
- Pemphigus
- Pityriasis subra pilaris
- Bullous pemphigoid

SYSTEMIC DISEASES
- Dermatomyositis
- Lupus erythematosus
- Sarcoidosis
- Graft versus host disease
- HIV

MALIGNANCY
- Lymphomas
- Leukemias
- Prostate
- Lung
- Thyroid

DRUGS
- Allopurinol
- Amiodarone
- Aztreonam
- Cefoxitin
- Chlorpromazine
- Antimalarials
- Aspirin
- Lithium

Modified from Balasubramaniam P, Berth-Jones J. Erythroderma: 90% skin failure. *Hosp Med.* 2004;65:100; and Rothe MJ, Bernstein ML, Grant-Kels JM. Life-threatening erythroderma: diagnosing and treating the "red man." *Clin Dermatol.* 2005;23:206, with permission.

Clinical Presentation. Erythroderma usually affects middle-aged men. When erythroderma is related to drugs, the disorder appears suddenly, with rapid and progressive inflammation. When caused by a dermatologic disease, progression of the erythroderma is slower, presenting as a generalized erythema in which scaling and desquamation are very variable; pruritus may be noted. If the itching is intense, one should suspect lymphoma as the underlying disease.

Systematically, there is an increase in capillary permeability with a rise in cardiac output, resulting in a distributive shock-like state. There is also an alteration in the fluid and electrolyte balance due to the cutaneous loss of fluids, electrolytes, and proteins.

Diagnosis. Laboratory findings are not particularly helpful in making the diagnosis of erythroderma. Clinical signs, together with a cutaneous biopsy, are what actually yield the data for the diagnosis. Interestingly, in one third of cases, an etiologic diagnosis is not made. A peripheral blood analysis is necessary to look for potential malignant hematologic problems.

Management. The main objective is the control of systemic problems derived from the loss of cutaneous function. Parallel to this, it is necessary to investigate the disease responsible for erythroderma in order to establish a specific treatment regimen. The fundamental pillar of this treatment is the restoration of fluid and electrolyte balance to obtain hemodynamic stability. With regard to the skin, potent topical agents are not recommended due to the risk of systemic effects.

A warm, humid environment improves patient comfort and prevents hypothermia. Apart from localized measures, systemic treatment should be established according to the suspected underlying disease. In the case where the underlying disease is not known, we evaluate the use of corticosteroids and cyclosporine (26).

Severe Drug Eruptions

Toxic Epidermal Necrolysis

Toxic epidermal necrolysis (TEN), described by Lyell, is a dermatologic disease caused by an idiosyncratic reaction to drugs (27). It most often starts with a nonspecific febrile picture, followed by mucocutaneous lesions, and later develops epidermal detachment, which affects more than 30% of the body's surface area (28); the mortality rate ranges between 30% and 50%. Sulfonamides are the drugs most frequently associated with TEN, followed by cephalosporins, quinolones, imidazoles, and anticonvulsants such as phenytoin. The list of drugs implicated continues to increase, including groups as diverse as antibiotics, analgesics, nonsteroidal anti-inflammatory agents, and sedatives (29).

Clinical Presentation. Following the febrile presentation, an eruption spreads symmetrically over the face and down the trunk, eventually covering the entire body. The lesions start as erythematous macules, followed by flaccid blisters that are easily ruptured, producing necrosis and weeping from the epidermis; the Nikolsky sign is positive. The eroded surface usually composes between 30% and 80% of the cutaneous surface. In most cases, there is mucous membrane involvement with painful erosions. On occasion, an extensive epithelial detachment occurs in the trachea, bronchi, and also in the gastrointestinal tract, resulting in respiratory failure and accompanying gastrointestinal symptoms.

Diagnosis. TEN lesions are characterized by a massive apoptosis of the epidermis that induces epidermal necrosis with the development of subepidermal blisters, with an underlying sparse mononuclear cell infiltration. The immunohistochemistry shows tumor necrosis factor-α deposits in the epidermis, with a predominance of T lymphocytes (30).

Management. After making the diagnosis, the first therapeutic response is the rapid withdrawal of potentially culpable medications from the patient, along with general supportive therapy; the latter therapy usually requires a burn or intensive care unit. Treatment is supportive, as there is no specific therapy available. Although corticosteroids have been used extensively, they have not demonstrated obvious beneficial effects and, in some series, result in an increase in mortality. Thus, these agents are not recommended in TEN. Notwithstanding this lack of positive effect of steroids, severe TEN may be treated with cyclosporine at a dose of 3 to 5 mg/kg/day; this regimen has resulted in promising results. Other therapies, such as zinc, plasmapheresis, and immunoglobulins, although promising, require more study (31,32).

Stevens-Johnson Syndrome

Stevens-Johnson syndrome (SJS) is a mucocutaneous disease caused by a drug-induced reaction, sharing etiologic, histologic, and therapeutic characteristics with TEN (33). Classically, SJS was considered a severe variant of erythema multiforme. Today, however, these are considered to be two different entities. Erythema multiforme is postinfectious in origin (seen especially after herpes and mycoplasma), and the lesions are, morphologically, target lesions with symmetric and mainly acral distribution and, histologically, have a more mononuclear infiltrate and a lesser degree of epidermal necrosis—different than SJS. Additionally, to further point out the differences, the mortality is low—5% to 15%—compared to the 30% to 50% seen with SJS (34).

The clinical presentation of SJS is the same as that of TEN but usually involves less than 10% of the total body surface area. The mucous membranes are involved, and a disseminated cutaneous eruption with discrete, dark-red maculae—sometimes with a necrotic center—followed by epidermal necrosis, are seen. This might be considered a TEN variant, but with a lesser cutaneous detachment and lower (5%–15%) mortality. Treatment involves withdrawal of causal drugs, supportive measures, and the avoidance of steroids (35).

Infectious Dermatologic Disorders

Staphylococcal Scalded Skin Syndrome

Staphylococcal scalded skin syndrome (SSSS) is a severe blistering disease caused by exfoliative exotoxin produced by *Staphylococcus aureus*. The exotoxin provokes subcorneal separation of the cornea stratum through interaction with desmoglein 1, essential for maintaining the integrity of the epidermis (36). This disorder predominantly affects children younger than

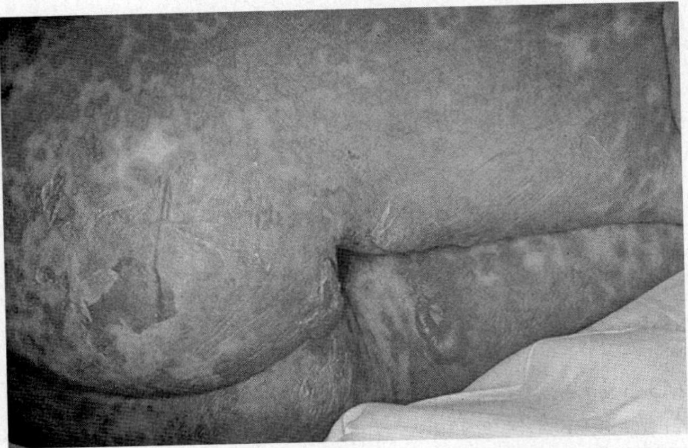

FIGURE 168.3. Widespread blistering and erosions over the limbs with staphylococcal scalded syndrome. (Courtesy of J.M. Casanova, M.D.: http://www.dermatoweb.net.)

5 years of age, although older children and adults may also suffer intoxication, especially when there are predisposing factors such as renal failure, immunosuppression, malignancy, or alcohol abuse. In such cases, the mortality rate may exceed 60%. Bullous impetigo (see section below, Cutaneous Infection) is a localized form of cutaneous staphylococci infection that normally appears during the first years of life, although occasionally it may be seen later, especially when associated with immunosuppression. For example, bullous impetigo may commonly be the first manifestation of HIV infection.

Clinical Presentation. SSSS is produced in the context of staphylococcal septicemia. The primary infection is usually not found cutaneously, but in the nasopharyngeal mucous membrane, in the urinary tract, or at the conjunctival level. Flaccid bullae form predominantly in the folds of the skin and around natural orifices. The blisters grow and break easily, leaving a wet erythematous base that gives the appearance of scalded skin (Fig. 168.3). At resolution, there is no scarring, and very rarely are the mucous membranes involved. The Nikolsky sign is positive in this disorder.

Diagnosis. The diagnosis is initially based on the clinical picture, with the presence of erythroderma, desquamation, and bullae. Microbiologic study, with the isolation of an exotoxin producing *S. aureus*, confirms the diagnosis. Histologic study reveals a subcorneal separation in the granular layer due to intraepidermal acantholysis. As with the isolation of *S. aureus*, the histologic study—showing no epidermal necrosis—permits the exclusion of TEN, as these two entities can be indistinguishable clinically (37).

Management. The resolution of the cutaneous lesions is swift after the initiation of an adequate antibacterial regimen, often with a beta-lactamase–resistant penicillin. As the cutaneous desquamation is superficial, there usually is no serious loss of fluids or electrolytes through the skin.

Summary

As we have seen, dermatologic disorders that are life threatening can be divided into two large groups. The first consists of autoimmune diseases that are usually diagnosed before the patient is admitted to the ICU; the prognosis can be modified if immunosuppressive agents are administered as treatment. The second group is made up of disorders that may start during the patient's stay in the ICU from toxic or infectious causes. Differentiating these disorders in critically ill patients receiving multiple medications often presents a diagnostic challenge. Among these disorders, those that carry the highest mortality are the vesiculobullous disorders, followed by TEN (38).

SYSTEMIC DISEASES PRESENTING AS DERMATOLOGIC-LIKE DISORDERS

Some dermatologic alterations are not signs of a life-threatening cutaneous disorder. However, they are expressions of potentially serious systemic diseases. Sometimes these lesions are subtle and may pass unnoticed by the patient and/or his or her physician; however, their recognition may be the key to obtaining early diagnosis and treatment (Table 168.5).

Peripheral Vascular Disorder–Related Systemic Infection

In some infectious systemic diseases, an alteration to the blood vessels is produced, secondary to direct vascular damage or, on occasion, due to a hypersensitivity reaction whereby immune-complex deposits give rise to characteristic cutaneous lesions.

Necrotic Purpuric Rash

Necrotic purpuric rash is typical in acute systemic infection by *Neisseria meningitidis*. Generally, early recognition of these lesions helps in the diagnosis of this severe systemic disease. Petechiae and ecchymoses are the most common lesions, usually localized on the trunk and the extremities (Fig. 168.4) although, on occasion, they may affect mucous membranes. Initially, the lesions are small, irregular, and slightly raised, but in some patients the lesions quickly become confluent, giving rise to large ecchymotic areas—a bad prognostic sign.

TABLE 168.5

DERMATOLOGIC DISORDERS THAT ARE MANIFESTATIONS OF A SYSTEMIC DISEASE

PERIPHERAL VASCULAR DISORDER–RELATED SYSTEMIC INFECTION
- Necrotic purpuric rash
- Ecthyma gangrenosum
- Septic microemboli

CONNECTIVE TISSUE DISORDERS
- Scleroderma
- Systemic lupus erythematosus
- Dermatomyositis

CUTANEOUS VASCULITIS

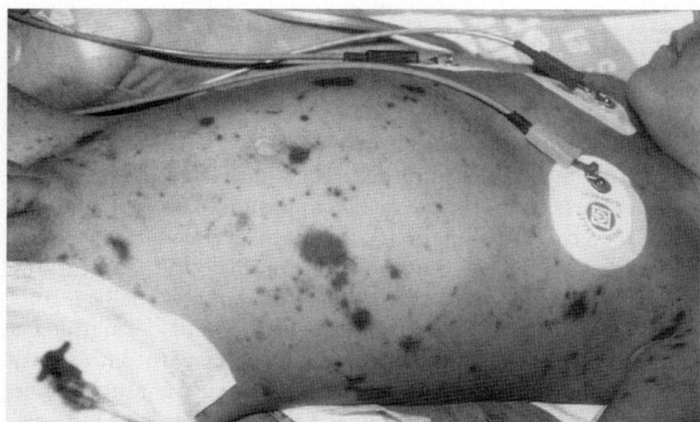

FIGURE 168.4. Necrotic purpuric rash in meningococcal septicemia.

In the most serious cases, these ecchymotic areas become necrotic, requiring amputation if the patient survives (39). Histologic study of the lesions reveals endothelial, damage, with areas of thrombosis and hemorrhage in the vascular wall, and containing nuclear "dust" and neutrophils in, and around, the vessels. The Gram stain and culture of the skin lesion biopsy may show meningococci.

When diagnosing a patient with fever and hemorrhagic eruption, especially in the presence of meningeal signs, meningococcemia should be suspected. Early diagnosis is crucial for establishing a cause and administering life-saving treatment for an illness with high mortality that affects mainly young people (37).

Ecthyma Gangrenosum

Ecthyma gangrenosum (EG) is an infectious vascular occlusive disease normally associated with *Pseudomonas aeruginosa* bacteremia, although, on rare occasions, it has been described with other bacterial infections such as *Chromobacterium violaceum* (40). Normally, EG is seen in immunologically compromised patients, such as those with diabetes mellitus, neutropenia, hematologic malignancies, organ transplantation, AIDS, or other severe chronic diseases in immunocompetent patients (41). The lesions of ecthyma gangrenosum are characterized by cutaneous macules or papules, with central vesicle, that progress into hemorrhagic bullae. These break, leaving ulcerations with a black necrotic center, surrounded by narrow, pink to violaceous halos. Perhaps most important, these lesions appear on the extremities and buttocks.

Histologic studies show invasion of the adventitial and medial layers of the small vessel walls by Gram-negative bacilli, resulting in a necrotizing and hemorrhagic vasculitis. Cultures of blood and of the vesicular contents will show *Pseudomonas aeruginosa* (42). Early treatment with intravenously administered antipseudomonal antibiotics is essential.

Septic Microemboli

Septic microemboli result in the eponymic Janeway lesions and Osler nodules, often associated with bacterial endocarditis. Janeway lesions are painless, irregular, and hemorrhagic macules that are found on the palms and soles (Fig. 168.5). Histologically, they show dermal neutrophilic microabscesses and vessel thrombosis without vasculitis. Gram stain of the tissue is usually positive for organisms (43).

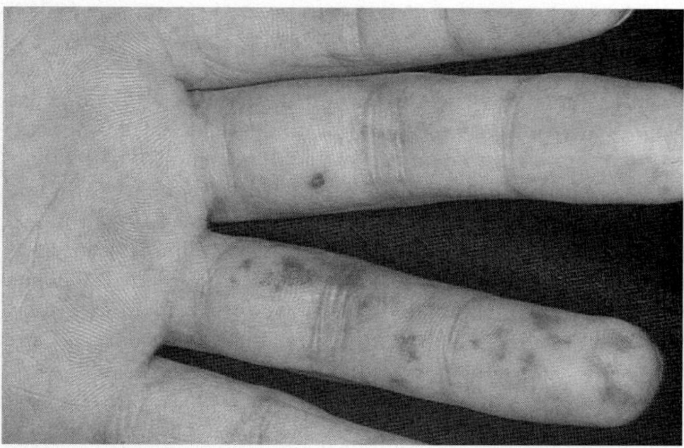

FIGURE 168.5. Multiple Janeway lesions on the fingers. (Courtesy of J.M. Casanova, M.D.: http://www.dermatoweb.net.)

Osler nodes are small, painful erythematous nodules—normally found in the pads of fingers or toes—that resolve without ulceration. Histologic evaluation shows endothelial swelling, inflammation, and thrombosis, with obliteration of the superficial arteriolar lumina. On occasion, a positive culture may be obtained from biopsy of the node (44).

Connective Tissue Disorders

Connective tissue diseases—such as scleroderma, lupus erythematosus, and dermatomyositis—are autoimmune disorders of unknown origin, which can affect various organs and show characteristic skin damage that can assist in making the diagnosis. It is the severity of the systemic manifestations of these disorders that is of prime significance for prognosis. These three diseases sometimes require admission to ICU, either because of their impact on vital organs or due to the secondary infectious complications related to the immunosuppressive treatment.

Scleroderma, a disorder characterized by widespread disruption of the microcirculation with intense fibrosis of the blood vessels, manifests with integumentary lesions with symmetrical fibrosis that usually affects the distal extremities and is often limited to the fingers and face, although a widespread form may affect the distal and proximal extremities and, often, the trunk and face (45).

Systemic lupus erythematosus (SLE) affects the skin, kidneys, lungs, central nervous system, and joints. The most frequent manifestations are arthralgia and/or arthritis in the muscles and bones, most commonly in the interphalangeal and metacarpophalangeal joints and in the knees, with interarticular bleeding or edema of the periarticular tissue. In the skin, a characteristic "butterfly" blush (erythema over the malar eminences of the face and bridge of the nose) is seen. When especially severe, acute cutaneous lupus erythematous produces vesiculobullous skin lesions (46).

Dermatomyositis is an inflammatory, degenerative myopathy of striated muscle with concomitant characteristic cutaneous manifestations. Noted on the integument is a heliotropic rash, which may or may not be accompanied by periorbital edema and violet Gottron papules on the extensor surfaces of the joints; these are pathognomonic of the disease (47).

Cutaneous Vasculitis

Vasculitis includes a varied group of diseases with different degrees of systemic manifestations, and common characteristic of inflammation and necrosis of the blood vessels.

The skin and subcutaneous tissues are frequently affected and often show the initial manifestation of vasculitis. Although the impact of the systemic vasculitis on the integument does not result in great risk, *per se*, its importance lies in the fact that it is suggestive of the type of vasculitis with which the patient is presenting and, because of the characteristics of damage and the skin's accessibility to diagnostic study, may assist in the generation of an appropriate differential diagnoses list.

Cutaneous manifestations of vasculitis include urticaria, purpura, papules, ulcer, livido reticularis, nodules, and digital gangrene. The skin injuries are not specific but provide a guide to the size of the blood vessel affected. Vasculitis affecting small vessels is noted as palpable purpura, above all on the lower extremities. This usually develops in crops of lesions, initially with reddish macules, turning into erythematous papules that develop into plaques. On the other hand, nodules are typical lesions of vasculitis affecting the larger blood vessels. They are usually hot, inflamed, red, and surrounded by a halo of *livido reticularis* (48). The classification most often used for vasculitis combines clinical and histologic data, the size of the affected vessel with distinguishing vasculitis of large, medium, and small blood vessels.

The variability in presentation, added to the general low index of suspicion in these cases, makes the diagnosis of vasculitis extremely difficult, and skin lesions may be crucial in the diagnostic evaluation (49). The systemic vasculitis presenting as skin lesions that most often require ICU admission are polyarteritis nodosa, microscopic polyangiitis, Wegener granulomatosis, and Churg-Strauss syndrome, and are discussed in another chapter. Leukocytoclastic angiitis is the most common cutaneous vasculitis, affecting small vessels and characterized by palpable purpura in the lower extremities (Fig. 168.6). The disease is generally restricted to the skin, and the prognosis tends to be good.

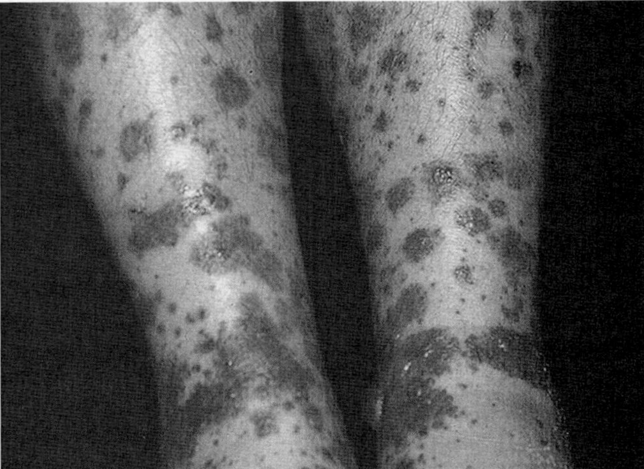

FIGURE 168.6. Palpable purpura affecting the lower legs in leukocytoclastic angiitis. (Courtesy of J.M. Casanova, M.D.: http://www.dermatoweb.net.)

DEPARTMENT OF DERMATOLOGIC DISORDERS DURING ICU STAY

Intensive care units are characterized by the use of invasive monitoring techniques and therapeutic procedures that, sometimes, represent an assault on the anatomic barrier of the patient. The critically ill patient's skin is also affected by a series of local factors such as immobility, humidity, and maceration, as well as more general factors such as diabetes mellitus and the use of corticosteroids that may compound dermatologic problems. The skin is in continuous contact with pathogens, and the alteration of its protective function and characteristics allows bacterial, viral, and fungal agents to more easily penetrate this barrier. On the other hand, ICU patients often receive many drugs that may result in cutaneous drug reactions.

The most common dermatologic problems in the ICU as a result of polypharmacy and a patient's prolonged length of stay are noted in Table 171.6. Although these dermatopathies do not usually increase patient mortality, they may require specific treatment.

Cutaneous Infection

Bacterial Infection

Superficial bacterial infections are usually produced by *Staphylococci aureus* and *Streptococci pyogenes*. The most frequent form of infection is impetigo (Fig. 168.7). This is an infection of the superficial layers of the epidermis that exists in two clinical varieties, bullous impetigo—caused exclusively by *Staphylococcus aureus*, a producer of an exotoxin—and impetigo contagiosa.

Impetigo contagiosa is the most common form, and is caused by either or both streptococci and staphylococci. It is characterized by discrete thin-walled vesicles that rapidly become pustular and then rupture. The exudates dry to form

TABLE 168.6

DERMATOLOGIC DISORDERS DEVELOPED DURING ICU STAY

CUTANEOUS INFECTION
Bacterial infection
Bullous impetigo
Impetigo contagiosa
Viral infection
Herpes simplex virus type 1 (HSV-1) and 2
Perioral/genital herpes
Eczema herpeticum
Varicella-zoster virus 3 (VZV)
Chickenpox (varicella)
Shingles (zoster)
Fungal infection (Candida *species*)
REACTIONS TO INTENSIVE THERAPY
Morbilliform reactions
Urticaria and angioedema
Contact dermatitis
Skin necrosis induced by drugs

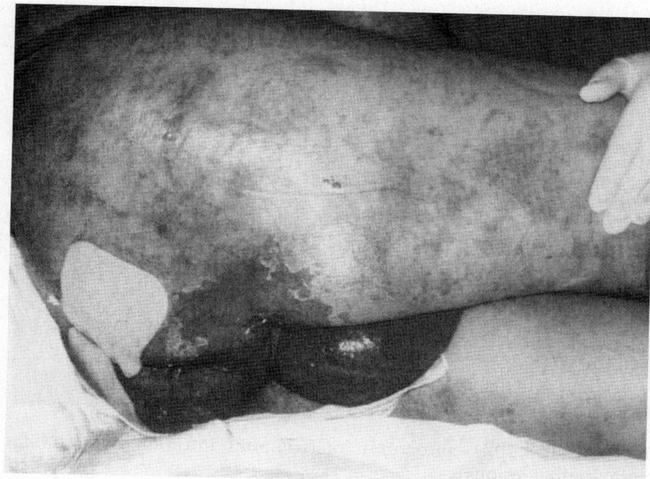

FIGURE 168.7. Subcorneal bullae followed by an exudative erosive lesion in impetigo.

loosely stratified golden yellow crusts, which usually appear on exposed areas of the body such as the face, nose, and extremities; they also appear in areas that have suffered trauma, erosion, or burn (50). In ICU patients, these lesions usually appear on areas of skin damaged by pressure, wounds, or trauma. For bacteriologic diagnosis, a culture of the lesion is required, as the exanthem resultant from *S. aureus* and group A streptococci are clinically indistinguishable. Although the therapeutic options include diverse oral and topical antimicrobials, as well as disinfectants, one should note that topical antibiotic treatment with mupirocin or fusidic acid is at least as effective—and perhaps more so—as oral antibiotics, without the side effects of the latter (51). With a localized skin infection, the procedure is to wash the area, remove the scabs, and then apply the topical antibiotic ointment. When the skin infection is extensive or there is systemic involvement, we use systemic antimicrobials, such as a beta-lactamase–resistant penicillin, amoxicillin/clavulanic acid, vancomycin, or linezolid.

Viral Infection

The herpes virus family, of which there are eight human serotypes, may produce significant skin lesions. In critically ill patients, viral skin lesions are almost always due to herpes virus types 1 and 2, and the varicella-zoster virus 3 (52).

Herpes Simplex Virus Types 1 (HSV-1) and 2 (HSV-2). Skin eruptions caused by HSV-1/2 are common dermatoses usually localized around the lips (HSV-1) or on the genitalia (HSV-2). Most often, the initial infection goes unnoticed; after the first infection, the virus moves through the peripheral sensory nerves and becomes latent in the posterior root ganglion.

HSV-1 is the most common of these virus types, affecting the perioral area and lips, although occasionally it can affect other areas of the body. After an initial, usually subclinical, infection in infancy, the organism may be reactivated. This presents as painful skin lesions around the lips, accompanied by a burning sensation and the formation of small vesicles grouped in bunches on an erythematous base. These vesicles become umbilicated and rupture quickly, forming a scab that heals after 7 to 10 days, without a scar. The reactivation of the labial herpes is aided by diverse factors such as hormonal alterations, febrile processes, or stressful situations frequent in the intensive care environment. The association of perioral herpes with bacterial infection is typical, especially that caused by *Streptococcus pneumoniae*. This demonstrates the phenomenon of the virus reactivation behaving as an indicator of underlying Gram-positive bacterial infection (53,54). Reactivation is also a frequent complication associated with immunosuppression (55), organ transplantation (56), dermatoses (57), and burn patients (58). Although the diagnosis is fundamentally clinical, the Tzanck test can show the presence of multinucleated giant cells, and direct immunofluorescence and polymerase chain reaction (PCR) techniques confirm the diagnosis. Topical treatment, begun as soon as possible after diagnosis, with 5% acyclovir or 1% peniclovir applied 5 times a day, is effective in reducing the duration and severity of symptoms. In extensive viral infections, systemic treatment is with acyclovir or famciclovir (59).

A serious variant of a skin infection by HSV is eczema herpeticum or Kaposi varicelliform eruption (60). This emerges in patients with previous dermopathy, generally atopic dermatitis, and is characterized by vesicular lesions in areas of dermatitis that grow into large erosive areas covered in honey-like crusts. This is accompanied by signs of systemic implications, and requires systemic treatment with acyclovir (10 mg/kg every 8 hours).

Varicella-zoster Virus 3. Varicella-zoster virus (VZV) 3 causes chickenpox (varicella) and shingles (zoster). Varicella is the most common form of the initial presentation of VZV. This is a contagious disease, generally benign and typically seen during infancy. It is rare among adults, but when present, is associated with severe complications such as varicella pneumonia, the most common complication occurring in 15% to 50% of cases with 10% to 35% mortality (61,62). The skin rash is quite characteristic: each spot starts as a 2- to 4-mm-diameter red papule, developing an irregular outline (rose petal) as a small vesicle appears. The vesicle quickly develops into a pustule, which becomes umbilicated and results in a pruritic scab in less than a day. One will observe multiple lesions in different evolutionary periods with this disorder (Fig. 168.8), as opposed to the lesions of smallpox, which develop in uniform "crops."

Varicella pneumonia normally emerges within 1 to 6 days of the skin rash. Patients who smoke tobacco, have a severe VZV rash, are pregnant, and/or are immune compromised or with a chronic obstructive pulmonary disease all have a higher risk of developing varicella pneumonia (63). The typical skin lesions, with respiratory symptoms and radiologic findings of interstitial pneumonitis (Fig. 168.9), are suggestive of the diagnosis. Optimal treatment is intravenous acyclovir at a dose of 10 mg/kg every 8 hours. Use of corticosteroids has demonstrated a significant improvement in oxygenation and shortening of the duration of mechanical ventilation in preliminary studies (64).

Herpes zoster is an acute radiculitis accompanied by a vesicular eruption grouped over an erythematous base localized in the corresponding dermatome on the affected ganglion (65). It is produced by a reactivation of the VZV that is latent in the ganglions of the nerve roots (66). The thoracic and trigeminal nerves are the most frequently affected dermatomes. Initially, a prodrome of hyperesthesia, dysesthesias, itching, or pruritus throughout the affected dermatome presents; later, the typical

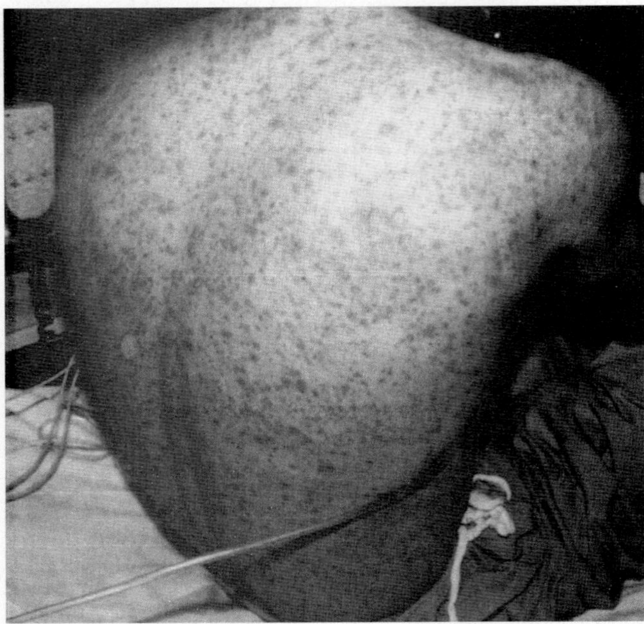

FIGURE 168.8. Adult with varicella. The rash is in different stages of evolution, with some vesicles, macules, and papules.

lesions appear with a maculopapular rash that evolves into vesicles grouped in bunches, distributed along the affected dermatome. The most common chronic complication of this acute radiculitis is postherpetic neuralgia, which can be debilitating.

Immunosuppressed patients may present with disseminated herpes zoster that starts by affecting contiguous dermatomes and later extends to larger areas of involvement. The treatment is focused on control of the infection and the pain of the acute phase, and the presentation of postherpetic neuralgia. Famciclovir, valganciclovir, and acyclovir are effective treatments for herpes zoster (67); in the most severe cases, intravenous agents are used. The use of corticosteroids to help with pain is of doubtful utility; gabapentin and the tricyclic antidepressants are recommended for postherpetic neuralgia (68).

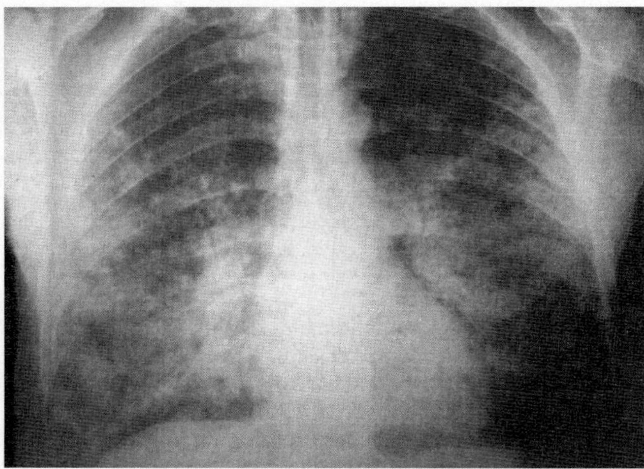

FIGURE 168.9. Chest radiograph showing bilateral interstitial infiltrates of a patient presenting with severe varicella pneumonia.

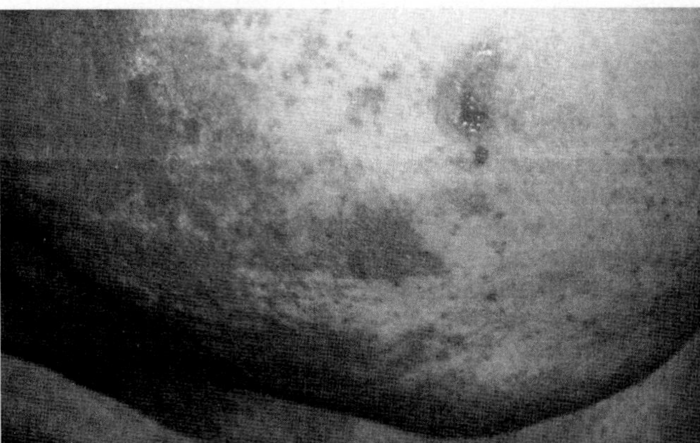

FIGURE 168.10. Genitocrural intertriginous infection by *Candida* with satellite lesions.

Fungal Infection (*Candida* species)

Cutaneous candidiasis is a superficial infection that emerges in damp and macerated areas of skin, usually in the folds of the axillae and the submammary area (69). Cutaneous candidiasis is a frequent problem in long-stay critically ill patients who have most often received broad-spectrum antibiotic therapy and have very limited mobility. The infection is characterized by intense shiny erythema with scarce whitish exudates and satellite papules and pustules (Fig. 168.10). Patients may have pruritus, burning, and pain in the affected areas.

Diverse factors assist in the candidal infection's initiation and progression. On the one hand, maintaining hygiene is important but, on the other hand, drying the skin of critically ill patients with limited movement—in some cases, with the added complication of obesity which involves deeper and more numerous skin folds—aids the infection (70). Other factors, such as diabetes mellitus, thermal injuries, and immunosuppression also predispose patients to candidal infections. On the local pulmonary level, use of inhaled corticoids helps the emergence of mucosal candidiasis (71).

The diagnosis can be supported by potassium hydroxide (KOH) exam of skin scrapings. Treatment includes hygiene, the avoidance of abrasion, and topical treatment with potassium permanganate, followed by topical clotrimazole or nystatin. Neutropenia and immunosuppression are risk factors in disseminated candidiasis, which may be seen as papules and pustules that extend over the entire body surface area. In these cases, systemic antifungal treatment—such as amphotericin B, fluconazole, voriconazole, or caspofungin—is advisable (72).

Reactions to Therapy in the ICU

ICU patients require multiple drug therapies, many of which are capable of inducing adverse reactions (73,74). Cutaneous involvement is the adverse reaction most frequently attributed to drugs (Table 168.7). Because the drugs have an antigenic potential determined by their physicochemical properties, there may be one of a number of immune reactions: Type I hypersensitivity reaction is defined as a fast-developing immunologic reaction that occurs in individuals having been previously sensitized by an antigen–antibody interaction. Urticaria

TABLE 168.7

DRUGS MOST COMMONLY ASSOCIATED WITH ACUTE ADVERSE DRUG REACTIONS

DRUGS MOST COMMONLY ASSOCIATED WITH ACUTE ADVERSE DRUG REACTIONS
PENICILLIN AND OTHER BETA-LACTAMS
■ Natural and semisynthetic penicillins
■ Cephalosporins
■ Monobactams
■ Carbapenems
NONSTEROIDAL ANTI-INFLAMMATORY
■ Salicylates
■ Indolacetics (indomethacin)
■ Aylacetic (diclofenac)
■ Propionic acid (ibuprofen)
■ Pyrazolones (metamizole)
■ Oxicams (piroxicam)
ANTIBIOTICS NON–BETA-LACTAMS
■ Tetracyclines
■ Sulfonamides
■ Levofloxacin
■ Azithromycin
■ Erythromycin
ANTICONVULSANTS
■ Phenytoin
■ Carbamazepine
■ Pentobarbital
■ Lamotrigine
ANTIHYPERTENSIVES
■ Angiotensin-converting enzyme inhibitors (ACEI)
■ Angiotensin II receptor antagonist (ARA II)
■ Thiazides
■ Diltiazem
OTHER
■ Contrast agents
■ Antiviral (acyclovir)
■ Antifungals (amphotericin B)
■ Steroids

and angioedema are the chemical expressions for these types of hypersensitivity reactions, with a morbilliform rash that is of unclear cause. Contact dermatitis is produced by a type IV hypersensitivity reaction through lymphocytes in skin that has been previously sensitized. In some cases, contact dermatitis is due to the direct irritative action of the external agent. However, secondary cutaneous necrosis to drugs is not an immunologic problem, but is attributed to direct toxicity of the exposed agent.

TEN and Stevens-Johnson syndrome also appear as a reaction to drugs, but, due to their seriousness and specific characteristics, these diseases are considered in their own right and are dealt with in a previous section.

Morbilliform Reactions

A morbilliform rash is the most common form of secondary rash caused by drugs, representing 40% of all drug reactions. With a rather unclear cause, it is characterized by erythematous macules and papules, generally symmetrically distributed,

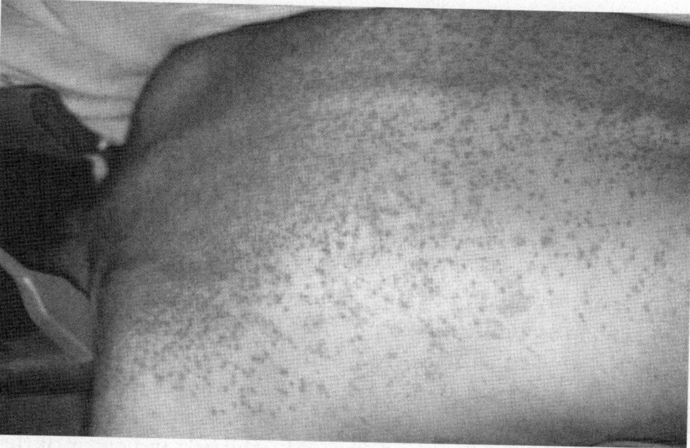

FIGURE 168.11. Maculopapular drug eruption. (Courtesy of J.M. Casanova, M.D.: http://www.dermatoweb.net.)

which can become confluent (Fig. 168.11). The rash usually begins on the trunk and in pressure-prone areas, subsequently extending to the extremities, and may include the mucous membranes, palms, and soles, although it does not usually affect the face. The morbilliform reaction usually appears about a week after starting the causative medication, and may last 1 to 2 weeks. The drugs most often associated with this rash are penicillin and its derivatives, sulfonamides, anticonvulsants, and allopurinol, although further exposure to the drug does not always cause a reappearance of the damage.

Urticaria and Angioedema

Urticaria is a skin lesion characterized by the emergence of wheals, defined as a confined elevation of the skin, erythematous or pale in the center, surrounded by an erythematous halo of variable size. In approximately half of all cases, urticaria is accompanied by angioedema that consists of edema of the deep dermis, the subcutaneous tissue, and the mucous membranes, including the respiratory and intestinal tract.

Multiple drugs are implicated in the emergence of urticaria/angioedema such as penicillin and other beta lactams, as well as nonsteroidal anti-inflammatory drugs that produce a type I urticarial eruption mediated by IgE. Codeine, morphine, other narcotics, and the iodine contrast agents can induce urticaria by nonimmunological degranulation of the mastocytes, independent of the IgE (75). Drug-induced urticaria produces a sudden benign and transitory eruption that normally disappears in less than 24 hours, and is characterized by the emergence of multiple erythematous papules and edema in any part of the body's surface, although it normally does not affect mucous membranes. It is normally pruritic, affecting mostly the scalp, palms, and soles. The lesions of angioedema have a variable coloration, from off-white to erythematous, are normally not painful, and usually last less than 24 hours. They are localized in areas where the dermis is thinnest, such as the face, and respiratory, gastrointestinal, and genitourinary mucous membranes. When it affects the oropharynx, it can produce acute compromise of the respiratory tract, creating a life-threatening situation that may require an urgent tracheostomy (76). Normally, angioedema accompanies the urticaria, although it may appear isolated as in cases of angioedema secondary to angiotensin-converting enzyme inhibitors or angioedema secondary to a deficit of C1 inhibitor (77,78).

Histologically, there are no differences between urticaria and angioedema. Edema of the dermis, vascular dilatation, and inflammatory perivascular infiltrate appear in both. The fundamental diagnosis is made clinically, and the treatment is based on the detection and withdrawal of the drugs that may be responsible, paying special attention to drugs administered within approximately the past 7 days. Treatment includes antihistamines (chlorpheniramine, 0.1 mg/kg), corticosteroids (methylprednisolone, 1 to 2 mg/kg), and, in case of respiratory tract compromise, epinephrine.

Angioedema due to C1 inhibitor deficiency, whether hereditary or acquired, is characterized by recurring episodes of peripheral angioedema associated with abdominal pain with variable clinical expression (79). The diagnosis is made through the evaluation of C4, which is decreased—the first indicator of the disease. Confirmation is noted by observing low levels of C1 inhibitor or a reduction of its functional activity. It is necessary to note that episodes of hereditary angioedema do not respond to normal treatment with epinephrine, antihistamines, and corticosteroids. The optimum treatment is the administration of concentrated C1 inhibitor (80).

Contact Dermatitis

Contact dermatitis is an eczematous disease attributed to an inflammatory reaction of the skin to external agents, irritants, or allergens. Irritative contact dermatitis is due to the direct action of a substance that provokes an inflammatory skin reaction without the intervention of an immunologic mechanism. Most cases of irritative dermatitis in the ICU are associated with hygienic body soap, iodine-based antiseptics, chlorhexidine (81), and the autoadhesive electrodes of continuous electrocardiographic monitoring (Fig. 168.12). Allergic contact dermatitis (ACD) is a delayed hypersensitivity reaction that is produced in skin previously sensitized to an allergen. There is a diverse range of topical drugs used commonly in the ICU that are capable of producing ACD—for example, transdermal nitroglycerin patches. It has also been related to antibiotics such as penicillin and sulfonamides, antihistamines, and corticosteroids (82).

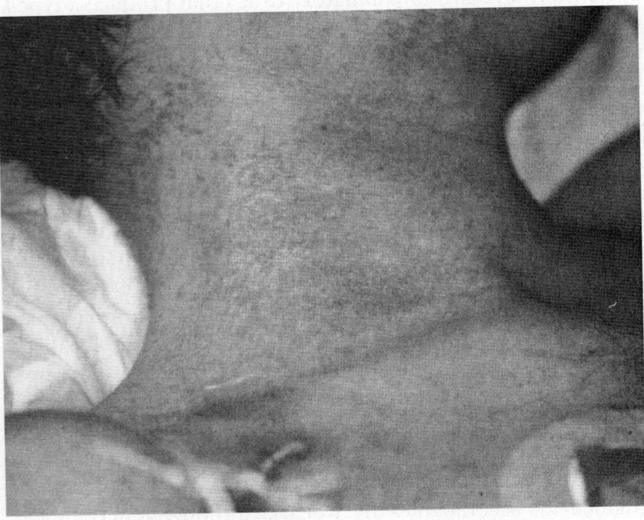

FIGURE 168.12. Irritant contact dermatitis associated with povidone-iodine.

Differentiation should be made between contact dermatitis and other eczematous disorders such as atopic dermatitis. Both are mediated by inflammatory mechanisms that provoke infiltrative inflammatory deposits in the dermis and epidermis, clinically expressed as erythema, with or without edema and vesicles (83). Typically, patients with contact dermatitis have an eczematous reaction with papules or vesicles over erythematous plaques and localized edema in areas exposed to the exogenous substance; intense pruritus is the most frequent symptom. Recent immunohistochemical studies show similar findings in both types of dermatitis, with similar morphologic characteristics, which is why distinguishing between the two can be difficult. Patch testing for ACD and a careful clinical history usually is the key to the diagnosis and allows it to be distinguished from other eczematous disorders (84). The treatment includes, first, withdrawal of the agent responsible, and symptomatic treatment with topical antihistamines and corticosteroids (85).

Skin Necrosis Induced by Drugs

Oral anticoagulants and intravenous vasopressor drugs can produce skin necrosis through alteration of blood circulation. Skin necrosis secondary to oral anticoagulants usually appears early, and is produced in areas rich in adipose tissue, such as the breast, buttocks, and thighs (86). It is characterized by pain and paresthesias, followed by erythema and purpuric lesions that quickly progress to extensive ecchymotic areas that are well circumscribed and blue-black in color with erythematous halos. The lesions can evolve into painful ulcers covered by necrotic eschar. Generally, skin necrosis is associated with congenital or acquired deficiency of protein C and/or S (87,88). The deficiency of these proteins generates a state of initial transitory hypercoagulability that provokes local thrombosis of the veins of the dermis and the subcutaneous cell tissue.

Skin necrosis can also appear as a complication of the infusion of vasopressor drugs, requiring, in some cases, amputation of the affected extremity. Classically, it is related to the use of high doses of dopamine and norepinephrine, but other associated factors—apart from the vasoconstriction provoked by the drug—have been considered to provoke tíssue necrosís. The existence of disseminated intravascular coagulation and hypovolemia are risk factors for the development of gangrene related to vasopressors (89–91). Vasopressin, useful in the treatment of catecholamine-resistant vasodilatory shock, may also provoke cutaneous ischemia, due to its vasoconstrictor action on the arteriolar level. This is particularly true in patients with preexisting peripheral arteriopathy and in the presence of septic shock (92). The ischemic skin lesions are normally localized in the distal area of the extremities and the trunk; interestingly, approximately 20% of patients may develop lingual ischemia. When the administration of vasopressin is by a peripheral vein, it may provoke local cutaneous ischemia if it infiltrates into the subcutaneous tissue. To avoid the potential for ischemic lesions, administration of vasopressin should be by central venous catheter, and careful monitoring of the extremities to detect ischemic changes should be carried out (93). The application of topical nitroglycerin, in addition to decreasing the dose of the vasopressor, may improve the symptoms and signs of ischemia (94).

DERMATOLOGIC DISORDERS IN SPECIFIC SITUATIONS

Graft Versus Host Disease

The allogenic transplant of hematopoietic stem cells is a procedure used to treat various malignant diseases, above all those of hematologic origin. Graft versus host disease (GVHD) is the most important complication in stem cell transplantation and occurs because of the introduction of immunologically competing cells into an immunodepressed host. It is the main cause of morbidity and death in transplant patients. GVHD is termed chronic or acute, depending on the time of appearance—before or after 100 days from the stem cell transplant (95).

Acute GVHD usually occurs between days 10 and 40 following the transplant. Its main manifestations are in the skin, liver, and gastrointestinal tract, secondary to damage to the epithelial cells of these areas. The integumentary effect is the most frequent dysfunction. This involvement begins with pain or itching, followed by a maculopapular rash resembling measles. The initial involved areas are the cheeks, neck, ears, palms, and soles and, later, the upper back. The early injuries can be folliculocentric blanching erythematous macules or papules, which are suggestive of GVHD, accompanied by very painful mouth ulcers. If not serious, the injuries can resolve spontaneously or after increasing the immune suppressant treatment. The most severe cases progress to generalized erythroderma, which, in some cases, develops into desquamative bullae similar to TEN with a positive Nikolsky sign. Apart from integumentary involvement, GVHD is accompanied by an effect on the liver, with abdominal pain and a pattern of cholestasis with associated elevated bilirubin and alkaline phosphate. In the gastrointestinal tract, GVHD is characterized by abdominal pain, secretory diarrhea, and, sometimes, intestinal bleeding.

Chronic GVHD often appears in patients who have previously suffered the acute form of GVHD. Other risk factors are advanced age of the donor, high level of histo-incompatibility, and previous total body irradiation. Chronic GVHD is characterized by its effect on the skin, oral mucous membranes, eyes, and salivary glands. The respiratory and gastrointestinal tract and the liver may also be affected. The skin lesions are characterized by an early lichenoid phase and a late sclerodermiform phase. Cutaneous biopsy confirms the diagnosis.

Treatment must be directed toward preventing GVHD by depleting lymphocytes in the graft donor and using immunosuppressants such as cyclosporin combined with methotrexate and corticosteroids (96). If, in spite of this treatment, the patient develops GVHD, an augmented dose of systemic steroids, cyclosporine, and azathioprine may be attempted to gain control. If it persists, photochemotherapy with psoralen and UV-A irradiation has been shown to be beneficial (97). Thalidomide and extracorporeal photopheresis have also been shown to be effective (98).

Acquired Immunodeficiency Syndrome

Infection with the human immunodeficiency virus (HIV) and the acquired immunodeficiency syndrome are related to many integumentary and mucous membrane manifestations. This damage is due to disrupted immunologic function, and may often be the first sign of the disease or a mark of its progress.

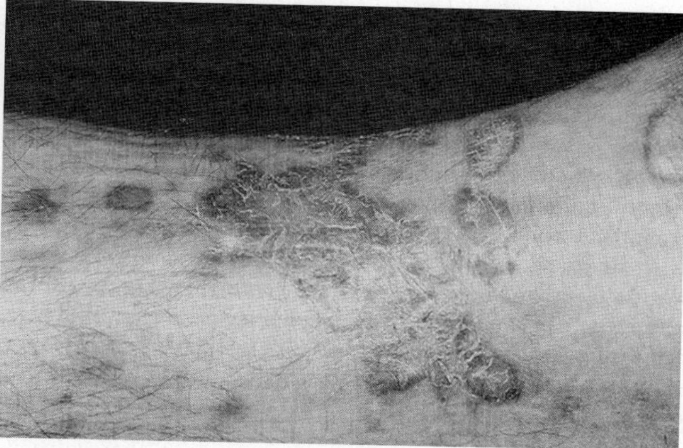

FIGURE 168.13. Cutaneous Kaposi sarcoma associated with acquired immunodeficiency syndrome. (Courtesy of J.M. Casanova, M.D.: http://www.dermatoweb.net.)

The severity and extent of the skin disorders related to HIV depends on the degree of immunodeficiency. During the asymptomatic phase of the infection, the immunologic response, although disrupted, maintains a dynamic balance against the activity of the virus, and is also capable of defending itself against opportunistic intruders. In this state, the main cutaneous manifestations are seborrheic dermatitis, psoriasis, xeroderma, and pruritic papular rashes. As the infection advances and the immunologic response diminishes, these skin diseases tend to become more chronic and severe, and opportunist infections appear, along with other more unusual disorders such as oral hairy leukoplakia, chronic herpes simplex, cryptococcosis, Kaposi sarcoma, etc. (Fig. 168.13).

The variety of integumentary disorders during the course of the infection is a consequence of the progressive immunodeficiency and of the underlying disease (99). The adoption of combined antiretroviral therapy in the treatment of HIV infection has changed the course of the disease, reducing the levels of viral proliferation and allowing a partial reconstitution of immunity. With combined antiretroviral treatment, the frequency of opportunist infections has significantly decreased and greater control of other dermatologic processes, such as psoriasis and seborrheic dermatitis, has been achieved (100).

PRIOR DERMATOLOGIC DISORDERS

Skin disorders are frequent in the general population. Patients with chronic skin disorders may require admission to the ICU for a life-threatening disease that has nothing to do with the skin, but we must also take the latter into account, along with other comorbidities, such as atrial fibrillation, diabetes mellitus, hypertension, and so forth, as some skin disorders may require specific care.

The diagnosis of a previous dermatologic disorder is optimally made with the clinical history, although sometimes, due to the severity of illness or sedation, the patient cannot assist with the history, and the definitive diagnosis can be verified with a dermatologist consultant.

Some chronic skin diseases, including psoriasis and diseases of the connective tissue, because of their development in outbreaks, can become acute during admission to the ICU and require specific treatment. Other common processes, such as lichen planus and atopic eczema, may require symptomatic treatment. Some chronic processes need prolonged treatment with antibiotics, corticosteroids, and/or immunosuppressive agents. These previous and ongoing treatments may require an alteration of our standard ICU guidelines or protocols. There are some processes, however, such as diabetic dermopathy, skin tumors, altered pigmentation, etc., that do not require specific care.

References

1. Vicent JL, Baltopoulos G, Bihari D, et al. Guidelines for training in intensive care medicine. *Intensive Care Med.* 1994;20:80.
2. Badia M, Trujillano J, Gasco E, et al. Skin lesions in the ICU. *Intensive Care Med.* 1999;25:1271.
3. Peter RU. Cutaneous manifestations in intensive care patients. *Intensive Care Med.* 1998;24:997.
4. Haake AR, Holbrook K. The structure and development of skin. In: Freedberg IM, Eisen AZ, Wolff K, et al., eds. *Dermatology in General Medicine.* 5th ed. New York, NY: McGraw-Hill; 1999:70.
5. Vaishampayan SS, Sharma YK, Das AL, et al. Emergencies in dermatology: acute skin failure. *MJAFI.* 2006;62:56.
6. García-Patos Briones V. Cuidados intensivos en dermatología. *Piel.* 1992;7: 277–285.
7. Irvine C. "Skin failure"—a real entity: discussion paper. *J Royal Soc Med.* 1991;84:412.
8. Herti M, Eming R, Veldman C. T cell control in autoimmune bullous skin disorders. *J Clin Invest.* 2006;116:1159.
9. Brenner S, Sasson A, Sharon O. Pemphigus and infections. *Clin Dermatol.* 2002;20:114.
10. Badia M, Trujillano J, Casanova JM, et al. Pénfigo de evolución fatal. Concepto de insuficiencia cutánea. *Med Intensiva.* 1994;2:85.
11. Scully C, Challacombe SJ. Pemphigus vulgaris: update on etiopathogenesis, oral manifestations, and management. *Crit Rev Oral Biol Med.* 2002;13:397.
12. Ruocco E, Baroni A, Wolf R, et al. Life-threatening bullous dermatoses: pemphigus vulgaris. *Clin Dermatol.* 2005;23:223.
13. Sánchez-Pérez J, García-Díez A. Pemphigus. *Actas Dermasifiliogr.* 2005;96: 329.
14. Fellner MJ, Sapadin AN. Current therapy of pemphigus vulgaris. *Mount Sinai J Med.* 2001;68:268.
15. Tirado-Sánchez A, León-Dorantes G. Treatment of pemphigus vulgaris. An overview in Mexico. *Allergol Immunolpathol.* 2006;34:10.
16. Harman KE, Albert S, Black MM. Guidelines for the management of pemphigus vulgaris. *Br J Dermatol.* 2003;149:926.
17. Bystryn JC, Rudolph JL. Pemphigus. *Lancet.* 2005;366:61.
18. Pitarch G, Sánchez-Carazo JL, Pardo J, et al. Treatment of severe refractory pemphigus vulgaris with rituximab. *Actas Dermosifiliogr.* 2006;97:10.
19. McCuin JB, Hanlon T, Mutasim DF. Autoimmune bullous diseases: diagnosis and treatment. *Dermatol Nurs.* 2006;18:20.
20. Stanley JR. Bullous pemphigoid. In: Freedberg IM, Eisen AZ, Wolff K, et al., eds. *Dermatology in General Medicine.* 5th ed. New York, NY: McGraw-Hill; 1999:666.
21. Khumalo NP, Murrell DF, Wojnarowska F, et al. A systematic review of treatments for bullous pemphigoid. *Arch Dermatol.* 2002;138:385.
22. Mengesha YM, Bennett ML. Pustular skin disorders. Diagnosis and treatment. *Am J Clin Dermatol.* 2002;3:389.
23. Sharkey MP, Muir JB. Staphylococcal scalded skin syndrome complicating acute generalized pustular psoriasis. *Australas J Dermatol.* 2002;43: 199.
24. Umezawa Y, Ozawa A, Kawasima T, et al. Therapeutic guidelines for the treatment of generalized pustular psoriasis (GPP) based on a proposed classification of disease severity. *Arch Dermatol Res.* 2003;295:S43.
25. Balasubramaniam P, Berth-Jones J. Erythroderma: 90% skin failure. *Hosp Med.* 2004;65:100.
26. Rothe MJ, Bernstein ML, Grant-Kels JM. Life-threatening erythroderma: diagnosing and treating the "red man." *Clin Dermatol.* 2005;23:206.
27. Lyell A. Toxic epidermal necrolysis: an eruption resembling scalding of the skin. *Br J Dermatol.* 1956;68:355.
28. Bachot N, Roujeau JC. Differential diagnosis of severe cutaneous drug eruptions. *Am J Clin Dermatol.* 2003;4:561.
29. Wolf R, Orion E, Marcos B, et al. Life-threatening acute adverse cutaneous drug reactions. *Clin Dermatol.* 2005;23:168.
30. Letko E, Papaliodis DN, Papaliodis GN, et al. Stevens-Johnson syndrome and toxic epidermal necrolysis: a review of the literature. *Ann Allergy Asthma Immunol.* 2005;94:419.
31. Chave TA, Mortimer NJ, Sladden MJ, et al. Toxic epidermal necrolysis: current evidence, practical management and future directions. *Br J Dermatol.* 2005;153:241.
32. de Juan Martín F, Bouthelier Moreno M, Marín Bravo MC, et al. Toxic epidermal necrolysis treated with intravenous immunoglobulin [in Spanish]. *An Esp Pediatr.* 2002;56:370.
33. García Doval I, Roujeau JC, Cruces Prado MJ. Toxic epidermal necrolysis and Stevens-Johnson syndrome: new issues in classification and therapy. *Actas Dermosifiliogr.* 2000;91:541.
34. Auquier-Dunant A, Mockenhaupt M, Naldi L, et al. Correlations between clinical patterns and causes of erythema multiforme majus, Stevens-Johnson syndrome, and toxic epidermal necrolysis. *Arch Dermatol.* 2002;138:1019.
35. Ghislain PD, Roujeau JC. Treatment of severe drug reactions: Stevens-Johnson syndrome, toxic epidermal necrolysis and hypersensitivity syndrome. *Dermatol Online J.* 2002;8:5.
36. Payne AS, Hanakawa Y, Amagai M, et al. Desmosomes and disease: pemphigus and bullous impetigo. *Curr Opin Cell Biol.* 2004;16:536.
37. Ramos-e-Silva M, Cardozo Pereira AL. Life-threatening eruptions due to infectious agents. *Clin Dermatol.* 2005;23:148.
38. Nair PS, Moorthy PK, Yogiragan K. A study of mortality in dermatology. *Indian J Dermatol Venerol Leprol.* 2005;71:23.
39. Welch SB, Nadel S. Treatment of meningococcal infection. *Arch Dis Child.* 2003;88:608.
40. Brown KL, Stein A, Morrell DS. Ecthyma gangrenosum and septic shock syndrome secondary to *Chromobacterium violaceum*. *J Am Acad Dermatol.* 2006;54:S224.
41. Asumang A, Goldsmith AL, Dryden M. Subcutaneous nodules with *Pseudomonas septicaemia* in an immunocompetent patient. *Anaesth Intensive Care.* 1999;27:213.
42. Solowski NL, Yao FB, Agarwal A, et al. Ecthyma gangrenosum: a rare cutaneous manifestation of a potentially fatal disease. *Ann Otol Rhinol Laryngo.*2004;113:462.
43. Vinson RP, Chung A, Elston DM, et al. Septic microemboli in a Janeway lesion of bacterial endocarditis. *J Am Acad Dermatol.* 1996;35:984.
44. Cardullo AC, Silvers DN, Grossman ME. Janeway lesions and Osler's nodes: a review of histopathologic findings. *J Am Acad Dermatol.* 1990;22:1088.
45. Chung L, Lin J, Furst DE, et al. Systemic and localized scleroderma. *Clin Dermatol.* 2006;24:374.
46. Rothfield N, Sontheimer RD, Bernstein M. Lupus erythematosus: systemic and cutaneous manifestations. *Clin Dermatol.* 2006;24:348.
47. Callen JP, Wortmann RL. Dermatomyositis. *Clin Dermatol.* 2006;24:363.
48. Carlson JA, Cavaliere LF, Grant-Kels JM. Cutaneous vasculitis: diagnosis and management. *Clin Dermatol.* 2006;24:414.
49. Semple D, Keogh J, Forni L, et al. Clinical review: casculitis on the intensive care unit, 1: diagnosis. *Crit Care.* 2005;9:92.
50. Matz H, Orion Wolf R. Bacterial infections: uncommon presentations. *Clin Dermatol.* 2005;23:503.
51. George A, Rubin G. A systematic review and meta-analysis of treatments for impetigo. *Br J Gen Pract.* 2003;53:480.
52. Rebora A. Life-threatening cutaneous viral diseases. *Clin Dermatol.* 2005; 23:157.
53. Pineda V. Aspectos clinicoepidemiológicos de la neumonía neumocócica. Diagnóstico diferencial. *An Pediatr, Monogr.* 2003;1:14.
54. Stevens JG, Cook ML, Jordan MC. Reactivation of latent herpes simplex virus after pneumococcal pneumonia in mice. *Infect Immun.* 1975;11:635.
55. Moloney FJ, Keane S, O'Kelly P, et al. The impact of skin disease following renal transplantation on quality of life. *Br J Dermatol.* 2005;153:574.
56. Griffiths WJH, Wreghitt TG, Alexander GJ. Reactivation of herpes simplex virus after liver transplantation. *Transplantation.* 2005;80:1353.
57. Hashizume H, Yagi H, Ohshima A, et al. Comparable risk of herpes virus infection between topical treatments with tacrolimus and corticosteroids in adults with atopic dermatitis. *Br J Dermatol.* 2006;154:1204.
58. Pruitt BA, McManus AT, Kim SH, et al. Burn wound infections: current status. *World J Surg.* 1998;22:135.
59. Arduino PG, Porter SR. Oral and perioral herpes simplex virus type 1 (HSV-1) infection: review of its management. *Oral Dis.* 2006;12:254.
60. Paradisi A, Capizzi R, Guerriero G, et al. Kaposi's varicelliform eruption complicating allergic contact dermatitis. *J Am Acad Dermatol.* 2006;54:732.
61. Peña L, Izaguirre D, Aguirrebengoa K, et al. Varicella pneumonia in adults: review of 22 cases. *Enferm Infecc Microbiol Clin.* 2000;18:493.
62. Gregorakos L, Myrianthefs P, Markou N, et al. Severity of illness and outcome in adult patients with primary varicella pneumonia. *Respiration.* 2002;69:330.
63. Mohsen AH, McKendrick M. Varicella pneumonia in adults. *Eur Respir J.* 2003;21:886.
64. Adhami N, Arabi Y, Raees A, et al. Effect of corticosteroids on adult varicella pneumonia: Cohort study and literature review. *Respirology.* 2006;11:437.

65. Stankus SJ, Dlugopolski M, Packer D. Management of herpes zoster (shingles) and postherpetic neuralgia. *Am Fam Physician.* 2000;61:2437.
66. Cohen JI, Brunell PA, Straus SE, et al. Recent advances in varicella-zoster virus infection. *Ann Intern Med.* 1999;130:922.
67. Shen MC, Lin HH, Lee SS, et al. Double-blind, randomized, acyclovir-controlled, parallel-group trial comparing the safety and efficacy of famciclovir and acyclovir in patients with uncomplicated herpes zoster. *J Microbiol Immunol Infect.* 2004;37:75.
68. Mounsey A, Matthew LG, Slawson DC. Herpes zoster and postherpetic neuralgia: prevention and management. *Am Fam Physician.* 2005;72:1075.
69. Janniger CK, Schwartz RA. Intertrigo and common secondary skin infections. *Am Fam Physician.* 2005;72:833.
70. Scheinfeld NS. Obesity and dermatology. *Clin Dermatol.* 2004;22:303.
71. Guillot B. Adverse skin reactions to inhaled corticosteroids. *Expert Opin Drug Saf.* 2002;1:325.
72. Huang DB, Ostrosky-Zeichner L, Wu JJ. Therapy of common superficial fungal infections. *Dermatol Ther.* 2004;17:517.
73. Vargas E, Terleira A, Hernando F, et al. Effect of adverse drug reactions on length of stay in surgical intensive care units. *Crit Care Med.* 2003;31:694.
74. Campos-Fernández Mdel M, Ponce-de-León-Rosales S, Archer-Dubon C, et al. Incidence and risk factors for cutaneous adverse drug reactions in an intensive care unit. *Rev Invest Clin.* 2005;57:770.
75. Nigen S, Knowles SR, Shear NH. Drug eruptions: approaching the diagnosis of drug-induced skin diseases. *J Drugs Dermatol.* 2003;2:278.
76. Lipozencic J, Wolf R. Life-threatening severe allergic reactions: urticaria, angioedema, and anaphylaxis. *Clin Dermatol.* 2005;23:193.
77. Sondhi D, Lippmann M, Murali G. Airway compromise due to angiotensin-converting enzyme inhibitor-induced angioedema. *Chest.* 2004;126:400.
78. Kaplan AP, Greaves MW. Angioedema. *J Am Acad Dermatol.* 2005;53:373.
79. Sánchez-Morillas L, Reaño Martos M, González Sánchez L, et al. Hereditary angioedema of delayed onset. *An Med Interna.* 2004;21:84.
80. Fay A, Abinum M. Current management of hereditary angio-oedema (C'1 esterase inhibitor deficiency) *J Clin Pathol.* 2002;55:266.
81. Garland JS, Alex CP, Mueller CD, et al. A randomized trial comparing povidone-iodine to a chlorhexidine gluconate-impregnated dressing for prevention of central venous catheter infections in neonates. *Pediatrics.* 2001; 107:1431.
82. Goh CL. Nonoccupational contact dermatitis. *Clin Dermatol.* 1998;16:119.
83. Akhavan A, Cohen SR. The relationship between atopic dermatitis and contact dermatitis. *Clin Dermatol.* 2003;21:158.
84. Rietschel RL. Clues to an accurate diagnosis of contact dermatitis. *Dermatol Ther.* 2004;17:224.
85. Cohen DE, Heidary N. Treatment of irritant and allergic contact dermatitis. *Dermatol Ther.* 2004;17:334.
86. Argaud L, Guerin C, Thomas L, et al. Extensive coumarin-induced skin necrosis in a patient with acquired protein C deficiency. *Intensive Care Med.* 2001;27:1555.
87. Muniesa C, Marcoval J. Coumarin induced skin necrosis. *Piel.* 2004;19:255.
88. Valdivielso M, Longo I, Lecona M, et al. Cutaneous necrosis induced by acenocoumarol. *J Eur Acad Dermatol Venereol.* 2004;18:211.
89. Hayes MA, Yau EH, Hinds CJ, et al. Symmetrical peripheral gangrene: association with noradrenaline administration. *Intensive Care Med.* 1992; 18:433.
90. Winkler MJ, Trunkey DD. Dopamine gangrene. Association with disseminated intravascular coagulation. *Am J Surg.* 1981;142:588.
91. Kaul S, Sarela AI, Supe AN, et al. Gangrene complicating dopamine therapy. *J R Soc Med.* 1997;90:80.
92. Düsner MW, Mayr AJ, Tür A, et al. Ischemic skin lesions as a complication of continuous vasopressin infusion in catecholamine-resistant vasodilatory shock: incidence and risk factors. *Crit Care Med.* 2003;31:1394.
93. Kahn JM, Kress JP, Hall JB. Skin necrosis after extravasation of low-dose vasopressin administered for septic shock. *Crit Care Med.* 2002;30:1899.
94. Anderson ME, Moore TL, Hollis S, et al. Digital vascular response to topical glyceryl trinitrate, as measured by laser Doppler imaging, in primary Raynaud's phenomenon and systemic sclerosis. *Rheumatology.* 2002;41: 324.
95. Vargas-Díez E, García-Díez A, Marín A, et al. Life-threatening graft-vs-host disease. *Clin Dermatol.* 2005;23:285.
96. Ruocco V, Sacerdoti G, Farro P, et al. Adverse drug reactions and graft-versus-host reaction: unapproved treatments. *Clin Dermatol.* 2002;20: 672.
97. Pinton PC, Porta F, Izzi T, et al. Prospects for ultraviolet A1 phototherapy as a treatment for chronic cutaneous graft-versus-host disease. *Haematologica.* 2003;88:1169.
98. Wu JJ, Huang DB, Pang KR, et al. Thalidomide: dermatological indications, mechanisms of action and side-effects. *Br J Dermato.* 2005;153:254.
99. Rigopoulos D, Paparizos V, Katsambas A. Cutaneous markers of HIV infection. *Clin Dermatol.* 2004;22:487.
100. Chang YC, Tyring SK. Therapy of HIV infection. *Dermatol Ther.* 2004;17: 449.

CHAPTER 169 ■ PREVENTION OF PRESSURE INJURIES IN THE INTENSIVE CARE UNIT

MATTHEW JAMES PETERSON • KATHLEEN E. FITZGERALD • LAWRENCE J. CARUSO

Pressure ulcers are painful, debilitating, and severely compromise an individual's health by increasing morbidity in terms of increased length of stay, risk of infection, and the need for additional surgical procedures. Also known as pressure sores, decubitus ulcers, and bedsores, pressure ulcers are a common problem in hospitals and nursing homes alike. They increase the nursing workload by 50% (1), and, in patients with clinically relevant pressure ulcers, the length of hospital stay increases by an average of 11 days (2). Generally, pressure ulcers are thought to be preventable, making this an important patient safety and risk management issue. It is a concern for patients, but also for hospitals and caregivers alike, as the incidence of pressure ulcers is used as an indicator of quality of care (3). Unfortunately, there are few objective data regarding methods of prevention, and current recommendations are based largely on expert opinion (4,5).

THE PRESSURE ULCER PROBLEM: INCIDENCE AND COSTS

The prevalence of pressure ulcers can range anywhere from 0% to over 33%, depending on the sector—from general or university hospitals to home care to nursing homes (3,6–14). Among ICU patients, prevalence has been reported to be roughly 14% (15). At our institution, Shands Hospital at the University of Florida, most hospital-acquired pressure ulcers documented in 2005 through September 2006 occurred in intensive care unit (ICU) patients (16). Not only are pressure ulcers a serious health threat to the patient, but they are extremely costly to the patient and the hospital or caregiver as well. It has been estimated that $11 billion* is spent on pressure ulcer treatment each year in the United States alone (13), with similar costs seen around the globe (8,9,11,17,18). The cost to manage one full-thickness ulcer can be as much as $70,000 (13).

In addition to the costs, pressure ulcers are considered preventable and have become a liability for hospitals and caregivers (6,17). The incidence of pressure ulcers is an indicator of quality of care as outlined by programs conforming to U.S. national Medicare and Medicaid requirements (3,6). Lawsuits have been filed against hospitals and caregivers by patients who have developed pressure ulcers. The verdicts in many of these lawsuits have been in favor of the afflicted plaintiffs under the claim of malpractice or negligence (7,11). In the 15-year span from 1983 to 1997, award settlements in the United States ranged from $2,200 to $65 million, with an average award of $250,000 (6,7).

ETIOLOGY AND RISK FACTORS OF PRESSURE ULCERS

By definition from the National Pressure Ulcer Advisory Panel (NPUAP) (19), a pressure ulcer is localized injury to the skin and/or underlying tissue usually over a bony prominence, as a result of pressure, or pressure in combination with shear and/or friction. Several contributing or confounding factors are also associated with pressure ulcers; the significance of these factors is yet to be elucidated.

High pressures can lead to ischemia of the affected tissue (20), resulting in a lack of oxygen transport and nutrients to the tissue. Oxygen delivery is compromised when the pressure applied over an area is greater than the capillary-closing pressure. Normal capillary pressures in the body range from about 10 to 30 mm Hg (21). Lower capillary-closing pressure values have been observed in unhealthy patients (22). When interface pressures, the pressure between the patient's body and his or her supporting surface—exceed these limits, reduced blood flow, accumulation of metabolites via lymphatic occlusion, and impairment of tissue reperfusion may occur, all of which can damage tissue (23–25).

It should be acknowledged that the measurement of interface pressures is not the direct measurement of the internal pressures experienced by the various internal tissues and vessels of the body (26). However, interface pressure mapping is the best method to noninvasively measure pressures exerted on the skin. Although not internal, these pressure measurements give the clinician investigator a good idea of the pressures exerted on the tissue just below the surface of the skin. Qualitatively, it should be recognized that increasing or decreasing interface pressures will consequently raise or lower the resulting internal pressures felt by the various internal tissues.

Not only is the magnitude of the pressure a factor, but its duration as well (20,27). The longer pressure is applied to one area, the more likely pressure ulcers will develop. One of the first studies demonstrating that pressure and time affects pressure ulcer formation was that of Kosiak in 1961 (28). This phenomenon was further studied by Reswick and Rogers in 1976. By measuring skin–cushion interface pressures on human volunteers and patients, they demonstrated an inverse relationship between pressure and time (28,29); the greater the pressure, the less time needed for pressure ulcer formation. Additional contributing factors for pressure ulcer formation are shear and frictional forces. Rubbing that occurs between a patient and his or her mattress sheets is a frictional force that can lead to additional undesired effects on underlying tissues. Shearing forces occur when the patient's skin sticks to the support surface and results in underlying tissue movement. This motion confers additional stresses on the underlying tissue, making it more susceptible to damage. In a porcine study carried out by Dinsdale in 1974, the presence of friction significantly increased the formation of pressure ulcers; the studies of Goldstein and Sanders in 1998 confirmed that skin breakdown occurred more rapidly as shear was increased (30).

Consequently, individuals who are at risk for pressure ulcers are those who have an altered state of consciousness and/or are physically unable to reposition themselves. Groups of patients immediately and obviously at risk are those with spinal cord injuries, paralysis, and significant thermal injuries (31), as well as those mechanically ventilated, and, in some instances, the weak or elderly. Patients with high pain thresholds or on pain medication may also be at risk, as they may not feel the need to periodically reposition themselves. More detailed pressure ulcer assessments are presented below.

PRESSURE ULCER LOCATIONS OF OCCURRENCE AND STAGES OF DEVELOPMENT

As we note, pressure sores are caused by unrelieved pressure (25,27). Pressure ulcers are most commonly found over and around bony prominences, locations where interface pressures are the greatest (20,27). Most pressure sores are found in the gluteal and sacral regions (30,32,33), notably around the sacrum, coccyx, and ischial tuberosities. The next most prevalent locations of pressure ulcers are found in the lower extremity, primarily the back of the heel, with the remaining found elsewhere on the body such as on the back, upper extremities, or the head (32,33).

According to the NPUAP, there are now six stages of pressure ulcer classification—an alteration from the traditionally four—ranging from suspected injury and initial redness to full-thickness tissue loss and necrosis. Despite the numbered stages of severity, the development and the healing of pressure ulcers do not necessarily pass consecutively from one stage to the next. All six stages are defined as follows (19):

Suspected deep tissue injury: Purple or maroon localized area of discolored intact skin or blood-filled blister due to damage of underlying soft tissue from pressure and/or shear. The area may be preceded by tissue that is painful, firm, mushy, boggy, and either warmer or cooler as compared to adjacent tissue.

Stage I: Intact skin with nonblanchable redness of a localized area usually over a bony prominence. Darkly pigmented skin may not have visible blanching; its color may differ from the surrounding area.

*Figures are in U.S. dollars.

Stage II: Partial-thickness loss of dermis presenting as a shallow open ulcer with a red pink wound bed, without slough. May also present as an intact or open/ruptured serum-filled blister.

Stage III: Full-thickness tissue loss. Subcutaneous fat may be visible but bone, tendon, or muscle are not exposed. Slough may be present but does not obscure the depth of tissue loss. May include undermining and tunneling.

Stage IV: Full-thickness tissue loss with exposed bone, tendon, or muscle. Slough or eschar may be present on some parts of the wound bed. Often includes undermining and tunneling.

Unstageable: Full-thickness tissue loss in which the base of the ulcer is covered by slough (yellow, tan, gray, green, or brown) and/or eschar (tan, brown, or black) in the wound bed.

PREVENTION OF PRESSURE ULCERS

As noted above, there are many contributing factors that tend to make a patient more susceptible to pressure ulcers. By noting these factors, several assessment tools, besides age, have been developed to try to prioritize those patients at higher risk. The Braden and Norton scales are widely used scales for pressure ulcer prevention (6,34). The Braden scale assesses six parameters: activity, dietary intake, mobility, sensory perception, friction, and skin moisture; the Norton scale assesses five parameters: activity, physical condition, mobility, mental status, and incontinence (6). These tools can be good predictors of at-risk patients, but have not been proved to be any more effective than clinical judgment (18) and are by no means fail-safe.

Once at-risk patients have been identified, there are several options to help provide the best possible care for these individuals. A wide variety of devices and methods are used to prevent pressure ulcers—from pressure-reducing and alternating air pressure mattresses to turning practices—which are described below (22).

Devices

Starting with the air support systems, various devices include mattresses, beds, and overlays. Alternating pressure air systems are the most common, and consist of a dynamic pressure-relieving system that alternates inflation among a variable number of cells of a mattress or overlay. Some systems are also sensitive to the patient's weight and adjust accordingly. Other pressure-reducing or support systems besides air include fiber, foam, gel, and water. The fiber support systems are overlays made from silicon hollow-core fiber that look like a duvet (i.e., a down comforter) and are divided into diagonal segments. The foam support systems are either overlays or mattresses that are made of multiple layers of foam with various densities that allow the patient to sink into the foam to distribute his or her weight. The gel systems are overlays that contain thick polymer gels or mattresses that consist of a gel that flows from cell to cell. Last, the water support systems consist of beds and overlays that use the buoyant effect of water to reduce pressures.

Methods

An alternative to pressure-relieving or -reducing devices is manual turning or repositioning of patients. Turning patients regularly every 2 hours to relieve interface pressures is one of the most common and reasonably effective pressure ulcer prevention methods and is considered a standard of care (10,20,34–37). However, in a study that implemented a turn-team with the goal of lowering pressure ulcer incidence rates, there was no statistically significant reduction in incidence despite a statistically significant decrease in average length of stay in the intensive care unit (3). Recent turning studies have attempted to determine the effectiveness of turning frequency. One demonstrated that turning every 4 hours on a viscoelastic foam mattress was better than turning every 2 or 3 hours on a standard mattress (36). Another study showed that unequal time intervals, 2-hour lateral and 4-hour supine versus 4-hour turning, showed fewer—although not a statistically significant difference—pressure ulcers in the more frequently turned group (37). Despite the research efforts, it is still unclear what turning protocols are safest for the patient and yet time- and cost-effective for caregivers.

RESEARCH

Preliminary research has addressed the interface pressures in healthy volunteers. The interface pressure between volunteers and an ICU bed was studied as the head of bed (HOB) was incrementally elevated from 0 to 75 degrees. Additionally, the interface pressure was studied as the volunteers were laterally turned every 2 hours; this standard of care was thought to prevent ulcer formation.

Effects of Elevating the Head of Bed

ICU patients are at particular risk for both pressure ulcers and ventilator-associated pneumonia (VAP) due to multiple predisposing factors. Current guidelines for mechanically ventilated patients recommend that they be kept in a semirecumbent position, with the HOB elevated 30 to 45 degrees to prevent aspiration and VAP (38). Although there is good evidence that the semirecumbent position has pulmonary benefits, its effect on pressure ulcer risk has not been defined.

Our group has assessed the effects of elevating the HOB on interface pressures over the buttocks and sacrum. Nine healthy volunteers were dressed in hospital scrubs and positioned supine on a modern ICU bed (Total Care, Hill-Rom, San Antonio, TX). A 48 by 48 array of half-inch sensors (2,304 total sensors) constituting a 2 foot by 2 foot square pad was positioned under the sacrum. A calibrated interface-pressure profile was acquired for each subject in the supine position, followed by progressive elevation of the head of the bed to 10, 20, 30, 45, 60, and 75 degrees, using the Xsensor (Calgary, Canada) interface pressure system (39).

Figure 169.1 presents the averaged subject data as the area over which an interface pressure greater than 30 mm Hg was obtained. Figure 169.2 presents the averaged subject peak-pressure data. A Wilcoxon rank sum test showed significant differences between the supine and the elevated HOB positions of greater than or equal to 45 degrees for both the peak interface

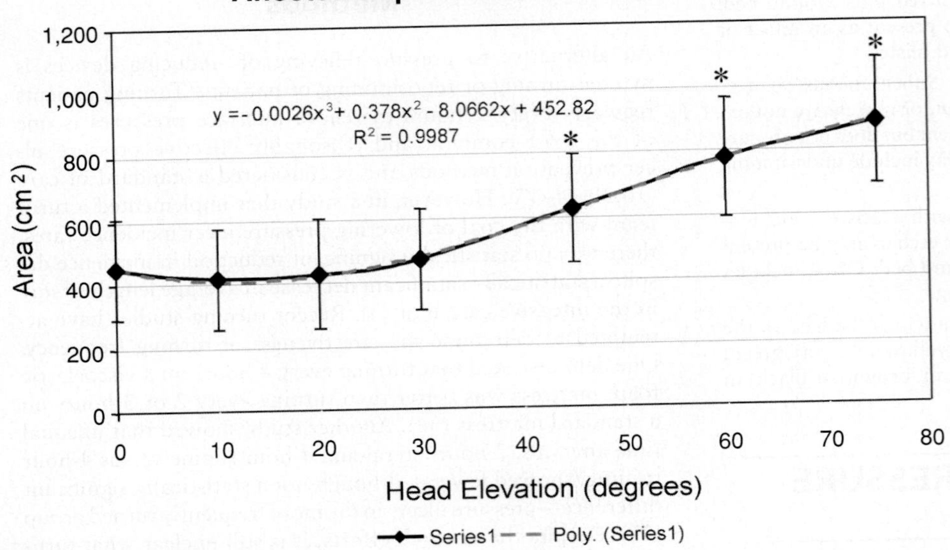

FIGURE 169.1. Affected supine area over 30 mm Hg. *p <0.05 compared to supine.

pressure and the affected area with a pressure greater than 30 mm Hg (p <0.05, two-tailed test). Figure 169.3 presents, visually, how the interface pressure and the affected area over 30 mm Hg increase over the sacral region when the HOB is elevated. It was found that raising the HOB to 45 degrees or higher to prevent pulmonary complications increases the interface pressure and the affected area between the skin and support surface, and may therefore increase the risk of pressure ulcers attributed to a skin–ICU bed interface pressure greater than 30 mm Hg.

Effects of Side Turning

Frequent turning of the patient from side to side is used routinely to decrease the risk of pressure ulcers by unloading pressure from at-risk areas. Minimizing the skin–support surface interface pressure below 30 mm Hg is thought to be beneficial, but the effectiveness of this technique is yet unclear.

Our group studied nine healthy volunteers dressed in hospital scrubs and positioned supine on a modern ICU bed (Total Care, Hill-Rom). A 48 by 48 sensor array constituting a 2 foot by 2 foot square pad was positioned under the sacrum. The subjects were positioned supine (S), turned left (L), and turned right (R) by an experienced ICU nurse. A calibrated interface-pressure profile was acquired at each position using the Xsensor interface pressure system.

Figure 169.4 shows a typical L, S, and R pressure profile. The legend denotes the interface pressure in mm Hg. All subjects exhibited some areas of skin that manifested an interface pressure greater than or equal to 30 mm Hg at each positions (average area per subject: 84.1 cm^2; range

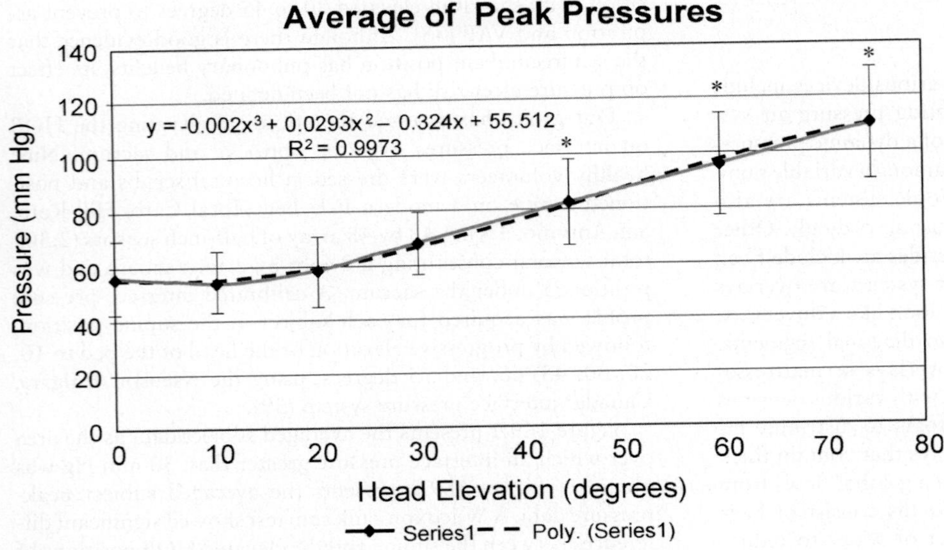

FIGURE 169.2. Average of peak pressures. *p <0.05 compared to supine.

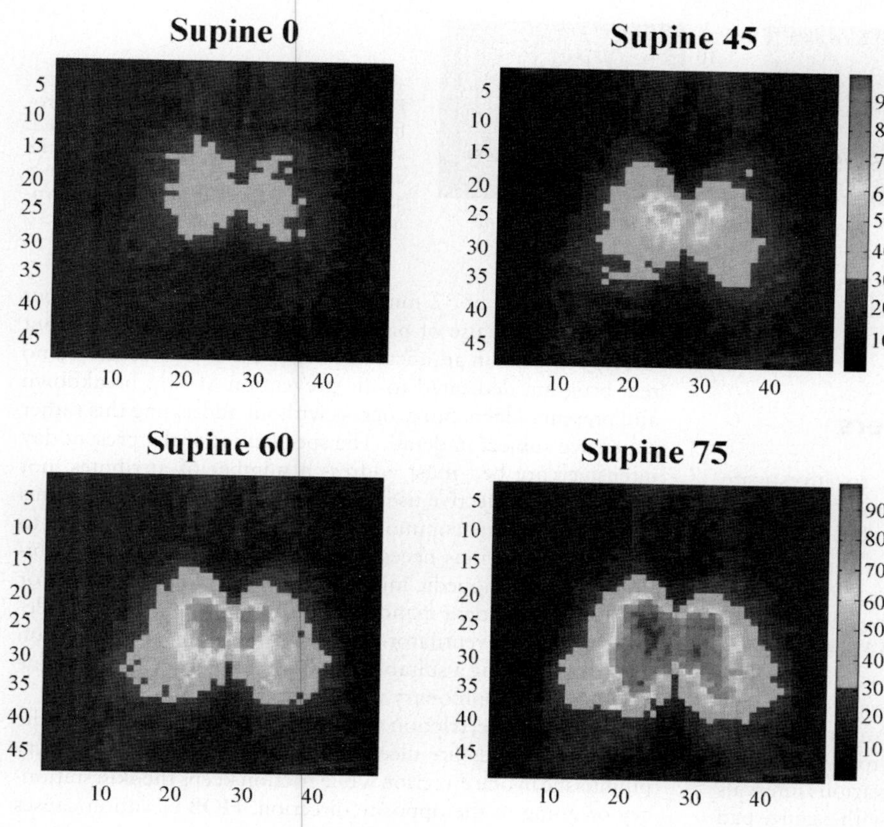

FIGURE 169.3. Interface pressure profiles (from **top left**): Supine, head of bed (HOB) 45 degrees, HOB 60 degrees, HOB 75 degrees. *Shading* denotes the area where the skin–bed interface pressure exceeds 30 mm Hg.

19.4 cm^2–229.0 cm^2); hence, the pressure was never relieved as intended (Fig. 169.5). Thus, it appears that standard turning by experienced ICU nurses does not unload all areas of high skin–bed interface pressure. These areas are at risk for skin breakdown, which may help explain why pressure ulcers still occur despite using the standard preventive measure of turning every 2 hours.

These data, although preliminary, suggest that side-to-side turning does not completely unload the at-risk skin. In the small sample of nine volunteers, there were some areas always at risk, regardless of the position, suggesting that the turning process is not enough to unload high pressures. We have called this at-risk area, the *triple jeopardy area*, because the skin is at risk in all three positions: supine, left, and right. Additionally *double jeopardy areas* are areas that are at risk in any two of the three positions. More data need to be collected on volunteers and/or patients to verify this conclusion. Also, in addition to analyzing the double and triple jeopardy areas, other parameters require investigation for the turned positions, including, but not limited to (a) maximum pressures, (b) average pressures, (c) pressure gradient, and (d) interface pressures in relation to the type and degree of turn. Area analysis should include (a) skin area at risk, (b) how at-risk skin area changes with turning, and (c) how sensitive the at-risk skin areas are to various pressure thresholds. Time duration analysis needs to be investigated as to how time is a factor in pressures and/or areas.

Support Apparatus

It should be noted that when nurses turn their patients, the patients must be supported to keep them correctly positioned. The equipment used at our institution (Shands Hospital at the University of Florida) is either foam pillows or wedges. Depending on the nurse's preference or material availability, patients are supported with these devices. Data need to be collected on patients and/or volunteers to analyze whether or not there is a difference between these devices in regard to patient safety. The parameters noted above, additionally, need to be analyzed comparing pillows to wedges in regard to turning. Moreover, the physical placement of the pillow/wedge in relation to the patient's anatomy could prove to be important, as well as the nurse's individual technique. Pillow/wedge placement and nurse variability (using different nurses) is, thus,

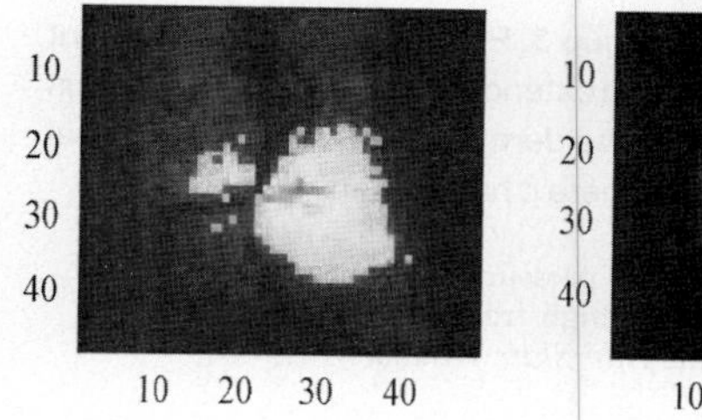

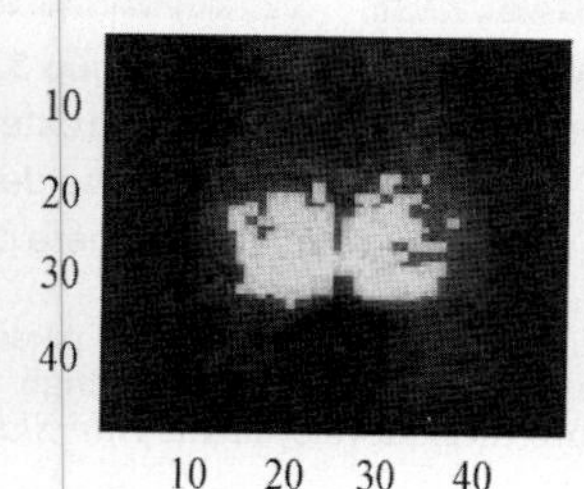

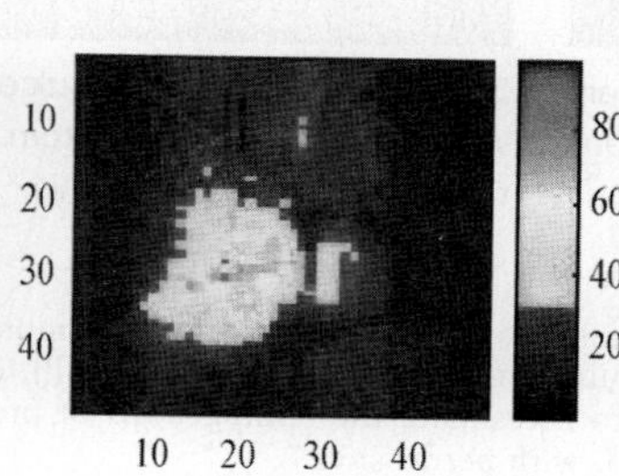

FIGURE 169.4. Interface pressure profiles (from **left to right**): Left turned, supine, right turned. *Shading* denotes the area where the skin–bed interface pressure exceeds 30 mm Hg.

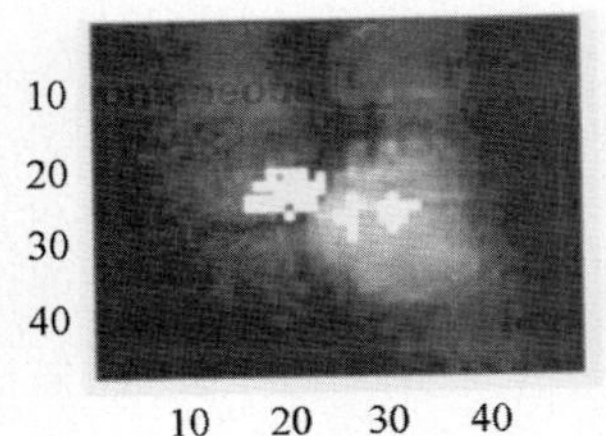

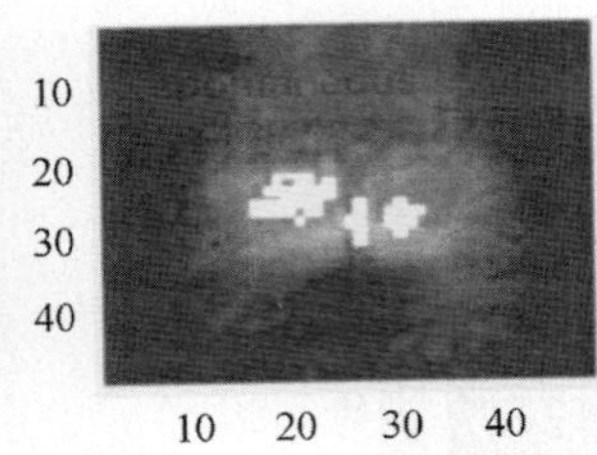

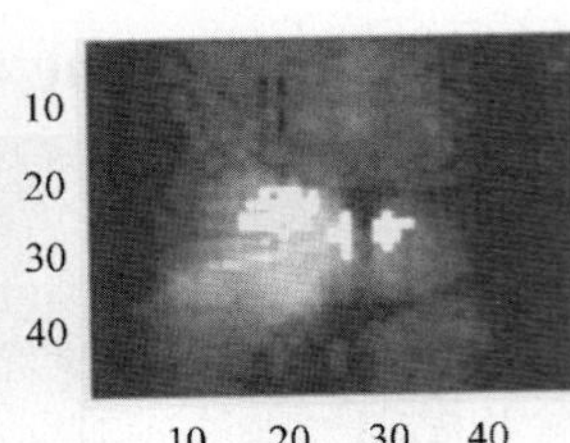

FIGURE 169.5. Interface pressure profiles (from **left** to **right**): Left turned, supine, right turned. *White* denotes the area where the skin–bed interface pressure exceeded 30 mm Hg throughout all turning positions.

another aspect requiring study, as well as nursing experience and length of shift.

Etiology of Pressure Ulcers

Work by Quintavalle et al. (12) continues to investigate the cause of pressure ulcers. These investigators used high-frequency ultrasound (HFUS) to image the skin of at-risk patients (Braden score 18 or less) in comparison to those of healthy volunteers. They obtained 1,139 readable images from 119 long-term residents. Their results showed that 630 (55.3%) of these images were abnormal, with 541 (47.5%) images showing evidence of deep subdermal edema and 89 (7.8%) images with superficial edema just below the epidermis. Due to apparent different causes for deep versus superficial pressure ulcers, a healthy volunteer was subjected to two forms of preulceration, and was imaged prior to and at various intervals during the intervention. One area was rubbed with a gauze pad for 7 minutes, and another area was subjected to lying on a hard object for 1 hour. The friction (gauze) demonstrated superficial edema with none in the deep tissue. The pressure demonstrated pockets of deep edema with no superficial edema. Of the images demonstrating deep edema, they were further divided into three subgroups that suggest three phases of pressure ulcer development, as can be seen in Figure 169.6. Their results also suggest that many pressure ulcers are in the process of formation before erythema is observed—the standard of care for skin assessment—as 79.3% of images showed tissue changes without any clinical signs of erythema.

To summarize, in patients at risk for skin breakdown, common wisdom is to reduce tissue pressures below the capillary-closing pressure of 32 mm Hg. Turning every 2 hours is not enough, and the use of passive turning devices can assist but clearly are only an adjunct. The bed is the actual issue, and no real program dedicated to the prevention of skin breakdown and pressure ulcers can progress without addressing this rather expensive subject in detail. The specificities of the present day intensive care bed must address a number of attributes, not limited to the effective use of the low-air-loss pressure systems that are now quite common. The ICU beds must also adjust to the proper positions necessary for patients who are immobilized due to orthopedic injuries. Pulmonary support alone for the intubated patient mandates a HOB position of 30 to 45 degrees to prevent ventilator-acquired pneumonia and aspiration while maintaining a suitable sacral pressure at the mattress line and enhanced pulmonary perfusion.

To summarize, friction and shearing forces contribute to the formation of pressure ulcers. Shearing is caused when gravity pulls tissue in one direction while friction keeps the skin stationary or going in the opposite direction. HOB elevation causes and enhances shearing forces.

SPECIAL CARE CONSIDERATIONS

Traumatic Brain Injury Patients

Patients with traumatic brain injuries (TBI) generally need a more upright position for several days, with little or only a gentle variation in the lateral position; they also require minimal stimulation due to management of potentially elevated intracranial pressure. This 30-degree head-up position subjects

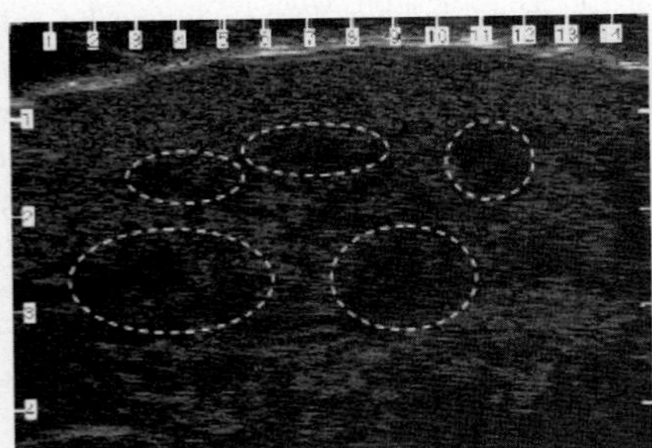

3A. Subgroup 1. Pressure ulcer development with pockets of edema in the subcutaneous tissue but with no dermal involvement.

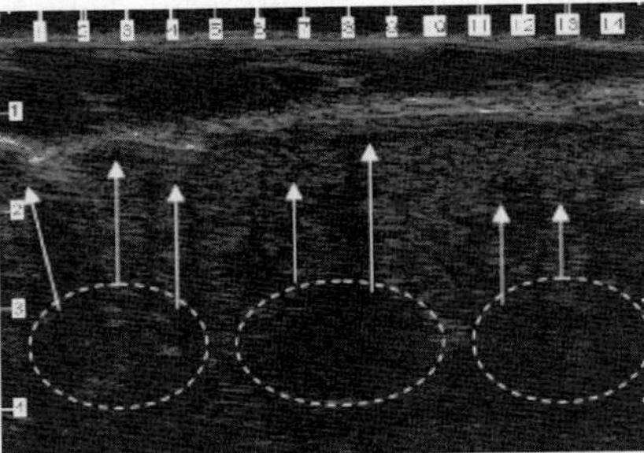

3B. Subgroup 2. Pressure ulcer development with edema extending from the subcutaneous tissue into the dermis.

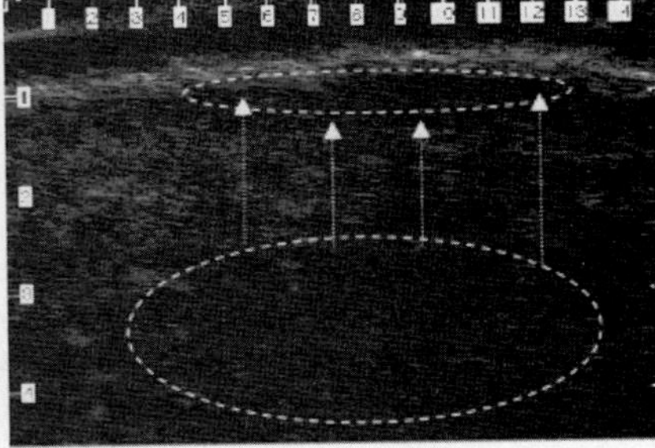

3C. Subgroup 3. Pressure ulcer development with edema extending from the subcutaneous tissue via the dermis to the dermal/epidermal junction where it has pooled.

FIGURE 169.6. High-resolution ultrasound images demonstrating the three phases of pressure ulcer development. (From Quintavalle PR, Lyder CH, Mertz PJ, et al. Use of high-resolution, high-frequency diagnostic ultrasound to investigate the pathogenesis of pressure ulcer development. *Adv Skin Wound Care*. 2006;19:498–505, with permission.)

these patients in particular to excess shearing and friction injury due to the persistent position and of the body during repositioning. The placement of these patients on appropriate beds, starting as soon after admission as possible, is critical for the prevention of pressure ulcers. Pressure damage to the areas around Aspen collars and tracheotomy sites are also influenced by the combination of rotation, friction, and moisture due to poor control of drainage or fluid resuscitation.

Obese Patients

The increasing weight and girth of the general ICU population has added to the problems with pressure ulcers, and is an additional consideration for ICU bed manufacturers and an added burden for both medical and nursing management of the ICU patient. The average ICU bed needs to support a patient who weighs from 200 kg to—not infrequently—more than 300 kg. The use of fluid bolus and massive replacements may cause the patient's dry weight to double. The tension on the skin not only adds to the weight and girth issue, but causes damage to the skin surface integrity which increases the tendency for skin tears and damage due to shearing forces and friction. A mattress surface covering that eases or facilitates patient movement during repositioning and that minimizes shearing and tearing forces on patient skin is clearly of decisive importance. The bed's ability to rotate laterally contributes to enhanced skin care, dermal perfusion, and increased pulmonary perfusion. Ease in attaining Trendelenburg and reverse Trendelenburg positions during procedures is obvious. Equally important to the management of the critically ill patient is the ability to transport (for example, to radiology) in the same bed and minimization of the need to transfer the patient more than is necessary, thereby decreasing the exposure to friction and shear. All of these beds need to have some degree of mobility, and, as our population increases in size, it seems reasonable to mechanize the bed's traveling mode for staff safety, speed, and convenience.

OTHER FACTORS AND INDICATORS

Pressure ulcers may, indeed, be a sign of inadequate nursing care, but they may also be an indicator of critical illness, significant comorbidities, and the intensive battle waged for the acutely ill patients that we see in our intensive care units today.

Some pressure ulcers are inevitable even with the very best of care, particularly in patients in whom immobilization is necessary or inevitable, and where sepsis, vasogenic shock, vasoactive drugs, and a myriad of other agents—while necessary for life-saving—are a detriment to skin perfusion and general skin integrity. Ischemic changes to skin surfaces that are weight-bearing are the primary cause of pressure ulcers. The ischemia caused by drugs used to treat shock due to sepsis and other life-threatening disease states is compounded by other relatively controllable events. Keeping the skin protected from contact with wet agents that irritate, due to either the acidic or basic nature of the liquid, is essential, and all patients should be checked for wetness every 2 hours, at a minimum. The use of effective barrier creams and ointments cannot be overstressed. The control of urine and bowel contamination is a must, and adequate appliances are available for the management of these problems, although it does require expert care to keep this seemingly simple requirement under control.

Friction and shear can also add to the damage of pressure over a bony prominence and, coupled with wetness, provide an environment that, if left unmanaged, can lead to devastating injury. Wetness does not directly cause pressure ulcers, but it does soften or macerate skin, which makes it more susceptible to damage from friction and shearing. The control of moisture is imperative and cannot be underestimated. Whether the moisture is caused by incontinence, wound drainage, or just a diaphoretic patient, it must be contained and managed.

When bed selection for the intensive care patient is completed, all patients should be assessed for risk factor identifiers using one of the generally accepted scales. The Braden scale used in our facility evaluates the following:

- The patient's nutritional status
- The ability of the patient to sense skin damage
- The ability of the patient to change position (mobility)
- The degree to which the patient is subjected to shearing forces and friction
- The degree of exposure to wetness or moisture

Once assessed, beginning on admission, each patient should be reassessed daily. As risk factors are identified, a plan of care is established and followed. It is imperative that a surveillance system be formulated to identify areas of weakness and areas for improvement be designed for any program to be successful. The surveillance system helps all staff members focus on the important issues and ensures that a steady decrease in the occurrence rate of pressure ulcers is seen within the unit. An aggressive, proactive approach is needed to address pressure ulcers in the acute care setting and should include a multidisciplinary team composed of nutritional, nursing, medical, and management personnel to develop programs, protocols, procedures, and practices that will continue to support and influence the best outcomes.

References

1. Barratt E. Pressure sores. Putting risk calculators in their place. *Nurs Times.* 1987;83:65–70.
2. Lapsley HM, Vogels R. Cost and prevention of pressure ulcers in an acute teaching hospital. *Int J Qual Health Care.* 1996;8:61–66.
3. Hobbs BK. Reducing the incidence of pressure ulcers: implementation of a turn-team nursing program. *J Gerontol Nurs.* 2004;11:46–51.
4. Agency for Healthcare Policy and Research. *Panel for the Prediction and Prevention of Pressure Ulcers in Adults. Clinical Practice Guideline Number 3.* Rockville, MD: U.S. Department of Health and Human Services, Public Health Service; 1992. AHCPR Publication No. 92-0047.
5. Wound Ostomy and Continence Nurses Society. Guideline for Prevention and Management of Pressure Ulcers. WOCN Clinical Practice Guideline Series, 2003.
6. Agostini JV, Baker DI, Bogardus ST. Prevention of pressure ulcers in older patients. In: Shojania KG, Duncan BW, McDonald KM, et al., eds. *Making Health Care Safer: A Critical Analysis of Patient Safety Practices.* UCSF; 2000:301–306.
7. Bennett RG, O'Sullivan J, DeVito EM, et al. The increasing medical malpractice risk related to pressure ulcers in the United States. *J Am Geriatr Soc.* 2000;48(1):73–81.
8. Haalboom J. Medical perspectives in the 21st century. In: Bader D, Bouten C, Colin D, et al., eds. *Pressure Ulcer Research: Current and Future Perspectives.* Berlin, Germany: Springer, 2005:11–21.
9. Hofman A, Geelkerken RH, Wille J, et al. Pressure sores and pressure-decreasing mattresses: controlled clinical trial. *Lancet.* 1994;343:568–571.
10. Lyder CH. Pressure ulcer prevention and management. *JAMA.* 2003;289:223–226.
11. Milne J, Pagnamenta F. An online ordering system for therapy beds and mattresses. *Br J Nurs.* 2004;13(19):S38–S42.

12. Quintavalle PR, Lyder CH, Mertz PJ, et al. Use of high-resolution, high-frequency diagnostic ultrasound to investigate the pathogenesis of pressure ulcer development. *Adv Skin Wound Care.* 2006;19:498–505.
13. Reddy M, Gill SS, Rochon PA. Preventing pressure ulcers: a systematic review. *JAMA.* 2006;296:974–983.
14. Stimler C, Pryor V. Impact results of a statewide effort to improve pressure ulcer prevention in New York state. 1999. IPRO HCQIP Publication No. 99–05.
15. Westrate JT, Bruining HA. Pressure sores in an intensive care unit and related variables: a descriptive study. *Intensive Crit Care Nurs.* 1996;12:280–284.
16. Shands Hospital, University of Florida. Decubitus ulcer events (all Shands heathcare facilities). 2005 and 2006.
17. Clark M, Price PE. Is wound healing a true science or a clinical art? *Lancet.* 2004;364:1388–1389.
18. Gebhardt KS. Pressure ulcer research: where do we go from here? *Br J Nurs.* 2004;13(19):S14–18.
19. National Pressure Ulcer Advisory Panel. Updated pressure ulcer staging. 2007. http://www.npuap.org/pr2.htm. Accessed May 7, 2007.
20. Colin D, Abraham P, Preault L, et al. Comparison of 90 degrees and 30 degrees laterally inclined positions in the prevention of pressure ulcers using transcutaneous oxygen and carbon dioxide pressures. *Adv Wound Care.* 1996;9(3):35–38.
21. Guyton AC, Hall JE. *Textbook of Medical Physiology.* 10th ed. Philadelphia, PA: WB Saunders; 2000:163–174.
22. Dealey C. Mattresses and beds. *J Wound Care.* 1995;4(9):409–412.
23. Gebhardt KS. Research in biomedical engineering: an overview of recent literature. *J Tissue Viability.* 2005;15(1):17–18.
24. Reddy NP. Effects of mechanical stresses on lymph and interstitial fluid flows. In: Bader DL, ed. Pressure Sores: Clinical Practice and Scientific Approach. London, England: Macmillan; 1990:203–220.
25. Rithalia SVS, Gonsalkorale M. Assessment of alternating air mattresses using a time-based interface pressure threshold technique. *J Rehabil Res.* 1998;35(2):225–230.
26. Bouten CV, Oomens CW, Baaijens FP, et al. The etiology of pressure ulcers: skin deep or muscle bound? *Arch Phys Med Rehabil.* 2003;84:616–619.
27. Rithalia SVS, Gonsalkorale M. Quantification of pressure relief using interface pressure and tissue perfusion in alternating pressure air mattresses. *Arch Phys Med Rehabil.* 2000;81:1364–1369.
28. Swain I. The measurement of interface pressure. In: Bader D, Bouten C, Colin D, et al., eds. *Pressure Ulcer Research: Current and Future Perspectives.* Berlin, Germany: Springer; 2005:51–71.
29. Stekelenburg A, Oomens C, Bader D. Compression-induced tissue damage: animal models. In: Bader D, Bouten C, Colin D, et al., eds. *Pressure Ulcer Research: Current and Future Perspectives.* Berlin, Germany: Springer; 2005:187–204.
30. Wang YN, Sanders J. Skin model studies. In: Bader D, Bouten C, Colin D, et al., eds. *Pressure Ulcer Research: Current and Future Perspectives.* Berlin, Germany: Springer; 2005:263–285.
31. Still JM, Wilson J, Rinker C, et al. A retrospective study to determine the incidence of pressure ulcers in burn patients using an alternating pressure mattress. *Burns.* 2003;29:505–507.
32. Amlung S, Miller W, Bosley L. The 1999 National Pressure Ulcer Prevalence Survey: a benchmarking approach. *Adv Skin Wound Care.* 2001;14(6):297–301.
33. Dealey C. The size of the pressure-sore problem in a teaching hospital. *J Adv Nurs.* 1991;16:663–670.
34. Bergstrom N. Patients at risk for pressure ulcers and evidence-based care for pressure ulcer prevention. In: Bader D, Bouten C, Colin D, et al., eds. *Pressure Ulcer Research: Current and Future Perspectives.* Berlin, Germany: Springer; 2005:35–50.
35. Defloor T, De Bacquer D, Grypdonck MHF. The effect of various combinations of turning and pressure reducing devices on the incidence of pressure ulcers. *Int J Nurs Stud.* 2005;42:37–46.
36. Dini V, Bertone M, Romanelli M. Prevention and management of pressure ulcers. *Dermatolog Ther.* 2006;19:356–364.
37. Vanderwee K, Grypdonck MHF, De Bacquer D, et al. Effectiveness of turning with unequal time intervals on the incidence of pressure ulcer lesions. *J Adv Nurs.* 2007;57(1):59–68.
38. American Thoracic Society, Infectious Diseases Society of America. Guidelines for the management of adults with hospital-acquired, ventilator-associated, and healthcare-associated pneumonia. *Am J Resp Crit Care Med.* 2005;171(4):388–416.
39. Xsensor. http://www.xsensor.com.

SECTION XIX ■ HEMATOLOGIC AND ONCOLOGIC DISEASE AND DYSFUNCTION

CHAPTER 170 ■ COAGULATION DISORDERS IN THE INTENSIVE CARE UNIT

ROBERT I. PARKER

This chapter focuses on various pathophysiologic conditions associated with abnormal hemostasis or abnormal laboratory measurements of hemostasis. However, to understand how to approach a patient with a bleeding problem, one must first have a basic understanding of the processes involved in regulating blood coagulation. Consequently, we will start with a brief overview of our current understanding of coagulation, including a brief discussion of the interactions of coagulation and inflammation.

The coagulopathic conditions frequently encountered in the intensive care unit (ICU) can be arbitrarily divided into three categories: (i) those associated with serious bleeding or a high probability of bleeding, (ii) thrombotic syndromes or conditions associated with a higher probability of thrombosis, and (iii) systemic diseases associated with acquired selective coagulation factor deficiencies. In addition, there are a few conditions associated with abnormal coagulation screening tests that represent laboratory phenomena not associated with an increased bleeding risk. A topical listing of these conditions is included for review in Table 170.1. The order in which these categories are listed suggests their relative importance to the critical care practitioner. This chapter will end by noting future directions in research and care of the critically ill patient with hemostatic abnormalities. Although space limitation will not allow for a comprehensive discussion of all aspects of pathophysiology, clinical presentation, and management of hemorrhagic and thrombotic disorders encountered in the ICU, I hope to provide a framework that will allow the reader to garner a basic understanding of the issues and direct him or her toward additional sources of information.

OVERVIEW OF COAGULATION

For years, medical students have been taught that the process of blood clotting is divided into the intrinsic, extrinsic, and common pathways (Fig. 170.1), and students have come away with the thought that clotting occurs as the result of an orderly sequential process. Although this arbitrary segmentation of the clotting process may allow for a basic level of understanding, it obscures the fact that once initiated, clot production and clot destruction (fibrinolysis) occur simultaneously, and also minimizes the role that platelets and the endothelium play in the overall process. This section of the chapter will try to clarify some of the newer thoughts on coagulation.

Whereas previously it was thought that the intrinsic pathway, beginning with the activation of factor XII (fXII) to activated factor XII (fXIIa) in contact with some biologic or foreign surface, was physiologically most important in the initiation of clot formation, we now know that the activation of fX to fXa through the action of the fVIIa/tissue factor (TF) complex is paramount in this regard (1,2). It is also evident that the various elements of the clotting cascade frequently act in concert; hence, the use of the term, *tenase*, to describe the action of fVIIa/TF complex along with the fIXa/fVIIIa complex on the activation of factor X to Xa, and the use of the term, *prothrombinase*, to describe the factor Xa/Va complex, which cleaves prothrombin (factor II) to form thrombin (factor IIa). In addition, we now know that there is cross talk between the two arms of the clotting cascade, with fVIIa being able to enhance the activation of fIX (to fIXa) and fXI (to fXIa), further pointing out the central role that fVIIa and TF play *in vivo* (Fig. 170.2). Furthermore, there are various positive feedback loops principally involving thrombin that enhance the upstream activation of the clotting process.

Tissue factor for the activation of coagulation is present not only in the subendothelial matrix, but is also found circulating freely in plasma as soluble tissue factor and contained on cellular elements such as monocytes. However, clotting does not occur in free-flowing blood but rather on surfaces. Platelets, endothelial cells, the subendothelial matrix, and biologic polymers—for example, catheters, grafts, stents, and so on—can provide these surfaces for clot formation, and all play a critical role in clot formation.

Platelets not only initiate clot formation through the formation of a platelet plug, but, more significantly, they bring specialized proteins that regulate the clotting response—for example, fVIII, inhibitors of fibrinolysis, and so on—to the area of bleeding, and provide a surface for the co-localization of clotting factors for efficient clot formation (Fig. 170.3). Platelets do not ordinarily adhere to the vascular endothelium, but when the endothelium is mechanically disrupted (e.g., cut) or activated by inflammation, platelets will bind to the endothelial cell or subendothelial matrix via a von Willebrand factor (vWf)-dependent mechanism. Once adherent, the platelets become activated and secrete various molecules that further enhance platelet adherence and aggregation, vascular contraction, clot formation, and wound healing (3).

The endothelium is a specialized organ that plays a central role in the regulation of clot formation (i.e., hemostasis) by presenting a nonthrombogenic surface to flowing blood and by enhancing clot formation when the endothelium is disrupted by trauma or injured by infection or inflammation (4,5) (Fig. 170.4). The normal endothelium produces

TABLE 170.1

OVERVIEW OF COAGULATION DISORDERS SEEN IN THE ICU

CONDITIONS ASSOCIATED WITH SERIOUS BLEEDING OR A HIGH PROBABILITY OF BLEEDING
Disseminated intravascular coagulation (DIC)
Liver disease/hepatic insufficiency
Vitamin K deficiency/depletion
Massive transfusion syndrome
Anticoagulant overdose (heparin, warfarin)
Thrombocytopenia (drug-induced, immunologic)
Acquired platelet defects (drug-induced, uremia)
THROMBOTIC CLINICAL SYNDROMES
Thrombotic thrombocytopenia purpura/hemolytic uremic syndrome
Deep venous thrombosis
Pulmonary embolism
Coronary thrombosis/acute myocardial infarction
LABORATORY ABNORMALITIES NOT ASSOCIATED WITH CLINICAL BLEEDING
Lupus anticoagulant
Reactive hyperfibrinogenemia
OTHER SELECTED CLINICAL SYNDROMES
Hemophilia (A and B)
Specific factor deficiencies associated with specific diseases
Amyloidosis, factor X; Gaucher, factor IX; nephrotic syndrome, factor IX, antithrombin III
Cyanotic congenital heart disease (polycythemia, qualitative platelet defect)
Depressed clotting factor levels (newborns)

inhibitors of blood coagulation and platelet activation, and modulates vascular tone and permeability. Endothelial cells also synthesize and secrete the components of the subendothelial extracellular matrix, including adhesive glycoproteins, collagen, fibronectin, and vWf. When the endothelium is disrupted, bleeding occurs. However, when *injured*, the endothelium often becomes a *pro*thrombotic rather than an antithrombotic organ, and unwanted clot formation may occur.

INTERACTION OF COAGULATION AND INFLAMMATION

There are multiple points of intersection between the biochemical events of inflammation and those of coagulation (6). Although a full discussion of these points is beyond the scope of this chapter, the cross talk between inflammation and coagulation likely takes place at the level of the endothelium, and is bidirectional wherein activation of either pathway affects the functioning of the other (6) (Fig. 170.5). While many different inflammatory cytokines have been identified as promoters of a procoagulant milieu, the interconnection of tissue factor (TF) and tissue necrosis factor-α (TNF-α) may potentially be the most important of these. During sepsis, tissue factor expression is up-regulated in activated monocytes and endothelial cells as a response to endotoxin, with the consequence being both the secretion of proinflammatory cytokines, such as interleukin-6 (IL-6) and TNF-α, from activated mononuclear cells, and the activation of coagulation. This results in increased thrombin production, which plays a central role in coagulation and inflammation through the induction of procoagulant, anticoagulant, inflammatory, and mitogenic responses (7). Thrombin

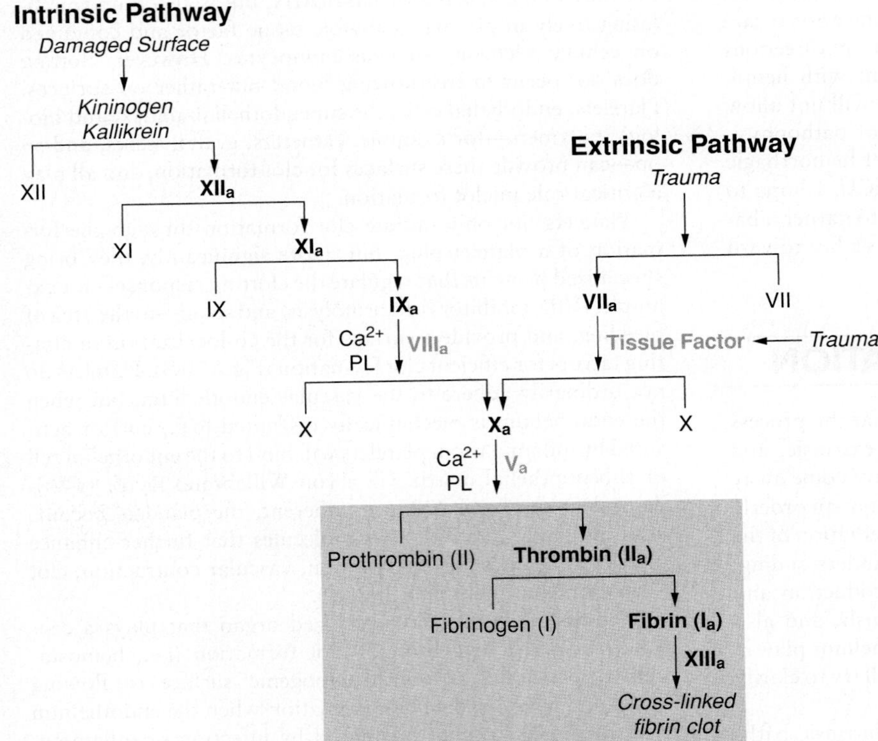

FIGURE 170.1. Coagulation is initiated either through the intrinsic pathway by activation of factor XII by the generation of high-molecular-weight kininogen and kallikrein, or through activation of the extrinsic pathway by tissue factor. Roman numerals indicate zymogen clotting factors; "a" indicates activated forms of the clotting factors.

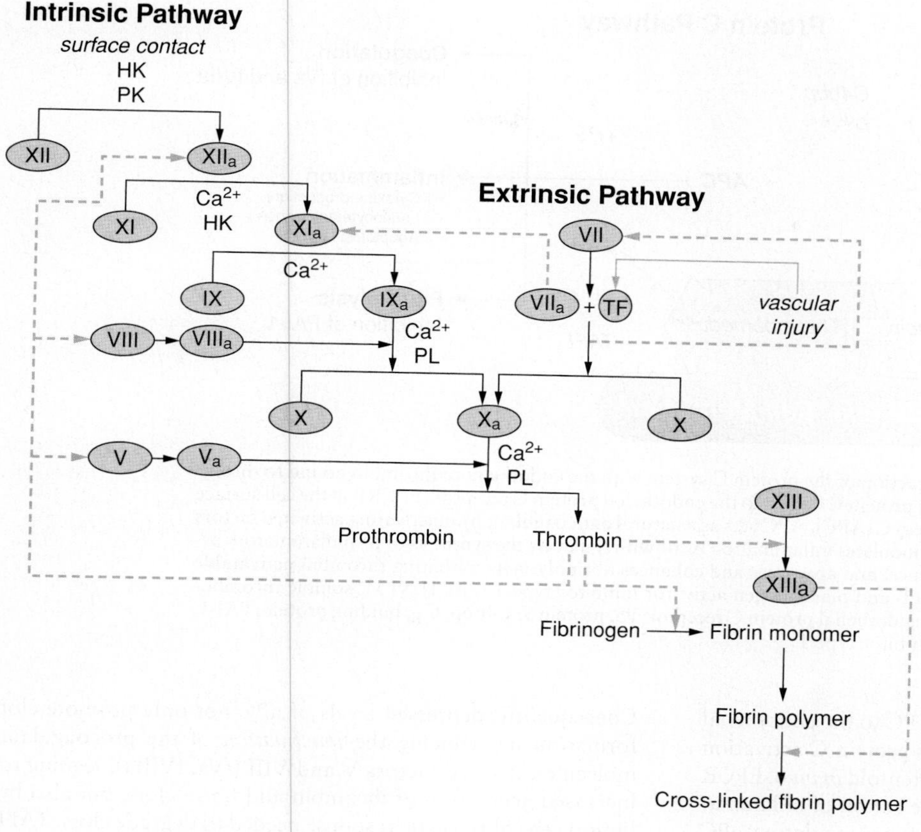

FIGURE 170.2. Modified clotting cascade indicating cross talk between the intrinsic and extrinsic pathways by the action of VIIa/tissue factor (TF) enhancing the conversion of factor XI to activated factor XI (XIa) (*dotted lines*). Ca^{2+}, calcium; HK, high-molecular-weight kininogen; PK, prekallikrein; PL, phospholipids.

results in the activation, aggregation, and lysis of leukocytes and platelets, and activation of endothelial cells, with resultant increase in proinflammatory cytokines IL-6 and TNF-α expression. The net result of thrombin generation is to produce a proinflammatory and procoagulant state, leading to the formation of fibrin and microvascular thrombosis. However, these proinflammatory effects of thrombin are counterbalanced by the anti-inflammatory effects of activated protein C (Fig. 170.4) (7).

A second important point of connection of coagulation and inflammation is through the protein C system (8–10). Although the anticoagulant effects of activated protein C (aPC) and its cofactor, protein S, are well known, only recently have the anti-inflammatory roles of these proteins been appreciated. In experimental models, aPC has been shown to increase the secretion of anti-inflammatory cytokines, reduce leukocyte migration and adhesion, and protect endothelial cells from injury. Additionally, the balance between the anticoagulant and anti-inflammatory roles of aPC may be mediated by the relative distribution of free and complement factor C_{4b} bound protein S (9,10). *In vitro*, aPC inhibits TNF-α elaboration from monocytes and blocks leukocyte adhesion to selectins, as well as having an influence on apoptosis (7). The protein C pathway is engaged when thrombin binds to thrombomodulin on the

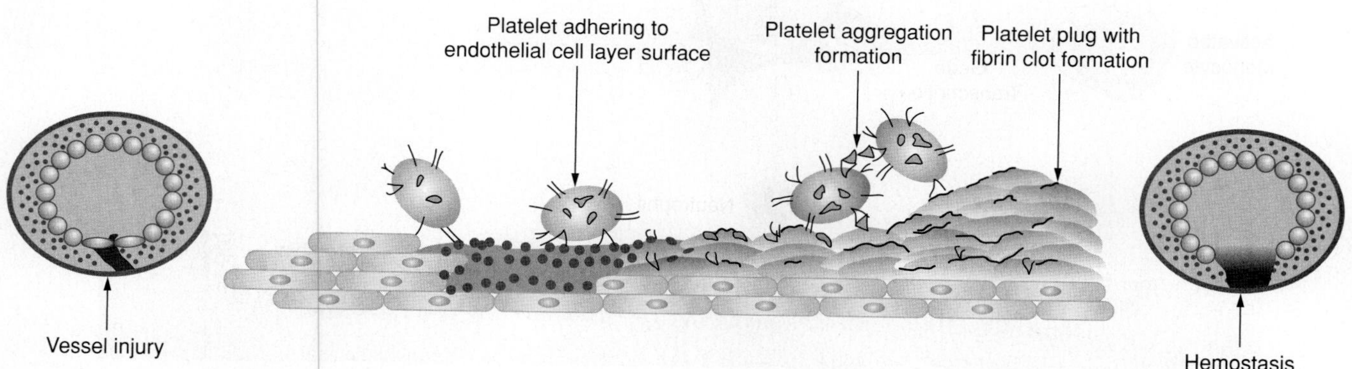

FIGURE 170.3. The role of platelets in mediating primary hemostasis at sites of vascular injury. Platelets are initially activated and express specific adhesion receptors on their surface, followed by adhesion to activated endothelial cells and exposed subendothelial components (e.g., collagen, von Willebrand factor). Subsequent platelet aggregation occurs with the development of a primary platelet plug. Coagulation occurs on the developing platelet plug with the creation of a fibrin clot.

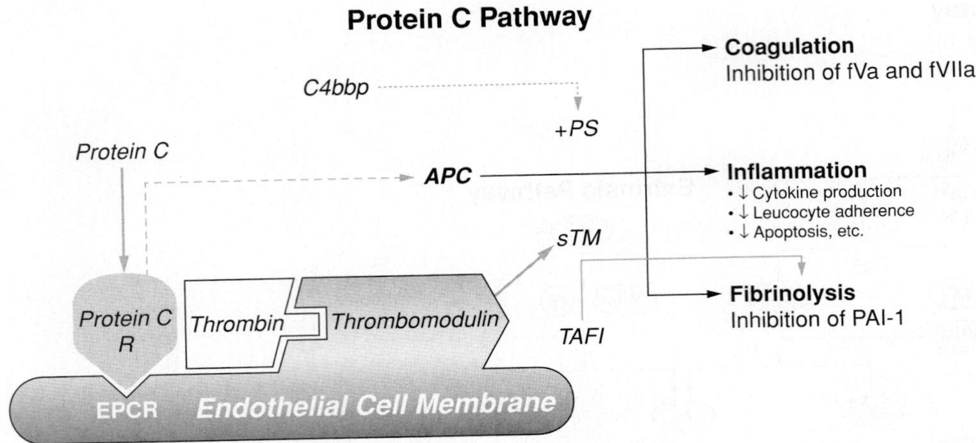

FIGURE 170.4. The interaction of the protein C system with the endothelium: thrombin bound to thrombomodulin (TM) modifies protein C bound to the endothelial protein C receptor (EPCR) on the cell surface to generate activated protein C (APC). APC acts as a natural anticoagulant by inactivating activated factors V (fVa) and VIII (fVIIa), modulates inflammation by down-regulating the synthesis of proinflammatory cytokines, leukocyte adherence, and apoptosis and enhances fibrinolysis by inhibiting thrombin-activatable fibrinolysis inhibitor (TAFI) and plasminogen activator inhibitor type-1 (PAI-1). sTM, soluble thrombomodulin; sEPCR, soluble endothelial protein C receptor; PS, protein S; C4bbp, C_{4b} binding protein; PAI-1, plasminogen activator inhibitor type 1.

surface of the endothelial cell. Binding of PC to the endothelial cell protein C receptor (EPCR) augments protein C activation by the thrombin–TM complex more than tenfold *in vivo*. EPCR is shed from the endothelium through the action of inflammatory mediators and thrombin, thereby down-regulating aPC generation in sepsis and inflammation.

The third important link between inflammation and coagulation occurs at the level of fibrinolysis and also involves the protein C system. Activated PC is capable of neutralizing the fibrinolysis inhibitors, *plasminogen activator inhibitor type-1* (PAI-1) and *thrombin activatable fibrinolysis inhibitor* (TAFI). Consequently, depressed levels of aPC not only promote clot formation by reducing the *inactivation* of the procoagulant molecule-activated factors V and VIII (fVa, fVIIIa), leading to increased generation of thrombin and fibrin clots, but also by limiting the fibrinolytic response needed to degrade clots. TAFI (also known as carboxypeptidase R) has also been shown to inactivate inflammatory peptides, such as complement factors C3a and C5a, which can play a role in the contact activation of coagulation. In addition, polymorphisms of the promoter region of the PAI-1 gene that lead to differences in PAI-1 production have been demonstrated to affect the prognosis

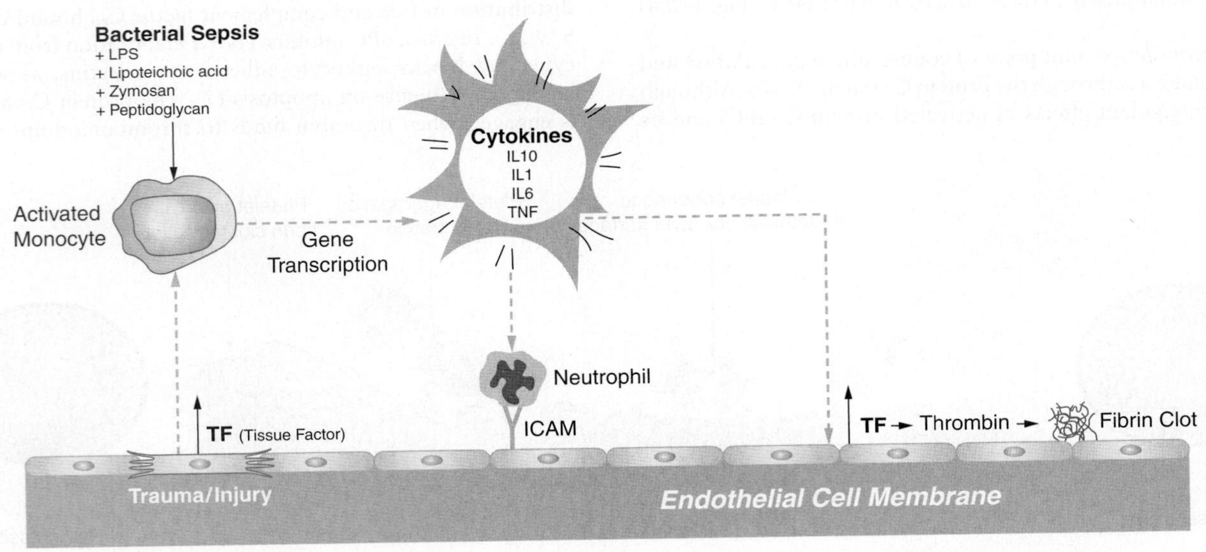

FIGURE 170.5. Inflammation enhances coagulation through the induction of proinflammatory cytokines, which induce tissue factor (TF) formation, which in turn decreases activated protein C (APC) formation, leading to enhanced thrombin and fibrin generation. In addition, the decrease in APC allows for greater inhibition of fibrinolysis through the action of plasminogen activator inhibitor type-1 (PAI-1). ICAM, intercellular adhesion molecule; IL, interleukin; LPS, lipopolysaccharide; TNF, tissue necrosis factor.

in meningococcal sepsis and multiple trauma, highlighting the important role of this regulatory system (11). This finding illustrates the significance of developing our knowledge of how common polymorphisms of genes that encode important molecules affect our response to infection and injury. A recent report, which demonstrated increased mortality and organ dysfunction and increased inflammation in patients who exhibited a specific polymorphism (1641AA) of the protein C gene (12), further reinforced the importance of the interactions between coagulation and inflammation and the central role of protein C, as well as the significant role that gene polymorphisms play in host responses and clinical outcomes.

AN APPROACH TO THE PATIENT WITH AN ACTUAL OR SUSPECTED COAGULATION DISORDER

Clinical History

Diagnostic assessment begins at the bedside. The medical history, both past and present, may lend some insight into the risk for significant bleeding (13,14). A prior history of prolonged or excessive bleeding, or of recurrent thrombosis, is a significant finding and should be ruled out. Specific questions regarding bleeding should investigate the occurrence of any of the following:

- Spontaneous, easy, or disproportionately severe bruising
- Intramuscular hematoma formation (either spontaneous or related to trauma)
- Spontaneous or trauma-induced hemarthrosis
- Spontaneous mucous membrane bleeding
- Prior problems with bleeding related to surgery (including dental extractions, tonsillectomy, and circumcision)
- The need for transfusions in the past
- Menstrual history
- Current medications

There are innumerable aspirin-containing medications available to the consumer, all of which can potentially interfere with platelet-mediated primary hemostasis. Many other drugs used in the ICU are also associated with bleeding abnormalities and are discussed below. In situations involving trauma (either surgical or accidental), it is imperative to determine the severity of injury relative to the magnitude of bleeding that followed. A prior history of significant thrombosis, such as deep venous thrombosis, pulmonary embolus, or stroke, also suggests the possibility that a hypercoagulable condition may be present. Given that thrombotic events are generally uncommon in younger adults, the occurrence of thrombotic events, particularly early cardiovascular events such as myocardial infarction, in young adult relatives should cause the clinician to consider the presence of a congenital thrombophilic abnormality in the patient. These include deficiencies of antithrombin-III, protein C or protein S, the presence of the factor V Leiden R506Q mutation, the prothrombin G20210A (or the newly described A19911G) (15,16) polymorphism/mutation, and the C677T mutation/polymorphism of the MTHFR (methylenetetrahydrofolate reductase) gene. In addition, vasculitis associated with an autoimmune disorder such as systemic lupus erythematosus (SLE) must always be considered in the evaluation of an individual with an unexplained pathologic clot. In all cases, the family history is essential in trying to separate congenital from acquired disorders.

In a general sense, one can segregate defects into those involving primary or secondary hemostasis according to the nature of the bleeding. Patients with primary hemostatic defects tend to manifest platelet or capillary type bleeding—oozing from cuts or incisions, mucous membrane bleeding, or excessive bruising. In women, this may manifest as menorrhagia. This type of bleeding is seen in patients with quantitative or qualitative platelet defects or von Willebrand disease. In contrast, patients with dysfunction of secondary hemostasis tend to display large vessel bleeding, characterized by hemarthroses, intramuscular hematomas, and the like. This type of bleeding is most often associated with specific coagulation factor deficiencies or inhibitors.

Physical Examination

Development of generalized bleeding in critically ill ICU patients presents a special problem. Such bleeding is often associated with severe underlying multiple organ system dysfunction and, thus, correction of the coagulopathy usually requires improvement in the patient's overall clinical status. Supportive evidence or physical findings of other concurrent organ system dysfunction, such as oliguria or anuria, respiratory failure, or hypotension, often are readily apparent. With the exception of massive transfusion syndrome (see below), generalized bleeding in critically ill patients is often caused by sepsis-related disseminated intravascular coagulation (DIC) (17,18). However, the clinician must also consider the coagulopathy of severe liver dysfunction, undiagnosed hemophilia, or, in the elderly or debilitated, vitamin K deficiency in the differential diagnosis (17–19).

The physical examination of the patient with a bleeding disorder should answer several basic questions. Is the process localized or diffuse? Is it related to an anatomic or surgical lesion? Is there mucosal bleeding? And finally, when appropriate, are there signs of either arterial or venous thrombosis? These answers may give clues to the cause of the problem as being a primary versus secondary hemostatic dysfunction, or anatomic bleeding versus generalized coagulopathy.

During the course of the examination, particular attention should be paid to the presence of several specific physical findings that may be helpful in determining the cause of a suspected hemostatic abnormality. For example, the presence of an enlarged spleen coupled with thrombocytopenia suggests that splenic sequestration may be a contributor to the observed thrombocytopenia. Furthermore, evidence of liver disease, such as portal hypertension and ascites, points to decreased factor synthesis as a possible cause of a prolonged PT or aPTT. When lymphadenopathy, splenomegaly, or other findings suggestive of disseminated malignancy are detected, acute or chronic DIC should be suspected as the cause of prolonged coagulation times, hypofibrinogenemia, and/or thrombocytopenia. Purpura that are palpable suggest capillary leak from vasculitis, whereas purpura associated with thrombocytopenia or qualitative platelet defects are generally not elevated and cannot be distinguished by touch. Finally, venous and arterial telangiectasia may be seen in von Willebrand disease and liver disease, respectively. When selective pressure is centrally applied to an arterial telangiectasia, the whole lesion fades, whereas a venous telangiectasia requires confluent pressure across the entire lesion, as with a glass slide, for blanching to occur.

Diagnostic Laboratory Evaluation

This section focuses on selecting appropriate tests to enable the clinician to sort out information from the history, physical examination, or previously obtained—and often confusing—laboratory data. Before we proceed, however, the importance of correct specimen collection for hemostatic evaluation must be emphasized. In the ICU, it is common for laboratory samples to be drawn through an indwelling arterial or central venous cannula, often because peripheral access is no longer available. Heparin-containing solution is, therefore, commonly present, either in the cannula flush medium to transduce a waveform or as a component of the intravenous infusion. Depending on the concentration of heparin in the infusing fluid and the volume of blood withdrawn, several tests can be influenced. Fibrin degradation products (FDPs) can be falsely elevated, and fibrinogen can be falsely low. Likewise, the prothrombin time (PT), activated partial thromboplastin time (aPTT), and thrombin time (TT) can be spuriously prolonged. A minimum of 20 mL of blood in adolescents and adults, and 10 mL of blood in younger children, should therefore be withdrawn through the cannula and either discarded or used for other purposes before obtaining a specimen for laboratory hemostasis analysis (20). This practice should minimize any influence of heparin on the results. In some clinical situations, it may not be reasonable to withdraw this volume of blood, and a peripheral venipuncture may be necessary. Because the aPTT is sensitive to the presence of small amounts of heparin, the presence of an unexpected prolonged aPTT obtained through a heparinized catheter should raise the suspicion of sample contamination. In this setting, the TT will also be prolonged, but will normalize if the contaminating heparin is neutralized (e.g., with toluidine blue or Hepasorb).

The presence of most suspected bleeding disorders can be confirmed using routinely available tests. These include evaluation of the peripheral blood smear, including an estimate of the platelet count and platelet and red blood cell morphologic features; measurement of the PT, aPTT, and the TT; and, finally, assays for fibrinogen or the presence of fibrin degradation products or the d-dimer fragment of polymerized fibrin. This latter test is more specific for the fibrinolytic fragment produced when polymerized fibrin monomer, produced through the action of thrombin on fibrinogen, is cleaved by the proteolytic enzyme, plasmin. In contrast to the older assays for fibrin degradation or fibrin split products (FDPs and FSPs), which will be positive even if fibrin is not produced—for example, the fragments are the result of proteolytic degradation of native fibrinogen—the d-dimer assay is positive only if fibrinogen has been cleaved to fibrin by the action of thrombin. Discretion should be used in determining which of these tests are most appropriate for assessment; they need not be ordered as a blanket panel on all patients with known or suspected bleeding disorders. Table 170.2 summarizes several major categories of hemorrhagic disorders and the tests that are characteristically abnormal in each. In most instances, measurement of the platelet count, fibrinogen

TABLE 170.2

HEMORRHAGIC SYNDROMES AND ASSOCIATED LABORATORY FINDINGS

Clinical syndrome	Screening tests	Supportive tests
DIC	Prolonged PT, aPTT, TT; decreased fibrinogen, platelets; microangiopathy	(+) FDPs, d-dimer; decreased factors V, VIII, and II (late)
Massive transfusion	Prolonged PT, aPTT; decreased fibrinogen, platelets ± Prolonged TT	All factors decreased; (–) FDPs, d-dimer (unless DIC develops); (+) transfusion history
Anticoagulant overdose		
Heparin	Prolonged aPTT, TT; ± prolonged PT	Toluidine blue/protamine corrects TT; reptilase time normal
Warfarin (same as vitamin K deficiency)	Prolonged PT; ± prolonged aPTT (severe); normal TT, fibrinogen, platelets	Vitamin K–dependent factors decreased; factors V, VIII normal
Liver disease		
Early	Prolonged PT	Decreased factor VII
Late	Prolonged PT, aPTT; decreased fibrinogen (terminal liver failure); normal platelet count (if splenomegaly absent)	Decreased factors II, V, VII, IX, and X; decreased plasminogen; ± FDPs unless DIC develops
Primary fibrinolysis	Prolonged PT, aPTT, TT; decreased fibrinogen ± platelets decreased	(+) FDPs, (–) d-dimer; short euglobulin clot lysis time
TTP	Thrombocytopenia, microangiopathy with mild anemia; PT, aPTT, fibrinogen generally WNL/ mildly abnormal	ADAMTS13 deficiency/inhibitor, unusually large vWf multimers between episodes; mild increase in FDPs or d-dimer
HUS	Microangiopathic hemolytic anemia, ± thrombocytopenia; PT, aPTT generally WNL	Renal insufficiency; FDPs and d-dimer generally (–)

DIC, disseminated intravascular coagulation; PT, prothrombin time; aPTT, activated partial thromboplastin time; TT, thrombin time; FDPs, fibrin degradation products; TTP, thrombotic thrombocytopenic purpura; WNL, within normal limits; vWf, von Willebrand factor; HUS, hemolytic uremic syndrome.

level, PT, aPTT, and TT should provide sufficient information for determining the correct diagnosis, or at least making an educated guess. By using these five screening tests and assessing other more specific tests only when an absolute diagnosis is necessary, inappropriate use of laboratory resources may be avoided.

Evaluation of Thrombosis

Patients who present with a thrombotic event will generally not display abnormalities of usual clotting studies—that is, their PT, aPTT, TT, and fibrinogen will usually be within normal ranges. Whereas hyperfibrinogenemia and persistent elevations of fVIII have been associated with an increased risk of thrombosis, both may be elevated by acute inflammation, and consequently, the finding of elevations of these clotting factors is generally not helpful in the evaluation of a thrombotic event in an acutely ill individual. Several inherited or acquired abnormalities that place an individual at increased risk for thrombosis have been identified, and determination of these factors should be undertaken when a thrombotic event is suspected or documented. Prior to the initiation of anticoagulation, plasma levels of protein C (antigen and activity), protein-S (antigen and activity), total and free, and antithrombin III (antigen and activity) should be obtained. In addition, PCR analysis for mutations in the factor V (factor V Leiden; [Arg]R506Q[Gln]), prothrombin ([Gly]G20210A[Ala], and [Ala]A19911G[Gly]) and methylenetetrahydrofolate reductase (MTHFR; [Cys]C677T[Thr]) genes should be performed. In addition, a baseline serum homocysteine may be obtained given that the thrombosis risk of the MTHFR mutation may be related to elevations of homocysteine caused by alterations in the metabolism of folic acid rather than the mutation *per se*. Acquired thrombotic risk factors include the presence of lupus anticoagulants, antiphospholipid, and anticardiolipin antibodies, which may be associated with underlying autoimmune disorders or with acute inflammation. In adult populations, approximately 40% of patients with thrombosis will not display one of the known thrombophilic risk factors. The intensivist must look for confounding clinical conditions such as severe dehydration with marked hemoconcentration—in the case of central venous sinus thrombosis, indwelling catheters, vascular compression—e.g., cervical ribs, type II heparin-induced thrombocytopenia (see below), and so forth, in their evaluation of a patient with thrombosis.

CONDITIONS ASSOCIATED WITH SERIOUS BLEEDING OR A HIGH PROBABILITY OF BLEEDING

Disseminated Intravascular Coagulation

Pathogenesis

Because it often occurs in conjunction with more serious, life-threatening disorders, DIC is one of the most serious hemostatic abnormalities seen in the ICU. The clinical syndrome itself results from the activation of blood coagulation, which then leads to excessive thrombin generation. The final result of this process is the widespread formation of fibrin thrombi in the microcirculation, with resultant consumption of certain clotting factors and platelets. Ultimately, this consumption generally results in the development of significant bleeding due to the rate of consumption outpacing the rate at which the clotting factors and platelets are produced (21). Table 170.3 reviews several specific conditions associated with the development of DIC. In general, the conditions associated with DIC are the same for either adult or pediatric populations. These include a wide variety of disorders that share as their common feature the ability to initiate coagulation to varying degrees. The mechanisms involved can generally be considered in two categories: those intrinsic processes that enzymatically activate procoagulant proteins, and those that cause the release of tissue factor, which then triggers coagulation. These are complex events that can lead to significant bleeding and often complicate the management of an already critically ill patient.

TABLE 170.3

UNDERLYING DISEASES ASSOCIATED WITH DISSEMINATED INTRAVASCULAR COAGULATION

- Sepsis
- Liver disease
- Shock
- Penetrating brain injury
- Necrotizing pneumonitis
- Tissue necrosis/crush injury
- Intravascular hemolysis
- Acute promyelocytic leukemia
- Thermal injury
- Freshwater drowning
- Fat embolism syndrome
- Retained placenta
- Hypertonic saline abortion
- Amniotic fluid embolus
- Retention of a dead fetus
- Eclampsia
- Localized endothelial injury (aortic aneurysm, giant hemangiomata, angiography)
- Disseminated malignancy (prostate, pancreatic)

Fibrinolysis invariably accompanies thrombin formation in DIC (21). Thrombin generation or release of tissue plasminogen activator usually initiates this process. Plasmin is generated, which in turn digests fibrinogen and fibrin clots as they form. Plasmin also inactivates several activated coagulation factors and impairs platelet aggregation. DIC represents an imbalance between the activity of thrombin, which leads to microvascular thrombi with coagulation factor and platelet consumption, and plasmin, which degrades these fibrin-based clots as they form. Therefore, thrombin-induced coagulation factor consumption, thrombocytopenia, and plasmin generation all contribute to the presence of bleeding.

In addition to bleeding complications, the presence of fibrin thrombi in the microcirculation also can lead to ischemic tissue injury. Pathologic data indicate that renal failure, acrocyanosis, multifocal pulmonary emboli, and transient cerebral ischemia may be related clinically to the presence of such thrombi. The fibrinopeptides A and B, resulting from enzymatic cleavage of fibrinogen, lead to pulmonary and systemic vasoconstriction, which can potentiate an existing ischemic injury. In a given patient with DIC, either bleeding or thrombotic tendencies may predominate; in most patients, bleeding is usually the predominant problem. In up to 10% of patients with DIC, however, the presentation is exclusively thrombotic—for example, pulmonary emboli with pulmonary hypertension, renal insufficiency, altered mental status, acrocyanosis—without hemorrhage. Whether the presentation of DIC is thrombotic, hemorrhagic, or compensated (that is, laboratory results consistent with DIC without overt bleeding), microthrombosis probably contributes to the development and progression of multiorgan failure.

Clinical Presentation and Diagnosis

The suspicion that DIC is present usually stems from one of two situations: unexplained generalized oozing or bleeding, or unexplained abnormal laboratory parameters of hemostasis. This usually occurs in the context of a suggestive clinical scenario or associated disease (Table 170.3). Although infection and multiple trauma are the most common underlying conditions associated with the development of DIC, certain other organ system dysfunctions predispose to DIC, including hepatic insufficiency and splenectomy (17,18). Both of these conditions are associated with impaired reticuloendothelial system function and consequent impaired clearance of activated coagulation proteins and fibrin/fibrin degradation fragments, which may inhibit fibrin polymerization and clot formation.

The clinical severity of DIC frequently has been assessed by the severity of bleeding and coagulation abnormalities. Recently, scoring tools using a panel of laboratory tests along with severity of illness scores to assess the likelihood and severity of DIC have been proposed in an attempt to determine the prognosis and direct initial therapy at the time of diagnosis. A list is found in Table 170.4. The use of these scoring systems for the early diagnosis and treatment of DIC does appear to have prognostic value, particularly in patients with sepsis (22–24). The systems suggested by Leclerc et al. (25) and Taylor et al. (26) are two of the more commonly used scoring systems and may serve as a template for the diagnosis of DIC; a qualitative score (3 out of tests positive) (Leclerc) or a quantitative score (Taylor) are strongly suggestive of a diagnosis of DIC. The combination of a prolonged PT, hypofibrinogenemia, and thrombocytopenia in the appropriate clinical setting is sufficient to suspect the diagnosis of DIC in most instances. Severe hepatic insufficiency, with splenomegaly and splenic sequestration of platelets, also can yield a similar laboratory profile and must be ruled out.

In addition to liver disease, several other conditions have presentations similar to DIC and must be considered in the differential diagnosis:

- Massive transfusion
- Primary fibrinolysis
- Thrombotic thrombocytopenic purpura/hemolytic uremic syndrome
- Heparin therapy
- Dysfibrinogenemia

With the exception of massive transfusion syndrome, these disorders generally have only two of the three characteristic laboratory findings of DIC; a comparison of the laboratory findings in these disorders is noted in Table 170.2. To confirm a diagnosis of suspected DIC, confirmatory tests indicating an increased fibrinogen turnover, such as elevated FDPs or d-dimer assay, may be necessary. The d-dimer assay for the D-D fragment of polymerized fibrin has been shown to be both highly sensitive and specific for proteolytic degradation of polymerized fibrin (fibrin clot that has been produced in the presence of thrombin). Consequently, this test is being used with increasing frequency in patients with suspected DIC. However, remembering that thrombin is produced whenever coagulation is activated in the presence of bleeding, the clinician must interpret a modest elevation of d-dimer in a postoperative or trauma patient with some degree of caution. The presence of a marked elevation of d-dimer in a nonbleeding patient essentially excludes primary fibrinogenolysis as the sole cause of measurable FDPs in the serum. The TT is a less sensitive test for DIC, but may be useful in cases of suspected heparin overdose because it will correct in the test tube with the addition of protamine sulfate or toluidine blue. Similarly, the euglobulin clot lysis time may not be sensitive to fibrinolysis associated with DIC but is significantly shortened in most cases of primary fibrinolysis. Other tests of purported value, such as soluble fibrin monomer or thrombin–antithrombin complex formation, either have problems with sensitivity or are impractical for widespread use outside of research settings.

TABLE 170.4

LABORATORY TESTS FOR THE DIAGNOSIS OF DIC

Test	Discriminator value
Platelet count	<80–100,000 cells/μL or a decrease of >50% from baseline
Fibrinogen	<100 mg/dL or a decrease of >50% from baseline
PT	>3 sec prolongation above ULN
FDPs	>80 mg/dL
d-Dimer	Moderate increase

PT, prothrombin time; FDPs, fibrin degradation products; ULN, upper limit of normal.

Thrombotic Thrombocytopenic Purpura (TTP) and Hemolytic Uremic Syndrome (HUS)

Specific mention of thrombotic thrombocytopenic purpura (TTP) and hemolytic uremic syndrome (HUS) should be made. Although neither generally produces a coagulopathic state, both are characterized by marked microangiopathy and microvascular thrombosis. Presently, these two diseases are felt to represent different ends of the spectrum of end organ dysfunction possible in microangiopathic states. HUS is more commonly seen in children, and is characterized by a prodrome of fever and diffuse, often bloody, diarrhea. Endemic cases of HUS are generally caused by verotoxin expressing enteropathic strains of *E. coli* (O157:H7) or Shiga toxin expressing strains of *Shigella*. Sporadic cases are generally not associated with diarrhea, and may represent variant TTP or familial defects in complement factor H. Therapy, including renal replacement measures, is supportive. Neither plasma infusion nor plasma exchange appears to be beneficial in the treatment of HUS. TTP is characterized by the pentad of microangiopathic hemolytic anemia (MAHA), thrombocytopenia, neurologic symptoms, fever, and renal dysfunction. Whereas only 40% of patients will display the full pentad, up to 75% will manifest a triad of MAHA, neurologic symptoms, and thrombocytopenia. This disorder is felt to be due to the absence or inhibition of a vWf cleaving protease (ADAMTS13), resulting in the circulation of unusually large vWf multimers, which can induce or enhance the pathologic adhesion of platelets to the endothelium. The therapy of choice for TTP is plasma exchange by apheresis. Platelet transfusions are generally not recommended except in the case of major bleeding.

Management

The primary treatment for DIC is correction of the underlying problem that led to its development. Specific therapy for DIC should not be undertaken unless (a) the patient has significant bleeding or organ dysfunction secondary to DIC, (b) significant thrombosis has occurred, or (c) if treatment of the underlying disorder—for example, acute promyelocytic leukemia—is likely to increase the severity of DIC.

Supportive therapy for DIC includes the use of several component blood products (27). Packed red blood cells are given according to accepted guidelines in the face of active bleeding. Fresh whole blood—that is, less than 24 to 48 hours old—also may be given to replete both volume and oxygen-carrying capacity, with the additional potential benefit of providing coagulation proteins, including fibrinogen, and platelets. Cryoprecipitate contains a much higher concentration of fibrinogen than does whole blood or fresh frozen plasma (FFP), and therefore is more likely to provide the quantity of fibrinogen needed to replete fibrinogen consumed during DIC. In this regard, FFP is of limited value for the treatment of significant hypofibrinogenemia because of the inordinate volumes required to produce any meaningful increase in plasma fibrinogen concentration. FFP infusions, however, may effectively replete other coagulation factors consumed with DIC such as protein C, although the increase in these proteins may be quite small unless large volumes of FFP are infused. The use of cryoprecipitate or FFP in the treatment of DIC has, in the past, been open to debate because of concern that these products merely provide further substrate for ongoing DIC and thus increase the amount of fibrin thrombi formed. However, clinical (autopsy) studies have failed to confirm this concern.

The goal of blood component therapy is not to produce normal numbers but rather to produce clinical stability. If the serum fibrinogen level is less than 75 to 50 mg/dL, repletion with cryoprecipitate to raise plasma levels to 100 mg/dL or higher is the goal. A reasonable starting dose is one bag of cryoprecipitate for every 10 kg body weight every 8 to 12 hours. As cryoprecipitate is not a standardized component (i.e., its content varies from bag to bag), one should recheck the fibrinogen level after an infusion to document the increase in fibrinogen level. The amount and timing of the next infusion is then adjusted according to the results. Platelet transfusions also may be used when thrombocytopenia is thought to contribute to ongoing bleeding. Many of the fibrin/fibrinogen fragments produced in DIC have the potential to impair platelet function by inhibiting fibrinogen binding to platelets. This may be clinically significant at the concentration of FDPs achieved with DIC. Platelet transfusions in patients with DIC should be considered to maintain platelet counts up to 40,000 to 80,000 cells/μL, depending on the clinical specifics of the patient.

Pharmacologic therapy for DIC has two primary aims: to "turn off" ongoing coagulation so that repletion of coagulation factors may begin, and to impede thrombus formation and ensuing ischemic injury. Two new recombinant blood products have been recently developed that have some usefulness in the treatment of DIC. The first is recombinant-activated protein C. This product has been shown to result in a 6% reduction in sepsis mortality in adults and possibly a reduction in the incidence of DIC (28). However, in older adults, its use was associated with an increase in intracranial bleeding. The second new agent for the treatment of severe bleeding, including DIC, is recombinant-activated factor VII (rhfVIIa). Although there are limited controlled trials of its use and none in the pediatric age range, with the exception of those patients with acquired inhibitors to fVIII, it has been proven to be a potent agent for the control of bleeding from several medical and surgical causes, including DIC and other consumptive coagulopathies (29–31). This agent has also been shown to correct the hemostatic defect caused by the antiplatelet agents aspirin and clopidogrel (32). There have been reports that use of rhfVIIa may result in an increase in thrombosis and thromboembolic events, although the incidence appears to be small and the severity of most events mild (33). In addition to activated protein C, other anticoagulant molecules such as heparin and antithrombin III and thrombolytic agents continue to be studied as therapy for DIC and sepsis (34,35).

Liver Disease and Hepatic Insufficiency

Abnormal Hemostasis in Liver Disease

Liver disease is a common cause of abnormal hemostasis in ICU patients, with abnormal coagulation studies or overt bleeding occurring in approximately 15% of patients with either clinical or laboratory evidence of hepatic dysfunction. It is a common cause of a prolonged PT or aPTT, often without any clinical sequelae. The hemostatic defect associated with liver disease is multifactorial, with multiple aspects of hemostasis affected (36,37).

In liver disease, the synthesis of several plasma coagulation proteins is impaired. These include factors II, V, VII, IX, and X. Fibrinogen synthesis by the liver usually can be maintained at levels that prevent bleeding until terminal liver failure supervenes. However, the function of fibrinogen synthesized by a diseased liver may not be normal, owing to an increased sialic acid content in its structure, which may result in a diminished ability to form clots (i.e., a dysfibrinogen). Factor XIII activity also is often decreased in the setting of hepatocellular disease. However, the clinical significance of this decrease in factor XIII is uncertain because levels as low as 3% provide normal fibrin clot stabilization. Although it is apparently synthesized by the liver, factor VIII (i.e., factor VIII coagulant protein [VIII:C], antihemophilic factor A [AHF]) synthesis seems to be independent of the state of hepatic function. Indeed, factor VIII levels may be increased in some types of liver disease. Plasma protein C and antithrombin III levels are low in many conditions of hepatic insufficiency, with variable effects.

In addition to these defects in plasma coagulation protein synthesis, many patients with liver disease, particularly cirrhosis, have increased fibrinolytic activity. The mechanism for this heightened fibrinolytic state is not clear, but may be related to the increased amounts of plasminogen activator often noted in these patients. It may be difficult to discern whether fibrinolysis occurs solely because of underlying severe liver disease or as a result of concurrent DIC, as patients with cirrhosis are at increased risk for the development of DIC. In liver disease, levels of FDPs can be increased by both increased fibrinolysis and by decreased hepatic clearance. Finally, clinically significant fibrinolysis is a frequent occurrence in patients who undergo portacaval shunt procedures. The clinical distinction between primary DIC and a secondary hemostatic defect resulting from liver disease can be virtually impossible to make if active bleeding is present.

Thrombocytopenia may be present to a variable degree in patients with hepatic dysfunction. This is usually ascribed to splenic sequestration. It is rarely profound and generally does not produce clinically significant bleeding as a solitary defect. *In vitro* platelet aggregation may also be affected, however. Increased plasma concentrations of FDPs are a possible cause of these qualitative platelet abnormalities. The thrombocytopenia of liver disease in conjunction with other coagulation or hemostatic defects secondary to liver disease may result in bleeding that is difficult to manage clinically, particularly if all aspects of the problem are not addressed.

Patients with hepatocellular disease may also exhibit decreased synthesis of the vitamin K–dependent anticoagulant proteins, protein C and protein S, as well as antithrombin-III (37). Decreased levels of these natural anticoagulants may increase the risk of thrombosis. Neither the PT, aPTT, nor TT will be affected by the levels of any of these naturally occurring anticoagulants.

Presentation

The hemostatic defect in liver disease is multifactorial, and each patient should be approached accordingly. The most common scenario is a patient with liver disease and a prolonged PT without overt bleeding in whom the potential for bleeding is a concern. In patients with liver disease and impaired synthetic capabilities, particularly those who are critically ill, factor VII activity levels are usually the first to decrease due to its short half-life—4 to 6 hours—and increased turnover. This results in a prolonged PT, and can be noted even when usual markers of hepatocellular injury or hepatic insufficiency remain relatively normal (36,37). A prolonged thrombin time in the setting of liver disease may indicate the presence of dysfibrinogenemia as a result of altered hepatic fibrinogen synthesis, or may indicate an acquired defect in fibrin polymerization (e.g., increased FDPs). As the severity of liver disease increases, the aPTT also may be affected, reflecting more severely impaired synthetic function. In this setting, plasma concentrations of the vitamin K–dependent coagulation proteins decrease, as does factor V, which is not vitamin K dependent. Although fibrinogen synthesis occurs in the liver, plasma levels of fibrinogen are generally maintained until the disease approaches end-stage. When fibrinogen levels are severely depressed, liver failure has typically reached the terminal phase. In contrast to the hypofibrinogenemia noted with consumptive coagulopathies, the synthetic hypofibrinogenemia of liver disease is not accompanied by a marked increase in either FDPs or d-dimers.

In more severe forms of liver disease, fibrinolysis may complicate clinical management. Differentiating between concomitant DIC and fibrinolysis attributable to liver disease alone may be difficult. The d-dimer assay result should be negative in the patient with liver disease and elevated FDPs, but no active bleeding. Further clinical distinction usually is not possible.

Management

If the patient is not actively bleeding, with certain provisos, no specific therapy is required. In patients with a prolonged PT who are in a postoperative state or are scheduled for an invasive procedure, correction of the PT may be attempted. FFP provides the most immediate source of specific coagulation factors (i.e., factor VII), and usually corrects an isolated mild PT prolongation. Cryoprecipitate is required only if fibrinogen levels are less than 50 to 100 mg/dL, or if there is documentation of a significant dysfibrinogenemia. Vitamin K deficiency also is relatively common in this patient population, and replacement may be needed. In contrast to patients with dietary vitamin K deficiency and normal liver function, correction of the PT in vitamin K–responsive critically ill patients typically requires longer than 12 to 24 hours. Patients with significant hepatic impairment may manifest a partial response or may not respond at all. The immediate use of FFP is therefore appropriate when rapid correction is necessary. Recombinant human-activated factor VII (rhfIIa) infusions have been shown to control the bleeding in severe liver disease, although this does not necessarily result in reduced mortality (38,39).

When the synthetic capability of the liver becomes more profoundly impaired, and the aPTT is also prolonged, greater volumes of FFP or more specific therapy may be needed. The use of factor IX concentrates (prothrombin complex concentrates) or rhfVIIa has been advocated, particularly if bleeding is present; however, their use remains controversial. Those products produced from plasma pooled from multiple donors carry a significant risk of both hepatitis B and C. In addition, they may provoke DIC and actually worsen hemostasis. The use of prothrombin complex concentrates or rhfVIIa should be reserved for patients with poorly controlled bleeding that is unresponsive to other more established therapeutic modalities such as infusion of FFP. Guidelines for the use of rhfVIIa are under development.

A comprehensive therapeutic approach is needed in the patient with active bleeding as a result of liver disease. Initially, FFP, 10 to 15 mL/kg body weight, may be given every 6 to 8 hours until bleeding slows significantly, and should then be continued at maintenance levels as dictated by clinical status and coagulation studies. Recombinant human-activated factor VII or prothrombin complex concentrates may be used in those patients unresponsive to FFP infusions (39). Cryoprecipitate should be infused for fibrinogen levels less than 50 to 100 mg/dL. Platelet transfusions also may be required if the platelet count is less than 40,000 to 80,000 cells/μL, depending on the clinical situation. Vitamin K should be empirically administered on the presumption that part of the synthetic defect may result from a lack of this cofactor. However, one must anticipate a poor response to vitamin K in the presence of severe liver disease. Transfusions of packed cells are given as deemed appropriate by the clinician.

Vitamin K Deficiency

The most common cause of a prolonged PT in the ICU is vitamin K deficiency. Vitamin K is necessary for the gamma-carboxylation of factors II, VII, IX, and X, without which these factors cannot bind calcium and are not efficiently converted into their activated forms. Factor VII has the shortest half-life of these coagulation proteins; accordingly, the PT is the most sensitive early indicator of vitamin K deficiency.

Vitamin K deficiency is relatively common in critically ill patients for several reasons, including the use of broad-spectrum antibiotics, poor nutrition preceding or subsequent to ICU admission, and the use of parenteral nutrition without vitamin K supplementation. Many of the second- and third-generation cephalosporins (e.g., ceftriaxone, cefpodoxime, cefepime, ceftazidime) may directly interfere with vitamin K absorption from the gut lumen. The metabolites of some of these antibiotics may even act as competitive inhibitors of vitamin K (i.e., cefamandole). In addition, these and other antibiotics may kill or inhibit the growth of gut bacteria, and thus limit the amounts of vitamin K that they normally produce and excrete into the gut lumen. Although malnutrition also may contribute to the development of vitamin K deficiency, this usually requires 1 to 2 weeks to develop in the complete absence of vitamin K intake. However, the use of parenteral alimentation without vitamin K supplementation, coupled with antibiotic use, may result in rapid vitamin K depletion; prolongation of the PT can occur within only 2 to 3 days. Finally, fat malabsorption states, including cystic fibrosis, may be associated with vitamin K deficiency. Vitamin K is fat soluble and is not absorbed well in some biliary tract and intrinsic small bowel disease. In the ICU, vitamin K deficiency usually results from the interaction of several of these factors, and is rarely limited to one of the conditions mentioned. It is the responsibility of the clinician to maintain an awareness of the potential for vitamin K deficiency and to treat accordingly.

The differential diagnosis of an isolated prolongation of the PT, with or without bleeding, includes both vitamin K deficiency and liver disease. The clinical presentation of these patients is often quite similar. In fact, the distinction sometimes can be made only on the basis of the response (or lack thereof) to empirical vitamin K therapy. Warfarin administration (either overt or covert) also should be excluded as a cause of a prolonged PT. Newer, long-acting vitamin K antagonist rodenticides (so-called *super-warfarin*), when ingested, produce a profound, prolonged, vitamin K–resistant reduction in vitamin K–dependent clotting factors and may produce an isolated prolongation of the PT initially. Treatment of poisoning with these agents requires the aggressive prolonged use of vitamin K and, in the bleeding patient, infusions of FFP or rhfVIIa. Confirmation of warfarin exposure as the cause of a prolonged PT is possible by toxicologic methods to detect the drug and/or its metabolites, or one can identify the presence of noncarboxylated forms of vitamin K–dependent clotting factors in plasma (*p*roteins *i*nduced by *v*itamin *K a*ntagonist; PIVKAs). In addition, the presence of a specific inhibitor or congenital deficiency of factor VII will also result in an isolated prolongation of the PT. Acquired inhibitors of factor VII are rare, and homozygous deficiency of factor VII has not been described. Individuals heterozygous for factor VII deficiency and those with certain polymorphisms of the promoter region of the factor VII gene tend to have factor VII levels in the 25% to 35% range, and do not appear to be at significant increased risk for bleeding. Lupus-like anticoagulants, resulting from inflammation, may also result in an isolated prolongation of the PT; these are generally of no clinical significance and are not associated with an increased risk of bleeding.

The laboratory findings of an isolated vitamin K deficiency, in addition to a prolonged PT, include a normal fibrinogen level, platelet count, and factor V level. Factor V is not a vitamin K–dependent protein, and should therefore be normal except in cases of DIC (consumption) or severe liver disease (decreased production). Prolongation of the aPTT from vitamin K deficiency, warfarin therapy, or from liver disease is a relatively late event, and occurs initially as a result of factor IX depletion.

Management

The management of vitamin K deficiency consists primarily of its repletion, usually by intravenous or subcutaneous routes in critically ill patients. Therapy should not await the development of bleeding or oozing, but should be administered when the PT abnormality is detected and vitamin K deficiency is thought to be responsible. As with other drugs administered subcutaneously (e.g., insulin), adequate blood pressure and subcutaneous perfusion are needed to ensure reliable absorption from the soft tissues. The possibility of anaphylactoid reactions with the intravenous use of vitamin K is of concern. This risk is markedly reduced when the drug is given as a piggyback infusion over 30 to 45 minutes in a small volume of fluid rather than as a bolus or slow-push dose (40); this is the preferred method of drug administration in hemodynamically unstable patients. However, incidences of anaphylaxis are still reported with this mode of infusion (41,42). The usual dose of vitamin K in adults is 10 to 15 mg intravenously or subcutaneously, 1 to 5 mg in young children, and up to 10 mg in larger children. In an otherwise healthy person, the PT should correct within 12 to 24 hours after this dose. Serial dosing of critically ill patients is often used, however, and the PT may require up to 72 hours to normalize. If the PT does not correct within 72 hours after three daily doses of vitamin K, intrinsic liver disease should be suspected. Further administration of vitamin K is of no additional benefit in this setting.

When the patient is actively bleeding, it is not sufficient to only provide vitamin K. A more immediate restoration of coagulation is required. FFP has traditionally been used in this setting. To restore hemostasis to an acceptable level, 30% to 50% of normal factor activity, 10 to 20 mL/kg body weight of FFP is typically required. A similar approach is used in patients previously given warfarin. Recombinant human-activated factor VII (rhfVIIa) has been used with success to reverse the bleeding noted in vitamin K deficiency and in warfarin overdose (39,43).

Massive Transfusion Syndrome

Transfusion of large quantities of blood can result in a multifactorial hemostatic defect. The genesis of this problem is related to the washout of plasma coagulation proteins and platelets, and it may be exacerbated by the development of DIC with consequent factor consumption, hypothermia, acidosis, or rarely, by citrate toxicity or hypocalcemia. These variables often act in combination to cause a coagulopathic state (44).

A washout syndrome can result from the transfusion of large amounts of stored blood products devoid of clotting factors and platelets. This develops exclusively in patients who receive large volumes of packed red blood cells (RBCs) (e.g., trauma victims, patients with massive gastrointestinal hemorrhage or hepatectomy, or those undergoing cardiopulmonary bypass) without also receiving FFP and platelets. Factors V and VII have short shelf half-lives and are often deficient in blood that has been banked longer than 48 hours. In addition, a qualitative platelet defect can be demonstrated in whole blood within hours of its storage, especially if an acid–citrate–dextrose solution is used. Consequently, transfusion of large quantities of stored whole blood may produce limited improvement of the bleeding resulting from decreased clotting factors and platelets. The development of a washout coagulopathy is directly dependent on the volume of blood transfused relative to the blood volume of the patient. As a general rule, residual plasma clotting activity after one blood volume exchange falls to 18% to 37% of normal, whereas after a two–blood volume exchange, residual activity is only 3% to 14%; and after a three–blood volume exchange, less than 5% of normal clotting function remains.

As previously discussed, DIC may develop in many clinical settings, including some associated with major hemorrhage or massive transfusion. In the presence of hypotension associated with hypovolemia or hemorrhagic shock, DIC is a common sequela. Major trauma itself, especially with the release of tissue factors into the plasma, also can result in the development of DIC. Exsanguinating hemorrhage sometimes requires blood replacement faster than a type-and-crossmatch of each unit can be performed, and unmatched blood is given as a lifesaving measure. Donor–recipient incompatibility—even when the mismatch is only of the minor blood group systems—can lead to DIC. Human error resulting in major incompatibility can produce severe hemolysis and be lethal. Finally, microaggregates of blood cells that form within stored blood products also can cause DIC. The advent of smaller pore, more effective filtering systems for blood product administration, however, has essentially eliminated this as a source of problems.

The patient who is bleeding as a consequence of massive transfusion or washout presents with diffuse oozing and bleeding from all surgical wounds and puncture sites. Laboratory abnormalities include prolonged PT, aPTT, and TT. Fibrinogen levels and platelet counts are typically decreased; FDPs are not usually increased unless concurrent DIC is present (Table 170.2). The likelihood that the clinico-laboratory picture is a direct result of the massive transfusion can be estimated from the amount of bleeding that has occurred and the blood volume administered relative to the patient's blood volume (i.e., the number of blood volume exchanges that have been given). The more stored blood (e.g., packed RBCs) transfused relative to the patient's blood volume, the greater the chance of the development of coagulopathy due to massive transfusion.

Management

The therapeutic approach to patients who develop a coagulopathy from massive transfusion is supportive. Platelets and FFP are given to replete the components of coagulation that are typically lacking (45). Platelet administration may help stem bleeding from anatomic wounds. Severe bleeding associated with thrombocytopenia alone is uncommon unless counts fall below 20,000 to 30,000 cells/μL of blood. Because of the complex nature of bleeding seen with massive transfusion, patients may benefit from platelet transfusion at counts even as high as 80,000 to 100,000 cells/μL. FFP is preferred over cryoprecipitate because it has a more complete coagulation protein composition. However, cryoprecipitate may be specifically given when fibrinogen depletion is thought to be a major contributor to the observed bleeding.

The prospective identification of those at risk of developing a coagulopathy from massive transfusion is critical. When the magnitude of the insult and the anticipated need for blood are large, both platelets and FFP should be given before a coagulopathy develops. In most patients (e.g., weight greater than or equal to 30 to 40 kg or body surface area [BSA] greater than or equal to 1.0 m^2), four units of platelets (or $\frac{1}{2}$ unit of apheresis-collected platelets) and one unit of FFP should be given for each five units of whole blood or packed cells transfused. This should prevent washout and its attendant bleeding. If the patient continues to bleed despite what should be adequate therapy for massive transfusion syndrome, other causes should be considered. Specifically, anatomic bleeding and the possibility of DIC should be investigated. Therapy in this setting may include rhfVIIa infusion (31).

Anticoagulant Overdose

Anticoagulant therapy is not unusual in the ICU, and the possibility of errors in administration exists. Methods of prophylactic anticoagulant use, systemic anticoagulation, and thrombolytic therapy are sometimes poorly standardized and can lead to overdose.

Heparin

Heparin is a repeating polymer of two disaccharide glycosaminoglycans, and is commercially prepared from either porcine intestinal mucosa or bovine lung. Heparin is currently found in two forms: unfractionated heparin (UH) and low-molecular-weight heparin (LMWH). It is important to understand the differences between these two forms of the drug, as they have different mechanisms of action and associated precautions. Unfractionated heparin has an immediate effect on coagulation that is mediated primarily through its interaction with antithrombin III. The resulting heparin–antithrombin III complex possesses a much greater affinity for thrombin than does AT-III alone and inactivates thrombin, thereby damping-down clot formation. In addition, heparin also has a direct effect of inhibiting activated factor X (fXa). This anticoagulant effect of UH is relatively minor. Consequently, achieving a therapeutic aPTT with UH is very difficult in the face of low levels of AT-III. The degree of anticoagulation produced by heparin is monitored by the prolongation of the aPTT.

In contrast, LMWH, produced by controlled enzymatic cleavage of heparin polymers, produces anticoagulation almost exclusively through inhibition of F.Xa. This produces a more stable degree of anticoagulation and, due to its longer half-life (approximately 3 to 5 hours) and biologic activity (approximately 24 hours), allows for intermittent bolus therapy every 12 or 24 hours while still maintaining a steady-state effect. However, LMWH does not produce consistent prolongation of the aPTT, and requires assay of anti-Xa activity for monitoring, if monitoring is desired.

Heparin is metabolized in the liver by the "heparinase" enzyme in a dose-dependent fashion, with excess heparin then being excreted through the kidneys. As the rate of heparin administration is increased, the half-life of the drug is prolonged due to the increase in the percentage of the drug being excreted by the kidney. For example, when a 10-unit/kg bolus of heparin is infused intravenously, the average half-life of the drug is 1 hour. If the bolus is increased to 400 or 800 units/kg, however, the half-life is prolonged to 2.5 and 5 hours, respectively. The nonlinear response results in greater drug effects on coagulation with smaller dosage increments. When one "reboluses" or increases a heparin infusion rate in response to insufficient anticoagulation (i.e., inadequate prolongation of the aPTT), a point will be reached when further small increments in the heparin infusion rate may result in a substantially greater prolongation of the aPTT. The risk of pathologic bleeding associated with heparin increases when the prolongation of the aPTT is beyond the therapeutic window, generally considered to be 1.5 to 2.5 times the patient's baseline aPTT and corresponding to a plasma heparin concentration of 0.2 to 0.4 units/mL. As a corollary, the administration of heparin as a continuous infusion rather than in an intermittent bolus dose regimen is less likely to be associated with pathologic bleeding.

Management. Serious bleeding associated with heparin overdose can be rapidly reversed by protamine sulfate. Protamine binds ionically with heparin to form a complex that lacks any anticoagulant activity. As a general rule, 1 mg of protamine neutralizes approximately 100 units of heparin (specifically, 90 USP units of bovine heparin or 115 USP units of porcine heparin). The dose of protamine needed is calculated from the number of units of active heparin remaining in the patient's system. This, in turn, is estimated from the original heparin dose and the typical half-life for that infusion rate. The aPTT is used to gauge the residual effects of heparin. Protamine itself potentially has anticoagulant effects, and precautions are necessary during its administration. The drug should be given by slow intravenous push over 8 to 10 minutes. A single dose should not exceed 1mg/kg, with a 50-mg maximum dose. This dose may be repeated, but no more than 2 mg/kg, to a 100-mg maximum dose, should be given as a cumulative dose without rechecking coagulation parameters. The dose of protamine should always be monitored by coagulation studies. Significant side effects are most commonly seen in situations of overly rapid drug administration, and include hypotension and anaphylactoid-like reactions. LMWH is not consistently neutralized by protamine, so invasive procedures should not be performed within 24 hours of administration. Bleeding following LMWH therapy has been treated effectively with rhfVIIa.

Warfarin

Warfarin and vitamin K are structurally similar in their respective 4-hydroxycoumarin nucleus and naphthoquinone ring. The mechanism of action of warfarin is through competitive binding at the vitamin K receptor site, where postribosomal modification, through γ-carboxylation of the vitamin K–dependent coagulation proteins—factors II, VII, IX, and X–occurs. This postsynthetic modification is necessary to produce a calcium-binding site on the molecule, which, when occupied, allows for the efficient activation of the zymogen clotting factor into its enzymatically active form. When warfarin is present in sufficient plasma concentrations, there is depletion of the active forms of vitamin K–dependent factors.

The PT, or more precisely the international normalized ratio (INR) calculated from the PT, is an accurate indicator of the effects of warfarin when its use has continued beyond 2 or 3 days. Factor VII has a half-life of only 4 to 6 hours, and the active form is rapidly depleted after one or two doses of warfarin. The remainder of the vitamin K–dependent factors may take up to a week to become depleted. The PT becomes prolonged and INR elevated with factor VII depletion alone, but does not reflect an overall state of anticoagulation until an equilibrium period of several days has passed. Over this time, the other vitamin K–dependent factors are depleted, and PT prolongation (INR elevation) can then be used to assess the anticoagulant effects of warfarin. In severe cases of warfarin overdose, the aPTT also becomes prolonged as a result of depletion of the active forms of factors II, IX, and X.

Several drugs and pathophysiologic conditions are associated with potentiation of warfarin's effects on coagulation. Table 170.5 lists many of the drugs known to prolong the effects of warfarin. These drugs have various mechanisms, which generally include either inhibition of function or competitive binding of the enzymes responsible for active warfarin metabolism. Aspirin does not seem to have any direct effect on warfarin metabolism, but can so profoundly influence qualitative platelet function that it must be considered as a potentiator of warfarin's anticoagulant effects. The same is true for clofibrate. Ingestion of large quantities of aspirin may also impair prothrombin (factor II) synthesis, further increasing the effects of warfarin administration. As warfarin is metabolized by the liver, conditions of acute and chronic hepatic dysfunction can alter warfarin metabolism and vitamin K–mediated γ-carboxylation of the vitamin K–dependent coagulation proteins. Broad-spectrum antibiotics also may limit vitamin K availability through their alteration of the gut flora, in addition to any direct effect on vitamin K metabolism. All of these factors may ultimately influence a patient's response to warfarin.

A clinical syndrome referred to as warfarin (Coumadin) necrosis has been noted during the initial stages of anticoagulation with a vitamin K antagonist. It is characterized clinically by the development of skin and subcutaneous necrosis, particularly in areas of subcutaneous fat, and pathologically by the thrombosis of small blood vessels in the fat and subcutaneous

TABLE 170.5

DRUGS THAT POTENTIATE THE ANTICOAGULANT EFFECTS OF WARFARIN

ANTIBIOTICS
Broad-spectrum antibiotics (especially cephalosporins)
Griseofulvin (oral)
Metronidazole
Sulfinpyrazone
Trimethoprim-sulfamethoxazole
ANTI-INFLAMMATORY DRUGS
Steroids (anabolic, in particular)
Acetylated salicylates
Phenylbutazone (oxyphenbutazone)
Sulfonamides
OTHER DRUGS
Cimetidine
Clofibrate
Disulfiram
Phenytoin
Thyroxine (both D- and L-isomers)
Tolbutamide

tissues. This syndrome is caused by the rapid depletion of the vitamin K–dependent anticoagulant protein C prior to achieving depletion of procoagulant proteins and occurs predominantly in individuals heterozygous for protein C deficiency. Whereas anticoagulation generally requires a decrease in procoagulant protein levels to approximately 20% to 25%, a prothrombotic milieu is created with protein C levels of 40% or less. Consequently, individuals who are heterozygous for protein C deficiency and have baseline protein C levels of 50% to 60% of normal may develop a prothrombotic environment during the first few days of warfarin therapy. The risk of developing warfarin necrosis appears to be greater when an initial dose of warfarin greater than 10 to 15 mg is administered. The development of this syndrome generally can be avoided if heparin and warfarin therapy are overlapped until "coumadinization" is complete and if large loading doses of warfarin are avoided.

Management. When overanticoagulation with warfarin presents with bleeding, immediate reversal is usually mandated (43). The treatment of choice is FFP, which provides prompt restoration of the deficient vitamin K–dependent coagulation proteins, along with restoration of hemostatic function. Ten to 15 mL/kg of FFP are usually sufficient to produce significant correction of the PT, although repeat infusions of FFP may be needed to effect continued correction of the PT due to the short half-life of factor VII (45). Vitamin K also may be administered, particularly in situations that are less acute (see above section Vitamin K Deficiency), although this will make it more difficult to "re-coumadinize" the patient afterwards. For severe bleeding or bleeding not controlled by FFP infusions, rhfVIIa has been used successfully.

Platelet Disorders

Platelets are necessary for efficient clot formation. They not only produce a physical barrier at the site of vascular injury, the so-called *platelet plug*, they also serve to focus the clotting process at the point of bleeding by delivering vasoconstrictors, clotting factors, and a surface on which clot development occurs to the bleeding site (Fig. 170.3). Quantitative and qualitative platelet disorders are a common cause of clinical bleeding

TABLE 170.6

PLATELET DISORDERS SEEN IN THE ICU

Quantitative	Qualitative
INCREASED DESTRUCTION	DRUGS
Immune	**Anti-inflammatory agents**
Idiopathic thrombocytopenic purpura	Aspirin (irreversible)
Systemic lupus erythematosus	Nonsteroidal anti-inflammatory agents
Acquired immunodeficiency syndrome	Corticosteroids
Drugs (gold salts, heparin, sulfonamides, quinidine, quinine)	**Antibiotics**
	Penicillins (e.g., ampicillin, carbenicillin, ticarcillin, penicillin-G)
Sepsis	
Nonimmune	Cephalosporins (e.g., cephalothin)
Thrombotic thrombocytopenic purpura/ hemolytic uremic syndrome	Nitrofurantoin
	Chloroquine, hydroxychloroquine
Mechanical destruction (e.g., cardiopulmonary bypass, hyperthermia)	**Phosphodiesterase inhibitors**
	Dipyridamole
	Methylxanthines (e.g., theophylline)
Consumption (i.e., DIC)	**Other drugs**
	Antihistamines
DECREASED PRODUCTION	Alpha-blockers (e.g., phentolamine)
Marrow suppression	Beta-blockers (e.g., propranolol)
Chemotherapy	Dextran
Viral illness (e.g., cytomegalovirus, Epstein-Barr virus, herpes simplex, parvovirus)	Ethanol
	Furosemide
	Heparin
Drugs (thiazides, ethanol, cimetidine)	Local anesthetics (e.g., lidocaine)
Marrow replacement	Phenothiazines
Tumor	Tricyclic antidepressants
Myelofibrosis	Nitrates (e.g., sodium nitroprusside, nitroglycerin)
Other conditions	
Splenic sequestration	
Dilution (see massive transfusion syndrome)	METABOLIC CAUSES
	Uremia
	Stored whole blood
	Disseminated intravascular coagulation (i.e., FDP-mediated inhibition)
	Hypothyroidism

DIC, disseminated intravascular coagulation; FDP, fibrin degradation product.

in the ICU. Table 170.6 presents an overview of platelet disorders based on this classification scheme.

Quantitative Platelet Disorders

A decrease in the number of circulating platelets reflects the presence of increased peripheral destruction/sequestration, decreased marrow production, or a combination of these factors. Examples of increased peripheral destruction include immune-mediated processes (both autoimmune and drug-induced), abnormal consumption (as in DIC), and mechanical destruction (e.g., cardiopulmonary bypass, hyperthermia). Autoimmune processes such as idiopathic thrombocytopenic purpura (ITP), SLE, or acquired immunodeficiency syndrome (AIDS) can result in increased peripheral destruction and increased splenic sequestration of platelets. Autoimmune destruction also may occur in conjunction with lymphocytic leukemia or lymphoma. The prototypic example of immune thrombocytopenia is ITP, in which immunoglobin—generally IgG—directed against specific platelet antigens is thought to be responsible for platelet destruction. Acute ITP is usually self-limited, with life-threatening bleeding occurring only rarely. In contrast, chronic ITP generally requires some sort of immunosuppressive therapy. Steroids, at a dose of 2 to 4 mg/kg/day of prednisone or its equivalent, may be given. High doses of intravenous gamma globulin at 1 to 2 g/kg and given over 2 to 5 days, and infusions of anti-RhD antigen antibody (WinRho) at 25 to 60 μg/kg, are equally efficacious in producing at least transient elevations in platelet counts. Agents such as vincristine/vinblastine, cyclophosphamide, and, most recently, rituximab (Rituxin; anti-CD20 monoclonal antibody) also have been used as immunosuppressants, with variable success, although responses are generally not immediate. Splenectomy may be required to avert serious bleeding complications in patients who do not respond to medical management, although this approach is chosen much less often in children than in adults. In ITP, the degree of bleeding attributed to the thrombocytopenia is generally less than that noted when thrombocytopenia results from decreased production. In general, severe bleeding is not noted until the platelet count is less than 10,000 cells/μL, although levels below 40,000 to 50,000 cells/μL may increase the risk of bleeding with an invasive procedure.

Drug-induced, immune-mediated platelet destruction is a cause of thrombocytopenia frequently considered in the thrombocytopenic ICU patient. Fortunately, when present, it is usually reversible; withdrawal of the offending drug prevents further immune-mediated platelet destruction. The exact mechanism of platelet destruction seems to be related to the binding of a drug to the platelet membrane, with subsequent binding to the platelet, platelet–drug complex, or both, of a specific antibody. The resulting platelet–drug–antibody complexes then are cleared by the reticuloendothelial system (e.g., the spleen), and thrombocytopenia develops. Drugs used in the ICU that are most commonly associated with this clinical picture include quinidine, quinine, heparin, gold salts, various penicillin and cephalosporin antibiotics, and the sulfonamides. The anticonvulsant valproic acid (Depakote, Depakene) frequently produces a dose-dependent thrombocytopenia that, at least in part, is immunologic in nature.

Various drugs are associated with a nonimmune mechanism of thrombocytopenia by bone marrow suppression. Most cancer chemotherapeutic agents produce thrombocytopenia as a consequence of marrow suppression. The thiazide diuretics, cimetidine, ethanol, and several of the cephalosporin and penicillin antibiotics may suppress platelet production. Generalized infection, such as bacterial sepsis, and many viral illnesses are also associated with bone marrow suppression and thrombocytopenia, even if there is an element of immune platelet destruction. Disorders such as Gaucher disease may produce a mild to moderate thrombocytopenia as a result of marrow replacement by nonhematopoietic cells.

Consumption of platelets also can cause thrombocytopenia. Mechanical destruction invariably occurs during the use of cardiopulmonary bypass machines, and it is not uncommon to note a 50% drop in platelet count postbypass when compared to preoperative platelet levels. Platelet counts may continue to decrease for 48 to 72 hours after bypass before recovering toward preoperative levels. Platelets may also be destroyed by the high body temperatures seen in severe hyperthermic syndromes, and are consumed during microvascular coagulation in DIC. In many of these circumstances, the thrombocytopenia may be the sole or a contributing cause of significant bleeding.

Heparin-induced Thrombocytopenia

The special problems associated with heparin merit emphasis. Heparin use is ubiquitous in the ICU, and the thrombocytopenia seen with its use may develop in one of two ways. Acute nonidiosyncratic heparin-induced thrombocytopenia is seen in approximately 10% to 15% of patients receiving heparin. The degree of thrombocytopenia is generally mild and usually remits despite continued use of the drug (type I HIT, or heparin-associated thrombocytopenia). The thrombocytopenia that develops has no clinical significance, and heparin need not be stopped in these patients.

Idiosyncratic heparin-induced thrombocytopenia is of much greater clinical consequence. Although it is a less frequent occurrence, typically being seen in fewer than 5% of patients receiving heparin, it has a much greater potential for clinical morbidity. Arterial thrombosis is the most significant risk of this form of heparin-induced thrombocytopenia (type II HIT) and may be life threatening, causing myocardial infarction, stroke, pulmonary embolism, or renal infarction. The mechanism of thrombosis is thought to be a consequence of the deposition of platelet aggregates in the microcirculation (46). Thrombocytopenia, like other immune-mediated drug reactions, seems to involve the formation of platelet aggregates mediated by the binding of specific antibody, directed against a heparin-platelet factor 4 complex, to platelets in the presence of heparin. This process requires minuscule amounts of heparin. Clinical bleeding is an infrequent problem in these patients in spite of the often marked thrombocytopenia observed.

From a practical perspective, the diagnosis of heparin-induced thrombocytopenia is usually one of exclusion. Diagnostic markers do exist (e.g., heparin-dependent platelet antibodies, aggregation or serotonin release), but these tests are best considered confirmatory and not exclusionary. An ELISA (enzyme-linked immunosorbent assay) for heparin-dependent platelet antibodies is the most common test obtained to investigate a possible diagnosis of HIT, but because of a relatively high false-positive rate, it is generally recommended that a more specific heparin-induced platelet injury assay, such as a serotonin release assay, be performed for confirmation. The diagnosis may be difficult to confirm because coexisting clinical illnesses with the potential to cause thrombocytopenia also may be present. Although heparin-induced thrombocytopenia is more likely to be associated with the use of bovine lung heparin, it can occur after exposure to porcine heparin or, much less commonly, to low-molecular-weight heparin. When type II HIT is suspected or confirmed, all exposure to heparin—including heparin flushes, heparin in total parenteral nutrition (TPN), and heparin-coated catheters—must be removed, and anticoagulation with an alternate agent must be initiated because of the risk of delayed thrombosis, which can occur up to 30 days after removal of heparin exposure (46). Patients with type II HIT should receive continued anticoagulation with direct thrombin inhibitors (argatroban, lepirudin) or with the heparinoid, Danaparoid. The direct thrombin inhibitors are preferred, as they carry no risk of cross-reacting with the heparin-dependent antibodies already present (47). Argatroban is cleared by the liver and lepirudin by the kidney. Consequently, the choice and dose of drug may be affected by the presence of hepatic or renal insufficiency. Warfarin alone is not adequate therapy for suspected type II HIT because of the risk of thrombosis from depression of protein C levels before the other factors are inhibited. However, warfarin can be used in conjunction with a direct thrombin inhibitor, and subsequently continued as a single agent once therapeutic suppression of vitamin K–dependent clotting factors has been achieved. Platelet transfusions are contraindicated in type II HIT due to the risk of inducing vascular thrombosis (46).

Qualitative Platelet Disorders

Many of the drugs frequently used in the ICU have the potential to impair platelet function. Frequently, the sicker the patient, the greater the likelihood that he or she will be exposed to one of these drugs. These patients often have other underlying pathophysiologic conditions that, in and of themselves, can predispose to bleeding. Table 170.6 provides an abbreviated list of the drugs that can affect at least *in vitro* platelet function.

Unnecessary drugs should always be viewed with a jaundiced eye and discontinued. These agents, as well as necessary drugs are, of course, suspect in patients with evidence or a strong suspicion of qualitative platelet dysfunction. In most cases, terminating the offending drugs usually results in a restoration of normal platelet functional activity. Aspirin is the notable exception, as it irreversibly inhibits platelet cyclooxygenase, resulting in a defect that lasts for the duration of the platelet life span—about 8 to 9 days. The effect is profound: a single 325-mg aspirin tablet results in a qualitative platelet defect that remains in 50% of the circulating platelets 5 days after its ingestion. Ideally, one would like to avoid all aspirin ingestion for at least 7 days prior to an elective invasive procedure.

Nonsteroidal anti-inflammatory agents (NSAIDs), such as ibuprofen or naproxen sodium, similarly inhibit platelet cyclooxygenase. However, their effects are reversible, and normal platelet function is usually restored within 24 hours of the last dose. Under most circumstances, the degree of platelet inhibition produced by NSAIDs is not clinically significant, and patients can receive these drugs for analgesia and fever control. It is reasonable, however, to minimize the use of NSAIDs in the bleeding, severely thrombocytopenic patient. Other antiplatelet agents, such as clopidogrel (Plavix) or dipyridamole (Persantine), can produce platelet inhibition that remains evident for several days after discontinuing the drug. The β-lactam antibiotics can sterically hinder the binding of the platelet aggregation agonist adenosine diphosphate (ADP) to its specific platelet receptor, thus resulting in impaired platelet aggregation under circumstances of normal physiologic stimulation. This, too, is reversed on removal of the drug. Fortunately, only a few patients exposed to these antibiotics will exhibit clinically significant platelet inhibition.

In the ICU, one must also always consider the possibility that a patient with bleeding suggestive of a platelet defect may have an inherited disorder of platelet function. Although rare, these disorders are encountered from time to time and include Glanzmann thrombasthenia (abnormal platelet GP IIb/IIIa), Bernard-Soulier syndrome (abnormal GP Ib/IX), Wiskott-Aldrich syndrome, platelet storage pool deficiency (abnormal platelet dense bodies), and the Gray platelet disorder (abnormal platelet-granules).

Management. Because many of the adverse drug-related platelet effects are reversible, unnecessary medications should *always* be discontinued promptly when platelet function seems impaired. In fact, as a general rule, it is never acceptable to leave a nonessential agent on the patient's medication list simply because it is benign; any drug in this category must be discontinued.

The more controversial issue is deciding whether platelet transfusions are warranted in a particular patient. The relationship of thrombocytopenia to clinical bleeding is relative; that is, it is difficult to identify a specific arbitrary platelet count (threshold) below which bleeding is likely to occur. Several conditions, such as massive transfusion syndrome and DIC, may respond to empirical platelet transfusion at counts as high as 80,000 or even 100,000 platelets/μL, although bleeding in the presence of a platelet count of 80,000 cells/μL (or greater) is unlikely to be a result of the thrombocytopenia. With other causes, such as thrombocytopenia seen with cancer chemotherapy and bone marrow aplasia, therapy may not be required until counts fall below 10,000 to 20,000 cells/μL. As previously stated, rhfVIIa has also been used to reverse the hemostatic defect caused by aspirin or clopidogrel (32).

The morbidity and mortality related to bleeding increase measurably in patients undergoing induction chemotherapy for acute leukemia when the platelet count falls below 10,000 to 20,000 cells/μL. The empirical administration of platelets to these patients significantly limits both morbidity and mortality. This finding, however, has been generalized to virtually all patients with platelet counts in this range; the appropriateness of this approach is unclear. A major concern that should temper the empirical use of platelet transfusion is the development of alloimmunization to transfused platelets, potentially negating any future benefit from platelet transfusion in a time of need. Patients with acute leukemia typically have self-limited marrow aplasia resulting from chemotherapy. Therefore, the need for platelet transfusion is also limited, and the chances for the development of antiplatelet antibodies are greatly decreased. Patients with aplastic anemia, however, have an ongoing need for platelet transfusion, so their risk of alloimmunization is high. Autoimmune disorders associated with increased peripheral platelet destruction, disorders of splenic sequestration, and drug-related thrombocytopenia are unlikely to benefit from platelet transfusion. An exception is related to a planned invasive procedure associated with an increased risk of bleeding. In this situation, empirical platelet transfusion immediately before the procedure may be reasonable. As previously noted, platelet transfusions in the presence of type II HIT are contraindicated.

Uremia

Uremia is commonly seen in the ICU and is associated with an increased risk of bleeding (48,49). Uremia has been shown to cause a reversible impairment of platelet function, although the "toxin" responsible for this defect is not well defined. Some studies have demonstrated an impairment of platelet–vessel wall interactions and suggest defects in von Willebrand factor. The degree of platelet impairment appears to be related to the severity of uremia for a given patient. In addition, thrombotic events are also increased in patients with uremia. These, too, appear to be multifactorial in cause but, in part, reflect the increased renal loss of antithrombin III and protein S in nephrotic-range proteinuria (50).

Several therapeutic approaches may modulate the qualitative platelet defect associated with uremia. The primary therapy in this setting is dialysis. Cryoprecipitate, 1-deamino-8-D-arginine vasopressin (DDAVP; 0.3 μg/kg maximum dose 21 mg), and conjugated estrogens (10 mg/day in adults) have been given to patients with severe uremia and an acquired defect in primary hemostasis with good results. The benefit derived by treatment with cryoprecipitate or DDAVP appears to be related to the consequent increase in the plasma concentration of the large multimeric forms of von Willebrand factor, thus greatly improving platelet adhesion. The duration of action of these agents, however, is limited, reaching their zenith between 2 and 6 hours. Additional doses of DDAVP during the same 24-hour period may result in a diminished response to the drug (tachyphylaxis) with little or no further benefit. Patients who exhibit tachyphylaxis to DDAVP may require 48 to 72 hours before again responding to this agent. The mechanism of action of the conjugated estrogens is not known. In contrast to the first two therapies described, the effect of estrogen is more protracted and does not diminish with repeat dosing, although a benefit is not noted for 3 to 5 days after starting therapy.

THROMBOTIC SYNDROMES

Thrombotic events may often be the cause of admission to an ICU, particularly if one includes acute coronary syndromes in this category. The noncardiac thrombotic syndromes frequently encountered in the ICU include the following:

1. Deep venous thrombosis (DVT) (specifically in association with a central venous catheter)
2. Heparin-induced thrombocytopenia
3. Pulmonary embolism syndrome
4. Thrombotic thrombocytopenic purpura/hemolytic uremic syndrome
5. Thrombotic DIC
6. Stroke
7. Central nervous system (CNS) venous sinus thrombosis (most commonly seen in infants and the elderly in association with marked dehydration)

Many of these conditions, particularly venous thromboembolic events, often develop while the patient is in the ICU and may be preventable. The intensivist should assess risk of DVT and risks of thromboprophylaxis in all patients and institute appropriate therapy on a case-by-case basis based on the assessed risk of thrombosis. In general, postoperative patients and those who will be immobilized for long periods of time are considered at risk, and should be candidates for some sort of thromboprophylaxis (51). Approximately 10% of ICU patients will develop DVT while in the ICU in spite of receiving a form of thromboprophylaxis, and up to 15% of these patients will experience a symptomatic pulmonary embolus (52,53). However, not all patients are at the same risk, and not all respond to prophylactic measures equally. Consequently, recognition of patient risk factors and initiation of effective prophylaxis measures is critical for the care of these patients.

Management

The initial management approach for a patient with a documented (or highly suspected) thrombotic event is generally anticoagulation with either UH or LMWH. The efficacy of either appears to be equivalent, although some studies suggest that the incidence of severe bleeding is less with LMWH (54). The use of LMWH may produce a more stable level of anticoagulation, which may result in fewer laboratory tests and dose adjustments. The choice of which agent to use is at the discretion of the intensivist. However, if repeated invasive procedures are anticipated, UH may be the preferred agent, owing to its shorter half-life. Most patients may be started on UH with a bolus dose of 50 units/kg, followed by a continuous infusion of 10 units/kg/hour; these doses may be reduced for the elderly or frail patient. Once initiated, anticoagulation is adjusted to keep the aPTT roughly 1.5 to 2.5 times baseline values (corresponding to a plasma heparin concentration of 0.2 to 0.4 units/mL). Dosing of LMWH is weight related. The dose of warfarin is titrated to maintain an INR of the PT between 1.5 and 4.0, depending on the intensity of anticoagulation desired.

SELECTED DISORDERS

Systemic Diseases Associated with Factor Deficiencies

Amyloidosis, Gaucher disease, and the nephrotic syndrome are occasionally seen in the ICU. Each may have one or more associated factor deficiencies that may complicate patient management and result in bleeding. Patients with either amyloidosis or Gaucher disease may develop factor IX deficiency. Factor X deficiency also has been associated with amyloidosis. These deficiencies generally result from the absorption of the specific clotting factor onto the abnormal proteins present with each disorder. In the nephrotic syndrome, factor IX deficiency also may develop. Although it was originally thought that proteinuria was responsible for the development of factor IX deficiency, this may not be the case. The deficiency typically remits with corticosteroid therapy. Finally, antithrombin III deficiency can be seen along with the nephrotic syndrome and may lead to thrombosis. The loss of antithrombin III does appear to be related to proteinuria.

Laboratory Disorders Not Associated with Bleeding

Lupus Anticoagulants

The lupus anticoagulant has received much attention as a potential cause of bleeding by virtue of its name and its associated laboratory abnormalities. As an isolated hemostatic defect, thrombosis is the more likely problem (25% incidence rate), with bleeding in one series occurring in only 1 of 219 patients with the lupus anticoagulant (55,56).

The PT and aPTT assays depend on the interaction of various coagulation factors with either a lipoprotein or phospholipid to activate coagulation efficiently. The lupus anticoagulant is an antiphospholipid antibody directed against these phospholipids or lipoproteins, and produces prolongation of the PT, aPTT, or the measured recalcification time of platelet-rich plasma. Prolongation of the aPTT occurs more commonly than prolongation of the PT, although an isolated prolongation of the PT can be seen. Twenty-five percent of patients with active SLE and the lupus anticoagulant also have associated thrombocytopenia or hypoprothrombinemia, and are therefore at risk for bleeding in contrast to those patients with the lupus anticoagulant alone who are not at increased risk for bleeding. Although the lupus anticoagulant was originally described in patients with SLE, it is not limited to this class of diseases. Indeed, lupus anticoagulants or anticardiolipin antibodies, or both, have been demonstrated in large percentages of patients with human immunodeficiency virus infection, hemophilia A, or both. Lupus anticoagulants also are observed in disorders accompanied by chronic and acute inflammation.

Thrombotic events in patients who exhibit a lupus anticoagulant may occur independent of the underlying disorder and can be directly related to the lupus anticoagulant itself. The likelihood of thrombosis associated with a lupus anticoagulant appears to be greatest when the lupus anticoagulant has specificity for β_2-glycoprotein I or phosphatidylserine. Some forms of the disorder, such as that associated with pregnancy, do respond to anti-inflammatory drugs such as aspirin or prednisone. Thrombosis, when it occurs, is equally likely to be venous or arterial. Venous thrombosis is more common in the extremities whereas arterial thrombosis is more common in the central nervous system. Placental infarcts are frequently seen in placental specimens in those patients with repeated fetal wastage. Stroke, myocardial infarction, and pulmonary embolization are also well described in patients with the lupus anticoagulant.

Reactive Hyperfibrinogenemia

Hyperfibrinogenemia is defined as a plasma fibrinogen concentration greater than 800 mg/dL. In the clinical laboratory, fibrinogen is measured using a functional assay in which time to fibrin clot formation is the end point. Plasma from the patient is allowed to clot in the presence of excess thrombin. The time to clotting in this setting is proportional to the amount of fibrinogen present in the sample. When excessive amounts of fibrinogen are present, clotting is incomplete, and fibrin fragments are formed that inhibit further fibrin clot formation. Other hematologic parameters, such as the aPTT, PT, and the TT, are consequently prolonged, suggesting a potential, although artifactual, risk for bleeding despite a high fibrinogen level. This can be evaluated by diluting the plasma to a normal fibrinogen concentration using saline or defibrinated plasma. These same clotting studies will now be normal. Bleeding is not seen unless the fibrinogen also is a dysfibrinogen, although even in these patients, bleeding remains an uncommon problem. In patients with dysfibrinogenemia, clotting studies fail to correct when either saline or defibrinated plasma dilutions are undertaken, thus distinguishing them from patients with reactive hyperfibrinogenemia.

FUTURE DIRECTIONS

Currently, much attention is being given to better understanding the interplay of coagulation and inflammation, and how the inflammatory state sets off a chain reaction resulting in microvascular thrombosis and multiorgan dysfunction/failure. Improving our grasp of these interactions requires that we increase our knowledge of the normal function of the endothelium, and how this function is disrupted in sepsis and severe acute illness. Other areas that need further research are the specific host factors that regulate the balance between too little and too much thrombosis, including how the numerous genetic polymorphisms of important regulatory protein genes affect the overall regulation of hemostasis. As our ability improves in treating the initial acute event that brings a patient to the ICU, we will gain a better understanding of all the processes and mechanisms that increase the risk of end-organ failure, which will allow us to treat them proactively. Newer, and old, drugs are being tested in the setting of sepsis to prevent DIC and microvascular thrombosis and, if successful, they may result in improved survival with decreased morbidity. Some of these strategies will involve ways to better regulate the coagulation process, but we also need to develop means by which to protect the endothelium. While waiting for these scientific and therapeutic advances, we, as clinicians, must also work to recognize disease processes earlier (e.g., DIC) so we can determine how to best use those treatments already available to us (e.g., activated protein C, thrombolytics, anticoagulants, and so on) more precisely, cost effectively, and safely.

References

1. Horne M. Overview of hemostasis and thrombosis; current status of antithrombotic therapies. *Thromb Res.* 2005;117:15.
2. Eilertsen KE, Osterud B. Tissue factor: (patho)physiology and cellular biology. *Blood Coagul Fibrinolysis.* 2004;15:521.
3. Hayward CP, Rao AK, Cattaneo M. Congenital platelet disorders: overview of their mechanisms, diagnostic evaluation and treatment. *Haemophilia.* 2006;12(Suppl 3):128.
4. Aird WC. The role of the endothelium in severe sepsis and the multiple organ dysfunction syndrome. *Blood* 2003;23:23.
5. Levi M, ten Cate H, van der Poll T. Endothelium: interface between coagulation and inflammation. *Crit Care Med.* 2002;30(Suppl):S220.
6. Dempfle CE. Coagulopathy and sepsis. *Thromb Haemost.* 2004; 91:213.
7. Esmon CT. Crosstalk between inflammation and thrombosis. *Maturitas.* 2004;47:305.
8. Liaw PCY. Endogenous protein C activation in patients with severe sepsis. *Crit Care Med.* 2004;32(Suppl):S214.
9. Joyce DE, Nelson DR, Grinnell BW. Leukocyte and endothelial cell interactions in sepsis: relevance of the protein C pathway. *Crit Care Med.* 2004;32(Suppl):S280.
10. Rigby AC, Grant MA. Protein S: a conduit between anticoagulation and inflammation. *Crit Care Med.* 2004;32(Suppl):S336.
11. Hermans PW, Hazelzet JA. Plasminogen activator inhibitor type 1 gene polymorphism and sepsis. *Clin Infect Dis.* 2005;41(Suppl 7):S453.

12. Walley KR, Russell JA. Protein C – 1641 AA is associated with decreased survival and more organ dysfunction in severe sepsis. *Crit Care Med.* 2007; 35:12.
13. Lillicrap D, Nair SC, Srivastava A, et al. Laboratory issues in bleeding disorders. *Hemophilia.* 2006;12(Suppl 3):68.
14. Khair K, Liesner R. Bruising and bleeding in infants and children—a practical approach. *Br J Haematol.* 2006;133:221.
15. Martinelli I, Battaglioli T, Tosatto A, et al. Prothrombin A19911G polymorphism and the risk of venous thromboembolism. *J Thromb Haemost.* 2007;4:2582.
16. Chinthammitr Y, Vos HL, Rosendaal FR, et al. The association of prothrombin A19911G polymorphism with plasma prothrombin activity and venous thrombosis. Results of the MEGA study, a large population-based case-control study. *J Thromb Haemost.* 2007;4:2587.
17. Oren H, Cingoz I, Duman M, et al. Disseminated intravascular coagulation in pediatric patients: clinical and laboratory features and prognostic factors influencing survival. *Pediatr Hematol Oncol.* 2005;22:679.
18. Chuansumrit A, Hotrakitya S, Sirinavin S, et al. Disseminated intravascular coagulation findings in 100 patients. *J Med Assoc Thai.* 1999;82(Suppl 1):S63.
19. Girolami A, Luzzatto G, Varvarikis C, et al. Main clinical manifestations of a bleeding diathesis: an often disregarded aspect of medical and surgical history taking. *Hemophilia.* 2005;11:193.
20. Barton JC, Poon MC. Coagulation testing of the Hickman catheter blood in patients with acute leukemia. *Arch Intern Med.* 1986;146:2165.
21. Bick RL, Arun B, Frenkel EP. Disseminated intravascular coagulation. Clinical and pathophysiological mechanisms and manifestations. *Haemostasis.* 1999;29:111.
22. Voves C, Wuillemin WA, Zeerleder S. International Society on Thrombosis and Haemostasis score for overt disseminated intravascular coagulation predicts organ dysfunction and fatality in sepsis patients. *Blood Coagul Fibrinolysis.* 2006;17:445.
23. Cauchie P, Cauchie Ch, Boudjeltia KZ, et al. Diagnosis and prognosis of overt disseminated intravascular coagulation in a general hospital—meaning of the ISTH score system, fibrin monomers, and lipoprotein-C–reactive protein complex formation. *Am J Hematol.* 2006;81:414.
24. Gando S, Iba T, Eguchi Y, et al. A multicenter, prospective validation of disseminated intravascular coagulation diagnostic criteria for critically ill patients: comparing current criteria. *Crit Care Med.* 2006;34:625.
25. Leclerc F, Hazelzet J, Jude B, et al. Protein C and S deficiency in severe infectious purpura of children: a collaborative study of 40 cases. *Intensive Care Med.* 1992;18:202.
26. Taylor FB Jr, Toh CH, Hoots WK, et al.; Scientific Subcommittee on Disseminated Intravascular Coagulation (DIC) of the International Society on Thrombosis and Haemostasis (ISTH). Towards definition, clinical and laboratory criteria, and a scoring system for disseminated intravascular coagulation. *Thromb Haemost.* 2001;86:1327.
27. Erber WN. Plasma and plasma products in the treatment of massive hemorrhage. *Best Pract Res Clin Haematol.* 2005;19:97.
28. Bernard GR, Vincent JL, Laterre PF, et al. Efficacy and safety of recombinant human activated protein C for severe sepsis. *N Engl J Med.* 2001;344:699.
29. Sallah S, Husain A, Nguyen NP. Recombinant activated factor VII in patients with cancer and hemorrhagic disseminated intravascular coagulation. *Blood Coagul Fibrinolysis.* 2004;15:577.
30. Scarpelini S, Rizoli S. Recombinant factor VIIa and the surgical patient. *Curr Opin Crit Care.* 2006;12:351.
31. Boffard KD, Riou B, Warren B, et al. Recombinant factor VIIa as adjunctive therapy for bleeding control in severely injured trauma patients: two parallel randomized, placebo-controlled, double blind clinical trials. *J Trauma.* 2005;59:8.
32. Altman R, Scazziota A, De Lourdes Herrera M, et al. Recombinant factor VIIa reverses the inhibitory effect of aspirin or aspirin plus clopidogrel on in vivo thrombin generation. *J Thromb Haemost.* 2006;4:2022.
33. O'Connell KA, Ward JJ, Wise RP, et al. Thromboembolic adverse events after use of recombinant human coagulation factor VIIa. *JAMA.* 2006; 295:293.
34. Davis-Jackson R, Correa H, Horswell R, et al. Antithrombin III (AT) and recombinant tissue plasminogen activator (R-TPA) used singly and in combination versus supportive care as treatment of endotoxin-induced disseminated intravascular coagulation (DIC) in the neonatal pig. *Thromb J.* 2006;4:7.
35. Jaimes F, de la Rosa G, Arango C, et al. A randomized clinical trial of unfractionated heparin for treatment of sepsis (the HETRASE study): design and rationale. *Trials.* 2006;7:19.
36. Al Ghumias AK, Gader A, Faleh FZ. Hemostatic abnormalities in liver disease: could some haemostatic tests be useful as liver function tests?: *Blood Coagul Fibrinolysis.* 2005;16:329.
37. Lisman T, Caldwell SH, Leebeck FWG, et al. Hemostasis in chronic liver disease. *J Thromb Haemost.* 2006;4:2059.
38. Ganguly S, Spengel K, Tilzer LL, et al. Recombinant factor VIIa: unregulated continuous use in patients with bleeding and coagulopathy does not alter mortality and outcome. *Clin Lab Haematol.* 2006;28:309.
39. Ramsey G. Treating coagulopathy in liver disease with plasma transfusions or recombinant factor VIIa: an evidence based review. *Best Pract Res Clin Haematol.* 2005;19:113.
40. American College of Chest Physicians. Sixth ACCP consensus conference on antithrombotic therapy. *Chest.* 2001;119:225.
41. Fiore LD, Scola MA, Cantillon CE, et al. Anaphylactoid reactions to vitamin K. *J Thromb Thrombolysis.* 2001;11:175.
42. Riegert-Johnson DL, Volocheck GW. The incidence of anaphylaxis following intravenous phytonadione (vitamin K1): a 5-year retrospective review. *Ann Allergy Asthma Immunol.* 2002;89:400.
43. Dentali F, Ageno W, Crowther M. Treatment of coumarin-associated coagulopathy: a systemic review and proposed treatment algorithms. *J Thromb Haemost.* 2006;4:1853.
44. Hardy JF, de Moerloose P, Samama CM; members of the Groupe d'Interet en Hemostase Perioperatoire. Massive transfusion and coagulopathy: pathophysiology and implications for clinical management. *Can J Anaesth.* 2006;53(6 Suppl):S40.
45. Hellerstern P, Muntean W, Schramm W, et al. Practical guidelines for the clinical use of plasma. *Thromb Res.* 2002;107(Suppl 1):S53.
46. Warkentin TE, Kelton JG. A 14-year study of heparin-induced thrombocytopenia. *Am J Med.* 1996;101:502.
47. Dager WE, White RH. Pharmacotherapy of heparin-induced thrombocytopenia. *Expert Opin Pharmacother.* 2003;4:919.
48. Sohal AS, Ganji AS, Crowther MA, et al. Uremic bleeding: pathophysiology and clinical risk factors. *Thromb Res.* 2006;118:417.
49. Boccardo P, Remuzzi G, Galbusera M. Platelet dysfunction in renal failure. *Semin Thromb Hemost.* 2004;30:579.
50. Molino D, DeLucia D, Gaspare de Santo N. Coagulation disorders in uremia. *Semin Nephrol.* 2006;26:46.
51. Geerts WH, Pineo GF, Heit JA, et al. Prevention of venous thromboembolism: the Seventh ACCP Conference on Antithrombotic and Thrombolytic Therapy. *Chest.* 2004;126(3 Suppl):338S.
52. Cook D, Crowther M, Meade M, et al. Deep venous thrombosis in medical-surgical critically ill patients: prevalence, incidence, and risk factors. *Crit Care Med.* 2005;33:1565.
53. Khouli H, Shapiro J, Pham VP, et al. Efficacy of deep venous thrombosis prophylaxis in the medical intensive care unit. *J Intensive Care Med.* 2006;21:352.
54. Kearon C, Ginsberg JS, Julian JA, et al. Comparison of fixed-dose weight-adjusted unfractionated heparin and low-molecular-weight heparin for acute treatment of venous thromboembolism. *JAMA.* 2006;296:935.
55. Galli M, Norbis F, Ruggeri L, et al. Lupus anticoagulants and thrombosis: clinical association of different coagulation and immunologic tests. *Thromb Haemost.* 2000;84:1012.
56. Bick RL, Ancypa D. The antiphospholipid and thrombosis (APL-T) syndromes: clinical and laboratory correlates. *Clin Lab Med.* 1995;15: 63.

CHAPTER 171 ■ TRANSFUSION THERAPY: WHEN TO USE IT AND HOW TO MINIMIZE IT

SAMIR M. FAKHRY • HANI SEOUDI

The ability to administer blood products is a critically important therapeutic modality in the care of patients with acute and chronic problems. When carried out with a thorough, up-to-date understanding of indications, risks, and benefits, blood transfusion is exceedingly safe and effective. Physicians encounter a large spectrum of medical and surgical conditions requiring transfusion therapy, including acute blood loss, catastrophic illness in the critical care setting, diseases associated with chronic anemia, and a variety of congenital and acquired bleeding disorders. The modern-day care of the critically ill requires a thorough knowledge of the pathophysiology of blood loss and anemia, as well as an understanding of normal hemostatic mechanisms and the sometimes complex disorders of coagulation encountered in these populations.

In this chapter, the basic concepts of acute blood loss are discussed, and the indications for and use of blood components, potential risks of blood products, and alternatives to blood transfusion are reviewed. Because blood products are a limited resource with potential serious adverse side effects, knowledge of appropriate indications, potential risks, and available alternatives should allow clinicians to exercise judgment in using this important resource. Based on the accumulating evidence, special emphasis will be placed on minimizing transfusion in the critical care setting.

HISTORY OF BLOOD TRANSFUSION

The ability to transfuse blood safely and successfully is a relatively recent medical advance. Early historical references to the use of bloodletting and phlebotomy were common, and were applied to many diseases and disorders. It is possible that salutary effects were realized in some situations, such as congestive heart failure, but the vast majority of these applications were based on medical ignorance and likely resulted in harm to unsuspecting patients.

In February 1666 in Oxford, England, Richard Lower demonstrated what is thought to be the first known successful transfusion on an animal. The technical details were published in the *Philosophical Transactions of the Royal Society* within a year of the experiment. Another Englishman, Francis Potter, may have preceded him with transfusions to animals, and possibly to humans, some years prior (1,2). Jean-Baptiste Denis is credited with the first transfusion to a human in 1667 performed in France. Denis gave 3 pints of sheep blood to a patient without ill effects. A subsequent attempt to give blood to the same man "to mollify his fiery nature" led to the patient's death shortly after the transfusion. A lawsuit resulted, and Denis went to trial but was ultimately exonerated. The Paris medical faculty then forbade blood transfusion, which led to bans on transfusion throughout Europe that lasted until modern times. An 1825 medical journal credited Dr. Philip Syng Physick of Philadelphia with blood transfusion to a patient, possibly the first record of successful transfusion of human blood (3). In 1828 in England, Blundell administered a small amount of human blood to a patient with postpartum hemorrhage, apparently small aliquots from himself, the husband, and another man (4). The patient reportedly felt better, but it is likely that the small-volume transfusion had little impact on her outcome. In fact, the patient was fortunate not to have suffered a serious transfusion reaction.

The routine, safe administration of blood products required several important scientific advances. The discovery of the A, B, and O blood types by Karl Landsteiner in 1900 and the AB blood type by Alfred Decastello and Adriano Sturli in 1902 began the era of modern blood transfusion. The first blood bank was established in 1932 in a Leningrad hospital. The first blood bank in the United States was established by Bernard Fantus in 1937 at Cook County Hospital in Chicago. By the 1940s, techniques of cross-matching, anticoagulation, and storage of blood, and the establishment of blood banks made routine blood transfusion a reality. The introduction of plastic storage containers in 1950 and the introduction of refrigerated centrifugation instruments in 1953 made component therapy possible (5).

BLOOD PRODUCT COLLECTION AND ADMINISTRATION

Approximately 14 million units of red blood cells (RBCs) (packed RBCs and whole blood), 9,875,000 units of platelets, and 4 million units of plasma are transfused annually in the United States (6,7). This represents an 11.8% increase since 1999 and a 56% increase since 1980 (8). The use of other components, especially platelets, has also increased. Because only about 5% of eligible donors ever donate blood, future increases may exacerbate shortages, especially as the U.S. population ages. Transfusion rates in the United States for 2001 have been estimated at 48.75 units of red cell transfusion per 1,000 population as compared to 44.93 units of red cell transfusion per 1,000 population in England, 28 units of red cell transfusion per 1,000 population in Australia, and in 54.8 units of red cell transfusion per 1,000 population in Denmark (9).

As anemia in critical care illness is common, 25% to 37% of patients receive at least one blood transfusion during their intensive care unit (ICU) stay (10–12). In one study (10), 85%

of patients with an ICU length of stay greater than 1 week received at least one blood transfusion. Notably, blood transfusion was not associated with acute blood loss in over two thirds of these cases. Phlebotomy and decreased production of blood cells have been implicated as significant contributors to anemia in the ICU. Since many studies have estimated daily blood loss from phlebotomy to be at least 40 mL/day (10,11,13), critical care practitioners should carefully consider the need for frequent blood draws in the ICU.

Collection and Preparation of Blood Products

Modern-day blood banks have adopted component therapy to optimize management of the blood supply. Blood is collected from donors and is then separated into its individual components—packed RBCs, plasma, platelets, and proteins—to maximize the benefits of each donated unit while minimizing the risk to recipients of blood products. Blood is collected from donors into plastic bags containing a citrate solution that binds calcium, thus preventing coagulation. These solutions include citrate phosphate dextrose (CPD), citrate phosphate double dextrose (CP2D), and citrate phosphate dextrose adenine (CPDA-1). Additional solutions are now available that extend the shelf life of packed RBCs, and contain dextrose, adenine, sodium chloride, and either phosphate (AS-3) or mannitol (AS-1 and AS-5). After collection, each unit is gently centrifuged to pack the RBCs, leaving approximately 70% of the platelets suspended in plasma; the platelet-rich plasma is removed and centrifuged again to sediment the platelets. All but a small amount of the resulting supernatant plasma is removed and rapidly frozen. The platelets are then resuspended, yielding a platelet concentrate. When the frozen plasma is stored at less than 18°C, it is referred to as fresh frozen plasma. If the frozen plasma is allowed to thaw at 4°C, the precipitate that remains can be collected to yield cryoprecipitate. Albumin and other proteins can then be extracted from the remaining plasma.

Another option for the collection of blood leukocytes, platelets, or plasma is through automated cell separators (apheresis). Blood is withdrawn from a donor and separated by centrifuge, and the desired component is removed. The remaining blood is returned to the donor. Using this technique, many units of leukocytes or platelets can be quickly removed, allowing blood banks to offer products such as single-donor platelet packs. The administration of a single-donor unit of platelets is advantageous since it exposes the recipient to only one person's antigens, whereas an equivalent dose of pooled platelet transfusion ("six pack" or "ten pack") exposes the patient to six or ten sets of antigens, respectively, making subsequent platelet transfusion less effective since antibodies are formed against the wide array of foreign antigens. In addition, bacterial contamination is less likely with single-donor apheresis platelets.

Storage Lesion

Storage and refrigeration create progressive changes in packed RBCs, known as the *storage lesion* (14). These changes include an increase in the concentration of potassium, phosphate, and ammonia; decrease in pH; altered affinity of hemoglobin for oxygen; changes in RBC deformability; hemolysis; development of microaggregates; release of vasoactive substances; and denaturation of proteins. In addition, the life span of RBCs becomes shorter the longer cells are stored. This is associated with a decrease in both intracellular 2,3-diphosphoglycerate (2,3-DPG) and adenosine triphosphate (ATP). The transfusion of large volumes of cold blood contributes to the development of hypothermia, one of the most clinically significant effects of storage on subsequent transfusion. With the exception of hypothermia, it is important to realize that many of these changes may be reversed shortly after transfusion, and may, in some cases, cause metabolic effects that are different from those predicted based on the above *ex vivo* observations. It is therefore critical not to empirically treat the theoretically anticipated effects of blood transfusions using "cookbook" approaches (such as giving one ampule of bicarbonate and one ampule of calcium with every "*x*" units of blood). Some of these treatments may, in fact, be harmful for the patient in hemorrhagic shock.

Administration of Blood Products

Transfusion based on sound physiologic principles and an understanding of relative risks and benefits should give maximal benefit to the patient, with efficient use of a valuable and finite resource. Utilizing data from recent studies, it is increasingly possible to base transfusion practice on scientific grounds. The most prominent example is the progressive abandonment of the "10/30" transfusion "trigger" for red cell transfusion in favor of lower transfusion triggers and, even more appropriately, transfusion practice based on patient physiology (10,15). The 10/30 transfusion trigger for red cell transfusion likely resulted from a recommendation in a 1942 publication that it was "wise" to maintain hemoglobin levels "between 8 and 10 grams per cubic centimeter" for patients who were poor surgical risks by giving a preoperative transfusion (16). No data were available to support this recommendation, but it stood relatively unchallenged for about 50 years. An expanding body of literature now suggests that arbitrary transfusion for a set transfusion trigger (e.g., the "10/30 rule") is ill-advised, and that purported cardiac risks with anemia are overemphasized (17). The following transfusion guidelines are presented based on the best evidence currently available. Given the active ongoing investigations in this area, it is likely that frequent updates will be forthcoming.

Whole Blood

There have been few widely accepted indications for whole blood in modern transfusion practice. Storage of whole blood precludes the extraction of components and, from a systems perspective, is highly inefficient. As such, whole blood is not available from most blood banks in the United States. In theory, the goals of oxygen delivery and volume expansion can be achieved with packed RBCs and crystalloid solutions. Recent experience with the use of whole blood by the U.S. military (18) has rejuvenated the cause of whole blood. This accumulating experience, especially with fresh whole blood having potentially beneficial effects on coagulopathy and hypothermia, may result in some modification of civilian practices in the future.

Red Blood Cells

Packed RBCs are the most commonly utilized blood product, providing oxygen-carrying capacity in cases of acute or chronic blood loss. The longest storage life currently allowed by the U.S. Food and Drug Administration (FDA) is 42 days. Longer storage times result in fewer than 75% of the RBCs remaining viable in circulation 24 hours after transfusion. Platelets degenerate at refrigerator temperatures, so refrigerated packed RBCs contain essentially no functioning platelets. The levels of factors V and VIII decrease significantly at 1°C to 6°C, while levels of other factors remain essentially unchanged. There are insignificant amounts of plasma in a unit of AS red cells.

Packed RBCs provide oxygen-carrying capacity and maintain oxygen delivery provided that intravascular volume and cardiac function are adequate. The decision to transfuse, and the amount of packed RBCs transfused, depend on the clinical situation. As noted previously, the use of a hematocrit of 30% (or a hemoglobin of 10 g/dL) as a transfusion trigger is no longer acceptable. One or more units of blood may be transfused with no predetermined number of units applicable. Each unit of packed RBCs typically raises the hematocrit 2% to 3% in a 70-kg adult, although this varies depending on the donor, the recipient's fluid status, the method of storage, and its duration.

With blood loss, oxygen delivery is maintained through a series of complex interactions and compensatory mechanisms. This includes increased cardiac output, increased extraction ratio, rightward shift of the oxyhemoglobin curve, and expansion of volume. Many anemic patients tolerate hemoglobin levels of 7 to 8 g/dL or less, as has been demonstrated in chronic renal failure and Jehovah's Witnesses (17). In general, cardiac output does not increase significantly until hemoglobin falls below approximately 7 g/dL. Young healthy patients tolerate acute anemia to hemoglobin levels of 7 g/dL or less through increases in cardiac output, provided they have a normal intravascular volume and high arterial oxygen saturation.

In a multicenter, randomized controlled study of transfusion in 838 patients in the critical care setting, a liberal transfusion strategy (transfusion for hemoglobin <10 g/dL) was compared with a restrictive strategy (transfusion for hemoglobin <7 g/dL). The restrictive strategy was found to be at least as effective as the liberal strategy, with the possible exception of patients with acute myocardial infarction and unstable angina (19). Suggested guidelines for RBC transfusion are listed in Table 171.1.

Leukocyte-reduced Red Blood Cells

The transfusion of RBCs has been associated with immunosuppression. This effect is thought to be related to exposure to leukocytes. Therefore, the use of leukocyte-reduced components has been proposed as a means of minimizing immunosuppression; the majority of red cells and platelet transfusions in the United States are currently leukocyte reduced. The efficacy of these preparations remains controversial, however, and compelling data are lacking. Recent recommendations for transfusion of leukocyte-reduced blood components are listed in Table 171.2 (20).

TABLE 171.1

GUIDELINES FOR TRANSFUSION OF PACKED RED BLOOD CELLS

- Ongoing bleeding with hemodynamic instability unresponsive (or incompletely responsive) to infusion of 2,000 to 3,000 mL crystalloid
- Hemoglobin <7 g/dL

TABLE 171.2

INDICATIONS FOR TRANSFUSION OF LEUKOCYTE-REDUCED BLOOD COMPONENTS

- To decrease the incidence of subsequent refractoriness to platelet transfusion caused by human leukocyte antigen (HLA) alloimmunization in patients requiring long-term platelet support
- To provide blood components with reduced risk for cytomegalovirus transmission
- To prevent future febrile nonhemolytic transfusion reactions (FNHTRs) in patients who have had a documented FNHTR
- To decrease the incidence of HLA alloimmunization in nonhepatic solid-organ transplant candidates.

Data from Ratko TA, Cummings JP, Oberman HA, et al. Evidence-based recommendations for the use of WBC-reduced cellular blood components. *Transfusion*. 2001;41:1310–1319.

Platelets

Platelet transfusions are indicated for patients who are at a significant risk of bleeding because of quantitative or qualitative platelet deficits. A unit of platelets can be prepared from individual (or "random") donors or by apheresis, whereby a donor provides the equivalent of 6 to 10 single "random" donor units. In selected cases, human leukocyte antigen (HLA)-matched platelets can be obtained by apheresis from HLA-matched donors. The efficacy of platelet transfusion may be assessed both by clinical parameters (improved hemostasis) and by following the platelet counts at 1 hour and 24 hours as an estimate of platelet survival. The platelet count at 1 hour post transfusion of a unit of platelets should increase by 5,000 to 10,000 platelets/μL. Less pronounced responses should be expected with repeated transfusion and the development of alloimmunization, or in the presence of fever, sepsis, or splenomegaly. If alloimmunization is thought to be the cause of a poor response, platelets from an HLA-matched donor may be needed.

The prophylactic transfusion of platelets in the absence of microvascular bleeding, a low platelet count in a patient undergoing a surgical procedure, or a platelet count that has fallen below 10,000 platelets/μL, in most medical patients, should be considered inappropriate. Disease state–specific triggers for platelet transfusion have been proposed and are listed in Table 171.3 (21). It is crucial to recognize that hypothermia depresses platelet function, and platelet transfusion is generally ineffective with depressed temperatures. Restoration of a normal temperature returns platelet function to normal and ameliorates microvascular bleeding.

Plasma

Plasma is used as a source of clotting factors in patients with coagulopathy and documented factor deficiency. This may occur with liver dysfunction, congenital absence of factors, and transfusion of factor-deficient blood products, or after the use of warfarin. A unit of plasma contains near-normal levels of all factors, including about 400 mg of fibrinogen, and generally

TABLE 171.3

INDICATIONS FOR TRANSFUSION OF PLATELETS

- Disseminated intravascular coagulation: 20,000–50,000 platelets/μL
- Major surgery in leukemia: 50,000 platelets/μL
- Thrombocytopenia with massive transfusion: 50,000 platelets/μL
- Invasive procedures in cirrhosis: 50,000 platelets/μL
- Cardiopulmonary bypass: 50,000–60,000 platelets/μL
- Liver biopsy: 50,000–100,000 platelets/μL
- Neurosurgical procedures: 100,000 platelets/μL

Data from Rebulla P. Platelet transfusion trigger in difficult patients. *Transfus Clin Biol.* 2002;9:249–254.

increases factor levels by about 3%. Adequate clotting can usually be achieved with factor levels greater than 30%, although higher levels are advisable in patients undergoing operative or invasive procedures. The prothrombin time (PT) and the activated partial thromboplastin time (aPTT) can be used to assess patients for plasma transfusion and to follow the efficacy of administered plasma. Recent experience suggests that the use of thromboelastography may provide advantages over the PT as a guide for the treatment of coagulopathy (22,23). Plasma can be frozen and stored for up to 1 year.

Plasma should not be given routinely or prophylactically by "cookbook" formula after RBC transfusion—for example, 2 units of plasma for every 5 units of packed RBCs—or "prophylactically" after cardiac bypass or other procedures. Plasma should not be used as a volume expander since crystalloids are cheaper, safer, and at least as effective. Broadly accepted guidelines for transfusion of plasma are listed in Table 171.4 (24).

Cryoprecipitate

Indications for the use of cryoprecipitate include factor deficiency (hemophilia A), von Willebrand disease, and hypofibrinogenemia (Table 171.5). Some patients with uremic bleeding may also benefit from cryoprecipitate transfusion. Cryoprecipitate is usually administered as a transfusion of 10 single units. Each 5- to 15-mL unit contains over 80 units of factor VIII and about 200 mg of fibrinogen. These relatively high concentrations allow the use of a smaller volume of cryoprecipitate than would be required if plasma were administered.

TABLE 171.4

INDICATIONS FOR TRANSFUSION OF PLASMA

- International normalized ratio (INR) >1.5 with an anticipated invasive procedure or surgery
- Massive hemorrhage (over one blood volume) with an INR >1.5
- Treatment of thrombotic thrombocytopenia purpura
- Inherited coagulopathies where a specific factor concentrate is not available
- Emergent reversal of anticoagulant therapy

Data from Toy P, Popovsky MA, Abraham E, et al., and the National Heart, Lung and Blood Institute Working Group on TRALI. Transfusion-related acute lung injury: definition and review. *Crit Care Med.* 2005;33:721–726.

TABLE 171.5

INDICATIONS FOR TRANSFUSION OF CRYOPRECIPITATE

- Hemophilia A
- von Willebrand disease
- Hypofibrinogemia
- Uremic bleeding
- As substitute for plasma if lower volume is desired

Risks of Blood Transfusion

Even though a blood transfusion is a potentially life-saving intervention, significant risks are still involved in the administration of these products. Risks range from minor febrile transfusion reactions to the transmission of viral infection to a potentially fatal transfusion of incompatible blood (Table 171.6). Blood banks in the United States generally conduct over ten individual tests or checks on donated units of blood in addition to the screening interview. Most (nine) are for infectious diseases. Screening of donors and the introduction of increasingly effective tests for hepatitis and human immunodeficiency

TABLE 171.6

RISKS OF BLOOD TRANSFUSION

- Transfusion-related acute lung injury
- Bacterial contamination of blood products
- Administrative error leading to transfusion of ABO-incompatible blood
- Viral infection transmission
  - Hepatitis B
  - Hepatitis C
  - Human immunodeficiency virus 1 and 2
  - Human T-cell leukemia virus 1 and 2
  - Epstein-Barr virus
  - Cytomegalovirus
  - Parvovirus B19
  - Human herpesvirus 8
  - Transfusion-transmitted virus
  - Mad cow disease (bovine spongiform encephalopathy)
  - West Nile virus
- Bacterial/protozoal infection transmission
  - Syphilis
  - Malaria
  - *Babesia microti*
  - *Trypanosoma cruzi*
  - *Yersinia enterocolitica*
  - *Serratia marcescens*
  - *Staphylococcus aureus*
  - *Staphylococcus epidermidis*
  - *Klebsiella pneumoniae*
  - *Trypanosoma cruzi*
- Transfusion reactions
  - Acute
  - Delayed
- Immunosuppression

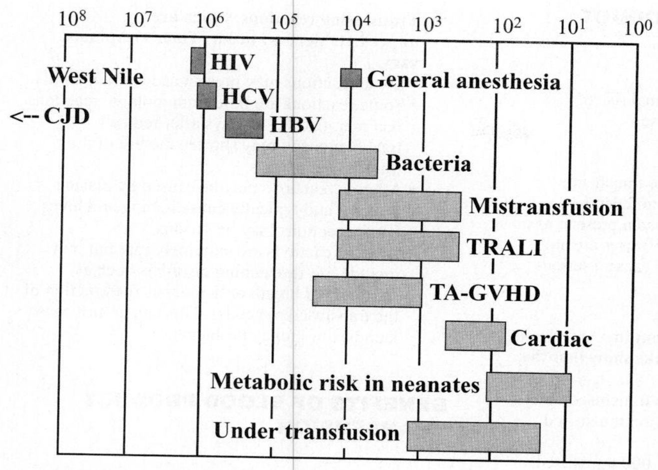

FIGURE 171.1. Estimates of the current risk per unit of blood transfusion. The vertical bars represent log risk estimates (1–10, 1–100, etc.). The dashed edges to lighter shaded horizontal bars signify that the upper and lower estimates of risk are uncertain. CJD, Creutzfeldt-Jacob disease; HIV, human immunodeficiency virus; HCV, hepatitis C virus; HBV, hepatitis B virus; TRALI, transfusion-related acute lung injury; TA-GVHD, transfusion-associated graft versus host disease. (From Dzik WH. Emily Cooley Lecture 2002: transfusion safety in the hospital. *Transfusion.* 2003;43:1190–1199.)

virus (HIV) have dramatically reduced the risks of transmission of these infections. The public has historically been most concerned about the transmission of HIV; however, recent data reveal that the leading causes of fatalities after blood transfusion continue to be administrative error, leading to transfusion of ABO-incompatible blood, bacterial contamination, and transfusion-related acute lung injury (TRALI). Overall, infectious risks of blood transfusion are far outweighed by noninfectious risks (Fig. 171.1). According to the FDA, TRALI was the leading cause of transfusion-related mortality in 2003 (24). An average of 11.7 deaths from bacterial sepsis per year in the United States was reported to the FDA from 2001 to 2003. This decreased to 7.5 deaths per year in 2004 and 2005, due at least in part to the mandating of bacterial screening of platelets, which began in 2004 (24,25). Transfusion of blood to the wrong person continues to be a serious threat to patients. In a review of a 10-year experience in New York State, Linden et al. estimated the risk of an ABO-incompatible transfusion at 1 in 38,000 units of red cells, with the risk of a fatal reaction at 1 in 1.8 million transfusions (26). A rate of ABO-incompatible transfusion of 1 in 12,000 units of red cells transfused has been reported from the hemovigilance program in Quebec, Canada (27).

Given the risks and benefits of blood transfusion, obtaining informed consent for transfusion of blood components is crucial in nonemergent situations. A summary of the rates of the more common, or more concerning, risks is provided in Table 171.7. These data may be useful for discussions with patients and their families, and may be incorporated into informational brochures addressing the risks and benefits of blood products (Fig. 171.2).

Transfusion Reactions

The classification of the American Association of Blood Banks for transfusion reactions is shown in Table 171.8. Hemolytic transfusion reactions can be categorized broadly into acute (<24 hours) and delayed (>24 hours) reactions. Hemolytic

TABLE 171.7

INFORMATION FOR PATIENTS: COMMONLY ASKED QUESTIONS ABOUT BLOOD TRANSFUSION

Complication	Risk from blood product transfusion	Comments
Febrile nonhemolytic transfusion reactions	Occurs in 0.5%–38% of all transfusions	Usually mild fever only More common with platelet transfusions
Severe acute hemolytic reaction	Fatal in 1 of 600,000 transfusions	Stop transfusion immediately and initiate supportive measures
Delayed hemolytic reaction	1 in 260,000 transfusions	Suspect when unexplained fever, fall in hematocrit, or jaundice occur
Bacterial contamination	1 in 15,000 platelet transfusions	Among leading causes of transfusion-related fatalities
Cytomegalovirus	Of concern in low-birth-weight infants and immunocompromised patients (e.g., transplant)	Between 50% and 85% of adults in the United States are carriers
Hepatitis B virus	<1 in 137,000	25% of carriers have active hepatitis and may progress to cirrhosis
Hepatitis C virus	<1 in 1 million	Most infected persons asymptomatic, but 80% become chronic
Human immunodeficiency virus	<1 in 1.9 million	Potentially fatal
Human T-cell leukemia virus 1 and 2	Very small	Rarely found in U.S. blood donors
West Nile virus	Very small when donors are properly screened	80% of those infected remain asymptomatic, 20% develop mild symptoms, and 1 in 150–200 infected people develop severe disease that may be fatal
Transfusion-related lung injury	1 in 5,000 units (estimated)	5%–10% fatal

Source: American Association of Blood Banks. www.aabb.org/content/About_Blood/Facts_About_Blood_and_Blood_Banking/fabloodtrans.htm. Accessed

BASIC INFORMATION...

YOUR PHYSICIAN FEELS THAT YOU MAY NEED A TRANSFUSION OF A BLOOD PRODUCT...

Please realize you will be given blood or blood products only if necessary. This brochure has been offered to help you understand the benefits, risks of, and alternatives to a blood transfusion and is not inclusive of all information. Your physician is the best source for additional information related to blood transfusions.

☞ **Blood products could include:**
- Red blood cells (known as "blood")
- Platelets
- Fresh frozen plasma (known as "plasma")
- Cryoprecipate (a specific part of plasma)

☞ **Blood products are prepared from carefully screened, healthy, human volunteers.**

Any treatment in medicine involves weighing the benefits and risks for each particular paitent. In your case, your physician has recommended that you receive a blood product. However, you need to understand the potential complications of transfusions, and also the consequences of NOT receiving that blood product.

RISKS OF BLOOD PRODUCT TRANSFUSION...

All blood products have a minimal risk of transmitting an infectious disease.

All blood products are tested for transfusion-transmitted diseases according to federal regulations. Yes, some risks remain present, as no screen can be 100% effective. Viruses are not commonly transmitted but may cause a serious disease.

☞ **March 2004 estimates from the American Association of Blood Banks show that the risk of getting:**
- HIV is <1 in 1.9 million transfused units
- Hepatitis C is <1 in million transfused units
- Hepatitis B is <1 in 137,000 transfused units

Source: www.aabb.org/All About Blood 3/25/04

☞ **Other risks include, but are not limited to:**
- Bacterial contamination of a unit of blood may occasionally occur and result in life-threatening infections.
- Transfusion errors, although rare, are also a potential risk of blood transfusion.

☞ **Transfusion reactions, which are unpredictable, may occur. Their symptoms vary.**
- Some reactions may present as fever and chills.
- Some reactions are mild immunologic reactions that manifest 10–14 days after red cell transfusion and may shorten the life of the transfused red cells.
- Allergic reactions may be caused by plasma proteins and typically cause itching and hives. Some reactions may be serious.
- Serious reactions are extremely rare but may include life-threatening disorders such as shortness of breath or hemolysis (destruction of the transfused red cells). This can in turn cause jaundice or kidney problems.

BENEFITS OF BLOOD PRODUCT TRANSFUSION...

Blood may be transfused to treat anemia or acute blood loss.
- Anemia: A deficiency in the oxygen-carrying material of the blood, also known as low blood count or low blood level.
- Symptoms that might improve after blood transfusion include weakness, shortness of breath, chest pain, or light headedness.
- Conditions that may be prevented with appropriate use of blood include strokes, heart attacks, kidney failure, and other serious problems, including death.
- Platelets, plasma, or cryoprecipitate may be prescribed for the prevention or treatment of bleeding problems.

FIGURE 171.2. Example of patient and family information booklet for blood transfusion. (Courtesy of Inova Fairfax Hospital, Falls Church, VA.)

TABLE 171.8

TRANSFUSION REACTIONS: AMERICAN ASSOCIATION OF BLOOD BANKS CLASSIFICATION

Type	Clinical features	Comments
Immunologic		
Hemolytic	Chills, fever, hypotension, renal failure, back pain, hemoglobinuria	Caused by red blood cell mismatch
Fever and/or chills, nonhemolytic	Temperature elevation >1°C, chills and/or rigors, headache, vomiting	
Urticarial	Pruritus, urticaria, flushing	
Anaphylactic	Hypotension, urticaria, bronchospasm, respiratory distress, wheezing, local edema, anxiety	Varies from isolated urticaria to fatal anaphylaxis
Transfusion-associated acute lung injury	Hypoxemia, respiratory failure, hypotension, fever	Leading cause of transfusion-associated mortality
Nonimmunologic		
Hypotension (associated with angiotensin-converting enzyme inhibition)	Flushing, hypotension	
Circulatory overload	Dyspnea, orthopnea, cough, tachycardia, hypertension, headache	
Nonimmune hemolysis	Hemoglobinuria	Caused by physical destruction of blood (heating, freezing, etc.)
Air embolus	Sudden dyspnea, cyanosis, chest pain, cough, hypotension, cardiac arrhythmia	
Hypocalcemia	Paresthesia, tetany, arrhythmia	
Hypothermia	Cardiac arrhythmia	
Transfusion-associated sepsis	Bacterial contamination of transfused blood	Consider in patients with fever >40°C and/or cardiovascular collapse

reactions occur when destruction of transfused RBCs occurs because of preformed antibodies, and is mediated by complement. The reaction varies from mild to severe, depending on the degree of complement activation and cytokine release (28). Severe acute hemolytic reactions are usually due to the transfusion of ABO-incompatible blood. Fatalities occur in 1 in 600,000 units, secondary to severe hemolytic transfusion reactions (29). Red cell destruction results in the release of peptides, which leads to hypotension, poor renal blood flow, an activated coagulation cascade, and, in more severe cases, disseminated intravascular coagulation (DIC). Clinical features include pain and redness along the vein used for infusion, chest pain, a feeling of doom, hypotension, oozing from wounds and intravenous sites, chills, fever, oliguria, and hemoglobinuria. In patients who are heavily sedated or unconscious, hypotension, hemoglobinuria, and diffuse oozing suggest the diagnosis of a severe, acute, hemolytic transfusion reaction. The diagnosis may be especially difficult in the patient under general anesthesia, and a high index of suspicion is needed in order to make a prompt diagnosis in such patients.

When a hemolytic or anaphylactic transfusion reaction is suspected, the infusion should be stopped immediately and the unit checked against the recipient's identification band to determine whether the wrong unit has been administered to the patient. The unit, including all intravenous solutions and tubing, should be sent promptly to the blood bank for examination. Blood should be drawn from a remote site and tested for free hemoglobin. The urine should also be tested for free hemoglobin. A direct antiglobulin test is indicated. Aggressive fluid resuscitation should be initiated, and urine output should be maintained at high levels. The early development of hypotension and DIC is associated with increased mortality.

Delayed hemolytic reactions tend to present 5 to 10 days after transfusion (28), with approximately 1 in 260,000 patients developing a significant hemolytic reaction (30). The degree of hemolysis may be significant in the patient whose total RBC mass has been replaced by massive transfusion. A transfused patient who develops an unexplained fall in hematocrit, fever, or jaundice should be evaluated for the possibility of a hemolytic reaction. The workup is similar to that for acute hemolytic reactions, and the need for clinical intervention is less likely.

Allergic nonhemolytic reactions are generally believed to be caused by recipient antibodies to infusing donor plasma proteins. The manifestations vary from a slight rash or urticaria to hemodynamic instability, with bronchospasm and anaphylaxis. Allergic reactions may be prevented by premedication with antihistamines (e.g., diphenhydramine). Recipient antibodies against antigens on donor leukocytes or platelets will produce febrile nonhemolytic reactions. Fevers and chills characterize these reactions shortly after the transfusion has started; thus, an acute hemolytic reaction and bacterial contamination of the unit should be ruled out. Treatment consists of antipyretics and transfusion of leukocyte-depleted blood components when pharmacotherapy fails.

Hypocalcemia rarely occurs in patients receiving 1 unit of blood at a time. The "prophylactic" use of calcium following blood transfusion is not evidence based. Patients receiving large volumes of citrated blood, especially if their liver function is compromised and/or they are hypothermic (e.g., liver transplant patients during their anhepatic phase in the operating room) are at greatest risk of hypocalcemia. In such unusual situations, treatment with calcium gluconate (not calcium chloride) may be needed, and ionized calcium determinations can help guide therapy.

Circulatory overload is a documented risk of blood transfusion, and thus, appropriate precautions should be taken in patients with borderline cardiac and/or renal function and the elderly. Particular care should be exercised in patients who require large volumes of plasma to rapidly correct coagulopathy associated with the use of warfarin. This should not be interpreted to mean that every patient who receives a blood transfusion should also be given a diuretic.

Transfusion-related Acute Lung Injury

The acute onset of pulmonary edema associated with transfusion and leading to death was first described in 1951 by Barnard (31). The term, *TRALI*, was introduced by Popovsky in 1983 (32). It is currently the leading cause of death after transfusion, with an estimated rate of 1 in 5,000 units transfused, although higher rates have been reported (33). Transfusion-related acute lung injury is likely underappreciated and underdiagnosed due to other more commonly recognized conditions (such as acute lung injury [ALI] and the acute respiratory distress syndrome [ARDS]) being often associated with blood transfusion, making the diagnosis of TRALI more difficult. The mortality rate associated with TRALI is in the range of 5% to 10% (34). These data suggest that all patients receiving blood products should be appropriately monitored, including pulse oximetry.

Transfusion-related acute lung injury occurs with the transfusion of all blood components, but especially platelets and plasma. The clinical syndrome is characterized by the acute onset of dyspnea, hypotension, hypoxemia, fever, and noncardiogenic pulmonary edema. The symptoms appear within 6 hours of transfusion, most often within 30 minutes. Since it is similar to many other conditions encountered in the critical care setting, the diagnosis of TRALI is made by exclusion. Like other etiologies of acute lung injury, TRALI causes an increase in pulmonary microvascular permeability with increased protein levels in the edema fluid. Two theories of the increased pulmonary microvascular permeability have been proposed in patients who develop TRALI. The first hypothesis suggests that leukocyte antibodies from the donor unit activate recipient leukocytes in the pulmonary circulation, leading to increased microvascular permeability and noncardiogenic pulmonary edema. Blood donations from multiparous women have been implicated as a contributing factor for TRALI, possibly because of increased leukocyte antibody levels. The second hypothesis assumes an initial predisposing event that primes the patient's neutrophils and sequesters them in the lung. Biologically active lipids and cytokines in the donor unit then further prime and activate the recipient's neutrophils, with resultant microvascular permeability and noncardiogenic pulmonary edema.

The treatment of TRALI is supportive and consists of appropriate hemodynamic and ventilatory support. Once TRALI is suspected, the transfusion should be terminated immediately and the blood bank notified. The donor unit can be tested for anti-HLA and/or antigranulocyte antibodies.

Transmission of Infection

Numerous viral and bacterial diseases may be transmitted by blood transfusion (Table 171.6). Since March 1999, pooled nucleic acid amplification testing (NAT) has been used to test for HIV and hepatitis C virus (HCV), which involves pooling of 16 to 24 individual blood samples and polymerase chain reaction or other amplification techniques to test for HIV and HCV nucleic sequences. Bacterial and protozoal diseases include syphilis, malaria, and infection with *Babesia microti, Trypanosoma cruzi, Yersinia enterocolitica, Serratia marcescens, Staphylococcus aureus, Staphylococcus epidermidis,* or *Klebsiella pneumoniae; Trypanosoma cruzi* causes Chagas disease, but transmission of this infection is very rare in the United States.

Bacterial Contamination

Bacterial contamination of blood is the most frequent cause of transfusion-transmitted infectious disease (35). After hemolytic reactions and TRALI, bacterial contamination is the most frequently reported cause of transfusion-related fatalities to the FDA (36). The agents most often implicated in packed RBC bacteremia were *Serratia* and *Yersinia*. For platelets, *S. aureus, Escherichia coli, Enterobacter,* and *Serratia* species were more frequently identified. Fever, chills, hypotension, tachycardia, and shock after transfusion should raise the suspicion of bacterial contamination, and blood cultures of the patient and unit should be obtained. Platelets, which are stored at 20°C to 24°C, are a good growth medium for bacteria. Platelets are now screened for bacterial contamination in the United States.

Hepatitis

Transmission of the infectious agents for hepatitis is among the most serious risks of blood transfusion. Past estimates of posttransfusion hepatitis were approximately 10%. Current data suggest that the infectious risk of hepatitis is <0.01% per unit transfused (30). All blood is screened for the hepatitis B virus (HBV), with tests for HB_SAg and anti-HB_C. In addition, blood is screened for HCV with anti-HCV testing. The risk of transfusion-associated HBV infection is approximately 1 in 30,000 to 1 in 250,000 per unit. With the development of pooled NAT tests for HCV, the window period has decreased, and the risk of HCV transmission is now as low as 1 in 1 million (37). No new case of transfusion-associated HCV has been detected by the Centers for Disease Control and Prevention Sentinel Counties Viral Hepatitis Surveillance System since 1994 in the United States.

Approximately half of the blood recipients who contract HBV infection develop symptoms; a much smaller percentage requires hospitalization. Approximately half of patients who contract posttransfusion HCV infection develop a chronic form of the disease. Many of those patients eventually develop significant liver dysfunction, including cirrhosis.

Human Immunodeficiency Virus

The risk of HIV transmission from blood transfusion has decreased dramatically since the early 1980s despite an increasing incidence of HIV infection in the general population. The window period from initial infection to the development of antibody to the virus poses a problem with the ability to detect all seropositive donors. With pooled NAT, the window period for detection of HIV has been reduced by 30% to 50%, and the risk of HIV transmission is estimated to be as low as 1 in 2 million units (37).

Human T-cell Leukemia Virus

In addition to the transmission of cytomegalovirus (CMV), hepatitis infection, and HIV, blood transfusion carries the risk of transmission of human T-cell leukemia virus (HTLV) 1 and 2 infection. Transmission of the virus, especially to immunocompromised patients, may cause illnesses such as T-cell leukemia, spastic paraparesis, and myelopathy, and has prompted routine screening of donors in the United States since 1989. The risk of HTLV 1 and 2 transmission is estimated to be 1 in 641,000 units.

Herpesviruses

CMV infection is endemic, so routine screening is not performed in the United States. About 20% of blood donors are infected with CMV by 20 years of age, and approximately 70% are infected by 70 years of age. The infection is carried in white blood cells (WBCs). Most patients who encounter problems with CMV are immunocompromised, especially transplant recipients on immunosuppressive drugs. Such patients require transfusion with CMV-reduced-risk—leukocyte-reduced or seronegative—blood products to avoid the transmission of this viral infection. Human herpesvirus 8 causes Kaposi sarcoma and lymphoma in patients with acquired immunodeficiency syndrome (AIDS) and other immunosuppressed states.

Graft Versus Host Reaction

Blood transfusion exposes the recipient to many cells and proteins from the donor. When immunologically competent lymphocytes are introduced into an immunocompromised patient, a graft versus host reaction can occur (28). The functional donor lymphocytes attack recipient tissues, notably the bone marrow, causing aplasia. Patients present with fever, rash, nausea, vomiting, diarrhea, liver function test abnormalities, and depressed cell counts. This complication is fatal in as many as 90% of the cases. The prevalence of this complication in the United States is not known but is thought to be rare. Rare cases have also been reported from familial directed donations and with HLA-matched platelets. γ-Irradiation of blood products eliminates this risk.

Immunomodulation

Allogeneic blood transfusion may alter the immune response in individuals and susceptibility to infection, tumor recurrence, and reactivation of latent viruses. It has been known since 1974 that the transfusion of packed RBCs depresses the immune response in patients undergoing renal transplantation; however, it is unclear to what extent these immunosuppressive effects exist in other recipients. Contradictory evidence exists concerning increased infections in patients given allogeneic blood transfusions. Similar controversy also exists regarding the exact relationship of blood transfusions to increased recurrence of tumor and poor prognosis. Early studies on colorectal cancer showed decreased survival and increased tumor recurrence in patients who were heavily transfused. Since then, studies on many tumors have been performed that have not yielded a decisive answer. The possibility exists that blood transfusion may represent a covariable, because very ill patients and those undergoing more difficult procedures for more extensive disease are more likely to receive blood transfusion. In light of the immunomodulating effects of allogeneic blood transfusion, leukocyte-depleted transfusions have been suggested as an alternative. In view of the data on immunosuppression from blood transfusion, it would seem reasonable to adopt a policy of blood conservation in the perioperative period in the absence of clear indications and acute symptoms. Leukocyte reduction of blood products is thought to decrease the risk of immunomodulation (38).

Decision Making in Blood Transfusion

Blood Transfusion in Hemorrhagic Shock

During World War I, it was believed that toxins caused vascular collapse in injured patients (39). Experiments in the 1930s by Dallas B. Phemister and Alfred Blalock showed that fluid was lost from the circulation into damaged tissues: the concept of fluid loss into a "third space." During World War II, plasma was the resuscitation solution of choice, as blood was rarely available. British forces in the North African campaign did utilize blood for casualties and noted improved outcome. Although solutions containing electrolytes were used for children with diarrhea, and advances in research had increased the understanding of metabolic and endocrine changes seen with injury, the use of plasma solutions prevailed until the Korean conflict. Subsequent experimental work indicated that extracellular fluids shifted into the intracellular space after significant hemorrhage with shock (40). Providing volume resuscitation in excess of shed blood became standard practice to maintain adequate circulation and to refill the "third space."

During World War II, acute tubular necrosis (ATN) was a common consequence of hypovolemic shock. As fluid resuscitation became more prevalent during the Korean and Vietnam conflicts, the incidence of ATN decreased. Yet, while posthypovolemic shock ATN became less common with better fluid resuscitation, the acute—initially termed the *adult*, to differentiate it from the neonatal syndrome—respiratory distress syndrome became increasingly common. The lung injury in ARDS was shown to be a function of the shock state rather than the resuscitation solution used.

The goal of resuscitation from shock is prompt restoration of adequate tissue and end-organ perfusion and oxygen transport. The American College of Surgeons Committee on Trauma developed a classification of hemorrhagic shock that permits useful guidelines for resuscitation (Table 171.9). Crystalloid is infused at a 3:1 ratio for every unit of RBCs administered, and therapy is monitored primarily by hemodynamic response. Because crystalloid solutions are universally available, and some delay is required to prepare blood products, crystalloid is the proper initial resuscitation fluid. Resuscitation proceeds with the use of blood products, depending on the patient's response. Although controversy existed in the past regarding the choice of a colloid solution (e.g., albumin, plasma) or a crystalloid solution (e.g., lactated Ringer [LR] solution or saline), recent evidence has confirmed that colloid solutions offer no advantages over crystalloids for fluid resuscitation in critically ill patients (41). Crystalloid solutions should be considered the solutions of choice because they are less expensive, need not be cross-matched, do not transmit disease, and probably result in less fluid accumulation in the lung. No experimental data indicate that using colloid rather than crystalloid solutions can prevent pulmonary edema. An updated review of randomized controlled trials of albumin resuscitation yielded no suggestion of a reduction in mortality when the colloid was used in hypovolemia or in critically ill patients with burns and hypoalbuminemia (42).

Several crystalloid solutions are available for resuscitation, but isotonic solutions should be used to avoid free water overload. While lactated Ringer solution is recommended as initial therapy, metabolic alkalosis is common after successful resuscitation with this solution and blood products because the lactate in LR solution and the citrate in banked blood are both converted to bicarbonate in the liver. LR solution contains calcium and, if it is mixed with a blood product, the blood may, in theory, clot in the bag. Normal (0.9%) saline solution is an acceptable alternative to LR solution, but large volumes can produce a hyperchloremic metabolic acidosis, which may complicate the use of base deficit in resuscitation. Since normal saline is compatible with all blood products, its use is sometimes preferred if transfusion is a possibility.

The decision to transfuse blood is highly dependent on the acuity of blood loss. Patients with acute, massive hemorrhage, such as those with trauma or gastrointestinal bleeding, show signs of hemodynamic instability early in their presentation. The clinical picture depends on the amount of blood loss (Table 171.9). For example, acute loss of 40% of the total blood volume (about 2,000 mL in a 70-kg patient) is associated with severe tachycardia, hypotension, depressed mental status, and

TABLE 171.9

CLASSES OF HEMORRHAGIC SHOCK

Class of hemorrhage	Blood volume loss	Characteristics	Treatment
I	15% (750 mL)	Vital signs essentially normal	No resuscitation generally needed
II	15%–30% (750–1,500 mL)	Tachycardia, decreased pulse pressure, anxiety, pallor, diaphoresis, acidosis	Crystalloid resuscitation needed. Blood transfusion given if no response to fluids (or if response is transient)
III	30%–40% (1,500–2,000 mL)	Hypotension, tachycardia, decreased mental status, oliguria	Blood transfusion generally needed, with crystalloids in 3:1 ratio
IV	>40% (>2,000 mL)	Severe tachycardia and hypotension, lethargy	Massive resuscitation with fluids and blood products needed

Adapted from the American College of Surgeons, Advanced Trauma Life Support.

oliguria. On the other hand, blood loss of up to 15% of the blood volume (750 mL) may not have any obvious physiologic effects.

It is important to remember that the diagnosis of hemorrhagic shock and the decision to administer blood transfusion should not be based solely on hypotension, tachycardia, or anemia. Hypotension does not generally occur until more than 30% of the blood volume has been lost. This is particularly the case in children who, due to very effective compensatory mechanisms, maintain their blood pressure despite severe blood loss. Conversely, elderly patients on β-blocking agents may not manifest significant tachycardia. Hemoglobin levels obtained early in the course of hemorrhagic shock do not reflect the severity of blood loss, as there has not been enough time for fluid shifts to occur. Therefore, blood transfusion should be based on a comprehensive assessment of the patient, including vital signs and estimation of the amount of blood loss, as well as clinical and laboratory evaluation of end-organ perfusion.

Acute, massive hemorrhage is managed initially with aggressive volume replacement using crystalloid solutions. After administering 2,000 to 3,000 mL of crystalloid solution, blood transfusion should be initiated in patients who continue to manifest unstable vital signs. This should occur concomitantly with expeditious surgical control of the bleeding sites. Cross-matched blood should be given as soon as it is available. If needed, type O negative blood can be given to women of childbearing age, and type O positive blood can be given to men of all ages and women older than 50 years of age until cross-matched blood is available. Correction of coagulopathy and hypothermia is paramount. A "damage control" surgical approach, aimed at rapid control of bleeding while delaying less urgent procedures, should be utilized. This helps reduce transfusion requirements and allows the patient to recover more quickly from shock.

Blood Transfusion in the Normovolemic Patient

Anemic patients with a normal blood volume, such as patients who have recovered from hemorrhagic shock and those with subacute or chronic anemia, are generally hemodynamically intact. Concerns regarding the diminished oxygen-carrying capacity of the blood may persist in some of these patients, especially those in the critical care setting. For many years, the standard of care dictated that a hematocrit level of at least 30% should be maintained; the rationale included faster recovery and prevention of myocardial ischemia, especially in patients with coronary artery disease. Recent data indicate that lower hematocrit levels are well tolerated, even in patients at risk for myocardial ischemia (10,43–47). Combined with the current understanding of blood transfusion risks, this has resulted in lowering the trigger level for transfusion.

There are now many reports demonstrating that blood transfusion is an independent risk factor for worse outcome, including increased mortality, especially in trauma patients (48–53). In a landmark study, Hébert et al. demonstrated that maintaining the hemoglobin at or above 10 g/dL (liberal strategy) in euvolemic critically ill patients—as compared to maintaining the hemoglobin at 7 g/dL, the conservative strategy—was not associated with any improvement in overall mortality (19). In fact, mortality was significantly lower with the conservative strategy (hemoglobin at 7 g/dL) among patients who were less acutely ill and in those who were younger than 55 years of age. Patients with active myocardial ischemia, defined as unstable angina and acute myocardial infarction, were excluded from the study. In the latter group of patients, maintaining the hemoglobin at or above 10 g/dL remains the standard of care, although there are conflicting data on that subject.

In a study of Medicare discharge records, elderly patients with acute myocardial infarction had a lower mortality if their hematocrit was 30% or higher (54). Another study suggested that a higher hematocrit upon admission to the ICU after coronary artery bypass grafting was associated with a higher rate of myocardial infarction (55). Despite the large body of evidence against empiric blood transfusion in normovolemic patients, physicians continue to transfuse patients with hematocrit levels between 21% and 30% (56). Finally, there have also been reports advocating a hematocrit level of 30% in septic patients (57), although these reports do not establish blood transfusion to a hematocrit of 30% as an independent factor contributing to improved outcome. The general trend, overall, appears to be that of an increasingly restrictive strategy of blood transfusion (11,12,58).

MINIMIZING TRANSFUSIONS IN THE INTENSIVE CARE UNIT

Immediate Concerns

Given the known risks and the costs associated with blood transfusions, a comprehensive strategy of blood conservation should be followed. The need to correct anemia should be assessed, sources of ongoing blood loss should be controlled, and measures to enhance erythropoiesis should be entertained.

Minimizing Unnecessary Blood Loss

A significant amount of blood can be lost with repeated phlebotomy in the ICU. This is particularly significant in children. Routine serial "blood draws" should be avoided. A policy of obtaining laboratory results only when clinically indicated should be followed. Microsampling techniques, including bedside point-of-care testing, limit the amount of blood lost with each blood draw. Since the estimated daily blood loss from phlebotomy is at least 40 mL/day (10,11,13), critical care practitioners should carefully consider the need for frequent phlebotomy in the ICU.

Optimization of Red Cell Production

Iron

Iron is essential for properly functioning hemoglobin, as it is the site of attachment of the oxygen molecule. Other oxygen-carrying proteins, such as myoglobin and cytochrome *a-a*3, also depend on iron. Many enzymes in the Kreb cycle contain iron in their functional groups. In the critically ill patient, iron deficiency anemia may be multifactorial, for example, poor gastrointestinal absorption, nutrient antagonism, and concomitant copper and vitamin A deficiencies (59).

Patients with the systemic inflammatory response syndrome (SIRS) have circulating cytokines that impair the release of iron stored in the reticuloendothelial system. This creates a situation where total body iron levels are normal but iron is not available for incorporation into red cell precursors (functional iron deficiency anemia).

Despite the central role that iron plays in oxygen delivery, it is still not known whether iron supplementation in critically ill anemic patients is beneficial (60). Perceived iron deficiency could be functional, rather than an absolute reduction in total body iron (61,62). In addition, iron supplementation has been implicated with an increased risk and severity of infection since free iron acts as a chelator of free radicals (63). There is currently no clear indication to administer supplemental iron to critically ill patients who are anemic.

Erythropoietin

Erythropoietin is a circulating glycoprotein secreted primarily by the kidneys in response to hypoxia. Its principal action is to stimulate the production and release of RBCs from the bone marrow (64). This hormone is now commercially available using recombinant DNA technology, and has been approved for use in anemic patients with end-stage renal disease. Its indications were extended to include anemic patients with chronic renal insufficiency, cancer, and AIDS. The indications for erythropoietin therapy are still being expanded. Patients undergoing elective surgical procedures that are typically associated with severe blood loss may benefit from preoperative erythropoietin therapy combined with autologous blood transfusion (65).

The potential therapeutic value of erythropoietin in anemia of critical illness is an area of intense research. Erythropoiesis in critically ill patients can be suppressed for a variety of reasons, including renal and hepatic failure. Circulating cytokines in SIRS suppress erythropoiesis both by blunting the response to and inhibiting the production of erythropoietin (66–72). Gabriel et al. noted that erythropoietin formation in patients with multiple organ dysfunction was inadequate to stimulate reticulocytosis in what was described as a relative erythropoietin deficit (73). In their study, high doses of recombinant human erythropoietin therapy did stimulate the erythropoietic system, as evidenced by a higher rate of reticulocytosis. There was, however, no increase in hematocrit or reduction in packed RBC transfusion during the 3 weeks of the study.

Studies have focused on the potential of human recombinant erythropoietin therapy to reduce transfusion requirements and improve outcome in critically ill patients (74). Corwin et al., in two randomized controlled trials (75,76), demonstrated a reduction of up to 19% in packed RBC units transfused and a greater increase in hematocrit in the group treated with erythropoietin; there were no differences in morbidity or mortality between the two groups. Georgopoulos et al. showed similar results, with the additional finding that the effects of erythropoietin therapy are dose dependent (77).

More recent studies have shown less favorable results. Another study by Corwin et al. noted that the use of erythropoietin alfa did not reduce the incidence of red cell transfusion among critically ill patients, and treatment with this agent was associated with an increase in the incidence of thrombotic events (78). A second study concluded that the use of a target hemoglobin level of 13.5 g/dL in chronic kidney disease was associated with increased risk and no improvement in quality of life (79). Several reports have also demonstrated adverse outcomes in cancer patients (80).

Adverse effects potentially attributable to erythropoietin therapy include hypertension, thrombotic complications, cardiovascular events, tumor progression in cancer patients, and increased risk of death. In November 2006, the FDA issued an alert to provide new safety information for erythropoiesis-stimulating agents (ESAs) (81). The alert was based on analyses of studies on cancer and orthopedic surgery patients who were found to have a higher chance of serious and life-threatening effects and/or death with the use of ESAs. The FDA recommends using the lowest dose possible to achieve a hemoglobin level that avoids the need for transfusion, and withholding the dose of the ESA if the hemoglobin level exceeds 12 g/dL or rises by 1 g/dL in any 2-week period.

Autotransfusion

Blood lost during surgical procedures can be retrieved, spun, washed, and filtered. The recovered RBCs are then reinfused back into the patient. Similarly, blood from drains such as thoracostomy tubes can be retrieved, collected in containers with citrate solutions to prevent clotting, and reinfused. Relative contraindications include contamination of blood with bacteria, malignant cells, or amniotic or ascitic fluids. Other strategies of blood conservation include preoperative autologous donation and acute normovolemic hemodilution (30).

Hemoglobin-based Oxygen Carriers

The search for a solution that can transport oxygen from the lungs to the tissues started in the early part of the 20th century and continues to the present day (82–84). These solutions are loosely termed "blood substitutes," although they should be more appropriately described as "oxygen carriers," since this is the only blood function for which they substitute. A variety of substances have been studied, including perfluorocarbons and porphyrins. Research on the latter two categories of oxygen carriers has been largely abandoned due to problems with manufacturing, ease of use, and adverse effects (85–87).

Current investigation is now focused on the hemoglobin-based oxygen carriers (HBOCs). Hemoglobin can be obtained from three sources: human blood from discarded units of packed RBCs, animal blood, and recombinant DNA technology.

Structure and Function of Normal Human Hemoglobin

Hemoglobin (Hb) is a large molecule made up of four polypeptide chains (two α- and two β-chains), with a molecular weight of 64,450. Each chain is conjugated with a heme moiety, an iron-containing porphyrin derivative to which oxygen attaches, forming oxyhemoglobin. When fully saturated, each Hb molecule has four oxygen molecules attached. Iron has to be in the ferrous state (Fe^{2+}) in order for oxygen to attach. When blood is exposed to various drugs and other oxidizing agents, ferrous iron is converted to ferric iron (Fe^{3+}), forming methemoglobin (met-Hb), which cannot bind oxygen. An enzyme within red cells, met-Hb reductase, converts met-Hb back to Hb.

The affinity of Hb for oxygen increases exponentially as more oxygen molecules attach, and hence the sigmoid nature of the oxygen–Hb dissociation curve. Factors that decrease the affinity of Hb to oxygen (i.e., making off-loading of oxygen easier) include acidosis and 2,3-DPG.

Characteristics of Cell-free Hemoglobin

Dissociation. When free in the plasma, the Hb tetramer dissociates into two $\alpha\beta$-dimers, which are filtered through renal glomeruli and can then precipitate in the renal tubules, causing obstruction. This adverse effect is further compounded by the decreased renal blood flow that results from the vasoconstrictive effect of Hb (88,89). Technologies were developed to produce large stable Hb polymers by cross-linking Hb molecules; the most commonly used cross-linking reagent is glutaraldehyde. This process results in the formation of polymers of varying sizes that do not filter through the glomeruli. Another strategy used to stabilize Hb was intramolecular cross-linking, whereby the cross-link was between α-chains of the same molecule so that neither polymerization nor subunit dissociation occurred; this product was abandoned due to intense vasoconstrictive features.

Viscosity. The lower viscosity of Hb solutions, compared to blood, was initially thought to be advantageous, as it provided less systemic vascular resistance. However, deeper insight into the physiology of the vascular endothelium revealed that the reduced shear stresses on the blood vessel wall were associated with decreased secretion of relaxing factors such as prostacyclin and endothelin, with a net vasoconstrictive effect. The resulting decrease in blood flow antagonizes the oxygen delivery function of Hb (90,91).

Vasoactivity. Most HBOCs have a systemic pressor effect (92,93), and some have the same effect on the pulmonary circulation as well (94). In addition to the above mechanisms of vasoconstriction, two other mechanisms are described: binding of nitric oxide and stimulation of catecholamine release; these effects have been associated with decreased cardiac output (95).

Affinity for Oxygen. Once released from the red cell, Hb loses its 2,3-DPG, and its affinity for oxygen increases. This causes a leftward shift of the oxygen–Hb dissociation curve, thus impairing the off-loading of oxygen. Strategies to decrease the affinity of Hb for oxygen include pyridoxalation and the use of bovine Hb. It is not clear whether decreasing the affinity of Hb for oxygen is beneficial. For example, higher levels of oxygen at the tissue level may trigger an autoregulatory response by the blood vessel wall, whereby there is decreased secretion of relaxing factors, resulting in vasoconstriction and decreased flow (96).

Oxidation. Deprived of the met-Hb reductase in red cells, free Hb is at higher risk of being oxidized into met-Hb. However, other antioxidants such as glutathione are available in the plasma to serve this function. Levels of met-Hb in patients receiving HBOCs do not appear to be physiologically significant (97).

Effects on the Inflammatory Response. HBOCs, unlike stored blood, lack the ability to stimulate neutrophils and incite an inflammatory response with its attendant systemic manifestations of multiple organ dysfunction (98).

Clinical Trials of Hemoglobin-based Oxygen Carriers

The most widely studied HBOC in clinical practice is a human polymerized hemoglobin product (PolyHeme, Northfield Laboratories, Evanston, IL). The first randomized trial in acute trauma and emergency surgery was published in 1998 (99), showing that PolyHeme maintained total hemoglobin in lieu of red cells despite the marked fall in RBC hemoglobin, and reduced the use of blood transfusion. The study concluded that PolyHeme appears to be a clinically useful blood substitute. A phase III trial involving 720 patients from 32 level I trauma centers was recently completed. The trial randomized trauma patients with evidence of hemorrhagic shock at the scene to either normal saline or PolyHeme. Treatment was started in the field and continued for up to 12 hours after injury. The primary end point was survival at 30 days. Preliminary results showed no statistically significant difference in survival between patients receiving PolyHeme without blood for up to 12 hours following injury and those receiving the standard of care, including early blood replacement. PolyHeme may, therefore, be useful when blood is needed but not available (100).

REFUSAL OF BLOOD TRANSFUSION

Critically ill patients with transfusion preferences present a challenging management problem. For example, Jehovah's Witnesses' refusal of blood and blood products is part of their religious beliefs (Genesis 9:3-4, Leviticus 17:10-11) (101). Honoring these beliefs requires modification of medical management strategies, and presents a unique opportunity to question transfusion guidelines and thresholds. The care of these patients requires early identification of transfusion preferences. All patients admitted to the critical care setting should have treatment preferences (including blood transfusion) discussed with them or their legal representative as soon as possible. Although transfusion may need to be administered in some emergent situations without the opportunity to obtain informed consent, in most circumstances the critical care practitioner should be able to discuss the risks, benefits, and potential complications of transfusion of various blood products with the patient or representative. Moreover, individual patients may have preferences—religious or otherwise—regarding some blood products but not others, so it is important to establish these preferences for each blood product available. Discussion with patients and family members should include a detailed explanation of each blood product, as the origin and technical aspects of these products may affect their acceptance. In the case of the Jehovah's Witness, or other groups with religious preferences, assistance from a church representative or other religious leaders may be extremely helpful to the family and the physician.

Although survival at lower levels of hemoglobin (>3 g/dL) have been reported, mortality rates exceed 50% when levels fall below 3 g/dL (102). A recent experience with an injured patient who was a Jehovah's Witness demonstrated that survival without neurologic impairment was possible even at extremely low hemoglobin and hematocrit levels (2.7 g/dL and 7.8%, respectively) (103). The implementation of blood conservation strategies, hormonal stimulation, and the use of red

TABLE 171.10

MANAGEMENT STRATEGIES FOR JEHOVAH'S WITNESSES WITH SEVERE ANEMIA

- **Blood conservation**
  - No routine blood draws
  - Consequential blood tests only
  - Use of capillary tubes for arterial blood gas analysis
  - Pediatric-size tubes for other tests
  - Decisive surgical interventions in cases of bleeding
  - Intraoperative and peri-procedure blood conservation
    - Hemostasis
    - Autologous transfusion (cell salvage device)
    - Normovolemic hemodilution
- **Maximization of oxygen delivery**
  - Maintain high oxygen saturation
  - Minimize oxygen demand
    - Sedation
    - Mechanical ventilation
    - Neuromuscular blockade
    - Allow permissive hypercapnia/metabolic acidosis
- **Hormonal stimulation**
  - High-dose recombinant erythropoietin
  - Iron supplementation
- **Red cell substitutes** (as they become available)

cell substitutes as they become available are options in the management of these patients. The use of high-dose erythropoietin (40,000 units subcutaneously every other day) and supplemental iron provide accelerated erythropoiesis under extreme circumstances. Table 171.10 lists potential strategies that may be useful in the management of the Jehovah's Witness and others who request that blood transfusion not be administered. A number of these strategies should be considered for all patients in the critical care setting to minimize the need for transfusion.

References

1. Webster C. The origins of blood transfusions: a reassessment. *Med Hist.* 1971;15:387–392.
2. Maluf NSR. A history of blood transfusion. *J Hist Med.* 1954;9:59–107.
3. Schmidt PJ. Transfusion in America in the eighteenth and nineteenth centuries. *N Engl J Med.* 1968;279:1319.
4. Blundell J. Successful case of transfusion. *Lancet.* 1828;1:431.
5. http ://www.aabb.org/Content/About Blood/Highlights_of_Transfusion_Medicine_History/highlights.htm. Accessed January 5, 2008.
6. American Association of Blood Banks for the United States Department of Health and Human Services. 2005 Nationwide Blood Collection and Utilization Survey Report. https://www.aabb.org/Content/Programs_and_Services/Data_Center/NBCUS/nbcus.htm. Accessed January 8, 2008.
7. Report on blood collection and transfusion in the United States in 2001. National Blood Data Resource Center; 2003.
8. Goodnough LT, Brecher ME, Kanter MH, et al. Blood transfusion. *N Engl J Med.* 1999;340:438–447, 525–533.
9. Cobain TJ, Vamvakas EC, Wells A, et al. A survey of the demographics of blood use. *Transfus Med.* 2007;17:1–15.
10. Corwin HL, Parsonnet KC, Gettinger A. RBC transfusion in the ICU. Is there a reason? *Chest.* 1995;108:767–771.
11. Vincent JL, Baron J-F, Reinhart K, et al. Anemia and blood transfusion in critically ill patients. *JAMA.* 2002;288:1499–1507.
12. Corwin HL, Gettinger A, Pearl RG, et al. The CRIT study: anemia and blood transfusion in the critically ill—current clinical practice in the United States. *Crit Care Med.* 2004;32:39–52.
13. Nguyen Ba V, Peres Bota D, Melot C, et al. Time course of hemoglobin concentrations in non-bleeding ICU patients. *Crit Care Med.* 2003;31:406–410.
14. Rutledge R, Sheldon GF, Collins ML. Massive transfusion. *Crit Care Clin.* 1986;2:791.
15. Vincent JL, Piagnerelli M. Transfusion in the intensive care unit. *Crit Care Med.* 2006;34(Suppl):S96–S101.
16. Adams RC, Lundy JS. Anesthesia in cases of poor surgical risk. *Surg Gynecol Obstet.* 1942;74:1011–1019.
17. Fakhry SM, Fata P. How low is too low? Cardiac Risks with Anemia. *Crit Care.* 2004;8(Suppl 2):S11–S14.
18. Holcomb JB. Damage control resuscitation. *J Trauma.* 2007;62:S36–S37.
19. Hebert PC, Wells G, Blajchman MA, et al. A multicenter, randomized, controlled clinical trial of transfusion requirements in critical care. *N Engl J Med.* 1999;340:409–417.
20. Ratko TA, Cummings JP, Oberman HA, et al. Evidence-based recommendations for the use of WBC-reduced cellular blood components. *Transfusion.* 2001;41:1310–1319.
21. Rebulla P. Platelet transfusion trigger in difficult patients. *Transfus Clin Biol.* 2002;9:249–254.
22. Kheirabadi BS, Crissey JM, Deguzman R, et al. *In vivo* bleeding time and *in vitro* thrombelastography measurements are better indicators of dilutional hypothermic coagulopathy than prothrombin time. *J Trauma.* 2007;62:1352–1361.
23. Clark P, Mintz PD. Transfusion triggers for blood components. *Curr Opin Hematol.* 2001;8:387–391.
24. Toy P, Popovsky MA, Abraham E, et al., and the National Heart, Lung and Blood Institute Working Group on TRALI. Transfusion-related acute lung injury: definition and review. *Crit Care Med.* 2005;33:721–726.
25. Blajchman MA, Vamvakas EC. The continuing risk of transfusion-transmitted infections. *N Engl J Med.* 2006;355:1303–1305.
26. Linden JV, Wagner K, Voytovich AE, et al. Transfusion errors in New York State: an analysis of 10 years' experience. *Transfusion.* 2000;40:1207–1213.
27. Robillard P, Itaj NK, Corriveau P. ABO incompatible transfusions, acute and delayed hemolytic transfusion reactions in the Quebec hemovigilance system—year 2000 (abstract). *Transfusion.* 2002;42(suppl):25S.
28. Snyder E. Transfusion reactions. In: Hoffman R, Benz EJ, Shattil SJ, et al., eds. *Hematology: Basic Principles and Practice.* 3rd ed. Philadelphia: Churchill Livingstone; 2000.
29. Goodnough LT. Erythropoietin therapy versus red cell transfusion. *Curr Opin Hematol.* 2001;8:405–410.
30. Goodnough LT, Brecher ME, Kanter MH, et al. Blood transfusion. *N Engl J Med.* 1999;340:438–447, 525–533.
31. Barnard R. Indiscriminate transfusion: a critique of case reports illustrating hypersensitivity reactions. *N Y State J Med.* 1951;51:2399–2402.
32. Popovsky MA, Abel MD, Moore SB. Transfusion-related acute lung injury associated with passive transfer of anti-leukocyte antibodies. *Am Rev Respir Dis.* 1983;128:185–189.
33. Toy P, Popovsky MA, Abraham E, et al., and the National Heart, Lung and Blood Institute Working Group on TRALI. Transfusion-related acute lung injury: definition and review. *Crit Care Med.* 2005;33:721–726.
34. Shander A, Popovsky MA. Understanding the consequences of transfusion-related acute lung injury. *Chest.* 2005;128:598S–604S.
35. Reading FC, Brecher ME. Transfusion-related bacterial sepsis. *Curr Opin Hematol.* 2001;8:380–386.
36. Kuehnert MJ, Roth VR, Haley NR, et al. Transfusion-transmitted bacterial infection in the United States, 1998 through 2000. *Transfusion.* 2001; 41:1493–1499.
37. Strong DM. Infectious risks of blood transfusions. *Am Blood Centers Blood Bull.* 2001;4(2).
38. Blajchman MA. Immunomodulation and blood transfusion. *Am J Ther.* 2002;9:389–395.
39. Rutherford EJ, Skeete D, Schooler WG, et al. Hematologic principles in surgery. In: Townsend CM, Beauchamp RD, Evers BM, et al., eds. *Sabiston Textbook of Surgery: The Biologic Basis of Modern Surgical Practice.* 17th ed. Philadelphia: Elsevier-Saunders; 2004:113–136.
40. Shires T, Coln D, Carrico J, et al. Fluid therapy in hemorrhagic shock. *Arch Surg.* 1964;88:688–693.
41. The SAFE Investigators. A comparison of albumin and saline for fluid resuscitation in the intensive care unit. *N Engl J Med.* 2004;350:2247–2256.
42. Alderson P, Bunn F, Lefebvre C, et al. Human albumin solution for resuscitation and volume expansion in critically ill patients. *Cochrane Database Syst Rev.* 2004;4:CD001208.
43. Hebert PC, Wells G, Berlin JA, et al. A Canadian survey of transfusion practices in critically ill patients. *Crit Care Med.* 1998;26:482–487.
44. Carson JL, Willett LR. Is a hemoglobin of 10 g/dl required for surgery? *Med Clin North Am.* 1993;77:335–347.
45. Sehgal LR, Zebala LP, Takagi I, et al. Evaluation of oxygen extraction ratio as a physiologic transfusion trigger in coronary artery bypass graft surgery patients. *Transfusion.* 2001;41:591–595.
46. Stehling L, Simon TL. The red blood cell transfusion trigger. Physiology and clinical studies. *Arch Pathol Lab Med.* 1994;118:429–434.
47. Greenburg AG. A physiologic basis for red blood cell transfusion decisions. *Am J Surg.* 1995;170:44S–48S.
48. Malone DL, Dunne J, Tracy JK, et al. Blood transfusion, independent of shock severity, is associated with worse outcome in trauma. *J Trauma.* 2003;54(5):898–907.
49. Robinson WP, Ahn J, Stiffler A, et al. Blood transfusion is an independent

predictor of increased mortality in nonoperatively managed blunt hepatic and splenic injuries. *J Trauma* 2005;58(3):437–445.

50. Hill GE, Frawley WH, Griffith KE, et al. Allogeneic blood transfusion increases the risk of postoperative bacterial infection: a meta-analysis. *J Trauma.* 2003;54(5):908–914.
51. Offner PJ, Moore EE, Biffl WL, et al. Increased rate of infection associated with transfusion of old blood after severe injury. *Arch Surg.* 2002;137:711–716.
52. Zallen G, Offner PJ, Moore EE, et al. Age of transfused blood is an independent risk factor for postinjury multiple organ failure. *Am J Surg.* 1999; 178:570–572.
53. Claridge JA, Sawyer RG, Schulman AM, et al. Blood transfusions correlate with infections in trauma patients in a dose-dependent manner. *Am Surg.* 2002;68:566–572.
54. Wu W, Rathore S, Wang Y, et al. Blood transfusion in elderly patients with acute myocardial infarction. *N Engl J Med.* 2002;345:1230–1236.
55. Spiess BD, Ley C, Body SC, et al. Hematocrit value on intensive care unit entry influences the frequency of Q-wave myocardial infarction after coronary artery bypass grafting. The Institutions of the Multicenter Study of Perioperative Ischemia (McSPI) Research Group. *J Thorac Cardiovasc Surg.* 1998;116:460–467.
56. Shapiro MJ, Gettinger A, Corwin HL, et al. Anemia and blood transfusion in trauma patients admitted to the intensive care unit. *J Trauma.* 2003;55(2):269–274.
57. Rivers E, Nguyen B, Havstad S, et al. Early goal directed therapy in the treatment of severe sepsis and septic shock. *N Engl J Med.* 2001;345:1368–1377.
58. Earley AS, Gracias VH, Haut E, et al. Anemia management program reduces transfusion volumes, incidence of ventilator-associated pneumonia, and cost in trauma patients. *J Trauma.* 2006;61(1):1–7.
59. Lynch SR. Interaction of iron with other nutrients. *Nutr Rev.* 1997;55:102–110.
60. Prelack K, Sheridan RL. Micronutrient supplementation in the critically ill patient: strategies for clinical practice. *J Trauma.* 2001;51(3):601–620.
61. Deitch EA, Sittig KM. A serial study of the erythropoietic response to thermal injury. *Ann Surg.* 1993;217:293–299.
62. Krantz SB. Pathogenesis and treatment of the anemia of chronic disease. *Am J Med Sci.* 1994;307:353–359.
63. Walter T, Olivares M, Pizarro F, et al. Iron, anemia, and infection. *Nutr Rev.* 1997;55:111–124.
64. Jelkmann W. Erythropoietin: structure, control of production, and function. *Physiol Rev.* 1992;72:449–489.
65. Goodnough LT, Monk TG, Andriole GL. Current concepts: erythropoietin therapy. *N Engl J Med.* 1997;336:933–938.
66. Means R Jr, Krantz SB. Progress in understanding the pathogenesis of the anemia of chronic disease. *Blood.* 1992;80:1639–1647.
67. Fuchs D, Hausen A, Reibnegger G, et al. Immune activation and the anaemia associated with chronic inflammatory disorders. *Eur J Haematol.* 1991;46:65–70.
68. Baer AN, Dessypris EN, Goldwasser E, et al. Blunted erythropoietin response to anaemia in rheumatoid arthritis. *Br J Haematol.* 1987;66:559–564.
69. Faquin WC, Schneider TJ, Goldberg MA. Effect of inflammatory cytokines on hypoxia-induced erythropoietin production. *Blood.* 1992;79:1987–1994.
70. Jelkmann W, Pagel H, Wolff M, et al. Monokines inhibiting erythropoietin production in human hepatoma cultures and in isolated perfused rat kidneys. *Life Sci.* 1992;50:301–308.
71. von Ahsen N, Muller C, Serke S, et al. Important role of nondiagnostic blood loss and blunted erythropoietic response in the anemia of medical intensive care patients. *Crit Care Med.* 1999;27:2630–2639.
72. Rogiers P, Zhang H, Leeman M, et al. Erythropoietin response is blunted in critically ill patients. *Intensive Care Med.* 1997;23:159–162.
73. Gabriel A, Kozek S, Chiari A, et al. High-dose recombinant human erythropoietin stimulates reticulocyte production in patients with multiple organ dysfunction syndrome. *J Trauma.* 1998;44(2):361–367.
74. Corwin HL. The role of erythropoietin therapy in the critically ill. *Transfus Med Rev.* 2006;20:27–33.
75. Corwin HL, Gettinger A, Rodriguez RM, et al. Efficacy of recombinant human erythropoietin in the critically ill patient: a randomized, double-blind, placebo-controlled trial. *Crit Care Med.* 1999;27:2346–2350.
76. Corwin HL, Gettinger A, Pearl RG, et al. Efficacy of recombinant human erythropoietin in critically ill patients: a randomized controlled trial. *JAMA.* 2002;288:2827–2835.
77. Georgopoulos D, Matamis D, Routsis C, et al. Recombinant human erythropoietin therapy in critically ill patients: a dose-response study. *Crit Care.* 2005;9:R508–515.
78. Corwin H, Gettinger A, Fabian T, et al. Efficacy and safety of epoetin alfa in critically ill patients. *N Engl J Med.* 2007;357:965.
79. Singh A, Szczech L, Tang K, et al. Correction of anemia with epoetin alfa in chronic kidney disease. *N Engl J Med.* 2006;355:2085.
80. Wright J, Ung Y, Julian J, et al. Randomized, double-blind, placebo-controlled trial of erythropoietin in non–small-cell lung cancer with disease-related anemia. *J Clin Oncol.* 2007;25:1027–1032.
81. FDA information for healthcare professionals. Erythropoietin-stimulating agents. http://www.fda.gov/cder/drug/InfoSheets/HCP/RHE2007HCP.pdf. Accessed January 15, 2008.
82. Sellards AW, Minot GR. Injection of hemoglobin in man and its relation to blood destruction, with special reference to the anemias. *J Med Res.* 1916; 34:469–494.
83. Winslow RM. Current status of oxygen carriers (blood substitutes): 2006. *Vox Sang.* 2006;91(2):102–110.
84. Stowell CP. Hemoglobin-based oxygen carriers. *Curr Opin Hematol.* 2002; 9:537–543.
85. Stowell CP, Levin J, Speiss BD, et al. Progress in the development of RBC substitutes. *Transfusion.* 2001;41:287–299.
86. Moore E. Blood substitutes: the future is now. *J Am Coll Surg.* 2003; 196(1):1–17.
87. Scott MG, Kucik DF, Goodnough LT, et al. Blood substitutes: evolution and future applications. *Clin Chem.* 1997;43:1724–1731.
88. Amberson WR, Jennings JJ, Rhode CM. Clinical experience with hemoglobin-saline solutions. *J Appl Physiol.* 1949;1:460–489.
89. Stavitsky JP, Doczi J, Black J, et al. A clinical safety trial with stroma-free hemoglobin. *Clin Pharmacol Ther.* 1978;23:73–80.
90. Intaglietta M, Johnson PC, Winslow RM. Microvascular and tissue oxygen distribution. *Cardiovasc Res.* 1996;32:632–643.
91. Karmaker N, Dhar P. Effect of steady shear stress on fluid filtration through the rabbit arterial wall in the presence of macromolecules. *Clin Exp Pharmacol Physiol.* 1996;23:299–304.
92. Keipert PE, Gonzales A, Gomez CL, et al. Acute changes in systemic blood pressure and urine output of conscious rats following exchange transfusion with diaspirin-crosslinked hemoglobin solution. *Transfusion.* 1993;33:701–708.
93. Przybelski RJ, Dailey EK, Birnbaum ML. The pressor effect of hemoglobin: good or bad? In: Winslow R, Vandegriff K, Intaglietta M, eds. *Advances in Blood Substitutes: Industrial Opportunities and Medical Challenges.* Boston: Birkhäuser; 1997:71–85.
94. Hess JR, Macdonald VW, Brinkley WW. Systemic and pulmonary hypertension after resuscitation with cell-free hemoglobin. *J Appl Physiol.* 1993;74:1769–1778.
95. Lamy ML, Dailey EK, Brichant JF, et al. Randomized trial of diaspirin cross-linked hemoglobin solution as an alternative to blood transfusion after cardiac surgery. *Anesthesiology.* 2000;92:646–656.
96. Intaglietta M. Microcirculatory basis for the design of artificial blood. *Microcirculation.* 1999;6:247–258.
97. Sprung J, Kindscher JD, Wahr JA, et al. The use of bovine hemoglobin glutamer-250 (Hemopure) in surgical patients: results of a multicenter, randomized single-blinded trial. *Anesth Analg.* 2002;94:799–808.
98. Johnson JL, Moore EE, Offner PJ, et al. Resuscitation with a blood substitutes abrogates pathologic postinjury neutrophil cytotoxic function. *J Trauma.* 2001;50:449–456.
99. Gould S, Moore E, Hoyt D, et al. The first randomized trial of human polymerized hemoglobin as a blood substitute in acute trauma and emergent surgery. *J Am Coll Surg.* 1998;187(2):113–120.
100. Moore EE, and the PolyHeme Study Group. Postinjury resuscitation with human polymerized hemoglobin: the U.S.A. multicenter trial. Papers Session, ACS 93rd Clinical Congress, New Orleans, LA, October 10, 2007.
101. The Bible. New International Version.
102. Cothren CC, Moore EE, Long JS, et al. Large volume polymerized haemoglobin solution in a Jehovah's Witness following abruptio placentae. *Transfus Med.* 2004;14(3):241–246.
103. Vaziri K, Roland J, Robinson L, et al. Extreme anemia in an injured Jehovah's Witness: a test of our understanding of the physiology of severe anemia and the threshold for blood transfusion. J Trauma Injury Infect Crit Care In press.

CHAPTER 172 ■ ANTITHROMBOTIC AND THROMBOLYTIC THERAPY

GOHAR H. DAR • STEVEN R. INSLER

The occurrence of venous and arterial thromboembolism has had a large impact on medical care and is a major cause of both morbidity and mortality. Arterial thromboembolism, commonly implicated in myocardial infarctions, stroke, and limb ischemia, is responsible for more deaths each year than the next seven leading causes of death combined (1,2). Venous thrombosis may lead to pulmonary embolism, right heart dysfunction, venous insufficiency, and the postthrombotic syndrome (3). The incidence of patients in the intensive care unit developing venous thromboembolism ranges from 5% to 33% (4–6). There are an estimated 2 million cases of venous thromboembolism each year in the United States alone, with an annual estimated mortality of about 60,000 from pulmonary embolism (7–9). The ability to rapidly diagnose and initiate effective therapy is paramount. This chapter will briefly review the formation of arterial and venous thrombi, regulation of the coagulation cascade, and current antithrombotic and thrombolytic therapies.

THROMBOGENESIS AND COAGULATION

Thrombosis can occur anywhere in the vascular system, in either the venous or arterial beds. Typically, deep venous thromboemboli are associated with many different clinical situations, and the stimulus for developing thrombi depends on the underlying clinical condition. A patient may have an underlying primary hypercoagulable predisposition to developing venous thrombosis secondary to decreased antithrombotic or increased prothrombotic proteins (thrombophilias) (10), increasing the relative risk of thrombosis up to tenfold. Deep venous thrombosis will form under conditions of low flow and are predominantly composed of fibrin and red blood cells. They usually originate in the muscular calf veins or in the valve cusps of the deep calf veins (1). Altered or low blood flow is commonly seen posttrauma, postoperatively, and in the critically ill patient. The risk factors for deep venous thrombosis are listed in Table 172.1.

In vivo, coagulation in the veins is initiated by a complex of tissue factor (TF, a type I transmembrane protein) and the serine protease factor VIIa. Low levels of factor VIIa circulate in plasma so that the system will respond efficiently if vessel injury occurs and tissue factor is exposed. The factor VIIa/tissue factor (TF) complex activates factors IX and X. Activated factor X cleaves small amounts of prothrombin to generate thrombin. The low concentrations of thrombin generated are sufficient to activate factors V and VIII, essential steps for the propagation of the coagulation cascade (11–13) (Fig. 172.1).

Arterial thrombi typically form under conditions of high flow (shear) conditions, and are made up primarily of platelet aggregates held together by fibrin strands. Most arterial thrombi are superimposed on ruptured atherosclerotic plaques. Plaque rupture exposes thrombogenic material in the lipid-rich core of the blood (14). When plaques rupture, subendothelial collagen and von Willebrand factor is exposed. Collagen and von Willebrand factor provide a substrate for platelet adhesion (15,16). Collagen binds to platelets' glycoprotein Ia/IIa receptor complex; von Willebrand factor binds to glycoprotein Ib/IX/V receptor complex; and other exposed extracellular matrix, such as fibronectin and laminin bind to glycoprotein VI. These actions cause the up-regulation of platelet glycoprotein IIb/IIIa receptor complex, which in turn results in platelet aggregation. Glycoprotein IIb/IIIa accelerates platelet adhesion to the subendothelium by binding to fibrinogen and von Willebrand factor (17,18). Additionally, plaque rupture causes TF release, which accelerates the extrinsic coagulation cascade (Fig. 172.2).

Once coagulation is initiated in either veins or arteries, and TF has activated factor VII, converting it to factor VIIa, the factor VIIa/TF complex activates factors IXa and Xa, respectively. Factor IXa binds to factor VIIIa on the membrane surfaces to form intrinsic tenase, which activates factor X. By feedback activation of factor VII, factor Xa initiates and amplifies coagulation (19,20).

Factor Xa propagates coagulation by binding with factor Va, and in turn activates prothrombin to thrombin and, ultimately, to fibrin clot formation. If the thrombus is of sufficient size to disrupt blood flow, shear increases and promotes additional platelet and fibrin deposition.

Regulation of the Coagulation Cascade

Three inhibitory systems are involved in the regulation of the coagulation cascade. The pathway of TF inhibition interferes with the initiation of coagulation. The protein C pathway regulates thrombin generation and inhibits the propagation of coagulation. Antithrombin blocks the generation of thrombin and, subsequently, thrombin activity. Additionally, the fibrinolytic system promotes fibrin degradation.

Tissue Factor Pathway Inhibitor

The factor VIIa/TF complex is inhibited by the TF pathway inhibitor, most of which is bound to endothelium, in two steps. First, the TF pathway inhibitor binds and then inactivates factor Xa. This complex in turn inactivates factor VIIa, which is bound to TF (21).

TABLE 172.1

POTENTIAL MECHANISMS BY WHICH VARIOUS CLINICAL CONDITIONS MAY FACILITATE DEEP VENOUS THROMBOSIS (DVT)

	Increased baseline propensity for thrombosis	Acute insult
Hypercoagulability	*Genetic* Increased coagulants Prothrombin mutation G20210A Decreased anticoagulants AT deficiency Protein C deficiency Protein S deficiency Factor V Leiden Acquired Malignancy Hyperhomocysteinemia HRT/OCT (?) Pregnancy (hormone-related) Nephrotic syndrome (loss of AT) Antiphospholipid syndrome Increased levels of clotting factors	*Increased Coagulants* Blood-borne tissue factor Malignancy (Trousseau syndrome) Congestive heart failure (?) Systemic infection (?) Exogenous administration of clotting factors rVIIa rVIII *Acute loss of anticoagulants* Nephrotic syndrome (loss of AT) Initial warfarin therapy without heparin
Direct Vessel Injury	Direct vessel injury most often represents an acute insult Examples of low-grade, chronic vessel injury that increase the baseline propensity for thrombosis may include: Endothelial injury secondary to chemotherapy Hyperhomocysteinemia Vasculitus Antiphospholipid syndrome	Intravascular catheters Trauma Surgery
Blood Stasis	More commonly functioning as an acute insult Precipitating thrombosis, rather than increasing the baseline propensity for thrombosis: Age Obesity Pregnancy (gradual immobility/stasis) Sedentarism	Hospitalization/bedridden Pregnancy (stasis) Limb paralysis (e.g., stroke, plaster casts) Right heart failure Long-haul flights Vein compression (e.g., enlarged lymph node)

AT, antithrombin; HRT/OCT,.
Risk factors or clinical conditions that increase the risk of DVT can be classified as either increasing the baseline propensity for thrombosis or precipitating the thrombotic event acutely. Thrombosis may occur by one of three major mechanisms: inducing hypercoagulability, directly injuring the vessel wall, or causing blood stasis (low flow).
From Lopez JA, Kearon,. Lee AY. Deep venous thrombosis. *Hematology.* 2004;1:442, with permission.

Protein C Pathway

The protein C pathway is initiated when thrombin binds to thrombomodulin, which is found on endothelium. Once bound to thrombomodulin, thrombin undergoes a conformational change at its active site, which converts it from a procoagulant enzyme to a potent activator of protein C. Activated protein C, a vitamin K–dependent protein, acts as an anticoagulant by proteolytically degrading and inactivating factors Va and VIIIa, thus blocking thrombin generation (22).

Antithrombin

Antithrombin inhibits thrombin, factor Xa, and other activated clotting factors, but in the absence of heparin, these reactions occur slowly. Heparin addition will increase the rate of inhibition of these reactions by 1,000-fold (23). Small amounts of the proteoglycan heparin sulfate located on the luminal surface may maintain intact endothelium in a nonthrombogenic state (24).

Fibrinolytic Degradation of Fibrin

This system is designed to remove intravascular fibrin and restore normal blood circulation. Fibrinolysis is initiated by plasminogen activators that convert plasminogen to plasmin, a trypsinlike protease. Plasmin degrades fibrin into soluble fibrin degradation products (25).

D-Dimers. D-dimers are a specific fibrin degradation product formed only by plasmin degradation of fibrin and not by plasmin degradation of intact fibrinogen (Fig. 172.3). Thus, its presence indicates that fibrin has been formed. D-dimer has been validated as a diagnostic tool to help in the exclusion of venous thrombosis and pulmonary embolism and is widely used in the emergency room setting for this purpose (26–28).

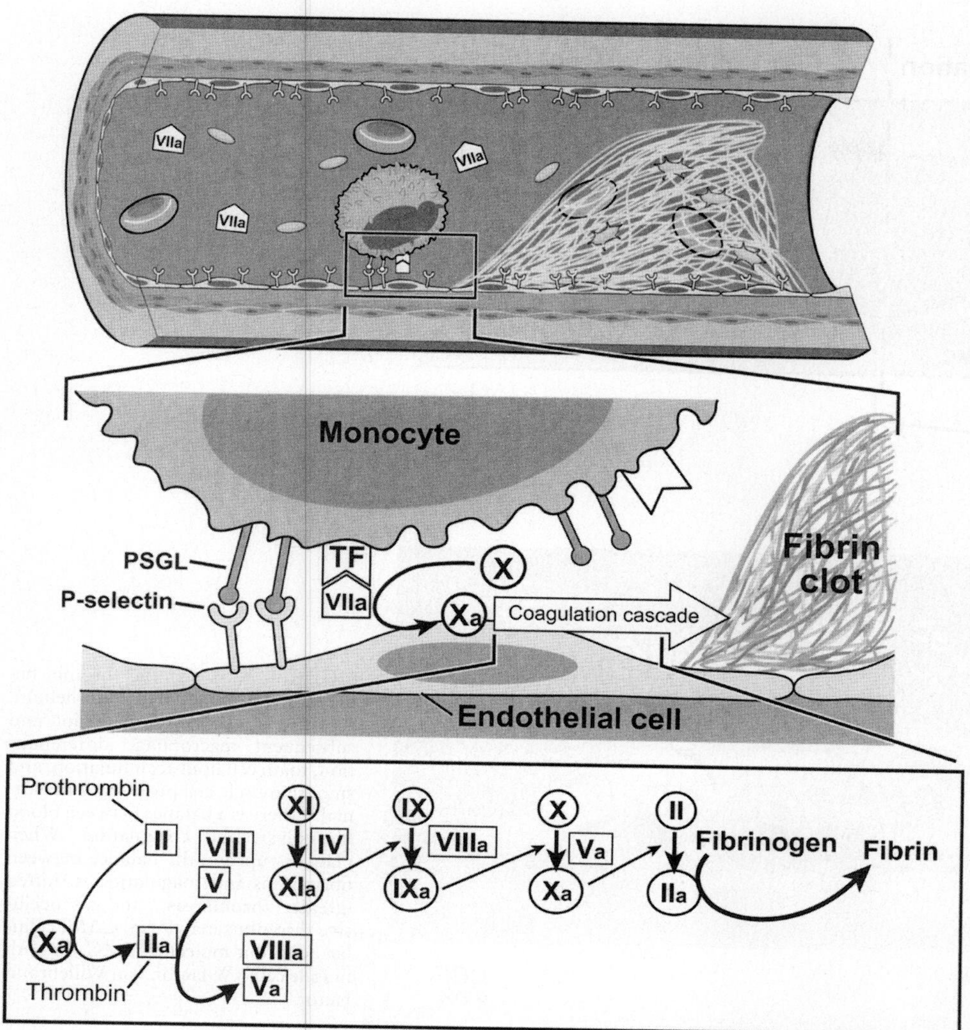

FIGURE 172.1. Model for venous thrombosis. Coagulation in veins is initiated by the tissue factor VIIa complex, which then activates factors IX and X. Factor II, prothrombin; factor IIa, thrombin; PSGL-1, p-selectin glycoprotein ligand-1; TF, tissue factor.

Elevated d-dimer levels have been reported as a marker of risk for both multiple organ failure and death in critically ill patients (29).

ANTIPLATELET AGENTS

Platelets are known to play a key role in the inflammatory and thrombotic cascade and are integral in the pathogenesis of arterial thrombosis, particularly in regions of high fluid shear stress including the coronary, cerebrovascular, and peripheral circulations. Platelet aggregation leading to a disruption of blood flow can have devastating outcomes, often causing permanent disability or death. The understanding of normal platelet function has led to the rational basis for development of antiplatelet agents.

Aspirin

Aspirin is the most widely used antiplatelet drug in the world. Although it has been used as an antipyretic agent since the mid-1800s, its antiplatelet effect was recognized only about 50 years ago. Activated platelets cleave phospholipids to generate arachidonic acid, which is converted to thromboxane-A2 through a series of reactions mediated by cyclo-oxygenase-1 (COX-1) and thromboxane-A2 synthase. There are three isoforms of cyclo-oxygenase enzyme, COX-1 being the major type and COX-3 being a variant of COX-1. COX-2 is the inducible form present in the cells at the site of inflammation.

Aspirin, acetylsalicylic acid, is an irreversible inhibitor of COX-1 and COX-3 at low concentrations. It has a rapid onset of action, approximately 30 minutes, and exerts its effect by acetylating the serine 529 site of platelet COX-1 enzyme (30). As the anucleate platelets are unable to synthesize new enzyme, a single daily dose of aspirin is sufficient to inhibit platelet function for the platelet life span. Restoration of normal aggregation on cessation of aspirin therapy results from young, newly released, nonacetylated platelets replacing the aspirin-treated ones. The dose of aspirin required to inhibit platelet function is relatively low compared with that required for an anti-inflammatory effect. The antithrombotic effect of aspirin saturates at doses of approximately 100 mg (31).

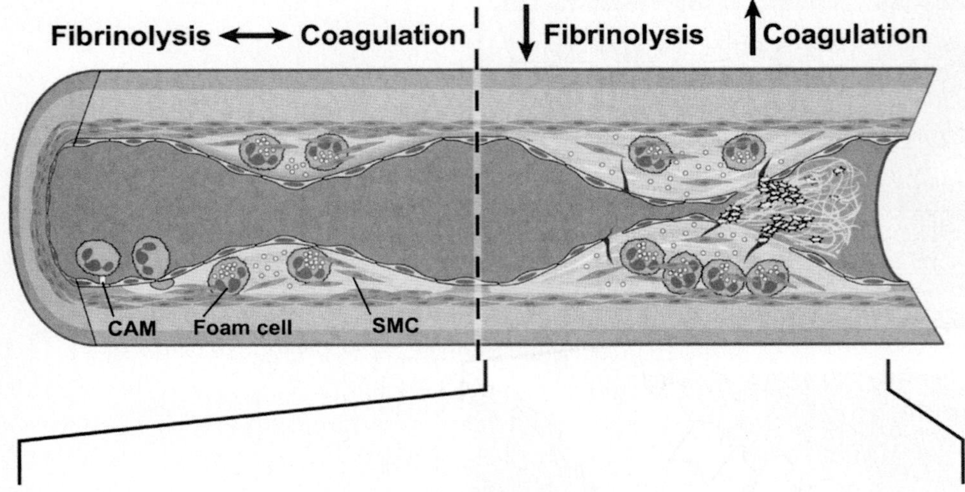

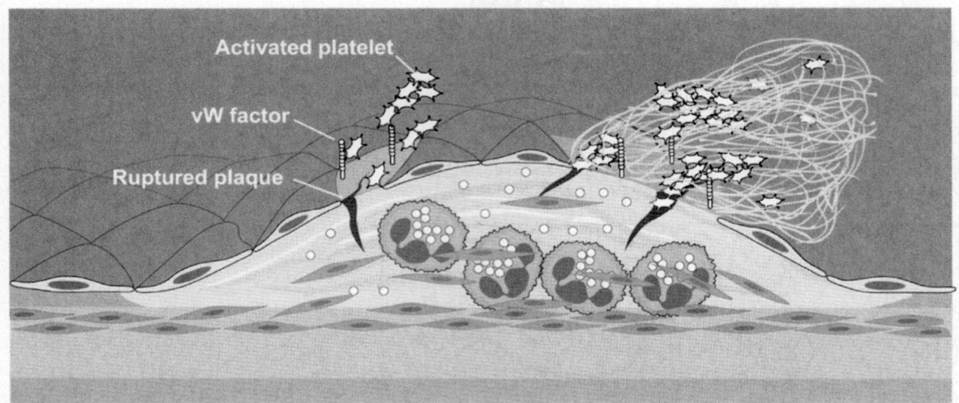

FIGURE 172.2. Arterial thrombi begin with a dysfunctional endothelium, resulting in monocyte infiltration and subsequent macrophage differentiation, foam cell lipid accumulation, and smooth muscle cell proliferation. Normally, there is a balance between blood fibrinolysis and coagulation. When plaques rupture, the balance between fibrinolysis and coagulation is shifted (greater thrombosis), and an occlusive thrombus may form. CAM, cellular adhesion molecule; SMC, smooth muscle cell; vW factor, von Willebrand factor.

The efficacy of aspirin in acute coronary syndrome has been established in numerous clinical trials. For example, the International Study of Infarct Survival (ISIS)-2 demonstrated that for acute myocardial infarction (MI), aspirin alone reduced mortality to a similar extent as did streptokinase alone, with an additive benefit when using both agents (32). A recent meta-analysis by the Antiplatelet Trialists' Collaboration found that aspirin reduced the risk of MI, stroke, or death from 13.3% to 8.0% in patients with unstable angina (33). The meta-analysis also found that the greatest risk reduction occurred with a dose of 75 mg to 150 mg per day; higher doses such as 325 mg per day did not appear to confer any added benefit. Aspirin therapy has, thus, become the standard for the secondary prevention of cardiovascular events in high-risk patients. The role of aspirin alone versus other antithrombotic agents in atrial fibrillation has been addressed in many studies, the results suggesting that the risk reduction of ischemic strokes associated with oral vitamin K–inhibiting anticoagulant therapy is greater than that provided by aspirin (34,35).

Aspirin Resistance

The efficacy of aspirin in the inhibition of platelet function differs between patients. Cardiovascular events occur preferentially in patients with low responses to aspirin therapy (36). This low response is referred to as *aspirin resistance*. The prevalence is reported to vary between 5% and 60%, depending on the laboratory studies used (37). Gum et al. (38), in a prospective study, followed 325 patients with stable coronary artery disease for 2 years, finding aspirin resistance in 5.5% of patients using optical platelet aggregability, and in 9.5% by using the Platelet Function Analyzer 100 (PFA-100). Aspirin-resistant patients were noted to have a 24% risk of death, MI, or stroke, as compared with a 10% risk for patients who were aspirin sensitive.

There are two aspects of resistance: biochemical and clinical. Biochemical resistance refers to the inability of aspirin to initiate platelet inhibition, whereas clinical resistance indicates an increased risk of cardiovascular events in patients receiving treatment with aspirin (39). Platelet receptor polymorphism is thought to be responsible for aspirin resistance (40).

The risk of hemorrhage, especially from the gastrointestinal tract, is a major concern when doses higher than 325 mg/day are used. The local effect of aspirin on the gastric mucosa is more prevalent with the higher doses, but patients with vascular malformations or mucosal lesions may bleed at lower doses, too. There is also a risk of cerebral hemorrhage in patients with prior stroke or with uncontrolled hypertension. In the event of hemorrhage, aspirin should be discontinued, and bleeding time should be measured and, if needed, treated with fresh platelet transfusion. For elective surgical procedures, aspirin should

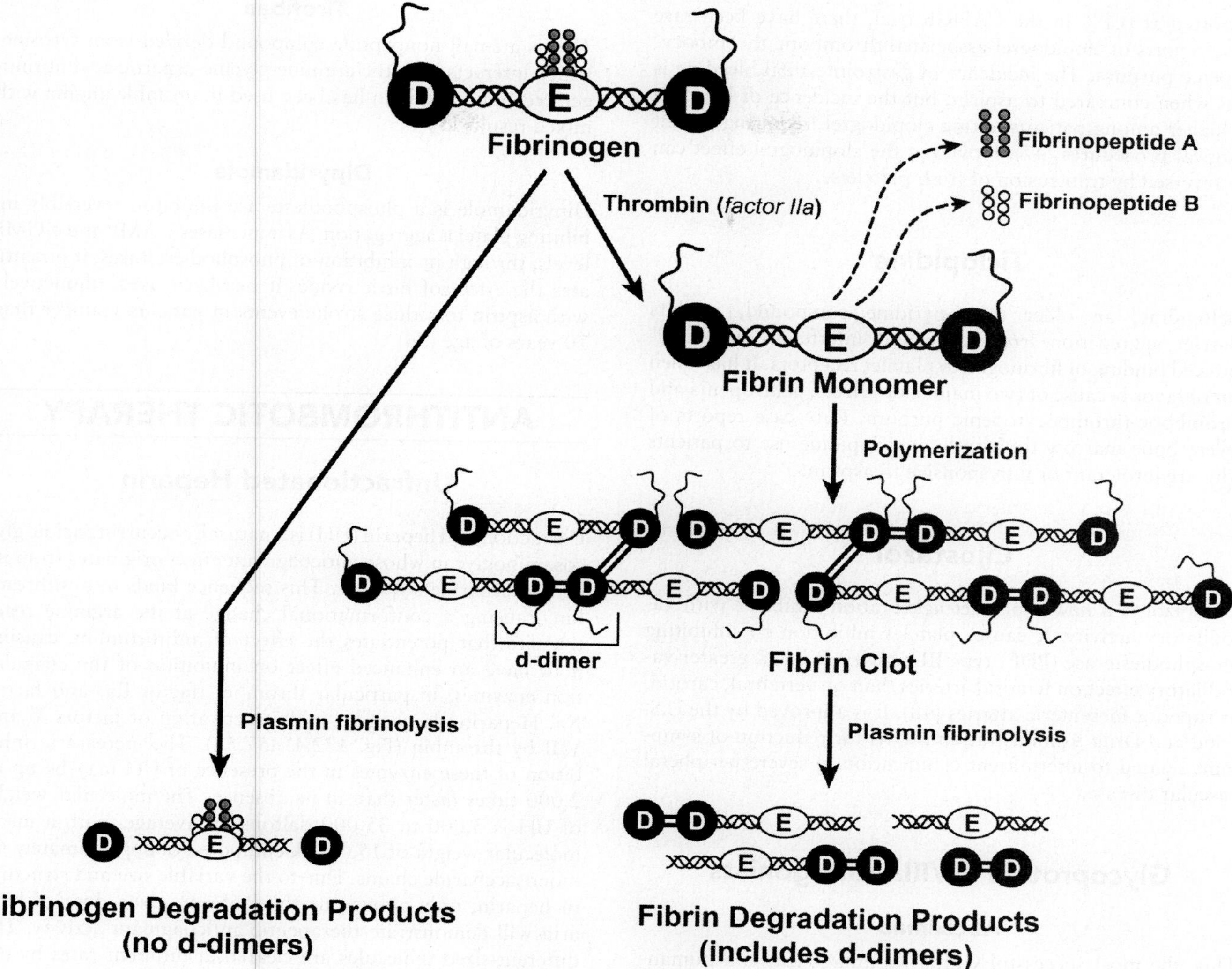

FIGURE 172.3. Fibrin clot formation and degradation. This figure shows the simplified conversion of fibrinogen into fibrin monomers called fibrinopeptides A and B. These monomers either polymerize to form fibrin clot or degrade into fibrinogen degradation products (without d-dimer formation). Fibrinolysis of a fibrin clot leads to formation of fibrin degradation products and d-dimers. Positive d-dimer assays are indicative of fibrin clot formation, followed by degradation by plasmin.

be stopped 5 days before surgery (41). Aspirin is not recommended for venous thromboembolic prophylaxis (42); other forms of standard venous thromboembolism prophylaxis—for example, subcutaneous heparin and pneumatic compression devices—are preferred.

Clopidogrel

Clopidogrel, a member of the thienopyridine family, is a potent platelet inhibitor, working by irreversibly binding to low-affinity adenosine diphosphate (ADP) receptors. It is rapidly absorbed and metabolized by the hepatic cytochrome P-450 enzyme system to an active metabolite that selectively and irreversibly inhibits ADP-induced platelet aggregation. This metabolite also impairs the activation of glycoprotein (GP) IIb/IIIa complex and prevents fibrinogen binding to the platelets. Platelets exposed to this drug are affected for the remainder of their life span. Dose-dependent platelet inhibition can be seen within 2 hours after a single oral dose. For maximum effect, patients may be given a loading dose of 300 to 600 mg, followed by 75 mg per day. With repeated doses of 75 mg per day, maximum platelet inhibition can be achieved within 3 to 7 days (43).

When steady state is achieved, platelet aggregation is inhibited by 40% to 60% (44). Prolongation of bleeding time is independent of age, renal impairment, or gender. Platelet aggregation and bleeding time generally return to baseline about 5 days after discontinuation of clopidogrel. The CAPRIE trial was among the first to establish that clopidogrel is more effective than aspirin in reducing atherosclerotic events—including peripheral vascular disease, myocardial infarction, and stroke—by 8.7% (45). The efficacy and safety of clopidogrel has been evaluated in acute coronary syndrome patients in the CURE trial, showing a 20% relative risk reduction in composite triple end points: nonfatal myocardial infarction, death, or stroke (46). Clopidogrel, like ticlopidine, prolongs the bleeding time. While there was an incidence of neutropenia reported at 0.1% in the CAPRIE trial, there have been rare case reports of clopidogrel-associated thrombotic thrombocytopenic purpura. The incidence of gastrointestinal bleeding is less when compared to aspirin, but the incidence of bleeding is higher among patients taking clopidogrel, requiring urgent surgical procedures (47). However, the clopidogrel effect can be reversed by transfusion of fresh platelets.

Ticlopidine

Ticlopidine, an older thienopyridine compound, inhibits platelet aggregation irreversibly and interferes with ADP-induced binding of fibrinogen to platelet receptors. It has fallen out of favor because of two major side effects: neutropenia and thrombotic-thrombocytopenic purpura. Rare case reports of severe bone marrow toxicity limit ticlopidine use to patients who are intolerant or unresponsive to aspirin.

Cilostazol

Cilostazol is a newer platelet aggregation inhibitor with vasodilatory activity. It causes platelet inhibition by inhibiting phosphodiesterase (PDE) type III activity. It has a greater vasodilatory effect on femoral arteries than on vertebral, carotid, or superior mesenteric arteries (48). It is approved by the U.S. Food and Drug Administration (FDA) for reduction of symptoms related to intermittent claudication in severe peripheral vascular disease.

Glycoprotein IIb/IIIa Antagonists

Abciximab

This, the most successful GPIIb/IIIa antagonist, is a human-murine Fab chimeric monoclonal antibody fragment to the GPIIb/IIIa binding site. It is a large protein with a rapid and prolonged response, causing the bleeding time to remain elevated for 12 hours after injection. Abciximab is used in combination with aspirin and heparin in patients with unresponsive unstable angina or undergoing percutaneous coronary intervention. It has been demonstrated to deliver a 60% relative risk reduction in triple end points: myocardial infarction, emergent revascularization, or cardiovascular deaths (49,50). The major complications of this agent include intracranial bleeding or a decrease in hemoglobin of more than 15%, reported as frequently as 10.5% (51). There is a high incidence of thrombocytopenia, which can be spurious (4%) due to platelet clumping, but true and severe thrombocytopenia may also develop, resulting in profound bleeding (52). In the event of profuse bleeding, platelet transfusions are required to normalize the platelet count. Desmopressin has been shown to normalize the bleeding time (53).

Eptifibatide

This is a disintegrin, derived from the southeastern pygmy rattlesnake. It is rapidly bound and rapidly reversed, with a normalization of the bleeding time within 1 to 4 hours. This drug has been shown to be more effective in milder forms of acute coronary syndromes (54).

Tirofiban

This is a small nonpeptide compound derived from tyrosine, which interacts with the arginine-glycine-aspartic acid fibrinogen receptor. Tirofiban has been used in unstable angina with mixed results (55).

Dipyridamole

Dipyridamole is a phosphodiesterase inhibitor, reversibly inhibiting platelet aggregation. As it increases c-AMP and c-GMP levels, through its inhibition of phosphodiesterases, it potentiates the effect of nitric oxide. It has been used adjunctively with aspirin to reduce stroke events in patients younger than 70 years of age (56).

ANTITHROMBOTIC THERAPY

Unfractionated Heparin

Unfractionated heparin (UH) is a naturally occurring acidic glycosaminoglycan whose anticoagulant effect originates from its pentasaccharide sequence. This sequence binds to antithrombin, causing a conformational change at the arginine reactive site that potentiates the effect of antithrombin, causing it to have an enhanced effect on inhibition of the coagulation enzymes, in particular thrombin (factor IIa) and factor Xa. Heparin also acts to inhibit activation of factors V and VIII by thrombin (Fig. 172.4) (57,58). The increase in inhibition of these enzymes in the presence of UH may be up to 2,000 times faster than in its absence. The molecular weight of UH is 3,000 to 35,000 daltons on average, with a mean molecular weight of 15,000 d, composed of approximately 45 monosaccharide chains. Due to the variable size and structure of heparin, only about one third of any given dose of heparin will demonstrate therapeutic anticoagulant activity. The different-sized molecules are cleared at different rates by the kidney, with the larger ones being cleared more rapidly. Thus, the combination of these factors leads to great variability in the anticoagulant effects on individuals, necessitating the need for monitoring with activated partial thromboplastin time (aPTT). Heparin is obtained from either bovine lung or porcine intestine and is available as a sodium or calcium salt.

The unit of heparin is measured in animals in a biologic assay, with the unit measurement being variable by as much as 50% on a weight basis. Therefore, UH is prescribed for patients on a unit basis per kilogram, not weight of medication (59). UH clearance involves a combination of rapid, saturable, and slower first-order mechanisms. The saturable phase of heparin clearance is via binding to receptors on endothelial cells and macrophages, where it becomes depolymerized, whereas the slower-phase first-order saturable mechanism is renal. At therapeutic doses, heparin is cleared predominantly through the rapid, saturable dose-dependent mechanism, and the anticoagulant effects are nonlinear, with both the intensity and duration of effect rising in disproportion to increasing dose.

Uses of Unfractionated Heparin

Heparin is indicated for prophylaxis of venous thromboembolism. It is used in the treatment of deep venous thrombosis (DVT) and pulmonary embolus, as well as for early treatment of patients suffering from acute coronary syndromes.

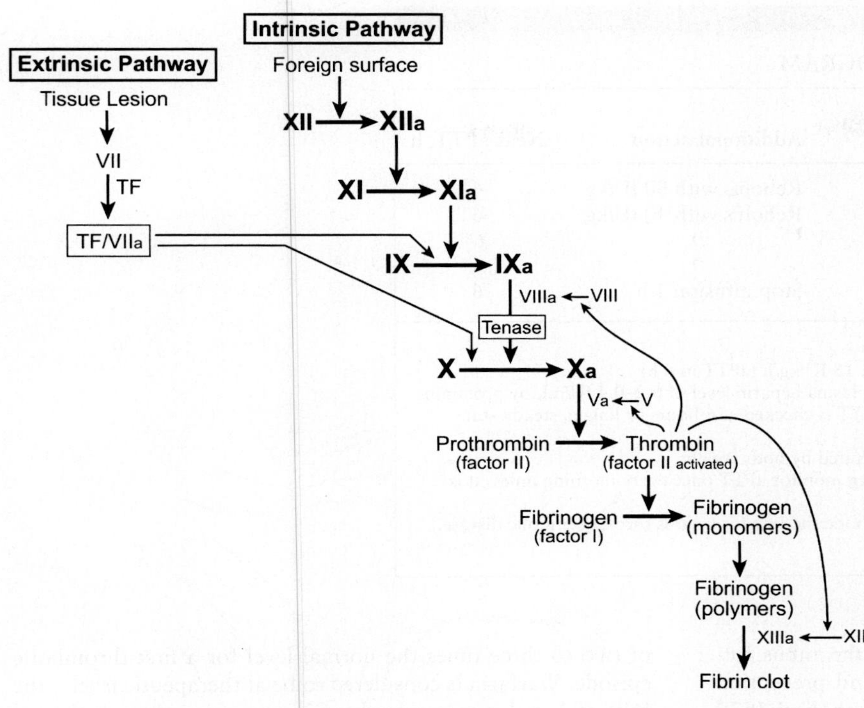

FIGURE 172.4. The coagulation cascade. The extrinsic pathway of coagulation is initiated by the factor VIIa/tissue factor complex, whereas the intrinsic pathway is initiated when factor XII contacts a foreign surface. Both pathways lead to factor IX and X activation. Activated factor IXa propagates coagulation by activating factor X in a reaction using activated factor VIIIa as a cofactor. Activated factor Xa combining with activated factor Va acts as a cofactor and converts prothrombin (factor II) to thrombin (factor IIa). Thrombin then converts fibrinogen to fibrin.

Prevention of Thromboembolism. Given the high rate of venous thromboembolism formation in critically ill patients, and the fact that clinical signs of DVT are unreliable, preventing the problem is an important strategy (60). Unfractionated heparin at a fixed low dose of 5,000 units, subcutaneously every 8 to 12 hours, results in a 60% to 70% relative risk reduction for DVT and fatal pulmonary embolus (42,61). In high-risk surgical and acutely ill medical patients, the use of low-molecular-weight heparin (LMWH) is becoming the standard for prevention of thrombosis (62,63).

In the patient who is unable to tolerate any type of anticoagulation, the use of compression stockings is useful as a mechanical means for preventing DVT by intermittently squeezing the patient's calves, which leads to increased blood flow through the venous system. Intermittent pneumatic compression may also stimulate fibrinolysis by stimulating the vascular endothelium (64).

Venous thromboembolism and pulmonary embolus. Therapy for treating proximal or symptomatic distal venous thromboembolism and pulmonary embolus is aimed at preventing extension of the clot with further embolization and recurrence; anticoagulation has long been an effective strategy for treatment of both conditions (65). Multiple studies have demonstrated the efficacy of heparin in reducing mortality in patients with venous thromboembolism (66,67), as well as the high mortality in patients with pulmonary embolus who did not receive anticoagulant therapy (68). More recent clinical studies further demonstrated the benefit of treating deep venous thrombosis with continuous intravenous heparin and, in some cases, preferably LMWH (69–71). Additionally, data show the effectiveness of using subcutaneous heparin as the initial treatment for deep venous thrombosis, as long as adequate doses are used and the activated partial thromboplastin time is prolonged into the therapeutic range (72–74). Recently, Kearon et al. (75) demonstrated that administration of a fixed dose, weight-adjusted, unfractionated heparin was as effective and safe as the administration of low-molecular-weight heparins in patients with acute deep venous thrombosis and may also be suitable for treatment in the outpatient setting.

Perhaps the most efficient and safe method for initiating intravenous heparin therapy is using weight-adjusted nomograms. In the first days of treatment, there is a weak association between a supratherapeutic aPTT and bleeding, which is in *marked contrast* to the significant relationship between subtherapeutic aPTT and recurrence of venous thromboembolism. The important consideration is to maintain a therapeutic range when heparin anticoagulation therapy is initiated, which is best achieved with frequent monitoring of plasma aPTT. Subtherapeutic dosing within the first 24 hours of a documented DVT resulted in a significantly greater frequency of venous thromboembolus recurrence when compared to those patients who reached a supratherapeutic threshold within 24 hours (76).

The weight-based method was developed by Raschke et al. (77) who found that a weight-based titration of unfractionated heparin resulted in a significant decrease in the time required to reach therapeutic levels as compared to a standard dosing scheme of heparin. These clinicians found that 97% of patients dosed using the weight-based nomogram achieve therapeutic levels within 24 hours of initiation as opposed to 77% in the standard dosing group (Tables 172.2 and 172.3).

Typically, the Raschke method of anticoagulation in the acute phase of venous thromboembolism is initiated with an intravenous loading dose of 80 units/kg, followed by 18 units/kg per hour. Subsequent doses should be adjusted using a standard nomogram to rapidly reach and maintain an aPTT that corresponds to therapeutic heparin levels of 1.5 to 2.5 times the baseline (77–82). Alternatively, therapeutic heparin anticoagulation is determined by achieving a plasma anti–factor Xa level of 0.35 to 0.7 units/mL (83,84). This therapeutic range is recommended based on animal studies (85), prospective studies and analysis of patients with established deep vein thrombosis

TABLE 172.2

WEIGHT-BASED HEPARIN DOSING NOMOGRAM

aPTT, s[b]	Dose change, U/kg/h	Additional action	Next aPTT, h
<35 (<1.2 × mean normal)	+4	Rebolus with 80 IU/kg	6
35–45 (1.2–1.5 × mean normal)	+2	Rebolus with 40 IU/kg	6
46–70[a] (1.5–2.3 × mean normal)	0	0	6[c]
71–90 (2.3–3.0 × mean normal)	−2	0	6
>90 (> × mean normal)	−3	Stop infusion 1 h	6

aPTT, activated prothrombin time.
Initial dosing: Loading 80 IU/kg; maintenance infusion: 18 IU/kg/h (aPTT in 6 h)
[a]Therapeutic range in seconds should correspond to a plasma heparin level of 0.2–0.4 IU/mL by protamine sulfate or 0.3–0.6 IU/mL by amidolytic assay. When aPTT is checked at 6 hours or longer, steady-state kinetics can be assumed.
[b]Heparin, 25,000 IU in 250 mL D_5W. Infuse at rate dictated by body weight.
[c]During the first 24 h, repeat aPTT every 6 h. Thereafter, monitor aPTT once every morning unless it is outside the therapeutic range.
From Hyers TM, Agnelli G, Hull RD, et al. Antithrombotic therapy for venous thromboembolic disease. *Chest.* 2001;119(Suppl):179S, with permission.

(84), and studies on the prevention of mural thrombus formation following myocardial infarction (86) and prevention of recurrent ischemia following coronary thrombolysis (87). Heparin anticoagulation should be continued for up to 5 days so that adequate anticoagulation is achieved. During this time, the aPTT should be monitored every 6 hours until the therapeutic range is achieved, and once daily thereafter. Preferably on day 1, the patient may be transitioned to long-term warfarin (5 mg), a vitamin K–antagonist agent that may be administered orally if the patient can tolerate enteral intake. The anticoagulation effect of warfarin is monitored by the international normalized ratio (INR) to achieve a therapeutic range of two to three times the normal level for a first thrombotic episode. Warfarin is considered to be at therapeutic level if the INR of 2 to 3 is maintained for 2 consecutive days. If the patient is unstable and unable to tolerate oral anticoagulation, intravenous heparin may need to be continued. It is important to keep in mind that warfarin interacts with many commonly used drugs in the intensive care unit, and its metabolism may be affected by hepatic and renal impairment. This may lead to erratic variation in the anticoagulant effect of warfarin and exposes the patient to increased risks of bleeding and thrombotic complications (7). The minimum recommended duration of warfarin therapy is 3 months (88,89), but further studies

TABLE 172.3

GUIDELINES FOR ANTICOAGULATION USING UNFRACTIONATED HEPARIN

Indication	Guidelines
VTE suspected	■ Obtain baseline aPTT, PT, CBC ■ Check for contraindication to heparin therapy ■ Order imaging study, consider giving heparin 5,000 IU IV
VTE confirmed	■ Rebolus with heparin 80 IU/kg IV and start maintenance infusion at 18 U/kg (see Table 172.2) ■ Check aPTT at 6 h to keep aPTT in a range that corresponds to a therapeutic blood heparin level (see text and Table 172.2) ■ Check a platelet count between days 3 to 5 ■ Start warfarin therapy on day 1 at 5 mg and adjust subsequent daily dose according to INR ■ Stop heparin therapy after at least 4–5 of combined therapy when INR is >2.0 ■ Anticoagulate with warfarin for at least 3 mo at an INR of 2.5; range: 2.0–3.0 (see Table 172.6)

aPTT, activated prothrombin time; PT, prothrombin time; CBC, complete blood count; IV, intravenously; INR, international normalized ratio.
For subcutaneous treatment with unfractionated heparin, give 250 IU/kg subcutaneously every 12 h to obtain a therapeutic aPTT at 6–8 h.
From Hyers TM, Agnelli G, Hull RD, et al. Antithrombotic therapy for venous thromboembolic disease. *Chest.* 2001;119(Suppl):180S, with permission.

have demonstrated that longer treatment is beneficial (90–92). In accordance with the American College of Chest Physicians Conference on Antithrombotic and Thrombolytic Therapy, it is now recommended that warfarin therapy be continued for at least 6 to 12 months after an acute thromboembolic episode arising from an idiopathic DVT. For those with recurrent events or who have permanent or long-term risk factors, the panel recommends indefinite therapy (89).

Acute Coronary Syndromes. The ACC/AHA updated guidelines (1999) for the management of patients with acute myocardial infarction (93) evaluated multiple trials comparing the use of LMWH with unfractionated heparin in non–ST elevation acute coronary syndrome (94–96). The studies cited demonstrate, as a whole, a clear benefit of LMWH over unfractionated heparin when it came to a lower event rate and relative risk reduction. These guidelines recommend using LMWH, as opposed to unfractionated heparin, due to its greater inhibition of factor Xa, the ability to administer the drug subcutaneously, and its high bioavailability. Other benefits of the drug are cited as well, such as the potential to prevent thrombin generation and inhibit thrombin, the lack of need to monitor coagulation, and the lower incidence of heparin-associated thrombocytopenia.

Monitoring UH

The most widely used test for evaluating the adequacy of heparin anticoagulation is the activated partial thromboplastin time (aPTT), a global coagulation test that is not always a reliable indicator of plasma heparin levels and/or the antithrombotic activity of heparin. The aPTT can be impacted by various acute phase reactant plasma proteins, including factor VIII. Additionally, the aPTT can be influenced by the coagulation timer and reagents used to perform the test (97). If a hospital is unable to measure plasma heparin levels directly, it is recommended that each laboratory standardize the therapeutic range of the aPTT to correspond to plasma levels of 0.3 to 0.7 IU/mL anti–factor Xa activity by an amidolytic assay.

Complications of Anticoagulation Therapy

Heparin Resistance

Some patients will require greater-than-average doses of heparin to achieve a therapeutic response. Patients are considered heparin resistant if their daily requirement of heparin exceeds 35,000 units per 24 hours; unfortunately, multiple studies demonstrate that at least 25% of patients with venous thromboemboli are heparin resistant. Heparin resistance may be associated with antithrombin deficiency, increased heparin clearance, increases in heparin-binding proteins, and increases in factor VIII, fibrinogen, and platelet factor 4. Aprotinin and nitroglycerin have been reported to cause drug-induced resistance, but the association with nitroglycerin remains controversial (98). Factor VIII and fibrinogen are elevated in response to acute illness or pregnancy. Elevation of factor VIII alters the response of the aPTT to heparin without decreasing the antithrombotic effect, as the anticoagulant effect is measured by the plasma aPTT and the antithrombotic effect is measured by anti–factor Xa activity become dissociated.

For those patients considered heparin resistant, the dose of heparin should be adjusted to maintain the anti–factor Xa heparin levels between 0.35 and 0.7 mIU/mL. In a randomized, controlled study by Levine and Hirsch (99), evaluating 131 patients with venous thromboembolism and manifesting heparin resistance, monitoring the aPTT was compared to anti–factor Xa activity; with no difference in clinical outcomes, it was found that the patient group monitored with anti–factor Xa heparin levels required significantly less heparin with no differences in bleeding.

Hemorrhagic Complications

The incidence of major hemorrhagic complications—defined as intracranial or retroperitoneal hemorrhage, hemorrhage requiring a transfusion, or hemorrhage directly related to death—from therapeutic anticoagulation is less than 5% (100). The risk increases with age, total dose of heparin per 24 hours, premorbid condition of the patient, concomitant use of aspirin, GPIIb/IIIa antagonists, or thrombolytic therapy. Intravenous (IV) heparin infusion appears to produce less marked bleeding complications than when the agent is administered subcutaneously; this may be due to a lower total dose of heparin via the IV, as compared to the subcutaneous, route (101).

The anticoagulant effect of UH can be neutralized rapidly by intravenous protamine. Protamine is a cationic protein derived from fish sperm that strongly binds to the anionic heparin compound in a ratio of approximately 100 units of UH/mg of protamine; for example, 50 mg of protamine would be required to neutralize 5,000 units of IV heparin. When heparin has been infused, only the heparin given over the prior 2 hours should be included in the calculation. If the heparin infusion was discontinued for more than 30 minutes but less than 2 hours, use one half of the calculated protamine dose. If the infusion was discontinued for greater than 2 hours, use one quarter of the calculated protamine dose; one should avoid giving 50 mg of protamine at one time, and, if given by infusion, it should not exceed 5 mg per minute to reduce the incidence of adverse reactions. Heparin neutralization can be confirmed by a fall in the aPTT.

The risks of severe adverse reactions to protamine, such as hypotension and bradycardia, are reduced with a slow administration of the drug over >3 minutes. Some clinicians will begin the protamine infusion following a 3- to 5-mg test dose administered over 1 minute (102). Allergic reactions including anaphylaxis are associated with a previous exposure to protamine-containing insulin—for example NPH-insulin (103)—fish hypersensitivity (104), and vasectomy. Patients at risk for developing antiprotamine antibodies can be pretreated with corticosteroid and antihistamine medications.

Heparin-associated (Induced) Thrombocytopenia

Heparin-associated thrombocytopenia (HIT) is an antibody-mediated adverse reaction to the administration of heparin and/or low-molecular-weight heparins (LMWH) and may lead to both arterial and venous thrombosis. The diagnosis is made both on clinical and serologic findings. HIT antibody formation, accompanied by an otherwise unexplained fall in platelet count by more than 50% from baseline and/or skin lesions at injection sites are the manifestations of HIT.

The incidence of HIT is less than 1% when heparin is given for less than 7 days; thereafter, when given to patients with an extended need for anticoagulation (such as intensive care unit patients), the incidence may rise to as much as 10% to 20% for the mild form (type 1) of HIT and to more than 5% for type 2, the more severe manifestation. The risk of developing HIT is increased by the use of heparin flush, prophylactic treatments, and increasing doses of heparin. HIT may occur more rapidly if the patient has had a recent exposure, within 100 days, to heparin, but it can also develop after more than 9 to 30 days following cessation of therapy, at which point it often goes undetected. A precipitous fall in platelet count from baseline platelet count is usually seen with the type 1 syndrome, and 50% to 75% of these patients may go on to develop the more ominous type 2 syndrome, which manifests with either the development of arterial, or more commonly, venous thrombotic complications.

Patients who develop HIT generate large amounts of thrombin. *In vivo*, platelet activation results from binding of the heparin PF4-IgG immune complexes to platelet factor IIa receptors. These increased levels of thrombin are demonstrated by elevated levels of thrombin–antithrombin complexes, which serve as an *in vivo* marker of thrombin generation, much higher than what is seen in control patients with deep venous thrombosis (105). The diagnosis can be confirmed with platelet function testing or the identification in the blood of the antibody to heparin-platelet factor 4 complex using an enzyme-linked immunoabsorbent assay (ELISA) (106) (Fig. 172.5).

Once the determination of HIT is made, it is not adequate simply to stop anticoagulation therapy with heparin or LMWH. Multiple studies document that patients continue to be at risk of thrombosis if no anticoagulation is given (107). Currently, alternative antithrombotic agents are being used and have been approved in many countries for the treatment of HIT. Three of the agents are direct thrombin inhibitors: argatroban, hirudin (lepirudin), and bivalirudin, and the other agent is a heparinoid, danaparoid (Table 172.4).

Argatroban is a small (MW 526) synthetic molecule derived from L-arginine that reversibly binds to thrombin. It is approved for prophylaxis and treatment of patients with HIT in both the United States and Canada. It reportedly has been associated with a lower thrombotic event rate in one prospective study. The half-life is less than 1 hour, and the drug is excreted normally, even in those with moderate renal failure. In the event of hepatic dysfunction, the dose of argatroban must be reduced. The anticoagulant effect is monitored by the aPTT.

Lepirudin is a recombinant polypeptide originally derived from the medicinal leech. It inhibits thrombin directly and is approved only for treatment of HIT. The anticoagulant effect

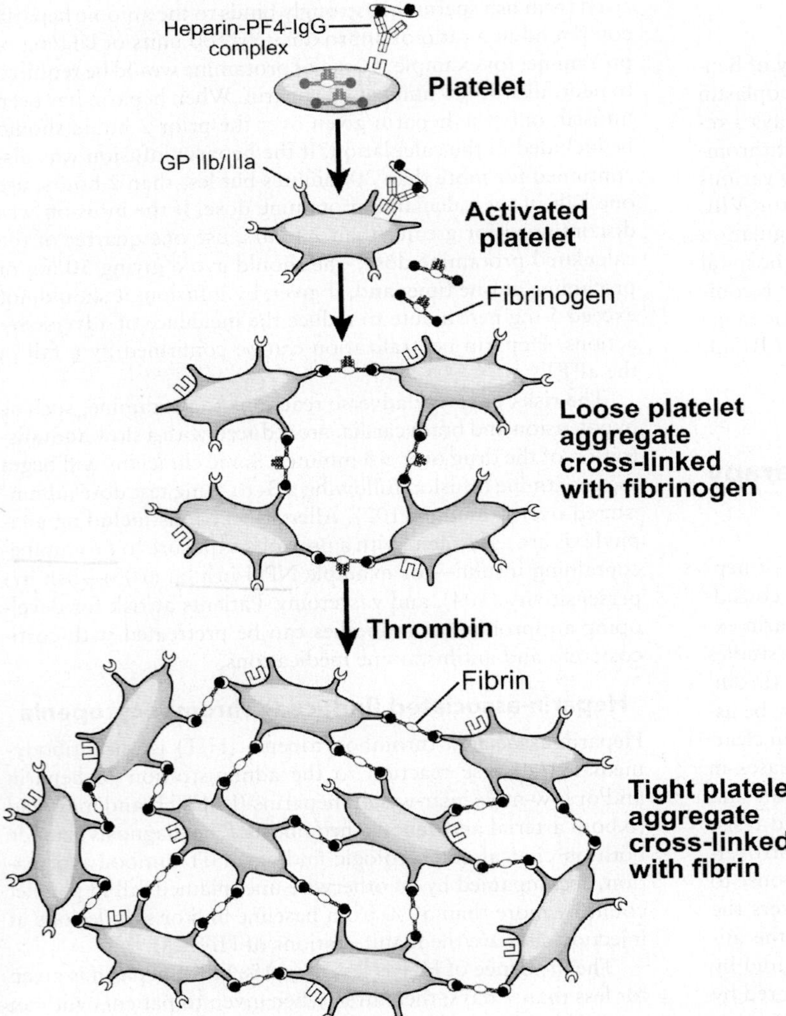

FIGURE 172.5. The immune-mediated platelet activation involves the binding of heparin–platelet factor 4–IgG complex to the platelets and brings about conformational changes, exposing GP11b/111a to fibrinogen. This complex leads to further platelet activation, cross-linking them into platelet aggregates. Thrombin plays a major role in the conversion of fibrinogen to fibrin, forming tight platelet aggregates. PF 4, platelet factor 4; IgG, immunoglobulin G; GP11b/111a, glycoprotein 11b/111a.

TABLE 172.4

ALTERNATIVES TO HEPARIN FOR THE TREATMENT OF HEPARIN-INDUCED THROMBOCYTOPENIA

Agent (direct thrombin inhibitors)	Clearance	Therapeutic dose	Therapeutic dose	Adverse effects
Lepirudin (Refludan, Berlex)[a]	Renal	IV, 0.4 mg/kg of body weight (up to 110 kg); IV bolus[b] followed by 0.15 mg/kg/h (up to 110 kg) (maximal initial infusion, 16.5 mg/h)	Measure aPTT 2 h after therapy started and after each dose adjustment; therapeutic range, 1.5–2.5 times the baseline value (optimal aPTT, <65 s); check baseline PT before switching therapy to warfarin[d]	Bleeding with therapeutic dose in 17.6% of patients; antilepirudin antibodies develop in 30% of patients
Argatroban (Novastan, GlaxoSmithKline)[a]	Hepatic	2 μg/kg/min continuous infusion (maximal infusion, 10 μg/kg/min)	Measure aPTT 2 h after therapy started and after each dose adjustment; therapeutic range, 1.5 to 2.5 times the beseline value (optimal aPPT; <65 s); check baseline PT before switching therepy to warfarin[d]	Bleeding with therapeutic dose in 17.6% of patients; antilepirudin antibodies develop in 30% of patients
Bivalirudin (Angiormax, The Medicines Company)[f]	Enzymatic (80%) and renal (20%)	2 μg/kg/min continuous infusion (maximal infusion, 10 μg/kg/min)	Measure aPTT 2 h after therapy started and after each dose adjustment therapeutic range, 1.5 to 2.5 times the baseline value (optimal aPTT, <65 s): check baseline PT before switching therapy to warfarin[d]	Bleeding with therapeutic dose in 17.6% of patients; antilepirudin antibodies develop in 30% of patients
Anti–factor Xa therapy Danaparoid (Orgaran, Diosynth)[g]	Renal	IV, 2,250 U bolus followed by 400 U/h for 4 h, then 150–200 U/h	Nor required, but if needed, maintain anti-factor Xa level, 0.5–0.8 U/mL	Bleeding with therapeutic dose in 8.1% of patients; cross-reactivity with PF4–heparin antibodies develop in 3.2% of patients

aPTT, activated partial thromboplastin time; PT, prothrombin time.
Except where indicated, the guidelines for dosing and monitoring are from the manufacturers of the drugs. Guidelines for therapeutic dosing are for intravenous (IV) infusion, except for bivalirudin, which is used in patients undergoing percutaneous coronary intervention (PCI). The guidelines of the American College of Chest Physicians recommend overlap use of direct thrombin inhibitor therapy and warfarin therapy for more than 5 days, whereas the Hemostasis and Thrombosis Task Force of the British Committee for Standards in Haemotology recommend overlap use of direct thrombin inhibitor therapy and warfarin therapy until the international normalized ratio (INR) is at a therapeutic level for at least 48 h.
[a]These drugs have been approved in the United States for the treatment of heparin-induced thrombocytopenia.
[b]Bolus therapy is not advised in older patients or patients with renal insufficiency.
[c]This value is the maximal aPTT recommended by Lubenow et al.
[d]Therapeutic lepirudin may prolong the baseline PT slightly, but it generally does not interfere with conversion from lepirudin to warfarin therapy. If the PT is prolonged by more than a few seconds, further evaluation should be undertaken before initiating warfarin.
[e]Combined anticoagulant therapy with argatroban and warfarin produces an INR response that is significantly greater than that obtained with warfarin alone. To change therapy from argatroban to warfarin for outpatient anticoagulant therapy, the INR should be monitored daily, and when the INR is greater than 4, the argatroban infusion should be withheld and the INR rechecked to determine whether it is therapeutic. An alternative strategy would be to use a chromogenic factor X assay to monitor warfarin therapy while the patient is also receiving argatroban.
[f]This drug has been approved in the United States for the treatment of patients undergoing percutaneous coronary intervention (PCI) who have heparin-induced thrombocytopenia or a history of heparin-induced thrombocytopenia.
[g]This drug is not available in the United States.
From Arepally GM, Ortel TL. Heparin-induced thrombocytopenia. *N Engl J Med.* 2006;355:814, with permission.

of lepirudin is monitored by the aPTT. It is renally excreted, and the risk for accumulation and bleeding is high in patients with renal failure; the half-life of lepirudin is 1.3 hours. Antibodies to lepirudin develop in approximately 30 percent of patients following their first exposure; this number may rise to 70 percent following repeat exposure. Serious anaphylactic reactions have occurred following initial and subsequent exposures to lepirudin, resulting in shock and death. Therefore, patients should not be treated with this agent more than one time. It has also been reported that a high percentage of patients who develop antihirudin antibodies may experience an increase in anticoagulant effect due to the delayed renal elimination of the lepirudin–antihirudin complexes, which still have activity. Thus, continued close monitoring of the aPTT is needed during the course of therapy, even when the initial anticoagulant effects appear stable, to avoid the risk of bleeding.

Danaparoid is a mixture of heparan sulfate, dermatan sulfate, and chondroitin sulfate; the drug reduces thrombin generation *in vivo* by the inhibition of factor Xa. Although no longer available in the United States, it is used for the treatment of HIT elsewhere. It is important to consider that cross-reactivity between heparin and danaparoid may occur in up to 30% of cases. In this case, a direct thrombin inhibitor should be used for treatment.

A third direct thrombin inhibitor, *bivalirudin*, is not approved for the treatment of HIT but has been successfully used and reported off-label for this use (107). An early transition from intravenous heparin or LMWH anticoagulation to warfarin (or an equivalent anticoagulant) has been standard therapy for most patients with acute venous and arterial thromboembolism. This approach may also help prevent HIT by limiting a patient's total dose-time exposure to these medications. One complication to be considered is that early transition has been associated with further thrombotic complications of venous limb gangrene and warfarin-induced skin necrosis (108,109). Warfarin and other equivalent vitamin K antagonists counter thrombin generation by slowly decreasing the plasma levels of the vitamin K factors (II, VII, IX, X) while concurrently decreasing the natural anticoagulant factors C and S. During the transition to oral vitamin K antagonist therapy in patients with HIT, thrombin is still being generated (warfarin having failed to control this). Due to their shorter half-lives, factors VII and protein C are reduced faster than the prothrombotic factors II, IX, and X. This results in a supratherapeutic INR secondary to factor VII depletion and a *transient hypercoagulable state* due to the decrease in protein C without a concurrent decrease in the prothrombotic levels of factors II and X. Throughout this process, there is still increased thrombin generation due to the HIT, and venous limb gangrene and/or warfarin-induced skin necrosis may develop as a result (107) (Table 172.5).

In these patients, it has been recommended to use the direct thrombin inhibitors available—argatroban, lepirudin, and bivalirudin or danaparoid—once HIT has been established and discontinue the use of heparin or LMWH. Anticoagulation needs to be ensured, and with use of these alternatives, there should be no interruption in anticoagulation therapy. Oral therapy with warfarin or an equivalent vitamin K–antagonist agent should be avoided until the patient's platelet count has recovered to near normal levels (greater than 150,000 platelets/μL). Thereafter, one may begin administering warfarin at modest doses (2.5–5.0 mg orally [PO]), titrating to and maintaining the target INR; warfarin should not be used as the initial treatment for HIT (107,110) (Table 172.6).

TABLE 172.5

HALF-LIVES OF THE VITAMIN K–DEPENDENT PROCOAGULANT AND NATURAL ANTICOAGULANT FACTORS

Factor	Half-life, h
VII	5–6
IX	24
X	30–50
II	96
Protein C	8–10
Protein S	42–60

From Bartholomew J. Transition to oral anticoagulants in patient with heparin-induced thrombocytopenia. *Chest*. 2005;127:31s, with permission.

TABLE 172.6

GUIDELINES FOR TRANSITION TO ORAL ANTICOAGULANT IN A PATIENT WITH HEPARIN-ASSOCIATED/INDUCED THROMBOCYTOPENIA (HIT)

Step	Description
1	Stop heparin or LMWH therapy
2	Ensure adequate levels of anticoagulation with a DTI or alternative anticoagulant
3	Avoid interruptions during treatment with a DTI or alternative anticoagulant
4	Wait until the platelet count has "cooled" or is near normal before beginning therapy with an oral anticoagulant
5	Initiate modest doses of an oral anticoagulant (2.5–5 mg warfarin)
6	Avoid overshooting the target INR[a]
7	Avoid using warfarin (or equivalent) as monotherapy

LMWH, low-molecular-weight heparin; DTI, direct thrombin inhibitor; INR, international normalized ratio.
[a]Recognize that cotherapy with a direct thrombin inhibitor prolongs the INR for a longer time than warfarin therapy alone.
From Bartholomew J. Transition to oral anticoagulants in patient with heparin-induced thrombocytopenia. *Chest*. 2005;127:32s, with permission.

Low-molecular-weight Heparin

Low-molecular-weight heparin (LMWH) is prepared from unfractionated heparin by controlled depolymerization of the parent drug into short segments. The molecular weight of LMWH ranges from 1,000 to 10,000, and about 20% of the LMWH chains contain pentasaccharide sequences that are needed for antithrombin binding.

Mechanism of Action

Unlike heparin, which binds to antithrombin and forms complexes with thrombin and factor Xa to produce anticoagulant effect, the LMWH chains are too short to bridge thrombin to antithrombin. Rather, it binds to antithrombin and brings about conformational changes that lead to inhibition of factor Xa. The ratio of inhibition of thrombin to factor Xa varies from 1:2 to 1:4 for different preparations of LMWH (111).

LMWH is being increasingly used for the treatment of venous thromboembolic disease in non-ICU patients. It can be administered as a subcutaneous injection once or twice daily and intravenously when a rapid anticoagulant effect is needed. It is as safe and effective as intravenous and subcutaneous unfractionated heparin (70).

TABLE 172.7

ADVANTAGES OF LOW-MOLECULAR-WEIGHT HEPARIN OVER UNFRACTIONATED HEPARIN

Advantage	Consequence
Better bioavailability and longer half-life after subcutaneous injection	Can be given subcutaneously once or twice daily for both prophylaxis and treatment
Dose-independent clearance	Simplified dosing
Predictable anticoagulant response	Coagulation monitoring is unnecessary in most patients
Lower risk of heparin-induced thrombocytopenia	Safer than heparin for short- or long-term administration
Lower risk of osteoporosis	Safer than heparin for extended administration

From Weitz JI. Anticoagulants and fibrinolytic drugs. In: Hoffman. *Hematology: Basic Principles and Practice*. 4th ed. Orlando, FL: Churchill Livingstone; 2005:2254, with permission.

The shorter chains of LMWH bind less avidly to endothelial cells, macrophages, and heparin-binding proteins and have better bioavailability (112). They tend to accumulate *in vivo*, leading to longer half-life, and have more predictable renal clearance and a greater ability to inactivate factor Xa compared to inactivation of thrombin and, consequently, have a negligible effect on the aPTT. The clearance of LMWH is dose independent and is accomplished almost exclusively by the kidneys; hence the drug can accumulate in renal insufficiency. LMWH has proved to be cost effective because of the reduced need for monitoring, and there are several advantages of LMWH over the UH (Table 172.7).

The disadvantages of LMWH, which may be more pertinent to the ICU, include the absence of an established dose for obese patients and impaired clearance in patients with renal failure. These can be overcome by monitoring anti–factor-Xa levels and adjusting the subsequent doses. Based on the anti–factor-Xa levels, LMWH has a plasma half-life of 4 hours. The therapeutic anti–factor Xa levels with LMWH range from 0.5 to 1.2 units/mL when measured 3 to 4 hours after drug administration. There is no rapid and complete antagonist to the anticoagulant effect of LMWH, which may complicate and hinder ICU and surgical procedures (7) (Table 172.8).

Dosing

The most commonly prescribed LMWHs are enoxaparin, dalteparin, and newer agents like tinzaparin.

Enoxaparin is primarily metabolized in the liver by desulfation and/or depolymerization to lower-molecular-weight species with much reduced biologic potency. Renal clearance of active fragments represents about 10% of the administered dose, and total renal excretion of active and nonactive fragments represents about 40% of the dose.

Prophylaxis of DVT following Abdominal Surgery in Patients at Risk for Thromboembolic Complications. Abdominal surgery patients at risk include those who are older than 40 years of age, obese, undergoing surgery under general anesthesia lasting longer than 30 minutes, or who have additional risk factors such as malignancy or a history of deep vein

TABLE 172.8

DOSAGE REGIMENS FOR PATIENTS WITH SEVERE RENAL IMPAIRMENT

Indication	Dosage regimen
Prophylaxis in abdominal surgery	30 mg administered SC once daily
Prophylaxis in hip or knee replacement surgery	30 mg administered SC once daily
Prophylaxis in medical patients during acute illness	30 mg administered SC once daily
Prophylaxis of ischemic complications of unstable angina and non–Q wave myocardial infarction when concurrently administered with aspirin	1 mg/kg administered SC once daily
In-patient treatment of acute deep vein thrombosis with or without pulmonary embolism when administered in conjunction with warfarin sodium	1 mg/kg administered SC once daily
Out-patient treatment of acute deep vein thrombosis without pulmonary embolism when administered in conjunction with warfarin sodium	1 mg/kg administered SC once daily

SC, subcutaneously.
From Hematological agents: anticoagulants: low molecular weight heparin. MD consult Core Service. St. Louis, MO: Elsevier; . (http://home.mdconsult.com/das/Pharm/view. Accessed)

thrombosis (DVT) or pulmonary embolism (PE) (113). The recommended dose of enoxaparin for this indication is 40 mg subcutaneously (SC) daily, beginning 2 hours preoperatively.

Treatment of DVT with or without PE. In patients with acute DVT with PE or patients with acute DVT without PE, but who are not candidates for outpatient treatment, the recommended dose of enoxaparin is 1 mg/kg every 12 hours administered SC (113).

Unstable Angina and Non–Q Wave Myocardial Infarction. In patients with unstable angina or non–Q wave myocardial infarction, the recommended dose of enoxaparin is 1 mg/kg administered SC every 12 hours in conjunction with oral aspirin therapy (100–325 mg daily) (113). Based on the currently available data on the efficacy and safety of LMWHs in the treatment of non–ST segment myocardial infarction and unstable angina, enoxaparin is the only LMWH to have consistently demonstrated both short- and long-term improvements in major ischemic outcomes compared with UH (95,96,114).

Hip or Knee Replacement Surgery. In patients undergoing hip or knee replacement surgery, the recommended dose of enoxaparin is 30 mg every 12 hours, administered by SC injection. Provided that hemostasis has been established, the initial dose should be given 12 to 24 hours after surgery. For hip replacement surgery, a dose of 40 mg once a day SC, given initially 12 (±3) hours prior to surgery, may be considered. Following the initial phase of thromboprophylaxis in hip replacement surgery patients, continued prophylaxis with enoxaparin 40 mg once a day administered by SC injection for 3 weeks is recommended. The usual duration of administration is 7 to 10 days.

Restricted Mobility. In medical patients at risk for thromboembolic complications due to severely restricted mobility during acute illness, the recommended dose of enoxaparin is 40 mg once a day administered by SC injection (113).

Mechanical Prosthetic Heart Valves. The use of enoxaparin has not been adequately studied for thromboprophylaxis or for long-term use in patients with mechanical prosthetic heart valves. Isolated cases of prosthetic heart valve thrombosis have been reported in patients with mechanical prosthetic heart valves who have received enoxaparin for thromboprophylaxis. Some of these patients were pregnant women in whom thrombosis led to maternal and fetal deaths. Insufficient data, issues related to the underlying disease state, and the possibility of inadequate anticoagulation complicates evaluation of these cases. Pregnant women with mechanical prosthetic heart valves may be at higher risk for thromboembolism (113).

Dalteparin. Like enoxaparin, dalteparin consists of small heparin molecules ranging from 2,000 to 9,000 daltons. It is administered subcutaneously and has better availability and a longer half-life than UFH. It has a similar mechanism of action as enoxaparin, selectively inhibiting factor Xa. The inhibitory activity is 2.7:1 compared to 1:1 for UH. The inhibition of factor Xa prevents the formation of fibrin clots. The elimination of the drug occurs via the renal route and is dose independent, with a plasma half-life of 3 to 5 hours. Dalteparin does not significantly affect the platelet activity, prothrombin time (PT), or aPTT and has been shown to be superior to warfarin in preventing DVT following total hip replacement surgery (115). The FRISC trial (Low-Molecular Weight Heparin [Fragmin] during Instability in Coronary Artery Disease) showed that dalteparin decreased the risk of death or acute myocardial infarction (AMI) by 36% as compared to aspirin alone (116).

In the FRIC trial (Fragmin in Unstable Coronary Artery Disease), dalteparin was found to be as effective as intravenous heparin in preventing death or AMI in the acute phase following unstable angina or non–Q wave myocardial infarction (114).

Tinzaparin. This is a relatively new drug with a similar mechanism of action and pharmacokinetic profile as enoxaparin and dalteparin. It was approved for treatment of symptomatic DVT in 2000.

Complications

Bleeding. The major complication of the LMWHs is bleeding and is as frequent as with UH. It is, of course, more common in patients receiving antiplatelet or antifibrinolytic therapy in addition to LMWH. Recent surgery, coagulopathy, or trauma also increases the risk of bleeding (117). Protamine sulfate can be used as an antidote, although it incompletely neutralizes the anticoagulant activity by binding only to the longer chains of LMWH. The longer chains are responsible for the antithrombin activity, but the short chains, which inhibit factor Xa activity, will not bind to protamine sulfate, resulting in the latter's ability to only partially reverse the effect of LMWH (118).

Thrombocytopenia. LMWH binds less avidly to platelets, causes less release of PF4, and has a reduced affinity for PF4. It is less likely to trigger the formation of antibodies. Therefore, the incidence of HIT is lower as compared to UH. Unfortunately, antibodies already formed in established HIT cases can exhibit cross-reactivity with LMWH and lead to thrombosis and other complications of this disorder (119,120), and for this reason LMWHs should not be used as a substitute for heparin in HIT patients.

Warfarin (Coumadin)

This is the most frequently prescribed oral anticoagulant, the fourth most prescribed cardiovascular agent, and overall, one of the most commonly prescribed drugs in the United States. Warfarin is well absorbed in the gut and transported in plasma bound to albumin.

Warfarin is an antagonist of vitamin K and is required for the posttranslational modification of clotting factors II, VII, IX, and X, as well as the naturally occurring endogenous anticoagulant proteins C and S. These factors are rendered biologically inactive without the carboxylation of selected glutamic acid residues, a process requiring reduced vitamin K as a cofactor. Antagonism of vitamin K, or a deficiency of this vitamin, reduces the rate at which these factors are produced, thereby creating a state of anticoagulation. Therapeutic doses of warfarin reduce the production of functional vitamin K–dependent clotting factors by 30% to 50%. A concomitant reduction in the carboxylation of secreted clotting factors yields a 10% to

40% decrease in the biologic activity of the clotting factors. As a result, the coagulation system becomes functionally deficient (121).

The prothrombin time (PT) is the primary assay used in monitoring warfarin therapy. Changes in the PT noted in the first few days of warfarin therapy are primarily due to the reduction in factors VII and IX, with the shortest half-lives, 6 and 24 hours respectively. Commercially available tissue thromboplastins differ in their sensitivity to the warfarin effect; hence, PTs performed with different thromboplastins are not always directly comparable, and for this reason, the international normalized ratio (INR) has been adopted using thromboplastins with international sensitivity index values near 1.0 (122).

Warfarin is used in patients with lower extremity DVT to prevent extension and to reduce the risk of pulmonary embolism. Patients with pulmonary embolism are treated with warfarin to prevent further thromboemboli. Warfarin is used in patients with atrial fibrillation and artificial heart valves to reduce the risk of embolic strokes. It is also helpful in preventing blood clot formation in certain orthopedic surgeries such as knee or hip replacements and in preventing thrombotic stenosis of coronary artery stents (Table 172.9).

The most common complication of warfarin therapy is bleeding, occurring in 6% to 39% of patients annually (123,124); the incidence of bleeding is related to the intensity of anticoagulation. As the need for intense anticoagulation has evolved and been reduced over the last 20 years, the incidence of bleeding has decreased significantly. Moderate bleeding (manifested by elevated INR) can be treated by adjusting down the warfarin dose. If severe bleeding is encountered, this can be adequately treated with fresh frozen plasma.

Alternative Therapies

Thrombin Inhibitors

Heparin, and subsequently LMWH, in addition to warfarin have been used effectively for the treatment of both venous and arterial thromboemboli, but these drugs have drawbacks. The biophysical limitations of heparin include the inability of the heparin/antithrombin complex to inhibit Factor Xa within the prothrombinase complex and thrombin bound to fibrin, clotting enzymes that are important triggers of thrombin growth (125). Direct thrombin inhibitors have properties that give them potential advantages over indirect thrombin inhibitors such as the heparins, including LMWH. This section will concentrate on these drugs.

Thrombin, a trypsinlike serine protease, is the enzyme that converts fibrinogen to fibrin; it may be inhibited either directly or indirectly. Indirect thrombin inhibitors act by catalyzing the reaction of antithrombin and/or heparin cofactor II. Thrombin has great substrate specificity secondary to its surface binding

TABLE 172.9

THERAPEUTIC GOALS AND DURATION OF WARFARIN ANTICOAGULATION

Indication	INR	Duration
Prophylaxis of venous thrombosis for high-risk surgery	2–3	Clinical judgment
Treatment of venous thrombosis		
First episode	2–3	3–6 mo[a]
High risk of recurrent thrombosis	2–3	Lifelong
Thrombosis associated with antiphospholipid antibody	3–4	Lifelong
Treatment of pulmonary embolism		
First episode	2–3	3–6 mo
High risk of recurrent embolism	2–3	Lifelong
Prevention of systemic embolism		
Tissue heart valves	2–3	3 mo
Acute myocardial infarction (to prevent systemic embolism)[b]	2–3	Clinical judgment
Valvular heart disease (after thrombotic event or dilated left)	2–3	Lifelong
Atrial fibrillation		
Chronic or intermittent	2–3	Lifelong
Cardioversion	2–3	3 weeks before and 4 weeks after atrial fibrillation if normal sinus rhythm is maintained
Prosthetic heart valves		
Aortic position		
Mechanical	2.5–3.5[c]	Lifelong
Bioprosthetic	2–3	Clinical judgment (3 mo optional)
Mitral position		
Mechanical	2.5–3.5[c]	Lifelong
Bioprosthetic	2–3	3 mo

INR, international normalized ratio.
[a]All recommendations are subject to modification by individual characteristics. First event with reversible or time limited risk factors (surgery, trauma, immobilization, estrogen use). Hyers TM, Agnelli G, Hull RD, et al. Antithrombotic therapy for venous thromboembolic disease. *Chest.* 2001; 119(Suppl):176s–193s.
[b]If oral anticoagulant therapy is elected to prevent recurrent myocardial infarction, an INR of 2.5–3.5 is recommended.
[c]Depending on the type of prosthetic valve and valve position (mitral), some patients may benefit from INR in upper therapeutic range.
From Horton JD, Bushwick BM, et al. Warfarin therapy: evolving strategies in anticoagulation. *Am Fam Physician.* 1999;59(4):636, with permission.

sites (e.g., exosite 1). Direct thrombin inhibitors directly bind thrombin (at the exosite 1 site or the other active site of thrombin) thereby blocking this procoagulant from reacting further. Direct thrombin inhibitors may be more advantageous over indirect thrombin inhibitors, such as heparin, because they do not bind plasma proteins and produce a more predictable response. Direct thrombin inhibitors do not bind PF4, and their anticoagulant activity is unaffected by the large quantities of PF4 released in the surrounding region of platelet-rich thrombi. Additionally, direct thrombin inhibitors inactivate fibrin-bound thrombin as well as fluid-phase thrombin (126).

Three parenteral direct thrombin inhibitors have been approved for limited use in the United States and Canada. Hirudin and argatroban are approved for treatment of patients diagnosed with heparin-associated thrombocytopenia. Bivalirudin has been approved as an alternative therapy for heparin-sensitive patients undergoing percutaneous coronary interventions.

Hirudin. This agent is a 65 amino acid polypeptide originally isolated from the salivary glands of the medicinal leech; it is now available in recombinant DNA technology (126). The recombinant form exhibits a, perhaps, tenfold reduced affinity for thrombin as compared to the native form of the drug (127). Hirudin directly inhibits thrombin in a bivalent manner in that the globular amino-terminal domain interacts with the active site of thrombin. The anionic carboxy-terminal tail binds to exosite 1 on thrombin, the substrate recognition site (126). The hirudin/thrombin complex is essentially irreversible. This may create a problem if significant bleeding should occur, as there is no specific antidote. Recombinant hirudins—for example, desirudin and lepirudin—have a leucine substituted for an isoleucine at the N-terminal end of the molecule. Lepirudin (Refludan) has been approved in North America for the treatment of heparin-induced thrombocytopenia subtypes 1 and 2 (128).

The plasma half-life of hirudin is approximately 60 minutes following intravenous injection and 120 minutes following subcutaneous administration (129). It is cleared via the kidneys and should be used with caution, if at all, in patients with renal insufficiency. The anticoagulant activity can be measured using the aPTT. Dose adjustment must be made to maintain the aPTT within a therapeutic range ratio of 1.5 to 2.0 approximately 4 hours after drug initiation. The correlation between plasma hirudin levels and the aPTT is nonlinear, and therefore the ecarin clotting time is the more preferable means of monitoring anticoagulation. Dose adjustments need to be made in those with renal impairment. Rarely, in the hirudin-treated patient, there may develop nonneutralizing hirudin antibodies that prolong its anticoagulant effect because of delayed hirudin–antibody complex clearance (125).

Hirudin has been successfully used, and is licensed for, the treatment of arterial or venous thrombosis complicating heparin-induced thrombocytopenia. It has also been used in patients with HIT undergoing cardiopulmonary bypass. Hirudin has been shown to be superior to heparin or LMWHs for thromboprophylaxis in patients undergoing elective hip arthroplasty, and it does not increase the risk of bleeding in this high-risk setting. Hirudin has been used extensively in patients with acute coronary syndromes and for venous thromboprophylaxis. However, because of its narrow therapeutic index and high risk of bleeding, it must be used with extreme caution and is not currently approved for this use (125).

Bivalirudin. This is a 20 amino acid synthetic polypeptide analogue of hirudin. The amino terminal D-Phe-Pro-Arg-Pro sequence, which binds to the active site of thrombin, is connected via four Gly residues to a carboxyl-terminal dodecapeptide that interacts with exosite 1 on thrombin (130,131). Bivalirudin differs from hirudin in that, once bound to thrombin, the Arg-Pro bond on the amino terminal extension of bivalirudin is cleaved, converting bivalirudin into a lower-affinity thrombin inhibitor, therefore producing only transient inhibition of the active site of thrombin and thereby allowing recovery of thrombin activity (132). The shorter half-life of bivalirudin, 25 minutes after intravenous injection, and the fact that only about 20% is renally excreted (133), may make bivalirudin a safer alternative to hirudin. In patients with a high risk of developing HIT, bivalirudin is typically administered as a weight-adjusted (1 mg/kg) bolus dose given prior to percutaneous coronary interventions and followed by a 4-hour infusion (0.2–0.5 mg/kg per hour); the dose is adjusted according to renal function. Robson et al. demonstrated that the plasma clearance of bivalirudin in patients with moderate or severe renal impairment is reduced by approximately 20% as compared to that in patients with normal or mild renal function, and suggests that bivalirudin infusion should be reduced by 20% in patients with moderate to severe renal impairment (134). The anticoagulant effect is monitored by the activated clotting time, and an additional bolus dose is given if the activated clotting time is less than 350 seconds.

Argatroban. This is a synthetic L-arginine derivative competitive inhibitor of thrombin. Argatroban binds noncovalently to the active site of thrombin to form a reversible complex (135). The plasma half-life of this agent is 45 minutes. It is monitored using the aPTT, and the dose is adjusted to maintain a therapeutic aPTT ratio of 1.5 to 3.0. It is metabolized in the liver and needs to be used with caution in patients with hepatic dysfunction (136). Argatroban is considered the drug of choice for patients with severe renal impairment. Therapy with this agent can prolong plasma INR more than the other direct thrombin inhibitors and may complicate overlap therapy with Vitamin K antagonists. Argatroban has been approved for use in patients with documented heparin-associated thrombocytopenia and for anticoagulation in heparin-induced thrombocytopenia patients undergoing percutaneous coronary intervention (128).

Melagatran/Ximelagatran. Melagatran is a dipeptide mimetic of the region of fibrinopeptide A that interacts with the active site of thrombin. This drug has poor oral bioavailability and must be given via the subcutaneous route. Ximelagatran is an uncharged lipophilic prodrug exhibiting about 20% bioavailability after oral administration. Once absorbed, ximelagatran is rapidly transformed to melagatran, which has a half-life of approximately 4 to 5 hours. The primary route of excretion for melagatran is the kidneys, where approximately 80% is eliminated. Dose adjustments may be needed in the elderly and in those patients with renal impairment. There appears to be no adverse food or drug interaction to influence the absorption of ximelagatran, and it therefore produces a predictable anticoagulant effect. The need for routine monitoring of this drug is usually unnecessary. Ximelagatran is under evaluation for thromboprophylaxis in orthopedic patients (137) and for treatment of venous thromboembolism and atrial fibrillation (138).

Factor Xa Inhibitors

Factor Xa is the rate-limiting step in the generation of thrombin. It is situated at the beginning of the common coagulation pathway, where both the intrinsic and extrinsic pathways converge. Drugs that block factor Xa are considered as either indirect or direct inhibitors. Indirect factor Xa inhibitors act by binding to and activating antithrombin, which then inhibits free factor Xa. Direct factor Xa inhibitors actually bind to and inhibit factor Xa without requiring antithrombin to be present.

Indirect Factor Xa Inhibitors. *Fondaparinux* and *idraparinux* are two relatively new parenteral indirect factor Xa inhibitors. They are synthetic analogues of the antithrombin-binding pentasaccharide sequence found in heparin and LMWH. However, these drugs are modified to increase their affinity for antithrombin as compared to both heparin and LMWH. The chain length of these molecules is too short to bridge thrombin to antithrombin; therefore, these agents act by catalyzing factor Xa inhibition by antithrombin. Their properties are quite different from those of LMWH (Table 172.10).

There are potential benefits of fondaparinux over LMWH. It is synthetically produced, has a longer half-life, and does not bind to plasma proteins other than antithrombin. Additionally, it does not bind to PF4 to form the heparin/PF4 complexes that serve as the antigenic target for the antibodies that cause heparin-induced thrombocytopenia, and may be safer to use in these patients (139,140). Fondaparinux has been extensively studied and has been found to be effective as an antithrombotic agent for the prevention and treatment of both venous and arterial disorders. It is currently approved as thromboprophylaxis following orthopedic procedures, as initial treatment for venous thromboembolism, and is being investigated as an antithrombotic agent in cardiac disease.

Idraparinux is a chemically modified analogue of fondaparinux that binds to antithrombin with such a high affinity that its half-life approximates that of antithrombin (141). This drug requires subcutaneous dosing only once a week. It is under evaluation for treatment of venous thromboembolism, as well as the long-term prevention of stroke in patients with chronic atrial fibrillation. Idraparinux may be useful in patients who cannot tolerate vitamin K–antagonist medications such as warfarin. One possible drawback to the use of this drug is its long half-life and lack of an antidote if bleeding occurs, although in one study, healthy volunteers had the anticoagulant effect reversed by recombinant factor VIIa (142).

Direct Factor Xa Inhibitors. Several synthetic direct factor Xa inhibitors are undergoing clinical trials. These drugs inhibit both free and activated platelet-bound factor Xa trapped within a thrombus as part of the prothrombinase complex. This property may offer an advantage over LMWH and the indirect factor Xa inhibitor agents. These drugs appear to inhibit thrombus formation while allowing time for sufficient thrombin to be generated to activate platelets. These agents may be associated with a lower incidence of major bleeding.

Thrombolytic Therapy

The fibrinolytic system of the body aids in dissolution of intravascular clots via the action of plasmin, which digests fibrin. Plasminogen, the inactive precursor, is converted to plasmin by the cleavage of a single peptide bond. Plasmin is a nonspecific protease, which acts by digesting fibrin clots as well as other proteins. Thrombolytic agents act as plasminogen-activating agents, catalyzing the conversion of endogenous plasminogen to plasmin. These agents will dissolve both fibrin deposits and pathologic thrombi at sites of vascular injury and, thus, may be associated with significant hemorrhage. When thrombolytic therapy is initiated, massive fibrinolysis may occur and potentially overwhelm the body's inhibitory controls. The use of thrombolytic therapy in the treatment of DVT and pulmonary embolus remains highly individual specific. The early use of thrombolytic therapy in the setting of DVT may decrease subsequent pain, swelling, and loss of venous valves, and has reportedly reduced the incidence of postphlebitic syndrome.

TABLE 172.10

PROPERTIES OF LOW-MOLECULAR-WEIGHT HEPARIN, FONDAPARINUX, AND IDRAPARINUX

Property	LMWH	Fondaparinux	Idraparinux
Source	Porcine mucosal heparin	Chemical synthesis	Chemical synthesis
Moecular weight (daltons)	Mean 5,000	1,728	1,727
SC bioavailability	~90%	100%	100%
Target(s)	Multiple: FXa > FIIa > FIXa, FXIa, FXIIa	FXa only	FXa only
Binding to proteins other than target	Yes	No	No
Anti-Xa:anti-lla	2–5:1	Anti-Xa only	Anti-Xa only
TFPI release from endothelium	Yes	No	No
Clearance	Renal primarily	Renal	Renal
Half life (SC route)	3–4 h	17–21 h	80–130 h
Effects of protamine	Partial neutralization	No effect	No effect
Potential for HIT	Low	Very low	Very low

LMWH, low-molecular-weight heparin; SC, subcutaneous; FXa, factor Xa; FIIa, factor IIa; FIXa, factor IXa; FXIa, factor XIa; FXIIa, factor XIIa; TFPI, tissue factor pathway inhibitor; HIT, heparin-induced thrombocytopenia.
From Weitz JI, Middeldorp S, Geerts W, et al. Thrombophilia and new anticoagulant drugs. *Hematology*. 2004;1:429, with permission.

In the treatment of pulmonary embolus, thrombolytic therapy followed by heparin administration has been shown to be more efficacious in thromboembolus dissolution as compared to heparin alone in the acute (first 24 hours) setting (143,144). These agents lead to a more rapid resolution of lung scan abnormalities and hemodynamic improvements, but the benefit over the longer term is questionable. Recent guidelines do not recommend thrombolysis for the treatment of deep vein thrombosis unless limb ischemia and limb loss is imminent (145).

Although beyond the scope of this review, thrombolytic therapy has become a standard treatment for patients presenting with acute ST-segment elevation myocardial infarction and new-onset left bundle branch block. Various clinical trials have demonstrated the importance and benefit of early and full reperfusion in improving clinical outcomes following an acute myocardial infarction (146–149). Thrombolytic therapy is also indicated in the treatment of ischemic stroke (150), cerebral vein and sinus thrombosis (151), thrombosed mechanical valves, and thrombosed arteriovenous shunts and catheters. These agents have evolved from the non–fibrin-selective first-generation agents to the more fibrin-selective third-generation agents. As there are still limitations with the currently available agents, work continues to achieve an ideal drug.

First-generation thrombolytic agents are not fibrin specific and convert circulating plasminogen to plasmin. There is constant equilibrium between circulating plasminogen and plasminogen that is in the thrombus. There is eventual depletion of plasminogen, therefore reducing clot lysis. Additionally, they are associated with increased risk of allergic reaction and have comparatively short half-lives.

Streptokinase is a single-chain polypeptide, with a molecular weight of 47 to 50.2 Kd, produced by group C β-hemolytic streptococci (152). It works by binding with circulating plasminogen to form an activator complex that converts plasminogen to plasmin by proteolytic cleavage, forming a streptokinase–plasmin complex (153). This 1:1 complex has increased catalytic activity compared with plasmin. The streptokinase–plasmin complex–mediated degradation of fibrin leads to stimulation of locally bound streptokinase–plasmin and streptokinase–plasminogen complexes, which results in an acceleration in plasminogen activation and clot dissolution. In addition, streptokinase can increase levels of activated protein C, enhancing clot lysis. The half-life of the streptokinase–plasminogen complex is approximately 23 minutes, with a lytic effect ranging from 82 to 184 minutes. There are no metabolites of streptokinase, and it is eliminated by the liver (154,155).

Adverse reactions include allergic reactions—rarely anaphylaxis and bleeding, which is, of course, common to all thrombolytics. Hypotension not related to bleeding or anaphylaxis may also be seen during streptokinase infusion in 1% to 10% of patients. When hypotension occurs, decreasing the infusion and close monitoring are recommended. For pulmonary embolus, the FDA recommends that streptokinase be given as a 1 million IU dose infusion over 24 hours. For acute myocardial infarction, the adult dose is 1.5 million IU in 50 mL 5% dextrose in water given intravenously over 5 minutes.

Urokinase is a two-chain serine protease containing 41 amino acid residues. It is isolated from human urine and fetal kidney cell cultures as a single-chain precursor, with a molecular weight of 54 kD. In plasma, the single-chain precursor is converted to the active two-chain urokinase plasminogen activator through limited hydrolysis by plasmin and kallikrein. The two-chain active form increases the efficacy of plasmin activation, which enhances further conversion of the single-chain precursor to the two-chain urokinase plasminogen activator form. Urokinase has a 15- to 20-minute half-life and is metabolized in the liver (156,157). Because it has a shorter half-life than streptokinase, urokinase produces a less sustained fibrinolysis. It has the same potential disadvantages of significant bleeding as do all thrombolytics. Human-derived urokinase is no longer available in North America and has been replaced by a recombinant product.

For pulmonary embolus, the FDA-approved regimen of urokinase is the administration of a 4,400 IU/kg body weight loading dose, followed by an infusion of 4,400 IU/kg for 12 to 24 hours. Urokinase for acute myocardial infarction is less well studied than other agents, but the most commonly used regimen is 2 million U given as an intravenous load, followed by 1 million U over the next 60 minutes.

Second-generation thrombolytics are fibrin selective and were developed with the intention to limit or avoid systemic thrombolysis. The present agents may cause a mild to moderate depletion in levels of circulation fibrinogen and plasminogen.

Tissue-type plasminogen activator (alteplase), a glycoprotein of 527 amino acids, was the first recombinant tissue-type plasminogen activator (rtPA) and is identical to the native form of the drug. Native tissue plasminogen activator (tPA) is naturally synthesized and made available by vascular endothelial cells. It is the enzyme that is responsible for most of the body's natural physiologic responses to clear and reduce excessive thrombus propagation. Tissue plasminogen activator binds fibrin with a greater affinity than streptokinase, converting plasminogen to plasmin once bound to a fibrin clot surface—hence the term "clot selective." Fibrin provides the platform for which tPA and fibrin may interact to enhance the catalytic efficiency of the plasminogen activation of tPA. Alteplase (rtPA) is rapidly cleared from plasma, primarily by the liver, having an initial half-life of less than 5 minutes. Heparin is usually administered with alteplase due to the very short half-life of this agent and to avoid reocclusion. This drug is not antigenic and is almost never associated with allergic reactions.

Alteplase is the lytic agent most commonly used for the acute treatment of myocardial ischemia (157), pulmonary embolism, and acute ischemic stroke. There are two different forms of tissue-type plasminogen activator based on the number of chains: the two-chain alteplase (recombinant) and the recombinant one-chain form.

For acute myocardial infarction, this drug may be given as an accelerated infusion (over 1.5 hours) or a long infusion (greater than 3 hours). It must be given in a 1 mg/mL concentration and be reconstituted with sterile water. The accelerated infusion of rtPA is 15 mg intravenously, followed by 0.75 mg/kg, up to 50 mg, intravenously over 60 minutes with a maximum total dose of 100 mg. This is the most common regimen used for acute myocardial infarction. Alternatively, the greater than 3-hour infusion begins as a 10-mg intravenous loading dose over 2 minutes, followed by a 50-mg infusion over the first hour, and by a 20-mg/kg infusion over the next 2 hours.

Alteplase is the only drug that has been studied and approved by the FDA for use in acute ischemic stroke with a well-established time of symptom onset of less than 3 hours. Once diagnosed, and within the defined time period, it is recommended that two peripheral intravenous lines—one for rtPA infusion and one for complications that may occur from therapy—be initiated. The recommended dose of alteplase for acute ischemic stroke is 0.9 mg/kg, to a maximum of 90 mg, infused over 60 minutes; 10% of the total dose is to be administered as an initial intravenous bolus over 1 minute (158).

The FDA-approved regimen for thrombolysis of pulmonary embolism is 100 mg of rtPA given as a continuous infusion over 2 hours: an initial 15-mg intravenous loading dose is followed by 85 mg over 2 hours. Heparin has been shown to improve the clinical course in hemodynamically stable patients with acute submassive pulmonary embolus when receiving rtPA. Given the short half-life of the drug, if the patient can tolerate it, it would seem beneficial to administer alteplase with heparin (159).

Third-generation thrombolytics are based on modifications of the tPA structure. These modifications may give the agents longer half-lives, increased resistance to plasma protease inhibitors, and/or cause more selective binding to fibrin.

Reteplase (rtPA) is a synthetic, nonglycosylated deletion-mutant form of tPA containing 355 of the 527 amino acids of native tPA; the drug is produced in *Escherichia coli* via recombinant technology. Reteplase binds fibrin five times less avidly than native tissue plasminogen activator, thus allowing the drug to diffuse through the clot rather than just binding to the surface as is the mechanism of tissue plasminogen activator. In high concentrations, reteplase does not compete with plasminogen for fibrin binding sites, but rather it allows plasminogen at the clot to be converted into plasmin. These reasons may explain why reteplase results in faster clot resolution in contrast to alteplase.

Reteplase is more rapidly cleared from plasma and has a somewhat extended half-life—11 to 19 minutes—than does alteplase. Reteplase undergoes primarily renal and some hepatic clearance; the agent is not antigenic and is rarely associated with allergic reactions. It must not be given with heparin due to physical incompatibility (160).

In the setting of acute myocardial infarction, the FDA has approved the adult dose of reteplase to be two intravenous loads of 10 U each. Each loading dose is to be given over 2 minutes, with the second loading dose given 30 minutes following the first (160). Although approved by the FDA only for use in the setting of acute myocardial infarction, reteplase has achieved wide off-label use for acute deep vein thrombosis and pulmonary embolism. The dosing schedule is the same as that approved for treatment of acute myocardial infarction.

Tenecteplase was approved as a fibrinolytic agent by the FDA in 2000. It is a genetically engineered mutation of tPA with a similar mechanism of action to alteplase. It is produced by recombinant technology using Chinese hamster ovary cells as a 527 amino acid glycoprotein, with several modifications in the amino acid sequence. As a result, tenecteplase has a decreased plasma clearance, a 15- to 19-minute half-life, a reduced sensitivity to plasminogen activator inhibitor (148), and greater fibrin specificity, which may lead to a reduction in hemorrhagic complications (160). Tenecteplase is administered as a 30- to 50-mg intravenous bolus over 5 seconds; the dose is calculated based on the patient's weight as follows: 0.5 mg/kg (149). The drug is currently under investigation for use in ischemic stroke.

Thrombolytic agents differ in their ability to cause clot lysis, as well as fibrin selectivity, and their ability to activate thrombosis and platelet aggregation. The clinical effectiveness of the same agent can be altered by dose, route of administration, and concomitant use of adjunctive agents. All thrombolytic agents are administered via the intravenous route in dosing regimens

TABLE 172.11

CHARACTERISTICS OF U.S. FOOD AND DRUG ADMINISTRATION–APPROVED THROMBOLYTIC AGENTS

	Streptokinase	Amistreplace	Alteplase	Reteplase	Tenecteplase
Molecular weight (daltons)	47,000	131,000	70,000	39,000	70,000
Half-life (min)	23	100	<5	13–16	20–24
Dose/time	1.5 MU × 30–60 min	30 mg × 5 min	100 mg × 90 min	10 + 10 U × 30 min	0.5 mg/kg × 5–10 s
Bolus administration	No	Yes	No	Yes	Yes
Metabolism	Hepatic	Hepatic	Hepatic	—	—
Allergic reactions	1–4%		<0.2%	No	<1%
Hypotension	Yes	Yes	No	No	No
Early heparin[a]	?Yes	?Yes	Yes	Yes	Yes
Fibrin selective	No	No	Yes	Yes	Yes
Systemic fibrinogen	Marked	Marked	Mild	Moderate	—
Fibrinogen breakdown	4+		1–2+	Unknown	4–15
Plasminogen binding	Indirect	Indirect	Direct	Direct	Direct
TIMI 3 flow (%)	32	43	54	60	66
≈90-min patency (%)	50	65	75	80	75
Intracerebral hemorrhage (%)	0.5	0.6	0.8	0.9	
Mortality rates (%)	7.3	10.5	7.2	7.5	

TIMI 3,
[a]The need for concomitant heparin has been formally tested with only streptokinase and alteplase.
From Khan IJ, Gowda RM. Clinical perspectives and therapeutics of thrombolysis. *Int J Cardiol.* 2003;91:117, with permission.

designed to achieve greater than 90% activation of the fibrinolytic system (161) (Table 172.11).

CLINICAL PEARLS

- Thrombosis may occur anywhere in the vascular system, either from primary hypercoagulable conditions (thrombophilias), acute vascular insult, or a combination of the two factors.
- The coagulation system depends on normal vascular endothelium to maintain antithrombotic activity and promote laminar fluid blood flow. When vascular injury occurs, it can immediately respond through thrombin generation and fibrin production at the site of vascular damage.
- Venous thrombi typically form under conditions of low flow and are mainly composed of fibrin and red blood cells. Arterial thrombi typically form under conditions of high flow and are predominantly composed of platelet aggregates held together by fibrin strands.
- The coagulation cascade is regulated by the tissue factor pathway inhibitor, the protein C pathway, and the fibrinolytic degradation of fibrin.
- Unfractionated heparin has been used in multiple clinical scenarios including prevention of venous thromboembolism, treatment of deep venous thrombosis and pulmonary embolism, and acute coronary syndromes. Until recently, it has been the most widely used antithrombotic agent, although it has several disadvantages.
- The most efficient and safe method for initiating intravenous heparin therapy is using weight-adjusted nomograms.
- A single dose of aspirin is sufficient to inhibit platelet function for the life span of the platelets (31).
- Clopidogrel is more effective than aspirin in reducing atherosclerotic events, including myocardial infarction, stroke, and peripheral vascular disease (45).
- The incidence of bleeding is higher among patients taking antiplatelet agents, requiring urgent surgical procedures (47).
- In the event of bleeding, the antiplatelet agent must be stopped, and platelet transfusion will be required to normalize platelet function.
- LMWH inhibits predominantly factor Xa to produce its anticoagulant effect. It can be administered as a subcutaneous injection once or twice a day.
- LMWH has proved to be cost effective as compared to unfractionated heparin because of reduced need for monitoring.
- LMWH tends to accumulate in patients with renal failure.
- There is no rapid and complete antagonist to the anticoagulant effects of LMWH, which may complicate ICU and surgical procedures (7).
- Direct thrombin inhibitors directly bind thrombin, thereby blocking its procoagulant effect. This class of drugs may be advantageous over indirect thrombin inhibitors such as heparin because they do not bind plasma proteins and produce a more predictable response.
- Drugs that block factor Xa are considered either indirect or direct inhibitors. Indirect agents act by binding to and activating antithrombin, which inhibits free factor Xa. Direct factor Xa inhibitors bind to and inhibit free factor and inactivate factor Xa bound to platelets.
- Thrombolytic agents act as plasminogen-activating agents, catalyzing the conversion of endogenous plasminogen to plasmin. These agents will dissolve both fibrin deposits and pathologic thrombi at sites of vascular injury and thus may be associated with significant hemorrhage.

References

1. Weitz JI, Hirsch J. New anticoagulant drugs. *Chest.* 2001;119:95s–107s.
2. Turpie A. State of the art—a journey through the world of antithrombotic therapy. *Semin Thromb Hemost.* 2002;28(3):3–11.
3. Puggioni A, Kalra M, Gloviczki P. Practical aspects of postthrombotic syndrome. *Dis Mon.* 2005;51:166–175.
4. Hirsch DR, Ingenito EP, Goldhaber SZ. Prevalence of deep venous thrombosis in patients in medical intensive care. *JAMA.* 1995;274:335–337.
5. Cade JF. High risk of the critically ill for venous thromboembolism. *Crit Care Med.* 1982;10:448–450.
6. Cook D, Attia J, Weaver B, et al. Venous thromboembolic disease: an observational study in medical-surgical intensive care unit patients. *J Crit Care.* 2000;15:127–132.
7. Williams MT, Phil NAM, Wallace MJ, et al. Venous thromboembolism in the intensive care unit. *Crit Care Clin.* 2003;19:185–207.
8. Schafer AI, Levine MN, Konkle BA, et al. Thrombotic disorders: diagnosis and treatment. *Hematology.* 2003;:520–539.
9. Hirsh J, Hoak J. Management of deep vein thrombosis and pulmonary embolism. A statement for healthcare professionals. Council on Thrombosis (in consultation with the Council on Cardiovascular Radiology), American Heart Association. *Circulation.* 1996;93:2212–2245.
10. Lopez J, Kearon C, Lee AYY. Deep venous thrombosis, *Hematology.* 2004;1:439–465.
11. Cumming AM, Shiach CR. The investigation and management of inherited thrombophilia. *Clin Lab Haematol.* 1999;25:207–210.
12. Broze GJ Jr. Tissue factor pathway inhibitor. *Thromb Haemost.* 1995;74:90–93.
13. Drake TA, Morrissey JH, Edgigton TS. Selective cellular expression of tissue factor in human tissues. Implications for disorders of hemostasis and thrombosis. *Am J Pathol.* 1989;134:1087–1097.
14. Fleck RA, Rao LV, Rapaport SI, et al. Localization of human tissue factor antigen by immunostaining with monospecific, polyclonal anti-human tissue factor antibody. *Thromb Res.* 1990;59:421–437.
15. Fuster V, Badimon L, Badimon JJ, et al. The pathogenesis of coronary artery disease and the acute coronary syndromes. *N Engl J Med.* 1992;326:310–318.
16. Eisenberg PR, Ghigliotti G. Platelet-dependent and procoagulant mechanisms in arterial thrombosis. *Int J Cardiol.* 1999;68(Suppl 1):S3–S10.
17. Ruggieri ZM. The role of von Willebrand factor and fibrinogen in the initiation of platelet adhesion to thrombogenic surfaces. *Thromb Haemost.* 1995;74:460–463.
18. Sakariassen KS, Fressinaud E, Girma JP, et al. Role of platelet membrane glycoproteins and von Willebrand factor in adhesion of platelets to subendothelium and collagen. *Ann N Y Acad Sci.* 1987;51:52–65.
19. Furie B, Furie BC. Molecular and cell biology of blood coagulation. *N Engl J Med.* 1992;326:800–806.
20. Gailani D, Broze GJ Jr. Factor XI activation by thrombin and factor XIa. *Semin Thromb Hemost.* 1993;19:396–404.
21. Broze GJ Jr. Tissue factor pathway inhibitor. *Thromb Haemost.* 1995;74:90–93.
22. Esmon CT, Ding W, Yasuhiro K, et al. The protein C pathway: new insights. *Thromb Haemost.* 1997;78:70–74.
23. Hirsch J. Heparin. *N Engl J Med.* 1991;324:1565–1574.
24. de Agostini AI, Watkins SC, Slayter HS, et al. Localization of anticoagulantly active heparan sulfate proteoglycans in vascular endothelium: antithrombin binding on cultured endothelial cells and perfused rat aorta. *J Cell Biol.* 1990;111:1293–1304.
25. Collen D. The plasminogen (fibrinolytic) system. *Thromb Haemost.* 1999;82:259–270.
26. Brown MD, Rowe BH, Reeves MJ, et al. The accuracy of the enzyme linked immunosorbent assay D-dimer test in the diagnosis of pulmonary embolism; a meta-analysis. *Ann Emerg Med.* 2002;40:133–144.
27. Perrier A, Desmarais S, Miron MJ, et al. Non-invasive diagnosis of venous thrombo-embolism in outpatients. *Lancet.* 1999;353:190–195.
28. Ohlmann P, Faure A, Morel O, et al. Diagnostic and prognostic value of circulating D-dimers in patients with acute aortic dissection. *Crit Care Med.* 2006;34(5):1358–1364.
29. Shorr AF, Thomas SJ, Alkins SA, et al. D-dimers correlates with proinflammatory cytokine levels and outcomes in critically ill patients. *Chest.* 2002;121:1262–1268.
30. Patrono C, Coller B, Fitzgerald GA, et al. Platelet-active drugs: the relationship among doses, effectiveness, and side effects: the Seventh

ACCP Conference on Antithrombotic and Thrombolytic Therapy. *Chest.* 2004;126:234S–64s.

31. Awtry EH, Loscalzo J. Aspirin. In: Michelson AD, ed. *Platelets.* Amsterdam, the Netherlands: Academic Press; 2002:745–768.
32. Randomised trial of intravenous streptokinase, oral aspirin, both, or neither among 17,187 cases of suspected acute myocardial infarction: ISIS-2. ISIS-2 (Second International Study of Infarct Survival) Collaborative Group. *Lancet.* 1988;2:349–360.
33. Antithrombotic Trialists' Collaboration. Collaborative meta-analysis of randomised trials of antiplatelet therapy for prevention of death, myocardial infarction, and stroke in high risk patients. *BMJ.* 2002;324:71–86.
34. Gullov AL, Koefoed BG, Petersen P, et al. Fixed minidose warfarin and aspirin alone and in combination vs adjusted-dose warfarin for stroke prevention in atrial fibrillation: Second Copenhagen Atrial Fibrillation, Aspirin, and Anticoagulation Study. *Arch Intern Med.* 1998;158:1513–1521.
35. Singer DE, Hughes RA, Gress DR. The effect of aspirin on the risk of stroke in patients with nonrheumatic atrial fibrillation. *Am Heart J.* 1992; 124:1567–1573.
36. Grotemeyer KH, Scharafinski, Husstedt IW. Two-year follow-up of aspirin responder and aspirin non responder. A pilot study including 180 post-stroke patients. *Thromb Res.* 1993;71:397–403.
37. Eikelboom JW, Hankey GJ. Aspirin resistance: a new independent predictor of vascular events? *J Am Coll Cardiol.* 2003;41:966–968.
38. Gum PA, Kottke-Marchant K, Poggio ED, et al. Profile and prevalence of aspirin resistance in patients with cardiovascular disease. *Am J Cardiol.* 2001;88:230–235.
39. Bhatt DL, Topol EJ. Scientific and therapeutic advances in antiplatelet therapy. *Nat Rev Drug Discov.* 2003;2:15–28.
40. Cambria-Kiely JA, Gandhi PJ. Aspirin resistance and genetic polymorphism. *J Thromb Thrombolysis.* 2002;14:51–58.
41. Ferraris VA, Ferraris SP, Joseph O, et al. Aspirin and postoperative bleeding after coronary artery bypass grafting. *Ann Surg.* 2002;235:820–827.
42. Clagett GP, Anderson FA, Levine MN, et al. Prevention of venous thromboembolism. *Chest.* 1992;102:391s.
43. Helft G, Osende JL, Worhtley SG, et al. Acute antithrombotic effect of a front load regimen of clopidogrel in patients with atherosclerosis on aspirin. *Arterioscler Thromb Vasc Biol.* 2000;20:2316–2321.
44. Curtin R, Cox D, Fitzgerald D, et al. Clopidogrel and ticlopidine. In: Michelson AD, ed. *Platelets.* Amsterdam, the Netherlands: Academic Press, 2002:787–801.
45. CAPRIE steering committee. A randomized, blinded, trial of Clopidogrel versus Aspirin in Patients at Risk of Ischemic Events. *Lancet.* 1996;348:1329–1339.
46. Clopidogrel in Unstable Angina to Prevent Recurrent Events Trial Investigators. Effects of clopidogrel in addition to aspirin in patients with acute coronary syndrome without ST-segment elevation. *N Engl J Med.* 2001;345:494–502.
47. Genoni M, Tavokoli R, Hofer C, et al. Clopidogrel before urgent coronary artery bypass graft. *J Thorac Cardiovasc Surg.* 2003;126:288–289.
48. Dawson DL, Cutler BS, Meissner MH, et al. Cilostazol has beneficial effects in the treatment of intermittent claudication. *Circulation.* 1998;98:678–686.
49. EPILOG Investigators. Platelet glycoprotein IIb/IIIa receptor blockade and low dose heparin during percutaneous coronary revascularization. *N Engl J Med.* 1997;336:1689–1696.
50. The EPISTENT Investigators. Randomized placebo controlled and balloon-angioplasty controlled trial to assess safety of coronary stenting with use of platelet glycoprotein IIb/IIIa blockade. Evaluation of platelet IIb/IIIa Inhibitor for stenting. *Lancet.* 1998:352:87–92.
51. The EPIC Investigators. Use of monoclonal antibody directed against the platelet gpIIb/IIIa receptor in high risk coronary angioplasty. *N Engl J Med.* 1994;330:956–61.
52. Sane DC, Damaraju LV, Topol E, et al. Occurrence and clinical significance of pseudothrombocytopenia during abciximab therapy. *J Am Coll Cardiol.* 2001;36:75–83.
53. Reiter RA, Mayr F, Blazicek H. Desmopressin antagonizes the in vitro platelet dysfunction induced by gpIIb/IIIa inhibitors and aspirin. *Blood.* 2003;102:4594–4599.
54. Ronner E, Boersma E, Akkerhuis KM, et al. Patients with acute coronary syndromes without persistent ST segment elevation undergoing percutaneous coronary intervention benefit most from early intervention with protection by a glycoprotein IIb/IIIa receptor blocker. *Eur Heart J.* 2002;23:239–246.
55. The Platelet Receptor Inhibition in Ischemic Syndrome Management (PRISM) study investigators. A comparison of aspirin plus tirofiban with aspirin plus heparin for unstable angina. *N Engl J Med.* 1998;339:1498–1505.
56. Sacco RL, Sivenius J, Diener HC. Efficacy of aspirin plus extended-release dipyridamole in prevention of stroke in high risk populations. *Arch Neurol.* 2005;62:403–408.
57. Beguin S, Lindhout T, Hemker HC. The mode of action of heparin in plasma. *Thromb Haemost.* 1988;60:457–462.
58. Ofosu FA, Hirsch J, Esmon CT, et al. Unfractionated heparin inhibits thrombin catalyzed amplification reactions of coagulation more efficiently than those catalyzed by factor Xa. *Biochem J.* 1989;257:143–150.
59. Hyers TM, Hull RD, Morris TA, et al. Antithrombotic therapy for venous thromboembolic disease. *Chest.* 2001;119:176S–193S.
60. Geerts W, Selby R. Prevention of venous thromboembolism in the ICU. *Chest.* 2003;124(Suppl):357S–363S.
61. Collins R, Scrimgoeour A, Yusuf S, et al. Reduction in fatal pulmonary embolism and venous thrombosis by perioperative administration of subcutaneous heparin. *N Engl J Med.* 1988;318:1162–1173.
62. Noble S, Peters DH, Goa KL. Enoxaparin: a reappraisal of its pharmacology and clinical applications in the prevention and treatment of thromboembolic disease. *Drugs.* 1995;49:388–410.
63. Samama MM, Cohen AT, Damon Jy, et al. A comparison of enoxaparin with placebo for the prevention of venous thromboembolism in acutely ill medical patients. *N Engl J Med.* 1999;341:793–800.
64. Jacobs DG, Piotrowski JJ, Hoppensteadt DA, et al. Hemodynamic and fibrinolytic consequences of intermittent pneumatic compression: preliminary results. *J Trauma.* 1996;40:710–716.
65. Barritt DW. Anticoagulant drugs in the treatment of pulmonary embolism: a controlled clinical trial. *Lancet.* 1960;1:1309–1312.
66. Kernohan RJ. Heparin therapy in thromboembolic disease. *Lancet.* 1966; 1:621–623.
67. Alpert JS. Mortality in patients treated for pulmonary embolism. *JAMA,* 1976;236:1477–1480.
68. Kanis JA. Heparin in the treatment of pulmonary thromboembolism. *Thromb Haemost.* 1974;32:517–527.
69. Levine M, Jent M, Hirsch J, et al. A comparison of low-molecular-weight heparin administered primarily at home with unfractionated heparin administered in the hospital for proximal deep-vein thrombosis. *N Engl J Med.* 1996;334:677–681.
70. Koopman MMW, Prandoni P, Piovella F, et al. Treatment of venous thrombosis with intravenous unfractionated heparin administered in the hospital as compared to subcutaneous low molecular weight heparin administered at home. *N Engl J Med.* 1996;334:682–687.
71. The Columbus Investigators. Low molecular weight heparin in the treatment of patients with venous thromboembolism. *N Engl J Med.* 1997; 337: 657–662.
72. Doyle DJ, Turpie AG, Hirsh J, et al. Adjusted subcutaneous heparin or continuous intravenous heparin in the treatment of deep venous thrombosis: a randomized trial. *Ann Intern Med.* 1987;107:441–445.
73. Pini M, Pattachini C, Quintavalla R, et al. Subcutaneous vs intravenous heparin for treatment of deep venous thrombosis: a randomized trial. *Thromb Haemost.* 1990;64:222–226.
74. Anderson G, Fagrell B, Holmgren K, et al. Subcutaneous administration of heparin: a randomized comparison with intravenous administration of heparin to patients with deep venous thrombosis. *Throm Res.* 1982;27:631–639.
75. Kearon V, Ginsberg JS, Julian JA, et al. Fixed-Dose Heparin (FIDO) Investigators. Comparison of fixed dose weight-adjusted unfractionated heparin and low-molecular-weight heparin for acute treatment of venous thromboembolism. *JAMA.* 2006;296:935–942.
76. Hull RD, Raskob GE, Brant RF, et al. Relation between the time to achieve the lower limit of the aPTT therapeutic range and recurrent venous thromboembolism during heparin treatment for deep vein thrombosis. *Arch Int Med.* 1997;157:2562–2568.
77. Raschke RA, Reilly BM, Guidry JR, et al. The weight-based heparin dosing nomogram compared with a "standard care" nomogram: a randomized controlled trial. *Ann Intern Med.* 1993;119:874–881.
78. Hull RD, Pineo GF. Heparin and low-molecular-weight heparin therapy for venous thromboembolism: will unfractionated heparin survive? *Semin Thromb Hemost.* 2004;30:11–23.
79. Anand SS, Bates S, Ginsberg JS, et al. Recurrent venous thrombosis and heparin therapy: an evaluation of the importance of early activated partial thromboplastin times. *Arch Intern Med.* 1999;159:2029–2032.
80. Cruikshank MK, Levine MN, Hirsch J, et al. A standard heparin nomogram for the management of heparin therapy. *Arch Int Med.* 1991;151:333–337.
81. Hollingsworth JA, Rowe BH, Brisebois FJ, et al. The successful application of a heparin nomogram in a community hospital. *Arch Int Med.* 1995;155:2095–2100.
82. Brown G, Dodek P. An evaluation of empiric vs nomogram based dosing of heparin in an intensive care unit. *Crit Care Med.* 1997;25:1534–1538.
83. Basu D, Gallus AS, Hirsh J, et al. A prospective study of value of monitoring heparin treatment with the activated partial thromboplastin time. *N Engl J Med.* 1972;287:324–327.
84. Hull RD, Raskob GE, Hirsh J, et al. Continuous intravenous heparin compared with intermittent subcutaneous heparin in the initial treatment of proximal vein thrombosis. *N Engl J Med.* 1986;315:1109–1114.
85. Chiu HM, Hirsh J, Yung WL, et al. Relationship between the anticoagulant and antithrombotic effects of heparin in experimental venous thrombosis. *Blood,* 1977;49:171–184.
86. Turpie AGG, Robinson JG, Doyle DJ, et al. Comparison of high dose with low subcutaneous heparin to prevent left ventricular mural thrombosis in patients with acute transmural anterior myocardial infarction. *N Engl J Med.* 1989;320:352–357.

87. Kaplan K, Davison R, Parker M, et al. Role of heparin after intravenous thrombolytic therapy for acute myocardial infarction. *Am J Cardiol.* 1987; 59:241–244.
88. Hyers TM, Agnelli G, Hull RD, et al. Antithrombotic therapy for venous thromboembolic disease. *Chest.* 2001;119(Suppl):176s–193s.
89. Buller HR, Agnelli G, Hull RD, et al. Antithrombotic therapy for venous thromboembolic disease: the seventh ACCP conference on antithrombotic and thrombolytic therapy. *Chest.* 2004;126(suppl):401s–428s.
90. Kearon C, Gent M, Hirsch J, et al. A comparison of three months of anticoagulation with extended anticoagulation for a first episode of idiopathic venous thromboembolism. *N Engl J Med.* 1999;340:901–907.
91. Schulman S, Rhedin AS, Lindmarker P, et al. A comparison of six weeks and six months of oral anticoagulant therapy after a first episode of venous thromboembolism. *N Engl J Med.* 1995;332:1661–1665.
92. Agnelli G, Prandoni P, Santamaria MG, et al. Three months versus one year of oral anticoagulant therapy for idiopathic deep venous thrombosis. *N Engl J Med.* 2001;345:165–169.
93. Ryan TJ, Antman EM, Brooks NH, et al. 1999 Update: ACC/AHA guidelines for the management of acute myocardial infarction. *J Am Coll Cardiol.* 1999;34:890–911.
94. Klein W, Buchwald A, Hillis SE, et al. A comparison of low molecular weight heparin with unfractionated heparin for 6 weeks in the management of unstable coronary artery disease: Fragmin in unstable heart coronary artery disease study (FRIC). *Circulation.* 1997;96:61–68.
95. Cohen M, Demers C, Gurfinkel EP, et al. A comparison of low-molecular weight heparin with unfractionated heparin for unstable coronary artery disease. Efficacy and safety of subcutaneous enoxaparin in non-q wave coronary events study. *N Engl J Med.* 1997;337:447–442.
96. Antman EM, McCabe CH, Gurfinkel EP, et al., for the TIMI 11B investigators. Enoxaparin prevents death and cardiac ischemic events in unstable angina/non-Q wave myocardial infarction: results of the TIMI 11B trial. *Circulation.* 1999;100:1593–1601.
97. Brill-Edwards P, Ginsberg JS, Johnston M, et al. Establishing a therapeutic range for heparin therapy. *Ann Intern Med.* 1993;119:104–109.
98. Raschke R, Guidry J, Laufer N. Heparin-nitroglycerin interaction [Letter]. *Am Heart J.* 1991;121:1849.
99. Levine MN, Hirsch J, Gent M, et al. A randomized trial comparing activated thromboplastin time with heparin assay in patients with acute venous thromboembolism requiring large daily doses of heparin. *Arch Intern Med.* 1994;154:49–56.
100. Levine MN, Raskob G, Beyth RJ, et al. Hemorrhagic complications of anticoagulant treatment: the Seventh ACCP Conference on Antithrombotic and Thrombolytic Therapy. *Chest.* 2004;126(Suppl):287S–310s.
101. Glazier RL, Crowell EB. Randomized prospective trial of continuous vs intermittent heparin therapy *JAMA.* 1976;236:520–526.
102. Horrow JC. Protamine: a review of its toxicity. *Anesth Analg.* 1985;64:348–361.
103. Stewart WJ, McSweeney SM, Kellet MR, et al. Increased risk of severe protamine reactions in NPH-Insulin-dependent diabetics undergoing cardiac catheterization. *Circulation.* 1984;70:788–792.
104. Caplan SN, Berkman EM. Protamine sulfate and fish allergy. *N Engl J Med.* 1976;295:172.
105. Warkentin TE, Elavathil LJ, Hayward CPM, et al. Multicentric warfarin induced skin necrosis complicating heparin induced thrombocytopenia. *Am J Hematol.* 1999;62:44–48.
106. Griffiths E, Dzik WH. Assays for heparin-induced thrombocytopenia. *Transfus Med.* 1997;7:1–11.
107. Bartholomew J. Transition to oral anticoagulants in patient with heparin-induced thrombocytopenia. *Chest.* 2005;127:27s–34s.
108. Warkentin TE, Elavathil LJ, Hayward CP, et al. The pathogenesis of venous limb gangrene associated with heparin-induced thrombocytopenia. *Ann Inten Med.* 1997;127:804–812.
109. Majerus PW, Broze GJ, Miletich JP, et al. Anticoagulant, thrombolytic, and antiplatelet drugs. In: Hardman JG, Limbird LE, eds. *Goodman and Gilman's The Pharmacological Basis of Therapeutics.* 9th ed. New York, NY: McGraw-Hill; 1996:1347–1351.
110. Srinivasan AF, Rice L, Bartholomew JR, et al. Warfarin-induced skin necrosis and venous limb gangrene in the setting of heparin-induced thrombocytopenia. *Arch Intern Med.* 2004;164:66–70.
111. Weitz JI. Low-molecular-weight heparins. *N Engl J Med.* 1997;337(10): 688–698.
112. Cosmi B, Fredenburgh JC, Rischke J, et al. Effect of nonspecific binding to plasma proteins on the antithrombin activities of unfractionated heparin, low-molecular-weight heparin, and dermatan sulfate. *Circulation.* 1997;95(1):118–124.
113. http://home.mdconsult.com/das/drug/view.
114. Klein W, Buchwald A, Hillis SE, et al. Comparison of low-molecular-weight heparin with unfractionated heparin acutely and with placebo for 6 weeks in the management of unstable coronary artery disease. Fragmin in unstable coronary artery disease study (FRIC). *Circulation.* 1997;96: 61–68.
115. Francis CW, Pellegrini VD, Totterman S, et al. Prevention of deep-vein thrombosis after total hip arthroplasty. Comparison of warfarin and dalteparin. *J Bone Joint Surg Am.* 1997;79:1365–1372.
116. Fragmin during Instability in Coronary Artery Disease (FRISC) study group. Low-molecular-weight heparin during instability in coronary artery disease. *Lancet.* 1996;347:561–568.
117. Levine MN, Raskob G, Landefeld S, et al. Hemorrhagic complications of anticoagulant treatment. *Chest.* 2001;119(Suppl):108s–121s.
118. Holst J, Linbald B, Berqvist D, et al. Protamine neutralization of intravenous and subcutaneous low-molecular-weight heparin. An experimental investigation in healthy volunteers. *Blood Coagul Fibrinolysis.* 1994;5(5):795–803.
119. Warkentin TE, Levine MN, Hirsh J, et al. Heparin-induced thrombocytopenia in patients treated with low-molecular-weight heparin or unfractionated heparin. *N Engl J Med.* 1995;332(20):1330–1335.
120. Newman PM, Swanson RL, Chong BH. Heparin-induced thrombocytopenia: IgG binding to PF4-heparin complexes in the fluid phases and cross reactivity with low molecular weight heparin and heparinoid. *Thromb Haemost.* 1998;80(2):292–297.
121. Routledge PA, Chapman DH, Davies DM, et al. Pharmacokinetics and pharmacodynamics of warfarin at steady state. *Br J Clin Pharmacol.* 1979; 8:243–7.
122. Hirsh J, Dalen JE, Deykin D, et al. Oral anticoagulants: mechanism of action, clinical effectiveness, and optimal therapeutic range. *Chest.* 1995;108(4 Suppl):231s–246s.
123. Levine MN, Raskob G, Landefeld S, et al. Hemorrhagic complications of anticoagulant treatment. *Chest.* 1995;108(4 Suppl):276s–290s.
124. Linkins LA, Weitz JI. New anticoagulants. *Semin Thrombos Hemost.* 2003; 29;619–631.
125. Weitz JI, Crowther M. Direct thrombin inhibitors. *Thromb Res.* 2002; 106:V275–V284.
126. Wallis RB. Hirudins: from leeches to man. *Semin Thromb Haemost.* 1996; 22:185–196.
127. Hofsteenge J, Stone SR, Donella-Deana A, et al. The effect of substituting phosphotyrosine for sulphotyrosine on the activity of hirudin. *Eur J Biochem.* 1990;188:55–59.
128. Weitz JI, Middledorp S, Geerts W, et al. Thrombophilia and new anticoagulant drugs. *Hematology.* 2004;1:424–438.
129. Lefevre G, Duval M, Gauron S, et al. Effect of renal impairment on the pharmacokinetics and pharmacodynamics of desirudin. *Clin Pharmacol Ther.* 1997;62:50–59.
130. Maraganore JM, Bourdon P, Jablonski J, et al. Design and characterization of hirulogs: a novel class of bivalent peptide inhibitors of thrombin. *Biochemistry.* 1990;29:7095–7101.
131. Skrrzypczak-Jankun E, Carperos VE, Ravichandran KG, et al. Structure of the hirugen and Hirulog 1 complexes of alpha-thrombin. *J Mol Biol.* 1991;221:1379–1393.
132. Witting JI, Bourdon P, Brezniak DV, et al. Thrombin-specific inhibition by and slow cleavage of Hirulog-1. *Biochem J.* 1992;283:737–743.
133. Robson R, White H, Aylward P, et al. Bivalirudin pharmacokinetics and pharmacodynamics: effect of renal function, dose, and gender. *Clin Pharmacol Ther.* 2002;71:433–439.
134. Hursting MJ, Alford KL, Becker JC, et al. Novastan (brand of argatroban): a small-molecule, direct thrombin inhibitor. *Semin Thromb Hemost.* 1997;23:503–516.
135. Hursting MJ, Alford KL, Becker JC, et al. Novastan (brand of argatroban): a small-molecule, direct thrombin inhibitor. *Semin Thromb Hemost.* 1997;23:503–516.
136. Francis CW, Berkowitz SD, Comp PC, et al. Comparison of ximelagatran with warfarin for the prevention of venous thromboembolism after total knee replacement. *N Engl J Med.* 2003;349:1703–1712.
137. O'Brien CL, Gage BF, et al. Costs and effectiveness of ximelagatran for stroke prophylaxis in chronic atrial fibrillation. *JAMA.* 2005;293:699–706.
138. Cohen AT, Davidson BL, Gallus AS, et al. Fondaparinux for the prevention of VTE in acutely ill medical patients. *Blood.* 2003;102:15a.
139. Linkins LA, Weitz JI. New anticoagulants. *Semin Thromb Hemost.* 2003; 29:619–631.
140. Herbert JM, Herault JP, Bernat A, et al. Biochemical and pharmacological properties of SANORG 34006, a potent and long-acting synthetic pentasaccharide. *Blood.* 1998;91:4197–4205.
141. Bijsterveld NR, Vink R, van Aken BE, et al. Recombinant factor VIIa reverses the anticoagulant effect of the long-acting pentasaccharide idraparinux in healthy volunteers. *Br J Haemotol.* 2004:124:653–658.
142. Levine M, Hirsh J, Weitz J, et al. A randomized trial of a single bolus dosage regimen of recombinant tissue plasminogen activator in patients with acute pulmonary embolism. *Chest.* 1990;98:1473–1479.
143. Dall-Volta S, Pall A, Santolacandro A, et al. PAIMS 2: alteplase combined with heparin versus heparin in the treatment of acute pulmonary embolism. *J Am Coll Cardiol.* 1992:20:520–526.
144. Garcia D, Ageno W, Libby E. Update on the diagnosis and management of pulmonary embolism. *Br J Haematol.* 2005;131:301–312.
145. ISIS-3 study group (third international study of infarct survival) Collaborative Group, ISIS-3: a randomized comparison of streptokinase vs. tissue plasminogen activator vs. anistreplase and of aspirin plus heparin vs. aspirin alone among 41,299 cases of suspected acute myocardial infarction. *Lancet.* 1992;339:753–770.

146. GUSTO Investigators. An international randomized trial comparing four thrombolytic strategies for acute myocardial infarction. *N Engl J Med.* 1993;329:673–682.
147. The Global Use of Strategies to open occluded Coronary Arteries (GUSTO III) Investigators. A comparison of reteplase with alteplase for acute myocardial infarction. *N Engl J Med.* 1997;337:1118–1123.
148. Assessment of the safety and efficacy of new thrombolytic (ASSENT-II) investigators. Single bolus tenecteplase compared with front loaded alteplase in acute myocardial infarction: the ASSENT-II double-blind randomized trial. *Lancet.* 1999;354:716–722.
149. Clark WM, Wissman S, Albers GW, et al. Recombinant tissue-type plasminogen activator (alteplase) for ischemic stroke 3 to 5 hours after symptom onset: the ATLANTIS study: a randomized controlled study. *JAMA.* 1999;282:2019–2026.
150. Stam J. Thrombosis of the cerebral veins and sinuses. *N Engl J Med.* 2005; 352:1791–1798.
151. Jackson KW, Tang J. Complete amino acid sequence of streptokinase and its homology with serine proteases. *Biochemistry.* 1982;21:6620–6625.
152. Reddy KN, Markus G. Mechanism of activation of human plasminogen by streptokinase. Presence of an active center I streptokinase-plasminogen complex. *J Biol Chem.* 1972;247:1683–1691.
153. Mentzer RL, Budzynski AZ, Sherry S. High dose, brief duration intravenous infusion of streptokinase in acute myocardial infarction: description of effects in the circulation. *Am J Cardiol.* 1986;57:1220–1226.
154. Col JJ, Col-De Beys CM, Renkin JP, et al. Pharmacokinetics, thrombolytic efficacy and hemorrhagic risk of different streptokinase regimens in heparin-treated acute myocardial infarction. *Am J Cardiol.* 1989;63:1185–1192.
155. Collen D, De Cock F, Lijnen HR. Biological and thrombolytic properties of proenzyme and active forms of human urokinase-II. Turnover of natural and recombinant urokinase in rabbits and squirrel monkeys. *Thromb Haemost.* 1984;52:24–26.
156. Kohler M, Sen S, Miyashita C, et al. Half-life of single-chain urokinase-type plasminogen activator (scu-PA) and two-chain urokinase-type plasminogen activator (tcu-PA) in patients with acute myocardial infarction. *Thromb Res.* 1991;62:75–81.
157. Clark W, Wissman S, Albers G, et al. Recombinant tissue-type plasminogen activator (alteplase) for ischemic stroke 3 to 5 hours after symptom onset: the ATLANTIS study: a randomized controlled trial. *JAMA.* 1999;282:2019–2026.
158. Konstantinides S, Geibel A, Heusel G, et al. Heparin plus alteplase compared with heparin alone in patients with submassive pulmonary embolism. *N Engl J Med.* 2002;347:1143–1150.
159. Verstraete M. Third-generation thrombolytic agents. *Am J Cardiol.* 2000; 109:52–58.
160. Bozeman WP, Kleiner DM, Ferguson KL. Empiric tenecteplase is associated with increased return of spontaneous circulation and short term survival in cardiac arrest patients unresponsive to standard interventions. *Resuscitation.* 2006;69:399–406.
161. Khan IJ, Gowda RM. Clinical perspectives and therapeutics of thrombolysis. *Int J Cardiol.* 2003;91:115–127.

CHAPTER 173 ■ HEMATOLOGIC CONDITIONS IN THE ICU

JAN S. MOREB

HEMATOPOIESIS

Cellular Components

Hematopoiesis is a polyclonal process that is responsible for the production and maintenance of blood and immune cells, thereby producing billions of new blood cells each day. Large numbers of blood and immune cells can be traced to a pool of hematopoietic stem cells (HSCs) from which these clones have originated. In the early 1960s, Till and McCulloch began analyzing the bone marrow to find out which components were responsible for regenerating blood. They defined what have remained the two hallmarks of an HSC: it can renew itself, and it can produce cells that give rise to all the different types of blood cells (1). Now it is also known that these cells can mobilize out of the bone marrow into circulating blood and can undergo programmed cell death, called *apoptosis*—a process by which cells that are detrimental or unneeded self-destruct, all for the purpose of maintaining homeostasis. The most primitive stem cell in the bone marrow is responsible for the production of all lymphoid (T, B, and natural killer lymphocytes), myeloid (granulocytes, monocytes), erythroid, and megakaryocytic (platelets) cell lineages, while maintaining sufficient numbers of pluripotent stem cells to sustain hematopoiesis throughout adult life. These cells can be found in a small population of cells characterized by the surface expression of CD34 molecule and by lack of markers of differentiation.

The production of differentiated blood cells is the real work of HSCs and progenitor cells. Progenitor or precursor cells are partly differentiated cells that divide and give rise to differentiated "specialized" cells. Such cells are usually regarded as "committed" to differentiating along a particular cellular development pathway. The HSC population supports a tremendous production of blood cells over an animal's life span, e.g., adult humans produce their body weight of red cells, white cells, and platelets every 7 years, whereas the mouse produces 60% of its body weight over a 2-year life span. Using DNA labeling data, investigators in the field have tried to characterize the HSC kinetics in the mouse. Based on such data, MacKey (2) was able to calculate that in the course of producing a mature, circulating blood cell, the original single hematopoietic stem cell will undergo between 17 and 19.5 divisions, providing a net output between approximately 170,000 and 720,000 blood cells.

A wide array of environmental factors, both humoral and cellular, regulate the quantity and behavior of these stem cells, including cytokines and chemokines, extracellular matrix components, as well as hematopoietic and nonhematopoietic cells such as natural killer (NK) cells, T cells, macrophages, fibroblasts, osteoblasts, adipocytes, and perhaps even neurons. In addition to this wide array of microenvironmental factors, several intrinsic genetic events are critical to hematopoiesis and are currently the subject of intense research (3). This complex interplay determines whether HSCs, progenitors, and mature blood cells remain quiescent, proliferate, differentiate, self-renew, or undergo apoptosis (4–6). Under normal conditions, most HSCs and many progenitors are quiescent in the G0 phase of the cell cycle; however, many of the more mature progenitors are proliferating and producing mature offspring (7). In the absence of any stresses, this is balanced by the rate of apoptosis in progenitors and mature cells (5).

In the event of stress, such as bleeding or infection, several processes occur. Stored pools of cells in the marrow or adherent to the endothelium are quickly released into the circulation to localize to the site of injury (8); additionally, fewer progenitors and mature cells undergo apoptosis (9,10). Furthermore, quiescent progenitors and HSCs are stimulated by various growth factors to proliferate and differentiate into mature white cells, red blood cells, and platelets. Finally, when the bleeding, infection, or other underlying stress ceases, the kinetics of hematopoiesis return to baseline levels. This process repeats itself innumerable times during the life span of an individual, and is seen in an exaggerated form following chemotherapy or bone marrow transplantation.

Humoral Mediators

Production of a specific type of differentiated blood cell from a stem cell is thought to occur randomly. Cytokines promote proliferation and survival of certain types of cells but do not affect which cell type is produced from a stem cell. As the progenitors differentiate, the phenotype-specific receptors evolve so that only certain cytokines can affect these new and more mature cells, while others maintain stem cell self-renewal and expansion (11). Cytokines are made and secreted mainly by helper T lymphocytes and macrophages, but also by other stroma cells such as fibroblasts and endothelial cells. A few of these cytokines have been synthesized and are FDA-approved for clinical use. These include erythropoietin (epoetin alfa, or long-acting darbepoetin alfa) for erythrocyte production, granulocyte colony-stimulating factor (G-CSF, filgrastim or long-acting pegfilgrastim), and granulocyte–macrophage colony-stimulating factor (GM-CSF, sargramostim) for neutrophil production, as well as stem cell harvest for transplantation and interleukin-11 (oprelvekin) for stimulation of megakaryocytes and production of platelets. The clinical development of other cytokines was complicated by either too many serious side effects (stem cell factor, ancestim) or the induction of neutralizing antibodies that cross-react with the endogenous molecule (thrombopoietin).

The term, *cytokine,* is a general one; other appropriate and more specific terms include: *lymphokine,* for cytokines made by lymphocytes; *monokine,* for cytokines made by monocytes; *chemokine,* for cytokines with chemotactic activities; and *interleukin,* for cytokines made by one leukocyte and acting on other leukocytes. Cytokines act on their target cells by binding specific membrane receptors through which they mediate their effect on inflammation, immunity, and hematopoiesis. Responses to cytokines include increasing or decreasing expression of membrane proteins—including cytokine receptors, proliferation, and secretion of effector molecules. Only a few cytokines are in clinical use today, mainly interferon-α and interferon-γ.

Cytokines are very important in critical care medicine, especially those proinflammatory cytokines released by monocytes/macrophages in response to infectious and noninfectious inflammation. The release of these cytokines results in whole body inflammation such as that seen in the systemic inflammatory response syndrome (SIRS). These patients also undergo an anti-inflammatory phase, which includes the release of cytokines with opposing—anti-inflammatory—biologic effects or naturally occurring cytokine antagonists, such as interleukin-1 receptor antagonist and tumor necrosis factor-α soluble receptors p55 and p75 (12,13). Clinical studies to intervene in the inflammatory response using these and other anticytokine therapy have been more than a little disappointing (14). On the other hand, many studies have shown that plasma concentrations of certain cytokines correlate with severity and outcome of sepsis (15,16).

DECREASED BLOOD COUNTS

Anemias

Anemia (hemoglobin concentration less than 12 g/dL) is present in 95% of patients to the intensive care unit, with about one third of those having upon admission concentration of less than 10 g/dL. In the assessment, particular attention should be paid to the time of onset, patient's ethnic origin, concurrent illness, procedures patient has undergone, drugs patient is receiving, and history of transfusions. One practical approach is to classify anemia into two major categories: anemia resulting from underproduction versus anemia due to increased destruction of red blood cells (RBC) (Table 173.1). These considerations will affect the type of laboratory tests and the need for transfusions.

Every effort should be exerted to obtain diagnostic tests prior to any transfusions. These should include a complete blood count, including hematocrit, hemoglobin, mean corpuscular volume (MCV) and hemoglobin (MCH), a reticulocyte count, and a stained blood smear. In addition, serum bilirubin and lactic acid dehydrogenase are useful to determine the presence of hemolysis. If immune hemolysis is suspected, direct Coombs test should be ordered (indirect Coombs test is done routinely with any cross-match request sent to the blood bank); or if hemoglobinopathy is suspected, hemoglobin electrophoresis should be obtained before transfusion.

TABLE 173.1

ANEMIA CLASSIFICATION

ANEMIAS SECONDARY TO MARROW UNDERPRODUCTION
■ **Decreased erythropoietin production**
Renal disease
Endocrine deficiency
Starvation
■ **Inadequate response to erythropoietin**
Iron deficiency
B_{12} deficiency
Folic acid deficiency
Anemia of chronic disease
Marrow infiltration
Sideroblastic anemia
Myelodysplastic syndrome
■ **Marrow failure**
Congenital dyserythropoietic anemia
Aplastic anemia
Pure red cell aplasia
Toxic marrow damage
ANEMIAS SECONDARY TO INCREASED DESTRUCTION
■ **Acquired**
Immune-mediated hemolytic anemia
Paroxysmal nocturnal hemoglobinuria
Hemolytic anemia due to red cell fragmentation (TTP, DIC)
Hemolytic anemia due to chemical or physical agents
Infections
Acquired hemoglobinopathies (methemoglobinemia)
■ **Hereditary**
Congenital hemoglobinopathies (sickle cell disease)
Enzyme deficiency (G6PD, pyruvate kinase)
Red cell membrane defects (spherocytosis, elliptocytosis)

TTP, thrombotic thrombocytopenic purpura; DIC, disseminated intravascular coagulation.

The physician in the ICU may be faced with the immediate decision of whether the patient requires transfusion with packed red blood cells (PRBC). For years, many physicians firmly believed that hemoglobin of 10 g/dL or hematocrit of 30% was desirable in anemic patients, especially those undergoing surgical procedures and/or with critical illness (17). This approach of using fixed transfusion triggers has been recognized as the main reason for high transfusion rates in ICU patients and is finally being replaced by a more physiologic approach in which the patient's intravascular volume and tissue oxygen needs are considered. A restrictive transfusion policy, in which hemoglobin concentration is maintained between 7 and 9 g/dL, has proved to be effective and yields decreased death rates in comparison to the liberal strategy (17–19). Indeed, in young traumatized patients, the hemoglobin is sometimes allowed to drift to as low as 5 g/dL, as long as there are no signs of oxygen delivery deficit such as elevated lactate levels, an unacceptable heart rate, or other symptoms. These patients are most often started on recombinant erythropoietin and have iron stores repleted, if necessary, to keep from undergoing transfusion.

Patients with acute myocardial infarction or unstable angina (17), and some cancer patients, may benefit from a higher hemoglobin level. Patients with a hemoglobin greater than or equal to 10 g/dL are unlikely to benefit from blood transfusion.

Anemia in Critical Illness

Anemia of hemoglobin less than or equal to about 8.5 g/dL is the most frequent type of anemia encountered in the ICU. As a result, more than 50% of these patients receive RBC transfusions during their ICU stay, as do more than 85% of patients with an ICU length of stay longer than 7 days. This trend was confirmed by two more recent studies: the CRIT study in the United States (20) and the ABC trial in Europe (21). Both studies also showed that the number of RBC transfusions a patient received was independently associated with longer ICU stay and increase in mortality. These and other similar epidemiologic studies have revealed some similarities. First, the vast majority of critically ill patients have anemia on admission to the ICU. Second, the most common indication for RBC transfusion in the ICU was treatment of the anemia. Third, the transfusion trigger in all these studies was hemoglobin of about 8.5 g/dL. Finally, RBC transfusions were increased in patients with prolonged ICU length of stay and increased age.

Possible mechanisms involved in anemia of acute critically ill patients include a blunted erythropoietin (EPO) response to anemia, with blood concentrations being inappropriately low in these patients; suppression of erythropoiesis by proinflammatory cytokines; possible blood loss from frequent phlebotomies; and blood loss from gastrointestinal bleeding as a result of gastric tubes, stress-induced mucosal ulcerations, acute renal failure, and frequent coagulation problems in ICU patients. This anemia shares characteristics with anemia of chronic inflammation such as high ferritin concentrations and low-to-normal transferrin saturation with functional iron deficiency (19).

Until recently, we understood little about the pathogenesis of anemia of chronic inflammation. It now appears that the inflammatory cytokine interleukin-6 (IL-6) induces the production of hepcidin, an iron-regulatory hormone that may be responsible for the hypoferremia and suppressed erythropoiesis (22). This discovery should lead to studies focused on the role of hepcidin in the anemia of the critically ill patient and better understanding of its pathogenesis.

The approach to treatment of this type of anemia should include measures to reduce blood loss, a restrictive blood transfusion policy, and possibly the use of recombinant human EPO (rh-EPO). Multiple studies have shown that the subcutaneous administration of rh-EPO at 40,000 units weekly, starting between days 3 and 7 of the ICU stay, resulted in a significant reduction in RBC transfusions and a higher hemoglobin level (23,24). Since iron is locked up in the phagocytic system and hardly available, the administration of intravenous iron, together with rh-EPO, may result in an enhanced rh-EPO effect. As only about 10% of oral iron is bioavailable, this route may not be appropriate in ICU patients. Additionally, because there have been anaphylactoid reactions reported with iron dextran, iron gluconate is the preferred formulation. Iron gluconate is administered at a dose of 125 mg diluted in 100 mL saline over 1 hour infusion or undiluted at a rate of 12.5 mg/minute daily for eight sessions, to a total cumulative dose of 1,000 mg.

Autoimmune Hemolytic Anemia

When a patient is critically ill from autoimmune hemolytic anemia (AIHA), the presenting signs and symptoms are those of normovolemic anemia, unless massive hemolysis is associated with hypotension, significant hemoglobinuria, and acute renal failure. Variable levels of jaundice may also be present in the nonmassive AIHA. Initial laboratory data may show an elevated reticulocyte index (greater than 2) identifying the mechanism of the anemia as hemolytic, an elevated indirect bilirubinemia and lactate dehydrogenase (LDH); the blood smear shows increased numbers of diffusely basophilic red cells, reflecting the increased reticulocytes, and variable numbers of microspherocytes and fragmented cells, indicative of the hemolysis (Fig. 173.1). In some instances, the urine may be discolored

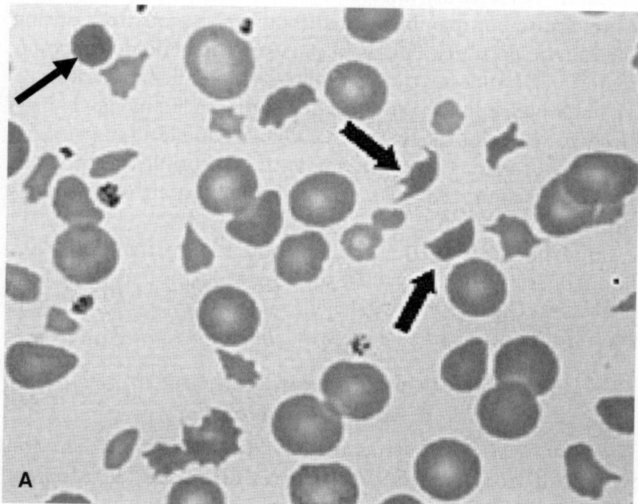

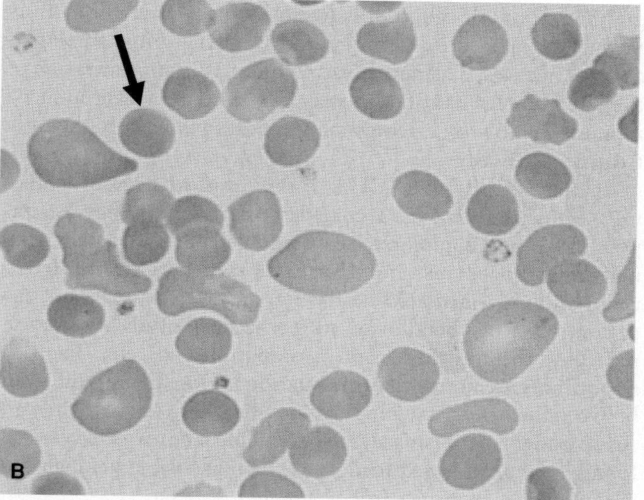

FIGURE 173.1. Microspherocytes (*thin arrows*) and schistocytes (fragmented cells, *thick arrows*) (**A**), spherocytes with increased reticulocytes (the large cells) (**B**) are usually seen in the peripheral blood smear of a patient with hemolytic anemia.

red, brown, or black if there has been sufficient intravascular hemolysis to produce hemoglobinuria. A positive result on direct antiglobulin (Coombs) test, indicating that immunoglobulin or complement is on the surface of the circulating red cells, identifies the immune etiology of the hemolysis. In the absence of recent transfusion, the diagnosis of AIHA is confirmed. This information may first become available when the blood bank attempts to cross-match the patient's blood for transfusion.

It is important to determine, by history and appropriate laboratory studies, whether the hemolysis could be related to a drug the patient is taking and whether it is caused by warm-reacting (usually IgG) or cold-reacting (usually IgM) antibodies. The mechanisms whereby drugs produce immune hemolysis are not absolutely clear, but evidence suggests an alteration of red cell surface antigens by the drug and production of antibodies that lead to hemolysis (25). In some instances, the drug must be present for hemolysis to occur (e.g., quinidine, penicillin); in others, hemolysis occurs even in the absence of the drug (e.g., methyldopa). Underlying diseases that may be associated with AIHA include infections, such as infectious mononucleosis and pneumonia caused by *Mycoplasma pneumonia;* collagen vascular diseases, especially systemic lupus erythematosus; and lymphoproliferative disorders such as chronic lymphocytic leukemia (26). In some instances, the AIHA may be the presenting manifestation of the underlying disease. In other instances, the AIHA may be associated with idiopathic thrombocytopenic purpura (ITP) as part of Evans syndrome.

The mainstay of treatment of AIHA caused by warm-reacting antibodies is the administration of corticosteroids, usually given in dosages equivalent to 60 to 80 mg/day of prednisone. In patients who do not respond to steroids, splenectomy, high-dose intravenous gamma globulin, rituximab chimeric anti-CD20 antibody, alemtuzumab humanized anti-CD52 antibody, or treatment with other immunosuppressive drugs may be useful.

Steroids are usually ineffective in AIHA caused by cold-reactive antibodies (cold agglutinin disease), but responses have been observed using larger doses. Patients with cold agglutinins may have symptoms related to impaired blood flow in acral parts where the blood temperature is low enough to permit agglutination of red blood cells by antibodies. Warming usually prevents or alleviates such symptoms; however, in a small percentage of cases, plasmapheresis to reduce the concentration of the offending IgM antibodies may be required. In drug-induced immune hemolysis, discontinuing the drug is usually the only treatment needed.

In the patient with AIHA with a critical degree of anemia, transfusion must be considered (27,28). It may be impossible to find compatible red blood cells by the usual cross-matching procedures, and transfused cells may be subject to rapid antibody-mediated destruction. On the other hand, the patient must not be allowed to die because of undue caution regarding the transfusion of incompatible red cells. The key to optimal care in this critical situation is close communication between the intensivist and the blood bank physician. When an AIHA patient is transfused, the patient must be observed closely for signs of accelerated hemolysis, such as visible hemoglobin in the plasma or urine.

Certain special considerations pertain to transfusion of patients with cold-reacting antibodies. Administered blood should be warmed to body temperature. Transfusion of plasma, which contains complement, should be avoided because hemolysis is complement mediated and may be limited by depletion of complement *in vivo*.

In massive hemolysis, therapeutic efforts should be directed at maintenance of blood pressure, renal blood flow, and urinary output. Intravenous fluids and diuretics such as furosemide should be used to maintain a urine flow of 100 mL/hour.

Hemolytic Anemia from G6PD Deficiency

Red blood cell glucose-6-phosphate dehydrogenase (G6PD) deficiency is inherited as an X-linked recessive disorder, affecting various population groups around the world. In the United States, African Americans are the group most often affected, with a gene frequency of about 11%. They have the G6PD A–variant of the enzyme and a mild to moderate deficiency. A recent study by the U.S. Army found that 2.5% of males and 1.6% of females were deficient. The highest rates of G6PD deficiency were in African American males (12.2%) and females (4.1%), along with Asian males (4.3%) (29). The red cell G6PD levels in affected men are 8% to 20% of normal. Clinically significant hemolysis occurs when red cells are subjected to an oxidative metabolic challenge, as may occur with exposure to certain drugs or with certain illnesses. Among drugs producing hemolysis are some sulfonamides, nitrofurantoins, and antimalarials such as primaquine. Illnesses most likely to trigger hemolysis are acute infections. Infectious hepatitis, in particular, has been associated with severe hemolytic episodes in G6PD-deficient patients.

Hemolysis in the G6PD-deficient patient may be sudden and massive, usually becoming apparent 1 to 3 days after the inciting stress, such as administration of an oxidant drug. Hemoglobinemia and hemoglobinuria may occur. The blood smear shows polychromatophilia within a few days, reflecting the developing reticulocytosis. Early in the course of the hemolytic episode, Heinz bodies may be identified in red cells by special staining methods. These precipitates of oxidatively denatured hemoglobin provide a useful diagnostic clue and should be sought if G6PD deficiency is suspected as a cause of acute hemolysis. However, the absence of Heinz bodies does not exclude this diagnosis. The red cell enzyme deficiency may be readily detected by laboratory assay when the patient is in a stable state but may be more difficult to demonstrate during a hemolytic episode. This is because the enzyme deficiency is greatest in the oldest red cells. These cells are the first destroyed in a hemolytic episode, and, as they are replaced by newly produced young cells, the overall red cell enzyme level may rise to the normal range. This replacement of susceptible erythrocytes by more resistant cells also tends to ameliorate the hemolysis with time.

If the diagnosis is suspected, any potentially offending drugs should be stopped. Otherwise, supportive care is usually all that is necessary. Although the deficiency is an X-linked trait, female heterozygotes may have hemolytic episodes.

Hemolytic Anemia from Red Cell Injury in the Circulation

Fragmentation and destruction of red cells in the circulation may result from increased shear stresses caused by turbulent blood flow. The two major categories of disease in which this kind of hemolysis occurs are malfunctioning intravascular prosthetic devices—for example, heart valves, vascular grafts, and shunts—and disorders affecting blood vessels that result in microangiopathic hemolytic disease, such as disseminated intravascular coagulation or thrombotic microangiopathy (TMA).

TMA encompasses the spectrum of thrombotic thrombocytopenic purpura (TTP) and hemolytic uremic syndrome. These forms of hemolytic disease are rarely of sufficient severity to require critical care. However, they can be seen in critically ill patients admitted to the ICU, and have been associated with various initiating factors such as severe infections, drug intake, malignancies, connective tissue diseases, and pregnancy (30). Because hemolysis is intravascular, hemoglobinemia and hemoglobinuria may be present. Characteristically, the blood smear shows red cell fragmentation producing micropoikilocytes (schistocytes, similar to that shown in Fig. 173.1). Typically, the TMA patients will also have thrombocytopenia, fever, and possibly neurologic and renal involvement.

Specific treatment is directed at the underlying disorder. Supportive measures may be required for the effects of hemolysis itself and to minimize any adverse renal consequences of hypotension and hemoglobinuria. These may include blood transfusion and hydration to ensure good urine flow. Occasionally, a badly malfunctioning prosthesis, such as an artificial heart valve, may require replacement, but this is more often necessary to correct a life-threatening hemodynamic abnormality than to alleviate severe hemolysis. The treatment of TMA with plasma administration, either infusion or plasmapheresis, is the only effective therapy that has dramatically improved the prognosis of these patients.

Sickle Cell Anemia

Sickle cell hemoglobin (hemoglobin S) is the result of a single nucleotide mutation in the sixth codon of the β globin gene (β^s). Heterozygous inheritance of hemoglobin S does not usually cause disease or symptoms but is detectable as sickle cell trait (31). Homozygous inheritance or compound heterozygous inheritance with another β globin gene results in disease. The discussion here is directed primarily toward homozygous sickle cell disease which includes those genotypes associated with chronic hemolytic anemia and vaso-occlusive pain: homozygous sickle cell disease (hemoglobin SS), hemoglobin SC disease (hemoglobin SC), sickle-β^0 thalassemia (hemoglobin Sβ^0), and sickle-β^+ thalassemia (hemoglobin Sβ^+), and other less common hemoglobin mutants. The clinical manifestations are related to the degree of intracellular polymerization of deoxyhemoglobin S (Table 173.2), and it is different among the various genotypes.

The clinical symptoms of sickle cell disease (SCD) affect multiple organs and may vary widely among patients. Chief among the clinical features are episodes of severe pain—namely, crises—in the chest, back, abdomen, or extremities. The acute chest syndrome, a frequent—and sometimes fatal—complication, affects more than 40% of all patients with SCD

TABLE 173.2

CLINICAL AND HEMATOLOGIC FINDINGS IN THE COMMON VARIANTS OF SICKLE CELL DISEASE AFTER THE AGE OF 5 YEARS

	Hemoglobin electrophoresis					Hematologic values			
Disease group	Clinical severity	S (%)	F (%)	A_2 (%)	A (%)	Hb g/dL	Retic (%)	MCV (fl)	RBC morphology
SS	Usually marked	>90	<10	<3.5	0	6–11	5–20	>80	Sickle cells-NRBC, normochromia, anisocytosis, poikilocytosis, target cells, Howell-Jolly bodies
Sβ° Thal	Marked to moderate	>80	<20	>3.5	0	6–10	5–20	<80	Sickle cells, NRBC, hypochromia, microcytosis, anisocytosis, poikilocytosis, target cells
Sβ^+ Thal	Mild to moderate	>60	<20	>3.5	10–30	9–12	5–10	<75	No sickle cells, hypochromia, microcytosis, anisocytosis, poikilocytosis, target cells
SC	Mild to moderate	50	<5	[a]	0	10–15	5–10	75–95	"Fat" sickle cells, anisocytosis, poikilocytosis, target cells
S HPFH	Asymptomatic	<70	>30	<2.5	0	12–14	1–2	<80	No sickle cells, anisocytosis, poikilocytosis, rare target cells

MCV, mean corpuscular volume; NRBC, nucleated red blood cells.
[a]50 percent Hb C.
Hematologic values are approximate. There is tremendous variability between disease groups and between individual patients of the same group, particularly regarding clinical severity.
For findings in younger children, see Brown AK, Sleeper LA, Miller ST, et al. Reference values and hematological changes from birth to five years in patients with sickle cell disease. *Arch Pediatr Adolesc.* 1994;48:796–804.
Adapted from NIH Publication No. 96-2117.

and can lead to acute and chronic respiratory insufficiency, including pulmonary hypertension. Its cardinal features are fever, pleuritic chest pain, referred abdominal pain, cough, lung infiltrates, and hypoxia. Other complications of SCD include recurrent strokes in young adults; parvovirus B19-induced aplastic crisis; hyperbilirubinemia from cholestatic syndrome or cholecystitis; liver disease; splenic infarctions; autosplenectomy with increased risk of fulminant septicemia caused by encapsulated organisms such as *Streptococcus pneumoniae* and *Haemophilus influenzae*; hematuria; priapism; bone infarctions with the risk of avascular necrosis; osteomyelitis and other musculoskeletal manifestations; leg ulcers; and spontaneous abortions (32). Despite the fact that some of these complications are fatal, many patients with SCD survive into their fifth and sixth decades in industrialized countries (33).

The goals of the SCD treatment are either to relieve symptoms of the complications or to prevent complications by using some of the new treatments targeting disease mechanisms. The treatment of the painful crisis is supportive. Dehydration, acidosis, infection, and hypoxemia all promote red cell sickling and should be prevented or corrected. Adequate relief of pain in the hospitalized patient usually requires parenteral administration of opioid analgesics at frequent fixed intervals. Sufficient analgesics should be used to relieve pain without worrying about addiction or side effects of opiates; patients can be given oral analgesics to take at home. Oxygen is often administered in sickle cell crisis, although its benefits are uncertain. Antibiotics that cover major pulmonary pathogens should be administered in patients with acute chest syndrome. Because there is no clear evidence that transfusion therapy shortens a simple painful crisis, and because the crisis is unpredictable and self-limited, transfusion is not a treatment for the uncomplicated painful crisis.

Transfusions are not needed for the usual anemia or episodes of pain. Urgent transfusions are needed when there is a severe sudden drop in hemoglobin, especially in children in whom splenic sequestration or aplastic crises present in this manner, and in severe acute chest syndrome with hypoxia. Chronic red cell transfusions have been shown to prevent strokes in patients with SCD, although the optimal duration of transfusion is unknown. However, the risks of transfusions must be weighed against the benefits. These risks include alloimmunization, infections, and iron overload. For patients undergoing general anesthesia, preoperative transfusion to a hematocrit above 30% reduced postoperative complications. Leukocyte-depleted red cells that are phenotypically matched for the antigens most frequently associated with immune response are preferred for transfusion. Exchange transfusion is the most rapid method to reduce the hemoglobin S concentration to less than 30% in urgent situations that arise from complications of SCD, such as stroke and severe acute chest syndrome, and in patients with striking cholestatic syndrome and signs of liver failure.

Preventive treatments should include early vaccinations against *S. pneumoniae* and *H. influenzae*; prophylactic penicillin in children until the age of 5 years; folic acid (1 mg daily) to all patients to prevent megaloblastic erythropoiesis; and hydroxyurea treatment to prevent complications. In a double-blind, placebo-controlled trial, hydroxyurea was shown to reduce the pain episodes, acute chest syndrome, blood transfusions, and hospitalizations (34). The improvements noted with hydroxyurea treatment correlate to increases in hemoglobin F levels and a decrease in granulocytes, monocytes, and reticulocytes (35). Hydroxyurea treatment should be reserved for patients with SCD who have severe complications. Other experimental treatments aimed at interrupting the disease mechanisms are in progress (36).

Specific Clinical Problems

1. If abdominal symptoms are present, the possibilities of cholecystitis and complications of cholelithiasis must be considered.
2. Rarely, bone marrow infarction may be extensive and may produce the syndrome of fat embolism. This syndrome is manifested by severe bone pain, fever, neurologic abnormalities, and respiratory distress. It may be fatal, and treatment by exchange transfusion can be life-saving. Fat embolism may be a cause of some cases of acute chest syndrome.
3. Hematuria occurs as a complication of the sickle cell diseases, including sickle cell trait, and may be severe. It is thought usually to result from sickling and vaso-occlusion in the renal medulla, but other causes unrelated to sickle disease must be excluded. Supportive treatment with hydration and, perhaps, urinary alkalinization is often sufficient for this self-limited complication.
4. Priapism, a frequent and painful complication of sickle cell disease, arises from the vaso-occlusion that produces congestion and sickling in the corpora cavernosa. It may resolve spontaneously, and initial conservative treatment with analgesics, hydration, and alkalinization is appropriate. Exchange transfusion and various surgical procedures have also been successful in terminating priapism.

Aplastic Crisis in Hemolytic Anemia

Sudden intensification of anemia in hemolytic disease resulting from a precipitous reduction in the rate of red cell production is known as *aplastic crisis*. It may occur in the course of any hemolytic disease but has been most commonly reported in congenital hemolytic disorders such as hereditary spherocytosis and sickle cell anemia. It is most common in children but also occurs in adults. Patients characteristically have fever, anorexia, nausea, and vomiting; abdominal pain and headache are common. Their anemia is usually severe and may be life-threatening; mild leukopenia and thrombocytopenia are often present. The aplastic nature of the anemia is demonstrated by an extremely low reticulocyte count and marked reduction in erythroid precursors in the bone marrow. The episode is self-limited, and recovery usually begins by 2 weeks. In the recovery phase, there is a return of vigorous erythropoiesis and often an outpouring of nucleated red cells and reticulocytes into the blood, frequently accompanied by leukocytosis and immature white blood cells. There is convincing evidence that parvovirus B19 is the cause of most aplastic crises (37).

Prompt recognition of this syndrome is important because of the suddenness and severity of the anemia. A low reticulocyte count in a patient with hemolytic disease is usually the main clue to the diagnosis. Treatment is via transfusion with red blood cells. The volume given should be sufficient to alleviate signs or symptoms of inadequate tissue oxygenation; that amount need not be exceeded, as episodes are self-limited, and the patient's hematocrit will return rapidly to its baseline level.

LEUKOPENIAS

The term, *leukopenia*, refers to a total white blood cell (WBC) count of less than 4,000 cells/μL, whereas granulocytopenia or neutropenia refers to a circulating granulocyte count below 1,500 cells/μL. WBC and granulocyte levels are lower in some ethnic groups, e.g., Africans, African Americans, and Yemenite Jews, without any clinical significance. The clinical importance of granulocytopenia relates to the associated increased risk of bacterial infection. If the absolute neutrophil count is less than or equal to 500 cells/μL, bacterial infection becomes the rule. Agranulocytosis implies severe neutropenia or a complete absence of granulocytes. Three patient groups are discussed as most pertinent to critical care situations: (a) Patients with neutropenia from primary bone marrow diseases or cytotoxic treatment; (b) patients in whom neutropenia exists alone or in combination with other cytopenias as an aplastic process; and (c) patients with neutropenia or agranulocytosis caused by immunologic mechanisms.

Primary Bone Marrow Diseases and Cytotoxic Treatment

This is the largest and most frequent entity that causes neutropenia. Bone marrow diseases such as leukemias, myelodysplastic syndrome, and marrow fibrosis frequently present with neutropenia. Chemotherapy-induced neutropenia is a common complication of the treatment of cancer. The risk of life-threatening infections increases with the increased severity of neutropenia and its duration, increasing patient age, and the coexistence of other severe illnesses. Many of these patients, whether inpatient or outpatient, end up in the ICU due to a rapid onset of septic shock. In current practice, the occurrence of neutropenic fever is an indication for hospitalization and prompt institution of intravenous wide-spectrum antibiotics. Before starting antibiotics, cultures of blood,* sputum, and urine should be obtained in all patients, and other sites should be cultured as indicated in individual patients. All patients should have chest radiographs taken as well. The common effects of bacterial infections—purulent sputum in pneumonia, pyuria in urinary tract infection, or abscess formation—are usually absent because of lack of granulocytes.

Many antibiotic regimens have been tested, and guidelines for a rational approach to therapy have been formulated (38). The choice of an antibiotic regimen should take into account any findings in the individual patient that suggest a specific site of infection and any knowledge of patterns of infection in a given institution. If cultures are positive, the antibiotic treatment should be adjusted accordingly. If cultures are negative, as is frequently the case, empirical therapy should be continued if the patient remains neutropenic and until counts recover. If, on the other hand, fever continues and the patient's general condition deteriorates with persistent neutropenia, it is appropriate in selected patients to prescribe empirical treatment with an antifungal agent, such as amphotericin B, because of the frequency of fungal infections in patients with prolonged neutropenia. Patients should be screened by obtaining a CT scan of sinuses, chest, abdomen, and pelvis for possible foci of invasive fungal infections. The galactomannan antigen test for aspergillus should be done routinely on blood and sputum (usually bronchoalveolar lavage) of immunosuppressed patients with neutropenia. If patients have central venous catheter, fungal and bacterial blood cultures should be obtained, and removal of catheters should be considered if blood cultures are positive for fungal infection or certain bacterial infections that are difficult to eradicate.

Various regimens of prophylactic antibiotics have been investigated for their efficacy in preventing infection in the neutropenic patient. The results have been too variable to justify blanket recommendations (39,40). The routine therapeutic use of colony-stimulating factors (such as G-CSF and GM-CSF) in febrile neutropenia to stimulate the proliferation and maturation of neutrophil progenitor cells was not recommended by the American Society of Clinical Oncology (ASCO). However, these factors should be considered in such patients at high risk for infection-related complications or who have prognostic factors that are predictive of poor clinical outcomes. High-risk features include expected prolonged (greater than 10 days) and profound (less than 0.1×10^3 cells/μL) neutropenia, age older than 65 years, uncontrolled primary disease, pneumonia, hypotension, multiorgan dysfunction, invasive fungal infection, or being hospitalized at the time of the development of the fever (41). On the other hand, colony-stimulating factors are recommended for primary and secondary prophylaxis used to prevent chemotherapy-induced neutropenia (41).

ICU physicians should be aware of respiratory status deterioration or acute respiratory distress syndrome (ARDS) during neutropenia recovery with or without the use of G-CSF (42,43). This could be related to the release of inflammatory cytokines by resident alveolar neutrophils and macrophages. Mortality can be as high as 62% in these patients, and therefore, immediate evaluation by bronchoscopy to rule out infection and early use of high-dose steroids could be critical for their survival.

Bone Marrow Aplasia

Neutropenia is part of the pancytopenia commonly present in aplastic anemia. Some cases of aplastic anemia seem to have an autoimmune basis; in others, a drug or chemical exposure may be suspected as a cause (44,45). No tests are available to prove an association in individual cases. Benzene and its derivatives are potentially toxic to the bone marrow, and many other chemicals, such as dichlorodiphenyltrichloroethane (DDT) and other insecticides, are suspect. Toluene exposure in glue sniffers may be associated with aplastic anemia. Many medications have been linked with aplastic anemia, which occurs as an idiosyncratic reaction in a small percentage of patients exposed to a given drug. Drugs for which an etiologic role seems likely include chloramphenicol, phenylbutazone, indomethacin, diphenylhydantoin, sulfonamides, and gold preparations. In at least half the cases of aplastic anemia, no cause is found or suspected.

The principles of treating infectious complications resulting from neutropenia in aplastic states are the same as those outlined earlier for neutropenia in malignant diseases. The treatment of aplastic anemia includes allogeneic bone marrow

*When blood cultures are drawn, there should never be any less than two full sets—four bottles—drawn. This routine is needed to prevent the possibility of a contaminated specimen being overtreated, or worse, undertreated.

transplantation in suitable patients, immunosuppressive therapy including antithymocyte globulin, and other supportive care measures such as antibiotic prophylaxis and colony-stimulating factors.

Immune and Drug-related Granulocytopenia

Neutropenia in adults often occurs as an isolated finding or in association with autoimmune disease such as rheumatoid arthritis, systemic lupus erythematosus, and other similar conditions. The evaluation should include the following: peripheral blood smear to seek out large granular lymphocytes (LGL); measurement of antinuclear antibodies, rheumatoid factor, and other autoantibodies; and possibly a bone marrow examination. Patients with chronic neutropenia, either idiopathic or autoimmune, usually do not require treatment. Patients with an absolute neutrophil count less than 500 cells/μL are prone to develop recurrent fevers and infections. In addition to antibiotics, G-CSF administration may improve the neutrophil count during the infection. Patients with LGL syndrome may not respond well to G-CSF, and may require immunosuppressive therapy, such as methotrexate or cyclosporine, alone or with G-CSF. Chronic neutropenia in association with rheumatoid arthritis, or Felty syndrome, is usually seen in severe cases with elevated rheumatoid factor. These patients who have recurrent fevers and infection require treatment similar to patients with LGL syndrome. Splenectomy should be considered in refractory cases.

Drug-induced agranulocytosis is a serious medical problem and occurs in 1% to 3% of patients treated with certain medications. The characteristic clinical syndrome includes high fever, chills, and severe sore throat (agranulocytic angina) caused by bacterial infection. Oral and pharyngeal ulcers, necrotizing tonsillitis, pharyngeal abscesses, and bacteremia may occur. The blood will demonstrate a virtual absence of granulocytes. The bone marrow may show absence of all granulocyte precursors or only the mature cells. The picture may superficially resemble acute leukemia, or a state of maturation arrest; the disease mechanism is often unclear. In some cases, it is an antibody against the drug acting as a hapten in association with endogenous antigen on neutrophil surface. Other drugs may impair production of neutrophils by direct toxic mechanism.

Serial blood counts are now recommended for patients on some drugs such as phenothiazines, clozapine, sulfasalazine, and antithyroid drugs because of the relatively high frequency of drug-induced neutropenia. Otherwise, management should include prompt withdrawal of all potentially offending drugs and the use of broad-spectrum antibiotics. Bone marrow examination is not usually indicated. The time to recovery may be proportional to the severity but is usually within about a week after withdrawal of the offending drug.

THROMBOCYTOPENIAS

Thrombocytopenia is a common laboratory abnormality in ICU patients that has been associated with adverse outcomes. The incidence of thrombocytopenia—defined as a platelet count of less than 150 × 10^3 cells/μL—has been reported to be 23% to 41.3%, with mortality rates up to 54% (46). The incidence of more severe thrombocytopenia—less than 50 × 10^3 cells/μL—is lower, about 10% to 17%, but is associated with greater mortality (46). The relationship between the time course of platelet counts and mortality in 1,449 critically ill patients was examined in a prospective multicenter observational study in 40 ICUs from Europe, the United States, and Australia (47). There was a documented increase in mortality in patients who had thrombocytopenia on day 4 of admission to the ICU and even higher mortality in those patients with documented thrombocytopenia by day 14.

TABLE 173.3

POTENTIAL CAUSES OF THROMBOCYTOPENIA

Sepsis, infections
Disseminated intravascular coagulation
Perioperative and postresuscitation hemodilution
Immune thrombocytopenias
Drug-induced thrombocytopenias
Liver disease/hypersplenism
Massive transfusion
Primary marrow disorder
Antiphospholipid antibody syndrome/lupus anticoagulant
Intravascular devices

Systematic evaluation of thrombocytopenia is essential to the identification of and management of the causes (46). There are numerous potential causes of thrombocytopenia in the ICU (Table 173.3). While sepsis is the most common cause, accounting for more than 48% of thrombocytopenia cases in the ICU, more than 25% of ICU patients have more than one cause (48). Drug-induced thrombocytopenia presents a diagnostic challenge inasmuch as many medications can cause thrombocytopenia, and critically ill patients often receive multiple drugs. One such drug is heparin, the most common cause of drug-induced thrombocytopenia due to immune mechanisms (46).

The first step in the diagnosis of true thrombocytopenia is to consider the mechanism (49). Is the thrombocytopenia caused by increased destruction, decreased production, or sequestration of platelets? As noted earlier, the presence of large platelets on the blood smear or by mean platelet volume (MPV) suggests active thrombopoiesis, though this finding may be equivocal. Therefore, examination of the bone marrow for the presence of megakaryocytes is often necessary to distinguish between increased destruction (presence of megakaryocytes) and decreased production (absence of megakaryocytes). The presence of splenomegaly raises the possibility of sequestration. Other laboratory tests are not necessary to evaluate the thrombocytopenia itself. The bleeding time is not useful in assessing thrombocytopenia. There is also the possibility of platelet clumping induced by the commonly used anticoagulant EDTA; platelet cold agglutinins; partial clotting of the blood sample; and platelet satellitosis, a disorder in which platelets cluster around white blood cells. When pseudothrombocytopenia is suspected, examining the peripheral blood smear and close communication with the laboratory is necessary.

Treatment of thrombocytopenia depends on the cause and is discussed below under the specific entities. First, some general principles of platelet transfusion are outlined (50). When thrombocytopenia is caused by destruction or sequestration of the patient's own platelets, transfused platelets are subject to the same fate. Thus, platelet transfusions most often are of little benefit, and are reserved for treatment of severe bleeding. When thrombocytopenia is caused by decreased platelet production, as in hematologic malignancies or during recovery from stem cell transplantation, serious hemorrhage can be prevented by regular transfusion of platelets. It is generally acceptable to use prophylactic transfusion to keep the platelet count greater than 10,000 to 20,000 cells/μL. Transfusion of one random donor platelet unit per 10 kg of recipient weight, or single-donor unit from apheresis, is usually used to achieve that goal, which can be confirmed by a repeat platelet count within an hour posttransfusion. The effectiveness of platelet transfusions is diminished in febrile, infected patients who may require larger and more frequent transfusions. Actively bleeding patients require more frequent transfusion and a higher target of platelet count, usually above 50,000 cells/μL. Chronically transfused patients may become refractory to platelet transfusions from random donors because of alloimmunization. Single-donor platelets limit exposure to foreign antigens and may delay immunization. Platelets obtained from family members by platelet apheresis may be considered in patients who are at risk for bleeding and refractory to random-donor platelets.

Thrombocytopenia with Infection

Mild and transient thrombocytopenia occurs with many systemic infections. The mechanism for this may be a combination of suppressed bone marrow production, increased destruction, and increased splenic sequestration. In bacteremia, platelets may be consumed because of disseminated intravascular coagulopathy, whereas in viral infection, platelet production may be suppressed. Thrombocytopenia is commonly associated with human immunodeficiency virus (HIV) infection, mainly due to decreased production, although sometimes an autoimmune mechanism is also involved. Thrombotic thrombocytopenic purpura (TTP) or thrombotic microangiopathy (TMA) may be associated with HIV as well as other infections such as streptococcal and *Escherichia coli* (51–53). Treating the underlying infection in most of these cases is usually adequate to correct the thrombocytopenia.

Drug-induced Thrombocytopenia

Drug-induced thrombocytopenia presents a diagnostic challenge because many medications can cause thrombocytopenia, and patients in ICU are often on multiple medications (54). The most commonly reported drugs with probable or definite relation to thrombocytopenia were quinidine, quinine, rifampin, and trimethoprim-sulfamethoxazole. Many other drugs can cause thrombocytopenia, including heparin, which is discussed in detail below, intravenous antibiotics, anticonvulsants, diuretics, and the platelet GP IIb-IIIa antagonists used in acute coronary syndrome. The underlying mechanism of drug-induced thrombocytopenia is usually immune, and at least three different types of antibodies appear to play a role: hapten-dependent antibodies, drug-induced platelet-reactive autoantibodies, and drug-dependent antibodies. Targets for drug-dependent antibodies are glycoproteins (GP) on the cell membrane of platelets, such as GP Ib/IX and GPIIb/IIIa. The diagnosis of drug-induced thrombocytopenia is usually supported by recovery to a normal platelet count within 5 to 7 days.

Treatment of drug-induced thrombocytopenia may require only withdrawal of the offending drug. Prednisone may be given if the diagnosis of idiopathic autoimmune thrombocytopenia (ITP) cannot be ruled out. Patients with severe thrombocytopenia caused by GP IIb-IIIa antagonists may require platelet transfusions because they are typically also receiving heparin and aspirin for their acute coronary syndrome. Although platelet serology tests are available, the results may not be available in a time frame that allows such information to be used in the decision-making process for drug-induced immune thrombocytopenia.

Heparin-induced Thrombocytopenia

Heparin-induced thrombocytopenia (HIT) is an anticoagulant-induced prothrombotic disorder caused by platelet activation of heparin-dependent antibodies of the immunoglobulin G class (46). The diagnosis of HIT should be considered when the platelet count falls to less than 150×10^3 cells/μL, or more than 50% decrease of the platelet count from baseline, between days 5 and 14 from start of heparin therapy (55). A high index of suspicion on the physician's part is key in making the diagnosis. The thrombocytopenia is usually moderate and resolves within a few days of discontinuing heparin. HIT without thrombosis is called *isolated HIT*, whereas *HIT thrombotic syndrome* (HITTS) denotes HIT complicated with thrombosis. The mortality rate associated with HIT ranges between 10% and 20% (46).

HIT is an immune-mediated hypersensitivity reaction to platelet factor 4 (PF4)/heparin complex. PF4 is a heparin-binding protein found naturally in platelet α granules, which undergoes conformational changes once bound to heparin. Anti-PF4/heparin antibodies are produced by many patients taking heparin, but only a few will develop thrombocytopenia (46). Anti-PF4/heparin antibodies are transient and usually become undetectable within a median of 50 to 85 days. If heparin is readministered to a patient with high levels of HIT antibodies, abrupt thrombocytopenia can occur. However, this likely will be more than 100 days after the last exposure to heparin (46). It is important to note that seroconversion can be found by ELISA (enzyme-linked immunosorbent assay) in up to 15% of patients on heparin; however, this does not constitute a diagnosis of HIT. In general, surgical patients, individuals exposed to higher doses of heparin for a longer time, and patients receiving unfractionated heparin (UFH), as opposed to low-molecular-weight heparin (LMWH), are more likely to develop HIT.

The frequency of HIT in ICU patients was examined in two major studies (56,57). The results suggested that only a small minority of ICU patients with thrombocytopenia receiving UFH have HIT, and that the PF4/heparin-reactive antibodies are more likely to be detected by ELISA assay than serotonin release assay (SRA), suggesting a possible *over*diagnosis—due to a high false-positive rate by ELISA—of HIT. The Complications After Thrombocytopenia Caused by Heparin (CATCH) registry is a recent attempt to achieve better understanding of the prevalence, consequences, and temporal relationship of HIT and thrombocytopenia among patients treated with anticoagulants. The thrombotic sequelae of HIT carry significant morbidity and may even be lethal. Some of the morbid events include deep venous thrombosis (DVT), pulmonary embolism, skin necrosis, limb ischemia, thrombotic stroke, and myocardial infarction (46). Venous thrombosis is the most common manifestation, with lower limb DVT predominating.

All strategies should be used to prevent HIT in ICU patients. Heparin locks for central venous catheters and hemodialysis catheters are commonly used in the ICU setting and may need to be reconsidered. Hemodialysis without heparin has been shown to be safe and effective. However, once the diagnosis of HIT is recognized, heparin should promptly be substituted with a direct thrombin inhibitor, such as argatroban or lepirudin, or the heparinoid danaparoid (not available in the United States) to reduce the risk of life-threatening thromboembolic events. Because warfarin can temporarily reduce the synthesis of protein C and S, causing a hypercoagulable state, it should never be used alone in the initial treatment of HIT, and its use should be postponed until substantial platelet recovery has occurred. Consultation with a hematologist in these situations should be considered in all critically ill patients. The argatroban dose is 2 μg/kg per minute in continuous infusion and dilution of 1 mg/mL. Dose adjustment is needed for hepatic impairment (use 25% of the dose), with the aim of a 1.5 to 3 times prolongation of activated prothrombin time (aPTT) in comparison to baseline. On the other hand, lepirudin treatment consists of a bolus 0.4 mg/kg (maximum of 44 mg), given over 10 to 15 seconds and followed by continuous infusion at 0.15 mg/kg per hour, with the goal of a 1.5 to 3 times prolongation of aPTT over baseline. The dose should be modified if creatinine is >1.5 mg/dL or clearance is <60 mL/minute. If given with Coumadin, discontinue lepirudin when an international normalized ratio (INR) of 2.0 is obtained.

In summary, the approach to patients with suspected or confirmed HIT includes the following:

1. Discontinuation of all heparin
2. Administration of alternative nonheparin anticoagulation, such as argatroban or lepirudin
3. Testing for anti-PF4/heparin antibodies, followed, if positive, by a serotonin release assay
4. Avoiding prophylactic platelet transfusions
5. Allowing platelet recovery before starting warfarin
6. Assessing for lower extremity DVT.

Patients with previous HIT who are antibody-negative and require cardiac surgery should receive UFH in preference to other anticoagulants, which are less validated for this purpose. Preoperative and postoperative anticoagulation should be handled with an anticoagulant other than UFH or LMWH. Patients with recent or active HIT should have surgery delayed until antibody is negative, if possible; otherwise, an alternative anticoagulant should be used (58).

Idiopathic Thrombocytopenic Purpura

Idiopathic thrombocytopenic purpura (ITP), also known as immune thrombocytopenic purpura, is a common cause of thrombocytopenia in both adults and children. Although it is usually in the differential diagnosis of thrombocytopenia, the diagnosis of ITP can usually be made only after exclusion of other causes of thrombocytopenia. When the history, physical examination, and blood count with peripheral smear are consistent with ITP and do not suggest other causes of thrombocytopenia, few diagnostic tests are necessary. Bone marrow examination may be important to rule out other primary marrow diseases such as myelodysplastic syndrome or lymphoproliferative disorders. In ITP, the marrow will show an increased number of megakaryocytes with immature forms and normal erythroid and myeloid lineages. A test for HIV is important in patients with risk factors for infection with this agent. Tests for platelet antibodies are not helpful because of lack of limited specificity and sensitivity. Thrombocytopenic purpura also may occur as one of the autoimmune complications of collagen vascular diseases such as systemic lupus erythematosus, or lymphoproliferative diseases such as chronic lymphocytic leukemia, and may even be the presenting manifestation of these disorders. ITP is categorized as acute, chronic, and refractory.

Many forms of treatment have demonstrated effectiveness in ITP. Because of the numerous therapeutic options, individualization of therapy is possible. Platelet transfusions are used only in the case of severe, life-threatening hemorrhage. Initial therapy is usually with corticosteroids in a dosage equivalent to 1 mg/kg per day of prednisone. If the platelet count does not rise substantially within 2 to 3 weeks, splenectomy is usually the next step. Splenectomy produces prolonged remissions in two thirds of cases, with additional partial remission in 15% of patients. Splenectomy also may be necessary in patients who have responded to steroids but cannot be weaned from the drug without the recurrence of thrombocytopenia. The 10% to 20% of patients who fail to respond to splenectomy may benefit from treatment with vincristine or immunosuppressive agents such as cyclophosphamide. The anabolic steroid, danazol, when given for periods of several months, also has been effective in some cases of ITP. Large doses of intravenous gamma globulin also may increase the platelet count in ITP, perhaps through blockage of reticuloendothelial sites of platelet destruction. The high cost of this therapy and the short duration of responses—usually 2 to 3 weeks—limit its use to certain specific circumstances such as active bleeding or prior to surgery. Anti-D therapy is effective only in Rh(D)+ patients and is not effective in splenectomized patients. Rituximab, a chimeric anti-CD20 monoclonal antibody, has been shown to be effective in chronic ITP (59). The overall goal in treating chronic/refractory ITP is to maintain a safe platelet count, defined as greater than about 10,000 to 20,000 cells/μL, and minimal therapy to minimize the morbidity and mortality associated with treatment.

When ITP occurs during pregnancy, there is an additional concern that the IgG autoantibody may cross the placenta and produce thrombocytopenia in the fetus and newborn. The lowest platelet count is usually seen several days after birth. The current practice is to use standard obstetric management of pregnancy and delivery. ITP should be differentiated from gestational thrombocytopenia that occurs in about 5% of normal women with uncomplicated pregnancies. The most important clue to differentiating the two is a history of previous thrombocytopenia when the woman was not pregnant. Also, more severe thrombocytopenia occurring before the third trimester is more likely to be ITP.

Thrombotic Thrombocytopenic Purpura

Thrombotic thrombocytopenic purpura (TTP) and its closely related disorders—hemolytic-uremic syndrome (HUS), thrombotic microangiopathy (TMA), and peripartum HELLP (hemolysis, elevated liver enzymes, and low platelets) syndrome—may be catastrophic and rapidly fatal. This disease entity was discussed in the first section of this chapter in regard to microangiopathic hemolytic anemia. TTP was defined by a pentad of abnormalities: thrombocytopenia from increased platelet destruction; microangiopathic hemolytic anemia caused by mechanical damage to red cells as a result of the vascular lesions; neurologic abnormalities; renal abnormalities; and fever. With the advent of curative plasma exchange in the 1970s, the urgency to establish a diagnosis and start treatment has resulted in using limited diagnostic criteria. Now only thrombocytopenia and microangiopathic hemolytic anemia are sufficient to begin plasmapheresis.

The clinical presentation is variable, but the thrombocytopenia and hemolytic anemia are often severe. A wide variety of fluctuating neurologic abnormalities may be present, including seizures, altered consciousness, delirium, and paresis. Renal abnormalities may include uremia, hematuria, and proteinuria. The reasons for fever are unclear.

The typical presentation for young children is to have a prodrome of bloody diarrhea caused by the Shiga toxin-producing enterohemorrhagic strain of *E. coli*. The laboratory findings in TTP are basically those related to the above features: thrombocytopenia, hemolytic anemia with red cell fragmentation, and renal dysfunction. Elevation of serum lactic acid dehydrogenase from intravascular hemolysis, and perhaps also damage to other tissues, is an index of activity of the disease. Coagulation tests are usually normal.

The basic pathogenic mechanism behind these syndromes is most likely related to the vascular endothelial cells. A role for ultralarge von Willebrand factor (vWF) multimers has been identified and is linked to endothelial damage and the occurrence of disseminated platelet thrombi. Recently, a specific metalloprotease (ADAMTS13) that rapidly cleaves these multimers has been identified (60,61). Deficiency of this metalloprotease activity appears to be associated with many, but not all, TTP cases (62).

Plasma exchange has dramatically changed TTP-HUS prognosis and outcome. Plasma infusion is less effective in adults, but it could be adequate in congenital TTP caused by ADAMTS13 deficiency. The duration of plasma exchange is unpredictable. Long durations, up to several months, may be required in patients with repeated relapses. The efficacy of additional treatments such as prednisone, platelet aggregation inhibitors, and splenectomy is unknown (see http://moon.ouhsc.edu/jgeorge).

Alcoholism-associated Thrombocytopenia

Platelet counts less than 100,000 cells/μL are present in over one fourth of critically ill alcoholic patients (63). There are many possible causes for thrombocytopenia in such patients, including hypersplenism and folic acid deficiency. However, it is important to recognize that reversible severe thrombocytopenia may occur as a direct effect of alcohol ingestion in some patients. Studies of the mechanism have demonstrated elements of both decreased effective platelet production and shortened platelet survival. Abnormalities of platelet function have been noted as well. Recovery begins 2 to 3 days after cessation of alcohol ingestion, and maximum platelet counts are reached in 1 to 3 weeks. There is often an overshoot to abnormally high platelet counts, which then return to baseline levels. Therapy consists of having the patient discontinue alcohol ingestion and providing appropriate supportive measures.

Thrombocytopenia Associated with Bone Marrow Disorders

Severe thrombocytopenia from impaired platelet production is a frequent concomitant of bone marrow disorders, such as aplastic anemia, leukemia, or other malignancies metastatic to the bone marrow, as well as cytotoxic chemotherapy of such disorders. Treatment is directed at the underlying disease.

INCREASED BLOOD COUNTS

Erythrocytosis

Erythrocytosis, defined as an abnormally increased red cell mass, may require critical care due to complications of blood hyperviscosity or because of hemorrhagic or thromboembolic complications that threaten some of these patients. The initial clue to the presence of erythrocytosis is usually a high value for hematocrit or hemoglobin concentration. Such values may be present without true erythrocytosis—that is to say, in the presence of a normal red cell mass—if the plasma volume is contracted. This circumstance is usually apparent, although it is often advisable to quantify the red cell mass (RCM) by direct measurement using radioisotopic red cell labels. The RCM is usually increased when the hematocrit is above 60% in a man or 57% in a woman.

True erythrocytosis results from one of two general mechanisms:

1. Polycythemia vera (PV) is a clonal abnormality of bone marrow stem cells resulting in autonomous overproduction of red cells and often of granulocytes and platelets.
2. Secondary erythrocytosis results from excess erythropoietin production in response to hypoxemia, abnormalities of oxygen release from hemoglobin, or autonomous hormone production (e.g., by renal or other tumors).

When the RCM is expanded and the hematocrit increased, blood viscosity is increased, and diminished blood flow, stasis, thrombosis, and tissue hypoxia may ensue. On the other hand, hemorrhagic tendency is also increased, particularly in PV, where elevated platelet counts and abnormalities of platelet function may also be present.

Polycythemia Vera

Criteria for the diagnosis of PV have been modified multiple times since the first criteria were published by Modan and Lilienfeld (64) in 1965; modified diagnostic criteria are shown in Table 173.4 (65). The detection by PCR of Janus kinase 2 (JAK2) tyrosine kinase in up to 97% of patients with PV increases the sensitivity and specificity of early diagnosis. The JAK2 V617F point mutation makes hematopoietic progenitors hypersensitive to the different growth factors, resulting in proliferation of all lineages (66). Risks in uncontrolled PV are primarily hyperviscosity and thromboembolic or hemorrhagic events. Patients at highest risk are those whose disease has shown particularly active cell proliferation requiring extensive therapy, those with a prior history of complications, and

TABLE 173.4

PROPOSED MODIFIED CRITERIA FOR THE DIAGNOSIS OF POLYCYTHEMIA VERA (PV)

A1 Raised red cell mass
Greater than 25% above mean normal predicted value, or a hematocrit value greater than 60% in males or 56% in females
A2 Absence of causes of secondary erythrocytosis
A3 Palpable splenomegaly
A4 Clonality marker, i.e., acquired abnormal marrow karyotype
B1 Thrombocytosis
Platelet count greater than 400×10^3 cells/μL
B2 Neutrophil leukocytosis
Neutrophil count greater than 10×10^3 cells/μL, or greater than 12.5×10^3 cells/μL in smokers
B3 Splenomegaly demonstrated on isotope or ultrasound scanning
B4 Characteristic BFU-E growth or reduced serum erythropoietin
A1 + A2 + A3 or A4 establishes PV
A1 + A2 + two of B establishes PV

BFU-E, erythroid burst-forming units.
Adapted from Pearson TC, Messinezy M, Westwood N, et al. A Polycythemia Vera updated: diagnosis, pathobiology, and treatment. *Hematology Am Soc Hematol Educ Program.* 2000;51.

the elderly. The level of the hematocrit or platelet count is not a reliable predictor. Symptoms resulting from decreased cerebral flow, such as headache, dizziness, and changes in vision are the most common manifestations of hyperviscosity. Hemorrhage or thrombosis can affect almost any body part. Peptic ulcer disease with bleeding is common. Thromboses may be arterial or venous. Fatigue, plethora, pruritus particularly with hot bath, excessive sweating, paresthesias (erythromelalgia), fullness in the left upper abdomen (splenomegaly), and shortness of breath are also some manifestations of PV. Surgery poses an enormous risk in the patient with uncontrolled PV because of a high incidence of thrombotic or hemorrhagic complications.

Patients with uncontrolled PV may present as medical emergencies requiring ICU care and urgent therapy. The mainstay of such therapy is phlebotomy to reduce hematocrit to less than 45%. This may be done as rapidly as 1 unit of blood every other day in young adults. Electrolyte solutions or plasma expanders should be administered with phlebotomy, as necessary, to avoid circulatory instability from sudden changes in blood volume. Elderly patients may tolerate phlebotomy less well, so that removal of volumes of 200 to 300 mL at less frequent intervals may be necessary. Because of the clinical observations of increased thrombosis with aggressive phlebotomy, the simultaneous use of cytotoxic chemotherapy is recommended as part of the initial therapy of patients older than 60 years of age, as well as in younger patients with thrombotic risk factors or a history of thrombosis. Hydroxyurea is often used for this purpose in an initial dose of 15 to 30 mg/kg per day. Long-term treatment with hydroxyurea may be linked with increased risk of transformation to acute leukemia. Emergency plateletpheresis may also be considered in such emergencies to lower an elevated platelet count.

Other treatment options include low-dose aspirin (81 mg/day), interferon-α, and anagrelide; these may be used together with phlebotomy as needed. In general, patients with PV should avoid practices and habits that augment hypercoagulability such as smoking, use of oral contraceptives, or hormone replacement therapy. Aggressive antithrombotic prophylaxis should be given postoperatively in addition to maintaining normal hematocrit and platelet counts.

Secondary Erythrocytosis or Polycythemia

The diagnosis of secondary erythrocytosis is made in a patient with an increased RCM in whom the criteria for PV are not met. These patients could either have physiologically appropriate increased RCM (for example, secondary to tissue hypoxemia) or inappropriately increased RCM (for example, secondary to increased erythropoietin production). Additional studies are needed to differentiate the diverse causes of polycythemia. Indications for phlebotomy in secondary erythrocytosis are less clear than in PV. The best current advice is to individualize therapy so as to maximize the patient's exercise tolerance and overall sense of well-being.

Thrombocytosis

With the availability of a platelet count as part of a routine blood count, an elevated platelet count, or thrombocytosis, has become an important clinical problem in hospitalized patients. Unlike thrombocytopenia, the literature dealing with thrombocytosis in ICU patients is very scant. Furthermore, unlike thrombocytopenia, the presence of thrombocytosis predicts a favorable outcome in ICU patients, whereas a blunted rise in platelet count may be associated with worse outcome. Thrombocytosis in hospitalized patients is classified according to its origin into primary (or clonal) and secondary (or reactive) forms. Primary thrombocytosis refers to a persistent elevation of platelet count due to clonal thrombopoiesis, as it occurs in myeloproliferative disorders including essential thrombocythemia (ET), PV, myelodysplastic syndrome, chronic myelogenous leukemia, and myelofibrosis. Secondary thrombocytosis is due to various conditions, some of them short-lived, such as acute bleeding, infection, trauma or other tissue injury, and surgery; other causes, such as malignancy, post splenectomy, chronic infection, iron deficiency, or chronic inflammatory disease may persist for a longer time. Multiple studies have been conducted on adult and pediatric hospitalized patients (67–71) with an elevated platelet count (more than 500×10^3 cells/μL), and the main conclusions suggest that whereas most patients have secondary thrombocytosis, a higher platelet count and increased thromboembolic complications are significantly associated with primary thrombocytosis. In one study, even when using greater than or equal to $1{,}000 \times 10^3$ cells/μL as the basis for defining extreme thrombocytosis, 82% of 231 patients analyzed were found to have an elevated platelet count due to reactive (secondary) thrombocytosis (72). In this study, the risk of bleeding and/or thrombosis was 56% in primary thrombocytosis, but only 4% in the secondary type. Unless additional risk factors are present, secondary thrombocytosis is not associated with an increased risk of thromboembolic events.

The treatment for primary thrombocytosis, such as ET, is based on risks for thrombosis or bleeding in the presence of vasomotor symptoms. Patients at increased risk—age older than 60 years, history of thromboembolism, a platelet count greater than 1,500,000 cells/μL—should receive platelet-lowering agents such as hydroxyurea, anagrelide, or interferon-α (IFN-α). Low-dose aspirin can be used for the relief of vasomotor symptoms, but if there is no relief, platelet-lowering agents should be added. Hydroxyurea is the recommended drug in patients 60 years of age or older, whereas IFN-α is the cytoreductive agent of choice for childbearing women. The aim should be to lower the platelet count to less than 400,000 cells/μL. Arterial or venous thrombosis should be treated with heparin and, possibly, thrombolysis in some arterial events; plateletpheresis may be indicated in both types of events. Low-dose aspirin may be useful in arterial thrombosis. In hemorrhage, it is appropriate to stop antiplatelet agents and transfuse platelets if the bleeding is persistent. Some patients with uncontrolled thrombocytosis (greater than 1,500,000 cells/μL) were found to have an acquired defect of von Willebrand factor, which contributes to the risk of bleeding. Thus, DDAVP, cryoprecipitate, or factor VIII concentrate may be indicated to treat hemorrhage in these patients.

Leukocytosis

As in thrombocytosis, leukocytosis can be due to primary bone marrow disorders or secondary disorders in response to acute infection or inflammation. Secondary leukocytosis is physiologic and transient, resolving after treating the underlying cause. *Leukemoid reaction* refers to a persistent leukocytosis of more than 50,000 cells/μL, with shift to the left. The major causes for such a reaction include severe infections, severe hemorrhage, acute hemolysis, hypersensitivity, and malignancies (paraneoplastic syndrome).

hyperleukocytosis syndrome. This occurs in leukemic states when the white blood cell count is high. Signs and symptoms are most commonly related to the central nervous system, eyes, and lungs. They include stupor, altered mentation, dizziness, visual blurring, retinal abnormalities, dyspnea, tachypnea, and hypoxia. Intracranial and pulmonary infarction or hemorrhage and sudden death may occur. Priapism and peripheral vascular insufficiency have also been linked with the syndrome. Although the pathogenesis is incompletely understood, autopsies have shown white cell aggregates, microthrombi, and microvascular invasion (leukostatic tumors) (73). The syndrome occurs more commonly in acute (AML) and chronic myelogenous leukemia (CML) than in acute lymphoblastic leukemia, and occurs rarely, if ever, in chronic lymphocytic leukemia. The level of the white blood cell count at which the syndrome appears is variable, depending perhaps on the maturity and size of the white blood cells present and the degree of coexisting anemia. A white count exceeding 100,000 cells/μL in acute myelogenous leukemia or the accelerated phase of CML is usually an alarming sign and an indication for prompt treatment. If there are signs or symptoms attributable to the hyperleukocytosis syndrome, then leukopheresis is indicated to rapidly and safely decrease the white count. At the same time, chemotherapy should be initiated, and treatment with allopurinol and intravenous hydration with urine alkalinization should be started in anticipation of the hyperuricemia. Hydroxyurea (6 g by mouth) is frequently used initially to produce rapid leukemic cell kill.

OTHER HEMATOLOGIC DISORDERS

Plasma Cell Dyscrasias

The presenting symptoms for these malignant disorders may include severe infection, spinal cord compression, or hyperviscosity syndrome that can lead to admission to the ICU. Total serum protein will be abnormally high on routine chemistry blood test. Subsequent evaluation will reveal monoclonal gammopathy of IgM in Waldenstrom macroglobulinemia or IgG/IgA in multiple myeloma. Hyperviscosity syndrome is rare and less frequent when IgG or IgA, respectively, are the abnormal proteins. The most common manifestations of the hyperviscosity syndrome are neurologic and include headache, visual disturbances, hearing loss, vertigo, altered consciousness (ranging from stupor to coma), paresis, seizures, and peripheral neuropathy. A bleeding tendency may exist because of the associated thrombocytopenia or interference by the abnormal protein with the function of platelets or plasma coagulation factors. The most rapidly effective form of therapy for hyperviscosity from serum protein abnormalities is plasmapheresis. At the same time, hydration and specific therapy for the underlying disease should be started.

STEM CELL TRANSPLANTATION

Patients after stem cell transplantation (SCT)—mainly allogeneic—constitute a large proportion of those with hematologic disorders who are admitted to the ICU. These patients are usually admitted with respiratory distress requiring mechanical ventilation, multiorgan failure, or septic shock, and have the highest mortality among cancer patients admitted to the ICU (74). Because of the generally poor outcome, especially for patients requiring mechanical ventilation, the utility of such support has been questioned (75,76). It is generally accepted that patients admitted to the ICU during the engraftment period should be fully supported because of better outcome (77). These patients may have the *engraftment syndrome*, which can result in cytokine-induced capillary leak syndrome with multiorgan failure or alveolar hemorrhage; early high-dose steroids can dramatically reverse the downhill course. These patients should also undergo bronchoscopy to rule out infection while receiving the steroid therapy. Early intervention and transfer to ICU in septic shock will result in improved outcome. After autologous SCT, patients usually have better survival in the ICU than after allogeneic SCT, even those requiring mechanical ventilation.

Admission to the surgical ICU is less frequent for patients after SCT, but some of the most frequent reasons include intestinal perforation and intracranial bleeding. This topic is dealt with in more detail elsewhere in this text.

SUMMARY

Benign and malignant hematologic disorders are frequently encountered in patients admitted to the intensive care units. Some of these disorders develop while patients are in the ICU for other reasons, such as anemia, HIT, TTP, and other drug-induced cytopenias. Other disorders are the primary reason for admission to the ICU and include neutropenic fever and septic shock, respiratory distress, serious life-threatening bleeding, and other disease-specific and chemotherapy-related complications. Familiarity with these problems and the early involvement of the hematology service in the evaluation and treatment of these specific entities are essential for better outcome and improved survival.

References

1. Till JL, McCulloch EA, Siminovitch L. A stochastic model of stem cell proliferation, based on the growth of spleen colony-forming cell. *Proc Natl Acad Sci U S A.* 1964;51:29.
2. MacKey MC. Cell kinetic status of haematopoietic stem cells. *Cell Prolif.* 2001;34:71.
3. Smith C. Hematopoietic stem cells and hematopoiesis. *Cancer Control.* 2003; 10:9.
4. Domen J, Weissman IL. Self-renewal, differentiation or death: regulation and manipulation of hematopoietic stem cell fate. *Mol Med Today.* 1999;5:201.
5. Domen J, Cheshier SH, Weissman IL. The role of apoptosis in the regulation of hematopoietic stem cells: overexpression of Bcl-2 increases both their number and repopulation potential. *J Exp Med.* 2000;191:253.
6. Orkin SH, Zon LI. Hematopoiesis and stem cells: plasticity versus developmental heterogeneity. *Nat Immunol.* 2002;3:323.
7. Hao QL, Thiemann FT, Petersen D, et al. Extended long-term culture reveals a highly quiescent and primitive human hematopoietic progenitor population. *Blood.* 1996;88:3306.
8. Rogowski O, Sasson Y, Kassirer M, et al. Down-regulation of the CD62L antigen as a possible mechanism for neutrophilia during inflammation. *Br J Haematol.* 1998;101:666.
9. Koury MJ, Sawyer ST, Brandt SJ. New insights into erythropoiesis. *Curr Opin Hematol.* 2002;9:93.
10. Endo T, Odb A, Satoh I, et al. Stem cell factor protects c-kit+ human primary erythroid cells from apoptosis. *Exp Hematol.* 2001;29:833.
11. Zhu J, Emerson SG. Hematopoietic cytokines, transcription factors and lineage commitment. i. 2002;21:3295.
12. Arend WP, Malyak M, Bigler CF, et al. The biological role of naturally-occurring cytokine inhibitors. *Br J Rheumatol.* 1991;30(Suppl 2):49–52.
13. Moldawer LL. Interleukin-1, TNF alpha and their naturally occurring antagonists in sepsis. *Blood Purif.* 1993;11:128.
14. Blackwell TS, Christman JW. Sepsis and cytokines: current status. *Br J Anaesth.* 1996;77:110.
15. Kox WJ, Volk T, Kox SN, et al. Immunomodulatory therapies in sepsis. *Intensive Care Med.* 2000;26(Suppl 1):S124.
16. Osuchowski MF, Welch K, Siddiqui J, et al. Circulating cytokine/inhibitor profiles reshape the understanding of the SIRS/CARS continuum in sepsis and predict mortality. *J Immunol.* 2006;177:1967.
17. Fakhry SM, Fata P. How low is too low? Cardiac risks with anemia. *Crit Care.* 2004;8(Suppl 2):S11.
18. Napolitano LM. Scope of the problem: epidemiology of anemia and use of blood transfusions in critical care. *Crit Care.* 2004;8(Suppl 2):S1.
19. van de Wiel A. Anemia in critically ill patients. *Eur J Int Med.* 2004;15: 481.
20. Corwin HL, Gettinger A, Pearl RG, et al. The CRIT study: anemia and blood transfusion in the critically ill–current clinical practice in the United States. *Crit Care Med.* 2004;32:39.
21. Vincent JL, Baron JF, Reinhart K, et al. Anemia and blood transfusion in critically ill patients. *JAMA.* 2002;288:1499.
22. Andrews NC. Anemia of inflammation: the cytokine-hepcidin link. *J Clin Invest.* 2004;113:1251.
23. Corwin HL, Gettinger A, Pearl RG, et al. Efficacy of recombinant human erythropoietin in critically ill patients: a randomized controlled trial. *JAMA.* 2002;288:2827.
24. Silver M, Corwin MJ, Bazan A, et al. Efficacy of recombinant human erythropoietin in critically ill patients admitted to a long-term acute care facility: a randomized, double-blind, placebo-controlled trial. *Crit Care Med.* 2006;34:2310.
25. Salama A, Mueller-Eckhardt C. On the mechanisms of sensitization and attachment of antibodies to RBC in drug-induced immune hemolytic anemia. *Blood.* 1987;69:1006.
26. Gehrs BC, Freidberg RC. Autoimmune hemolytic anemias. *Am J Hematol.* 2002;69:258.
27. Jeffries LC. Transfusion therapy in autoimmune hemolytic anemia. *Hematol Oncol Clin North Am.* 1994;8:1087.
28. Reardon JE, Marquea MB. Laboratory evaluation and transfusion support of patients with autoimmune hemolytic anemia. *Am J Clin Pathol.* 2006;125(Suppl 1):S71.
29. Chinevere TD, Murray CK, Grant E Jr, et al. Prevalence of glucose-6-phosphate dehydrogenase deficiency in U.S. Army personnel. *Mil Med.* 2006;171:905.
30. Coppo P, Adrie C, Azoulay E, et al. Infectious diseases as a trigger in thrombotic microangiopathies in intensive care unit (ICU) patients? *Intensive Care Med.* 2003;29:564.
31. Sears DA. Sickle cell trait. In: Embury SH, Hebbel RP, Mohandas N, et al., eds. *Sickle Cell Disease: Basic Principles and Clinical Practice.* New York: Raven Press; 1994:381.
32. Steinberg MH. Management of sickle cell anemia. *N Engl J Med.* 1999; 340:1021.
33. Platt OS, Brambilla DJ, Rosse WF, et al. Mortality in sickle cell disease: life expectancy and risk factors for early death. *N Engl J Med.* 1994;330:1639.
34. Charache S, Terrin ML, Moore RD, et al. Effect of hydroxyurea on the frequency of painful crises in sickle cell anemia. *N Engl J Med.* 1995;332: 1317.
35. Charache S. Mechanism of action of hydroxyurea in the management of sickle cell anemia in adults. *Semin Hematol.* 1997;34(Suppl 3):15.
36. Buchanan GR, DeBaun MR, Quinn CT, et al. Sickle cell disease. *Hematology Am Soc Hematol Educ Program.* 2004:35.
37. Lefrere JJ, Courouce AM, Bertrand Y, et al. Human parvovirus and aplastic crisis in chronic hemolytic anemias: a study of 24 observations. *Am J Hematol.* 1986;23:271.
38. Hughes WT, Armstrong D, Bodey GP, et al. 2002 guidelines for the use of antimicrobial agents in neutropenic patients with cancer. *Clin Infect Dis.* 2002;34:730.
39. van de Wetering MD, de Witte MA, Kremer LC, et al. Efficacy of oral prophylactic antibiotics in neutropenic afebrile oncology patients: a systematic review of randomised controlled trials. *Eur J Cancer.* 2005;41:1372.
40. Gafter-Gvili A, Fraser A, Paul M, et al. Meta-analysis: antibiotic prophylaxis reduces mortality in neutropenic patients. *Ann Intern Med.* 2005;142:979.
41. Smith TJ, Khatcheressian J, Lyman GH, et al. 2006 update of recommendations for the use of white blood cell growth factors: an evidence-based clinical practice guideline. *J Clin Oncol.* 2006;24:3187.
42. Azoulay E, Darmon M, Delclaux C, et al. Deterioration of previous acute lung injury during neutropenia recovery. *Crit Care Med.* 2002;30:781.
43. Karlin L, Darmon M, Thiery G, et al. Respiratory status deterioration during G-CSF-induced neutropenia recovery. *Bone Marrow Transplant.* 2005; 36:245.
44. International Agranulocytosis and Aplastic Anemia Study. Risks of agranulocytosis and aplastic anemia: a first report of their relation to drug use with special reference to analgesics. *JAMA.* 1986;256:1749.
45. Kaufman DW, Kelly JP, Jurgelon JM, et al. Drugs in the aetiology of agranulocytosis and aplastic anaemia. *Eur J Haematol Suppl.* 1996;60:23.
46. Napolitano LM, Warkentin TE, Almahameed A, et al. Heparin-induced thrombocytopenia in the critical care setting: diagnosis and Management. *Crit Care Med.* 2006;34:1.
47. Akca S, Haji-Michael P, de Mendonca A, et al. Time course of platelet counts in critically ill patients. *Crit Care Med.* 2002;30:753.
48. Vanderschueren S, De Weerdt A, Malbrain M, et al. Thrombocytopenia and prognosis in intensive care. *Crit Care Med.* 2000;28:1871.
49. Rutherford CJ, Frenkel EP. Thrombocytopenia. Issues in diagnosis and therapy. *Med Clin North Am.* 1994;78:555.
50. Heal JM, Blumberg N. Optimizing platelet transfusion therapy. *Blood Rev.* 2004;18:149.
51. Drews RE, Weinberger SE. Thrombocytopenic disorders in critically ill patients. *Am J Respir Crit Care Med.* 2000;162(2 Pt 1):347.
52. Coppo P, Adrie C, Azoulay E, et al. Infectious diseases as a trigger in thrombotic microangiopathies in intensive care unit (ICU) patients? *Intensive Care Med.* 2003;29:564.
53. Morrin MJ, Jones FG, McConville J, et al. Thrombotic thrombocytopenic purpura secondary to Streptococcus. *Transfus Apher S.* 2006;34:153.
54. Drews RE. Critical issues in hematology: anemia, thrombocytopenia, coagulopathy, and blood product transfusions in critically ill patients. *Clin Chest Med.* 2003;24:607.
55. Warkentin TE, Chong BH, Greinacher A. Heparin-induced thrombocytopenia: towards consensus. *Thromb Haemost.* 1998;79:1.
56. Verma AK, Levine M, Shalansky SJ, et al. Frequency of heparin-induced thrombocytopenia in critical care patients. *Pharmacotherapy.* 2003;23: 745.
57. Crowther MA, Cook DJ, Meade MO, et al. Thrombocytopenia in medical-surgical critically ill patients: prevalence, incidence, and risk factors. *J Crit Care.* 2005;20:348.
58. Keeling D, Davidson S, Watson H. Haemostasis and thrombosis task force of the British committee for standards in haematology. The management of heparin-induced thrombocytopenia. *Br J Haematol.* 2006;133:259.
59. Giagounidis AA, Anhuf J, Schneider P, et al. Treatment of relapsed idiopathic thrombocytopenic purpura with the anti-CD20 monoclonal antibody rituximab: a pilot study. *Eur J Haematol.* 2002;69:95.
60. Tsai HM. Physiologic cleavage of von Willebrand factor by a plasma protease is dependent on its conformation and requires calcium ion. *Blood.* 1996;87:4235.
61. Furlan M, Robles R, Galbusera M, et al. von Willebrand factor-cleaving protease in thrombotic thrombocytopenic purpura and the hemolytic-uremic syndrome. *N Engl J Med.* 1998;339:1578.

62. Dlott JS, Danielson CF, Blue-Hnidy DE, et al. Drug-induced thrombotic thrombocytopenic purpura/hemolytic uremic syndrome: a concise review. *Ther Apher Dial.* 2004;8:102.
63. Peltz S. Severe thrombocytopenia secondary to alcohol use. *Postgrad Med.* 1991;89:75.
64. Modan B, Lilienfeld AM. Polycythemia vera and leukemia. *Medicine.* 1965; 44:305.>
65. Pearson TC, Messinezy M, Westwood N, et al. A Polycythemia Vera updated: diagnosis, pathobiology, and treatment. *Hematology Am Soc Hematol Educ Program.* 2000;:51.
66. Bellucci S, Michiels JJ. The role of JAK2 V617F mutation, spontaneous erythropoiesis and megakaryocytopoiesis, hypersensitive platelets, activated leukocytes, and endothelial cells in the etiology of thrombotic manifestations in polycythemia vera and essential thrombocythemia. *Semin Thromb Hemost.* 2006;32(4 Pt 2):381.
67. Santhosh-Kumar CR, Yohannan MD, Higgy KE, et al. Thrombocytosis in adults: analysis of 777 patients. *J Intern Med.* 1991;229:493.
68. Griesshammer M, Bangerter M, Sauer T, et al. Aetiology and clinical significance of thrombocytosis: analysis of 732 patients with an elevated platelet count. *J Intern Med.* 1999;245:295.
69. Chen HL, Chiou SS, Sheen JM, et al. Thrombocytosis in children at one medical center of southern Taiwan. *Acta Paediatr Taiwan.* 1999;40:309.
70. Gurung AM, Carr B, Smith I. Thrombocytosis in intensive care. *Br J Anaesth.* 2001;87:926.
71. Valade N, Decailliot F, Rebufat Y, et al. Thrombocytosis after trauma: incidence, aetiology, and clinical significance. *Br J Anaesth.* 2005;94:18.
72. Buss DH, Cashell AW, O'Connor ML, et al. Occurrence, etiology, and clinical significance of extreme thrombocytosis: a study of 280 cases. *Am J Med.* 1994;96:247.
73. McKee LC Jr, Collins RD. Intravascular leukocyte thrombi and aggregates as a cause of morbidity and mortality in leukemia. *Medicine.* 1974;53: 463.
74. Staudinger T, Stoiser B, Mullner M, et al. Outcome and prognostic factors in critically ill cancer patients admitted to the intensive care unit. *Crit Care Med.* 2000;28:1322.
75. Naeem N, Reed MD, Creger RJ, et al. Transfer of the hematopoietic stem cell transplant patient to the intensive care unit: does it really matter?. *Bone Marrow Transplant.* 2006;37:119.
76. Kew AK, Couban S, Patrick W, et al. Outcome of hematopoietic stem cell transplant recipients admitted to the intensive care unit. *Biol Blood Marrow Transplant.* 2006;12:301.
77. Pene F, Aubron C, Azoulay E, et al. Outcome of critically ill allogeneic hematopoietic stem-cell transplantation recipients: a reappraisal of indications for organ failure supports. *J Clin Oncol.* 2006;24:643.

CHAPTER 174 ■ ONCOLOGIC EMERGENCIES

S. ANJANI D. MATTAI • JEFFREY S. GROEGER

Cancer is the second leading cause of death in the United States, surpassed only by heart disease. Approximately one million new cases of squamous and basal skin cancers and 1,445,000 new cases of all other cancers (excluding carcinoma *in situ*, with the exception of *in situ* bladder carcinoma) are likely to be diagnosed this year. When adjusted for normal life expectancy, a 5-year relative survival rate of 66% has been calculated for all cancers diagnosed between the period of 1996 and 2002, compared to 51% between 1975 and 1977 (1). New chemotherapeutic regimens, stereotactic radiosurgery (2), hematopoietic stem cell transplantation, including cord transplantation (3), and the expansion of biologic therapy with monoclonal antibodies (4) offer hope but may lead to complications rarely seen in the nononcologic patient. It is beyond the scope of this chapter to discuss all aspects of cancer that warrant admission to an intensive care unit, and such topics as infection in the immunocompromised host, shock, coagulation abnormalities, and multisystem organ failure are discussed elsewhere in this book. Herein, we focus on clinical conditions that arise either as a direct result of a neoplasm or antineoplastic therapies.

HYPERCALCEMIA

Hypercalcemia is the most common of the paraneoplastic syndromes, developing in 10% to 30% of all patients with malignancy at some time during their disease course (5–7). Breast cancer, lung cancer, and multiple myeloma represent the most common malignancies associated with hypercalcemia (5). The presence of hypercalcemia in a patient with cancer portends an extremely poor prognosis, particularly when elevated parathyroid hormone-related protein (PTHrP) levels are detected (8,9); approximately 50% of cancer patients with hypercalcemia will die within 30 days (10).

Pathophysiology

Hypercalcemia of malignancy results from increased bone resorption and subsequent release of calcium from bone into the extracellular fluid (11). Classification is based on the mechanism by which the elevated calcium is generated, of which there are four recognized types:

1. Humoral hypercalcemia of malignancy (HHM)
2. Local osteolytic hypercalcemia
3. Tumor production of the active form of vitamin D
4. Ectopic parathyroid hormone (PTH) secretion (5)

Humoral Hypercalcemia of Malignancy (HHM)

This is the most common cause of cancer-induced hypercalcemia, seen in 80% of cases (7,12). The mechanism is mediated by parathyroid hormone-related protein (PTHrP), which is secreted into the systemic circulation by malignant tumors (12)—most frequently squamous cell carcinoma, renal cell carcinoma, ovarian and endometrial carcinomas, human T-cell lymphoma/leukemia virus (HTLV)-associated lymphomas, and breast carcinoma (5). Normally, PTHrP is expressed in many nonneoplastic adult and fetal tissues where it is involved in cell growth and differentiation but is not systemically secreted in significantly detectable levels. Because of its structural homology with parathyroid hormone at the amino terminal end, humoral PTHrP binds to PTH receptors in bone and kidney, causing an increase in bone resorption and distal tubular calcium resorption (5,13).

Local Osteolytic Hypercalcemia

Seen in about 20% of cases of malignant hypercalcemia, this form occurs when tumor cells present in bone metastases induce osteoclastic bone resorption by secreting cytokines—for example, tumor necrosis factor, interleukin-1, interleukin-6, macrophage inflammatory protein, and lymphotoxin—which, in turn, stimulate local macrophages within the tumor to differentiate into osteoclasts. Local osteolytic hypercalcemia occurs frequently in breast cancer, non–small cell lung cancer, and multiple myeloma (9).

Tumor Production of the Active Form of 1,25-dehydroxyvitamin D

Occurring in less than 1% of cases, this entity is seen in some lymphomas. The hypercalcemia is mediated by enhancement of both osteoclastic bone resorption and intestinal resorption of calcium.

Ectopic Parathyroid Hormone (PTH) Secretion

The final mechanism of hypercalcemia of malignancy is ectopic PTH secretion, which has been adequately described in only eight patients (5).

Differential Diagnosis

Malignancies and primary hyperparathyroidism account for approximately 90% of all cases of hypercalcemia and may coexist in the critically ill cancer patient (14). Among hospitalized patients, neoplastic disease is the most common cause, accounting for more than 65% of cases (15,16). Renal failure, thyrotoxicosis, granulomatous diseases such as sarcoid and tuberculosis, adrenal insufficiency, immobilization, vitamin A or D intoxication, milk alkali syndrome, familial hypocalciuric hypercalcemia, and medications such as thiazide diuretics, lithium, estrogens, and tamoxifen are also included in the differential diagnosis of hypercalcemia (16,17).

Clinical Presentation

There are multiple symptoms of hypercalcemia (Table 174.1), which are nonspecific and often attributed to coexisting chronic or terminal illness (9). In general, the symptoms correlate with the absolute concentration and the rapidity in rise of the serum calcium (18). Neurologic, gastrointestinal, renal, cardiac, and bone-related manifestations may be present. Neurologic symptoms may be mild at lower serum calcium levels or when the hypercalcemia has developed slowly. Mild drowsiness or fatigue may progress to weakness, lethargy, stupor, and eventually coma in hypercalcemic crisis or in acutely rising hypercalcemia (11). Psychotic behavior, visual and speech abnormalities, hypotonia, and occasionally localizing signs on neurologic exam, often thought to be secondary to metastatic disease, may be exhibited, and may resolve with therapy that lowers serum calcium (16,19). In older patients, neurologic dysfunction may be more pronounced even at lower concentrations of serum calcium (5).

TABLE 174.1

CLINICAL MANIFESTATIONS IN HYPERCALCEMIA

NEUROLOGIC
Drowsiness, weakness, lethargy
Stupor, coma
Psychosis
Visual and speech impairment
Focal neurologic deficits
GASTROINTESTINAL
Anorexia
Nausea, vomiting
Constipation
Abdominal pain
Peptic ulcer disease
Pancreatitis
RENAL
Nephrogenic diabetes insipidus
Acute renal failure
CARDIAC
PR interval prolongation
QRS complex widening
QT interval shortening
T wave changes
Bradyarrhythmias
Bundle branch block
AV nodal block
Cardiac arrest
BONE
Pain
Pathologic fractures

Data from Stewart AF. Hypercalcemia associated with cancer. *N Engl J Med.* 2005;352:373; Halfdanarson TR, Hogan WJ, Moynihan TJ. Oncological emergencies: diagnosis and treatment. *Mayo Clin Proc.* 2006;81(6):835; Hypercalcemia. *CancerMail from the National Cancer Institute.* http://cancerweb.ncl.ac.uk. Accessed December 11, 2006; Germano T. The parathyroid gland and calcium-related emergencies. *Top Emerg Med.* 2001;23(4):51; Bushinsky DA, Monk RD. Calcium. *Lancet.* 1998;352:306; Cogan MG, Covey GM, Arieff AL, et al. Central nervous system manifestations of hyperparathyroidism. *Am J Med.* 1978;65:963; 2005 American Heart Association Guidelines for Cardiopulmonary Resuscitation and Emergency Cardiovascular Care. *Circulation.* 2005;112(24 Suppl):IV1–121; and Berensen JR. Treatment of hypercalcemeia with bisphosphonates. *Semin Oncol.* 2002:29(6 Suppl 21):12.

Gastrointestinal symptoms are related to smooth muscle hypotonicity and include anorexia, nausea, vomiting, constipation, and abdominal pain (11). Infrequently, hypercalcemia may present as peptic ulcer disease (18) and pancreatitis (20).

Renal manifestations result from the impairment of renal water-concentrating ability because antidiuretic hormone (ADH) secretion is inhibited by hypercalcemia. Subsequent dehydration decreases the glomerular filtration rate and reduces renal excretion of excess serum calcium. To expand the extracellular volume, compensatory proximal tubular resorption of sodium and calcium occurs, leading to a paradoxical increase in serum calcium (21). Frank renal failure may ensue, particularly in the patient with multiple myeloma (11). In contradistinction to primary hyperparathyroidism, hypercalcemia of malignancy is rarely associated with nephrolithiasis and nephrocalcinosis, because hypercalciuria must be chronic for these renal manifestations to occur (11,14).

Cardiovascular symptoms of hypercalcemia are marked by increased myocardial contractility and irritability (11). Electrocardiographic changes include a PR-interval prolongation, QRS-complex widening, QT-interval shortening, and T-wave changes (16). At increasing serum calcium levels, patients may experience bradyarrhythmias and bundle branch block, with progression to AV nodal block and cardiac arrest at serum concentrations of 18 mg/dL (11).

Finally, the bone symptoms of hypercalcemia, which include pathologic fractures and pain, can be attributed to osteolytic metastases or humorally mediated bone resorption (11).

Diagnosis

Calcium is present in the extracellular fluid (ECF) in three fractions: (i) 50% is the ionized free fraction, (ii) 40% is protein bound (primarily to albumin) and is not renally filtered, and (iii) 10% is complexed to anions (18). Hypercalcemia is diagnosed by measuring the ionized calcium level, as this is the biologically active level that correlates with the signs and symptoms of hypercalcemia. Except in the presence of hypoalbuminemia, the ionized calcium level can be inferred from the total plasma calcium. In cancer patients, hypoalbuminemia is common, and the total plasma calcium must be corrected to reflect the calcium level that would have been measured as if the albumin were in the normal range. In general, for each 1 g/dL decrease in serum albumin, there is a 0.8 mg/dL decrease in serum calcium. This method of calculation is inaccurate in the presence of calcium-binding immunoglobulins, as seen in multiple myeloma. This circumstance warrants measurement of the ionized calcium level because the total serum calcium level may significantly overestimate the ionized fraction (11). Although ionized calcium concentrations increase with acidosis and decrease with alkalosis, these changes are relatively small and do not lead to clinically significant events (22).

Once the diagnosis of hypercalcemia is confirmed by obtaining corrected calcium levels, measurement of the intact PTH level—suppressed in hypercalcemia of malignancy and elevated in primary hyperparathyroidism—is often necessary to differentiate among the mechanisms of hypercalcemia. PTH lowers serum phosphate and increases serum chloride concentrations (14). A low serum chloride (less than 100 mEq/L) suggests hypercalcemia of malignancy, whereas elevation of serum chloride is caused by hyperchloremic acidosis resulting from PTH-induced renal bicarbonate loss seen in hyperparathyroidism (9). Ectopic hyperparathyroidism is an extremely rare cause of malignant hypercalcemia, and elevations in PTH levels are more likely to indicate concomitant primary hyperparathyroidism in cancer patients with hypercalcemia (21). In contrast to PTH level measurement, determination of the serum PTHrP concentration is not routine. However, it may be useful in identifying the mechanism of hypercalcemia. For example, PTHrP levels are low in patients with primary hyperparathyroidism but high in patients with either HHM alone or concomitant primary hyperparathyroidism and malignant hypercalcemia (12,23). PTHrP has also been used in evaluating the response to bisphosphonate therapy; patients with PTHrP levels above 12 pmol/L were reported to be less responsive to pamidronate and more likely to develop recurrent hypercalcemia within 14 days (24).

Treatment

The only effective long-term means of reversing malignancy-associated hypercalcemia is reduction in tumor burden (Table 174.2); antihypercalcemic therapy is a temporizing measure that does not affect survival (5). The aggressiveness of the therapeutic approach depends on the potential for palliation and cure. When all antitumor strategies have failed, or in patients who do not wish to pursue further treatment of their cancer, an ethical, humane, and appropriate approach may involve withholding antihypercalcemic treatment (5,9). Stewart (5) has classified hypercalcemia based on serum calcium levels into mild hypercalcemia (10.5–11.9 mg/dL), moderate hypercalcemia (12.0–13.9 mg/dL), and severe hypercalcemia (14.0 mg/dL or greater) as a guide to therapeutic interventions. In addition to the magnitude of hypercalcemia, the severity of symptoms and the cause of hypercalcemia are other important factors in formulating an appropriate treatment strategy. In general, severe hypercalcemia requires emergent, aggressive treatment in the presence or absence of symptoms, whereas interventions in mild to moderate hypercalcemia are contingent on the severity of the symptoms. Prior to initiating therapy, the clinician should assess the patient for correctable factors that may contribute to hypercalcemia. Exogenous sources of calcium such as calcium-containing intravenous fluids, parenteral nutrition, and oral calcium supplements should be removed. In addition, thiazide diuretics, vitamins A and D, calcitriol, lithium, and estrogens or antiestrogens used as therapy for breast carcinoma should be discontinued (11). Immobilization is a well-established cause of hypercalcemia, and weight-bearing ambulation is recommended whenever possible (25). Finally, in the presence of hypophosphatemia, hypercalcemia becomes more difficult to treat. Hypophosphatemia is frequently observed in cancer patients for multiple reasons including poor nutrition, saline diuresis, PTHrP effects, use of antacids and loop diuretics, and hypercalcemia itself. Oral or nasogastric phosphate supplementation should be administered to keep the calcium-phosphate product between 30 and 40. Intravenous phosphorous replacement may precipitate hypocalcemia, seizures, and acute renal failure, and is reserved for patients in whom oral or nasogastric administration cannot be performed (5).

Fluids and Diuretics

The initial intervention in the treatment of hypercalcemia is the administration of isotonic saline at a rate of 200 to 500 mL/hour based on the degree of hypovolemia and renal and cardiovascular dysfunction (5). Once the fluid deficit is replaced, the infusion rate should be decreased to 100 to 200 mL/hour in patients without cardiac or renal impairment (20). The patient must be carefully monitored to prevent fluid overload. Saline hydration reduces serum calcium level by increasing the glomerular filtration rate and increasing calcium delivery to the proximal tubule where urinary calcium excretion is augmented by the calciuric effects of saline (5).

TABLE 174.2

TREATMENT OF HYPERCALCEMIA OF MALIGNANCY

DEFINITIVE TREATMENT	
Antitumor therapy to reduce tumor burden	
INITIAL TREATMENT	
Removal of exogenous calcium sources:	
Intravenous fluids parenteral nutrition, oral calcium supplements, thiazide diuretics, vitamins A and D, calcitriol, lithium, estrogens, antiestrogens	
Weight-bearing ambulation	
Phosphate repletion	
Fluids and diuresis	
Saline hydration	
Loop diuretics	Judicious use in euvolemic or hypervolemic patients; now less favorable because of hypokalemia, hypomagnesemia, volume depletion
PHARMACOLOGIC TREATMENT	
Bisphosphonate therapy	
Principal agents in hypercalcemic treatment	
Zoledronate	15-min infusion
Pamidronate	2-h infusion
	Bisphosphonate adverse effects: Acute and chronic renal failure, fever arthralgias, ocular inflammation, electrolyte imbalance, osteonecrosis of the jaw
Other Agents	
Calcitonin	Useful in congestive heart failure or renal failure
Glucocorticoids	Used in lymphomas with elevated levels of 1, 25-vitamin D
Mithramycin	Use limited by adverse effects: Thrombocytopenia, anemia, leukopenia, renal failure
Gallium nitrate	Use limited by 5-day continuous infusion, nephrotoxicity
DIALYSIS	
For patients with renal failure or congestive heart failure	

Data from Stewart AF. Hypercalcemia associated with cancer. *N Engl J Med.* 2005;352:373; Halfdanarson TR, Hogan WJ, Moynihan TJ. Oncological emergencies: diagnosis and treatment. *Mayo Clin Proc.* 2006;81(6):835; Hypercalcemia. *CancerMail from the National Cancer Institute.* http://cancerweb.ncl.ac.uk. Accessed December 11, 2006; Germano T. The parathyroid gland and calcium-related emergencies. *Topics in Emerg Med.* 2001;23(4):51; Bushinsky DA, Monk RD. Calcium. *Lancet* 1998;352:306; Cheng C, Chou C, Lin S. An unrecognized cause of recurrent hypercalcemia: immobilization. *South Med J.* 2006;99(4):371; Body JJ. Hypercalcemia of malignancy. *Semin Nephrol.* 2004;24:48; Berenson JR, Lipton A. Bisphosphonates in the treatment of malignant bone disease. *Annu Rev Med.* 1999;50:237; and Tanveyanon T, Stiff PJ. Management of the adverse effects associated with intravenous bisphosphonates. *Ann Oncol.* 2006;(17):897.

Loop diuretics inhibit calcium reabsorption at the loop of Henle, and, hence, also increase calciuresis. These agents should be used judiciously and only after euvolemia is achieved in hypovolemic patients or in patients who present with volume overload (5,9,16). Because of ensuing complications such as hypokalemia, hypomagnesemia, and volume depletion, and because of the availability of bisphosphonates, loop diuretics are used less favorably in clinical practice (26).

Bisphosphonate Therapy

Bisphosphonates inhibit osteoclastic bone resorption and are the principal agents used in the management of hypercalcemia of malignancy (27). When compared to saline and diuretics alone, and other antiresorptive agents including calcitonin, bisphosphonates are superior in treating hypercalcemia of malignancy (5). Because only 1% to 2% of oral bisphosphonates are absorbed, these drugs are administered intravenously (7). Pamidronate, and zoledronate are the most commonly used bisphosphonates, and are the two agents that have been approved by the Food and Drug Administration (FDA) for the treatment of hypercalcemia of malignancy. Clodronate and ibandronate are available in Europe and other countries. Patients respond to bisphosphonate therapy within 2 to 4 days, with a nadir in serum calcium occurring within 4 to 7 days; normocalcemia may persist for 2 to 4 weeks (5,18). Compared to pamidronate, zoledronate is 850 times more potent and is more efficacious, although this increased efficacy is of unclear clinical significance (9,28). In a pooled analysis of two randomized controlled trials comparing a single 4-mg dose of zoledronic acid to a 90-mg dose of pamidronate, serum calcium concentrations normalized within 10 days in 88% versus 70% of patients, respectively, and the duration of response was 32 days versus 18 days, respectively, within the two groups (28). Although pamidronate may be the less expensive of the two agents, zoledronate can be administered over a shorter interval of 15 minutes, making it advantageous in the outpatient setting; pamidronate requires a 2-hour infusion. Both zoledronate and pamidronate have been associated with acute and chronic renal failure, with more adverse events reported with zoledronate. Dose reduction of zoledronate is recommended in patients with a creatinine clearance between 30 and 60 mL/minute; however, the American Society of Clinical Oncology does not recommend changing the dose or infusion rate of pamidronate in patients with a serum creatinine of less than 3 mg/dL (5,29). Other complications of bisphosphonates include acute systemic inflammatory reactions such as fever and arthralgias, as well as ocular inflammation, electrolyte imbalance, and osteonecrosis of the jaw (29).

Other Agents

Calcitonin is a well-tolerated synthetic polypeptide analogue of salmon calcitonin, which reduces serum calcium levels by inhibiting bone resorption. When administered subcutaneously or intramuscularly, it produces a rapid but transient decrease in serum calcium levels within 12 to 24 hours (5,9). This agent is useful in patients with congestive heart failure or renal failure where saline, diuresis, and bisphosphonates may be contraindicated. Tachyphylaxis may occur with continued use (7). Glucocorticoids are effective in decreasing serum calcium in hypercalcemia of malignancy associated with some lymphomas, particularly Hodgkin lymphoma. Elevated levels of 1,25-vitamin D are present in Hodgkin's lymphoma (7); glucocorticoids, in addition to increasing renal calcium excretion, block vitamin D–mediated calcium absorption in the gastrointestinal tract (11). These agents have limited utility in the acute setting because a reduction in serum calcium may not be observed for 1 to 2 weeks (11). Mithramycin, an inhibitor of osteoclast RNA synthesis and formerly a first-line hypocalcemic agent, has serious adverse effects including thrombocytopenia, anemia, leukopenia, and renal failure (5). Gallium nitrate has the disadvantage of requiring continuous infusion over 5 days and has potential nephrotoxicity. Finally, dialysis may be used to treat patients with hypercalcemia complicated by renal failure or congestive heart failure (5,18).

ACUTE TUMOR LYSIS SYNDROME

Definition

Acute tumor lysis syndrome (ATLS) occurs as a consequence of the rapid and massive destruction of tumor cells resulting in the release of intracellular metabolites into the circulation in quantities sufficient to exceed renal excretory capacity (30,31). The four biochemical disturbances generated by this process that characterize the syndrome are life threatening (32):

1. Hyperkalemia
2. Hyperphosphatemia
3. Hypocalcemia
4. Hyperuricemia

These metabolic abnormalities have widespread adverse effects on the cardiac, musculoskeletal, nervous, and renal systems.

Acute tumor lysis syndrome is most frequently observed after the administration of cytotoxic chemotherapy in patients with high-grade hematologic malignancies—classically, Burkitt's lymphoma and acute lymphocytic leukemia (ALL) (7,33,34). The incidence of clinically significant ATLS in non-Hodgkin's lymphoma and ALL has been reported as 6% (35) and 5.2% (7), respectively. Metabolic derangements in these patients may develop within a few hours to a few days after initiating chemotherapy (7,36). Other malignancies in which ATLS has been described include chronic leukemia, low-grade lymphoma, and, rarely, multiple solid tumors such as metastatic breast carcinoma, lung carcinoma, seminoma, thymoma, medulloblastoma, ovarian carcinoma, rhabdomyosarcoma, melanoma, vulvar carcinoma, and Merkel cell carcinoma (31). The syndrome can also occur after radiation therapy, immunotherapy (rituximab and interferon), and endocrine therapy (corticosteroids and tamoxifen) (7,31,33). Spontaneous tumor lysis syndrome (STLS) is a rare entity that develops primarily in Burkitt's lymphoma and leukemia in the absence of any treatment. The increased purine metabolism from high tumor cell turnover rates in these malignancies leads to hyperuricemia and consequent uric acid nephropathy (37,38). Prompt recognition of STLS is essential because it is associated with poor outcomes and high mortality rates (38). Predisposing factors for developing ATLS include large tumor burdens (33), bulky lymphadenopathy (7), extensive bone marrow involvement (33), rapid tumor cell proliferation, leukocytosis (more than 50×10^3 cells/μL) (31), elevated lactate dehydrogenase (LDH) (more than 1,500 IU) (33), and high tumor chemosensitivity (7,32). Pretreatment hyperuricemia, renal dysfunction, and hypovolemia, as well as treatment with nephrotoxic agents, also confer an increased risk of ATLS (31).

Pathophysiology

Rapid dissolution of cells with aggressive cytotoxic therapy results in an increase in plasma uric acid, potassium, and phosphorus levels. The hyperphosphatemia, in turn, precipitates secondary hypocalcemia. Hyperkalemia occurs 6 to 72 hours after the administration of chemotherapy (36). Associated manifestations include lethargy, nausea, vomiting, diarrhea, muscle weakness, paresthesias, and electrocardiographic abnormalities such as peaked T waves, PR-interval prolongation, and QRS-complex widening. Ventricular arrhythmias may lead to sudden death (7,31).

Hyperphosphatemia is seen 24 to 48 hours following chemotherapy (36). Malignant cells may contain up to four times more phosphorous than nonneoplastic cells, and, as plasma phosphorous increases with cell lysis, the normal renal mechanism that excretes excess phosphate and prevents distal tubular reabsorption becomes overwhelmed, leading to hyperphosphatemia (39). Signs and symptoms of acute hyperphosphatemia are manifestations of secondary hypocalcemia, and range from no symptoms to anorexia, vomiting, confusion, neuromuscular irritability, tetany, carpopedal spasm, seizures, dysrhythmias, and cardiac arrest (7,31). Secondary hypocalcemia occurs in association with hyperphosphatemia because when the calcium phosphate product exceeds 60, calcium phosphate precipitates into tissues, including the renal interstitium and tubules, resulting in nephrocalcinosis (32). However, hypocalcemia may persist even after correction of hyperphosphatemia when an inappropriately low plasma calcitriol level is present (40). Hypocalcemia itself causes a rise in serum parathyroid hormone, which, in turn, increases phosphate resorption in the proximal tubule, leading to nephrocalcinosis and acute renal failure (7).

Hyperuricemia occurs 48 to 72 hours after chemotherapy (36). Patients may exhibit nonspecific symptoms such as nausea, vomiting, anorexia, and lethargy. Acute renal failure with associated oliguria, edema, hypertension, and altered sensorium will be seen in untreated patients (33). Uric acid is generated from purine metabolism in the liver. Adenosine and guanosine nucleotides are degraded to hypoxanthine and xanthine, respectively, and xanthine oxidase converts these products to uric acid (7). Rapidly proliferating neoplastic cells have high turnover rates with accelerated purine catabolism from DNA and RNA degradation (41), and these cells contain large amounts of purine nucleotides; consequently, with cytotoxic therapy, there is a rapid rise in plasma uric acid (33). Uric acid is excreted by the kidneys through the processes of glomerular filtration, partial proximal tubular reabsorption, and distal tubular secretion (32). The clearance of uric acid is independently proportional to intravascular volume status (31) and the urinary flow rate (32), and may be significantly reduced in the presence of dehydration or tubular obstruction from acute nephrocalcinosis or uric acid nephropathy. Uric acid nephropathy develops when uric acid crystals deposit in the renal tubules and collecting ducts because of acidic conditions. The urinary pKa of uric acid is 5.4, and the luminal pH of the distal tubules and collecting ducts is 5.0, resulting in the poor solubility of uric acid in acidic urine (7). This poor solubility, coupled with the marked hyperuricosuria present in ATLS, leads to uric acid precipitation, intraluminal obstruction, oliguria, and acute renal failure (7,42). Acute renal failure (ARF) in ATLS may also be mediated by renal calculi from phosphate and uric acid precipitation (31), as well as from ischemic acute tubular necrosis caused by renal hypoperfusion (33). Drug toxicity, sepsis, and tumor-associated obstructive uropathy or renal parenchymal infiltration may exacerbate ATLS-induced ARF (39).

Classification

Although no widely accepted definition of ATLS currently exists, Hande and Garrow (35) first classified ATLS into laboratory TLS and clinical TLS. Cairo and Bishop (39) have modified and further developed this classification system into the Cairo-Bishop definition, which uses laboratory and clinical data in conjunction with a grading scale to assess the severity of ATLS. Laboratory TLS (LTLS) is defined as two or more of the following metabolic abnormalities occurring 3 days before or 7 days after chemotherapy: uric acid 8 mg/dL or greater, potassium 6 mg/dL or greater, phosphorous 6.5 mg/dL or greater, or a 25% increase in baseline levels of these metabolites, and calcium 7 mg/dL or less, or a 25% decrease from baseline level. Clinical tumor lysis syndrome is defined as LTLS in addition to one or more of the following findings: increased serum creatinine (1.5 times the upper limit of normal), cardiac arrhythmia/sudden death, or seizure. The grading of ATLS from 0 through 5 is determined by the presence or absence of LTLS, the degree of serum creatinine elevation, and the presence and severity of the cardiac arrhythmia and seizure (39).

Prevention and Treatment

Early recognition of patients at high risk for ATLS is an essential component of the management strategy so that appropriate prophylactic interventions can be instituted.

Fluids and Alkalinization

Except in patients at risk for congestive heart failure, aggressive intravenous hydration with isotonic or hypotonic saline (42) is the single most important intervention for both prevention and treatment of ATLS. Cytotoxic therapy should be delayed whenever possible to administer appropriate hydration (7,42). Intravenous hydration should commence 2 days before and for 2 to 3 days after chemotherapy (31,33) at a rate of 3,000 mL/m^2 per day (7,9,39), or two to four times the daily fluid maintenance requirement to achieve a urine output of 100 mL/m^2/hr or greater (31,39). Aggressive administration of intravenous fluid increases the intravascular volume, renal blood flow, glomerular filtration rate, and urinary flow rate, resulting in correction of electrolyte derangements by dilution of the extracellular fluid and prevention of phosphate and uric acid precipitation by increasing urinary excretion of these metabolites (31,33,39). Volume expansion alone may be insufficient to maintain adequate urine output, necessitating the administration of diuretics. Once euvolemia is achieved, and no signs of acute obstructive uropathy are present, a dose of furosemide—0.5 to 1 mg/kg or 2 to 4 mg/kg for severe oliguria or anuria—may induce or improve urine output (35). The effectiveness of furosemide is diminished in the setting of uric acid precipitation in the renal tubules; in this circumstance, mannitol, at a dose of 0.5 mg/kg, may be administered.

Alkalinization of the urine to a pH 7.0 or greater remains controversial (7,9,39). This practice is based on the biochemical properties of uric acid, that is, uric acid is 13 times more soluble at pH 7.0 than at pH 5.0 (32), maximal solubility of uric acid is attained at pH 7.5, and urine alkalinization (pH 6.5 or greater) enhances renal excretion of uric acid (39). What limits this approach is that calcium phosphate precipitation increases with systemic alkalinization, exacerbating nephrocalcinosis (7,31). Additionally, hypoxanthine and xanthine solubility are substantially reduced, leading to xanthine nephropathy with concurrent allopurinol therapy (9,31,39).

Management of Hyperuricemia

Allopurinol reduces the risk of ATLS when administered 2 to 3 days prior to chemotherapy by inhibiting the production of uric acid (9). Allopurinol is both a synthetic structural analogue of the purine base, hypoxanthine, and a competitive inhibitor of xanthine oxidase (33), and, therefore, in the presence of allopurinol, xanthine oxidase cannot catalyze the conversion of hypoxanthine to xanthine and xanthine to uric acid (31). Allopurinol is administered orally at 300 to 800 mg daily (10 mg/kg per day or up to 400 mg/m^2 per day) in one to three divided doses, and should be titrated to uric acid level. Intravenous allopurinol was approved by the FDA in 1999 and can be administered in doses of 200 to 400 mg/m^2 per day (maximum 600 mg/day) in patients unable to tolerate oral medications, although the cost per day ranges between $400 and $1,000 (7,43). Dose adjustment of allopurinol is required for reduced creatinine clearance (7,43). There are several limitations with allopurinol therapy:

1. A reduction in serum uric acid level is not seen before 48 to 72 hours after initiating allopurinol because the drug inhibits the synthesis of uric acid but does not affect the pretreatment uric acid concentration (7).

2. Inhibition of xanthine oxidase by allopurinol leads to increased plasma levels of xanthine and hypoxanthine, which may precipitate in the renal tubules (33).
3. Three percent of patients develop hypersensitivity reactions, including Stevens-Johnson syndrome.
4. Allopurinol intevracts with many drugs, including chemotherapeutic agents such as cyclosporine and azathioprine (42).

Another agent that lowers uric acid concentration is urate oxidase. Urate oxidase converts uric acid to allantoin, which is five to ten times more soluble in urine than uric acid. Present in many mammalian species, urate oxidase is not expressed in human beings as a result of a nonsense mutation in the coding region during hominoid evolution (44). A nonrecombinant form of urate oxidase was first obtained from *Aspergillus flavus* and has been used in France (1975) and Italy (1984) for treatment of hyperuricemia. Subsequently, a recombinant urate oxidase, rasburicase, was developed because of the 4.5% of hypersensitivity reactions that occurred with the nonrecombinant form (7,31,33,42). Rasburicase was FDA approved in 2002 for use in pediatric patients at risk for ATLS (44). An injectable dose of 0.15 to 0.20 mg/kg normalizes uric acid levels within 4 hours of administration in children and adults (7,42). This dose may be repeated daily for a total of 5 days, and chemotherapy should be initiated 4 to 24 hours after the first dose. In addition to being more effective than allopurinol in reducing pretreatment and posttreatment uric acid levels, rasburicase does not generate increased xanthine and hypoxanthine levels, thereby minimizing the risk of uric acid nephropathy that may be seen with allopurinol use (7,31,42). Of note, rasburicase is contraindicated in patients with glucose-6-phosphate dehydrogenase (G6PD) deficiency. Bronchospasm and anaphylaxis may rarely occur with rasburicase therapy (45). There is insufficient evidence that rasburicase reduces the incidence of dialysis in ATLS, and because a 5-day course of therapy is approximately 2,000 to 3,000 times more expensive than a 5-day course of oral allopurinol (7,43), cost-effectiveness must be considered in formulating a treatment plan.

Correction of Electrolyte Abnormalities

Because of the potential for life-threatening arrhythmias, prompt recognition of electrolyte derangements is imperative. Laboratory monitoring should be performed every 4 to 6 hours in the first 24 hours of chemotherapy in patients at high risk for ATLS, and then every 6 to 8 hours thereafter (42). A baseline electrocardiogram (ECG) should be obtained to assess for cardiac effects related to electrolyte abnormalities. Hyperkalemia is treated with calcium gluconate to stabilize the cardiac membrane and with intravenous insulin/dextrose and inhaled $beta_2$ agonists to facilitate intracellular shift of potassium. Although sodium bicarbonate may also shift potassium intracellularly by improving the metabolic acidosis, its use may result in inappropriate volume expansion. Potassium binding resins such as sodium polystyrene sulfate increase potassium elimination in the gastrointestinal (GI) tract and have a delayed hypokalemic effect. Diuretics can be administered to reduce serum potassium in patients without renal failure. When acute renal failure occurs, dialysis may be required to emergently reduce serum potassium. Asymptomatic hypocalcemia should be left untreated to preclude calcium phosphate precipitation; however, symptomatic hypocalcemia is managed with intravenous calcium gluconate. Treatment of hyperphosphatemia with oral phosphate binders such as aluminum hydroxide or aluminum carbonate will usually concurrently correct the hypocalcemia (7,31).

Dialysis

Dialysis is indicated in patients with marked elevations in serum uric acid, phosphate, and potassium that do not respond to aggressive treatment, and in patients with ARF with volume overload, severe uremia, or acidosis (31,33,39). Hemodialysis is used in ATLS because it is superior to peritoneal dialysis in the clearance of both uric acid and phosphorous (31,39).

OBSTRUCTIVE SYNDROMES

Superior Vena Cava Syndrome

Definition

Superior vena cava syndrome (SVCS) describes the set of signs and symptoms associated with obstruction of the superior vena cava, which may be caused by extrinsic compression, vascular invasion, or intraluminal thrombosis of the vein (46–48). The SVC is a thin-walled, compliant, low-pressure middle mediastinal vessel, rendering it easily vulnerable to disease processes in the adjacent right lung, the paratracheal and perihilar lymph nodes, the mainstem bronchi, the esophagus, and the thoracic spinal cord (48,49).

First described by William Hunter (50) in 1757 in a patient with an aortic aneurysm secondary to syphilis, SVCS was—prior to the widespread use of antibiotics—primarily a complication of infectious diseases, as seen in syphilitic aortitis, histoplasmosis-induced fibrosing mediastinitis, and tuberculous mediastinitis (51,52). Currently, malignancy is the most common cause of SVCS. The percentage of cases attributable to cancer varies widely in the literature from 78% (48,53) to as high as 90% to 97% (54–57). A more recent retrospective study, reviewing the outcome of 78 patients over 5 years, reported malignancy as the cause of SVCS in 60% of the patients, with an increasing proportion of benign causes related to the presence of intravascular devices, e.g., central venous catheters and pacemaker wires (71%) (58). Other benign causes of SVCS include fibrosing mediastinitis from prior irradiation or histoplasmosis, aortic dissection, and complications of surgery, such as aortic dissection repair (54,58). Bronchogenic carcinoma accounts for 85% to 90% of the malignancies in which SVCS presents (54,57). Overall, SVCS develops in 2% to 10% of lung malignancies (47,52,56,59,60), and the risk of SVCS is higher in small cell lung cancer, with an incidence of 6.6% to 12% (59) because it involves the central mediastinal structures. In addition, because of the anatomic location of the SVC, right-sided lung cancers cause SVCS four times as often as left-sided lung cancers (56). Other neoplasms include malignant lymphomas; although Hodgkin's lymphoma more often involves the mediastinum, it rarely causes SVCS (48,54). Primary germ cell cancers, thymoma, mesothelioma (60), and metastatic disease (primarily breast carcinoma) constitute a small proportion of SVCS cases (54,58,60).

Clinical Presentation

SVCS may be the initial presentation of bronchogenic carcinoma and lymphoma, or may arise in patients with previously documented malignancy (53,58). The severity of signs and symptoms depends on the extent, location, and rapidity of onset of the SVC occlusion (55). In general, obstruction within or below the azygos vein results in more dramatic symptoms. Normally, azygos venous capacity increases from 11% to 35% to augment drainage of the head and neck (47), but impedance of flow from obstruction precludes this auxiliary function (47,54,60). With slowly developing SVCS, collateral vessels in the chest wall and upper extremities are recruited as a diversion for the existing SVC engorgement; hence, SVCS in this population is of insidious onset, as in fibrosing mediastinitis (55). The most commonly reported symptom in SVCS is dyspnea followed by head and facial swelling (48,58). Other cardiopulmonary symptoms include cough, orthopnea, and chest pain. Associated signs are neck and arm vein distention, plethora or cyanosis of the head and neck (48), venous collateralization in the arms and upper chest wall (54), and chronic pleural effusions (54,55). More extensive airway or vascular obstruction is predicted when positional maneuvers such as lying supine or leaning forward exacerbate respiratory or cardiac symptoms; for example, respiratory insufficiency in the supine position worsens as the weight of the mediastinal structures impinges on the tracheobronchial tree. In the substantially compromised patient with SVCS, cardiopulmonary arrest may ensue simply with the administration of sedatives and general anesthesia (54). Other head and neck signs and symptoms range from conjunctival and periorbital edema, nasal congestion, dysphagia, and hoarseness due to laryngeal nerve compression (61) to proptosis, glossal edema, stridor secondary to laryngeal edema, and tracheal obstruction (54,55). Patients with central nervous system (CNS) manifestations may exhibit mild headaches, dizziness, and lethargy with progression to syncope (in rapidly developing or complete SVC obstruction) seizures, or coma (from cerebral edema and increased intracranial pressure) (47,54). Bleeding complications such as epistaxis, hemoptysis (54), and gastrointestinal hemorrhage from esophageal varices (in long-standing SVC) (55) may occur.

Diagnostic Investigations

Imaging. Once the clinical diagnosis of SVC syndrome is suspected, confirmation can be obtained using both radiologic and nuclide techniques. Chest radiography reveals widening of the superior mediastinum in approximately 60% of patients (53,54,56) and pleural effusions, most frequently right-sided, in up to 25% of patients (48,54). A normal chest radiograph does not exclude the diagnosis. Contrast-enhanced helical computed tomography (CT) accurately delineates the site, extent, and cause of the occlusion (56,60), as well as any associated thrombus and collateral vessel development (60). The radiologic diagnosis of SVCS is made by demonstrating both decreased or absent venous opacification below the level of obstruction and prominent collateral vessel opacification (56). MRI is an alternative imaging method in patients with iodinated contrast allergy or without adequate venous access for contrast administration, but offers no distinct advantage over CT (48,54,62). Venography is most useful when planning bypass or stenting procedures (48,60). Although venography is superior to CT in identifying the site and extent of obstruction and in mapping the collateral circulation, it does not elucidate the underlying cause of the SVCS (62), unless SVC thrombosis alone is the causative factor (52,56,60). Radionuclide ^{99m}technetium venography is a less invasive alternative to standard venography but lacks the image resolution of the latter (48). Although not a well-established diagnostic modality in clinical practice, helical CT phlebography, which involves simultaneous bilateral antecubital vein injection with intravenous contrast, produces both detailed CT images of the mediastinum and a CT venogram that correlates well with digital venography. Flow artifact (inhomogeneous contrast opacification) created by physiologic mixing of contrast-opacified and nonopacified blood may mimic intraluminal filling defects in patent vessels and remains the major limitation of this technique (62).

Histiologic Diagnosis. Sputum cytology, thoracentesis, percutaneous needle biopsy, bronchoscopy, mediastinoscopy, or thoracotomy are all methods used to obtain pathologic specimens. The diagnostic yields are as follows: bronchoscopy, 50% to 70%; transthoracic needle aspiration biopsy, 75%; mediastinoscopy or mediastinotomy, greater than 90% (63). Historically, the treatment practice was to administer emergent radiotherapy for SVCS without establishing a histiologic diagnosis. This strategy was predicated on the following beliefs: SVCS was a life-threatening emergency necessitating immediate intervention; invasive diagnostic procedures were associated with a high risk of morbidity, including bleeding and anesthetic complications; and unresectable lung malignancy was the most probable cause of the SVCS (46,56,59). Presently, it is well established that in the absence of tracheal obstruction or severe laryngeal or cerebral edema, SVCS itself results in no life-threatening complications (59,60,64–66); that invasive investigative procedures such as percutaneous needle biopsy, bronchoscopy, mediastinoscopy, and thoracotomy can be performed safely and with minimal bleeding risk; and that forgoing a pathologic diagnosis is unjustified, except in severe airway obstruction or cerebral edema (56,58,67,68), because identification of the underlying condition guides appropriate treatment of the SVCS in both benign and malignant disease.

Treatment

The primary goals of treatment are symptom relief and eradication or palliation of the underlying malignancy. Initial symptomatic management involves bed rest, head elevation to reduce venous pressure, and supplemental oxygen administration. Diuretics and sodium restriction may decrease edema, but reports are anecdotal. Use of glucocorticoids to minimize inflammatory responses to tumor or radiotherapy (XRT) is controversial (48,56), but steroids are a mainstay of treatment in non-Hodgkin lymphoma (NHL) (54,56).

Endovascular Stenting. If these conservative measures are ineffectual in controlling symptoms, a percutaneously placed endovascular stent can be inserted with or without balloon angioplasty (56). In recent studies, relief of symptoms occurred immediately after stent placement in 80% to 95% of patients with few complications (69,70). A systematic review of the literature found that morbidity increased with stent insertion if thrombolytics were administered. One group advocates stent insertion as a first-line therapy for symptom relief because, after placement, symptoms were rapidly alleviated in 18/18 patients, enabling all to begin XRT the following day (71). In a study involving 52 patients with non–small cell lung cancer (NSCLC) and SVCS, immediate symptom relief permitted patients to receive the appropriate hydration required with full doses of platinum therapy (69). Recurrence of SVCS occurs in 10% to 30% of patients after primary therapy with chemotherapy and/or radiation, and, in these cases, stent placement may be used for palliation (56,72).

Thrombolysis. With the increased use of intravascular devices, thrombus now accounts for a larger proportion of the benign causes of SVCS (58). When SVC syndrome is attributable to thrombosis of a central venous catheter, and catheter preservation is desired, thrombolytic therapy given within 5 days of symptom onset is associated with an 88% success rate versus 25% after 5 days (56,72).

Radiotherapy and Chemotherapy. The treatment modality selected should be individualized to the type of malignancy, stage, and performance status of each patient (52,60). Primary management of solid tumors and NSCLC involves XRT. NSCLC associated with SVCS carries a poor prognosis, with 1-year survival in one series 17% (48,73), and a review of 1,635 patients showed a median survival of 5 months (74). The treatment of choice in NSCLC is XRT and possible stent insertion (48). Within 72 hours of XRT, patients have relief of symptoms, and within 2 weeks, 70% to 90% of patients are symptom free (56). In a large systematic review, 60% of the NSCLC patients had relief of SVCS after chemotherapy and/or radiotherapy, and SVCS recurred in 19% (60).

Chemotherapy prolongs survival and improves quality of life in patients with small cell lung cancer (SCLC), and addition of thoracic irradiation may reduce the recurrence risk of SVCS. In the aforementioned systematic review, SVCS was relieved in 77% of patients receiving chemotherapy and/or radiation, with relapse in 17% of patients (60). Lymphoma and germ cell tumors are usually treated with chemotherapy based on the histiologic type, grade, and stage of the disease. In Hodgkin's lymphoma, chemotherapy followed by XRT to areas of bulky disease may be indicated (56). In non-Hodgkin's lymphoma, XRT alone may be used in early-stage disease, and chemotherapy is the treatment for higher-stage tumors. Whether to irradiate areas of bulky disease in NHL after chemotherapeutic remission is less clear; however, with residual tumor or progression of disease after chemotherapy, radiotherapy is administered (56).

Surgery. Surgical bypass of the obstruction with vein grafts or prosthetic grafts may be appropriate in patients with benign causes of SVCS. In patients with malignancy, surgical intervention, when no further treatment options are possible, at best, is a palliative measure with poor long-term survival (56,55).

ACUTE AIRWAY OBSTRUCTION

Oropharyngeal and Tracheal Obstruction

Sudden upper airway obstruction (UAO) of the larynx, pharynx, or extrathoracic trachea is uncommon with cancers of the head and neck. Tumors of the larynx, pharynx, base of tongue, and thyroid are primarily slow growing and, as they progressively enlarge, obvious signs and symptoms of airway compromise are usually evident prior to the development of acute obstruction (75); tracheal masses, which take years to be discovered, first become symptomatic when the airway lumen is narrowed by 75% (76). Mechanisms of UAO include direct tracheal invasion as well as extrinsic tracheal compression (77).

In the head and neck, direct tracheal invasion is seen with locally advanced oropharyngeal tumors, laryngeal neoplasms associated with bulky or supraglottic lesions, and rarely, thyroid cancer and primary tracheal tumors (75). In thyroid cancer, tracheal invasion develops in 1% to 6.5% of patients, and UAO is the most common cause of death in this group (78). Bilateral thyroid cancer may cause glottic obstruction from bilateral laryngeal nerve paralysis and resultant bilateral vocal cord paralysis (75). Direct tumor extension into the trachea from adjacent structures by malignancies of the lung, esophagus, and mediastinum occurs more frequently than metastatic disease spread (79).

Tracheal impingement in lung cancer occurs when there is tracheal ingrowth of the primary tumor originating in a mainstem bronchus or from enlarging paratracheal or subcarinal lymph nodes. Bilateral vocal cord paralysis with recurrent laryngeal nerve paralysis may also be associated with lung malignancies (75,80). Extrathoracic malignancies may metastasize to mediastinal and endobronchial lymph nodes, causing airway obstruction. Renal cell carcinoma, sarcomas, breast cancer, and colon cancer are most commonly involved (81). Melanoma may arise as a primary tracheal tumor but more often is a metastatic lesion (79).

Tracheal compression, which is usually attributable to benign disease, is a secondary mechanism of UAO in neoplastic disease and is often the initial presentation of mediastinal tumors and extensive lymphoma (82).

Clinical Presentation

Patients may present with dysphagia, hoarseness, intractable cough, hemoptysis, dyspnea, or stridor (54,75). Important goals during physical examination are to determine whether impending airway obstruction is present and to localize the site of the lesion. Once stridor is apparent, the airway caliber has profoundly narrowed to approximately 6 mm, and without intervention, complete UAO is imminent. Inspiratory stridor implies an extrathoracic lesion at the level of the glottis or above, whereas expiratory stridor suggests an intrathoracic lesion. Biphasic stridor may be indicative of a subglottic or tracheal mass. Voice alteration, such as muffling and hoarseness, accompanies subglottic lesions and unilateral vocal cord paralysis, respectively (47).

Diagnostic Investigations

A chest radiograph may identify an obstructive neck mass and consequent tracheal deviation. Flexible oropharyngeal or nasopharyngeal endoscopy can be performed to assess the airway. Once the airway is stabilized, high-resolution CT of the head and neck provides comprehensive evaluation of the sites of narrowing and the size and extent of the tumor in relation to adjacent structures. Spirometry demonstrates a plateau in the inspiratory limb of the flow-volume loop if there is a fixed obstructive lesion in the extrathoracic trachea (83).

Treatment

Initial management includes head elevation and administration of cool humidified oxygen. Case reports have demonstrated that inhalation of a helium–oxygen mixture, consequent to its lower density compared to oxygen supplementation alone, reduces the work of breathing (54,84,85). Airway obstruction in patients with bulky oropharyngeal, laryngeal, or thyroid carcinomas will require emergent or elective tracheostomy. Endotracheal intubation is not recommended for patients with bulky, friable, laryngeal, and/or pharyngeal disease, as it may exacerbate existing airway edema and hemorrhage (75). For intraluminal tracheal lesions, bronchoscopy with interventions such as laser therapy (86,87), brachytherapy, photodynamic therapy, or stenting may be performed to rapidly alleviate symptoms (87). Stents are also useful in palliating symptomatic extrinsic compression (54,88). Endotracheal intubation or stenting may be used to maintain the airway when there is extrinsic compression from lymphoma (88) or other highly radiosensitive or chemosensitive tumors with anticipation of rapid reduction of tumor mass. Surgical resection is indicated for primary airway tumors (54,89) and for lung cancers without mediastinal lymph node involvement. In lung and thyroid cancers that directly invade the trachea, surgery may be curative (79); metastatic disease to the trachea requires palliative treatment.

Intrathoracic Obstruction

Intrathoracic airway obstruction may be present with intrinsic primary endobronchial tumors such as bronchogenic carcinoma and carcinoid, with metastatic tumors or their associated lymphadenopathy (lung, renal, breast, thyroid, and colon cancers, and sarcoma or melanoma), or with bulky disease causing airway compression. Symptoms often progress slowly over time, and patients may complain of dyspnea, wheezing, or chest discomfort, leading to the misdiagnosis of asthma or bronchitis prior to the development of fulminant airway obstruction (90). Postobstructive pneumonia may be a finding on initial presentation. With impending obstruction, patients may exhibit hypertension, tachycardia, tachypnea, and significant pulsus paradoxus. Poor air movement, use of accessory muscles, and mental status changes are indicators of severe obstruction. Progressive symptoms may result in negative pressure pulmonary edema and anoxic brain injury (83). Chest examination may reveal a prolonged expiratory time and wheezing. Respiratory symptoms are unilateral with lesions below the carina (90), and the chest radiograph reveals asymmetric lung fields, particularly on end-expiration. Stable patients should have a flow-volume loop performed. An intrathoracic, mobile tracheal lesion above the carina will demonstrate airway compression during the expiratory phase, producing flattening of the expiratory limb of the flow-volume loop, whereas a plateau in both inspiratory and expiratory limbs will be observed with fixed obstructive lesions (83). Chest CT defines tumor extent and location, but rigid bronchoscopy is usually necessary to evaluate the airway in impending obstruction. When airway obstruction is severe, flexible bronchoscopy is hazardous because this technique does not permit ventilatory support, and, additionally, the bronchoscope may obstruct the already narrowed airway lumen (90).

Treatment proceeds with the general measures of oxygen or helium/oxygen supplementation and, possibly, steroids. If endotracheal intubation is required, the clinician must recognize the potential for hemodynamic compromise associated with asymmetric obstruction and significant increases in airway pressure distal to the obstruction (83). Bronchoscopy with various interventions, including debridement, dilation, endotracheal stent placement, laser ablation, photodynamic therapy, and placement of brachytherapy catheters may relieve symptoms (90). External beam radiotherapy may also play a role. In lung cancer, tracheal and carinal resection is indicated in patients without mediastinal lymph node involvement for a potential cure (54).

NEUROLOGIC SYNDROMES

Spinal Cord Compression

Etiology and Pathophysiology

Malignant spinal cord compression (MSCC) is a profoundly debilitating, but usually nonfatal, manifestation of metastatic cancer, occurring in 5% to 10% of cancer patients (91–93). The term, *MSCC*, refers to epidural, intramedullary, and leptomeningeal disease; however, the focus of this section is on epidural spinal cord compression (ESCC) because the literature primarily discusses this population (93). Although any malignancy capable of metastatic spread may give rise to MSCC, prostate, breast, and lung cancers are most commonly involved, with each accounting for 15% to 20% of cases (91,94) or, in combination, 60% of cases (93,95). The cumulative incidence of MSCC is specific to tumor type, with the highest rates occurring in multiple myeloma (8%), prostate cancer (7%), and nasopharyngeal cancer (6.5%) (95). Other tumors include non-Hodgkin's lymphoma and renal cell carcinoma, with each representing 5% to 10% of cases (96), and gastrointestinal cancers, sarcoma, melanoma, thyroid cancer (92,93), and unknown primary carcinoma (95,96). Enlarging meningiomas, nerve sheath tumors, and leptomeningeal metastases may also compress the spinal cord. Nonmalignant causes of MSCC in the cancer patient are epidural abscesses in the presence of immune compromise and hematoma with bleeding diatheses (97).

MSCC has a proclivity for the thoracic spine (92,96,98–100) and is estimated to occur in this location in approximately 60% to 66% of cases (97,99). Twenty percent of cases involve the lumbar spine (92,97), and MSCC: in the cervical spine is uncommon in 7% to 10% of cases (99,100). Prostate and colorectal carcinomas favor the lumbosacral spine (97). MSCC is the initial manifestation of malignancy in 20% of patients. One series found that carcinomas of the lung and unknown primary, multiple myeloma, and non-Hodgkin's lymphoma accounted for 78% of patients with MSCC presenting with malignancy compared to 26% in patients with previously established malignancy (100).

The mechanisms by which MSCC occurs include vertebral body invasion by tumor with possible vertebral collapse causing encroachment on the anterior spinal cord (85%); direct extension into the intervertebral space by paraspinal lymphoma, sarcoma, or lung cancer, seen in 10% to 15% of cases (9,92); and epidural or intramedullary space invasion, seen in less than 5% of cases (92). The mechanism of injury to the spinal cord is mediated by white matter vasogenic edema and axonal swelling that result from cord compression. Venous hypertension, decreased spinal cord blood flow, and cord infarction ensue, resulting in ischemic hypoxic neuronal injury. Vascular endothelial growth factor (VEGF) is generated in association with spinal cord hypoxia, and it is thought that dexamethasone may down-regulate VEGF expression, resulting in the beneficial actions of steroids in MSCC (96).

Clinical Presentation

Pain, which may be characterized as localized, radicular, or referred, is the primary presenting symptom in MSCC, occurring in 83% to 95% (96,98,101) of patients for a median of 8 weeks prior to diagnosis (96,98). Focal bony pain is typically localized, dull or aching, and constant. Direct tenderness of the involved vertebral body may be evident with periosteal destruction (102). With time, radicular pain occurs in the dermatome of the affected nerve root and is severe, deep, and lancinating. Radicular symptoms occur most often in the lumbosacral spine and may be unilateral or bilateral, the latter more frequent with thoracic spine involvement (97,103). Referred pain does not radiate, but appears in a region distal to the area of pathology; for example, sacroiliac pain may result from L1 compression (103). The pain of MSCC is typified by worsening with recumbency secondary to distention of the epidural venous plexus (96,97). Coughing, sneezing, or Valsalva maneuvers will also exacerbate the pain (103). Straight-leg raising identifies a lumbosacral radiculopathy, and neck flexion reproduces symptoms of thoracic radiculopathy (97,101,103).

Motor weakness is present in 60% to 85% of patients on diagnosis of MSCC. Although only one third of patients complain of lower extremity weakness on initial presentation (97), two thirds are not ambulatory at the time of diagnosis (96,97). Motor deficits at the level of the conus medullaris or above generally have a symmetric distribution. Paresis is usually seen in the extensors of the upper extremities or the flexors of the lower extremities, depending on the location of the lesion in the spine. Upper motor neuron signs such as spasticity, hyperreflexia, and Babinski responses, may be present. Cervical lesions may lead to quadriplegia and respiratory collapse (102).

Sensory deficits, reported as varying degrees of paresthesias, are less common than motor deficits but can be found in 40% to 90% of patients. The level of hypesthesia on examination occurs one to five levels below the actual anatomic level of cord compression (96). The sensation of an electric shock radiating through the spine and extremities with neck flexion, termed the *Lhermitte's sign* is seen infrequently with cervical or thoracic neoplasms. Perineal paresthesias may occur with cauda equina lesions. Gait ataxia may follow sensory loss impairment, but in the absence of sensory findings, impairment of the spinocerebellar tract should be considered.

Bowel and bladder dysfunction reflects autonomic dysfunction and is a late manifestation of MSCC (103). Patients report urinary hesitancy and frequency, and both incontinence of urine, from poor sphincter tone or overflow of urine, and urinary retention may ensue. At the time of diagnosis, 50% of patients are incontinent or catheter-dependent (101). Patients may also exhibit erectile dysfunction and impotence. Constipation and incontinence of stool with diminished sphincter tone may be present (103). Narcotics are widely used in cancer patients and are capable of precipitating urinary retention and constipation; however, spinal lesions must be excluded in these patients before narcotic use is implicated.

Diagnostic Investigation

The imaging study of choice in evaluating MSCC is magnetic resonance imaging (MRI) because it is a noninvasive test that provides high resolution of the soft tissues, including bony metastases and intramedullary pathology. One study found that MRI had a sensitivity, specificity, and overall accuracy of 93%, 97%, and 95%, respectively, in detecting MSCC in patients with known malignancies, excluding primary CNS tumors (104). It is fundamental to recognize that when the entire spine is imaged beyond the area of clinically determined cord compression, multiple epidural metastases (MEMs) are found in 30% of patients. Because the presence of MEMs may alter treatment strategy, several studies have purported using whole-spine MRI in all patients undergoing imaging (94,104,105). With the relative paucity of cervical spine metastases, if the clinical presentation does not suggest cervical disease, it may be acceptable to image the thoracolumbar spine alone (106). Myelography with or without CT myelogram is a more invasive tool than MRI and is used in imaging MSCC when MRI is contraindicated. CT alone does not adequately define the soft tissues and spinal cord, and plain radiographs and radionuclide testing have low sensitivity and specificity for demonstrating MSCC. Plain films detect vertebral metastases at the site of known cord compression only 80% of the time (9,97), and many metastases are missed because the ability to visualize these lesions requires that 30% to 40% of the bone be eroded (107). Bone scintigraphy is the most cost-effective and sensitive technique in imaging vertebral metastases.

Treatment

The goals of therapy are pain control and preservation of neurologic function to improve quality of life. Narcotic and corticosteroids administration, XRT, and surgery may all be used.

Corticosteroids. In a randomized trial that established the efficacy of corticosteroids in cord compression, patients were assigned to XRT with or without dexamethasone. At the conclusion of the study, 81% of those receiving corticosteroids and XRT versus 63% of those receiving XRT alone remained ambulatory. At 6 months, the percentages were 59% and 33% in the two groups, respectively (108). There are less well established data regarding the use of high-dose dexamethasone regimens because, although higher doses (100-mg versus 10-mg boluses) may have greater clinical efficacy in improving posttreatment ambulation, they are associated with a higher proportion of adverse effects. Typical regimens include a 10-mg bolus, followed by 16 mg divided four times daily, tapered over 2 weeks. High-dose regimens (100-mg bolus, then 96 mg divided four times daily, tapered over 2 weeks) (93) may be reserved for patients with paresis or paraplegia. In ambulatory patients who are asymptomatic and undergoing XRT, corticosteroids may be withheld (93,94,109).

Surgery and Radiation. A recent randomized trial demonstrated that direct decompressive surgery followed by radiotherapy is superior to radiotherapy alone for patients with MSCC. Patients were assigned to either surgery followed by XRT or to XRT alone. The study was stopped early because the primary end point had been satisfied, and a therapeutic advantage of surgery plus XRT was observed: 84% of the surgery group versus 57% of the XRT group were ambulatory after therapy. Additionally, those in the surgery group were ambulatory for 122 days compared to 13 days in the XRT group after treatment. Furthermore, of the patients unable to ambulate on entering the study, 62% of those receiving surgery and radiation versus 19% receiving XRT alone regained the ability to ambulate (110). Therefore, radiotherapy alone should be used for patients who are not surgical candidates. Radiotherapy may also be useful in preserving neurologic function in subclinical MSCC (94). Most tumors causing MSCC are not chemosensitive.

Prognosis

The median survival in MSCC patients receiving XRT is 3 to 6 months (96). Patients who initially present with paralysis or become paralyzed after treatment have a shorter life expectancy than those who are ambulatory (94). Multiple studies have shown that the ambulatory function on diagnosis of MSCC is the most important predictor of outcome of ambulatory function after irradiation. This finding underscores the need for education of both the clinician and the patient to enable prompt recognition of MSCC. In one study, delay in diagnosis was attributed to the patient's failure to identify symptoms and diagnostic delays by the generalist and hospital practitioner, leading to deterioration in motor or bladder function (111).

CARDIAC TAMPONADE

Primary neoplasms of the myocardium and pericardium are uncommon, but metastatic disease to the pericardial space is frequently seen (112). Primary pericardial tumors, of which mesothelioma represents the largest proportion, are 40 times less common than metastatic disease. Secondary malignancies include, most frequently, lung, breast, and ovarian carcinomas, and melanoma, lymphoma, and leukemia (113). Malignancy is a primary cause of pericardial effusion in the United States (114), and pericardial tamponade resulting from malignant pericardial effusion (MPCE) represents at least 50% of reported cases of pericardial fluid collection requiring intervention (115,116). Autopsy series have reported, with varying estimates, that MPCE is seen in 2% to 22% of cancer patients (47,114,115,117), and that these effusions are clinically quiescent, remaining unrecognized (47). In some patients, MPCE may be the initial presentation of cancer, but in any patient, it signifies a dismal prognosis, with most patients dying within 1 year (118). Pericardial effusions in some cancer patients may be attributable to comorbid conditions rather than to malignant disease, and other causes must be considered, such as radiation-induced pericarditis, infection, uremia, myocardial infarction, congestive heart failure, and pneumonia (113).

Pathophysiology

The pericardium is a fibroserous sac, composed of two layers that surround the heart. The outer layer is the fibrous pericardium, which attaches to the diaphragm and securely anchors the heart within the thoracic cavity. The serous pericardium is a single layer of mesothelial cells and its underlying connective tissue, which lines the fibrous pericardium. During embryonic development, the heart invaginates the walls of the serous pericardium, creating a potential space between an inner serous layer that is adherent to the heart (visceral pericardium) and an outer serous layer that lines the fibrous pericardium (parietal pericardium). The pericardial space is formed between the two serous layers, and it normally contains 15 to 50 mL of fluid for lubrication. The fluid is drained from the right pleural space into the right lymphatic duct, and from the parietal pericardium into the thoracic duct (119,120). Any interruption in this flow will result in accumulation of fluid and pericardial effusion. The mechanisms by which malignant disease generates MPCEs include direct invasion of the pericardium or myocardium, and disruption of lymphatic flow from lymph node metastases or from prior radiotherapy to the chest or mediastinum (115,117). The tumors that invade the pericardium directly or hematogenously are most often lung cancer, followed by lymphoma and breast cancer (47,115).

With either of the aforementioned mechanisms, pericardial fluid accumulates and inhibits passive diastolic filling of the normally low-pressure right heart structures, producing jugular and abdominal venous hypertension (115). As the pericardial effusion expands, the heart is further compressed, leading to reduced diastolic compliance, decreased diastolic filling, and, ultimately, decreased stroke volume, cardiac output, and blood pressure. Right atrial and right ventricular collapse ensues, resulting in frank tamponade, which, untreated, will lead to shock (121). *Pericardial reserve volume* is approximately 10 to 20 mL, and is defined as the volume that will just distend the pericardium. As the pericardial effusion enlarges, capacity for stretch is exceeded. Therefore, when fluid accumulates rapidly, the pericardium cannot stretch rapidly enough to accommodate the added volume, and the heart becomes compressed (120). Under these circumstances, acute tamponade may occur with as little as 50 mL of fluid (121). When effusions develop chronically, the pericardium is able to compensate by stretching slowly over time—the phenomenon of stretch relaxation (120–122). In cancer patients, the MPCE develops slowly, and as much as 2 L of pericardial fluid may be present before critical symptoms occur (121).

Clinical Presentation

Patients may be asymptomatic with small pericardial effusions (9,113) and, in general, symptoms correlate with the compressive effect of the effusion on surrounding structures, including the lung, trachea, and esophagus. Symptoms include dyspnea, cough, chest pain, hoarseness, hiccups, and dysphagia (120). The most commonly reported physical sign is distension of the jugular veins. The classic finding of the Beck's triad of hypotension, increased jugular venous pressure, and quiet heart sounds may be present in addition to the Kussmaul's sign, which is paradoxical jugular venous distention and increased jugular venous pressure on inspiration. Sinus tachycardia, hepatomegaly, and peripheral edema may all be apparent. On cardiac examination, dullness beyond the apical impulse and rales can be detected, and in patients with inflammatory effusions, a pericardial rub is often heard. A narrow pulse pressure is frequently noted, and pulsus paradoxus, a decrease in systolic blood pressure greater than 10 mm Hg, is observed in 77% of patients with acute tamponade; patients may report a feeling of uneasiness (121). When low-output shock results from failure of compensatory mechanisms to maintain cardiac output, the patient exhibits cold, clammy skin, cyanosis, oliguria, and altered mental status (122).

Diagnostic Investigations

Chest radiograph reveals a water bottle–shaped heart with widening of the cardiac silhouette and, occasionally, pericardial calcifications (121). Pleural effusions will be present in one third of cases (115). The electrocardiogram may demonstrate a low-voltage QRS or nonspecific ST-T wave changes (9).

Electrical alternans in the P wave and QRS complex is a rare finding, noted in 0% to 10% of patients (120), in which every other QRS complex has a lower voltage and/or reversed polarity (121). The echocardiogram precisely localizes the pericardial fluid, discerns the quality of the effusion (homogeneous versus heterogeneous), determines whether loculations or bulky tumor are present, assesses right and left ventricular function, and ascertains whether right atrial and right ventricular diastolic collapse are present. On echocardiography, the heart may be seen to swing in a pendular fashion within the pericardial fluid. Right heart catheterization is the definitive standard for further defining the pericardial effusion. Classically, there will be equalization of diastolic pressures across all cardiac chambers (115).

Treatment

Treatment strategy should be individualized to each patient based on age, comorbid conditions, malignancy type, and overall prognosis (114). Cardiac tamponade is a class I indication, as designated by the European Society of Cardiology Task Force, for performing pericardiocentesis, and the initial emergent intervention in malignant cardiac tamponade is to drain the effusion, usually in conjunction with echocardiographic guidance (113). Fluid should be sent for chemical analysis, microbiology, and cytology; the effusion is removed successfully in 97% of patients (123). The guidelines recommend that in the absence of tamponade, systemic chemotherapy be administered as baseline treatment (113), thereby precluding recurrences in 67% of cases (123). Systemic chemotherapy is effective in controlling malignant effusions when the tumors are chemosensitive, as in lymphoma, leukemia, and breast cancer. Notably, XRT is highly effective (93%) in controlling malignant pericardial effusions in patients with lymphoma and leukemia, although radiation myocarditis or pericarditis is, in itself, a complication of radiotherapy (123). Pericardiocentesis should be performed in MPCE, especially when these are large, for symptomatic relief and to establish a cause. Because fluid reaccumulates within 48 hours of the initial pericardiocentesis (124), intrapericardial sclerosing or cytostatic agents, selected according to tumor type, should be administered to prevent recurrence. The mechanism of action of sclerosing agents is to effect symphysis of the visceral and parietal pericardia (113). A surgical approach to MPCE management is subxiphoid pericardiotomy to create a pericardial window. An advantage of this technique is that it is performed using local anesthesia and has a low recurrence rate. Additionally, tissue can be obtained for pathologic review. However, there is a small risk of myocardial laceration, pneumothorax, and mortality with this procedure. One study showed a 12% recurrence at 1 year and a 4% reoperation rate for subxiphoid pericardiotomy (114). Pleuropericardiotomy and pericardiectomy, which require general anesthesia, have higher morbidity and mortality rates, and are rarely used in MPCE management (113). Percutaneous balloon pericardiotomy may become the procedure of choice in the future. Requiring only local anesthesia, it facilitates passage of pericardial fluid into the left pleural or peritoneal spaces, which have greater resorptive capacity. The major side effect is asymptomatic pleural effusion in most patients (47,125). Percutaneous balloon pericardiotomy appears to be a safe and effective technique in patients with large MPCEs and recurrent tamponade (90% to 97%) (125,126). Reaccumulation rates with this method are 0% to 6%. Reaccumulation rates for other therapies that are administered after initial pericardiocentesis is performed are radiotherapy, 33%; systemic chemotherapy, 30%; sclerotherapy with tetracycline, 15% to 30%; and mechanical therapies, including indwelling pericardial catheter placement, balloon pericardiotomy, and thoracotomy with pericardiostomy, 0% to 15% (47).

Even if there is no reaccumulation of fluid, cardiac function may remain impaired in the presence of epicardial infiltration by tumor. Diastolic dysfunction occurs because of the constrictive effect of a diseased epicardium surrounding the heart. Effusive-constrictive pericarditis results in a combination of tamponade and cardiac restriction. This entity must be considered in the differential diagnosis when a patient develops hemodynamic collapse a few days after pericardiocentesis. Pericardiectomy may be useful in alleviating the constrictive component; irrespective of this procedure, mortality is extremely high (47,127,128).

Prognosis

Survival after the development of a malignant pericardial effusion is extremely poor (124,128). The pericardial lesions either contribute to or directly cause death in 86% of untreated patients with symptomatic MPCE (128). In one series of 275 patients with MPCE, the median survival was 135 days, and the chance of surviving the first year was 26%. The findings of male gender, lung cancer, positive fluid cytology for malignant cells, and the clinical presentation of cardiac tamponade or hemodynamic collapse were independently associated with poor survival (124). In another series, which concluded that a poor prognosis was associated with positive fluid cytology, median survival was 7.3 weeks versus 29.7 weeks in the positive cytology and negative cytology groups, respectively. MPCE and abnormal cytology were found to be independent predictors of death (129). Taken together, these prognostic factors can be used to make practical and realistic treatment decisions.

GASTROINTESTINAL EMERGENCIES

Neutropenic Enterocolitis

Neutropenic enterocolitis (NE) is also known as necrotizing enteropathy, ileocecal syndrome, or typhlitis (130), from the Greek derivation of the word "typhlon," or cecum (131). Necrotizing enteropathy was first described in adult patients with leukemia and lymphoma more than four decades ago (132), and typhlitis was recognized as an equivalent entity involving the cecum in children undergoing induction therapy for acute leukemia in 1970 (133). The disorder is a life-threatening inflammatory syndrome in the immunocompromised patient that involves the terminal ileum, ascending colon, and cecum (134). Because the disease affects both the small and large bowel, the term, *neutropenic enterocolitis*, is most commonly used (135). The cardinal features that define the syndrome are fever, abdominal pain, and bowel wall thickening in a patient with neutropenia (134,136), where *neutropenia* is defined as a neutrophil count of either less than 500 neutrophils/μL, or less than 1,000 neutrophils/μL with an expected precipitous decline to below 500 neutrophils/μL (137,138). In its natural history, the disease may progress to bowel ulceration, necrosis, and perforation, and ultimately, sepsis and death (133).

Neutropenic enterocolitis (NE) occurs primarily in patients following aggressive cytotoxic therapy for acute leukemia (134,139) and other hematologic malignancies such as lymphoma (134,136), chronic leukemia (134), multiple myeloma (134–136), and rarely in solid tumors, such as colon, breast, testicular, lung (130,140), and pancreatic cancer (140). In leukemia, administration of drugs toxic to the bowel mucosa, such as cytosine arabinoside (141), which cause cellular atypia to frank ulceration, increases the risk of NE (140). Other agents include cytarabine, cisplatin, fluorouracil, vincristine, doxorubicin, 5-fluorouracil, thioguanine, and mercaptopurine (141). NE is rare in solid tumors, but there are case reports identifying the syndrome in breast cancer patients receiving taxanes (142–144). Interestingly, there are also case reports of acute leukemia patients presenting with NE in the absence of chemotherapy (136), indicating that drug toxicity is a predisposing factor rather than a prerequisite in the disease pathogenesis (136). Other immunocompromised patients in whom NE occurs include cases of aplastic anemia (134,136,139,145), cyclic neutropenia (146,147), agranulocytosis (148), Felty syndrome, thalassemia minor, systemic lupus erythematosus (134), and HIV disease (134,149). Patients receiving immunosuppressive therapy for bone marrow (150) or renal transplantation (151) are also at risk.

The incidence of NE in adults varies widely in the literature, ranging from 0.8% to 26%. In a recent systematic review, the pooled incidence rate for adults hospitalized for treatment of hematologic malignancies and solid tumors and for aplastic anemia was 5.3%. The incidence of NE in the acute leukemia group receiving myelosuppressive therapy, with the exclusion of transplant patients, was 5.6%. Extrapolating from these findings, the authors concluded that neutropenia rather than acute leukemia is the primary risk factor for NE (134). In another study, 88 (6%) of 1,450 consecutive patients treated for leukemia had clinical manifestations of NE (152). Although the incidence may be low, it is the high mortality rate associated with NE that underscores its designation as an oncologic emergency. Initial studies reported mortality rates ranging from 50% to 100% (153). The above systematic review stated that several authors observed a rate of 50% or higher, with other published figures ranging between 40% and 50% (154).

Pathogenesis

NE has a predilection for the terminal ileum, cecum, and appendix (154). One factor that may explain this predisposition is the overall decreased blood supply to the colon (136). Also, inherent to the cecum is decreased vascularity and increased distensibility compared to other colonic segments (140,142), and progressive distention in the cecum may cause increasing intraluminal pressure and exacerbation of submucosal edema (140). The pathogenesis of NE is multifactorial and remains unclear (130,136). Drug-induced cytotoxic mucosal injury (130,131,140) initiates the process by limiting cellular proliferation and generating glandular epithelial atypia and necrosis (cytosine arabinoside), and by producing myenteric plexus degeneration (vincristine) (140). Subsequently, mucosal barrier integrity is breached because cells cannot rapidly regenerate to repair the damaged surface (140). Once mucosal damage develops, bacterial translocation occurs, resulting in microbial infection and sepsis (130,140). Marked neutropenia impairs host defense and promotes further microbial invasion; bowel flora becomes altered (136). Blood cultures are often positive for *Clostridium septicum*, *C. difficile*, *Escherichia coli*, *Pseudomonas*, *Klebsiella*, *Enterobacter*, and *Staphylococcus* (135,140). Candidiasis, primarily *Candida albicans,* which colonizes mucosal surfaces, is the most common fungal infection in neutropenic patients and is associated with a high morbidity and mortality (155). These microbial infections lead to inflammation and edema. With sustained profound neutropenia, bacterial invasion is unconstrained, resulting in transmural necrosis, hemorrhage, ulceration, and perforation (135,136,140,156). In addition to drug-induced mucosal injury, infiltration of mucosa with leukemic and lymphoproliferative cells and mucosal ischemia from sepsis-related hypotension may also participate in initiating and perpetuating mucosal injury (140,154).

Symptoms

The onset of NE is 7 to 10 days after treatment when neutropenia is evident. The clinical presentation includes fever, occurring in 90% of all hospitalized neutropenic patients at any time (140), nausea and vomiting, abdominal pain, and watery or bloody diarrhea. Physical examination may reveal stomatitis with diffuse mucositis, abdominal tenderness, abdominal distention, and peritoneal signs suggestive of bowel perforation (140,141,157). In 60% to 80% of patients, right lower quadrant (RLQ) tenderness is elicited. Palpation of a mass in the RLQ usually indicates a thickened, dilated, fluid-filled cecum (140).

Differential Diagnosis

Neutropenic enterocolitis must be included in the differential diagnosis whenever a neutropenic patient presents with fever and abdominal pain, particularly RLQ pain. Other entities that may mimic NE are pseudomembranous colitis, acute appendicitis, acute cholecystitis, acute pancreatitis (152), diverticulitis (158), ischemic colitis, Ogilvie's syndrome (colonic pseudo-obstruction) (159), chemotherapy-induced abdominal pain (130), and ileus secondary to vincristine toxicity (152). Gastrointestinal bleeding may occur in 35% of typhlitis cases, and hemorrhage should suggest NE rather than appendicitis (157).

Diagnostic Investigation

On laboratory analysis, in addition to neutropenia, thrombocytopenia may be seen. Blood cultures are positive in 50% to 82% of cases for bowel organisms as described above (135). Stool studies may be notable for absence of *C. difficile* toxin A because *C. difficile* is not the primary pathogen in NE (134,142).

Plain radiographs of the abdomen are usually normal or nonspecific. Findings may include a decrease in right lower quadrant gas with dilated small bowel loops and air fluid levels consistent with a distal bowel obstruction. Free intraperitoneal air after perforation, pneumatosis coli, or localized or diffuse "thumb-printing" characteristic of mucosal edema may be exhibited (130,140).

Sonography assists in confirming the diagnosis of NE and in excluding other differential diagnoses by detecting bowel wall thickening. Additionally, ultrasound is useful in following the clinical course of the disease (136,152). Sonographic manifestations of NE include a rounded mass with dense central echoes and a wider hyperechoic periphery (130), pseudopolypoid changes of the cecal mucosa, and pericolic fluid collections (140). One study of neutropenic enterocolitis demonstrated that patients with sonographically detected bowel wall thickness of greater than 10 mm had a significantly higher mortality rate (60%) than did those with bowel wall thickness less than or equal to 10 mm (4.2%) (152).

Computed tomography is a more accurate modality for assessing cecal wall thickening and evaluating the extent of the colitis (130,136). It also has utility in differentiating NE from appendicitis, appendiceal abscess, or pseudomembranous colitis (159). CT findings include diffuse submucosal thickening and edema of the terminal ileum and ascending colon, mural hemorrhage, pericolic fluid collections, abscess formation, pneumatosis coli, and intraperitoneal free air (136). The false-negative rates in identifying NE for CT, ultrasound, and plain radiographs are 15%, 23%, and 48%, respectively (139).

Barium enema is unsafe because it may result in bowel perforation in the presence of severely damaged, necrotic bowel (131,160). Endoscopic evaluation is generally avoided because it involves a high risk of perforation in addition to hemorrhagic and infectious complications, and it may precipitate fulminant mural necrosis (130). Colonoscopy has been performed in a paucity of patients and will reveal irregular nodular mucosa, ulcerations, hemorrhagic friability, and a masslike lesion resembling carcinoma (131).

Histopathology

With the difficulty of obtaining biopsy specimens, a tissue diagnosis is not required to confirm NE. On gross examination, striking bowel wall thickening is evident. Scattered serosal ecchymoses give the bowel a dusky appearance. Microscopy demonstrates pronounced transmural submucosal edema, vasculitis, stromal hemorrhage, and patchy or complete epithelial necrosis, resulting in mucosal ulceration and pseudomembrane formation. With further damage, transmural necrosis leads to muscularis propria degeneration. Vascular injury effects intramural and intraluminal hemorrhage, and fibrin thrombi may be seen in the submucosal vessels. Polymicrobial infiltration with bacteria and fungi is observed in 53% of postmortem cases (154). Very few inflammatory cells are observed, and rarely, leukemic or lymphoproliferative infiltrates invade the bowel wall. Neutrophils are absent, and aneutrophilia in the setting of marked cell injury is pathognomonic for NE (134,154).

Management

Prospective trials or case control studies evaluating therapeutic interventions in NE are lacking (134). Management strategy remains controversial regarding the decision to proceed with early surgical intervention versus a conservative approach (161). Conservative management of NE involves bowel rest, intravenous fluid and blood product resuscitation, broad-spectrum antibiotics, granulocyte colony-stimulating factor (G-CSF), and frequently, parenteral nutrition (130,141). Use of omeprazole and gastric decompression is not advocated by some authors because these interventions facilitate bacterial migration from the bowel into the respiratory tract, predisposing the patient to pneumonia (134). Medications that inhibit bowel motility, such as antidiarrheal and narcotic agents should be avoided since they perpetuate ileus and promote bacterial overgrowth (141). Patients with chemotherapy-induced NE may suffer from repeated episodes with future treatment; therefore, further chemotherapy should be withheld until NE has completely resolved. Bowel decontamination may be helpful before subsequent chemotherapy, although this is not well-studied (131).

Selection of broad-spectrum antibiotics should incorporate the Infectious Diseases Society of America (ISDA) 2002 recommendations for febrile neutropenia (137) as well as the 2003 ISDA guidelines for complicated intra-abdominal infections (162). Without prompt antibiotic therapy, neutropenic patients with Gram-negative bacteremia have a mortality rate approaching 40% (163). The antibiotic(s) of choice in NE must demonstrate activity against both Gram-negative and anaerobic organisms. Options include the following: monotherapy with a carbapenem or piperacillin–tazobactam; duotherapy with another antipseudomonal β-lactam plus an aminoglycoside; or duotherapy with cefepime or ceftazidime plus metronidazole (134,141,162). Antifungal therapy with amphotericin B therapy should be considered for empiric therapy in profoundly neutropenic patients whose fevers persist beyond 5 days despite receiving appropriately dosed broad-spectrum antibiotics (137).

Granulocyte colony-stimulating factor (G-CSF) increases cell division in myeloid precursor cells, decreases bone marrow transit time, and modulates activity and function of developing and mature neutrophils (156). The current American Society of Clinical Oncology (ASCO) guidelines recommend G-CSF administration in febrile neutropenic patients with a high risk for infection-associated complications and poor prognostic factors, such as profound neutropenia (less than 100 cells/μL), sepsis, pneumonia, hypotension, invasive fungal infection, and uncontrolled primary disease (164); NE undisputedly meets these criteria. G-CSF administration in chemotherapy-related febrile neutropenia reduces hospitalization time and time to neutrophil recovery, and may have an impact on infection-related mortality that warrants further study (165). Clinical improvement in NE patients is usually seen after normalization of the neutrophil count with discontinuation of chemotherapy. It has been observed that symptoms commence as the white blood cell count (WBC) declines after chemotherapy, and recovery begins after the nadir when the WBC is increasing (130).

There are no standard recommendations, but rather, general guidelines in the literature regarding surgical intervention in NE; however, most patients are unlikely to be surgical candidates. Early reports recommended aggressive and early surgical resection of involved bowel, anticipating that in the natural history of NE, bowel perforation is inevitable (134). Recent series demonstrate successful nonsurgical management (134,161,166). More recent publications support surgery with laparotomy alone for patients with perforation and ileus (134). Some advocate that patients who fail to improve or develop bowel perforation and peritonitis after 2 or 3 days of conservative therapy warrant consideration for surgery (142,167). Several authors recommend surgery for severe complications such as abscess, necrotic bowel, and obstruction (136). In general, definitive indications for surgery include intraperitoneal free air/perforation, generalized peritonitis, and persistent bleeding in spite of correction of coagulopathy (130,140). Important considerations that must influence the decision to surgically intervene are the patient's prognosis and comorbidities because postoperative morbidity and mortality is greater in individuals with coexistent diseases (140). If surgery is warranted, the procedure of choice is colectomy with ileostomy and mucous fistula; a primary anastomosis is used in very few patients (168). Of note, the extent of mucosal necrosis may be underestimated by the appearance of the serosa. A surgeon must ensure complete resection of edematous bowel, even in the absence of necrosis and inflammation, to preclude a fatal outcome (140).

TOXICITY OF CHEMOTHERAPY

Most antineoplastic agents exert their therapeutic actions by targeting rapidly proliferating malignant cells. Because these agents interrupt fundamental cellular processes such as DNA, RNA, and protein synthesis, they are not completely specific to malignant cells and will also act on normal tissues, causing multiple toxicities. Rapidly regenerating cells, such as the hematopoietic lineage, gastrointestinal mucosa, spermatogonia, and hair follicles may suffer transient toxicity compared to cells that have limited regenerative capacity, including those of the myocardium, and nerves (169–171). This section focuses on the major life-threatening toxicities that occur with commonly used chemotherapeutic agents.

Pulmonary Toxicities

Pulmonary toxicity, both acute and chronic, is seen increasingly with numerous antineoplastic agents (172). Chemotherapy-induced lung disease (CLD) describes lung injury with multiple etiologic agents and varying pathophysiologic mechanisms. These major mechanisms include direct lung toxicity, immunologic response, and increased capillary permeability. The corresponding clinical presentations are interstitial pneumonitis/fibrosis, hypersensitivity syndrome, and capillary leak syndrome, respectively, and each may eventuate in fulminant respiratory failure. Symptoms can appear immediately or months after termination of therapy (173).

Antitumor Antibiotics

Bleomycin. Bleomycin is an antitumor antibiotic used in the treatment of lymphoma, germ cell tumors, cervical carcinoma, and head and neck squamous cell carcinoma. The absence of bleomycin hydrolase in the skin and lungs prevents deactivation of the drug, accounting for its selective toxicity. Bleomycin interstitial pneumonitis is the most ominous toxicity, associated with a 3% mortality rate (174) and occurring in 0% to 46% of patients receiving bleomycin-containing regimens, either during treatment or up to 6 months after discontinuation (175). Toxicity is mediated by the mechanism of direct lung injury via generation of cytokines and free radicals, the sequelae of which are endothelial damage, inflammatory cell infiltration, fibroblast activation, and fibrosis (173,175). There is conflicting evidence in the literature as to whether perioperative oxygen supplementation exceeding a concentration of 24% fractional inspired oxygen causes synergistic toxicity with bleomycin through the production of free radicals (176,177).

Mitomycin C. This is an antibiotic used in treating solid tumors, primarily breast and lung carcinomas. The mechanism of injury is alkylation of endothelial cell DNA, precluding cell division. This agent is associated with the development of an interstitial pneumonitis/fibrosis (178,179), usually 3 to 12 months after therapy (179,180), with a 3% to 14% incidence. Mortality is as high as 14% to 50% (178,179,181). Risk factors include oxygen exposure, prior irradiation, and other cytotoxic drug administration, such as bleomycin, cisplatin, the vinca alkaloids, cyclophosphamide, and doxorubicin. Drug withdrawal, steroids, and avoidance of supplemental oxygen may be helpful (180).

Mitomycin–vinca alkaloid syndrome is a unique entity occurring with a 6% incidence after the vinca alkaloid is administered to patients receiving combination therapy with mitomycin and vinblastine but not with the vinca alkaloid alone. Severe hypoxemia ensues with development of interstitial infiltrates on chest radiograph. Most patients show acute improvement within 24 hours with oxygen, diuretics, and occasionally, mechanical ventilation, although chronic lung damage occurred in 60% of patients in one study (178).

Alkylating Agents

Carmustine (BCNU). This is a nitrosourea used in the management of central nervous system tumors and in induction therapy for bone marrow transplantation (BMT). Its cytoxicity is mediated by alkylation of guanine in DNA (172). Carmustine causes dose-dependent pulmonary fibrosis and carries the highest incidence of fibrosis among the nitrosoureas. The mortality rate ranges from 24% to as high as 90% in some reports (180,181). In 1% and 30% of the patients receiving high- and low-dose carmustine, respectively, early-onset fibrosis and alveolitis will occur. In up to 40% of the patients undergoing induction for BMT, pulmonary fibrosis will develop within 2 years. Late fibrosis can be observed up to 17 years after exposure. Concomitant radiotherapy, chronic obstructive pulmonary disease (COPD), and pneumoconioses increase the risk of carmustine toxicity. Sixty percent of patients will respond dramatically to steroids (180).

Microtubule-targeting Agents

Taxanes. Paclitaxel inhibits microtubule disassembly (182), and has activity against solid tumors such as non–small cell lung carcinoma, breast carcinoma, and ovarian carcinoma (173); it is prepared in Cremophor, a castor oil-based solution (173,182). A type I hypersensitivity reaction, characterized by urticaria, bronchospasm, angioedema, and hypotension, occurs within 2 to 10 minutes of infusion of paclitaxel (182,183) with a 3% to 10% incidence (180), and is attributable to the Cremophor vehicle rather than paclitaxel itself (173). Premedication with steroids and H_1 and H_2 blockers can curtail this reaction (182).

Antimetabolites

Cytosine Arabinoside. Ara-C is a substituted nucleoside antimetabolite that disrupts DNA replication and is used in the therapy of leukemia and non-Hodgkin's lymphoma. One of its toxicities is the abrupt onset of endothelial inflammation and capillary leak syndrome (173), causing noncardiogenic pulmonary edema, acute dyspnea, and a diffuse interstitial and alveolar pattern. Management is supportive and includes oxygen, diuretics, and mechanical ventilation when needed (180).

Gemcitabine. This is a pyrimidine analogue, structurally similar to ara-C (183), that has activity against tumors of the pancreas, lung (NSCLC), breast, and ovaries. Recent large series report an incidence of lung toxicity of less than 1% to 1.4% (184). The proposed mechanism of injury involves pulmonary endothelial cell damage resulting in capillary leak syndrome (173,183). The symptoms of gemcitabine pulmonary toxicity range from mild dyspnea to a fatal acute respiratory distress syndrome. Increasing age, pulmonary neoplasm, and prior radiotherapy may be contributing risk factors (173,185). Patients respond rapidly to corticosteroids (173), but fatalities do occur (173,181,183,185,186).

Differentiation Agents

All-*trans*-Retinoic Acid. ATRA is a differentiation agent used for the treatment of acute promyelocytic leukemia (APL). It is associated with retinoic acid syndrome, developing in 20% to 50% of APL patients receiving ATRA (187) a median of 7 days (range 0–35 days) after induction therapy (188). The clinical presentation includes fluid retention, weight gain, fever, and musculoskeletal pain, with progression to respiratory distress, pulmonary infiltrates, pleural (187) and pericardial effusions (180), renal insufficiency, skin infiltrates, hypotension, and death (187). Corticosteroids are highly effective when the syndrome commences but have limited utility once pulmonary symptoms are apparent. The putative mechanism of the pulmonary toxicity of ATRA is a capillary leak syndrome (180).

Monoclonal Antibodies

Trastuzumab. This is a humanized monoclonal antibody that targets the epidermal growth factor type 2 (HER2) receptor (189). In approximately 25% of breast cancers, the HER2 receptor is overexpressed (183) and is associated with a poor prognosis (190), a finding that provides the rationale for use of trastuzumab in HER2 receptor–positive metastatic breast cancer. A retrospective analysis of 25,000 patients identified bronchospasm as the only manifestation of pulmonary toxicity. Nine cases (0.04%) attributable to trastuzumab infusion were fatal; most serious reactions commenced within 2 hours of infusion, and most fatalities were observed in patients with poor performance status and severe underlying pulmonary disease (191).

Bevacizumab. This is a recombinant humanized monoclonal antibody directed against vascular endothelial growth factor (VEGF) that inhibits binding of VEGF to its receptors, hence impairing angiogenesis. The drug is approved for first-line treatment of advanced colorectal cancer in combination therapy (183). In a phase II randomized trial of 99 patients with advanced or recurrent NSCLC, the incidence of hemoptysis in patients with NSCLC was demonstrably higher in patients treated with bevacizumab, carboplatin, and paclitaxel (20%) than in those treated with carboplatin and paclitaxel alone (6%). Four patients in the bevacizumab group had severe hemoptysis, which occurred with an incidence of 9.1% and was associated with squamous cell pathology, tumor necrosis and cavitation, and centrally located tumors in close proximity to major blood vessels (192). A recent study excluded patients with pre-existing hemoptysis and squamous cell pathology based on the premise that squamous carcinomas, as a consequence of their location and ability to cavitate, are more prone to bleeding. With these exclusions, a 1.9% incidence of life-threatening hemorrhage with bevacizumab was observed (193).

Alemtuzumab. This is a monoclonal antibody to the lymphocyte and monocyte cell surface antigen CD52 and is used as a salvage therapy for chronic lymphocytic leukemia (194). In a series of 16 patients with B-cell chronic lymphocytic leukemia (B-CLL), the associated pulmonary toxicity in one patient was severe bronchospasm that responded to corticosteroids (195).

Cardiac Toxicities

Antitumor Antibiotics

Anthracyclines. These are red-pigmented antibiotics (rhodomycins), which include doxorubicin, daunorubicin, idarubicin, and epirubicin (196). They are active against a broad spectrum of tumors, such as breast and esophageal carcinomas, Hodgkin's and non-Hodgkin's lymphomas, osteosarcomas, Kaposi's sarcoma, and soft-tissue sarcomas. Three mechanisms that lead to oxidative stress (197) contribute to the cardiac toxicity of these agents: mitochondrial dysfunction and consequent adenosine triphosphate depletion; free radical lipid peroxidation by iron–doxorubicin complexes; and glutathione peroxidase depletion (196). Histopathology demonstrates myofibril dropout, vacuolization of myocardial cells, and necrosis (196,197). Acute cardiotoxicities include nonspecific ST-T wave changes (198), supraventricular tachycardia (SVT), ventricular arrhythmias, myopericarditis, cardiomyopathy, and sudden death. The cardiomyopathy is dose dependent, and is classified as subacute and late. Subacute cardiomyopathy presents within 8 months of therapy, with a peak onset of 3 months, whereas late cardiomyopathy is observed after 5 or more years. A continual decline in left ventricular function results in congestive heart failure (CHF) (196); liposomal doxorubicin may play a role in reducing cardiotoxicity (199). Dexrazoxane, an iron chelator with cardioprotective properties, has been demonstrated to substantially reduce toxicity (197,200). Toxic effects may be compounded by other therapies, including trastuzumab, cyclophosphamide, dactinomycin, mithramycin, mitomycin, etoposide, melphalan vincristine, bleomycin, dacarbazine (196), and taxanes (201,202).

Mitoxantrone. This agent has structural similarity to the anthracyclines, and is used in managing metastatic breast cancer, acute myeloid leukemia, and non-Hodgkin's lymphoma (202). The mechanism of cardiac injury, like that of the anthracyclines, may involve iron chelation complexes (203); arrhythmias and dose-dependent heart failure are toxicities. The incidence of a moderate to severe decrease in left ventricular ejection fraction (LVEF) and of CHF is 13% and 2.6%, respectively, with a cumulative dose of less than or equal to 140 mg/m^2. Doses below 110 mg/m^2 decrease the incidence of heart failure, whereas incidence increases with doses greater than 160 mg/m^2 (196).

Mitomycin C. In addition to its lung toxicity, mitomycin is cardiotoxic, resulting in an increased incidence of cardiac failure with cumulative doses exceeding 30 mg/m^2 (196,204). Additive cardiotoxicity occurs when mitomycin is used in conjunction with anthracyclines (204); superoxide free radicals may mediate this toxicity (198).

Alkylating Agents

Cyclophosphamide. This agent is a nitrogen mustard alkylating agent effective in treating leukemia, lymphoma, multiple myeloma, mycosis fungoides, neuroblastoma, and ovarian cancer. Acute cardiotoxicity may develop with doses of 120 mg/kg to 170 mg/kg given over 1 to 7 days in preparation for bone marrow transplantation. Electrocardiogram may reveal decreased QRS amplitude, nonspecific T-wave abnormalities, poor R-wave progression, supraventricular and ventricular tachyarrhythmias, and second-degree atrioventricular block (203). Acute fulminant CHF may occur in up to 28% of patients treated with high-dose cyclophosphamide (196), but CHF is usually short lived and reversible (203). The drug is metabolized to its active form in the liver by the cytochrome P-450, and more rapid metabolism amplifies the risk of CHF (205). Another cyclophosphamide-related cardiotoxicity is hemorrhagic myocarditis, putatively mediated by endothelial capillary injury, which results in pericardial effusion, tamponade, and death; most effusions are treatable with corticosteroids and analgesics. When the purine analogue pentostatin (198) is used in bone marrow conditioning regimens in combination with cyclophosphamide, there is an increased incidence of fatal cardiac toxicity (196) that includes myocardial infarction, CHF, and arrhythmias (198). There may be an additive effect of cyclophosphamide and anthracycline-induced cardiomyopathy, but the data are conflicting (196).

Iphosphamide. This is an alkylating agent, with similar properties to cyclophosphamide, used to treat lymphoma, leukemia, and testicular and bladder tumors. Arrhythmias and transient, reversible, dose-dependent CHF—as with cyclophosphamide—may be seen (203,206).

Cisplatin. This agent cross-links interstrand DNA. It is used in treating cancers of the testes, bladder, ovaries, and other tumors. Bradycardia, supraventricular tachycardia (196), acute ischemia (207), myocardial infarction, and ischemic cardiomyopathy may be observed (196). Acute chest pain and palpitations may be associated with cisplatin infusion. Late complications can occur 10 to 20 years after therapy. Hypomagnesemia and hypokalemia generated by cisplatin-induced tubular defects (196) may exacerbate arrhythmias (198).

Microtubule-targeting Agents

Vinca Alkaloids. Vinca alkaloids include vincristine and vinblastine, which are used for management of hematologic malignancies and solid tumors, and vinorelbine, a semisynthetic derivative used in NSCLC therapy. These agents exert their toxicity by inhibiting microtubule assembly, and all possess vasoconstrictive properties. Hypertension, vasospastic myocardial ischemia, and myocardial infarction may be seen (198). Vinorelbine toxicity is more common in women than men (208).

Taxanes. (See also Pulmonary Toxicities, above.) Hypertension (196) and cardiac arrhythmias, most commonly transient asymptomatic bradycardia (182), are observed with paclitaxel. In a large series, the incidence of more significant bradyarrhythmias—Mobitz type I and II heart block and complete heart block—was 0.1% (209). Rarely, atrial and ventricular tachycardias, myocardial ischemia, and myocardial infarction occur, often in patients with underlying cardiac disease or electrolyte derangements (196). Docetaxel may lead to the potentiation of anthracycline cardiomyopathy (202).

Antimetabolites

5-Fluoruracil and Capecitabine. 5-Fluoruracil (5-FU) is a synthetic pyrimidine antimetabolite used in regimens for managing multiple solid tumors including gastrointestinal, breast, ovarian, and head and neck malignancies. Myocardial ischemia, possibly triggered by coronary vasospasm, is a well-known cardiac toxicity that occurs with increased frequency in combination with cisplatin. In one study, silent ischemic ECG changes were identified during 24 hours of observation in up to 68% of patients receiving a continuous 5-FU infusion (210). Other cardiac manifestations include chest pain, angina, atrial and ventricular arrhythmias, myocardial infarction, persistent ventricular dysfunction, sudden death, and cardiogenic shock (196,203) requiring inotropic support (196). Pre-existing cardiac morbidity significantly increases the risk of cardiotoxicity compared to no prior cardiac disease (15.1% vs. 1.5%) (203). Given the potential for severe cardiotoxicity, infusions should be terminated when chest pain occurs. The oral equivalent of infused 5-FU is capecitabine, which exhibits a similar cardiotoxicity profile to 5-FU (211).

Topoisomerase Inhibitors

Etoposide. This agent is a topoisomerase II inhibitor used primarily for treatment of refractory testicular tumors and small cell lung carcinoma. Hypotension is the most common side effect (198). Myocardial infarction (198,212) and vasospastic angina (196) may also occur. Prior chemotherapy or mediastinal irradiation may increase the risk of myocardial infarction after etoposide therapy (196).

Biologic Response Modifiers

Interferons. These are glycoprotein biologic response modifiers classified according to their respective derivations: interferon-*alfa* (leukocytes), interferon-*beta* (fibroblasts), and interferon-*gamma* (lymphocytes) (196). They are used to treat various tumors including renal cell carcinoma, metastatic melanoma, multiple myeloma, Kaposi sarcoma, and some leukemias and lymphomas. Cardiovascular toxicities include hypertension or hypotension (198), ischemia in patients with coronary artery disease, myocardial infarction, arrhythmias (20% incidence) (213), sudden death, and cardiomyopathy characterized by resolution with termination of the infusion (214).

Interleukin-2 (IL-2). This is a glycoprotein biologic response modifier derived from helper T-lymphocytes, and is approved for the treatment of metastatic renal cell cancer. Most patients develop capillary leak syndrome and hypotension associated with decreased peripheral vascular resistance necessitating vasopressors (196). In a study of 423 treatment courses with IL-2, 65% required pressor support for hypotension (215). In patients with coronary artery disease, direct myocardial toxicity precipitates ischemia, myocardial infarction, arrhythmias, and death. IL-2 may also predispose patients to ventricular and supraventricular arrhythmias, which are seen in 14% to 21% of patients (196).

Differentiation Agents

All-*trans*-Retinoic Acid. (See also Pulmonary Toxicities.) Pericardial effusions, cardiac tamponade, myocardial ischemia (196), fatal infarction, and thrombosis (198), in addition to pulmonary toxicity, may occur with the retinoic acid syndrome as described above (196).

Arsenic Trioxide. Arsenic trioxide is a differentiation agent effective in treating relapsed acute promyelocytic leukemia. Like all-*trans*-retinoic acid, it may also cause the retinoic acid syndrome. Prolongation of the QT interval is another complication seen in up to 63% of patients, leading to torsades de pointes (196) and sudden death. The degree of QT prolongation is higher in the presence of hypokalemia (216); therefore, careful monitoring of electrolytes and maintaining levels in the high normal range is prudent.

Monoclonal Antibodies

Trastuzumab. (See also Pulmonary Toxicities.) There is an increased risk of cardiotoxicity associated with trastuzumab, which is highest in patients receiving concurrent anthracycline plus cyclophosphamide (27%) compared to concomitant trastuzumab and paclitaxel (13%) or trastuzumab alone (3%–7%) (217). The mechanism of cardiac toxicity of trastuzumab is not well understood, but cardiac erbB2 is essential for myocyte function, and trastuzumab targets both HER2 and erbB2 receptors (203,218). Early following initial treatment, there may be an asymptomatic decline in LVEF with late progression to dilated cardiomyopathy (203). Risk factors for cardiovascular toxicity include older age, cumulative doxorubicin dosage 400 mg/m^2 or greater, (217), and concurrent anthracycline and trastuzumab administration, rather than temporally separated dosing (218).

Rituximab. The CD20 antigen, present on normal and malignant B cells, is the target of the chimeric murine/human monoclonal antibody rituximab, which is used to treat leukemias and lymphomas, as well as benign diseases. Cardiac toxicity involves arrhythmias and angina in less than 1% of infusions (196). Most adverse effects with rituximab are infusion related, usually occurring within 2 hours of the first infusion (219). Acute infusion-related deaths have been reported in 0.04% to 0.07% of cases. The clinical presentation in these patients includes hypoxia, pulmonary infiltrates, adult respiratory distress syndrome, myocardial infarction, ventricular fibrillation, and cardiogenic shock (196). Hypersensitivity reactions, including hypotension, angioedema, hypoxia, or bronchospasm, may occur in up to 10% of cases. Management is supportive, using intravenous fluids, antihistamines, acetaminophen, bronchodilators, and vasopressors (198).

Cetuximab. This agent is a human/mouse chimeric monoclonal antibody designed to target the human epidermal growth factor receptor. It is used alone or in combination therapy with irinotecan to treat metastatic colorectal cancer. Life-threatening infusion reactions occur in 3% of patients with bronchospasm, urticaria, and hypotension (220). Interstitial pneumonitis with noncardiogenic pulmonary edema is a rare toxicity (198).

Bevacizumab. (See also Pulmonary Toxicities.) This agent is associated with CHF, hypertension, and arterial thromboembolism. With bevacizumab monotherapy, 2% of patients developed moderate to life-threatening (grades 2 to 4) left ventricular dysfunction (221). CHF developed in 14% of patients concurrently receiving anthracyclines, and in 4% of patients who had previously received anthracyclines or left chest wall irradiation (196,198). Clinical trials have also documented hypertension in 5% of patients, with reports of hypertensive crisis, hypertensive encephalopathy, and subarachnoid hemorrhage (198). The FDA has issued a warning to health care providers announcing that bevacizumab has demonstrated an increased risk of arterial thromboembolic events, which include cerebrovascular accident, transient ischemic attack, myocardial infarction, and angina (222). In addition, the risk of fatal arterial thrombotic events is doubled to 5% in patients receiving intravenous 5-FU and bevacizumab (222,223).

Hematologic Toxicities

Thalidomide

Thalidomide is a sedative-hypnotic agent with anti-inflammatory properties, used in multiple myeloma patients to treat advanced and chemotherapy-refractory disease (224,225). Its mechanism of action is unclear, but immune modulation, antiangiogenesis, and tumor necrosis factor-*alpha* may play a role (226). There is an increased risk of venous thromboembolism (VTE) associated with thalidomide, occurring at a mean of 2 months of therapy (227). Lower extremity deep venous thrombosis (DVT) is the most frequent thrombotic complication occurring with thalidomide treatment, and approximately 50% of these patients will develop PE. The mechanism of thalidomide-induced DVT is not well defined. Thalidomide may exert a direct effect on endothelial cells that have been injured by other chemotherapy agents such as doxorubicin (226). In one study, VTE rates with thalidomide monotherapy, thalidomide–dexamethasone, thalidomide–doxorubicin, and thalidomide–dexamethasone–doxorubicin were less than 5%, 9%, 12%, and 22%, respectively (228). These findings suggest a role for VTE prophylaxis, and further investigation is warranted.

Hormones

Estramustine. Estramustine phosphate has hormonal properties because it contains nor-nitrogen mustard linked to 17 beta-estradiol. It is used in the treatment of prostate cancer. In up to 10% of patients receiving estramustine, venous thrombosis, pulmonary emboli, and myocardial and cerebrovascular ischemia may occur (196).

Tamoxifen and Aromatase Inhibitors. Tamoxifen and the aromatase inhibitors—anastrozole, letrozole, and exemestane—are used as adjuvant therapy for early-stage estrogen receptor–positive breast carcinoma (229). It is well known that there is an increased risk of VTE with tamoxifen. The following data clearly quantifies the risk: the incidence of VTE in the general population is 0.12% per year and 0.09% per year in women. In women with early-stage breast cancer and no adjuvant treatment, compared to those receiving tamoxifen, the incidence increases to 0.4% over 5 years and 1.4% to 1.7% over 5 years, respectively. This incidence escalates to 10.8% over 5 years in the same population of women who receive concurrent tamoxifen and chemotherapy. Aromatase inhibitors (AI) are generally associated with a lower risk of VTE than tamoxifen. In the ATAC trial (Arimidex, Tamoxifen, Alone, or in Combination) at 5 years, the incidence of VTE with anastrazole was 1.6% versus 2.4% with tamoxifen (230).

Gastrointestinal Toxicities

Bevacizumab

This agent is associated with both bowel perforation and gastrointestinal hemorrhage. In a randomized controlled trial in patients with metastatic colon cancer, subjects received either irinotecan, fluorouracil, and leucovorin (IFL) plus bevacizumab, or IFL alone. Gastrointestinal perforation was observed in six patients (1.5%) treated with IFL plus bevacizumab with one fatality compared to no patients in the control group (231). A more recent phase II trial adding bevacizumab to bolus 5-FU and leucovorin reported bowel perforation in 2% of cases (223). In a phase II trial of bevacizumab in combination with fluorouracil and leucovorin in advanced refractory colorectal cancer, severe to life-threatening gastrointestinal hemorrhage (grades 3 and 4) was seen in 3.8% of patients (232).

Genitourinary Toxicities

Cyclophosphamide and Ifosfamide

Cyclophosphamide and ifosfamide induce an early (within 72 hours of administration) hemorrhagic cystitis via their metabolite, acrolein, that causes denudation of the bladder mucosa and bleeding (233,234). In the past, early hemorrhagic cystitis was observed in over 40% of bone marrow transplants, but that rate has dramatically declined to 5% with aggressive hydration regimens and administration of the thiol mesna. Mesna is a type of thiol that inactivates acrolein in the bladder after itself being converted to the active form in the kidney. It must be administered prior to cyclophosphamide infusion and continued after the infusion is terminated consequent to its shorter half-life. In cases of hemorrhagic cystitis that have progressed to intractable or profuse bleeding, bladder irrigation and cystoscopy with clot extraction and fulguration may be necessary to achieve hemostasis (234). Cystectomy, vascular ligation, or hyperbaric therapy (233) may be required in recalcitrant cases. Late occurring hemorrhagic cystitis commences 72 hours after administration of preparatory regimens in bone marrow transplantation, with risk factors including viral infections, busulfan use, pelvic irradiation, older age at transplantation, allogenic transplantation, and graft versus host disease (235).

Mitomycin C

Mitomycin C has been discussed with reference to its pulmonary and cardiac toxicities. Another life-threatening manifestation associated with mitomycin is the thrombotic thrombocytopenic purpura-hemolytic uremic syndrome (TTP-HUS). This entity is a distinct multiorgan disorder distinguished by thrombocytopenia, microangiopathic hemolytic anemia (MAHA), and tissue ischemia precipitated by platelet agglutination in the arterial microvasculature (236). The classic pentad—fever thrombocytopenia, MAHA, renal failure, and neurologic dysfunction—is no longer required to make the diagnosis. Instead, the new definition encompasses a broad spectrum of conditions in which unexplained thrombocytopenia and MAHA are present (237). Of the chemotherapeutic agents associated with TTP-HUS, mitomycin is the most common, but bleomycin, cisplatin, and gemcitabine are also causes of the syndrome (236). The pathogenic mechanism of mitomycin C–induced TTP-HUS may involve chemotherapy-induced endothelial cell injury (238,239) and circulating immune complexes against tumor-related antigens (239). In some cancer patients, it may be difficult to attribute TTP-HUS to mitomycin, because malignancy-induced TTP-HUS is clinically indistinguishable from mitomycin-induced disease. TTP-HUS is typically seen 4 to 8 weeks following the final dose of mitomycin. Patients usually present with dyspnea from noncardiogenic pulmonary edema, which may progress to adult respiratory distress syndrome, and may mimic mitomycin lung toxicity. Renal failure is generally present, whereas neurologic symptoms are infrequent (237). Unfortunately, patients with mitomycin-induced TTP-HUS do not respond to plasmapheresis. Immunoadsorption of plasma over a staphylococcal protein A column to remove immune complexes may be effective in these patients (240). The prognosis of mitomycin-induced TTP-HUS is poor, with most patients succumbing to pulmonary or renal failure or to their underlying malignancy within 4 months (237).

References

1. *Cancer Facts & Figures 2007*. Atlanta, GA: American Cancer Society; 2007: 1–51.
2. Copelan EA. Hematopoietic stem-cell transplantation. *N Engl J Med.* 2006;354:1813–1826.
3. Hazard LJ, Jensen RL, Shrieve DC. Role of stereotactic radiosurgery in the treatment of brain metastases. *Am J Clin Oncol.* 2005;28(4):403–410.
4. Scappaticci, FA. Mechanisms and future directions for angiogenesis-based cancer therapies. *J Clin Oncol.* 20(18):3906–3927.
5. Stewart AF. Hypercalcemia associated with cancer. *N Eng J Med.* 2005; 352:373.
6. Rosol TJ, Capen CC. Mechanisms of cancer-induced hypercalcemia. *Lab Invest.* 1992; 67:680.
7. Fojo AT. Oncologic emergencies: metabolic emergencies. In: DeVita VT, Hellman S, Rosenberg SA, eds. *Cancer: Principles and Practice of Oncology.* 7th ed. Philadelphia, PA: Lippincott Williams & Wilkins; 2005:2297–2299.
8. Pecherstorfer M, Schilling T, Blind E, et al. Parathyroid hormone-related protein and life expectancy in hypercalcemic patients. *J Clin Endocrinol Metab.* 1994;78:1268.
9. Halfdanarson TR, Hogan WJ, Moynihan, TJ. Oncological emergencies: diagnosis and treatment. *Mayo Clin Proc.* 2006;81(6):835.
10. Ralston SH, Gallagher SJ, Patel U, et al. Cancer-associated hypercalcemia: morbidity and mortality: clinical experience in 126 treated patients. *Ann Intern Med.* 1990;112:499.
11. Hypercalcemia. *CancerMail from the National Cancer Institute.* http://cancerweb.ncl.ac.uk. Accessed December 11, 2006.
12. Dunbar ME, Wysolmerski JJ, Broadus AE. Parathyroid hormone-related protein: from hypercalcemia of malignancy to developmental regulatory molecule. *Am J Med Sci.* 1996;312(6):287.
13. Rizzoli R, Ferrari SL, Pizurki L, et al. Actions of parathyroid hormone and parathyroid hormone-related protein. *J Endocrinol Invest.* 1992;15(9 Suppl 6):51.
14. Zaharani AA, Levine ML. Primary hyperparathyroidism. *Lancet.* 1997; 349:1233.
15. Walls J, Ratcliffe WA, Howell A, et al. Parathyroid hormone and parathyroid hormone-related protein in the investigation of hypercalcaemia in two hospital populations. *Clin Endocrinol.* 1994;41(4):407.
16. Germano T. The parathyroid gland and calcium-related emergencies. *Top Emerg Med.* 2001;23(4):51.
17. Potts JT. Diseases of the parathyroid gland and other hyper- and hypocalcemic disorders. In: Kasper DL, Braunwald E, Fauci AS, et al., eds. *Harrison's Principles of Internal Medicine*; 16th ed. 2005:332.

18. Bushinsky DA, Monk RD. Calcium. *Lancet.* 1998;352:306.
19. Cogan MG, Covey GM, Arieff AL, et al. Central nervous system manifestations of hyperparathyroidism. *Am J Med.* 1978;65:963
20. 2005 American Heart Association Guidelines for Cardiopulmonary Resuscitation and Emergency Cardiovascular Care. *Circulation.* 2005;112(24): IV1–121.
21. Berenson JR. Treatment of hypercalcemia with bisphosphonates. *Semin Oncol.* 2002:29(6 Suppl 21):12.
22. Wang S, McDonnell EH, Sedor FA, et al: pH effects on measurements of ionized calcium and ionized magnesium in the blood. *Arch Pathol Lab Med.* 2002;126:947.
23. Bilezekian JP, Silverberg SJ. Asymptomatic primary hyperparathyroidism. *N Engl J Med.* 2004:350:1746.
24. Gurney H, Grill V, Martin TJ. Parathyroid hormone-related protein and response to pamidronate in tumour induced hypercalcemia. *Lancet.* 1993;341:1611.
25. Cheng C, Chou C, Lin S. An unrecognized cause of recurrent hypercalcemia: immobilization. *South Med J.* 2006;99(4):371.
26. Body JJ. Hypercalcemia of malignancy. *Semin Nephro.l* 2004;24:48.
27. Berenson JR, Lipton A. Bisphosphonates in the treatment of malignant bone disease. *Annu Rev Med.* 1999;50:237.
28. Major P, Lortholary A, Hon J, et al. Zoledronic acid is superior to pamidronate in the treatment of hypercalcemia of malignancy: a pooled analysis of two randomized, controlled clinical trials. *J Clin Oncol.* 2001; 19:558.
29. Tanveyanon T, Stiff PJ. Management of the adverse effects associated with intravenous bisphosphonates. *Ann Oncol.* 2006;(17):897.
30. Silverman P, Distelhorst CW. Metabolic emergencies in clinical oncology. *Semin Oncol.* 1989;16(6):504–515.
31. Rampello E, Fricia T, Malaguarnera M. The management of tumor lysis syndrome. *Nat Clin Pract Oncol.* 2006;3(8):438–447.
32. Chasty RC, Liu-Yin JA. Acute tumor lysis syndrome. *Br J Hosp Med.* 1993;49(70):488–492.
33. Davidson MD, Thakkar S, Hix JK, et al. Pathophysiology, clinical consequences, and treatment of tumor lysis syndrome. *Am J Med.* 2004;116:546–554.
34. Cohen LF, Balow JE, Magrath IT, et al. Acute tumor lysis syndrome: a review of 37 patients with Burkitt's lymphoma. *Am J Med.* 1980;68:486–491.
35. Hande KR, Garrow GC. Acute tumor lysis syndrome in patients with high-grade non-Hodgkin's lymphoma. *Am J Med.* 1993;94:133.
36. Flombaum CD. Metabolic emergencies in the cancer patient. *Semin Oncol.* 2000;27:322–334.
37. Jasek AM, Day HJ. Acute spontaneous tumor lysis syndrome. *Am J Hematol.* 1994;47:129–131.
38. Hsu H, Chan Y, Huang C. Acute spontaneous tumor lysis presenting with hyperuricemic acute renal failure: clinical features and therapeutic approach. *J Nephrol.* 2004;17:50–56.
39. Cairo MS, Bishop M. Tumour lysis syndrome: new therapeutic strategies and classification. *Br J Haematol.* 2004;127:3–11.
40. Dunlay RW, Camp MA, Allon M, et al. Calcitriol in prolonged hypocalcemia due to the tumor lysis syndrome. *Ann Intern Med.* 1989;110:162–164.
41. Altman A. Acute tumor lysis syndrome. *Semin Oncol.* 2001;28(Suppl 5): 3–8.
42. Navolanic PM, Pui C-H, Larson RA, et al. Elitek-rasburicase: an effective means to prevent and treat hyperuricemia associated with tumor lysis syndrome, a Meeting Report, Dallas, Texas, January 2002. *Leukemia.* 2003;17(3):499–514.
43. Ueng S. Rasburicase (Elitek): a novel agent for tumor lysis syndrome. *Proc (Bayl Univ Med Cent).* 2005;18(3):275–279.
44. Yeldani AV, Yeldani V, Kumar S, et al. Molecular evolution of the urate oxidase- encoding gene in hominoid primates: nonsense mutations. *Gene.* 1991;109:281–284.
45. Rasburicase US FDA Drug Approval: News: Micromedex. www.micromedex.com/pressroom/news_feeds/fdaapprovals/fda rasburicase.html. Accessed April 14, 2007.
46. Abner A. Approach to the patient who presents with superior vena cava obstruction. *Chest.* 1993;103(4 Suppl):394S.
47. Lamont EB, Hoffman PC. Oncologic emergencies. In: Hall JB, Schmidt GA, Wood LDH, eds. *Principles of Critical Care.* 3rd ed [book online]. New York, NY: McGraw-Hill, 2005. http://www.accessmedicine.com/resourceTOC.aspx?resourceID=76. Accessed April 21, 2007.
48. Yahalom J. Oncologic emergencies: superior vena cava syndrome. In: DeVita VT, Hellman S, Rosenberg SA, eds. *Cancer: Principles and Practice of Oncology.* 7th ed. Vol 2. Philadelphia, PA: Lippincott Williams & Wilkins; 2005:2274–2280.
49. Duwe BV, Sterman DH, Musani AI. Tumors of the mediastinum. *Chest.* 2005;128(4):2893.
50. Hunter W. The history of an aneurysm of the aorta with some remarks on aneurysms in general. *Med Observ Inq.* 1757;1:323.
51. Schechter MM. The superior vena cava syndrome. *Am J Med Sci.* 1954; 227:46.
52. Reed ED. Superior vena cava syndrome. *UpToDate* [serial online]. http://www.uptodateonline.com. Accessed April 21, 2007.
53. Parish JM, Marschke RF, Dines DE, et al. Etiologic considerations in superior vena cava syndrome. *Mayo Clin Proc.* 1981;56(7):407.
54. Gucalp R, Dutcher J. Oncologic emergencies. In: Kasper D, Braunwald E, Fauci A, et al. *Harrison's Internal Medicine.* 16th ed [book online]. New York, NY: McGraw-Hill; 2005. http://www.accessmedicine.com/resourceTOC.aspx?resourceID=4. Accessed April 21, 2007.
55. Lochridge SK, Knibbe WP, Doty DB. Obstruction of the superior vena cava. *Surgery.* 1979; 85:14.
56. Ostler PJ, Clarke DP, Watkinson AF, et al. Superior vena cava obstruction: a modern management strategy. *Clin Oncol.* 1997;9:83–89.
57. Theodore PR, Jablons D. Thoracic wall, pleura, mediastinum, and lung. In: Doherty GM, Way LW, eds. *Current Surgical Diagnosis and Treatment* [book online]. New York, NY: McGraw-Hill, 2005. http://www.accessmedicine.com/resourceTOC.aspx?resourceID=23. Accessed April 21, 2007.
58. Rice TW, Rodriguez R, Michael R, et al. Superior vena cava syndrome: clinical and evolving etiology. *Medicine.* 2006;85(1):37.
59. Ahmann F. A reassessment of the clinical implications of the superior vena cava syndrome. *J Clin Oncol.* 1984;2:961.
60. Rowell NP, Gleeson FV. Steroids, radiotherapy, chemotherapy and stents for superior vena caval obstruction in carcinoma of the bronchus: a systematic review. *Clin Oncol (R Coll Radiol).* 2002;14(5):338.
61. Crausman RS, De Palo VA, Sid RL. Diseases of the mediastinum. In: Hanley ME, Welsh CH, eds. *Current Diagnosis & Treatment in Pulmonary Medicine.* 1st ed. [book online]. New York, NY: McGraw-Hill, 2003. http://www.accessmedicine.com/resourceTOC.aspx?resourceID=37. Accessed April 21, 2007.
62. Qanadli SD, El Hajjam M, Bruckert F, et al. Helical CT phlebography of the superior vena cava: diagnosis and evaluation of venous obstruction. *AJR Am J Roentgenol.* 1999;172(5):1327.
63. Wilson LD, Detterbeck FC, Yahalom J. Superior vena cava syndrome with malignant causes. *N Engl J Med* 2007;356:1862.
64. Escalante CP. Causes and management of superior vena cava syndrome. *Oncology. (Williston Park).* 1993;7:61.
65. Schraufnagel DE, Hill R, Leech JA, et al. Superior vena caval obstruction. Is it a medical emergency? *Am J Med.* 1981;70(6):1169.
66. Gauden SJ. Superior vena cava syndrome induced by bronchogenic carcinoma: is this an oncological emergency? *Australas Radiol.* 1993;37(4):363.
67. Yellin A, Rosen A, Reichert N, et al. Superior vena cava syndrome: the myth—the facts. *Am Rev Respir Dis.* 1990;141(5):1114–1990.
68. Porte H, Metois D, Finzi L, et al. Superior vena cava syndrome of malignant origin. Which surgical procedure for which diagnosis? *Eur J Cardiothorac Surg.* 2000;17(4):384.
69. Urruticoechea A, Mesia R, Dominguez J, et al. Treatment of malignant superior vena cava syndrome by endovascular stent insertion. Experience on 52 patients with lung cancer. *Lung Cancer.* 2004;43(2):209.
70. Courtheoux P, Alkofer B, Al Refaï M, et al. Stent placement in superior vena cava syndrome. *Ann Thorac Surg.* 2003;75(1):158.
71. Chatziioannou A, Alexopoulos T, Mourikis D, et al. Stent therapy for malignant superior vena cava syndrome: should be first line therapy or simple adjunct to radiotherapy. *Eur J Radiol.* 2003;47(3):247.
72. Gray BH, Olin JW, Graor RA, et al. Safety and efficacy of thrombolytic therapy for superior vena cava syndrome. *Chest.* 1991;99(1):54.
73. Armstrong BA, Perez CA, Simpson JR, et al. Role of irradiation in the management of superior vena cava syndrome. *Int J Radiat Oncol Biol Phys.* 1987;13:531.
74. Martins SJ, Pereira JR. Clinical factors and prognosis in non-small cell lung cancer. *Am J Clin Oncol.* 1999;22(5):453.
75. Strong EW. Head and neck emergencies. *Curr Probl Cancer.* 1979;4:36.
76. McCarthy MJ, Rosado-de-Christenson ML. Tumors of the trachea. *J Thorac Imag.* 1995;10:180.
77. Noppen M, Poppe K, D'Haese J, et al. Interventional bronchoscopy for treatment of tracheal obstruction secondary to benign or malignant thyroid disease. *Chest.* 2004;125:723.
78. Muehrcke DD. Surgical treatment of thyroid cancer invading the airway. *Surg Rounds.* 1994;:669.
79. Lau CL, Patterson GA. Diagnosis and management of tracheal neoplasms. In: Cummings CW, Flint PW, Haughey BH, et al., eds. *Otolaryngology: Head & Neck Surgery.* 4th ed. [book online]. Philadelphia, PA: Elsevier Mosby; 2005. http://www.mdconsult.com/about/book/70835644-4/instruct.html?DOCID=1263. Accessed April 29, 2007.
80. Balkissoon RC, Baroody FM, Togias A. Disorders of the upper airways. In: Mason RJ, Murray JF, Broaddus VC, et al., eds. *Textbook of Respiratory Medicine.* 4th ed. [book online]. Philadelphia, PA: Elsevier Saunders; 2005. http://www.mdconsult.com/about/book/71527034-3/instruct.html?DOCID=1288. Accessed April 29, 2007.
81. Wood DE. Management of malignant tracheobronchial obstruction. *Surg Clin North Am.* 2002;82:621.
82. Yu KCY. Airway management and tracheostomy. In: Lalwani AK, ed. *Current Diagnosis & Treatment in Otolaryngology—Head & Neck Surgery.* [book online]. New York, NY: McGraw-Hill; 2004. http://www.accessmedicine.com/resourceTOC.aspx?resourceID=39. Accessed April 22, 2007.
83. Gehlbach B, Kress JK. Upper airway obstruction. In: Hall JB, Schmidt GA, Wood LDH, eds. *Principles of Critical Care.* 3rd ed. [book

online]. New York, NY: McGraw-Hill; 2005 http://www.accessmedicine.com/resourceTOC.aspx?resourceID=76. Accessed April 22, 2007.
84. Boorstein JM, Boorstein SM, Humphries GN, et al. Using helium-oxygen mixtures in the emergency management of acute upper airway obstruction. *Ann Emerg Med.* 1989;18(6):688–690.
85. Jaber S, Carlucci A, Boussarsar M, et al. Helium-oxygen in the postextubation period decreases inspiratory effort. *Am J Respir Crit Care Med.* 2001;164:633.
86. Lund ME, Garland R, Ernst A. Airway stenting: applications and practice management considerations. *Chest.* 2007;131:579.
87. Wood DE, Liu Y, Vallières E, et al. Airway stenting for malignant and benign tracheobronchial stenosis. *Ann Thorac Surg* 2003;76:167.
88. Fan AC, Baron TH, Utz JP. Combined tracheal and esophageal stenting for palliation of tracheoesophageal symptoms from mediastinal lymphoma. *Mayo Clin Proc.* 2002;77(12):1347.
89. Regnard JF, Fourquier P, Levasseur P. Results and prognostic factors in resections of primary tracheal tumors: a multicenter retrospective study. *J Thorac Cardiovasc Surg.* 1996;111(4):808.
90. Ernst A, Feller-Kopman D, Becker HD, et al. Central airway obstruction. *Am J Respir Crit Care Med.* 2004;169:1278.
91. Helweg-Larsen S, Sorensen PS, Kreiner S. Prognostic factors in metastatic spinal cord compression: a prospective study using multivariate analysis of variables influencing survival and gait function in 153 patients. *Int J Radiat Oncol Biol Phy.s* 2000;46:1163.
92. Klimo P Jr, Schmidt MH. Surgical management of spinal metastases. *Oncologist.* 2004;9(2):188.
93. Loblaw DA, Laperriere NJ. Emergency treatment of malignant extradural spinal cord compression: an evidence-based guideline. *J Clin Oncol.* 1998;16:161.
94. Loblaw DA, Perry J, Chambers A, et al. Systematic review of the diagnosis and management of malignant extradural spinal cord compression: the Cancer Care Ontario practice guidelines initiative's Neuro-Oncology Disease Site Group. *J Clin Oncol.* 2005;23(9):2028.
95. Loblaw DA, Laperriere NJ, Mackillop WJ. A population-based study of malignant spinal cord compression in Ontario. *Clin Oncol (R Coll Radiol).* 2003;15:211.
96. Prasad D, Schiff D. Malignant spinal-cord compression. *Lancet Oncol.* 2005;6(1):15.
97. Baehring JM. Spinal cord compression. In: DeVita VT, Hellman S, Rosenberg SA, eds. *Cancer: Principles and Practice of Oncology.* 7th ed. Vol 2. Philadelphia, PA: Lippincott Williams & Wilkins; 2005:2288.
98. Helweg-Larsen S, Sorensen PS. Symptoms and signs in metastatic spinal cord compression: a study of progression from first symptom until diagnosis in 153 patients. *Eur J Cancer.* 1994;30A(3):396.
99. Schiff D, O'Neill BP, Wang CH, et al. Neuroimaging and treatment implications of patients with multiple epidural spinal metastases. *Cancer.* 1998;83:1593.
100. Schiff D, O'Neill BP, Suman VJ. Spinal epidural metastasis as the initial manifestation of malignancy: clinical features and diagnostic approach. *Neurology.* 1997;49(2):452.
101. Bach F, Larsen BH, Rohde K, et al. Metastatic spinal cord compression. Occurrence, symptoms, clinical presentations and prognosis in 398 patients with spinal cord compression. *Acta Neurochir (Wien).* 1990;107(1–2):37.
102. Willson JKV, Masaryk TJ. Neurologic emergencies in the cancer patient. *Semin Oncol.* 1989;16:490.
103. Portenoy RK, Lipton RB, Foley KM. Back pain in the cancer patient: an algorithm for evaluation and management. *Neurology.* 1987;37:134.
104. Li C, Poon PY. Sensitivity and specificity of MRI in detecting malignant spinal cord compression and in distinguishing malignant from benign compression fractures of vertebrae. *Magn Reson Imaging.* 1988;6:547–556.
105. Cook AM, Lau TN, Tomlinson MJ, et al. Magnetic resonance imaging of the whole spine in suspected malignant spinal cord compression: impact on management. *Clin Oncol (R Coll Radiol).* 1998;10(1):39.
106. Schiff D, O'Neill BP, Wang CH, et al. Neuroimaging and treatment implications of patients with multiple epidural spinal metastases. *Cancer.* 1998;83(8):1593.
107. Ecker RD, Endo T, Wetjen NM. Diagnosis and treatment of vertebral column metastases. *Mayo Clin Proc.* 2005;80(9):1174.
108. Sorensen S, Helweg-Larsen S, Mouridsen H, et al. Effect of high-dose dexamethasone in carcinomatous metastatic spinal cord compression treated with radiotherapy: a randomised trial. *Eur J Cancer.* 1994;30A(1):22.
109. Maranzano E, Latini P, Beneventi S, et al. Radiotherapy without steroids in selected metastatic spinal cord compression patients: a phase II trial. *Am J Clin Oncol.* 1996;19:179.
110. Patchell RA, Tibbs PA, Regine WF, et al. Direct decompressive surgical resection in the treatment of spinal cord compression caused by metastatic cancer: a randomised trial. *Lancet.* 2005;366(9486):643.
111. Husband DJ. Malignant spinal cord compression: prospective study of delays in referral and treatment. *Br Med J.* 1998;317(7150):18.
112. Pierri MK. Heart disease. In: Groeger JS, ed. *Critical Care of the Cancer Patient.* St. Louis, MO: Mosby-Year Book; 1991:64.
113. Maisch B, Seferovi PM, Risti AD. Guidelines on the diagnosis and management of pericardial diseases executive summary: the task force on the diagnosis and management of pericardial diseases of the European Society of Cardiology. *Eur Heart J.* 2004;25:587.
114. Campbell PT, Van Trigt P, Wall TC. Subxiphoid pericardiotomy in the diagnosis and management of large pericardial effusions associated with malignancy. *Chest.* 1992;101:938.
115. Decamp MM, Mentzer SJ, Swanson SJ, et al. Malignant effusive disease of the pleura and pericardium. *Chest.* 1997;112(4 Suppl):291S.
116. Nguyen DM, Schrump DS. Treatment of metastatic cancer: malignant pleural and pericardial effusions. In: DeVita VT, Hellman S, Rosenberg SA, eds. *Cancer: Principles and Practice of Oncology.* 7th ed. Vol 2. Philadelphia, PA: Lippincott Williams & Wilkins; 2005:2382–2392.
117. Cullinane CA, Paz IB, Smith D, et al. Prognostic factors in the surgical management of pericardial effusion in the patient with concurrent malignancy. *Chest.* 2004;125:1328.
118. Garcia-Riego A, Cuinas C, Vilanova JJ. Malignant pericardial effusion. *Acta Cytol.* 2001;45:561.
119. Gray H. In: Louis WH, ed. *Gray's Anatomy of the Human Body.* 20th ed. [book online]. Philadelphia, PA: Lea & Febiger, 1918; New York, NY: Bartleby.com, 2000. http://www.bartleby.com/107. Accessed April 21, 2007.
120. Stouffer GA, Sheahan RG, Lenihan D, et al. Diagnosis and management of chronic pericardial effusions. *Am J Med Sci.* 2001;322:79.
121. Fiedler M, Nelson LA. Cardiac tamponade. *Int Anethes Clin.* 200543(4):33.
122. Spodick DH. Acute cardiac tamponade. *N Engl J Med.* 2003;349:684.
123. Vaitkus PT, Herrmann HC, LeWinter MM. Treatment of malignant pericardial effusion. *JAMA.* 1994;272:59.
124. Tsang TS, Seward JB, Barnes ME, et al. Outcomes of primary and secondary treatment of pericardial effusion in patients with malignancy. *Mayo Clin Proc.* 2000;75(3):248.
125. Galli M, Politi A, Pedretti F, et al. Percutaneous balloon pericardiotomy for malignant pericardial tamponade. *Chest.* 1995;108:1499.
126. Ziskind AA, Pearce AC, Lemmon CC, et al. Percutaneous balloon pericardiotomy for the treatment of cardiac tamponade and large pericardial effusions: description of technique and report of the first 50 cases. *J Am Coll Cardiol.* 1993;21:1.
127. Sagristà-Sauleda J, Angel J, Sànchez A, et al. Effusive-constrictive pericarditis. *N Engl J Med.* 2004;350:469.
128. Wang HJ, Hsu K, Chiang FT, et al. Technical and prognostic outcomes of double- balloon pericardiotomy for large malignancy-related pericardial effusions. *Chest.* 2002;122:893.
129. Gornik HL, Gerhard-Herman M, Beckman J. Abnormal cytology predicts poor prognosis in cancer patients with pericardial effusion. *J Clin Oncol.* 2005;23(22):5211.
130. O'Connor K, Dijkstra B, Kelly L, et al. Successful conservative management of neutropenic enterocolitis: a report of two cases and review of the literature. *ANZ J Surg.* 2003;73(6):463.
131. Wong Kee Song L, Marcon NE. Necrotising enterocolitis (typhlitis) in adults. *UpToDate* [serial online]. http://www.uptodate.com. Accessed April 29, 2007.
132. Amromin GD, Solomon RD. Necrotizing enteropathy: a complication of treated leukemia or lymphoma patients. *JAMA.* 1962;182:23.
133. Wagner ML, Rosenberg HS, Fernbach DJ, et al. Typhlitis: a complication of leukemia in childhood. *Am J Roentgenol Radium Ther Nucl Med.* 1970;109:341.
134. Gorschlüter M, Mey U, Strehl J, et al. Neutropenic enterocolitis in adults: systematic analysis of evidence quality. *Eur J Haematol.* 2005;75(1):1.
135. Bibbo C, Barbieri RA, Deitch EA, et al. Neutropenic enterocolitis in a trauma patient during antibiotic therapy for osteomyelitis. *J Trauma.* 2000;49:760.
136. Hsu T, Huang H-H, Yen D H-T. ED presentation of neutropenic enterocolitis in adult patients with acute leukemia. *Am J of Emerg Med.* 2004; 22(4):276.
137. Hughes WT, Armstrong D, Bodey GP, et al. 2002 guidelines for the use of antimicrobial agents in neutropenic patients with cancer. *Clin Infect Dis.* 2002;34:730.
138. Segal BH, Walsh TJ, Gea-Banacloche JC, et al. Infections in the cancer patient. In: DeVita VT, Hellman S, Rosenberg SA, eds. *Cancer: Principles and Practice of Oncology.* 7th ed. Vol 2. Philadelphia, PA: Lippincott Williams & Wilkins; 2005:2460–2514.
139. Sloas MM, Flynn PM, Kaste SC, et al. Typhlitis in children with cancer: a 30-year experience. *Clin Infect Dis.* 1993;17:484.
140. Williams N, Scott ADN. Neutropenic colitis: a continuing surgical challenge. *B J Surg.* 1997;84(9):1200.
141. Cappell MS. Colonic toxicity of administered drugs and chemicals. *Am J Gastroenterol.* 2004;99(6):117.
142. Kouroussis C, Samonis G, Androulakis N, et al. Successful conservative treatment of neutropenic enterocolitis complicating taxane-based chemotherapy: a report of five cases. *Am J Clin Oncol.* 2000;23(3):309.
143. Ibrahim NK, Sahin AA, Dubrow RA, et al. Colitis associated with docetaxel-based chemotherapy in patients with metastatic breast cancer. *Lancet.* 2000;355:281.
144. Pestalozzi BC, Sotos GA, Choyke PL, et al. Typhlitis resulting from treatment with Taxol and doxorubicin in patients with metastatic breast cancer. *Cancer.* 1993;71:1797.
145. Weinberger M, Hollingsworth H, Feuerstein IM, et al. Successful surgical management of neutropenic enterocolitis in two patients with severe

aplastic anemia. Case reports and review of the literature. *Arch Intern Med.* 1993;153:107.
146. Geelhoed GW, Kane MA, Dale DC, et al. Colon ulceration and perforation in cyclic neutropenia. *J Pediatr Surg.* 1973;8:379.
147. Gorschluter M, Glasmacher A, Hahn C, et al. Severe abdominal infections in neutropenic patients. *Cancer Invest.* 2001;19:669.
148. Ryan ME, Morrissey JF. Typhlitis complicating methimazole-induced agranulocytosis. *Gastrointest Endosc.* 1983;29:299.
149. Cutrona AF, Blinkhom RJ, Crass J, et al. Probable neutropenic enterocolitis in patients with AIDS. *Rev Infect Dis.* 1991;13:828.
150. Mehta J, Nagler A, Or R, et al. Neutropenic enterocolitis and intestinal perforation associated with carboplatin-containing conditioning regimen for autologous bone marrow transplantation. *Acta Oncol.* 1992;31: 591.
151. Frankel AH, Barker F, Williams G, et al. Neutropenic enterocolitis in a renal transplant patient. *Transplantation.* 1991;52:913.
152. Cartoni C, Dragoni F, Micozzi A, et al. Neutropenic enterocolitis in patients with acute leukemia: prognostic significance of bowel wall thickening detected by ultrasonography. *J Clin Oncol.* 2001;19:756.
153. Shamberger RC, Weinstein HJ, Delorey MJ, et al. The medical and surgical management of typhlitis in children with acute nonlymphocytic (myelogenous) leukemia. *Cancer.* 1986;57:603.
154. Mourra N, Nion-Larmurier I, Parc R, et al. Neutropenic enterocolitis in acute myeloblastic leukaemia. *Histopathology.* 2005;46(3):353.
155. Guiot HFI, Fibbe WE, van't Wout JW, et al. Risk factors for fungal infection in patients with malignant hematologic disorders: implications for empirical therapy and prophylaxis. *Clin Infect Dis.* 1994;18:525.
156. Lord BI, Bronchud MH, Owens S, et al. The kinetics of human granulopoiesis following treatment with granulocyte colony-stimulating factor in vivo. *Proc Natl Acad Sci U S A.* 1989;86:9499.
157. Katz JA, Wagner ML, Gresik MV, et al. Typhlitis: an 18-year experience and postmortem review. *Cancer.* 1990;65:1041.
158. Daniele B, Rossi GB, Losito S. Ischemic colitis associated with paclitaxel. *J Clin Gastroenterol.* 2001;33(2):159.
159. de Brito D, Barton E, Spears KL, et al. Acute right lower quadrant pain in a patient with leukemia. *Ann Emerg Med.* 1998;32:98.
160. Kaste SC, Flynn PM, Furman WL. Acute lymphoblastic leukemia presenting with typhlitis. *Med Pediatr Oncol.* 1997;28(3):209.
161. Gandy W, Greenberg BR. Successful medical management of neutropenic enterocolitis. *Cancer.* 1983;51:1551.
162. Solomkin JS, Mazuski JE, Baron EJ, et al. Guidelines for the selection of anti-infective agents for complicated intra-abdominal infections. *Clin Infect Dis.* 2003;37(8):997.
163. Viscoli C. Planned progressive antimicrobial therapy in neutropenic patients. *Br J Haematol.* 1998;102(4):879.
164. Ozer H, Armitage JO, Bennett CL, et al. 2000 update of recommendations for the use of hematopoietic colony-stimulating factors: evidence-based, clinical practice guidelines. American Society of Clinical Oncology Growth Factors Expert Panel. *J Clin Oncol.* 2000;18:3558.
165. Clark OAC, Lyman GH, Castro AA, et al. Colony-stimulating factors for chemotherapy-induced febrile neutropenia: a meta-analysis of randomized controlled trials. *J Clin Oncol.* 2005;23:4198.
166. O'Brien S, Kantarjian HM, Anaissie E. Successful medical management of neutropenic enterocolitis in adults with acute leukemia. *South Med J.* 1987;80:1233.
167. Wade DS, Nava HR, Douglass HO. Neutropenic enterocolitis. Clinical diagnosis and treatment. *Cancer.* 1992;69:17–23.
168. Moir CR, Scudamore CH, Benny WB. Typhlitis: selective surgical management. *Am. J Surg.* 1986;151:563.
169. Small EJ. Chemotherapy of urologic tumors. In: Tanagho EA, McAninch JW, eds. *Smith's General Urology.* 16th ed. [book online]. New York, NY: McGraw-Hill; 2004. http://www.accessmedicine.com/resourceTOC.aspx?resourceID=21. Accessed May 1, 2007.
170. Chu E. Pharmacology of cancer chemotherapy: drug development. In: DeVita VT, Hellman S, Rosenberg SA, eds. *Cancer: Principles and Practice of Oncology.* 7th ed. Vol 1. Philadelphia, PA: Lippincott Williams & Wilkins, 2005:307–316.
171. Floyd JD, Nguyen DT, Lobins RL, et al. Cardiotoxicity of cancer therapy. *J Clin Oncol.* 2005;23:7685.
172. White DA, Orenstein M, Godwin TA, et al. Chemotherapy-associated pulmonary toxic reactions during the treatment of breast cancer. *Arch Intern Me.* 1984;144:953.
173. Vander Els NJ, Stover DE. Chemotherapy-induced lung disease. *Clin Pulm Med.* 2004;11(2):84.
174. Simpson AB, Paul J, Graham J, et al. Fatal bleomycin pulmonary toxicity in the west of Scotland 1991-95: a review of patients with germ cell tumours. *Br J Cancer.* 1998;78(8):1061.
175. Sleijffer S. Bleomycin-induced pneumonitis. *Chest.* 2001;120:617–624.
176. Donat SM, Levy DA. Bleomycin associated pulmonary toxicity: is perioperative oxygen restriction necessary? *J Urol.* 1998;60(4):1347.
177. Goldiner PL, Schweizer O. The hazards of anesthesia and surgery in bleomycin-treated patients. *Sem Oncol.*1979;6:121.
178. Rivera MP, Kris MG, Gralla RV, et al. Syndrome of acute dyspnea related to combined mitomycin plus vinca alkaloid chemotherapy. *Am J Clin Oncol.* 1995;18:245.
179. Castro M, Veeder MH, Mailliard JA. A prospective study of pulmonary function in patients receiving mitomycin. *Chest.* 1996;109:939.
180. Abid SH, Malhotra V, Perry MC. Radiation-induced and chemotherapy-induced pulmonary injury. *Curr Opin Oncol.* 2001;13(4):242.
181. Stover DE, Kaner RJ. Adverse effects of treatment: pulmonary toxicity. In: DeVita VT, Hellman S, Rosenberg SA, eds. *Cancer: Principles and Practice of Oncology.* 7th ed. Vol 2. Philadelphia, PA: Lippincott Williams & Wilkins; 2005:2536–2545.
182. Rowinsky EK, Donehower RC. Paclitaxel (Taxol). *N Engl J Med.* 1995; 332:1004.
183. Dimopoulou I, Bamias A, Lyberopoulos P, et al. Pulmonary toxicity from novel antineoplastic agents. *Ann Oncol.* 2006;17(3):372.
184. Aapro MS, Martin C, Hatty S. Gemcitabine—a safety review. *Anticancer Drugs.* 1998;9:191.
185. Gupta N, Ahmed I, Steinberg H, et al. Gemcitabine-induced pulmonary toxicity: case report and review of the literature. *Am J Clin Oncol.* 2002; 25(1):96.
186. Pavlakis N, Bell DR, Millward MJ, et al. Fatal pulmonary toxicity resulting from treatment with gemcitabine. *Cancer.* 1997;80:286.
187. Camacho LH, Soignet SL, Chanel S, et al. Leukocytosis and the retinoic acid syndrome in patients with acute promyelocytic leukemia treated with arsenic trioxide. *J Clin Oncol.* 2000;18:2620.
188. De Botton S, Dombret H, Sanz M. Incidence, clinical features, and outcome of all trans- retinoic acid syndrome in 413 cases of newly diagnosed acute promyelocytic leukemia. The European APL group. *Blood.* 1998;92 (8):2712.
189. Vogel CL, Franco SX. Clinical experience with trastuzumab (Herceptin). *Breast J.* 2003;9(6):452.
190. Slamon DJ, Clark GM, Wong SG, et al. Human breast cancer: correlation of relapse and survival with amplification of the HER-2/neu oncogene. *Science.* 1987;235:174.
191. Cook-Bruns N. Retrospective analysis of the safety of Herceptin immunotherapy in metastatic breast cancer. *Oncology.* 2001;61(Suppl 2):58–66.
192. Johnson DH, Fehrenbacher L, Novotny WF, et al. Randomized phase II trial comparing bevacizumab plus carboplatin and paclitaxel with carboplatin and paclitaxel alone in previously untreated locally advanced or metastatic non-small cell lung cancer. *J Clin Oncol.* 2004;22:2184.
193. Sandler A, Gray R, Perry MC, et al. Paclitaxel-carboplatin alone or with bevacizumab for non-small-cell lung cancer. *N Eng J Med.* 2006;355(24): 2542.
194. Wierda WG, Kipps TJ, Keating MJ. Novel immune-based treatment strategies for chronic lymphocytic leukemia. *J Clin Oncol.* 2005;23:6325.
195. Rieger K, Von Grünhagen U, Fietz T, et al. Efficacy and tolerability of alemtuzumab (CAMPATH-1H) in the salvage treatment of B-cell chronic lymphocytic leukemia—change of regimen needed?. *Leuk Lymphoma.* 2004;45(2):345.
196. Floyd JD, Nguyen DT, Lobins RL, et al. Cardiotoxicity of cancer therapy. *J Clin Oncol.* 2005;23:7685.
197. Singal PK, Iliskovic N. Doxorubicin-induced cardiomyopathy. *N Engl J Med.* 1998;339:900.
198. Yeh ETH, Tong AT, Lenihan DJ, et al. Cardiovascular complications of cancer therapy: diagnosis, pathogenesis, and management. *Circulation.* 2004;109(25):3122.
199. Batist G, Ramakrishnan G, Rao CS, et al. Reduced cardiotoxicity and preserved antitumor efficacy of liposome-encapsulated doxorubicin and cyclophosphamide compared with conventional doxorubicin and cyclophosphamide in a randomized, multicenter trial of metastatic breast cancer. *J Clin Oncol.* 2001;19:1444.
200. Swaim S, Whaley FS, Gerber M, et al. Cardioprotection with dexrazoxane for doxorubicin-containing therapy in advanced breast cancer. *J Clin Onco.* 1997;15:1318.
201. Gehl J, Boesgaard M, Paaske T, et al. Combined doxorubicin and paclitaxel in advanced breast cancer: effective and cardiotoxic. *Ann Oncol.* 1996;7(7):687.
202. Malhotra V, Dorr VJ, Lyss AP, et al. Neoadjuvant and adjuvant chemotherapy with doxorubicin and docetaxel in locally advanced breast cancer. *Clin Breast Cancer.* 2004;5(5):377.
203. Shenkenberg TD, VonHof DD. Mitoxantrone: a new anticancer drug with significant clinical activity. *Ann Intern Med.* 1986;105:67.
204. Yahalom J, Portlock CS. Adverse effects of treatment: cardiac toxicity. In: DeVita VT, Hellman S, Rosenberg SA, eds. *Cancer: Principles and Practice of Oncology.* 7th ed. Vol 2. Philadelphia, PA: Lippincott Williams & Wilkins, 2005:2546–2555.
205. Verweij J, Funke-Kupper AJ, Teule GJ, et al. A prospective study on the dose dependency of cardiotoxicity induced by mitomycin C. *Med Oncol Tumor Pharmacother.* 1988;5:159.
206. Ayash LJ, Wright JE, Tretyakov O, et al. Cyclophosphamide pharmacokinetics: correlation with cardiac toxicity and tumor response. *J Clin Oncol.* 1992;10(6):995.
207. Quezado ZM, Wilson WH, Cunnion RE, et al. High-dose ifosfamide is associated with severe, reversible cardiac dysfunction. *Ann Intern Med.* 1993;118(1):31.
208. Talcott JA, Herman TS. Acute ischemic vascular events and cisplatin. *Ann Intern Med.* 1987;107:121.

209. Lapeyre-Mestre M, Gregoire N, Bugat R, et al. Vinorelbine-related cardiac events: a meta—analysis of randomized clinical trials. *Fundam Clin Pharmacol.* 2004;18:97.
210. Arbuck SG, Strauss H, Rowinsky E, et al. A reassessment of the cardiac toxicity associated with Taxol. *Monogr Natl Cancer Inst.* 1993;15: 117.
211. Rezkalla S, Kloner RA, Ensley J, et al. Continuous ambulatory ECG monitoring during fluorouracil therapy: a prospective clinical study. *J Clin Oncol.* 1989;7:509–514.
212. Van Cutse ME, Hoff PM, Blum JL, et al. Incidence of cardiotoxicity with the oral fluoropyrimidine capecitabine is typical of that reported with 5-fluorouracil. *Ann Oncol.* 2002;13:484.
213. Airey CL, Dodwell DJ, Joffe JK, et al. Etoposide-related myocardial infarction. *Clin Oncol.* 1995;7:135.
214. Martino S, Ratanatharathorn V, Karanes C, et al. Reversible arrhythmias observed in patients treated with recombinant alpha 2 interferon. *J Cancer Res Clin Oncol.* 1987;113:376.
215. Sonnenblick M, Rosemann D, Rosin A. Reversible cardiomyopathy induced by interferon. *BMJ.* 1990;300:1174.
216. Lee RE, Lotze MT, Skibber JM, et al. Cardiorespiratory effects of immunotherapy with interleukin-2. *J Clin Oncol.* 1989;7:7.
217. Barbey J, Pezzullo J, Soignet S. Effect of arsenic trioxide on QT interval in patients with advanced malignancies. *J Clin Oncol.* 2003;21:3609.
218. Seidman A, Hudis C, Pierri MK, et al. Cardiac dysfunction in the trastuzumab clinical trials experience. *J Clin Oncol.* 2002;20:1215.
219. Keefe DL. Trastuzumab-associated cardiotoxicity. *Cancer.* 2002;95(7): 1592.
220. Pettengell R, Linch D. Position paper on the therapeutic use of rituximab in CD20-positive diffuse large B-cell non-Hodgkin's lymphoma. *Br J Haematol.* 2003;121(1):44.
221. Saltz LB, Meropol NJ, Loehrer PJ Sr, et al. Phase II trial of cetuximab in patients with refractory colorectal cancer that expresses the epidermal growth factor receptor. *J Clin Oncol.* 2004;22:1201.
222. Cobleigh MA, Langmuir VK, Sledge GW, et al. A phase I/II dose-escalation trial of bevacizumab in previously treated metastatic breast cancer. *Semin Oncol.* 2003;30:11.
223. US Food and Drug Administration 2005 safety alerts for drugs, biologics, medical devices and dietary supplements: update: Avastin (bevacizumab). January 6, 2005 http://www.fda.gov/medwatch/SAFETY/2005/safety05.htm#Avastin.
224. Kabbinavar FF, Schulz J, McCleod M, et al. Addition of bevacizumab to bolus fluorouracil and leucovorin in first-line metastatic colorectal cancer: results of a randomized phase II trial. *J Clin Oncol.* 2005;23:3697.
225. Osman K, Comenzo R, Rajkumar SV. Deep venous thrombosis and thalidomide therapy for multiple myeloma [Letter]. *N Engl J Med.* 2001;344: 1951.
226. Mehta J, Desikan R, Ayers D, et al. Antitumor activity of thalidomide in refractory multiple myeloma. *N Engl J Med.* 1999;341:1565.
227. Rajkumar SV. Thalidomide therapy and deep venous thrombosis in multiple myeloma [Editorial]. *Mayo Clin Proc.* 2005;80(12):1549.
228. Bennett CL, Schumock GT, Desai AA, et al. Thalidomide-associated deep vein thrombosis and pulmonary embolism. *Am J Med.* 2002;113(7):606.
229. Bennett CL, Angelotta C, Yarnold PR, et al. Thalidomide- and lenalidomide-associated thromboembolism among patients with cancer. *JAMA.* 2006;296:2558.
230. Pritchard KI, Paterson AH, Paul NA, et al. Increased thromboembolic complications with concurrent tamoxifen and chemotherapy in a randomized trial of adjuvant therapy for women with breast cancer. National Cancer Institute of Canada Clinical Trials Group Breast Cancer Site Group. *J Clin Oncol.* 1996;4:2731.
231. Lycette JL, Luoh S, Beer TM, et al. Acute bilateral pulmonary emboli occurring while on adjuvant aromatase inhibitor therapy with anastrozole: cases report and review of the literature. *Breast Cancer Res Treat.* 2006;99:249–255.
232. Hurwitz H, Fehrenbacher L, Novotny W, et al. Bevacizumab plus irinotecan, fluorouracil, and leucovorin for metastatic colorectal cancer. *N Engl J Med.* 2004;350:2335.
233. Chen HX, Mooney M, Boron M, et al. Phase II multicenter trial of bevacizumab plus fluorouracil and leucovorin in patients with advanced refractory colorectal cancer: an NCI treatment referral center trial TRC-0301. *J Clin Oncol.* 2006;24:3354.
234. Walker RD. Cyclophosphamide induced hemorrhagic cystitis. *J Urol.* 1999; 161(6):1747.
235. Desai AA, Fleming G. Toxicities of chemotherapy in critical care. In: Hall JB, Schmidt GA, Wood LDH, eds. *Principles of Critical Care.* 3rd ed. [book online]. New York, NY: McGraw-Hill; 2005. http://www.accessmedicine.com/resourceTOC.aspx?resourceID=76. Accessed May 1, 2007.
236. Yamamoto R, Kusumi E, Kami M, et al. Late hemorrhagic cystitis after reduced-intensity hematopoietic stem cell transplantation (RIST). *Bone Marrow Transplant.* 2003;32:1089.
237. Elliott MA, Nichols WL. Thrombotic thrombocytopenic purpura and hemolytic uremic syndrome. *Mayo Clin Proc.* 2001;76(11):1154–1162.
238. Medina PJ, Sipols JM, George JN. Drug-associated thrombotic thrombocytopenic purpura-hemolytic uremic syndrome. *Curr Opin Hematol.* 2001;8(5):286–293.
239. Verweij J, van der Burg M, Pinedo H. Mitomycin C-induced hemolytic uremic syndrome: six case reports and review of the literature on renal, pulmonary and cardiac side effects of the drug. *Radiother Oncol.* 1987;8:33.
240. Gordon LI, Kwaan HC. Cancer- and drug-associated thrombotic thrombocytopenic purpura and hemolytic uremic syndrome. *Semin Hematol.* 1997;34:140.
241. Snyder HW Jr, Mittelman A, Oral A, et al. Treatment of cancer chemotherapy-associated thrombotic thrombocytopenic purpura/hemolytic uremic syndrome by protein A immunoadsorption of plasma. *Cancer.* 1993;71:1882.

CHAPTER 175 ■ MASS CASUALTY INCIDENTS: ORGANIZATIONAL AND TRIAGE-MANAGEMENT ISSUES THAT IMPACT CRITICAL CARE

FREDERICK M. BURKLE, JR. • MICHAEL D. CHRISTIAN • LEWIS RUBINSON

Mass casualty incidents (MCIs) are characterized by such high numbers (hundreds to tens of thousands), severity, and diversity of injuries and illnesses that they can overwhelm the ability of local medical resources to deliver comprehensive and definitive medical care to all victims (1). Recent experience with large-scale natural disasters, bombings, threats of weapons of mass destruction, and pandemics suggest that modern-day mass casualty events would compromise the ability of all local, regional, or national health systems to deliver services consistent with established standards of care while rapidly overwhelming both the medical and public health systems. Yet no one recent event revealed the dangers and opportunities posed by potential MCIs more than the severe acute respiratory syndrome (SARS) pandemic that spread from rural China to 40 countries in 10 days (2,3). SARS exposed severe international political and legal impediments that not only prevented an effective and efficient local-to-international response but also contributed to the transmission of the disease. Only when emergency actions by the World Health Assembly gave the World Health Organization (WHO) unprecedented authority to overcome national sovereignty restrictions in favor of international protection was the pandemic controlled (4,5). Clearly, what happens locally, as a potential global threat, has immediate international implications. Over a prolonged period of time, local capability and capacity to optimize services, such as those of critical care, requires unprecedented collaboration, communication, and cooperation of state, national, and international resources (2).

Victims in the developed world are not prepared for the sudden challenges posed by an MCI that limits resources. Nowhere is this more evident than in countries that enjoy everyday critical care that provides highly advanced and technologically dependent medical, surgical, monitoring, and care to victims in a critical or unstable condition. Arguably, critical care is the most expensive high technology and resource-intensive area of medical care, and the pressure to respond in like-minded fashion to any MCI with unlimited resources is immense (6). MCIs, in particular, the 1995 Tokyo Subway sarin attack, the 2001 anthrax letter attacks, and the 2003 SARS outbreaks, have transformed the requirements for health care facilities (HCFs), and in the process, made the critical community more aware of how devastating the potential expectations and risks of their roles and responsibilities are. The greatest challenge for HCFs, already overwhelmed on a daily basis with high acuity, declining bed capacity, and health care worker (HCW) shortages, will be the sudden presentation of large numbers of severely critical victims (7). HCFs are expected to increase their capacity (staffing, equipment, and prioritization of care) by 110% to 120% to cope with a major MCI (8). Depending on the cause of the MCI, the patient mix may range from primarily "walking wounded" or those with minimal illnesses (i.e., influenza pandemic), to the vast majority of those requiring hospital admission for critical care (i.e., inhalational plague, anthrax, mutational avian influenza).

Organization science research challenges communities to continuously maintain effective, high-quality, and competent working conditions despite disasters that "fluctuate widely and are extremely hazardous and unpredictable" (9). New organizational systems that achieve flexibility and a degree of reliability under turbulent conditions have in common: standardization, specialization, formalization, and hierarchical authority. One community level system is the National Incident Management System (NIMS) and its Incident Command System (ICS), designed and used by many public safety professions. The NIMS has shown consistent capacity of reliability in conventional disaster conditions along with the ability to structure and restructure on a moment-to-moment basis to respond to unforeseen complications provoked by large, complex, and dynamic emergencies and disasters (9).

This chapter will focus first on the description of established disaster management schemes under the NIMS that address the integration of multidisciplinary local, national, regional, and international assets required for effective management of MCIs; schemes that also have responsibility to address issues of critical care decision making and communications. Knowledge of these schemes will allow the critical care community to be a more effective player at the emergency response table (7). At no time in the care of a population will critical care be more responsive to and its success dependent on other agencies and organizations than during an MCI. Second, this chapter will address critical care decision making, including the inevitable triage management of limited resources, which under the rubric of surge capacity requirements, should ensure the greatest good for the greatest number (2,10).

THE ORGANIZATION FOR MASS CASUALTY MANAGEMENT

The coordinated response to large-scale disasters by local communities, nation-states, regions, and international organizations such as the WHO is no longer an *ad hoc* process derived from local disaster plans. Emergencies are typically divided into three phases (pre-event, event, and postevent) with particular activities occurring during each phase (11). The medical and public health planning requirements that support critical care will first occur at a local level and within health care facilities responsible for those services (7). As the planning process evolves and the MCI escalates, it is necessary to integrate both planning and operational activities at county, state, national, and even international levels. At regional and national levels, governmental jurisdictions have adopted NIMS for achieving unified interagency and intra-agency management during operations for any large-scale and MCI disaster. The NIMS goal is to ensure that there is a comprehensive national framework to support efficient and effective incident management regardless of size, nature, or complexity of the incident. The NIMS framework provides for a seamless interface and standardization of emergency organizational structures, emergency plan training, emergency response equipment, communication, and other technologies (Fig. 175.1) (12,13). However, health care and public health must still work to standardize their terminology for resources (people, equipment, etc.).

Within this NIMS scheme is the *Incident Command System* (ICS), the *Unified Command System* (UCS), and the *Emergency Operations Center* (EOC) concept that facilitates the policy and operational processes at the local level. To ensure that ongoing services remain a viable and credible option when practice and resources are constrained, critical care services must understand the larger system in which they will need to work. Health care workers will be required to make uncomfortable but real decisions that are often population based and are not part of their daily routine. Understanding the system in which management of an MCI occurs is a first step in that process (12–16).

Incident Command System

Traditionally, disaster management has involved integration of local fire, police, and emergency medical services. However, modern responses to MCIs involve services from many different agencies and organizations including public health. The more complex the disaster, the more agencies will participate. By definition, MCIs require unprecedented coordination, collaboration, and cooperation of disparate organizations and jurisdictions to ensure operational success. In the 1970s, the

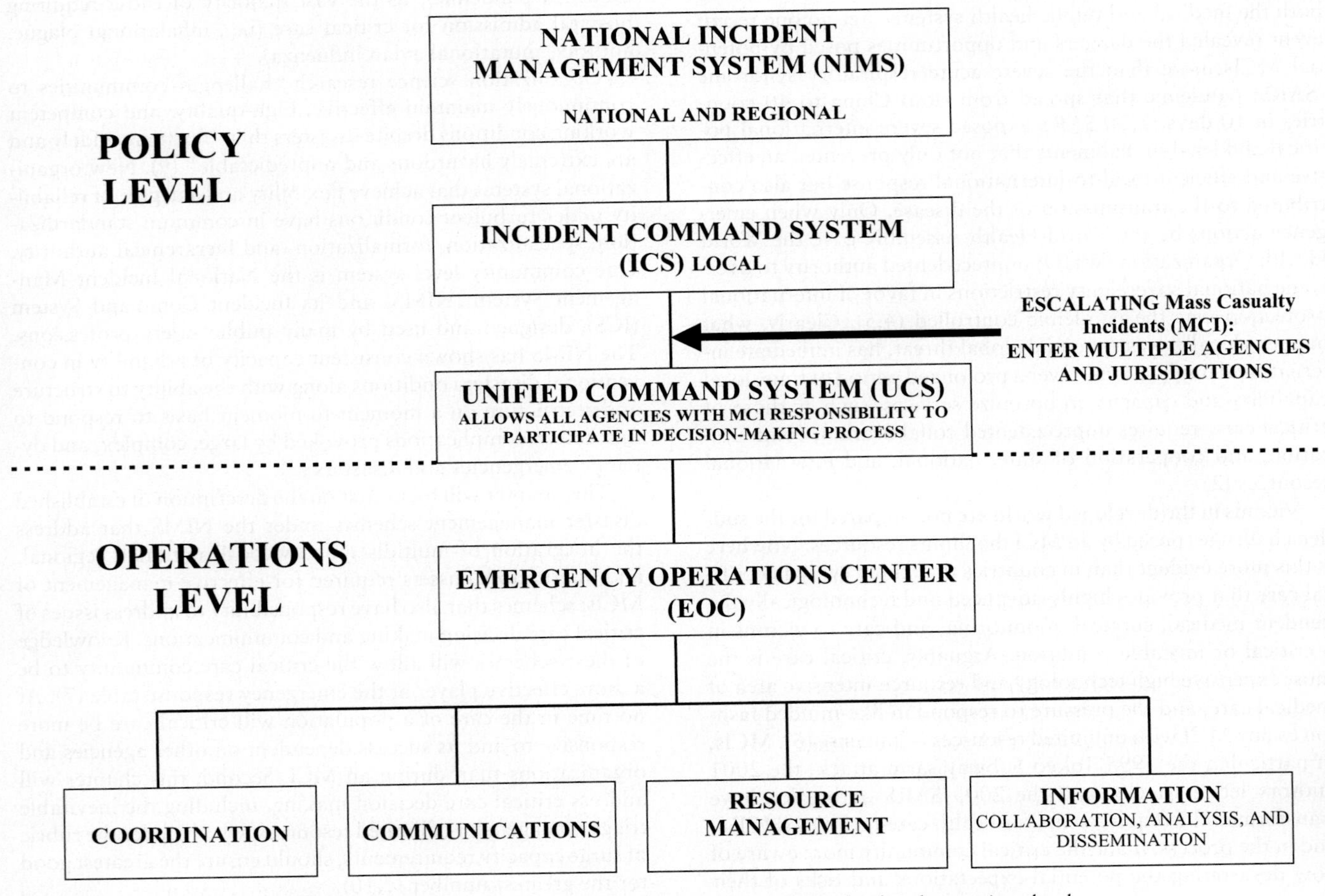

FIGURE 175.1. National Incident Management System: Policy level and operations level.

Incident Command System (ICS) was created to provide a common organizational structure and language to coordinate and simplify communication and establish clear lines of authority with a seamless command structure. For more than 30 years, disaster management resources in North America, the United Kingdom, and parts of New Zealand and Australia have continued to use the ICS as the accepted standard for all disaster response (12,13,16,17).

The ICS is organizationally flexible to meet the needs of disasters of any kind and size, yet is based on consistent and common features seen in all disasters. The ICS structure is based on common functional requirements, not titles (Fig. 175.1). All participants must adhere to the structure of the ICS to integrate successfully into the disaster management response. The basic organizational structure of ICS has five major *functional* management activities (11,12,15):

1. The *Incident Commander* maintains overall responsibility for disaster response and the Incident Action Plan (IAP), which defines the response activities and resource use for a specific period of time
2. The *Operations* Section is responsible for the following:
   - Directing and coordinating all operations
   - Ensuring the safety of Operations Section personnel
   - Assisting the Incident Commander in developing response goals and objectives
   - Implementing the Incident Action Plan
   - Requesting (or releasing) resources through the Incident Commander
   - Updating the Incident Commander on status of the situation and resources
3. The *Planning* Section is responsible for the following:
   - Collection, evaluation, dissemination, and use of information about the development of the incident and status of resources
   - Creation of the Incident Action Plan, which develops action plans and collects/evaluates information
4. The *Logistics* Section is responsible for the following:
   - Provision of facilities, services, and materials for the incident, including essential personnel to meet incident needs
   - Long-term or extended operations (i.e., the Medical Unit in the Logistics Section provides care for the incident responders, not civilian victims)
5. The *Finance and Administration* Section is responsible for monitoring costs

Under the ICS, only those management sections and positions that are needed are activated, but the responsibilities for each function falls to the Incident Commander if the section is not activated. Any ICS sections or positions may be opened, closed, expanded, or contracted depending on need. To ensure universality and transparency, the common position titles remain no matter how large or small the ICS structure (15,16). Briggs (14) emphasizes that the structural basis for ICS continuity is found in familiar basic and public health terminology. The functional basis of the ICS is analogous to the ABC (airway, breathing, circulation) approach to trauma care. Like the changing severity of presentation of individual trauma cases, the ICS structure based on functional elements allows expressions of the differences seen in multiple MCIs while ensuring that the ABCs of disaster response are universally heeded.

Medical concerns related to conventional MCIs are as follows:

- Search and rescue
- Triage and initial stabilization
- Definitive medical care
- Evacuation

Public health consequences of MCIs involve the following:

- Water
- Food
- Shelter
- Sanitation
- Security and safety
- Transportation
- Communication
- Disease surveillance
- Endemic and epidemic diseases

Unified Command System

The ICS structure is modular and generic (12–17). For disasters of a minor nature, all functional elements may not be used. However, when a new service enters the ICS (which is common as the MCI escalates, intensifies, and becomes more complex), a Unified Command System (UCS) is formed (Fig. 175.1). The Unified Command guarantees a *single* command structure when there is overlap of jurisdictional (e.g., county, state, national) or functional responsibilities (agencies with different or competing legal, geographic, and functional responsibilities that need to work together). In the case of a hospital scenario, Unified Command would dictate that many different hospital departments may work in cooperation. All responding agencies/departments will work together to develop a common goal for responding to the MCI. This is referred to as the *Incident Action Plan* (IAP), which determines the allocation of scarce resources and assistance under a common goal. This is illustrated in a pandemic when coordination among local, national, regional, and international organizations is critical to managing rapidly constrained resources while preventing secondary infections by impeding transmission of disease across geographic boundaries.

Emergency Operations Centers

Mignone and Davidson define the Emergency Operations Center (EOC) as a "location from which personnel representing various organizations, both public and private, come together during an emergency or disaster event to: (1) coordinate response and recovery actions; (2) conduct strategic decision-making; and (3) manage resource allocation" (18). The EOC is the location where the Emergency Control Group (ECG) meets (Fig. 175.1). The ECG is responsible for various actions, in general the management of "big picture" decisions of community-wide resources and response (15–17). Whereas the Incident Commander runs the incident, the EOC/ECG is responsible for organizational continuity and maintaining this at all times. Examples of EOC activities:

- Requesting mutual aid resources
- Locating requested resources and directing them to the ICS staging area

- Managing a wide-scale evacuation
- Establishing shelters and coordinating social services
- Coordinating messages with the ICS Information Officer
- Transmitting information over the Emergency Alert System (EAS)
- Resolving policy issues

In any large urban area, many EOCs may exist in every organization, agency, and hospital and are generally institution specific (19). In public health emergencies, such as pandemics where the incident is ubiquitous rather than geographically defined, the lead agency EOC may, in effect, be that of the jurisdictional Department of Health that expands as needed with ethicists, legal consultants, and specialists in infectious disease, critical care, and other areas. Still, a major challenge facing health care providers used to individual-based care lies in their capacity and capability to make an operational shift to population-based triage management including the necessity for a health-inclusive EOC (2,10).

Hospital Emergency Incident Command System

For many hospitals in the United States, the Hospital Emergency Incident Command System (HEICS) has become the adaptation of ICS to hospital emergency functions (20,21). The HEICS uses a similar ICS management structure that incorporates defined responsibilities, clear reporting channels, and common nomenclature. The HEICS identifies positions designed to facilitate expanding or contracting requirements as needs dictate, such as the demand for multidisciplinary medical specialists to support existing critical care assets. Both the ICS and the HEICS have been modified based on emerging needs such as adding expert advice in chemical, biological, radiologic, and nuclear (CBRN) emergencies, critical care, more robust mental health consultation, mass fatality and expectant triage category experts, and leadership to coordinate the massive requirements for information technology services and systems (21). Representatives from other hospital HEICS may be called on to serve as ICS consultants to provide expertise, especially on the coordinated and collaborative sharing of scarce resources (19).

THE INCIDENT COMMAND SYSTEM AND CRITICAL CARE MANAGEMENT

The ICS methodology addresses the inherent inabilities of disaster managers to adjust (expand or contract) their agencies, organizations, or services to shifting situational demands, nonstandard terminology, and communications procedures among responding agencies (11,13). To have a voice in MCI decision making and resource allocation, the responding critical care community must have a clear understanding of the ICS. This includes ability to optimize available critical care resources and ensure that requested requirements are both realistic and well understood; and in framing the request one must appropriately use supporting legal, logistic, administrative, and operational resources supplied under ICS policies and structure.

Mass casualty incident decision making must ensure justice and equity while maintaining the greatest good for the greatest number. These triage-management decisions require a strong and coordinated public health workforce and leadership to ensure a smooth integration of multidisciplinary assets. No one agency, organization, or authority possesses the total expertise and resources to address and manage all population-based requirements (2,10). The ICS addresses the problems of adjusting through action planning protocols and guidelines that include requirements for critical care resource allocation and surge capacity. The ICS structure provides the coordinated opportunity for policy discussion and decision making to occur that guarantee that such expanded services are operationally available to the EOC. Specific Job Action Sheets, which should be written before any disasters, large or small, describe the specific duties of each team member from the ICS to the EOC, and indicate steps to be taken throughout the stages of the MCI (15).

In an illness-dominated mass casualty incident, such as a pandemic, the central jurisdictional EOC becomes the operations center providing a decision-making hub (2,10,22,23) for the following:

- Broad evidence-based situational awareness of the MCI
- Local linkages for regional resources
- Ongoing development and maintenance of strategic alliances with local to international agencies and organizations
- Facilitation and integration of resources
- Communication and health information system content and management
- Just-in-time training of volunteers to meet surge capacity requirements
- Development of communitywide triage protocols and the analysis of triage outcomes of resources and strategic decision making under surge capacity requirements.

This strategic triage decision-making function within the EOC is critical in establishing lines of authority to eliminate competition for resources among providers and health facilities (10). To optimize outcomes, the EOC or its equivalent at regional, national, and international levels must possess a timely and accurate evidence-based situational awareness capacity to coordinate daily, if not hourly, triage-management decisions which are immediately passed on to hospitals, ambulatory health care facilities, and other public and private agencies and organizations with health care responsibilities (2). Situational awareness includes data regarding present system demands and resource availability as well as forecasted demands and resources availability. Daily outcome data analyses seed the situational awareness information and allow the EOC to maintain an overall status of the MCI's impact on the population base and redirect resources where needed. Analysis of outcome data and subsequent revision of triage protocols based on this information is necessary to prevent either over- or under-triage, both of which decrease overall survival (2,10,24).

CRITICAL CARE TRIAGE MANAGEMENT

In normal circumstances and on a daily basis, critical care is offered only to those whose condition is potentially reversible and who have a good chance of surviving with intensive care support (25–27). Since the critically ill are close to dying, the outcome of this intervention is difficult, if not impossible, to predict. Many patients still die in the critical care unit. A prime requisite for admission is that the underlying condition is reversible. Therefore, treatment is merely meant to support the patient, during which time treatments or the natural history of the acute affliction will lead to resolution. Rubinson and Toole suggest that a major challenge of MCIs is "to determine when, and on what basis, traditional standards of critical care are modified to accommodate emergency conditions, and when modified standards to focus on key interventions" (28). This model of care is referred to as mass critical care (29). In an MCI, mass critical care is implemented when usual surge response code orange/disaster protocols such as canceling elective surgery, discharging or transferring patients as possible, and opening up alternative care areas will be insufficient to meet the demands placed on the health care system. Coordination of affected hospitals to facilitate implementation of similar measures in triage management is required (2,28). Furthermore, Farmer and Carlton suggest that shortfalls in critical care that will impact services are as follows (30):

- Insufficient coordination between hospitals and civil/government response agencies (e.g., the NIMS/ICS)
- Insufficient on-site critical care capability
- A lack of portability of acute care processes (e.g., patient transport)
- Education and training shortfalls
- The inability of hospitals to align disaster requirements with other competing priorities

TRIAGE

International law precedence requires an equitable, fair, and transparent triage process that provides the best opportunity to survive for as many victims as possible (2,10,31–34). All patients will be cared for, every human life must be valued, and every human being deserves respect, caring, and compassion (34). However, triage does not guarantee survival, only the best opportunity to survive within the constraints of the available resources (10). In an MCI, especially where there is a scarcity of resources, assistance shifts to population-based care. Decision criteria requires that those selected to receive the limited resources must have a likelihood of medical success, yet the selection must not impede the conservation of scarce resources for those equally in need (35). In an MCI, both individual care and population requirements impact each and every triage decision.

Conventional Mass Casualty Incident Triage

The vast majority of MCIs have been dominated by patients with traumatic injuries, most of whom are not critically injured. These MCIs do not generate large numbers of casualties with respiratory failure, septic shock, or coma, and those that do usually receive rescue, transportation, stabilization, and definitive critical care using existing local or regional capabilities (36–39). The National Disaster Medical System (NDMS) designates the simple triage and rapid treatment (START) as the uniform method for initial field triage in conventional MCIs and disasters (40). START evaluates respiratory, circulatory, and neurologic function and provides four care categories (nonsalvageable or dead, major injury, minor injury, and walking wounded). Field emergency care is restricted to the ABCs (airway, breathing, and circulation procedures) (40). A second-phase triage process termed secondary assessment of victim end point (SAVE) further assesses injuries on the basis of trauma survival statistics to direct limited resources, triage tags, and tracking to victims expected to derive the most benefit from treatment (41). Both methodologies remain the basis for point-of-contact (i.e., prehospital or the emergency department) initial evaluation for all-hazards disaster planning documents, and in basic and advanced disaster life-support training aimed primarily at managing traumatic MCIs (2,40).

Restrictive resource limitations and a worsening case definition in a conventional MCI, or an explosive or nuclear event, may require further EOC triage decisions based on inclusion and exclusion criteria and minimal qualifications for survival (MQS) (2,10,42–44).

- *Inclusion criteria* are the expected management standards that health care providers are trained to meet based on a resource-complete environment. Examples of inclusion criteria are the universally accepted standards for the use of resources for resuscitation and management that are traditionally found in courses for advanced cardiac, trauma, and pediatric life support.
- *Exclusion criteria* conversely refer to situations where expected resources are limited or lacking and care must proceed without all standards of care and equipment being met.
- *Minimum qualifications for survival* represent a ceiling on the amount of resource expenditures that will be allocated to any one case definition, ensuring that a maximum benefit of available resources is realized to ensure a population-based best opportunity for survival. Examples are the EOC determining that resource limitations would dictate that high resource maintenance cardiac or respiratory arrest interventions might be limited, as would restrictions on transfusions for traumatic injuries, or in the implementation of criteria protocols for ventilator use in those with unlikelihood of survival. Each MQS diagnosis is subject to change on arrival of surge capacity resources.

The operational level EOC must balance available resources against the best opportunity to survive. The impact of this triage-management practice and decisions may not be fully known until the end of the MCI when outcome analyses are performed.

Bioevent Triage Management

Bioevents include both naturally occurring and the deliberate release of a biologic agent in a population resulting in a mass illness incident (epidemic or pandemic). Whereas these bioevents have similarities with other MCIs, there are also major differences, especially in the approach to triage management of surge capacity resources (2). Bioevents are characterized by massive numbers of individuals seeking health care (2). Unique to the planning of bioevents is that only 40% to 50% of health care providers are expected to respond or be available, in contrast to conventional MCIs where health care facilities are often inundated with health care volunteers (45). A population-based approach requires a shift from the individual care role of clinicians to a population-based decision-making approach of patients. This does not minimize the importance of clinical tasks, but rather adds the dimension of new public health and surge capacity interventions that improve *access and availability* of limited health resources for the entire population. Individuals within a population experiencing a bioevent share the following (2,46):

- Most have either the same condition or are susceptible to it.
- All have shared health care needs.
- Everyone in the population requires some intervention, which ranges from education to critical care.
- Large-scale bioevents may require a sustained operational response lasting 12 to 24 months.
- Especially with long-term bioevents, operational continuity of the health care system to manage medical issues other than those related to the involved biologic agent must remain a focus.

Severity, as indicated by rising case fatality rates, occurs dramatically as disease transmission increases and resources become limited. What at first appears to be a static, well-controlled local event can quickly become a regional, national, or international disaster of paralytic proportions (2,10,47).

The central jurisdictional EOC will determine surge capacity requirements for five population categories: those susceptible but not exposed (Susceptible category), those exposed but not yet infectious (Exposed category), the infectious (Infectious category), those removed by death or recovery (Removed category), and those protected by vaccination or prophylactic medication (Vaccinated category), termed the SEIRV methodology (2,48,49). The unique requirements and demands of each triage category may mandate that professionals with specific category expertise be assigned to the medical component of the ICS or centralized EOC (21). In turn, the EOC

- Determines surge capacity requirements for each SEIRV category
- Determines triage criteria, including minimal qualifications for survival (MQS) and exclusion criteria
- Enforces compliance measures
- Ensures data collection, analysis, and measures of effectiveness using this information as the basis of daily reports and determination of effectiveness of triage-management

Conventional triage methodologies, such as START and SAVE, risk impeding control of transmission by not recognizing those most in need of care in a bioevent MCI. The START and SAVE triage methodologies are based on severity of presentation and have limited application in bioevents in which point-of-contact decisions must be based on exposure, duration, or infectiousness (2,10). Decisions at every level are influenced by bioagent lethality, dose-dependent onset and duration, illness severity profiles, time to death or recovery, and surge capacity requirements and resources (2).

Within the community, the initial point of contact (POC) for potential victims comes through established hotlines and 911 calls. A simple series of questions can determine whether the caller is probably exposed or infectious, versus probably not exposed or infectious. A series of questions concerning transport capacity and self-assisted care would follow, pointing the caller to one of three options: ambulatory clinic, designated influenza hospital, or home (self or assisted) care. A similar hotline approach was successfully used by Toronto during SARS and has become the first level of triage in future outbreaks (2). Current CDC guidelines recommend phone triage with pre-established criteria for emergency transport and plans for coordination with other transport organizations for delivery of large numbers of victims at the height of the pandemic, the transport of multiple patients on a single run, and use of vehicles other than those designed for medical transport (e.g., buses) (50). The EOC may consider systemwide exclusion criteria that would limit emergency medical services (EMS) transport to only noninfectious cases. EMS providers in Hong Kong experienced a higher attack rate for SARS, a risk dependent on the use of personal protective equipment, type of transfer, and decision to intubate (51). Such population-based triage decisions underscore the importance for a central EOC management authority.

CRITICAL CARE MANAGEMENT

In contrast to the availability of trauma capacity to implement interventions in conventional MCIs, resource implementation for bioevents vary considerably from jurisdiction to jurisdiction. This is especially evident in critical care. The developing situational awareness process within the EOC will identify gaps, limitations, and the surge capacity requirements gained from disaster managers, health care facilities, volunteer agencies and organizations, and others with specific roles and responsibilities for each triage category. Because it is possible that fewer health care providers than expected will report to work in a major bioevent, the EOC must provide means to include provisions for just-in-time training, personal and family support, immunization or prophylactic antibiotics and antivirals, and bioagent-specific protective equipment to these workers and potential volunteers (2,45,52).

A full list of items that would compromise the triage-management process in a bioevent MCI is beyond the scope of this chapter; however, a partial list of resources commonly triaged includes

- Antivirals/antibiotics
- Vaccines
- Mechanical ventilators and ancillary equipment
- Pulse oximeters
- Medical oxygen
- Protective masks and equipment
- Nursing staff
- Laboratory support
- Acute care/ICU beds
- Housekeeping staff
- Morgue services
- Trained volunteers

Critical Care Beds

Guidelines suggest that 20% of general hospital beds are available within 24 hours during conventional disasters, and a severalfold increase can be realized if acute care patients are admitted preferentially (39). Theoretically, if personnel and equipment are available, most of a general hospital can be modified for a semblance of critical care delivery. The lessons of SARS have resulted in decisions to purchase countrywide ventilator resources in anticipation of a more aggressive and lethal influenza pandemic.

Personnel

Workforce shortages are already prevalent on a daily basis where staffing is a critical triage issue for most hospitals, and 12% of ICUs have been forced to close beds due to nursing shortages (39). Critical shortages also exist in trained respiratory care specialists, pharmacists, and physicians. This will be the major barrier to the provision of critical care should an MCI occur. A two-tiered staffing model using care teams calls for non–critical care trained personnel to work collaboratively with specialized health care professionals (23). This model is also supported by the Society of Critical Care Medicine Hospital Disaster management course, which trains in core critical care knowledge and skills to non–critical care personnel. For example, teams of dentists, a profession comfortable with the airway and who, in the past, have been trained by the military to be anesthetists during all-out war, can be trained in intubation and manual ventilation while being supervised by a respiratory therapist who assumes the role of team respiratory supervisor.

The goal of all triage management in a large-scale bioevent is to prevent secondary infections (2,10). The risk of secondary infections may be higher in the critical care setting in part due to the number of interventions (e.g., endotracheal intubation, suctioning, manual ventilation) causing aerosolization of infectious material (53,54). Studies support the efficacy of correct personal protective equipment (PPE). Unfortunately, compliance among health care providers is as low as 56% to 67%.

Mechanical Ventilation

Since the SARS epidemic of 2002–2003, and the threat of an influenza pandemic, specific attention has been focused on how to plan for and implement a large-scale bioevent approach that does require triage management of large numbers of survivable and nonsurvivable respiratory failure cases where evacuation is not an option (39). The demand for positive pressure ventilation will likely far exceed conventional ICU capabilities, and without careful predisaster planning, hundreds or thousands of victims may have to forgo potentially life-saving critical care. Whereas most of these MCIs would occur in chemical inhalation disasters, radiation exposures, and tsunamis causing aspiration pneumonia and septic shock, it is bioevent public health emergencies that many believe have the greatest likelihood of causing mass respiratory failure.

Thousands of ventilators will be required for a mass illness response event such as an influenza pandemic. However, studies suggest that full-feature ventilators currently available for use range in number from 53,000 to 105,000. The Strategic National Stockpile (SNS) maintains 4,100 ventilators for deployment to disaster areas; however, the U.S. Department of Health and Human Services in 2006 revealed intentions to purchase an additional 6,000. A full listing of alternate positive pressure ventilation (PPV) equipment for mass casualty care designed for short-term PPV in non-ICU locations is found elsewhere. (See recommended readings below.)

The stockpiling of full-feature ventilators by hospitals, hospital systems, or states is cost prohibitive. Rubinson et al. (29) suggest that stockpiling of sophisticated portable ventilators, which provide only a basic mode of ventilation, should be easy and safe to use for both adult and pediatric patients, especially if large numbers of patients are monitored by single respiratory providers or small teams that may include health care providers with EOC-directed just-in-time training. Because pulse oximetry devices may also be in short supply, this training would also include frequent checking of vital signs with attention to respiratory rate and use of accessory muscles (39).

Hick and O'Laughlin (55) provide a sample concept of operations for the development of triage criteria for restriction of mechanical ventilation in epidemic situations. Christian et al. (56) and Melnychuk and Kenny (57) provide an expanded critical care pandemic triage protocol for assessment of admission to critical care units during an influenza pandemic. This triage protocol uses the Sequential Organ Failure Assessment score (SOFA), and specifically addresses the importance of a centrally placed province or state EOC-level triage committee to implement critical inclusion, exclusion, and MQS criteria. Also stressed is the central jurisdictional EOC's "absolute command and control over critical care resources in order to ensure accountability" (56). The EOC must support the critical care triage issues by authoritatively implementing the protocols in all hospitals when appropriate, and then monitoring its effectiveness though maintaining and analyzing outcome indicators. Both studies emphasize ethical principles and potential pitfalls of their approaches (55,56). Triage for critical care begins in the prehospital setting and extends to the emergency department. *Given the complexity of triage for critical care, this coordinated triage process should be performed under the guidance of a trained critical care triage officer.* These triage decisions are only as accurate as the knowledge concerning what is operationally current and the resources available in each triage category. Ultimately, each triage level decision will have a direct effect on clinical decisions at the critical care level (2).

Medical Oxygen

Triage management will be limited by the availability of medical-grade oxygen, which is not supplied through the Strategic National Stockpile (39). Bulk liquid is the main source of oxygen for hospitals and remains the best option for supporting mass mechanical ventilation. The large majority of nonventilated patients will be maintained outside the hospital setting with oxygen supplies using reservoir cannulas or pulsed-dose technology.

Infection Control

Infection control is a key component of any MCI involving an infectious bioagent. As mentioned earlier, SARS revealed that health care workers and patients in the critical care environment are particularly vulnerable to nosocomial transmission of infectious agents, due to invasive procedures such as intubation, suctioning, and central line insertion (53,54,58,59). This highlights the need for infection control to be incorporated into all disaster planning (60). The basic approach to infection control in critical care units should consider administrative controls, environmental engineering, protective equipment, and quality control (53). The primary goal is to prevent transmission to health care workers and other patients. Cohorting of patients who are likely or unlikely to be infectious is an important first step in containing the spread of illness and is facilitated through use of the SEIRV protocol discussed above. During a biologic disaster involving an infectious agent, separate ICUs should be developed to deal with infectious and noninfectious patients. For example a hospital with a single medical-surgical ICU and a coronary care unit (CCU) could designate its medical-surgical ICU as the infectious ICU, and then use its postanesthetic care unit (PACU) to manage noninfectious surgical patients and the CCU for all noninfectious medical patients requiring critical care. Although cohorting should not be relied on as a foolproof method of infection control, it does significantly decrease the exposure of highly susceptible critically ill patients to potential infection. When planning alternative critical care locations during a surge, infection control issues must also be considered. One option includes the use of portable HEPA (high-efficiency particulate air) filters to create negative pressure units (61). As discussed earlier, some procedures in the ICU require higher levels of personal protection given they have the potential to generate aerosols, thus increasing the risk of airborne transmission even for infectious agents that would otherwise typically be transmitted only via droplets. Additional precautions and possibly the use of special procedure rooms should be considered for high-risk procedures. A full discussion of infection control practices in critical care is beyond the scope of this chapter, and interested readers should refer to comprehensive articles discussing the transmission of respiratory pathogens (62,63).

A common theme that has been revisited throughout this chapter is the need for real-time data to guide decision making and responses. This is also true for infection control as was demonstrated during SARS. In Toronto, we learned that during a biologic disaster, even more important than the initiation of the response was the transition from response to recovery. Simply put, how to detect and respond to an outbreak was well understood, but how to end an outbreak was not. The failure to detect an ongoing chain of SARS transmission in a hospital led to a second large wave of infections and deaths after infection control precautions were discontinued. Appropriate surveillance data could have detected and prevented this second wave of illness (64,65).

SUMMARY

Mass critical care requires modification to standards of critical care interventions, personnel staffing, equipment, and triage management to provide an acceptable level of care. At a minimum, hospitals must plan to deliver to critically ill patients a basic mode of the following:

- Mechanical ventilation
- Hemodynamic support
- Antibiotic or other disease-specific countermeasure therapy (i.e., thrombolysis in myocardial infarctions)
- A small set of prophylactic interventions that are recognized to reduce the serious adverse consequences of critical illness

Clearly, the management of an MCI is best undertaken by strengthening local capacity. All intensivists should take the Society for Critical Care Medicine Fundamentals of Disaster Management course or a similar program. Critical care professionals must raise public awareness, advocate for better education and training, and take the lead in planning and preparing to care for large numbers of critically ill patients that far exceed available ICU beds. This must include issues of health care rationing and the decision process on who will receive mechanical ventilation and other life-saving treatments. As a first step, one needs to understand the organizational system that drives the policy and operational components of triage management. Only then will the critical care community be able to optimize resource allocation, establish legitimate triage protocols and criteria, and ensure a process that provides the greatest good for the greatest number.

Recommended Readings for Critical Care Response Planning

- Rubinson L, Nuzzo JB, Talmor DS, et al. Augmentation of hospital critical care capacity after bioterrorist attacks or epidemics: recommendation of the Working Group on Emergency Mass Critical Care. *Crit Care Med.* 2005;33:2393–2403.
- Rubinson L, Toole T. Critical care during epidemics. *Crit Care.* 2005; 9:. http://ccforum.com/inpress/cc3533.
- Rubinson L, Branson RD, Resik N, et al. Positive-pressure ventilation quipment for mass casualty respiratory failure. *Biosecur Bioterror.* 2006;4:183–194.
- Burkle FM. Population-based triage management in response to surge-capacity requirements during a large-scale bioevent disaster. *Acad Emerg Med.* 2006 Nov;13(11):1118–1129.
- Society of Critical Care Medicine. Guidelines for ICU Admission, Discharge, and Triage. *Crit Care Med.* 1999 Mar;27(3):633–638.
- Agency for Healthcare Research and Quality. Altered Standards of Care in Mass Casualty Events. Health Systems Research, Inc. AHRQ Publication No. 05-0043, April 2005.
- Christian MD, Hawryluck L, Wax RS, et al. Development of a triage protocol for critical care during an influenza pandemic. *CMAJ* 2006;175(11):1377–1381.
- Christian MD, Kolleck D, Schwartz B. Emergency preparedness: what every health care worker needs to know. *CJEM.* 2005;7(5);330–337.

References

1. Statement on Disaster and Mass Casualty Management. American College of Surgeons Ad Hoc Committee on Disaster and Mass Casualty Management, Committee on Trauma. *Bull Am Coll Surg.* 2003;88(8):14–15.
2. Burkle FM. Population-based triage management in response to surge-capacity requirements during a large-scale bioevent disaster. *Acad Emerg Med.* 2006;13(11):1118–1129.
3. Christian MD, Poutanen SM, Loutfy MR, et al. Severe acute respiratory syndrome. *Clin Infect Dis.* 2004;38(10):1420–1427.
4. Heymann DL, Rodier B. SARS: a global response to an international threat. *Brown J World Aff.* 2004; Winter/Spring: 185–197.
5. Burkle FM. Integrating international responses to complex emergencies, unconventional war, and terrorism. *Crit Care Med.* 2005;33(1 Suppl):S7–12.
6. Halpern NA, Pastores SM, Greenstein RJ. Critical care medicine in the United States 1985–2000: an analysis of bed numbers, use, and costs. *Crit Care Med.* 2004;32:1254–1259.
7. Macintyre AG, Christopher GW, Eitzen E, et al. Weapons of mass destruction events with contaminated casualties: effective planning for health care facilities. *JAMA.* 2000;283:242–249.
8. Sullivan MG. With planning, hospitals can manage mass casualties. *ACEP News.* 2006:21.
9. Bigley GA, Roberts KH. The Incident Command System: high reliability organizing for complex and volatile task environments. *Acad Manage J.* ;44:1281–1300.
10. Burkle FM. Mass casualty management of a large-scale bioterrorist event: an epidemiological approach that shapes triage decisions. *Emerg Med Clin North Am.* 2002;20(2):409–436.
11. Christian MD, Kolleck D, Schwartz B. Emergency preparedness: what every healthcare worker needs to know. *Can J Emerg Med.* 2005;7(5):330–337.
12. Stumpf J. Incident Command System: the history and need. *Internet J Rescue Disaster Med.* 2001;2(1). http://www.ispub.com/ostia/index.php?xmlPrinter=true&xmlFilePath=journals/ijrdm/vol2n. Accessed July 4, 2006.
13. National Incident Command System (NIMS). http://www.fema.gov/emergency/nims/index.shtm. Accessed October 12, 2006.

14. Briggs SM. Disaster management teams. *Curr Opin Crit Care.* 2005;11(6): 585–589.
15. Hospital Emergency Incident Command System. http://www.emsa.ca.gov?Dms2?heics3.htm. Accessed October 12, 2006.
16. The Federal, Provincial and Territorial Network on Emergency Preparedness and Response (Canada). National Framework for Health Emergency Management: guideline for program development. 26-11-2004.
17. Center for Emergency Preparedness and Disaster Response. National Incident Command System (ICS) for Health Care. Yale New Haven Health: Online Education and Training. http://ynhhs.emergencyeducation.org/courses/em140nims/sec2_nims.asp. Accessed–October 12, 2006.
18. Mignone AT, Davidson R. Public health response actions and the use of emergency operations centers. *Prehosp Disast Med.* 2003;18(3):217–218.
19. Cook L. The World Trade Center attack. The paramedic response: an insider's view. *Crit Care.* 2001;5(6):301–303.
20. Zane RD, Prestipino AL. Implementing the hospital incident command system: an integrated delivery system's experience. *Prehosp Disaster Med.* 2004;19(4):311–317.
21. Arnold JL, Dembry LM, Tsai MC, et al. Recommended modifications and applications of the hospital incident command system for hospital emergency management. *Prehosp Disaster Med* 2005;20(5):290–300.
22. Barbisch D. Regional responses to bioterrorism and other medical disasters: developing sustainable surge capacity. In: Johnson JA, Ledlow GR, Cwiek MA, eds. *Community Preparedness and Response to Terrorism.* Westport, CT: Praeger Press, 2005:77–88.
23. Christian MD, Wax R, Lazar N, et al. Critical care during a pandemic: Final Report of the Ontario Health Plan for an influenza pandemic. Working group on adult critical care admission, discharge, and triage criteria. Toronto, ON, CAN: Ontario Health System, 2006:2–25.
24. Frykberg ER. Medical management of disasters and mass casualties from terrorist bombings: how can we cope? *J Trauma* 2002;53:201–212.
25. Consensus statement on the triage of critically ill patients. Society of Critical Care medicine Ethics Committee. *JAMA.* 1994;271(15):1200–1203.
26. Guidelines for intensive care unit admission, discharge, and triage. Task Force of the American College of critical care medicine. Society of Critical Care Medicine. *Crit Care Med.* 1999;27(3):633–638.
27. Sinuff T, Kahnamoui K, Cook DJ, et al. Rationing critical care beds: a systematic review. *Crit Care Med.* 2004;32(7):1588–1597.
28. Rubinson L, Toole T. Critical care during epidemics. *Crit Care.* 2005; 9(4):311–313. http://ccforum.com/inpress/cc3533. Accessed October 9, 2006.
29. Rubinson L, Nuzzo JB, Talmor DS, et al. Augmentation of hospital critical care after bioterrorist attacks or epidemics: Recommendations of the Working Group on Emergency Mass Critical Care. *Crit Care Med.* 2005;33:2393–2403.
30. Farmer JC, Carlton PK. Providing critical care during a disaster: the interface between disaster response agencies and hospitals. *Crit Care Med.* 2006;34(3):S56–59.
31. Smith GP. Triage: endgame realities. *J Contemp Health Law Policy.* 1985; 1:143–152.
32. Domres B, Koch M, Manger A, et al. Ethics and triage. *Prehosp Disaster Med.* 2001;16:53–58.
33. Orr RD. Ethics issues in bioterrorism. University of Vermont College of Medicine, Bioterrorism e-mail Module #2, August 4, 2003:1–7.
34. Singer PA, Benatar SR, Berstein M, et al. Ethics and SARS: lessons from Toronto. *BMJ.* 2003;327:1342–1344.
35. Burkle FM. Triage. In: Burkle FM, Sanner PH, Wolcott BW, eds. *Disaster Medicine.* New York, NY: McGraw-Hill; 1984:45–80.
36. Mallonee S, Shariat S, Stennies G, et al. Physical injuries and fatalities resulting from the Oklahoma City bombing. *JAMA.* 1996;276:382–387.
37. Guha-Sapir D, Parry L, Degomme O, et al. Risk factors for mortality and injury: post-tsunami epidemiological findings from Tamil Nadu. Brussels, Belgium: CRED; 2006. http://www.em-dat.net/documents/Publication/RiskFactorsMortalityInjury.pdf. Accessed October 18, 2006.
38. Schultz CH, Koenig KL, Noji EK. A medical disaster response to reduce immediate mortality after an earthquake. *N Engl J Med.* 1996;334:438–444.
39. Daugherty EL, Branson R, Rubinson L. Mass casualty respiratory failure. *Curr Opin Crit Care.* 2007;13(1):51–56.
40. Disaster Medical System. Triage Systems and methods. Element 7.2. Available at: http://mvemsa.com/disaster/DMS%20Grant%20Proj/templates/triage_system.htm. Accessed June 3, 2005.
41. Benson M, Koenig KL, Schultz CH. Disaster triage: START, then SAVE–a new method of dynamic triage for victims of a catastrophic earthquake. *Prehosp Disaster Med.* 1996;11:117–124.
42. Winslow GR. *Triage and Justice.* Berkeley, CA: University of California Press; 1982:1–23.
43. Pledger HG. Triage of casualties after nuclear attack. *Lancet.* 1986; 2(8508):678–679.
44. Coupland RM. Epidemiological approach to surgical management of casualties of war. *BMJ.* 1994;308:1693–1697.
45. Qureshi K, Gershon RR, Sherman MF, et al. Health care worker's ability and willingness to report to duty during catastrophic disasters. *J Urban Health.* 2005;82:378–388.
46. Halpern R, Boulter P. Population-based health care: definitions and applications. https://www.thci.org/downloads/topic11_00.PDF. Accessed June 27, 2006.
47. Koenig KL, Dinerman N, Kuehl AE. Disaster nomenclature—a functional impact approach: The PICE system. *Acad Emerg Med.* 1996;3:723–727.
48. Bombardt JN. Contagious disease dynamics for biological warfare and bioterrorism casualty assessments. West Point, NY. Institute for Defense Analysis paper P-3488. February 2000:3–33.
49. Bombardt JN. Summary of smallpox and pneumonic plague casualty estimates. Alexandria, VA: Institute for Defense Analysis briefing report. July 10, 2000:1–35.
50. Centers for Disease Control and Prevention. Emergency medical services and non-emergent (medical) transport organizations pandemic influenza planning checklist. http://www.pandemicflu.gov/plan/emgncymedical.html. Accessed October 17, 2006.
51. Sapsin JW, Gostin LO, Vernick JS, et al. SARS and international legal preparedness. *Temple Law Rev.* 2004;77:155–174.
52. Alexander GC, Wynia M. Ready and willing? Physicians' sense of preparedness for bioterrorism. *Health Aff.* 2003;22(5):189–197.
53. Christian MD, Loutfy M, McDonald LC, et al. Possible SARS coronavirus transmission during cardiopulmonary resuscitation. *Emerg Infect Dis.* 2004;10(2):287–293.
54. Fowler RA, Guest CB, Lapinsky SE, et al. Transmission of severe acute respiratory syndrome during intubation and mechanical ventilation. *Am J Respiratory Crit Care Med.* 2004;169(11):1198–1202.
55. Hick JL, O'Laughlin DT. Concept of operations for triage of mechanical ventilation in an epidemic. *Acad Emerg Med.* 2006;13:223–229.
56. Christian MD, Hawryluck L, Wax RS, et al. Development of a triage protocol for critical care during an influenza pandemic. *CMAJ.* 2006;175(11):1377–1381.
57. Melnychuk RM, Kenny NP. Pandemic triage: the ethical challenge. *CMAJ.* 2006;175(11):1393–1394.
58. Ofner M, Lem M, Sarwal S, et al. Cluster of severe acute respiratory syndrome cases among protected health care workers-Toronto, April 2003. *Can Commun Dis Rep.* 2003;29(11):93–97.
59. Scales DC, Green K, Chan AK, et al. Illness in intensive care staff after brief exposure to severe acute respiratory syndrome. *Emerg Infect Dis.* 2003;9:1205–1210.
60. Hawryluck L, Lapinsky S, Stewart T. Clinical review: SARS - lessons in disaster management. *Crit Care.* 2005;9(4):384–389.
61. Rosenbaum RA, Benyo JS, O'Connor RE, et al. Use of a portable forced air system to convert existing hospital space into a mass casualty isolation area. *Ann Emerg Med.* 2004;44(6):628–634.
62. Muller MP, McGeer A. Febrile respiratory illness in the intensive care unit setting: an infection control perspective. *Curr Opin Crit Care.* 2006; 12(1):37–42.
63. Karwa M, Currie B, Kvetan V. Bioterrorism: preparing for the impossible or the improbable. *Crit Care Med.* 2005;33(1 Suppl):S75–S95.
64. Wallington T, Berger L, Henry B, et al. Update: severe acute respiratory syndrome–Toronto, 2003. *Can Commun Dis Rep.* 2003;29(13):113–117.
65. Wong T, Wallington T, McDonald LC, et al. Late recognition of SARS in nosocomial outbreak, Toronto. *Emerg Infect Dis.* 2005;11(2):322–325.

CHAPTER 176 ■ BIOTERRORISM

EDGAR JIMENEZ • F. ELIZABETH POALILLO

IMMEDIATE CONCERNS

Hospitals and, in particular, emergency departments (ED) should maintain a high level of suspicion for syndromes that may represent potential terrorist activities. Routine surveillance can range from the training of personnel in the recognition of specific conditions to participation in electronic networks that may detect deviations from the routine and seasonal presentations among several area hospitals. The ED is the key component in protecting the hospital from contamination. Areas for isolation and decontamination of early suspicious cases should be set up and readily available in order to prevent dissemination throughout the facility and the community.

Depending on the type of agent released, the affected population may present acutely, with a large number of simultaneous cases, or insidiously over a period of days to weeks. This latter presentation is far more dangerous, as it may not trigger hospital defense systems, resulting in a severe compromise of the facility. All hospitals in the United States, as a condition for accreditation from the Joint Commission on the Accreditation of Health Care Organizations (JCAHO), should have a response plan with clearly identified triggers of when it will be implemented. All plans must be tested and adjusted in advance with routinely scheduled drills (1). The plan should have enough flexibility so the intensity of the response is appropriate for the magnitude of the event. Still, there are key components that need to be addressed in any plan:

- Implementation of the Hospital Incident Command System (2) (Fig. 176.1)
- Notification and coordination with public and other authorities (Fig. 176.2)
- Delineation of perimeters and facility access
- Deployment of decontamination equipment, first receivers, and personal protective equipment (PPE)
- Distribution of surge teams, equipment, and medications
- Establishment of patient flows to designated surge areas, including discharge and transfer of patients

Critical care resources—equipment, designated areas, and personnel—are a crucial part of the response, as a large number of these patients will require a high level of support, in particular; airway management, mechanical ventilation, and hemodynamic interventions (3).

HISTORICAL PERSPECTIVE

The lessons learned throughout ancient—and recent—history involving chemical, biologic, and radiologic events have challenged medical professionals to develop interventions aimed at minimizing the impact of such incidents. Knowledge, coupled with detailed preparation plans, is requisite for the successful resolution of such a crisis. Current recommendations emphasize the requirement of not only planning, but also the value of practicing the institution's response to a biologic incident through simulations and drills. Additionally, the development of all plans and their drills need be coordinated with external entities that would interface with the hospital if an event occurred.

In many instances, one aspect of planning is the approach to triage. The concept of triage requires a careful examination in light of a major biologic event or pandemic, and a review of existing resources. Furthermore, "surging" patient volumes in conjunction with potentially less appropriately trained personnel may require a planned degradation of standard of care.

Some relevant episodes of humankind's history include epidemics and pandemics that affected Athens (in 430 BC, likely smallpox) and the Roman Empire (such as malaria around 300 BC and smallpox, first described by Galen in 165 AD) (4), the "Black Death" epidemics of the Middle Ages (5), the influenza epidemics of the 20th century and, more recently, the severe acute respiratory syndrome (SARS) outbreak (6).

Centuries of warfare have resulted in the development of weapons with the aim of causing mass casualties within the enemy lines, known currently as *weapons of mass destruction* (WMD). The practice of catapulting corpses and dead animals is described as a tactic of the Roman Empire when they besieged cities. In 1346, the Tatar forces were catapulting plague-ridden corpses in what is now the Ukraine (7). Boiling oil was used as a deterrent to offensive troop actions on fixed fortifications throughout the Middle Ages. These actions can be considered early biologic and chemical attempts at warfare. In 1941, after a decade of experimentation with several agents, cholera was used in Changteh during the invasion of China by Japan. During the Iran–Iraq war of the 1980s, the world witnessed the utilization of more sophisticated chemical weapons that had been developed throughout the "Cold War" years (8).

More recently, terrorist activity has been associated with conventional bombings and destruction of societal infrastructure. Some of the most well-known terrorist activities have been the bombings of the World Trade Center in 1993; the Murrah Federal Building, Oklahoma City, in 1996; the U.S. Embassies in Lebanon, Saudi Arabia, Kenya, and Tanzania; the events of September 11, 2001, which targeted the World Trade Center and the Pentagon; the railway stations in Madrid, which were bombed on March 11, 2004; the mass transit bombings in London in 2005; and the repetitive bombings

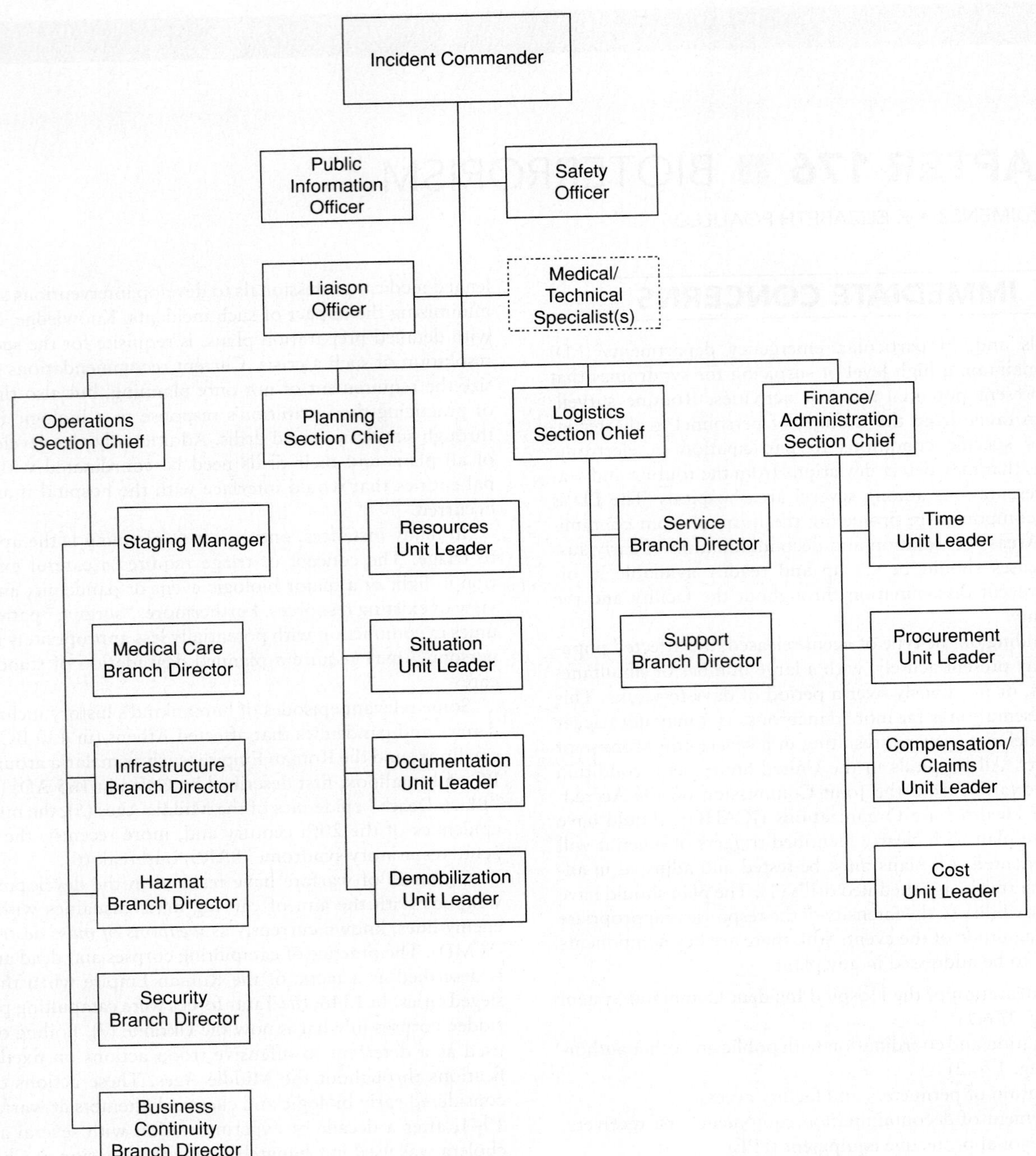

FIGURE 176.1. Basic elements of the Hospital Incident Command System (HICS). (From *HICS Guide Book* 2006:21. http://www.emsa.ca.gov/HICS/files/Guidebook_Glossary.pdf. Accessed October 27, 2008.)

and suicide bombings in Sri Lanka, Israel, Saudi Arabia, Lebanon, Pakistan, and Iraq (9,10).

Other recent terrorist activities also include biochemical attacks, such as the tainting of salad bars at The Dalles, Oregon, in 1984 with *Salmonella typhimurium* by the Rajneeshee cult (11); the release of anthrax in Tokyo in 1993 by the Aum Shunrikyo; and the distribution of anthrax in the U.S. mail in 2001, which affected postal workers, the news media, and politicians and their staff. Aum Shunrikyo also claimed responsibility for the release of sarin gas in the subway system in Tokyo in 1995 (12).

At the present time, there are significant concerns that bombing activities may evolve into improvised radiologic dispersal devices (RDDs)—a conventional bomb contaminated

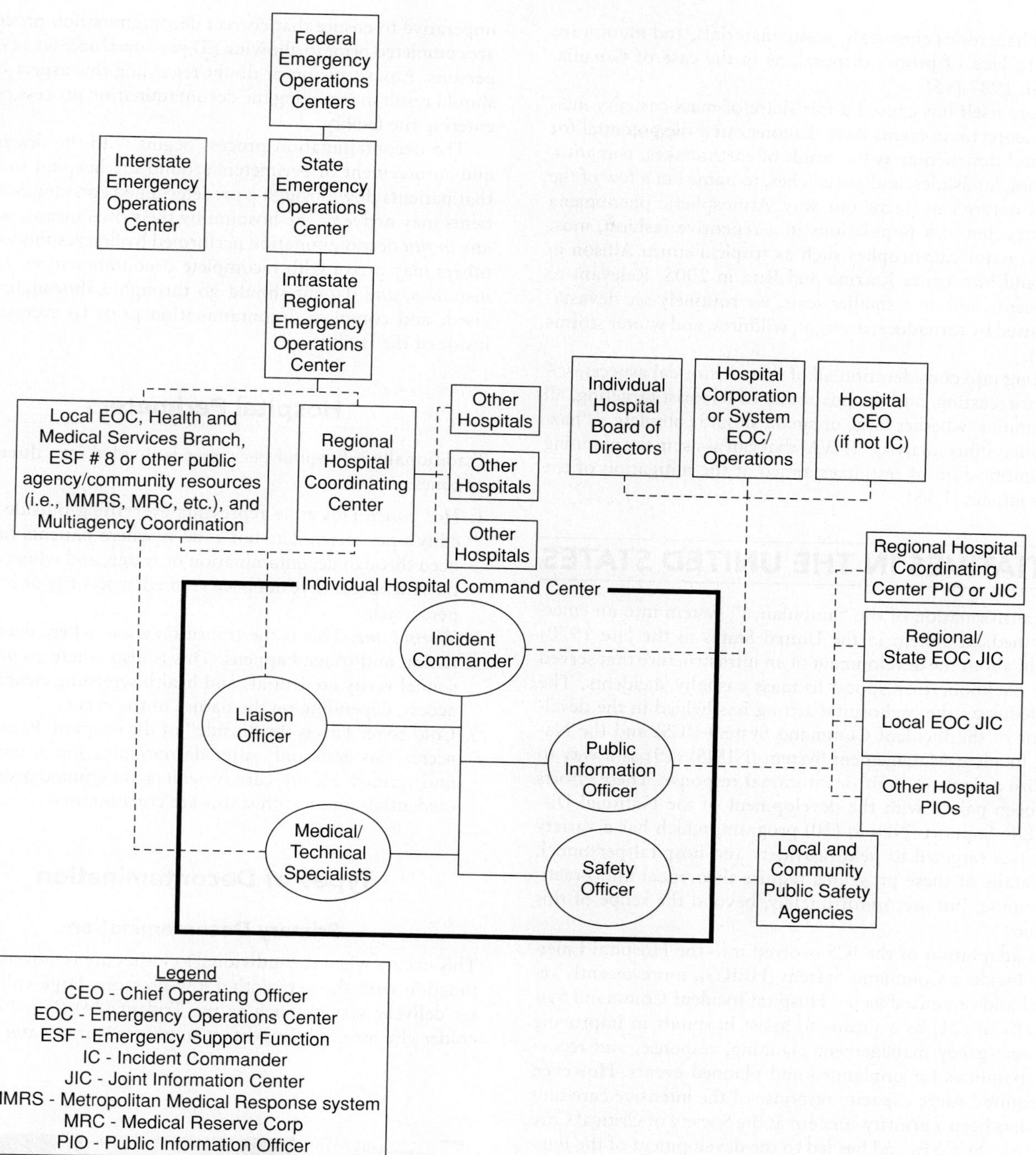

FIGURE 176.2. Diagram illustrating the potential coordination of the Hospital Incident Command System (HICS) with organizations to the facility. (From HICS Guidebook 2006:21. http://www.emsa.ca.gov/HICS/files/Guidebook_Glossary.pdf. Accessed October 27, 2008.)

with radioactive waste material, also known as a "dirty bomb" (13)—as well as the release of biologic or chemical agents.

Accidental releases of chemical agents have been an unfortunate result of industrialization and are ever-present threats of which governments and the population at large must be aware. One of the most devastating events of this nature was the accidental release of methylisocyanate gas in Bhopal, India, in 1984 (14), resulting in the deaths of more than 3,000 people with over 500,000 injured. Similarly, the quest for energy through nuclear reactors resulted in the radiologic accidents of Chernobyl in the Ukraine in 1986, and Three Mile Island, Pennsylvania, in 1979. Although these events occurred in stationary structures and threatened surrounding communities, one must keep in mind that this type of risk may be transported over the railway or highway systems through any area in the form of hazardous chemicals, waste materials, and munitions, or due to lack of proper disposal, as in the case of Goiania, Brazil, in 1987 (15).

Nature itself has caused a fair share of mass casualty incidents. Geotectonic events have demonstrated the potential for chaos and destruction as the result of earthquakes, tsunamis, volcanoes, landslides, and avalanches, to name but a few of the hazards nature can throw our way. Atmospheric phenomena have impacted vast populations in a repetitive fashion, most recently major catastrophes such as tropical storm Allison in 2002, and hurricanes Katrina and Rita in 2005. Relevant to these events, but on a smaller scale, we routinely see devastation caused by tornadoes, drought, wildfires, and winter storms (16,17).

Taking into consideration all of these historical aspects, scientific forecasting, and the possibility of terrorist targeting, all communities, whether large or small, should complete a "hazard vulnerability analysis" (HVA) that can assist in the planning and identification of resources aimed at the mitigation of the event's impact (1,18).

INITIATIVES IN THE UNITED STATES

The transformation of the "ambulance" system into an emergency medical system in the United States in the late 1970s brought about the development of an infrastructure that served as the backbone to respond to mass casualty incidents. The early focus on the prehospital setting has helped in the development of the Incident Command System (ICS) and the National Incident Management System (NIMS) (19) as a way to organize a single or multi-institutional response. These efforts have been paired with the development of the National Disaster Life Support (NDLS) (20) program, which has a variety of courses targeted to field providers and hospital personnel. The details of these programs require theoretical and practical training, but are, unfortunately, beyond the scope of this chapter.

An adaptation of the ICS evolved into the Hospital Emergency Incident Command System (HEICS), more recently renamed and organized as the Hospital Incident Command System (HICS) (21) as a means to assist hospitals in improving their emergency management planning, response, and recovery capabilities for unplanned and planned events. However, the required surge capacity response of the intensive care unit (ICU) has been a priority concern at the Society of Critical Care Medicine (SCCM), and has led to the development of the Fundamentals of Disaster Management (FDM) course (22). This course includes didactic and hands-on development of skills to utilize equipment provided by the Strategic National Stockpile (SNS), and targets intensivists and hospital staff.

DECONTAMINATION AND FIRST RECEIVERS

Education of proper decontamination techniques for various agents must be included in any plan for a hospital to respond to a multiple casualty incident (MCI). Improper technique, or lack of deployment, may lead to exposure of the ED personnel and the facility in general, as was experienced in 1995 in Tokyo with the release of sarin in the subway system (12,23). Thus, it is imperative to ensure that correct decontamination procedures are completed prior to allowing ED personnel access to exposed persons. Any suspicion or doubt regarding this aspect of care should result in repeating the decontamination process prior to entering the facility.

The decontamination process begins with the designation and enforcement of perimeters around the hospital to ensure that patients flow through a predetermined corridor. Some patients may arrive to the hospital by their own means, without any *in situ* decontamination performed by first responders, and others may arrive with incomplete decontamination. In most instances, *any* patient should go through a thorough, supervised, and complete decontamination prior to accessing the inside of the facility.

Hospital Perimeters

Traditionally a hospital perimeter is divided into three areas, or zones:

1. *Hot zone:* This zone represents everything outside the facility's perimeter. The hot zone is where patients have not been through decontamination or triage, and where credentials for access have not been verified by security or screening personnel.
2. *Warm zone*: This is the transition zone, where decontamination and triage happens. This is also where security personnel verify credentials and health screening clearance for access, depending on the nature of the event.
3. *Cold zone*: This is the "inside" of the hospital. Patients will access this zone only after decontamination is completed and verified. Health care providers are granted access after credentials and health status are corroborated.

Types of Decontamination

Primary Decontamination

This occurs when the individual's clothes are removed, in conjunction with showers with a low-pressure, large-volume water delivery system, such as the Trident (24) (Fig. 176.3). In colder climates, it is important to ensure warm water delivery

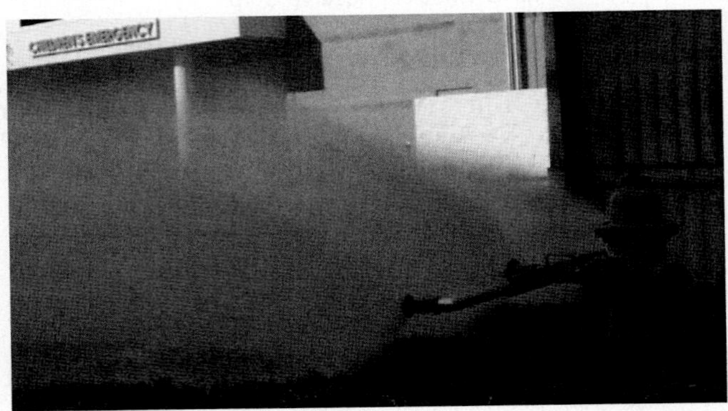

FIGURE 176.3. Low-pressure high-volume expanded triple system deployed with fire hydrant connection. (Courtesy of Orlando Regional Medical Center.)

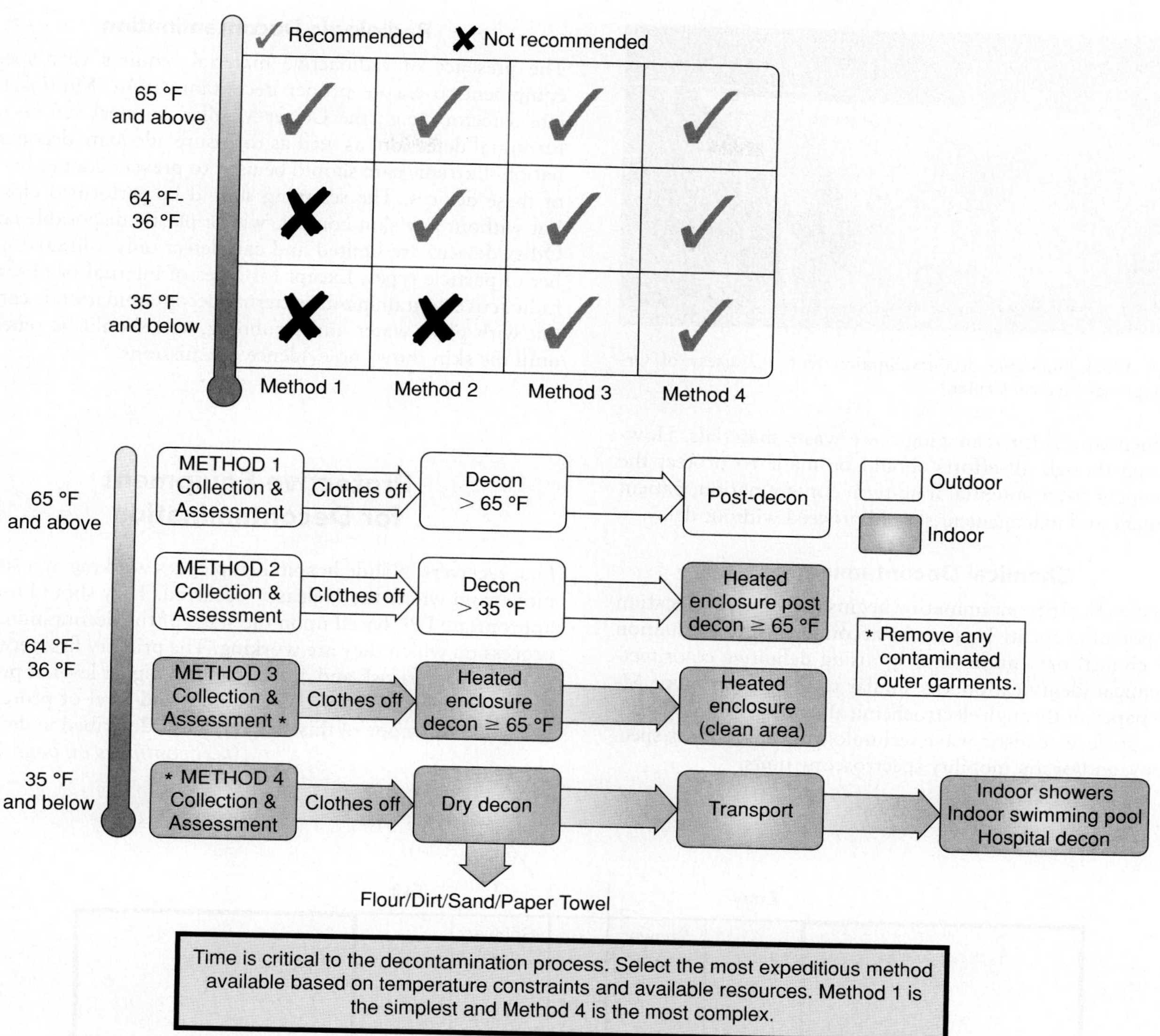

FIGURE 176.4. Decontamination (Decon) methods based on ambient temperatures (From U.S. Army Soldier and Biological Chemical Command (SBCCOM). Guidelines for cold weather mass decontamination during a terrorist chemical incident. 2003:5. http://www.ecbc.army.mil/downloads/cwirp/ECBC_cwirp_cold_weather_mass_decon.pdf. Accessed October 27, 2008.)

systems, as well as consideration of indoor or pool decontamination techniques (25) (Fig. 176.4), in order to minimize exposure and improve compliance. Privacy is another major consideration that will help improve compliance by the establishment of corridors and barriers installed to protect patients' dignity after clothing has been removed for decontamination.

Secondary Decontamination

This is performed by either health care workers following specific guidelines for nonambulatory patients or by the ambulatory patients themselves following clearly written and pictorially explicit instructions made available in the most common regional languages to accomplish self-decontamination. This latter group would then only require minor supervision from health care workers to ensure proper compliance.

Although many solutions have been proposed for use during this stage of decontamination, it is now recommended that plain water, in conjunction with scrubbing, be used. This can usually be implemented very quickly in order to expedite the removal of the agent and decrease any possible absorption. In some instances, the application of mild soapy solutions can be used for oily residues; however, the decontamination process should not be delayed to add soap (26).

Some hospitals have incorporated permanent decontamination areas, such as showers and rooms, within their architectural façade design at the emergency department entry; others rely on the quick deployment of tents (Fig. 176.5) or temporary decontamination corridors with low-pressure, high-volume expanded shower triple system (Fig. 176.3), or via water hoses from fire engines (Fig. 176.6).

The contaminated water is ideally pumped from the containment pools to bladders and cisterns that will require special disposal. The Environmental Protection Agency and the Occupational Safety and Health Administration (OSHA) have

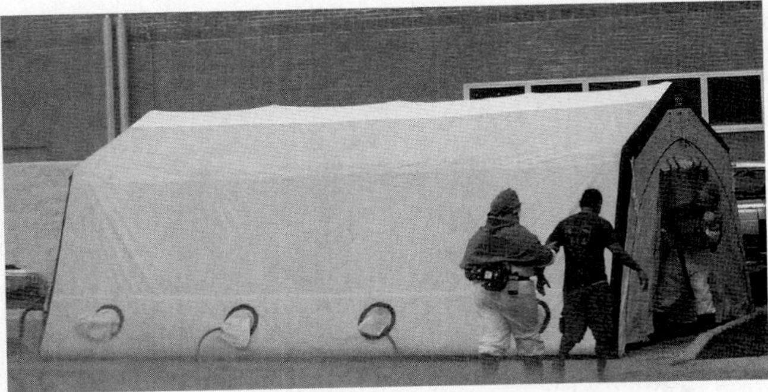

FIGURE 176.5. Inflatable decontamination tent. (Courtesy of Orlando Regional Medical Center.)

recommendations for managing these waste materials. However, even though all efforts should be made to protect the environment from potential long-term contamination, patient assessment and management should proceed without delay.

Chemical Decontamination

Proper chemical decontamination begins with the identification of the potential agent. This can be accomplished by evaluation of the clinical presentation, or by using definitive colorimetric chemical identification kits similar to the military type M-8/M-9 paper, or through electrochemical sensors, radiologic detectors, surface acoustic wave technology, infrared mass spectroscopy, and/or ion mobility spectroscopy units.

Radiologic Decontamination

The presence of radioactive material requires very specific equipment to ensure proper decontamination. Multiparticulate detectors (e.g., the Geiger-Mueller counter) can be used for initial detection, as well as to ensure adequate decontamination. Extreme care should be used to prevent contamination of these devices. The scanning should be performed close to but without any skin contact, with a plastic disposable cover. Other devices are limited and can detect only a limited number of particle types. Except for cases of internal or absorbed radioactive contaminants, external decontamination is carried out with plain water and scrubbing, and should be repeated until the skin shows no evidence of emissions.

Protective Equipment for Decontamination

First receivers include hospital employees working at a site remote from where the "release" occurred. They should use the appropriate PPE based upon the stage of the decontamination process on which they are working. The primary first receivers have the highest risk and, thus, require a higher level of protection. The delineation of their training and level of protection is beyond the scope of this chapter, but is described in detail in

(*text continues on page 2622*)

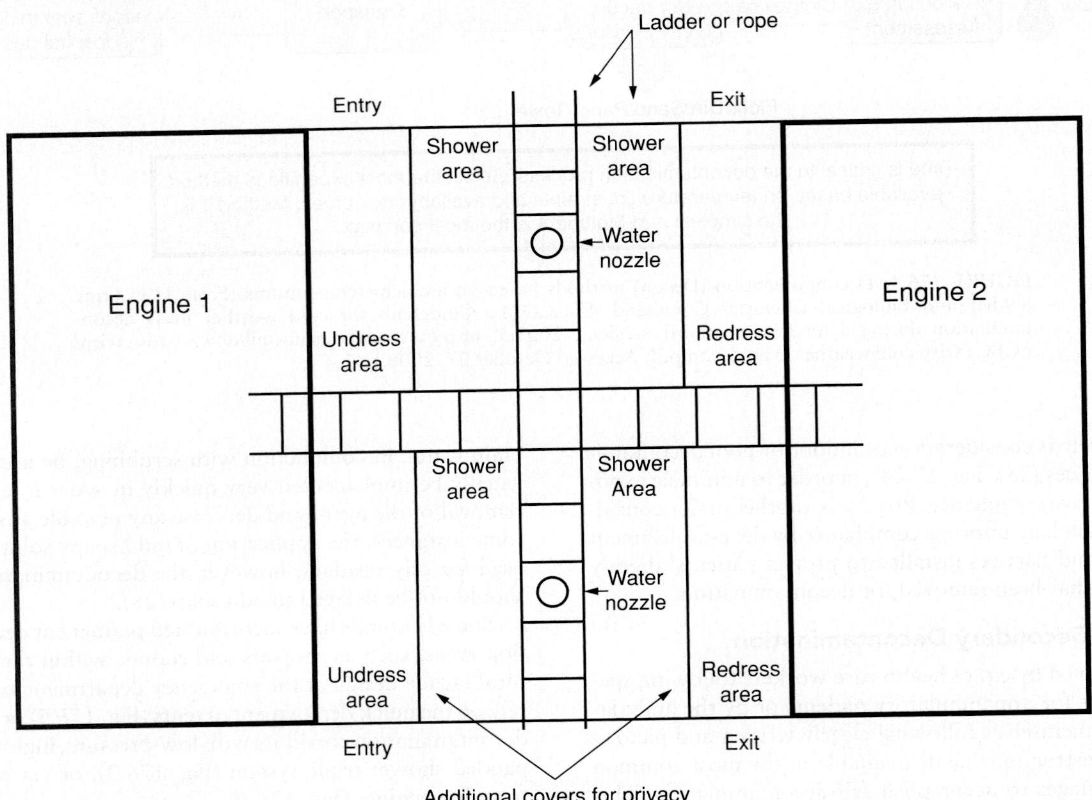

FIGURE 176.6. Emergency decontamination corridor system with fire engines and ladders. (From U.S. Army Soldier and Biological Chemical Command (SBCCOM). Guidelines for mass casualty decontamination. 2000:10. http://www.chem-bio.com/resource/2000/cwirp_guidelines_mass.pdf. Accessed October 27, 2008.)

TABLE 176.1

PLANNING ASSUMPTIONS AND RECOMMENDATIONS FOR MASS CRITICAL CARE

Planning assumptions regarding the current critical care medicine response capacity for bioterrorism

1. Future bioterrorist attacks may be covert and could result in hundreds, thousands, or more critically ill victims.
2. Critical care will play a key role in decreasing morbidity and mortality rates after a bioterrorist attack.
3. Mass critical care could not be provided without substantial planning and new approaches to providing critical care.
4. A hospital would have limited ability to divert or transfer patients to other hospitals in the aftermath of a bioterrorist attack.
5. Currently deployable medical teams of the federal government would have a limited role in increasing a hospital's immediate ability to provide critical care to large numbers of victims of a bioterrorist attack.
6. Hospitals may need to depend on nonfederal sources or reserves of medications and equipment necessary to provide critical care for the first 48 hrs following discovery of a bioterrorist attack.

Recommendations for hospital planning and response for emergency mass critical care

Modifying usual standards of care

1. Hospitals should develop a set of emergency mass critical care practices that could be implemented in the event critical care capacity of that hospital is exceeded.

Decisions regarding which critical care interventions should be provided: Essential elements of critical care

2. To ensure the availability of essential critical care interventions, the Working Group recommends that hospitals give priority to interventions that fulfill the following criteria: a) interventions that have been shown or are deemed by critical care experts' best professional judgment to improve survival, and without which death is likely; b) interventions that do not require extraordinarily expensive equipment; and c) interventions that can be implemented without comsuming extensive staff or hospital resources.
3. Hospitals should plan to be able to deliver the following during emergency mass critical care: basic modes of mechanical ventilation, hemodynamic support, antibiotic or other disease-specific countermeasure therapy, and a small set of prophylactic interventions that are recognized to reduce the serious adverse consequences of critical illness.
4. Hospitals should plan to be able to administer intravenous fluids resuscitation and vasopressor to large numbers of hemodynamically unstable victims and should stockpile sufficient equipment to do this without relying on external resources for at least the first 48 hrs of the hospital medical response.
5. Hospitals should plan to provide at least two widely accepted prophylactic interventions that are used every day in critical care: maintaining the head of a mechanically ventilated patient's bed at 45 degrees to prevent ventilator-associated pneumonia and thromboembolism prophylaxis.

Decisions regarding who receives critical care services

6. If there are limited hospital resources and many critically ill patients in need, triage decisions regarding the provision of critical care should be guided by the principle of seeking to help the greatest number of people survive the crisis. This would include patients already receiving ICU care who are not casualties of an attack.

Who should provide emergency mass critical care

7. In the event that critical care needs in a hospital cannot be met by intensivists and critical care nurses, usual ICU staffing should be modified to include nonintensivist clinicians and noncritical care nurses, using a two-tiered staffing model.
8. When there are inadequate numbers of intensivists, hospitals should plan for nonintensivists to manage approximately six critically ill patients and to have intensivists coordinate the efforts of up to four nonintensivists.
9. If a hospital has insufficient numbers of critical care nurses to appropriately manage patients, noncritical care nurses should be assigned primary responsibility for patient assessment, nursing care documentation, administration of medications, and bedside care (e.g., head of bed at 45 degrees, moving patient to prevent pressure ulcers), and critical care nurses should advise noncritical care nurses on critical care issues such as vasopressor and sedation administration.
10. If possible, a noncritical care nurse should be assigned to no more than two critically ill patients, and up to three noncritical care nurses would work in collaboration with one critical care nurse.
11. Bioterrorism training for noncritical care practitioners should include basic principles of critical care management.

Infection control for emergency mass critical care

12. Hospitals should develop pre-event plans to augment usual or modified-airborne infection isolation capacity for critically ill victims of a bioattack with a contagious pathogen.
13. Hospitals should stockpile enough PPE to care for mass casualties of a bioterrorist attack for up to 48 hrs. Also, all hospital clinical staff should receive initial and periodic training on principles of health care delivery using PPE.

Where emergency mass critical care should be located

14. When traditional critical care capacity is full, additional critically ill patients should receive care in non-ICU hospital rooms that are concentrated on specific hospital wards or floors.
15. Hospitals should plan to be able to measure oxygen saturation, temperature, blood pressure, and urine output for the victims of bioattacks in emergency mass critical care conditions.

Learning during emergency mass critical care

16. Hospitals should have information technology capabilities for analyzing clinical data for patients receiving emergency mass critical care and for quickly sharing new observations with a broader clinical community.

Medications for emergency mass critical care

17. Hospitals should develop a list of drugs to stockpile for up to a 48-hr response to a mass casualty event using selection criteria that include likelihood the drug would be required for care of most patients, proven or generally accepted efficacy by most practitioners, cost, ease of administration, ability to rotate into the hospital's formulary prior to expiration, and resources required for medication storage.

ICU, intensive care unit; PPE, personal protective equipment.
From Rubinson L, Nuzzo J, Talmor D, et al. Augmentation of hospital critical care capacity after bioterrorist attacks or epidemics: recommendations of the Working Group on Emergency Mass Critical Care. *Crit Care Med.* 2005;33(Suppl.):E2393.

TABLE 176.2

GUIDELINES FOR IDENTIFICATION OF A BIOTERRORISM EVENT

- Unusual temporal or geographic clustering of illness
- Unusual age distribution of common disease (e.g., an illness that appears to be chickenpox in adults but is really smallpox)
- Large epidemic, with greater caseloads than expected, especially in a discrete population
- More severe disease than expected
- Unusual route of exposure
- A disease that is outside its normal transmission season, or is impossible to transmit naturally in the absence of its normal vector
- Multiple simultaneous epidemics of different diseases
- A disease outbreak with health consequences to humans and animals
- Unusual strains or variants of organisms or antimicrobial resistance patterns

A. SENTINEL CLUES FOR A CATEGORY A BIOLOGIC AGENT

Pneumonia or influenzalike syndromes

- Chest pain, dry cough, possible nausea, and abdominal pain, followed by sepsis, shock, widened mediastinum, hemorrhagic pleural effusions, and respiratory failure
  Gram-positive bacillus may be isolated.
  Consider inhalation anthrax.
- Pneumonia associated with mucopurulent sputum, chest pain, and hemoptysis, particularly in an otherwise normal host
  Gram-negative bacillus isolated
  Consider pneumonic plague.
- Bronchopneumonia associated with pleuritis and hilar lymphadenopathy, particularly in an otherwise normal host
  Gram-negative coccobacillus isolated
  Consider tularemia.

Cutaneous ulcer or ulceroglandular syndromes

- Painless ulcer covered by a black eschar, surrounded by extensive nonpitting edema that is out of proportion to the size of the ulcer. Fever and regional lymphadenopathy may be present.
  Consider cutaneous anthrax.

Fever and rash syndromes

- An abrupt, influenzalike illness with fever, dizziness, myalgias, headache, nausea, abdominal pain, diarrhea, and prostration. Evidence of "leaky capillary syndrome" with edema or signs of bleeding ranging from conjunctival hemorrhage, mild hypotension, flushing, petechiae, and ecchymoses to shock and generalized mucous membrane hemorrhage and evidence of pulmonary, hematopoietic, renal, and neurologic dysfunction
  Consider viral hemorrhagic fevers.
- Febrile illness with myalgias, followed in 2 to 3 days by a generalized macular or papular-vesicular-pustular eruption, with greatest concentration of lesions on the face and distal extremities, including the palms. On any one part of the body (face, arms, chest), all lesions are at the same stage of development (all papules, vesicles, pustules, or scabs).
  Consider smallpox.

Paralytic syndromes

- Paralytic illness characterized by symmetric, descending flaccid paralysis of motor and autonomic nerves, usually beginning with the cranial nerves
  Consider botulism.

B. REPORTING PROTOCOLS IF BIOTERRORISM IS SUSPECTED AS RESPONSIBLE FOR AN ILLNESS

- Establish isolation and personnel protection level.
- Contact local public health department immediately.
- Do not wait for confirmation.
- Record data and order tests.
- Alert clinical laboratory.
- Arrange for consultations.
- Follow hospital protocol.
- Notify hospital epidemiologist/infection control specialist.
- Discuss findings with all involved parties.

From *The American College of Physicians Guide to Bioterrorism Identification.* http://www.acponline.org/bioterro/bio_pocketguide.pdf. Accessed October 27, 2008.

TABLE 176.3

BIOLOGICAL AGENTS CATEGORY A

Entity	Agent	Transmission	Minimum PPE (ideal PPE)	When to suspect	Presentation	Diagnosis	Treatment	Alternative treatment	Prophylaxis	Vaccine
Anthrax	*Bacillus anthracis*	Direct contact—Cutaneous anthrax Airborne—Inhalational anthrax (consider terrorist activity) Ingestion—Gastrointestinal anthrax and Oropharyngeal NO person to person	Standard precautions	Characteristic skin lesions Rapidly progressive pneumonia CXR: Widened mediastinum (lymphadenopathies) & pleural effusions	Pustule that progresses to a skin ulcer with black necrotic center Respiratory failure Septic shock Diarrhea	Gram Stain Cultures	Ciprofloxacin (1)	Doxycycline (2) + 1 or 2 additional antimicrobials	Ciprofloxacin (3) or Doxycycline (4) or Amoxicillin (if pregnant and sensitive strain)	Yes
Botulism	Neurotoxin of *Clostridium botulium* (BoNT)	Ingestion of toxin (consider terrorist activity—water supply) Inhalation of toxin Infection with toxin production NO person to person	Standard precautions **(Droplet if meningitis supected)**	Occulobulbar paralysis	Symmetric descending paralysis	Clinical BoNT detection (Days) (CDC)	Supportive Antitoxin (early)		Antitoxin Monoclonal Ab (Limited supply)	No
Plague	*Yersinia pestis*	Vector (Rodent fleas) (Bubonic plague) Inhalation (Pneumonic plague) (consider terrorist activity) PERSON TO PERSON	Droplet **(Airborne)**	Large inguinal and axillary lymphadenopathies (bubonic) Sepsis Unusual number of patients with a fulminant course of productive cough and pneumonia. Sepsis.	Buboes DIC, Sepsis Respiratory failure Pneumonia, Sepsis	Gram Stain Cultures Immunofluorescence	Streptomycin (5) or Gentamicin (6)	Doxycycline (2) or Chloramphenicol (7) or Ciprofloxacin (1)	Doxycycline (4) or Ciprofloxacin (3)	No

(*continued*)

TABLE 176.3

(CONTINUED)

Entity	Agent	Transmission	Minimum PPE (ideal PPE)	When to suspect	Presentation	Diagnosis	Treatment	Alternative treatment	Prophylaxis	Vaccine
Smallpox	Variola virus	Direct contact Fomites Airborne PERSON TO PERSON	Airborne (PAPR)	Papulo-pustular rashes	Progression from: (duration) No symptoms—Incubation (7–14 d.) Enanthema (2–4 d.)—Contagious Early rash—Maculo-papular (4 d.) Umbillicated centrifugal rash ALL lesions AT SAME STAGE Scabs (5 d.) Pustules (5 d.) Scabs resolve—Noncontagious	Clinical PCR (CDC)	<3 days of exposure: Vaccinia vaccine Vaccinia Immune Globuline (VIG) (8) Vaccinia Immune Globuline IV (VIGIV) (9) Cidofovir (10) >3 days of exposure: Supportive		See Treatment	Yes
Tularemia	*Francisella tularensis*	Direct contact with infected animal carcasses (rabbits, hares, rodents) Arthropod bites (tick, deerfly) Ingestion of contaminated food or water Inhalation (consider terrorist activity) NO person to person	Standard precautions	Unusual number of patients with respiratory or systemic illnesses.	Ulceroglandular Oculoglandular Oropharyngeal Pneumonic Sepsis	Gram Stain Direct Fluorescent Antibody Culture requires special media Serology only retrospective value	Streptomycin (5) or Gentamicin (6)	Doxycycline (2) or Chloramphenicol (7) or Ciprofloxacin (1)	Doxycycline (4) or Ciprofloxacin (3)	No

VHF (Viral Hemorrhagic Fevers)	Ebola Marburg Lassa Machupo Rift Valley	Direct contact Airborne (Hypothetical) PERSON TO PERSON	Droplet (**Airborne**) (**PAPR**)	Unusual number of patients with fever, myalgias, conjunctivitis in a severely ill patient with either a purpuric or hemorrhagic maculopapular rash.	Maculopapular rash, purpuric or hemorrhagic Bleeding diathesis: Epistaxis, hematemesis, hematochezia Pneumonitis	Clinical CDC		Supportive Ribavirin (11) (not effective against Ebola or Marburg) Specific Immune Globuline (difficult to obtain)		Ribavirin (12) (in needle sticks)	No

Adapted from:
1- Pandemic Point-of care Guide. Joint Commission Resources. 2007
2- Fundamentals of Disaster Management. 2nd Edition. Society of Critical Care Medicine. 2004
3- Centers for Disease Control and Prevention—Bioterrorism, available at: http://www.bt.cdc.gov/agent/agentlist-category.asp (Accessed 1-5-08)
PPE: Personal Protective Equipment, PAPR: Powered Air-Purifying Respirator
BoNT detection: DEFINE

TABLE 176.4

BIOLOGICAL AGENTS CATEGORY B & C

Entity	Agent	Transmission	Minimum PPE	When to suspect	Presentation	Diagnosis	Treatment	Alternative treatment	Prophylaxis	Vaccine
Brucellosis	*Brucella sp.*	Direct Contact Ingestion (consider terrorist activity) PERSON TO PERSON (Extremely rare)	Standard precautions	Unusual number of patients with: Fever, myalgias, malaise, sweats, sepsis	Nonspecific	Gram stain Blood cultures Anti-O Antibody titer (≥1:160)	Doxycycline (2) plus Rifampin (13)	Trimethoprim/ Sulfamethoxazole (14, 15) plus Gentamicin (6)	Doxycycline (4) plus Rifampin (13)	No
Ricin toxin	Toxin from Castor bean plant *Ricinnus communis*	Direct Contact Ingestion Inhalation (consider terrorist activity)		Unusual number of patients with: Nausea, vomiting, abdominal pain, diarrhea Dyspnea, ALI, ARDS	Gastrointestinal symptoms Hypovolemic shock Respiratory failure	Difficult Urinary ricinine (CDC) Environmental specimens to CDC for immunoassays and PCR				
Cholera	*Vibrio cholerae*	Ingestion	Standard precautions	Abrupt, copious watery diarrhea	Abrupt, copious watery diarrhea Very rare abdominal pain or fever		Rehydration, aggressive Doxycycline 300 mg PO—1 dose or Ciprofloxacin 1 gm PO—1 dose or Azithromycin 1 gm PO—1 dose			Yes
Foodborne Infections	*Escherichia coli* (O157:H7, enterotoxigenic) *Campylobacter sp.* *Salmonella typhi & non-typhi* *Shigella sp* *Giardia lamblia* *Listeria monocytogenes* *Entamoeba histolytica* *Yersinia enterocolitica* *S. aureus* (enterotoxin B) Others.	Ingestion	Standard precautions	Diarrhea, nausea, vomiting, fever, chills	Diarrhea, nausea, vomiting, fever, chills	Direct smear Stool cultures Blood cultures	Azythromycin (16) or ciprofloxacin (3) Azythromycin (16) Ciprofloxacin (3) Ciprofloxacin (3) Metronidazole 500–750 mg PO TID Ampicillin 2 gm IV Q 6 h Metronidazole 500–750 mg PO TID Trimethoprim/ Sulfamethoxazole (15) Supportive Various other antibiotics	Ceftriaxone (16) Azythromycin (16) Paramomycin (16) Paramomycin (16)		No

Glanders	*Burkholderia mallei*	Direct contact Ingestion Inhalation PERSON TO PERSON	Standard precautions Droplet in pulmonary cases	Massive numbers of patients with similar clinical presentation	Localized Infection Pulmonary Infection Bloodstream Infection Chronic Infection (Extremities, spleen or liver)	Skin cultures Sputum cultures Blood cultures Urine cultures	Trimethoprim/ Sulfamethoxazole (14)	Tetracyclines (16) Ciprofloxacin (16) Streptomycin (16) Imipenem (16) Ceftazidime (16)	No
Melioidosis	*Burkholderia pseudomallei*	Direct contact Ingestion Inhalation PERSON TO PERSON	Standard precautions Droplet in pulmonary cases	Massive numbers of patients with similar clinical presentation	Acute localized Infection Pulmonary Infection Acute Bloodstream Infection Chronic Suppurative Infection	Skin cultures Sputum cultures Blood cultures Urine cultures	Trimethoprim/ Sulfamethoxazole (14) or Ceftazidime (16)	Imipenem (16) Meropenem (16) Chloramphenicol (16)	No

Adapted from:
1- Pandemic Point-of care Guide. Joint Commission Resources. 2007
2- Fundamentals of Disaster Management. 2nd Edition. Society of Critical Care Medicine. 2004
3- Centers for Disease Control and Prevention—Bioterrorism, available at: http://www.bt.cdc.gov/agent/agentlist-category.asp (Accessed 1-5-08)
PPE: Personal Protective Equipment

TABLE 176.5

TREATING AGENTS

Agent	Dose
1. Ciprofloxacin	
Adults	400 mg IV Q 12 h
Pregnancy	400 mg IV Q 12 h
2. Doxycycline	
Adults	100 mg IV Q 12 h
Pregnancy	100 mg IV Q 12 h
3. Ciprofloxacin	
Adults	500 mg PO BID
Pregnancy	500 mg PO BID
4. Doxycycline	
Adults	100 mg PO BID
Pregnancy	100 mg PO BID
5. Streptomycin	
Adults	1 gm IM Q 12 h
6. Gentamicin	
Adults	5 mg/kg IM or IV Q 24 h
Pregnancy	5 mg/kg IM or IV Q 24 h
7. Chloramphenicol	
Adults	25 mg/kg IV Q 6 h
8. VIG	
Adults	0.6 mL/kg IM
9. VIGIV	
Adults	100 mg/kg IV at rate: 1 mL/kg/h for 30 min, then 2 mL/kg/h for 30 min, then 3 mL/kg/h for 30 min
10. Cidofovir	
Adults	5 mg/kg IV over 1 h
11. Ribavirin	
Adults	30 mg/kg IV loading dose 16 mg/kg IV Q 4 h for 4 days, then 8 mg/kg IV Q 4 h for 6 days
12. Ribavirin	
Adults	500 mg PO Q 6 h for 7 days

Note: These are starting doses for adults only; for length of therapy, pediatric therapies and further indications, consult with health authorities or infectious disease specialists

the OSHA publication, *Best Practices for Hospital-based First Receivers* (27).

Levels of PPE include class A, B, and C ensembles. Level A ensembles include the highest level of respiratory protection—a self-contained breathing apparatus that is worn inside vapor-protective chemical clothing. Level B ensembles involve heavy-splash chemical protective clothing with the use of self-contained breathing apparatus (some PPE in this level may be encapsulated but should not be confused with the garment rating of vapor protective). Level C ensembles involve light-splash chemical clothing in conjunction with either a filter cartridge face mask or powered air-purifying respirator (PAPR) in which the appropriate filter that provides respiratory protection must be used for the specific product involved within a qualified atmosphere containing an appropriate level of oxygen. Due to the dynamics involved, level C ensembles are usually suitable for hospital first receivers (based upon the specifics of the substances involved), and consist of:

- A chemical resistant suit
- Two layers of gloves
- Chemical-resistant boots
- A breathing device

In most cases, more complex systems requiring compressed air are not warranted at the hospital, and are usually reserved for first responders at the area of the primary event. Efforts toward establishing a relationship with the local hazardous materials team will provide the following benefits: recognition of jurisdictional capabilities, improved communication between on-scene first responders and the emergency department first receivers, and established trust for accuracy of relayed chemical hazard information and/or personnel protective equipment selection criteria.

The donning of this equipment represents a significant added physical and emotional stressor for first receivers. In order to minimize potential complications, a set of minimal physical conditions are required prior to its utilization. Periodic checks and a "buddy system" are recommended (27). First receivers should have scheduled training sessions in order to don and doff their gear properly. They should also follow clear guidelines for adequate rotations, rehydration, and monitoring. First receivers have an average effective time of about 20 minutes, which can be significantly shortened due to weather conditions. Cooling vests with packaged dry ice or water-recirculation suits have been used in warm climates and may triple the effective time, but close monitoring is still required.

Once decontaminated, the patient may require placement in isolation areas with or without negative environmental pressure. All personnel in the cold zone that come in contact with patients exposed to a potential biologic agent should wear, at minimum, gear consisting of a liquid-proof disposable gown (Tyvek or similar material), gloves, goggles, and surgical mask. Depending on the agent, higher levels of respiratory protection may be required.

ROLE AND EXPECTATIONS OF THE INTENSIVIST

Intensivists play a key role in preparing the hospital for these types of events. The SCCM has already developed the FDM to provide this type of education to ICU practitioners. Within their individual facilities, the intensivist should partner with ED personnel, hospital administrators, pharmacists, engineers, local first responders, area hazardous materials teams, and community services leaders in order to develop a plan that includes triggers, communications, personnel distribution, equipment and medication stocks, surge areas and facilities, and ongoing education and drills.

PLANNING AND AUGMENTING RESPONSES

As this textbook goes to press, in the United States, most medical facilities are functioning at full or near-full capacity during routine operations (3). This is further complicated by ongoing health care worker staff deficits; therefore, staffing and personnel should be a major focus in the planning of a "surge" response during a multiple casualty incident (MCI). In order to increase the capacity to respond, a group of 34 North American experts led by Rubinson published their recommendations in 2005 (3); these are summarized in Table 176.1.

(*text continues on page 2626*)

TABLE 176.6

CHEMICAL AGENTS

Type	Acronym	Other name	Military detection	Classic findings	Other signs and symptoms	Decontamination	Treatment	Miscellaenous
Nerve	GA GB GD GF VX	Tabun Sarin Soman Cyclohexyl sarin Methylphosphonothioic acid	M256A1 CAM M8 paper M9 paper M8A1 alarm M8 alarm	Miosis Sialorrhea Rhinorrhea Fasciculation	Blurred vision Headache Nausea & vomiting Sialorrhea Diaphoresis Diarrhea Seizures Dyspnea	Remove clothing Gentle skin wash (avoid abrading skin) Flush eyes with water or saline	Atropine 2 mg IV / IM every 5 min Repeat as needed based on symptoms Pralidoxime 600–1800 mg IM or 1 gm IV (max 2 g/hour) MARK-I kit contents: AtroPen—atropine sulfate 2 mg in 0.7mL ComboPen—pralidoxime chloride (2-PAM) 600 mg in 2 mL Benzodiazepines for seizures Oxygen Ventilatory support	In high exposures: Unconsciousness Flaccid paralysis
Blood/ Asphyxi-ant	AC CK	Arsine Hydrogen cyanide Cyanogen chloride	M256A1 Ticket NOT—M8A1 NOT—CAM	Cherry red skin or Cyanosis or Frostbite (when applied in liquid form)	Few: Giddiness Palpitations Dizziness Nausea & vomiting Gasping Hyperventilation Drowsiness Seizures (terminal)	Remove clothing (if no frostbite) Gentle skin wash (avoid abrading skin) Flush eyes with water or saline	Oxygen ANTIDOTES: Amyl Nitrate by inhalation 1 amp (0.2 mL) every 5 min Sodium Nitrate 300 mg IV over 5–10 min Sodium thiosulfate 12.5 gm IV over 10–20 min Repeat Sodium nitrate base on patient's weight and hemoglobin level	Metabolic aciosis Venous oxymetry above normal Arsine and cyanogen may cause delayed pulmonary edema

(continued)

TABLE 176.6

(CONTINUED)

Type	Acronym	Other name	Military detection	Classic findings	Other signs and symptoms	Decontamination	Treatment	Miscellaneous
Pulmonary/ Choking	Chlorine Phosgene Diphosgene Chloropicrin	CL CG DP PS	No detection	Odor of newly mown hay or grass or corn	Eye irritation Airway irritation Dyspnea Wheezing Coughing Laryngeal edema Pulmonary edema ALI & ARDS	Fresh air Oxygen Remove clothing Gentle skin wash (avoid abrading skin) Flush eyes with water or saline	Termination of exposure No antidote Supportive treatment	
Blistering/ Vesicant	Phosgene Oxime Mustard gas Sulfur mustard Nitrogen mustard Lewisite	CX H HD HN L	**CX:** M256A1 M8 alarm **Mustards:** M256A1 CAM M8 paper M9 paper M8 alarm **NOT** - M8A1 alarm **L:** M256A1 **ONLY**	CX Odor: Pungent or pepperish HD Odor: Garlic or horseradish L Odor: Geranium	Eye edema and tearing Skin erythema and blistering Airway sloughing Dyspnea Coughing Pulmonary edema	Remove clothing Gentle skin wash (avoid abrading skin) Flush eyes with water or saline	Termination of exposure Supportive treatment **Mustards:** No antidote **Antidote for Lewisite (L): British Anti-Lewisite (BAL)** or Dimercaprol	Bone marrow suppression
Riot Control Agents	Chloroacetophenone Ortho-chlorobenzylidene malononitrile	CN or MACE CS	No detection	Lacrimation Rhinorrhea Erythema	Dyspnea Tachypnea Wheezing	Flush eyes with water or saline Flush skin with water Decontamination is usually not indicated	Supportive treatment	Usual: Self-limiting Unsual: Pulmonary edema

Adapted from references 22 & 26.
amp = ampule
mg = milligram
gm = gram
mL = milliliter
IV = Intravenous
IM = Intramuscular
min = minutes

TABLE 176.7

PERSONAL PROTECTIVE EQUIPMENT (PPE): DONNING AND DOFFING AND ENHANCED AIRBORNE PRECAUTIONS WITH POWERED AIR-PURIFYING RESPIRATOR (PAPR)[a]

PRIOR TO ENTERING THE ROOM
(For leaving the room, proceed to step VI.)

Step I
The following articles must be put on in the ANTE room. If there is no ANTE room, they should be donned prior to entering the intensive care unit (ICU).
1. Properly fitted N-95 mask (minimum)
2. Impervious isolation gown
3. Gloves (place two strips of tape onto the glove and the gown, one anterior and one posterior)

Step II
Routine care PPE (second layer)
The following articles are to be worn in addition to PPE in step I, prior to entering the patient's room for **routine** patient care.
WARNING: If you anticipate aerosolization of secretions (e.g., endotracheal intubation, cardiac arrest, tracheostomy, bronchoscopy, endotracheal tube exchange, and so forth), skip this section and **proceed to steps III, IV, and V** prior to entering the room.
1. Disposable goggles (place a strip of tape onto goggles and forehead)
2. Second impervious isolation gown (see pix 2 on PAPR sheet)
3. Second set of gloves (place two strips of tape onto the glove and the gown, one anterior and one posterior; see pix 3A,B on PAPR sheet)
4. Hair net or hat (optional)

YOU MAY NOW ENTER THE ROOM FOR ROUTINE CARE

Step III
Testing the HEPA filter and electric pump battery efficiency
1. Attach breathing tube (black) to the air pump/filter/battery (PAPR) assembly box (gray) with a twist-and-lock motion.
2. Turn the power switch ON.
3. Check air flow by inserting floater cone inside the free end of the black tube. Floater device should remain suspended, with the lower indicator line *not* touching the tube's end. This indicates proper functioning of the unit. If cone does not float, **DO NOT USE** THIS UNIT AND SEND FOR SERVICING.
4. Turn the power switch OFF and set unit aside.

Step IV
Donning the hood (REQUIRES ASSISTANCE)
1. Secure long hair.
2. Put on a hair cover (optional).
3. Peel off protective layer from face shield.
4. Attach breathing tube to the top of the hood; a snap should be heard.
5. Place the pump/filter/battery assembly (gray) (PAPR) box around waist and adjust belt. Leave the box in the back.
6. Turn the power switch ON.
7. Ensure the breathing tube is free from twists, kinks, or damage.
8. With assistance, put hood on, face first. Ensure that the elasticized edge of the face seal is under the chin and along the cheeks. Ensure the N-95 mask remains securely in place (4).
9. Center inner headband around forehead and verify that straps on top of the hood are in contact with the top of the head.

Step V
PAPR PPE (second layer)
1. Lift the outer shroud of the hood.
2. Put on a second impervious isolation gown, ensuring that it covers the inner shroud ONLY (5).
3. Allow the outer shroud to cover the top portion of the isolation gown.
4. Apply second pair of gloves (place two strips of tape onto the glove and the gown, one anterior and one posterior).

You may now enter the room to perform procedures where aerosolization of secretions are anticipated.

PRIOR TO LEAVING THE ROOM

Step VI
Removal of routine care PPE
1. Grasp front of second isolation gown (top layer) with both hands, and pull forward to remove from shoulders.
2. Remove second isolation gown with taped gloves as one unit, as you roll inside out, prior to discarding.
3. Remove disposable goggles, grasping above the ear. DO NOT touch the frame area around the eyes. Discard goggles.

Step VII
Removal of PAPR PPE (REQUIRES ASSISTANCE)
1. Second person detaches breathing tube from the assembly unit and turns OFF unit.
2. From the outside, grasp the hood at the top of the head and under chin simultaneously, and remove hood.
3. Dispose of hood respirator and breathing tube.
4. Second person unties second isolation gown (top layer).
5. Grasp front of second isolation gown with both hands, and pull forward to remove from shoulders.
6. Remove second isolation gown with taped gloves as one unit, as you roll inside out, prior to discarding.
7. Remove air pump/filter/battery assembly box and place inside double plastic bags while in the room.
8. Exit the room, maintaining the first PPE layer (N-95 mask, hair net, goggles, and gown); bring the double-bagged air pump/filter/battery assembly box for processing.

[a]The following guidelines are intended to illustrate a suggested donning and doffing sequence for Enhanced Airborne precautions, using the 3M BE-10 Series PAPR. They are not intended to substitute the recommendations of the Infection Control or Critical Care Groups of your institution. Please refer to the manufacturer's instructions for further details of assembly, handling, and cleaning.

Classification and Initial Treatment for Bioterrorism Agents

The bioterrorism agents are classified as category A, B, or C based on their availability, potential for dissemination and infectivity, and their ability to cause events of large magnitude; category A agents are the most severe. Table 176.2 summarizes early warnings of a bioterrorism event, signs and symptoms of syndromes caused by biologic agents, and initial steps to take if an illness is suspected to be related to a bioterrorism activity. Tables 176.3 and 176.4 enumerate the clinical presentations, diagnostic tests, and available treatments for category A and categories B and C, respectively; Table 176.5 details dosing of drugs for treatment of potential bioterrorism agents.

Classification and Initial Treatment for Chemical Agents

The chemical agents are divided in five different groups:

1. Nerve agents: Anticholinesterase activity
2. Asphyxiants or blood agents: Cyanide based
3. Choking or pulmonary-damaging agents: Direct airway cytotoxicity
4. Blistering or vesicant agents: Direct skin cytotoxicity; may also affect airway
5. Incapacitating agents: For riot control

The details on agents, symptoms, detection, and basic treatment are listed in Table 176.6.

PERSONAL PROTECTIVE EQUIPMENT IN THE INTENSIVE CARE UNIT

As was evidenced during the SARS epidemic in 2003, in spite of following the recommendations for using personal protective equipment in the ICU, several health care workers contracted the illness when they were present during an endotracheal intubation of a patient. Based on the experience from Toronto, Canada, and the work of Zamora et al. (28), it appears that the current recommendations (29) for use of PPE may be flawed, particularly in the case of probable aerosolization of secretions. The SCCM and the World Federation of Societies of Intensive and Critical Care Medicine have adopted new recommendations for PPE that are included in the SCCM course of FDM (22); these are described in the following paragraphs.

If possible, the area designated in the ICU should be turned into a negative pressure environment. Patient rooms should function as negative pressure areas as well, either by design or by installing portable negative pressure units.

The entire ICU is considered a "warm" zone, where all staff—including medical, nursing, respiratory therapy, secretarial, and housekeeping—wear a basic layer of PPE that includes:

- Scrubs
- Gown
- Gloves, with longitudinal taping
- N-95-type mask
- Nonabsorbent material shoes

The donning and doffing of PPE should follow a checklist to ensure that the steps are followed in the recommended sequence, and none is skipped or missed.

If a patient's room needs to be accessed for routine care (e.g., monitoring, titration of IV treatments, positional changes, adjustment of ventilator settings, or blood sampling) that would not result in the generation and dispersion of aerosols, a second layer of PPE is recommended that includes:

- Eye protection (taped goggles)
- Hair-covering device (hair net or hat)
- A second gown
- A second layer of gloves, with longitudinal taping

If the patient's room needs be accessed for airway manipulation, where there is a high risk for aerosolization of secretions (e.g., the use of bag-valve-mask, endotracheal intubation, open circuit suctioning, bronchoscopy, or disconnection from

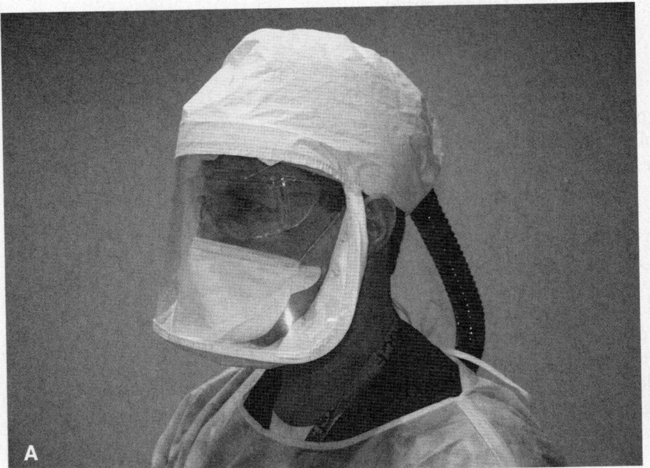

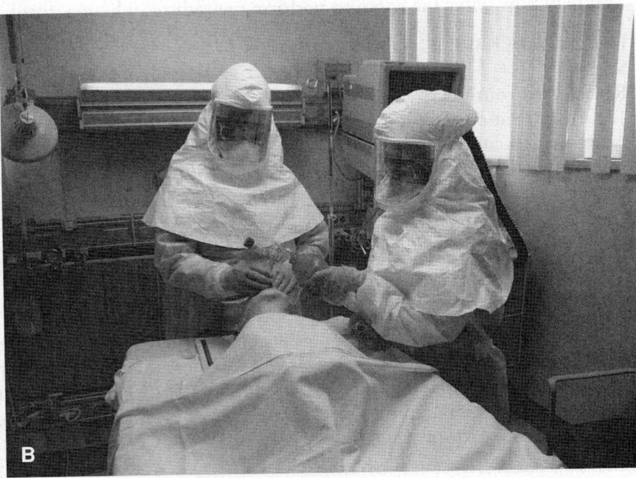

FIGURE 176.7. **A:** Face shield powered air-purifying respirator (PAPR). **B:** Medical personnel with full hood PAPR in an isolation room simulation. (Courtesy of Orlando Regional Medical Center.)

ventilator), a higher level of PPE should be used, including a PAPR, as well as the second layer noted above (Table 176.7). The PAPR used indoors in the ED or ICU should be of a light material, and should not be confused with the PAPR used in decontamination lines at the entrance of the hospital.

This "indoor" PAPR offers high-level protection for biologic agents only, and is available as a face shield (higher chance of neck contamination with aerosols) or as a full hood (preferable) (Fig. 176.7A,B).

The doffing (removal) of the PPE is probably—and remarkably—the most important phase, as the likelihood of contamination increases significantly if procedures are not properly followed. Again, a checklist is recommended (Table 176.7). All materials should be disposed, and the PAPR unit placed in a double-bag system in order to be taken to the processing area. In a biologic event, all mechanical ventilators should have a HEPA filter on the exhalation circuit.

TABLE 176.8

VENTILATOR AND INTENSIVE CARE TRIAGE TOOL

INCLUSION CRITERIA

The patient must meet one of criteria A or B

A. Requirement for invasive ventilatory support:
- Refractory hypoxemia (SpO_2 <90% on nonrebreather mask/FiO_2 >0.85)
- Respiratory acidosis with pH <7.2
- Clinical evidence of impending respiratory failure
- Inability to protect or maintain airway

B. Hypotension:

Hypotension (systolic blood pressure [SBP] <90 or relative hypotension) with clinical evidence of shock (altered level of consciousness, decreased urine output, or other end-organ failure) refractory to volume resuscitation requiring vasopressor/inotrope support *that cannot be managed on the ward.*

EXCLUSION CRITERIA

The patient is excluded from admission/transfer to critical care if ANY of the following (*) are present:

*Severe trauma (defined by each center based on their experience with the Injury Severity Score [ISS], Trauma and Injury Severity Scoring system [TRISS] or similar)

*Severe burns

A patient with any two of the following:
- i. Age >60 years old
- ii. Total body surface area (TBSA) >40%
- iii. Inhalation injury

*Cardiac arrest:

Unwitnessed cardiac arrest

Witnessed cardiac arrest not responsive to electrical therapy (defibrillation, cardioversion, or pacing)

Recurrent cardiac arrest

*Severe cognitive impairment

*Advanced untreatable neuromuscular disease

*Metastatic malignancy

*Advanced and irreversible immunocompromise

*Severe and irreversible neurologic event/condition

*End-stage organ failure meeting following criteria

*Cardiac:
- i. New York Heart Association (NYHA) class III or IV heart failure

*Lung:
- i. Chronic obstructive pulmonary disease (COPD) with force expiratory volume in 1 second (FEV_1) <25% predicted, baseline PaO_2 <55 mm Hg, or secondary pulmonary hypertension
- ii. Cystic fibrosis with postbronchodilator FEV_1 <30% or baseline PaO_2 <55 mm Hg
- iii. Pulmonary fibrosis with vital capacity (VC) or total lung capacity TLC <60% predicted, baseline PaO_2 <55 mm Hg, or secondary pulmonary hypertension
- iv. Primary pulmonary hypertension with NYHA class III to IV heart failure, or right atrial pressure >10 mm Hg, or mean pulmonary arterial pressure of >50 mm Hg

Liver
- i. Child Pugh score ≥7

*Age >85 years old

*Requirement for transfusion of >6 units packed red blood cells within 24-h period

*Elective palliative surgery

Adapted from Christian M, Hawryluck L, Wax R, et al. Development of a triage protocol for critical care during an influenza pandemic. *CMAJ.* 2006;175(11); 1377.

TABLE 176.9

THE SOFA SCALE

Variable	Value 0	1	2	3	4
PaO_2/FiO_2, mm Hg	>400	≤400	≤300	≤200	≤100
Platelets (×1,000/μL)	>150	≤150	≤100	≤50	≤20
Bilirubin, mg/dL (μmol/L)	<1.2 (<20)	1.2–1.9 (20–32)	2.0–5.9 (33–100)	6.0–11.9 (101–203)	>12 (>203)
Hypotension	None	MAP <70 mm Hg	Dop ≤5[a]	Dop >5[a] Epi ≤0.1[a] Norepi ≤0.1[a]	Dop >15[a] Epi >0.1[a] Norepi >0.1[a]
Glasgow coma score	15	13–14	10–12	6–9	<6
Creatinine, mg/dL (μmol/L)	<1.2 (<106)	1.2–1.9 (106–168)	2.0–3.4 (269–300)	3.5–4.9 (301–433)	>5 (>434)

[a] μg/kg/min.
Dop, dopamine; Epi, epinephrine; Norepi, norepinephrine.

VENTILATOR TRIAGE

Another area that deserves attention is the distribution of mechanical ventilators when demand exceeds availability. It is imperative that well-defined, objective criteria be used for their assignment (Table 176.8). In a major MCI, where the number of patients far exceeds the available resources, it is imperative to utilize a protocol with easy-to-follow tools, with clear definitions based on objective criteria. Christian et al. (30) have published a protocol that uses the Sequential Organ Failure Assessment (SOFA) as the base for the initial classification of patients, with follow-up at 48 and 120 hours. Once the patient has passed the inclusion and exclusion criteria, the SOFA-based (Table 176.9) initial (Table 176.10) evaluation is performed. There are repeat evaluations at 48 (Table 176.11) and 120 hours (Table 176.12).

TABLE 176.10

INITIAL ASSESSMENT

Critical care triage tool (initial assessment)		
Color	**Criteria**	**Priority/action**
Blue	Exclusion Criteria or SOFA > 11	Medical Management ± Palliate D/C from CC
Red	SOFA ≤ 7 or Single Organ Failure	Highest
Yellow	SOFA 8-11	Intermediate
Green	No significant organ failure	Defer or D/C Reassess as needed

D/C–Discharge
CC–Critical Care
Adapted from reference 30.

SUMMARY

Health care institutions across the globe should recognize that they must be prepared to provide services for potentially massive numbers of casualties. While sociopolitical events—terrorist activities—are presently foremost in our thoughts, increasing industrialization, environmental hazards, and globalization pose equal threats to society. Emerging communicable diseases are perhaps the most insidious threats to anticipate, but if the response is inadequate, these may result in the collapse not only of health care institutions, but of governmental infrastructure as well.

TABLE 176.11

48-HOUR ASSESSMENT

Critical care triage tool (48-hour assessment)		
Color	**Criteria**	**Priority/action**
Blue	Exclusion Criteria or SOFA > 11 or SOFA 8-11 no Δ	Palliate and D/C from CC
Red	SOFA < 11 and decreasing	Highest
Yellow	SOFA < 8 no Δ	Intermediate
Green	No longer ventilator dependent	D/C from CC

D/C–Discharge
CC–Critical Care
Δ–change
Adapted from reference 30.

TABLE 176.12

120-HOUR ASSESSMENT

Critical care triage tool (120-hour assessment)		
Color	**Criteria**	**Priority/action**
Blue	Exclusion Criteria or SOFA > 11 or SOFA < 8 no Δ	Palliate and D/C from CC
Red	SOFA < 11 and Decreasing progressively	Highest
Yellow	SOFA < 8 minimal decrease (<3 points in past 72 h)	Intermediate
Green	No longer ventilator dependent	D/C from CC

D/C–Discharge
CC–Critical Care
Δ-change
Adapted from reference 30.

An effective response to an event of significant magnitude requires planning, which includes coordination with local and federal authorities, communication, education, and practice. It is our hope that this chapter serves as a basic tool to elucidate some of the larger concepts in preparing a response to these disasters; it will not replace an in-depth planning and training program.

References

1. Joint Commission on Accreditation of Healthcare Organizations. *Comprehensive Accreditation Manual for Hospitals: The Official Handbook*. Oakbrook Terrace, IL: Joint Commission Resources; 2006:EC-4.10.
2. The Hospital Incident Command System. Emergency Medical Services Authority, California. http://www.emsa.ca.gov/hics/hics.asp. Accessed October 27, 2008.
3. Rubinson L, Nuzzo J, Talmor D, et al. Augmentation of hospital critical care capacity after bioterrorist attacks or epidemics: recommendations of the Working Group on Emergency Mass Critical Care. *Crit Care Med.* 2005; 33(Suppl.):E2393.
4. McNeill WH. *Plagues and Peoples*. New York: Bantam Doubleday Dell Publishing Group, Inc.; 1976.
5. Hays J. *Epidemics and Pandemics: Their Impacts on Human History*. Santa Barbara, CA: ABC-Clio; 2005.
6. Centers for Disease Control. SARS website. http://www.cdc.gov/ncidod/sars/. Accessed October 27, 2008.
7. Jacobs M. The history of biologic warfare and bioterrorism. *Dermatol Clin.* 22(3):231.
8. Ali J. Chemical weapons and the Iran-Iraq war: a case study in non-compliance. *The Non-proliferation Review*. Center for Non-proliferation Studies; 2001:43. http://cns.miis.edu/pubs/npr/vol08/81/81ali.pdf. Accessed.
9. U.S. designated foreign terrorist organizations. Infoplease http://www.infoplease.com/ipa/A0908746.html. Accessed October 27, 2008.
10. U.S. Department of State, Country Reports on Terrorism. http://www.state.gov/s/ct/rls/crt/2006/82738.htm. Accessed October 27, 2008.
11. Torok TJ, Tauxe RV, Wise RP, et al. A large community outbreak of salmonellosis caused by intentional contamination of restaurant salad bars. *JAMA.* 1997;278(5).
12. Kisala R, Mullins MR. *Religion and Social Crisis in Japan: Understanding Japanese Society through the Aum Affair*. New York: Palgrave; 2001.
13. Occupational Health and Safety Administration (OSHA). U.S. Department of Labor: Radiological Dispersal Devices(RDD)/Dirty Bombs. http://www.osha.gov/SLTC/emergencypreparedness/rdd_tech.html. Accessed October 27, 2008.
14. 1984: Hundreds die in Bhopal chemical accident. BBC News website. http://news.bbc.co.uk/onthisday/hi/dates/stories/december/3/newsid_2698000/2698709.stm. Accessed October 27, 2008.
15. McKenna T, Buglova E, Kutkov V, et al. Lessons learned from Chernobyl and other emergencies: establishing international requirements and guidance. *Health Physics.* 2007;93(5):527.
16. Noji EK. Public health in the aftermath of disasters. *BMJ.* 2005;330:1379.
17. Spiegel PB. Differences in world responses to natural disasters and complex emergencies. *JAMA.* 2005;293:1915–1918.
18. Kaiser Permanente. Medical Center Hazard and Vulnerability Analysis. http://www.gnyha.org/22/File.aspx. Accessed October 27, 2008.
19. National Incident management System (NIMS) website. http://www.fema.gov/emergency/nims/. Accessed October 27, 2008.
20. National Disaster Life Support Foundation (NDLS) website. http://www.bdls.com/common/content.asp. Accessed October 27, 2008.
21. Emergency Medicine System Agency, California: The Hospital Incident Command System, HICS Guide Book 2006. http://www.emsa.ca.gov/hics/hics%20guidebook%20and%20glossary.pdf. Accessed October 27, 2008.
22. Society of Critical Care Medicine (SCCM). Fundamentals of Disaster Management course. http://www.sccm.org/FCCS_and_Training_Courses/FDM/Pages/default.aspx. Accessed October 27, 2008.
23. Okumura T, Hisaoka T, Yamada A, et al. The Tokyo subway sarin attack -10 lessons learned *Toxicol. Appl. Pharmacol.* 2005;207(2; Suppl 1):471.
24. By Hydro-Therm, Inc. http://www.tridentone.com/. Accessed October 27, 2008.
25. U.S. Army Soldier and Biological Chemical Command (SBCCOM). Guidelines for cold weather mass decontamination during a terrorist chemical incident. 2003. http://www.ecbc.army.mil/downloads/cwirp/ECBC_cwirp_cold_weather_mass_decon.pdf. Accessed October 27, 2008.
26. U.S. Army Soldier and Biological Chemical Command (SBCCOM). Guidelines for mass casualty decontamination. 2000. http://www.chem-bio.com/resource/2000/cwirp_guidelines_mass.pdf. Accessed October 27, 2008.
27. Occupational Safety and Health Administration. OSHA Best practices for hospital-based first receivers of victims from mass casualty incidents involving the release of hazardous substances. January 2005. http://www.osha.gov/dts/osta/bestpractices/firstreceivers_hospital.pdf. Accessed October 27, 2008.
28. Zamora J, Murdoch J, Simchison B, et al. Contamination: a comparison of 2 personal protective systems. *CMAJ.* 2006;175(3):249.
29. Center for Disease Control. Donning and removing sequences for personal protective equipment (PPE). http://www.cdc.gov/ncidod/sars/pdf/ppeposter1322.pdf. Accessed October 27, 2008.
30. Christian M, Hawryluck L, Wax R, et al. Development of a triage protocol for critical care during an influenza pandemic. *CMAJ.* 2006;175(11); 1377.

CHAPTER 177 ■ EMERGENT PANDEMIC INFECTIONS AND CRITICAL CARE

LENNOX K. ARCHIBALD

The prevalence or incidence rate of infection, or the presence of an infectious agent that is usually present in a community, defined population, or institution is the baseline or expected level of that infection. If this level is approximately constant at a low incidence or prevalence rate over a defined time period, then the infection or agent is regarded as *endemic*. Infections that occur irregularly over a period of time are deemed *sporadic*. If the infection is persistent at high incidence or prevalence rates, then it is regarded as *hyperendemic*. A level of infection in a defined population in excess of the expected or baseline level over a given time period is regarded as an *epidemic* or *outbreak*; the period of time over which this excess occurs is known as the *epidemic period*. An epidemic of communicable infection that becomes very widespread, affects a whole region or continent, or spreads over several countries and affects many people is termed a *pandemic*. A disease or illness is not a pandemic merely because it is widespread or kills a large number of people; it must also be infectious.

Three key factors set the conditions for a pandemic:

1. The emergence of a new strain of micro-organism
2. The ability of that strain to infect humans and cause serious illness; i.e., the capacity of the organism to cause disease in an infected host (its pathogenicity) and the severity of the disease produced (its virulence)
3. The ability of the micro-organism to spread easily among humans

Infectious disease pandemics proceed until the number of susceptible hosts in the population at risk falls below the number at which the probability of contact, transmission, and infection becomes too low for the process to continue. In the modern era of rapid air travel to any geographic area on the globe, variations in population demographics, and changing or unpredictable human behavior, the interactions of the factors that determine whether a pandemic will occur are complex and have to be analyzed using sophisticated statistical modeling techniques. These same factors and their interactions, however, have made statistical models less successful in predicting onset, size, and duration of epidemics, especially those that occur in complex environments like intensive care units (ICU) in tertiary care hospitals. Within the ICU, factors that decrease transmission of communicable infection—such as the distance between individuals (i.e., reducing the likelihood of contact through isolation), adherence to infection control guidelines, immunization, herd immunity, increasing levels of natural immunity following infection, depression of agent reservoirs, and viability by control programs or seasonal climatic change—are offset by the ICU environment, in which there are patients with a relatively high severity of illness, increased use of medical devices, fluctuating nurse-to-patient ratios, varying degrees of immunization or vaccination, and exposure to health care personnel who move freely among other patients and health care personnel within the institution.

The relevance and importance of pandemic preparedness in critical care medicine is underscored by the reality that, while there has been a general decrease in the total number of beds in United States hospitals during the 1990s, the number of ICU beds has increased during the same period (1). This increase in the numbers of ICU beds suggests that hospitals in the United States are now admitting a larger number of critically ill patients to these units, where there are relatively high rates of medical device and antimicrobial use. Furthermore, crowding is likely to become a factor when there is a high patient census, along with a parallel increase in numbers of health care personnel required to staff these units. As hospitals become more and more specialized, the possibility of multiple hospital outbreaks becomes a greater concern. This occurs most commonly by interhospital spread or movement of patients from long-term care facilities to hospitals. In the case of a pandemic event, emergency rooms of tertiary care hospitals become the natural aggregating and triage centers for symptomatic patients. However, the ability of emergency rooms to triage or handle large numbers of symptomatic patients is limited by the ever-present risk of person-to-person transmission in the waiting room, the limited space to evaluate people, and insufficient personnel to handle a high patient load.

At some juncture, individuals with a relatively high severity of illness resulting from the pandemic will require some form of critical care management that warrants ICU admission, provided sufficient beds and ancillary equipment such as ventilators are available. In the wake of a pandemic, those tertiary care hospitals with large numbers of ICU beds will, by default, have to provide critical care management for greater numbers of patients. The implications of this scenario are serious and complex, and include the following:

- The increased human and material resources that would be required to manage very sick patients during a pandemic
- The difficulties in triaging patients with vague or mild symptoms, who do not meet the case definition for the infection yet who might be potentially infectious
- The limited availability of designated areas for cohorting patients who need to be isolated
- The logistics of implementing and maintaining infection control practices and procedures in the ICU during a pandemic and consequently, the inevitable transmission of the pandemic agent among patients and health care workers,

notwithstanding the institution of infection control practices and procedures

- The risk of further transmission of the micro-organism by ICU personnel who also work or are "floated" in other areas of the hospital

This chapter addresses five true or potentially emergent pandemic infections:

1. The severe acute respiratory syndrome (SARS)—A true pandemic caused by a previously unrecognized corona virus
2. Avian influenza—Not yet a true pandemic but one that infectious diseases experts believe is imminent and long overdue
3. Dengue fever and dengue hemorrhagic fever—A mosquito-borne infection that has spread insidiously across the globe and is now considered a pandemic by many experts
4. Tuberculosis—A pandemic caused by *Mycobacterium tuberculosis* and largely attributable to the nearly three-decade-long human immunodeficiency virus (HIV) pandemic
5. Infections caused by *Staphylococcus aureus* resistant to methicillin group penicillins (MRSA)—Perhaps the only bacterial micro-organism that has reached pandemic proportions in health care settings around the world

Patients who acquire any of these five infections not infrequently require management in ICUs. The SARS pandemic of 2002 emerged suddenly and unexpectedly, and affected health care workers but was successfully controlled through the application of basic infection control principles and guidelines that had already been established, validated, and ratified. The expected emergence of the impending avian influenza pandemic has underscored the importance of preparedness for an event that is oftentimes decried as "crying wolf" by some, while at the same time characterized as "a matter of when, rather than if" by others. The fact remains that, should an influenza pandemic occur, substantial numbers of infected patients would almost certainly require critical care management, underscoring the need for preparedness from diagnostic, management, control, and preventive perspectives. The third viral pandemic—dengue fever—is a zoonotic infection caused by an arbovirus that is endemic in countries across the globe and whose occurrence is still on the increase. Aiding this transmission is the unpredictable pattern of global warming affecting the breeding sites of mosquitoes, flooding resulting from hurricanes, increasing urbanization, ease of travel across the globe, and dynamic movements of immigrants from endemic to nonendemic regions. Although public health preparedness will be alluded to, the focus of this chapter will be on the epidemiology, clinical features, and manifestation of these infections. In addition, the chapter reflects some of the issues pertinent to preparedness, interventions, and obstacles that must be addressed by critical care personnel in tertiary care centers for the diagnosis, management, control, and prevention of these infections.

SEVERE ACUTE RESPIRATORY SYNDROME (SARS)

In November 2002, the Centers for Disease Control and Prevention (CDC) and the World Health Organization (WHO) reported an investigation of a multicountry outbreak of unexplained pneumonia referred to as SARS—officially, the first pandemic of the 21st century (2–4). SARS began as an outbreak of atypical pneumonia among patients in the Guangdong province of China. A Chinese physician, who had taken care of patients with SARS, subsequently traveled to Hong Kong and transmitted the infection to guests at the Metropole Hotel. These guests, in turn, unwittingly became the index cases for SARS outbreaks in Canada, Hong Kong, Singapore, Vietnam, and Taiwan (5–9). Subsequently, the condition was reported in more than 8,400 people globally and resulted in over 800 deaths (5,7,10). The case-fatality rate was estimated at 13% for patients younger than 60 years of age and 43% for those older than 60 years of age (11).

SARS is caused by a novel strain of coronavirus (SARS-CoV) that was first identified in Canada in early March 2003 (12). The origin of SARS-CoV is unclear; however, because genetic changes occur frequently in these viruses, it is thought that the outbreak might have been facilitated by cross-species transmission of the virus from animals to humans (13). Sequence analyses of the genome suggest that SARS-CoV is a new virus that is distinct from all other known human coronaviruses (14,15). Indeed, the plausibility of cross-species transmission of a recombinant animal virus was substantiated by the observation and documentation of the close proximity of humans to animals in the Guangdong province in southern China, where the first outbreak occurred and SARS is believed to have emerged (2,9). During the latter part of 2003 and early 2004, sporadic outbreaks of SARS were documented and investigated in the region of China where the first outbreaks had originated (16). Subsequent studies have since confirmed that the SARS-CoV strains in these later outbreaks were different from those isolated during 2002–2003 (17). In a recent review, Wang et al. (18) concluded that these findings support the existence of independent species-crossing of SARS-CoV, and that SARS epidemics could likely recur in the future at different times and regions, depending on the distribution of reservoirs and transmitting hosts.

Before the SARS pandemic, coronaviruses already were known to be ubiquitous, and were recognized as the underlying cause of illness in various animals, including pigs, cattle, dogs, cats, and chickens. Indeed, coronaviruses had long been found to be associated with upper respiratory infections and, sometimes, pneumonia in humans (19). Although the natural reservoir of SARS-CoV remains uncharacterized, the virus has been isolated from all of the above animals as well as civet cats, a delicacy in the Far East (20–22).

Mode of Transmission

The primary mode of transmission of SARS-CoV is largely through direct or indirect contact of mucous membranes (eyes, nose, or mouth) with large infectious respiratory droplets (23–25). This mode of transmission suggests that the major risk factor for acquisition of infection by susceptible persons is intimate direct contact with one or more individuals who are already infected or colonized. However, the unusually rapid transmission of SARS-CoV suggests that airborne transmission through droplet nuclei (i.e., droplets less than 10 μm in diameter) might play a significant role in transmission. Droplet nuclei, the mode of transmission of influenza, measles, and tuberculosis, theoretically would enable SARS-CoV to reach the lung alveoli in at-risk contacts (26). This may explain why aerosol-producing procedures, such as bronchoscopy or nebulized medication in health care facilities, have been implicated as independent risk factors in SARS-CoV transmission and outbreaks (27–29). Although SARS-CoV is shed in large quantities in stool, and the fecal-oral route represents the principal mode of transmission among many animals (18), reports of foodborne or waterborne transmission among humans have not been substantiated (30). Nonetheless, SARS-CoV survives for many days in feces, and when dried on environmental surfaces, it is plausible that fomites could potentially play a role in transmission of the virus (31). However, the exact role of fomites in person-to-person transmission of SARS-CoV in health care settings or the community remains uncharacterized (30). To date, there have been no documented instances of SARS-CoV isolation from asymptomatic persons.

The phenomenon of "superspreading events" plays an important role in the transmission of SARS-CoV in health care settings (25,32–34). In the mechanism of superspreading events, SARS-CoV is transmitted from one individual to several secondary cases (32,35–37). Risk factors found to be associated with superspreading events include a high severity of illness scores, greater age, and increased numbers of secondary contacts (37). Superspreading has facilitated the transmission of SARS-CoV within health care settings in Singapore (12,27) and Toronto (12). The hospital in-patient environment provides an efficient site for the transmission of SARS-CoV infection and superspreading events (35–37).

Signs and Symptoms

SARS is characterized by rapid onset of high fever, malaise, myalgia, chills, rigors, and sore throat, followed by shortness of breath, cough, and radiographic evidence of pneumonia (12,38,39). The median incubation period range is generally between 4 and 7 days (range: 2 to 10 days) (2). Some patients develop profuse watery diarrhea, although, as stated above, the role of fecal-oral transmission remains uncharacterized (39). After 1 week of illness, patients with SARS frequently develop respiratory failure, which often requires critical care management for respiratory support and mechanical ventilation (30,39). Chest radiographs frequently show nonspecific patchy opacification but may be normal during the early stages of the infection (40). Because of the nonspecific clinical manifestations at presentation, a precise diagnosis of SARS might not be possible, compounded by the difficulty in differentiating SARS from other clinical syndromes (37). Thus, all diagnoses of community-acquired pneumonia become suspect during a SARS pandemic, and a history of exposure to a patient with probable SARS or travel to SARS-affected geographic areas should heighten clinical suspicion and increase the likelihood of the diagnosis (41). In patients with suspected SARS or in patients who develop respiratory symptoms during a putative or true SARS pandemic, the workup for known causes of community-acquired pneumonia should certainly be performed, and appropriate specimens should be sent to the designated State Health Department or CDC for viral identification and serologic analysis.

Laboratory Features

Laboratory features include lymphopenia, thrombocytopenia, and elevated levels of lactate dehydrogenase, aspartate aminotransferase, and creatinine kinase (12). SARS-CoV can be detected by the polymerase chain reaction (PCR) in respiratory secretions and other body fluids; however, PCR is not sensitive during the early stages of the illness. Specific SARS-CoV antibodies are detectable but play little or no role in making a diagnosis during the acute stages of the pneumonia, especially during a pandemic. However, detection of antibodies provides a retrospective diagnosis as part of clinical confirmation or surveillance activities. The presence of underlying disease, elevated initial C-reactive protein levels, and positive SARS-CoV in nasopharyngeal aspirate samples are associated with an increased risk of respiratory failure and mortality (41).

Prevention and Control of SARS

In Canada, transmission of the SARS-CoV occurred predominantly among health care workers within the health care setting, presumably through close contact with symptomatic persons (12,42). Health care workers made up a large proportion of cases, accounting for 37% to 63% of suspected SARS cases in highly affected countries (23,43–45). Thus, the fundamental tenets of prevention and control should include the institution and implementation of basic infection control practices and procedures, early detection and prompt isolation of affected patients, contact tracing, and quarantine of putative contacts (34,46,47). Because SARS-CoV is generally not identified before recommended infection-control precautions for SARS are implemented, and unrecognized cases are a significant source of transmission, the primary strategy to reduce transmission in health care settings is early recognition and isolation of patients who *might* have the syndrome, as well as the institution of triage algorithms for practices in hospitals and ambulatory care settings (47–51). In Vietnam and Canada, the pandemic was brought under control through the institution of a constellation of interventions that included (i) early detection and prompt isolation of case-patients; (ii) implementation of traditional infection control practices, such as scrupulous hand-washing and environmental decontamination, and use of personal protective equipment where deemed necessary; (iii) initiation of surveillance activities for patients with SARS; and (iv) education and training of patients, relatives, and caregivers (52,53).

Control of Transmission Measures

Transmission of SARS-CoV may occur on an aircraft when infected persons fly during the symptomatic phase of illness (54). Thus, in the event of a possible pandemic, airline travelers need to be screened before leaving for and after arriving from SARS-endemic regions. In a retrospective cohort study of nurses who worked in ICUs in Toronto, practices such as assisting during intubation, suctioning before intubation, and manipulation of oxygen masks were found to be risk factors for acquiring SARS (34). This study also found that consistently wearing a mask, regardless of type (i.e., either surgical or particulate respirator type N-95), was protective for nurses and resulted in an 80% reduction in risk of infection (34). Of note, the risk of SARS-CoV transmission and infection among nurses who consistently wore N-95 masks was approximately half that for the surgical mask; however, this difference was not statistically significant (34). These data concur with the findings of Seto et al. (25), who established that both surgical masks and N-95 masks were protective against SARS among health care workers in Hong Kong, and with anecdotal reports from Bach Mai hospital in Hanoi, Vietnam, where SARS was controlled and contained largely through adherence to basic infection control principles, use of surgical masks, and quarantine of close contacts (unpublished personal communication, Infection Control Department, Bach Mai Hospital, Hanoi, Vietnam). Finally, Loeb et al. (34) established unequivocally that use of personal protective equipment (i.e., use of N-95 masks, gowns, gloves, and goggles) were important preventive measures when caring for SARS patients. Ultimately, improvement in the outcomes of patients with SARS is dependent on heightened levels of clinical suspicion, rapid case detection and isolation, strict attention to infection control practices and procedures, use of masks when providing care for putative SARS, and development and use of reliable diagnostic tests and effective antiviral and immunomodulatory agents and vaccines (41).

INFLUENZA

Influenza is an acute febrile illness caused by a group of respiratory viruses primarily infecting the columnar cells of the upper respiratory tract. Humans are the major hosts of these viruses, which are the most important cause of wintertime respiratory morbidity throughout the world. Despite vaccines and antiviral therapies, influenza epidemics still occur every year. The magnitude of influenza outbreaks during the winter is dictated by the interaction between agent and host, and the environment in which this interaction occurs.

Agent factors include the degree of molecular change in the virus compared with the previous year, and the pathogenicity and virulence of the new winter strain. Host factors that determine the size of the outbreak for a particular year include the numbers of susceptible individuals and the proportion of individuals who received that year's influenza vaccine. Important environmental factors that facilitate transmission include crowding in health care institutions, day care centers, schools, waiting rooms, barracks, and other places where people aggregate.

Severe influenza pandemics have been recorded since the days of Hippocrates, and, over the past 300 years, at least 10 pandemics have been recorded at irregular intervals. The pandemic of 1580 started in Asia and spread to Africa, Europe, and the Americas. Within 6 weeks, all of Europe was affected, resulting in high mortality rates. For example, 9,000 of 80,000 residents died in Rome during one 10-day period, and some Spanish cities were described as "nearly depopulated by the disease." In the 1918–1919 Spanish influenza epidemic, an estimated 50 to 100 million persons (a disproportionate number of them healthy young adults) died worldwide—over 500,000 in the United States alone (55). The 1957–1958 Asian and the 1968–1969 Hong Kong pandemics caused substantial morbidity, although mortality estimates were lower compared with 1918: two million for the 1957 pandemic (70,000 excess U.S. deaths) and one million (34,000 excess U.S. deaths) in 1968 (56). The occurrence of these three influenza pandemics during the 20th century was not an aberration, but rather a manifestation of the continuing emergence of virulent strains of a virus that has adapted to efficient human transmission, and which continues to undergo point mutations and genetic exchange or reassortment (56).

Influenza viruses belong to the orthomyxovirus family. These viruses are enveloped, pleomorphic, and contain negative, single-stranded RNA, which is organized into eight gene segments that code for ten proteins. They are classified into three major serotypes—influenza A, B, and C—based on differences in a stable internal ribonucleoprotein antigen. Two surface glycoproteins—hemagglutinin (HA) and neuraminidase (NA)—constitute the major antigens and are therefore the prime targets of the protective host immune response and vaccine prophylaxis. HA is so named because of its ability to agglutinate red blood cells from chickens or guinea pigs *in vitro* and facilitates viral attachment to the host respiratory epithelial cells. Antibodies to HA are protective. The NA glycoprotein is involved in viral entry into the host cell by helping release virions from cells, and is important in the process of the viral envelope fusion with the host cell membrane as a prerequisite to viral entry into the human cell. Antibodies to NA appear to modify disease severity by inhibiting the spread of virus in the infected host and limiting the amount of virus released from host cells.

Influenza Types

Influenza A is the most extensively studied of the three types; influenza B is more antigenically stable and usually occurs in more localized outbreaks; influenza C appears to be a relatively minor cause of disease and differs considerably from A and B types, possessing only seven RNA segments and no NA. The structure and function of influenza viruses are directly associated with the pathogenesis of infection and disease, and with diagnosis. Only influenza A and B cause epidemic infections and disease in humans.

Among the 16 known HA subtypes (H1–H16) and nine NA glycoprotein subtypes (N1–N9) of influenza A viruses, three major subtypes of hemagglutinins (H1, H2, and H3) and two subtypes of neuraminidases (N1 and N2) are known to cause infection in humans (H1N1, H1N2, H3N2). The three 20th century pandemics were caused by strains of avian influenza A viruses classified as H1N1 for 1918, H2N2 for 1957, and H3N2 for the 1968 pandemic virus. The 1968 H3N2 strain had the same NA glycoprotein as the 1957 H2N2 strain. Influenza viruses are named on the basis of the following nomenclature: type/geographic source/strain number/year isolated (specific H and N subtypes). Thus, for the 2006/2007 influenza season, the vaccine included A/New Caledonia/20/1999 (H1N1)-like, A/Wisconsin/67/2005 (H3N2)-like, and B/Malaysia/2506/2004-like antigens (CDC, Atlanta, GA). These viruses were used because they are representative of influenza viruses that were anticipated to circulate in the United States during the 2006/2007 influenza season and have favorable growth properties in eggs (CDC, Atlanta, GA).

Influenza A

A key feature of influenza A viruses is their ability to undergo periodic antigenic change more commonly and to a much greater degree than other respiratory viruses. These antigenic changes occur through two completely different mechanisms: antigenic drift and antigenic shift (57,58). In antigenic *drift*, point mutations in the HA or NA genes cause minor antigenic changes to the main surface glycoproteins, resulting in strain variants. Antigenic drift within major subtypes can involve either the HA or NA antigen or the genes encoding nonstructural proteins, and can result from a single mutation on the viral RNA. Antigenic drift is a continuous process that leads to emergence of strain variants, most of which form evolutionary dead ends. Eventually, however, a strain becomes predominant worldwide—1 to 3 years on average. Immunity against one strain might be limited, and antibodies formed to older viruses gradually lose their ability to protect against newer strains. As a result, people recurrently become susceptible to influenza, and, thus, vaccine strains must be updated annually. According to the CDC, antigenic drift causes seasonal epidemics in the United States, resulting each year in over 200,000 hospitalizations and approximately 36,000 deaths; more than 90% of these deaths occur in persons older than 65 years of age. Only antigenic drifts in the hemagglutinins have been described for influenza B viruses.

Antigenic *shift* is the emergence of a novel human influenza virus subtype through genetic reassortment between human and animal viruses or through direct animal- or poultry-to-human transmission, resulting in a virus bearing new HA or NA antigens. Basically, reassortment occurs when an avian or animal virus and human-adapted virus "swap genes" in a coinfected cell of an animal or human, and a third virus results that can be readily transmitted by and between humans. Antigenic shift is relatively infrequent; however, because there is little or no immunity to a novel virus, it remains the initiating event for pandemics that occur if there is efficient and sustained virus transmission among humans. Compared with regular seasonal epidemics, the emergence of a novel influenza virus through antigenic shift will result in more infections and more serious illness among those infected, with the ever-present possibility of global spread if the virus is sufficiently transmissible among humans. Antigenic shifts are associated with epidemics and pandemics of influenza A, whereas antigenic drifts are associated with more localized outbreaks. Genetic analysis of the 1957 H2N2 and 1968 H3N2 pandemic virus strains indicate that these strains emerged by genetic reassortment between avian viruses and seasonal human viruses. The emergent virus strains adapted genetic material from the human strains that enabled growth in humans; however, the genes for the hemagglutinins that induce a humoral response were acquired from the avian viruses. Before 1997, there was no evidence or documentation that influenza A (H5N1) subtype could cause infections and severe disease in humans (59–61).

The mean incubation time from exposure to and infection with the influenza A virus to the onset of symptoms is about 2 days. Symptoms characteristically begin with the abrupt onset of fever (greater than 37.8°C), chills, headache, myalgia, and malaise, anorexia, sore throat, coughing, sneezing, and shortness of breath. Fever peaks within 24 hours of onset and lasts 1 to 5 days. Within 6 to 12 hours, the illness reaches maximum severity, and a dry nonproductive cough develops. Symptoms may range from afebrile respiratory illnesses, similar to the common cold, to systemic involvement with relatively little involvement of the respiratory system. In uncomplicated influenza, physical findings are generally few or nonspecific and may improve over 2 to 5 days, followed by gradual improvement, although the illness may last for 1 week or more. Some patients develop persistent weakness or easy fatigability that may last for several weeks. The clinical outcome is directly dependent on the viral load, which peaks at about 48 hours after exposure. The larger the infecting doses of virus, the more severe the course of illness. Viral shedding begins 24 to 48 hours before the onset of symptoms and continues for about a week after the onset of the illness.

Complications Associated with Influenza A. Influenza can result in multiple significant complications, such as progressive infection involving the tracheobronchial tree and lungs (e.g., acute viral or bacterial pneumonia) and extrapulmonary complications. Patients with chronic medical conditions, such as chronic obstructive pulmonary disease, chronic cardiovascular disease, cirrhosis of the liver, chronic renal failure, diabetes mellitus, or long-standing rheumatoid arthritis, immunocompromised patients, and the elderly are particularly susceptible to these complications. When the respiratory tract is involved, the respiratory epithelium becomes damaged within 24 hours of infection, rendering the patient susceptible to secondary bacterial pneumonia.

At-risk patients who are infected with the influenza virus usually develop bacterial pneumonia 4 to 14 days after the onset of influenza symptoms. Bacterial pathogens that commonly cause superinfection include *Streptococcus pneumoniae*, *S. aureus*, *Haemophilus influenzae*, or group A streptococcus. Bacterial superinfection can develop at any time in the acute or convalescent phase of the infection, and is often characterized by an abrupt worsening of the patient's condition after initial stabilization. Although acute viral pneumonia is relatively uncommon, patients with significant underlying cardiovascular disease appear to be most commonly affected. Mortality rates among patients with bacterial pneumonia and acute viral pneumonia tend to be relatively high in the elderly. The clinician must be alert because patients with viral pneumonia usually present with the typical features of influenza but then develop an exacerbation of respiratory symptoms, hemoptysis, and respiratory failure. Chest radiographs in patients with viral pneumonia generally have a reticular interstitial pattern rather than radiologic characteristics of consolidation; blood gases reflect severe hypoxemia; and cultures of the blood and respiratory tract are generally negative for bacterial growth.

Extrapulmonary complications include musculoskeletal abnormalities, such as myositis and rhabdomyolysis; neurologic sequelae such as encephalopathy, encephalitis, transverse myelitis, or Guillain-Barré syndrome; myocarditis; and, rarely, Reye syndrome (62). The latter is almost never seen nowadays with the decreased use of aspirin as an antipyretic and analgesic in children. Mortality rates attributable to influenza in patients with underlying chronic medical conditions are probably underestimated because many of these patients die ostensibly through exacerbation of the underlying chronic respiratory or cardiovascular condition which, in fact, rendered them susceptible to the influenza virus in the first place.

Avian Influenza A. Influenza A viruses naturally infect avian and mammalian species, although wild aquatic birds are considered the prime reservoir. In these natural hosts, the viruses show minimal evolution at the amino acid level over extended periods, suggesting the influenza–bird association is ancient (61). Through antigenic shift, influenza A viruses that are naturally resident in wild waterfowl (e.g., aquatic ducks, geese, and swans) acquire the potential for transmission to humans. Viruses are shed in respiratory secretions and feces of birds, and can survive at low temperatures and low humidity for days to weeks. Reassortment possibilities include the emergence and spread of avian strains through permutations and combinations of any of the 16 HA glycoprotein and 9 NA subtypes.

Avian influenza A viruses are classified in one of the following two categories: low pathogenic or highly pathogenic forms. The criteria for high pathogenicity among these viruses include one or more of the following: (i) any avian influenza A virus that is lethal for 4-week-old chickens; (ii) any H5 or H7 virus that has a multibasic amino acid sequence at the HA cleavage site; or (iii) any non-H5 or H7 that kills one to five of eight inoculated chickens and grows in cell culture without trypsin (63). Highly pathogenic avian influenza viruses are usually H5 or H7 subtypes, which are associated with high mortality in domestic poultry but do not cause illness in wild birds. Although low pathogenic avian influenza viruses do not usually cause illness in wild birds, they may cause mild illness in domestic poultry, can cause outbreaks worldwide, and can evolve into highly pathogenic strains. During infections of domesticated poultry, some influenza strains of the H5 or H7 subtypes mutate to highly pathogenic and infectious strains.

Two factors increase the probability of the emergence of H5N1 viruses with the potential to directly infect humans: (i) the continued spread of the H5N1 strain in birds increases the opportunities for direct human contact, which in turn facilitates the selection of strains that are able to efficiently recognize human receptors; and (ii) the more frequently humans become infected with H5N1 strains, the higher the probability that these strains would get the chance to interact with the current seasonal influenza virus strains, leading to genetic reassortment and swapping of genes in a coinfected cell that results in H5N1 strains, or a third virus that is readily transmitted by and between humans or has adapted for growth in humans.

The first indication that a highly pathogenic H5N1 avian influenza virus can cause significant human disease occurred in early 2004, when this strain was implicated as the cause of viral pneumonia in a series of patients hospitalized with respiratory symptoms in Hanoi, Vietnam (64,65). Other recent outbreaks of highly pathogenic avian influenza strains in poultry in Canada (H7N3) and the Netherlands (H7N7), and their subsequent transmission to humans, have intensified concern over the emergence of a novel strain of influenza with pandemic potential (66–69). Overall, however, influenza A (H5N1) in humans is still poorly understood. Moreover a lack of autopsy data has limited the understanding of the pathogenesis and disease progression in humans infected with the H5N1 strain.

Published reports indicate that the clinical course of influenza A (H5N1) infection in humans is characterized by rapid deterioration and high mortality rates. A recent case-control study identified the presence in the household, and the handling, of dead or sick poultry in an H5N1-affected area and lack of access to an indoor water source as risk factors for H5N1 infection (70). Although limited human-to-human transmission has been documented (71), some studies suggest that exposure alone to persons who might be a source of H5N1 infection might not necessarily be a risk factor for this mode of transmission (70,72). These data suggest two possible mechanisms for transmission: inhalation or conjunctival deposition of large infectious droplets that could travel short distances, or the presence or consumption of infected poultry in the home (73).

The incubation period for human avian influenza A (H5N1) infection is 2 to 8 days but may be as long as 17 days (62). More recently, a study of patients with influenza A (H5N1) infection showed that disease progression is associated with elevated viremic levels and development of intense inflammatory responses—a finding that had already been established for seasonal influenza A virus strains (74). Early symptoms of influenza A (H5N1) include a high fever, diarrhea, vomiting, abdominal pain, chest pain, and bleeding from the nose and gums (62). Pneumonia that did not respond to antimicrobials is a common complication, suggesting that the process is likely a viral pneumonia, usually without bacterial superinfection at the time of hospitalization (62). Data from Vietnam suggest that multifocal consolidation involving at least two lung zones was the most common radiographic abnormality at the time of admission (62). In severe cases, respiratory failure occurs within 3 to 5 days after onset of symptoms, and may progress to the acute respiratory distress syndrome within a week from the time of onset of illness (75). Other documented complications include the reactive hemophagocytic syndrome, extensive hepatic central lobular necrosis, acute renal tubular necrosis, rhabdomyolysis, pancytopenia, cardiac dilatation and dysrhythmias, ventilator-associated pneumonia, pulmonary hemorrhage, pneumothorax, and the systemic inflammatory response syndrome without documented bacteremia (62,75–78). The mortality rate among patients with influenza A (H5N1) infection is high; since 2003, over 50% of persons who have been treated for avian H5N1 infection have died, with the highest death rates among persons younger than 15 years of age in Thailand (62). The most common cause of death is progressive respiratory failure.

Laboratory Diagnostic Tests

Common laboratory findings include leukopenia (especially lymphopenia), thrombocytopenia, raised aminotransferase levels, and elevated creatinine levels (62). Diagnosis of influenza requires collection of appropriate clinical specimens. For example, respiratory viruses grow in the epithelial lining of the nasal mucosa. Thus, a nasal wash is the optimal specimen for recovering respiratory viruses. Because the influenza virus is enveloped, it is less stable and may become nonviable during specimen collection and processing. Thus, the specimen, ideally, should be transported immediately to the laboratory in a sterile container; specimens that cannot be delivered immediately to the laboratory should be refrigerated until transported. Dry nasal swabs, throat swabs, or calcium alginate swabs are not appropriate for recovering respiratory viruses and should be discouraged. Unlike human influenza A infection, avian influenza (H5N1) is more commonly detected in, and has higher viral RNA levels in, pharyngeal versus nasal specimens (62).

Rapid enzyme immunoassay (EIA) testing of nasal washes for influenza A and B are available and are useful in the outpatient clinic or the emergency room. In these settings, physicians may use the EIA test results to discharge patients or to initiate prompt therapy and infection control measures. Recently, a food and drug administration (FDA)-approved EIA that distinguishes influenza A and influenza B antigens became available. The EIA test is approved for nasopharyngeal swabs, although nasal washes afford the best sensitivity. Rapid antigen tests are less sensitive in detecting influenza A (H5N1) infections compared with real-time PCR assays (75).

Rapid inpatient diagnosis is achievable through use of fluorescent antibody to directly detect the influenza antigen. This immunofluorescence testing of properly procured specimens for influenza A and B is usually performed with a respiratory viral battery that includes adenovirus; influenza A and B; parainfluenza 1, 2, and 3; and respiratory syncytial virus. The fluorescent antibody test has a relatively high sensitivity and specificity, and turnaround time is approximately 2 hours. Fluorescent antibody-negative specimens should be cultured for the above respiratory viruses; influenza cell cultures take between 5 and 7 days to grow. As with respiratory syncytial virus, viral culture is the gold standard for laboratory diagnosis of influenza A.

Serologic testing requires testing of paired serum specimens, the first taken during the acute phase and the second taken 2 to 4 weeks later. The diagnosis is made by demonstrating a fourfold or greater increase in complement-fixing or hemagglutination inhibition antibody titers in the paired serum specimens. However, serologic testing for influenza A and B has a low sensitivity. For these reasons, serologic testing is not useful for diagnosis in the acute phase of influenza; however, it may be used for establishing a retrospective diagnosis and for surveillance activities and epidemiologic studies.

Therapy

Medical management of influenza A infection comprises three essential components: (i) symptomatic, supportive therapy—rest, fluid replacement (oral or intravenous as deemed appropriate), and cautious use of analgesics, keeping in mind the association between salicylate use and Reye syndrome in children; (ii) initiation of antiviral therapy; and (iii) timely anticipation of complications, such as bacterial superinfection. Antimicrobial prophylaxis has not been shown to increase or reduce the risks for developing bacterial superinfection. Moreover, there is always a putative risk that empiric antimicrobial therapy could increase the emergence of antimicrobial resistance among micro-organisms in the respiratory tract.

Antiviral therapy is available for influenza viruses. Adamantine drugs, such as amantadine and rimantadine, are M2 protein blockers that are both active against influenza A. These M2 protein blockers cause a loss in ion channel function and inhibition of ribonucleoprotein release and of the uncoating process. For human influenza A infection, 4 to 5 days of amantadine or rimantadine therapy initiated within 24 to 48 hours of symptoms can lead to reduction in fever, systemic complaints, and viral shedding. Rimantadine is approved for persons aged 13 years and older. NA inhibitors, such as oseltamivir and zanamivir, are also available as antiviral therapy and act by inhibiting the cleavage of the virus from sialic acid, which blocks the release of new virus, thereby preventing the propagation of infection. Oseltamivir is FDA-approved for patients ages 2 years and older, and therapy should be started within 24 to 48 hours of symptoms. NA inhibitors are active against both influenza A and B.

Both adamantine and NA inhibitors are effective in prophylaxis against seasonal influenza, do not promote resistance among the pandemic strains, and have been shown to reduce the duration of symptoms, severity of illness, and the number of days confined to bed and of functional respiratory involvement (79). The utility of antiviral therapy in noncomplicated influenza infection remains a highly debatable issue. Moreover, there is a paucity of data on the utility of these agents in patients who have already developed complications, such as viral pneumonia or bacterial superinfection. Antiviral drugs can be used early in a pandemic, and do not require specific production and formulation (79). Patients with suspected influenza A (H5N1) should promptly receive a NA inhibitor pending the results of diagnostic laboratory testing (62); early treatment provides the greatest clinical benefit (75). NA inhibitors are efficacious in preventing febrile illness, although systemic infection can still occur; they also provide a degree of protection against the next wave of the pandemic virus (79). The roles played by corticosteroids and immunomodulators, such as interferon-alpha, in the management of influenza A (H5N1) infection remain uncharacterized.

Infection Control within the Health Care Setting

Transmission of influenza in health care settings is well documented and can occur between patients and health care personnel, or health care workers can transmit the virus to patients or other health care workers (73,80,81). During a pandemic, control and prevention of influenza A (H5N1) transmission in the inpatient setting requires institution of current guidelines for the prevention of transmission in health care settings (82): scrupulous attention to infection control practices and procedures, including strict attention to hand-washing and hygienic practices in conjunction with established guidelines for the prevention of hospital-acquired pneumonia (51,62,82). As recommended for the control of SARS, use of N-95 masks has been shown to be effective in reducing person-to-person transmission. However, surgical masks are acceptable if the N-95 varieties are not available.

The best prevention for influenza is to avoid the illness, although this is largely unattainable and difficult during a pandemic. Annual influenza vaccination is recommended for all high-risk patients (e.g., those with chronic lung or cardiac disease) and their close contacts, including medical personnel and household members, and universal vaccination of all children is recommended (83). It is widely appreciated that should an avian influenza A pandemic occur, a vaccine against the pandemic strain will not be immediately available. Moreover, since the major determinant of protection afforded by the influenza vaccine recipient is the generation of HA antibodies that provide protection approximately 2 weeks after administration, immediate benefit will not be rendered to vaccine recipients. Chemoprophylaxis with oseltamivir once daily for 7 to 10 days has been suggested for persons who might have had an unprotected exposure to avian influenza H5N1 (62,84,85). Although there is a paucity of published data regarding the utility of pre-exposure prophylaxis, a recent review suggested that it might warrant consideration if there is evidence that the influenza A (H5N1) strain is being transmitted person-to-person with increased efficiency or if there is a likelihood of a high-risk exposure (62).

DENGUE FEVER

Dengue fever is the most common arbovirus disease in the world, and although most cases have been reported in Asia, the number of countries with endemic dengue activity has increased dramatically in recent decades (86). The dengue fever

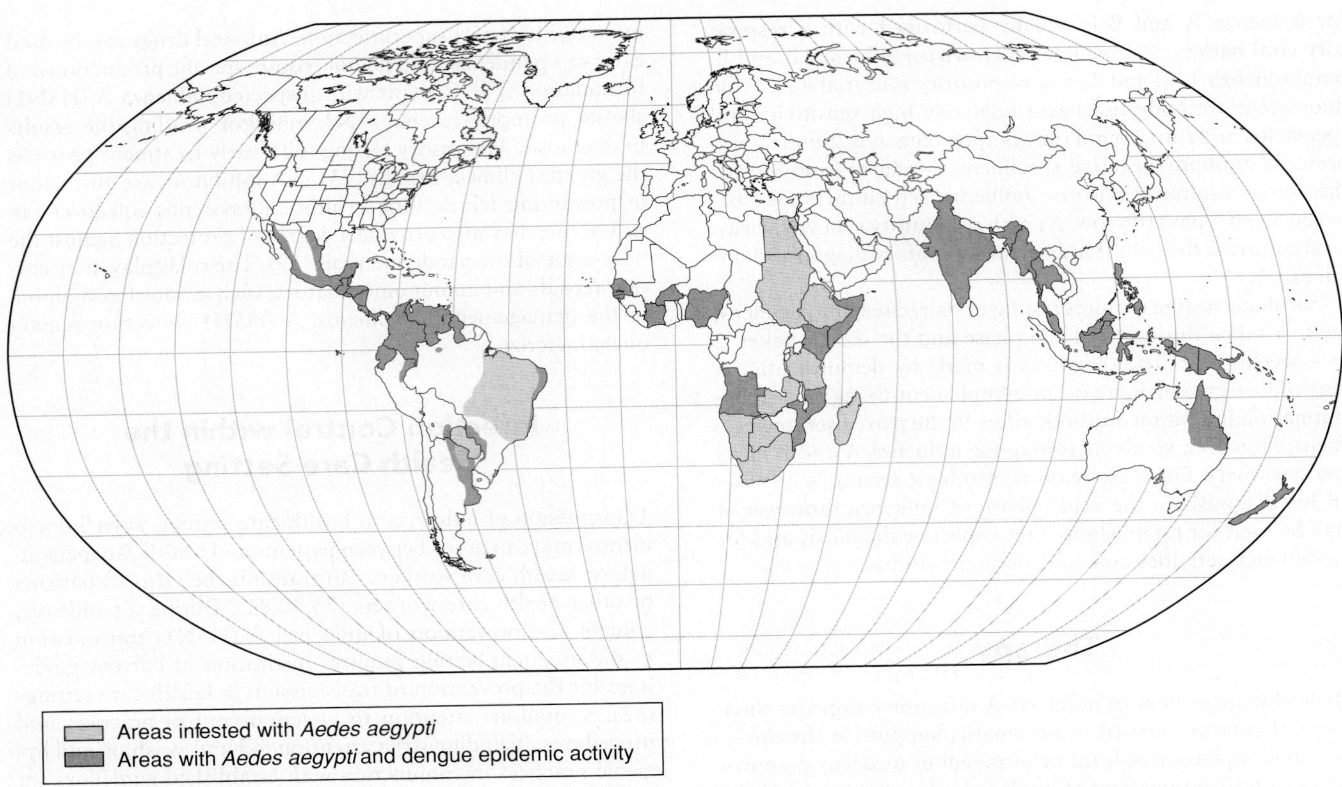

FIGURE 177.1. World distribution of dengue viruses and their mosquito vector, *Aedes aegypti*, in 2005. (Courtesy: Centers for Disease Control and Prevention, Atlanta, GA.) (From http://www.cdc.gov/NCIDOD/dvbid/dengue/map-distribution-2005.htm.)

virus is now endemic in over 100 tropical and subtropical countries in Southeast Asia, Africa, the Western Pacific, Africa, the Americas, the Caribbean, and the Eastern Mediterranean (Fig. 177.1) (87). The annual occurrences of dengue fever and its serious sequelae—dengue hemorrhagic fever—are estimated at about 100 million and 250,000 cases, respectively, with an estimated mortality rate of 25,000 per year (86–88). Because many of the countries where the virus is endemic remain popular tourist areas, and international travelers can both acquire and spread dengue virus infection, the public and clinical implications of this infection remain pertinent to critical care specialists in developed countries (87).

The dengue fever virus is a small mosquito-borne virus that belongs to the virus family Flaviviridae, genus *Flavivirus*, and contains a single strand of nonsegmented, positive sense RNA enclosed in a tight envelope. Disease is caused by four closely related but antigenically distinct serotypes: DENV types 1 to 4 (89). Worldwide, the virus is transmitted person-to-person primarily by the female *Aedes aegypti* mosquito (86–89); in the continental United States, two major dengue vectors, *Ae. aegypti* and *Ae. albopictus* mosquitoes, are widely distributed, and are likely to play important roles in transmission of the virus in North America during a dengue fever pandemic (90). These are day-biting species well adapted to urban settings and found inside and around houses, particularly in places where clean stagnant water has collected in receptacles, such as tires, domicile rainwater tanks, empty oil drums, discarded plastic containers and soft drink cans, or plant pots. Humans are the principal reservoir for the dengue virus and are able to sustain a viremia for up to 10 days after acquiring the infection; there is no known natural animal reservoir of infection. After it takes a blood meal from an infected human, the mosquito vector transmits the virus to new hosts during subsequent blood feeds.

Global warming has been associated with changes in the environment in regions across the globe, which has led to increased flooding in urban areas and facilitated the breeding of mosquitoes (91,92). In addition, warmer and wetter weather have extended the range of major mosquito vectors, especially the species that transmit the dengue virus. However, there are no firm data that unequivocally link global warming with the current dengue pandemic. In truth, the increasing occurrence of dengue virus infection is more likely a result of a complex interplay of multiple factors that encompass climate changes and natural disasters, urbanization, lack of or ineffective vector control programs, virus evolution, and increasing ease of global air travel (87,93,94). Transmission of the dengue virus infection in patient care settings and among laboratory personnel has been described, and is attributed largely to mucocutaneous contact with infected blood from travelers, needle stick injury, or blood transfusion (95–98).

Signs and Symptoms

The incubation period of dengue fever ranges from 3 to 14 days during which the virus multiplies in lymph nodes. Infection with any of the four serotypes can cause disease ranging from mild infection (dengue fever) with complete recovery to severe disease (i.e., dengue hemorrhagic fever and dengue shock syndrome) that may result in substantial morbidity and mortality. "Typical" dengue fever has an abrupt onset and is characterized by high fever; headache; retro-orbital pain worsened by eye movement; pain in the joints, limbs, and muscles (breakbone fever); and a rash that resembles a sunburn. Other symptoms may include abdominal pain and vomiting, sore throat, altered taste sensation, and general depression; cough is particularly common in children. On examination, the face is usually flushed, the eyes congested, and cervical lymph nodes enlarged. The high fever may be sustained for about a week, but often falls to normal after 2 to 4 days, returning after another 24 hours, giving rise to the so-called "saddle-back fever" curve. During the second fever phase, the patient often develops a characteristic maculopapular rash over the entire body except the face, and the pulse tends to be disproportionately slow. Uncomplicated dengue fever is a mild form of the condition with the characteristic clinical features of fever, joint ache, severe headaches, weakness, and skin rashes. This form of dengue fever is not fatal, rarely affects children, and usually lasts just 3 to 4 days.

Through a mechanism known as *immune enhancement*, previous or sequential infection with the dengue virus increases the risk for progression to dengue hemorrhagic fever and dengue shock syndrome in subsequent infections, which are also more likely on reinfection with a different serotype (99). *Hemorrhagic dengue* was first described in the Philippines in 1953, and during the 1960s, large outbreaks occurred in South East Asia. The immunologic response is an anamnestic reaction, with IgG antibodies persisting from the previous infection. Dengue hemorrhagic fever is characterized by high fever, alteration in microvascular permeability leading to plasma leakage, hepatomegaly, and circulatory failure—the key feature of *dengue shock syndrome* (100). The face is pale or mottled and cyanosed, skin is clammy and cold, and pulse is thready. In addition, the palms and soles become red and edematous, and the patient may develop petechiae and purpuric lesions. Bleeding varies from these skin lesions to epistaxis, bleeding from the gums or gastrointestinal tract, or hematuria. Unless urgently treated, death ensues from profound shock, severe bleeding, or both, within a few hours of presentation.

Plasma leakage is a result of damage to endothelial cells during the course of dengue infection; this damage is attributable to cytokine release rather than a cytopathic effect of the virus itself on the endothelium (90,101). Progression to the dengue hemorrhagic syndrome is not uniform among persons infected with the dengue virus. Several factors determine whether or not an infected person will develop the syndrome: (i) HLA gene linkage or ethnicity have been shown to make a person susceptible or resistant to the virus; for example, persons of African ethnicity harbor a gene that proffers resistance, and dengue hemorrhagic fever appears to occur rarely in European travelers (90,102–104); (ii) vascular permeability is age related, with very young children and the elderly most susceptible (105); and (iii) differences in the intrinsic virulence of various virus strains explain the ability of some strains over others to cause progression of dengue fever to dengue hemorrhagic fever and the dengue shock syndrome (90).

Vascular Permeability

Vascular permeability is the key feature in dengue hemorrhagic fever; however, as Halstead (90) pointed out, at its onset, vascular permeability exhibits only subtle changes, which can make early diagnosis difficult. The sphygmomanometer cuff tourniquet test has been widely used to screen children for vascular permeability, and though a positive test is an early correlate of dengue hemorrhagic fever (90), the test itself has a sensitivity of only 42% and a specificity of 94% (106). Thus, a negative tourniquet test alone does not necessarily exclude an ongoing dengue infection (90). A better screening test for incipient dengue hemorrhagic fever and early evidence of vascular permeability is detection of protein or heparin sulfate in acute-phase urine (90,107). The diagnosis is made principally on epidemiologic and clinical grounds but may be confirmed by serologic testing. A large proportion of asymptomatic infection is found in travelers to endemic regions (108,109). In addition, Wichmann et al. (104) point out that substantial underdiagnosis persists largely because the condition and its clinical features are not well known or familiar to medical practitioners in industrialized countries.

Treatment

There are no specific therapies for dengue fever, dengue hemorrhagic fever, or dengue shock syndrome, which has to be differentiated from the toxic shock syndrome. Treatment is directed against the shock and hemorrhage rather than against the infection. Clinical outcomes are largely dependent on careful history and physical examination, and a high index of suspicion among physicians for the diagnosis, especially among travelers who present with symptoms (87). Dengue fever, dengue hemorrhagic fever, and dengue shock syndrome cause substantial morbidity; death rates can be as high as 30% if these complications are not managed properly (110,111). Although vaccines for flaviviruses, such as yellow fever and Japanese encephalitis, are available, a dengue vaccine is still under development, made complicated by the need to incorporate all four virus serotypes into a single preparation (110). Thus, until a safe and effective tetravalent vaccine becomes available, prevention will be attained only through vector control programs and avoidance of mosquito bites through protective gear and insect repellent.

Summary

In summary, dengue fever and dengue hemorrhagic fever have reached pandemic proportions in countries across the globe, and dengue has become one of the most important tropical diseases in the first decade of the 21st century (88). The resurgence has been linked to population growth, urbanization, air travel, and changes in the environment that have all favored extension of the ranges of the mosquito vector or its ability to thrive (88). Unfortunately, lack of or inadequate existing surveillance activities have resulted in reduced ascertainment of the early stages of epidemic transmission, with gross underreporting of cases until the epidemic is recognized as dengue (88,112). Travelers returning from endemic regions are at particular risk of acquiring dengue fever. Persons who travel repeatedly to countries with high dengue endemicity put themselves at risk of becoming reinfected with a different serotype of the dengue virus, thereby predisposing themselves to dengue hemorrhagic fever. In the characterization of fever in the tropics or among returning travelers, clinicians need to have a high degree of suspicion and maintain dengue high on their list of differential diagnoses following a thorough history and physical examination.

TUBERCULOSIS: FALLOUT OF THE HUMAN IMMUNODEFICIENCY VIRUS PANDEMIC

By definition, HIV infection reached pandemic proportions years ago with over 40 million persons infected in Southeast Asia, sub-Saharan Africa, and the Indian subcontinent, and over 25 million deaths since the emergence of the retrovirus in the late 1970s (113). In the United States alone, approximately one million persons are infected with HIV, and 40,000 new infections occur yearly (114). Since 1981, more than a half million persons in the United States have died from HIV infection (115). However, most HIV transmission and infection are inextricably linked with changes in human ecologic and social behavior rather than the inevitability of eventual infection associated with, for example, a large influenza pandemic. Moreover, because primary HIV infection is asymptomatic in 10% to 50% of individuals, acute infection with the HIV virus generally does not warrant critical care management unless the patient presents with opportunistic or nonopportunistic infections as a direct result of immunosuppression, or is admitted for investigation of undifferentiated febrile or respiratory illnesses, neurologic syndromes, or gastrointestinal symptoms. Certainly, there is already a vast amount of published literature on the epidemiology of the HIV pandemic, the management of HIV-infected patients, and the opportunistic infections associated with the acquired immune deficiency syndrome (AIDS). Institution of highly active antiretroviral therapy (HAART) regimens that target different proteins involved in HIV pathogenesis has reduced rates of death and illness in North America, Western Europe, and other industrialized countries (115,116). Unfortunately, HAART is not routinely available to HIV-infected persons in many of the poorer nations where mortality rates still remain unacceptably high.

What the HIV pandemic has wrought in less-developed countries is the emergence of a true pandemic of tuberculosis. Before the HIV pandemic, *M. tuberculosis* infection and disease was already endemic in many less developed countries, although not at pandemic proportions. With the onset of the HIV pandemic, there has been a dramatic parallel increase in rates of tuberculosis among HIV-infected patients in less developed countries, especially sub-Saharan Africa, Southeast Asia, and increasingly, the Indian subcontinent—greater than 80% of all patients with tuberculosis live in sub-Saharan Africa and Asia (117). It is now estimated that tuberculosis is prevalent in one third of the world's population, and from this reservoir, there are over 9 million new cases of tuberculosis worldwide each year, resulting in an annual death toll of approximately 2 million infected persons (114,117). Indeed, *M. tuberculosis* has now been established as the first or second most common cause of bloodstream infections in febrile adults who present to emergency rooms in sentinel hospitals in Tanzania, Malawi, Uganda, and Thailand (118–123).

Although comparative rates of *M. tuberculosis* infections are relatively lower among HIV-infected patients in North America and Western Europe, the WHO generally considers *M. tuberculosis* infections a true pandemic that is unequivocally linked with immunosuppression resulting from HIV infection. This problem, however, has certainly been compounded by other factors associated with poverty, such as overcrowding, malnutrition, lack of access to health care, and poor sanitation, made particularly worse in refugee camps resulting from natural and man-made disasters and war (117). The fact remains that going into the latter part of the first decade in the 21st century, tuberculosis is still the leading cause of death among HIV-infected patients worldwide. Moreover, one of the biggest treatment dilemmas is how to manage tuberculosis and HIV infection at the same time. For HIV-infected patients from developed countries, risk factors for tuberculosis include travel to regions of the world with high endemic rates of *M. tuberculosis* infection or contact with an individual with active tuberculosis.

Major Issues

The major issues regarding tuberculosis within the critical care setting include (i) the ability of clinicians to recognize active or disseminated tuberculosis; (ii) the need to have a high level of suspicion for active tuberculosis when interpreting sputum smear results and abnormal chest radiographs, especially for at-risk patients or individuals who resided in HIV-endemic regions; (iii) the importance of collecting appropriate sputum specimens for screening smears and cultures, and rational interpretation of results; (iv) the utility and interpretation of tuberculin skin tests; (v) the timely institution of infection control measures for the prevention of transmission of the tubercle bacillus from infected patients or health care personnel to other individuals in the unit by isolating of patients with active disease or positive smears in properly designed rooms maintained at negative pressure differentials; (vi) collection of appropriate sputum specimens for follow-up smears and cultures per CDC recommendations (124); (vii) involvement of infection control and occupational health personnel in preventive decision making for patients and staff who might have been exposed inadvertently to persons with active tuberculosis (82,124); and (viii) awareness by all health care personnel of the basic tenets of guidelines published by CDC for the prevention of tuberculosis in health care settings (82,124).

Resistant Strains

Perhaps the most insidious occurrence resulting from the tuberculosis pandemic is the emergence of strains of *M. tuberculosis* resistant to standard antituberculous agents (Fig. 177.2). During the 1990s, multidrug-resistant (MDR); tuberculosis—defined as resistance to at least both isoniazid and rifampin—emerged as a threat to therapy, control, and prevention of tuberculosis both in the United States and worldwide (Fig. 177.2) (125–127). MDR-tuberculosis is almost certainly associated with the ready availability and overprescribing of antituberculous agents. For example, MDR-*M. tuberculosis* was less frequent in Malawi, where antituberculous agents were significantly less likely to be prescribed because of reduced availability compared with Thailand, where these agents were more readily available (118). The treatment of MDR-tuberculosis has clinical and public health implications—largely related to the fact that therapy requires the use of alternative second-line

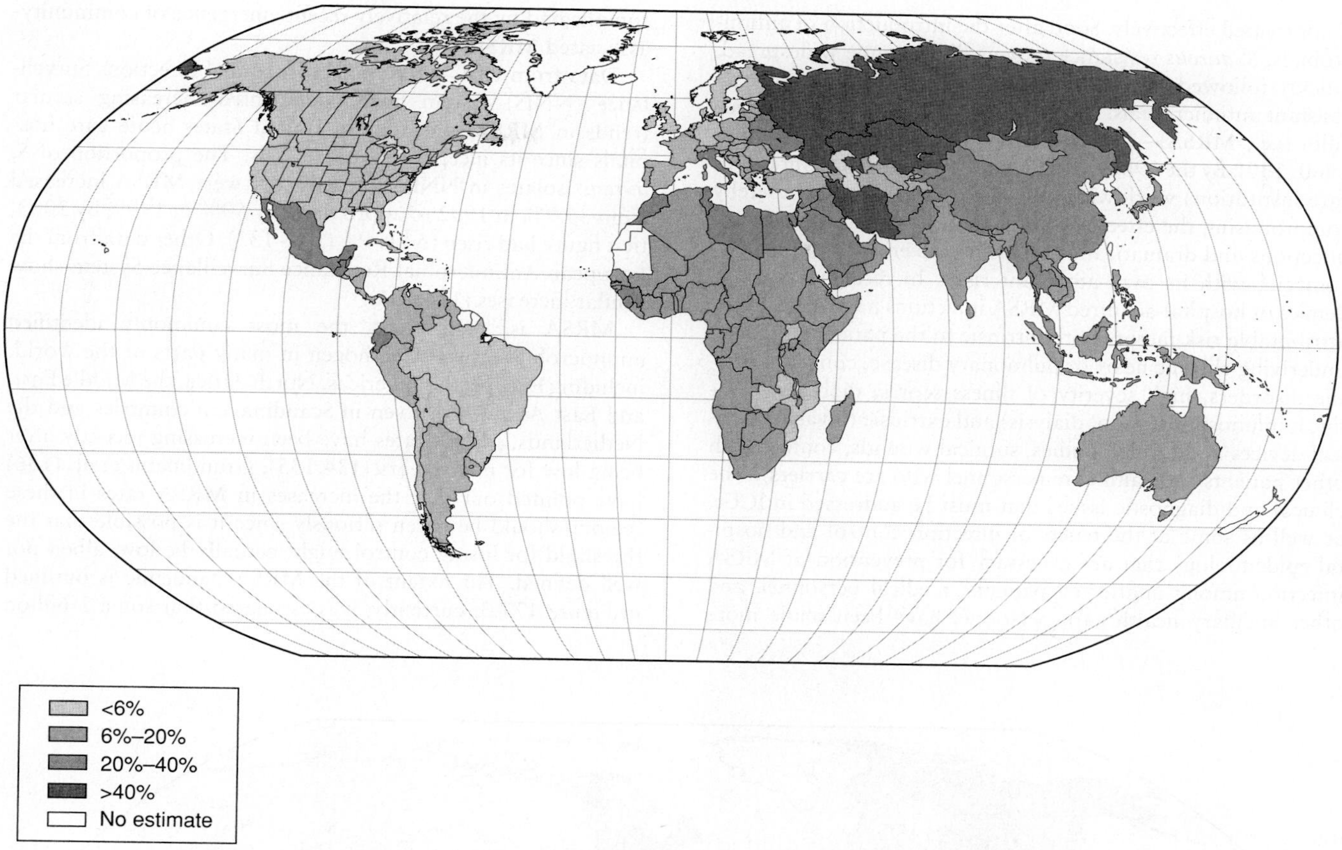

FIGURE 177.2. 2006 Global distribution of multidrug-resistant tuberculosis (MDR-TB) among previously treated cases. (From Zignol M, Hosseini MS, Wright A, et al. Global incidence of multidrug-resistant tuberculosis. *J Infect Dis.* 2006;194:479–85, with permission.)

drugs that are more expensive, toxic, and less effective than first-line isoniazid- and rifampin-based regimens (128).

In 2000, a committee was created to address the accessibility and availability of second-line drugs worldwide, while ensuring their proper use to prevent increased drug resistance (126,127). During this endeavor, the Committee ascertained numerous reports of tuberculosis caused by extensively drug-resistant (XDR) strains of *M. tuberculosis* (i.e., strains resistant to practically all second-line agents) (127). To assess the frequency and distribution of XDR-tuberculosis, CDC and WHO carried out a survey of an international network of tuberculosis laboratories from 1993 through 2004 (127). Of 17,690 *M. tuberculosis* isolates characterized, 20% were MDR and 2% were found to be XDR. In addition, the study found that 4% of MDR tuberculosis cases in the United States were, in fact, caused by XDR-*M. tuberculosis* (127). In October 2006, the WHO Global Task Force on XDR-tuberculosis met in Geneva, Switzerland, to review available information on the emergence of XDR-tuberculosis and to recommend measures to prevent and control this serious international public health threat (129). The Task Force concluded that: (1) XDR-tuberculosis stems from poor general tuberculosis control and the consequent development of MDR-tuberculosis; (2) it is associated with high mortality rates; (3) HIV-infected patients are particularly vulnerable; and (4) since many countries do not have laboratory capacity to diagnose drug-resistant tuberculosis, information on its distribution and magnitude is incomplete; treatment is difficult; and appropriate second-line drugs are not universally available (129). The Task Force also approved the following revised laboratory case definition for XDR-tuberculosis: "XDR-tuberculosis is tuberculosis showing resistance to at least rifampin and isoniazid, which is the definition of MDR-tuberculosis, in addition to any fluoroquinolone, and to at least one of the three following injectable drugs used in anti-tuberculosis treatment: capreomycin, kanamycin and amikacin" (129).

CDC and WHO have deemed XDR-tuberculosis a serious emerging public health threat, raising the specter of a pandemic of untreatable tuberculosis (127). Both agencies have identified a need for more population-based surveillance data to characterize the magnitude and trends of XDR-tuberculosis worldwide, expansion of activities to detect drug-resistant tuberculosis accurately and rapidly, and a need for algorithms to treat the infection effectively (127,129).

METHICILLIN-RESISTANT *STAPHYLOCOCCUS AUREUS* (MRSA)

S. aureus is an important cause of infections of the skin, soft tissue, wounds, respiratory tract, urinary tract, central nervous system, and the bloodstream, and can be rapidly fatal if not treated effectively. Soon after the introduction of antimicrobials, *S. aureus* resistance to penicillin became widespread, quickly followed by resistance to semisynthetic penicillinase-resistant antimicrobials, such as methicillin, oxacillin, and nafcillin (i.e., MRSA)—first detected in the United Kingdom in 1960 (130). By the 1980s, MRSA had spread throughout health care institutions worldwide and in the United States, thereby compromising the effectiveness of therapy for staphylococcal infections and dramatically increasing the empiric use of vancomycin, with its own attendant risks. In recent years, epidemics of hospital-acquired MRSA infections have highlighted attributable risk factors both intrinsic to the patient (e.g., age, underlying chronic heart or pulmonary disease, connective tissue disorders, high severity of illness scores, diabetes mellitus, immunosuppression, dialysis) and extrinsic (invasive medical devices and foreign bodies, surgical wounds, contact with other patients or health care personnel who are carriers). The clinical and diagnostic issues that must be addressed in ICUs, as well as some of the tenets of infection control and hospital epidemiology that are necessary for prevention of MRSA infection among unaffected patients, medical personnel, and other ancillary health care personnel have been made more complicated by the relatively recent emergence of community-associated MRSA.

Data from CDC's National Nosocomial Infections Surveillance (NNIS) system have documented increasing secular trends in MRSA infections in United States acute care hospitals since its inception in the 1970s. The proportion of *S. aureus* isolates in NNIS hospitals that were MRSA increased from 35.9% in 1992 to approximately 50% in 1999; by 2003, that figure had risen to 64.4% (131–133). Other data from the European Antimicrobial Resistance Surveillance System show similar increases (134,135).

MRSA is, at present, the most commonly identified antimicrobial-resistant pathogen in many parts of the world, including Europe, the Americas, North Africa, the Middle East, and East Asia (136). Even in Scandinavian countries and the Netherlands, MRSA rates have been increasing recently after being low for many years (134,135); Grundmann et al. (136) have pointed out that the increases in MRSA rates in these regions should be taken seriously since it is possible that the threshold for losing control might actually be low, albeit not well defined. The extent of the MRSA pandemic is outlined in Figure 177.3; currently, it is estimated that some 2 billion

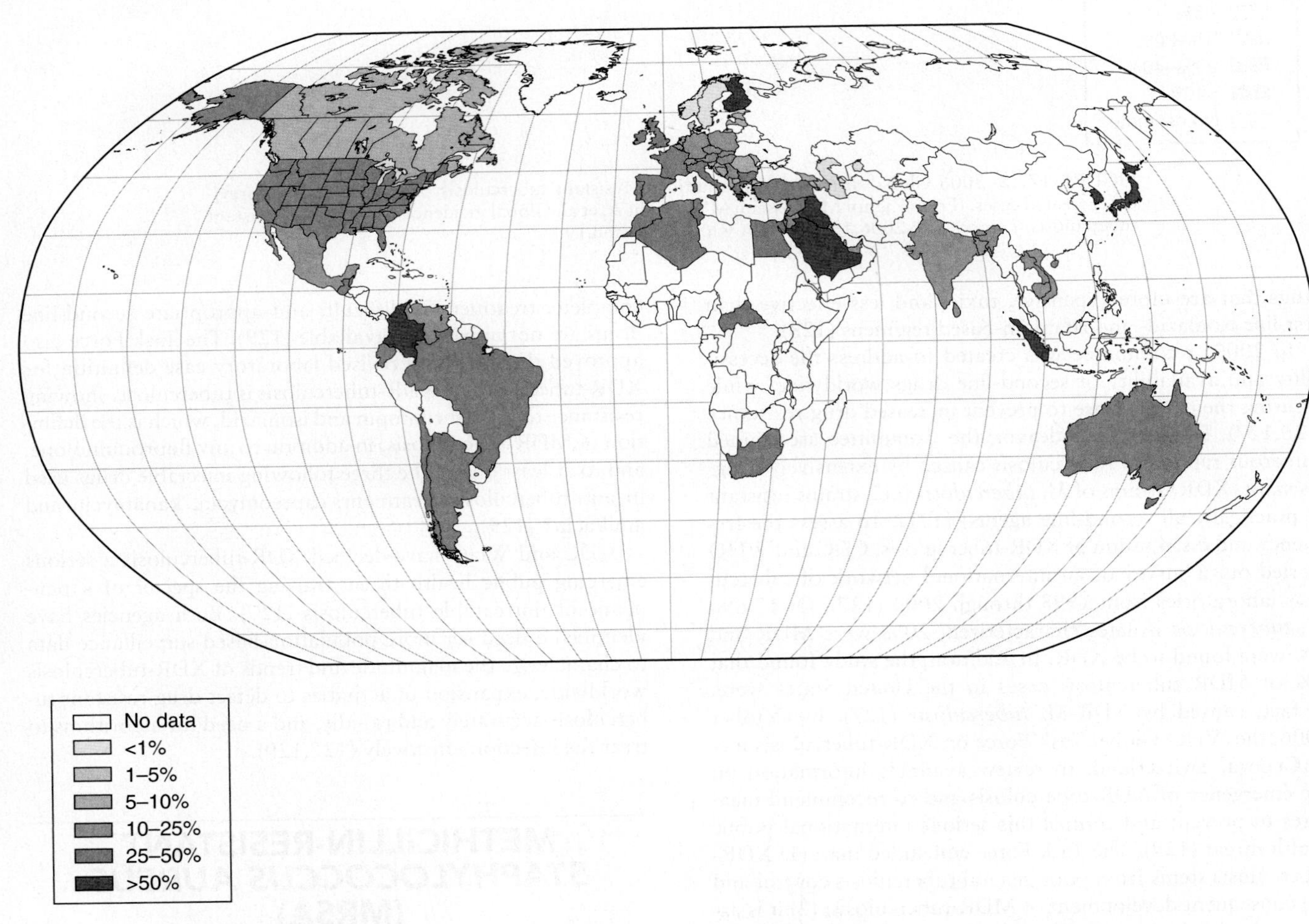

FIGURE 177.3. Worldwide prevalence of methicillin-resistant *Staphylococcus aureus* (MRSA) displayed by country. (From Grundmann H, Aires-de-Sousa M, Boyce J, et al. Emergence and resurgence of methicillin-resistant *Staphylococcus aureus* as a public-health threat. *Lancet*. 2006;368:874–885, with permission.)

individuals are carrying *S. aureus* worldwide and between 2 million and 53 million people carry MRSA across the globe (137,138). Other national data suggest that, despite more awareness among health care professionals of the adverse implications associated with MRSA colonization and infection, and despite more attention being paid to implementation of infection control guidelines, the prevalence rate of health care-associated MRSA infections in United States acute care hospitals is still on an upward trend (133).

Antimicrobial resistance among MRSA isolates is linked to a large mobile genetic element known as the staphylococcal cassette chromosome *mec* (SSC*mec*) gene that has been introduced into methicillin-susceptible *S. aureus* strains (the origin of this *mec* element remains unknown). The SCC*mec* element carries a methicillin-resistance determinant—*mecA*—that encodes for an additional penicillin-binding protein (PBP2A) with reduced affinity for β-lactam antimicrobials, in addition to the regulatory genes (*mec I* and *mecRI*) of *mec A* (136,139). Five types of SCC*mec* (SCC*mec* I–V) have been described: most health care-associated strains carry one of types I, II, or III, whereas community-acquired MRSA tend to be predominantly type IV and less commonly type V. Pulsed-field gel electrophoresis (PFGE) characterization of 3,000 MRSA isolates from hospitals in Southern and Eastern Europe, Latin America, and the United States has identified five major MRSA clones (140). These five pandemic clones were found to have evolved from two distinct and completely different ancestral backgrounds: one traced back to methicillin-susceptible *S. aureus* strains circulating in Danish hospitals during the 1950s; the other to MRSA strains recovered in Japan and the United States (140).

Risk Factors for Infection/Colonization

Individuals colonized with MRSA in their anterior nares can function as reservoirs for the organism over long periods (141). Recognition of colonized individuals is important because such persons may become infected; in the critical care setting, these persons may be a source of infection or colonization to other patients or health care personnel. Various epidemiologic studies have shown that the risk factors for MRSA carriage are similar to those for MRSA infection and include hospitalization (particularly in ICUs, surgery wards, other nursing units with documented high prevalence rates), invasive medical device use, the elderly, open wounds, underlying debilitation, proximity to other patients infected or colonized with MRSA, prior detection of MRSA, diabetes mellitus, treatments by injection, prior antimicrobial therapy, long inpatient stays, prior nursing home stays, visits at home by a nurse, or long periods of antimicrobial therapy (142–145). Health care personnel caring for MRSA-infected or MRSA-colonized patients with risk factors may themselves become colonized with MRSA and subsequently transmit the organism to noncolonized at-risk patients. Recent work by Huang et al. (146,147) has established that approximately 29% of newly detected MRSA carriers develop invasive disease within 18 months. There is now ample evidence that MRSA does not simply replace methicillin-susceptible *S. aureus* as a cause of health care-associated infection, but rather adds to the burden of infections caused by *S. aureus*.

In 2006, population-based estimates of nasal carriage of *S. aureus*, MRSA, and identification of risk factors for carriage were carried out by two groups that independently analyzed the 2001–2002 National Health and Nutrition Examination Survey (NHANES) data for the noninstitutionalized U.S. population, including children and adults (137,148). The findings of both groups were similar: (i) close to 90 million persons (i.e., 32% of the U.S. population) were colonized with *S. aureus*; and (ii) the prevalence of MRSA among *S. aureus* isolates was 2.6%, for an estimated population carriage of MRSA of 0.8% or 2.2 million persons (137,148). One of the studies also found that *S. aureus* colonization prevalence was highest in participants 6 to 11 years old whereas MRSA colonization was associated with age 60 years of age or older, but not necessarily with recent health care exposure (137).

Prevention

Standard approaches to preventing MRSA transmission include implementing CDC guidelines that recommend isolation of patients colonized or infected with MRSA in a private or dedicated room, and use of gowns, gloves, and masks when appropriate by all personnel entering the room (i.e., contact isolation). Many hospitals actively screen all patients when they are admitted to high-risk hospital areas (i.e., ICUs, transplant units, or surgical wards) and implement appropriate contact isolation for those identified as carriers. This approach, referred to as active screening and isolation, minimizes the possibility of transmitting MRSA between patients via the hands or clothes of healthcare workers, and has been effective in some centers (149,150). The major criticism of active screening and isolation programs is that it takes an average of 3 days from the time a nasal screening swab is obtained from a patient and is logged in the microbiology laboratory specimen-receiving station to the time the patient is confirmed as a MRSA carrier and gets reported to those who need to know in the inpatient service. Person-to-person MRSA transmission may occur during those 3 days. Therefore, decreasing the time it takes to identify a patient as a MRSA carrier will eliminate this delay, and may provide a rational strategy for reducing the transmission of MRSA in the inpatient setting. Recently, there has been an increasing body of literature regarding new methods for rapid identification of MRSA from clinical specimens (151–153). However, there are very few published data regarding the utility of rapid MRSA identification in reducing MRSA transmission and infection in the critical care setting (151,154).

Community-associated Strains

In 1993, new strains of MRSA were identified among people in Western Australia who had not been in contact with the health care system (155). Since then, there has been worldwide recognition of the emergence of community-associated MRSA strains. The incidence of community-associated MRSA is increasing in various populations across the United States (156). Previously healthy young adults are particularly affected, and several outbreaks of community-associated MRSA have been reported involving children, prison inmates, Alaskan Natives, Native Americans, Pacific Islanders, intravenous drug abusers, the homeless, children in day care, athletes who participate in contact sports, and military personnel, although infections are by no means restricted to these populations (157–165). Contact sports associated with outbreaks of community-associated MRSA include football, soccer, rugby, basketball, volleyball, wrestling, and cross-country running; skin breaks, a result of inadvertent trauma, commonly facilitate transmission of the pathogen among participants in these sports (160,164). Other risk factors found to be associated with community-associated MRSA infection in athletes include turf and grass burns sustained during play, gridiron playing position, sharing of soap bars and towels in the playing field and training areas, and nasal carriage of MRSA (159,160). A single toxin, Panton-Valentine leukocidin (PVL), has been linked by epidemiologic studies to community-associated MRSA infection (166–168). Recently, however, it was established that MRSA strains lacking PVL are just as likely to be virulent and to cause severe infection as PVL-positive strains, suggesting that PVL is not the major virulence determinant of community-associated MRSA (166).

Approximately 85% of community-associated MRSA infections involve the skin and subcutaneous tissues, with the most common presentations being an abscess or folliculitis in otherwise healthy individuals who do not have MRSA-associated risk factors (157,165). A predominant clone of community-associated MRSA, the USA 300 clone, appears to be the predominant cause of community-onset *S. aureus* skin and soft-tissue infection (169). Also, the presence of unique virulence factors may be responsible for potentially lethal necrotizing pneumonia and other invasive infections in both immunocompetent and immunosuppressed individuals (157,165,170–174).

Community-associated MRSA isolates are generally susceptible to multiple classes of antimicrobials other than β-lactams, and infections can be treated with trimethoprim–sulfamethoxazole, doxycycline, or clindamycin (170,175); for severe infections, vancomycin, daptomycin, quinupristin/dalfopristin, or linezolid can be used, though delay in initiating appropriate antimicrobial therapy for severe infections can cause substantial morbidity or even be life threatening (175).

Surveillance Measures

The diversity of strain types involved in epidemiologically clear outbreaks of MRSA suggests the spread of genetic information among different strains with strong predispositions for causing infections in hospital patients. Alternatively, the association could be due merely to the fact that resistance provides a dramatic marker that increases the likelihood that an epidemic will be recognized and investigated. If so, as infection control personnel in hospitals initiate surveillance activities and develop more sensitive means for recognizing outbreaks and clusters of infections, and more effectively share surveillance data with their counterparts in other local hospitals (e.g., through areawide surveillance systems supported by local health departments), interhospital transmission of infection will likely be more readily recognized and controlled. The main obstacle to endeavors that properly and comprehensively address the clinical and public health challenges of MRSA infections both in hospitals and the community remains the changing face of health care in the United States. Adding to the complexity of the issue are the uncharacterized confounding variables of long-term care facilities, freestanding medical clinics and surgery centers, and home care, where substantial amounts of patient care are now provided or delivered.

Control and Prevention

That endemic and epidemic health care–associated infections are preventable has periodically been reaffirmed by the myriad of single-center studies published over the past two decades dealing with the unequivocal effect of hand-washing with soap and water; proper care of urinary catheters, respirators, intravascular catheters, and surgical wounds; numerous evidence-based infection control guidelines published by the CDC; and position papers issued by the Society of Healthcare Epidemiology of America (SHEA), the Association of Practitioners of Infection Control, and the Infectious Diseases Society of America (82,176–178). However, according to CDC data, although overall rates of health care–associated infections at the main anatomic sites (i.e., bloodstream, respiratory tract, wounds, urine) have been falling, infections caused by MRSA have been increasing in hospitals across the United States. The seriousness of the problem was underscored in a recent editorial by Muto (179), who made the point that "for as long as CDC has measured the prevalence of hospital-acquired infections caused by multidrug-resistant organisms, it has been increasing."

There is little doubt that we would not be where we are today had more attention been paid to the published evidence-based data regarding which interventions have been effective in controlling the transmission of health care–associated, antimicrobial-resistant pathogens. After decades of discussing control of antimicrobial-resistant, health care–associated pathogens in the medical literature, there is actually very little evidence of success either in the control of the infections caused by these pathogens or in halting the increasing incidence of resistance among isolates. The myriad articles published have, in effect, helped explain this failure because much of the published data on health care–associated infections have been carried out in hospitals that had implemented untried control programs or had substantially ineffective programs. Moreover, despite all the resources expanded in surveillance programs for health care-associated infections in facilities across the country, there remains substantial variation in surveillance practices from one medical center to another, as well as the inconsistent use of effective control measures (e.g., surveillance cultures not being performed as recommended) or failure of hospitals to use these measures due to lack of commitment by health care companies and administrators alike to initiate and enforce them. In addition, there appears to be moderate compliance with goals to optimize antimicrobial use and to detect, report, and control the spread of antimicrobial-resistant pathogens.

In the Netherlands and some Scandinavian countries, rates of health care–associated MRSA infections have been maintained at less than 3% through programs that include screening of patients and exposed health care workers in aggressive "search and destroy" MRSA prevention programs (180,181). Recent American guidelines are advocating an approach similar to the search and destroy paradigm (176). The value of obtaining screening cultures in areas with high MRSA endemicity, however, remains controversial (136).

Numerous reports presented at the SHEA annual meetings for each of the years 2003–2005 have repeatedly shown control of endemic or epidemic MRSA infections through implementation of the SHEA guidelines, with more emphasis on contact precautions and less on standard precautions (25 such reports in the past two SHEA annual meetings). In fact, CDC has not provided any evidence-based data that show standard precautions and passive surveillance have begun to bring the spread of MRSA under control (182).

The tenets of the SHEA guidelines are based on identification and containment of spread through the following:

1. Active surveillance cultures to identify the reservoir for spread
2. Routine hand hygiene
3. Barrier precautions for patients known or suspected to be colonized or infected with MRSA
4. Implementation of an antimicrobial stewardship program
5. Decolonization or suppression of colonized patients (176)

There is increasing evidence that screening of high-risk patients combined with a comprehensive prevention program consisting of contact precautions and scrupulous hand hygiene can reduce transmission of MRSA (136,142,143, 183,184). Grundmann et al. (136,142,185–189) recently pointed out that virtually all published analyses comparing the costs of screening patients on admission and using contact precautions with colonized patients, with the cost savings made by preventing health care–associated MRSA infections, have concluded that the combination of surveillance cultures and barrier precautions results in substantial cost savings for health care facilities.

In summary, active surveillance cultures for MRSA in the critical care setting and isolation of colonized persons is a highly effective strategy for control of MRSA. Isolation purely on the basis of history of previous detection, at least for MRSA, appears to be of little benefit. Standard precautions and isolation of the occasional patient recognized to be colonized through routine clinical cultures are minimally effective. The onus is now on health care professionals and health care administrators to invest intelligently in prevention programs and enhance existing surveillance activities in targeted areas, as well as to avoid viewing death and morbidity attributable to MRSA as inevitable. However, it must be equally understood and appreciated by relatives, patients, lawyers, administrators, and health care workers alike that the following types of patients are particularly susceptible to or likely to acquire health care–associated MRSA infections: those born very prematurely or the elderly; those who are debilitated or have severe congenital abnormalities; patients with diabetes mellitus, connective tissue disorders, or end-stage respiratory, liver, renal, or cardiac disease; and patients with numerous invasive medical devices or who have undergone one or more major surgical procedures or other invasive procedures.

The challenge that faces us now is controlling the transmission of strains of community-associated MRSA that become endemic within the inpatient setting, especially in ICUs. New MRSA clones have emerged in the community that combine antimicrobial resistance with easy transmissibility and virulence (136,168). The worry is that these could take hold in hospitals where patients are particularly vulnerable.

SUMMARY

We have highlighted five infections that either have emerged into pandemics or, in the case of avian influenza, has a high potential to do so. Patients with any of these five infections may require management in an ICU. Knowledge of these infections is important for ICU personnel if appropriate management, as well as infection control and preventive measures, is to be instituted in a timely manner. The common threads running through these five pandemic infections include the need for physicians to have high indices of clinical suspicion and, early on, consider these diagnoses and the importance of infection control, surveillance, and education for staff and patients alike.

SARS was controlled largely through early detection and implementation of traditional infection control practices, environmental decontamination, use of personal protective equipment, surveillance activities, and education and training of patients, relatives, and caregivers. Avian influenza, where there have been outbreaks, has largely been controlled through early recognition, scrupulous attention to infection control practices and procedures, institution of established guidelines for the prevention of hospital-acquired pneumonia, and annual influenza vaccination for all high-risk patients and their close contacts—including medical personnel as well as household members. Dengue must be considered in the characterization and workup of fever among returning international travelers, and clinicians in critical care need to have a high degree of suspicion for the associated clinical syndromes. Preventing the transmission of tuberculosis in the in-patient setting is made all the more imperative because of the limited therapeutic options available once a patient has acquired infection caused by MDR and, especially, XDR strains. Compounding the risk of tuberculosis in the in-patient setting is the looming possibility of transmission of untreatable XDR strains to previously healthy humans, including health care personnel. Control and prevention of MRSA infections, too, have been made especially difficult since the emergence of community-associated strains that have insidiously crept into the in-patient setting, raising the possibility of transmission of MRSA to healthy personnel with no obvious risk factors. For further information, the reader may wish to refer to the references to seek additional information on the epidemiology, clinical and therapeutic issues, immunology, and specific infection control guidelines for each of the five infections.

References

1. Archibald L, Phillips L, Monnet D, et al. Antimicrobial resistance in isolates from inpatients and outpatients in the United States: increasing importance of the intensive care unit. *Clin Infect Dis.* 1997;24:211.
2. Centers for Disease Control and Prevention. Outbreak of severe acute respiratory syndrome—worldwide, 2003. *MMWR Morb Mortal Wkly Rep.* 2003;52:226.
3. Centers for Disease Control and Prevention. Update: severe acute respiratory syndrome–United States, May 14, 2003. *MMWR Morb Mortal Wkly Rep.* 2003;52:436.
4. Centers for Disease Control and Prevention. Update: outbreak of severe acute respiratory syndrome–worldwide, 2003. *MMWR Morb Mortal Wkly Rep.* 2003;52:241.
5. Ksiazek TG, Erdman D, Goldsmith CS, et al. A novel coronavirus associated with severe acute respiratory syndrome. *N Engl J Med.* 2003;348:1953.
6. Berger A, Drosten C, Doerr HW, et al. Severe acute respiratory syndrome (SARS)-paradigm of an emerging viral infection. *J Clin Virol.* 2004;29:13.
7. Drosten C, Gunther S, Preiser W, et al. Identification of a novel coronavirus in patients with severe acute respiratory syndrome. *N Engl J Med.* 2003;348:1967.
8. Kuiken T, Fouchier RA, Schutten M, et al. Newly discovered coronavirus as the primary cause of severe acute respiratory syndrome. *Lancet.* 2003;362:263.
9. World Health Organization. Acute respiratory syndrome. China, Hong Kong Special Administrative Region of China, and Viet Nam. *Wkly Epidemiol Rec.* 2003;78:73.

10. Peiris JS, Guan Y, Yuen KY. Severe acute respiratory syndrome. *Nat Med.* 2004;10(Suppl):S88.
11. Donnelly CA, Ghani AC, Leung GM, et al. Epidemiological determinants of spread of causal agent of severe acute respiratory syndrome in Hong Kong. *Lancet.* 2003;361:1761.
12. Poutanen SM, Low DE, Henry B, et al. Identification of severe acute respiratory syndrome in Canada. *N Engl J Med.* 2003;348:1995.
13. Lingappa JR, McDonald LC, Simone P, et al. Wrestling SARS from uncertainty. *Emerg Infect Dis.* 2004;10:167.
14. Marra MA, Jones SJ, Astell CR, et al. The genome sequence of the SARS-associated coronavirus. *Science.* 2003;300:1399.
15. Rota PA, Oberste MS, Monroe SS, et al. Characterization of a novel coronavirus associated with severe acute respiratory syndrome. *Science.* 2003; 300:1394.
16. Liang G, Chen Q, Xu J, et al. Laboratory diagnosis of four recent sporadic cases of community-acquired SARS, Guangdong Province, China. *Emerg Infect Dis.* 2004;10:1774.
17. Song HD, Tu CC, Zhang GW, et al. Cross-host evolution of severe acute respiratory syndrome coronavirus in palm civet and human. *Proc Natl Acad Sci U S A.* 2005;102:2430.
18. Wang LF, Shi Z, Zhang S, et al. Review of bats and SARS. *Emerg Infect Dis.* 2006;12:1834.
19. Weiss SR, Navas-Martin S. Coronavirus pathogenesis and the emerging pathogen severe acute respiratory syndrome coronavirus. *Microbiol Mol Biol Rev.* 2005;69:635.
20. Fouchier RA, Kuiken T, Schutten M, et al. Aetiology: Koch's postulates fulfilled for SARS virus. *Nature.* 2003;423:240.
21. Martina BE, Haagmans BL, Kuiken T, et al. Virology: SARS virus infection of cats and ferrets. *Nature.* 2003;425:915.
22. Weingartl HM, Copps J, Drebot MA, et al. Susceptibility of pigs and chickens to SARS coronavirus. *Emerg Infect Dis.* 2004;10:179.
23. Varia M, Wilson S, Sarwal S, et al. Investigation of a nosocomial outbreak of severe acute respiratory syndrome (SARS) in Toronto, Canada. *CMAJ.* 2003;169:285.
24. Yu IT, Sung JJ. The epidemiology of the outbreak of severe acute respiratory syndrome (SARS) in Hong Kong—what we do know and what we don't. *Epidemiol Infect.* 2004;132:781.
25. Seto WH, Tsang D, Yung RW, et al. Effectiveness of precautions against droplets and contact in prevention of nosocomial transmission of severe acute respiratory syndrome (SARS). *Lancet.* 2003;361:1519.
26. Tang JW, Li Y, Eames I, et al. Factors involved in the aerosol transmission of infection and control of ventilation in healthcare premises. *J Hosp Infect.* 2006;64:100.
27. Centers for Disease Control and Prevention. Severe acute respiratory syndrome—Singapore, 2003. *MMWR Morb Mortal Wkly Rep.* 2003;52: 405.
28. Centers for Disease Control and Prevention. Cluster of severe acute respiratory syndrome cases among protected health-care workers—Toronto, Canada, April 2003. *MMWR Morb Mortal Wkly Rep.* 2003;52:433.
29. Centers for Disease Control and Prevention. Update: severe acute respiratory syndrome–Toronto, Canada, 2003. *MMWR Morb Mortal Wkly Rep.* 2003;52:547.
30. Peiris JS, Chu CM, Cheng VC, et al. Clinical progression and viral load in a community outbreak of coronavirus-associated SARS pneumonia: a prospective study. *Lancet.* 2003;361:1767.
31. Dowell SF, Simmerman JM, Erdman DD, et al. Severe acute respiratory syndrome coronavirus on hospital surfaces. *Clin Infect Dis.* 2004;39:652.
32. Christian MD, Loutfy M, McDonald LC, et al. Possible SARS coronavirus transmission during cardiopulmonary resuscitation. *Emerg Infect Dis.* 2004;10:287.
33. Ofner M, Lem M, Sarwal S, et al. Cluster of severe acute respiratory syndrome cases among protected health care workers—Toronto, April 2003. *Can Commun Dis Rep.* 2003;29:93.
34. Loeb M, McGeer A, Henry B, et al. SARS among critical care nurses, Toronto. *Emerg Infect Dis.* 2004;10:251.
35. Wong RS, Hui DS. Index patient and SARS outbreak in Hong Kong. *Emerg Infect Dis.* 2004;10:339.
36. Wong TW, Lee CK, Tam W, et al. Cluster of SARS among medical students exposed to single patient, Hong Kong. *Emerg Infect Dis.* 2004;10:269.
37. Shen Z, Ning F, Zhou W, et al. Superspreading SARS events, Beijing, 2003. *Emerg Infect Dis.* 2004;10:256.
38. Tsang KW, Ho PL, Ooi GC, et al. A cluster of cases of severe acute respiratory syndrome in Hong Kong. *N Engl J Med.* 2003;348:1977.
39. Peiris JS, Yuen KY, Osterhaus AD, et al. The severe acute respiratory syndrome. *N Engl J Med.* 2003;349:2431.
40. Lapinsky SE, Hawryluck L. ICU management of severe acute respiratory syndrome. *Intensive Care Med.* 2003;29:870.
41. Hsueh PR, Yang PC. Severe acute respiratory syndrome (SARS)—an emerging infection of the 21st century. *J Formos Med Assoc.* 2003;102:825.
42. Poutanen SM, McGeer AJ. Transmission and Control of SARS. *Curr Infect Dis Rep.* 2004;6:220.
43. Chen KT, Twu SJ, Chang HL, et al. SARS in Taiwan: an overview and lessons learned. *Int J Infect Dis.* 2005;9:77.
44. Twu SJ, Chen TJ, Chen CJ, et al. Control measures for severe acute respiratory syndrome (SARS) in Taiwan. *Emerg Infect Dis.* 2003;9:718.
45. Masur H, Emanuel E, Lane HC. Severe acute respiratory syndrome: providing care in the face of uncertainty. *JAMA.* 2003;289:2861.
46. Srinivasan A, Jernign DB, Liedtke L, et al. Hospital preparedness for severe acute respiratory syndrome in the United States: views from a national survey of infectious diseases consultants. *Clin Infect Dis.* 2004;39:272.
47. Srinivasan A, McDonald LC, Jernigan D, et al. Foundations of the severe acute respiratory syndrome preparedness and response plan for healthcare facilities. *Infect Control Hosp Epidemiol.* 2004;25:1020.
48. Ho PL, Tang XP, Seto WH. SARS: hospital infection control and admission strategies. *Respirology.* 2003;8(Suppl):S41.
49. Lateef F. SARS changes the ED paradigm. *Am J Emerg Med.* 2004;22:483.
50. Chow CB. Post-SARS infection control in the hospital and clinic. *Paediatr Respir Rev.* 2004;5:289.
51. Tablan OC, Anderson LJ, Besser R, et al. Guidelines for preventing health-care–associated pneumonia, 2003: recommendations of CDC and the Healthcare Infection Control Practices Advisory Committee. *MMWR Recomm Rep.* 2004;53(RR-3):1.
52. Shaw K. The 2003 SARS outbreak and its impact on infection control practices. *Public Health.* 2006;120:8.
53. McDonald LC, Simor AE, Su IJ, et al. SARS in healthcare facilities, Toronto and Taiwan. *Emerg Infect Dis.* 2004;10:777.
54. Olsen SJ, Chang HL, Cheung TY, et al. Transmission of the severe acute respiratory syndrome on aircraft. *N Engl J Med.* 2003;349:2416.
55. Taubenberger JK, Morens DM. 1918 Influenza: the mother of all pandemics. *Emerg Infect Dis.* 2006;12:15.
56. Kilbourne ED. Influenza pandemics of the 20th century. *Emerg Infect Dis.* 2006;12:9.
57. Cox NJ, Subbarao K. Influenza. *Lancet.* 1999;354:1277.
58. Cox NJ, Subbarao K. Global epidemiology of influenza: past and present. *Annu Rev Med.* 2000;51:407.
59. Webster RG. Influenza: an emerging disease. *Emerg Infect Dis.* 1998;4: 436.
60. Webster RG. Wet markets—a continuing source of severe acute respiratory syndrome and influenza? *Lancet.* 2004;363:234.
61. Webster RG, Peiris M, Chen H, et al. H5N1 outbreaks and enzootic influenza. *Emerg Infect Dis.* 2006;12:3.
62. Beigel JH, Farrar J, Han AM, et al. Avian influenza A (H5N1) infection in humans. *N Engl J Med.* 2005;353:1374.
63. Pearson JE. International standards for the control of avian influenza. *Avian Dis.* 2003;47(Suppl 3):972.
64. Nguyen HL, Saito R, Ngiem HK, et al. Epidemiology of influenza in Hanoi, Vietnam, from 2001 to 2003. *J Infect.* 2007; Epub ahead of print Jan 11, 2007.
65. Tran TH, Nguyen TL, Nguyen TD, et al. Avian influenza A (H5N1) in 10 patients in Vietnam. *N Engl J Med.* 2004;350:1179.
66. Hirst M, Astell CR, Griffith M, et al. Novel avian influenza H7N3 strain outbreak, British Columbia. *Emerg Infect Dis.* 2004;10:2192.
67. Tweed SA, Skowronski DM, David ST, et al. Human illness from avian influenza H7N3, British Columbia. *Emerg Infect Dis.* 2004;10:2196.
68. Fouchier RA, Schneeberger PM, Rozendaal FW, et al. Avian influenza A virus (H7N7) associated with human conjunctivitis and a fatal case of acute respiratory distress syndrome. *Proc Natl Acad Sci U S A.* 2004;101: 1356.
69. Koopmans M, Wilbrink B, Conyn M, et al. Transmission of H7N7 avian influenza A virus to human beings during a large outbreak in commercial poultry farms in the Netherlands. *Lancet.* 2004;363:587.
70. Dinh PN, Long HT, Tien NTK, et al. Risk factors for human infection with avian influenza A H5N1, Vietnam, 2004. *Emerg Infect Dis.* 2006;12:1841.
71. Ungchusak K, Auewarakul P, Dowell SF, et al. Probable person-to-person transmission of avian influenza A (H5N1). *N Engl J Med.* 2005;352:333.
72. Areechokchai D, Jiraphongsa C, Laosiritaworn Y, et al. Investigation of avian influenza (H5N1) outbreak in humans—Thailand, 2004. *MMWR Morb Mortal Wkly Rep.* 2006;55(Suppl 1):3.
73. Bridges CB, Kuehnert MJ, Hall CB. Transmission of influenza: implications for control in health care settings. *Clin Infect Dis.* 2003;37:1094.
74. de Jong MD, Simmons CP, Thanh TT, et al. Fatal outcome of human influenza A (H5N1) is associated with high viral load and hypercytokinemia. *Nat Med.* 2006;12:1203.
75. Chotpitayasunondh T, Ungchusak K, Hanshaoworakul W, et al. Human disease from influenza A (H5N1), Thailand, 2004. *Emerg Infect Dis.* 2005; 11:201.
76. To KF, Chan PK, Chan KF, et al. Pathology of fatal human infection associated with avian influenza A H5N1 virus. *J Med Virol.* 2001;63:242.
77. Chan PK. Outbreak of avian influenza A(H5N1) virus infection in Hong Kong in 1997. *Clin Infect Dis.* 2002;34(Suppl 2):S58.
78. Yuen KY, Chan PK, Peiris M, et al. Clinical features and rapid viral diagnosis of human disease associated with avian influenza A H5N1 virus. *Lancet.* 1998;351:467.
79. Monto AS. Vaccines and antiviral drugs in pandemic preparedness. *Emerg Infect Dis.* 2006;12:55.
80. Salgado CD, Farr BM, Hall KK, et al. Influenza in the acute hospital setting. *Lancet Infect Dis.* 2002;2:145.
81. Arden NH. Control of influenza in the long-term-care facility: a review of established approaches and newer options. *Infect Control Hosp Epidemiol.* 2000;21:59.

82. Sehulster L, Chinn RY. Guidelines for environmental infection control in health-care facilities. Recommendations of CDC and the Healthcare Infection Control Practices Advisory Committee (HICPAC). *MMWR Recomm Rep.* 2003;52(RR-10):1.
83. Centers for Disease Control and Prevention. Influenza and pneumococcal vaccination coverage among persons aged > or = 65 years—United States, 2004–2005. *MMWR Morb Mortal Wkly Rep.* 2006;55:1065.
84. Hayden FG, Belshe R, Villanueva C, et al. Management of influenza in households: a prospective, randomized comparison of oseltamivir treatment with or without postexposure prophylaxis. *J Infect Dis.* 2004;189: 440.
85. Welliver R, Monto AS, Carewicz O, et al. Effectiveness of oseltamivir in preventing influenza in household contacts: a randomized controlled trial. *JAMA.* 2001;285:748.
86. Gibbons RV, Vaughn DW. Dengue: an escalating problem. *BMJ.* 2002;324: 1563.
87. Wilder-Smith A, Schwartz E. Dengue in travelers. *N Engl J Med.* 2005;353: 924.
88. Gubler DJ. Epidemic dengue/dengue hemorrhagic fever as a public health, social and economic problem in the 21st century. *Trends Microbiol.* 2002; 10:100.
89. Gubler DJ. Dengue and dengue hemorrhagic fever: its history and resurgence as a global public health problem. In: Gubler DJ, Kuno G, eds. *Dengue and Dengue Hemorrhagic Fever.* Oxford UK: CABI Publishing;1997:1.
90. Halstead SB. More dengue, more questions. *Emerg Infect Dis.* 2005;11: 740.
91. Khasnis AA, Nettleman MD. Global warming and infectious disease. *Arch Med Res.* 2005;36:689.
92. Reiter P. Climate change and mosquito-borne disease. *Environ Health Perspect.* 2001;109(Suppl 1):141.
93. Rodriguez-Roche R, Alvarez M, Holmes EC, et al. Dengue virus type 3, Cuba, 2000–2002. *Emerg Infect Dis.* 2005;11:773.
94. Guzman MG, Kouri G. Dengue: an update. *Lancet Infect Dis.* 2002;2:33.
95. Chen LH, Wilson ME. Nosocomial dengue by mucocutaneous transmission. *Emerg Infect Dis.* 2005;11:775.
96. Nemes Z, Kiss G, Madarassi EP, et al. Nosocomial transmission of dengue. *Emerg Infect Dis.* 2004;10:1880.
97. Wagner D, de With K, Huzly D, et al. Nosocomial acquisition of dengue. *Emerg Infect Dis.* 2004;10:1872.
98. de Wazieres B, Gil H, Vuitton DA, et al. Nosocomial transmission of dengue from a needlestick injury. *Lancet.* 1998;351:498.
99. Halstead SB, O'Rourke EJ. Dengue viruses and mononuclear phagocytes, I: infection enhancement by non-neutralizing antibody. *J Exp Med.* 1977; 146:201.
100. Halstead SB. Pathogenesis of dengue: challenges to molecular biology. *Science.* 1988;239:476.
101. Jessie K, Fong MY, Devi S, et al. Localization of dengue virus in naturally infected human tissues, by immunohistochemistry and in situ hybridization. *J Infect Dis.* 2004;189:1411.
102. Stephens HA, Klaythong R, Sirikong M, et al. HLA-A and -B allele associations with secondary dengue virus infections correlate with disease severity and the infecting viral serotype in ethnic Thais. *Tissue Antigens.* 2002;60:309.
103. Guzman MG, Kouri GP, Bravo J, et al. Dengue hemorrhagic fever in Cuba, 1981: a retrospective seroepidemiologic study. *Am J Trop Med Hyg.* 1990;42:179.
104. Wichmann O, Lauschke A, Frank C, et al. Dengue antibody prevalence in German travelers. *Emerg Infect Dis.* 2005;11:762.
105. Guzman MG, Kouri G, Bravo J, et al. Effect of age on outcome of secondary dengue 2 infections. *Int J Infect Dis.* 2002;6:118.
106. Cao XT, Ngo TN, Wills B, et al. Evaluation of the World Health Organization standard tourniquet test and a modified tourniquet test in the diagnosis of dengue infection in Viet Nam. *Trop Med Int Health.* 2002;7: 125.
107. Wills BA, Oragui EE, Dung NM, et al. Size and charge characteristics of the protein leak in dengue shock syndrome. *J Infect Dis.* 2004;190: 810.
108. Potasman I, Srugo I, Schwartz E. Dengue seroconversion among Israeli travelers to tropical countries. *Emerg Infect Dis.* 1999;5:824.
109. Cobelens FG, Groen J, Osterhaus AD, et al. Incidence and risk factors of probable dengue virus infection among Dutch travellers to Asia. *Trop Med Int Health.* 2002;7:331.
110. Ooi EE, Goh KT, Gubler DJ. Dengue prevention and 35 years of vector control in Singapore. *Emerg Infect Dis.* 2006;12:887.
111. Nimmannitya S. Dengue hemorrhagic fever: diagnosis and management. In: Gubler DJ, Kuno G, eds. *Dengue and Dengue Hemorrhagic Fever.* Oxford, UK: CABI Publishing; 1997:133.
112. Gubler DJ. *Aedes aegypti* and *Aedes aegypti*-borne disease control in the 1990s: top down or bottom up. Charles Franklin Craig Lecture. *Am J Trop Med Hyg.* 1989;40:571.
113. UNAIDS. 2004 report on the global AIDS epidemic: 4th global report. http://unaids.org/bangkok2004/reprt.html. Accessed February 9, 2007.
114. Fauci AS, Touchette NA, Folkers GK. Emerging infectious diseases: a 10-year perspective from the National Institute of Allergy and Infectious Diseases. *Emerg Infect Dis.* 2005;11:519.
115. Centers for Disease Control and Prevention. HIV/AIDS surveillance report, 2005. Vol. 17. Atlanta, GA: U.S. Department of Health and Human Services, Centers for Disease Control and Prevention; 2006.
116. UNAIDS. AIDS epidemic update: special report on HIV/AIDS: December 2006. UNAIDS/World Health Organization. http://data.unaids.org/pub/EpiSlides/2007/2007_epiupdate_en.pdf. Accessed August 23, 2008.
117. World Health Organization. *Global tuberculosis control: surveillance, planning, financing: WHO report 2006.* Geneva, Switzerland: World Health Organization; WHO/HTM/TB/2006.362.
118. McDonald LC, Archibald LK, Rheanpumikankit S, et al. Unrecognised *Mycobacterium tuberculosis* bacteraemia among hospital inpatients in less developed countries. *Lancet.* 1999;354:1159.
119. Archibald LK, den Dulk MO, Pallangyo KJ, et al. Fatal *Mycobacterium tuberculosis* bloodstream infections in febrile hospitalized adults in Dar es Salaam, Tanzania. *Clin Infect Dis.* 1998;26:290.
120. Archibald LK, McDonald LC, Rheanpumikankit S, et al. Fever and human immunodeficiency virus infection as sentinels for emerging mycobacterial and fungal bloodstream infections in hospitalized patients >/=15 years old, Bangkok. *J Infect Dis.* 1999;177:87.
121. Archibald LK, McDonald LC, Nwanyanwu O, et al. A hospital-based prevalence survey of bloodstream infections in febrile patients in Malawi: implications for diagnosis and therapy. *J Infect Dis.* 2000;181:1414.
122. Bell M, Archibald LK, Nwanyanwu O, et al. Seasonal variation in the etiology of bloodstream infections in a febrile inpatient population in a developing country. *Int J Infect Dis.* 2001;5:63.
123. Ssali FN, Kamya MR, Wabwire-Mangen F, et al. A prospective study of community-acquired bloodstream infections among febrile adults admitted to Mulago Hospital in Kampala, Uganda. *J Acquir Immune Defic Syndr Hum Retrovirol.* 1998;19:484.
124. Centers for Disease Control and Prevention. Guidelines for preventing the transmission of *Mycobacterium tuberculosis* in health-care settings, 2005. *MMWR Morb Mortal Wkly Rep.* 2005; 54(RR-17):1.
125. Dooley SW, Jarvis WR, Martone WJ, et al. Multidrug-resistant tuberculosis. *Ann Intern Med.* 1992;117:257.
126. Pablos-Mendez A, Raviglione MC, Laszlo A, et al. Global surveillance for antituberculosis-drug resistance, 1994–1997. World Health Organization—International Union against Tuberculosis and Lung Disease Working Group on Anti-Tuberculosis Drug Resistance Surveillance. *N Engl J Med.* 1998;338:1641.
127. Centers for Disease Control and Prevention. Emergence of *Mycobacterium tuberculosis* with extensive resistance to second-line drugs—worldwide, 2000–2004. *MMWR Morb Mortal Wkly Rep.* 2006;55:301.
128. Gupta R, Kim JY, Espinal MA, et al. Public health. Responding to market failures in tuberculosis control. *Science.* 2001;293:1049.
129. World Health Organization. Extensively drug-resistant tuberculosis (XDR-TB): recommendations for prevention and control. *Wkly Epidemiol Rec.* 2006;81:430.
130. Jevons MP. Celbenin-resistant staphylococci. *BMJ.* 1961;1:124.
131. Boyce JM, Jackson MM, Pugliese G, et al. Methicillin-resistant *Staphylococcus aureus* (MRSA): a briefing for acute care hospitals and nursing facilities. The AHA Technical Panel on Infections within Hospitals. *Infect Control Hosp Epidemiol.* 1994;15:105.
132. Centers for Disease Control and Prevention. National Nosocomial Infections Surveillance (NNIS) system report, data summary from January 1992 through June 2003, issued August 2003. *Am J Infect Control.* 2003;31:481.
133. Klevens RM, Edwards JR, Tenover FC, et al. Changes in the epidemiology of methicillin-resistant *Staphylococcus aureus* in intensive care units in US hospitals, 1992-2003. *Clin Infect Dis.* 2006;42:389.
134. Tiemersma EW, Bronzwaer SL, Lyytikainen O, et al. Methicillin-resistant *Staphylococcus aureus* in Europe, 1999–2002. *Emerg Infect Dis.* 2004;10:1627.
135. Tiemersma EW, Monnet DL, Bruinsma N, et al. *Staphylococcus aureus* bacteremia, Europe. *Emerg Infect Dis.* 2005;11:1798.
136. Grundmann H, Aires-de-Sousa M, Boyce J, et al. Emergence and resurgence of methicillin-resistant *Staphylococcus aureus* as a public-health threat. *Lancet.* 2006;368:874.
137. Kuehnert MJ, Kruszon-Moran D, Hill HA, et al. Prevalence of *Staphylococcus aureus* nasal colonization in the United States, 2001–2002. *J Infect Dis.*2006;193:172.
138. Beretta AL, Trabasso P, Stucchi RB, et al. Use of molecular epidemiology to monitor the nosocomial dissemination of methicillin-resistant *Staphylococcus aureus* in a university hospital from 1991 to 2001. *Braz J Med Biol Res.* 2004;37:1345.
139. Hartman B, Tomasz A. Altered penicillin-binding proteins in methicillin-resistant strains of *Staphylococcus aureus. Antimicrob Agents Chemother.* 1981;19:726.
140. Oliveira DC, Tomasz A, de Lencastre H. Secrets of success of a human pathogen: molecular evolution of pandemic clones of methicillin-resistant *Staphylococcus aureus. Lancet Infect Dis.* 2002;2:177.
141. Marschall J, Muhlemann K. Duration of methicillin-resistant *Staphylococcus aureus* carriage, according to risk factors for acquisition. *Infect Control Hosp Epidemiol.* 2006;27:1206.
142. Troillet N, Carmeli Y, Samore MH, et al. Carriage of methicillin-resistant *Staphylococcus aureus* at hospital admission. *Infect Control Hosp Epidemiol.* 1998;19:181.

143. Lucet JC, Chevret S, Durand-Zaleski I, et al. Prevalence and risk factors for carriage of methicillin-resistant *Staphylococcus aureus* at admission to the intensive care unit: results of a multicenter study. *Arch Intern Med.* 2003;163:181.
144. Hidron AI, Kourbatova EV, Halvosa JS, et al. Risk factors for colonization with methicillin-resistant *Staphylococcus aureus* (MRSA) in patients admitted to an urban hospital: emergence of community-associated MRSA nasal carriage. *Clin Infect Dis.* 2005;41:159.
145. Kenner J, O'Connor T, Piantanida N, et al. Rates of carriage of methicillin-resistant and methicillin-susceptible *Staphylococcus aureus* in an outpatient population. *Infect Control Hosp Epidemiol.* 2003;24:439.
146. Huang SS, Yokoe DS, Hinrichsen VL, et al. Impact of routine intensive care unit surveillance cultures and resultant barrier precautions on hospital-wide methicillin-resistant *Staphylococcus aureus* bacteremia. *Clin Infect Dis.* 2006;43:971.
147. Huang SS, Platt R. Risk of methicillin-resistant *Staphylococcus aureus* infection after previous infection or colonization. *Clin Infect Dis.* 2003;36:281.
148. Mainous AG, III, Hueston WJ, Everett CJ, et al. Nasal carriage of *Staphylococcus aureus* and methicillin-resistant *S. aureus* in the United States, 2001–2002. *Ann Fam Med.* 2006;4:132.
149. Clancy M, Graepler A, Wilson M, et al. Active screening in high-risk units is an effective and cost-avoidant method to reduce the rate of methicillin-resistant *Staphylococcus aureus* infection in the hospital. *Infect Control Hosp Epidemiol.* 2006;27:1009.
150. Khoury J, Jones M, Grim A, et al. Eradication of methicillin-resistant *Staphylococcus aureus* from a neonatal intensive care unit by active surveillance and aggressive infection control measures. *Infect Control Hosp Epidemiol.* 2005;26:616.
151. Harbarth S, Masuet-Aumatell C, Schrenzel J, et al. Evaluation of rapid screening and preemptive contact isolation for detecting and controlling methicillin-resistant *Staphylococcus aureus* in critical care: an interventional cohort study. *Crit Care.* 2006;10:R25.
152. Huletsky A, Lebel P, Picard FJ, et al. Identification of methicillin-resistant *Staphylococcus aureus* carriage in less than 1 hour during a hospital surveillance program. *Clin Infect Dis.* 2005;40:976.
153. Jonas D, Speck M, Daschner FD, Grundmann H. Rapid PCR-based identification of methicillin-resistant *Staphylococcus aureus* from screening swabs. *J Clin Microbiol.* 2002;40:1821.
154. Struelens MJ. Rapid identification of methicillin-resistant *Staphylococcus aureus* (MRSA) and patient management. *Clin Microbiol Infect.* 2006; 12(Suppl 9):23.
155. Turnidge JD, Bell JM. Methicillin-resistant *Staphylococcus aureus* evolution in Australia over 35 years. *Microb Drug Resist.* 2000;6:223.
156. Levison ME, Fung S. Community-associated methicillin-resistant *Staphylococcus aureus*: reconsideration of therapeutic options. *Curr Infect Dis Rep.* 2006;8:23.
157. Cohen PR. Cutaneous community-acquired methicillin-resistant *Staphylococcus aureus* infection in participants of athletic activities. *South Med J.* 2005;98:596.
158. Nguyen DM, Mascola L, Brancoft E. Recurring methicillin-resistant *Staphylococcus aureus* infections in a football team. *Emerg Infect Dis.* 2005;11:526.
159. Kazakova SV, Hageman JC, Matava M, et al. A clone of methicillin-resistant *Staphylococcus aureus* among professional football players. *N Engl J Med.* 2005;352:468.
160. Begier EM, Frenette K, Barrett NL, et al. A high-morbidity outbreak of methicillin-resistant *Staphylococcus aureus* among players on a college football team, facilitated by cosmetic body shaving and turf burns. *Clin Infect Dis.* 2004;39:1446.
161. Lindenmayer JM, Schoenfeld S, O'Grady R, et al. Methicillin-resistant *Staphylococcus aureus* in a high school wrestling team and the surrounding community. *Arch Intern Med.* 1998;158:895.
162. Centers for Disease Control and Prevention. Community-associated methicillin-resistant *Staphylococcus aureus* infections in Pacific Islanders-Hawaii, 2001–2003. *MMWR Morb Mortal Wkly Rep.* 2004;53:767.
163. Centers for Disease Control and Prevention. Methicillin-resistant *Staphylococcus aureus* infections among competitive sports participants—Colorado, Indiana, Pennsylvania, and Los Angeles County, 2000–2003. *MMWR Morb Mortal Wkly Rep.* 2003;52:793.
164. Barr B, Felkner M, Diamond PM. High school athletic departments as sentinel surveillance sites for community-associated methicillin-resistant staphylococcal infections. *Tex Med.* 2006;102:56.
165. Elston DM. Community-acquired methicillin-resistant *Staphylococcus aureus. J Am Acad Dermatol.* 2007;56:1.
166. Voyich JM, Otto M, Mathema B, et al. Is Panton-Valentine leukocidin the major virulence determinant in community-associated methicillin-resistant *Staphylococcus aureus* disease? *J Infect Dis.* 2006;194:1761.
167. Seybold U, Kourbatova EV, Johnson JG, et al. Emergence of community-associated methicillin-resistant *Staphylococcus aureus* USA300 genotype as a major cause of health care-associated blood stream infections. *Clin Infect Dis.* 2006;42:647.
168. Robinson DA, Kearns AM, Holmes A, et al. Re-emergence of early pandemic *Staphylococcus aureus* as a community-acquired methicillin-resistant clone. *Lancet.* 2005;365:1256–1258.
169. King MD, Humphrey BJ, Wang YF, et al. Emergence of community-acquired methicillin-resistant *Staphylococcus aureus* USA 300 clone as the predominant cause of skin and soft-tissue infections. *Ann Intern Med.* 2006;144:309.
170. Miller LG, Perdreau-Remington F, Rieg G, et al. Necrotizing fasciitis caused by community-associated methicillin-resistant *Staphylococcus aureus* in Los Angeles. *N Engl J Med.* 2005;352:1445.
171. Drews TD, Temte JL, Fox BC. Community-associated methicillin-resistant *Staphylococcus aureus*: review of an emerging public health concern. *WMJ.* 2006;105:52.
172. Dehority W, Wang E, Vernon PS, et al. Community-associated methicillin-resistant *Staphylococcus aureus* necrotizing fasciitis in a neonate. *Pediatr Infect Dis J.* 2006;25:1080.
173. Frazee BW, Salz TO, Lambert L, Perdreau-Remington F. Fatal community-associated methicillin-resistant *Staphylococcus aureus* pneumonia in an immunocompetent young adult. *Ann Emerg Med.* 2005;46:401.
174. McAdams RM, Mazuchowski E, Ellis MW, et al. Necrotizing staphylococcal pneumonia in a neonate. *J Perinatol.* 2005;25:677.
175. Lu D, Holtom P. Community-acquired methicillin-resistant *Staphylococcus aureus*, a new player in sports medicine. *Curr Sports Med Rep.* 2005;4:265.
176. Muto CA, Jernigan JA, Ostrowsky BE, et al. SHEA guideline for preventing nosocomial transmission of multidrug-resistant strains of *Staphylococcus aureus* and enterococcus. *Infect Control Hosp Epidemiol.* 2003;24:362.
177. Larson EL. APIC guideline for handwashing and hand antisepsis in health care settings. *Am J Infect Control.* 1995;23:251.
178. Boyce JM, Pittet D. Guideline for hand hygiene in health-care settings: recommendations of the Healthcare Infection Control Practices Advisory Committee and the HICPAC/SHEA/APIC/IDSA Hand Hygiene Task Force. *Infect Control Hosp Epidemiol.* 2002;23(Suppl 12):S3.
179. Muto CA. Why are antibiotic-resistant nosocomial infections spiraling out of control? *Infect Control Hosp Epidemiol.* 2005;26:10.
180. Verhoef J, Beaujean D, Blok H, et al. A Dutch approach to methicillin-resistant *Staphylococcus aureus. Eur J Clin Microbiol Infect Dis.* 1999;18:461.
181. Salmenlinna S, Lyytikainen O, Kotilainen P, et al. Molecular epidemiology of methicillin-resistant *Staphylococcus aureus* in Finland. *Eur J Clin Microbiol Infect Dis.* 2000;19:101.
182. McGeer A. News in antimicrobial resistance: documenting the progress of pathogens. *Infect Control Hosp Epidemiol.* 2004;25:97.
183. Jernigan JA, Titus MG, Groschel DH, et al. Effectiveness of contact isolation during a hospital outbreak of methicillin-resistant *Staphylococcus aureus. Am J Epidemiol.* 1996;143:496.
184. Lucet JC, Paoletti X, Lolom I, et al. Successful long-term program for controlling methicillin-resistant *Staphylococcus aureus* in intensive care units. *Intensive Care Med.* 2005;31:1051.
185. Jernigan JA, Clemence MA, Stott GA, et al. Control of methicillin-resistant *Staphylococcus aureus* at a university hospital: one decade later. *Infect Control Hosp Epidemiol.* 1995;16:686.
186. Chaix C, Durand-Zaleski I, Alberti C, et al. Control of endemic methicillin-resistant *Staphylococcus aureus*: a cost-benefit analysis in an intensive care unit. *JAMA.* 1999;282:1745.
187. Papia G, Louie M, Tralla A, et al. Screening high-risk patients for methicillin-resistant *Staphylococcus aureus* on admission to the hospital: is it cost effective? *Infect Control Hosp Epidemiol.* 1999;20:473.
188. Vriens M, Blok H, Fluit A, et al. Costs associated with a strict policy to eradicate methicillin-resistant *Staphylococcus aureus* in a Dutch University Medical Center: a 10-year survey. *Eur J Clin Microbiol Infect Dis.* 2002; 21:782.
189. Karchmer TB, Durbin LJ, Simonton BM, et al. Cost-effectiveness of active surveillance cultures and contact/droplet precautions for control of methicillin-resistant *Staphylococcus aureus. J Hosp Infect.* 2002;51:126.

CHAPTER 178 ■ DISASTER RESPONSE

W. CRAIG FUGATE • DONALD R. SESSIONS

The response to major emergencies resulting from natural, technologic, biologic, or societal causes begins with preparation. For the purpose of this discussion, the term, *incidents*, will refer to unexpected occurrences, whereas *events* pertain to planned or foreseen activities. *Natural disasters* or incidents include exogenous events (hurricanes, floods, tornados) and endogenous events (volcanoes, earthquakes). *Biologic disaster* refers to events that present the potential to adversely affect the health of living organisms via the spread of disease by toxins or pathogenic organisms. *Technologic disasters* usually involve man-made infrastructures such as chemical plant explosions, mining accidents, or train derailments resulting in the spill and/or release of hazardous cargo. *Societal disasters* generally refer to incidents involving crime or civil disorder, terrorism, and/or war. They are often precipitated by a group, community, culture, or region's inability to meet the needs of its citizens. Although disasters themselves may be accompanied by outbreaks of civil unrest, societal disasters are usually a form of protest against current sociopolitical issues.

The vulnerabilities of a given geographic area must be identified and contingency plans developed. This type of planning is designed to address potential or forecasted consequences that may occur associated with specific hazard(s). Awareness of the potential for one type of hazard to become the catalyst for related emergencies that, collectively, may become a catastrophic incident is paramount.

Within the United States, assessment of the potential for natural disaster identifies the West Coast as having the highest probability for catastrophic seismic disturbances, mudslides, and wildfire. The entire Gulf and Eastern coastlines maintain the potential for experiencing the effects of hurricanes, wildfire, and tropical storms. Although not limited to this area by any means, the Midwest hosts a geographic environment conducive to the spawning of tornados associated with severe weather. Obviously, northern areas of the United States have experienced cold weather events such as blizzards and ice storms. Phenomena such as these are, of course, seen in our sister countries. For example, over the past several years, there have been severe flooding and mudslides in Switzerland, Germany, Austria, Moldova, Slovenia, Romania, and Bulgaria (2005) (1); extreme temperatures with attributable deaths in France (2003) as well as other parts of Europe (2); and the effects of the Indian Ocean tsunami in December of 2004 (3).

Although the potential for technologic, environmental, societal, and biologic-related disasters may be assessed as presenting a higher or lower probability for occurrence in specific areas, there are no areas truly free from the risk of these hazards.

Although in the United States it is recognized that all disasters fall under the immediate command and control of the local authority having jurisdiction in the area of the incident, a framework does exist for accessing additional resources through regional mutual aid agreements, and through state and federal assistance. The reality, however, is—and this is a critical issue—that at times, requested resources may take 3 to 5 days to initiate field operations in the disaster area and, depending on the type and severity of the event, the requested resources may have been affected by the same disaster. Thus, the need to identify regional resources and develop and review contingency plans, as well as being willing and able to anticipate consequences associated with various disasters, is of utmost importance to the disaster response planner/manager.

For the purpose of emergency response, a *disaster* is basically defined as an incident that either immediately overwhelms, or is expected to exhaust, available community resources. The goals of emergency management are to stop the loss, meet the needs of the disaster survivors, support the responders, and aid in moving from a mode of emergency response to that of recovery. To meet these goals, the basic planning components for managing a disaster are as follows:

- Identify the type of incident.
- Identify the areas of vulnerability.
- Be aware of the forecasted occurrence rate.
- Be ready for the anticipated consequences.

These will be discussed in detail below.

ISSUES TO CONSIDER WHEN EVALUATING AND RESPONDING TO A DISASTER

Disaster Behavioral Health

In disaster situations, survivors experience emotions such as feelings of being at risk of death, in fear or panic, helplessness, despair, and depression associated with separation from loved ones. Efforts to relocate these individuals to safety if possible; calm their fears; rebuild their sense of safety, community, and self-sufficiency, which aids in rekindling hope; provide for their basic needs; and attempt to reunite them with family will aid in beginning the emotional recovery process. Behavioral health issues, including depression, fear, anxiety, and feelings of separation, can occur for days, weeks, months, and in some cases, years. Having a finger on the pulse of the community will allow the responders to gauge the requirement for specialized mental health services to address the needs of the surviving population.

In general terms, disasters often bring out the best and worst in human nature. Episodes of civil disorder often occur as a result of some type of triggering issue, be it economic, political, or related to a volatile community. Although it may be possible, at times, to anticipate the potential for civil disorder in the setting of contentious political or economic events, such events may also be associated with any significant emergency that disrupts the infrastructure of a community. Early efforts to ensure restoration of the citizens' basic needs will go far to avoiding this consequence.

Jurisdictional Authority

Most emergency management personnel recognize and embrace the philosophy that all disasters are local. With this in mind, the need for communities and regional organizations to work together to ensure an appropriate jurisdictional response pending the arrival of state and/or federal resources should be obvious. A solid relationship between, and with, local emergency managers not only results in acquiring knowledge of the community's capabilities and established contingency plans, but also presents stakeholders (fire departments, emergency medical services, law enforcement, public health, educational institutions, and so on) the opportunity to integrate into the local emergency planning process. It is precisely the collaboration and focusing of local and regional organizations on the "big picture" of disaster management that underscores the need for the proactive organization and early activation, of the emergency operations center (EOC) to support the community and emergency responders.

The efforts coordinated by an EOC to manage the overall disaster response will benefit from the preparatory work accomplished through community contingency planning. Areas addressed through these plans should include, but not be limited to, continuity of operation of critical facilities, mass casualty care, provision of food and water, care for persons with special needs, resource support, and utilities and energy supply. Because of the potential for disruption in the normal supply chain, personnel assigned logistic support responsibilities should be involved in all contingency planning discussions to ensure that supplies anticipated to be needed immediately are identified in advance, and are either on hand or accessible to support critical facilities.

Critical facilities are defined as those whose function and operations are essential to the needs of the community. Included within this designation are hospitals, law enforcement, fire stations, emergency medical services, public health departments, emergency management, communications, utilities, and their supporting organizations. Within each critical facility or support organization, efforts to establish and practice the National Incident Management System (NIMS)-compatible command and control procedures are key to enabling a coordinated local/ state/federal response.

Along with comprehensive emergency management plans, there should be specific operational guidelines outlining the steps required to rapidly return a critical facility to its operational capability following an adverse event related to the impact of a disaster. These types of plans are referred to as *continuity of operations plans* (COOP) (4). Within this plan, information outlining an agency's mission, essential functions, delegations of authority, lines of succession, employee specialized skills, emergency contact information, and basic procedural guidelines for re-establishing operational control of the organization at a secondary location are addressed.

Along with emergency planning, response and recovery programs, and/or continuity of operations planning, efforts directed to ensure the welfare of employees* required to remain at a given facility in support of operations, must be addressed (5). In addition, the identification of safe routes of travel for employees summoned to work during times of community emergencies must be addressed; this becomes extremely critical during concurrent communitywide evacuation directives. Finally, managers of personnel required for incident response and/or support should encourage their employees to complete family planning checklists (6), ensuring their availability to respond in times of need.

Through communication with local emergency management personnel, exploration of the community's resources, and capabilities of the jurisdiction's first-response personnel, construction of appropriate contingency plans and procedures may be performed in advance of a disaster and made available for implementation when the need arises. For example, many large metropolitan areas maintain first responders trained to handle emergencies involving building collapse, trench collapse, confined space rescue, elevated rescue, heavy vehicle and machinery extrication, and hazardous materials. In the absence of these resources, specialty teams may need to be summoned to respond and address incidents involving the need for these types of services. Although many states in the United States possess resources with various levels of response capability, federal urban search and rescue teams are available to support local needs through a Governor's declaration of a state of emergency and subsequent request of federal resources.

Under the Federal Stafford Act (Robert T. Stafford Disaster Relief and Emergency Management Assistant Act, Public Law 93-288, as amended), only the state governor may request federal assistance through the president. With this declaration, channels are open to localities to receive the many types of specialty teams and resources available through state and federal emergency management authorities. Several examples of specialty resources listed within the national response framework (7) are found in Table 178.1.

An active, factual, and rational public education campaign promoting citizen disaster preparedness is critical to ensuring that citizens are best prepared to survive the adverse impact of a disaster on the community.

Resource Typing

Common terminology relating to resource needs is essential to ensuring that emergency managers receive the proper "tool" for the task at hand. A resource typing system (8) database has been included within the framework of the National Incident Management System (NIMS) for this specific purpose. Groups representing specialists from emergency management, emergency medical services (EMS), fire and hazardous materials, law enforcement, health and medical services, public works, search and rescue, and animal health at local, state, and federal levels provide input for the construction of this list of accessible resources.

*For example, what might the response be of (EMS) workers who were expected to stay on the job during an epidemic outbreak of severe avian influenza if welfare of their families were not considered?

TABLE 178.1

EXAMPLES OF SPECIALTY RESOURCES LISTED WITHIN THE NATIONAL RESPONSE FRAMEWORK

Damage assessment teams
Urban search and rescue teams (USAR)
Disaster medical assistance teams (DMAT)
Disaster mortician assistance teams (DMAT)
Incident management teams (IMT)
Military and National Guard units
Nuclear incident response teams (NIRT)
Veterinarian medical assistant teams (VMATs)
National medical response teams (NMRTs)
Domestic emergency response teams (DERTs)
Scientific and technologic advisory and response teams (START)
Domestic animal and wildlife emergency response teams and mitigation assessment teams

Data from Department of Homeland Security. National response framework, p. 41, with permission. http://www.dhs.gov/xprepresp/committees/editorial_0566.shtm. Accessed April 18, 2007.

Within each category, numeric classification (typing) levels are assigned, indicating the general degree of capability that a given resource possesses, with type I being the greatest, followed by type II, type III, and so on. The specific capabilities each asset type offers—the number of personnel, type of apparatus, specific training levels, equipment, personal protective equipment, etc.—are addressed within each category.

The need to use common terminology becomes apparent when considering disaster response management on a global level. For example, when fire agencies in the eastern part of the United States have requested tanker support, they have, historically, received a truck capable of ferrying hundreds of gallons of water to the scene. On the other hand, when the same request is made by an agency on the West Coast, the result may be the deployment of an aircraft carrying thousands of gallons of fire retardant. Similar concern has arisen in EMS, where one area of the country requested a rescue unit and was provided an ambulance, whereas in a different geographic region the same request resulted in the provision of a nontransport unit equipped with extrication and basic medical equipment. Within the public works services, without capability and resource typing, a piece of heavy equipment might be requested and arrive being either too small or too large for the desired task. The requirement to specifically identify and relay the precise needs of those overseeing the response is critical to the cohesive overall management of the incident and deployment of available resources.

THE INCIDENT MANAGEMENT SYSTEM

In March, 2004, within the United States, Presidential Directive No. 5 (6) was promulgated that established the National Incident Management System (NIMS) (10) as the model for effectively commanding and controlling the response to significant emergencies or disasters. This model identifies organizational branches that an Incident Commander (IC) may employ to coordinate emergency response.

The Incident Command System (ICS) has been likened to a tool box containing the organizational tools that may be used to manage any incident regardless of the level of complexity or size. The IC maintains the responsibility of ensuring that all elements are addressed to achieve an effective response. Through the use of the ICS, an incident can be managed by a group of individuals overseeing resources within a reasonable span of control.

The NIMS may be used by any level of authority, be it the on-scene commander; a municipal, county, or state emergency manager; or federal agencies providing additional resources and assistance. In fact, the organizational concepts are not limited to the management of emergencies.

Incident Command Structure

Incident management involves basic functions required to oversee and coordinate the response to a major emergency event. The command structure begins with the IC and his or her general staff branches: operations, planning, finance, and logistics. The roles of each position and the manner in which delegated tasks may be organized are identified below.

Incident Commander

The IC is responsible for the overall coordination of resources and strategy to address the emergency event. The IC may also create command staff positions that could include the following:

- A *liaison officer* whose job is to aid in coordinating activities with outside agencies
- A *safety officer* who monitors and anticipates hazardous conditions or unsafe situations, developing and recommending measures for ensuring responder safety
- A *public information officer* who manages media responding to the event and, under direction from the IC, releases information regarding the event

Operations Branch

The operations branch is responsible for coordinating the tactics of the response elements so that the strategic initiatives are supported. Operating under the operations branch, one may find functional branches such as public works, health, fire, urban search and rescue, hazardous materials, and law enforcement. There may also be multijurisdictional branches such as local, state, or federal; or geographic branches such as Division 1/Division 2, or East/West.

Reporting to these branches of operations are the specific groups assembled to carry out the strategic initiatives established with the Incident Action Plan (IAP). Examples include, but are certainly not limited to, suppression, search, triage, treatment, surveillance, debris removal, perimeter control, and so on.

Planning Branch

As one might presume, the planning branch is responsible for developing the IAP, which uses incident-specific information in support of the IC's strategic initiatives. For example, the IAP may add detail to the IC's outline of goals and objectives

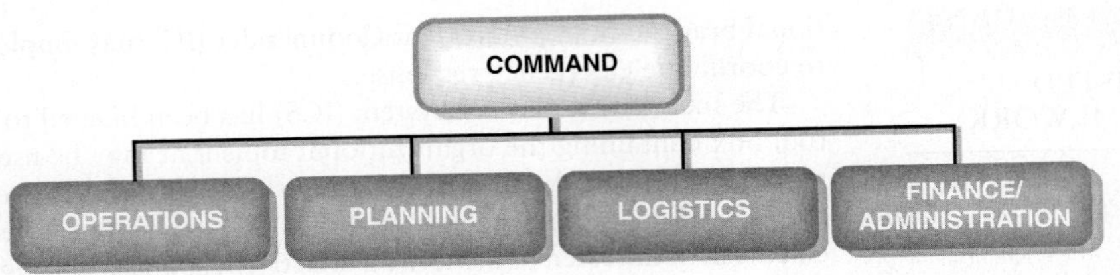

FIGURE 178.1. The basic incident command system (ICS) model. (From NIMSOnline.com. Basic ICS graphics, with permission. http://www.nimsonline.com/download_center/nims_ics_graphics.htm. Published October 1, 2004. Accessed April 18, 2007.

by analyzing damage assessment data, resource availability, weather conditions, etc. Reporting to the planning branch are functional groups, such as those listed below:

- The *resource unit*, which ensures that all assigned personnel and resources at an incident are categorized by capability and that their status is tracked
- The *situation unit* collects, processes, and organizes situation information, prepares situation summaries, forecasts, and develops projections of future events related to the incident
- The *demobilization unit* develops the demobilization plan, including specific instructions for all personnel and resources released from the incident
- The *documentation unit* maintains complete files of the incident, including a record of all important decisions taken to resolve the incident for legal, analytic, and historical purposes
- *Technical specialists* or subject matter experts may be required to provide technically specific information to aid mitigation efforts

The IAP is defined as a written† plan containing general objectives reflecting the overall strategy for management of the incident. It may include identification of operational resources and assignments, along with specific direction and key information for the management of the incident for one or more operational periods. Common examples of IAP components include the following:

- Incident name
- Operational period and mitigation strategy
- Identification of ICS organization
- Resources on scene
- Strike team or unit leaders and staff
- Communications plan and assignments
- Special instructions (weather, hazards, and so on)
- Plan author and approving authority

Finance Branch

This branch is responsible for the facilitation of contractual agreements and documentation of allocated resources to ensure reimbursement for supplies and services required to execute the IAP. Reporting to this group are functional groups such as the following:

- The *compensation claims unit* handles injury compensation and claims
- The *procurement unit* handles all financial matters pertaining to vendor contracts, identifies sources for equipment, and executes equipment rental agreements and supply contracts
- The *cost unit* maintains and provides cost analysis data for the incident
- The *time unit* is responsible for recording of personnel time of all relevant agencies

Logistics Branch

As one might expect from the name given this branch, it is responsible for the acquisition of needed equipment and supplies to support the IAP. This branch is essentially the backbone of the response, as the strategic initiatives are greatly dependent on having the necessary tools, supplies, equipment, and resources to implement the IAP. Reporting to this group may be functional groups such as the following:

- The *supply unit* is responsible for ordering, receiving, storing, and processing all incident-related resources, personnel, and supplies.
- The *ground support unit* is responsible for maintaining primary tactical apparatus and vehicles, fuel supplies, provision of transportation, usage documentation of all ground equipment, and development of the incident traffic plan.
- The *facilities unit* assembles, maintains and, ultimately, demobilizes all facilities used to support incident operations.
- The *communications unit* assembles and tests all communications equipment; operates the incident communications center; distributes, repairs, and recovers communications equipment assigned to incident personnel; and develops the incident communications plan for effective use of deployed communications equipment.
- The *medical unit* is responsible for development of the incident medical plan, identifying procedures for managing medical emergencies, and planning for continuity of medical care, including vaccinations, vector control, occupational health, prophylaxis, and mental health services for incident personnel.

The strength of the ICS is its expandability. Any incident, regardless of type, can be effectively managed by augmenting managerial and support positions as required. Although many day-to-day operations are managed with one IC absorbing all previously discussed roles, the ability to expand the management structure as an incident grows in size and/or complexity, while using a uniform system, is key to a successful outcome.

The basic ICS model identifying the IC and command staff is presented in Figure 178.1 (8), with an expanded operations multijurisdictional ICS model identifying the potential for build-out of managerial branches shown in Figure 178.2 (9). Included within the ICS framework is the ability to establish a

†The IAP may be oral in small incidents.

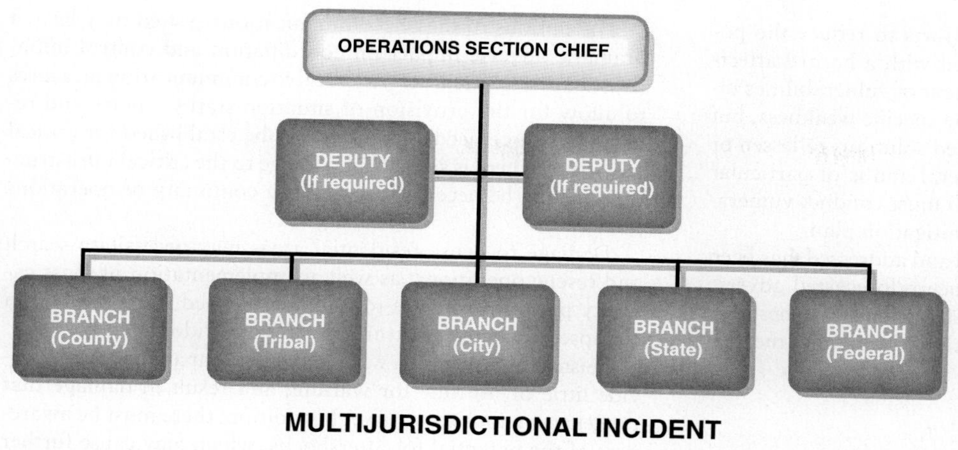

FIGURE 178.2. The expanded operations branch multijurisdictional incident command system (ICS) model. (From NIMSOnline.com. Expanded ICS graphics, with permission. http://www.nimsonline.com/download_center/nims_ics_graphics.htm. Published October 1, 2004. Accessed April 18, 2007.

unified command. The unified command structure allows for shifting of responsibility to seamlessly take place as the modes of managing the incident progress from crisis to consequence response.

Establishing a unified command involves managerial representatives from the various agencies, or "stakeholders," having significant involvement in the mitigation effort, being present at the command post to provide direct input to the IC. In the setting of a terrorist event, law enforcement officials may initially take the command position, as crisis management activities are paramount, with an eventual passing of command to fire rescue, public works, and/or health department managers for consequence management. Although there is only one IC in charge of the overall response at any given time, as the expertise needed to respond to a given phase of an event shifts, the type of IC required will change; with the ICS, such a handoff of responsibility is easily possible.

EMERGENCY MANAGEMENT

As previously mentioned, the main elements for managing an emergency or disaster begin with an analysis of the hazards that may affect a given area, the vulnerabilities that exist within that area, the frequency of occurrence of specific hazards, and the anticipated consequences of those hazards in the specific area.

Hazard Considerations

In preparation for the coordination of emergency response efforts relating to specific emergencies, the types of hazards that may occur in an area must be considered. These may include but are, of course, not limited to those listed in Table 178.2.

Any of these hazard types may affect a given area coinciding with the local events taking place, such as ongoing special ceremonies or celebrations, mass gatherings, major repairs or renovations to critical infrastructure, and/or localized supply shortages to note only a few possibilities. In other words, the emergency/disaster does not occur out of context, and that context consists of the actual conditions on the ground (at the site) where the event occurs. If, for example, the area infrastructure has been degraded by years of neglect, this element would alter the way the emergency/disaster plays out in the affected area.

Although each incident is unique in its presentation and development, there are common needs associated with all hazard types, which include, but are not limited to, the need for warning systems, communications, sheltering, management of the injured, provision of security, and debris removal.

Vulnerability Assessment

Vulnerability assessments should highlight a community's weaknesses in the context of specific hazards. Vulnerabilities may include communications and technologic systems, the lack of and need for hardening of critical facilities, flood- or storm surge–prone areas, special needs populations, security issues, operational policies and procedures, etc.

An assessment of a community's vulnerabilities in the face of a hazard—that is, an emergency/disaster—becomes the

TABLE 178.2

HAZARDOUS INCIDENTS THAT MAY REQUIRE EMERGENCY RESPONSE EFFORTS

Transportation incidents
Severe weather-related events
- Flooding and storms
- Hurricanes
- Mudslides
- Droughts

Earthquakes
Large urban fires (conflagrations) and wildfires
Communications systems disruptions
Power system disruptions
Civil disorders
Hazardous materials incidents
Maritime emergencies (oil spills and hazardous cargo)
Nuclear power plant emergency
Terrorism
Pandemic infections

blueprint for predisaster mitigation efforts to reduce the potential adverse consequences associated with a hazard affecting an identified vulnerability. Assessment of vulnerabilities involves not only the identification of the specific weakness, but also must include one or more suggested solutions to lessen or eliminate the risk. This is true in general and is of particular importance for critical facilities, which must conduct vulnerability assessments to determine their mitigation plan.

If the vulnerability, once recognized and addressed, has been dealt with properly, the identified concern/forecasted adverse consequence should be eliminated. Efforts such as these are geared to ensuring continuity of operations throughout the hazard's impact.

Frequency of Occurrence

There are geographic regions in any country more susceptible to specific hazards during specific times than are other areas. Each hazard must be evaluated in the context of the geographic and historical probability of its occurrence and/or reoccurrence.

Some basic assumptions apply to assessing the frequency of occurrence:

- Tropical systems with the potential to become hurricanes form in the Atlantic waters and the Gulf of Mexico between June 1 and November 30 of each year.
- Seasonal weather events are the primary cause associated with floods.
- Seismic disturbances may occur at any moment, often with little or no warning.
- Each day, hundreds of thousands of gallons and/or pounds of potentially hazardous materials are transported through communities via road, sea, air, and railways.

When assessing the likelihood of occurrence of an incident, many data sources exist in local, state, or federal emergency response records or archived weather data, which will allow the statistical quantification of the risk of any given area that may experience a specific hazard. Comparisons may be drawn with other geographic areas possessing similar characteristics—the hypothesis being, if it happened there, why not here? In contingency planning, the viewpoint is not that it has not happened here, but rather, that it has not happened here *yet*. Notwithstanding this apparent truism, planning efforts should be greatest in preparation for incidents having the highest potential of occurrence in a given area, with emphasis on the consequences that are expected to occur.

Consequences of the Hazard

Associated with any hazard exposure is the potential for consequences to an area or jurisdiction. Although these consequences may be unique to a specific type of hazard, more often there are common consequences seen in all disasters regardless of the specific type. For example, a tornado touchdown, hurricane landfall, ice storm, or other severe weather incidents may all result in power outages, disruptions in communications systems, injuries, and debris removal, as well as the mandate to provide citizens with shelter and immediate basic needs.

Disruptions to the telecommunications system may have a dramatic adverse impact on coordination and control initiatives for critical facilities. Alternative communication measures to allow for the provision of situation status reports and relaying resource needs requests must be established for critical facilities. If there is significant damage to the critical infrastructure, it may be necessary to activate continuity of operations plans.

Damage to dense residential areas may necessitate search and rescue operations, as well as implementation of mass casualty plans in response to multiple trapped survivors within collapsed structures or transportation corridors.

Seismic disturbances, which may occur at any moment, provide little or no time for warning and result in damage that ranges from none to massive. In addition, there must be awareness of the potential for aftershocks, which may cause further damage to compromised or collapsed structures where rescue operations may be underway or may affect locations used for mass care and shelter. Geologic disturbances may also trigger associated events such as a tsunami, the most recently seen in Thailand in December of 2004. In deep bodies of water, waves spawned by a precipitating event, such as an earthquake, may travel at speeds over 600 miles per hour and rise to as high as 50 to 100 feet when approaching the coastal shallows (13). With advance warning, citizens can seek high ground and take other protective actions.

Tropical storm systems are usually seasonal and divided into three categories based on sustained wind speed.

- *Tropical depressions*: Sustained winds up to 38 miles per hour
- *Tropical storms*: Sustained winds between 39 and 73 miles per hour
- *Hurricanes*: Sustained winds above 74 miles per hour

Winds associated with a major hurricane and/or tornadoes occurring before, during, and immediately after the hurricane threat has passed can destroy mobile homes, damage or destroy buildings and trees, and disrupt electrical and gas utilities. Similar consequences are also associated with earthquakes, floods, and wildfire. Slower-moving storms generally produce the greatest rainfall totals (14).

Contingency and emergency plans should take into account areas vulnerable to flooding and identify evacuation routes for citizens, as well as transportation corridors for the delivery of additional supplies. Environmental concerns may be associated with damaged infrastructure and/or contamination of potable water supply. There may also be a need to establish decontamination corridors at medical facilities not only for arriving survivors, but for support personnel as well.

Maritime accidents have the potential to become widespread disasters, as they may lead to hazardous materials spills that can potentially destroy a bay's ecosystem, fishing, tourism, and area industry. A recent example of such an incident is the 900 foot cargo ship *Cosco Busan*'s collision with one of the Bay Bridge support towers in San Francisco Bay, California. The collision caused a breach in the ship's hull, releasing approximately 58,000 gallons of fuel into the Bay, fouling 40 miles of shoreline from Oakland to Bolinas.

Major fires and wildfires present the potential to threaten life, adversely affect health, and destroy residential, commercial, industrial, agricultural, and specific critical infrastructure. For populations within the general area of a wildfire or major building fire, smoke can easily affect those with respiratory sensitivity who are not imminently threatened by the advancing flames. These types of incidents may also result in the release and/or spread of hazardous materials.

Hazardous materials may be released from their containers due to fire, severe weather, or road, rail, or marine transportation accidents. A significant release of hazardous materials may trigger mass evacuations, result in shelter-in-place directives, or a combination of both strategies. Long-term evacuations may involve providing citizens with shelter options and meeting basic needs.

Radiologic and nuclear jurisdictional consequences should be identified. Current estimates indicate that, in the United States, nearly 3 million people reside within 10 miles of an operating nuclear power plant. Local, state, and federal agencies maintain emergency response plans in the event of a nuclear plant emergency. These generally involve two emergency planning zones, one covering a 10-mile radius from the plant and the second expanded to a radius of 50 miles. Within the 10-mile radius, depending on the specific type of incident, individuals could be harmed through direct radiation exposure. By way of comparison, outside this initial zone and extending to a 50-mile radius, individuals could be subjected to radioactive contamination of food, water, crops, and livestock (15).

The effects of any disaster can either be minimized or exacerbated by the presence or absence of available energy supply within the impacted area. Energy is required for daily operations, such as the functioning of hospitals, police and fire stations, preservation of perishable food items and medications, lighting and transportation signaling devices, domestic fuel commerce, structural heating and cooling, lift stations to pump sewage, and water treatment and distribution systems.

Another risk requiring consideration, brought about through technologic enhancements in medical and nursing care, is the increased use of residential-stationed medical life support equipment—for example, a ventilator-dependent quadriplegic patient with a home ventilator. The identification of special needs populations within a community allows for the development of contingency plans to address specific requirements, be they special services, sheltering, provision of specialized medical care, priority power restoration, or general transportation. However, again we point out that only with appropriate preincident planning and resource stockpiling/designation will it be possible to properly care for these individuals. Hurricane Katrina, in 2005, highlighted the consequences of inadequate planning and resource availability in the face of a severe weather event.

Power and telecommunications outages may also disrupt all electronic forms of payments, such as debit and credit card payments. Customers and employees remaining in, or evacuating from, affected areas may need unexpectedly large amounts of cash to pay for critical goods or services or to comply with evacuation orders.

Contingency plans, as previously noted, must include procedures and arrangements for ensuring the operation of facilities deemed critical to supporting the community. As an example, in anticipation of hurricanes or other disasters with advance warning, some financial institutions have included within their contingency plans guidelines for ordering large shipments of cash and enhanced security precautions prior to the expected onset of the hazard.

If generators are to be relied on to provide emergency power, procedures for a continued supply of fuel must be developed. Plans identifying additional supplies that are accessible through regional vendors and/or commercial trucking firms should involve memorandums of understanding, which *must* include backup procedures for ensuring the acquisition of critical supplies during worst case scenarios.

In summary, for each jurisdiction, identifying common consequences experienced by the community via an assessment of various hazards will aid in the construction of an all-hazards comprehensive emergency management plan. Every emergency involves, to some degree, the need for public warning or information systems, communications capability, sheltering provisions, management capability for the injured, ensuring security, and debris removal. Thus there is much that can be standardized in the planning and preparation for these disparate occurrences. Emergency managers must focus on the primary rules for dealing with disasters, which will enable them to minimize losses and steer the incident from a response mode to the recovery mode. Efforts to pursue predisaster mitigation projects to lessen, or eliminate, the consequences of an event or hazard should be part of all strategic planning sessions and discussions.

RULES FOR MANAGING DISASTER RESPONSE

The Incident Commander should use the concept of unified command in which there is one plan and one team working collectively—and using the same rules—in pursuit of the same common set of goals.

The primary rules for dealing with a forecasted or real-time disaster include the following:

- *Meet the needs of the disaster survivors.*
  Those responsible for managing any emergency will benefit greatly from monitoring the needs of those for whom they are attempting to provide direct services, as well as the needs of their responders. The requirement to engage in an ongoing needs analysis is paramount and must consider the following:
  - ☐ Basic medical and mental health support
  - ☐ Provision of food and water
  - ☐ Security presence
- *Meet the needs of the responders*
  If forward incident management teams—incident management planning groups traveling ahead of specific resources—have arrived and completed a preliminary damage assessment, and identified areas to be searched and staging and base of operations locations for responding resources, the following additional immediate needs should be recognized:
  - ☐ Security for staging, base of operations, and urban search and rescue (USAR) missions
  - ☐ Emergency fuel for equipment and apparatus
  - ☐ Sanitation facilities

Many specialty resources—for example, USAR teams—deploy into these areas with the capability to literally be self-sufficient for a specified period of time. Identification of any requested resource needs in advance will ease the burden on the logistics branch and ensure the ability of that specific resource to perform commensurate with its capability.

GOALS FOR MANAGING DISASTER RESPONSE

The responsibility to manage any incident begins with defining pre-established goals that will lead to the successful management of the emergency, resolution of consequences, and mitigation of the incident itself. The following basic goals outline the steps to surviving the first 72 hours of a disaster:

- *Establish communications with areas impacted.*
  Communication with the emergency operations center in the impacted area should occur within 1 hour. This includes the ability to speak with those overseeing emergency management in the impacted area, as well as being able to reach them physically. There may be times when, because of the level of damage and/or destruction of infrastructure, one is limited to verbal communication with those in the impacted area, and resources cannot get to those in need.
- *Secure the area.*
  Security in the impacted area must be such that the general safety of first responders and disaster workers can be reasonably ensured within the first 12 hours of the event. One of the most recent examples of situations that prevented emergency crews from deploying to target areas was seen associated with the response into some of the areas of New Orleans immediately after Hurricane Katrina. The need for establishing a secured presence also aids in calming surviving populations.
- *Search the area.*
  Within our State of Florida, the goal to complete search and rescue operations is set at 24 hours after crews are able to enter the impacted area(s). We point out that this is not a national or international goal—at least at this point—but should be considered for inclusion in any guidelines.

In trauma management, the term, the *golden hour*, has been used to identify the desired time frame for delivery of trauma survivors to an appropriate medical facility for surgical intervention. The activities involved in the management of the trauma victim must all be accomplished within the golden hour to allow the patient the best chance for survival. In disaster response, the first 24 hours identifies the *golden day*. Within this time frame, trapped and injured survivors must be accessed, treated, and relocated to appropriate facilities. The reality is that those surviving the first 24 hours without advanced life support and/or rescue services will generally be able to help meet their own needs in the following days.

For this reason, in forecasted hazards such as hurricanes, USAR assets are usually pre-positioned in hardened locations so they may advance to targeted areas as winds subside after the hurricane landfall. This practice affords the ability to initiate search and rescue operations within hours following the event. The trauma victim has to survive the golden hour to make it to intensive care. The comparison can be made that the disaster victim has to make it past the golden day to transition to recovery.

With more advanced technology, USAR crews are beginning to integrate the use of the U.S. national grid system (USNG), which establishes a nationally consistent map and spatial grid reference system. The ability to provide accurate mapping based on precise geopositioning allows for better deployment of resources to achieve rapid primary search and rescue. This system dramatically reduces the potential for duplicative efforts in covering targeted areas.

- *Meet basic human needs.*
  Private sector retailers are often the best resource in meeting most needs in the aftermath of disaster. Where retailers are unable to open due to damage or lack of resources, emergency managers will need to fill the gaps. Pre-positioned cargo transport vehicles containing caches of bottled water, ready-to-eat meals (MREs, or shelf-stable meals composed of both standard and special diet menus), and shelter supplies are extremely beneficial in maintaining a healthy mental outlook and behavior in disaster survivors. Following the restoration of primary communications, these supplies can be moved into impacted areas, providing aid and comfort to those in need. The basic human needs caches include the following:
  - ☐ Medical supplies
  - ☐ Water
  - ☐ Food (MREs)
  - ☐ Shelter
  - ☐ Emergency fuel
  - ☐ Ice—a distant sixth unless the temperature is excessively hot
- *Restore critical infrastructure.*
  The restoration of critical infrastructure is an intrinsic component clearly affecting the survivability of those involved in the incident. The benefits of moving quickly toward a recovery mode, regardless of the timeline for completion, will go a long way to ensuring citizens do not abandon the area. Once a community's population, or a portion of it, retreats and begins to rebuild their lives at alternate locations, they often opt not to return. Through an effective presence of security and observed efforts to restore critical infrastructure, chances of geographic abandonment by large portions of the affected community may be averted. Key elements of critical infrastructure include the following:
  - ☐ Communications
  - ☐ Roadways and primary access routes
  - ☐ Utilities and fuel depots
  - ☐ Sewer and water systems
  - ☐ Support for critical facilities:
    - Assistance to local governmental organizations
    - Assistance in implementing their continuity of operations plans

  Upon restoration of power and return to normal protocols for the delivery and sales of commodities, citizens may begin to assist in their own migration to the recovery mode. It is imperative during this time that public safety messages are released to the public outlining safety-related practices and hazards. They may include issues such as carbon monoxide safety, generator use, emergency fuel storage, downed power line safety, drinking water guidelines, and wildlife advisories.
- *Open schools and local business.*
  The return to normal activities for children and adults within the impacted area rekindles faith that the event is in transition and efforts to restore their community are underway. Additionally, keeping the schools open will ensure there are no gaps in attaining the educational objectives, that is, finishing the academic year.

Local businesses returning to normal operation is a matter of necessity both for the owners and the community. The longer local businesses remain inoperable, the smaller the chances for a prosperous return of the commercial infrastructure; without the re-establishment of businesses, the community cannot begin to return to a self-sustaining mode.

- *Begin the recovery.*
  The goal of stabilization after the incident should occur within the first 72 hours following impact. It must be apparent to onlookers and survivors that the pendulum is beginning to shift toward recovery.
  Stabilization includes the completion of search and rescue activities, provision of basic health and mental health services, and the transfer of patients requiring further treatment to appropriate medical facilities—that is, functioning hospitals, dialysis centers, nursing homes, and so forth. The establishment of an adequate supply of potable water for drinking, cooking, and basic sanitation needs, as well as sufficient shelter and feeding capability for those affected, should be accomplished. Arrangements for sustained emergency fuel supplies and power generating equipment should be in place to provide for the continued operation of critical and/or targeted facilities complementing ongoing recovery operations.

EMERGENCY SUPPORT FUNCTIONS

Emergency managers within emergency operations centers (EOC) use emergency support functions (ESF) to organize, coordinate, and support the overall response effort (16). The expansion or customization of these ESFs to meet a community's organizational needs is appropriate.

The intent associated with the grouping of ESFs is to enhance efficiency and reduce redundancy or duplication of efforts, allowing agencies to focus on their respective mission-essential functions. For example, if throughout a given jurisdiction, all vehicles of law enforcement, fire rescue, public works, and disaster support staff and generators powering critical facilities required fuel, it is more efficient to place one call to meet all needs rather than having each agency contract and compete for separate deliveries within the impacted area.

Although not limited to the following, the list below identifies ESFs used in the National Response Framework.

ESF 1: Transportation

This ESF is responsible for the coordination of the following:

- Federal and civil transportation support
- Transportation safety
- Restoration and recovery of transportation infrastructure
- Movement restrictions
- Damage and impact assessment

ESF 2: Communications

This ESF is responsible for the following:

- Coordination with telecommunications industry
- Restoration and repair of telecommunications infrastructure
- Protection, restoration, and sustainment of national cyber and information technology resources

ESF 3: Public Works and Engineering

This ESF is responsible for the following:

- Infrastructure protection and emergency repair
- Infrastructure restoration
- Engineering services and construction management
- Critical infrastructure liaison

ESF 4: Firefighting

This ESF is responsible for coordination of the following:

- Firefighting activities on federal lands
- Resource support to urban and rural firefighting operations

ESF 5: Emergency Management

This ESF is responsible for the following:

- Coordination of incident management efforts
- Issuance of mission assignments
- Resource and human capital
- Incident action planning
- Financial management

ESF 6: Mass Care, Housing, and Human Services

This ESF is responsible for coordinating the following:

- Mass care
- Disaster housing
- Human services

ESF 7: Resource Support

This ESF is responsible for functions including, but not limited to, the provision of facility space, office equipment, and supplies, and securing contracting services.

ESF 8: Public Health and Medical Services

ESF 8 is responsible for coordinating the following:

- Public health
- Medical services
- Mental health services
- Mortuary services

ESF 9: Urban Search and Rescue

This ESF's responsibilities include searching for, locating, and effecting the rescue of disaster survivors in urban, suburban, and rural environments.

ESF 10: Oil and Hazardous Materials Response

The responsibilities of ESF 10 include coordination of the following:

- Oil and hazardous materials (chemical, biologic, radiologic, and so on) response
- Environmental and short- and long-term clean-up

ESF 11: Agriculture and Natural Resources

Responsibilities for this ESF include the following:

- Nutrition assistance
- Animal and plant disease/pest response
- Food safety and security
- Natural and cultural resources and historic properties protection and restoration

ESF 12: Energy

This ESF is responsible for coordinating the following:

- Energy infrastructure assessment, repair, and restoration
- Energy industry utilities coordination
- Energy forecast

ESF 13: Public Safety and Security

The responsibilities of ESF 13 include the following:

- Facility and resource security
- Security planning and technical and resource assistance
- Public safety and security support
- Support to access, traffic, and crowd control

ESF 14: Long-Term Community Recovery and Mitigation

This ESF is responsible for the following:

- Social and economic community impact assessment
- Long-term community recovery assistance to states, local government, and the private sector
- Mitigation analysis and program implementation

ESF 15: External Affairs

The responsibilities of this ESF include the following:

- Emergency public information and protective action guidance
- Media and community relations
- Congressional and international affairs
- Tribal and insular affairs

THE NATIONAL RESPONSE FRAMEWORK

The goal of the National Response Framework (NRF) is generation of a template that all agencies, stakeholders, and response partners may use to effectively communicate, manage, and function in response to a catastrophic disaster.

The National Response Framework, as required by Presidential Homeland Security Directive (PSD) No. 5, establishes a uniform all-hazards approach to organizing the management and federal response to major disasters. The NRF is indicated for all incidents requiring a coordinated federal, state, local, tribal, private, and nongovernmental entity response. The National Incident Management System (NIMS) is the framework on which all communication, command, and control will occur to cohesively integrate requested federal resources by a given state.

The use of the Incident Command System (specifically NIMS) was established within PSD No. 5 and applies to all federal, state, local, tribal, private, and nongovernmental public service entities. Eligibility for the receipt of federal funding is contingent on each state's adoption of NIMS.

Training

Federal, state, local, tribal, private sector, and nongovernmental personnel with direct roles in emergency management or response must complete Incident Command System (ICS) and National Incident Management System (NIMS) training. Included within this targeted group are emergency services disciplines such as public health, hospitals, emergency medical services, fire service, law enforcement, and emergency management. Additionally, public works, utilities, and support and volunteer personnel all fall into this comprehensive response group.

The identified training levels, segregated by roles and responsibilities, are outlined below‡. Specific training opportunities may be accessed via the internet through the Federal Emergency Management Agency (FEMA) Incident Command System Resource Center or local emergency management.

‡Entry-level responders:

- FEMA IS-700; NIMS, An Introduction
- ICS-100; Introduction to the Incident Command System or equivalent

First-line, single resource, field supervisors:

- ICS-700; ICS-100; and ICS-200, Basic Incident Command System or equivalent

Middle management: strike team leaders, division supervisors, EOC staff, and so on:

- ICS-700; ICS-800, National Response Framework; ICS-100; ICS-200; and ICS-300

Command and general staff; area, emergency, and emergency operations center (EOC) managers:

- ICS-700; ICS-800, National Response Framework; ICS-100; ICS-200; ICS-300; and ICS-400

SUMMARY

Recognizing that our primary goals are saving lives, providing aid, and stopping the loss associated with natural disasters and/or catastrophic incidents, the unfortunate reality with many response efforts is that, even with the best funded and most competently led response, we are able to make an impacted area merely tolerable. It is only in the months to years following an event that recovery operations and efforts are directed at and—with luck, hard work, and adequate resources—able to restore the community to a predisaster status. If one considers the quality of life survivors had before the disaster, depending, of course, on the scale of the incident, it may be several years until the recovery mode is truly completed. Psychological trauma is often long-lasting not only for those surviving the disaster, but for those involved in the response as well. To date, there exist areas within South Florida that have still not returned to August 1992 pre-Hurricane Andrew status. As of mid-2007, no qualified dates have been released targeting the expected completion date for recovery efforts following Hurricane Katrina's landfall in late August of 2005.

Contingency planning, preparedness, and disaster mitigation efforts are critical elements that affect the overall management and response to disasters. Those placed in charge of managing specialty services must plan activities to ensure, at a minimum, that

- Critical and key personnel are available to respond in support of the emergency through the creation of family emergency plans and identified methods of emergency communication
- Vulnerabilities that exist are identified and either mitigated or have contingency plans associated with each issue to ensure continuity of operations
- An adequate supply of expendable supplies exists within the organization or is readily available through mutual aid agreements or contractual services
- A relationship exists with local emergency management agencies for the timely provision of situation status reports and for accessing additional supplies and/or resources
- Basic needs are available for personnel, including food, rest periods, security, housekeeping practices, and other protective measures, which enable response and support personnel to focus on their respective responsibilities during crisis periods
- Familiarization with basic principles of incident command, the National Incident Management System (NIMS), and the National Response Framework (NRP) is accomplished.

Failure to focus on the global picture of managing the overall response may end up narrowing one's view to issues that may appear significant but, in retrospect, were secondary to the primary goals. This can be equated to avoiding focus on an angulated arm fracture when managing the emergency care of the multisystem trauma patient. Akin to the airway, breathing, and circulation (ABCs) principles of basic life support, adhering to the three basic rules for disaster response management will keep the focus on the global picture:

Rule 1: Meet the needs of the disaster survivors.
Rule 2: Meet the needs of the responders.
Rule 3: See rule 1.

After any significant incident or disaster, the need for a thorough critique, identifying practices and procedures that had successful results, as well as those practices and procedures in need of modification for improvement, are critical elements in the path to preparation for the next response, then and the next response is *when*, not if.

References

1. Federal Emergency Management Agency. Continuity of operations programs. http://www.fema.gov.governmental/coop/index.shtm#0. Accessed April 18, 2007.
2. Federal Emergency Management Agency. Emergency management guide for business and industry. http://www.fema.gov/business/guide/index.shtm. Accessed April 18, 2007.
3. Federal Emergency Management Agency. Emergency planning and checklists. http://www.fema.gov/areyouready/emergency_planning.shtm. Accessed April 18, 2007.
4. Department of Homeland Security. National Response Plan, p. 41. http://www.dhs.gov/xprepresp/committees/editorial_0566.shtm. Accessed April 18, 2007.
5. NIMSOnline.com. Resource typing system. http://www.nimsonline.com/resource_typing_system/index.htm. Published October 1, 2004. Accessed April 27, 2007.
6. Department of Homeland Security. Presidential Directive No. 5. http://www.dhs.gov/xnews/releases/press_release_0105.shtm. Accessed April 18, 2007.
7. Federal Emergency Management Agency. National Incident Management System. http://www.fema.gov/emergency/nims/index.shtm. Accessed April 16, 2007.
8. NIMSOnline.com Published October 1, 2004. Basic ICS graphics. http://www.nimsonline.com/download_center/nims_ics_graphics.htm. Accessed April 18, 2007.
9. NIMSOnline.com. Expanded ICS graphics. http://www.nimsonline.com/download_center/nims_ics_graphics.htm. Published October 1, 2004. Accessed April 18, 2007.
10. National Oceanic and Atmospheric Association. West coast and Alaska tsunami warning center. http://wcatwc.arh.noaa.gov/subpage1.html. Accessed April 18, 2007.
11. National Hurricane Center. Hurricane flooding; a deadly inland danger. http://www.nws.noaa.gov/om/hurricane/pdfs/InlandFlooding.pdf. Accessed April 22, 2007.
12. United States Nuclear Regulatory Commission. Frequently asked questions about preparedness and response. http://www.nrc.gov/about-nrc/emerg-preparedness/faq.html. Accessed April 22, 2007.
13. Department of Homeland Security. National Response Plan, p. 12. http://www.dhs.gov/xprepresp/committees/editorial_0566.shtm. Accessed April 18, 2007.
14. BBC. Floods sweep across Switzerland. http://news.bbc.co.uk/2/hi/europe/4175944.stm#graphic. Published 23 August, 2005.
15. Bernard EN, Mofjeld HO, Titov VV, et al. Tsunami: scientific frontiers, mitigation, forecasting, and policy implications. *Proc Roy Soc London.* 2006;364(1845):1989–2007.
16. National Climatic Data Center. Global hazards/events. http://lwf.ncdc.noaa.gov/oa/climate/research/2003/aug/hazards.html. Published August 2003.

APPENDICES ■ CRITICAL CARE CATALOG

JOSEPH VARON, MD, FACP, FCCP, FCCM • SANTIAGO HERRERO, MD, FCCP

APPENDIX A: PREFIXES AND CONVERSIONS

TABLE A.1

METRIC PREFIXES

Multiple	Prefix	Abbreviation
10^{12}	tera-	T
10^{9}	giga-	G
10^{6}	mega-	M
10^{3}	kilo-	k
10	deca-	da
10^{-1}	deci-	d
10^{-2}	centi-	c
10^{-3}	milli-	m
10^{-6}	micro-	μ
10^{-9}	nano-	n
10^{-12}	pico-	p
10^{-15}	femto-	f
10^{-16}	atto-	a

TABLE A.2

FAHRENHEIT AND CELSIUS TEMPERATURE CONVERSIONS

Celsius scale (°C): Degree of Celsius (or centigrade) equals 1/100th of the difference in temperature of melting ice and boiling water at the atmospheric pressure of 760 mm Hg.

Fahrenheit scale (°F): The interval between freezing and boiling is divided into 180°.

°C = (5/9°F) – 32

°F = (9/5°C) + 32

°C	°F	°C	°F
45	113.0	32	89.6
44	111.2	31	87.8
43	109.4	30	86.0
42	107.6	29	84.2
41	105.8	28	82.4
40	104.0	27	80.6
39	102.2	26	78.8
38	100.4	25	77.0
37	98.6	24	75.2
36	96.8	23	73.4
35	95.0	22	71.6
34	93.2	21	69.8
33	91.4	20	68.0

APPENDIX B: DUBOIS BODY SURFACE AREA NOMOGRAM

Body surface area = ([Height in cm]$^{0.718}$) ([Weight in kg]$^{0.427}$) (74.49)

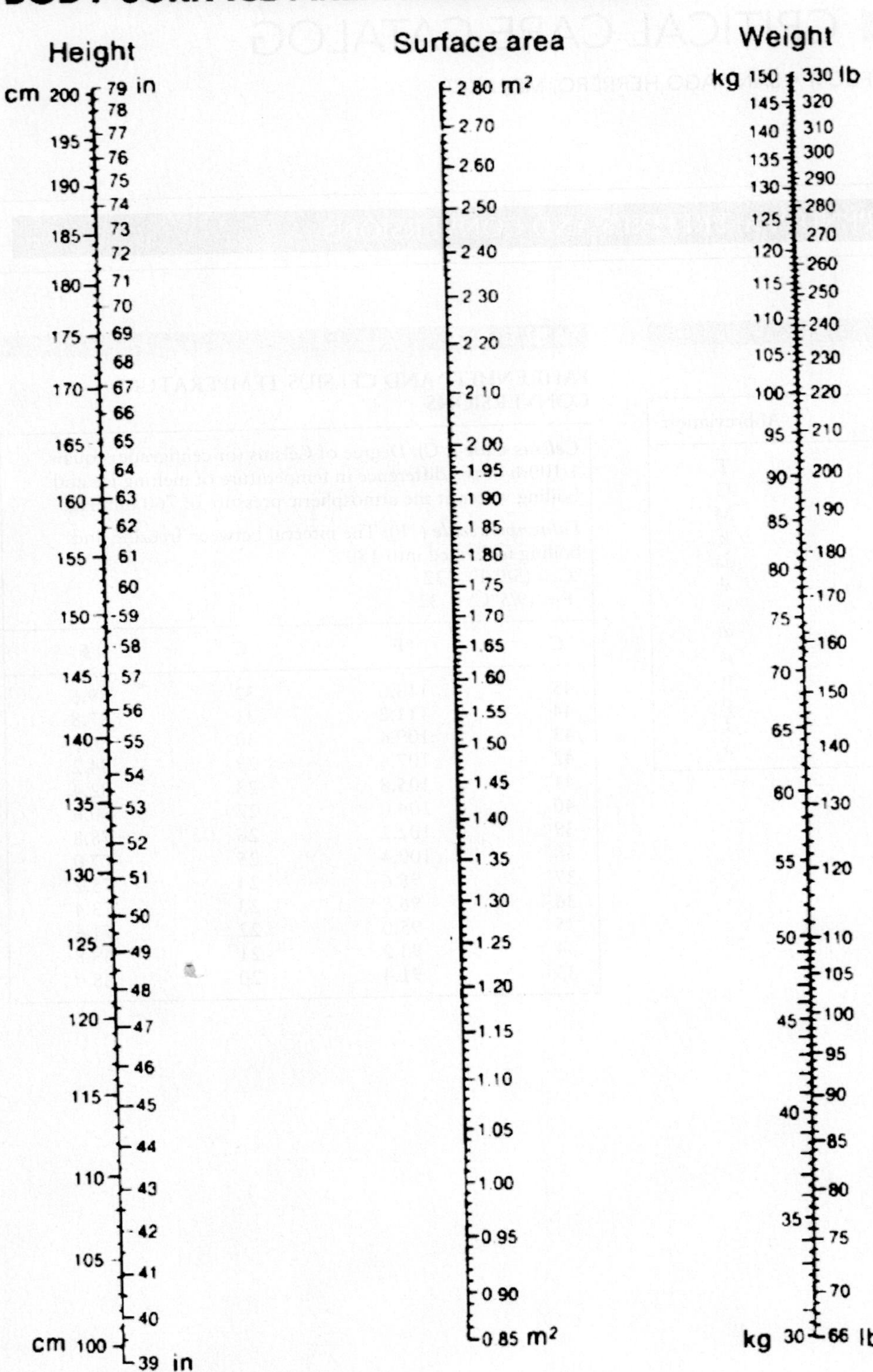

FIGURE B.1. Nomogram for determination of body surface area in adults. A straight edge is placed so that it connects the patient's height (*left column*) with his or her weight (*right column*) crossing the center column at the point indicating the body surface area. (From DuBois D, DuBois EF. A formula to estimate the approximate surface area if height and weight be known. *Arch Intern Med.* 1916;17:863, used by permission.)

APPENDIX C: FLUIDS AND ELECTROLYTES

TABLE C.1

INTRAVENOUS FLUIDS

Solution			Na	Cl	K	Ca	Mg	Acetate	Gluconate	Albumin	Lactate	Dextrose
Units	mOsm/L	pH	mmol/L			mg/dL				g/L		
5% Dextrose (D_5W)	250–253	5	—	—	—	—	—	—	—	—	—	50
0.45% NaCl (½ NS)	155	5–5.6	77	77	—	—	—	—	—	—	—	—
0.9% NaCl (NS)	308	5.7	154	154	—	—	—	—	—	—	—	—
0.45% NaCl + D_5W (D_5 ½ NS)	406	4–4.4	77	77	—	—	—	—	—	—	—	50
0.9% NaCl + D_5W (D_5NS)	561	4–4.4	154	154	—	—	—	—	—	—	—	50
Ringer solution	309	6	147	156	4	4–4.5	—	—	—	—	—	—
Lactated Ringer (LR)	275	6.7	130	109	4	3	—	—	—	—	28	—
5% Dextrose + lactated Ringer (D_5LR)	525–530	4.7–5	130	109	4	3	—	—	—	—	28	50
Plasma protein fractions 5%	294	6.7–7.3	130–160	90	0–5	—	0–3	0–27	0–23	0–12.5	—	—
3% NaCl	1,026	5.8	513	513	—	—	—	—	—	—	—	—
5% NaCl	1,710	5–6	855	855	—	—	—	—	—	—	—	—
Mannitol 5%	275	6										
Mannitol 1.0%	550	6										
Mannitol 15%	825	6										
Mannitol 20%	7.100	6										
Mannitol 25%	1,375	6										
Fresh frozen plasma	31.0–33.0		7.68	76	3.2	3.2	8.2	—	—	—	—	—
Dextran–40 in NS	310	5–5.5	154	154	—	—	—	—	—	—	—	—
Dextran–70 in D_5W	287	3.5–7										50
5% Albumin	300	6.9	145	145						50		
25% Albumin		6.9	145	145						250		
Hydroxyethyl starch 6% (Hetastarch)	310	5.5	1.54	154								

Na, sodium; Cl, chloride; K, potassium; Ca, calcium; Mg, magnesium; D_5W, 5% dextrose in water; NaCl, sodium chloride; NS, normal saline.

TABLE C.2

ELECTROLYTE COMPOSITION OF VARIOUS BODY FLUIDS

Fluid (mMoL/L)	Na^+	K^+	Cl^-	HCO_3^-	Volume (L/d)
Saliva	30	20	35	15	1–1.5
Gastric fluid (pH <4)	60	10	90	—	2.5
Gastric fluid (pH >4)	100	10	100	—	2
Bile	145	5	110	40	1.5
Duodenum	140	5	80	50	—
Pancreas	140	5	75	90	0.7–1.0
Ileum	130	10	110	30	3.5
Cecum	80	20	50	20	—
Colon	60	30	40	20	—
Sweat	50	5	55	—	0–3
New ileostomy	130	20	110	30	0.5–2.0
Adapted ileostomy	50	5	30	25	0.4
Colostomy	50	10	40	20	0.3

OSMOLALITY

Calculated serum osmolality

$$= 2[Na^+] + \frac{[glucose]}{18} + \frac{[BUN]}{2.8} + \frac{[mannitol]}{18} + \frac{[EtOH]}{4.6} + \frac{[ethylene\ glycol]}{6.2} + \frac{[methanol]}{3.2}$$

[Normal 275–290 mmol/kg]

Osmolar gap =
Measured serum osmolality − Calculated serum osmolality
[0–5 mOsm/kg]

Sodium (Na^+)
Pseudohyponatremia with hyperglycemia
Each 100-mg/dL increase in serum glucose (above 100 mg/dL) decreases Na^+ by 1.6 mmol/L

Free water deficit in hypernatremia

$$= (0.6)\,(\text{body weight in kg})\left(\frac{[Na^+]}{140} - 1\right)$$

Free water excess in hyponatremia

$$= (0.6)\,(\text{body weight in kg})\left(1 - \frac{[Na^+]}{140}\right)$$

POTASSIUM (K^+)

$[K^+]$ increases 0.6 mmol/L for each 0.1-unit decrease in pH

APPENDIX D: ACID-BASE

TABLE D.1

ANTICIPATED CHANGES IN SIMPLE DISTURBANCES

Primary disorder	Primary	Secondary	Compensation	Limit	Net effect
Metabolic acidosis	↓ $[HCO_3]$	↓ $PaCO_2$	$\Delta\ PaCO_2 = 1.0–1.4 \times \delta\ [HCO_3]$	10 mm Hg	↑ $[H^+]$(↓ pH)
Metabolic alkalosis	↑ $[HCO_3]$	↑ $PaCO_2$	$\Delta\ PaCO_2 = 0.5–1.0 \times \delta\ [HCO_3]$	55 mm Hg No hypoxia	↓ $[H^+]$(↑ pH)
Respiratory acidosis	↑ $PaCO_2$	↑ $[HCO_3]$	Acute: $\Delta\ [H^+]\ 0.75\ \delta\ PaCO_2$ $\Delta\ [HCO_3] = 1$ mmol/L ↑ /10 mm Hg ↑ $PaCO_2$ $\Delta\ [HCO_3] = 0.1 \times \delta\ PaCO_2$ Chronic: $\Delta\ [HCO_3] = 0.35 \times PaCO_2$ $\Delta\ [HCO_3] =$ mmol/L ↑ /10 mm Hg ↑ $PaCO_2$	30 mmol/L HCO_3 45 mmol/L HCO_3	↑ $[H^+]$(↓ pH)
Respiratory alkalosis	↓ $PaCO_2$	↓ $[HCO_3]$	Acute: $\Delta\ [HCO_3] = 0.2 \times \delta\ PaCO_2$ $\Delta\ [HCO_3] = 1$ mmol/L ↓ /10 mm Hg ↓ $PaCO_2$ $\Delta\ [H^+]\ 0.75\ \delta\ PaCO_2$ Chronic: $\Delta\ [HCO_3] = 0.5 \times \delta\ PaCO_2$ $\Delta\ [HCO_3] = 2–5$ mmol/L ↓ /10 mm Hg ↓ $PaCO_2$	18 mmol/L 12–15 mmol/L	↓ $[H^+]$(↑ pH)

CAUSES OF SIMPLE ACID-BASE DISTURBANCES

A. Metabolic acidosis
   1. Increased anion gap (usually decreased chloride)
      a. Acidosis
         1. Alcoholic ketoacidosis
         2. Diabetic ketoacidosis
         3. Starvation ketoacidosis
         4. Ethylene glycol ingestion
         5. Paraldehyde
         6. Methanol ingestion
         7. Lactic acidosis
         8. Uremic acidosis
         9. Hyperosmolar nonketotic coma
      b. Nonacidosis
         1. Hypokalemia
         2. Hypocalcemia
         3. Hypomagnesemia
         4. Hyperalbuminemia
         5. Nitrate usage
         6. Penicillin/carbenicillin
         7. Pseudohypernatremia
         8. Pseudohypochloremia
         9. False decrease in serum HCO_3^-
   2. Normal anion gap (usually increased chloride)
      a. Acidosis
         1. Carbonic anhydrase inhibitors
         2. Ureterosigmoidostomy
         3. Ileostomy
         4. Diarrhea
         5. Pancreatic fistula
         6. Parenteral nutrition
         7. Ingestion of NH_4Cl
         8. Ingestion of HCl or other acid
         9. Renal tubular acidosis
         10. Dilutional acidosis
         11. Following respiratory alkalosis
         12. Cholestyramine
         13. Normal saline infusions
      b. Nonacidosis
         1. Hyperkalemia
         2. Hypocalcemia
         3. Hypomagnesemia
         4. Hypoalbuminemia
         5. IgG
         6. Lithium
         7. Pseudohyponatremia
         8. Pseudohyperchloremia
         9. False increase in serum HCO_3^-

B. Metabolic alkalosis
   1. Loss of H^+
      a. Gastrointestinal loss
         1. Vomiting, nasogastric suction
         2. Antacids
         3. Chloride-depleting diarrhea
      b. Renal loss
         1. Diuretics

2. Excess mineralocorticoid
3. Postchronic hypercapnia
4. Decreased chloride intake
5. High-dose penicillins
6. Hypercalcemia

c. Intracellular H^+ shift
1. Hypokalemia
2. Refeeding

2. HCO_3^- retention
a. Massive transfusions
b. $NaHCO_3$ therapy
c. Milk-alkali syndrome

3. Volume contraction
a. Diuretics
b. Gastrointestinal losses in patients with achlorhydria
c. Sweat losses in cystic fibrosis

C. Respiratory acidosis
1. Central nervous system (CNS) depression
2. Chronic obstructive lung disease
3. Severe asthma
4. Pneumothorax
5. Abdominal distention
6. Pulmonary edema
7. Mechanical underventilation
8. Idiopathic hypoventilation
9. Neuromuscular disease

D. Respiratory alkalosis
1. Salicylate toxicity
2. Hepatic failure
3. Psychogenic hyperventilation
4. Pulmonary edema
5. Asthma
6. Systemic inflammatory response syndrome
7. Restrictive lung disease
8. Primary CNS disease
9. Mechanical overventilation
10. Hypoxemia

APPENDIX E: FORMULAS

CEREBRAL/NEUROLOGIC FORMULAS

Intracranial pressure (ICP)
[<20 cm H_2O, <15 mm Hg]

$$\text{Cerebral perfusion pressure (CPP)} = \text{MAP} - \text{ICP}$$

[70–100 mm Hg]

Cerebral vascular resistance (CVR)
[1.5–2.1 mm Hg/100 g/min/mL]

$$\text{Cerebral blood flow (CBF)} = \text{CPP/CVR}$$

[75 mL/100 g gray matter/min]
[45 mL/100 g white matter/min]

Jugular bulb saturation ($S_{jv}O_2$)
[55%–70%]

$$\text{Cerebral metabolic rate } (\text{CMRO}_2) = (\text{CBF})(\text{CaO}_2 - \text{C}_{jv}\text{O}_2)$$

[3–3.5 mL/100 g/min]

$$\text{Cerebral oxygen extraction} = \frac{\text{CMO}_2}{(\text{CBF})(\text{CaO}_2)} = \frac{\text{CaO}_2 - \text{C}_{jv}\text{O}_2}{\text{CaO}_2}$$

HEMODYNAMIC FORMULAS

$$\text{Pulse pressure} = \text{systolic BP} - \text{diastolic BP}$$

$$\text{Mean arterial pressure (MAP)} = \frac{\text{SBP} + 2(\text{DBP})}{3}$$

[70–105 mm Hg]

Central venous pressure (CVP)
[0–8 mm Hg]

Mean pulmonary artery pressure ($\overline{\text{PA}}$)
[10–20 mm Hg]

Pulmonary artery occlusion pressure (PAOP)
[4–12 mm Hg]

$$\text{Cardiac output (CO)} = \text{Stroke volume (SV)} \times \text{Heart rate (HR)}$$

[4–8 L/min]

$$\text{Cardiac index (CI)} = \frac{\text{CO}}{\text{BSA}}$$

[2.5–4.0 L/min/m^2]

$$\text{Pulmonary vascular resistance (PVR)} = \frac{(\overline{\text{PA}} - \text{PAOP})80}{\text{CO}}$$

[150–250 dyne/s/cm^{-5}]

$$\text{Pulmonary vascular resistance index (PVRI)} = \frac{(\overline{\text{PA}} - \text{PAOP})80}{\text{CI}}$$

[100–240 dyne/s/cm^{-5}/m^2]

$$\text{Systemic vascular resistance (SVR)} = \frac{(\text{MAP} - \text{CVP})80}{\text{CO}}$$

[800–1,200 dyne/s/cm^{-5}]

$$\text{Systemic vascular resistance index (SVRI)} = \frac{(\text{MAP} - \text{CVP})80}{\text{CI}}$$

[1,300–2,900 dyne/s/cm^{-5}/m^2]

$$\text{Stroke volume index (SVI)} = \frac{\text{CI}}{\text{HR}}$$

[40 ± 7 mL/beat/m^2]

Right ventricular stroke work index (RVSWI)

$$= SVI(\overline{PA} - CVP)(0.0136)$$

[6–10 g · meter/m^2 per beat]

Left ventricular stroke work index (LVSWI)

$$= SVI(MAP - PAOP)(0.0136)$$

[43–56 g · meter/m^2 per beat]

Arterial O_2 content (CaO_2) = O_2 combined with hemoglobin + O_2 dissolved in the plasma

[1 g Hb binds 1.36 mL O_2]

$$= (1.36)(Hb)(SaO_2) + 0.0031(PaO_2)$$

[20 mL O_2/dL]

Mixed venous O_2 saturation ($S\bar{v}O_2$)
[75%]

$$\text{Mixed venous } O_2 \text{ content } (C\bar{v}O_2) = (1.36)(Hb)(S\bar{v}O_2) + 0.0031(PvO_2)$$

[15 mL O_2/dL]

$$O_2 \text{ delivery } (\dot{D}O_2) = CO \times CaO_2 \times 10$$

[600–1,000 mL O_2/min]

$$\text{Oxygen delivery indexed } (DO_2I) = CI \times CaO_2 \times 10$$

[500–600 mL/min/m^2]

$$O_2 \text{ consumption } (\dot{V}O_2) = CI(CaO_2 - C\bar{v}O_2)$$

[110–150 mL/min/m^2]

$$O_2 \text{ extraction ratio} = \frac{(CaO_2 - C\bar{v}O_2)}{CaO_2}$$

[25%]

RESPIRATORY FORMULAS

Oxygenation

Fraction of inspired O_2 (FIO_2)
[0.21–1.0]

$$\text{Respiratory quotient } (R) = VCO_2 \text{ expired}/VO_2 \text{ inspired}$$

[Normal: 0.8]

Barometric pressure (PB)
[760 mm Hg at sea level]

Partial pressure of H_2O (PH_2O)
[47 mm Hg at 37°C]

$$\text{Partial pressure of inspired } O_2 \ (PIO_2) = FIO_2 \ (PB - PH_2O)$$

[150 mm Hg at sea level]

Partial pressure of alveolar O_2 (PAO_2) (alveolar gas equation)

$$PAO_2 = FIO_2\,(PB - PH_2O) - \frac{PaCO_2}{R}$$
$$= (FIO_2 \times 713) - (PaCO_2/0.8) \text{ (at sea level)}$$
$$= 150 - (PaCO_2/0.8) \text{(at sea level on room air)}$$

[Range: 100 mm Hg on room air; 673 mm Hg on 100% O_2]

Partial pressure of arterial O_2 (PaO_2)
[70–100 mm Hg]

Increased: hyperventilation, increased FIO_2, contaminated sample

Decreased: hypoventilation, decreased FIO_2, $\dot{V}/\dot{Q}$ mismatch, intrapulmonary or anatomic R → L shunt, diffusion abnormalities

$$\text{Alveolar–arterial } O_2 \text{ gradient } (P(A - a)O_2) = PAO_2 - PaO_2$$

[3–16 mm Hg on room air; 25–65 mm Hg on 100% O_2]

Ventilation

Partial pressure of arterial CO_2 ($PaCO_2$)
[46 mm Hg]

Partial pressure of alveolar (expired) CO_2 ($P\bar{E}CO_2$)

Dead-space ventilation (VD): Portion of VT that does not participate in gas exchange

$$VD = \text{anatomic dead space} + \text{physiologic dead space}$$

[150 mL]

Engelhoff modification of the Bohr formula for dead space

$$\frac{VD}{VT} = \frac{PaCO_2 - PECO_2}{PaCO_2}$$

$$\text{Minute ventilation (VE)} = \text{respiratory rate} \times VT$$

Pulmonary capillary blood O_2 content (CcO_2)

$$= 1.36\,(Hb)\,(SaO_2)\,(FIO_2) + 0.003\,(PBH_2O - PaCO_2)\,(FIO_2)$$

$$\text{Shunt fraction } (\dot{Q}s/\dot{Q}t) = \frac{CcO_2 - CaO_2}{CcO_2 - CvO_2}$$

Lung Volumes

Tidal volume (VT): Volume inspired/expired with each breath
[500 mL; 6–7 mL/kg lean body weight]

Inspiratory reserve volume (IRV): Maximal inspired volume end-tidal inspiration
[25% of vital capacity (VC)]

Inspiratory capacity (IC): Maximal volume inspired from resting expiratory level

$$IC = IRV + VT$$

[1–2.4 L]

Expiratory reserve volume (ERV): Maximal expired volume from end-tidal inspiration

[25% of vital capacity (VC)]

Residual volume (RV): Volume remaining in lungs after maximal expiration

[1–2.4 L]

Functional residual capacity (FRC): Volume remaining in lungs at end-tidal expiration

$$FRC = ERV + RV$$

[1.8–3.4 L]

Vital capacity (VC): Maximal volume expelled by forceful effort after maximal inspiration

$$VC = IRV + ERV + VT$$

[3–5 L; 50–60 mL/kg lean body weight in females; 70 mL/kg lean body weight in males]

Total lung capacity (TLC): Volume in lungs at end of maximal inspiration

$$TLC = VC + RV$$

[4–6 L]

LUNG MECHANICS

Plateau pressure (Pplat)
Peak inspiratory pressure (PIP)
Positive end-expiratory pressure (PEEP)

Compliance = change in volume/change in pressure

$$\text{Static compliance (Cst)} = \frac{VT}{\text{Pplat} - \text{PEEP}}$$

[70–160 mL/cm H_2O (paralyzed/anesthetized and supine)]

$$\text{Dynamic compliance (Cdyn)} = \frac{VT}{\text{PIP} - \text{PEEP}}$$

[50–80 mL/cm H_2O (paralyzed/anesthetized and supine)]

RENAL FORMULAS

$$\text{Creatinine clearance } (Cl_{Creat}) = \frac{(U_{Creat})(\text{urine volume})}{P_{Creat}}$$

Fractional excretion of sodium ($FeNa^+$)

$$= \frac{\text{urine } [Na^+]}{\text{plasma } [Na^+]} \times \frac{\text{plasma [creatinine]}}{\text{urine [creatinine]}} \times 100$$

Free water clearance

$$= \text{urine vol} - \frac{\text{urine osmolality}}{\text{plasma osmolality}} \times \text{urine vol}$$

TABLE E.1

DAILY RENAL EXCRETION OF CATIONS AND ANIONS IN NORMALS

Electrolyte	Urinary excretion (mmol/d)
CATIONS	
Na	127 ± 6
K	49 ± 2
Ca	4 ± 1
Mg	11 ± 1
NH_4	28 ± 2
Total	219 ± 3
ANIONS	
Cl	135 ± 5
SO_4	34 ± 1
PO_4	20 ± 1
Organic anions	29 ± 1
Total	221 ± 6

Na, sodium; K, potassium; Ca, calcium; Mg, magnesium; NH_4, ammonia; Cl, chloride; SO_4, sulfate; H_2PO_4, phosphate.
From Goldstein MB, Bear R, Richardson RMA, et al. The urine anion gap: a clinically useful index of ammonium excretion. *Am J Med Sci.* 1986;292:198, with permission.

TABLE E.2

USE OF URINE ELECTROLYTES

Diagnostic problem	Urinary value	Primary diagnostic possibilities
Volume depletion	Na = 0–10 mmol/L	Extrarenal sodium loss
	Na >10 mmol/L	Renal salt wasting or adrenal insufficiency
Acute oliguria	Na = 0–10 mmol/L	Prerenal azotemia
	Na >30 mmol/L	Acute tubular necrosis
Hyponatremia	Na = 0–10 mmol/L	Severe volume depletion, edematous
	Na >dietary intake	Inappropriate antidiuretic hormone secretion; adrenal insufficiency
Hypokalemia	K = 0–10 mmol/L	Extrarenal K loss
	K >10 mmol/L	Renal K loss
Metabolic alkalosis	Cl = 0–10 mmol/L	Cl-responsive alkalosis
	Cl = dietary intake	Cl-resistant alkalosis

Na, sodium; K, potassium; Cl, chloride.

TABLE E.3

INTERPRETATION OF URINE ELECTROLYTES

Electrolyte	Normal response	Patient response	Potential pitfalls
Na^+	Reflects diet and ECF volume; <10 mmol if ECF vol contracted	>20 mmol in ECF vol contraction suggests renal tubular damage	Diuretic use No reabsorbed anions Recent vomiting, drugs
Cl^-	Reflects diet and ECF volume; <10 mmol if ECF vol contracted	>20 mmol with ECF vol contraction suggests renal damage	Diuretic Diarrhea
K^+	Reflects diet, plasma [K], aldosterone action	If hypokalemia and urine [K] >20 mM or rate of K excretion >30 mmol/d then K excretion too high	K-sparing diuretics Low urine [Na] Water diuresis
pH	Depends on acid-base status Useful for bicarbonaturia	Useful once low NH_4^+ excretion confirmed to define cause of low NH_4^+	Unreliable for urine NH_4^+ Urinary tract infection
HCO_3^-	Depends on diet and acid-base status; >10 mM indicates HCO_3^- load 0 in acidemia	High urine HCO_3^- with chronic metabolic alkalosis indicates vomiting or HCO_3^- input High urine HCO_3 with acidemia in pRTA	Urinary tract infection Carbonic anhydrase inhibitors
(Na^+, K^+, Cl^-)	Depends on diet and acid-base status	Na + K > Cl = low urine NH_4^+ Cl > Na + K = high urine NH_4^+	Ketonuria Drug anions Alkaline urine

Na^+, sodium; Cl, chloride; K^+, potassium; HCO_3^-, carbonate; NH_4, ammonia; ECF, extracellular fluid; pRTA, partial renal tubular acidosis; vol, volume.
From Halperin ML, Goldstein MB. *Fluid, Electrolyte and Acid-Base Emergencies.* Philadelphia: WB Saunders; 1988, with permission.

TOXICOLOGY FORMULAS

Serum methanol concentration [MeOH] in mg/dL
$= 3.2(\text{Osm}_s - (2 \times [\text{Na}^+]) - ([\text{BUN}]/2.8) - ([\text{glucose}]/18) - ([\text{ETOH}]/4.6) - 10)$

Ethylene glycol concentration $= 6.2(\text{Osm}_s - (2 \times [\text{Na}^+]) - ([\text{BUN}]/2.8) - ([\text{glucose}]/18) - ([\text{EtOH}]/4.6) - 10)$

INFECTIOUS DISEASES FORMULAS

Antibiotic kinetics:

The *volume of distribution* (V_D) of an antimicrobial is calculated as:

$$V_D = \frac{A}{C_p}$$

where A = total amount of antibiotic in the body and C_p = antibiotic plasma concentration.

Repetitive dosing of antibiotics depends on the principle of *minimal plasma concentrations* (C_{min}):

$$C_{min} = \frac{D}{(V_D)(2^n - 1)}$$

where D = dose and n = dosing interval expressed in half-lives.

The *plasma concentration at steady state* (C_{ss}) of an antimicrobial can be estimated utilizing the following formula:

$$C_{ss} = \frac{\text{Dose per half-life}}{(0.693)(V_D)}$$

Antibiotic adjustments:
Renal dysfunction in critically ill patients is common. In those patients receiving aminoglycosides, dosage modification is required according to the *aminoglycoside clearance:*

$$\text{Aminoglycoside clearance} = (C_{cr})(0.6) + 10$$

where C_{cr} = creatinine clearance in mL/minute.

In order to estimate the *creatinine clearance*, the *Cockcrof and Gault formula* is utilized:

$$C_{cr}\,(\text{mL/min}) = \frac{(140 - \text{age}) \times \text{weight}}{\text{Cr} \times 72}$$

where Cr = serum creatinine in mg/dL. Another modification to this formula is the *Spyker and Guerrant method*:

$$C_{cr}\,(\text{mL/min}) = \frac{(140 - \text{age}) \times (1.03 - 0.053 \times \text{Cr})}{\text{Cr}}$$

APPENDIX F: PHARMACOLOGY

DRUG FORMULAS

Drug clearance $= V_d \times K_{el}$

Drug half-life $(T_{1/2}) = 0.693/K_{el}$

Drug elimination constant $(K_{el}) = \dfrac{\ln([\text{peak}]/[\text{trough}])}{t_{\text{peak}} - t_{\text{trough}}}$

Drug loading dose $= V_d \times [\text{target peak}]$

Drug dosing interval

$$= (-1/K_{el}) \times \ln([\text{desired trough}]/[\text{desired peak}]) + \text{infusion time (h)}$$

TABLE F.1

DRUG DOSAGE ADJUSTMENTS IN RENAL FAILURE

	Dose adjustment	GFR (mL/min)			Removed By	
		>50	10–50	<10	Hemodialysis	Peritoneal dialysis
Aminoglycosides						
Gentamicin	D	60–90	30–70	20–30	Yes	Yes
	I	8–12	12	24		
Tobramycin	D	60–90	30–70	20–30	Yes	Yes
	I	8–12	12	24		
Antifungals						
Amphotericin B	I	24	24	24–36	No	No
Flucytosine	I	6	12–24	24–48	Yes	Yes
Antituberculous						
Ethambutol	I	24	24–36	48	Yes	Yes
Isoniazid	D	100	100	66–75	Yes	Yes
Rifampin	I	None	None	None	No	No
Antivirals						
Acyclovir	I	8	24	48	Yes	—
Amantadine	I	12–24	48–72	168	No	No
Cephalosporins						
Cefamandole	I	6	6–8	8	Yes	—
Cefazolin	I	6	12	24–48	Yes	—
Cefotaxime	I	6–8	8–12	12–24	Yes	—
Cefoxitin	I	8	8–12	24–48	Yes	—
Cephalothin	I	6	6	8–12	Yes	Yes
Chloramphenicol	D	None	None	None	Yes	No
Clindamycin	D	None	None	None	No	No
Erythromycin	D	None	None	None	No	No
Metronidazole	I	8	8–12	12–24	Yes	No
Nitrofurantoin	D	100	Avoid	Avoid	Yes	—
Penicillins						
Amoxicillin	I	6	6–12	12–16	Yes	No
Ampicillin	I	6	6–12	12–16	Yes	No
Carbenicillin	I	8–12	12–24	24–48	Yes	Yes
Dicloxacillin	D	None	None	None	No	—
Nafcillin	D	None	None	None	No	—
PCN G	I	6–8	8–12	12–16	Yes	No
Piperacillin	I	4–6	6–8	8	Yes	—
Ticarcillin	I	8–12	12–24	24–28	Yes	Yes
Sulfas/trimethoprim						
Sulfamethoxazole	I	12	18	24	Yes	No
Trimethoprim	I	12	18	24	Yes	No
Tetracyclines						
Doxycycline	I	12	12–18	18–24	No	No
Minocycline	D	None	None	None	No	No
Vancomycin	I	24–72	72–240	240	No	No

(*continued*)

TABLE F.1

(CONTINUED)

	Dose adjustment	GFR (mL/min) >50	GFR (mL/min) 10–50	GFR (mL/min) <10	Removed by Hemodialysis	Removed by Peritoneal dialysis
Antihypertensives						
Atenolol	D	None	50	25	Yes	—
Captopril	D	None	None	50	Yes	—
Clonidine	D	None	None	50–75	No	—
Hydralazine	D	8	8	12–24	No	No
Methyldopa	I	6	9–18	12–24	Yes	Yes
Metoprolol	D	None	None	None	Yes	—
Minoxidil	D	None	None	None	Yes	
Nadolol	D	None	50	25	Yes	—
Nitroprusside	D	None	None	None	Yes	—
Prazosin	D	None	None	None	No	No
Propranolol	D	None	None	None	No	—
Antiarrhythmics						
Bretylium	D	None	25–50	Avoid	?	—
Disopyramide	I	None	12–24	24–40	Yes	—
Lidocaine	D	None	None	None	No	—
Procainamide	I	4	6–12	8–24	Yes	—
Quinidine	I	None	None	None	Yes	Yes
Calcium blockers						
Diltiazem	D	None	None	None	—	—
Nifedipine	D	None	None	None	—	—
Verapamil	D	None	None	None	No	—
Digoxin	D	100	25–75	10–25	No	No
	I	24	36	48		
H_2 bockers						
Cimetidine	D	800/d	600/d	400/d	No	No
Ranitidine	D	None	150/d	150/d	No	—
Nizatidine	D	None	150/d	150 qod	—	—
Famotidine	D	None	None	20/d or (40 qod)	—	—

GFR, glomerular filtration rate; PCN G, penicillin G; D, dosage reduction method of dosage adjustment; I, interval extension method of dosage adjustment; qod, every other day; H_2, histamine.
From Bennett WM, Aronoff GR, Golper TA, et al. *Drug Prescribing in Renal Failure*. Philadelphia: American College of Physicians; 1987, with permission.

DRUGS COMMONLY USED IN THE INTENSIVE CARE UNIT (IN ALPHABETICAL ORDER), EXCLUDING ANTIBIOTICS

Adenosine

a. Action: Slows atrioventricular (AV) nodal conduction; produces short-term (seconds) high-degree AV blockade
b. Indications: Antiarrhythmic; useful for diagnosing supraventricular tachycardias and effective for terminating reentrant AV tachyarrhythmias
c. Loading dose: 6- or 12-mg intravenous (IV) bolus followed with a rapid saline flush
d. Dose interval/infusion: Wait 1–2 min between doses; no continuous infusion
e. Comments: Give through central venous catheter; contraindicated in heart block; sick sinus syndrome (except if pacemaker present), ventricular arrhythmias

Alfentanil

a. Action: Potent opiate receptor ligand; produces decreases in heart rate; respiratory depressant; may produce skeletal muscle rigidity
b. Indications: Opioid analgesia
c. Loading dose: 5–150 μg/kg used, depending on additional anesthetic agents used; lower dose required in the elderly
d. Dose interval/infusion: Maintenance of anesthesia usually with 0.5–3.0 μg/kg/min
e. Comments: $^1/_5$ to $^1/_3$ as potent as fentanyl; more rapid onset of action with shorter duration than other opioids

Aminophylline

a. Action: Bronchodilator, improves diaphragm contractility; positive inotrope and chronotrope; natriuretic and diuretic
b. Indications: Bronchoconstriction
c. Loading dose: 5–6 mg/kg lean body weight over 20 min (if patient already taking aminophylline/theophylline then check level, begin infusion, and then adjust dose based on baseline value)

d. Dose interval/infusion: 0.2–0.8 mg/kg/min (use increased dosage with smokers; decreased dosage with the elderly, patients with heart or liver disease)
e. Comments: Produces increased irritability, agitation, tachycardia, arrhythmias, nausea, and vomiting

Amrinone/milrinone

a. Action: Inhibit cellular phosphodiesterase, producing extracellular to intracellular calcium shift; increased contractility but with arterial and venous dilatation
b. Indications: Positive inotrope
c. Loading dose: Amrinone 0.75–3.0 mg/kg over 2–3 min; milrinone 50 μg/kg over 10 min
d. Dose interval/infusion: Amrinone 5–10 μg/kg/min continuous infusion; milrinone 0.375–0.75 μg/kg/min
e. Comments: Synergistic with dobutamine (because of receptor down-regulation in congestive heart failure); hepatic metabolism; renal excretion; rapid onset of action; dose-related thrombocytopenia with prolonged use of amrinone

Atracurium

a. Action: Nondepolarizing neuromuscular blocker; minimal dose-dependent histamine (H_2) release; no vagal activity
b. Indications: Intermediate-acting neuromuscular blockade
c. Loading dose: 0.4–0.5 mg/kg intubating dose
d. Dose interval/infusion: 4–12 μg/kg/min continuous infusion
e. Comments: Titrate to effect in intensive care unit (ICU) patients (monitor with train-of-four testing); onset within 3–5 min; 25–35 min duration; 40–60 min recovery; no dose adjustment in hepatorenal dysfunction

Bumetanide

a. Action: Acts at loop of Henle to prevent chloride and sodium uptake; diuretic
b. Indications: Decreased urine output, mobilize edema fluid, pulmonary edema, treat hypercalcemia
c. Loading dose: 0.5–1.0 mg over 1–2 min
d. Dose interval/infusion: Repeat dose every 2–3 h; up to 10 mg/d
e. Comments: Observe for secondary electrolyte disturbances (hyponatremia, hypokalemia)

Calcium chloride/gluconate

a. Action: Required for wide variety of cellular functions
b. Indications: Ionized hypocalcemia; vasopressor; hypermagnesemia/hyperkalemia (stabilizes cell membrane); calcium channel blocker overdose
c. Loading dose: 90 mg Ca IV bolus (chloride: 1 g = 272 mg [13.6 mmol] Ca) (gluconate: 1 g = 90 mg [4.65 mmol] Ca)
d. Dose interval/infusion: 0.5–2.0 mg/h adjust to ionized calcium value
e. Comments: Monitor for hypercalcemia, hypophosphatemia, and decreased sensorium

Clonidine

a. Action: Central α_2-receptor agonist
b. Indications: Hypertension; withdrawal syndromes (opiates, nicotine); modulate sympathetic hyperactivity of closed head injury
c. Loading dose: 0.1 mg transdermal weekly (may require 2–3 d for response); for hypertensive urgencies use 0.2–0.3 mg orally every 20 min until target blood pressure is reached (maximum 0.9 mg)
d. Dose interval/infusion: Usually twice daily when taken orally, no intravenous formulation
e. Comments: Usual maximum dose 2.4 mg/d; rebound hypertension with acute withdrawal

dDAVP

a. Action: Synthetic vasopressin; decreased excretion of free water; increases factor VIII levels
b. Indications: Central (neurogenic) diabetes insipidus (DI); bleeding in patients with decreased factor VIII levels
c. Loading dose: 2–4 μg IV or subcutaneously (SQ) for DI; 0.3 μg/kg IV over 15–30 min for bleeding
d. Dose interval/infusion: Twice daily
e. Comments: Dose for central DI by following urine output/osmolarity and serum sodium/osmolarity

Diazepam

a. Action: Benzodiazepine
b. Indications: Sedation, anxiety, agitation; ethanol withdrawal; seizures
c. Loading dose: 5 mg
d. Dose interval/infusion: Begin at 5 mg/h and titrate to effect
e. Comments: Central nervous system (CNS) depression

Diltiazem

a. Action: Calcium channel blockade; negative inotrope and peripheral vasodilator; depresses sinoatrial (SA) and AV node
b. Indications: Hypertension, angina; rate control in atrial fibrillation/flutter
c. Loading dose: 0.25 mg/kg IV over 2 min
d. Dose interval/infusion: 5–15 mg/h
e. Comments: Maximum dose 360 mg/d

Dobutamine

a. Action: Positive inotrope, peripheral vasodilator, increases automaticity of SA node and enhances conduction through AV node and ventricles
b. Indications: Low cardiac output states, especially with increased systemic vascular resistance
c. Loading dose: 2.5–20.0 μg/kg/min
d. Dose interval/infusion: Titrate to effect
e. Comments: No dopaminergic effects on renal vessels; tachycardia may be a problem; contraindicated in idiopathic hypertrophic subaortic stenosis; tolerance may develop

Dopamine

a. Action: Dose-dependent vasopressor acting at multiple receptor sites
b. Indications: Hypotension; increases renal blood flow and subsequently urine output
c. Loading dose: None
d. Dose interval/infusion: Dopaminergic 0.5–2.0 μg/kg/min; β plus dopaminergic 2–10 μg/kg/min; α, β, and dopaminergic at >10 μg/kg/min
e. Comments: Tachycardia may be significant; necrosis at injection site with extravasation (treat with phentolamine)

Epinephrine

a. Action: α- and β-receptor agonist; vasopressor, positive inotrope and chronotrope; bronchodilatation; increased glycogenolysis

b. Indications: Bronchoconstriction; allergic reactions; advanced cardiac life support; refractory hypotension
c. Loading dose: 1-mg bolus IV
d. Dose interval/infusion: 1–4 μg/min titrated to effect
e. Comments: Increased myocardial oxygen consumption with arrhythmias and ischemia; hypertension; hyperglycemia; poor renal perfusion

Esmolol

a. Action: short-acting β-blockade ($\beta_1 > \beta_2$)
b. Indications: Supraventricular tachyarrhythmias; hypertension
c. Loading dose: 0.5–1.0 mg/kg over 1 min
d. Dose interval/infusion: 10–300 μg/kg/min
e. Comments: Hypotension; bradycardia; bronchospasm; may prolong neuromuscular blockade effects of succinylcholine; contraindicated in bradycardia, heart block, cardiogenic shock

Fentanyl

a. Action: Potent opiate receptor ligand; produces decreases in heart rate, blood pressure, and cardiac index; respiratory depressant; may produce skeletal muscle rigidity
b. Indications: Opioid analgesia
c. Loading dose: 1–3 μg/kg, depending on additional anesthetic agents used
d. Dose interval/infusion: 0.01–0.3 μg/kg/h
e. Comments: Approximately 100 times as potent as morphine; no histamine release

Flumazenil

a. Action: Benzodiazepine antagonist; acts centrally at benzodiazepine receptors
b. Indications: Complete or partial reversal of sedative effects of benzodiazepines; reversal effects occur within 1 min of intravenous dose
c. Loading dose: 0.2 mg IV over 15–30 s
d. Dose interval/infusion: Can repeat 0.2 mg every 60 s up to total dose of 1 mg; may use up to 3 mg in suspected benzodiazepine overdose; no continuous infusion
e. Comments: Effective reversal of benzodiazepine effects lasts 20 min, so repeated dosing with flumazenil may be necessary; liver metabolism

Furosemide

a. Action: Inhibits chloride and sodium reabsorption in ascending loop of Henle, producing a diuretic effect
b. Indications: Decreased urine output, acute oliguric renal failure, mobilize edema fluid, pulmonary edema, hypercalcemia
c. Loading dose: 10–200 mg, depending on the clinical situation
d. Dose interval/infusion: Begin at 5 mg/h and titrate to effect
e. Comments: Hepatic metabolism, renal excretion; up to 6 g/d has been given by continuous infusion; observe for electrolyte disturbances (hyponatremia, hypomagnesemia, hypokalemia)

Glucagon

a. Action: Increases glycogenolysis and gluconeogenesis producing hyperglycemia; increases lipolysis; positive inotrope; decreases gastrointestinal (GI) motility and secretions
b. Indications: Hypoglycemia; β-blocker and calcium channel blocker overdoses; hypotension
c. Loading dose: 0.5–1.0 mg SQ/IV/intramuscularly (IM)
d. Dose interval/infusion: Repeat loading dose every 15 min; 1–20 mg/h as continuous infusion
e. Comments: Hyperglycemia; tachycardia; hypokalemia

Haloperidol

a. Action: Dopaminergic blockade acting as an antipsychotic
b. Indications: Agitation; acute psychosis
c. Loading dose: 0.5–5.0 mg IV/IM
d. Dose interval/infusion: Can be given hourly; 1–20 mg/h as continuous infusion
e. Comments: Decrease dose in hepatic dysfunction; observe closely for dystonic reactions and sedative effects; α-blockade

Heparin

a. Action: Anticoagulant acting through antithrombin III complexes
b. Indications: Deep venous thrombosis (acute and prophylaxis); pulmonary embolism; acute myocardial infarction; hemodialysis; catheter patency
c. Loading dose: Wide variety, depending on clinical situation
d. Dose interval/infusion: Adjusted to desired anticoagulant effect, usually based on following serial activated partial thromboplastin time (aPTT)
e. Comments: Side effects include hemorrhage, thrombocytopenia, fever

H_2 blockers (cimetidine, famotidine, ranitidine)

a. Action: H_2 receptor competitive antagonist decreasing gastric acid secretion
b. Indications: Prophylaxis for stress ulcer GI bleeding, acute/chronic peptic ulcer disease, acid hypersecretory diseases, reflux disease
c. Loading dose for stress ulcer prophylaxis: Cimetidine 300 mg IV every 6 h; famotidine 20 mg IV every 12 h; ranitidine 50 mg IV every 8 h
d. Dose interval/infusion: Total daily dose divided into continuous infusion, may be placed in parenteral nutritional formulas
e. Comments: Adjust dose based on creatinine clearance

Isoproterenol

a. Action: Nonspecific β-agonist; positive inotrope and chronotrope; bronchodilator
b. Indications: Bronchoconstriction; symptomatic bradycardia; β-blocker overdose
c. Loading dose: 0.02–0.06 mg IV
d. Dose interval/infusion: 2–20 μg/min
e. Comments: Tachycardia; arrhythmias (torsade de pointes); myocardial ischemia; anxiety

Labetalol

a. Action: α_1- and nonspecific β-blocker
b. Indications: Hypertension
c. Loading dose: 5–20 mg IV
d. Dose interval/infusion: Boluses can be repeated every 5 min; continuous infusion of 1–2 mg/min titrated to effect
e. Comments: Observe for bronchospasm, bradycardia

Levosimendan

a. Action: Calcium sensitization for positive inotrope effect and activation of adenosine triphosphate (ATP)-dependent potassium channels for vasodilation and cardioprotective effect

b. Indication: Decompensated low-output heart failure (cardiac index <2.5 L/min/m^2 or pulmonary capillary wedge pressure [PCWP] >16 mm Hg or left ventricular ejection fraction [LVEF] <0.4)
c. Dose infusion/interval: Infusion 0.05–0.2 μg/kg/min for 24 h
d. Comments: Most common adverse reaction is headache and hypotension (both 5%); caution in renal, hepatic impairment, severe hypotension, severe tachycardia, history of torsades de pointes; correct hypovolemia

Lidocaine

a. Action: Antiarrhythmic and local anesthetic
b. Indications: Local anesthesia; ventricular arrhythmias; prophylaxis in acute myocardial infarction
c. Loading dose: 1.0–1.5 mg/kg bolus IV (maximum load, 3 mg/kg)
d. Dose interval/infusion: Bolus repeated in 20 min; 1–4 mg/min continuous infusion
e. Comments: Observe for metabolic acidosis, altered mental status (including seizures), and myocardial depression; hepatic metabolism; methemoglobinemia

Lorazepam

a. Action: Benzodiazepine
b. Indications: Agitation; seizures; supplemental sedation with neuromuscular blockade
c. Loading dose: 2-mg bolus IV
d. Dose interval/infusion: Begin at 1 mg/h and titrate to effect
e. Comments: CNS depression

Magnesium

a. Action: Coenzyme; muscular contractility; nerve conduction; membrane stabilization; antiseizure; inhibits uterine contractility
b. Indications: Hypomagnesemia; arrhythmias; pre-eclampsia and eclampsia
c. Loading dose: 1–4 g over 15 min (infuse over 4 h for treatment of asymptomatic hypomagnesemia)
d. Dose interval/infusion: Subsequent dosing based on desired clinical effect and serum levels
e. Comments: Observe for hypotension and heart block; respiratory and CNS depressant (primarily in patients with renal dysfunction)

Metocurine

a. Action: Nondepolarizing neuromuscular blocker; moderate H_2 release; some bradycardia
b. Indications: Long-acting neuromuscular blockade
c. Loading dose: 0.2–0.4 mg/kg for intubation
d. Dose interval/infusion: 5–10 mg/h
e. Comments: Titrate to effect in ICU patients (monitor with train-of-four testing); onset within 1.5–10 min; 70–90 min duration of action; 90–180 min recovery; partial renal excretion

Midazolam

a. Action: Short-acting benzodiazepine
b. Indications: Sedation, anxiety, agitation; ETOH withdrawal; seizures
c. Loading dose: 1–4 mg
d. Dose interval/infusion: 1–20 mg/h titrated to effect
e. Comments: CNS depression; active metabolites; respiratory depression when used in combination with narcotics; three to four times the potency of diazepam

Mivacurium

a. Action: Nondepolarizing neuromuscular blocker; minimal to moderate H_2 release; minimal tachycardia
b. Indications: Short-acting neuromuscular blockade
c. Loading dose: 0.1–0.25 mg/kg intubating dose
d. Dose interval/infusion: 5–15 μg/kg/min continuous infusion; onset in 2–4 min; 13–40 min duration of action; 6–14 min recovery
e. Comments: Titrate to effect in ICU patients (monitor with train-of-four testing)

Morphine

a. Action: Opioid analgesia; venodilation
b. Indications: Analgesia, sedation; pulmonary edema
c. Loading dose: 1–5 mg IV
d. Dose interval/infusion: Rebolus every 2–3 h; 1–10 mg/h continuous infusion titrated to effect
e. Comments: CNS disturbances; hypotension (especially if intravascular volume depletion is present); respiratory depression; histamine release

Nicardipine

a. Action: Noncardiosuppressive calcium channel antagonist
b. Indications: Postoperative hypertension, prevention of vasospasm from subarachnoid hemorrhage; angina
c. Loading dose: 5 mg/h and increase by 2.5 mg/h every 15 min
d. Dose interval/infusion: 1–15 mg/h; 20–40 mg orally three times daily
e. Comments: Hypotension; reflex tachycardia

Nifedipine

a. Action: Calcium channel blocker; minimal myocardial depression with slowing of conduction; smooth muscle relaxation
b. Indications: Angina, hypertension
c. Loading dose: 10–20 mg orally or sublingually
d. Dose interval/infusion: Hourly as needed, no intravenous preparation; maximum dose 180 mg/d
e. Comments: Hypotension and reflex tachycardia

Nimodipine

a. Action: Calcium channel antagonist; minimal cardiovascular effect
b. Indications: Prevention of vasospasm due to subarachnoid hemorrhage
c. Loading dose: None, no IV formulation available
d. Dose interval/infusion: 60 mg orally or sublingually every 4 h for 21 d
e. Comments: Hypotension may occur

Nitroglycerin

a. Action: Smooth muscle relaxation through nitric oxide pathway; pulmonary vasculature and venous vasodilator; decreased preload; improved coronary blood flow
b. Indications: Myocardial ischemia; hypertension; congestive heart failure; esophageal spasm

c. Loading dose: None necessary in intravenous dosing
d. Dose interval/infusion: 10–400 μg/min titrated to effect
e. Comments: Liver metabolism; renal excretion; tolerance; rare methemoglobinemia; increased cerebral blood flow (CBF); hypotension

Nitroprusside

a. Action: Arterial and venous vasodilatation through nitric oxide pathway; coronary vasodilatation; increased CBF and volume with subsequent increased intracranial pressure
b. Indications: Hypertension; acute left ventricular failure
c. Loading dose: Not indicated
d. Dose interval/infusion: 0.5–10 μg/kg/min and titrate to effect
e. Comments: Coronary steal (angina) possible with coronary vasodilatation; metabolic acidosis; follow thiocyanate levels if toxicity suspected (toxicity: Amyl nitrate and sodium nitrite converts hemoglobin to methemoglobin; methemoglobin binds cyanide; sodium thiosulfate converts cyanide to thiocyanate)

Norepinephrine

a. Action: α- and β_1-agonist; arterial and venous vasoconstriction; minimal chronotropic effect
b. Indications: Hypotension
c. Loading dose: Not indicated
d. Dose interval/infusion: 2–40 μg/min titrated to effect
e. Comments: Decreased renal perfusion; peripheral vasoconstriction; arrhythmias; tissue necrosis with extravasation

Octreotide

a. Action: Mimics effects of somatostatin; increases GI motility while decreasing GI and pancreatic secretions; decreases splanchnic blood flow
b. Indications: Gut neuroendocrine tumors, diarrhea, excess GI/pancreatic secretions; variceal hemorrhage
c. Loading dose: 250-μg bolus
d. Dose interval/infusion: 25–100 μg three times daily or 50–250 μg/h infusion
e. Comments: Total dose, 50–1,500 μg/d; both hypoglycemia and hyperglycemia

Pancuronium

a. Action: Nondepolarizing neuromuscular blocker; no histamine release, modest to marked vagal block with tachycardia
b. Indications: Long-acting neuromuscular blockade
c. Loading dose: 0.1-mg/kg intubating dose
d. Dose interval/infusion: 1–2 μg/kg/min continuous infusion
e. Comments: Titrate to effect in ICU patient (monitor with train-of-four testing); onset within 2–4 min and duration of action of 60–100 min; recovery within 120–180 min; primarily renal excretion

Phentolamine

a. Action: α-blocker; vasodilatation
b. Indications: Hypertension; pheochromocytoma
c. Loading dose: 5 mg IV/IM to effect
d. Dose interval/infusion: No continuous infusion
e. Comments: Monitor for hypotension

Phenylephrine

a. Action: α-agonist; arterial and venous vasoconstriction; vasopressor with reflex decrease in heart rate
b. Indications: Hypotension
c. Loading dose: Not indicated
d. Dose interval/infusion: 10–40 μg/min titrated to effect
e. Comments: Hypertension, bradycardia, myocardial ischemia, decreased renal perfusion

Procainamide

a. Action: Antiarrhythmic; vasodilatation
b. Indications: Supraventricular and ventricular arrhythmias; recurrent atrial fibrillation/flutter
c. Loading dose: 50 mg/min to effect or total dose of 17 mg/kg
d. Dose interval/infusion: 2–6 mg/min continuous infusion
e. Comments: Observe for conduction disturbances (including torsade) and myocardial depression

Propofol

a. Action: Alkylphenol
b. Indications: Short-acting sedative
c. Loading dose: 1.5–3 mg/kg
d. Dose interval/infusion: Titrate to effect; usual dose is 10–50 μg/kg/min
e. Comments: No analgesic properties; very short duration of action (2–3 min); reduce dosage in the elderly; monitor triglyceride values

Propranolol

a. Action: Nonspecific β-blockade; decreased heart rate and contractility; antiarrhythmic
b. Indications: Supraventricular tachyarrhythmias, angina, hypertension, acute myocardial infarct
c. Loading dose: 0.5–1.0 mg bolus IV
d. Dose interval/infusion: Repeat bolus every 5 min to effect
e. Comments: Bradycardia, hypotension, bronchospasm

Protamine

a. Action: Heparin antagonist (complexes with heparin)
b. Indications: Reverse the effects of heparin
c. Loading dose: 1 mg/90 IU bovine heparin; 1 mg/115 IU porcine heparin over 1–3 min
d. Dose interval/infusion: Titrate to aPTT
e. Comments: Maximum dose of 50 mg in any 10-min period; observe for bleeding after large dosages; hypotension

Rocuronium

a. Action: Nondepolarizing neuromuscular blocker; minimal H_2 release; minimal to moderate vagal blockade
b. Indications: Intermediate-acting neuromuscular blockade
c. Loading dose: 0.4–1.2 mg/kg intubating dose
d. Dose interval/infusion: 10–12 μg/kg/min continuous infusion
e. Comments: Titrate to effect in ICU patients (monitor with train-of-four testing); 1–3 min onset of action; 22–67 min duration of action; recovery in 10–20 min

Succinylcholine

a. Action: Depolarizing neuromuscular blocker; no H_2 release, some vagal stimulation
b. Indications: Rapid onset of paralysis; short-acting neuromuscular blockade
c. Loading dose: 0.3–1.5 mg/kg

d. Dose interval/infusion: Continuous infusion of 7.1–142 μg/kg/min
e. Comments: Onset in 0.5–5 min with duration of action of 2–3 min and recovery within 10 min; hyperkalemia; prolonged blockade in patients with atypical pseudocholinesterase; increased intracranial pressure (ICP)

Sufentanil

a. Action: Potent opiate receptor ligand; produces decreases in heart rate, blood pressure, and cardiac index; respiratory depressant; may increase ICP in patients with compromised intracranial compliance; may produce skeletal muscle rigidity
b. Indications: Opioid analgesia
c. Loading dose: 1–30 μg/kg, depending on other anesthetic agents used
d. Dose interval/infusion: As needed, no infusion
e. Comments: Five to ten times as potent as fentanyl with a shorter duration of action; muscle rigidity

Thiopental

a. Action: Barbiturate with hypnotic and anesthetic properties
b. Indications: General anesthesia, seizures, increased ICP
c. Loading dose: 3–5 mg/kg for induction of anesthesia; 75–125 mg for treatment of seizures
d. Dose interval/infusion: Additional doses as clinically indicated; no continuous infusion
e. Comments: Observe clinically and use blood levels as necessary; respiratory depression

Thrombolytics (streptokinase, urokinase, tissue plasminogen activator)

a. Action: Plasminogen activators; plasmin produced; plasmin degrades fibrinogen and fibrin, dissolving pre-existing thrombi
b. Indications: Pulmonary embolism, acute myocardial infarction, venous thrombosis, graft thrombosis, catheter occlusion
c. Loading dose: Varies, depending on agent used and clinical condition
d. Dose interval/infusion: Variable
e. Comments: Bleeding (about 5% of patients); absolute contraindications include active hemorrhage, recent (2 mo) neurologic injury/surgery/tumor

Vasopressin

a. Action: Decreases hepatic blood flow and portal pressure; increased clotting; decreased free water excretion; increases gut motility
b. Indications: Central (neurogenic) DI; bleeding esophageal varices, septic shock, and cardiopulmonary resuscitation
c. Loading dose: Central DI–aqueous vasopressin 5–10 IU IM/SQ
d. Dose interval/infusion: Central DI—two to four times daily dosing (follow polyuria and serum sodium); GI bleeding—aqueous vasopressin 0.2–1.0 U/min IV
e. Comments: CNS disturbances, hypertension, angina, hyponatremia; metabolic acidosis

Vecuronium

a. Action: Nondepolarizing neuromuscular blocker; no H_2 release; no vagal activity or tachycardia
b. Indications: Intermediate-acting neuromuscular blockade
c. Loading dose: 0.08 mg/kg intubating dose
d. Dose interval/infusion: 1–2 μg/kg/min continuous infusion
e. Comments: Titrate to effect in ICU patients (monitor with train-of-four testing); onset within 2.5–4.5 min; 35–45 min duration; recovery within 45–60 min; renal and hepatic excretion

Verapamil

a. Action: Antiarrhythmic; calcium channel blockade
b. Indications: Treatment of angina, hypertension, hypertrophic cardiomyopathy, and supraventricular tachyarrhythmias (SVTs) (slows ventricular response in atrial fibrillation or flutter and may convert SVT to sinus rhythm)
c. Loading dose: 0.075–0.15 mg/kg (5–10 mg) IV over 2–3 min; may repeat bolus in 10 min
d. Dose interval/infusion: Continuous infusion of 5 mg/h titrated to effect
e. Comments: May produce hypotension: Bradycardia and AV block in patients treated with concomitant β-blockers

APPENDIX G: DERMATOMES

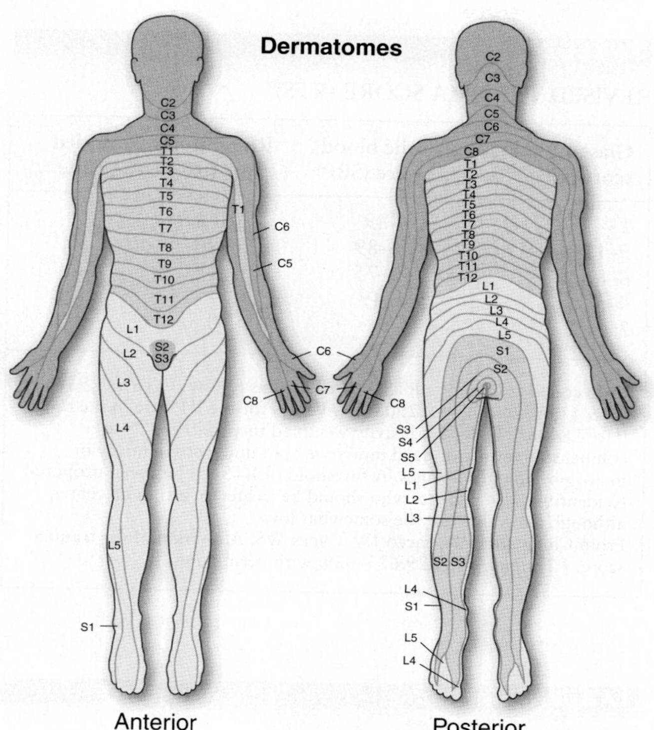

FIGURE G.1.

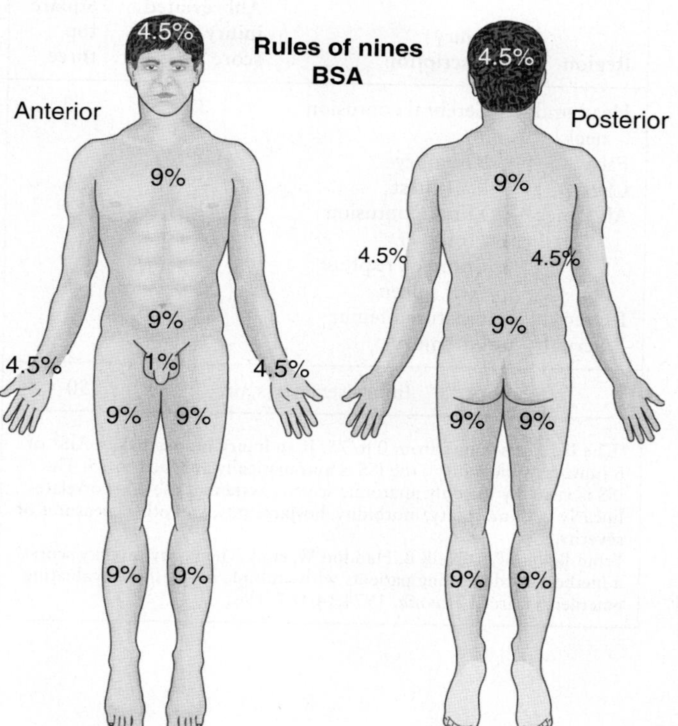

FIGURE G.2. BURNS: To estimate the extent of burn, the *rule of nines* for body surface area (BSA) is commonly used: Children: arms 9 percent each; legs 9 percent each; head 13 percent; trunk 18 percent anterior, 18 percent posterior; genitalia 1 percent. Lund and Browder chart for estimation of burn extent. (From Artz CP and Yarbrough DR III. Burns: including cold, chemical, and electric injuries. In: Sabiston CC Jr, editor: *Textbook of Surgery: the biological basis of modern surgical practice*, Ed 11, WB Saunders: Philadelphia, 1977. (With permission)

APPENDIX H: ORGAN INJURY SCALING, TRAUMA SCORING SYSTEMS

TRAUMA SCORING SYSTEMS

TABLE H.1

ABBREVIATED INJURY SCORE (AIS)

Score	Injury[a]
1	Minor
2	Moderate
3	Serious
4	Severe
5	Critical
6	Unsurvivable

[a]Injuries are ranked on a scale of 1 to 6, with 1 being minor, 5 severe, and 6 an unsurvivable injury. This represents the "threat to life" associated with an injury and is not meant to represent a comprehensive measure of severity.
From Copes WS, Sacco WJ, Champion HR, et al. Progress in characterizing anatomic injury. In *Proceedings of the 33rd Annual Meeting of the Association for the Advancement of Automotive Medicine, Baltimore*, with permission.

TABLE H.2

GLASGOW COMA SCORE (GCS)[a]

Score[b]	Best eye response (E)
1	No eye opening
2	Eye opening to pain
3	Eye opening to verbal command
4	Eyes open spontaneously
Score[b]	**Best Verbal Response (V)**
1	No verbal response
2	Incomprehensible sounds
3	Inappropriate words
4	Confused
5	Orientated
Score[b]	**Best Motor Response (M)**
1	No motor response
2	Extension to pain
3	Flexion to pain
4	Withdrawal from pain
5	Localizing pain
6	Obeys commands

[a]Note that the phrase "GCS of 11" is essentially meaningless, and it is important to break the figure down into its components, such as E3V3M5 = GCS 11.
[b]A coma score of 13 or higher correlates with a mild brain injury, 9–12 is a moderate injury, and 8 or less a severe brain injury.
From Teasdale G, Jennett B. Assessment of coma and impaired consciousness. *Lancet*. 1974;ii:81–83, with permission.

TABLE H.3

REVISED TRAUMA SCORE (RTS)[a]

Glasgow coma score (GCS)[b]	Systolic blood pressure (SBP)	Respiratory rate (RR)	Coded value
13–15	>89	10–29	4
9–12	76–89	>29	3
6–8	50–75	6–9	2
4–5	1–49	1–5	1
3	0	0	0

[a]The coded form of the RTS is calculated as follows: RTS = 0.9368 GCS + 0.7326 SBP + 0.2908 RR. Values for the RTS are in the range 0 to 7.8408. The RTS is heavily weighted toward the GCS to compensate for major head injury without multisystem injury or major physiologic changes. A threshold of RTS <4 has been proposed to identify those patients who should be treated in a trauma center, although this value may be somewhat low.
From Champion HR, Sacco JW, Copes WS. A revision of the trauma score. *J Trauma*. 1989;29:623–629, with permission.

TABLE H.4

INJURY SEVERITY SCORE (ISS)[a]

Region	Injury description	Abbreviated injury score (AIS[b])	Square top three
Head and neck	Cerebral contusion	3	9
Face	No injury	0	
Chest	Flail chest	4	16
Abdomen	Minor contusion of liver	2	25
	Complex rupture of spleen	5	
Extremity	Fractured femur	3	
External	No injury	0	
	Injury severity score:		50

[a]The ISS takes values from 0 to 75. If an injury is assigned an AIS[b] of 6 (unsurvivable injury), the ISS is automatically assigned to 75. The ISS is virtually the only anatomic scoring system in use and correlates linearly with mortality, morbidity, hospital stay, and other measures of severity.
From Baker SP, O'Neill B, Haddon W, et al. The injury severity score: a method for describing patients with multiple injuries and evaluating emergency care. *J Trauma*. 1974;14:187–196.

APPENDIX I: SEDATION SCORES

TABLE I.1

RAMSAY SCALE

Level	Characteristics[a]
1	Patient awake, anxious, agitated, or restless
2	Patient awake, cooperative, orientated, and tranquil
3	Patient drowsy, with response to commands
4	Patient asleep, brisk response to glabella tap or loud auditory
5	Patient asleep, sluggish response to stimulus
6	Patient has no response to firm nailbed pressure or other noxious stimuli

From Ramsay MAE, Savege TM, Simpson BRJ, et al. Controlled sedation with alphaxolone/alphadolone. *BMJ.* 1974;ii:656–659, with permission.

TABLE I.2

RICHMOND AGITATION-SEDATION SCALE (RASS)

Score	Term	Description
+4	Combative	Overtly combative or violent; immediate danger to staff
+3	Very agitated	Pulls on or removes tube(s) or catheter(s) or has aggressive behavior toward staff
+2	Agitated	Frequent nonpurposeful movement or patient–ventilator dyssynchrony
+1	Restless	Anxious or apprehensive but movements not aggressive or vigorous
0	Alert and calm	
−1	Drowsy	Not fully alert, but has sustained (>10 seconds) awakening, with eye contact, to voice
−2	Light sedation	Briefly (<10 seconds) awakens with eye contact to voice
−3	Moderate sedation	Any movement (but no eye contact) to voice
−4	Deep sedation	No response to voice, but any movement to physical stimulation
−5	Unarousable	No response to voice or physical stimulation

From Sessler CN, Gosnell MS, Grap MJ, et al. The Richmond agitation-sedation scale: validity and reliability in adult intensive care unit patients. *Am J Respir Crit Care Med.* 2002;166:1338–1344, with permission.

APPENDIX J: SEVERITY SCORING SYSTEMS

TABLE J.1

ACUTE PHYSIOLOGIC AND CHRONIC HEALTH EVALUATION (APACHE II)

A: Acute physiological score (APS; 12 variables)

Physiologic variable	High abnormal range +4	+3	+2	+1	0	Low abnormal range +1	+2	+3	+4
Temperature rectal (°C)	≥41	39–40.9		38.5–38.9	36–38.4	34–35.9	32–33.9	30–31.9	≤29.0
Mean arterial pressure (mm Hg)	≥160	130–159	110–129		70–109		50–69		≤49
Heart rate—ventricular response	≥180	140–179	110–139		70–109		55–69	40–54	≤39
Respiratory rate—nonventilated or ventilated	≥50	35–49		25–34	12–24	10–11	6–9		≤5
Oxygen: A-a DO_2 or PaO_2 (mm Hg)									
a. $FiO_2 \geq 0.5$ record A-a DO_2	≥500	350–499	200–349		≤200				
b. $FiO_2 < 0.5$ record only PaO_2					PO_2 >70	PO_2 61–70		PO_2 55–60	PO_2 <55
Arterial pH	≥7.7	7.6–7.69		7.5–7.59	7.33–7.49		7.25–7.32	7.15–7.24	<7.15
Serum HCO_3—only if no ABGs	≥52	41–51.9		32–40.9	23–31.9		18–21.9	15–17.9	<15
Serum sodium (mmoL/L)	≥180	160–179	155–159	150–154	130–149		120–129	111–119	≤110
Serum potassium (mmoL/L)	≥7	6–6.9		5.5–5.9	3.5–5.4	3–3.4	2.5–2.9		≤2.5
Serum creatinine (μmoL/L)	≥350	200–340	150–190		60–140		<60		
Hematocrit (%)	≥60		50–50.9	46–49.9	30–45.9		20–29.9		≤20
White blood cell count (×1,000/mm³)	≥40		20–39.9	15–19.9	3–14.9		1–2.9		<1
Glasgow coma score (GCS) Score = 15 minus actual GCS									

B: Age points: Age (years)	Points	C: Chronic health points: History	Points for elective surgery	Points for emergency surgery	Apache II score: Sum of A + B + C
≤44	0	**Liver:** Biopsy-proven cirrhosis and documented portal hypertension or prior episodes of hepatic failure	2	5	A: APS
45–54	2	**Cardiovascular:** NYHA Class IV	2	5	B: Age points score
55–64	3	**Respiratory:** e.g., severe COPD, hypercapnia, home O_2, pulmonary hypertension	2	5	
65–74	5	**Immunocompromised**	2	5	C: Chronic health points score
≥75	6	**Renal:** Chronic dialysis	2	5	Total:

ABG, arterial blood gas; NYHA, New York Heart Association; COPD, chronic obstructive pulmonary disease.
From Knaus WA, et al. APACHE II: a severity of disease classification system. *Crit Care Med.* 1985;13:818–829, with permission.

TABLE J.2

SIMPLIFIED ACUTE PHYSIOLOGY (SAPS II) (SCORE

Variable	26	13	12	11	9	7	6	5	4	3	2	0	1	2	3	4	6	7	8	9	10	12	15	16	17	18
Age in years												<40						40–59				60–69	70–74	75–79		≥80
Heart rate (beat/min)				<40							40–69	70–119				120–159		≥160								
Systolic blood pressure (mm Hg)		<70						70–99				100–199		≥200												
Body temperature (°C)												<39°C			≥39°C											
PaO_2/FiO_2 (mm Hg) only if VENT or CPAP				<100	100–199	≥200																				
Urinary output (L/d)				<0.500					0.500–0.999			≥1.000														
Blood urea (mmol/L) (g/L)												<10.0 <0.60					10.0–29.9 0.60–1.79				≥30.0 ≥1.80					
WBC count (10^3/mL)			<1.0									1.0–19.9		≥20.0												
Serum K^+ (mEq/L)										<3.0		3.0–4.9		≥5.0												
Serum Na^+ (mEq/L)								<125				125–144	≥145													
Serum HCO_3 (mEq/L)							<15			15–19		≥20														
Bilirubin (if jaundice μmol/L) (mg/L)												<68.4 <40.0				68.4–102.4 40.0–59.9				≥102.5 ≥60.0						
Glasgow coma score (points)	<6	6–8				9–10		11–13				14–15														
Chronic diseases																				Met. Cancer	Hem. Mal				AIDS	
Type of admission												Elective surgery					Medical		Surgery emergency							

VENT, ventilator; CPAP, continuous positive airway pressure; WBC, white blood cell; Met Cancer, metastatic carcinoma; Met, metastatic; hem mal, hematologic malignancy; AIDS, acquired immunodeficiency syndrome.
The SAPS II score registers the worst value of selected variables, within the first 24 hours after admission.
From Le Gall JR, Lemeshow S, Saulnier F, et al. A new simplified acute physiology score (SAPS II) based on a European/North American multicenter study. *JAMA*. 1993;270:2957–2963, with permission.

TABLE J.3

SEQUENTIAL ORGAN FAILURE ASSESSMENT (SOFA) SCORE

Organ system		Score 0	Score 1	Score 2	Score 3	Score 4
Respiration	Lowest PaO_2/FiO_2 (mm Hg) or (Kpa) Respiratory support (yes/no)	>400 >53.33	≤400 40–53.33	≤300 26.67–40	≤200 13.33–26.67 and yes	≤100 ≤13.33 and yes
Coagulation	Lowest platelet ($10^3/mm^3$)	>150	≤150	≤100	≤50	≤20
Hepatic	Highest bilirubin (mg/dL) or (μmol/L)	<1.2 <20	1.2–1.9 20–32	2.0–5.9 33–101	6.0–11.9 102–204	≥12 >204
Circulatory	Lowest mean arterial pressure (mmHg)	>70	<70			
	Highest dopamine dose (μg/kg/min)			≤5	>5	>15
	Highest epinephrine dose (μg/kg/min)				≤0.1	>0.1
	Highest norepinephrine dose (μg/kg/min)				≤0.1	>0.1
	Dobutamine (yes/no)			Any dose[a]		
Neurologic	(GCS, see Table H-2)	15	13–14	10–12	6–9	<6
Renal	Highest creatinine level (mg/dL) or (μmol/L) Total urine output (mL/24 h)	<1.2 <110	1.2–1.9 110–170	2.0–3.4 171–299	3.0–4.9 300–440 <500	≥5.0 >440 <200

GCS, Glasgow Coma Score.
SOFA total (Σ **6 items**). The SOFA score assesses the function of 6 different organ systems: respiratory (partial arterial oxygen pressure (PaO_2)/fraction of inspired oxygen [FiO_2]), cardiovascular (blood pressure, vasoactive drugs), renal (creatine and diuresis), hepatic (bilirubin), neurological (Glasgow Coma Score), and hematological (platelet count).
From Vincent JL, Moreno R, Takala J, et al. The SOFA (Sepsis-related Organ Failure Assessment) score to describe organ dysfunction/failure. On behalf of the Working Group on sepsis-related problems of the European Society of Intensive Care Medicine. *Intensive Care Med.* 1996;22:707–710, with permission.

TABLE J.4

MULTIPLE ORGAN DYSFUNCTION SCORE (MODS)

Variables	Points 0	1	2	3	4
PaO_2/FiO_2	<300	226–300	151–225	76–150	≤75
Creatinine serum	≤100	101–200	201–350	351–500	≥500
Bilirubin	≤20	21–60	61–120	121–240	>240
Heart rate	≤10	10.1–15	15.1–20	20.1–30	>30
Platelet count	>120	81–120	51–80	21–50	≤20
Glasgow coma score	15	13–14	10–12	7–9	≤6

From Marshall JC, Cook DJ, Christou NV, et al. Multiple organ dysfunction score: a reliable descriptor of a complex clinical outcome. *Crit Care Med.* 1995;23:1638–1652, with permission.

APPENDIX K: ANTIBIOTICS

TABLE K.1

AMINOPENICILLINS

Drug	Drug class	Adults (usual dose[a])	Actions, interactions, and others	Spectrum of activity, indications, and active against most strains of	Route, reduce dose, and contraindications
Ampicillin	Aminopenicillin	Usual dose: IV: 2.0 g IV q4h PO: 500 mg q6h	Allopurinol (increased frequency of rash) Warfarin (increased INR)	*Streptococcus pneumoniae; Staphylococcus aureus* (penicillinase and nonpenicillinase producing); *Haemophilus influenzae*, and group A β-hemolytic *Streptococci* Bacterial meningitis caused by *Escherichia coli*, group B *Streptococci*, and other Gram-negative bacteria (*Listeria monocytogenes, Neisseria meningitidis*) Endocarditis caused by susceptible Gram-positive organisms including *Streptococcus* sp., penicillin G–susceptible *Staphylococci*, and *Enterococci*. Endocarditis due to enterococcal strains usually respond to intravenous therapy Gram-negative sepsis caused by *E. coli, Proteus mirabilis*, and *Salmonella* sp. Gastrointestinal infections caused by *Salmonella typhosa* (typhoid fever), other *Salmonella* sp., and *Shigella* sp. Urinary tract infections caused by *E. coli* and *Proteus mirabilis*	Primary mode of elimination: Renal Reduce dose in moderate to severe renal impairment
Amoxicillin	Aminopenicillin	Usual dose: IV: 500 mg–1 g tds (higher doses: 2 g 4 hourly in endocarditis PO: 1 g q8h	Bactericide Some Gram-negative activity	■ *Streptococcus pneumoniae* ■ *Haemophilus influenzae* (except COPD patients) ■ β-Hemolytic *Streptococci* ■ *Streptococcus pyogenes* do not produce β-lactamase ■ *Enterococcus faecalis*	■ Primary mode of elimination: Renal ■ Reasonable oral absorption (oral preparation) ■ Reduce dose in moderate to severe renal impairment
Amoxicillin/ clavu-lanate	Aminopenicillin/β-lactam inhibitor combination	Usual dose: 500/125 mg (PO) q8h or 875/125 mg (PO) q12h for severe infections or respiratory tract infections		**Aerobic Gram-positive micro-organisms** *Streptococcus pneumoniae* (including isolates with penicillin MICs ≤ 2 μg/mL) **Aerobic Gram-negative micro-organisms** *Haemophilus influenzae* (including β-lactamase–producing isolates) *Moraxella catarrhalis* (including β-lactamase–producing isolates) The following *in vitro* data are available, but their clinical significance is unknown. **Aerobic Gram-positive micro-organisms** *Staphylococcus aureus* (including β-lactamase–producing isolates) NOTE: *Staphylococci* that are resistant to methicillin/ oxacillin must be considered resistant to amoxicillin/clavulanic acid *S. pyogenes*	■ Primary mode of elimination: Renal ■ Reduce dose in moderate to severe renal impairment ■ 875/125 mg formulation should not be used in patients with CrCl <30 mL/min

(continued)

TABLE K.1

(CONTINUED)

Drug	Drug class	Adults (usual dose[a])	Actions, interactions, and others	Spectrum of activity, indications, and active against most strains of	Route, reduce dose, and contraindications
Ampicillin/ sulbactam	Aminopenicillin/β-lactam inhibitor combination	Usual dose: IV: 1.5–3.0 g q6h Remember: Na^+ content = 4.2 mEq/g Total dose of sulbactam should not exceed 4 g/day	Bactericide Broad-spectrum antibiotic and a β-lactamase inhibitor For mild or moderate infection, 1.5 g IV q6h Pseudoresistance with *E. coli*/ *Klebsiella* (*in vitro*)	**Gram-negative bacteria** *Haemophilus influenzae* (β-lactamase and non–β-lactamase producing); *Moraxella* (Branhamella) *catarrhalis* (β-lactamase and non–β-lactamase producing); *Escherichia coli* (β-lactamase and non–β-lactamase producing); *Klebsiella* spp. (all known strains are β-lactamase producing); *Proteus mirabilis* (β-lactamase and non–β-lactamase producing); *Proteus vulgaris*; *Providencia rettgeri*; *Providencia stuartii*; *Morganella morganii*; *Neisseria gonorrhoeae* (β-lactamase and non–β-lactamase producing). **Anaerobes** *Clostridium* sp.; *Peptococcus* sp.; *Peptostreptococcus* sp.; *Bacteroides* sp., including *B. fragilis*	■ Primary mode of elimination: Renal and hepatic ■ Ampicillin and sulbactam for injection may be administered by either the IV or the IM routes ■ In patients with impairment of renal function, the elimination kinetics of ampicillin and sulbactam are similarly affected

INR, international normalized ratio; COPD, chronic obstructive pulmonary disease; MIC, minimum inhibitory concentration; CrCl, creatinine clearance.
Cunha BA. *Antibiotic Essentials*. 5th ed. Royal Oak, MI: Physicians Press; 2006.
From website http://www.drugs.com (drug information online). Revised from November 2006.

TABLE K.2

ANTIPSEUDOMONAL PENICILLINS

Drug	Drug class	Adults (usual dose[a])	Actions, interactions, and others	Spectrum of activity, indications, and active against most strains of	Route, reduce dose, and contraindications
Piperacillin	Antipseudomonal penicillin	Usual dose: IV: 34 g q48h	Drug interaction with aminoglycosides in renal failure	Prophylaxis: Piperacillin is indicated for prophylactic use in surgery including intra-abdominal (gastrointestinal and biliary) procedures, vaginal hysterectomy, abdominal hysterectomy, and cesarean section. Piperacillin should only be used to treat or prevent infections that are proven or strongly suspected to be caused by susceptible bacteria. **Indications and use** Intra-abdominal infections including hepatobiliary and surgical infections caused by *E. coli, Pseudomonas aeruginosa, Enterococci, Clostridium* spp., anaerobic cocci, or *Bacteroides* spp., including *B. fragilis.* Urinary tract infections caused by *E. coli, Klebsiella* spp., *P. aeruginosa, Proteus* spp. including *P. mirabilis*, or *Enterococci* Gynecologic infections including endometritis, pelvic inflammatory disease, pelvic cellulitis caused by *Bacteroides* spp. including *B. fragilis*, anaerobic cocci, *Neisseria gonorrhoeae*, or *Enterococci (E. faecalis)* Septicemia including bacteremia caused by *E. coli, Klebsiella* spp., *Enterobacter* spp., *Serratia* spp., *P. mirabilis, S. pneumoniae, Enterococci, P. aeruginosa, Bacteroides* spp., or anaerobic cocci. Lower respiratory tract infections caused by *E. coli, Klebsiella* spp., *Enterobacter* spp., *P. aeruginosa, Serratia* spp., *H. influenzae, Bacteroides* spp., or anaerobic cocci. Skin and skin structure infections caused by *E. coli, Klebsiella* spp., *Serratia* spp., *Acinetobacter* spp., *Enterobacter* spp., *P. aeruginosa, Morganella morganii, Providencia rettgeri, Proteus vulgaris, P. mirabilis, Bacteroides* spp. including *B. fragilis*, anaerobic cocci, or *Enterococci* Bone and joint infections caused by *P. aeruginosa, Enterococci, Bacteroides* spp., or anaerobic cocci	■ Primary mode of elimination: Renal ■ Reduce dose in moderate to severe renal impairment
Piperacillin/ tazobactam	Antipseudomonal penicillin	Usual dose: IV: 4.5 g q8h Pneumonia nosocomial, use 4.5 g (IV) q6h	Drug interaction with aminoglycosides and vecuronium	Indicated for nosocomial pneumonia (moderate to severe) caused by piperacillin-resistant, β-lactamase–producing strains of *Staphylococcus aureus* and by piperacillin/tazobactam-susceptible *Acinetobacter baumannii, Haemophilus influenzae, Klebsiella pneumoniae*, and *Pseudomonas aeruginosa* (nosocomial pneumonia caused by *P. aeruginosa* should be treated in combination with an aminoglycoside) Community-acquired pneumonia (moderate severity only) caused by piperacillin-resistant, β-lactamase–producing strains of *H. influenzae* Appendicitis (complicated by rupture or abscess) and peritonitis caused by piperacillin-resistant, β-lactamase–producing strains of *Escherichia coli* or the following members of the *Bacteroides fragilis* group: *B. fragilis, B. ovatus, B. thetaiotaomicron*, or *B. vulgatus*	■ Mode of elimination: 20% in bile, 80% unchanged in urine ■ Reduce dose in moderate to severe renal impairment

(continued)

TABLE K.2

(CONTINUED)

Drug	Drug class	Adults (usual dose[a])	Actions, interactions, and others	Spectrum of activity, indications, and active against most strains of	Route, reduce dose, and contraindications
				Uncomplicated and complicated skin and skin structure infections, including cellulitis, cutaneous abscesses, and ischemic/diabetic foot infections caused by piperacillin-resistant, β-lactamase–producing strains of *S. aureus* Infections caused by piperacillin-susceptible organisms for which piperacillin has been shown to be effective are also amenable to piperacillin tazobactam content. Postpartum endometritis or pelvic inflammatory disease caused by piperacillin-resistant, β-lactamase–producing strains of *E. coli*	
Ticarcillin disodium	Antipseudomonal penicillin	Usual dose: IV: 3 g q6h	Drug interaction with aminoglycosides in renal failure	Ticarcillin is a semisynthetic antibiotic with a broad spectrum of bactericidal activity against many Gram-positive and Gram-negative aerobic and anaerobic bacteria. Ticarcillin is, however, susceptible to degradation by β-lactamases, and therefore, the spectrum of activity does not normally include organisms that produce these enzymes.	■ Primary mode of elimination: Renal ■ Reduce dose in moderate to severe renal impairment
Ticarcillin/ clavulanate	Ticarcillin disodium (Antipseudomonal penicillin) + β-lactamase inhibitor clavulanate potassium (the potassium salt of clavulanic acid), for intravenous administration	Usual dose: IV: 3.1 g q4–6h (3.1 g vial containing 3 g ticarcillin and 100 mg clavulanic acid) Moderate infections 200 mg/kg/d in divided doses every 6 h Severe infections 300 mg/kg/d in divided doses every 4 h For patients weighing <60 kg, the recommended dosage is 200–300 mg/kg/d, based on ticarcillin content, given in divided doses every 4–6 hours.	Drug interaction with aminoglycosides in renal failure	Ticarcillin is a semisynthetic antibiotic with a broad spectrum of bactericidal activity against many Gram-positive and Gram-negative aerobic and anaerobic bacteria. Ticarcillin is, however, susceptible to degradation by β-lactamases, and therefore, the spectrum of activity does not normally include organisms that produce these enzymes. **Gram-positive aerobes** *Staphylococcus aureus; Staphylococcus epidermidis* **Gram-negative aerobes** *Citrobacter* sp.; *Enterobacter* sp., including *E. cloacae; Escherichia coli; Haemophilus influenzae; Klebsiella* sp. including *K. pneumoniae; Pseudomonas* sp. including *P. aeruginosa; Serratia marcescens* **Anaerobic bacteria** *Bacteroides fragilis group; Prevotella* (formerly *Bacteroides*) *melaninogenicus* **Gram-positive aerobes** *Staphylococcus saprophyticus; Streptococcus agalactiae* (group B); *Streptococcus bovis; Streptococcus pneumoniae* (penicillin-susceptible strains only); *Streptococcus pyogenes; Viridans group streptococci* **Gram-negative aerobes** *Acinetobacter baumannii; Acinetobacter calcoaceticus; Acinetobacter haemolyticus; Acinetobacter lwoffi; Moraxella catarrhalis; Morganella morganii; Neisseria gonorrhoeae; Pasteurella multocida; Proteus mirabilis; Proteus penneri; Proteus vulgaris; Providencia rettgeri; Providencia stuartii; Stenotrophomonas maltophilia* **Anaerobic bacteria** *Clostridium* sp. including *C. perfringens, C. difficile, C. sporogenes, C. ramosum,* and *C. bifermentans; Eubacterium* sp.; *Fusobacterium* sp. including *F. nucleatum and F. necrophorum; Peptostreptococcus* sp.; *Veillonella* sp.	■ Primary mode of elimination: Renal ■ Reduce dose in moderate to severe renal impairment

Cunha BA. *Antibiotic Essentials.* 5th ed. Royal Oak, MI: Physicians Press; 2006.
From website http://www.drugs.com (drug information online). Revised from November 2006.

TABLE K.3

CARBAPENEMS

Drug	Drug class	Adults (usual dose[a])	Actions, interactions, and others	Spectrum of activity, indications, and active against most strains of	Route, reduce dose, and contraindications
				Aerobic and facultative Gram-positive micro-organisms *Staphylococcus aureus* (methicillin-susceptible isolates only); *Streptococcus agalactiae; Streptococcus pneumoniae* (penicillin susceptible isolates only); *Streptococcus pyogenes* Note: Methicillin-resistant *Staphylococci* and *Enterococcus* spp. are resistant to ertapenem.	
Ertapenem	Carbapenem	Usual dose: IV/IM: 1 g q24h	Not a substrate/inhibitor of cytochrome P450 enzymes Probenecid (decrease clearance of ertapenem)	**Aerobic and facultative Gram-positive micro-organisms** *Escherichia coli; Haemophilus influenzae* (β-lactamase negative isolates only); *Klebsiella pneumoniae; Moraxella catarrhalis; Proteus mirabilis* **Anaerobic micro-organisms** *Bacteroides fragilis; Bacteroides distasonis; Bacteroides ovatus; Bacteroides thetaiotaomicron; Bacteroides uniformis; Clostridium clostridiiforme; Eubacterium lentum; Peptostreptococcus* sp.; *Porphyromonas asaccharolytica; Prevotella bivia*	Primary mode of elimination: Renal Reduce dose in moderate to severe renal impairment.
Imipenem/ cilastatin	Carbapenem	Usual dose: IV: 1000 mg q6h (4 g) only in severe life-threatening infections (mainly in some Pseudomonas species) no more than 50 mg/kg/24h IV: 250 mg q6h in mild infections IV: 500 mg q8h (1.5 g) or q6h (2.0 g) in moderate infections Total dose of sodium 37.5 mg (1.6 mEq) by 500 mg Imipenem	The bactericidal activity of imipenem results from the inhibition of cell wall synthesis	**Conditions:** Bacterial septicemia. Lower respiratory tract infections. Urinary tract infections (complicated and uncomplicated). Nosocomial pneumonia, peritonitis, sepsis. Gynecologic infections. Bone and joint infections. Skin and skin structure infections. Endocarditis. Polymicrobic infections. **Gram-positive aerobes** *Enterococcus faecalis* (formerly *S. faecalis*) (NOTE: Imipenem is inactive *in vitro* against *Enterococcus faecium* [formerly *S. faecium*]); *Staphylococcus aureus* including penicillinase-producing strains; *Staphylococcus epidermidis* including penicillinase-producing strains; *Streptococcus agalactiae* (group B streptococci); *Streptococcus pneumoniae; Streptococcus pyogenes* **Gram-negative aerobes** *Acinetobacter* spp.; *Citrobacter* spp.; *Enterobacter* spp.; *Escherichia coli; Gardnerella vaginalis; Haemophilus influenzae; Haemophilus parainfluenzae* *Klebsiella* spp.; *Morganella morganii; Proteus vulgaris; Providencia rettgeri; Pseudomonas aeruginosa* (NOTE: Imipenem is inactive *in vitro* against *Xanthomonas [Pseudomonas] maltophilia* and some strains of *P. cepacia*); *Serratia* spp., including *S. marcescens*	Central nervous system adverse experiences such as confusional states, myoclonic activity, and seizures have been reported during treatment with imipenem. Reduce dose in moderate to severe renal impairment. For patients on hemodialysis, imipenem is recommended only when the benefit outweighs the potential risk of seizures.

(*continued*)

TABLE K.3

(CONTINUED)

Drug	Drug class	Adults (usual dose[a])	Actions, interactions, and others	Spectrum of activity, indications, and active against most strains of	Route, reduce dose, and contraindications
				Gram-positive anaerobes *Bifidobacterium* spp.; *Clostridium* spp.; *Eubacterium* spp.; *Peptococcus* spp.; *Peptostreptococcus* spp.; *Propionibacterium* spp. **Gram-negative anaerobes** *Bacteroides* spp., *including B. fragilis; Fusobacterium* spp. **Gram-positive aerobes** *Bacillus* spp.; *Listeria monocytogenes; Nocardia spp.; Staphylococcus saprophyticus;* group C *streptococci;* group G *streptococci; Viridans group streptococci* **Gram-negative aerobes** *Aeromonas hydrophila; Alcaligenes* spp.; *Capnocytophaga* spp.; *Haemophilus ducreyi; Neisseria gonorrhoeae* including penicillinase-producing strains *Pasteurella* spp.; *Providencia stuartii.* **Gram-negative anaerobes** *Prevotella bivia; Prevotella disiens; Prevotella melaninogenica; Veillonella* spp. *In vitro* tests show imipenem to act synergistically with aminoglycoside antibiotics against some isolates of *Pseudomonas aeruginosa.*	
Meropenem	Carbapenem	Usual dose: IV: 500 mg q8h	Pneumonia, urinary tract infection, gynecologic infections, skin and skin structure infections	Meropenem is a broad-spectrum carbapenem antibiotic. It is active against Gram-positive and Gram-negative bacteria. Meropenem has significant stability to hydrolysis by β-lactamases of most categories, both penicillinases and cephalosporinases produced by Gram-positive and Gram-negative bacteria. Meropenem should not be used to treat methicillin-resistant *staphylococcus aureus* (MRSA). *In vitro* tests show meropenem to act synergistically with aminoglycoside antibiotics against some isolates of *Pseudomonas aeruginosa.*	Reduce dose in moderate to severe renal impairment.
		Usual dose: IV: 1 g q8h	Nosocomial pneumonia, peritonitis, neutropenic patients, sepsis		
		Usual dose: IV: 2 g q8h	Meningitis and cystic fibrosis		

Cunha BA. *Antibiotic Essentials*. 5th ed. Royal Oak, MI: Physicians Press; 2006.
From website http://www.drugs.com (drug information online). Revised from November 2006.

TABLE K.4

MONOBACTAMS

Drug	Drug class	Adults (usual dose[a])	Actions, interactions, and others	Spectrum of activity, indications, and active against most strains of	Route, reduce dose, and contraindications
Aztreonam	Monobactam It was originally isolated from *Chromobacterium violaceum.*	Usual dose: IV: 1–2 g q8h Usual dose: IV: 2 g q6h	■ Synthetic bactericidal antibiotic ■ Synthetic bactericidal antibiotic ■ Meningeal dose	Aerobic Gram-negative microorganisms: *Citrobacter* spp., including *C. freundii; Enterobacter* spp., including *E. cloacae; Escherichia coli; Haemophilus influenzae* (including ampicillin-resistant and other penicillinase-producing strains); Klebsiella, Proteus, and Serratia species.	Reduce dose in moderate to severe renal impairment.

Cunha BA. *Antibiotic Essentials*. 5th ed. Royal Oak, MI: Physicians Press; 2006.
From website http://www.drugs.com (drug information online). Revised from November 2006.

TABLE K.5

CEPHALOSPORINS (PARENTERAL)

Drug	Drug class	Adults (usual dose[a])	Actions, interactions, and others	Spectrum of activity, indications, and active against most strains of	Route, reduce dose, and contraindications
Cefazolin	First-generation cephalosporin	Usual dose: IV: 1 g q8h Remember: Na^+ content = 46 mg per g cefazolin	*In vitro* tests demonstrate that the bactericidal action of cephalosporins results from inhibition of cell wall synthesis **Drug interactions** None	*Staphylococcus aureus* (including penicillinase-producing strains); *Staphylococcus epidermidis;* Methicillin-resistant staphylococci are uniformly resistant to cefazolin. Group A β-hemolytic *Streptococci* and other strains of streptococci (many strains of enterococci are resistant) *Streptococcus pneumoniae; Escherichia coli; Proteus mirabilis; Klebsiella* sp.; *Enterobacter aerogenes; Haemophilus influenzae*	Reduce dose in moderate to severe renal impairment.
Cefuroxime	Second-generation IV/oral cephalosporin	Usual dose: IV: 1.5 g q8h PO: 500 mg q12h Remember: Na^+ content = 2.4 mEq/g	Cefuroxime has *in vitro* activity against a wide range of Gram-positive and Gram-negative organisms, and it is highly stable in the presence of β-lactamases of certain Gram-negative bacteria. The bactericidal action of cefuroxime results from inhibition of cell wall synthesis.	**Aerobes, Gram-positive** *Staphylococcus aureus; Staphylococcus epidermidis; Streptococcus pneumoniae; Streptococcus pyogenes* (and other streptococci) NOTE: Most strains of enterococci (e.g., *Enterococcus faecalis* [formerly *Streptococcus faecalis*]), are resistant to cefuroxime. Methicillin-resistant staphylococci and *Listeria monocytogenes* are resistant to cefuroxime. **Aerobes, Gram-negative** *Citrobacter* spp.; *Enterobacter* spp.; *Escherichia coli; Haemophilus influenzae* (including ampicillin-resistant strains); *Haemophilus parainfluenzae; Klebsiella* spp. (including *Klebsiella pneumoniae*); *Moraxella* (*Branhamella*) *catarrhalis* (including ampicillin- and cephalothin-resistant strains); *Morganella morganii* (formerly *Proteus morganii*); *Neisseria gonorrhoeae* (including penicillinase- and non–penicillinase-producing strains); *Neisseria meningitidis; Proteus mirabilis; Providencia rettgeri* (formerly *Proteus rettgeri*); *Salmonella* spp.; *Shigella* spp.	Reduce dose in moderate to severe renal impairment. Do not use for meningitis prophylaxis.
Cefotaxime	Third-generation cephalosporin	Usual dose: 2 g IV q6h	Administer by IV injection or infusion or by deep IM injection.	**Lower respiratory tract infections,** including pneumonia, caused by *Streptococcus pneumoniae* (formerly *Diplococcus pneumoniae*), *Streptococcus pyogenes*[b] (group A streptococci) and other streptococci (excluding enterococci, e.g., *Enterococcus faecalis*), *Staphylococcus aureus* (penicillinase and nonpenicillinase producing), *Escherichia coli, Klebsiella* sp., *Haemophilus influenzae* (including ampicillin-resistant strains), *Haemophilus parainfluenzae, Proteus mirabilis, Serratia marcescens,*[b] *Enterobacter* sp., indole- positive *Proteus* and *Pseudomonas* sp. (including *P. aeruginosa*).	Reduce dose in moderate to severe renal impairment.

Genitourinary infections

Urinary tract infections caused by *Enterococcus* sp., *Staphylococcus epidermidis, Staphylococcus aureus*[b] (penicillinase and nonpenicillinase producing), *Citrobacter* sp., *Enterobacter* sp., *Escherichia coli, Klebsiella* sp., *Proteus mirabilis, Proteus vulgaris,*[b] *Providencia stuartii, Morganella morganii,*[b] *Providencia rettgeri,*[b] *Serratia marcescens*, and *Pseudomonas* sp. (including *P. aeruginosa*). Also, uncomplicated gonorrhea (cervical/urethral and rectal) caused by *Neisseria gonorrhoeae*, including penicillinase-producing strains.

Gynecologic infections, including pelvic inflammatory disease, endometritis, and pelvic cellulitis caused by *Staphylococcus epidermidis, Streptococcus* sp., *Enterococcus* sp., *Enterobacter* species,[b] *Klebsiella* sp.,[b] *Escherichia coli, Proteus mirabilis, Bacteroides* sp. (including *Bacteroides fragilis*[b]), *Clostridium* sp., and anaerobic cocci (including *Peptostreptococcus* sp. and *Peptococcus* sp.) and *Fusobacterium* sp. (including *F. nucleatum*[b])

Bacteremia/septicemia caused by *Escherichia coli, Klebsiella* sp., *Serratia marcescens, Staphylococcus aureus,* and *Streptococcus* sp. (including *S. pneumoniae*)

Skin and skin structure infections caused by *Staphylococcus aureus* (penicillinase and nonpenicillinase producing), *Staphylococcus epidermidis, Streptococcus pyogenes* (group A streptococci) and other streptococci, *Enterococcus* sp., *Acinetobacter* species,[b] *Escherichia coli, Citrobacter* species (including *C. freundii*[b]), *Enterobacter* sp., *Klebsiella* sp., *Proteus mirabilis, Proteus vulgaris,*[b] *Morganella morganii, Providencia rettgeri,*[b] *Pseudomonas* sp., *Serratia marcescens, Bacteroides* sp., and anaerobic cocci (including *Peptostreptococcus*[b] sp. and *Peptococcus* sp.)

Intra-abdominal infections including peritonitis caused by *Streptococcus* sp.,[b] *Escherichia coli, Klebsiella* sp., *Bacteroides* sp., and anaerobic cocci (including *Peptostreptococcus*[b] sp. and *Peptococcus*[b] sp.) *Proteus mirabilis,*[b] and *Clostridium* species[b]

Bone and/or joint infections caused by *Staphylococcus aureus* (penicillinase- and nonpenicillinase-producing strains), *Streptococcus* sp. (including *S. pyogenes*[b]), *Pseudomonas* sp. (including *P. aeruginosa*[b]), and *Proteus mirabilis*[b]

(continued)

TABLE K.5

CONTINUED

Drug	Drug class	Adults (usual dose[a])	Actions, interactions, and others	Spectrum of activity, indications, and active against most strains of	Route, reduce dose, and contraindications
				Central nervous system infections (e.g., meningitis and ventriculitis), caused by *Neisseria meningitidis*, *Haemophilus influenzae*, *Streptococcus pneumoniae*, *Klebsiella pneumoniae*,[b] and *Escherichia coli*[b]	
Ceftazidime	Third-generation cephalosporin	Usual dose: 2 g IV q8h	Ceftazidime is bactericidal in action, exerting its effect by inhibition of enzymes responsible for cell wall synthesis.	**Lower respiratory tract infections, including pneumonia, caused by** *Pseudomonas aeruginosa* and other *Pseudomonas* spp.; *Haemophilus influenzae*, including ampicillin-resistant strains; *Klebsiella* spp.; *Enterobacter* spp.; *Proteus mirabilis; Escherichia coli; Serratia* spp.; *Citrobacter* spp.; *Streptococcus pneumoniae;* and *Staphylococcus aureus* (methicillin-susceptible strains). **Skin and skin structure infections caused by** *Pseudomonas aeruginosa; Klebsiella* spp.; *Escherichia coli; Proteus* spp., including *Proteus mirabilis* and indole-positive *Proteus; Enterobacter* spp.; *Serratia* spp.; *Staphylococcus aureus* (methicillin-susceptible strains); and *Streptococcus pyogenes* (group A β-hemolytic streptococci). **Urinary tract infections, both complicated and uncomplicated, caused by** *Pseudomonas aeruginosa; Enterobacter* spp.; *Proteus* spp., including *Proteus mirabilis* and indole-positive *Proteus; Klebsiella* spp.; *and Escherichia coli* **Bacterial septicemia caused by** *Pseudomonas aeruginosa, Klebsiella* spp., *Haemophilus influenzae, Escherichia coli, Serratia* spp., *Streptococcus pneumoniae*, and *Staphylococcus aureus* (methicillin-susceptible strains) **Bone and joint infections caused by** *Pseudomonas aeruginosa, Klebsiella* spp., *Enterobacter* spp., and *Staphylococcus aureus* (methicillin-susceptible strains) **Gynecologic infections**, including endometritis, pelvic cellulitis, and other infections of the female genital tract caused by *Escherichia coli* **Intra-abdominal infections, including peritonitis caused by** *Escherichia coli, Klebsiella* spp., and *Staphylococcus aureus* (methicillin-susceptible strains) and polymicrobial infections caused by aerobic and anaerobic organisms and *Bacteroides* spp. (many strains of *Bacteroides fragilis* are resistant)	Reduce dose in moderate to severe renal impairment.

				Central nervous system infections, including meningitis, caused by *Haemophilus influenzae* and *Neisseria meningitidis*. Ceftazidime has also been used successfully in a limited number of cases of meningitis due to *Pseudomonas aeruginosa* and *Streptococcus pneumoniae*.	
Cefepime	Fourth-generation cephalosporin	Usual dose: 1–2 g IV q12h For proven serious systemic *P. aeruginosa* infections, febrile neutropenia, or cystic fibrosis: 2 g (IV) q8h (max dose) Meningeal dose: 2 g (IV) q8h (max dose)	Local intolerances to IV or IM administration of cefepime were not statistically different from those of ceftazidime administration	*In vitro*, activity against **Gram-positive organisms** including *Streptococcus agalactiae*, *Streptococcus pneumoniae*, *Streptococcus pyogenes*, and penicillin-susceptible *Staphylococcus aureus* **The broad range of Gram-negative organisms sensitive to include** family Enterobacteriaceae, *Klebsiella pneumoniae*, *Haemophilus influenza*, *Neisseria meningitidis*, *Neisseria gonorrhoeae*, and *Pseudomonas aeruginosa*	Reduce dose in moderate to severe renal impairment

[b]Usual dose, assumes normal renal/hepatic function.
Cunha BA. *Antibiotic Essentials*. 5th ed. Royal Oak, MI: Physicians Press; 2006.
From website http://www.drugs.com (drug information online). Revised from November 2006.

TABLE K.6

GLYCOPEPTIDES

Drug	Drug class	Adults (usual dose[a])	Actions, interactions, and others	Spectrum of activity, indications, and active against most strains of	Route, reduce dose, and contraindications
Vancomycin	Glycopeptide	The initial dose should be no <15 mg/kg, even in patients with mild to moderate renal insufficiency Usual dose IV: 1 g q12h	The bactericidal action of vancomycin results primarily from inhibition of cell wall biosynthesis. In addition, vancomycin alters bacterial cell membrane permeability and RNA synthesis. Concomitant administration of vancomycin and anesthetic agents has been associated with erythema and histaminelike flushing and anaphylactoid reactions.	Indicated for the treatment of serious or severe infections caused by susceptible strains of methicillin-resistant (β-lactam–resistant) staphylococci. It is indicated for penicillin-allergic patients; for patients who cannot receive or who have failed to respond to other drugs, including the penicillins or cephalosporins; and for infections caused by vancomycin-susceptible organisms that are resistant to other antimicrobial drugs. Also indicated for initial therapy when methicillin-resistant staphylococci are suspected, but after susceptibility data are available, therapy should be adjusted accordingly. Effective in the treatment of *staphylococcal endocarditis*. Its effectiveness has been documented in other infections due to staphylococci, including septicemia, bone infections, lower respiratory tract infections, and skin and skin structure infections. Effective alone or in combination with an aminoglycoside for endocarditis caused by *S. viridans or S. bovis*. For endocarditis caused by *enterococci* (e.g., *E. faecalis*), vancomycin hydrochloride has been reported to be effective only in combination with an aminoglycoside. Effective for the treatment of *diphtheroid* endocarditis Has been used successfully in combination with rifampin, an aminoglycoside, or both, in early-onset prosthetic valve endocarditis caused by *S. epidermidis* or *diphtheroids* The parenteral form of vancomycin may be administered orally for treatment of antibiotic-associated pseudomembranous colitis produced by *C. difficile* and for staphylococcal enterocolitis	Dosage adjustment must be made in patients with impaired renal function. Vancomycin dosage schedules should be adjusted in elderly patients Dosage table for vancomycin (adapted from Moellering et al.)[b] Creatine Clearance/ Dose mL/min—mg/24 h 100—1,545 90—1,390 80—1,235 70—1,080 60—925 50—770 40—620 30—465 20—310 10—155

Cunha BA. *Antibiotic Essentials*. 5th ed. Royal Oak, MI: Physicians Press; 2006.
From website http://www.drugs.com (drug information online). Revised from November 2006.

TABLE K.7

CHLORAMPHENICOL, CLINDAMYCIN, ERYTHROMYCIN GROUP, KETOLIDES

Drug	Drug class	Adults (usual dose[a])	Actions, interactions, and others	Spectrum of activity, indications, and active against most strains of	Route, reduce dose, and contraindications
Chloramphenicol	Chloramphenicol sodium succinate	Chloramphenicol sodium succinate is intended for intravenous use only. It has been demonstrated to be ineffective when given intramuscularly. 0.25–1 g IV q6h (max. of 4 g/d) Administration of 50 mg/kg/d in divided doses will produce blood levels of the magnitude to which the majority of susceptible micro-organisms will respond.	The most serious adverse effect of chloramphenicol is bone marrow depression. Serious and fatal blood dyscrasias (aplastic anemia, hypoplastic anemia, thrombocytopenia, and granulocytopenia) are known to occur after the administration of chloramphenicol.	Chloramphenicol must be used only in those serious infections for which less potentially dangerous drugs are ineffective or contraindicated: 1. Acute infections caused by *Salmonella typhi* 2. Serious infections caused by susceptible strains: ■ *Salmonella* sp. ■ *H. influenzae*, especially meningeal infections ■ *Rickettsia* ■ Lymphogranuloma-psittacosis group ■ Various Gram-negative bacteria causing bacteremia, meningitis, or other serious Gram-negative infections ■ Other susceptible organisms that have been demonstrated to be resistant to all other appropriate antimicrobial agents 3. Cystic fibrosis regimens	Total urinary excretion of chloramphenicol in these studies ranged from a low of 68% to a high of 99% over a 3-d period. From 8% to 12% of the antibiotic excreted is in the form of free chloramphenicol
Clindamycin	Clindamycin phosphate	IV or IM: 600–900 mg q8h PO: 0.15–0.45 g q6h	Pseudomembranous colitis has been reported with nearly all antibacterial agents, including clindamycin, and may range in severity from mild to life threatening.	**Aerobic Gram-positive cocci**, including: *Staphylococcus aureus* (penicillinase- and nonpenicillinase-producing strains); *Staphylococcus epidermidis* (penicillinase- and nonpenicillinase-producing strains); *Streptococci* (except *Enterococcus faecalis*); *Pneumococci* **Anaerobic Gram-negative bacilli**, including *Bacteroides* sp. (including *Bacteroides fragilis* group and *Bacteroides melaninogenicus* group) and *Fusobacterium* species **Anaerobic Gram-positive non–spore-forming bacilli**, including *Propionibacterium, Eubacterium,* and *Actinomyces* sp. **Anaerobic and microaerophilic Gram-positive cocci**, including *Peptococcus* sp., *Peptostreptococcus* sp., *Microaerophilic streptococci,* and *Clostridia*	The elimination half-life of clindamycin is increased slightly in patients with markedly reduced renal or hepatic function. Hemodialysis and peritoneal dialysis are not effective in removing clindamycin from the serum.

(*continued*)

TABLE K.7
(CONTINUED)

Drug	Drug class	Adults (usual dose[a])	Actions, interactions, and others	Spectrum of activity, indications, and active against most strains of	Route, reduce dose, and contraindications
Clarithromycin	Semi-synthetic macrolide antibiotic	Usual dose: PO: 0.5 g q12h	**Drug Interactions:** Patients who are receiving single doses of clarithromycin and theophylline or carbamazepine may be associated with an increase of serum theophylline and carbamazepine concentrations.	**Aerobic Gram-positive micro-organisms** *Staphylococcus aureus; Streptococcus pneumoniae; Streptococcus pyogenes* **Aerobic Gram-negative micro-organisms** *Haemophilus influenzae; Haemophilus parainfluenzae; Moraxella catarrhalis* **Other micro-organisms** *Mycoplasma pneumoniae; Chlamydia pneumoniae* **Mycobacteria** *Mycobacterium avium* complex consisting of *Mycobacterium avium* and *Mycobacterium intracellulare* β-Lactamase production should have no effect on clarithromycin activity. Most strains of methicillin-resistant and oxacillin-resistant staphylococci are resistant to clarithromycin. **Helicobacter** *Helicobacter pylori*	Contraindications: Any of the following drugs: cisapride, pimozide, astemizole, terfenadine, and ergotamine or dihydroergotamine. If clarithromycin is coadministered with cisapride, pimozide, astemizole, or terfenadine resulting in cardiac arrhythmias (QT prolongation, ventricular tachycardia, ventricular fibrillation, and torsades de pointes), this is most likely due to inhibition of metabolism of these drugs.
Linezolid	Oxazolidinone	Usual dose: PO or IV dose: 600 mg q12h all indications except 400 mg q12h for uncomplicated skin infections	**Reversible myelosuppression** including anemia, leukopenia, pancytopenia, and thrombocytopenia has been reported in patients. In cases where the outcome is known, when linezolid was discontinued, the affected hematologic parameters have risen toward pretreatment levels. **Lactic acidosis** has been reported with the use of linezolid. Spontaneous reports of **serotonin syndrome** associated with the coadministration of linezolid and serotonergic agents, including antidepressants **Peripheral and optic neuropathy** have been reported in patients treated with Linezolid	**Aerobic and facultative Gram-positive micro-organisms** *Enterococcus faecium* (vancomycin-resistant strains only); *Staphylococcus aureus* (including methicillin-resistant strains); *Streptococcus agalactiae; Streptococcus pneumoniae* (including multidrug-resistant isolates); *Streptococcus pyogenes* **Aerobic and facultative Gram-positive micro-organisms** *Enterococcus faecalis* (including vancomycin-resistant strains); *Enterococcus faecium* (vancomycin-susceptible strains); *Staphylococcus epidermidis* (including methicillin-resistant strains); *Staphylococcus haemolyticus; Viridans group streptococci* **Aerobic and facultative Gram-negative micro-organisms** *Pasteurella multocida*	Linezolid is primarily metabolized by oxidation of the morpholine ring, which results in two inactive ring-opened carboxylic acid metabolites: The aminoethoxyacetic acid metabolite (A) and the hydroxyethyl glycine metabolite (B). Nonrenal clearance accounts for approximately 65% of the total clearance of linezolid. Under steady-state conditions, approximately 30% of the dose appears in the urine as linezolid, 40% as metabolite B, and 10% as metabolite A.

Cunha BA. *Antibiotic Essentials*. 5th ed. Royal Oak, MI: Physicians Press; 2006.
From website http://www.drugs.com (drug information online). Revised from November 2006.

TABLE K.8

TETRACYCLINES

Drug	Drug class	Adults (usual dose[a])	Actions, interactions, and others	Spectrum of activity, indications, and active against most strains of	Route, reduce dose, and contraindications
Doxycycline	Derived from oxytetracycline	Usual dose: PO: 0.1 g q12h IV: 0.1 g q12h	The tetracyclines are primarily bacteriostatic and are thought to exert their antimicrobial effect by the inhibition of protein synthesis.	Wide range of Gram-positive and Gram-negative micro-organisms **Aerobic Gram-positive micro-organisms** *Bacillus anthracis; Listeria monocytogenes; Staphylococcus aureus* **Aerobic Gram-negative micro-organisms** *Bartonella bacilliformis; Brucella* sp.; *Calymmatobacterium granulomatis; Campylobacter fetus; Francisella tularensis; Haemophilus ducreyi; Haemophilus influenzae; Neisseria gonorrhoeae; Vibrio cholerae; Yersinia pestis.* **Anaerobic micro-organisms** *Actinomyces israelii; Fusobacterium fusiforme; Clostridium* sp. **Other micro-organisms** *Borrelia recurrentis; Chlamydia psittaci; Chlamydia trachomatis; Mycoplasma pneumoniae; Rickettsiae; Treponema pallidum; Treponema pertenue*	Can be used in patients with renal failure Hemodialysis does not alter serum half-life.
Oxytetracycline	Tetracycline	Usual dose: PO: 0.25–0.5 g q6h IV: 0.5–1.0 g q12h	Primarily bacteriostatic	Wide range of Gram-positive and Gram-negative micro-organisms, similar to other tetracyclines	Contraindicated in pregnancy, hepatotoxicity in mother, transplacental to fetus. Intravenous dosage over 2.0 g/d may be associated with fatal hepatotoxicity

Cunha BA. *Antibiotic Essentials*. 5th ed. Royal Oak, MI: Physicians Press; 2006.
From website http://www.drugs.com (drug information online). Revised from November 2006.

TABLE K.9

FLUOROQUINOLONES

Drug	Drug class	Adults (usual dose[a])	Actions, interactions, and others	Spectrum of activity, indications, and active against most strains of	Route, reduce dose, and contraindications
Ciprofloxacin	Fluoroquinolone	Usual dose: IV: 400 mg q8–12h (infusion over a period of 60 min) PO: 500–750 mg q12h	Inhibition of bacterial topoisomerase IV and DNA gyrase (both of which are type II topoisomerases), enzymes required for DNA replication, transcription, repair, and recombination **Drug interactions** with theophylline, caffeine, warfarin phenytoin, sulfonylurea glyburide, metronidazole, probenecid, piperacillin sodium, and cyclosporine	**Aerobic Gram-positive micro-organisms** *Enterococcus faecalis* (many strains are only moderately susceptible); *Staphylococcus aureus* (methicillin-susceptible strains only); *Staphylococcus epidermidis* (methicillin-susceptible strains only); *Staphylococcus saprophyticus; Staphylococcus pneumoniae* (penicillin-susceptible strains); *Staphylococcus pyogenes* **Aerobic Gram-negative micro-organism** *Citrobacter* (*diversus, freundii*); *Enterobacter cloacae; Escherichia coli; Haemophilus* (*influenzae, parainfluenzae*); *Klebsiella pneumoniae; Moraxella catarrhalis; Morganella morganii; Proteus* (*mirabilis, vulgaris*), *Providencia* (*rettgeri, stuartii*); *Pseudomonas aeruginosa; Serratia marcescens.* Also ciprofloxacin has been shown to be active against *Bacillus anthracis* both *in vitro* and by use of serum levels as a surrogate marker.	Contraindications: Concomitant administration with tizanidine Patients with impaired renal function: Creatinine clearance (mL/min): ■ >30 (see usual dose) ■ 5–29 (200–400 mg q18–24h)

Levofloxacin	Fluoroquinolone	Usual dose: 250–750 mg qd PO or IV	Inhibition of bacterial topoisomerase IV and DNA gyrase (both of which are type II topoisomerases), enzymes required for DNA replication, transcription, repair, and recombination **Drug interactions** with theophylline, caffeine, warfarin, phenytoin, sulfonylurea glyburide, metronidazole, probenecid, piperacillin sodium, and cyclosporine	**Acute bacterial sinusitis** due to *Streptococcus pneumoniae, Haemophilus influenzae*, or *Moraxella catarrhalis* **Acute bacterial exacerbation of chronic bronchitis** due to *Staphylococcus aureus, Streptococcus pneumoniae, Haemophilus influenzae, Haemophilus parainfluenzae*, or *Moraxella catarrhalis*. **Nosocomial pneumonia** due to methicillin-susceptible *Staphylococcus aureus, Pseudomonas aeruginosa, Serratia marcescens, Escherichia coli, Klebsiella pneumoniae, Haemophilus influenzae*, or *Streptococcus pneumoniae*. Adjunctive therapy should be used as clinically indicated. Where *Pseudomonas aeruginosa* is a documented or presumptive pathogen, combination therapy with an antipseudomonal *β*-lactam is recommended. **Community-acquired pneumonia** due to *Staphylococcus aureus, Streptococcus pneumoniae* (including multidrug-resistant strains [MDRSP]),[a] *Haemophilus influenzae, Haemophilus parainfluenzae, Klebsiella pneumoniae, Moraxella catarrhalis, Chlamydia pneumoniae, Legionella pneumophila*, or *Mycoplasma pneumoniae* **Complicated skin and skin structure infections** due to methicillin-susceptible *Staphylococcus aureus, Enterococcus faecalis, Streptococcus pyogenes*, or *Porteus mirabilis*. **Uncomplicated skin and skin structure infections** (mild to moderate) including abscesses, cellulites, furuncles, impetigo, pyoderma, and wound infections, due to *Staphylococcus aureus* or *Streptococcus pyogenes* **Chronic bacterial prostatitis** due to *Escherichia coli, Enterococcus faecalis*, or *Staphylococcus epidermidis* **Complicated urinary tract infections** (mild to moderate) due to *Enterococcus faecalis, Enterobacter cloacae, Escherichia coli, Klebsiella pneumoniae, Proteus mirabilis*, or *Pseudomonas aeruginosa* **Acute pyelonephritis** (mild to moderate) caused by *Escherichia coli* **Uncomplicated urinary tract infections** (mild to moderate) due to *Escherichia coli, Klebsiella pneumoniae*, or *Staphylococcus saprophyticus*	Clearance of levofloxacin is substantially reduced and plasma elimination half-life is substantially prolonged in patients with impaired renal function (creatinine clearance <50 mL/min), requiring dosage adjustment in such patients to avoid accumulation. Neither hemodialysis nor continuous ambulatory peritoneal dialysis (CAPD) is effective in removal of levofloxacin from the body, indicating that supplemental doses of levofloxacin are not required following hemodialysis or CAPD. Adverse reactions: Opiate screen false positives; photosensitivity; QTc interval prolongation and tendinopathy
Moxifloxacin	Fluoroquinolone	Usual dose: 400 mg PO or IV qd	The bactericidal action of moxifloxacin results from the interference with topoisomerase II and IV.	Community-acquired pneumonia (CAP), including CAP caused by multidrug-resistant *Streptococcus pneumoniae*[b] Complicated skin and skin structure infections, including diabetic foot infections Complicated intra-abdominal infections, including polymicrobial infections such as abscesses	Similar to other fluoroquinolones

[a]MDRSP (multidrug-resistant *Streptococcus pneumoniae*) are strains resistant to two or more of the following antibiotics: penicillin (minimum inhibitory concentration [MIC] = 2 μg/mL), second-generation cephalosporins (e.g., cefuroxime, macrolides, tetracyclines, and trimethoprim/sulfamethoxazole).
[b]Multidrug-resistant *S. pneumoniae* includes isolates previously known as PRSP (penicillin-resistant *S. pneumoniae*), and are strains resistant to two or more of the following antibiotics: Penicillin (MIC $\geq$2 mg/mL), second-generation cephalosporins (e.g., cefuroxime), macrolides, tetracyclines, and trimethoprim/sulfamethoxazole.
Cunha BA. *Antibiotic Essentials*. 5th ed. Royal Oak, MI: Physicians Press; 2006.
From website http://www.drugs.com (drug information online). Revised from November 2006.

TABLE K.10

POLYMYXINS

Drug	Drug class	Adults (usual dose[a])	Actions, interactions, and others	Spectrum of activity, indications, and active against most strains of	Route, reduce dose, and contraindications
Polymyxin B	Phospholipid cell membrane-altering antibiotic	0.75–1.25 mg/kg (IV) q12 h (1 mg = 10,000 units)	Colistin is polycationic and has both hydrophilic and lipophilic moieties. These interact with the bacterial cytoplasmic membrane, changing its permeability. This effect is bactericidal. The main toxicities described with intravenous treatment are nephrotoxicity and neurotoxicity. At a dose of 160 mg colistimethate IV q8h, very little nephrotoxicity is seen. (Conway SP, Etherington C, MundayJ, et al. (2000). “Safety and tolerability of bolus intravenous colistin in acute respiratory exacerbation in adults with cystic fibrosis”. Ann Pharmacother 34: 1238-42.)	Colistin is effective against Gram-negative bacilli, except Proteus and Burkholderia cepacia, and is used as a polypeptide antibiotic. Multidrug-resistant Acinetobacter baumanii, even in Acinetobacter meningitis with intrathecal polymyxin E Mycobacterium aurum was susceptible to the antibiotic colistin (polymyxin E),which had an MIC of 5 micrograms/ml and an apparent bactericidal effect at concentrations above 50 micrograms/ml. Cited from David HL, Rastogi N. Antibacterial action of colistin (polymyxin E) against Mycobacterium aurum. Antimicrob Agents Chemother. 1985 May; 27(5): 701-707	Usage in pregnancy: The safety of this drug in human pregnancy has not been established.
Polymyxin E	Colistin (Polymyxin E) is a polymyxin antibiotic produced by certain strains of Bacillus polymyxa var. colistinus. There are 2 forms of colistin available commercially: colistin sulfate and colistimethate sodium (colistin methanesulfonate sodium, colistin sulfomethate sodium).	Colomycin 1,000,000 units is 80 mg colistimethate Coly-mycin M 150 mg “colistin base” is 360 mg colistimethate or 4,500,000 units	Polymyxins bind to the cell membrane and alters its structure making it more permeable. The resulting water uptake leads to cell death. They are cationic, basic proteins that act like detergents. Intereactions: Anphotericin B, amikacin, gentamicin, tobramycin, vancomycin. Adeverse effects: Renal failure (tubular necrosis). Neurotoxicity associated with very prolongued or high serum levels; neuromuscular blockade with renal failure and or neuromuscular disorders	Bactericidal for gram-negative; little to no effect on gram-positive since cell wall is too thick to permit access to membrane	Colistin sulfate and colistimethate sodium are eliminated from the body by different routes.

Cunha BA. *Antibiotic Essentials*. 5th ed. Royal Oak, MI: Physicians Press; 2006.
From website http://www.drugs.com (drug information online). Revised from November 2006.

TABLE K.11

AMINOGLYCOSIDES

Drug	Drug class	Adults (usual dose[a])	Actions, interactions, and others	Spectrum of activity, indications, and active against most strains of	Route, reduce dose, and contraindications
Gentamicin	Aminoglycoside antibiotic, derived from *Micromonospora purpurea*, an actinomycete	Usual dose: Gentamicin sulfate 3 mg/kg/d q8h In patients with life-threatening infections: 5 mg/kg/d q24h (preferred over q8h dosing) Intravenous use only for gentamicin sulfate in 0.9% sodium chloride.	Bactericidal antibiotic that acts by inhibiting normal protein synthesis in susceptible micro-organisms **Drug interactions:** Amphotericin B, cephalothin, cyclosporine, enflurane, methoxyflurane, polymyxin B, radiographic contrast, vancomycin (increase nephrotoxicity), cisplatinum, etc. (see specifications of the product)	*Escherichia coli; Proteus* sp. (indole-positive and indole-negative); *Pseudomonas aeruginosa*; species of *Klebsiella-Enterobacter-Serratia* group; *Citrobacter* sp.; and *Staphylococcus* sp. (including penicillin and methicillin-resistant strains) Gentamicin is also active *in vitro* against species of *Salmonella* and *Shigella.*	To adjust the doses for patients with renal impairment Adverse reactions: Nephrotoxicity: Adverse renal effects have been reported. They occur more frequently in patients with a history of renal impairment and in patients treated for longer periods or with larger dosages than recommended. Others such as neurotoxicity (serious adverse effects on both vestibular and auditory branches of the eighth nerve), peripheral neuropathy, or encephalopathy, including numbness, skin tingling, muscle twitching, convulsions, and a myasthenia gravis-like syndrome, have been reported. (see specifications of the product).
Amikacin	Semi-synthetic aminoglycoside antibiotic, derived from kanamycin	Usual dose: Amikacin sulfate IV: 15 mg/kg or 1 g q24h (preferred to q12h dosing)	**Drug interactions:** See gentamicin sulfate.	**Gram negative** Amikacin is active *in vitro* against *Pseudomonas* sp., *Escherichia coli, Proteus* sp. (indole-positive and indole-negative), *Providencia* sp., *Klebsiella-Enterobacter-Serratia* sp., *Acinetobacter* (formerly Mima-Herellea) sp., and *Citrobacter freundii* When strains of the above organisms are found to be resistant to other aminoglycosides, including gentamicin, tobramycin, and kanamycin, many are susceptible to amikacin *in vitro.* **Gram positive** Amikacin is active *in vitro* against penicillinase and nonpenicillinase-producing *Staphylococcus* sp. including methicillin-resistant strains. However, aminoglycosides in general have a low order of activity against other Gram-positive organisms.	See gentamicin sulfate.
Tobramycin	Aminoglycoside antibiotic, derived from the actinomycete *Streptomyces tenebrarius*	Usual dose: Tobramycin sulfate: IV: 5 mg/kg q24h or 240 mg q24h (preferred over q8h dosing). The dosage should be reduced to 3 mg/kg/d as soon as clinically indicated.	Tobramycin acts by inhibiting synthesis of protein in bacterial cells. For **drug interactions** see gentamicin sulfate.	**Gram-positive aerobes** *Staphylococcus aureus* **Gram-negative aerobes** *Citrobacter* sp., *Enterobacter* sp., *Escherichia coli, Klebsiella* sp., *Morganella morganii, Pseudomonas aeruginosa, Proteus mirabilis, Proteus vulgaris, Providencia* sp., *Serratia* sp. Aminoglycosides have a low order of activity against most Gram-positive organisms, including *Streptococcus pyogenes, Streptococcus pneumoniae,* and *Enterococci*	See gentamicin sulfate.

Cunha BA. *Antibiotic Essentials.* 5th ed. Royal Oak, MI: Physicians Press; 2006.
From website http://www.drugs.com (drug information online). Revised from November 2006.

TABLE K.12

MISCELLANEOUS

Drug	Drug class	Adults (usual dose[a])	Actions, interactions, and others	Spectrum of activity, indications, and active against most strains of	Route, reduce dose, and contraindications
Metronidazole	Nitroimidazole antiparasitic/ antibiotic	Usual dose: IV: 1 g q/24h PO: 500 mg q12h	Metronidazole is a synthetic antibacterial compound. **Drug interactions:** Warfarin and other oral coumarin anticoagulants, phenytoin or phenobarbital, cimetidine, and disulfiram	**Anaerobic Gram-negative bacilli**, including *Bacteroides* sp., including the *Bacteroides fragilis* group *(B. fragilis, B. distasonis, B. ovatus, B. thetaiotaomicron, B. vulgatus); Fusobacterium* sp. **Anaerobic Gram-positive bacilli**, including *Clostridium* sp. and susceptible strains of *Eubacterium* **Anaerobic Gram-positive cocci**, including *Peptococcus* sp.; *Peptostreptococcus* sp.	Primary mode of elimination: Hepatic
Trimethoprim (TMP)/sulfamethoxazole (SMX) or cotrimoxazole	Synthetic folate antagonist/ sulfonamide	Usual dose: IV or PO: 2.5–5 mg/kg q6h	Sulfamethoxazole is bacteriostatic and trimethoprim is bactericidal **Drug interactions:** Warfarin (monitoring carefully); phenytoin (folate deficiencies when is used concomitantly); thiazides increased incidence of thrombocytopenia with purpura in elderly patients; cyclosporine (nephrotoxicity reversible); digoxin; indomethacin; pyrimethamine; tricyclic antidepressants; amantadine; methotrexate; and oral hypoglycemic agents	Primary agent in the treatment of *Pneumocystis carinii pneumonia* (PCP), an opportunistic infection in patients with HIV/AIDS, and as secondary prophylaxis of PCP in patients who have already had at least one episode of PCP. Also is indicated for the treatment of chronic bronchitis, enterocolitis caused by strains of *Shigella (flexneri and sonnei)*, acute otitis media in children, traveler's diarrhea caused by enterotoxigenic *Escherichia coli* and *Shigella* sp., and bacterial urinary tract infections	SMX-TMP is metabolized in the liver. Urinary concentrations of both active drugs are decreased in patients with impaired renal function. Only small amounts of trimethoprim are excreted in feces via biliary elimination. Trimethoprim and active sulfamethoxazole are moderately removed by hemodialysis.

Cunha BA. *Antibiotic Essentials*. 5th ed. Royal Oak, MI: Physicians Press; 2006.
From website http://www.drugs.com (drug information online). Revised from November 2006.

TABLE K.13

ANTIFUNGALS

Drug	Drug class	Adults (usual dose[a])	Actions, interactions, and others	Spectrum of activity, indications, and active against most strains of	Route, reduce dose, and contraindications
Amphotericin B	Antifungal Polyene macrolide antibiotic produced by soil bacteria *Streptomyces nodosus*	Usual dose: IV: 0.5–0.8 mg/kg q24h	Amphotericin B is the gold standard for the treatment of serious and invasive systemic mycosis as well as for Kala-Azar. **Drug interactions:** Avoid concomitant administration of nephrotoxic drugs and bone marrow suppressants.	Amphotericin B has useful activity against candidiasis, cryptococcosis, histoplasmosis, blastomycosis, paracoccidioidomycosis, coccidioidomycosis, aspergillosis, extracutaneous sporotrichosis, zygomycosis (mucormycosis), penicilliosis (*Penicilliosis marneffei*) pseudallescheriasis, hyalohyphomycosis (including infection due to *Acremonium, Fusarium, Penicillium,* etc.) and phaeohyphomycosis (including infection due to *Alternaria, Bipolaris, Cladosporium, Cladophialophora, Curvularia, Exophiala, Exserohilum, Fonsecaea, Phialophora, Wangiella,* etc.). Empirical antifungal therapy is useful to granulocytopenic patients with persistent or recurrent fever.[a]	Primary mode of elimination: Metabolized The most common cause for withdrawal of or failure to continue amphotericin B therapy is its severe renal toxicity in nearly half of all the patients. The second problem, which is a major one, is the nephrotoxicity of amphotericin B.
Liposomal amphotericin B	Antifungal Polyene macrolide antibiotic True liposomal preparation of amphotericin B in which lipid complex of liposomes is constituted of lecithin and cholesterol	Usual dose: IV: 3–6 mg/kg q24h	Is the most effective and affordable drug for treatment of both **systemic mycosis** and Kala-Azar. **Drug interactions:** As with conventional amphotericin B, avoid concomitant administration of nephrotoxic drugs and bone marrow suppressants, only and in patients with hypokalemia.	Amphotericin B shows a high order of *in vitro* activity against many species of fungi *viz. Histoplasma capsulatum, Cryptococcus immitis, Candida* sp., *Blastomyces dermatitidis, Rhodotorula, Cryptococcus neoformans, Sporothrix schenckii, Mucor* sp., *Aspergillus fumigatus, Malassezia furfur, Trichosporon beigelii, Saccharomyces cerevisiae, Scedosporium* sp., *Paecilomyces* sp., *Penicillium* sp., *Fusarium* sp., *Bipolaris* sp., *Exophiala* sp., *Cladophialophora* sp., *Absidia* sp., *Apophysomyces* sp., *Cunninghamella* sp., *Rhizomucor* sp., *Rhizopus* sp., *and Saksenaea* sp. These fungi are inhibited by concentrations of amphotericin B ranging from 0.03 to 1 μg/mL *in vitro*. Amphotericin B also has activity against species of *Leishmania* and is found to be effective in the treatment of Kala-Azar.	Primary mode of elimination: Metabolized

[a]Walsh TJ, Lee J, Lecciones J. Empiric therapy with amphotericin B in febrile granulocytopenic patients. *Rev Infect Dis*. 1991;13:496–503.

(continued)

TABLE K.13

(CONTINUED)

Drug	Drug class	Adults (usual dose[a])	Actions, interactions, and others	Spectrum of activity, indications, and active against most strains of	Route, reduce dose, and contraindications
Fluconazole	Triazole antifungal agent	Usual dose: 400 mg (IV/PO) × 1 dose, then 200 mg (IV/PO) q24h Usual dose for candidemia: 400 mg (IV/PO) q24h after loading dose of 800 mg (IV/PO) Meningeal dose: 400 mg (IV/PO) q24h	Fluconazole is a highly selective inhibitor of fungal cytochrome P450 sterol C-14 α-demethylation. **Drug interactions:** Oral contraceptives, cimetidine, antacid, hydrochlorothiazide, rifampin, warfarin, phenytoin, cyclosporine, zidovudine, theophylline, terfenadine, oral hypoglycemic agents, tolbutamide, glipizide, glyburide, rifabutin, tacrolimus, cisapride, midazolam, azithromycin (not significant)	**Prophylaxis** Fluconazole is also indicated to decrease the incidence of candidiasis in patients undergoing bone marrow transplantation who receive cytotoxic chemotherapy and/or radiation therapy. Fluconazole exhibits *in vitro* activity against *Cryptococcus neoformans* and *Candida* spp. Fungistatic activity has also been demonstrated in normal and immunocompromised animal models for systemic and intracranial fungal infections due to *Cryptococcus neoformans* and for systemic infections due to *Candida albicans.* **Fluconazole is indicated for the treatment of:** 1. Vaginal candidiasis (vaginal yeast infections due to *Candida*) 2. Oropharyngeal and esophageal candidiasis. In open noncomparative studies of relatively small numbers of patients, fluconazole was also effective for the treatment of *Candida* urinary tract infections, peritonitis, and systemic *Candida* infections including candidemia, disseminated candidiasis, and pneumonia. 3. Cryptococcal meningitis	Primary mode of elimination: Renal Contraindications: Terfenadine and cisapride Fluconazole has been associated with rare cases of serious hepatic toxicity.
Voriconazole	Triazole antifungal agent	Usual dose: **IV dosing:** Loading dose of 6 mg/kg (IV) q12h × 1 day, then maintenance dose of 4 mg/kg (IV) q12h. It is possible to switch to weight-based PO maintenance IV dose. **PO dosing:** 1. If weight ≥40 kg: Loading dose of 400 mg (PO) q12h × 1 day, then maintenance dose of 200 mg (PO) q12h. If response is inadequate, increase dose to 300 mg (PO) q12h. 2. If weight <40 kg: Loading dose of 200 mg (PO) × 1 day, then maintenance dose of 100 mg (PO) q12h. If response is inadequate, increase dose to 150 mg (PO) q12h. In patients with chronic and/or non life-threatening infections, loading dose may be given PO.	**Mode of action** of voriconazole is the inhibition of fungal cytochrome P450-mediated 14 α-lanosterol demethylation, an essential step in fungal ergosterol biosynthesis. **Drug interactions:** Benzodiazepines, vinca alkaloids, carbamazepine, ergo alkaloids, rifampin, rifabutin, sirolimus, long-acting barbiturates (see contraindications), cyclosporine, omeprazole, tacrolimus, phenytoin, warfarin, statins, dihydropyridine, calcium channel blockers (low arterial pressure), sulfonylureas (hypoglycemia). Potential hepatotoxicity risk	**Invasive aspergillosis** Indicated for the primary treatment of acute invasive aspergillosis (*Aspergillus* spp.) Also with *Fusarium* spp. and *Scedosporium* spp. **Other disease-causing agents** Voriconazole was shown to be effective against both *Scedosporium apiospermum* and *Fusarium* spp. For *Scedosporium apiospermum*, a successful response to Vfend was reported in 15 of 24 subjects (63%). In those with *Fusarium* spp., 9 of 21 (43%) were successfully treated with voriconazole.	Primary mode of elimination: Hepatic Contraindications: Long-acting barbiturates

Itraconazole	Antifungal agent	Usual dose: 200 mg (IV/PO) q24h 200 mg capsule/solution (PO) q24h. Begin itraconazole for acute/severe infections with a loading regimen of 200 mg (IV) q12h × 2 days (4 doses), then give 200 mg (IV or PO) q24h maintenance dose. Each IV dose should be infused over 60 minutes.	**Drug interactions:** Coadministration of cisapride, pimozide, quinidine, *dofetilide,* or levacetylmethadol (levomethadyl) with itraconazole.	**Itraconazole exhibits *in vitro* activity against** *Blastomyces dermatitidis, Histoplasma capsulatum, Histoplasma duboisii, Aspergillus flavus, Aspergillus fumigatus, Candida albicans,* and *Cryptococcus neoformans.* **Itraconazole also exhibits varying *in vitro* activity against** *Sporothrix schenckii, Trichophyton species, Candida krusei,* and other *Candida* species. Fungistatic activity has been demonstrated against disseminated fungal infections caused by *Blastomyces dermatitidis, Histoplasma duboisii, Aspergillus fumigatus, Coccidioides immitis, Cryptococcus neoformans, Paracoccidioides brasiliensis, Sporothrix schenckii, Trichophyton rubrum,* and *Trichophyton mentagrophytes.*	Primary mode of elimination: Hepatic; metabolized predominantly by the cytochrome P450 3A4 isoenzyme system (CYP3A4) Patients with impaired hepatic function should be carefully monitored when taking itraconazole. If signs or symptoms of congestive heart failure appear during administration of itraconazole, monitor carefully and consider other treatment alternatives. **Contraindications:** Cisapride, oral midazolam, pimozide, quinidine, dofetilide, triazolam, and levacetylmethadol (levomethadyl) are contraindicated with itraconazole.
Caspofungin	Echinocandin antifungal	Usual dose: 70 mg (IV) × 1 dose, then 50 mg (IV) q24h In patients weighing more than 80 kg it is recommended that 70 mg/d is given rather than 50 mg/d. Patients with moderate liver insufficiency should receive a dose of 35 mg/d.	Caspofungin is not an inhibitor and is a poor substrate for cytochrome people P450 enzymes. **Drug interactions:** Cyclosporine, tacrolimus, carbamazepine, rifampin, dexamethasone, efavirenz, nelfinavir, nevirapine, phenytoin	Caspofungin is active against all species of *Candida*. It is extremely active against all species except *Candida parapsilosis, Candida guilliermondii,* and *Candida lusitaniae,* against which it is moderately active. Caspofungin is also very active against all *Aspergillus* sp. It does not kill *Aspergillus* completely in test tubes. There is a very limited amount of activity against *Coccidioides immitis, Blastomyces dermatitidis, Scedosporium* sp., *Paecilomyces variotii,* and *Histoplasma capsulata* but it is likely that the activity is not sufficient for clinical use.	Primary mode of elimination: Hepatic

From Cunha BA. *Antibiotic Essentials*. 5th ed. Royal Oak, MI: Physicians Press; 2006, with permission.
From website http://www.drugs.com (drug information online). Revised from November 2006.

INDEX

Page numbers followed by *f* and *t* denote figure and table, respectively.